CECIL
TEXTBOOK
of
MEDICINE

CECIL
TEXTBOOK
19th edition
of
MEDICINE

Edited by

JAMES B. WYNGAARDEN, M.D.

Professor of Medicine and
Associate Vice-Chancellor for Health Affairs,
Duke University School of Medicine,
Durham, North Carolina

LLOYD H. SMITH, Jr., M.D.

Professor of Medicine and
Associate Dean,
University of California, San Francisco,
School of Medicine,
San Francisco, California

J. CLAUDE BENNETT, M.D.

Professor and Chairman,
Department of Medicine,
University of Alabama at Birmingham,
School of Medicine,
Birmingham, Alabama

W. B. SAUNDERS COMPANY
HARCOURT BRACE JOVANOVICH, INC.
Philadelphia London Toronto Montreal Sydney Tokyo

W. B. SAUNDERS COMPANY
Harcourt Brace Jovanovich, Inc.

The Curtis Center
Independence Square West
Philadelphia, PA 19106

Library of Congress Cataloging-in-Publication Data

Cecil textbook of medicine / edited by James B. Wyngaarden,
Lloyd H. Smith, Jr., J. Claude Bennett.—19th ed.

p. cm

Rev. ed. of: Textbook of medicine / [edited by] Cecil. 18th ed.
1988.

Includes bibliographical references and index.

ISBN 0–7216–2928–8 (single v.).—ISBN 0–7216–2929–6 (v. 1).—
ISBN 0–7216–2930–X (v. 2).—ISBN 0–7216–2931–8 (set)

1. Internal medicine   I. Cecil, Russell L. (Russell La Fayette),
   1881–1965.   II. Wyngaarden, James B.   III. Smith,
   Lloyd H.   IV. Bennett, J. Claude.   V. Title: Textbook
   of Medicine.

[DNLM: 1. Medicine. WB 100 C3888]

RC46.C423 1992

616—dc20

DNLM/DLC   91–31268

Editor: John Dyson
Designer: Lorraine B. Kilmer
Production Manager: Frank Polizzano
Manuscript Editors: Donna Walker and Bonnie Boehme
Illustration Coordinator: Matt Andrews
Indexer: Donna Walker

ISBN 0–7216–2928–8   Single Volume
ISBN 0–7216–2929–6   Volume 1
ISBN 0–7216–2930–X   Volume 2
ISBN 0–7216–2931–8   Set

CECIL TEXTBOOK OF MEDICINE

DOSAGE NOTICE

ALSO ASSOCIATED WITH THE *CECIL TEXTBOOK OF MEDICINE*

Review of General Internal Medicine: A Self-Assessment Manual, 5th Edition, 1992
Editors: J. Allen D. Cooper, Jr., M.D.; Peter G. Pappas, M.D.

The fifth edition of this self-assessment book contains approximately 1200 questions covering all the specialty areas of internal medicine. The answers are linked to this edition of the *Cecil Textbook of Medicine*, to the *Cecil Essentials of Medicine*, and to other readily available sources.

Available from W. B. Saunders Company
The Curtis Center
Independence Square West
Philadelphia, PA 19106

Material in the chapters listed below is in the public domain:

PREFACE

The 19th edition of the *Cecil Textbook of Medicine* appears on the one-hundredth anniversary of the publication of William Osler's influential *The Principles and Practice of Medicine*, a monumental single-authored volume notable for its comprehensive clinical coverage, authoritative pathologic descriptions, and literary qualities. Microbiology was then the newest medical science. A tone of therapeutic nihilism was the book's most salutary contribution. At least two generations of physicians would fall under its influence. The textbook ushered in a period of increasingly exact diagnosis, especially in infectious diseases, and an ever more critical evaluation of drugs, remedies, and nostrums in the practice of medicine. It also led to the establishment of the Rockefeller Institute, founded to address the pervasive ignorance of the pathophysiology of disease so abundantly displayed in Osler's textbook, avant garde though it was for its day.

Thirty-five years later, in 1927, Russell Cecil introduced "*A Text-book of Medicine* by American authors." Single-authored textbooks had largely given way to books jointly authored by a small number of writers, but the idea of an edited textbook compiled by multiple authors, each writing on topics of personal interest and experience, was new. Basic biologic sciences were making increasingly important contributions to clinical medicine, and these were to be accorded substantial attention. The maturing sciences were physiology, pharmacology, and biochemistry. With succeeding editions, Cecil's philosophy became more explicit. Cecil believed that ". . . in terms of biological processes, fragmentation of the discussion of disease is artificial" (Preface, 10th edition, 1959). Each chapter was a treatise in which clinical description, pathologic information, pathophysiologic knowledge, diagnostic criteria, and therapeutic measures were well integrated, so that students and physicians consulting the text could secure the most authoritative information available and find it in one place (Beeson and McDermott, Preface, 11th edition, 1963).

Cecil's inaugural philosophy continues into the 19th edition of the *Cecil Textbook*, 65 years later, appropriately adapted to ever-changing circumstances. By 1992, several generations of physicians have learned medicine with the help of *Cecil*. The series spans a period of remarkable progress in biomedical and behavioral sciences, and each new edition has incorporated new insights on disease causation, prevention, and treatment. The pace has quickened as we approach the twenty-first century. New technologies have revolutionized molecular genetics, neurobiology, immunology, cell biology, and structural biology; the application of these disciplines to all branches of the traditional biomedical sciences proceeds apace. The structure of DNA was elucidated less than 40 years ago, and recombinant DNA technology was discovered less than 20 years ago. Today, the leitmotif of biologic science, regardless of its disciplinary name, is increasingly cell and molecular biology. This theme is now permeating medicine and prefiguring the developments of the next few decades. Beyond these contributions from the biologic sciences, applications of the physical and mathematical sciences, especially in diagnostic imaging (CT, MRI, PET, and sonography) and in the information sciences, continue to alter medical practice. In such a climate of change, medical competence itself is fragile. It must be constantly renewed or else it will erode.

To reflect the best in medical practice, a major textbook of medicine must also be constantly renewed. In that spirit, this edition of the *Cecil Textbook of Medicine* has been thoroughly revised. As before, approximately one third of the book is "new" in that different authors have been selected, in this way assuring that their chapters have been completely recast. All other chapters have been revised and updated by their current authors, carefully chosen authorities in their respective subjects. The editors are deeply grateful to all retiring authors for the high standards of their contributions. We have retained the two-color presentation of figures and charts, so well received in the 18th edition, and have expanded the color plates from 8 to 16 pages.

The most extensive change in the 19th edition is the further expansion of space devoted to the acquired immunodeficiency syndrome (AIDS), a still unfolding epidemic. This condition now commands a part of its own (Part XXI, HIV and Associated Disorders), comprising 13 newly written chapters: "Immunology Related to AIDS" (B. D. Walker); "Biology of Human Immunodeficiency Viruses" (G. M. Shaw); "Epidemiology of HIV Infection and AIDS" (J. W. Curran); "Prevention of HIV Infection" (M. S. Saag); "Neurologic Complications of HIV-1 Infection" (R. W. Price); "Pulmonary Manifestations of AIDS: Special Emphasis on Pneumocystosis" (F. R. Sattler); "Gastrointestinal Manifestations of AIDS" (J. G. Bartlett); "Cutaneous Signs of AIDS" (N. S. Penneys); "Ophthalmologic Manifestations of AIDS" (M. A. Jacobson); "Hematology/Oncology in AIDS" (J. E. Groopman and D. T. Scadden); "Renal, Cardiac, Endocrine, and Rheumatologic Manifestations of HIV Infection" (M. S. Saag); "Treatment of AIDS and Related Disorders" (R. Yarchoan and S. Broder); and "Chronic Management and Counseling for Persons with HIV Infection" (J. A. Bartlett). In addition, related chapters on AIDS dementia and on opportunistic infections associated with AIDS, found elsewhere in the book, have been thoroughly updated.

A new chapter, "Human T Cell Lymphotropic Virus Type I–Associated Myelopathy and Tropical Spastic Paraparesis" (R. W. Price), reflects the growing appreciation of other retroviruses as causes of human disease. Oncology (Part XIII) has been strengthened by the addition of two new chapters: "Oncologic Emergencies" (S. M. Hahn and A. Russo) and "Metastatic Cancer, Source Unknown" (D. C. Ihde). In addition, a new chapter, "Ovarian Carcinoma" (H. W. Jones), is included in Part XVI, Endocine and Reproductive Diseases. Part XXIII, Neurology, has been reorganized to increase the depth of focus on problems of the elderly. New chapters include "Neurologic Problems Associated with Aging" (F. Plum) and "Disturbances of Memory and Language" and "Alzheimer's Disease and Related Dementias" (both by A. R. Damasio). Also, "Brief Loss of Consciousness," "Sustained Impairments of Consciousness," and "Brain Death" (all by F. Plum) are now full chapters.

New chapters have also been added elsewhere, including "Zoonoses" (B. McLain), "Liver Transplantation" (J. P. Roberts), and "Erythromelalgia" (E. V. Ball). Part IV, Principles of Diagnosis and Management, is now expanded by a new chapter, "NSAID's: Aspirin and Aspirin-like Drugs" (G. Weissmann), in response to the need for an authoritative discussion of the nature, use, and side effects of these widely employed agents. Also, in this edition "Antimicrobial Therapy" (L. S. Young) and "Antiviral Therapy" (a new chapter by M. Middlebrooks) have been transferred from Part IV to be associated more closely with chapters on specific bacterial and viral diseases in Part XX, Infectious Diseases. As in recent editions of *Cecil*, each chapter lists a limited number of carefully selected, recent references to research or review articles in accessible journals, or to books, that may be consulted for additional information. The particular value of each entry is briefly described in an annotation. Finally, a new chapter entitled "Internal Medicine and Today's Internist" has been contributed by our co-editor, J. Claude Bennett, whom the continuing editors warmly welcome to the task of shepherding the 19th edition of *Cecil*, with its attendant high honor and immense responsibility.

Cecil not only stands alone; it is also the senior member of a trilogy. *Cecil Essentials of Medicine* (edited by T. E. Andreoli, C. C. J. Carpenter, F. Plum, and L. H. Smith, Jr.), now in its 2nd edition, offers a more concentrated guide to what every doctor should know about internal medicine. It is designed primarily for the medical student, for whom the authoritative compendium of *Cecil* may sometimes seem formidable. Nevertheless, it serves in general as a useful point of entry guide. *Cecil Review of General Internal Medicine* (edited by J. A. D. Cooper, Jr., and P. G. Pappas) appears in a 5th edition in parallel with this 19th edition of *Cecil*. As before, its 1200 questions and answers are designed to be of general educational benefit as well as to reinforce the value of *Cecil* as a reference text.

Editing a major textbook is a complex task, as one attempts to balance content, format, style, integration, and innovation. The editors have been privileged to work with an admirable group of colleagues in this shared responsibility. Fred Plum has continued in his role as Editor for Neurology. We welcome two new Consulting Editors: Gerald L. Mandell for Infectious Diseases and Robert K. Ockner for Digestive Diseases. They join a seasoned team of fellow Consulting Editors: Thomas E. Andreoli (Renal Diseases), John F. Murray (Respiratory Diseases), David G. Nathan (Hematologic and Hematopoietic Diseases), and Thomas W. Smith (Cardiovascular Diseases). We thank our retiring Consulting Editors, Robert Lefkowitz, William Paul, and Marvin Sleisenger, for extraordinary contributions to *Cecil*, in one case (M. Sleisenger) extending over eight editions. The Consulting Editors continually review their respective sections of this complex book and bring us their ideas and expertise concerning modifications. Our special gratitude is extended to the 360 contributors who have written the 534 chapters that collectively constitute this 19th edition. The ultimate value and authenticity of *Cecil* lie not with the editors but with the scholarship and experience that these individual physicians and scientists have brought to this joint enterprise.

"Language is the armoury of the human mind; and at once contains the trophies of its past, and the weapons of its future conquests." The weaponry of language, in Coleridge's image above, does not always come fully burnished in submitted manuscripts. As in the 18th edition, we have been most fortunate to work with seasoned editorial assistants in Washington (Margaret Quinlan), San Francisco (Judith Serrell), and Birmingham (Carolyn Thomley), without whose dedication and skill this large project could not have been completed. At W. B. Saunders Company, Lorraine Kilmer, Donna Walker, Frank Polizzano, and Faith Voit carried out with experienced professionalism the intricate task of formatting, editing, and assembling the book. The overall editor at the W. B. Saunders Company for this 19th edition of *Cecil* was again John Dyson, who has been an invaluable guide, colleague, and good friend. We are deeply indebted to him for his extensive contributions in bringing to completion this 19th edition of a venerable book.

JAMES B. WYNGAARDEN, M.D.
LLOYD H. SMITH, JR., M.D.
J. CLAUDE BENNETT, M.D.

CONTRIBUTORS

ROBERT H. ALLEN, M.D.

Professor of Medicine and of Biochemistry and Director, Division of Hematology, University of Colorado Health Sciences Center School of Medicine. Staff Physician, University Hospital, Denver, Colorado.

Megaloblastic Anemia

DAVID H. ALPERS

Professor of Medicine and Chief, Division of Gastroenterology, Washington University School of Medicine. Physician, Barnes Hospital, and Consultant, Jewish Hospital of St. Louis and St. Louis Children's Hospital, St. Louis, Missouri.

Principles of Nutritional Support: Enteral Nutritional Therapy

DAVID F. ALTMAN, M.D.

Professor of Clinical Medicine and Associate Dean, University of California, San Francisco, School of Medicine, San Francisco, California.

Food Poisoning

KARL E. ANDERSON, M.D.

Professor, University of Texas Medical School at Galveston. Full-time Active Member of the Medical Staff, The University of Texas Medical Branch Hospitals, Galveston, Texas.

The Porphyrias

W. FRENCH ANDERSON, M.D.

Adjunct Professor, Graduate Genetics Program, George Washington University School of Medicine and Health, Washington, D.C.; Faculty, Department of Medicine and Physiology, National Institutes of Health Graduate Program. Chief, Molecular Hematology Branch, National Heart, Lung, and Blood Institute, National Institutes of Health, Bethesda, Maryland.

Expectations from Recombinant DNA Research

THOMAS E. ANDREOLI, M.D.

Professor and Chairman, Department of Internal Medicine, University of Arkansas College of Medicine. Chief of Medicine, University Hospital of Arkansas, Little Rock, Arkansas.

Approach to the Patient with Renal Disease; Disorders of Fluid Volume, Electrolyte, and Acid-Base Balance; The Posterior Pituitary

VINCENT T. ANDRIOLE, M.D.

Professor of Medicine, Yale University School of Medicine. Attending Physician, Yale–New Haven Hospital, New Haven, Connecticut.

Urinary Tract Infections and Pyelonephritis

FREDERICK R. APPELBAUM, M.D.

Professor of Medicine, University of Washington School of Medicine. Member, Fred Hutchinson Cancer Research Center, Seattle, Washington.

The Acute Leukemias

FRANK C. ARNETT, M.D.

Professor of Internal Medicine. University of Texas Medical School at Houston. Chief, Division of Rheumatology, Hermann Hospital and Lyndon B. Johnson General Hospital, Houston, Texas.

Rheumatoid Arthritis

WILLIAM J. ARNOLD, M.D.

Clinical Professor of Medicine, University of Chicago Pritzker School of Medicine, Chicago. Chairman, Department of Internal Medicine, Lutheran General Hospital, Park Ridge, Illinois.

Specialized Procedures in the Management of Patients with Rheumatic Diseases

DENNIS A. AUSIELLO, M.D.

Associate Professor of Medicine, Harvard Medical School. Chief, Renal Unit, Massachusetts General Hospital, Boston, Massachusetts.

Natriuretic Hormones

BERNARD M. BABIOR, M.D., Ph.D.

Adjunct Professor of Medicine, University of California, San Diego, School of Medicine. Member and Head, Division of Biochemistry, Department of Molecular and Experimental Medicine, Research Institute of Scripps Clinic. Staff Physician, Division of Hematology/Oncology, Scripps Clinic and Research Foundation, La Jolla, California.

Function of Neutrophils and Mononuclear Phagocytes; Disorders of Neutrophil Function

GROVER C. BAGBY, Jr., M.D.

Professor of Medicine and Medical Genetics, Oregon Health Sciences University School of Medicine. Section Head, Hematology and Medical Oncology, Veterans Affairs Medical Center, Portland, Oregon.

Leukopenia; Leukocytosis and Leukemoid Reactions

EUGENE V. BALL, M.D.

Professor of Medicine, University of Alabama School of Medicine. Staff Physician, University of Alabama Hospital, Birmingham, Alabama.

Behçet's Disease; Systemic Diseases in Which Arthritis Is a Feature; Miscellaneous Forms of Arthritis; Nonarticular Rheumatism; Articular Tumors; Erythromelalgia

ROBERT W. BALOH, M.D.

Professor of Neurology and Surgery (Head and Neck), University of California, Los Angeles, UCLA School of Medicine. Director, Neurotology Laboratories, University of California at Los Angeles Medical Center, Los Angeles, California.

The Special Senses

MURRAY G. BARON, M.D.

Professor and Associate Chairman, Department of Radiology, Emory University School of Medicine. Associate Chairman, Radiology Department, Emory University Hospital; Attending Neurologist, Grady Memorial Hospital and Henrietta Egleston Hospital for Children, Atlanta, Georgia.

Radiology of the Heart

ROBERT B. BARON, M.D., M.S.

Associate Professor of Clinical Medicine, University of California, San Francisco, School of Medicine. Director, Primary Care Internal Medicine Residency Program, and Continuing Medical Education, Department of Medicine, University of California San Francisco Medical Center, San Francisco, California.

Protein-Energy Malnutrition

WILLIAM H. BARRY, M.D.

Nora Eccles Harrison Professor of Cardiology, University of Utah School of Medicine. Attending Cardiologist, University of Utah Hospital and Clinics, Salt Lake City, Utah.

Cardiac Catheterization and Angiography

JOHN A. BARTLETT, M.D.

Assistant Professor of Medicine, Duke University Medical Center, Durham, North Carolina.

Chronic Management and Counseling for Persons with HIV Infection

JOHN G. BARTLETT, M.D.

Professor of Medicine, Johns Hopkins University School of Medicine. Chief, Division of Infectious Diseases, Johns Hopkins Hospital, Baltimore, Maryland.

Lung Abscess; Clostridial Diseases; Gastrointestinal Manifestations of AIDS

NATHAN M. BASS, M.D., Ph.D.

Associate Professor of Medicine, University of California, San Francisco, School of Medicine. Attending Physician, University of California San Francisco Medical Center, San Francisco, California.

Toxic and Drug-Induced Liver Disease

STEPHEN G. BAUM, M.D.

Professor of Medicine, Mount Sinai School of Medicine of the City University of New York. Director, Department of Medicine, Beth Israel Medical Center, New York, New York.

Mycoplasmal Infections; Adenovirus Diseases

JOHN D. BAXTER, M.D.

Professor of Medicine and Director, Metabolic Research Unit, University of California, San Francisco, School of Medicine. Chief, Division of Endocrinology, Moffitt Hospital, San Francisco, California.

Disorders of the Adrenal Cortex

STEPHEN B. BAYLIN, M.D.

Professor of Oncology and Medicine, Johns Hopkins University School of Medicine. Active Staff Member, Johns Hopkins Hospital, Baltimore, Maryland.

Endocrine Manifestations of Tumors: "Ectopic" Hormone Production

CHARLES E. BECKER, M.D.

Professor of Medicine, University of California, San Francisco, School of Medicine. Director, Center for Occupational and Environmental Health, University of California, San Francisco. Chief, Occupational Medicine and Toxicology, San Francisco General Hospital Medical Center, San Francisco, California.

Principles of Occupational Medicine

MICHAEL D. BENDER, M.D.

Associate Clinical Professor of Medicine, University of California, San Francisco, School of Medicine. Director of Medical Education and Attending Physician, Mills-Peninsula Hospitals, Burlingame, and Seton Medical Center, Daly City, California.

Diseases of the Peritoneum, Mesentery, and Omentum

PAUL E. BENDHEIM, M.D.

Associate Professor of Neurology, State University of New York Health Science Center at Brooklyn College of Medicine. Head, Laboratory of Neurodegenerative Diseases, Institute for Basic Research, Staten Island, New York.

Creutzfeldt-Jakob Disease

J. CLAUDE BENNETT, M.D.

Professor and Chairman, University of Alabama School of Medicine. Physician-in-Chief, University of Alabama Hospital, Birmingham, Alabama.

Internal Medicine and Today's Internist;
The Immune System: Introduction

EDWARD J. BENZ, Jr., M.D.

Professor of Internal Medicine and Genetics; Chief, Section of Hematology; and Vice Chairman, Department of Internal Medicine, Yale University School of Medicine. Attending Physician and Chief of Hematology, Yale–New Haven Hospital, New Haven, Connecticut.

Structure, Function, and Synthesis of the Human Hemoglobins;
Classification and Basic Pathophysiology of the Hemoglobinopathies;
Hemoglobinopathies with Altered Solubility or Oxygen Affinity

PAUL D. BERK, M.D.

Lillian and Henry M. Stratton Professor of Molecular Medicine; Professor of Medicine and Biochemistry; and Chief, Division of Liver Diseases (Department of Medicine), Mount Sinai School of Medicine of the City University of New York. Attending Physician, Mount Sinai Medical Center, New York, New York.

Erythrocytosis and Polycythemia; Myeloproliferative Disorders

BRUCE BEUTLER, M.D.

Associate Professor of Internal Medicine, University of Texas Health Science Center at Dallas Southwestern Medical School. Attending Physician, Parkland Memorial Hospital, Dallas, Texas.

The Pathogenesis of Fever

STEVEN M. BEUTLER, M.D.

Clinical Assistant Professor of Medicine, University of California, Irvine, California College of Medicine, Irvine. Director, Division of Infectious Diseases, San Bernadino County Medical Center, and Assistant Chairman, Department of Medicine, St. Bernadine Medical Center, San Bernadino, California.

The Pathogenesis of Fever

J. THOMAS BIGGER, Jr., M.D.

Professor of Medicine and of Pharmacology, Columbia University College of Physicians and Surgeons. Attending Physician and Director, Arrhythmia Control Unit, Presbyterian Hospital in the City of New York, New York.

Cardiac Arrhythmias

DANIEL D. BIKLE, M.D., Ph.D.

Associate Professor, University of California, San Francisco, School of Medicine. Attending Physician, University of California San Francisco Medical Center; Co-Director, Special Diagnostic and Treatment Unit, Department of Veterans Affairs Medical Center, San Francisco, California.

Vitamin D; Osteomalacia and Rickets

J. MICHAEL BISHOP, M.D.

Professor, Microbiology and Immunology, Biochemistry and Biophysics; and Director, The G. W. Hooper Research Foundation, University of California, San Francisco, School of Medicine, San Francisco, California.

Oncogenes

ALAN L. BISNO, M.D.

Professor of Medicine, University of Miami School of Medicine. Chief, Medical Service, Veterans Administration Medical Center, and Attending Physician, Jackson Memorial Hospital, Miami, Florida.

Rheumatic Fever

WILLIAM A. BLATTNER, M.D.

Chief, Viral Epidemiology Section, Environmental Epidemiology Branch, Epidemiology and Biostatistics Program, Division of Cancer Etiology, National Cancer Institute, National Institutes of Health, Rockville, Maryland.

Retroviruses That Cause Human Disease

WILLIAM J. BLOT, Ph.D.

Chief, Biostatistics Branch, National Cancer Institute, National Institutes of Health, Bethesda, Maryland.

The Epidemiology of Cancer

ROGER BONE, M.D.

The Ralph Crissman Brown Professor and Chairman, Department of Internal Medicine, Rush Medical College of Rush University. Chief, Section of Pulmonary and Critical Care Medicine, Rush-Presbyterian-St. Luke's Medical Center, Chicago, Illinois.

Bronchiectasis; Cystic Fibrosis

THOMAS D. BOYER, M.D.

Professor of Medicine and Director, Division of Digestive Diseases, Emory University School of Medicine, Atlanta, Georgia.

Cirrhosis of the Liver and Its Major Sequelae

CHARLES B. BRENDLER, M.D.

Associate Professor of Urology, Johns Hopkins University School of Medicine. Active Full-time Staff Member, Department of Urology, Johns Hopkins Hospital, Baltimore, Maryland.

Diseases of the Prostate

SAMUEL BRODER, M.D.

Director, National Cancer Institute; Attending Physician, Clinical Center, National Institutes of Health, Bethesda, Maryland.

Treatment of AIDS and Related Disorders

PHILIP A. BRUNELL, M.D.

Professor of Pediatrics in Residence, University of California, Los Angeles, UCLA School of Medicine. Director, Pediatric Infectious Diseases, Cedars-Sinai Medical Center, Los Angeles, California.

Measles; Rubella; Varicella

JOHN D. BRUNZELL, M.D.

Professor of Medicine, Division of Metabolism, University of Washington School of Medicine, Seattle, Washington.

The Hyperlipoproteinemias

REBECCA H. BUCKLEY, M.D.

J. Buren Sidbury Professor of Pediatrics and Professor of Immunology, Duke University School of Medicine. Chief, Division of Pediatric Allergy and Immunology, Duke University Hospital, Durham, North Carolina.

Primary Immunodeficiency Diseases

WARD E. BULLOCK, M.D.

Arthur Russell Morgan Professor of Medicine and Director, Division of Infectious Diseases, University of Cincinnati College of Medicine. Attending Physician, University Hospital; Consulting Physician in Infectious Diseases, Department of Veterans Affairs Medical Center and Children's Hospital Medical Center, Cincinnati, Ohio.

Actinomycosis; Nocardiosis

PAUL A. BUNN, Jr., M.D.

Professor of Medicine; Director, University of Colorado Cancer Center; and Head, Division of Medical Oncology, University of Colorado Health Sciences Center School of Medicine. Staff Physician, University Hospital, Denver, Colorado.

Paraneoplastic Syndromes; Tumor Markers

DAVID M. BURNS, M.D.

Associate Professor of Medicine, Department of Medicine, Pulmonary and Critical Care Division, University of California, San Diego, School of Medicine, La Jolla. Medical Director, Department of Respiratory Therapy, University of California San Diego Medical Center, San Diego, California.

Tobacco and Health

THOMAS BUTLER, M.D.

Professor, Texas Tech University Health Sciences Center School of Medicine. Attending Physician, University Medical Center, Lubbock, Texas.

Typhoid Fever; Shigellosis; Yersinia *Infections; Nonsyphilitic Treponematoses; Relapsing Fever*

JOEL N. BUXBAUM, M.D.

Professor of Medicine, New York University School of Medicine. Chief, Rheumatology Section, Veterans Administration Medical Center; Attending Physician, Bellevue Hospital Center, New York, New York.

The Amyloid Diseases

PETER H. BYERS, M.D.

Professor, Departments of Pathology and Medicine, University of Washington School of Medicine, Seattle, Washington.

The Marfan Syndrome; Ehlers-Danlos Syndrome

ANDREI CALIN, M.D., F.R.C.P.

Consultant Rheumatologist, Royal National Hospital for Rheumatic Diseases, Bath, Ireland.

The Spondylarthropathies

BARTOLOME R. CELLI, M.D.

Associate Professor, Boston University School of Medicine. Chief, Pulmonary Section, Veterans Administration Medical Center; Director, Respiratory Care Center, University Hospital, Boston, Massachusetts.

Diseases of the Diaphragm, Chest Wall, Pleura, and Mediastinum

JOHN P. CELLO, M.D.

Professor of Medicine, University of California, San Francisco, School of Medicine. Attending Physician, Moffitt-Long Hospitals; Chief of Gastroenterology, San Francisco General Hospital Medical Center, San Francisco, California.

Gastrointestinal Hemorrhage

BRUCE A. CHABNER, M.D.

Director, Division of Cancer Treatment, National Cancer Institute, National Institutes of Health, Bethesda, Maryland.

Oncology: Introduction

ROBERT M. CHANOCK, M.D.

Laboratory of Infectious Diseases, National Institute of Allergy and Infectious Diseases, National Institutes of Health, Bethesda, Maryland.

Respiratory Syncytial Virus; Parainfluenza Viral Diseases

SANDY F. S. CHUN, M.D.

Staff Physician, Kaiser Foundation Hospital, Santa Clara, California.

Zygomycosis

LINDA HAWES CLEVER, M.D., F.A.C.P.

Clinical Professor of Medicine, University of California, San Francisco, School of Medicine. Chairman, Department of Occupational Health, and Active Staff Member, California Pacific Medical Center, San Francisco, California.

The Health of the Physician

RAY E. CLOUSE, M.D.

Associate Professor of Medicine, Washington University School of Medicine. Associate Physician, Barnes Hospital; Consulting Physician, The Jewish Hospital of St. Louis and The John Cochran Veterans Administration Medical Center, St. Louis, Missouri.

Parenteral Nutrition

C. GLENN COBBS, M.D.

Professor of Medicine and Vice Chairman for Veterans Affairs, University of Alabama School of Medicine. Chief, Medical Service, Veterans Administration Medical Center, Birmingham, Alabama.

Bartonellosis

MARTIN G. COGAN, M.D.

Professor of Medicine, University of California, San Francisco, School of Medicine. Chief, Nephrology Section, Department of Veterans Affairs Medical Center, San Francisco, California.

Specific Renal Tubular Disorders

JORDAN J. COHEN, M.D.

Dean and Professor of Medicine, State University of New York at Stony Brook Health Sciences Center School of Medicine. President, Medical Staff, and Attending Physician, Department of Medicine, University Hospital, Stony Brook, New York.

Vascular Disorders of the Kidney

LAWRENCE S. COHEN, M.D.

The Ebenezer K. Hunt Professor of Medicine, Yale University School of Medicine. Attending Physician, Yale–New Haven Hospital, New Haven, Connecticut.

Surgical Treatment of Coronary Artery Disease; Diseases of the Aorta

SIDNEY COHEN, M.D.

Chairman, Department of Medicine, and Richard Laylord Evans Professor of Medicine, Temple University School of Medicine, Philadelphia, Pennsylvania.

Diseases of the Esophagus

ZANVIL A. COHN, M.D.

Professor, Laboratory of Cellular Physiology and Immunology, Rockefeller University. Senior Physician, Rockefeller University Hospital, New York, New York.

Leprosy—Hansen's Disease

WILLIAM G. COUSER, M.D.

Professor of Medicine, University of Washington School of Medicine. Head, Division of Nephrology, University of Washington Medical Center, Seattle, Washington.

Glomerular Disorders

PHILIP E. CRYER, M.D.

Professor of Medicine and Director, Division of Endocrinology, Diabetes and Metabolism, Washington University School of Medicine. Physician, Barnes Hospital, St. Louis, Missouri.

The Adrenal Medullae; The Carcinoid Syndrome

RONALD G. CRYSTAL, M.D.

Chief, Pulmonary Branch, National Heart, Lung and Blood Institute, National Institutes of Health, Bethesda, Maryland.

Interstitial Lung Disease

JAMES W. CURRAN, M.D., M.P.H.

Director, Division of HIV/AIDS, Center for Infectious Diseases, Centers for Disease Control, Atlanta, Georgia.

Epidemiology of HIV Infection and AIDS

JOHN J. CURTIS, M.D.

Professor of Medicine, University of Alabama School of Medicine. Staff Physician, University of Alabama Hospital, Birmingham, Alabama.

Treatment of Irreversible Renal Failure: Renal Transplantation

DAVID C. DALE, M.D.

Professor of Medicine, University of Washington School of Medicine. Attending Physician, University of Washington Medical Center, Seattle, Washington.

The Febrile Patient

ANTONIO R. DAMASIO, M.D., Ph.D.

Professor, University of Iowa College of Medicine. Head, Department of Neurology, University of Iowa Hospitals and Clinics, Iowa City, Iowa.

Diagnosis of Regional Cerebral Dysfunction; Disturbances of Memory and Language; Alzheimer's Disease and Related Dementias

TROY E. DANIELS, D.D.S., M.S.

Professor and Chair, Division of Oral Pathology, School of Dentistry, University of California, San Francisco. Attending Dentist, Moffitt-Long Hospitals and University of California San Francisco Medical Center, San Francisco, California.

Diseases of the Mouth and Salivary Glands

MICHAEL DECK, M.B., B.S., F.R.A.C.R., F.R.C.R.

Professor of Radiology, Cornell University Medical College. Attending Radiologist, New York Hospital, New York, New York.

Radiologic Imaging Techniques

LEONARD J. DEFTOS, M.D.

Professor of Medicine, University of California, San Diego, School of Medicine, La Jolla. Staff, Laboratory of Bone and Mineral Research, Department of Veterans Affairs Medical Center, San Diego, California.

Calcitonin and Medullary Thyroid Carcinoma

ANDREW DEISS, M.D.

Associate Professor of Medicine, University of Utah School of Medicine. Associate Chief of Staff for Research and Development, Veterans Affairs Medical Center, Salt Lake City, Utah.

Wilson's Disease

VINCENT W. DENNIS, M.D.

Professor of Medicine and Chief, Division of Nephrology, Duke University School of Medicine, Durham, North Carolina.

Investigations of Renal Function

ROBERT J. DESNICK, Ph.D., M.D.

Arthur J. and Nellie Z. Cohen Professor of Pediatrics and Genetics and Chief, Division of Medical and Molecular Genetics, Mount Sinai School of Medicine of the City University of New York. Attending Physician, Mount Sinai Medical Center, New York, New York.

Fabry's Disease

IVAN DIAMOND, M.D., Ph.D.

Professor and Vice Chairman, Department of Neurology, and Professor of Pediatrics and Pharmacology, University of California, San Francisco, School of Medicine. Director, Ernest Gallo Clinic and Research Center. Attending Neurologist, University of California San Francisco Medical Center, San Francisco General Hospital, and Department of Veterans Affairs Medical Center, San Francisco, California.

Alcoholism and Alcohol Abuse; Nutritional Disorders of the Nervous System

EUGENE P. DIMAGNO, M.D.

Professor of Medicine, Mayo Medical School. Consultant in Internal Medicine and Gastroenterology, Mayo Clinic; Director of GI Diagnostic Unit, Saint Mary's Hospital, Rochester, Minnesota.

Carcinoma of the Pancreas

CHARLES A. DINARELLO, M.D.

Professor of Medicine, Tufts University School of Medicine. Staff Physician, New England Medical Center, Boston, Massachusetts.

The Acute Phase Response

WILLIAM E. DISMUKES, M.D.

Director, Division of Infectious Diseases, and Professor and Vice-Chairman for Educational Programs, Department of Medicine, University of Alabama School of Medicine. Attending Physician, University of Alabama Hospital, Birmingham, Alabama.

The Mycoses: Introduction; Histoplasmosis; Blastomycosis; Paracoccidioidomycosis; Cryptococcosis; Sporotrichosis; Candidiasis

R. GORDON DOUGLAS, Jr., M.D.

Clinical Professor of Medicine, Cornell University Medical College. Attending Physician, New York Hospital, New York, New York.

Introduction to Viral Diseases; Influenza; Arthropod-Borne Viral Encephalitides

JEFFREY M. DRAZEN, M.D.

Parker B. Francis Professor of Medicine, Harvard Medical School. Chief, Combined Pulmonary and Critical Care Divisions, Beth Israel and Brigham and Women's Hospitals, Boston, Massachusetts.

Asthma

DOUGLAS A. DROSSMAN, M.D.

Professor of Medicine and Psychiatry, Division of Digestive Diseases, University of North Carolina at Chapel Hill School of Medicine. Attending Physician, University of North Carolina Hospitals, Chapel Hill, North Carolina.

The Eating Disorders

RICHARD J. DUMA, M.D., Ph.D.

Professor of Medicine, Microbiology, and Pathology, Virginia Commonwealth University Medical College of Virginia School of Medicine. Chairman, Division of Infectious Diseases, Department of Internal Medicine, Medical College of Virginia Hospitals, Richmond, Virginia.

Pneumococcal Pneumonia

DAVID T. DURACK, M.B., D.Phil.

Professor of Medicine and of Microbiology and Immunology, Duke University School of Medicine. Chief, Division of Infectious Diseases, Duke University Hospital, Durham, North Carolina.

Infective Endocarditis

PAUL H. EDELSTEIN, M.D.

Associate Professor of Pathology and Laboratory Medicine and of Medicine, University of Pennsylvania School of Medicine. Director of Clinical Microbiology and Attending Physician in Infectious Diseases, Hospital of the University of Pennsylvania, Philadelphia, Pennsylvania.

Legionellosis

THEODORE C. EICKHOFF, M.D.

Professor of Medicine, University of Colorado Health Sciences Center School of Medicine. Director of Internal Medicine, Presbyterian–Saint Luke's Medical Center, Denver, Colorado.

Colorado Tick Fever

RONALD J. ELIN, M.D., Ph.D.

Clinical Professor of Pathology, Uniformed Services University of the Health Sciences F. Edward Hebert School of Medicine. Pathologist, Clinical Center, National Institutes of Health, Bethesda, Maryland.

Laboratory Reference Interval Values of Clinical Importance

EDWARD A. EMMETT, M.B., S.

Worksafe Australia, National Occupational and Health Safety Commission, Sydney, Australia.

Occupational Diseases of the Skin

ANDREW G. ENGEL, M.D.

William L. McKnight 3M Professor of Neuroscience, Mayo Medical School. Attending Physician, Saint Mary's and Rochester Methodist Hospitals, Rochester, Minnesota.

Diseases of Muscles (Myopathies) and Neuromuscular Junction

JEROME ENGEL, Jr., M.D., Ph.D.

Professor of Neurology and Anatomy and Cell Biology, University of California, Los Angeles, UCLA School of Medicine. Attending Neurologist and Chief of Epilepsy and Clinical Neurophysiology, University of California at Los Angeles Medical Center, Los Angeles, California.

The Epilepsies

DOUGLAS V. FALLER, Ph.D., M.D.

Associate Professor, Harvard Medical School. Staff Physician, Dana Farber Cancer Institute and Children's Hospital, Boston, Massachusetts.

Diseases of the Lymph Nodes and Spleen

BARRY L. FANBURG, M.D.

Professor of Medicine, Tufts University School of Medicine. Chief, Pulmonary Division, New England Medical Center, Boston, Massachusetts.

Sarcoidosis

W. EDMUND FARRAR, M.D.

Professor of Medicine and Microbiology, Infectious Diseases Division, Medical University of South Carolina College of Medicine. Staff Physician, Medical University of South Carolina Hospital, Charleston Memorial Hospital, and Veterans Administration Medical Center, Charleston, South Carolina.

Erysipeloid

MARK FELDMAN, M.D.

Professor and Vice Chairman, Department of Internal Medicine, University of Texas Health Science Center at Dallas Southwestern Medical School. Chief, Medical Service, Department of Veterans Affairs Medical Center, Dallas, Texas.

Peptic Ulcer: Complications

DAVID W. FERGUSON, M.D.

Associate Professor of Medicine, Cardiovascular Division, Department of Internal Medicine, University of Iowa College of Medicine. Director, Cardiovascular Intensive Care Unit, Clinical Cardiovascular Physiology Laboratory, and Heart Failure Clinic, University of Iowa Hospitals and Clinics, Iowa City, Iowa.

Shock

ALFRED P. FISHMAN, M.D.

William Maul Measey Professor of Medicine, University of Pennsylvania School of Medicine. Attending Physician, Hospital of the University of Pennsylvania, Philadelphia, Pennsylvania.

Pulmonary Hypertension

GARRET A. FITZGERALD, M.D.

Professor of Medicine and of Pharmacology; The William Stokes Professor of Experimental Therapeutics; Chief, Division of Clinical Pharmacology, Vanderbilt University School of Medicine. Attending Physician, Hypertension and Clinical Pharmacology, Vanderbilt University Medical Center, Nashville, Tennessee.

Prostaglandins and Related Compounds

SUZANNE W. FLETCHER, M.D.

Adjunct Professor, University of Pennsylvania School of Medicine, Philadelphia, Pennsylvania.

Clinical Approach to the Patient

KATHLEEN M. FOLEY, M.D.

Professor of Neurology and Pharmacology, Cornell University Medical College. Chief, Pain Service, Department of Neurology, Memorial Hospital, New York, New York.

Pain and Its Management

BERNARD G. FORGET, M.D.

Professor of Medicine and Human Genetics, Yale University School of Medicine. Attending Physician, Yale–New Haven Hospital, New Haven, Connecticut.

Sickle Cell Anemia and Associated Hemoglobinopathies

MICHAEL M. FRANK, M.D.

Professor and Chairman, Department of Pediatrics, and Professor, Department of Medicine, Duke University School of Medicine. Staff Physician, Duke University Hospital, Durham, North Carolina.

Urticaria and Angioedema

WILLIAM T. FRIEDEWALD, M.D.

Vice-President and Chief Medical Director, Metropolitan Life Insurance Company, New York, New York.

Epidemiology of Cardiovascular Disease

GARY D. FRIEDMAN, M.D., M.S.

Assistant Director for Epidemiology and Biostatistics, Division of Research, Kaiser Permanente Medical Care Program, Oakland. Associate Clinical Professor of Medicine and of Family and Community Medicine, University of California, San Francisco, School of Medicine, San Francisco; Lecturer in Epidemiology, School of Public Health, University of California, Berkeley, California.

The Preventive Health Examination

JAMES F. FRIES, M.D.

Associate Professor of Medicine, Stanford University School of Medicine. Staff Physician, Stanford University Hospital, Stanford, and Veterans Administration Medical Center, Palo Alto, California.

Approach to the Patient with Musculoskeletal Disease

LAWRENCE A. FROHMAN, M.D.

Professor of Medicine and Director, Division of Endocrinology and Metabolism, University of Cincinnati College of Medicine. Director of Endocrinology, University of Cincinnati Hospital, Cincinnati, Ohio.

Neuroendocrine Regulation and Its Disorders; The Anterior Pituitary

PATRICIA A. GABOW, M.D.

Professor, University of Colorado Health Sciences Center School of Medicine. Director of Medical Services, Denver General Hospital, Denver, Colorado.

Cystic Disease of the Kidney

JOHN N. GALGIANI, M.D.

Professor of Medicine, University of Arizona College of Medicine. Chief, Section of Infectious Diseases, Department of Veterans Affairs Medical Center, Tucson, Arizona.

Coccidioidomycosis

RENATE E. GAY, M.D.

Research Associate Professor of Medicine, University of Alabama School of Medicine, Birmingham, Alabama.

Connective Tissue Structure and Function

STEFFEN GAY, M.D.

Professor of Medicine, University of Alabama School of Medicine, Birmingham, Alabama. Director, WHO Collaborating Centre for the Biochemical Classification and Diagnostic Criteria of Rheumatoid Arthritis and Allied Diseases.

Connective Tissue Structure and Function

GORDON N. GILL, M.D.

Professor of Medicine and Co-Director, Division of Endocrinology and Metabolism, University of California, San Diego, School of Medicine, La Jolla. Attending Physician, University of California San Diego Medical Center, San Diego, California.

Principles of Endocrinology

JOHN W. GITTINGER, Jr., M.D.

Professor of Surgery and Neurology and Chairman, Division of Ophthalmology, University of Massachusetts Medical School. Chief of Ophthalmology, University of Massachusetts Medical Center, Worcester, Massachusetts.

Eye Diseases

JOHN H. GLICK, M.D.

Professor of Medicine and Madlyn and Leonard Abramson Professor of Clinical Oncology, University of Pennsylvania School of Medicine. Director, University of Pennsylvania Cancer Center; Attending Physician, Hospital of the University of Pennsylvania, Philadelphia, Pennsylvania.

Hodgkin's Disease

JOHN W. GNANN, Jr., M.D.

Assistant Professor of Medicine and Microbiology, University of Alabama School of Medicine. Attending Physician, Division of Infectious Diseases, University of Alabama Hospital, Birmingham, Alabama.

Foot-and-Mouth Disease; Mumps

CLEON W. GOODWIN, M.D.

Associate Professor, Department of Surgery, Cornell University Medical College. Associate Attending Surgeon and Director, Burn Center, New York Hospital; Associate Attending Surgeon, Jamaica Hospital, New York, New York.

Electrical Injury

SHERWOOD L. GORBACH, M.D.

Professor of Community Health, Medicine, and Microbiology and Immunology, Tufts University School of Medicine. Attending Physician, New England Medical Center and St. Elizabeth's Hospital, Boston, Massachusetts.

Diseases Caused by Non–Spore-Forming Anaerobic Bacteria

JARED J. GRANTHAM, M.D.

Professor of Medicine, University of Kansas Medical Center School of Medicine. Director of Nephrology, University of Kansas Medical Center, Kansas City, Kansas.

Acute Renal Failure

BRUCE M. GREENE, M.D.

Professor of Medicine and Director, Division of Geographic Medicine, Department of Medicine, University of Alabama College of Medicine. Staff Physician, University of Alabama Hospital and Veterans Administration Medical Center, Birmingham, Alabama.

Advice to Travelers; Enteric Infections: Introduction; Onchocerciasis

HARRY L. GREENE, M.D.

Professor of Pediatrics and Associate Professor of Biochemistry, Vanderbilt University School of Medicine. Director, Clinical Nutrition Center, and Associate Director, Vanderbilt Hospital, Nashville, Tennessee.

The Glycogen Storage Diseases; Fructose Intolerance

JOSEPH C. GREENFIELD, Jr., M.D.

James B. Duke Distinguished Professor, Duke University School of Medicine. Chairman, Department of Medicine, Duke University Hospital, Durham, North Carolina.

Electrocardiography

WILLIAM B. GREENOUGH, III, M.D.

Professor of Medicine and of International Health, Johns Hopkins University School of Medicine. Attending Physician, Francis Scott Key Medical Center and Johns Hopkins Hospital, Baltimore, Maryland.

Cholera

JAMES H. GRENDELL, M.D.

Associate Professor of Medicine and Physiology, University of California, San Francisco, School of Medicine. Chief, Gastroenterology Section, Department of Veterans Affairs Medical Center, San Francisco, California.

Vascular Diseases of the Intestine

JEROME E. GROOPMAN, M.D.

Associate Professor of Medicine, Harvard Medical School. Chief of Hematology/Oncology, New England Deaconess Hospital, Boston, Massachusetts.

Langerhans Cell (Eosinophilic) Granulomatosis; Hematology/Oncology in AIDS

CARL GRUNFELD, M.D., Ph.D.

Associate Professor of Medicine, University of California, San Francisco, School of Medicine. Co-Director, Special Diagnostic and Treatment Unit, Department of Veterans Affairs Medical Center, San Francisco, California.

Pancreatic Islet Cell Tumors

RICHARD L. GUERRANT, M.D.

Thomas H. Hunter Professor of International Medicine and Head, Division of Geographic Medicine, University of Virginia School of Medicine. Attending Physician, University of Virginia Hospital, Charlottesville, Virginia.

Campylobacter *Enteritis; Enteric* Escherichia coli *Infections*

STEPHEN M. HAHN, M.D.

Junior Attending Physician, Medicine/Radiation Oncology Branches, National Cancer Institute, National Institutes of Health, Bethesda, Maryland.

Oncologic Emergencies

JOHN L. HAMERTON, D.Sc.

Professor, Department of Human Genetics, University of Manitoba Faculty of Medicine, Winnipeg, Manitoba, Canada.

Chromosomes and Their Disorders

STEPHEN B. HANAUER, M.D.

Associate Professor of Medicine, University of Chicago Pritzker School of Medicine. Co-Director, Outpatient Gastroenterology Clinic, University of Chicago Hospitals, Chicago, Illinois.

Inflammatory Bowel Disease

WILLIAM L. HASKELL, Ph.D.

Professor of Medicine, Stanford University School of Medicine, Stanford, California.

Exercise and Health

BARTON F. HAYNES, M.D.

Chief, Division of Rheumatology and Immunology and Frederic M. Hanes Professor of Medicine, Duke University School of Medicine. Chief, Division of Rheumatology and Immunology, Duke University Hospital, Durham, North Carolina.

Glucocorticosteroid Therapy; Wegener's Granulomatosis and Midline Granuloma

JOHN P. HAYSLETT, M.D.

Professor of Medicine, Yale University School of Medicine. Attending Physician, Yale–New Haven Hospital, New Haven, Connecticut.

Renal Disease in Pregnancy

BERNADINE P. HEALY, M.D.

Director, National Institutes of Health, Bethesda, Maryland.

Miscellaneous Conditions of the Heart: Tumor, Trauma, and Systemic Disease

DONALD A. HENDERSON, M.D., M.P.H.

Edgar Berman Professor, Johns Hopkins School of Hygiene and Public Health, Baltimore, Maryland.

Variola and Vaccinia

ERIK L. HEWLETT, M.D.

Professor of Medicine and of Pharmacology, University of Virginia School of Medicine. Staff Physician, University of Virginia Hospital, Charlottesville, Virginia.

Diphtheria

EDWARD W. HOLMES, M.D.

Chairman, Department of Medicine, Hospital of the University of Pennsylvania, Philadelphia, Pennsylvania.

Other Disorders of Purine Metabolism

LEWIS B. HOLMES, M.D.

Professor of Pediatrics, Harvard Medical School. Pediatrician and Chief, Embryology-Teratology Unit, Children's Service, Massachusetts General Hospital; Director of Genetic and Birth Defects Evaluation and Counseling, Antenatal Diagnostic Test Center, Brigham and Women's Hospital, Boston, Massachusetts.

Congenital Malformations

PHILIP C. HOPEWELL, M.D.

Professor of Medicine, University of California, San Francisco, School of Medicine. Chief of Chest Service, San Francisco General Hospital Medical Center, San Francisco, California.

Critical Care Medicine

DONALD R. HOPKINS, M.D., M.P.H.

Senior Consultant, Global 2000/Carter Center, Chicago, Illinois.

Dracunculiasis

RICHARD B. HORNICK, M.D.

Clinical Professor of Medicine, University of Florida College of Medicine, Gainesville. Vice President of Medical Education, Orlando Regional Medical Center, Orlando, Florida.

Tularemia; Rickettsial Diseases

DAVID S. HOWELL, M.D.

Professor of Medicine and Director, Arthritis Division, University of Miami School of Medicine. Staff Physician, Jackson Memorial Hospital, Miami, Florida.

Osteoarthritis; The Painful Shoulder; The Painful Back

STEPHEN B. HULLEY, M.D., M.P.H.

Professor and Chief, Division of Clinical Epidemiology, Department of Epidemiology and Biostatistics, University of California, San Francisco, School of Medicine, San Francisco, California.

Principles of Preventive Medicine; Control of Unintended Injuries and Those Due to Violence

GENE HUNDER, M.D.

Professor of Medicine, Mayo Medical School. Chairman, Division of Rheumatology, and Consultant in Internal Medicine and Rheumatology, Mayo Clinic, Rochester, Minnesota.

Polymyalgia Rheumatica and Giant Cell Arteritis

DANIEL C. IHDE, M.D.

Professor of Medicine, Uniformed Services University of the Health Sciences F. Edward Hebert School of Medicine. Deputy Chief, Navy Medical Oncology Branch, National Cancer Institute, National Institutes of Health, Bethesda, Maryland.

Approach to the Patient with Metastatic Cancer, Primary Site Unknown

ROBERT W. IKE, M.D.

Instructor of Internal Medicine, University of Michigan Medical School. Attending Physician, University of Michigan Hospital, and Consultant, Department of Veterans Affairs, Veterans Administration Medical Center, Ann Arbor, Michigan.

Specialized Management Procedures for Rheumatic Diseases

JULIANNE IMPERATO-McGINLEY, M.D.

Associate Professor of Medicine, Cornell University Medical College. Associate Attending Physician in Medicine, New York Hospital–Cornell University Medical Center, New York, New York.

Disorders of Sexual Differentiation

MARK A. JACOBSON, M.D.

Assistant Professor of Medicine in Residence, University of California, San Francisco, School of Medicine. Director, Clinical Research Section, AIDS Program, San Francisco General Hospital Medical Center, San Francisco, California.

Ophthalmologic Manifestations of AIDS

JOSEPH JANKOVIC, M.D.

Professor of Neurology and Director of Parkinson's Disease Center and Movement Disorders Clinic, Baylor College of Medicine. Senior Attending Physician, Methodist Hospital and Texas Medical Center, Houston, Texas.

The Extrapyramidal Disorders

WALDEMAR G. JOHANSON, Jr., M.D.

Professor, Department of Internal Medicine, University of Texas Medical School at Galveston, Galveston, Texas.

Introduction to Pneumonia; Pneumonia Caused by Aerobic Gram-Negative Bacilli; Recurrent Aspiration Pneumonia

RICHARD B. JOHNSTON, Jr., M.D.

William H. Bennett Professor of Pediatrics, University of Pennsylvania School of Medicine. Senior Physician, Children's Hospital of Philadelphia, Philadelphia, Pennsylvania.

Whooping Cough

HOWARD W. JONES, III, M.D.

Professor, Obstetrics and Gynecology, and Director of Gynecologic Oncology, Vanderbilt University School of Medicine. Staff Physician, Vanderbilt University Hospital and Metropolitan Nashville General Hospital, Nashville, Tennessee.

Ovarian Carcinoma

ANTHONY KALES, M.D.

Professor and Chairman, Department of Psychiatry, Pennsylvania State University College of Medicine. Director, Sleep Research and Treatment Center, Milton S. Hershey Medical Center, Hershey, Pennsylvania.

Sleep and Its Disorders

JOHN P. KANE, M.D., Ph.D.

Professor of Medicine and of Biochemistry and Biophysics, University of California, San Francisco, School of Medicine. Attending Physician, Moffitt-Long Hospitals, San Francisco, California.

The Judicious Diet

ALBERT Z. KAPIKIAN, M.D.

Head, Epidemiology Section, Laboratory of Infectious Diseases, National Institute of Allergy and Infectious Diseases, National Institutes of Health, Bethesda, Maryland.

The Common Cold; Viral Gastroenteritis

ALLEN P. KAPLAN, M.D.

Chairman, Department of Medicine, State University of New York at Stony Brook Health Sciences Center School of Medicine. Staff Physician, University Hospital, Stony Brook, and Veterans Administration Medical Center, Northport, New York.

Anaphylaxis

GILLA KAPLAN, Ph.D.

Associate Professor, Laboratory of Cellular Physiology and Immunology, Rockefeller University, New York, New York.

Leprosy—Hansen's Disease

MANUEL E. KAPLAN, M.D.

Professor of Medicine, University of Minnesota Medical School. Chief of Hematology/Oncology, Department of Veterans Affairs Medical Center, Minneapolis, Minnesota.

Hemolytic Disorders: Introduction; Acquired Hemolytic Disorders

SAMUEL KAPLAN, M.D.

Professor of Pediatrics (Cardiology), University of California, Los Angeles, UCLA School of Medicine. Attending Physician, University of Califonia at Los Angeles Medical Center, Los Angeles, California.

Congenital Heart Disease

DONALD KAYE, M.D.

Professor and Chairman, Department of Medicine, Medical College of Pennsylvania. Chief of Medicine, Hospital of the Medical College of Pennsylvania; Consultant, Veterans Affairs Medical Center, Philadelphia, Pennsylvania.

Salmonella Infections Other Than Typhoid Fever

JAMES W. KAZURA, M.D.

Professor of Medicine and International Health, Case Western Reserve University School of Medicine. Physician, University Hospitals of Cleveland, Cleveland, Ohio.

Nematode Infections

MICHAEL J. KEATING, M.B., B.S., F.R.A.C.P.

Professor of Medicine, University of Texas Medical School at Houston. Associate Vice President for Clinical Investigation, University of Texas M. D. Anderson Cancer Center, Houston, Texas.

The Chronic Leukemias

ELLIOT D. KIEFF, M.D., Ph.D.

Albee Professor of Medicine and of Microbiology and Molecular Genetics, Harvard Medical School. Director, Infectious Disease Division, Brigham and Women's Hospital, Boston, Massachusetts.

Infectious Mononucleosis

CHARLES H. KING, M.D.

Associate Professor of Medicine, Case Western Reserve University School of Medicine. Assistant Physician, University Hospitals of Cleveland, Cleveland, Ohio.

Cestode Infections

SAULO KLAHR, M.D.

Joseph Friedman Professor of Renal Disease and Director, Renal Division, Washington University School of Medicine. Physician, Barnes Hospital; Staff Physician and Consultant in Nephrology, Jewish Hospital of St. Louis, St. Louis, Missouri.

Structure and Function of the Kidneys; Obstructive Uropathy

JAMES P. KNOCHEL, M.D.

Professor of Internal Medicine, University of Texas Health Science Center at Dallas Southwestern Medical School. Chairman, Department of Internal Medicine, Presbyterian Hospital; Senior Attending Physician, Parkland Memorial Hospital, Dallas, Texas.

Disorders Due to Heat and Cold

EDWIN H. KOLODNY, M.D.

Professor of Neurology, Harvard Medical School. Associate Neurologist, Massachusetts General Hospital, Boston, Massachusetts.

Gaucher Disease; Niemann-Pick Disease

HERMES A. KONTOS, M.D., Ph.D.

Professor of Medicine; Chairman, Division of Cardiology; and Vice-Chairman, Department of Internal Medicine, Virginia Commonwealth University Medical College of Virginia School of Medicine, Richmond, Virginia.

Vascular Diseases of the Limbs

RICHARD M. KRAUSE, M.D.

Senior Scientific Advisor, Fogarty International Center, National Institutes of Health, Bethesda, Maryland.

Streptococcal Diseases

GUENTER J. KREJS, M.D.

Professor and Chairman, Department of Medicine, Karl-Franzens-Universitat, Graz, Austria.

Diarrhea

WILLIAM L. KRINSKY, M.D., Ph.D.

Associate Clinical Professor of Epidemiology, Section of Medical Entomology, Yale University School of Medicine, New Haven, Connecticut.

Arthropods and Leeches

DONALD J. KROGSTAD, M.D.

Associate Professor of Pathology and Medicine, Washington University School of Medicine. Staff Physician, Barnes Hospital and Jewish Hospital of St. Louis, St. Louis, Missouri.

Malaria

JAMES P. KUSHNER, M.D.

Maxwell M. Wintrobe Professor of Medicine and Chief, Division of Hematology-Oncology, University of Utah School of Medicine. Attending Physician, University of Utah Hospital and Veterans Affairs Medical Center, Salt Lake City, Utah.

Normochromic, Normocytic Anemias; Hypochromic Anemias

ROBERT A. KYLE, M.D.

Professor of Medicine and of Laboratory Medicine, Mayo Medical School. Chair, Division of Hematology and Internal Medicine, Mayo Clinic and Mayo Foundation, Rochester, Minnesota.

Plasma Cell Disorders

DAVID J. LANG, M.D.

Vice-Chair, Department of Pediatrics, University of California, Irvine, California College of Medicine, Irvine. Pediatrician-in-Chief and Director of Medical Education, Research, and Infectious Disease, Children's Hospital of Orange County, Orange, California.

Cytomegalovirus Infection

P. REED LARSEN, M.D.

Professor of Medicine, Harvard Medical School. Chief, Thyroid Division, and Senior Physician, Brigham and Women's Hospital, Boston, Massachusetts.

The Thyroid

ROBERT B. LAYZER, M.D.

Professor of Neurology, University of California, San Francisco, School of Medicine, San Francisco, California.

Degenerative Diseases of the Nervous System

GERALD S. LAZARUS, M.D.

Hartzell Professor and Chairman, Department of Dermatology, University of Pennsylvania School of Medicine. Chief, Department of Dermatology, Hospital of the University of Pennsylvania, Philadelphia, Pennsylvania.

Panniculitis and Disorders of the Subcutaneous Fat

E. CARWILE LeROY, M.D.

Professor of Medicine, Medical University of South Carolina College of Medicine. Attending Physician, Medical University Hospital, Charleston, South Carolina.

Systemic Sclerosis

BERNARD LEVIN, M.D.

Professor of Medicine, University of Texas Medical School at Houston, and Clinical Professor, Baylor College of Medicine. Chief, Section of Gastrointestinal Oncology and Digestive Diseases, University of Texas M. D. Anderson Cancer Center, Houston, Texas.

Neoplasms of the Large and Small Intestine

DAVID E. LEVY, M.D.

Clinical Associate Professor of Neurology, Cornell University Medical College. Associate Attending Neurologist, New York Hospital, New York, New York.

Cerebrovascular Diseases

BRIAN J. LEWIS, M.D.

Clinical Professor of Medicine, University of California, San Francisco, School of Medicine. Staff Physician, The Permanente Medical Group, San Francisco, California.

Breast Cancer

ALFRED J. LEWY, M.D., Ph.D.

Professor of Psychiatry, Ophthalmology, and Pharmacology, Oregon Health Sciences University School of Medicine. Director, Sleep and Mood Disorders Laboratory and Mass Spectrometry Laboratory, Oregon Health Sciences University, Portland, Oregon.

The Pineal Gland

LAWRENCE M. LICHTENSTEIN, M.D.

Professor of Medicine, Johns Hopkins University School of Medicine, Baltimore, Maryland.

Insect Sting Allergy

JOHN LINDENBAUM, M.D.

Professor of Medicine and Acting Chairman, Department of Medicine, Columbia University College of Physicians and Surgeons. Attending Physician and Acting Director, Medical Service, Presbyterian Hospital in the City of New York, New York.

An Approach to the Anemias

IRIS F. LITT, M.D.

Professor of Pediatrics, Stanford University School of Medicine. Director, Division of Adolescent Medicine, Stanford University Hospital and Children's Hospital at Stanford, California.

Adolescent Medicine

JOHN N. LOEB, M.D.

Professor of Medicine, Columbia University College of Physicians and Surgeons. Attending Physician, Presbyterian Hospital in the City of New York, New York.

Polyglandular Disorders

DONALD B. LOURIA, M.D.

Professor and Chairman, Department of Preventive Medicine and Community Health, University of Medicine and Dentistry of New Jersey–New Jersey Medical School, Newark, New Jersey.

Trace Metal Poisoning

JOHN M. LUCE, M.D.

Associate Professor of Medicine and Anesthesia, University of California, San Francisco, School of Medicine. Associate Director, Medical-Surgical Intensive Care Unit, San Francisco General Hospital Medical Center, San Francisco, California.

Critical Care Medicine

ROBERT G. LUKE, M.D.

Chairman, Department of Internal Medicine, University of Cincinnati College of Medicine. Physician-in-Chief, University of Cincinnati Hospital, Cincinnati, Ohio.

Treatment of Irreversible Renal Failure: Dialysis

SAMUEL E. LUX, M.D.

Professor of Pediatrics, Harvard Medical School. Chief, Division of Hematology/Oncology, Children's Hospital, Boston, Massachusetts.

Hereditary Defects in the Membrane or Metabolism of the Red Cell

ADEL A. F. MAHMOUD, M.D., Ph.D.

Chairman, Department of Medicine, Case Western Reserve University School of Medicine. Physician-in-Chief, University Hospitals of Cleveland, Cleveland, Ohio.

Introduction to Protozoan and Helminthic Diseases; Schistosomiasis

STEPHEN E. MALAWISTA, M.D.

Professor of Medicine, Department of Internal Medicine, Yale University School of Medicine. Attending Physician, Yale–New Haven Hospital, New Haven, and Veterans Affairs Medical Center, West Haven, Connecticut.

Infectious Arthritis; Lyme Disease

PETER F. MALET, M.D.

Associate Professor of Medicine, University of Pennsylvania School of Medicine. Director, Gallstone Evaluation and Treatment Center, Hospital of the University of Pennsylvania, Philadelphia, Pennsylvania.

Diseases of the Gallbladder and Bile Ducts

GERALD L. MANDELL, M.D.

Professor of Internal Medicine; Owen R. Cheatham Professor of the Sciences; Head, Division of Infectious Diseases, University of Virginia School of Medicine, Charlottesville, Virginia.

Introduction to Microbial Disease; Introduction to Bacterial Disease

HENRY J. MANKIN, M.D.

Edith M. Ashley Professor of Orthopaedic Surgery, Harvard Medical School. Chief of the Orthopaedic Service, Massachusetts General Hospital, Boston, Massachusetts.

Bone Tumors

DOUGLAS J. MARCHANT, M.D.

Professor of Surgery and of Obstetrics and Gynecology, Tufts University School of Medicine. Senior Gynecologist, New England Medical Center, Boston, Massachusetts.

Nonmalignant Diseases of the Breast

ANDREW M. MARGILETH, M.D.

Professor of Pediatrics, University of Virginia School of Medicine. Attending Associate Consultant in Pediatric Dermatology and Infectious Diseases, University of Virginia Hospital, Charlottesville, and Mary Washington Hospital, Fredericksburg, Virginia.

Cat Scratch Disease

ALEXANDER R. MARGULIS, M.D.

Professor of Radiology, University of California, San Francisco, School of Medicine. Staff Radiologist, Moffitt-Long Hospitals; Consultant, San Francisco General Hospital Medical Center, Mt. Zion Hospital, Department of Veterans Affairs Medical Center, and Letterman Army Medical Center, San Francisco, California.

Overview of Imaging Techniques and Projection for the Future

LAWRENCE F. MARSHALL, M.D.

Professor of Surgery, University of California, San Diego, School of Medicine, La Jolla. Chief, Neurosurgical Services, University of California San Diego Medical Center, San Diego, California.

Injury to the Head and Spinal Cord

STEPHEN J. MARX, M.D.

Chief, Mineral Metabolism Section, National Institute of Diabetes and Digestive and Kidney Diseases, National Institutes of Health, Bethesda, Maryland.

Mineral and Bone Homeostasis

HENRY MASUR, M.D.

Clinical Professor of Medicine, George Washington University School of Medicine and Health Sciences, Washington, D.C. Chief, Critical Care Medicine Department, Clinical Center, National Institutes of Health, Bethesda, Maryland.

Toxoplasmosis

ALVIN M. MATSUMOTO, M.D.

Associate Professor of Medicine, University of Washington School of Medicine. Attending Physician, Geriatric Research, Education and Clinical Center, Veterans Administration Medical Center, Seattle, Washington.

The Testis and Male Sexual Function

RICHARD A. MATTHAY, M.D.

Professor and Associate Chairman, Department of Medicine, Yale University School of Medicine. Associate Director, Winchester Chest Clinic, Yale–New Haven Hospital, New Haven, Connecticut.

Chronic Airways Diseases; Abnormalities of Lung Aeration

JAMES R. McARTHUR, M.D.

Professor of Medicine and Hematology, University of Washington School of Medicine. Director, American Society of Hematology Slide Bank. Attending and Consulting Physician, University of Washington Medical Center, Seattle, Washington.

Selection and Preparation of Slides for Hematology Color Plates

J. BRUCE McCLAIN, M.D.

Associate Professor of Medicine, Uniformed Services University of the Health Sciences F. Edward Hebert School of Medicine, Bethesda, Maryland. Staff Physician, Department of Bacterial Diseases, Walter Reed Army Institute of Research, Washington, D.C.

Leptospirosis; Zoonoses

T. DWIGHT McKINNEY, M.D.

Professor of Medicine and Director, Nephrology Section, Indiana University School of Medicine. Staff Physician, Indiana University Medical Center, Richard L. Roudebush Veterans Administration Medical Center, and Wishard Memorial Hospital, Indianapolis, Indiana.

Tubulointerstitial Diseases and Toxic Nephropathies

JAY E. MENITOVE, M.D.

Clinical Associate Professor of Medicine, Medical College of Wisconsin and University of Wisconsin Medical School. Medical Director, Blood Center of Southeastern Wisconsin, Milwaukee, Wisconsin.

Blood Transfusion

DEAN D. METCALFE, M.D.

Head, Mast Cell Physiology Section, Laboratory of Clinical Investigation, National Institute of Allergy and Infectious Diseases, National Institutes of Health. Staff Physician, Clinical Center, National Institutes of Health, Bethesda, Maryland.

Mastocytosis

MARK MIDDLEBROOKS, M.D.

Associate/Fellow, Department of Medicine, Division of Infectious Diseases, University of Alabama School of Medicine. Staff Physician, University of Alabama Hospital, Birmingham, Alabama.

Antiviral Therapy; Herpes Simplex Virus Infections

DEANE F. MOSHER, M.D.

Professor of Medicine and Physiological Chemistry and Head, Section of Hematology, University of Wisconsin Medical School. Consultant, University of Wisconsin Hospital and Clinics, Madison, Wisconsin.

Disorders of Blood Coagulation

ARNO G. MOTULSKY, M.D., D.Sc.

Professor of Medicine and Genetics, University of Washington School of Medicine. Attending Physician, University of Washington Medical Center, Seattle, Washington.

Hemochromatosis; Hereditary Syndromes Involving Multiple Organ Systems

BALFOUR M. MOUNT, C.M., M.D., F.R.C.S.C.

Professor of Surgery and Director, Division of Palliative Care, McGill University Faculty of Medicine. Attending Physician, Royal Victoria Hospital, Montreal, Quebec, Canada.

Care of Dying Patients and Their Families

S. HARVEY MUDD, M.D.

Guest Worker, Laboratory of General and Comparative Biochemistry, National Institute of Mental Health, National Institutes of Health, Bethesda, Maryland.

Homocystinuria

MAURICE A. MUFSON, M.D.

Professor of Microbiology and Professor and Chairman, Department of Medicine, Marshall University School of Medicine. Associate Chief of Staff for Research, Veterans Administration Medical Center; Staff Physician, Cabell Huntington Hospital and St. Mary's Hospital, Huntington, West Virginia.

Viral Pharyngitis, Laryngitis, Croup, and Bronchitis

JOHN F. MURRAY, M.D.

Professor of Medicine, University of California, San Francisco, School of Medicine. Former Chief of the Chest Service, San Francisco General Hospital Medical Center, San Francisco, California.

Respiratory Diseases: Introduction; Respiratory Structure and Function; Respiratory Failure

BRYAN D. MYERS, M.B., Ch.B., M.R.C.P.(UK)

Professor of Medicine and Chief, Division of Nephrology, Stanford University School of Medicine. Chief of Nephrology, Stanford University Medical Center, Stanford, California.

Diabetes and the Kidney

DAVID G. NATHAN, M.D.

Robert G. Stranahan Professor of Pediatrics, Harvard Medical School. Physician-in-Chief, Children's Hospital, Boston, Massachusetts.

Introduction to Hematologic Diseases

FRANKLIN A. NEVA, M.D.

Chief, Laboratory of Parasitic Diseases, National Institute of Allergy and Infectious Diseases, National Institutes of Health. Attending Physician, Clinical Center, National Institutes of Health, Bethesda, Maryland.

American Trypanosomiasis; Leishmaniasis

ARTHUR W. NIENHUIS, M.D.

Chief, Clinical Hematology Branch, National Heart, Lung and Blood Institute, National Institutes of Health, Bethesda, Maryland.

The Thalassemias

ALAN S. NIES, M.D.

Professor of Medicine and Pharmacology and Head, Division of Clinical Pharmacology, University of Colorado Health Sciences Center School of Medicine. Attending Physician, University Hospital, Denver, Colorado.

Principles of Drug Therapy; Interactions Between Drugs; Adverse Reactions to Drugs

CHARLES P. O'BRIEN, M.D., Ph.D.

Professor and Vice-Chairman of Psychiatry, University of Pennsylvania School of Medicine. Chief of Psychiatry, Veterans Affairs Medical Center, Philadelphia, Pennsylvania.

Drug Abuse and Dependence

ROBERT K. OCKNER, M.D.

Professor of Medicine and Director, Liver Center, University of California, San Francisco, School of Medicine. Attending Physician, Moffitt-Long Hospitals, San Francisco, California.

Introduction to Gastrointestinal Diseases; Clinical Approach to Liver Disease; Acute Viral Hepatitis; Chronic Hepatitis

JERROLD M. OLEFSKY, M.D.

Professor of Medicine, University of California, San Diego, School of Medicine, La Jolla. Staff Member, Medical Research Service, Department of Veterans Affairs Medical Center, San Diego, California.

Diabetes Mellitus

SUZANNE OPARIL, M.D.

Professor of Medicine and Associate Professor of Physiology and Biophysics, University of Alabama School of Medicine. Director, Hypertension Program, Division of Cardiovascular Diseases, and Attending Cardiologist, University Hospital, Birmingham, Alabama.

Arterial Hypertension

WALTER A. ORENSTEIN, M.D.

Director, Division of Immunization, Centers for Disease Control, Atlanta, Georgia.

Immunization

ERIC A. OTTESEN, M.D.

Attending Physician, Clinical Center, National Institutes of Health, Bethesda, Maryland, and Children's Hospital National Medical Center, Washington, D.C.

Filariasis: Introduction; Lymphatic Filariasis; Tropical Eosinophilia; Loiasis; Other Filarial Infections

MICHAEL N. OXMAN, M.D.

Professor of Medicine and Pathology, University of California, San Diego, School of Medicine, La Jolla. Staff Physician, Infectious Diseases Section, Department of Veterans Affairs Medical Center, San Diego, California.

Enteroviral Diseases; Epidemic Pleurodynia; Myocarditis and Pericarditis Caused by Enteroviruses; Mucocutaneous Syndrome Caused by Enteroviruses; Acute Hemorrhagic Conjunctivitis

CHARLES Y. C. PAK, M.D.

University Distinguished Chair in Mineral Metabolism, University of Texas Health Science Center at Dallas Southwestern Medical School, Dallas, Texas.

Renal Calculi

FRANK PARKER, M.D.

Professor and Chairman, Department of Dermatology, Oregon Health Sciences University School of Medicine. Staff Physician, Oregon Health Sciences University Hospital, Portland, Oregon.

Cutaneous Manifestations of Internal Malignancy; Skin Diseases

STEPHEN G. PAUKER, M.D.

Professor of Medicine, Tufts University School of Medicine. Chief, Division of Clinical Decision Making, Department of Medicine, New England Medical Center, Boston, Massachusetts.

Clinical Decision Making

NEAL S. PENNEYS, M.D., Ph.D.

Professor of Dermatology, University of Miami School of Medicine. Attending Physician, Jackson Memorial Hospital, Miami, Florida.

Cutaneous Signs of AIDS

JOSEPH K. PERLOFF, M.D.

Streisand/American Heart Association Professor of Medicine and Pediatrics, University of California, Los Angeles, UCLA School of Medicine, Los Angeles, California.

Diseases of the Myocardium

WALTER L. PETERSON, M.D.

Professor of Medicine, University of Texas Health Science Center at Dallas Southwestern Medical School. Chief of Digestive Diseases, Department of Veterans Affairs Medical Center, Dallas, Texas.

Peptic Ulcer: Medical Therapy

THEODORE L. PHILLIPS, M.D.

Professor and Chairman, Department of Radiation Oncology, University of California, San Francisco, School of Medicine. Attending Physician, Long-Moffitt Hospitals, San Francisco; Chief, Section of Radiation Oncology, University of California Davis Hospital, Davis, California.

Radiation Injury

CLAUDE A. PIANTADOSI, M.D.

Associate Professor of Medicine, Duke University School of Medicine. Attending Physician, Duke University Hospital, Durham, North Carolina.

Physical, Chemical, and Aspiration Injuries of the Lung

F. XAVIER PI-SUNYER, M.D.

Professor of Clinical Medicine, Columbia University College of Physicians and Surgeons. Chief, Division of Endocrinology, Diabetes, and Nutrition; Director, Obesity Research Center, St. Luke's–Roosevelt Hospital Center, New York, New York.

Obesity

PHILIP A. PIZZO, M.D.

Professor of Pediatrics, Uniformed Services University of the Health Sciences F. Edward Hebert School of Medicine. Chief of Pediatrics and Head, Infectious Disease Section, National Cancer Institute, National Institutes of Health, Bethesda, Maryland.

The Compromised Host

FRED PLUM, M.D.

Anne Parrish Titzell Professor and Chairman of Neurology and Neuroscience, Cornell University Medical College. Neurologist-in-Chief, Department of Neurology, New York Hospital–Cornell Medical Center, New York, New York.

Clinical Neurologic Diagnosis; Neurologic Problems Associated with Aging; Disturbances of Consciousness and Arousal; Sustained Impairments of Consciousness; Brain Death; Brief Loss of Consciousness; Disorders of Motor Function

RICHARD L. POPP, M.D.

Professor of Medicine, Stanford University School of Medicine. Associate Chairman, Department of Medicine, Stanford University Hospital, Stanford, California.

Echocardiography

CAROL S. PORTLOCK, M.D.

Associate Professor of Clinical Medicine, Cornell University Medical College. Acting Chief, Lymphoma Service, Memorial Sloan-Kettering Cancer Center, New York, New York.

Introduction to Neoplasms of the Immune System; The Non-Hodgkin's Lymphomas

JEROME B. POSNER, M.D.

Professor of Neurology and Neuroscience, Cornell University Medical College. Attending Neurologist, Memorial Sloan-Kettering Cancer Center, New York, New York.

Nonmetastatic Effects of Cancer on the Nervous System; Clinical Neurologic Diagnosis; Episodic Loss of Motor Function; Disorders of Sensation; Mechanical Lesions of the Spine and Related Structures

RICHARD W. PRICE, M.D.

Professor and Head, Department of Neurology, University of Minnesota Medical School. Chief of Neurology Service, University of Minnesota Hospital, Minneapolis, Minnesota.

Neurologic Complications of HIV-1 Infection; Viral Infections of the Nervous System

WILLIAM A. PULSINELLI, M.D., Ph.D.

Professor of Neurology and Neuroscience, Cornell University Medical College. Attending Neurologist, New York Hospital, New York, New York.

Cerebrovascular Diseases

THOMAS C. QUINN, M.D.

Senior Investigator, National Institute of Allergy and Infectious Diseases, National Institutes of Health; Associate Professor of Medicine and International Health, Johns Hopkins Medical Institutions. Staff Physician, Johns Hopkins Hospital, Baltimore, and Clinical Center, National Institutes of Health, Bethesda, Maryland.

African Trypanosomiasis

CHARLES E. RACKLEY, M.D.

Anton and Margaret Fuisz Professor of Medicine and Director, Lipid Disorder Center, Georgetown University School of Medicine. Attending Physician, Department of Medicine, Georgetown University Medical Center, Washington, D.C.

Valvular Heart Disease

JONATHAN I. RAVDIN, M.D.

Professor and Vice Chairman, Department of Medicine, Case Western Reserve University School of Medicine. Chief, Medical Service, Department of Veterans Affairs Medical Center, Cleveland, Ohio.

Amebiasis

ROBERT W. REBAR, M.D.

George B. Riley Professor and Chairman, Department of Obstetrics and Gynecology, University of Cincinnati College of Medicine. Clinical Director, Department of Obstetrics and Gynecology, University of Cincinnati Hospital, Cincinnati, Ohio.

The Ovaries

CHARLES E. REED, M.D.

Professor of Internal Medicine, Mayo Medical School. Staff Physician, Saint Mary's and Methodist Hospitals, Rochester, Minnesota.

Drug Allergy

ROBERT R. RICH, M.D.

Professor of Microbiology and of Immunology and Medicine and Vice President and Dean of Research, Baylor College of Medicine. Attending Physician, Veterans Affairs Medical Center; Medical Staff Member, Methodist Hospital, Houston, Texas

Immune Complex Diseases

CHARLES T. RICHARDSON, M.D.

Clinical Professor of Internal Medicine, University of Texas Health Science Center at Dallas Southwestern Medical School. Attending Physician, Baylor University Medical Center, Dallas, Texas.

Peptic Ulcer: Pathogenesis; Zollinger-Ellison Syndrome

B. LAWRENCE RIGGS, M.D.

Purvis and Roberta Tabor Professor of Medical Research, Mayo Medical School, Rochester, Minnesota.

Osteoporosis

ROGER S. RITTMASTER, M.D.

Associate Professor, Dalhousie University Faculty of Medicine. Active Staff Member, Camp Hill Medical Center, Halifax, Nova Scotia, Canada.

Hirsutism

RICHARD S. RIVLIN, M.D.

Professor of Medicine, Cornell University Medical College. Head, Nutrition Research Program, Memorial Sloan-Kettering Cancer Center; Chief, Nutrition Division, New York Hospital–Cornell Medical Center; Visiting Physician, Rockefeller University Hospital, New York, New York.

Disorders of Vitamin Metabolism: Deficiencies, Metabolic Abnormalities, and Excesses

JOHN PAUL ROBERTS, M.D.

Assistant Professor of Surgery, University of California, San Francisco, School of Medicine, San Francisco, California.

Liver Transplantation

WILLIAM O. ROBERTSON, M.D.

Professor of Pediatrics, University of Washington School of Medicine. Medical Director, Washington Poison Network, Children's Hospital and Medical Center, Seattle, Washington.

Common Poisonings

WILLIAM J. ROGERS, M.D.

Professor of Medicine, University of Alabama School of Medicine. Director of Coronary Care Unit, University of Alabama Hospital, Birmingham, Alabama.

Angina Pectoris

JOHN ROSS, Jr., M.D.

Professor of Medicine, University of California, San Diego, School of Medicine, La Jolla. Head, Division of Cardiology, University of California San Diego Medical Center, San Diego, California.

Cardiac Function and Circulatory Control

RUSSELL ROSS, Ph.D.

Professor and Chairman of Pathology, University of Washington School of Medicine, Seattle, Washington.

Atherosclerosis

DAVID A. ROTTENBERG, M.D.

Director, PET Imaging Service, and Chief, Neurology Service, Veterans Administration Medical Center, Minneapolis, Minnesota.

Disorders of Intracranial Pressure

DAVID W. ROWE, M.D.

Professor of Pediatrics, University of Connecticut School of Medicine. Attending Physician, John Dempsey Hospital and University of Connecticut Health Center, Farmington, Connecticut.

Osteogenesis Imperfecta

JOHN W. ROWE, M.D.

President and Professor of Medicine and Geriatrics, Mount Sinai School of Medicine of the City University of New York. President, Mount Sinai Medical Center, New York, New York.

Aging and Geriatric Medicine

ROBERT M. RUSSELL, M.D.

Professor of Medicine and Nutrition, Tufts University Schools of Medicine and Nutrition. Staff Physician, New England Medical Center, Boston, Massachusetts.

Nutrient Requirements; Nutritional Assessment

ANGELO RUSSO, M.D., Ph.D.

Senior Investigator, National Cancer Institute, National Institutes of Health. Staff Physician, Clinical Center, National Institutes of Health, Bethesda, Maryland.

Oncologic Emergencies

MICHAEL S. SAAG, M.D.

Assistant Professor of Medicine, Division of Infectious Diseases, University of Alabama School of Medicine, and Director, University of Alabama AIDS Outpatient Clinic. Associate Director, General Clinical Research Center, and Assistant Chief, Medical Service, Veterans Administration Medical Center, Birmingham, Alabama.

Mycetoma; Dematiaceous Fungal Infections; HIV and Associated Disorders: Introduction; Prevention of HIV Infection; Renal, Cardiac, Endocrine, and Rheumatologic Manifestations of HIV Infection

R. BRADLEY SACK, M.D., Sc.D.

Professor, Department of International Health, Johns Hopkins University School of Hygiene and Public Health. Staff Physician, Department of Medicine, Johns Hopkins Hospital, Baltimore, Maryland.

The Diarrhea of Travelers

ROBERT A. SALATA, M.D.

Assistant Professor of Medicine and International Health, Case Western Reserve University School of Medicine. Attending Physician and Consultant, University Hospitals of Cleveland, Cleveland, Ohio.

Brucellosis

SYDNEY E. SALMON, M.D.

Regents Professor of Medicine, University of Arizona College of Medicine. Director, Arizona Cancer Center; Attending Physician, University Medical Center, Tucson, Arizona.

Principles of Cancer Therapy

JOHN E. SALVAGGIO, M.D.

Henderson Professor of Medicine and Vice Chancellor, Tulane University School of Medicine. Active Staff Member, Tulane University Hospital; Visiting Physician, Charity Hospital and Department of Veterans Affairs Medical Center, New Orleans, Louisiana.

Allergic Rhinitis

JAY P. SANFORD, M.D.

Professor of Medicine Emeritus and Dean Emeritus, Uniformed Services University of the Health Sciences F. Edward Hebert School of Medicine, Bethesda. Attending Physician (Infectious Diseases), Walter Reed Army Medical Center, Washington, D.C., and National Naval Medical Center, Bethesda, Maryland.

Dengue; West Nile Fever; Phlebotomus Fever; Rift Valley Fever; Alphaviruses Associated with Polyarthritis; Snake Bites

CLIFFORD B. SAPER, M.D.

William D. Mabie Professor of Neuroscience and Neurology, University of Chicago Pritzker School of Medicine. Staff Physician, University of Chicago Hospitals, Chicago, Illinois.

Autonomic Disorders and Their Management

FRED R. SATTLER, M.D.

Associate Professor of Medicine, University of Southern California School of Medicine. Coordinator, Interdisciplinary AIDS Service, Los Angeles County–University of Southern California Medical Center, Los Angeles, California. Chairman, Opportunistic Infections Committee, AIDS Clinical Trials Group, Division of AIDS, National Institutes of Allergy and Infectious Disease, National Institutes of Health.

Pulmonary Manifestations of AIDS: Special Emphasis on Pneumocystosis

DAVID T. SCADDEN, M.D.

Instructor in Medicine, Harvard Medical School. Active Staff, New England Deaconess Hospital, Boston, Massachusetts.

Hematology/Oncology in AIDS

WILLIAM SCHAFFNER, M.D.

Professor and Chairman, Department of Preventive Medicine, and Professor of Medicine (Infectious Diseases), Vanderbilt University School of Medicine. Hospital Epidemiologist, Vanderbilt University Hospital, Nashville, Tennessee.

Prevention and Control of Hospital-Acquired Infections

BRUCE F. SCHARSCHMIDT, M.D.

Professor of Medicine and Director, Division of Gastroenterology, University of California, San Francisco, School of Medicine. Attending Hematologist, Liver Transplant Service, and Attending Physician, University of California San Francisco Medical Center, San Francisco, California.

Bilirubin Metabolism and Hyperbilirubinemia; Inherited, Infiltrative, and Metabolic Disorders Involving the Liver; Acute and Chronic Hepatic Failure; Hepatic Tumors

HERBERT H. SCHAUMBURG, M.D.

Professor and Chairman, Department of Neurology, Albert Einstein College of Medicine of Yeshiva University. Director of Neurology, Montefiore Medical Center, Bronx, New York.

Diseases of the Peripheral Nervous System

LAWRENCE R. SCHILLER, M.D.

Clinical Assistant Professor of Internal Medicine, University of Texas Health Science Center at Dallas Southwestern Medical School. Director of Gastrointestinal Physiology Laboratory and Attending Physician, Baylor University Medical Center, Dallas, Texas.

Peptic Ulcer: Epidemiology, Clinical Manifestations, and Diagnosis

STEPHEN C. SCHIMPFF, M.D.

Professor of Medicine, Pharmacology, and Oncology, University of Maryland School of Medicine. Executive Vice President, University of Maryland Medical System, Baltimore, Maryland.

Diseases Caused by Pseudomonads

THEODORE R. SCHROCK, M.D.

Professor of Surgery, University of California, San Francisco, School of Medicine, San Francisco, California.

Diseases of the Rectum and Anus

H. RALPH SCHUMACHER, Jr., M.D.

Professor of Medicine and Acting Chief, Rheumatology Section, University of Pennsylvania School of Medicine. Director, Arthritis-Immunology Center, Veterans Affairs Medical Center, Philadelphia, Pennsylvania.

Crystal Deposition Arthropathies; Relapsing Polychondritis; Multifocal Fibrosclerosis

BENJAMIN D. SCHWARTZ, M.D., Ph.D.

Professor of Medicine (Rheumatology), Washington University School of Medicine. Chief, Division of Rheumatology, Jewish Hospital of St. Louis; Associate Attending Physician, Barnes Hospital, St. Louis, Missouri.

The Major Histocompatibility Complex and Disease Susceptibility

CHARLES H. SCOGGIN, M.D.

President, Somatogen, Broomfield, Colorado.

Pulmonary Neoplasms

CHARLES R. SCRIVER, M.D.C.M., F.R.S.C.

Professor of Biology, Human Genetics, and Pediatrics, McGill University Faculty of Medicine. Physician and Director, DeBelle Laboratory for Biomedical Genetics, Montreal Children's Hospital, Montreal, Quebec, Canada.

Hyperaminoaciduria; The Hyperphenylalaninemias

S. K. K. SEAH, M.D., Ph.D.

Associate Professor of Medicine, McGill University Faculty of Medicine. Attending Physician, Montreal General Hospital, Montreal, Quebec, Canada.

Hermaphroditic Flukes

MARGRETTA R. SEASHORE, M.D.

Professor of Human Genetics and Pediatrics, Yale University School of Medicine. Attending Physician, Yale–New Haven Hospital, New Haven, Connecticut.

Genetic Counseling

STANTON SEGAL, M.D.

Professor of Pediatrics and Medicine, University of Pennsylvania School of Medicine. Director, Division of Biochemical Development and Molecular Diseases, Children's Hospital of Philadelphia, Philadelphia, Pennsylvania.

Galactosemia

ROBERT M. SENIOR, M.D.

Dorothy R. and Hubert C. Moog Professor of Pulmonary Diseases in Medicine, Department of Medicine, Washington University School of Medicine. Director, Respiratory and Critical Care Division, Department of Medicine, Jewish Hospital of St. Louis, St. Louis, Missouri.

Pulmonary Embolism; Fat Embolism Syndrome

F. JOHN SERVICE, M.D., Ph.D.

Professor of Medicine, Mayo Medical School. Consultant, Division of Endocrinology and Metabolism, Department of Internal Medicine, Mayo Clinic, Rochester, Minnesota.

Hypoglycemic Disorders

RALPH SHABETAI, M.D., F.R.C.P.(Edin)

Professor of Medicine, University of California, San Diego, School of Medicine, La Jolla. Chief of Cardiology, Department of Veterans Affairs Medical Center, San Diego, California.

Diseases of the Pericardium

GEORGE M. SHAW, M.D., Ph.D.

Associate Professor of Medicine, Division of Hematology and Oncology, University of Alabama School of Medicine, Birmingham, Alabama.

Biology of Human Immunodeficiency Viruses

JOHN N. SHEAGREN, M.D.

Professor of Medicine, University of Illinois College of Medicine at Chicago. Chairman, Department of Internal Medicine, Illinois Masonic Medical Center, Chicago, Illinois.

Shock Syndromes Related to Sepsis; Staphylococcal Infections

DEAN SHEPPARD, M.D.

Associate Professor of Medicine, University of California, San Francisco, School of Medicine. Attending Physician, Chest Service, San Francisco General Hospital Medical Center, San Francisco, California.

Occupational Pulmonary Disorders

ROBERT E. SHOPE, M.D.

Professor of Epidemiology, Yale University School of Medicine, New Haven, Connecticut.

Arthropod-Borne Viral Diseases: Introduction; Viral Hemorrhagic Fevers

JONAS A. SHULMAN, M.D.

Professor of Medicine (Infectious Diseases), Emory University School of Medicine. Chief of Medicine, Crawford Long Hospital of Emory University, Atlanta, Georgia.

Anthrax

MARC SHUMAN, M.D.

Professor of Medicine and Associate Director, Cancer Research Institute, University of California, San Francisco, School of Medicine. Attending Physician, Moffitt-Long Hospitals, San Francisco, California.

Hemorrhagic Disorders: Abnormalities of Platelet and Vascular Function

MARK SIEGLER, M.D.

Professor of Medicine, University of Chicago Pritzker School of Medicine; Director, Center for Clinical Medical Ethics, University of Chicago. Attending and Consulting Physician, University of Chicago Hospitals, Chicago, Illinois.

Clinical Ethics in the Practice of Medicine

DONALD H. SILBERBERG, M.D.

Professor and Chairman, Department of Neurology, University of Pennsylvania School of Medicine. Chief of Service, Department of Neurology, Hospital of the University of Pennsylvania, Philadelphia, Pennsylvania.

The Demyelinating Diseases

ROGER P. SIMON, M.D.

Professor, Department of Neurology, University of California, San Francisco, School of Medicine. Chief, Neurology Service, San Francisco General Hospital Medical Center, San Francisco, California.

Parameningeal Infections; Neurosyphilis

FREDERICK R. SINGER, M.D.

Professor of Medicine in Residence, University of California, Los Angeles, UCLA School of Medicine. Director, Bone Center, Cedars-Sinai Medical Center, Los Angeles, California.

Paget's Disease of Bone

PETER A. SINGER, M.D., F.R.C.P.C.

Assistant Professor of Medicine and Associate Director, Centre for Bioethics, University of Toronto Faculty of Medicine. Attending Physician, Toronto Hospital (Toronto Western Division), Toronto, Ontario, Canada

Clinical Ethics in the Practice of Medicine

EDUARDO SLATOPOLSKY, M.D.

Professor of Medicine, Washington University School of Medicine. Director, Chromalloy American Kidney Center; Attending Physician, Barnes Hospital; Consultant in Nephrology, Jewish Hospital of St. Louis, St. Louis, Missouri.

Renal Osteodystrophy

MARVIN H. SLEISENGER, M.D.

Professor of Medicine and Director, Cancer Research Institute, University of California, San Francisco, School of Medicine. Attending Physician, Moffitt-Long Hospitals; Consulting Physician, Department of Veterans Affairs Medical Center, San Francisco, California.

Miscellaneous Inflammatory Diseases of the Intestine

WILLIAM S. SLY, M.D.

Professor and Chairman, Edward A. Doisy Department of Biochemistry and Molecular Biology, St. Louis University School of Medicine. Active Staff Member, Cardinal Glennon Children's Hospital, St. Louis, Missouri.

The Mucopolysaccharidoses

LLOYD H. SMITH, Jr., M.D.

Professor of Medicine and Associate Dean, University of California, San Francisco, School of Medicine, San Francisco, California.

Medicine as an Art; Primary Hyperoxaluria; The Hyperprolinemias and Hydroxyprolinemia; Diseases of the Urea Cycle; Branched-Chain Aminoaciduria; Disorders of Pyrimidine Metabolism; Phosphorus Deficiency and Hypophosphatemia; Disorders of Magnesium Metabolism

THOMAS W. SMITH, M.D.

Professor of Medicine, Harvard Medical School. Chief, Cardiovascular Division, Brigham and Women's Hospital, Boston, Massachusetts.

Approach to the Patient with Cardiovascular Disease; Heart Failure

WILLIAM J. SNAPE, Jr., M.D.

Professor of Medicine, University of California, Los Angeles, UCLA School of Medicine. Chief of Gastroenterology, Harbor-UCLA Medical Center, Los Angeles, California.

Disorders of Gastrointestinal Motility

ROSEMARY SOAVE, M.D.

Assistant Professor of Medicine and Public Health, Cornell University Medical College. Associate Attending Physician, New York Hospital–Cornell Medical Center, New York, New York.

Cryptosporidiosis

BURTON E. SOBEL, M.D.

Tobias and Hortense Lewin Distinguished Professor in Cardiovascular Disease, Washington University School of Medicine. Director, Cardiovascular Division, Washington University School of Medicine and Barnes and Wohl Hospitals, St. Louis, Missouri.

Acute Myocardial Infarction

ANDREW H. SOLL, M.D.

Professor of Medicine, University of California, Los Angeles, UCLA School of Medicine. Chief of Gastroenterology, Wadsworth Veterans Administration Medical Center, Los Angeles, California.

Gastritis

ROGER D. SOLOWAY, M.D.

Marie B. Gale Professor of Medicine and Acting Chairman, Department of Internal Medicine, University of Texas Medical School at Galveston, Galveston, Texas.

Diseases of the Gallbladder and Bile Ducts

P. FREDERICK SPARLING, M.D.

Professor and Chairman, Department of Medicine, University of North Carolina at Chapel Hill School of Medicine. Chair, Department of Medicine, University of North Carolina Hospitals, Chapel Hill, North Carolina.

Sexually Transmitted Diseases

ALLEN M. SPIEGEL, M.D.

Chief, Molecular Pathophysiology Branch, National Institute of Diabetes and Digestive and Kidney Diseases, National Institutes of Health, Bethesda, Maryland.

The Parathyroid Glands, Hypercalcemia, and Hypocalcemia

ALAN M. STAMM, M.D.

Associate Professor of Medicine, University of Alabama School of Medicine. Attending Physician, University of Alabama Hospital, Birmingham, Alabama.

Listeriosis

WALTER E. STAMM, M.D.

Professor of Medicine, University of Washington School of Medicine. Head, Infectious Disease Division, Harborview Medical Center, Seattle, Washington.

Diseases Caused by Chlamydiae

ALFRED D. STEINBERG, M.D.

Chief, Cellular Immunology, Arthritis and Rheumatism Branch, National Institute of Arthritis and Musculoskeletal and Skin Diseases, National Institutes of Health. Attending Physician, Clinical Center, National Institutes of Health, Bethesda, Maryland.

Systemic Lupus Erythematosus

WILLIAM M. STEINBERG, M.D.

Professor of Medicine, George Washington University School of Medicine and Health Sciences. Staff Physician, Division of Gastroenterology, George Washington University Hospital, Washington, D.C.

Pancreatitis

DAVID A. STEVENS, M.D.

Professor of Medicine, Stanford University School of Medicine, Stanford. Chief, Division of Infectious Diseases, Department of Medicine, Santa Clara Valley Medical Center, San Jose. Principal Investigator, Infectious Disease Research Laboratory, California Institute for Medical Research, San Jose, California.

Aspergillosis; Zygomycosis

DAVID P. STEVENS, M.D.

Scott R. Inkley Professor of General Internal Medicine and Vice Chairman, Department of Medicine, Case Western Reserve University School of Medicine. Chief, Division of General Internal Medicine, University Hospitals of Cleveland, Cleveland, Ohio.

Giardiasis; Other Protozoan Diseases

DANIEL P. STITES, M.D.

Professor and Vice Chairman, Department of Laboratory Medicine, University of California, San Francisco, School of Medicine. Staff Physician, University of California San Francisco Medical Center, San Francisco, California.

Diseases of the Thymus

RAINER STORB, M.D.

Professor of Medicine, University of Washington School of Medicine. Head, Program in Transplantation Biology, and Member, Fred Hutchinson Cancer Research Center, Seattle, Washington.

Bone Marrow Transplantation

GORDON J. STREWLER, M.D.

Associate Professor of Medicine, University of California, San Francisco, School of Medicine. Chief, Endocrine Unit, Department of Veterans Affairs Medical Center, San Francisco, California.

Osteonecrosis, Osteosclerosis, and Other Disorders of Bone

WADI N. SUKI, M.D.

Professor of Medicine and of Molecular Physiology and Biophysics, and Chief, Renal Section, Department of Medicine, Baylor College of Medicine. Senior Attending Physician and Chief, Renal Service, Methodist Hospital, Houston, Texas.

Hereditary Chronic Nephropathies

MORTON N. SWARTZ, M.D.

Professor of Medicine, Harvard Medical School. Chief, James Jackson Firm Medical Services; Member, Infectious Disease Unit, Massachusetts General Hospital, Boston, Massachusetts.

Bacterial Meningitis; Meningococcal Disease; Infections Caused by Haemophilus Species

NORMAN TALAL, M.D.

Professor of Medicine and Microbiology and Head, Division of Clinical Immunology, University of Texas Medical School at San Antonio. Head, Division of Clinical Immunology, Medical Center Hospital; Chief, Division of Clinical Immunology, Audie L. Murphy Veterans Hospital, San Antonio, Texas.

Sjögren's Syndrome

CLIFFORD TASMAN-JONES, M.B., Ch.B., F.R.C.P., F.R.A.C.P.

Head, Section of Gastroenterology and Human Nutrition, University of Auckland Medical School. Senior Physician and Gastroenterologist, Auckland Hospital, Auckland, New Zealand.

Disturbances of Trace Mineral Metabolism

RICHARD C. THIRLBY, M.D.

Clinical Assistant Professor of Surgery, University of Washington School of Medicine. Attending Surgeon, Virginia Mason Medical Center, Seattle, Washington.

Peptic Ulcer: Surgical Therapy

PHILLIP P. TOSKES, M.D.

Professor of Medicine, University of Florida College of Medicine. Director, Division of Gastroenterology, Hepatology and Nutrition, Shands Hospital of the University of Florida College of Medicine; Chief, Gastroenterology Section, Veterans Administration Medical Center, Gainesville, Florida.

Malabsorption

GARY J. TUCKER, M.D.

Professor and Chairman, Department of Psychiatry and Behavioral Sciences, University of Washington School of Medicine. Staff Physician, University of Washington Medical Center, Seattle, Washington.

Psychiatric Disorders in Medical Practice

J. BLAKE TYRRELL, M.D.

Clinical Professor of Medicine and Associate Director, Metabolic Research Unit, University of California, San Francisco, School of Medicine. Director, Endocrine Clinic, Moffitt-Long Hospitals, San Francisco, California.

Disorders of the Adrenal Cortex

JOUNI UITTO, M.D., Ph.D.

Professor and Chairman, Department of Dermatology, Jefferson Medical College of Thomas Jefferson University. Staff Physician, Thomas Jefferson University Hospital, Philadelphia, Pennsylvania.

Pseudoxanthoma Elasticum

JACK A. VENNES, M.D.

Professor of Medicine, University of Minnesota Medical School. Staff Physician, University of Minnesota Hospitals and Clinics, Minneapolis, Minnesota.

Gastrointestinal Endoscopy

NICHOLAS A. VICK, M.D.

Professor of Neurology, Northwestern University Medical School, Chicago. Head, Division of Neurology, Evanston Hospital, Evanston, Illinois.

Intracranial Tumors and States of Altered Intracranial Pressure

JONATHAN D. VICTOR, M.D., Ph.D.

Professor of Neurology and Neuroscience, Cornell University Medical College. Attending Neurologist, New York Hospital, and Associate Attending Physician, Hospital for Special Surgery, New York, New York.

Neurologic Diagnostic Procedures

JOHN E. VOLANAKIS, M.D.

Anna Lois Wares Chair of Medicine in Rheumatology and Professor of Medicine, Microbiology, and Pathology, University of Alabama School of Medicine, Birmingham, Alabama.

Complement

FRANCIS A. WALDVOGEL, M.D.

Professor of Medicine, University of Geneva. Chairman, Department of Medicine, and Physician-in-Chief, Clinique Medical Therapeutique, University Hospital, Geneva, Switzerland.

Osteomyelitis

BRUCE D. WALKER, M.D.

Assistant Professor of Medicine, Harvard Medical School. Attending Physician, Infectious Disease Unit, Massachusetts General Hospital, Boston, Massachusetts.

Immunology Related to AIDS

SUSAN D. WALL, M.D.

Associate Professor of Radiology, University of California, San Francisco, School of Medicine. Assistant Chief of Radiology, Department of Veterans Affairs Medical Center, San Francisco, California.

Diagnostic Imaging Procedures in Gastroenterology

DAVID C. WARNOCK, M.D.

Professor of Medicine and Physiology, University of Alabama School of Medicine, Birmingham, Alabama.

Chronic Renal Failure

STANLEY J. WATSON, Ph.D., M.D.

Professor of Psychiatry, Mental Health Research Institute, University of Michigan, Ann Arbor, Michigan.

The Endorphin Family of Opioid Peptides: Biochemistry, Anatomy, and Physiology

RICHARD A. WEISIGER, M.D., Ph.D.

Associate Professor, Department of Medicine and Liver Center, University of California, San Francisco, School of Medicine. Staff Physician, University of California San Francisco Medical Center and Moffitt Hospital, San Francisco, California.

Hepatic Metabolism in Liver Disease; Laboratory Tests in Liver Disease

GERALD WEISSMANN, M.D.

Professor of Medicine and Director, Division of Rheumatology, New York University School of Medicine. Attending Physician in Medicine, Tisch and Bellevue Hospitals, and Consulting Physician, Veterans Administration Medical Center, New York, New York.

NSAID's: Aspirin and Aspirin-like Drugs; Tissue Injury in Rheumatic Diseases

PETER F. WELLER, M.D.

Associate Professor of Medicine, Harvard Medical School. Associate Physician, Beth Israel and Brigham and Women's Hospitals, Boston, Massachusetts.

Eosinophilic Syndromes

RICHARD J. WHITLEY, M.D.

Professor of Pediatrics, Microbiology, and Medicine, University of Alabama School of Medicine. Staff, Children's Hospital, Birmingham, Alabama.

Antiviral Therapy; Herpes Simplex Virus Infections

RICHARD D. WILLIAMS, M.D.

Professor and Chairman, Department of Urology, University of Iowa College of Medicine. Chairman, Department of Urology, University of Iowa Hospitals and Clinics, Iowa City, Iowa.

Anomalies of the Urinary Tract; Tumors of the Kidney, Ureter, and Bladder

T. FRANKLIN WILLIAMS, M.D.

Director, National Institute on Aging, National Institutes of Health, Bethesda, Maryland.

Management of Common Problems in the Elderly

JOHN WILLIAMSON, B.Sc., M.B., B.S., D.A.(Melb)

Senior Lecturer, Department of Anaesthesia and Intensive Care, and Hyperbaric Medicine, Adelaide University Medical School. Director of Hyperbaric Medicine, Royal Adelaide Hospital, Adelaide, South Australia.

Venomous and Poisonous Marine Animals

SIDNEY J. WINAWER, M.D.

Professor of Clinical Medicine, Cornell University Medical College. Chief, Gastroenterology Service; Head, Laboratory for Gastrointestinal Cancer Research and World Health Organization Collaborating Center for the Prevention of Colorectal Cancer, Memorial Sloan-Kettering Cancer Center, New York, New York.

Neoplasms of the Stomach

SHELDON M. WOLFF, M.D.

Endicott Professor and Chairman, Department of Medicine, Tufts University School of Medicine. Physician-in-Chief, New England Medical Center, Boston, Massachusetts.

The Vasculitic Syndromes; Polyarteritis Nodosa Group

EMANUEL WOLINSKY, M.D.

Professor Emeritus, Medicine and Pathology, Case Western Reserve University School of Medicine. Head, Division of Microbiology, and Physician, Infectious Disease Division, Department of Medicine, Metropolitan Medical Center, Cleveland, Ohio.

Tuberculosis; Other Mycobacterioses

JERRY S. WOLINSKY, M.D.

Professor of Neurology, University of Texas Medical School at Houston. Attending Neurologist, Hermann Hospital, Houston, Texas.

Neurologic Disorders Associated with Altered Immunity or Unexplained Host-Parasitic Alterations

ROBERT L. WORTMANN, M.D.

Professor and Vice Chairman, Department of Medicine, Medical College of Wisconsin. Chief of Medical Service, Clement J. Zablocki Veterans Administration Medical Center, Milwaukee, Wisconsin.

Polymyositis

DANIEL G. WRIGHT, M.D.

Professor of Medicine, Uniformed Services University of the Health Sciences F. Edward Hebert School of Medicine, Bethesda, Maryland. Chief, Department of Hematology, Walter Reed Army Institute of Research, Washington, D.C.

Familial Mediterranean Fever

TERESA L. WRIGHT, B.M., B.S.

Assistant Professor of Medicine, University of California, San Francisco, School of Medicine. Staff Physician, Department of Veterans Affairs Medical Center; Attending Physician, University of California San Francisco Medical Center, San Francisco, California.

Parasitic, Bacterial, Fungal, and Granulomatous Liver Disease

JAMES B. WYNGAARDEN, M.D.

Professor of Medicine and Associate Vice-Chancellor for Health Affairs, Duke University School of Medicine. Physician, Duke University Hospital, Durham, North Carolina.

Medicine as a Science; The Use and Interpretation of Laboratory-Derived Data; Human Heredity; Inborn Errors of Metabolism; Metabolic Diseases: Introduction; Alcaptonuria; Gout

ROBERT YARCHOAN, M.D.

Senior Investigator, Medicine Branch, National Cancer Institute, National Institutes of Health. Attending Physician, Clinical Center, National Institutes of Health, Bethesda, Maryland.

Treatment of AIDS and Related Disorders

LOWELL S. YOUNG, M.D.

Clinical Professor of Medicine, University of California, San Francisco, School of Medicine. Chief, Division of Infectious Diseases, Pacific Presbyterian Medical Center, San Francisco, California.

Antimicrobial Therapy

NEAL S. YOUNG, M.D.

Chief, Clinical Services, and Head, Cell Biology Section, Clinical Hematology Branch, National Heart, Lung, and Blood Institute, National Institutes of Health, Bethesda, Maryland.

Aplastic Anemia and Related Bone Marrow Failure Syndromes

BARRY L. ZARET, M.D.

Robert W. Berliner Professor of Medicine, Professor of Diagnostic Radiology, and Chief of Cardiovascular Medicine, Yale University School of Medicine. Chief of Cardiology, Yale–New Haven Hospital, New Haven, Connecticut.

Nuclear Cardiology

ELIZABETH J. ZIEGLER, M.D.

Professor of Medicine, University of California, San Diego, School of Medicine, La Jolla. Attending Physician, University of California San Diego Medical Center, San Diego, California.

Extraintestinal Infections Caused by Enteric Bacteria

DOUGLAS P. ZIPES, M.D.

Professor of Medicine, Indiana University School of Medicine. Attending Physician, Indiana University Medical Center, Wishard Memorial Hospital, and Richard L. Roudebush Veterans Administration Medical Center, Indianapolis, Indiana.

Sudden Cardiac Death

CONTENTS

(Detailed table of contents begins on page xxxi.)

PART XX INFECTIOUS DISEASES

Section One   Introduction

Section Two   Bacterial Diseases

Streptococcal Diseases

Endocarditis

Staphylococcal Infections

Bacterial Meningitis, Morton N. Swartz

Osteomyelitis

Whooping Cough

Diphtheria

Clostridial Diseases, John G. Bartlett

Anaerobic Bacteria

Enteric Infections

Other Bacterial Infections

Diseases Due to Mycobacteria

Sexually Transmitted Diseases, P. Frederick Sparling

Spirochetal Diseases Other Than Syphilis

Diseases Caused by Chlamydiae, Walter E. Stamm

Rickettsial Diseases, Richard B. Hornick

Zoonoses

Section Three   Viral Diseases

Viral Infections of the Respiratory Tract

PART XXI   HIV AND ASSOCIATED DISORDERS

PART XXII   DISEASES CAUSED BY PROTOZOA AND METAZOA

PART XXIII   NEUROLOGY

COLOR PLATES

The hematology color photomicrographs (which are used with permission) are from the American Society of Hematology Slide Bank, third edition. This edition is supported in part by an educational grant from Ortho Biotech. Specific contributors to these four plates are:

James R. McArthur, *Director*   Marion Dugdale   Mudite Petersons
John R. Bolles, *Assistant Director*   Eugene P. Ewing   Jean Shafer
Marguerite Candler Ballard   Joseph Fanning   Claud Sultan
Ann Bell   N. Frickhofen   Marilyn Winkler
Yvonne Betson   Elaine Jaffe   M. M. Wintrobe
Richard Brunning   Charles L. Johnston   Rose Yoda
L. W. Diggs   Pamela Kidd   Neal S. Young
                                                               Dorothea Zucker-Franklin

Information about slide orders can be obtained from Dr. James R. McArthur.

The following code refers to the approximate magnification of the hematology color photomicrographs.

(L.P.) = Low-power magnification (dry)

(H.P.) = High-power magnification (dry)

(L.O.) = Low oil immersion magnification ($\sim$800–1000$\times$)

(H.O.) = High oil immersion magnification ($\sim$1500$\times$)

(V.H.O.) = Very high oil magnification (significantly in excess of 1500$\times$)

CECIL
TEXTBOOK
of
MEDICINE

PART I
MEDICINE AS A LEARNED AND HUMANE PROFESSION

As originally conceived by Russell Cecil in the 1920's, this textbook aims to provide both an overview of internal medicine and an encyclopedic and up-to-date reference that incorporates recent research. Its audience has grown over the years, ranging from medical students to seasoned practitioners. Although the essays that follow are addressed primarily to the former group, the editors hope that all our readers may find them worthy of at least passing attention. All readers of this book deserve a broader perspective of medicine than is offered by its subject matter alone.

1 Internal Medicine and Today's Internist

J. Claude Bennett

QUESTIONS/PLEAS OF THE PATIENT

"How can I find a good doctor?"

"How can I find a good doctor whom I can afford?"

"How can I find a good doctor who cares about me as a person?"

"How can I find a good doctor who will take the time to listen and understand?"

People who need medical care ask these questions throughout the world every day. They ask them because they face a health care system that is scientifically complex, organizationally over-loaded, and generally not oriented to the patient as a *person*. When an individual first becomes ill, regardless of the symptoms, he or she needs most someone who seems to say, "I am a good doctor; I charge a reasonable amount for my services; I care about you, the patient; and I will take the time to listen and understand."

A prominent teacher/physician in a major medical center taught his students to "listen to the patient and he will tell you what is wrong, and he will tell you what he needs." Having found a physician who answers so profoundly to their needs, some patients are extremely grateful—but most are utterly over-whelmed. With the discovery of that relationship, the difference between a superb technician and a true physician really becomes evident to the patient. That physician/teacher was a scholarly gentleman with deep scientific insight and an active and stimulating clinical and research practice. Unfortunately, he developed crippling rheumatoid arthritis in the midst of his career. Beyond question, his own disease sensitized him to the complex mix of expectations, needs, fears, and appreciation that patients feel when facing a physical-mental trial while at the same time looking for that perfect physician to help them. Patients flocked to this doctor—not just for his accurate diagnoses, his correct therapies, or even his warmth, but for the intellect he expressed and the sheer joy of living that he extended in every encounter with another human being. He had a Shakespearean grasp of the qualities of being human and an uncommon ability to transmit love and respect for his fellow human beings. He exhibited the ideal all physicians should emulate. Many readers know a phy-

sician with these characteristics; all should seek to know one and to develop their own professional persona so that human qualities are not lost to technical acumen.

THE SCIENTIFIC AND TECHNOLOGIC BACKGROUND OF A "GOOD DOCTOR"

Since Flexner issued his famous report in 1910, American medical education has striven toward the development of a strong scientific base. This intellectual prerequisite, therefore, has become an integral part of premedical, undergraduate, graduate, and, indeed, continuing medical education. Biomedical science is fundamental to understanding disease, making diagnoses, developing new therapies, and appreciating the complexities and contributions of new technologies. Physicians cannot be satisfied with simply knowing that a certain form of therapy works 80 to 90 per cent of the time. They must understand the basic physiology and pharmacology of any approach they use. They must possess the intellectual tools to follow reports of current research in medical journals so that they can continue to grasp the newest and latest approaches, no matter how complicated the field may become. That is why, in a textbook of medicine like this, strong emphasis is given to how things work, what goes amiss when pathologic processes ensue, and what effect a given therapy has in correcting that defect. We seek to create within the minds of our readers a yearning for a greater depth of understanding and a continuing commitment to stay at the frontier of scientific knowledge. These are, in fact, among the hallmarks of a professional in any scientific field.

We are moving into an era when pharmacotherapeutic agents are no longer merely wonders of organic chemistry, but increasingly often are biologic products. Some of these are isolated from nature; others are developed by recombinant DNA technology. On the horizon is the availability of a true replacement or supplement for defective or deficient biochemical constituents of the body. No physician can with intellectual honesty use these new classes of agents without fully understanding their action, their meaning, and their potential side effects. The diagnostic and therapeutic contributions and potential, in clinical situations, of biocompatible prosthetic devices, nuclear magnetic resonance spectroscopy, high-frequency laser beams, and so on through developments not yet conceived, can be appreciated only by the mind that is disciplined in fundamental science.

THE ORGANIZATION AND FINANCING OF TODAY'S MEDICINE

Patients, as well as their representatives in government, industry, and managed-care organizations, are concerned about the rising cost of medical care. The total bill for health care in America now rises at a rate of about 10 per cent per year, an increase that seems to continue unabated. Federal legislation instituting diagnosis-related groups (DRG's) has clearly moderated the rise of hospital costs, but physician costs continue to rise at an ever-increasing rate. Every student of medicine should ask if this is realistic. Is it sustainable? Is it defensible? What will be the limits? Patients already ask, "Can I really afford the best doctors in the most prestigious practices, in the most famous medical centers?" "Can I afford to be referred to a subspecialist?" "Can I afford to be out of work and in the hospital?" "Can I afford to pay my rising insurance premiums?" "How much deductible on my insurance can I afford?" Worse yet, an increasing number of patients have to make choices between seeking medical and dental care and getting food, clothing, shelter, and other essentials of daily living. These issues have become major concerns in American households and clearly represent one of the most disturbing weaknesses in our economy, of which now nearly 12 per cent (by annual gross national product) is devoted to health care, up from 8 per cent in 1975.

Over the last two to three decades it has been a goal of our nation to promote ever-increasing quality and cost-effectiveness of health care for all. Unfortunately, we have failed miserably. The United States spends more per capita on health care than any other nation in the world. Yet in the major indices of health our population ranks nineteenth! At the same time we continue to see a wasteful maldistribution of physicians both by specialty and geographically and a growing number of medically indigent and medically uninsured people in our nation. Somehow, the costs of what we are trying to achieve—even though the goal is commendable—are not being placed in proper perspective by the medical profession, health-care managers, and representatives of the people in order to provide suitable care for all. Unfortunately, in the present system the real needs of the populace are not always met by affordable services. At the same time, over-utilization of medical services may be the very engine that drives up the total cost of health care delivery. With the passage of the Medicare program for the elderly and the Medicaid plan for the poor by Congress in 1965, we had hoped as a nation that we were moving toward a more just and efficient system. In fact, the opposite has been the trend. This societal goal must now be readdressed, reformulated, and restructured in terms of modern needs, reflecting fairly and fully measured cost/benefit ratios for every form of medical service.

Medical professionals often attribute overutilization to patient behavior. In fact, however, physicians control 70 per cent of health expenditures. A few patients with hypochondriasis, for example, may visit physicians too often, and many older patients may seek medical help at times when a friendly, reassuring chat is their real desire, but in the final analysis utilization of the health care system is in the hands of physicians. Ironically, although physician competence is often equated to mastery of expensive techniques and technologies, physicians are actually at their professional best when listening to the patient and respond-ing to what they hear and see with medicine's most comprehen-sive armamentarium. Overutilization, when it occurs, is thus most likely to be our fault as physicians. Our responsibility as professionals is to be absolutely certain that our errors in this direction are driven by well-founded concern for the health of our patients, not by the financial interests of our practices or the hospitals where we work.

Individual physicians, then, must take a personal and profes-sional interest in the control of health care costs—not only because it is right for the nation, but because it is right for the patient. In our litigious society, a legalistically defensive approach to medical practice has become too prevalent. The conditions that engender this tendency must be altered. Physicians must use all of their diagnostic skills to focus on the very best approach to medical diagnosis and therapy and to steer away from unnec-essary use or repetition of expensive procedures such as computed tomography, magnetic resonance imaging, and cardiac catheter-ization. The physician must use intellect—scientific knowledge and analytical skills—to best serve the patient without inundating the system with unnecessary costs and the patient with a financial burden he simply cannot continue to bear.

Costs can be controlled only if physicians are convinced of the need and are willing to participate in providing this vital service. One aspect of this control is attention to various possible means of health care finance, including prepaid plans, preferred provider organizations, health maintenance organizations, and other man-aged care systems. All of these must be carefully explored with a view to making health care accessible where it is most needed. Clearly, multiple tools and programs may be necessary, but they should not be thrust upon the patient simply to satisfy doctrines of free enterprise. To provide the best health care in a finite economy we need systems that provide such care in the most efficient way, regardless of the payment scheme.

Another aspect of our cost-control job is to support and participate in research on outcomes, aiming toward systematic evaluation of cost-effectiveness of the medical procedures we choose in the light of *all* the interests of our patient. For example, we do not know why treatment of prostatic hypertrophy is more commonly medical in some parts of the nation, surgical in others. Why does the incidence of caesarean sections vary so widely? The costs and benefits of coronary angioplasty versus bypass surgery remain obscure. Every year *billions* of dollars are spent as a result of clinical decisions that may hinge on these or similar issues. Physicians must involve themselves in the processes of change with an eye first to the individual patient and then to society.

THOSE WHO CARE

"How can I find a good doctor who cares about me as a person?"

When speaking of caring, one has to define specifically what is meant. A physician can diagnose and prescribe in a technically correct and scientific but insensitive way, and the patient may be made better—even cured. On the other hand, when the patient asks the question, "Does my physician really care?" the patient means, "Does it matter to the physician what happens to me? Does my doctor show sensitivity and compassion beyond the mere technical qualities of medicine?" It is in this sense that we address ourselves to the nature of those who care.

It may seem odd to talk about caring as a skill, but in a real sense it is just that. Those involved in the education of students realize that at least some forms of compassion have to be learned. The developing physician must see such traits in action in order to acquire and apply them in interaction with patients and their families. Sometimes this involves *learning how* to demonstrate compassion. Kahlil Gibran has taught us, "You give but little when you give of your possessions—it is when you give of yourself that you truly give." Giving of ourselves—with ease, with grace, and with meaning—is for most of us an acquired skill. Sometimes it involves a deep sense of reawakening within, to bring out an innate sensitivity and compassion that perhaps has not expressed itself since childhood. At other times, learning to care may involve a complete transformation of behavior and attitudes toward people, particularly those who are not from our own cultural background. Many believe that the greatest responsibility in medical education today is to foster compassion within the student of medicine.

To receive medical care, patients must trust their bodies and their very lives to physicians, and so to be in an honest position to give medical care, physicians must earn such radical trust. Mere technical treatment of disease does not suffice. Patients must be able reasonably to believe that their physicians care about them in an extraordinarily personal way. This exchange of care for trust, while not identical to friendship or love, is equally binding. From it develops an interdependence that is far from unwholesome; rather, it potentiates care and promotes healing. Our late twentieth century sophistication and technologic orien-tation have too often cost us warmth, humor, and humanity, leaving us in social isolation. We do far better as professionals to err on the side of being human with our patients than to try to play *deus ex machina*, the god from the machine.

THE SOCIAL RESPONSIBILITIES AND HUMANISTIC QUALITIES OF "THE GOOD DOCTOR"

The patient says, "Take charge, make me well, help me feel comfortable, show me compassion, listen to my problems and I will give you trust." Dag Hammarskjöld reminds us of "the humility which comes from others having faith in you" (*Markings*, 1965). The natural outcome of this giving and receiving of trust is that the physician must accept some degree of obligation to the patient. Of course, the patient, if able, keeps some respon-sibility for the healing process, but the physician must be willing to answer the patient's needs, however demanding, however changing, however at times unreasonable or falsely perceived. Generalists in internal medicine undertake a long-term commit-ment to a patient's care. They are reminded daily that this commitment continues beyond a particularly insightful diagnosis or the completion of an endoscopic procedure: that the patient still needs care when the numbers are back from the most recent cardiac catheterization or when the final stitch is completed in a complex procedure and the patient is rolled from the operating suite. The internist continues to care for and nurture the patient through the whole process of healing in a way that requires enormous skill in close personal interaction.

Help with Family Interactions

The woman who comes into her physician's office with a history of fatigue, listlessness, inability to sleep, and irritability may be describing the early symptoms of a morbid disease. She may, however, be showing signs of depression secondary to her inability to cope any longer with an alcoholic husband, with a teenage son addicted to cocaine, or with an elderly mother for whom she must care. The wise physician considers organic pathology but also realizes that presenting symptoms may be only part of what is really troubling the patient. This requires an unusual sensitivity and an ability to pursue in a cautious, understanding, and careful way and to listen to the concerns and needs the patient describes—traits, again, that can and must be developed and practiced. The physician's role is to help the patient understand the connections between unpleasant situations, emotional disturbances, and organic symptoms. Sometimes patients are helped simply by understanding those relationships and being aware that the doctor appreciates them and reassures, listens with a sympathetic ear, and seldom advises in a direct way, but does express concern. In earlier days, when most medical care was delivered at home, the physician was quickly made aware of living situations and family interactions—if he or she did not already know the entire family and their circumstances. Today when the patient comes to the office, generally alone and certainly out of socioeconomic context, it is much more difficult to perceive what is going on. The physician must exercise a much greater degree of skill and understanding in exploring family interrelationships during a history and physical examination or in an even shorter visit.

Help with Obtaining Necessary Additional Professional Services

The warm and intimate relationship that any patient seeks is not one that a typical patient can have with many physicians at the same time. The internist must demonstrate a variety of skills, attitudes, and abilities and a store of diverse information that allows him or her to be the patient's health care *manager* as well as his confidant, keeping in mind that the average patient does not understand the system of medical referrals for subspecialty consultation.

An oncologist/internist recently described for me how she weaves the fabric of health care management for a patient who has been referred with a positive biopsy for a malignant disease. In this situation the oncologist has to view herself as the captain of a rather complicated ship. She has to talk with the referring physician, obtain the biopsy slides, have them re-read by her own consulting pathologist, and review them herself. She then has to review the chart and the radiographs with a consulting radiologist and decide, given all the data, how best to institute therapy. This may require interaction with the surgeon, with the radiation oncologist, and with additional specialists with the skills for exploration, including various techniques for interventional radiology or endoscopy. Having decided on the course to take, she then has to become the patient's advocate and interact with the surgeon, the radiation oncologist, or other consultants on the patient's behalf and with the patient's best interests in mind. It is then necessary to spend time with the patient to explain the disease and what is to be expected and with the family to answer their questions and as much as possible to enlist them as allies for the hard times to come. Further, she has to commit herself to the long-term counseling, reassurance, and constant caring needed by a patient with a chronic and possibly fatal disease. This physician's role is much different from that of a physician-technician who performs a procedure and then sends the patient back to the doctor who will care for the long-term needs. While technicians' roles in this process are often crucial, their interactions with the patient are brief. The health care manager, in this case the oncologist, knits the technical information together and confers with her patient about the best way to proceed.

The physician who takes responsibility for the total oversight of the patient's needs as related to the disease is the one who really must captain the ship and with whom the patient needs a very special, trusting relationship. Too often in modern medicine, with its exquisitely developed technologies, a degree of impersonal behavior creeps in. The skilled cardiac surgeon, the superb master of angioplasty, the excellent endoscopist, the impressive neurosurgeon all touch "our" patients from time to time, exercise their skills in their one intervention, and then go on to the next patient. The general internist must define the need for the procedural intervention, give support during its execution, and most importantly continue to care following the procedure. When the consulting surgeon or specialist is no longer available, the one-on-one interaction between the patient and the internist, "*his or her* doctor," must remain inviolate.

Help with Suffering

Most chronic diseases involve physical, mental, and emotional suffering to some degree during their courses. Some patients do beautifully because of their own intrinsic personalities, strong wills, or deep convictions. Others have great difficulty and sometimes even the toughest break under the severe suffering of a chronic illness. Physicians must develop skills of interpersonal relationship based on familiarity with all sides of life and especially with suffering. They need to *participate* in suffering. They need to be able to relate it to a broad range of experience so that they can deal with an enormous variety of patients at many different stages of coping with their suffering. Students sometimes get a glimpse of this in dealing with patients on inpatient services, but most often in outpatient clinics where they treat chronic diseases that continue unabated for many years. Often the physician has little specific therapy to offer except a kind touch, a gentle presence, and a knowing acknowledgment. Students of medicine learn through experience with patients as their own involvement in the practice of medicine grows through the years. The best physicians are always learning, because each patient teaches something new about the way in which a particular kind of suffering must be considered and ameliorated.

In the last two decades, patient support groups have become more numerous and more widely sought by patients. Many are now associated with major medical centers. These groups play a vitally important role in allowing patients to express their concerns and fears and to hear other patients in similar situations share their concerns and frustrations. As important as these are, as constructive as they are, and as meaningful as they have become in the overall care of patients, physicians still must understand the circumstances and the degree of suffering of each patient. Each one's needs are unique. Merely sharing them does not make them go away, and merely knowing that someone else also carries burdens does not solve the problem. The physician must be both interactive and supportive—even when the ways to change the physical situation may be sadly limited.

Help with Aging

The past several decades have seen a remarkable increase in the proportion of the population over 65, over 75, and even over 85 years of age—the last being the fastest-growing of all age groups. These proportions will continue to increase significantly (Fig. 1–1). Already the average age of the practice population in the offices of many general internists exceeds 70 years. This demographic shift has been accompanied by increasing awareness of the general field of geriatric medicine and expanding knowledge of the biologic processes involved in aging. Projected population trends indicate that every general internist must become experienced in the needs of the geriatric population, as the aging process involves essentially every organ system. However, there are at least two—the nervous system and the musculoskeletal system—with which essentially every person reaching the seventh, eighth, and ninth decades of life will experience trouble to an increasing degree. Much of this is discussed in Ch. 442 and in the chapters involving rheumatologic diseases, especially osteoarthritis.

Memory loss of some degree is essentially universal in the elderly, although it clearly is more pronounced in some than others and may or may not be associated with the true clinical syndrome of Alzheimer's disease. Memory loss affects the individual's self-perception, ability to interact with friends and family,

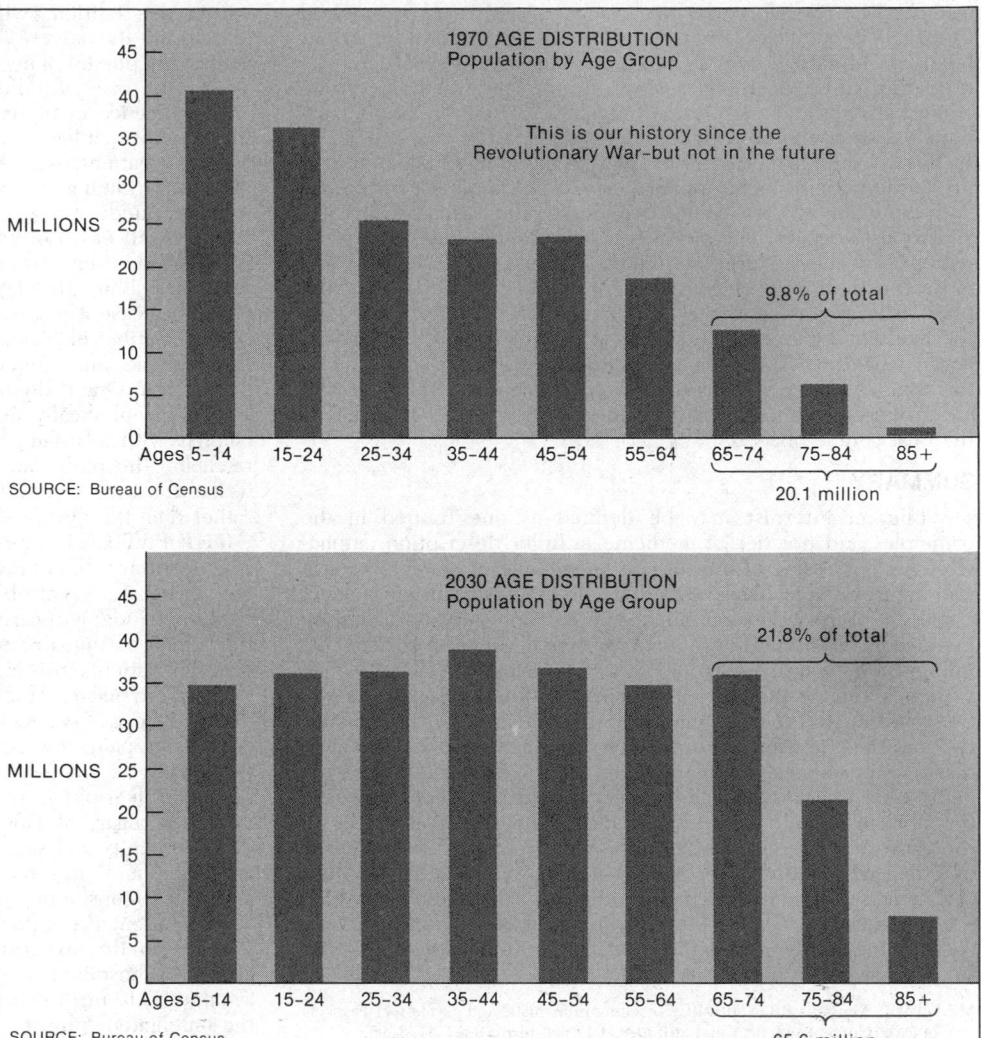

FIGURE 1–1. The Aging of the American population. (From Numbers that make you think. Retirement Systems of Alabama Advisor XV (9):3, 1990; with permission.)

and ability to accommodate to the pressures of our changing world. It can put barriers between the individual and those he or she most needs. This is true even for the very lucky individual who is able to maintain work activities, friends, and family as he or she did in his prime. The same situation develops with osteoarthritis, as gait problems, muscle fatigue, and weakness become more prevalent with advancing age. These effectively limit the individual's ability to get away from home and sustain a normally active lifestyle. Physical difficulties simply prohibit him or her from doing the things he or she likes to do. Much of the focus of the general internist, therefore, is to keep the elderly individual as physically and mentally active and as personally and emotionally interactive with others as possible.

Loneliness, despair, chronic illness, and depression are all prevalent in the geriatric population. Our effort must be to treat individual symptoms and organ system failure as they appear—but, most important, to help aging individuals develop an overall lifestyle that gives them a sense of well-being—of being useful, of being appreciated, and of having meaning in their lives. The internist must devote increasing time and effort to aging patients and must be particularly sensitive to subtle changes in their environments, including the loss of a loved one, shrinking income relative to cost of living, dislocation from their homes, and the despair that comes from being unable to adjust to new surroundings such as a retirement center or nursing home. Each of these profoundly affects the way a patient reacts to physical diseases. The responsibility of the internist extends beyond the usual in this situation and requires a very special integration of medical knowledge and knowledge of how people adjust to their changing needs.

Help with Dying

Rarely does an individual really wish to die, but when the time does come patients want to die with dignity. What most of us desire above all is not just life, but a satisfactory quality of life, and we may sometimes quite rationally risk death to escape an unacceptable life. Issues surrounding dying patients and even the realistic definition of death are topics frequently encountered by today's internist.

It is an often if sometimes faintly praised triumph for modern medicine that we now have the technologic skills and instrumentation to keep essential body functions such as circulation and respiration operating almost indefinitely. The ability to continue these functions regardless of the expected outcome for the patient has produced considerable ethical conflict for many who deal with patients in critical life support areas and intensive care units.

Young people in medical training must make an effort to become "comfortable" with the process and the event of dying. The problems of when to withdraw life support mechanisms or to withhold resuscitation may present deep emotional conflicts for medical students—as well as for many very experienced physicians. Although medical ethics touches almost every aspect of health and the practice of medicine (see Ch. 4), the particular problems related to dying patients, stemming in part from legal considerations and from highly publicized special cases, put the physician in an especially difficult position. Only recently have objective conclusions begun to emerge from clinical investigation of outcomes from intensive care units. Although striking successes do occur, the survival rate with a high quality of life upon discharge from intensive care units is less than one would hope (see Ch. 71). Therefore, the physician frequently may be required to make difficult decisions for or with the patient and his or her family. Ultimately, society at large will have to make policy regarding those decisions, using information based on careful clinical studies and analyses of the costs of sustaining life in truly hopeless situations. But that policy has not yet been established. In this area the skilled internist plays a uniquely personal role in preparing patients for terminal situations, becoming their teacher and confidant as they come to understand the disease process and what to expect. The physician is also called upon to help the patient's loved ones prepare for the outcome.

Each patient must be considered individually, keeping in mind previously expressed wishes, the nature of the terminal illness, the likelihood of recovery with an acceptable quality of life, and family wishes and interactions. Although these factors are difficult to weigh in the care of dying patients, objective evaluation and an unswerving concern for the patient will lead the physician to the best course of action.

SUMMARY

While an internist may be defined as one trained in the principles and practice of medicine, a fuller description emphasizes his possession of uncommon knowledge of biologic science ranging from molecular events to whole organ system physiology, a special appreciation for human life and the needs of suffering people, and a comprehensive perspective on modern society—its influence on our lives and its stresses on our social structure. Although this chapter has emphasized patient/physician interaction, we must recognize that basic biomedical science provides the infrastructure for our profession. We must first and foremost master our science if we are to be good physicians. We must know what is best to offer to correct the disease; then we weave the fabric of the physician's social and ethical responsibilities into the context of current medical care organization. Few physicians function well merely as knowledgeable scientists or talented technicians, but none functions well simply as a crutch on which the patient can lean. The good physician—the one patients seek—must combine working scientific techniques with compassion and social responsibility.

Merkel WT, Margolis RB, Smith RC: Teaching humanistic and psychosocial aspects of care: Current practices and attitudes. J Gen Intern Med 5:34, 1990.

Scherr L, Farber SJ, Hildreth EA, et al.: American College of Physicians Ethics Manual. Part 1: History; the patient; other physicians. Ann Intern Med 111:145, 1989.

Smedira NG, Evans BH, Grais LS: Withholding and withdrawal of life support from the critically ill. N Engl J Med 322:309, 1990.

2 Medicine as an Art

Lloyd H. Smith, Jr.

What is medicine? "Medicine is not a science but a learned profession, deeply rooted in a number of sciences and charged with the obligation to apply them for man's benefit." In this eloquent statement from an earlier edition of this book, Walsh McDermott defined medicine as a human activity undertaken for the benefit of others whether in the area of public health, "statistical compassion," or in the care of the individual patient.

Medicine can also be defined in other terms. It is a mutable body of knowledge, skills, and traditions applicable to the preservation of health, the cure of disease, and the amelioration of suffering. The boundaries of medicine blend into psychology, sociology, economics, and even cultural heritage. Disease may be encoded in the genome; disease may also be encoded by the deprivations of poverty and ignorance. Medicine must therefore be concerned not only with an abnormal molecule but also with an abnormal childhood. As such it is open ended in a way that is both humbling and exhilarating to those who pursue it as a career.

Medicine is continually changing. The honored verities of one generation become the shopworn shibboleths of the next. Much of what we now so confidently espouse, including that compressed within this edition, will amuse our successors as remarkably bizarre in its naiveté. Medical competence is based on the continuing pursuit of ever-changing concepts. It must be renewed as the substance of medicine itself is transformed.

The practice of medicine is far more than the application of scientific principles to a particular biologic aberration. Its focus is on the patient, whose welfare is its continuing purpose. That purpose of medicine is self evident in theory, but more difficult to sustain under the pressures of medical practice. For example, it is tragically easy for the patient to become merely the repository in which a disease or a syndrome has chosen to manifest its particular silhouette. During the training years every physician has subconsciously participated in what might be termed the personification of disease. A case of meningitis is admitted through the emergency room; a pheochromocytoma will be discussed at Grand Rounds. It is perhaps inevitable that a disease becomes symbolically an entity to the physician who must become familiar with all of its manifestations and guises. In the art of medicine the physician must be the advocate of the patient as well as the adversary of disease. It is the patient who is personified rather than the disease.

THE PATIENT. The description of a patient is simply that of a fellow human being in need of help. The patient comes seeking help because of a problem relating to his or her health. This subjective judgment carries with it disquieting concerns, although these may be unexpressed. Anxiety is present even in the most stoical of patients; this fact must never be forgotten or disregarded by the physician. The patient's anxiety may be specific—for example, fear of cancer with all that implies in the public mind concerning pain, degradation, and inexorable death. More often the anxiety is amorphous: fear of loss of independence or employment; fear of failure to meet obligations to one's family or to retain the regard of a loved one; or fear of an inability to maintain a life of dignity and significance. In the rush to crystallize a chief complaint and present illness the physician too often brushes aside these considerations.

The patient presents to the physician on alien and unfamiliar ground—in the structured and artificial setting of an office, a clinic, or a hospital bed. This form of health care of the individual, as opposed to health care in the aggregate, is often described by the unfelicitous phrase "the personal encounter system." Unfortunately it often seems distressingly like confrontation to the patient, who comes after all for comfort, not for encounter. Each human being is unique within a life that is enormously complex—in heredity, early experiences, cultural and psychological environment, education, opportunities, successes, failures, fantasies, emotional commitments, motivations, and in the adjustments and compromises that serve to cripple or to mature. Living, therefore, is the ultimate personal encounter system. With an extensive and diverse experience the patient comes to the physician with "a problem." A chief complaint is requested. Defenses must be lowered and the emotions that spill out may be distressing. The patient's response must be selective and brief; as a result it is not infrequently distorted, perhaps even misleading.

What does the patient want when coming to see a physician? There are certain common hopes and expectations. Patients want to be listened to, so that their fears and concerns can be fully expressed and the burden shared. They want physicians to be interested in them as fellow human beings in a compassionate but nonjudgmental fashion. They expect professional competence incorporating the best in medical science and technology. They want to be reasonably informed as to the probable cause of their concerns and what the future is likely to hold. They want not to be abandoned. To each patient these desires and expectations vary in relative importance. It is notable that not all patients expect to be cured. These expectations are further discussed in the light of how the physician should endeavor to meet them.

TRADITIONAL EXPECTATIONS OF PATIENTS. *Patients want to be listened to and understood.* This has been well expressed by Wilfred Trotter, a great English neurosurgeon:

". . . As long as medicine is an art, its chief and characteristic instrument must be human faculty. We come therefore to the very practical question of what aspects of human faculty it is necessary for the good doctor to cultivate. . . . The first to be named must always be the power of attention, of giving one's whole mind to the patient without the interposition of oneself. It sounds simple but only the very greatest doctors ever fully attain it. It is an active process and not either mere resigned listening or even politely waiting until you can interrupt. Disease often tells its secrets in a casual parenthesis. . . ."

Eventually the medical record must be organized in a logical and consistent fashion. But a history rarely unfolds that way. Patients do not divulge their fears in neat paragraphs or in direct responses to a cascade of queries. It is important to let patients tell their own stories. The manner of formulation and expression of symptoms and anxieties may be as informative as the medical data transmitted. The good physician is an attentive listener, with an ear for Trotter's "casual parenthesis."

Patients want physicians to be interested in them as fellow human beings. This interest cannot be that of the unusual "case" of the carcinoid syndrome or of hairy cell leukemia; the center of interest must be the patient as a person. It is difficult for the physician to feign such an interest, for patients are very perceptive, especially during the vulnerability that illness induces. In the practice of medicine the physician encounters all of the virtues and vices to which mankind is heir. The physician need not be morally neutral in personal judgments, but these must be stringently excluded from professional activities. The response of the physician to human frailty and fallibility should be that of compassion rather than cynicism, of interest in the infinite variety of human experience rather than of repulsion from its aberrations.

Patients expect professional competence in medical science and technology. The physician must be a scholar both to attain professional competence and to sustain it during times of revolutionary changes in science and technology. All of the other attributes of the good physician are of little avail in the absence of sound scholarship. Compassion is no substitute for knowing what should be done. The education of the physician and the role of the physician as a scientist will be discussed more fully below.

Patients want to be kept informed. The physician must listen to and communicate with the patient. Time must be set aside for this. Failure to do so is a serious error, for silence is a form of communication that is usually adverse. The physician should voluntarily answer questions of concern to the patient. The physician must also inform the patient concerning the illness and what it implies. A number of books have been developed to assist in patient education and are often quite effective in translating medical terminology into lay terms. Furthermore, clubs for mutual support and education have been formed by patients who share their common experiences with such chronic disabilities as ileostomies or amputations. Admirable and important as these are, they do not obviate the need for patients to learn from their own physicians about their particular illnesses and what they may mean in and for their future lives. This need extends beyond the legal confines of informed consent, which is now an important issue in medical practice.

Patients want not to be abandoned. Death comes to everyone. There are finite limits to what can be accomplished by medical science and technology in the alleviation of suffering and the prolongation of life. This fact is well known to both patients and physicians. When that limit is reached, the physician often feels powerless and even guilty that no more can be done. As a consequence there is a tendency to withdraw attention and direct it elsewhere. Nothing could be a greater mistake. It is at the margins of medical science that the role of the physician is enhanced. It is here that the art of medicine comes to the forefront in the care of the patient, whether it be by emotional support, relief of pain, small adjustments in medicines or diet, daily conversation and examination, or other methods to show that the patient is still someone of dignity and worth in whom interest has not been lost and for whom hope has not been abandoned. And when no more can be done for the patient, it is time to care for the family. At this stage, as Walsh McDermott has written, "it is up to each of us to follow to the fullest measure the charge laid down long ago for the physician to become himself the treatment."

THE PHYSICIAN. The physician has both chosen and been chosen to enter an arduous and demanding profession, the origins of which stretch back to antiquity. Part priest, part shaman, part mystic, part alchemist, the physician of the past reflected the beliefs and expectations of the time and met a perceived need of fellow men. The history of medicine is part of the heritage of every physician and reflects the cultural history of each society.

The physician enters a profession with established values and traditions of ethical conduct and responsibilities. But each physician, like each patient, is unique. The physician is not a disembodied instrument that can be passively shaped by the profession, but rather a human being with innate strengths and weaknesses that must be recognized in order to meet the expectations of patients and of the profession, not least of which are those standards established for oneself. The qualities of the ideal physician are easy to state but difficult to attain: compassion, sincere interest in one's fellow man, knowledge of human nature, tact, equanimity, sustained scholarship, curiosity, and high ethical standards. Physical and mental vigor might be added to those traits, for the life of the physician is not for the languid or the disengaged. No one has been endowed with or ever fully achieves excellence in all of these qualities. One must first know oneself and judge how one can most closely approach those ideals in one's professional life.

THE EDUCATION OF THE PHYSICIAN. Barriers are encountered at the very beginning in the initial selection for medical school as many seek entry for few positions. Undergraduate education is sometimes distorted and breadth of personal experience curtailed in a grim and often distasteful race for competitive acceptance. This inadvertent feedback inhibition not infrequently results from erroneous conceptions of what may or may not impress admission committees of medical schools. Nevertheless, the phenomenon remains a concern to all who are interested in the future of our profession. Admission committees of medical schools too often exercise allosteric control over the higher education of those destined to enter our profession.

The Basic Science Years. In the standard curriculum of medical school in the United States two years are largely devoted to the sciences basic to medicine and two years to clinical training. Fortunately there are a number of interesting variations on this thematic progression which diminish its rigidity and permit the student to re-explore basic science after an introductory clinical experience.

In the United States students usually arrive at medical school after an intensive four-year experience at a college or a university. They anticipate a scholarly atmosphere of a graduate school which will prepare them to enter the practice of a profession for which they hold idealistic expectations. Instead they are immediately assailed with a formidable array of "basic sciences" linked to the structure and function of the human organ systems. New facts constitute not so much an intellectual feast as an engorgement. Each discipline is attended by devotees who are passionately persuaded of the seminal role of their segment of science in the future of the profession. This commitment is translated into the basic academic commodity, curricular time, in which these cluttered wares are exhibited. Awed by the dimensionless task, students struggle with uneven success to assimilate and survive, conscious always that their receptor mechanisms are overloaded and of a continuing sense of high output failure. They look forward in hope that subsequent years will reward their endurance in the more congenial atmosphere of the clinic.

This is patently a caricature, as all will recognize. It can be said, as Mark Twain said of Wagner's music, "it is not as bad as it sounds." The quality of basic science in medical schools is often superb; the substance of modern science has a certain grandeur; many faculty members are gifted in imparting a sense of intellectual adventure to their students; finally, many students now arrive at medical school with a mature understanding of one or more of the fundamental disciplines of biology. Nevertheless this caricature contains elements of truth as seen from the perspective of medical students. The central question is not whether basic science is necessary for medical research, since few would deny its importance there, but whether it is relevant in the education of every physician to the degree to which it is currently emphasized. In the real world of patient care, public health, and medical economics, should the student have to struggle with the intricacies of post-transcriptional modifications of messenger RNA, or is this merely a rite of passage prescribed by a science-obsessed faculty? This is a reasonable question and calls for a response other than a simple reference to flexnerian orthodoxy.

A knowledge of the scientific underpinnings of medicine is clearly necessary in order to marshal the basic information required to understand a patient's illness and to be able to reason logically about the problems of diagnosis and therapy. If there were any doubt on that point, it would be quickly dispelled by random perusal of this book. Much of the basic science which seems abstruse and irrelevant today will find its way into clinical practice in the not too distant future. Medical research is only one step removed from patient care.

Beyond the assimilation of scientific information, there is an even more important consideration. Many of you will have most of your professional experience in the twenty-first century. The changes in medical science and technology will be enormous and largely unpredictable. Only the scientific method will remain unaltered as an invaluable instrument with which fallible man can acquire new knowledge and, equally important, discard that which proves fallacious. It is imperative that students learn the scientific method as part of their education if they are to participate critically and effectively in a changing profession. How can this be done? Perhaps the best method is to participate personally, even for a relatively brief period of time, in a research project so that learning comes from first-hand experience. If that does not prove practical, one can pursue some scientific topic in depth and write a critical analysis of it. It is important to learn one area of inquiry in great detail, even though it may have to be a limited area, in order to penetrate to its frontier. It is only there that science can be understood as a process rather than as a repository.

The Clinical Years. Most students enter the clinical years with a sense of relief, but it is relief lined with anxieties. Some of these anxieties cluster around the following questions:

How can I cope with the uncertainties of clinical medicine?

What are the boundaries of clinical medicine? How much and what am I supposed to learn?

How will I function in my interactions with patients?

How will I measure up to the expectations of my colleagues?

How will I be able to maintain my own identity as an individual in a profession that so obsessively dominates my time and energy?

Other questions could be formulated. Each student possesses a unique idiotype of anxieties that cannot be purged by platitudes. Each will arrive at personal answers, or more likely at personal accommodations, through experience.

The Uncertainty Principle of Clinical Medicine. There is an "uncertainty principle" in medicine as there is in physics. The practice of medicine is inexact and will remain so. If it were not, it would be a science or a technology rather than an art. The measuring instrument is personal and unique. Subjective mensuration defies precision. Who can quantify nausea or the severity of pain? Symptoms may be forgotten, suppressed, or amplified when filtered through the grid of personality. Available data are often indirect, incomplete, or even contradictory. Patients respond in varying fashions to treatment across the range from simple reassurance (which is rarely simple) to surgical or pharmaceutical interventions. Clinical medicine is often based on experience and judgment—which are largely euphemisms for a knowledge of probabilities.

The process of formulating a diagnosis or selecting a therapy is not as arbitrary as it first seems. There are rational means for narrowing the range of diagnostic possibilities: a precise description of symptoms; an accurate and thorough characterization of physical findings; selective laboratory studies to evaluate the functions of organ systems; a synthesis of information to define syndromic patterns; a marshaling of information on etiology and pathogenesis. All of this requires attention to detail, consistency of work habits, and good intellect.

Hypotheses are formed and algorithms branch away from various entry points as new data are obtained which support or fail to support a working diagnosis. This process of clinical reasoning is often best displayed in the clinicopathologic conference (CPC). In the absence of certainty, best guesses must be utilized and in making informed guesses, generally dignified as judgments, the clinician actually relies upon subliminal statistics.

Medical decisions based on probabilities are necessary but also perilous. Even the most astute physician is occasionally wrong. The wise physician often recognizes that a decision is erroneous and discards or modifies the hypothesis on which it is based. The best decision may be approached only by successive approximations. Action may have to be taken despite lack of confirmation of a hypothesis (working diagnosis). Chester M. Jones, a noted clinical teacher, used to say: "If you cannot make a diagnosis, make a decision." Despite the remarkable contributions of science and technology, clinical medicine is frequently inexactitude in action. The student entering the clinical years quickly realizes the dangers to the welfare of the patient of dogmatism in clinical practice. The ambiguities and errors that you encounter in your own experience and observe in the work of others should be an antidote to arrogance. Some errors are inevitable and should not humiliate you, but they should teach humility.

What is the role of the *Cecil Textbook of Medicine* in the learning process? This book attempts to provide the student or the physician with succinct but authoritative summaries about diseases or groups of diseases. Essays written by more than 250 acknowledged experts in their respective fields represent collectively a systematic approach to internal medicine. The chapters are designed to give a basic, lucid, and up-to-date consensus concerning the state of the art in our understanding of specific diseases, but they cannot be all inclusive. Many of the topics discussed within a few pages have received more extended treatment elsewhere as separate monographs. Each of the subspecialty areas (cardiology, gastroenterology, endocrinology, etc.) is the subject of textbooks similar in size to this one. The student should therefore cultivate the habit of consulting at least some of the carefully selected references that extend the information supplied in this basic text.

In general it is also wise for students to begin reading medical journals early in their study of clinical medicine. In this way a start can be made toward the regular study of current medical literature and also the foundations of one's own medical library can be laid. Each student may have a personal preference. The most frequently read medical jounal by students and practitioners is the *New England Journal of Medicine.* It is particularly useful for the student with its CPC, surveys of medical progress, editorial comments on current topics, original articles, and lively correspondence. In this manner the student establishes an early acquaintance with the frontiers of medicine and with its issues, uncertainties, and controversies.

The Student and the Patient. One of the student's earliest concerns on entering clinical medicine is how to interact with patients and how to assume the traditional role of a physician. The student is concerned that personal insecurities will impair effective communication with patients in whose care he or she is now called upon to participate. Rarely does this turn out in practice to be a serious problem. The expectations of most patients in the physician-patient interaction, discussed above, are realistic ones. Patients are usually aware of the progression of assigned responsibilities in the student-house staff-faculty team and do not expect omniscience or authoritarianism from the student. Not infrequently the patient forms a special attachment to the student, especially if the student has been perceptive enough to listen in the sense described above by Wilfred Trotter. If the student respects the personal dignity of the patient as a fellow human being, and listens in a sensitive manner, the patient responds with gratitude and returns that respect. Even when patients are initially perceived as hostile or belligerent, the student must maintain equanimity and try to understand the sources of these reactions. Do not allow yourself to be drawn into the flippant cynicism that sometimes passes for sophistication in the subculture of student and house staff training. Francis Peabody's sentient summary is still most apt, "for the secret of the care of the patient is in caring for the patient."

Students and Their Colleagues. Beginning in the clinical years the relationships of students with their colleagues in medicine undergo a subtle change. No longer are they merely the passive recipients of data and concepts supplied by the faculty through lectures, conferences, syllabi, or laboratories. They are participating with graduated responsibilities in the practice of medicine. A point in the medical history or a question asked by the student may prove decisive in arriving at the solution of a clinical problem. Frequently the most effective teachers of students are the house staff or more advanced students. Students will find many residents to be splendid teachers who not only make them feel at home in the service but also take the extra time to include them in all of the discussions. On most teaching services there is a certain amount of badinage or gamesmanship which enlivens interactions. If this is recognized as such, and not taken too seriously, it can serve to enhance rather than demean the learning experience. As a student you must not hesitate to ask questions or bring up new points of view and must not be intimidated by your current position in this shifting hierarchy. Even the chief medical resident faced similar qualms only a few years ago. But above all, remember that it is the patient's welfare, and not your own ego, that is paramount.

The Physician as a Nonphysician. Beginning in the basic science years but exacerbated in the clinical years, students often become concerned about the level of commitment demanded of them. How much of a life that is finite in time and energy must be devoted to medicine? What is the boundary between dedication and obsession? After all, one does not really become a physician; one remains a human being who has acquired certain knowledge and skills that allow one to function as a physician during specific periods of time. What should those times be? How and when does one shift roles from being a physician to being a "nonphysician"? This is, of course, a generic question that is as applicable to science, art, business, or any other human activity as it is to medicine.

The student will not readily find an all-embracing answer to this question. Each student will most likely evolve a personal answer and it will be an operational one representing the integral of microcompromises and adjustments made throughout one's subsequent career. The "complete physician," narrowly construed, would be a very poor physician if he were merely an observer rather than a participant in the pageantry of his time. Physicians owe it to themselves, to their families, to society, and to their patients not to become simply skilled but detached automatons. On the other hand, the practice of medicine is not a job but a profession that cannot be sealed off into convenient hours for earning one's living. To attempt to do so smacks of dilettantism. Between these extremes one must decide for oneself where the compromises will be made along the varying border between personal and professional life. Tensions will remain, but properly channeled they can be creative and rewarding.

3 Medicine as a Science

James B. Wyngaarden

It is not my purpose in this chapter to contend that medicine is itself a science, much less merely the application of scientific knowledge to the diagnosis and treatment of human diseases. Rather it is to accord the scientific base of the profession of medicine its proper recognition as the foundation of the intellectual and professional competence that enables a skillful physician to serve other human beings in the preservation of health and the prevention, diagnosis, and amelioration or cure of disease.

In the interactions of physicians with people of extraordinary diversity, whether throughout the full life cycle or in a single encounter, it is difficult to imagine any form of knowledge that does not prove useful at one time or another in the practice of medicine. Yet it is knowledge of humans, in all their biologic, behavioral, and social complexity, and the ability to base one's decisions and actions on that knowledge that distinguish physicians from other professionals. The particular training of the individual physician and extent of his or her knowledge, judgment, wisdom, compassion, and humanity distinguish the truly great physician from others. But the effectiveness of a physician begins with professional competence, without which compassion and humanity are ineffectual. And a major portion of professional competence depends on understanding the scientific principles of the branch or segment of medicine practiced.

I say "branch or segment of medicine practiced" to acknowledge that medicine is far too vast and complex a field to be mastered in all its specialties and techniques by any one physician. Nevertheless, all physicians need a considerable breadth of scientific knowledge of the type acquired during a lengthy primary and secondary education, a liberal arts college experience, and a medical school curriculum. In addition, each physician needs to acquire a profound understanding of the particular science base of his or her specialty and a comfortable familiarity with it. The neurologist and ophthalmologist must delve deeply into the neurosciences, the rheumatologist into immunology and connective tissue biology, and the psychiatrist into behavioral and social sciences.

The *Cecil Textbook of Medicine* is a comprehensive general textbook of medicine, principally of diseases of young, mature, or aging adults, which stresses medical as contrasted with surgical approaches. It addresses the full expanse of what is usually termed general internal medicine, but with sufficient detail that each part also defines the scope of a major medical subspecialty, albeit in considerably less detail than corresponding subspecialty texts provide. It is intended to speak to the needs of advanced medical students and graduate physicians in training as well as practicing physicians. Accordingly, the *Textbook* extends its taproots into a remarkably large and rich garden of biologic and behavioral science. The practitioners of medicine of the scope addressed in this book thus have need for a broader grasp of scientific principles and specific information than almost any other subgroup of physician. And given the pace of scientific advances and the extraordinary potential of the new biology to explicate life processes and their aberrations, and of the biotechnology industry to develop new agents of remarkable specificity and complexity, the need for continuing scientific currency becomes a daunting challenge to maintaining and extending one's professional competence. Only through continuing attention to one's scientific education can the physician be a critical and independent participant in medical progress and avoid the pitfall of becoming a passive purveyor of medical fashion.

Advances in biologic science and accompanying technologic developments underlie most of the medical progress of the past half century, which has so remarkably advanced the ability of the physician to intervene in illness. Much of this progress has been in fundamental or "basic" science, conducted in the pursuit of understanding for its own sake. Significant progress has also resulted from research conducted by physician-scientists with a specified clinical goal in mind—for example, the elucidation of a disease mechanism or the critical evaluation of a therapeutic practice. Advances in medicine also continue to occur through serendipity or by astute clinical observations concerning patients or groups of patients and their illnesses. Nevertheless, the only rational approach to finding new methods for prevention or treatment is based on scientific explanations of the causes and mechanisms of disease. As Sir William Osler has said of the ambitions of medicine, "To wrest from nature the secrets which have perplexed philosophers in all ages, to track to their sources the causes of disease."[*]

Some years ago, Comroe and Dripps[†] traced the origins of ten major clinical innovations in cardiovascular and pulmonary medicine in an effort to identify the antecedents of these advances. Over 60 per cent of the enabling discoveries were in the category of basic science; over 40 per cent were the result of research carried out without any particular clinical application in mind. These observations are probably representative of medical progress in general.

The ability to control infections with antibiotics, hypertension with antihypertensive agents, and inflammatory reactions with glucocorticoids represents remarkable advances that have contributed to a lengthening of life expectancy. But the agenda is far from being fulfilled. The major health care problems of our time lie in the continued existence of diseases for which we can as yet do little. We have no definitive answers for cancer,

---

*Bean WB: Sir William Osler Aphorisms. Springfield, Ill., Charles C Thomas, pp 61–62. Quoted by Jackson CE, Norum RA: N Engl J Med 321:1040, 1989.

†Comroe JH, Dripps RD: The top ten clinical advances in cardiovascular-pulmonary medicine and surgery between 1945 and 1975: How they came about. Bethesda, Md., Public Inquiries and Reports Branch, National Heart, Lung, and Blood Institute, National Institutes of Health, 1977.

rheumatoid arthritis, schizophremia, and many other diseases, the descriptions of which constitute the substance of this book —or else we have what Lewis Thomas has called a "halfway technology," measures capable of modifying and ameliorating illness but not of preventing or curing it. Medicine as a science is incomplete and will remain so, for science itself is by its nature incomplete.

The present bioscientific character of medical practice is a relatively recent development. Throughout most of recorded history, medicine was anything but scientific. Diagnoses were inexact, causes of diseases poorly understood, and therapies frivolous and haphazard. Interventions by physicians consisted of myriads of procedures with no scientific foundation. Nor could there be such a foundation, for the scientific base did not yet exist.

Harbingers of change emerged slowly in the early nineteenth century, as new principles of physics and chemistry were applied to medicine. Physiologists stressed functions of organs and tissues. Its exemplars, especially Claude Bernard (1813–1878), emphasized the experimental method in establishing biologic knowledge and the necessity of basing medical practice in such knowledge. Pathologists, led by Virchow (1821–1902), stressed the critical study of normal and abnormal tissues and the correlation of features of disease with precise anatomic observations. Bacteriologists, with Pasteur (1822–1895) and Koch (1843–1910) in the vanguard, began to identify the microorganisms and to implicate specific organisms in specific diseases—the anthrax bacillus in anthrax, the tubercle bacillus in consumption, the pneumococcus in lobar pneumonia, the streptococcus in puerperal fever. The groundwork for future therapies was being laid by these great Western European scientists, but physicians could do relatively little about most illnesses at the time. Their major contributions were diagnostic, prognostic, and supportive. By correct diagnosis they could advise concerning outcome. By common-sense supportive measures they could provide comfort and maximize opportunities for recovery. But interventions were as likely as not to make things worse. The first edition of Osler's *Textbook of Medicine* in 1892 was revolutionary for its skepticism and its therapeutic nihilism, as this outstanding physician and teacher condemned the majority of nostrums and remedies as useless, even harmful.

Slowly, specific therapies—insulin for diabetes, liver extract for pernicious anemia—or specific immunizations—diphtheria antitoxin, pneumococcic antisera—appeared. But it was not until the decade of 1935 to 1945 that the entry of sulfonamides and penicillin into clinical medicine made curable a large number of previously lethal and untreatable diseases. It is customary to date the beginnings of modern medicine from these relatively recent events.

The language of contemporary biologic science has become increasingly biochemical. The compositions of organs, tissues, cells, organelles, and membranes have been defined. The biosynthesis and catabolism of hundreds of compounds have been elucidated. The regulation of body processes has been described at progressively finer levels and in chemical language. Many pharmacologic agents are now understood in terms of specific loci and mechanisms of action. The expansion of new knowledge continues at a pace that is bewildering to all but experts in a given field. Current advances are particularly rapid in immunology, virology, molecular and cellular biology, peptide research, and structural biology. A beginning has been made in explaining human behavior in mechanistic terms, as more and more chemical mediators and pharmacologic modifiers are discovered.

We are in a molecular age of basic biologic science. The molecular influence pervades all the traditional disciplines underlying clinical medicine. Approximately 375 inborn errors are now understood in terms of specific missing or abnormal enzymes or other proteins. There are more than 575 known abnormal human hemoglobins, and for each of these the precise structural defect in the DNA of the mutant gene can be defined. Membrane, cytoplasmic, and nuclear receptors for hormones and drugs are exploding upon us, and old as well as new diseases are being defined in terms of receptor abnormalities—for example, type II hypercholesterolemia and nephrogenic diabetes insipidus. Recognition of opiate receptors has led to the discovery of endogenous peptides (endorphins) with analgesic activity. Their localization gives promise of further understanding of the limbic system, affective states, and addictions. The number and function of neurotransmitters have greatly increased, and these and other advances in neuroscience portend exciting developments in understanding how the brain works. DNA sequencing techniques and restriction endonucleases now permit precise identification of the exact structural alteration of the gene in an increasing number of hereditary diseases. The complete sequencing of the human genome is now technically possible and is being undertaken. A coordinated international program is being organized in the hope of accomplishing this goal in about 15 years. About 0.5 per cent of it has already been done. Gene therapy—both pharmacologic modification of specific gene action and physical replacement of damaged genetic segments—is now possible in experimental systems (see Ch. 32).

Much of the recent fundamental information in science has been obtained by the process of reductionism—the belief that all living processes can ultimately be explained in biochemical terms. The scientists responsible for our evolving understanding of biologic systems know that the reductionist approach must often precede reconstitutive endeavors. Scientific progress rests on myriads of small observations, tedious measurements, and the findings of investigators asking humble, answerable questions. Instead of reaching for the whole truth, the scientist examines small, defined, and clearly separable phenomena. The pattern of science is a stepwise extension of what came before, with an occasional giant leap forward through great discovery.

The examples of advances in medical science mentioned above have been largely drawn from the areas of ultrastructure, biochemistry, and molecular biology. In biology these disciplines have arbitrary and porous boundaries: physiology, pharmacology, neurosciences, cell biology, molecular biology, biochemistry, immunology, biophysics—all are in a phase of confluence, and the common language is chemistry. Medicine is not only a branch of applied biology, however. It also subsumes many aspects of psychology, sociology, anthropology, and economics. These disciplines, too long neglected or denigrated as "soft science," are now increasingly recognized as germane to medicine as a discipline and the practice of medicine as a profession.

However, not all observers of the evolution of modern medicine are in agreement with the current emphasis on scientific discovery as the motive force of medical advance. Critics of the bioscientific strategy of medicine, especially Ivan Illich, have claimed that the great advances that have dramatically reduced mortality rates consist in the improvement of the environment, the correction of malnutrition, and the control of infectious diseases through immunizations and antimicrobial agents, and that the relevant medical breakthroughs largely occurred before the prodigious expansion of federal support of biomedical science begun in the early 1950's. They contend that the enormous expenditures that have made the United States pre-eminent in biomedical research have produced too little in the way of medical advance to justify their continuation and have instead fostered the development of an extremely costly technology that has had only a minimal effect upon mortality statistics. They propose that the bioscientific strategy of medicine be replaced by an ecologic strategy for health.

No doubt safe water supplies, better sewage disposal, improved nutrition, immunizations, and improved standards of living deserve considerable credit for health improvements. In addition, the current public concern with the environment—with air, water, and food safety—will probably result in further health improvements. These are part of a new ecologic strategy for health. But one does not need to denigrate science in order to support a concomitant environmental concern. A scientific strategy for medicine and an ecologic strategy for health are not mutually exclusive. Furthermore, the medical advances of the past few decades—for example, in the treatment of Hodgkin's disease, childhood leukemias, Parkinson's disease, Wilson's disease, and AIDS, and, more recently, relief of an impending worldwide insulin shortage with rDNA-derived insulin, replacement of potentially virus-contaminated growth hormone with rDNA-derived growth hormone, and production of erythropoietin for treatment of anemia of end-stage renal disease—have all depended on a deeper and clearer understanding of biologic mechanisms and application of basic scientific knowledge to clinical problems.

The list of human diseases for which there are as yet no definitive measures for prevention or cure is still formidable. Fresh insights into the nature of these diseases are needed, insights that can come only from continued basic research. But the expansion of the knowledge bank of the past quarter century justifies great optimism for the eventual control and cure of major diseases and the possible elimination of premature death from illness. The science and the art of medicine must remain intimately linked if physicians are to be maximally effective.

THE PHYSICIAN AS A SCIENTIST. Since medicine is derived from a number of sciences relevant to the health of individuals or of groups, physicians must be trained as scientists to utilize these complex disciplines effectively.

To be a scientist, the physician must be conversant with the processes of scientific inquiry—how data are obtained and evaluated; how hypotheses are framed, modified, or discarded; the uses and limitations of inductive reasoning. In short, they must understand science as an intellectual instrument that has been slowly improved over centuries. Only in this way can they remain attentive to medical progress. Both the spirit and rigor of science are necessary for the physician to become and remain a scholar in medicine. Medical practice itself contains many of the elements of scientific inquiry in the pursuit and evaluation of data (history, physical examination, laboratory studies) and in framing a hypothesis (tentative clinical diagnosis).

As a scientist the physician is the beneficiary of both the fruits of scientific research and the mental discipline of the scientific method. To a greater or lesser degree the physician also has the opportunity to contribute personally to medical progress. Most medical research is now carried out by teams of participating investigators in elaborately equipped laboratories that utilize the advanced instrumentation and technology of modern science. There is still room, however, for scientific contributions made by inquiring physicians based on their own experiences in patient care. Much of medical progress has derived from this kind of curiosity in the past. In addition, this form of clinical research, on whatever modest scale it may be engaged in, adds excitement and zest to professional life. As Thomas Hobbes has written: "Desire to know why, and how, curiosity, which is a lust of the mind, that by a perseverance of delight in the continued and indefatigable generation of knowledge, exceedeth the short vehemence of any carnal pleasure."

---

4 Clinical Ethics in the Practice of Medicine

Mark Siegler and Peter A. Singer

Clinical medical ethics (CME) is a practical discipline that aims to improve patient care and patient outcomes. It focuses on the doctor-patient relationship and takes explicit account of the ethical and legal issues that patients, physicians, and health care institutions must address in reaching the best decisions for individual patients. CME emphasizes that in practicing good clinical medicine physicians must combine scientific and technical abilities with ethical concerns for the personal preferences and values of the patient who seeks their help. CME also provides a structured approach to decision making that can assist physicians to identify, analyze, and resolve clinical ethical dilemmas.

CME begins with the encounter between patient and physician, an encounter that both establishes the doctor-patient relationship and imposes stringent moral requirements on the physician, including the need for honesty, competence, compassion, and respect for the patient. Beyond these fundamental moral requirements, CME assists physicians to address a wide range of specifically ethical problems—for example, informed consent, end-of-life decisions, allocation of scarce resources, confidentiality, and third party interference with the autonomy of both patients and physicians—problems that arise with increasing frequency in the practice of modern high technology medicine.

For the foreseeable future, the critical problem facing concerned patients and conscientious physicians will be to balance the rights and responsibilities of patients and physicians at a time when societal values and expectations are changing rapidly and relations between patients and physicians are increasingly regulated and legislated. In the light of such changes, CME may assist patients, physicians, and society to achieve an ethically acceptable new arrangement because CME emphasizes the moral dimensions of the encounter between patient and physician, an encounter that remains the central and unchanging event in medicine.

This chapter aims to introduce students and practicing physicians to the field of clinical ethics by describing a framework for approaching ethical problems in clinical practice. The framework proposes that three sets of considerations be taken into account in analyzing ethical problems in clinical medicine: (1) clinical circumstances, (2) patient preferences, and (3) socioeconomic constraints.

DECISION MAKING STRATEGY FOR CLINICAL ETHICAL PROBLEMS

Every aspect of medical practice involves ethical considerations, but during the past 20 years certain issues have become recognized as specifically ethical "issues" or "problems." In recent years, investigators have begun to describe the epidemiology of these ethical problems in clinical practice. A 1981 study found that the incidence of ethical dilemmas recognized in a medical inpatient service was 17 per cent when an internist-ethicist participated on ward rounds. The ethical problems, in order of decreasing frequency, included withholding tests or treatment, informed consent, truth telling, and allocation of limited resources. A 1988 study found that important ethical problems were noted in 30 per cent of patients in an internal medicine office practice. The most common ethical problems in this outpatient study were costs of care, psychological factors that influence patient preferences, competence and capacity to choose, and informed consent.

Experienced clinicians who have faced each of these problems many times before often can respond to them appropriately without analyzing and dissecting each case. Students of medicine, however, may find it useful to consider explicitly three sets of issues when confronted with an ethical problem. These three levels of consideration are (1) the clinical circumstances presented by the patient's case, (2) the patient's wishes regarding treatment, and (3) the socioeconomic factors that tend to constrain individual patient-doctor decision making at levels 1 and 2.

CLINICAL CIRCUMSTANCES

Both the ethical and medical evaluations of a patient's case begin from precisely the same point: an accurate assessment of the patient's clinical circumstances. Data concerning the patient's clinical situation are collected through the traditional methods of history taking, physical examination, and laboratory investigations. From these data, the physician reaches a diagnosis and prognosis and develops options for therapy. Finally, the physician makes a specific recommendation to the patient after taking account of the nature of the medical problem, the values and goals of the patient, and the risks and benefits of various alternative treatment approaches for the particular patient. The physician informs and educates the patient about the anticipated benefits from the clinical recommendation and encourages the patient to accept the proposed treatment or a reasonable alternative. This is usually the critical step in the doctor-patient encounter. In general, patients accept the physician's recommendation because the physician and patient share the same goal—improvement of the patient's health status—and because patients usually trust and have confidence in both the physician's technical abilities and his or her concern for the patient as an individual.

Prior to making recommendations to a patient, the physician is obligated to consider two clinical issues that may influence the process of clinical-ethical decision making: (1) Is the patient competent? (2) Is the treatment proposal "futile"? If the patient is incompetent, the focus of decision making broadens to incorporate the patient's family or other surrogate decision maker (see below, "Incompetent Patients"). If the proposed treatment is futile, the focus of decision making may be narrowed to clinical circumstances alone.

Competency Assessment

The assessment of competency plays a pivotal role in patient care. Whether a doctor finds a patient competent or incompetent often determines whether or not the doctor accepts the patient's stated wishes about treatment or takes steps to review or override the patient's decision. Respect for the ethical and legal rights of patients means that competent patients may accept or reject treatment even if it may result in their death. On the other hand, doctors are obligated to question or even overrule requests to forego treatment made by incompetent patients because they are expected to protect patients from serious harm that the patient would not intend if he or she were competent. With so much at stake, it would be desirable to have well-developed clinical standards for the determination of competency. Unfortunately, at present, there are no clearly stipulated criteria for the determination of competency at the bedside.

The President's Commission for the Study of Ethical Problems in Medicine and Biomedical and Behavioral Research identified three elements of competency: possession of a set of values and goals, the ability to communicate and understand information, and the ability to reason and deliberate about one's choices. The Commission also noted that competency was specific to "the person's actual functioning in situations in which a decision about health care was to be made." More recently, Appelbaum and Grisso have suggested that the competent patient should be able to communicate choices, understand relevant information, appreciate the situation and its consequences, and manipulate information rationally. An effective clinical index of patient competency, however, would require a list of specific questions for the physician to ask the patient, clearly stipulated criteria for the appraisal of patient responses, and a mechanism for combining the responses on individual questions into an overall assessment. Until such an index has been developed and evaluated, physicians and consultants must continue to rely on ad hoc assessments of competency.

At the extremes, doctors can usually establish whether a patient is competent or incompetent. Moreover, the clinician can sometimes restore patients to a state of competency by treating reversible causes of cognitive dysfunction, correcting a wide range of metabolic encephalopathies, or discontinuing psychoactive drugs. If uncertainty remains about the patient's competency, the physician should consult with colleagues, such as psychiatrists, neurologists, institutional ethics committees, ethics consultation services, and hospital attorneys.

Futility

The claim that a treatment is futile is often used to justify a shift in the physician's ethical obligations to patients. In clinical situations in which nonfutile treatments are available, the physician has an obligation to discuss therapeutic alternatives with the patient and to encourage patient choice. By contrast, a physician is under no obligation to offer, or even to discuss, futile therapies. This shift in obligation is supported by moral reasoning in ancient and modern medical ethics, by public policy, and by case law.

Given this shift in ethical obligations, one might expect that physicians would have unambiguous criteria for determining when a therapy is futile. Unfortunately, this is not the case. Ambiguity in determining futility arises from disagreements about the goals of therapy and uncertainty about the probability of attaining those goals. Given the importance of futility claims in clinical practice, physicians must try to separate these two components of futility determinations: the goals of therapy and the chances of attaining them.

In some situations, physicians may acknowledge that therapy is effective but believe that the goals that can be achieved with therapy are not desirable or not compatible with adequate quality of life. Examples are prolonged nutritional support for patients in a persistent vegetative state and the treatment of pneumonia in a patient dying of untreatable pancreatic cancer. In such situations, physicians should acknowledge that potentially achievable goals exist. Since quality-of-life judgments are best made by the patient, these treatment decisions should be discussed with the patient or the patient's surrogate or be based on the patient's previously expressed goals.

In other situations, physicians may regard the likelihood of therapeutic success as quite remote, for example, cardiopulmonary resuscitation for elderly patients with cancer or sepsis and further chemotherapy for a patient with advanced metastatic cancer. It is not clear exactly how such probability considerations should be factored into clinical decision making, how low a probability (? 10%, 5%, 0.5%) constitutes "futility," or whether determination of probable futility should be made by the patient, the physician, or society (e.g., third-party payers).

"Futility" is an important clinical concept, but physicians should use it with precision. Physicians should stipulate whether they consider the goals of treatment undesirable or the chance of success too low. Unless the specific circumstances are explicitly recognized as "futile" by professional consensus or by legal-administrative guidelines, the physician should review his conclusions with the competent patient or the incompetent patient's surrogate decision maker.

PATIENT PREFERENCES

How patient preferences are incorporated into clinical decision making depends on whether the patient is competent or incompetent; decision making for competent and incompetent patients is the focus of the first two parts of this section. The third part examines the situation that arises when the patient's and physician's preferences conflict.

Competent Patients

Given the medical facts (as organized and presented by the physician), what course of action does the competent patient wish to pursue? This is the pivotal question in the therapeutic alliance between doctor and patient. The doctor should educate the patient regarding clinical condition, prognosis, and therapeutic options. The patient may then choose a course of management based on his preferences, values, and goals.

In the doctor-patient relationship, the doctor has both objective and subjective roles. In conveying the clinical circumstances to the patient, the doctor must be reasonably objective so as not to bias the patient's choice. After this objective information has been presented, however, physicians are entitled to offer their subjective opinion to the patient about which treatment choice the physician would prefer. Such personal opinions should be clearly identified as such, and, whenever possible, the physician should also explain why a particular choice of treatment seems preferable.

The patient's right to participate in treatment decisions is well recognized in law, philosophy, public policy, and clinical practice. Perhaps the clearest *legal* statement of this right was enunciated in 1914 by Justice Cardozo: "Every human being of adult years and sound mind has the right to determine what shall be done with his own body." The *philosophical* right of patients to control their own medical care is based on the principle of individual autonomy. In the 1980's, a Presidential Commission clearly stated that respect for patient preferences should be the basis of *public policy* in medical ethics. Moreover, there is evidence from *clinical* research that empowering patients to participate in their own health care may actually lead to improved functional outcomes in chronic diseases.

Incompetent Patients

As a practical matter, competent adult patients can discuss their treatment preferences directly with their physician; incompetent patients cannot. Since the 1976 Quinlan case, judges and legislators have increasingly permitted others to make decisions on behalf of incompetent patients. Forty states have enacted laws recognizing the authority of "living wills," and 17 states have laws about durable powers of attorney for health care. Since only 15 per cent of Americans have executed a formal advance directive, court opinions in many states also permit a process called surrogate decision making, in which another person known as a surrogate decision maker can make decisions on behalf of an incompetent patient.

Surrogate decision making is a method that physicians can use to care for incompetent patients who lack advance directives. Such decision making relies on two standards: substituted judgment and best interests. The goal of substituted judgment, the preferred standard, is "to reach the decision that the incapacitated person would make if he or she were able to choose." Substituted judgment relies upon a knowledge of the patient's attitudes, values, and aspirations; such information must be supplied by the family or friends of the patient. Recent empiric data that show low rates of agreement between patients and their surrogates in resuscitation and end-of-life decisions raise troubling questions about the adequacy of the substituted judgment approach and argue for broader use of advance directives. In the *Cruzan* decision, the United States Supreme Court ruled that in applying the substituted judgment approach, states may establish standards of evidence for determining a patient's prior wishes.

The best interests test is applied in situations in which the patient's attitudes and values are not known to the physician and cannot be learned in the future because of the patient's irreversible cognitive impairment. The best interests approach encourages a surrogate to balance the benefits and burdens of treatment for a particular patient by applying "objective, societally shared criteria." Since such criteria are difficult to agree upon in a pluralistic society, the best interests standard should be used only as a last resort in reaching decisions for incompetent patients who lack advance directives and whose prior attitudes and preferences are not known.

Conscientious Objection

Sometimes the patient or surrogate chooses a treatment option to which the physician is morally opposed. Examples of such treatment plans might include elective abortion, discontinuation of tube feeding, or the request for physician-assisted euthanasia. The right of individual health care providers to refuse to participate in treatment plans that they find morally objectionable has been well established. The President's Commission noted that a health care professional is not "obligated to accede to the patient in a way that violates . . . the provider's own deeply held moral beliefs." (The health care professional may not refuse to provide emergency care.) If the provider refuses, on grounds of personal conscience, to participate in a patient's legal treatment (or nontreatment) request, he should usually arrange for an alternative source of care for the patient. The prerogative of health care facilities or of the entire medical profession to refuse to participate in a morally objectionable treatment plan is more complex and has been discussed elsewhere (see Miles et al., 1989).

SOCIOECONOMIC CONSIDERATIONS

Many factors influence and constrain the individual decisions made by doctors and patients. These factors include family wishes, institutional policies, laws, scarce resources, and economic costs. Because in the 1990's economic considerations are likely to become increasingly important in individual decisions, we focus here on potential conflicts between medical ethics and medical economics.

The cost of health care raises challenging ethical issues at several levels. At the national and state level, the 12 per cent of gross national product ($661 billion in 1990) spent on health care must be balanced against other priorities such as defense, education, and housing. Moreover, priorities must be set between different health programs, as exemplified by the 1988 decision in Oregon to cut funding for organ transplantation in favor of prenatal care. At the institutional level, health care facilities must choose to emphasize some services, such as burn care or cardiac surgery, at the expense of others. It is, however, at the level of the individual patient-physician relationship that economic-ethical conflicts are of greatest concern to the practicing physician.

From the perspective of individual physicians, the essential ethical dilemma is how to incorporate considerations of costs into the traditional decision making framework that places priority on clinical circumstances and patient preferences. Specifically, is it ethically acceptable for physicians to recommend a "less than optimal" management strategy to a patient because of the cost concerns of third parties such as insurance companies, federal or state payers, or HMO's?

Conflict arises between the physician's obligation to serve the patient's "good" and his obligation to serve the public "good" by controlling health care costs. This conflict admits no easy resolution. Some argue that the physician's obligation to control cost may, at times, outweigh his obligation to the patient. We agree that the physician is not obliged to provide inappropriate or ineffective health services (even at the patient's request). We believe, however, that physicians should not withhold medically indicated and desired services on grounds of cost control.

The physician should serve as the patient's advocate (and not as the payer's gatekeeper) for health services that are likely to benefit the patient. Conversely, in a world of limited resources, the physician has the duty to not expend resources that are medically inappropriate or that the patient does not want. For example, researchers at RAND have found that 14 per cent of coronary artery bypass procedures and 32 per cent of carotid endarterectomies are performed for inappropriate reasons, and the National Leadership Commission on Health Care has estimated that the United States could save as much as $22 billion per year by eliminating inappropriate care. There are, of course, many areas of uncertainty in which solid outcome data do not exist or in which marginal benefits and marginal costs must be given serious consideration. The principles of clinical ethics suggest that such decisions be based primarily on clinical circumstances and patient preferences.

The limitation of health services for reasons of cost is a political decision that a society may choose to make. The principle of justice requires, however, that such decisions not be made capriciously in the context of individual patient-physician relationships, but rather as the openly debated public policy of a democratic society.

CONCLUSIONS

In the last decade, clinical medical ethics has emerged as a new and useful component of medical practice. CME emphasizes that technical and ethical concerns are inseparable in the practice of medicine. CME focuses on the continuing centrality of the doctor-patient relationship and on how patients and physicians work within existing administrative structures to reach mutual agreement on clinical decisions that affect the patient. In addition, CME offers a language of discourse that attempts to broaden the medical model from one that is narrowly technical to one that takes serious account of the needs and wants of individual patients. The language and content of clinical ethics have been adopted not only by patients, physicians, and medical educators, but also by health economists, hospital administrators, legislators, and judges. In this regard, ethical considerations in medicine are likely to remain an important component of medical education, clinical practice, and the political evolution of our health system.

After a century of extraordinary scientific achievements, unparalleled in the history of medicine, medical educators and political leaders have come to acknowledge the importance of combining technical excellence with ethical sensitivity to the individual patient's goals. Plato recognized the importance of this 2500 years ago when, in Book IV of *The Laws*, he described the excellent physician as one who ". . . treats disease by going into things thoroughly from the beginning in a scientific way and takes the patient and family into confidence. Thus he learns something from the sufferer . . . He does not give prescriptions until he has won the patient's support, and when he has done so, he steadfastly aims at providing complete restoration to health by persuading the sufferer into compliance. . . ." The best clinical medicine, Plato tells us, is achieved when patient and physician have established a relationship in which technical and personal aspects of care are integrated. The practice of ethical medicine in the twenty-first century will require nothing more but demand nothing less.

Appelbaum PS, Grisso T: Assessing patients' capacities to consent to treatment. N Engl J Med 319:1635–1638, 1988. *A review of the four factors to consider in assessing patients' decision-making capacity.*

Connelly JE, DalleMura S: Ethical problems in the medical office. JAMA 260:812–815, 1988. *An empirical study of the epidemiology of outpatient clinical-ethical problems.*

Emanuel LL, Emanuel EJ: The medical directive. A new comprehensive advance care document. JAMA 261:3288–3293, 1989. *An expanded version of the "living will" which may prove more useful clinically.*

Ethics Committee, American College of Physicians: American College of Physicians Ethics Manual, 2nd edition. Ann Intern Med 111:245–252, 327–335, 1989. *An official consensus statement by the American College of Physicians on a wide range of ethical issues that relate to internal medicine practice, including decisions to forego life-sustaining treatments and economic-ethical conflicts.*

Jonsen AR, Siegler M, Winslade WJ: Clinical Ethics: A Practical Approach to Ethical Decisions in Clinical Medicine. 3rd ed. New York, Pergamon Press, 1990. *A practical guide to help clinicians deal with ethical problems that occur frequently in medical practice.*

Lantos JD, Singer PA, Walker RM, et al.: The illusion of futility in clinical practice. Am J Med 87:81–84, 1989. *An analysis of how the powerful concept of "futility" is used and misused in clinical medicine.*

Lo B, Schroeder SA: Frequency of ethical dilemmas in a medical inpatient service. Arch Intern Med 141:1062–1064, 1981. *An empirical study of the epidemiology of inpatient clinical-ethical problems.*

Miles SH, Singer PA, Siegler M: Conflicts between patients' requests to forego treatment and the policies of health care facilities. N Engl J Med 321:48–50, 1989. *An approach for resolving conflicts that arise when patient preferences conflict with institutional policy.*

President's Commission for the Study of Ethical Problems in Medicine and Biomedical and Behavioral Research: Making Health Care Decisions: The Ethical and Legal Implications of Informed Consent in the Patient-Practitioner Relationship, Vol. 1. Washington, D.C., U.S. Government Printing Office, 1982. *This important report concluded that ethically valid consent is a process of shared decision making between physicians and patients.*

Siegler M, Singer PA, Schiedermayer DL: Medical Ethics: An Annotated Bibliography. Philadelphia, American College of Physicians, 1988. *A clinically oriented annotated bibliography of the medical ethics literature through July 1988; designed to accompany the second edition of the American College of Physicians Ethics Manual.*

Singer PA, Siegler M: Elective use of life-sustaining treatments. *In* Stollerman GH (ed.): Advances in Internal Medicine, Vol. 36. New York, Year Book, 1991. *Reviews empirical data and provides a clinical approach to the elective use of life-sustaining treatments in internal medicine.*

PART II

HUMAN GROWTH, DEVELOPMENT, AND AGING

5 Adolescent Medicine

Iris F. Litt

The teenager is a psychosocially and physically unique individual, and this uniqueness has important implications for health and health care. In addition to the age-specific features of this period of life, there are significant differences among adolescents, based upon their rates of pubertal development as well as their psychosocial development. The view of the adolescent from the physical standpoint reveals the importance of stage of pubertal development, rather than chronologic age, as an organizing principle, owing to the wide variability in timing of pubertal events. From a psychosocial perspective, early adolescents, middle adolescents, and late adolescents have many psychosocial and cognitive characteristics shared with others in their own age groups. There is a growing tendency to combine these vantage points and recognize the areas of interaction between pubertal and psychosocial development.

PSYCHOSOCIAL DEVELOPMENT

During adolescence, certain tasks must be mastered if the child is going to evolve into a successful adult in our society. These include the "tasks of adolescence": the process of separation from the protective milieu of the family and, with it, development of independence; incorporation of the physical and emotional effects of pubertal hormonal changes into one's self-concept; development of a clear sexual identity and a sense of sexual adequacy; educational and vocational decision making; and achievement of the capacity for intimacy. Accomplishing these goals may, in actuality, take a lifetime, but the physician caring for adolescents may encounter opportunities to assist in the psychosocial development of the adolescent.

The physician may foster development of independence by encouraging the adolescent to make his or her own appointments, by promising confidentiality when appropriate, by handing the prescription directly to the adolescent patient rather than to the parent, and so on. Encouraging the parent of a chronically ill adolescent to assign household chores, to provide an allowance, and to allow going to friends' houses for "overnights" may prevent infantilization at the time when adolescents must be allowed to experience their emerging maturity. Failure to do so often results in "acting-out" behavior. One consequence of the stereotype of adolescents as rebellious patients is that physicians may expect them to be noncompliant with prescribed medication. When this stereotype is examined, however, it is found that the incidence of noncompliance is no different among adolescents than among adult patients, in the range of 40 to 50 per cent. The factors associated with noncompliance among adolescents are, however, different. Self-concept is the single most important predictor of compliance: The teenager who has a positive self-image is likely to follow the physician's advice. Moreover, the risk of noncompliance is great with any medication that affects appearance adversely, such as a systemic corticosteroid. The patient's satisfaction, a valid predictor of compliance for adult patients, is also important for the adolescent patient, but here again its determinants are different. The satisfied adolescent patient is the one whose privacy is respected, who is afforded the courtesy of confidentiality, and who is informed about the reasons for laboratory testing. Self-concept is also related to the risk of pregnancy during adolescence. Poor self-concept may place the young adolescent girl at increased risk of an exploitative relationship or cause her to lack the confidence to set limits within a sexual relationship. Low self-concept is also associated with poor compliance with oral contraceptives, further contributing to pregnancy risk.

Among the many causes of poor self-concept is the timing of pubertal maturation. For males, maturing earlier than the peer group appears to be an advantage, associated with popularity and athletic prowess, whereas a late-maturing male is predisposed to poorer educational performance and lower self-image. For females, the effects vary with the environmental context; for example, early maturers who remain in a kindergarten–through–eighth grade school exhibit no apparent ill effect from being out of synchrony with their peer group, whereas those early maturers who move to a junior high school have a higher incidence of poor self-image, have a lower grade-point average, and date more. Timing of pubertal development may also influence selection of sports involvement. Early-maturing females tend to have more adipose tissue, are more buoyant, and therefore may be channeled into swimming. The late-maturing girl, on the other hand, with her shorter upper to lower body ratio and leaner body may be more likely to become a ballet dancer or runner. An increase in body fat accompanies normal pubertal development in females, who often have difficulty reconciling it with our society's idealized female form of a skinny fashion model. Their dissatisfaction may result in dieting and the risk of nutritional deficiencies. This puberty-associated dieting may be the forerunner of anorexia nervosa in the predisposed individual (see Ch. 12).

The physician may assist the adolescent's development of a healthy sense of sexual identity and adequacy by offering reassurance about the normality of secondary sex characteristics and genitalia during the course of a routine physical examination. This is particularly important when gynecomastia is observed, as this common phenomenon often causes concern to the adolescent male, who is unlikely to have the courage to inquire about it. The female adolescent with asymmetry of her breasts or one who has not gotten pregnant despite having had unprotected intercourse, or the male teenager who has never impregnated his sexual partner, all may be questioning their sexual adequacy and normality. Even more problematic is the male adolescent who has a renal or urologic condition. The separation of reproductive from excretory function and structure may not be known or apparent to the apprehensive patient, although this is often assumed by his physician. A useful method for allaying such fear may be concrete explanations about anatomy and pathogenesis of the condition, prefaced by a comment like the following: "Some other boys who have had this operation have been worried that it may interfere with their ability to have sex. I don't know if you have had this worry, but I want to reassure you that it will not."

COGNITIVE DEVELOPMENT

The issues of counseling and confidentiality in the context of health care delivery to adolescents are complicated by the developmental differences in cognition among them. Piaget classified children and adolescents on the basis of discrete stages of cognitive development (Table 5–1). According to this schema, most early adolescents are at the stage of concrete operational thinking, whereas middle and late adolescents are more likely to have progressed to the highest stage of development, that of formal operations. This stage is distinguished by the ability to generate hypotheses that may be tested without their actual enactment. Moreover, the person in the stage of formal operations can think abstractly, entertain multiple contingencies simultaneously, generalize from one situation to another, and consider potential behavioral consequences logically without actually having to experience them. Piaget's static, categoric approach to cognitive development has been challenged. Newer research in the field stresses "trends" in domain-specific development. For example, the thinking of the younger individual is now regarded as more "empirico-deductive" than that of the older adolescent, who is viewed as more "hypothetico-deductive." Whatever the system used to evaluate cognition, it is important for the physician working with the adolescent patient to be able to assess his or her capacity for understanding the information conveyed and using it in a manner conducive to improving health status. For example, the adolescent female who is not able to think abstractly may have difficulty adhering to a regimen of oral contraceptives designed to prevent pregnancy. Similarly, truly informed consent to participate in a research project may not be obtainable from an adolescent subject unable to consider hypothetic consequences of his or her decision to participate or not.

PUBERTAL DEVELOPMENT

The Endocrinology of Puberty

The signal that initiates puberty remains elusive but it is known that just prior to puberty there is decreasing sensitivity of the hypothalamus and pituitary to circulating estrogen and testosterone and to the restraining influence of the hypothalamic arcuate neuron gonadotropin-releasing hormone. The latter is a pulsatile secretion augmented by sleep. The onset of puberty is marked by increased secretion of luteinizing hormone (LH) by the pituitary during sleep in a pulsatile fashion. The amplitude and frequency of LH pulses increase as puberty progresses. In late puberty, the adult pattern of approximately 12 pulses, evenly distributed over the course of a 24-hour period, is reached. There is a sex difference in gonadotropin secretion during puberty: A dramatic increase in LH levels occurs during early puberty in boys and later in girls. Follicle-stimulating hormone (FSH), on the other hand, rises gradually throughout puberty in boys and manifests an early rise in girls. The effect of the gonadotropin rise in males is to stimulate testicular production of testosterone. In females, the gonadotropin rise (predominantly involving FSH) stimulates the ovary to produce estradiol, with serum levels rising incrementally as puberty progresses. This is manifested by the development of secondary sex characteristics (see p. 17). Cyclic fluctuations in estradiol levels are noted around the time of menarche. Estrone, derived from conversion of estradiol and adrenal androstenedione, reaches its peak at sex maturity rating (SMR) 2 in girls. In boys, both estrone and estradiol (derived from conversion of adrenal and testicular testosterone and androstenedione) contribute to the frequent occurrence (in 30 to 50 per cent) of gynecomastia during SMR 2 and 3. Circulating sex hormones exert a constant or tonic negative feedback effect upon the hypothalamus in both sexes. The female also experiences a cyclic positive feedback loop by which increasing levels of circulating estrogens in the follicular phase cause a surge in LH. Sex

TABLE 5–1. PIAGET'S ERAS AND STAGES OF LOGICAL AND COGNITIVE DEVELOPMENT

Era I	(ages 0–2): The era of sensorimotor intelligence
Era II	(ages 2–5): Symbolic, intuitive, or prelogical thought
Era III	(ages 6–10): Concrete operational thought
Era IV	(ages 11–adulthood): Formal operational thought

hormone binding globulin levels fall in males during puberty. As only unbound sex hormones are physiologically active, this results in levels of free testosterone that are more than twice the female levels. Prolactin secretion by the pituitary is augmented by estrogen, resulting in higher levels in females than males, peaking between SMR 2 and 3. Prolactin response to thyrotropin-releasing hormone (TRH) stimulation, however, peaks at SMR 4 to 5.

Growth Hormone and Somatomedin-C

Growth hormone is also produced in a pulsatile fashion, during sleep stages 3 and 4 in early puberty. Somatomedins are responsible for the anabolic activity of growth hormone. Somatomedin-C (IGF-1) levels are age dependent and rise in conjunction with advancing development of secondary sex characteristics during puberty. Accordingly, their levels correlate better with stage of sexual maturation than chronologic age.

Physical Growth During Puberty

During puberty, a growth spurt is experienced by every organ system in the body, with the exception of the central nervous system, which remains stable in size, and the lymphoid system, which undergoes involution. The most noticeable changes produced by the pubertal growth spurt are in height, weight, and the secondary sex characteristics.

The pubertal height spurt occurs during midpuberty (SMR 3 to 4) in most individuals, with its peak occurring at an average age of 12 years in girls and 14 years in boys. During this height spurt, males gain 10.3 ± 1.54 cm per year and females gain 9.0 ± 1.03 cm per year. The growth velocity is greater the earlier it occurs. There is an orderly pattern of linear growth, beginning with the foot, followed within 6 months by the lower leg and then the thigh. Growth of the upper extremity and of the trunk occurs after that of the lower extremity. The later onset of the growth spurt in males than in females results in a longer period of prepubertal growth and hence longer legs in males. Assessment of height during puberty should be undertaken using a height velocity curve, which records increments in height per year (Fig. 5–1).

Approximately 4 months after the peak of leg-length acceleration, there is an increase in the biacromial and biiliac diameters, the former of greater magnitude in males and the latter in females, resulting in characteristic sex differences in adult physiques. At about the same time, the cranial bones undergo a growth spurt, particularly the jaw, which becomes more prominent, especially in boys. Elongation of the pharynx causes lowering of the hyoid bone. Dentition is another reflection of pubertal development. The cuspids (canines) and first molars of the primary dentition are shed by early adolescence, at which time the permanent cuspids and the first and second premolars erupt in their place. The timing of appearance of the second permanent molar correlates well with that of menarche. The third molars, "wisdom teeth," erupt during late adolescence.

Bone age can be determined from a roentgenogram of the hand, which is compared with standards in an atlas. During puberty, there is close correlation between bone age and stage of sexual maturation (SMR—see below).

Although both sexes experience a weight spurt during puberty, its origin is different in males and females. In males, it is due to increase in muscle mass, and in females, to fat tissue. Eight per cent of body composition is about average fat content in both sexes throughout childhood. At puberty, males experience a loss in fat tissue, whereas it begins to increase in females and reaches approximately 22 per cent when pubertal growth is complete (SMR 5).

Secondary Sex Characteristics

Estrogen and testosterone have a profound effect on a variety of tissues and organs during puberty. These effects are collectively referred to as secondary sex characteristics and include voice change, body and facial hair in males, breast development in females, and axillary and pubic hair in both sexes. Of these changes, those most consistent in pattern and timing are pubic hair in both sexes and breast development in females. Accordingly, these traits have formed the basis for categorization of the

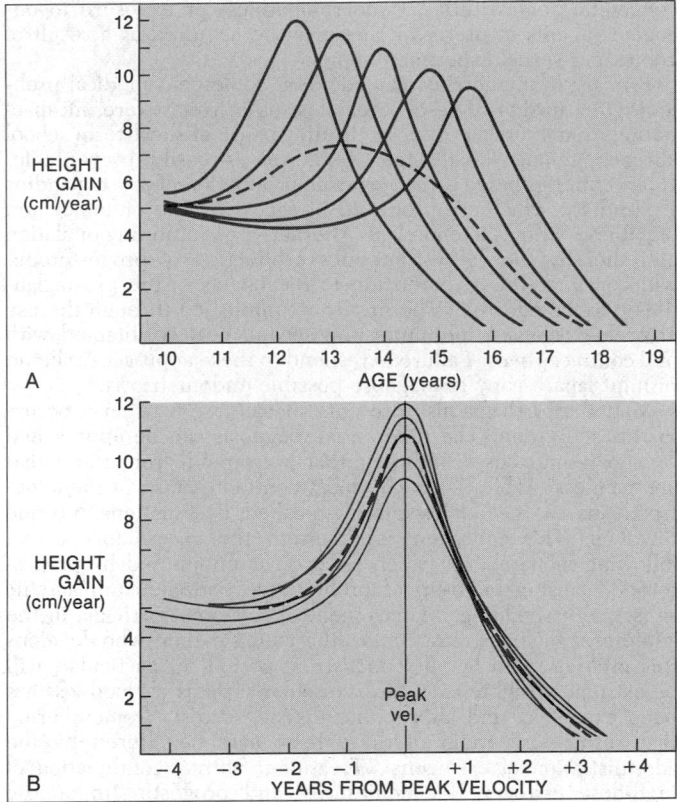

FIGURE 5–1. The relation between individual and mean velocities during the adolescent spurt. *A,* The individual height velocity curves of five boys of the Harpenden Growth Study (solid lines) with the mean curve (dashed) constructed by averaging their values at each age. *B,* The same curves all plotted according to their peak height velocity. (Adapted by permission of the publishers from *Fetus into Man* by J. M. Tanner, Cambridge, Mass.: Harvard University Press, copyright © 1978 by J. M. Tanner.)

stages of pubertal development, generally referred to as sex maturity ratings (SMR's).

STAGES OF PUBERTAL DEVELOPMENT (SMR's): BREAST

SMR 1: Childlike. No breast development.
SMR 2: Appearance of a breast bud.
Increase in diameter of the areola. Average age is 11.2 ± 1.6 years.
SMR 3: Enlargement of the breast. Average age is 12.15 ± 1.09 years.
SMR 4: The areola and papilla enlarge to form a mound above the underlying breast tissue. Average age is 13.11 ± 1.15 years.
SMR 5: Adult configuration with areola and underlying breast tissue in same plane. Average age is 14.5 ± 1.6 years.

STAGES OF PUBERTAL DEVELOPMENT (SMR's): PUBIC HAIR

SMR 1: Childlike. No pubic hair.
SMR 2: Hair is fine, long, silky, and lightly pigmented. Distributed in the midline, along the separation of the labia majora in females and the base of the phallus in males. Average age is 11.9 ± 1.5 years in females and 12.3 ± 0.8 years in males.
SMR 3: Hair is darker and coarser and begins to curl. It extends upward and laterally. Average age is 12.7 ± 0.5 years in females and 13.9 ± 1.04 years in males.
SMR 4: Adult texture and distributed to cover the mons pubis. Average age is 13.4 ± 1.2 in females and 14.36 ± 1.08 years in males.
SMR 5: Adult texture. Distributed beyond the mons to the medial aspect of the thighs. Average age is 14.6 ± 1.1 years in females and 15.3 ± 0.8 years in males.

STAGES OF PUBERTAL DEVELOPMENT (SMR's): MALE GENITALIA

SMR 1: Childlike. Testes average 2 ml in volume.
SMR 2: Scrotal skin begins to redden and thin. Scrotum narrows proximally, testes enlarge, and left testis lowers. Penis begins to lengthen. Mean age is 11.64 ± 1.07 years.
SMR 3: Testes continue to enlarge. Growth of corpora cavernosa penis contributes to widening, as well as lengthening, of penis. Mean age is 12.85 ± 1.04 years.
SMR 4: Further enlargement of testes and penis. Scrotum darkens. The glans becomes prominent. Average age is 13.7 ± 1.02 years.
SMR 5: Testes have reached adult size of approximately 25 ml and weight of 20 gm. Full reproductive capability by this stage. Average age is 15.1 ± 1.1 years.

"Primary" Sex Characteristics

The sine qua non of puberty is attainment of reproductive function. To this end, there is considerable growth of the reproductive organs. As indicated above, this process in the male commences with enlargement of the testes as a result of the growth in size of their seminiferous tubules and the number of Leydig and Sertoli cells. The epididymis, seminal vesicles, and prostate enlarge as well. The capacity for ejaculation is achieved approximately 1 year after testicular growth begins, coincident with appearance of pubic hair (SMR 2). For most, the first ejaculatory episode occurs in the context of masturbation, followed about 1 year later by nocturnal emissions. The median age for appearance of sperm in the first morning urine sample is 13.5 to 14.5 years. The timing of spermarche is asynchronous with other manifestations of puberty, occurring at any SMR from 1 to 5 and antedating the peak height velocity. Although complete reproductive capability is not reached until SMR 5, it is possible for impregnation to occur earlier. Accordingly, anticipatory guidance about pregnancy prevention should commence during early to middle adolescence for males.

Increasing levels of estrogen during pubertal development lead to endometrial thickening, enlargement of the corpus, and increase in cellular content of actomyosin, creatine phosphokinase (CPK), and adenosine triphosphate (ATP). Menarche occurs at a mean age of 13.3 ± 1.3 years, although its timing corresponds better with developmental than chronologic age. Ten per cent of girls have menarche at SMR 2, 20 per cent at SMR 3, 60 per cent at SMR 4, and the remaining 10 per cent at SMR 5. In addition, there is close concordance between menarche and the peak of the weight velocity curve, which follows by approximately 6 months the peak of the height velocity curve. The interrelationships of timing of pubertal events are shown in Figures 5–2

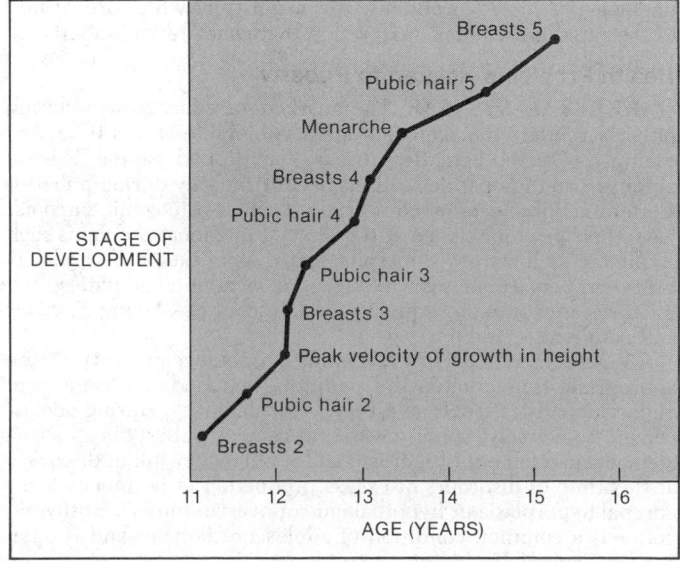

FIGURE 5–2. Sequence of breast and pubic hair development in adolescent girls.

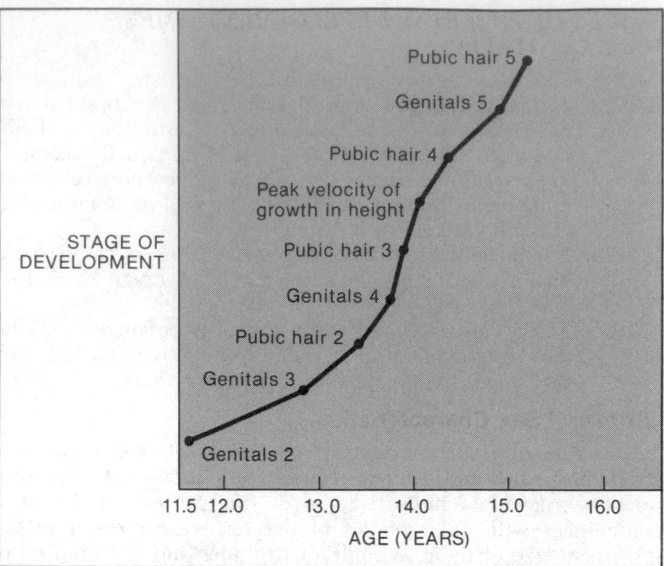

FIGURE 5–3. Sequence of genital and pubic hair development in adolescent boys.

and 5–3. These interrelationships are useful in the clinical assessment of the young adolescent who is concerned about her failure to begin to menstruate. Regardless of her chronologic age, she should be further evaluated if she is more than 1 year older than her mother or siblings at the time they experienced menarche, if she is at SMR 5, or if her bone age is 14.5 years or greater. In addition, failure to begin pubertal development by the age of 11 years should be cause for concern. Menarche occurs earlier in the obese than the lean adolescent female. Moreover, weight loss of as little as 10 per cent of body weight may result in cessation of menstruation, as can vigorous athletic training with or without weight loss. Full reproductive capability is typically reached within a year following menarche, but some adolescents ovulate regularly from the time of menarche, underscoring the need for timely education about pregnancy risk.

HEALTH PROBLEMS OF ADOLESCENTS

The image of adolescents as healthy and therefore not in need of health care has been fostered by a number of factors. Among them is the fact that this age group contributes only 11 per cent of office visits to physicians, the majority for gynecologic or obstetric care or acute injuries. However, data from the National Health Examination Survey of 1966 to 1970 reveal that 20 per cent of presumably healthy 12- to 17-year-olds have previously undiagnosed health problems, the majority of which are related to the rapid growth and maturation that characterize puberty.

Health Problems Related to Puberty

SKELETAL SYSTEM. The marked osseous growth during puberty renders the skeletal system vulnerable at this time. For example, Osgood-Schlatter disease or slipped capital femoral epiphysis and idiopathic scoliosis occur primarily during puberty. Certain neoplasms of osseous origin, such as osteogenic sarcoma, have their peak incidence at this time. Functional problems such as pitcher's elbow or "shin splints" are manifestations of adolescents' propensity for overinvolvement in athletic activities, and fractures are common sequelae of adolescent risk-taking behavior and resultant accidents.

ENDOCRINE SYSTEM. Failure to achieve puberty at the appropriate time is often the symptom that leads to diagnosis of endocrinopathies, such as pituitary insufficiency, during adolescence. Conversely, syndromes of precocious puberty or exaggerated adrenarche (e.g., hirsutism and acne) may result in discovery at this time of disorders of excess production of hormones (e.g., adrenal hyperplasia or hypothalamic or ovarian tumor). Euthyroid goiter is a common condition of adolescent females and is often the first sign of Hashimoto thyroiditis.

GYNECOLOGIC. Gynecologic problems are common during this age period. They may be the result of previously undiagnosed

congenital abnormalities, endocrinopathies, or exposure to oncogenic agents in utero, or they may be acquired as a result of adolescent sexual experimentation.

Primary dysmenorrhea is a common adolescent medical problem. One third of adolescent females suffer from severe, incapacitating dysmenorrhea. It is the leading cause of short-term school absence among female teenagers, yet is easily preventable. Intervention is based on suppressing production of prostaglandins $F_{2\alpha}$ and E_2, which are produced in excess by the endometrium of patients with dysmenorrhea. Alternatively, inhibiting ovulation and thereby the corpus luteum's production of progesterone, which primes the myometrium to the effects of the prostaglandins, will be effective. The first is accomplished through the use of cyclo-oxygenase inhibitors; the second goal is obtained with oral contraceptives. Failure to respond to these approaches should prompt laparoscopy to diagnose possible endometriosis.

Menometrorrhagia also presents special issues when it occurs in this age group. The differential diagnosis can be approached by separating those conditions that are painful from those that are painless (Table 5–2). The most common cause of menometrorrhagia in the adolescent is so-called dysfunctional uterine bleeding. This condition results from the anovulatory cycles following menarche in which estrogen is unopposed by progesterone, causing build-up of proliferative endometrium and its subsequent shedding. Management of menometrorrhagia in the adolescent includes reassurance (the young patient who develops this problem with her first menstrual period, in particular, will be extremely frightened), cardiovascular support if blood loss has been excessive, and appropriate diagnostic tests (remembering that results of certain of these tests may be altered by the administration of estrogens). Treatment with a combination of high-dose estrogen (for hemostasis) and progestin (to oppose endogenous estrogen effect), as may be found in Enovid (mestranol and norethynodrel), is effective except in cases of pregnancy, trauma, or infection.

Another menstrually associated condition of particular importance in adolescents is toxic shock syndrome (see Ch. 300). Forty-two per cent of cases reported during its peak years of 1980 to 1982 were in this age group.

A number of other gynecologic conditions of adolescents result from sexual experimentation. The reported prevalence of sexual intercourse among American girls between 13 and 19 years of age increases from 10 to 50 per cent and sexually transmitted diseases and pregnancy increase correspondingly.

Pregnancy during adolescence continues to be a major problem in the United States, which has the highest rate of any of the developed countries. Close to one-half million 15- to 19-year-olds become pregnant yearly. In addition, over the past two decades, there has been nearly a 200 per cent rise in the rate of out-of-wedlock births in this age group, as well as an increase in the number of unmarried adolescents who elect to keep their babies rather than place them for adoption. Among those under the age

TABLE 5–2. DIFFERENTIAL DIAGNOSIS OF MENOMETRORRHAGIA

Painless	Painful
Systematic	Trauma
Coagulopathy	Threatened abortion
Congenital	Salpingitis
von Willebrand disease	Intrauterine device
Acquired	
Aspirin sensitivity	
Aplastic anemia	
Anticoagulant treatment	
Neoplasm–bone marrow infiltration	
Idiopathic thrombocytopenia	
Endocrine	
Hypothyroidism	
Oral contraceptives–used improperly	
Local	
Gynecologic	
Dysfunctional uterine bleeding	
Neoplasm	

From Litt IF: Menstrual problems during adolescence. Reproduced by permission of Pediatrics in Review, Vol. 4, page 203, copyright 1983.

of 15 years, the pregnancy rate continues to rise, with 31,000 births last year. In addition to the psychosocial sequelae of adolescent births (such as adverse educational, vocational, economic, and marital outcomes), those who become pregnant under the age of 15 years are generally at increased risk for obstetric and perinatal complications such as toxemia, postpartum hemorrhage, postpartum infection, and small-for-gestational age and stillborn infants.

SEXUALLY TRANSMITTED DISEASE (STD). Adolescents have the highest rate of sexually transmitted disease of any age group. The most common of the STD's are gonorrhea, chlamydial and human papilloma virus (HPV) infections. Physicians should routinely test for the presence of other STD's when one is discovered, treat with the shortest effective methods, including parenteral antibiotics when feasible, and extend confidentiality to contacts.

Violence

Accidents, homicides, and suicides together are responsible for 70 per cent of adolescent deaths. Anticipatory guidance, prevention, and identification and referral of the youngster at risk are therefore important interventions by the physician.

ACCIDENTS. Although athletic injuries and accidental drowning contribute significantly to morbidity and mortality, the greatest toll among adolescents is taken by accidents involving motor vehicles. Sixteen- to 19-year-olds constitute 8 per cent of the United States population yet account for 17 per cent of vehicular fatalities. Passengers in cars driven by adolescents account for 63 per cent of automotive deaths. More male than female adolescents are involved as drivers in fatal accidents, and most of these occur between the hours of 8 P.M. and 4 A.M. Aside from failure to use seatbelts in cars and to wear helmets on motorcycles, alcohol abuse is the leading cause of most motor vehicular fatalities. Lowering the drinking age to 18 years has been associated with a 5 per cent increase in fatal automotive accidents. Talking with adolescent patients about their use of automotive safety devices and alcohol use prior to driving should be a routine part of health care. Moreover, physicians may act to improve the well-being of their teenaged patients by influencing legislative efforts such as those directed at requiring seatbelts in school buses and use of motorcycle helmets, raising the drinking age, and imposing late-night curfews for adolescent drivers.

SUICIDE. Suicide currently ranks as the third leading cause of death among the 15- to 19-year-old cohort in the United States. Completed suicides are more likely to occur in males, whereas female adolescents are more likely to make uncompleted attempts. Sex differences also exist regarding the method used in the attempt; males are more likely to use violent methods, such as shooting, hanging, or wrist slashing, whereas females are more prone to ingestion of drugs. Chronically ill adolescents are at high risk for suicide, and their own medication may be ingested in the suicide attempt. Alternatively, the medication is often that of the parent with whom the teenager is in conflict. Assessment of the seriousness of the adolescent's suicide attempt becomes crucial to planning following such an act. The physician may be surprised to learn that the youngster who ingested a bottle of antibiotics was actually expecting to die as a result or, conversely, that the one who took a bottle of acetaminophen resulting in admission to the intensive care unit had erroneously thought the substance harmless and was only trying to get some attention from his or her parents. The adolescent who fails in an initial suicide attempt is at increased risk for a subsequent serious one, if the crisis has not been adequately addressed in the interim. Simply attending to the pharmacologic or surgical sequelae of the attempt does little to resolve the underlying conflict. Short-term hospitalization is often effective in providing a secure setting for the teenager and impressing parents with the need to seek help for the contributing problems.

Identification of the adolescent at risk for suicide prior to an attempt presents an even greater challenge to the physician. Mood swings from deep despair to the heights of elation are not uncommon during adolescence, but persistence of the depressed mood should be regarded as a sign of potential trouble. According to Puig-Antich, depression should be considered persistent if it lasts for at least 3 consecutive hours for three or more periods

TABLE 5–3. THE WELL-ADOLESCENT VISIT: EARLY ADOLESCENCE (TANNER 2)

	Females	Males
Screening		
Physical	Hematocrit	—
	Urine culture screen	—
	Tuberculin test	Tuberculin test
Psychosocial	Self-image	Self-image
	Depression	Depression
	Peer interaction (including sexuality)	Peer interaction (including sexuality)
	School performance	School performance
	Substance abuse	Substance abuse
Health promotion	Self-examination of breasts	Self-examination of scrotum
	Nutrition counseling	Nutrition counseling
Prevention	Smoking	Smoking
	Cycle safety	Cycle safety
	Automotive passenger safety	Automotive passenger safety
	Immunization update	Immunization update
Anticipatory guidance	Developing independence	Developing independence
	Dealing with peer pressure	Dealing with peer pressure
	Confidentiality	Confidentiality
	Variations in growth and development	Variations in growth and development
	Dating	Dating
	Preparation for menarche	
Physical examination with special attention to:	Blood pressure	Blood pressure
	Height, weight	Height, weight
	Skinfold thickness	Skinfold thickness
	—	Grip strength
	Stage of sexual development	Stage of sexual development
	Scoliosis	—
	Goiter	—
	Acne	Acne
	—	Gynecomastia
	Tibial tubercle	Tibial tubercle
	Gait	
Symptomatic treatment (anything revealed by the above +)	Acne	Acne
	Dysmenorrhea	—

From Litt IF: Adolescent health care. *In* Green M, Haggarty RJ (eds.): Ambulatory Pediatrics IV. Philadelphia, W. B. Saunders Company, 1989.

TABLE 5–4. THE WELL-ADOLESCENT VISIT: MID-ADOLESCENCE (TANNER 3–4)

	Females	Males
Screening		
Physical	Vision testing	Vision testing
	Hearing testing	Hearing testing
If sexually active	Pap smear	—
	VDRL	VDRL
	Gonorrhea culture	Gonorrhea culture
Prevention	Automotive safety	Automotive safety
	STD prevention	STD prevention
	Pregnancy prevention	Pregnancy prevention
	Vocational/educational planning	Vocational/educational planning
	Obesity/inactivity	Obesity/inactivity
Physical examination	Breast masses	Gynecomastia
	—	Testicular tumor
	Vaginal discharge	Urethral discharge
	Pregnancy	—

From Litt IF: Adolescent health care. *In* Green M, Haggarty RJ (eds.): Ambulatory Pediatrics IV. Philadelphia, W. B. Saunders Company, 1989.

each week. Expressions of hopelessness and helplessness are also serious signs of depression. Disturbance of eating or sleeping may or may not be found in the depressed adolescent. A family history of depression is a useful predictor of seriousness. Some depressed adolescents may, alternatively, appear perpetually euphoric and may engage in socially self-destructive behavior such as drug use or sexual promiscuity. In evaluating the adolescent suspected of depression, it may be useful to inquire about plans for the future. When none are expressed or when the response is "what does it matter, I won't be here much longer," serious depression is obvious. When there is a suggestion of depression, the physician should not hesitate to inquire if the teenager has ever felt so sad that death was viewed as preferable. If the answer is affirmative, the existence of a suicide plan should be sought and such a patient should be immediately evaluated by a psychiatrist. Such questioning will not prompt suicidal thoughts in a youngster who has not already had them and will be greeted with relief by the one who has.

Substance Abuse

Experimentation with drugs serves a variety of purposes for adolescents in our society. It may symbolize attainment of adult maturity or rejection of parental values, facilitate peer acceptance, reduce stress, and, for some, provide an opportunity to explore the limits of new cognitive abilities through hallucinogenic effects. Intervention strategies for preventing or stopping drug use by adolescents must consider these various developmentally adaptive implications. Since more than 90 per cent of adolescents have experimented with either alcohol or marijuana by the time of high school graduation, the focus of the physician's involvement should be on the functional and physical implications of use rather than on the simple ascertainment of use or non-use.

Overall use of illicit drugs by high school seniors has decreased from a peak of 54 per cent in 1978 to 42 per cent in 1987 (Johnston et al.). Decline of daily marijuana use to 3.0 per cent is largely responsible for this finding. Declines have also been recorded for use of amphetamine, methaqualone, LSD (lysergic acid diethylamide), barbiturates, tranquilizers, heroin, inhalants, and phencyclidine. By contrast, however, cocaine use has doubled and smokeless tobacco is now used by approximately 20 per cent of male adolescents. Other sex differences include the increase in smoking by adolescent females and their 45 per cent lifetime incidence of use of diet pills. Alcohol is the most widely abused substance by this age group, with 93 per cent reporting use at some time and 5.5 per cent citing daily use. The time of greatest risk for initiation of cigarette smoking and alcohol and marijuana use is prior to the age of 20 years. Follow-up studies of adolescent "problem" drinkers demonstrated that one half of the males and one quarter of the females continued to have drinking problems as young adults.

Pubertal growth and development may be adversely affected by the use of drugs during this period of life. That the incidence of menstrual dysfunction resulting from drugs is higher in adolescent than adult women suggests greater vulnerability of the hypothalamic-pituitary-ovarian axis in the young. Heroin appears to block gonadotropin-releasing hormone. Amphetamines interfere with stage 4 sleep and may thus impair secretion of gonadotropins in early puberty. Induction of smooth endoplasmic reticulum of the liver by a variety of abused substances, such as opiates, barbiturates, and tobacco smoke, has the potential for accelerating metabolism of hormones important for pubertal development, such as estrogens.

Regular use of any drug will eventually diminish the youngster's ability to function appropriately in school, to hold a job, or to operate a motor vehicle. An "amotivational" syndrome has been described in chronic marijuana users who lose interest in age-appropriate behavior.

The "infectious disease" model of prevention has little relevance to the problem of adolescent drug or alcohol abuse, nor are "scare" techniques effective. A more realistic approach is one that anticipates that most adolescents will experiment with some drug at some point and is designed to delay that event as long as possible, to limit the extent of use, and to prevent its use in conjunction with operating a motor vehicle. Presentation of

TABLE 5–5. THE WELL-ADOLESCENT VISIT: LATE ADOLESCENCE (TANNER 5)

	Females	Males
Screening		
Physical	Genetically transmitted diseases	Genetically transmitted diseases
If sexually active	Pap smear	—
	VDRL	VDRL
If homosexual or bisexual	Gonorrhea culture	Gonorrhea culture, HIV
	—	
Prevention	Automotive safety	Automotive safety
	STD prevention	STD prevention
	Pregnancy prevention	Pregnancy prevention
	Obesity/inactivity	Obesity/inactivity
Anticipatory guidance	Planning for marriage	Planning for marriage
	Vocational/educational planning	Vocational/educational planning
	Cults	Cults
	Becoming a health care consumer	Becoming a health care consumer
	Leaving home	Leaving home
	Moving into work force/college	Moving into work force/college
	Entering military	Entering military
	Health insurance	Health insurance
Physical examination	Breast masses	Testicular tumor
	Vaginal discharge	Urethral discharge
	Pregnancy	—
Treatment	Corrective surgery (after growth complete)	Corrective surgery (after growth complete)

From Litt IF: Adolescent health care. *In* Green M, Haggarty RJ (eds.): Ambulatory Pediatrics IV. Philadelphia, W. B. Saunders Company, 1989.

factual information about medical complications of drug use by health professionals appears to have some positive impact. Strategies that enable young adolescents to resist peer pressure to smoke, by the use of trained peer counselors using role-playing techniques, have significantly reduced the onset of smoking in a number of studies.

The content of the medical evaluation of the adolescent is outlined in Tables 5–3 to 5–5.

General

Litt IF: Evaluation of the Adolescent Patient. Philadelphia, Hanley and Belfus, 1990. *A symptom-focused guide to assessment of the adolescent patient.*

Growth and Development

Grumbach MM: The neuroendocrinology of puberty. *In* Krieger DT, Hughes JC (eds.): Neuroendocrinology. Sunderland, Mass., Sinauer Associates, 1980. *The intricacies of neuroendocrine pathways and developmental interrelationship are presented in an easily understood manner.*

Kagan J, Coles R (eds.): Twelve to Sixteen: Early Adolescence. New York, W. W. Norton and Company, 1972. *A series of papers on various psychosocial aspects of adolescent development.*

Litt IF: Adolescent health care. *In* Green M, Haggerty RJ (eds.): Ambulatory Pediatrics. IV. Philadelphia, W. B. Saunders Company, 1989. *Useful information and suggestions for approaching and screening adolescents in an ambulatory setting.*

Litt IF: Menstrual problems during adolescence. Pediatr Rev 4:203, 1983. *A review of special issues in care of adolescents with menstrual disorders.*

Litt IF, Martin JA: Development of sexuality and its problems. *In* Levine MD, Carey WB, Crocker AC, et al. (eds.): Developmental-Behavioral Pediatrics. Philadelphia, W. B. Saunders Company, 1983. *Development of sexuality begins at birth and is influenced by a variety of social, psychological, and physical factors thereafter. This article reviews the process.*

Marshall WA, Tanner JM: Puberty. *In* Davis JA, Dobbing J (eds.): Scientific Foundations of Pediatrics. 2nd ed. Baltimore, University Park Press, 1974. *A concise review of the physiology and endocrinology of puberty with excellent charts and tables.*

Vaughan VC III, Litt IF: Child and Adolescent Development: Clinical Implications. Philadelphia, W. B. Saunders Company, 1990. *A comprehensive review and synthesis of biologic, psychosocial, and cognitive development.*

Zacharias L, Wurtman RJ: Age at menarche. N Engl J Med 280:868, 1969. *The multifactorial influences on menarcheal timing are chronicled.*

Depression (Suicide)

Beck AT, Beck R, Kovacs M: Classification of suicidal behaviors: Quantifying intent and medical lethality. Am J Psychiatry 132:285, 1975. *Useful in the assessment of seriousness of a suicidal attempt in patients of any age.*

Mattsson A: Adolescent depression and suicide. *In* Friedman SB, Hoekelman RA (eds.): Behavioral Pediatrics. New York, McGraw-Hill Book Company, 1980. *Useful categorization of manifestations of depression in the adolescent.*

Pugh-Antich J, Rabinovich H: Major child and adolescent psychiatric disorders. *In* Levine MD, Carey WB, Crocker AC, et al. (eds.): Developmental-Behavioral Pediatrics. Philadelphia, W. B. Saunders Company, 1983. *A summary of the psychobiology of adolescent behavioral disorders and their management.*

Adolescent Pregnancy

Alan Guttmacher Institute: Teenage Pregnancy: The Problem That Hasn't Gone Away. New York, Alan Guttmacher Institute, 1981. *Summary of statistics relating to adolescent sexual activity, pregnancy, abortion, and contraceptive use.*

Substance Abuse

Jessor R, Jessor SL: Adolescence to young adulthood: A twelve-year prospective study of problem behavior and psychosocial development. *In* Mednick S, Hornway M (eds.): Longitudinal Research in the United States. New York,

Praeger, 1984. *A comprehensive prospective assessment of early psychosocial predictors of drug use during adolescence as well as its implications for adult behavior.*

Johnston LD, O'Malley PM, Bachman JG: Illicit Drug Use, Smoking and Drinking by America's High School Students, College Students and Young Adults, 1975–1987. U. S. Dept. of Health and Human Services, Public Health Service, Alcohol, Drug Abuse and Mental Health Administration, 1988. *A longitudinal study of trends in adolescent drug use.*

Kandel DB, Logan JA: Patterns of drug use from adolescence to young adulthood: 1) Periods of risk for initiation, continued use, and discontinuation. Am J Public Health 74:660, 1984.

6 Aging and Geriatric Medicine

John W. Rowe

THE DEMOGRAPHIC IMPERATIVE

The Longevity Revolution

Over the next several decades, the practice of medicine in North America will be increasingly influenced by the health care needs of our rapidly enlarging elderly population. The portion of our population over age 65 years has grown from 4 per cent in 1900 to its current level of approximately 12.7 per cent. As members of the post–World War II "baby boom" age, projections call for a steady rise in the number of elderly in the United States from 25.5 million in 1980 to 64 million in 2030, when one of every five Americans will be 65 years or older. These changes reflect decreased death rates not only in youth and middle age but also in old age: Life expectancy at age 65 has risen from 11.9 years in 1900 to 16.9 years in 1987.

A second demographic shift of major importance is hidden within the general increase in the number of older persons. The elderly population itself is aging rapidly (Fig. 6–1). The longevity revolution has even affected the very old, as the past three decades have brought a 26 per cent reduction in mortality rates in individuals over age 80 in the United States. This trend will continue and, in fact, accelerate, as the number of persons over age 85 is projected to triple by the year 2020.

Coupling Longevity with Health

These remarkable improvements in life expectancy have focused attention on improving health span and maintaining functional ability in old age. The general health status of older persons is substantially better than is often assumed. Objective health data show a pattern in which vigorous old age predominates. Dependency and institutionalization are the exception rather than the rule, since only 5 per cent of America's elderly reside in nursing homes at any one time. Most community-dwelling older Americans are cognitively intact and fully independent in their activities of daily living.

However, as individuals age they accumulate disabilities and

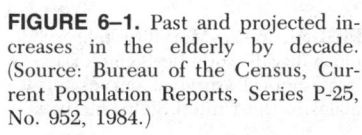

FIGURE 6–1. Past and projected increases in the elderly by decade. (Source: Bureau of the Census, Current Population Reports, Series P-25, No. 952, 1984.)

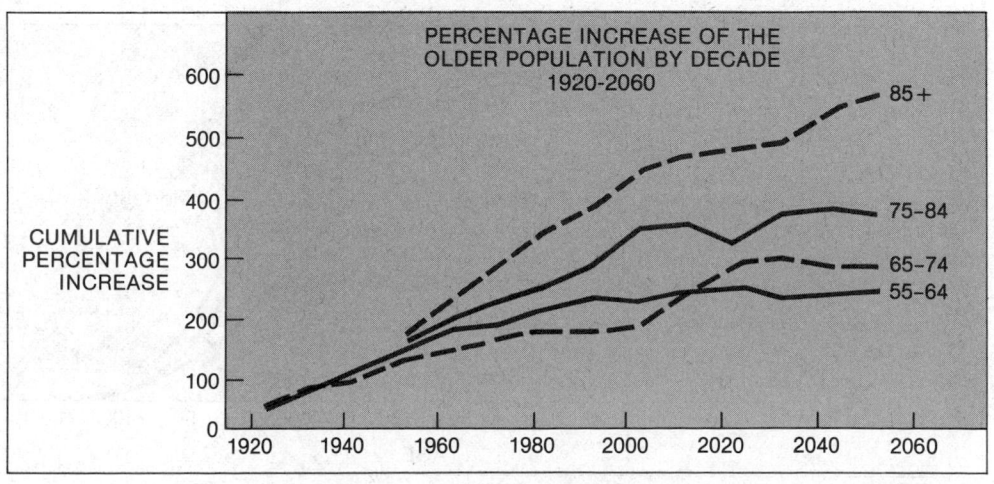

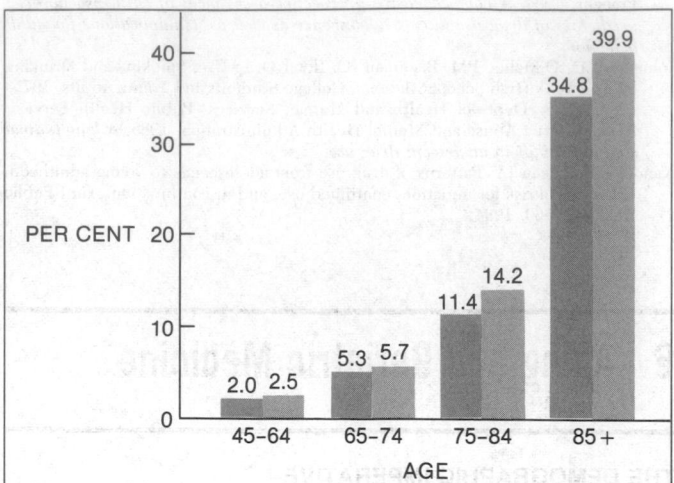

FIGURE 6–2. Percentages of community-dwelling adults, by age group, requiring assistance in basic activities (walking, bathing, dressing, using the toilet, transferring from bed to chair, eating, going outside) and in home-management activities (shopping, chores, meals, handling money) because of chronic disease. Colored bars denote basic activities and gray bars home-management activities.

diseases, and doctor visits increase. A substantial portion of community-dwelling elderly report major activity limitations due to chronic conditions. These functional impairments are clearly age related. The proportion of community-dwelling elderly that requires assistance with basic activities increases from approximately 5 per cent at ages 65 to 74 to nearly 12 per cent at ages 75 to 84 to approximately 35 per cent above the age of 85 (Fig. 6–2). Even if one maintains functional independence into old age, the risk of prolonged frailty is still high. For independent persons between the ages of 65 and 70 years, about 60 per cent of the remaining years will be characterized by independence; this proportion falls to 40 per cent at age 85.

Prolongation of Morbidity

The now familiar mortality curve for a modern aging population (Fig. 6–3C) has beneath it two additional clinically relevant curves, one describing the effect of age on the portion of the population in good health (i.e., morbidity curve, Fig. 6–3A) and another describing the transition of diseased aging individuals from the asymptomatic to the symptomatic or functionally impaired state (disability curve, Fig. 6–3B).

A major health policy issue relates to the relationship between future changes in morbidity and disability in an aging population. The question is whether we will see a prolongation of dependency (i.e., widening of gap between curves of Fig. 6–3B and C) or whether active life expectancy will increase (i.e., compression of morbidity), as health promotion and disease prevention strategies

become increasingly effective and curve 6–3B shifts rightward toward the mortality curve. The initial hope that as mortality declined, morbidity would also decline, has recently been challenged by studies suggesting that the increased lifespan of the oldest old is not accompanied by decreased morbidity and may actually result in more dramatic increases in the need for health care services, unless our understanding of disease in old age, and our capacity to treat it, improve substantially.

BIOLOGIC THEORIES OF AGING

Theories Relating to Alterations in Proteins

ERROR IN PROTEIN SYNTHESIS

This theory holds that age-associated impairments in cellular function result from an accumulation of errors in protein synthesis. It is reasoned that random errors in DNA, transcription, or translation accumulate with aging to a level that markedly impairs cell function. Substantial basic research in aging over the past two decades has shown that both transcription and translation maintain their fidelity with advancing age and that aging is characterized by a remarkable constancy of the composition of a variety of physiologically important proteins. Specific findings inconsistent with the error catastrophe theory include the facts that aged fibroblast cultures infected with viruses do not have a decreased virus yield, that newly synthesized enzymes from tissues in the aged are found to contain no synthetic errors, that experimentally induced errors fail to produce an error catastrophe, and that there is no increase in the infidelity of tRNA's with age and no age-related differences in the accuracy of poly(U)-directed protein synthesis. Thus, the error theory is considered by many to be disproven.

POST-TRANSLATIONAL MODIFICATIONS (CROSS-LINKAGE THEORY)

This theory is based on findings that although transcription and translation are intact with age, *altered* proteins accumulate with advancing age. Thus, post-translational modifications may be important in mediating age-related losses in cell and organ function. A number of physiologically critical enzymes have been shown to undergo post-translational modifications with age, although these changes are by no means universal. One important post-translational modification—glycosylation—appears to be important in age-related development of increasing opacification in crystalline lens protein and eventual development of cataracts. Another modification, increased cross-linking, is central to the major aging modifications in collagen and might have direct clinical consequences for arteriosclerosis and other diseases. Cross-links should not be considered important only in extracellular tissues, since an age-related increase in cross-links has also been shown to occur in DNA. There are a number of criticisms of this theory, including the lack of evidence for varied rates of post-translational change in the same class of molecules in different species despite the remarkable diversity in species specificity of lifespan. Although it is unlikely that post-translational modifications are central to all aging-related biologic decrements, there is general agreement that they may play an important role in the emergence of some clinical consequences of aging.

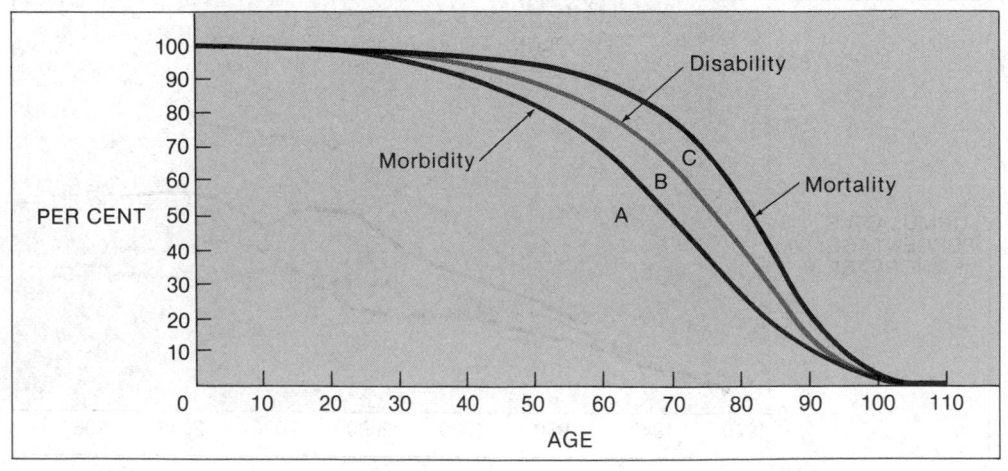

FIGURE 6–3. Mortality (observed), morbidity (hypothetical), and disability (hypothetical) survival curves for females in the United States in 1980.

Another aspect of protein chemistry that has attracted substantial gerontologic attention is alteration with age in the *rate* of protein biosynthesis. Although there appears to be no missynthesis of proteins with age, many proteins are *produced more slowly* in aged cells than in their younger counterparts. Delays have been identified in all of the four major stages of protein synthesis, including amino acylation of tRNA, initiation, elongation, and termination.

In addition, lysosomal pathways for *elimination* of proteins are substantially altered with age, with some proteins being degraded more quickly than in younger cells and others more slowly. Future experiments involving recombinant DNA techniques to correct modifications in these lysosomal pathways may permit evaluation of the impact of these changes on cell aging.

DNA DAMAGE AND REPAIR THEORY

The intact fidelity of protein synthesis with age does not exclude major age-related alterations in DNA, since a substantial portion of DNA is responsible for regulatory rather than synthetic activities. The DNA damage and repair theory focuses on the facts that, throughout life, DNA is constantly damaged and that age-related impairments in the repair mechanisms might be expected to be associated with progressive declines in cellular function. Although modifications in DNA repair capacity with age have been identified, these have generally not been well correlated with lifespan, suggesting either that DNA repair defects are not important in aging or that, to date, investigations have not focused on the critical repair mechanisms.

Free Radical Theory

Free radicals are highly reactive atoms or molecules bearing an unpaired electron, which can cause random damage to structural proteins, enzymes, informational macromolecules, and DNA. In mammals the most important source of free radicals is the reduction of oxygen, with subsequent development of hydrogen peroxide. The free radical theory holds that advancing age is associated with an accumulation of low-level free radical damage, which leads to the physiologic and clinical consequences associated with aging. Normal defense mechanisms against free radical damage include a number of endogenous antioxidants, including selenium-containing glutathione peroxidase, superoxide dismutase, DNA repair mechanisms, and alpha-tocopherol. Preliminary support for this theory rests in studies which indicate that animals whose oxygen consumption is high in proportion to their size have shorter lifespans and that administration of antioxidants results in modest increases in life expectancy. Within primates, the levels of the cellular antioxidant superoxide dismutase correlate well with lifespan. In addition, in lower forms of life, mutations leading to defects in production of free radical quenching enzymes are associated with shorter lifespan.

Organ System Theory (Pacemaker Theory)

This theory holds that certain organs or organ systems decline with advancing age and their loss of function drives the systemic aging process. The organs that have attracted the most attention as the "pacemakers" of aging are the immune system and the neuroendocrine system, particularly the hypothalamus.

With regard to immunosenescence, aging is associated with declines of over 75 per cent in T lymphocyte function as well as a progressive development of autoantibodies, with obvious potential clinical ramifications, such as increased morbidity from infections, increased risk of cancer, and perhaps autoimmune damage as well. Support for the importance of these changes in the aging process is found in studies of mice identical except for the major histocompatibility complex (MHC), which show a close relation between MHC and lifespan.

The neuroendocrine system is another central control complex in which marked age-related changes have been identified and which has been targeted as a possible aging pacemaker. Sympathetic nervous system responsiveness is increased with age, and it has been postulated that this increase might be responsible for a number of age-related changes, such as hypertension, impaired carbohydrate tolerance, and altered sleep architecture. Investigators have also sought to identify the presence of a "death hormone," a substance that is produced in increasing amounts with advancing age and that might regulate the aging process, or perhaps a "Methuselah hormone," which is present in decreasing amounts with advanced age. To date, no firm data are available to support the presence of such substances.

These theories focusing on individual organ systems as major regulators of systemic aging suffer from the weaknesses that not all organisms known to age have well-developed immune or neuroendocrine systems and that such theories would fail to explain the origin of the changes in the pacemaker system itself.

GENETIC ASPECTS OF AGING

Despite the apparent lack of evolutionary value to increases in lifespan beyond the reproductive years, gerontologists have long been attracted to the notion that just as growth and development are clearly regulated by a systematic turning on and off of various genes, so aging might represent a process in which systematic modifications in gene expression result in age-related physiologic and pathologic changes. Several of the theories of aging discussed above are linked by the likelihood that the basic mechanisms of aging—whether they be decreases in the production of antioxidants, impairments in DNA structure or repair, or age-related modifications of protein disposal systems or T lymphocyte function—may all have a genetic basis.

Substantial information exists to support the view that genetic factors are important to the aging process. There is a remarkable species specificity to lifespan. Within an individual species, the life expectancy of identical twins is more similar than that of nonidentical twins, which in turn is more similar than that of siblings. On a more basic level, recent studies in *Caenorhabditis elegans*, a nematode, have identified mutant varieties with lifespans that exceed normal lifespans by 50 per cent. In some of these strains, the lifespan extension appears to be due to a single gene change. These findings suggest that more intensive genetic approaches are promising avenues for future research in aging.

CLINICAL IMPACT OF THE AGING PROCESS
Distinction Between Successful and Usual Aging

A thorough understanding of age-related physiologic changes that occur in humans, in the absence of disease, is critical to diagnosis and management of disease in old age. These physiologic changes influence the presentation of disease, its response to treatment, and the complications that ensue. Cross-sectional and longitudinal studies in carefully screened, community-dwelling groups across the adult age range indicate that increasing age is accompanied by inevitable physiologic changes that are separate from the effects of disease. Growth and development, characterized by rapid increases in many physiologic functions, generally continue into early adulthood, peaking in the late twenties or early thirties. In those variables that change with age after adulthood, and not all do, a linear decline begins at the end of the growth and development phase and continues into old age. There is generally no pleasant plateau during the middle years, during which physiologic function is stable, but rather a progressive age-related reduction in the function of many organs.

The elderly population is characterized by substantial variability in the severity of age-related physiologic changes, as rates of organ aging vary substantially among healthy elderly individuals. Physiologically, it seems that as individuals become older, they become less like each other. For many organs the physiologic losses that accompany "normal" aging now appear to be significantly less than was previously assumed. Thus, the differences between older persons may be due, in part, to lifestyle differences that confound the effects of aging. For instance, although maximal oxygen consumption has repeatedly been shown to decline with age, studies also indicate that oxygen consumption increases in response to exercise training in older persons, with older master athletes achieving levels higher than those seen in normal young adults. As greater attention is paid to the potential beneficial effects of exercise, diet, smoking cessation, moderation in alcohol intake, and so forth, we may encounter increasing numbers of robust elders who demonstrate *successful aging*, i.e., not only lack of disease, but also physiologic performance only moderately below that of healthy young adults. However, the fact remains that most older adults exhibit another syndrome, that of usual aging, in which the effects of aging per se are mixed with adverse effects of confounding environmental, dietary, or lifestyle factors.

Distinction Between Aging and Disease

Since age has an important influence on numerous physiologic variables, and since detection of disease depends upon the determination that an individual is different from what would be expected by virtue of his age, it is important to establish age-adjusted criteria for clinically relevant variables to facilitate differentiation of the physiologic consequences of usual aging from those of concomitant diseases. Such criteria have been in wide clinical use for many years for several clinically important functions. For example, spirometric measures of pulmonary function are commonly expressed as "per cent of expected" for age and body size. Similarly, the validity of an exercise tolerance test as a suitable stress for detection of ischemic heart disease is judged on the basis of age-adjusted achievements of maximum heart rates. Standardized criteria are also available for age-related changes in glomerular filtration rate (GFR) and oral glucose tolerance, although variability of these functions is great among the elderly and individual determinations are required to guide diagnosis or therapy. If measurement of GFR is not available, application of age-related standards of renal function is facilitated by the fact that the age-related decline in creatinine clearance (approximately 10 ml per minute per decade) is balanced by a similar reduction in endogenous creatinine production. Thus, serum creatinine levels remain unchanged in spite of substantially lower GFR's in older patients. Familiarity with age changes in renal function and the hepatic oxidizing system is of particular importance in guiding drug therapy in the elderly (see below).

Interaction of Aging and Disease

There is a wide spectrum of interaction between aging processes and diseases, ranging from a lack of interaction at one extreme to age changes that have direct adverse clinical sequelae. Several specific clinically relevant points along this continuum can be identified.

PHYSIOLOGIC VARIABLES THAT DO NOT CHANGE WITH AGE

Perhaps the most important phenomenon seen in the aged, from a clinical standpoint, is no age-related change at all. Too frequently, clinicians attribute a disability or abnormal physical or laboratory finding to "old age," when the actual cause may be a specific disease process. Often there is no influence of age on the specific variable being evaluated. For example, old patients with low hematocrit values may be incorrectly characterized as

having "anemia of old age" and be assured that no diagnostic evaluation or treatment is warranted. Data from several sources clearly indicate that in healthy, community-dwelling elders, there is no age-related change in hematocrit. Thus, a low hematocrit level in an elderly individual cannot be ascribed to normal aging and requires prompt investigation and treatment. Other common clinical measures not strongly influenced by age include fasting blood glucose level, serum electrolyte concentrations, blood pH and carbon dioxide content, and numerous hormone levels, including those of insulin, cortisol, thyroxine, and parathyroid hormone.

IMPAIRED HOMEOSTASIS IN THE ELDERLY

This category encompasses age-related reductions in the function of numerous organs that place the elderly person at special risk of increased morbidity from coincident pathologic changes in those organs. Although usual age-related declines in physiologic function are not so severe as to result in impairments in function under basal circumstances, these declines are of sufficient magnitude to reduce physiologic reserve and thus to move old individuals closer to the clinical threshold for the emergence of symptoms. Declines in basal immune, renal, and pulmonary function and the declines in glucose tolerance and cardiac function during physiologic stress all place the elderly at risk for earlier emergence or greater severity of clinical disease. This fact can be illustrated with several clinically relevant examples:

1. Aging is associated with significant progressive reductions in the dopamine content of the substantia nigra. These decreases may interact with pathophysiologic changes to account for the increasing prevalence of Parkinson's disease in late life and are also consistent with the well-recognized enhanced susceptibility of older individuals to extrapyramidal side effects of neuroleptic agents.

2. Age-related reductions in pulmonary function are so substantial that healthy individuals in the ninth decade of life frequently have only one half of the pulmonary function of their 30-year-old counterparts. Thus, acute bacterial pneumonias of equal initial severity are much more likely to induce a serious clinical manifestation in the elderly. In addition, the marked decline in immune function with age will also be expressed as an impaired capacity to respond to the infecting agent and a subsequent worsening of the clinical picture.

3. Since usual renal function in older persons may be as much as 40 per cent less than in healthy younger adults, the loss of one kidney due to ureteral obstruction, vascular occlusion, or trauma is more likely to result in a clinically significant reduction in overall renal function in an old patient than in a healthy younger individual.

4. The mortality associated with severe burns increases dra-

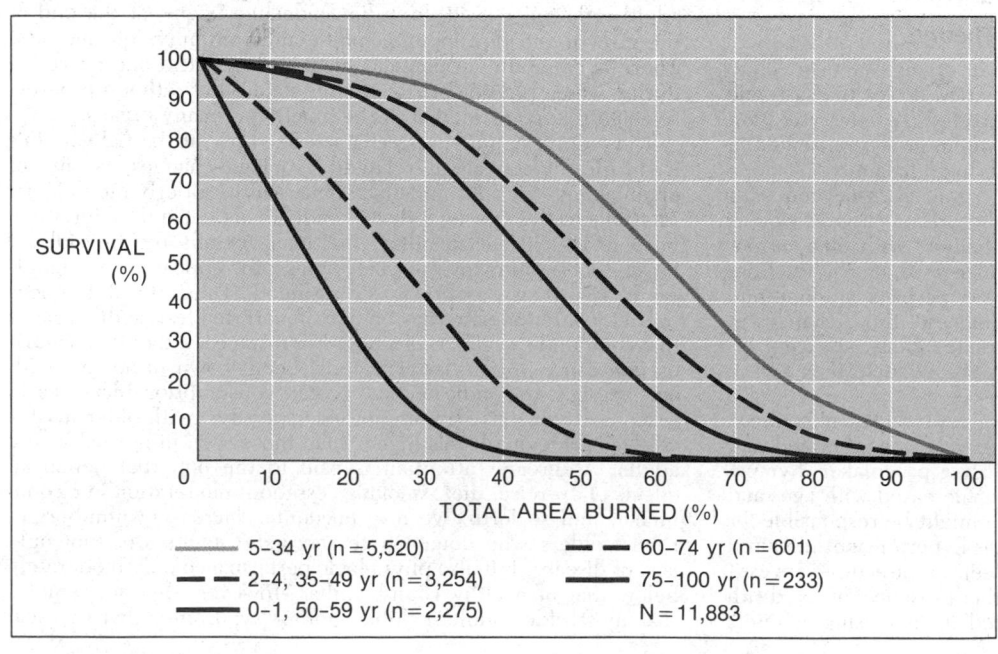

FIGURE 6–4. Survival of patients as a function of the total percentage of body surface burned and age.

matically with advancing age throughout adulthood (Fig. 6–4). This effect, which reflects the multiple parallel reductions in physiologic function during middle age and early senescence, is apparent well before diseases become highly prevalent and exemplifies the impaired homeostasis associated with the physiologic changes with age.

ALTERED PRESENTATION OF DISEASE IN THE ELDERLY

Age-related alterations in disease presentation have long been recognized as being of major importance to the practice of geriatric medicine. Many diseases occurring in both young and old adults have manifestly different clinical presentations and natural histories, depending upon the age of the individual. These disorders should not be regarded as being either more or less severe in the elderly, but just different. One example is hyperthyroidism. Young individuals often present with agitation, anxiety, an elevated heart rate and blood pressure, hyperactive deep tendon reflexes, complaints of weight loss and irritability, hyperkinesis, and a palpable goiter. In the older person with thyroid hormone levels equally elevated, irritability and hyperkinesis are infrequent and goiter is rare. In addition, deep tendon reflexes may be normal or even hypoactive, and the older patient may present a deactivated clinical picture ("apathetic thyrotoxicosis"). Physicians not familiar with presentation of thyroid hormone excess in the elderly may miss the diagnosis early on, thus permitting the adverse sequelae to persist.

Another disorder that is revealed differently in different age groups is uncontrolled diabetes mellitus. In children and young adults, uncontrolled diabetes is generally manifested as diabetic ketoacidosis. By contrast, the elderly with uncontrolled diabetes frequently present with hyperosmolar nonketotic coma, with blood glucose levels markedly higher than in ketoacidosis and a relative or absolute lack of circulating ketones. Thus, the elderly may present with obtundation or in coma secondary to markedly high blood osmolality, whereas younger individuals are more likely to present with severe metabolic acidosis, polyuria, or volume depletion or any combination. The physiologic mechanisms underlying these major effects of age on presentation of common diseases remain unexplained.

HEALTH PROMOTION AND DISEASE PREVENTION IN THE ELDERLY

Not many years ago, it would have seemed paradoxical to discuss health promotion and disease prevention for the elderly. Recently, however, this has become an important theme in geriatrics in view of both the remarkable increases in longevity and the awareness that the physiologic and pathophysiologic changes associated with advancing age may be much more reversible than was previously appreciated. This *plasticity* of the aging process is reflected in findings that moderate exercise (30 minutes three times weekly) retards age-related loss of bone mineral content in elderly women, including individuals in their ninth decade of life living in long-term care facilities. Similarly, even though elderly smokers have a much higher risk of cardiac mortality than nonsmokers, quitting smoking late in life is associated with a rapid and sustained reduction in mortality from coronary disease. Clearly, one should not assume that risk factors are necessarily cumulative in their impact or that little is to be gained by altering long-term habits or treating longstanding disorders in the elderly. This perspective not only is relevant for healthy older persons but can help limit disability and dependence in those suffering from one or more chronic conditions.

A note of caution is required concerning health promotion and disease prevention strategies in the elderly population. Attempts to improve the quality of old age require an understanding of the risk factors for common diseases in the elderly and the efficacy of strategies to decrease the risk of morbidity. Simplistic generalizations of findings in young and middle-aged groups to the elderly are fraught with difficulty. The elderly clearly represent a select group of survivors with physiologic alterations that may influence pathophysiologic processes.

Another aspect of prevention in the care of the elderly is recognition that physiologic or pathologic changes so common in advancing age as to be considered "normal aging" should not be considered to be without risk. Thus, although systolic blood pressure increases with advancing age, it is also clear that rises in systolic pressure are associated with marked increase in the risk of stroke and coronary heart disease. Elevations in blood sugar represent another potentially harmful aging change that is usually considered harmless.

Finally, it should be noted that remarkable beneficial effects can be gained by modest delays in the onset of age-related disorders. For instance, the increase with age in the incidence of hip fracture among the very old is so steep that if preventive strategies, such as calcium supplementation or exercise, delayed clinical expression of osteoporosis for 5 years, without increasing lifespan, the result would be a 50 per cent reduction in the number of hip fractures.

MEDICATION USE IN OLDER PERSONS

Numerous studies have documented that old people have more trouble with medications than do the adult population in general. The aged use an excessive proportion of the prescription and over-the-counter drugs consumed in the United States. Although the elderly represent less than 12 per cent of our population, they purchase 25 per cent of the drugs sold in America. This excess consumption of medications is accompanied, not surprisingly, by higher rates of side effects. Of equal importance is that when older people consume the same drugs with the same frequency as the young, toxicity is still more frequent and severe in the elderly. Often, standards for the use of current therapeutic agents were developed in young adults, and simplistic application of these guidelines to the elderly is often hazardous. Rates of adverse drug reaction rise steadily after age 50, and patients over 60 years old are twice as likely to suffer an adverse drug reaction as younger patients. Those over 80 years have a one in four risk of drug intoxication, twice the rate seen in patients under 50 years. Hospital stays are prolonged for all patients with adverse reactions, but older patients remain hospitalized the longest.

This increased toxicity of medication use in the elderly has three components: special vulnerability due to the physiologic effects of aging (drug-age interaction); modification of drug effects by multiple diseases often present in frail elders (drug-disease interaction); and the interactions of a given pharmacologic agent with the other medications, over the counter or prescribed, that the individual is taking (drug-drug interaction).

With regard to drug-age interactions, the changes with aging that occur in hepatic drug oxidation systems and in renal function have their major clinical impact on alterations in the pharmacokinetics of many medications. Several very commonly used medications such as digitalis and aminoglycoside antibiotics are excreted primarily via renal mechanisms and thus have prolonged half-lives in many elderly compared with younger adults, necessitating an adjustment in treatment schedules. These pharmacokinetic considerations are frequently compounded by parallel changes in pharmacodynamics, inasmuch as the tissues of elderly individuals, especially the central nervous system, become more sensitive to some agents with advancing age. Older persons are more sensitive than younger adults to the sedative effects of benzodiazepines and to the analgesic effects of narcotics. The combination of alterations in pharmacokinetics and pharmacodynamics is often further influenced by changes in body composition in the elderly. The average old individual has more fat and less lean body mass per kilogram of body weight than the younger adult. Thus, the volumes of distributions of many agents, such as diazepam, are altered in the elderly. Similarly, circulating levels of serum albumin fall moderately with age and influence free circulating levels of medications that are highly protein bound, such as phenytoin.

Drug-disease interactions are particularly common in the elderly. It is not uncommon to have five or six major diagnoses exist in as many organ systems of a frail elderly patient. The resulting frequent worsening of one illness by treatment of another leads to disproportionately longer hospital stays and increased frequency of complications. Drug-drug interactions are clearly more common in the elderly in view of the polypharmacy noted above.

Andres R, Bierman EL, Hazzard WR: Principles of Geriatric Medicine. New York, McGraw-Hill Book Company, 1985. *A detailed comprehensive textbook of geriatrics.*

Schneider EL, Rowe JW: Handbook of the Biology of Aging. 3rd ed. San Diego, Academic Press, 1990. *An encyclopedic reference text, very detailed and well referenced, covering all aspects of aging from plants and nematodes through detailed system-by-system discussions of human aging.*

Greenblatt DJ, Seller EM, Shader RI: Drug therapy: Drug disposition in old age. N Engl J Med 306:1081, 1982. *A useful review of the principles of geriatric pharmacology.*

Hayflick L: Theories of biological aging. *In* Andres R, Bierman EL, Hazzard WR (eds.): Principles of Geriatric Medicine. New York, McGraw-Hill Book Company, 1985, pp 9–22. *This chapter provides a detailed review of the major current biologic theories of aging, with a good historical review and balanced perspectives of the evidence for and against each theory.*

Katz S, Branch LG, Branson MH, et al.: Active life expectancy. N Engl J Med 309:1218, 1983. *This important paper coined the phrase "active life expectancy" and provides information on the functional capacity of the elderly.*

Rowe JW: Health care of the elderly. N Engl J Med 312:827, 1985. *A detailed, heavily referenced review of the physiologic changes with age and their clinical influence, with additional updates on several geriatric diseases, including dementia, incontinence, and osteoporosis.*

Rowe JW, Besdine RW: Geriatric Medicine. Boston, Little, Brown and Company, 1988. *A concise, practical textbook of geriatric medicine for students and practitioners. Emphasis on both normal aging and age-related diseases.*

Rowe JW, Kahn RL: Human aging: Usual versus successful. Science 237:143, 1987. *A review of the importance of distinguishing between the effects of intrinsic aging processes and extrinsic, often preventable factors that complicate "normal" aging.*

Salzman C: Clinical Geriatric Psychopharmacology. New York, McGraw-Hill, 1984. *A very concise, practical clinical guide to use of psychotropic medications in the elderly with numerous references and instructive clinical vignettes.*

Schneider EL, Brody JA: Aging, natural death, and the compression of morbidity—another view. N Engl J Med 309:854, 1983. *A detailed update of evidence for and against the compression of morbidity hypothesis.*

7 Management of Common Problems in the Elderly

T. Franklin Williams

A physician must approach the care of elderly persons with an informed, comprehensive, balanced perspective about aging itself and about the diseases and disabilities that commonly occur in older people. The previous chapter has described the physiologic changes that normally occur with aging. From the clinical perspective it is important to keep in mind that most older people are in reasonably good health and, despite some decline in maximum functional ability, can still function well at all ordinary activities. There are many persons in their eighties and nineties who can and do carry on all usual living activities, take long walks, are intellectually sharp with good memories, continue to be sexually active, and most of the time are symptom free. Thus when someone, no matter how old, comes to a physician with a complaint of discomfort or dysfunction, the complaint should not be dismissed as being simply "old age," but should be investigated and treated appropriately.

At the same time, a physician must understand that with increasing age people do accumulate chronic diseases and disabilities. Over the age of 65, 80 per cent have one or more chronic conditions; among the most common are some form of arthritis (present in 40 per cent in national surveys), hearing impairment (30 per cent), and chronic cardiac conditions (20 per cent). One in five persons over the age of 75 may be expected to have diabetes. In those 75 or older, four or more identifiable chronic problems are commonly present.

In addition to recognizing and treating the acute and chronic *diseases* that occur, the physician must give attention to the functional losses, the *disabilities* that are present, and attempt to reverse or minimize them no matter what can or cannot be done about underlying chronic diseases. The ultimate goal of care for elderly persons should be to restore or maintain as much function as possible—to help the patient to maintain as much independence of living, as much of a preferred lifestyle, as possible. Such a rehabilitative approach is an essential part of the therapy.

In those elderly patients who have some irreversible functional losses and thus need regular assistance, an additional part of the plan for care must be identification of who will provide the needed help and where. The extent and quality of family support and the potentials for community or institutional support services must be determined and worked into the overall, ongoing therapeutic program.

SPECIAL FEATURES OF THE WORKUP OF ELDERLY PATIENTS

HISTORY TAKING. Special attention should be given to the history of other (chronic) conditions in addition to the immediate chief complaint and to obtaining additional historical information from close relatives and previous records. An older person, like any patient consulting a physician, is most interested in having the immediate problem addressed and may tend to downplay past history and other chronic but less troubling conditions. It is the interaction of multiple diseases, the necessity to deal simultaneously with these multiple problems, that is one of the distinguishing characteristics of geriatric medicine. A closely related necessity is to obtain complete information on all drugs the patient is taking, both prescribed and over-the-counter medications. The number and variety are often astounding, and unfavorable drug interactions commonly contribute to the patient's discomfort and dysfunctions. A good technique is to have the patient (or responsible family member) bring in all the medications the patient is taking, for review, on each office visit.

Certain common functional problems should be explicitly inquired about: any history of falling; any episodes of urinary incontinence; any disturbances in sleep; and any difficulties with vision, hearing, or sexual function.

One must keep in mind the atypical presentations of common acute problems: pneumonia presenting as confusion, acute myocardial infarction as sudden weakness, or an acute abdomen as refusal to eat.

It is a good practice whenever possible to talk with one or more close family members to obtain their observations on the patient's functional status, mood, and daily routines, including intake of food and medicines. Such additional information is absolutely essential if there is evidence of dementia or depression in the patient—in such circumstances the patient may give quite a misleading story. If the patient is living alone (as a third or more of older women are), then it may be desirable or even necessary to have the benefit of observations from a home visit by the physician or by a visiting nurse or social worker.

The physician should obtain summaries or copies of all previous records, including results of all diagnostic tests. Such information should help both in managing current problems and in reducing the extent of further diagnostic tests that are needed. In particularly complex or unclear situations, there should be direct discussion with physicians who have previously seen the patient.

PHYSICAL EXAMINATION. As part of a regular complete physical examination of an older patient, certain features should receive special attention, depending in part on clues from the history. These include evaluation of mobility, mental status, mood, vision, hearing, and performance of usual activities of daily living. In recent years considerable attention has been given to developing simple, reliable, objective procedures and instruments for assessing these characteristics which may be used practically in physicians' practices. Applegate et al. (1990) provide a summary of such instruments; Lachs et al. (1990) describe a simple sequence for detecting potential problems which should then lead to more thorough investigations.

In light of the frequency of poor eating practices by older persons, particularly those living alone, special attention should be given to any indications of poor nutrition—weight loss, anemia, vitamin deficiency. A careful oral examination is important.

ADDITIONAL DIAGNOSTIC TESTS. The same general principles for choosing diagnostic tests for younger patients should apply in the workup of older patients. The aim is to obtain any information that will help in clarifying the cause of disease or the functional loss, *if* this information will likely lead to effective therapy. Decisions should be weighed in consultation with the patient and close family before diagnostic procedures are embarked on. If the treatment plans will not be changed by the outcome of the procedure, then it should not be done. However, because of the tendency, referred to earlier, to dismiss treatable problems of elderly patients as simply the concomitants of old age, it is important to identify any potentially reversible condition and to use relevant diagnostic aids.

ASSESSMENT OF FAMILY AND COMMUNITY SUPPORTS. A final essential element in the workup of a frail, elderly person, i.e., a patient who may face the necessity of ongoing help with daily activities, is the collection of information about the home environment, the family relationships, the degree of supporting services potentially available, the degree of "burn-out" or exhaustion that may have already occurred, and the availability of home care services and institutional services in the community. A visiting nurse or social worker can be very helpful in obtaining some of these services and in helping to integrate them into an overall plan.

DIAGNOSIS AND MANAGEMENT OF MAJOR COMMON PROBLEMS OF ELDERLY PATIENTS

EPISODES OF ACUTE ILLNESS. Older people with diminished reserves and chronic diseases are more prone to injuries, acute infections (especially respiratory), and other acute illnesses than are younger people, and are also more likely to decompensate at such times. It is a common observation that an old person, previously mentally competent at home, may become quite confused on admission to the strange environment of a hospital under the stresses of an acute illness. Careful attention must be given to every aspect of the patient's status, looking for the appearance of heart failure, overt diabetes, delirium, or increased risk of falling. Drug regimens should be kept simple and the possibility of deleterious effects of overdosage or drug interactions should be continuously reviewed.

Recovery from an acute illness will also take longer than in a younger person, and there is real risk that the previous functional level may not be regained. As early as possible in an episode of acute illness the older patient should be helped to be up and about, to keep joints supple and muscular strength as intact as possible, to retain or regain urinary continence through use of regular toilet facilities, to dress and feed oneself, and to engage in social exchanges in usual ways, i.e., out of bed and dressed, and to return home as quickly as possible. Convalescent and rehabilitative efforts should be continued as long as any progress is being made.

DEMENTIA. The loss of mental competence is one of the most common and most distressing of functional disabilities in older persons, affecting up to 40 to 45 per cent of those over age 80. We now know that dementia is *not* a feature of normal aging but instead is due to one or another of several disease processes. The most common form of dementia in old people is that of the Alzheimer's type, accounting for 50 per cent or more of cases. This is a (usually) progressive dementia associated with considerable cerebral atrophy and characteristic pathologic changes in selected regions of the brain, with neurofibrillary tangles within the neurons and amyloid plaques at end-plates. These damaged neurons are producing far less of the neurotransmitter acetylcholine (and possibly other neurotransmitters also) than normal. Research at an accelerating pace is providing promising clues to causes (both genetic and environmental) and to potentially effective interventions including nerve growth factors and drugs aimed at increasing the supply or persistence of acetylcholine. Thus far, results are inconclusive.

Other causes of dementia in older people include damage from multiple small infarcts or one or more larger infarcts secondary to cerebrovascular disease, metabolic or endocrine disorders such as hypothyroidism and vitamin B_{12} deficiency, brain tumors, brain injury (such as late dementia in professional boxers, which has the same pathologic changes as Alzheimer's disease), Korsakoff's dementia of chronic alcoholism, and the condition known as normal-pressure hydrocephalus. Most importantly, severe depression can present as dementia, reversible with successful treatment of the depression. Indeed, a number of the possible causes are potentially reversible or treatable. Thus it is essential, when confronted by an older person with any signs of dementia, to conduct a thorough differential diagnostic evaluation. This should include comprehensive mental testing to define the extent of the dementia, specific tests for all of the treatable causes, and in most instances, a scan—computed tomographic (CT) or magnetic resonance imaging (MRI)—which can usually identify or exclude infarcts and tumors and can help diagnose normal-

pressure hydrocephalus. Evidence of cerebral atrophy alone would be consistent with, but not diagnostic of, dementia of Alzheimer's type, inasmuch as a significant degree of atrophy occurs in the normal aging process without loss of mental function. However, unequivocal progression in such atrophy, as seen in a repeated scan within 6 to 24 months, does not occur in normal older persons and is strong diagnostic confirmation of Alzheimer's disease.

The physician should be sensitive to the alarm older patients and family members may have at the least sign of any aberration in mentation and should be able to reassure them that "benign forgetfulness" is a common trait at all ages. Benign forgetfulness characteristically is the inability to recall a name or some specific element of a prior experience, when one thinks one should be able to do so. The person can recall many related features of the person or episode and knows precisely what element or name is not being recalled. Usually recall of that element will occur later, unexpectedly. In contrast, a person with progressive dementia will have no recollection of the entire episode, as if it never happened, or can make only feeble, ineffective efforts to reconstruct the identity of the forgotten subject.

If the final diagnosis is dementia of the Alzheimer's type or one of the other irreversible dementias, the physician, nurses, and social workers must treat the family as well as the patient and help them to make the best of a distressing situation. The long-established daily activities of the patient in familiar surroundings should be maintained as much as possible, with avoidance of surprises or new and different decisions to be made. Family members should be helped to accept the services of home support personnel to assist in the care of the patient—housekeeper, personal care aide, home health aide, or nurse—as needed to help prevent "burn-out" on their part; to accept respite care for the patient (day programs or temporary full-time care given in the home or a temporary nursing home admission) so that the family members may get away for a vacation or a special occasion; and to accept permanent nursing home care for the patient if this becomes best for everyone. They should be informed of support groups like the Alzheimer's Association, chapters of which now exist in most larger communities, and should be put in touch with social agencies and legal resources if necessary to help in making various legal and financial arrangements. The physician's involvement in all of these aspects may seem to some to be peripheral to the practice of medicine but in fact is central to the physician's primary goals of maintaining the health and functioning of the patient and the patient's family to the maximum extent possible. In working with problems like these the physician needs the close participation of well-informed nurses and social workers who can take the lead in management of many aspects.

The physician should keep in mind (and the family should be reminded) that any sudden worsening of dementia is not consistent with Alzheimer's disease and is likely a sign of some complicating acute illness.

DEPRESSION. Depressive reactions of varying degrees of severity are more common in elderly persons than has been recognized and warrant more attention in diagnosis and treatment. As a person lives into later years, losses are inevitable—death of family members and friends, usually "loss" of job through retirement, usually less income, often loss of some degree of health, less vigor, possibly loss of familiar home environment through moving. Some degree of grief and reactive depression is to be expected in response to such losses, but emotionally healthy older persons work through such grief and return to their usual level of mood, outlook, and activity. Persistence of depressive symptoms may represent activation of a longer-standing depressed state or appearance of a new disorder.

If depression is suspected, it should be thoroughly evaluated with psychiatric consultation and perhaps treated by therapeutic trials of antidepressant drugs. In severe instances not responsive to drugs, electroshock therapy has been found to be successful in many elderly patients.

FALLS. Falling is common as people become older, occurring as often as once a year or more in half of those over age 75. In addition to the accompanying risk of injury—with up to 5 per cent of falls there may be fracture of the hip or arm—one or more falls may lead to such a fear of further falling that an older person severely limits mobility and activities. Falls are often also a harbinger of other diseases or disabilities.

A number of risk factors contribute to the likelihood of falling, and it is typically the multiplicity of such risk factors in the same person that makes falling highly likely, rather than any one of them. These include diminished distant vision, deafness, disturbances in balance, abnormal gait, weakness in the lower extremities, decreased mental status, orthostatic hypotension, depression, and effects of drugs on alertness. All such factors should be searched for and as many as possible corrected as a part of regular preventive care and especially at the time of any fall.

Environmental hazards also contribute to the risk. A home visit by at least one of the professionals should include observation and recommendations for correcting such environmental hazards as poor lighting, rugs that can slide, objects blocking usual walkways, lack of nonslipping strips and handgrips in bath tubs, and lack of handrails on stairs.

A person who has fallen should be thoroughly examined for subtle signs of injury or fracture and for any underlying or associated disease condition, including a new febrile illness, painless myocardial infarction, and stroke.

URINARY INCONTINENCE. Lack of control of urination is far more common than generally recognized; some studies suggest that up to 30 per cent of older women have this problem. It has been referred to as the "closet disease" of old age because of the high frequency of denial of its presence—out of embarrassment or the mistaken view that nothing can be done about it. Older persons living alone may become oblivious to its presence, unaware of the odors that are obvious to visitors. Frequent urinary incontinence, particularly night-time incontinence, by a person living with family is a major cause of caregiver exhaustion and the precipitating reason for their seeking institutional care.

For all of these reasons it is important for the physician, in evaluating any older patient, to determine (from patient, family, or visiting nurse) whether the patient has any problem with urinary incontinence and, if so, to conduct a thorough diagnostic workup and, based on the findings, to undertake appropriate treatment. In most instances the problem can be eliminated or controlled.

A good first step in evaluating reported or suspected urinary incontinence is to arrange to have an "incontinence diary" kept by the patient or caregiver—a daily record for several days of just when episodes of incontinence occur, roughly how much urine is spilled, the circumstances—while up and about or in bed or while on the way to the bathroom but "didn't quite make it"—and whether the patient is aware of the episode. In some instances simply keeping such a diary leads a previously careless person to achieve satisfactory control. The diary provides information on the magnitude of the problem and clues to possible causes.

Further workup of the incontinence should proceed from simple to more complex tests, as needed. Urinalysis and culture may indicate a urinary tract infection that, if eliminated, will result in restoration of continence. Observing whether there is any urinary spillage with coughing or straining in the upright position (after adequate hydration) may point to stress incontinence. Catheterization after the patient has attempted to void completely can provide evidence for an obstructed or atonic bladder and overflow incontinence.

The most common cause of urinary incontinence in older people is instability of the detrusor system of the bladder—the loss of normal neurologic inhibiting influences as the bladder fills. The detrusor muscle, if uninhibited, will begin to contract spontaneously when filling has reached relatively small volumes, 150 ml or less, and the patient will find it difficult or impossible to suppress the tendency to void. Unequivocal diagnosis of this condition requires cystometric studies and such should be done when needed; some physicians who are thoroughly familiar with the differential diagnosis of incontinence may choose to use first a trial of therapy for the presumptive diagnosis of instability, once other causes such as those referred to above have been eliminated.

In persons with stress incontinence or detrusor instability, the use of biofeedback and other training exercises has been found to help a number of patients to control this problem. Assuring quick access to a toilet, such as use of a bedside toilet at night, can help a person with detrusor instability reach the toilet in time. If stress incontinence in women is associated with major anatomic changes, e.g., severe uterine prolapse, or when prostatic obstruction in men is the apparent cause, surgical intervention may be indicated.

Drugs with anticholinergic effects are successful in decreasing detrusor instability in some patients; their use is often limited by undesirable anticholinergic effects in other organ systems, such as dry mouth and disturbances in gastrointestinal function. At least theoretically, anticholinergic drugs could worsen dementia of the Alzheimer's type (see above). Efforts have been made to identify drugs of this type whose effects are mainly on the bladder. Oxybutynin has smooth muscle-relaxing as well as anticholinergic effects, and imipramine has at least theoretically useful sympathomimetic and anticholinergic actions.

When overflow incontinence is secondary to a distended, atonic bladder (as with diabetic neuropathy), cholinergic drugs may be helpful.

Even if none of the above approaches is effective, acceptable management of the incontinence may be achieved through use of special waterproof pants with absorbent liners, the use of special absorbent pads on the bed, specially fitted collecting devices in women, and in selected patients the use of intermittent straight catheterization. The use of chronic indwelling catheters is rarely indicated.

PRESSURE ULCERS AND CONTRACTURES. These are unfortunate and for the most part preventable common complications of chronic illness in frail older people. Even a few hours of total immobility, as after a stroke or in the recovery period following surgery, will likely result in pressure damage to the skin and subcutaneous tissues; as little as a day or two of immobility in a joint may lead to contracture formation. Once these problems develop, correcting them is a long, tedious, and expensive process.

Preventive measures for any patient at risk of developing pressure (decubitus) ulcers or contractures should include regular, frequent passive or active movement of joints and turning, assiduous skin care, careful attention to avoiding potential damage from wrinkled bed clothes, and care in lifting, not pulling, a patient while changing his or her position.

Ulcers should be kept clean, with scrubbing and soaking three to four times a day; mild antiseptic cleansing solutions such as half-strength providone are better than stronger agents, which may cause further tissue damage. A good practice is to leave wet-to-dry gauze dressings on the wound. Surgical debridement of any necrotic tissue should be done.

As important as local care of the wound is attention to adequate general nutrition and to the treatment of any systemic disease that may cause a general catabolic response. With good wound care in a patient who is adequately nourished and otherwise well or recovering, ulcers will heal rapidly; the presence of chronic infection elsewhere, or poor nutrition, can thwart the effectiveness of even the best wound care. With large ulcers, once the wound surface is thoroughly healthy, skin grafting may be indicated.

Minor degrees of contractures can often be corrected with regular, frequent, careful stretching exercises, following a regimen established for the patient by a physical therapist. More severe and unresponsive contractures may require surgical correction. Such a step can be valuable and justified if it helps to restore mobility and independence or significantly eases nursing care burdens.

DECISIONS ABOUT LONG-TERM CARE. Elderly persons who acquire chronic, irreversible functional losses must have appropriate ongoing supportive services. The goal should be to substitute help only to the extent necessary, thus preserving the maximum possible degree of independence for the patient.

Often the need for decisions arises at a time of crisis. Already borderline functional capabilities of the older person may have further deteriorated owing to a new condition, e.g., injury, stroke, and so on, or the caregiving spouse or child may become ill or unable to continue the previous extent of care. The physician, in collaboration with other professionals (e.g., visiting nurse, social worker) and the patient and family, must weigh the relative merits and feasibility of maintaining the patient at home with support services or arranging care in a nursing home or intermediate care facility. Most older people strongly prefer to continue living in their familiar home settings, and most families desire to help the patient to stay there. Through thoughtful use of various supportive services—Meals on Wheels, housekeeper, personal care or home health aides, day programs—it is possible to maintain many such patients at home whose care needs would have equally well justified nursing home admission.

These features are discussed here because with the continually growing numbers of very elderly persons in our society there will be major increases in the pressures on our long-term care systems, and physicians will continue to be involved at the critical points of decision making where careful efforts to help stabilize and maintain many patients at home will be most important. Comprehensive geriatric evaluation services are becoming available, as ambulatory or inpatient units, in many settings. They have been shown to be valuable for consultative help at these critical points in the lives of many older people and their families.

CARE OF TERMINALLY ILL ELDERLY PERSONS. "Aging" and "dying" are so often thought of as almost synonymous that the problems of how to approach terminal care and how far to go in heroic or extraordinarily expensive diagnosis and treatment are considered by many to be issues that primarily appear in the care of the aged. The actual picture is somewhat different. Almost all of the circumstances in which inevitable death can be predicted in a fairly short time occur in patients with advanced cancer, at any age. For elderly patients with terminal cancer the same principles of care apply as for younger patients: When patient, family, and the responsible physician have agreed that no further efforts at curative therapy are warranted, the primary goal should be comfort care, avoiding heroics.

Similar decisions can be made in instances in which an older person has had such irreversible loss of mental function that he or she has little, if any, remaining apparent contact with surroundings and communication with others, especially family or nursing personnel. If those who are closest to the patient agree on the hopelessness of further curative or extraordinary treatment, including their view that this is also what the patient would say for himself or herself (or perhaps did say earlier, verbally or in writing, such as in a "living will"), then comfort care should be the practice.

The precise details of comfort care will vary with the condition of each individual patient. Overall, the physician should be concerned to see that pain is relieved, that the patient's own preferences for daily routines and activities are respected, including preferred foods, cleanliness, comfortable positioning, visits by family or friends, and outings, and that no diagnostic or treatment efforts are undertaken that may be unpleasant or painful or that will not contribute to comfort. These guidelines do not eliminate all ambiguity. For example, what should the physician decide when confronted with a new infection such as pneumonia in a patient in whom comfort care is the primary goal? If no treatment is given, the patient will likely have several days of very uncomfortable respiratory distress and may or may not survive. Comfort care in this instance would probably include respiratory therapy to help clear the airway and use of an oral antibiotic, avoiding painful injections or intravenous therapy.

Applegate WB, Blass JP, Williams TF: Instruments for the functional assessment of older patients. N Engl J Med 322:1207, 1990. *A good summary of clinically useful instruments for assessing physical, cognitive, and emotional functions.*

Blazer DG: Depression in Late Life. St. Louis, C. V. Mosby, 1982. *A thorough and practically useful presentation of this topic, including information on incidence and prevalence, diagnosis and differential diagnosis, and effective modes of therapy.*

Katzman R: Alzheimer's disease (medical progress). N Engl J Med 314:964, 1986. *An excellent summary of current knowledge of pathophysiology, possible causes, diagnosis, and management of this condition, including references to useful screening tests for dementia.*

Lachs MS, Feinstein AR, Cooney LM Jr, et al.: A simple procedure for general screening for functional disability in elderly patients. Ann Intern Med 112:699, 1990. *A useful guide to detecting evidence for such disabilities as a routine part of the workup.*

NIH Consensus Conference: Urinary incontinence in adults. JAMA 261:2685, 1989. *A careful summary of evidence and recommendations on recognition, evaluation, and treatment of this condition. The background papers (and summary) are published in J Am Geriatr Soc 38:263–386, 1989.*

Radebaugh TS, Hadley E, Suzman R (eds.): Symposium on falls in the elderly: Biological and behavioral aspects. Clin Geriatr Med 1 (3), August, 1985. *This NIH symposium covers the many interrelated risk factors contributing to this major cause of disability among older people.*

Rubenstein LZ, Campbell LJ, Kane RL (eds.): Geriatric assessment. Clin Geriatr Med 3 (1), February, 1987. *With increasing recognition of the value of comprehensive geriatric assessment, this volume provides information on when, where, how, and by whom such assessment may best be done.*

8 Care of Dying Patients and Their Families

Balfour M. Mount

Death calls into question our competence, our unconscious premises regarding the omniscience of modern medical science, and the nature of our role as caregivers. It raises questions concerning meaning, life, death, and immortality. It may undermine communication with our patients and their family members, resulting in increased isolation and despair. It presents us with a therapeutic paradox, since it is both the time when it is said that "nothing more can be done" and a time to relieve suffering and promote reconciliation and growth. The physician has an unparalleled opportunity to act as a catalyst to enable comfort, communication, integration, and healing.

DEFINITION AND GOALS OF PALLIATIVE CARE

Palliative care aims at improving the quality of life when treatment aimed at cure and prolongation of life is no longer appropriate. It offers services designed to address the physical, psychological, social, and spiritual needs of dying patients and their families. Its goals are to relieve suffering, to attain patient comfort without iatrogenic somnolence or change in affect, to assist patient and family in making the most of decreasing resources, and to support those involved in a search for meaning.

SYMPTOM CONTROL

Elimination of pain and the control of other symptoms are the foundation on which competent care of the dying rests. Chapter 26 provides a detailed review of pain and its management.

Table 8–1 offers guidelines for symptom control. Because symptoms may change rapidly, frequent re-evaluation is an essential component of effective care of the dying. Norms of care are redefined in this setting. Only investigations which may lead to a treatment that will improve quality of life are considered. Blood pressure, pulse, and temperature are not routinely monitored, whereas the frequency of bowel movements is!

Skill must be developed in the management of symptoms commonly encountered in terminal care, including insomnia, confusion, anorexia, dry or sore mouth, altered taste, nausea and vomiting, constipation, diarrhea, bowel obstruction, dyspnea, cough, pruritus, decubitus ulcers, and urinary frequency and incontinence.

Attention to detail is required for both assessment and care planning. For one very weak patient, use of a bedside commode or a bedpan and simple acceptance of occasional incontinence of urine and stool enabled conservation of scant energy reserves for eagerly anticipated daily visits with his family. Bowel care for the equally weak, fiercely independent man in the next bed involved planned nonintervention while he laboriously struggled unaided to the toilet some 15 feet from his bed. A gentle offer of assistance was given ("When you wish, just let us know"), and a discussion of his need for autonomy was held with family members. Thus, radically different approaches to the details of bowel care were used for two dying men with divergent needs.

Competent care of the dying involves compulsive care of skin, mouth, and eyes; adaptation of activities of daily living, furniture, and utensils to accommodate progressive weakness (a favorite chair raised on blocks, a padded and raised toilet seat, a spoon with a padded handle to accommodate a weak grip); clean smooth sheets; quiet music, flowers, and a few cherished belongings; the reassuring glow of soft lighting at night; and the reliable availability of both skilled nursing and an interested physician.

TABLE 8–1. GUIDELINES FOR SYMPTOM CONTROL

1. "Nothing matters more than the bowels" (Saunders). Daily assessment needed.
2. Control of one symptom improves control of all symptoms.
3. Most symptoms are caused by multiple factors. Psychological distress may augment all symptoms.
4. "Assessment must precede treatment" (Twycross).
5. Rule out correctable factors underlying each symptom.
6. Clarify who is bothered by symptom: patient, family, or staff.
7. Give simple explanation for each symptom to patient and family. Diagrams helpful.
8. Consider anticipated prognosis, functional status, and the patient's goals in determining appropriate treatment.
9. Discuss treatment options with patient and family and involve them in treatment planning where practical.
10. Determine what was helpful in the past.
11. Use a total-care approach employing nondrug, environmental, and other supportive measures.
12. If needed, utilize combinations of pharmacologic agents when differing mechanisms of action and toxicity permit.
13. Prescribe drugs prophylactically in individually optimized, regular doses for persistent symptoms.
14. Never say "Nothing more can be done." Consult or refer if comfort is not achieved.

Fears and misunderstandings about existing or anticipated symptoms and the effects of medication are common. They are minimized if patient and family are involved in both planning and providing care. Clear explanations of symptoms and treatment options give reassurance that "the doctor understands what's going on" and "there is a plan."

COMMUNICATION ISSUES

Giving bad news is always difficult. The physician should bring to discussions of prognosis not a set of fixed rules concerning whether "to tell" or "not to tell," but an openness to examining with the patient the reality at hand. Communication that is insensitive in the interest of "telling all" or evasive, falsely optimistic, or otherwise misleading in the interest of "protecting" the patient generally risks seriously undermining long-range physician credibility. Studies suggest that the majority of patients with a serious illness sense the possibility of death, whether or not they have been told. Fears are usually diminished if they can be named.

For the patient, integration of "bad news" is usually a process, not an event. Grave tidings are often repressed and simply "not heard" at the first airing. The physician should follow the pace of disclosure set by the patient, being sensitive to all forms of communication: plain language ("I fear I may be dying"), symbolic language ("I keep dreaming of a long tunnel with a candle at the end and I am afraid someone is going to blow the candle out"), and nonverbal communication (depressed facial expression, excessive muscle tension). It has been estimated that 80 per cent of communication is nonverbal. The absence of questions does not mean that questions do not exist for the patient. The physician who says "I never tell patients they have cancer unless they ask me" risks leaving the responsibility of broaching the most sensitive and awesome questions to the one who is most vulnerable, the patient.

Discussions should be positive yet reality oriented. "Am I dying? How long do I have?" may be responded to by "I don't know how long any of us have to live. If you are asking if it is serious enough to warrant getting your affairs in order, I would say yes, get your house in order. While you're doing that, you and I will deal with the medical problems you're experiencing."

Discussions focused on the goals of treatment minimize uncertainty and foster confidence. Involving the family in these discussions facilitates their subsequent mutual support. Sitting together, patient, family, and doctor examine what is still possible rather than what has been lost.

"There are only three aims we can have in treating any illness, Bill. We are not going to be able to cure your tumor, in the sense of making it go away permanently. But, you know, there are many medical problems we can't cure—including diabetes,

arthritis, and most types of heart disease—yet many people with these conditions live meaningful lives, sometimes for longer periods than we expect.

"So 'cure' isn't an option. What about the next goal, 'to prolong life'? You could undergo surgery, but there is no sense putting you through something that wouldn't be helpful." (Surgery is often used as the first example, since it presents a concrete, easily grasped image of futility.) "With treatments as they now stand, the same would be said for chemotherapy, radiotherapy, and immunotherapy." (The phrasing focuses on the limitations of current therapy, not the hopelessness of the illness.)

"Does this mean nothing more can be done?" (thus naming the worst fear). "Not at all! It simply means we are at the third goal—that of focusing on the quality of life. How can we make the best of this? Let's examine that. If I understand you, the three complaints you have right now are your backache, that cough, and your loss of appetite. Let's see what we can do about each of these. . . ."

The patient and family are left with a clear understanding that the issue is not "to treat or not to treat," but an appropriate shifting in therapeutic goals by a physician who is interested, involved, and undaunted by the specter of this illness. Hope is contagious. Hope is a way through, not a way out.

Specific estimates of survival should never be given, since they are based on data relevant to populations of patients with the same illness, not to the patient in question. No matter how carefully phrased, such pronouncements always unsheathe a sword of Damocles that heightens anxiety and drains ability to live fully in the moment. "I have only 2 more months."

Acceptance of the present reality, including the increasing weakness, dependence, uncertain future, and impending loss, frees the patient to choose from available options. Acceptance of that kind is not born out of despair and resignation. It is the transcendant alternative to denial. It is a path to meaning which is possible even in the face of physical deterioration and advancing disease.

FAMILY AS THE UNIT OF CARE

Terminal illness is a pressure cooker of family stress. Grief, fear, anger, and guilt abound. Longstanding interpersonal tensions tend to be accentuated. Brief family meetings to discuss treatment plans and identify problems and fears are a time-efficient tool highly effective in preventing impending crises, clarifying misunderstandings, and building bridges of mutual support.

Table 8–2 presents a checklist of areas of inquiry useful in family assessment. Ensure that children and the elderly are informed and involved. Their exclusion often leaves them ill-prepared for loss.

The bereaved are a high-risk population with an increased incidence of impaired function, medical illness, psychological distress, and even death. Some who have been found to have an increased risk of bereavement morbidity are listed in Table 8–3. Referral to programs offering bereavement support may be beneficial.

DYING AT HOME

Death has been moved from the home to the institution in industrial nations, and family members often feel ill-prepared to care for dying loved ones. With careful planning, family education, mobilization of community resources, and continuing support, however, both family and patient may benefit from experiencing this last time together in the home.

TABLE 8–2. FAMILY ASSESSMENT ISSUES

1. Identity of nuclear family, extended family, and social network.
2. Characteristics of family system: roles, relationships, communication patterns.
3. Presence of concurrent life crises.
4. History of coping with past crises.
5. Values and beliefs about death.
6. Response to current illness: changes in roles and relationships.
7. Family resources: physical, emotional, financial, social, spiritual.
8. Immediate family needs.
9. Long-range family needs.

TABLE 8–3. SELECTED BEREAVEMENT RISK INDICATORS

1. Parental grief.
2. Social isolation.
3. Timid, dependent personality; poorly developed coping skills.
4. Short preparation time (duration of illness).
5. Ambivalent or charged relationship with deceased.
6. Concurrent life crisis.
7. Pining and clinging in final illness.
8. Grief expression repressed by cultural or family norms.
9. Disenfranchised grief: mistress, lover, divorcée, loss of a secret relationship.

Home care of the dying begins with careful home assessment performed by an experienced home care team able to direct the family to needed community resources and to recommend modifications in living arrangements and furnishings to simplify care. "You will find it much easier if you rent a hospital bed. They are inexpensive. Try placing it in the living room where she can be quiet, close to the family, and able to see the children passing in the street.

"She is weaker now. You will need a handrail and small bench for the bath tub and a walker. I think you would find a commode for the bedside helpful as well."

An effective palliative home care program implies the involvement of a team. Regularly scheduled nursing visits are supplemented by emergency visits as required. A trusted physician is available to consult in the home when the need arises. A social worker, occupational therapist, chaplain, and volunteers may all play a role. Simple, clear routines for medications and treatments are established. A sense of order and safety is fostered by round-the-clock availability of telephone consultation with experienced staff who are aware of recent changes in the patient's condition and medications. Brief respite admissions before family exhaustion sets in may serve to prolong capability of home care.

A sensitive discussion with the family about what to do when their loved one dies may promote a sense of confidence and preparedness. Acknowledgment of a job well done ("You certainly have done well to keep her at home this long") helps to allay feelings of inadequacy and guilt should admission to hospital become necessary.

AS DEATH APPROACHES

During the final days or weeks of a terminal illness, frequent changes in clinical status may occur. Eventualities such as the need for parenteral or rectal medications should be foreseen and planned for. Common crises include progressive weakness, inability to swallow and aspiration of oral intake, inability or refusal to take medications, changing levels of consciousness and orientation, restlessness, and urinary or fecal incontinence. Careful planning and prompt response to the request for emergency assistance can avoid unnecessary admission to hospital.

Decreasing requirements for most medications are encountered as death approaches. Individualized reductions in dose can prolong an alert, interactive, comfortable state, often to the moment of death.

Noisy upper airway secretions ("death rattle") are troubling to the family, who will need reassurance, but they are generally not troubling to the patient. They may be reduced by early intervention with hyoscine 0.4 mg given subcutaneously at intervals of 2 to 4 hours as needed.

Questions and fears the patient and family have about death should be gently explored. The will, funeral arrangements, and a "life review" may be discussed as a means of completing unfinished business and facilitating closure.

Encourage family members, including the young, the elderly, and those from out of town, to visit earlier rather than later. Assess bereavement risks and arrange follow-up support if indicated.

Decathexis, a protective "separating off" or "turning in" by the patient, is sometimes seen as death approaches. A simple explanation may reassure the concerned family that this is not depression or rejection but a normal protective mechanism. "He doesn't need you to say much now, but your presence will help."

Take premonitions of death seriously, and watch for the need for family members to give their lingering loved one permission to die. "It's all right, John. You can let go. You've taken care of everything. We'll miss you, but thanks to you we'll be O.K."

AT THE TIME OF DEATH

The hours that surround the death of a family member are charged with meaning for the bereaved and are usually remembered for years to come. Caregivers may use this to therapeutic advantage by establishing guidelines for patient and family care that facilitate subsequent grief work.

Endeavor to have someone sitting at the bedside of the imminently dying person. If the bedside companion is a family member, be sensitive to his or her need either for support or for time to be alone with the loved one. Encourage available family members to view the body before it has been moved to the funeral home. Seeing the body facilitates acceptance of the fact of death.

When family members arrive, offer support and quiet hospitality, including a handkerchief, a cup of tea, a listening ear. Acknowledge the support given by the bereaved to the deceased during the illness.

Allow sufficient time with the body for active grieving. It is a helpful role model for a caregiver to unobtrusively touch the body, indicating that there is nothing frightening about physical contact with the body—an experience that may be highly effective in promoting closure.

Discuss whether the family wishes to have an autopsy. Many find the documentation of reality that it provides helpful in the months and years to come.

When death occurs in a hospital, ask the family if they would prefer to collect and pack their loved one's personal effects, particularly if a child has died. A memento of the event such as a lock of hair or a picture may be an aid to bereavement, especially in parental grief.

Respect cultural differences in the expression of acute grief. Mediterranean peoples, some Asian nationalities, and others may be extremely vocal and demonstrative in their grieving. Wails, screams, fainting attacks, and highly dramatic gestures such as throwing themselves across the body of the deceased have therapeutic value for many and may be followed in a remarkably short period of time by a sense of composure and evident relief.

Acknowledge the mystery of death without offering "answers" concerning the unknowable. Honor religious rites and prayers meaningful to the bereaved.

The presence at the death or funeral service of the physician who was involved during the illness assists review of the illness, emphasizes the value of the deceased, underscores respect for the family, and assists the physician's own grief work.

THE PHYSICIAN AND DEATH

In caring for the dying, physicians are challenged in each dimension of their personhood. William James termed death "the worm at the core of man's pretensions to happiness," while La Rochefouchauld observed: "Death and the sun are not to be looked at steadily." What do we do with our accumulated losses as caregivers? How do we establish a new balance in our emotional economy when an important investment has been lost? At what cost? To whom? Do our professional encounters with death leave a need for thicker defensive shells, emotional distancing, intellectualization, and acting out? The risk is minimized if we accept relief of suffering as our mandate rather than the narrower goal of fighting disease and if we attend to our own physical, psychosocial, and spiritual needs. Indeed, confrontation with death may foster insight and enrich life. It has been said that to live is to suffer and to survive is to find meaning in the suffering; that having a "why" to live can enable living with any "how"; that our last freedom, when all others have been stripped away, is the ability to choose our response in a given set of circumstances. It is a privilege to be able to assist our patients in their growing toward an understanding of the truth of these observations. It is a source of personal growth when we recognize their truth ourselves.

Cassel E: The nature of suffering and the goals of medicine. N Engl J Med 306:639, 1982. *A classic examination of the components of personhood and their impact on the experience of illness.*

Doyle D: Palliative Care: The Management of Far Advanced Illness. Philadelphia, The Charles Press, 1984. *Comprehensive review of management strategies in both nonmalignant and malignant advanced disease.*

Frankl V: Man's Search for Meaning. New York, Simon and Schuster, 1963. *A psychiatrist and Auschwitz survivor reflects on motivation, meaning, and quality of life. Moving. Insightful. A classic.*

Saunders C: The Management of Terminal Malignant Disease. 2nd ed. Baltimore, Edward Arnold, 1984. *The principles and practice of palliative medicine by the pioneering founder of the modern hospice movement.*

Twycross RG, Lack SA: Therapeutics in Terminal Cancer. 2nd ed. New York, Churchill Livingstone, 1990. *A useful and authoritative guide to the care of patients with advanced cancer. Pragmatic. Organized for easy reference at the bedside.*

Walsh TD: Symptom Control. Cambridge, Mass., Blackwell Scientific Publications, 1989. *Detailed consideration of symptom control from angina to xerostomia! Additional chapters on ten specific areas of clinical concern including the elderly, stoma care, menopause, multiple sclerosis, pregnancy, and speech disorders.*

Worden JW: Grief Counselling and Grief Therapy. A Handbook for the Mental Health Practitioner. New York, Springer Publishing, 1982. *Mechanisms of grief and approaches to helping the bereaved accomplish the "tasks of mourning." Lucid and informative. An excellent resource for the general physician.*

PART III

PERSONAL HEALTH CARE AND PREVENTIVE MEDICINE

9 PRINCIPLES OF PREVENTIVE MEDICINE

Stephen B. Hulley

In the early part of this century the efforts of preventive medicine were focused on the predominant cause of illness and death at the time, infectious disease. In western countries, governmental provisions to control the spread of disease with modern water and sewage systems complemented the success of the medical profession in the developing science of immunization. These programs combined with improved nutrition, better medical care, and other factors to make death from infectious disease an uncommon event by 1980. Despite a small reversal of this trend in the next decade caused by the AIDS epidemic, life expectancy has risen to unprecedented levels and the noninfectious and chronic diseases have become the major cause of death and disability (Table 9–1). A new set of strategies has evolved to prevent the chief causes of mortality today: coronary heart disease, cancer, stroke, and injury.

Preventive medicine is based on epidemiologic studies that have identified risk factors for these conditions. Many of these risk factors are aspects of individually chosen lifestyles: cigarette smoking (the most important single cause of preventable death), substance abuse, and unhealthy eating and exercising habits. This has changed the nature of the therapeutic relationship. The patient must take on the larger responsibility of making the necessary lifestyle changes, and the physician must now add the role of health counselor to his clinical duties.

RISK MODIFICATION

The process of guiding lifestyle change *begins* with serving as a model. A physician who has healthy habits and provides an appropriate environment (prohibiting smoking in the waiting room, for example) has set the stage for successful intervention. The *second step* is to identify the individual characteristics of the patient, testing for the presence of risk factors and exploring motivations for changing, and for not changing, unhealthy habits. The *third step* is to provide a clear message about the scientific facts on the relationship between risk factors and disease, specifying, for example, the nature and extent of the adverse health consequences of cigarettes.

The *fourth step* is to formulate and apply recommendations that will lead to behavior change. These include (1) involving the patient as a partner in choosing attainable objectives and in making a firm commitment (a written contract may be helpful); (2) adjusting the environment to promote the desired behavior (by discarding ashtrays and not keeping unhealthy food in the home, for example); (3) establishing and rehearsing new behaviors step by step (first eating a healthier breakfast, then incorporating a 10-minute walk in commute, etc.); (4) positively reinforcing desired behavior (through praise, rewards, and risk factor feedback); and (5) involving the family and other social supports. Many clinics include staff with special skills in behavioral medicine, but even in the absence of formal training, physicians can accomplish a great deal just by addressing and lending importance to these activities. In addition to serving as health counselors themselves, physicians can guide the patient's access to other resources for lifestyle changes by providing pamphlets (obtained free from organizations like the American Heart Association) and by referral to appropriate books, support groups, and health professionals.

Whatever the intervention approach, the *fifth step* is a sustained effort to follow up on the risk factor levels. Habits are difficult to change, and health counselors need the tenacity and imagination to try a variety of approaches over the years. This does not mean harassing an unwilling or unsuccessful patient. The best health counselors are sensitive to the preferences of their patients and make wise decisions about when to promote recommendations for change and when to leave the patient alone.

IMPLICATIONS OF CHRONIC DISEASE PREVENTION

If the entire population were fully successful in the lifestyle changes proposed in this second wave of twentieth century preventive medicine efforts, the chief causes of premature death in western countries might become far less common. In addition to further extending life expectancy, the potential reward of fully effective lifestyle intervention is the possibility that most people could live their full lifespan without major illness or disability.

Speculation of this sort is based, in part, on the remarkable decline in mortality observed in the United States over the past

TABLE 9–1. ANNUAL MORTALITY RATES AND YEARS OF LIFE LOST PREMATURELY IN THE UNITED STATES IN 1900 AND IN 1986

Causes of Death*	1900 Annual Mortality (rate/100,000)	1986 Annual Mortality (rate/100,000)	Years of Potential Life Lost Before Age 65 by Persons Dying in 1986
Diseases of the heart	137	319	1,600,000
Malignant neoplasms	64	196	1,800,000
Cerebrovascular disease	107	62	200,000
Injuries	83	61	3,700,000
All others	1330	237	4,700,000
Total	1721	873	12,000,000

*The causes of death are the four most common in 1986. The statistics, which are not age adjusted, are subject to the usual inaccuracies of death certificate attribution. The top three causes of death in 1900 were pneumonia and influenza (202/100,000), tuberculosis (194/100,000), and diarrhea and enteritis (143/100,000).

TABLE 9–2. FIFTEEN AREAS OF ENDEAVOR FOR PREVENTIVE MEDICINE ESTABLISHED BY THE U.S. DEPARTMENT OF HEALTH AND HUMAN SERVICES

Topics that Are Covered in Chapters of this Section
Smoking and health
Injury prevention
Control of stress and violent behavior
Nutrition
Physical fitness and exercise
Misuse of alcohol and drugs
Immunization

Topics that Are Addressed Elsewhere in this Book
High blood pressure
Sexually transmitted diseases
Toxic agents
Occupational safety and health
Infectious diseases

Topics that Are the Concern of Other Specialties
Family planning
Pregnancy and infant health
Fluoridation and dental health

20 years. The chief component of the decline is coronary heart disease, which has decreased more rapidly in the United States (2 per cent per year) than in any other nation. It seems reasonable to attribute this, at least in part, to the changes in lifestyle that are occurring in this country: the substantial decline in the national prevalence of smoking and of inadequately treated hypertension, the decrease in the mean serum cholesterol level, and the movement to become more physically fit.

The extent and thrust of preventive medicine today have been established by formal health goals in 15 areas of endeavor, created by the U.S. Department of Health and Human Services (Table 9–2). For each of these topics, there are specific objectives for the nation to achieve by the year 2000 that address health status, risk factor levels, public and professional awareness, provision of health services, and mechanisms for evaluation. This section of *Cecil Textbook of Medicine* addresses 7 of these 15 topics that are part of personal health care.

SUMMARY

The emergence of chronic and noninfectious disease as the predominant cause of death and disability in western nations has been accompanied by a growing importance of lifestyle factors as causal agents in health and disease. Among these, cigarette smoking is the single most important modifiable health hazard; abuse of alcohol and other substances, sedentary lifestyle, and improper diet are also important. The clinician's role in preventive medicine still begins with immunization and treatment of such medical conditions as hypertension, but it now extends to health counseling: examining a patient's risk factors, educating the patient, listening to preferences for changing (or not changing) lifestyle, implementing the appropriate behavioral interventions, and following up on these personal health care strategies over the years.

Higgins M, Thom T: Trends in coronary heart disease in the U.S. Int J Epidemiol 18(Suppl 1):S58, 1990. *Recent update on the remarkable 20-year decline in CHD mortality.*
Martin AR, Coates TJ: A clinician's guide to helping patients change. West J Med 146:751, 1987. *Practical guidelines in helping patients modify their risks.*
McGinnis JM, Hamburg MA: Opportunities for health promotion and disease prevention in the clinical setting. West J Med 149:468, 1988. *Practical and concise summary of prevention approaches for clinicians.*
Public Health Service, U.S. Dept of Health and Human Services: The 1990 Objectives for the Nation: A mid course review. 1986. *Update on progress in achieving the 1990 objectives for 15 areas of preventive medicine.*
U.S. Dept. of Health, Education and Welfare: Healthy People: The Surgeon General's Report on Health Promotion and Disease Prevention. DHEW Publication No. 79–55071, 1979. *Summary of trends in illness and death rates from 1900 to the 1970's.*
U.S. Preventive Services Task Force: Guide to clinical preventive services. Baltimore, Williams and Wilkins, 1989. *Most comprehensive set of prevention guidelines.*

10　Tobacco and Health
David M. Burns

Cigarette smoking is the largest preventable public health problem in the United States. An estimated 390,000 deaths per year, one sixth of the total mortality in the United States, occur prematurely secondary to the smoking habits of the American population.

Tobacco use, both oral and smoking, was introduced to European settlers by the American Indian, and tobacco was one of the main cash crops in revolutionary America. The invention of a cigarette-making machine in the 1880's and, around the turn of the century, of matches that could be carried safely resulted in a marked shift in tobacco consumption from predominantly pipes, cigars, and chewing tobacco to predominantly cigarettes. Per capita cigarette consumption in the United States increased from 54 in 1900 to a peak of 4336 in 1963. This dramatic switch to cigarette use was followed some 20 to 25 years later by an equally dramatic rise in deaths from lung cancer. The risks associated with tobacco smoking appear to be closely related to the amount of smoke inhaled. Smokers who have used only pipes or cigars tend not to inhale, and therefore the majority of the health risks are correlated with cigarette consumption (Table 10–1).

In the early part of the century, cigarette smoking was largely a male habit, but in the late 1930's and early 1940's women began to smoke in large numbers. Currently, smoking habits in young adults are similar for the two sexes. The prevalence of cigarette smoking is declining in both men and women in the United States population. In contrast, a new marketing effort for smokeless tobacco has led to a major resurgence of snuff use, particularly among adolescent males.

CIGARETTE SMOKE

Tobacco smoke is a complex mixture of some 4000 individual constituents. The smoke is a combination of pyrolysis and distillation products distributed between a particulate phase and a gas phase. Tar, the total particulate matter of the smoke once the water vapor and nicotine have been removed, is the major carcinogen of whole smoke. The gas phase of the smoke has a number of irritating and ciliotoxic agents, as well as high levels of carbon monoxide.

FACTORS DETERMINING RISK

The risks due to cigarette smoking vary with differences in individual smoking habits and with the presence of other risk factors. The risk increases with increasing number of cigarettes

TABLE 10–1. INCREASED RISKS FOR CIGARETTE SMOKERS

Cardiovascular Disease
Coronary artery disease
Peripheral vascular disease
Aortic aneurysm
Stroke

Cancer
Lung
Larynx, oral cavity, esophagus
Bladder, kidney
Pancreas

Lung Disorders
Cancer (as noted above)
Chronic bronchitis with airflow obstruction
Emphysema

Complications of Pregnancy
Infants—small for gestational age, higher perinatal mortality
Maternal complications—placenta previa, abruptio placentae

Gastrointestinal Complications
Peptic ulcer
Esophageal reflux

Other
Altered drug metabolism

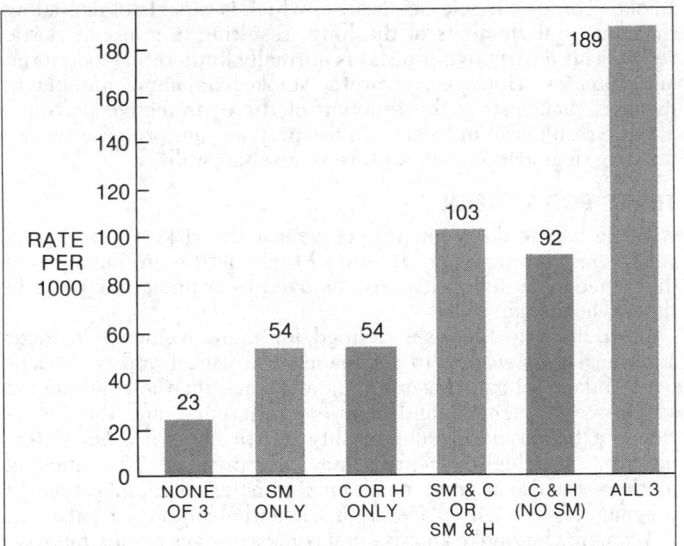

FIGURE 10–1. Major risk factor combinations, 10-year incidence of first major coronary events, men age 30 to 59 at entry, Pooling Project. Risk factor status at entry: Definitions of the three major risk factors and their symbols are hypercholesterolemia (C) = ≥ 250 mg/dl; elevated blood pressure (H) = diastolic pressure ≥ 90 mm Hg; cigarette smoking (SM) = any current use of cigarettes at entry.

smoked per day, depth of inhalation, and duration of the smoking habit. The risk also increases with the younger age at which regular smoking is begun.

A given dose of smoke exposure may interact with other personal characteristics or environmental exposures to magnify the risk of disease greatly. Thus, the risks incurred by cigarette smoking in someone with elevated blood pressure or high levels of asbestos exposure are much larger than the risks for smokers without those characteristics. In addition, the presence of smoking-induced disease in one organ system (e.g., chronic obstructive lung disease) may alter the ability to treat or survive a second disease process (e.g., lung cancer).

CARDIOVASCULAR DISEASE

Cigarette smokers have almost twice the risk of nonsmokers of developing a myocardial infarction or dying of coronary heart disease. This relative risk of heart disease is even greater at younger ages, when the incidence of disease would otherwise be very low. The relative risks for sudden death from coronary disease, peripheral vascular disease, and aneurysm of the aorta are even higher. In contrast, cigarette smokers have only a slightly greater risk of developing angina pectoris.

The magnitude of the risk of coronary heart disease associated with cigarette smoking is equivalent to the risks associated with elevated blood pressure or elevated serum cholesterol. The per cent of the population with smoking as a risk factor is substantially larger than the percentage with either elevated blood pressure or elevated serum cholesterol. As a result, *smoking ranks as the largest avoidable cause of coronary heart disease in the American population.*

Cigarette smoking acts as an independent risk factor for coronary heart disease; that is, its effect is not explained by levels of other risk factors. When more than one risk factor is present, however, smoking interacts with the other major risk factors to increase the risk synergistically (Fig. 10–1). The presence of smoking, or of either of the other risk factors, increases the risk by 31 per 1000, compared with the risk of someone with none of the risk factors. The presence of a second risk factor in someone who smokes results in an increase in risk of 49 per 1000 over the risk when only one risk factor is present, and the addition of a third risk factor increases the risk by 86 per 1000. The actual risk is always greater than the sum of the risks measured independently, suggesting that when multiple risk factors are present, they interact to create more disease. This interaction may occur by accelerating the development of atherosclerosis or by increasing the likelihood or severity of a myocardial infarction for any given level of atherosclerosis.

Smokers have more atherosclerosis than nonsmokers, particularly in the aorta. Smoking a cigarette raises heart rate and blood pressure, necessitating a greater myocardial oxygen delivery, while the carbon monoxide in the smoke increases the blood's carboxyhemoglobin level, thus decreasing its oxygen-carrying capacity. Cigarette smoking also increases platelet adhesiveness and lowers the threshold for ventricular fibrillation and may thereby play a role in the acute events surrounding some thrombotic myocardial infarctions.

Cigarette smoking has a more profound effect on the peripheral vascular bed than on the coronary or cerebral vessels. Over 90 per cent of patients with atherosclerotic peripheral vascular disease are cigarette smokers. Cessation of cigarette smoking is critical to treatment of these patients. In those who fail to quit, there is a higher incidence of amputation, and surgical therapy is dramatically less successful.

The risk of coronary heart disease due to smoking is present at all ages beyond 30, but smoking is responsible for a greater proportion of coronary deaths in younger age groups than in older age groups. This risk declines dramatically with the cessation of cigarette smoking. By 5 years after the last cigarette, the risk in those who had smoked less than one pack per day approximates the risk in lifelong nonsmokers. For those who had smoked more than one pack per day, a small residual risk of coronary heart disease may persist.

CANCER

Lung cancer is the largest cause of death from cancer in men and women (Ch. 68). *Approximately 85 per cent of mortality due to lung cancer is causally attributed to cigarette smoking and is therefore potentially preventable.*

Cigarette smokers are ten times more likely to develop lung cancer than nonsmokers. This risk is proportional to the number of cigarettes smoked per day, increasing to 20 to 25 times the risk of the nonsmoker in those who smoke two or more packs of cigarettes per day. The risk is also increased in those who inhale more deeply or began smoking at a younger age. Lung cancer death rates begin to increase rapidly after age 35 (Fig. 10–2). Cigarette smoking causes all of the major types of lung cancer, including squamous cell, adenocarcinoma, oat cell, and large cell

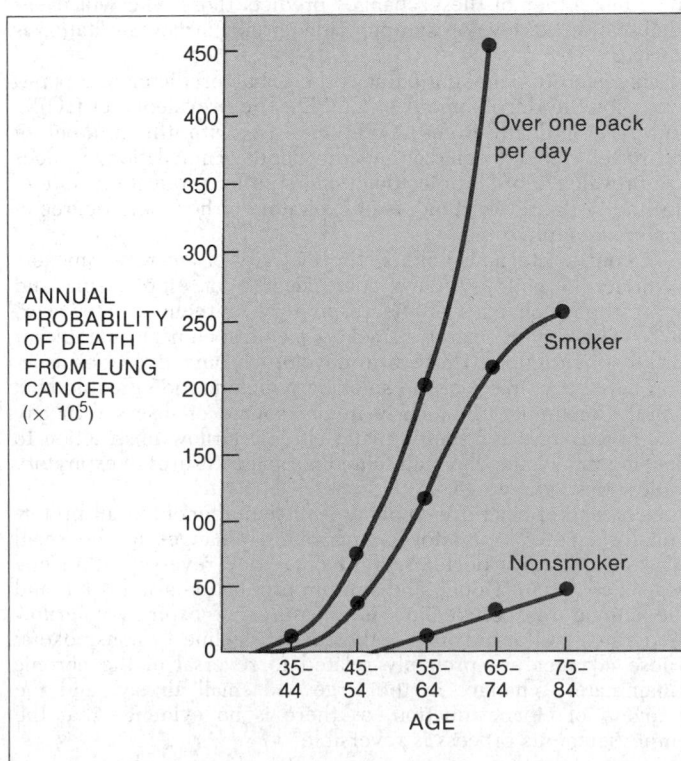

FIGURE 10–2. Annual death rate from lung cancer in nonsmokers, smokers in general, and those who smoke more than one pack per day.

carcinoma. Asbestos exposure and uranium mining interact with cigarette smoking to increase the risk of lung cancer dramatically.

The relative risks of developing *laryngeal cancer* for the cigarette smoker closely track those of lung cancer, but the total number of cases is smaller and the survival better. Cigarette smokers are five times more likely to develop *cancer of the oral cavity and esophagus*, and there appears to be a synergistic interaction between cigarette smoking and alcohol consumption for cancer of the larynx, oral cavity, and esophagus. Cigarette smoking is also a major contributing factor in *cancers of the bladder, kidney, and pancreas*, and an association between cigarette smoking and *gastric and cervical cancers* has been noted. The use of chewing tobacco or snuff can cause cancers of the cheek or gum. Overall, tobacco consumption is responsible for approximately 30 per cent of the total United States cancer mortality.

Cigarette smoking induces changes in the respiratory epithelium that progress from hyperplasia to dysplasia and even to carcinoma in situ. Tobacco smoke contains a variety of tumorigenic agents, including several that can act as complete carcinogens. The impact of these tumorigenic agents may be magnified by the ciliotoxic agents in the smoke that interfere with the normal clearance mechanisms of the lung and result in a prolonged retention of the carcinogenic agents in the lung.

Cessation of cigarette smoking results in a lessening of the risk of cancer in comparison with the risk to the continuing smoker. The risk for light smokers approximates the risk of the nonsmoker by 10 to 15 years after cessation. Heavy smokers have a residual two- to threefold increased risk that is proportional to their lifetime exposure to smoke.

CHRONIC OBSTRUCTIVE PULMONARY DISEASE (COPD)

Cigarette-induced lung injury is characterized by three overlapping syndromes: cough and mucus hypersecretion, bronchitis with airflow obstruction, and emphysema (see Ch. 58). By age 60 most cigarette smokers have changes in the airways and some degree of pathologic emphysema, but only the minority have symptomatic ventilatory limitation. The prevalence of cough increases in cigarette smokers by the early teens, and the small airways are abnormal in many smokers by early adulthood. Whether either of these changes predicts those who will eventually go on to develop symptomatic chronic airflow limitation is unclear.

The cigarette smoking habit is the major predictor in a population for the development of COPD. The prevalence of COPD and risk of death from COPD increase with the number of cigarettes smoked per day and the depth of inhalation, as does the prevalence of chronic cough and sputum production, rate of decline in the measurements of expiratory airflow, and degree of anatomic emphysema.

In contrast to nonsmokers, the majority of cigarette smokers examined at autopsy have some degree of emphysema and hypertrophic changes of the respiratory epithelium. However, only a minority of cigarette smokers manifest clinically significant airflow obstruction. Those who develop chronic airflow obstruction may be a subset of the smoking population identifiable by a rapidly declining FEV_1 early in the course of disease. In any event, it is rare for symptomatic chronic airflow obstruction to develop in anyone who maintained normal measures of expiratory airflow through age 45.

Cessation of cigarette smoking is of some benefit at all preterminal stages of ventilatory impairment. Changes in the small airways and early declines of FEF_{25-75} may reverse within one year of cessation. Cough and sputum production also lessen, and the annual rate of decline in measures of expiratory airflow moderates and approximates the rate of decline in nonsmokers. These changes are probably related to reversal of the chronic inflammatory changes in the large and small airways and the recovery of ciliary function, as there is no evidence that the emphysematous process is reversible.

Lungs of smokers contain increased numbers of alveolar macrophages and polymorphonuclear leukocytes, probably drawn there as part of the inflammatory response to the irritants in the smoke. These cells release elastase, which is capable of degrading the structural elements of the lung, resulting in a loss of elastic recoil. This destructive process is normally limited by bloodborne antiproteases. However, cigarette smoke contains a number of oxidants that destroy the function of these protective proteins, and the result is an imbalance in the protease-antiprotease system favoring degradation and rupture of alveolar walls.

RISKS FOR WOMEN

Being female does not protect against the risks of developing cancer or chronic lung disease. Much of the premenopausal difference in cardiovascular risk enjoyed by women disappears in those who smoke.

In addition to the risks defined for men, women also incur additional risks related to pregnancy and use of oral contraceptives. Infants of smoking mothers are small for their gestational age in weight, length, and head circumference, and they experience a higher perinatal mortality, particularly if other determinants of a high-risk pregnancy are present. The smoking mothers are also at greater risk for the maternal complications of pregnancy, especially placenta previa and abruptio placentae.

Women who smoke and use oral contraceptives greatly increase their risk of cardiovascular disease. They are over 30 times more likely to develop a myocardial infarction, and about 20 times more likely to have a subarachnoid hemorrhage, than their nonsmoking peers who do not use oral contraceptives.

INVOLUNTARY SMOKING

Environmental tobacco smoke contains most of the toxic and carcinogenic compounds identified in mainstream smoke; and therefore the question is not whether these agents can cause disease, but rather whether the dose and mode of exposure experienced in involuntary smoking carry a measurable risk. Absorption of smoke constituents from the environment has been documented in both infants and adults, and a number of epidemiologic studies have demonstrated health effects in humans.

Involuntary smoking can cause lung cancer in nonsmokers. The risk is small in comparison to active smoking but is large in comparison to other carcinogenic exposures experienced by the general population. From 500 to 5000 lung cancers per year have been estimated to result from involuntary smoking.

The majority of nonsmokers express annoyance and experience eye and respiratory tract irritation on exposure to smoke. Individuals with pre-existing disease may become more symptomatic on exposure to smoke, particularly those with allergies, and possibly those with chronic heart and lung disease. Nonsmokers with long-term exposure to environmental tobacco smoke may develop changes in the small airways of the lung.

Infants of smoking parents have a higher incidence of bronchitis and pneumonia in the first year of life, and the children of smoking mothers experience a developmental lag in lung growth.

CIGARETTES WITH LOW TAR AND NICOTINE

The machine-measured yield of tar and nicotine for the average cigarette smoked by the American population has been steadily declining. Smokers of lower yield cigarettes have a slightly lower risk of lung cancer than smokers of the high-yield cigarette, but this benefit disappears if they increase the number of cigarettes they smoke per day. There is also a lower prevalence of cough and phlegm, but probably no major impact on the risk of developing cardiovascular disease or chronic airflow obstruction. There are two major reasons why the decline in machine-measured tar and nicotine yield has not been accompanied by a concomitant reduction in biologic effect: (1) Many smokers may compensate for the decline in yield by increasing the number of cigarettes smoked per day, or by inhaling more deeply, thereby negating any possible reduction in smoke exposure "dose." (2) The machine-measured yield may not correspond to the yield when the cigarette is actually smoked. This is particularly true for the very low-yield cigarettes that have vents or channels designed into the filter so that the machine draws very little smoke through the filter. These vents can be occluded by the smoker, or the volume of the puff increased, with a resultant dramatic rise in the yield. For these cigarettes, the measured tar and nicotine yields have almost no relation to either actual yield or biologic potency.

An additional concern is the wide variety of flavoring and other additives that have been used to compensate for the decline in tobacco content. These additives are considered trade secrets and may be added to the cigarette without informing the public of their presence and without any review for toxic effects. These additives represent a major gap in the understanding of the disease risks associated with smoking the modern cigarette.

OTHER EFFECTS

Cigarette smokers have a greater incidence of gastric and duodenal ulcers and delayed healing of these ulcers. Smoking also relaxes the esophageal sphincter and may contribute to esophageal reflux.

Several of the constituents of tobacco smoke are capable of inducing hepatic microsomal systems, which then alter the metabolism of other drugs. Theophylline, phenacetin, antipyrine, caffeine, and imipramine are metabolized more rapidly by smokers, and adjustment in the dosage may be required with cessation. Smokers have lower blood levels of vitamins C and B_{12}. Hematocrit and hemoglobin levels, as well as carboxyhemoglobin levels, are elevated in smokers; and smoking is one cause of an elevated red cell volume. Smokers also have small alterations in the other diagnostic tests, including a higher leukocyte count, but these differences are not usually clinically significant for an individual patient.

Pipe and cigar smokers who have never smoked cigarettes have a lower risk of cardiovascular disease, lung cancer, and chronic airflow obstruction than do cigarette smokers. They have similar risks of cancer of the upper respiratory tract. These differences are due to the tendency of pipe and cigar smokers not to inhale the more irritating smoke of these forms of tobacco. Cigarette smokers who switch to pipes and cigars do tend to inhale, however, and so it is not clear that switching to a pipe or cigars results in a lowering of the risks for the cigarette smoker.

The re-emergence of oral snuff use among male adolescents in the last several years has generated substantial public health concern. Smokeless tobacco use can cause cancer of the cheek and gum and gingival recession. It may also increase the risk of other oral cancers, and regular use of snuff can lead to nicotine addiction.

SMOKING BEHAVIOR AND CESSATION

Regular cigarette smoking begins almost exclusively during adolescence; 90 per cent of smokers begin before age 20. The availability and relatively low cost of cigarettes coupled with peer pressure and the desire to model adult behavior are determinants of adolescent smoking. Tobacco advertising may also influence the initiation of regular smoking by creating an image of the smoker as a secure, confident, successful, in control, and attractive individual. By smoking, adolescents are able to superimpose this positive image created by advertising on their own inadequate self-image and thereby feel better. Those adolescents with the least external validation of their self worth (through academic, athletic, or social achievements) are the ones most in need of manipulation of their internal self-image and, correspondingly, most susceptible to the images presented by advertising.

Addiction to cigarettes depends on nicotine. Beyond the pharmacologic stimulus of nicotine, however, the smoker usually creates a series of learned responses that reduce stress and alter mood. The pattern of tobacco use therefore merges into the way that the smoker learns to deal with the world. Cessation of smoking requires that the smoker give up a major coping mechanism.

Smoking cessation clinics have long-term success in 30 to 40 per cent of the smokers who persevere in their programs, but comparatively few smokers are willing to participate in these clinics. Current tobacco control strategies emphasize altering the environment in which the smoker lives by making smoking socially unacceptable, by increasing the cost of cigarettes, and by limiting the locations in which it is permissible to smoke.

Physicians can effect sustained cessation of smoking in a substantial number of patients if they are willing to treat smoking as a potentially serious medical problem. This requires obtaining information, defining a therapeutic plan, and following the results of that therapy. The information to be obtained includes the smoking status, a history of past cessation attempts and the

methods used, as well as the current interest in quitting. In addition, the time from awakening to first cigarette is a measure of the strength of the addiction and may be useful in deciding whether to prescribe pharmacologic aids to the cessation attempt. In their offices physicians can ask the patient to quit, can motivate the attempt, and can negotiate a date for quitting. No smoking patient should leave the office without understanding that his or her smoking is a major health problem. The responsibility of the physician is not to get all patients to quit on a single visit, but to move each smoking patient closer to cessation on each visit. Those who have not thought about quitting should think about it; those who are thinking about it should try; and those who have tried and failed should be motivated to try again. Smokers should be encouraged to quit "cold turkey" rather than tapering down. The follow-up of cessation advice is also critical, not only because it reinforces the importance of cessation for the patient, but also because it improves the likelihood of successful cessation. A simple letter of encouragement from the physician 2 weeks following the quit date may substantially improve patient motivation and success.

The use of nicotine gum increases the chance of successful short-term cessation when utilized with an appropriate behavioral intervention program. Clonidine, particularly when used as a patch, has shown promise as a means of reducing the withdrawal symptoms but remains an investigational drug for this purpose.

Effective smoking intervention by the physician can be delivered in 3 to 5 minutes using the above approach. Physicians should refer patients who need more extensive assistance to programs designed to provide this assistance. A variety of community organizations provide cessation assistance, both in groups and as self-help materials, and these organizations can be located in the telephone directory or by contacting the local heart, lung, or cancer societies.

Fielding JE: Smoking: Health effects and control. N Engl J Med 313:491, 555, 1985. *An overall review of smoking issues.*

Glynn TJ, Manley MW, Pechacek TF: Physician-initiated smoking cessation program: The National Cancer Institute Trials. *In* Engstrom P (ed.): Advances in Cancer Control. New York, Alan R. Liss, in press. *A review of the current state of our knowledge on effective office-based smoking interventions.*

Health and Public Policy Committee, American College of Physicians: Methods for stopping cigarette smoking. Ann Intern Med 105:281, 1986. *A review of smoking cessation methods.*

Janerick DT, Thompson D, Varela LR, et al.: Lung cancer and exposure to tobacco smoke in the household. N Engl J Med 323:632, 1990. *These studies suggest that 17 per cent of lung cancer among nonsmokers may be secondary to exposure to cigarette smoke during childhood and adolescence.*

U.S. Dept. of Health and Human Services: The Health Consequences of Smoking Cessation: A Report of the Surgeon General. Sept., 1990, in press. *A complete review of the benefits of cessation.*

U.S. Dept. of Health and Human Services: The Health Consequences of Smoking: Cardiovascular Disease. DHHS Publication No. (PHS) 84–50204, 1983. *A review of the evidence on smoking and cardiovascular disease.*

U.S. Dept. of Health and Human Services: The Health Consequences of Smoking: Chronic Obstructive Lung Disease. DHHS Publication No. (PHS) 84–50205, 1984. *A review of the evidence on smoking and lung disease.*

U.S. Dept. of Health and Human Services: The Health Consequences of Smoking: Involuntary Smoking. DHHS Publication (CDC) 87–8398, 1986. *A review of the evidence on involuntary smoking.*

U.S. Dept. of Health and Human Services: The Health Consequences of Using Smokeless Tobacco. DHHS Publication No. (PHS) 86–2874, 1986. *A review of the health effects of using snuff.*

11   Control of Unintended Injuries and Those Due to Violence

Stephen B. Hulley

Deaths from injury are the fourth most common cause of death in the United States; they number more than 150,000 each year and are the leading cause of death for young and middle-aged people in the age range 1 to 45. The problem is even larger if *nonfatal* injuries, some of which cause permanent disability, are considered: There are several hundred injury-related emergency room visits for every death from injury. One third of all injury deaths are due to motor vehicles, one third result from other forms of unintended injury (falls are the most common, followed by drowning, fires, and poisoning), and the remaining third are due to violence (homicide and suicide).

Each of these causes of death and disability has risk factors that identify high-risk groups and that are susceptible to physician-mediated efforts to prevent occurrence or recurrence. Yet until recently, injury control has been largely ignored by the medical and public health establishment; it is the sleeping giant of preventive medicine.

THE EPIDEMIOLOGY OF UNINTENDED INJURIES

Motor vehicle fatality rates decreased by one third in the 1970's after automobile safety regulations and the 55 mile per hour national speed limit were instituted, but most of the benefit has since been lost as average speeds have returned to higher levels and smaller cars (which have a twofold higher crash fatality rate) have become more prevalent. Deaths due to motor vehicles rise to alarmingly high levels among young adults, particularly males (Fig. 11–1). The impact of this is brought home by the current projection that 1.4 per cent of all 15-year-old boys in the United States will die of an injury before age 25. The most important modifiable risk factors are excessive alcohol intake, which plays a role in half of all fatal crashes, and the failure to observe speed limits and to use seatbelts.

Half of all deaths from unintended injury are unrelated to traffic. Falls are the most common cause (27 per cent), followed by drowning (15 per cent), fire (12 per cent), poisoning (6 per cent), adverse effects of medical care (5 per cent), unintended firearm use (4 per cent), aspiration of food (4 per cent), airplane crashes (3 per cent), machinery accidents (3 per cent), aspiration other than food (3 per cent), electric current (2 per cent), and other less common causes. These deaths tend to have a common pattern of risk factors, including male sex, old age, low income, and alcohol intake.

Implications for Medical Practice

Injury prevention has assumed an important role in the practice of medicine only in the field of pediatrics. Perhaps it has not received more attention in internal medicine because the term "accident" connotes an event that has occurred by chance and is therefore unavoidable. This is far from the case; there are many lifestyle risk factors for injuries that are suitable for intervention with various behavioral techniques. (For this reason, the term "unintended injury" is now preferred over "accident," and the term "motor vehicle crash" over "motor vehicle accident.") The potential for preventing premature death and disability is substantial, and injury prevention advice should become as important in the general practice of medicine as the more familiar interventions on risk factors for cardiovascular disease and cancer.

Advice on preventing *motor vehicle injuries* begins with widely known precepts such as observing the speed limit and using a diagonal-lap or other well-designed seatbelt. From the medical viewpoint, patients should be warned when drugs that impair performance are prescribed, especially those like diazepam that may interact with alcohol. But the most important concern is alcohol itself. The knowledge that a particular patient drinks heavily should prompt a clinician to point out the danger to that individual and to others. Intervention can include counseling on ways to alter alcohol habits and on the use of other drivers, alternative forms of transportation, or different locations for drinking. The alarming motor vehicle crash rate among teenagers can be approached by counseling parents on the rules that they can establish for when and how their teenage children may drive (e.g., curfews for use of the family car). Society plays an important role in these areas—for example, in setting the penalties for drunken driving and for the minimum age for licensing—and physicians can be an important force behind social legislation of this sort.

Injuries due to *falls* in the elderly can be prevented by designing an environment that makes falls less likely (e.g., by providing handrails and night lights and by removing loose rugs) and that reduces the extent of injury should a fall occur (e.g., through avoiding sharp corners and selecting a home without stairs). The clinician should undertake regular tests and appropriate correction of problems with vision and should identify and treat diseases that impair mobility and balance, advising against heavy alcohol use and not prescribing drugs that contribute to these problems. Hip fracture has received less attention than it deserves (there are more than 200,000 each year, involving one of every three women who reach extreme old age, and half of these die or are permanently disabled). White women are at the greatest risk and should receive treatment to retard osteoporosis (Ch. 238). This may include postmenopausal estrogens for some and should always include advice about calcium intake (1000 to 1500 mg per day in the diet or as calcium carbonate supplements), about not smoking (cigarettes are a risk factor for hip fracture), and about being physically active.

Many of the other causes of unintentional injury can be controlled by discussing the role of excess alcohol and other specific risk factors with patients. *Drowning*, for example, can be made less likely by fencing in swimming pools where there are small children and by instruction in water safety rules. Injury due to *fires* can be reduced by counseling on the dangers of smoking (cigarettes are the most common cause of fire-related deaths) and on the value of smoke detectors and fire extinguishers.

THE EPIDEMIOLOGY OF INJURY DUE TO VIOLENCE

The homicide rate in the United States has doubled in recent years and now exceeds 20,000 per year. One third of all homicides are between family members, and another third involve people

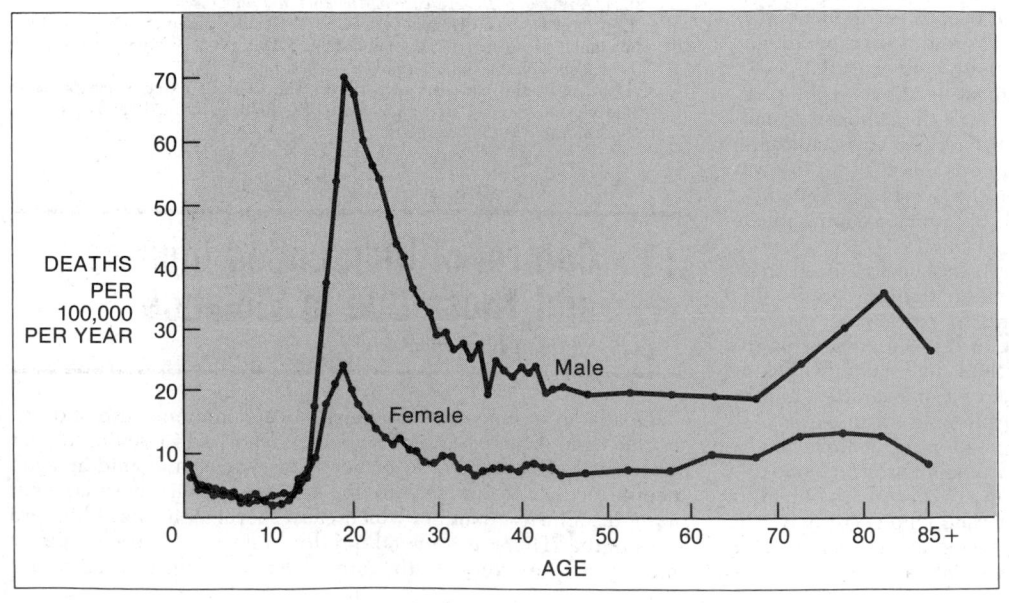

FIGURE 11–1. Age-specific death rates of motor vehicle occupants in the United States in 1976. The very high rates in 16- to 30-year-old males are a major component of the premature loss of life in this country. (From Haddon W, Baker SP: Injury control. *In* Clark D, MacMahon B [eds.]: Preventive and Community Medicine. Boston, Little, Brown & Co, 1981, pp 109–140.)

who know each other. In the United States, more than half of all homicides are carried out with handguns. Countries like England, Sweden, and Japan that have strict handgun ownership laws have handgun homicide rates that are 100-fold lower; these countries also have much lower overall rates of homicide. It is difficult to estimate the rates of nonfatal injury due to violence (assault, wife beating, rape, and child abuse), but each is undoubtedly far more common than homicide. Suicide rates have increased slightly in recent years, particularly in young men. Almost all forms of violent injury are more common in the male sex and in the socioeconomically disadvantaged, and all are commonly associated with excessive alcohol intake.

Implications for Medical Practice

The medical profession's role in dealing with the death and disability that result from violent behavior begins at an individual level. One focus is on preventing the occurrence (primary prevention) or recurrence (secondary prevention) of violent episodes, and the other is on providing medical, psychiatric, and social service care for the victims. Victims of assault and rape may present themselves for treatment of the injury, but those involved in violence within the family, such as wife beating, child abuse, or self-destructive behavior, often do not volunteer the information. The existence of a problem can sometimes be discovered by gentle probing about clues such as unexplained bruises or depressed affect. Interventions to prevent future episodes include psychiatric and social service referral, notification of police and public health authorities (when appropriate), and counseling by the clinician. The management of such problems is a major challenge to a physician's wisdom, courage, and skill.

The medical profession's most effective avenue for preventing violence may be in guiding the evolution of society and its rules. Doctors are important opinion leaders, and their comments on the medical and epidemiologic facts can help mold public opinion and legislation directed at such things as handgun control and violence in the media.

Approaches of this sort are probably the only way that the medical profession can have an effect on the most serious injury control issue of our age: the prevention of nuclear war. In addition to their general civic responsibility to express their views on this problem, some physicians regard it as a professional responsibility to educate community leaders and acquaintances on medical realities such as the false security of civil defense plans that would be inoperable in the event of a nuclear attack.

SUMMARY

Injuries are the most important cause of premature death and disability in western countries. One third of all deaths from injury are due to motor vehicle crashes, one third to other unintended causes (especially falls), and one third to intentional violence. Interventions designed to prevent each of these sources of injury are a useful and neglected focus for preventive medicine.

Physicians can play a major role in counseling individual patients about lifestyle factors that prevent motor vehicle crash injuries (e.g., avoiding alcohol in excess, using seatbelts, and setting curfews for teenage drivers) and about those that prevent other forms of unintended injuries (e.g., avoiding alcohol in excess and various medical and environmental strategies to prevent osteoporosis, falls, drowning, and fire in the home). Physicians need to take a greater role in the primary and secondary prevention of injury due to violence. In addition, medical professionals can contribute to the emergence of societal measures dealing with hazards to health that range from drunken driving to nuclear war.

Baker SP, O'Neill B, Karpf RS: The Injury Fact Book. Lexington, Mass., D. C. Heath & Company, 1984. *A fascinating and readable book that comprehensively describes the epidemiology of injury: who is especially at risk and what are the potentially modifiable risk factors.*
Cassel C, McCally M, Abraham H: Nuclear Weapons and Nuclear War: A Source Book for Health Professionals. New York, Praeger Publishers, 1984. *Reports on the medical, biologic, psychologic, and ethical implications by many of the major medical writers on this topic.*
Lowenstein SR, Hunt D: Injury prevention in primary care. Ann Intern Med 113:261, 1990. *Recent review of the issues and literature.*
National Committee for Injury Prevention and Control: Injury prevention: Meeting the challenges. Am J Preventive Med 5 (Suppl 3), 1989. *Recent and well-balanced review of this developing field.*

Riggs BL, Melton LJ: Involutional osteoporosis. N Engl J Med 314:1676, 1986. *Good review of strategies for preventing osteoporosis.*
Tinetti ME, Speechley M: Prevention of falls among the elderly. N Engl J Med 320:1055, 1989. *Review of causes of falls and practical approaches to prevention.*

12 The Judicious Diet

John P. Kane

The composition of an individual's diet and its relationship to his or her energy needs and to special requirements for growth, repair, or response to stress are among the important variables in the maintenance of health or the advent of disease. In Part XV of this book, there is an extensive discussion of nutritional requirements for calories, amino acids, essential fatty acids, minerals, and vitamins. Obviously, a judicious diet is one that meets these requirements for the individual. An excess of calories leads to obesity, one of the most prevalent nutritional disorders found in the developed countries of the world. This is discussed in detail in Ch. 203. Undernutrition can also produce serious impairment of health (Ch. 201). Deficits or excesses of other nutrients lead to a wide variety of specific disorders. In this chapter, however, we shall be concerned with variables within what would ordinarily be considered an adequate diet but that may influence the susceptibility of the individual to four major classes of disease: atherosclerosis, hypertension, cancer, and urolithiasis.

In few areas relevant to health is there so much misinformation and faddism as surrounds the subject of diet. Billions of dollars are spent in this major national industry to promote an astonishing variety of nostrums and dietary aberrations alleged to promote holistic health, vitality, and attractiveness or to reverse the process of disease. By and large, these programs are ingenious but harmless instruments to defraud the credulous. In some cases, however, they either produce harmful dietary imbalances or delay the patient's seeking effective medical care. Physicians need to be informed about the dimensions of this cultism in order to be able to advise their patients and to participate effectively in the development of controlling public policy.

DIET AND ARTERIOSCLEROSIS

In current models of atherogenesis, cholesterol and its esters enter the artery wall via plasma lipoproteins. These lipoproteins include low density lipoproteins (LDL), intermediate density lipoproteins (IDL), and, perhaps to a lesser extent, very low density lipoproteins (VLDL). More extensive descriptions of these lipoproteins and of their metabolism are given in Ch. 172. Elevated levels of LDL and IDL are strongly associated epidemiologically with accelerated atherogenesis. For instance, the risk of coronary heart disease in the United States, where the average level of serum cholesterol in an adult male is approximately 215 mg per deciliter, is several-fold higher than that in rural Japan, where the average is about 160 mg per deciliter. An inverse relationship between plasma levels of high density lipoprotein (HDL) cholesterol and risk of coronary heart disease has been noted in a number of epidemiologic surveys. This may reflect the efficiency of mechanisms involved in the centripetal (retrieval) pathways of cholesterol transport.

The risk of coronary heart disease correlates with levels of cholesterol as low as 180 mg per deciliter in plasma. The majority of individuals in industrialized Western nations would therefore be expected to benefit from reduction of levels of serum cholesterol, primarily reflecting changes in the content of LDL in plasma. The results of several intervention studies lend support to this contention. Increasing the levels of HDL in plasma in order to increase the mobilization and retrieval of cholesterol might be equally attractive, but no studies have been reported of the effect of such an intervention on heart disease independent of changes in other lipoproteins. The rationale for prevention of atherosclerosis and guidelines for management of hyperlipidemia with diet and drugs have been set forth by a panel of experts in the National Cholesterol Education Program. This program recommends that all patients with LDL cholesterol levels over 159 mg per deciliter be treated and that those with levels between 130 and 159 mg per deciliter be treated if coronary disease or at least two of a group of defined risk factors are present.

A single pattern of dietary modification is appropriate for individuals with nearly all types of primary hyperlipidemia (excepting only primary chylomicronemia), as well as for those individuals in the population at large who have less striking elevations of levels of atherogenic lipoproteins. The elements of this "universal" diet are considered individually.

1. *Reduce body weight to the ideal.* This primarily induces a marked reduction in elevated VLDL levels. It also effects a modest reduction in LDL cholesterol levels and may increase HDL cholesterol levels slightly. Maintenance of ideal body weight is the most effective means of forestalling the appearance of type II diabetes, itself a risk factor for atherosclerosis.

2. *Decrease the intake of saturated fat.* This change effects a potent and uniform lowering of LDL cholesterol. The typical American diet contains approximately 40 per cent or more of calories as fat (15 per cent saturated fat). Levels of 30 per cent of calories as fat (less than 10 per cent saturated fat) can be achieved easily, and an intake of less than 7 per cent saturated fat is attainable with major changes in food selection. To achieve the 30 per cent level of dietary fat, fat-rich meats, dairy products, and items such as certain baked goods must be restricted. To achieve the 20 per cent level, major substitution of vegetable protein sources for meats must be made.

When the intake of saturated fats is decreased, there are several possible sources of replacement calories: polyunsaturated fats, monounsaturated fats, and carbohydrates. Major substitution with polyunsaturated fat may result in lower levels of HDL cholesterol and of the principal HDL protein, apolipoprotein A-I. Furthermore, polyunsaturated fatty acids are susceptible to hydroperoxidation, which could lead to generation of free radical chains and perhaps to carcinogenesis. Monounsaturated fats, abundant in certain vegetable oils such as olive oil, do not increase LDL levels and do not hydroperoxidize readily. HDL cholesterol levels are somewhat higher with use of monounsaturates than with diets that are low in total fat. Trans fatty acids formed during catalytic hydrogenation or prolonged heating exert effects similar to those of saturated fats. Major substitution of carbohydrate for fat is associated with modest elevations of plasma triglyceride levels in the short term, but these levels return to normal after a period of several months. Strict vegetarians tend to have lower levels of both LDL and HDL than individuals on a typical American diet, but the changes in LDL levels are of much greater magnitude. Furthermore, potentially important differences in composition of HDL are seen, with an increased ratio of phospholipid to cholesterol. Vegetarian diets appear to be compatible with good health, provided that the foods selected supply all essential amino acids and adequate amounts of vitamin B$_{12}$.

Omega-3 fatty acids contained in marine fish oils, appear to have a unique ability to reduce elevated levels of VLDL and chylomicrons in plasma at doses of 15 to 20 grams per day. Plasma levels of LDL may be decreased modestly in some individuals with normal or moderately elevated levels of plasma cholesterol and even increased in some, accompanied by some decrease in HDL cholesterol levels. The marked decreases in plasma triglycerides that occur are due at least in part to inhibition of VLDL secretion. Omega-3 fatty acids moderately reduce formation of thromboxane B$_2$ in platelets, inhibiting aggregation and adhesion, an effect that may account in part for the low incidence of arteriosclerotic heart disease in populations for whom cold-water marine fish are a major food source.

Overall, a major reduction of saturated fat should be made from levels found in Western diets, and complex carbohydrate should be used to provide the requisite caloric replacement. Small amounts of polyunsaturated fats from plant sources should be used to provide essential fatty acids. The use of fish oils might be considered if hypertriglyceridemia is present.

3. *Decrease the intake of cholesterol.* Reduction of dietary saturated fats automatically eliminates much cholesterol; however, rich sources such as organ meats and egg yolks should be restricted specifically. The effect of restriction of cholesterol on LDL levels varies widely among individuals. This variation appears to reflect two factors: (a) There is an approximately fourfold difference among individuals in the fraction of dietary cholesterol that is absorbed. (b) There are differences in the degree to which dietary cholesterol is capable of suppressing endogenous cholesterogenesis. It is reasonable to presume, however, that reduction of dietary cholesterol is likely to be of benefit. The typical American diet provides 400 mg or more of cholesterol per day, but an intake of 250 to 300 mg per day is relatively easily achieved, and intakes of 100 mg per day can be achieved with more rigorous mixed diets. Strict vegetarian diets contain no cholesterol.

4. *Restrict alcohol.* Alcohol should be limited in all cases to maintain ideal body weight. VLDL secretion is increased dramatically by even limited use of alcohol. Therefore, alcohol should always be restricted in the diet of individuals with elevated serum triglycerides. Increased alcohol intake may be associated with elevated levels of HDL cholesterol, but it is not yet clear whether this change represents subspecies of HDL that participate in centripetal cholesterol transport. No categorical presumption of beneficial effects of alcohol on HDL can yet be made.

5. *Other factors.* Increased dietary fiber appears to have a marginal effect on serum lipoprotein levels, although certain sources of fiber, such as oat or wheat bran, appear to reduce LDL levels slightly. In addition, saponins in foodstuffs such as oats may decrease absorption of cholesterol. The ingestion of lecithin, which is widely suggested by health food advocates, lacks significant effect, as do a number of vitamins and minerals that have been similarly recommended.

Individuals adhering to this regimen may show reductions of plasma cholesterol levels of 10 or even 15 per cent on the basis of reduction of saturated fats. An additional reduction of 1 to 10 per cent may be achieved by restriction of cholesterol. At least a twofold reduction in risk of coronary disease would be expected in the American population if such modifications of lipid levels were uniformly achieved.

DIET AND HYPERTENSION

Essential hypertension has been assumed to result from a constitutional inability to excrete sodium chloride efficiently, because of which calcium ions accumulate in arteriolar smooth muscle cells, increasing tonicity. Indeed, evidence from cross-transplantation studies in animals and from human renal transplants lends credence to the existence of such a mechanism. Cross-cultural studies also have shown, in the aggregate, convincing positive correlation between blood pressure and intake of salt. Patient populations with essential hypertension are heterogeneous with respect to renin levels, plasma calcium concentrations, response to individual antihypertensive drugs, and sensitivity to dietary salt. Normotensive individuals and perhaps half of American patients with hypertension do not show a pressor response to increased dietary salt. Thus, justification for the prescription of reduced salt intake appears to be limited to individuals with salt-sensitive hypertension and members of their kindreds. Most Americans consume 10 to 20 grams of salt per day; an intake of 4 grams is a more reasonable goal for individuals in such kindreds. Increasing calcium intake has been reported to reduce blood pressure. If true, this effect will probably be restricted to a subset of patients. Furthermore, indiscriminate increase in calcium intake could increase urinary calcium excretion in individuals with absorptive hypercalciuria (Ch. 88). Thus, increasing calcium intake to prevent or treat hypertension cannot be recommended as a general measure at this time.

DIET AND CANCER

The consumption of certain major food components is epidemiologically correlated with an increased incidence of some types of cancer. Although the mechanisms of these associations are still largely unknown, a judicious diet at this time involves changes that would be expected to minimize these risks. A number of components that occur in foods naturally or are formed or added during processing are mutagens in bacterial test systems (Ames test) or carcinogens or promoters of carcinogenesis in whole animals. Prudence would dictate elimination of these from human consumption to whatever extent is practicable, because definitive studies demonstrating specific risks of these agents in humans may emerge only slowly.

DIETARY FAT. In multinational studies, the prevalence of cancer of the breast, colon, and prostate correlates with dietary fat intake. Within cultures, however, breast cancer correlates poorly, whereas colon cancer continues to show a positive correlation with fat intake in many, but not all, studies. Also, the incidence of breast cancer changes slowly when women immigrate to countries with a high incidence and high-fat diets, whereas that of colon cancer accommodates within a few years. Enhancement of chemical carcinogenesis by dietary fat occurs in several animal models. Total fat intake correlates best with carcinogenesis at high levels, but polyunsaturated fats appear to be most important at lower levels of intake. Polyunsaturated fats are substrates for hydroperoxidative reactions initiating free radical chains, and therefore they probably should not constitute a major component of the diet. Reduction of total fat intake, with an increased content of complex carbohydrates, is completely compatible with the "prudent" diet for prevention of arteriosclerotic heart disease.

FIBER. Carcinogens formed in the bowel may play a role in the development of carcinoma of the colon. Increased fiber in the diet would decrease the duration of contact of carcinogens with the mucosa and therefore might reduce the risk of cancer. Only minimal epidemiologic support for this view exists. With the possible exception of pentosans from wheat, fiber has not been proven effective in animal models. In many studies, a reduced risk of cancer is more closely correlated with the intake of fruits and vegetables than with fiber per se.

ALCOHOL. Alcohol consumption has long been known to correlate with risk of carcinoma of the mouth, pharynx, and esophagus. Several studies have also shown a strong correlation with risk of breast cancer. Alcohol also appears to be teratogenic in humans and causes congenital malformations, mental dysfunction, and growth retardation in infants born to alcohol-abusing mothers. Alcohol metabolism produces acetaldehyde, which is both mutagenic and carcinogenic, in addition to other mutagenic and carcinogenic compounds.

POSSIBLE RISKS ASSOCIATED WITH LOW LEVELS OF CHOLESTEROL IN PLASMA. An increased risk of cancer has been associated epidemiologically with very low levels of serum cholesterol. When present such an association is always weak and tends to occur only in the lowest range of cholesterol levels. Further, in nearly 20 prospective population studies, half have shown no such correlation, especially in those in which sufficient time elapsed between measurement of serum lipids and detection of cancer to minimize the number of pre-existing cancer cases. Because many cancers reduce levels of LDL, the association may be completely an epiphenomenon. Furthermore, the risk of colon and rectal cancer is positively correlated with serum cholesterol levels. In view of the strong correlation of higher levels of cholesterol in plasma with risk of coronary disease, dietary modifications directed at lowering the risk of coronary disease should not be abandoned on the premise that a significant increase in the risk of cancer would ensue. Two studies have yielded a weak association between extremely low levels of serum cholesterol (less than 130 mg per deciliter) and cerebral hemorrhage, especially when hypertension is present. This suggests that reduction of total cholesterol levels below 150 to 160 mg per deciliter may be contraindicated.

FOOD PREPARATION AND PRESERVATION. Exposure of meats to high temperatures, as in charcoal broiling, may be important in oncogenesis because compounds with very high carcinogenic potential are formed. In addition to benzo(a)pyrene, several mutagenic pyrolysates are formed from amino acids. Components of wood smoke in smoked foods have been linked epidemiologically and from animal studies to carcinoma of the gastrointestinal tract. Nitrites, used as preservatives in meats, react with a number of natural amines and even certain medications to form nitrosamines, which are mutagenic. This reaction is favored by low pH; hence it proceeds readily in the stomach. Clinical observations tend to link nitrites with carcinogenesis of the stomach and esophagus. Vitamin C inhibits the formation of nitrosamines in vitro. Increased intake of this vitamin by the public may account in part for decreases in the incidence of

gastric carcinoma observed in recent years. At this time, restriction of nitrites and nitrosamines in the diet would appear reasonable. This is complicated by the presence of large amounts of nitrates, which can be reduced to nitrites, in certain vegetables that have been overfertilized by growers. The average American ingests about 75 mg of nitrate, 0.8 mg of nitrite, and 1 μg of preformed nitrosamines daily.

NATURALLY OCCURRING CARCINOGENS AND MUTAGENS. Several species of *Aspergillus* molds produce aflatoxins, which are among the most potent natural carcinogens. These agents are carcinogenic in a number of animals, chiefly causing carcinoma of the liver. Induction of tumors of colon, lung, and kidney has also been observed. Aflatoxins have been linked strongly to human hepatocellular carcinoma in Africa and Asia, acting in concert with the hepatitis B virus. Aflatoxins have been found chiefly in peanuts, apple products, and grains stored under moist conditions. Efforts to reduce the intake of these agents center on proper storage of foods. Emerging awareness of other naturally occurring mutagens and carcinogens may be expected to lead to an evaluation of their importance in human carcinogenesis. Among these agents are allyl isothiocyanate found in many plant sources; hydrazine derivatives found in many mushrooms; safrol of sassafras; the methyl xanthines of coffee, tea, and cocoa; and phorbol esters and pyrrolizidine alkaloids found in herbal teas.

NATURAL INHIBITORS OF CARCINOGENESIS. Some naturally occurring compounds appear to inhibit carcinogenesis by certain agents. Tocopherols, which interrupt free radical chains, are capable of reducing the carcinogenicity of doxorubicin (Adriamycin) and daunomycin and are protective against oxygen radical damage to tissues. Certain indoles found in cruciferous vegetables (broccoli, cabbage, cauliflower, and the like) inhibit the carcinogenicity of benzo(a)pyrene, and substituted isothiocyanates found in these plants inhibit the carcinogenesis induced by polycyclic aromatic hydrocarbons. Higher intakes of beta-carotene and perhaps other carotenoids have been correlated with reduced risk of cancer of the lung in several studies. Weaker correlations with other tumor types have also been observed. Selenium, a cofactor in the reduction of hydroperoxides, also may confer resistance to free radical-mediated carcinogenesis.

DIET AND UROLITHIASIS

Certain measures that should reduce the risk of urolithiasis are applicable to the general population (also see Ch. 88). Sufficient intake of water to ensure a daily urine volume of 2 to 3 liters is a most important preventive measure and is useful in all forms of urolithiasis. Restriction of dietary purine intake is also desirable because uricosuria can enhance the crystallization of calcium oxalate as well as uric acid. Restriction of the intake of animal proteins reduces the "acid ash" residue of urine, diminishing the urinary excretion of calcium, a stratagem that may also be of value in prevention of osteoporosis.

Moderate restriction of oxalate intake is reasonable in view of the prevalence of oxalate stones. More stringently reduced intake should be advised for individuals who have had one or more oxalate stones, if urinary oxalate is elevated. The oxalate content is particularly high in rhubarb, spinach, chard, beets, citrus pulp, pecans, peanuts, sweet potatoes, and a number of berries and fruits. Citrate appears to inhibit the crystallization of calcium with oxalate. Some patients with calcium oxalate urolithiasis have low levels of citrate in urine. Regular intake of citrate-rich, pulp-free fruit juices appears to be a reasonable intervention. In general, restriction of dietary calcium should be limited to patients with hypercalciuria.

SUMMARY

The following recommendations for dietary modifications can be made for the general population. Caloric intake should be adjusted to achieve and maintain ideal body weight. Fat intake should be reduced to 30 per cent of total calories (7 to 10 per cent as saturated fat) or less, and cholesterol intake to 150 mg, or less, per day. Even moderate use of alcohol should be avoided in individuals with hypertriglyceridemia. Complex carbohydrates should be used to make up the caloric deficits resulting from these changes. Individuals with a predisposition to hypertension should limit salt intake to 4 grams per day. Prudence also suggests reasonable limitation of charcoal-broiled and smoked foods and foods rich in nitrites or nitrates.

Ames BN: Dietary carcinogens and anticarcinogens: Oxygen radicals and degenerative diseases. Science 221:1256, 1983. *A comprehensive review of mutagens and carcinogens in the diet.*

Ames BN: Food constituents as a source of mutagens, carcinogens, and anticarcinogens. *In* Knudsen I (ed.): Genetic Toxicology of the Diet. New York, Alan R. Liss, Inc, 1986, pp 3–32. *A discussion of mechanisms by which food constituents can promote or retard the formation of tumors.*

Committee on Diet, Nutrition, and Cancer. Assembly of Life Sciences, National Research Council: Diet, Nutrition and Cancer. National Academic Press, 1982. *A comprehensive evaluation of the roles of dietary components and additives in carcinogenesis.*

The Expert Panel: Report of the National Cholesterol Education Program Expert Panel on detection, evaluation, and treatment of high blood cholesterol in adults. Arch Intern Med 148:36, 1988. *Guidelines for the detection of hyperlipidemia and its treatment with diet and drugs, proposed by a consensus panel appointed by the National Heart, Lung, and Blood Institute.*

Menkes MS, Comstock GW, Vuilleumier JP, et al.: Serum beta-carotene, vitamins A and E, selenium, and the risk of lung cancer. N Engl J Med 315:1250, 1986. *Epidemiologic evidence relating beta-carotene and vitamin E to a reduced risk of lung cancer.*

Mensink RP, Katan MB: Effect of dietary trans fatty acids on high-density and low-density lipoprotein cholesterol levels in healthy subjects. N Engl J Med 323:439, 1990. *New evidence on the impact of trans fatty acids on plasma lipoproteins.*

Nordy A, Goodnight SH: Dietary lipids and thrombosis. Relationships to atherosclerosis. Arteriosclerosis 10:149, 1990. *A review of the role of diet and thrombogenesis.*

Trock B, Lanza E, Greenwald P: Dietary fiber, vegetables and colon cancer: Critical review and meta analysis of the epidemiologic evidence. J Natl Cancer Inst 82:650, 1990. *A review of dietary factors related to colon cancer.*

Willett WC, Stampfer MJ, Colditz GA, et al.: Moderate alcohol consumption and the risk of breast cancer. N Engl J Med 316:1174, 1987. *Observations on the association of alcohol with breast cancer.*

Willett W: The search for the causes of breast and colon cancer. Nature 338:389, 1989. *A comprehensive review of the relationships of a number of dietary factors to the risk of developing breast or colon cancer.*

13 Exercise and Health

William L. Haskell

The biologic and psychologic benefits ascribed to exercise are extremely diverse and vary substantially with regard to scientific documentation. Some of these benefits have been definitively established and are achievable by anyone who exercises appropriately. Other benefits, frequently promoted by exercise advocates, usually do not occur, and at times inappropriate advice has been given that has placed patients at undue risk for exercise-caused morbidity or mortality. As with many other areas of health promotion, enthusiasm to help others by encouraging them to exercise can easily outstrip the scientific basis for such actions. While the idea that exercise promotes health is not new, many of the details regarding specific health benefits and exercise requirements are still much debated and under investigation.

EXERCISE AND PHYSICAL WORKING CAPACITY

The most effective method of achieving an increase in physical working capacity or "physical fitness" is through a systematic increase in habitual exercise (exercise training). This increase in capacity is an adaptative response by the body to the stress placed on various tissues and biologic functions by the increased metabolic or physical demands of the exercise. If the appropriate type of exercise is performed at the proper intensity, duration, and frequency, sedentary individuals of all ages will achieve significant improvements in physical working capacity. After training, they will be able to exercise at a greater intensity and for a longer duration than before. Also, at the same submaximal exercise intensity they will experience less fatigue. This increase in functional capacity is due to enhanced metabolic capacity and efficiency of skeletal muscle, increased capacity for substrate and oxygen delivery to the muscle, and changes in autonomic nervous system regulation during exercise.

Increases in physical working capacity often are equated inappropriately with improvements in health status or disease prevention. This is an important and often difficult distinction to make: that while a very high level of physical fitness usually requires good health, an improvement in fitness does not ensure an increase in resistance to disease or a reduction in clinical manifestations. For example, patients with disorders such as emphysema, diabetes, or hypertension can significantly increase their working capacity through exercise without necessarily changing the severity of their disease or their medical prognosis. Becoming more physically fit and improving health status are interrelated but not synonymous.

HEALTH BENEFITS OF EXERCISE

Most of the health-related benefits of exercise appear to result from the increase in metabolism required to provide the energy needed for skeletal muscle contraction. This increase in demand for energy triggers a number of adaptations designed to enhance the efficiency and capacity of the skeletal muscle to perform work and minimize fatigue. Adaptations also occur in those systems that support the increased energy requirements of skeletal muscle, including the nervous, endocrine, cardiovascular, respiratory, and skeletal systems.

CORONARY HEART DISEASE. The area of greatest scientific inquiry regarding the health benefits of exercise has been its potential role in the prevention of coronary heart disease (CHD). In classic studies of a generation ago the conductors on double-decker buses in London were shown to develop fewer manifestations of CHD than did the less active bus drivers. Most subsequent studies have confirmed that men and women who select more active jobs or leisure-time pursuits tend to experience fewer fatal and nonfatal CHD events. These studies do not rigorously demonstrate a cause and effect relationship, but the direction of the association is positive and quite consistent, the magnitude of the differences in CHD events is clinically meaningful, and the amount of exercise performed during leisure time associated with lower CHD risk is well within the capacity of most healthy adults. As of yet no randomized trial of adequate design has been performed to determine if an increase in exercise by sedentary adults free of clinically evident CHD on entry into the study would significantly reduce future CHD events.

Patients with ischemic heart disease enrolled in exercise-based cardiac rehabilitation programs experience a significantly lower cardiovascular and all-cause mortality rate than do nonparticipants one to three years following hospitalization. Although other risk factors were also altered in some studies, exercise training appears to have been the essential ingredient. Exercise training also improves clinical status (less angina, shortness of breath, fatigue) and functional capacity. In general, appropriate exercise enhances both the clinical and psychological status of these patients and should be included in a comprehensive treatment program.

There are several mechanisms by which exercise can reduce CHD risk. Exercise may maintain or increase oxygen supply to the myocardium by decreasing the progression of atherosclerosis, increasing coronary collateralization, or enlarging the diameter of proximal coronary arteries, but these changes have not been clearly documented to occur in humans. Potentially beneficial changes in blood clotting–fibrinolysis activity and in plasma lipoprotein profiles often follow training and may improve the coronary blood flow in some individuals.

Endurance exercise training decreases myocardial oxygen demand, primarily by a decrease in heart rate at rest, and decreases in heart rate and systolic blood pressure during submaximal exercise. These changes are most likely produced by a modification in central nervous system regulation of cardiovascular function (decreased sympathetic and increased parasympathetic drive) and an increase in blood volume, with little, if any, change occurring in intrinsic myocardial function.

CARBOHYDRATE METABOLISM. A frequently unrecognized health benefit of exercise is its effect on carbohydrate metabolism. During large-muscle, dynamic exercise of moderate intensity, the glycogen stored in skeletal muscle is used for the production of energy and becomes partially depleted. For the next 24 to 72 hours this glycogen is replaced by the uptake of glucose from the blood. In addition to this acute effect of increased glucose removal, the insulin receptors in skeletal muscle and adipose tissue increase in sensitivity and thus remove glucose more effectively at any given concentration of plasma insulin. This "insulin-sparing" effect of endurance exercise training decreases insulin production and may reduce the risk of insulin deficiency developing with increasing age.

OSTEOPOROSIS. The bone mineral loss that occurs with aging is accelerated by inactivity, especially bed rest (Ch. 238). Exercise will blunt but not prevent all of this loss. For example, in a survey of postmenopausal women, level of habitual activity was one of the major determinants of bone mass as measured by computed tomography. In the more active women, arm and leg bone mass was greater after accounting for the effects of age, body weight, and calcium intake. Also, when a cohort of elderly women exercised three times per week for 30 minutes each session, an increase in bone mineral content was observed (2.3 per cent), while 12 women who remained sedentary during this time showed a decrease of 3.3 per cent ($p < 0.005$). These experiences support the use of moderate intensity exercise requiring the movement of body weight against gravity as part of a comprehensive program of osteoporosis prevention. One note of caution is that young women who become amenorrheic in conjunction with vigorous exercise training experience loss of bone mass that may last for several years after return of normal menstrual function.

WEIGHT CONTROL. More physically active individuals tend to weigh less than their sedentary counterparts and at any given body weight have a greater muscle mass. Even though calorie consumption frequently goes up when sedentary people exercise substantially more, they usually lose adipose tissue. Not only are more calories expended during exercise, but the *resting metabolic rate* may be increased for an extended period after exercise. *Basal metabolic rate* at any given body weight may also increase. People who include exercise as part of their weight loss program are more successful in maintaining optimal weight. For these reasons, exercise, along with proper nutrition, can improve health status by contributing to the maintenance of optimal body composition.

PSYCHOLOGICAL STATUS. Many physically active people state that the major health benefit that keeps them exercising is their improved psychological status. They report less anxiety and depression, more self-confidence, and an increased ability to cope with at-home and job-related stress. How frequently such benefits occur when sedentary people take up exercise is not known, nor is there any understanding of how to design an exercise program to maximize the positive psychological effects. Whether or not this perceived improvement in psychological status has a biologic basis has not been established. Proposed explanations for a biologic basis are the decrease in circulating catecholamines produced by exercise training and the acute increase in beta-endorphins that occurs during and following vigorous exercise. Regardless of the mechanism, consideration should be given to getting sedentary people up and away from chronic stress-producing environments and having them participate in an exercise of their choice.

OTHER DISORDERS. There are a number of other situations in which selected patients with an established disease tend to show some clinical improvement if they exercise properly, but there is no good evidence that exercise prevents these disorders. Diseases included in this category are chronic obstructive lung disease (emphysema and bronchitis), mild or labile hypertension, osteoarthritis, and intermittent claudication. Exercise has not been shown to prevent any infectious disease.

A Comment on Safety

When recommending exercise for health promotion, one does battle with the proverbial two-edged sword. Inappropriate exercise literally can pose dangers to life and limb. Most commonly musculoskeletal discomfort or injury is caused by trauma or overuse. Much less frequently, a major cardiac event is precipitated, usually ventricular fibrillation, but the likelihood that exercise will cause a cardiac arrest in individuals without underlying cardiac disease is remote.

Other health risks of exercise are usually limited to individuals with established disease (e.g., diabetes, asthma, or renal failure) or occur with very extended or competitive exercise. The most important of these risks is the development of severe heat injury (Ch. 532). These injuries cannot be totally prevented if adults increase their exercise, but the risks can be reduced by proper medical evaluation, individualized exercise recommendations, and improved public education.

MEDICAL EVALUATION

Guidelines vary regarding the type of medical evaluation recommended prior to initiating a health-oriented exercise program. Advice depends on the specific exercise to be undertaken, as well as on the person's age and clinical status. For sedentary people who plan to undertake a low-level program such as brisk walking, no special medical examination is recommended unless they currently are under treatment for cardiopulmonary, metabolic, or musculoskeletal disorders. Such patients should be evaluated by a physician prior to an increase in exercise. For persons under age 40 who are free of clinically evident cardiopulmonary, metabolic, or musculoskeletal disorders, no special medical evaluation is considered necessary if they also are free of major cardiopulmonary disease risk factors (hypertension, hypercholesterolemia, or cigarette smoking). All persons under age 40 with disease or increased cardiopulmonary risk or over age 40 should have a medical examination prior to beginning vigorous exercise. An electrocardiographic and blood pressure–monitored exercise tolerance test should be included in the medical evaluation of all patients with cardiopulmonary disorders. Such tests should be symptom limited and monitored by a physician. Similar tests are recommended but not required for clinically healthy persons.

IMPLICATIONS FOR MEDICAL PRACTICE

The *type* of exercise that provides the greatest health benefits and permits the greatest increase in energy expenditure with the least fatigue consists of performing rhythmic contractions of large muscles to move the body over a distance or against gravity. Such exercise frequently is referred to as being endurance or "aerobic," since, if it is performed at an intensity that is moderate relative to the person's capacity, most of the resynthesis of high-

TABLE 13–1. THE EXERCISE PRESCRIPTION

Type of Exercise
Primarily aerobic
Stretching for flexibility
Resistance exercise for muscle tone

Intensity
Moderate relative to capacity (50%–75%)
Target heart rate = 60%–85% MHR
Maximum heart rate (MHR) = 220 − age

Duration
25–45 minutes per session
Target of 300 kilocalories per session

Frequency
Daily if intensity <65% MHR and duration <30 minutes
Every other day if intensity >65% and duration >30 minutes

Session
Warm-up, 3 to 5 minutes
Conditioning, 15 to 40 minutes
Cool-down, 2 to 5 minutes

Progression
Use exercise log
Keep pulse in target range
Evaluate every 2–4 weeks or each visit

Warning Signs
Severe musculoskeletal pain
Claudication
Chest pressure/pain, discomfort
Unusual shortness of breath
Dizziness, nausea, vomiting

energy compounds in the muscle is performed in the presence of oxygen. Examples of this type of exercise are walking, hiking, jogging or running, cycling, cross-country skiing, swimming, active games and sports, selected calisthenics, and vigorous at-home or on-the-job chores. While very specific activities may be required when training for athletic competition, for health purposes any exercise of this type seems to be of benefit if performed frequently enough at the proper intensity (Table 13–1).

The exercise-induced changes that contribute to health are achieved when the exercise *intensity* is somewhat greater than that usually performed by the individual. This increased intensity or overload causes adaptations that allow the metabolic needs of the muscles during exercise to be more readily met. While exercise intensities even slightly greater than usual will produce changes, the usual recommendation is that exercise for optimizing health should be performed at 50 to 75 per cent of the individual's oxygen transport (aerobic) capacity or at 60 to 85 per cent of maximal achievable heart rate during exercise. Using these guidelines, exercise training heart rates for individuals 30 years of age would range from 114 to 162 beats per minute, whereas at age 60 the range would be from 86 to 137 beats per minute. For most people this recommendation produces a substantial intensity overload, since they usually do not exercise at more than about 40 per cent of their aerobic capacity during everyday activities.

The exercise *duration* to be recommended depends on the person's health or fitness goals and exercise capacity as well as on the type of exercise being performed. People who do even a little bit of exercise on a regular basis are better off than those who do almost nothing. A reasonable goal for a sedentary person is an energy expenditure over usual activities of approximately 300 kilocalories per session with a *frequency* of at least every other day. Most clinically healthy adults have the capacity to expend from 400 to 700 kilocalories per hour while performing activity of moderate intensity; thus they can expend 300 kilocalories in 25 to 45 minutes. Activities meeting this goal include walking or jogging 4 kilometers, cycling or swimming for 30 minutes, or playing several sets of singles tennis lasting for 45 minutes. Lower intensity exercise such as walking or gardening will not produce a large increase in exercise capacity, but if performed for longer periods or more frequently, it seems to provide many of the health benefits derived from more vigorous exercise.

SUMMARY

Inactivity does not appear to be the sole cause of any major disease, but a physically active lifestyle improves general health status and retards many of the functional impairments that frequently occur with aging. Success in initiating and maintaining an exercise program is most likely to occur when it is individually designed and takes into account the person's goals, interests, skills, and exercise opportunities, as well as exercise capacity. Patients should be advised to set aside a time for exercise and to fill it with a variety of activities, rather than selecting a single activity as the sole basis for increasing exercise for health purposes. The exercise plan should be convenient to perform, fit within the general lifestyle of the individual, and be considered fun or at least enjoyable. Success at exercise is increased when the individual has acquired the *knowledge* of what is to be done and why, the *confidence* that success can be achieved, and the *patience* to wait for the benefits to accrue.

American College of Sports Medicine: Guidelines for Graded Exercise Testing and Exercise Prescription. 4th ed. Philadelphia, Lea & Febiger, 1990. *Comprehensive guidelines for the exercise testing and training of healthy persons and patients.*
Horton ES: Role and management of exercise in diabetes mellitus. Diabetes Care 11:201, 1988. *A comprehensive review of the biochemical effects of exercise on carbohydrate metabolism and the implication of these data for the use of exercise in the prevention and treatment of diabetes mellitus.*
Oldridge NB, Guyatt GH, Fischer ME, et al.: Cardiac rehabilitation after myocardial infarction: Combined experience of randomized clinical trials. JAMA 260:945, 1988. *Review of major studies of exercise rehabilitation following myocardial infarction demonstrating an overall reduction in cardiovascular and all-cause mortality in program participants.*
Powell KE, Thompson PD, Caspersen CJ, et al.: Physical activity and the incidence of coronary heart disease. Ann Rev Public Health 8:253, 1987. *A critical review of the relationship of habitual physical activity and ischemic heart disease mortality as established by epidemiologic observations.*

14 Alcoholism and Alcohol Abuse
Ivan Diamond

EPIDEMIOLOGY

Nearly two thirds of Americans over age 14 drink alcoholic beverages. Their per capita consumption is the equivalent of 9.7 gallons of whiskey, 89 gallons of beer, or 31 gallons of wine per year. Heavy drinkers, who constitute 10 per cent of the drinking population in the United States (7 per cent of the total adult population), account for half of the alcohol consumed and nearly all of the socioeconomic and medical complications of alcoholism and alcohol abuse. In 1990 the estimated annual cost of these problems to American society was $136 billion. Alcoholism and alcohol abuse are encountered in all socioeconomic classes and cultural groups; it is estimated that the prevalence of alcohol-related problems among hospitalized patients is 25 per cent.

DEFINITIONS

Alcoholism is characterized by addiction to ethanol. Although there are behavioral and socioeconomic definitions of alcoholism, in a medical setting alcoholism refers to a chronic disease in which the alcoholic craves and consumes ethanol without satiation, becomes increasingly *tolerant* to the intoxicating effects of the drug, and, when drinking is discontinued, exhibits the symptoms and signs of withdrawal as evidence of *physical dependence* on ethanol. Alcoholism with ethanol dependence can also develop as a secondary complication of depression, bipolar affective disorder, or schizophrenia, but 80 per cent of alcoholics have alcoholism without prior evidence of major psychiatric problems (*primary alcoholism*). Individuals who drink prodigiously without evidence of physical dependence are considered to have *alcohol abuse*. They often continue excessive drinking, sometimes episodically (*binge drinking*), despite significant personal socioeconomic hardship and medical complications.

GENETIC FACTORS

While environmental conditions influence drinking habits and the prevalence of alcoholism and alcohol abuse, there is also persuasive evidence that many individuals are at risk to develop alcoholism because of genetic factors. Alcoholism tends to run in families, and studies of alcoholism in identical twins, alcoholic parents and children, and offspring from alcoholic parents adopted into nondrinking families consistently suggest a genetically transmitted susceptibility for alcoholism. This is particularly evident for "male-limited" alcoholism in fathers and sons with antisocial, impulsive, novelty-seeking behavior, who become alcoholics in teenage years; they usually cannot abstain from drinking throughout life. Adoption studies indicate that this type of alcoholism in the biologic father is a much greater predictor for alcoholism in the son than is the environment in which the boy is raised. This is in contrast to other types of familial and nonfamilial alcoholism in which individuals may begin drinking as teenagers but become alcoholic later in life without an apparent genetic predisposition.

Such patients appear to have less difficulty in abstaining from alcohol once they develop motivation to stop drinking.

PHARMACOLOGY OF ETHANOL

ETHANOL ABSORPTION, DISTRIBUTION, AND ELIMINATION. Ethanol is absorbed rapidly and completely from the gastrointestinal tract and is detected in the blood within minutes of ingestion. Clinically significant amounts of vaporized alcohol can also be absorbed directly through the lungs. About 25 per cent of ethanol enters the bloodstream from the stomach and 75 per cent from the intestine, but many factors modify gastrointestinal absorption. These include food, the rate of drinking, the concentration, amount, and type of alcoholic beverage, and variations in gastrointestinal motility. For example, most foods in the stomach delay gastric absorption of ethanol, and pylorospasm due to high concentrations of alcohol in the stomach can slow gastric emptying and retard intestinal absorption. By contrast, rapid gastric emptying or gastrectomy causes increased rates of alcohol absorption from the small intestine.

Because of its solubility properties, ethanol readily crosses biologic membranes and equilibrates rapidly into total body water. Ninety to 98 per cent is removed by metabolism in the liver, and the remainder is excreted by the kidneys, lungs, and skin. Elimination follows zero-order kinetics and is independent of concentration; a 70-kg man can metabolize 5 to 10 grams of ethanol per hour. Since the average drink contains 12 to 15 grams of ethanol, blood alcohol levels continue to rise when an individual drinks at a rate greater than metabolism, but when drinking is discontinued, blood levels fall about 10 to 25 mg per deciliter per hour.

ETHANOL METABOLISM. Ethanol oxidation to acetaldehyde by alcohol dehydrogenase in the liver is the most clinically significant rate-limiting step, accounting for more than 90 per cent of ethanol metabolism in vivo. When blood alcohol concentrations are high, a microsomal ethanol oxidizing system can also generate acetaldehyde. Moreover, this second enzyme system mediates ethanol effects on drug metabolism in the liver (Ch. 118). Acetaldehyde is converted to acetate by aldehyde dehydrogenase, a metabolic step with important clinical ramifications. For example, 50 per cent of Japanese and other Asian people have a mutation in an aldehyde dehydrogenase isoenzyme which results in reduced enzyme activity in vivo. Shortly after drinking alcohol, affected individuals develop increased blood acetaldehyde levels and experience an *alcohol-flush* reaction, characterized by vasodilatation with facial flushing, hot sensations, tachycardia, and hypotension. These unpleasant experiences can act as a deterrent to drinking, and in Japan people with this mutation have a lower rate of alcoholism. Pharmacologic inhibition of aldehyde dehydrogenase causes even more severe aversive symptoms after drinking alcohol and is the reason why disulfiram (Antabuse) has been used to help discourage drinking. Disulfiram inhibits aldehyde dehydrogenase (and other sulfhydryl-containing enzymes), but it is not ordinarily toxic when taken therapeutically without ethanol. After drinking alcohol, however, patients on prophylactic disulfiram therapy have large increases in blood acetaldehyde levels and develop a more severe *acetaldehyde syndrome.* They can experience dysphoria, intense palpitations, sweating, thirst, throbbing headache, dyspnea, nausea and vomiting, weakness, vertigo, and syncope. Disulfiram does not cure alcoholism and is not widely used.

In peripheral tissues, acetate derived from acetaldehyde is converted to acetyl coenzyme A and subsequently to CO_2 and water. Complete oxidation of ethanol yields 7.1 kcal per gram, and some estimate that ethanol accounts for 10 per cent of the total caloric intake in the United States. Alcoholics often obtain 50 per cent of their calories from ethanol, and some develop serious nutritional deficiencies, particularly for protein, thiamine, folate, and pyridoxine (Table 14–1) (Ch. 204). Moreover, as a consequence of ethanol metabolism, alcoholics can develop hypoglycemia (Ch. 219), lactic acidosis (Ch. 75), hyperuricemia (Ch. 183), hypertriglyceridemia (Ch. 172), and ketoacidosis (Ch. 75) (Table 14–1).

ACUTE AND CHRONIC TOLERANCE TO ETHANOL. Tolerance develops after prolonged exposure to ethanol and is characterized by a reduced response to ethanol. When blood

TABLE 14–1. ALCOHOL-RELATED MEDICAL DISORDERS

Affected Organ or System	Disorder
Nutrition	Deficiencies of:
	Folate, thiamine, pyridoxine, niacin, and riboflavin
	Magnesium, zinc, calcium
	Protein
Brain	Hepatic encephalopathy
	Wernicke-Korsakoff syndrome
	Cerebral atrophy
	Amblyopia
	Central pontine myelinolysis
	Marchiafava-Bignami disease
Nerve	Neuropathy
Muscle	Myopathy
Liver	Fatty liver
	Hepatitis
	Cirrhosis
	Hepatoma
Heart	Hypertension
	Cardiomyopathy
	Arrhythmia
Blood	Anemia
	Leukopenia
	Thrombocytopenia
	Macrocytosis
Gut	Esophagitis and gastritis
	Pancreatitis
Metabolite and electrolytes	Hypoglycemia
	Hyperlipidemia
	Hyperuricemia
	Ketoacidosis
	Hypomagnesemia
	Hypophosphatemia
Endocrine	Pseudo-Cushing's syndrome
	Testicular atrophy
	Amenorrhea
Bone	Osteopenia

alcohol levels are no longer rising several hours after a drinking episode, normal subjects can appear to be sober at even higher alcohol concentrations that caused intoxication hours earlier. This phenomenon is known as *acute tolerance.* Similarly, chronic alcoholics have increased resistance to the intoxicating effects of ethanol and can even appear to be sober at blood alcohol levels of 400 to 500 mg per deciliter, concentrations known to produce stupor, coma, or death in naive individuals. This is known as *chronic tolerance.* Indeed, some chronic alcoholics can be so tolerant to ethanol as to survive blood alcohol concentrations as high as 1500 mg per deciliter. Thus, despite legal definitions of intoxication at blood alcohol levels above 100 mg per deciliter, a single blood ethanol determination may not accurately measure the extent of drunkenness.

ACUTE ETHANOL INTOXICATION

There is virtually no blood-brain barrier to ethanol; uptake into the brain is limited primarily by cerebral blood flow and capillary perfusion. Therefore, within a short period of time after drinking, the concentration of ethanol in the brain is nearly the same as the level of alcohol in the blood. In nonalcoholics, rising blood alcohol levels to 50 to 150 mg per deciliter are associated with increasing symptoms of intoxication (Table 14–2). Symptoms vary directly with the rate of drinking and are more severe when the blood alcohol concentration is rising than when it is falling. Most individuals feel euphoric, lose social inhibitions, and manifest expansive, sometimes garrulous behavior, whereas others may become gloomy, belligerent, or even explosively combative. Some people do not experience euphoria but instead become sleepy after moderate drinking; they rarely abuse alcohol. Neurologic signs of intoxication include impaired cognition, slurred

TABLE 14–2. BLOOD ETHANOL LEVELS AND SYMPTOMS

Blood Ethanol Levels (mg/dl)	Symptoms	
	Sporadic Drinkers	Chronic Drinkers
50–100	Euphoria Gregariousness Incoordination	Minimal or no effect
100–200	Slurred speech Ataxia Labile mood Drowsiness Nausea	Sobriety or incoordination Euphoria
200–300	Lethargic Combative Stuporous Incoherent speech Vomiting	Mild emotional and motor changes
300–400	Coma	Drowsiness
>500	Respiratory depression Death	Lethargy Stupor Coma

speech, incoordination, mild truncal ataxia, and slow or irregular eye movements. Signs of increased sympathetic activity include mydriasis, tachycardia, and skin flushing. The findings of central nervous system (CNS) depression predominate at higher blood alcohol concentrations. Cerebellar and vestibular function deteriorates, and drunkenness is characterized by dysarthria, more severe ataxia, nystagmus, and diplopia. Patients may become lethargic with bradycardia, reduced blood pressure, and diminished respirations, sometimes complicated by vomiting and pulmonary aspiration. In nonalcoholics, stupor and coma may develop at 400 mg per deciliter, and fatalities ensue at 500 mg per deciliter usually because of respiratory depression with ventilatory acidosis and hypotension. The LD_{30} for ethanol is approximately 450 mg per deciliter.

Alcoholic blackouts sometimes complicate acute alcohol intoxication during consumption of large amounts of ethanol. These episodes, which can occur in alcoholics or sporadic drinkers, are characterized by several hours of amnesia without impaired consciousness during the event. The patient reports an inability to remember new events but has no difficulty with long-term memory or immediate recall. These symptoms resemble the syndrome of transient global amnesia (Ch. 469).

EVALUATION AND MANAGEMENT. Severe acute alcohol intoxication can be fatal and is a medical emergency. The immediate history should include information about the quantity of alcohol consumed, the rate of drinking, use of other drugs including methanol, complicating medical and psychiatric disorders, and prior alcohol abuse or alcoholism. If the patient is stuporous and unable to walk, the airway must be evaluated immediately. Indications for endotracheal intubation and assisted ventilation include marked hypoventilation, accumulating secretions, and coma. In such patients, complications such as hypoglycemia, meningitis, and subdural hematoma must be considered. Evidence of head trauma or focal or lateralizing neurologic signs suggests urgent intracranial pathology, and a computed tomography (CT) scan should be performed immediately. Otherwise, routine CT scans for alcohol intoxication are not indicated. Gastric lavage may be performed if obtundation is due to recent and massive alcohol consumption, but only after endotracheal intubation. Hemodialysis should be considered if the blood ethanol level exceeds 600 mg per deciliter.

After a history and physical examination, patients with adequate vital signs, acceptable mental status, and no evidence of other disorders can be kept under observation until sobriety returns. However, medical information is usually incomplete, and it is often necessary to anticipate complications commonly associated with severe alcohol intoxication or alcoholism (see Table 14–1). Routine blood counts and chemistries will uncover anemia (Ch. 122), hypokalemia, hypophosphatemia, and hypomagnesemia (Ch. 75, 194, and 195). Alcoholic hypoglycemia (Ch. 219) can be evaluated rapidly by a bedside blood glucose determination. If laboratory results are delayed, 12.5 to 25 grams of glucose should be given intravenously. Alcoholic ketoacidosis (Ch. 75) will be improved by infusion of 5 per cent dextrose in 0.5N saline. Elevated serum ammonia levels support the diagnosis of hepatic encephalopathy (Ch. 123). If the blood alcohol level is too low to account for the patient's obtundation or if improvement does not occur as expected, it is necessary to search for other causes of stupor and coma (Ch. 443).

ETHANOL WITHDRAWAL SYNDROME

Ethanol is a CNS depressant. In alcoholics, the nervous system appears to adapt to chronic ethanol exposure by increasing the activity of neural mechanisms that counteract alcohol's depressant effects. When drinking is abruptly reduced or discontinued, these stimulatory neural mechanisms are left unrestrained by ethanol, and a hyperexcitable *ethanol withdrawal syndrome* develops. This is evidence of *physical dependence* on ethanol. The ethanol withdrawal syndrome consists of several characteristic abnormalities that vary in severity. These include tremulousness, disordered perceptions, seizures, and delirium tremens (Table 14–3).

The general medical evaluation and management are as described for acute ethanol intoxication. One hundred milligrams of thiamine should be given parenterally to all patients undergoing ethanol withdrawal to prevent or treat Wernicke's encephalopathy (Ch. 456), followed by daily multivitamins. It is important to search for evidence of alcohol-related medical disorders (see Table 14–1) and the associated complications of alcohol abuse, as described earlier. The alarming symptoms of ethanol withdrawal are best managed by substituting another CNS depressant. However, alcoholics undergoing withdrawal are very resistant to sedatives (*cross-tolerance*), and large doses are often required to calm their agitation. The more specific forms of treatment are listed under the individual manifestations below.

TREMULOUSNESS. Tremor, the earliest, most common, and most apparent symptom, begins about 6 to 8 hours after the last drink, usually the morning after an overnight abstinence ("morning shakes"). Tremor is generalized, coarse, and rapid and is often accompanied by irritability, nausea, and vomiting. The patient usually senses an inner tremulousness even when tremor is not severe. Self-treatment commonly consists of a morning drink to "quiet the nerves," after which drinking is continued for the rest of the day. If the alcoholic does not resume drinking, tremor becomes much more intense by 24 to 36 hours and is exacerbated by motor activity or stress. It can be so severe as to interfere with walking, eating, or speech. Accompanying symptoms and signs of sympathetic hyperactivity are also apparent. The patient is increasingly anxious and easily startled by minor stimuli and complains of insomnia and anorexia. Increased sweating, facial flushing, mydriasis, tachycardia, and mild hypertension occur. Although most abnormalities subside in a few days, increased arousal and anxiety may persist for 2 weeks.

DISORDERED PERCEPTIONS. Disordered perceptions also accompany the development of tremor and sympathetic hyperactivity in approximately 25 per cent of tremulous patients. These symptoms similarly become most pronounced at 24 to 36 hours, before clearing in a few days. The patient frequently experiences vivid nightmares that interfere with sleep; ordinary visual, auditory, and tactile experiences may become distorted and misinterpreted during waking hours.

Sometimes alcoholics undergoing withdrawal develop isolated and more prolonged auditory hallucinations (*alcoholic hallucinosis*), despite being alert, oriented, and without memory loss. Hallucinations may continue for weeks even though other signs of ethanol withdrawal have improved and the patient is less agitated and tremulous. In the absence of sympathetic hyperactivity, persistent auditory hallucinations may be confused with acute schizophrenia (Ch. 456). However, alcoholic hallucinosis is

TABLE 14–3. ETHANOL WITHDRAWAL SYNDROME

8 hours	Tremulousness, anxiety, irritability, nausea, and vomiting
24 hours	Hyperexcitability, insomnia, disordered perceptions, convulsions
2–5 days	Delirium tremens

closely associated with ethanol withdrawal and usually subsides in weeks to months.

Benzodiazepines are widely used to manage tremulousness and disordered perceptions during ethanol withdrawal. The goal is to suppress symptoms and produce mild sedation, and drug dosage is adjusted to the severity of the withdrawal reaction. Patients with mild tremulousness and few associated symptoms usually respond to oral diazepam, 5 to 10 mg every 4 to 6 hours. Dosage is then reduced by 20 to 25 per cent on successive days, or increased if symptoms of ethanol withdrawal return. Diazepam is used intravenously if symptoms are severe, and some patients may require extraordinarily high doses to achieve mild sedation. Once the symptoms of ethanol withdrawal are suppressed, it is necessary to avoid oversedation and the danger of respiratory depression by carefully titrating the dose of diazepam to just keep the patient calm.

ETHANOL WITHDRAWAL SEIZURES. Five to 33 per cent of alcoholics develop generalized tonic-clonic convulsions, most often within 12 to 24 hours after reducing or discontinuing alcohol consumption. Ethanol withdrawal seizures characterize ethanol dependence in experimental animals, and mice have been bred to be genetically prone to develop convulsions during withdrawal, suggesting that genetic factors could be important in humans. An alternate view is that the first seizure in alcoholics may be a consequence of ethanol toxicity. Ethanol withdrawal seizures are usually associated with a history of chronic daily drinking, but 5- to 7-day episodes of binge drinking can also be followed by convulsions. Seizures may be one to six in number and usually occur within a 6-hour period. Alcoholics who have seizures during one episode of ethanol withdrawal are likely to have convulsions again when alcohol withdrawal is repeated. Focal seizures are less common and should always suggest a focal lesion and an additional diagnosis. Status epilepticus occurs in about 3 per cent of cases, and ethanol withdrawal accounts for about 15 per cent of all patients who present with status epilepticus (Ch. 483).

Most ethanol withdrawal convulsions are brief and self-limited. However, a complete evaluation for a convulsive disorder is indicated (Ch. 483) if there is a clinical suspicion of other CNS disorders, if the patient has focal seizures, if there are more than six seizures, if the convulsions persist beyond 6 hours, or if the postictal state is prolonged. Typical ethanol withdrawal seizures do not require specific anticonvulsant therapy; phenytoin does not prevent recurrent seizures in these patients. However, status epilepticus from any cause is a medical emergency and requires immediate treatment with anticonvulsants as described in Ch. 483.

DELIRIUM TREMENS. Delirium tremens, the most alarming manifestation of the ethanol withdrawal syndrome, occurs in about 5 per cent of such patients. It is characterized by agitated arousal, global confusion and disorientation, insomnia, and vivid, often threatening hallucinations and delusions. Signs of sympathetic hyperactivity include tremor, mydriasis, tachycardia, fever, and intense diaphoresis. In contrast to tremulousness, disordered perceptions, and seizures, which appear earlier after withdrawal, delirium tremens begins abruptly within 2 to 4 days of abstinence, often as a surprising development in unrecognized alcoholics who have been admitted to the hospital for other reasons. These patients are terrified by their hallucinations and can be combative, destructive, and very dangerous. Episodes of delirium tremens last from one to three days and end as abruptly as they begin. However, relapses can occur and the disorder may continue for days to weeks with intervening periods of lucidity.

Delirium tremens requires hospitalization and vigorous emergency treatment. When there are no signs of sympathetic hyperactivity, it may be difficult to distinguish delirium tremens from an acute psychosis. However, the diagnosis is usually suggested by the evolution of symptoms in a chronic alcoholic undergoing withdrawal. The differential diagnosis includes alcoholic hypoglycemia, overdose with anticholinergic agents, intoxication with amphetamines, cocaine, and phencyclidine (PCP), encephalitis, meningitis, thyrotoxicosis, and withdrawal from other sedating drugs. Seizures are unusual in delirium tremens and should be evaluated promptly because of the possibility of meningitis or other diagnoses. Mortality can reach 15 per cent, primarily because of injuries or associated medical disorders complicated by hyperthermia and dehydration. Volume depletion accompanying delirium tremens may cause circulatory collapse, and fluid losses can require replacement of 4 to 10 liters in the first day. The goal of treatment is to control behavior and suppress symptoms without danger to the patient. Five to 10 mg or more of diazepam is given intravenously every 5 to 15 minutes until the patient is calm, and maintenance therapy is continued every 1 to 4 hours, as needed. Initially, as much as 200 mg of diazepam may be required before agitation subsides, and some patients may need up to 1200 mg in the first 3 to 4 days of treatment to keep calm.

RECOGNITION AND REHABILITATION OF ALCOHOLICS

Most alcoholics rarely admit to problem drinking and are often not recognized by their primary care physicians. Instead, alcoholics are usually identified because of the adverse socioeconomic consequences of heavy drinking or the development of medical complications and the alcohol-related disorders (see Table 14–1) which bring them to medical attention. After several days of detoxification under medical supervision, the patient should be referred to a rehabilitation program because alcoholism and alcohol abuse can rarely be treated by the physician alone. The patient needs encouragement to develop a high level of motivation to stop drinking and to adjust to a life without alcohol. The most successful treatment usually requires active participation of family members, friends, and peers, and the prognosis is best for alcoholics who enter treatment programs before the onset of associated medical disorders. Many patients and families find local support groups such as Alcoholics Anonymous and Al-Anon to be very helpful, and about 50 to 70 per cent of socially stable, middle-class alcoholics can achieve abstinence. However, this success rate is not attributable to a specific kind of rehabilitation scheme.

Adinoff B, Bone GHA, Linnoila M: Acute ethanol poisoning and the ethanol withdrawal syndrome. Med Toxicol 3:172, 1988. *An extensive discussion of the presentation and management of ethanol intoxication and withdrawal.*

Goldstein DB: Pharmacology of Alcohol. New York, Oxford University Press, 1983. *An excellent introduction to the principles of ethanol pharmacology.*

Kiianmaa K, Tabakoff B, Saito T (eds.): Genetic Aspects of Alcoholism. Helsinki, The Finnish Foundation for Alcohol Studies, 1989. *This book includes a series of brief presentations about the major issues concerning the genetics of alcoholism and the characteristics of low-risk and high-risk individuals.*

Porter R, Mattson R, Kramer J, et al. (eds.): Alcohol and Seizures: Basic Mechanisms and Clinical Concepts. Philadelphia, F.A. Davis, 1990. *This book focuses on the pathogenesis and management of ethanol withdrawal seizures.*

Seventh Special Report to the U.S. Congress on Alcohol and Health. U.S. Dept. of Health and Human Services. Rockville, Md., National Institute on Alcohol Abuse and Alcoholism, 1990. *An excellent comprehensive discussion of the major socioeconomic and biomedical problems of alcoholism and alcohol abuse.*

15 Drug Abuse and Dependence

Charles P. O'Brien

In the 1990's substance abuse is found in all strata of American society. The average physician is likely to encounter many patients exhibiting behavioral or medical complications of licit or illicit drug use, but the relationship of the symptoms to drugs often goes unrecognized. Early diagnosis, which is critical for effective treatment, is difficult because at an early stage patients rarely fit the addict stereotype.

Clinicians have been mainly concerned with tolerance and physical dependence. *Tolerance* is the result of a homeostatic process in which the body adapts to the repeated effects of a drug. This adaptation tends to compensate for the pharmacologic effects of the drug with the result that higher doses are required to achieve a drug effect. With daily dosing, tolerance increases and a state of physical dependence can occur. *Physical dependence* is diagnosed by the presence of a rebound known as a *withdrawal syndrome* that follows interruption of dosing. Withdrawal phenomena tend to be opposite to the effects of the drugs themselves. Thus a drug that produces sedation is marked by hyperreflexia and irritability during withdrawal, and a stimulant drug is followed by weakness and depression during withdrawal.

Changes in *behavior* are the pivotal diagnostic criteria for drug dependence. While tolerance and physical dependence have been emphasized in the past, *intermittent* use that does not cause tolerance or a withdrawal syndrome may produce behavioral or social consequences urgently requiring treatment. *Drug abuse* is therefore defined as a maladaptive pattern in the use of any substance which persists despite adverse social, psychological, or medical consequences. The pattern of abuse may be intermittent and the condition does not meet the criteria for dependence. *Drug dependence* is a behavioral syndrome that involves compulsive drug-taking, neglect of constructive activities, and adverse social effects and *may* include pharmacologic tolerance and physical dependence.

RECOGNITION. Since early diagnosis is so important, the physician should have a low threshold for including drug abuse in the differential diagnosis of any patient. The abuse pattern that presents the most difficulty is that of a successful middle-class adult whose substance abuse is detected incidental to a routine physical examination or during treatment of an unrelated disorder. Invariably the patient denies that drug or alcohol abuse is a problem. Physicians must be aware that denial of problems and minimizing of the drug or alcohol use are fundamental aspects of the syndrome. These patients usually do not admit to a problem until it becomes so severe that there is no alternative, by which time treatment is much more difficult.

The diagnosis of drug abuse or dependence is basically a clinical diagnosis. The physician should use all available information, including the patient's history, information from relatives or employer, physical examination, and laboratory tests. Blood or urine tests showing the presence of drugs or their metabolites can be useful but also misleading. The toxicologic tests, when properly done and confirmed, indicate use within a varying period of time depending on the drug and its dose. Such tests do not disclose pattern of use or the presence of dependence. Metabolites of some drugs, such as marijuana or cocaine, remain in the urine for at least several days following a single dose. Thus the tests require interpretation and integration with other clinical information.

Clues discovered on the physical examination include the presence of scars from numerous intravenous injections ("tracks") or edema of the arms and veins that are difficult to find. Chronic sinusitis or a scarred and perhaps perforated nasal septum suggests "snorting" of cocaine, a powerful vasoconstrictor. Frequent injuries due to falls or auto accidents are seen in sedative abusers as well as alcoholics. Infections such as abscesses, hepatitis, respiratory infections, and endocarditis are well-known risks of drug abuse. The most devastating disease associated with drug abuse is acquired immunodeficiency syndrome (AIDS), and intravenous drug users now represent more than 25 per cent of cases of HIV infection.

Physicians must also be alert to the signs of drug abuse in order to avoid unwittingly prescribing medication that will perpetuate the dependence. Patients taking sleeping medications, pain medications, or antianxiety agents on a chronic basis may visit several physicians in order to obtain a larger drug supply. Others deliberately feign illness, particularly pain syndromes. Some will have read textbooks and recite classic descriptions of acute renal calculus, migraine headache, or pancreatitis. Physicians should be particularly wary of patients who ask for a specific medication or who claim to have an "allergy" to non-narcotic pain medication.

American Psychiatric Association: Diagnostic and Statistical Manual of Mental Disorders, 3rd ed. rev. Washington, D.C., American Psychiatric Association, 1987, pp 165–186. *Clear summary of the new diagnostic criteria for dependence on alcohol and other drugs.*

Jaffe J: Drug addiction and drug abuse. *In* Gilman AG, Goodman LS, Rall TR, et al. (eds.): The Pharmacological Basis of Therapeutics. 8th ed. New York, Pergamon Press, 1990. *Thorough discussion of pharmacologic and clinical aspects of drug abuse.*

Smith DE (ed.): Addiction medicine. West J Med 152:499, 1990. *A special issue that contains 21 articles covering many general topics relating to drug abuse and dependence.*

SEDATIVES

Examples of sedatives include the following:
Ethanol
Barbiturates
Diazepam (Valium)
Alprazolam (Xanax)
Flurazepam (Dalmane)
Lorazepam (Ativan)
Meprobamate (Miltown)
Glutethimide (Doriden)

These drugs are central nervous system depressants and all are capable of producing abuse, tolerance, and physical dependence. Their withdrawal syndromes are generally similar, although the sedatives come from different chemical categories (e.g., alcohol, barbiturate, benzodiazepine). Their effects are additive, and they are often used in combination. This aspect is particularly important in considering interactions with alcohol (Ch. 14) and in treating patients who are dependent on multiple sedatives with different durations of action.

Patterns of Abuse

There are two basic patterns of sedative drug abuse other than that with alcohol: One is produced inadvertently by taking prescription sedatives without proper concern for their potential to produce dependence, and the second involves deliberate use of sedatives to obtain a "high."

PRESCRIPTION SEDATIVES. The problem of improper use of prescription sedatives is a concern to all physicians because they are among the most widely prescribed of all drugs throughout the world. They have legitimate medical uses in the short-term treatment of insomnia or anxiety and in the long-term treatment of seizure disorders. The chronic use of medication for insomnia, however, often leads to problems because insomnia is merely a symptom. It may signal the presence of an underlying illness, or it may simply require a change in activity patterns, but the chronic use of sedatives simply adds a new problem. After daily use for several weeks, tolerance develops and sleep difficulties may return, often in a modified form. The patient may have become dependent, however, on the daily ingestion of the sedative. If the drug is stopped, a rebound occurs, with the appearance of symptoms worse than those experienced prior to treatment. Sedatives are not equal in their tendency to produce this iatrogenic insomnia. Long-acting benzodiazepines, for example, are unlikely to produce rebound effects at usual doses. Other liabilities are associated with their use, however, such as "hangover" effects, which produce subtle neuropsychological deficits and may mimic dementia in older persons. On balance, insomnia should not be treated with drugs except for brief periods of time.

Another pattern associated with the prescription of sedatives is that found in the treatment of anxiety. Benzodiazepines (e.g., diazepam, alprazolam) are the most effective medications available for the treatment of anxiety, and they produce relatively less sedation than older medications used for this purpose, such as meprobamate or phenobarbital. Symptoms of anxiety are widespread; one survey found that about 15 per cent of all Americans received a prescription for one of these drugs in a single year. While some argue that this suggests overprescribing, it is not out of line with experiences in other western countries.

Approximately 6 per cent of the population take benzodiazepines chronically, and this leads to *tolerance* and *physical dependence*. This does not imply a similar prevalence of *abuse* because the patient may be taking the benzodiazepine for a legitimate anxiety disorder. It does mean, however, that since the patient perceives less sedation, there may be a tendency to increase the dose. It also implies that the patient should be warned about withdrawal symptoms if the drug is terminated abruptly. Occasionally, a patient who allows a prescription for a short-acting benzodiazepine to run out is brought to an emergency room because of benzodiazepine withdrawal seizures. Some of these patients are mislabeled "addicts," even though the patient has never used more of the antianxiety medication than was prescribed. Others, however, become deliberate abusers of sedatives after beginning treatment for anxiety under a doctor's care and may purposely increase their dose while obtaining medication from several different physicians. Benzodiazepines in general have a relatively low abuse potential, but their use should be avoided or severely limited in patients with a history of alcoholism or other forms of drug abuse.

DELIBERATE SEDATIVE ABUSE. Sedatives are used at parties by groups of abusers, usually adolescents and young adults, to obtain a "high." The "high" appears to be a form of disinhibition or release and depends partially on the setting in which the drug is taken. As with alcohol, increasing the dose produces depression and eventual loss of consciousness. A dangerous aspect of sedative abuse is that tolerance to the sought-after subjective effects rapidly develops, but tolerance to the depressant effects on the brain stem remains low. As the experienced user increases the dose to obtain a "high," he or she may unexpectedly reach the dose that depresses vital functions and threatens survival.

Abstinence Syndrome

The withdrawal syndrome following sedative dependence is similar to alcohol withdrawal (described in Ch. 14). Among the sedatives, the syndrome varies in onset, duration, and severity with the dose and duration of action of the drug used and the duration of daily use. The long-acting benzodiazepines, such as diazepam, may have a withdrawal syndrome whose onset is delayed for several days following the termination of the drug. At doses within the therapeutic range, withdrawal symptoms may consist of only mild irritability, complaints of peculiar sensations, diaphoresis, and sleep disturbance accompanied by rebound increases in rapid eye movement (REM) sleep. The symptoms may be similar to the anxiety symptoms for which the drug was initially prescribed. At higher doses, the sedative withdrawal syndrome is more severe and can be life-threatening. Major abnormalities include paroxysmal electroencephalographic (EEG) abnormalities, generalized seizures, and a toxic psychosis similar to delirium tremens. Restlessness, anxiety, tremulousness, and weakness occur, often accompanied by orthostatic hypotension, nausea, cramps, and vomiting. Irritability, anxiety, photophobia, depressive symptoms, and neuropsychological deficits may persist for weeks or months.

Treatment

The acute withdrawal syndrome should be considered a serious medical illness usually requiring inpatient treatment. Close monitoring for cardiac arrhythmias or seizures is necessary. Several detoxification techniques are available, each requiring the substitution of a prescribed sedative with cross-tolerance for the drug on which the patient is dependent. The physician should not simply accept the history but rather determine the level of dependence by giving a test dose of a known sedative, such as diazepam or pentobarbital. If the patient shows no evidence of slurred speech or sedation after a test dose of 20 to 40 mg of diazepam, a higher level of dependence is indicated, and the daily sedative dose should be adjusted accordingly. Gradual detoxification using diazepam can be accomplished over 1 to 3 weeks, although in some treatment centers where diazepam is the object of much drug-seeking behavior and manipulation by patients, phenobarbital is preferred. Patients dependent on both a short-acting sedative, such as alcohol, and a long-acting drug, such as diazepam, should be watched for a biphasic withdrawal. The alcohol withdrawal peaks and subsides during the first week, but the diazepam withdrawal may not be evident until early in the second week. Patients dependent on both an opioid, such as heroin, and a sedative should be maintained on a low dose of methadone until the sedative withdrawal is completed. After detoxification, the patient must be put in a treatment program to prevent recurrence, as described at the end of this chapter.

American Psychiatric Association: Benzodiazepine Dependence, Toxicity and Abuse, APA Task Force Report. Washington, D.C., American Psychiatric Association, 1990. *Excellent review of the data concerning the use and risks of benzodiazepines with practical prescribing guidelines.*

O'Brien CP, Woody GE: Sedative hypnotic and anti-anxiety agents. In Frances AJ, Hales R (eds.): American Psychiatric Association Annual Review, Vol 5, Washington, D.C., APA Press, 1986, pp 186–199. *Review of diagnosis, treatment, and prevention of sedative abuse.*

STIMULANTS

Examples of stimulants include the following:
Cocaine
Dextroamphetamine
Methamphetamine
Methylphenidate (Ritalin)
Phenmetrazine (Preludin)
Diethylpropion (Tepanil)

Patterns of Abuse

Cocaine became the major drug of abuse in the United States, excluding alcohol, during the 1980's. At present, attitudes toward the use of cocaine have become more negative among high school seniors, but overall use has not yet significantly declined. Despite increased efforts at federal interdiction, cocaine supplies in the United States have increased so rapidly that the price has become low. Not only is cocaine available to a wider market, especially children, but its sellers have developed clever new and efficient ways to administer cocaine, increasing its potency and danger.

Until recently, cocaine hydrochloride was available as a white powder through illicit channels in an adulterated form and at a cost so high that only the affluent could afford to use it regularly. The typical mode of administration was "snorting," which consists of application of the powder to the nasal mucous membranes. Intravenous injection of an aqueous solution was also used, resulting in a more rapid onset and greater likelihood of seizures. Inhalation of the "free base" alkaloid form of cocaine has more recently been found to be the most convenient and efficient system for delivering the drug to the brain. During the mid-1980's, dealers began supplying a mass-produced solid form of "free base" called "crack." "Crack" is produced by sodium bicarbonate extraction of cocaine hydrochloride; the agent can be sold in small yellow-white lumps for as little as $5 to $10 per dose. When heated in a small pipe, the resulting cocaine vapor can be inhaled, producing a brief and very intense "high." This drug is clearly the *most addicting substance* yet encountered by clinicians. Dependence in the behavioral sense can be produced very rapidly, perhaps in days and certainly in weeks. Users may administer the drug continuously for several days without eating or sleeping. The widespread availability of "crack," its cheap price, and its tendency to produce dependence have led to problems in all strata of society.

The sought-after effect of cocaine is an intense "high" or euphoria, which is often described in sexual terms but is claimed to be "better than sex." The euphoria may last only a few minutes, depending on the dose and mode of administration. The aftereffect is one of depression and craving for more cocaine. During a period of regular cocaine use, the person becomes irritable and suspicious. High doses may result in persecutory delusions or hallucinations, but these are more common with longer-acting stimulants such as amphetamines. Families and friends of chronic cocaine users often note personality changes not observed by the users themselves. Alcohol, sedatives, opioids, and marijuana are often taken concurrently to combat the anxiety and irritability experienced by those using cocaine regularly. Users deprived of cocaine experience intense craving, depression, apathy, fatigue, and sleepiness.

Amphetamines and related drugs have a longer duration of action than cocaine, but many of the effects are similar. Dextro-amphetamine has been used by physicians for a variety of conditions, including weight reduction, narcolepsy, and attention deficit disorder. Amphetamines have not been shown to be of value in weight reduction programs, and their use for all purposes has been curtailed by legal restrictions. In the early 1990's, a new street drug consisting of crystalline methamphetamine ("ice") has been reported. Like "crack," this drug can be heated and inhaled, thus producing a longer-lasting and potentially more dangerous state of intoxication. Because stimulants produce effects that are mostly pleasant, patients have a tendency to increase the dose and to take them longer than the prescribing physician intended. Tolerance develops rapidly to the stimulant effects of amphetamines, but with higher doses, toxic effects are common. These effects can resemble acute paranoid schizophrenia with delusions and hallucinations. Cessation of use of amphetamines produces a withdrawal syndrome similar to that after cocaine use and depressive symptoms that may continue for several months.

The milder stimulants, such as methylphenidate and phenmetrazine, rarely are associated with abuse problems, but they should be prescribed only when specifically indicated and with awareness of their abuse potential.

Pharmacology

Cocaine has several effects, but the critical action for abuse potential appears to be the blocking of reuptake of dopamine at central synapses, thus increasing the effects of synaptic dopamine. Systemic effects of cocaine and amphetamine include increased cardiac contraction, increased blood pressure and heart rate, dilated pupils, constriction of peripheral blood vessels, rise in body temperature, relaxation of the bronchial musculature, and increases in central venous pressure, pulmonary arterial pressure, and renal blood flow. Cocaine is an effective topical local anesthetic and vasoconstrictor of mucous membranes. Low doses of stimulants increase alertness and physical and cognitive ability. Stimulants do reduce appetite, but significant tolerance develops to this effect. When stimulants are discontinued, a rebound increase in weight often leaves the person heavier than before the drug was taken.

Heavy users report acute tolerance to the euphorigenic effects of cocaine when the drug is used repeatedly at a single occasion. However, a day or two later, a "high" can again be obtained at approximately the same dose as previously. Tolerance to the respiratory and cardiac stimulatory effects of cocaine does occur. Although abrupt cessation of stimulant use produces a distinct withdrawal syndrome as described above, it is generally limited to *behavioral* evidence of brain dysfunction rather than reflected in the presence of physical signs. During the excessive periods of sleep seen during withdrawal, the EEG shows a significant increase in the proportion of REM sleep and nightmares may occur. Rarely, withdrawal has been marked by headaches, profuse sweating, muscle cramps, disorientation, and confusion.

Adverse Effects

The most common adverse effect of cocaine use is loss of control, so that a severe dependence syndrome occurs with neglect of all constructive activities. *Acute cocaine toxicity* is dose related and is characterized by sympathomimetic effects, including tachycardia, hypertension, hyperthermia, and arrhythmias, and is followed by seizures, brain stem depression, and cardiorespiratory collapse. Stroke, coma, intracranial vasculitis, myocardial infarction, and sudden death have each occasionally occurred as complications of cocaine binges. At lower doses the acute toxic effects may be marked by a brief period of paranoid behavior with hallucinations. *Acute amphetamine toxicity* is also characterized by excessive sympathomimetic stimulation. There may be stereotyped compulsive behavior, tactile hallucinations consisting of "bugs" crawling under the skin, and visual or auditory hallucinations.

Chronic use of intranasal cocaine commonly causes ulceration or perforation of the nasal septum. Chronic users are typically debilitated and subject to infections as a result of neglect of hygiene, lack of sleep, and poor nutrition. There is evidence of neuronal degeneration in dopamine-rich areas of the brains of animals treated chronically with amphetamine. This raises the possibility of an increased risk for later development of Parkinson's disease. Schizophrenic disorders have been reported to be increased in chronic stimulant users. Chronic cocaine use among pregnant women results in a high incidence of premature, low birth weight, and neurologically abnormal infants.

Treatment

Treatment of the anxiety reactions and irritability produced by cocaine or amphetamines can be accomplished with benzodiazepines. Acute psychotic reactions may require haloperidol if amphetamines are involved, but reactions produced by cocaine are usually self-limiting. Withdrawal from stimulant dependence requires a supportive environment and protection from the supply of cocaine. Intense craving for cocaine is the most prominent of the withdrawal symptoms, although severe fatigue and depression may occur. The most difficult aspect of treatment is to prevent relapse when the patient returns to his or her normal environment and is confronted with opportunities to re-establish the habit. This aspect of treatment is discussed at the end of this chapter.

Gawin FH, Ellinwood EH: Cocaine and other stimulants. N Engl J Med 318:1173, 1988. *Review of clinical and pharmacologic aspects of stimulant abuse.*

Lange RA, Cigarroa RG, Yancy CW Jr, et al.: Cocaine-induced coronary-artery vasoconstriction. N Engl J Med 321:1557, 1989. *Excellent study of the effects of cocaine on cardiac function.*

OPIOIDS

Examples of opioids include the following:

Agonists

Morphine
Methadone
Meperidine (Demerol)
Oxycodone (Percodan)
Propoxyphene (Darvon)
Heroin
Hydromorphone (Dilaudid)
Fentanyl (Sublimaze)
Codeine

Mixed agonist-antagonists

Pentazocine (Talwin)
Nalbuphine (Nubain)
Buprenorphine (Buprenex)
Butorphanol (Stadol)

Antagonists

Naloxone (Narcan)
Naltrexone (Trexan)

Opiates are derivatives of the opium poppy plant, which contains more than 20 alkaloids. Heroin, morphine, and codeine are examples of commonly used *opiates*. Synthetic drugs that act via opiate receptors in the body are called *opioids*. The body also produces peptides that act at these receptors as neurohormones or neurotransmitters and are called *endogenous opioids* (Ch. 209).

Patterns of Abuse

Opioid abuse has been a problem in the United States for well over 100 years. The patterns have changed considerably since the turn of the century, when most opium-dependent persons were either Civil War veterans or users of patent medicines. Currently two abuse patterns exist in this country. The smaller group by far involves those patients initially treated by a physician for a legitimate pain problem with opioid drugs. The pain may become chronic and the dose is increased, usually at the patient's demand. The treatment may have begun with a relatively weak medication, such as propoxyphene or pentazocine, but it tends to progress through to the more potent opioids, such as oxycodone or hydromorphone. Prescriptions may be refilled excessively, and patients may visit more than one physician for medication or frequent emergency rooms. Such individuals vehemently deny being addicts; they are just seeking relief of pain. On closer examination, however, they are usually found to have symptoms of anxiety or depression that are temporarily relieved by opioids.

The second pattern is that of intentional misuse of opioids for their euphoria-producing ability. Intermittent heroin use, primarily among males in the inner city, typically begins during adolescence, and dependence ensues within a year or two of first use. Development in all areas—educational, social, occupational, and even psychosexual—is curtailed by use of heroin. It is not known how many people begin experimenting with heroin and stop using it. Those who continue to use heroin develop tolerance to its euphorigenic effects, continue to increase the dose, and soon find that they must use the drug daily to avoid withdrawal symptoms even while chasing that elusive first "high."

Older users tend to introduce younger ones to heroin and to techniques of crime required to support the "habit." Street heroin available in the United States tends to be diluted many times so that there may be an average of only 4 to 10 mg of heroin in a typical 100-mg bag. Furthermore, the heroin on the street at any given time may be more or less potent, depending on the supply and the pressure from law enforcement agencies. Most street heroin users have relatively mild degrees of physical dependence in terms of number of milligrams of heroin or its equivalent in morphine or methadone per day. Heroin-dependent persons, although they insist that they are seeking a "high," actually fear withdrawal and go to great lengths to obtain sufficient drug to inject themselves one to three times per day.

Some heroin users discover that prescription medications are more reliable than street drugs because the latter have no quality control. Hydromorphone, a very potent opioid, cannot be distinguished from heroin even by experienced users under double-blind conditions. Addicts may visit physicians or emergency rooms and feign pain syndromes to obtain opioids. Occasionally, unscrupulous physicians may simply sell prescriptions for whatever the addict requests. A few addicts have had prescription pads printed with their own name and a false Drug Enforcement Agency (DEA) number in an effort to trick pharmacists. Some of the prescription drugs prized on the street are not even the more potent ones.

In recent years heroin dependence has spread from inner-city to middle-class populations. The same supply system that distributes cocaine and marijuana also makes heroin available. Some educated and employed persons seeking a "thrill" prefer the effects of heroin. Others learn to use heroin to combat some of the unpleasant anxiety and irritability produced by chronic cocaine use.

Pharmacology

Opioids act at specific receptors that are widely distributed throughout the body in virtually all major organ systems. Since these receptors are heavily represented in the endocrine, cardiovascular, gastrointestinal, and nervous systems (Ch. 209), the effects of opioids are many and varied. The potency of individual drugs appears to depend on receptor affinity as well as metabolism. Heroin, for example, is diacetylmorphine, which has high lipid solubility and enters the brain rapidly. It is hydrolyzed to morphine, which is the form active at opiate receptors. Other opioids have similar systemic effects but reach brain receptors less rapidly. The mixed agonist-antagonist drugs, such as pentazocine, butorphanol, and nalbuphine, appear to act as agonists at kappa opiate receptors, but they also act as antagonists at mu (morphine) receptors. Thus, pentazocine can relieve pain on its own but, if given to someone already receiving morphine, displaces the morphine and precipitates withdrawal symptoms. Pure antagonists, such as naloxone and naltrexone, have no opiate-like effects, but they can reverse overdose and precipitate withdrawal if given *after* an opioid and prevent opiate effects if given *before* the opioid.

After heroin injection, traces of morphine can be found in the urine for about 12 to 48 hours, depending on the dose and the laboratory detection technique. Quinine, a common adulterant of street heroin, persists longer, but it is also found in legal substances such as tonic water. Parenteral injections of morphine or methadone have equal analgesic effects and persist for 4 to 6 hours, whereas heroin is three times as potent, and meperidine and codeine are one tenth as potent as morphine. Codeine, meperidine, and methadone remain active when taken orally, and the duration of action of methadone is extended considerably when taken orally. For prevention of withdrawal in dependent persons, methadone remains active for 24 to 30 hours, far longer than its analgesic effect.

Opioids appear to produce a state in which the patient can still feel pain but is less bothered by it. This state is produced, at least in part, by activation of an endogenous pain control system mediated via opiate receptors. Inhibition of pain sensation occurs at the spinal level as well as within the brain. Opioids are much more effective for clinical pain with anxiety than for experimental pain in research subjects. Opioids produce a reduction in anxiety, some sedation, and a feeling of well-being or euphoria. This effect seems important to both their clinical usefulness and their abuse potential. It is this euphoria that is sought by street addicts and that probably leads some medical patients to abuse prescribed opioids.

Tolerance to the euphoric effects of opioids develops rapidly, resulting in a tendency for users to increase their dose if possible. Only partial tolerance develops to other effects, such as pupillary constriction, inhibition of gastrointestinal contractions, and suppression of anterior pituitary function.

Adverse Effects

Acute opioid overdose occurs when a user inadvertently injects a much higher dose than expected. This also can be seen when a previously tolerant person returns to opioid use after a long interval, so that most of his tolerance has been lost. Many of the "overdoses" found with street heroin are now thought to have been due to a reaction to some of the adulterants rather than to the opiate. Acute reactions to adulterants including quinine, allergic reactions, and synergistic interactions among several drugs used simultaneously may produce the *acute heroin reaction.* The syndrome is marked clinically by the rapid development of cyanosis, pulmonary edema, respiratory distress, and altered levels of consciousness progressing to coma. Increased intracranial pressure and occasionally seizures are seen. Fever to 40°C may occur initially and persist for 48 hours in association with leukocytosis. The pupils are usually pinpoint, although dilated, nonreactive pupils may occur with hypoxia or use of multiple drugs. The pathologic picture includes pulmonary congestion and edema and frequently cerebral edema.

Opioids themselves are surprisingly nontoxic even when used in substantial daily doses for many years. Partial tolerance develops to their pharmacologic effects on the endocrine system. Thus females on methadone initially are amenorrheic, but the cycle usually returns in 6 to 12 months. Cortisol, luteinizing hormone, and testosterone are depressed while the patient is on methadone. Sexual response may be delayed; sperm count and ejaculate volume are reduced. Since street heroin users tend to have frequent periods of partial withdrawal, their endocrine systems are in turmoil. In contrast, a level dose of methadone induces some order, and the effects are reversible when the opioid is terminated. Chronic constipation may persist throughout opioid use.

The major adverse effects of opioid use come from the adulterants found in street drugs and the nonsterile practices typically followed by users. Skin abscesses, cellulitis, and thrombophlebitis are the most frequent complications. Pentazocine injection causes chronic ulcers and sclerosis of muscle in the area of injection. Septicemia and bacterial endocarditis with involvement of either or both sides of the heart are seen. *Staphylococcus aureus* is frequently the causative agent in right-sided endocarditis. Peripheral and pulmonary embolic phenomena occur.

Viral hepatitis has long been common among intravenous drug abusers owing to the practice of sharing needles during an injection session. More recently this illness has been overshadowed by the appearance of AIDS. In 1990, up to 60 per cent of patients in methadone programs in some large cities tested positive for HIV antibodies, and it has been suggested that this group is particularly susceptible to the infection because the drugs may suppress host resistance. Intravenous drug abusers tend to persist in high-risk practices such as needle-sharing and unprotected sex despite knowledge of the danger.

Among applicants for drug abuse treatment, 75 to 80 per cent of heroin users have significantly abnormal liver function tests. These findings may be related to persistent chronic hepatitis, but alcohol, malnutrition, allergic phenomena, and the toxic effects of adulterants may contribute. Pulmonary complications include pneumonia, abscess, infarct, and tuberculosis. Disseminated extrapulmonary tuberculosis has been reported. Angiothrombotic pulmonary hypertension and granulomatosis result from the intravenous injection of foreign bodies, including talc or cotton. Other complications include nephropathy, local arterial occlusion, phlebitis, mycotic aneurysms, and necrotizing angiitis.

Neurologic complications of street heroin use include transverse myelitis, acute inflammatory polyneuropathy, peripheral nerve lesions, toxic amblyopia secondary to quinine, and muscle disorders, including acute rhabdomyolysis with myoglobinuria and a fibrosing chronic myopathy. Septic states may lead to bacterial meningitis and brain, subdural, and epidural abscesses. Tetanus may result from dirty needles.

Pregnant addicts have a high incidence of toxemia and premature deliveries. About 50 per cent of their newborns require treatment of withdrawal symptoms.

Treatment

More distinctly different kinds of treatment are available for dependence on opioid drugs than for any other type of drug dependence. As with other drugs, the prevention of relapse to drug-seeking behavior is the most difficult aspect, as described later. The treatment of *acute overdose* is effective and straightforward. In any emergency situation in which opioid overdose is suspected, naloxone should be administered, preferably intravenously. The patient will have constricted pupils, and a dose of 0.4 mg naloxone should cause an increase in pupil size, respiratory rate, and alertness within several minutes. Repeated doses may be necessary if the patient does not respond within several minutes to the first dose. Absence of a response to naloxone excludes the diagnosis of opioid overdose.

There is virtually no risk in giving naloxone, but the potential benefits mean that it should be tried even in doubtful cases. Two pitfalls should be mentioned, however. One is that naloxone not only reverses the overdose but also goes beyond mere reversal and actually precipitates *withdrawal* symptoms in opioid-dependent persons. To avoid this, the dose of naloxone should be titrated according to the level of consciousness and respiratory rate. The second risk is that the more rapid metabolism of naloxone than that of a long-acting drug, such as methadone, may result in a later recurrence of the overdose symptoms. Naloxone should be titrated via an intravenous drip or repeated every 2 to 3 hours with careful monitoring of vital signs for at least 24 hours.

The opioid withdrawal syndrome varies in severity and duration, depending on the specific drug, dose, and duration of use. The typical heroin-dependent person notes the onset of withdrawal 6 to 10 hours after the last injection. Feelings of drug craving, anxiety, restlessness, irritability, sweating, rhinorrhea, and yawning develop early. These are followed by dilated pupils, sneezing, piloerection, anorexia, nausea, vomiting, diarrhea, abdominal cramps, bone pain, myalgias, tremors, sleep disturbance, and, very rarely, convulsions or cardiovascular collapse. Untreated, these symptoms peak at 36 to 48 hours and gradually subside over 5 to 10 days. Withdrawal is generally not life-threatening, and it has been compared with a severe case of the "flu." There is also a protracted abstinence syndrome consisting of mild symptoms of anxiety, sleep disturbance, and autonomic nervous system instability, which may persist for 6 months after acute withdrawal. Longer-acting opioids, such as methadone, produce an abstinence syndrome that develops more slowly and with less intensity but persists much longer.

Medically assisted withdrawal is usually accomplished using methadone, beginning with a test dose of 20 mg. If 20 mg has no appreciable effect on the signs and symptoms within 1 hour, an additional 20 mg can be given. The methadone can be gradually reduced over 7 to 10 days. An alternative is clonidine, an alpha$_2$-adrenergic agonist/partial agonist, which produces complex central effects that result in reduced central adrenergic outflow. Developed for the treatment of hypertension, clonidine has also been found to reduce many of the signs of autonomic hyperactivity during opioid withdrawal. Thus clonidine can be useful in situations in which methadone is not available. Beginning with low doses of 0.1 to 0.2 mg to minimize the possibility of postural hypotension, clonidine can be increased to 1 to 1.5 mg daily in divided doses over 4 to 10 days and then tapered over the next 5 days.

CANNABIS (Marijuana and Hashish)

Cannabis is not a single drug, but a complex preparation containing many biologically active chemicals. Δ-9-Tetrahydrocannabinol (Δ-9-THC) accounts for most of the pharmacologic effects of the complex.

Patterns of Abuse

Cannabis has long been used in many societies as a form of folk medicine and for relaxation. Throughout the 1970's, its use increased explosively in the United States. Surveys indicate that use peaked in 1979 when more than 50 million Americans reported using the drug at least once, and 9 per cent of high school seniors reported daily use. In the 1980's, the popularity of this drug declined, partially due to decreased availability and increased price. Domestic sources of marijuana have recently increased and use is still common, but significantly less than in the past. The vast majority of users smoke marijuana cigarettes or hashish pipes in groups in which the ritual of preparation and sharing is part of the social interaction. Others demonstrate a compulsive pattern of daily use, with lives dominated by the acquisition and use of cannabis.

Pharmacology

Cannabis preparations are three to four times more potent when smoked than when taken orally. After inhalation, effects begin within 3 minutes and peak within 1 hour, and the subject reports feeling "normal" within 3 hours. Psychomotor effects, however, such as impairment on eye-tracking and vigilance tasks, may be evident for up to 11 hours after a single dose.

The acute physiologic effects of cannabis are dose related and include an increase in heart rate, conjunctival vascular congestion, decreased intraocular pressure, bronchodilation, increased airway conductance, and peripheral vasodilation. Dryness of mouth, fine tremors, ataxia, nystagmus, nausea, and vomiting have been noted. Sleep patterns are altered, and orthostatic hypotension occurs infrequently.

Delta-9-tetrahydrocannabinol is the main psychoactive factor in marijuana. A cannabinoid receptor has been located and characterized in rat brain, but no endogenous cannabinoid-like factor has yet been identified. Psychoactive effects depend on the dose, route of administration, personality and experience of the user, and environment in which the drug is used. Enhanced perceptions of colors, sounds, and tastes have been reported. Time seems to pass slowly, and the ability to learn new facts is impaired. There is often some drowsiness and inattentiveness, which may account for some of the poor performance on driving simulators. *Motor vehicular driving performance is definitely impaired by cannabis*, and this impairment may persist for several hours after the period of obvious intoxication. Tolerance and physical dependence have been experimentally demonstrated with regular cannabis use. This is not relevant to the occasional user, but daily heavy users show clinical evidence of withdrawal when deprived of access to cannabis.

Cannabis contains chemicals with unusually high lipid solubility and thus a high affinity for brain tissue. Metabolites may persist for several weeks, although their biologic significance is unknown. Urine tests for marijuana can remain positive for more than a week after a dose and even longer in chronic users. Positive urine tests have also been experimentally demonstrated in subjects who simply sat for several hours in a room where marijuana was being smoked.

Cannabis derivatives have been investigated for their therapeutic potential in several illnesses. The antiemetic effect is useful for some patients in reducing the nausea produced by cancer chemotherapy. The accompanying psychological effects have so far limited its usefulness. Glaucoma, convulsive seizures, asthma, and muscle spasticity are other conditions in which cannabis or a synthetic analogue may eventually prove useful.

Adverse Effects

Most clinicians believe that regular cannabis use by adolescents impairs maturation and often results in poor social and scholastic adjustment. Although there is no way to experimentally demonstrate causality, cannabis use is associated with poor academic performance. Occasional users have fewer problems, but acute panic, paranoid reactions, and frightening distortions of body image are sometimes experienced. Rarely, these reactions are severe enough to require emergency room treatment. Such reactions seem to be more common with higher doses and with oral administration rather than with smoking, which is easier to titrate. Patients with a history of schizophrenia may be particularly sensitive to adverse consequences of cannabis and should be warned to avoid it.

The cardiac stimulatory effects of cannabis may pose a threat to patients with cardiovascular disease. Chronic smoking of cannabis produces inflammatory changes in the bronchi and sinusitis. Experimentally cannabis is carcinogenic, but clinical studies are confounded by the concurrent use of tobacco by virtually all regular cannabis smokers.

Treatment

The acute anxiety reactions produced by cannabis are seldom severe enough to warrant medical attention. Treatment should be supportive and reassuring with frequent reminders of the drug-induced nature of the symptoms. Benzodiazepines may be indicated in more severely agitated states. For the chronic heavy user, treatment is much more difficult. Such patients typically insist that treatment is not necessary, and they feel no need to stop using cannabis on a daily basis. Meanwhile, they are failing in school or employment. Psychotherapy is unlikely to be of value unless the cannabis consumption can be interrupted. Hospitalization or entrance into a therapeutic community may be indicated, if the patient can be so persuaded. Medication is usually not required to treat withdrawal, and the drug-free patient clears mentally over several weeks. Psychotherapy is often necessary in addition to removing the cannabis.

Marijuana and Health. Report of a study by a Committee of the Institute of Medicine: Division of Health Sciences Policy. Washington, D.C., National Academy Press, 1982. *Critical review of the published reports of marijuana's effects on organ systems and behavior.*

PSYCHEDELICS

Psychedelic drugs include the following:
Lysergic acid diethylamide (LSD)
Mescaline
Phencyclidine (PCP)
5-Methoxy-3,4-methylene dioxyamphetamine (MDMA; "ecstasy")
Dimethyltryptamine (DMT)
Psilocybin

Many drugs at some dose produce hallucinations, but the drugs classified here reliably produce distortions in perception or thinking as a primary effect, even at low dose. This category represents several chemical classes and different mechanisms of action. Phencyclidine in particular is quite different from the others in that it produces, in addition to hallucinations, analgesia and amphetamine-like stimulation.

Patterns of Abuse

Hallucinogenic drugs are among the oldest known psychoactive drugs, having long been used as adjuncts to religious practices in some societies. During the 1960's they became well known on college campuses, where they were used in an effort to "gain insight" or to experiment in expanding the potential of the mind. Physicians in emergency rooms were frequently called upon to treat young people suffering from "bad trips" or adverse reactions to these substances. One of the problems with the use of illicit supplies of these drugs is their gross mislabeling. Chemical analyses of samples obtained from street purchases show that phencyclidine ("angel dust," PCP) and by-products of phencyclidine are often the active ingredient in LSD or psilocybin purchases. Thus users often get unexpected and severe effects. Use of phencyclidine as a veterinary anesthetic has been discontinued, and it is now available only from clandestine laboratories where purity is quite variable. The toxic by-products produced during phencyclidine synthesis may cause severe toxic symptoms.

The use of psychedelics declined in the late 1970's and early 1980's, but the use of PCP continues to be a significant problem in some areas. The typical pattern of psychedelic drug use involves intermittent rather than daily use. Recently there has been great interest in MDMA, known as "ecstasy." This drug has been reported to facilitate insight and maturation and thus enhance the effects of psychotherapy. The drug has never been studied rigorously for this use, however, and thus there is no evidence to support these claims. Similar claims were made for LSD in the past and all attempts to demonstrate a beneficial effect failed. Both MDMA and the closely related MDA are toxic to serotonergic nerve cells.

Pharmacology

LSD is the most potent psychedelic drug known. It has marked effects on serotonergic systems in the CNS, but it affects other systems as well; the mechanism for its psychoactive effects is unknown. The usual street dose of LSD is around 200 μg, but doses as low as 20 μg produce psychological effects in susceptible individuals. Central sympathomimetic stimulation occurs within 20 minutes of oral ingestion and is characterized by mydriasis, hyperthermia, tachycardia, elevated blood pressure, piloerection, increased alertness, and facilitation of monosynaptic reflexes. Nausea and vomiting occasionally occur.

Psychoactive effects of LSD, developing within 1 to 2 hours, vary with the subject, dose, setting, expectation, and mood of the subject. Perceptions are heightened and may become overwhelming. Afterimages are prolonged and may overlap with ongoing perceptions. There may be a sense of unusual clarity, and one's thoughts may assume extraordinary importance. Time seems to pass slowly, and body distortions are commonly perceived. True hallucinations, usually visual, may occur in susceptible individuals. Mood is highly variable and labile and may range from expansive reactions characterized by euphoria and self-confidence to a constricted reaction marked by depression and panic.

The syndrome begins to clear after 10 to 12 hours, but fatigue and tension may persist for an additional 24 hours. The duration of action of mescaline is about 12 hours and that of psilocybin 4 to 6 hours. Tolerance develops to repeated daily doses of LSD within 3 to 4 days, but recovery is rapid and weekly use of the same dose is possible.

Phencyclidine comes in various forms (powder, liquid, capsule, tablet) and often is taken inadvertently when the user is expecting something else. It produces a prompt stimulant effect similar to that of amphetamine and usually a feeling of euphoria. Ataxia, slurred speech, nystagmus, and feelings of numbness are commonly observed. At higher doses, frightening and bizarre visual hallucinations can arise. There may be hostile or aggressive behavior and amnesia for the episode. With still higher doses, catatonia and coma occur, with the patient's eyes open and the pupils partially dilated. Heart rate and blood pressure are elevated. Tolerance to the stimulant effects occurs, and some mild withdrawal symptoms have been observed in daily users.

Adverse Effects

The acute reactions such as panic or psychosis ("bad trip") most commonly complicate psychedelic use. With LSD, these reactions vary in intensity and occasionally have led to self-injury or suicide. Phencyclidine is more likely to produce a severe reaction that results in suicide, often by drowning. Assaults and murders have been attributed to the effects of phencyclidine, and aggressive behavior can occur during the psychotic episode.

Prolonged psychotic episodes sometimes occur after psychedelic use. It is not known whether these can occur only in individuals who have pre-existing tendencies toward psychosis. Many clinicians believe that chronic or high-dose use of psychedelics, especially phencyclidine, can produce prolonged psychosis even in healthy individuals. Overdose resulting in death can occur with phencyclidine. The syndrome can progress rapidly from aggressive psychotic behavior to coma with elevated blood pressure, dilated pupils, muscular rigidity, arrhythmias, and seizures.

Another adverse effect of psychedelic use is known as "flashbacks." These are brief reappearances of the hallucinations or distortions experienced during the acute ingestion occurring days or weeks after the last psychedelic dose. "Flashbacks" appear to be more common with heavy use, and they eventually disappear without treatment.

Treatment

The use of medication in an emergency situation with a patient suffering from an unknown drug reaction can be dangerous owing to progression of the street drug effect with further absorption from the gut and to possible drug interactions with any prescribed medications. Thus treatment of acute panic reactions is best accomplished, when possible, by a supportive environment, observation, and reassurance. In severely agitated patients, intramuscular lorazepam or haloperidol can be used. Prolonged psychosis requires hospitalization and treatment with neuroleptics.

Treatment of phencyclidine overdose may require support of vital signs. Gastric lavage with activated charcoal may prevent further absorption of the drug. To enhance the excretion of phencyclidine, acidification of the urine may be accomplished acutely by intravenous ammonium chloride, 75 mg per kilogram per day in four divided doses, or ascorbic acid, 500 mg every 4 hours, with repeated monitoring of blood pH, blood gases, blood urea nitrogen (BUN), blood ammonia, and electrolytes. If symptoms are mild, cranberry juice and 1 or 2 grams of ascorbic acid given orally four times per day may be sufficient.

ANTICHOLINERGIC COMPOUNDS

Effects in some ways similar to those of psychedelic drugs may be produced by ingestion of the alkaloids *atropine, hyoscyamine,* and *scopolamine* in their natural plant forms. These are found in "herbal teas" and a variety of proprietary medications, and several deaths have occurred. Excessive use of *antihistaminic* compounds with anticholinergic effects also occurs. Psychoactive effects are those of an acute toxic delirium with confusion, visual or tactile hallucinations, and amnesia for the episode. Symptoms of the potent peripheral effects of the intoxication include dilated pupils, tachycardia, dry mouth, flushing, and hyperthermia. Treatment is symptomatic and consists of protecting the patient from self-injury, providing fluids, and reducing the fever. Administration of cholinesterase inhibitors and lorazepam intramuscularly may be indicated in severe cases. Phenothiazines are contraindicated because of their anticholinergic effects. Anticholinergic drugs are sometimes sold as hallucinogenics, thus creating a potentially dangerous additive interaction if a phenothiazine is administered in the emergency room to treat a "bad trip."

INHALANTS

Examples of inhalants include the following:

Toluene (airplane glue)
Kerosene
Gasoline
Carbon tetrachloride
Amyl nitrite
Nitrous oxide

Chemicals that are volatile at room temperatures and that produce perceptible changes in brain function when inhaled have been popular among certain groups as a means of producing altered states of consciousness. There are characteristic patterns for each chemical.

Organic solvents, such as toluene, are typically used by children beginning at about age 12. The material is usually placed in a plastic bag, and the vapors are inhaled. Dizziness and intoxication are described after several minutes of inhalation. Inhalant abuse also involves the use of aerosol sprays containing fluorocarbon propellants. Prolonged exposure or daily use may result in toxic effects on several organ systems, including cardiac arrhythmias, bone marrow depression, cerebral degeneration, and damage to liver, kidney, and peripheral nerves. Death has occasionally been attributed to inhalant abuse, probably via the mechanism of cardiac arrhythmias, especially accompanying exercise or associated with upper airway obstruction.

Amyl nitrite is a yellowish, volatile, inflammable liquid with a fruity odor. It produces dilation of smooth muscle and has been used in the past for treatment of angina. In recent years, amyl nitrite has been used to enhance orgasm, particularly by male homosexuals. It is sold in the form of room deodorizers and can produce a feeling of "rush," flushing, and dizziness. Adverse effects include palpitations, postural hypotension, and headache progressing to loss of consciousness.

Nitrous oxide, alone or in combination with oxygen, and *halothane* are sometimes used as intoxicants by medical personnel. Compulsive use and chronic toxicity have not been reported, but there are obvious acute dangers in the unauthorized use of such potent agents.

Treatment

Since the effects of solvents are brief, specific acute treatments are generally not indicated. When inhalant use is chronic or associated with other psychiatric diagnoses, specific psychiatric treatment and measures to prevent relapse are indicated.

Sharp CW, Brehem ML: Review of Inhalants: From Euphoria to Dysfunction. NIDA Research Monograph Series No. 15, National Institute on Drug Abuse, Rockville, MD 20857. *Good review of clinical and toxicologic aspects of the spectrum of inhalant problems.*

NICOTINE

The medical consequences of smoking tobacco products are covered in many chapters of this book because the effects are so widespread. As the dangers of smoking have become so well known, it has become more apparent that smoking cigarettes can produce a very powerful dependence on nicotine, which is clearly an addicting drug. Cessation of smoking may be very difficult even in patients who strongly desire to remain abstinent (see Ch. 10).

ILLICIT SYNTHETIC DRUGS (Designer Drugs)

The so-called designer drugs are produced in clandestine laboratories, and they vary in their composition and purity. Fentanyl analogues have been produced that have extremely potent opioid actions and have resulted in overdose deaths. Other attempts at synthesis of opioids have resulted in toxic compounds. An example is MPTP, a toxic by-product of botched attempts to synthesize a meperidine (Demerol) analogue, which produces an irreversible Parkinson's syndrome in those who have taken it intravenously. Other chemicals found in street samples are phenethylamines, which are analogues of amphetamine, and various analogues of phencyclidine. In evaluating the drug history of any patient, the physician must remember that those who purchase drugs on the street have no way of knowing what they actually take.

TREATMENT OF DRUG DEPENDENCE

The treatment of drug dependence involves four stages (Table 15–1): acknowledgment, detoxification, pharmacotherapy, and psychotherapy.

ACKNOWLEDGMENT OF THE PROBLEM. Rarely does a patient in the early and most treatable phase of drug dependence spontaneously volunteer for treatment. Friends or relatives who observe the signs of a drug problem must confront the patient. Often the family physician is in a good position to notice the problem early and to convince the patient to enter treatment. Confrontation is best accomplished when several concerned people approach the patient together in a firm but supportive way. Even when confronted with evidence of a substance abuse problem, the patient usually continues to deny its existence, making persistence necessary.

DETOXIFICATION. The pharmacologic aspects of detoxification were described in the discussions of specific drug categories. In some cases, hospitalization is mandatory, particularly when there is a large degree of physical dependence. If, however, the drug taking can be interrupted while the individual remains an outpatient, this can be far less expensive and just as effective. "Treatment programs" that advertise a 28-day inpatient treatment of drug dependence are misleading, because the heart of effective treatment is continued therapy, usually lasting months or years, designed to prevent relapse after the patient returns to work or school. Frequently, the patient has so much cognitive impairment during the detoxification period that he or she retains little of therapy or education provided during this first phase.

PHARMACOTHERAPY. This mode of therapy has been dis-

TABLE 15–1. TREATMENT OF DRUG DEPENDENCE

	Confrontation	Detoxification	Pharmacotherapy	Psychotherapy
Sedatives	S	Diazepam or phenobarbital	Antidepressants as needed	S
Stimulants	I	Not usually needed	Antidepressants or neuroleptics	I
Opioids	M	Methadone or clonidine	Methadone, naltrexone, or antidepressants	M
Cannabis	I	None	Antidepressants, as needed	I
Psychedelics	L	None	Neuroleptics as needed	L
Inhalants	A	None	None	A
Nicotine	R	Nicotine gum	None	R

cussed under specific drug categories. For the most part, pharmacotherapy involves treatment of specific psychiatric disorders, such as affective disorders or psychosis commonly associated with a particular form of drug dependence. It must be remembered that patients who have abused one drug have a strong likelihood of abusing a prescribed psychoactive drug. For this reason, antianxiety agents or sedatives should rarely if ever be prescribed in the rehabilitation of drug-dependent persons.

Certain pharmacotherapies are directed at the drug-seeking behavior rather than an associated psychiatric disorder. The use of disulfiram (Antabuse) in the treatment of alcoholics is discussed in Ch. 14. Opioid-dependent patients who have repeatedly relapsed after detoxification can be transferred from the use of illicit drugs to methadone maintenance. The patient can then be maintained on a steady dose of methadone as a substitute for his opioid drug of choice. The advantage is that the patient is stabilized owing to the long duration of action of methadone and, if properly managed, experiences no "highs" or "lows." Patients are able to function well on methadone and perform complex tasks competently. Methadone may enable the patient to participate effectively in a rehabilitation program, including psychotherapy. Methadone may involve several years of maintenance and must be used only in authorized programs in which staff have received specialized training.

Naltrexone (Trexan) is a relatively long-acting opioid antagonist. Before receiving this medication, the patient must be thoroughly detoxified or the naltrexone will precipitate withdrawal. Since naltrexone blocks opiate receptors, the effects of impulsive opioid use are prevented while naltrexone is in the body. This treatment has been successful in conjunction with a comprehensive rehabilitation program, including a wide range of psychotherapies. Naltrexone must be taken at least two or three times per week to protect against relapse, so it requires strong motivation on the part of the patient to remain opioid free.

PSYCHOTHERAPY. Psychotherapy is generally similar across all classes of drugs. It should be started as early as possible in the treatment program, but it is of little value when the patient is still intoxicated or confused. This treatment is, however, completely compatible with pharmacotherapy such as psychoactive medication, methadone, naltrexone, disulfiram, or nicotine chewing gum. Such psychotherapy is broadly defined and involves counseling regarding job-finding or legal problems, family therapy, group therapy, individual therapy, all types of behavioral treatments, and self-help programs such as Narcotics Anonymous. The purpose of these treatments is to teach the patient alternate behaviors to drug ingestion and to enable him or her to deal more effectively with problems of living. The general physician often can convince patients to join a specialized treatment program and can collaborate in the medical aspects of the treatment. Severe forms of drug dependence, however, are best managed by a treatment team specially trained in this area of medicine.

Hayashida M, Alterman A, McLellan AT, et al.: Comparative effectiveness of inpatient and outpatient detoxification of patients with mild to moderate alcohol withdrawal syndrome. N Engl J Med 320:358, 1989. *Controlled study demonstrating that outpatient detoxification is approximately as effective as inpatient detoxification for the majority of alcoholics.*

Woody GE, McLellan AT, Luborsky L, et al.: Psychotherapy for opiate dependence: A twelve-month follow-up. Am J Psychiatry 144:590, 1987. *This study of 112 opiate addicts demonstrated that psychotherapy is effective when combined with methadone treatment.*

16 Immunization

Walter A. Orenstein

Immunization is one of the most cost-effective means of preventing morbidity and mortality from infectious diseases. Routine immunization, particularly of children, has resulted in decreases of 90 per cent or more in reported cases of measles, mumps, rubella, congenital rubella syndrome, polio, tetanus, diphtheria, and pertussis.

General Characteristics of Immunizations

Immunization protects against disease or the sequelae of disease through administration of an immunobiologic: vaccines, toxoids, immune globulin preparations, and antitoxins. Protection induced by immunization can be active or passive.

ACTIVE IMMUNIZATION. Administering a vaccine or toxoid causes the body to produce an immune response against the infectious agent or its toxins. Vaccines consist of suspensions of live (usually attenuated) or inactivated microorganisms or fractions thereof. Toxoids are modified bacterial toxins that retain immunogenic properties but lack toxicity. Active immunization generally results in long-term immunity, although onset of protection may be delayed because it takes time for the body to respond. With live attenuated vaccines small quantities of living organisms multiply within the recipient until an immune response cuts off replication. In contrast, inactivated vaccines and toxoids contain large quantities of antigen. Live vaccines generally induce immune responses more closely paralleling natural infection and are more likely to induce long-term immunity. Most induce active immunity in the majority of recipients after a single dose; killed vaccines, in contrast, often require multiple doses.

PASSIVE IMMUNIZATION. Temporary immunity is provided through administration of preformed antibodies as immune globulins or antitoxins. Immune globulins (IG), obtained from human blood, may contain antibodies to a variety of agents depending on the pool of human plasma used in preparation. Specific immune globulins are made from plasma from donors with high levels of antibodies to specific antigens, such as tetanus immune globulin (TIG). Most immune globulins must be injected intramuscularly. A special preparation for intravenous use is also available. Antitoxins are solutions of antibodies derived from animals immunized with specific antigens (e.g., diphtheria antitoxin). Table 16–1 gives the major indications for currently available immune globulins and antitoxins. Passive immunization is usually used to protect individuals immediately prior to an anticipated exposure or shortly after a known or suspected exposure to an infectious agent.

ROUTE AND TIMING OF VACCINATION. Each immunobiologic has a preferred site and route of administration. Vaccines containing adjuvants should be injected intramuscularly (IM). For adults, most IM injections should be given in the deltoid. Use of the buttocks is discouraged except when large volumes are required both because of the potential for damage to the sciatic nerve and because of diminished immune response to some vaccines such as hepatitis B. Subcutaneous vaccines are also usually administered in the deltoid area, and intradermal vaccines are usually given on the volar surface of the forearm. Many immunobiologics can be given simultaneously to reduce the number of health care visits required for full immunization. In general, inactivated vaccines and toxoids can be given simultaneously at different sites. With vaccines that frequently cause side effects, such as cholera and parenterally administered typhoid vaccines, it may be best to separate administration by at least a week. With the exception of cholera and yellow fever vaccines, which should ideally be administered at least 3 weeks apart, live and inactivated vaccines can be administered at the same time. Measles, mumps, and rubella (MMR) vaccine can be administered with oral polio vaccine (OPV); OPV can be administered with yellow fever vaccine. For theoretical reasons, live vaccines not delivered on the same day should be separated by at least 1 month. Immune globulin may interfere with the take of live vaccines such as measles. Ideally, such vaccines should be administered at least 2 weeks prior to IG or 3 months after IG. IG does not appear to interfere with the response to OPV.

ADVERSE REACTIONS. Hypersensitivity to vaccine components can lead to local and systemic reactions ranging from mild to severe. Responsible components may include animal proteins, antibiotics, preservatives, and stabilizers. Egg proteins, contained in vaccines grown in chicken eggs or chick embryo tissue culture, are common allergens in measles, mumps, influenza, and yellow fever vaccines. In general, persons without anaphylactic type allergies to eggs can be given these vaccines safely. Persons with anaphylactic reactions to eggs, however, should receive these vaccines only with extreme caution under established protocols (see Greenberg and Birx, 1988).

TABLE 16-1. PASSIVE IMMUNIZATIONS FOR ADULTS

Disease	Name of Material	Comments and Use
Tetanus	Tetanus immune globulin human (TIG)	Management of tetanus-prone wounds and treatment of tetanus
Diphtheria	Diphtheria antitoxin equine	Treatment of established disease, high frequency of reactions to serum of nonhuman origin
Rabies	Rabies immune globulin human (RIG) Antirabies, serum equine (ARS)	Postexposure prophylaxis of animal bites
Measles	Immune globulin, human (IG)	Prevention or modification of disease in contacts of cases; not for control of epidemics
Hepatitis A	Immune globulin, human (IG)	Protection of household contacts; control of epidemics; pre-exposure prophylaxis for travelers
Hepatitis B	Hepatitis B immune globulin, human	For needle stick or mucous membrane contact with HBsAG-positive persons; for sexual partners with acute hepatitis B or hepatitis B carriers; for infants born to mothers who are HBsAg-positive; for infants whose mother or primary caregiver has acute hepatitis B
Varicella zoster	Varicella zoster immune globulin (VZIG)	Persons under 15 years of age with underlying disease who have not had varicella and who are exposed to varicella; may be given to known susceptible adults, particularly if antibody-negative
Erythroblastosis fetalis	Rh immune globulin (RIG)	Rh-negative women who give birth to Rh-positive infants or who abort
Hypogammaglobulinemia	Immune globulin, intravenous	Maintenance therapy
Idiopathic thrombocytopenic purpura	Immune globulin, intravenous	Therapy of acute episodes
Botulism	Trivalent A, B, and E antitoxin, equine	Treatment of botulism
Snakebite	Antivenin, equine (North American coral snake antivenin)	Specific for North American coral snake, *Micrurus fulvius*
	Antivenin, equine Crotalidae, polyvalent	Effective for viper and pit viper, including rattlesnakes, copperheads, moccasins
Spider bite	Antivenin, equine	Specific for black widow spider, *Latrodectus mactans*, and other members of the genus

No vaccine is completely safe or completely effective. Recommendations for use are based on an evaluation of the risks and benefits. Two major bodies make recommendations regarding immunization of adults: (1) the Task Force on Adult Immunization of the American College of Physicians, which publishes the *Guide for Adult Immunization*, and (2) the Immunization Practices Advisory Committee (ACIP) of the U.S. Public Health Service. The latter group publishes its information in the *Morbidity and Mortality Weekly Report*. The reader is referred to these sources for comprehensive information on vaccines, including indications, contraindications, precautions, and side effects.

ADVERSE EVENTS. Prior to licensure, vaccines are evaluated in prospective, randomized double-blind, placebo-controlled trials that are capable of detecting common adverse reactions attributable to vaccine. Uncommon and rare adverse events must usually be evaluated in postmarketing studies. Physician reporting of serious events temporally related to vaccination forms the basis for assessing whether such events are actually caused by the vaccine. Such events are usually called "adverse events" as opposed to "adverse reactions," which imply in advance that the vaccine produced the illness. It must be determined whether the clinical syndrome is distinctive from events not caused by vaccine and, if not, whether the frequency of the illness following vaccination is significantly greater than that expected from chance alone.

GENERAL CONSIDERATIONS. Immunizations for adults depend on age, lifestyle, occupation, and medical conditions. All adults should have a primary series of tetanus and diphtheria toxoids with boosters of combined toxoids (Td) every 10 years. Persons born in or after 1957 should have evidence of immunity to measles and mumps. Rubella vaccine is especially indicated for susceptible females of childbearing age. Pneumococcal vaccine and annual vaccination against influenza are indicated for all adults 65 years of age and older. Health care workers exposed to blood or blood products should receive hepatitis B vaccine. Those caring for patients at high risk of complications from influenza should receive annual vaccination. Health care workers likely to come in contact with persons transmitting measles, mumps, or rubella should be immune to those diseases.

IMMUNOCOMPROMISE. Patients with conditions that compromise their immune systems should not receive live attenuated vaccines. Such patients include those with immunodeficiency diseases, leukemia, lymphoma, and generalized malignancy and those who are immunosuppressed from therapy with corticosteroids, alkylating agents, antimetabolites, and radiation. An exception is infection with human immunodeficiency virus (HIV). Asymptomatic patients should receive MMR vaccine. MMR should be considered for symptomatic patients with HIV. Because of the availability of enhanced potency inactivated polio vaccine (eIPV), all patients known to be infected with HIV should receive eIPV instead of OPV. Patients with leukemia in remission who are off all chemotherapy for at least 3 months may receive live-virus vaccines. Short-course therapy (< 2 weeks) with corticosteroids, alternate-day regimens with low to moderate doses of short-acting corticosteroids, and topical applications or tendon injections do not ordinarily contraindicate live vaccines.

Immunocompromised patients can receive inactivated vaccines and toxoids, although the efficacy of such preparations may be diminished. Patients with known HIV infection should receive pneumococcal vaccine. Those with symptomatic infection should receive annual vaccination against influenza.

PREGNANCY. In general, live vaccines should not be given to pregnant women because of the theoretical concern that such vaccines could adversely affect the fetus. No significant adverse events attributable to vaccination with MMR of pregnant women have been documented, but pregnant women should not receive MMR, and women who do receive MMR should wait 3 months before becoming pregnant. Polio and yellow fever vaccines should not usually be given to pregnant women unless there is substantial risk of disease. Td is especially indicated for pregnant females who are not appropriately vaccinated to prevent neonatal tetanus in their infants. Vaccination is best performed after the first trimester. All pregnant women should be screened for hepatitis B surface antigen (HBsAg). Offspring of carrier mothers should receive HBV and hepatitis B immune globulin (HBIG).

INDIVIDUAL IMMUNOBIOLOGIES (Table 16-2)

Tetanus and Diphtheria (Ch. 310 and 306)

Tetanus toxoid is one of the most effective immunizations, with over 95 per cent protection following a primary series. The adsorbed is preferred over the fluid preparation because it induces protective levels of antitoxin that persist longer after fewer doses. In persons 7 years of age or older, it should always be used in combination with Td, which is more than 85 per cent effective in preventing disease. A primary series consists of three doses (Table 16–2). There is no need to repeat doses if the schedule is interrupted. Boosters are recommended every 10 years. An easy way to remember is to schedule immunization at the middle of each decade (e.g., 25 years, 35 years, etc.).

Following a wound, persons of unknown immunization status or those who have received fewer than three doses of tetanus toxoid should receive a dose of Td regardless of the severity of the wound. Td is also indicated for those who previously received three or more doses if more than 10 years have elapsed, in the case of clean, minor wounds, and if more than 5 years have elapsed for all other wounds. TIG should be administered simultaneously at a separate site to persons who have not received at least three doses of toxoid and who have wounds that are not clean and minor.

Measles (Ch. 367)

Measles immunization is recommended for all persons born in or after 1957 who lack evidence of immunity to measles: prior physician-diagnosed measles, laboratory evidence of immunity, or appropriate vaccination. Prior to 1989, appropriate vaccination consisted of a single dose of live vaccine administered on or after the first birthday. Now, a routine two-dose schedule is recommended: the first dose, which is 95 to 98 per cent effective, at 15 months of age and the second dose either at entry to primary school or at entry to middle or junior high school, depending upon local policy. Most adults are considered to have been appropriately vaccinated if they received one dose of vaccine administered on or after their first birthday. Some adults, however, who are at increased risk of measles (health care workers with direct patient contact, students in colleges, international travelers, etc.) should ideally receive a second dose of vaccine unless they have documentation of prior physician-diagnosed measles or serologic evidence of immunity. Persons embarking on foreign travel should ideally have received two doses or have other evidence of measles immunity. Persons born before 1957 are usually immune as a result of natural infection and do not require vaccination, although there is no contraindication if they are believed to be susceptible.

During outbreaks of measles in institutions, all persons at risk who have not received two doses or who lack other evidence of measles immunity should be vaccinated. Measles vaccine is usually administered as combined measles, mumps, and rubella vaccine (MMR) to ensure immunity against all three diseases. There is no harm if individuals are already immune to one or more of the components.

Measles vaccine is contraindicated for pregnant women on theoretical grounds, for persons with moderate to severe acute febrile illnesses, and for persons with altered immunocompetence except those with HIV infection (Table 16–2). Patients with anaphylactic reactions to eggs should be vaccinated only with caution under established protocols.

Approximately 5 to 15 per cent of susceptible recipients of measles vaccine develop fever of 39.4°C or higher with onset between 5 and 12 days after vaccination and lasting 1 to 2 days. About 5 per cent develop transient rashes. The overall rate of reactions following the second dose of a measles-containing vaccine is substantially lower than after the first dose. Encephalopathy or encephalitis following measles vaccines has been reported at a rate lower than the background or expected rate.

Rubella (Ch. 368)

Rubella vaccine is indicated for adults, particularly women of childbearing age, without a prior history of rubella, vaccination on or after the first birthday, or laboratory evidence of immunity. A single dose of vaccine is 95 per cent or more effective. Many persons receive two doses of rubella vaccine via the two-dose schedule of MMR.

Follow-up of 305 susceptible women who received rubella vaccines within 3 months of the estimated date of conception has failed to reveal any evidence of defects compatible with congenital rubella syndrome in their offspring. Nevertheless, vaccine is contraindicated in pregnant women on theoretical grounds.

Reactions occur only in susceptible persons. Up to 40 per cent of susceptible adults develop arthralgia, usually of the small peripheral joints, and 10 to 20 per cent develop frank arthritis. Joint symptoms usually begin 1 to 3 weeks following vaccination and persist for 1 day to 3 weeks. Very rarely patients have developed chronic recurrent or persistent joint symptoms following vaccination. In fact, such symptoms are considerably more common after the disease than after the vaccine. Other rare adverse events include transient peripheral neuritis and pain in the arms and legs. Rubella vaccine is contraindicated for persons with moderate to severe acute febrile illnesses and for persons with reduced immunocompetence. When given with measles vaccine, it may be administered to those with asymptomatic HIV infection and considered for those with symptomatic infection. Rubella vaccine is grown in human diploid cells and can be administered without problems to persons with allergy to eggs.

Mumps (Ch. 370)

Mumps vaccine is indicated for all persons, especially susceptible males, without a prior history of vaccination on or after the first birthday, physician-diagnosed mumps, or laboratory evidence of immunity. Most persons born prior to 1957 can be considered immune as a result of natural infection, although there is no contraindication if such persons are thought to be susceptible. In clinical trials, a single dose of vaccine has induced seroconversion in more than 90 per cent of recipients.

Adverse events following mumps vaccine are uncommon—fever, parotitis, and allergic manifestations. Mumps vaccine is contraindicated for pregnant women on theoretical grounds, for persons with moderate to severe acute febrile illnesses, and for persons with altered immunocompetence. Combined with measles vaccine, it may be given to those with asymptomatic HIV infection and considered for those with symptomatic infection. Patients with anaphylactic reactions to eggs should be vaccinated only with caution under established protocols.

Hepatitis B

Hepatitis B vaccine is the first vaccine that can prevent cancer (an estimated 800 persons die annually in the United States from hepatitis B–related liver cancer; many times more die in the Third World). It can also prevent acute and chronic complications of hepatitis B, including an estimated 4000 deaths annually from cirrhosis and 250 deaths annually from fulminant hepatic disease in the United States. The original hepatitis vaccine in the United States consisted of purified, inactivated, alum-adsorbed, 22-nm hepatitis B surface antigen (HBsAg) particles obtained from human plasma. Currently produced vaccines are derived from insertion of the gene for HBsAg into *Saccharomyces cerevisiae*. Hepatitis B vaccine, the first licensed vaccine made using recombinant techniques, produces adequate antibody responses in more than 90 per cent of normal adults and more than 95 per cent of normal infants, children, and adolescents when administered in a three-dose series. Dosage depends on the product, the age group, and the underlying clinical condition and can be determined by consulting the package insert. The duration of vaccine-conferred immunity is not known, although follow-up of vaccinees within 7 years indicates persistence of protection against clinically significant infections (i.e., detectable viremia and clinical disease). Booster doses are not currently recommended. Vaccine must be injected intramuscularly, preferably in the deltoid.

Current strategy targets vaccine use to high-risk populations (Table 16–2). Such targeted vaccination has not had a significant impact on hepatitis B incidence, and strategies of universal vaccination are now being considered. Universal infant vaccination is now recommended for populations with highly endemic hepatitis B, including Alaskan natives, Pacific islanders, and infants of mothers born in countries with high endemicity of hepatitis B (e.g., eastern Asia). Universal screening for HBsAg is recommended for all pregnant women, with administration of three doses of vaccine and one dose of HBIG recommended for infants of carrier mothers. Universal vaccination of all infants and/

TABLE 16–2. SELECTED IMMUNIZING AGENTS INDICATED FOR ADULTS*

Disease	Immunizing Agent	Indications	Schedule	Major Contraindications	Comments
Immunizations Indicated for All Adults					
Diphtheria	Tetanus and diphtheria toxoids combined (Td)	All adults	2 doses 4 wk apart; 3rd dose 6–12 mo after 2nd dose; booster every 10 yr; no need to repeat if schedule is interrupted	History of neurologic or severe hypersensitivity reaction following a previous dose	—
Tetanus	Tetanus and diphtheria toxoids combined (TD)	All adults	3 doses needed for primary series; 2 doses 4 wk apart; 3rd dose 6–12 mo after the 2nd dose; booster every 10 yr; no need to repeat if schedule is interrupted.	History of neurologic or severe hypersensitivity reaction following a previous dose	Special recommendations for wound treatment (see text)
Immunizations Recommended for Many Adults					
Influenza	Inactivated influenza virus vaccine	All adults ≥65 yr; other adults with high-risk conditions; adults caring for persons with high-risk conditions, including medical personnel (see text)	Annual vaccination; see annual ACIP recommendation	Anaphylactic hypersensitivity to eggs	—
Pneumococcal disease	23-valent polysaccharide vaccine	Adults with cardiovascular disease, pulmonary disease, diabetes mellitus, alcoholism, cirrhosis, cerebrospinal fluid leaks, splenic dysfunction or anatomic asplenia, Hodgkin's disease, lymphoma, multiple myeloma, chronic renal failure, nephrotic syndrome, immunosuppression, HIV infection; high-risk populations, such as certain native Americans and *all* adults ≥65 yr	1 dose; a second dose should be considered 6 or more years later for adults at high risk of disease (e.g., asplenic patients) as well as those who lose antibody rapidly (e.g., nephrotic syndrome, renal failure, transplant recipients)		—
Measles	Live-virus vaccine	All adults born after 1956 without history of live vaccine on or after 1st birthday, physician-diagnosed measles, or detectable measles antibody; persons born before 1957 can generally be considered immune	1 dose sufficient for most adults; 2 doses at least 1 month apart indicated for persons entering college, medical facility employment, traveling abroad, or at risk of measles during outbreaks	Altered immunity (e.g., leukemia, lymphoma, generalized malignancy, congenital immunodeficiency, immunosuppressive therapy); immune globulin within prior 3 mo; untreated tuberculosis; anaphylactic hypersensitivity to neomycin; pregnancy	May be administered combined with mumps and rubella vaccines for persons who might be susceptible to these other diseases. Persons with anaphylactic allergies to eggs may be vaccinated with extreme caution using established protocols (see text). Vaccine should be administered to persons with asymptomatic HIV infection and should be considered for symptomatic HIV patients.
Rubella	Live-virus vaccine	Adult women of childbearing age who lack history of rubella vaccine and detectable rubella-specific antibodies in serum; both males and females in institutions where rubella outbreaks may occur, such as hospitals, the military, and colleges	1 dose	Pregnancy, altered immunity (e.g., leukemia, lymphoma, generalized malignancy, congenital immunodeficiency, immunosuppressive therapy), immune globulin within the 3 mo prior to vaccination, anaphylactic hypersensitivity to neomycin; administration of blood products should not contraindicate postpartum vaccination; however, in this instance, serologic testing 6–8 wk after vaccination should be performed	Women should be counseled to avoid pregnancy for 3 mo following vaccination; available data on previous and current rubella vaccines indicate that the risk, if any, of causing defects compatible with congenital rubella syndrome is small. The ACIP believes that, although a final decision rests with the patient and her physician, vaccination of a pregnant woman should not ordinarily indicate that an abortion is necessary.
Mumps	Live-virus vaccine	All adults born after 1956 without history of live vaccine on or after 1st birthday, physician-diagnosed mumps, or detectable mumps antibody; persons born before 1957 can generally be considered immune	1 dose	Altered immunity (e.g., leukemia, lymphoma, generalized malignancy, congenital immunodeficiency, immunosuppressive therapy); immune globulin within prior 3 mo; anaphylactic hypersensitivity to neomycin; pregnancy	Although persons born before 1957 are generally immune, vaccine can be given to adults of all ages and may be particularly indicated for postpubertal males, who are thought to be susceptible. Persons with anaphylactic allergies to eggs may be vaccinated with extreme caution using established protocols (see text).

TABLE 16–2. SELECTED IMMUNIZING AGENTS INDICATED FOR ADULTS* *Continued*

Disease	Immunizing Agent	Indications	Schedule	Major Contraindications	Comments
Hepatitis B	Inactivated virus vaccine	Health care and public safety workers potentially exposed to blood; clients and staff of institutions for the developmentally disabled; hemodialysis patients; sexually active homosexual men; users of illicit injectable drugs; recipients of clotting factors; household and sexual contacts of HBV carriers; inmates of long-term correctional facilities; heterosexuals treated for sexually transmitted diseases or with multiple sexual partners; and travelers with close contact for ≥6 mo with populations with high prevalence of hepatitis B carriage	IM; 3 doses at 0, 1, and 6 mo	—	Pregnancy should not be considered a contraindication if the woman is otherwise eligible. All pregnant women should be screened for hepatitis B surface antigen (HB$_s$Ag), and infants of carrier mothers should be vaccinated at time of delivery with hepatitis B immune globulin and vaccine. Do not administer vaccine subcutaneously.

Immunizations Recommended for Special Situations

Disease	Immunizing Agent	Indications	Schedule	Major Contraindications	Comments
Poliomyelitis	e-IPV (inactivated), OPV (live attenuated)	Certain adults who are at greater risk of exposure to wild poliovirus than the general population, including travelers to countries where polio is epidemic or endemic; members of community or specific population groups with disease caused by wild polioviruses; laboratory workers handling specimens that may contain polioviruses; health care workers in close contact with patients who may be excreting wild polioviruses	For unvaccinated adults, e-IPV is preferred: 2 doses, 4 wk apart; a 3rd dose 6–12 mo after the 2nd; if less than 4 wk available before protection is needed, a single dose of OPV or e-IPV. For incompletely immunized adults, a complete primary series with either vaccine is used; primary series consists of three doses of e-IPV or OPV; no need to restart interrupted series. A single dose of OPV or e-IPV can be given to adults who previously completed a primary series.	For OPV, immunodeficiency diseases; patients with altered immune status (e.g., leukemia); household contacts of immunodeficient patients; household contacts in whom there is a family history of immunodeficiency until the immune status of individuals is established. On theoretical grounds, pregnant women should not receive e-IPV or OPV. However, if immediate protection is needed, OPV can be used.	Adults who have not been adequately immunized against polio are at a very small risk of polio when their children are vaccinated with OPV. The child can be vaccinated with OPV regardless of the immune status of the parents. An acceptable alternative, provided the full immunization of the child is not compromised, is to vaccinate the parents first with e-IPV.
Rabies	Inactivated vaccine; human diploid cell rabies vaccine (HDCV); or rabies vaccine adsorbed (RVA)	High-risk persons, including animal handlers, selected laboratory and field workers, and persons traveling for ≥1 mo to areas at high risk of rabies	Pre-exposure *prophylaxis*: 3 doses of 1.0 ml IM for HDCV or RVA on days 0, 7, and 28; for HDCV only, 3 doses of 0.1 ml ID on days 0, 7, and 21 or 28	History of severe hypersensitivity reaction	Further doses needed after exposure. If to be given concurrently with chloroquine, only the IM route should be used.
Meningococcal disease	Polysaccharide vaccine containing tetravalent A, C, W135 and Y	Terminal complement component deficiencies; anatomic or functional asplenia; and travelers who will live in areas with hyperendemic or epidemic disease; may be useful during localized outbreaks	1 dose	—	—
Typhoid fever	Heat-phenol inactivated vaccine; live attenuated Ty2IA oral vaccine	Travelers to areas where the risk of prolonged exposure to contaminated food and water is high; may be considered for family and intimate contacts of carriers and laboratory workers who work with *Salmonella typhi*	*Inactivated vaccine:* two 0.5-ml doses SC 4 or more wk apart; boosters of 0.5 ml SC or 0.1 ml ID every 3 yr *Oral vaccine:* 4 doses on alternate days; boosters every 4 yr	Severe local or systemic reaction to a prior dose	Efficacy only 50–77%; food and water precautions essential
Yellow fever	Live attenuated virus (17 D strain)	Persons living or traveling in areas where yellow fever exists	1 dose; boosters every 10 yr	Immunocompromised persons; history of anaphylactic allergies to eggs; pregnancy on theoretical grounds, although may be given if risk is high	—
Cholera	Inactivated vaccine	Meeting international travel requirements	Two 0.5-ml doses SC or IM or two 0.2-ml doses ID 1 wk to 1 mo apart; booster doses every 6 mo		

*See text and package inserts for further details, particularly regarding indications, dosage, mode of administration, side effects, and adverse reactions and contraindications. ACIP = Immunization Practices Advisory Committee; e-IPV = enhanced potency inactivated polio vaccine; OPV = live-virus trivalent oral polio vaccine. Adapted with permission from JAMA 248:1607, 1982. Copyright 1982, American Medical Association.

or all adolescents is now being discussed as a means of substantially reducing and even eliminating the considerable health burden of hepatitis B in the United States.

The major side effect is soreness at the injection site. Guillain-Barré syndrome (GBS) among adults following receipt of the plasma-derived vaccine shows borderline statistically significant increased risk after the first dose; however, the overall risk, if real, is very small and is outweighed by the substantial benefits of vaccination. Information about GBS and recombinant vaccines is not available. There is no risk of acquiring HIV infection from either vaccine.

Influenza (Ch. 364)

Annual influenza vaccination is indicated for adults at high risk of complications from the disease: (1) persons with chronic cardiopulmonary disorders, (2) residents of nursing homes or other chronic care facilities, (3) persons 65 years of age or older, (4) patients with other chronic diseases such as metabolic disorders (e.g., diabetes mellitus), kidney dysfunction, hemoglobinopathies, and immunosuppression, and (5) children on long-term aspirin therapy. In addition, transmission of influenza to high-risk patients can be reduced by annual vaccination of health care workers in institutions, offices, and homes who have contact with high-risk patients and immunization of household contacts of such patients.

The efficacy of influenza vaccine varies with host condition and the degree to which antigens in the vaccine match viruses in circulation the following season. Current vaccines contain whole or split inactivated viruses of three major antigenic types—A (H3N2), A (H1N1), and B. Provided that there is a good match, vaccine efficacy is usually 70 to 90 per cent among normal healthy young adults. Efficacy is substantially lower, however, among the institutionalized elderly, often between 20 and 40 per cent. Nevertheless, despite low efficacy at preventing illness, the vaccine appears to protect against pneumonia and death on the order of 60 to 90 per cent. Ideally, vaccines should be administered during November of each year, although earlier in the fall suffices if circumstances require.

Persons with anaphylactic allergies to eggs should not be vaccinated. The most common side effect is soreness at the injection site. Fever, malaise, and myalgia may begin 6 to 12 hours after vaccination and persist for 1 to 2 days, although such reactions are most common in children exposed to vaccine for the first time. Severe allergic reactions are rare. GBS has not been associated with any vaccines used since A/New Jersey (swine flu) in 1976.

Pneumococcal Vaccine (Ch. 292)

Pneumococcal vaccine consists of the purified polysaccharide capsular antigens from the 23 types of *Streptococcus pneumoniae* that are responsible for 88 per cent of the bacteremic disease in the United States. Most healthy adults, including the elderly and patients with alcoholic cirrhosis and diabetes mellitus, develop a twofold or greater rise in type-specific antibodies within 2 to 3 weeks of vaccination. Although serologic response is generally acceptable, estimates of vaccine efficacy in preventing disease vary widely. Efficacy may be lower in some patients, such as those with alcoholic cirrhosis or Hodgkin's disease. Evidence regarding efficacy against pneumonia among high-risk populations is not clear. Regardless, the preponderance of information supports use of pneumococcal vaccine in high-risk populations. Indications for vaccine are shown in Table 16–2.

Immunity may decrease 6 or more years following initial vaccination; boosters should therefore be considered at that time for adults at highest risk of fatal infection (e.g., asplenic patients) as well as for those who lose antibody rapidly such as patients with nephrotic syndrome or renal failure.

Local reactions are frequent. Fewer than 1 per cent of vaccinees experience severe local reactions or systemic illness such as fever and malaise. Severe events such as anaphylaxis are rare.

Special efforts should target hospitalized patients. Approximately two thirds of patients later admitted with pneumococcal disease had been hospitalized for other reasons within the preceding 5 years.

Poliomyelitis (Ch. 475)

The last documented cases of indigenously acquired poliomyelitis caused by wild polio viruses in the United States were reported in 1979. All indigenous cases since 1981, approximately eight per year, have been linked epidemiologically and/or via laboratory tests to OPV exposure. Between 1973 and 1984, the overall risk of vaccine-associated polio was one case for every 2.6 million doses distributed. The risk is higher for immunodeficient persons; an estimated 0.5 per cent of these recipients develop polio. Vaccine polioviruses may spread from recipients to contacts, and cases among the latter account for over half of the total vaccine-associated cases.

Adults are at increased risk of paralytic disease from receipt of OPV; their routine vaccination is not warranted, therefore, given the small risk of exposure to wild virus in the United States. The major indication for adult vaccination is travel to areas where wild polio viruses are endemic or epidemic. For children, OPV is the vaccine of choice; for previously unvaccinated adults, however, eIPV is indicated. Travelers who have histories of partial vaccination should complete a primary series (three doses) of either eIPV or OPV. Persons who formerly completed a primary series should receive a booster of OPV or eIPV. Health care personnel who come in contact with wild viruses should be immune to polio. EIPV is the vaccine of choice in such persons to protect both the recipient and any immunocompromised persons with whom the health care worker has contact from exposure to OPV. Parents of children to be vaccinated with OPV may elect to receive eIPV prior to vaccination of their child. Most providers administer OPV to the child regardless of the parent's immune status.

A primary series of both OPV and eIPV consists of three doses (Table 16–2). There are no known serious side effects of eIPV. OPV should never be given to immunocompromised individuals or to a child living in a household with immunocompromised persons.

Meningococcal Polysaccharide Vaccine (Ch. 302)

A quadrivalent meningococcal polysaccharide vaccine containing serogroups A, C, Y, and W135 is now available. These groups account for approximately 40 to 50 per cent of meningococcal disease in the United States. Serogroups A and C vaccines have had 85 to 95 per cent efficacy in epidemic settings, whereas vaccines for the other groups have documented good immunogenicity in adults. The duration of immunity is unknown, although protection in older children and adults probably persists at least 3 years. Protection in preschool children may be shorter. Routine vaccination is not recommended in the United States because of the low risk of infection. A single dose is indicated for high-risk persons (Table 16–2). Vaccination may also be useful during localized epidemics of serogroups in the vaccine. Meningococcal vaccine may be offered to travelers and persons who will live in areas with hyperendemic or epidemic disease, e.g., the "meningitis belt" of sub-Saharan Africa stretching from Mauritania to Ethiopia.

Booster doses are not currently recommended for adults. The major side effects are local reactions lasting 1 to 2 days.

Rabies (Ch. 477)

Rabies vaccine is indicated for pre-exposure prophylaxis of high-risk persons, including animal handlers, selected laboratory and field workers, and persons traveling for more than 1 month to areas where rabies is a constant threat. The pre-exposure regimen consists of either three 1.0-ml intramuscular injections on days 0, 7, and 28 for all rabies vaccines or, for the human diploid cell vaccine (HDCV) only, three 0.1-ml intradermal injections on days 0, 7, and 21 or 28. Testing for serum antibody or a booster every 2 years is indicated for persons with continuing risk. Postexposure treatment depends on prior exposure to vaccine and is discussed in detail in Ch. 477.

Vaccines Intended Primarily for International Travelers (Ch. 290)

YELLOW FEVER (Ch. 391). Yellow fever now occurs only in areas of South America and Africa. Vaccination with a single dose of the live attenuated 17D strain of virus confers protection to almost all recipients for at least 10 years. Boosters are recommended every 10 years for those at risk. Side effects are uncommon. Yellow fever vaccine should not be given to immunocompromised persons or those with anaphylactic allergies to eggs. The vaccine is contraindicated in pregnant women on theoretical grounds, although if such women must travel to a high-risk area, they may be vaccinated.

TYPHOID VACCINE (Ch. 313). Two types of vaccines, a live attenuated Ty21a oral vaccine and a parenteral heat-phenol–inactivated vaccine, appear to be of comparable efficacy (50 to 77 per cent). Typhoid vaccine is indicated primarily for travelers to areas where the risk of prolonged exposure to contaminated food and water is high. The vaccine is not optimally effective; food and water precautions are still essential. The vaccine may also be considered for family or other intimate contacts of typhoid carriers and for laboratory workers who work with *Salmonella typhi*. For adults and children 6 years of age and older, either vaccine may be used. For Ty21a, one enteric-coated capsule is taken every other day for four doses. Alternatively, two doses of inactivated vaccine separated by 4 or more weeks may be given. The duration of protection with Ty21a is not known; the manufacturer recommends a repeat primary series every 4 to 5 years for persons at risk. Boosters every 3 years are recommended for recipients of the inactivated vaccine if they continue to be at risk.

The parenteral vaccine is often associated with local reactions and fever. Reactions to the oral vaccine appear to be rare.

CHOLERA (Ch. 317). Cholera vaccines offer only about 50 per cent protection after completion of a primary series of two doses 1 week to 1 month apart. Peak protection appears about 2 months after the last dose, and protection wanes by 3 to 6 months. Vaccination often results in significant local reactions accompanied by fever. Neurologic reactions are rare. The major indication is to meet requirements imposed by some countries for entry.

Other Vaccines

A number of other vaccines, used in selected circumstances, include (1) smallpox vaccine, which is used by the military and laboratory workers who handle orthopox viruses; (2) BCG vaccine, a vaccine used to prevent tuberculosis, which has very limited use in the United States; (3) oral adenovirus vaccines types 4 and 7 for use in the military; (4) anthrax vaccine, which is indicated in selected high-risk worker populations; and (5) plague vaccine, which may be considered for workers at risk and for some travelers. In addition, trivalent botulism antitoxin (ABE) is available from the CDC for treatment of suspected cases of botulism. Japanese encephalitis vaccine (with a protective efficacy of greater than 95 per cent) is available in Canada, Australia, and various European and Asian countries. Although not currently licensed in the United States, the vaccine is indicated for persons who live in endemic areas or will travel to rural endemic areas during transmission season.

Although not available today, a number of vaccines are under development and may be licensed in the future. Extensive field trials have occurred with varicella vaccine, which is probably the closest to completing development. Because of the biotechnology revolution, it is likely that many more vaccines will become available in the future.

ACP Task Force on Adult Immunization, Infectious Diseases Society of America. Guide for Adult Immunization, 2nd ed. Philadelphia, American College of Physicians, 1990, pp 1–188. *An excellent comprehensive guide covering all aspects of adult immunization. A must for the physician who cares for adults, whether in primary, secondary, or tertiary care.*

Centers for Disease Control: Adult Immunization. Recommendations of the Immunization Practices Advisory Committee (ACIP). MMWR 33:1S, 1984. *A compendium of ACIP statements on immunizations for adults as well as valuable information on other aspects of immunization. This version is currently being revised. ACIP statements on individual vaccines are published as available in the* Morbidity and Mortality Weekly Report.

Committee on Infectious Diseases, American Academy of Pediatrics: Report of the Committee on Infectious Diseases. 21st ed. Elk Grove Village, Ill., American Academy of Pediatrics, 1988, pp 1–566. *The "Red Book" is published every 2 to 3 years and addresses in a comprehensive manner vaccination of children and adolescents as well as other issues relating to prevention, control, and treatment of infectious diseases.*

Centers for Disease Control: Health Information for International Travel. Washington, D.C., U.S. Government Printing Office, 1989. *A complete guide for the international traveler, including required and recommended vaccinations. Revised annually.*

Centers for Disease Control: Measles prevention: Recommendations of the Immunization Practices Advisory Committee (ACIP). MMWR 38 (S-9):1, 1989. *A thorough review of the current measles situation and the new recommendations for a routine two-dose schedule.*

Centers for Disease Control: Protection against viral hepatitis: Recommendations of the Immunization Practices Advisory Committee (ACIP). MMWR 39 (RR-2):1, 1990. *An extensive document covering all aspects of hepatitis B prevention and control.*

Greenberg MA, Birx DL: Safe administration of mumps-measles-rubella vaccine in egg-allergic children. J Pediatr 113:504, 1988. *A protocol for vaccinating persons with anaphylactic allergies to eggs. Also reviews other protocols.*

17 The Preventive Health Examination

Gary D. Friedman

The primary purpose of preventive health examinations is to maintain or improve health. The rationale is that early detection of disease or of high risk of subsequent disease can lead to treatment or remedial measures that will prevent or postpone morbidity, disability, or mortality.

An "annual physical" for asymptomatic adults was once accepted as good medical practice. In recent years periodic health examinations have become controversial: (1) The costs of a thorough medical history, physical examination, and standard laboratory tests would be enormous if these procedures were annually and universally applied. (2) Many elements of traditional check-ups have not been shown to benefit asymptomatic persons. On the other hand, certain simple procedures and screening tests have the potential of prolonging life and preventing disability.

ROUTINE TESTS AND PROCEDURES OF PROVEN OR PROBABLE VALUE IN PREVENTIVE CARE FOR ADULTS. A test is suitable for routine use if it can detect a serious and relatively common disease at an early stage, or at a predisease high-risk stage, when treatment or intervention would be more effective. Furthermore, the test should be relatively economical in terms of both money and professional time. A few tests or procedures meet these criteria; a few others are of probable value but less universally accepted (Table 17–1). Doubts about tests of probable value revolve primarily around the benefits of treatment compared with the harm of labeling (e.g., mild asymptomatic diabetes mellitus), the high relative frequency and high cost of evaluating false-positive results (e.g., occult blood in the stool), and the low yield of significant disease in the asymptomatic patient (e.g., palpating the abdomen).

Some previously accepted tests are no longer advised. A good example is the routine chest radiograph, which has not proved effective in reducing mortality from lung cancer. Additional tests currently recommended for pregnant women, such as screening for bacteriuria or hepatitis B surface antigen, are discussed in the *Guide to Clinical Preventive Services* (see references). Evidence concerning the efficacy in preserving health and the cost-effectiveness of screening tests is slow to accumulate. As it does, current recommendations may be expected to change.

ADDITIONAL BENEFITS OF PREVENTIVE HEALTH APPRAISALS. Detecting disease or abnormalities is not the only benefit of the preventive health examination. Negative findings are also of value because of the reassurance they provide to the patient, especially if the patient has received what he or she perceives to be a thorough examination. In contemplating cuts in the content of routine checkups, physicians and health care planners must weigh the immediate economic gains against the possible decrease in this reassurance if patients perceive the examinations to be abbreviated or cursory.

A lengthy and thorough examination when a patient is first seen permits collection of baseline data that may be useful when symptoms or findings develop later. Also, the additional time spent in obtaining a medical and social history, examining the patient, and discussing the patient's concerns helps to establish a good doctor-patient relationship. Further, certain valuable information can be obtained during a thorough first examination

TABLE 17–1. STANDARD CONTENT OF THE PREVENTIVE HEALTH EXAMINATION FOR ASYMPTOMATIC, NONPREGNANT ADULTS

Of Accepted Value	Of Probable Value, Especially in High-Risk Individuals
Medical History	
1. Smoking, particularly cigarettes	1. Postmenopausal bleeding
2. Drinking alcohol to excess	2. Immunization status
3. Failure to wear seat belts in cars and safety helmets on motorcycles or bicycles	3. Use of nonmedical drugs other than alcohol, tobacco, and caffeine
4. Unsafe sexual practices	4. Lack of regular physical activity
5. Excessive sun exposure	5. Excessive saturated fat consumption
Physical Examination	
1. Assessment of obesity	1. Search for cancers or precancerous lesions of the skin, mouth, pharynx, thyroid, testes, uterus, prostate, and rectum
2. Measurement of blood pressure	
3. Detection of suspicious breast lumps	2. Palpation of the abdomen for aortic aneurysms in men at least 60 years of age
Laboratory or Diagnostic Studies	
1. Mammography in women at least 50 years of age	1. Mammography in women age 35 or 40 to 49 years
2. Papanicolaou test for cervical cancer	2. Test of stool for occult blood
3. Serum cholesterol concentration	3. Fasting blood glucose (in persons at high risk for diabetes mellitus)
4. Serologic test for latent syphilis, cervical culture for gonorrhea, and serologic test (with counseling) for HIV infection (for persons at high risk)	4. Tuberculin skin test (in high-risk individuals)
	5. Sigmoidoscopy in persons at least 50 years of age
	6. Testing for *Chlamydia* infection (in high-risk individuals)

and need not be sought routinely again. A good example is rheumatic heart disease detected by history and cardiac auscultation.

MULTIPHASIC AND SELECTIVE SCREENING. Screening tests aimed at early disease detection are sometimes offered singly, as in special programs to detect tuberculosis, diabetes mellitus, or breast cancer. Clearly, it is more economical and efficient to test for several diseases at a single visit than for single diseases at several visits. Multiphasic screening provides several tests comparatively economically at one patient visit and can be used as part of a periodic health examination. Components of health screening or health examinations may be used for some patients and not others, depending on previous findings, risk characteristics, medical history, or current symptoms of the patient. This use of screening tests is known as selective or discriminate screening.

FREQUENCY OF EXAMINATIONS. It is not clear how frequently preventive health examinations, either basic or thorough, should be performed. The physician must strike a balance between excessive costs and low yield of too frequent examinations, and the chance that an important and controllable condition will develop and become irreversible if examinations are not provided often enough. Several sets of recommendations have been made recently based on available evidence and "prudent" judgment (see references). A common theme is that the incidence of most disabling and fatal diseases increases with age. Thus, basic examinations containing essential tests such as blood pressure measurement and breast palpation should increase in frequency from once in several years in the patient's twenties to annually in the fifties or sixties and older. As age advances it is advisable to observe the patient for losses in hearing, vision, and mental functioning as well. Even if losses are irreversible, knowledge of these limitations aids in advising the patient and his or her family. Clearly, in our present state of knowledge, clinical

judgment must play an important role both in deciding on the frequency of examinations and in selecting examination components for individual patients based on their age, sex, medical history, and current risk status. Many of the preventive maneuvers can, of course, be incorporated into visits for care of illness.

NEED FOR APPROPRIATE FOLLOW-UP. A *health examination is of little value without appropriate follow-up*, including treatment of early disease if indicated and counseling to encourage favorable changes in risk factors and a healthier lifestyle. For many physicians the latter may require a change in orientation. The training of the physician, particularly the internist, tends to emphasize disease and treatment rather than health and prevention, diseases with complex pathogenesis rather than simple injuries, and technical procedures rather than simple observation and conversation. Time spent detecting and correcting unhealthy habits, such as failure to use seat belts in cars, may in the long run do more for the health of the patient than routinely performing panels of biochemical tests. Complementary changes are required, not only in the system of providing and paying for care, but also in the orientation of many patients. They must be made aware that much of the responsibility for staying healthy is theirs.

American Cancer Society: Report on the cancer-related health checkup. CA 30:194, 1980. *A critical evaluation of methods of early detection of cancer.*

Breslow L, Somers AR: The lifetime health-monitoring program: A practical approach to preventive medicine. N Engl J Med 296:601, 1977. *This review of health examinations contains recommendations that emphasize a changing approach for different age groups and the need for cost-effective preventive measures.*

Canadian Task Force on the Periodic Health Examination (Spitzer W, chairman): The periodic health examination. Can Med Assoc J 121:1193, 1979; 130:1276, 1984; 134:721, 1986; 138:617, 1988. *A summary of various components of preventive health examinations and preventive care. The need for a selective rather than a routine approach is emphasized.*

Council on Scientific Affairs, Division of Scientific Activities, American Medical Association: Medical evaluation of healthy persons. JAMA 249:1626, 1983. *A brief compilation of recommendations concerning health examinations at all ages, reviewed in the context of current and previous positions of the American Medical Association.*

Frame PS: A critical review of adult health maintenance. J Fam Pract 22:341, 417, 511; 23:29, 1986. *An updated and very readable review of major elements of the adult health examination with specific recommendations.*

Guide to clinical preventive services: An assessment of the effectiveness of 169 interventions. Report of the U.S. Preventive Services Task Force, Baltimore, Williams and Wilkins, 1989. *A thorough, well-organized review of a large number of preventive maneuvers in the context of the doctor's office or clinic.*

Medical Practice Committee, American College of Physicians: Periodic health examination: A guide for designing individualized preventive health care in the asymptomatic patient. Ann Intern Med 95:729, 1981. *A diagrammatic summary of recommendations that are considered minimal preventive measures for apparently well asymptomatic individuals at low medical risk.*

Oboler SK, LaForce FM: The periodic physical examination in asymptomatic adults. Ann Intern Med 110:214, 1989. *An up-to-date evaluation of the usefulness in periodic health appraisals of components of the physical examination.*

18 The Health of the Physician

Linda Hawes Clever

Physicians are a singular lot. In some areas, their health habits and health are exemplary, yet in others they are dangerous to themselves and patients. The purpose of this chapter is to review available data about the lives, deaths, and personal health practices of physicians and to make recommendations about health maintenance activities for them.

PHYSICIANS' WORK

Physicians work harder than most people. They work 15 hours per week longer than other professionals; take less vacation time (4 weeks per year versus 8 weeks per year for most other professionals); and work more years than the general population and therefore have a shorter retirement (3.1 years versus 7.8 years). They also have unique responsibilities and duties.

Demands of Training and Practice

Tensions develop early in medicine. Students and house officers may have to contend with information overload, sleep deprivation, sexual harassment and other abuse, time limitations, health risks, lack of faculty support, and chemical dependency. They, and physicians in practice, also cite special pressures generated by patients and patients' families. These include unwarranted but firmly held expectations of cure, relief, or certainty. Physicians are disturbed by inflicting pain during diagnostic tests, coping with their own minor or grievous errors, and dealing with dying patients. Physicians feel angry or guilty about working with "difficult" patients or being unable to answer questions. They dislike medical politics, paperwork, and committee work. Public policy changes spawn concerns about preserving the quality of patient care, competition from other physicians and health practitioners, independence, the funding of both research and graduate medical education, and income maintenance. Professional liability casts a long shadow, with a 10 per cent increase per year in medical malpractice suits. The world changes rapidly; morale wavers.

Family and Lifestyle Tensions and Pleasures

It has been said that physicians have one of the few socially acceptable reasons for abandoning a family. The rigors of being "on call" can interfere with family plans. Intensive focus on professional responsibilities leads to muddled values, constricted relationships, and stunted personal growth. Taxing schedules can clash with parenting and constrict creativity. Even reading for pleasure, attending church, and exercise may be squeezed out by professional pressures. Women face particular demands as they juggle family and work exigencies.

Fairness requires comments on the "other" side. There are numerous intrinsic pleasures in the medical profession. Making precision diagnoses, teaching, counseling, providing support and motivation, ameliorating suffering, treating disease, and saving lives are particularly satisfying. Developing personal relationships with patients and their families and earning a reasonable living have appeal. Working with people during crises and dealing with the most private aspects of their lives and bodies provide staggering yet exhilarating experiences.

PHYSICIANS' HEALTH

Overall Mortality

Unfortunately, data about the health status of physicians are scattered and rarely provide comparisons with other professionals. Despite the complexities and challenges of physicians' work and lives, *they are at least as healthy as the general population in most respects.*

For both male and female physicians in the United States, age-adjusted mortality is less than for their counterparts in almost every 5-year grouping from age 20 to over 85. Life expectancy for male and female physicians is greater by over 3 years and over 1 year respectively, than for the general American population from ages 25 to 80. Firm conclusions about the relative longevity of specialists and nonspecialists await further studies.

Disease-Specific Mortality

TOBACCO-RELATED ILLNESS. About one third of Americans smoke; fewer than 10 per cent of physicians smoke; and fewer than 5 per cent of physicians under 30 years of age smoke. It is not surprising that *smoking-related mortality among physicians is plummeting.* Deaths from lung cancer in male physicians in California halved between 1950 to 1959 and 1970 to 1979; other smoking-related diseases had striking declines (bronchitis, chronic obstructive pulmonary disease, and cancers of the esophagus and mouth). Although the incidence of fatal arteriosclerotic cardiovascular disease among physicians *was* higher than in the general population, it is now lower.

SUICIDES. On the darker side, *early death from suicide* appears to be excessive among physicians. Male physicians probably commit suicide twice as often as the United States white male population. Female physicians take their own lives at a rate slightly more than triple that of white American women. Differences in suicide rates by specialty have not been verified. Professionals in other health sciences such as dentistry and pharmacy have strikingly higher suicide rates than physicians. Overall, however, data are marred by incorrect reporting or underreporting, small numbers, and inadequate comparison groups by age, sex, and profession. It is not surprising that physicians may have the same sorts of characteristics that drive others to suicide. These include a variety of family-related markers such as (1) death of a close relative during childhood or thereafter, (2) being single, and (3) excessive or incomplete integration into a family unit. Depression is an important element (Ch. 451). Other psychiatric diagnoses such as severe personality disorder or psychosis may also lead to suicide. A history of a prior suicide attempt is a warning of high suicide risk. Financial problems, poor health, and substance abuse often contribute as well. Special problems that may incline physicians toward suicide include professional isolation, the tensions of training or practice, unrealistic expectations, rifts in relationships, and the exhaustion and emotional burdens of patient care.

Morbidity

The age-adjusted death rate of physicians is lower than that of other Americans, but it might be even lower except for several factors. For example, most physicians *do not have their own doctor* who can provide health promotion and surveillance. Fortunately, two thirds of physicians over 50 have routine health examinations. Self-treatment, curbstone consultations, and delays because of embarrassment about professional courtesy can impede diagnosis and treatment. Fear and denial may slow care. A pathologic extension of denial is the "physician invulnerability syndrome," which is characterized by the conviction that the personal and family problems, the aggravations, and the diseases that affect others cannot or will not affect the physician.

Substance Abuse

There is reason for concern about alcohol and drug abuse among physicians. Reliable, recent statistics are scarce, however. Current literature suggests parity between physicians and the general public in the prevalence of alcoholism. Drug abuse may be somewhat more common among physicians than other Americans. Regardless of population comparisons, of course, *substance abuse is a deadly problem for physicians, their families, and their patients.* Damage to patients resulting from confusion, inattention, poor judgment, unavailability, or psychomotor deficits often occurs before the physician seeks, or is forced, into care. Automobile and private plane accidents are associated with intoxication, as are family dissolution and substance abuse in children of abusers (see Ch. 15). Although denial plays a major role at the inception of addiction and denial makes therapy more challenging, physicians seem to have a better prognosis, with treatment, than other middle-class substance abusers.

PERSONAL HEALTH PRACTICES OF PHYSICIANS

Many health promotion efforts for adults target smoking cessation, good nutrition, exercise, moderation of alcohol intake, immunization, and seatbelt use. The regular use of low-dose aspirin to counter cardiovascular disease may become indicated. As with other health care workers, universal precautions for infectious diseases and hazardous chemicals are being emphasized. The exceptional record of physicians in smoking avoidance has already been described, but other health habits seem to be less exemplary. For example, although most physicians report that they are careful about dietary fat, calories, and/or salt, 29 to 58 per cent acknowledge that they are overweight. Thirty-seven to 73 per cent of physicians do not engage in weekly vigorous exercise. Although most are moderate in the frequency and volume of alcohol consumption, 13 to 24 per cent of physicians drink daily, and 20 per cent have at least two drinks when they do drink. Up to 10 per cent of physicians are problem drinkers.

Immunization

By and large, physicians have an abysmal record of immunization for diseases that can affect them or that they can transmit. For example, only 10 to 31 per cent of rubella antibody–negative physicians who work with children, pregnant women, and other patients receive rubella vaccine. At least 84 per cent of physicians are susceptible to hepatitis B (and, therefore, delta hepatitis), but very few house officers or attending physicians receive hepatitis B vaccine. The prevalence of immunization of physicians for tetanus/diphtheria, polio, and influenza is unknown. Since health risks and costs are low, results are favorable, and the professional liability of not being vaccinated is high, wise physicians get vaccinated.

AIDS and Hepatitis B

AIDS is causing widespread tragedy. Among physicians, it can engender fear, dislike, exhaustion, avoidance, a sense of helplessness, and skewed experience (in medical training and practice). It can also bring the distinct satisfactions of making difficult diagnoses, providing treatment and comfort, solving research challenges, and working with respected colleagues. The causative agent, human immunodeficiency virus (HIV), can be transmitted during medical procedures, especially by punctures with hollow needles when visible blood is injected into the health care worker. The risk of transmitting HIV during a needle stick has been estimated at 0.4 per cent. This is small compared to the risk of transmitting hepatitis B virus (HBV) during a similar accident: 25 per cent. To avoid disease and death, it is imperative for physicians and other health care workers to use universal precautions. That is, assume that all patients are infected with all agents. Whenever a procedure may be damp or wet or fluids may fly, gloves, goggles, and masks, as indicated, must be worn. Hepatitis B vaccine and AIDS vaccine (if and when available) must be taken.

Other important measures during the AIDS catastrophe include continuing education, examination of prejudices, and provision of support groups and grief counseling for caregivers.

TABLE 18–1. SUGGESTIONS TO PHYSICIANS ABOUT GOOD HEALTH

Do:
1. Get help when you need it. Don't deny; don't delay.
2. Fasten your seatbelt—always.
3. Get antibody screening and appropriate vaccination for hepatitis B, tetanus/diphtheria, influenza, rubella, pneumonia, polio, and measles.
4. Practice moderation in diet and alcohol intake.
5. Exercise regularly and sensibly.
6. Engage fully in the pageantry of living in activities with your family, friends, and community.
7. Cultivate your creativity; be interested, not just interesting, and use your sense of humor.
8. Start planning for your retirement 25 to 30 years before your goal.
   a. Feel free to relish your profession, and if you don't, consider important changes.
   b. Get reputable, professional help with financial planning.

Do not:
1. Smoke.
2. Use nonprescribed drugs.
3. Ignore your family and friends while serving others or meeting their demands.
4. Ignore your own needs for personal and intellectual growth.

Seatbelt Use

Seatbelt use by physicians is the least well-documented good health habit. One might extrapolate from other factors that correlate with seatbelt use (such as educational level, regular visits to a dentist, and nonsmoking) that physicians buckle up more often than others. Such a practice would be felicitous, since (1) many physicians drive hundreds of miles per week; (2) each American has a one in three chance of being disabled by an automobile injury during his or her lifetime; (3) always using a seatbelt can reduce the risk of serious injury or death by greater than one half.

Effects on Others of Good Health Habits by the Physician

Good health practices not only improve the health and lives of physicians themselves but also can affect others as well. As implied above, moderation of alcohol use and eschewing of drug use by physicians can prevent direct harm to patients. Vaccination of physicians can prevent transmission of infectious diseases. Of great importance is the observation that *physicians' personal health habits help determine the advice that they give to patients.* Physicians with good health habits (regarding smoking, weight, exercise, and alcohol) are far more likely to counsel primary prevention than are others.

RECOMMENDATIONS

Physicians, in concert with their own physicians and families, need to analyze their own health and health behavior (Table 18–1). They need to assess pain and pleasure, risks and benefits. If change is necessary or desirable, a plan needs to be developed. Barriers need to be removed, incentives and rewards incorporated, and progress documented and celebrated.

Hayward RA, Shapiro MF: A national study of AIDS and residency training: Experiences, concerns, and consequences. Ann Intern Med 114:23, 1991. *A cross-sectional, self-administered questionnaire sent to senior internal medicine and family medicine residents revealed their experiences with AIDS patients, plans for providing primary care to them, and impressions about the adequacy of training as well as their concerns about contracting human immunodeficiency virus infection.*

Koran LM, Litt IF: House staff well-being. West J Med 148:97, 1988. *A large number of house officers at a university medical center were surveyed. Results include the incidence of anxiety or depression, drug and alcohol use, and comparisons of men and women as well as married and unmarried house officers by departments.*

Lewis CE, et al.: The counseling practices of internists. Ann Intern Med 114:54, 1991. *This paper combines an analysis of physicians' health education advice to their patients with their own health promotion activities. Areas covered include smoking, seat belt use, alcohol use, and exercise.*

McAuliffe WE, Rohman M, Santangelo S, et al.: Psychoactive drug use among practicing physicians and medical students. N Engl J Med 315:805, 1986. *This well-referenced research paper shows that physicians' use of psychoactive drugs is not very different from that of other professionals. High drug use by younger physicians and poor education of most physicians about drugs and alcohol are danger signals, however.*

Roy A: Suicide in doctors. Psychiatry Clin North Am 8:377, 1985. *Its important topic, incisive commentary, and 44 references make this short paper especially useful.*

PART IV

PRINCIPLES OF DIAGNOSIS AND MANAGEMENT

19 Clinical Approach to the Patient

Suzanne W. Fletcher

When a patient sees a doctor, whether in the office, the hospital ward, the emergency room, or the nursing home, almost always the patient is seeking help—to regain or retain physical, emotional, and/or mental health. The physician's task is to work for the health of the patient. The doctor does so by trying to prevent, cure or ameliorate disease; relieve discomforts such as pain or nausea; help the patient to be as functional as possible; prevent untimely death; and maximize contentment and satisfaction. (Some have summarized these activities as tackling "the five D's" of health— disease, discomfort, disability, death, and dissatisfaction.) Sometimes there is success in all these areas; in the best of circumstances, the doctor is able to prevent disease and help the patient remain healthy. In other cases, disease and death will triumph, and it is possible only to make the patient more comfortable. In some cases, none of the goals is achieved. Regardless of success, it is important that the physician work on the five D's in every encounter with a patient. By doing so, the doctor learns to focus on health outcomes of the patient and to test the myriad activities of clinical medicine against these outcomes.

In most clinical encounters the patient presents one or more basic questions to the doctor: Am I sick? If so, what is causing my sickness? Will it go away? Will it kill me? Can you make me well, or at least better? If I am not sick, can you help me stay well?

The patient's questions set the stage for the clinical activities of making a diagnosis, determining prognosis, carrying out treatment, promoting health, and preventing disease. These activities make up the bulk of daily clinical work. Although young physicians learn them one at a time, the master clinician blends them so skillfully that often it is difficult to discern which is occurring at a given moment. For instance, when obtaining a history or performing a physical examination to determine a diagnosis, the master clinician all the while is considering prognosis and is treating the patient with appropriate attention, words, empathy, and therapeutic and preventive information, thus ensuring that the patient feels and is better just for having been with the doctor.

DIAGNOSIS

Diagnosis is accomplished with history, physical examination, and laboratory tests. Modern medicine has shifted attention toward the laboratory, but even today most of the diagnosis is accomplished by the history and physical examination, which narrow the diagnostic possibilities before laboratory tests are used. Also, through taking the medical history and conducting the physical examination, the doctor humanizes the medical encounter for the patient and sets the stage for successful treatment.

Medical History

There are standard sections to a complete medical history (Table 19–1). It is usually appropriate to obtain the complete history when a physician and patient meet for the first time.

During follow-up visits active medical problems are the focus. If the patient's presenting complaint is urgent, it may not be feasible to obtain a complete medical history—for example, when a patient is admitted to the intensive care unit or is seen in the emergency room or walk-in clinic. In all cases, the doctor should start with what is most important in the history (the present illness), and according to circumstances, adjust the rest of the history taking. The patient's medical history can and should be augmented at each subsequent doctor-patient encounter.

HISTORY OF THE PRESENT ILLNESS. The present illness is like a newspaper story. For each major symptom, the doctor must determine *what* (pain, nausea, weakness, etc.), *where* (part of body), *when* (continuous, intermittent, time of day, etc.), *how much* (severity), *chronologic course* (beginning of symptom, end, improvement, worsening), and what makes the symptom *better or worse*. It is important to determine what medical care the patient has already received for the problem, including laboratory tests previously done, their results, the diagnosis reached, the treatment given, whether the patient adhered to the treatment, and results of the treatment. Finally, the physician must seek answers to questions that narrow the diagnostic possibilities. This step, the most difficult part of obtaining an understanding of the present illness, requires a great deal of diagnostic skill and knowledge. Skilled clinicians form diagnostic hypotheses early in the patient's story and are able to ask specific questions, the answers to which confirm or exclude a given diagnostic possibility. Parts of the history of the present illness (description of symptoms and treatment compliance) are best obtained from the patient, whereas others (details about previously performed laboratory tests and treatment) are best acquired from medical sources.

TABLE 19–1. THE PATIENT'S MEDICAL HISTORY

Description of patient
  Age, gender, race, occupation, and, for women, parity
Chief Complaint
  Four or five words, preferably quoting the patient, stating the purpose of the visit and the duration of the complaint. Occasionally the patient states a request (e.g., "I need a flu shot") instead of a complaint.
Other physicians involved in the patient's care
  Name, address, telephone number, and relationship to the patient
History of the present illness
  For each major symptom, what, where, when, how much, chronologic course, what makes the symptom better or worse, past medical care, questions to narrow diagnostic possibilities
Past medical history
  Previous illnesses and hospitalizations, immunizations, medications the patient takes, allergies, and alcohol, tobacco, and drug habits
Social and occupational history
  Description of a typical day in the patient's life and how the present illness affects it, social supports (family, friends, and colleagues) available to the patient, and occupational history
Family history
  History of genetically related diseases in the patient's family and longevity and cause of death of family members
Review of systems
  Systematic review of major organ systems: skin, hematopoietic system (including lymph nodes), head, eyes, ears, nose, mouth, throat, neck, breasts, and respiratory, cardiovascular, gastrointestinal, genitourinary, musculoskeletal, nervous, endocrine and psychiatric systems

THE CLINICAL INTERVIEW TECHNIQUE. The interaction of a doctor and patient during the medical interview is, at its best, a marvelous mixture of art and science. The art is the interaction of two unique human beings; the science is from both the biologic and behavioral sciences.

Each physician must develop an interviewing technique that is comfortable and true to his or her own personality. The interview style must also vary according to the particular patient. Some patients are incredibly long-winded; others, right to the point; and still others, mute. Some patients want to control the encounter, some are passive, some are downright hostile. The doctor should adjust the interview accordingly. At all times, however, the patient must be treated with courtesy and dignity.

Certain principles are emerging from scientific study of the doctor-patient interview. It is the physician's job to manage the pace and direction of the interview. At the beginning, the doctor should introduce himself or herself and address the patient by name. It is reasonable to indicate how long the encounter is likely to last, thereby setting the stage for subsequent activities. The physician should communicate total attention toward the patient. Usually, this is best done by sitting down and looking the patient in the eye. Even a few minutes of full attention are worth 30 minutes of distracted interaction.

Most patients do not follow the order the physician wants in the medical history. A patient may include bits and pieces of social and family history while describing the current complaint. It is the physician's job to fashion order out of the story, while still allowing the patient a chance to tell the story in his or her own way. Giving the patient this chance increases the likelihood of patient satisfaction with the clinical encounter as well as the patient's willingness to follow the doctor's advice about treatment. In addition, many doctors enjoy listening to their patients. Over a lifetime, a physician will meet patients from almost every class, race, educational level, profession, moral persuasion, and personality type. The rich variety of humanity can be gleaned by listening to patients' stories told in their own ways.

After introductions, the physician asks why the patient has come. Then the doctor should listen. If questions are needed to help the patient along, they should be open-ended and nonspecific. After a few minutes, the doctor should begin to direct the interview more actively, by facilitating the patient's story with more directed questions. Often, it helps to summarize the history during the interview. Finally, the doctor must narrow the diagnostic possibilities with appropriate questions.

If time is short, the doctor must take charge of the interview more quickly, but in almost all circumstances, the patient should be given a chance to tell his or her story. If the physician takes charge too quickly, not only does patient satisfaction and cooperation decrease, but the chances for a missed diagnosis increase. This is especially true when the patient is afraid or uncomfortable to speak openly, as with teenage pregnancies or cases of sexual abuse.

PAST MEDICAL HISTORY, SOCIAL HISTORY, FAMILY HISTORY, AND REVIEW OF SYSTEMS. These sections (Table 19–1) are far more rote than the history of the present illness, and the questions in each section are best memorized. The doctor should explain briefly each new section so that the patient understands the shift in topic ("Now I would like to ask you about other illnesses you may have had in the past") and start with general questions ("Have you ever been sick before?").

Usually, the social history is least relevant for diagnosis and therefore is most frequently shortened or omitted by physicians. However, learning about a patient's daily life, how the current illness is affecting it, and what social supports the patient can call on for assistance are particularly important when trying to fashion an effective treatment for the patient.

Because most questions in the latter sections of the medical history are standard, in some cases answers can be obtained by giving the patient a printed questionnaire or by using a computerized questionnaire. Both can be set up in a branching manner, so that affirmative answers can be explored further.

Physical Examination

The physical examination is accomplished with the eyes, ears, hands, and sometimes the nose. Physicians in training should practice the complete physical examination on as many patients as possible to master all parts thoroughly. A complete examination, with a thorough neurologic and pelvic examination, takes even skillful examiners a good deal of time. Sometimes, because of time and setting restraints, or because the visit is a follow-up, the doctor conducts only a partial examination.

Several principles are important every time a physician performs a physical examination. The physician must demonstrate respect for the patient and the patient's modesty, making sure to expose private parts of the body only for as long as necessary for a careful examination. The physical examination should follow a standard order and be carried out in a systematic manner. It should be as comfortable as possible for the patient and require a minimum amount of shifting and changing of position. The more uncomfortable parts of the examination, such as the rectal and pelvic examinations, generally should be performed last.

The physical examination starts with inspection, begun during the interview, and obtaining the vital signs. The physician always should examine carefully those parts of the body that are related or potentially related to the reason for the patient's visit. Whenever possible, objective measurements, such as number and size of nodes, breadth of the liver, or the circumference of the calf, should be taken and recorded, not only for accurate assessment of the clinical course of a medical condition but also for more precise communication with other clinicians who may see the patient. In most cases there is time to perform at least a cursory complete examination as well. The less time spent on the examination, the more intently the physician should use his or her eyes to pick up every possible cue.

Physicians should strive to improve their physical examination skills throughout their careers. One way to do this is to pick out different parts of the examination and practice it on every patient seen during a given period. For example, a few weeks of extra attention to the thyroid will solidify and improve that examination, even if none of the patients so examined has thyroid disease.

Questioning and examining the patient are types of diagnostic tests, subject to scientific investigation just as laboratory tests are. Some questions and examination techniques are more valid than others in making diagnoses. For example, the many different ways of examining the breast are not equally good at detecting lumps. As research develops improved examination techniques, clinicians should master them.

Laboratory Tests

Although laboratory tests have become a standard part of the doctor-patient encounter, their correct use is complex and subject to a number of scientific principles (see Ch. 21). One of the modern physician's most important tasks is to learn these principles and use laboratory tests appropriately. The physician must also explain clearly to the patient the purpose and use of tests, as described below. Although generally used for diagnosis or screening, occasionally a laboratory test is ordered as a therapeutic maneuver. For example, a patient with chest pain may be reassured by a normal chest radiograph.

PROGNOSIS

It is important to tell the patient the diagnosis (writing it down often helps) and discuss what to expect from the clinical course of the condition. For many patients, the prognosis of the illness is their greatest concern. If it is likely that the illness will resolve without sequelae, reassurance is often all that is needed.

The most difficult prognoses to discuss are those for lethal illnesses, especially for most cancers. Most patients want to know even bad prognoses, but how much a physician tells a given patient should be determined primarily by the patient, not the physician. The physician has the duty to make the patient aware of his or her willingness to discuss prognosis. Often detailed discussions are best conducted at follow-up visits, after the two have had a chance to get to know each other. The best physicians blend honest fact and hope together, helping the patient through the complicated steps of shock, denial, depression, and acceptance of a fatal illness. Most importantly, they make it clear that they will not abandon the patient.

Doctors should educate themselves about the clinical course of the medical illnesses they encounter. No matter the import of the disease, they should learn how long, on average, the pain of herpes zoster continues, the headache of sinusitis persists, and the patient with class IV congestive heart failure lives.

TREATMENT AND PREVENTION

Increasingly, patients visit doctors not for diagnosis but for treatment of ongoing medical problems. Even when a doctor must make the diagnosis, it is important to remember that making a diagnosis alone cannot improve the health of the patient. Only treatment and prevention can.

Two general principles should be kept in mind about treatment. First, the physician should treat the patient as well as the disease. With every clinical encounter, the physician should strive to ensure that the patient feels better just for having been with the doctor. When prescribing specific treatment, alleviation of symptoms, especially pain and nausea, is often as important to the patient as, say, antibiotics for an infection. Second, successful treatment for an illness, especially outside the hospital, usually requires the active participation of the patient.

Therapeutic Procedures

Therapeutic procedures like surgery, radiation, angioplasty, and chemotherapy (as well as invasive diagnostic tests) must be explained thoroughly to the patient; in most cases, signed consent must be obtained. The physician must help the patient understand what will happen during the procedure, the hoped-for outcome and its probability, and adverse effects of the procedure and their probabilities. Informed consent is a medical-legal requirement, but just as important, it is a requirement of excellent clinical care. Technologic advances in medicine are complicated, rarely without the potential for adverse complications, and often costly. True informed consent requires a great deal of clinical skill on the doctor's part. The physician should act as the patient's advocate. The patient should be given the necessary facts, but not overwhelmed with incomprehensible technical details or a long list of terrifying yet improbable adverse effects of a procedure. The physician should freely give professional advice but clearly communicate that the final decision is the patient's. If the patient remains undecided about a procedure after a thorough discussion, in most cases it is best to delay the decision. A patient who feels pressured by the doctor to undergo a risky procedure may be particularly upset if complications arise.

Medications

The physician's medication order will usually be carried out in the hospital regardless of the patient's understanding or cooperation, but this is certainly not true outside the hospital. With ambulatory patients it is especially important to explain the medication to the patient, its purpose in simple terms, its dosage schedule, and how long the patient should continue the medicine.

It is useful to ask the patient to bring all medicines to each follow-up visit. Many patients do not know the names of their medicines; discussing pills in bottles is easier than abstract medication names. Often the doctor can make a rough estimate of medication compliance by the level of pills in the bottle (although for ongoing prescriptions patients may combine bottles or refill prescriptions before beginning to take the medication in a particular bottle, thus making accurate compliance measurement impossible). Sometimes the physician discovers that the patient does not have one of the prescribed medicines. The doctor may discover that the patient is taking medication prescribed by another physician. For each medicine discussed, the doctor should ask how often the patient is taking it and if there are any problems. If the patient is taking the medicine incorrectly, the physician can determine whether the problem is misunderstanding of the dosage schedule, forgetfulness, an adverse side effect, the cost of the drug, or some other reason.

To help the patient take prescribed medication, the physician should follow a few common sense rules. The most important determinant of medication compliance is the number of medicines prescribed, so parsimony is key. In general, and especially for a patient on multiple medications, the doctor should strive for simple (once or twice daily) dosage schedules of the least expensive effective medication. At follow-up visits, the fewer the medication changes the better. For patients who have trouble remembering to take their medicines, written instructions or pill containers with alarms can help. Sometimes the physician can

refer the patient to special pharmacy or nursing programs for help with medication compliance.

Prevention

Preventive activities (performing a breast examination and ordering a mammogram on an asymptomatic 55-year-old nurse, administering influenza vaccine to an 80-year-old retired janitor with congestive heart failure, or counseling a 45-year-old truck driver to stop smoking) are periodically performed according to an algorithm based on the patient's age, gender, and clinical status. Prompting systems, such as a prevention checklist, help incorporate appropriate preventive activities into the doctor-patient encounter. If there is no checklist or other system in place, the doctor should briefly consider what preventive activities are indicated in a patient of the given age and sex (see Ch. 17) and perform them.

Doctors perform three types of preventive activities: screening examinations to identify asymptomatic disease or risk factors, immunizations to prevent subsequent disease, and lifestyle counseling to stop harmful habits and promote healthful ones. Physician counseling, especially for smoking cessation and dietary changes, is beginning to receive serious scientific study.

It is much more difficult to get a patient to change daily habits than to agree to screening tests. Physicians who counsel patients to make lifestyle changes should expect many failures. Before beginning counseling, the patient's motivation for change should be determined. If the patient is motivated, and most are, counseling should concentrate on the actual steps the patient should take. Follow-up is key. Most patients fail the first few times they attempt to make a lifestyle change. If that happens, the doctor should encourage the patient to keep trying and avoid being judgmental. Success with even a small percentage of patients can lead to substantial health benefits. If doctors succeed in helping only 10 per cent of their patients who smoke to break the habit, it has been estimated that over 1 million American lives would be saved.

WRAP-UP

After taking the medical history, performing the physical examination, reviewing what laboratory tests are being ordered and why, and discussing recommended treatment and preventive activities, the doctor and patient should discuss follow-up plans and what to do if a problem occurs before the scheduled follow-up visit. The patient should be given the physician's name, *in writing*, and should know how to contact the doctor if the need arises. These steps are particularly important in the practice of internal medicine, in which most patient care involves chronic medical problems rather than episodic illness. The patient should be given a chance to ask any questions he or she may have. At the end of the visit, the doctor should indicate that it was good to see the patient.

CONCLUSION

A successful doctor-patient encounter requires a great deal of work on the doctor's part. The physician must be thinking of many different things at once, not only the diagnostic possibilities, but also the prognostic implications, how and what to communicate to the patient, how to help the patient feel as comfortable as possible, what laboratory tests and therapy to choose, and how to explain them clearly to the patient. These questions must be addressed and updated constantly throughout the interview, often simultaneously. The doctor must translate all the above thought processes into effective interactions with the patient and must work to develop a partnership with the patient so that medically indicated diagnostic tests and treatments that are acceptable to the patient are identified and used. Overriding all of these activities, the doctor must keep asking how to improve and enhance the health of the patient, how to change the five D's.

Paradoxically, modern medicine, with its powerful technologies for diagnosis and treatment, requires more than ever that the physician emphasize one of medicine's most ancient activities, that of being a teacher. Fittingly, society requires that the doctor work with, not on, the patient. Although physicians may come to have a good deal of influence with some of their patients, the best carefully avoid trying to have power over their patients. Like great physicians of old, they know the truth of the classic maxim that the secret of the care of the patient is caring for the patient. By doing so skillfully, the modern physician can help each patient maximize the chances for better health.

Fletcher RH, Fletcher SW, Wagner EH: Clinical Epidemiology—The Essentials. Baltimore, Williams and Wilkins, 1988. *This text outlines the clinical-epidemiologic principles that underlie all doctor-patient encounters.*

Haynes RB, Taylor DW, Sackett DL (eds.): Compliance in Health Care. Baltimore, Johns Hopkins University Press, 1979. *A text with many useful chapters, this book summarizes much of the theory, research findings, and clinical applications of the compliance literature.*

Kottke TE, Battista RN, DeFriese GH, Brekke ML: Attributes of successful smoking cessation interventions in medical practice: A meta-analysis of 39 controlled trials. JAMA. 259:2883–2889, 1988. *The article reviews the techniques found to be effective in physician counseling for smoking cessation.*

Lipkin M, Quill TE, Napadano RJ: The medical interview: A core curriculum for residencies in internal medicine. Ann Intern Med 100:277–284, 1984. *The result of the Working Group on the Model Curriculum of the Task Force on the Medical Interview and Related Skills of the Society for Research and Education in Primary Care Internal Medicine, the curriculum outlines objectives, knowledge, and skills clinicians should master in four areas of the medical interview: (1) patient-centered interviewing and treatment, (2) biopsychosocial approach to clinical reasoning and patient care, (3) personal development of humanistic values, and (4) psychosocial and psychiatric medicine.*

Morgan WL, Engel GL: The Clinical Approach to the Patient. Philadelphia, W. B. Saunders Company, 1969. *This classic text and guide to the medical interview and physical examination is especially good for medical students but has useful insights for physicians at all stages.*

Schneiderman H: Bedside Diagnosis: An Annotated Bibliography of Recent Literature on Interviewing and Physical Examination. Philadelphia, American College of Physicians, 1988. *This annotated bibliography lists references on the medical history and physical diagnosis, collected from a computerized search of the medical literature from 1974 through 1987 and other materials collected by the author.*

20 Clinical Decision Making

Stephen G. Pauker

The primary role of the physician is to make decisions—about what tests to order, what test results mean, what drugs to administer, whether or not to perform surgery. Virtually all medical decisions are made beneath a cloak of uncertainty—about diagnosis, the effectiveness of therapeutic alternatives, prognosis. Classic medical education has rarely included a formal approach to decision making in an uncertain world, despite its central position in medical practice. Over the past two decades, normative prescriptive techniques, borrowed from the military and business worlds, have been applied increasingly to medicine.

The benefits of these approaches rest on their explicit nature, on their unyielding requirements for information, and on the ability to ask "What if?" What if this disease were more likely? What if surgery were more effective but also engendered a higher risk? What if the patient is an octogenarian? What if the optimal time for diagnostic testing has passed and the test's sensitivity has therefore diminished? Of course, these approaches also carry significant cost: They are unfamiliar to most physicians, sometimes require extra effort, and always require the decision maker to confront uncertainty and to be explicit about his or her assumptions and data base.

Clinical decision analyses are often confused with clinical algorithms or flow charts, which have gained increasing popularity as media for representing and communicating management strategies. The latter are compact schemata for summarizing a set of rules of "if-then" statements that can lead the clinician down an established management pathway. It would be possible, for example, to translate many of the management strategies in this book into flow charts. Unfortunately, algorithms do not provide a process for creating such rules; they are most often the implicit product of singular or communal experience, although algorithms are sometimes annotated to describe the rationale that underlies them. Indeed, some investigators have used the decision analytic techniques described in this chapter to help formulate algorithms.

THE INTERPRETATION OF DATA

In making a diagnosis, the physician moves continually between two tasks: data gathering and data interpretation. The former task involves identifying potential data elements and deciding which elements to select. The latter task involves modifying a set of hypotheses based on new data elements; those new elements might be drawn from the patient's history, from the physical examination, from laboratory tests, or from the patient's response to diagnostic or therapeutic maneuvers. In each case, however, the new data may suggest new diagnostic hypotheses and almost always will modify the clinician's strength of belief in existing hypotheses. Those beliefs can be most conveniently represented as *probabilities*, the likelihood of each diagnosis on a scale from 0 to 1, which can be manipulated by several basic rules:

1. The probability of a diagnosis being false ($P_{no\ dis}$) equals ($1 - P_{dis}$) where P_{dis} is the probability of the diagnosis.
2. The list of alternative diagnoses must be exhaustive, and the probabilities must sum to 1.0 (thus, one often includes a category "other" in the list of diagnoses).
3. The various hypotheses must be mutually exclusive (thus, if one hypothesis is that diseases a and b coexist, then the explicit hypothesis "diseases a and b" must be included).
4. Among these mutually exclusive diagnoses, the probability that the patient has at least one of several diagnoses equals the sum of their probabilities [thus, $P_{a\ or\ b}$ equals ($P_a + P_b$)].
5. If events are independent, then their joint probability equals the product of the probabilities (thus, $P_{a\ and\ b}$ equals $P_a \times P_b$).
6. If events are dependent, then their joint probability equals the product of the probability of the first (P_a) and the conditional probability of the second, given the first ($P_{b/a}$).

Bayes' Rule

In this context, data are interpreted using Bayes' rule, a relation among probabilities that allows the clinician to modify his or her level of belief in each hypothesis based on incremental data. The technique begins with the probability of each disease before knowledge of the incremental finding. These probabilities are called the *prior probabilities* and are often estimated by the prevalence of each disease. Next, for each disease the conditional *probability* of the incremental finding ($P_{finding/dis_i}$) is specified. Although these probabilities can be combined using the equation for Bayes' rule

$$P_{dis/finding} = \frac{P_{dis_i} \times P_{finding/dis_i}}{\sum_{i=1}^{n} P_{dis_i} \times P_{finding/dis_i}}$$

it is almost always easier to use the tabular form of the technique (Table 20–1) or the cohort flow form (Fig. 20–1).

In the simplest case, the physician considers a single disease and interprets a diagnostic test result, which is either positive or negative. In that situation, the probability of a positive test result

TABLE 20–1. USING BAYES' RULE TO INTERPRET A SPUTUM CYTOLOGIC STUDY DEMONSTRATING ATYPICAL CELLS IN A NONSMOKER WITH A PULMONARY NODULE

A Diagnosis	B Prior Probability	C Conditional Probability of Observed Test Result	D Product (Col B times Col C)	E Revised or Posterior Probability (Col E/Sum)
Cancer	0.01	0.40	0.004	0.04
No Cancer	0.99	0.10	0.099	0.96
			Sum = 0.103	

Step 1: List diagnoses in Column A.
Step 2: List prior probabilities in Column B.
Step 3: List conditional probabilities of finding in Column C.
Step 4: Multiply Columns B and C and place products in Column D.
Step 5: Divide each entry in Column D by sum of Column D and place quotients in Column E.

in a patient who has the disease, $P_{\text{positive test/dis}}$, is called the *sensitivity* of the test, and the probability of a negative test result in a patient who does not have the disease, $P_{\text{negative test/no dis}}$, is called *specificity* of the test. The examples in Table 20–1 and Figure 20–1 demonstrate common settings in which implicit test interpretation is fraught with error: (1) In the setting of a low prior probability of disease, a positive finding often does not suggest a very high probability of disease unless the test is extremely specific; and (2) in the setting of a high prior probability of disease, a negative finding often does not suggest a very low probability of disease unless the test is extremely sensitive. Especially in these situations, it would be important to interpret the finding in an explicit and formal manner, using probabilities as described here.

When interpreting several findings, the calculated posterior or revised probabilities based on the first finding become the prior probabilities for interpreting the next finding in a sequential application of Bayes' rule. In such circumstances, the several findings may not be conditionally independent of one another. For example, in the diagnostic evaluation of a patient suspected of having a pulmonary embolism, the chest radiograph and the lung scan are not conditionally independent: In the setting of a normal chest film, a perfusion scan with a segmental defect is far more suggestive of pulmonary embolism than the same scan result in a patient with the radiologic findings of chronic pulmonary disease. In such situations, the probability of the finding must be conditioned on both disease and on the other dependent findings ($P_{\text{finding/dis and other findings}}$).

Many findings are innately continuous in nature, e.g., a serum creatine kinase level, the size of the liver, and the size of the left atrium. For a given finding to be positive or negative, one must first establish a *criterion* for defining a positive result. Furthermore, to determine the conditional probabilities of a given finding, one needs a separate *gold standard* to define the presence or absence of each disease. Changing either the gold standard or the test criterion changes the conditional probabilities of the findings. For example, if a positive exercise tolerance test is defined as one with $\geq$ 1 mm ST depression, then the sensitivity for the diagnosis of coronary disease would be 81 per cent and the specificity would be 85 per cent (see data in Fig. 20–1). On the other hand, if a positive result were defined as > 2 mm ST depression, then the sensitivity would be only 23 per cent but the specificity would be 99 per cent. In general, a more strict criterion (e.g., > 2 mm compared with $\geq$ 1 mm of ST depression) increases specificity and decreases sensitivity; a more lax criterion increases sensitivity and decreases specificity. The relations among sensitivity, specificity, and the definition of a positive finding are summarized by a *receiver operator characteristic (ROC) curve*, which plots the sensitivity, $P_{\text{positive result/dis}}$, on the vertical axis against (1 − specificity), $P_{\text{positive result/no dis}}$, on the horizontal axis for a variety of criteria for a positive result.

DECIDING WHICH STRATEGY IS BEST

Whenever the physician manages a patient, he or she must choose among alternative plans. Such decisions often involve balancing risks and benefits. These choices often can be made more explicit and consistent by employing formal *decision analysis*. The technique involves seven basic steps: (1) frame the question; (2) structure the problem; (3) determine the probability of the possible outcomes; (4) assign a value or utility to each possible outcome; (5) calculate the best strategy; (6) vary the assumptions and data over reasonable ranges to see whether the apparently optimal strategy changes; and (7) interpret the analysis.

As an example, consider a 54-year-old man with acute myelogenous leukemia complicating longstanding lymphoma. The patient is immunosuppressed by chemotherapy and develops a persistent fever, pulmonary infiltrates, and respiratory distress

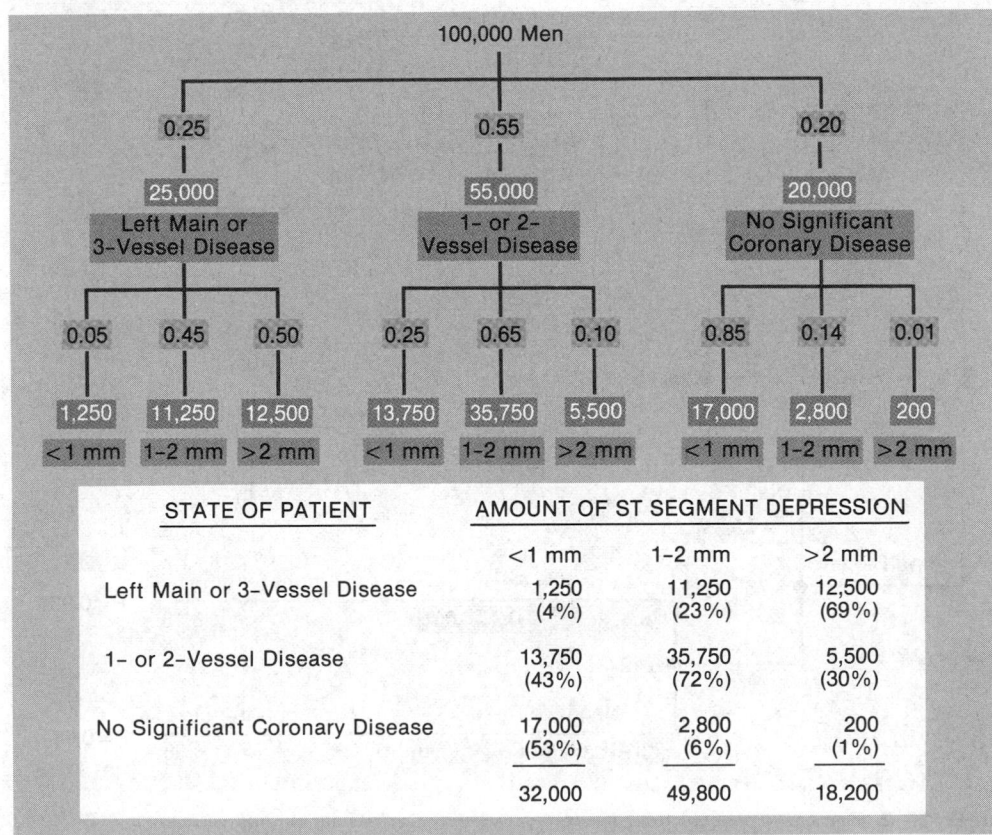

STATE OF PATIENT	AMOUNT OF ST SEGMENT DEPRESSION		
	<1 mm	1–2 mm	>2 mm
Left Main or 3-Vessel Disease	1,250 (4%)	11,250 (23%)	12,500 (69%)
1- or 2-Vessel Disease	13,750 (43%)	35,750 (72%)	5,500 (30%)
No Significant Coronary Disease	17,000 (53%)	2,800 (6%)	200 (1%)
	32,000	49,800	18,200

FIGURE 20–1. Cohort flow model of Bayes' rule used to interpret an exercise tolerance test in a 50-year-old man with typical angina. Consider a cohort of 100,000 such men: 25 per cent have left main or 3-vessel disease, 55 per cent have 1- or 2-vessel disease, and 20 per cent are free of significant coronary disease. If the conditional probabilities of <1 mm, 1–2 mm, and >2 mm of ST depression are as shown and determine how many men from each diagnostic subgroup will have each finding, then of the 1,250 + 13,750 + 17,000 (or 32,000) men with <1 mm of ST depression, 17,000, or 53 per cent, will have no significant coronary disease, 43 per cent will have 1- or 2-vessel disease, and 4 per cent will have left main or 3-vessel disease.

without clear etiology and despite empiric treatment with antibiotics and antituberculosis drugs. The possibilities of empiric therapy with amphotericin and open lung biopsy are raised.

Framing the Question

Formal decision analysis is designed to answer specific questions by evaluating well-specified alternatives and choosing the best. Rather than asking "How should this patient be managed," we shall ask which of three alternatives is best: (1) empiric therapy with amphotericin, (2) conservative therapy, or (3) open lung biopsy with the amphotericin decision being based on the biopsy results.

Structuring the Problem

The typical decision tree contains three basic elements: (1) decision nodes depicting choices, (2) chance nodes depicting events or diagnostic alternatives not under the control of the decision maker, and (3) outcome or terminal nodes summarizing events not explicitly occurring within the time horizon of the decision tree. This problem can be represented by the decision tree shown in Figure 20–2. The three choices are depicted by the decision node at the left. In both the "No Amphotericin" and "Amphotericin" strategies, prognosis is determined by whether or not a fungal infection is present and by the probability of short-term survival, conditioned on the presence or absence of fungal infection and on whether or not specific antifungal therapy is given. In the "Lung Biopsy" strategy, initially there is a chance of dying during the procedure. The biopsy may be either positive or negative, with the likelihood being determined by the prior probability of fungal infection and the sensitivity and specificity of the biopsy. If the biopsy result is positive, then the probability

of fungal infection will increase (the revised probability being calculated by Bayes' rule) and amphotericin will be administered. If the biopsy is negative, then the probability of fungal infection will decrease and amphotericin will be withheld.

Determining the Probabilities

In a decision tree, probabilities describe the present state of the patient (e.g., whether or not fungal disease is present) and the patient's prognosis. In both cases, these estimates can be based on the literature or on expert opinion. In either case, the physician uses descriptions of the past experience of other similar patients to predict the current and future state of the patient at hand.

In this case, we estimated the probability of fungal infection to be 30 per cent; we estimated the chance of dying from untreated fungal infection to be 95 per cent and the chance of dying from treated fungal infection to be 45 per cent. If fungal disease is not present, we estimated that the probability of death during this hospitalization to be 20 per cent. We estimated that, in this setting, lung biopsy would be associated with a 5 per cent mortality, a sensitivity of 80 per cent in diagnosing fungal infection, and a specificity of 98 per cent.

Assigning Utilities

The relative value of each possible outcome is summarized on a single consistent scale by a utility. Such scales can be arbitrary (e.g., 0 being the worst outcome and 100 being the best) or can describe the outcomes in identifiable units (e.g., 5-year survival, years of life, years of disease-free survival, or even dollars spent). One useful metric can be *quality-adjusted life expectancy*, in which average survival is depreciated by long- and short-term morbidities. If such a metric is used, it is sometimes possible for

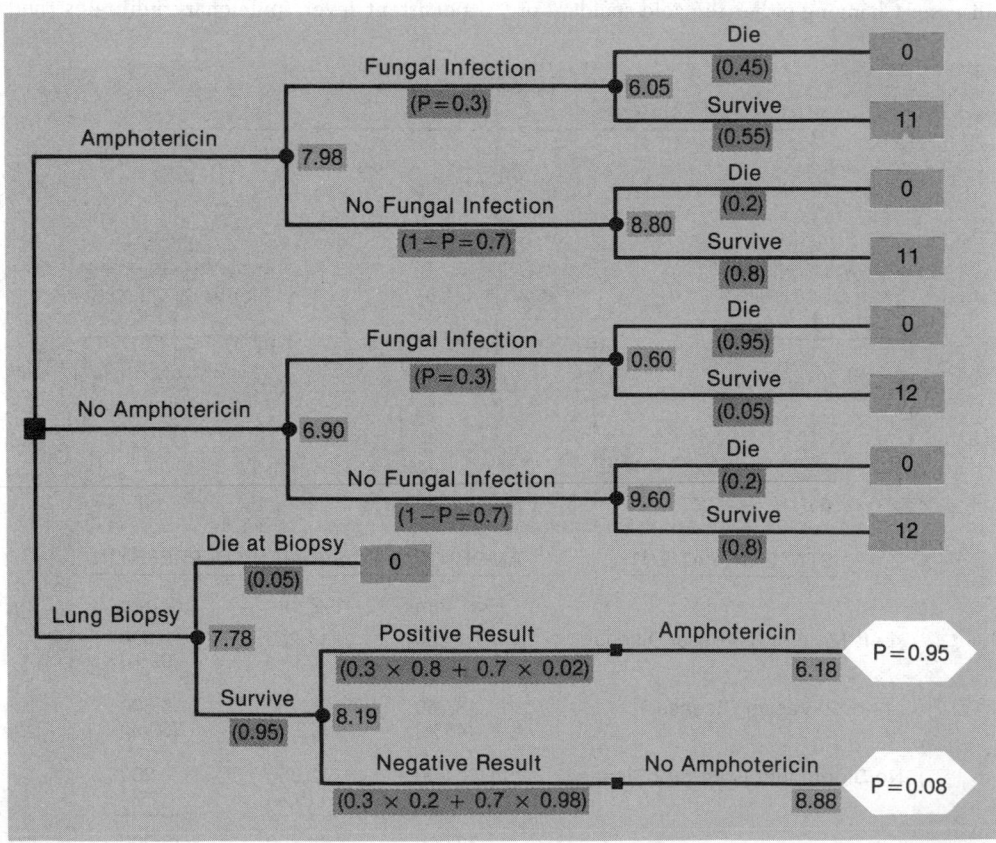

FIGURE 20–2. Decision tree depicting management choices in an immunosuppressed man with fever and pulmonary infiltrates. Decision nodes appear as squares. Chance nodes appear as circles. Outcome or terminal nodes appear as rectangles that contain the assigned utilities (in this case as quality-adjusted months of survival). Probabilities are shown (shaded red) within parentheses on each branch of each chance node. The hexagons at the end of the "Lung Biopsy" strategy represent the use of the "No Amphotericin" and "Amphotericin" subtrees (which are used in the first two branches of the main decision node) with the probability of fungal infection being modified to 0.95 and 0.08 after a positive and negative biopsy, respectively, by the application of Bayes' rule. Calculated expected utilities are shown solid red to the right of each chance node. The sensitivity of the biopsy is taken as 0.8; the specificity is taken as 0.98. P = Probability of fungal infection.

the patient or the patient's family to contribute to the decision by expressing their attitudes about quality of life.

In this case, we shall use average survival modified by the short-term morbidity of amphotericin therapy. We estimated that survival would be 18 months if the patient achieves a remission of his leukemia but only 3 months if he does not. Because we assumed the chance of remission to be 60 per cent, the average survival for this man, if he survived the acute event, would be 60 per cent × 18 plus 40 per cent × 3, or 12 months. Although many physicians are very conservative in using amphotericin, the literature suggests that death and permanent renal failure are extremely rare complications of that drug; most side effects involve short-term toxicity. We assumed that the average duration of amphotericin therapy would be 2 months and that short-term morbidity would, on average, diminish quality of life during that period to half of what it otherwise would have been. Thus, we subtracted 1 month from the life expectancy to account for this morbidity, yielding a quality-adjusted survival of 11 months if amphotericin is administered. We assigned a utility of 0 to death during this acute illness.

Calculating the Expected Utility

In evaluating a tree, the decision maker follows two basic rules: (1) When facing a choice, select the option with the highest utility or expected utility; (2) when evaluating a chance event, the expected utility is the weighted average of the utilities of its outcomes, with the weights being the respective probability of each outcome. In applying these rules, the decision maker begins at the distal outcome nodes of the tree and sequentially calculates the average or expected utility of each node, moving toward the proximal decision node.

In this case, consider first the top branch of the decision node, the "Amphotericin" strategy. The highest distal chance node describes the short-term consequences of a fungal infection treated with specific antifungal therapy. There is a 0.45 probability of dying (utility 0) and 0.55 probability of surviving (utility 11 quality-adjusted months). Thus, the average or expected utility of this chance node is 0.45 × 0 plus 0.55 × 11, or 6.05 quality-adjusted months. Similarly, the expected utility of amphotericin in the absence of a fungal infection (the second distal chance node) is 0.2 × 0 plus 0.8 × 11, or 8.8 quality-adjusted months. The expected utility of the "Amphotericin" strategy is the weighted average of these two expected utilities: 0.3 × 6.05 plus 0.7 × 8.8, or 7.98 quality-adjusted months. In a similar fashion, we calculated the expected utility of "No Amphotericin" to be 6.9 quality-adjusted months.

Next we consider the lowest branch of the main decision node: the "Lung Biopsy" strategy. As depicted at the end of the "Positive" result branch, the expected utility is calculated using the "Amphotericin" subtree, with the probability of fungal infection being increased to 0.95. In that case, the expected utility is 0.95 × 6.05 plus 0.05 × 8.8, or 6.18 quality-adjusted months. Similarly, the expected utility of the "Negative" result branch is calculated with the "No Amphotericin" subtree, with the probability of fungal infection being decreased to 0.08, yielding 0.08 × 0.6 plus 0.92 × 9.6, or 8.88 quality-adjusted months. The weighted average of these expected utilities depends on the probability of a positive result (0.3 × 0.8 plus 0.7 × 0.02, or 0.25). The expected utility of the entire strategy is a weighted average of this result (8.19 quality-adjusted months) and the 5 per cent chance of a procedure-related death (utility 0), providing an expected utility of 7.78 quality-adjusted months.

Performing Sensitivity Analyses

Having calculated the expected utility in the baseline case, we next examine various central assumptions to determine whether reasonable variations in those assumed values will change the conclusions. Such sensitivity analyses initially examine variables one at a time, usually beginning with the "softest" data. Such analyses are often called *one-way sensitivity analyses* (see Fig. 20-3).

Typically, one strategy will be best for all values of the variable below a certain cutoff, and another strategy will be best for all values above that cutoff. The value at which the strategies have equal expected utility is called the *threshold* value for that variable. In addition to finding relevant threshold values, it is

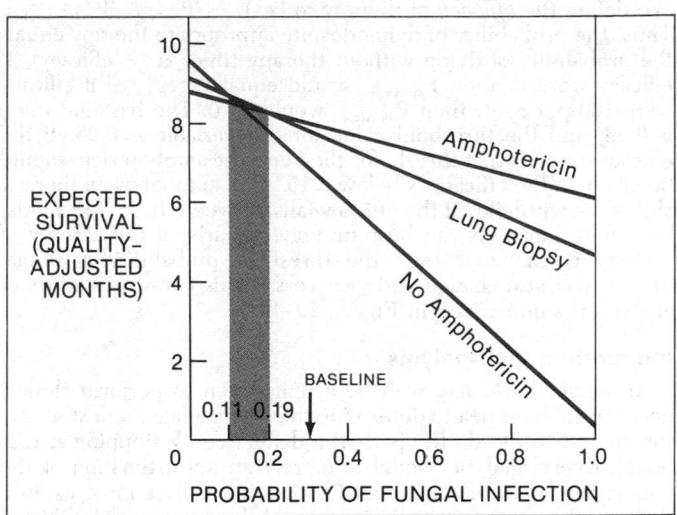

FIGURE 20–3. One-way sensitivity analysis of the effect of changing the probability of fungal infection in the decision tree shown in Figure 20–2. If the probability of fungal infection is zero, then the "No Amphotericin" strategy is best. If the probability of fungal infection is 100 per cent, then empiric amphotericin therapy is best. Lung biopsy is the optimal strategy in the narrow region between the two thresholds (vertical color bar) at 0.11 and 0.19. The baseline value of 0.3 is shown by the arrow.

often important to examine the magnitude of the differences in expected values of the various strategies. If those differences are very small and potentially clinically insignificant, then the decision may well be a *close call*, and there may be relatively little to gain or lose in selecting one management plan over another. With sufficient time and energy or with adequate computational support, the clinician also can examine the effect of simultaneous changes in two or more variables. Such multiway sensitivity analyses are often summarized by decision diagrams that specify the best strategy for each combination of values (see Fig. 20–4).

In this case, the softest piece of data is the likelihood that this patient has a fungal infection. The one-way sensitivity analysis of this variable is summarized in Figure 20–3. Another central variable is the effectiveness of amphotericin in enhancing survival in an immunosuppressed patient known to have fungal disease.

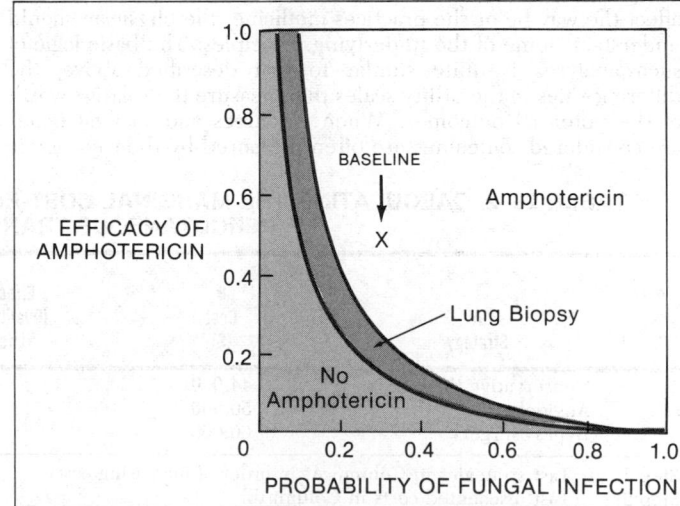

FIGURE 20–4. Two-way sensitivity analysis of the relation between the probability of fungal infection (horizontal axis) and the efficacy of amphotericin (vertical axis). Each combination of values corresponds to a unique point on the graph. All combinations falling in the lighter shaded area correspond to settings in which "no amphotericin" is the best strategy. All combinations falling in the darker shaded area correspond to settings in which "lung biopsy" is best. The baseline values correspond to the bold X, which lies within the settings in which amphotericin is best.

We define the *efficacy* of therapy to be $1 - (P_{die/Ampho}/P_{die/No\ Ampho})$. Thus, the probability of dying despite appropriate therapy equals the probability of dying without therapy times $(1 - efficacy)$. If efficacy were 0, then $P_{die/Ampho}$ would equal $P_{die/No\ Ampho}$; if efficacy were 100 per cent, then $P_{die/Ampho}$ would be 0. The baseline value is 0.53, and the threshold value for this variable is 0.28. If the efficacy exceeds that threshold, then empiric amphotericin should be given. If the efficacy is below 0.15, then amphotericin therapy should be withheld. If the efficacy falls between these thresholds, then lung biopsy is the best strategy. Clearly, if the efficacy of therapy is changed, then the threshold probability of fungal disease will also change and vice versa. This two-way sensitivity analysis is summarized in Figure 20–4.

Interpreting the Analysis

Although there may well be a temptation to perform clinical decision analyses just to determine the best management strategy, the analyst would do the patient a disservice by stopping at that point. Every analytic model is merely an approximation of the underlying medical dilemma. The careful analyst must explore the model to discover its limitations. Only then can the clinician have reasonable confidence in its conclusions. One of the central benefits of a clinical decision analysis should be a better understanding of the clinical problem and a delineation of the settings in which the planned strategy is proper.

In this analysis, we see that empiric therapy with amphotericin is appropriate for any patient who has at least a moderate likelihood (over 20 per cent) of fungal infection. Therapy based on the results of lung biopsy is best only for the narrow wedge of patients falling in the darker shaded region of Figure 20–4. This region would be broadened if lung biopsy had a lower complication rate but would still be limited by the imperfect sensitivity of the test: Some patients with potentially treatable fungal infections would be denied therapy if their biopsy yielded falsely negative results. The major driving force is the surprisingly benign characteristics of amphotericin. Although patients receiving the drug have significant short-term morbidity, very few develop permanent renal insufficiency and even fewer die.

COST-BENEFIT AND COST-EFFECTIVENESS ANALYSES

The practice of medicine in a world of limited resources sometimes leads physicians to consider not only what is "best" for the patient but also the resources that such medical care will use. In such contexts, cost-benefit and cost-effectiveness analyses can be used to establish policies. Because those policies may affect the way he or she practices medicine, the physician should understand some of the underlying principles. The basic logic of such analyses is quite similar to that described above; the difference lies in the utility scales that measure the relative worth of the potential outcomes. When resources and societal issues are considered, outcomes are often measured by their economic

impact. Economists argue that the magnitude of a cost depends on, among other things, *when* that cost is incurred. Money saved or spent immediately is worth more than money saved or spent in the future. This principle is called the *discounting* of future benefits and costs: Future costs and benefits are diminished by a fixed proportion for each year into the future when such cost and benefits occur. When several different utilities are considered (e.g., survival and economic costs), some analysts argue that all utility scales should be discounted at the same rate; other analysts argue that discounting should be restricted to monetary factors. When considering the economics of medical care, we should be careful to distinguish actual *costs* from *charges*, which may be quite distorted by particular billing practices or insurance plans. We also should consider *indirect costs* (e.g., heating and cleaning in the hospital and even malpractice insurance) and *induced costs* (e.g., the diagnostic evaluation of patients with falsely positive screening test results and even the medical care for treating cancer that develops years later in a patient who is "saved" from tuberculous pneumonia). Even among true direct costs, we must distinguish between *average* costs and *variable* costs (e.g., if a new policy eliminates the need for 30 creatine phosphokinase tests each day, the hospital may not be able to decrease its laboratory personnel and thus may save only part of the cost of the tests).

In a *cost-benefit analysis*, economic impact is the only utility scale used: All benefits are measured in those terms. Thus, if a strategy increases survival, that benefit is translated into its monetary equivalent: Each year of life saved would be associated with a societal worth, perhaps based on economic productivity. If the benefits minus the costs of a given strategy are positive, the program contributes in the net to society. Presumably, the bigger the difference, the larger the contribution. If the costs of a strategy exceed its benefits, the program should not necessarily be rejected. Society might well wish to underwrite such a program. For example, extending the life of a disabled, elderly nursing home resident might not provide net economic benefit to society, but our ethical values argue strongly against withdrawing care from such individuals.

Because the economic value of life and improved quality of life are difficult to quantify, we often turn to *cost-effectiveness analyses*, in which two separate utility measures are analyzed simultaneously, e.g., monetary costs and years of life saved. The results are expressed as the *ratio* of cost to benefits. That ratio does not measure the overall worth of a single strategy; rather, it is used to compare strategies. Often the strategy that engenders greater resource costs is also the strategy that provides the greater effectiveness. Thus, one usually examines the ratio of the difference in costs to the difference in effectiveness (the *marginal cost-effectiveness ratio*), which might be expressed as additional dollars spent per additional year of life saved or even as additional dollars spent per additional cancer detected (Table 20–2). Such analyses rarely tell the decision maker in an absolute sense which strategy is best: They provide only a measure of cost per unit of gain. Some external standard, perhaps established by society, must be applied to decide how much money is too much to spend to gain

TABLE 20–2. CALCULATING THE MARGINAL COST-EFFECTIVENESS OF CORONARY BYPASS SURGERY AND PERCUTANEOUS TRANSLUMINAL ANGIOPLASTY*

A Strategy	B Cost ($)	C Effectiveness (Quality-Adjusted Life Years)	D Marginal Cost ($)	E Marginal Effectiveness (QALY)	F Marginal C/E Ratio ($/QALY)
Conservative therapy	44,000	5.8			
Angioplasty	50,000	6.7	6,000	0.9	6,667
Bypass surgery	60,000	7.2	10,000	0.5	20,000

Step 1:   List strategies in Column A, in order of increasing cost.
Step 2:   List discounted costs in Column B.
Step 3:   List discounted effectivenesses in Column C.
Step 4:   Calculate marginal (additional) cost of each strategy compared to next least expensive alternative (a strategy pair) and record in Colmun D.
Step 5:   For each strategy pair, calculate marginal (additional) effectiveness achieved for that marginal cost and record in column E.
Step 6:   If entry in Column E is negative, then that next least expensive strategy has higher effectiveness and this strategy is dominated and eliminated from consideration.
Step 7:   Divide each value in Column D by corresponding value in Column E and record marginal cost-effectiveness ratio in column F.

*For a 55-year-old man with chronic stable angina in terms of additional cost per quality-adjusted life year gained (three-vessel disease and depressed ejection fraction)

a year of life. Such analyses can also help when we must choose among alternate uses for a fixed amount of resource, i.e., a budget. When we have only another $100,000 to spend, should we "buy" one heart transplant, five coronary bypass operations, or a year of therapy for 1000 hypertensive men? These are difficult decisions, but physicians must now contribute to the discussion, hopefully in a logical, explicit, and useful way.

Diamond GA, Forrester JS: Analysis of probability as an aid in the clinical diagnosis of coronary-artery disease. N Engl J Med 300:1350, 1979. *Provides data and techniques for the interpretation of exercise testing in the context of various clinical presentations of coronary disease.*

Gottlieb JE, Pauker SG: Whether or not to administer amphotericin B to an immunosuppressed patient with hematologic malignancy and undiagnosed fever. Med Decision Making 1:75, 1981. *The detailed clinical decision analysis that forms the basis for the amphotericin decision model.*

Griner PF, Mayesski RJ, Mushlin AI, et al.: Selection and interpretation of diagnostic tests and procedures. Ann Intern Med 94:553, 1981. *Primer on Bayes' rule with many examples.*

Kassirer JP: The principles of clinical decision making: An introduction to decision analysis. Yale J Biol 49:149, 1976. *Conversational introduction to building decision trees for professional football and medicine.*

Kassirer JP, Moskowitz AJ, Lau J, et al.: Decision analysis: A progress report. Ann Intern Med 106:275, 1987. *Review of the literature and classification of techniques and clinical questions.*

Lusted LB: Introduction To Medical Decision Making. Springfield, Ill., Charles C Thomas, 1968. *One of the first monographs suggesting how probability theory could be applied to medicine.*

McNeil BJ, Keeler E, Adelstein SJ: Primer on certain elements of medical decision making. N Engl J Med 293:211, 1975. *General introduction to Bayes' rule, ROC analysis, and information theory.*

Pauker SG, Kassirer JP: Medical progress: Decision analysis. N Engl J Med 316:250, 1987. *A tutorial about new techniques.*

Plante DA, Kassirer JP, Zarin DA, et al.: A clinical decision consultation service. Am J Med 80:1169, 1986. *Description of experience using clinical decision analysis in the care of individual patients.*

Raiffa H: Decision Analysis: Introductory Lectures on Choices Under Uncertainty. Reading, Mass., Addison-Wesley, 1968. *The classic introduction to decision theory for business students.*

Sox HC, Blatt MA, Higgins MC, et al.: Medical Decision Making. Boston, Butterworths, 1988. *Very readable compact introduction for students and practitioners.*

Wong JB, Sonnenberg FA, Salem DN, et al.: Myocardial revascularization for chronic stable angina: An analysis of the role of percutaneous transluminal coronary angioplasty based on data available in 1989. Ann Intern Med (in press). *A detailed cost-effectiveness analysis of revascularization for chronic stable angina.*

Weinstein MC, Fineberg HV, Elstein AS, et al.: Clinical Decision Analysis. Philadelphia, W.B. Saunders Company, 1980. *Overall introduction replete with examples.*

21 The Use and Interpretation of Laboratory-Derived Data

James B. Wyngaarden

The basic workup of a patient begins with the acquisition of information. The experienced clinician will acquire a discerning and sensitive history and perform a thorough physical examination and such laboratory tests as may be necessary to evaluate the general health of the patient, to arrive at a specific diagnosis, to assess the functional status of involved organs, or to provide a basis for monitoring effectiveness of therapy.

Until two decades ago only a few laboratory tests were performed routinely in the workup of a patient. When screening was practiced, the panel of tests was usually limited to hemoglobin (or hematocrit) determination, blood cell counts, urinalysis, stool examination for occult blood, and perhaps a chest radiograph and an electrocardiogram, particularly in adults. Additional tests were ordered only when suggested by the clinical assessment. In this setting an attending physician could evaluate the reasoning process that led a physician in training to order a serum calcium determination or a serum alkaline phosphatase assay. The ordering of laboratory procedures was a consequence of the intellectual discipline of constructing a logical differential diagnosis or of the need to monitor the progress of a patient, e.g., one in diabetic ketoacidosis. Thus it was a vital component of the educational process itself.

In 1966 Thiers published a provocative study comparing the results of a screening battery of 11 tests run by an automated multichannel analyzer with those of tests specifically ordered on the same patients by physicians as part of the admission workup. The screening battery detected twice as many abnormal test results as were uncovered by selective ordering. The most common findings were elevated glucose and uric acid concentrations. Ensuing developments were rapid. Ingenious automated analyzers brought an increasing number and variety of tests within the reach of all practitioners. The cost of such a screening battery fell rapidly until soon one could obtain 12 to 18 test results for no more than the cost of 3 or 4 selected tests run manually a decade earlier.

The inclusion of a panel of chemical tests or enzyme assays of blood (or urine) became a routine component of a basic medical workup. For more than a decade, medical students and resident physicians have been brought up with a dependency upon such screening batteries of chemical measurements. Only a few hospitals resisted the temptation to institute such screening procedures and continued the traditional practice of letting the intellectual evaluation of the patient determine the indications for further laboratory procedures. The pendulum has now begun to swing back, as the limited utility of large panel testing has become more generally recognized. Only a small number of "screening tests" (history, physical examination, stool guaiac test, and blood pressure measurement) have actually been shown to improve the health outcome of asymptomatic outpatients. Admission screening tests, such as a "Chem 12," complete blood count, and sedimentation rate, have a relatively low yield: Fewer than 1 per cent lead to a "new" diagnosis. In fact, fewer than 10 per cent of Chem 12 data are ever used clinically, and as few as 40 per cent of "abnormal" results initiate a follow-up. Furthermore, unnecessary hospitalization has occurred when one laboratory test result of a screening panel was "abnormal" by chance on a statistical basis alone. Whenever 20 procedures are done, whose "normal" range is defined as the central 95 per cent segment, one test result will, on the average, fall outside this range on the basis of chance alone, in 64 per cent of instances $[1 - (0.95^{20} = 0.36) \times 100]$. Statistically, 46 per cent of all Chem 12 panels performed on healthy individuals will result in one "abnormal" result. Repetition of tests showing such aberrant results contributes to the high cost of medical care, but only rarely to the detection of significant dysfunction or disease. As a consequence of this additional experience, some large teaching hospitals have discontinued screening panels. This movement has been accelerated by the exclusion of routine screening procedures from the list of reimbursable expenditures by some third-party payers of medical services.

In order to utilize the results of laboratory tests intelligently (and economically), the physician must be able to evaluate the validity of the test result, understand principles of variation and distribution of values, and integrate the data received from the laboratory with the information acquired from the patient. If the test result deviates from values found in a healthy control population, is the difference trivial, or is it indicative of important dysfunction? Should the test be repeated? How often need a particular measurement be followed up? What additional tests or studies are indicated on the basis of these leads?

The more information the physician has, the more effective the physician should be in caring for the patient. To ensure that this is the result requires knowledge of science and medicine, clinical judgment, and a profound respect for the limitations of the laboratory. One of the best ways of acquiring the constructively critical attitude so essential to the proper evaluation of laboratory data is to work in a laboratory for a while. There is a paradox in the present pattern of medical education: At a time of increasing reliance upon an expanding array of laboratory tests in the practice of medicine, learning experiences in the laboratory have largely been eliminated from the medical curriculum!

SOME LIMITATIONS OF THE LABORATORY

CRITERIA FOR EVALUATION OF LABORATORY METHODS. A trustworthy laboratory test must pass critical evaluations of analytic specificity, sensitivity, accuracy, and precision.

Specificity refers to the detection of the substance in question and no other. It is doubtful that any test is absolutely specific for the substance being measured. There is always some other substance around that is capable of reacting. In biochemical analyses this limitation is most serious in tests dependent upon color development, less in the case of assays dependent upon degradation of the analyte by purified enzymes, and perhaps least in such procedures as atomic absorption spectroscopy.

Sensitivity refers to the ability of the test to detect the substance in question at the required concentrations, namely, those at which the compound exists in body fluids.

Accuracy refers to the quantitative detection of the correct amount of the substance being measured. This property rests upon both specificity and sensitivity. A test may be accurate in the absence of certain interfering drugs, and only in a certain range of values. It may fail this criterion under other conditions.

Precision embodies *repeatability*, the obtaining of the same result on samples analyzed in replicated fashion, and *reproducibility*, representing quality control over time.

THE "LAW OF ERRORS." Early in the nineteenth century, the German mathematician and physicist Johann C. F. Gauss introduced the "law of errors." This law states that in repeated measurements of the *same* object or substance, the random component on the errors will be distributed about the mean as a frequency function. This distribution, which is bell shaped, is often called "normal" or "gaussian." Note that the law applies to repeated measurements of the same item. Its extension to a population of those items is justifiable only under certain circumstances, for not all distributions are bell shaped, and not all bell-shaped distributions are gaussian. The matter of distributions will be discussed further below, when we consider the topic of "normal range" of a biologic variable.

SOURCES OF VARIANCE

These include some factors under the control of the clinician, such as the dietary preparation of the patient and the techniques of collection and handling of samples. Reduction of variance to an acceptable minimum requires compulsive attention to every detail of the process.

LABORATORY ERRORS. There is imprecision in every measurement. In tests run by hand, pipetting, timing, reading, and recording errors occur. They are more frequent when technicians are overworked or fatigued. It is common to find greater scatter of results of replicate tests at the end of the day than at the beginning. Technician fatigue can be largely eliminated by automation, but there will always remain the technical limitations of machines and the human error in the preparation of reagents, in the standardization of instruments, and in the copying of test results. Quality control varies widely from laboratory to laboratory. Split samples submitted to different laboratories may show surprising disparities in results.

DRUG INTERFERENCE. According to Osler, humans are distinguished from all other members of the animal kingdom by their desire to take drugs. Since many patients do not regard proprietary pain remedies or vitamins as drugs, the physician may obtain a negative drug history unless questions are appropriately phrased. Drugs have great potential for interference with laboratory tests. High-resolution chromatography of urine yields about 300 peaks of ultraviolet-absorbing materials. Two hundred and fifty of these disappear when the "normal subject" abstains from salicylates and vitamins for a few days. Salicylates, vitamins, and many other drugs or their metabolites also produce chromogens that interfere with certain analytic methods employed in automated tests, particularly of the urine.

DISTRIBUTIONS OF VALUES

There is widespread belief among medical students and physicians that when the sample of test results from a healthy population is large enough, the distribution will be "normal" (gaussian); that on this assumption one may justifiably determine a mean value ($\bar{x}$) and its standard deviation (s); that the value, $\bar{x} \pm 2s$, will include the central 95 per cent of all measurements; that this segment of the distribution is the "normal range"; and that values that fall outside this range are by definition "abnor-

mal." These assumptions are erroneous in many instances, particularly in the case of organic analytes. The experimental fact is that for about one half of the methods of clinical chemistry, the distribution is smooth, unimodal, and skewed and that $\bar{x} \pm 2s$ does not cut off the desired central 95 per cent. For example, among the distributions of serum calcium, inorganic phosphorus, magnesium, alkaline phosphatase, total proteins, albumin, uric acid, and blood urea, only that of albumin is gaussian. All others are skewed, leptokurtic, or both. In such situations, the value $\pm 2s$ will cut off many more measurements in one tail of the distribution than the other. The uncritical application of principles of normal distributions in situations in which variables are not normally distributed sometimes leads to values of $\bar{x} - 2s$ that are negative, surely a biologic absurdity (see Fig. 21-1).

One can avoid the question of gaussian distribution by use of *nonparametric* methods for estimating the reference range, that is, methods that do not involve any a priori assumption regarding the parental distribution shape except that it is continuous. Two nonparametric methods of normal range estimation are the method of *percentile estimates* with associated nonparametric confidence intervals and the method of nonparametric *tolerance intervals*, which include a specified proportion of the population with a specified probability.

Physicians are familiar with the percentile method of expressing interindividual variation through the use of pediatric growth charts of height and weight. The method avoids the arbitrary distinction of normal and abnormal. It also removes the aura of precision of the standard deviation.

From every laboratory test for which a good normal-value study has been done, the laboratory can report not only the result but also the percentile corresponding to that result and appropriate to the age and sex of the patient under study. With this information the clinician can appreciate just how common or how unusual the test result is. The percentile method is superior to an arbitrary definition of a normal range, such as $\bar{x} \pm 2s$, even in those few cases in which a distribution is gaussian because it indicates for each test result the relationship of that result to the healthy population. The percentile method is also superior to the definition of the normal range as the range of all observed values in a healthy sample population because the latter method seriously underestimates any selected segment, e.g., the central 95 per cent, in small samples.

With the percentile method, if one wishes to cut off the lowest and highest 2.5 per cent, or 5 per cent, one simply orders all values and finds the value that cuts off the desired percentage of observations at either tail of the distribution. Obvious outlier values are discarded. The complete percentile range is readily defined. No assumptions are required about distribution shape except that it is continuous. From the size of the healthy population represented in the distribution, the confidence limits of a given percentile may be ascertained, with known probability, by reference to standard tables.

REFERENCE INTERVALS. From this discussion, it is clear

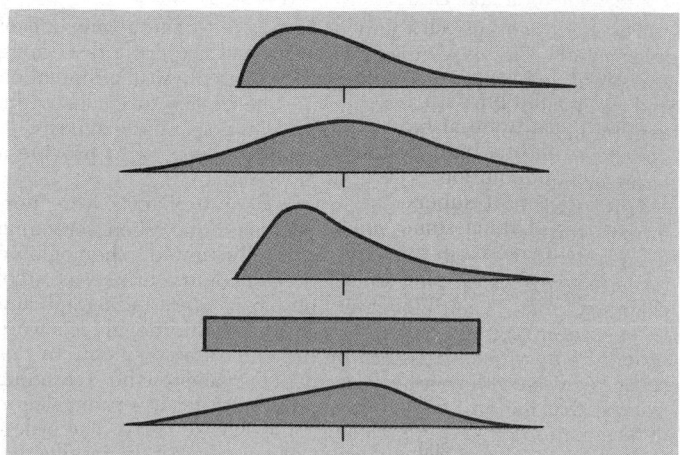

FIGURE 21-1. Five distributions with the same mean and standard deviation ($\bar{x} = 4$, s = 2.83). From top to bottom: χ_4^2, normal, lognormal, rectangular, and mixture of two normals. (From Elveback LR: Mayo Clinic Proc 47:93, 1972; with permission.)

that "normal range" is an arbitrary and potentially misleading term. By whatever method it is defined, the normal range excludes observations of the parental distribution of healthy subjects and very likely includes some values of other distributions. What the clinician desires is cut-off points at either end of a distribution that includes nearly all values of healthy individuals in the central segment, and very few values of other distributions, i.e., that the numbers of false-positive and false-negative values are both minimized. Ingrained habits will probably lead us to select the central 95 per cent of the parental distribution as "clinical limits," even though there is no magic in this number. Some clinical investigators advocate use of the central 90 per cent.

The term "normal range" has come in for substantial criticism. The connotation of a sharp demarcation between normal and abnormal values is unfortunate and usually erroneous. A value may fall outside the range, $\bar{x} \pm 2s$, or the central 95 per cent segment, on the basis of chance alone one time in 20 for each test! The present consensus is that laboratory results should be interpreted in relationship to "reference intervals" rather than normal ranges. In the case of inorganic analytes (sodium, potassium, etc.), the quoted reference intervals for a given laboratory test result are about the same as the previously published normal ranges. In the case of organic analytes (glucose, cholesterol, uric acid, bilirubin, etc.), the reference intervals differ considerably from $\bar{x} \pm 2s$ values. The term "reference intervals" emphasizes the manner in which such intervals are determined and avoids an assumption of normality or abnormality of the test result. The newer terminology requires the laboratory to describe what it is using as a reference population to generate the interval values.

Influence of Age. The distributions of values of many plasma constituents vary with age in the apparently healthy population. For example, plasma cholesterol concentrations in men, 90 per cent limits, are 216 mg per deciliter in the 20- to 29-year age group and 258 mg per deciliter in the over 50-year age group.

Influence of Sex. Distributions in men may differ from those in women. For example, in women, cholesterol values analogous to those cited above for men are 208 and 281 mg per deciliter, respectively. Plasma urate concentration values, mean and 90 per cent limits, are 4.9 (2.7 to 7.2) mg per deciliter in men and 4.0 (2.5 to 6.3) mg per deciliter in premenopausal women. Mean serum calcium values in normal men decline 0.0068 mg per deciliter per year from age 20 to age 80. Those of women show no regression against age. This is an important point in the diagnosis of hyperparathyroidism, which is chiefly a disease of the older age group.

Other Influences. These include weight (creatinine values), diet (triglycerides), drugs (diuretics), environment (altitude—hemoglobin), lifestyle (vegetarian diet), habits (alcohol), and the analytic methods themselves.

BIOLOGIC REFERENCE INTERVALS. In a few instances, sufficient data are available to set reference intervals on the basis of risk assessments. For example, Table 21–1 shows reference intervals for total and LDL cholesterol in plasma selected on the basis of low, moderate, and high risk for coronary heart disease, as determined by epidemiologic studies.

Another example concerns urate concentration values. An electrolyte solution with the sodium concentration of plasma is saturated with urate at 6.4 to 6.8 mg per deciliter. In addition, proteins of plasma bind urate equivalent to about 4 per cent of the amount in solution. Values above 7.0 (perhaps 7.2) mg per deciliter represent supersaturation and are associated with increased risk of renal stone and clinical gout. The magnitude of the risk factor increases as urate concentration values rise above

7.0 mg per deciliter. The 95 per cent limits of serum urate values in "healthy" male New Zealand Maoris are 4 to 10 mg per deciliter, and 10 per cent of adult males develop gout. Surely values of serum urate above 7.0 mg per deciliter in this male population cannot be considered "normal," even though they fall within the reference interval as selected by the usual criteria.

DISCONTINUOUS DISTRIBUTIONS. Some traits may be distributed bimodally or trimodally. Such relationships are most likely in families in which there is a monogenetic disease characterized by a chemical abnormality. For example, measurements of galactose-1-phosphate uridyltransferase activity in the families of patients with transferase deficiency galactosemia are distributed trimodally. The effects of two and of one mutant allele are clearly distinguishable from the normal and from each other. Assay values in the three modes are zero, 7.5 to 13.5 units, and 19.5 to 32 units. The intermediate enzyme assay values are found in subjects who are presumed heterozygotes by pedigree analysis. It is common to hear the term "heterozygote value" applied to an enzyme activity value approximately one half of normal. This practice is justifiable only when assay data are combined with pedigree data, for there may be other reasons for a reduced enzyme assay value that have nothing to do with genetics.

An apparently continuous distribution with marked skewing may at times be dissected into two or even three distribution modes by appropriate clinical and pedigree studies. For example, the distribution of plasma cholesterol concentrations in familial hypercholesterolemia displays marked overlap between subjects who are clinically normal and those who are heterozygotes by pedigree analysis. Similarly, there is considerable overlap between heterozygotes and abnormal homozygotes. Only a complete family pedigree permits adequate definition of the range of values in each distribution mode.

THE PHYSICIAN AND THE LABORATORY TEST RESULT

The tables at the end (Part XXVI) of this book contain values that define the reference intervals for a large number of substances commonly measured in clinical medicine. They represent the best data currently available but are subject to all the uncertainties discussed above. In some instances more selective data of an age- and sex-matched control population will need to be consulted by the physician.

Clinical judgment will always be required in the interpretation of laboratory data. For example, a blood urea nitrogen (BUN) concentration of 22 mg per deciliter is not a normal value for a patient on a very low protein diet. Also, electrolyte values of sodium at 145 mEq per liter, potassium at 3.5 mEq per liter, chloride at 98 mEq per liter, and CO_2 at 30 mEq per liter may indicate metabolic alkalosis even though all individual values fall within published reference intervals.

Laboratory tests are critical to the diagnosis of disease and management of patients. The physician must know the limits of reliability and usefulness of each test result in the clinical setting of the individual patient. This is particularly true when all deviant test results have returned to normal but the patient is not improving. It is especially when laboratory data provide little or no help that the patient needs a doctor.

Dales LG, Friedman GD, Collen MF: Evaluating periodic multiphasic health checkups: A controlled trial. J Chronic Dis 32:385, 1979. *Only a limited number of screening tests (history or physical examination, stool test for occult blood, and blood pressure) actually improve health outcome of asymptomatic outpatients.*

TABLE 21–1. CLASSIFICATION OF TOTAL AND LDL-CHOLESTEROL LEVELS AMONG AMERICAN ADULTS ACCORDING TO RISK FOR CORONARY HEART DISEASE

Classification Based on Total Cholesterol	Classification Based on LDL-Cholesterol
<200 mg/dl (<5.17 mmol/L) Desirable blood cholesterol 200–239 mg/dl (5.17–6.18 mmol/L) Borderline high blood cholesterol ≥240 mg/dl (≥6.21 mmol/L) High blood cholesterol	<130 mg/dl (<3.36 mmol/L) Desirable LDL-cholesterol 130–159 mg/dl (3.36–4.11 mmol/L) Borderline high-risk LDL-cholesterol ≥160 mg/dl (≥4.14 mmol/L) High-risk LDL-cholesterol

Source: National Institutes of Health Publication No. 90–2964, 1990.

Dixon RH, Laszlo J: Utilization of clinical chemistry services by medical house staff. Arch Intern Med 134:1064, 1974. *Less than 10 per cent of data obtained from a panel of 12 tests were used clinically.*

Elveback LR, Guillier CL, Keating FR: Health, normality, and the ghost of Gauss. JAMA 211:69, 1970. *Of eight distributions evaluated, only that of serum albumin was "normal" or gaussian.*

Korvin CC, Pearce RH, Stanley J: Admissions screening: Clinical benefits. Ann Intern Med 83:197, 1975. *Admission screening tests have a relatively low benefit. Fewer than 1 per cent lead to new diagnoses of significance to the patient.*

Mainland D: Remarks on clinical "norms." Clin Chem 17:267, 1971. *An excellent article explaining the use of nonparametric methods for establishing reference intervals.*

Parkerson GR, Eisenson HJ: Association of patient and physician characteristics with follow-up of abnormal laboratory results. J Fam Pract 11:943, 1980. *As few as 40 per cent of abnormal results initiate clinical follow-up.*

Recommendations for Improving Cholesterol Measurement. U.S. Department of Health and Human Services, Public Health Service, National Institutes of Health Publication No 90–2964, February, 1990. *This publication presents new reference intervals for serum cholesterol values in adults (total and LDL-cholesterol) based on risk for coronary heart disease.*

Valenstein PN: Evaluating diagnostic tests with imperfect standards. Am J Clin Pathol 93:252, 1990.

Young DS, Pestaner LC, Gibberman V: Effects of drugs on clinical laboratory tests. Clin Chem 21:1D–432D, 1975.

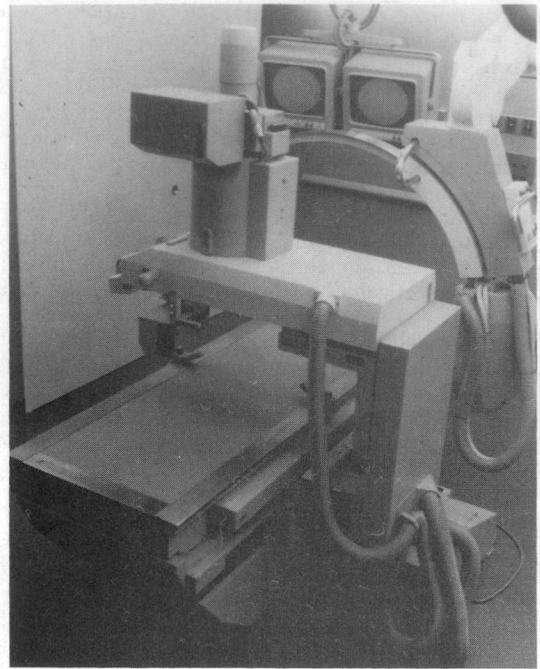

FIGURE 22–1. Photograph of a bi-plane fluoroscopic and radiographic multipurpose room with digital fluoroscopy. Multiple types of procedures are performed in this room: interventional, angiography, biliary procedures (including gallstone removal), gastrointestinal examinations, myelography, etc. Machines of this type, although expensive, are cost efficient because they are in constant use.

22 Overview of Imaging Techniques and Projection for the Future

Alexander R. Margulis

HISTORICAL PERSPECTIVE

Radiology has undergone tremendous changes in the post–World War II decades. Progress in technologic developments related to medical imaging has been continuously accelerating, making diagnostic radiology one of the most exciting areas of diagnostic medicine during the last few years. Diagnostic imaging has been and continues to be the direct beneficiary of some of the areas of technology that are most heavily subsidized by governments and industry. Space exploration provided miniaturization of imaging equipment components. Extremely high-resolution television techniques used for space exploration and photographing of the earth's surface and advances in computers and techniques of storage of information have contributed to the development of digital radiography, highly advanced x-ray computed tomography (CT) machines, positron emission tomography, and magnetic resonance imaging (MRI). These modalities, although expensive, are eventually cost effective because they significantly reduce invasiveness and permit the performance of many procedures on an outpatient basis. Because of this they have found ready acceptance and have rapidly proliferated, not only in the United States, but throughout the Western world and Japan.

PRESENT STATUS OF RADIOLOGIC IMAGING

Conventional Radiography

The term "conventional radiography" is a misnomer today. Equipment that was considered advanced in the early 1970's is today hopelessly obsolete. Although there have been no breakthroughs in x-ray tube design, the generators and controls have been computerized; the television cameras are smaller and more reliable; and the equipment as a whole has grown more functional and often multipurpose. The highly specialized, extremely expensive rooms used in the past for angiography only are changing, particularly in small hospitals, into rooms that can be used for many different procedures, including digital subtraction fluoroscopy (Fig. 22–1). Even conventional darkrooms are being replaced by daylight developing facilities, which save space, time, and personnel. These trends of saving space, time, and personnel will become even more evident in the future as departments of radiology will have to become smaller and more intensively active

and will have to serve inpatients and outpatients with the same equipment over longer hours each day.

As computers improve and the capacity to store data increases, the present halide film will be replaced by laser discs or other similar devices that will significantly reduce the size of filing areas and permit rapid and reliable access to images projected on television monitors. Hard copies from laser cameras will be instantly available in multiple formats similar to CT and MRI.

As videotaping improves and better resolution is obtained, fluoroscopic information will be recorded on tape and diagnostic frames will be recorded on multiformatted hard copy as the only record. This will result in reduced radiation exposure and eventually in cost saving.

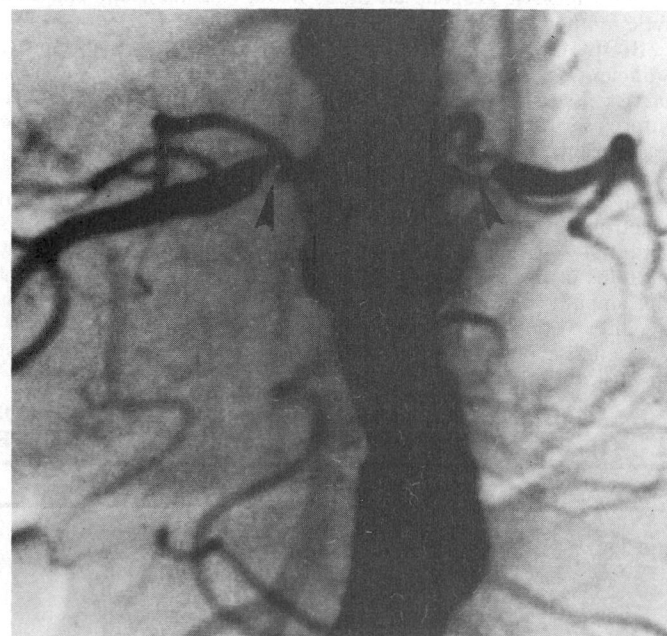

FIGURE 22–2. Intra-arterial digital subtraction aortogram showing bilateral renal artery stenoses (*arrowheads*).

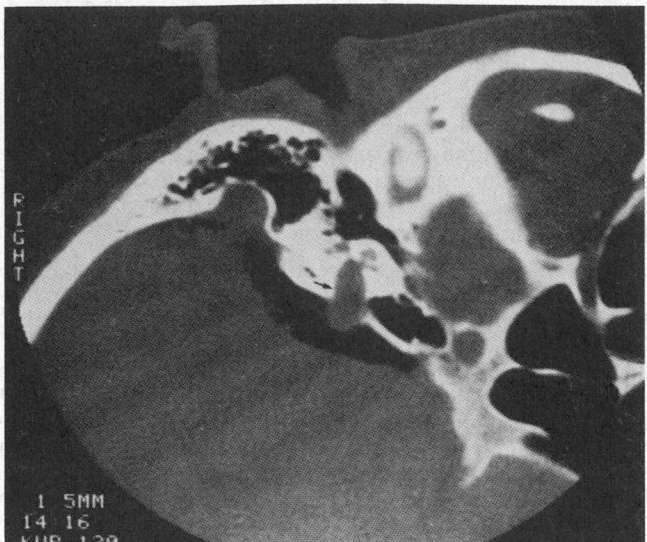

FIGURE 22–3. High-resolution axial view computed tomogram showing an acoustic neuroma widening the internal acoustic meatus. The lesion itself (*arrow*) is seen with outstanding detail.

Digital Radiography and Fluoroscopy

Digital subtraction fluoroscopy did not fulfill all the expectations that greeted its introduction at the end of the 1970's. It was expected then that all arteriography would be performed intravenously, noninvasively, with images showing excellent detail. This has not occurred, and angiography still requires that large amounts of iodine-containing contrast media be injected intravenously through catheters advanced into large veins. Even then, owing to breathing or involuntary motion, blurring detracts from the quality of the images. At this time intra-arterial injections of small amounts of contrast medium appear to be the best method for performing digital subtraction angiography (Fig. 22–2). Further improvements in digital subtraction fluoroscopy will probably occur, but as even digital subtraction angiography is invasive, it is probable that duplex ultrasonography and/or magnetic resonance angiography (MRA) will be the accepted mode of diagnostic angiography as their spatial resolution improves. Digital subtrac-

tion angiography, however, will continue to be indispensable for the performance of vascular interventional radiologic procedures.

Computed Tomography

CT has become an indispensable diagnostic tool in a modern hospital as well as in sophisticated outpatient centers throughout the United States, Canada, most of Western Europe, and particularly Japan. For the last 10 years there has been a steady improvement in the quality of images. The speed of scanning, which indirectly also results in better spatial resolution, has come down to 1 second for conventional CT scanners and is in the 20 msec range for the ultrafast CT scanner, an advanced scanner with no moving parts. CT is still considered an acceptable method for the examination of the brain (Fig. 22–3) and spine. CT is still the modality of choice for the examination of the mediastinum and chest, as well as the upper abdomen and peritoneal cavity. It is a tomographic examination in the axial plane, but it also allows redisplay of images in any plane (Fig. 22–4), and with newer napiol scanners, scans without gaps can be obtained, providing three-dimensional data that can then create images in any plane, including curved oblique planes of the spine. CT numbers accurately reflect the average density of small tissue volume elements and can be used to identify various tissues, fluids, and lesions. CT is of great advantage in showing tumors, abscesses, ruptures of organs, and accumulation of fluid, with high accuracy. Since the introduction of MRI, CT has remained the examination of choice for organs in the peritoneal cavity and the alimentary tube, with MRI rapidly replacing it in most other areas. CT is also the preferred procedure for the guidance of needle biopsies and introduction of tubes for drainage of abcesses. Ultrasound guidance is an alternate approach. A recent application of ultrafast CT has been examination for the detection of coronary arterial calcifications. This test is significantly more sensitive than image-intensified fluoroscopy and appears to be valuable in predicting obstructive coronary disease in the third, fourth, and fifth decades of life.

Ultrasonography

Diagnostic ultrasonography uses a pulse echo device to record reflected waves of a sound beam in two dimensions. The resolution of sonographic images is inferior to the image obtained from CT or MRI, predominantly because of noise in the images. The great advantages of this modality, however, are (1) it is relatively

FIGURE 22–4. Coronal sections through spine showing nerve bundles in the canal. These are computer-generated images obtained with a modern, ultrafast CT scanner generating thin slices without gap. The three-dimensional information can yield direct images in any plane.

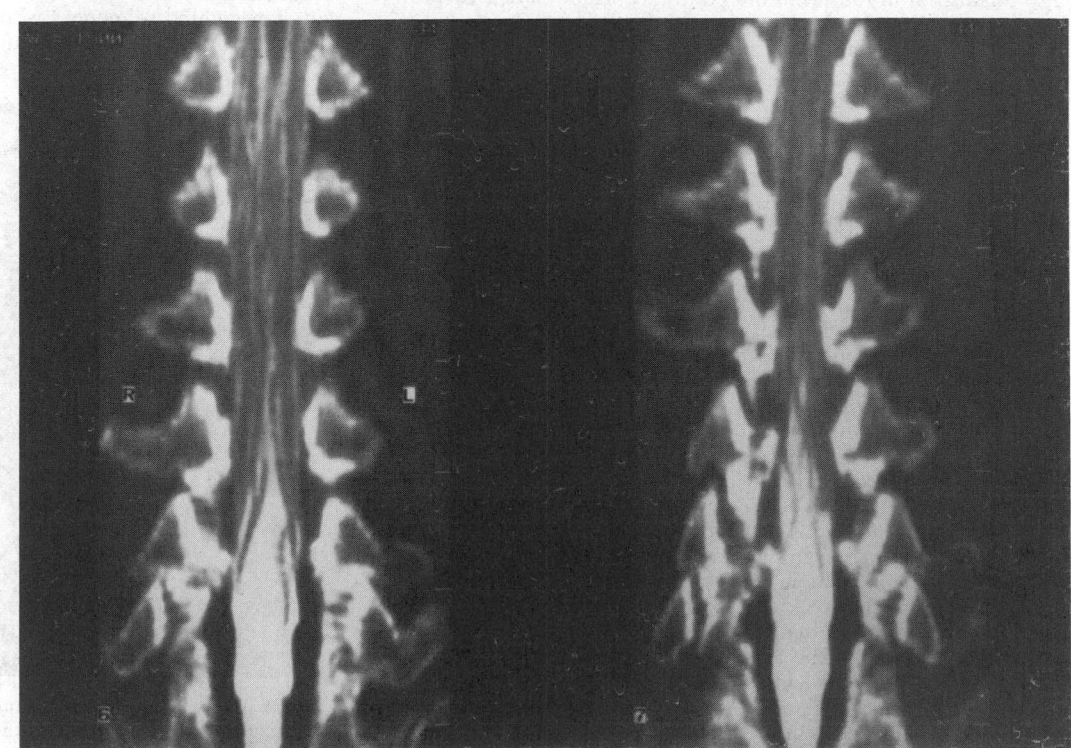

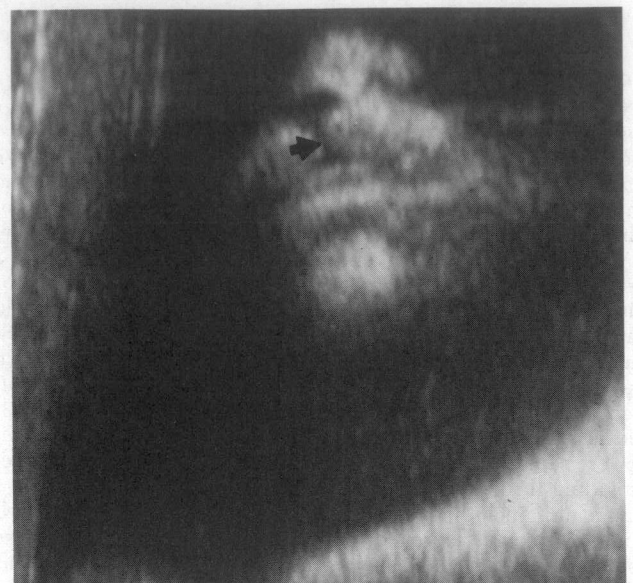

FIGURE 22–5. Ultrasonogram of fetus in uterus showing a cleft palate (*arrow*). Such detail is obtainable only with highly sophisticated equipment.

inexpensive, (2) it is rapid, (3) it can produce images in real time, (4) it can obtain images in any plane without revision of format, (5) because of its speed it is ideal for directing certain interventional procedures, and (6) no biologic hazards have been demonstrated within the diagnostic range. It does not depend on ionizing radiation. The disadvantages of the method are that (1) it is highly dependent on operator skill, (2) its spatial resolution and resolving power lag behind those of CT and MRI, and (3) no good contrast media are available at present. In the diagnostic range, ultrasonography is of no use in examining the lungs, the brain through the intact skull of an adult, the spine, or areas where there is a great deal of gas. Ultrasound images, however, exceed the quality of CT in asthenic or cachectic individuals. It is currently the method of choice in examining the female pelvis, particularly in obstetrics. An entire field of intrauterine diagnosis of fetal abnormalities by ultrasonography has developed, leading also to surgical intrauterine interventions, again guided by ultrasonography (Fig. 22–5). Ultrasonography is also of great use in diagnosis of abnormalities of the neonatal brain through the intact skull and in the intraoperative diagnosis of brain abnormalities through open skull flaps.

Within the last 5 years, intracavitary ultrasonographic procedures have become among the most commonly used examinations, particularly transrectal ultrasonography for the staging and needle biopsy guidance of carcinoma of the prostate. The transrectal approach is also useful in the staging of carcinoma of the rectum. Endovaginal ultrasonography is an excellent procedure for the staging of pelvic malignancies in the female. Transesophageally introduced ultrasound transducers have been used for the study and staging of neoplasms of the esophagus and stomach and are also of value in echocardiography. A more detailed discussion of echocardiography is found in Ch. 39. Ultrasound guidance of needle biopsies and introduction of drainage catheters is in common use and is competing there with CT. Ultrasonography is also used in guiding the introduction of nephrostomy tubes for the direct drainage of the renal pelves or ureters in obstruction.

Duplex ultrasonography, a combination of Doppler and imaging ultrasonography, is becoming a common method for the screening of major vessels for patency and evaluation of flow. It is particularly valuable in the neck and extremities, but it is increasingly applied for the determination of patency of the vessels of transplanted organs and in the follow-up of repair of aneurysms of the aorta and its major branches. Color Doppler ultrasonography, assigning different colors to the vessels according to the direction of flow, is rapidly receiving acceptance.

The many uses of ultrasonography are responsible for the presence of a vast array of equipment varying from relatively simple, inexpensive hand-held units that permit only gross screening and serve as an adjunct to the physical examination, to highly sophisticated, very precise, versatile duplex units capable of rendering excellent images with high spatial resolution. The cost of such equipment can be 10 to 20 times higher than that of the simplest clinical ultrasound apparatus.

Magnetic Resonance Imaging

MRI is an imaging modality that has been derived from chemical magnetic resonance. For imaging, hydrogen protons give the best images. The strength of the signal will indicate the amount of hydrogen modified by tissue relaxation parameters, T1 and T2. T1, also known as the spin lattice parameter, is dependent on the interaction of other nuclei with hydrogen. T2 depends on the influence of protons on each other. It is also referred to as the spin-spin parameter. Other parameters such as diffusion, magnetic susceptibility, and chemical shift also affect the image characteristics and sequences can be devised to enhance, for each, the differences between normal and abnormal tissues. The techniques of MRI are so numerous that it is possible to individualize them according to the problem investigated. By applying the right sequence, a great deal of information about the nature of normal and abnormal tissues can be obtained. MRI has several advantages over other imaging modalities. MRI offers superb resolving power. This is due to contrast resolution that is considerably better than that of CT, with spatial resolution often comparable to that of CT.

MRI is already superior to any other imaging modality in the examination of the brain (Fig. 22–7), spinal cord (Fig. 22–9), cancellous bone, the male and female pelvic organs (Figs. 22–6 and 22–8), and the urinary bladder. With the use of surface or specially designed coils, it is the best method for the examination of large joints (Fig. 22–10). It has in general replaced arthrography of the knee, hip, shoulder, and temporomandibular joint. MRI has been very successful in the examination of the spine. With respiratory suppression techniques, electrocardiographic (ECG) gating, and fast cines sequences, it is providing outstanding images of the heart (Fig. 22–11). Studies of the mediastinum of quality unsurpassed by other modalities are also being obtained. MRI is valuable in the examination of the liver, particularly in the search for metastases, hepatocellular carcinomas, and hemangiomas. With the intravenous injection of gadolinium DTPA (0.5 μmol per kilogram) it has advantages over other techniques in the examination of the kidneys.

Gadolinium-DTPA (gadopentetate dimeglumine, Gd-DTPA) with T_1 weighted sequences is also very useful in improving the sensitivity of MRI in the examination of the brain, particularly

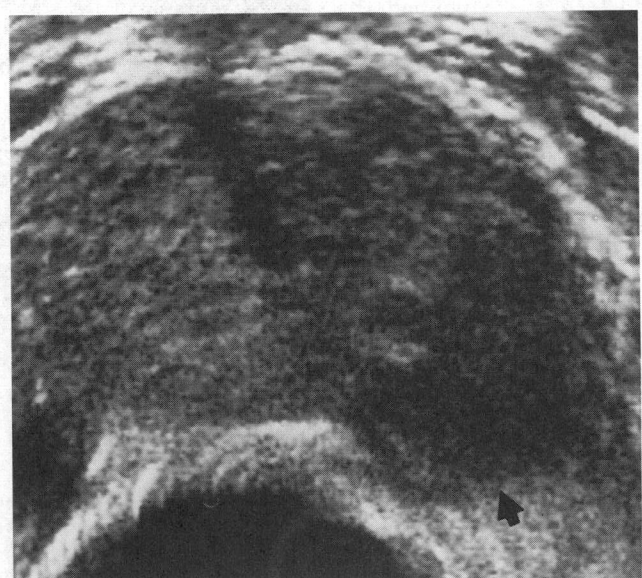

FIGURE 22–6. Transrectal ultrasonogram of prostate showing a carcinoma (*arrow*) that has penetrated through the capsule.

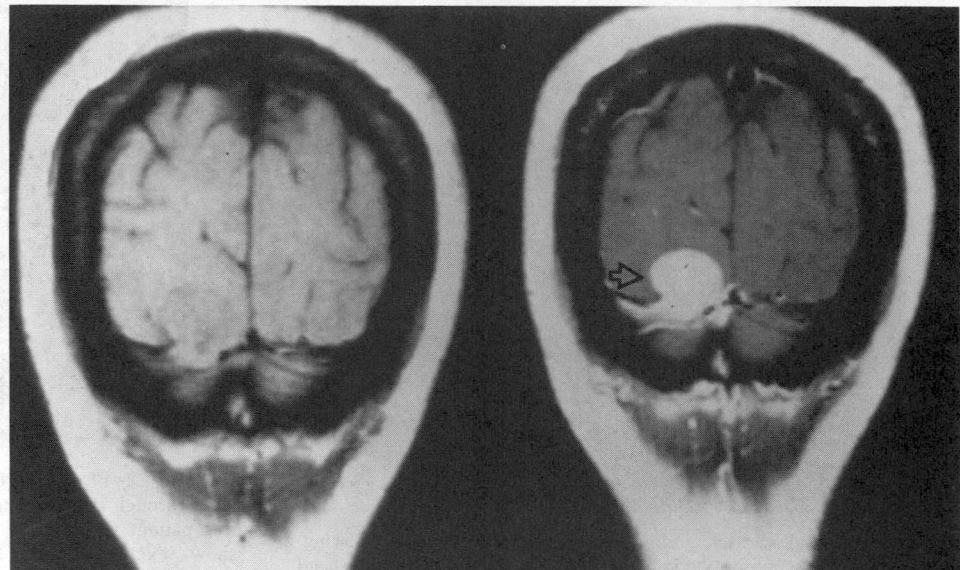

FIGURE 22–7. Coronal MR images of head showing a meningioma before and after gadolinium-DTPA (gadopentetate dimeglumine) injection (*arrow*).

for meningiomas and acoustic neurinomas and for lesions of the spinal cord. Gd-DTPA is also valuable in improving the staging of pelvic tumors. Other contrast media, generally employing firmly chelated paramagnetic metals, are being developed to improve the diagnostic capabilities of MRI in focal diseases of the liver, spleen, and pancreas. Contrast media that would permit MR lymphangiography are also being developed and tested. The drawbacks of paramagnetic contrast media are their cost and the occasional necessity to use sequences before and after contrast media enhancement.

MR angiography, a method of studying vessels and flow through magnetization of the moving column of blood in one direction while the signal of the blood moving in the opposite direction is suppressed by a saturation radiofrequency pulse above the field of view, is evolving very rapidly. It is already a noninvasive screening procedure for vessel patency, and it possesses better spatial resolution than Doppler ultrasonography. It cannot, however, compete with Doppler in price and will need further improvements in spatial resolution before it replaces contrast x-ray digital subtraction selective arteriography. MRI does not show calcifications. It is currently of no value in the examination of the small bowel and its mesentery and has only limited applications in the examination of the pancreas. In the staging of tumors of the rectum and esophagus it is not superior to CT. Further drawbacks are relatively slow scanning (in minutes at present), the expense of the equipment and siting, the large

amounts of space necessary for the facility, and the danger of loose metallic objects flying into the machine. Other disadvantages are the inability to examine patients with cardiac pacemakers, metallic particles in the eyes, or vascular metallic clips in brain vessels. The drawback of slow scanning by MRI is being eliminated by the development of rapid scanning sequences (in seconds), which use different pulses, resulting in reduced flip angles of protons, and imaginative handling of data by the computer. It appears, however, that echoplanar techniques permitting real time imaging by rapid acquisition of data are rapidly improving the quality of images and may become the most useful technique of the future. The use of MRI in the United States has increased by 41 per cent between 1989 and 1990. It is estimated that there are 1500 MR imagers operating clinically in the United States at the start of 1990.

Although MRI has greatly improved the sensitivity of cross-sectional imaging in many areas of the body and the rapid scanning techniques that are being developed promise to make MRI the universal tomographic imaging modality, it has not fulfilled the expectations of significantly improving diagnostic specificity. These expectations may still be met with improvements in localized magnetic resonance spectroscopy (LMRS) and spectroscopic imaging (MRSI). LMRS of ^{31}P has the disadvantages that ^{31}P is not very sensitive for MR and is present in only small quantities in the body. As ^{31}P is very important in energy transfer, it is particularly useful in the study of diseases of muscle and

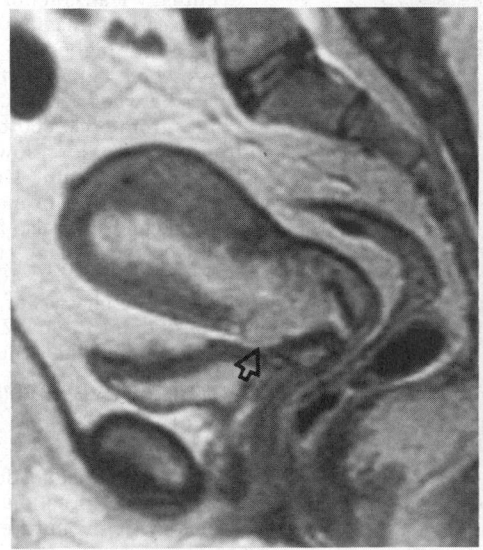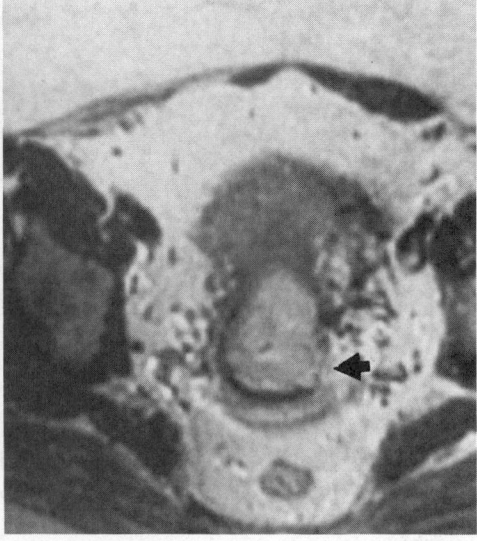

FIGURE 22–8. Sagittal and transverse MR images of the pelvis showing an endometrial carcinoma that has broken through the myometrium anteriorly and laterally (*arrows*) and invaded the left parametrium.

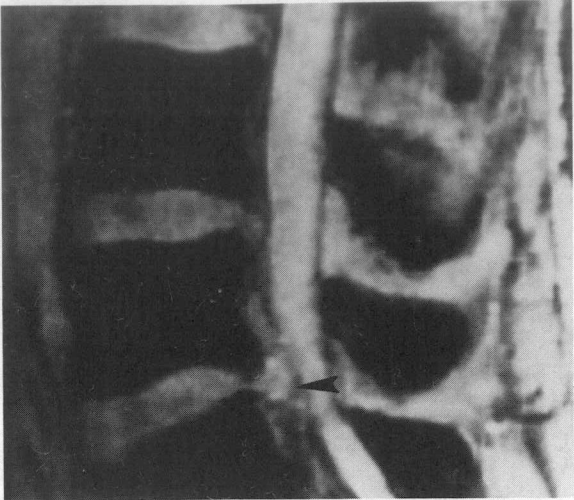

FIGURE 22–9. A sagittal gradient-echo image of the spine showing a ruptured nucleus pulposus compressing the cauda equina (*arrowhead*). With this technique, the vertebral bone marrow is dark (signal void).

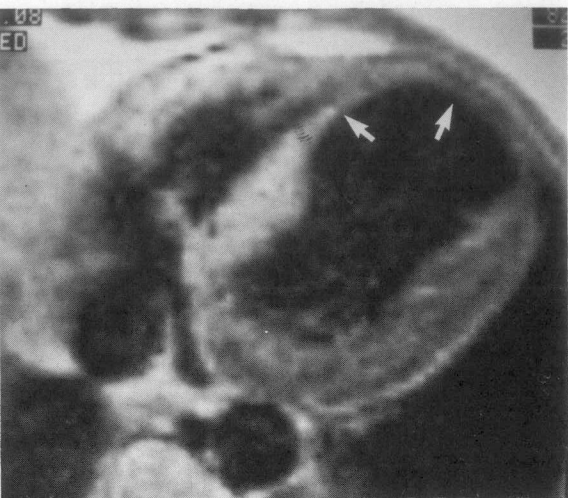

FIGURE 22–11. Gated (ECG) magnetic resonance image at a transverse level through the left ventricle sharply displays the myocardial walls. In this patient with a prior anteroseptal myocardial infarction, the image shows severe thinning of the anterior septum and anterior wall of the left ventricle (*arrows*).

brain, but the voxels (volume elements from which signal emanates) are relatively large (2 to 3 cu cm). ^{1}H (protons) LMRS is more promising. The voxels can be 10 times smaller than for ^{31}P, it is most MR-sensitive and is present in all tissues, and it is involved in all physiologic processes. ^{13}C is natively present in only small quantities but can be introduced into the body as a tracer.

The greatest promise for spectroscopy, however, lies in spectroscopic imaging. Data from multiple voxels in one area of the body are acquired simultaneously. Certain peaks are isolated and can either form separate images or can be superimposed in color over a proton image of the same area. An example for the future would be superimposing an image of lactate in red over the gray-scale proton image, showing the ischemic area localized in the myocardium. Spectroscopic MR imaging has the highest potential of combining images of abnormal physiology with abnormal morphology.

The Algorithmic Approach

With many different radiologic modalities, the physician is often in a dilemma as to which examination is indicated and, if several are to be requested, in what order they should be performed. The algorithmic approach offers a logical sequence in which one examination follows the previous one, depending on

its results, in order to provide a definitive diagnosis. This approach relies very much on the equipment available as well as on the skills of the operators. It is often linked with local experience and sometimes is tinged with prejudice. The best approach for selecting the proper procedures results from a continuing dialogue between the clinician and radiologist in which the two familiarize each other with the newest developments and experiences.

Financial Considerations

The cost of radiologic equipment has soared; in most hospitals modern imaging equipment has overwhelmed equipment budgets. The sophistication and expense of the equipment necessitate an organized referral system to prevent duplication of equipment and to allow utilization of imaging systems to their best advantage. Noninvasive imaging procedures can result in shorter hospital stays, in avoidance of hospitalization altogether, and in almost complete elimination of exploratory surgery. When surgery is necessary, precise preoperative diagnosis shortens the procedure and reduces the number of complications. Properly utilized and properly distributed imaging systems can enhance outpatient diagnostic capabilities, thus shortening hospital stays and greatly reducing the number of acute care hospitals needed. Interventional radiologic procedures are relatively less invasive than surgical procedures. Their advances have already served to avoid or shorten hospitalizations and to reduce significantly the number of complications and expense of open surgery. The elimination of hospital beds resulting from all these procedures should eventually lead to enormous cost savings.

The cost of imaging equipment is still very high and, unit for unit, is the highest in all of the health industry. The price of a fluoroscopic radiography room without siting but with installation varies between $300,000 and $400,000. The cost of a CT scanner ranges from $600,000 to $1.5 million, and MR scanners can cost from $850,000 for a low field permanent magnet to $2.25 million for a 1.5-tesla unit with spectroscopic and advanced imaging options. The cost of magnetic shielding and siting of a 1.5- or 2-tesla magnet may also be a million dollars or more. The cost of a sophisticated biplane computerized angiographic unit with high-resolution (1024 × 1024) TV screens can exceed 1.5 million dollars. The charges of some often-ordered radiologic procedures are listed in Table 22–1. Although costs vary somewhat from hospital to hospital, they are fairly typical.

FUTURE DEVELOPMENTS IN IMAGING

With the continuous advances in the development of computers and television systems, combining increased versatility and decreased cost, diagnostic imaging can expect to make progress in several new directions. It is certain that the departments of radiology of the future in the industrialized world will become

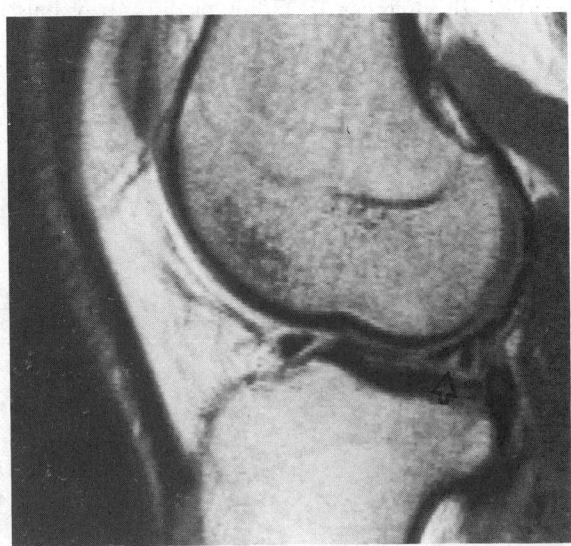

FIGURE 22–10. Sagittal MR image of knee showing a torn posterior meniscus (*arrow*).

TABLE 22–1. TYPICAL CHARGES OF SOME COMMONLY ORDERED RADIOLOGIC PROCEDURES

Procedure	Technical and Professional
Chest, posteroanterior and lateral	$135.00
Barium enema	$319.00
Upper GI	$314.00
Small bowel	$439.00
Head CT	
without contrast	$756.00
with contrast	$841.00
Abdominal CT	
without contrast	$1004.00
with contrast	$1087.00
MRI: head, abdomen, pelvis	
1 sequence	$907.00
2 sequences	$1054.00
3 sequences	$1202.00
3+ sequences	$1347.00
MRI: lower extremity or upper extremity	
1 sequence	$840.00
2 sequences	$976.00
3 sequences	$1112.00
3+ sequences	$1248.00
Ultrasonography	
Pelvic	$285.00
Abdominal	$314.00
Transrectal	$220.00

totally computerized, integrating into the hospital's general computer system. This means that images themselves as well as reports will be instantly available on television monitors on wards along with laboratory information and information from medical records and pathologic studies. These systems will be expensive but at the same time will be cost effective, saving on personnel, communication, and duration of hospital stay of the patient. Computers will also help to store data correlating clinical information and allowing the most efficient and most rational algorithmic approaches for reaching the correct diagnosis. Computers will therefore help physicians, surgeons, and radiologists to reach the correct, least invasive, and most time-saving sequence of diagnostic studies. Similarly, artificial intelligence based on clinical experience and previous imaging results will also help in selection of the proper techniques for rapid diagnoses. This again will not only improve clinical results but will also make the use of equipment more cost effective and less traumatic for patients.

These remarkable advances in imaging will increasingly attract the interest and collaboration of other physicians (such as internists, neurologists, ophthalmologists, obstetricians, neurosurgeons, and surgeons) with the radiologist in the field of diagnostic imaging in order to optimize progress through the exchange of experience and ideas.

Historical and General References

Grigg ERN: The Train of the Invisible Light. Springfield, Ill., Charles C Thomas, 1965. *An extensive, well-illustrated review of the development of roentgenology from its earliest days.*

Digital Radiography and Fluoroscopy

Carmody RF, Yang PJ, Seeger JF, Capp MP: Digital subtraction angiography: Update 1986. Invest Radiol 21:899–905, 1986. *Good review.*
Enzmann DR, Djang WT, Riederer SJ, et al.: Digital subtraction angiography: Current status and use of intra-arterial injection. Radiology 146:669, 1983. *A clever technical review of two approaches to digital angiography.*
Foley WD, Milde MW: Intra-arterial digital subtraction angiography. Radiol Clin North Am 23:293, 1985. *A clear, objective view of the subject.*
Riederer SJ, Kruger RA: Basic Concepts of Digital Subtraction Angiography. Boston, G. K. Hall Medical Publisher, 1984. *More extensive and more basic discussion of the subject.*
Riederer SJ, Kruger RA: Intravenous digital subtraction: A summary of recent developments. Radiology 147:633, 1983. *An extensive summary of multiple approaches with the advantages and disadvantages of each.*

Computed Tomography

Agatston AS, Janowitz WR, Hildner F, et al.: Quantification of coronary artery calcium using ultrafast CT. J Am Coll Cardiol 15:827–832, 1990. *An excellent article on the importance of coronary artery calcification as shown by ultrafast CT.*

Lee JKT, Sagel SS, Stanley RJ (eds.): Computed Body Tomography with MRI Correlations. 2nd ed. New York, Raven Press, 1989. *A well-illustrated, modern, complete textbook on computed tomography of the body. Particularly good sections on kidney and liver.*
Moss AA, Gamsu G, Genant HK (eds.): Computed Tomography of the Body. Philadelphia, W.B. Saunders Company, 1983. *Still the best.*

Ultrasonography

Callen PW (ed.): Ultrasonography in Obstetrics and Gynecology. 2nd ed. Philadelphia, W. B. Saunders Company, 1988. *Even better than the first edition; a well-illustrated and organized textbook on modern ultrasound applications in the field of obstetrics and gynecology.*
Sarti DA, Sample WF (eds.): Diagnostic Ultrasound. Text and Cases. 2nd ed. Chicago, Year Book Medical Publishers, Inc., 1987. *Still one of the best-illustrated books on ultrasonography, with exquisite illustrations.*

Magnetic Resonance

Higgins CB, Hricak H: Magnetic Resonance Imaging of the Body. New York, Raven Press, 1987. *Superb treatise of MR body imaging. Easily understandable.*
James TL, Margulis AR (eds.): Biomedical Magnetic Resonance. San Francisco, Radiology Research and Education Foundation, 1984. *Multiauthored, still valid.*
Margulis AR, Crooks LE: Present and future status of MR imaging. AJR 150:487–492, 1988. *A good review of the state of MR imaging.*
Pykett IL: NMR imaging in medicine. Sci Am 246:78, 1982. *An imaginative, clear, and well-illustrated explanation of the physics and techniques of NMR.*
Rothschild P, Crooks LE, Margulis AR: Direction of MR imaging. Invest Radiol 25(1):275–281, 1990. *An up-to-date discussion of MRI.*
Stark DD, Bradley WG Jr.: Magnetic Resonance Imaging. St. Louis, The C. V. Mosby Company, 1988. *The most complete update on MR imaging. The physics is simply worded for physicians.*

Economic Data and Benefits

Margulis AR, Shea WJ Jr: Advances in Imaging Technology and Their Impact on Medicine. Mackenzie Davidson Memorial Lecture, April 1986. Br J Radiol 59:309–315, 1986. *A review of the status of imaging.*
Newton DR, Witz S, Norman D, et al.: Economic impact of CT scanning on the evaluation of pituitary adenomas. Am J Neurol Radiol 4:57, 1983. *A carefully designed study showing the economic benefits of computed tomography in one selected condition where controls were available.*
Norman D, Ulloa N, Brant-Zawadzki M, et al.: Intraarterial digital subtraction imaging cost considerations. Radiology 156:33, 1985. *Irrational handling of new technology.*
Sox H, Stern S, Owens D, Abrams HL: Assessment of Diagnostic Technology in Health Care: Rationale, Methods, Problems, and Directions. Washington, D.C., National Academy Press, 1989. *A complete multiauthored review of approaches to diagnostic technology assessment.*

Interventional Radiology

Kadir S: Diagnostic Angiography. Philadelphia, W.B. Saunders, 1986. *Detailed textbook on angiography.*
Castaneda-Zuniga W, Tadavarthy SF: Interventional Radiology. Baltimore, Williams and Wilkins, 1988. *A complete, innovative treatment of the subject.*
Johnsrude IS, Jackson DC, Dunnick NR: A Practical Approach to Angiography. Boston, Little, Brown and Company 1987. *A pratical book.*

23 Principles of Drug Therapy

Alan S. Nies

Because all patients respond differently to drugs, individualization of drug dosages is required so that therapy will be effective and nontoxic. A basic tenet of clinical pharmacology is that a closer relationship exists between the concentration of drug in the blood and the drug's effect than between drug dose and effect. The relationship between drug concentration and effect has fostered the study of the factors influencing drug movement in the body, a science called pharmacokinetics (Fig. 23–1). Rational drug therapy requires a basic understanding of pharmacokinetic principles that can be applied to patient care. In this way the amount of drug delivered to the target tissue can be controlled within a definable and safe range.

ABSORPTION. When a drug is administered, it must first be absorbed into the systemic circulation to produce its effects. In the simplest case, the drug is given intravenously, and absorption is obviously complete and immediate. For all other routes of administration, there is a delay before the drug reaches the circulation, and the absorption may be incomplete. Most drugs

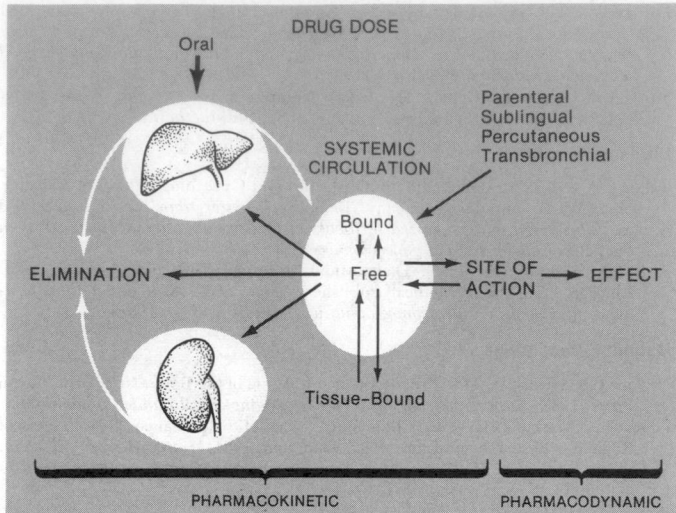

FIGURE 23–1. Drug movement in the body. The variation in effects following a given dose is related to pharmacokinetic and pharmacodynamic factors. The systemic circulation can be sampled to determine the pharmacokinetics.

are absorbed by passive diffusion into the circulation from their site of administration. Since the process of diffusion is dependent upon the concentration of drug contacting the absorbing surface, the rate of absorption can be influenced by affecting the rate of dissolution of the dosage form. Depot intramuscular preparations of some drugs (e.g., penicillin, progesterone) slowly release the active drug into tissue fluids, from which it can be absorbed into the circulation. In this way, drug levels in the blood can be maintained by a continuous absorption process for many hours or days even though the drug may be rapidly eliminated from the body. A similar technique can be used for oral drug administration by producing a dosage form that slowly releases active drug. The duration of sustained absorption from an oral preparation, however, is limited by the gastrointestinal transit time. Drugs that are slowly absorbed from the intestine may be affected by alterations in gut transit time more than drugs that are rapidly absorbed. An increase in gut motility leads to a decrease in the extent of absorption of slowly absorbed drugs (such as digoxin or sustained release preparations of several drugs), whereas a decrease in motility may increase the extent of absorption.

Depending on the drug, absorption can occur from the skin or through the nasal, oral, or bronchial mucous membranes. Nitro-

glycerin can be absorbed percutaneously, buccally, and sublingually. When given as a sublingual tablet or sprayed into the mouth, nitroglycerin is rapidly absorbed into the systemic circulation and produces a transient effect. When applied to the skin, nitroglycerin has a slow but sustained absorption lasting up to 24 hours with a sustained release patch. The transdermal route also can be used for scopolamine, estradiol, and clonidine. However, most drugs are not absorbed well from the skin or oral mucous membrane because of the limited surface utilized for absorption and the solubility characteristics of the drug. Occasionally, unwanted systemic effects follow the absorption of topically applied drugs from the skin (e.g., corticosteroids) or eye (e.g., timolol).

Parenteral, sublingual, transbronchial, and percutaneous routes of absorption have the advantage of delivering the drug directly into the systemic circulation. By contrast, when absorbed by the intestine, the drug enters the portal circulation and is presented to the liver, where a portion of the drug can be eliminated before reaching the systemic circulation (Fig. 23–1). Thus, nitroglycerin can be absorbed readily from the intestine but is rapidly destroyed by the liver so that only a fraction of the orally administered dose reaches the circulation. A similar situation exists for propranolol, in which over half of an orally administered dose is removed by the liver. Hepatic removal during absorption of drug from the gut is called "first-pass" or "presystemic" elimination and, along with poor absorption from the intestine, accounts for the need to give larger oral than parenteral doses of some drugs to achieve equivalent pharmacologic effects. "Bioavailability" is the fraction of the dose that reaches the systemic circulation. Bioavailability ranges from 0 (no drug reaches the systemic circulation) to 1 (all of the ingested dose reaches the systemic circulation). For some drugs, such as lidocaine and morphine, the oral bioavailability is sufficiently low to preclude oral administration. Formulation of oral preparations can affect bioavailability. There are well-documented examples of differences in bioavailability for different brands of the same drug. In addition, sustained-release preparations often show greater interpatient variation in bioavailability than do standard formulations of the same drug. For all pharmacokinetic calculations utilizing the oral dosage, the dosage must be corrected for less than complete bioavailability.

DISTRIBUTION. Once absorbed into the systemic circulation, the drug distributes throughout the body. If the drug is injected intravenously, it is first delivered to the well-perfused tissues and only more slowly distributed to less well-perfused tissues. By measuring drug concentrations in plasma at various times after a drug is administered, a curve can be described from which distribution and elimination can be quantified. For example, if 100 mg of lidocaine is given as an intravenous bolus to an adult, the curve in Figure 23–2 results. This curve of lidocaine concentration versus time can be separated into an early distribution

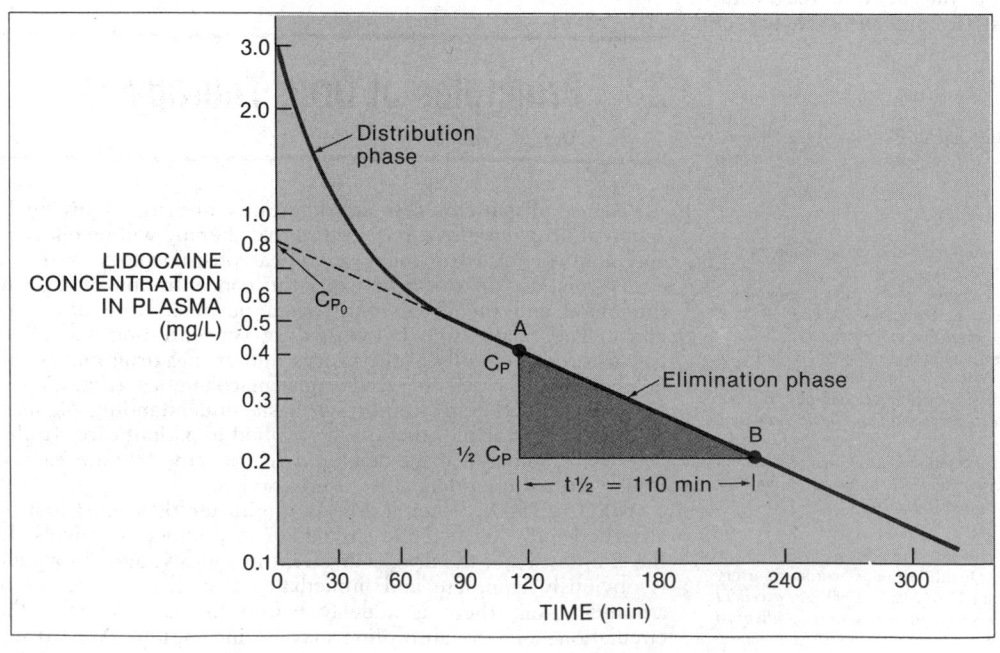

FIGURE 23–2. Lidocaine concentrations on a log scale plotted against time in minutes following a 100-mg bolus given intravenously to a 70-kg person. The C_{P_0} is the concentration of lidocaine in plasma that would be achieved if the dose were distributed instantaneously to the tissues. C_P at point A is twice the concentration of lidocaine at point B. The time between point A and point B is the half-life ($t\frac{1}{2}$).

TABLE 23–1. PHARMACOKINETIC PARAMETERS FOR SOME COMMONLY USED DRUGS

	Cl_r* (ml/min)	Cl_{nr}† (ml/min)	Per Cent‡ Nonrenal	V_D (liter/kg)	t½ (hours)	Per Cent** Bound
Aminoglycosides	70	3	5	0.3	2–3	<10
Carbamazepine	0	70	100	1.3	15	75
Digitoxin	0	3	100	0.6	165	97
Digoxin§	110	40	30	7	36	25
Disopyramide	60	40	40	0.8	6	20–70
Flecainide	100	400	80	9	15	50
Lidocaine	60	800	95	1.7	1.7	70
Lithium	30	0	0	0.6	15	0
Mexiletine	50	400	90	6	11	65
Penicillin G	350	35	10	0.2	0.5	65
Phenobarbital	1.5	4	70	0.6	86	50
Procainamide	330	120	30	1.6	3	65
Quinidine	100	200	65	2.5	7	75
Theophylline¶	0	55	100	0.5	7	55
Tocainide	70	110	60	3.1	14	10
Valproic Acid	0	8.5	100	0.15	14	93

*Cl_r = renal clearance for an adult with a creatinine clearance of 100 ml per minute.
†Cl_{nr} = nonrenal clearance for an adult.
‡Per cent nonrenal is the nonrenal clearance as a percentage of the total clearance.
§The oral bioavailability of digoxin is 0.7 from the tablet and 0.95 from the capsule.
¶Aminophylline is 85 per cent theophylline.
**Per cent bound to plasma proteins.

phase, during which the drug rapidly disappears from the circulation, and a later elimination phase, during which drug in the blood is in equilibrium with drug in the tissues (Fig. 23–2). The effects of most drugs are related to the plasma concentration during the elimination phase. However, whether the plasma concentration of the drug during the distribution phase is predictive of drug effects depends on the particular drug. For a drug such as lidocaine that quickly reaches its sites of action, the initial concentrations shortly after a bolus of drug can produce therapeutic antiarrhythmic effects and toxic effects on the heart or brain. On the other hand, digoxin requires time to equilibrate with its cardiac receptors. When given intravenously, digoxin does not produce maximal cardiac effects for 4 to 8 hours, during which time the blood levels are falling as the drug equilibrates with tissues. After the equilibration period of 8 hours, digoxin concentrations fall more slowly, and only then does the digoxin concentration correlate with the drug's effects.

Apparent Volume of Distribution. The relationship between the amount of drug in the body and the concentration of drug in the plasma is defined as the "apparent volume of distribution" (V_D) of the drug:

$$V_D = \frac{\text{amount of drug in the body}}{\text{concentration of drug in plasma}}$$

The V_D is the "apparent" volume needed to contain the entire amount of drug if the drug were everywhere at the same concentration as in the plasma. The apparent volume of distribution of a drug during the elimination phase can be determined from a semi-log plot of the plasma drug concentration versus time by extrapolating the elimination phase back to zero time, giving the C_{P_0} (plasma concentration at time 0), an estimate of the concentration of drug in the plasma that would have been achieved by the intravenous dose of drug if the drug had been distributed throughout the tissues instantaneously. Thus:

$$V_D = \frac{\text{IV dose}}{C_{P_0}}$$

In Figure 23–2, the C_{P_0} for lidocaine is 0.84 mg per liter following a 100-mg dose. The V_D for lidocaine, therefore, is 100 mg ÷ 0.84 mg per liter = 119 liters. The V_D for several drugs are shown in Tables 23–1 and 23–2.

The V_D is an empirically determined constant that allows one to relate the plasma concentration to the amount of drug in the body and should not be given a physiologic interpretation relating to real body volumes. For many drugs the V_D is larger than the entire body. For example, digoxin has a V_D of 7 liters per kilogram or about 500 liters in a 70-kg person. Such a large apparent volume of distribution indicates that most of the drug in the body is not in the plasma but is bound to the tissues at a greater concentration than in the plasma.

LOADING DOSES. A major use of the apparent volume of distribution is to calculate the loading dose required to achieve a desired plasma drug concentration (Table 23–3). From Figure 23–2 the V_D of lidocaine is 119 liters in a 70-kg person. In order to establish rapidly a therapeutic plasma lidocaine concentration of 2 mg per liter, a loading dose of 238 mg (desired concentration × V_D) must be given. After the distribution phase, the loading dose (238 mg) will be contained in an apparent volume of 119 liters, resulting in a plasma concentration of 2 mg per liter. However, because lidocaine and many other drugs can produce toxic effects during the distribution phase, the entire loading dose should not be given in a single bolus; to do so would produce lidocaine concentrations during the distribution phase that would be potentially toxic. The initial high concentrations can be avoided by giving the desired amount of drug in divided doses or as an infusion rather than a bolus. This also allows the loading process to be aborted if early signs of drug toxicity occur. If the drug can be given orally, high initial concentrations are less of a problem after a loading dose because gradual absorption from the intestine allows time for the drug to distribute to the tissues during the absorption process. As an example, the V_D of phenytoin is 0.6 liter per kilogram or 40 liters in a 70-kg adult. To achieve a low therapeutic plasma concentration of 10 mg per liter requires a loading dose of 400 mg. Since phenytoin has an oral bioavailability of 0.8, an oral loading dose of 500 mg (400 ÷ 0.8) will deliver 400 mg to the systemic circulation. Because of its slow absorption the 500 mg of phenytoin can be given safely as a single oral dose even though the 400-mg loading dose given as a bolus intravenously could cause a cardiac arrest. A loading dose also can be used to boost an inadequate drug concentration into the therapeutic range. A patient with a phenytoin level of 5 mg per liter

TABLE 23–2. DRUGS SHOWING DOSE-DEPENDENT KINETICS

	Maximal Metabolic Rate	Volume of Distribution
Salicylate	4000 mg/day	0.2–0.6 liter/kg*
Ethanol	8000 mg/hour	0.6 liter/kg
Phenytoin†	700 mg/day‡	0.6 liter/kg

*The volume of distribution of salicylate increases with increasing dose.
†The oral bioavailability of phenytoin is 0.8.
‡Some individuals have a lower maximal metabolic rate.

TABLE 23–3. CLINICALLY USEFUL EQUATIONS

Loading

$$\text{Dose} = \frac{\text{Desired Concentration} \times V_D}{\text{Bioavailability}}$$

Maintenance

$$\text{I or Dose/t} = \frac{\text{Steady-state Concentration} \times \text{Clearance}}{\text{Bioavailability}}$$

Half-life

$$t_{1/2} = \frac{0.693 \times V_D}{\text{Clearance}} = \frac{0.693 \times V_D \times \text{Steady-state Concentration}}{\text{I or Dose/t}}$$

Renal Function
Creatinine Clearance =
(ml/min in males)

$$\frac{(140 - \text{Age}) \times \text{Weight (kg)}}{72 \times \text{Serum Creatinine (mg/dl)}}$$

or

$$0.81 \times \text{Serum Creatinine } (\mu\text{mol/liter})$$

(For females multiply calculated value by 0.85)

V_D = Apparent volume of distribution.
t = Dosing interval.
I = Infusion rate.

can be given a 400-mg phenytoin load (or 500 mg orally) to increase his level to 15 mg per liter.

ELIMINATION. *Drug Clearance.* Once in the circulation, drugs are eliminated from the body by two major processes: hepatic metabolism-biliary excretion and renal filtration-secretion into the urine. With a few important exceptions, the rates of hepatic and renal elimination are directly proportional to the concentration of the drug in the plasma, a process mathematically described as "first order." The pharmacokinetic parameter best describing the efficiency of the elimination processes is drug clearance. Drug clearance is defined as the volume of a fluid (usually plasma or blood) from which all drug is removed per unit of time. Clearance is familiar to clinicians defining renal function. Creatinine clearance is the volume of plasma that is completely cleared of creatinine per minute and can be directly determined by relating the rate of creatinine excretion into the urine to the plasma creatinine concentration. *Renal drug clearances* can be determined in the same way by dividing renal excretory rate of the drug by the plasma drug concentration. *Hepatic drug clearance* is, by analogy to renal clearance, the volume of blood or plasma entirely cleared of drug by the liver and is therefore the rate of drug removal by the liver divided by the drug concentration in blood or plasma. *Total drug clearance* (Cl) is the sum of all the individual organ clearances, which consists of renal (Cl_r) and nonrenal (Cl_{nr}) clearances. Total drug clearance is the rate of drug elimination by all processes (R) divided by the plasma concentration (C_p):

$$Cl = \frac{\dot{R}}{C_p}$$

Drug clearance can be influenced by the blood flow to the clearing organ, the binding of drug to plasma proteins, and the activity of the processes responsible for drug removal, such as hepatic enzyme activity, glomerular filtration rate, and renal secretory processes. In physiologic terms, drug clearance by an organ is the product of organ blood flow (Q) and the fraction of the drug in the blood extracted on a single passage through the organ (E): Cl = QE. The extraction ratio, E, is calculated by dividing the arteriovenous difference in drug concentration ($C_a - C_v$) by the arterial drug concentration (C_a):

$$E = \frac{C_a - C_v}{C_a}$$

Clearance is *independent* of the distribution of drugs in the body (i.e., the V_D), since the eliminating organs "see" and can remove only the drug present in the blood.

Drug Half-Life. Both the clearance and the distribution of drug in the body influence the amount of time necessary to eliminate drug from the body. The proportion of the apparent volume of distribution cleared of drug per unit of time is a constant called the "first-order elimination rate constant," or k_e:

$$k_e = \frac{Cl}{V_D}$$

This constant describes the exponential disappearance of drug from the plasma with time during the elimination phase. When plotted on semi-log graph paper, as in Figure 23–2, the exponential elimination phase is a straight line with a slope of K_e. A conceptually more useful term describing the time required to eliminate drug is the drug's elimination half-life ($t\frac{1}{2}$), which is the time required to reduce the plasma concentration of drug (and hence the body load of drug) to half the initial concentration. For drugs with first-order elimination, the $t\frac{1}{2}$ is independent of drug concentration. The $t\frac{1}{2}$ is frequently determined graphically as in Figure 23–2, and mathematically the half-life is the natural logarithm of 2 (indicating a reduction of drug concentration by half) divided by the elimination rate constant: $t\frac{1}{2} = \ln 2/K_e = 0.693/K_e$. Since the elimination rate constant is related to both clearance and volume of distribution as independent variables, it can be appreciated that half-life must also be related to these two variables:

$$t\frac{1}{2} = \frac{0.693 \, V_D}{Cl}$$

As the apparent volume of distribution increases, the half-life is prolonged for any given drug clearance, since a greater "volume" must be cleared of drug; as clearance increases, half-life shortens for any given V_D. A change in half-life frequently is used as an index of a change in efficiency of drug elimination, but this is true only when the apparent volume of distribution is unchanged. Disease can alter the apparent volume of distribution as well as drug clearance. Half-life, being affected by both V_D and Cl, may be affected to a greater or lesser extent than drug clearance, and therefore $t\frac{1}{2}$ may not indicate the degree of abnormality in drug elimination. For example, patients with congestive heart failure have a 50 per cent reduction in the clearance of lidocaine and may, in addition, have a similarly contracted volume of distribution of the drug. Since both Cl and V_D can be reduced by a similar magnitude, the half-life may be unchanged and may not give any clue to the abnormal lidocaine clearance and the need for reduced infusion rates to avoid toxicity. (See "Maintenance Doses" below for discussion of the relationship of clearance to steady-state blood concentration.)

With first-order drug elimination, half the drug is eliminated in the first half-life, half the remaining drug eliminated in the second half-life, and so forth. Thus, by starting with an effective blood level, which we shall call 100 per cent, 50 per cent will be present after one half-life, 25 per cent after two half-lives, 12.5 per cent after three half-lives, 6.25 per cent after four half-lives, and 3.125 per cent after five half-lives, as shown in Figure 23–3 for lidocaine. For practical purposes, most drugs can be considered to have been eliminated completely when less than 10 per cent of the effective concentration remains in the body, requiring three to four half-lives. For lidocaine (Fig. 23–3) this time is about 6 hours.

DRUG ACCUMULATION. When drug is given as a sustained infusion or in repeated doses, drug accumulates in the body until a steady state is achieved, at which time the amount of drug being administered is equal to the amount of drug eliminated so that body stores and plasma levels remain constant. The time course of drug accumulation, like the time course of elimination, is determined by the drug's elimination half-life, these processes being mirror images of each other (Fig. 23–3). Thus, accumulation to half the ultimate steady state occurs in one half-life, 75 per cent in two half-lives, 87.5 per cent in three half-lives, and 93.75 per cent in four half-lives. For practical purposes, the steady state is considered to have been achieved when 90 per cent of the ultimate accumulation occurs, requiring three to four half-lives. For drugs with short half-lives, accumulation occurs rapidly. However, for drugs with long half-lives, accumulation occurs slowly, and loading doses are frequently required to achieve a prompt therapeutic effect. Regardless of whether a loading dose

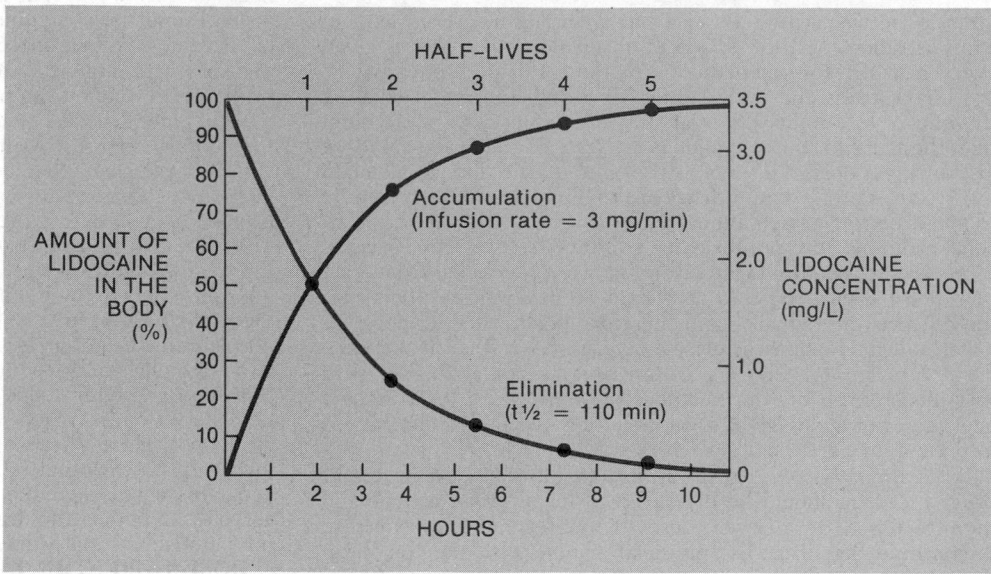

FIGURE 23–3. The accumulation of lidocaine during an infusion of 3 mg per minute and the elimination of lidocaine after the drug is discontinued. Time is indicated in hours and in half-lives and concentration in milligrams per liter. The amount of lidocaine in the body is the percentage remaining after discontinuation of the drug (elimination curve—red) or the percentage of the ultimate steady-state value achieved by the chronic infusion (accumulation curve). The two curves are mirror images of each other.

is given, the ultimate steady-state concentration achieved depends only on the maintenance dose and drug clearance. Figure 23–3 shows the accumulation of lidocaine to a steady state during a constant intravenous infusion of 3 mg per minute. The ultimate steady-state plasma level is approached with a half-life of 110 minutes. A loading dose would be required to achieve therapeutic concentrations more quickly.

When a drug is given intermittently, such as procainamide, illustrated in Figure 23–4, the average concentration approaches steady state with the same time course as during a constant infusion. The more frequently doses are given, the smaller the differences between peak and trough plasma concentrations, and the closer the intermittent dosing approximates an intravenous infusion.

Whenever the drug doses or infusion rates are changed, a new steady state will be achieved. The approach to the new steady state also is dependent on the half-life so that three to four half-lives are required before the plasma concentrations and body stores of drug are at 90 per cent of the new steady state. Therefore, the effects of a dosage adjustment are not immediate and are not fully expressed for a time that is dependent on the drug's half-life.

MAINTENANCE DOSES. Steady state is achieved when the rate of drug administration equals the rate of drug elimination. The rate of drug administration is either the infusion rate (I) or the dose per unit time (D/t), and the rate of drug elimination is the product of drug clearance (Cl) and the drug concentration (C_p). Therefore, during a steady-state infusion, $I = ClC_p$, and during intermittent dosing, $D/t = ClC_p$. Note that there is a direct, linear relationship between the dose and the resulting steady-state plasma concentration, which is independent of the distribution of the drug (Fig. 23–5). The equations for steady state can be used to calculate the infusion rate or the intermittent dose required to achieve a desired plasma concentration, and, conversely, the plasma concentration at steady state produced by a known infusion rate can be used to calculate drug clearance (Table 23–3). With the value for V_D (see Table 23–1), half-life can also be calculated from the steady-state data as $0.693 V_D/Cl$ (Table 23–3). For procainamide with a clearance of 450 ml per minute, an infusion rate of 2 mg per minute will achieve and maintain a steady-state concentration of 4.4 µg per milliliter: $I = 450$ ml per minute $\times$ 4.4 µg per milliliter $= 2$ mg per minute. The half-life of procainamide in this patient is 0.693 (1.6 liters per kilogram $\times$ 70 kg)/0.45 liters per minute $= 172$ minutes, or about 3 hours. If procainamide is given intermittently, the same average concentration will be achieved if 360 mg is infused over 3 hours, is given as a single dose every 3 hours, or is given as 180 mg every 90 minutes (see Fig. 23–4). Obviously, drug concentrations fluctuate when a drug is given intermittently, and the degree of fluctuation depends on the

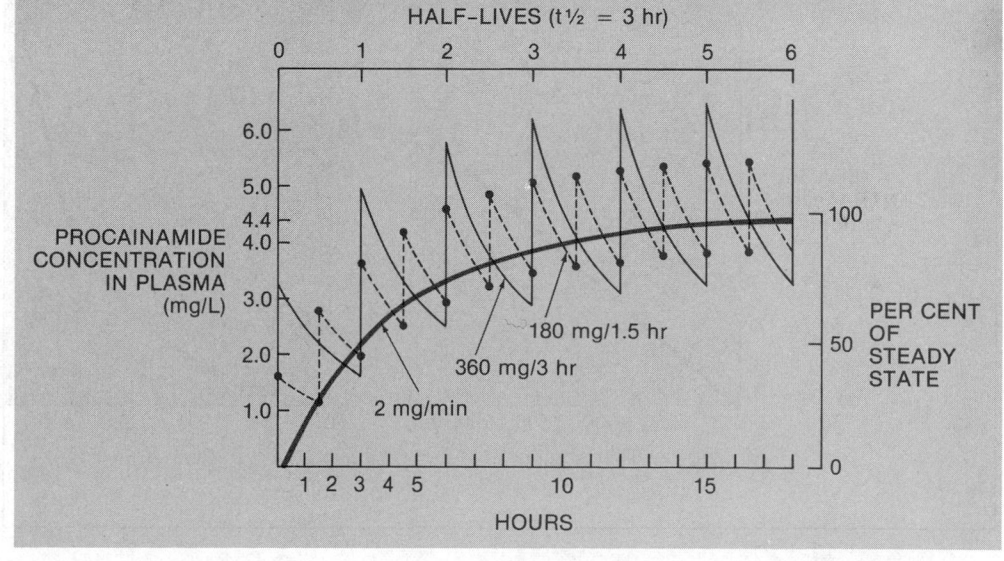

FIGURE 23–4. The accumulation to steady state of procainamide given as an infusion of 2 mg per minute (smooth red curve) or intermittent doses of 180 mg per 1.5 hours (dashed line) or 360 mg per 3 hours (solid line). Regardless of the method of administration, the accumulation follows the same time course and requires three to four half-lives to reach 90 per cent of steady state.

interval between drug doses, the drug half-life, the route of administration, and the speed of absorption. If a dose is given every half-life, the fluctuation is at most 100 per cent; that is, the blood levels and body stores fall to half the initial level by the end of the dosage interval. If the drug is given more often than the half-life, the fluctuations are less. In each case, the drug lost during a dosage interval is replaced by the dose to maintain the steady state. Usually drugs are given at least every half-life to avoid extreme fluctuations of blood levels. Only if very high concentrations are nontoxic or continuously effective plasma levels are not required can a drug be given much less frequently than one half-life. When a dose is given orally, absorption from the gut occurs gradually, and therefore peak concentrations are lower and fluctuations in plasma levels are less than if the same dose were administered as an intravenous bolus. In fact, with sustained-release oral formulations, absorption can be sustained over most of the dosage interval, resulting in minimal fluctuations in plasma levels.

If a patient becomes toxic during an infusion of a necessary drug, the drug should be discontinued for a period of time and then resumed at a lower dose. To determine how long to discontinue the drug, the physician should estimate the $t\frac{1}{2}$ in the individual patient rather than assume an average value. For instance, suppose a patient becomes toxic during an infusion of aminophylline at 0.8 mg per kilogram per hour and is found to have a plasma theophylline concentration of 36 mg per liter. If this is a steady-state concentration, the drug should be discontinued for one half-life and then resumed at an infusion rate of 0.4 mg per kilogram per hour, which should achieve a steady-state plasma theophylline concentration of 18 mg per liter. Since $t\frac{1}{2}$ = 0.693 V_D/Cl and Cl = I/Cp_{ss} (Table 23–3) and aminophylline is 85 per cent theophylline, the $t\frac{1}{2}$ in this patient is 15.6 hours, assuming a normal V_D. This relatively long half-life is due to the low clearance in this patient. It would be inappropriate to discontinue the drug for only 7 hours (the average half-life) because this would prolong the toxicity.

DRUG REMOVAL FOLLOWING OVERDOSE. The principles described above can be used to predict the efficacy of hemodialysis or hemoperfusion in removing drug following an overdose. To be a valuable addition to the therapy of overdose, the drug removal process must make a substantial contribution to overall clearance of the drug and the amount of drug removed must be a significant portion of the body load. Consider the case of a digoxin overdose in an adult producing a plasma digoxin level of 8 ng per milliter. The body load of digoxin is $V_D \times C_p$ or 500 liters $\times$ 8 µg per liter = 4 mg. At a clearance of 100 ml per minute with the hemoperfusion apparatus, the rate of drug removal with a C_p of 8 ng per milliliter is Cl $\times$ C_p = 100 ml per

minute $\times$ 8 ng per milliliter = 800 ng per minute = 48 µg per hour, or only 1 per cent of the body load. Therefore, hemoperfusion cannot be of significant value in reducing the body stores of digoxin. The reason so little drug is removed is related to digoxin's very large V_D, so that very little drug is present in the plasma from which it can be cleared. Recently, digoxin antibodies (Fab fragment) have become available for the treatment of life-threatening digoxin toxicity. These antibodies have such a high affinity for digoxin that the drug is removed from tissue sites, including those areas responsible for toxicity, and becomes trapped as an inactive digoxin-antibody complex in the plasma. This shift of drug from tissue to plasma results in a reduction of the V_D for digoxin by a factor of 10 or more. Thus not only is digoxin reduced by binding to the antibody, but much more digoxin is present in the plasma, from which it can be cleared by normal renal excretory processes. In theory this technique could also be applied to other drugs with a large V_D.

The other circumstance that limits the benefit to be gained by hemoperfusion is when the drug normally has a very large clearance. The clearance of the tricyclic antidepressants, for instance, is in the range of 1000 ml per minute. If a hemoperfusion apparatus could clear the drug at 100 ml per minute, it would add only 10 per cent to the normal clearance and would therefore not be of substantial value.

DOSE-DEPENDENT PHARMACOKINETICS. For a few drugs, the pharmacokinetics do not follow the rules outlined above, and such drugs are said to have dose-dependent, nonlinear, or saturation kinetics (see Table 23–2). For those drugs the amount of drug eliminated is not directly related to the drug concentration (first order), but as the concentration of drug is increased, the relative amount of drug eliminated decreases (i.e., clearance decreases) until a maximal rate of drug metabolism is achieved that is independent of drug concentration, at which point drug elimination is termed zero order. With such drugs, the relationship of maintenance dose to the steady-state plasma concentration is not linear, and a small increment in dose can result in a very large increase in plasma concentration (Fig. 23–5).

Phenytoin is the most important example of a therapeutic agent with dose-dependent kinetics. A dose of 300 mg of phenytoin daily may give a plasma level of 8 mg per liter, and a dose of 400 mg per day, a plasma level of 25 mg per liter. Since patients differ in their ability to eliminate phenytoin, proper dosage adjustments are difficult to predict for an individual patient, and plasma concentration measurements (see below) must be used to establish a proper maintenance dose. High-dose salicylate therapy also behaves in a dose-dependent manner, as does ethanol. However, ethanol is eliminated by zero-order kinetics at all doses, and therefore its elimination is much more predictable than that of phenytoin and salicylate, for which the elimination changes from first order to zero over the therapeutic range.

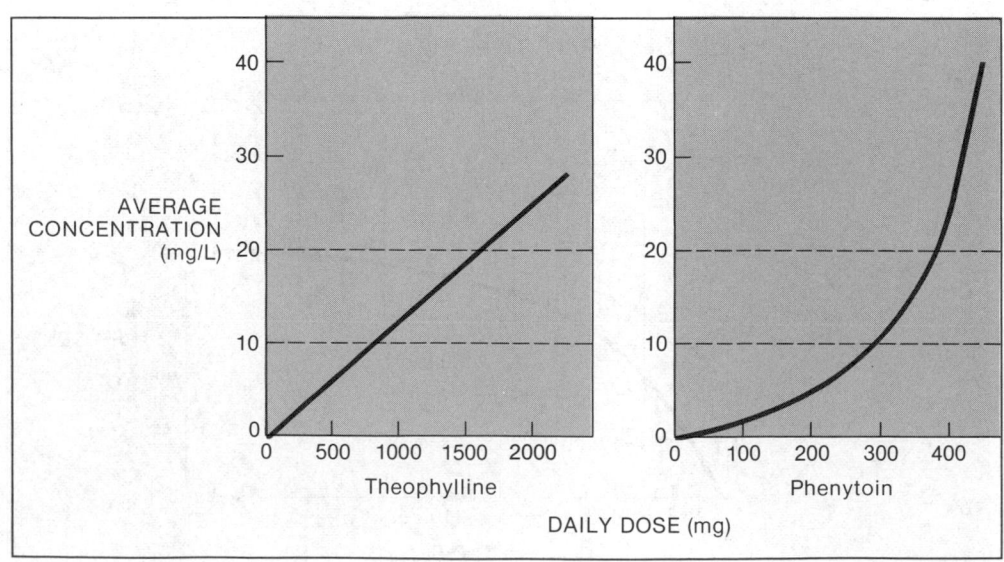

FIGURE 23–5. Average steady-state concentration of theophylline and phenytoin as a function of daily dose. The data for theophylline are from a patient with a metabolic clearance of 55 ml per minute. The data for phenytoin are from a patient with a maximum metabolic rate of 550 mg per day and a half-maximum rate of metabolism occurring at a plasma concentration of 9 mg per liter. The therapeutic ranges are 10 to 20 mg per liter for both drugs as shown. Note that the increase of theophylline concentration is linear with dose, indicating first-order pharmacokinetics. However, the increase of phenytoin dose is not linear except at very low doses. As the plasma concentration of phenytoin approaches the therapeutic range, small increments in dose result in large increases in plasma concentration characteristic of substances that have dose-dependent pharmacokinetics.

USE OF PLASMA DRUG CONCENTRATION TO GUIDE THERAPY. The principles outlined above allow the clinician to choose a loading and maintenance dose based on the desired plasma concentration to achieve therapeutic effects and minimize the risk of toxicity. The underlying premise is that following distribution of a dose, the concentration of drug in plasma is in equilibrium with drug at the site of action and therefore is a direct reflection of the drug at the target site (see Fig. 23–1).

However, the published pharmacokinetic data on which initial dosage recommendations are based are averages for a population and usually need modification for the individual patient. Dosage adjustment is best accomplished when the therapeutic effects of the drug are readily quantifiable, such as with antihypertensive drugs and oral anticoagulants. For many drugs, however, the desired endpoint is difficult to assess clinically, either because there is no readily quantifiable measurement to assess drug effect or because the disease being treated has an intermittent expression so that the clinician cannot be certain that a therapeutic effect has been achieved. Two good examples are epilepsy and sporadic cardiac arrhythmias, in which drug dosage adjustments are difficult to make from clinical observation. Frequently, therefore, patients with sporadic arrhythmias or epilepsy receive doses of drugs based on the average patient, and if these doses are ineffective or toxic, the drug is deemed a failure and the patient is "resistant" or "intolerant" to the therapy, in which case other drugs are tried.

Dosage adjustment can be aided by using the plasma concentration when there are no other easily quantifiable endpoints by which the drug's therapeutic effects can be gauged. In order for the plasma concentration to have therapeutic meaning, the drug in plasma must be in equilibrium with the drug at the site of action and the effects must be reversible. If a drug has irreversible effects, such as the effect of aspirin to inhibit platelet aggregation, the plasma level will not correlate with effect. Fortunately, such situations are uncommon.

The sources of variation in drug effects can be divided into pharmacokinetic and pharmacodynamic factors. Those factors that alter the plasma drug concentration resulting from a given dose are the pharmacokinetic variables—absorption, distribution, and clearance. Those factors that alter the response to a given plasma level are the pharmacodynamic variables. If the pharmacodynamic variation among patients is very large, then plasma drug concentrations will not be a helpful guide for therapy. Fortunately, pharmacokinetic factors account for the major variation in response among patients for many drugs, and this variability can be managed with the use of plasma drug level monitoring.

Therapeutic Window. For plasma levels to be a useful guide to therapy, the range of drug concentrations required for optimal therapeutic effects with minimal toxicity must be established. This range is called the "therapeutic window" and is determined experimentally for each drug in a group of patients who are carefully observed for desired and toxic drug effects (Fig. 23–6). The width of the therapeutic window relates to the steepness of the concentration-effect curve and is an index of the pharmacodynamic variability in the population being treated. For procainamide, illustrated in Figure 23–6, the therapeutic window is 4 to 8 mg per liter. The separation between the therapeutic and toxic concentration-effect curves is an index of the toxicity of the drug frequently referred to as the "therapeutic index," which is the toxic dose divided by therapeutic dose. For procainamide the therapeutic index is ~3. With all drugs there is overlap between the therapeutic and toxic ranges. In addition, since the therapeutic window is based on a population of patients, one cannot be certain of the optimal drug concentration for a given patient. Although most patients achieve a therapeutic effect within the therapeutic range, a few patients require concentrations below or above the range. Similarly, toxicity begins to occur in some patients within the therapeutic window, but the incidence of side effects increases sharply as the therapeutic range is exceeded. Therefore, the plasma concentration cannot be an infallible guide to safe and effective therapy, since it controls only the pharmacokinetic variability and not the pharmacodynamic variability. It is undoubtedly better, however, than the use of a standard dose that allows for no variability.

Table 23–4 lists some drugs for which therapeutic windows have been established. These drugs have several common characteristics: First, their pharmacologic effects are not readily quantifiable; second, they are used for therapy of serious or life-threatening illness so that therapeutic inefficacy cannot be tolerated; and third, their toxicity is serious, and the therapeutic index is small. Therapeutic windows are not required for drugs that have a very large therapeutic index and are used for therapy of diseases that do not have serious consequences if undertreated.

Interpretation of Plasma Drug Concentration. **Timing.** Several problems exist in interpretation of plasma drug concentrations. If the blood sample is drawn during the distribution phase shortly after drug administration, the plasma drug concentration is high, may not reflect drug at the site of action, and certainly does not indicate the steady-state drug concentration. The data on which the therapeutic windows are based are concentrations obtained after the distribution phase and frequently are minimal or trough concentrations. Therefore, the best time to draw blood for drug assay is just prior to a dose, during a steady-state infusion, or, for drugs given once or twice daily, at least 8 hours after a dose.

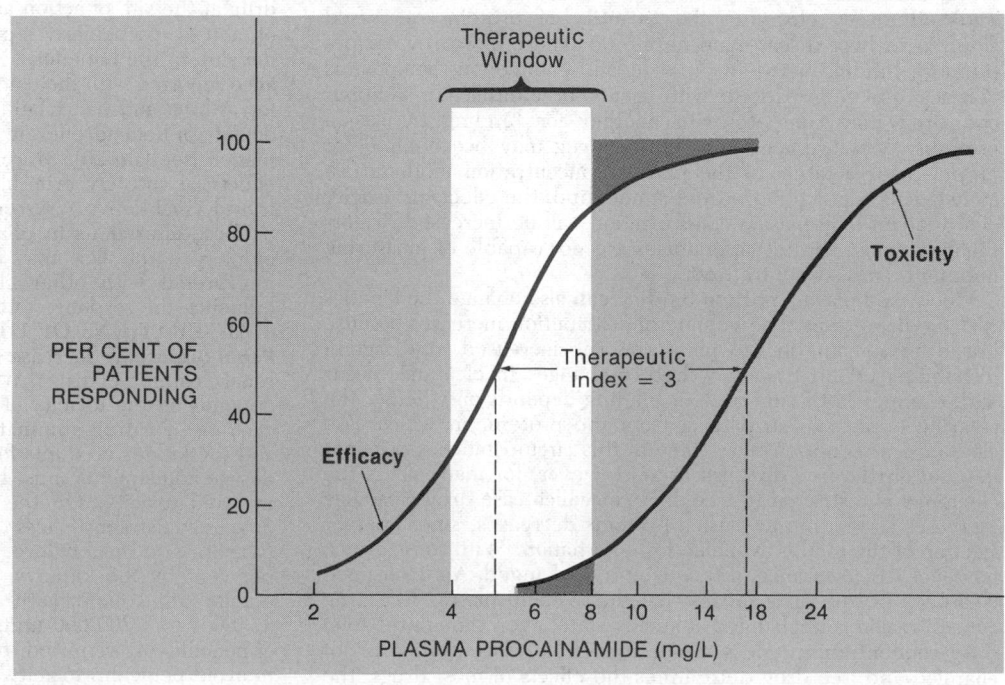

FIGURE 23–6. Population dose-response curves for the antiarrhythmic and acute toxic effects of procainamide. The therapeutic window is the range encompassing most of the therapeutic dose-effect curve and includes less than 10 per cent of the toxic dose-effect curve. The toxic dose divided by the therapeutic dose is the therapeutic index, here shown for 50 per cent of the population. Individual patients may lie anywhere on these curves.

TABLE 23–4. THERAPEUTIC WINDOWS

Drug	Therapeutic Range
Cardiovascular Drugs:	
Digitoxin	10–25 µg/liter
Digoxin	0.8–2 µg/liter
Disopyramide	2–6 mg/liter
Flecainide	0.2–1 mg/liter
Lidocaine	1.5–5 mg/liter
Mexiletine	0.5–2 mg/liter
Procainamide	4–8 mg/liter
Quinidine	2–6 mg/liter
Theophylline	8–20 mg/liter
Tocainide	4–12 mg/liter
Antiseizure Drugs:	
Carbamazepine	6–12 mg/liter
Ethosuximide	40–80 mg/liter
Phenobarbital	15–30 mg/liter
Phenytoin	10–20 mg/liter
Valproic acid	50–100 mg/liter
Antibiotics:*	
Amikacin‡	20–40 mg/liter
Carbenicillin	100–300 mg/liter
Gentamicin‡	5–10 mg/liter
Penicillin G†	1–25 mg/liter
Tobramycin‡	5–10 mg/liter
Others:	
Lithium	0.5–1.5 mEq/liter
Nortriptyline	50–150 µg/liter
Salicylate	<300 mg/liter

*Actual concentration required related to minimal inhibitory concentration for infecting bacterium.

†1 mg of penicillin = 1.6×10^6 units.

‡Peak levels.

Protein Binding. A second potential problem in interpretation of plasma drug concentration is abnormal binding of drugs to plasma proteins. Many drugs are highly bound (> 80 per cent) to plasma protein, and routine assays of plasma for drug concentrations include total (bound plus free) drug. However, only the free drug is in equilibrium with the tissues and the site of action. If the fraction bound is constant, then total drug concentration is an accurate index of the free drug concentration. If binding is altered by other drugs or by disease, then the meaning of a given total concentration of drug is changed, since a greater proportion of the drug is unbound. Both liver and kidney disease can alter the protein binding of some drugs (phenytoin, digitoxin, clofibrate, diazoxide, some sulfonamides, valproic acid, and salicylic acid) either by changing the quantity of protein (decreased albumin in liver disease and nephrotic syndrome) or by competition for binding between the drug and endogenous compounds that accumulate in patients with uremia or jaundice. In addition, one drug may compete with another for binding to plasma proteins. Measurement of unbound drug may be required for proper interpretation of the plasma concentration in these circumstances, since if more drug is unbound, the effects or toxicity of any given total plasma concentration will be increased. Unfortunately, most clinical laboratories are not capable of measuring unbound drug concentrations.

Decreased plasma protein binding can also change the kinetics of drug disposition. The volume of distribution increases because less drug remains in the plasma as the increased free fraction distributes to the tissues. Whether changes in clearance occur with changes in plasma protein binding depends on whether the clearing organ can strip drug from the protein, in which case clearance does not change, since in this circumstance it does not depend on the free drug fraction. However, for many drugs the clearance is restricted to free drug, in which case drug clearance increases as binding to plasma proteins decreases, since a larger fraction of the total is available for elimination. With these drugs, however, the clearance of *free* drug is unchanged. An unchanged clearance of free drug means that the average plasma free drug concentration is unchanged at steady state, even though the total drug concentration is less. Since free drug concentration is not changed and free drug determines the effects of most drugs, the daily dose of drug need not be changed. The best-studied example is that of phenytoin, which is normally >90 per cent bound to plasma albumin. In patients with uremia, phenytoin binding can decrease to 70 per cent so that the unbound fraction increases from 10 to 30 per cent. As a consequence of the increase in free fraction, both the apparent volume of distribution and the clearance increase. The plasma concentration of total phenytoin falls as a result of the increased clearance, but the average free concentration at steady state is unchanged. A therapeutic phenytoin level with 90 per cent protein binding is 10 to 20 mg per liter, corresponding to an unbound drug concentration of 1 to 2 mg per liter. With 30 per cent unbound, the corresponding therapeutic level of total phenytoin would be 3.3 to 6.7 mg per liter to achieve the same free drug concentration. Obviously, if the goal were to attain a total concentration of 10 to 20 mg per liter with 30 per cent unbound phenytoin, toxicity would result, since the free drug concentration would be threefold higher than therapeutic.

Active Metabolites. A third pitfall in interpretation of the plasma concentration of some drugs is the presence of unmeasured but active or toxic drug metabolites. Procainamide is metabolized to acecainide (formerly called N-acetylprocainamide), which has antiarrhythmic activity. The importance of active metabolites depends on their intrinsic activity and toxicity and the extent to which they accumulate relative to the parent compound. In situations in which a metabolite accounts for a significant portion of the drug's activity or toxicity, the metabolite must be measured along with the parent drug for proper interpretation.

Optical Isomers. The majority of drug molecules have an asymmetric center and can exist as two isomers called enantiomers, which are mirror images of each other. Most of these drugs are administered as racemic (equimolar) mixtures of the isomers. Although the enantiomers frequently have different pharmacologic effects, pharmacokinetics, and/or toxicity, clinically available drug assays do not distinguish between them. This leads to a number of potential problems that are only beginning to be appreciated but will be of increasing relevance to the design and testing of new drugs and the interpretation of plasma concentration data.

Pharmacodynamic Changes. A final factor altering the interpretation of plasma levels is a physiologic change that alters the response to a given plasma concentration. For instance, a change in serum potassium, magnesium, or calcium concentration alters the toxic concentration-effect relationship for digoxin such that concentrations not usually associated with adverse effects may now be toxic. The development of tolerance to a drug also distorts the relationship of plasma concentration to effect. Tolerance can be defined as a reduction in response to a given concentration of drug at the site of action and was originally recognized for drugs of abuse, particularly opiates. However, tolerance may also develop to the beneficial effects of therapeutic drugs. The tolerance reported with the continuous use of beta-adrenergic agonists for asthma and heart failure may be due to a reduction in the density of beta-adrenergic receptors during chronic agonist stimulation (see Ch. 25). More recently, tolerance to the therapeutic effects of nitroglycerin has been described with the 24-hour transdermal delivery systems.

These alterations in pharmacodynamics of the drug response emphasize the fact that plasma drug concentrations must be interpreted with other clinical and laboratory data that may influence the response to the drug.

ALTERATIONS OF DRUG DOSES IN DISEASE STATES.

Renal Disease. A decrease in renal function results in a decreased renal clearance of drugs. Whether a dosage adjustment is required depends on the toxicity of the drug and the importance of renal clearance for drug elimination. If the drug has significant toxicity and the kidney accounts for most of the drug's elimination, then dosage adjustments must be made in patients with renal disease to avoid toxicity. On the other hand, if the drug is nontoxic, dosage adjustment is less critical even if the drug accumulates in patients with renal failure. For instance, penicillin is cleared >90 per cent by the kidneys, but because it is relatively nontoxic, dosage adjustments are not required for low-dose therapy (600,000 to 1,200,000 units per day). However, if massive doses of pencillin are required, then dosage adjustments must be made to avoid penicillin toxicity.

TABLE 23–5. THE RENAL ELIMINATION RATE CONSTANTS (k_r), NONRENAL ELIMINATION RATE CONSTANTS (k_{nr}), AND PER CENT NONRENAL ELIMINATION IN A NORMAL INDIVIDUAL FOR SELECTED DRUGS

	k_r (per hour)	k_{nr} (per hour)	Per Cent Non-renal
Group A (>80% renal)			
Acyclovir	0.2	0.02	10
Amantadine	0.05	0.005	10
Amikacin	0.3	0.01	5
Amoxicillin	0.6	0.1	10
Ampicillin	0.5	0.06	10
Atenolol	0.10	0.005	5
Bretylium	0.07	0.01	15
Carbenicillin	0.5	0.05	10
Cefamandole	0.84	0.04	5
Cefazolin	0.3	0.02	5
Cefoxitin	1.0	0.05	5
Cephalexin	0.7	0.03	5
Cephalothin	1.4	0.03	5
Cephradine	0.5	0.05	10
Colistin	0.3	0.02	10
Flucytosine	0.24	0.01	5
Gentamicin	0.3	0.02	5
Kanamycin	0.3	0.01	5
Methicillin	1.2	0.15	10
Methotrexate	0.07	0.007	10
Moxalactam	0.3	0.02	5
Oxypurinol*	0.03	0.003	10
Penicillin G	1.3	0.1	10
Polymyxin B	0.13	0.02	10
Streptomycin	0.24	0.01	5
Tetracycline	0.07	0.01	10
Ticarcillin	0.6	0.06	10
Tobramycin	0.3	0.01	5
Vancomycin	0.12	0.003	5
Group B (50–80% renal)			
Cefotaxime	0.6	0.28	30
Cephapirin	0.9	0.3	25
Cimetidine	0.27	0.09	25
Dicloxacillin	0.6	0.6	50
Erythromycin	0.30	0.15	35
Ethambutol	0.09	0.09	50
Isoniazid (slow acetylators)	0.12	0.12	50
Lincomycin	0.1	0.06	40
Nadolol	0.03	0.01	25
Nafcillin	0.7	0.5	40
Oxacillin	1.1	0.35	25
Oxytetracycline	0.065	0.015	20
Ranitidine	0.25	0.08	25
Trimethoprim	0.03	0.03	50
Group C (<50% renal)			
Amphotericin B	0.01	0.02	70
Chloramphenicol	0.02	0.3	80
Clindamycin	0	0.25	100
Doxycycline	0.005	0.03	80
Flecainide	0.013	0.03	80
Isoniazid (fast acetylators)	0.1	0.4	80
Mexiletine	0.006	0.06	90
Minocycline	0	0.06	100
Rifampin	0	0.25	100
Sulfamethoxazole	0.01	0.06	85
Tocainide	0.02	0.03	60

*Oxypurinol is the major active metabolite of allopurinol.

Fortunately, renal drug clearance is closely correlated with the clearance of creatinine even for those drugs that are eliminated by tubular secretion. For this reason, an adjustment of the average drug dose can be calculated from the creatinine clearance. The process is simple: The calculated renal drug clearance is reduced by the same proportion as the reduction from 100 ml per minute in the creatinine clearance (see Table 23–3). If the drug is cleared by nonrenal (usually hepatic) mechanisms as well

as by renal mechanisms, only the renal clearance (Cl_r) is adjusted; the nonrenal clearance (Cl_{nr}) is assumed to remain normal. The dose is then adjusted in direct proportion to the change in total clearance, since $Cl \times C_p$ = dose/time. Renal and nonrenal clearances for some drugs are listed in Table 23–1. Consider as an example the alteration of digoxin dosage in renal failure. The average renal clearance of digoxin is 110 ml per minute at a creatinine clearance of 100 ml per minute; the nonrenal clearance is 40 ml per minute. If the measured creatinine clearance is 50 ml per minute, or half normal, then the renal clearance of digoxin is reduced by a similar fraction; thus, Cl_r(digoxin) = 55 ml per minute in this patient. If the nonrenal clearance is assumed to be unchanged, the total digoxin clearance is $Cl_{nr} + Cl_r = 40 + 55 = 95$ ml per minute in the patient with a creatinine clearance of 50 ml per minute, versus a total digoxin clearance of 150 ml per minute in a patient with normal renal function. The total digoxin clearance is therefore reduced by the fraction $95/150$ and the dose should be adjusted using the same fraction. If the average dose is 0.25 mg per day, this would be decreased to $95/150 \times 0.25$ mg = 0.16 mg per day. These calculations can give only a first approximation of the appropriate dose for an individual patient, since they are based on the average dose for the average patient. In practice, a dose conveniently close to the calculated dose is administered to the patient, and the patient's response and/or plasma drug concentrations are monitored. With the information provided by either the plasma drug concentrations or clinical observations, the dosage can be adjusted.

If the desired plasma concentration is known, one can calculate the dosage directly from the drug clearance (see Table 23–3). For example, an average procainamide concentration of 5 μg per milliliter is desired in a patient with a creatinine clearance of 50 ml per minute. The total procainamide clearance is $50/100 \times 330$ (Cl_r) + 120 (Cl_{nr}) = 285 ml per minute. An infusion of 1.4 mg per minute ($Cl \times C_p$) or a dose of 250 mg every 3 hours will achieve and maintain the desired plasma concentration.

Although drug clearance is the best way to calculate doses for drugs, clearance data are not available for many drugs. For a few drugs, published nomograms are available to guide dosage. It would be preferable, both from a practical and from an intellectual standpoint, to be able to use a more generally applicable method to calculate proper dosage. Two such methods are outlined in the next two paragraphs.

For many drugs, the elimination rate constant (k_e) is known. If the apparent volume of distribution is unchanged in renal disease, then the k_e and Cl are proportional ($k_e = Cl/V_D$) and the change in k_e can be used to adjust the dose in a manner entirely analogous to the use of changes in clearance to adjust dose. Like clearance values, the elimination rate constant can be expressed as the sum of the rate constants for the separate eliminating organs; thus $k_e = k_{renal} + k_{nonrenal}$. Values for k_r and k_{nr} are listed in Table 23–5. To use these values to adjust dosage in renal insufficiency, the procedure is exactly the same as with the clearance calculations used above. Thus, k_e for amikacin in a patient with normal renal function is 0.31, which is made up of $k_r = 0.3$ and $k_{nr} = 0.01$. The dose alteration in a patient with a creatinine clearance of 25 ml per minute is calculated as follows: The k_r for the patient is $25/100 \times 0.3 = 0.08$. The k_e therefore is $k_r + k_{nr} = 0.08 + 0.01 = 0.09$ versus the normal k_e of 0.31. The dose of amikacin must therefore be reduced to 0.09/0.31 or 30 per cent of the usual dose per unit time. As can be readily appreciated, the dose of amikacin is reduced almost in proportion to the reduction in creatinine clearance, since the nonrenal elimination is negligible until creatinine clearance is reduced to very low values (i.e., <15 ml per minute). Several other drugs that are like amikacin in this regard are in Group A in Table 23–5. For all these drugs, dosage adjustment can be made by multiplying the usual dose by the fraction of the creatinine clearance remaining in the patient. When the patient has essentially no renal function, then the small k_{nr} may be used to calculate doses as illustrated above. For drugs that have nonrenal elimination that is a substantial fraction (e.g., 20 to 50 per cent) of the total elimination, the dosage reduction in renal insufficiency is less than the reduction in creatinine clearance and can be calculated as illustrated above. These drugs are in Group B in Table 23–5. If the nonrenal elimination is greater than 50 per cent of the k_e, then the dosage usually does not need to be adjusted for changes in renal function. In all cases, the calculations adjust only the average dose, and blood level determinations are required to make final dosage adjustments. This is particularly true if nonrenal elimination may also be reduced, as in liver or cardiac disease.

A final method for estimating the average dose in patients with renal failure is to use the per cent nonrenal elimination determined in normal individuals. These values are listed in Tables 23–1 and 23–5 and are frequently available for drugs even if clearances or elimination rate constants are not. This method uses the nomogram in Figure 23–7, in which creatinine clearance is plotted against the drug clearance as a per cent of normal. The black lines intersecting the black ordinate are for drugs that have a nonrenal elimination of 0 to 50 per cent in a normal individual. The nomogram is used by drawing a perpendicular line to the creatinine clearance until it intersects the black line corresponding to the drug of interest. The per cent drug clearance can then be read directly from the red ordinate and the dosage adjusted accordingly. For instance, consider the amikacin example calculated above. Since the per cent nonrenal elimination in a normal individual is ~5 per cent, the clearance values for amikacin fall on the line intersecting the ordinate at 5 per cent in Figure 23–7. The drug clearance as a percentage of normal for a creatinine clearance of 25 ml per minute is ~30 per cent (as indicated by the dotted line), and the dose of this drug in the patient with a creatinine clearance of 25 ml therefore must be 30 per cent normal.

The reduction in dose per unit time can be applied to patient care by giving either the reduced dose at the usual interval or the same dose at a longer interval. The average plasma level is the same by both methods, but the fluctuations in plasma concentration are less when the reduced dose is given at the usual intervals.

Loading doses for most drugs used in patients with renal failure need not be adjusted for creatinine clearance because V_D is usually close to normal. However, since the $t\frac{1}{2}$ of renally cleared drugs is prolonged in these patients, drug accumulation during initiation of therapy with maintenance doses is slower. Because of the slower accumulation, a loading dose may be required in patients with renal failure in order to achieve a therapeutic blood concentration rapidly, whereas patients with normal renal function may not need a loading dose for the same drug. Digoxin, for example, with a half-life of 1.5 days in a patient with normal renal function accumulates to 90 per cent of steady-state levels in 5 days (three to four half-lives), and many patients need not be loaded, since this accumulation is sufficiently rapid to produce the desired therapeutic effects. On the other hand, in a patient without renal function, digoxin half-life increases to 5 days. If the anephric patient is begun on the appropriately reduced maintenance dose of digoxin, accumulation to the same steady-state level takes more than 15 days to occur. In this case, a loading dose may be desired to achieve a more rapid effect without waiting for drug accumulation. However, whether or not a loading dose is given, the ultimate steady-state drug concentration is the same and, as always, depends only on drug dose and drug clearance.

Patients with end-stage renal disease are usually supported with hemodialysis. Dialysis can remove some therapeutic drugs from the circulation and necessitate supplemental dosing to maintain a therapeutic effect. The most important characteristics of the drug that determine the ability of dialysis to remove a significant amount of drug from the body are the V_D, drug binding to plasma proteins, and the nonrenal clearance of the drug. Of these, V_D is the most important parameter, and only if it is less than 1 liter per kilogram can significant amounts of drug be removed by dialysis. Dialysis is also more effective in drug removal if the drug is not highly bound to plasma proteins. Since clearance of drugs by hemodialysis is limited to a maximum of ~ 100 ml per minute, drugs that have a relatively small extrarenal clearance (< 400 ml per minute) may have a significant increment in their removal rate during hemodialysis even if they are not normally cleared by the kidney. For instance, aminoglycosides have a small V_D, low binding to plasma protein, and mostly renal clearance and are therefore removed to a significant extent by hemodialysis. Theophylline, although not normally cleared by the kidneys, has a relatively small V_D, a nonrenal clearance of 55 ml per minute, and moderate protein binding and therefore may be sufficiently removed during a 3- to 6-hour hemodialysis session to require a modest supplemental dosage. For most drugs that require supplemental therapy after hemodialysis to maintain a therapeutic effect, blood level determinations are available as a guide.

Some drugs form metabolites that are active or toxic and are eliminated by the kidneys. In patients with renal insufficiency, these metabolites may accumulate and produce effects. As an example, procainamide is in part excreted unchanged and in part metabolized to acecainide, which has antiarrhythmic effects and can produce toxicity. The metabolite may achieve concentrations in renal failure that are many-fold higher than the parent drug and can contribute to the antiarrhythmic effects and toxicity of procainamide. Drugs with renally excreted active or toxic metabolites include (in addition to procainamide) meperidine, propoxyphene, allopurinol, acetohexamide, clofibrate, nitrofurantoin, and nitroprusside. If alternative drugs are available for the

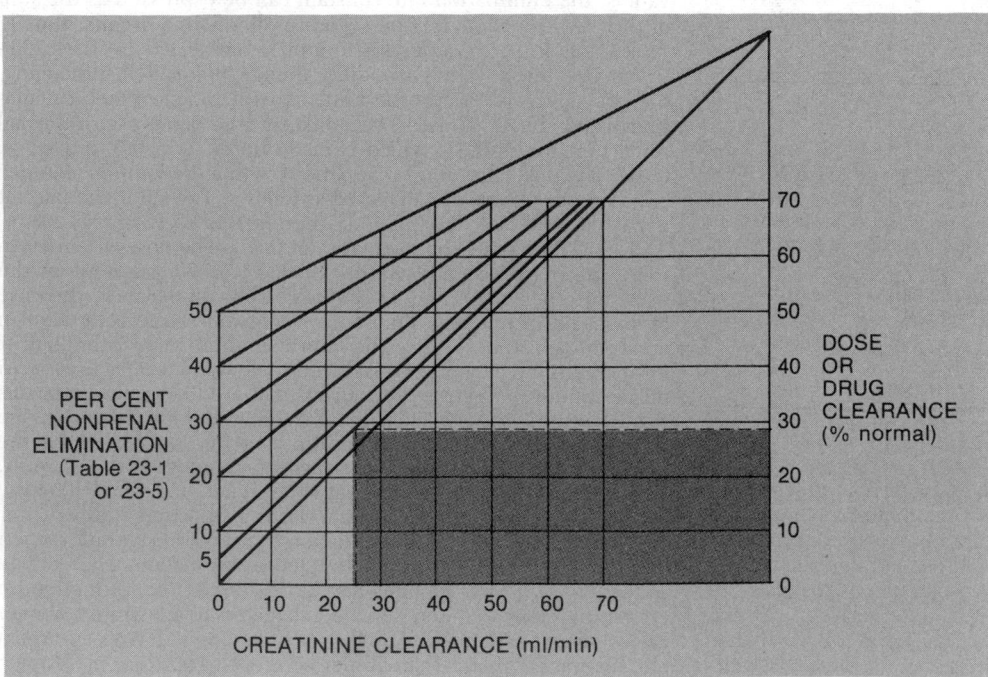

FIGURE 23–7. Nomogram for calculation of drug doses in patients with renal disease. The dose of any drug in a patient with renal disease (as a per cent of normal) is determined by connecting a line from the measured or calculated creatinine clearance to the black line that corresponds to the per cent nonrenal elimination for the drug of interest (from Table 23–1 or 23–5). The point of intersection is then extended to the red axis, where the dose per unit time as a per cent of normal is read directly. The dotted line indicates that in a patient with a creatinine clearance of 25 ml per minute the dose of amikacin, which normally has 5 per cent nonrenal elimination, must be reduced to approximately 30 per cent of normal.

treatment of patients with renal insufficiency, it is probably best to avoid the former drugs when active or toxic metabolites may accumulate.

Hepatic Disease. Although many drugs are biotransformed by the liver, no quantitive predictor of the degree of abnormality in drug metabolism is available for patients with liver disease. If the indices of the liver's capacity to form proteins (serum albumin level and prothrombin time) are abnormal, then it is probable that the clearance of drugs metabolized by the mixed function oxidase (P450) system will be reduced. However, the elimination of drugs metabolized by hepatic conjugation mechanisms is much less affected by chronic liver disease. Acute liver disease has an inconstant and unpredictable effect on drug metabolism, but, in general, drug metabolism is not so abnormal as with chronic liver disease.

With chronic liver disease, portacaval anastomoses may develop. Not only does this decrease the blood flow to the liver with consequent reduction in clearance of some drugs, but the portacaval shunting can allow drug absorbed by the gut to pass directly into the systemic circulation and bypass the liver, thereby avoiding the "first-pass" or "presystemic" elimination. For those drugs that are largely extracted from the blood by the liver (e.g., propranolol, metoprolol, lidocaine), portacaval shunting allows a much greater fraction of an orally administered dose to reach the systemic circulation.

Hemodynamic Disorders. Pharmacokinetics can be affected in several ways by disorders of the circulation. Hypotension and poor cardiac output reduce renal blood flow, glomerular filtration rate, and hepatic blood flow. As with primary renal disease, the impairment in renal drug excretion may be estimated by the change in creatinine clearance and dosage adjustments made accordingly. The effects of reduced hepatic blood flow on drug metabolism are highly dependent on the drug. For drugs that are essentially completely cleared from the blood on a single passage through the liver, i.e., when the extraction from the blood is close to 100 per cent, a reduction in liver blood flow reduces hepatic drug clearance proportionately. On the other hand, many drugs that are metabolized are extracted poorly by the liver, and for these drugs a reduction in liver blood flow has relatively little influence on their hepatic clearance. A complicating factor is that circulatory abnormalities also can result in hepatic congestion or tissue hypoxia that can impair hepatocellular function, so that drug metabolism may be reduced during hypotensive states independent of the effects of blood flow on drug delivery to the liver. Therefore, it is difficult to predict the proper dosage of hepatic metabolized drugs in individual patients with circulatory abnormalities. Certainly a drug such as lidocaine that has a very high hepatic clearance is cleared less well in congestive heart failure or shock, and the maintenance infusion rates must be reduced by about half in these situations to avoid toxicity.

The distribution of some drugs is also affected by hemodynamic changes. For several drugs with large distribution volumes (lidocaine, quinidine, and procainamide), the apparent volume of distribution is decreased in heart failure and shock, and loading doses should also be reduced to avoid toxic plasma concentrations. However, for theophylline, a drug with a relatively small volume of distribution, the apparent volume of distribution is not changed by heart failure. Since data are not available for most drugs, we advise a conservative approach to loading and maintenance doses of toxic drugs in the setting of congestive heart failure or shock, with careful monitoring of the clinical status and plasma levels to guide further dosage adjustments.

USE OF DRUGS IN THE ELDERLY. Elderly persons (over 65 years) comprise 11 to 12 per cent of the United States population, but over 30 per cent of all prescriptions are written for this group of patients, and the trend is for an increased prescribing rate in the elderly in contrast to a decreased rate in younger patients. As an individual ages, changes occur that may affect drug kinetics and drug action. These age-related changes accentuate the normal interindividual variation in drug effects, thus making the elderly the most diverse segment of the adult population in terms of their drug responses. Because of the changes that occur with aging, the number of illnesses present, and the large numbers of drugs used in this population, the elderly are also highly susceptible to serious adverse drug effects and drug interactions.

The pharmacokinetic changes that occur in the elderly are related to changes in body composition as well as to changes in function of pharmacokinetically important organs. In spite of a decrease in gastric acid secretion, a decrease in mucosal absorptive surface of the small bowel by about 30 per cent, and a decrease in splanchnic blood flow by about 40 per cent, very few studies have shown an effect of aging on drug absorption.

The distribution of drugs may change markedly with aging, probably because lean body mass and total body water decrease as the percentage of total body fat increases. In addition, the plasma concentration of albumin decreases, probably as a result of decreased albumin production by the liver, and this may affect those drugs that are bound to plasma albumin. Alpha$_1$-acid glycoprotein, the major plasma protein that binds basic drugs, is not diminished with aging. Because of the changes in body composition, water-soluble drugs that are not bound to plasma proteins may have a reduced apparent volume of distribution. However, for lipid-soluble drugs, such as many psychotropic agents, the volume of distribution relative to body weight may be increased, probably because of the increased percentage of body weight as fat. For water-soluble, albumin-bound drugs, the changes in distribution with aging are not predictable.

The clearance of many drugs is diminished in the elderly. Cardiac output and blood flow to the kidneys and liver may decrease by 30 to 40 per cent with aging, and glomerular filtration rate may be reduced by as much as 50 per cent. However, since older persons have a decreased muscle mass, they have a decreased rate of creatinine production so that a reduced creatinine clearance can coexist with an apparently normal serum creatinine concentration. As a general rule, one should consider that renal elimination of drugs is reduced by 50 per cent in elderly patients without evidence of renal disease and make dosage adjustments accordingly.

Both hepatic blood flow and the intrinsic ability of the liver to metabolize some drugs may be reduced in the elderly, but the interindividual variability in the metabolism of drugs is so large as to preclude any useful predictions. The reduction in hepatic blood flow influences the hepatic elimination of drugs with high extraction ratios, such as lidocaine. The reduction in mixed function oxidase activity in some elderly patients may reduce the clearance of drugs with a low hepatic extraction ratio as well as reduce the presystemic (first-pass) elimination of those drugs with a high hepatic extraction ratio. However, conjugation reactions usually are unaffected by aging.

Elimination half-life of many drugs is increased with aging as a consequence of a larger apparent volume of distribution and/or a smaller metabolic or renal clearance. Frequently, elimination half-life can be prolonged even without changes in drug clearance. This is true with diazepam, which has an increased apparent volume of distribution with no change in metabolic clearance, and this combination of changes produces a prolonged elimination half-life.

Age-related changes in target-organ responsiveness are also important. The antianxiety agents and sedative hypnotic agents produce greater degrees of depression of central nervous system function in the elderly than in the young even at the same plasma levels. The hypotensive side effects of many psychotropic drugs are greater in the elderly because of reduced functioning of baroreceptor reflexes. Hemorrhage with anticoagulants is more common in the elderly even with good control of the clotting parameters. These changes in pharmacodynamics require the use of smaller doses of drugs in the elderly, even if the kinetics of the drug are not altered.

The following general principles derive from studies of drugs in the elderly: (1) Drugs that are eliminated by the kidneys very likely have a reduced clearance, and the doses required to achieve a therapeutic blood concentration may be 50 per cent of those required in a young population. (2) Drugs that are eliminated by the liver may be less affected, but for parenterally given drugs such as lidocaine that have high hepatic clearances, the reduction in liver blood flow would be expected to decrease the clearance of the drug. In addition, some individuals have a reduction in hepatic drug metabolism, and enzyme induction may not occur as readily in the elderly. (3) The sensitivity of target organs to drugs is increased for central nervous system depressants and probably for other drugs as well. Thus, the elderly constitute a population in whom drug use is likely to be marred by enhanced toxicity, and physician awareness of the possibility of altered drug disposition or effects is mandatory. It is a population in which drugs should be used in the lowest effective doses and only in individuals in whom they are absolutely necessary. That this is not commonly done is indicated by the increasing numbers of prescriptions written for elderly patients, frequently without well-defined endpoints or even well-defined therapeutic indications. Frequent reviews of the patient's drug history, including over-the-counter medications, and discontinuation of those drugs that are not necessary would greatly improve medical care for the elderly population.

Benet LZ, Williams RL: Design and optimization of dosage regimens: Pharmacokinetic data. *In* Gilman AG, Rall TW, Nies AS, Taylor P (eds.): Goodman and Gilman's Pharmacological Basis of Therapeutics. 8th ed. New York, Pergamon Press, 1990, pp 1650–1735. *This series of tables lists the pharmacokinetic parameters of over 150 drugs with references to the literature. This represents the most concise and complete listing currently available and is the source for some of the data in Table 23–5.*

Bennett WM, Aronoff GR, Golper TA, et al.: Drug Prescribing in Renal Failure. Dosing Guidelines for Adults. Philadelphia, American College of Physicians, 1987. *A useful paperback manual that recommends dosage adjustments for many drugs in patients with varying degrees of renal dysfunction and those on dialysis.*

Bjornsson TD: Nomogram for drug dosage adjustment in patients with renal failure. Clin Pharmacokin 11:164, 1986. *This review of drug elimination in renal disease uses an approach to dosage adjustment similar to the nomogram in this chapter. There is an extensive compilation of over 130 drugs that can be used as a reference for those drugs not in Table 23–1 or Table 23–5.*

Cartwright A, Smith C: Elderly People, Their Medicines and Their Doctors. London, Routledge, 1988. *A landmark community-based study of medication use by the elderly in the United Kingdom. The findings indicate that although many elderly would rather not take drugs, patient compliance and knowledge of the purpose of their medications are quite good. However, there is a need for additional physician effort to avoid contraindicated and duplicated drugs, to improve the labeling and written instructions for patients, and to review the medications at each visit and discontinue those that are no longer needed.*

Montamat SC, Cusack BJ, Vestal RE: Management of drug therapy in the elderly. N Engl J Med 321:310, 1989. *A review of the use of drugs in the elderly that summarizes the relevant literature.*

Wilkinson GR, Shand DG: A physiological approach to hepatic drug clearance. Clin Pharmacol Ther 18:377, 1975. *This article discusses hepatic drug clearance in relation to blood flow, enzyme activity, and plasma protein binding. The concepts are valuable for physiologically oriented individuals.*

24 Interactions Between Drugs

Alan S. Nies

Good medical practice frequently demands treatment with multiple drugs for a single disease in an attempt to maximize therapeutic effects and minimize side effects. When one is treating multiple diseases, the number of co-administered drugs increases, as does the possibility of undesirable interactions occurring between the drugs. Entire textbooks have been written in an attempt to list all possible drug interactions. It is obviously impossible for a clinician to remember such lists, and frequently the *clinically important* drug interactions are lost in the midst of large listings of interactions that are based on undocumented case reports, animal experimentation, or theory.

Not all drug interactions that occur are clinically important because (1) many drugs have such large therapeutic indices that toxicity does not result when there are moderate increases in drug concentration; (2) the disease being treated may not be serious so that a change of drug concentration to less than therapeutic levels may not be easily recognized; (3) many drugs are given without well-defined therapeutic endpoints, making the drug effect difficult to assess, and therefore changes in drug effect are not recognized; (4) there is a large intersubject variability due to genetic, environmental, and disease factors that may obscure many drug interactions. These comments are not to imply that drug interactions are not important. Drug interactions are important if the drug has easily recognizable toxicity and a low therapeutic index such that small increases in amount of drug

in the body produce significant toxicity. Second, drug interactions are recognized and important if the diseases that are being controlled with the drug are serious or potentially fatal when undertreated. Third, drug interactions are recognized if the therapeutic endpoints for the drug are clearly defined or if drug levels are used to maximize therapy for a given drug. Thus major interactions have been reported with anticoagulants and oral hypoglycemics, both of which have easily recognizable toxicity with low therapeutic indices. Drug interactions are reported with antiseizure medication and antiarrhythmic drugs; not only do these drugs have recognized toxicity, but also the diseases being treated become clinically manifest if the amount of drug is inadequate. Drug interactions have been recognized with cardiac glycosides when blood levels are used to maximize efficacy in some patients.

Clinically important drug interactions are related to (1) changes in the amount of drug or active metabolite available at the site of action, the so-called pharmacokinetic drug interactions, or (2) changes in drug effect without a change in pharmacokinetics, the pharmacodynamic drug interactions. These latter interactions may result from interactions at a receptor site, from independent actions of two drugs either adding to or counteracting the effects of each other, or from one drug altering the cellular milieu, thus changing the effects of another drug.

PHARMACOKINETIC DRUG INTERACTIONS

These interactions involve the processes of absorption, distribution, and elimination such that there is a change in the amount of a drug (or an active metabolite) at the site of action and a corresponding change in drug effect.

Interactions Resulting in Less Drug Available at the Site of Action

DECREASED ABSORPTION. Since drug absorption generally occurs across the gastrointestinal mucosa by passive diffusion, one drug would not be expected to compete with another for absorption. However, drugs may physically interact in the lumen of the gastrointestinal tract so as to cause decreased absorption. Cholestyramine and colestipol, resins used to bind bile acids and to lower serum cholesterol, can also bind a number of drugs if they are simultaneously present in the gastrointestinal lumen. Thus cholestyramine can diminish the absorption of thyroid hormones, cardiac glycosides, warfarin, and corticosteroids. It is likely that other drugs also bind to the steroid-binding resins, so one is advised to separate the administration of the resin from that of other drug doses by at least 2 hours.

Tetracyclines are potent chelating agents that form insoluble complexes with metal ions such as magnesium, calcium, and aluminum, commonly found in antacids, as well as with iron, with the result that the absorption of tetracycline is reduced. Sucralfate used for peptic ulcer disease has been reported to reduce the absorption of warfarin and phenytoin. Kaolin used to halt diarrhea effectively inhibits the absorption of some drugs such as lincomycin and digoxin. In addition, drug products may contain "inert" substances that can interact with other drugs. For instance, para-aminosalicylic acid (PAS) contains bentonite (a kaolin-like substance), which can hamper the absorption of co-administered rifampin.

If a drug is susceptible to degradation at acid pH, anything that delays emptying of the stomach, such as a drug with anticholinergic properties, can result in more degradation of the co-administered acid-sensitive drug, e.g., penicillin G or L-dopa, and thus a decrease in the amount of drug absorbed. Conversely, a drug that speeds gastric emptying, such as metoclopramide, can increase the absorption of acid-unstable drugs. With most other drugs only the time course of absorption is changed so that drug absorption is faster if gastric emptying is enhanced or slower if gastric emptying is delayed, but the total amount of drug absorbed is unchanged. Whether a change in rate of absorption results in any important clinical effects depends on whether rapid absorption is necessary for drug effect, in which case drug effect is diminished. Usually, if total absorption is unchanged, there is no important interaction, particularly during chronic administration of drugs.

The pH of the gastrointestinal fluid can affect the dissolution of drug from the dosage form. Ketoconazole, a weak base, is most soluble in acidic gastric fluid. If gastric pH is increased by antacids or H_2-antihistamines, the dissolution and hence the absorption of ketoconazole are reduced.

ALTERED DISTRIBUTION. A few drugs reach their site of action via active transport. In this case, drugs can compete with each other for the transport mechanism. In order to produce blockade of adrenergic activity, the antihypertensive drugs guanethidine, guanadrel, and bethanidine must be actively transported by an amine transport system into adrenergic neurons. This transport system can be interfered with by tricyclic antidepressants, high doses of phenothiazines, and some sympathomimetic amines. Thus co-administration of guanethidine with one of these other compounds effectively blocks the antihypertensive effects of guanethidine. This is an undesirable interaction with guanethidine; however, with the antiarrhythmic drug bretylium, sympathetic blockade produces orthostatic hypotension as an unwanted side effect. Bretylium also gains access to adrenergic neurons via the same amine transport system used by guanethidine. Therapeutic advantage can be taken of a drug interaction that blocks access of bretylium to its antiadrenergic site of action. Thus tricyclic antidepressants or ephedrine reverses bretylium's sympathetic blocking effects but does not affect the direct antiarrhythmic effects of bretylium.

ENHANCED METABOLISM. Several drugs can increase the ability of the liver to metabolize other drugs by the mixed function oxidase (P450) system. Phenobarbital, other barbiturates, phenytoin, rifampin, glutethimide, griseofulvin, ethanol, phenylbutazone, chronic smoking, certain chlorinated hydrocarbons such as lindane and DDT, carbamazepine, and primidone have all been associated with induction of hepatic microsomal, drug-metabolizing enzymes. The amount of enzyme induction that occurs appears to be under genetic control, and not all individuals experience quantitatively similar effects when taking an inducing agent.

Induction of hepatic metabolizing enzymes can affect many drugs. The effects are greatest when the drugs are given orally, because all of the drug must pass through the liver prior to reaching the systemic circulation. Therefore, even for drugs that have a systemic clearance largely dependent upon hepatic blood flow, the amount of drug that escapes metabolism on the first pass is influenced by enzyme-inducing drugs. Some examples of drugs that can have their metabolism induced are oral anticoagulants, quinidine, digitoxin, corticosteroids, low-dose oral contraceptives, cyclosporine, some beta-adrenergic blockers, mexiletine, and theophylline. The induction of corticosteroid metabolism has produced some interesting effects, including (1) inappropriate interpretation of low-dose dexamethasone suppression tests in which the enhanced metabolism of dexamethasone produced by enzyme induction resulted in too low a dexamethasone concentration to inhibit normal steroidogenesis; (2) exacerbation of steroid-dependent asthma; (3) rejection of a renal transplant by individuals who required steroids and received an enzyme-inducing agent; (4) nonresponsiveness of the nephrotic syndrome to steroid therapy; and (5) increased adrenal corticosteroid replacement dosage in patients with Addison's disease.

Frequently the most critical time occurs when the inducing agent is discontinued. At this time the drug-metabolizing activity gradually decreases, and drug toxicity can occur if dosage adjustments of other co-administered drugs are not made. This phenomenon has been described most frequently with induction of warfarin metabolism and resultant warfarin toxicity when the inducing agent is discontinued.

Interactions Resulting in More Drug Available at the Site of Action

ENHANCED ABSORPTION. In general, absorption is not a common process in which drugs can interact to enhance efficacy. One exception is with acid-unstable drugs and enhanced gastric emptying mentioned above. Another potential interaction is with relatively poorly absorbed drugs, such as tablet formulations of digoxin, with which absorption occurs throughout the gastrointestinal tract. With such a drug a decrease in intestinal motility could enhance the degree of absorption by prolonging contact with the absorbing mucosa.

ALTERED DISTRIBUTION. Many drugs are bound to plasma proteins, and drug so bound is not available for action at

receptors or for distribution throughout the body. In addition, for many compounds only the free drug is available for metabolism or excretion. The drug bound to plasma protein, therefore, acts as an inactive reservoir of drug in the blood. Since drugs can compete with each other for binding to plasma proteins, a potential for interactions exists. Pure plasma protein–binding interactions, however, rarely are clinically significant. The one probable exception to this is the displacement of albumin-bound bilirubin by sulfonamides or salicylates, thus allowing the bilirubin to distribute into the tissues and cause kernicterus in jaundiced infants. However, when a drug is displaced from plasma protein binding, it very rapidly distributes into the apparent volume of distribution so that the increase in free drug concentration in the plasma is always considerably less than suggested by experiments in vitro. The larger the apparent volume of distribution, the less of an impact a displacement from protein binding has. Following the immediate displacement and redistribution of the drug, the free fraction generally is readily available for metabolism or excretion, and the clearance processes in the body reduce the free drug concentration to that which existed prior to the protein-binding interaction (Fig. 24–1). Therefore the effect of such an interaction is small and transient. The relationship of free drug to total drug, however, is changed by such drug interactions, and therefore the interpretation of plasma drug assays that measure total drug in blood may have to be altered (see Ch. 23).

DECREASED METABOLISM. Inhibition of drug metabolism can have a profound effect on drug disposition, resulting in drug toxicity. Inhibition of the metabolism of one drug by another occurs rapidly, and the enhanced effect or toxicity therefore often occurs shortly after the interaction takes place. Some drugs seem to be rather specific for inhibiting the metabolism of other individual drugs. However, there are a few drugs that can inhibit the metabolism of many drugs. The most commonly used such drug is cimetidine, which can inhibit the metabolism of theophylline, warfarin, diazepam, phenytoin, lidocaine, chlordiazepoxide, propranolol, carbamazepine, digitoxin, imipramine, quin-

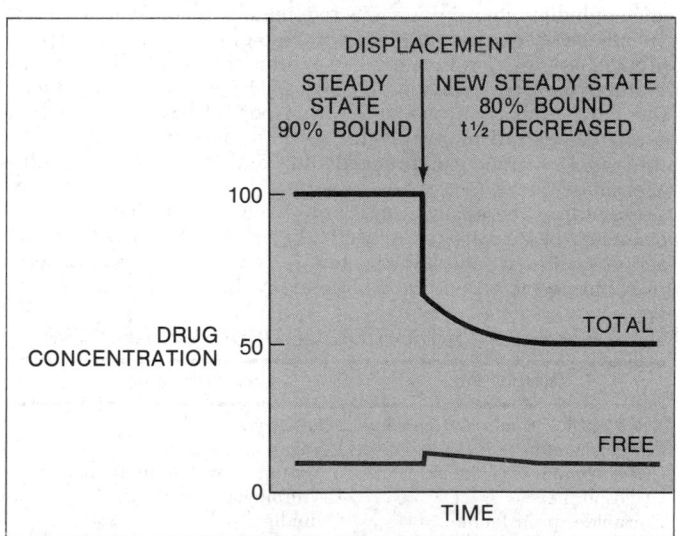

FIGURE 24–1. The effects of altered plasma drug binding on total and free plasma concentrations of the drug. The drug is assumed to be bound 90 per cent to albumin, not bound to tissues, and to have a V_D of 8.5 liters. At the arrow an agent is given that displaces the drug from albumin such that binding is reduced to 80 per cent. The expected changes are an immediate increase in free drug concentration by only 40 per cent, with a fall of total concentration to 70 per cent of the initial value. Since the free drug clearance is not altered by this interaction, a new steady state is achieved with the same free drug concentration and a reduction of total concentration to 50 per cent. For drugs with larger volumes of distribution, i.e., more tissue binding, the immediate increase of free concentration is even less than in this example, but the ultimate steady-state condition of unchanged free drug concentration and a halving of the concentration of total drug is the same. (Adapted from Shand et al.: *In* Handbook of Experimental Pharmacology. Vol 28, No 3, pp 272–314, 1975.)

idine, flecainide, calcium channel blockers, and probably others. The antiarrhythmic drug amiodarone also appears to be a potent inhibitor of the metabolism of many other drugs, including warfarin, phenytoin, flecainide, calcium channel blockers, and quinidine. Since amiodarone has a half-life of 1 to 2 months, inhibition of enzyme activity produced by amiodarone may persist for several months after the drug is discontinued. Other important interactions resulting from decreased metabolism are listed in Table 24–1. As with other interactions resulting in an increased amount of drug at the sites of action, the most important examples are drugs that have a low therapeutic index and easily recognized, serious toxicity.

In addition to inhibition of hepatic drug metabolism via mixed function oxidase, inhibition of metabolism at other enzyme sites can be important. Thus nonselective monoamine oxidase inhibitors can inhibit the metabolism of catecholamines and tyramine at multiple sites, allowing for build-up of these substances and the so-called cheese reaction due to enhanced catecholamine release with the ingestion of tyramine-containing foods. The new MAO inhibitor selegiline (deprenyl), which is selective for the B isozyme of MAO, does not produce this type of interaction at low doses (< 20 mg per day). Allopurinol inhibits xanthine oxidase, which can be important for the metabolism of azathioprine and 6-mercaptopurine. If allopurinol is given, much less azathioprine or 6-mercaptopurine is needed for equivalent effects. As discussed above, ethanol can induce hepatic microsomal drug-metabolizing enzymes. However, if ethanol is present, it can also act as an inhibitor of drug metabolism. Thus drugs given to an individual who is intoxicated may have an enhanced effect, whereas drugs given to an individual who has been drinking chronically but is no longer intoxicated may have diminished effect.

DIMINISHED RENAL EXCRETION. Some important drug interactions occur when active transport of one drug across the renal tubule is inhibited by another drug. Most of the reported interactions occur at the acid transport site. Thus probenecid is given to decrease penicillin clearance and thereby increase penicillin blood levels. Phenylbutazone can inhibit the renal clearance of hydroxyhexamide, an active metabolite of acetohexamide, and thereby increase its hypoglycemic effect. Salicylates, phenylbutazone, and probenecid can inhibit the renal elimination of methotrexate and enhance its effect. Drugs can also interact at the renal tubular site for active transport of bases, which is the probable mechanism by which cimetidine and amiodarone reduce the renal clearance of procainamide and its active metabolite, acecainide.

Quinidine, verapamil, and amiodarone can reduce the renal clearance of digoxin. The exact tubular site at which this interaction occurs is not known, but it is a significant interaction resulting in increased digoxin blood levels and effects.

TABLE 24–1. INHIBITION OF DRUG METABOLISM

Metabolism of	Inhibited by
Azathioprine, 6-mercaptopurine	Allopurinol
Carbamazepine	Verapamil, isoniazid
Catecholamines, tyramine	Monoamine oxidase inhibitors
Cyclosporine	Erythromycin, ketoconazole
Encainide, propafenone, propranolol	Quinidine
Phenobarbital	Valproic acid
Phenytoin	Isoniazid (in slow acetylators), chloramphenicol, cimetidine, clofibrate, phenylbutazone, disulfiram, dicumarol, amiodarone, valproic acid
Theophylline	Cimetidine, erythromycin, troleandomycin
Tolbutamide	Chloramphenicol, phenylbutazone, clofibrate, sulfaphenazole, dicumarol
Warfarin	Phenylbutazone, alcohol, disulfiram, allopurinol, cimetidine, disopyramide, sulfinpyrazone, trimethoprim-sulfamethoxazole, metronidazole, amiodarone

Decreased renal excretion of lithium occurs when proximal tubular reabsorption is enhanced. Since lithium and sodium are handled similarly in the proximal tubule, anything that results in more proximal tubular sodium reabsorption also affects lithium in the same way. Thus dietary salt restriction, salt depletion due to diarrhea, and diuretics acting at more distal segments of the nephron can reduce renal lithium excretion, requiring a reduction in lithium dose. Indomethacin and other nonsteroidal anti-inflammatory drugs also reduce lithium clearance, probably by enhancing proximal tubular reabsorption of the ion.

PHARMACODYNAMIC DRUG INTERACTIONS

Numerous drugs interact with each other at receptor sites or have additive effects by acting at separate sites on cells. Thus vitamin K can inhibit the effects of warfarin. Propranolol can interact with epinephrine by blocking the beta-adrenergic receptors and thus allowing the alpha-adrenergic effects of epinephrine to be unopposed, which can result in severe hypertension. Clonidine has been shown to have its antihypertensive effects in humans inhibited by tricyclic antidepressants. The mechanism for this is not entirely worked out but might be an interaction at an alpha-adrenergic receptor in the brain.

Additive effects of drugs are common. Additive negative cardiac inotropic effects of disopyramide, beta-adrenergic blockers, and calcium channel blocking drugs can produce heart failure. Similarly, the additive negative chronotropic and dromotropic effects of amiodarone, digoxin, beta-adrenergic blockers, and calcium channel blocking drugs can produce bradycardia, sinus arrest, or atrioventricular block. Two drugs that may affect the eighth cranial nerve, such as ethacrynic acid and aminoglycosides, may produce additional ototoxicity if given together. Drugs such as curare have an enhanced effect if given with aminoglycosides, lincomycin, clindamycin, quinidine, or quinine, which also affect neuromuscular function.

One drug may alter the normal homeostatic mechanisms, resulting in a change in the internal milieu and thereby enhancing or diminishing the effect of another drug. The best-studied example of this type of interaction is the effect of diuretics to produce hypokalemia, which enhances the toxicity of cardiac glycosides.

Some drug interactions have not been well characterized, although the interaction is clearly significant. This is true for the interaction of warfarin with clofibrate. Clofibrate has a marked effect to increase the efficacy of warfarin, but sufficient pharmacokinetic changes to account for this effect do not occur even though clofibrate may displace warfarin from plasma protein.

When viewed in perspective, drug interactions are only one of many factors that can alter the response of patients to drugs. Clinicians must be aware of the serious interactions and have well-defined therapeutic goals so that altered amounts or effects of drugs become evident. The only way to accomplish this is to individualize therapy using effects or plasma drug levels when appropriate, particularly for drugs with low therapeutic indices or during treatment of serious illnesses. Care must be used when a drug regimen is changed in any major way. If an interaction is appreciated, dosage adjustments can be made, and the two drugs often can be used together effectively. Drug interactions are an accepted fact of modern medical practice and should not be ignored, nor should they be overly feared.

Hansten PD, Horn JR: Drug Interactions. 6th ed. Philadelphia, Lea and Febiger, 1989. *This frequently revised text is a useful compilation of known drug interactions. The interactions listed are referenced, and an estimate of probable clinical significance of the interaction is given. The 6th edition is available in a loose-leaf format that can be updated periodically with inserts sent by the publisher.*

McInnes GT, Brodie MT: Drug interactions that matter. A critical reappraisal. Drugs 36:83, 1988. *There is no dearth of reviews on this topic trying to sort the clinically important from the unimportant drug interactions. This review is recent and well referenced.*

Shand DG, Mitchell JR, Oates JA: Pharmacokinetic drug interactions. *In* Gillette JR, Mitchell JR (eds.): Handbook of Experimental Pharmacology. Vol 28, No 3. Concepts in Biochemical Pharmacology. New York, Springer-Verlag, 1975, pp 272–314. *This is a thorough review of pharmacokinetic mechanisms whereby drugs can interact. It is not a complete listing of potential drug interactions, although many illustrative examples for the various mechanisms are given.*

25 Adverse Reactions to Drugs

Alan S. Nies

Although difficult to quantify, adverse reactions to drugs constitute an inevitable consequence of modern therapeutics. No drug is devoid of the potential to do harm, and benefit-versus-risk decisions are made with every decision to start drug therapy. Frequently it is difficult to be certain that an adverse effect is due to an individual drug because of the confounding effects of the underlying disease and the use of multiple drugs.

The overall incidence of significant adverse drug reactions is probably quite low, in the range of 1 to 5 per cent. Nevertheless, adverse drug reactions account for 2 to 10 per cent of admissions to hospital medical departments. An inpatient has a 10 to 20 per cent chance of experiencing a major adverse drug reaction, which is the most common iatrogenic illness in the hospital. Patients at highest risk are those who are receiving the most drugs and who have the most complicated illnesses. Drugs most commonly associated with serious adverse reactions include cardiovascular drugs (especially digitalis), steroidal and nonsteroidal anti-inflammatory drugs, diuretics, theophylline, anticoagulants, CNS active drugs, and antimicrobials.

Recent studies do not indicate that the incidence of adverse drug reactions is decreasing. On the contrary, the risk may be increasing as the number of potent drugs available increases. It is impossible to make a quantitative statement of risk versus benefit of medical therapy. Adverse reactions cannot be completely prevented even under the best of circumstances. Nonetheless, it is important to continue investigation into ways to assess the risk and to reduce both the incidence and severity of these adverse reactions.

MECHANISMS OF ADVERSE DRUG REACTIONS

Unwanted effects of drugs are due to (1) exaggerated responses to the known desired or unwanted pharmacologic effects of the drug; (2) immunologic reactions to the drug or its metabolites; and (3) toxic effects of a drug or its metabolites. "Idiosyncratic" effects may be due to any of these mechanisms. The extension of the normal pharmacology accounts for most adverse drug effects. However, since these effects are predictable, they often may be avoided or treated by careful dosage adjustment without necessarily discontinuing drug treatment. The immunologically mediated and toxic adverse effects of drugs are less predictable and may be so severe as to require discontinuation of the offending drug. These latter effects are the least well understood, but mechanisms of some of the toxic drug effects have been discovered. Any organ system can be affected by drugs, and drug-induced disease should be a consideration in the differential diagnosis of most syndromes that present to an internist.

EXAGGERATED RESPONSES TO DRUGS

Excessive drug effects result from altered pharmacokinetics or altered target-organ response, as discussed in the previous chapters. Thus adverse drug effects are more common in the elderly, in patients with abnormal renal or hepatic function, and in patients receiving other drugs that may result in pharmacokinetic or pharmacodynamic interactions.

An example of a disease exaggerating the unwanted effects of a normally innocuous drug is the reduction in glomerular filtration rate produced by nonsteroidal anti-inflammatory drugs in patients who have activation of their sympathetic nervous system and/or increased plasma renin activity as a result of hepatic, renal, or cardiovascular disease. This adverse effect is a consequence of the same pharmacologic action responsible for the salutary effects of the drug, namely, inhibition of cyclo-oxygenase activity with a reduction in prostaglandin synthesis.

In addition, patients may have genetic abnormalities that make them susceptible to one or another effect of a drug. These genetic differences may be quantitative deviations from the norm or qualitative abnormalities. An example of such quantitative differences is the variability in hepatic drug oxidation that is described by a unimodal frequency distribution. Twin studies have indicated that genetic differences account for much of the variation between

individuals in the metabolism of phenytoin, phenylbutazone, warfarin, ethanol, nortriptyline, and salicylate. In addition, an increasing number of drug metabolic processes are now recognized to be controlled by genes at a single locus, such as slow acetylation of isoniazid, some sulfonamides, and procainamide; deficient parahydroxylation of phenytoin; deficient hydroxylation of debrisoquin, or mephenytoin; deficient N-glucosidation of amobarbital; and deficient hydrolysis of succinylcholine. The excessive drug effects resulting from the genetically determined slow metabolic processes reflect an increased concentration of unmetabolized drug available at the site of action.

In addition to these quantitative differences in drug metabolism, genetic abnormalities may result in qualitatively different responses to drugs. These reactions are due to known properties of the drug that are usually not important but become markedly exaggerated owing to the genetic defect. Thus individuals with a deficiency of the enzyme activity of glucose-6-phosphate dehydrogenase (G6PD) are unable to cope with the oxidative stress produced by some drugs, and hemolysis results. Drugs having this effect include primaquine, aspirin, sulfonamides, nitrofurantoin, sulfones, vitamin K, probenecid, quinidine, and quinine. In a similar manner, genetic deficiency of methemoglobin reductase results in inability to maintain hemoglobin in the ferrous form, resulting in methemoglobinemia upon exposure to some oxidizing drugs such as sulfones, sulfonamides, and nitrites. Likewise certain genetically abnormal hemoglobins may be unstable and result in drug-induced hemolysis or methemoglobinemia. Frequently patients with these "pharmacogenetic" syndromes are unaware of any abnormality until they are challenged with a drug that produces the adverse effect.

TOXIC AND IMMUNOLOGIC REACTIONS

Adverse drug reactions in these categories are often lumped together because it is frequently difficult to be certain of the etiology of an individual reaction (Table 25–1). Toxic reactions include direct effects of a drug on a target organ, such as the nephrotoxicity and ototoxicity produced by aminoglycosides. In other cases drugs are metabolized to reactive intermediates that can covalently bind to cellular components, often near the site of metabolism, and produce toxicity. This mechanism is well established for the hepatotoxicity produced by overdoses of acetaminophen. During therapeutic use of acetaminophen the small amount of reactive metabolite formed by oxidative metabolism is rapidly detoxified by interacting with reduced glutathione. With overdose, however, glutathione is depleted, and the reactive metabolite attacks hepatic macromolecules, resulting in liver damage. Sulfhydryl-containing compounds such as N-acetylcysteine or cysteamine can protect the liver by reducing the amount of toxic metabolite that remains unreacted with a sulfhydryl-containing compound. Other drugs may produce liver disease by somewhat similar mechanisms. Isoniazid-induced hepatitis may result from acetylation to acetylisoniazid that can be hydrolyzed to acetylhydrazine, which can be oxidized by the hepatic mixed function oxidase system to a reactive metabolite. One might expect from this theory that individuals who rapidly acetylate isoniazid would be more susceptible to the hepatotoxicity. However, the opposite may be true. This apparent discrepancy may be related to observations that rapid acetylators not only form acetylisoniazid rapidly but also quickly convert this metabolite to diacetylisoniazid, which is nontoxic. Slow acetylators, on the other hand, form acetylisoniazid gradually but are much less able to convert it to diacetylisoniazid. Consequently, more of the acetylisoniazid is available for hydrolysis to acetylhydrazine and subsequent oxidation to the reactive metabolite. However, considerable controversy remains regarding the relevance of this theory to the clinical hepatitis that results from isoniazid, and other factors, such as the patient's age, are also important.

Hepatocellular damage, such as that produced by methyldopa or halothane, is frequently considered to be immunologically produced. However, reactive metabolites could be important for these as well as a variety of other drugs that produce hepatotoxicity on occasion.

Immunologic reactions to drugs account for only 5 to 10 per cent of all adverse drug reactions and probably result from the

TABLE 25–1. "ALLERGIC" DRUG REACTIONS

Type of Reaction	Example (not inclusive)
Definite Immunologically Mediated Syndromes	
1. Immediate hypersensitivity (IgE-mediated) reactions	Penicillin-induced anaphylaxis Insulin-induced wheal and flare
2. Cytotoxic reactions	Drug-induced destruction of formed elements in the blood: Penicillin-induced hemolytic anemia Quinidine- or quinine-induced thrombocytopenia Phenylbutazone-induced granulocytopenia
3. Immune complex–induced vasculitis	Serum sickness–like reactions to penicillin, sulfonamides, and other drugs presenting as fever, rash, palpable purpura, arthralgia, and/or lymphadenopathy
4. Delayed hypersensitivity reactions	Contact dermatitis from topically applied drugs
Possible Immunologically Mediated Syndromes but with Unknown Mechanism	
1. Skin rashes of various types	Many drugs and a variety of skin eruptions
2. Stevens-Johnson syndrome	Sulfonamides, penicillins, phenytoin, phenylbutazone
3. Fever	Antibiotics, quinidine, methyldopa, procainamide, phenytoin, antineoplastic drugs
4. Pneumonitis	Löffler's syndrome
5. Lupus erythematosus–like condition	Procainamide, hydralazine, isoniazid
6. Hepatic dysfunction	Chlorpromazine-induced cholestasis ? Methyldopa-induced hepatitis ? Halothane-induced hepatitis
7. Renal dysfunction	Interstitial nephritis from methicillin, furosemide, allopurinol
8. Lymphadenopathy	Phenytoin, sulfonamides

drug or a reactive metabolite combining with a protein to form an antigenic drug-protein complex that stimulates the immune response. Without such a reaction, most drugs, which have a molecular weight less than 1000, would not be able to elicit an immunologic response. The typical immunologic reaction requires a latent period of 10 to 20 days for stimulation of the production of antibodies and activated immune effector cells that cause the allergic reaction. After the initial exposure, however, the allergic reaction occurs with a much shorter or no latent period after re-exposure to the drug. Drug hypersensitivity can produce mediator release, initiate cell lysis, activate the complement system, or activate cellular hypersensitivity reactions.

The most dramatic allergic reaction is anaphylaxis, or IgE-mediated hypersensitivity. Penicillin is the most common drug to produce anaphylaxis, but many other drugs or diagnostic agents (such as Bromsulphalein) can produce this life-threatening reaction. Although oral therapy is least sensitizing, once sensitization has occurred, anaphylaxis may occur with any route of administration. A history of penicillin allergy increases the risk of this reaction occurring, but most (75 per cent) of the 100 to 300 patients dying of penicillin-induced anaphylaxis each year have no history of penicillin allergy. Skin testing with penicilloyl-polylysine, penicillin G, and penicilloic acid is the best method to identify patients at risk for anaphylaxis and should be used if penicillin therapy is considered mandatory in a patient with a history of penicillin allergy. Patients with a negative skin test can be given penicillin therapy cautiously. Patients with a positive skin test should be desensitized prior to receiving penicillin

therapy. Unfortunately, a negative assay in vitro to detect penicilloyl-specific IgE is less specific than skin testing to rule out the possibility of penicillin anaphylaxis, but a positive test in vitro has the same implications as a positive skin test.

Cytotoxic allergic reactions occur when a drug binds to the surface of a cell and is then attacked by antibody. Penicillin-induced hemolytic anemia is of this type. Immune complexes of drug and antibody may become adsorbed to the cell membrane, resulting in complement-mediated cytotoxicity. Thrombocytopenia and hemolytic anemia due to quinine or quinidine are examples of immune complex–mediated cytotoxicity. Methyldopa-induced Coombs' positivity occurs in up to 20 per cent of patients on therapy for over 6 months and results in antibodies directed at the Rh loci of the red cell. However, the continued presence of methyldopa is not necessary for the immune reaction to continue, and the Coombs' positivity only gradually resolves upon discontinuation of the drug.

Circulating immune complexes of drug and antibody can produce serum sickness (see Ch. 245 and 256), a vasculitic syndrome produced by deposition of immune complexes. Penicillin, sulfonamides, thiouracil, cholecystographic dyes, phenytoin, and other drugs can cause serum sickness.

Drug-induced lupus syndromes as caused by procainamide, hydralazine, and isoniazid may be associated with circulating immune complexes. In this case the drug or a reactive metabolite may interact with nuclear material to allow formation of antinuclear antibodies. The drug-induced systemic lupus erythematosus (SLE) (see Ch. 261) differs from spontaneous lupus by being uncommon in blacks and by only rarely causing nephritis. The acetylator phenotype also is important in drug-induced lupus. Hydralazine-induced lupus is very uncommon in fast acetylators. Procainamide-induced lupus occurs with smaller cumulative doses of drug in slow acetylators, although fast acetylators are also at risk.

In addition to the immune phenomena outlined above, many other syndromes are attributed to drug allergy (Table 25–1). These include a variety of skin rashes, drug fever, pulmonary reactions, hepatocellular or cholestatic reactions, interstitial nephritis, and lymphadenopathy. For most of these reactions, the exact immune mechanism is unknown. One interesting syndrome that is sometimes classified as immune but may involve other mechanisms as well is that of aspirin sensitivity. In some patients this syndrome resembles IgE-mediated allergy with rhinitis, sinusitis, nasal polyps, and asthma. However, other cyclo-oxygenase inhibitors, such as indomethacin and meclofenamate, also produce asthma in many of these patients, suggesting a possible etiologic role for an arachidonic acid metabolite, such as a leukotriene, rather than an immunologic mechanism. It seems likely that several syndromes of aspirin sensitivity exist.

Some adverse drug reactions mimic anaphylactic reactions but are not immune mediated. Such reactions are due to direct release of mediators by drugs and are called anaphylactoid reactions. Reactions to radiocontrast dyes are of this type. The risk of re-exposure to the dye is unpredictable and skin testing is of no value. If re-exposure is absolutely necessary, pretreatment with steroids and H_1-antihistamines is the current practice. Since the newer, low-osmolality radiocontrast media appear to produce fewer anaphylactoid reactions, their use is preferable in patients who give a history of reaction to the older agents.

RECOGNITION AND IDENTIFICATION

Adverse drug effects must first be suspected to be recognized. In some situations, the adverse effect mimics the illness being treated (for instance, arrhythmias caused by antiarrhythmic drugs or antibiotic-induced fever). In other instances, the reaction is more obviously drug induced, as is the case with characteristic skin rashes or anticoagulant-induced bleeding. The first confirmation of an adverse reaction is its disappearance with drug withdrawal. In some cases cautious readministration of the putative offending drug may be warranted if the drug is likely to be required again for therapy. In the case of serious allergic or toxic reactions, however, this may be too dangerous. Tests in vitro are occasionally helpful for drug-induced thrombocytopenia or hemolytic anemia but are not useful for most drug reactions. Skin testing is of value with penicillin, insulin, and horse serum.

Adverse reactions will continue to occur as long as potent drugs are available. Most of the reactions are predictable. The unexpected toxic and immunologic reactions remain a problem that continues to stimulate discussions as to how to detect rare adverse effects. During the process of drug development, reactions occurring less often than 1 per 1000 patients are not detected. In addition, drugs are developed by testing in patients who have well-defined diseases, are not on many other drugs, are not pregnant, and are usually neither in the pediatric nor the geriatric population. After approval, however, all patient populations may be exposed to the drug. Therefore, the adverse effects of a new drug frequently are not discovered until after marketing. Different systems exist for early detection of drug reactions after marketing. A major mechanism is an early warning that results from anecdotal reports by practicing physicians to pharmaceutical companies or drug regulatory agencies or letters published in general medical journals. Following the first alerts, a verification mechanism is required. It is in this area that much remains to be learned. Postmarketing surveillance of patients taking drugs will not be effective for uncommon drug reactions unless sample sizes of more than 100,000 patients are followed. Surveys of patients with certain diseases to determine the incidence of use of the drug suspected to have caused the illness (case-control study) may be a more efficient way to detect drug-induced illness for rare adverse effects. A controversial but promising and potentially powerful new method for detecting or verifying adverse events after drug marketing is the technique of automated record linkage, whereby computerized data bases are used to link prescription records with the medical records of individual patients. However, the alert practitioner has been and will continue to be the primary individual who makes the initial important observation that often provides the first clue to an unsuspected adverse drug reaction.

Anderson J, Adkinson NF Jr: Allergic reactions to drugs and biologic agents. JAMA 258:2891, 1987. *Part of the "primer on allergic and immunologic diseases," this short review outlines the mechanisms of immunologic reactions to drugs. The authors provide relevant references and distinguish between allergic reactions for which the immune mechanisms are established and those that are only conjectured to be immunologically mediated.*

Davies DM (ed.): Textbook of Adverse Drug Reactions. 3rd ed. Oxford, Oxford University Press, 1985. *This well-referenced book is organized by specific syndromes, with a discussion of the drugs that may cause the syndrome. General problems of detecting and verifying adverse reactions are also discussed.*

Edlavitch SA: Adverse drug event reporting. Improving the low US reporting rates. Arch Intern Med 148:1499, 1988. *This editorial discusses the importance of spontaneous reports of drug reactions by physicians in providing an early warning of previously unsuspected drug risks. It accompanies a study indicating that nearly half of the physicians in the United States are unaware of the existence of the FDA reporting system for adverse drug events, and those that are aware report only a low percentage of such events. Suggestions for improving the system are discussed.*

Lewis JH, Zimmerman HJ: Drug-induced liver disease. Med Clin North Am 73:775, 1989. *This is an update discussing the spectrum, pathology, and possible mechanisms of drug-induced liver disease and serves as an entry to the extensive literature on this important adverse drug effect.*

Steel K, Gertman PM, Crescenzi C, et al.: Iatrogenic illness on a general medical service at a university hospital. N Engl J Med 304:638, 1981. *This study of a medical service indicates a 36 per cent incidence of iatrogenic illness, of which 42 per cent were drug related.*

26 Pain and Its Management

Kathleen M. Foley

INTRODUCTION

Pain is the most common symptom for which patients seek medical assistance. To manage pain, the physician must understand its nature—the relationship between its medical, psychologic, and social aspects—and must establish a relationship of mutual trust with the patient. The physician's therapeutic task is twofold: to discover and treat the cause of the pain and to treat the pain itself, whether or not the underlying cause is treatable. Advances in knowledge of the physiology, pharmacology, and psychology of pain perception have led to improved care of

patients with both acute and chronic pain (see also Ch. 455), but a lack of generally agreed-upon definitions and classification of pain has hampered communication among physicians. To provide a more common ground for the evaluation and treatment of patients with pain, the International Association for the Study of Pain (IASP) has proposed a working definition: Pain is "an unpleasant sensory and emotional experience associated with either actual or potential tissue damage, or described in terms of such damage." The IASP has also developed a taxonomy of pain syndromes that serves as a universal classification of pain syndromes (see references).

TYPES OF PAIN

Clinically, pain can be classified *temporally* as acute or chronic, *physiologically* as somatic, visceral, or neuropathic, and *etiologically* as medical or psychogenic.

TEMPORAL CHARACTERISTICS. Patients with severe *acute pain* can usually give a clear description of its location, character, and timing. Furthermore, objective signs, particularly of autonomic nervous system hyperactivity, with tachycardia, hypertension, diaphoresis, mydriasis, and pallor are present. The pain is usually self-limited (e.g., postoperative pain, acute traumatic pain). The patient's ability to tolerate acute pain is influenced by the setting of the pain, its duration, and its psychologic significance. Treatment of both the cause of acute pain and the pain itself is usually possible. Pain lasting longer than 3 months is usually considered *chronic*. In patients with chronic pain, the localization, character, and timing of the pain are often more vague, and because the autonomic nervous system adapts, signs of autonomic hyperactivity disappear. Significant changes occur in the psychologic, social, and functional status of patients with chronic pain, often requiring a multidisciplinary approach to treatment, including pharmacologic, behavioral, and rehabilitative therapeutic approaches.

PHYSIOLOGIC CHARACTERISTICS. *Somatic pain* results from activation of peripheral receptors and somatic efferent nerves, without injury to the peripheral nerves or central nervous system. The pain can be either sharp or dull but is typically well localized and intermittent. *Visceral pain* results from activation of visceral nociceptive receptors and visceral efferent nerves and is characterized as a deep aching, cramping sensation, often referred to cutaneous sites. *Neuropathic pain* results from direct injury to peripheral receptors, nerves, or central nervous system. It is typically burning and dysesthetic and often occurs in an area of sensory loss (e.g., postherpetic neuralgia). The autonomic nervous system plays a significant modulatory role in all three types of pain but is most prominent in visceral and neuropathic pain. The somatic and visceral types of pain are readily managed with a wide variety of nonopioid or opioid analgesics, anesthetic blocks, and neurosurgical approaches. In contrast, neuropathic pain has a variable response to nonopioid and opioid analgesics and to anesthetic and neurosurgical procedures.

ETIOLOGIC CHARACTERISTICS. Patients with chronic pain can generally be classified into one of three major etiologic groups, allowing for some overlap. The first group includes patients with chronic pain associated with *structural disease*. Such pain occurs, for example, with rheumatoid arthritis, metastatic cancer, and sickle cell anemia and is usually characterized by prolonged episodes of pain alternating with pain-free intervals or by unremitting pain waxing and waning in severity. Successful treatment of the pain is closely allied with treatment of the disease, but in certain instances treatment of the pain is the only therapeutic goal, e.g., the dying cancer patient with pain. Psychological factors may play an important role in exacerbating or relieving pain, but analgesic drug therapy is the mainstay of therapy while attempting to treat the underlying disease.

The second group comprises patients who suffer from *psychophysiologic disorders* causing pain. In these patients, structural disease such as a herniated disc or torn ligaments may once have been present but psychological factors have caused chronic physiologic alterations, such as muscle spasm, which produce pain long after the underlying defect has healed. Typically, such patients are physically inactive and spend much of their time thinking and talking about their pain, often leading to social and emotional isolation. Patients are more impaired by their "chronic illness behavior" than by a defined pathologic condition. They usually respond poorly to analgesic drugs and often suffer from iatrogenic complications, such as adverse drug reactions and ineffective surgical procedures. They use health care resources excessively. Successful treatment can be expected only through a structured rehabilitation program designed to modify pain behaviors and not through medical intervention designed to correct pathologic conditions. Multidisciplinary pain clinics that diagnose and treat intractable pain exist in many centers and should be utilized to evaluate and treat such patients.

Patients of the third group complain of pain that appears to have neither a structural nor a physiologic basis. These patients probably suffer from *somatic delusions*. Such patients usually have serious psychiatric disorders, and the history of the pain is so vague and bizarre and its distribution so unanatomic as to suggest the diagnosis. These patients respond only to psychiatric therapy.

ASSESSMENT OF PAIN

No objective tests (except observing patient behavior) assess the severity of pain or even its presence. Therefore, the physician must accept the patient's report, taking into consideration his or her age, cultural background, environment, and psychological circumstances known to alter reaction to pain.

A thorough history, general physical examination, and careful neurologic examination are imperative in any patient complaining of pain. The description of the nature and distribution of the pain may be so characteristic (e.g., trigeminal neuralgia or tabetic lightning pains) that it allows no other diagnosis. Inquiry should be made concerning (1) the temporal pattern of pain, (2) its distribution, (3) exacerbating factors, (4) relieving factors, and (5) its meaning to the patient. For example, headache beginning early in the morning before arising suggests increased intracranial pressure, whereas headache occurring late in the day is more suggestive of tension. Back pain and sciatica made worse by sitting or walking suggest disc disease, whereas back pain and sciatica that are worse while the person is in bed indicate intraspinal tumor. All pain is relieved to some extent by distraction and a pleasurable environment and is exacerbated by anxiety or psychological stress. Postoperative pain has positive meaning for the patient undergoing hip replacement but negative meaning for the patient who has been diagnosed with metastatic bone disease to the hip. Clarifying the patient's concept of what the pain implies can improve the physician's understanding of the psychological factors associated with the pain.

A careful psychiatric history, looking particularly for signs and symptoms of depression, should be elicited from all patients. The distinction between pain and suffering should be made by both the physician and the patient. Specifically, physicians should inquire about the degree to which pain has interfered with the patient's activities, whether he or she is having difficulty sleeping, and whether there is a change in appetite or bowel habits. Early morning awakening, anorexia, and constipation are somatic manifestations of depression and may either be caused by chronic pain or exacerbate the effects of the pain. Patients should be questioned about suicidal thoughts associated with the severity and chronicity of the pain.

A general physical examination must be performed. Both the physical and the laboratory examination should begin with the assumption that the site of pathologic change is at the site of pain. The painful areas should be examined for swelling and redness as well as for any obvious deformity. (The pain of herpes zoster usually precedes the rash, and occasionally on examination one may note the faintest reddening of the skin in a dermatomal distribution.) The areas reported as painful should be palpated, the temperature estimated, and points of tenderness sought. (If the site of pain is in a soft tissue, bone, or joint, it should be tender to palpation as well as spontaneously painful.) Joints should be taken through a full range of motion, and the effect of movement on the pain assessed. Nerve trunks going to the extremities should be palpated and stretched by movement of that member (e.g., straight-leg raising, abduction and extension of the arm). Inflamed and compressed nerve roots and nerve plexuses are more painful when stretched. A careful neurologic examination must also be performed. If there are neurologic abnormalities (e.g., weakness, sensory loss, and reflex changes) in the painful part, one can infer that nervous system disease is responsible for the pain. However, the absence of neurologic abnormalities on first examination does not guarantee that the nervous system is free of disease, because the process may simply not have advanced beyond the stage of selectively involving pain pathways. For example, a Pancoast's tumor may cause shoulder and arm pain before other signs of neural involvement, such as Horner's syndrome or motor or sensory loss, appear.

Finally, laboratory examinations are performed. If the site of disease appears to be in bones or joints, radiographs, computed tomography (CT) scans, magnetic resonance imaging (MRI), or radioisotope scans may localize it. First attention should be paid to the local site of pain, but the physician should be familiar with the common referred patterns of pain (e.g., hip disease commonly causes knee pain, cardiac pain is frequently referred to the ulnar aspect of the arm and forearm, the pain of renal colic may be felt primarily in the groin and testicle, and pain resulting from disease of the throat may be referred to the ear).

Referred pain is pain perceived at a site remote from the source of the disturbance. Usually, referred pain is perceived as cutaneous and is evoked by disease of deep structures innervated by the same dermatome. Referred pain may be associated with cutaneous hyperalgesia and even relieved by procaine injection into the area of referral. When pain is referred to the same dermatome or myotome that innervates the diseased structure (e.g., pain down the medial aspect of the arm [T1-T2] produced by myocardial infarction or angina pectoris), it is often helpful in diagnosis. However, pain is sometimes referred a great distance from the primary site to segments not similarly innervated, and in such cases the mechanism is perplexing (e.g., anginal pain referred to the jaw). Various theories, such as division of the same nerve into deep and superficial branches, release of chemical mediators into the nervous system, and convergence of cutaneous and visceral nerves into a common synaptic pool at the spinal cord, all explain the dermatomal referral of pain but fail to explain pain at remote sites.

MANAGEMENT OF PAIN

Recent advances in pain research provide a scientific rationale that has improved treatment. These include better and more effective use of standard drug therapy (non-narcotic, narcotic, and adjuvant analgesic drugs), the development of new drugs and the use of novel routes of drug administration, more selective anesthetic and neurosurgical approaches, and the integration of behavioral approaches to pain control.

General Principles (Table 26–1)

1. Pain is best managed by treating the underlying disorder (e.g., steroids for giant cell arteritis relieve headache; radiation therapy for bone pain caused by cancer is often helpful), but in many patients the pain is chronic and the physician is able neither to treat the underlying disturbances nor to offer specific therapy for that type of pain.

2. Pain should be treated early and promptly. The persistence of untreated pain results in significant psychological morbidity, most commonly anxiety and depression with a sense of loss of control and hopelessness. Early treatment that provides prompt and continuous pain relief is crucial to prevent further compromise of the patient's emotional resources.

3. Multiple therapeutic approaches, often delivered simultaneously, should be utilized because different treatment modalities may be additive or synergistic when used together rather than separately. For example, combinations of narcotic and non-narcotic analgesics provide greater analgesia than either alone. Nonpharmacologic methods, such as relaxation techniques and cognitive coping skills, coupled with physical therapy and vocational rehabilitation, can often help in selected patients with chronic pain, especially when added to judicious drug therapy.

4. Narcotic drugs should be used with discrimination, but they should not be withheld if alternative therapy is ineffective. Long-term use of narcotics produces tolerance and physical dependence. Tolerance is the term used to describe increasing dose requirements to maintain analgesia. *Physical dependence* means

TABLE 26–1. GUIDELINES FOR THE USE OF ANALGESICS IN PAIN MANAGEMENT

1. Tailor drugs to nature and severity of pain
2. Know the pharmacology of the drug prescribed
   a. Know the duration of the analgesic effect
   b. Know the pharmacokinetic properties of the drug (duration of action and half-life)
   c. Know the equianalgesic doses for the drug and its route of administration (Table 26–2)
3. Adjust the route of administration to the patient's needs using oral, rectal, subcutaneous, intramuscular, intravenous, epidural, and intrathecal routes
4. Administer the analgesic on a regular basis after initial titration of the dose
5. Use drug combinations to provide additive analgesia and reduce side effects, e.g., nonsteroidal anti-inflammatory drugs, antihistamine (hydroxyzine), amphetamine (dextroamphetamine)
6. Avoid drug combinations that increase sedation without enhancing analgesia, e.g., benzodiazepine (diazepam) and phenothiazine
7. For narcotics, anticipate and treat side effects
   a. Sedation
   b. Respiratory depression
   c. Nausea and vomiting
   d. Constipation
   e. Multifocal myoclonus and seizures
8. When using narcotics, watch for the development of tolerance
   a. Switch to an alternate narcotic analgesic
   b. Start with one half of the equianalgesic dose and titrate to pain relief
   c. Use adjuvant analgesics and anesthetic and neurosurgical approaches
9. Prevent acute withdrawal
   a. Taper drugs slowly
   b. Use diluted doses of naloxone (0.4 mg in 10 ml of saline) to reverse narcotic-induced respiratory depression in the physically dependent patient and administer cautiously
10. Do not use placebos to assess pain

that the signs and symptoms of withdrawal appear if the narcotic drug is abruptly discontinued. These effects should not be confused with psychological dependence or *"addiction,"* which implies both a craving for the drug for effects other than analgesia and drug abuse behavior. The percentage of patients who actually become psychologically dependent on narcotics when they are given to treat medical illness is unknown, but recent data suggest that psychological dependence is unusual in patients treated for pain when the pain is later relieved by other means.

5. Psychological factors play a major role in chronic pain and must be carefully assessed. However, no patient should be diagnosed as having "psychogenic" pain until an exhaustive examination has ruled out structural disease. Depression should be identified and treated, and since the tricyclic antidepressants have analgesic properties as well, they are useful adjuvant analgesic drugs, particularly in patients with neuropathic pain.

6. Placebo effects are important. A positive analgesic response from intramuscular saline indicates only that the patient is a placebo responder. It does not suggest that the pain is unreal or less severe than reported by the patient. Misuse of placebo creates distrust between the patient and the physician and interferes with adequate pain assessment and management. In most clinical studies, up to one third of patients report relief of pain when given a placebo.

Drug Therapy

Analgesic drugs can be divided into three groups: Group I—the non-narcotic analgesics, such as aspirin and acetaminophen and the nonsteroidal anti-inflammatory drugs (NSAID's), act peripherally, probably on pain receptors; Group II—the narcotic agonist and antagonist drugs activate opiate receptors in the central and peripheral nervous systems; and Group III—the adjuvant analgesic drugs are designed for management of symptoms other than pain but produce relief in certain pain states (carbamazepine for trigeminal neuralgia) or potentiate narcotic analgesics. These three groups represent the mainstay of therapy for patients with acute and chronic pain. Effective use of these drugs requires an understanding of their pharmacologic characteristics and selection of a particular drug and dose geared to the needs of the individual patient.

NON-NARCOTIC ANALGESICS (Table 26–2). Aspirin, acetaminophen, and the NSAID's are the first-line agents for the management of mild to moderate pain, and in patients with severe pain these drugs potentiate the effects of narcotic analgesics. Non-narcotic analgesics have a ceiling effect, and their long-term use is limited by gastrointestinal and hematologic side effects. The choice and use of these drugs must be individualized, with the patient receiving maximal levels of one drug before another is tried. If pain control is ineffective or the non-narcotic agents are poorly tolerated, the use of narcotic analgesics is indicated. In general, the use of narcotics is limited to acute structural or chronic, irreversible structural pain, as in cancer.

NARCOTIC ANALGESICS (Table 26–3). The narcotic analgesics vary in potency, efficacy, and adverse effects. They are classified as agonist or antagonist drugs, depending on their ability to bind to the opiate receptors and produce analgesia. The narcotic *agonist* drugs, such as morphine, bind to specific opiate receptors, resulting in analgesia. These agents are commonly used in the management of chronic pain of structural cause, such as cancer pain. The narcotic *antagonist* drugs block the effect of morphine at its receptor. Included in this category is a group of drugs with analgesic properties referred to as the mixed agonist-antagonist drugs. These drugs are often used in acute postoperative pain management but are of limited use in chronic pain management for several reasons: They produce psychotomimetic effects with increasing doses; only pentazocine is available in oral form and only in combinations with naloxone, aspirin, or acetaminophen; they precipitate withdrawal in narcotic-dependent patients. Effective use of narcotic analgesics requires balancing of the desirable effect of pain relief with the undesirable side effects of nausea, vomiting, mental clouding, sedation, tolerance, and physical dependence. These undesirable effects impose a practical limit on the dose one can give a particular patient.

Much of the difficulty encountered with the clinical use of narcotics arises from individual variation, consisting of differences in response of specific patients to the same drug dose. Thus, although Tables 26–2 to 26–4 can serve as reference points, individualization of drug treatment is the cardinal rule of management. Drugs should be given in sufficient amounts and at close enough intervals to achieve adequate pain relief. "Weak"

TABLE 26–2. ORAL NON-NARCOTIC ANALGESIC DRUGS

Drug	Indications	Equianalgesic Dose	Starting Dose (mg), Range/24 hr	Comments
Aspirin	Often used in combination with narcotics	650	650	Contraindicated in hepatic and renal dysfunction; avoid during pregnancy, in hemolytic disorders, and in combination with steroids
Acetaminophen	Like aspirin	650	650	
Ibuprofen	Higher analgesic potential than aspirin	ND	200–400	Like aspirin
Fenoprofen	Like ibuprofen	ND	200–400	Like aspirin
Diflunisal	Longer duration of action than ibuprofen; higher analgesic potential than aspirin	ND	500–1000	Like aspirin
Naproxen	Like diflunisal	ND	250–500	Like aspirin

ND = not documented.

narcotics, such as codeine, propoxyphene, and oxycodone, are selected to treat moderate pain. If the pain remains unrelieved, the "strong" narcotic analgesics, such as morphine, hydromorphone, levorphanol, and methadone, should be employed. To ensure adequate dosing schedules, one must know the clinical pharmacology of the narcotic analgesics, including their duration of analgesic effect, their half-lives, and the equianalgesic doses for both oral and parenteral routes of administration. For example, the plasma half-lives of the narcotics vary widely and do not correlate with their analgesic time courses. Both methadone, with a half-life of 15 to 30 hours, and levorphanol, with a half-life of 12 to 16 hours, produce analgesia for only 4 to 6 hours. With repeated doses, these drugs accumulate in plasma and can result in excessive sedation and respiratory depression. It is necessary to adjust the dose and schedule, considering both the patient's degree of pain relief and the plasma half-life of the drug when it is introduced.

Knowledge of the equianalgesic doses when a switch is made from one medication to another or from one route of administration to another prevents undermedication. However, cross-tolerance is not complete, and patients tolerant to the analgesic effects of one narcotic can often be given another to provide better analgesia. The usual rule is to begin with one half of the calculated equianalgesic dose of the new drug and increase as required.

Medication should be administered on a regular basis, with the interval between doses based on the duration of the analgesic effect. The pharmacologic objective is to maintain the plasma level of the drug above the "minimal effective concentration for pain relief." The time required to reach steady state after repeated administration depends on the half-life of the drug; full assessment of the analgesic efficacy of a drug regimen may take 24 hours for a drug such as morphine or up to 5 to 7 days for methadone.

Combinations of drugs enable the physician to improve pain relief without escalation of the narcotic dose. Several combinations have been proven effective, including a narcotic plus a non-narcotic (aspirin, acetaminophen, or ibuprofen), a narcotic plus an amphetamine (dextroamphetamine, 10 mg), and a narcotic plus an antihistamine (100 mg of hydroxyzine given intramuscularly). Other drugs such as diazepam and chlorpromazine do not provide additive analgesia and may produce additive sedative effects.

Oral administration of drugs is the most practical route, but the choice must be made according to the needs of the patient. Several alternate methods of drug administration have been developed to maximize pharmacologic effects and minimize the undesirable effects associated with standard methods. The approaches that are most useful in the management of acute or chronic pain with chronic medical illness include slow-release morphine preparations effective for 8 to 12 hours, enabling a full night's rest; continuous subcutaneous and intravenous infusions for patients who are unable to tolerate oral analgesics because of gastrointestinal obstruction or malabsorption and in whom repeated parenteral dosing is difficult because of limited muscle mass or a bleeding diathesis; and epidural and intrathecal narcotic administration via temporary catheters or implanted pumps. This last approach minimizes the distribution of drugs to receptors in the brain stem and cerebral hemispheres, avoids the side effects of systemic administration, and is effective in selected patients with cancer pain who are unable to tolerate the excessive sedation or mental clouding associated with an oral or parenteral route.

Patient-controlled analgesia (PCA) has developed as a useful approach to treat both acute postoperative and chronic cancer-related pain. Parenteral infusion (intravenous or subcutaneous) of opioids can be self-administered by the patient using specially designed computerized pumps that can be set to deliver specific amounts of drugs on demand or by continuous infusions. These devices allow patients control in their own pain management. Studies demonstrate that patients using PCA use less medication than patients who must relay on standard postoperative or chronic pain management approaches.

Side Effects of Narcotics. Side effects of the narcotic analgesics should be anticipated and treated. *Sedation and drowsiness* vary with the drug dose and may occur after either single or repeated

TABLE 26–3. NARCOTIC ANALGESIC DRUGS

Class	Drug	Indications	IM/PO Equianalgesic Dose (mg)*	Starting Dose (mg) Range/24 hr	Comments
Morphine-like agonist, mild to moderate pain	Codeine	Often used in combination with non-narcotic analgesics	32/65	32–65	Commonly used as first drug
	Oxycodone	Shorter acting; combination with non-narcotic analgesics limits dose escalation	5/30	5–10	Fewer side effects than codeine, available alone
	Meperidine	Shorter acting; biotransformed to normeperidine, a toxic metabolite	75/300	50–100	Normeperidine accumulates with repetitive dosing, causing CNS excitation; not for use in patients with renal dysfunction or receiving monoamine oxidase inhibitors
	Proproxyphene hydrochloride (Darvon)	Used in combination with non-narcotic analgesics; long half-life; biotransformed to potentially toxic metabolite (norproproxyphene)	65 PO	65–130	Proproxyphene and metabolite accumulate with repetitive dosing; overdose complicated by convulsions
Mixed-agonist antagonist	Pentazocine	In combination with non-narcotics, in combination with naloxone to discourage parenteral abuse	50 IM	50–100	May cause psychotomimetic effects; may precipitate withdrawal in narcotic-dependent patients
Morphine-like agonists, moderate to severe pain	Morphine	Used for chronic cancer pain, available in oral liquid and tablets and slow-release preparations	10/60	30–60	Standard of comparison for narcotic-type analgesics; morphine-6-glucuronide, active metabolite, accumulates in renal failure
	Hydromorphone (Dilaudid)	Like morphine	1.5/8.0	4–8	Slightly shorter acting, high-potency IM dosage form available for tolerant patients
	Methadone (Dolphine)	Like morphine; may accumulate with repetitive dosing, causing excessive sedation	10/20	10–20	Good oral potency; long plasma half-life
	Levorphanol (Levo-Dromoran)	Like methadone	2/4	2–4	Like methadone

*Dose given intramuscularly or by mouth.
IM = intramuscular; CNS = central nervous system.
Equianalgesic doses are based on single-dose controlled analgesic studies.

administration. Reducing the individual dose and prescribing it more frequently, switching to a drug with a short plasma half-life (hydromorphone), using an amphetamine (dextroamphetamine, 2 to 5 mg) in combination with the narcotic twice daily, and discontinuing all other sedative drugs are useful approaches to counteract the sedative effects.

Respiratory depression is the most serious adverse effect, but tolerance develops rapidly, allowing prolonged use of narcotics for chronic pain. If respiratory depression occurs, it can be reversed by administering the specific narcotic antagonist naloxone in a dose of 0.4 mg per milliliter. In patients who receive narcotics for prolonged periods and develop respiratory depression, diluted doses of naloxone (0.4 mg in 10 ml of saline) should be infused slowly to reverse the respiratory depression but prevent precipitation of severe withdrawal symptoms. The occurrence of *nausea and vomiting* with one drug does not mean that all narcotics will produce similar symptoms. Changing to an alternate narcotic or using an antiemetic in combination commonly obviates this effect. Tolerance rapidly develops to the emetic effect of narcotics so that after a few days antiemetics often are unnecessary. *Constipation* should be prevented by the provision of a regular bowel regimen, including cathartics, stool softeners, and careful attention to diet. *Multifocal myoclonus* may occur with toxic doses of any narcotic. The most common offender is meperidine because of the accumulation of the active metabolite normeperidine, which can cause seizures. Since the half-life of normeperidine is 16 hours, it may take several days for toxic side effects to clear. Patients should be switched to morphine to control their pain and managed symptomatically for seizures.

Tolerance is common when patients receive narcotic analgesics chronically for pain. The earliest sign is a decrease in the duration of effective analgesia. Increasing the frequency of drug administration of the dose provides improved pain relief. There is no limit to tolerance, and the dose of drug should not be the major concern of the prescribing physician. Adjuvant drugs and anesthetic and neurosurgical methods sometimes help to manage pain in the tolerant patient. These guidelines notwithstanding, the management of pain with narcotic analgesics is difficult and requires meticulous attention by the physician.

ADJUVANT ANALGESICS (Table 26–4). The adjuvant analgesics include several different categories of drugs, including anticonvulsants, phenothiazines, tricyclic antidepressants, antihistamines, amphetamines, and steroids (see Table 26–4). Carbamazepine and phenytoin are useful in the management of patients with some neuropathic pain syndromes, e.g., trigeminal neuralgia. The mechanism of action is suppression of the spontaneous neuronal firing that commonly occurs with nerve injury. For both drugs, the minimal effective concentration for analgesia is unknown.

Certain phenothiazines have potent analgesic effects. Methotrimeprazine (Levoprome) has an analgesic potential close to that of morphine (15 mg given intramuscularly is equivalent to 10 mg of morphine given intramuscularly). This drug helps manage severe pain in patients tolerant to narcotic analgesics. The tricyclic antidepressants both enhance the analgesic effects of morphine and have independent analgesic properties. Doses of 10 to 75 mg administered orally are used to treat postherpetic neuralgia. The analgesic effects of these drugs occur independently of their antidepressant properties. The antihistamine hydroxyzine and the amphetamine dextroamphetamine are also sometimes helpful adjuvants. Steroids produce analgesia in patients with acute inflammatory diseases and in patients with tumor infiltration of bone or nerve or both. A series of drugs from other drug classes has been reported to be useful in specific pain states. Baclofen and pimozide in patients with trigeminal neuralgia have demonstrated efficacy in patients refractory to tegretol. Mexiletine, an antiarrhythmic cardiac drug, has analgesic effects in managing patients with painful diabetic neuropathy.

Alternate Methods of Pain Control

A variety of nonpharmacologic therapeutic approaches can be used alone or in combination with the analgesic drugs. These include physical therapy, trigger point injections, transcutaneous nerve stimulation, and certain behavioral approaches, all of which should be familiar to general physicians. Technically demanding anesthetic and neurosurgical approaches require consultation with pain experts. Certain guidelines apply to these procedures:

1. Evaluate thoroughly the nature of the pain and the prognosis of the patient's primary disease. Neurolytic nerve blocks and neuroablative and neurostimulatory surgical procedures often yield only temporary relief in patients with chronic pain and are not useful for neuropathic pain. In contrast, patients with cancer pain of somatic origin who are not expected to live for more than several months are excellent candidates for such procedures.

2. Nondestructive procedures, such as transcutaneous electrical stimulation or temporary blocks with local anesthetics, should be tried first.

3. Start with the least destructive procedure. For example, try

TABLE 26–4. ADJUVANT ANALGESIC DRUGS

Class	Drug	Indications	Starting Dose (mg) Range/24 hr	Comments
Anticonvulsants	Phenytoin (Dilantin)	Neuropathic pain, acute lancinating type (tic)	100, 100–300	Start with low doses; titrate slowly
	Carbamazepine (Tegretol)	Acute lancinating type (tic)	100, 200–800	Useful in paroxysmal nerve pain
Antidepressants	Amitriptyline, imipramine	Neuropathic pain, e.g., postherpetic neuralgia	10, 10–150	Start at low dose and titrate slowly; have analgesic properties
Stimulants	Dextroamphetamine	Somatic and visceral pain, e.g., postoperative	2.5, 10	Additive analgesia in combination with narcotics; reduces sedative effects
Antihistamine	Hydroxyzine	Somatic and visceral pain	25, 100	Additive analgesia in combination with narcotics; antiemetic, antianxiety properties
Phenothiazine	Methotrimeprazine (Levoprome)	Somatic and visceral pain; useful in narcotic-tolerant patients with GI obstruction and pain	10 (IM), 10–40 (IM)	Has antianxiety and antiemetic effects; available only in IM preparation
Steroids	Prednisone	Somatic and neuropathic pain, e.g., inflammatory pain, reflex sympathetic dystrophy	5, 5–60	Anti-inflammatory, antiemetic, analgesic effects
	Dexamethasone		0.5, 0.5–16	Same as prednisone
Miscellaneous	Baclofen	Paroxysmal pain of trigeminal neuralgia and central pain states	10, 10–80	May be used with tegretol
	Pimozide	Refractory trigeminal neuralgia	2, 4–12	Adverse effects include acute dystonia and akathisias
	Mexiletine	Neuropathic pain; useful in diabetic neuropathy	150, 150–600	Dose-response studies have not been done

continuous epidural local anesthetics to manage perineal pain before initiating an intrathecal neurolytic block.

4. Evaluate patients psychologically. If psychological factors play a major role in the pain, such procedures will not help and will often exacerbate the condition.

5. Inform the patient fully of the potential risks and benefits of the planned procedure.

PHYSICAL THERAPY. Chronic pain is commonly associated with reduced physical activity and splinting or immobilization of the injured body part. A graded exercise program with appropriate use of splints and braces and reactivation of the injured part plays a pivotal role in re-establishing the functional status of the patient. Local rubbing and transcutaneous electrical stimulation for "counterirritation" may help to mobilize the patient with a localized pain. Trigger point injections with either saline or a local anesthetic provide dramatic relief of painful muscle spasm.

BEHAVIORAL THERAPY. Behavioral approaches that often improve the patient's coping mechanism include breathing exercises to increase relaxation, coping strategies to integrate pain symptoms into a functioning lifestyle, and improving control over psychological factors of anxiety, fear, and demoralization associated with chronic pain.

ANESTHETIC PROCEDURES (Table 26–5). Local anesthetics and injectable neurolytic agents are sometimes useful in managing both acute and chronic pain that occupies a well-defined anatomic site. Sympathetic blocks, for example, often predict the relief that can be expected from sympathectomy in treating causalgia due to peripheral sensory nerve damage. Blocking nerves with short- or long-acting anesthetics determines in a reversible manner whether semipermanent nerve blocks will be effective and what side effects they might have. In some patients, particularly when muscle spasm plays a major role in pain production, repeated temporary blocks produce long-lasting relief of pain. If an anesthetic nerve block has been effective temporarily and then begins to lose its efficacy, neurolytic agents, such as phenol, alcohol, and freezing (cryoanesthesia), can be used to destroy nerve structures. The principal pathologic effect produced by these neurolytic agents is demyelination with secondary nerve degeneration. Because peripheral nerves and roots have overlapping sensory functions, multiple nerves and roots must be blocked to yield adequate pain control. Since such blocks may paralyze as well as anesthetize, they have a limited role in extremity pain and are most useful to treat thoracic and abdominal pain or perineal and sacral pain in patients with cancer.

Neurolytic agents can be injected into the epidural or intrathecal space as well as into peripheral nerves or roots. However, the limitations of motor weakness and autonomic dysfunction make this technique suitable for only a limited number of patients. Neurolytic blocks find their best use in the management of well-defined localized pain caused by cancer. Their role in managing pain of nonmalignant origin is controversial because they work for only a limited period of time. There is a real risk of adding morbidity without providing pain relief, and they are not effective in managing neuropathic pain.

Blocks of the cervical (stellate ganglion) and lumbar sympathetic chains are most useful in managing limb pain and swelling associated with vascular or peripheral nerve injury, as occurs in diabetic peripheral vascular disease and reflex sympathetic dystrophy. Celiac plexus block is the procedure of choice to manage visceral pain from pancreatic carcinoma.

Intermittent or continuous epidural infusions of local anesthetics are useful for temporary relief of chronic pain involving the lumbosacral plexus and sacrum. This approach is most useful to treat an acute exacerbation of chronic cancer pain. The technique does not result in cross-tolerance with opiate analgesia, and it can be appropriately titrated to provide anesthesia without interruption of motor or autonomic function.

An anesthetic approach to manage diffuse pain is intermittent inhalation therapy with nitrous oxide. It is administered in oxygen through a non-rebreathing face mask with concentration ranging from 25 to 75 per cent.

NEUROSURGICAL PROCEDURES (Table 26–6). Pharmacologic procedures requiring neurosurgery include placement of intraventricular, epidural, or intrathecal catheters and implanted reservoirs or pumps to infuse agents used to manage selected patients with pain and cancer in whom systemic drugs are either ineffective or associated with excessive side effects. These approaches are not useful in managing non-cancer-related chronic pain problems.

Neurostimulatory procedures are performed by implanting electrodes in or on the desired portion of the nervous system and leading the electrodes to an implanted conductive receiver attached to an external transmitter. The technique allows the patient to control the timing and intensity of the stimulation. Electrical stimulation of the dorsal columns of cervical or thoracic spinal cord sometimes controls bilateral or midline neuropathic pain. Unfortunately, tolerance to the analgesic effect alters long-term usefulness of this procedure. Electrodes are usually placed in the epidural space over the dorsal column rather than directly on the spinal cord, thus reducing the risk of cord damage. Electrical stimulation of the periventricular gray matter of the brain stem also has been used for chronic neuropathic pain, especially if dorsal column stimulation or neurolytic blocks fail. Stimulation is delivered for no longer than 20 to 25 minutes at a time, three or four times a day. Tolerance develops more rapidly with increased use of the stimulator. Both animal studies and observations of human beings indicate that periventricular stimulation is associated with total body analgesia but without a

TABLE 26–5. TYPES OF ANESTHETIC PROCEDURES COMMONLY USED IN CHRONIC PAIN

I. Nerve Blocks	
Peripheral	Pain in discrete dermatomes in chest and abdomen
Epidural	Unilateral lumbar or sacral pain
	Midline perineal pain
	Bilateral lumbosacral pain
Intrathecal	Midline perineal pain
	Bilateral lumbosacral pain
Autonomic	Reflex sympathetic dystrophy, e.g.,
Stellate ganglion	frozen shoulder
	Arm pain
Lumbar sympathetic	Reflex sympathetic dystrophy
	Lumbosacral plexopathy
	Vascular insufficiency of the lower extremity
Celiac plexus	Midabdominal pain
II. Continuous Epidural	Unilateral and bilateral lumbosacral
Infusion with Local	pain
Anesthetic	Midline perineal pain
III. Inhalation Therapy	Generalized pain
	Incident pain
IV. Trigger Point Injection	Focal muscle pain

TABLE 26–6. NEUROABLATIVE, NEUROSTIMULATORY, AND NEUROPHARMACOLOGIC PROCEDURES

Site	Neurostimulatory	Neuroablative	Neuropharmacologic
Peripheral nerve	Transcutaneous and percutaneous electrical nerve stimulation	Neurectomy	Local anesthetics
Nerve root		Rhizotomy	Local anesthetics Neurolytic agents*
Spinal cord	Dorsal column stimulation	Dorsal root entry zone lesions Cordotomy Myelotomy	Epidural and intrathecal opiates*
Brain stem	Periaqueductal stimulation	Mesencephalic tractotomy	Intraventricular opiates*
Thalamus	Thalamic stimulation	Thalamotomy	
Cortex		Cingulumotomy Frontal lobotomy	
Pituitary		Trans-sphenoidal hypophysectomy*	Chemical hypophysectomy*

*Procedures restricted for the treatment of chronic cancer-related pain.

decrease in sensory or motor function. This procedure is available in only a few specialized centers.

Medial thalamic stimulation is used to manage chronic but unilateral intractable pain. Electrodes are placed stereotactically in medial thalamus contralateral to the pain. Stimulation results in localized analgesia. This procedure is used to manage the thalamic pain syndrome, phantom limb pain, and peripheral nerve injury pain, particularly when pain involves the head or neck. About 50 per cent of patients with localized neuropathic pain respond to thalamic stimulation.

In addition to neurostimulatory procedures, portions of the nervous system from peripheral nerves to the cerebral cortex can be lesioned to relieve pain. The most commonly used procedure is cordotomy. Other procedures have had only limited success and are marked by significant neurologic morbidity. Cordotomy is the most useful neurosurgical procedure for relief of chronic somatic pain and the most commonly used procedure for the management of patients with localized cancer pain. Cordotomy can be performed as a percutaneous stereotactic radiofrequency procedure or as an open surgical ablation. Because the spinothalamic tract is selectively interrupted, only pain and temperature sensation are lost (on the contralateral side of the body). Cutaneous sensation and motor power remain intact, although some ipsilateral weakness or ataxia occurs transiently in about 20 per cent of patients. Cordotomy is most useful to manage unilateral pain below the neck. Initial pain relief occurs in 90 per cent of patients. This figure drops to 50 per cent at 6 months and about 40 per cent at the end of 1 year. One to 2 per cent of postcordotomy patients develop burning dysesthesias (anesthesia dolorosa), which are often as distressing as the original pain. Because of both the limited duration of its effectiveness and the risk of producing neuropathic pain, cordotomy is not indicated for management of chronic nonmalignant pain. Bilateral cordotomy can be performed to manage midline or perineal pain associated with cancer. If performed in the cervical area, bilateral cordotomy risks producing sleep-induced apnea. The second risk of bilateral cordotomy is bladder dysfunction. With unilateral cordotomy, 7 to 10 per cent of patients develop mirror pain on the opposite side of the body even when the original pain is relieved. Mirror pain can occur in the absence of a definable lesion in the affected area, and its pathogenesis is unknown. Other neuroablative procedures are rarely used.

Management of Cancer Pain

Figure 26–1 provides an algorithm for the management of cancer pain. It attempts to integrate assessment techniques, drug therapy, and anesthetic, neurosurgical, and behavioral approaches and stresses continuity of care. Treatment of cancer pain must begin with a careful diagnostic assessment that addresses not only the medical nature of pain but also its psychological and social components. At the time of assessment, a plan is developed to treat both the cancer, if possible, and the pain itself. If the anticancer treatment is effective, pain relief usually occurs, and the drugs used for analgesia can be discontinued without difficulty. Pain relief begins with analgesic drugs. Incorporated in Figure 26–1 is the World Health Organization's Cancer Pain Relief Program. It proposes an analgesic drug ladder moving from nonopioid drugs alone or in combination with adjuvant drugs through weak opioids to strong opioids. If pain relief is achieved with this program, no further therapy is necessary. In patients with severe, persistent pain not responsive to analgesic drugs or in whom the side effects of the drugs are not tolerated, physicians should first try switching to alternate analgesics or changing the route or timing of drug administration. For example, intrathecal opioids are indicated for relief of pain in patients in whom systemic analgesics produce confusion or excessive sedation.

If the pain is unresponsive to analgesic drugs and is localized (e.g., intercostal pain from tumor infiltration of the chest wall), neurolytic blocks are indicated. If the pain is unilateral and below the waist, cordotomy should be considered. For more diffuse pain unresponsive to analgesics, neurostimulatory procedures, including nitrous oxide inhalation and chemical hypophysectomy, may be considered. Behavioral approaches, which include relaxation techniques, breathing exercises, and cognitive control of pain, serve as adjuvants and should be integrated into the management of patients with chronic pain.

As the algorithm indicates, whatever the techniques of pain management used in patients with cancer, the physician is responsible for delivering continuing care, constantly reassessing both the diagnosis and the treatment to achieve optimum relief of pain and suffering for both patient and family.

Bonica JJ (ed): The Management of Pain. 2nd ed. Philadelphia, Lea & Febiger, 1989. *This two-volume text provides detailed descriptions of acute and chronic pain syndromes with excellent anatomic graphics.*

Cousins M, Bridenbaugh P (eds.): Neural blockade. *In* Clinical Anesthesia and Management of Pain. 2nd ed. Philadelphia, J.B. Lippincott Co, 1988. *This text describes the commonly used anesthetic procedures in acute and chronic pain management.*

International Association for the Study of Pain: Classification of chronic pain, descriptions of chronic pain syndromes and definitions of pain terms. Pain (Suppl) 3:S1–S225, 1986. *This useful volume contains descriptions of chronic pain syndromes and definitions of pain terms.*

Payne R, Foley KM (eds.): Current Therapy in Pain. Philadelphia, B.C. Decker, 1987. *This paperback pocket book provides short, well-summarized practical management approaches for common pain disorders.*

Loeser JD, Egan KJ (eds.): Managing the Chronic Pain Patient. New York, Raven Press, 1989. *This concise book provides practical guidelines for the evaluation and treatment of patients with chronic pain.*

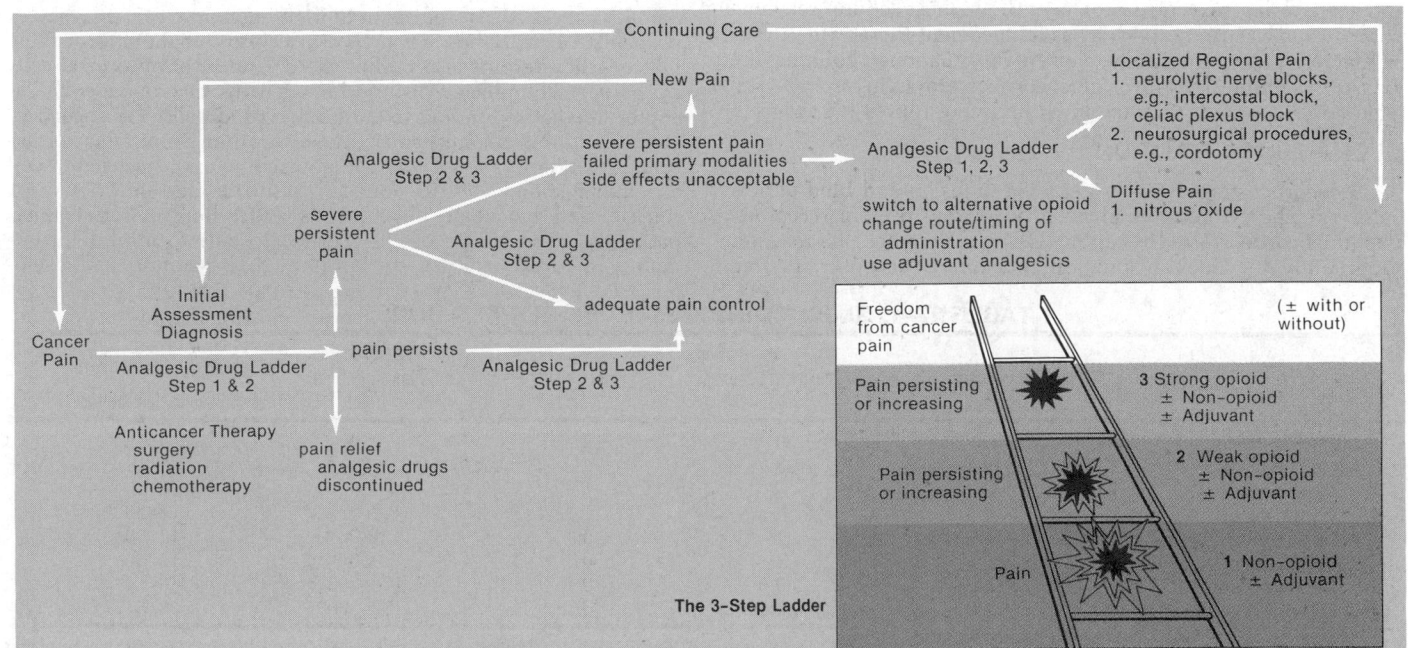

FIGURE 26–1. Algorithm for the management of cancer pain.

27 Glucocorticosteroid Therapy

Barton F. Haynes

In 1949, demonstration that the symptoms of rheumatoid arthritis could be treated with adrenal glucocorticosteroids ushered in a new era of therapy for immune-mediated diseases. With the introduction of glucocorticosteroids into clinical medicine has come the ability to cure adrenal insufficiency (Addison's disease) and to treat a wide spectrum of previously untreatable inflammatory conditions. However, glucocorticosteroid therapy is a double-edged sword with serious and often devastating side effects associated with its use. Understanding the mechanisms of action as well as the advantages and disadvantages of different glucocorticosteroids and their treatment regimens is essential for the physician to use appropriate clinical judgment in glucocorticosteroid administration.

BIOCHEMISTRY AND PHARMACOLOGY

Glucocorticosteroids are one of the three classes of steroids, the others being mineralocorticosteroids and the sex hormones, that are synthesized by the adrenal cortex. Glucocorticosteroids are endogenously synthesized from cholesterol to cortisol (hydrocortisone) via pregnenolone and progesterone. Cortisol is the principal circulating glucocorticosteroid in humans. The existence of glucocorticosteroid activity depends on the presence of a hydroxyl group at carbon 11 of the steroid molecule. Cortisol and prednisone are 11-ketocorticosteroids and therfore lack glucocorticosteroid activity until converted in the liver to the corresponding 11-beta-hydroxyl compounds, cortisol and prednisolone. All glucocorticosteroid preparations marketed for topical or local use are 11-beta-hydroxyl steroids, which do not require bioconversion for activity. Hydrocortisone has an approximate plasma half-life of 90 minutes (Table 27–1) and is metabolized in a number of tissues, particularly the liver. Glucocorticosteroids are irreversibly reduced and conjugated with glucuronic acid in the liver, thus enhancing excretion by the kidney. Ninety-five per cent of circulating endogenous cortisol is bound to plasma proteins—the majority to corticosteroid-binding globulin (transcortin). Adrenal cortisol production is regulated by hypothalamic production of corticotropin-releasing hormone that induces anterior pituitary production of ACTH (see Ch. 217).

The common synthetic glucocorticoids used clinically are listed in Table 27–1. These drugs differ in their plasma half-life, relative anti-inflammatory potency, and salt-retaining potency. Cortisone and cortisol (hydroxycortisone) have the highest sodium-retaining potency and are used especially as replacement therapy in adrenal insufficiency but are rarely chosen in situations requiring the long-term administration of glucocorticosteroids in supraphysiologic doses as anti-inflammatory or immunosuppressive agents.

MECHANISMS OF ACTION

Glucocorticosteroids enter cells via diffusion and bind to hormone-specific cytoplasmic glucocorticosteroid protein receptors. The glucocorticosteroid receptor (GR) is a member of a receptor superfamily to which belong the vitamin D receptor, thyroid hormone receptor, and retinoic acid receptor. Intracellular GR is present in an inactivated form in the cytosol of most mammals. Upon interaction of the GR with corticosteroids, a binding region for DNA is exposed on the GR. The activated GR is translocated to the nucleus, binds to glucocorticosteroid-response elements on DNA and, in doing so, induces subsequent transcription of specific mRNA's.

FACTORS THAT AFFECT RESPONSES TO GLUCOCORTICOSTEROIDS. In general, the potency of a steroid (Table 27–1) is correlated with the binding affinity of the molecule for intracellular GR. In addition, plasma protein concentrations influence glucocorticosteroid bioavailability; when patients with hypoalbuminemia are treated with glucocorticosteroids, they have an increased incidence of steroid side effects. In patients with severe liver disease, the conversion of glucocorticosteroids to the 11-beta-hydroxyl (active) form may not be efficiently made. Another factor that affects bioavailability of steroids is the rate of steroid metabolic degradation. For example, concomitant administration of phenobarbital or phenytoin enhances the rate of glucocorticosteroid clearance by the liver by increasing the activity of liver microsomal enzymes.

Two mechanisms of resistance to glucocorticosteroid effects have been described. First, certain leukemias and tumors have been shown to be resistant to steroid lytic effects owing to lack of or decreased numbers of GR. Second, one study has suggested that the presence of autoantibodies to lipocortins (a family of steroid-inducible proteins) can be responsible for poor responses to glucocorticosteroids in patients with autoimmune diseases.

ANTI-INFLAMMATORY EFFECTS. The effects of glucocorticosteroids following receptor binding are complex and can be manifested at both the molecular and cellular levels. One family of proteins that mediates anti-inflammatory activities of glucocorticosteroids is the lipocortins. Lipocortins inhibit synthesis of the inflammatory molecules (leukotrienes, thromboxanes, prostaglandins, and platelet-activating factor) by inhibition of the activity of phospholipase A_2. In general, glucocorticosteroids act via suppression of the production and/or function of many mediators of the inflammatory response (Table 27–2).

EFFECTS ON CELLS THAT MEDIATE INFLAMMATORY AND IMMUNE RESPONSES. Glucocorticosteroids exert profound effects on neutrophil differentiation, migration, and function (Table 27–2). Administration of glucocorticosteroids in vivo causes a redistribution of bone marrow neutrophils as well as increased production of neutrophils resulting in a peripheral neutrophilia, preventing ingress of neutrophils to areas of inflammation. Glucocorticosteroids inhibit neutrophil adherence to endothelium, neutrophil chemotaxis, neutrophil plasminogen activator production, and neutrophil superoxide generation.

Glucocorticosteroids redistribute monocytes out of the peripheral circulation with the peak effect 4 to 6 hours following steroid administration. This redistribution of mononuclear phagocytes prevents extravasation of monocytes into inflammatory sites. Glucocorticosteroids also inhibit the clearance of opsonized cells by tissue macrophages by interferring with macrophage Fc receptor–mediated binding to antibody-coated cells. Glucocorticosteroids inhibit all mechanisms necessary for granuloma formation, including monocyte chemotaxis, monocyte giant cell formation, monocyte plasminogen activator and interleukin 1 release, and monocyte phagocytosis and killing of intracellular pathogens. The ability of glucocorticosteroids to inhibit inflammatory mediator release by both the lipoxygenase and cyclo-

TABLE 27–1. GLUCOCORTICOSTEROID PREPARATIONS

	Anti-inflammatory Potency	Equivalent Dose (mg)	Sodium-retaining Potency	Approximate Plasma Half-life (min)	Biologic Half-life (hr)
Hydrocortisone	1	20	2+	90	8–12
Cortisone	0.8	25	2+	30	8–12
Prednisone	4	5	1+	60	12–36
Prednisolone	4	5	1+	200	12–36
Methylprednisolone	5	4	0	180	12–36
Triamcinolone	5	4	0	300	12–36
Betamethasone	20–30	0.6	0	100–300	36–54
Dexamethasone	20–30	0.75	0	100–300	36–54

From Garber EK, Targoff C, Paulus HE: *In* Paulus HE, Furst DE, Droomgoole SH (eds.): Drugs for Rheumatic Diseases. New York, Churchill Livingstone, 1987, pp 446; with permission.

TABLE 27–2. GLUCOCORTICOSTEROID EFFECTS ON IMMUNE CELLS AND HUMORAL FACTORS

Glucocorticoid effects on leukocyte movement

Lymphocytes

Circulating lymphocytopenia 4–6 hours following drug administration secondary to redistribution of cells to other lymphoid compartments

Depletes recirculating lymphocytes

Selectively depletes T lymphocytes (especially CD4 subset) more than B lymphocytes and natural killer cells

Monocyte-Macrophages

Circulating monocytopenia 4–6 hours following drug administration, probably secondary to redistribution

Inhibits accumulation of monocyte-macrophages at inflammatory sites

Neutrophils

Circulating neutrophilia

Accelerated release of neutrophils from the bone marrow

Blocks accumulation of neutrophils at inflammatory sites, probably secondary to reduced adherence

Eosinophils

Circulating eosinopenia, probably secondary to redistribution

Decreased migration of eosinophils into immediate hypersensitivity skin test sites

Glucocorticoid effects on leukocyte function

Lymphocytes

Delayed hypersensitivity skin testing suppressed by inhibition of recruitment of monocyte-macrophages

Lymphocyte proliferation to antigens suppressed more easily than proliferation to mitogens

Mixed leukocyte reaction proliferation suppressed

High concentrations in vitro suppress T lymphocyte–mediated cytotoxicity

Antibody-dependent cell-mediated cytotoxicity not depressed

Natural killer cell cytotoxicity suppressed

Regulatory effects on helper and suppressor cell populations

Decrease in T cell interleukin 2, gamma interferon, and colony stimulation factor production

Lysis of cortical thymocytes and activated peripheral T cells

Monocyte-Macrophages

Cutaneous delayed hypersensitivity suppressed by inhibition of lymphocyte effect on the macrophage

Probable blockade of Fc receptor binding and function

Depressed bactericidal activity

Possible decrease in monocyte chemotaxis

Decrease in monocyte interleukin 1 release

Neutrophil

Probably no effect of phagocytic and bactericidal capability

Antibody-dependent cellular cytotoxicity increased

Probably decreased lysosomal release but little effect on lysosomal membrane stabilization at pharmacologic concentrations

Chemotaxis inhibited only by suprapharmacologic concentrations

Glucocorticoid effects on humoral factors

Mild decrease in immunoglobulin levels but no decrease in specific antibody production

Complement metabolism probably unaffected

Decreased reticuloendothelial clearance of antibody-coated cells

Effects on kinins and prostaglandins

Inhibits plasminogen activator release

Potentiates the actions of catecholamines

Possibly antagonizes histamine-induced vasodilatation

Adapted, with permission, from the Annual Review of Pharmacology and Toxicology, Vol. 19, © 1979 by Annual Reviews, Inc.

oxygenase pathways leads to decreased production of prostaglandin E_2, thromboxane B_2, and leukotriene B_4 by tissue macrophages.

Eosinophils and basophils, like monocytes, are redistributed out of the circulation following glucocorticosteroid administration in vivo. Eosinophil adherence, chemotaxis, and killing are inhibited by glucocorticosteroids, correlating with the observed efficacy of corticosteroid therapy in clinical syndromes characterized by tissue or peripheral eosinophilia such as *idiopathic hypereosinophilic syndrome* (see Ch. 150) and *eosinophilic fasciitis* (see Ch. 262). Basophil histamine and leukotriene release is also inhibited by glucocorticosteroids.

As with other immune cell types, glucocorticosteroids exert profound effects on both lymphocyte traffic and lymphocyte cell function. Glucocorticosteroid administration in vivo induces a rapid redistribution of T cells out of the circulation with CD4+ T cells preferentially decreased over CD8+ T cells. B cells are only minimally redistributed out of the circulation, whereas natural killer cells are spared the lymphopenic effect and remain in the circulation following glucocorticosteroid administration in vivo. Although glucocorticosteroids do not lyse normal circulating T cells, they do lyse cortical thymocytes and activated mature T cells.

Functionally, corticosteroids administered in vivo (high divided-dose therapy) result in suppression of B cell immunoglobulin production after 2 to 4 weeks of therapy. Similarly, while natural killer cells (CD16+ large granular lymphocytes bearing Fc receptors for IgG) are not depleted from the circulation, glucocorticosteroids markedly inhibit the ability of natural killer cells to kill other cell types. In general, most of the recognized lymphocyte functions—proliferation, mediator production, response to mediators, and cytotoxic effector function—have been shown to be decreased by corticosteroids. However, among immune cells, some lymphocyte functions are more resistant to corticosteroids than others (Table 27–2).

Both T cells and monocytes participate in granuloma formation. Thus, granulomatous hypersensitivity diseases such as *sarcoidosis* are generally responsive to steroid therapy. By contrast, infectious diseases such as *tuberculosis* that are held in check by granulomatous inflammation are prone to exacerbation or relapse during high-dose glucocorticosteroid therapy, owing to glucocorticosteroid-induced inhibition of granuloma formation.

EFFECTS ON CONNECTIVE TISSUE. Glucocorticosteroids reduce bone formation and increase bone resorption rates as well. Parathyroid hormone levels are elevated by glucocorticosteroid administration, most likely reflecting glucocorticosteroid-mediated inhibition of calcium absorption from the gastrointestinal tract. Glucocorticosteroids inhibit wound healing by suppressing prostaglandin synthesis and fibroblast collagen synthesis. Glucocorticosteroids inhibit connective tissue glycoaminoglycan biosynthesis and promote abnormal small blood vessel formation. During chronic administration of corticosteroids, these effects can lead to osteopenia, loss of connective tissue in skin and tendons, skin striae, and telangiectasia.

PRINCIPLES OF THERAPY

The modern principles of clinical use of glucocorticosteroids were established in 1966 by George Thorn, who emphasized that the following considerations were necessary. Prior to use of glucocorticosteroids as pharmacologic agents, the physician should ask: How serious is the underlying disorder? How long will therapy be required? What is the anticipated effective steroid dose? Is the patient predisposed to any of the known hazards of glucocorticosteroid therapy (such as glucose intolerance, osteoporosis, peptic ulcer disease, tuberculosis, hypertension, or psychiatric difficulties)? Which glucocorticosteroid preparations should be used? Can other modes of therapy be used to minimize either steroid dosage or steroid side effects? Is an alternate-day glucocorticosteroid regimen indicated?

INDICATIONS FOR USE. Glucocorticosteroids are most often used for their anti-inflammatory and immunosuppressive effects and for replacement therapy in adrenal insufficiency (see Ch. 217). The use of glucocorticosteroids as antitumor agents is described in Ch. 164. Steroids have been used to stabilize the cardiovascular system in hypotensive states such as septic shock, although recent large clinical trials have not demonstrated any efficacy for glucocorticosteroids in decreasing mortality in septic shock. Glucocorticosteroids are administered in the treatment of brain and spinal edema, particularly in the setting of primary tumors or metastases to the brain or spinal cord. Steroids have been postulated to work in brain edema by decreasing sodium in edema fluid, by stabilizing vascular permeability, and by decreasing production of CSF. In some cases, an antitumor effect by high-dose steroids may occur. Glucocorticosteroids are given for hypercalcemia associated with sarcoidosis or certain tumors. In this setting the therapeutic effect is related to an increase in renal excretion of calcium and a decrease in calcium absorption from the gastrointestinal tract.

Steroid effects on monocytes, neutrophils, lymphocytes, eosinophils, and basophils (Table 27–2) make glucocorticosteroids effective anti-inflammatory and immunosuppressive agents in many rheumatic diseases. For instance, glucocorticosteroids are the mainstay of therapy for *polymyalgia rheumatica, temporal arteritis* (see Ch. 267), and severe manifestations of *systemic lupus erythematosus* (see Ch. 261).

Immunosuppressive regimens that include glucocorticosteroids have been used to inhibit T cell– and monocyte-mediated allograft rejection such as occurs in heart and renal transplantation. Although many antibody- and immune complex–mediated diseases are treated with glucocorticosteroids, antibody-forming cells (B lymphocytes and plasma cells) are relatively resistant to the suppressive effects of steroids such that very high doses of steroids are needed to suppress B cell immunoglobulin production. Thus, the beneficial effects of glucocorticosteroids in immune complex–mediated diseases are likely mediated by the immune system subsequent to immune complex formation. It has been suggested, for example, that glucocorticosteroids are effective in autoimmune hemolytic anemias and other cytopenias by inhibiting the binding of antibody-coated cells to Fc receptors of macrophages in the reticuloendothelial system, thus preventing cell clearance and destruction.

Glucocorticosteroids are extensively used in the treatment of asthma and immediate hypersensitivity allergic conditions. Although the precise mechanisms of action are undefined, steroids are thought to work in asthma and other allergic reactions by inhibition of prostaglandin and leukotriene formation, by suppression of expression of lymphocyte surface receptors for IgE, and by depletion of intracellular histamine. Other specific actions of glucocorticosteroids relevant to asthma include prevention and reversal of late-phase reactants, reduction in mucus secretion, and augmentation in beta-adrenergic responsiveness.

Other clinical situations in which glucocorticosteroids have been used include a wide range of dermatologic and ophthalmologic conditions and prevention of reactions to intravenous contrast material.

LOCAL CORTICOSTEROID ADMINISTRATION. In some situations, local glucocorticosteroid therapy that delivers a concentrated dose of drug only to the affected site is preferable to systemic therapy. Examples of effective local therapy include topical glucocorticosteroid cream for contact dermatitis, administration of glucocorticosteroids for various ocular inflammatory conditions, and injection of microcrystalline preparations of corticosteroids intra-articularly or in bursae to control local joint or bursal inflammation. In each of these situations, if sufficient topical therapy is administered for a long enough time, systemic absorption of steroids occurs and predisposes the patient to systemic side effects and toxicities of glucocorticosteroids. An important advance in the treatment of asthma and severe allergic rhinitis has been the use of inhaled (for asthma) or intranasal (for rhinitis) glucocorticosteroids (see Ch. 57 and 246).

SYSTEMIC THERAPY. Several factors should be considered in the choice of a particular glucocorticosteroid preparation. For anti-inflammatory and immunosuppressive regimens, a steroid drug that possesses little or no mineralocorticosteroid activity is preferred to minimize salt retention and hypertension (see Table 27–1). Cortisol (hydrocortisone) has the greatest degree of mineralocorticosteroid activity, and this preparation is frequently used as replacement therapy in adrenocortical insufficiency (see Ch. 217.6).

There is a direct correlation between plasma and biologic half-life, potency, and toxic side effects of glucocorticosteroid preparations (see Table 27–1). Dexamethasone, betamethasone, and triamcinolone are longer acting, more potent, and associated with more deleterious side effects than the shorter-acting prednisone and methylprednisolone. Thus, prednisone is used more commonly in daily and alternate-day regimens, whereas dexamethasone is routinely used only when continuous glucocorticosteroid effects are needed, e.g., to control brain edema. The shorter-acting glucocorticosteroids such as prednisone are essential for constructing regimens for patients to ensure that the shortest duration of steroid effect needed to control the immune process being treated is used.

DAILY GLUCOCORTICOSTEROID THERAPY. For most of the immunologic diseases that require glucocorticosteroid therapy, the most common regimen is administration of prednisone orally in a single daily morning dose or in divided doses throughout the day. Divided-dose therapy is more potent therapeutically than daily or alternate-day glucocorticosteroids, and likewise, divided-dose therapy is more toxic than either daily or alternate-day regimens, particularly with regard to predisposition to infections and suppression of the hypothalamic-pituitary-adrenal (HPA) axis. Thus, for immune-mediated diseases, the shorter-acting prednisone is generally used in a manner that closely mimics the normal diurnal cortisol cycle. Prednisone is optimally given early in the morning (6 to 8 A.M.) such that exogenously administered steroid levels peak early in the day and then fall later in the evening to allow endogenous ACTH secretion to occur. Given that the diseases for which steroids are used are heterogeneous in etiology, treatment response, and severity, no single set of strict guidelines is available for glucocorticosteroid use. Nonetheless, general guidelines exist that pertain to most situations.

Once the decision has been made that glucocorticosteroid therapy is appropriate (such as for severe manifestations of *systemic lupus erythematosus* or in combination therapy with cyclosphosphamide for *systemic necrotizing vasculitis*), glucocorticosteroid therapy should be initiated with prednisone, 1 to 2 mg per kilogram body weight in three to four divided doses (Fig. 27–1). Since divided-dose therapy is a potentially toxic regimen as well as the most anti-inflammatory and anti-immunosuppressive, divided-dose therapy should be tapered to single-dose daily therapy once clinical remission has been achieved. To change from divided-dose daily therapy to single-dose daily therapy, the divided dose (e.g., 20 mg prednisone three times a day) is consolidated to one dose orally in the morning with the same total (e.g., 60 mg prednisone once a day). The single daily dose can then be gradually tapered until the lowest single daily dose that can control the disease is reached or glucocorticosteroid

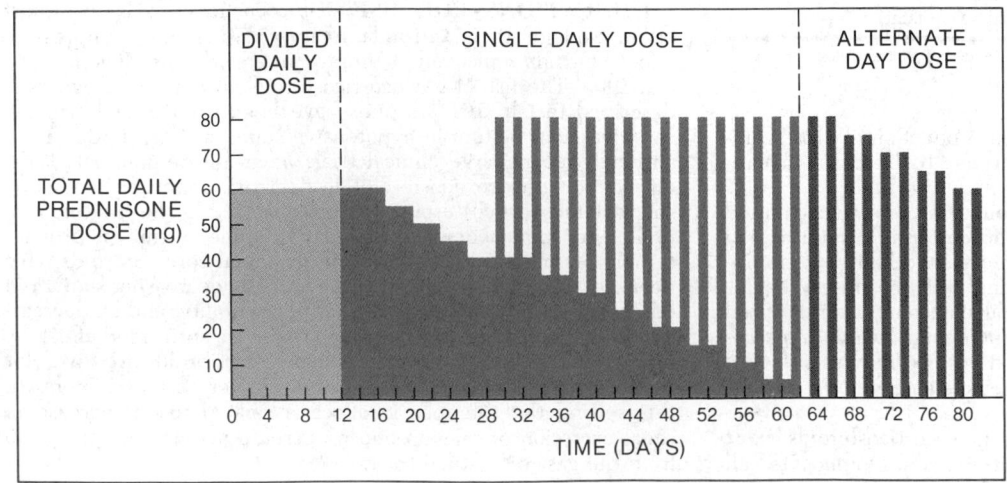

FIGURE 27–1. Schematic method of tapering oral glucocorticosteroids from divided-dose therapy to daily single dose to an alternate-day dose regimen.

TABLE 27–3. TOXIC SIDE EFFECTS OF GLUCOCORTICOSTEROID ADMINISTRATION

Cardiovascular and fluid balance
  Hypertension
  Sodium and fluid retention
  Hypokalemic alkalosis
Dermatologic
  Vascular fragility
  Inhibition of fibroblast collagen synthesis, striae, impaired wound
    healing
Endocrine-metabolic
  Suppression of HPA axis
  Negative balance of nitrogen, potassium, calcium
  Hyperglycemia
  Hyperlipoproteinemia
  Nonketotic hyperosmolar states
  Suppression of growth in children
  Secondary amenorrhea, acne, virilization
  Truncal obesity, moon facies, mediastinal and spinal canal lipomatosis
  Fatty infiltration of the liver
Gastrointestinal
  Peptic ulcer disease
  Pancreatitis
  Intestinal perforation
Immunologic
  Alteration of immune cell number and function
  Opportunistic infections
  Suppression of delayed hypersensitivity skin tests
  Rare hypersensitivity reactions
Musculoskeletal
  Osteopenia, osteoporosis, bone fractures
  Aseptic necrosis of bone, bone pain
  Myopathy
Neuropsychiatric
  Pseudotumor cerebri
  Psychiatric symptoms (psychosis, personality changes)
  Psychological dependence on glucocorticoids
Ophthalmic
  Glaucoma
  Posterior subcapsular cataracts

therapy can be stopped altogether. Adjunctive nonsteroidal therapy for the disease in question, such as nonsteroidal anti-inflammatory agents for connective tissue diseases, is important for facilitating the ease of steroid tapering. Single-dose daily therapy (particularly the lower doses, less than 40 mg daily) provides for some normal HPA function in some individuals and also provides for periods of normal immune cell function to prevent opportunistic infections. After initiating glucocorticosteroid therapy, since most inflammatory diseases often are self-remitting illnesses, one should always seek to taper and, if possible, discontinue corticosteroids to prevent or limit toxic side effects.

The decision to reduce the daily steroid dosage is reached when (a) the disease activity is controlled, (b) other steroid-sparing drugs are added to the patient's regimen and the disease is controlled, or (c) the side effects due to glucocorticosteroids are so severe that dose reduction is mandatory. Collapsed vertebral bodies due to severe osteoporosis and opportunistic infections are two consequences of glucocorticosteroid therapy which dictate a reduction in steroid dosage as soon as possible.

ALTERNATE-DAY GLUCOCORTICOSTEROID THERAPY. One effective regimen for tapering glucocorticosteroid therapy is to convert the regimen from a daily divided dose to a single daily dose and then to a single dose on alternate days. The eventual goal in most disease states is to taper off therapy altogether if possible. In many inflammatory diseases such as *polyarteritis nodosa*, *Wegener's granulomatosis*, and *sarcoidosis*, it is relatively easy to taper glucocorticosteroid therapy to an alternate-day regimen; in others, such as *temporal arteritis* and *systemic lupus erythematosus*, it is more difficult. Nonetheless, if the patient can be tapered to an alternate-day regimen, a considerable service is done for the patient, as the level of unwanted side effects on alternate-day steroids is markedly reduced compared with equivalent-dose daily regimens.

Figure 27–1 illustrates one method of tapering corticosteroids when they are used to induce remission in a steroid-sensitive immune-mediated disease. This is a stylized example, and the

tempo and increments of drug tapering need to be modified according to the clinical setting and the severity and degree of response of each individual patient. In this example, therapy is begun to induce remission of clinical symptoms at a dose of prednisone of 20 mg orally three times daily. After 2 weeks, the divided dose is consolidated to one 60-mg daily oral dose. After tapering the single daily dose of prednisone to 30 mg daily, and if the disease remains in remission, a conversion to alternate-day therapy can be attempted. The rationale for alternate-day glucocorticosteroid therapy is to administer a dose of a short-acting steroid at regular 48-hour intervals which will maintain suppression of disease activity while avoiding the toxic side effects associated with daily regimens. There are many ways to convert from a daily to an alternate-day glucocorticosteroid regimen. It is important to go slowly to prevent disease relapse and to make the patient as comfortable as possible with nonsteroidal anti-inflammatory drug supplements on the days off prednisone.

Another common pitfall is to give too little glucocorticosteroid on the "on" day. One effective way to convert to alternate-day therapy is initially to double one of the daily doses of steroids and to maintain the other prednisone dose on the second day (Fig. 27–1). The daily dose of 30 mg is doubled to 60 mg and kept there while the alternate daily dose is gradually tapered to zero and becomes the "off" day. After the dose has been converted to an alternate-day regimen of prednisone 60 mg on the "on" day and 0 mg on the "off" day, the level of the prednisone dose on the "on" day can begin to be tapered. In most instances both the speed and the amount of decrements shown in the example in Figure 27–1 will have to be modified (usually speed decreased and intervals between doses increased) to accommodate each patient's disease severity and clinical course. Specifically, when tapering the "off" day steroid from 20 mg to 0 mg, it frequently is necessary to use 2.5-mg or 1-mg decrements to get to 0 mg. Also, after the "off" day dose has been tapered to 0 mg, it is usual to hold the "on" day at its current level (in the example, 60 mg per day) for 1 to 2 weeks prior to beginning to taper the "on" day to lower doses. Finally, when the "on" day reaches 20 mg, small decrements (1 to 2.5 mg) are usually indicated to reach the lowest allowable dose or to taper off completely.

The regimen shown in Figure 27–1 would be most typical of a 2-month prednisone taper in a patient with uncomplicated *systemic necrotizing vasculitis* who was also being treated with a cytotoxic agent. On the basis of the plasma half-life of prednisone, the highest single dose that one could administer on an alternate-day basis without suppressing the HPA axis on the "off" day is 80 to 120 mg. A short-acting glucocorticosteroid is essential for an alternate-day regimen. For example, using dexamethasone or betamethasone in an alternate-day regimen defeats the purpose of the alternate-day schedule in that these long-acting glucocorticosteroids have biologic half-lives longer than 24 hours.

BURST OR INTERMITTENT-PULSE GLUCOCORTICOSTEROID THERAPY. For some clinical situations, short courses or bursts of corticosteroid therapy, either alone or in combination with other drugs, control the clinical symptoms. Severe poison ivy or poison oak contact dermatitis is an example of a common disease in which "burst" therapy is used. Patients are usually given 60 mg of prednisone or methylprednisolone orally for 2 or 3 days; then the dose is rapidly tapered by 10-mg decrements per day until the drug is completely discontinued. On this type of "burst" regimen, there is little danger of glucocorticosteroid-induced side effects. High-dose "burst" or "pulse" intravenous glucocorticosteroids came into widespread use in the early 1970's for the management of acute renal allograft rejection. Intravenous pulse glucocorticosteroid therapy has been used in progressive rheumatic diseases such as *systemic lupus erythematosus* and in nonrheumatic diseases such as *idiopathic rapidly progressive glomerulonephritis* and in *Goodpasture's syndrome*. Although efficacy in many clinical situations remains controversial, in certain situations such as acute allograft rejection and recent-onset renal failure in *lupus nephritis*, clinical efficacy has been demonstrated.

Methylprednisolone is generally employed for "pulse" regimens because of its high potency and low salt-retaining activity. Intravenous pulse regimens are theoretically desirable in order to obtain a rapid and prolonged therapeutic effect with fewer glucocorticosteroid side effects. While most anti-inflammatory and immunosuppressive effects of glucocorticosteroids that occur with intravenous pulse doses of methylprednisolone also occur at lower doses, certain effects have been seen only at high doses of glucocorticosteroids. These effects include inhibition of granulocyte aggregation, inhibition of T cell interleukin 2 receptor expression, and prolonged suppression of natural killer cell activity. Recently, intravenous pulse methylprednisolone therapy has been suggested to improve monocyte Fc receptor function in patients with *systemic lupus erythematosus*. It is important to administer large doses of intravenous methylprednisolone slowly over 1 hour to avoid abrupt potassium and fluid shifts, which can lead to acute cardiac dysfunction.

A question is frequently asked regarding the use of ACTH versus glucocorticosteroids. There is no convincing evidence that ACTH is superior to glucocorticosteroids in the treatment of any disease. ACTH administration has several drawbacks. ACTH can be given only parenterally, and response to ACTH depends on an induced adrenal glucocorticosteroid response, the magnitude of which is variable.

SIDE EFFECTS OF GLUCOCORTICOSTEROID THERAPY

Suppression of the HPA Axis. Although precise criteria are not available to establish the minimal dose of glucocorticosteroid that can cause suppression of the HPA axis, in some individuals short courses of oral glucocorticosteroid therapy (the equivalent of 30 mg per day for 1 week) can be associated with abnormal HPA function for as long as 12 months. Thus, prophylactic glucocorticosteroids should be considered during times of maximal stress (trauma or major surgical procedures) in the following patients: (a) those with a known diagnosis of primary or secondary adrenal insufficiency, (b) those currently treated with exogenous steroids for chronic diseases, (c) those treated daily with exogenous steroids (prednisone 30 mg daily) for a period exceeding 1 week during the past 12 months, (d) those with signs or symptoms suggestive of hypoadrenalism and an abnormal rapid ACTH stimulation test (see Ch. 217.5), and (e) those scheduled to undergo, or with a history of, bilateral adrenalectomy or hypophysectomy.

If patients who are suspected of HPA axis suppression are to be subjected to severe stress such as a major surgical procedure, they should receive parenteral hydrocortisone in doses of 100 mg every 4 to 6 hours during surgery and for several days thereafter, depending on recovery period (see Ch. 217.6).

To determine suppression of the HPA axis in a person who has recently received glucocorticosteroid therapy, a rapid ACTH stimulation test can be performed (see Ch. 217.5 for procedures). Recovery of HPA function once glucocorticosteroids have been discontinued is a slow process. As yet there are no proven therapies to hasten the process.

OTHER SIDE EFFECTS

Other toxic side effects of glucocorticosteroid administration are listed in Table 27–3. The side effects involve many organ systems and can be devastating. The frequency and severity of toxic side effects in most cases are directly related to the dose and duration of therapy. Unfortunately there are no proven regimens for limiting the complications and side effects of glucocorticosteroid therapy other than treating the patient with the lowest dose of steroid that will control the disease and discontinuing the drug as soon as the disease warrants doing so.

To minimize steroid-induced osteopenia and associated fractures, it has been suggested that the 24-hour urine calcium output be measured after 1 to 3 months of glucocorticosteroid therapy and oral calcium and possibly vitamin D be given based on the level of urinary calcium excretion.

Infections represent the most serious and potentially life-threatening complication of corticosteroid therapy. In patients on long-term daily doses of glucocorticosteroids, the index of suspicion should be high for occult infections. For example, joint inflammation that persists or develops in the rheumatoid arthritis patient on oral corticosteroid therapy should be suspected of

being infectious and the possibility excluded by arthrocentesis. The best method of preventing infectious complications of glucocorticosteroid therapy is always to taper the drug to the lowest possible dose and to attempt either to taper the dose to an alternate-day regimen or to stop steroid therapy completely. One common mistake in the management of glucocorticosteroid therapy is to leave the patient on the dose of the drug that induced remission in the disease instead of tapering the dose to the lowest level possible. During or after tapering of glucocorticosteroids, patients may develop symptoms of glucocorticosteroid withdrawal, such as myalgias and arthralgias, that in some cases may mimic symptoms of the underlying disease.

Camussi G, Tetta C, Bussolino F, Baglioni C: Anti-inflammatory peptides (antiflammins) inhibit synthesis of platelet-activating factor, neutrophil aggregation and chemotaxis, and intradermal inflammatory responses. J Exp Med 171:913–927, 1990. *Recent article describing mechanism of action of lipocortins at a molecular level.*

Flower RJ: Lipocortin and the mechanisms of action of the glucocorticosteroids. Br J Pharmacol 94:987–1015, 1988. *In-depth review of the role that lipocortins play in mediating the anti-inflammatory effects of glucocorticosteroids.*

Garber EK, Targoff C, Paulus HE: Corticosteroids in the rheumatic disease: Chronic low doses, chronic high doses, "pulses," intra-articular. In Paulus HE, Furst DE, Dromgoole SH (eds.): Drugs for Rheumatic Diseases. New York, Churchill Livington, 1987, pp 443–476. *Comprehensive review of steroid use in rheumatic diseases, including intra-articular glucocorticosteroid administration.*

Haynes BF, Fauci AS: The differential effect of in vivo hydrocortisone on the kinetics of subpopulations of human peripheral blood T lymphocytes. J Clin Invest 61:703, 1978. *Original paper describing the effect of glucocorticosteroids on subsets of human T cells, with detailed kinetic studies.*

Kaliner M: Mechanism of glucocorticosteroid action in bronchial asthma. J Allergy Clin Immunol 76:321–329, 1985. *Review article with in-depth analysis of effect of steroids on allergic reactions, including asthma.*

Kerhl J, Fauci AS: The clinical use of corticosteroids. Ann Allergy 50:2, 1983. *An outstanding review article on the theoretical and practical aspects of glucocorticosteroid use.*

Napolitano LM, Chernow B: Guidelines for corticosteroid use in anesthetic and surgical stress. Int Anesthesiol Clin 26:226, 1988. *Excellent review article with guidelines for perioperative treatment with glucocorticosteroids of patients suspected of having HPA suppression.*

Thorn GW: Clinical considerations in the use of corticosteroids. N Engl J Med 274:775, 1966. *The classic paper on clinical use of corticosteroids.*

28 Common Poisonings

William O. Robertson

DEFINITION. Man's chemical environment was recognized as a threat to health long before the birth of Christ. Well-documented outbreaks of occupational mercury and lead "poisonings" had been recorded and preventive measures implemented by 200 B.C. The Middle Ages saw arsenic poisoning employed as a political weapon. More recent times have seen increasing recognition of industrial toxins, "accidental poisoning" in childhood, purposeful overdoses in adults, adverse reactions to drugs, and environmental hazards for us all. The common theme is entrance of an exogenous chemical into an organism and subsequent disruption of its metabolism. The term "poison" has undergone quantitative redefinition so that now such ubiquitous substances as table salt and drinking water are firmly established as being "poisonous." Recall that more than 400 years ago, Paracelsus cautioned "All substances are poisons: There is none that is not a poison. The right dose differentiates a poison and a remedy." Finally, the host-organism itself has contributed to a better comprehension of the word "poison," as genetic variability has been recognized to determine the impact of a given molecule in such hereditary disorders as phenylketonuria, glucose-6-phosphate dehydrogenase deficiency, and others. As man's understanding of life has expanded, the connotation of poisoning has undergone substantial evolution.

ETIOLOGY. Approximately 1.2 million chemical entities had been identified and coded by 1950; the number had risen to more than 4.3 million by 1976. By 1992, the number will exceed 11 million. Although not all of these compounds have been marketed, many new organic compounds have appeared in the home and the workplace. For example, available formulations of pesticides have increased 50-fold over the past 30 years. Moreover, manufacturing processes have released additional compounds into the workplace or the environment with capabilities of serving as poisons. Currently employed methods to determine carcinogenicity, mutagenicity, and teratogenicity indict chemicals as dangerous when simultaneous epidemiologic data from humans fail to support such contentions—e.g., formaldehyde, fluorides, dioxins. Since proving a negative remains so ephemeral, it appears likely that "scare incidents" that eventually prove groundless—e.g., cranberries in the 1960's, sturgeon (Hg) in the 1970's, and Agent Orange (dioxins) in the 1980's—will be even more commonplace.

New chemical techniques have permitted prompt and complete identification of poisonings and have uncovered the causes of such diverse entities as Minamata disease (teratogenesis consequent to methyl mercury), an outbreak of ascending paralysis affecting more than 4000 with more than 400 deaths in Iraq (also caused by methyl mercury), the "gray syndrome" in premature infants (caused by chloramphenicol), mesotheliomas induced by asbestos, and an epidemic of angiosarcoma of the liver among industrial workers (caused by vinyl chloride). Nevertheless, many unknowns remain and justify careful prospective monitoring of industry, of the home, and of the environment. Unfortunately, the combination of more "synthetic chemicals," vastly more precise testing techniques, a press far more devoted to Rachel Carson's *Silent Spring* than to Dupont's "better living through chemistry," and an increasingly litigious society has created an era of "toxic torts" and its consequences, plus a very anxious and concerned public and profession. As a consequence, primary care physicians are bound to be involved in disputes stemming from industrial, occupational, and environmental origins.

INCIDENCE. Over the past 25 years progressively more reliable data have been gathered about deaths from poisonings, the leading agents, and the number of such deaths attributable to each among children less than five years old and among the overall population (Table 28–1). Although concern for infants and toddlers prompted the creation of our nation's Poison Center Network, deaths from poisoning among that group have plummeted over the past 30 years; these children were, fortunately, greatly underrepresented in 1984, accounting for only 2.2 per cent of poisoning deaths despite the fact that their "accidental ingestions" account for 62 per cent of the 1,368,000 human exposures summarized by the National Data Collection System of the American Association of Poison Control Centers in 1988. By 1989, the percentage had fallen still further; viewed over time, some 450 deaths occurred nationwide among children less than 5 years of age in 1962 from accidental poisoning due to household products and prescription items, compared to only 31 in 1989—a remarkable decline in mortality. Among adults precise data are more difficult to retrieve. Incomplete data attest that a minimum of 12,000 deaths occur annually as a result of suicide by poisoning.

EPIDEMIOLOGY. There are significant differences in the epidemiology of poisonings among children under 5 years of age compared with the remainder of the population. With adults, occupational and industrial exposures, suicide gestures or attempts, and homicides depend upon host factors and environmental settings as well as involved chemicals. In contrast, among children under 5, host and environmental factors are less variable. In the United States, occurrences peak at 24 to 32 months of age, and more male than female children are involved; poisonings happen most frequently between 11 A.M. and 12 noon or between 5 and 6 P.M. and in places of easiest exposure—the kitchen, the bedroom, and the bathroom. In addition, illness in the family or "life stress situations" increase the likelihood of accidental ingestion.

PREVENTION. Avoiding exposure to the toxin is the ultimate precaution; among adults, a variety of approaches have been employed—some with obvious effectiveness, others without. For example, the use of mercury in the felting process of hats has been outlawed since 1941; that source of mercury poisoning has disappeared in the hatting industry. Beryllium has been excluded from fluorescent light bulbs, and that source of exposure no longer exists. Similarly, where arsenic has been eliminated from pesticidal preparations and where naphthylamine has been eliminated from the rubber industry, human illness has been avoided. Some of these steps have resulted from legislative processes; others are the result of voluntary activity on the part of industry or an aware public.

Among children some approaches have also proved effective; others are without much evidence of success. For example, efforts directed at altering toddlers' exploratory behaviors in family settings have not proved effective. In contrast, the use of safety caps on medicine bottles had important consequences. For the 10-year period between 1959 and 1969, almost 100 deaths occurred annually from accidental salicylate poisoning in children under 5; in 1988, only one such death was reported. Several variables have been cited as definitely contributory: (1) the manufacturers' voluntary reduction of the number of tablets as well as of the amount of aspirin per bottle; (2) the introduction of a favorable flavor to the "baby aspirin" as an attractive alternative to larger tablets; (3) programs of professional and public education; (4) the appearance of acetaminophen as a rival to aspirin, with its subsequent capture of 30 per cent of the analgesic-antipyretic market, and more recently, their replacement by still newer nonsteroidal anti-inflammatory drugs (NSAID's) attempting to avoid Reye's syndrome; and (5) the mandated use of safety caps or child-resistant containers. All have had an impact, but current professional opinion holds that safety caps have contributed approximately 60 per cent of the variance. As safety caps have subsequently been applied to other prescription products and dangerous household items such as petroleum distillates and caustics, their impact has been felt there also. Unfortunately, safety caps may have a negative effect among the geriatric population, among whom as many as 50 per cent cite them as contributing to their lack of compliance in taking prescribed medications.

Since 1953, more than 500 poison centers have been established across the country to provide professionals and patients with ingredient information, toxic potentials, and treatment alternatives. Initially, the FDA's National Clearinghouse of Poison Control Centers was intended to serve as the coordinating unit; it also provided technical information to centers. In recent years, several microfiche systems—particularly "Poisondex" (Micromedex, Denver) which has evolved to a CD-ROM system—have been developed to catalogue product information and to outline management approaches; they are capable of storing information on more than 400,000 products in a limited space and in an easily retrievable manner. Moreover, such systems avoid filing errors and permit updating of information on a quarterly basis.

Over the years the American Association of Poison Control Centers has served to produce educational material aimed at preventing poisoning, to establish standards for the operation of poison centers, to conduct self-assessment examinations for those staffing poison centers, and to implement a nationwide program aimed at regionalizing the poison center network. More recently, the American Academy of Clinical Toxicology and the American Board of Medical Toxicology have been developed to serve as the specialty society and certifying body, respectively, to further

TABLE 28–1. DEATHS DUE TO "ACCIDENTAL" POISONING IN THE UNITED STATES IN 1985

	All Ages	Under 5 Years	5–44 Years	45+ Years
Total solids and liquids	4091	55	2835	1201
Medications	3612	32	2618	962
Analgesics, antipyretics	1209	4	1016	189
Opiates	867	2	779	86
Sedatives, hypnotics	32	1	22	9
Psychotropic drugs	267	5	160	101
Other CNS drugs	448	6	400	42
Other drugs	1560	11	981	563
Nondrugs	479	23	217	239
Alcohol	305	2	137	166
Paints, solvents, cleaners	85	8	52	25
Pesticides	21	6	5	10
Corrosives, caustics	11	1	1	9
Foods, plants	6	0	2	4
Other	51	6	20	25
Gases and vapors	1079	25	608	446
Carbon monoxide	880	14	518	348

Data from National Safety Council Accident Facts. Chicago, National Center for Health Statistics, 1988.

the academic and professional goals of physicians involved in such programs.

DIAGNOSIS. The diagnosis of an accidental (or a purposeful) poisoning can be made only if considered; this is true for either the adult or child with unexplained signs or symptoms. Once the possibility of poisoning is entertained, a careful search is made for a possible container and its label or for a solid medication form and its drug-identifying imprint; next, the toxic potential of the substance can be verified from existing information or by contacting the nearest poison center. Often the presenting clinical signs and symptoms are so characteristic as to permit diagnosis—e.g., the hyperventilation (following vomiting) of acute salicylism, the extrapyramidal manifestations of phenothiazine reactions. Sometimes diagnostic confirmation can be established by the patient's response to a specific antidote, e.g., naloxone. On other occasions, analysis of specimens of body fluids—blood, urine, vomit, gastric contents, or stool—is necessary for diagnosis. As a generalization, "routine toxic screens" have proved to be of relatively little value in the child and are decried by many experts as inaccurate, confusing, and not helpful in the adult. Where the history or the environment provides a lead to the potential toxins, modern technology is proving increasingly useful. In the absence of such leads, helpful results are admittedly scarce.

Particularly helpful to toxicologists have been the Consumer Product Act of 1970 and the Commission Coordinating Safety Packaging Regulations, which have promulgated adequate labeling of hazardous substances across the country. *The label on the container is the single most useful information in accidental poisonings.* In the absence of a label, generic information about ingredients of household, industrial, and pharmaceutical products is available from a poison center or from a particularly useful textbook: *Clinical Toxicology of Commercial Products.* The information on the prescription bottle, on the package insert, or from the imprint of the solid medication form (such imprints exist on virtually all tablets and capsules) is equally important and ought to be diligently pursued.

Once the ingested poison has been identified, the problem remains to determine its potential for harm in the particular patient. That potential depends upon the amount and form ingested, the toxicity of the agent, the time lapse involved, and a variety of host factors. The amount ingested can sometimes be estimated by observers or by determining the amount of material remaining in the container. The toxicity of a particular poison can be assessed by reference to known data on human experiences, to animal LD_{50}'s, and to derivative "minimal lethal doses." One must be particularly cautious about overinterpreting LD_{50}'s or animal studies; in many instances the results are not transferable to the human. A toxicity rating has proved useful in estimating the degree of risk to the patient (Table 28–2).

In recent years, toxicologic analysis of body fluids has assumed an increasingly significant role in the diagnosis and management of poisoning, but it remains a relatively small one. Technical developments perfecting chemical analysis by mass spectrophotometry, gas-liquid chromatography, and spin resonance now allow toxic screening for a variety of poisons from minuscule amounts of body fluids. Commercial laboratories as well as a number of hospital, public health, and university laboratories provide qualitative and quantitative analyses for sedatives, narcotics, psychotropics, heavy metals, pesticides, and other compounds, all of which enable a speedy and accurate diagnosis. Nevertheless, such determination (i.e., specifying the type and

TABLE 28–2. TOXICITY RATING

Rating	Probable Lethal Dose	
	mg/kg	For 70-kg Man
6—Supertoxic	<5	A taste <7 drops
5—Extremely toxic	5–50	7 drops to 1 tsp
4—Very toxic	50–500	1 tsp to 1 oz
3—Moderately toxic	500 mg–5 grams	1 oz to 1 pint
2—Slightly toxic	5–15 grams	1 pint to 1 quart
1—Practically nontoxic	>15 grams	>1 quart

From Gosselin RE, Hodge HC, Smith RP: Clinical Toxicity of Commercial Products. 5th ed. © 1984, The Williams & Wilkins Company, Baltimore.

amount of barbiturate in the blood) often does not alter management of the patient. Thus, in instances of barbiturate overdose, measurements of blood gases and pH prove more effective in coping with the clinical problem than does the quantitative determination of barbiturate level. Notable exceptions occur when specific quantification is critical in deciding on therapy—e.g., the use of acetaminophen blood levels and the Matthews-Rumack nomogram in deciding on the use of its antidote (N-acetylcysteine) before clinical signs or symptoms of illness appear, or the use of the serum salicylate concentration and the Done nomogram in determining the need for therapy in acute salicylate ingestion; and the value of the serum iron concentration along with clinical signs and symptoms in contemplating chelation therapy with desferrioxamine for iron poisoning. So too, identifying the presence of methyl alcohol or ethylene glycol can be critical in therapeutic management. Regardless of these several exceptions, the point remains that historical and clinical features plus the routinely available laboratory tests are usually paramount. Assisting the physician are a number of texts listed at the end of this chapter.

TREATMENT. Even before the ingested (or inhaled) substance has been identified and its toxic potential determined, first aid measures and supportive care ought to be initiated. Subsequent efforts are directed toward (1) preventing absorption of the substance; (2) curtailing its conversion in the body to its active form or hastening its conversion to an inactive one; (3) neutralizing or counteracting its clinical effect; and (4) enhancing its excretion from the body. In the majority of instances instituting measures to enable the patient to tolerate the temporary impact of the toxin and then to recuperate on his or her own remains the most effective course of action and often prevents subsequent poisonings as a result of overzealous treatment.

Supportive Measures. Prompt attention to supportive measures before a crisis has arisen, is, in fact, usually the single most critical element in managing the overdosed patient. The airway must be maintained, ventilation assured, cardiac output sustained, peripheral vascular collapse avoided, convulsions controlled, and hypertension and increased intracranial pressure lowered. Physical and chemical options ought to be carefully reviewed in advance of the patient's arrival if possible. Life support mechanisms can tide the patient over a period of compromised function as a result of anesthesia, an accidental overdose, or the purposeful induction of "barbiturate coma." But those measures must be carefully planned, carried out by skilled personnel, and monitored in detail if optimal benefit is to be achieved.

Prevention of Absorption. This is best accomplished in the conscious child or adult by *induction of emesis* as opposed to gastric lavage. Although gastric lavage has a tradition in emergency medicine, its yield of ingested material falls short of the returns by emesis. Moreover, despite improved emergency transport systems, there are significant time delays in delivering the patient to a health care facility where lavage can be undertaken. During that time, significant absorption takes place. By contrast, efforts to induce vomiting can be initiated in the home—particularly if syrup of ipecac is available there. If not, it is readily obtained from local pharmacies, 24-hour corner groceries, emergency vehicles, and neighbors. One should administer 15 ml to a child or 15 to 30 ml to an adult together with 200 to 300 ml of any fluids—water, soft drinks, milk, or juices—and wait 10 to 15 minutes with an appropriate receptacle for vomiting to occur. If no vomiting ensues in 20 minutes, one should repeat the initial dose of syrup of ipecac and administer more fluids. If no syrup of ipecac is available, one should try gagging the patient but should be prepared for failure; one should then encourage the patient to drink 30 to 45 ml of liquid dishwashing detergents (anionic or nonionic but *not* cationic detergents) together with 240 ml of fluid. If the patient has already arrived in the emergency room, apomorphine can be used. It proves effective in 4 to 5 minutes but results in a drowsy patient despite use of naloxone. In all circumstances one should avoid table salt as an emetic agent; its use can compound the problem with acute hypernatremia. One should always avoid emesis in the comatose or convulsing patient or in the patient who has ingested a caustic. Syrup of ipecac proves effective in acute phenothiazine ingestions, but not in the face of chronic overdose; any form of emesis is maximally effective in the first 1 to 1.5 hours after ingestion; seldom is it useful after 2 hours' delay.

Gastric lavage, using a large-bore tube and 1000 to 3000 ml of half-strength saline as the rinse, together with terminal instillation of activated charcoal, is the only option for the unconscious patient. In patients over 2 years of age, concomitant use of a cuffed endotracheal tube is indicated to avoid aspiration. Despite the fact that most toxins are absorbed rapidly and thus escape delayed evacuation efforts, on occasion substantial portions of ingested agents have been recovered, especially in suicidal patients who have consumed poisons that delay gastric emptying, slow intestinal motility, or depress overall body function. In those instances attempts at evacuation are recommended but cannot be expected to be effective in more than one of five patients.

Activated charcoal can be used to complement either of the measures discussed above, but not with syrup of ipecac until after emesis has occurred. Since the mid-1980's, increasing numbers of emergency physicians are resorting to exclusive use of activated charcoal in overdose patients who make it to the emergency room, avoiding both induction of emesis and gastric lavage; a substantial data base supports their contention. The large surface area of charcoal permits significant adsorption of the toxin, precluding its absorption from the gut. Given by mouth or via nasogastric tube in amounts of 5 to 15 times the amount of the ingested toxin, activated charcoal has diminished absorption by as much as 50 per cent with significant therapeutic benefits. Recent pharmacologic research supports the contention that absorption may be prevented by early intervention with charcoal but, equally importantly, finds that excretion of those compounds that are recycled via the gastrointestinal tract can be significantly increased by repetitive oral instillation of activated charcoal.

Cathartics, laxatives, enemas, and *colonic irrigations* are "heroic" measures devoid of evidence of effectiveness; in fact, cathartics can increase the rate of absorption of some barbiturates.

Inhibition of metabolism of a potential toxin to its active form or conversion to an inactive form is an option and, when feasible, may prove beneficial. For example, methyl alcohol becomes active only after it is converted to formaldehyde and formic acid; administering ethyl alcohol to the patient takes advantage of substrate competition (it is favored over methyl alcohol by the enzymatic processes involved), permitting significant reduction in the rate of metabolism of methyl alcohol and resulting in diminished formation of formaldehyde and formic acid, which in turn can be more easily scavenged by existent metabolic processes.

In other instances, enhancement of enzymatic activity may *activate* a toxin. For example, pretreatment of the pregnant woman and fetal liver with phenobarbital enhances conjugation of bilirubin, but such pretreatment augments the conversion of carbon tetrachloride to its deleterious metabolite.

Chelating agents also limit the entry of certain toxins into metabolic pathways and augment excretion of the inactivated material. This approach has been particularly useful in poisonings by heavy metals—treatment of arsenic, mercury, and lead with dimercaprol (BAL), D-penicillamine, and edetate (EDTA), respectively. Similarly, desferrioxamine is useful in both acute and chronic iron poisoning.

Specific antidotes to counteract the effects of specific toxins are limited to a few compounds, but when one exists its usefulness is great. Paramount is the example of naloxone, an opiate derivative, which, when administered in adequate amounts (often *considerably more* than the recommended 0.4 mg) to a patient with heroin overdose, results in the patient's sitting up and talking within 20 seconds! Administered to the nonoverdosed patient, naloxone is devoid of any action, thus constituting a unique example of an antagonist drug without any agonist effects. Most other antidotes have agonist as well as antagonist effects. Common examples of such antidotes include atropine for organophosphate and carbamate insecticide poisoning, methylene blue for methemoglobinemia, nitrites plus thiosulfate for cyanide ingestion, N-acetylcysteine for acetaminophen overdoses, pyridoxine for isoniazid toxicity and diphenhydramine for phenothiazine-induced extrapyramidal reactions. In addition, recent advances in immunology have resulted in the use of portions of antibodies ("Fab" fragments) to "neutralize" the clinical effects of overwhelming digoxin poisonings. Introduced as Digibind, this antidote has established itself as a remarkably successful remedy for dangerously moribund overdosed patients, reversing cardiac arrhythmias in minutes. Moreover, monoclonal antibodies to various toxins are being developed for possible clinical use—either via injection into the patient or by being affixed to perfusion columns.

Enhancing elimination of a toxin can be accomplished by several mechanisms. For example, in carbon monoxide poisoning, use of 100 per cent oxygen by ventilatory mask has both theoretical and practical benefit. In instances of phencyclidine ingestion, continuous gastric lavage, taking advantage of "ion trapping" of the recycled phencyclidine via the gastric mucosa, is reported to be effective. Ion trapping is also employed in acute salicylate poisoning via alkalinization of the urine. In the kidney tubule, free salicylate molecules ionize in the presence of an alkaline medium and are not resorbed, thus being "captured" in the urine and excreted into the bladder. In contrast, amphetamine (a weak base) is captured in the kidney tubule by acidifying the urine with ascorbic acid or ammonium chloride. In general, forced osmotic diuresis, particularly chemical diuresis with common diuretics (e.g., furosemide), is of little or no benefit in enhancing the excretory processes.

By contrast, *dialysis* and *hemoperfusion* have proved to be effective therapeutic tools, although not as effective as had been initially believed. For example, a decade ago many patients with barbiturate overdose were subjected to extracorporeal or peritoneal dialysis; today, fewer than 1 in 300 such patients are so treated. If renal shutdown has occurred, as in mercury poisoning, dialysis will prove lifesaving, although it is unlikely to augment excretion of the mercury molecule. Exceptions do exist, as in dialysis for ethylene glycol overdoses. Hemoperfusion and lipid dialysis both serve as effective mechanisms in eliminating specific offending substances from the body, e.g., ethchlorvynol. To be effective, a significant proportion of the total body toxin must be present in the blood and must not be tightly bound to serum protein. For many compounds, such as digoxin, tricyclic antidepressants, and phenothiazines, these conditions are not met, and dialysis and hemoperfusion do little to reduce the total body burden of toxin. Knowledge of the "apparent volume of distribution" of a compound permits prediction of the usefulness of dialysis or hemoperfusion (see Ch. 78.1).

Occasionally, still other techniques, such as *exchange transfusions* in boric acid or iron poisoning, may be useful. So-called *gut lavage*, a virtually continuous through-and-through rinse of the bowel via instillation of large amounts of physiologic fluids into the intestine through a nasogastric tube, has been reported effective in paraquat overdoses when no alternatives exist. Careful consideration of the metabolic pathways of the involved substance combined with empiric evidence of previous outcomes serves as the best guide for management.

Treatment of Specific Common Poisonings. In addition to the general principles of treatment discussed above, a few common poisonings warrant specific mention.

Aspirin (salicylate) poisoning formerly accounted for 20 per cent of ingestions among children under 5 years of age; today, it is responsible for only 1 to 2 per cent. However, it remains a concern for all age groups—particularly because of its widespread use as a potential suicidal agent among the elderly. Acute ingestions in excess of 100 mg per kilogram of body weight deserve induction of emesis; aspirin leads to rapid metabolic acidosis in children under 4 years of age and to initial respiratory alkalosis in the adult. Both groups vomit; this permits early detection and helps in differentiation from acetaminophen ingestion. Alkalinizing the urine proves remarkably effective with the single acute ingestion; one should consult the Done nomogram for prognosis. The administration of intravenous $NaHCO_3$ (3 mEq per kilogram of body weight) to young children usually proves effective in raising urine pH above 7.0. A later second or third dose of approximately one half of that amount may be necessary to sustain alkalinization of the urine and thereby promote ionization and reduce reabsorption of salicylate. The use of acetazolamide to alkalinize the urine should be avoided; its mechanism of action also accelerates transport of salicylate into the central nervous system (CNS). Urinary elimination of the salicylate moiety removes the cause of the acidosis—a far more effective approach to therapy than treatment of the systemic acidosis itself. In the adult, initial blood pH may be elevated; nonetheless, it is the urine pH that is critical to monitor. In general, additional potassium administration is necessary only for the chronically intoxicated patient or later in the course of acute intoxications in adults. Occasionally dialysis may be warranted, but ordinarily general supportive measures prove sufficient. Chronic overdoses are far less responsive to any specific interventions, but supportive treatment can be crucial.

Acetaminophen has captured 30 per cent of today's analgesic-antipyretic market; liquid formulations are being augmented by solid preparation forms, some of which are in "extra strength" dosages. In Britain, acetaminophen has been a particularly popular suicidal substance; management is often complicated by the fact that no significant symptoms may appear until after irreversible liver damage has occurred. If recognized early—preferably less than 8 hours and certainly less than 16 hours after ingestion—determination of the serum level and comparison of it against standards on the Matthews-Rumack nomogram permit an appropriate decision about the possible use of an antidote, either N-acetylcysteine or methionine (both sulfhydryl donors). Both appear to enter into metabolic pathways via glutathione mechanisms and to preclude the formation of an epoxide derivative of acetaminophen that binds covalently to liver macromolecules, resulting in liver cell destruction. An intravenous preparation of the antidote is available that is strongly favored and widely used in Britain; it ought to be available in the United States soon. Currently, only an oral form is available in the United States, and its use presents difficulties because of associated emesis. Of special note is the apparent diminished susceptibility to toxicity in the preadolescent compared with the adult.

Significant overdoses of *anticholinergic substances* in various forms (e.g., tricyclic antidepressants, atropine, antihistamines, phenothiazines, jimson weed) produce fever, flushing, widely dilated pupils, and CNS signs and symptoms varying from somnolence and coma to delirium and seizures. Each of these specific drugs may also produce additional specific symptoms by other mechanisms—e.g., diphenhydramine hydrochloride (Benadryl) occasionally results in extrapyramidal reactions; tricyclic antidepressants cause cardiac arrhythmias. For this class of drugs, physostigmine is available both as a diagnostic agent and as a therapeutic substance; because administration of physostigmine may itself induce seizures in 15 to 20 per cent of treated patients, its use has declined significantly. The dose is 0.5 mg administered slowly intravenously for the child under 5 and 1 to 2 mg for the adult, repeated as often as necessary to control seizures. Today, however, most centers rely on diazepam treatment instead. In all instances atropine should be immediately available during physostigmine infusion, and Valium also ought to be available should a convulsion occur. Tricyclic antidepressant overdoses are now numerically the most serious of prescription medicine hazards. These are best approached by using diazepam (Valium) or phenobarbital to control seizures, by maintaining a blood pH above 7.45 to prevent tachyarrhythmias either by administering $NaHCO_3$ or by controlled ventilation in the obtunded patient, and by use of conventional cardiac drugs should arrhythmias ensue.

Acute petroleum distillates (hydrocarbons) cause their most significant damage as a function of their initial action on the lungs via aspiration; such aspiration occurs at the time of ingestion or inhalation. Both in laboratory animals and in humans, large amounts of various petroleum distillates have been consumed and retained without development of any signs or symptoms save for odoriferous eructations ("smelly burps") and diarrhea. As a general rule, neither lavage nor induction of emesis is indicated in such ingestions unless some additional toxin (e.g., parathion) has been dissolved in the hydrocarbon. When such is the case, induction of emesis has supplanted gastric lavage as the treatment of choice. When pulmonary aspiration has occurred, supportive measures are introduced; antibiotics and steroids are widely used but without much evidence of effectiveness.

Use patterns of anticonvulsants have changed in recent years with the advent of valproic acid and the increased use of carbamazepine (Tegretol). Valproic acid overdoses are similar to those of other sedatives and, in fact, are often less severe. However, valproic acid interacts with other drugs, particularly other sedatives, potentiating their actions. The greatest concerns are hepatic necrosis and a Reye-like syndrome. Valproic acid should be avoided during pregnancy because it is associated with an increase in fetal neural tube defects. Carbamazepine, also a potential teratogen, is noted for its propensity to induce seizures in the overdosed patient, who otherwise appears to be heavily sedated. No specific antidote is available; routine supportive therapy is used. Techniques aimed at enhancing excretion, other than use of repetitive doses of oral activated charcoal, have not been proven satisfactory and are thus not advised.

Carbon monoxide (see Ch. 528) ranks high as a contributor to common poisonings, suicides, and accidental deaths. The mechanism of action involves acute interruption of both oxygen transport and oxygen metabolism, with a rapid cessation of life functions. Prompt recognition of exposure and removal of the patient from the contaminated environment are essential. Hastening of excretion of carbon monoxide by administration of oxygen and consideration of hyperbaric oxygen treatment are currently the hallmarks of management.

Caustic compounds, including acids and alkalis, appear to exert their toxic effects largely via alterations of pH and their consequences on the gastrointestinal tract. Experimental evidence suggests that the damage done by alkalis is complete within 30 seconds after exposure; that done by acids may be somewhat slower to appear. Current recommendations for management are avoidance of major efforts to empty the gastrointestinal tract, neutralization of the offending compound by the administration of a protein-containing substance (such as milk), and careful assessment of the esophagus for the possibility of acute burns. This last point frequently necessitates esophagoscopy because the presence or absence of burns in the mouth proves nonpredictive of the status of the esophagus. In addition to concerns about the acute situation—managed by dilatation, steroids, and antibiotics—much interest now focuses on follow-up for 20 to 40 years because of a significantly increased risk of carcinoma of the esophagus.

Cyanide has gained its deserved reputation for toxicity by its ability to inhibit oxygen utilization at the level of the cell via cytochrome oxidase inhibition; severe metabolic acidosis can occur almost instantaneously. Most exposures are occupational; occasional exposures are the result of homicidal efforts, particularly associated with capsule tampering, and rare consequences are found subsequent to l-mandelonitrile-β-glucuronic acid (Laetrile) administration or nitroprusside overdose. As soon as cyanide poisoning is suspected, administration of nitrite—via a 3 per cent solution intravenously or amyl nitrite inhalation—is crucial. It converts hemoglobin to methemoglobin, which selectively binds cyanide. This is followed by administration of sodium thiosulfate to convert cyanide to the less toxic thiocyanate. Recent experience in Europe suggests the use of dicobalt edetate may be even more effective—but avoidance is the goal.

Drugs of abuse haunt the profession, the emergency room, and our society. Were the offending agent easily identified with certainty—e.g., heroin—the immediate remedy would be obvious—naloxone. Such instances are almost nonexistent; more than 90 per cent of what is bought and sold "on the street" is not what it has been represented to be. Even imprinted capsules have been counterfeited in efforts to "con" the buyer. In other instances the basic ingredient has been "cut" with an inert substance or "laced" with some other psychoactive substance. Enormous geographic variations seem to exist across the country, with phencyclidine ("angel dust," PCP) being particularly popular in Los Angeles and Detroit, Ritalin in Seattle, and heroin and cocaine ("crack") in New York.

The laboratory may be helpful in instances of opiate overdose but is of virtually no value for lysergic acid diethylamide (LSD) or PCP (see Ch. 15). As a consequence, symptomatic management predominates; the unconscious or convulsing adult may routinely be approached as a potential heroin addict, an alcoholic, or a hypoglycemic individual; the hyperactive, "spacey" patient prompts consideration of PCP, LSD, and related sympathomimetic agents (amphetamine, phenylpropanolamine, etc.), as well as recreational cocaine or psychosocial decompensation. Supportive measures may include monitoring, restraints, sedatives (diazepam is "customary"), succinylcholine, hydration, and ventilatory and cardiac measures. As a generalization, the acute management proves far more successful than treatment of the underlying problem, but efforts ought to be directed at the latter, as it provides the only true solution to the basic problem.

Ethyl alcohol (see Ch. 14) is mentioned here to stress its ubiquity and the epidemiologic point that it is remarkably prevalent as a cause of admission to hospital for children, with both purposeful and accidental ingestions, as well as a cause of birth defects among newborns. Also, ethyl alcohol augments the potential toxicity of a number of other compounds, such as diazepam.

Halogenated hydrocarbons (including chlorinated insecticides such as chlorophenothane, or DDT) serve as a source of a myriad of occupational, industrial, and pharmacologic exposures. Almost invariably lipid soluble, most are readily absorbable by the gastrointestinal tract, the respiratory epithelium, or the skin. Fortunately, most are metabolically rather stable compounds within the human organism; thus reproduction of still more hazardous metabolites is minimized. Nonetheless, many of the compounds gain access to fat storage deposits or neural tissue and cause both central and peripheral nervous system symptoms. For some (e.g., 2,3,7,8-tetrachlorodibenzodioxin, or dioxin) there are concerns about long-term toxicity and teratogenicity. Treatment modes include elimination of subsequent exposures, attempts to retrieve unabsorbed quantities from the gastrointestinal tract, and general supportive measures in response to symptoms.

Iron salts ($FeSO_4$, Fe gluconate) represent a hazard confined almost exclusively to children who "accidentally" consume prenatal tablets. Recently increasing numbers of iron poisoning have been recognized in adults. While initial reports of a 50 per cent mortality rate were greatly inflated (instead it hovers at approximately 1 per cent), iron poisoning typifies the problem of the "unsuspected toxin" about which parents, parent surrogates, and physicians may be uninformed. When ingestions are known to exceed 50 to 60 mg per kilogram or when serum levels (taken 3 to 6 hours after ingestion) exceed 400 to 500 µg per deciliter, observation and chelation with desferrioxamine ought to be seriously considered, particularly if clinical symptoms such as upper abdominal pain, nausea, and vomiting are present. Management of the acute ingestion calls for prompt gastric emptying and efforts to minimize absorption of the iron salts. More serious overdoses have prompted heroic measures, including surgical extirpation of ingested tablets and attempts at exchange transfusion. To date, studies have documented no serious consequences from ingestion of iron as a component of children's chewable vitamin preparations despite predictions to the contrary.

Methanol and *ethylene glycol* present significant problems of metabolic acidosis in clinically poisoned patients. Diagnosis is often considered following discovery of an unexplained anion gap. These compounds both depend upon alcohol dehydrogenase for their metabolism. The current approach to therapy takes advantage of this situation and provides ethanol (5 to 10 grams per hour intravenously) as a competitive inhibitor of toxin metabolism—thus slowing the formation of toxic metabolites, formaldehyde, and formic acid from methanol, or glycoaldehyde and glycolic, glyoxylic, and oxalic acids from ethylene glycol, to rates of formation permitting these products to be disposed of by ordinary metabolic or excretory pathways. For emphasis, an alternative approach currently employed in Europe involves 4-methyl-pyrazole administered to block alcohol dehydrogenase activity, thus accomplishing the same objective as that sought with ethyl alcohol. It is likely to be available in the United States soon. In the meantime, for large overdoses hemodialysis may be required to eliminate the offending toxin.

Organophosphate and carbamate insecticides can both prove exquisitely toxic in minute amounts. The mechanism of action involves inhibition of acetylcholine metabolism via cessation of cholinesterase function. Prompt recognition of symptoms secondary to acute exposure can prove lifesaving. Detecting symptoms secondary to chronic exposure (e.g., peripheral neuropathy) can serve to eliminate much patient distress and employee unhappiness. In general, acute distress is ushered in via excessive secretions in the upper airway, with respiratory distress, diffuse muscular weakness, nausea, vomiting, and collapse. Treatment requires prompt and repeated administration of large amounts of atropine for both types of poisoning. Pralidoxime (2PAM) is also strongly recommended to assist in the rejuvenation of cholinesterase levels. Introduced in large measure as a "safer" replacement for DDT, these compounds have been responsible for large numbers of acute poisonings but, as far as can be determined, are yet to be implicated in carcinogenicity, teratogenicity, or chronic liver disease.

Paraquat (and its associated congeners) is a particularly popular and effective herbicide. While controversy rages about the consequences of environmental exposures, no controversy exists on the issue of acute, purposeful overdoses; they are devastating. Paraquat is a harsh gastrointestinal irritant that also inhibits renal function; its most destructive impact is on the respiratory tract, where it inhibits superoxide dismutase and kills via "oxygen toxicity." Current approaches to therapy favor such dramatic efforts as "gut lavage," with some suggestion that hemoperfusion might be warranted. However, overdoses are likely to be lethal.

Theophylline and its congeners have been recognized as inducing seizures, cardiac arrhythmias, and occasional deaths in overdose situations. More recently, "therapeutic misadventures" have been recognized; inadvertent overdoses, alterations of theophylline metabolism by viral infections and nutritional variations, and the tendency to use theophylline in large quantities for relatively minor illnesses all increase the likelihood of such occurrences. Beta blockers can be used in managing the clinical symptoms of overdose—particularly the associated anxiety and tachycardia—but should not be used in asthmatic individuals. Children seem more resistant to the serious side effects than do adults, but occasionally both groups may have to be considered for hemoperfusion. Peritoneal and extracorporeal hemodialysis have both been reported to be ineffective.

Although ingestions of *plants and plant elements* constitute the single most frequent reason for telephoning poison centers, the overall problem is best put in perspective by Fraser's analysis of Britain's most recent 20-year experience with poisonings:

> Plants are the most overrated poisons of childhood. In earlier decades there were occasional deaths, most caused by the umbelliferae (particularly hemlock water dropwort) and the solanaceae (various nightshades). From 1958 to 1977 there were three deaths, and in one the role of the ingestion in the child's demise is doubtful. The others were caused by hemlock and by *Amanita phalloides* (death cup), both in children aged five and nine. Laburnum is frequently cited as the most toxic and commonly fatal poisonous plant in both children and adults, but there appears to be no report this century of childhood poisoning death. One adult death in unusual circumstances has been recorded.

Confirming this observation is the fact that the more than 90,000 plant ingestions reported to poison centers in 1988 led to but a single death—of an adult who ate water hemlock.

CONCLUSION. Chemical hazards have always been a way of life. Today their numbers continue to escalate. But modern technology permits both identification and quantification of minuscule amounts of some toxins—uncovering, for example, tamperings with cyanides. At the same time, "media hype" may distort risks—for example, with regard to the purported dangers of methamphetamine laboratories—to such an extent that the prudent physician is overcome with frustration. As a consequence, while the physician is well advised to add possible poisoning to the differential diagnosis for any unexplained collection of signs or symptoms in a patient of any age, unless he or she is confident of the timeliness and completeness of his or her understanding about a specific item, additional consultation is strongly advised.

Arena J, Drew RH: Poisoning: Chemistry, Symptoms and Treatment. 5th ed. Springfield, Ill., Charles C Thomas, 1986. *Derived from years of experience and leadership in the poisoning field, this book is well organized, carefully edited, and readable, with a remarkable collection of cases and common sense.*

Bryson PD. Comprehensive Review in Toxicology. Rockville, Md., Aspen Publishers, 1989. *Authored by an experienced practicing medical toxicologist, this remarkably thorough text clarifies a number of significant clinical concerns.*

Dreisbach RH, Robertson WO: Handbook of Poisoning. 12th ed. Los Altos, Calif., Lange Publishing Company, 1987. *This pocket-sized book is both comprehensive and concise. Up-to-date and always helpful to review for omissions in one's approach, it proves particularly valuable to the primary care physician.*

Ellenhorn MJ, Barceloux DG: Medical Toxicology: Diagnosis and Treatment of Human Poisoning, New York, Elsevier, 1988. *The latest and by far most comprehensive and complete human toxicology text; lucidly written, particularly well indexed, and appropriately clinical in its management recommendations.*

Goldfrank LR, Flomenbaum N, Lewin N, et al.: Toxicologic Emergencies. 4th ed. Norwalk, CT, Appleton-Century-Crofts, 1990. *Probably the most clinically relevant and readable of all the texts available, it summarizes a remarkable amount of experience in readily retrievable form—and in a format aimed at anticipating the reader's needs.*

Gosselin RE, Hodge HC, Smith RP: Clinical Toxicology of Commercial Products.

5th ed. Baltimore, Williams & Wilkins Company, 1984. *Long established as the "bible" of the field, this compendium provides a concise overview of poisoning issues, as well as a thorough and well-edited clinical description of approximately 50 generic poisonings. It has a comprehensive listing of trade-name entities and generic items in household and commercial product fields. Authoritative the world over.*

Haddad LM, Winchester JF: Clinical Management of Poisoning and Drug Overdose. 2nd ed. Philadelphia, W. B. Saunders Company, 1990. *A recent book with contributions chiefly by American experts, this is currently a most comprehensive text for the recognition and clinical management of poisoning.*

Klaassen CD, Amdur MD, Doull J: Toxicology: The Basic Science of Poisons. 3rd ed. New York, Macmillan, 1986. *This text constitutes the "compleat" basic science approach for the toxicologist. With 42 contributors and critical editing, the final product covers the field from salt to water to radiation.*

Journals: Virtually any clinical journal may prove the source of a fascinating case report or a valuable review in the field of poisoning. Lancet, JAMA, N Engl J Med, and the traditional medical and pediatric specialty journals are particularly valuable resources. In the more limited field of clinical toxicology the following are of note: (1) Veterinary and Human Toxicology: The official journal of the American Association of Poison Control Centers and the American Academy of Clinical Toxicology, always updating the clinical field. (2) The American Journal of Emergency Medicine, published by W. B. Saunders Company, whose September issue annually provides nationwide incidence data from the American Association of Poison Control Centers (AAPCC). (3) Clinical Toxicology: A blend of industrial, environmental, and accidental cases appears here, together with results of bench research. (4) Emergency Medicine: A controlled circulation journal particularly noted for "The Toxic Emergency," a periodic contribution of Donald Kunkel. (5) The Annals of Emergency Medicine, focusing on many acute toxic episodes.

29 NSAID's: Aspirin and Aspirin-like Drugs

Gerald Weissmann

HISTORY

Salicylates as Antipyretics and Analgesics

On June 2, 1763, the Royal Society received a communication from Reverend Edmund Stone of Chipping Norton in Oxfordshire. Its opening lines are probably unmatched in clinical pharmacology:

> Among the many useful discoveries which this age has made, there are very few which better deserve the attention of the public than what I am going to lay before your Lordship. There is a bark of an English tree, which I have found by experience to be a powerful astringent and very efficacious in curing aguish and intermittent disorders.

The tree was the willow (*Salix alba*), the astringent bark of which contains salicin, the glycoside of salicylic acid. Stone had discovered that salicylates reduced the fever and aches produced by a variety of acute, shiver-provoking illnesses, or agues.

In 1990, the salicylate most commonly used is acetylsalicylic acid, aspirin. At over-the-counter doses (1 to 3 grams per day) aspirin is *analgesic* and *antipyretic*. In addition, at lower doses (80 to 325 mg per day) aspirin is used to prevent coronary and cerebral thrombosis by virtue of its *antiplatelet* effect. And for 100 years very high doses (4 to 8 grams per day) have been used to reduce the redness and swelling of joints in rheumatic fever, gout, and rheumatoid arthritis.

Salicylates also have a wide variety of other biologic effects, only some of which are related to their current use in clinical medicine. Salicylates can dissolve corns on the toes, a *keratolytic* effect; provoke loss of uric acid from the kidneys, their *uricosuric* property; and kill bacteria in vitro, their *antiseptic* action. Aspirin inhibits the formation of prostaglandins and thereby inhibits the clotting of blood, induces peptic ulcers, and promotes fluid retention by the kidney. Cell biologists use aspirin and salicylates to inhibit anion transport across cell membranes, to interfere with the activation of white cells, and to uncouple oxidative phosphorylation by isolated mitochondria. Botanists use salicylates to induce flowering of *Impatiens*; indeed, the function of salicylates in plants such as the voodoo lily or skunk cabbage is to induce temperature rises of 12 to 16°C in the course of efflorescence. Salicylates therefore not only reduce fever but also produce it! Finally, molecular biologists use salicylates to activate genes that code for heat-shock proteins in the lampbrush chromosomes of *Drosophila*.

"About six years ago," wrote Stone in his letter to the Royal Society, "I accidentally tasted [the willow bark], and was surprised at its extraordinary bitterness; which immediately raised in me a suspicion of its having the properties of the Peruvian bark." Peruvian bark (*cinchona*) was a venerable remedy for the ague. Stone proceeded to offer a skillful rationale for the use of willow bark in febrile disorders: the traditional doctrine of signatures—i.e., that "many natural maladies carry their cures along with them, or their remedies lie not far from their cause." Since moist shires, like those drained by the Avon or Isis, abound in both fevers and willows, Rev. Stone set out to test whether the former might be cured by the latter. Six years of careful clinical observation and the treatment of 50 patients with willow extracts prepared in water, tea, or beer culminated in his letter to the Royal Society. The eighteenth century had found a predictable remedy for fever.

Hippocrates (fourth century B.C.) had advocated the chewing of willow leaves for relief of the pains of childbirth, and there are references by Pliny (first century) and Galen (second century) to the *analgesic* property of willow, but it remained for Stone to put extract of willow bark into our pharmacopoeia as an effective *antipyretic* agent.

By 1828, at the Pharmacologic Institute of Munich, Buchner isolated a tiny amount of the active glycoside, salicin, in the form of bitter-tasting, yellow, needle-like crystals. Two years later, Leroux in Paris improved on the extraction procedure and obtained 1 ounce of salicin from 3 pounds of the bark. By 1838, Raffaele Pira of Pisa, writing in the *Comtes Rendu de l'Academie de Science*, described how he obtained a pure substance from salicin by hydrolyzing the glycoside in a CrO_3-mediated oxidation via an aldehyde intermediate. He gave it the name by which we know it today: "*l'acide salicylique*," or salicylic acid. Willow bark was not alone in providing a rich natural source of salicylates. Meadowsweet (*Spireae ulmaria*) yielded ample quantities of an ether-soluble oil from which a *Spirsäure* was crystallized in 1835 by the Swiss chemist Karl Jakob Lowig. In 1839 Dumas demonstrated that the *Spirsäure* of Lowig was nothing else than the *acide salicylique* of Piriâ. Another Gallic pharmacologist, Auguste Andre Thomas Cahours (1843), showed that oil of wintergreen—a traditional remedy for aguish disorders—contained the methyl ester of salicylic acid and prepared *acide salicylique* from it.

As was to be the case in much of nineteenth century chemistry, French and British scientists were slightly ahead of the Germans in the study of natural products, whereas Germans held the edge in synthetic know-how. Forced to compete with the French and British dye industries which supplied their textile mills with pigments imported from overseas colonies, the Germans replied by inventing cheap aniline dyes, creating in their train such giant enterprises as I. G. Farben. By 1833, the pharmacist E. Merck of Darmstadt had obtained a clean preparation of salicin which was cheaper by half than the impure willow extracts used as antipyretics, but a cheap, pure, acceptable remedy was not available until 1860, when Kolbe and his students at Marburg succeeded in the first synthesis of salicylic acid and its sodium salt from phenol, CO_2, and sodium. Using industrial variations of the Kolbe synthesis, one of his students, Friedrich von Heyden, established in 1874 the first large factory in Dresden devoted to the production of synthetic salicylates. The availability of cheap salicylic acid spread its clinical use far and wide.

Salicylates as Anti-inflammatory Drugs

The first successful treatment of acute rheumatism was reported in 1876 by Stricker and Ries in the *Berliner Medizinische Wochenschrifft* and by Maclagan writing in *The Lancet*. Stricker and Ries reported the complete cure of acute "polyarthritis rheumatica" by sodium salicylate at doses of 5 to 6 grams per day. Almost simultaneously, Maclagan reported his results with salicylic acid and salicin at similar dosage levels; he paid tribute to the still prevalent doctrine of signatures, pointing out that cases of acute rheumatism were most abundant in moist areas where the willow grows.

Stricker and Ries and Maclagan had demonstrated a clinical property of high-dose salicylates that was not to be tested in the laboratory until the 1930's: They found that salicylates reduce not only fever and pain but also redness and swelling. That anti-inflammatory property was next used to advantage by the Parisian, Germain See, who in 1877 introduced salicylates (both *acid salicylique* and *salicin*) as effective treatments for gout and "chronic poly-arthritis." See had great success among his well-off clientele with the use of salicylates in acute and chronic gout, so great indeed that the *British Medical Journal*, in an editorial note, called him to task for charging up to 80 pounds sterling to treat a patient with gout by means of 6 to 8 grams of sodium salicylate per day, when the price of the drug was but 5 pence per gram! There the matter rested, with high doses of sodium salicylate more or less accepted as a new treatment in many rheumatic diseases, while lower doses (1.5 to 2.0 grams per day) seemed to relieve aches and pains.

Aspirin

In 1898 a new chapter was written: Felix Hofmann was an aniline dye chemist at the Friedrich Bayer–Eberfeld division of the I. G. Farben cartel when his father complained to him of gastric irritation from the sodium salicylate he was taking for "rheumatism." Hofmann searched the chemical literature for less acidic derivatives and hit upon acetyl derivatives of sodium salicylate first described by G. Von Gilm in 1859 and 10 years later by a certain H. Kraut (sic). Although von Gilm and Kraut had outlined synthesis of the compound, they had no notion of what its biologic effects might be. Hofmann repeated the synthesis (via acetic anhydride) and tried acetylsalicylic acid first on himself and then on his father: It proved more palatable, less irritating to the stomach, and—he claimed—more effective. Hofmann took the material to his supervisor, Heinrich Dreser, head of Bayer's laboratory of pharmacology, who reported that aspirin performed better both in laboratory and in clinic and called the new drug *aspirin*, the *a* from *acetyl* and the *spirin* from the German *Spirsäure*.

The Aniline Derivatives as Analgesics and Antipyretics

Competitors entered the field as the markets expanded for other drugs that could reduce fever and pain. Based on anecdotal accounts from the Alsace that a product formed from aniline treated with vinegar made a useful febrifuge, Karl Morner in 1889 synthesized the material—acetanilide—and isolated its metabolites. Acetanilide itself, unfortunately, caused bone marrow depression and anemias in a distinct number of patients, so other derivatives were sought. Acetanilide and the widely used phenacetin are metabolized to *N-acetyl-p-aminophenol*, which by various anagramatic combinations yields the generic names *acetaminophen* in the United States and *paracetamol* in the United Kingdom. In 1955 acetaminophen acquired a tradename in the United States that was to make it famous: *Tylenol*—also from ac*etyl*-p-aminoph*enol*.

NSAID's vs. Cortisone

Neither acetanilide nor phenacetin proved as useful as aspirin in the treatment of rheumatic fever or rheumatoid arthritis: They were not anti-inflammatory. For half a century (1900–1950) clinicians appreciated that there was something unique about high-dose salicylates. At levels over 4 grams per day, only salicylates—of all the analgesics—were anti-inflammatory. They also brought under control the erythrocyte sedimentation rate and levels of C-reactive protein in serum. Indeed, when James Reid in 1948 demonstrated an inverse relationship between plasma salicylate levels and signs of rheumatic inflammation, he asked "Does sodium salicylate cure rheumatic fever?" The answer came from well-controlled and definitive studies in the 1950's that were prompted by the discovery of ACTH and cortisone, the most potent anti-inflammatory compounds ever described.

Each of over two dozen studies concluded that neither steroids (cortisone and its derivatives) nor salicylates (aspirin or sodium salicylate) actually cure rheumatic fever or rheumatoid arthritis—and that in the short run both types of agents are equally effective at suppressing acute inflammation. Since the course of acute rheumatic fever is easier to document than that of rheumatoid arthritis, it is worth paying attention today to the back-to-back trials of steroids versus aspirin and sodium salicylate. These were performed by the Medical Research Council of Britain and the American Heart Association (reported in 1955) and the Combined Rheumatic Fever Study Group of the United States (reported in 1961) and showed that salicylates at doses high enough to yield plasma levels of 25 to 35 mg per deciliter (6 to 9 grams per day) were as effective anti-inflammatory agents as cortisone or prednisone in rheumatic fever.

NSAID MODE OF ACTION: INHIBITION OF PROSTAGLANDIN SYNTHESIS

Unfortunately, until 1971 no useful hypothesis had emerged as to how salicylates exert their various effects. Pharmacologists had shown that salicylate analgesia was due to a peripheral effect—as opposed to morphine's central action. In contrast, physiologists maintained that salicylates did not reduce fever by peripheral action but worked directly on the fever centers of the hypothalamus. Renal physiologists found that low doses of salicylates raised uric acid in the blood by blocking tubular secretion by the kidney while, paradoxically, high doses of salicylates lowered uric acid by blocking its tubular absorption. Clinicians found that the latter property explained the utility of salicylates in both acute and chronic gout. It was more difficult to explain how aspirin inhibited platelet function, caused salt and water retention, and provoked severe dyspepsia. And why did some patients develop nasal polyps, with sniffles and wheezes: aspirin "hyper-sensitivity"?

The most important recent contribution to the story of aspirin-like drugs was made by John Vane (now Sir John) at the Royal College of Surgeons in London in 1971. Vane had been impressed that many forms of tissue injury are followed by release of prostaglandins, the oxidation products of arachidonic acid. Prostaglandins E_1 and F_2 had been shown to be associated with acute vasodilation and fever. Vane and his colleagues found that aspirin-like drugs inhibited the biosynthesis of prostaglandins E_2 and $F_2\alpha$ from radiolabeled arachidonic acid in studies in vitro. Moreover, they found that platelets taken from volunteers given aspirin and indomethacin 1 hour before venipuncture failed to make prostaglandins in response to thrombin, and that catecholamine-induced release of prostaglandins from canine spleens could be inhibited by indomethacin—albeit less consistently than by aspirin or sodium salicylate.

All that remained was to show how and when prostaglandins caused redness and swelling with heat and pain and to study the exact means whereby aspirin-like drugs inhibited the enzyme that transformed arachidonic acid to the stable prostaglandins E_1 and E_2, etc. The enzyme has been found to be a 70-kDa homodimer localized to microsomal membranes; it has been cloned and sequenced and was first called "prostaglandin synthase," then "cyclo-oxygenase," and today is known as "prostaglandin H synthase" (Fig. 29–1). This single enzyme catalyzes two reactions: the bis-deoxygenation of arachidonic acid to form prostaglandin H_2 (cyclo-oxygenase activity) and the reduction of hydroperoxides to the corresponding alcohols. This enzyme therefore produces stable prostaglandins of the E and F series via the unstable *endoperoxide* intermediates, PGG_2 and PGH_2. The endoperoxides, which are critical for platelet function, are transformed by platelets to a most potent vasoconstricting and platelet-aggregating substance, thromboxane B_2. Meanwhile, Vane had isolated a potent vasodilator, prostacyclin (prostaglandin I_2), which was also made from arachidonate by the cyclo-oxygenase of endothelial cells. Since platelets make thromboxane B_2, which constricts the smooth muscle of blood vessels, and since blood vessel walls make prostacyclin I_2, which powerfully relaxes blood vessels and inhibits platelet aggregation, the hunt was on for ways of inhibiting the synthesis of thromboxane but not prostacyclin.

Vane and his associates in the 1970's had amassed convincing evidence that the prostaglandin hypothesis of aspirin action was largely correct. They pointed out that almost all aspirin-like drugs (by then generally called "nonsteroidal anti-inflammatory drugs," or NSAID's) inhibited prostaglandin synthetase and that the potency of these drugs (ID_{50}) in this regard pretty much paralleled their clinical potency or their effect in experimental animals; e.g., aspirin was anywhere from one fortieth to one two-hundredth as active as indomethacin and from one fifth to one fiftieth as active as ibuprofen. Indeed, by 1990, over 40 NSAID's had reached the clinic and each of them at one dose or another inhibits the synthetase. It should also be noted, however, that since 1971, inhibition of PG synthetase has been a sine qua non for their introduction! Only NSAID's, but not central analegesics such as morphine or codeine, inhibited PG synthetase, nor did antihistamines, antiserotonin drugs, cortisone, and its analogues. Moreover, concentrations of NSAID's that could be achieved in the circulation (allowing for protein binding) were in excess of those required to inhibit the enzyme in disrupted cell preparations.

Vane and his colleagues argued that stable prostaglandins not only were produced at sites of inflammation, but alone or in concert with other mediators could provoke all the cardinal signs of inflammation. Indeed, prostaglandins E_1 and E_2 *do* induce vasodilation; they promote edema when dilated blood vessels have been made leaky by histamine; they produce fever when injected either into the cerebral ventricles or directly into the anterior hypothalamus; and they sensitize pain receptors of the skin to such other pain-provoking humors as bradykinin and histamine. Sound explanations were offered for a few troubling discrepancies. Acetaminophen was ineffective at inhibiting prostaglandin synthesis by enzyme preparations from a variety of tissues but was effective against the synthetase from brain. And although nonacetylated salicylates were roughly one tenth as potent as aspirin in vitro, studies of urinary prostaglandin metabolites showed that sodium salicylate effectively diminished excretion of these metabolites in man. Sodium salicylate also effectively reduced prostaglandin release in models of experimental inflammation in animals.

NSAID SIDE EFFECTS

Perhaps the most persuasive aspect of the prostaglandin hypothesis was its explanation of the clinical side effects of NSAID's. A major problem with NSAID's at anti-inflammatory doses is that they provoke stomach irritation and sometimes ulceration. Aspirin is the worst offender in this regard. This irritative property is due to the need for endogenous prostaglandins by the gastric mucosa in order to regulate its overproduction of acid and to synthesize the mucous barrier that prevents its self-digestion. But now an *exogenous* prostaglandin E_1 analogue (misoprostol) has been approved for the prevention and treatment of NSAID-induced ulcers.

Moreover, most NSAID's prevent the body from excreting salt and water properly, especially when heart or liver disease compromises renal blood flow. NSAID's block the formation of the vasodilator PGI_2 by kidney cells, and renal blood supply is reduced even further. Another side effect of NSAID's—but not sodium salicylate—is induction of the aspirin sensitivity syndrome in those genetically susceptible: wheezing, sneezing, and polyp formation. Nowadays, thanks to the elucidation of arachidonic acid metabolism, we attribute these consequences to the diversion of arachidonate from blocked PGH synthase to the 5-lipoxygenase pathway which is not inhibited by NSAID's. It is by means of the lipoxygenase pathways that leukotrienes C, D, and E are formed, and these have been implicated in aspirin hypersensitivity.

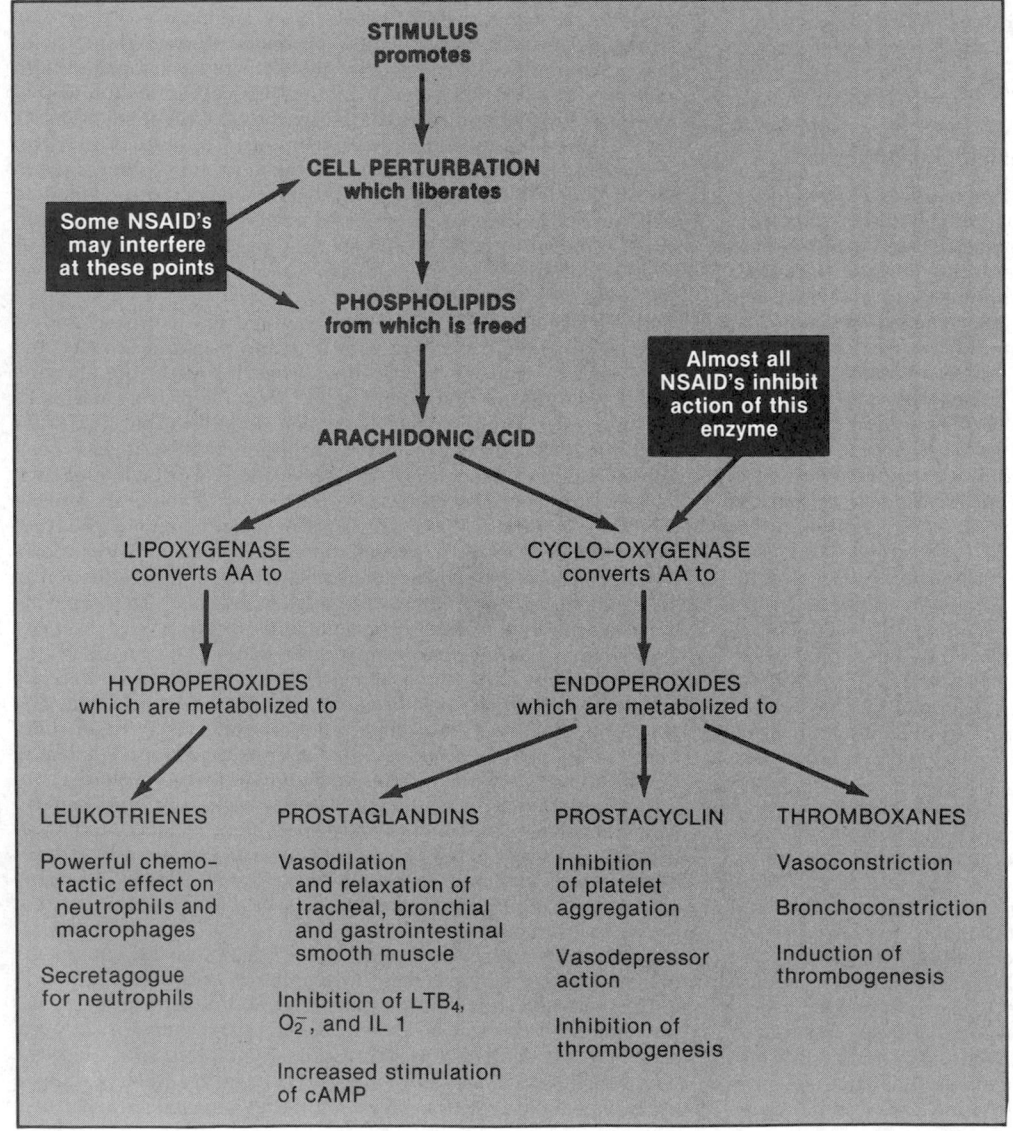

FIGURE 29–1. The inflammatory cascade. LTB_4 = leukotriene B_4; O_2^- = super-oxide anion; IL 1 = interleukin 1; cAMP = cyclic adenosine monophosphate.

Finally, the most common side effect of NSAID's, and especially of aspirin, is their interference with platelet function. Patients on these drugs sometimes suffer from untoward bleeding after tooth extraction, minor surgery, or trauma. Weiss and Aledort in 1967 showed that aspirin inhibits normal platelet aggregation both in vitro and in vivo. All NSAID's that inhibit PGH synthase—again with the exception of sodium salicylate—inhibit platelet function by blocking formation of endoperoxides and thromboxane A_2, which are intermediates in platelet stimulus-response coupling.

INHIBITION OF PGH$_2$ SYNTHASE

The interaction of NSAID's with the PGH synthase has been studied in detail at the molecular and physiologic levels. Lands and Kulmacz have shown that aspirin and indomethacin interact in a complex, biphasic fashion with the enzyme, whereas other NSAID's such as ibuprofen, naproxen, and meclofenamate simply interfere with binding of arachidonate to its oxidation site. Aspirin and indomethacin bind rapidly, in a reversible, competitive manner to the arachidonate-binding site, and then go on to inactivate the synthase irreversibly. Aspirin, moreover, acetylates serine residue 506 of the enzyme. When the PGH synthase is that of the platelet, it remains inactivated for the life of the cell, and thromboxane cannot be made. However, in endothelial cells, which can synthesize new enzyme, prostacylin synthesis is inhibited no more than a few days. Indeed, Fitzgerald has showed that low oral doses of aspirin (less than 325 mg per day) can irreversibly block the PGH synthase activity of a pool of platelets in the portal circulation *before* salicylate appears in the general circulation. These two observations explain why it is possible, by means of low-dose aspirin, to inhibit formation of the endoperoxides (PGG_2, PGH_2) and thromboxane A_2—all of which promote clotting and vasoconstriction—without inhibiting synthesis of prostacyclin (PGI_2), which inhibits platelet function and dilates blood vessels.

NSAID ACTIONS NOT DEPENDENT ON PROSTAGLANDINS

The hypothesis that the local production of prostaglandins leads to *inflammation* has been only partly substantiated. Whereas Vane's proposal that all NSAID's inhibit the transformation of arachidonic acid to stable prostaglandins (i.e., PGE_2 and PGI_2) has turned out to be largely correct, we lack sufficient evidence to generalize this proposition to all products of the arachidonic acid cascade and to all NSAID's at all dosages. The three major antipyretic, analgesic drugs exert diverse effects on prostaglandin biosynthesis. When used to treat rheumatic diseases in dosages of 4 to 8 grams, aspirin has antipyretic, anti-inflammatory, and analgesic effects and can inhibit the synthesis of prostaglandins in disrupted cell preparations. At the intermediate dosage indicated for analgesia (650 mg every 3 to 4 hours), aspirin has antipyretic and analgesic but not anti-inflammatory activity. And at its lowest clinical dosage (80 to 325 mg per day), aspirin exerts only its antiplatelet effect. Levels of salicylate in the plasma of individuals given intermediate, analgesic doses of aspirin are sufficient to inhibit prostaglandin biosynthesis in vivo by kidneys, platelets, and vascular endothelium, whereas the low levels of aspirin given to prevent thrombosis affect only prostaglandin synthesis by platelets. By contrast, rheumatologists have known since the 1950's that higher plasma concentrations (18 to 30 mg per deciliter) are required to achieve an anti-inflammatory effect. Those observations suggest two possibilities: Either the PGH synthase of cells that provoke inflammation is relatively insensitive to aspirin or aspirin at higher concentrations has a mode of action beyond its capacity to inhibit prostaglandin biosynthesis to which it owes its anti-inflammatory property.

Further evidence that aspirin-like drugs exert clinical effects that do not depend on inhibiting prostaglandin biosynthesis can be drawn from the properties of sodium salicylate and acetaminophen. Although sodium salicylate shares many of the properties of aspirin, it fails to inhibit prostaglandin biosynthesis in disrupted cell preparations at concentrations that may be achieved in plasma (approximately 5 mM). Moreover, clinical studies show that since nonacetylated salicylates do not inhibit platelet function in vitro or ex vivo, they do not cause bleeding. Indeed, acetaminophen, which also fails to inhibit prostaglandin biosynthesis, does not affect platelet aggregation, nor is it by any means anti-inflammatory. We must therefore conclude that pain and fever can effectively be reduced without inhibiting the synthesis of prostaglandins at all (Table 29–1).

PRO- AND ANTI-INFLAMMATORY PROPERTIES OF PROSTAGLANDINS

The Vane hypothesis is further weakened by findings from many laboratories, including our own, that stable prostaglandins (PGE_1, PGE_2, PGI_2) possess not only proinflammatory but also anti-inflammatory properties. It has been well appreciated that these compounds produce vasodilation, act in synergy with complement component C5a or leukotriene B4 to produce edema, mediate fever and myalgia in response to interleukin 1, and act in synergy with bradykinin to provoke pain. They also inhibit the function of T-suppressor cells. All of these are *proinflammatory* effects of prostaglandins.

On the other hand, Zurier and others had shown that high doses of these stable prostaglandins inhibit inflammation in animal models of arthritis, and much lower doses inhibit inflammation induced by local skin irritants. Since the early 1970's we have known that PGI_2 and stable prostaglandins of the E type inhibit the activation in vitro of neutrophils, platelets, and mononuclear phagocytes by interfering with their stimulus-response coupling. NSAID's increase cellular cAMP in these cells, levels of which are regulated via prostaglandin receptors. The relevance in vivo of these data obtained in vitro is supported by the observation that one can reduce experimental arthritis or glomerulonephritis in rats by treatment with systemic PGE_1. These are *anti-inflammatory* effects of prostaglandins.

As a class, NSAID's are planar, organic anions that partition across the lipid bilayers of plasma membranes in accordance with the Nernst equation. The more acidic the pH (as at inflammatory sites) the greater the lipophilicity of NSAID's, which subsequently interfere with cell function, including assembly of a superoxide anion–generating system by a cell-free, membrane-rich preparation from neutrophils, the activity of phospholipase C in mononuclear cells, the 12-hydroperoxyeicosatetraneonic acid peroxidase in platelets, and signal transduction in neutrophils and lymphocytes.

The first effect of aspirin-like drugs on cell metabolism was found to be the uncoupling of oxidative phosphorylation by isolated mitochondria; until Vane's work in 1971 this was held to be their major mode of action! More recent studies have shown that aspirin (but not acetaminophen) alters the uptake of precursor arachidonate and its insertion into the membranes of cultured human monocytes and macrophages. Salicylates also inhibit anion transport across a variety of cell membranes, including those of

TABLE 29–1. EFFECTS OF COMMONLY USED ANALGESIC AND ANTIPYRETIC AGENTS

| | Acetylsalicylic Acid | | | | | |
	Low Dose*	Intermediate Dose*	High Dose*	Sodium Salicylate	Newer NSAID's†	Acetaminophen
Antipyretic	0	+	+	+	+	+
Analgesic	0	+	+	+	+	+
Anti-inflammatory	0	0	+	+	+	+
Inhibit PG synthesis of platelets	+	+	+	0	+	0
Inhibit PG synthesis systemically	0	+	+	±	+	0

*Low dose, 80 to 325 mg per day; intermediate dose, 650 mg to 3 grams per day; high dose, >3 grams per day.
†Includes indomethacin, ibuprofen, naproxen, diclofenac, piroxicam.

the mammalian red cell and rabbit choroid plexus and renal tubular epithelium. Again, the capacity of salicylates to inhibit anion movements is not shared by acetaminophen. Finally, NSAID's inhibit synthesis of cartilage proteoglycan and bone metabolism (both in vitro and in vivo) by mechanisms that do not depend on the inhibition of the PGH synthase. It is a matter of clinical concern that some classes of NSAID's (e.g., salicylates), but not all (e.g., piroxicam), inhibit proteoglycan synthesis, thereby promoting loss of cartilage matrix.

NSAID's INTERFERE WITH NEUTROPHIL FUNCTIONS

Recent work has shown that aspirin-like drugs affect stimulus-response coupling in the most abundant cells of acute inflammation: neutrophils. Neutrophils injure tissues by releasing proteases, inflammatory peptides, reactive oxygen species such as O_2^- and H_2O_2, and lipid irritants such as platelet-activating factor and leukotriene B_4. Activation of the neutrophil in response to soluble stimuli (chemoattractants) or to immune complexes follows general pathways of stimulus-response coupling of secretory cells and is inhibited by all NSAID's studied so far.

NSAID's—indomethacin, piroxicam, diclofenac, and ibuprofen (at micromolar concentrations)—inhibit the cell-cell aggregation of human neutrophils induced by chemoattractants and mediated by the cell surface adhesion molecule CD11b/CD18. Although *all* NSAID's inhibit aggregation, only some inhibit enzyme release and/or O_2^- generation. Millimolar concentrations of sodium salicylate and aspirin alike (levels achieved in the treatment of rheumatoid arthritis or rheumatic fever) are required to inhibit the aggregation of neutrophils. However, at these concentrations sodium salicylate *does not* interfere with the activation of platelets or synthesis of thromboxane A_2. In contrast, aspirin at one tenth to one hundredth of these concentrations inhibits platelet aggregation and completely inhibits thromboxane biosynthesis via its effect on PGH synthase. It is therefore likely that the shared anti-inflammatory effects of aspirin and sodium salicylate are related to their common inhibition of neutrophil activation rather than to their divergent actions on prostaglandin biosynthesis. In contrast to aspirin and sodium salicylate, acetaminophen has no effect on neutrophil aggregation.

Inhibitory effects of NSAID's on neutrophil activation in vitro can also be demonstrated in the clinic. Indeed, neutrophils derived from the synovial fluid of patients with rheumatoid arthritis produced less superoxide anion following 10 days of therapy with piroxicam, whereas cells from normal volunteers given ibuprofen or piroxicam for 3 days failed to aggregate normally in response to chemoattractants. Sodium salicylate, an ineffective inhibitor of PGH synthase in vitro, is as effective as aspirin at inhibiting neutrophil activation.

It is somewhat paradoxical that both NSAID's and prostaglandins of the E series have similar *inhibitory* effects on the activation of such inflammatory cells as the neutrophil or platelet. Addition of PGE_1 or PGE_2 to human neutrophils at nanomolar to micromolar concentrations fails to override the inhibition by piroxicam of superoxide generation induced by chemoattractants. In the presence of piroxicam, superoxide anion generation was diminished by a factor of approximately 10 to 40 nmoles per liter of cytochrome c reduced per 10^6 cells. Recent studies, with the clinically useful PGE_1 derivative misoprostol, also show additive or synergistic rather than antagonistic effects between NSAID's and prostaglandins.

At anti-inflammatory concentrations, NSAID's appear to uncouple receptors with their effector molecules in the plasmalemma, including those regulated by at least one guanine nucleotide–binding (G) protein. Pertussis toxin, via its capacity for ADP-ribosylation of the alpha subunit of some plasma membrane G proteins, interferes with signal transduction in a variety of cells, including the neutrophil. Compared to pertussis toxin, sodium salicylate alone inhibits only modestly the production of superoxide induced by chemoattractants while inhibiting aggregation to a far greater extent. However, sodium salicylate blocks the inhibitory effect of pertussis toxin on neutrophils: Cells coincubated with both pertussis toxin and sodium salicylate regained their pertussis toxin–inhibited capacity to generate superoxide anion. This paradoxical effect of salicylate suggests that salicylates interfere with the action of pertussis toxin near the site of its interaction with the alpha subunit of the G protein. NSAID's (salicylate, piroxicam, and indomethacin) block the pertussis toxin–dependent ADP-ribosylation of the G protein in purified neutrophil membranes, and salicylates and piroxicam inhibit, in part, the pertussis toxin–sensitive formation of diacylglycerol that follows cell activation.

THE PHYLOGENY OF NSAID STUDIES

A final blow to the generality of the prostaglandin hypothesis comes from the sea. The cell biology of marine sponges, such as *Microciona prolifera*, was first examined by Robert Hooke, who in 1685 suggested in *Microcosmographica* that all living creatures contained a commonality of substructure that under the microscope resembled the "cells of monks." We may recall that the name "cell" derives from Hooke's studies of onion root tips and sponges. *M. prolifera*, which is both the most primitive and most ancient of animal creatures (10^9 years in ancestry), offers a unique model for investigating the anti-inflammatory effects of NSAID's. The activation of sponge cells in the course of cell-cell aggregation is not influenced by stable prostaglandins, nor do sponge cells contain cyclo-oxygenase activity. Nevertheless, aggregation of marine sponge cells is inhibited by NSAID's—either by aspirin or sodium salicylate and by 12 other NSAID's tested, but not by acetaminophen. After dispersion of the cells by treatment with EDTA and removal of the chelator with calcium, cell-cell aggregation of the *M. prolifera* cells is rapidly induced by phorbol esters or by addition of an inophore that raises cytosolic calcium. They are also aggregated by a species-specific aggregation factor called MAF, a 20×10^6 MW proteoglycan, and by arachidonic acid. Both aspirin and sodium salicylate—at millimolar concentrations—inhibit aggregation of these cells in response to MAF. Ibuprofen, piroxicam, and diclofenac—at micromolar concentrations—but not acetaminophen, also inhibit aggregation of these primitive cells. Since the concentrations of NSAID's that inhibit aggregation of marine sponges are the same as those that inhibit neutrophil aggregation, and since marine sponges *cannot* make prostaglandins, we may conclude that these effects—like those of NSAID's on insects (*Drosophila* chromosomes) or plants (voodoo lilies) or human cells (neutrophils)—are unlikely to result from their inhibition of prostaglandin synthesis.

Abramson S, Weissmann G: The mechanisms of action of nonsteroidal antiinflammatory drugs. Arthritis Rheum 32:1–9, 1989. *The physicochemical properties of NSAID's may alter the fluidity of the plasma membrane and thereby disrupt molecular interactions required for normal signal transduction across the lipid bilayer. The alternative hypothesis to J.R. Vane's.*

Clinch D: Why not have definitive trials of gastrointestinal safety for non-steroidal anti-inflammatory drugs? Proc R Soc Med 81:158–160, 1988. *A discussion of gastric inflammation and ulceration associated with NSAID's, which also shows that 74 per cent of NSAID-associated ulcers occur within 6 months of treatment.*

Ferreira SH, Vane JR: New aspects of the mode of action of nonsteroid antiinflammatory drugs. Ann Rev Pharm 14:57–73, 1974. *This review surveys work between 1973 and 1974 on the possible mode of action and on the clinical effects of that group of drugs variously known as non-narcotic analgesics, non-steroidal anti-inflammatory drugs, aspirin-like drugs, or antiphlogistic acids.*

Graham GG: Pharmacokinetics and metabolism of nonsteroidal antiinflammatory drugs. Med J Aust 147:597–602, 1987. *This review of the few controlled studies shows that plasma levels of NSAID's, when in the therapeutic range, correlate with response.*

Hennekens CH, et al.: Final report on the aspirin component of the ongoing physicians' health study. N Eng J Med 321:129–135, 1989. *Aspirin at low doses prevents myocardial infarction.*

Kulmacz RJ: Topography of prostaglandin H synthase. Antiinflammatory agents and the protease-sensitive arginine 253 region. J Biol Chem 264:14136–14142, 1989. *The best recent review of how NSAID's work on inhibition of the enzyme.*

Pedersen AK, FitzGerald GA: Dose-related kinetics of aspirin: Presystemic acetylation of platelet cyclooxygenase. N Eng J Med 311:1206–1210, 1984. *How aspirin affects platelets in vivo.*

Raskin I, Ehmann A, Melander WR, Meeuse BJ: Salicylic acid: A natural inducer of heat production in arum lilies. Science 237:1601–1602, 1987. *How salicylates work in plants.*

Ritossa F: A new puffing pattern induced by temperature shock and DNP in Drosophila. Exp XII:571–573, 1962. *Sodium salicylate induces heat shock proteins in Drosophila.*

Rodnan GP, Benedek TG: The early history of antirheumatic drugs. Arthritis Rheum 13:145–165, 1970. *A superb review of NSAID's before the days of prostaglandins.*

Tainter ML, Ferris AJ: Aspirin in Modern Therapy. New York, Bayer Company Division of Sterling Drug, Inc., 1969. *A review of NSAID history, with a discussion of their mode of action before the prostaglandin hypothesis.*

Vane JR: Inhibition of prostaglandin synthesis as a mechanism of action for aspirin-like drugs. Nature (London) New Biol 231:232–235, 1971. *The classic.*

PART V
PRINCIPLES OF HUMAN GENETICS

30 Human Heredity

James B. Wyngaarden

The appreciation of genetic factors as arbiters of human disease is a relatively recent development in medical history. Scattered references to inheritance of biologic characteristics may be found in the records of several millenia, including the frequently cited Talmudic exemption from circumcision of males born into families of bleeders, but discernible patterns of hereditary transmission were recognized first in the eighteenth and nineteenth centuries. In the 1750's Maupertuis described the autosomal dominant inheritance of polydactyly. The essential features of X-linked inheritance of hemophilia were described in the early 1800's by several writers and the pattern was formally outlined by Nasse in 1820. The pattern of inheritance now recognized as autosomal recessive was described by Adams in 1814, and the biologic consequences of consanguinity first reported by Bemiss in 1857. In 1876, Galton introduced the twin method of separating effects of heredity from those of environment; later he initiated quantitative studies of polygenic inheritance.

Genetics as an experimental science owes its origins to Gregor Mendel and his cross-breeding of garden peas, tall and short, yellow seed and green seed, round seed and wrinkled seed. From these studies Mendel derived concepts of dominant and recessive traits, hereditary factors (which we now call *genes*), alternative factors (*alleles*), true breeding plants with two identical factors (*homozygotes*), and non–true breeding plants with alternative factors (*heterozygotes*). His experiments led to the formulation of laws of *unit inheritance* (that "factors" retain their identity from generation to generation and do not blend in the hybrid), of *segregation* (that two members [alleles] of a single pair of factors [genes] are never found in the same gamete but always segregate), and of *independent assortment* (that members of different pairs of genes [nonalleles] assort to gametes independent of one another). These laws, formulated in 1865, had almost no immediate impact on biologic thought, but they are now cornerstones of genetics. They were rediscovered about 1900 by several workers independently and first applied to human disease by Sir Archibald Garrod in his concept of "inborn errors of metabolism" in 1908.

DNA AS GENETIC MATERIAL

In 1944 Avery and his associates at the Rockefeller Institute established that the hereditary information in the transforming principle of pneumococci resided in its deoxyribonucleic acid (DNA). From that date onward DNA has been considered the basic material of the gene. In 1953 Watson and Crick proposed a molecular model for the structure of DNA, consisting of two polynucleotide strands twisted together in a double helix with the purine and pyrimidine bases facing inward and attached to each other, binding the two chains. This model offered a rational structure for replication of DNA and for storage of hereditary information within sequences of purine and pyrimidine bases. This structure has since been established by x-ray crystallography. The genetic code, namely the precise triplet sequences of purine and pyrimidine bases in the structural gene that specify the individual amino acids of a polypeptide chain, was discovered by Nirenberg in 1961.

The amount of DNA in each human cell is sufficient to code for approximately 1 million polypeptides of average length. Estimates of the number of structural genes in humans range from 50,000 to 100,000; large amounts of DNA constitute noncoding sequences whose function is as yet obscure. Only a small number of structural genes has been identified. In the most recent update of his catalogue of *Mendelian Inheritance in Man*, McKusick lists phenotypic variations or diseases of 2656 established genetic loci, plus of an additional 2281 loci not yet fully validated, thus implying that at least 4937 genes have undergone mutation so as to cause human disease or polymorphism. In humans, hereditary information is distributed in 23 pairs of chromosomes—22 pairs of autosomes and one pair of sex chromosomes (X + Y, male; X + X, female)—plus the unpaired "mitochondrial chromosome" (see below).

THE GENE AND PROTEIN SYNTHESIS

In specifying the amino acid sequence of a polypeptide, a structural gene first transfers its information to a complementary strand of messenger RNA (mRNA), which in turn governs the order of amino acids in a polypeptide. The transfer of information from DNA to RNA involves no change of language (nucleotide → nucleotide) and is called *transcription;* the transfer of information from RNA to polypeptide involves a new language (nucleotide → amino acid) and is called *translation*. Almost all protein synthesis takes place in ribosomes, cytoplasmic bodies composed of another type of RNA (ribosomal RNA) and protein. An exception is a small amount of specific protein synthesis that takes place in mitochondria.

MUTATION

Broadly defined, a mutation is a stable, heritable alteration in the structure of DNA which can be passed from cell to progeny. From the standpoint of evolution, mutations are essential for the generation of sufficient genetic diversity to permit species to adapt to their environment through the mechanism of natural selection

Mutations may involve millions of base pairs in the structure of a chromosome, as in duplications, deletions, and translocations of a portion of one chromosome to another. Mutations can involve an entire human genome of 3 billion base pairs, as in triploidy, in which a third copy of the entire chromosomal apparatus occurs. At the other extreme, a mutation can be minute and involve a small deletion or insertion, or a replacement of only a single base pair *(point mutation)*. If deletions or insertions occur in a coding region, they give rise to *frame-shift* mutations because they alter the reading frame distal to the mutation. Thus frame-shift mutations alter the protein sequence and frequently result in peptide chain termination through generation of a stop codon.

Point mutations, replacement of one base by another in a coding region, may be of three types: (1) a *synonymous* mutation (about 23 per cent of random base substitutions in coding regions), in which the base replacement does not lead to a change in the amino acid but only to a different codon for the same amino acid; (2) a *missense* mutation (about 73 per cent of base substitutions in coding regions), in which the base change results in substitution of one amino acid for another; and (3) a *nonsense* mutation (about

4 per cent of base substitutions in coding regions), in which the base change generates one of the termination codons.

Large deletions may interrupt a coding region and cause an absence of a protein product. Or, if the deletion removes a bridge between two coding regions, the result may be a fusion or hybrid protein containing the initial sequence of one protein and the terminal portion of the other. Such deletions may result from unequal crossing over between homologous genes. In addition, there are complex mutations involving transcriptional, splicing, and RNA processing mutations.

THE GENETIC DIVERSITY OF MAN

The cause of genetic heterogenicity, i.e., of differences between members of homologous gene pairs, is *mutation* of gene structure. Variations of chromosome content are introduced by *recombination*, a process in which genetic material is exchanged between homologous chromosomes during the pairing that takes place in meiosis, and by *translation*, a process in which chromosomal breakage and reunion result in the insertion of whole segments of chromosomes in new locations within the same or another chromosome. Additional variations in genetic constitution, or genotype, result from the *random distribution* ("independent assortment") of one member of each paired chromosome into daughter cells during reductive division of the germ cells. The interplay of all these forces provides each human being except monovular twins with a unique inheritance.

POLYMORPHISM

Many proteins exist in two or more forms in the normal population. These multiple forms are due to the presence in the population of multiple genes (alleles) at the same genetic locus coding for the same protein. If the most common allele at a given locus accounts for fewer than 99 per cent of the alleles in the population, *polymorphism* is said to occur. By definition, when polymorphism exists at a genetic locus, at least 2 per cent of the population must be heterozygous at that locus. Table 30–1 lists selected proteins for which polymorphism has been demonstrated electrophoretically. Most of these genetically determined variations in protein structure are unassociated with clinical disease.

As many as 28 per cent of human genetic loci show multiple alleles in the population. Moreover, the average individual is detectably heterozygous at 7 per cent of his or her loci. Since most detection methods require a change in the charge of the protein, they can detect only about one third of the actual base changes that are possible, because only one third of point mutations result in a substitution of an amino acid with a different charge. Thus, all individuals may actually be heterozygous at as many as 20 per cent of their loci.

At most genetic loci (e.g., the gene for β-globin) one standard allele accounts for the vast majority of alleles in the population, and alternative alleles are rare. At other loci, no single allele occurs with sufficient frequency to be designated standard or normal. The α-chain of haptoglobin, a plasma protein, represents one such extreme example of genetic polymorphism. In this instance all polymorphic forms of haptoglobin appear to function equally in hemoglobin binding. Polymorphisms represent conspicuous examples of human biochemical diversity.

THE HUMAN GENE MAP

About 2500 autosomal loci are known and another 2100 are strongly indicated on the basis mainly of characteristic patterns of inheritance of alternative forms of a given trait. At least 3000 of these are associated with a disease phenotype. This implies that at least 3 to 6 per cent of the 50,000 to 100,000 human genes have undergone mutation so as to cause human disease. The chromosomal locations are known for over 2100 of these loci. In addition, over 160 loci have been assigned to the X-chromosome.

HUMAN GENETIC DISEASE

Genetics is concerned with the study of hereditary variations. When variations are extreme and impair the health, fitness, or reproductive capacity of the individual, we consider them diseases. These extreme variations are of three principal types: (1) chromosomal aberrations, (2) single-gene differences that exhibit

TABLE 30–1. SOME PLASMA PROTEINS AND CELLULAR ENZYMES THAT EXHIBIT ELECTROPHORETICALLY DETECTABLE POLYMORPHISMS

Protein	Locus Name
Plasma proteins	
Haptoglobin (α-chain)	Hp α
Transferrin	Tf
Vitamin-D binding protein	Gc (for group-specific component)
Ceruloplasmin	Cp
α-1-Antitrypsin	Pi (for protease inhibitor)
α-1-Acid glycoprotein	Oro (for orosomucoid)
β-2-Glycoprotein I	—
Properdin factor B	Bf
Complement	
Second component	C2
Third component	C3
Fourth component	C4
Sixth component	C6
Enzymes	
Pancreatic amylase	AMY_2
Cholinesterase	E_2
Red blood cell enzyme	
Acid phosphatase 1	ACP_1
Adenosine deaminase	ADA
Adenylate kinase	AK_1
Carbonic anhydrase 2	CA_2
Diaphorase (NADPH-dependent)	DIA_2
Esterase D	ESD
Galactose-1-uridyltransferase	GALT
Glucose-6-phosphate dehydrogenase	Gd
Glutamic pyruvic transaminase	GPT
Glutathione peroxidase	GPX
Glutathione reductase	GSR
Glyoxalase I	GLO
Peptidase A	PEPA
Peptidase C	PEPC
Peptidase D	PEPD
Phosphoglucomutase 1	PGM_1
Phosphoglucomutase 2	PGM_2
Phosphogluconate dehydrogenase	PGD
Uridine monophosphate kinase	UMPK
White blood cell enzymes	
Aconitase (soluble)	$ACON_8$
Cytidine deaminase	CDA
α-L-Fucosidase	αFUC
α-Glucosidase	αGLUC
Glutamic-oxaloacetic transaminase (mitochondrial)	GOT_M
Hexokinase 3	HK_3
Malic enzyme (mitochondrial)	ME_M
Phosphoglucomutase 3	PGM_3

mendelian patterns of inheritance, and (3) polygenic disorders, in which two or more, often multiple, genes each contribute to the characteristic in question. Examples of the first two categories are relatively easy to recognize. They are discussed in Ch. 31 and 33. Many genetic diseases are dependent upon environmental factors for their expression, e.g., phenylalanine ingestion in phenylketonuria or milk ingestion in galactosemia. Other hereditary diseases are kept in abeyance by specific environmental factors: Scurvy is an inborn error of metabolism (absence of the hepatic enzyme that converts L-gulonolactone to L-ascorbic acid in man, monkey, and guinea pig) kept in remission by vitamin C; metabolic cretinism is foiled in its expression by the administration of thyroid hormone. The greatest difficulty in sorting out the relative importance of genetic and environmental influences is encountered with common diseases. In disorders such as rheumatoid arthritis, essential hypertension, and coronary artery disease, genetic influences are important but hard to identify in specific biochemical terms. In most polygenic disorders, genetic factors are multiple and still beyond definition.

The pace of genetic advance across the full spectrum of molecular biology to human heredity is currently very rapid. The revolution in biology of the past three decades is increasingly molding medical science and practice. New insights into the genetic control of the immune response (see Ch. 250) are explaining disease susceptibilities and facilitating organ and tissue transplantation. Susceptibility to cancer is being explained by the interplay between oncogenes, anti-oncogenes, and environmental exposures (see Ch. 157). As additional genetic mechanisms are disclosed, they will illuminate more and more human diseases and from time to time suggest new avenues of therapy.

THE FAMILY HISTORY. A careful family history is indispensable in the assessment and understanding of hereditary disease. The interviewer should ascertain whether anyone in the family has had a condition similar to that of the patient, and whether this condition or any other "runs in the family." Particularly in the case of rare disorders one should inquire whether the parents are related, and, if this is not known, whether they or their families came from the same village or community and whether their forebears may have intermarried. Since some disorders are more common in certain ethnic groups than in others, the ethnic origin of the parents should also be elicited.

The rarer the recessive disorder in a specific population, the greater is the likelihood of parental consanguinity. Tay-Sachs disease is relatively rare in non-Jews, in whom the gene frequency is low, but a high proportion of non-Jewish parents of Tay-Sachs children are consanguineous. By contrast, Tay-Sachs disease is relatively common in Jews of eastern European origin, in whom the gene frequency is relatively high. In parents of Jewish children with Tay-Sachs disease in the United States the frequency of consanguinity is only slightly higher than in the general population.

Certain ethnic backgrounds increase the likelihood of certain diagnostic possibilities while decreasing that of others. Thalassemia is chiefly a disorder of people of the Mediterranean region and of Southeast Asia, familial Mediterranean fever is a disorder of Armenians and Sephardic Jews, acatalasia is a disease of Japanese and Koreans, and gout is very common among the Maori. By contrast, cystic fibrosis is rare in blacks, phenylketonuria is uncommon in Jews, and sickle cell anemia does not occur in Caucasians.

PEDIGREE ANALYSIS. The chief method of study of an inherited disease in humans is the observation of its pattern of distribution in kindreds, i.e., of its pedigree pattern. The construction of a pedigree pattern begins with the individual first detected, who is referred to as the proband, index case, or propositus (female = proposita). The pedigree pattern allows one to judge whether the distribution conforms to mendelian principles of segregation and assortment and thus represents single-factor inheritance. Patterns that do not conform to mendelian principles may represent polygenic traits in which a number of genes each contributes a minor effect. Valid pedigrees depend on accurate and extensive information about the kindred. This information is likely to be more reliable when based on observer detection than when based on memory.

MONOGENIC DISORDERS. Disorders caused by single mutant genes show one of four simple (mendelian) patterns of inheritance: (1) autosomal dominant, (2) autosomal recessive, (3) X-linked dominant, or (4) X-linked recessive. Dominant traits are those expressed in the heterozygote (as well as in the homozygote or hemizygote). Recessive traits are those expressed in the homozygotes (or hemizygotes) but silent in the heterozygote. The terms *dominant* and *recessive* refer to the phenotypic expression of the trait, not to the expression of the gene. Thus it is incorrect to speak of a dominant or recessive gene. A gene is either expressed or not expressed. Whether the trait is considered dominant or recessive often depends upon the level of observation. Sickle cell anemia is a recessive trait; i.e., it requires a double dose of the abnormal gene for expression at the clinical level. Nevertheless, the sickle gene is expressed in single dose as well, giving rise to carriers with SA hemoglobin. Recessive traits are *codominant* when viewed biochemically at the level of the gene product.

With few exceptions, each of the approximately 5000 mendelian diseases is rare. The overall population frequency of monogenic disorders is about 10 per 1000 live births, comprising about 7 per 1000 dominants, about 2.5 per 1000 recessives, and about 0.4 per 1000 X-linked conditions (see Table 30–2).

If a particular disease shows a mendelian pattern of inheritance, its pathogenesis, no matter how complex, must be due to a single abnormal protein molecule. For example, in sickle cell disease, such seemingly unrelated disturbances as hemolytic anemia,

TABLE 30–2. PREVALENCE OF SELECTED MONOGENIC DISORDERS AMONG LIVEBORN INFANTS*

Disorder	Estimated Prevalence
Autosomal Dominant	
Familial hypercholesterolemia	1 in 500
Polycystic kidney disease	1 in 1250
Huntington disease	1 in 2500
Hereditary spherocytosis	1 in 5000
Marfan syndrome	1 in 20,000
Autosomal Recessive	
Sickle cell anemia	1 in 625 (U.S. blacks)
Cystic fibrosis	1 in 2000 (Caucasians)
Tay-Sachs disease	1 in 3000 (U.S. Jews)
Cystinuria	1 in 7000
Phenylketonuria	1 in 12,000
Mucopolysaccharidoses (all types)	1 in 25,000
Glycogen storage disease (all types)	1 in 50,000
Galactosemia	1 in 57,000
Homocystinuria	1 in 200,000
X-linked	
Duchenne muscular dystrophy	1 in 7000
Hemophilia	1 in 10,000

*Data assembled from Galjaard, Carter, and Motulsky.

painful crises, nephropathy, vascular occlusions, and *Salmonella* osteomyelitis are all physiologic consequences of a single missense mutation, resulting in a single amino acid substitution in the β-globin chain. When two or more phenotypic characters are controlled by a single gene, that gene is said to have *pleiotropic* effects.

AUTOSOMAL DOMINANT TRAITS. Autosomal genes are those genes situated on chromosomes other than the X or Y. When there are two alleles, A and a, at a locus, three possible genotypes exist: AA, Aa, and aa. Genotypes AA and aa are *homozygotes;* Aa is a *heterozygote.*

Dominant traits are fully manifest in the presence of a gene in the heterozygous state, i.e., when only one abnormal gene (*mutant allele*) is present and the corresponding partner allele on the homologous chromosome is normal. Figure 30–1 shows a typical pedigree of transmission of an autosomal dominant trait. The following features are characteristic: (1) Each affected individual has an affected parent (unless the condition arose by a new mutation in a germ cell that formed the individual); (2) an affected individual will bear, on average, an equal number of affected and unaffected offspring; (3) males and females will be affected in equal numbers; (4) each sex can transmit the trait to male and female offspring (i.e., male-to-male transmission is possible); (5) normal children of an affected individual will have only normal

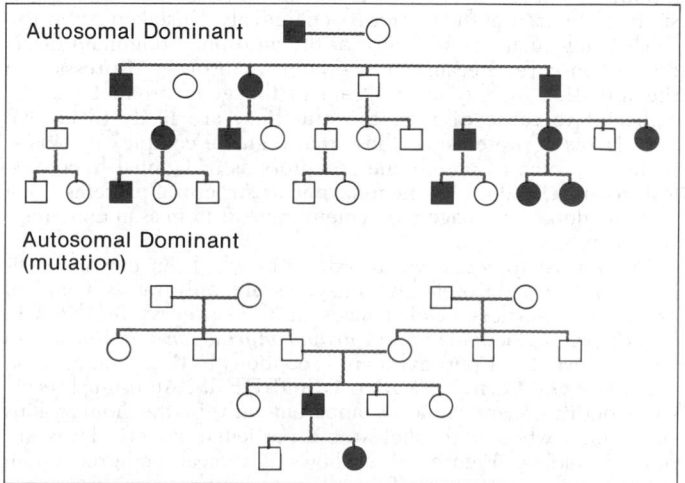

FIGURE 30–1. Pedigrees of autosomal dominant traits. In the lower pedigree the normal parents of the affected individual suggest the possibility of a new mutation. Solid symbols indicate those affected. (For details see text.)

offspring; and (6) when the trait does not impair viability or reproductive capacity, there will be *vertical* transmission of the trait through successive generations.

Most autosomal dominant disorders show two additional characteristics that are not seen in recessive disorders: (1) marked variability in severity, or *expressivity*, and (2) delayed age of onset. Dominant traits in humans often exert only mild effects. Occasionally the expression of the abnormal gene is so weak that a generation appears to be skipped because the carrier of the abnormal gene is clinically normal. When this is the case, the trait is said to be *nonpenetrant*. When a gene of a dominant trait exists in the homozygous state, the effect may be very severe, perhaps lethal. Examples are common in animals in which experimental matings can be constructed, but rare in humans, because matings of two affected heterozygotes are exceptional. One example is homozygous familial hypercholesterolemia. Others possibly include achondroplasia and Osler-Weber-Rendu syndrome. Delayed age of onset is seen in Huntington's disease and adult polycystic kidney disease. These disorders do not become manifest clinically until adult life, even though the mutant gene has been present since conception.

In every autosomal dominant disease some affected persons owe their disorder to a new mutation rather than to an inherited allele. Since a reasonable estimate of the frequency of mutation is of the order of 5×10^{-6} mutations per gene per generation, and since a dominant trait requires a mutation in only one of the parental gametes, one would expect that about 1 in 100,000 newborn persons would possess a new mutation at any given genetic locus. Many mutations will be silent or will involve a recessive function and not be manifest in a single gene dose. However, others will cause a defective gene product that gives rise to a dominant trait.

The percentage of patients with dominant disorders that represents a new mutation is inversely proportional to the effect of the disease upon *biologic fitness*, i.e., survival to adult life, and reproductive capacity. If a dominant mutation produces early death or absolute infertility, genetic transmission is impossible, and all cases represent new mutations. In tuberous sclerosis, the severe mental retardation reduces biologic fitness to about 20 per cent of normal, and the proportion of cases due to new mutations is about 80 per cent. In dominant conditions such as familial hypercholesterolemia, in which there is no reduction in biologic fitness, virtually all cases have a family pedigree showing classic vertical transmission

New mutations appear to be more frequent in the germ cells of fathers of relatively advanced age. Both Marfan syndrome and achondroplastic dwarfism display such "paternal age effect." Fathers of sporadic cases of both conditions are an average of 5 to 7 years older than the general population of fathers or than fathers who transmit these syndromes because of an inherited mutation. Diagnosis of a new mutation must exclude low expressivity of the trait in the carrier parent and also mistaken paternity.

The molecular basis of most of the autosomal dominant disorders is obscure. Because in a dominant disorder expression of the mutation in only 50 per cent of the gene product may be sufficient to cause disease, the mutations are likely to involve two classes of proteins: (1) those that regulate complex metabolic pathways, such as membrane receptors as in familial hypercholesterolemia, and (2) key nonenzymic or structural proteins, such as hemoglobin or collagen, or a membrane protein as in hereditary spherocytosis.

In contrast to recessive disorders, in which an enzyme deficiency is the rule, defective enzymes are only rarely found in dominant disorders. Deficiencies of *C-1–esterase inhibitor* in hereditary angioedema and of *uroporphyrinogen-1 synthetase* in acute intermittent porphyria are exceptions to this general rule.

AUTOSOMAL RECESSIVE DISORDERS. Autosomal recessive conditions are clinically apparent only in the homozygous state, i.e., when both alleles at a particular genetic locus are mutant alleles. Figure 30–2 shows a typical pedigree of an autosomal recessive trait. The following features are characteristic: (1) The parents are clinically normal; (2) only siblings are affected; (3) males and females are affected in equal proportions; (4) if an affected individual marries a homozygous normal person, none of the children will be affected but all will be heterozygous

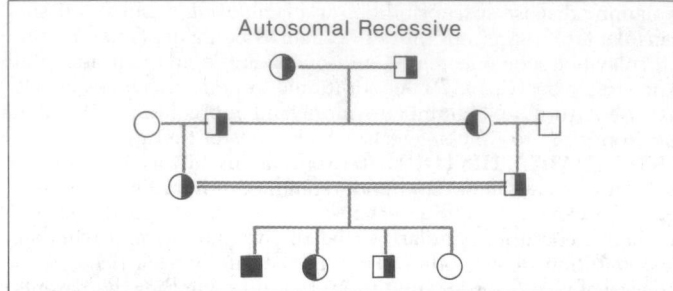

FIGURE 30–2. Pedigree of autosomal recessive trait. Note that both parents are heterozygous. One sib is affected, two are carriers, and one is normal. Double line (===) indicates that parents are related by descent (first cousins).

carriers; (5) if an affected individual marries a heterozygous carrier, one half of the children will be affected, and the pedigree pattern will superficially suggest a dominant trait; (6) if two individuals who are homozygous for the same mutant gene marry, all of their children will be affected; (7) if both parents are heterozygous at the same genetic locus, one fourth of their children will be homozygous affected, one fourth will be homozygous normal, and one half will be heterozygous carriers of the same mutant gene; and (8) the less frequent the mutant gene is in the population, the greater is the likelihood that the affected individual is the product of consanguine parents.

In actual practice, unless the kinship is very large, the ratio of affected to unaffected sibs is frequently greater than one in four. Inclusion of probands in the enumeration loads the results in favor of the trait. In a sibship of 100 or even 10 the loading factor is not pronounced. However, in all ascertainable one-child sibships the involvement is 100 per cent, in two-child sibships it is 67 per cent (when the fundamental probability is 50 per cent), in three-child sibships it is 57 per cent, and so on. In small sibships a correction must be made for *bias of ascertainment*. The simplest method is to exclude the proband from the calculation and to determine the proportion of affected children among the remaining sibs.

In most autosomal recessive conditions the clinical presentation tends to be more uniform than in dominant diseases, and the onset is often early in life. Recessive disorders are commonly diagnosed in childhood. Approximately 630 well-established recessive traits have been recognized in humans, and in over 300 of these the mutant enzyme or other protein has been identified.

A *completely* recessive disease is one in which the heterozygote is clinically normal. When some features of the disease are detectable in the heterozygote, the disease is sometimes said to show *intermediate inheritance*, or to be *incompletely recessive* or *incompletely dominant*. The ambiguity of these terms from classic genetic studies of phenotypes is further emphasized by results of different methods of detection of gene effects. In many instances of completely recessive inheritance, refined biochemical observations enable the recognition of the trait in the clinically normal heterozygote. An example is Tay-Sachs disease, in which clinically normal parents and some sibs can be shown to be heterozygotes by assay of hexosaminidase A in leukocytes. Because of its importance in genetic counseling, the detection of healthy heterozygous carriers of genes that in the homozygous state cause overt disease is one of the most significant aspects of medical genetics. Since by definition a dominant trait is one that is detectable in the heterozygous state, Tay-Sachs disease (and many others) is recessive when the clinical phenotype is considered and dominant when the biochemical phenotype is determined.

In pure form a recessive disease requires the inheritance of identical mutant genes from both parents. When the mutant genes are rare, the likelihood that any two unrelated parents are carriers for the same defect is small. Inheritance of two different mutant genes derived from the same locus gives rise to *heterollelic compounds*. Individuals with Hb SC disease are genetic compounds who have inherited a different abnormal β-globin gene from each parent. Genetic compounds are also known in cystinuria, phenylketonuria, certain of the mucopolysaccharidoses, "homozygous" familial hypercholesterolemia, and several other disorders.

If the parents of a child with a recessive disorder have a common ancestor who carried a mutant gene, then the likelihood that two of the descendants would each have inherited the gene becomes relatively great. The less frequent the gene, the stronger is the likelihood that an affected individual has resulted from a consanguine mating. First cousins share, on the average, one eighth of their genes. When two first cousins marry, an offspring has, on the average, one sixteenth of the loci homozygous for a gene derived from a common ancestor. In general, offspring of first-cousin mating are slightly more likely to have congenital malformations, as well as mental defects and metabolic diseases, than are children born to unrelated parents.

Increased frequency of consanguinity is not observed if the recessive disease is common. Sickle cell anemia, phenylketonuria, cystic fibrosis, and Tay-Sachs disease are examples in which the carrier (heterozygote) state is frequent in certain populations and in which consanguinity is usually not present in the parents. Increase in consanguinity would also not be expected in dominant or X-linked traits or genetic compounds.

A high percentage of recessive disorders involves abnormalities of enzyme proteins. In most reactions the normal maximal enzyme activity is greatly in excess of catalytic requirements; i.e., the concentration of a substrate is usually maintained at a point well below saturation for the enzyme that metabolizes it. Hence a reduction to 50 per cent of normal activity in a heterozygote does not impair the health of the carrier, whereas a total or nearly total deficiency may result in a serious inborn error of metabolism. These conditions are discussed in Ch. 31.

X-LINKED INHERITANCE. Diseases or traits that result from genes located on the X chromosome are termed X-linked. Since the female has two X chromosomes, she may be either heterozygous or homozygous for the mutant gene, and the trait may exhibit recessive or dominant expression. The male has only one X chromosome and therefore is *hemizygous* for X-linked traits. Males can be expected to express X-linked traits regardless of their recessive or dominant behavior in the female. Thus, the terms X-linked dominant or X-linked recessive refer only to expression of the trait in females.

Since males transmit their X chromosome only to daughters, an important feature of X-linked inheritance is the absence of male-to-male transmission. Affected males transmit the trait to all of their daughters and none of their sons.

Since the female carries two X chromosomes in each cell, it might be expected that the concentrations of proteins determined by genes on the X chromosome would be twice that of males who carry only one X chromosome per cell. This is not the case, and the explanation is provided by the process of X-inactivation first proposed by Mary Lyon, and often termed the *Lyon hypothesis*. In all adult female cells only one of the X chromosomes is genetically active. Early in differentiation one of the X chromosomes becomes inactive and forms the *Barr body*. Inactivation is random so that for each cell there is an equal probability that the paternally or maternally derived X chromosome will be inactivated. Once one of the two X chromosomes is inactivated, the same X chromosome remains inactive throughout all subsequent cell divisions. Thus, on the average one half of the cells of a female will express the X chromosome of her father, and one half of her mother: In this respect the normal female is a mosaic. If one of the X chromosomes carries a mutant gene, the probability is that the mutant phenotype will be expressed in one half of her cells. However, this statistical probability may be disturbed in at least two ways: (1) Since inactivation of one of the X chromosomes occurs early in development and is random, some females may by chance have many more cells that carry an active X chromosome derived from one parent than from the other; and (2) if one of the X chromosomes carries a mutant gene that confers a metabolic disadvantage upon cells with that mutation, these cells may survive less frequently during development, and the female offspring may have cells that carry predominantly or exclusively the active X chromosome without the mutation.

Over 160 loci have been identified on the human X chromosome, and many have been mapped to specific regions on the long or the short arm of the chromosome.

X-Linked Dominant Traits. This mode of inheritance (Fig. 30–3) is uncommon. Its characteristic features are as follows: (1)

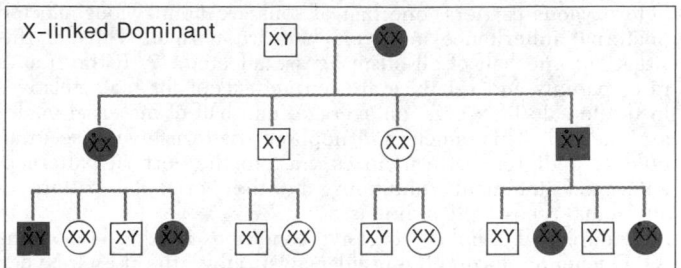

FIGURE 30–3. Pedigree of dominant X-linked trait. The X chromosome bearing the abnormal gene is designated by a small dot.

Females are affected about twice as often as males, (2) heterozygous females transmit the trait to both sexes with a frequency of 50 per cent, (3) hemizygous affected males transmit the trait to all of their daughters and none of their sons, and (4) the expression is more variable and generally less severe in heterozygous females than in hemizygous affected males. Examples of X-linked dominant inheritance include the $Xg(a^+)$ blood group, vitamin D-resistant (hypophosphatemic) rickets, and pseudohypoparathyroidism.

Some rare X-linked dominant disorders occur only in the heterozygous female, because the condition is lethal in the hemizygous affected male. Additional characteristics of this form of inheritance are as follows: (1) An affected mother transmits the trait to one half of her daughters (heterozygotes), and (2) an increased frequency of abortions occurs in affected women, the abortions representing affected male fetuses. Examples of disorders that appear to fit this mode of inheritance include incontinentia pigmenti, focal dermal hypoplasia, orofaciodigital syndrome, and hyperammonemia caused by ornithine transcarbamylase deficiency.

X-Linked Recessive Traits. This mode of inheritance (Fig. 30–4) is relatively common. Its characteristic features are as follows: (1) The disorder is fully expressed only in the hemizygous affected male. (2) Heterozygous females are usually normal; occasionally they may exhibit mild features of the disorder; rarely they may be almost as severely affected as the hemizygous affected male (this variability is attributed to the probability that a disproportionate percentage of *normal* X chromosomes of the heterozygous female may have been inactivated early in development [see "Lyon hypothesis," above]). (3) On average, a heterozygous female transmits the trait to one half of her sons (hemizygous affected), but the other half are normal. (4) On average, one half of daughters of a heterozygous female are carriers and one half are normal. (5) All daughters of an affected male married to a normal female are carriers, and no sons of such a union are affected (no father-to-son transmission). (6) In the rare event of the union of an affected male and a heterozygous female, one half of daughters are homozygous affected and one half are

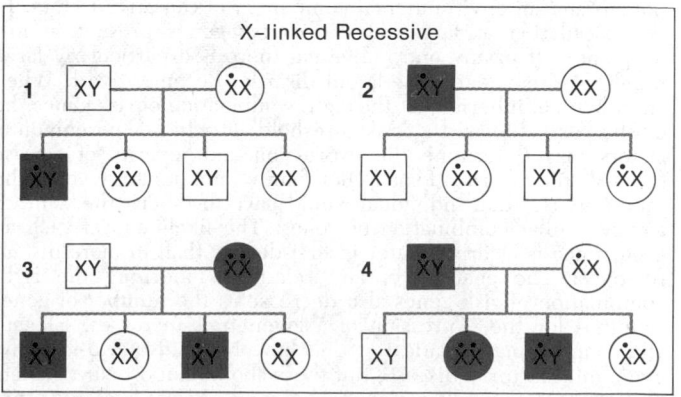

FIGURE 30–4. Pedigrees of X-linked recessive trait. The X chromosome bearing the abnormal gene is designated by a small dot. Affected individuals are indicated by solid squares (males) and circles (females). Pedigree 1 is commonly observed; pedigree 4 is rare.

heterozygous carriers; one half of sons are hemizygous affected (maternal inheritance) and one half are normal. Thus in this situation, one half of all offspring are affected. (7) If the trait is rare, parents and relatives are normal except for male relatives in the female line; e.g., on average, one half of maternal uncles are affected. This "uncle and nephew" pattern gives rise to an *oblique* pedigree pattern, in contrast to the vertical pattern of autosomal dominant conditions and the horizontal pattern of autosomal recessive conditions.

Examples of X-linked recessive conditions include hemophilia A, Duchenne form of muscular dystrophy, the Lesch-Nyhan syndrome, glucose-6-phosphate dehydrogenase deficiency, and Fabry's disease. In several of these, e.g., Duchenne muscular dystrophy and Fabry's disease, heterozygous females may exhibit mild or even moderately severe forms of the disease. Color blindness is also an X-linked inherited trait, but it is sufficiently frequent (occurring in about 8 per cent of Caucasian males) that the occurrence of homozygous color-blind females is not rare.

It is important to distinguish between X-linked inheritance and *sex-influenced autosomal dominant inheritance*. Baldness and hemochromatosis are examples of autosomal dominant traits that are sex influenced. Heterozygous females express the gene for baldness only when a source of testosterone becomes available (e.g., a masculinizing tumor of the ovary). Heterozygous females rarely develop clinical hemochromatosis because menstruation and pregnancy mitigate the accumulation of iron.

Y-LINKED INHERITANCE. A gene on the Y chromosome is transmitted through the father to all of his sons and none of his daughters. The only genes currently known to be located on the Y chromosome are those that determine "maleness" and an antigen that influences graft rejection. The maleness gene (testes determining factor) has been cloned.

POLYGENIC INHERITANCE. Most phenotypic traits are determined by the collaboration of many genes at different loci rather than by single gene effects. Polygenic inheritance is suggested for traits that show continuous variation in the form of a normal distribution curve. Height and intelligence are examples of polygenic traits in which the extremes of the distribution are not necessarily considered abnormal. Parents and offspring, and on average siblings also, have 50 per cent of their genes in common. Second-degree relatives share on average one fourth of all genes ($\frac{1}{2}$)², and third-degree relatives (cousins) share one eighth ($\frac{1}{2}$)³. Thus as the degree of relation becomes more distant, the probability of inheriting the same combination of genes is reduced, and the degree of resemblance is likely to be less.

Many of the common chronic diseases of adults (such as essential hypertension, diabetes mellitus, hyperuricemia, hypercholesterolemia, coronary artery disease, and schizophrenia) and the common birth defects of children (such as cleft palate and lip and congenital heart disease) that tend to run in families fit best into the category of *multifactorial genetic disease*. This category should be suspected when the pedigree of a disease does not support inheritance in a simple dominant or recessive manner. In multifactorial genetic disease there is both a polygenic component and an environmental component of causative factors. In the population at large there are *risk* genes present in low frequency. If in any one individual there is a particularly large number of risk genes, the latent disorder becomes overt. When an individual inherits just the right combination of risk genes, he or she passes beyond a "risk threshold" at which environmental factors may determine the expression and severity of disease (Fig. 30–5). In order for another family member to develop the same disease, that individual would have to inherit the same or a very similar combination of genes. The likelihood of such an occurrence is clearly greater in first-degree than in more distant relatives. The chances of any relative's inheriting the right combination of risk genes also decrease as the number of genes required for the expression of a given trait increases. Elegant and complex mathematical models have been advanced for polygenic-multifactorial disease, but these should not obscure the fact that each of the risk genes must express itself, like any other gene, by way of a specific biochemical product. Eventually the vague concept of genetic susceptibility of polygenic inheritance must yield to the basic premise that genes control the synthesis of specific proteins with specific functions. We may anticipate

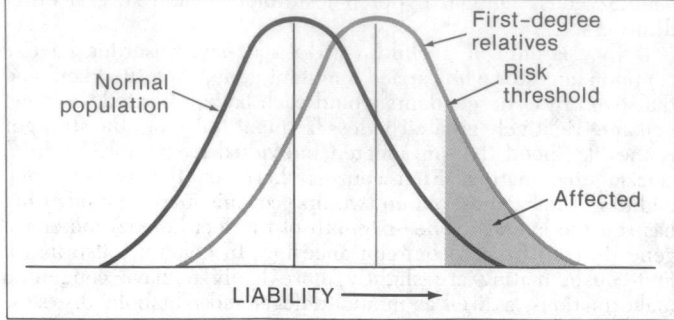

FIGURE 30–5. Diseases that conform to a polygenic multifactorial model of inheritance lead to an increased prevalence of disease among the relatives of affected individuals. This increased prevalence is most evident among first-degree relatives.

that risk genes will be identified in the future using restriction fragment length polymorphism (RFLP) and complex linkage analysis models.

To date the genetic loci most prominently associated with disease susceptibility are those composing the major histocompatibility (MHC) locus or human leukocyte antigen (HLA) system. There are seven internationally recognized, highly polymorphic components of the human MHC: HLA-A, -B, and -C, collectively known as class I antigens, are formed on most nucleated cells; HLA-DR, -DQ, and -DP, collectively known as class II antigens, are restricted primarily to B lymphocytes, monocytes, macrophages, activated T cells, and endothelial cells; and HLA-D, a functional activity recognized through the complex proliferative responses to allogeneic cells in mixed lymphocyte cultures. The products of these genes are proteins that are found on the surface of body cells and that enable an individual's immune system to distinguish its own cells (self) from those of someone else (nonself). Each HLA locus in the population consists of multiple alleles, each of which produces an immunologically distinct protein. HLA-A has at least 24 alleles, HLA-B has at least 52, C has at least 11, D has at least 26, DR has at least 20, DQ has at least 9, and DP has at least 6. The inheritance of certain alleles predisposes to the development of certain diseases, in some instances when the individual is exposed to a particular environmental challenge. For example, the frequency of B27 allele in the white population is approximately 8 per cent. In patients with ankylosing spondylitis the frequency of B27 is over 90 per cent. In Australian aborigines and black Africans the B27 antigen is virtually absent and the frequency of ankylosing spondylitis is sharply reduced. A Caucasian with the B27 antigen is approximately 120 times more likely to develop ankylosing spondylitis than one who does not posses the antigen; the increased liability among Japanese with the B27 antigen is 300 times. Reiter's syndrome may follow an infection of the bowel or urinary tract with *Shigella*, *Salmonella*, or *Yersinia* organisms. No less than 20 per cent of B27-positive individuals with *Shigella* infections develop Reiter's syndrome. Other examples include the association of HLA-DR and -DQ with type 1 insulin-dependent diabetes mellitus, HLA-DR3 with endocrine disorders, HLA-DR2 with narcolepsy, and HLA-A3 with hemochromatosis.

Multifactorial or polygenic inheritance must not be confused with *genetic heterogeneity*. Hypercholesterolemia and hyperuricemia behave as multifactorial traits when viewed at the population level. At the family level, however, it is sometimes possible to identify a single locus that is mainly responsible for the disease in that family. Examples include familial hypercholesterolemia, an autosomal dominant trait present in about 5 per cent of subjects with premature myocardial infarctions, which in single-gene dosage produces atherosclerosis in the absence of any extraordinary environmental factor; or hypoxanthine-guanine phosphoribosyltransferase deficiency, an X-linked recessive trait present in about 0.5 per cent of subjects with gout, which in the hemizygous state produces marked purine overproduction without any relationship to obesity or alcohol consumption.

MITOCHONDRIAL INHERITANCE. Each mitochondrion contains several circular chromosomes that code for certain ribosomal and transfer ribonucleic acids (RNA's) and for 13 polypeptides involved in oxidative phosphorylation, the chief function of the mitochondrion. The mitochondrial code differs from that of nuclear DNA and that of any contemporary prokaryote; it is similar to that of bacteria. Mitochondrial inheritance is exclusively matrilineal. Diseases that are thought to involve mitochondrial mutations include Leber hereditary optic atrophy, infantile bilateral striatal necrosis, and myoclonic epilepsy with "ragged red fibers."

GENE FREQUENCY. The distribution of a mutant gene in the general population may be calculated on the basis of the Hardy-Weinberg equation. If the frequency of a particular gene A is p, then that of its alternative allele is $(1 - p) = q$. There will be three genotypes in the population: Those who are homozygous AA, those who are heterozygous Aa, and those who are homozygous aa. In a randomly mating population the frequencies of these genotypes will be in the proportion p^2(AA), $2pg$(Aa), and q^2(aa). An important consequence of this distribution is that irrespective of the initial frequency of the genes A and a in the population, the proportion of the three genotypes will tend to remain constant in succeeding generations, provided that there is no difference in biologic fitness of any of the genotypes. If there is unequal viability or fertility among the three genotypes, or if mating is not random, the frequency calculations require considerable correction, and in small populations major changes in gene frequency can occur on the basis of chance alone.

If the frequency of a recessive disease in a particular population is known, the frequency of heterozygous carriers and of the abnormal gene can be calculated. Thus for a recessively inherited disease aa (q^2) with a frequency of 1 per 10,000 (e.g., albinism), the frequency of the gene a (q) will be 1 per 100, and that of heterozygous carriers will be $2 \times p \times q = 2 \times 99/100 \times 1/100$ = approximately 1 in 50. Thus, in this particular example there will be 200 clinically unaffected carriers of the abnormal gene for every affected individual. Table 30–2 lists the frequency of several inherited diseases. Cystic fibrosis, a recessively inherited disease, has a prevalence in the white population of about 1 per 2500 (q^2); thus the frequency of the gene (q) is 1 in 50 and of heterozygous carriers is approximately 1 in 25, or 4 per cent of the white population. A similar calculation with respect to sickle cell anemia among United States blacks ($q^2 = 1/625$) yields a frequency of heterozygous carriers of 1 in 12.5, or 8 per cent of the United States black population.

The frequency of most genes in the population is relatively stable. When a gene is rare and severely disadvantageous, the rate of its introduction into a population by spontaneous mutation is balanced by the rate of elimination of the disadvantageous gene by natural selection. The frequency of the disadvantageous gene, however, can be stabilized at a high level if the heterozygotes are slightly favored (increased biologic fitness) and leave a greater number of progeny than either homozygote. When a rare form of a species is present at a frequency that cannot be maintained by recurrent mutation alone, a *balanced polymorphism* is said to exist. Usually this means that the rarer of two allelic forms occurs with a frequency of at least 1 per cent of the population. When this is found, *heterozygote advantage* should be suspected. An example of such a balanced polymorphism is the increased resistance of individuals heterozygous for the sickle cell trait to falciparum malaria. Although persons with sickle cell disease (homozygotes, SS hemoglobin) often die before they can reproduce, and thus remove the sickle cell gene from the population, the prevalence of heterozygotes (SA hemoglobin) may nevertheless reach 40 per cent in certain West African populations. Death from falciparum malaria is much less frequent in carriers of the sickle cell trait than in noncarriers, and thus the heterozygote does have an advantage. Whether the extraordinary frequency of heterozygotes for the sickle cell gene in West Africa is due entirely to differential mortality or in part to differential fertility is uncertain, but this example suffices to illustrate that the effects of genes can be assessed only in relation to a particular environment. In most instances, however, a distinct advantage for the heterozygote of a polymorphic trait (of which there are many; see Ch. 31) cannot be demonstrated, and the possibility exists that certain polymorphic traits are genetically neutral.

The term *genetic load* has been used to describe the total genetic disability of a population. It comprises both a *mutational load*, based on recurrent mutation of a normal gene to a lethal or sublethal gene, and a *segregational load*, resulting from segregation of the harmful gene from advantaged heterozygotes, as in the example of sickle cell heterozygotes discussed above. Each individual has been estimated to have three to eight genes, which, if homozygous instead of heterozygous, would be lethal. The relative contribution of the segregational and mutational loads to the total genetic load is uncertain.

Beaudet AL, Scriver CR, Sly WS, et al.: Introduction to Human Biochemical and Molecular Genetics. New York, McGraw-Hill Book Company, 1990. *A concise, historical perspective and summation of what we know about basic principles of human genetics, which emphasizes causes (mutations), pathogenesis, and therapy.*

Cavalli-Sforza LL, Bodmer WF: The Genetics of Human Populations. 2nd ed. San Francisco, W.H. Freeman and Company, 1978. *An authoritative textbook of human genetics.*

Galjaard H: Genetic Metabolic Diseases. Early Diagnosis and Prenatal Analysis. Amsterdam, Elsevier/North Holland Biomedical Press, 1980. *An 850-page book on hereditary disorders, about one third of which is devoted to methods and results of prenatal diagnosis.*

McKusick VA: Mendelian Inheritance in Man. 9th ed. Baltimore, Johns Hopkins University Press, 1990. *A catalogue of autosomal dominant, autosomal recessive, and X-linked phenotypes, with brief descriptions and literature references for each.*

Scriver CR, Beaudet AL, Sly WS, et al.: The Metabolic Basis of Inherited Disease. 6th ed. New York, McGraw-Hill Book Company, 1989. *Authoritative discussions of all inborn errors of metabolism for which there is a substantial body of metabolic or biochemical information.*

Vogel F, Motulsky AG: Human Genetics: Problems and Approaches. 2nd ed. Berlin, Springer-Verlag, 1986. *A superb and up-to-date treatment of human genetics.*

31 Inborn Errors of Metabolism

James B. Wyngaarden

The inspired concept of inborn errors of metabolism, developed by Archibald Garrod in the first decade of this century, marks the birth of biochemical genetics. Garrod's studies of alcaptonuria, pentosuria, albinism, and cystinuria led to the proposal of a new category of diseases in which a block in a metabolic pathway arises from an inherited deficiency of a specific enzyme. This concept was proved in 1948 when Gibson found a deficiency of NADH-dependent methemoglobin reductase in recessive methemoglobinemia. This was soon followed by the discovery in 1952 by Cori and Cori of a deficiency of glucose-6-phosphatase in von Gierke's disease, in 1953 by Jervis of phenylalanine hydroxylase deficiency in phenylketonuria, and in 1956 by LaDu of homogentisic acid oxidase deficiency in alcaptonuria as originally predicted by Garrod. By 1990 deficiencies of over 300 different enzymes have been associated with hereditary disease. Of even greater importance in the history of genetics was the remarkable insight in Garrod's hypothesis that the primary action of a gene is to control the synthesis of a specific enzyme. Decades later Beadle (1945) independently proposed the one gene–one enzyme hypothesis anticipated by Garrod.

In 1949 Pauling, Itano, and associates observed that sickle cell hemoglobin exhibited abnormal electrophoretic behavior and introduced the concept of *molecular disease*, in which a structural alteration in a macromolecule accounted for a specific functional change that was responsible for a disease state. In 1953 Ingram demonstrated the substitution of a single amino acid residue in the β-chain of sickle cell hemoglobin, confirming the concept of molecular disease and initiating an ever-lengthening series of findings of structural alterations in macromolecules that result from gene mutations. For a time "missing" enzyme diseases and hemoglobinopathies were thought to represent distinct categories of disease, perhaps representing defects of control and structural genes, respectively. More sensitive techniques have disclosed low levels of residual activity of the deficient enzyme in many inborn errors of metabolism. In some cases the mutation has affected a critical portion of the enzyme, radically reducing its catalytic activity; in others the mutation has rendered the enzyme highly unstable. In the case of erythrocytes that lack a nucleus and cannot continue to synthesize new protein, enzyme lability results in low enzyme activity values in the older cells. In several instances amino acid sequence studies of enzymes have disclosed single amino acid substitutions analogous to the defect in sickle hemoglobin. Thus many inborn errors of metabolism are molecular diseases in which the *primary* defect lies in the genetic specification of the protein.

INBORN ERRORS AND MUTANT PROTEINS

Although most of the well-defined inborn errors of metabolism are inherited as recessive conditions, in principle any human phenotype showing mendelian genetics must be based on a specific variant or missing protein. Thus not only autosomal and X-linked recessive but also autosomal and X-linked dominant conditions may be expressed through abnormal proteins. Examples in which a mutant protein has been identified include autosomal recessive, alcaptonuria (homogentistic acid oxidase); X-linked recessive, Lesch-Nyhan syndrome (hypoxanthine-guanine phosphoribosyltransferase); autosomal dominant, acute intermittent porphyria (uroporphyrinogen I synthetase). No example of an X-linked dominant condition in which the mutant protein has been identified can be cited as yet. In one condition of this category, X-linked familial hypophosphatemic rickets, a defect in Na-dependent phosphate transport is suspected but the membrane carrier has not been identified. The concept of inborn errors of metabolism has broadened considerably since first propounded by Garrod. A reasonable definition would include any condition of clinical significance that shows a mendelian mode of inheritance, but in practice the term is restricted to conditions that have recognizable biochemical manifestations.

A mutant protein that cannot be detected by functional assay may nevertheless retain immunologic reactivity. However, in some instances no protein can be detected by functional or immunologic means. In the terminology of microbial genetics, the former class of mutants is frequently called CRM(+) ("krim" positive) and the latter CRM(−). The presence of CRM(−) material suggests that the genetic defect is due to a missense mutation with a consequent amino acid substitution that destroys the activity but not the antigenicity of the mutant enzyme. In most cases in which mutant enzymes have been studied, cross-reactive material has been detected. However, in the Lesch-Nyhan syndrome only 1 CRM(+) mutant has been found among 14 studied. At the pseudocholinesterase locus, 17 CRM(+) mutants and 18 CRM(−) mutants have been recognized. A CRM(−) reaction does not prove that no protein is present; the protein may be so altered that both enzyme function and immunologic reactivity have been lost.

Mutation does not necessarily result in loss of enzyme activity. Several examples of increased activity are known. The best examples are three types of phosphoribosylpyrophosphate synthetase overactivity associated with purine overproduction and gout. In one there is a 2.5-fold increase in enzyme activity per molecule; in another, excessive activity is a reflection of diminished affinity for normal intracellular nucleotide inhibitors; in a third, the overactivity results from an increased affinity for ribose 5-phosphate, a substrate of the reaction. All of these changes reflect alterations of enzyme structure. Some of the clinical conditions in which an abnormality of a specific protein has been observed are listed in Tables 31–1 and 31–2. Others include deficiencies of peptide hormones, abnormalities of binding proteins (receptor diseases) and of epidermal proteins, and defects in transmembrane transport (e.g., cystinuria). Chromosome mapping data exist for many inborn errors.

GENETIC HETEROGENEITY

When two or more mutations produce identical or closely similar clinical syndromes, *genetic heterogeneity* is said to exist. In some instances the mutations may be at different loci (*nonallelic* genes), whereas in others they may occur in different portions of the same locus (*allelic* genes). Hemophilia can be caused by a mutation at either of two distinct loci on the X-chromosome, one leading to a deficiency of Factor VIII (classic hemophilia) and the other to a deficiency of Factor IX (Christmas disease). By contrast, the multiple variants of G6PD, over 315 as of 1990, represent different structural gene mutations at a single locus. A striking example of both allelic and nonallelic heterogeneity is hereditary methemoglobinemia, which can be produced by at least ten different mutations at three distinct loci: two at the locus for the α-chain of hemoglobin, three at the locus for the β-chain, and at least five at the locus for NADH methemoglobin reductase.

One of the most stunning developments of the last decade is the recognition that many genetic diseases present in many variant forms, and that the same disease entity can be caused by an array of mutations affecting the structural gene in different potentially large series of allelic variations. Duchenne muscular dystrophy can result from deletions, translocations, duplications, and point mutations of the dystrophin gene, all resulting in apparent absence of dystrophin in skeletal muscle. In the allelic but milder condition, Becker muscular dystrophy, dystrophin is present but is of altered size or quantity.

In view of the multiple alleles that occur at many genetic loci (genetic polymorphism, see Ch. 30), persons who appear to be homozygous for a genetic trait may actually have inherited different abnormal alleles from each parent. Such individuals are said to be *genetic compounds*. The clinical syndrome in a genetic compound may be intermediate in severity and manifestations between the syndromes produced by homozygosity for either allele. A classic example is hemoglobin SC disease, which results when an offspring inherits a Hb S gene (beta-6$^{glu \to val}$) from one parent and a Hb C gene (beta-6$^{glu \to lys}$) from the other. Another is the mucopolysaccharide storage disease resulting from inheritance of one gene for Hurler's disease (severe) and one for Scheie's disease (mild). In both these examples the severity is intermediate between the diseases associated with the respective homozygous states. Table 31–3 lists selected inherited diseases for which genetic compounds have been demonstrated.

ETIOLOGY. The etiology of an inborn error of metabolism is a mutant gene. If the amino acid sequence of the mutant protein is known, it is possible to deduce the nature of the mutation from the genetic code. For example, the human variant of glucose-6-phosphate dehydrogenase, G6PD Hektoen, differs from normal G6PD in a single amino acid substitution, HIS→TYR. This substitution corresponds to a mutation from GTA(or G) to ATA(or G) in a codon in the structural gene for G6PD. The G6PD locus emerges as the locus of the human genome with the greatest apparent extent of genetic polymorphism. Nevertheless, extensive tests carried out with numerous endonuclease probes within the gene and flanking regions of the gene, covering over 300 restriction sites, have surprisingly revealed only one restriction fragment length polymorphism (RFLP). Most of the amino acid sequence information of human mutant proteins has been obtained from studies of red blood cell proteins, such as hemoglobin and G6PD. At least four types of mutations can be discerned by this approach: deletions, duplications, missense mutations, and frame-shift mutations.

Another type of mutation, the nonsense mutation, has also been demonstrated in humans, using DNA restriction enzyme analysis and DNA sequencing techniques. The partial nucleotide sequence of β-globin mRNA isolated from a unique patient with homozygous β°-thalassemia disclosed a replacement of an adenine by a uracil in the codon for position 17. This changed the RNA codon from AAG to AUG, a termination codon. As a result a nonfunctional partial β-chain, only 16 amino acids long, was synthesized. Hb McKees-Rock represents another example of mutation of an amino acid codon to a terminator codon, but in this case the β-globin is shortened by only two amino acids and is functional.

DNA cloning techniques permit direct study of the altered DNA sequence in many human mutations, even those that involve genes that code for quantitatively minor proteins, such as most enzymes. The new technique of polymerase chain reaction (PCR) permits amplification of very minute quantities of DNA and, together with use of suitable restriction enzymes and gene probes, enables investigators to produce quantities of DNA adequate for sequence analysis in situations in which this would previously have been impossible. These techniques are greatly accelerating the precise definition of genetic errors at the DNA level.

In addition, the discovery of an array of restriction endonucleases, enzymes capable of cleaving DNA at precise sites characterized by specific short recognition sequences, has permitted identification of RFLP's as genetic markers of human disease.

TABLE 31–1. DISORDERS IN WHICH DEFICIENT ACTIVITY OF A SPECIFIC ENZYME HAS BEEN DEMONSTRATED IN HUMAN BEINGS*

Condition	Enzyme with Deficient Activity	Condition	Enzyme with Deficient Activity
Acatalasia	Catalase	Gout, primary	PP-ribose-P synthetase (increased)
Acid phosphatase deficiency	Acid phosphatase	Granulomatous disease, X-linked	NADPH oxidase
Acyl CoA dehydrogenase deficiency	Acyl CoA decarboxylase	Hemolytic anemia	Adenosine deaminase
Adrenal hyperplasia	Cholesterol desmolase	Hemolytic anemia	Aldolase A
Adrenal hyperplasia	3-β-Hydroxysteroid dehydrogenase	Hemolytic anemia	Diphosphoglycerate mutase
Adrenal hyperplasia	21-Hydroxylase	Hemolytic anemia	γ-Glutamylcysteine synthetase
Adrenal hyperplasia	11-β-Hydroxylase	Hemolytic anemia	Glucose phosphate isomerase
Adrenal hyperplasia	17-α-Hydroxylase	Hemolytic anemia	Glutathione peroxidase
Albinism	Tyrosinase	Hemolytic anemia	Glutathione reductase
Alcaptonuria	Homogentisic acid oxidase	Hemolytic anemia	Glutathione synthetase
Aldosterone deficiency I	18-Hydroxylase (corticosterone methyl oxidase I)	Hemolytic anemia	Hexokinase
		Hemolytic anemia	Phosphofructokinase, muscle M.
Aldosterone deficiency II	18-OH-Dehydrogenase	Hemolytic anemia	Phosphoglycerate kinase
Alpha-methylacetoaceticaciduria	β-Ketothiolase	Hemolytic anemia	Pyrimidine 5'-nucleotidase
Anemia, megaloblastic	Dihydrofolate reductase	Hemolytic anemia	Pyruvate kinase
Apnea, drug-induced	Pseudocholinesterase	Hemolytic anemia	Triosephosphate isomerase
Argininemia	Arginase	Histidinemia	Histidine:ammonia lyase
Argininosuccinic aciduria	Argininosuccinate lyase	HMG-CoA lyase deficiency	3-Hydroxy-3-methylglutarate-CoA lyase
Aspartylglycosaminuria	Aspartyl glycosaminidase		
Ataxia, intermittent	Pyruvate decarboxylase	Homocystinuria I	Cystathionine beta-synthase
Cerebrotendinous xanthomatosis	Mitochondrial 26-hydroxylase	Homocystinuria II	N(5,10)-Methylenetetrahydrofolate reductase
Cholesteryl ester deficiency (Norum-Gjone disease)	Lecithin cholesterol acyltransferase (LCAT)	4-Hydroxybutyricaciduria	Succinic semialdehyde dehydrogenase
Citrullinemia	Argininosuccinate synthetase	3-Hydroxy-3-methylglutaryl-CoA lyase deficiency	3-Hydroxy-3-methylglutaryl-CoA lyase
Coproporphyria	Coproporphyrinogen III oxidase		
Crigler-Najjar syndrome	Glucuronyl transferase	Hydroxyprolinemia	Hydroxyproline oxidase
Cystathioninuria	γ-Cystathionase	Hyperalaninemia	β-Alanine-α-ketoglutarate aminotransferase
2,8-Dihydroxyadenine nephrolithiasis	Adenine phosphoribosyl transferase		
		Hyperammonemia I	Ornithine transcarbamylase
Disaccharide intolerance I	Invertase	Hyperammonemia II	Carbamyl phosphate synthetase
Disaccharide intolerance II	Invertase, maltase	Hyperammonemia III	N-Acetylglutamate synthetase
Disaccharide intolerance III	Lactase	Hyperglycerolemia	ATP:glycerol phosphotransferase
Ehlers-Danlos syndrome, type VI	Collagen lysyl hydroxylase	Hyperglycinemia, ketotic I	Propionyl CoA carboxylase, α subunit
Ehlers-Danlos syndrome, type VII	Procollagen peptidase		
Epidermolysis bullosa	Collagenase	Hyperglycinemia, ketotic II	Propionyl CoA carboxylase, β subunit
Ethanolaminosis	Ethanolamine kinase		
Fabry's disease	α-Galactosidase A	Hyperglycinemia, nonketotic form	Glycine formiminotransferase
Farber's lipogranulomatosis	Ceramidase	Hyperlysinemia	Lysine-α-ketoglutarate reductase
Formiminotransferase deficiency	Formiminotransferase	Hyperphenylalaninemia: DHPR-deficient form	Dihydropteridine reductase (DHPR)
Fructose intolerance	Fructose-1-phosphate aldolase "B"		
Fructose-1,6-diphosphatase deficiency	Fructose-1,6-diphosphatase	Hyperphenylalaninemia: GTP-CH-deficient form	Guanosine-triphosphate cyclohydrolase (GTP-CH)
Fructosuria	Hepatic fructokinase	Hyperphenylalaninemia: 6-PTS-deficient form	6-Pyruvoyl tetrahydropterin synthase (6-PTS)
Fucosidosis	α-L-Fucosidase		
Galactokinase deficiency	Galactokinase	Hyperprolinemia I	Proline oxidase
Galactose epimerase deficiency	Galactose epimerase	Hyperprolinemia II	δ-1-Pyrroline-5-carboxylate dehydrogenase
Galactosemia	Galactose-1-phosphate uridyl transferase		
		Hypoglycemia	Glycogen synthase
Gangliosidosis, G$_{M1}$	β-Galactosidase A,B	Hypophosphatasia	Alkaline phosphatase
Gangliosidosis, G$_{M2}$ (Tay-Sachs disease)	β-Hexosaminidase A	I-cell disease	UDP-N-acetylglucosamine: lysosomal enzyme N-acetyl glucosaminyl-1-phosphotransferase
Gangliosidosis, G$_{M2}$	β-Hexosaminidase A		
Gangliosidosis, G$_{M2}$ (Sandhoff's disease)	β-Hexosaminidase B	Ichthyosis, X-linked	3-β-Hydroxy steroid sulfatase
Gangliosidosis, G$_{M3}$	UDP-N-acetyl-galactosaminyl transferase	Immunodeficiency disease	Adenosine deaminase
		Immunodeficiency disease	Purine nucleoside phosphorylase
Gaucher's disease	Glucocerebrosidase	Immunodeficiency disease	Uridine monophosphate kinase
G6PD deficiency (favism, primaquine sensitivity, etc.)	Glucose-6-phosphate dehydrogenase	Intestinal lactase deficiency (adult)	Lactase
		Isovaleric acidemia	Isovaleryl CoA dehydrogenase
Glutaric aciduria I	Glutaryl-CoA dehydrogenase	Ketoacidosis, infantile	Succinyl CoA:3-ketoacid CoA-transferase
Glutaric aciduria II	Acyl-CoA dehydrogenase, multiple		
Glutathionemia	γ-Glutamyl transferase	Krabbe's disease	Galactocerebroside β-galactosidase
Glycogen storage disease Ia	Glucose-6-phosphatase	Lactic acidosis, congenital	Dihydrolipoyl dehydrogenase
Glycogen storage disease Ib	Glucose-6-phosphate translocase	Lactosyl ceramidosis	Neutral β-galactosidase
Glycogen storage disease II	α-1,4-Glucosidase	Leigh's necrotizing encephalomyelopathy	Pyruvate carboxylase
Glycogen storage disease III	Amylo-1, 6-glucosidase		
Glycogen storage disease IV	Amylo-(1,4 to 1,6)-transglucosidase	Lesch-Nyhan syndrome	Hypoxanthine-guanine phosphoribosyl transferase
Glycogen storage disease V	Muscle phosphorylase		
Glycogen storage disease VI	Liver phosphorylase or phosphorylase kinase	Lipase deficiency, congenital	Lipase (pancreatic)
		Lipoprotein lipase deficiency (type I hyperlipoproteinemia)	Lipoprotein lipase
Glycogen storage disease VII	Muscle phosphofructokinase	Lysine intolerance	L-Lysine:NAD-oxidoreductase
Gout, primary	Hypoxanthine-guanine phosphoribosyl transferase	Male pseudohermaphroditism	Testicular 17,20-desmolase

Table continued on following page

TABLE 31–1. DISORDERS IN WHICH DEFICIENT ACTIVITY OF A SPECIFIC ENZYME HAS BEEN DEMONSTRATED IN HUMAN BEINGS* Continued

Condition	Enzyme with Deficient Activity	Condition	Enzyme with Deficient Activity
Male pseudohermaphroditism	Testicular 17-ketosteroid dehydrogenase	Myopathy	Myoadenylate deaminase
Male pseudohermaphroditism	Steroid 5α-reductase	Myopathy, lipid	Carnitine palmitoyl transferase I or II
Mannosidosis	α-Acid-mannosidase	Niemann-Pick disease	Sphingomyelinase
Maple sugar urine disease	Branched-chain keto acid decarboxylase	Ornithinemia with gyrate atrophy	Ornithine-δ-aminotransferase
		Orotic aciduria I	Orotate phosphoribonyl transferase and orotidine-5' phosphate decarboxylase
Metachromatic leukodystrophy I	Arylsulfase A (cerebroside sulfatase)		
Methemoglobinemia	Cytochrome b_5 reductase		
Methionine adenosyl transferase deficiency (hypermethioninemia)	Methionine adenosyl transferase	Orotic aciduria II	Orotidylic decarboxylase
		Oxalosis I (glycolic aciduria)	Alanine: glyoxylate aminotransferase
2-Methylacetoacetyl-CoA thiolase deficiency	2-Methylacetoacetyl-CoA thiolase	Oxalosis II (glyceric aciduria)	D-Glyceric dehydrogenase
		5-Oxoprolinuria (pyroglutamic aciduria)	Glutathione synthetase
β-Methyl crotonyl glycinuria I	β-Methyl crotonyl-CoA carboxylase		
Methylene tetrahydrofolate reductase deficiency	Methylene tetrahydrofolate reductase	Pentosuria	L-Xylulose reductase
		Phenylketonuria	Phenylalanine hydroxylase
Methylmalonic aciduria I (vitamin B_{12}-unresponsive)	Methylmalonic CoA mutase	Phosphoglycerate mutase deficiency	P-glycerate mutase
		Porphyria, acute hepatic	Porphobilinogen synthetase
Methylmalonic aciduria II (vitamin B_{12}-responsive)	ATP: cobalamine adenosyl transferase	Porphyria, acute intermittent	Uroporphyrinogen I synthetase
		Porphyria, congenital erythropoietic	Uroporphyrinogen III cosynthase
Mevalonic aciduria	Mevalonate kinase	Porphyria cutanea tarda	Uroporphyrinogen decarboxylase
Mitochondrial myopathy	NADH-CoA reductase	Porphyria variegata	Protoporphyrinogen oxidase
Mucolipidoses II and III	N-Acetylglucosamine-1-phosphotransferase	Prolidase deficiency	Prolidase (Peptidase D)
		Propionic aciduria	Propionyl-CoA carboxylase
Mucolipidosis IV	Ganglioside neuramindase	Protoporphyria	Heme synthetase (ferrochelatase)
Mucopolysaccharidosis IH (Hurler's)	α-L-Iduronidase	Pulmonary emphysema, or cirrhosis	α-1-Antitrypsin
		Pyridoxine-dependent infantile convulsions	Glutamic acid decarboxylase
Mucopolysaccharidosis IS (Scheie's)	α-L-Iduronidase		
Mucopolysaccharidosis II (Hunter's)	Iduronate sulfatase	Pyrimidinemia	Dihydropyrimidine dehydrogenase
Mucopolysaccharidosis IIIA (Sanfilippo's)	Heparan sulfate sulfatase	Pyruvate carboxylase deficiency	Pyruvate carboxylase
		Refsum's disease	Phytanic acid α-hydroxidase
Mucopolysaccharidosis IIIB (Sanfilippo's)	N-Acetyl-α-D-glucosaminidase	Renal tubular acidosis with deafness	Carbonic anhydrase B
		Rickets, vitamin D dependent	25-Hydroxycholecalciferol 1-hydroxylase
Mucopolysaccharidosis IIIC	Acetyl-CoA:alpha glucosaminide N-transferase		
Mucopolysaccharidosis IIID	N-Acetyltransglucosamine-6-sulfate sulfatase	Saccharopinuria	Saccharopine dehydrogenase
		Sarcosinemia	Sarcosine dehydrogenase complex
Mucopolysaccharidosis IVA (Morquio's)	Galactose-6-sulfatase	Sialidosis	α-Neuraminidase
Mucopolysaccharidosis IVB	β-Galactosidase	Sulfite oxidase deficiency	Sulfite oxidase
Mucopolysaccharidosis VI (Maroteaux-Lamy)	Arylsulfatase B	Sulfite oxidase and xanthine dehydrogenase deficiency	Molybdenum cofactor
Mucopolysaccharidosis VII	β-Glucuronidase	Trypsinogen deficiency	Trypsinogen
Multiple carboxylase deficiency, late-onset	Biotinase	Tyrosinemia A	Fumarylacetoacetate hydrolase
		Tyrosinemia II (Richner-Hanhart syndrome)	Tyrosine transaminase
Multiple carboxylase deficiency (several forms)	Holocarboxylase synthetase		
		Urocanic acidemia	Urocanase
Muscle lactate dehydrogenase deficiency	Muscle-specific subunit of LDH	Valinemia	Valine transaminase
		Wolman's disease	Acid lipase
Myeloperoxidase deficiency with disseminated candidiasis	Myeloperoxidase	Xanthinuria	Xanthine oxidase
		Xanthurenic aciduria	Kynureninase
		Xylosidase deficiency	Xylosidase

*Based upon McKusick VA: In Scriver CR, Beaudet AL, Sly WS, et al. (eds.): The Metabolic Basis of Inherited Disease. 6th ed. New York, McGraw-Hill, 1989, with modifications.

Polymorphisms result from mutational events that either alter an existing or create a new recognition site, thus generating fragments of either greater or lesser lengths than are found in the case of normal individuals. Linkage maps of the human genome are made possible by the RFLP technique, and genetic linkage analysis can identify DNA markers close to human disease loci. This in turn permits the strategy of mapping and cloning genes prior to the identification of their products, a process called "reverse genetics." This approach has led to cloning of the genes for chronic granulomatous disease, Duchenne muscular dystrophy, and hereditary retinoblastoma and to mapping of the genes for Huntington disease, adult polycystic kidney disease, neurofibromatosis, von Hippel–Lindau disease, polyposis of the colon, and cystic fibrosis to specific sites in the human genome. Members of the last group of genes are likely to be cloned in the foreseeable future. The cloned gene can be inserted into an organism or cell in which it can be expressed, and the synthesized protein can then be identified. These approaches have led to the identification of dystrophin, the protein absent in Duchenne muscular dystrophy, as the prototype of reverse genetics. Duchenne muscular dystrophy is the first disorder in which the sequence of analysis proceeding from mapping of the gene, through identification and characterization of mRNA and cDNA, to the recognition of the protein, has run its full course. These recent developments are discussed in Ch. 32.

PATHOGENESIS OF GENETIC DISEASE. The consequence of a mutation depends on the function normally served by the product of the gene. Mutations in genes for rRNA or tRNA would very likely affect protein synthesis generally and might be incompatible with life. No such mutations have been identified in mammalian systems, although they are known in bacteria.

Defects involving nonenzymic proteins undoubtedly account for a large number of genetic diseases, but relatively few have been defined biochemically. The hemoglobinopathies are an exception. Over 580 hemoglobin variants are now known. Many additional examples exist of mutations affecting nonenzymic proteins, and more are being discovered with increasing frequency.

TABLE 31–2. SOME DISORDERS IN WHICH A DEFICIENCY OF A PLASMA PROTEIN HAS BEEN DEMONSTRATED IN HUMAN BEINGS

Condition	Plasma Protein
Afibrinogenemia	Fibrinogen
Agammaglobulinemia, X-linked	IgA, IgG
Agammaglobulinemia, selective IgA	IgA
Agammaglobulinemia, selective IgG	IgG
Analbuminemia	Albumin
Atransferrinemia	Transferrin
Complement deficiency states, selective C1q, C1r, C1s, C2, C3, C4, C5, C6, C7, C8	C1q, C1r, C1s, C2, C3, C4, C5, C6, C7, C8
Factor VII deficiency	Factor VII
Factor X (Stuart factor) deficiency	Factor X
Fibrin-stabilizing factor deficiency	Factor XIII
Hageman trait	Factor XII
Hemophilia A	Factor VIII
Hemophilia B	Factor IX
Hereditary angioedema	C1-inhibitor
Hypoprothrombinemia	Factor II
Parahemophilia	Factor V
PTA deficiency	Factor XI

PTA = plasma thromboplastin antecedent.

In one of these, the ZZ variant of α-1-antitrypsin deficiency, two amino acid substitutions (missense mutations) in α-1-antitrypsin lead to the production of a modified protein that is not susceptible to normal post-translational processing. As a consequence carbohydrate residues are not added to the protein in the normal manner, and the defective glycoprotein accumulates in liver cells, possibly because the altered molecule cannot be secreted. Other examples in which a specific mutant protein has been identified include various lipoproteins, the abnormal plasma membrane receptor in familial hypercholesterolemia, the abnormal cytoplasmic androgen receptor in the complete form of testicular feminization, an abnormal insulin in familial hyperproinsulinemia, and an abnormal protein called dynein in the microtubules of cilia in Kartagener's syndrome.

The largest number of known inborn errors of metabolism involves deficiencies of enzymes that catalyze discrete steps in biosynthetic or catabolic sequences. The consequences of metabolic blocks depend upon the function of the affected sequence and the properties of the affected substrates. In some conditions the disease is manifested by the inability to form a specific product, as in the failure of melanin production in one form of albinism. In others, accumulation of the precursor of a blocked reaction results in toxicity or in a storage disease. In phenylketonuria the block in phenylalanine hydroxylase results in accumulation of phenylalanine and overproduction of toxic phenylketone products. Deficiencies of various catabolic enzymes explain the progressive tissue accumulations in the mucopolysaccharidoses and sphingolipidoses. In some enzyme deficiencies,

TABLE 31–3. INHERITED METABOLIC DISEASES FOR WHICH GENETIC COMPOUNDS HAVE BEEN DEMONSTRATED

α-1-Antitrypsin deficiency
Cystinosis
Cystinuria
"Homozygous" familial hypercholesterolemia (LDL receptor-internalization defect)
Galactosemia (galactose-1-phosphate uridyltransferase deficiency)
Gaucher's disease (glucocerebrosidase deficiency)
Glucosephosphate isomerase deficiency
Hemoglobin α-chain variants
Hemoglobin β-chain variants
Hurler-Scheie syndrome (α-L-iduronidase deficiency)
Iminoglycinuria
Metachromatic leukodystrophy (cerebroside sulfatase deficiency)
Hereditary methemoglobinemia (NADH dehydrogenase deficiency)
Phenylketonuria (phenylalanine hydroxylase deficiency)
Pseudocholinesterase deficiency
Pyruvate kinase deficiency

LDL = low density lipoprotein; NADH = reduced form of nicotinamide adenine dinucleotide.

disease results from failure to modify another protein. For example, in some types of Ehlers-Danlos syndrome collagen polypeptide synthesis is normal but enzymes essential in cross-linking are deficient, with the result that fragile collagen is produced.

TREATMENT OF INBORN ERRORS OF METABOLISM. Treatment of the patient with an inherited disorder depends upon accurate diagnosis and an understanding of the pathophysiology of the disease, including an appreciation of the interaction of genetic and environmental factors. Well-known examples are phenylketonuria, which predisposes to toxic reactions to dietary phenylalanine, and G6PD deficiency, which predisposes to hemolysis following ingestion of fava beans, during the course of acute viral hepatitis and infectious mononucleosis, or after administration of certain drugs, including aspirin and phenacetin. In such instances control of environmental factors may mitigate or neutralize the effect of the genetic change.

The balance of this chapter is devoted to a discussion of forms of treatment of value in specific hereditary disorders.

Treatment at the Metabolite Level. This approach usually involves nutritional or pharmacologic measures, or both.

Dietary Restriction of Substrate. Dietary restriction often reduces the excessive substrate that accumulates behind a metabolic block. A general reduction in protein intake prevents brain damage in disorders of the urea cycle associated with ammonia intoxication, including argininosuccinicaciduria and citrullinemia. A diet low in phenylalanine is effective in preventing growth and mental retardation in phenylketonuria, if started soon after birth. A fructose-free diet controls the symptoms of hereditary fructose intolerance resulting from deficiency of fructose-1-phosphate aldolase. Similarly, a diet that is virtually galactose free averts brain damage and cataract formation in children with galactokinase or galactose-1-phosphate uridyl transferase deficiency.

Replacement of the Deficient End-Product. A metabolic block may also result in a critical shortage in the product of the reaction or later products of the sequence. Replacement may alleviate the deficiency state. Goiter resulting from a block in thyroxine production can be treated and cretinism prevented by replacement of thyroid hormone. In the adrenogenital syndromes, corticosteroid administration supplies the missing hormone, corrects the disordered steroidal secretory pattern, and leads to remission of the clinical manifestations. In orotic aciduria, administration of uridine supplies the pyrimidines needed for hematopoietic functions and corrects the macrocytic anemia, and also suppresses orotic acid synthesis and urolithiasis.

Depletion of Storage Substances. In some hereditary disorders the clinical consequences result from accumulation of stored materials in the tissues, and removal of the excess material may ameliorate the effects of the genetic lesion. Removal of stored copper in Wilson's disease by penicillamine and of excess iron in hemochromatosis by frequent phlebotomy illustrates this approach. Use of uricosuric agents to deplete the body of uric acid in tophaceous gout and of cholestyramine to reduce serum cholesterol levels in familial hypercholesterolemia are additional examples. The use of cysteamine to help eliminate cystine in cystinosis is a recently introduced example.

Use of Metabolic Inhibitors. When a toxic metabolite accumulates because of a metabolic error, it may be possible to control its production by use of an appropriate metabolic inhibitor. Allopurinol inhibits xanthine oxidase and controls uric acid production in gout and 2,8-dioxyadenine production and renal stone formation in patients with homozygous adenine phosphoribosyl-transferase deficiency. Clofibrate, which inhibits synthesis or release of glyceride from the liver, reduces blood lipid levels to normal in type III hyperlipoproteinemia. Use of mevinolin, a potent inhibitor of 3-hydroxy-3-methylglutaryl-CoA reductase, in patients with hypercholesterolemia who are heterozygous for mutations at the LDL receptor locus, is a recent example. This drug reduces the rate of synthesis of cholesterol.

Treatment at the Level of the Dysfunctional Protein

Amplification of Enzyme Activity. Many enzyme proteins require cofactors for biologic activity. In some inborn errors the mutation affects the ability of the apoenzyme to combine with its cofactor. In other genetic disorders there is a metabolic defect in the conversion of a precursor vitamin to its active cofactor form.

In both situations administration of the appropriate cofactor may increase the catalytic activity of the apoenzyme. Pyridoxine (vitamin B_6) is a cofactor for cystathionine synthetase. In more than one half of patients with homocystinuria caused by deficient synthetase activity, administration of large doses of pyridoxine partially overcomes the block in homocysteine metabolism. Similarly the ketoacidosis of some patients with methylmalonicaciduria is corrected by treatment with pharmacologic doses of vitamin B_{12}, and the clinical and hematologic abnormalities of patients with hereditary dihydrofolate reductase deficiency are corrected by administration of small doses of 5-formyltetrahydrofolate, which bypasses the metabolic block (replacement of deficient end-product).

Phenobarbital and certain other drugs increase production of smooth endoplasmic reticulum and of certain of its enzymes, including NADPH-cytochrome C reductase, cytochrome P-450, and several drug-hydroxylating enzymes. Administration of phenobarbital to patients with unconjugated hyperbilirubinemia in a variant of the Crigler-Najjar syndrome or with Gilbert's syndrome may reduce plasma bilirubin levels following induction of hepatic glucuronyl-transferase.

Replacement of Mutant Protein. Direct replacement of the missing protein is an attractive approach to the treatment of recessively inherited diseases. Greater success has been achieved in deficiencies of nonenzymic than of enzymic proteins. Examples include replacement of gamma globulin in agammaglobulinemia, of albumin in analbuminemia, and of Factor VIII in hemophilia. In each of these cases, the deficient gene product is a plasma protein. The metabolic and immunologic defects of patients with adenosine deaminase deficiency are transiently corrected by infusion of irradiated erythrocytes containing normal levels of adenosine deaminase.

Much less success has attended efforts to replace missing enzymes that normally function within cells. Enzyme infusions have been attempted in the mucopolysaccharidoses, Gaucher's disease, Tay-Sachs disease, and Pompe's disease, but therapeutic benefits are unproved. The lysosomal storage diseases are perhaps the best candidates for treatment by administration of exogenous enzyme, for cells have highly specific mechanisms for taking up exogenous proteins and delivering them to lysosomes. However, the exogenous protein must bind to a specific recognition site on the plasma membrane of the target cell so that it can be selectively internalized. Enzymes have been coupled covalently to other molecules for which tissues contain receptors, on the theory that in this manner the enzyme might be conveyed to the lysosomes along with the primary ligand. Recently bovine adenosine deaminase cross-linked to polyethylene glycol (PEG) has been administered by intravenous infusion to patients with adenosine deaminase deficiency and severe combined immunodeficiency disease. PEG treatment of the enzyme confers both stability and immunologic neutrality to the enzyme. Weekly injections have resulted in sustained blood adenosine deaminase levels and gradual improvement in immunologic function over several months.

Modifying the Mutant Protein. Many proteins can be modified by the addition of subgroups. For example, sickle cell hemoglobin can be carbamylated by cyanate at the valine in position 1 of the β-chain, which then blocks the hydrophobic bonding of the normal val-1 to the mutant val-6 of β-globin of Hb S, thereby preventing sickling in vitro. Severe toxic reactions, such as peripheral neuropathy, sharply limit the clinical usefulness of cyanate therapy in patients with sickle cell disease. Nevertheless, this approach holds promise for the future.

Organ Transplantation. Allotransplantation of organs has been attempted in a variety of inherited diseases. In some instances, transplantation is done strictly to supply the recipient with a tissue that can provide a missing protein; in others, the transplant also (or only) replaces a damaged organ. Examples of the former include bone marrow transplants for a number of immunodeficiency states, such as lymphopenic hypogammaglobulinemia, (Swiss type), Wiskott-Aldrich syndrome, and severe combined immunodeficiency disease, as well as for lysosomal storage diseases and β-thalassemia; and liver transplants for type I glycogen storage disease, ornithine transcarbamylase deficiency, and homozygous familial hypercholesterolemia. Examples of the latter include liver transplants for hepatic failure from Wilson's disease, α-1-antitrypsin deficiency, and hepatorenal tyrosinosis; and heart transplants for hereditary cardiomyopathy. The greatest experience has involved renal transplantation, which has been performed in Alport's syndrome, renal amyloidosis, cystinosis, Fabry's disease, Gaucher's disease, oxalosis, and some other conditions. The results in most instances have paralleled those of renal transplantation for other forms of end-stage renal disease. There has been no evidence of reactivation of the renal lesion in patients with Alport's syndrome, or of development of cystinosis or Fabry's disease in the transplanted kidneys. Amyloidosis has recurred in the graft on rare occasions. By contrast severe recurrent oxalosis has developed in a number of transplanted kidneys. Patients with Fabry's disease have developed measurable levels of the missing enzyme, ceramide trihexosidase, in plasma following renal transplantation, and there have been a few long-term survivals. Nevertheless, renal transplantation in patients with inborn errors of metabolism should be limited to replacement of failed kidneys. Results do not warrant use of renal transplantation primarily for enzyme replacement.

Other Surgical Procedures. Surgical removals also play a role in certain hereditary disorders. Examples include splenectomy in hereditary spherocytosis and colectomy in preventing neoplastic transformation in polyposis of the colon. Also, surgery offers a quick and permanent cure for polydactyly as well as for certain other dominantly inherited defects.

Genetic Engineering. The use of recombinant DNA technology in the diagnosis and treatment of inborn errors is discussed in Ch. 32.

McKusick VA: Phenotypic diversity of human diseases resulting from allelic series. Am J Hum Genet 25:446, 1973. *An analytical review of different disorders that can result from series of mutations involving the same gene.*

Scriver CR, Beaudet AL, Sly WS, et al. (eds.): The Metabolic Basis of Inherited Disease. 6th ed. New York, McGraw-Hill Book Company, 1989. *Authoritative discussions of all inborn errors of metabolism for which there is a substantial body of metabolic or biochemical information.*

32 Expectations from Recombinant DNA Research

W. French Anderson

Over the past 15 years, a revolution has occurred in DNA research, variously referred to as recombinant DNA technology, genetic engineering, molecular cloning, gene splicing, or biotechnology. The new DNA research is making a major impact on clinical medicine in four areas: (1) understanding of the molecular basis of human (particularly genetic) diseases, (2) prenatal diagnosis, (3) production of human biologic products, and (4) gene therapy. Categories 1 to 3 are already a reality, and human gene therapy is fast approaching that status.

THE MOLECULAR BASIS OF HUMAN DISEASES

Although the human diseases studied by recombinant DNA techniques at present are the genetic diseases, the power of this technology is beginning to be felt in many other areas of human physiology and pathophysiology. All living processes are ultimately controlled by genes. Therefore, as genes are "cloned" (i.e., isolated) and as their products (which can be obtained in large amounts once the gene is cloned; see below) are studied both in vitro and in vivo, more is learned about the reactions that the genes govern. The result is that the normal physiology of a process becomes better understood. An example is the regulation of the hematopoietic system. As the genes for various growth factors and cytokines are obtained and their products made available for study (e.g., granulocyte-macrophage colony-stimulating factor [GM-CSF], erythropoietin, interleukin 2 [IL2], and so forth), a much clearer understanding is emerging on how proliferation and differentiation are controlled in the bone marrow. Another example is the immune system, in which the genes for the various cell surface receptors (e.g., IL2 receptor, T cell receptor, and so on) are being cloned and analyzed.

It is the genetic diseases, however, that have primarily benefited from the recombinant DNA revolution. Most studied are the thalassemias and hemoglobinopathies (see Ch. 136). A dozen years ago the genetics of β-thalassemia was extremely confusing. There were various clinical classifications to account for the range of severity seen. It was assumed that there must be different genotypes and that many patients were probably genetic compounds. Now, most of the genes that can produce β-thalassemia have been sequenced, and the mechanisms underlying the various β-zero and β-plus thalassemias have been elucidated (see Ch. 136). Not only has this information led to a better comprehension of the thalassemia syndromes, but also it has made prenatal diagnosis and genetic counseling much more accurate. Similar progress in the understanding of a number of other genetic diseases is under way.

PRENATAL DIAGNOSIS

Prenatal diagnosis can be used for the detection of a number of genetic diseases; see, for example, Ch. 36, and also the discussion in the chapter on sickle cell anemia (Ch. 136). Recombinant DNA technology has greatly expanded the accuracy, range, and safety of this procedure. Previously, it was necessary to obtain the gene product in sufficient amounts to be detectable by biochemical methods. For example, in the prenatal diagnosis of β-thalassemia, fetal blood would be sampled at around 18 weeks of gestation (either by fetoscopy or placental aspiration), with a 5 per cent fetal mortality rate. Globin chains would then be fractionated. Analysis of fetal DNA, on the other hand, can be carried out on a small number of amniotic cells (with a fetal mortality rate of only 0.3 per cent) or from chorionic villi (with a fetal loss of 4 per cent but with the distinct advantage of making a diagnosis as early as 9 to 10 weeks of gestation).

There are a number of techniques that can be used to analyze fetal DNA for single-gene disorders. First is the straightforward method of restriction endonuclease mapping. A restriction enzyme cuts DNA at a specific short (4- to 6-nucleotide) sequence. If a genetic disorder alters the sequence recognized by a restriction enzyme, digestion of the fetal DNA with that enzyme provides an immediate diagnosis. Unfortunately, there are only a few situations in which this technique is applicable (e.g., sickle cell anemia). A second procedure is to make a linkage analysis with a restriction fragment length polymorphism (known as RFLP) (see Ch. 31). This approach has become increasingly valuable as sufficient RFLP's have been located to make a roadmap of the entire human genome. Finally, a procedure that promises to be extremely valuable is the use of oligonucleotide probes that are specific for individual mutations. In theory, every genetic disease could be detected directly by hybridizing a normal and "mutant" oligonucleotide probe to a sample of fetal DNA.

It is clear that the new technology will revolutionize prenatal diagnosis. What is uncertain is how long it will take to transfer these sophisticated procedures from research laboratories to routine clinical use.

HUMAN BIOLOGICS PRODUCED BY BIOTECHNOLOGY

Genetic engineering is currently being used by biotechnology companies to produce large quantities of previously unavailable human biologics (usually peptides or proteins). What products are being made? Why these products? How are they being made? How good are they?

A number of human proteins produced by the new technology are now used clinically. Insulin, growth hormone (GH), and α and β interferon were the first ones licensed by the United States Food and Drug Administration (FDA). Examples of other biologics made by recombinant DNA technology are gamma interferon, interleukin 2 (IL2), tumor necrosis factor (TNF), erythropoietin, and hepatitis B vaccine. In each case, the biologic was chosen because of the importance of the protein in treating specific human disease states (either established: insulin, GH; or postulated), the commercial market expected for the compound, and the ability to apply recombinant DNA techniques to synthesize large quantities of the human protein in bacteria (or in yeast or other cells) inexpensively.

The Technology

A gene is a sequence of nucleotides in DNA which codes for a product. In order to get a bacterium (the most common biologic "factory" in use at present) to produce a human protein, it is necessary to obtain a DNA copy of the protein—in other words, to obtain a piece of double-stranded DNA that carries the precise sequence of nucleotides that codes for the protein. This DNA is then inserted into a bacterial plasmid—a circle of naturally occurring nonchromosomal DNA that replicates freely in the cytoplasm of a bacterium. Any gene (bacterial, plant, animal, or human) that is inserted into the plasmid with the correct control signals can, in theory, be transcribed and translated into protein within the bacterium. The synthesized protein can then be purified from the bacterial cells.

There are a number of ways to acquire a human gene suitable for engineered protein production in bacteria. One procedure is to sequence a portion of the human protein of interest and then, by using the genetic code, determine the DNA sequence that would give the known amino acid sequence. Then a segment of DNA one and one half to several dozen nucleotides long is chemically synthesized so as to be exactly complementary to a portion of the expected sequence of the messenger RNA (mRNA). "Exactly complementary" means that the DNA "probe" has T (thymine) where the mRNA has an A (adenine), a C (cytosine) where the mRNA has a G (guanine), and so forth. This DNA probe can be tagged with radioactivity and then used to find (by hybridization) the desired mRNA in extracts of the appropriate human cells. The mRNA is isolated, purified, and shown to be capable of being translated in vitro to give the predicted human protein. This mRNA is then transcribed into full-length complementary (or copy) DNA, called cDNA, by the enzyme reverse transcriptase. The resulting DNA is an exact code of the mRNA for the human protein. It can now be made double stranded (by the action of other enzymes) and inserted into a bacterial plasmid along with the appropriate control signals.

Several requirements must be met in order to obtain large quantities of human proteins in bacteria. The human gene must be attached within the plasmid to a bacterial control signal that will be switched on at a high level. Several such "promoter" regions are used, including those from the lactose operon, from the bacteriophage lambda, and so on. Second, other regulatory signals (for example, a binding site so that the transcribed RNA will attach to and be translated by ribosomes) must be present adjacent to the human gene. Third, any hard-to-handle portion of DNA (for example, nucleotides producing a leader sequence of amino acids or an intervening sequence) should be removed, since bacteria are not equipped to carry out many of the post-transcriptional and post-translational modifications that eukaryotic cells can perform. Fourth, the human protein must be protected from proteinases within the bacterium.

How good are these biologically engineered human proteins? They should be perfectly acceptable for administration to patients. In most cases, they should be pure and contain no infectious contaminants or animal antigenic material. However, unless purified extensively, they might contain clinically relevant amounts of bacterial antigenic substances. In addition, since some products isolated directly from the body have a number of biologic compounds bound to them, the clinical effect of a "pure" engineered product (e.g., albumin) might be somewhat different from that of the natural product.

The Next Products

What human biologics are now under development? Those being prepared for human trials fall into four broad categories: vaccines, blood components, neurohormones, and diagnostics.

VACCINES. The first recombinant DNA vaccine approved by the FDA (July 1986) for clinical use was that for hepatitis B. Specific vaccines for influenza and malaria are in clinical trials. Potential vaccines for a number of other diseases are currently in preparation, e.g., leprosy, tuberculosis, typhoid, acquired immunodeficiency syndrome (AIDS), and so forth. This new generation of vaccines should be superior to those in use today. A precise portion of the antigenic surface of a virus or a parasite can be selected and the DNA complement to this moiety prepared. Since a bacterial control signal will transcribe any sequence of DNA attached to it, the DNA coding for just the antigenic site desired can be inserted into bacteria for large-scale production of material. Or the DNA could be inserted into, for example, vaccinia in order to take advantage of a well-characterized vaccination agent. It appears to be possible to prepare highly specific vaccines by this approach.

BLOOD COMPONENTS. Several different types of blood components are being prepared for clinical trials.

Clotting Factors. The genes for factor VIII, von Willebrand's factor, and factor IX have been obtained. Human protein C has also been cloned.

Albumin. The great demand for albumin as a plasma expander has resulted in a major effort to produce human albumin by genetic engineering techniques. The advantage of engineered albumin (besides increased availability and decreased cost) should be that there will be no risk of hepatitis, AIDS, or other infectious contamination.

Thrombolytic Agents. Blood clots are a major cause of death and disabling diseases in the United States. Consequently, readily available clot-specific thrombolytic agents would be clinically useful. Biotechnology is being employed to isolate the genes for, and to engineer the production of, tissue-type and urokinase-type plasminogen activators. These proteins should be superior to the currently available agents, urokinase and streptokinase. Tissue plasminogen activator is now in clinical use.

Biologic Response Modifiers. The family of interferons, the family of interleukins, several colony-stimulating factors (GM-CSF, G-CSF, M-CSF), TNF, and other molecules are under active clinical investigation. Considerable effort is being expended to identify other factors, particularly a molecule that would stimulate the earliest pluripotent stem cell. Major advances in clinical manipulation of the immune system are expected when the genes of the major histocompatibility complex and the immunoglobulin gene families are more fully understood.

NEUROHORMONES. This complex group includes a large number of hormones, various neuropeptides, and the neurotransmitters with their receptors. Insulin and growth hormone are already used clinically.

DIAGNOSTICS. Since viruses consist of sequences of DNA or RNA with a coat, diagnostic techniques that would rapidly and accurately identify the presence of specific viruses in body tissues or fluids by using DNA probes are being developed. Polymerase chain reaction (PCR) is a new technology that greatly enhances the sensitivity of these diagnostic tests.

OTHER AREAS. Finally, two other areas need to be mentioned. A further understanding of oncogenes, tumor suppressor genes, and antimetastasis genes and their roles in cancer should lead to the development of drugs or antibodies that could be used to inhibit specific steps in the pathway leading from a normal to a malignant cell. Second, the tremendous potential of recombinant DNA research to produce useful new agricultural plants and improved farm animals should have a large effect on the food supply of the world.

GENE THERAPY

By gene therapy is meant the insertion of a normal gene into the appropriate cells of a patient in such a way that the exogenous gene produces a product that will cure, or at least ameliorate, the genetic defect. For some genetic conditions (specifically those caused by a single gene mutation that produces a defective product that can be isolated), gene therapy should be a beneficial therapeutic procedure in the future.

The Technology of Gene Therapy

It is now possible by the use of recombinant DNA technology to isolate specific normal genes from the DNA of human tissue. A gene can be isolated if it can be recognized, and it can be recognized if the protein product that it makes can be isolated. The defective product in many genetic diseases is a protein (e.g., an enzyme in many of the inborn errors of metabolism; β-globin in sickle cell anemia or Cooley's anemia). In a manner similar to that described above in the section on human biologics, a DNA probe can be synthesized. With this probe it is possible to locate the gene in human DNA, isolate (i.e., clone) it, and purify it. Any gene can be cloned once a probe for the gene exists.

The cloned gene can be inserted into cells in any one of a number of ways. The three most commonly used techniques are (1) microinjecting directly into a cell's nucleus, (2) forming a calcium phosphate precipitate of the DNA and then incubating tissue culture cells with this precipitate, and (3) inserting the gene into a nonpathogenic virus and infecting cells with this recombinant virus. All three procedures have been used successfully to insert cloned genes into cells growing in tissue culture. By far, the most efficient procedure at present is the use of retrovirus-based vectors carrying exogenous genes.

Vectors derived from retroviruses possess several advantages as a gene delivery system. First, up to 100 per cent of cells can be infected and can express the integrated viral (and exogenous) genes. Second, as many cells as desired can be infected simultaneously. Third, under appropriate conditions, the DNA can integrate as a single copy at a single, albeit random, site. Finally, the infection and long-term harboring of a retroviral vector usually do not harm cells. Several retroviral vector systems have been developed; those projected for human use are constructed from the Moloney murine leukemia virus. Evidence obtained from studies with experimental animals and in tissue culture indicates that retroviruses can be used as a reasonably efficient delivery system.

The next question is, what target cell to use? At present, the only human cells that can be used effectively for gene transfer are blood cells. No other cells (except, perhaps, skin cells) can be extracted from the body, grown in culture to allow insertion of exogenous genes, and then successfully reimplanted into the patient from whom the tissue was taken. In the future, as more is learned about how to package the DNA and to make it tissue specific, the intravenous route would be the simplest and most desirable. However, attempting to give a foreign gene by injection directly into the bloodstream is not advisable with our present state of knowledge, since the procedure would be enormously inefficient and there would be little control over the DNA's fate.

Ethics

The ethics of gene therapy in humans has been discussed for many years. Essentially all observers have stated that they believe that it would be ethical to insert genetic material into a human being for the sole purpose of medically correcting a severe genetic disorder in that patient—in other words, somatic cell gene therapy. Attempts to correct a patient's reproductive cells (i.e., germ line gene therapy) or to alter or improve a "normal" person by gene manipulation (i.e., enhancement or eugenic genetic engineering) are controversial areas. However, somatic cell gene therapy for a patient suffering a serious genetic disorder would be ethically acceptable if carried out under the same strict criteria that cover other new experimental medical procedures. The techniques now being developed by clinical investigators for human application are for somatic cell, not germ line, gene therapy.

What criteria should be satisfied prior to the time that somatic cell gene therapy is tested in a clinical trial? Three general requirements are that it should be shown in animal studies that (1) the new gene can be put into the correct target cells and will remain there long enough to be effective; (2) the new gene will be expressed in the cells at an appropriate level; and (3) the new gene will not harm the cell or, by extension, the recipient. These criteria are very similar to those required prior to the use of any new drug, therapeutic procedure, or surgical operation. The requirements simply state that the new treatment should get to the area of disease, correct it, and do more good than harm.

Although retroviruses have many advantages for gene transfer, they also have disadvantages, which leads to questions about safety. One problem is that they can rearrange their own structure, as well as exchange sequences with other retroviruses. There is a built-in safety feature with the mouse retroviral vectors now in use, however; these mouse structures have a very different sequence from known primate retroviruses, and there appears to be little or no homology between the two. Therefore, it has been possible to build a relatively safe retroviral vector.

Even with a "safe" vector, however, the problem of insertional mutagenesis remains. Since a retroviral vector incorporates into the genome randomly, it may inactivate an important gene or, worse, activate an oncogene. It is uncertain how great a danger this problem poses but it is thought to be small. As with any new clinical protocol, the total expected benefit for the patient must be weighed against potential risks. Ultimately, local institutional review boards and the National Institutes of Health Recombinant DNA Advisory Committee (RAC) together with its Human Gene Therapy Subcommittee, as well as the FDA, must decide if a given protocol is ready for human application.

Present Capabilities

The first human gene transfer clinical protocol was approved by the NIH and the FDA on January 19, 1989, after several months of extensive public review. The protocol was as follows:

A retroviral vector was built that carried a bacterial marker gene. The vector, called N2, was constructed from the Moloney murine leukemia retrovirus. The marker gene was NeoR (standing for resistance to neomycin), a bacterial gene that makes an enzyme (neomycin phosphotransferase) that inactivates one subclass of neomycin-like antibiotics. The objective was to use the marker gene as a means of acquiring information about a new form of cancer therapy called TIL adoptive immunotherapy.

Tumor-infiltrating lymphocytes (TIL) are cells from tumor suspensions cultured in IL2 that can mediate cancer regression when adoptively transferred back into the patient. About 40 per cent of patients with malignant melanoma or renal cell carcinoma have an objective response. The mechanism of this anticancer action is not known. It was postulated that if the TIL could be marked by the N2 vector, then the survival and traffic of these cells in vivo could be monitored. To accomplish this objective an aliquot of TIL from each patient received the NeoR gene via retrovirus-mediated gene transfer ex vivo. The gene-modified cells were then grown in parallel with the nontransduced TIL. Both populations were returned to the patient, and the marked cells were monitored by analyzing blood and tumor biopsies over time.

Five patients with advanced malignant melanoma were each given a single infusion of autologous gene-marked TIL between May 22 and July 21, 1989. The data from these patients demonstrated that TIL can be identified in the bloodstream for 3 weeks in all patients, and then in occasional blood samples at very low levels at later times. Marked TIL could be isolated from tumor specimens, in one patient at 2 months after infusion. No side effects or other problems resulted from the administration of the gene-modified TIL in the five patients.

The success of the human gene transfer clinical protocol has opened the door for attempts at gene therapy itself. A human gene therapy clinical protocol was approved by the NIH RAC on July 31, 1990, and the first patient was treated on September 14, 1990. The protocol calls for inserting a normal human adenosine deaminase (ADA) gene into autologous T lymphocytes of children suffering from ADA deficiency and returning these gene-corrected T cells to the patient. ADA deficiency is one cause of severe combined immunodeficiency (SCID), a rare genetic disease that often is fatal in the first years of life. The primary defect is in the T lymphocytes, so the correction of the patient's T cells should be beneficial.

Clinical protocols are being prepared which are designed to treat other genetic diseases (e.g., hemophilia, thalassemia, Gaucher's disease), cancer (e.g., insertion of cytokines that possess antitumor activity into TIL), viral diseases (e.g., insertion of a soluble CD4 gene into autologous cells of AIDS patients), and cardiovascular diseases (e.g., insertion of the tissue plasminogen activator gene into vascular endothelial cells seeded onto vascular grafts in order to attempt to reduce clot formation).

Overview

It now appears that effective delivery-expression systems are available that will allow reasonable attempts at somatic cell gene therapy. The first clinical trials have begun.

Gene therapy is a procedure with enormous potential. It should, in the future, provide a treatment for many types of serious diseases. Some claims made about the potential of genetic engineering in humans are highly unlikely. Patients with multigenic diseases, in which the genes as well as the intracellular products involved are unknown, will not be candidates for gene therapy for a long time to come, if ever. Likewise, characteristics such as personality and intelligence are probably outside the realm of this technique's potential. Only traits produced by identifiable single genes can be approached by genetic engineering.

The power to cure a genetic defect is an awesome one. But the goal of biomedical research is, and has always been, to alleviate human suffering. Gene therapy, with proper safeguards imposed by society, is a logical part of that effort.

Eglitis MA, Anderson WF: Retroviral vectors for introduction of genes into mammalian cells. BioTechniques 6:608, 1988. *This review explains the technology of retrovirus-mediated gene transfer.*

Friedmann T: Progress toward human gene therapy. Science 244:1275, 1989. *This recent review covers the whole field of human gene therapy.*

33 Chromosomes and Their Disorders

John L. Hamerton

Cytogenetics is the study of the chromosomes and their behavior as it relates to transmission of the genetic material from parent to offspring. Errors in chromosome behavior and structure are the cause of a wide range of clinical syndromes.

Humans have 46 chromosomes, which consist of 22 pairs of homologous chromosomes (identical in regard to morphology and constituent gene loci) and one pair of sex chromosomes (X and Y), one partner of each pair being derived from the mother and one from the father. The genes are arranged along the chromosomes in linear order, each gene having a precise position or *locus*. Genes that have their loci on the same chromosome are said to be *linked*, or more precisely, to be *syntenic*. Alternate forms of a gene that occupy the same locus are called *alleles*. Any one chromosome bears only a single allele at a given locus, although in the population as a whole there may be multiple alleles, any one of which can occupy that specific locus.

CELL DIVISION

The number of chromosomes found in somatic cells is constant and is termed the diploid (2n) number. Each gamete, however, has only half the *diploid* number and is said to be *haploid* (n). In order to maintain this regularity two types of cell division occur: *mitosis*, which is the cell division occurring in somatic tissues during growth and repair, and *meiosis*, which is the specialized form of cell division occurring during the formation of the gametes.

MITOSIS. The function of mitosis is the distribution and maintenance of the continuity of the genetic material in every cell of the body. This process consists of a number of different phases, which results in an equal distribution of the chromosomes to the two daughter cells. The cell cycle has four stages: mitosis or M, G_1, S, and G_2. The G_1 phase follows mitosis, during which RNA and protein synthesis occurs. S is the period during which DNA replication takes place and the DNA content of the cell doubles, and G_2 is the period during which energy requirements for cell division are built up and any repair of errors in DNA synthesis takes place.

MEIOSIS (Fig. 33–1). This process occurs only during the formation of the gametes and results in four daughter cells, each with the haploid number of chromosomes. In males each primary spermatocyte forms four functional spermatids that develop into sperm, while in females each oocyte forms only one ovum, the remaining products of meiosis being nonfunctional polar bodies.

The first division of meiosis consists of an extremely long and complex *prophase* during which DNA replication occurs. This is divided into a number of stages during which crossing over and reassortment of genetic material occur. Initially the chromosomes are apparently single threads that begin to shorten and thicken. This is followed by the commencement of pairing of homologous chromosomes (*synapsis*). After pairing is completed, the chromosomes continue to shorten and are now known as *bivalents*, which are held together only at specific points (*chiasmata*). At this stage of prophase each homologous chromosome can be seen to be visibly doubled (two chromatids) so that each bivalent, which continues to shorten and thicken, consists of four chromatids.

The end of prophase is marked by the disappearance of the nuclear membrane and the formation of a spindle, heralding entry into *metaphase* of the first meiotic division. The bivalents are arranged on the equatorial plate of the spindle as a result of a series of complex chromosome movements. The homologous centromeres are undivided at this point and lie opposite each other on the equatorial plate (co-orientation). As soon as this process is complete, the paired homologues separate and move to opposite poles (*anaphase*). The cell then proceeds to the second meiotic division. This is essentially a mitotic division in which the chromosomes have already doubled so that there is no need for DNA synthesis. In addition, the genetic material has undergone exchange at meiosis I so that the sister chromatids are not genetically identical.

The major consequences of meiosis are threefold: (1) the halving of the chromosome number; (2) the co-orientation of the bivalents on the metaphase plate, which ensures the regular distribution of the chromosomes to the daughter cells; and (3) the independent assortment of genetic material that results both from genetic crossing over and from the random assortment of the maternal and paternal homologues to the two daughter cells in meiosis I.

Two processes are fundamental to meiosis: chromosome pairing, which results in formation of the bivalents, and chiasma formation. Chiasmata have two main functions: They are the points on the chromosomes at which genetic crossing over takes place, and they serve to maintain bivalent association throughout the prophase and metaphase. Meiosis thus ensures genetic variability as a result of random segregation of the parental homologous chromosomes and the exchange of genetic material by crossing over between nonsister chromatids.

METHODS FOR THE PREPARATION OF CHROMOSOMES

Since nondividing chromosomes cannot be analyzed, dividing cells are required for chromosome analysis. The cell type most commonly used is the mitogenically stimulated peripheral blood lymphocyte. Skin fibroblasts, bone marrow cells, amniotic fluid cells, and chorion villus cells are also used for special tests. Dividing cells are accumulated at metaphase. In order to accomplish this, colcemid, a drug that destroys the mitotic spindle, is added to the culture medium toward the end of the culture period. The cells are then subjected to hypotonic treatment, followed by fixation and spreading on microscope slides. The slides are then stained.

Staining techniques may result in either a nonbanded or a banded appearance of the chromosomes. Most laboratories today use one of several banding techniques, since this results in a great deal of additional information. These methods provide a means for the precise identification of an extra or missing chromosome and the precise localization of breakpoints in chromosome rearrangements (Fig. 33–2).

Recent developments have resulted in the expansion of the number of visible bands from between 200 and 300 to between 1000 and 2000. This allows the recognition of small deletions and duplications. Most laboratories today work with chromosomes in which between 400 and 800 bands can be recognized.

HUMAN CHROMOSOME NOMENCLATURE

The 46 human chromosomes consist of three types designated by the position of the centromere or primary constriction. These are metacentric, submetacentric, and acrocentric, depending upon whether the position of the centromere is median, submedian, or terminal. Now that each individual chromosome pair can

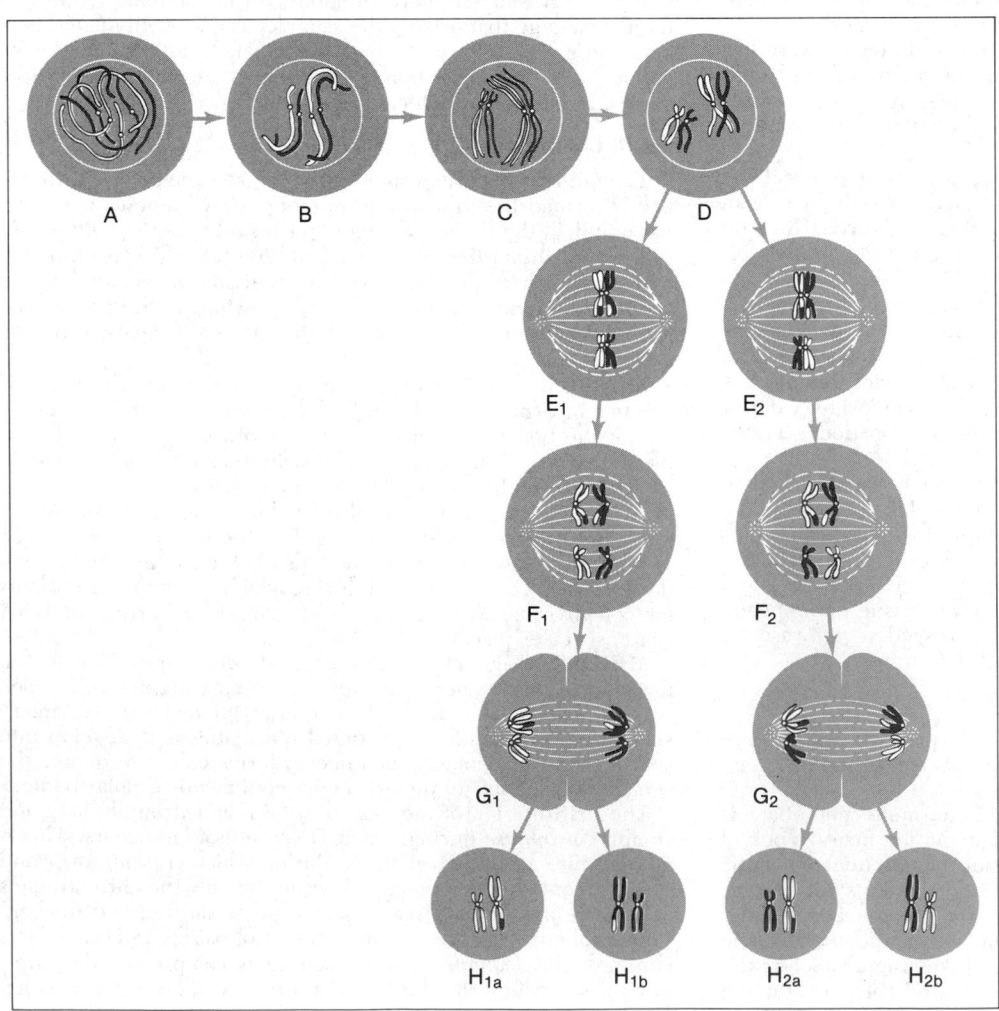

FIGURE 33–1. The stages of the first division of meiosis. Paternal and maternal chromosomes are shown in red and white, respectively. A to D, Stages of prophase. E to G, Metaphase 1 to anaphase 1. H_1 to H_2, Daughter cells with haploid number of chromosomes prior to entering the second division of meiosis. Note the chromosome exchanges that have taken place.

be recognized, the chromosomes are numbered from 1 to 22 in descending order of length. In the female the two sex chromosomes, designated X chromosomes, are identical, while in the male the two sex chromosomes, designated X and Y, are morphologically different.

Chromosome Variants

This term refers to consistent minor chromosome changes often involving the short arms of the acrocentric chromosomes, the long arm of the Y chromosome, or the constitutive heterochromatin near the centromere of chromosomes 1, 9, and 16. These have little obvious clinical significance but may be useful as genetic markers. They occur much more frequently in the population than do major chromosome abnormalities, and they often segregate in families in a mendelian manner. Recent studies suggest that about 70 per cent of newborn infants carry one or more variant chromosomes.

Nomenclature

The nomenclature used to describe the chromosomes, chromosome bands, chromosome variants, and chromosome rearrangements is given in detail in an International System of Human Cytogenetic Nomenclature (ISCN) (1985). A shorthand notation is used to describe the chromosome complement of an individual. In this notation the number of chromosomes is specified first, followed by the listing of the sex chromosomes. Thus a normal female karyotype is designated 46,XX and a normal male karyotype 46,XY. Any deviations from a normal karyotype are written after the sex chromosomes. An individual autosome is referred to by its number, its short arm by the letter "p," and its long arm by the letter "q." A "+" or "−" sign written after the p or q indicates an increase (+) or decrease (−) in the length of the arm. When written before a designated chromosome the sign indicates that the chromosome is extra (+) or missing (−).

Examples: 46,XY,18q− describes a male with 46 chromosomes, including one chromosome 18 whose long arm is diminished in length.

47,XX, +21 describes a female with 47 chromosomes, including an extra chromosome 21 in addition to the 46 chromosomes of the normal karyotype.

A diagrammatic representation of the human chromosome 1 showing differing degrees of chromosome banding is given in Figure 33–3.

CHROMOSOME ABNORMALITIES

Chromosome abnormalities can be divided into two classes: abnormalities of number and of structure.

Abnormalities of Chromosome Number. These arise from nondisjunction, that is, from *the failure of two homologous chromosomes in the first division of meiosis or of two sister chromatids in mitosis or the second division of meiosis to pass to opposite poles of the cell* (Fig. 33–4). Nondisjunction results in cells with abnormal chromosome numbers. If these cells are gametes, fertilization will result in a zygote with an abnormal chromosome number. If nondisjunction occurs during an early cleavage division of a zygote, then a chromosome mosaic may result. This is an individual with two or more cell lines differing in chromosome complement. Table 33–1 gives examples of chromosome abnormalities resulting from nondisjunction.

Abnormalities of Chromosome Structure. These result from chromosome breakage and reunion. When a chromosome breaks it can rejoin in its old form (restitution) or it can rejoin with another broken chromosome (reunion). Reunion leads to a structural rearrangement that can be *balanced* or *unbalanced*. If it is balanced the amount of genetic material is presumed to be identical to that found in a normal cell, and there is a simple rearrangement of the distribution of this material. Types of balanced rearrangements include the balanced reciprocal translocation, robertsonian translocations, and inversions. Balanced chromosome rearrangements do not usually lead to any clinical change. If the rearrangement is unbalanced this indicates loss or gain of chromosome material. Loss includes a deficiency or a deletion. Gain includes a duplication. Such unbalanced rearrangements usually result in changes in the clinical phenotype.

CHROMOSOME DELETION. Deletion is the loss of a chromosome segment following chromosome breakage. Deletions may be terminal or interstitial or result in ring chromosomes (Fig. 33–5A, B, and E).

INVERSIONS (Fig. 33–5C and D). These result from two chromosome breaks and inversion of the intervening segment and can be detected only by chromosome banding studies that show a changed banding sequence. Inversions result in disturbances in chromosome pairing and in the formation of unbalanced as well as balanced gametes.

BALANCED RECIPROCAL TRANSLOCATION (Fig. 33–6). This results from exchange of chromosome segments between

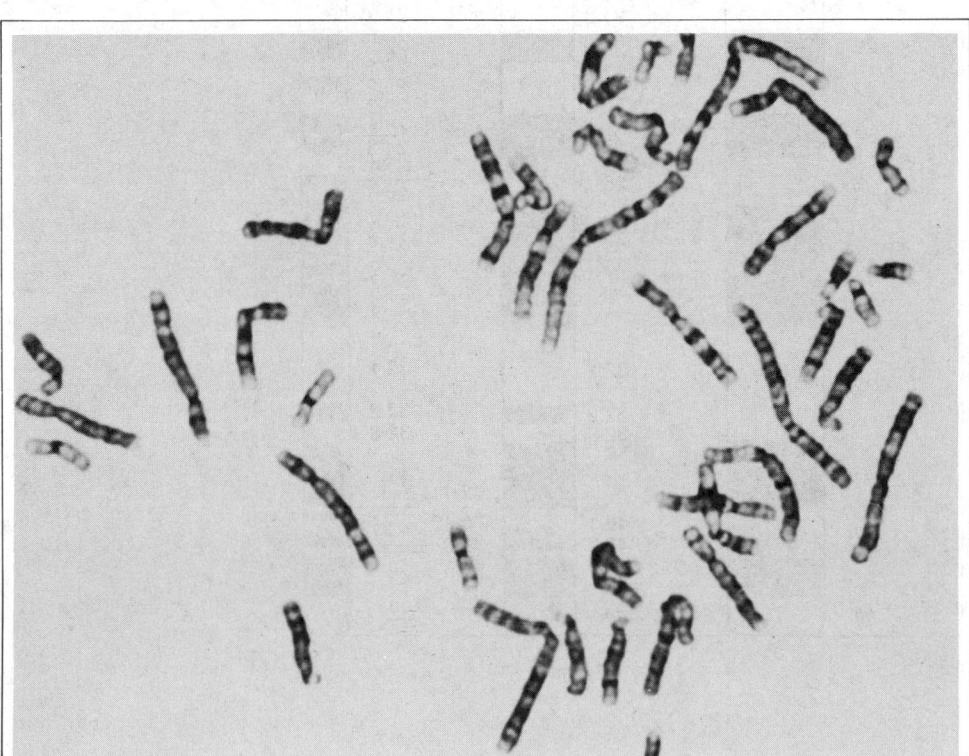

FIGURE 33–2. Human chromosomes at mitotic metaphase. G-banding, approximately 550-band stage. (Courtesy of Dr. H. S. Wang.)

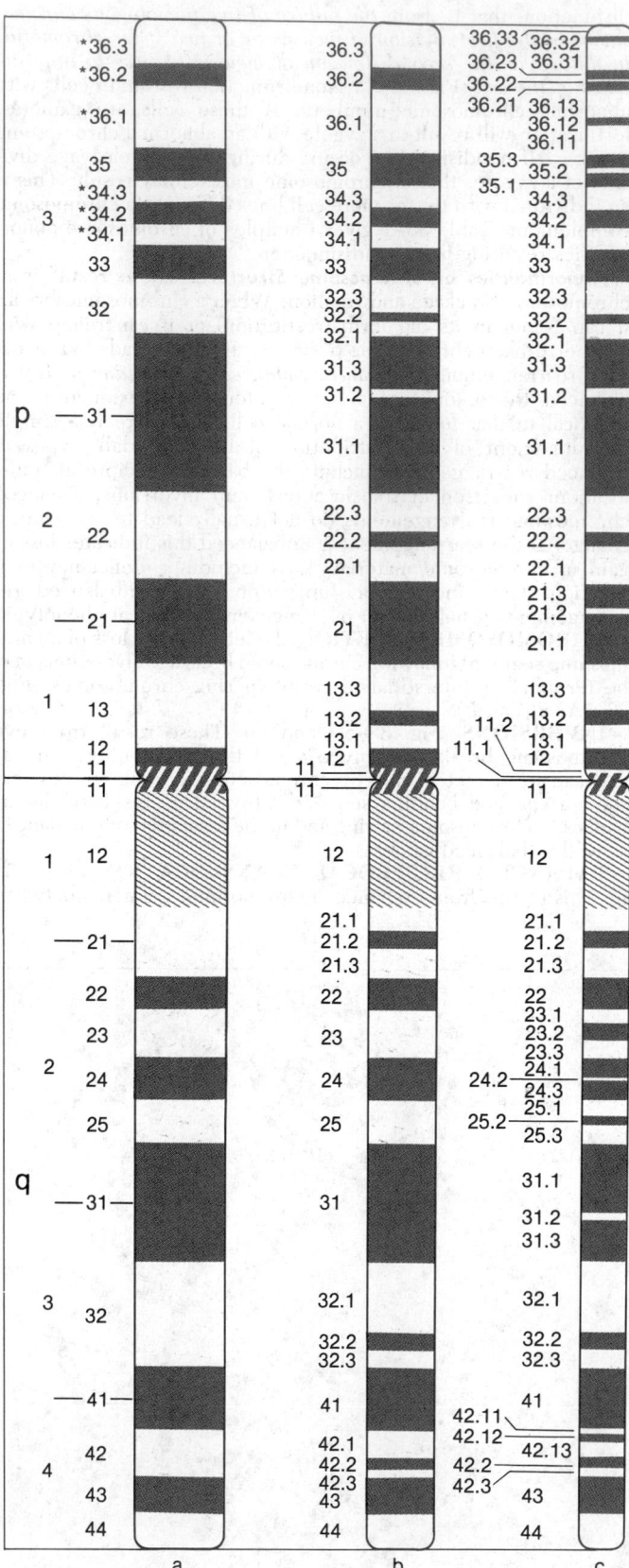

FIGURE 33–3. Human chromosome 1. Idiogram showing chromosome bands at different resolutions. *a*, Approximately 400 bands; *b*, 550 bands; *c*, 850 bands. The band nomenclature and subdivision are according to the internationally agreed upon system (ISCN 1985).

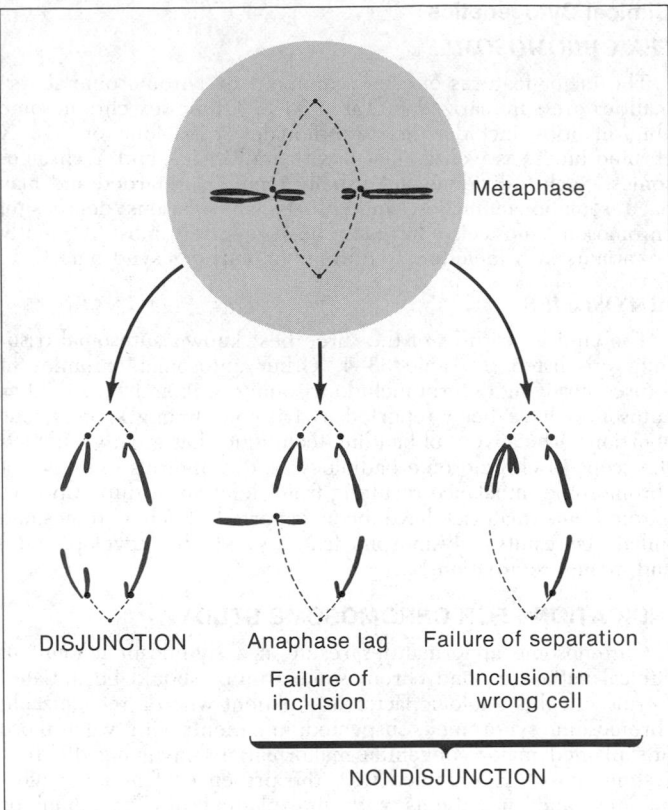

FIGURE 33–4. Diagram illustrating chromosome disjunction and two types of nondisjunction—anaphase lagging and failure of separation. (From Hamerton JL: Human Cytogenetics. Vol 1. New York, Academic Press, 1971.)

nonhomologous chromosomes. An individual carrying such a rearrangement has a higher frequency of abnormal gametes as the result of a disturbance in chromosome pairing at meiosis. Such individuals themselves have a balanced chromosome complement and are clinically normal, but they may have a high risk of having congenitally malformed children and/or spontaneous abortions. Normal children may also be born, and such persons require careful genetic counseling.

ROBERTSONIAN TRANSLOCATION. This is a specific type of unequal reciprocal translocation that occurs between acrocentric chromosomes, resulting in the formation of a new metacentric chromosome from two acrocentric chromosomes. Such rearrangements may be important in the transmission of Down's syndrome when one of the chromosomes involved is chromosome 21, the other usually being chromosome 14.

POPULATION CYTOGENETICS

Chromosome abnormalities form a significant component of the deleterious genetic load carried by the human population.

TABLE 33–1. EXAMPLES OF CHROMOSOME ABNORMALITIES DUE TO NONDISJUNCTION IN HUMANS

Sex Chromosomes	Autosomes†
47,XXY (Klinefelter's syndrome) *46,XY/47,XXY	21-trisomy (47,XX or XY, +21)
47,XYY	13-trisomy (47,XX or XY, +13)
47,XXX	18-trisomy (47,XX or XY, +18)
45,X (Turner's syndrome) *45,X/46,XX (ovarian dysgenesis)	21-monosomy (45,XX or XY, −21)

*Examples of chromosome mosaics due to nondisjunction or chromosome loss during an early cleavage division.

†In describing a chromosome abnormality the words "trisomy" and "monosomy" refer simply to an additional or missing chromosome.

About 6 per 1000 newborn babies have a major chromosome abnormality that may result in some degree of morbidity or mortality at some time during life. The frequency of the different types of chromosome abnormalities found when large numbers of newborn infants are screened is shown in Table 33–2.

Chromosome abnormalities found among infants at birth are, however, only a very small proportion of the total load of chromosome abnormalities seen at conception. The majority of these are lethal or sublethal and are lost during gestation as either very early abortions or failures of implantation (monosomies, and so on), or as recognized abortions and perinatal deaths. This group includes most trisomies, triploids (3n), and tetraploids (4n). A significant proportion of infants dying in the perinatal and neonatal periods have been shown to have a major chromosome abnormality. About 50 per cent of all embryos and fetuses spontaneously aborted have a chromosome abnormality, and about 6 per cent of stillborn infants and those dying in the perinatal period have abnormal chromosomes.

In addition to the large number of data on newborn babies and spontaneous abortions, there are now data on large numbers of mothers who have received amniocentesis because of a maternal age of 35 and over. A recent study of over 50,000 amniocenteses shows that, overall, about 2 per cent of the fetuses in midtrimester pregnancies in mothers aged 35 and above have a chromosome abnormality.

X CHROMOSOME INACTIVATION

In 1961 Mary Lyon proposed an hypothesis to account for dosage compensation for X-linked genes between males and females in humans and mammals. She based her hypothesis on observations of the mosaic patterns created by X-linked coat color genes in female mice and the observation by Barr and Bertram of a condensed chromatin mass in neurons of female cats. These observations have subsequently been extended to other tissues and species, including humans. The Lyon hypothesis states that

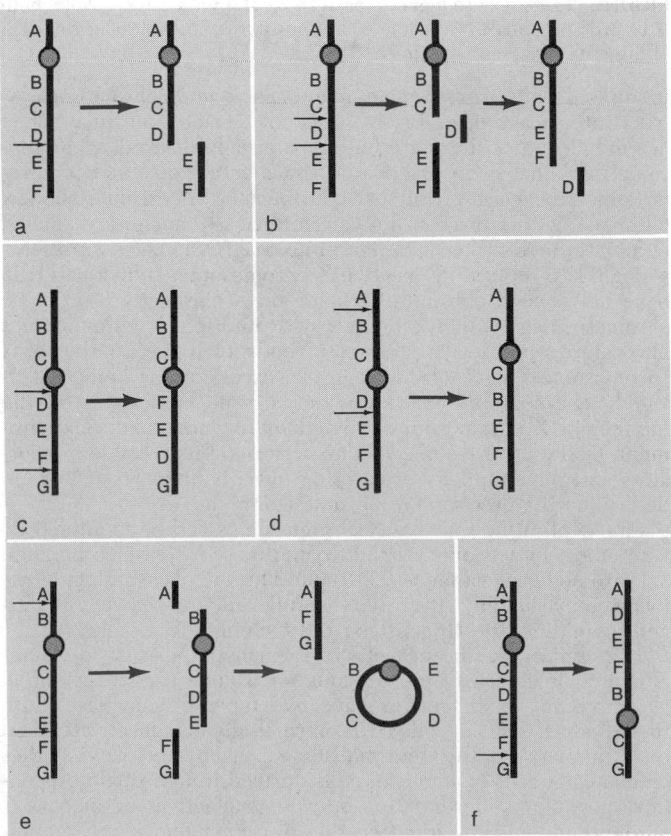

FIGURE 33–5. Types of chromosome rearrangement: *a,* terminal deletion; *b,* interstitial deletion; *c,* paracentric inversion; *d,* pericentric inversion; *e,* ring chromosome; *f,* segmental shift. (From Hamerton JL: Human Cytogenetics. Vol 1. New York, Academic Press, 1971.)

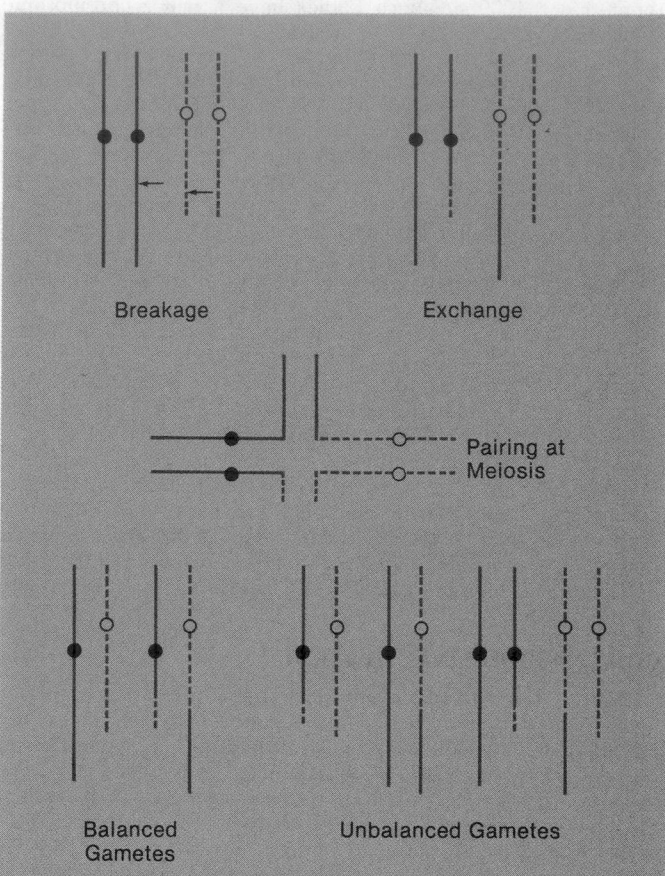

FIGURE 33–6. Consequences of reciprocal translocation. Note both balanced and unbalanced gametes are possible as a result of segregation of the exchanged chromosomes.

in diploid cells from female mammals, one X chromosome is inactivated early in embryogenesis; that inactivation may affect at random either the maternal or paternally derived X chromosome; and that once inactivated, inactivation of either X chromosome remains fixed in that cell lineage. The visible manifestation of X inactivation in the interphase nucleus is the X chromatin or Barr body, which in normal XX females represents a single late replicating inactive X chromosome. Individuals who have only one X chromosome have no X chromatin (said to be chromatin negative). Individuals with multiple X chromosomes have always one less X chromatin body than the number of X chromosomes, all X chromosomes in excess of one being inactivated. The sex chromatin provides a rapid clinical test of the number of X chromosomes carried by an individual. Sex chromatin testing is rarely used today because of its possible inaccuracies and the simplicity of carrying out a lymphocyte culture to determine the precise chromosome complement.

Late-replicating inactive X chromosomes can be identified by autoradiography using tritiated thymidine or by the incorporation of 5-bromodeoxyuridine (BUDR) into DNA in place of thymidine, followed by staining with a dye that differentiates between BUDR and thymidine (the Hoechst-BUDR technique).

The clinical significance of the Lyon hypothesis is best demonstrated in females heterozygous for a gene carried by the X chromosome. Such females have two types of somatic cells in their bodies, one in which the normal allele is inactivated and the other in which the abnormal allele is inactivated. Thus studies on clones of cells (colonies of cells derived from a single progenitor) may allow differentiation between the active and inactive X chromosome and the identification of carrier females. Examples of diseases in which carrier detection has been based on this phenomenon include the Lesch-Nyhan syndrome, Fabry's disease, testicular feminization syndrome, and mucopolysaccharidosis type II (Hunter's syndrome).

Clinical Cytogenetics

SEX CHROMOSOMES

The major features of a few common sex chromosome abnormalities are summarized in Table 33–3. Other sex chromosome abnormalities include the rare females with four or five X chromosomes, as well as males with multiple X and Y chromosomes. Such individuals are usually mentally retarded and may have somatic anomalies. Individuals with various degrees of chromosome mosaicism have also been reported, most frequently as variants in Klinefelter's syndrome or Turner's syndrome.

AUTOSOMES

The clinical features of the three best known autosomal trisomies are listed in Table 33–4. Other autosomal trisomies in fetuses surviving to term include trisomies 8, 9, and 22. All other autosomes have been reported as trisomic among spontaneous abortions. The advent of banding techniques has greatly widened the scope of chromosome pathology, and numerous examples of chromosome imbalance resulting from deletion or duplication of chromosome material have been reported. Such chromosome imbalance results in dysmorphic features and often developmental and mental retardation.

INDICATIONS FOR CHROMOSOME STUDY

Chromosome abnormalities result in a significant amount of clinical pathology, and chromosome studies should be initiated to rule out this etiologic factor in a patient when a recognizable chromosome syndrome is suspected; in patients with two or more unexplained major congenital malformations involving different systems possibly combined with the presence of minor malformations; and in patients with unexplained developmental or mental retardation. Certain cases of abnormal sexual development, leukemia, and certain solid tumors associated with congenital malformations and known to be associated with specific chromosome abnormalities (aniridia, Wilms' tumor, retinoblastoma) require chromosome studies. Chromosome banding is mandatory to identify the chromosome involved as well as to rule out possible structural changes not detectable by other means.

Chromosome Breakage Syndromes

Three diseases are commonly associated with unrepaired chromosome breaks. These are Fanconi's anemia (FA), ataxia-telangiectasia (AT), and Bloom's syndrome (BS). These are so characterized because in addition to their typical clinical features they share the propensity to chromosome breakage that can be seen in cultured cells and that commonly occurs with several times the frequency observed in normal individuals. Each of these diseases is inherited as an autosomal recessive condition. Two of these conditions are associated with congenital malformations (BS and FA), and all three have an increased frequency of malignancy.

TABLE 33–2. FREQUENCY OF CHROMOSOME ABNORMALITIES AMONG LIVE BIRTHS*

Sex Chromosomes	Frequency
Male	
47,XYY	1:1022
47,XXY	1:1022
Other	1:1277
Female	
45,X	1:9586
47,XXX	1:958
Other	1:2739
Autosomal trisomics	
+D	1:18984
+E	1:8136
+G	1:802
Balanced structural	1:517
Unbalanced structural	1:1675
Total	1:167

*Based on 54,952 babies: 35,779 males, 19,173 females.

TABLE 33–3. COMMON SEX CHROMOSOME ABNORMALITIES

Chromosome Complement	Eponym	X Chromatin	Frequency (live birth)	Phenotype
Males				
47,XXY	Klinefelter's syndrome	Positive	1:1000	Often tall, eunuchoid males with hypogonadism, feminine distribution of hair, gynecomastia, testicular atrophy after puberty with hyalinized tubules, Leydig cell hyperplasia, often low IQ. May have psychosocial difficulties (see Ch. 222).
47,XYY	None	Negative	1:1000	Often no phenotype abnormalities; usually tall to very tall. May have psychosocial problems.
Females				
45,X and other variants of the X chromosome and mosaics	Turner's syndrome or ovarian dysgenesis	Negative or positive	1:10,000	These patients have ovarian dysgenesis with webbing of neck, short stature (< 153 cm). Often congenital heart disease, skeletal defects, and renal anomalies. This is Turner's syndrome. Other patients may have ovarian dysgenesis without webbing of the neck and with much less frequent somatic anomalies. Invariably they are of short stature (< 153 cm) (see Ch. 224).
47,XXX	None	Double	1:1000	This is extremely variable. Often no phenotypic abnormalities but may be mentally retarded or may have psychosocial problems. Often fertile although may be infertile.

TABLE 33–4. THREE BEST-KNOWN AUTOSOMAL TRISOMIES

Chromosome Complement	Eponym	Frequency (live birth)	Phenotype
21-Trisomy (47,XX, +21 47,XY, +21)	Down's syndrome Mongolism	1:700	Typical facial appearance, epicanthic folds, upslanting palpebral fissures, broad bridge of the nose, protruding tongue, open mouth, hypoplastic superior helices, flattened facial profile. Invariable mental retardation, muscular hypotonia, and often congenital heart disease (Fig. 33–7).
18-Trisomy (47,XX, +18 47,XY, +18)	Edwards' syndrome	1:8000	Full-term infants of low birth weight with severe mental and motor retardation. Usually have a prominent occiput and frequently occurring facial abnormalities, including micrognathia, a Grecian nose, low-set and malformed ears, cleft lip and palate. The facial appearance is disproportionately small for the size of the cranium, which itself is small. Flexion deformities of fingers are often severe. Mental retardation is often severe. Congenital heart defect is common. Survival for more than a few months is rare.
13-Trisomy (47,XX, +13 47,XY, +13)	Patau's syndrome	1:20,000	Usually low birth weight infants of full-term gestation with a typical facial appearance, including a broad nose, hypertelorism, microphthalmia, anophthalmia, often with coloboma, and micrognathia. They are usually microcephalic, ears are low-set and malformed, and there is a large broad and bulbous nose. There are often flexion deformities and frequent polydactyly and syndactyly. Survival is usually very short.

TABLE 33–5. PHENOTYPES ASSOCIATED WITH SMALL CHROMOSOME ABNORMALITIES AND THEIR INHERITANCE

Phenotype	Chromosome Abnormality	Origin
Cri du chat	5pter–p15 (del)	Paternal
Aniridia/Wilms tumor (WAGR)	11p13 (del)	Maternal in sporadic cases
Retinoblastoma (RB1)	13q14.2 (del)	?
Prader-Willi syndrome (PWCR)	15q11.2–13 (del or dup)	Paternal
Angelmann syndrome (ANCR)	15q11.2–13 (del)	Maternal
Cat-eye syndrome	22pter–q11 (dup)	Maternal
DiGeorge malformation complex	22pter–q11 (del)	Maternal
Trichorhinophalangeal syndrome II	8q13–22 (del)	Maternal; maternally transmitted when inherited
Miller-Dieker syndrome	17p13 (del)	Paternal
Beckwith-Wiedemann syndrome	11p15.5 (dup)	Paternal

Data primarily from Hall, 1990.

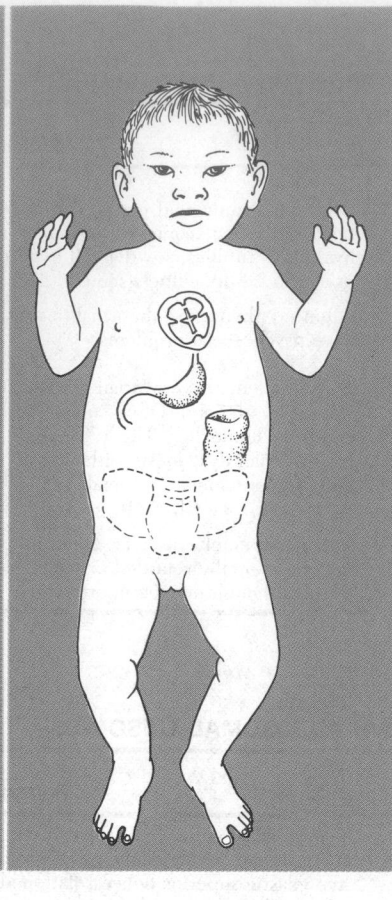

Growth failure

Mental retardation

Flat occiput

Dysplastic ears

Many "loops" on finger tips

Simian crease

Medial axial triradius

Unilateral or bilateral absence of one rib

Intestinal stenosis

Umbilical hernia

Dysplastic pelvis

Hypotonic muscles

Big toes widely spaced

Broad flat face

Slanting eyes

Epicanthus

Short nose

Small and arched palate

Big wrinkled tongue

Dental anomalies

Short and broad hands (clinodactyly)

Congenital heart disease

Megacolon

FIGURE 33–7. Clinical findings in trisomy 21. (From Vogel F, Motulsky AG: Human Genetics: Problems and Approaches. Berlin, Springer-Verlag, 1986.)

This may be the consequence of alterations in DNA repair process.

Sister chromatids can be differentially stained by a modification of the Hoechst-BUDR technique. This permits the identification of exchanges between sister chromatids. Such sister chromatid exchanges (SCE) occur with an increased frequency in BS and in normal individuals may be increased as the result of exposure to chromosome-damaging agents.

New Chromosomal Syndromes—Microcytogenetics

The advent of high-resolution chromosome banding has allowed a much greater definition of banding patterns and has thus allowed the recognition of smaller deletions and duplications of chromosome material. This has led to the development of "microcytogenetics" and the observation that several hereditary syndromes of uncertain etiology and involving multiple systems have been shown to be associated with small chromosome deletions (Table 33–5). Particularly interesting is the observation that both the Prader-Willi and Angelmann syndromes are apparently caused by very similar small chromosome deletions involving 15q11.2–13. In the case of the Prader-Willi syndrome the deleted chromosome is invariably inherited from the father, whereas in the Angelmann syndrome the abnormal chromosome is inherited from the mother. It has been suggested that the differences between these two conditions are due to the imprinting of the abnormal chromosome, which varies with its origin. The nature of such imprinting is at present unknown, but it has been suggested that DNA methylation may play a role. Recently it has been suggested that both chromosome 15's are maternal in origin (maternal isodisomy or heterodisomy) and that there is no paternal contribution in some cases of Prader-Willi syndrome in which there is no evidence of a chromosome abnormality. Other studies have shown that this observation does not apply to all such families lacking a detectable abnormality, and the final determination of the nature of the defect in Prader-Willi syndrome must await further molecular studies.

Heritable Fragile Sites

Chromosome breakage is usually random; however, some individuals may exhibit breakage or a nonstaining chromosome region (chromosome gap) at a specific site in a significant proportion of metaphases. In many cases such sites may be induced by the use of folate-deficient culture medium, although a few sites are folate insensitive. These specific sites, known as fragile sites, may represent alterations in the DNA and are often heritable. While most fragile sites are not associated with disease or other clinical problems, the fragile site at Xq28 is known to be associated with one common form of X-linked mental retardation among males.

PRENATAL DIAGNOSIS

The diagnosis of chromosome abnormalities at midtrimester gestation is now a routine procedure for certain pregnancies. It involves the aspiration of a small sample of amniotic fluid (amniocentesis), culturing of the fetal cells contained in the fluid, and determination of the karyotype of these cells and thus of the fetus. The major indications for the use of this technique for the detection of chromosome abnormalities are (1) maternal age—usually offered to all mothers over the age of 35 at the time of delivery; (2) presence of a parental chromosome abnormality—if one parent is a balanced translocation carrier and particularly if the translocation was detected as the result of the previous birth of a clinically abnormal infant; (3) previous trisomy—those cases in which the mother has previously had a trisomic infant or possibly in which she is known to have had a previous instance of spontaneous abortion in which the abortus was karyotyped and shown to be trisomic; and (4) abnormal levels (high or low) of α-fetoprotein.

The safety and reliability of amniocentesis as a diagnostic technique have now been well established by numerous studies, and it is generally accepted that amniocentesis increases the risk of miscarriage by 0.5 to 1 per cent above the inherent risk for that individual without intervention. Other risks of the test, including fetal and maternal morbidity, are negligible. In competent hands the test has been shown to have nearly 100 per cent reliability for the detection of chromosome abnormalities.

Recently, direct transcervical and transabdominal aspiration of the chorionic villus (chorionic villus sampling, or CVS) has been used both for the prenatal diagnosis of chromosome abnormalities and for the isolation of DNA for the diagnosis of several different genetic diseases. Clinical trials have shown that CVS results in only a slightly higher risk to the fetus than genetic amniocentesis (GA). Because of the nature of the tissue obtained by CVS, the frequency of confined mosaicism is greater in cells obtained by CVS than in cultured amniocytes derived directly from the fetus. This may present greater interpretive problems to the cytogenetic laboratory. With improved ultrasonographic resolution it may be possible to perform GA earlier in pregnancy, at around the thirteenth week of gestation. Clinical trials of early GA are needed to determine its safety and accuracy.

These newer techniques hold promise of being able to perform a genetic diagnosis at the end of the first or early in the second trimester of pregnancy.

DeGrouchy J, Turleau C: Clinical Atlas of Human Chromosomes. 2nd ed. New York, John Wiley & Sons, 1984. *A review of chromosomal syndromes with numerous illustrations and references.*

Evans JA, Hamerton JL: Chromosomal anomalies. *In* Clarke AM, Clarke ADB, Berg JM (eds.): Mental Deficiency, The Changing Outlook. 4th ed. London, Methuen, 1985. *A review of chromosome abnormalities and their relationship to mental retardation.*

Hall JG: Genomic imprinting: Review and relevance to human diseases. Am J Hum Genet 46:857–873, 1990. *A review of a possible new mechanism of genetic regulation and its relationship to human disease.*

Hamerton JL: Population cytogenetics: A perspective. *In* Adonolfi M, Baron P, Giarnelli F, et al. (eds.): Pediatric Research: A Genetic Approach. London, Heineman Medical Books, 1982. *Deals with frequency of chromosome abnormalities in populations.*

ISCN: An International System of Human Cytogenetic Nomenclature. Birth Defects Original Article Series 21:1–116. New York, March of Dimes, 1985. *The basic handbook of nomenclature rules for human chromosomes including high-resolution banding.*

Vogel F, Motulsky AG: Human Genetics: Problems and Approaches. 2nd ed. Berlin, Springer-Verlag, 1986. *A detailed treatise on human genetics from both a basic and a clinical viewpoint. Numerous references. Chapter 2 deals extensively with human cytogenetics.*

34 Congenital Malformations

Lewis B. Holmes

INCIDENCE

Two per cent of newborn infants have serious malformations, most of which are compatible with survival. Many additional malformations, such as genitourinary, vertebral, and heart defects, are identified during childhood and the teenage years. Many adults with congenital malformations are unaware of the significance of these problems for their health or the potential significance for their unborn children.

ETIOLOGIES

The recognized causes of malformations include genetic abnormalities, environmental factors, and the combined effects of mutant genes and environmental factors, i.e., multifactorial inheritance (Table 34–1). Multifactorial inheritance is the most common of these etiologies. However, the cause of at least 40 per cent of all malformations is not known. One example of a cause that is neither environmental nor genetic is a vascular abnormality. Occlusion of blood vessels during development has been postulated to cause intestinal atresia and hydranencephaly; absence of vessels and abnormal persistence of vessels have been observed in absence of the radius and absence of the tibia.

A few hereditary malformations have been shown to be due to biochemical abnormalities, such as a deficiency of 5α-reductase in individuals with pseudovaginal perineoscrotal hypospadias, an autosomal recessive disorder characterized by ambiguous genitals. An abnormal α-2 chain in type I collagen has been identified in skin fibroblasts from a woman with type I osteogenesis imperfecta, a skeletal dysplasia inherited as an autosomal dominant trait (see Ch. 189).

In multifactorial inheritance, clinical studies of human and

TABLE 34–1. RECOGNIZED ETIOLOGIES OF MALFORMATIONS PRESENT IN ADULTS

	Examples
1. Genetic abnormalities	
a. Single mutant gene	
i. Autosomal dominant trait	Polycystic kidney disease, adult type Polysyndactyly
ii. Autosomal recessive trait	Mohr's syndrome (oro-facial-digital syndrome, type II)
iii. X-linked dominant trait	Telecanthus-hypospadias (BBB) syndrome
iv. X-linked recessive trait	Metacarpal 4-5 fusion
b. Chromosome abnormalities	
i. Trisomy of autosomes	Down's syndrome
ii. Interstitial deletion	Aniridia-Wilms' tumor
iii. Sex chromosome abnormalities	45,X (Turner's syndrome); 47,XXY (Klinefelter's syndrome)
2. Environmental factors	
a. Uterine facts	Amniotic band syndrome
b. Intrauterine infection	Congenital rubella syndrome
c. Drugs	Fetal hydantoin syndrome
3. Genetic plus environmental factors (multifactorial inheritance)	Heart defects Cleft lip and/or palate Hypospadias Pyloric stenosis Hirschsprung's disease

laboratory examples have shown that several genes (including major genes) are involved, as well as environmental factors such as maternal influences, uterine factors, the season of the year, and socioeconomic class. Most individuals with a malformation attributed to multifactorial inheritance are the only affected members of their families. However, affected individuals have an increased risk of having affected sibs or affected children. The recurrence risk is usually between 1 and 10 per cent, which is 10 to 40 times greater than the incidence of the malformation in the general population.

About 0.6 per cent of newborn infants have a major chromosome abnormality, but many do not survive to the adult years. Down's syndrome results from the most common trisomy, and survival of most affected newborns to the adult years is now expected. Down syndrome is due to trisomy 21 in 95 per cent of cases, with the other 5 per cent due to translocation or other unusual chromosome abnormalities. In trisomy 21, the extra chromosome comes from the mother 75 per cent of the time. Since women over age 35 now are having a smaller portion of all pregnancies, 80 per cent of the infants with Down's syndrome are being born to women of less than 35 years.

Common sex chromosome abnormalities, such as 47,XYY and 47,XXX, are usually not associated with any congenital malformations. Boys with 47,XXY (Klinefelter's syndrome) may have abnormal physical features that are evident in the teenage years. Girls with the 45,X (Turner's) syndrome are usually recognized in infancy because of associated lymphedema, webbed neck, heart defects, and short stature or in the teenage years because of failure of puberty to occur spontaneously.

CLINICAL RELEVANCE

The following examples illustrate the potential significance of a malformation to the affected adult and his or her children.

Relevance to the Health of the Affected Person

CONGENITAL ABSENCE OF ONE KIDNEY. About 1 in 700 infants has unilateral renal agenesis. Most affected individuals are asymptomatic. However, they have an increased risk of structural malformations of the ureter, such as ureteropelvic junction stricture, and associated infections, hypertension, and so forth. The affected female may have a bicornuate uterus or absence of the half of the uterus on the same side as the renal aplasia. Affected males may have absence of the vas deferens on the same side. Parents with unilateral renal agenesis have an increased risk of having infants with either the same malformation or bilateral renal agenesis, which is fatal.

BRACHYDACTYLY, TYPE E. Owing to premature closure

of epiphyses, persons with this autosomal dominant disorder have short hands and feet with a variable pattern of shortening of the first, fourth, and fifth metacarpals and metatarsals and distal phalanges of the thumb and great toe. They also have a mild-to-moderate degree of shortness of stature. Severe hypertension is often a problem in the affected teenager and young adult. The cause of the hypertension has not been determined.

BRANCHIO-OTO-RENAL SYNDROME. The person with this autosomal dominant disorder has a pattern of malformations that includes malformed ears, preauricular tags, preauricular sinus, and branchial cleft sinus. The mildly affected adult is often not diagnosed until a more severely affected child is born. The affected adult may have significant hearing loss or renal hypoplasia.

KLIPPEL-FEIL SYNDROME. The person with fusion or hemivertebrae of one or more cervical vertebrae usually has a short neck, limited rotation of the head, a low hairline, and a webbed neck. Common associated problems include hearing loss, heart defects, Sprengel's deformity, and genitourinary anomalies, such as aplasia of müllerian structures.

POLYCYSTIC KIDNEY DISEASE. The affected individual with the adult form has an increased risk of having cerebral aneurysms and pancreatic cysts. Prenatal diagnosis using DNA probes is now possible in some families; recent studies show at least two genes can cause this type of polycystic kidney disease (see Ch. 89).

Relevance to Increased Risk of Having Affected Children

MULTIFACTORIAL INHERITANCE. The adult with one of the common malformations attributed to this process has an increased risk of having an affected child. For malformations that show an altered sex ratio, the sex of the affected parent is important in determining the risk of having an affected child (Table 34–2). In general, the parent of the less frequently affected sex has a greater risk of having affected children. For example, *intestinal aganglionosis* (Hirschsprung's disease) is much more common in males than females, but the affected female has a much greater risk of having affected children (Table 34–2).

With early surgical closure and better treatment of the associated hydrocephalus and urinary tract infections, males and females with *spina bifida* (myelomeningocele) are surviving to adult years and usually have normal intelligence. Both affected males and affected females may be fertile. The affected adult has an increased risk of about 3 per cent that each child will have a neural tube defect.

HYPERTELORISM. The mother who has a broad bridge of the nose and hypertelorism* has an increased risk of having severely malformed sons. For example, the female who carries the X-linked gene for the telecanthus-hypospadias (BBB) syndrome shows only hypertelorism, but sons who inherit this gene have a severe malformation syndrome that may include hypertelorism, broad nasal bridge, cleft lip and palate, heart defects, imperforate anus, hypospadias, and mental deficiency. Mothers with the autosomal dominant disorder known as the Opitz-Frias (or G) syndrome also have hypertelorism and a broad bridge of the nose. Their affected sons and daughters have at birth aspiration due to a laryngotracheoesophageal cleft, stridor, and associated malformations such as cleft lip, heart defects, hypospadias (males), and imperforate anus. Unfortunately, the physical features of broad nasal bridge and hypertelorism are nonspecific, and the risk for the woman with no affected children cannot be determined.

MENTAL RETARDATION. There are many causes of mental retardation. The mildly retarded woman without striking physical abnormalities may be a carrier of significant and relatively common genetic abnormalities that give her an increased risk of having severely affected sons. Two examples are the fragile-X syndrome and the Coffin-Lowry syndrome. The fragile-X syndrome is a common cause of mental retardation, mild facial abnormalities, and sometimes macro-orchidism in males. The

---

*Hypertelorism can be determined most precisely from an anteroposterior radiograph that shows an increased bony interorbital distance.

TABLE 34–2. RISK OF AFFECTED CHILDREN FOR PARENT WITH MALFORMATION ATTRIBUTED TO MULTIFACTORIAL INHERITANCE

Malformation	Risk of Affected Child (per cent)	Prevalence of Condition in General Population (per cent)
1. Intestinal aganglionosis (Hirschsprung's disease)	2.0	0.02
2. Hypospadias	6.0	0.8
3. Club foot	1.4	0.13
4. Congenital hip dislocation	4.3	0.8
5. Ventricular septal defect	4.0	0.2
6. Pyloric stenosis	4 (affected father) 13 (affected mother)	
7. Cleft palate	6.2	0.3
8. Spina bifida (meningomyelocele)	2.0	0.14

affected female may show mosaicism for the marker X chromosome, an abnormality of the distal portion of the long arm of the X chromosome that can be identified in cytogenetic studies only if special media and processing are used. The woman who has the X-linked gene for the Coffin-Lowry syndrome shows only mild mental retardation, short stature, short and hyperextensible hands, and tufted distal phalanges. The affected male is much more severely affected, with severe mental deficiency, short stature, stiff joints, coarse facial features, pectus carinatum, and large, soft hands.

PRENATAL DIAGNOSIS

The techniques used most often for diagnosing malformations in the fetus are cell culture of amniocytes removed at 16 to 18 weeks of gestation, assay for α-fetoprotein (AFP) in the amniotic fluid and maternal serum, and ultrasound imaging. Early amniocentesis is now offered at 12 to 14 weeks of pregnancy at some medical centers. Parents who have previously had a child with trisomy 21 have a 1 per cent risk of having a second child with trisomy 21 regardless of the mother's age. For the woman who has previously had a child with anencephaly or spina bifida, prenatal diagnosis includes amniocentesis to measure the level of AFP and ultrasound imaging for hydrocephalus, the cranial defect in anencephaly, and the spinal defect in meningomyelocele. A neural tube defect is confirmed by an increase in the level of AFP and acetylcholinesterase in the amniotic fluid. Both the amniocytes removed at amniocentesis and the chorionic villi removed transcervically at 9 to 11 weeks of gestation can be used to identify chromosome abnormalities, hemoglobinopathies, and metabolic disorders in the fetus. Limb malformations, diaphragm defects, ventral abdominal wall defects, hydrocephalus, and renal agenesis can be investigated with ultrasound imaging. However, the accuracy of prenatal diagnosis varies with the quality of the equipment used and the experience of the sonographer.

Prenatal screening for neural tube defects and chromosome trisomies is now available as an option in prenatal care. Serum AFP is measured in the mother at 15 to 17 weeks of pregnancy. Errors in diagnosis result from incorrect gestational age and alterations in the range of normal values in obese women with diabetes mellitus. The pregnant woman with an elevated serum level of AFP should have ultrasound imaging and if no abnormality is seen, amniocentesis for AFP and acetylcholinesterase. Elevations in AFP also occur in twin pregnancies, intrauterine death, and other malformations such as esophageal atresia, omphalocele, and hereditary nephrosis. A skin-covered neural tube defect, such as a lumbar meningocele, will be missed in prenatal screening with serum AFP. Measuring maternal serum levels of AFP, estriol, and hCG identifies 60 per cent of the infants with trisomy 21 (low AFP and estriol and high hCG). In general, prenatal AFP screening is most effective if carried out by individuals who are experienced in identifying the causes of false-positive and false-negative values and who educate the parents initially about the steps involved and the benefits and accuracy of the testing.

FETAL SURGERY

Catheters have been introduced to relieve malformations that cause obstruction of the flow of urine or of cerebrospinal fluid.

This approach is experimental. One major problem is to identify an abnormality early enough to permit intervention before the fetus has suffered irreversible lung hypoplasia, the usual cause of death in infants with oligohydramnios from urinary tract obstruction. Another problem is that the fetus in whom only hydrocephalus or urinary tract obstruction is visible by ultrasonography may have multiple malformations that become apparent only after birth.

PREVENTION OF MALFORMATION

Pregnant women with several different medical diseases or exposures have an increased risk of having children with birth defects. If the patient is informed of this risk before conception or soon after conception, these risks can be either lessened or eliminated. These efforts at prevention require special efforts in education, as most women receive routine prenatal care too late to benefit from counseling. Specific opportunities in prevention include the following:

CHRONIC ALCOHOLISM. Exposure of the fetus to high maternal levels of alcohol causes growth retardation before and after birth, microcephaly, brain malformations, mental deficiency, and a characteristic pattern of craniofacial features (fetal alcohol syndrome). The lower the level of exposure, the less the risk of damage to the fetus. If the pregnant woman decreases her alcohol consumption at any time in pregnancy, it is beneficial to the fetus, although a decrease before or soon after conception is the most beneficial.

DIABETES MELLITUS. The woman with insulin-dependent diabetes mellitus is two to three times more likely to have a child with serious malformations than the nondiabetic woman. The malformations include spina bifida, anencephaly, heart defects, vertebral and genitourinary malformations, and multiple malformations. The risk of having a malformed infant correlates inversely with the quality of control of her disease, glucose metabolism in particular, very early in pregnancy. The lower the level of glycosylated hemoglobin before or soon after conception, the lower her risk of having a malformed child.

MATERNAL PHENYLKETONURIA (PKU). Children with PKU identified at birth through neonatal screening for metabolic diseases will have normal development and intelligence if the dietary treatment (low phenylalanine, low protein) is begun soon after birth. The diet is usually discontinued in the early school years. However, successfully treated females with PKU who are no longer on the diet have a risk of over 90 per cent that any pregnancy will either end in a spontaneous abortion or result in a child with microcephaly and mental deficiency, and often heart defects as well. The risk of damage to the fetus correlates with the blood level of phenylalanine in the mother. If the woman with PKU resumes the low-phenylalanine diet before conception she has her best chance of having a normal child. If the diet is resumed in the first trimester, as soon as she knows she is pregnant, the child is less severely damaged than if no dietary treatment is used during pregnancy. Unfortunately, many young women with PKU are not aware of their risk of having children with serious birth defects.

Ardinger HH, Buetow KH, Bell GI, et al.: Association of genetic variation of the transforming growth factor-alpha gene with cleft lip and palate. Am J Hum Genet 45:348, 1989. *A new finding that shows how DNA technology may help clarify the genetic aspects of multifocal inheritance.*

Hanley WB, Clark JTR, Schoonheyt W: Maternal phenylketonuria (PKU)—a review. Clin Biochem 20:149, 1987. *A thorough review of the teratogenic effects of PKU in the pregnant woman and efforts at preventing these effects.*

Jones KL: Smith's Recognizable Patterns of Human Malformation. 4th ed. Philadelphia, W. B. Saunders Company, 1988. *A thorough tabulation of recognized malformation syndromes.*

Kimberling WJ, Fain PR, Kenyon JB, et al.: Linkage heterogeneity of autosomal dominant polycystic kidney disease. N Engl J Med 319:913, 1988. *Shows that more than one gene causes this type of polycystic kidney disease.*

Nelson K, Holmes LB: Malformations due to presumed spontaneous mutations in newborn infants. N Engl J Med 320:19, 1989. *The first clinical assessment of the apparent etiology of all congenital malformations in a large, unselected population of newborn infants.*

Roodhooft AM, Birnholz JC, Holmes LB: Familial nature of congenital absence and severe dysgenesis of both kidneys. N Engl J Med 310:1341, 1984. *Shows the potential genetic significance of unilateral renal agenesis in an adult.*

Shepard TH: Catalog of Teratogenic Agents. 6th ed. Baltimore, The Johns Hopkins University Press, 1989. *A summary of experimental and clinical intervention on the potential teratogenic effects of common drug and other environmental exposures.*

Wald NJ, Cuckle HS, Densem JW, et al.: Maternal serum unconjugated oestriol

as an antenatal screening test for Down's syndrome. Br J Obstet Gynecol 95:344, 1988. *Shows the basis for expanded prenatal screening with three maternal serum constituents: α-fetoprotein, hCG, and estriol.*

35 Genetic Counseling
Margretta R. Seashore

Genetic counseling can be defined as a process in which an individual or family obtains information about a genetic condition that may affect them. The purpose of genetic counseling is to enable individuals and families to make important decisions about marriage, reproduction, and health management based on the facts of the genetic situation for which a risk is perceived. This process is part of a thorough genetic evaluation in which the diagnosis is made or confirmed, the genetic model is developed, the information is communicated, the options are discussed, and psychosocial support is offered. Any breakdown in this progression may lead to information being misunderstood, misinterpreted, or misused.

DIAGNOSIS

The first step in genetic counseling is to confirm the diagnosis. The worst error that can be made is to provide an elegant and sophisticated analysis for the wrong disorder. The importance of this step cannot be overemphasized. Many persons have been given general diagnoses, such as mental retardation, for which there can be a multitude of genetic as well as nongenetic explanations. The increasing definition of the molecular pathology of many disorders has heightened the importance of recognizing genetic heterogeneity. For example, at least 20 different forms of muscular dystrophy have been identified which are clinically similar. Both X-linked and autosomal recessive forms are known. At least two, Becker and Duchenne dystrophy, are X-linked conditions that are allelic but clinically quite distinct. Differentiations of this kind must be made with as much accuracy as possible if the patient and family are to be given the most precise answers.

The confirmation of the diagnosis uses five medical tools, four of which are very familiar to all clinicians. These are medical records, medical history, physical examination, conventional laboratory tests, and molecular genetic analysis. The importance of reviewing medical records seems obvious, yet it can be a difficult task to accomplish completely. Validation of the rate of progression of symptoms and signs, the development of the present physical findings, and the results of prior laboratory tests are all best determined from the medical records. In addition, the status of family members can sometimes be assessed from examination of their medical records. Often the medical geneticist has been told of a relative who "had the same problem" only to learn from that individual's medical records that the relative's problem was entirely different.

The medical history provides clues to the beginnings and progression of symptoms and signs which may provide valuable hints to diagnosis. The pattern of progression in the degenerative neurologic disorders provides important diagnostic information. A history of more than two spontaneous miscarriages may suggest a chromosomal translocation in one parent. Early death of infants in the pedigree may suggest an inborn error of intermediary metabolism.

The physical examination again provides the opportunity to consider genetic heterogeneity. For example, there are many genetic causes of short stature. The details of the physical examination may provide the information on which the correct genetic diagnosis depends. Precise measurement of anthropometric features can be compared with values in the literature and the diagnostic considerations narrowed.

Conventional laboratory tests often provide helpful diagnostic information to complete the genetic diagnosis. Radiographic appearance of bones is often the critical information in diagnosing

TABLE 35–1. MOLECULAR DIAGNOSTIC TOOLS IN GENETIC COUNSELING: CONDITIONS FOR WHICH DNA-BASED DIAGNOSIS HAS BEEN ACCOMPLISHED

Adult polycystic kidney disease
Duchenne muscular dystrophy
Cystic fibrosis
Fragile-X syndrome
Hemophilia A
Huntington disease
Multiple endocrine neoplasia
Myotonic dystrophy
Neurofibromatosis type 1
Neurofibromatosis type 2
Ornithine transcarbamoylase deficiency
Phenylketonuria
Tay-Sachs disease
Thalassemias
Sickle cell anemia
Wiskott-Aldrich syndrome

the chondrodystrophies, for example. Measurement of proteins, such as α_1-antitrypsin, can demonstrate the most important feature of a condition.

The development of molecular diagnostic tools that can provide precise definition of the mutation or utilize linkage to a specific genetic marker has revolutionized genetic counseling. In the past, the chromosomal location of specific genes was inferred from pedigree information for the X chromosome and linkage to specific protein markers for autosomes. Now the chromosomal location of many more genes is known, linkage to specific DNA markers has been established, and many genes of clinical importance have been cloned and sequenced. It is likely that within the next two decades, the entire human genome will be mapped and entirely sequenced. More than 1500 genes have now been mapped to specific locations in the human genome. Many of these comprise specific genes or linkage markers for some of the 2000 single-gene conditions that appear in the McKusick catalog of mendelian phenotypes. The number of conditions that show linkage to known genetic markers or to anonymous DNA probes grows daily. These new tools can be used to enhance the precision of genetic diagnosis and counseling (see Ch. 32 for molecular methods). Table 35–1 lists examples of many of the genetic conditions that can be diagnosed using these molecular tools. This list is being expanded at a rapid rate and should not be taken to be complete. At least one disease has been mapped to each chromosome (Table 35–2). Any condition mapped to a specific chromosomal location can theoretically be diagnosed

TABLE 35–2. EXAMPLES OF ONE CONDITION MAPPED TO EACH CHROMOSOME

Genetic Condition	Map Location
Charcot-Marie-Tooth neuropathy 1	1q
von Hippel–Lindau syndrome	3p
Huntington disease	4pter–p16
Familial polyposis of the colon	5q21–p22
Congenital adrenal hyperplasia	6p21.3
Cystic fibrosis	7q31–q32
Langer-Gideon syndrome	8q24
Friedreich ataxia	9q13–q21
Multiple endocrine neoplasia IIB	10pter–q11
Wilms' tumor–aniridia syndrome	11p13
Stickler syndrome	12q14
Wilson disease	13q14–q21
Variegate porphyria	14q
Xeroderma pigmentosum (comp group F)	15
Adult-type polycystic kidney disease	16p13
Neurofibromatosis	17q11.2
Kidd blood group	18q11–q12
Myotonic dystrophy	19q13.3–q13.3
Alagille syndrome	20p12–p11
Alzheimer disease 1	21pter–q21
NF2 (bilateral acoustic neuroma)	22q11–q13.1
Duchenne muscular dystrophy	Xp21.3–p21.1

using molecular methods, given the appropriate molecular probes and informative family members.

THE GENETIC MODEL

The next essential step to be taken before the genetic counseling visit with the patient and family can take place is the development of the genetic model. The patient has come with the question "what is it and is it inherited?" Arrival at a diagnosis leads to the answer to the first part of the question. The second part is crucial to the process of genetic counseling. The development of the genetic model requires use of the family history, the precise diagnosis, and knowledge of the possible genetic mechanisms. The diagraming of the pedigree from the family history may fit such an obvious genetic model that further analysis is simple. When the physical examination and laboratory studies are typical of a recognized genetic condition such as Duchenne muscular dystrophy and the pedigree demonstrates a clear pattern of X-linked inheritance, the development of the genetic model is straightforward. More often, however, the pedigree is less clear. Where there is familial aggregation without an obvious mendelian pattern or the individual is the only affected member of the family at present, all possible genetic mechanisms must be considered and excluded or confirmed. The genetic model must then be used to identify those at risk for the condition.

Three general genetic mechanisms must be considered: chromosomal, mendelian, and multifactorial. The chromosomal disorders should be considered as a possible explanation for multiple anomalies, mental retardation, recurrent miscarriages, and unexplained stillbirths. These are considered in detail in Ch. 33. Empiric figures must be used to predict the recurrence of chromosomal abnormalities in a family. These range between 1 and 10 per cent, and the literature must be consulted with reference to the specific situation.

When a clear mendelian pattern is seen and the disorder is a recognized mendelian condition, counseling is based on that pattern. When the family history fails to demonstrate a mendelian pattern, the diagnosis is reviewed and the medical literature consulted to determine the inheritance pattern for the specific disorder. With autosomal recessive conditions the birth of an affected child may be the first signal that a set of parents is heterozygous for a rare recessive condition. Here the genetic model depends on the correct diagnosis and the known inheritance pattern for that disorder. For X-linked conditions, the decision must be made whether the affected individual represents a new mutation or inheritance from a heterozygous mother who by chance has no affected relatives. In the past, Bayesian calculations based on the pedigree have been the mainstay of this kind of analysis. Today, however, molecular diagnostic tools have refined the ability to determine heterozygosity in this situation. For dominantly inherited conditions, the literature must be consulted to determine the proportion of patients who represent new mutations, a figure that can approach 50 per cent. When a new mutation is the explanation, others in the family are not at risk, but each offspring of the affected individual has a 50 per cent risk of inheriting the gene. Variability in expression can confound the analysis of a family demonstrating an autosomal dominant condition. The possibility of gonadal mosaicism, although rare, can never be eliminated. In general, however, the absence of the condition in any other family member makes the likelihood high that the patient represents a new mutation. Frequently no mendelian hypothesis can be sustained, yet there is familial aggregation of the disorder. Many conditions, such as neural tube defects and cleft lip and palate, appear to be multifactorial in origin with both genetic and environmental components. Genetic counseling for these conditions must rely on empiric figures for the specific condition.

THE COUNSELING PROCESS

Once the genetic model has been established, the process of communicating this information to the patient and family must begin.

The process of genetic counseling itself has the following components: transferring information about the genetic risks, putting the risks in perspective, providing a summary of the disorder, and discussing the options. It must begin with the individual who brought the original question. An explanation of the genetic risks requires imparting factual information using scientific concepts that are not familiar to everyone. It is important that the facts which form the basis of the development of the genetic model be clearly explained. However, it is neither possible nor desirable to present an entire course in medical genetics to the anxious patient and family. Therefore, the relevant facts must be carefully culled from the counselor's knowledge store and communicated clearly. It is important to remember that persons may be very anxious and find it difficult to absorb complex material, especially if they are fearful about the implications of the information. The strategy of first presenting a brief summary of the conclusions and their implications, stating that the evidence for this conclusion will presently be discussed, can allay some fears and relieve some of the distraction that prevents families from hearing this kind of information.

If the condition is a chromosome disorder, the structure and ways of identifying chromosomes must be mentioned and the specific disorder illustrated. Using teaching aids such as diagrams and photographs of chromosomes is helpful, the normal situation providing a frame of reference. When the condition is a mendelian disorder, the basic concepts of single-gene inheritance must be discussed briefly, but the discussion should center on the mode of inheritance involved in the particular family and not be clouded with a great deal of extraneous material about other modes of inheritance. Families without a prior family history of the disorder may have difficulty with the fact that the disorder has never been seen in their family. An explanation of heterozygosity may help clarify autosomal recessive inheritance. Autosomal dominant inheritance is easy to understand when there are other affected individuals and the pedigree demonstrates a clear vertical pattern. Of more difficulty to the family is the new mutation. Careful examination of other family members must be performed before the presence of the condition can be excluded. As with the chromosome disorders, the use of such teaching aids as gene diagrams, sample pedigrees, and other models may be extremely valuable.

A second important component of genetic counseling is putting the risk in perspective. Many workers in the field (see Hsia) have noted that perception of risk may be of more importance in family decision making than the actual numerical value of the risk. This perception depends on at least two factors: risk compared to background risk, and overall burden, a combination of risk and severity. A risk of 1 in 4 of recurrence in a second child, in the case of PKU for example, is very much greater than a risk of 1/10,000 in the general population. Conversely, a risk of 1/10,000 may sound high to a couple who believe that the chances of something being wrong with an unborn child is 1 in a million. The presentation of such risk figures can change the perception of that risk. For example, a 1 in 4 chance of recurrence of PKU is also a 3 to 1 chance against recurrence. The judgment of burden, first put forth by C.O. Carter, is a very personal one. Physical handicap may be a severe burden for one family, whereas another may find that tolerable but mental handicap unacceptable. Helping families to think about risks in these ways is an important component of genetic counseling.

Genetic counseling also includes a description of the disorder. Many persons go to their local library in an attempt to find literature about the disorder or ask medical friends to do so. Often this results in misinformation or information that is out of date. Providing written material about the disorder is often helpful. Many genetic counseling clinics have pamphlets, booklets, and other literature to provide. The family should also be furnished with a written report of the counseling summarizing the important points.

REPRODUCTIVE OPTIONS AND PRENATAL DIAGNOSIS

If risk to future unborn children is at issue, as it so often is, the family in whom a risk for genetic disease has been identified must be told about the reproductive options available to them. Aside from refraining from having children at all, the options can enhance the chances of having healthy children for the family at risk. Adoption should be discussed. Reproductive technologies such as in vitro fertilization with a donor egg or artificial insemination by donor should be addressed. The risk of the same genotype in a donor must be excluded. Appropriate referral to experts in those areas of alternative reproductive options must be made.

Prenatal diagnosis is an important reproductive option for families that are at high risk for the birth of a child with a genetic disorder. Indications for prenatal diagnosis are summarized in Table 35–3.

Prenatal diagnosis is also used to address pregnancies at risk because of maternal disease or maternal exposure to a potential teratogen. The concern is not necessarily genetic, but there is a risk for a condition that can be diagnosed during fetal life.

The methods in prenatal diagnosis depend on the following: imaging the fetus; examination of DNA in cells of fetal origin; analysis of chromosomes in fetal cells; examination of proteins from cells of fetal origin; examination of proteins, metabolites, and other small molecules of fetal origin; and direct visualization of the fetus.

Imaging of the fetus is largely performed using ultrasonography. Estimation of fetal age and assessment of fetal growth can be readily performed. Fetal anatomy and organ function can be evaluated. Anatomic abnormalities such as spina bifida, anencephaly, hydrocephalus, limb malformations, cardiac malformations, and renal anomalies can be visualized.

The genetic material of the fetus, both chromosomes and specific DNA segments, can be analyzed using cells of fetal origin obtained either at amniocentesis or by chorionic villus sampling (CVS). The major autosomal and sex chromosomal aneuploidies can be diagnosed in this way, along with chromosomal rearrangements, deletions, insertions, and the like. Any DNA-based diagnosis that can be performed on cells can be performed on fetal cells. Cells of fetal origin obtained either at amniocentesis or by CVS can also be used to measure enzyme activity, characterize proteins, look for stored material, or perform other biochemical studies specific to the disorder being diagnosed. In most cases, such studies will have been preceded by family studies that have characterized the disorder and demonstrated the informativeness of the methods to be used.

Enzymes, proteins, and other chemicals of biologic importance can be measured in amniotic fluid. Such analyses include measurement of α-fetoprotein and acetylcholinesterase in the evaluation of neural tube defects and 17-OH progesterone in congenital adrenal hyperplasia.

No risk to the unborn fetus has been recognized as a complication of ultrasonography. Midtrimester amniocentesis (15 to 20 weeks' gestation) is associated with a less than 0.5 per cent risk of miscarriage incident to the procedure. Direct trauma to the fetus is very rare in experienced hands, and other risks such as respiratory difficulties, hip dislocation, and club foot are controversial. CVS (9 to 11 weeks' gestation) has a slightly higher risk than amniocentesis, estimated at about 2 per cent or less. Both the transcervical and the transabdominal approaches are being used, and the procedures continue to be critically evaluated. The timing of both amniocentesis and CVS is also being studied, with later CVS and earlier amniocentesis as possibilities.

Fetoscopy is infrequently performed and normally is done only when other diagnostic avenues have failed. It can be used to visualize fetal anatomy and to obtain fetal blood samples, for example to confirm a chromosomal or biochemical diagnosis. Occasionally biopsy of fetal tissues such as liver or skin can be performed to look for a specific condition.

Prenatal diagnosis performed for a pregnancy determined to

TABLE 35–3. INDICATIONS FOR PRENATAL DIAGNOSIS

Advanced parental age (usually maternal)
Family history of inherited disease
Risk of chromosome disorder
   Previous child with chromosomal abnormality
   Parent with known chromosomal translocation
Heterozygote screening based on ethnicity
   Tay-Sachs (Ashkenazi Jews; French Canadians)
   Thalassemias (Mediterraneans, Arabs, Indo-Pakistanis)
   Sickle cell anemia (Blacks, Mediterraneans, Arabs, Indo-Pakistanis, Turks, Southeast Asians)
Pregnancy screening
   Maternal serum α-fetoprotein

TABLE 35–4. CONDITIONS THAT HAVE BEEN DIAGNOSED PRENATALLY*

Disorder	Diagnostic Method
All defined chromosomal disorders	Cytogenetic analysis
Adrenoleukodystrophy	DNA and long-chain fatty acid
Cystinosis	Cystine uptake
Cystic fibrosis	DNA analysis
Duchenne muscular dystrophy	DNA analysis
Ectodermal dysplasia	Fetoscopy, skin biopsy
Fabry disease	α-Galactosidase A
Gaucher disease	β-Glucosidase
GM$_2$-gangliosidosis I (Tay-Sachs)	Hexosaminidase A
Hemoglobinopathies	DNA analysis
Hemophilia A	DNA analysis
Metachromatic leukodystrophy	Aryl-sulfatase A
Mucopolysaccharidosis I (Hurler)	α-L-Iduronidase
Neural tube defects	α-Fetoprotein, ultrasonography, amniotic fluid acetylcholinesterase
Omphalocele	α-Fetoprotein, ultrasonography
Osteogenesis imperfecta	Ultrasonography
Phenylketonuria	DNA analysis

*See Milunsky for more information.

be at risk following heterozygote or pregnancy screening tests is specific to the disorder being sought. Tay-Sachs disease and the hemoglobinopathies are the major examples of heterozygote states being identified in at-risk populations. Since the gene for cystic fibrosis has been mapped and the mutation associated with about 70 per cent of the cases identified, there has been much discussion of population screening for that gene. At present, the limitations in identifying the other mutations have made population screening difficult. However, in a family that already has an individual affected with cystic fibrosis, prenatal diagnosis can be done using DNA-based analysis of fetal cells. Table 35–4 lists some conditions that can be diagnosed prenatally.

Pregnancy screening, usually done by measuring α-fetoprotein in maternal serum, identifies fetuses at risk for open body wall defects, including spina bifida, anencephaly, omphalocele, and gastroschisis. More specific diagnosis is usually attempted using fetal imaging and measurement of proteins such as α-fetoprotein and acetylcholinesterase in amniotic fluid. Recent studies have suggested that maternal serum α-fetoprotein concentration is low in a percentage of pregnancies in which the fetus has trisomy 21. The biologic explanation for this observation is lacking, but the association has allowed refinement of the risk assessment for fetal aneuploidy based on maternal age and maternal serum α-fetoprotein concentration, and amniocentesis can be offered to the woman whose new risk assessment warrants it.

It is of utmost importance that the pregnant woman for whom prenatal diagnosis is performed be given extremely clear counseling. Spelling out the expectations and limitations of the testing prior to any procedures is critical. The diagnoses that are being sought must be explained. It is very easy for the woman to conclude that a normal test result shows that the baby will be "normal," when in fact only a short list of pathologic conditions has been excluded. Normalcy is never completely assured. It is helpful to point out that a condition or conditions have been sought for which the patient had a risk higher than that of the general population. The result after these conditions have been excluded is that the pregnancy stands at the same risk for many other potential problems as others in the general population.

Much more difficult is the situation in which the result of the test is not normal. Although it is best that this possibility be discussed beforehand and the options considered, it is no longer considered necessary that the woman make a decision prior to learning the test results. The implications of the diagnosis must be reviewed with care, sensitivity, and accuracy. The options for the woman are to terminate the pregnancy or to carry it to term. The decision to terminate must be made in collaboration with the obstetrician who will perform the procedure so that the process can be described and possible complications reviewed. The choice of procedure depends on the stage of pregnancy, and the complications are specific to the particular procedure. In general, a second-trimester termination is a more complicated procedure than a first-trimester termination. Psychosocial support after the procedure is crucial. Most families who elect to terminate a pregnancy go through a period of grieving for the loss of the hoped-for normal child. Many such pregnancies were planned and wanted. The family should be offered the chance to visit with the genetic counselor to discuss their normal feelings of sadness and loss and to join a support group if one is available. There is no evidence for long-term psychological sequelae of genetic pregnancy termination.

Thoughtful genetic counseling challenges the skills of the physician in diagnosis, analysis, communication, and support. Rarely is it the province of only one person, but rather it requires the collaborative efforts of an experienced team. From the initial evaluation through the development of the genetic model and identification of those at risk to the completion of the transfer of information, the use of these skills serves to enable patients and their families to make intelligent, informed, and reasoned decisions for their futures.

Collins FS, Gelehrter TD: Principles of Medical Genetics. Baltimore, Williams & Wilkins, 1989. *A new and good general human genetics textbook, up-to-date in molecular material.*

Frets P, Duivenvoorden H, et al.: Factors influencing the reproductive decision after genetic counseling. Am J Med Genet 35:496–502, 503–509, 1990. *Others in the series of articles on the psychodynamics of genetic counseling.*

Hsia YE, Silverberg R, et al.: Counseling in Genetics. New York, Alan R. Liss, 1979. *Thorough discussion of all aspects of genetic counseling by several very experienced geneticists and counselors.*

Lippman-Hand A, Fraser F-C: Genetic counseling—the post-counseling period. II. Making reproductive choices. Am J Med Genet 4:73, 1979. *The third in a series of articles on the psychodynamics of genetic counseling.*

McKusick V: Mendelian Inheritance in Man. 9th ed. Baltimore, Johns Hopkins University Press, 1990. *Exhaustive catalog of mendelian phenotypes.*

Milunsky A: Genetic Disorders and the Fetus: Diagnosis, Prevention and Treatment. 2nd ed. New York, Plenum Press, 1986. *Extensive textbook on prenatal diagnosis.*

Weatherall DG: The New Genetics and Clinical Practice. Oxford, Oxford University Press, 1985. *Details about modern methods of molecular diagnosis of genetic disorders.*

36 Approach to the Patient with Cardiovascular Disease

Thomas W. Smith

Common to the care of all patients with cardiovascular disease is a data base on which sound diagnostic and therapeutic decisions can be made. This chapter outlines an approach to cardiovascular data collection that emphasizes general principles and strategies and is intended to complement the more specific consideration of disease entities in the chapters that follow. One of the endlessly fascinating aspects of medicine is that each patient presents to the physician a unique story of his or her past history and present illness. Textbook descriptions of disease therefore convey at best a set of findings that the author regards as typical but that never quite fit in detail the findings present in any one individual patient. Hence, an open mind is essential during the evaluation of each patient so that diagnostic possibilities are not overlooked or prematurely discarded.

A dazzling array of diagnostic tests is now available for the evaluation of patients with evident or suspected cardiovascular disease. Sensitivity and specificity are known, or can be estimated, for each method under a given set of clinical circumstances. Redundancy must be avoided to achieve a favorable cost:benefit ratio (e.g., radionuclide ventriculography often yields information regarding ventricular function that can be obtained from a two-dimensional echocardiogram, and both methods may be superfluous if the patient undergoes left ventriculography as part of a cardiac catheterization procedure). The emerging discipline of decision analysis (see Ch. 20), with emphasis on the proper application of Bayes' theorem, should help in formulating strategies for the development of an adequate cardiovascular data base.

Although accurate diagnosis is a key element in patient care, prognosis is also vitally important to the patient and often to the physician, who must formulate a program of treatment. Information over and above that needed to establish a diagnosis is typically required to allow an accurate prediction of outcome. This exercise in probability statistics is challenging and deserves careful attention as an essential component of the comprehensive care of the patient.

COMPONENTS OF THE CARDIOVASCULAR WORKUP

The three essential components of the clinical data base are the history, physical examination, and laboratory studies. Although this sequence of data acquisition is typically followed, the value of returning to the bedside (often repeatedly) to refine the assessment of historical information and physical findings as the workup progresses cannot be overstated.

History

The cardinal symptoms of cardiovascular disease are listed in Table 36–1. *Dyspnea* (an abnormally uncomfortable awareness of breathing) and the related items in the first line are discussed in detail in Ch. 40. Historical information is particularly important in distinguishing among heart failure, pulmonary disease (including pulmonary emboli), metabolic disturbances producing aci-

dosis, and anxiety as factors causing dyspnea. The nature of onset and duration of symptoms, relation to position, and precipitating and alleviating factors all provide important clues to the underlying pathophysiologic process.

Fatigue and *weakness* are common to many physical and emotional disease states and are nonspecific; nevertheless, it is important to record quantitative information in the history (e.g., flights of stairs or distance on level ground that the patient can manage) for current and future reference. *Cough*, initially dry and irritative, is a common early manifestation of elevated left-heart filling (and hence pulmonary venous) pressures. *Hemoptysis* should be characterized in regard to color and nature of admixture of blood and sputum to help distinguish between pulmonary (e.g., bronchitis, pulmonary infarction) and cardiac causes (e.g., pulmonary edema, hemorrhage from loss of bronchial vein integrity, as in mitral stenosis). *Cyanosis* is discussed in Ch. 40.

Chest pain or discomfort should be characterized in terms of location, quality, course of onset and offset, duration, and precipitating and alleviating factors. Pain due to ischemic heart disease is considered in Ch. 48, but one should remember that the original meaning of the term angina is *choking* rather than pain, and it is often described by the patient with words such as "pressure" or "squeezing" discomfort. Pericardial pain is more likely to be left sided, sharp in character, and related to breathing and position. Pleuritic pain also tends to be localized and sharp and is related to breathing or coughing. Chest wall pain is often long lasting and associated with tenderness to pressure applied at the trigger area.

Palpitation refers to an awareness of the heart beat, usually occurring in response to a change in cardiac rhythm or rate or by increased contractile force. It is a common anxiety-related symptom in patients without heart disease. Awareness of irregularity of the heart beat is more closely correlated with cardiac rhythm disturbances. *Dizziness* and *syncope* are frequent manifestations of cardiac arrhythmias and demand careful evaluation, often with 24-hour electrocardiographic (ECG) monitoring. These symptoms also occur as a consequence of orthostatic hypotension due to reduced blood volume, vasodilator drugs, or autonomic dysfunction. Obstruction to venous return from any cause also predisposes to these symptoms. *Claudication* refers to pain or an uncomfortable sensation of tiredness, usually in calf and/or thigh muscles, that occurs in response to exertion and is relieved by rest. This common symptom of peripheral arterial insufficiency is further discussed in Ch. 54.

TABLE 36–1. CARDINAL SYMPTOMS OF CARDIOVASCULAR DISEASE

Dyspnea, orthopnea, paroxysmal nocturnal
  dyspnea, wheezing
Fatigue, weakness
Cough, hemoptysis
Cyanosis
Chest pain or discomfort
Palpitations, dizziness, syncope
Edema
Pain in extremities with exertion
  (claudication)

Edema refers to swelling, usually of a dependent part of the body, due to retention of excess fluid. It is typically maximal in the feet at the end of the day and resolves, at least partially, by morning. Local factors such as deep venous disease predispose to unilateral edema. Patients confined to bed usually accumulate fluid in the sacral area.

The Physical Examination

Five elements constitute the cardiovascular physical examination. These are

1. Physical appearance
2. Venous pressure and pulse contours
3. Arterial pressure and pulse contours
4. Movement of the heart
5. Auscultation

PHYSICAL APPEARANCE. This is important in assessing the nature and severity of heart disease and also in providing clues to systemic diseases that affect the heart. Important cardiac problems are frequently encountered in patients with Marfan's syndrome, Turner's syndrome, Down's syndrome, the pickwickian syndrome, scleroderma, and thyroid disease, all of which are often recognizable on the basis of careful inspection of the patient's appearance. The funduscopic examination yields important information with regard to hypertension, diabetes mellitus, and sometimes infective endocarditis (Roth's spots). Cheyne-Stokes respirations are often seen in patients with advanced heart failure. Sometimes a highly specific cardiac diagnosis can be made on the basis of the physical appearance, such as the association of atrial septal defect with the bony abnormalities of the upper extremity that constitute the Holt-Oram syndrome. Cyanosis and clubbing of the fingertips indicate right-to-left shunting in patients with congenital heart disease.

VENOUS PRESSURE AND PULSE. Both external and internal jugular veins require careful inspection: external for estimation of mean right atrial pressure and internal for wave form as well as pressure. Figure 36–1 illustrates the typical features of the normal jugular venous pulse and indicates the terminology applied to the various aspects of this wave form. The A wave reflects right atrial contraction and occurs immediately prior to the carotid arterial pulse and first heart sound. The X descent occurs with right atrial relaxation and continues with early right ventricular contraction. The C wave, often superimposed on the beginning of the A wave, coincides with the carotid pulse itself.

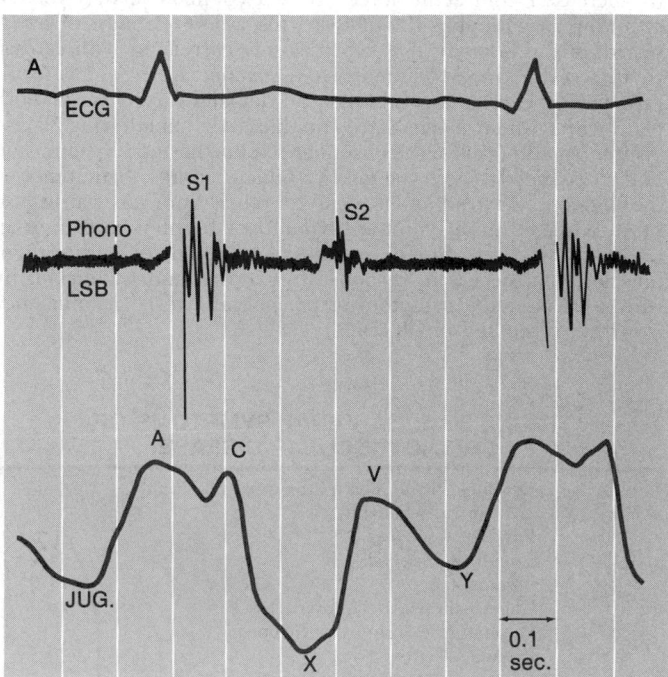

FIGURE 36–1. Normal jugular venous pulse.

The V wave in the normal jugular venous pulse represents passive right atrial filling behind a closed and competent tricuspid valve. The Y descent reflects sudden termination of the V wave with right ventricular relaxation and opening of the tricuspid valve. The X descent is normally the more evident of the two declining phases of the jugular venous pulse. These phenomena are best noted with the patient so positioned that the top of the venous column can be observed throughout the cardiac cycle. Estimation of the central venous pressure is accomplished by estimating its height in centimeters above the sternal angle of Louis, adding 5 cm to allow for the normal relation of the right atrium to the external chest wall. Normal venous pressure varies from 5 to 10 cm of H_2O. The A wave tends to be accentuated in disease states characterized by reduced right ventricular compliance, tricuspid stenosis, or rhythm disturbances in which the atrium contracts against a closed tricuspid valve ("cannon" A waves). Tricuspid insufficiency produces systolic or regurgitant waves that obliterate the normal jugular venous V waves. Abnormalities associated with pericardial disease are discussed in Ch. 51.

ARTERIAL PRESSURE AND PULSE. Examination of the arterial pulse yields critically important information regarding the cardiovascular system. Arterial pressure should always be measured in both arms because of the unexpected discrepancies that are encountered in disease states or that are occasionally due to congenital anomalies. Use of a cuff of appropriate size is essential, and the arterial blood pressure should be recorded in both supine and standing position to assess volume status and the adequacy of reflex vasoconstrictor responses. Pulsus paradoxus refers to a decrease in systolic blood pressure of greater than 10 mm Hg on inspiration and is a typical feature of pericardial tamponade.

The carotid arteries provide the most direct reflection of cardiac activity because of their central location in proximity to the left ventricle and aorta. The amplitude of the carotid pulse is typically increased under circumstances associated with higher cardiac output, including fever, anemia, hyperthyroidism, and arteriovenous fistulas. The regularity (or lack thereof) indicates disturbances of rhythm or hemodynamics as in pulsus alternans. The wave form of the arterial pulse yields clues regarding runoff from the aorta, as in aortic insufficiency or arteriovenous fistula; a bisferious quality is often present in aortic insufficiency and should be distinguished from the spike-and-dome contour encountered in patients with hypertrophic cardiomyopathy with obstruction (i.e., hypertrophic subaortic stenosis). The volume of the carotid pulse is typically reduced in heart failure and in mitral or aortic stenosis. Peripheral arterial pulses other than the carotid pulses should be felt and compared, with particular attention to a pulse delay at the femoral artery as a manifestation of coarctation of the aorta. Patients with claudication should have their lower extremity pulses examined both at rest and with exercise, since the latter maneuver often accentuates asymmetries.

MOVEMENT OF THE HEART. Observation, palpation, and percussion are the traditional means for physical examination of cardiac movements. Inspection of the precordium reveals asymmetries that serve as clues to chronic cardiac hypertrophy, particularly in congenital disease. The partial left lateral decubitus position is optimal for observation as well as palpation of the left ventricle in most patients. Diffuse left parasternal cardiac movement is often best appreciated with the heel of the palm, whereas higher frequency events (S_1, ejection clicks, S_2, opening snap, and thrills) are best felt with firm pressure and the tactile use of the fingertips. Precordial movements should be described at the apex, left parasternal area, and the right and left second intercostal spaces. The normal tapping impulse of the left ventricular apex is replaced by a more diffuse and sometimes dyskinetic impulse in patients with cardiac enlargement from a variety of causes. Displacement of the left ventricle is typically downward and to the left with cardiomegaly. Systolic overload with concentric hypertrophy increases the duration of the apex impulse and can be distinguished from the hyperdynamic impulse accompanying volume overload lesions, such as mitral or aortic insufficiency. Right ventricular enlargement produces a left parasternal systolic lift that is occasionally mimicked by the anterior motion of the heart with systolic expansion of the left atrium in the presence of severe mitral insufficiency. Pulmonary hypertension may be accompanied by a palpable pulmonary artery segment in the second left interspace and by a palpable pulmonic component of the second sound (P_2). Prominent third or fourth heart sounds can often be palpated as well as heard.

Thus, with the data gleaned from physical appearance, the venous and arterial pulse characteristics, and cardiac motion properties, the experienced clinician is armed with substantial information about cardiac anatomy and physiology before employing the stethoscope.

AUSCULTATION. Satisfactory cardiac auscultation requires a stethoscope that fits the ears snugly but comfortably and has the shortest tubing consistent with convenient use. The examination should be carried out in a quiet area, which sometimes requires moving the patient to a more suitable place when ambient noise levels are excessive. A systematic approach, as in all facets of physical examination, is important. Apart from the most obvious and dramatic auscultatory events, one generally hears only what one listens for. Beginning at the apex, the timing and nature of the first and second heart sounds are determined. Separable components of these events should be carefully noted. If the first sound has more that one component, S_4, asynchronous closure of mitral and tricuspid valves, and ejection clicks must be distinguished. Higher frequency transient systolic and diastolic sounds are listed in Table 36–2 and should be listened for explicitly. Murmurs should be identified and characterized, using the diaphragm to distinguish high-frequency events and the bell for lower frequency sounds. The examination should include listening with the patient sitting and leaning forward, supine, and in the left lateral decubitus position. Position may have a particularly marked effect on the character and loudness of pericardial friction rubs. Standing, exercising, isometric handgrip, and the Valsalva maneuver are important in specific circumstances, as outlined in the chapters that follow.

The plethora of sophisticated laboratory examinations now available should refine, rather than render obsolete, physical diagnostic skills. Every opportunity should be taken to review physical findings with the additional insights provided by noninvasive and invasive laboratory studies.

Laboratory Studies

Laboratory studies of patients with cardiovascular disease run the gamut from routine examinations (chest radiograph, electrocardiogram) that should be performed on virtually every patient being evaluated to highly sophisticated techniques that would be appropriate for specific individual subsets of patients. Remarkable progress in the past decade in noninvasive techniques now permits adequate evaluation of many patients without need for cardiac catheterization. Nevertheless, catheterization and angiography are essential components of the cardiovascular workup in most patients with advanced valvular or coronary artery disease.

ELECTROCARDIOGRAM. The standard 12-lead electrocardiogram remains a cornerstone of the clinical cardiologic evaluation. Although vectorcardiography and other more sophisticated approaches have their proponents, the standard 12-lead ECG

remains a highly cost-effective screening test. It is reviewed in detail in Ch. 39.4. Detailed clinicopathologic correlations accumulated over more than two generations provide a wealth of background information. The most important applications are in assessment of cardiac arrhythmias, in which analysis of the P wave and the QRS complex, and their temporal relation to each other, forms the basis for the definition and clinical diagnosis of rhythm disturbances. Existence and location of myocardial ischemia and infarction represent other important components of the information inherent in the ECG. Right and left ventricular hypertrophy patterns, as well as right and left atrial abnormalities, are well described. Characteristic electrocardiographic findings are frequently important in the assessment of congenital heart disease.

The 12-lead electrocardiogram augmented with a standard exercise protocol is important in the assessment of ischemic heart disease (see Ch. 48.1). Both establishment of coronary artery obstructive disease and useful prognostic information are available from this study. Risk stratification in patients who have had myocardial infarctions is heavily dependent upon the exercise ECG. The predictive accuracy of the exercise ECG examination for coronary artery disease in specific patient subsets is well defined. It is important not only to classify ST-segment depression but also to assess duration of exercise, maximum heart rate achieved, blood pressure response, time of onset of ST-segment depression, and time of resolution. A decrease in blood pressure during exercise correlates closely with advanced three-vessel or left main coronary artery obstructive disease. As in all such examinations, the diagnostic and predictive accuracy is dependent on the population of patients studied, and false-positive exercise ECG results are relatively commonly encountered in women, especially from populations with a low predicted incidence of obstructive coronary artery disease.

Assessment of symptoms of palpitations, dizziness, and syncope now rests heavily on the 24-hour (Holter) ECG. This approach is essential in the evaluation of cardiac arrhythmias and of response to antiarrhythmic drug regimens. Recent technical advances permit the assessment of transient ST-segment and T-wave changes reflecting myocardial ischemia, findings of particular value in the assessment of patients with variable threshold or "silent" ischemia.

CHEST RADIOGRAPHY. Posteroanterior and lateral views are a component of virtually every cardiovascular evaluation. Important findings are reviewed in Ch. 39.1. Chest radiography always supplements, rather than replaces, physical examination, since the two approaches yield complementary information. Echocardiography yields more accurate and specific information regarding individual chamber sizes. Evidence of calcification of cardiac structures should be sought on the chest radiograph, although fluoroscopic examination and echocardiography both tend to be more sensitive for this purpose.

ECHOCARDIOGRAPHY. This noninvasive technique uses high-frequency sound waves that reflect from cardiac structures, permitting the imaging of cardiac anatomy and motion. The technique is considered in detail in Ch. 39.3. Two-dimensional echocardiography has largely replaced the M-mode display, although the latter provides superior quantitative details regarding wall thickness and chamber dimensions. This examination is now standard in the assessment of ventricular function and valvular abnormalities.

The Doppler method is the standard technique for assessment of intracardiac blood flow, shunts, and valvular stenosis and regurgitation. In selected patients, echocardiographic information, together with full clinical assessment, permits valvular surgery without prior cardiac catheterization. Echocardiography is diagnostic in cases of left atrial myxoma, mitral valve prolapse, and hypertrophic cardiomyopathy. It is frequently useful for visualization of vegetations on heart valves in patients with infective endocarditis. Pericardial fluid and tamponade are routinely assessed by echocardiography, which is also useful in guiding pericardiocentesis.

Transesophageal echocardiography is available in most referral centers and gives particularly high-resolution images of the heart and proximal great vessels.

TABLE 36–2. SYSTOLIC AND DIASTOLIC SOUNDS

Systolic
  Early
    Ejection sounds (aortic, pulmonary)
    Systolic ejection clicks (mitral apparatus)
    Opening click of aortic valve mechanical prosthesis
  Mid to late
    Mitral valve clicks (prolapse)

Diastolic
  Early
    Opening snaps
    Early third sound of pericardial constriction or mitral regurgitation
    Opening click of mitral valve mechanical prosthesis
    "Tumor plop" of atrial myxoma
  Mid
    Third heart sound or gallop (S_3)
    Summation gallop ($S_3 + S_4$)
    Pericardial knock
  Late (presystolic)
    Fourth heart sound (S_4)

High-resolution B-mode ultrasonography with color Doppler imaging is of substantial value in the noninvasive diagnosis of both peripheral arterial (including carotid) and venous disease.

RADIONUCLIDE STUDIES. These tests involve injection of radioisotopes into the circulation with detection by special instrumentation. One of the most useful of these techniques is radionuclide ventriculography, also referred to as gated blood pool scanning. Technetium 99m (^{99m}Tc) bound to albumin stays in the blood pool and permits imaging of the size and contractile function of cardiac chambers. Special applications include detection of intracardiac shunts by "first pass" methods. Most commonly, the technique is used to assess left and right ventricular function by measurement of end-systolic and end-diastolic dimensions, permitting evaluation of regional wall motion and the derivation of values for right and left ventricular ejection fractions.

Scanning with radioactive thallium (^{201}Tl) permits assessment of myocardial perfusion. The radioisotope is injected at maximum exercise and localizes in cardiac muscle as a function of coronary flow; areas of diminished myocardial perfusion are visualized as "cold" spots on the myocardial image. Viable but ischemic myocardium subsequently fills in with more homogeneous ^{201}Tl distribution, whereas previous infarction produces a persistent cold spot.

Scanning with ^{99m}Tc pyrophosphate can be used to visualize areas of myocardial necrosis and is occasionally useful in evaluation of patients with suspected myocardial infarction when other studies are equivocal.

CLINICAL APPLICATION. The safety of noninvasive techniques tempts the clinician to overutilize them, since no physical harm is likely to result and some incremental information is often obtained. Cost-effectiveness considerations must be kept in mind, however, and the use of these tests must be orchestrated so that the essential clinical decisions can be made without unnecessary cost and inconvenience to the patient. Some elements of noninvasive test information are superfluous if the patient is destined to undergo complete evaluation by cardiac catheterization and angiography. Newer noninvasive techniques including fast computed tomographic (CT) scanning and magnetic resonance imaging (MRI) need to be incorporated into cost-effective diagnostic strategies as these methods become more widely available.

CARDIAC CATHETERIZATION. This invasive approach provides information on intracardiac and vascular pressures and flows. Gradients across stenotic valves and great vessels can be measured and systemic and pulmonary blood flows quantified. Contrast agents can be injected selectively to define the anatomy of cardiac chambers, coronary vessels, and pulmonary and peripheral vessels. The technique of cardiac catheterization and angiography is considered in detail in Ch. 39.5. This diagnostic approach is usually employed when a cardiac surgical or catheter-based interventional procedure is under consideration.

Other applications of cardiac catheterization include electrophysiologic studies with pacing and mapping procedures to evoke and localize the source of cardiac rhythm disturbances. Endomyocardial biopsy is a standard technique for the assessment of transplant rejection, unexplained cardiomyopathy, suspected myocarditis, suspected infiltrative diseases such as cardiac amyloidosis, or doxorubicin cardiotoxicity.

Cardiac catheterization procedures form the basis for therapeutic interventions, including percutaneous transluminal coronary angioplasty, or ablative procedures, such as those for the management of patients with Wolff-Parkinson-White syndrome refractory to drug therapy.

Although cardiac catheterization involves substantial expense and a small but finite risk of morbidity and mortality, this approach remains indispensable in the assessment of a wide array of cardiac problems that remain unsolved after complete noninvasive assessment. A frequent problem is the adult patient with a chest pain syndrome consistent with angina pectoris but with a negative or equivocal exercise electrocardiogram. Such patients may be severely disabled by these symptoms and attendant anxiety. Even though coronary artery surgery may not loom as a likely therapeutic approach, coronary arteriography can be of substantial value, especially when normal coronary anatomy is found, directing the diagnostic evaluation in more productive directions and restoring a previously incapacitated patient to full activity.

TABLE 36–3. A COMPARISON OF THREE METHODS OF ASSESSING CARDIOVASCULAR DISABILITY

Class	New York Heart Association Functional Classification	Canadian Cardiovascular Society Functional Classification	Specific Activity Scale
I	Patients with cardiac disease but without resulting limitations of physical activity. Ordinary physical activity does not cause undue fatigue, palpitation, dyspnea, or anginal pain.	Ordinary physical activity, such as walking and climbing stairs, does not cause angina. Angina with strenuous or rapid or prolonged exertion at work or recreation.	Patients can perform to completion any activity requiring ≥7 metabolic equivalents, e.g., can carry 24 lb up eight steps; carry objects that weigh 80 lb; do outdoor work (shovel snow, spade soil); do recreational activities (skiing, basketball, squash, handball, jog/walk 5 mph).
II	Patients with cardiac disease resulting in slight limitation of physical activity. They are comfortable at rest. Ordinary physical activity results in fatigue, palpitation, dyspnea, or anginal pain.	Slight limitation of ordinary activity. Walking or climbing stairs rapidly, walking uphill, walking or stair climbing after meals, in cold, in wind, or when under emotional stress, or only during the few hours after awakening. Walking more than two blocks on the level and climbing more than one flight of ordinary stairs at a normal pace and in normal conditions.	Patient can perform to completion any activity requiring ≥5 metabolic equivalents but cannot and does not perform to completion activities requiring ≥7 metabolic equivalents, e.g., have sexual intercourse without stopping, garden, rake, weed, roller skate, dance fox trot, walk at 4 mph on level ground.
III	Patients with cardiac disease resulting in marked limitation of physical activity. They are comfortable at rest. Less than ordinary physical activity causes fatigue, palpitation, dyspnea, or anginal pain.	Marked limitation of ordinary physical activity. Walking one to two blocks on the level and climbing more than one flight in normal conditions.	Patient can perform to completion any activity requiring ≥2 metabolic equivalents but cannot and does not perform to completion any activities requiring ≥5 metabolic equivalents, e.g., shower without stopping, strip and make bed, clean windows, walk 2.5 mph, bowl, play golf, dress without stopping.
IV	Patient with cardiac disease resulting in inability to carry on any physical activity without discomfort. Symptoms of cardiac insufficiency or of the anginal syndrome may be present even at rest. If any physical activity is undertaken, discomfort is increased.	Inability to carry on any physical activity without discomfort—anginal syndrome *may be* present at rest.	Patient cannot or does not perform to completion activities requiring ≥2 metabolic equivalents. *Cannot* carry out activities listed above (Specific Activity Scale, Class III).

Reproduced by permission of the American Heart Association, Inc., from Goldman L, et al.: Comparative reproducibility and validity of systems for assessing cardiovascular functional class: Advantages of a new specific activity scale. Circulation 64:1227, 1981.

ELEMENTS OF A COMPLETE CARDIOVASCULAR DIAGNOSIS

Coordinated use of the history, physical examination, and laboratory studies permits a full diagnosis to be established in nearly all patients, including the following five elements:

1. Etiology of the cardiovascular problem
2. Anatomic abnormalities, including quantification to the extent possible
3. Physiologic status, including pressures, flows, and relevant gradients
4. Functional capacity (see Table 36–3)
5. Prognosis

Diagnostic Strategies

The most appropriate approach to a patient with suspected cardiovascular disease depends on the age and clinical presentation of the patient. A systolic ejection murmur at the base in a healthy teenager with an otherwise normal clinical evaluation, including ECG and chest radiograph, should ordinarily constitute adequate grounds for reassurance and avoidance of more elaborate studies. In an elderly patient with a systolic ejection murmur at the base, slow-rising carotid arterial pulses, and symptoms suggesting possible aortic stenosis, however, the chest radiograph, electrocardiogram, and echocardiogram with Doppler study are necessary, at a minimum, to determine whether further and more aggressive evaluation is warranted.

Since prevention is a highly desirable goal in cardiovascular medicine, certain diagnostic tests may be warranted in individual patients even in the absence of specific symptoms. In addition to careful history and physical examination, serum cholesterol measurements are appropriate in most patients, especially those with a family history of coronary artery disease, to assess risk and to guide therapeutic intervention. Use of exercise electrocardiography in sedentary, middle-aged individuals who are contemplating an exercise program remains controversial; many physicians would advocate this procedure, especially if the patient has risk factors for coronary artery disease.

There is no simple formula for defining the data base that is adequate for clearance of patients for noncardiac surgery. A simple, informal stress test of walking up one or more flights of stairs to observe the presence or absence of dyspnea or chest discomfort often obviates the need for more expensive and elaborate formal exercise testing. When extensive procedures such as peripheral vascular surgery or abdominal aortic aneurysm resection are contemplated in older patients with known or suspected coronary artery disease, aggressive diagnostic work-up, sometimes including cardiac catheterization and coronary arteriography, may be necessary because of limitations imposed by vascular disease on exercise electrocardiography or other approaches to assessment of cardiac reserve requiring exercise stress.

Perloff JK: Physical Examination of the Heart and Circulation. 2nd ed. Philadelphia, W. B. Saunders Company, 1990. *A pocket-sized compendium of up-to-date information, well illustrated and referenced.*

---

37 Epidemiology of Cardiovascular Disease

William T. Friedewald

Cardiovascular diseases have been the major health problem and the leading cause of death in the United States for several decades. The various statistics defining the magnitude of the problem are staggering. Estimates suggest that over 60 million people have some form of cardiovascular disease. In 1987, 977,000 people died of cardiovascular disease, which accounted for 46.0 per cent of all deaths. This problem also ranks as the leading reason for social security disability, limitation in physical activity, and hospital bed use, accounting for 46 million bed days in 1984. In 1986 it was estimated that cardiovascular diseases carried a direct health expenditure cost of $62 billion and additional indirect costs of $65 billion.

COMPONENTS OF CARDIOVASCULAR DISEASE

Cardiovascular disease is a general diagnostic category consisting of several separate diseases. One component, congenital heart disease, occurs at a rate of approximately 7 per 1000 live births, leading in 1986 to 5800 deaths, 3300 of which occurred before the age of 1 year. Another component, rheumatic heart disease, has had a dramatic 90 per cent decline over the last 40 years in the age-adjusted death rate (Table 37–1). Although 1.9 million people still have the disease, with approximately 6300 deaths in 1987, it has become a minor contributor to the overall cardiovascular disease problem. Coronary heart disease and cerebrovascular disease continue to be the major components of cardiovascular disease. Each year an estimated 1.25 million heart attacks occur (of which 800,000 are first attacks), leading to 512,000 deaths in 1987. Eight and one-half per cent of men and 3.7 per cent of women aged 45 to 64 years have overt coronary heart disease, and over the age of 65, these percentages increase to 17.8 in men and 12.0 in women. Cerebrovascular disease is found in 2.0 per cent of men (1.8 per cent of women) between the ages of 45 and 64 and 6.3 per cent of men (5.5 per cent of women) aged 65 and older, with 150,000 deaths due to this cause in 1987.

CARDIOVASCULAR DISEASE MORTALITY

These diseases have not always been the major health problem of the United States. In 1900 the five leading causes of death were (1) pneumonia and influenza combined, (2) tuberculosis, (3) diarrhea, enteritis, and ulceration of the intestines, (4) diseases of the heart, and (5) intracranial lesions of vascular origin. These categories all had rates greater than 100 per 100,000 population. By 1940, only two disease categories still had rates greater than 100 per 100,000: diseases of the heart and cancer and other malignant tumors. The infectious diseases had, to a large extent, been controlled, and their mortality rates have continued to fall. The "epidemic" of cardiovascular disease, especially coronary heart disease, had begun. By 1963, the mortality rate from coronary heart disease reached a peak; there has been a progressive and steady decline since then (Fig. 37–1). Despite the continued magnitude of the coronary heart disease problem, the focus recently has been on this dramatic reversal. Not only is the percentage of decline large, but also the impact on the total number of deaths in the United States is large and has led to an increase in life expectancy. In fact, the recent rate of improvement in life expectancy compares with that seen in the 1940's,

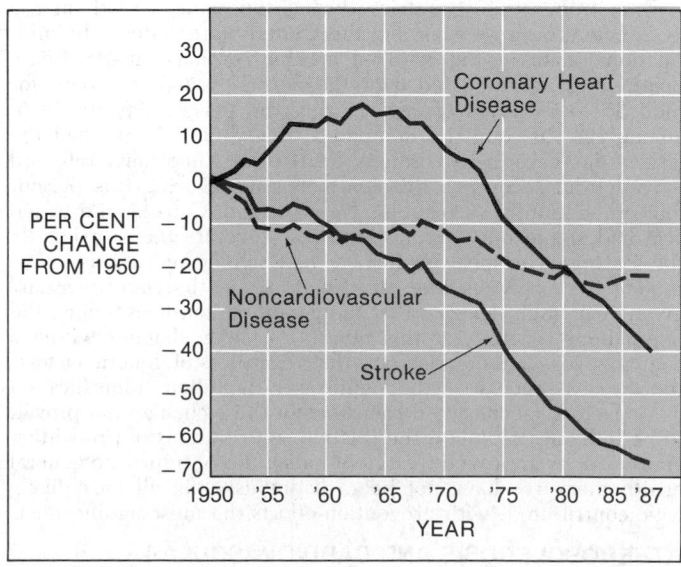

FIGURE 37–1. Per cent change in age-adjusted death rates in the United States, 1950 to 1987. (Source: Vital Statistics of the United States, National Center for Health Statistics.)

TABLE 37–1. AGE-ADJUSTED DEATH RATES* FOR MAJOR CARDIOVASCULAR DISEASES AND ALL OTHER CAUSES OF DEATH COMBINED IN THE UNITED STATES, 1905 TO 1987

Year	All Causes	All Causes Except Cardiovascular Diseases	Cardiovascular Diseases			
			Total	Coronary Heart Disease	Cerebrovascular Disease	Rheumatic Heart Disease
1905	1673.5	1315.9	357.6	NA	134.4	NA
1915	1443.4	1072.6	370.8	NA	123.3	NA
1925	1299.9	920.5	379.4	NA	114.2	NA
1935	1165.8	777.9	387.9	NA	94.4	NA
1945	947.4	556.9	390.5	NA	85.4	18.4
1955	764.6	368.5	396.1	200.0	83.0	11.2
1960	760.9	367.4	393.5	214.6	79.7	9.6
1965	739.0	364.8	374.2	215.8	72.7	7.4
1970	714.3	368.0	346.3	200.4†	66.3	6.3
1975	630.4	337.0	293.4	170.1†	53.7	4.8
1980	585.8	325.4	260.4	149.8	40.8	2.6
1985	546.1	318.5	227.6	125.5	32.3	1.9
1987	536.2	321.8	214.4	114.0	30.1	1.7

*Rate per 100,000 population age adjusted to the United States population, 1940.
†Comparability ratio applied to convert rate to level comparable to rates for 1980 and 1987.
NA = Not available.

when tuberculosis and other infectious diseases were being controlled. In 1987 a 45-year-old person could, on the average, expect to live 3.3 years longer than would have been expected in 1965. Estimates suggest that 45 per cent of this declining total mortality rate is due to the decline in coronary heart disease. The decline in death due to cerebrovascular disease, although even more impressive with a 66 per cent decrease since 1950, has been less of a contributing factor because cerebrovascular disease is less prevalent.

Declines in coronary heart disease mortality have been greater in young adults, but there has been a remarkable uniformity among blacks and whites and among men and women. Despite some early doubts when the reversal in rates was beginning, this decline in coronary mortality is real and not artifactual. It cannot be explained by (1) problems in trend measurement, such as a shift in classifying deaths as due to some other disease, (2) the waning of periodic respiratory epidemics that can contribute to the deaths of many patients with coronary heart disease, or (3) the depletion of the pool due to other causes of death in people expected to be susceptible to coronary heart disease. In addition, the decline has been too steep and long lasting to be reasonably explained by a simple random, temporary downturn. Determining precisely when the true decline began is complicated by these factors, but the increasing rate most likely changed to a decline in the mid 1960's, perhaps somewhat earlier in women.

Data from other countries during the same period offer a perspective on understanding the United States rates. The multinational data in Figure 37–2 are for coronary heart disease death rates age adjusted over the four 10-year age groups for men 35 to 74 years of age. During the period 1969 to 1985, among the 29 countries compared, the United States had the largest decrease in its coronary heart disease mortality rate and moved from second to thirteenth in rank. During this period, four other countries (Australia, New Zealand, Canada, and Israel) also had significant declines, whereas several others, primarily the Eastern European countries, had significant increases. Although the large absolute difference in rates by country in any given year might suggest that the genetic differences among the populations account for this range, the large changes within a country over time demonstrate that regardless of genetic factors, the disease process can be significantly modified. Identification of the factors specifically responsible for these changes has proved to be difficult. Although the relative contributions of prevention efforts versus improved treatment modalities or improved general health measures have not been distinguishable, all most likely have contributed, with prevention efforts the most significant.

ATHEROSCLEROSIS AND CARDIOVASCULAR DISEASE

The major pathologic process leading to disease of the heart and blood vessels is atherosclerosis, with hypertension either a contributing or a primary problem. Atherosclerosis in its most malignant and rare form begins in early childhood and becomes rapidly manifest as clinical coronary heart disease or sudden death in adolescence. The more common and highly prevalent form begins to develop in adolescence and slowly progresses over several decades, gradually occluding the arterial lumen and eventually manifesting clinically as a stroke, angina pectoris, claudication, myocardial infarction, or, most devastatingly, sudden death. Although the factors that may lead to an acute clinical event, such as arterial spasm, acute thrombosis, or embolism, are not completely understood, the underlying, if not immediate, problem is predominantly atherosclerosis.

Laboratory and clinical research efforts continue in the search for the underlying cause or causes of atherosclerosis, examining those factors that may initiate the process as well as those that may cause the milder, highly prevalent, presumed early forms of the disease (i.e., fatty streaks on the arterial surface) to progress in many individuals to the more serious, complicated, and obstructing form of the disease. Other research efforts are concentrating on the later, but still preclinical, stages of the process, searching for improved and more quantitative diagnostic techniques. Meanwhile, epidemiologic research efforts have made and continue to make major contributions to both prevention and treatment approaches to the cardiovascular disease problem through identification of personal and environmental characteristics that markedly increase an individual's probability of developing specific cardiovascular diseases.

RESEARCH IN CARDIOVASCULAR DISEASE

The research approach that has been repeatedly used in several large observational studies of cardiovascular disease is exemplified by the Framingham Heart Study, begun in 1948 in a relatively small town in Massachusetts. A sample (5209 men and women aged 30 to 62) of the total population agreed to be part of this study, undergoing thorough examinations every 2 years, with intense follow-up for the development of both fatal and nonfatal diseases. This population has remained under close scrutiny continuously since originally recruited and examined over the 2-year period from 1948 to 1950. Similar studies have been performed in other groups in the United States, as well as around the world. In Tecumseh, Michigan, 8624 men and women; in Evans County, Georgia, 3102 men and women; in Albany, New York, 1913 male civil servants; and in Chicago, Illionis, 1264 male gas company employees and 1983 male employees of the Western Electric Company were recruited and observed over several years. The critical elements of these studies have been the (1) inclusion of relatively large numbers of people to allow for important and sufficiently powerful subsample analyses, (2) enrollment of participants by methods that would make them reasonably representative of the total population from which they were recruited, (3) careful determination of all the variables (such

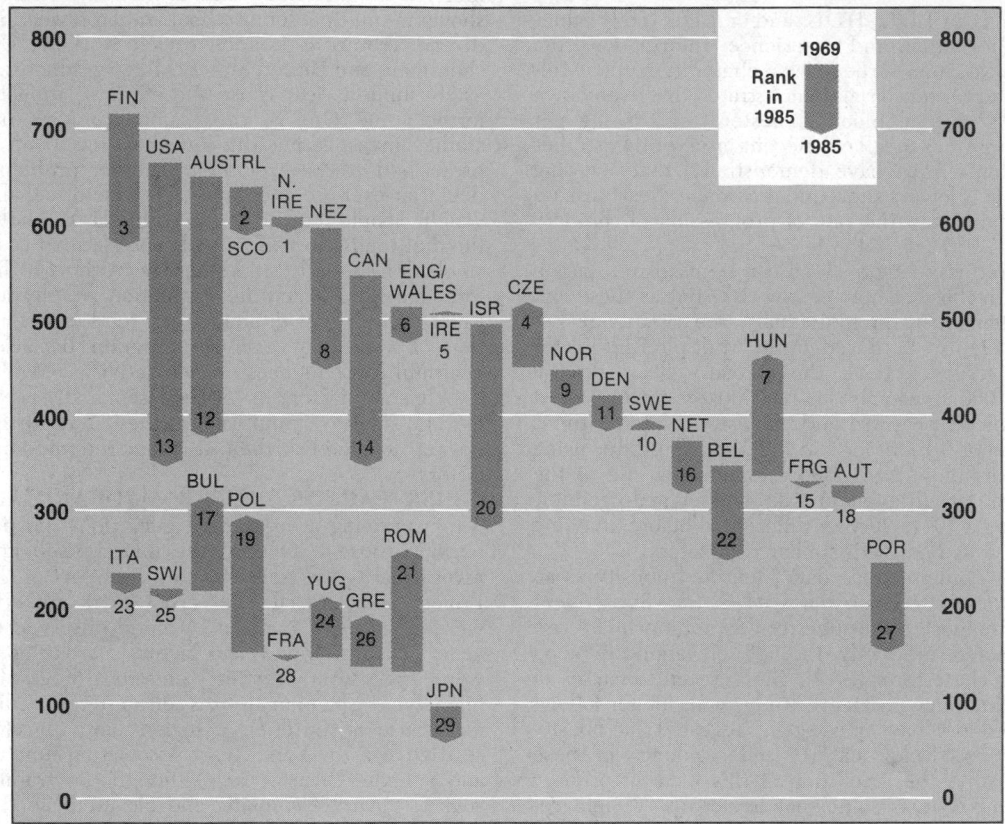

FIGURE 37–2. Age-adjusted coronary heart disease mortality rates per 100,000 population for men, ages 35 to 74, by country, 1969 to 1985. (Source: World Health Organization, World Health Statistics Annual.)

as height, blood pressure, smoking and dietary histories, and blood chemical determinations) in a standardized, reproducible manner, and (4) meticulous follow-up of all the participants for the development of fatal and nonfatal events recorded and defined in a predetermined and standardized fashion.

RISK FACTORS IN CARDIOVASCULAR DISEASE

From these United States studies and others worldwide, a consistent list of so-called risk factors for subsequent cardiovascular disease has been identified. These risk factors can be grouped into two broad categories: *unmodifiable* (such as older age, male gender, and family history of premature heart disease) and potentially *modifiable* (such as cigarette smoking, high blood pressure, high blood cholesterol level, diabetes, and the less prognostic factors of overweight, physical inactivity, and psychological factors). These factors can be used to identify clearly those in the population who are at especially high risk of developing cardiovascular disease.

CIGARETTE SMOKING. Cigarette smoking is established as a risk factor not only for lung cancer, emphysema, and bronchitis but also for coronary, cerebral, and peripheral vascular disease. This association has been seen in many countries, among widely diverse ethnic groups, in both sexes, and across various adult age groups. In addition, the risk increases with heavier cigarette use and the longer one has smoked. Equally important has been the observation that this increased risk falls rapidly over time when people quit smoking. For coronary heart disease, approximately 40 per cent of the increased risk is removed within 5 years of quitting, although it takes several more years of nonsmoking to achieve the level associated with someone who has never smoked.

HIGH BLOOD PRESSURE. High blood pressure is a powerful risk factor for cerebrovascular disease as well as for coronary heart disease and the atherosclerotic process directly. An estimated 58 million people have high blood pressure, defined as a level equal to or greater than 140 mm Hg systolic or 90 mm Hg

diastolic or as being on a regimen of antihypertensive medication. An important result of the epidemiologic studies was the observation that the relationship between blood pressure and cardiovascular risk was not only a positive one (a higher blood pressure resulted in a higher disease rate) but also a smooth one (there was no sharp breakpoint in the curve such that below a certain blood pressure level the risk remained constant or became nonexistent) Thus, the lower the blood pressure, within reasonable physiologic limits, the lower the level of risk. These observations prompted several important intervention trials, which have now clearly established the value of aggressively treating elevated blood pressure.

BLOOD CHOLESTEROL LEVELS. A clear and positive relationship between cholesterol levels and subsequent coronary heart disease has repeatedly been demonstrated. Later information refined the nature of this association but did not weaken it. Cholesterol in the plasma is transported by the lipoproteins. The cholesterol level associated with the low density lipoprotein (LDL) fraction was seen to be positively correlated with coronary heart disease, whereas the cholesterol associated with the high density lipoprotein (HDL) was negatively correlated (the higher the level, the lower the risk). These initial observations have been verified in several different populations and have been shown to be independent of each other, as well as of other known risk factors. As with blood pressure and cardiovascular disease risk, for both LDL cholesterol and HDL cholesterol, the curve is smooth (in the populations studied, there was no breakpoint in the curve observed). The evidence regarding HDL, although more recent than that for LDL, supports a powerful role for HDL in coronary heart disease risk and may explain some of the difference in risk between men and women, with women having higher average levels of HDL than do men. This ratio of LDL to HDL, an efficient method of combining the information from the two separate measures, has been shown to be more predictive than either measure alone. The appropriate clinical use of the mix of LDL, HDL, and/or LDL:HDL values must await more information and experience. Information from over 350,000 American men screened for eligibility in the Multiple Risk Factor Intervention Trial demonstrated that even down to and below levels of total blood cholesterol of 182 mg per deciliter, the risk continues to fall off. Recent intervention studies in hypercholesterolemic men have demonstrated that lowering blood cholesterol levels lowers subsequent coronary heart disease morbidity and mortality and the rate of progression of coronary atherosclerosis.

Each of these three risk factors alone can be used to separate groups of people into those at high or low risk. But as these risk factors occur simultaneously in individuals, the risk range becomes even larger (Fig. 37–3). Based on the Multiple Risk Factor Intervention Trial screenee data, the coronary heart disease mortality rate (1.6/1000 screenees) for nonsmokers in the lowest tertile of diastolic blood pressure and cholesterol is nine times lower than the rate (14.6/1000) for the highest risk group, using only these three variables. Age uniformly remains one of the most powerful factors at all levels of risk, as does male gender, with women realizing a 10- to 20-year differential before attaining the same level of risk as men with similar risk factors.

OBESITY. Initial epidemiologic data identified obesity as an important risk factor for coronary heart disease. Subsequent analyses, however, suggested that obesity was not a primary risk factor but rather acted indirectly through elevation of blood pressure and blood cholesterol levels. More recent analyses of the data from the Framingham Heart Study, with longer follow-up of people in the cohort, have once again suggested that obesity is indeed a primary risk factor that acts independently of these other factors. Clinically, the resolution of this issue of primary versus secondary causation is somewhat irrelevant. Weight reduction should lower the risk of coronary heart disease, whether it acts through a lowered blood pressure and/or cholesterol level or as a lowered risk factor itself.

DIABETES. Diabetes is a powerful and independent risk factor for cardiovascular disease, which remains the major cause of death in diabetic persons. An important remaining issue is whether an elevated blood glucose level is responsible for the observed higher rate of cardiovascular disease and, if it is, whether lowering or, preferably normalizing the glucose level will lower the risk. Regardless of the answers, for the present the important observation is that diabetic individuals are at higher risk of cardiovascular disease, and thus careful attention should be paid not just to the blood glucose level and its control but also to the other risk factors that may coexist in a given patient and additionally elevate the risk.

PHYSICAL INACTIVITY. An association between a less active lifestyle and increased risk of coronary heart disease has been shown in multiple longitudinal and cross-sectional studies in such diverse groups as London transit workers, United States longshoremen, and United States college graduates. However, studies establishing a clear cause-and-effect relationship have not been forthcoming. One of the major problems in the randomized studies investigating this question has been adherence to the prescribed exercise regimen. Another problem is that as people begin an exercise program, other factors change as well. Overweight people tend to lose weight, HDL cholesterol levels rise, the diet tends to change, and those individuals who are cigarette smokers frequently stop smoking. Although these covarying factors make the scientific evaluation of physical exercise as an isolated risk factor difficult, they tend to favor the recommendation of a prudent exercise program because of the multiple healthful consequences of such activity.

Other risk factors for cardiovascular disease have been identified in single or multiple studies, but further information is needed to establish them as independent, important prognostic factors.

RISK FACTORS AFTER MYOCARDIAL INFARCTION. After surviving a myocardial infarction, the primary risk factors become those related to the infarct itself and the damage to myocardial tissue (see Ch. 48.2). As part of the Coronary Drug Project clinical trial, 2789 post–myocardial infarction patients were given usual medical care and observed over a period of 5 years. The most powerful factors increasing risk in this group were persistent resting electrocardiographic abnormalities (namely ST segment depression and ventricular conduction defects), use of diuretics, a higher (and therefore more activity-restrictive) New York Heart Association functional classification, and a higher heart rate. Although the traditional risk factors, such as cigarette smoking and elevated blood cholesterol levels and blood pressure, remained prognostic, they were weaker factors overshadowed now by primary damage to the myocardium. In addition, with sudden death as the initial clinical presentation of cardiovascular disease in approximately one quarter of patients, it is obviously important to establish effective prevention modalities before the onset of clinical disease. Much current myocardial infarction research is focusing on therapeutic approaches that seek to minimize the extent of myocardial damage or even prevent the development of the infarct entirely. Nonetheless, the greatest potential for continuing and accelerating the decline in cardiovascular disease rates rests with prevention or treatment of the factors that lead to clinical presentation of disease and more profoundly of the factors that lead to or accelerate the atherosclerotic process.

CHANGES IN RISK FACTORS. Significant changes have

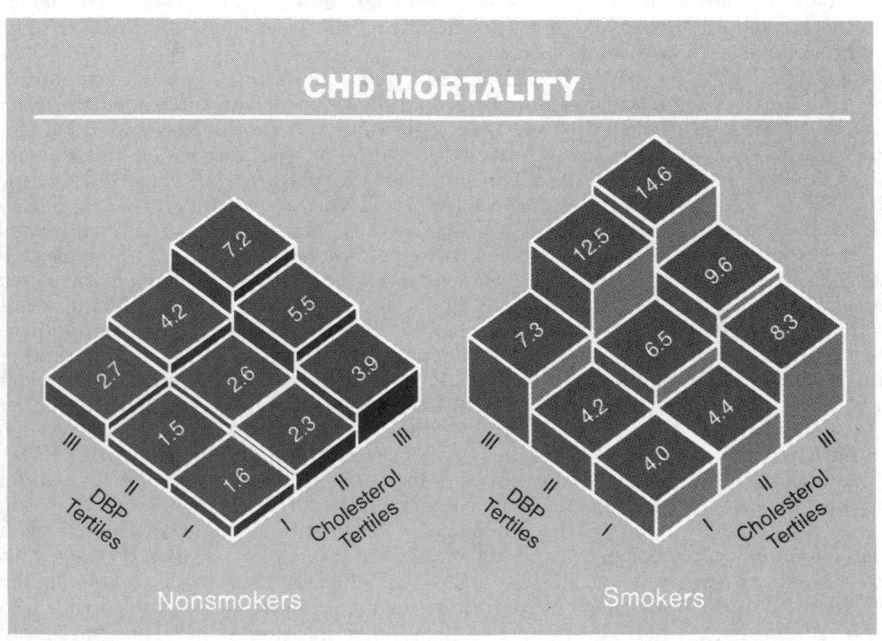

FIGURE 37–3. Age-adjusted CHD mortality rates per 1000 screenees for the Multiple Risk Factor Intervention Trial among smokers and nonsmokers for cholesterol tertiles (I = ≤ 196, II = 197–228, III = ≥ 229) and diastolic blood pressure (DBP) tertiles (I = ≤ 79, II = 80–87, III = ≥ 88).

occurred nationally in the major modifiable risk factors. In 1965, 50 per cent of men aged 20 or greater were cigarette smokers. In 1987 that figure had dropped to 32 per cent. For women the change has been modest, falling from 32 per cent in 1965 to 27 per cent in 1987. From 1965 to 1983, consumption of tobacco fell from 11.5 to 6.6 pounds per capita. In 1971 and 1972 only 16.5 per cent of people with high blood pressure (defined as a level equal to or greater than 160 mm Hg systolic or 95 mm Hg diastolic or as being on a regimen of antihypertensive medication) were effectively controlled. By the late 1970's, this figure had increased to 34 per cent nationally, and by the mid 1980's to 57 per cent in a sample from seven states. During this same period, visits to a physician for high blood pressure increased by 58 per cent. In addition, salt sales fell from 2.2 pounds per capita in 1972 to 1.4 in 1985. Average blood cholesterol levels in men fell from 217 mg per deciliter in the period between 1960 and 1966 to 211 in the late 1970's. Additional decline is suspected, but later national blood levels are not available. Annual food availability surveys, which serve as estimates of actual food consumption data (which are not routinely collected), show some dramatic changes between 1965–67 and 1983–85. The annual per capita availability in pounds of whole milk fell from 240 to 125, of eggs from 40 to 33, of meat from 124 to 121, and of animal fats and oils from 17 to 13. The availability in pounds of low-fat milk rose from 42 to 111, of poultry from 31 to 48, of fresh fruits from 79 to 88, and of vegetable fats and oils from 35 to 51. These impressive changes clearly demonstrate that the United States public can and will modify lifestyle behavior and suggest that additional gains in the prevention of the cardiovascular diseases can be made.

Goldman L, Cook EF: The decline in ischemic heart disease mortality rates: An analysis of the comparative effects of medical interventions and changes in lifestyle. Ann Intern Med 101:825, 1984. *An interesting attempt at quantification of the relative contribution of lifestyle and treatment factors to the decline in coronary heart disease mortality.*

Gordon T, Garcia-Palmieri MR, Kagan A, et al.: Differences in coronary heart disease in Framingham, Honolulu and Puerto Rico. J Chronic Dis 27:329, 1974. *A valuable comparison of the relationship between risk factors and subsequent coronary heart disease in three geographically and ethnically diverse populations.*

Health, United States, 1990. U.S. Department of Health and Human Services, Public Health Service, National Center for Health Statistics. DHHS Publication No. (PHS) 89–1232, March, 1989. *A frequently updated report presenting national data on morbidity and mortality, health delivery costs, and prevention programs with detailed tables.*

The Joint National Committee on Detection, Evaluation, and Treatment of High Blood Pressure: The 1984 Report of the Joint National Committee on Detection, Evaluation, and Treatment of High Blood Pressure. Arch Intern Med 144:1045, 1984. *A succinct and still authoritative review of the major clinical issues involving high blood pressure with a list of key references.*

Proceedings of the Conference on the Decline in Coronary Heart Disease Mortality. U.S. Department of Health, Education, and Welfare, Public Health Service. DHEW Publication No. (NIH) 79–1610, 1979. *A careful review of the issues bearing on the decline, with a useful appendix.*

Report of the Expert Panel on Detection, Evaluation, and Treatment of High Blood Cholesterol in Adults. U.S. Department of Health and Human Services, Public Health Services, National Institutes of Health. NIH Publication No. 89–2925, January, 1989. *A concise review of the major issues involving blood cholesterol and health risks, with a list of key references.*

The Surgeon General's Report on Nutrition and Health, 1988. U.S. Department of Health and Human Services, Public Health Service (PHS) Publication No. 88–50210, 1988. *A remarkably complete and reasonably concise summary of the relationship between major nutrients and disease.*

World Health Statistics Annual 1970–1990. World Health Organization. *International vital statistics and population data in tabular form by country.*

38 Cardiac Function and Circulatory Control

John Ross, Jr.

FUNCTIONAL ANATOMY OF THE HEART

The right ventricle is thin walled (3 to 4 mm) and somewhat irregular in shape, with the interventricular septum being largely formed by the left ventricle. The right ventricle is more compliant than the left, the upper limit of normal for right ventricular end-

diastolic pressure being 6 mm Hg (Table 38–1). The left ventricle has a thicker wall (8 to 9 mm), and the upper limit of normal for the left ventricular end-diastolic pressure is higher (12 mm Hg, Table 38–1). The left ventricle has an ellipsoidal shape, shortens more in its short axis, and normally empties about two thirds of its contents during ejection (see "ejection fraction," Table 38–1, average normal ejection fraction 65 per cent).

In addition to its four muscular chambers with accompanying valves, the heart has an electrical activation and conduction system, an autonomic neural supply, and a coronary circulation. The three main coronary arteries divide into lesser branches and eventually send small, penetrating vessels directly into the myocardium to supply a very dense capillary network. During coronary vasodilation, approximately one capillary per muscle cell provides a rich blood supply to the heavily working myocardium.

The electrical subsystem includes the sinoatrial (SA) node, comprising special pacemaker cells with continuous phase 4 depolarization, and the atrioventricular (AV) node, which exhibits delayed or decremental conduction, allowing atrial depolarization to precede ventricular depolarization by approximately 140 msec and atrial contraction thereby to serve as a "booster pump" for filling the ventricles. From the AV junction (or node) the electrical impulse rapidly spreads through the specialized His-Purkinje conduction system in approximately 40 msec to reach the ventricles, which contract slightly out of phase (left before right), left ventricular contraction beginning about 50 msec after the onset of the QRS complex.

The nervous subsystem supplying the heart consists of sympathetic and parasympathetic divisions. There is a rich network of sympathetic nerve terminals containing norepinephrine distributed throughout the atria and ventricles, which allows reflex regulation of the contractility of the myocardium via β-adrenergic receptors on the myocardial cells, which also are accessible to circulating catecholamines. Sympathetic nerves also innervate the coronary arteries. The sympathetic nerves also heavily innervate the SA node and AV junction, where increases in sympathetic tone increase the heart rate (enhanced rate of phase 4 depolari-

TABLE 38–1. PRESSURES AND VOLUMES IN THE NORMAL HEART

Pressures
Left sided
1. Left atrial pressure (normal mean pressure ≤ 12 mm Hg)
2. Left ventricular pressure
  a. Peak systolic pressure (same as aorta)
  b. Maximum dP/dt (1200–3500 mm Hg/sec)
  c. Left ventricular end-diastolic pressure (normal ≤ 12 mm Hg)
3. Aorta
  a. Systolic pressure (wide normal range, usually 100–150 mm Hg in adults)
  b. Diastolic pressure (wide normal range, usually 60–90 mm Hg in adults)
Right sided
1. Right atrial pressure (normal mean pressure ≤ 6 mm Hg)
2. Right ventricular pressure
  a. Peak systolic pressure (normal 15–30 mm Hg)
  b. Right ventricular end-diastolic pressure (normal ≤ 6 mm Hg)
3. Pulmonary artery
  a. Systolic pressure (normal 15–30 mm Hg)
  b. Diastolic pressure (normal 4–12 mm Hg)

Volumes
Left sided (at rest)
1. Left ventricular end-diastolic volume (normal 70–100 ml/m²)
2. Left ventricular end-systolic volume (normal 25–35 ml/m²)
3. Stroke volume (wide normal range, usually 40–70 ml/m²)
4. Ejection fraction (stroke volume divided by end-diastolic volume [normal 0.55–0.80])

Time-related measurements
1. Heart rate (wide normal range, usually 60–100 beats/minute)
2. Cardiac index (2.5–4.2 liters/min/m²)

Resistances
1. Systemic vascular resistance (770–1500 dynes sec cm⁻⁵)
2. Pulmonary vascular resistance (20–120 dynes sec cm⁻⁵)

zation), improve conduction velocity through the AV junction, and enhance synchronicity of the ventricular muscle. Enhanced strength of muscle contraction and increased velocity of both muscle contraction and relaxation accompany the increased heart rate during sympathetic stimulation, as with excitement or exercise. Parasympathetic fibers from the vagus nerves containing acetylcholine provide heavy innervation to the right and left atria, the SA node, and the AV junction, but there are few parasympathetic nerve terminals in the ventricles or the conduction system below the AV junction. Activation of the parasympathetic system has a slowing effect on the SA node (reduced rate of phase 4 polarization) and slows conduction through the AV junction, providing reciprocal neural control with the sympathetic nervous system. The contractility of atrial muscle is depressed by parasympathetic stimulation, but there is minimal effect on the ventricles because of their sparse innervation by vagal fibers.

Unlike skeletal muscle, cardiac muscle can regulate its contractility, or inotropic state. The force of cardiac muscle contraction, as well as its velocity, is normally regulated to a large degree by the amount of free calcium (Ca^{++}). Ca^{++} enters the cell when the calcium "gate" is open during phase 2 of the action potential (Fig. 38–1). This provides some of the activating Ca^{++}, but the action potential (and the increasing Ca^{++} itself) triggers much more Ca^{++} release from the sarcoplasmic reticulum (Fig. 38–1). Ca^{++} then binds to a subunit of troponin on the actin filament, causing a conformational change that uncovers the active site, and allows a tension-generating bond to occur between actin and myosin. More Ca^{++} allows more sites to bind. *Between* contractions, the sarcoplasmic reticulum rapidly and actively sequesters Ca^{++} (Fig. 38–1), so that the level at the myofilaments falls below that required for the actin-myosin interaction. Ca^{++} is also extruded more slowly against an electrical and chemical gradient. One important mechanism is a 3:1 sodium for calcium exchange across the sarcolemma (Fig. 38–1), which is driven mainly by the sodium gradient generated by the sodium/potassium ATPase membrane pump. Myocardial contractility is normally increased by catecholamines, which stimulate the β receptors and augment intracellular cyclic adenosine monophosphate (AMP), which leads to phosphorylation of the calcium channel and increased Ca^{++} influx during the action potential. Increasing extracellular calcium also augments myocardial contractility. Increased rate of Ca^{++} reuptake by the sarcoplasmic reticulum also occurs, leading to more rapid relaxation.

A variety of other mechanisms stimulate myocardial contractility in the normal and failing heart. Digitalis, by inhibiting membrane sodium/potassium ATPase, causes an increase of intracellular sodium, which decreases the sodium gradient, thereby leading to increased intracellular Ca^{++} and enhanced contractility (Fig. 38–1). β-Adrenergic agonist drugs such as dobutamine are used to treat the acutely failing heart as well. Some newer positive inotropic agents (e.g., amrinone and milrinone) act largely by inhibiting phosphodiesterase, leading to increased intracellular cyclic AMP, and other new drugs are under study that may increase the sensitivity of the myofilaments to Ca^{++}.

DIASTOLIC PROPERTIES OF THE HEART. A major feature of relaxed cardiac muscle is its intrinsic stiffness while at rest. Skeletal muscle, when isolated from its bony supports, can be overstretched easily, but cardiac muscle at first stretches readily but then, when stretched further, reaches an elastic limit, giving a much steeper relation between length and resting tension at long muscle lengths. Thus, within the walls of the ventricles, particularly the left ventricle, there is an extracellular network of collagen fibers which prevent overdistention with sudden changes in the venous return to the heart.

This property of heart muscle results in a nearly exponential relation between cardiac volume and pressure wherein small changes in volume produce large pressure changes as the ventricle is further filled beyond the upper limit of normal for left ventricular end-diastolic pressure (Fig. 38–2). Thus, the slope of this relation or chamber stiffness ($\Delta P/\Delta V$) increases as the ventricle is filled, and compliance ($\Delta V/\Delta P$) falls. Of course, when an abnormal chamber, such as a hypertrophied left ventricle, is compared with a normal chamber at the same cardiac volume, the entire diastolic pressure-volume relationship is shifted upward and steepened (Fig. 38–2), and the abnormal chamber is said to be stiffer or less compliant than normal. Even in chronically dilated hearts (as in the normal heart), it does not appear possible to stretch sarcomere lengths much beyond 2.2 μm, the optimum sarcomere length, so that the heart never appears to operate on a descending limb of the relation between resting sarcomere length and the active tension developed after muscle stimulation.

A thick, hypertrophied ventricle with decreased compliance causes increased resistance to filling, which can lead to diastolic cardiac dysfunction even when systolic function is maintained. In this setting atrial dilation and hypertrophy occur in order to maintain the atrial contribution to ventricular filling. The importance of this contribution is apparent in patients with severe hypertrophy caused, for example, by aortic stenosis or hypertrophic obstructive cardiomyopathy. Loss of an appropriately timed atrial contraction often results in marked exacerbation of dyspnea and left heart failure. In these patients, during sinus rhythm the left ventricular end-diastolic pressure is markedly elevated owing to a large A wave, whereas mean diastolic pressure, which is reflected back through the pulmonary veins

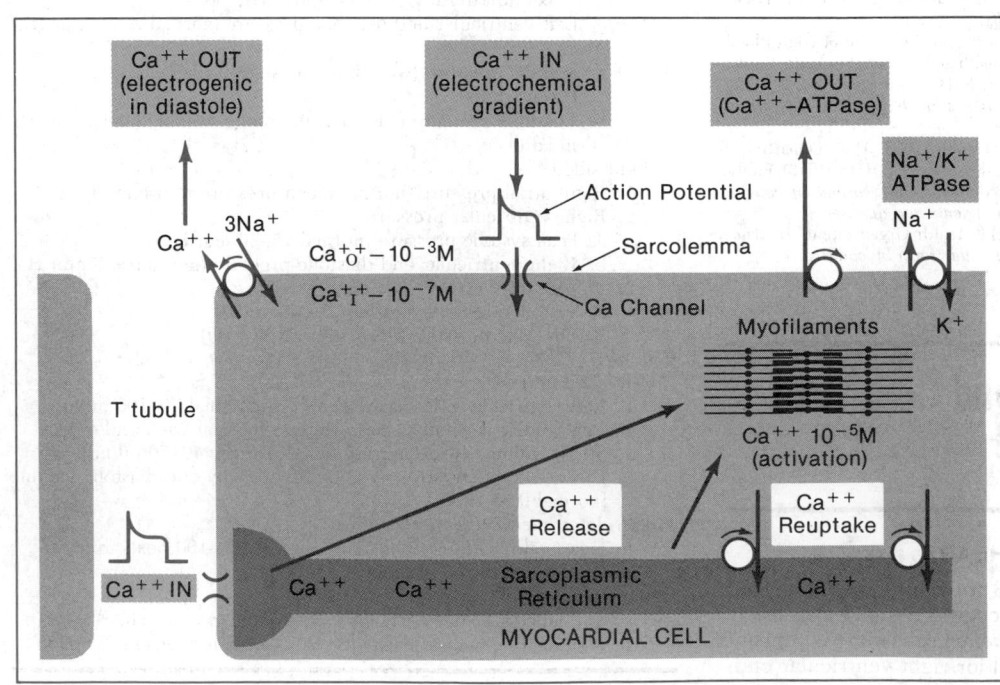

FIGURE 38–1. Movements of Ca^{++} during the cardiac cycle in a myocardial cell. Inward movement occurs across the sarcolemma during the action potential and also triggers Ca^{++} release from the sarcoplasmic reticulum. Free Ca^{++} is rapidly removed from the cytoplasm by the sarcoplasmic reticulum and slower extrusion across the sarcolemma occurs by Na^+-Ca^{++} exchange and by an active Ca^{++} pump (Ca^{++}-ATPase). (Adapted from West JB (ed.): Best and Taylor's Physiological Basis of Medical Practice. 11th ed. © 1985, the Williams & Wilkins Co., Baltimore.)

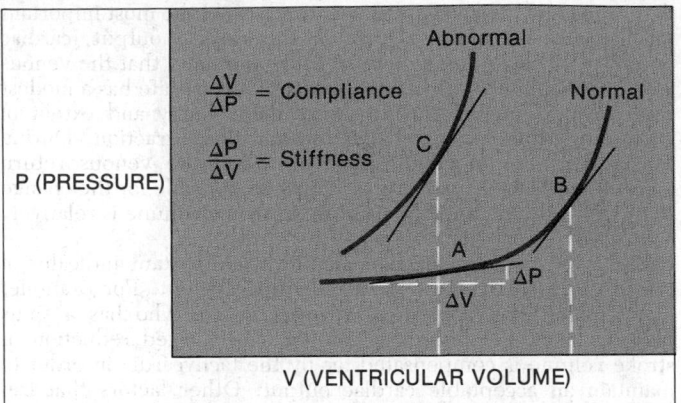

FIGURE 38–2. Diastolic pressure-volume curves of left ventricle under normal conditions and in the presence of severe ventricular hypertrophy (abnormal). Note the nearly exponential shape of the curves. The stiffness at any point on the normal curve ($\Delta P/\Delta V$) is shown by a tangent. Notice that ventricular stiffness increases (tangent A to tangent B) with ventricular filling to a larger ventricular volume. The stiffness of two ventricular chambers can be compared at a common volume, and comparison of the stiffness of the normal with that of the abnormal (hypertrophied) ventricle shows that the latter is markedly increased (tangent A versus tangent C). Compliance is the inverse slope ($\Delta V/\Delta P$) of the curve, and therefore the abnormal ventricle has a markedly reduced compliance. (Adapted from West JB (ed.): Best and Taylor's Physiological Basis of Medical Practice. 11th ed. © 1985, the Williams & Wilkins Co., Baltimore.)

into the lungs, is maintained at a lower level. When atrial contraction and the A wave "kick" are lost, as in atrial fibrillation, there is an increase in mean left atrial pressure in an attempt to maintain the same level of end-diastolic pressure and cardiac output.

CARDIAC CONTRACTION AND ITS REGULATION

DETERMINANTS OF CARDIAC PERFORMANCE. There are four major determinants of the performance of both ventricles. These factors are interrelated but considered separately for convenience.

1. Preload
2. Afterload
3. Contractility
4. Heart rate

The Preload. This refers to the loading condition on the heart at the end of diastole, which is primarily set by the venous return to the heart. In isolated heart muscle, it is defined as the force stretching the resting muscle to a given length prior to contraction. In the intact heart, it is less easily defined. Estimates of preload include measurements of the ventricular end-diastolic volume or the end-diastolic pressure (although the two are not linearly related, Fig. 38–2), and in acutely ill patients, it may be convenient to measure the ventricular "filling pressure" (the mean right or left atrial pressure, or the pulmonary artery wedge pressure) as an index of the preload. Within limits, as the preload increases, there is an increase in cardiac performance manifested by an increase in systolic pressure development or the volume of blood ejected. This represents the ascending limb of the familiar Frank-Starling relationship.

This overall relationship is often referred to as a ventricular function curve (Fig. 38–3). Some measure of cardiac performance, such as the stroke volume or stroke work (stroke volume × arterial pressure), is plotted as a function of some measure of the preload, such as the filling pressure or the end-diastolic pressure. The concept of the ventricular function curve is important, since it allows an objective assessment of the contractility of the ventricles. For example, the normal ventricle has a steep function curve, relatively small changes in end-diastolic pressure producing large changes in performance, whereas the failing ventricle has a downwardly displaced and flattened curve (Fig. 38–3). Such curves can permit a comparison between subjective signs or symptoms and objective measurements. Since the failing left ventricle operates near the peak of its ventricular function curve, the combination of a high filling pressure and low cardiac output

(Fig. 38–3, point D) explains the clinical picture of dyspnea and fatigue (see Ch. 40).

An important distinction must be made between the right atrial pressure, which represents the filling pressure of the right ventricle and can be estimated from the jugular veins, and the left atrial pressure, which is the filling pressure of the left ventricle. The mean left atrial pressure can be assessed from the mean pulmonary artery (or "capillary") wedge pressure, often measured by a flow-directed balloon catheter. In manipulating the volume status of the acutely ill patient, except in cases of isolated right ventricular failure, it is preferable to measure the left ventricular filling pressure, because the failing left ventricle usually has a more important role in determining arterial pressure and the forward cardiac output.

The Afterload. Afterload refers to the load against which the ventricle must contract when it ejects blood. In isolated heart muscle, it can be accurately defined as the load (or force) resisting shortening after the muscle is stimulated to contract and lift a load. In the intact heart, afterload is often estimated as the systolic arterial pressure. A better measure of the afterload is the systolic wall stress, which can be related to the systolic pressure, heart size, and wall thickness through the simplified Laplace relation:

$$\sigma = \frac{PR}{2h}$$

in which σ = wall stress or force/cross-sectional area, P = intraventricular pressure, R = radius of chamber (radius of curvature of the wall), and h = wall thickness.

The effect of afterload on performance is relatively straightforward. As arterial pressure is increased, the stroke volume tends to fall because the ventricle has greater difficulty in ejecting blood against a higher load. Such an effect is seen most clearly in experimental preparations when the preload is held constant (and cannot compensate for changes in afterload), and an inverse relation between the afterload (or systolic ventricular pressure) and the stroke volume is observed. In the intact circulation, changes in preload and afterload are closely related. For example, as the arterial pressure is increased in the normal heart, the left ventricle has greater difficulty in ejecting blood, which results in larger end-systolic and end-diastolic volumes, and the increasing preload then tends to restore the stroke volume.

Another way of representing ventricular function is the pressure-volume loop and the end-systolic pressure-volume relation (Fig. 38–4). (The slope of the latter relation has been used as a

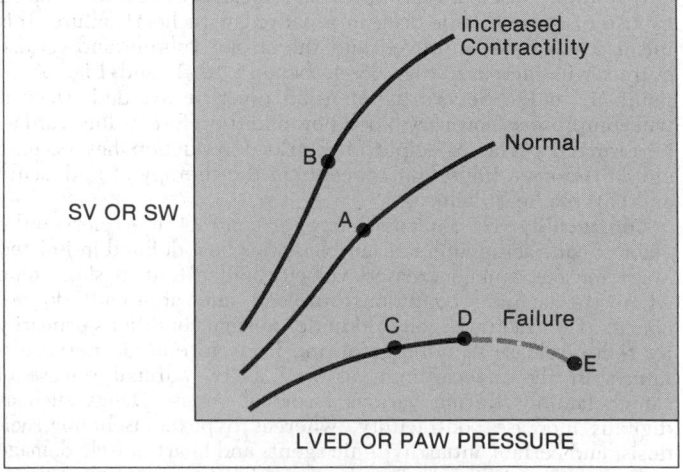

FIGURE 38–3. Left ventricular function curves relating the left ventricular filling pressure to ventricular performance expressed as stroke volume (SV) or stroke work (SW). The filling pressure can be expressed as either the left ventricular end-diastolic (LVED) pressure or the pulmonary artery wedge (PAW) pressure. Curves indicate normal, increased, or depressed ventricular contractility. Points A and B show the effects of a positive inotropic drug, which increases ventricular performance while reducing the filling pressure. See text for further discussion.

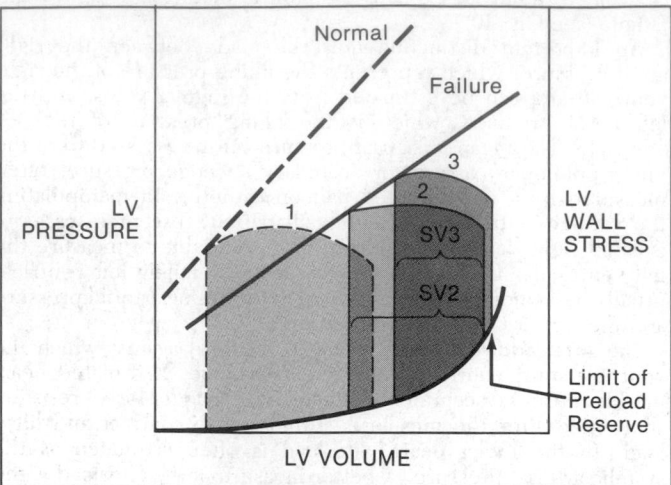

FIGURE 38–4. Left ventricular (LV) diastolic and end-systolic pressure-volume relations together with pressure-volume loops under normal conditions (*dashed lines*) and during heart failure when the linear end-systolic pressure-volume relation is shifted downward and to the right (failure). Beat 2 to beat 3 shows the effect of acutely increasing the left ventricular systolic pressure with a pure vasoconstrictor when there is little or no preload reserve; the stroke volume drops (SV2 to SV3). In chronic heart failure, the dilated left ventricle may be operating under basal conditions similar to beat 3, and left ventricular wall stress (right-hand ordinate) may be elevated despite a normal left ventricular systolic pressure. Under these circumstances use of a vasodilator drug may relieve this "afterload mismatch" and allow the ventricle to improve the stroke volume by lowering the wall stress (beat 3 to beat 2). (Adapted from West JB (ed.): Best and Taylor's Physiological Basis of Medical Practice. 11th ed. © 1985, the Williams & Wilkins Co., Baltimore.)

load-independent measure of contractility.) The end-systolic pressure-volume relation is shifted upward by enhanced contractility and downward by depressed contractility on heart failure (Fig. 38–4). The failing left ventricle exhibits enhanced sensitivity to afterload (decreased slope of the end-systolic pressure-volume relation), and when it reaches the limit of its preload reserve, any further increase in afterload (expressed as pressure or wall stress in Figure 38–4), such as by increased systemic vascular resistance and/or progressive heart failure, causes the stroke volume to fall (Fig. 38–4, beat 2 to beat 3, and Fig. 38–3, point E). This condition has been termed "afterload mismatch."

If systemic vascular resistance and arterial pressure are reduced by use of a vasodilator drug in a patient with heart failure, this mismatch will be improved and the stroke volume and cardiac output will increase (Fig. 38–4, beats 3 to 2, and Fig. 38–3, points E to D). Severe hypotension must be avoided, since it will compromise coronary blood flow and therefore reduce cardiac performance. The principle of afterload reduction has become one of the most important concepts in the therapy of both acute and chronic heart failure.

Contractility. The inotropic state, or contractility, refers to the vigor of contraction of heart muscle and is best defined in isolated heart muscle as an increased velocity and extent of shortening when the loading conditions (preload and afterload) do not change. Contractility is altered under normal conditions primarily by reflex release of norepinephrine from adrenergic nerve terminals in the myocardium, as well as by adrenal release of catecholamines during various forms of stress. Drugs such as digitalis increase contractility, whereas hypoxia, ischemia, acidosis, and certain antiarrhythmic agents and heart muscle damage reduce contractility. In terms of ventricular function curves, drugs that increase contractility shift the curve upward and to the left, increasing stroke volume or stroke work at a given end-diastolic pressure (Fig. 38–3, points A to B). With depression of contractility, the ventricular function curve shifts down and to the right, with a reduction in stroke volume at a given left ventricular end-diastolic pressure (Fig. 38–3).

Heart Rate. The frequency of contraction is an important

determinant of cardiac performance and one of the most important mechanisms available to increase the cardiac output (cardiac output = stroke volume × heart rate), provided that the venous return is increased (see below). Increased heart rate has a modest positive inotropic effect, increasing the velocity and extent of shortening while reducing the duration of contraction. During the response to moderate exercise, when the venous return increases, a higher heart rate is mainly responsible for the change in cardiac output, since the increase in stroke volume is relatively small.

The level of the heart rate may be an important indicator of the cardiovascular status of an individual patient. For example, in a patient with acute severe heart failure who has a sinus tachycardia of 140 beats per minute, the marked reduction in stroke volume is compensated for by the tachycardia in order to maintain an acceptable cardiac output. Other factors that can raise the resting heart rate must also be considered, including fever, anemia, thyrotoxicosis, and anxiety.

ASSESSMENT OF CARDIAC PERFORMANCE. Quantitative indices of cardiac performance can be measured in the cardiac catheterization laboratory or in critical care units. For reference, normal pressures, cardiac volumes, cardiac output, and vascular resistance are listed in Table 38–1. Volume measurements are normalized to allow interpatient comparison by dividing by the body surface area (square meters), obtained from a standard table based on height and weight. The maximum value of the first derivative of left ventricular pressure during isovolumetric systole (dP/dt) is sometimes used as a measure of contractility. One very useful index of ventricular function is the ejection fraction, which is the stroke volume divided by the end-diastolic volume. A normal ejection fraction of the left ventricle is 0.55 or greater, and in severe heart failure the ejection fraction may be reduced to less than 0.20.

As discussed above, *ventricular function curves* (Fig. 38–3) are often employed to demonstrate changes in inotropic state, whereas changes in preload move the ventricle up and down on a *single* curve. Experimentally, they are produced by progressive infusions of fluid, whereas in the clinical setting often only two points on a curve are available, before and after an intervention.

When two ventricular function curves are compared, they generally are compared at the same level of mean arterial pressure, since, as discussed above, the stroke volume of the ventricle is changed by altered afterload. Hence, decreased afterload would shift the relation between stroke volume and filling pressure upward, and increased afterload would shift the relation downward. In heart failure, such an effect is sometimes represented as an apparent "descending limb" of function. As discussed earlier, in such a setting, the preload reserve is exhausted and lowering the afterload would improve the stroke volume and cardiac performance (Figs. 38–3 and 38–4).

Venous return and cardiac output curves can be used to represent cardiocirculatory responses under experimental conditions, and although venous return curves cannot be performed in humans, they allow insight into the highly important role of the venous return. The heart behaves as a demand pump, ejecting whatever blood is returned to it under normal conditions, and only in heart failure or when filling is impaired (as in constrictive pericarditis) does the heart itself become the limiting factor for cardiac output. Therefore, the return of blood to the heart (the venous return), which is regulated by a number of mechanical, neural, and humoral factors, through its influence on preload is a key determinant of cardiac performance under normal conditions.

In A.C. Guyton's analysis, cardiac function is represented by a cardiac output curve that intersects a venous return curve at any given-state condition (Fig. 38–5). Noncardiac factors that influence the venous return include the volume of blood in the vascular bed (transfusion shifts the venous return curve upward, whereas bleeding shifts it downward). The position of the venous return curve is also affected by neurohumoral factors, increased sympathetic tone shifting the venous return curve upward and to the right and vice versa; venoconstriction produced by increased sympathetic tone also displaces blood from the peripheral circulation toward the central (cardiopulmonary) circulation, whereas decreased tone to the veins causes pooling of blood in the peripheral circulation. With this framework, changes in *both*

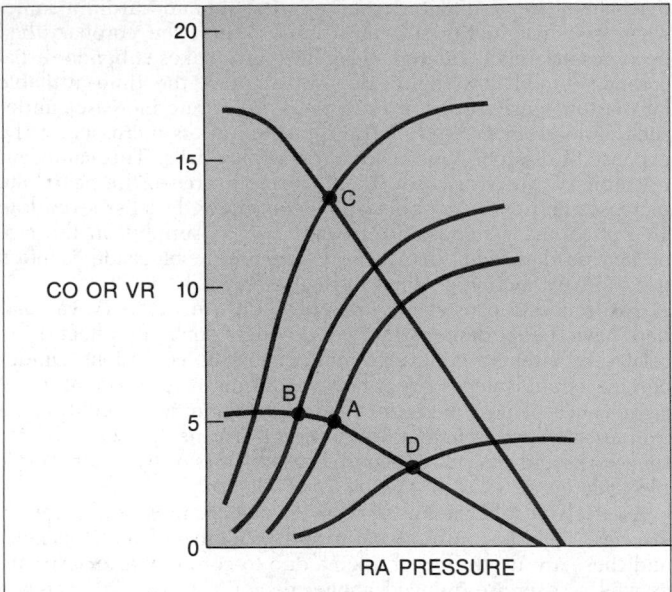

FIGURE 38–5. Relationship between the filling pressure of the heart, expressed as the right atrial (RA) pressure, and either cardiac output (CO) or venous return (VR). Venous return curves are represented as an inverse relation between the cardiac output or venous return and the right atrial pressure; the lower curve represents normal conditions and the upper curve shows the effect of marked sympathetic stimulation during exercise. The series of cardiac output curves shows a positive relation between right atrial pressure and cardiac function. Any steady-state condition is represented by the intersection of these two curves. Shown are normal conditions (A), electrical pacing of the heart (B), severe exercise (C), and heart failure (D). See text for further discussion.

cardiac performance and peripheral circulatory regulation (venous return) can be represented as they influence the cardiac output. Positive inotropic interventions, decreased afterload, and other factors shift the cardiac output curve upward, and opposite effects, including heart failure, shift it downward (Fig. 38–5).

The importance of venous return can be illustrated by the response to electrical cardiac pacing to increase the heart rate, a response in which myocardial contractility is increased. Since no significant effects on the peripheral circulation occur, no change in the cardiac output is observed. This response occurs because the normal heart operates near the flat portion of the normal venous return curve (near the point of venous collapse), and therefore even though the cardiac output curve is shifted upward, the venous return curve is unchanged, and there can be no alteration of the cardiac output (Fig. 38–5, points A to B). The response to exercise using this diagram is discussed subsequently under integrated responses.

REGULATION OF MYOCARDIAL OXYGEN CONSUMPTION

The heart is almost entirely supplied with energy from ATP and creatine phosphate produced by aerobic metabolism, and for practical purposes, the total energy expenditure of the normal heart can be equated with its oxygen consumption. The myocardial oxygen consumption (MVO_2) of the left ventricle can be determined using the Fick principle as the product of its coronary blood flow and the arteriovenous oxygen difference, calculated using blood samples from an artery and from the coronary sinus. Since the heart is a continuously active organ, its oxygen consumption is high relative to other organs, and the MVO_2 of the normal human left ventricle at rest is approximately 6 to 8 ml per minute per 100 grams.

The determinants of the MVO_2 of the heart (most of which is used by the left ventricle) consist of the basal oxygen consumption, which supplies energy for cell maintenance processes including the calcium and sodium pumps, protein synthesis, and so on. The remainder of the oxygen expenditure is controlled by the type of activity that the heart is called upon to perform. The determinants of MVO_2 are

1. Basal oxygen requirements
2. Systolic pressure (or wall stress)
3. Heart rate
4. Myocardial contractility (inotropic state)
5. Wall shortening against a load (related to cardiac work)

Systolic pressure, heart rate, and *contractility* are the major determinants of MVO_2, whereas shortening of the wall utilizes relatively less oxygen. There is a nearly linear relation between systolic pressure development by the left ventricle and MVO_2, and with the Laplace equation, this relation can also be expressed as systolic wall stress versus MVO_2. Thus, as systolic pressure doubles, the MVO_2 of the left ventricle approximately doubles. There is also a nearly linear relationship between heart rate and the MVO_2 and, again, an approximate doubling of the MVO_2 occurs as the heart rate increases twofold. If the heart rate and systolic pressure are held constant and a positive inotropic agent is administered, a rather marked increase in MVO_2 can be demonstrated, associated with a pronounced increase in the velocity of shortening and some increase in the extent of myocardial fiber shortening. It is possible that this extra energy expenditure is related, at least in part, to increased oxygen use by the calcium sequestration mechanism of the sarcoplasmic reticulum. Decreased contractility of the myocardium has been shown to cause a reduction of MVO_2.

The oxygen cost of myocardial fiber shortening against a load is relatively low. This is exemplified by experiments in which the systolic arterial pressure was elevated while the cardiac output and heart rate were held constant, and a marked stimulation of MVO_2 was produced, whereas if the cardiac output was increased over a wide range while the arterial pressure and heart rate were constant, only small changes in MVO_2 occurred. These findings indicate a high oxygen cost of "pressure work" and a relatively low oxygen cost of "volume work." The importance of heart rate and systolic pressure has resulted in the use of simplified indices of MVO_2, such as the heart rate × blood pressure (the "double product"). In clinical studies, this provides a means of estimating the effect of an antianginal drug (such as a beta blocker) on cardiac oxygen requirements during exercise.

The fact that myocardial energy expenditure, expressed as MVO_2, is closely linked to mechanical cardiac performance carries important implications in various disease states. For example, in valvular heart disease, chronic mitral regurgitation places a large volume overload on the heart due to the low impedance backward leak into the left atrium. In this condition, the systolic left ventricular pressure is not elevated, and since the left ventricle is performing extra "volume work," the MVO_2 of the left ventricle is not significantly increased. Therefore, in the absence of coronary artery disease, oxygen supply-demand imbalance and angina pectoris are rarely seen in chronic mitral regurgitation. In contrast, in patients with aortic stenosis, the high left ventricular systolic pressure with elevated MVO_2 of the entire chamber can lead to reduction of coronary vasodilator reserve. Therefore, subendocardial ischemia with angina pectoris is quite common in aortic stenosis, particularly during exercise or when left ventricular failure is beginning to occur, even in the absence of coronary artery disease. Of course, in chronic coronary artery disease, during exercise virtually all of the major determinants of MVO_2 are augmented, and in the presence of a stenosed coronary artery with impaired vasodilator reserve, coronary blood flow cannot keep pace with enhanced oxygen demands, and regional myocardial ischemia with angina pectoris occurs (see Ch. 48.1).

REGULATION OF CORONARY BLOOD FLOW

In keeping with the high energy requirements of the normal myocardium, coronary blood flow is relatively high, averaging 60 to 90 ml per minute per 100 grams in the normal human left ventricle when an individual is at rest. Extraction of oxygen by the heart is the highest of any organ, so that little additional oxygen extraction can occur during stress. This means that changes in oxygen demand of the heart are met chiefly by alterations in oxygen supply through changes in coronary blood flow, reflected by a nearly linear positive relation between the MVO_2 and the coronary blood flow. Although cardiac metabolism is the main determinant of coronary blood flow, several additional factors can be of importance:

1. MV_{O_2}
2. Coronary perfusion pressure
3. Systolic compression
4. Alpha-adrenergic tone to the coronary arteries (or exogenous vasoconstrictors)
5. Vasodilators (epinephrine, exogenous vasodilator substances)

Since the MV_{O_2} is influenced by each of the major determinants of cardiac performance, coronary blood flow is altered in the appropriate direction. There is evidence that release of the ATP metabolite adenosine, a potent coronary vasodilator, is involved in some of the responses of the coronary blood flow to altered cardiac performance and metabolism, although a number of other stimuli to vasodilation (such as decreased P_{O_2}, decreased pH, and increased K^+ during enhanced metabolic activity) may also be important.

Under normal conditions, the mean coronary perfusion pressure is not a major determinant of coronary blood flow, except as it affects the systolic arterial pressure and therefore the MV_{O_2}. Of course, on a moment-to-moment basis, the phasic pattern of coronary blood flow to the left ventricle shows a slow fall during diastole as the aortic pressure falls, as well as a sharp drop during systole as the squeezing action of the left ventricular wall compresses the intramural vessels and shuts down coronary blood flow, particularly to the subendocardial layers. However, the mean flow has been shown to be independent of the mean coronary perfusion pressure within certain limits, a phenomenon termed "autoregulation." Studies in which the coronary arteries are perfused *separately* from the aorta show that between mean coronary perfusion pressures of about 60 and 150 mm Hg coronary blood flow is maintained constant, provided that the MV_{O_2} of the heart does not change (Fig. 38–6). When the coronary perfusion pressure drops below 60 mm Hg, the coronary bed reaches the limit of autoregulation and tends to become fully dilated; at that point, perfusion pressure becomes the major determinant of coronary blood flow, and flow drops as pressure falls below that value with an exponential relation between pressure and flow typical of a passive blood vessel (Fig. 38–6). Obviously, in coronary artery disease the coronary perfusion pressure can become extremely important, since the perfusion pressure beyond an area of stenosis may be relatively low.

Systolic compression of coronary vessels in the inner (subendocardial) left ventricular wall almost entirely shuts off coronary blood flow during systole, but this does not occur in the outer wall (subepicardium). During diastole, flow to the subendocardium becomes slightly higher than in the outer wall, in order to compensate for the loss of flow during systole, a phenomenon

that makes the vasodilator reserve in the subendocardium somewhat *less* than in the subepicardium. When the coronary bed becomes maximally dilated, this effect also makes subendocardial coronary blood flow highly dependent upon the time available for diastolic perfusion. For example, if heart rate increases under such circumstances, systolic time per minute is increased at the expense of diastolic time, and coronary flow falls. This can occur in coronary artery disease, when, during exercise, the heart rate increases and coronary blood flow consequently falls beyond an area of coronary stenosis (decreased oxygen supply), in the face of increased oxygen demands. β-adrenergic blockade is often used to treat angina pectoris in this setting (Ch. 48.1).

α-Adrenergic constrictor influences on the coronary vascular bed have been demonstrated. Although such an effect is of relatively minor significance under normal conditions, under certain circumstances of reflex activation it can be of great significance. There is recent evidence that under conditions of exercise-induced ischemia, α-adrenergic coronary vasoconstrictor tone exists and can be reduced by vasodilators or by α-adrenergic blockade.

A variety of substances can relax the smooth muscle of coronary arteries, including nitroglycerin and calcium channel blockers, and these are used to treat angina due to coronary artery spasm, as well as exercise-induced angina pectoris. Certain prostaglandins and agents such as vasopressin and ergonovine are coronary vasoconstrictors, and ergonovine is used as a diagnostic test to evoke coronary spasm in patients with variant angina.

Recently, endothelium-derived relaxing factor (EDRF) has been established as an important endogenous mediator of large artery dilation in response to increased flow, and its release also is responsible for the coronary vasodilator properties of several substances, including acetylcholine and bradykinin. The absence of the endothelium (as in certain coronary atherosclerotic lesions) can alter the vascular responses to such stimuli.

REGULATION OF THE PERIPHERAL CIRCULATION

The heart pumps blood sequentially through the pulmonary and systemic circulations. Throughout the circulation, the small arterioles provide the main site for vascular resistance regulation. There is a wide variability in cardiac output distribution and in oxygen extraction by various organs; for example, the kidneys have a high blood flow (20 per cent of the cardiac output) and a low oxygen extraction, whereas the coronary circulation has a lower flow but a much higher oxygen extraction. The large conduit arteries have a high velocity of blood flow (aorta = 31 cm per second), whereas in the capillaries, the enormous total cross-sectional area results in marked slowing of blood flow (0.05 cm per second), allowing exchange of metabolites. The veins contain 75 to 80 per cent of the total blood volume in the circulation and serve a capacitance function, i.e., as a blood volume reservoir.

The general organization of the systemic circulation is such

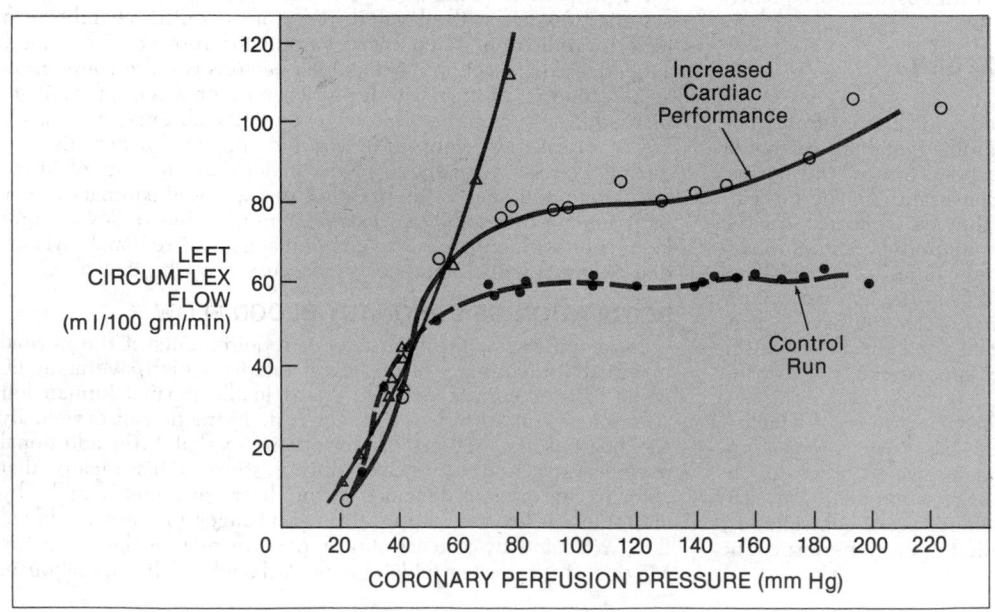

FIGURE 38–6. Autoregulation in the coronary circulation. When the left ventricular work is held constant and the coronary perfusion pressure is altered (coronary artery separately perfused from a controlled pressure source), coronary blood flow remains relatively constant over a wide range (*closed circles*, control run). At a coronary perfusion pressure below approximately 60 mm Hg, the limit of vasodilator reserve is reached, autoregulation is lost, and coronary flow is directly determined by the coronary perfusion pressure. The pressure-flow relation then falls on a curve of maximum vasodilation (passive pressure-flow curve of a distensible blood vessel, *open triangles*). Coronary blood flow is regulated at a higher level when cardiac performance and hence MV_{O_2} are increased (*open circles*, increased cardiac performance). (Adapted from West JB (ed.): Best and Taylor's Physiological Basis of Medical Practice. 11th ed. © 1985, the Williams & Wilkins Co., Baltimore.)

that the arterial bed serves as a pressure reservoir from which the circulations to the various organs operate in parallel. Thus, each organ takes the blood supply that it requires by regulating its *local* vascular resistance primarily on the basis of metabolic needs (autoregulation, as discussed earlier for the coronary circulation), whereas the *total* peripheral vascular resistance (TPVR) is primarily controlled by cardiovascular reflexes and maintains the pressure in the arteries. Thus, blood pressure = cardiac output × TPVR, and it is protected by the reflexes. For example, during tilting or standing abruptly, venous return and cardiac output fall (venous pooling), but a reflex increase in TPVR prevents a marked drop in the blood pressure.

REFLEX NEURAL CONTROL. The autonomic nervous system and certain neurohumoral factors maintain circulatory homeostasis through regulation of the heart rate, myocardial contractility, vascular tone in the arterioles and small veins, and the blood volume.

The high-pressure baroreceptors, which sense stretch in the walls of arteries, are located in the carotid sinuses and aortic arch. They increase their afferent impulse traffic when the blood pressure rises, and vice versa, and these nerve impulses affect the cardiovascular regulatory centers in the medulla. For example, as arterial pressure is increased, the enhanced impulse traffic stimulates the vagus to slow the heart rate and simultaneously inhibits the cardioaccelerator center. Simultaneously, the vasoconstrictor center is also inhibited, reducing sympathetic tone to the peripheral arterioles and also lowering venous tone. Thus, the reduced peripheral vascular resistance and venous return, together with the slowed heart rate, lower the increased blood pressure toward its previous level. With a decrease in blood pressure, as with moderate bleeding, opposite effects would occur, tending to restore the lowered blood pressure. With a significant drop in blood pressure, reflex release of catecholamines from the adrenal glands also occurs.

Reflex control of the heart and circulation is also under the influence of higher brain centers, as when marked emotional stress activates the sympathetic nervous system. Such central stimulation, as well as reflex activation of the sympathetic nervous system via receptors in the exercising skeletal muscle, produce the marked sympathetic stimulation of exercise. At rest, there appears to be little sympathetic tone affecting heart rate or myocardial contractility, and the heart rate is primarily under the control of parasympathetic influences.

Low-pressure baroreceptors (stretch receptors) are also located in the heart, particularly in the atria and the pulmonary veins, with fewer in the ventricles (see also blood volume regulation). Increased stretch of the atrial receptors can induce tachycardia (the Bainbridge reflex). More marked stretch of these low-pressure receptors produces a depressor reflex, with withdrawal of sympathetic tone and a fall in peripheral vascular resistance, which contributes to high-pressure baroreceptor regulation of the blood pressure. Syncope in some patients with aortic stenosis and high intracardiac pressure may be due to sudden activation of these intracardiac receptors.

REGULATION OF BLOOD VOLUME. The magnitude of blood volume is an important factor affecting cardiovascular function, and it is important in long-term regulation of the blood pressure. Loss of fluid volume occurs primarily through the kidneys, whereas sweating, respiratory, and gastrointestinal losses are less important (except during extreme conditions). Since approximately 20 per cent of the resting cardiac output passes through the kidneys, they provide an ideal location for regulating sodium and water balance. In addition, the hypothalamic osmoreceptors that regulate thirst and antidiuretic hormone (ADH) secretion are of great importance. Since these subjects are discussed in detail in Ch. 75, only selected cardiovascular factors are mentioned here.

An increase in blood volume, as might occur by increased intake of salt and water, would increase the diastolic volume of the cardiac chambers and the cardiac output. Atrial receptors sensitive to stretch activate vasodilating reflexes to the kidneys, increasing renal blood flow, and atrial receptors also reflexly stimulate the central nervous system to diminish the secretion of ADH. These factors would tend to increase the output of urine and sodium excretion, restoring the blood volume toward normal. A decrease in effective blood volume would have opposite effects.

Also, a peptide called atrial natriuretic factor (ANF) has been isolated which causes renal sodium loss and is also a vasodilator. It is released by the atria upon stretch, and ANF levels rise with acute and chronic circulatory congestion.

An additional highly important control mechanism for the regulation of arterial pressure and blood volume is the renin-angiotensin system (see Ch. 44). Reduction in renal perfusion (reduced pressure and flow) is sensed by the juxtaglomerular apparatus, which releases renin, whereas increased effective blood volume shuts off the stimulus for renin release. Renin enzymatically promotes the formation of angiotensin I from a precursor in the bloodstream, which is then converted to angiotensin II by the converting enzyme. Angiotensin II is a powerful vasoconstrictor, but small subpressor doses of angiotensin II also increase aldosterone secretion. Aldosterone, in turn, acts on the kidney to promote retention of salt and water, thereby counteracting the original stimulus of decreased effective blood volume.

With congestive heart failure, there is increased retention of salt and water, which leads to edema formation and increased blood volume. There may be increased aldosterone levels in severe heart failure secondary to reduced renal perfusion and activation of the renin-angiotensin system. Diuretics are used in this setting, and in severe heart failure with hyponatremia that is unresponsive to diuretics, use of an angiotensin-converting enzyme inhibitor may reverse this process by lowering angiotensin II and aldosterone levels, as well as by lowering vascular resistance and afterload on the left ventricle.

INTEGRATED CARDIOVASCULAR RESPONSES

It is important to emphasize the significance of interactions between the peripheral circulation and the heart in considering integrated responses. Certain peripheral circulatory factors, including the total peripheral vascular resistance and the venous capacitance, affect two important mechanical determinants of cardiac performance, the preload and the afterload. Venous return, of course, primarily determines the cardiac output. In addition, feedback control by neurohumoral reflex mechanisms simultaneously regulates both the heart and the peripheral circulation.

CHANGES IN VENOUS RETURN. Venous return to the right heart varies with normal respiration. It increases during inspiration as intrathoracic pressure falls (thereby increasing the pressure gradient for right heart filling), and moment-to-moment operation of the Frank-Starling mechanism in both ventricles to vary the stroke volume keeps the output per minute of the two sides of the heart in equilibrium.

A more marked stimulus, the Valsalva maneuver, which is useful in the physical diagnosis of heart murmurs, causes a marked decrease in the venous return to the heart because of the abrupt elevation of intrathoracic pressure, and after 15 to 20 seconds the associated drop in blood pressure produces reflex tachycardia and increased myocardial contractility. During this phase of the maneuver, cardiac murmurs associated with blood flow across a narrowed valve, such as that of aortic stenosis, diminish in intensity because of the reduced cardiac output, whereas the murmur associated with hypertrophic cardiomyopathy increases owing to the effect of reduced heart size and increased contractility to narrow the left ventricular outflow tract.

Vasodilator drugs that have a considerable venodilating effect, such as nitroglycerin, nitroprusside, and captopril, can have different effects on the cardiac output in the normal circulation and in congestive heart failure. Thus, in the normal circulation the cardiac output falls with nitroprusside, since the venous return curve is shifted downward as blood volume is displaced from the central circulation and pooled in the peripheral veins (decreased effective blood volume), whereas during cardiac failure, the associated unloading of the left ventricle by the arteriole-dilating action of this drug releases blood from the central circulation, which counterbalances the drug's venodilator effect; therefore, the venous return curve is not shifted downward, and the marked shift upward of the cardiac output curve due to reduced afterload results in an increased cardiac output (Fig. 38–5, points D to A).

It is also important to note that certain chronic cardiac conditions can limit the venous return to the heart because of impaired cardiac filling. These include chronic constrictive pericarditis and restrictive cardiomyopathy.

CHANGES IN HEART RATE. The lack of effect on cardiac output of changing heart rate by electrical pacing over a wide range has been previously discussed. But the usual increases in heart rate that occur as a component of cardiocirculatory reflex responses are ordinarily accompanied by increased myocardial contractility, venoconstriction, and an increased cardiac output. Below a certain level of heart rate, as in complete heart block with a ventricular rate of 40 beats per minute, the resting cardiac output may not be maintained, since the stroke volume is maximal (preload reserve fully utilized) and the ventricular output becomes rate limited. In addition, with marked resting tachycardia (approaching 200 beats per minute or more), as in paroxysmal atrial or ventricular arrhythmias, the available diastolic filling time is shortened because of the increased number of contractions per minute, and inadequate ventricular filling leads to a fall in the cardiac output. The loss of an appropriately timed atrial contraction in some dysrhythmias may further contribute to inadequate cardiac filling.

EXERCISE. Many mechanisms can come into play to cause the increased cardiac output that accompanies normal exercise. In nonsedentary individuals during low levels of exercise, increased stroke volume, combined with a mild increase in heart rate, augments the cardiac output. With marked exercise, as sympathetic stimulation and circulating catecholamine levels increase, the increased venous return causes further utilization of the Frank-Starling mechanism, and the stroke volume is further enhanced as increased myocardial contractility augments the ejection fraction. However, the stroke volume reserve is relatively small. The most important cardiac mechanism allowing a very high cardiac output during intense exercise in such individuals is augmented heart rate, which may reach 180 beats per minute or higher. Increased myocardial contractility also combines with decreased total peripheral vascular resistance (caused by marked vasodilation in the exercising muscles) to shift the cardiac output curve upward. In addition, increased sympathetic tone shifts the venous return curve upward (decreased venous capacitance), and it is steepened by decreased venous and arteriolar resistance. Therefore, the intersection of the venous return and cardiac output curves occurs at a markedly increased cardiac output, with only a mild elevation of the right atrial pressure (Fig. 38–5, points A to C). Thus, *both* peripheral and circulatory adaptations are involved in the exercise response.

Braunwald E (ed.): Heart Disease: A Textbook of Cardiovascular Medicine. 3rd ed. Philadelphia, W.B. Saunders Company, 1988, pp 383–425. *Up-to-date review of cardiac performance from the cellular level to the intact heart. Also includes the pathophysiology of heart failure.*

Ross J Jr: Assessment of cardiac function and myocardial contractility. *In* Hearst JW (ed.): The Heart. New York, McGraw-Hill Book Company, 1986, pp 265–298. *Current concepts concerning left ventricular function under normal and abnormal loading conditions, including heart failure and valvular heart disease.*

West JB (ed.): Best and Taylor's Physiological Basis of Medical Practice. 11th ed. Baltimore, Williams & Wilkins Company, 1985, pp 207–262, 284–307. *Basic physiology text that assumes little advanced knowledge. Pathophysiologic examples are concerned with cardiac function, circulatory control, myocardial oxygen consumption, coronary circulation, and heart failure.*

39 Specialized Diagnostic Procedures

39.1 RADIOLOGY OF THE HEART

Murray G. Baron

The heart casts a homogeneous shadow on the chest film. No internal detail can be seen within its contours because the radiodensities of blood, myocardium, and other cardiac tissues are so similar that one cannot be distinguished from the others. Only the two borders of the silhouette, where the heart contacts the radiolucent, air-containing lung, can be clearly discerned in any one projection. Changes in the size and/or shape of the cardiac chambers and great vessels usually alter the shape of the heart and its contours. However, because the heart is a three-dimensional structure and all of the cardiac chambers do not form borders in any one projection, multiple views are required to accurately evaluate its image. With the advent of echocardiography, the routine need for this "cardiac series" has disappeared. However, a remarkable amount of information regarding the heart can be gleaned from the standard frontal and lateral projections. As they are a part of most routine medical examinations, they are a useful screening tool for the detection of heart disease as well as for evaluating the severity of known disease, documenting the natural history of the disease, and assessing the efficacy of treatment.

ROENTGEN ANATOMY (Fig. 39–1)

Radiographic examination of the chest consists of at least a posteroanterior film. The right cardiac border in this projection has two components: a straight, vertical upper half formed by the superior vena cava and a gently convex lower half representing the lateral wall of the right atrium. Some patients are able to lower their diaphragms sufficiently during inspiration to uncover a small, straight segment of the inferior vena cava between the diaphragm and the right atrium.

The left cardiac border is composed of four distinct curves. The uppermost bulge represents the aortic knob. This is formed by the most distal portion of the aortic arch, beyond the left subclavian artery, where it turns downward to become the descending aorta. The prominence below the knob is formed by the main pulmonary artery and the subvalvular portion of the outflow tract of the right ventricle. The lowermost third of this border represents the anterolateral wall of the left ventricle. Between this and the outflow tract of the right ventricle is a short, flat or slightly concave segment where the left atrial appendage reaches the border of the heart.

In the lateral view (Fig. 39–1C), the anterior border of the cardiac silhouette is formed by the body and outflow tract of the right ventricle. The heart lies in the anterior portion of the chest, and the right ventricle abuts on the lower third of the sternum. The outflow tract and pulmonary artery slope posteriorly, and air-containing lung is interposed between the heart and the anterior chest wall, forming the "retrosternal clear space." The upper half of the posterior border of the cardiac silhouette, beginning at the carina and extending downward, is formed by the posterior wall of the left atrium and the lower half by the posterior wall of the left ventricle. The left atrial contour is usually not well visualized because it blends with the shadows of the posterior mediastinum. The shadow of the inferior vena cava can usually be seen extending obliquely and anteriorly from the diaphragm. The lowermost portion of normal left ventricular margin crosses the shadow of the cava about 2 cm above the left leaf of the diaphragm.

Alterations in the contour of the heart usually reflect dilatation and/or hypertrophy of the chambers, changes secondary to some underlying lesion. Many times, the pattern of these changes together with the appearance of the pulmonary vasculature points to the specific primary abnormality. Chest films are not sensitive or accurate as a detector of cardiac hypertrophy because the thickened myocardium often encroaches more on the chamber lumen rather than extending outward and enlarging the heart (Fig. 39–2). With severe hypertrophy, as in hypertrophic cardiomyopathy, the heart enlarges to the left and the apex becomes blunted and rounder than usual. However, this is not a pathognomonic appearance. On the other hand, dilatation of one or more chambers tends to alter the cardiac silhouette in a characteristic and recognizable manner.

HEART SIZE

A normal cardiac silhouette is no guarantee that the heart is normal. Angina, for example, no matter how severe, does not affect heart size unless there is also decompensation of the left ventricle. Similarly, the patient with restrictive cardiomyopathy may be in severe congestive failure with a normal-appearing

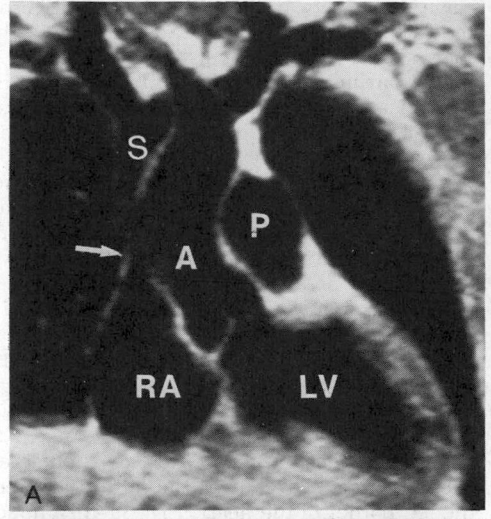

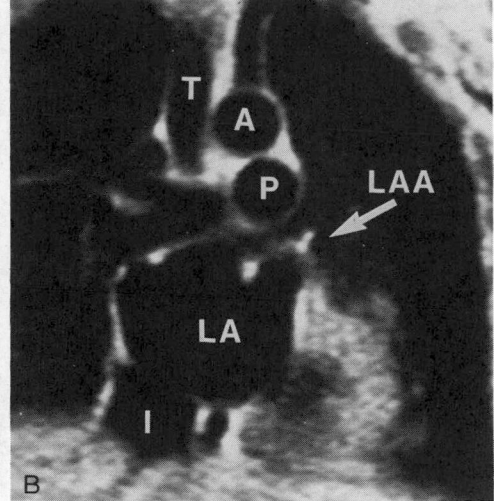

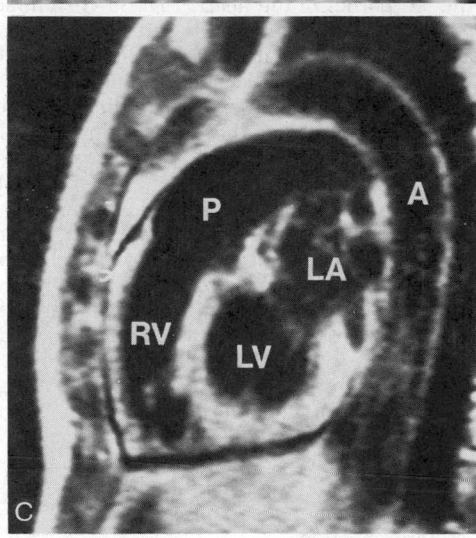

FIGURE 39–1. Normal roentgen anatomy. Magnetic resonance images. *A*, Coronal section at level of aortic valve. The right border of the cardiac silhouette is formed by the superior vena cava (S) and the right atrium (RA). The arrow indicates the caval-atrial junction. The lower portion of the left cardiac border is formed by the left ventricle (LV). A = Ascending aorta; P = main pulmonary artery. *B*, Coronal section at level of left atrium. The upper portion of the left cardiac border is formed by the aorta (A), main pulmonary artery (P), and left atrial appendage (LAA). LA = Left atrium; I = inferior vena cava; T = trachea. *C*, Sagittal section near midline. The right ventricle (RV) forms the anterior surface of the heart, abutting the sternum. The pulmonary artery (P) extends upward and posteriorly from the ventricle. The posterior border of the heart is formed by the left atrium (LA) and left ventricle (LV).

heart. Conversely, enlargement of the heart always indicates the presence of cardiac or pericardial disease. Therefore, accurate evaluation of heart size is important.

Over the years, various measurements have been proposed as objective means for assessing heart size. The simplest of these is the transverse cardiac diameter. This has proved to be of little value because the normal range is so great and its size varies with the age, sex, and body habitus of the patient. However, when the transverse cardiac diameter is considered together with the patient's body surface area, a satisfactory distinction can be made between normal and abnormal. This is not a practical solution, as the data needed to calculate body surface area are usually not available when reviewing chest films. An approximation of body habitus can be gained from the size of the patient's chest. The cardiothoracic ratio is measured by dropping a vertical line through the heart and measuring the greatest distance to the right and left cardiac borders (Fig. 39–2). The sum of the two is the transverse cardiac diameter. The transverse thoracic diameter is the greatest width of the chest, measured from inner surfaces of the ribs. Dividing this into the transverse cardiac diameter gives the cardiothoracic ratio. A ratio of less than 0.6 can be considered within the limits of normal. Setting this value at 0.5, as is often done, produces many false-positive results.

In most cases, accurate measurements of the cardiac silhouette are not necessary, and a reasonably experienced observer can achieve a similar degree of accuracy by visually estimating heart size. Regardless of the method used, several cautions must be observed if overreading of abnormality is to be avoided. The single factor having the greatest effect on apparent cardiac size is the degree of inspiration. The volume of the heart is essentially constant throughout the cardiac cycle. With expiration, as the diaphragm moves up, the vertical diameter of the heart is

shortened and there is a compensatory increase in its transverse diameter. Because of the increase in width, the heart appears larger on expiratory films. The degree of inspiration can be gauged from the relationship of the diaphragm to the ribs. On a properly positioned frontal chest film, a reasonable degree of inspiration is indicated if the diaphragm is pulled down below the posterior portion of the ninth rib.

When the anteroposterior diameter of the chest is small, the heart may be compressed between the sternum and the spine so that it splays to one or both sides. For this reason, the heart often appears enlarged in patients with a straight back syndrome or with a pectus excavatum deformity of the sternum. An epicardial fat pad (actually it is truly extrapleural fat, outside of the pericardium) can occur in one or both cardiophrenic angles and makes the heart appear larger than it actually is. However, the fat often causes the cardiophrenic angle to appear abnormally obtuse or makes the cardiac apex indistinct. In addition, on a properly exposed film, the slightly more radiolucent image of the fat can usually be distinguished from the greater density of the heart.

A change in the size of the cardiac silhouette can also occur between systole and diastole. This is important because chest films are exposed at random with reference to the phase of the cardiac cycle and so may be misleading when comparing the heart size on two films of the same patient made at different times. This usually does not create a problem, as in the majority of cases the difference in the transverse cardiac diameter between the two phases is small, measuring no more than several millimeters. However, in younger patients, especially the more athletic ones, with a slow heart rate and large stroke volume, phasic change in the cardiac diameter can be as much as 2 cm.

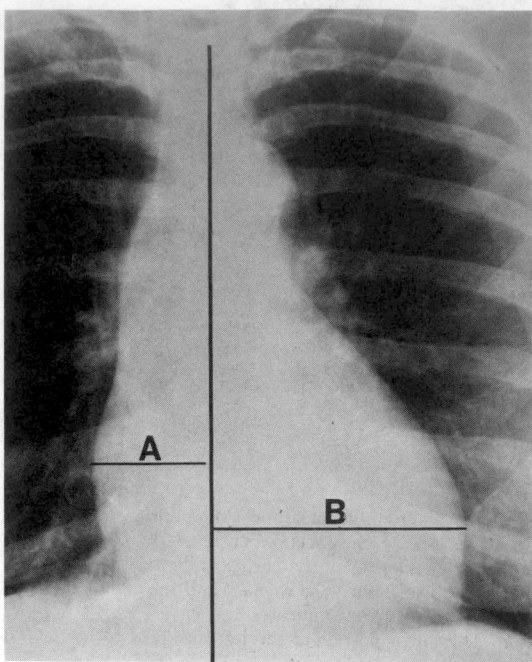

FIGURE 39–2. Measurement of the transverse cardiac diameter. Severe aortic stenosis with a 95-mm systolic gradient across the valve. The heart, although considerably hypertrophied, is normal in size and configuration. A vertical line is drawn through the heart. The greatest distance to the right cardiac border (A) and to the left cardiac border (B) are then measured. Transverse cardiac diameter = A + B.

CHAMBER ENLARGEMENT

Left Atrium

Dilatation of the left atrium alone, in the absence of a left-to-right shunt, is most often due to disease of the mitral valve, although it can also result simply from atrial fibrillation. The two "popular" roentgen signs of left atrial enlargement, a double contour within the right cardiac border and elevation of the left main bronchus, are both accurate when present but are insensi-

tive and not seen in about half of the cases of significant mitral valve disease. In order to produce a discernible margin within the cardiac silhouette, the thickness of the heart must increase sharply at some point. This occurs in mitral valve disease when the left atrium enlarges and protrudes posteriorly from the back of the heart. The right border of the left atrium is then silhouetted against the lung, and its contour is seen within the right side of the cardiac silhouette (Fig. 39–3A). This is not apparent with lesser degrees of left atrial enlargement. When the right atrium enlarges, as is common in longstanding mitral disease, it blends in with the enlarged left atrium and the double contour is lost. Thus, the double contour is not present with mild left atrial enlargement or in severe cases of mitral disease. Furthermore, the radiologic technique used for chest films is chosen to provide optimal images of the lungs. If the heart is enlarged, it will be underexposed and a double contour may not be seen within its opaque silhouette. For the same reason, the position of the left main bronchus often cannot be clearly visualized through the mediastinal shadow.

The most sensitive sign of left atrial enlargement in the frontal chest film is a convexity of the left atrial appendage segment on the left border of the heart (Fig. 39–3). The left atrial appendage extends anteriorly along the left border of the heart. When the appendage dilates, it forms a bulge on the left cardiac contour immediately below the main pulmonary artery segment. As the left atrium enlarges, it extends to the right and can form a portion of the right border of the cardiac silhouette (Fig. 39–3B).

Left Ventricle

The appearance of the dilated left ventricle depends to a large extent on the underlying cause. When it is due to insufficiency of the aortic or mitral valve, the ventricle elongates and its apex is displaced downward, to the left and posteriorly (Fig. 39–4). When the dilatation is due to coronary artery disease or primary myocardial disease, the ventricle tends to assume a more globular shape; thus, the apex is still displaced to the left. In the lateral view, the downward extension of the enlarged left ventricle covers more of the inferior vena caval shadow than normally. Thus, the crossing of the left ventricular margin with that of the cava occurs nearer to the diaphragm. Unfortunately, the practical usefulness of this sign is limited because a factitious appearance often results if the patient is rotated only slightly from a true lateral projection.

Enlargement of the left ventricle produces a smoothly curved dilatation of the lower left portion of the cardiac silhouette. A localized bulge in this contour most often represents a ventricular aneurysm (Fig. 39–5). Dilatation of the left ventricle is usually

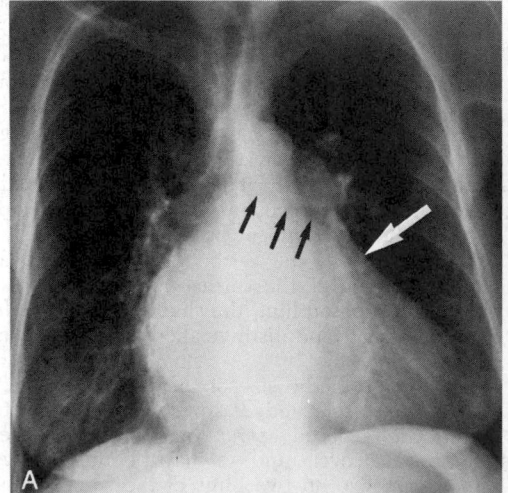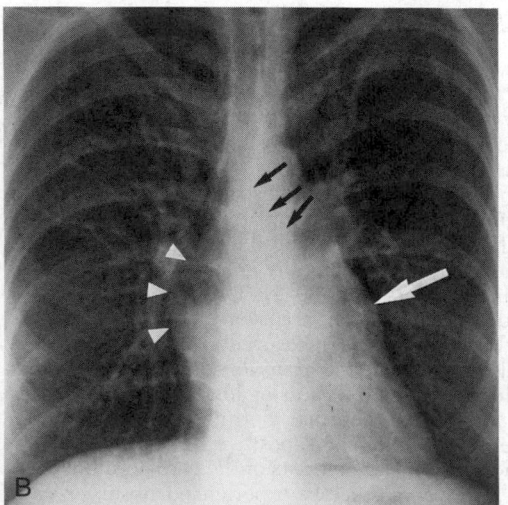

FIGURE 39–3. Left atrial enlargement in mitral valve disease. *A*, Patient 1: The enlarged left atrium causes the central portion of the cardiac silhouette to be abnormally dense. The right border of the atrium is seen within the right side of the cardiac silhouette. The left main bronchus (*small arrows*) is elevated. The region of the left atrial appendage (*white arrow*) is slightly concave because this structure was resected at the time of previous mitral commissurotomy. *B*, Patient 2: The enlarged left atrial appendage bulges from the left side of the heart (*white arrow*) while the body of the atrium (*arrowheads*) extends beyond the right atrium to form a part of the right heart border. There is no double density seen within the heart, and the left main bronchus (*small arrows*) is not elevated.

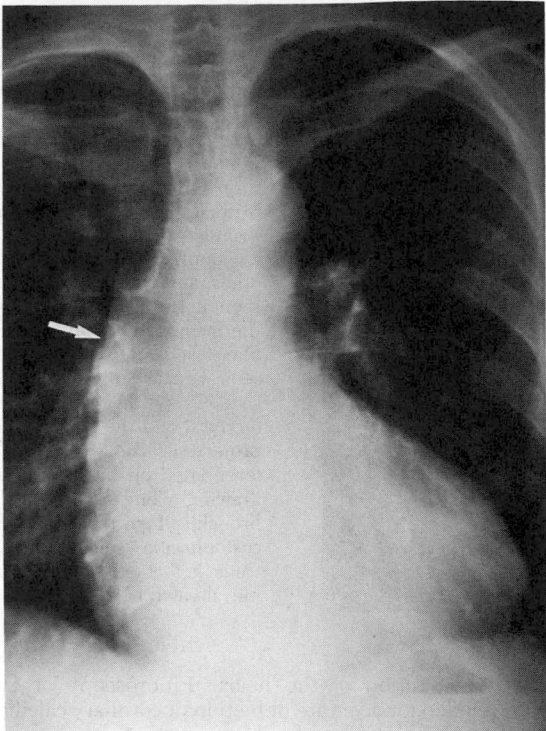

FIGURE 39–4. Left ventricular dilatation, aortic insufficiency. The apex of the heart is displaced downward and to the left. The ascending aorta (*arrow*) is diffusely dilated. The pulmonary vasculature is normal.

associated with elevation of left ventricular end-diastolic pressure. This increases the resistance to left atrial emptying and can result in dilatation of the atrium. Thus, left atrial enlargement in the presence of a large left ventricle does not necessarily indicate the presence of mitral valve disease.

Right Atrium

Enlargement of the right chambers of the heart alone is uncommon in adults. When seen, it is usually due to subacute bacterial endocarditis of the tricuspid and/or pulmonic valves, most often in drug addicts. Cardiac lesions involving the right

side of the heart also occur with the carcinoid syndrome. Dilatation of the right atrium causes an accentuation and outward bowing of its curvature on the lower half of the right cardiac contour. With greater degrees of dilatation, the cardiac silhouette enlarges to the right (Fig. 39–6).

Right Ventricle

The right ventricle is the most difficult of the four cardiac chambers to evaluate on chest films. Except for a small area in the subpulmonic region, the chamber does not form a border in the frontal projection. Even moderate right ventricular enlargement may produce no abnormality in this view other than some elevation of the main pulmonary artery. As right ventricular size increases, the transverse diameter of the heart enlarges to the left, and the cardiac apex may become elevated (Fig. 39–6). Thus, enlargement of either or both ventricles displaces the apex of the heart to the left. It is often not possible to distinguish between biventricular enlargement or dilatation of one or the other of the ventricles.

As the right ventricle enlarges, its area of contact with the sternum, seen in the lateral projection, extends upward and tends to obliterate the retrosternal clear space. This is a nonspecific sign, as it depends on the shape of the chest and the size of the left ventricle as well as the size of the right ventricle.

CALCIFICATION

Calcium deposits, because they have a greater radiodensity than the cardiac soft tissues, can be seen within the cardiac silhouette. Valvular calcification most often involves the mitral and aortic valves, and is consistent with significant stenosis. This is particularly true of the mitral valve. The calcium is deposited in irregular clumps, near the valve commissures. The two valves insert on a common fibrous tendon and are in contact with each other. They lie within the midportion of the cardiac silhouette in the frontal projection, just to the left of the spine (Fig. 39–7A). Determination of which valve is calcified may be difficult. They can be separated on fluoroscopy because the motion of the aortic valve approaches the vertical, whereas the orbit of mitral motion is oriented nearer to the horizontal. The distinction can also be made on films in the lateral view. If a line is drawn from the left main bronchus (seen as a circular shadow superimposed on the

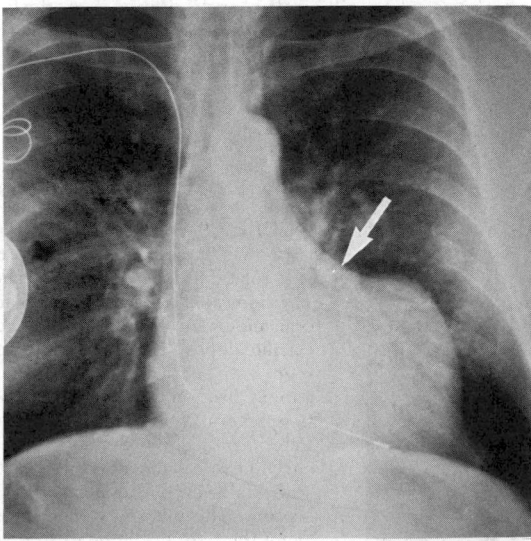

FIGURE 39–5. Left ventricular aneurysm. A bulge on the lower portion of the left cardiac border, formed by the anterolateral wall of the left ventricle, represents a ventricular aneurysm. The patient had suffered a myocardial infarct 1 year previously. The left atrial appendage segment (*arrow*) is normal. A transvenous pacemaker has been inserted through the right subclavian vein. The electrode tip is situated in the apex of the right ventricle.

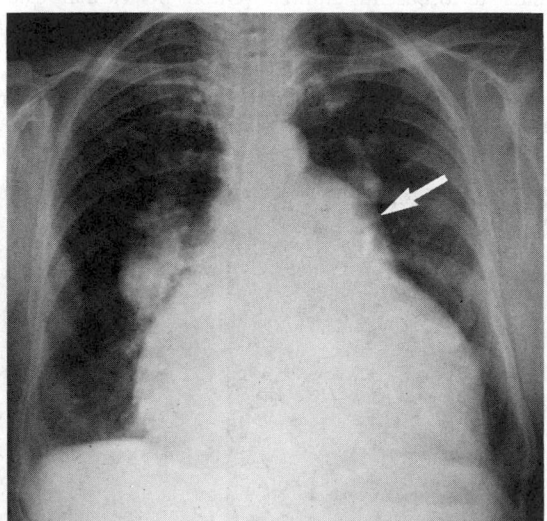

FIGURE 39–6. Right ventricular enlargement. Resistive pulmonary hypertension, secondary to atrial septal defect. The main pulmonary artery (*arrow*) and the right pulmonary artery are markedly dilated. The left pulmonary artery was also dilated but is hidden by the heart in this view. There is a sudden "cutoff" of the vascular shadows just beyond the hila. This is characteristic of resistive pulmonary hypertension. The right ventricle is enlarged, elevating the cardiac apex and displacing it to the left. The accentuation of the curvature of the lower right cardiac border and enlargement of the cardiac silhouette to the right are caused by dilatation of the right atrium.

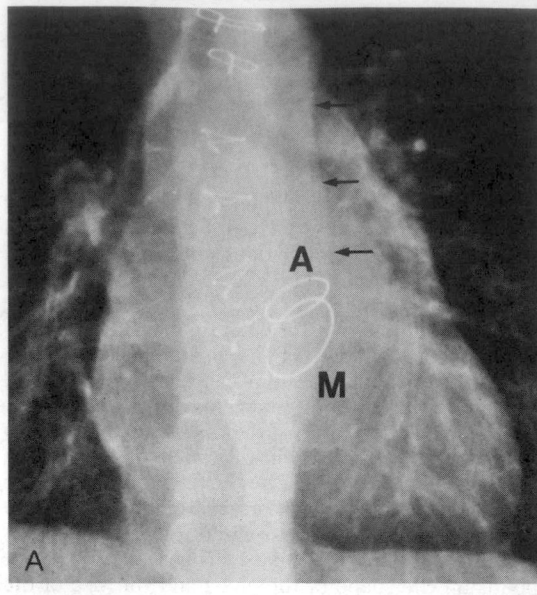

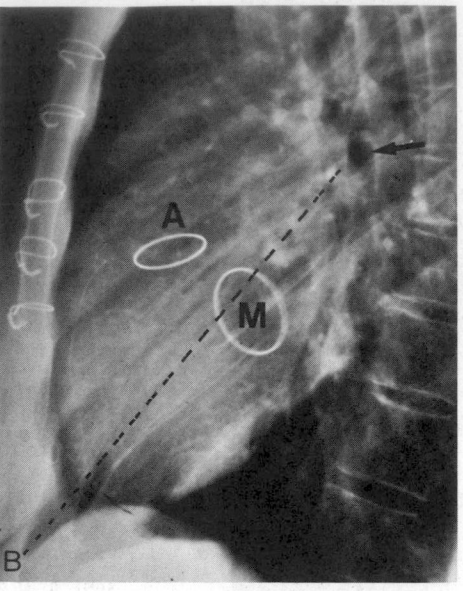

FIGURE 39–7. Location of the mitral and aortic valves. Both mitral and aortic valves have been replaced by porcine heterografts. The circular stents indicate the location and tilt of each valve. M = Mitral valve; A = aortic valve. *A,* Frontal projection. The two valves are normally in contact with each other, and it is difficult to separate them in the frontal projection. Furthermore, on a routinely exposed film, calcific deposits are not easily seen because of the overlapping shadows of the descending aorta (*arrows*) and the spine. *B,* Lateral projection. The valves can be differentiated on the lateral view by drawing a line from the left main bronchus (*arrow*) to the anterior costophrenic sulcus. The aortic valve lies above this line and the mitral valve below it.

lowermost part of the trachea) to the anterior costophrenic angle, the mitral valve is below this line and the aortic valve is above it (Fig. 39–7*B*).

Calcification of the mitral annulus, most often occurring in elderly females, can be distinguished from valvular calcification because it forms a heavy, relatively smooth curvilinear shadow in the form of an O or a C. Calcification of the wall of the left atrium, although rare, is virtually pathognomonic of rheumatic heart disease. It appears as fine, linear calcific shadows seen through the cardiac silhouette outlining the contour of the left atrium.

Calcification of the myocardium in coronary artery disease indicates a previous transmural infarct and frequently a ventricular aneurysm. The calcified scar is visualized as a fine, curvilinear density, most often on the anterolateral aspect of the heart, seen best in the frontal view (Fig. 39–8*A*), or in the lower portion of the interventricular septum, seen best in the lateral projection (Fig. 39–8*B*). Calcification of the pericardium is usually coarser and tends to occur in clumps. Often pericardial calcium is distributed in the interventricular sulcus and the atrioventricular grooves but when extensive, the deposits may coalesce and completely surround the heart (Fig. 39–9).

It is uncommon to see calcification of the coronary arteries on chest films because the deposits are thin and their shadows are blurred by the motion of the heart. Fluoroscopy or fast CT scanning is needed for accurate detection of coronary calcification. Although a high percentage of patients with significant coronary stenosis show coronary artery calcification, in individual patient assessment this is not a particularly meaningful statistic. Most of these data come from cardiac catheterization laboratories and are based on a highly selected patient population. The incidence of coronary artery calcification without significant accompanying stenosis increases with age, and calcification in asymptomatic individuals over 75 is of questionable significance. On the other hand, its occurrence below the age of 55 is highly significant. A search for coronary calcification is indicated in those younger patients with atypical symptoms that, in themselves, are not sufficient to justify coronary arteriography.

PERICARDIAL EFFUSION

The pericardium is a serosal lined sac containing a small amount of fluid. It completely invests the heart, except for a small area on its posterior surface between the entrances of the pulmonary veins and the superior and inferior venae cavae. When fluid accumulates in the pericardium, the sac distends smoothly, enlarging the cardiac silhouette and giving it a flask-shaped appearance. This shape can also be seen with a dilated, failing heart. Differentiation of the two conditions is readily made from

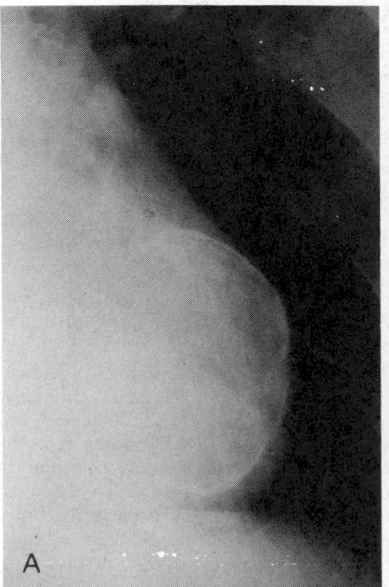

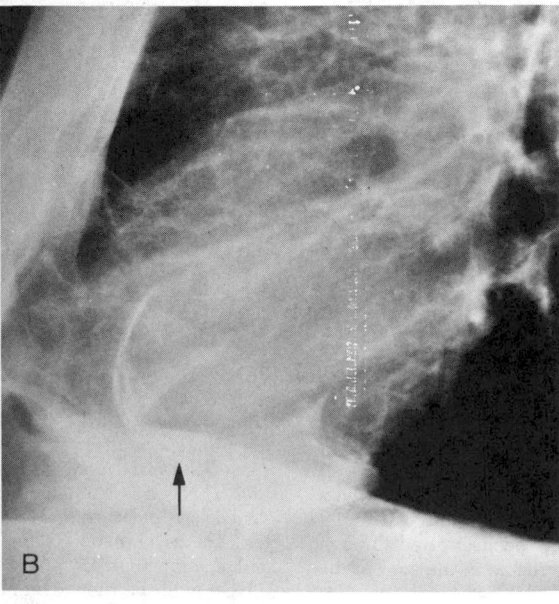

FIGURE 39–8. Calcified myocardial infarcts. *A,* Patient 1: Frontal projection. Anterolateral left ventricular aneurysm. The fine calcific line outlines an anterolateral aneurysm of the left ventricle. The calcific deposit is much finer than that seen with pericardial calcification. The patient had suffered a myocardial infarction several years earlier. *B,* Patient 2: Lateral projection. Septal infarction. The curvilinear calcific deposit is within the scarred lower portion of the ventricular septum. The infarct extended posteriorly along the base of the heart to involve the diaphragmatic wall of the left ventricle (*arrow*).

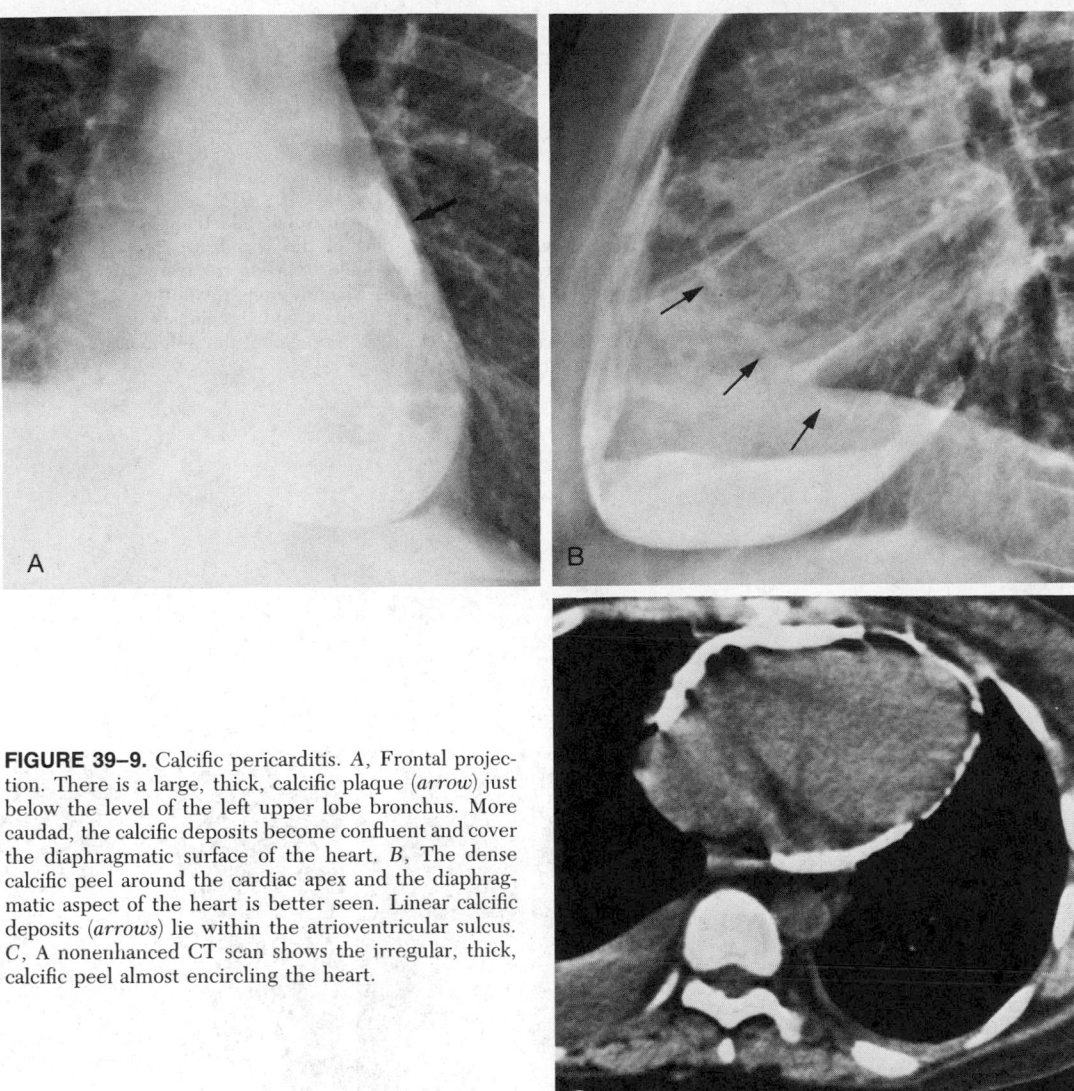

FIGURE 39–9. Calcific pericarditis. *A,* Frontal projection. There is a large, thick, calcific plaque (*arrow*) just below the level of the left upper lobe bronchus. More caudad, the calcific deposits become confluent and cover the diaphragmatic surface of the heart. *B,* The dense calcific peel around the cardiac apex and the diaphragmatic aspect of the heart is better seen. Linear calcific deposits (*arrows*) lie within the atrioventricular sulcus. *C,* A nonenhanced CT scan shows the irregular, thick, calcific peel almost encircling the heart.

the appearance of the pulmonary hila on the chest film and usually is apparent by echocardiography.

The pericardial sac extends onto the great vessels reaching to, or slightly above, the level of the bifurcation of the main pulmonary artery (Fig. 39–10). As the sac distends it tends to overlap and obscure the hilar vessels. On the other hand, as the heart fails, the vessels become congested and appear more prominent than normal (Fig. 39–11).

Posterior displacement of the epicardial fat line provides a second reliable sign of pericardial effusion. In adults, fat is often insinuated between the myocardium and the visceral pericardium (the epicardium). This is sometimes seen in the lateral projection as a curvilinear, radiolucent shadow outlining the anterior aspect of the heart. The outer surface of the parietal pericardium borders on the mediastinal fat behind the sternum. The soft tissue density between these two fat lines, therefore, represents the pericardium, the epicardium, and the fluid between them. When normal, this stripe is no more than 1 to 2 mm thick. As fluid accumulates in the pericardial sac, the epicardial fat line is displaced posteriorly and the pericardial stripe widens (Fig. 39–12).

PULMONARY VASCULATURE

Almost all of the linear shadows in the lung are cast by the pulmonary arteries and veins. The terminal branches of the vessels are too small to be visualized as individual structures. The same is true of the interstitial tissues that support the alveoli and form the primary and secondary interlobular septae. However, the summation of their shadows does give the pulmonary field an overall grayish cast. The large vessels are seen because they are set off against the surrounding air-containing alveoli.

INTRACARDIAC SHUNTS

The caliber of the pulmonary vessels reflects the volume of blood flow into the lungs. When this volume is diminished because of a right-to-left shunt, the pulmonary vessels become smaller and, as a result, the lungs appear more radiolucent. This occurs only when blood from the right side of the heart can bypass the lungs. Thus, even in severe isolated pulmonary vascular stenosis, the pulmonary vascularity is within normal limits. Increased size and prominence of the pulmonary vessels, both central and peripheral, usually reflect the increased pulmonary blood flow secondary to a left-to-right shunt (Fig. 39–13A). The vessels in the lower as well as the upper lung fields are dilated. Although the pulmonary arteries and veins become abnormally prominent when there is congestive failure, there are usually additional signs of pulmonary venous hypertension or interstitial edema which distinguish the appearance from that of shunt vasculature.

The vessels to the lower lobes carry about 60 to 70 per cent of

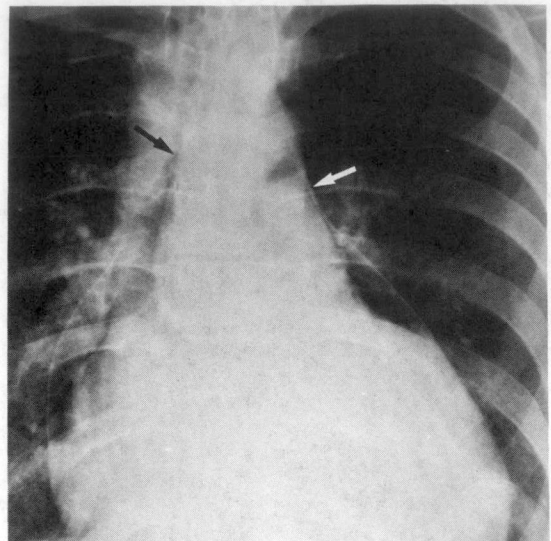

FIGURE 39–10. The superior pericardial reflection. Pericardial effusion following tap. During pericardiocentesis, some of the withdrawn fluid was replaced with air. The normal pericardium is now outlined between the intrapericardial air and the air in the lungs and is seen as a thin linear shadow along the outer border of the cardiac silhouette. The film is made in the erect position and the air has risen to the highest point of the pericardial cavity (*arrows*), above the level of the pulmonary hila and almost reaching to the aortic arch.

FIGURE 39–11. Hilum overlay sign. *A*, Pericardial effusion. The heart is diffusely enlarged. Its silhouette extends outward and obscures the hilar shadows in each lung. *B*, Dilated cardiomyopathy. The heart is diffusely enlarged. The failing left ventricle has caused congestion of the hilar vessels and they are more prominent than normal.

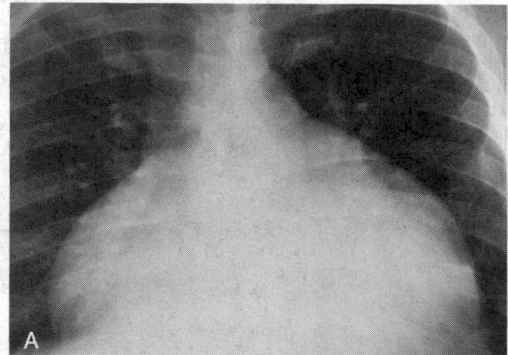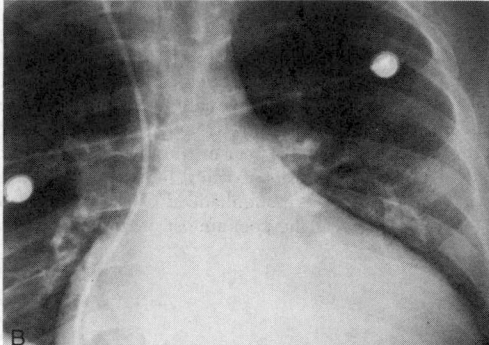

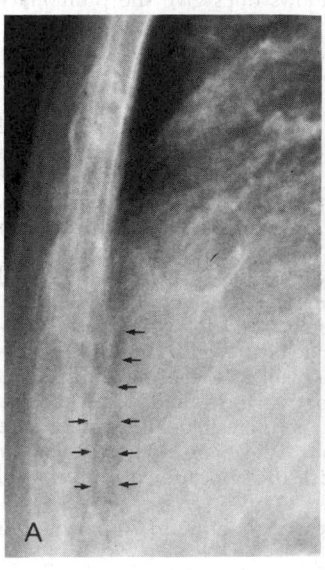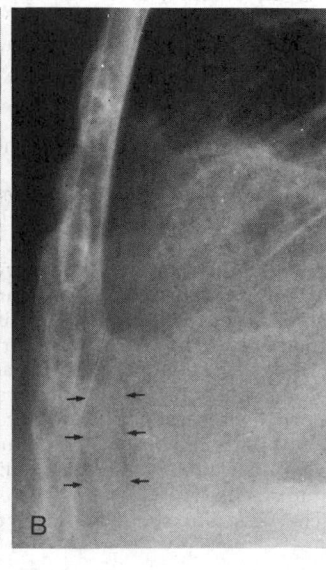

FIGURE 39–12. Pericardial effusion. Posterior displacement of epicardial fat line. The two lines of arrows point to the substernal fat and the subepicardial fat layers. *A*, Normal. The fine line of soft tissue density between the fat layers represents the epicardium, the pericardium, and the fluid between them. *B*, Same patient with a pericardial effusion. The epicardial fat line is displaced posteriorly, and the pericardial stripe is abnormally wide.

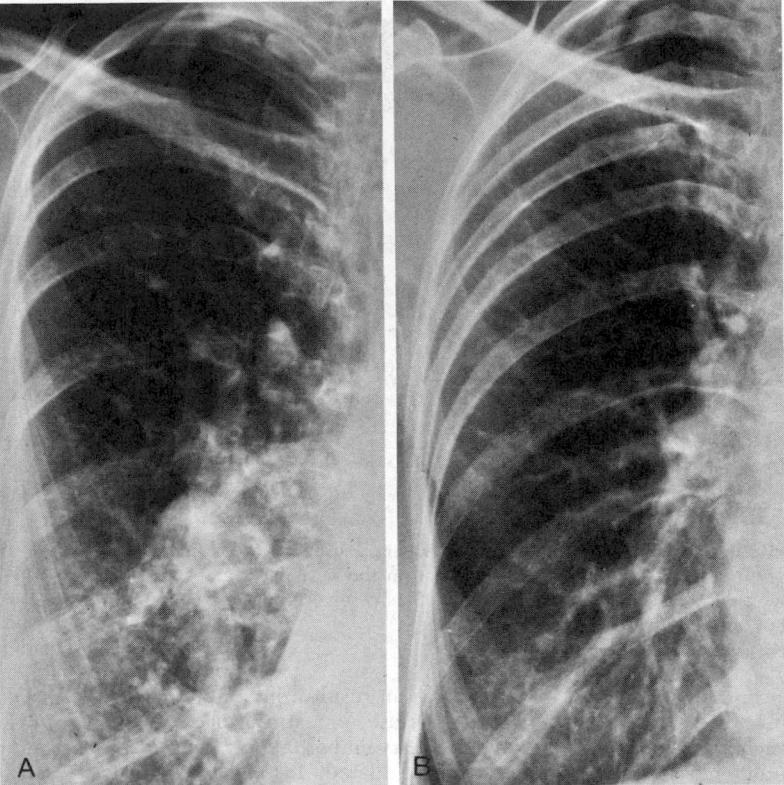

FIGURE 39–13. Pulmonary vasculature. *A*, Atrial septal defect, left-to-right shunt. All pulmonary vessels, to the lower lobes as well as the upper lobes, are dilated, indicating increased blood flow. *B*, Mitral stenosis, pulmonary venous hypertension with redistribution of the pulmonary vasculature. The lower lobe vessels are constricted and the upper vessels, which now carry more blood, are of greater caliber.

the pulmonary blood flow and normally are of greater caliber than the vessels to the upper lobes. As pulmonary venous pressure increases, the lower lobe vessels tend to constrict. This increases resistance to blood flow, resulting in blood being shunted to the upper lungs and dilatation of the upper lobe vessels. This redistribution of pulmonary vasculature is a reliable sign of pulmonary venous hypertension (Fig. 39–13*B*). With sufficient further increase in the venous pressure, interstitial pulmonary edema develops.

PULMONARY EDEMA

Normally, there is a constant circulation of fluid from the capillaries through the interstitium and back to the bloodstream by way of the lymphatics. As pulmonary venous pressure increases, more and more fluid leaks from the capillary bed, the capacity of the lymphatics is exceeded, and the interstitium becomes waterlogged. Because the interlobular septae at the

outer bases of the lungs are oriented parallel to the x-ray beam on an erect film, when thickened, they can be seen as parallel, short, horizontal lines in the lung, above the costophrenic sulci (Kerley B lines). Kerley A lines also represent interlobular septae that are longer and usually are seen in the upper lung fields. They are within the depth of the lung and usually do not reach the pleural surface. Most of the other septae, although thickened, cannot be identified as individual structures, but their summation pattern creates random "noise" on the film that tends to obscure the shadows of the pulmonary vessels (Fig. 39–14). Edema of the bronchial walls and the peribronchial connective tissues causes the shadows of the bronchial walls to become thickened and less distinct. This "peribronchial cuffing" is most often seen in the superior portion of the pulmonary hilum, where the anterior segmental bronchus of the upper lobe is viewed on end. When the interstitium can no longer accommodate the excess fluid, it spills into the alveoli (Fig. 39–15). At this point, the typical auscultatory findings of pulmonary edema appear.

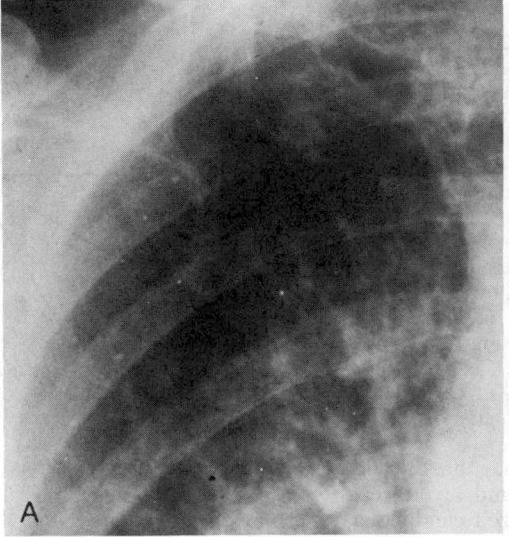
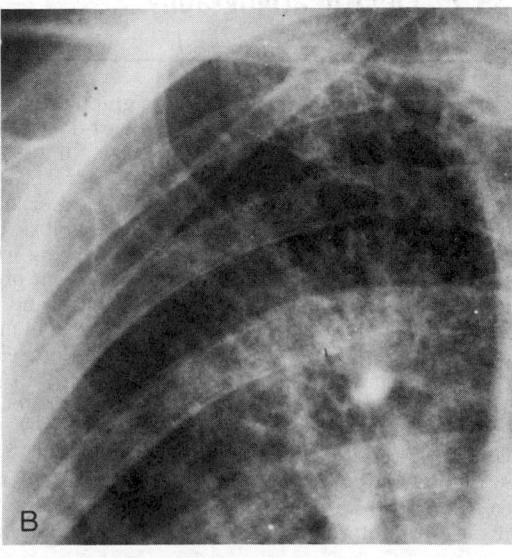

FIGURE 39–14. Interstitial pulmonary edema. *A*, Close-up of the right upper lobe. Portable film of a patient with acute myocardial infarct. The pulmonary vessels are well outlined. *B*, Two days later, the patient became tachypneic. There were no abnormal auscultatory findings in the lungs. Radiographically, the lung fields are noisy, with numerous, random shadows obscuring the outline of the pulmonary vessels. The appearance and the time sequence of the changes are characteristic of interstitial pulmonary edema.

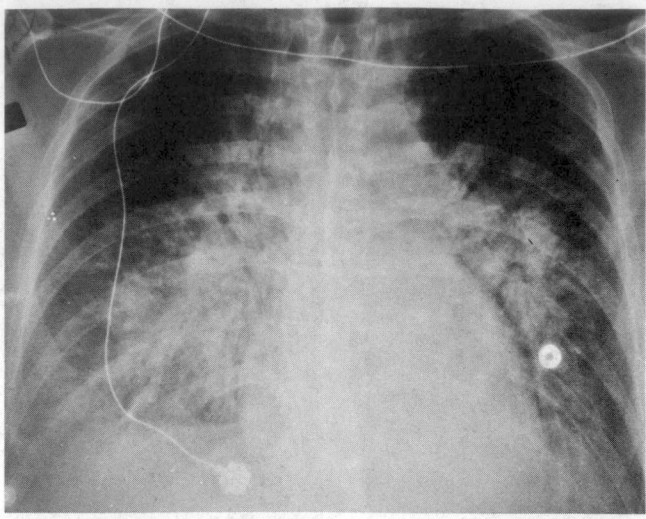

FIGURE 39–15. Alveolar pulmonary edema, acute myocardial infarction. There are patchy areas of consolidation in the perihilar regions of both lungs. Dilatation of the heart after a massive myocardial infarction may not be seen for the first 24 to 48 hours.

Pulmonary arterial hypertension can result from a left-to-right intracardiac shunt, mitral valve disease, or extracardiac disease such as repeated episodes of pulmonary embolization. The central pulmonary arteries become grossly dilated. Instead of gradual tapering as they bifurcate, there is a sudden, sharp change in the caliber of the vessels. The size and number of the smaller arterial branches decrease, creating an appearance that has been likened to a "pruned tree" (Fig. 39–6). With severe pulmonary hypertension, the right heart chambers may dilate. Once this picture of resistive pulmonary hypertension develops, it is difficult to determine whether the original cause was cardiac or extracardiac. The radiographic appearance of pulmonary hypertension is relatively specific but not sensitive. Clinically significant hypertension can be present with a normal-appearing pulmonary vascular bed.

Baron MG: Radiology and Angiocardiography. *In* Onkman FFY (ed.): The Ciba Collection of Medical Illustrations. Vol. 5: The Heart. Summit, N.J., CIBA Publications Department, 1969.

Chen JT: The plain radiograph in the diagnosis of cardiovascular disease. Radiol Clin North Am 21:609, 1983.

Felson B: The mediastinum. Semin Roentgenol 4:41, 1969.

Lane EJ Jr, Carsky EW: Epicardial fat: Lateral plain film analysis in normals and in pericardial effusion. Radiology 91:1, 1968.

Meszaros WT: Lung changes in left heart failure. Circulation 47:859, 1973.

39.2 Electrocardiography

Joseph C. Greenfield, Jr.

The electrocardiogram (ECG) is a graphic representation of the electrical activity generated by the heart during the cardiac cycle and is recorded from the body surface. In 1903, Wilhelm Einthoven used a string galvanometer to record the first EKG (Elektrokardiogramm, Ger.) Shortly thereafter, a clinically useful instrument was manufactured by the Cambridge Scientific Instrument Company. Following the pioneering work of Frank N. Wilson and his associates in the development of lead systems in the 1930's, the ECG became standardized and now consists of 12 leads. The recorders currently in use obtain at least three leads simultaneously, and many use digital processing to improve recording characteristics. At present, the ECG is the most commonly employed noninvasive diagnostic tool in cardiology. Approximately 90 million ECG's are recorded each year in the United States alone.

ELECTROPHYSIOLOGY. Cardiac muscle may be divided conveniently into specialized conducting tissue and myocardial tissue for contraction. Some cells of the specialized conducting

TABLE 39–1. POSITION OF CHEST LEADS

V_1	Fourth intercostal space (ICS) at the right sternal border
V_2	Fourth ICS at the left sternal border
V_3	Halfway between V_2 and V_4
V_4	Fifth ICS at the left midclavicular line
V_5	Fifth ICS at the left anterior axillary line
V_6	Fifth ICS at the left axillary line

When several sequential ECG's are to be obtained, e.g., in the coronary care unit, it is important to mark the location of the chest electrodes to minimize changes in the waveform resulting from variation in electrode placement.

A similar configuration on the right chest can aid in the diagnosis of right ventricular infarction.

tissue possess the potential for spontaneous depolarization, a process termed automaticity. The electrical activity of all myocardial cells is made possible by the presence of ionic gradients maintained across the membranes of individual cells.

Myocardial activation normally begins with the spontaneous calcium-dependent depolarization of cells within the sinoatrial (SA) node located at the junction of the right atrium and superior vena cava. The impulse propagates in a wavelike fashion through the atrial myocardium to the atrioventricular (AV) node located in the lower portion of the interatrial septum. Conduction through the AV node primarily involves the calcium-dependent process of depolarization and is delayed owing to membrane properties of nodal cells. The membrane properties in the proximal and distal segments of the AV node vary such that conduction in the proximal segment is slow and may occur with decrement, whereas conduction in the distal segment is more rapid.

The impulse is rapidly transmitted through the bundle of His, which bifurcates into the narrow right bundle branch (RBB) and the fibers that become the left bundle branch (LBB). The LBB divides further into two main collections of fibers forming the anterior (superior) and posterior (inferior) fascicles. The distal portion of the specialized conducting system is a network of smaller fibers, the Purkinje system, which delivers the propagated impulse to the remaining ventricular tissue, resulting in a synchronized myocardial contraction.

LEAD SYSTEMS. Ten electrodes are used in the standard ECG lead system. One is placed on each of the four limbs and six at different locations on the anterior chest wall (Table 39–1). The right leg electrode functions as a ground lead. In recording the standard frontal plane limb leads, I, II, and III, the right arm, left arm, and left leg are used as follows: Lead I measures the potential difference between the right arm (−) and the left

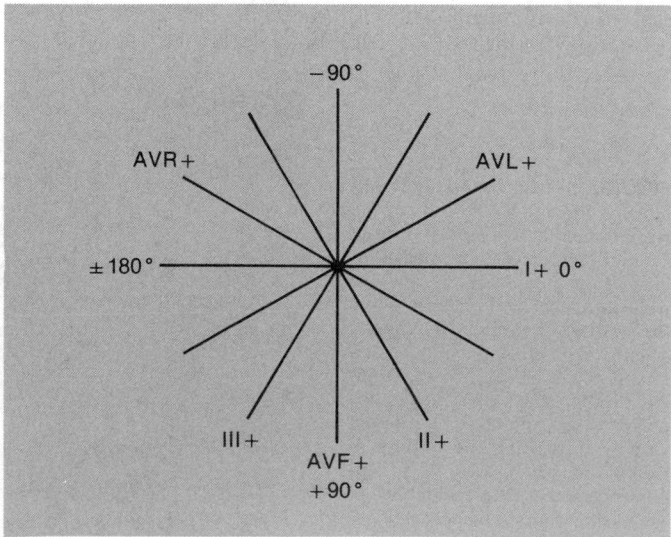

FIGURE 39–16. The limb leads are used to form a hexaxial reference system for the frontal plane. The axis of each lead is separated by approximately 30 degrees from the axes of the two adjacent leads.

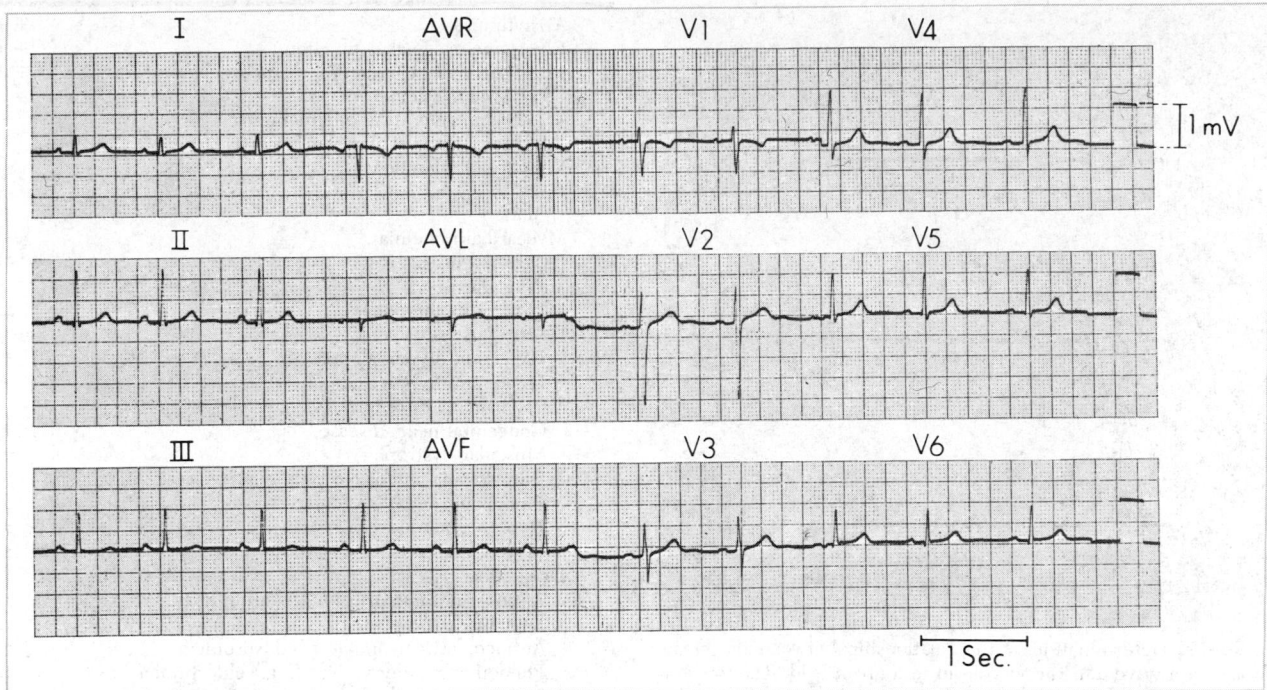

FIGURE 39–17. Normal electrocardiogram; the three leads in each column or lead set are recorded simultaneously.

arm (+). Lead II measures the potential difference between the right arm (−) and the left leg (+). Lead III measures the potential difference between the left arm (−) and the left leg (+). This is the original bipolar lead configuration designed by Einthoven. The other three frontal plane leads—aV_R, aV_L, aV_F—are constructed using a modified central terminal of Wilson, which augments the voltage output, hence the prefix aV. The exploring electrode, placed on the right arm (aV_R), left arm (aV_L), and left leg (aV_F), functions as a positive unipolar lead. The relationship among the six frontal plane leads is shown in Figure 39–16. The six chest leads also function as positive unipolar leads, using the central terminal as the reference point. The ECG leads are displayed in sequence, beginning with lead I, II, and III, followed by aV_R, aV_L, and aV_F, and then the chest leads from V_1 through V_6. A normal ECG recorded in this manner is illustrated in Figure 39–17.

Normally the ECG is recorded on a graph, using a standard paper speed of 25 mm per second. The paper is marked with a light vertical line every millimeter (0.04 second) and a heavy vertical line every 5 mm (0.20 second). The paper also has horizontal lines separated by 1 mm and a dark horizontal line every 5 mm. Vertical deflection is calibrated in terms of voltage, so that 10 mm equals 1.0 mV.

WAVEFORMS. The waveforms and intervals of the ECG are shown in Figure 39–18. The P wave reflects the electrical activity recorded during atrial depolarization and, in the normal ECG, precedes ventricular depolarization. The QRS complex occurs during ventricular depolarization. The Q wave is the initial downward deflection, the R wave is the initial upward deflection, and the S wave is the second downward deflection. A second upward deflection or a third downward deflection is defined as R′ or S′, respectively. A Q, R, and S may not be present in each lead; e.g., if the entire lead is negative, it is termed a QS wave. The time from the onset of the P wave to the beginning of QRS is the PR interval; normally the range is 0.12 to 0.20 second. The QRS duration normally is less than 0.10 second. The T wave is inscribed during the period of ventricular repolarization. The electrical activity during atrial repolarization usually is masked by the QRS complex. The interval from the end of QRS to the beginning of the T wave is termed the ST segment. The interval from the onset of QRS to the end of the T wave is the QT interval and is a function of rate. A small deflection following the T wave is the U wave; the precise origin of this waveform is unknown.

LEARNING ELECTROCARDIOGRAPHY. There are two general approaches to learning electrocardiography: (1) the pattern recognition method and (2) the spatial vector approach. In the former, the student memorizes the multiple normal and abnormal waveforms for each lead and gains the necessary expertise through experience in interpreting a large number of ECG's with clinical correlation. This technique is used by all experienced electrocardiographers, and illustrations of this approach are provided in the legends of Figures 39–21 to 39–25. In the spatial vector approach, popularized by R. P. Grant, the waveform is reduced to a vector representing the magnitude and direction of the mean electrical forces of P, QRS, and T. Using this technique, the student can quickly learn to define the normal ECG and the major abnormalities. This approach is based on the fact that the magnitude of a wave in any lead is a function of the relationship between the electrical axis of the heart and that lead (Fig. 39–19). From the hexaxial reference system of the six frontal plane leads illustrated in Figure 39–16, the spatial vector approach can be used to obtain the mean frontal plane axis for the normal electrocardiogram (Fig. 39–17). The QRS complex is

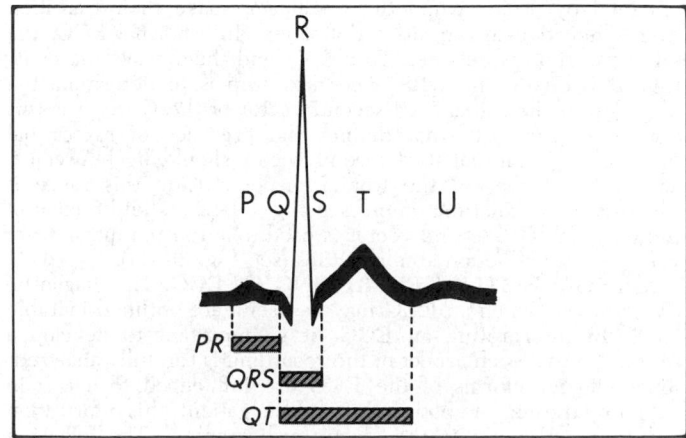

FIGURE 39–18. The ECG waveforms and intervals (horizontal bars) are illustrated. For description, see text.

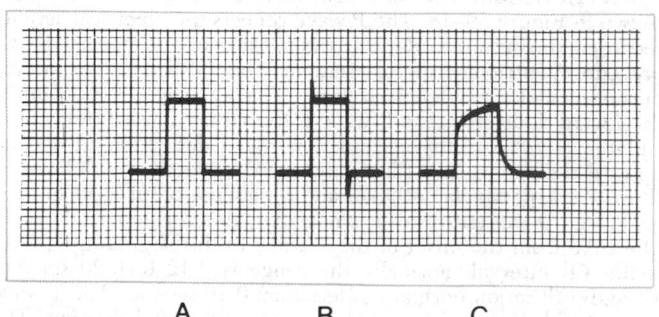

FIGURE 39–19. Determination of the relationship between the mean electrical axis of a wave and the waveform in a given lead. The top row depicts an entirely positive waveform; thus, the axis is parallel to the lead. In the second row the waveform is biphasic and the summation of the positive and negative parts is zero. In this instance, the mean electrical axis of the wave is perpendicular to the lead. (Note that the arrow could be drawn in the opposite direction and still be perpendicular to the lead.) In the third row, a biphasic waveform is shown in which the majority of the area is positive. The mean electrical axis is roughly at a 45-degree angle to the lead.

upright (positive) in lead I; thus the mean axis must be between +90 degrees and −90 degrees, i.e., on the positive side of a line perpendicular to lead I. Since the QRS complex is also positive in leads II and III, the axis must be between +30 and +90 degrees. Since the mean QRS complex is slightly negative in lead aV_L, the mean QRS vector is approximately +70 degrees. A similar determination then can be made for P and T waves. In the frontal plane, the mean P vector should be between 0 and +80 degrees, and the mean QRS and T vectors should lie between −30 and +90 degrees. A mean QRS vector more negative than −30 degrees is considered left-axis deviation and more positive than +100 degrees is defined as right-axis deviation. The angle between the mean QRS and T vectors in the frontal plane should be less than 80 degrees. Application of the spatial vector technique to the transverse plane is somewhat more difficult, since the six percordial leads do not define a precise reference system. An estimate of the vector can be obtained by noting when the waveforms make their transition from a negative to a positive deflection. In a normal ECG, the QRS transition is between V_2 and V_5, and the T wave makes its transition before the QRS. The next step is to determine the direction of the initial 0.04-second vector of the QRS. It is this portion of the QRS that defines the presence of myocardial infarction. The initial 0.04-second vector should lie between 0 and +90 degrees in the frontal plane; outside this range it suggests myocardial infarction (see Fig. 39–22). The direction of the terminal 0.04-second vector is used to aid in the diagnosis of ventricular conduction abnormalities (see Fig. 39–24).

APPROACH TO INTERPRETING AN ECG. The diagnostic categories in which an ECG may be useful are outlined in Table 39–2. In interpreting an ECG, it is important to develop a routine so that each aspect of the recording is carefully analyzed. Since the waveforms of the ECG are influenced to a certain extent by the age and body habitus of the patient, this information should be available to the electrocardiographer. The following eight sequential steps are useful for proper ECG interpretation.

1. *Quality of the ECG recording.* This includes proper stan-

TABLE 39–2. DIAGNOSTIC CATEGORIES IN WHICH AN ECG IS USEFUL

Arrhythmias	+ +
Electronic pacemaker function	+ +
Intraventricular conduction disturbances	+ +
Chamber enlargement	
Left and right atrial enlargement	+
Left and right ventricular hypertrophy	+
Myocardial infarction	
Old	+
Acute	+
Myocardial ischemia	+
Pericardial disease	
Pericarditis	±
Pericardial tamponade	±
Electrolyte disturbances	
Hypo- and hyperkalemia	+
Hypo- and hypercalcemia	+
Miscellaneous disorders	
Congenital heart disease	±
Muscular dystrophy	±
Emphysema and/or cor pulmonale	±
Pulmonary emboli	±
Hypothermia	±
Myxedema	±
Drug effects	
Antidysrhythmic drugs (e.g., quinidine)	±
Digitalis	±
Antineoplastic agents (e.g., doxorubicin)	±
Phenothiazine derivatives (e.g., chlorpromazine)	±
Antidepressant drugs (e.g., amitriptyline)	±
Antiparasitic compounds (e.g., emetine)	±

The symbols indicate the necessity for ECG to establish diagnosis:
  + + ECG is essential for diagnosis.
    + ECG is important for diagnosis.
    ± ECG may be useful for diagnosis.

dardization (Fig. 39–20), lead placement (Fig. 39–21), and identification of significant artifacts. The student must learn to evaluate the quality of the recording. Serious misdiagnosis can result if the quality of the ECG is ignored.

2. *Measurements.* The heart rate can be estimated adequately by employing the method outlined in Table 39–3. The amplitude, duration, and intervals of the various waveforms are measured in the standard frontal plane limb leads. Abnormality of the QRS duration, PR interval, and QT interval also is determined in these leads. Proper measurement of the waveforms is enhanced by simultaneous recording of three leads, since the interrelationships between the waveforms can be easily seen. The QT interval must be corrected for heart rate. The corrected QT interval (QT_c) is given by Bazet's formula:

$$QT_c = \frac{QT}{\sqrt{RR \text{ interval (seconds)}}}$$

and should be between 0.33 and 0.47 second.

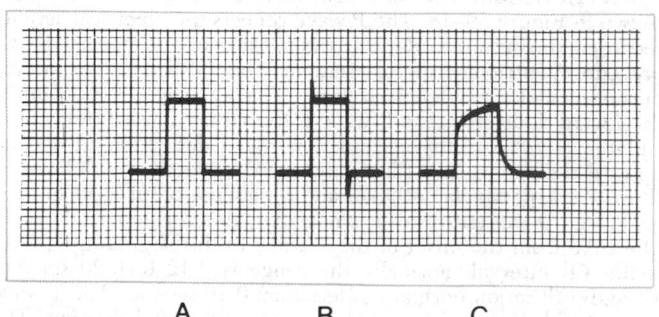

A   B   C

FIGURE 39–20. In *A,* a correct standardization having a true square wave response is illustrated. *B* represents a standardization obtained from an instrument in which the response is underdamped; the amplitude of the waves will be spuriously enhanced. In *C,* the recorder is overdamped, resulting in both a spuriously decreased amplitude and an increased width of the waveform.

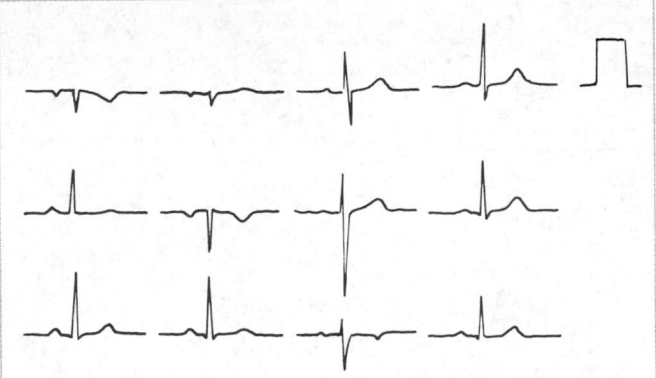

FIGURE 39–21. Two examples of incorrect lead placement from the same patient illustrated in Figure 39–17. Both the left and right arm leads and chest leads V1, 2, 3 are reversed. Reversal of the arm lead results in a mirror image recording of lead I and is easily recognized, since the P wave is negative. If missed, a spurious diagnosis of lateral wall infarction may be made. Reversal of the right precordial leads may result in an incorrect diagnosis of either right ventricular hypertrophy or posterior wall infarction.

3. *Determination of rhythm.*
4. *Examination of P wave.* Determine if atrial enlargement (see Fig. 39–23) or intra-atrial block is present.
5. *Examination of QRS.* Determine if myocardial infarction (Fig. 39–22), ventricular hypertrophy (Fig. 39–23), or ventricular conduction defect (Fig. 39–24) is present.
6. *Examination of ST segment.* Determine if abnormal displacement of the ST segment is present; depression is termed subendocardial (Fig. 39–25) and elevation subepicardial (Fig. 39–22) injury. The ST segment is shortened in hypercalcemia and prolonged in hypocalcemia.
7. *Examination of T wave.* Defining the significance of T-wave abnormalities is the most difficult aspect of electrocardiography. In general, marked T-wave abnormalities that occur either without other ECG abnormalities or with myocardial infarction are defined as ischemic or primary T-wave changes (Fig. 39–22). T-wave abnormalities that occur with conduction defects or ventricular hypertrophy are spoken of as secondary (Fig. 39–23). The T waves also are important in the diagnosis of drug effects and electrolyte abnormalities.
8. *Comparison with patient's previous ECG's.* It is extremely important to compare a new tracing with a previous electrocardiogram for two reasons: (1) Although the ECG may still be within the normal range, significant changes may have occurred; and (2) a comparison allows the electrocardiographer to date specific abnormalities that may have important therapeutic implications.

COMPUTER INTERPRETATION OF THE ECG. The development of algorithms to process and interpret ECG's has progressed to the point that, at present, there are several acceptable programs available for routine clinical use. Although these programs are important in decreasing processing time and enhancing storage, they must be viewed as an assist device to the electrocardiographer and not as a replacement.

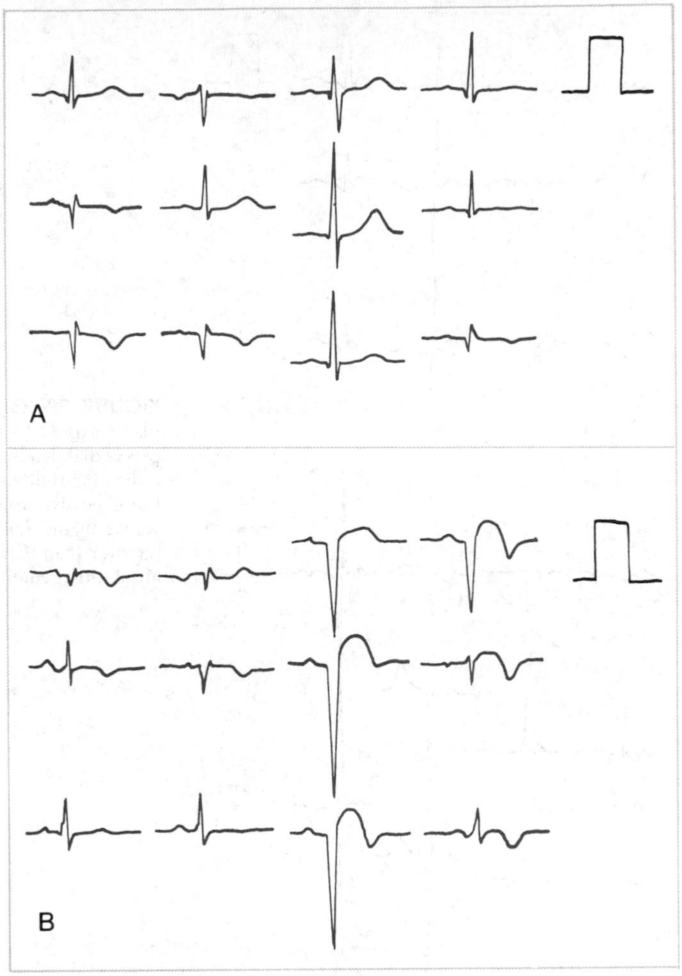

A

B

FIGURE 39–22. The ECG lead sets are recorded in the same sequence as in Figure 39–17. *A,* Inferior and posterior infarction. Note the abnormal superiorly and anteriorly directed initial forces, i.e., significant Q waves in leads II, III, and AVF, and a broad R wave in V1. Note the concomitant negative T waves in the same frontal plane leads (inferior ischemia). *B,* Anterolateral myocardial infarction. The initial forces are posterior and to the right, i.e., extensive Q waves in leads I, AVL, and V1 through V4. Also note the concomitant ST segment elevation (epicardial injury) and T wave inversion (anterior ischemia) in the precordial leads, indicating that the myocardial infarction is probably acute.

OTHER RECORDING TECHNIQUES. Several of the other ECG recording techniques and uses are described in Table 39–4.

The vectorcardiogram (VCG) is used to obtain a true orthogonal lead system (XYZ leads) so that the cardiac dipole is in the center of the chest. Since it is time consuming to record a VCG properly, it is not generally used. The VCG is primarily beneficial in

TABLE 39–3. DETERMINATION OF HEART RATE

Interval in Large Boxes Between Two Complexes	Heart Rate (beats/min)
1	300
2	150
3	100
4	75
5	60
6	50

The ECG recording paper is marked vertically by light lines; every fifth line is heavily marked. The time increment separating two heavy lines (one large box) is 0.02 second. To determine the rate rapidly, note the interval between two complexes and estimate the rate from this table.

TABLE 39–4. DIAGNOSTIC USES OF OTHER ECG RECORDING TECHNIQUES

Vectorcardiograms: old myocardial infarction, ventricular hypertrophy, ventricular conduction abnormalities
Body surface mapping: precise definition of instantaneous depolarization and repolarization—primarily experimental at present
Signal-averaged ECG: prediction of serious ventricular arrhythmias
Exercise electrocardiography: transient subendocardial or transmural injury
Ambulatory monitoring: arrhythmias, transient subendocardial injury
Transtelephone monitoring: arrhythmias, pacemaker function
His bundle recordings: arrhythmias and conduction defects
Esophageal leads: arrhythmias

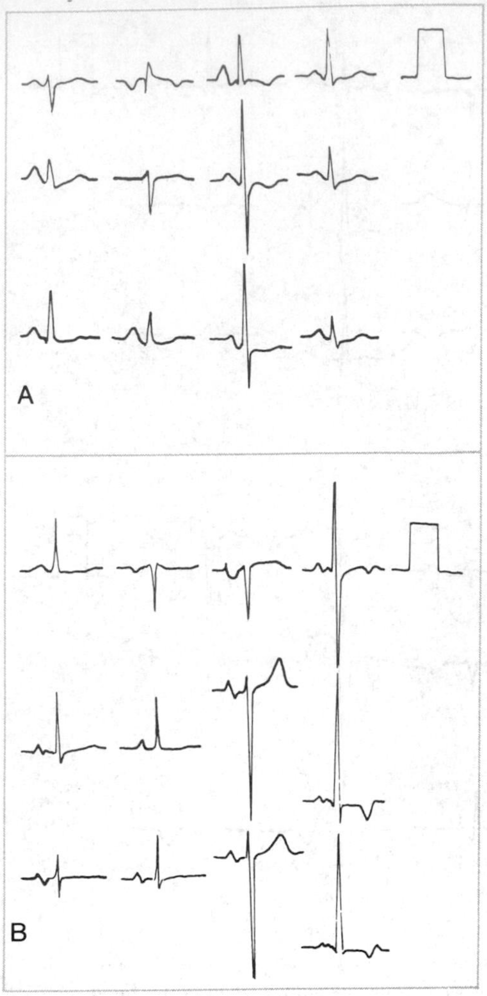

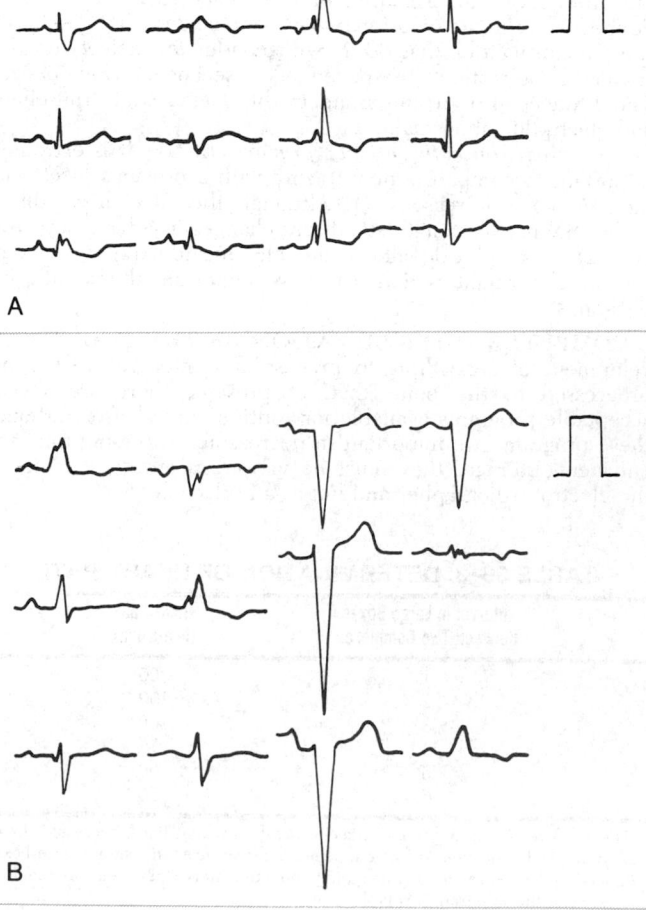

FIGURE 39–23. *A*, Right ventricular hypertrophy. The mean frontal plane axis is to the right, and there is excessive voltage in the right precordial leads. Also note the tall symmetrical P wave in lead II, indicating right atrial enlargement. *B*, Left ventricular hypertrophy. Note the excessive voltage in the lateral precordial leads and the inverted T waves in the same leads, indicating abnormal repolarization. The wide (greater than 0.12 second) biphasic P wave in lead V$_1$ is indicative of left atrial enlargement.

FIGURE 39–24. *A*, Right bundle branch block. The QRS duration is greater than 0.12 second, and the axis of the terminal 0.04 second of the QRS is to the right and anterior. *B*, Left bundle branch block. The QRS duration is greater than 0.12 second, and the terminal 0.04 second of the QRS is to the left and posterior. Note the secondary T wave changes in leads I and V$_6$.

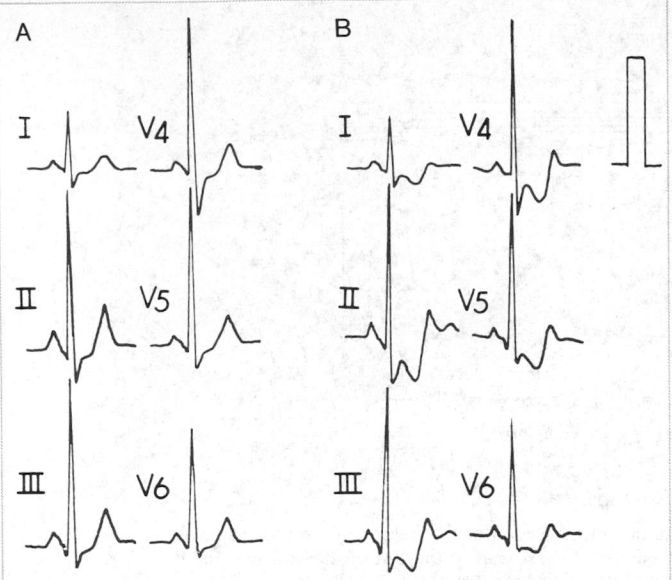

FIGURE 39–25. Recording obtained (*A*) prior to and (*B*) during an exercise test. Note the depression and downward sloping of the S-T segment wave during exercise. This is a typical pattern of subendocardial injury.

teaching electrocardiography and in enhancing the diagnosis of myocardial infarction, conduction defects, and ventricular hypertrophy.

A further refinement is body surface mapping, in which multiple precordial leads are obtained and a computer is utilized to generate a continuous body surface map of the change in electrical potential during depolarization and repolarization.

These techniques are still in the experimental stage, but ultimately may prove to be important in obtaining maximal information on the electrical activity of the heart. Low amplitude signals from the terminal part of QRS and the ST segment can be detected by signal averaging techniques and represent fractional conduction in infarcted regions. Current data suggest that the signal-averaged ECG may be useful in predicting patients with a high likelihood of having serious ventricular arrhythmias.

The ECG stress test is a widely used technique designed to assess the ability of the coronary circulation to deliver oxygen at a rate commensurate with the metabolic needs of the myocardium. Because myocardial metabolism is almost entirely aerobic, an inadequate increase in coronary flow quickly results in ischemia of the inner layers of the heart. The characteristic ST segment response is flat (square wave) or downward sloping. An abnormal ST segment is 0.1 mV or greater, measured 0.08 second after the end of the QRS complex (Fig. 39–25).

Chou TC, Helm RA: Clinical Vectorcardiography. 2nd ed. New York, Grune & Stratton, 1974. *Complete coverage of vectorcardiography.*

Lipman, BS, Massie E, Kleiger RE: Clinical Scalar Electrocardiography. 7th ed. Chicago, Year Book Medical Publishers, 1984. *Excellent general text covering all phases of electrocardiography.*

Marriott HJL: Practical Electrocardiography. 8th ed. Baltimore, Williams & Wilkins Company, 1983. *A comprehensive description of electrocardiography.*

39.3 Echocardiography

Richard L. Popp

PULSED REFLECTED ULTRASOUND

Echocardiography includes a family of diagnostic procedures that use ultrahigh-frequency sound waves to record the structure of the heart, and the blood flow velocities within the heart, throughout the cardiac cycle. Sound frequencies in the range of 1 to 10 million cycles per second, or megaHertz (MHz), are transmitted from a piezoelectric crystal along a carefully defined path within the thorax. A transducer is placed on the chest wall,

and a short burst of ultrasound is transmitted through the chest and into the underlying cardiac structures. The transducer then acts as a sound receiver until the next pulse. At each interface of materials with differing acoustic impedance, part of the sound is reflected or refracted and the remaining sound energy is further transmitted for subsequent acoustic reflection. The acoustic reflecting interfaces oriented perpendicular to the path of sound travel produce reflected sound that is received by the transducer on the chest wall as an "echo" of the transmitted sound. The location of each reflecting surface relative to the transducer can be calculated from the known velocity of sound in tissue and the elapsed time between sound transmission and reception of the echo. This series of depth readings is displayed on an oscilloscope for each pulse of sound, as shown in Figure 39–26. The strength of each echo is indicated by the brightness of the signal on the display device. Blood within the heart chambers usually gives signals of low amplitude that are not displayed. This "brightness-modulated" (B-mode) record of the reflecting interfaces is the building block for both two-dimensional (2D) and time-motion (M-mode) echocardiography.

One thousand pulses per second are created with typical instruments used clinically. A high sampling rate facilitates tracking motion of cardiac structures, yet there is usually enough time for the sound to return from even the most distant reflectors before the next pulse. Sequentially directing the sound beam along a given path, usually a pie-shaped sector of a circular plane, for each successive pulse produces a two-dimensional map of the structures underlying the transducer, called a 2D echocardiogram (Fig. 39–26). Clinical instruments sweep the sound beam through an arc of 60 to 90 degrees, by electronic or mechanical means, to create an imaging plane for visualizing a cross-section of the heart. Thus each 2D ultrasonic image is made up of multiple individual lines of sound reflection information. Depending on the basic pulse repetition rate, the time required for a single sound pulse to travel round trip through the thorax, and the number of such pulses per 2D image, 15 to 60 individual 2D image frames per second are available for interpretation. The images usually are presented on a digital scan converter that interpolates data between the scan lines and gives the impression of watching the heart in motion. The standardized examination provides multiple 2D cross-sectional planes through all parts of the heart using specific transducer locations, as shown in Figure 39–27. The dynamic three-dimensional structure of the heart can be understood by mentally assembling these multiple slices. An electrocardiogram is included as a reference signal in these studies.

A single direction of the sound beam, within the 2D image, may be selected for special attention and very high sampling rate. In this case, a given sound beam direction is repeatedly sampled, and the motion along the path of the sound beam is displayed with respect to time. The usual display is on an oscilloscope or strip chart recorder and is called a time-motion, T-M, or M-mode echocardiogram (right panel, Fig. 39–26). This method of recording is especially useful for identifying precise timing of motion of cardiac structures, such as valves, with respect to the electrocardiogram, phonocardiogram, or Doppler echocardiogram (to be described below). Historically, the M-mode echocardiogram was the first to be used.

Normal or abnormal patterns of cardiac chamber size and connection, wall thickness, wall motion, valve structure, and valve motion all are well assessed by echocardiographic study (Figs. 39–28 and 39–29). It is the method of choice for visualizing many abnormal structures, such as vegetations of infective endocarditis, intracardiac tumors, mural thrombi, and pericardial fluid.

During acute and chronic ventricular ischemia and acute infarction, the echocardiographic images accurately show the extent of myocardial thinning and segmental akinesis or dyskinesis. Exercise-induced segmental abnormalities may be observed as well. The acute complications of myocardial infarction that may be detected by imaging and Doppler echocardiography include pericardial effusion with or without cardiac tamponade, flail mitral leaflet (ruptured papillary muscle), acute mitral regurgitation of papillary muscle dysfunction, acute ventricular septal

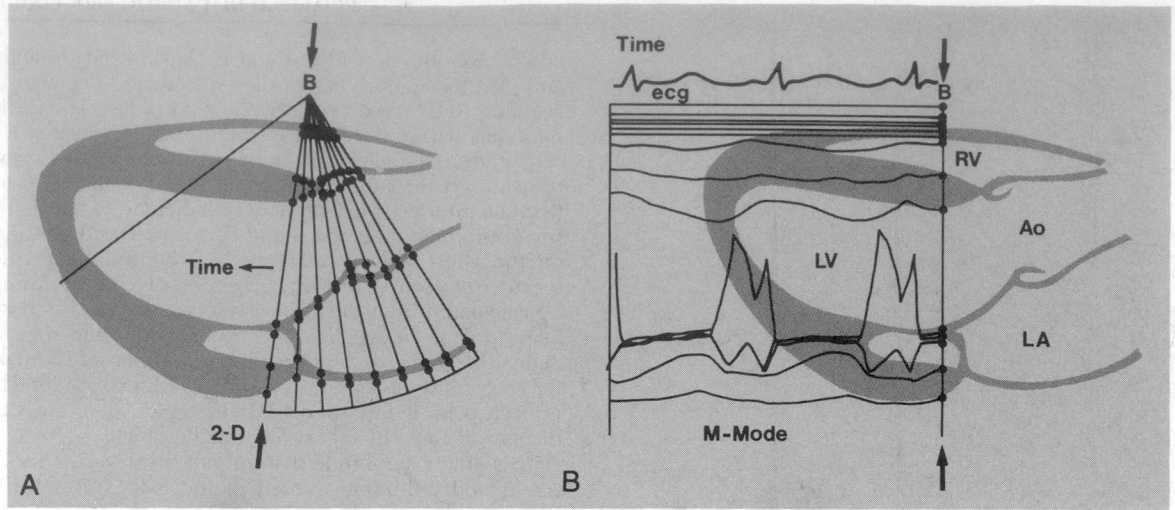

FIGURE 39–26. *A*, A schematic two-dimensional (2D) image of a cross-section of the heart oriented as displayed by echocardiography. The sound transducer is located on the anterior chest wall to the left of the sternum, at B. Sequential sound pulses and the returning echoes from reflecting interfaces are displayed as individual lines (*large arrows*), with dots of light defining the loci of reflectors. B = Brightness-modulated display. Many such lines, accumulated over 1/60 to 1/15 second, make up a single 2D image. *B*, A schematic time-motion (M-mode) echocardiogram produced by tracing out the location of structures moving during the cardiac cycle under a stationary sound transducer. As in *A*, the transducer on the chest wall creates a B-mode (B, *arrows*) display of sequential pulses and traces the motion pattern of each echo-producing interface. The M- and W-shaped patterns represent the anterior and posterior mitral valve leaflets, respectively. Ao = Aorta; ecg = electrocardiogram; LA = left atrium; LV = left ventricle; RV = right ventricle. (Modified from Popp RL, Rubenson DS, Tucker CR, et al.: Echocardiography: M-mode and two-dimensional methods. Ann Intern Med 93:844, 1980.)

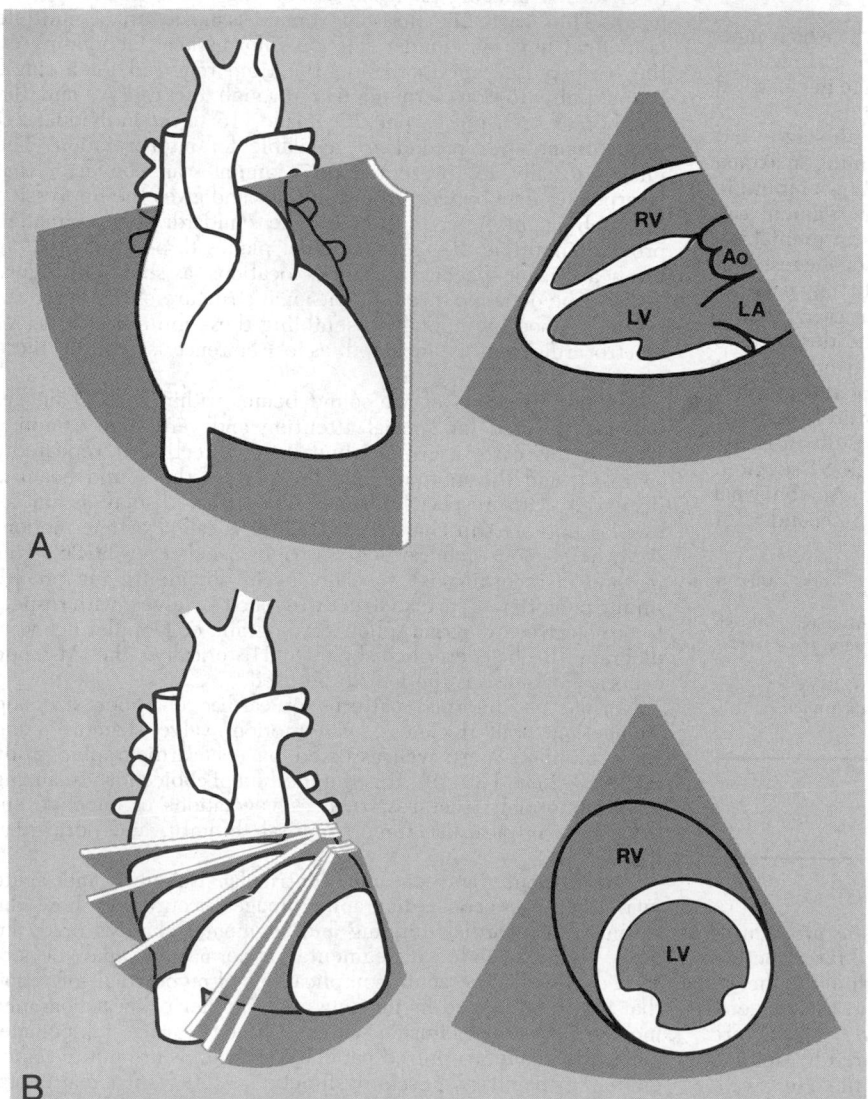

FIGURE 39–27. Schematic illustration of some standard 2D imaging planes used for clinical cardiac studies. *A*, Parasternal transducer position, with the imaging plane oriented parallel to the long axis of the left ventricle (LV) and intersecting a portion of the right ventricular outflow tract (RV), aortic root (Ao), and left atrium (LA). *B*, Transducer position as in *A*, but the imaging planes (six illustrated) are oriented parallel to the left ventricular short axis.

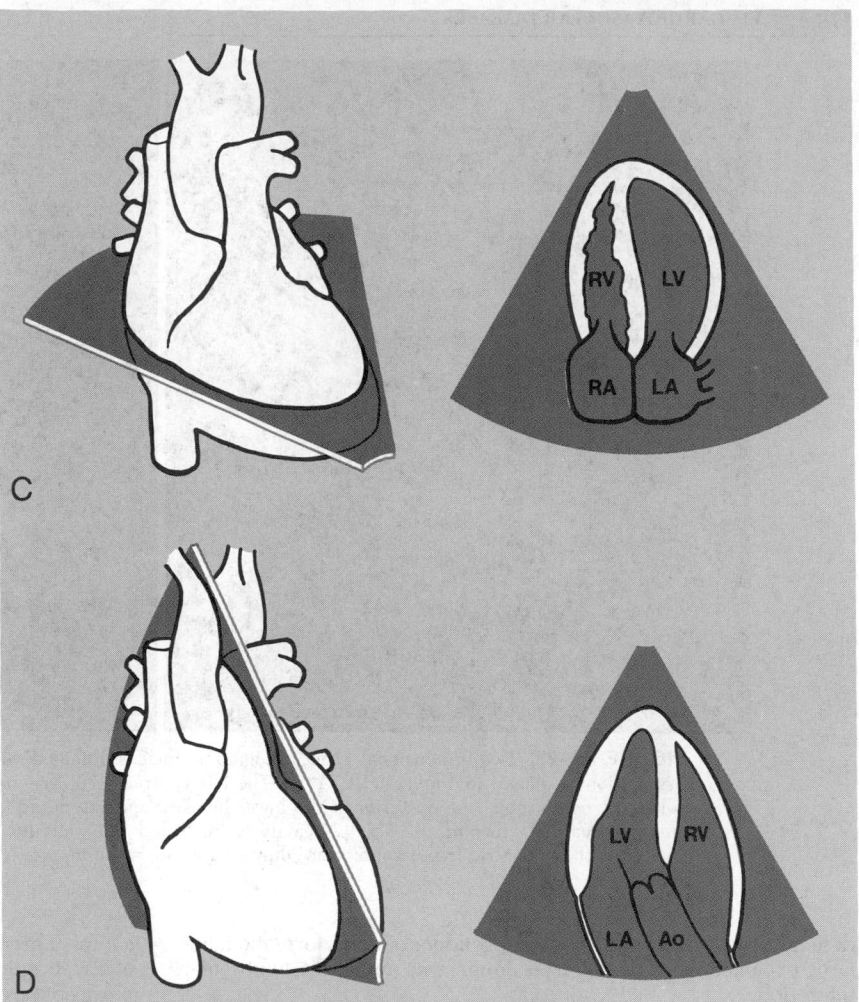

FIGURE 39–27 *Continued C,* Apical transducer position, with the imaging plane oriented to show the four main chambers of the heart (4-chamber view). The 2D image is displayed relative to the transducer so that the cardiac apex is shown near the transducer. RA = right atrium. *D,* Transducer position as in *C,* but the imaging plane is oriented parallel to the left ventricular long axis, as in panel *A.* (Redrawn from Popp RL, Fowles RE, Coltart DJ, et al.: Cardiac anatomy viewed systematically with two-dimensional echocardiography. Chest 75:579, 1979.)

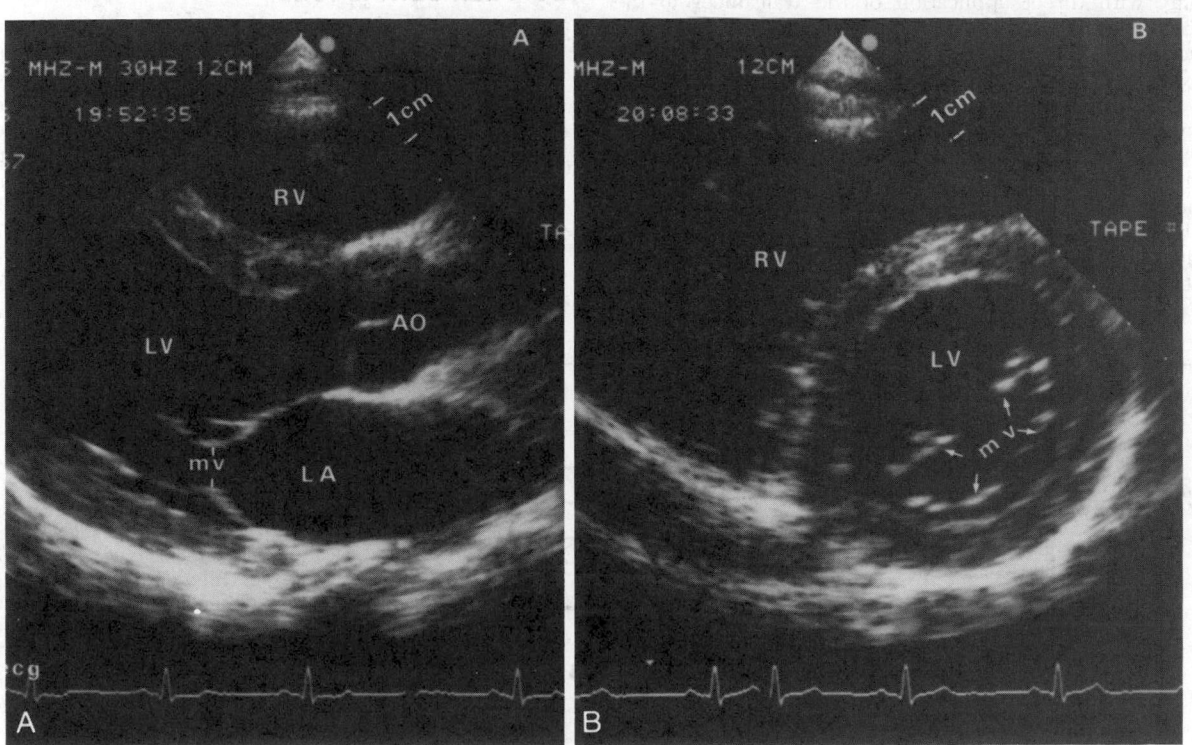

FIGURE 39–28. Two-dimensional echocardiographic images of a normal heart. Panels *A* and *B* were obtained with transducer positions and imaging plane orientations as shown in Figure 39–27*A* and *B,* respectively. Abbreviations as in Figure 39–27. mv = Mitral valve leaflets. (Note depth calibration scale at 1-cm intervals along right margin of each image.) The electrocardiograms (ecg) at the bottom of the panels are interrupted to indicate the timing of each image frame (late diastole in *A,* early diastole in *B*).

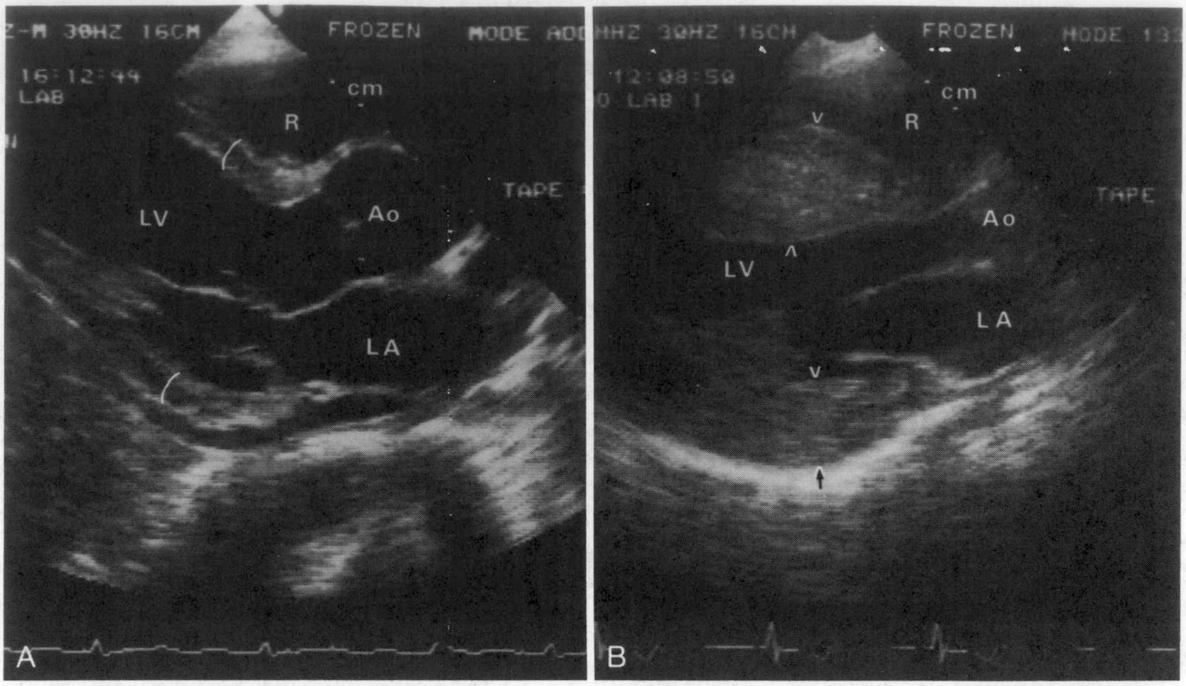

FIGURE 39–29. Two-dimensional echocardiographic images obtained with transducer position and image plane orientation as shown in Figure 39–27A. *A*, The left ventricle (LV) has normal wall thickness (white brackets). A relatively echo-free space posterior to the lower bracket, and extending toward the left atrium (LA), represents a small pericardial effusion. *B*, The LV cavity is small and the walls (*arrowheads*) are massively thickened in a patient with concentric hypertrophic cardiomyopathy. Ao = Aorta; cm = centimeter scale; R = right ventricle.

defect, myocardial rupture with pseudoaneurysm formation, infarct expansion producing true aneurysm, and right ventricular infarction.

Echocardiographic imaging also may be performed "invasively," as when transesophageal transducers are used or during thoracotomy with direct application of the transducer to the epicardium. These approaches produce superb images owing both to lack of sound scattering in the thorax and to the feasibility of using very high-frequency (5 to 10 MHz) ultrasound, which has high physical resolution but poor soft tissue penetration. Intravenous injections of many fluids, such as physiologic saline solution, contain myriad microbubbles of gas, which may be visualized by echocardiography as they travel through the right side of the heart. The gas does not pass through the pulmonary capillary bed, so if microbubble echoes are seen immediately in the left side of the heart, one may assume an intracardiac shunt is present, and a delayed appearance implies an intrapulmonary

shunt. Direct intra-aortic or intracoronary injection of various contrast agents has been used in attempts to visualize coronary perfusion areas of the left ventricle and experimentally to assess washout rates with altered coronary flow.

DOPPLER ULTRASOUND

Sound energy is transmitted as a series of compression-rarefaction waves with a given periodicity or wave frequency. Sound reflected from stationary surfaces has the same basic frequency as the transmitted sound, as shown in Figure 39–30. However, if the reflector or reflectors are moving relative to the direction of sound transmissions, the sequential interaction of the compression-rarefaction waves with the reflector results in a change in the frequency of the sound, as shown in Figure 39–30. This frequency shift is the Doppler effect, and it enables calculation of the velocity of the reflector if one knows the originally transmitted frequency, the received frequency, the speed of

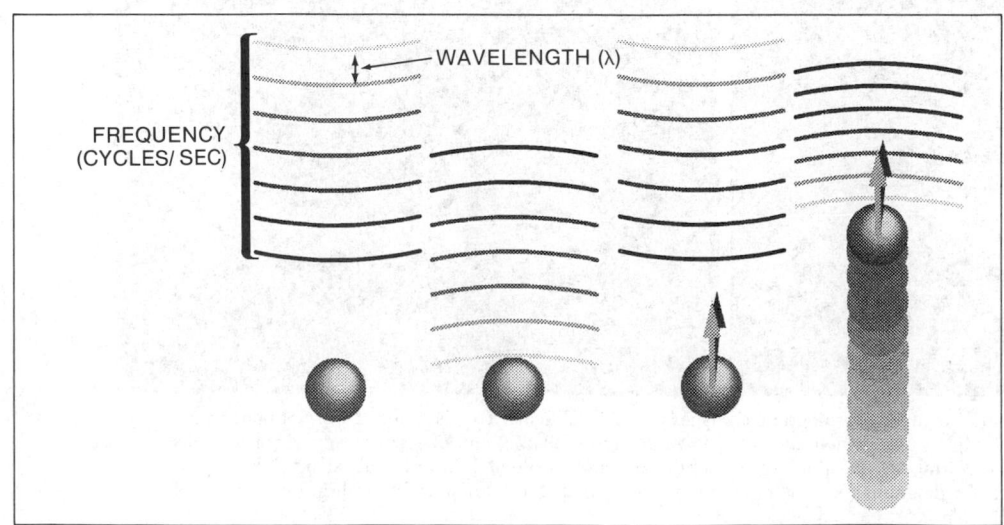

FIGURE 39–30. Schematic diagram of the Doppler principle as applied in echocardiography. From left to right: Sound waves of a given frequency (cycles/sec) and wave length (λ) are transmitted into the chest. Sound reflected from a stationary target has the same frequency as that transmitted. Sound directed toward a moving target interacts with the reflector and alters the frequency of the returning sound by a factor related to the speed of the moving target, the original sound frequency, and the angle of interception of the two.

sound in the medium (soft tissues), and the angle between the sound beam and the direction of the moving reflectors. The moving column of blood, with its cells and fluctuations in spatial distribution of cells, is the source of the Doppler frequency shift measured by echocardiography. An indicator of the beam direction undergoing Doppler frequency analysis is superimposed on the 2D image to help orientation and facilitate placing the beam in the general direction of flow. Fortunately, the change in frequency obtained with clinical instruments is in the audible range, so one may optimally match the direction of the sound beam with the direction of the blood flow by adjusting the transducer while listening to the signal. A beam-to-flow angle of zero degrees is desirable, since the calculated velocity is a function of the cosine of this angle (cos 0° = 1), but an angle of up to 20 degrees produces underestimation of velocities of up to only 6 per cent.

Blood flow toward or away from the transducer produces an increase or decrease in sound frequency, respectively, so both the velocity and the direction of the blood are measurable. These signals are usually displayed with velocities calculated from received Doppler shifted frequencies plotted versus time. The velocity spectrum is arranged above or below a baseline to convey information on flow direction, as shown in Figures 39–31 and 39–32.

Pulsed wave (PW) Doppler echocardiography is performed with pulses of ultrasound as described above, and frequency analysis is possible for sound returning from any given distance from the transducer. Thus, a signal received during systole from the left atrium and indicating high-velocity flow directed into the atrium from the ventricle signifies mitral regurgitation. This technique has proved especially valuable in locating intracardiac shunts, such as atrial or ventricular septal defects (Fig. 39–31) and patent ductus arteriosus. Since the product of the mean flow velocity (centimeters per second) and cross-sectional flow area (square centimeters) is volumetric flow (cubic centimeters per

second), flow within the pulmonary artery or left ventricular outflow tract, or across the tricuspid or mitral valves, can be estimated. Comparison of flows across the pulmonary artery and aorta gives an estimate of shunt flow across the septal defects, for example. Measurement of cardiac output by this method is useful clinically; however, the procedure is technically demanding.

PW methods provide spatial resolution but have limited velocity resolution because of the physical-mathematical constraints of sampling periodically. This trade-off is the opposite of that with continuous wave (CW) Doppler echocardiography, which uses one transducer to transmit, and another to receive, reflected sound continuously. CW Doppler methods have no spatial resolution within the path of the beam but can display frequency shifts corresponding to very high flow velocities. A major series of applications of Doppler echocardiography derives from the relationship of measured velocities to corresponding drops in pressure within the heart or vascular system. A cardiac valve stenosis presents an obstacle to flowing blood, which results in an increased velocity through the area of obstruction. This convective acceleration is the major factor producing a drop in pressure (ΔP, or pressure gradient) across the stenosis. The pressure difference can be accurately estimated instantaneously by CW Doppler echocardiography from the maximum flow velocity (V) achieved ($\Delta P = 4V^2$), as first shown by Holen and co-workers (1976). The ability to obtain intracardiac and intravascular pressure information noninvasively has been a significant advance in the capabilities of echocardiography. Many patients with aortic or mitral stenosis or both now have adequate preoperative hemodynamic assessment on the basis of clinical features and echocardiography only. The method for calculating instantaneous and mean pressure drops across a stenotic aortic valve is shown in Figure 39–32.

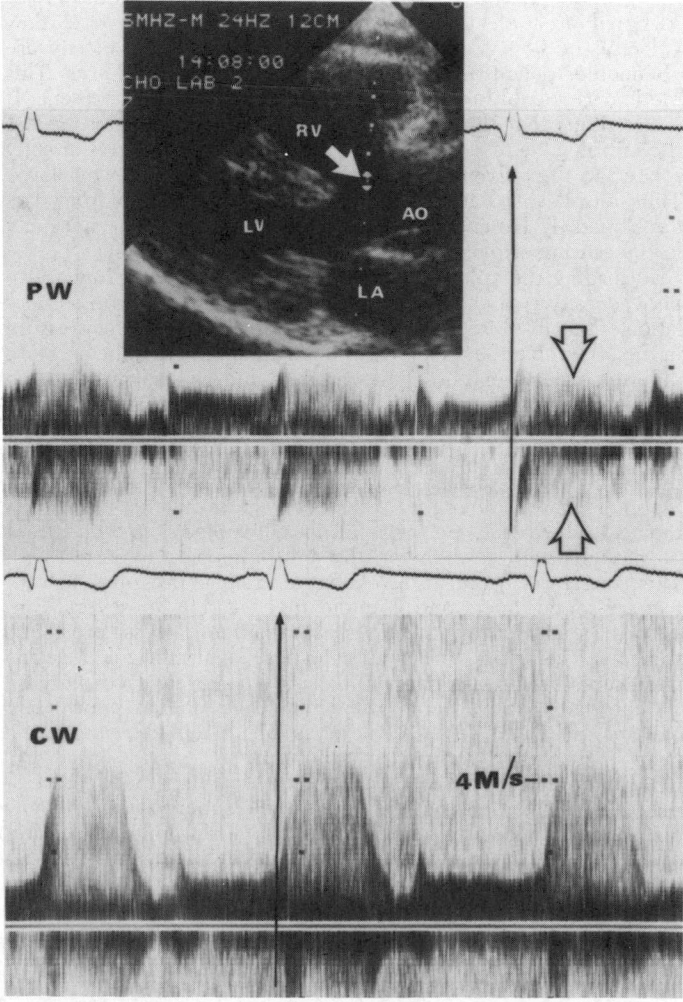

FIGURE 39–31. Methods of displaying a Doppler echocardiographic study in a patient with ventricular septal defect. The black panel above is a 2D image taken with transducer position and image plane orientation as in Figure 39–27A. The white arrow points to the sample volume indicator for pulsed-wave (PW) Doppler ultrasound analysis. This illustration is from a patient with a large defect of the septum between the right ventricle (RV) and left ventricle (LV). The white panels below are spectral displays of the Doppler ultrasound signals in a patient with a small ventricular septal defect. The PW record indicates a frequency shift (*open arrows*) from the area of the sample volume (above), which occurs in systole after the onset of the electrocardiographic QRS (*long arrow*). The continuous-wave (CW) record indicates high-velocity (>4 M/s) flow somewhere along the dotted line shown above. The systolic pressure difference between the right and left ventricles can be calculated from the CW signal as shown in Figure 39–32. The location of the signal origin is defined by PW, while the CW signal defines high-flow velocity quantitatively but is ambiguous regarding signal locus. Other abbreviations as in Figure 39–26.

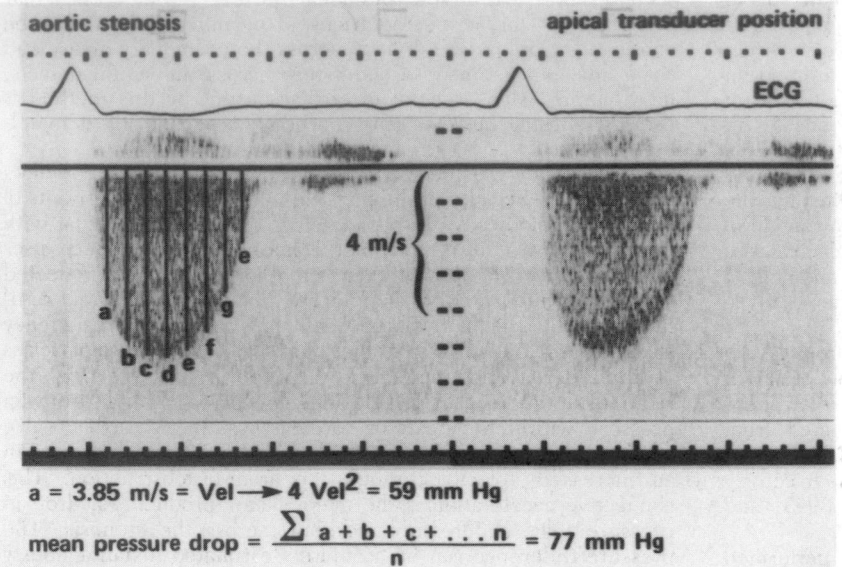

aortic stenosis   apical transducer position

ECG

4 m/s

$a = 3.85 \text{ m/s} = Vel \longrightarrow 4\, Vel^2 = 59 \text{ mm Hg}$

$$\text{mean pressure drop} = \frac{\sum a + b + c + \ldots n}{n} = 77 \text{ mm Hg}$$

FIGURE 39–32. Continuous-wave Doppler ultrasound recording of aortic outflow velocities from a patient with aortic stenosis. The transducer is at the apex, so flow toward the aorta is registered below the baseline in this spectral display of velocity (M/s) versus time. The systolic signal occurs after each QRS of the electrocardiogram (ECG). Instantaneous (vertical lines a through e) maximum velocities (Vel) are assumed to occur in the most narrow part of the stenosis and to correspond to instantaneous pressure drops across the stenosis. The formulae for calculating the instantaneous and mean pressure drops in mm Hg are given below. n = Number of samples.

The pressure drop across a stenotic valve is dependent on both the valve area and the blood volume crossing the valve per unit of time. Aortic valve area is accurately estimated by applying the Gorlin formula (see Ch. 39.5) using Doppler ultrasound–derived values for ejection time, stroke volume, and pressure gradient. Alternatively, one may calculate the flow per beat (see above) from the mean flow velocity and cross-sectional area of the left ventricular outflow tract immediately below the stenotic valve and assume that this same flow is represented by the product of the mean flow velocity within, and the cross-sectional area of, the stenotic valve. The outflow tract flow velocity, outflow tract area, and aortic valve flow velocity are obtainable, permitting calculation of the aortic valve area. This method is reliable even when aortic regurgitation is present. It is fortuitous that the time required for the pressure drop across the mitral valve to reach one half of the maximum level is directly related to the valve area at virtually all clinically relevant flows. Thus mitral valve area may be accurately calculated from data developed by Holen and colleagues (1977) without the necessity for measuring stroke volume.

Recording the velocity of blood flowing across a narrow orifice between any two chambers or cardiovascular loci permits calculation of the absolute pressure level in one chamber if the pressure in the other chamber is known. For example, the systolic pressure difference between the right ventricle and right atrium can be calculated from the velocities recorded from tricuspid regurgitant flow. The sum of jugular venous or right atrial pressure and the atrioventricular pressure difference is the right ventricular systolic pressure. The prevalence of tricuspid regurgitation detectable by Doppler echocardiography sufficient to perform this calculation ranges from over 70 per cent (in normal subjects) to 80 per cent (in patients with cardiomyopathy and pulmonary hypertension). This concept is useful in assessing ventricular pressures in ventricular septal defect and is under investigation for several conditions. Quantitating the pressure gradient across prosthetic valves and assessing the central or perivalvular origin of regurgitant prosthesis leaks noninvasively are major advances because the alternative of catheter placement to get similar information may require trans-septal catheterization of the left side of the heart or direct left ventricular puncture.

Advancing microprocessor technology for high-speed processing of ultrasonic echoes has permitted superposition of flow direction and velocity information, obtained from Doppler frequency shift analysis throughout the imaging field, upon the 2D image itself. The velocity data are coded in color and shade for direction and velocity, respectively, and are presented as a color velocity map within the cardiac chambers of the 2D image at frame rates of 12 to 30 per second. This flow velocity tomographic image is similar to angiographic projectional images in that it gives the appearance of blood moving normally or abnormally across the valves and within the chambers (see Color Plate 4A and B). Clinical instruments generally provide standard 2D, M-mode, PW, and CW Doppler audio and spectral displays as well as the color flow velocity images.

Echocardiography has some advantages over competing imaging technologies. These include no risk from ionizing radiation, portability of equipment, noninvasive imaging, high imaging rate, no requirement for contrast injection, and generally low cost for the study. Its disadvantages include poor-quality images in 5 to 20 per cent of various patient groups and lack of complete quantitative data from most clinical laboratories.

Feigenbaum H: Echocardiography. 3rd ed. Philadelphia, Lea & Febiger, 1986. *This encyclopedic text is useful for the neophyte as well as the advanced student. Its strength in discussion of M-mode and 2D methods is not quite matched in areas discussing Doppler ultrasonography.*

Hatle L, Angelsen B: Doppler Ultrasound in Cardiology. 2nd ed. Philadelphia, Lea & Febiger, 1985. *The most authoritative text on this subject. The chapters on the physics of blood flow and Doppler analysis are excellent. The comprehensive illustrations of pathologic and normal flow velocity patterns are superb. Much of the information included is not published elsewhere.*

Holen J, Aaslid R, Landmark K, et al.: Determination of pressure gradient in mitral stenosis with a non-invasive ultrasound Doppler technique. Acta Med Scand 199:455, 1976. *The classic work describing the clinical use of the relationship between maximum blood velocity detected by Doppler ultrasonography and pressure gradient calculated from the velocity.*

Holen J, Aaslid R, Landmark K, et al.: Determination of effective orifice area in mitral stenosis from non-invasive ultrasound Doppler data and mitral flow rate. Acta Med Scand 201:83, 1977. *Original description of the pressure half-time method for estimation of mitral orifice area using Doppler ultrasonography.*

Popp RL: Echocardiography (Part 1). N Engl J Med 323:101, 1990. Echocardiography (Part 2). N Eng J Med 323:165, 1990. *A recent review of the clinically accepted uses of echocardiography.*

Popp RL, Macovski A: Ultrasonic diagnostic instruments. Science 210:268, 1980. *A more detailed discussion of the instrumentation for producing ultrasonic images than given in this chapter.*

39.4 Nuclear Cardiology

Barry L. Zaret

Nuclear cardiology is based upon the ability of externally placed instruments to detect, define, and quantify radiation emanating from cardiac structures following injection of a radioisotope. The utility of nuclear procedures for defining pathophysiologic, prognostic, and diagnostic phenomena in cardiac patients has been established. The procedures can be safely repeated and are suitable for both imaging and biodistribution studies. Changes in cardiac function, ventricular volume, myocardial perfusion, viability, and metabolism can be evaluated in appropriate clinical circumstances.

At present, a major clinical application of nuclear cardiology is in the assessment of global and regional cardiac performance. This is achieved with radionuclides that remain within the intravascular space during the period of study. Computer technology is critical for such measurement. Cardiac performance can be assessed in two general ways: during the first pass of the isotope through the central circulation or following its equilibration in the cardiac blood pool. First-pass radionuclide angiocardiography is completed within 30 seconds following intravenous injection of a technetium–99m (^{99m}Tc) compound. There is temporal and anatomic segregation of the radioactive bolus during its first transit through the central circulation. Thus it is possible to make concomitant measurements of right and left ventricular function without concern that radioactivity present in one ventricle is interfering with the analysis of the other. Analysis of time-activity curves generated from the respective ventricular regions allows determination of ventricular ejection fraction (Fig. 39–33). Count rates emanating from a cardiac chamber are proportional to the volume of the chamber. In addition to analysis of ejection fraction, rates of ventricular filling and emptying, and ventricular volumes, quantitative and qualitative assessments of regional wall motion can be made from the same data.

The alternative and much more widely used approach to assessing cardiac performance involves equilibration radionuclide studies. Physiologic signals are introduced that convert the conventional static imaging procedure into a dynamic assessment of cardiac function. To obtain this goal, ^{99m}Tc is bound to the patient's own erythrocytes. The ^{99m}Tc label remains evenly distributed throughout the intravascular blood volume for several hours. With the use of the electrocardiogram, nuclear data are segregated according to the time of their occurrence within the cardiac cycle. Data are summed over several hundred cardiac cycles, and composite data are quantified and displayed as sequential 10- to 50-msec points, which together define a representative cardiac cycle. The ventricular volume curve derived from these data is suitable for direct measurement of ejection fraction, rates of filling and ejection, and ventricular volumes. The data are also displayed as a series of images that, when projected in cinematic format, provide a direct visual assessment of the regional contraction patterns of the heart (Fig. 39–34). Computer techniques, particularly regional ejection fraction, now make it possible also to quantify regional function motion accurately. With the regional ejection fraction technique, the left ventricular blood pool in the left anterior oblique position is divided into five discrete areas corresponding to septal, apical, and lateral regions. Individual time-activity curves are obtained from each of these regions, thereby providing quantitative regional analysis.

Both first-pass and equilibrium techniques can be employed to study cardiac performance under conditions of rest and exercise. Data may be accumulated during supine, semisupine, or upright bicycle exercise. Often critical data emerge only when the patient is evaluated during stress. The normal response to exercise involves an augmentation in the pump function of both ventricles, generally defined as an increase in ejection fraction of at least 5 per cent (in absolute ejection fraction units) and the presence of normal regional wall motion. Abnormal exercise ventricular reserve may be encountered in a variety of pathophysiologic conditions involving coronary artery disease and intrinsic myocardial, valvular, and congenital heart disease.

The study of cardiac performance employing nuclear techniques has been particularly useful in coronary artery disease. The ejection fraction is the single best clinical indicator of global ventricular pump performance. The index is of major prognostic importance in patients with coronary artery disease, either immediately following myocardial infarction or in the chronic or subacute phases of disease. Analysis of the ventricular ejection fraction is based upon radioactivity counts. It is not dependent upon geometric assumptions concerning ventricular shape or ventricular volume. In coronary artery disease, particularly following myocardial infarction, asymmetric contraction patterns are common. In these ischemic ventricles, cavitary shapes frequently cannot be approximated by idealized geometric models. Consequently, in coronary artery disease, ejection fraction is measured most accurately by the nuclear approach. Using portable equipment, it is possible to study cardiac performance at the bedside of the acutely ill. Such studies have demonstrated substantial abnormalities in the functioning of the ischemic left ventricle during the acute phase of myocardial infarction. Right ventricular infarction occuring in the course of inferior wall infarction has been identified and further defined. The important negative prognostic impact of functional left ventricular aneurysm formation during acute anterior infarction has been defined. Assessment of regional and global function also is an important means of evaluating the effect of thrombolytic therapy for acute infarction.

Abnormalities of ventricular performance are found in approximately 85 per cent of patients with coronary artery disease studied during exercise stress. Myocardial ischemia is reflected in abnormal ventricular reserve. Abnormal responses of the ejection fraction may be encountered in a variety of conditions, but the development of new regional abnormalities of wall motion is quite specific for coronary artery disease. Abnormal exercise performance has important prognostic implications, particularly following infarction.

In addition, recent technical advances now make it possible to

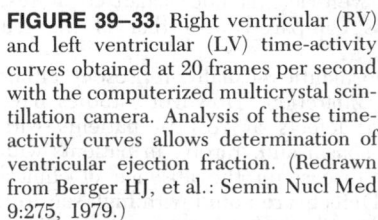

FIGURE 39–33. Right ventricular (RV) and left ventricular (LV) time-activity curves obtained at 20 frames per second with the computerized multicrystal scintillation camera. Analysis of these time-activity curves allows determination of ventricular ejection fraction. (Redrawn from Berger HJ, et al.: Semin Nucl Med 9:275, 1979.)

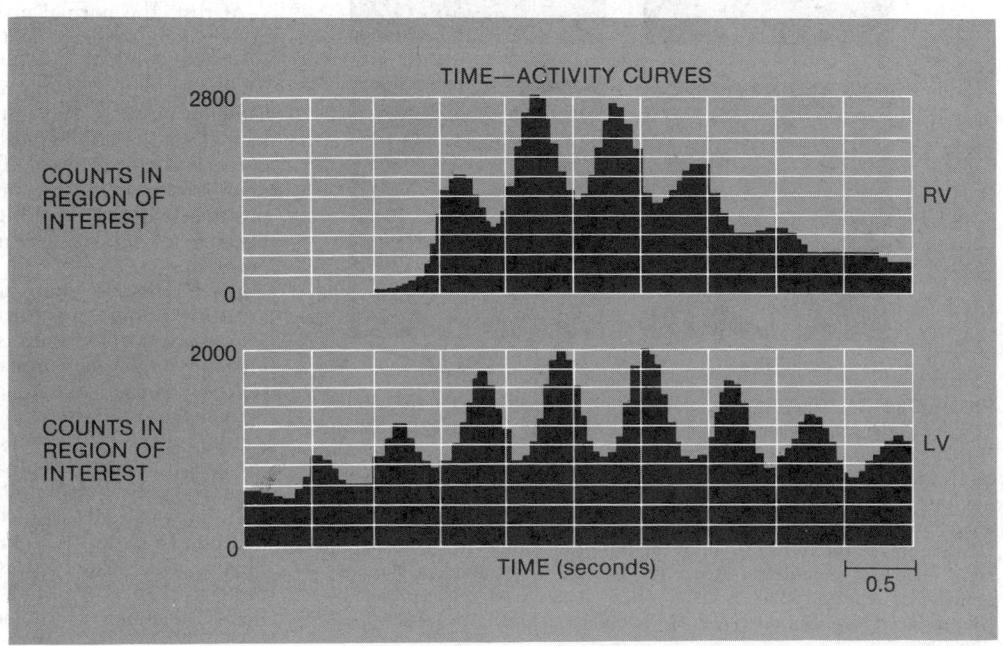

monitor ventricular function in ambulatory patients using a miniaturized detector system employing the principles of equilibrum radionuclide angiocardiography. With this approach, abnormalities of ventricular performance have been noted during routine activities in patients with coronary disease. This new technique, still under active investigation, offers promise for the study of silent myocardial ischemia.

Radionuclide assessment of ventricular performance may also be employed in the evaluation of patients with valvular disease at rest or exercise. Resting measurement of cardiac function provides important preoperative prognostic data and may also be of value in defining the physiologic significance of valvular lesions such as mitral regurgitation. For example, normal left ventricular function in a patient with severe mitral regurgitation would imply a primary valvular problem, whereas severe ventricular dysfunction would suggest secondary mitral regurgitation resulting from diffuse myocardial disease. Assessment of performance under hemodynamic stress may help define the advent of irreversible damage in valvular heart disease. This is particularly important in aortic regurgitation, in which irremediable change in left ventricular function is frequently present by the time valve surgery is considered.

Assessment of ventricular performance and ventricular volumes is critical to the understanding and treatment of congestive heart failure. Knowledge of the degree of impairment in ventricular performance has prognostic and therapeutic relevance. In addi-

tion, an important group of patients with primary diastolic dysfunction (normal systolic function and impaired measures of diastolic filling) has been defined well with nuclear techniques. This group may involve as much as 20 to 40 per cent of patients presenting for evaluation of clinical congestive heart failure. It is highly important to define such patients, since routine heart failure therapy is not effective. These patients appear to respond to calcium channel blocking agents.

Radionuclide studies also have been employed in the evaluation of myocardial function in patients with lung disease in which the major hemodynamic burden falls on the right ventricle. Right ventricular performance can probably be evaluated best with the first-pass technique. Abnormalities in right ventricular performance have been noted at rest and during exercise in patients with chronic obstructive pulmonary disease. Pharmacologic interventions may modify abnormal right ventricular performance.

These techniques also have been utilized for long-term studies assessing cardiac therapy. A prototype example has been the application of radionuclide angiocardiography for the serial assessment of ventricular function in patients receiving the antineoplastic agent doxorubicin. Use of this agent has been limited by the frequent development of a drug-induced cardiomyopathy. Serial measurement of cardiac ejection fraction during the course of therapy has led to a set of dosage guidelines that help avert cardiotoxicity.

MYOCARDIAL PERFUSION IMAGING

Myocardial perfusion imaging utilizes radionuclides that traverse the myocardial capillary system and enter the myocardial cell. The radionuclide currently employed for these studies is thallium-201 (^{201}Tl). This tracer is considered a potassium analogue, since its distribution generally mirrors that of intracellular potassium. Thallium-201 is produced in the cyclotron and has a physical half-life of approximately 72 hours. After intravenous injection it is rapidly extracted and distributed within the myocardium according to regional myocardial blood flow and regional cellular viability. Recently, a new group of ^{99m}Tc perfusion tracers, the isonitriles, has been developed. These radiopharmaceuticals, although currently still experimental, should be in the clinical arena shortly. They offer several potential advantages over ^{201}Tl. These include better imaging characteristics, ability to administer a higher dose, better suitability for tomographic studies, and biologic properties that involve lack of major washout following administration. This latter property allows for delayed imaging following administration, particularly in the acute situation, thereby allowing definition of risk zones in acute ischemic syndromes. The ability to administer a ^{99m}Tc bolus intravenously allows for measurement of ejection fraction prior to perfusion imaging. The isonitrile images may also be ECG gated, allowing for better image resolution as well as potential quantification of regional function.

At rest, the normal myocardial perfusion image demonstrates homogeneous uptake in the left ventricular wall with a central area of decreased activity corresponding to the left ventricular cavity. In approximately 20 per cent of normal persons, there is a region of decreased uptake at the cardiac apex corresponding to a normal relative apical thinning. Abnormal image patterns of decreased myocardial perfusion demonstrate a region of relatively decreased radionuclide uptake. Images are obtained in multiple positions. The normal right ventricle is not visualized at rest because of its smaller mass compared with that of the left ventricle.

In the resting state, abnormalities usually represent either acute or remote myocardial infarction. However, studies have also demonstrated perfusion defects at rest in patients with unstable angina or coronary spasm and, rarely, in patients with severe obstructive coronary disease in the absence of clinical evidence of acute ischemia. Defects are noted with high sensitivity during the early hours of acute myocardial infarction. Within the first 6 hours, virtually all infarcts may be identified. After 24 hours, sensitivity falls to 80 to 90 per cent.

In most patients with coronary artery disease without previous infarction, myocardial perfusion patterns appear normal at rest. This is to be expected, since coronary blood flow is relatively uniform at rest, even in the presence of severe coronary obstruction. The major physiologic abnormality in coronary disease is

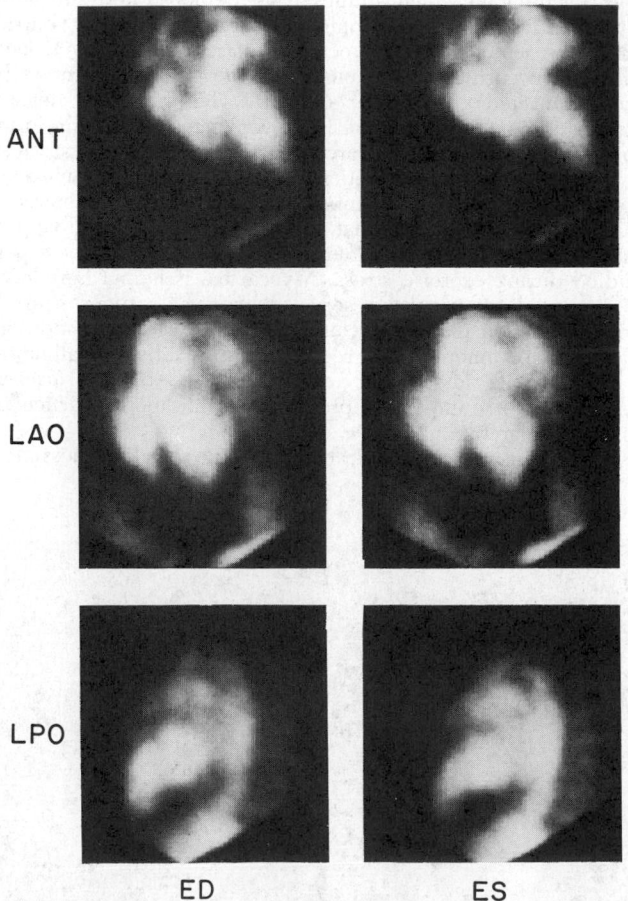

ANT

LAO

LPO

ED   ES

FIGURE 39–34. Gated cardiac blood pool studies obtained in the anterior (ANT), 45-degree left anterior oblique (LAO), and left posterior oblique (LPO) positions. End-diastolic images (ED) are shown on the left and end-systolic (ES) on the right. Note that radioactivity is present throughout the entire cardiac blood pool. A large anteroapical left ventricular aneurysm is appreciated in all three positions. Note that in the LAO position image the left ventricle is the posterior cardiac structure and the right ventricle the anterior structure. These are separated by the interventricular septum, which is displayed as an area devoid of radioactivity. (Reproduced from Berger HJ, et al.: Radiol Clin North Am 18:441, 1980.)

diminished coronary vascular reserve. Therefore, to detect perfusion abnormalities in coronary disease it is necessary to study patients under conditions of increased myocardial blood flow. Most work has employed exercise as an appropriate stress. Thallium-201 is injected at peak exercise, and imaging is begun within 10 minutes after injection. Since thallium is rapidly extracted by myocardium, it can be injected during the period of maximal heterogeneity of regional myocardial blood flow, and its distribution reflects this heterogeneity. Comparison of images obtained immediately following exercise with those obtained following a redistribution phase 2 to 4 hours after exercise allows definition of transiently ischemic zones (Fig. 39–35). Defects present on exercise but not at redistribution are most consistent with transient ischemia; defects that are unchanged are most consistent with previous infarction and scar; and defects that are present at redistribution but are markedly increased during exercise are most consistent with transient ischemia superimposed upon the scar. Recently, it has been recognized that delayed imaging may be important for detecting viable yet ischemic myocardium that appears as a fixed defect on the initial stress and redistribution images. For this purpose 24-hour imaging studies, with or without a second injection of radioisotope, have been employed. In this manner, up to 40 per cent of fixed defects have been demonstrated to have some reversibility. The overall sensitivity of this technique for detecting significant ischemic disease is approximately 80 per cent. The specificity of the technique is excellent. This technique is of greatest value diagnostically in patients with equivocal exercise electrocardiograms, abnormal baseline electrocardiograms, or suspected false-positive or false-negative conventional exercise tests. Both imaging with the patient at rest and exercise/redistribution studies have been of value in evaluating thrombolysis and reperfusion. Exercise studies also are of major value in assessing prognosis following infarction in stable coronary disease and in evaluating patients after coronary angioplasty. In addition to the magnitude of the perfusion defect, increased lung uptake has been demonstrated to be a potent prognostic index in coronary disease patients.

An alternative means of stress perfusion imaging involves use of the coronary vasodilator, dipyridamole. Thallium myocardial distributions following dipyridamole provide data comparable to those noted with exercise. However, with pharmacologic stress, evaluation is based upon differences in flow without implying ischemia, whereas with exercise, evaluation is based upon heterogeneity of flow, generally associated with ischemia. Dipyridamole studies are of particular value in patients unable to exercise.

This type of study has been of particular value in identifying myocardial ischemia in peripheral vascular disease patients undergoing preoperative cardiac evaluation.

Thallium planar imaging is now increasingly quantitative. Computer techniques provide objective definition of the presence and extent of defects as well as quantification of regional tracer washout kinetics. Contemporary evaluation of thallium imaging data should include quantitative interpretation of visual data.

Single photon emission computed tomography (SPECT) thallium studies are currently employed widely. In comparative studies with planar imaging, SPECT has been shown to have similar diagnostic accuracy. A major current use involves definition of multiple vascular bed involvement in coronary disease. Although its clinical role has not been completely defined, it is anticipated that SPECT studies involving the isonitriles will prove to be a significant diagnostic advance.

INFARCT-AVID IMAGING

An additional radionuclide approach involves definition of acute myocardial infarction and regions of acute myocardial necrosis. This is performed with "infarct-avid" radiotracers, which bind selectively to regions of acute infarction. The current agent for this procedure is ^{99m}Tc stannous pyrophosphate. Acute infarcts are visualized as regions of increased radionuclide uptake. The mechanism of abnormal pyrophosphate accumulation appears to be related to regional calcium deposition, as well as binding to denatured proteins. Pyrophosphate uptake also is dependent upon sufficient residual blood flow to allow entry of the radioactive tracer.

The infarct zone can be visualized within 24 to 48 hours of the onset of infarction. Maximal visualization generally occurs from 48 to 72 hours after the infarct. Images usually are not positive within the first 24 hours unless thrombolysis has occurred. Images generally are no longer positive 7 to 10 days after the infarct. Pyrophosphate infarct imaging is most valuable in patients presenting several days after infarction when other studies are equivocal or nondiagnostic.

Radiolabeled antimyosin antibody has recently been proposed as an alternative means of infarct-avid imaging. Initial trials with this agent have been quite promising with respect to infarct definition and prognostic impact. In addition, antimyosin imaging studies have been employed for defining acute myocarditis in patients with heart failure and for defining cardiac transplant rejection.

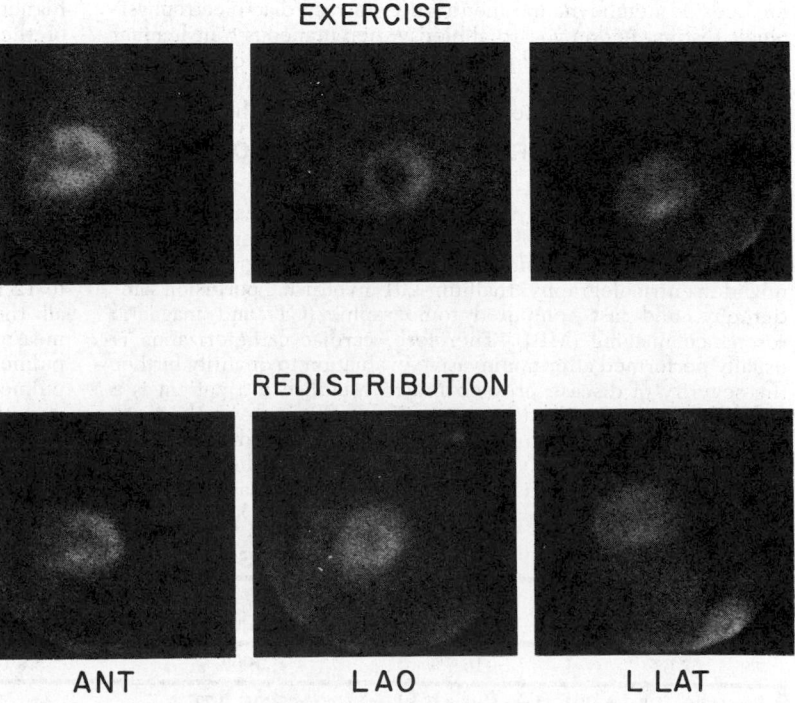

EXERCISE

REDISTRIBUTION

ANT   LAO   L LAT

FIGURE 39–35. Exercise (upper panels) and redistribution (lower panels) thallium-201 myocardial perfusion images in a patient with significant coronary artery disease. Anterior position (ANT) images are shown in the left panels, left anterior oblique (LAO) images in the middle panels, and left lateral (L LAT) images in the right panels. Note a significant perfusion defect present in the anteroseptal wall seen in the LAO image and in the anteroapical wall seen in the L LAT image during exercise, with substantial redistribution and filling in of the perfusion defect on the redistribution images. This study is consistent with transient myocardial ischemia and coronary artery disease involving at least the left anterior descending coronary artery.

POSITRON TOMOGRAPHY (PET)

This technique involves imaging and quantification of the intracardiac distribution of positron-emitting radionuclides. By virtue of the types of radionuclides available and the instrumentation employed, this technique has provided new insight into metabolism and coronary flow. Since carbon–11 is a positron emitter, a variety of biologically active compounds can be radiolabeled and used for imaging. These include fatty acids, metabolites, receptor ligands, and neurotransmitters.

There has been great interest recently in PET studies of myocardial metabolism and perfusion. Of most immediate clinical impact has been the demonstration that increased regional glucose accumulation in areas that are hypoperfused represents viable tissue with a substantial likelihood of improved function with revascularization. This has been demonstrated using fluorodeoxyglucose as the radiopharmaceutical. This "glucose-perfusion mismatch" offers major opportunities for evaluating stunned and hibernating myocardium in ischemic heart disease as well as ischemic cardiomyopathy. Recent additional comparative studies have also involved radiolabeled acetate, palmitate, and glucose. Finally, tomographic perfusion imaging involving positron-emitting rubidium, water, and nitrogen-labeled ammonia has also shown promise, although experience is currently somewhat limited.

Gerson MC: Cardiac Nuclear Medicine. New York, McGraw-Hill Book Company, 1987. *This multiauthored text contains 11 chapters devoted to nuclear cardiology and provides an excellent overview of technical aspects of the field as well as appropriate clinical applications.*

Wackers FJ: Myocardial perfusion imaging. *In* Gottschalk A, Hoffer PB, Pochen EJ (eds.): Diagnostic Nuclear Medicine. Baltimore, Williams & Wilkins Company, 1988, pp 291–354. *An excellent overview of myocardial perfusion imaging. This review contains 218 references.*

Zaret BL, Berger HJ: Nuclear cardiology. *In* Hurst JW (ed.): The Heart. 7th ed. New York, McGraw-Hill Book Company, 1990, pp 1899–1950. *A comprehensive review of all aspects of nuclear cardiology, with 309 individual references cited.*

39.5 Cardiac Catheterization and Angiography

William H. Barry

Cardiac catheterization provides a unique, comprehensive, and quantitative assessment of cardiac structure and function and is frequently utilized in the diagnosis and management of patients with heart disease. With the further application of this procedure for bedside hemodynamic monitoring, intracardiac electrophysiologic testing, endomyocardial biopsy, percutaneous transluminal coronary angioplasty, and percutaneous balloon valvotomy, it has become increasingly important for the internist to understand the indications, capabilities, and risks of cardiac catheterization.

INDICATIONS FOR CARDIAC CATHETERIZATION AND ANGIOGRAPHY

The accuracy of noninvasive evaluation has increased remarkably recently, because of the greatly improved sensitivity and specificity of two-dimensional Doppler echocardiography, radionuclide ventriculography, thallium-201 myocardial perfusion scintigraphy, and fast computed tomographic (CT) and magnetic resonance imaging (MRI). Therefore, cardiac catheterization is usually performed after noninvasive evaluation to quantify further the severity of disease present and to establish if a patient is a candidate for surgical intervention. Table 39–5 shows the diagnoses of a typical series of patients referred for cardiac catheterization. The vast majority of patients undergoing this procedure have coronary artery disease, with valvular disease a distant

second. Table 39–6 lists the usual indications for cardiac catheterization and coronary angiography in patients with coronary artery disease or valvular heart disease.

TECHNIQUES AND THEIR HAZARDS

ARTERIAL AND VENOUS ACCESS. Two basic approaches are used for insertion of catheters into arteries and veins. The first involves incision of the skin overlying the vessel, dissection of the vessel free of surrounding tissue, and incision of the vessel with direct insertion of the catheter. The advantage of this method, usually reserved for the brachial artery or antecubital vein, is that it provides direct access to the vessels, so that they may either be tied off (vein) or repaired (brachial artery) after completion of the catheterization procedure, decreasing the likelihood of hematoma formation. The disadvantages of the technique are that an incision is required in the skin, increasing the patient's discomfort in the postcatheterization period; and there is a significant (2 to 3 per cent) incidence of thrombosis of the brachial artery. However, this approach is usually preferred in patients with severe atherosclerotic disease of the aorta or iliofemoral arteries.

In the Seldinger technique, an artery or vein is punctured percutaneously with a needle, and by means of a thin, flexible guide wire, an arterial or venous sheath or a catheter is inserted into the vessel. The percutaneous technique is employed most frequently for the femoral artery and vein, the axillary artery, or the subclavian or internal jugular vein. This technique is relatively simple, and no sutures are required. The disadvantage is that one does not have direct control of the vessels after withdrawal of the catheters or sheaths, and control of postcatheterization bleeding may be more difficult than with the direct approach. Patients must therefore be relatively immobile for at least 4 to 6 hours. At present, the percutaneous femoral approach in which the femoral artery and femoral vein are punctured is most commonly utilized for cardiac catheterization and coronary angiography.

Catheterization and angiography can cause stroke or myocardial infarction due to vessel occlusion by clot from the tip of the catheter, dislodgment of atherosclerotic material, or dissection of the vessel wall, although the incidence of these complications is low (Table 39–7). Catheterization of the left side of the heart generally carries a much higher risk than that of the right because of the ability of the lung vascular bed to filter out thrombi. To decrease the risk of thrombosis and embolization, heparin is usually administered prior to catheterization of the left side of the heart. The anticoagulant effect of heparin is usually reversed with protamine at the termination of the procedure, before the final withdrawal of the sheath or catheter. Angiography carries a higher risk than simple pressure measurements of the left side of the heart because of the additional catheter manipulation, selective placement of the catheters within the coronary arteries, and use of angiographic contrast solution, especially in patients with more severe cardiac diseases. In addition, risk is increased in patients over 60 years of age, in patients with severe heart failure, and in patients with significant valvular heart disease.

PRESSURE MEASUREMENTS. Measurement of intracardiac pressures, by attaching the end of the fluid-filled catheter to an external pressure transducer, is an essential part of the cardiac catheterization procedure. Phasic pressure waveforms up to 12 Hz may be recorded with this technique (Fig. 39–36), and all the pressures within the cardiac chambers are routinely measured, with the exception of the left atrial pressure. The pulmonary capillary "wedge" pressure, in which a segment of the pulmonary arterial tree is occluded either with the catheter tip or with a small balloon attached to the end of a catheter (a flow-directed Swan-Ganz type of catheter), is recorded to approximate the true left atrial pressure (Fig. 39–36). The normal values for intracardiac pressures are given in Ch. 38.

TABLE 39–5. DIAGNOSES OF 562 PATIENTS CONSECUTIVELY STUDIED

Coronary Artery Disease (CAD)	Valvular Disease	CAD and Valvular Disease	Cardiomyopathy	Normal Persons	Congenital Heart Disease	Miscellaneous
62.6%	16.7%	6.0%	5.9%	6.4%	1.4%	0.9%

Adapted from Barry WH, et al.: Cathet Cardiovasc Diagn 8:401, 1979.

TABLE 39–6. POSSIBLE INDICATIONS FOR CARDIAC CATHETERIZATION AND ANGIOGRAPHY

Suspected Coronary Artery Disease	Suspected Valvular Disease

1. Angina, especially if:
   unstable
   refractory to treatment
   strongly positive treadmill
      ECG
   young person with positive
      family history
	1. Aortic stenosis if:
	   angina
	   syncope
	   CHF

2. After acute myocardial
   infarction (including patients
   who have received
   thrombolytic
   therapy) if:
   angina
   positive treadmill ECG
	2. Aortic regurgitation if:
	   CHF
	   angina
	   progressive cardiac
	      enlargement

3. In selected patients suspected
   to have "silent" ischemia:
   occupational hazards
   strong family history of
      infarction/sudden death
	3. Mitral stenosis* if:
	   CHF refractory to digitalis
	      and diuretics
	   recurrent emboli with atrial
	      fibrillation

4. Patients with ischemic
   cardiomyopathy and
   congestive heart failure
   (CHF)
	4. Mitral regurgitation if:
	   CHF
	   progressive cardiac
	      enlargement

5. In patients with high risk (age,
   diabetes, lipid disorder) prior
   to major noncardiac surgery; in
   patients at risk for coronary
   artery disease in whom cardiac
   surgery is planned	

Additional Miscellaneous Indications:
Congenital heart disease
Pericardial disease
Percutaneous transluminal coronary angioplasty
Electrophysiologic study
Biopsy
Hemodynamic monitoring
Balloon valvotomy

*Operation may be performed without catheterization if diagnosis is certain.

The shape as well as the magnitude of the intracardiac pressure waveforms contains diagnostic information. For example, in mitral regurgitation there is a large v wave in the left atrial or pulmonary artery wedge pressure recording (Fig. 39–37). A large v wave in the right atrial pressure tracing indicates tricuspid insufficiency. Simultaneous pressures are usually measured in the pulmonary wedge position and left ventricle to quantitate mitral valve function. A pressure gradient in diastole between the pulmonary wedge pressure and left ventricular diastolic pressure is seen, for example, in mitral stenosis (Fig. 39–38). Left ventricular and aortic pressures are measured simultaneously to assess aortic valve function.

Comparison of pressures in different chambers can also be very

TABLE 39–7. COMPLICATIONS OF CARDIAC CATHETERIZATION AND ANGIOGRAPHY*

	Per Cent Incidence in	
Complication	Patients with CAD†	Patients with Valvular‡ Heart Disease
Death	0.10	0.1
Myocardial infarction	0.06	0.2
Cerebrovascular accident	0.07	0.4
Arrhythmia	0.47	2.0
Vascular complications	0.46	1.7
Other	0.58	2.4
TOTAL	1.74	6.8

*Adapted from The Registry of Society for Cardiac Angiography and Interventions. Cathet Cardiovasc Diagn 17:5–21, 1989.
†Data on 222,553 patients.
‡Data on 1483 patients.

useful. In patients with pericardial constriction, there is equalization of the right atrial and pulmonary artery wedge pressures, and the mean right atrial pressure is greater than one third of the right ventricular systolic pressure. Measurement of intracardiac pressures during exercise or pacing stress may provide useful information as well. For example, patients with mitral stenosis or mitral insufficiency may have relatively normal resting pressures but abnormally high pulmonary artery wedge pressures with exercise. Patients with coronary artery disease may have normal left ventricular diastolic pressures at rest, which elevate markedly during angina produced by pacing tachycardia, reflecting ischemic left ventricular dysfunction.

MEASUREMENT OF CARDIAC OUTPUT. The most accurate way to measure cardiac output is by the Fick method, in which oxygen consumption is measured by determining the oxygen content in expired air collected over a 3-minute period. This allows determination of oxygen consumption in milliliters per minute. Collection of samples from the pulmonary artery (mixed venous sample) and a systemic artery allows determination of the arteriovenous (AV) oxygen difference. If the value for hemoglobin concentration in the blood is known, this allows calculation of the milliliters of blood that had to flow through the lungs to acquire the amount of oxygen consumed.

$$\text{Cardiac output (liters/min)} = \frac{\text{oxygen consumption (ml } O_2/\text{min)}}{\text{A-V } O_2 \text{ difference (ml } O_2 / \text{liter blood)}}$$

$$\text{A-V } O_2 \text{ difference (ml } O_2 / \text{liter blood)} = 13.9 \times \text{hemoglobin (gm/dl)} \times (\% \text{ sat A} - \% \text{ sat V})$$

Cardiac output may be normalized by dividing by body surface area (m^2) and expressed as cardiac index. In patients with intracardiac shunts, correction for the shunt must be made. This occurs most commonly in adult patients with atrial septal defects or ventricular septal defects with a left-to-right shunt. The pulmonary artery saturation in these conditions is elevated relative to the true mixed venous saturation, which is most closely approximated by the superior vena cava saturation. Standard methods exist for quantification of left-to-right and right-to-left intracardiac shunts.

Another method commonly used for measurement of cardiac output is dye dilution, in which indocyanine green dye is injected into a peripheral vein, with continuous sampling of the dye concentration in blood drawn from a peripheral artery.

The cardiac output is calculated as $\dfrac{i}{c \times t}$ where i is the quantity of indicator injected, c is the average arterial concentration of the indicator during its first pass, and t is the total duration of the dye concentration curve. The product of c and t is easily determined by planimetry of the area under the first-pass curve. Cardiac output determined by dye dilution may be inaccurate in patients with extremely low outputs or with mitral or aortic regurgitation. The dye curve is also distorted by the presence of intracardiac shunts and in fact may be used in certain circumstances to diagnose the presence and direction of an intracardiac shunt.

With the "thermodilution" method the indicator is not dye, but cold saline injected into the right atrium. Temperature changes are detected with a thermistor in the pulmonary artery. The advantages of the thermodilution method are that it is relatively unaffected by mitral and aortic regurgitation and it may be repeated frequently to measure serial outputs. It is influenced by respiration, by the presence of shunts that increase pulmonary flow, and by the presence of tricuspid regurgitation. At the present time, the Fick method is most commonly employed in the cardiac catheterization laboratory, and the thermodilution method is most commonly utilized in intensive care unit settings where patients are being monitored with catheters in the right side of the heart.

From measurements of cardiac output and pressure gradients across vascular beds, the systemic and pulmonary vascular resistances may be calculated. Elevations in systemic vascular resis-

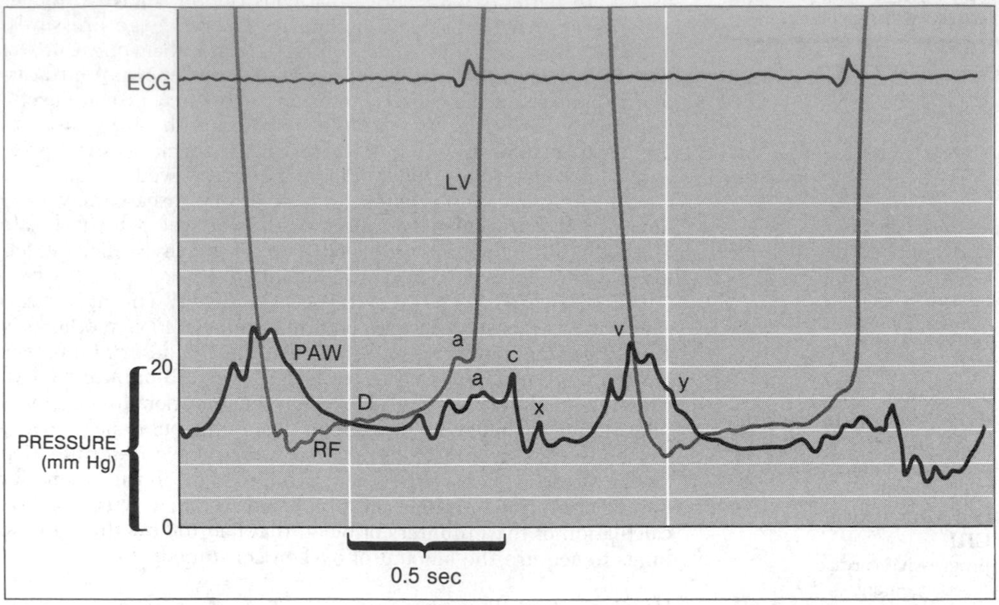

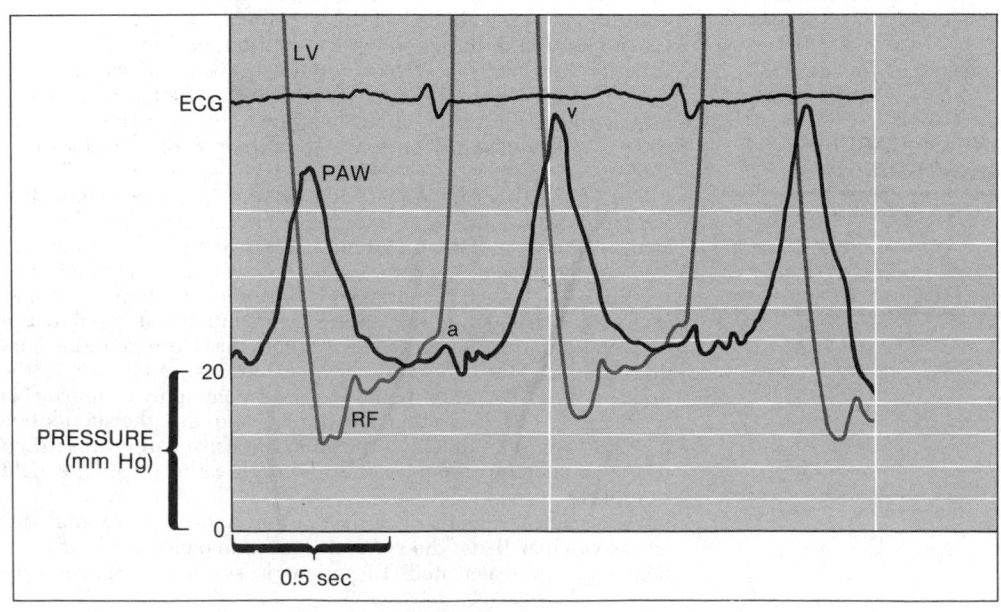

FIGURE 39–36. Simultaneous pulmonary artery wedge (PAW) pressure and left ventricular pressure (LV) in a normal patient. RF = Rapid LV filling; D = diastasis of LV filling; a = atrial contraction pressure wave. Note the delay of the PAW pressure relative to LV pressure.

tance are important in patients with chronic congestive heart failure and may identify those patients who will respond favorably to vasodilator therapy. Pulmonary vascular resistance is frequently elevated in patients with severe left ventricular failure and elevated pulmonary venous pressures, in patients with mitral valve disease, in patients with left-to-right shunts, and always in patients with primary pulmonary hypertension. Measurement of changes in pulmonary and systemic vascular resistances and in cardiac outputs and pressures before and after administration of vasodilator drugs may be helpful in guiding treatment of patients with specific disorders and is frequently employed in the catheterization laboratory setting.

Determination of cardiac output simultaneous with measurement of pressure gradients across the aortic, mitral, tricuspid, or pulmonic valve allows estimation of valve area by use of the Gorlin formula (see Fig. 39–38). The calculated valve area may differ significantly from the true valve area, particularly in the presence of very low cardiac output or valvular insufficiency. Nevertheless, this measurement is often useful in guiding surgical interventions.

ANGIOGRAPHY. During routine cardiac catheterization, left ventriculography and coronary angiography are commonly performed. For left ventriculography, contrast material is injected into the left ventricular chamber and cineangiographic filming is performed at 30 to 60 frames per second. Ejection fraction is determined as the fraction of end-diastolic ventricular volume ejected each systole. In patients with mitral regurgitation, the degree of regurgitation is usually graded on a simple 1+ to 4+ scale. In patients with coronary artery disease, segmental contraction abnormalities are frequently present, and these may be quantified by a variety of regional indices of left ventricular performance.

Injection of dye into the aortic root allows assessment of the degree of aortic insufficiency, and right ventricular contrast injection allows assessment of the tricuspid valve. Pulmonary angiography may also be performed to assess the pulmonary vasculature and to detect presence of pulmonary emboli.

Adverse effects of cardiac angiography include a negative inotropic effect due to calcium binding by the contrast agent and an intravascular volume-expanding effect due to hyperosmolality of the contrast material. The myocardial depressant effects of contrast agents are usually not a problem unless ventricular function is severely compromised. In these patients, the risks of left ventriculography may be reduced by using newer nonionic,

FIGURE 39–37. Simultaneous PAW and LV pressures in a patient with severe mitral regurgitation. Note large v wave with rapid y descent.

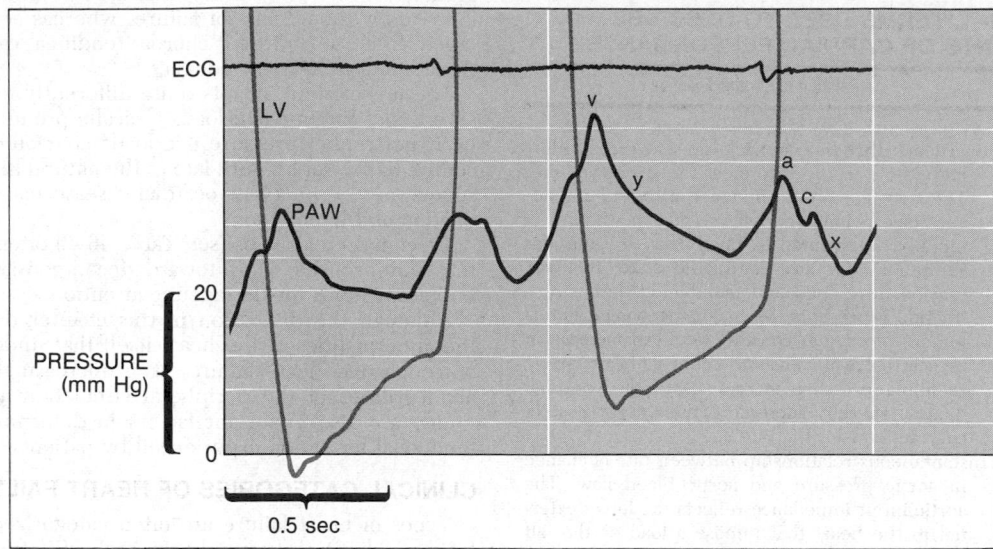

FIGURE 39–38. Simultaneous PAW and LV pressures in a patient with mitral stenosis. Note the slow y descent and the large gradient throughout diastole between PAW and LV diastolic pressures. The actual mitral valve area (M.V.A.) may be estimated as:

$$\text{M.V.A.} = \frac{\text{diastolic mitral flow (ml/sec)}}{38 \ \sqrt{\text{diastolic pressure gradient}}}$$

Thus, for a given M.V.A., the pressure gradient across the valve goes up as the *square* of mitral valve flow. This explains why the PAW pressure rises so markedly with increased cardiac output and hence increased mitral valve flow. Increased heart rate shortens diastolic time, and hence increases the mitral valve flow rate per unit of diastolic time at any given cardiac output.

non–calcium-binding contrast agents or digital image enhancement techniques that permit use of a small volume of contrast material.

Coronary cineangiography is performed by injecting a contrast agent selectively into the right or left main coronary ostia and filming at 30 frames per second. The degree of coronary artery obstruction in multiple views is assessed by measuring the percentage of narrowing of the artery at the site or sites of obstruction or by determining the percentage of area of stenosis by video-densitometric measurements. The presence and location of collateral vessels in relationship to partially or totally occluded coronary artery narrowings are also determined. In patients with no or only minor coronary artery narrowings, but with a suggestive history of chest pain, ergonovine may be infused intravenously to precipitate coronary artery spasm, which then can be documented angiographically.

Descriptions of the indications, techniques, and risks of newer procedures that also involve cardiac catheterization and angiography, such as coronary angioplasty, endomyocardial biopsy, balloon valvotomy, and electrophysiologic study, are beyond the scope of this brief summary but may be found in the selected references included.

Detre K, Holubkov R, Kelsey S, et al.: One year follow-up results of the 1985–1986 National Heart, Lung, and Blood Institute's percutaneous transluminal coronary angioplasty registry. Circulation 80:421–428, 1989. *Representative report of current success rate and complications.*

Grossman W: Cardiac Catheterization and Angiography. 3rd ed. Philadelphia, Lea & Febiger, 1986. *Excellent comprehensive text on catheterization and angiography.*

Latac B, Cribier A, Koning R, Lefelsure E: Aortic stenosis in elderly patients aged 80 or older: Treatment by percutaneous balloon valvuloplasty in a series of 92 cases. Circulation 80:1514–1520, 1989. *Summary of results of percutaneous balloon aortic valvotomy.*

Mason JW, O'Connell JB: Clinical merit of endomyocardial biopsy. Circulation 75:972–980, 1989. *Summary of indications for endomyocardial biopsy.*

Palacios I, Block PC, Wilkins GT, Weyman AE: Follow-up of patients undergoing percutaneous mitrial balloon valvotomy. Circulation 79:573–579, 1989. *Summary of current results of percutaneous balloon mitral valvotomy.*

Registry Committee of the Society for Cardiac Angiography and Interventions: Complications of cardiac catheterization. Cath Cardiovasc Diagn 17:5–21, 1989. *Excellent current description of type and incidence of complications associated with cardiac catheterization and coronary angiography.*

40 Heart Failure

Thomas W. Smith

The heart generates the motive force to satisfy the metabolic needs of tissues by delivery of blood containing oxygen and nutrients. The minute-to-minute adjustments in the distribution of the cardiac output according to physiologic priorities (e.g., muscular exercise, heat loss, and digestion) require a complex regulatory system that must also serve to protect vital organs such as the heart and brain when cardiac output is compromised.

The normal or failing heart, in terms of its structure and function, may be examined as a pump, as a muscle, or as a component of the circulatory system. This chapter addresses aspects of heart failure common to the various disease entities discussed in subsequent chapters.

GENERAL ASPECTS

Textbooks commonly define heart failure as a condition in which the heart cannot pump an adequate supply of blood at normal filling pressures to meet the metabolic needs of the body. Clinicians and clinical investigators, however, define heart failure operationally as a syndrome in which ventricular dysfunction is accompanied by reduced exercise capacity. Table 40–1 provides explanations of terms commonly used to describe determinants of cardiac performance.

Heart failure is encountered with increasing frequency, the number of hospital discharges in the United States with this diagnosis having more than doubled in the period from 1973 to 1986. Most of this increase is attributable to an aging population with a high incidence of cardiovascular disease; heart failure is now the most common DRG throughout the United States for patients aged 65 and above.

Despite advances in the medical and surgical management of cardiovascular disease, the prognosis for patients with overt heart failure remains quite limited. About half of patients die within 4 years after this diagnosis; among the group with advanced heart

TABLE 40–1. TERMS USED TO DESCRIBE DETERMINANTS OF CARDIAC PERFORMANCE

Term	Relation to Cardiac Function
Afterload	Resistance that the ventricle must overcome during systole in order to eject the stroke volume. The two major determinants are aortic impedance (see below) and left ventricular volume.
Energetics	Generally determined as myocardial oxygen consumption. For any contractile state, the wall tension developed and maintained during contraction represents the major mechanical determinant of oxygen consumption. An increase in myocardial wall tension occurs in heart failure as filling pressure increases and the ventricle dilates, thereby increasing the energy cost of contraction (see Fig. 40–3).
Impedance (during ejection)	Instantaneous relationship between rate of change in aortic pressure and aortic blood flow. The aortic input impedance reflects the forces external to the heart that impose a load on the left ventricle, including stiffness of aortic wall. Determined primarily, but not exclusively, by total peripheral vascular resistance to runoff from the arterial tree. Normal peripheral resistance is approximately 1500 dynes • sec/cm^{-5} or 15 peripheral resistance units (also known as Wood's units).
Inotropic state	A measure of contractility.
Preload	Rigorously, stretch of myocardial fibers at end-diastole; commonly used as a synonym for venous return to the heart or end-diastolic volume.

failure, 50 per cent or more die within 1 year. Several factors have been shown to be independent predictors of survival in patients with heart failure. The extent of impairment of ventricular function, usually judged by left or right ventricular ejection fraction, is correlated with prognosis, as are reduced cardiac index and elevated ventricular filling pressures. Exercise capacity, as well as peak O_2 consumption and New York Heart Association functional class, are valid predictors of survival. Neurohumoral activation as evidenced by elevated plasma norepinephrine levels, basal plasma renin activity, or plasma atrial natriuretic factor has adverse prognostic significance, as does hyponatremia. The occurrence of either ventricular or supraventricular arrhythmias is predictive of shorter survival. Of note, about 40 to 50 per cent of deaths among heart failure patients occur suddenly and are thought to be due in large part to ventricular arrhythmias, occurring at times when patients are relatively compensated and out of hospital. Antiarrhythmic drug therapy has not yet been shown to alter this situation, but the automatic implantable cardioverter/defibrillator shows promise.

Given the limited outlook despite application of all available treatment modalities for patients with heart failure, the clinician must do everything possible to *prevent* progression of heart disease to the point where cardiac reserve and compensatory mechanisms are exhausted and the syndrome of overt congestive heart failure supervenes.

The term *heart failure* is often used as a synonym for myocardial failure, emphasizing the impaired performance of the heart as a muscle and as a pump. It also provides a rationale for medical treatment. Subsequent chapters deal with syndromes in which the cause of circulatory compromise lies elsewhere, such as in abnormalities of the heart valves or pericardium or inappropriate heart rates.

Imbalance between circulatory demands and cardiac response sets the stage for the syndrome of heart failure. Volume overload is generally tolerated better than pressure overload. Aortic or mitral insufficiency produces *volume* overload that may be tolerated for years without overt heart failure; *pressure* overload from aortic stenosis, in contrast, usually results in earlier onset and more rapid progression of heart failure. Gradually developing

overloads are accommodated better than acute overloads. Thus, gradually developing chronic mitral regurgitation is often present for years without signs of failure, whereas acute mitral regurgitation from a ruptured chorda tendinea can precipitate life-threatening pulmonary edema.

The myocardium adapts quite differently to volume and pressure loads. Volume overloads typically produce dilation followed by hypertrophy; pressure overloads characteristically elicit concentric hypertrophy until late in the natural history when dilation supervenes. Primary myocardial disease usually results in both dilation and hypertrophy.

Precipitating stresses (see Table 40–2) often tip the balance of the compromised heart toward decompensation and constitute important items for therapeutic attention.

Although the discussion in this chapter deals primarily with the abnormalities of the heart itself that underlie the syndrome of congestive heart failure, it is increasingly recognized that abnormalities of the peripheral circulation and neurohormonal milieu are also important factors in determining the degree of functional limitation experienced by patients with heart failure.

CLINICAL CATEGORIES OF HEART FAILURE

Types of heart failure are often categorized according to five features: duration (acute or chronic), initiating mechanisms, the ventricle primarily affected, the clinical syndrome, and the underlying physiologic derangements.

Acute Versus Chronic Heart Failure

The clinical manifestations of heart failure often begin insidiously and progress gradually into a chronic state. Alternatively, onset may be abrupt, as after acute myocardial infarction or chorda tendinea rupture.

Compensatory mechanisms in both acute and chronic heart failure include increased systemic vascular resistance and redistribution of blood flow. However, these adaptive mechanisms in acute and chronic heart failure differ quantitatively and sometimes also in direction. For example, *acute* distention of the left atrium generally promotes a sodium-poor diuresis, whereas *chronic* distention of the left atrium elicits salt and water retention.

Initiating Mechanisms

Each initiating mechanism has its own distinctive characteristics. For example, the symptoms and signs that evolve in rheumatic heart disease differ from those of hypertensive heart

TABLE 40–2. PRECIPITATING OR EXACERBATING FACTORS IN CONGESTIVE HEART FAILURE

Increased demand:
Anemia
Fever
Infection
Fluid overload
Increased dietary salt intake
High environmental temperature
Renal failure
Hepatic failure
Thyrotoxicosis
Arteriovenous (AV) shunt (Paget's disease of bone)
Respiratory insufficiency
Emotional stress
Pregnancy
Obesity
Arrhythmias
Pulmonary embolism
Ethanol ingestion
Thiamine deficiency
Uncontrolled hypertension
Poor compliance with therapeutic regimen
Drugs
Beta-adrenergic blockers
Antiarrhythmic drugs (e.g., disopyramide)
Salt-retaining drugs
Steroids
Nonsteroidal anti-inflammatory agents

disease, whereas both have a different natural history from that of cor pulmonale. Even a single etiology, arteriosclerosis, may have distinctly different consequences, depending on the size and location of affected vessels. Progressive narrowing and gradual occlusion of distal branches of the coronary arteries may be so covert that shortness of breath and fatigue may be misinterpreted as the general physical decline of advancing age. In contrast, abrupt closure of a major coronary artery may result in myocardial necrosis followed by an acute low output state or by progressive chronic heart failure.

Left Versus Right Heart Failure

One ventricle bears the brunt of many disease processes and fails before the other. Because of the prevalence of cardiac disorders that overload or damage the left ventricle, heart failure most often begins with that ventricle. Breathlessness is the most common presenting symptom and is a direct consequence of elevated left ventricular filling pressure and pulmonary congestion. When the right ventricle fails, systemic venous congestion and peripheral edema predominate. Left ventricular failure is the most common cause of right ventricular failure, and breathlessness may improve as right ventricular output falls and pulmonary congestion diminishes.

The mechanism by which left ventricular failure causes the right ventricle to fail is not clear. Pulmonary hypertension secondary to left ventricular failure may contribute, but the degree of pulmonary hypertension is often insufficient to constitute a formidable burden on the right ventricle. Interdependence of the two ventricles, with failure of shared muscle in the ventricular septum, may also contribute. Right ventricular failure is an uncommon cause of left ventricular failure, but there is a relatively high frequency of independent left ventricular disease in elderly patients with right ventricular failure.

The combination of left and right ventricular (biventricular) failure, with elevated filling pressures of both ventricles causing pulmonary and systemic venous hypertension, results in the syndrome known as "congestive heart failure." This term implies reduced effort tolerance, breathlessness, distended neck veins, hepatic engorgement, and peripheral edema.

Backward Versus Forward Heart Failure

"Backward failure" refers to elevated cardiac filling pressures and attributes to the consequent venous congestion a critical role in the evolution of the syndrome of heart failure. "Forward failure" refers to decreased cardiac output and inadequate perfusion of organs. This distinction has limited clinical usefulness and has largely been replaced by more specific consideration of ventricular filling pressures and cardiac output.

High Versus Low Output Failure

The separation into "high" and "low" output failure distinguishes certain clinical manifestations, rather than causes, of myocardial failure. It serves (1) to distinguish a type of myocardial failure ("high output failure") in which the circulation remains brisk and the extremities tend to remain warm despite elevated venous pressures and a lower cardiac output than existed prior to the onset of heart failure; (2) to emphasize that the cardiac output and the circulatory adjustments during heart failure are conditioned by the state that existed prior to heart failure; and (3) to relate etiology to typical clinical features of heart failure. In regard to this last point, the more common causes—arteriosclerosis, myocardial disease, valvular disease, hypertension, and pericardial disease—tend to produce low output states; other, less common causes, including hyperthyroidism, Paget's disease of bone, anemia, beriberi, and arteriovenous fistula, tend to be associated with high output states. The essence of cardiac failure, however, remains the inability of the heart to increase its output appropriately in relation to demand.

Congestive Failure Versus Congested State

Elevated volume of the circulation, with preserved ventricular function, characterizes the "congested state." It is commonly encountered in intensive care facilities, where vigorous volume infusions are often used to combat systemic hypotension. It is encountered on a chronic basis in severe anemia and chronic renal insufficiency and less often in Paget's disease or beriberi.

In these situations, venous hypertension results from expanded intravascular volume, rather than from impaired myocardial contractile state.

In time, myocardial failure may supervene, with an inadequate increase in cardiac output for the increment in oxygen uptake during exercise. Correction of inciting factors and administration of diuretics are effective in both the "congested state" and in "congestive heart failure."

Systolic Versus Diastolic Failure

Recent studies indicate that up to one third of patients evaluated for symptoms and signs of heart failure have normal or nearly normal left ventricular ejection fractions, but because of the low compliance of the chamber they require substantially elevated filling pressures to maintain an adequate forward stroke output. These patients with diastolic dysfunction usually suffer from one (or more) of three underlying problems: (1) left ventricular hypertrophy (e.g., due to hypertension, aortic stenosis, or hypertrophic cardiomyopathy); (2) myocardial ischemia, which impairs ventricular relaxation; and (3) infiltrative disease (most commonly amyloidosis). Much of the discussion that follows focuses on the "classic" syndrome of congestive heart failure that accompanies a dilated heart with impaired systolic function. It is essential to distinguish these patients from those with predominant diastolic dysfunction, who require a distinctly different therapeutic approach (see below). Echo-Doppler study usually provides definitive information distinguishing these patient subsets, as does radionuclide ventriculography.

SUBCELLULAR BASIS FOR CONTRACTION

Cardiac contraction is initiated by depolarization of the sarcolemmal membrane, which activates slow calcium channels that undergo a transient increase in calcium permeability. The resulting calcium influx triggers the release of a much larger amount of calcium from the sarcoplasmic reticulum with consequent sarcomere shortening; the sarcoplasmic reticulum then resequesters calcium to turn off myofilament interaction, permitting myocardial relaxation.

Contractile force in heart muscle is generated by interactions among contractile proteins in repeating units (sarcomeres) that compose the individual muscle fibers (myofibrils). Within each sarcomere, the contractile proteins are arranged in thick filaments consisting of myosin and thin filaments consisting of actin and the modulator proteins troponin and tropomyosin. Interaction of calcium with one of three proteins composing troponin initiates the contractile process by removing a troponin-tropomyosin–induced inhibition of thick and thin filament interaction.

Changes in the length of heart muscle during contraction and relaxation are explained by the sliding filament hypothesis. During contraction, the thin actin filaments are propelled past the myosin thick filaments by force generated by ATP-dependent movement of cross-bridges consisting of the head portion of the myosin molecule. As the muscle shortens, the cross-bridges disengage and then engage other sites with a ratchet-like action. Depending on the number of cross-bridges that interact at a given time, different tensions are developed. Energy-dependent uptake of cytosolic calcium by the sarcoplasmic reticulum allows cross-bridge disengagement and relaxation to occur. Abundant mitochondria generate energy for the contractile machinery by oxidative phosphorylation fueled by free fatty acids and, to a lesser extent, glucose.

For the sarcomere, as for the whole heart (see Preload, below, and Table 40–1), the tension developed during contraction is directly related to its end-diastolic length. Stretching to permit optimal thick and thin filament overlap increases the ability of individual contractile elements to develop force. There are still many uncertainties regarding molecular details of the contractile process, and much is still to be learned about cardiac "success" as an essential background against which to examine basic mechanisms in cardiac "failure."

PATHOPHYSIOLOGIC INTERPLAY

Because of their location, structure, and function, the heart and lungs operate as a functional unit. The continuity of the muscle that surrounds the ventricular chambers, the shared ventricular septum, and the encasing pericardium ensure coordinate function, yet each ventricle functions as a separate muscular pump with its own atrial booster pump. In the normal heart, at least 50 per cent of the ventricular end-diastolic volume is ejected with each beat. Although many properties of ejection are inherent in the architecture and physiology of cardiac muscle, adaptability to changing metabolic needs is provided by a superimposed set of neurohumoral adjustments that modulate cardiac rate, loading, and contractility.

Each ventricle has its own capacity to withstand and repair the stresses imposed by normal and abnormal function. The two ventricles also have different designs in keeping with their different physiologic functions. Before birth, both ventricles bear similar pressure loads. After birth, the right ventricular workload decreases as pulmonary arterial pressure falls. The greater workload of the mature left ventricle, together with the greater prevalence of diseases that compromise the left side of the heart and its blood supply, result in the preponderance of left over right ventricular dysfunction in groups of patients in whom ischemic disease and hypertension are common.

ASSESSMENT OF CARDIAC PERFORMANCE

In terms of its performance, the heart may be assessed as a pump, as a muscle, or as a component of the circulatory system. Hemodynamic pressure and flow measurements characterize its behavior as a pump. Principles of muscle mechanics are used to describe its behavior as a muscle. Its adequacy as a component of the circulatory system is reflected in the consequences of reduced cardiac output, redistribution of blood flow, organ hypoperfusion, and pulmonary or systemic venous congestion.

Heart as a Pump: Hemodynamics

By the time overt heart failure is apparent, the large functional reserve of the normal heart is compromised and a variety of mechanisms operate to compensate for its diminished performance. Despite an inappropriately low cardiac output, the blood pressure at rest tends to remain normal or even increases, albeit with frequent reduction in pulse pressure.

CARDIAC OUTPUT. In response to peripheral demands, a complex set of control mechanisms modulates heart rate and the extent of stretch and shortening of myocardial fibers and, hence, the stroke volume and the cardiac output (stroke volume times heart rate). Three principal variables determine the stroke volume (Table 40–1): preload, afterload (resistance to ventricular emptying during systole), and the contractile state of the heart. For practical purposes, three of the principal determinants of cardiac output—preload, afterload, and heart rate—are readily measured. Contractile (inotropic) state remains difficult to assess in formal quantitative terms, but noninvasive (echo-Doppler) and minimally invasive (radionuclide ventriculography) methods yield the requisite data for most clinical decision making. Ejection fraction is commonly used as a clinically useful index (albeit impure) of contractile state, and the maximum rate of pressure rise during the isovolumetric phase of systole (dP/dt) is a useful measure in invasive hemodynamic investigations.

Relationships among these determinants vary with the state of the heart and circulation. Thus when contractility is impaired, stroke output and cardiac output tend to be maintained by ventricular dilation (Frank-Starling mechanism), limiting the value of cardiac output as a measure of inotropic state to experimental circumstances in which preload, afterload, and heart rate can be held constant.

Indicator-dilution techniques can be used in the ICU or cardiac catheterization laboratory for determination of cardiac output. In resting adults, the normal range is between 2.5 and 3.6 liters per minute per square meter of body surface area. Decreased cardiac output at rest occurs only in advanced stages of cardiac impairment. A blunted cardiac output response to exercise occurs much earlier. Supine exercise in normal subjects should increase the cardiac output by at least 600 ml per minute for each 100-ml increment in oxygen consumption; lower values indicate reduced cardiac performance. In heart failure the arteriovenous oxygen difference is abnormally wide, resulting chiefly from the low

oxygen content of venous blood returning to the heart. Oxygenation of blood in the lungs remains nearly normal until pulmonary vascular congestion becomes sufficiently severe to create ventilation-perfusion mismatch with effective shunting, or abnormal diffusion barriers to oxygen transport.

During exercise, cardiac output normally increases as a linear function of oxygen consumption, although for any level of exercise the cardiac output tends to be lower in the upright position. Increases in cardiac output in the upright posture are accomplished principally by increases in heart rate rather than in stroke volume. In heart failure, cardiac output is particularly dependent on heart rate, both at rest and during exercise.

VENTRICULAR END-DIASTOLIC PRESSURE AND VOLUME. Impaired systolic ventricular emptying leads to an increase in the end-systolic residual volume of blood in the ventricle, predisposing to an increase in end-diastolic volume. Since this is inconvenient to measure or monitor, ventricular end-diastolic pressure is customarily followed for clinical purposes on the premise that a change in pressure is effected by a change in ventricular volume. Exceptions occur, however, including structural changes in the myocardium (fibrosis, edema, and hypertrophy) and pericardial constriction that cause disproportionate rises in end-diastolic pressure relative to volume. Acute ischemia also produces transient reduction in left ventricular compliance. Conversely, in some states of chronic volume overload, compliance increases so that increased volumes are accommodated at end-diastole with relatively modest pressure increases.

A left ventricular end-diastolic pressure greater than 12 to 15 mm Hg is abnormal. The corresponding upper limit for the right ventricle is 6 to 10 mm Hg. It is straightforward to estimate the right ventricular end-diastolic pressure by measuring the central venous pressure. In the absence of mitral obstruction or increased pulmonary vascular resistance, pulmonary arterial diastolic pressure approximates left ventricular end-diastolic pressure. Pulmonary capillary wedge pressure or diastolic pressure measured with a Swan-Ganz catheter is widely used in ICU settings to monitor left ventricular filling pressures.

To summarize, the performance of heart muscle depends on two essential components: fiber length (Frank-Starling mechanism) and inherent contractility (inotropic state). The normal heart autoregulates to maintain cardiac output. The variables involved are preload, afterload, contractility, and heart rate. With chronic overloading, the heart undergoes dilation, hypertrophy, or both.

PRELOAD. According to the Frank-Starling mechanism, an increase in end-diastolic volume (preload) results in more forceful contraction with enhancement of ventricular emptying and stroke volume. A unique ventricular function curve exists for each state of contractility (Fig. 40–1). The curve for a failing ventricle is shifted downward and flattened such that stroke volumes are reduced despite abnormally high end-diastolic volumes or pressures. The elevated filling pressures are responsible for congestion and edema in the venous beds leading to the failing ventricle.

In the normal heart, the Frank-Starling mechanism serves to match the stroke outputs of the two ventricles. In heart failure, this mechanism plays the additional role of helping to support the cardiac output.

AFTERLOAD. Afterload refers to the resistance that the ventricle must overcome during systole in order to eject the stroke volume. It incorporates all factors that oppose shortening of the ventricular fibers. In practice, it is estimated for the left heart either from the arterial blood pressure or from calculation of systemic vascular resistance (ratio of blood pressure to flow, expressed in units of dynes · sec/cm^{-5} or in peripheral resistance units). Right ventricular afterload (pulmonary artery pressure) can be estimated satisfactorily in most patients by echo-Doppler measurements.

In the assessment of patients, the relationship of blood pressure to cardiac output and peripheral resistance (P/Flow = R) is quite useful. Interventions that cause an increase in cardiac output without changing systemic blood pressure must cause vasodilation, thereby decreasing peripheral vascular resistance or afterload. Improved emptying of the left ventricle is usually accompanied by a decrease in its filling pressure (pulmonary capillary wedge or pulmonary artery diastolic pressure).

If preload and contractility remain constant, increasing after-

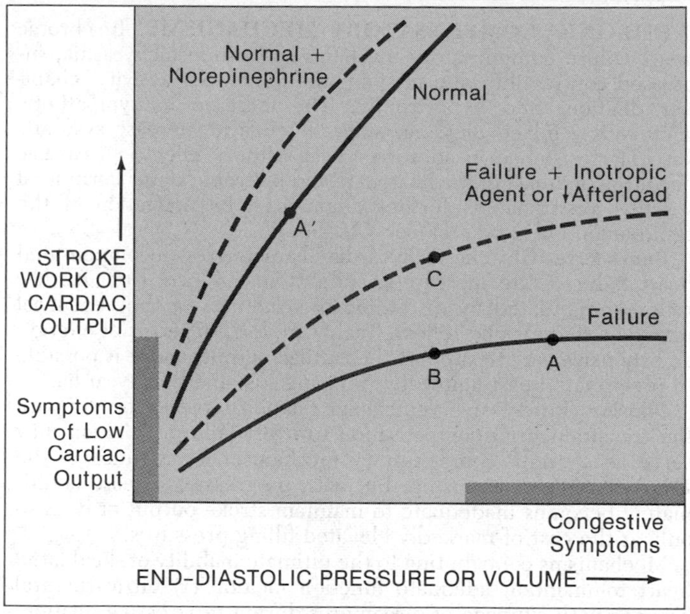

FIGURE 40–1. Schematic diagram demonstrating the relationship between ventricular end-diastolic pressure or volume and cardiac index in a normal and a failing heart. The normal left ventricle increases its stroke output as preload (often measured clinically as pulmonary capillary wedge pressure) increases, moving up the ascending limb of the curve until reserve is exhausted. In heart failure, the ventricular function curve is displaced downward and to the right. An increase in contractility, as after administration of norepinephrine or digitalis, displaces the curve to the left; i.e., a larger stroke output is accomplished at any given filling pressure. A and A′ represent the operating points at rest of a hypothetical patient with heart failure and of a normal person, respectively. Reduction of physical activity allows the failing heart to meet the demands of the metabolizing tissues. Treatment of heart failure by a reduction in preload (e.g., with a diuretic or a vasodilator acting predominantly on the venous bed) causes a shift from point A to B on the same ventricular function curve. Administration of a positive inotropic agent or a vasodilator producing afterload reduction shifts the curve as shown, resulting in improvement of the circulatory state in the direction shown by a shift from point A to C.

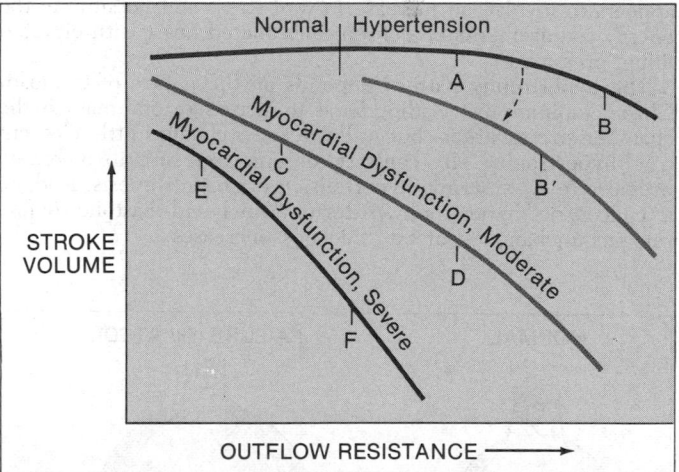

load in the normal heart tends to decrease both the extent and the speed of contraction to a minor extent. Reduction in afterload has the opposite effects. Within broad physiologic limits, the normal ventricle maintains a relatively constant stroke volume as afterload is increased (Fig. 40–2). The impaired ventricle responds quite differently, with progressive diminution in its ability to eject blood against a given afterload as the severity of myocardial dysfunction advances. Figure 40–2 illustrates the rationale for afterload reduction in the management of heart failure.

CONTRACTILITY (INOTROPIC STATE). Modulation of sympathetic nervous activity provides the major component of short-term adjustment of contractile state in the normal heart and also mediates increases in heart rate and venous tone. Unlike the Frank-Starling mechanism, the increase in force and velocity of contraction is accomplished without any increase in fiber length (end-diastolic volume). Contractility does not limit the output of the normal heart. By contrast, the failing heart is limited in its myocardial performance, indicated by displacement of the ventricular function curve as shown in Figure 40–1.

An objective index of myocardial contractility that could be measured independent of myocardial fiber length would be useful (1) to assess the effects on the myocardium of interventions such as the administration of digitalis or other inotropic agents; (2) to determine serial changes in inotropic state in an individual during the evolution of heart failure and in response to treatment; and (3) to compare the inotropic state in different individuals. However, distinction between the effects of loading conditions and intrinsic contractility is difficult because of the strong influence of loading on hemodynamic measurements. Changes in preload or afterload can modify ventricular performance greatly without affecting intrinsic inotropic state. Since conventional hemodynamic measurements do not take heart size into account, comparisons of contractility in hearts of different size are difficult to interpret.

Ejection Fraction. This term denotes the fraction of the right or left ventricular end-diastolic volume ejected per beat. It is useful as an integrative measure of contractility and is determined by contrast ventriculography, by gated blood pool radionuclide imaging, or by echocardiography. The normal left ventricular ejection fraction ranges from 0.56 to 0.78. A reduced ejection fraction in a patient with normal valves and a dilated ventricle strongly suggests decreased contractility, particularly in the absence of increased afterload. Abnormalities of regional myocardial function are often evident in the pattern of ventricular contraction demonstrated by these techniques and suggest focal ischemic disease, but may also be observed in primary cardiomyopathic disorders.

Other Techniques. Simultaneous graphic recording of the electrocardiogram, phonocardiogram, and carotid arterial pulse contour provides another noninvasive means of assessing cardiac function but has been almost entirely supplanted by the more clinically useful echo-Doppler assessment. Accurate measurement of ventricular dP/dt can be accomplished at cardiac catheterization and provides a measure of contractile state less subject to the influence of loading conditions than most other approaches; its use is largely confined to research applications.

FIGURE 40–2. Relation of left ventricular stroke volume to systemic outflow resistance in normal and diseased hearts. A family of curves may be described, depending on the severity of the myocardial disease. If cardiac function is normal, a rise in resistance results in hypertension, since cardiac output remains fairly constant. Heart failure in a hypertensive patient could be shown by a move to either point B, a high resistance with normal function, or point B′, which represents a shift to a slightly depressed ventricular function curve. When myocardial dysfunction is more severe, as shown by the lower two curves, blood pressure is no longer directly determined by resistance, since stroke volume and resistance are inversely related. Consequently, arterial pressure may be similar at points E and F despite marked differences in cardiac output and resistance. It is also apparent that a reduction in outflow resistance does not affect significantly the stroke volume of the normal ventricle. However, it can produce a marked increase in the stroke volume of the failing ventricle (F→E). (Adapted from Cohn JN, Franciosa JA: Vasodilator therapy of cardiac failure. N Engl J Med 297:27, 1977. By permission of the New England Journal of Medicine.)

CHRONIC COMPENSATORY MECHANISMS. In chronic heart failure compensatory mechanisms include tachycardia, increased contractility due to sympathetic nervous activity, chamber dilation, and hypertrophy. The increase in sympathetic activity is a mixed blessing, since it tends to increase systemic vascular resistance in addition to its salutory effects on cardiac output by increasing the heart rate and inotropic state. Peripheral vascular resistance is further augmented by activation of the renin-angiotensin system (see Ch. 44).

Heart Rate. Chronic tachycardia characterizes decompensated heart failure. The increase in rate stems in part from cardiac reflexes stimulated by distention of structures at the venoatrial junctions (Bainbridge reflex). Tachycardia is, in terms of energy, an expensive way to support the cardiac output, and it is possible to precipitate heart failure by inducing sustained tachycardia.

Dilation. Progressive ventricular dilation typically occurs with the transition from compensation to overt failure. Dilation may serve as a useful compensatory mechanism for a time via the Frank-Starling relationship, but with progressive disease it ultimately becomes inadequate to maintain stroke output or does so only at the cost of markedly elevated filling pressures.

Mechanisms contributing to the ultimate inability of the dilated heart to maintain adequate function include (1) ultrastructural changes with slippage of sarcomeres during progressive dilation; as a result, they are not stretched to generate optimal contractility; and (2) increased wall tension (law of Laplace, Fig. 40–3) resulting in increased myocardial oxygen consumption; a corollary is that in contrast to the normal heart, in which the wall tension decreases in the course of systole, wall tension tends to remain high throughout contraction in the dilated heart. Thus chronic dilation has important limitations as a compensatory mechanism in cardiac failure.

Hypertrophy. Sustained abnormal pressure or volume loads lead to an increase in ventricular mass. This involves changes in gene expression and increased protein synthesis. Decreased protein degradation rates may occur as well in response to mechanical overload or dilation. The stimulus for hypertrophy appears to involve an increase in wall stress and possibly in the energy requirements of a chronically dilated heart with elevated filling pressures.

The hypertrophy pattern depends on the nature of the load. Chronic volume overloading leads to increased total mass as the chamber size enlarges, but wall thickness changes little ("eccentric" hypertrophy). By contrast, chronic exposure to increased pressure (e.g., systemic hypertension or aortic stenosis) leads to a "concentric" hypertrophy pattern in which end-diastolic volume remains unchanged but wall thickness increases.

Abnormal electrical conduction patterns can interfere with the normal, smoothly coordinated contraction pattern of the normal heart, as can myocyte loss with focal or diffuse fibrosis. Ischemic myocardial damage tends to cause hypertrophy and remodeling of residual muscle because the geometry of the abnormal ventricle causes it to operate at a mechanical disadvantage and also because normal muscle must work, and expend energy, in moving and stretching adjacent damaged muscle or scar.

In early or mild hypertrophy, muscle mass and capillary vessels increase proportionately, preserving the nutritive and contractile properties of the myocardium. With progressive hypertrophy (in the absence of ventricular dilation), additional sarcomeres are laid down, wall thickness increases, and ventricular wall stress tends to be maintained at a normal level despite increased cavity pressure, as indicated in Figure 40–3. This process ultimately exacts a price, however, since increased wall thickness often leads to increased wall stiffness (reduced compliance), thus necessitating a disproportionate rise in filling pressure to maintain adequate end-diastolic ventricular volume. The increasingly recognized syndrome of diastolic ventricular dysfunction, which occurs relatively commonly in the presence of a preserved ventricular ejection fraction, leads to elevated pulmonary or systemic venous pressures, which contribute to symptoms of dyspnea or peripheral edema. In addition, beyond a certain point, coronary flow reserve diminishes and contractile function declines. Thus, once unremitting hypertrophy begins, the myocardium has embarked on the road to overt failure.

Despite the depressed contractile state associated with later stages of hypertrophy, circulatory function is maintained for a time by the combination of increased muscles mass, dilation, and augmented sympathetic drive. With continuing loss of myocardial contractility, or loss of muscle cells (e.g., from ischemic or inflammatory processes), circulatory compensation can no longer be maintained. The typical clinical and hemodynamic manifestations of congestive heart failure then emerge as cardiac output fails to meet demands and filling pressures increase.

Heart as a Muscle

Consideration of the ventricular performance of the failing heart usually centers on the contraction phase. Events during diastole, however, influence ventricular compliance and hence filling pressures, as well as the subsequent contraction and the energy supply for contraction and relaxation.

RELAXATION AND DISTENSIBILITY. Diastolic filling of the ventricle depends on the time available (a function of heart rate), the timing and properties of atrial systole, and the diastolic properties of the ventricle. Relaxation of cardiac muscle is an energy-requiring process (see above) that is quite vulnerable to adenosine triphosphate (ATP) depletion caused by ischemia. Although heart failure per se does not necessarily impair ventricular relaxation, associated processes of hypertrophy, fibrosis, and ischemia often reduce chamber distensibility and further increase filling pressures to levels producing pulmonary edema. This problem can be particularly severe in hypertrophic cardiomyopathy and in diseases such as amyloidosis that markedly reduce left ventricular diastolic compliance. Elderly patients with hypertension and diabetes mellitus seem especially prone to diastolic ventricular dysfunction. Management of the subset of patients with predominant diastolic dysfunction is discussed below.

ENERGETICS. The heart depends on aerobic metabolism for its supply of energy, the bulk of which is spent to support contraction. The major determinants of oxygen consumption of the heart include the interrelated components of rate, ventricular pressure, volume, work, wall tension, and contractile state. The time integral of systolic tension relates closely to myocardial oxygen consumption, whereas fiber shortening has a minor effect on myocardial oxygen consumption.

The cellular and biochemical basis for heart failure remains unsettled. It is generally agreed that there are no consistent defects in energy metabolism or in protein synthesis and turnover. Current investigation is centered on excitation-contraction coupling and mechanisms that control calcium homeostasis.

Compensatory mechanisms in advanced heart failure tend to increase myocardial oxygen requirements by several mechanisms, including increased preload due to salt and water retention and

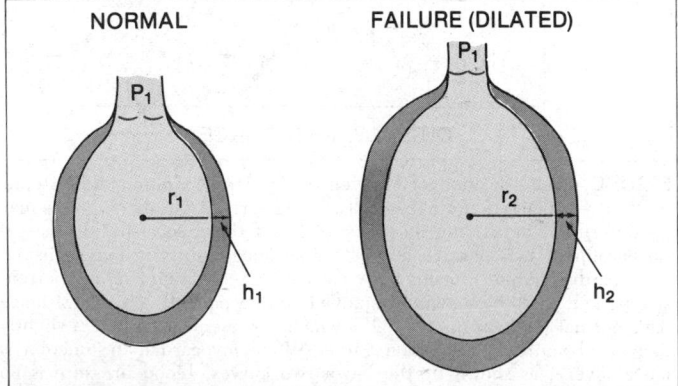

FIGURE 40–3. Laplace relationship applied to the dilated heart. The tension developed in the wall of the heart during systole (T) is a directional force that is proportional to the product of the mean pressure that the wall is supporting (P) and the mean radius (r). To a first approximation, $T = \dfrac{Pr}{2}$. Dilation of the heart ($r_2 > r_1$) at the same pressure ($P_1 = P_2$) increases wall tension ($T_2 > T_1$). Should the wall become thinner during dilatation, the wall stress would increase as the cross-sectional area of myocardium (h) decreased.

enhanced sympathetic drive with consequently increased afterload, contractility, and heart rate. Increased preload and afterload are also the result of activation of the renin-angiotensin-aldosterone system.

Heart as Component of the Circulatory System

With loss of cardiac reserve and onset of overt heart failure, peripheral mechanisms are called upon to sustain blood pressure and to distribute the limited cardiac output to vital beds.

VENOUS HYPERTENSION. As the ejection fraction falls and the ventricle fails to empty properly during systole, the volume of unexpelled blood increases with an accompanying increase in diastolic pressure in the ventricles and in the atria and proximal veins. Other elements that contribute to the venous hypertension include (1) increased tone in venous capacitance vessels; (2) blood volume expansion as a consequence of renal sodium and water retention; and, on occasion, (3) incompetence of mitral or tricuspid valves with regurgitation of blood from ventricle to atrium as the valve becomes incompetent from intrinsic valvular disease, papillary muscle dysfunction, ventricular dilation, or inadequate closure during an arrhythmia.

PERIPHERAL MECHANISMS TO SUSTAIN BLOOD PRESSURE AND CARDIAC OUTPUT. To sustain and distribute the cardiac output, and to maintain systemic arterial pressure, important peripheral mechanisms are activated.

In the normal circulation, the cardiac output doubles in response to a four- or fivefold increase in total body oxygen consumption. When functional impairment is such that the cardiac output cannot keep pace with peripheral demands, blood flow is redistributed to defend vital areas such as the brain and heart. The autonomic nervous system participates in this modulation of the circulation and contributes also to activation of mechanisms that mediate the retention of sodium and water.

Peripheral vasoconstriction and tachycardia characterize the common forms of heart failure. However, despite a generalized increase in sympathetic nervous activity, norepinephrine stores in the heart muscle are depleted because of its enhanced turnover rate. Pharmacologic agents such as reserpine or guanethidine further deplete cardiac catecholamine stores and can aggravate heart failure, as can β-adrenergic antagonists such as propranolol and the many other drugs of this class.

The contribution of the parasympathetic nervous system to the control of heart rate and baroreceptor activity is impaired in heart failure, but therapeutic implications of these phenomena are not yet clear.

Peripheral Vasoconstriction. Peripheral arteriolar and venous constriction, mediated in large part by increased sympathetic nervous and renin-angiotensin system activity, is an important compensatory mechanism in heart failure that has both positive and negative consequences, as noted earlier. The extent to which accumulation of sodium and water in the arteriolar wall contributes to increased arteriolar resistance is as yet unclear.

Venoconstriction augments venous return by facilitating the return of blood to the central veins, increasing central venous pressure and hence preload. The principal determinant of elevated filling pressures, however, is the inability of the failing ventricle to eject the venous return.

Redistribution. Maintenance of oxygen and substrate delivery to brain and myocardium during states of limited cardiac output requires diversion of flow from skin, kidneys, splanchnic viscera, and skeletal muscle. This redistribution of blood flow initially occurs during activity or stress as cardiac output fails to increase sufficiently to meet the increment in metabolism; in severe heart failure, redistribution operates also at rest. The redistribution of blood flow to essential beds depends on the balance among sympathetic and renin-angiotensin system activities and local metabolism. The vasculature of skin, kidney, splanchnic beds, and skeletal muscle is richly innervated. Furthermore, these tissues have relatively low metabolic rates at rest, permitting sympathetic nervous and angiotensin II–mediated vasoconstriction to override local vasodilator effects of metabolites. By contrast, the circulations to brain and myocardium are less subject to α-adrenergically mediated vasoconstrictor influences because these organs, with their high oxygen consumption, produce metabolic dilator substances that offset increased sympathetic tone.

Under normal physiologic circumstances, exercise with the attendant need for heat dissipation induces an increase in cutaneous blood flow. Patients in heart failure, by contrast, fail to increase cutaneous flow despite this increased need for heat loss. Thus the patient in heart failure preserves systemic arterial pressure and flow to vital organs by suffering the consequences of impaired heat loss as well as limitation of blood flow to exercising muscle groups.

THE VALSALVA MANEUVER. An abnormal response to the Valsalva maneuver, in which intrathoracic pressure is maintained at approximately 40 mm Hg for 10 to 12 seconds, is characteristic of left ventricular failure. In normal subjects there is a characteristic decrease in blood pressure and pulse pressure and increase in heart rate; at cessation of straining, the blood pressure, pulse pressure, and bradycardia tend to overshoot. By contrast, in the presence of left ventricular failure there is a "square wave" response in which normal reflex responses are blunted. Hence blood pressure increases at the onset of straining, stays elevated throughout the maneuver, and decreases abruptly to baseline after the maneuver with no overshoot; tachycardia is absent.

SALT AND WATER RETENTION. As overt heart failure develops, there is typically a decrease in renal blood flow and glomerular filtration rate, with an associated redistribution of renal blood flow. These changes contribute to the sodium and water retention that characterizes heart failure, but the nature and extent of the response differ according to the severity of heart failure, as discussed subsequently under diuretics. Hemodynamic abnormalities are undoubtedly involved in activating the renin-angiotensin-aldosterone system both via direct effects on the kidney and via indirect effects stemming from activation of mechanoreceptors in the distended left atrium. Recognition of the role of hyperaldosteronism in the genesis of sodium and water retention has resulted in the development of aldosterone antagonists as useful adjuncts in the therapy of heart failure.

Sweat and saliva are sodium poor in patients with decompensated heart failure. Antidiuretic hormone (arginine vasopressin) levels tend to be elevated in heart failure and may contribute to elevated systemic vascular resistance, but probably are not important in salt or water retention.

An increase of about 10 to 20 per cent in circulating blood volume contributes to maintenance of cardiac output and perfusion of vital organs in moderate-to-severe heart failure, augmenting ventricular end-diastolic volume and thereby tending to improve pump performance. The resulting elevation of filling pressure, however, promotes edema formation by raising venous and capillary pressures proximal to the failing ventricle. By the time the circulating blood volume has increased by 20 per cent, the extravascular fluid volume may well have increased by a factor of two.

Exercise Testing

Graded treadmill or bicycle exercise testing has been used investigatively to determine maximum total body oxygen uptake (aerobic capacity). The endpoint of fatigue generally coincides with the point at which aerobic metabolism can no longer meet tissue demands and lactate production begins (anaerobic threshold). This approach has also been used to assess quantitatively the effects of therapeutic interventions for the treatment of heart failure.

CLINICAL MANIFESTATIONS OF HEART FAILURE

The signs and symptoms of heart failure depend on which ventricle has failed and the severity and duration of failure. The clinical picture in left ventricular failure is dominated by *symptoms* of pulmonary congestion and edema. By contrast, right ventricular failure is dominated by *signs* of systemic venous congestion and peripheral edema. Weakness, fatigue, and effort intolerance are common to right or left ventricular failure as well as biventricular failure.

Left Ventricular Failure

The symptom of breathlessness predominates in patients with left ventricular failure and varies with position and activity. Noteworthy physical signs are most evident in the heart, lungs, or respiratory control mechanisms.

DYSPNEA. Dyspnea (breathlessness) during limited exertion is typically the earliest symptom of left heart failure and is usually associated with an increased rate of breathing (tachypnea). Although many details of the physiologic basis for the sensation of dyspnea remain unclear, some aspects of the etiology of respiratory symptoms from pulmonary congestion deserve consideration. Since the bronchial capillaries drain for the most part via the pulmonary veins, congestion tends to develop in alveolar and bronchial vascular networks simultaneously. Interstitial edema surrounding pulmonary capillaries appears to stimulate juxtacapillary receptors known as J-receptors, which in turn elicits a reflexly mediated pattern of rapid and shallow breathing. At the same time, bronchial congestion stimulates mucus production, and the distended bronchial capillaries may rupture, with resulting cough and hemoptysis. Bronchial mucosal edema causes increased resistance in small airways, producing wheezing and respiratory distress known as cardiac asthma. The increased work of moving fluid-laden, noncompliant lungs must be accomplished in the face of decreased blood flow to respiratory muscles and also increased diffusion barriers to oxygen exchange across the alveolar-capillary interface, contributing to respiratory muscle fatigue and the sensation of dyspnea.

Thus, the symptom of dyspnea in left heart failure clearly relates to the increase in blood volume and interstitial fluid content of the lungs at the expense of air. Ventilation increases, and the awareness of dyspnea becomes more severe as minute ventilation approaches the maximal ventilatory capacity.

ORTHOPNEA. Dyspnea that occurs soon after lying flat (and is relieved by sitting up) is known as orthopnea. The pathophysiologic basis for orthopnea is the increase in venous return from the lower extremities and splanchnic bed to the lungs in the recumbent position, together with the reabsorption of peripheral edema that accumulates during the day. Orthopnea is a relatively reliable marker for left ventricular failure, whereas the dyspnea associated with chronic lung disease or musculoskeletal disorders is typically less aggravated by lying flat. Patients usually learn to avoid dyspnea of this sort by sleeping with the head and thorax on two or more pillows. In advanced heart failure, orthopnea may be so severe as to cause the patient to sleep upright in a chair. An orthopneic cough has the same significance as orthopnea and is presumably the consequence of venous congestion and edema. Patients with left heart failure may also complain of precordial distress in the supine position that is difficult to distinguish from symptoms caused by myocardial ischemia.

NOCTURIA. In early heart failure, limitation of renal blood flow with upright activity during the day gives way to more normal renal perfusion and diuresis while supine at night. This causes nocturia, a common early symptom of incipient heart failure.

PAROXYSMAL NOCTURNAL DYSPNEA. Severe respiratory distress may arouse the patient from sleep. Relief is urgently sought by sitting up and often by finding an open window. In addition to exacerbation of pulmonary vascular congestion and edema during supine sleep, blunting of the respiratory center response to sensory input from the lungs during sleep, together with increased venous return, allows pulmonary venous congestion and edema to accumulate and trigger the alarming episode of breathlessness.

ACUTE PULMONARY EDEMA. In an episode of acute left ventricular failure, pulmonary venous and capillary pressure can increase abruptly to levels exceeding plasma oncotic pressure, with consequent rapid accumulation of edema fluid in the interstitial spaces and alveoli. Interstitial pulmonary edema leads to an increase in respiratory rate (see foregoing discussion) and tends to produce alveolar hyperventilation and respiratory alkalosis. However, when free fluid enters the alveoli and bronchioles, respiratory acidosis may occur owing to an intolerable increase in the work of breathing. Hypoxemia also occurs commonly because of imbalances between alveolar ventilation and alveolar blood flow (ventilation-perfusion mismatch or "shunting").

Symptoms of pulmonary edema may begin with a nonproductive cough, with wheezing, or with frank dyspnea. Apart from tachypnea and possibly evidence of underlying heart disease on physical examination, few physical signs may be present initially. Later, as free fluid accumulates in distal airways, rales become audible at the lung bases and extend upward accompanied by rhonchi as the episode progresses. In severe acute pulmonary edema, the patient is typically pale, sweating, cyanotic, gasping for breath, and sometimes producing pink or blood-tinged frothy sputum.

HEMOPTYSIS. Rust-colored sputum containing heart failure cells (alveolar macrophages containing hemosiderin) sometimes occurs in severe chronic left heart failure and is seen with particular frequency in patients with advanced mitral stenosis. Frankly bloody sputum should suggest the possibility of pulmonary infarction, but expectoration of substantial quantities of blood can also occur as a consequence of rupture of engorged bronchial capillaries in patients with chronic left heart failure, including that caused by uncorrected mitral stenosis.

CHEYNE-STOKES RESPIRATION. Advanced heart failure may be accompanied by periodic breathing with alternate periods of apnea and hyperventilation. Because of slowing of the circulation time from lungs to brain, the arterial Po_2 reaches its peak and the arterial Pco_2 its nadir during apnea. At this time alveolar gas tensions are exactly opposite. During hyperpnea the alveolar Po_2 reaches its peak and the alveolar Pco_2 its nadir. Thus, changes in arterial blood gases are responsible for the cyclic ventilation, which in turn causes the changes in alveolar gas tensions. As would be expected from this delay of the normal negative feedback loop, the longer the circulation time, the longer are the cycles of hyperventilation and apnea. The neurologic changes of advanced age predispose to Cheyne-Stokes breathing, as does cerebrovascular disease.

Physical and Laboratory Signs of Left Heart Failure

The patient with decompensated left heart failure is generally tachypneic, pale, dusky, and sweaty. The handshake is cold because of peripheral vasoconstriction, and tachycardia is present. The pulse pressure is usually narrow, often with a modest increase in diastolic pressure. The neck veins are not distended if the left ventricle alone has failed.

THE HEART. Cardiac enlargement is often evident upon inspection, percussion, and palpation of the apical impulse and is confirmed by radiographic and echocardiographic examination. This finding is more typical of valvular or primary myocardial disease than of ischemic heart disease. With increased left heart filling pressure, pulmonary venous pressure increases and the pulmonary arterial pressure must also increase. The pulmonic component of the second heart sound (P_2) therefore tends to increase in intensity. In the presence of left ventricular dilation, papillary muscle dysfunction, or both, the mitral valve leaflets may fail to appose properly, resulting in mitral incompetence.

Gallop Rhythm. The presence of a protodiastolic third heart sound (S_3 gallop) in an adult with heart disease usually signifies the presence of ventricular failure. The timing of the normal first and second sounds and the abnormal third sound, in conjunction with an increased heart rate, results in the characteristic cadence of the gallop rhythm. The third heart sound occurs in early diastole coincident with rapid ventricular filling. The S_3 gallop appears to be produced by vibrations of the ventricular walls as the rapidly inflowing blood is abruptly arrested. A third heart sound is a normal finding in children and in young adults.

Presystolic gallop rhythms result from the atrial contribution to ventricular filling. The atrial or S_4 gallop is characteristic of decreased ventricular compliance and typically results from left ventricular hypertrophy or ischemia rather than from myocardial dysfunction or failure, although an S_4 gallop is typically present in patients with symptoms and signs of heart failure due predominantly to diastolic dysfunction. When a patient with an audible fourth heart sound develops overt heart failure, a third sound may appear, causing a quadruple rhythm. If the heart rate is sufficiently rapid or the PR interval is prolonged, S_3 and S_4 may merge, producing a summation gallop. The presence of a summation gallop has the same clinical implication as other protodiastolic (S_3) gallop rhythms.

Pulsus Alternans. The presence of alternating strong and weak beats (the fundamental rhythm remaining regular) usually signifies advanced heart failure. Pulsus alternans can be detected by palpation or by sphygmomanometry and often follows an atrial or ventricular premature beat for several cycles. Mechanical alternans of this sort is only rarely associated with electrical alternans. Pulsus alternans has been attributed to a severe disturbance of excitation-contraction coupling, the detailed pathophysiology of which is unclear.

THE LUNGS. The sequence of pulmonary findings with advancing left heart failure has been described in the foregoing section on acute pulmonary edema.

THE ELECTROCARDIOGRAM. Electrocardiographic abnormalities result from underlying cardiac disease, therapeutic agents (e.g., digitalis), or both and yield little information regarding the functional status of the heart.

RADIOLOGIC ASPECTS. The chest radiograph is usually quite helpful in the diagnosis and assessment of left ventricular failure (see Ch. 39.1). The cardiac silhouette is typically, but not invariably, enlarged and may assume telltale configurations that are determined by the underlying disease process. In contrast to normal, the pulmonary vasculature is prominent in the upper lung zones, reflecting pulmonary venous hypertension and redistribution of blood flow because of encroachment upon the lower lung vessels by edema and possibly fibrosis. Enlarged hilar shadows and prominent septal lines, particularly near the costophrenic angles (Kerley's B lines), are typical findings. Alveolar edema results in a generalized clouding of the lung fields but can occur in focal or patchy distributions that are difficult to distinguish from pneumonia. Pleural effusions sometimes occur in predominantly left-sided heart failure but are more characteristic of biventricular failure. Interstitial and alveolar edema may lessen or disappear with onset of right ventricular failure. A widened superior vena cava shadow suggests right ventricular failure and systemic venous congestion.

NONINVASIVE ASSESSMENT. Echocardiographic study constitutes a cost-effective approach to the evaluation of patients with heart failure, and together with Doppler study in most instances is advisable at an early stage in the workup of this group of patients (see Ch. 39.3). Valuable information can be obtained in every etiologic class of patients, including those with ischemic disease, cardiomyopathy, valvular disease, hypertensive disease, congenital disease, and cor pulmonale. Echo study is of particular value in making the important distinction between predominant systolic and diastolic ventricular dysfunction.

CARDIAC CATHETERIZATION. Invasive evaluation is usually appropriate in patients who are candidates for cardiac surgery or catheter-based interventional procedures such as coronary angioplasty or valvuloplasty, as discussed in Ch. 39.5. Right ventricular endomyocardial biopsy is valuable in patients suspected of having inflammatory or infiltrative disease and for assessment of myopathic effects of certain antineoplastic drugs (e.g., doxorubicin). Endomyocardial biopsy is routinely done using a percutaneous jugular approach at intervals following cardiac transplantation for assessment of the adequacy of immunosuppressive therapy.

PULMONARY FUNCTION TESTS. The course of left ventricular failure, including the response to treatment, can be followed by consecutive determinations of vital capacity, although this practice has been largely supplanted by other approaches in recent years. With interstitial pulmonary edema, expiratory flow rates at low lung volumes are reduced and distal airways tend to close prematurely during expiration, trapping gas within the lungs and disturbing the normal relation of ventilation to perfusion. This produces a widening of the alveolar-arterial Po_2 difference and a decrease in arterial Po_2 due to venous admixture. Arterial oxygen saturation is typically nearly normal, however, unless intrinsic lung disease is present. The arteriovenous oxygen content difference increases with decreasing cardiac outputs as tissue extraction of oxygen becomes more complete. Systemic arterial Pco_2 remains normal or low unless ventilation is compromised in the course of pulmonary edema. Endotracheal intubation and assisted ventilation may be indicated if progressive carbon dioxide retention is documented by serial blood gas measurements.

Right Ventricular and Biventricular Failure

CLINICAL MANIFESTATIONS. Isolated right ventricular failure is uncommon in adults and is usually a consequence of cor pulmonale secondary to intrinsic lung disease or, on occasion,

chronic volume overload from a congenital intracardiac left-to-right shunt (e.g., atrial septal defect). Right ventricular failure is encountered most often as a complication of left ventricular failure. In the presence of elevated right heart filling pressures, neck veins are distended and fill from below. Hepatic enlargement and tenderness to gentle palpation result from passive congestion, and manual compression over the liver causes further distention of the neck veins (hepatojugular reflux). In the presence of biventricular failure, signs of right ventricular failure may dominate, but the presence of dyspnea and rales should suggest additional left ventricular failure. Accompanying low cardiac output results in signs of increased sympathetic nervous activity and of organ hypoperfusion. It should be remembered that a critically lowered cardiac output from any cause sufficient to produce metabolic acidosis occasions hyperventilation in defense of acid-base balance, and this must be distinguished from the tachypnea of left heart failure. Advanced right-sided or biventricular failure may be associated with anorexia, weight loss, and malnutrition ("cardiac cachexia").

Cyanosis. Cyanosis is caused by 5 or more grams per 100 ml of unoxygenated hemoglobin in the subpapillary venous plexus of the skin. This occurs in right heart failure because the congested venules contain blood from which considerable oxygen has been extracted because of the slow flow. This is typically accompanied by relatively normal arterial Po_2 values unless intrinsic lung disease or intracardiac shunting is present. Cyanosis is usually absent in left heart failure unless caused by a complication (e.g., pneumonia) or by pulmonary edema.

Abnormal Heart and Lungs. Although dyspnea accompanying left ventricular failure may be partially relieved by onset of right ventricular failure, some dyspnea usually persists, together with tachypnea and basal rales. Tricuspid valvular insufficiency commonly accompanies severe right ventricular dilation and failure and contributes to systemic venous engorgement. The murmur of tricuspid insufficiency is distinguished from that of mitral insufficiency by its location (lower left border of sternum), by its tendency to increase during inspiration, and by associated physical signs, such as hepatic pulsation and systolic waves in the jugular venous pulse. Doppler echocardiography greatly assists in the assessment of this problem. Pleural effusion, often unilateral, is more common in right-sided or biventricular than in isolated left ventricular failure.

Systemic Venous Congestion. Elevation of systemic venous pressure is a sine qua non of right heart failure. Responsible mechanisms include (1) the inability of the failing ventricle to eject the venous return without abnormally high filling pressures, causing (2) an increase in the volume of blood in the large systemic veins; and (3) increased venomotor tone resulting from increased sympathetic nervous system activity. Increased systemic venous pressure is responsible for the hepatomegaly, occasional splenomegaly, and peripheral edema that characterize decompensated right ventricular failure. Usually less apparent are the associated congestion and edema of the gastrointestinal tract.

Pressure in the jugular venous system, a useful index of right atrial pressure, may be estimated from the height of the column of blood distending the cervical veins. The cervical veins are normally flat in the upright posture in the absence of raised intrathoracic pressure, whereas in right heart failure they are prominent and distended. The wave form of venous pulsation is usually best appreciated from inspection of the right internal jugular vein, adjusting the angle of the patient's upper body to bring out the top of the venous pressure column. Tricuspid insufficiency distorts the normal venous pulse by producing a systolic or C-V wave that has no counterpart in the normal jugular venous pulse. Occasionally, compression over the liver is necessary to display the increased blood volume in the venous system, but the examiner must avoid being misled by venous distention from involuntary expiration against a closed glottis (the Valsalva maneuver).

Liver. The liver is typically enlarged and tender in right heart failure. If the onset is acute, right upper quadrant pain may result from constraint of the swollen liver by its tight capsule. Splenomegaly is uncommon except in prolonged passive congestion of the liver, and pain or tenderness of the spleen should raise the question of superimposed systemic embolization and splenic infarction.

Early congestion of the liver may cause modest increases in the concentrations of hepatic enzymes such as alkaline phosphatase in serum, and increases in serum bilirubin may occur. Hyperbilirubinemia from this cause usually consists of a combination of conjugated and unconjugated bilirubin. Frank jaundice is uncommon unless hepatic congestion is associated with longstanding pulmonary congestion or pulmonary infarction.

Hypoglycemia may occur if cardiac output is severely compromised and hepatic congestion is marked and protracted. This is attributed to depletion of liver glycogen stores and increased formation of lactic acid from glucose induced by hypoxia.

Repeated and prolonged episodes of right heart failure with reduced hepatic blood flow and elevated venous pressures can cause atrophy and centrilobular necrosis of liver cells and can lead to extensive fibrosis ("cardiac cirrhosis") that is difficult to distinguish from posthepatitic cirrhosis. Hepatic failure with precoma or coma is a rare, preterminal complication of this sequence of events.

Extracellular Fluid Compartments. The fluid compartments of the body are normally maintained constant by neurohormonally mediated interplay among intake (governed by thirst and appetite), exchanges of fluid and electrolytes (governed by passive and active transport mechanisms), and excretion (regulated primarily by the kidneys). In heart failure, excessive retention of sodium and water by the kidneys results in an isosmotic expansion of extracellular fluid, including the circulating blood volume. In mild heart failure, retention of sodium and water may serve to expand the blood volume to sustain venous return and the forward output of the failing heart through the Frank-Starling mechanism. However, retention of salt and water only exacerbates pulmonary and systemic congestion and edema when the myocardium can no longer respond positively to increased filling pressure and volumes.

The distribution of excess extracellular ("third space") fluid varies among patients. Under the influence of gravity, edema accumulates in the feet and ankles of ambulatory patients but shifts to the sacral region in the bedridden patient. Localization occurs in areas of low tissue pressure, such as the back of the ankle. Colloid osmotic pressure and the integrity of the lymphatic system also influence extracellular fluid distribution.

Peripheral Edema. Dependent edema developing over the course of the day and subsiding by morning is a characteristic feature of right heart failure. It is a direct consequence of elevated systemic venous pressure and is typically preceded by a gain in weight. Persistent edema is accompanied relatively frequently by complications such as low-grade cellulitis, and the combination of edema and sluggish venous flow predisposes to deep venous thrombosis and pulmonary embolism.

Pleural Effusion. The infrequency of hydrothorax in isolated right ventricular failure dictates that the association of pleural effusion and cor pulmonale should lead one to search for another cause, such as pulmonary infarction. It is, however, common in biventricular failure. Hydrothorax results from impaired removal of isotonic fluid from the pleural space because of elevated venous pressures in both the pulmonary and the systemic circulations, compromising transcapillary exchange of water at the pleural surface and also impeding lymphatic drainage. Hydrothorax contributes to dyspnea reflexly, probably by stimuli from lungs and chest wall, as well as by displacing ventilated lung tissue from the relatively fixed volume of the thoracic space. Pulmonary embolism and infarction may contribute to pleural effusion in two ways: by transit of fluid from the infarcted area of the lung to the pleural space or by aggravation of heart failure.

Ascites. The presence of free fluid in the abdominal cavity is a late manifestation of right heart failure, usually associated with systemic venous hypertension, peripheral edema, and hydrothorax. It is commonly encountered in the setting of tricuspid valve disease or chronic constrictive pericarditis. Elevated pressures in portal and hepatic veins and in the systemic veins draining the peritoneum contribute to the formation of ascites, but renal retention of sodium and water is a prerequisite. It may

contribute to anorexia and can cause abdominal discomfort or pain in patients with severe right ventricular failure.

Pericardial Effusion. Patients with chronic heart failure commonly have increased amounts of fluid in the pericardial sac that can be demonstrated echocardiographically. Only rarely, however, does it accumulate to an extent that produces further hemodynamic compromise (tamponade).

Anasarca. Advanced and protracted right ventricular failure without adequate treatment can cause edema fluid to accumulate throughout the body, most conspicuously in subcutaneous tissues as well as abdominal and thoracic cavities. Face and arms are typically spared until the preterminal stages of failure. This clinical picture occurs rarely in the present era of potent diuretics.

Gastrointestinal Tract. Systemic venous hypertension leads to edema of the bowel wall. These changes interfere with absorption of drugs or foods only when heart failure is severe, but reduced bioavailability of furosemide and perhaps other drugs can occur under these circumstances. In severe congestive heart failure, anorexia, nausea, and vomiting may occur from reflex, central, local, or drug-induced causes. Protein-losing enteropathy can occur in the setting of severe right heart failure.

Brain. Nonspecific complaints, including headache and insomnia, are common in heart failure and are usually attributable to some diminution of cerebral blood flow and triggering mechanisms such as dyspnea that contribute to insomnia. Neurologic or behavioral aberrations are more frequent when the burdens of a limited cardiac output are superimposed on antecedent neurologic disease (e.g., cerebrovascular disease or prior stroke) or on personality disorder. Irritability, restlessness, and limited attention span are associated with severe congestive heart failure. Stupor and coma supervene when cardiac output is critically reduced.

Kidney. Oliguria occurs with decompensation in isolated right or left heart failure but is more prominent in the latter or in biventricular failure. The urine is sodium poor but has a relatively high specific gravity (1.020 to 1.030). Prerenal azotemia is common, particularly in the presence of intrinsic renal disease or after vigorous diuresis. Azotemia with high urine specific gravity is characteristic of heart failure (and dehydration) and stands in contrast to the low specific gravity expected with renal insufficiency due to intrinsic renal disease. Blood urea nitrogen is typically elevated out of proportion to serum creatinine. Proteinuria is common but does not usually exceed 1 gram per day.

Other Manifestations. In chronic severe congestive heart failure, weakness and gradual loss of tissue mass are frequent concomitants and may progress to cachexia. At this late stage, the patient is usually suffering from anorexia and often gastrointestinal symptoms and electrolyte disturbances as well. Although organ hypoperfusion and congestion play an important part in this syndrome, the physician must maintain vigilance to avoid additional contributions from overvigorous use of digitalis and diuretics.

Anxiety. This is a common feature of cardiac disease by the time the heart fails. Manifestations of anxiety may be difficult to distinguish from symptoms of the underlying cardiac disorder because of the nonspecific nature of complaints such as breathlessness. Symptoms related to hyperventilation as well as palpitations may contribute to the patient's anxiety by reinforcing the impression that organic heart disease is present. The physician must proceed with the separate assessment of organic and psychosomatic aspects of the disease process, recognizing that a careful history and physical examination, together with judicious use of noninvasive diagnostic methods, help to establish the extent to which organic heart disease is responsible for the patient's symptoms.

CLINICAL MANAGEMENT OF HEART FAILURE
General Approaches

The management of congestive heart failure includes three general types of approaches. The first is removal of the underlying cause. This deserves top priority in all cases and includes measures such as surgical correction of valvular lesions or congenital malformation. It also includes medical treatment of hypertension or infective endocarditis when present.

The second approach consists of removal of precipitating causes of heart failure. Frequently the initial development or exacerba-

TABLE 40–3. MEASURES IN THE MANAGEMENT OF CONGESTIVE HEART FAILURE

A. Improve pump performance of the failing ventricle
  1. Cardiac glycosides (digoxin)
  2. Sympathomimetic drugs (dopamine, dobutamine)
  3. Other positive inotropic drugs (amrinone)
  4. Pacemaker for bradycardia or loss of atrioventricular synchrony
B. Reduction of cardiac work load
  1. Rest (physical and emotional)
  2. Correction of obesity
  3. Vasodilator drugs
  4. Assisted circulation (e.g., intra-aortic balloon counterpulsation)
C. Control salt and water retention
  1. Limit dietary sodium intake
  2. Diuretics
  3. Mechanical removal of fluid
    a. Thoracentesis
    b. Paracentesis
    c. Dialysis
    d. Phlebotomy

tion of heart failure is related not to worsening of the underlying cardiac condition but rather to a superimposed stress. Typical factors that can precipitate overt congestive heart failure, apart from changes in the status of the heart itself, are listed in Table 40–2.

The third set of measures, treatment of clinical manifestations of heart failure, occupies the remainder of this chapter. This approach may in turn be divided into three categories, as summarized in Table 40–3:

1. Measures to improve the contractile performance of the heart.
2. Measures to reduce cardiac work.
3. Measures to control excessive retention of salt and water.

As listed in Table 40–3, several therapeutic entities are available in each category. Cardiac glycosides and sympathomimetic agents constitute the principal drugs that enhance the pumping performance of the failing heart. In addition, placement of a pacemaker may improve pumping performance either by supporting a more appropriate heart rate or by restoring atrial augmentation of ventricular filling if synchronous atrioventricular contraction can be achieved (see Ch. 42).

Reduction of the work load of the failing heart can be accomplished by physical and emotional rest, by appropriate treatment of obesity, and by vasodilator therapy. Under specific circumstances, assisted circulation with the intra-aortic balloon pump can usefully contribute to this goal.

Finally, control of the excessive retention of salt and water is approached by instituting a low-sodium diet and the use of diuretic drugs. Under some circumstances, mechanical removal of fluid is of value.

These measures are customarily applied in a stepwise fashion, as outlined in detail in Table 40–4.

Strategy of Heart Failure Management

The many etiologies and degrees of severity of heart failure demand an individualized approach to each patient. Nevertheless, certain general principles apply to the management of various subsets of patients. The comments that follow are relevant to patients with *systolic* ventricular dysfunction (i.e., reduced ejection fraction). In the past, it has not been considered appropriate to institute specific therapeutic measures until symptoms of overt heart failure occur—that is, until the patient makes the transition from functional class I to class II. This recommendation could change, depending on the outcome of current therapeutic trials of vasodilator administration to patients with ventricular dysfunction but without overt heart failure. The first approach (see Table 40–4) in all instances includes judicious limitation of activity, advising the patient to avoid physical exertion that produces undue dyspnea or exhaustion. The degree of restriction should be tailored to the severity of heart failure. It is important not to limit activity so severely that skeletal muscle deconditioning, rather than the underlying cardiac problem, becomes the limiting factor in the patient's activity. Physical activity should, however, be markedly restricted in the setting of acute decompensation of chronic heart failure, a situation in which hospitalization is generally advisable.

PHARMACOTHERAPY. A diuretic, a vasodilator (usually an angiotensin converting enzyme inhibitor), or a cardiac glycoside may be added in early class II, with the choice of one or more based on the balance between risk and expected benefit. In many cases, modest doses of a mild diuretic such as a thiazide restore the patient to an essentially asymptomatic state. A vasodilator such as captopril or enalapril should be used if there is evidence of elevated peripheral vascular resistance (systemic hypertension) and no contraindications exist (e.g., postural hypotension or renal impairment, especially in the presence of bilateral renal artery stenosis). Dietary sodium restriction may be limited to avoidance of heavily salted foods and the use of the salt shaker at the table.

TABLE 40–4. STEPS IN THE MANAGEMENT OF CHRONIC CONGESTIVE HEART FAILURE

| Steps | Functional Class | | |
	II	III	IV
A	*Restrict physical activity:* Limit competitive sports and heavy labor	Reduce work schedule; rest periods during day	Limit to house and finally to bed and chair
B	*Dietary sodium restriction:* Eliminate salt shaker and heavily salted foods	Eliminate salt in cooking and at table (Na intake ~ 1.2 to 1.8 grams)	As in III, plus low-sodium foods (Na intake <1 gram)
C	*Diuretics:* Thiazide or low-dose loop diuretic	Loop diuretic (progressive doses); consider adding distally acting (K-sparing) diuretic	Loop diuretic with distally acting (K-sparing) and/or thiazide diuretic
D	*Vasodilators:* Hydralazine and isosorbide dinitrate *or* an ACE inhibitor (captopril or enalapril) ————————————————————→		Intravenous nitroprusside
E	*Digitalis glycosides:* Conventional maintenance doses ————————————————————→		Dose to maintain serum level in 1.5 ng/ml range
F			*Other inotropic drugs (intravenous):* Dopamine, dobutamine, amrinone
G			*Consider cardiac transplantation* *Thoracentesis, paracentesis* *Hemodialysis; extracorporeal ultrafiltration* *Assisted circulation (e.g., intra-aortic balloon pump)*

Special low-sodium foods are expensive and can be so unpalatable as to impair nutrition.

When symptoms persist or evolve on the simple regimen outlined above, combination therapy with diuretics, vasodilators, and cardiac glycosides should be considered. Intensification of the diuretic regimen is often necessary. Problems such as mitral regurgitation are particularly amenable to treatment with vasodilators, as discussed below.

As the severity of heart failure advances, increased restriction of physical activity is usually necessary, and patients often require rest periods during the day as class III symptoms evolve. When patients remain symptomatic during ordinary activity on a program that includes loop diuretics, digitalis, and vasodilators, detailed evaluation is advisable to search for precipitating causes and to consider the possibility of more aggressive approaches. In patients who have progressed to functional class IV, hospitalization is often advisable and the use of intravenous sympathomimetic agents can be considered, in addition to optimization of the vasodilator, diuretic, and cardiac glycoside regimens. In patients who meet appropriate criteria, cardiac transplantation should also be considered at this time if not earlier.

During episodes of decompensation, the hazards of deep venous thrombosis and pulmonary embolism must be guarded against, and the use of minidose heparin (see Ch. 54) is a relatively safe and effective approach during hospitalization. At these times, emotional as well as physical rest is important, and anxiety-provoking situations should be carefully avoided. Marked anxiety or insomnia may be treated with benzodiazepines such as diazepam or the shorter-acting agent triazolam.

DIET. Rigid salt restriction can usually be avoided until diuretics are no longer capable of controlling the accumulation of salt and water. Water intake does not, in general, require specific restriction unless dilutional hyponatremia supervenes.

OXYGEN. Patients with hypoxia, and certainly those with pulmonary edema, benefit from oxygen inhalation, conveniently given by nasal prongs at 4 to 6 liters per minute. In general, supplemental oxygen is worthwhile whenever the arterial oxygen saturation falls below 90 per cent. This is a particularly effective way of reducing right ventricular afterload, since oxygen is a potent pulmonary arteriolar vasodilator.

PHYSICAL REMOVAL OF FLUID. The availability of potent diuretics limits the need for thoracentesis or paracentesis, but these procedures may be important diagnostically when the accumulation of fluid in serous cavities is not readily explained on the basis of heart failure alone. Pulmonary embolism, for example, is a relatively common cause of pleural effusion, and a diagnostic thoracentesis often provides critically important information leading to this diagnosis. Drainage of pleural or ascitic fluid should be carried out slowly, at a rate of not more than about 1500 ml per hour, and the total quantity of fluid removed on any single occasion should not exceed about 1500 ml because of the risk of fluid shifts from the vascular to the extravascular compartment, with consequently inadequate ventricular filling pressures. Particular caution is required in patients (such as those with aortic stenosis or hypertrophic cardiomyopathy) who have reduced ventricular compliance and require high ventricular filling pressures to maintain adequate stroke volume.

Acute Pulmonary Edema

Acute pulmonary edema is a medical emergency in which the immediate therapeutic goals are to (1) improve oxygenation; (2) reduce venous return (preload); (3) reduce anxiety; and (4) treat causal and precipitating factors. Placement of flow-directed pulmonary artery (Swan-Ganz) and arterial lines for monitoring of pressures and arterial blood gases is often advisable. The patient is placed in a trunk-up, legs-down posture and given humidified 100 per cent oxygen, by positive pressure mask if possible. Vital signs are monitored frequently, and an intravenous cannula is inserted for secure intravenous access. Arterial blood gas, blood urea nitrogen (BUN) or creatinine, electrolyte, and complete blood count measurements are obtained at once. An electrocardiogram and chest radiograph (taken with a portable machine if necessary) should also be obtained, and electrical conversion of supraventricular or ventricular tachyarrhythmias should be con-

sidered if present and if not due to digitalis excess. Ultrasound (echocardiographic) study is indicated at the earliest opportunity if the nature and extent of underlying cardiac disease are not entirely clear.

Morphine given intravenously (2 to 10 mg, repeated every 10 to 15 minutes) reduces venous return and allays anxiety; naloxone should be available in case of respiratory depression. Nitroglycerin given sublingually or intravenously further reduces venous return; nitroprusside given intravenously may be used if the blood pressure is adequately maintained and afterload reduction is desirable. Furosemide should be given intravenously in a 20- to 40-mg dose and repeated in increasing doses as necessary to achieve a diuresis. Aminophylline, 250 to 500 mg given slowly intravenously (5.6 mg per kilogram), may be useful to relieve bronchospasm and promote diuresis but can exacerbate sinus or ectopic tachycardias.

If severe respiratory distress persists, tourniquets applied to three of four extremities and rotated every 15 to 20 minutes may be of value. If respiratory acidosis (pH of 7.10 or less) or severe hypoxemia ($Po_2 < 50$ mm Hg) persists, endotracheal intubation and controlled positive-pressure ventilation should usually be instituted. Phlebotomy and hemodialysis deserve consideration in refractory cases. Digitalis has a secondary role in this clinical setting, except occasionally in the management of supraventricular tachyarrhythmias. Superimposed hypotension and low cardiac output states are considered in Ch. 41. Concurrently, vigorous attention should be directed to the identification and management of precipitating factors (see Table 40–2).

Diuretics

Salt and water retention with consequent expansion of the intravascular and interstitial compartments is a sine qua non of chronic congestive heart failure and accounts for many of the common signs and symptoms. Elimination of excess salt and water is an essential goal in management of heart failure.

Two stages characterize diuretic use: first, the elimination of accumulated excess fluid; and second, maintenance of optimal "dry" weight. Care of patients in the hospital typically focuses on elimination of excess fluid, which is facilitated by the controlled salt intake and limited activity of hospitalized patients. Maintenance of optimal fluid balance out of hospital requires adjustments in the context of the individual patient's diet and activity. A sound approach is the use of the mildest diuretic program that is consistent with maintenance of appropriate fluid balance and a salt intake that promotes a nutritious diet. Severe sodium restriction is usually unnecessary except in very severe congestive heart failure. Overly rigorous restriction of sodium intake, together with use of potent diuretics, is a well-known formula for impaired renal function, oliguria, and prerenal azotemia, particularly in the elderly.

CONTROL OF SODIUM BALANCE. The key role of diuretics in management of heart failure relates to the central role of the kidney as a target of many of the neurohumoral and hemodynamic changes that occur in heart failure. Reduced cardiac output causes activation of the renin-angiotensin system in the kidney, with consequent reduction in renal blood flow and increased glomerular filtration fraction, leading to increased resorption of salt and water by the proximal tubule. Elevated plasma angiotensin II levels contribute to increased systemic vascular resistance and increase aldosterone release from the adrenal. Increased renal sympathetic nerve activity also tends to reduce renal blood flow and to release renin from the macula densa, as well as directly augmenting sodium resorption along other segments of the nephron. Intrarenal blood flow redistribution contributes to the formation of relatively concentrated urine (Fig. 40–4). Plasma vasopressin levels are frequently elevated in patients with heart failure, causing further limitation of free water clearance. Together with the increase in thirst of patients with advanced heart failure, this leads to a hyponatremic state that is a particularly ominous prognostic sign in heart failure.

Diuretics intervene in the pathophysiology of heart failure by reducing the reabsorption of sodium and its accompanying anions, as well as water, by the renal tubule. The four major classes of diuretics in current clinical use are summarized in Table 40–5. Each of these agents affects renal tubular function in a distinct way, and each tends to produce a characteristic set of abnormal-

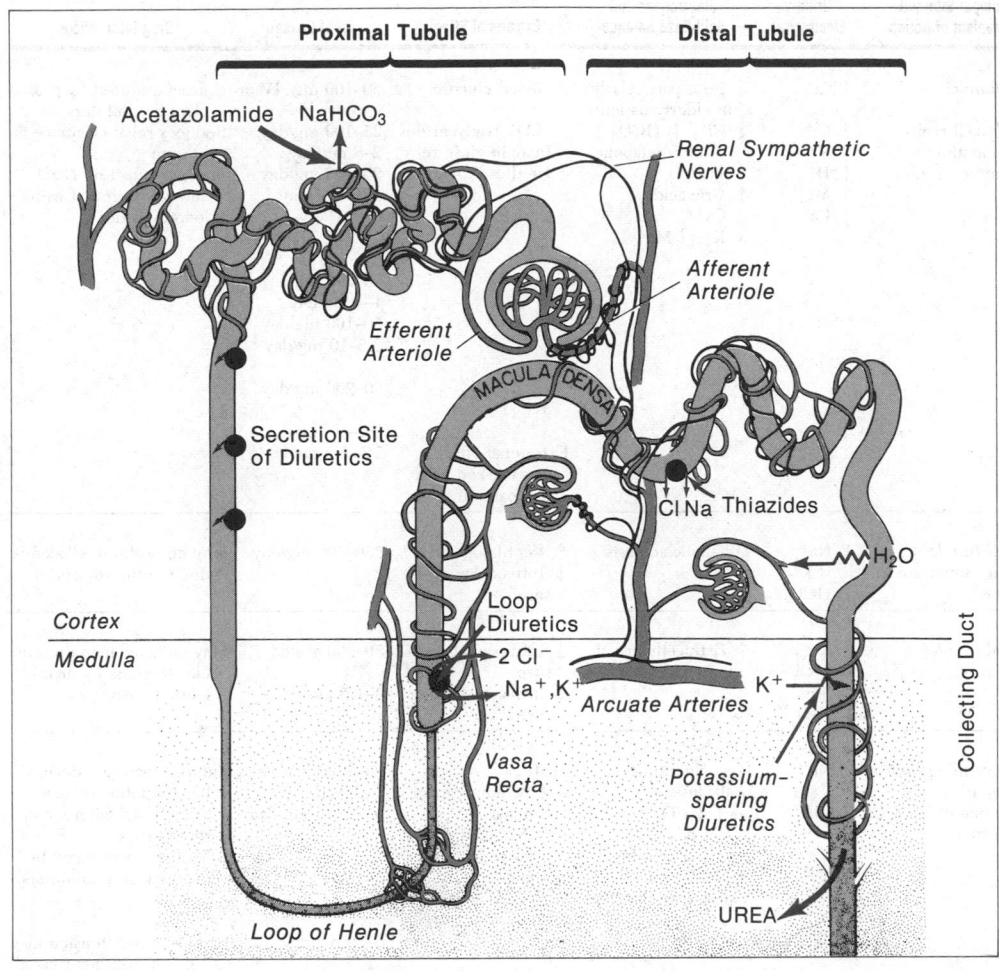

Proximal Tubule   **Distal Tubule**

Acetazolamide NaHCO₃

Renal Sympathetic
Nerves

Afferent
Arteriole

Efferent
Arteriole

MACULA DENSA

Secretion Site
of Diuretics

Cl Na Thiazides

H₂O

Cortex
Medulla

Loop
Diuretics

2 Cl⁻

Na⁺,K⁺   Arcuate Arteries   K⁺

Vasa
Recta

Potassium-
sparing
Diuretics

Collecting Duct

UREA

Loop of Henle

FIGURE 40–4. Sites of diuretic action in the mammalian nephron. Fluid resorption across the proximal tubule accounts for approximately two thirds of the resorption of filtered sodium and H_2O. Neuronal, hormonal, and hemodynamic factors, both extrinsic and intrinsic to the kidney, affect the volume and content of urine formation by altering the rate of formation of glomerular filtrate, thereby altering the balance of Starling forces between the proximal tubule and postglomerular peritubular capillaries. Agents that alter the rate of formation of glomerular filtrate, such as ACE inhibitors, may enhance the delivery of solute and water to more distal segments of the nephron that are sensitive to diuretics. Nonsteroidal anti-inflammatory drugs may diminish the glomerular filtration rate, thus reducing the flow of urine to distal diuretic-sensitive portions of the nephron. A reduction in systemic blood pressure, or in renal artery pressure distal to the stenotic arterial lesion, below that necessary for formation of glomerular filtrate renders the kidney refractory to any diuretic. With the exception of the osmotic diuretics that are freely filtered at the glomerulus, most diuretics reach their site of action along the nephron after being secreted into the tubular lumen by the organic anion secretory transport system of the straight proximal tubule (pars recta).

About one third of the glomerular filtrate arrives at the descending limb of Henle's loop; no active transport of solute occurs here, although the tubular epithelium is highly permeable to water, which leaves the nephron for the increasingly hyperosmotic medullary interstitium. Most of the solute transport responsible for maintaining the hypertonicity of the medullary interstitium occurs in the water-impermeable thick ascending limb of Henle's loop. Here, a NaK cotransport system in the luminal membrane is coupled to the uptake of two chloride ions, a process dependent upon the electrochemical driving force for sodium generated by the NaK-ATPase on the basolateral membrane of these cells. This Na/K/2 Cl cotransport system on the luminal membrane of the tubular cells is the site of action for the loop diuretics (furosemide, bumetanide, and ethacrynic acid). Inhibition of cation transport by loop diuretics prevents the normal generation of the hypertonic medullary interstitium, thus reducing the osmotic gradient for free water clearance of ADH-sensitive tubular cells in the collecting duct, and also delivers large amounts of solute and water to the distal nephron, thus overwhelming distal Na⁺ and Cl⁻ resorption sites.

The thick ascending limb approaches its own glomerulus as it re-enters the cortex and passes between the afferent and efferent arterioles to form the juxtaglomerular apparatus (JGA), the tubular contribution to which is termed the macula densa. Loop diuretics may directly stimulate the release of renin by the JGA, an action that may contribute to the extrarenal vascular effects of these drugs. The distal convoluted tubule begins beyond the macula densa. Na⁺ and Cl⁻, as well as other ions (e.g., Ca⁺⁺), are resorbed in this segment. The thiazide diuretics and related drugs inhibit NaCl resorption in this segment, although the mechanism is unknown; they also enhance Ca⁺⁺ resorption by tubular cells in this segment. Salt resorption by this distal, water-impermeable portion of the nephron allows the formation of a dilute urine, hence the term "cortical diluting segment." Thiazide-induced inhibition of NaCl resorption in this segment therefore may lead to hyponatremia, particularly when accompanied by elevated ADH levels and increased thirst.

The cortical collecting duct actively resorbs NaCl via an aldosterone-sensitive mechanism. This leads to increased net resorption of Na⁺ into cells and hence to a lumen negative potential difference that favors the secretion of K⁺ and H⁺ ions. This is why increased Na⁺ concentrations and high flow rates in the cortical collecting duct, as after loop or thiazide diuretic administration, lead to enhanced passive K⁺ secretion. Anti-aldosterone drugs, such as spironolactone, competitively inhibit aldosterone's binding to its receptor, thereby limiting Na⁺ permeability by the apical membrane and reducing K⁺ secretion.

As illustrated, the blood supply to each nephron is derived from several sources. The afferent arteriole that enters the glomerulus is richly innervated with sympathetic nerve endings, particularly as it enters the glomerulus at its vascular pole within the juxtaglomerular apparatus. Increased sympathetic discharge to the kidney results in increased net NaCl resorption even in the absence of changes in glomerular hemodynamics. Elevated efferent sympathetic activity, as is often seen in decompensated congestive heart failure, would be expected to result in avid retention of solute due to reduced renal perfusion, increased renin release, and enhanced tubular resorption of solute. Dopamine is a potent renal vasodilator and may directly affect tubular epithelia to reduce NaCl resorption, thus acting as a natriuretic agent. Exogenously administered dopamine, particularly when infused at rates of 2 to 3 μg per minute, may be a useful adjunct to diuretic therapy in selected with advanced CHF.

TABLE 40–5. DIURETICS: ACTION, DOSAGE, AND DRUG INTERACTIONS

Diuretic	Brand Name	Principal Site and Mechanism of Action	Effects on Urinary Electrolytes	Effects on Blood Electrolytes and Acid-Base Balance	Extrarenal Effects	Usual Dosage*	Drug Interactions
Thiazides and Related Compounds							
Chlorothiazide	Diuril	*Distal tubule:*	$\uparrow$ Na$^+$	$\downarrow$ Na$^+$, particularly in elderly patients	$\uparrow$ Blood glucose	50–100 mg, IV or p.o.	Efficacy reduced by prostaglandin inhibitors
Hydrochlorothiazide	Hydro-Diuril	Inhibit NaCl reabsorption and	$\uparrow$ Cl$^-$	$\downarrow$ Cl$^-$, $\uparrow$ HCO$_3^-$ —mild metabolic	$\uparrow$ LDL/triglycerides (may be dose related)	25–100 mg/day	Reduces renal clearance of lithium
Trichlormethiazide			$\uparrow$ K$^+$	alkalosis		2–8 mg/day	
Chlorthalidone	Metahydrin Hygroton	$\uparrow$ Ca^{2+} excretion	$\uparrow$ H$^+$	$\uparrow$ Uric acid		25–100 mg/day	Additive effect on NaCl and K$^+$ excretion with
Metolazone	Zaroxolyn		$\uparrow$ Mg^{2+} $\downarrow$ Ca^{2+}	$\uparrow$ Ca^{++} $\downarrow$ K$^+$, $\downarrow$ Mg^{2+}		5–10 mg/day	loop diuretics
Cyclothiazide	Anhydron					2–6 mg/day	
Hydroflumethizide	Diucardin					25–200 mg/day	
Polythiazide	Renese					1–4 mg/day	
Quinethazone	Hydromox					50–100 mg/day	
Methyclothiazide	Enduron Aquatensen					2.5–10 mg/day	
Benzthiazide	Aquatag Exna					50–200 mg/day	
Bendroflumethiazide	Naturetin					2.5–30 mg/day	
Indapamide	Lozol	Vasodilator			Extrarenal effects less marked with indapamide	2.5–5 mg/day	
Carbonic Anhydrase Inhibitor							
Acetazolamide	Diamox	*Proximal tubule:* Carbonic anhydrase inhibitor	$\uparrow$ Na$^+$, $\uparrow$ K$^+$ $\uparrow$ HCO$_3^-$	Metabolic acidosis	$\uparrow$ Ventilatory drive $\downarrow$ Intraocular pressure	250–500 mg/day	May be useful in alkalemia due to other diuretics
Osmotic Diuretics							
Mannitol	Osmitrol	*Proximal tubule* (primarily)	$\uparrow$ Na$^+$, $\uparrow$ Cl$^-$	$\uparrow$ Extracellular volume transiently	$\downarrow$ Intracranial pressure	50–200 gm/day, IV	May enhance loop diuretic effectiveness by maintaining GFR
Glycerol	Glyrol		$\uparrow$ H$_2$O		$\downarrow$ Intraocular pressure	1–1.5 gm/kg	
Loop Diuretics							
Furosemide	Lasix	*Thick ascending limb of loop of Henle:*	$\uparrow\uparrow$ Na$^+$	Hypochloremic alkalosis ($\uparrow$ HCO$_3^-$)	Acute: $\uparrow$ Venous capacitance	20–1000 mg/day, p.o./IV	Tubular secretion delayed by competing organic acids (renal failure) and
Bumetanide	Bumex	Inhibition of Na/K/Cl cotransport	$\uparrow\uparrow$ Cl$^-$	$\downarrow$ K$^+$, $\downarrow$ Na$^+$ $\downarrow$ Cl$^-$, $\downarrow$ Mg^{2+} $\uparrow$ Uric acid (less than thiazide)	$\uparrow$ Systemic vascular resistance Chronic: $\downarrow$ Cardiac preload	0.5–20.0 mg/day	some drugs Effectiveness reduced by prostaglandin inhibitors
Piretanide†	Arelix Diumax Tauliz					6–20 mg/day	Excessive hypotension may occur in patients treated chronically with a loop diuretic when begun on an ACE inhibitor
Ethacrynic acid	Edecrin				Ototoxicity	50–200 mg/day, IV	Additive ototoxicity with aminoglycosides
Mefruside†	Baycaron Mefiusal	Similar to thiazides				25–50 mg/day	Longer duration of action than furosemide
Muzolamine† Torasemide†		Less K$^+$ wasting				2.5–5 mg/day	
Potassium-Sparing Diuretics							
Spironolactone	Aldactone	*Collecting duct:* Aldosterone antagonist	$\downarrow$ K$^+$ $\uparrow$ Na$^+$	$\uparrow$ K$^+$, particularly in patients with	Gynecomastia	25–100 mg/day	Useful adjunct to therapy with K$^+$-wasting diuretics; triamterene with in-
Canrenoate† (potassium)			$\uparrow$ Cl$^-$	$\downarrow$ GFR; metabolic acidosis			domethacin may cause abrupt $\downarrow$ GFR
Triamterene	Dyrenium	Inhibit apical membrane Na$^+$ conductance	$\uparrow$ HCO$_3^-$			100–300 mg/day	
Amiloride	Midamor					5–10 mg/day	

*Route of administration is p.o. except as noted.
†Not yet licensed for use in the United States.
GFR = glomerular filtration rate; LDL = low density lipoproteins; ACE = angiotensin-converting enzyme.

ities in electrolyte patterns, fluid balance, and acid-base homeostasis. The more potent the diuretic, the greater the potential risk for severe and sometimes life-threatening disturbances of electrolyte and acid-base balance.

THIAZIDES. Because of their effectiveness by oral administration, their predictable effects, and their relative freedom from toxicity, thiazide diuretics are very commonly used in the management of heart failure. The thiazide diuretics include several agents with chemical and pharmacologic similarities. The prototype is chlorothiazide. Chlorthalidone and metolazone are heterocyclic compounds that share the basic benzothiadiazine nucleus. All of these drugs inhibit sodium chloride reabsorption in the distal tubule. This effect is not dependent upon the weak carbonic anhydrase inhibitory activities common to most of these drugs. By inhibiting sodium chloride transport in the distal tubule, dilution of tubular fluid is prevented and delivery of solute and water to the hydrogen- and potassium-secreting sites in the collecting duct is enhanced. Calcium reabsorption is also promoted by the thiazides, probably by enhancement of calcium entry into epithelial cells of the distal tubule and perhaps by mild volume depletion as well.

The thiazides are useful in the initial management of mild to moderate congestive heart failure. Their utility is limited, however, by avid solute reabsorption in the more proximal nephron segments. Thiazides are largely ineffective when the glomerular filtration rate is less than 30 ml per minute. They are often useful in the treatment of refractory edema in combination with loop diuretics, as discussed subsequently.

Potentially troublesome side effects include potassium depletion, hyperuricemia, glucose intolerance, and plasma lipid elevations, as discussed below. Care must be taken to avoid gastric and small bowel irritation from the potassium chloride supplements that are often required in conjunction with thiazide diuretics.

CARBONIC ANHYDRASE INHIBITORS. Related to the thiazides are the carbonic anhydrase inhibitors, of which acetazolamide is the only agent currently available. This drug results in urinary sodium and bicarbonate losses until the plasma bicarbonate level falls to the point at which renal tubular bicarbonate reabsorption (both proximal and distal) exceeds the filtered load of bicarbonate. Thus, these agents tend to have a transient effect. The sodium and potassium loss accompanying bicarbonate excretion is moderate, but acetazolamide may be of value in patients with high serum bicarbonate levels, as may occur in cor pulmonale or metabolic alkalosis. The presence of metabolic acidosis, e.g., from renal failure or hepatic failure, constitutes a contraindication to its use.

LOOP DIURETICS. These agents are the most potent diuretics in common clinical use and are capable of inducing a natriuresis of up to 20 per cent of the filtered load of sodium for limited periods. They are of particular value in three situations: in acute pulmonary edema, used intravenously; in severe or refractory heart failure; or when renal function is impaired. Ethacrynic acid is chemically different from furosemide and its analogues but appears to share a similar set of pharmacologic properties. These diuretics act to inhibit the Na/K/2 Cl transport system that is responsible for solute reabsorption in the thick ascending limb of the loop of Henle. Each of these drugs is secreted into the tubular lumen by the organic acid secretory pathway, and their effects may therefore be delayed or decreased by exogenous (e.g., probenecid) or endogenous (organic anion accumulation in uremia) competitive inhibitors of the transporter.

Gastrointestinal absorption of furosemide, the most commonly used of the loop diuretics, is variable, with an average bioavailability of 60 per cent. This is substantially diminished when the drug is given with meals. Congestive heart failure can decrease absorption rates of both furosemide and bumetanide. The nonsteroidal anti-inflammatory drugs, including aspirin, tend to blunt the natriuretic response to all of the loop diuretics.

The loop diuretics in general produce systemic hemodynamic changes that precede and are presumably unrelated to the degree and extent of diuresis they induce. Acute administration of furosemide causes a rapid increase in venous capacitance, with a consequent decline in cardiac filling pressures. This effect is accompanied by an increase in plasma renin activity that can produce an appreciable rise in systemic vascular resistance. These effects on the peripheral vasculature tend to plateau in the lower dose range at about a 20-mg intravenous dose of furosemide. Although the loop diuretics are potent inhibitors of Na/K/2 Cl cotransport, this process is not clinically important outside the kidney, except in the cochlea, where it is thought to account for the eighth nerve toxicity that is seen with loop diuretics, particularly ethacrynic acid. The ototoxicity of loop diuretics is synergistic with that of aminoglycoside antibiotics.

Bumetanide and piretanide tend to have higher bioavailability and greater potency than furosemide and may be slightly less ototoxic. Other differences among these closely related compounds appear to be small and probably clinically unimportant.

An important advantage of the loop diuretics is their rapid onset of action, with a diuretic response typically appearing within a few minutes of intravenous administration.

POTASSIUM-SPARING DIURETICS. Two groups of drugs fall into this class: (1) the aldosterone antagonist and (2) the direct inhibitors of sodium permeability in the collecting duct. The aldosterone antagonist most frequently used is spironolactone, although canrenoate and canrenone have essentially identical effects. The aldosterone antagonists compete with the native hormone for cytoplasmic receptors in responsive cells, ultimately

reducing sodium reabsorption. Therapeutic efficacy of these agents is limited when used alone, but they are often useful in combination with other potent diuretics.

Amiloride and triamterene are structurally related compounds that inhibit sodium uptake in collecting duct epithelial cells by inhibiting sodium conductance. A principal effect of these drugs is to reduce renal potassium secretion, which may be useful in concert with the action of potassium-wasting compounds such as the thiazides and loop diuretics but which may lead to clinically important hyperkalemia, particularly in patients with renal failure. The potassium-sparing diuretics tend to cause a mild metabolic acidosis. In patients with chronic obstructive pulmonary disease, these agents may be preferred to diuretics that enhance renal hydrogen losses and secondarily reduce ventilatory drive. Apart from causing hyperkalemia, these drugs are relatively benign. Spironolactone can cause troublesome gynecomastia.

OSMOTIC DIURETICS. These agents are rarely of use in the management of heart failure, but it should be remembered that radiographic contrast dyes are filtered by the glomerulus and act as osmotic diuretics, increasing urinary loss of salt and water. This volume-contracting effect can be important in fragile patients, such as those with severe aortic stenosis. An important characteristic of osmotic diuresis is its ability to maintain urine flow even at very low glomerular filtration rates, as occur in hypotension or dehydration.

COMBINED DIURETIC REGIMENS. Combined use of diuretics in patients with heart failure is usually considered for two main reasons: to avoid electrolyte disturbances that occur with the isolated use of a powerful agent such as a loop diuretic, especially in chronic therapy, and to augment salt and water excretion in the face of refractory edema. A third possible indication is the avoidance of ototoxicity from large doses of loop diuretics.

Combined use of potassium-sparing diuretics with a more proximally acting agent such as a thiazide or a loop diuretic constitutes a common practice. The potassium-sparing diuretics limit potassium and hydrogen ion loss induced by diuretics that act more proximally.

The combination of a loop diuretic with a thiazide or metolazone often results in a synergistic augmentation of salt and water excretion. This combination of agents is capable of producing marked intravascular volume depletion and electrolyte disturbances. Potassium wasting can be severe, and serum potassium levels require close monitoring. In general, this combination of diuretics should be initiated in a hospital setting, with careful regulation of the regimen on an outpatient basis with weight measurements taken daily and frequent checks of serum electrolyte and creatinine levels.

COMPLICATIONS OF DIURETIC THERAPY. Problems complicating diuretic therapy include intravascular volume depletion and hypotension from overly vigorous diuresis; hyponatremia, often due to prolonged diuretic therapy with inadequate sodium intake and often with excessive water intake; hypokalemia from the use of thiazides or loop diuretics, or both, with inadequate potassium supplementation, predisposing to cardiac arrhythmias with or without concomitant digitalis excess; hyperkalemia from potassium-sparing diuretic administration and potassium supplements; metabolic alkalosis with or without potassium depletion; hyperuricemia secondary to thiazide or loop diuretic administration; magnesium depletion, often occurring in parallel with potassium depletion; and increased serum low density lipoprotein and triglyceride levels in patients receiving thiazides.

As a final comment, many patients treated for congestive heart failure spend a period of weeks developing the excessive fluid accumulation that characterizes this disease state; there is little virtue and much potential harm in attempting to correct this problem in an unduly short period of time. In general, in the absence of acute pulmonary edema, a reasonable goal (even in the era of DRG's) is about 1 kg of fluid loss per day.

Digitalis Glycosides

Cardiac glycosides have been used in the management of heart failure for more than 200 years and remain the only drugs currently available for long-term ambulatory use that have a positive inotropic effect. The relatively narrow therapeutic-toxic ratio of cardiac glycosides renders them particularly difficult to use, and the clinician should have a detailed understanding of the actions and pharmacokinetics of one drug of this class, such as digoxin. Because digoxin has supplanted almost entirely the use of other cardiac glycosides in the United States, the discussion focuses on this agent.

BASIC MECHANISM OF CARDIAC GLYCOSIDE ACTION. A consensus exists that the sequence of events leading to the positive inotropic effect of digitalis on both normal and failing cardiac muscle is as summarized in Figure 40–5. The digitalis glycosides bind to a site on the extracellular facing aspect of NaK-ATPase, the enzyme constituting the "sodium pump" that moves sodium and potassium across cell membranes against their respective concentration gradients. The complete amino acid sequences of the alpha and beta subunits of the enzyme are known. When a cardiac glycoside binds to the alpha subunit, that individual sodium pump unit is completely inhibited. When a fraction of NaK-ATPase sites on a cardiac myocyte are occupied, intracellular sodium concentration tends to rise. Through the mechanism of sodium-calcium exchange, this leads in turn to augmentation of the intracellular calcium content. Since calcium constitutes the trigger that leads to the contractile event, the increase of intracellular calcium stores (up to a point) enhances the contractile state of both normal and failing myocardium.

The electrophysiologic toxicity commonly observed with excessive doses of digitalis is probably due to the same fundamental mechanism of sodium pump inhibition. At higher doses and myocardial concentrations of the drug, impairment of sodium and potassium transport leads to characteristic disturbances of impulse formation and conduction, as discussed below. It is likely that intracellular calcium overload contributes to the cardiotoxicity of the digitalis glycosides, at least under circumstances that have been studied experimentally.

ELECTROPHYSIOLOGIC EFFECTS. Most of the antiarrhythmic effects of digitalis are the results of its actions at the level of the atria and atrioventricular junction. Conduction velocity is increased by cardiac glycosides in atrial and ventricular myocardium, but it is decreased in the AV conduction system and His-Purkinje system. Similarly, the effective refractory period is shortened in atrial and ventricular myocardium but tends to be lengthened in specialized conduction tissues. These effects are largely mediated by increased vagal tone, rather than by direct effects of cardiac glycosides, although the latter can be documented at the upper end of the dose range. Of particular importance in the management of supraventricular tachyarrhythmias is the tendency of digitalis to lengthen the refractory period and to slow conduction in the atrioventricular node. At toxic doses and blood levels, digitalis enhances sympathetic nerve traffic to the heart, thus increasing the propensity to ectopic impulse formation at atrial, atrioventricular junctional, and ventricular levels.

HEMODYNAMIC EFFECTS. The positive inotropic action is a direct effect of digitalis on cardiac myocytes. Endogenous norepinephrine stores are not necessary to permit expression of this effect. A useful way to appreciate the effect of digitalis on the intact circulation is by consideration of the ventricular function curves shown in Figure 40–1. In contrast to diuretics, which reduce preload and shift the circulatory state to the left along a given ventricular function curve, a positive inotropic agent shifts the entire curve upward and to the left toward the normal curve. Since contractility does not limit cardiac output in the normal circulation, digitalis would not be expected to change output in normal subjects. This is the case. As soon as the contractile state becomes limiting, however, digitalis increases cardiac output and lowers filling pressures of both the right and the left ventricles. Thus, cardiac glycosides are of clinical value in patients with congestive heart failure in the presence or absence of supraventricular tachyarrhythmias such as atrial fibrillation or atrial flutter. Although opinion is less uniform regarding patients in sinus rhythm, recent studies have documented benefit in the majority of patients who have dilated, failing ventricles with poor systolic function. These patients must be carefully distinguished from those with predominant diastolic dysfunction (noncompliant ventricles and elevated filling pressures but normal ejection fractions) who are unlikely to benefit. Thus, patients who are most likely to benefit are those having cardiomegaly with impaired systolic contraction, often accompanied by S_3 gallops. There is no convincing evidence of desensitization or tolerance to the cardiac effects of digitalis, and the positive inotropic effects are sustained over periods of months and years in patients with congestive heart failure.

To summarize, as pathologic processes such as ischemia, volume or pressure loads, or primary myocardial disease lead to reduced contractility, compensatory mechanisms emerge. Elevated end-diastolic pressure and volume augment ventricular performance through the Frank-Starling mechanism. Sympathetic tone tends to increase, thus enhancing contractile state, and the process of ventricular hypertrophy generates additional contractile elements. Each of these mechanisms, however, exacts a price. Excessive elevation of filling pressures results in pulmonary or peripheral edema. Excessive sympathetic tone results in tachycardia and, together with elevated renin-angiotensin system activity, in increased peripheral vascular resistance as well as increased myocardial oxygen consumption. With the progression of underlying cardiac disease, the compensatory mechanisms ultimately fail, or the consequences of these mechanisms become limiting (for example, with emergence of pulmonary edema). Administration of cardiac glycosides under these circumstances enhances myocardial contractility, decreasing the dependence of the circulation on compensatory mechanisms and providing improved cardiac reserve. Improved ventricular function yields a higher cardiac output at any given ventricular filling pressure. With the alternative therapeutic modalities now available, there is little virtue in giving cardiac glycosides to the brink of toxicity. Rather, conventional doses (see below) resulting in serum digoxin concentrations not exceeding 1.5 to 1.7 ng per milliliter appear to yield the best risk-benefit ratio.

PHARMACOKINETICS, BIOAVAILABILITY, AND DOSAGE CONSIDERATIONS. Summarized in Table 40–6 are the important pharmacokinetic variables and dosage ranges for cardiac glycosides in current clinical use. The values cited are averages, and individual variation is to be expected.

Digoxin. This is the most widely used preparation, particularly in hospitalized patients. Its virtues include flexibility of route of administration and intermediate duration of action. Digoxin is excreted exponentially (i.e., first-order kinetics) with a half-life of about 36 hours in young, healthy, normal subjects. In older patients with cardiac disease but without elevated BUN or serum creatinine levels, a half-life of 48 hours represents a more appropriate first approximation. Such patients excrete approximately one third of body stores daily, for the most part in unchanged form, although about 10 per cent of patients excrete substantial quantities of the inactive metabolite dihydrodigoxin, which arises through bacterial biotransformation in the gut lumen. The excretion of digoxin by the kidney is directly proportional to glomerular filtration rate (and hence creatinine clearance) and is relatively independent of the rate of urine flow in patients with intact renal function. Clearance may decrease somewhat in patients with prerenal azotemia. There is also evidence for some secretion of the drug at the renal tubular level.

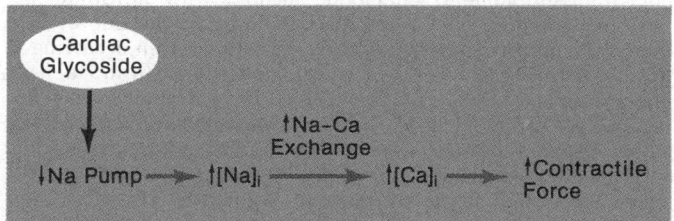

FIGURE 40–5. Schematic representation of the mechanism of inotropic action of cardiac glycosides. Binding of digitalis to NaK-ATPase inhibits this enzyme and hence the active outward transport of Na^+ across the myocardial cell membrane. Na^+ pump inhibition leads to increased intracellular Na^+ ($[Na]_i$) content and activity, which in turn alters Na-Ca exchange with consequent increase in Ca influx, decrease of Ca efflux, or both. The resulting increase in intracellular Ca ($[Ca]_i$) is presumed to mediate the observed increase in myocardial contractile force.

TABLE 40–6. PHARMACOLOGY OF CARDIAC GLYCOSIDES

Agent	Gastrointestinal Absorption	Onset of Action* (minutes)	Peak Effect (hours)	Average Half-Life†	Principal Metabolic Route (Excretory Pathway)	Average Digitalizing Dose		Usual Daily Oral Maintenance Dose‖
						Oral‡	Intravenous§	
Digoxin	55%–75%¶ (Lanoxicaps 90%–100%)	15–30	1½–5	36–48 hours	Renal; some gastrointestinal excretion	1.25–1.50 mg	0.75–1.00 mg	0.25–0.50 mg**
Digitoxin	90%–100%	25–120	4–12	4–6 days	Hepatic#; renal excretion of metabolites	0.70–1.20 mg	1.00 mg	0.10 mg

Modified from Smith TW: Drug therapy: Digitalis glycosides. N Engl J Med 288:719, 1973. By permission of the New England Journal of Medicine.

*For intravenous dose.
†For normal subjects (prolonged by renal impairment with digoxin and probably by severe hepatic disease with digitoxin).
‡Divided doses over 12 to 24 hours at intervals of 6 to 8 hours.
§Given in increments for initial subcomplete digitalization, to be supplemented by further small increments as necessary.
‖Average for adult patients without renal or hepatic impairment; varies widely among individual patients and requires close medical supervision.
¶For tablet form of administration (may be less in malabsorption syndromes and in formulations with poor bioavailability).
#Enterohepatic cycle exists.
**Approximately 20 per cent lower maintenance doses are required if gel solution in capsules (Lanoxicaps) is used. Maintenance dose must be reduced in patients with renal impairment (see text).

Therapy can be instituted in patients without urgent indications by starting the daily maintenance dose without a loading dose. This results in stable plateau concentrations of the drug in four to five excretory half-lives, or about 1 week. In patients with severe renal impairment, the half-life of the drug is prolonged to as much as 4 to 5 days, and steady-state levels are reached on a daily maintenance regimen only after 3 to 4 weeks.

Digoxin is extensively bound to tissues (large volume of distribution), and the drug is consequently not effectively removed from the body by hemodialysis. Lean body mass should be used for purposes of dosage calculation. Infants and children absorb and excrete digoxin much as do adults, although secretion at the renal tubular level may be somewhat more important in prepubertal patients.

An important interaction between digoxin and quinidine has been described, leading to a substantial increase in steady-state serum digoxin levels (averaging about twofold) when conventional quinidine doses are added to a maintenance digoxin regimen. Increases in the serum digoxin level are also observed when verapamil or amiodarone is given concurrently.

Bioavailability of digoxin in the standard tablet formulation is 55 to 75 per cent. The higher estimate is usually used in converting oral to intravenous doses. A preparation in which digoxin is dissolved in an encapsulated gel gives higher bioavailability, requiring a slight adjustment in the standard maintenance doses, as noted in Table 40–6. Previously marketed preparations with poor bioavailability properties are no longer available in the United States, thanks to action by regulatory agencies.

The maintenance digoxin dose required to replace daily losses varies from about 37 per cent of the body content in patients with normal renal function to 14 per cent in patients with essentially no renal function. The latter figure is an average, however, and some patients require substantially more or less than the maintenance dose that would be predicted by the 14 per cent figure. A useful approximation of daily per cent of loss of digoxin from the body is given by the following expression:

$$\text{Per cent daily loss} = 14 + \frac{C_{Cr} \text{ in ml/min}}{5}$$

Useful nomograms have been developed for loading and maintenance doses of digoxin, but it is important that these be used only as first approximations and that the patient be followed closely until a stable steady state is reached. Adjustments subsequently are required with changes in renal function, related either to intrinsic renal disease or to altered renal perfusion due to cardiac disease.

Digitoxin. This cardiac glycoside is the least polar and the most slowly excreted of the cardiac glycosides in current use. It is the principal constituent of the whole leaf of the digitalis plant. Gastrointestinal absorption of digitoxin is virtually complete. The drug binds avidly to serum albumin, and only about 3 per cent of the drug circulates in the free, pharmacologically active state at conventional doses and serum levels. It thus differs substantially from digoxin, which is only about 23 per cent bound to plasma proteins at usual doses. Because of the high degree of serum protein binding, renal clearance of digitoxin is minimal and the drug is metabolized to a variety of poorly defined derivatives, presumably in the liver. Some enterohepatic cycling occurs in the case of digitoxin but is not important for digoxin. The half-time for digitoxin excretion averages about 5 to 6 days and is not appreciably affected by altered renal function.

Standard pharmacology texts give details of pharmacokinetics of other glycosides such as deslanoside and ouabain, which are rarely if ever used clinically at present in the United States.

DIGITALIS USE IN CONGESTIVE HEART FAILURE. The therapeutic use of digitalis in patients with normal sinus rhythm is complicated by the lack of any easily measurable therapeutic endpoint, such as that provided by the ventricular rate in patients with atrial fibrillation. Digitalis is of value in patients with symptoms and signs of heart failure due to ischemic cardiomyopathy, valvular disease, hypertensive heart disease, many types of congenital heart disease, and dilated cardiomyopathies and in some patients with cor pulmonale and overt right ventricular failure. The drug is of no demonstrated benefit in isolated mitral stenosis with normal sinus rhythm unless right ventricular failure is present. Similarly, little benefit can be expected in patients with pericardial tamponade or constrictive pericarditis. The latter disease states are all characterized by mechanical limitations to cardiac function, rather than by impairment of myocardial contractility. In hypertrophic cardiomyopathy with an obstructive element, digitalis may in fact be deleterious if left ventricular contractility increases and produces greater outflow obstruction. As noted previously, patients with symptoms of dyspnea on exertion due to high diastolic filling pressure from decreased ventricular compliance, but with well-preserved ejection fractions, are unlikely to benefit from digitalis if sinus rhythm is present.

The prophylactic use of digitalis in patients with diminished cardiac reserve who are expected to undergo a major stress such as surgery remains controversial. Many clinicians prefer to withhold digitalis until a specific indication arises.

The use of digitalis in the management of supraventricular rhythm disturbances is considered in Ch. 42. The drug is potentially dangerous in patients with Wolff-Parkinson-White syndrome.

INDIVIDUAL SENSITIVITY TO DIGITALIS. Table 40–7 lists factors that influence the sensitivity of individual patients to digitalis. These are factors intrinsic to the patient, rather than factors that influence *apparent* sensitivity, such as alterations in drug bioavailability or in the excretion pattern of the drug.

Electrolyte and Acid-Base Disturbances. Potassium depletion increases the likelihood that patients will develop digitalis toxic-

TABLE 40–7. FACTORS INFLUENCING INDIVIDUAL SENSITIVITY TO DIGITALIS

Type and severity of underlying cardiac disease
Serum electrolyte derangement
    Hypokalemia or hyperkalemia
    Hypomagnesemia
    Hypercalcemia
    Hyponatremia
Acid-base imbalance
Concomitant drug administration
    Anesthetics
    Catecholamines and sympathomimetics
    Antiarrhythmic agents
Thyroid status
Renal function
Autonomic nervous system tone
Respiratory disease

ity. Hypokalemia has a primary arrhythmogenic effect of its own and also tends to increase cellular binding of digitalis glycosides. Potassium depletion must be guarded against carefully in patients on potassium-wasting diuretics. Magnesium depletion also predisposes to digitalis toxicity and is a common concomitant of diuretic therapy. Elevated serum calcium levels may enhance ventricular automaticity and may also predispose to digitalis toxicity.

Acid-base disturbances appear to exert their effects largely through shifts in serum potassium concentration, and the acid-base disturbances per se usually have little effect within the range commonly encountered clinically.

Drug Interactions. Several drugs, including cholestyramine, colestipol, and neomycin, decrease absorption of orally administered digoxin, as do nonabsorbable antacids and Kaopectate. Quinidine, verapamil, and amiodarone all increase steady-state serum digoxin levels.

Type and Severity of Underlying Heart Disease. The most important factor influencing individual digitalis sensitivity is the type and severity of underlying heart disease. Otherwise healthy subjects are remarkably tolerant of large doses of digitalis, and toxicity typically manifests itself as disturbances of atrioventricular conduction rather than life-threatening tachyarrhythmias. In patients with advanced heart failure or severe focal ischemia, however, the therapeutic ratio of digitalis is remarkably low, and these patients may experience potentially life-threatening toxicity at doses and serum levels no more than twice the optimal amount.

Digitalis and Ischemic Heart Disease. The effects of digitalis on myocardial oxygen consumption, and therefore its use in patients with ischemic heart disease, depend primarily on the prior state of the ventricle. In the normal-size ventricle, the enhanced contractile state may modestly increase oxygen consumption. If failure and ventricular dilation are present, however, digitalis administration tends to reduce cardiac dimensions and thereby reduces wall tension (Laplace's relation) such that myocardial oxygen consumption may not increase or may even be reduced. It is important, therefore, to assess carefully the state of ventricular function prior to instituting digitalis therapy in patients with ischemic disease.

The role of digitalis therapy in acute myocardial infarction is limited. Other measures are generally preferable in the management of mild congestive heart failure in this setting. When symptoms and signs of overt left ventricular failure persist despite optimal use of diuretics and vasodilators, digitalis may be added at about 75 per cent of the usual loading dose. The loading dose should be given over a period of 18 to 24 hours with close monitoring of cardiac rhythm. It is customary to use digoxin in the presence of atrial fibrillation, which is typically a manifestation of heart failure in patients with acute myocardial infarction.

Some evidence suggests that patients may experience excess mortality when maintained on digitalis long-term following acute myocardial infarction, but most studies indicate that the mortality trends are accounted for by baseline variables such as greater severity of heart failure, rather than a deleterious effect of conventional doses of digoxin.

Advanced Age. It is unlikely that advanced age per se has an independent adverse effect on digitalis tolerance, but the reduced renal and pulmonary functions that attend advanced age require appropriate consideration.

Renal Failure. Factors influencing digitalis absorption and elimination, as well as rapid shifts in electrolytes with hemodialysis, predispose to digitalis toxicity. It is wise to leave an extra margin of safety in digitalis doses in managing these patients.

Thyroid Disease. Hyperthyroidism tends to reduce the response of patients to digitalis, whereas hypothyroidism increases the likelihood of digitalis toxicity. The failure of a patient with atrial fibrillation to respond to standard doses of digoxin with appropriate slowing of the heart rate should raise the question of occult thyrotoxicosis.

Pulmonary Disease. It is generally agreed that patients with chronic pulmonary disease, and especially with acute respiratory insufficiency, experience an increased frequency of digitalis intoxication. This may be related both to the underlying lung disease and hypoxia and to the sympathomimetic drugs that these patients often receive. It should be assumed that patients with a variety of pulmonary diseases may be sensitive to the arrhythmogenic effects of conventional doses and serum levels of cardiac glycosides.

SERUM DIGITALIS CONCENTRATIONS. Assay of serum digoxin concentration is routinely performed in most clinical laboratories, usually with the radioimmunoassay technique. There is a relatively constant ratio of serum or plasma to myocardial digoxin concentration, and thus the clinical effect of digoxin is directly related to the serum level. Nevertheless, there is considerable overlap in serum levels between patients with and without evidence of toxicity. Thus, serum concentration data must always be interpreted in the overall clinical context. Mean serum digoxin concentrations in groups of patients without evidence of toxicity, and with an expected therapeutic effect, average 1.4 ng per milliliter. Doubling the digoxin dose in a patient on a steady-state regimen can be expected to double the serum concentration when a new steady state is reached.

Serum digitoxin concentrations average about 10-fold higher than those of digoxin because of the binding of digitoxin to serum proteins.

The upper limit of the "therapeutic" range for digoxin is usually taken as about 2.0 ng per milliliter, but patients with supraventricular tachyarrhythmias, including atrial fibrillation and atrial flutter, may require appreciably higher levels to gain adequate control of the ventricular response and may tolerate these higher levels with no evidence of toxicity. Conversely, unusually sensitive patients may experience toxicity at serum levels as low as 1.0 ng per milliliter. It is not necessary to monitor serum digoxin levels routinely in patients who are doing well on standard maintenance doses of the drug. Serum levels may be of use, however, in the assessment of unexpected responses to therapy, including lack of the expected therapeutic response (Is the patient taking the drug?) or in situations in which digitalis toxicity is suspected (for example, multifocal ventricular premature beats in a patient with overt congestive heart failure who is taking digoxin).

DIGITALIS TOXICITY. At the cellular level, exposure to excessive levels of cardiac glycosides causes increased automaticity and decreased conduction. These abnormalities are reflected in a broad array of rhythm disturbances that are often difficult to distinguish from those caused by underlying heart disease. Commonly encountered rhythm disturbances, in decreasing order of incidence, include ventricular ectopic rhythms, AV block, atrial arrhythmias, sinoatrial arrhythmias, AV dissociation, and accelerated AV junctional rhythms.

Sinus Node and Atrium. Slowing of the sinus rate in patients with congestive heart failure is largely mediated by improved cardiac function and withdrawal of elevated sympathetic tone. Sinus rate is not a very useful indicator of digitalis effect, since it tends to remain rapid in the presence of fever, infection, anemia, thyrotoxicosis, or a variety of other conditions that predispose to sinus tachycardia. At high toxic doses, digitalis can cause direct depression of sinus node automaticity, or more likely sinoatrial exit block, which produce bradyarrhythmias.

Atrioventricular Node. The effective refractory period of the atrioventricular (AV) node is prolonged by digitalis, chiefly through increased vagal activity. In addition, the conduction velocity through the AV junction is reduced. As digoxin doses are increased, first-degree block (PR interval > 0.20 second) may appear, followed by second-degree AV block of the Mobitz type I or Wenckebach variety (see Ch. 42). With still higher doses, complete AV dissociation and third-degree block can occur. A typical manifestation of digitalis toxicity in the presence of atrial fibrillation is AV dissociation, often accompanied by increased automaticity of pacemakers in the AV junction. This causes regularization of a previously irregular ventricular rate.

His-Purkinje System. Digitalis-induced increase in the automaticity of cells in the His-Purkinje system is a relatively common manifestation of digitalis excess and is responsible for rhythm disturbances, including ventricular premature beats, ventricular bigeminy, and ventricular tachycardia.

Clinical Manifestations of Digitalis Toxicity. Gastrointestinal Symptoms. Anorexia, nausea, and vomiting are common consequences of digitalis toxicity. Unfortunately, these are present prior to the onset of rhythm disturbances in only about 50 per cent of cases.

Neurologic Symptoms. Headache, fatigue, malaise, disorientation, confusion, delirium, and seizures can occur, and visual symptoms, including disturbances of color vision, are well known. In fact, the gastrointestinal symptoms actually arise from the effects of digitalis on the chemoreceptor trigger zone in the medulla rather than as a result of direct irritation of the gastrointestinal system.

Massive Cardiac Glycoside Overdose. Suicidal or accidental digitalis overdose can produce the entire array of typical cardiac arrhythmias, including refractory ventricular fibrillation. In addition, hyperkalemia is sometimes encountered owing to interference with sodium and potassium transport across cell membranes throughout the body. This must be taken into account in considering the use of potassium supplements in cases in which massive toxicity may occur.

Treatment of Digitalis Intoxication. The most important element of successful treatment is early recognition that a cardiac rhythm disturbance is due to digitalis toxicity. For many of the most common manifestations, such as occasional ventricular premature beats, first-degree AV block, or atrial fibrillation with a slow ventricular response, temporary withdrawal of the drug with electrocardiographic monitoring (if indicated) until the arrhythmia has disappeared constitutes adequate management. The maintenance dose should then be adjusted to prevent recurrence. Arrhythmias that impair cardiac function because of rates that are too rapid or too slow, or those that suggest the possibility of progression to more malignant arrhythmias, require more aggressive management. Ventricular tachycardia due to digitalis toxicity requires immediate vigorous treatment. Bradyarrhythmias, including sinus bradycardia, sinoatrial arrest, or exit block, and atrioventricular block of second or third degree can sometimes be treated effectively with atropine, 0.5 to 1.0 mg given intravenously. Pervenous electrical pacing should be instituted if atropine is not rapidly effective.

Potassium. Potassium repletion is useful in the treatment of ectopic tachyarrhythmias when hypokalemia is present or when the serum potassium level is in the low normal range. Potassium must be given with caution in other circumstances because of the risks of hyperkalemia, particularly in the presence of renal impairment or of conduction disturbances.

Lidocaine and Phenytoin. These are the most useful drugs in the treatment of ectopic rhythm disturbances caused by digitalis. They tend to have minimal adverse effect on sinoatrial or AV conduction. Lidocaine is given intravenously in 100-mg bolus doses every 3 to 5 minutes, followed by a maintenance intravenous infusion of 15 to 20 µg per kilogram of body weight per minute, as required to maintain control of the rhythm disturbance and to avoid neurologic signs and symptoms. Phenytoin* is given in a dose of 100 mg by slow intravenous infusion, repeated every 5 minutes until onset of toxicity or control of the arrhythmia, followed by an oral maintenance dose of 400 to 600 mg per day if control of the rhythm disturbance is achieved.

---

*This use is not listed in the manufacturer's directive.

Beta-Adrenergic Blocking Drugs. Beta blockade has been useful in the treatment of some arrhythmias caused by digitalis excess but tends to decrease conduction as well as myocardial contractility and therefore is not widely used in this setting.

Quinidine and Procainamide. These drugs carry a risk of depression of sinoatrial and atrioventricular node function and can also depress myocardial contractility. Other agents are usually preferable for use in digitalis toxicity.

Direct Current (DC) Countershock (also see Ch. 42). This is generally inadvisable in the presence of digitalis intoxication because it may evoke severe arrhythmias in this setting. However, it must occasionally be used when other methods have been ineffective in the presence of a life-threatening arrhythmia. Risk is decreased when lower energy levels are employed, and careful titration is essential. Cardioversion is generally a benign procedure in patients without digitalis-induced rhythm disturbances.

Steroid-Binding Resins, Hemodialysis, and Hemoperfusion. These techniques have not been demonstrated to be effective in the management of advanced digitalis intoxication and are not recommended. Hemodialysis may be of value in controlling the serum potassium level in patients with refractory hyperkalemia.

Digoxin-Specific Antibodies. Purified Fab fragments of digoxin-specific antibodies are available for treatment of advanced digitalis toxicity of sufficient severity to be potentially life threatening. More than 2000 patients have now been treated, with a high degree of efficacy and with adverse side effects largely limited to those expected from withdrawal of digitalis effects. This approach is recommended for patients in whom conventional measures are not rapidly effective.

Vasodilators

Cardiac loading has a strong dependence on the resistance and capacitance properties of the peripheral vascular bed. Thus, vasodilator therapy in heart failure is designed to reduce the preload or afterload, or both, of a failing ventricle by relaxing vascular smooth muscle in the periphery. Vasodilators have been shown to improve survival in patients with continuing symptoms of heart failure who are taking digitalis and diuretics.

PRINCIPLES OF VASODILATOR THERAPY. As summarized in Figure 40–2, the normal ventricle is able to respond to increased afterload with an increase in the force of contraction such that there is little, if any, change in stroke volume until extreme elevations in afterload are encountered. As the ventricle fails, the relationship between afterload and stroke volume shifts downward and to the left so that a relatively modest change in outflow resistance causes a substantial alteration in stroke volume. This constitutes both a pathophysiologic problem and a therapeutic opportunity. The opportunity follows from the uniform increase in peripheral vascular resistance observed in untreated patients with decompensated congestive heart failure. Activation of the sympathetic nervous system and of the renin-angiotensin system accounts for most of the increase in peripheral resistance. These responses of the peripheral vascular system to a perceived decrease in cardiac output have survival value under conditions of hemorrhage or dehydration by redirecting the cardiac output to essential beds, including the brain and coronary circulation. Since congestive heart failure was presumably not an evolutionary pressure, it is not surprising that these primitive mechanisms for the defense of blood flow to vital organs prove maladaptive in the patient with chronic congestive heart failure.

As illustrated in Figure 40–1, the failing heart responds to a reduction in afterload by shifting its ventricular function curve toward normal, although the inotropic state remains unchanged. An attractive feature of afterload reduction is the ability to increase cardiac output without increasing preload or myocardial oxygen consumption.

VASODILATOR AGENTS. In the following discussion, primary consideration is given to vasodilator therapy for left ventricular failure, although the failing right ventricle also benefits from reduced pulmonary vascular resistance. The most potent afterload-reducing agent in the pulmonary circulation is oxygen; there is, as yet, no drug that reliably exerts a preferential afterload-reducing effect in the pulmonary circulation.

The action of vasodilator drugs is described in terms of effects on the venous bed (preload) or the arteriolar bed (afterload). Table 40–8 summarizes data on the vasodilators in current clinical use in the management of heart failure.

Venous Dilators. These reduce the vascular smooth muscle tone in the systemic venous bed, increasing its capacitance and shifting blood volume from the arterial to the venous side of the circulation. Thus, patients with pulmonary vascular congestion and edema due to high left heart filling pressures obtain symptomatic relief, limited only by the necessity to maintain a level of preload that results in an adequate forward cardiac output. The most selective agents for this purpose are the nitrates, including nitroglycerin and the longer-acting orally administered compounds such as isosorbide dinitrate. Many investigators believe that much or most of the clinical benefit of vasodilator use derives from the venous dilator component. In chronic congestive heart failure, administration of agents that preferentially dilate the arteriolar bed without a preload-reducing component, such as minoxidil and hydralazine, fails to show sustained benefit.

Arteriolar Dilators. These reduce left ventricular afterload and tend to redistribute blood flow among organ beds in ways that are, unfortunately, not always predictable. The improvement in blood flow to exercising skeletal muscle is relatively limited. Nevertheless, the forward stroke output of the left ventricle is delivered with a lower wall tension, such that myocardial oxygen consumption is favorably affected. The most selective agent routinely used in obtaining an afterload-reducing effect is hydralazine.

Balanced Vasodilators. The balanced vasodilators exert an effect on both preload and afterload through a generalized relaxing effect on vascular smooth muscle. The prototype short-acting agent of this kind is nitroprusside. This agent has found widespread application in the management of acute heart failure states, including acute pulmonary edema. Used with care, it can also improve the circulatory state of patients with combined hypotension and low forward output, provided that adequate arterial pressure can be maintained by the use of volume loading or inotropic drugs or both. The tendency of nitroprusside to reduce systemic arterial pressure is offset to a considerable extent by the increased stroke output. The unloading effect of nitroprusside is most helpful when the left ventricular filling pressures are maintained in the vicinity of 15 mm Hg, which may require administration of intravenous fluids. An important advantage of nitroprusside in intensive care unit settings is its short duration of action, permitting minute-to-minute titration of the circulatory state.

A regimen yielding a balanced vasodilator effect is hydralazine and nitrates, the latter often given as the long-acting oral preparation isosorbide dinitrate. In an important multicenter study (Cohn, 1986), the protocol randomly assigned patients taking digitalis and diuretics to hydralazine with isosorbide dinitrate, to prazosin, or to placebo. The group treated with hydralazine and nitrates showed a 38 per cent mean reduction in mortality during the initial year of treatment, and the improved survival was sustained to the 3-year point. The prazosin-treated group showed no significant difference from the placebo group. An analogous, albeit smaller, study in Scandinavia in class IV patients demonstrated a similar improvement in survival in patients on diuretics and digoxin randomized to receive in addition the ACE inhibitor enalapril. The hydralazine-nitrate combination is now being compared to enalapril in a multicenter randomized trial (VHeFT-II) with survival as the primary endpoint.

The ACE inhibitors captopril and enalapril are available as balanced vasodilators for the management of patients with heart failure. Multicenter trials have demonstrated sustained improvement in symptoms and exercise tolerance, and large-scale therapeutic trials with survival endpoints are currently in progress in several subsets of patients. Many clinicians find that captopril and enalapril provide a relatively simple and controllable approach to vasodilator therapy, and hence constitute vasodilators of choice in many centers. Special caution and the use of very small initial doses of these drugs, which can produce severe hypotension and renal failure, are required. An irritating, persistent dry cough is a class effect of ACE inhibitor drugs that occurs in up to 10 per cent of patients.

Not all patients who appear to be reasonable candidates for vasodilator use in advanced heart failure can tolerate the drugs initially, and not all of the group that initially tolerates the regimen still show demonstrable benefit at the end of 3 months. Although results can be optimized by careful selection of patients and judicious use of available agents, the fact remains that some patients with advanced heart failure are unable to tolerate vasodilators, chiefly because of postural hypotension.

Combined Drug Therapy

Although patients with mild heart failure (early class II symptoms) can often be managed with a single class of drugs, accumulating evidence indicates that combination therapy with all

TABLE 40–8. MAJOR VASODILATOR DRUGS*

Drug	Mechanism of Action	Venous Dilating Effect (Preload Reduction)	Arteriolar Dilating Effect (Afterload Reduction)	Usual Dosage	Comments
Nitroglycerin	Direct	+ + +	+	10–100 μg/min, IV 5–20 mg, transdermal 0.4 mg, s.l.	Tolerance may be a problem with sustained continuous use. May be used sublingually to control acute increases in left atrial pressure.
Isosorbide dinitrate	Direct	+ + +	+	5–20 mg q. 2 hr, s.l. 10–60 mg q. 4 hr, p.o.	Improved survival shown in chronic CHF when used with hydralazine.
Nitroprusside	Direct	+ + +	+ + +	5–150 μg/kg/min IV; usual dose, 50–75 μg/kg/min	Used IV only. Drug is light sensitive. Hazard of thiocyanate or cyanide toxicity with prolonged high doses.
Hydralazine	Direct	0	+ + +	10–75 mg q. 6 hr p.o.	Sustained benefit in heart failure not shown when used as sole vasodilator.
Prazosin†	Alpha-adrenergic blockade (alpha₁ selective)	+ + +	+ +	1–5 mg q. 6 hr p.o.	Extra caution required with initial doses. Tolerance requires dosage adjustments and complicates use in heart failure.
Captopril	Angiotensin converting enzyme (ACE) inhibitor	+ + +	+ +	6.25–25.0 mg q. 6–8 hr, p.o.	Approved by F.D.A. for use in chronic CHF. Acute renal failure can occur with initial doses; initiate use with extra caution.
Enalapril	ACE inhibitor	+ + +	+ +	2.5–10 mg q. 12 hr p.o.	Approved by F.D.A. for use in chronic CHF. Acute renal failure can occur with initial doses; initiate use with extra caution. Avoid potassium-sparing diuretics.

*All of these agents may cause severe hypotension, and special caution is required with initial use, particularly in patients with severe congestive heart failure. Heart rate changes with all agents listed are usually minor unless a hypotensive response elicits reflex tachycardia; prazosin can cause bradycardia with initial use. Calcium channel blocking drugs (verapamil, diltiazem, and dihydropyridines including nifedipine) are effective vasodilators but are not recommended for management of heart failure with systolic dysfunction because of their potential negative inotropic effects on the heart.

†Prazosin was not found to improve survival compared to placebo when added to diuretics and digoxin in patients with class II and III chronic heart failure (Cohn, 1986).
CHF = congestive heart failure; F.D.A. = Food and Drug Administration.

three major classes of drugs tends to keep heart size and wall stress as well as symptoms at a minimum while allowing the patient maximal effort tolerance within the limits imposed by the underlying cardiac problem. Implicit in the scheme outlined in Table 40–4 is the working hypothesis that in patients with compromised contractile function, combination therapy with a diuretic, vasodilator, and digitalis yields optimal benefit while allowing each drug to be used at a dose level as far as possible from its toxicity threshold. There is substantial evidence documenting the additive beneficial hemodynamic effects of a vasodilator and a positively inotropic drug such as digoxin, as well as additive effects of combined use of digoxin and an ACE inhibitor on exercise tolerance. The experienced clinician usually elects to add these classes of agents to the regimen one at a time to permit assessment of the incremental response at each step, but in most cases evaluates the response to combined treatment with all three classes in patients who remain symptomatic at levels of activity they wish to maintain.

Treatment of Diastolic Ventricular Dysfunction

The elements of therapy in patients with predominant diastolic dysfunction differ in certain important ways from those in patients with "classic" congestive heart failure accompanying a dilated ventricle with impaired systolic function. Pulmonary congestion is appropriately treated in both subsets of patients with diuretics and other means of preload reduction, including venodilators. Nitroglycerin taken sublingually can be used effectively by patients to forestall or slow the progression of episodes of elevated left ventricular filling pressures that might otherwise progress to frank pulmonary edema. It is important to avoid excessive preload reduction in the predominant diastolic dysfunction patient, however, in order to avoid symptoms and signs of low cardiac output. Anti-ischemic and antihypertensive treatment should be pursued aggressively when these disorders and their attendant pathophysiology underlie diastolic ventricular dysfunction, with removal of ischemia and regression of hypertrophy as the goals of therapy. Atrial augmentation of ventricular systole is particularly important in these patients, and every effort should be made to maintain or restore normal sinus rhythm or pacemaker-induced AV synchrony. Calcium channel blocking drugs may be of benefit in some patients with predominant diastolic dysfunction but are generally to be avoided in the presence of severe systolic dysfunction because of their potential negative inotropic effects. Finally, positively inotropic agents such as digoxin have no established role in the management of patients with predominant diastolic dysfunction and are contraindicated in patients with hypertrophic cardiomyopathy and dynamic outflow tract obstruction.

Refractory Heart Failure

Therapeutic advances have left in their wake a subset of patients with marked impairment of ventricular function (often with left ventricular ejection fractions in the 10 to 20 per cent range) who survive but are severely symptomatic on maximal tolerated doses of diuretics, digitalis, and vasodilators. Those who meet additional relevant criteria (including preserved function of other organ systems, no elevation of pulmonary vascular resistance, no active infection) may be referred for consideration of heart transplantation after detailed explanation of the potential risks and benefits of this procedure. This procedure now has relatively widespread application since the advent of cyclosporine for immunosuppression, and more than 150 centers in the United States now have active programs. Survival exceeds 60 per cent in transplanted patients at 5 years in larger series, compared with an expected mortality well in excess of 50 per cent at 12 months in patients treated by conventional means, and functional recovery is often gratifying. Expectations must be tempered by the very limited availability of donor hearts, however, which has recently plateaued in the 1500 to 2000 per year range in the United States.

Treatment of acute decompensation using intravenous β-adrenergic or dopaminergic agonists, or the phosphodiesterase inhibitor amrinone, is covered in Ch. 41. Longer-term use of orally active β-adrenergic agonist drugs has proved disappointing, in part because of rapid development of tolerance, and cannot be recommended. Several phosphodiesterase inhibitor drugs are under continuing clinical study, including amrinone, milrinone,* and enoximone.* These agents have both vasodilator and positive inotropic properties related to enhancement of cyclic adenosine monophosphate levels in vascular smooth muscle and myocardium. Although symptoms appear to be improved in some patients treated chronically with these investigational agents, statistically compelling evidence of sustained efficacy or improved survival is lacking. The artificial heart has been developed sufficiently for placement in several patients, but results to date have been disappointing because of unsolved thromboembolic problems, and mechanical assist devices are in current investigational use mainly to provide a bridge to heart transplantation in potentially suitable candidates.

---

*Investigational drug.

ACKNOWLEDGMENT: Ralph A. Kelly, M.D., has made major contributions to the coverage of diuretics, including Figure 40–4.

Berger BE, Warnock DG: Clinical uses and mechanisms of action of diuretic agents. *In* Brenner BM, Rector FC (eds.): The Kidney. Philadelphia, W. B. Saunders Company, 1986, pp 433–455. *A compact summary of clinically relevant information as stated in the title.*

Captopril Multicenter Research Group: A placebo-controlled trial of captopril in refractory congestive heart failure. J Am Coll Cardiol 2:755, 1983. *A well-designed controlled trial demonstrating improved clinical state and effort tolerance among 92 patients with heart failure refractory to digitalis and diuretics randomized to additional treatment with placebo or the ACE inhibitor captopril, which was subsequently approved by the United States Food and Drug Administration for the indication of congestive heart failure. Results are typical of a number of similar clinical trials with ACE inhibitors.*

Cohn JN, et al.: Effect of vasodilator therapy on mortality in chronic congestive heart failure: Results of a VA cooperative study. N Engl J Med 314:1547, 1986.

CONSENSUS Trial Study Group: Effects of enalapril on mortality in severe congestive heart failure. Results of the Cooperative North Scandinavian Enalapril Survival Study. N Engl J Med 316:1429–1435, 1987. *The above two studies establish the role of balanced vasodilator therapy in improving survival when added to diuretics and digoxin (which were continued) in patients with chronic congestive heart failure. At a mean follow-up of 2.3 years, the study of Cohn et al showed improved survival (risk reduction of 34 per cent) among patients treated with hydralazine and nitrates. Mortality in the prazosin-treated group was indistinguishable from that in the group receiving placebo. Overall mortality, as expected, was high (36 to 47 per cent at 3 years) and was higher still in the CONSENSUS trial, which enrolled class IV heart failure patients. Mortality was reduced by 31 per cent at 1 year by addition of enalapril to the regimen in the CONSENSUS trial.*

Packer M (ed.): Physiologic determinants of survival in congestive heart failure. Circulation 75:IV-1–IV-111, 1987. *This supplement to Circulation contains 14 papers reviewing the various factors influencing prognosis in heart failure and current aspects of vasodilator, inotropic, and antiarrhythmic therapy and their potential impact on survival.*

Pouleur H (ed.): Diastolic function in heart failure: Clinical approaches to its understanding and treatment. Circulation 81:III-1–III-158, 1990. *This supplement to Circulation contains 21 papers covering virtually all clinically relevant aspects of diastolic dysfunction, including pathophysiology, role in heart failure, and therapeutic implications.*

Smith TW (ed.): Digitalis Glycosides. Orlando, Fla., Grune & Stratton, 1986. *This 348-page book summarizes available information on all aspects of the basic and clinical pharmacology, clinical use, and toxicity problems related to the cardiac glycosides.*

Smith TW, Braunwald E, Kelly RA: The management of heart failure. *In* Braunwald E (ed.): Heart Diseases. 4th ed. Philadelphia, W. B. Saunders Company, 1991. *A detailed consideration of general and specific aspects of congestive heart failure management with more than 500 references.*

---

41 Shock

David W. Ferguson

Shock—a rude unhinging of the machinery of life.
SAMUEL GROSS, 1972

Rather than a specific disease, shock is a complex clinical syndrome, the successful treatment of which requires vigilant medical attention, precise hemodynamic monitoring, and a thorough understanding of the basic principles of circulatory physiology and the pharmacology of cardiac and vasoactive medications. This chapter reviews the basic principles of circulatory control as they relate to the shock syndrome, the systemic and cellular mechanisms involved in the pathogenesis of the shock state, the differential diagnosis of shock, and the clinical characteristics of specific shock syndromes and provides general and specific recommendations pertaining to current therapy of this disorder.

DEFINITION. The term "shock" (Fr. *choc*), first used by the French physician LeDran in 1773 to describe the clinical characteristics of patients after severe gunshot trauma, is a nonspecific term now used to describe complex pathophysiologic syndrome(s) arising from any of a multitude of etiologies. Common to all of these syndromes of shock is a failure of the circulatory system to maintain cellular perfusion and function. Shock usually results from a critical impairment of blood flow to vital organs and tissues and/or the inability of those tissues to utilize essential nutrients. The common denominator in all forms of shock is microcirculatory insufficiency, which may arise from a wide variety of causes. Nevertheless, the end result of irreversible shock is cellular membrane dysfunction, abnormal cellular metabolism, and eventually cellular death. Shock is inferred from clinical evidence of major organ hypoperfusion in the setting of hemodynamic instability usually associated with relative or absolute hypotension. An understanding of the pathophysiology and treatment of shock requires a firm foundation in normal circulatory control mechanisms.

MECHANISMS OF CIRCULATORY CONTROL— NORMAL AND DURING SHOCK

The basic underlying abnormality in all forms of shock is a state of disordered cellular metabolic support. Shock of any etiology is associated with reduced or insufficient cellular oxygen consumption. Since all cellular functions depend upon adequate tissue perfusion, an understanding of the pathophysiology of shock requires an understanding of the normal determinants of tissue perfusion.

Major Determinants of Tissue Perfusion

The basic functions of the circulation are the delivery of oxygen and essential nutrients to peripheral tissues and the removal of metabolic wastes from those tissues. In most cases of shock, there is either insufficient delivery or inappropriate distribution of oxygen and nutrients. These disorders account to a large extent for the impairment of tissue metabolic consumption that characterizes the shock syndrome.

The major determinants of normal tissue perfusion are listed in Table 41–1. Perfusion of peripheral tissues depends upon cardiac, vascular, and microcirculatory factors. Perfusion of any organ depends upon systemic arterial pressure (the driving force for blood flow through the organs), the resistance offered by the vasculature of that organ, and the patency of nutritional capillaries within the organ.

Systemic arterial pressure is determined by cardiac output and the resistance of the total vascular tree:

$$\text{Arterial Pressure} = \text{Cardiac Output} \times \text{Total Vascular Resistance}$$

Vascular resistance is predominantly a function of the radius or caliber of blood vessels, which is influenced by neurogenic, humoral, and myogenic factors that regulate the tone of vascular smooth muscle. Thus, blood flow to any one organ depends on cardiac function, vascular muscle tone, and the caliber of resistance beds both in the systemic arterial tree and within the organ itself. The determinant of exchange of substrates and metabolites within the tissue is the microcirculation. A patent nutritional capillary network is the critical interface between the circulation and the cell. The following discussion reviews the critical cardiac, vascular, and microcirculatory determinants of tissue perfusion which are important in understanding the pathophysiology and treatment of shock.

CARDIAC FACTORS. Cardiac Output. Cardiac output is the product of heart rate and stroke volume. When averaged over time, the cardiac output of the right ventricle equals that of the left ventricle.

$$\text{Cardiac Output} = \text{Heart Rate} \times \text{Stroke Volume}$$

In normal resting adults, a heart rate of 70 beats per minute and a stroke volume of 70 to 75 ml per beat produce a cardiac output

TABLE 41–1. MAJOR HEMODYNAMIC DETERMINANTS OF TISSUE PERFUSION

I. **Systemic arterial pressure**
  A. Total vascular resistance
    1. Total arteriolar resistance, vascular muscle tone
      a. Tissue metabolites
      b. Neurohumoral factors
      c. Toxins
    2. Blood viscosity
  B. Cardiac output
    1. Heart rate: Bradyarrhythmias and tachyarrhythmias
    2. Stroke volume
      a. Preload (cardiac filling pressure and volume)
        1) Total circulating blood volume
          a) External loss
          b) Internal loss or sequestration
          c) Red blood cell mass
          d) Capillary hydrostatic pressure
          e) Capillary permeability
          f) Oncotic pressure
        2) Distribution of blood volume
          a) Body position (gravity)
          b) Intrapericardial pressure
          c) Intrathoracic pressure
          d) Venous tone
          e) Skeletal muscle pump
        3) Atrial contraction
          a) Contractile state
          b) Timing (AV synchrony)
        4) Diastolic filling time (heart rate)
      b. Inotropic state
        1) Total functioning ventricular muscle mass
        2) Intrinsic (myocardial) control mechanisms
          a) Adrenergic receptors
          b) Excitation-contraction coupling
        3) Extrinsic (noncardiac) neurocirculatory control mechanisms
          a) Circulating catecholamines
          b) Autonomic nervous system
          c) Myocardial depression
        4) Myocardial perfusion (oxygen supply)
          a) Aortic diastolic pressure
          b) Fixed and nonfixed coronary obstructions
          c) Metabolic coronary vasodilation
          d) Neurogenic control mechanisms
        5) Myocardial oxygen demand
          a) Heart rate
          b) Cardiac size
          c) Afterload
          d) Contractility
          e) Pharmacologic agents
        6) Physiologic depressants
          a) Acidosis
          b) Hypoxemia
          c) Alkalosis (severe)
        7) Pharmacologic depressants
        8) Humoral agents
          a) Catecholamines
          b) Myocardial depressant factors
      c. Afterload
        1) Aortic diastolic pressure
          a) Systemic vascular resistance
          b) Arterial viscoelasticity
          c) Aortic root blood volume
        2) Ventricular size (law of Laplace)
        3) Impedance
II. **Organ vascular resistance**
  A. Occlusive vascular disease
  B. Local arteriolar and venular resistance
    1) Neurogenic factors
    2) Humoral factors
    3) Local autoregulation
  C. Blood viscosity
III. **Nutritional microcirculatory patency**
  A. Precapillary sphincter tone
  B. Postcapillary venular tone
  C. Intracapillary aggregation of blood components
  D. Capillary endothelial integrity

of approximately 5 liters per minute. A decrease in cardiac output to less than 2 liters per minute per square meter of body surface area (cardiac index) may result in severe shock, particularly if imposed over a short time interval.

Heart Rate. Normal individuals tolerate a wide range of heart rates, from approximately 30 to 180 beats per minute, assuming underlying normal cardiac function. An increase in heart rate is one of the earliest physiologic responses to a fall in arterial pressure and is modulated by the autonomic nervous system. Physiologic ranges of tachycardia usually increase cardiac output, but marked increases in heart rate may limit cardiac diastolic filling time and thereby result in a low cardiac output and a fall in arterial blood pressure. The tolerable limits for heart rate decrease with underlying cardiovascular impairment. For example, ventricular tachycardia or rapid atrial fibrillation in a patient with recent myocardial infarction produces a reduction in cardiac output and arterial pressure that, if uncorrected, may result in cardiogenic shock. Immediate treatment to restore normal cardiac rate and rhythm is essential in such a patient.

However, management of the patient in shock who is noted to be tachycardic requires an appreciation of the differential diagnosis of the tachycardia. In the setting of sinus tachycardia, the clinician needs to realize that a "compensatory tachycardia" is often seen in patients with fever, anemia, sepsis, hemorrhage, or severe hypovolemia. In these settings, sinus tachycardia is an appropriate reflex circulatory adjustment to maintain cardiac output. It would therefore be deleterious to attempt to treat the tachycardia alone (e.g., with β-adrenergic or calcium channel blocking agents) without determining the underlying etiology of the tachycardia (e.g., hypovolemia) and correcting the primary defect rather than its physiologic compensatory response.

Marked bradycardia may also cause a reduction in cardiac output and result in hypotension. In many situations, bradycardia is vagally mediated and responds to anticholinergic maneuvers (e.g., atropine). Many commonly utilized medications (e.g., β-adrenergic and calcium channel blockers) may aggravate bradycardia in patients with acute circulatory insults or may attenuate normal sympathetically mediated tachycardic responses. Sinus bradycardia and atrioventricular (AV) block are often seen immediately following myocardial infarction and should be reversed if they contribute to hypotension.

Stroke Volume. Stroke volume is the amount of blood ejected by the ventricle with each cardiac contraction and is determined by cardiac preload, inotropic state, and afterload. A decrease in stroke volume may be caused by (1) a decrease in cardiac filling (preload), (2) a decrease in myocardial contractility (inotropic state), or (3) an increase in cardiac afterload (Figs. 41–1 and 41–2).

Preload is defined as the stretch or tension on an individual sarcomere just prior to the onset of fiber shortening. Clinically, preload refers to the volume of blood filling the ventricle at the end of diastole (presystole). Ventricular preload regulates the subsequent force of cardiac contraction as described by Starling's law of the heart. Preload is often assessed clinically as ventricular

filling pressure rather than volume. The clinician must remember that it is the *compliance* (distensibility) of the ventricle that determines the relationship between pressure and volume:

Compliance = Change in Volume / Change in Pressure

Thus, the "optimal" preload (as assessed by filling pressure) for an individual patient may vary significantly with alterations in the compliance of the ventricle.

The most important determinant of cardiac preload is the total circulating blood volume. A reduction in blood volume may be either absolute or relative to the capacity of the vascular tree. Absolute reduction in blood volume is apparent when blood or fluids are lost, causing a hypovolemic state leading to hypovolemic shock, as seen in such clinical disorders as hemorrhage (internal or external), excessive vomiting, diarrhea, burns, renal loss of fluid (diabetes mellitus or diabetes insipidus), excessive diuresis, and excessive perspiration without fluid replacement. Internal losses of fluid occur with disorders such as peritonitis, pancreatitis, intestinal obstruction with extravasation of fluid, splanchnic ischemia with bowel necrosis and gangrene, fractures with extensive muscle trauma, hemothorax, and hemoperitoneum.

However, total blood volume must be not only adequate but also appropriately distributed for preload to be sufficient to maintain stroke volume. The chief determinants of the distribution of preload include body position (gravity), venous tone, intrathoracic and intrapericardial pressure, and the skeletal muscle pump. Compression of the heart may prevent its filling, as in pericardial tamponade or tension pneumothorax. Mechanical obstruction to blood flow may cause hypotension and shock in patients with atrial myxoma, a ball-valve thrombus, or pulmonary embolism. Positive-pressure ventilation may also decrease venous return and cardiac filling. Relative decreases in blood volume occur when there is loss of vascular tone because of the administration of anesthetics or ganglionic blockers, after spinal cord injury or surgery, and in patients with neuropathy or autonomic insufficiency. Pooling of blood thus results in a decrease in cardiac filling pressure.

Another important determinant of ventricular preload is atrial contraction and the rate of diastolic filling of the ventricle. Although atrial contraction in a normal heart may determine only 5 to 10 per cent of the subsequent ventricular stroke volume, in a diseased heart the contribution of atrial contraction to the subsequent ventricular stroke volume may be as great as 40 to 50 per cent. This is the primary reason that patients with hypertrophic cardiomyopathy, critical aortic stenosis, or acute myocardial infarction undergo rapid hemodynamic decompensation with the onset of atrial fibrillation and loss of an organized atrial component to ventricular preload.

Inotropic state refers physiologically to the magnitude and rate of myocardial fiber contraction under a given set of loading conditions. From the clinical standpoint, inotropic state refers to the contractile strength of the heart and is determined by a number of factors. These include the total mass of functioning

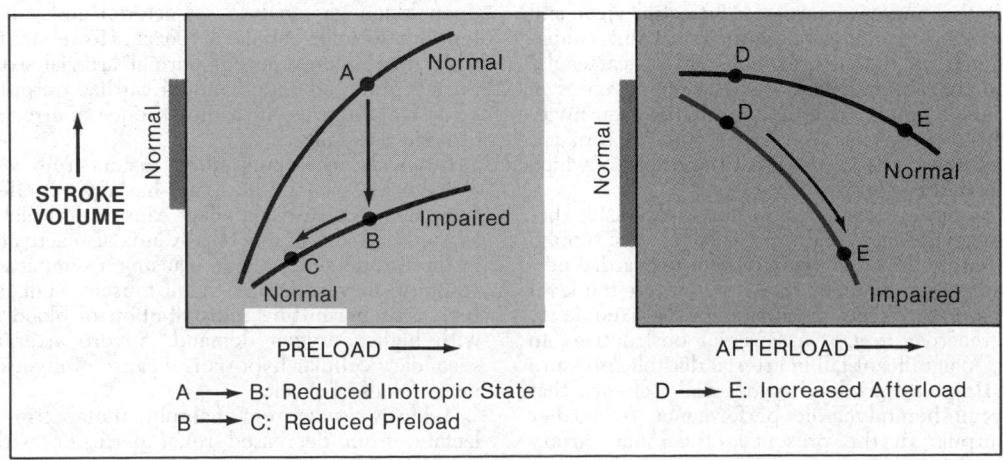

FIGURE 41–1. Effects on stroke volume of alterations in preload, afterload, and contractility.

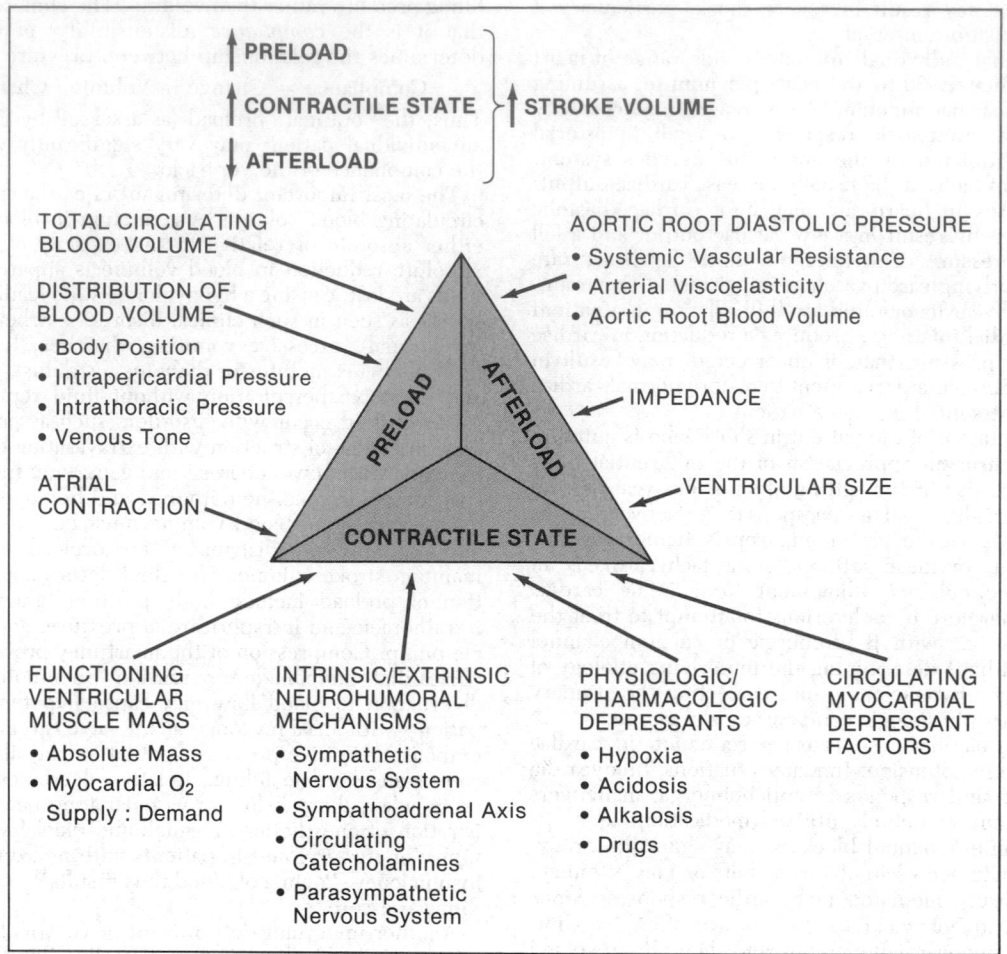

FIGURE 41–2. Determinants of stroke volume.

ventricular muscle, myocardial perfusion, intrinsic and extrinsic neurocirculatory control mechanisms, and the presence or absence of physiologic and pharmacologic stimulants or depressants. In addition, certain shock states may be associated with circulating "myocardial depressant factors" that impair cardiac performance.

Detailed autopsy studies in patients dying of cardiogenic shock following myocardial infarction have demonstrated that loss of greater than 30 to 35 per cent of functioning left ventricular muscle mass results in marked impairment of cardiac inotropic performance to a degree that is usually incompatible with maintenance of an effective cardiac output.

An important determinant of cardiac contractile performance is the sympathetic nervous system via activation of β-adrenoreceptors in the heart that increase cardiac contractile vigor and heart rate. These effects are mediated both by efferent sympathetic nerves impinging on the myocardium and by catecholamines released from the adrenal medulla. The effectiveness of such cardiac stimulants depends upon the number and sensitivity of cardiac β-adrenergic receptors. These receptors in turn are modified by various disease states, the most important of which is underlying chronic heart failure.

Myocardial performance depends upon the relationship between myocardial oxygen demand and myocardial oxygen supply. Myocardial oxygen supply depends primarily on myocardial perfusion, which is determined to a significant extent by the level of arterial diastolic pressure and the presence of fixed (e.g., atherosclerotic) or reactive (e.g., vasospastic) obstructions to coronary blood flow. A significant fall in arterial diastolic pressure (e.g., to <60 mm Hg) may produce myocardial ischemia that further impairs overall hemodynamic performance by further reducing cardiac output. In the presence of coronary artery disease, resistance to flow is due largely to structural changes in

the coronary vessel wall, and maximal vasodilation tends to occur distal to the site of coronary stenosis because of excessive accumulation of vasodilator metabolites. In this setting, arterial pressure becomes the determinant of perfusion to the ischemic segment through collateral vessels or across a coronary narrowing.

Among the pathophysiologic depressants common in shock are *hypoxia* and *acidosis*. Tissue hypoxia is a cellular diagnosis that is clinically inferred by evidence of organ dysfunction in the setting of cardiovascular abnormalities known to be associated with impairment of tissue perfusion. Hypoxemia, on the other hand, is a laboratory diagnosis based upon an arterial blood gas determination of reduced oxygen tension (P_{O_2}) and/or increased alveolar-arterial oxygen tension gradient. The clinician often relies upon blood gas analyses of arterial and mixed venous oxygen tensions to infer cellular hypoxia. However, tissue hypoxia may occur in the presence of normal arterial oxygen tension (e.g., during profound reductions of cardiac output), and cellular hypoxia may be present in the absence of arterial hypoxemia (e.g., cyanide poisoning).

In shock, hypoxemia often results from ventilation-perfusion abnormalities in the lung and has several effects on the circulation. A direct vascular effect causes vasodilation in organs such as the heart and brain. Hypoxemia also activates chemoreceptors in the carotid sinus region, causing a sympathetic vasoconstrictor response in vessels of skeletal muscle, skin, and the splanchnic bed, thus permitting redistribution of blood to the vital organs with higher oxygen demand. Severe arterial hypoxemia with secondary cellular hypoxia is a cause of myocardial depression in many forms of shock.

Acidosis results from anaerobic metabolism with the release of lactate, from decreased renal perfusion with accumulation of organic acids, and from hypoventilation with secondary respiratory acidosis. Acidosis reduces myocardial contractility and the vasoconstrictor response to various endogenous and exogenous neurohumoral agents.

Finally, a number of pharmacologic agents utilized in the treatment of critically ill patients have direct or indirect depressant effects on the myocardium and should be avoided if at all possible. These include sedative hypnotic agents, anesthetic agents, antiarrhythmic agents, β-adrenergic blocking agents, and calcium channel antagonists.

Afterload is best understood as the sum of forces that the ventricle must overcome in order to eject blood. Afterload is determined primarily by the diastolic arterial pressure at the root of the aorta, ventricular size (law of Laplace), and vascular impedance. The diastolic pressure at the root of the aorta is determined primarily by total systemic vascular resistance, arterial viscoelasticity, and the volume of blood present in the root of the aorta at the onset of ventricular contraction. Impedance is the sum of factors opposing blood flow from the ventricle and is determined by inertial, viscous, resistance, and compliance components. Impedance relates to the dynamic relation of changes in pressure and flow. In general, clinicians cannot accurately measure impedance and therefore rely upon a *calculated resistance*, derived from measurement of the ratio of pressure gradient to flow across a circulation, for assessment of afterload (i.e., calculated systemic vascular resistance = [mean arterial pressure − mean right atrial pressure] / [systemic cardiac output]).

VASCULAR FACTORS. These determine the resistance to blood flow and the transcapillary exchange of gases and nutrients within tissue beds. Resistance to flow of blood through an organ bed is determined by the viscosity of the blood and by the length and cross-sectional area of the blood vessels perfusing that organ. The cross-sectional area is the most important component, as vascular resistance is inversely proportional to the fourth power of the radius of the vessel. The radius is in turn determined by the tone of vascular smooth muscle in the wall of the vessel. Vascular smooth muscle tone is modulated by neurogenic influences mediated primarily through the sympathoadrenal system and by circulating humoral and local metabolic factors.

Neurogenic Control. Sympathoadrenal discharge to the circulatory system is regulated by medullary neurons in the vasomotor centers of the brain stem. Activity of these neurons is modulated by afferent neural impulses originating in various peripheral sensory receptors located in strategic areas throughout the body. Important among these receptors are the arterial (sinoaortic) and cardiopulmonary baroreceptors, chemoreceptors, and somatic receptors in skeletal muscle. Activities originating in higher portions of the central nervous system also impinge upon the brain stem vasomotor centers and thereby centrally modulate sympathetic and parasympathetic output.

The heart functions both as a muscle pump and as a peripheral sensory and endocrine organ. *Cardiopulmonary baroreceptors*, located primarily in the posterior wall of the left ventricle, are tonically active mechanoreceptors that are activated by expansion and stretch of the myocardium. When activated by an increase in cardiac preload, these "low pressure" receptors exert an afferent inhibitory influence on brain stem cardiovascular centers and thereby decrease efferent sympathetic outflow from these centers. Conversely, reduction in the stretch of these ventricular receptors, as during hypovolemia or assumption of upright posture, results in a lessening of their tonic afferent inhibition on brain stem centers and releases efferent sympathetic activity to cause reflex vasoconstriction, tachycardia, and the release of renin.

The *arterial baroreceptors*, located in the carotid sinus and aortic arch regions, are "high-pressure" mechanoreceptors that are activated by an increase in arterial pressure. When activated, these receptors exert an afferent inhibition on the brain stem vasomotor centers, thereby decreasing efferent sympathetic drive and resulting in vasodilation and bradycardia. Conversely, when deactivated by a fall in arterial pressure, the afferent inhibitory arterial baroreceptor input to the brain stem is decreased, resulting in an increase in sympathetic efferent tone with compensatory vasoconstriction and tachycardia.

In addition to inhibitory receptors such as the cardiac and arterial baroreceptors, peripheral excitatory afferent mechanisms also exist which contribute importantly to reflex control of the circulation. Severe hypoxia, often found in association with shock, activates excitatory *chemoreceptors* located in the carotid sinus region. This exerts an excitatory afferent influence on the brain stem centers, resulting in an increase in efferent sympathetic tone and vasoconstriction. *Somatic receptors* are metabolic receptors in exercising muscle that are activated by metabolic products of exercise and produce an afferent excitatory influence on the brain stem cardiovascular centers. This effect results in an increase in efferent sympathetic discharge to nonexercising muscles, with resultant vasoconstriction and increase in blood pressure to compensate for metabolic vasodilation occurring in exercising muscle beds.

During circulatory perturbations, synergistic and/or antagonistic activation of these multiple reflex pathways may occur. The net effect on cardiovascular homeostatic mechanisms depends upon the relative influence of these various regulatory pathways, along with a number of other neurohumoral responses not discussed here. For example, during moderate acute hemorrhage, the reduction of central cardiopulmonary blood volume and decrease in blood pressure simultaneously deactivate the cardiopulmonary baroreceptors and the arterial baroreceptors. These two baroreflex pathways synergistically produce an increase in sympathetic efferent outflow from the brain stem vasomotor centers. Similarly, in certain shock states, the combined deactivation of arterial baroreceptors by hypotension and the activation of the chemoreceptor reflex by hypoxia results in a significant synergistic effect on the ventilatory response as well as the circulatory sympathetic drive.

Conversely, there may be situations in which reflex responses have competing effects. This may occur, for example, when cardiac receptors are activated following acute myocardial infarction by the dyskinetic bulge of the left ventricle, while the arterial baroreceptors are deactivated because of hypotension. In the experimental preparation, the inhibitory influence of the bulging left ventricular wall on the sympathetic outflow predominates and overrides the arterial baroreflex, preventing vasoconstriction and thus causing a decrease in the afterload on the damaged left ventricle. Teleologically, this effect may be beneficial, as it tends to decrease left ventricular work following such an acute myocardial insult.

HUMORAL FACTORS. A number of circulating humoral agents play important roles in cardiovascular homeostasis. The release of hormones such as renin, vasopressin, adrenal steroids, prostaglandins, kinins, atrial natriuretic factor, and catecholamines is partially mediated through the autonomic nervous system and partly through direct and indirect cellular effects of toxins, ischemia, and antigens in various organs. These hormones have direct cardiovascular and renal effects and indirect effects on central and/or peripheral adrenergic transmission.

Renin-Angiotensin. The release of renin, synthesized primarily in the juxtaglomerular apparatus of the kidney, is regulated by various stimuli, including renal afferent arteriolar pressure, sodium concentration within the macula densa, stimulation of renal sympathetic nerves, circulating angiotensin II, and electrolyte concentration in circulating plasma. A fall in arterial blood pressure or an increase in sympathoadrenal discharge to the kidney results in the release of renin. Renin functions as a proteolytic enzyme, resulting in the conversion of inactive angiotensinogen to angiotensin I, which is further converted to angiotensin II by angiotensin-converting enzyme, primarily in the lung. Angiotensin II is a very potent direct-acting vasoconstrictor that also facilitates the release of norepinephrine from sympathetic nerve terminals. The net result is peripheral vasoconstriction in an attempt to maintain arterial pressure. In addition, the increase in angiotensin II causes an increase in release of aldosterone with consequent retention of sodium and water.

Vasopressin. This important osmolality-regulating and vasoconstrictor hormone is released from the posterior pituitary primarily in response to increases in osmolality as well as in response to hypovolemia. Vasopressin appears to play a role in the circulatory control response to shock, both through its antidiuretic effect and through its vasoconstrictor action. In addition, vasopressin stimulates release of ACTH and cortisol. Release of vasopressin is reduced by stretch of left atrial receptors during hypervolemia and by stretch of the arterial baroreceptors during hypertension; conversely, during hemorrhage and systemic hypotension, or when patients are on cardiopulmonary bypass, blood levels of vasopressin increase significantly. Vasopressin may be released by as little as a 10 per cent reduction in blood volume. Thirst and the release of vasopressin may be induced by a central nervous system action of angiotensin. From the standpoint of managing the shock patient, it is important to realize that vasopressin secretion is stimulated by nausea, morphine, and hypoxia and may be inhibited by catecholamines and alcohol.

Kinins. A variety of potent vasodilator polypeptides are formed by the action of certain proteolytic enzymes on plasma protein precursors. Bradykinin serves as the prototype for this class of endogenous peptides. Their major physiologic role may be the local regulation of blood flow and function of such organs as the salivary gland, pancreas, and kidney. In pathophysiologic states, kinins are believed to play a part in the hyperemia associated with inflammation and as vasodilators in hypotension produced by anaphylactic reactions. Renal kinins may cause diuresis and natriuresis.

Serotonin and Histamine. Serotonin released from platelets and histamine released from mast cells during anaphylaxis or during complement activation in shock may play an important role in regulating local vascular tone and capillary permeability.

Prostacyclin and Thromboxane A$_2$. Prostaglandins may be released in various organs during ischemia and may contribute to reactive hyperemia and vasodilation. The prostaglandin endoperoxides formed in platelets and in blood vessels are pivotal in the synthesis of two potent substances with opposing effects on the formation of thrombi. Prostacyclin, a powerful vasodilator and inhibitor of platelet aggregation, is synthesized in the vascular wall, mostly in the endothelial layer, from endoperoxides. In the platelets, however, endoperoxides are converted to thromboxane A$_2$, which causes vasoconstriction and platelet aggregation. In shock, damage to endothelial cells may inhibit synthesis of prostacyclin; in addition, platelets may release thromboxane A$_2$, causing intravascular platelet aggregation, clumping, and vasoconstriction.

Neuropeptides. Recent experimental and clinical studies in shock have emphasized the potentially important role of certain neuropeptides in regulating cardiovascular adjustments to shock and trauma. Among these important mediators are endogenous opioids (e.g., β-endorphin), thyrotropin-releasing hormone (TRF), and adrenocorticotropin (ACTH). β-Endorphin and adrenocorticotropin are stored in the pituitary gland and secreted concomitantly under stress. These agents appear to modulate autonomic function through central nervous system action, and they may play a role in the peripheral integration of autonomic nervous system activity. The β-endorphins, in particular, may play an important role in the pathophysiology of certain types of shock, most notably hemorrhagic, endotoxic (septic), and spinal shock. β-Endorphins may contribute directly or indirectly to myocardial depression during shock states. Experimental and limited clinical studies have suggested that pharmacologic blockade of the action of such endogenous opiates, by the use of specific antagonists such as naloxone, may improve cardiovascular stability in certain shock states. However, the precise role of these agents and such therapy remains to be defined (see Management).

Thyrotropin-releasing hormone (TRF) is a neuropeptide with potent central cardiovascular actions. Although frequently thought of primarily as a hypothalamic hormone with specific endocrinologic actions (e.g., stimulating release of thyroid-stimulating hormone from the pituitary), a major fraction of TRF is found outside of the hypothalamus in the brain and spinal cord. Experimental studies have suggested that exogenously administered TRF improves cardiorespiratory function in certain shock states, possibly through antagonism of adverse physiologic effects of endogenous opioids. The clinical importance of TRF in shock states in humans remains to be defined.

Atrial Natriuretic Factors. These biologically active peptides are released from specific granules in atrial myocytes and to a lesser extent from ventricular myocytes. These peptides bind to specific high-affinity receptors located in adrenal, renal, and vascular beds. These peptides produce direct vasorelaxant effects on vascular smooth muscle and natriuretic effects in the kidney. In addition, atrial natriuretic factor inhibits the action of renin and the production of aldosterone. Animal studies have suggested that these agents may alter the sensitivity of baroreceptors. While atrial natriuretic factor has been found to be elevated in pathophysiologic states such as severe heart failure, the exact role of these peptides in severe hemodynamic disorders such as shock remains unclear.

Catecholamines. The catecholamines norepinephrine and epinephrine are potent modulators of cardiovascular homeostasis. Released primarily from sympathetic nerve terminals, norepinephrine increases myocardial contractility and heart rate through activation of β-adrenoceptors and therefore increases cardiac output. In addition, norepinephrine has potent α-adrenergic actions and produces vasoconstriction, although the magnitude of this effect varies from tissue to tissue. Norepinephrine is a potent vasoconstrictor in skin, muscle, and splanchnic beds, whereas it may produce vasodilation in coronary vascular beds through a β$_2$-adrenergic mechanism. Epinephrine is released primarily from the adrenal glands, where the ratio of its release to that of norepinephrine is 10:1. Epinephrine has α, β$_1$, and β$_2$ effects and produces a modest increase in cardiac output through β$_1$ effects. However, epinephrine redistributes cardiac output away from the kidney and splanchnic circulation toward skeletal muscle, where its β$_2$ effect predominates with vasodilation. In other beds, epinephrine has significant α-vasoconstricting effects. Epinephrine may also effect release of norepinephrine from adrenergic nerve terminals through a prejunctional action.

Local Autoregulatory Mechanisms. Blood vessels have an intrinsic ability to autoregulate vascular tone and thereby maintain blood flow over a wide range of perfusion pressures. This property is independent of systemic neurogenic influences or humoral factors. Different vascular beds vary with respect to their ability to maintain blood flow. The cerebral, coronary, and renal circulations have the most developed autoregulatory mechanisms. Thus, during a fall in arterial pressure, vasodilation in these vascular beds maintains blood flow and oxygen delivery to the brain and heart and helps to preserve sodium and water balance. Although a myogenic response intrinsic to the smooth muscle may partially explain the phenomenon, accumulation of tissue metabolites following a transient period of ischemia may also cause vasodilation and restore blood flow. The specific mediator of metabolic vasodilation is not known, but it is likely that a combination of changes in oxygen, carbon dioxide, hydrogen ions, and other cations, in osmolality, in the amount of adenosine compounds, and in Krebs cycle intermediates and other metabolites released in the immediate environment of blood vessels contributes to adjustments in vascular tone.

Finally, apart from neural and humoral influences, the presence of occlusive vascular disease may play an important role in determining resistance to flow through regional circulations. This effect depends upon both fixed physical obstruction to the cross-sectional area of the perfusion bed and abnormalities in vascular reactivity induced by atherosclerotic changes in the vascular endothelium.

MICROCIRCULATION AND TRANSCAPILLARY EXCHANGE. The most critical aspect of the pathogenesis of shock takes place at the level of the microcirculation. In essence, all shock can be considered a form of microcirculatory failure. Delivery of a significant amount of blood to an organ does not guarantee that all the segments of that organ and all capillaries are perfused appropriate to the regional metabolic demand.

Intraorgan Blood Flow Distribution. Adequate tissue perfusion depends upon blood flow through vascular channels in which diffusion between the blood and tissues can occur. These channels are referred to as nutritional capillaries, as contrasted to nonnutritional vessels that do not permit capillary exchange. The latter are referred to as arteriovenous shunts. An example of the importance of the intraorgan redistribution of blood flow is observed in myocardial infarction, in which an increase in coronary blood flow may not increase perfusion to the infarcted segment. Under some circumstances, a coronary vasodilator may redistribute flow away from ischemic into nonischemic regions (e.g., administration of a potent intravenous vasodilator to a patient with severe fixed coronary obstruction with consequent induction of a coronary steal phenomenon). Similarly, the pattern of intraorgan blood flow may be critical in the kidney. Acute tubular necrosis associated with shock may reflect a reduction in glomerular filtration in the outer cortex because of a localized increase in vascular resistance in this region and a selective reduction in blood flow. Interventions that alter total renal blood flow can produce significant redistribution of flow within the kidney; for example, renal vasoconstriction following adrenergic discharge tends to shunt blood away from the outer cortex, whereas renal vasodilators (including the loop diuretic furosemide) shunt blood toward the outer cortical nephrons.

Pre- and Postcapillary Resistance. The precapillary sphincters regulate the patency of nutritional or "exchange" capillaries. The tone of these sphincters may be modulated by neurohumoral factors that contribute to the circulatory adjustments in shock. The metabolic products at the local tissue level are important determinants of the tone of these sphincters, which regulate the total functional capillary surface area and in turn determine the potential capillary area available for intravascular-to-extracellular fluid and solute exchange. The capillary hydrostatic force driving fluid out of the capillaries into the extracellular space depends on the ratio of post- to precapillary resistances. In hypovolemic or hemorrhagic shock, the fall in arterial pressure causes activation of the sympathoadrenal system, constriction of precapillary resistance vessels, and a fall in capillary hydrostatic pressure, facilitating movement of fluids from the extracellular to the intravascular space. This partially restores intravascular volume. Hematocrit, viscosity of blood, and plasma oncotic pressure fall. With persistent hypotension and ischemia, the vasoconstrictor response of precapillary resistance vessels becomes less pronounced because of tissue acidosis while resistance of postcapillary vessels (venules) increases. This creates a situation in which more fluid is lost from the vascular to the interstitial space. Thus, venular resistance and the reactivity of venules to the various vasoactive agents involved in shock become important. Venules may even be relatively more reactive than precapillary resistance vessels to catecholamines, which activate α-vasoconstrictor receptors. This differential effect in favor of postcapillary vasoconstriction also further increases hydrostatic pressure and intravascular fluid loss.

Capillary Permeability and Oncotic Pressure. Colloid osmotic pressure is a major determinant of intravascular volume. Albumin is the main osmotically active protein in plasma. The balance between colloid osmotic pressure and capillary hydrostatic pressure determines the balance between intravascular and extracellular fluid spaces. A significant degree of hypovolemia and hemoconcentration may take place either because of excessive capillary hydrostatic pressure from an increase in the ratio of post- to precapillary resistance or because of a reduction in plasma protein and consequent reduction of plasma oncotic pressure. Reduction of circulating plasma proteins may occur as a result of increased capillary permeability and loss of plasma proteins from the intravascular to the extracellular space. The balance between oncotic and hydrostatic pressures is also an important determinant of the level of pulmonary edema and is critical in the management of the shock lung syndrome. An appreciation of the important interplay between hydrostatic and colloid pressures is crucial to the selection of appropriate intravenous volume replacement in the therapy of many types of shock. Similarly, nutritional support of the critically ill patient is important in the effort to maintain adequate production of albumin.

Shock resulting from increased vascular permeability, as in anaphylactic shock or snake venom poisoning, is characterized by a dramatic reduction of plasma volume. Hematocrit rises sharply and oncotic pressure drops. This increase in capillary permeability may be partly related to release of histamine, metabolites, or humoral factors that alter endothelial permeability.

Intravascular Hemagglutination and "Blood Sludging." Erythrocytes, leukocytes, and platelets undergo agglutination to a variable degree in association with the shock syndromes in thermal burn, sepsis, trauma, and perhaps even hemorrhage. These aggregates may cause obstruction of nutritional capillaries as well as arterioles. The precipitating events are numerous. They may include platelet aggregation by catecholamines; damage to endothelial lining of small blood vessels and capillaries with subsequent fibrin deposition and accumulation of microthrombi; hypoxia increasing the rigidity of red blood cells; oxygen free radicals generated by endothelial cells or neutrophils; and release of vasoactive peptides and anaphylatoxins as a result of complement activation. These may cause additional damage to endothelial cells and increase the tone of precapillary sphincters, leading to further reduction in tissue perfusion and cellular injury.

PATHOPHYSIOLOGY AND STAGES OF SHOCK

From a conceptual standpoint, shock can be considered to progress through stages of lesser to greater severity and from reversible to irreversible derangements of metabolic processes. This conceptual framework involves stages of compensated, decompensated, and irreversible shock as summarized in Figure 41–3 and Table 41–2.

STAGE I—COMPENSATED SHOCK. In early shock, hypotension may arise from either a fall in cardiac output or peripheral vasodilation. The fall in cardiac output and arterial pressure

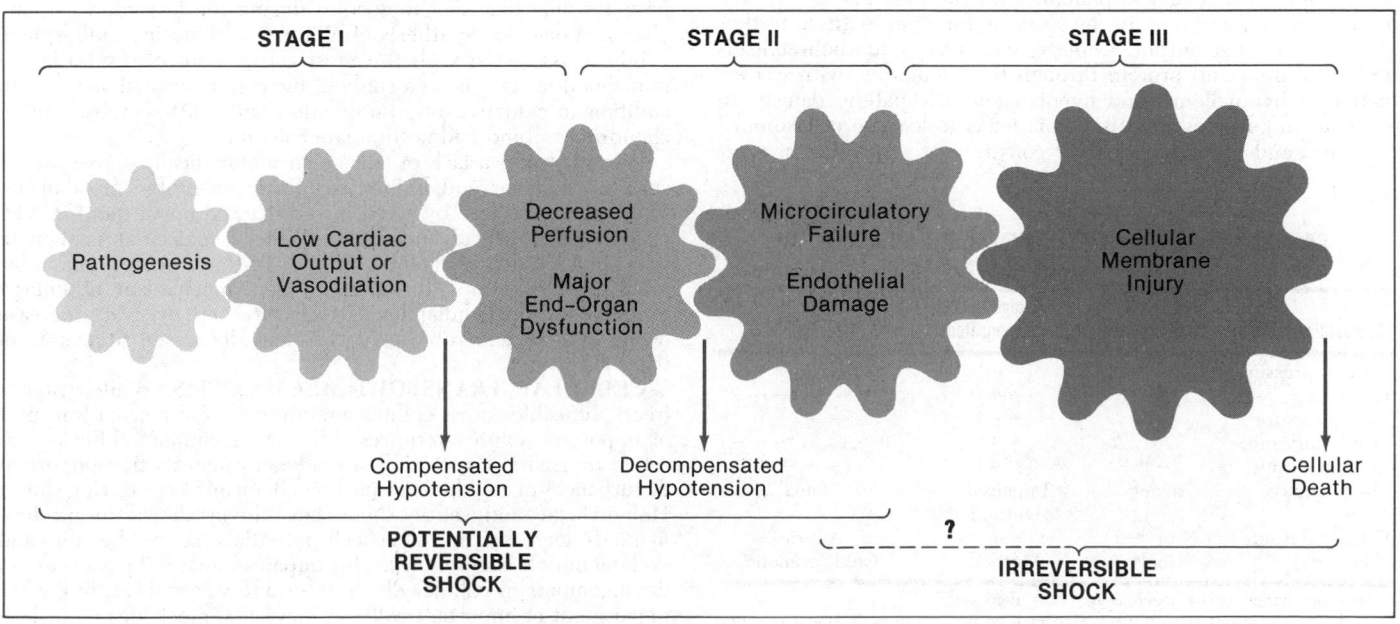

FIGURE 41–3. Pathophysiology of shock.

triggers compensatory mechanisms, which attempt to restore arterial pressure and blood flow to vital organs such as the brain and heart. At this stage, symptoms and signs of hemodynamic impairment are often subtle, and a high degree of clinical suspicion is required to identify early signs of hemodynamic compromise. Arterial pressure is usually maintained or mildly reduced; there is an increase in heart rate and a narrowing of pulse pressure; and there may be mild anxiety and early peripheral vasoconstriction. If shock is identified and vigorously treated at this stage, the syndrome may be successfully reversed in many cases.

STAGE II—DECOMPENSATED SHOCK. At this stage in the progression of shock, the compensatory mechanisms invoked during stage I to maintain perfusion of vital organs are insufficient to compensate for the hemodynamic insult. Patients may demonstrate impairment of major organ perfusion as manifested by altered mental state (impaired cerebral perfusion), reduced urine output (renal hypoperfusion), and myocardial ischemia (coronary flow impairment). The patient in this stage demonstrates the classic clinical picture of shock with hypotension, tachycardia, tachypnea, and narrowed pulse pressure (rapid, weak, and thready pulse). The external appearance of the patient reflects excessive sympathetic drive with acrocyanosis, peripheral vasoconstriction, and diaphoresis (cold and clammy extremities). Rapid aggressive intervention is required to restore cardiac output and perfusion of the tissues in this stage, prior to the onset of irreversible shock.

STAGE III—IRREVERSIBLE SHOCK. Excessive and prolonged reduction of tissue perfusion leads to significant alterations in cellular membrane function, aggregation of blood cells in the microcirculation, and "sludging" in the capillaries. The vasoconstriction that has taken place in the less vital organs in order to maintain blood pressure is now excessive and has reduced perfusion to such a point that cellular damage occurs. In this stage of shock, arterial pressure continues to fall progressively to a critical level at which vital organ perfusion is reduced and a vicious circle of further impairment ensues. Critical impairment of renal perfusion leads to acute tubular necrosis. Ischemia of the gastrointestinal tract leads to necrotic damage of the mucosa with a breakdown of this natural barrier and the subsequent absorption into the circulation of bacteria and their toxins with secondary detrimental effects on other organs. A generalized endothelial damage and disseminated intravascular coagulation may occur. Bacterial toxins may react with neutrophils and cause the release of vasodilator polypeptides that contribute to the fall in arterial pressure. Severe acidosis results from anaerobic metabolism as peripheral organs fail to receive nutrients sufficient to maintain aerobic metabolic pathways. Decreased perfusion of the coronary circulation, particularly in patients with coronary disease, results in further impairment of myocardial function with a further decline in cardiac output. Damage to capillary endothelium leads to loss of fluid and protein through the capillaries, with exacerbation of hypovolemia and hypotension. Ultimately, damage to cellular membranes from ischemia leads to leakage of lysosomal enzymes and other intracellular constituents, to progressive reduction in high-energy phosphate levels, and to cellular destruction. This terminal stage of shock is characterized by irreversible impairment of subcellular machinery, as discussed in the following section.

CELLULAR AND BIOCHEMICAL FACTORS IN SHOCK

MITOCHONDRIAL FUNCTION. Mitochondrial electron transport–linked mechanisms provide greater than 95 per cent of the body's energy needs under normal resting conditions. To do this, mitochondria utilize more than 90 per cent of the available cellular oxygen. The delivery of this essential oxygen depends upon maintenance of adequate tissue perfusion and the integrity of the capillary-interstitial-cellular interface. Shock of many diverse etiologies has been shown to result in progressive defects in mitochondrial metabolism.

Hypoxia alone may reduce the rate of adenosine triphosphate (ATP) synthesis by mitochondria, but it does not cause significant damage to mitochondrial membrane functions unless it is severe, sustained, or associated with ischemia, which also reduces the availability of other substrates. In fact, adaptation to hypoxia appears to take place such that when mitochondria are isolated from animal tissues after the animals have been exposed to brief periods of hypoxia, their capacity to respire and synthesize ATP in vitro is enhanced. During ischemia or shock, mitochondria cannot respond to increased energy needs by normal increases in oxidative phosphorylation.

Possible mechanisms involved in mitochondrial abnormalities during shock include structural changes (e.g., swelling), alterations of enzyme systems secondary to loss of critical cofactors, decreases in mitochondrial magnesium levels, increases in mitochondrial calcium concentration, alterations in mitochondrial sodium and potassium content, inhibition of mitochondrial function by agents such as free fatty acids, and free radical oxidation of phospholipids in the mitochondrial membranes.

It is unclear whether the degree of mitochondrial damage is a uniform feature in all tissues of the patient with shock or is manifested to a greater degree in some organs than in others. In experimental models, hepatic mitochondrial damage appears to dominate, whereas cerebral mitochondrial function appears to be preserved until very late in the experimental shock state. Experimental studies suggest that mitochondrial dysfunction may be reversed by interventions in the very early stages of shock, but the limits of this critical period of reversibility are unknown at present.

METABOLIC ALTERATIONS. Survival of aerobic cells depends on the availability of substrates and oxygen to the mitochondria, which provide most of the high-energy phosphate needs of the cell and utilize most of the available oxygen in the process. During oxidative phosphorylation, 36 moles of ATP are produced per mole of glucose, whereas in the anaerobic state, glycolysis provides only two ATP molecules during the breakdown of one glucose molecule. Synthesis of ATP from adenosine diphosphate (ADP) is associated with the most active state of respiration in mitochondria and is determined by cell energy demands. In addition to oxidative phosphorylation and ATP synthesis, mitochondria can bind and accumulate calcium.

During shock, a lack of oxygen in metabolically active organs such as the liver and kidney results in anaerobic metabolism. This is demonstrated by an early and marked impairment in ATP production. With advanced shock, this impairment is seen in other organs such as skeletal muscle. In these organs, anaerobic metabolism becomes the predominant mechanism of energy production, and cellular levels of lactate and pyruvate increase owing to both anaerobic glycolysis and decreased utilization of these substrates.

CELLULAR TRANSPORT MECHANISMS. While water is freely diffusible across cellular membranes, the normal transport of important solutes requires diffusion, facilitated diffusion, or active transport. Experimental evidence suggests that important disturbances in cellular transport mechanisms occur during shock. Hemorrhagic and septic shock have been shown to produce marked decreases in electrical potentials across hepatic and skeletal muscle membranes. This impairment and the consequent derangements in cellular electrolytes and water result in further impairment of important cellular enzymatic mechanisms, including glycolytic and gluconeogenic pathways.

TABLE 41–2. PATHOPHYSIOLOGIC STAGES OF SHOCK—CLINICAL SIGNS

Clinical Parameters	Stage I (Compensated)	Stage II (Decompensated)	Stage III (Irreversible)
Arterial pressure	N or (−)	(− −)	(− − −)
Heart rate	(+)	(+ +)	(+ + +) to (− − −)
Pulse pressure	(−)	(− −)	(− − −)
Respiratory rate	N	(+ +)	(+ + +) to (− − −)
Cardiac output	(−)*	(− −)	(− − −)
Mental status	Anxiety	Impaired/Obtunded	Coma
Urinary output	N or (−)	(− −)	Anuric
Skin	Cool*	Mottled	Cold, cyanotic

N = no change; (−) = decreased; (+) = increased.

*A high cardiac output and warm skin may be present in early stages of septic shock.

RETICULOENDOTHELIAL DYSFUNCTION. The reticuloendothelial system functions to remove foreign protein and particulate matter from the circulation. An important relationship between reticuloendothelial integrity and function, phagocytic activity, and survival has been suggested in experimental models of shock. Shock results in depression of this system, probably due to impairment of perfusion of the liver and spleen. While the precise abnormalities in reticuloendothelial function in shock remain to be defined, evidence suggests that at least part of the abnormality is due to impairment of opsonization activity resulting in impaired phagocytosis. This may result in the accumulation of toxic substances such as endotoxin, cellular aggregates, and immunologic complexes.

INSULIN RESISTANCE. Circulatory failure and shock are associated with hyperglycemia and abnormal glucose tolerance. While insulin levels often increase in shock, tissue response to insulin appear to be impaired, although the mechanism(s) responsible for this abnormality are not well defined.

OXYGEN-HEMOGLOBIN AFFINITY. Delivery of oxygen to the tissues depends upon the cardiac output and the oxygen carrying capacity of blood:

$$O_2 \text{ Delivery} = \text{Cardiac Output} \times \text{Blood } O_2\text{-Carrying Capacity}$$

Over 98 per cent of oxygen in the circulating blood is bound to hemoglobin. The oxygen-carrying capacity of blood is thus critically dependent upon the amount of hemoglobin and the saturation of the hemoglobin with oxygen. Normal hemoglobin, when 100 per cent saturated, carries 1.38 ml of oxygen per gram of hemoglobin. Thus, 100 ml of arterial blood with normal hemoglobin content (e.g., 15 grams), which is 96 to 98 per cent saturated (e.g., Po_2 = 95 to 100 mm Hg), carries 20 ml of oxygen to the tissues. Mixed venous blood returning to the right heart has an oxygen saturation of 75 per cent at a Po_2 of 40 mm Hg and contains 15 ml of oxygen per deciliter. The normal arteriovenous (AV) oxygen content difference is therefore 5 ml per deciliter of blood. The extraction of oxygen from hemoglobin by the tissues is not complete and depends to a large extent on the affinity of hemoglobin for oxygen, i.e., the shape of the oxygen-hemoglobin dissociation curve.

Hydrogen ions (Bohr effect), carbon dioxide, and 2,3-diphosphoglyceric acid (2,3-DPG) cause greater dissociation of oxygen from hemoglobin because of their preferential affinity for reduced hemoglobin. The concentration of 2,3-DPG in red cells results from a side reaction of glycolysis and increases during anemia, hypoxia, and acidosis. A drop in hemoglobin, hypoxemia, and acidosis may thus be partly compensated for by a shift of the oxygen dissociation curve to the right, favoring greater delivery of oxygen to the tissues at the same Po_2. This compensatory mechanism, in addition to the increase in cardiac output, provides for better oxygenation as extraction of oxygen increases at the expense of the oxygen reserve in venous blood. In certain tissues, however, such as the myocardium, extraction of oxygen at rest is already large, and any additional oxygen demand or a decrease in oxygen-hemoglobin dissociation such as in alkalosis requires greater delivery of oxygen, i.e., higher coronary blood flow.

In shock, the pH, carbon dioxide, and 2,3-DPG levels are changing, and one cannot calculate oxygen extraction from values of arterial Po_2 because the shape of the oxyhemoglobin dissociation curve cannot be predicted accurately. It is preferable to measure oxygen content or saturation of venous and arterial blood; if saturation is lower than predicted from values of Po_2, one can deduce that there is a shift of the dissociation curve to the right, and vice versa. Overzealous correction of acidosis with bicarbonate may, through the Bohr effect on hemoglobin affinity for oxygen, actually reduce oxygen delivery to the tissues. Hypophosphatemia (reported during hyperalimentation) may decrease 2,3-DPG and oxygen delivery.

LYSOSOMAL ABNORMALITIES. While present in most tissues, the higher concentrations of lysosomes in the body are found in the liver, kidney, and spleen. Lysosomes are cytoplasmic vesicles that contain a variety of potent hydrolytic enzymes bound in a latent form. These enzymes are capable of hydrolyzing a wide variety of intra- and extracellular macromolecules. When released from organelles as a consequence of certain forms of cellular injury, these enzymes may contribute to the pathogenesis or the propagation and perpetuation of shock. They are most active at an acid pH, which makes them potentially more destructive in the setting of hypoxia and shock.

Numerous morphologic and biochemical observations implicate the lysosomal enzymes in the perpetuation of shock, but at this time the evidence for their primary involvement is unclear. In organs such as the liver, spleen, and intestine, the lysosomes enlarge during the early phases of shock. This is associated with a decrease in the total activity of lysosomal hydrolases in tissues and a corresponding increase in activity in the soluble fraction of the tissue homogenate. This indicates a loss of lysosomal membrane integrity in vivo. The lysosomes obtained from animals in shock demonstrate an enhanced release of enzymes in vitro. A reduction in lysosomal membrane integrity has also been observed in animals after administration of endotoxin. In several animal studies, the levels of hydrolases found in blood, lymph, or serum seem to correlate with severity of shock.

MYOCARDIAL DEPRESSANT FACTOR(S). Initially described in 1966 in the plasma of cats following hemorrhagic shock, myocardial depressant factor (MDF) is an incompletely understood factor associated with almost all forms of shock. Experimental and clinical studies have described elevated plasma levels of MDF in cases of hemorrhagic, septic, cardiogenic, traumatic, and burn shock. An apparent common denominator in these various shock states that is related to the plasma level of MDF is the degree of splanchnic hypoperfusion that occurs. A critical component appears to be marked impairment of pancreatic perfusion, which is believed to result in pancreatic ischemia and acidosis leading to lysosomal disruption. The release of lysosomal enzymes and activation of zymogenic enzymes (e.g., conversion of trypsinogen to trypsin and chymotrypsinogen to chymotrypsin) appear to be related to the formation of MDF. MDF is believed to be released from leaky acinar cells in the pancreas and carried to peripheral sites of the circulation. MDF has been demonstrated in both intact animals and isolated tissue preparations to exert a potent negative inotropic action. The resulting impairment in cardiac output leads to further pancreatic hypoperfusion, and a positive feedback loop is believed to result in further release of this agent. In addition to the cardiodepression, MDF appears to produce vasoconstriction in splanchnic resistance vessels and impairs function of the reticuloendothelial system.

A number of agents have been demonstrated to be effective in preventing the formation of MDF in various shock states. These include the synthetic glucocorticoids, the protease inhibitor aprotinin, angiotensin-converting enzyme (ACE) inhibitors, angiotensin receptor antagonists, thromboxane antagonists, thromboxane synthetase inhibitors, lipoxygenase inhibitors, opiate receptor antagonists, and vasodilator prostaglandins. In addition, agents that have been shown to significantly counteract the negative inotropic actions of MDF include digitalis glycosides, glucagon, isoproterenol, dopamine, amrinone, and calcium ion. The precise role played by MDF in the pathogenesis of clinical shock syndromes remains to be defined.

COMPLEMENT ACTIVATION. The complement system consists of a series of discrete plasma proteins that are present as inactive precursors until they are activated by highly specific biochemical reactions. Activation of the complement system results in the cleavage of several low molecular weight vasoactive peptides from the complement molecules. These peptides in turn have a wide variety of significant biologic effects. For example, during the activation of C2, a cleavage product occurs that has kinin-like activity, which then can significantly influence capillary permeability. Two other activation peptides, C3a and C5a, release histamine from mast cells, have chemotactic activity, and constrict vascular smooth muscle. Another fragment, C3B, acts as an opsonin and facilitates phagocytosis. Polymorphonuclear leukocytes may be attracted chemotactically through activation of esterases on their surface and may release their lysosomal enzymes if the concentration of the complement reaction product C5a is large enough. Platelets may have an increase in their procoagulant activity. In addition to the direct and indirect effects of the fragments of activated complement on cells, their aggregation as complexes on the surface of cell membranes causes cellular destruction. The expressions of all these effects are increased capillary permeability, increased leukocyte accumulation and infiltration, release of lysosomal enzymes, and activation of intravascular coagulation factors. Clinically, these result in such entities as glomerulitis, necrotizing vasculitis, the Schwartzmann reaction, thrombocytopenia, and other manifestations of microcirculatory collapse and intravascular plugging seen in prolonged shock and endotoxemia.

Although the side effects of complement activation in shock are detrimental, leading to cellular death, the fundamental biologic activities of the complement components are beneficial in enhancing phagocytosis and mediating the inflammatory response to local infection or irritation, in the neutralizing of viruses, and, finally, in modulating the immune response.

EICOSANOIDS. These lipid substances, derived from arachidonic acid (eicosatetraenoic acid), have recently been implicated as important mediators of ischemic and circulatory shock. During ischemic and shock states, a variety of these substances are produced, the most important of which are the vasoconstrictor prostaglandins (PG), thromboxanes (TX), and leukotrienes (LT).

PGF_2-α has been found to be increased in animals with hemorrhagic, endotoxic, cardiogenic, and burn shock and has been identified as a potent vasoconstrictor of coronary, mesenteric, and renal vessels and is believed to play some role in the pathogenesis of circulatory shock. TXA_2 is believed to play three important roles in shock: (1) induction of vasoconstriction, (2) aggregation of circulating platelets, and (3) induction of leakage in lysosomal membranes. It is believed to play a role in myocardial ischemia, sudden death, and circulatory shock. Recent experimental evidence suggests that thromboxane synthetase inhibitors may play a protective role in certain types of myocardial ischemia, trauma, and endotoxic shock.

Leukotrienes (LTs) are the major biologically active products of the lipoxygenase pathway of arachidonic acid metabolism and are produced by pulmonary parenchymal cells, macrophages, mast cells, white blood cells, and connective tissue cells. These agents appear to be potent vasoconstrictors and bronchoconstrictors. The exact role, if any, that these agents play in the pathogenesis of shock remains to be defined experimentally.

OXYGEN FREE RADICALS. Oxygen free radicals may be generated in tissues during shock states. The unpaired electron in these radicals may react with any cellular component, but particularly with unsaturated fatty acids and sulfhydryl amino acids, and cause cellular damage. The clinical documentation of the relative importance of these factors and the effectiveness of their elimination awaits further experimentation in humans.

TUMOR NECROSIS FACTOR. Tumor necrosis factor (TNF, cachectin) is a recently recognized endogenous mediator of shock and inflammation. TNF is derived from mononuclear phagocytes on exposure to lipopolysaccharide endotoxin, and TNF appears to be responsible for many of the deleterious effects of endotoxin. TNF appears to be one of the primary mediators of experimental septic shock, with many of the lethal cytotoxic effects of endotoxin being due to host cell effects mediated by this agent. Biologic effects attributed experimentally to TNF include the suppression of lipoprotein lipase biosynthesis by adipocytes, induction of antigenic determinants on fibroblasts and endothelial cells, stimulation of products of prostaglandin E_2 and collagenase, and activation of neutrophils. This latter effect appears responsible for many of the inflammatory changes seen in sepsis that lead to tissue damage. TNF also exerts a catabolic effect on bone and cartilage and is an endogenous pyrogen. TNF appears to share many of the same bioactivities of other inflammatory cytokines such as interleukin-1. The precise role of TNF in clinical shock is under active investigation.

ETIOLOGY OF SHOCK—CLASSIFICATION

While the end result of most shock syndromes involves irreversible deterioration of cellular and subcellular metabolic processes and structural integrity, it is clinically useful to consider the differential diagnosis of shock from a functional standpoint. This classification scheme emphasizes potential initiating pathogenic mechanisms. Most cases of shock can be considered to arise from one of four basic abnormalities: (1) hypovolemia, (2) cardiac functional impairment, (3) obstruction of major vascular conduits, and (4) inappropriate distribution of cardiac output

secondary to abnormal vasodilation. These functional etiologies of shock are outlined in Table 41–3. Common clinical syndromes representative of the functional types of shock are discussed below.

HYPOVOLEMIC SHOCK. Perfusion of major organs and peripheral tissues depends upon the integrity of a vascular pump (heart), a capacitance vascular tree, and an intravascular blood volume. Hypovolemic shock is the most common type of shock seen clinically and is due to an absolute and often sudden reduction in circulating blood volume relative to the capacity of the vascular system. The classic hemodynamic features of this type of shock include tachycardia, hypotension, reduced cardiac filling pressures, and peripheral vasoconstriction (see Table 41–2). An important aspect of this type of shock is the *rapidity* with which hypovolemia occurs. A sudden reduction in circulating blood volume of 10 per cent in previously healthy individuals results in mild reduction in arterial pressure and moderate reduction in cardiac output. A sudden reduction in blood volume of 20 per cent produces moderate hypotension and moderately severe reductions in cardiac output. The loss of 40 per cent of circulating blood volume produces profound reductions in arterial pressure and cardiac output. These hemodynamic consequences are accentuated in patients with pre-existing cardiovascular,

TABLE 41–3. ETIOLOGIC CATEGORIES OF SHOCK

I. Hypovolemic shock
  A. Hemorrhagic (e.g., trauma, gastrointestinal hemorrhage)
  B. Hypovolemic, nonhemorrhagic
    1. External fluid loss (e.g., vomiting, diarrhea, polyuria, burns)
    2. Internal extravascular sequestration (e.g., peritonitis, pancreatitis)

II. Cardiogenic shock
  A. Acute myocardial infarction
    1. Loss of critical muscle mass (e.g., large anterior wall infarction)
    2. Acute mechanical lesion (e.g., ventricular septal rupture, mitral insufficiency)
    3. Acute right ventricular infarction
    4. Left ventricular free wall rupture
    5. Left ventricular aneurysm
  B. Valvular heart disease
    1. Critical valvular stenosis (e.g., aortic or mitral stenosis)
    2. Severe valvular insufficiency (e.g., acute aortic or mitral insufficiency)
  C. Nonvalvular obstructive cardiac lesions
    1. Atrial myxoma or ball-valve thrombus
    2. Cardiac tamponade
    3. Restrictive cardiomyopathy (e.g., amyloid)
    4. Constrictive pericardial disorder
  D. Nonischemic myopathic processes
    1. Fulminant myocarditis
    2. Physiologic depressants (e.g., acidosis, hypoxia)
    3. Pharmacologic depressants (e.g., calcium channel blockers)
    4. Pathophysiologic depressants (e.g., myocardial depressant factor)
  E. Dysrhythmias
    1. Severe bradyarrhythmias (e.g., high-degree AV block)
    2. Tachyarrhythmias
      a. Ventricular (e.g., ventricular tachycardia)
      b. Supraventricular (e.g., atrial fibrillation or flutter with rapid ventricular response)

III. Vascular obstructive shock
  A. Massive pulmonary embolism
  B. Tension pneumothorax
  C. Excessive positive-pressure ventilation
  D. Aortic dissection

IV. Distributive shock and miscellaneous
    1. Sepsis
    2. Anaphylaxis
    3. Massive tissue injury (e.g., crush)
    4. Prolonged ischemia/hypoxia
    5. Neurogenic shock
    6. Endocrine disorders
      a. Addisonian crisis
      b. Profound hypothyroidism
    7. Drug or toxin induced

pulmonary, renal, or cerebrovascular disorders. In contrast, a similar degree of volume loss occurring over a longer period of time (days to weeks) may not be accompanied by the same magnitude of hemodynamic impairment.

Hypovolemia may occur as a result of loss of blood volume secondary to hemorrhage (internal or external) or may arise as a result of the loss of fluid and electrolytes. This latter form of hypovolemia may occur following severe loss of gastrointestinal fluids (e.g., diarrhea, vomiting), renal losses (e.g., polyuria), external losses of fluids secondary to impairment of surface tissue integrity (e.g., burns), or internal losses of fluids without a change in total body water (e.g., third-space sequestration of fluids).

As previously noted, hypovolemia usually results in the induction of neurohumoral compensatory mechanisms that produce the characteristic features of shock (e.g., tachycardia, tachypnea, and peripheral vasoconstriction). However, it has been known for some time, although poorly appreciated by clinicians, that profound exsanguinating hemorrhage may present as paradoxical bradycardia (or absence of tachycardia) due to activation of cardiac mechanoreceptors in the setting of vigorous contraction of a "volume-depleted" ventricle. Recent observations in normal humans have demonstrated that abrupt decreases in cardiac filling pressures can result in sympathetic inhibition with profound hypotension and bradycardia. This afferent inhibition from ventricular receptors may override the hypotension-induced deactivation of arterial baroreceptors. Thus, the presentation of a patient with obvious hypovolemic hypotension in the absence of tachycardia should alert the clinician to the possibility of massive volume loss and the need for vigorous volume resuscitation.

CARDIOGENIC SHOCK. Cardiogenic shock may arise from a number of underlying etiologies, the usual common denominator of which is inadequate stroke volume. A strict hemodynamic operational definition, based upon invasive hemodynamic monitoring, is necessary to differentiate cardiogenic from hypovolemic shock.

Cardiogenic shock most commonly presents as an acute deterioration of cardiac function, although this may be superimposed on chronic impairment. The most common etiology of cardiogenic shock is acute myocardial infarction. Cardiogenic shock in this setting carries a mortality of 50 to 90 per cent, varying according to the mechanism of the hemodynamic insult and the aggressiveness of treatment. Shock following myocardial infarction is more common in the setting of anterior infarctions than inferior infarctions. However, large inferoposterior infarctions or inferior infarctions with significant right ventricular involvement may produce cardiogenic shock. Detailed anatomic studies of patients succumbing to cardiogenic shock following acute infarction, in the absence of mechanical lesions, have demonstrated that impairment of 30 to 35 per cent or more of functioning ventricular muscle usually accompanies this syndrome.

In addition to large losses of functioning ventricular muscle mass, cardiogenic shock may arise from the development of intracardiac mechanical defects. These include acute ventricular septal rupture, acute mitral insufficiency (papillary muscle dysfunction or rupture), and left ventricular free wall rupture. The frequency of shock due to acute mitral insufficiency and ventricular septal rupture is evenly divided between anterior and inferior infarctions.

Non–infarct-related etiologies of cardiogenic shock include critical valvular heart disease, disorders of pericardial restraint, obstructive myopathic cardiac disorders, acute cardiomyopathies of diverse etiologies, and marked disorders of cardiac rate and rhythm. In addition, an element of myocardial depression may be a significant factor in the pathogenesis of shock from sepsis and severe hemorrhage. These noninfarction etiologies are outlined in Table 41–3.

VASCULAR OBSTRUCTIVE SHOCK. The most common example of shock secondary to acute obstruction of the vascular tree is acute cardiac tamponade with resultant impairment of diastolic ventricular filling. This may arise as a result of trauma, infection, neoplasm, or cardiac rupture. It is the rapidity of accumulation of pericardial volume, rather than the absolute volume, that is the critical determinant of the hemodynamic impairment in cardiac tamponade. Rapid accumulations of as little as 100 to 200 ml of blood in the pericardium may produce tamponade. Similarly, therapeutic removal of small amounts of

fluid (e.g., 50 to 100 ml) may be all that is required to relieve tamponade and allow diastolic ventricular filling to resume and cardiac output to rise.

Other examples of obstructive shock include massive pulmonary embolism with obstruction of the right ventricular outflow or main pulmonary artery, tension pneumothorax, and abrupt aortic occlusion due to dissection or massive thromboembolism.

DISTRIBUTIVE SHOCK. This functional classification involves shock syndromes manifested by decreased vascular resistance that is not adequately compensated for by alterations in cardiac output. The classic example of distributive shock is endotoxin sepsis.

The incidence of septic shock in the hospital setting appears to have increased over the past several decades, probably as a consequence of multiple medical advances in other areas. It is estimated that 1 per cent of hospital admissions are complicated by gram-negative sepsis, and the mortality from septic shock ranges from 30 to 80 per cent. Rather than a primary community-acquired phenomenon, septic shock more commonly arises in hospitalized patients and is one of the most common causes of mortality in intensive care unit patients.

Septic shock is most commonly associated with gram-negative infections, and approximately 40 per cent of gram-negative bacteremias are complicated by shock. Gram-negative septic shock is most often an example of an opportunistic infection. The most common gram-negative organisms associated with septic shock include *Escherichia coli, Klebsiella, Enterobacter,* and *Pseudomonas* species. The most common sources for these infectious agents are the genitourinary and gastrointestinal tracts, followed by respiratory tract, wounds, and sites of indwelling vascular access. Important non–gram-negative organs associated with septic shock include some gram-positive *Staphylococcus* and *Streptococcus* species and fungal organisms such as *Candida.*

Host factors important in the propensity for development of septic shock include advanced age, diabetes, debilitation and malnutrition, chronic alcohol or intravenous drug use, neoplastic diseases, immunocompromised state (especially granulocytopenia), and multiple organ failure.

Septic shock often follows a trimodal pattern of hemodynamic presentation: "warm" shock, "cold" shock, and multisystem organ failure. Early sepsis is often associated with a decrease in systemic vascular resistance, due most likely to the release of vasodilatory mediators such as bradykinin and histamine, and an increase in cardiac output ("warm" shock). The early stages of sepsis are characterized hemodynamically by low cardiac filling pressures, increased cardiac output, tachycardia, fever, and decreased whole-body oxygen consumption. This latter effect is likely due to impaired mitochondrial oxygen utilization and deficient oxygen delivery to cells despite an increase in overall cardiac output (maldistribution of cardiac output). Late in the sequence of septic shock, there is a decline in cardiac output and profound hypotension with severe acidosis, hypoxemia, and hypoxia ("cold" shock). Recent evidence suggests that the initial increase in cardiac output is often followed by a decrease in ventricular ejection fraction, possibly due to a myocardial depressant factor, myocardial edema, or altered responsiveness to adrenergic stimuli.

Lipopolysaccharide endotoxin appears to be a common etiologic factor in septic shock, as previously reviewed in this chapter (Cellular and Biochemical Factors in Shock). The end stages of septic shock are often associated with multiple organ system failure with profound derangements in cardiovascular, pulmonary, and renal systems. The adult respiratory distress syndrome is a common complication of septic shock and is discussed below.

COMMON COMPLICATIONS OF SHOCK

DISSEMINATED INTRAVASCULAR COAGULATION. Disseminated intravascular coagulation (DIC) is a syndrome often seen in shock, particularly that due to gram-negative septicemia, and is associated with a high mortality rate. The clinical hallmark of DIC is the simultaneous occurrence of intravascular clotting and fibrinolysis, although bleeding dominates the clinical picture in most cases. The syndrome causes renal cortical necrosis, generalized ischemic damage of multiple organs, consumption of coagulation factors, and bleeding and may also contribute to the pathogenesis of shock lung.

ADULT RESPIRATORY DISTRESS SYNDROME. The adult respiratory distress syndrome (ARDS), previously known as "shock lung," is a common complication of various shock syndromes and emphasizes the disastrous complications of microcirculatory failure. ARDS is defined physiologically as the presence of severe hypoxemia ($PaO_2/F_{IO_2} < 150$ torr), chest roentgenographic evidence of generalized pulmonary infiltrates, reduced lung compliance, absence of significant elevations of pulmonary venous pressures as confirmed by invasive hemodynamic monitoring (e.g., pulmonary capillary wedge pressure < 18 mm Hg), and absence of alternative explanations for the clinical presentation.

ARDS is most commonly seen in association with sepsis but may also complicate major trauma, aspiration of gastric contents, multiple blood transfusions, drug overdose, and primary pneumonic infections. The onset of ARDS may be extremely rapid (e.g., within 1 to 2 hours) but more often follows the initiating event by 24 to 48 hours. In most series, the mortality associated with ARDS is greater than 50 per cent and as great as 90 per cent in patients with combined ARDS and sepsis. The presence of other shock-associated disorders, such as multiple organ failure or severe infections, increases the mortality.

Three pathologic phases of ARDS have been described. An early exudative phase (24 to 96 hours) is characterized by death of alveolar type I cells, regional microatelectasis, and accumulation of protein-rich edema and fibrin with endothelial cell swelling. Complement-mediated neutrophil activation is a prominent early feature and likely contributes to endothelial damage. A second proliferative phase is characterized by the formation of hyaline membranes and rapid proliferation of type II alveolar cells. A chronic or late proliferative phase is characterized by widespread fibrosis. ARDS appears to produce inhomogeneous lesions in the lung, with the dependent portions being affected to a greater extent.

The physiologic consequences of ARDS include severe hypoxemia, reduced lung compliance, reduced functional residual lung capacity, increased dead space ventilation, pulmonary hypertension, and a nidus for superimposed pulmonary infection. The cause of death in patients who develop ARDS in the setting of shock is usually not respiratory failure. Early deaths are usually due to the underlying illness, and late deaths are related to complications of the treatment of this type of patient. Secondary lung infection is a common complication of ARDS. In those patients surviving ARDS, approximately one third have persistent pulmonary symptoms.

ACUTE RENAL FAILURE. Acute renal failure is a common complication of shock, regardless of primary etiology, and is responsible for considerable morbidity and mortality in this syndrome. Current mortality rates for acute renal failure developing in all hospitalized patients average 40 to 60 per cent. The most common causes of acute renal failure in hospitalized patients include decreased renal perfusion (of particular concern in the shock patient), administration of radiographic contrast agents, and administration of nephrotoxic drugs, particularly the aminoglycoside antibiotics.

The most common mechanism of acute renal failure in the setting of shock is probably acute tubular necrosis, otherwise known as vasomotor nephropathy. The pathogenesis of this disorder usually involves severe reductions in renal cortical blood flow due to marked preglomerular vasoconstriction. Vasomotor nephropathy is usually manifested by oliguria but can occasionally present as total anuria, persists for 1 to 3 weeks, and can be followed by a recovery phase associated with marked diuresis. In most patients, the serum creatinine rises 1 to 4 mg per deciliter per day, and the mortality increases with total increases of 3 mg per deciliter or more.

In the management of the shock patient, close attention needs to be paid to monitoring urine output and ensuring that cardiac preload and cardiac output are adequate to maintain renal perfusion. The onset of anuria requires that postrenal obstructive etiologies be excluded rapidly. In the case of trauma, consideration must be given to vascular insults (renal artery or renal vein occlusion) and to rhabdomyolysis as possible etiologies of renal failure.

CLINICAL PRESENTATION

The classic clinical presentation of shock is a patient who is hypotensive (systolic arterial pressure less than 90 mm Hg or more than 60 mm Hg less than baseline); has a tachycardia with a weak and thready pulse; is hyperventilating; has cold, clammy, cyanotic skin; and has a dulled sensorium ranging from agitation to stupor or coma. The patient is frequently oliguric (urine output less than 30 ml per hour) or anuric.

This classic shock pattern of presentation is not always present, and the recognition of the subtle or early presentation of shock may be crucial. For example, a patient may have a "normal" blood pressure (e.g., 110/70), but this may actually represent "relative hypotension" if the patient has a history of severe hypertension. Early shock may be indicated only by unexplained agitation or tachycardia in the absence of cardiovascular collapse. Some patients with septic or neurogenic shock may present with peripheral vasodilation and warm hyperperfused extremities (so-called warm shock).

Finally, the clinical manifestations of the patient may be altered by pre-existing disease or by chronic pharmacologic agents. If possible, rapid assessment of medical history and medication regimens should be obtained during the initial assessment of the patient.

Assessment of the Shock Patient

GENERAL PRINCIPLES. There are five major goals in the management of the patient in shock: (1) rapid recognition of the shock state; (2) correction of the initial insult, (3) correction of the secondary consequences of the shock state, (4) maintenance of the function of vital organs, and (5) identification and correction of aggravating factors. All five goals are approached simultaneously in an organized and methodical way so as to ensure optimal therapy (Fig. 41–4). The prognosis of a patient in shock is determined in part by the etiology of the shock state (e.g.,

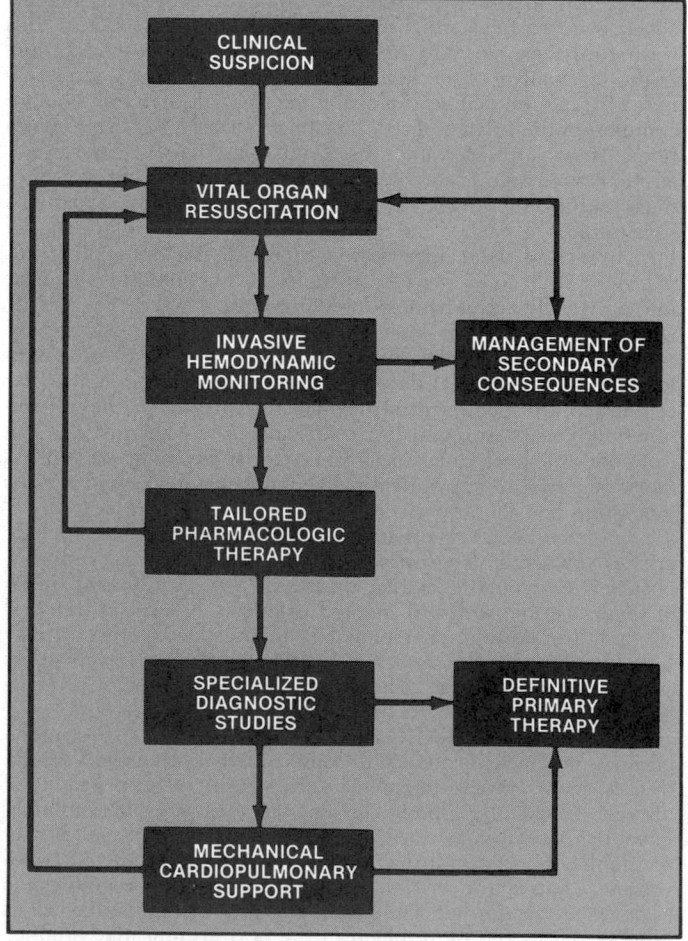

FIGURE 41–4. Strategy for management of the shock patient.

hypovolemic traumatic shock in a young, healthy adult carries a mortality of less than 20 per cent in many centers, whereas cardiogenic shock due to massive anterior wall myocardial infarction carries a mortality of greater than 70 per cent even in the most aggressive medical center). Prognosis is also affected by the duration of shock and consequent secondary organ dysfunction and by the speed of recognition and appropriateness of medical intervention. Finally, the prognosis of the patient in shock is also affected by the preshock status of the patient with respect to pre-existing medical conditions.

CRITICAL CARE TEAM. Successful and sophisticated management of a patient in shock requires an integrated team approach that begins to function upon initial contact with the patient and extends through periods of resuscitation, early stabilization, diagnostic evaluation, definitive therapy, and recovery phases of treatment. In addition to a primary physician knowledgeable in critical care who is responsible for the overall coordination of patient-care efforts, the management of these patients requires a number of other highly motivated, well-trained, and objective but empathetic professionals. Such a team includes critical care nurses, respiratory therapists, hemodynamic monitoring technicians, special procedure and diagnostic technicians, nutrition/dietetic consultants, and physical therapists. Finally, the immediate availability of multiple surgical and medical subspecialty consultants is essential for the care of these complexly and critically ill patients.

MEDICAL HISTORY AND PHYSICAL EXAMINATION. A rapid but thorough medical history and a complete but directed physical examination should be performed during the initial assessment and early management of the shock patient. Particular attention should be directed to the recent medical history and the details of the present illness in an effort to rapidly identify precipitating or causative factors of shock. Pertinent medical history should be obtained with emphasis placed on pre-existing cardiopulmonary, renal, hepatic, neurologic, and hematologic disorders. A complete listing of current medications and known allergies should be obtained from the patient, medical record, or closest relative.

A systematic and complete "head-to-toe" physical examination should be performed, consistent with the patient's clinical condition. During the examination, particular attention should be directed to assessment of the patient's airway, ventilation, circulation, and neurologic status. In the case of trauma, the patient's axial skeleton should be appropriately splinted until critical injuries to the head, spine, pelvis, and extremities have been excluded.

Sinus tachycardia is one of the earliest compensatory mechanisms for a fall in arterial pressure or cardiac output, and the differential diagnosis of this increase in heart rate includes the seven H's of hypovolemia, hypotension, heart failure, hypoxemia, hyperthermia, hyperthyroidism, and reflex hyperadrenergic state (e.g., reflex tachycardia seen in some cases of anterior wall myocardial infarction). Other important possible causes of tachycardia include anxiety and pulmonary embolism. The clinician must remember that unexplained tachycardia may be one of the earliest indications of impending cardiovascular collapse and therefore must not be ignored or inappropriately treated until the differential diagnosis is appropriately addressed.

The most important initial assessment of the patient should be directed to the patency and adequacy of the airway. If the patient is unable to ventilate or cannot adequately protect the airway, endotracheal intubation is indicated. Initial assessment of circulatory reserve can be obtained by palpation of central arteries (e.g., femoral) and by sphygmomanometric measurement of blood pressure. Particular attention should be focused on the pulse pressure, as a narrow pulse pressure suggests marked impairment of stroke volume.

INTRAVENOUS ACCESS. At least two large-bore intravenous catheters (16 gauge or larger) should be inserted in peripheral extremities, and at least one central venous sheath (8 Fr or greater) should be inserted under optimal sterile conditions as rapidly as possible. During placement of these venous access catheters, blood can be obtained for essential hematologic and chemical studies and for blood typing and cross-matching. In most circumstances, isotonic fluids (e.g., normal saline or Ringer's lactate) should be infused through these catheters pending further assessment of the patient.

INITIAL HEMATOLOGIC/BIOCHEMICAL DETERMINATIONS. Essential initial laboratory determinations should include those that may alter immediate therapy. These include complete blood count, serum electrolytes (sodium, potassium, calcium, magnesium), and arterial blood gases. Additional laboratory parameters should be obtained as indicated by the patient's presentation and the most likely etiologies for the shock state (e.g., blood culture; toxicology screen; cardiac enzyme panels).

A key element in the therapy of a patient in shock is hemodynamic monitoring.

Patient Monitoring

Management of the patient in shock requires accurate and serial measurements of heart rate and rhythm, respiratory rate and adequacy of gas exchange, systemic arterial pressure and cardiac filling pressures, tissue perfusion, and end-organ function. A reference for normal hemodynamic parameters in adults is provided in Table 41–4.

ELECTROCARDIOGRAPHIC MONITORING. Continuous electrocardiographic monitoring permits assessment of cardiac rate and rhythm and allows prompt detection of serious cardiac arrhythmias such as ventricular tachyarrhythmias, atrial fibrillation, high-degree AV block, and marked sinus bradycardia. The use of a monitoring lead, or preferably several leads, that provides adequate assessment of atrial as well as ventricular rhythms (e.g., MCL_1) is essential. Serial standard 12-lead electrocardiograms permit indirect assessment of myocardial ischemia and may be required for analysis of complex rhythm disorders.

ARTERIAL PRESSURE MONITORING. An indwelling arterial catheter is essential for continuous on-line assessment of arterial pressure and also provides a convenient access for obtaining blood samples. Assessment of arterial pressure by sphygmomanometry is not adequate for most patients with shock, is often an unreliable indicator of true core blood pressure in the hypotensive patient, and fails to provide continuous on-line assessment of blood pressure in patients with rapidly changing cardiovascular states. The choice of insertion site for arterial line placement depends upon the status of the patient being monitored, the presence and severity of peripheral vascular disease, and the expertise of the critical care team. In general, the more severe the shock state, the more central should the arterial catheter be placed in order to assess core blood pressure. In contrast, the

TABLE 41–4. NORMAL RESTING ADULT HEMODYNAMIC PARAMETERS

Parameter	Wave	Range (mm Hg)
Hydrostatic pressures		
Systemic arterial pressure		
Systemic arterial	Systolic	100–140
	Diastolic	60–90
	Mean	70–105
Right heart pressures		
Right atrial	"a"	2–10
	"v"	2–10
	Mean	2–8
Right ventricular	Systolic	15–30
	Diastolic	2–8
Pulmonary arterial	Systolic	15–30
	Diastolic	4–12
	Mean	9–18
Pulmonary capillary wedge	"a"	3–15
	"v"	3–15
	Mean	2–10
Cardiac output determinations		
Cardiac index (L/min/m²)		2.6–4.2
Arterial–mixed venous oxygen content difference (ml/dl)		3.0–5.0

From Grossman W: Cardiac Catheterization and Angiography. 3rd ed. Philadelphia, Lea and Febiger, 1986.

more central the placement, the higher the complication rate with long-term use of these catheters. The clinician must therefore assess the risk-benefit ratio of arterial cannulation sites in each individual patient. In patients with intense endogenous adrenergically medicated vasoconstriction or under the influence of potent vasoconstricting drugs, monitoring of pressure in small peripheral arteries such as the radial may be inadequate owing to vessel constriction. In the most severely ill patient, rapid insertion of a femoral arterial catheter under optimal sterile conditions provides the most accurate means of monitoring blood pressure. This catheter can always be removed and replaced with a more distal one as the patient's hemodynamic status improves. Alternative sites for arterial pressure monitoring include the radial, brachial, axillary, and dorsalis pedis arteries.

Complications associated with arterial pressure monitoring include bleeding, arterial thrombosis, vasospasm, infection, aneurysm or pseudoaneurysm formation, embolization (distal and proximal), limb ischemia, and pain. Appropriate care must be taken to ensure adequate collateral circulation prior to insertion of the arterial line, if possible, and to follow the patient closely for early signs of ischemia, infection, or embolization at or distal to the insertion site. These catheters should be changed to a new site, under sterile conditions, at least every 72 hours.

CARDIAC FILLING PRESSURE ASSESSMENT. Cardiac preload may need to be assessed invasively in patients with shock, as the physical examination is often not sensitive enough to determine accurately the state of cardiac filling, much less to monitor rapidly changing trends in this important determinant of cardiac output and blood pressure. The relative risk-benefit ratio of invasive hemodynamic monitoring must be assessed in each individual patient. In those patients requiring invasive monitoring, the assessment of central venous pressure (e.g., superior vena caval pressure) alone is inadequate for most patients in shock, as this pressure reflects only diastolic filling of the right ventricle. Central venous pressure monitoring alone may be adequate for the young patient who clearly has no underlying cardiac or pulmonary impairment, is not on a mechanical ventilator, and suffers only from clearly identified hypovolemic shock secondary to trauma. In the critically ill shock patient, the use of a flow-directed pulmonary artery catheter with cardiac output capability is often required for optimal management.

A flow-directed pulmonary artery balloon catheter (Swan-Ganz catheter) is an essential component of the monitoring of most patients in shock. This catheter can be inserted either peripherally from a median antecubital vein or through more central venous access sites such as the percutaneous internal jugular, external jugular, subclavian, or femoral venous approach. Such a catheter can be inserted "blindly" by pressure waveform analysis or under fluoroscopic guidance. During initial catheter insertion, measurements should be obtained of right atrial, right ventricular, pulmonary arterial, and pulmonary capillary wedge pressures during held end-expiration without a Valsalva maneuver. These measurements provide assessment of the preload of the right ventricle (right atrial and right ventricular end-diastolic pressures) and of the left ventricle (pulmonary arterial diastolic and pulmonary capillary wedge pressures). In the absence of significant vascular obstruction between the pulmonary artery and the left ventricle (e.g., severe fixed pulmonary arteriolar hypertension, pulmonary venous occlusive disease, mitral stenosis), the pulmonary capillary wedge pressure should reflect left ventricular end-diastolic pressure and thereby provide an index of left ventricular preload. In the presence of very rapid heart rates or acute severe aortic insufficiency, the pulmonary capillary wedge pressure may not reflect true left ventricular filling pressure.

The clinician must remember, however, that the left ventricular volume is the critical determinant of preload, and the relation between this volume and the left heart filling pressure depends upon the compliance (distensibility) of the ventricle. At the bedside, the clinician can determine in vivo Starling curves in the individual patient by assessing cardiac output at various levels of cardiac filling pressure during incremental volume loading. This also allows an assessment of the compliance of the ventricle by relating the volume infused to the resulting filling pressure. By obtaining measurements of heart rate, blood pressure, cardiac output, pulmonary capillary wedge pressure, and arterial oxygen tension, the optimal preload in an individual patient can be determined which provides adequate perfusion without compromising ventilation.

In selected patients, a series of oximetry blood samples should be obtained during the initial insertion of the pulmonary artery catheter. This is most important in the patient with presumed cardiogenic shock in the setting of a new systolic murmur in whom the differential diagnosis includes ventricular septal rupture (diagnosed by step-up in oxygen saturation from the right atrium to the pulmonary artery) versus mitral insufficiency. It is essential to obtain blood samples from the superior vena cava, right atrium, pulmonary artery, and systemic artery to perform an oximetry series. As a rule of thumb, there should be no greater than a 7 per cent step-up in oxygen saturation from the superior vena cava to the pulmonary artery in the absence of a left-to-right intracardiac shunt.

In general, only right heart catheters that have the added capability for assessment of cardiac output should be utilized in the monitoring of the shock patient. A proximal lumen for right atrial injection, coupled with an in-line thermistor for assessment of temperature at the tip of the catheter in the pulmonary artery, permits bedside assessment of cardiac output by the thermodilution technique. This indicator-dilution technique utilizes injection of cold saline into the right atrium and the time-dependent appearance of the "cold" indicator in the pulmonary artery to construct an indicator-dilution curve for assessment of cardiac output.

In addition, the Swan-Ganz catheter provides a distal monitoring port in the pulmonary artery which can be utilized for drawing pulmonary artery blood samples for chemical determinations. Important among these is the assessment of mixed venous oxygen saturation and content. Simultaneously obtaining arterial and mixed venous (pulmonary arterial blood in the absence of a left-to-right intracardiac shunt) blood samples permits assessment of arterial–mixed venous oxygen content difference, where O_2 content difference (ml/dl) = hemoglobin (grams) × saturation difference × 1.38 (ml O_2 per gram hemoglobin that is 100 per cent saturated). This provides an inverse assessment of cardiac output by the Fick principle and is complementary to the thermodilution technique for measurement of cardiac output. As cardiac output increases, arterial–mixed venous oxygen content difference should narrow, and vice versa, assuming constant hemoglobin content and oxygen consumption. The normal arterial–mixed venous oxygen content difference is 3.0 to 5.0 ml per deciliter and is a clinically useful reflection of oxygen extraction as well as an indicator of the adequacy of cardiac output in relation to systemic metabolic demand.

Newer modifications of the pulmonary artery catheter with an in-line fiberoptic system permit continuous assessment of pulmonary artery saturation (mixed venous saturation), based upon reflectance spectrophotometry. The mixed venous oxygen saturation is determined by the relationship between oxygen delivery and oxygen consumption in the systemic circulation and can be considered a reflection of "oxygen reserve." In general, mixed venous oxygen saturations greater than 65 per cent represent adequate reserves, whereas those less than 35 per cent indicate severe impairment of tissue oxygenation (assuming an arterial $F_{I_{O_2}} = 0.21$, room air).

Continuous monitoring of mixed venous oxygen saturation with fiberoptic catheters provides another complementary continuous assessment of a patient's hemodynamic status. A reduction in mixed venous oxygen saturation may be produced by a decrease in cardiac output, decrease in arterial oxygen saturation, decrease in hemoglobin, or increase in oxygen consumption (e.g., hyperthermia, pain, seizures). Conversely, an increase in mixed venous oxygen saturation may indicate an increase in cardiac output, an increase in inspired oxygen concentration, a decrease in oxygen consumption (e.g., hypothermia, pharmacologic paralysis, anesthesia), a decrease in peripheral tissue oxygen extraction (e.g., sepsis), a left-to-right shunt, or an artifactual increase in mixed venous saturation due to a wedged catheter.

A reduction of mixed venous oxygen saturation to less than 50 per cent is frequently associated with the development of anaerobic metabolism. An important exception to this generalization is sepsis, in which a decrease in tissue oxygenation is associated with an increase in mixed venous oxygen saturation, probably due at least in part to peripheral AV shunting.

Finally, the assessment of pulmonary arterial blood gases permits analysis of pH, P_{CO_2}, and P_{O_2} in the systemic venous return and may have important applications for monitoring the success of cardiopulmonary resuscitation in certain patients.

Further modifications of the Swan-Ganz catheter have permitted monitoring of intracardiac electrocardiograms and the passage of temporary pacing wires into the right ventricle for external electrical pacing of patients with hemodynamically significant bradyarrhythmias.

The clinician must remember that the Swan-Ganz catheter is expensive to insert and monitor, and complications such as arrhythmias, infection, and pulmonary infarction may accompany its use. Rigorous attention to detail and expertise in the use of this catheter are essential to ensure an optimal risk-benefit ratio during its use. These catheters should be inserted only by physicians adequately trained in the use of these devices who possess extensive knowledge pertaining to indications, potential complications, and analysis of the information they provide. The patient with indwelling Swan-Ganz and arterial catheters requires continuous monitoring of pressure waveforms to detect catheter migration or occlusion. Rigorous attention to sterile technique should be employed in the care of the patient with such catheters.

URINARY CATHETER. An indwelling bladder catheter permits hourly assessment of urinary output, a reflection of effective renal perfusion. A decline in urinary output to less than 20 ml per hour is often an indication of inadequate renal perfusion. The most frequent cause of oliguria in the setting of shock is hypovolemia. Fluid deficits are often underestimated, particularly in the presence of sepsis. If oliguria persists despite adequate administration of volume expanders, as confirmed by left heart filling pressures, then additional therapies such as dopamine may be required. The diagnosis of anuria should be made only once it is confirmed that the bladder catheter is patent and there is no obstruction from the renal pelvis to the catheter.

PHYSIOLOGIC SCORING SYSTEMS. Potentially beneficial prospective data acquisition and management systems for evaluating patients requiring admission to critical care environments for shock and other conditions have been under development for over 10 years. These systems have utilized commonly obtained clinical and laboratory data to formulate a prognostic score soon after a patient's admission and thereby attempt to predict a "seriousness-of-illness" index and projected mortality. The goal behind such systems is to guide appropriateness of therapy and utilization of intensive care resources. These attempts to define the extent of physiologic derangements at the time of patient presentation may provide important information relative to management of patients with shock. At present, however, no universally accepted scoring system has been developed.

SPECIALIZED DIAGNOSTIC STUDIES

In addition to the standard diagnostic studies (e.g., electrocardiogram, chest roentgenogram, hematologic and biochemical blood studies) employed in the management of shock patients, certain auxiliary specialized studies may be of benefit in the management of these patients.

ECHOCARDIOGRAPHY. Two-dimensional echocardiography with Doppler capability provides a rapid, noninvasive, and sensitive bedside tool for the evaluation of the patient with unexplained shock. The echocardiogram is particularly useful for providing the following: (1) rapid assessment of generalized and regional myocardial systolic function, (2) evaluation for intrapericardial fluid accumulation and echocardiographic suggestion of tamponade physiology (diastolic right ventricular collapse), (3) assessment of cardiac valves for stenosis, regurgitation, and vegetations, (4) evaluation for intracardiac shunts (e.g., ventricular septal rupture) and left ventricular aneurysm, (5) assessment of prosthetic valve function, and (6) assessment for aortic dissection (transesophageal echocardiography). Noncardiac ultrasound examinations are invaluable for assessment of certain intra-abdominal, pelvic, retroperitoneal, intrathoracic, and other deep masses and fluid accumulations. Identification of abdominal aortic aneurysms, deep venous thromboses, and fetal-uterine abnormalities is an additional feature of ultrasonography that may play an important role in the management of the shock patient.

NUCLEAR MEDICINE STUDIES. A variety of isotope imaging studies may be of benefit in the management of the shock patient. Ventilation-perfusion lung scans may be useful in the diagnosis or exclusion of massive pulmonary emboli. Renal perfusion studies may be of benefit in the differential diagnosis of acute renal failure. First-pass radionuclide ventriculograms provide important information about systolic and diastolic function of the right and left ventricles. Labeled red cell and white cell scans may be of benefit in identifying localized sites of bleeding or abscesses, respectively. Brain flow studies may be of benefit in assessing neurologic status in the shock patient and may help in identifying potential central nervous system pathology.

COMPUTED TOMOGRAPHY AND NUCLEAR MAGNETIC RESONANCE IMAGING. These techniques provide noninvasive anatomic detail of most major regions of the body and can often be very useful in the evaluation of selected patients in shock (e.g., suspected aortic dissection, retroperitoneal hemorrhage, brain stem stroke).

INTERVENTIONAL CARDIOVASCULAR RADIOLOGY STUDIES. Cardiac catheterization is an essential component in the initial evaluation and management of the patient with cardiogenic shock. In addition to providing necessary anatomic diagnosis as a guide to definitive surgical therapy in some patients, cardiac catheterization may provide the route for definitive nonsurgical therapy in certain forms of cardiogenic shock. This includes the use of percutaneous transluminal balloon coronary angioplasty for reperfusion therapy in cardiogenic shock following myocardial infarction, and balloon valvuloplasty as therapy for cardiogenic shock in high surgical risk patients with critical aortic stenosis. Other noncardiac vascular diagnostic procedures are often required for localization of vascular trauma (e.g., aortic dissection), confirmation of suspected massive pulmonary embolism, and definitive therapy in certain cases (e.g., percutaneous insertion of inferior vena cava filter in survivors of submassive pulmonary emboli despite adequate anticoagulation).

Techniques under development for further specialized monitoring of shock patients include transcutaneous monitoring of arterial oxygen and carbon dioxide tensions, tissue electrodes for direct measurement of tissue oxygenation, measurement of respiratory muscle strength by assessment of maximum airway pressures, assessment of respiratory muscle fatigue by measuring tension-time index of the diaphragm, continuous monitoring of end-tidal P_{CO_2} by capnography for assessment of arterial P_{CO_2}, thermal dye techniques for measurement of extravascular lung water, and double-indicator dilution techniques for evaluation of pulmonary endothelial integrity.

THERAPEUTIC GUIDELINES IN SHOCK MANAGEMENT

Management of the patient in shock consists of primary therapy directed at the underlying insult and secondary therapy directed at the consequences of the shock state. Primary therapy depends upon identification of the etiology of the shock state. Examples of primary therapy are surgical repair of a ruptured abdominal aortic aneurysm, pericardiocentesis for cardiac tamponade, and antibiotic therapy for sepsis. Major efforts in the initial management of patients with shock are simultaneously directed at identification and reversal of the primary etiology while at the same time managing the secondary consequences of the shock state (Fig. 41–4). Selected aspects of this management are reviewed.

PAIN CONTROL. Patients in shock are often in pain and may be frightened or agitated. Care must be taken to avoid approaches to these problems that can worsen the underlying hemodynamic instability of the patient. Essentially all pharmacologic measures for pain control or anxiolysis produce some degree of hemodynamic compromise and must therefore be carefully titrated with close observation of the patient's hemodynamic and ventilatory status. In the setting of shock, all medications must be administered via the intravenous route, as absorption of intramuscular or subcutaneous medication is unpredictable and therefore unreliable.

In general, severe pain can be most easily managed by judicious administration of a reversible narcotic such as morphine sulfate (2 to 4 mg IV increments). Potential side effects following morphine include vasodilation with hypotension (mediated by histamine release, direct vasodilation, and neurogenic mechanisms), vagally mediated bradyarrhythmias, respiratory depression, nausea and vomiting, and biliary spasm. The primary route of morphine metabolism is hepatic glucuronic acid conjugation. Patients with hepatic dysfunction, common in shock states, may be very sensitive to the effects of morphine, as may be the elderly. An advantage of morphine and similar opioid agonists is the capacity for rapid pharmacologic antagonism with agents such as naloxone, should adverse effects follow their administration. Naloxone may have additional benefits in shock, as discussed below.

OXYGEN ADMINISTRATION. Oxygen is a drug, and its use should be guided by considerations applicable to the use of other drugs in the treatment of shock. In general, oxygen should be administered initially to most patients in shock, in view of the likelihood of impaired peripheral oxygen delivery. However, the administration should be performed via a high-flow system (one that delivers the entire inspired oxygen atmosphere), so that the fraction of inspired oxygen administered to the patient (FI_{O_2}) is controlled. This permits bedside assessment of the degree of arterial hypoxemia (defined by the alveolar-arterial oxygen gradient), as the calculation of alveolar Po_2 depends upon a known FI_{O_2}. Clinically useful high-flow systems include Venturi masks in the nonintubated patient and ventilators in the intubated patient. An attempt should be made to provide sufficient oxygen to achieve an arterial oxygen saturation of 90 per cent or higher. In the patient requiring positive-pressure ventilation, an attempt should be made to achieve this with an FI_{O_2} of 0.60 or less, in order to reduce the incidence of pulmonary oxygen toxicity. This may be facilitated by the judicious use of positive end-expiratory pressure (PEEP). Continuous assessment of arterial oxygen saturation can be guided by the use of pulse oximetry, but significant alterations in management must be based upon direct assessment of arterial blood gases.

Mechanical ventilation is indicated in the management of the shock patient for the following: (1) apnea or ventilatory failure (acute respiratory acidosis), (2) failure to adequately oxygenate with high-flow system, (3) mechanical splinting of the flail chest wall, (4) relief of the metabolic stress of the work of breathing in selected patients, and (5) adjunctive therapy for other interventions. During mechanical ventilation, careful attention must be paid to the hemodynamic effects of positive intrathoracic pressure. This requires an indwelling pulmonary artery catheter and close assessment of cardiac filling pressure, cardiac output, and arterial blood gases.

CORRECTION OF HYPOVOLEMIA. Hypovolemia is the most common cause of shock seen clinically and may occur in any type of shock, whether or not it is associated with external signs of blood or fluid loss. If there is no evidence of actual fluid or blood loss, there may be significant volume shifts from the intravascular to extracellular spaces because of increased capillary permeability and endothelial damage. This may occur in any vascular bed but is most common in the splanchnic and pulmonary beds. In any shock syndrome associated with decreased tissue perfusion, fluid may also shift intracellularly because of changes in cellular membrane permeability.

The effective and sustained maintenance of cardiac output is critically dependent upon an adequate preload (ventricular filling pressure). The administration of potent inotropic and vasopressor agents in the presence of hypovolemia may be ineffective and often aggravates the clinical condition rather than improves it. As previously discussed, the accurate assessment of cardiac filling pressures often requires the use of invasive hemodynamic monitoring with an indwelling Swan-Ganz catheter. Attempts should be made to provide adequate left heart filling pressures, based upon assessment of the pulmonary capillary wedge pressure and cardiac output. This usually requires maintaining the true (e.g., pulmonary capillary wedge–intrathoracic pressures) filling pressures at or above 10 to 12 mm Hg, but even higher filling pressures (e.g., 18 to 20 mm Hg) may be required in the presence of a noncompliant left ventricle (e.g., acute myocardial infarction shock). These concerns must be balanced by the relative risk of

pulmonary hydrostatic toxicity in some patients with high filling pressures, particularly in the setting of ARDS.

In most cases of shock presenting as profound hypotension and in the absence of obvious acute pulmonary edema, initial management includes positioning the patient in reverse Trendelenburg position (unless head or chest injury contraindicates this position) to permit gravitational return of lower limb blood volume to the central circulation. This should be followed by rapid insertion of large-bore intravenous catheters and the initiation of volume resuscitation with warmed crystalloid solutions. Intravenous infusion volumes of up to 200 ml per minute may be required in some patients and usually require pressurized volume infusion systems. Initial assessment of the adequacy of volume resuscitation can be based upon examination of neck veins, blood pressure, state of consciousness, and clinical signs of tissue perfusion such as color, warmth, capillary refill, and urine volume. In those patients who fail to respond to rapid volume resuscitation, consideration should be given to instituting assessment of cardiac filling pressures with invasive hemodynamic monitoring.

If the patient has cardiogenic shock or signs of pulmonary edema, one should insert a Swan-Ganz catheter prior to administration of volume expanders. If, as frequently happens, the physical examination is misleading and the patient's pulmonary artery diastolic or capillary wedge pressures are less than 12 to 15 mm Hg, one should administer 250 to 500 ml of a crystalloid to the patient every 10 to 15 minutes until achieving a steady left heart filling pressure of 15 to 20 mm Hg. If perfusion of tissues fails to improve or worsens and filling pressures remain above 15 to 20 mm Hg or if true pulmonary edema supervenes, then volume infusion should be stopped and inotropic therapy initiated.

PNEUMATIC ANTI-SHOCK GARMENTS. Lower body external compression garments may be of benefit in certain cases of hypovolemic shock, particularly those involving major trauma. The prototype device is the military anti-shock trouser (MAST) garment. Although controversial, the MAST garment appears to offer potential beneficial effects in certain patients. The MAST suit has been found to increase arterial pressure in hypovolemic shock patients, control certain forms of hemorrhage (e.g., lower abdominal or pelvic), improve carotid and upper body blood flow, and improve the ability of prehospital personnel to start intravenous lines. The mechanisms of action of the garment remain controversial but probably involve decreasing radius of blood vessels compressed by the suit, decreasing the volume of compressed compartments, and increasing venous return. However, potential adverse effects of this device have been identified. These include restriction of blood flow to compressed extremities with increased ischemia, restriction of ventilation, profound hypotension following excessively rapid deflation, renovascular insufficiency, lower extremity compartmental syndromes, arterial thrombosis, and increased bleeding from some vascular injuries. The MAST garment may be of limited short-term benefit for out-of-hospital resuscitation of the traumatic shock patient but should be used only by personnel experienced in the differential diagnosis of shock and familiar with the complications of this device. Prophylactic placement of a noninflated MAST garment should be considered in certain shock patients prior to transport from the scene of trauma to a medical facility, or between medical facilities, especially when the mode of transport (e.g., helicopter) may limit resuscitation techniques.

VOLUME-EXPANDING AGENTS. Debate continues regarding the ideal agent for intravascular volume repletion. In general, this depends upon the etiology of the hypovolemia. Crystalloids are usually the initial agents used for volume resuscitation. Proposed advantages of crystalloids include the argument that the key problem in shock is often shrinkage of the extracellular fluid compartment, which is more appropriately repleted with crystalloid; excessive increases in pulmonary vascular pressures are less likely with crystalloids than colloids; crystalloids are free of the potential for anaphylaxis seen with some colloids; crystalloids can provide safe and effective restoration of circulating blood volume for short periods of time; crystalloids improve microcirculatory flow by reducing blood viscosity; and crystalloids are generally less expensive than colloids.

Selected patients may benefit from colloid administration. Potential advantages of colloids include the finding that smaller volumes of colloids are required to achieve volume repletion because these agents remain in the circulation because of their higher oncotic pressure; greater maintenance of plasma oncotic pressure with colloid than with crystalloid repletion; and the potential metabolic advantages of certain colloid preparations. Obviously, loss of massive amounts of blood in the setting of major trauma should be managed with administration of blood products in combination with crystalloids.

Commonly utilized crystalloids include isotonic normal saline and Ringer's lactate solution. Normal saline contains 140 mEq of sodium and 140 mEq of chloride, whereas Ringer's lactate solution contains 130 mEq of sodium, 4 mEq of potassium, 108 mEq of chloride, and 28 mEq of lactate. When large volumes of fluid are administered, isotonic saline can produce a dilutional acidosis, which can be avoided if Ringer's lactate is used. In contrast, large infusions of Ringer's lactate may produce hyperkalemia in the renal failure patient, and some patients with severe shock may have difficulty metabolizing lactate. In general, initial crystalloid resuscitation of the hypovolemic trauma patient should be given at a ratio of 3:1 per unit of estimated whole blood loss. Crystalloid infusions should be delivered through large-bore catheters with pressure infusion bags if needed, and every effort should be made to infuse solutions previously warmed to normal core body temperature.

Commonly utilized colloids in the management of shock include whole blood, plasma, serum albumin, gelatin preparations, and plasma substitutes such as dextran and hydroxyethyl starch (Hetastarch). Whole blood requires cross-matching and carries the potential risk of disease transmission. However, in cases of massive hemorrhage, whole blood is the preferred agent for volume repletion. Alternative procedures include the administration of packed red blood cells together with crystalloid or colloid volume expanders. Considerations for the use of colloid volume expanders such as albumin or hydroxyethyl starch include major volume resuscitations in which the patient is estimated to have circulating blood volume deficits of 30 per cent or more. In these patients, additional blood component therapy is dictated by the coagulation profile, hemoglobin concentration, and platelet count.

Fresh frozen plasma is a readily available source of biologically active coagulation factors and may therefore be appropriate in some cases of shock. However, other volume expanders may be as effective. In addition, fresh frozen plasma should be considered as an important reserve of coagulation factors and administered when needed for these functions.

Albumin is available as purified albumin, salt-poor purified albumin, and plasma protein fraction albumin. Although it is true that albumin remains in the intravascular space for a longer period than do crystalloids, this is a time-dependent phenomenon and the plasma half-life of exogenously administered albumin is approximately 16 hours. Albumin is clinically available as 5 per cent and 25 per cent solutions in isotonic saline. Potential disadvantages of albumin include potential for lowering serum ionized calcium levels, risk of anaphylaxis, the potential for exacerbating interstitial edema in shock conditions associated with capillary leak (e.g., sepsis, ARDS, intestinal obstruction), and the cost of these preparations. Albumin preparations should not be used indiscriminately.

Dextran is a large polymer of glucose and is commercially available as preparations with average molecular weights of 40,000 and 70,000 (dextran-40 and dextran-70). Both dextran preparations remain in the intravascular space for a significant period of time, longer for dextran-70 (up to 24 hours) than for dextran-40 (several to 12 hours). These agents are eliminated by renal clearance. Theoretically, dextran is an ideal volume expander because of its long "dwell time" in the intravascular space and its biodegradability. Dextran increases plasma volume to a degree equal to or greater than that infused, although this effect is limited by the induced diuresis. The effective volume expansion of dextran-40 is significantly greater than that achieved with 5 per cent albumin and much less expensive. However, the potential advantages of dextran are significantly counterbalanced by serious side effects. The side effects associated with dextran include platelet dysfunction and coagulation abnormalities, anaphylactic reactions, and renal failure. In addition, obligate diuresis occurs following dextran infusion, and therefore urine output cannot be used as an indicator of the sufficiency of volume repletion. Finally, dextran may interfere with cross-matching of blood, can falsely elevate some determinations of blood glucose levels, and may interfere temporarily with the immune function of the reticuloendothelial system.

A newer synthetic colloid used in volume expansion is hydroxyethyl starch (Hetastarch), which resembles glycogen. This agent is available in a 6 per cent solution with average molecular weight of particles being 69,000. Hetastarch has a long half-life in the plasma of greater than 2 weeks. The blood volume expansion achieved with Hetastarch is equal to or greater than that achieved with dextran or albumin, and the side effects appear less. Minor alterations in laboratory coagulation parameters are seen with Hetastarch infusion, but clinical bleeding is rare in doses of less than 1500 ml per day. Hetastarch is not immunogenic, does not produce histamine release, and has a very low incidence of anaphylactic reactions. Serum amylase levels are increased following Hetastarch administration, but no clinical evidence of pancreatic dysfunction is noted.

Hetastarch, as well as the other volume expanders discussed, does not carry oxygen and therefore must be administered in association with blood in patients with massive hemorrhage. During the use of all volume expanders, patients must be carefully monitored for signs of volume overload, especially pulmonary edema.

Limited experimental and clinical trials are currently investigating the potential role of red blood cell substitutes for resuscitation of patients with severe hemorrhagic shock. The use of fluorocarbon red blood cell substitutes, capable of transporting small quantities of oxygen, appears interesting and of potential benefit in selected patients. However, the dilutional effect of these agents and the need for high levels of oxygen administration in such patients may limit the efficacy of this therapy.

CORRECTION OF ACIDOSIS. A significant secondary complication in shock of any etiology is the development of metabolic acidosis as a consequence of tissue ischemia. Severe acidosis impairs metabolic processes, impedes normal neurovascular interactions, and may prevent effective pharmacologic actions of various vasopressor and inotropic agents administered to the shock patient.

The differential diagnosis of metabolic acidosis is aided by calculation of the anion gap, where the anion gap = $[Na^+]$ − $([Cl^-] + [HCO_3^-])$ and should be approximately 12 to 16 mEq per liter. Increases in the anion gap are due to increased endogenous acid production (e.g., lactic acidosis, diabetic ketoacidosis, alcoholic ketoacidosis, starvation), increased exogenous acids (e.g., aspirin toxicity, methanol, ethylene glycol, paraldehyde), or decreased acid excretion (e.g., renal failure). A metabolic acidosis with normal anion gap is usually due to gastrointestinal or renal loss of bicarbonate or may be a complication of parenteral hyperalimentation.

If arterial pH is less than 7.00 and respiratory acidosis has been excluded as the etiology, intravenous sodium bicarbonate should be administered and titrated to maintain a pH in the range of 7.30 or higher. Care must be taken to avoid overcorrection and the induction of metabolic alkalosis, as this may also impair cardiac function and decrease oxygen delivery to the tissues by shifting the oxyhemoglobin dissociation curve to the left. In addition, inappropriate administration of sodium bicarbonate may produce sodium and water overload, can induce hypokalemia, and may worsen central nervous system acidosis.

TREATMENT OF ARRHYTHMIAS. In general, the physician managing the patient in shock should treat disturbances of cardiac electrical activity only if these disturbances produce hemodynamic instability (e.g., hypotension, heart failure, myocardial ischemia) or if the specific rhythm is of clear prognostic significance (e.g., high-degree AV block in the setting of an anterior wall myocardial infarction). It must be remembered that all of the currently available antiarrhythmic agents possess known adverse side effects, and many of them have negative inotropic properties to some degree. Thus, an attempt to "abolish" the appearance of premature ventricular complexes on the monitor in an otherwise electrically stable patient is not appropriate. It is the patient and not the monitor which must be evaluated and treated.

Ventricular fibrillation is managed with nonsynchronized electrical countershock, delivered as rapidly as possible. Standard cardiopulmonary resuscitation may be required until a shock can be delivered or during intervening periods between defibrillation attempts.

Sustained ventricular tachycardia with profound hemodynamic instability should be treated with synchronized electrical countershock. An initial electrical dose of 100 joules should be applied, and repeated if necessary, prior to increasing energy dose. If the ventricular tachycardia is sustained and causes severe hemodynamic compromise, the patient may be treated with intravenous lidocaine, with an initial bolus of 1.0 to 1.5 mg per kilogram, followed by initiation of a continuous infusion at 2 mg per minute and a repeat bolus of 0.5 to 0.75 mg per kilogram 10 to 15 minutes later. Patients who are prone to serious complications following lidocaine are those 65 years of age or older, those in severe heart failure, and those with compromised hepatic function. These are important factors to consider in the management of the shock patient. In particular, care must be taken to follow plasma drug levels in those patients who require sustained infusions. Every effort should be made to discontinue these drugs as soon as possible once the patient has been stabilized, in order to avoid drug-related toxicity. Alternative agents for management of sustained ventricular tachycardia include bretylium and procainamide.

Accelerated idioventricular rhythm is seen frequently in patients with acute myocardial infarction. This is usually a benign rhythm that does not require treatment.

Sinus tachycardia is often an initial autonomically mediated compensatory response to a fall in arterial pressure and cardiac output. Particularly in the young patient, rapid rates of sinus tachycardia must be distinguished from other forms of supraventricular tachycardia in order to avoid inappropriate attempts at conversion of this rhythm. Sinus tachycardia should be considered a diagnostic sign rather than a dysrhythmia.

Supraventricular tachyarrhythmias (atrial tachycardias, atrial flutter, atrial fibrillation) that are associated with marked hemodynamic compromise are best treated with synchronized electrical cardioversion. Atrial flutter may respond to energies as low as 10 to 20 joules, whereas atrial fibrillation may require 100 to 200 or more joules. Medical therapy of these arrhythmias includes the use of digitalis glycosides, calcium channel blockers, and/or β-adrenergic blockers. However, these latter two classes of drugs are relatively contraindicated in the shock patient. Inappropriate administration of potent intravenous calcium channel blockers for treatment of supraventricular tachycardias in patients with underlying shock has been associated with adverse outcomes, including death.

Sinus bradycardia may be a manifestation of rapid, profound, exsanguinating hemorrhage as previously discussed. Other mechanisms of sinus bradycardia include vagally mediated responses to local (e.g., cardiac receptor) or generalized (e.g., pain) noxious stimuli. Sinus bradycardia is commonly seen following inferior wall myocardial infarction, owing to activation of cardiac afferents and inhibitory cardiac reflexes. Sinus bradycardia usually responds to atropine (0.6 to 1.0 mg IV). Care must be taken to avoid too small a dose of atropine (e.g., ≤0.4 mg), as this may induce a centrally mediated vagal response that paradoxically worsens the bradycardia. An adult patient should not be considered "atropine-resistant" until he or she has received a total intravenous dose of 3.0 mg atropine.

Conduction disturbances such as AV block carry a variable prognosis, and the approach to therapy depends on the underlying mechanism and clinical state. In the setting of acute inferior wall myocardial infarction, AV block is usually neurogenically mediated by afferent inhibitory cardiac reflexes, responds to atropine, and has a good prognosis. In contrast, AV block in the setting of anterior wall infarction is usually due to ischemic impairment of the AV node or His bundle, frequently does not respond to atropine, and has a poor prognosis, as it reflects a large infarction. If atropine fails to counteract and reverse the hemodynamic compromise of AV block, external (transthoracic)

or internal (transvenous) electrical pacing can be employed. In general, it is preferred to re-establish organized AV synchrony, with associated atrial loading of ventricular preload, rather than to rely on ventricular pacing alone. This may occasionally require the use of combined atrial and ventricular synchronized electrical pacing modalities.

CORTICOSTEROIDS. The potential beneficial effect of steroids has been suggested to relate primarily to their action on cellular membranes, with stabilization of lysosomal membranes thought to be a primary focus of their effect. Steroids may also prevent the release of β-endorphin, which can cause myocardial depression. The use of steroids in clinical shock remains controversial. At present, there are no well-controlled trials supporting the routine use of steroids in most forms of shock, and several trials have shown no benefit of steroids in the management of septic shock. One of the most controversial areas in critical care medicine is the role of supraphysiologic doses of corticosteroids in the management of septic shock and ARDS. Despite initial enthusiasm for the use of steroids in septic shock in the 1970's, no conclusive data in humans are currently available to support the widespread use of corticosteroids in septic shock. This applies to other nonendocrine forms of shock as well. Similarly, there are no well-accepted data to support the routine use of corticosteroids in patients with ARDS, regardless of the underlying etiology. This applies to ARDS following aspiration and drowning as well as to that occurring in the setting of sepsis. While controversial, recent data from multicenter sepsis studies suggest that steroids may actually worsen the prognosis of patients with sepsis-related ARDS.

The one clear indication for corticosteroid administration in human shock is acute adrenal crisis with cardiovascular collapse. In this setting, prompt therapy with steroids is lifesaving. In addition to steroids, these patients also require vigorous volume repletion and careful monitoring and repletion of serum glucose.

OPIOID ANTAGONISTS. As previously discussed, shock of various etiologies has been associated with an increase in circulating levels of endogenous opioid substances, the most common of which appears to be β-endorphin. Experimental studies in animals with septic shock have suggested that this agent plays an important role in mediating the hypotensive and cardiodepressant effects of sepsis. Experimental studies of hypovolemic and septic shock in animals have suggested that acute antagonism of endogenous opiates with naloxone may produce beneficial hemodynamic effects.

Limited clinical trials since 1981 have suggested that pharmacologic antagonism of these opioids by the administration of the narcotic antagonist naloxone may produce beneficial hemodynamic effects in patients with septic shock. However, these studies have not been conclusive, and contradictory reports of no benefit have been published. A major area of potential concern relates to the most appropriate dose of naloxone to be administered, and in what types of shock this agent might be beneficial. At the present time, this appears to be an area of intense interest, but detailed prospective trials in large numbers of patients need to be performed to resolve the question of benefit. Reports of potential adverse effects following naloxone administration to patients with shock include reversal of opiate analgesia, pulmonary edema, ventricular arrhythmias, and unexpected hypotension.

SYMPATHOMIMETIC AMINES. These drugs are used to increase cardiac output through their inotropic action and to redistribute blood flow to vital organs by their selective vasoconstricting action. The net desired effect of these agents is therefore an increase in arterial pressure and/or cardiac output with improved perfusion of ischemic regions. Unfortunately, no single agent appears to produce the effects desired in all forms of shock, which is not surprising in view of the various mechanisms of the shock state. There are also two potential problems associated with the use of these types of agents. If arterial pressure is elevated significantly, the hypertension can cause a detrimental increase in cardiac afterload and increase myocardial oxygen demand (see Fig. 41–1). Thus, judicious elevation of arterial pressure to levels adequate for peripheral perfusion is the goal, while avoiding excessive hypertension. The blood pressure range needed to meet these criteria varies with each patient. Reasonable guidelines are to achieve a systolic arterial pressure of 110 to 130 mm Hg and to maintain diastolic arterial pressure in the 60- to 80-mm Hg range. The second and related potential problem associated with these agents is their vasoconstricting effect. While some degree of vasoconstriction is desired in nonessential organ beds, it should be avoided in critical organs. Thus, the proper use of sympathomimetic amines requires a thorough knowledge of their cardiovascular effects. These effects depend primarily upon the affinity of the individual agent for various types of adrenergic receptors.

ADRENERGIC RECEPTORS. The adrenergic receptors are classified as α or β receptors with respect to their cardiac and vascular actions. Over the past 10 years, both prejunctional and postjunctional adrenergic receptors have been identified, and various subtypes of receptors have been characterized. Several have been cloned and their primary structure has been defined. However, from a practical clinical standpoint, the catecholamines utilized to treat shock can be understood by considering three specific types of postsynaptic adrenergic receptors. The α receptors are located primarily in blood vessels and mediate vasoconstriction. The β receptors are present in the blood vessels as well as the myocardium. Activation of β_1 receptors in the heart produces an increase in myocardial contractility and heart rate. Activation of β_2 receptors in blood vessels produces vasodilation. The same catecholamine may activate both α and β receptors, depending on the dose and the organ in which it is acting. The net effect depends to a large extent on the relative distribution of the various receptor subtypes in the organ. The sympathomimetic amines that are commonly used clinically in the management of the patient in shock include dopamine, dobutamine, epinephrine, norepinephrine, and isoproterenol. The relative actions and potencies of these agents are summarized in Table 41–5.

Administration of each of these catecholamines to patients carries the potential for adverse side effects. Common to all of these agents are the potential complications of cardiac arrhythmias, nausea, vomiting, ischemia of major organs with prolonged infusions of potent vasoconstrictors, and localized skin necrosis with inadvertent extravasation of these agents.

INOTROPIC AND VASOPRESSOR AGENTS. *Norepinephrine.* Norepinephrine is the primary neurotransmitter of the sympathetic nervous system. It increases myocardial contractility by activating β_1 receptors and thus may increase cardiac output. In blood vessels, it activates primarily α receptors, thereby producing vasoconstriction. The magnitude of its effect on blood vessels varies from one organ to another. Norepinephrine is a very potent vasoconstrictor in skin, muscle, and splanchnic beds, whereas in the coronary vessels it activates the β_2 receptors as well as the α receptors. Because there is a paucity of α receptors in the coronary vessels (in contrast to other vascular beds), norepinephrine causes vasodilation of the coronary arteries.

Norepinephrine offers several distinct advantages in the treatment of shock. It increases cardiac output and redistributes blood flow away from the extremities and toward the heart and brain and increases arterial pressure. This in turn increases coronary blood flow to ischemic myocardium. Because it is a potent peripheral vasoconstrictor, norepinephrine may be particularly useful in septic shock, a condition associated with significant peripheral vasodilation and resultant hypotension.

Norepinephrine should be administered intravenously through a secure catheter, preferably a centrally placed one, in order to diminish the risk of extravasation, which can result in severe

tissue necrosis. Norepinephrine should be initiated at a dose of approximately 0.050 μg per kilogram per minute and the infusion titrated to achieve the desired hemodynamic effect. Upper recommended limits of infusion are approximately 1.0 μg per kilogram per minute. Norepinephrine is rapidly cleared from the circulation with a half-life of 2 to 3 minutes, although this is variable. It is enzymatically degraded in the liver and kidney and is also cleared by regional reuptake into sympathetic nerve terminals.

If hypoxia, hypovolemia, and acidosis have been corrected, the lack of a response to norepinephrine is probably an indication of significant myocardial damage. Prolonged infusions of norepinephrine, or infusions of large doses, are associated with major end-organ (e.g., liver and kidney) ischemic necrosis. It is a potent vasoconstrictor of the pulmonary circulation and should be used with caution in patients with pulmonary hypertension.

Dopamine. This is one of the most commonly utilized drugs in the treatment of shock, probably related to its unique dose-dependent pharmacologic effects. Dopamine is the naturally occurring precursor of norepinephrine. When administered in low doses (1 to 3 μg per kilogram per minute), dopamine activates dopaminergic (DA) vasodilatory receptors in the renal, mesenteric, cerebral, and coronary circulations. DA-1 receptors are located on postsynaptic membranes and mediate vasodilation, and presynaptic DA-2 receptors prevent the release of endogenous norepinephrine, thereby potentiating the vasodilating effects in these circulations. In infusion ranges of 3 to 10 μg per kilogram per minute, dopamine activates β_1-adrenergic receptors and increases heart rate, myocardial contractility, and cardiac output. In doses greater than 20 μg per kilogram per minute, dopamine produces vasoconstriction through activation of α-adrenergic receptors in the arteries and veins of most vascular beds. Thus, at the upper infusion ranges, dopamine may distribute blood flow away from the extremities and toward the kidney, gut, heart, and brain. However, it is necessary to administer moderate to large doses to maintain arterial pressure and coronary blood flow, particularly following myocardial infarction. These larger doses oppose the dopaminergically mediated vasodilation in some vascular beds.

Epinephrine. Epinephrine is an endogenous catecholamine that is produced and released primarily from the adrenal medulla. Epinephrine activates myocardial β_1 receptors and vasoconstrictor α receptors in most vessels except in skeletal muscle and coronary vessels, where it activates β_2 receptors when administered in low doses. It increases cardiac output but redistributes blood flow away from the kidney and splanchnic circulations toward skeletal muscle. At low doses (0.005 to 0.02 μg per kilogram per minute in adults), epinephrine primarily stimulates β-adrenergic receptors and produces peripheral vasodilation and increases in heart rate and contractility. As the infusion rate is increased, α-vasoconstrictor effects become more prominent. Epinephrine also has important respiratory effects, with β_2 receptor–mediated bronchodilation and inhibition of mast cell degranulation. Epinephrine is a potent renal artery vasoconstricting agent in humans, even at low doses, and this limits its clinical utility.

Epinephrine is rapidly cleared from the circulation by the liver and kidney and has a half-life of approximately 2 minutes. Metabolism is via the enzymes catechol-O-methyl transferase and monoamine oxidase. Epinephrine is also well absorbed from the tracheobronchial tree, and this agent may be administered via injection through an endotracheal tube during initial resuscitation of patients in cardiac arrest or those in whom venous access is not yet available.

Isoproterenol. Isoproterenol is a synthetic nonselective β-adrenergic agonist that activates primarily vascular β_2 receptors, resulting in vasodilation, and myocardial β_1 receptors, resulting in an increase in heart rate, contractility, and cardiac output. The magnitude of the vasodilator effect of isoproterenol varies in different vascular beds, depending on the density of β_2 receptors and the affinity of the drug for them. The major vasodilator action of isoproterenol is in skeletal muscle beds.

Isoproterenol is *not* recommended for either cardiogenic or septic shock. In cardiogenic shock, it significantly increases myocardial oxygen demands, and despite the increase in coronary

TABLE 41–5. INITIAL HEMODYNAMIC EFFECTS OF CATECHOLAMINES

Catecholamine	Heart Rate	Arterial Pressure	Cardiac Output	Systemic Resistance
Norepinephrine	(+)	(+ +)	(+)/NC	(+ +)
Epinephrine	(+)	(+)	(+)	(+)/NC
Dopamine	(+)	(+)	(+)	(+)/NC
Isoproterenol	(+)	(−)/NC	(+ +)	(−)
Dobutamine	NC/(+)	NC	(+)	NC/(−)

Note: There may be marked regional variations in reactions of different vascular beds to these agents. (+) = increase; (−) = decrease; NC = no change.

blood flow, the ischemic region of the myocardium may be hypoperfused as indicated by increased lactate production. The use of isoproterenol for shock should probably be limited to the temporary treatment of hemodynamically significant, atropine-resistant high-grade AV block until a temporary pacemaker can be inserted. Even in this condition, the potential for inducing vasodilatory hypotension and increasing ventricular arrhythmias must be recognized. In addition, by overcoming hypoxia-induced pulmonary vasoconstriction in some patients, isoproterenol may increase intrapulmonary shunting of blood and result in a worsening of arterial oxygenation.

Dobutamine. This synthetic sympathomimetic amine has predominant β_1 activity. In contrast to dopamine, dobutamine has much less α-vasoconstricting activity but equal positive inotropic effects. Thus, in equal inotropic doses, dobutamine tends to lower the pulmonary capillary wedge pressure while dopamine tends to increase it. Dobutamine is reported to have a lower incidence of cardiac arrhythmias. In experimental models of myocardial infarction, the administration of dobutamine resulted in significantly smaller infarcts than did dopamine, possibly owing to the intracardiac release of norepinephrine produced by dopamine. Thus, especially in the setting of acute myocardial infarction with pump failure but without significant hypotension, dobutamine may be a preferred agent over dopamine for improving cardiac output.

Dobutamine is usually initiated at an infusion rate of 2 to 5 μg per kilogram per minute and titrated to desired hemodynamic effect. The usual infusion rate is 5 to 15 μg per kilogram per minute. The plasma half-life of dobutamine is approximately 2 to 3 minutes in patients with heart failure, with clearance achieved via catechol-O-methyl transferase.

Amrinone. Amrinone is a bipyridine that differs from the sympathomimetic amines and digitalis glycosides with respect to its mechanism of action. Amrinone has phosphodiesterase-inhibiting action that is thought to be (at least in part) the mechanism of its inotropic effect. It possesses positive inotropic and, to a lesser extent, chronotropic actions and is a potent vasodilator. In patients with heart failure, amrinone augments cardiac dP/dt without significant increases in heart rate or blood pressure and reduces left heart filling pressures as well as systemic vascular resistance. There is, however, wide variability in responses of individual patients to amrinone, which makes dosing guidelines difficult to apply.

The recommended dosage for amrinone is an initial intravenous loading dose of 0.75 mg per kilogram over 3 to 5 minutes, followed by a continuous infusion of 5 to 10 μg per kilogram per minute, and a second loading dose of equal magnitude 30 minutes after the initial load. The total daily dose of amrinone should not exceed 10 mg per kilogram.

Amrinone has a relatively long half-life. It is not approved for use in children. Intravenous amrinone has been associated with thrombocytopenia in approximately 4 per cent of patients, and elevation of liver enzymes is reported with long-term infusion. This agent may be considered as an alternative to dobutamine in patients with severe cardiogenic low output syndromes. In addition, the combined use of amrinone and dobutamine or dopamine may be considered in some patients who fail to respond to one agent alone.

Digitalis Glycosides. In general, digitalis glycosides are not indicated as inotropic agents in the management of shock. This is related to the narrow therapeutic-to-toxic ratio and the difficulty in titrating the dose. In addition, the vasoconstrictor actions of digitalis may exacerbate splanchnic ischemic in the shock patient. The one possible role of digitalis in the management of the shock patient may be heart rate control in patients with atrial fibrillation who cannot be successfully electrically cardioverted. However, even in this condition, digitalis must be given very carefully and the patient monitored closely for adverse effects, particularly if there is superimposed renal impairment.

VASODILATOR AGENTS IN SHOCK. While at first glance the administration of vasodilator agents to patients in shock may seem contradictory, the clinical utility of these agents in certain disorders of low cardiac output emphasizes the critical relationship between the contractile state of the ventricle and the afterload against which it must contract. In general, the beneficial effects of vasodilators are to (1) decrease myocardial metabolic demands by decreasing cardiac preload and cardiac size, (2) to decrease ventricular afterload and increase cardiac output without adversely affecting mean perfusion pressure, and (3) to dilate microcirculatory vessels. An important point that must be stressed is that the beneficial effects of vasodilator agents in the therapy of severe heart failure and/or shock depend upon the presence of adequate (e.g., not reduced) cardiac filling pressures and the ability of the ventricle to respond to changes in preload or afterload (e.g., absence of fixed obstructions to cardiac flow, such as is seen with critical aortic stenosis).

Reduction in Preload. Patients in cardiogenic shock may require a high preload and filling pressure to maintain an adequate stroke volume. However, an excessive elevation of filling pressure is detrimental because of pulmonary congestion and increased myocardial oxygen demand. A reduction in myocardial oxygen demand without a significant reduction in stroke volume can be achieved by decreasing ventricular volume and size in patients who have abnormally elevated cardiac filling pressures (e.g., pulmonary capillary wedge pressures of 18 mm Hg or greater) and evidence of pulmonary congestion. Reduction in cardiac size decreases myocardial wall tension, which is a major determinant of myocardial oxygen requirements. Preload may be reduced by the use of diuretic agents or venodilating drugs. The goal of venodilator therapy is to decrease cardiac preload and cardiac size without altering arterial blood pressure. As previously noted, the efficacy of such an approach depends upon the compliance of the ventricle. A reduction in excessively high cardiac preload may be of benefit not only in reducing myocardial oxygen demands, but also in relieving pulmonary venous congestion and pulmonary edema. In some patients with marked increases in preload, in association with marked impairment of contractile performance and borderline hypotension, it may be desirable and necessary to combine a vasodilator agent with an inotropic agent so as to maintain mean arterial pressure within acceptable bounds.

Reduction in Afterload. It is possible to reduce afterload on a failing ventricle without adversely altering mean arterial pressure, by nature of the increase in cardiac output that usually follows the reduction in afterload. However, such an approach requires close hemodynamic monitoring, and systemic hypotension is always a potentially catastrophic side effect of afterload reduction in patients with severely compromised hemodynamic status. During administration of afterload-reducing vasodilators, the systolic arterial pressure should not fall more than 10 mm Hg (unless the patient is being treated for hypertension), and the diastolic arterial pressure (coronary perfusion pressure) should be maintained at or above 60 to 65 mm Hg in most patients. Reduction in ventricular afterload is ideal in the patient with severe heart failure, marked pulmonary venous hypertension with pulmonary edema, and impaired cardiac output but without systemic arterial hypotension of significant degree.

Arteriolar vasodilators are particularly effective in the management of shock due to acute intracardiac left-to-right shunts or regurgitant lesions. Examples of these conditions include acute ventricular septal rupture, acute mitral insufficiency due to papillary muscle rupture, and acute aortic insufficiency due to flail aortic valve leaflet complicating bacterial endocarditis. By acutely reducing impedance to ventricular ejection, nitroprusside may limit the degree of left-to-right shunt in the setting of a septal defect or the degree of mitral insufficiency or aortic insufficiency by reducing resistance to ventricular ejection. However, this effect is frequently achieved at the expense of an increase in heart rate due to unloading of arterial baroreceptors by this agent.

Microcirculatory Vasodilation. In some patients, despite prolonged administration of dopamine or norepinephrine, tissue perfusion is not improved. The reason may be that extensive myocardial damage has occurred. It is also possible that constriction of microcirculatory vessels may prevent perfusion of exchange capillaries.

Nitroprusside. Nitroprusside is a cyanide-containing, direct-acting, smooth muscle–vasodilating agent that causes relaxation of both arteries and veins. It is the classic "balanced" vasodilator, with effects on both capacitance and resistance vessels. The mode of action of nitroprusside is believed to involve activation of soluble guanylate cyclase with consequent elevation of cGMP in vascular smooth muscle cells, leading to activation of cGMP-dependent protein kinase activity. It does not depend upon the sympathetic nervous system or adrenergic receptors. Its onset of action is within seconds of administration, and its duration of effect is 1 to 3 minutes. Nitroprusside can be initiated as an intravenous infusion at approximately 10 μg per minute, with the rate increased every 5 to 10 minutes by 10 μg per minute increments until the desired hemodynamic effect is achieved.

In the setting of power failure following myocardial infarction, nitroprusside should be administered only to patients who are instrumented with indwelling systemic and pulmonary arterial catheters, as the clinician needs to follow arterial and cardiac filling pressures closely during infusion of this very potent vasodilator.

The principal complications associated with nitroprusside infusion include the possibility of hypotension, thiocyanate/cyanide toxicity with prolonged (≥72 hour) infusions of high doses, and a reduction in arterial oxygen tension due to pulmonary vascular vasodilating effects and consequent increase in ventilation-perfusion mismatching.

Nitroglycerin. This is also a very effective vasodilator with predominant effects on the venous capacitance vessels and lesser effects on arteriolar resistance vessels. When therapy is initiated, nitroglycerin can be started as an intravenous infusion of 10 μg per minute, then titrated upward in 10 μg per minute increments every 3 to 5 minutes as indicated by hemodynamics. Nitroglycerin is particularly effective in the management of acute pulmonary edema complicating myocardial infarction. Adverse side effects include headache, hypotension, and occasional nausea and vomiting.

MECHANICAL AND ARTIFICIAL CARDIOPULMONARY ASSISTANCE IN SHOCK. Recent advances have made available various mechanical support devices for the temporary management of patients with medically refractory shock of various etiologies. While clinical experience is limited and controlled clinical trials often are not available, consideration of such devices is appropriate in certain subgroups of patients.

Intra-aortic Balloon Counterpulsation. The intra-aortic balloon pump (IABP) has been used for 15 years in the management of certain types of cardiogenic shock. Currently, the device can be inserted percutaneously through a femoral artery and advanced under fluoroscopic guidance to the thoracic aorta just distal to the left subclavian artery. The balloon is mechanically inflated with carbon dioxide or helium during diastole and rapidly deflated at the onset of ventricular systole. The primary effects of the balloon are therefore (1) an increase in diastolic aortic root (coronary perfusion) pressure, and (2) a mechanical reduction in aortic root blood pressure and volume (impedance) at the onset of systole. The desired hemodynamic effects of the intra-aortic balloon pump are an increase in coronary perfusion pressure, a reduction in ventricular afterload, an increase in forward cardiac ejection fraction, and a reduction in left-to-right or backward cardiac flow.

The IABP is most useful in the management of patients with cardiogenic shock due to acute ventricular septal rupture or acute papillary muscle rupture or dysfunction with mitral insufficiency. In contrast to similar afterload-reducing effects achieved with nitroprusside, the IABP can reduce impedance to ventricular ejection without causing an increase in heart rate (myocardial oxygen demand). At the same time, the mechanical increase in peak augmented diastolic arterial pressure provides an increase in myocardial oxygen supply. The IABP may also be of temporary benefit in patients with ischemia-induced ventricular depression in the setting of high-grade coronary artery lesions, until revascularization can be achieved (i.e., coronary angioplasty or coronary artery bypass surgery) or following cardiopulmonary bypass.

The IABP should be considered only a temporary support device and should be used only in patients who have a correctable cardiac lesion or reasonable likelihood of recovery from an acute cardiac insult. Despite optimal technique, a major complication rate of approximately 10 to 30 per cent is reported with the device, most notably secondary to distal limb ischemia, vascular damage, or infection. The IABP is contraindicated in patients with aortic insufficiency, severe peripheral vascular disease, or

inability to tolerate systemic anticoagulation. The IABP may be a useful support device for patients undergoing major surgery (cardiac or otherwise) in the presence of severe impairment of cardiac function.

Cardiac Assist Devices and Artificial Heart. Significant progress has been made over the past 33 years since the first heart-lung machine was used in 1957 to support a patient with cardiogenic shock following acute myocardial infarction. In selected patients with refractory cardiogenic shock, external left and/or right cardiac assist devices have been used to "bridge" patients to cardiac transplant or permit patient survival for a long enough period to allow recovery of intrinsic myocardial function (e.g., in certain patients with severe inflammatory myocarditis). These assist devices require surgical thoracotomy for insertion of large vascular conduits involving the great vessels or the atria and ventricles themselves. Major complications including infection, bleeding, and thrombosis with systemic embolization have been reported with these devices. However, they have been successfully used as a bridge to successful cardiac transplantation in selected patients.

Implantable mechanical heart devices have been reported in a small number of patients, but no long-term success has been achieved and major complications are associated with these devices. Implantable artificial hearts have been utilized for up to 243 days in patients awaiting cardiac transplantation.

Extracorporeal Membrane Oxygenator and Bedside Cardiopulmonary Bypass. Additional recent experience has been reported with emergent bedside initiation of full cardiopulmonary bypass via percutaneous femoral arterial and venous approaches, utilizing a portable cardiopulmonary bypass machine with membrane oxygenator. Limited experience has been reported with this technique in patients with refractory shock or cardiac arrest.

NUTRITIONAL SUPPORT OF THE SHOCK PATIENT

A frequently overlooked but extremely important aspect of the care of the shock patient is nutritional support. In many cases, wound healing, tissue repair, weaning from ventilator support, and therefore long-term survival may be adversely influenced by failure to appreciate the metabolic stresses of the shock state and to provide adequate nutritional support during the early as well as later phases of treatment. Time is a crucial element in the nutritional support of the shock patient. The physician must not allow his or her attention to other traditional details of management to prevent or delay attention to this important aspect of the patient's care. In general, most patients developing shock have suffered major metabolic insults and can rapidly develop catabolic states. This is particularly true of the intubated patient or the patient maintained NPO for extended periods of time following resuscitation. In the case of intubation, the placement of an endotracheal tube should routinely be followed by the placement of a nasogastric tube for initial gastric decompression and then conversion to a gastric feeding tube. Potential contraindications to nasogastric tube placement include midline craniofacial and head trauma, suspected or potential esophageal perforation, and known obstruction of the esophagus.

As soon as possible, patients should begin receiving nutritional support via enteral or parenteral routes. Close monitoring should be performed on a routine basis with daily determinations of calorie intake and biweekly determinations of serum albumin, electrolytes, total lymphocyte count, transferrin level, liver function studies, and prothrombin time. Estimations of carbohydrate, protein, and fat requirements should be based upon the patient's nitrogen balance, nature of insult, and associated medical problems. Continuing assessment of vitamin and essential trace metal levels is important in the long-term care of these patients.

Abboud FM, Heistad DD, Mark AL, Schmid PG: Reflex control of the peripheral circulation. Prog Cardiovasc Dis 18:371–403, 1976. *Review of the major factors of autonomic circulatory control operative in both healthy human subjects and under various disease states.*

Altura BM, Lefer AM, Schumer W: Historical perspective of shock. *In* Altura BM, Lefer AM, Schumer W (eds.): Handbook of Shock and Trauma. New York, Raven Press, 1983. *Provides historical review of the development of understanding of pathophysiology and treatment of shock.*

Bernton EW, Long JB, Holaday JW: Opioids and neuropeptides: Mechanisms in circulatory shock. Fed Proc 44:290–299, 1985. *Reviews potential roles of endogenous opioids, thyrotropin-releasing hormone, and other neuropeptides in central cardiovascular regulatory mechanisms during shock.*

Beutler B, Cerami A: Cachectin/tumor necrosis factor: An endogenous mediator of shock and inflammation. Immunol Res 5:281–293, 1986. *Provides a perspective on the biologic role of tumor necrosis factor as a mediator of the cellular toxicity associated with endotoxic shock.*

Bone RC, Fisher CJ, Clemmer TP, et al. and the Methylprednisolone Severe Sepsis Study Group: A controlled clinical trial of high-dose methylprednisolone in the treatment of severe sepsis and septic shock. N Engl J Med 317:653–658, 1987. *Report of a large, prospective, double-blind, placebo-controlled trial of methylprednisolone in management of patients with sepsis and septic shock, showing no benefit of this steroid and an increase in secondary infections in the steroid-treated patients.*

Chaudry IH: Cellular alteration in shock and ischemia and their correction. Physiologist 28:109–117, 1985. *Presents an overview of cellular and subcellular events in shock in a well-organized manner.*

Ellrodt AG: Sepsis and septic shock. Emerg Med Clin North Am 4:809–840, 1986. *Provides well-referenced overview of most important areas in etiology, pathophysiology, and treatment of septic shock.*

Goldberg LI, Rajfer SI: Dopamine receptors: Applications in clinical cardiology. Circulation 72:245–248, 1985. *Reviews the cardiovascular and renal actions of dopamine and emphasizes the unique effects of this agent on dopaminergic receptors.*

Lefer AM: Eicosanoids as mediators of ischemia and shock. Fed Proc 44:275–280, 1985. *Provides an overview of the variety and role of eicosanoids identified in ischemic and circulatory shock and discusses potential pharmacologic modulation of these mediators.*

Lefer AM: Interaction between myocardial depressant factor and vasoactive mediators with ischemia and shock. Am J Physiol 252 (Regulatory Integrative Comp. Physiol. 21):R193–R205, 1987. *This excellent review discusses a variety of vasoactive mediators produced in ischemia and shock states, with particular emphasis on myocardial depressant factor, and reviews new pharmacologic approaches to the blockade of these mediators.*

McSwain NE Jr.: Pneumatic anti-shock garment: State of the art 1988. Ann Emerg Med 17:506–525, 1988. *Provides exhaustive experimental and clinical information on the use of external pneumatic pressure trousers (MAST suit) in the management of hypotension and shock.*

Parrillo JE, Burch C, Shelhamer JH, et al: A circulating myocardial depressant substance in humans with septic shock. J Clin Invest 76:1539–1553, 1985. *Study of the cardiodepressant effect of serum extract from patients with septic shock and myocardial depression.*

Sanders JS, Ferguson DW: Profound sympathoinhibition complicating hypovolemia in humans. Ann Intern Med 111:439–441, 1989. *Reviews the potential mechanisms responsible for paradoxic autonomic response to acute hypovolemic hypotension in humans.*

Shapiro BA, Cane RD: Blood gas monitoring: Yesterday, today, and tomorrow. Crit Care Med 17:573–581, 1989. *Reviews the history of blood gas determination and provides an up-to-date assessment of new monitoring techniques.*

Suffredini AF, Fromm RE, Parker MM, et al.: The cardiovascular response of normal humans to the administration of endotoxin. N Engl J Med 321:280–287, 1989. *Report of careful hemodynamic measurements obtained in normal human subjects following administration of bacterial endotoxin, demonstrating left ventricular systolic depression independent of changes in ventricular volume or systemic vascular resistance.*

Tobin MJ: Respiratory monitoring in the intensive care unit. Am Rev Resp Dis 138:1625–1642, 1988. *Extensive review of recent advances in monitoring ventilation/respiration parameters in the intensive care environment.*

Zimmerman JJ, Dietrich KA: Current perspectives on septic shock. Pediatr Clin North Am 34:131–163, 1987. *Comprehensive overview of pathophysiology of septic shock.*

42 Cardiac Arrhythmias

J. Thomas Bigger, Jr.

Optimal management of cardiac arrhythmias requires knowledge of their (1) mechanism, etiology, and natural history and (2) effect on the hemodynamic state. Before selecting therapy, the physician should thoroughly assess the patient's physical, psychological, and biochemical state. The chosen treatment—whether drugs, devices, or surgery—must be monitored closely for its initial and continued effectiveness and for adverse effects. This chapter discusses mechanisms, electrocardiographic (ECG) recognition, and management of cardiac arrhythmias.

ANATOMIC CONSIDERATIONS

Normal Specialized Impulse-Generating and Conducting System

SINUS NODE. The sinus node is situated at the junction between the superior vena cava and the right atrium. The node surrounds a large central artery arising from the right (55 per cent) or left (45 per cent) circumflex coronary artery. Two types of special muscle fibers are found in the node: P (pacemaker) and T (transitional) cells. P cells are small (diameter of 5 to 10 μ) ovoid or stellate cells that have a low density of mitochondria, sarcoplasmic reticulum, and myofibrils, suggesting a lack of contractile function. P cells occur in tight clusters and attach only to other P cells or T cells; intercellular attachments are sparse, correlating with the slow conduction in the sinus node.

T cells are intermediate in size, structure, and cellular organization between P cells and ordinary atrial myocardium. T cells may attach either to P cells or to working myocardial cells. T cells surround the sinus node and presumably serve both to organize impulses leaving the node and to hinder access of premature ectopic atrial impulses.

INTERNODAL TRACTS. Three internodal tracts connecting the sinus node to the atrioventricular (AV) node have been described: anterior, middle, and posterior. The *anterior internodal tract* also connects to the left atrium via the interatrial bundle of Bachmann. The three internodal tracts are widely separated in the interatrial septum but converge above and behind the AV node.

Internodal tracts contain working atrial cells interspersed with large cells that resemble ventricular Purkinje cells. Because internodal pathways are difficult to trace by serial microscopic sections, some doubt their presence or functional significance. Internodal tracts continue to function in high extracellular K^+ concentrations, a property that has been used to demonstrate their functional continuity and preferential internodal conductivity.

ATRIOVENTRICULAR NODE. The AV node lies beneath the endocardium of the right atrium near the septal leaflet of the tricuspid valve and immediately anterior to the ostium of the coronary sinus. The AV nodal artery usually arises from the right coronary artery. In the central portion of the AV node, the myocytes form tangled swirls with ample interconnections. Ultrastructurally, cells in the mid-AV node resemble the sinus node T cells. Toward the distal end of the AV node, myocytes pallisade into linear arrays as they form the bundle of His.

The region between the ostium of the coronary sinus and the posterior margin of the AV node is richly supplied by cholinergic ganglia. Retronodal chemoreceptors may trigger vagal reflexes during ischemia of the posterior wall of the heart. These reflexes can produce marked bradycardia, peripheral vasodilatation, nausea, sweating, and salivation.

HIS-PURKINJE SYSTEM. The AV bundle (bundle of His) is a thick, cable-like structure about 15 mm in length that emerges from the anterior, inferior border of the AV node (Fig. 42–1). The bundle of His penetrates the central fibrous body and courses to the crest of the muscular interventricular septum, where it divides into left and right bundle branches. The His bundle is the only normal route for AV conduction. Damage to the AV bundle can cause AV conduction delay or block. The His bundle is generously supplied with arterial blood from the anterior and posterior descending coronary arteries; therefore, extensive coronary disease is required to produce ischemic damage.

The left bundle branch is a broad sheet of fibers that cascade under the noncoronary cusp of the aortic valve and down the left side of the interventricular septum. The left bundle branch connects first with myocardium in the septum and near the papillary muscles, causing early activation of these regions.

The right bundle branch emerges from the bundle of His and courses down the right side of the interventricular septum to make its first connections with ventricular myocardium near the base of the anterior papillary muscle. From here, peripheral branches spread up the interventricular septum and the free wall of the right ventricle.

The terminal Purkinje fibers form extensive interconnected lacy networks on the endocardium of both ventricles. In human hearts, no Purkinje fibers are found in the outer two thirds of the ventricular walls. Purkinje cells are large—15 to 30 mm in diameter and 20 to 100 mm in length—with a round, centrally located nucleus in the cell. Purkinje fibers contain fewer myofibrils and mitochondria than working ventricular muscle. External to the sarcolemmal basement membrane is a thick surface coat of negatively charged glycoproteins that function in Ca^{2+} binding

FIGURE 42–1. The anatomy and characteristic action potentials of the specialized impulse-generating and conducting system of the heart. A, A diagram of the conduction system of the heart. SAN = Sinoatrial node; AVN = atrioventricular node; HB = bundle of His; RBB = right bundle branch; LBB = left bundle branch; PF = Purkinje fiber. B, Typical action potentials from the sinus node (SN), atrium (AT), atrioventricular node (AVN), Purkinje fiber (PF), and ventricular muscle (VM). C, Relationship of deflections in the His bundle (HB) electrogram to depolarization of the sites shown in B and to the electrocardiographic deflections. Depolarization of the lower atrial septum (A), bundle of His (H), and ventricular septum (V) is recorded in the bipolar His bundle electrogram. The H deflection partitions the PR interval into two subintervals: the AH interval, representing atrioventricular nodal conduction, and the HV interval, which measures conduction to the His-Purkinje system. (From Braunwald E: Heart Disease: A Textbook of Cardiovascular Medicine. Philadelphia, W. B. Saunders Company, 1980.)

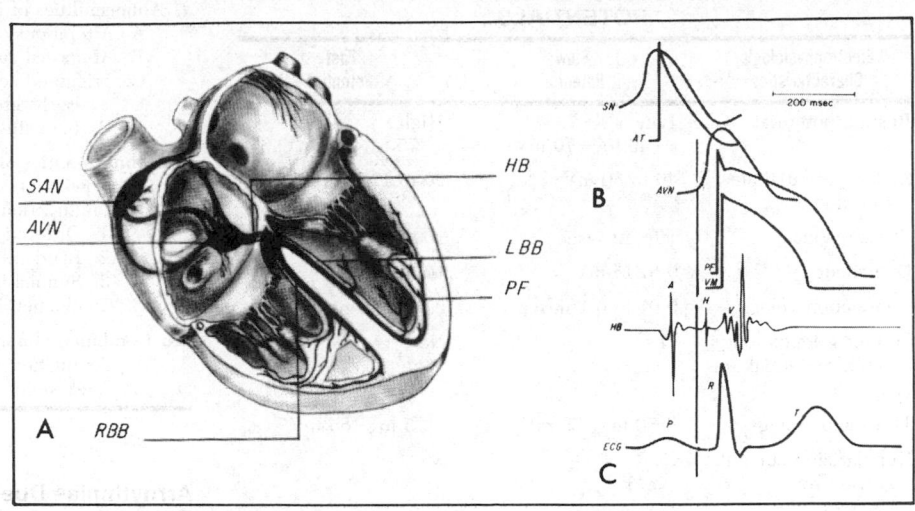

and exchange. Intercalated disks are well developed in Purkinje fibers and provide low-resistance pathways for current flow and for diffusion of ions and small molecules.

Function of the Specialized Impulse-Generating and Conducting System

The normal heartbeat begins in the sinus node and spreads slowly through perinodal fibers to reach specialized atrial tracts and ordinary atrial muscle (Fig. 42–1). Specialized atrial tracts transmit the cardiac impulse rapidly from the sinus node to the AV node and to the left atrium. The cardiac impulse slows dramatically in the AV node, accounting for most of the PR interval in the ECG. Conduction accelerates tremendously in the His bundle, and excitation of the bundle branches and peripheral Purkinje fibers occurs with blazing speed. The great mass of ordinary ventricular muscle is activated almost simultaneously over much of its endocardial surface. Then activation spreads to the epicardium to complete the cardiac excitation cycle.

BRIEF REVIEW OF CARDIAC CELLULAR ELECTROPHYSIOLOGY

RESTING POTENTIAL. The sarcolemma of cardiac cells is a hydrophobic phospholipid bilayer. Protein molecules that cross the entire width of the membrane provide hydrophilic channels and permit hydrated cations or anions to cross the sarcolemma. Ion-selective channels and energy-dependent ion pumping establish transmembrane gradients of Na^+ and K^+ that determine the resting voltage difference of about -80 to -90 mV across the sarcolemma, the *resting transmembrane voltage* (Vm).

ACTION POTENTIALS. When cardiac cells activate, a complex sequence of voltage changes occurs as a function of time and membrane ionic currents. Figure 42–2 diagrams the four phases of a Purkinje fiber *action potential*. Sinus and AV nodal cells have a slowly rising phase 0 and lack distinct phases 1, 2, and 3 (see Fig. 42–1). During phase 4, many cells have a steady transmembrane voltage, but automatic fibers in the sinus node and His-Purkinje system spontaneously depolarize and can initiate impulses that propagate to the rest of the heart.

OVERDRIVE SUPPRESSION. In the normal heart, P cells in the sinus node depolarize and overdrive subsidiary pacemaker cells in the atrial specialized tracts, coronary sinus region, or His-Purkinje system. The faster subsidiary pacemakers are overdriven, the more Na^+ centers the cell per unit of time. As the $[Na]_i$ increases, the activity of the Na^+/K^+ exchange pump becomes more electrogenic; i.e., the ratio of Na^+ out to K^+ in increases, hyperpolarizing the cell and counteracting pacemaker activity. If the dominant pacemaker stops, there is a pause in rhythm. However, as the $[Na]_i$ is pumped out, outward pump current declines until spontaneous depolarization resumes. As the pump current declines, the firing rate in the subsidiary pacemaker increases gradually—the "warm-up" phenomenon.

FAST AND SLOW RESPONSES. Cardiac action potentials are classified as *fast* or *slow* responses (Table 42–1). The *fast response* (Fig. 42–3) is generated by intense inward i_{Na}, has a large, fast-rising phase 0, propagates rapidly, and has a large safety factor for conduction. Working myocardial cells in the atria, ventricles, and Purkinje fibers have fast responses. The *slow response* has a slowly rising phase 0, propagates slowly, and has a low safety factor for conduction (Fig. 42–3). Cells in the sinus node, pectinate muscles, AV node, and AV rings have slow responses. Depolarization in slow response fibers is due to slow inward current (i_{si}) carried by Ca^{2+} and, to a lesser extent, Na^+ ions.

REFRACTORINESS. Refractoriness is involved in the pathogenesis of many arrhythmias and in the action of antiarrhythmic drugs. The effective refractory period (ERP), the minimum interval between two propagating responses, is closely linked to

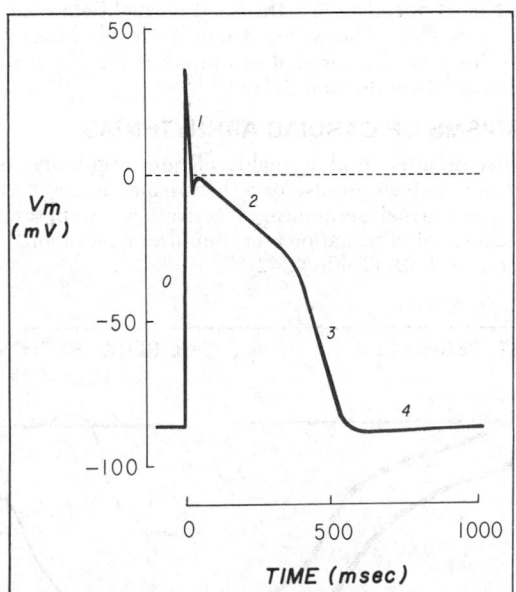

FIGURE 42–2. The cardiac action potential of a Purkinje fiber has five distinct phases: rapid depolarization (0), early repolarization (1), plateau (2), rapid repolarization (3), and diastole (4). (From Braunwald E: Heart Disease: A Textbook of Cardiovascular Medicine. Philadelphia, W. B. Saunders Company, 1980.)

TABLE 42–1. COMPARISON OF SLOW AND FAST ACTION POTENTIALS

Electrophysiologic Characteristics	Slow Potential	Fast Potential
Resting potential	Low (−40 to −70 mV)	High (−75 to −90 mV)
Action potential amplitude	40 to 80 mV	90 to 120 mV
Phase 0 Vmax	1 to 10 V/sec	200 to 800 V/sec
Overshoot	0 to 15 mV	10 to 30 mV
Conduction velocity	0.01 to 0.1 m/sec	0.5 to 3.0 m/sec
Stimulus-dependent action potential amplitude	Yes	No
Threshold voltage	−50 to −30 mV	−75 to −65 mV
Depolarizing current carried by	Ca^{2+} (Na^+)	Na^+
Ionic current activates	Slow (0.5 msec)	Fast (10 to 20 msec)
Ionic current inactivates	Slow (0.5 msec)	Fast (50 to 100 msec)
Channel blocked by	Mn^{2+}, LA^{3+}, verapamil diltiazem, nifedipine	Tetrodotoxin, class 1 antiarrhythmics

action potential duration (APD) in fast-response fibers because recovery from inactivation in the Na^+ channel closely parallels repolarization. However, in sinus and AV nodal cells (slow responses), refractoriness can outlast full repolarization so that the ERP is much longer than the APD.

RESPONSIVENESS AND CONDUCTION. The term *membrane responsiveness* applies to the response of a cardiac fiber to a stimulus. Changes in the maximum rate of depolarization during phase 0 (max) provide an index of changes in availability of the Na^+ current. In cardiac Purkinje fibers and other fast-response fibers, V_{max} is strongly dependent on Vm at the instant of excitation; as soon as the fiber is fully repolarized, it is fully responsive. In slow-response fibers, responsiveness does not return until well after repolarization is complete. There is a considerable safety factor for conduction in fast-response fibers; V_{max} must be reduced to less than half normal before conduction velocity decreases. The safety factor is much lower in slow-response fibers so that premature impulses are likely to experience substantial conduction delay or block.

MECHANISMS OF CARDIAC ARRHYTHMIAS

An arrhythmia is an abnormality of rate, regularity, or site of origin of the cardiac impulse or a disturbance in conduction that causes an abnormal sequence of activation. Arrhythmias may arise because of alternations in impulse generation, impulse conduction, or both (Table 42–2).

TABLE 42–2. MECHANISMS RESPONSIBLE FOR CARDIAC ARRHYTHMIAS

I. **Abnormalities of impulse generation**
  A. Alterations of normal automaticity
  B. Abnormal automaticity
  C. Triggered activity
    1. Early afterdepolarizations
    2. Late afterdepolarizations

II. **Abnormalities of impulse conduction**
  A. Slowing of conduction and block
  B. Unidirectional block and reentry
    1. Ordered reentry
    2. Random reentry
    3. Summation and inhibition
  C. Conduction block, electrotonus, and reflection

III. **Combined abnormalities of impulse generation and conduction**
  A. Conduction showed by phase 4 depolarization
  B. Parasystole

Arrhythmias Due to Abnormalities of Impulse Generation

Many arrhythmias arise because of either depressed or enhanced normal automaticity. Abnormal automaticity and triggered activity also are important mechanisms for arrhythmogenesis.

ALTERED NORMAL AUTOMATICITY. Only a few cardiac cell types develop normal automaticity: sinus node, internodal tracts, fibers near the ostium of the coronary sinus, distal AV node, and the His-Purkinje system.

Sinus Node. The rate of firing in the sinus node can be altered by autonomic activity or intrinsic disease. Increased vagal activity can slow or stop sinus node pacemakers by increasing membrane K^+ conductance of P cells. Increased sympathetic nerve traffic to the sinus node causes sinus tachycardia.

Purkinje Fibers. Augmented automaticity due to increased sympathetic nerve activity in the His-Purkinje system is a common cause of human arrhythmias. AV junctional pacemakers can fire faster than a normal sinus node because of selective traffic on sympathetic nerves, local release of catecholamines, or enhanced responsiveness of β-adrenergic receptors. Also, vagal and sympathetic activity can increase together; the vagus slows the sinus rate and AV conduction while sympathetic activity increases the firing rate in the His-Purkinje system.

In diseased hearts, automaticity in the His-Purkinje system may become reduced. In the sick sinus syndrome, it is typical for the ventricular escape pacemakers to be depressed, producing long pauses when the sinus node pacemaker fails. In AV block due to bundle branch disease, ventricular pacemakers also may be abnormally slow.

Abnormal Impulse Generation

Abnormal automaticity or triggered activity can generate impulses even in fibers that are incapable of normal automaticity, e.g., ordinary atrial or ventricular muscle cells.

ABNORMAL AUTOMATICITY. Abnormal automaticity refers to spontaneous diastolic depolarization in depolarized cells. Pur-

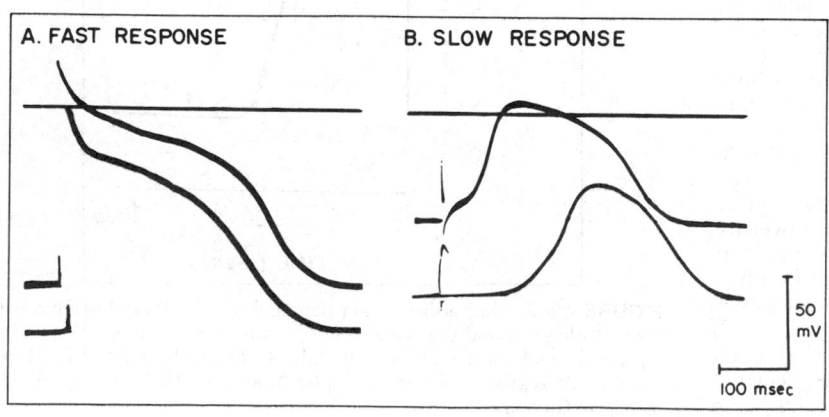

A. FAST RESPONSE B. SLOW RESPONSE

50 mV

100 msec

FIGURE 42–3. Two types of cardiac action potentials: (A) fast action potential, (B) slow action potential. (From Wit AL, Rosen MR, Hoffman BF: Electrophysiology and pharmacology of cardiac arrhythmias. II. Relationship of normal and abnormal electrical activity of cardiac fibers to the genesis of arrhythmias. Am Heart J 88:515–524, 1974. With permission of the publisher.)

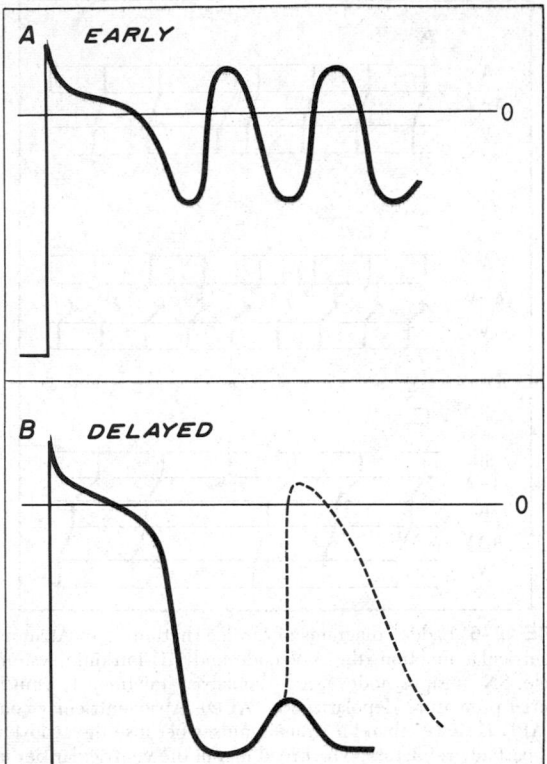

FIGURE 42–4. Afterdepolarizations and triggered activity. *A,* Early afterdepolarization. Repolarization of the Purkinje fiber is interrupted by two secondary depolarizations, which can activate adjacent fibers and cause arrhythmias, e.g., torsades de pointes. *B,* Delayed afterdepolarizations. After full repolarization, the Purkinje fiber depolarizes. If the afterdepolarization reaches threshold voltage, a propagating response can occur. (From Bigger JT: Electrophysiology for the clinician. Eur Heart J 5(Suppl B):1–9, 1984.)

kinje fibers, atrial cells, and ventricular cells can show spontaneous diastolic depolarization and repetitive automatic firing when their resting Vm is reduced to -60 mV or below. Abnormal automaticity is seen in Purkinje fibers depolarized by acute myocardial infarction. Abnormal automaticity and repetitive firing can be evoked in normal atrial or ventricular cells by applying depolarizing current. Abnormal automaticity is not readily suppressed by overdrive pacing.

TRIGGERED ACTIVITY. Repetitive firing in heart muscle can be caused by triggered activity. Triggered activity is *not* a form of automaticity but is capable of producing a sustained tachyarrhythmia. Two primary mechanisms can initiate triggered activity: early afterdepolarizations and delayed afterdepolarizations (Fig. 42–4).

Early Afterdepolarizations. Early afterdepolarizations are secondary depolarizations that occur before repolarization is complete, often from the action potential plateau (Fig. 42–4). Experimentally, early afterdepolarizations have been produced in cardiac Purkinje fibers by stretching or crushing, hypoxia, cooling, low [K]ₒ, high [Ca]ₒ, catecholamines, and chemicals and drugs (such as veratrine, aconitine, quinidine, sotalol, or *N*-acetyl procainamide). Torsades de pointes in humans is thought to be the counterpart of triggered activity due to early afterdepolarizations.

Delayed Afterdepolarizations. A delayed afterdepolarization is a secondary depolarization occurring after full repolarization has been achieved which is dependent on the previous action potential (Fig. 42–4). Delayed afterdepolarizations can reach threshold and cause a single premature depolarization or trigger a series of impulses. Delayed afterdepolarizations can be induced by digitalis, easily in the His-Purkinje system and with more difficulty in specialized atrial or ordinary ventricular cells. Some of the digitalis-induced ventricular tachycardias in humans behave like triggered activity produced by digitalis in isolated tissue preparations. In the atria, coronary sinus, and mitral valve, delayed

afterdepolarizations and triggered activity can be caused by catecholamines.

Arrhythmias Caused by Abnormalities of Impulse Conduction

Reentry seems to be a common cause of cardiac arrhythmias in humans, e.g., paroxysmal supraventricular tachycardia and constantly coupled ventricular premature complexes. Reentrant arrhythmias usually are started by an initiating premature complex; i.e., they are self-sustained but are not self-initiated. To start reentry, one-way conduction block must occur and there must be an anatomic or functional "barrier" that forms a circuit (Fig. 42–5). Also, the path length of the reentrant circuit must be greater than the wavelength of the cardiac impulse (wavelength = conduction velocity × refractory period). For reentry to occur, conduction must be very slow, refractoriness very short, or both. Reentry has been demonstrated in anatomic loops (e.g., rings of Purkinje fibers) or anatomic obstacles (e.g., scars). Reentry occurring in unbranched bundles or sheets of cardiac muscle has been given specialized names, e.g., reflection or leading-edge reentry.

Reentry can be subdivided into random and ordered forms. In random reentry, the cardiac impulse conducts over circuits that change their location and size as a function of time, e.g., atrial and ventricular fibrillation. In ordered reentry, the circuit for reentrant activity is relatively constant.

LEADING-EDGE REENTRY. Reentrant excitation can be initiated in vitro by premature stimulation in small, thin pieces of normal atrium that contain no anatomic obstacles or loops of tissue. Conduction is slowed because activation occurs when the tissue is partially refractory. Block occurs in some regions because of local differences in refractory periods. The pathway for reentrant activity can stabilize and be sustained.

Cranefield PF: The Conduction of the Cardiac Impulse. Mount Kisco, N.Y., Futura Publishing Company, 1975. *A monograph that reviews the concepts of fast and slow action potentials and their role in the genesis of reentrant cardiac arrhythmias.*

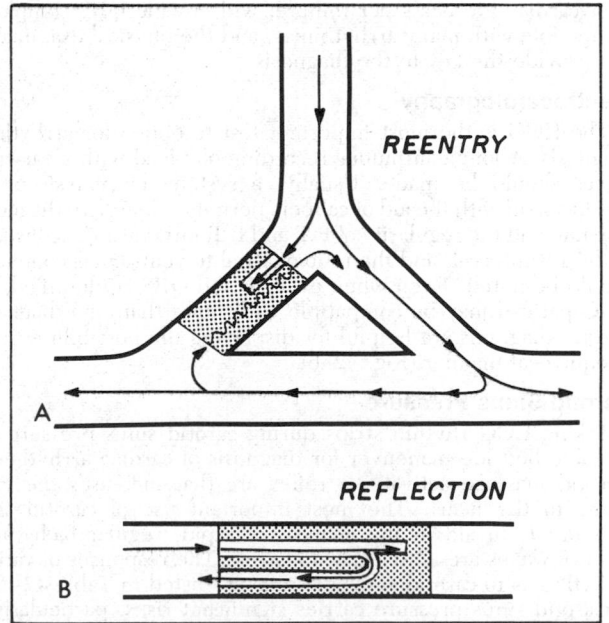

FIGURE 42–5. Two models of reentry according to Schmitt and Erlanger. *A,* Diagram showing a loop of cardiac fibers that could represent either a terminal branch of a Purkinje fiber ending on ventricular muscle or a loop of the Purkinje syncytium. In this case, one-way block and slow conduction permit reentry. *B,* A linear strand of cardiac muscle showing a depolarized zone in a portion of its cross-section. One-way block occurs in the depolarized zone, permitting the propagating impulse to reflect back in the direction from which it came. (From Braunwald E: Heart Disease: A Textbook of Cardiovascular Medicine. Philadelphia, W. B. Saunders Company, 1980.)

Fozzard HA, Haber E, Jennings RB, et al. (eds.): The Heart and Cardiovascular System, Scientific Foundations. New York, Raven Press, 1986. *The section of cardiac electrophysiology and arrhythmias contains detailed reviews of current knowledge and thought on the electrophysiology of the heart, the genesis of cardiac arrhythmias, and the epidemiology of human arrhythmias. Other sections contain excellent reviews of the embryology, anatomy, and pathology of the heart. Profusely illustrated and exhaustively referenced.*

Hackel DB: Anatomy and pathology of the cardiac conducting system. *In* Edwards JE, Lev M, Abell MA (eds.): The Heart. Baltimore, Williams & Wilkins Company, 1974, pp 232–247. *A concise description of the normal anatomy and pathology of the conduction system.*

Noble D: The Initiation of the Heartbeat. London, Oxford University Press, 1979. *An account of cardiac electrophysiology for medical students and clinicians who are unfamiliar with electronics and mathematics. Even the most difficult concepts of cardiac excitation are explained clearly and concisely. Selective references to the classic papers in electrophysiology.*

Noble D: The surprising heart: A review of recent progress in cardiac electrophysiology. J Physiol 353:1–50, 1984. *A detailed review of cellular electrophysiology of the heart. Amply referenced.*

DIAGNOSTIC APPROACHES TO CARDIAC ARRHYTHMIAS

The history, physical examination, 12-lead electrocardiogram, 24-hour continuous electrocardiographic recordings, exercise tests, intermittent electrocardiographic recordings, and clinical electrophysiologic studies are the primary tools used in the diagnosis of cardiac arrhythmias. Decisions about treatment may require other laboratory studies to define better the etiology of heart disease, other aspects of the functional status of the heart, e.g., left ventricular function or perfusion, or function of other organ systems.

History and Physical Examination

The primary purposes of the history are (1) to formulate a hypothesis about the presence and type of arrhythmia, (2) to detect factors that trigger the onset of the arrhythmia or intensify arrhythmic symptoms, (3) to establish the frequency and pattern of occurrence of the arrhythmia, and (4) to establish the functional consequences of the arrhythmia.

The physical examination provides information about the presence and type of heart disease and the degree of cardiac impairment. The physical examination in conjunction with the ECG can aid in the differential diagnosis of arrhythmias. A regular tachycardia, 150 beats per minute, with a wide QRS complex is compatible with many arrhythmias, and the physical examination can provide the key to the diagnosis.

Electrocardiography

The ECG is the most important test to obtain for arrhythmia diagnosis. A long continuous recording of a lead with clear-cut P waves should be made. Usually, a systematic analysis of the rhythm strip with the aid of calipers permits a definitive diagnosis. The rate and the regularity of P-P and R-R intervals, the constancy of the PR interval, and the ratio of atrial to ventricular complexes should be noted. Even when every P and QRS is identified, the ECG pattern may be compatible with more than one diagnosis. Ladder diagrams are helpful for displaying the possibilities in an unequivocal manner (Fig. 42–6).

Carotid Sinus Pressure

Taking ECG rhythm strips during carotid sinus pressure is a valuable bedside maneuver for diagnosis of cardiac arrhythmias. Carotid massage activates a reflex arc that increases the vagal traffic to the heart. The most important use of carotid sinus pressure is to aid in the analysis of rapid, regular tachycardia when P waves are not clearly apparent. The responses of various arrhythmias to carotid sinus massage are listed in Table 42–3.

Carotid sinus pressure carries significant risks, particularly in older patients, i.e., syncope, convulsions, stroke, prolonged asystole, or ventricular tachyarrhythmias. In patients with digitalis toxicity, carotid sinus pressure may provoke malignant ventricular arrhythmias.

Special Procedures to Detect Atrial Activation

All of the P waves must be identified to make rhythm analysis reliable. P waves can be detected using special lead placement, e.g., the Lewis lead, esophageal electrograms, or transvenous bipolar catheter electrodes.

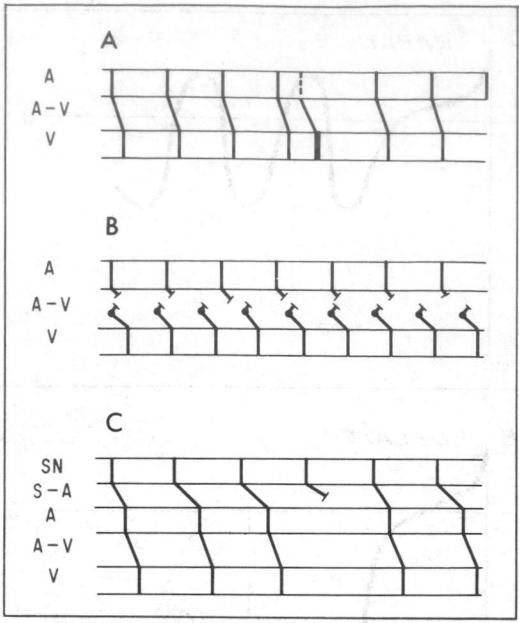

FIGURE 42–6. Ladder diagrams of cardiac rhythm. A = Atrium; A-V = atrioventricular junction (the A-V node and His-Purkinje system); V = ventricle; SN = sinus node; S-A = sinoatrial junction. *A*, Sinus rhythm with atrial premature depolarization (APD). Atrioventricular conduction of the APD is slower than for sinus impulses because the atrioventricular node is partially refractory. The broad line in the ventricular tier indicates aberrant ventricular conduction of the APD, which occurs because the premature impulse arrives during the relative refractory period of the His-Purkinje system. *B*, Atrioventricular junctional rhythm. The A-V junctional automatic rhythm captures the ventricles but shows retrograde block. The sinus node controls the atria, but the sinus impulse finds the A-V node refractory and is blocked; i.e., there is interference between the sinus and junctional rhythm. *C*, Type I (Wenckebach) sinoatrial block. The sinus impulse travels through the perinodal junctional tissues with increasing delay until block finally occurs. (From Braunwald E: Heart Disease: A Textbook of Cardiovascular Medicine. Philadelphia, W. B. Saunders Company, 1980.)

Ambulatory ECG Recording

In 1961, Holter described the technique of ambulatory ECG recording. A light, portable tape recorder continuously records the ECG for 24 hours while the patient performs his or her usual daily activities and records the activities and symptoms in a diary. The primary indications for ambulatory ECG recordings are listed in Table 42–4.

INTERMITTENT RECORDERS. When symptoms occur only occasionally, intermittent recorders permit monitoring lasting from a few days to many weeks even though the ECG recordings are brief (seconds to minutes). These recorders may be attached to patients continuously or intermittently.

Hard-wired Recorders. Intermittent recorders of the hard-wired type are continuously attached to the patient by electrodes and cables. Patients activate these recorders by pressing a switch. Some units have 40 to 100 seconds of electronic memory and sample the ECG continuously, replacing old data with new. When activated, 30 to 60 seconds of ECG prior to patient activation are recorded. Data are retrieved from hard-wired systems either by direct playback or by telephonic transmission.

Intermittently Attached Recorders, Telephonic Transmission. These devices are typically about the size and shape of a radio-paging unit. The patient applies ECG leads when symptoms occur. Units with memory can store one to three ECG samples for subsequent telephone transmission. Commercial services provide immediate evaluation of the ECG transmission. Transmissions are acted on in accordance with the instructions of the patient's physician.

Intracardiac Recording and Stimulation (*Endocardial Electrical Stimulation*)

Over the past 25 years, intracardiac recording and stimulation have developed as a diagnostic and therapeutic tool for the

TABLE 42-3. EFFECT OF CAROTID SINUS PRESSURE ON TACHYARRHYTHMIAS

Arrhythmia	Response to Carotid Sinus Pressure
Sinus tachycardia	1. Gradual slowing during massage, gradual speeding after massage
Paroxysmal supraventricular tachycardia (AV nodal)	1. No effect, or 2. Abrupt conversion to sinus rhythm, or 3. Slight slowing
Paroxysmal supraventricular tachycardia (anomalous AV connection)	1. No effect, or 2. Abrupt conversion to sinus rhythm, or 3. Slight slowing
Nonparoxysmal supraventricular tachycardia	1. No effect, or 2. AV block, slowed ventricular rate, or 3. Gradual slowing of ventricular rate
Atrial flutter	1. AV, slowed ventricular rate, or 2. No effect, or 3. Atrial fibrillation
Atrial fibrillation	1. AV block, slowed ventricular rate, or 2. No effect
Ventricular tachycardia	1. No effect, or 2. AV dissociation

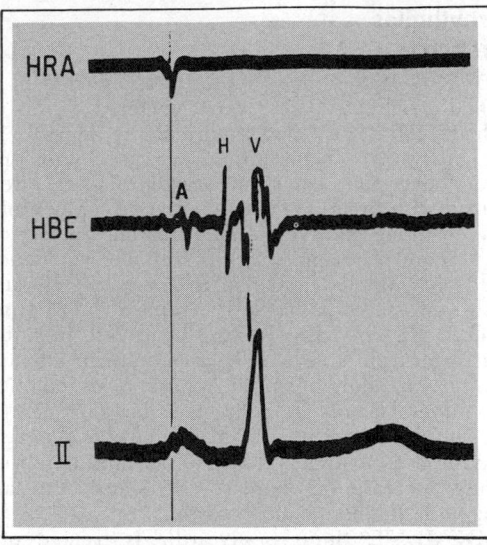

FIGURE 42-7. Intracardiac recordings. A high right atrial bipolar electrogram (HRA), His bundle bipolar electrogram (HBE), and tracing from lead II of the electrocardiogram. A = Atrial depolarization; H = depolarization of the His bundle; V = depolarization of the upper ventricular septum. The PA interval represents intra-atrial conduction time (upper to lower atrium); AH represents atrioventricular nodal conduction; and HV represents the His-Purkinje conduction time. The thin vertical line correlates the onset of atrial activation in the three recordings. (From Braunwald E: Heart Disease: A Textbook of Cardiovascular Medicine. Philadelphia, W. B. Saunders Company, 1980.)

management of human cardiac arrhythmias. Local electrical activity can be recorded from the portions of the heart that are electrically silent on the body surface ECG, e.g., sinus node, His bundle, right bundle branch, left bundle branch, selected sites in the right or left ventricle. The sequence and time of activation of atria and ventricles can be mapped, and AV conduction can be partitioned into AV nodal and His-Purkinje components (Fig. 42-7). Recordings from selected sites are used with pacing and programmed stimulation sequences to evaluate automaticity, conduction, refractoriness, and the causes of arrhythmias

TABLE 42-4. INDICATIONS FOR LONG-TERM CONTINUOUS ECG RECORDINGS

I. **Detect and quantify arrhythmias or conduction defects in patients with symptoms** (e.g., syncope or other central nervous system symptoms, palpitations, or angina pectoris)

II. **Quantify arrhythmias, conduction defects, or ischemia in patients with predisposing conditions**
  A. Sick sinus syndrome
  B. Pre-excitation syndromes
  C. AV conduction defects
  D. Pacemaker malfunction
  E. Mitral value prolapse
  F. Long QT syndrome
  G. After myocardial infarction
  H. Angina pectoris
  I. Hypertrophic or dilated cardiomyopathy
  J. Heart failure

III. **Evaluate activity**
  A. To detect exercise-related arrhythmias or conduction defects
  B. To detect ischemia during activity

IV. **Evaluate therapy**
  A. Antiarrhythmic drug treatment
  B. Fad diets
  C. Drugs with cardiac adverse effects
  D. Pacemakers
  E. Automatic implantable cardioverter/defibrillator
  F. Surgery
    1. Ischemia or arrhythmias after coronary artery bypass graft surgery
    2. Pre-excitation after division of anomalous AV connection
    3. AV conduction after surgical division or catheter ablation of the His bundle

in intact man. These techniques not only have enhanced our understanding of arrhythmias and conduction defects but also have improved our ability to select and evaluate therapy. Some of the major clinical uses of electrophysiologic studies are listed in Table 42-5.

Bigger JT Jr, Reiffel JA, Coromilas J: Ambulatory Electrocardiography. In Platia EV (ed.): Nonpharmacologic Management of Cardiac Arrhythmias. Philadelphia, J.B. Lippincott Company, 1986, pp 36–61. *A comprehensive review of the technology, indications, and clinical uses of ambulatory electrocardiography. Liberally illustrated and referenced.*

Horowitz LN, Josephson ME, Kastor JA: Intracardiac electrophysiologic studies as a method for the optimization of drug therapy in chronic ventricular arrhythmias. Prog Cardiovasc Dis 23:81, 1980. *Gives the details of electrophysiologic methods for evaluating drug therapy of malignant ventricular arrhythmias.*

Josephson ME, Seides SF: Clinical Cardiac Electrophysiology: Techniques and Interpretations. Philadelphia, Lea & Febiger, 1979. *A detailed description of the techniques of clinical electrophysiology and the interpretation of the findings. Intended for the internist and clinical cardiologist without an extensive background in cardiac electrophysiology.*

Morganroth J: Ambulatory Holter electrocardiography: Choice of technologies and clinical uses. Ann Intern Med 102:73, 1985. *A concise review of the current status of ambulatory electrocardiography.*

Wenger NK, Mock MB, Ringqvist I (eds.): Ambulatory Electrocardiographic Recording. Chicago, Year Book Medical Publishers, Inc., 1981. *Manuscripts from a workshop held at the National Heart, Lung, and Blood Institute. The topics of methodology, recording and analysis systems, quality control, and clinical, epidemiologic, and research applications are discussed thoroughly.*

SPECIFIC CARDIAC ARRHYTHMIAS

Clinically, cardiac arrhythmias are classified by their presumed site of origin, i.e., atrial, AV junctional, or ventricular, and as premature complexes, bradycardia, or tachycardia. It would be desirable to use the precise mechanism to classify clinical arrhythmias, but this is impossible because we do not know the precise mechanism of many cardiac arrhythmias. For some arrhythmias, e.g., the ventricular arrhythmias, prognostic significance can be assigned with reasonable precision. When this is the case, a prognostic classification is useful for guiding decisions about management. In this section, we use a classification based on the site of origin and rate as the framework within which to discuss the definition, pathophysiology, ECG diagnosis, significance, and management of each arrhythmia. The emergency and chronic treatments of cardiac arrhythmias are outlined in Tables 42-6 and 42-7.

Atrial Arrhythmias

SINUS RHYTHM

ECG DIAGNOSIS. Sinus rhythm is recognized in the ECG by a normal atrial rate and P wave vector, i.e., an upright P wave in leads III and aV$_f$ and a normal PR interval. In adults, sinus rates below 60 or 50 per minute are called sinus bradycardia and those above 100, sinus tachycardia. Heart rate changes synchronized with breathing are called sinus arrhythmia and are caused by changing parasympathetic nervous activity. Sinus arrhythmia is more pronounced in children and young adults than in the elderly. Marked sinus arrhythmia can be difficult to distinguish from sinoatrial block or ectopic atrial rhythms.

CLINICAL FEATURES. Resting heart rate in sinus rhythm varies with age: from 130 to 160 per minute in infants to 50 to 100 per minute in adults. Gender, temperature, emotion, effort, and neurohumoral factors also influence sinus rate. The maximum heart rate during exercise varies from almost 200 per minute in healthy young persons to less than 140 per minute in the elderly. Many drugs increase or decrease the sinus rate, usually by interacting with autonomic mechanisms.

MANAGEMENT. Sinus bradycardia is treated only when symptomatic. When acute and symptomatic sinus bradycardia is due to increased vagus nerve activity, heart rate can be increased by intravenous (IV) atropine injection. Rarely, IV isoproterenol infusion may be needed. Chronic symptomatic sinus bradycardia is an indication for an electronic pacemaker. Treatment of sinus tachycardia is based on the cause, usually extracardiac.

ATRIAL PREMATURE COMPLEXES

Atrial premature complexes (APC's) arise in the atria outside the sinus node. APC's occur in normal and diseased hearts. In heart disease, APC's herald sustained atrial arrhythmias such as flutter, fibrillation, or paroxysmal supraventricular tachycardia.

ECG DIAGNOSIS. APC's typically have premature P waves, abnormal P wave morphology, and a prolonged PR interval. Early APC's can be difficult to see because the P wave is superimposed on the T wave. Also, APC's can block in the AV node to produce pauses that can be misinterpreted as a sinus pause or sinoatrial block. Usually, APC's reset the sinus node so that the sum of the pre- and postextrasystolic P-P intervals is less than two sinus cycles (Fig. 42–8). If sinus reset does not occur because the APC occurs late or the perinodal refractory period is long, a compensatory pause occurs. An APC can conduct aberrantly, causing the QRS to be wide and bizarre like a VPC (Fig. 42–9). Aberrant conduction occurs when APC's activate one of the bundle branches, usually the right, during its relative refractory period. Left bundle branch block aberrancy implies an abnormality in the left bundle branch (Fig. 42–9).

MANAGEMENT. The objective of treating APC's is to control symptoms or prevent sustained symptomatic arrhythmias. In

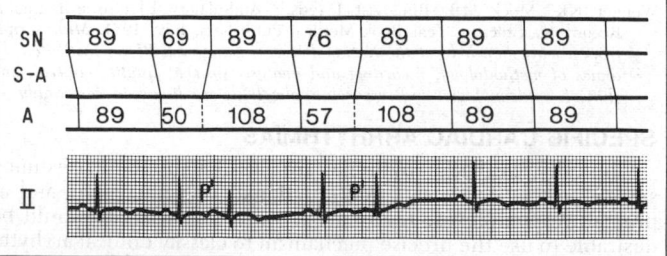

FIGURE 42–8. Atrial premature depolarization (APD). The ladder diagram correlates with the events in the lead II electrocardiographic strip below. SN = Sinus node; S-A = junctional tissues between sinus node and atrium; A = atrium. The time intervals in the ladder diagram are given in msec $\times 10^{-1}$ (e.g., 89 represents 890 msec). The third and fifth P waves are APD's (P'). These P' waves are premature and inverted. The P'R interval is prolonged, and QRS duration is normal. The APD's capture the sinus node and reset it; therefore, the pause following APD's is less than compensatory. (From Braunwald E: Heart Disease: A Textbook of Cardiovascular Medicine. Philadelphia, W. B. Saunders Company, 1980.)

TABLE 42–5. INDICATIONS FOR CLINICAL ELECTROPHYSIOLOGIC STUDIES—ENDOCARDIAL ELECTRICAL STIMULATION

I. To evaluate mechanism, site, and extent of arrhythmia and/or conduction defect
  A. Sick sinus syndrome
  B. Pre-excitation syndrome
  C. Supraventricular tachycardia
  D. Distinguish between supraventricular arrhythmias with aberration and ventricular arrhythmias
  E. Type I AV block with bundle branch block
  F. Type II AV block with normal QRS
  G. Bifascicular block occurring in acute myocardial infarction

II. To search for a cause for syncope
  A. Evaluate sinus node function
  B. Evaluate AV node function
  C. Evaluate function of His-Purkinje system
  D. Evaluate functional characteristics of anomalous AV connections
  E. Provoke arrhythmias
    1. Supraventricular tachycardia
    2. Atrial flutter or fibrillation
    3. Ventricular tachycardia

III. To evaluate therapy
  A. Drug therapy
    1. Prevent inducible arrhythmias
    2. Measure conduction and refractoriness in anomalous AV connections
    3. Evaluate adverse effects
      a. Sinus node function
      b. AV node function
      c. His-Purkinje system
      d. Effect on device function
  B. Surgical therapy
    1. Preoperative endocardial catheter mapping
      a. Location of anomalous AV connections
      b. Location of VT circuit
      c. Need for concomitant pacemaker implantation
    2. Postoperative evaluation
      a. Presence of anomalous AV connections
      b. Arrhythmia inducible
  C. AICD therapy
    1. Preoperative evaluation
      a. Determine that VT or VF is inducible
      b. Determine that VT or VF is drug resistant
      c. Determine need for concomitant pacemaker implantation
    2. Intraoperative evaluation
      a. Determine quality of rate-sensing electrograms
      b. Determine quality of patch electrograms
      c. Determine defibrillation thresholds
      d. Induce clinical arrhythmia to test sensing and termination of ventricular arrhythmias by the AICD
    3. Postoperative evaluation
      a. Induce VT or VF to test the performance of the AICD
      b. Acquaint the patient with the sensation of AICD discharge
  D. Pacemaker therapy
    1. Evaluate condition for suitability for pacemaker therapy
      a. Supraventricular tachycardia due to reciprocation in the AV node
      b. Supraventricular tachycardia due to reciprocation in anomalous AV connections
      c. Reentrant ventricular tachycardia
    2. Determine the information needed to select pacemaker type and parameters

IV. To apply ablation therapy
  A. Posterior septal anomalous AV connections (experimental)
  B. AV node or bundle of His
  C. Ventricular tachycardia (experimental)

AICD = Automatic implantable cardioverter defibrillator; VT = ventricular tachycardia; VF = ventricular fibrillation.

patients with normal hearts, treatment should be focused on general hygienic measures; rest and reducing the use of tobacco, alcohol, or caffeine often reduce the frequency of APC's. In some patients with intermittent, sustained atrial arrhythmias, APC's should be treated with digitalis or class I, II, or IV antiarrhythmic drugs to prevent sustained arrhythmias.

TABLE 42–6. EMERGENCY TREATMENT OF CARDIAC ARRHYTHMIAS

Arrhythmia	Usual First Treatment	Other Effective Treatments	Comments
Atrial fibrillation	Digitalis	Cardioversion; propranolol; acebutolol; verapamil	If hypotensive due to rapid ventricular rate, cardiovert. Avoid propranolol or verapamil in patients with heart failure or hypotension. Avoid digitalis or verapamil in Wolff-Parkinson-White syndrome.
Atrial flutter	Cardioversion	Digitalis; verapamil; propranolol; acebutolol; rapid atrial pacing	Very large doses of digitalis, e.g., 4–6 mg, often are required to achieve AV block in atrial flutter.
Paroxysmal supraventricular tachycardia (AV nodal)	Vagal maneuvers; adenosine; verapamil	Digitalis; propranolol; acebutolol; procainamide	Do not treat wide QRS complex tachycardia with verapamil unless the diagnosis of PSVT is certain. Use cardioversion for PSVT with hypotension.
Paroxysmal supraventricular tachycardia (anomalous AV connection)	Vagal maneuvers; adenosine; verapamil	Cardioversion	If the RP interval suggests anomalous AV connection, an electrophysiologic study should be considered.
Sick sinus syndrome	Pacemaker	Digitalis; pacemaker plus drug with class I antiarrhythmic action	Digitalis usually improves atrial tachyarrhythmias without aggravating sinus bradycardia or AV block.
Nonparoxysmal AV junctional tachycardia	Stop digitalis	Potassium; observation	If the arrhythmia is caused by digitalis toxicity and serum K^+ is low, digitalis should be stopped and potassium should be given.
Sustained ventricular tachycardia	Cardioversion	Lidocaine; procainamide	If VT is well tolerated, intravenous lidocaine or procainamide can be tried.
Ventricular fibrillation	Cardioversion	—	Lidocaine, bretylium tosylate, or propranolol may be helpful when ventricular fibrillation recurs several times immediately after cardioversion.
Digitalis-toxic atrial tachycardia with block or ventricular tachycardia	Lidocaine; phenytoin	Potassium	Avoid cardioversion or bretylium tosylate, which may precipitate ventricular fibrillation.
Digitalis-toxic asystole or AV block	Pacemaker	Fab fragments of digoxin-specific antibodies; dialysis	If associated with malignant hyperkalemia, these rhythms are always fatal unless treated promptly with Fab fragments of digoxin-specific antibodies.

TABLE 42–7. CHRONIC TREATMENT OF CARDIAC ARRHYTHMIAS

Arrhythmia	Usual First Treatment	Other Effective Treatments	Comments
Atrial fibrillation	Digitalis	Drug with class I antiarrhythmic action and digitalis; digitalis and propranolol; digitalis and verapamil	Drugs with class I antiarrhythmic action are used to maintain sinus rhythm; propranolol, acebutolol, or verapamil is used as adjunct to control ventricular rate in atrial fibrillation.
Atrial flutter	Drug with class I antiarrhythmic action	Digitalis; propranolol; verapamil	
Paroxysmal supraventricular tachycardia (AV nodal)	Digitalis	Drug with class IC antiarrhythmic action; propranolol	
Paroxysmal supraventricular tachycardia (anomalous AV connection)	Drug with class IC antiarrhythmic action	Drug with class IA antiarrhythmic action	Surgical ablation is preferable if patient also has atrial fibrillation with rapid ventricular response, if the anomalous AV connection has a short refractory period, or if the patient is noncompliant or has adverse effects from drugs.
Sick sinus syndrome	Pacemaker	Pacemaker and digitalis; pacemaker and drug with class I antiarrhythmic action	With the arrhythmias effectively treated, prognosis is determined by the severity of associated heart disease.
High-grade AV block	Pacemaker	—	No drugs are needed.
Symptomatic ventricular premature complexes or unsustained VT	β blocker	Drug with class I antiarrhythmic action	For benign and potentially malignant ventricular arrhythmias, β blockers are safest and often control symptoms. When heart failure is present, disopyramide and flecainide are relatively contraindicated.
Sustained ventricular tachycardia	Drug with class I antiarrhythmic action	Drug with class III antiarrhythmic action	Treatment must be guided by a method with high predictive accuracy, e.g., endocardial electrical stimulation. A common sequence of drugs is: class IA → class IA + class IB → class IC → class III. If drugs fail or are not evaluable, an implantable cardioverter/defibrillator usually is the best treatment. In selected cases, surgical excision of the arrhythmogenic tissue is the best choice.

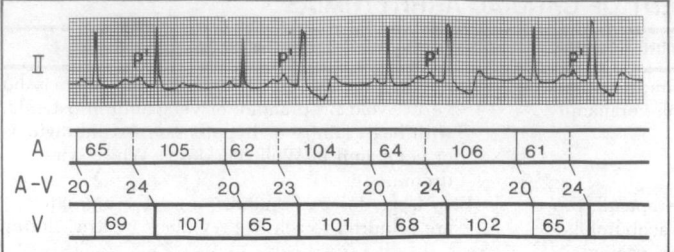

II								
A	65	105	62	104	64	106	61	
A-V	20	24	20	23	20	24	20	24
V		69	101	65	101	68	102	65

FIGURE 42–9. Atrial premature depolarizations (APD's) with aberrant conduction. The ladder diagram depicts the events in the lead II electrocardiographic strip above. A = Atrium; A-V = atrioventricular node and His-Purkinje system; V = ventricle. Time intervals are in msec $\times 10^{-1}$ (65 represents 650 msec). APD's are represented by dashed lines in the atrial tier; the wide QRS complexes are represented by a wide bar in the ventricular tier. APD's occur in a bigeminal pattern. The even (ectopic) P waves (P') are premature and have configurations slightly different from the odd P waves. Although the P-P' interval is relatively long (>600 msec), the P'-R interval is also prolonged, and the QRS complex following each P' is aberrant (left bundle branch block configuration)—a pattern of aberration suggesting bundle branch disease. Note that the QRS complex after the longest P-P' interval (second QRS) is least aberrant. (From Braunwald E: Heart Disease: A Textbook of Cardiovascular Medicine. Philadelphia, W. B. Saunders Company, 1980.)

PAROXYSMAL SUPRAVENTRICULAR TACHYCARDIA

ECG DIAGNOSIS. Typically, paroxysmal supraventricular tachycardia (PSVT), also known as paroxysmal atrial or nodal tachycardia and reciprocating AV nodal tachycardia, has the following electrocardiographic features: a regular, rapid rate of 150 to 230 per minute; QRS duration less than 100 msec; and an abnormal P wave in a fixed relationship to each QRS. The P wave often is superimposed on the T wave or the QRS complex. PSVT starts abruptly, usually initiated by an APC or VPC. Often, the atrial rate in PSVT is about 185 per minute. The rate of PSVT often is faster in infants and children, in the Wolff-Parkinson-White (WPW) syndrome, and in thyrotoxicosis. The rate of PSVT is likely to be slower when AV node disease or certain drugs are present. The R-R intervals in typical PSVT are extremely regular except for the first or last few cycles of an episode. Carotid sinus massage either has no effect on PSVT or terminates it. In the presence of AV nodal disease or drugs that depress nodal conduction, e.g., digitalis or verapamil, fixed 2:1 AV block or AV Wenckebach can occur during PSVT.

The QRS complexes may be wide, resembling ventricular tachycardia, due either to a pre-existing wide QRS or to aberrant conduction of the rapid atrial rhythm. If AV dissociation can be documented, the rhythm originates in a subatrial location and is not PSVT. His bundle recording can differentiate between PSVT and ventricular tachycardia (Fig. 42–10).

The mechanism of PSVT is often AV nodal reentry initiated by an APC. The PSVT in the WPW syndrome is reentrant using

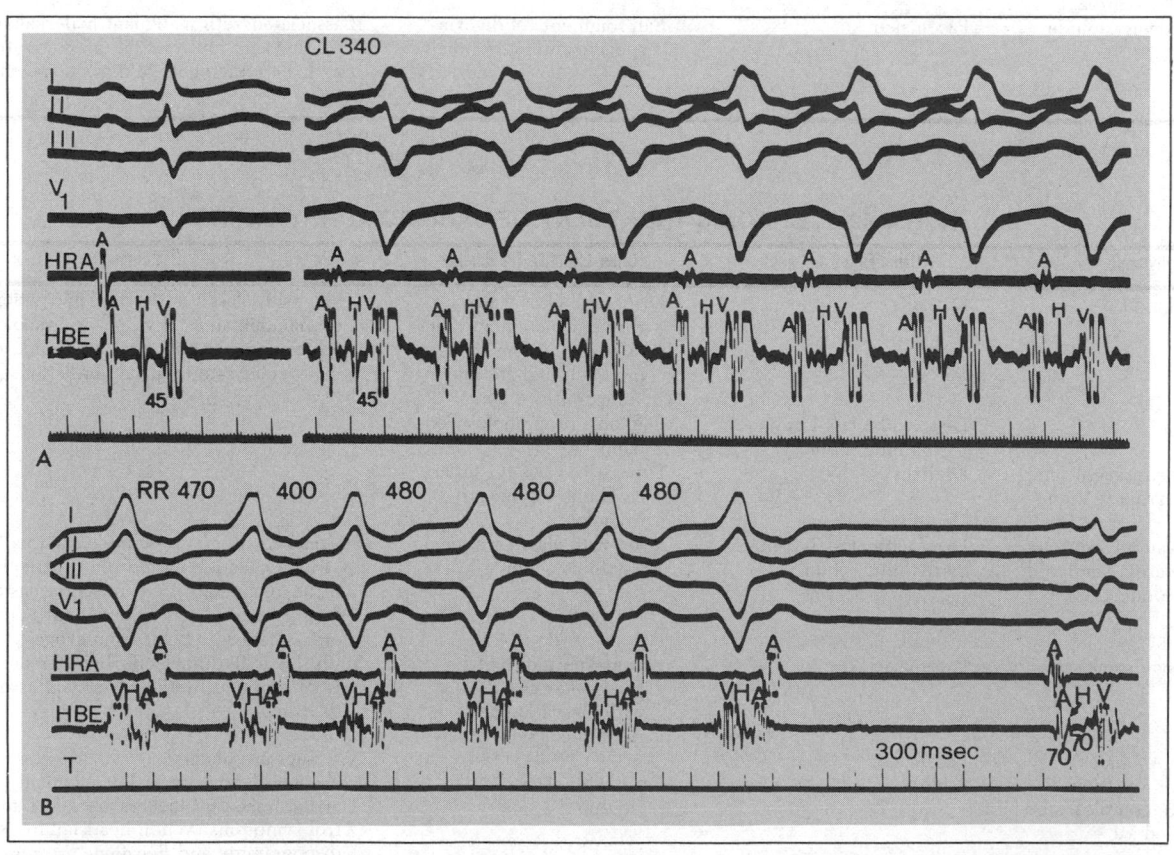

FIGURE 42–10. His bundle recording in regular tachycardia with a wide QRS complex. *A*, Supraventricular tachycardia. The left panel is a record taken during sinus rhythm; the QRS is normal. The right panel is a record taken during tachycardia; a left bundle branch block pattern is present. The normal HV interval in the His bundle electrogram (HBE) indicates that the rhythm is supraventricular tachycardia with aberrant conduction. *B*, Ventricular tachycardia. The last six depolarizations of a tachycardia and the first of sinus rhythm are shown. A left bundle branch block pattern is present during the tachycardia. In the His bundle electrogram, the ventricles depolarize (V) before the bundle of His (H), indicating that the rhythm is ventricular tachycardia. Ventriculoatrial conduction shows a stable 1:1 pattern. (From Caracta AR, Damato AN: Significance of His bundle electrocardiography. *In* Fowler NO (ed.): Cardiac Diagnosis and Treatment. 2nd ed. New York, Harper and Row, 1976, pp 979–1008.)

the anomalous AV connection in the retrograde direction and the AV node in the antegrade direction (Fig. 42–11).

Nonparoxysmal atrial tachycardia probably is due to ectopic automaticity or triggered activity in the atrium. Atrial tachycardia with AV block suggests digitalis toxicity, particularly if the atrial rate is slow, e.g., 140 beats per minute.

CLINICAL FEATURES. PSVT occurs in normal as well as diseased hearts. Attacks of PSVT begin abruptly, cause palpitations, and may also end abruptly. The patient may learn maneuvers that are likely to stop the tachycardia, e.g., cough, Valsalva maneuver, or facial immersion. The hemodynamic effects of PSVT vary tremendously and depend on rate and the severity of heart disease. When PSVT is rapid, e.g., 180 to 220 beats per minute, systemic arterial pressure often falls and diastolic pressure rises in both ventricles, even in persons without heart disease. Prolonged and rapid supraventricular tachycardia can cause marked salt and water retention.

MANAGEMENT. Vagal maneuvers (e.g., Valsalva maneuver or carotid sinus massage), adenosine, or verapamil is effective in about 90 per cent of the episodes. When PSVT causes hypotension or heart failure, DC cardioversion should be used. For prevention of recurrences of PSVT due to AV nodal reentry, digitalis usually is tried first. If digitalis fails, potent drugs with class I antiarrhythmic action are quite effective. Surgery may be preferred to drugs in the WPW syndrome with recurrent symptomatic tachyarrhythmias.

ATRIAL FLUTTER

ECG DIAGNOSIS. Typically, atrial flutter has the following ECG features: rapid atrial rate, 250 to 350 beats per minute, narrow QRS, and ventricular rate of 125 to 175 per minute, i.e., 2:1 AV conduction ratio (Fig. 42–12). In atrial flutter, the baseline of the ECG has a characteristic saw-toothed or undulating appearance best seen in leads II, III, and aV$_F$. Quinidine and other drugs with class I action can slow atrial flutter rate dramatically. In persons with a normal AV node, the AV conduction ratio usually is 2:1. Higher ratios suggest AV node disease or drug effect. Rarely, atrial flutter conducts to the ventricles with a 1:1 ratio, resulting in a ventricular rate of about 300 and hemodynamic collapse. The QRS complex usually is normal during atrial flutter but may be wide owing to pre-existing bundle branch block.

CLINICAL FEATURES. Atrial flutter usually signifies either intrinsic heart disease or adverse extrinsic influences on the heart. Atrial flutter is associated with scarred atria due to rheumatic heart disease, coronary heart disease, or primary myocardial disease. Also, atrial flutter is associated with atrial enlargement, e.g., interatrial septal defect, mitral or tricuspid stenosis/regurgitation, or chronic ventricular failure. Atrial flutter occurs in toxic or metabolic conditions that affect the heart, e.g., thyrotoxicosis, alcoholism, or beri-beri, or when the pericardium is inflamed or infiltrated, e.g., with pneumonia or bronchogenic carcinoma. In all these conditions, atrial flutter is much less common than atrial fibrillation. Atrial flutter tends to be unstable, either reverting to sinus rhythm or converting to atrial fibrillation. Probably because the atria contract vigorously in atrial flutter, systemic emboli are less common during atrial flutter than during atrial fibrillation.

MANAGEMENT. The best choice for the acute treatment of symptomatic atrial flutter is atrial pacing or DC cardioversion because digitalis usually fails to slow the ventricular rate and digitalis, verapamil, or drugs with class I antiarrhythmic action usually fail to convert atrial flutter to sinus rhythm. IV verapamil or β blockers can be useful temporizing measures to control heart rate while arrangements are made for DC cardioversion. A drug with class I antiarrhythmic action alone or with digitalis is the usual treatment to prevent recurrence of atrial flutter.

ATRIAL FIBRILLATION

ECG DIAGNOSIS. Atrial fibrillation has the following features: absence of P waves; irregular atrial activity at a rate of 350 to 600 per minute; and rapid, irregularly irregular ventricular rhythm (150 to 200 per minute). The cardinal feature is the presence of fibrillatory waves best seen in ECG leads II, III, aV$_F$, or V$_1$ and at slow ventricular rates. Conditions or drugs that shorten the AV nodal refractory period, e.g., exercise, fever, hyperthyroidism, or catecholamines, increase the ventricular rate. Conversely, factors that prolong AV nodal refractoriness slow ventricular rate.

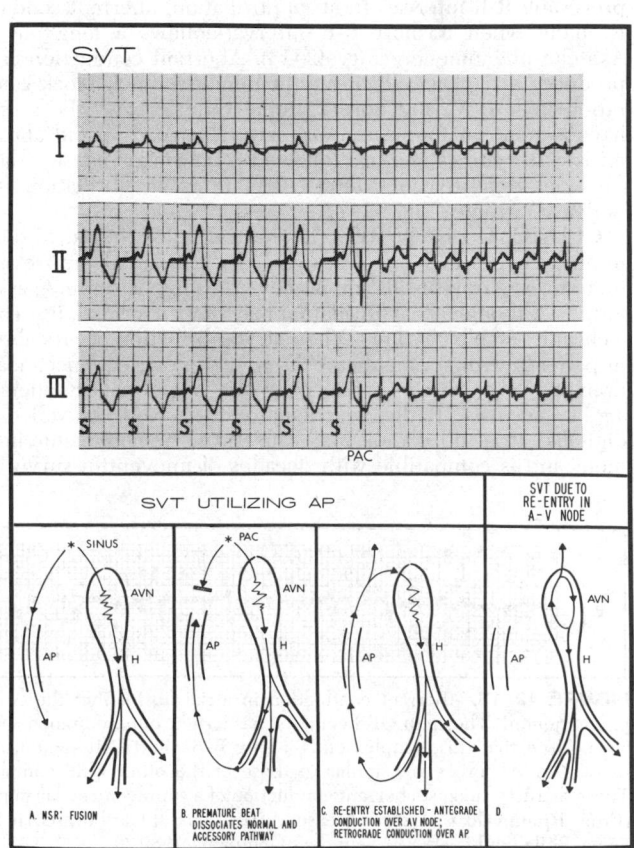

FIGURE 42–11. Mechanism of supraventricular tachycardia utilizing an accessory pathway. The upper panel demonstrates an electrocardiogram recorded in a patient with Wolff-Parkinson-White syndrome during straight atrial pacing and the introduction of a premature atrial beat. The first five beats are preceded by a stimulus artifact (S); a short PR interval and a wide QRS complex indicate the presence of pre-excitation. Following the introduction of a premature beat, a narrow QRS tachycardia is initiated. The events underlying this supraventricular tachycardia are diagrammatically shown in the lower panels. During sinus rhythm (A), fusion is present owing to conduction over the AV node (AVN) and the accessory pathway (AP). In B, an atrial premature depolarization blocks the accessory pathway and conducts with delay over the AV node, thus dissociating the activity of the normal and accessory pathways. In C, the impulse conducting through the ventricle travels retrograde over the accessory pathway and reenters the atrium, establishing a tachycardia. D demonstrates schematically the reentry circuit underlying supraventricular tachycardia resulting from reentry confined to the AV node.

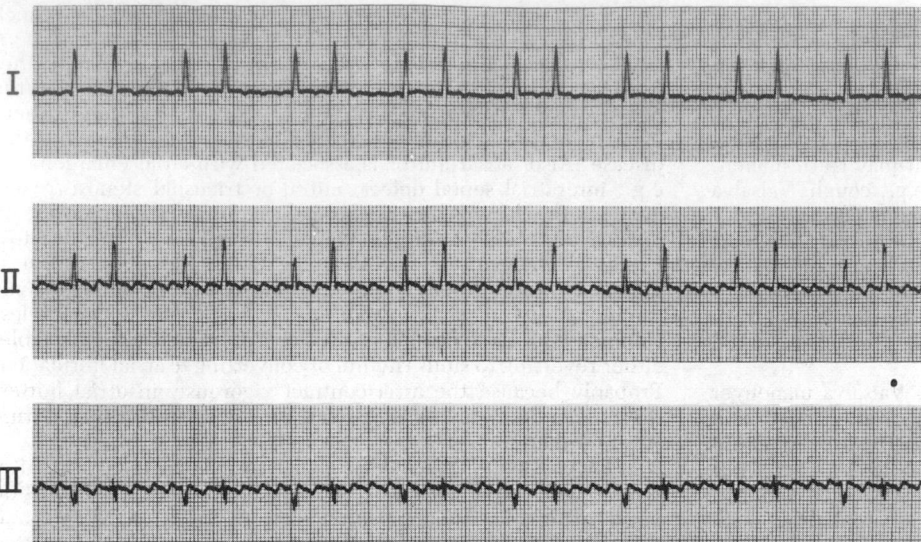

FIGURE 42–12. Atrial flutter with varying AV block. This electrocardiogram, recorded during a period of varying AV block induced by a vagal maneuver, demonstrates the characteristic "saw-toothed" appearance of P waves during atrial flutter.

Because atrial fibrillation is so common, this diagnosis should be entertained for any rapid rhythm that has irregularly irregular R-R intervals. Patients with the WPW syndrome may develop extremely rapid ventricular rates during atrial fibrillation.

Atrial fibrillation coexists with many other arrhythmias and conduction defects; two occur frequently and are critically important to diagnose correctly. The first is AV junctional arrhythmia caused by digitalis toxicity. As digitalis slows the ventricular rate, AV junctional automaticity increases. First, junctional escape complexes terminate long R-R intervals or the ventricular rate becomes regular at a slow rate. Then the junctional focus accelerates to produce nonparoxysmal AV junctional tachycardia. The second is aberrant conduction of supraventricular impulses that must be distinguished from VPC's. The duration of refractoriness in the His-Purkinje system is directly proportional to the preceding R-R interval. In atrial fibrillation, aberrant conduction is likely when a short R-R interval follows a long one—the Ashman phenomenon (Fig. 42–13). Aberrant conduction usually produces a triphasic (RSR') right bundle branch block configuration in lead V_1 and normal initial QRS forces. VPC's usually have a mono- or biphasic QRS pattern in lead V_1 and abnormal initial QRS forces and are followed by a longer pause. Another cause of repetitive aberrant QRS's in atrial fibrillation is the WPW syndrome (Fig. 42–14).

CLINICAL FEATURES. Like atrial flutter, atrial fibrillation implies myocardial or pericardial disease or adverse extrinsic influences. Atrial fibrillation is about 20 times as common as atrial flutter. Although atrial fibrillation may be paroxysmal, it is usually a chronic, stable rhythm. When atrial fibrillation occurs abruptly in patients with serious heart disease, the consequences may be dramatic, e.g., disconcerting palpitations, pulmonary edema, or angina pectoris. If the ventricular rate is well controlled with digitalis, atrial fibrillation may cause little hemodynamic impairment and is compatible with decades of uneventful survival. As

with atrial flutter, atrial fibrillation occurs in many etiologic forms of heart disease. Chronic atrial inflammation and lack of effective atrial contraction promote left atrial thrombi and increased risk for systemic emboli. Atrial fibrillation may occur as an isolated arrhythmia in patients without heart disease or any other systemic illness. This condition has been called "lone atrial fibrillation."

MANAGEMENT. The objective of treating acute atrial fibrillation is to slow the rate. For symptomatic hypotension, immediate cardioversion is indicated. Usually, rate is controlled with IV digoxin (see Table 42–11). Verapamil or β-blocking drugs are useful adjuncts for achieving rate control but can aggravate heart failure or cause hypotension. Digitalis and verapamil are best avoided in patients with WPW because they can increase the ventricular rate and trigger ventricular fibrillation. The objectives of chronic treatment of atrial fibrillation are to (1) control ventricular rate, (2) prevent thromboemboli, and (3) maintain sinus rhythm.

MULTIFOCAL ATRIAL TACHYCARDIA

ECG DIAGNOSIS. The ECG features of multifocal atrial tachycardia are frequent APC's, often occurring in runs that have dramatically different P wave morphology and marked variability in P-P interval.

CLINICAL FEATURES. This rhythm occurs in patients with decompensated or overtreated chronic obstructive pulmonary disease. These patients often have severe derangement of arterial blood gases and electrolytes and are being treated aggressively with theophylline and/or catecholamines.

MANAGEMENT. Multifocal atrial tachycardia is resistant to digitalis therapy. Therapy is directed at improving ventilation and eradicating infection to improve arterial blood gases. The dose of bronchodilators may need to be reduced as well. Verapamil can be used to control the arrhythmia while adjusting the other medications.

SINOATRIAL BLOCK

ECG DIAGNOSIS. Impulses generated in the sinus node may conduct slowly or block in the junction between the sinus node and atrium. First-degree SA block, i.e., a delay in conduction from sinus node to the atrium, cannot be recognized in the standard ECG but can be identified by electrophysiologic studies. Second-degree SA block can be diagnosed electrocardiographically. Type I second-degree SA block is recognized by Wenckebach periodicity of the P-P intervals (Fig. 42–15). In type II second-degree SA block, the P-P interval suddenly lengthens to a value almost precisely twice the usual P-P interval. Third-degree SA block causes atrial arrest.

CLINICAL FEATURES. SA block indicates intrinsic sinus node disease, electrolyte disturbance, or an adverse drug effect,

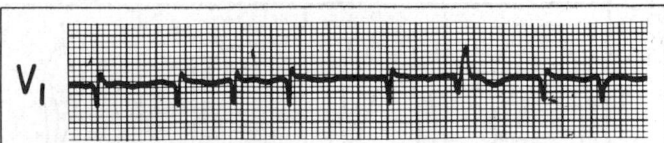

FIGURE 42–13. Aberrant conduction in atrial fibrillation (the Ashman phenomenon). The sixth QRS complex has a right bundle branch appearance. Note that this complex ends a long R-R–short R-R sequence and that its initial forces are similar to those of the other QRS complexes. These features suggest aberrant conduction of a supraventricular impulse. (From Braunwald E: Heart Disease: A Textbook of Cardiovascular Medicine. Philadelphia, W. B. Saunders Company, 1980.)

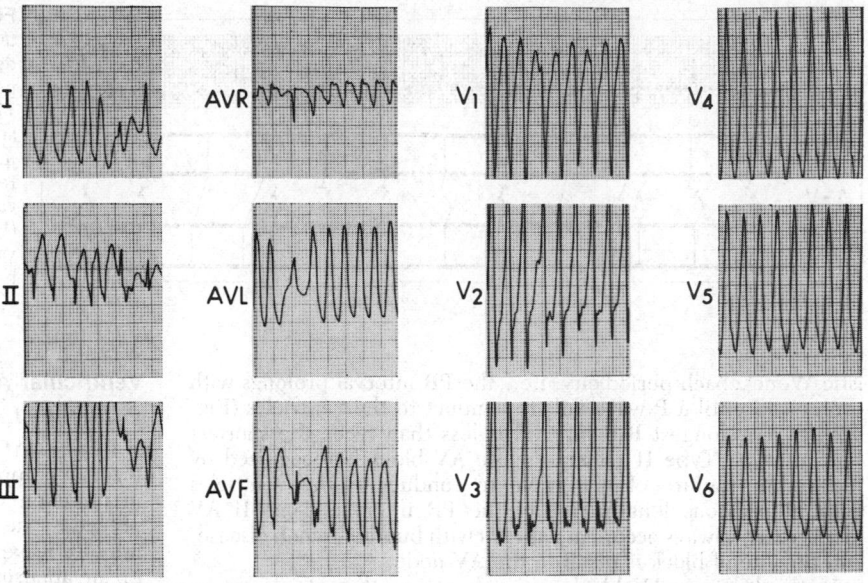

TG M79212

FIGURE 42–14. Atrial fibrillation in the Wolff-Parkinson-White syndrome. The electrocardiogram demonstrates the irregularly irregular response associated with anomalous-appearing QRS complexes resulting from atrial fibrillation with rapid conduction over the accessory pathway to the ventricle.

most often digitalis. Drugs with class I antiarrhythmic action can cause SA block in patients with pre-existing sinus node dysfunction.

Sick Sinus Syndrome. The sick sinus syndrome is characterized by intrinsic inadequacy of sinus node pacemaking and/or conduction failure between the sinus node and the rest of the atrium. In the bradycardia-tachycardia syndrome, recurrent supraventricular tachyarrhythmias alternate with sinus bradycardia and/or subatrial bradyarrhythmias. Conduction disturbances are common in the atria, AV node, bundle branches, and ventricles, but ventricular ectopic activity is rare.

Symptoms in sick sinus syndrome may be intermittent, varied, and difficult to correlate with ECG changes. Syncope, dizziness, and palpitations are common, probably because these symptoms are used for case finding and diagnosis. Congestive heart failure or angina can be aggravated. Cerebral thromboembolism is common in the bradycardia-tachycardia syndrome.

MANAGEMENT. Persistent, symptomatic sinus bradycardia is an indication for pacemaker therapy. Digitalis can be used to control the atrial tachyarrhythmis and, contrary to expectation, usually does not aggravate coexistent bradyarrhythmias. After pacemaker implantation, drugs with class I antiarrhythmic action can be used to control tachyarrhythmias. Symptoms can be improved with pacemaker therapy in the bradycardia-tachycardia syndrome, but cerebral thromboembolism continues. The prognosis of effectively treated sick sinus syndrome is determined by associated heart disease. Treatment of atrial fibrillation in the

sick sinus syndrome can cause severe bradycardia. A temporary ventricular pacemaker should be used when attempting to convert atrial fibrillation with slow ventricular rate to sinus rhythm.

AV Junctional Arrhythmias

AV JUNCTIONAL PREMATURE COMPLEXES

ECG DIAGNOSIS. AV junctional premature complexes are much less common than either APC's or VPC's. Typical ECG features are an abnormally premature or absent P wave and a premature QRS complex with a normal configuration. The position of the premature P wave (P') is critical to the diagnosis. The P' may occur 0.10 second or less before, during, or 0.20 second or less after the premature QRS. P' is inverted in leads II, III, and aV$_F$. The clinical significance of AV junctional premature complexes is similar to that of nonparoxysmal AV junctional tachycardia (see below).

NONPAROXYSMAL AV JUNCTIONAL TACHYCARDIA

ECG DIAGNOSIS. Nonparoxysmal AV junctional tachycardia is caused by enhanced automaticity in the AV junction. The junctional focus fires 70 to 130 per minute (Fig. 42–16). The QRS complex usually is normal or slightly aberrant. If the AV junctional focus captures the atria, the retrograde P may be positioned 0.10 second or less in front of the QRS, simultaneous with the QRS, or 0.20 second or less after the QRS. This arrhythmia often is associated with AV nodal conduction impairment and AV dissociation. The atrial rhythm may intermittently capture the junctional focus and ventricle (see Fig. 42–19).

CLINICAL FEATURES. Nonparoxysmal AV junctional tachycardia has great significance because it is associated with acute inferior myocardial infarction, digitalis toxicity, acute carditis (e.g., viral myocarditis or acute rheumatic fever), or surgical trauma.

MANAGEMENT. Treatment should be focused on the underlying condition, e.g., myocarditis or digitalis toxicity. In acute inferior myocardial infarction and after open heart surgery, nonparoxysmal AV junctional tachycardia is usually transient and requires no therapy. In digitalis toxicity, this arrhythmia should prompt intensive management of toxicity.

AV BLOCK

ECG DIAGNOSIS. AV block is classified as first-, second-, and third-degree. First-degree AV block, i.e., a prolonged PR interval, is caused by conduction delay in the AV node. Second-degree AV block is subdivided into type I (AV nodal) and type II (His-Purkinje). Type I second-degree AV block has character-

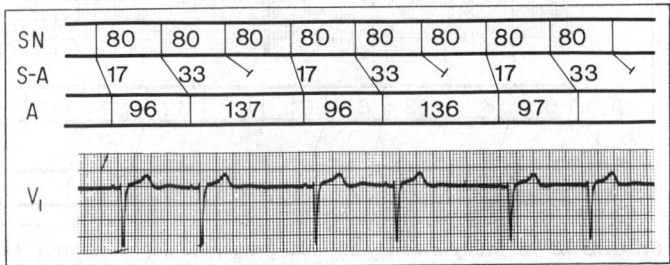

SN	80	80	80	80	80	80	80	80
S-A	17	33		17	33		17	33
A		96	137	96	136	97		

FIGURE 42–15. Second-degree sinoatrial block, type I (Wenckebach). The ECG shows periodicity of the P waves and QRS complex. The PR is constant. This pattern is consistent with a constant sinus node rate of 75 per minute (sinus cycle length = 800 msec) with 3:2 sinoatrial shock. The sinoatrial conduction times are assumed. (From Braunwald E: Heart Disease: A Textbook of Cardiovascular Medicine. Philadelphia, W. B. Saunders Company, 1980.)

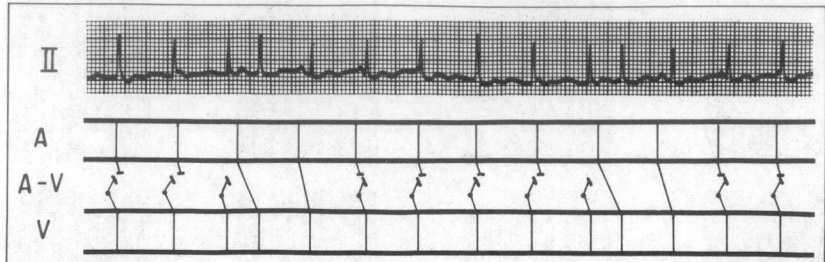

FIGURE 42–16. Nonparoxysmal atrioventricular junctional tachycardia with atrial capture of the ventricles. Two independent rhythms coexist: sinus tachycardia at 107 beats per minute and atrioventricular junctional tachycardia at 115 beats per minute. Sinus rhythm always controls the atria. The ventricles are usually controlled by the AV junctional focus, because its rate is faster. When time relationships are appropriate, atrial depolarizations propagate through the AV junction and capture the ventricles. (From Braunwald E: Heart Disease: A Textbook of Cardiovascular Medicine. Philadelphia, W. B. Saunders Company, 1980.)

istic Wenckebach periodicity; i.e., the PR interval prolongs with each cycle until a P wave fails to conduct to the ventricles (Fig. 42–17). The longest R-R interval is less than twice the shortest R-R interval. Type II second-degree AV block is recognized by the sudden failure of a P wave to conduct to the ventricles without previous lengthening of the PR interval. Type II AV block nearly always occurs in patients with bundle branch disease, and the site of block is distal to the AV node.

In third-degree AV block, sinus or some other atrial rhythm controls the atria while the ventricles are controlled by an independent AV junctional or ventricular pacemaker. The QRS usually is prolonged, and the ventricular rate is between 35 and 50.

CLINICAL FEATURES. First-degree AV block causes no symptoms but may cause the first heart sound to be soft because the AV valves almost close before ventricular contraction. Second-degree AV block usually causes no symptoms unless the ventricular rate becomes very slow. It may be possible to discern second-degree AV block by characteristic pulse intervals, intermittent prominent A waves, and changing intensity of the first heart sound. In complete heart block with sinus rhythm, the pulse is slow, full, and regular; intermittent cannon A waves occur in the jugular venous pulse; and the first heart sound varies markedly in intensity.

MANAGEMENT. First-degree AV block requires no treatment. Type I second-degree AV block usually resolves without the need for a temporary pacemaker. When type I block is caused by a chronic AV junctional disease, block can progress slowly to complete AV block. Type II second-degree AV block usually results from chronic bundle branch disease and often progresses to complete heart block. Chronic, symptomatic second- or third-degree AV block should be treated with an implanted pacemaker.

Ventricular Arrhythmias
VENTRICULAR PREMATURE COMPLEXES (VPC's)

ECG DIAGNOSIS. The QRS is premature, wide, and often bizarre in appearance; the ST segment and T wave are opposite in direction to the QRS complex; and no premature P wave precedes the premature QRS complex (Fig. 42–18). As the impulse leaves its ectopic site of origin, it activates the ventricle in an abnormal sequence, accounting for the striking QRS-T abnormalities. Typically, a VPC is followed by a fully compensatory pause, i.e., the RV interval plus the VR interval is equal to two R-R intervals in sinus rhythm (Fig. 42–18). VPC's may be *interpolated* between two successive sinus complexes. "Concealed" retrograde conduction of the interpolated VPC into the AV node causes the PR interval of the subsequent sinus complex to prolong. Certain patterns of VPC's have special names. When every other QRS is a VPC, the pattern is termed *bigeminy;* a VPC every third QRS is termed *trigeminy;* and two successive VPC's are termed a *pair* or a *couplet.*

CLINICAL FEATURES. Infrequent VPC's are commonly found even in young persons, and VPC frequency increases with age. While sporadic VPC's in persons with normal hearts do not seem to affect outcome adversely, VPC's confer significant risk of subsequent cardiac death in heart disease. When VPC's are caused by drug toxicity, e.g., digitalis, quinidine, or tricyclic antidepressants, lethal rhythm disturbances may ensue unless the drug is discontinued. A strong association exists between myocardial infarct size and the frequency of VPC's in acute myocardial infarction and a weak association between poor left ventricular function and frequency of VPC's during recovery.

MANAGEMENT. The most important issue in the treatment of VPC is the selection of patients for treatment. In general, only very symptomatic VPC's need treatment, and drugs with class II antiarrhythmic action (β-adrenergic blockade) are the first choices for treatment of benign and potentially malignant ventricular

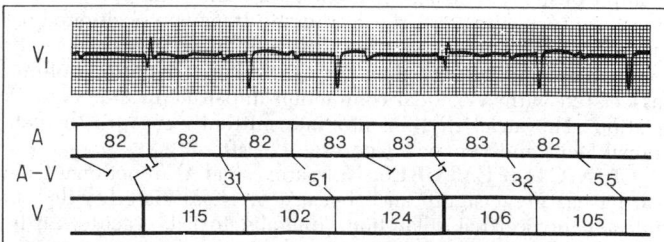

FIGURE 42–17. Sinus rhythm with type I second-degree atrioventricular block (Wenckebach) and junctional escape complexes. Sinus rhythm is regular at a rate of 73 beats per minute. The third P wave from the left begins a 3:2 Wenckebach cycle. The first PR interval of the cycle is quite long (0.31 sec), and the PR increment in the second cycle is large (an additional 0.20 sec). The third P wave of the cycle is blocked in the A-V node. The PR interval following the pause is short (0.10 sec), and the QRS complex is aberrant; this is a junctional escape complex. The tracing demonstrates both impaired conduction and enhanced automaticity in the A-V junction. Type I A-V block nearly always occurs in the A-V node, and A-V junctional escape complexes are presumed to arise in the bundle of His or the most proximal portions of the bundle branches. (From Braunwald E: Heart Disease: A Textbook of Cardiovascular Medicine. Philadelphia, W. B. Saunders Company, 1980.)

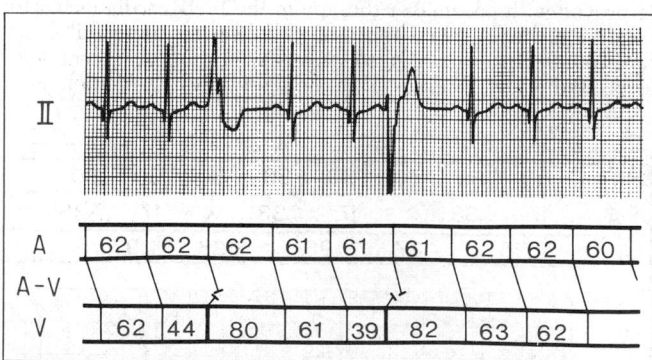

FIGURE 42–18. Multiformed ventricular premature depolarizations. The third and sixth QRS complexes are VPD's with strikingly different configurations. Also, the coupling interval of the two VPD's differs by 50 msec. Such a difference in configuration may be due either to a different site of origin or to a difference in the sequence of ventricular activation from the same site of origin. (From Braunwald E: Heart Disease: A Textbook of Cardiovascular Medicine. Philadelphia, W. B. Saunders Company, 1980.)

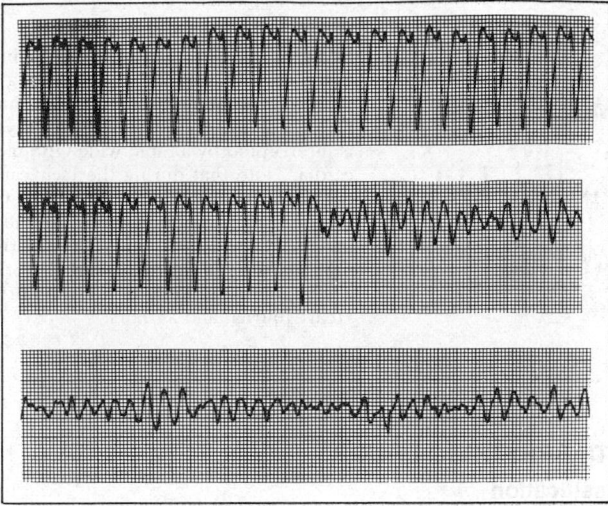

FIGURE 42–19. Ventricular tachycardia and ventricular fibrillation. Three continuous strips from lead V₄ of a Holter electrocardiograph. The top strip shows ventricular tachycardia at 214 cycles per minute—an unusually rapid rate for ventricular tachycardia. Ventricular fibrillation begins in the middle strip and continues on the bottom strip. Note the irregularity in amplitude and period of deflections recorded during ventricular fibrillation. (From Braunwald E: Heart Disease: A Textbook of Cardiovascular Medicine. Philadelphia, W. B. Saunders Company, 1980.)

arrhythmias. IV lidocaine or procainamide is usually used to treat VPC's occurring immediately after myocardial infarction or cardiac surgery.

VENTRICULAR TACHYCARDIA (VT)

ECG DIAGNOSIS. The most prevalent definition of ventricular tachycardia is three or more VPC's in succession at a rate of 100 per minute or greater. Ventricular tachycardia may be unsustained, i.e., last less than 15 to 30 seconds, or sustained (Fig. 42–19). In a tachycardia with wide QRS complexes, two findings strongly suggest VT: *ventricular captures* and *fusion complexes*. Sinus impulses may capture the ventricle during VT, producing either a normal QRS (ventricular capture) or a QRS intermediate in contour between normal and the QRS of ventricular tachycardia (fusion complex). Sustained VT can be difficult to distinguish from supraventricular arrhythmias with a wide QRS complex. A His bundle recording can easily distinguish between these two possibilities (see Fig. 42–10).

CLINICAL FEATURES. Unsustained VT nearly always occurs in patients with heart disease, most often in those with coronary heart disease. Two weeks after myocardial infarction, about 10 per cent of patients have VT detected by a single 24-hour continuous ECG recording. Patients with class III or IV heart failure have a 40 to 50 per cent prevalence of VT in a 24-hour ECG. Most episodes of VT in either setting are brief, i.e., three to five consecutive VPC's, and asymptomatic, yet increase the risk of dying two- to fourfold. Sustained VT is rare and has a poor prognosis. As with other tachyarrhythmias, the severity of symptoms in sustained VT is related primarily to the rate of the tachycardia and left ventricular function. Blood pressure and mental status are not useful for distinguishing between VT and PSVT with aberrant conduction. Sustained VT is prone to deteriorate into ventricular fibrillation.

MANAGEMENT. The management of symptomatic, unsustained VT is the same as that described above for VPC's. Sustained VT in chronic heart disease is treated acutely with IV lidocaine or procainamide, if the patient is hemodynamically stable, or by DC cardioversion if unstable (Fig. 42–19). Baseline studies should include 48 hours of continuous ECG recording, exercise testing, endocardial electrical stimulation, and cardiac catheterization with coronary angiography. The drug/dose finding and long-term management of these patients should be guided by rigorous methods with high predictive accuracy. The standard method is endocardial electrical stimulation. A programmatic noninvasive approach using 24-hour continuous ECG recordings

and exercise tests also can be used. The usual sequence for drug testing is class IA (e.g., quinidine or procainamide), IA plus IB (e.g., quinidine and mexiletine), and III (amiodarone), or an unapproved drug (e.g., dl-sotalol). If an effective drug is not found, an implantable defibrillator is usually the best treatment. In selected cases, surgery is the best choice.

ACCELERATED IDIOVENTRICULAR RHYTHM (AIVR)

ECG DIAGNOSIS. Accelerated idioventricular rhythm is defined as three or more consecutive QRS complexes of ventricular origin with a rate between 50 and 100 (Fig. 42–20). Fusion QRS complexes often begin or end an episode of AIVR.

CLINICAL FEATURES. AIVR occurs in about 30 per cent of patients with acute myocardial infarction, equally commonly in inferior or anterior infarcts. AIVR frequently follows coronary reperfusion. AIVR is usually asymptomatic and therefore needs no treatment. The incidence of ventricular fibrillation and hospital mortality is not increased in patients who have AIVR.

VENTRICULAR PARASYSTOLE

ECG DIAGNOSIS. Ventricular parasystole is an automatic rhythm in the His-Purkinje system that competes with sinus rhythm. Parasystole has two cardinal features: variable coupling of VPC's and a common denominator for interectopic intervals. Entrance block removes the parasystolic focus from the suppressant influence of the sinus impulses, permitting a stable automatic rhythm to emerge; the ectopic focus activates the ventricle every time it fires unless the ventricle is refractory (Fig. 42–20).

CLINICAL FEATURES. Parasystole often is resistant to antiarrhythmic drug therapy, and untreated patients seem to have a good prognosis.

VENTRICULAR FLUTTER AND FIBRILLATION

ECG DIAGNOSIS. The diagnosis of ventricular flutter is made when the ventricular tachyarrhythmia has large sinusoidal or zigzag QRS's and the rate is between 240 and 280 per minute. Multiform VT or torsades de pointes is recognized by the periodic twisting of the points of the QRS complexes (Fig. 42–21). Ventricular fibrillation is recognized in the ECG by the absence of QRS complexes and T waves and the presence of low-amplitude baseline undulations that are variable in both amplitude and periodicity (Fig. 42–19).

CLINICAL FEATURES. Ventricular flutter is rarely recorded because it is unstable and tends to convert to sinus rhythm or, more often, to ventricular fibrillation. Ventricular flutter or fibrillation is catastrophic. Cardiac pumping ceases instantly, the patient loses consciousness, and, if cardiopulmonary resuscitation is not started within a few minutes, the patient dies. Identifiable causes are acute myocardial ischemia or infarction; marked electrolyte disturbances, e.g., hypokalemia; marked hypothermia; electrocution; and drug toxicity. Most victims of ventricular fibrillation who are resuscitated do *not* have one of these condi-

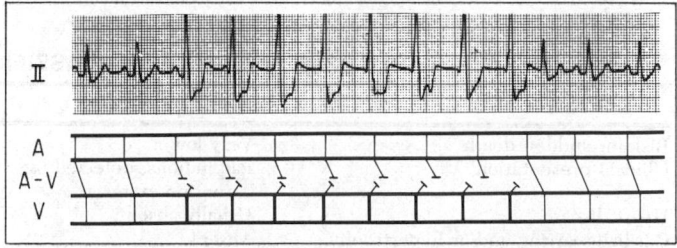

FIGURE 42–20. Accelerated idioventricular rhythm. Sinus rhythm at 88 cycles per minute is interrupted by a rhythm with wide QRS complexes at 95 cycles per minute. Note that the PR interval progressively shortens at the onset of the ventricular rhythm and that sinus rhythm continues unperturbed by the ventricular rhythm (atrioventricular dissociation). After eight QRS complexes of ventricular rhythm, sinus rhythm resumes. (From Braunwald E: Heart Disease: A Textbook of Cardiovascular Medicine. Philadelphia, W. B. Saunders Company, 1980.)

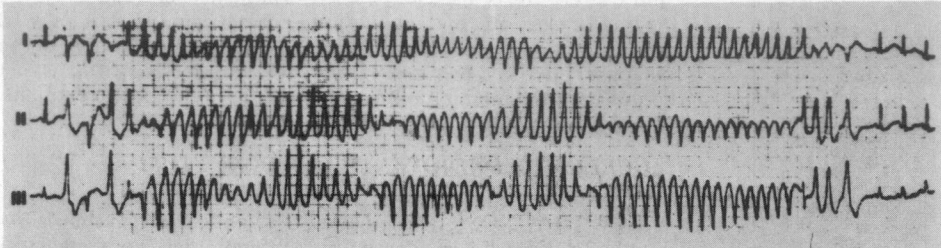

FIGURE 42–21. Torsades de pointes. Sinus rhythm associated with a long QT interval is present at the beginning and at the end of this rhythm strip. Sinus rhythm is interrupted by a rapid wide QRS tachycardia. Note that during the tachycardia, the direction of the points of the QRS complex appears to revolve around an imaginary isoelectric line. (From Krikler DM, Curry DVL: Br Heart J 38:118, 1976. With permission of the British Heart Journal and authors.)

tions but do have advanced coronary atherosclerosis and poor ventricular function.

MANAGEMENT. The only effective treatment for ventricular fibrillation is prompt defibrillation. In most cases, ventricular fibrillation does not recur after defibrillation. When it does, lidocaine, bretylium, or propranolol may help to stabilize the rhythm. When no transient or reversible cause for ventricular fibrillation is found (e.g., myocardial infarction, electrolyte abnormality, or drug toxicity), the process for evaluating long-term treatment is much the same as described above for sustained VT. Unfortunately, a smaller fraction of patients, about 60 to 70 per cent, have VT induced by programmed ventricular stimulation. Nevertheless, the uninducible patients have a high recurrence rate for ventricular fibrillation.

The management of multiform VT (torsades de pointes) is based on its pathophysiology: toxic drug effects, hypokalemia and/or hypomagnesemia, and slow heart rates. Treatment may include avoidance of drugs with class I antiarrhythmic action, ventricular pacing, reducing the level of the culprit drug, repletion of electrolytes, treatment with IV Mg^{2+}, or catecholamine infusion.

PROGNOSTIC CLASSIFICATION OF VENTRICULAR ARRHYTHMIAS. Table 42–8 outlines the classification of ventricular arrhythmias as determined by the presence of heart disease, left ventricular function, and arrhythmia characteristics. Prognosis is an important basis for deciding whom to treat and how to sequence the treatment choices.

Bigger JT Jr, Reiffel JA: Sick sinus syndrome. Ann Rev Med 30:91, 1979. *A comprehensive review of the human sinus node dysfunction. Liberally referenced.*

Marriott HJL: Practical Electrocardiography. 8th ed. Baltimore, Williams & Wilkins Company, 1988. *A textbook designed to emphasize the simplicities of the ECG, provide only those concepts that make everyday ECG interpretation more intelligible, and provide illustrations and discussion of all important ECG patterns. Excellent for learning or reviewing the ECG patterns of arrhythmias.*

Zipes DP: Specific arrhythmias: Diagnosis and treatment. In Braunwald E (ed.): Heart Disease. A Textbook of Cardiovascular Medicine. 3rd ed. Philadelphia, W. B. Saunders Company, 1988, pp 658–716. *Detailed description of the clinical features, electrocardiographic recognition, and treatment of cardiac arrhythmias. Contains 52 figures and 372 references.*

ANTIARRHYTHMIC DRUGS

Classification

Antiarrhythmic drugs have been classified according to their mechanisms of action into four classes (Table 42–9). One could think of digitalis as having class V drug action, i.e., a strong cholinergic action that can repolarize stretched or damaged atrial cells and thereby speed conduction. Digitalis glycosides slow conduction in the AV node, tending to slow or abolish reentrant rhythms that use the AV node.

Use-Dependent Block of Ionic Channels

Many antiarrhythmic drugs act on ionic channels in the sarcolemma. Drugs with class I antiarrhythmic action block the Na^+ channel so that ionic conductance falls to zero until the drug dissociates from the channel. Most drugs with class I antiarrhythmic action bind to open or inactivated channels; drug-associated channels have slow or incomplete reactivation. Drug binding and Na^+ channel blockade increase with rate, producing *use-dependent block.* If the association and dissociation of drug from the Na^+ channel both are rapid, use-dependent block attains a steady state after a few action potentials and, if the interval between action potentials is reasonably long, little block persists at the time of the next action potential upstroke. If dissociation is slow, use-dependent block requires many action potentials to develop fully as the degree of block increases with each depolarization.

Specific Antiarrhythmic Drugs

This section gives a brief summary of the pharmacology and indications for each antiarrhythmic drug. This information is supplemented by information given in tables; Table 42–10 gives pharmacokinetic data for the drugs and Table 42–11 gives information on contraindications, precautions, and adverse effects.

DRUGS WITH CLASS IB ANTIARRHYTHMIC ACTION

LIDOCAINE. Lidocaine is a local anesthetic used frequently to treat ventricular arrhythmias in intensive care units. It has

TABLE 42–8. PROGNOSTIC CLASSIFICATION OF VENTRICULAR ARRHYTHMIAS*

	Benign	Potentially Malignant	Malignant
Risk for sudden death	Very low	Low to moderate	High
Clinical presentation	Palpitations; detected by routine exam	Palpitations; detected by routine exam or screening	Palpitations; syncope; cardiac arrest
Heart disease	Usually absent	Present	Present
Cardiac scarring and/or hypertrophy	Absent	Present	Present
VPC frequency	Low to moderate	Moderate to high	Moderate to high
Paired VPC and/or unsustained VT	Absent	Common	Common
Sustained VT	Absent	Absent	Present
Hemodynamic effects of arrhythmia	Absent	Absent to mild	Moderate to severe

VPC = Ventricular premature complex(s); VT = ventricular tachycardia.
*The characteristics listed in this table are typical but do not represent the full range of observations. For example, benign ventricular arrhythmias can be frequent and occasionally repetitive. For potentially malignant or malignant ventricular arrhythmias, the risk within a class depends strongly on left ventricular ejection fraction.

TABLE 42–9. CLASSIFICATION OF ANTIARRHYTHMIC DRUGS ACCORDING TO THEIR MECHANISM OF ACTION

Class	Action	Drugs
I	**Sodium channel blockade**	
B	Minimal phase 0 depression Slow conduction 0 to 1+ Shorten repolarization	Lidocaine, mexiletine, tocainide
A	Moderate phase 0 depression Slow conduction 2+ Prolong repolarization*	Disopyramide, moricizine, procainamide, quinidine
C	Marked phase 0 depression Slow conduction 4+ Little effect on repolarization	Encainide, flecainide, indecainide, propafenone
II	**β-Adrenergic blockade**	Acebutolol, propranolol
II	**Prolong repolarization**	Amiodarone, bretylium, sotalol
IV	**Calcium channel blockade**	Diltiazem, verapamil

*Moricizine does not prolong repolarization.

two major advantages: It reaches a steady state rapidly after starting or changing the dose, and it lacks significant adverse hemodynamic effects.

Pharmacology. Lidocaine prevents reentrant rhythms, decreases automaticity in Purkinje fibers, and increases the ventricular fibrillation threshold. Lidocaine has an intense depressant action on depolarized tissues but almost none on normal cardiac cells. Lidocaine has a negligible effect on the ECG. Lidocaine shortens the ERP of the His-Purkinje system. Lidocaine has no significant effect on the autonomic nervous system.

Indications. Lidocaine is used only for ventricular arrhythmias, particularly those caused by acute myocardial infarction, open heart surgery, and digitalis intoxication. Lidocaine is relatively ineffective for ventricular arrhythmias in chronic coronary heart disease or cardiomyopathy.

Pharmacokinetics. Lidocaine is administered intravenously and, rarely, intramuscularly. Steady-state plasma lidocaine concentration depends strongly on hepatic blood flow. About 70 per cent of plasma lidocaine is bound to α_1 acid glycoprotein, an acute phase reactant. At a given total plasma concentration, the free concentration falls as the α_1 acid glycoprotein increases in the first few days after infarction or surgery.

MEXILETINE. Mexiletine is an orally active local anesthetic, available in the United States since 1986, that is similar to lidocaine chemically and electrophysiologically.

Pharmacology. Mexiletine has an antiautomatic effect on Purkinje fibers and depresses phase 0 of fast action potentials more than lidocaine. It shortens the action potential duration and ERP of Purkinje fibers and ventricular muscle. Mexiletine has little effect on the ECG.

Indications. Like lidocaine, this drug is not indicated for atrial arrhythmias. In chronic coronary heart disease or cardiomyopathy, the drug is about 60 per cent effective in controlling symptomatic, unsustained ventricular arrhythmias, less than drugs with class IA or IC antiarrhythmic action.

PHENYTOIN. Phenytoin is an anticonvulsant that has been used as an antiarrhythmic since the 1960's. Phenytoin is electrophysiologically similar to lidocaine and has no significant effect on the ECG. Phenytoin has complex central autonomic actions that decrease efferent traffic on cardiac sympathetic nerves during digitalis toxicity. Phenytoin has no peripheral cholinergic or β-adrenergic blocking activity.

Indications. Phenytoin is used to treat paroxysmal atrial flutter or fibrillation, supraventricular arrhythmias, and ventricular arrhythmias caused by digitalis but is ineffective for the common atrial arrhythmias, e.g., atrial flutter, atrial fibrillation, and PSVT. Phenytoin is effective against ventricular arrhythmias after acute myocardial infarction or open heart surgery, but lidocaine is easier to use. Plasma concentrations above 10 μg per milliliter are effective for reducing ventricular arrhythmias in the year after myocardial infarction. Phenytoin, like other drugs with class I antiarrhythmic action, is relatively ineffective against recurrent, sustained VT in patients with chronic coronary heart disease.

Pharmacokinetics. The enzymes that metabolize phenytoin can saturate at antiarrhythmic plasma concentrations, causing plasma concentration to rise sharply to toxic levels. Phenytoin should not be infused because its alkaline pH causes severe phlebitis.

TOCAINIDE. Tocainide is an orally effective analogue of lidocaine that was approved in 1984 for use in the United States. Tocainide has cardiac electrophysiologic effects almost identical

TABLE 42–10. PHARMACOKINETIC PROPERTIES OF ANTIARRHYTHMIC DRUGS

Drug	Volume of Distribution (L/kg)	Half-time of Elimination (Hours)	Bioavailability	Major Route of Elimination	Protein Binding (%)	Effective Plasma Concentration (μg/ml)
Digoxin	10.0	24–72	50–80	Kidney	25	>0.0008
Lidocaine	1.0	1–3	—	Liver	70	1–5
Mexiletine	9.5	8–14	80–90	Liver	60	0.7–2.0
Phenytoin	0.7	18–30	60–80	Liver	90	8–20
Tocainide	3.0	10–14	80–90	Kidney, liver	10	6–15
Disopyramide	0.8	7–9	75–90	Kidney	Dose-dependent	2–5
Moricizine	4.5	3–5	35–45	Liver	>90	—
Procainamide	2.0	3–6	75–85	Kidney, liver	15	4–20
Quinidine	2.5	5–9	70–80	Liver	90	2–6
Encainide	4.0	1–3	20–40	Liver	80	—
Flecainide	10	13–30	>90	Kidney, liver	40	0.2–1.0
Indecainide	5.0	7–9	>90	Kidney	50	0.4–1.0
Propafenone	3.5	3–10	3–40	Liver	95	—
Acebutolol	1.2	2–4	35–45	Kidney, liver	25	—
Propranolol	4.0	3–6	20–50	Liver	>90	0.04–0.9
Amiodarone	60.0	500–1000	30–40	Liver	>95	0.5–2.5
Bretylium	6.0	8–12	20–30	Kidney	5	—
dl-Sotalol	2.0	7–15	>90	Kidney	0	1.0–4.0
Diltiazem	5.5	2–6	40–50	Liver	75	0.5–2.0
Verapamil	4.0	4–10	10–35	Liver	90	0.1–0.2

TABLE 42–11. ADVERSE EFFECTS OF ANTIARRHYTHMIC DRUGS

	Contraindications	Precautions	Adverse Effects
Digoxin	Hypersensitivity to the drug	Reduce dose in renal insufficiency; hypokalemia, hypomagnesemia, and hypercalcemia predispose to digitalis toxicity; may accelerate the ventricular response to atrial flutter or fibrillation in Wolff-Parkinson-White syndrome; may worsen outflow obstruction in hypertrophic obstructive cardiomyopathy; serum digoxin concentration increased by quinidine and verapamil; absorption may be increased by some antibiotics; use cautiously with β blockers or calcium channel antagonists in atrial fibrillation	Ventricular arrhythmias, including ventricular tachycardia; accelerated junctional rhythms; atrial tachycardia with AV block; AV dissociation; progression of AV block Anorexia; nausea, vomiting; visual disturbances; weakness
Lidocaine	Known hypersensitivity to local anesthetics of the amide type; patients with Stokes-Adams syndrome, or with severe degrees of SA, AV, or intraventricular block in the absence of a pacemaker	Accumulation in heart failure or hepatic insufficiency or after prolonged infusions; reduce dosage in children and elderly patients; safety in malignant hyperthermia not established; cimetidine and propranolol increase plasma lidocaine concentration	Bradycardia, hypotension, and cardiovascular collapse Drowsiness, confusion, dizziness, respiratory depression, and arrest; vomiting; visual disturbances; convulsions; twitching; unconsciousness; allergic reactions secondary to lidocaine sensitivity
Mexiletine	Cardiogenic shock; pre-existing second- or third-degree AV block in the absence of a pacemaker	Patients with first-degree AV block, sinus node dysfunction, intraventricular conduction abnormalities; may worsen arrhythmias; mexiletine levels increased by cimetidine; use cautiously in patients with a history of seizures, hypotension, heart failure, or liver disease	GI distress, lightheadedness, tremor, coordination difficulties, diplopia, paresthesia, confusion
Phenytoin	History of hypersensitivity to hydantoin products; sinus bradycardia, SA block, second- or third-degree AV block; Stokes-Adams syndrome	Use cautiously in presence of hypotension and myocardial depression; may worsen arrhythmias; discontinue if skin rash develops; may cause hypoglycemia; multiple drug interactions; may be associated with congenital malformations	Hypotension and bradycardia with rapid IV injection Nystagmus, ataxia, slurred speech; Stevens-Johnson syndrome; sensory neuropathy; lymphadenopathy, pancytopenia; megaloblastic anemia, gingival hyperplasia, hyperglycemia, hypocalcemia
Tocainide	Hypersensitivity to this drug or to local anesthetics of the amide type; second- or third-degree AV block in the absence of a pacemaker	May cause blood dyscrasias, pulmonary fibrosis, pneumonitis; may aggravate heart failure or worsen ventricular arrhythmias; may accelerate the ventricular response in atrial fibrillation; accumulates in severe renal or hepatic insufficiency	Nausea, vomiting, lightheadedness, dizziness, tremor, diplopia, paresthesia, confusion, *agranulocytosis*, thrombocytopenia, hypoplastic anemia
Disopyramide	Cardiogenic shock; pre-existing second- or third-degree AV block in the absence of a pacemaker; congenital QT prolongation; known hypersensitivity to the drug	*Use cautiously with left ventricular dysfunction*, sick sinus syndrome, bundle branch block, or AV block; prior digitalization suggested for atrial flutter or fibrillation to prevent increase in ventricular rate. May precipitate myasthenic crisis, glaucoma, or urinary retention; may cause hypoglycemia; serum level may be lowered by phenytoin	*Heart failure;* worsening of arrhythmias; AV block; hypotension; may cause significant prolongation of QRS and QT intervals *Urinary retention;* dry mouth; constipation; blurred vision; impotence; cholestatic jaundice; fever; thrombocytopenia; granulocytopenia; gynecomastia
Procainamide HCl	Second- or third-degree AV block unless a pacemaker is present; torsades de pointes; lupus-like syndrome; hypersensitivity to the drug	Reduce dosage in renal insufficiency; may accelerate the ventricular response in atrial fibrillation or atrial flutter; may exacerbate myasthenia gravis	Hypotension; worsening of ventricular arrhythmias; myocardial depression; AV block *Lupus-like syndrome;* GI distress; *agranulocytosis;* hemolytic anemia; fever; thrombocytopenia; rash; myalgia; hallucinations; psychosis
Quinidine sulfate	Hypersensitivity to quinidine; complete AV block; complete bundle branch block or other severe intraventricular conduction defects exhibiting marked QRS widening; myasthenia gravis; arrhythmias due to digitalis toxicity	May accelerate the ventricular response to atrial flutter or atrial fibrillation; *concurrent use with digoxin increases plasma digoxin levels;* drugs that increase hepatic drug-metabolizing enzymes decrease the plasma concentration of quinidine; may worsen heart failure; test dose recommended because of idiosyncratic response; may require change in oral anticoagulant dose	Hypotension; worsening of ventricular arrhythmias; asystole; may increase AV or bundle branch block; may cause significant prolongation of QRS and QT intervals; *syncope; torsades de pointes* *Diarrhea;* nausea, *thrombocytopenia;* hemolytic anemia; granulocytopenia; fever; visual disturbances; hypersensitivity reaction; cinchonism; rash

TABLE 42–11. ADVERSE EFFECTS OF ANTIARRHYTHMIC DRUGS Continued

	Contraindications	Precautions	Adverse Effects
Encainide	Second- or third-degree AV block or right bundle branch block with associated hemiblock unless a pacemaker is in place; cardiogenic shock; known hypersensitivity; asymptomatic ventricular arrhythmias after myocardial infarction	May worsen sinus node dysfunction; increases pacing thresholds; may suppress ventricular escape rhythms; reduce dose with renal insufficiency; cimetidine increases encainide serum concentration	*New or worsened ventricular tachycardia or ventricular fibrillation;* second- or third-degree AV block; increases mortality when used to treat potentially malignant ventricular arrhythmias after myocardial infarction Dizziness; visual disturbances; headache; vertigo; leg cramps
Flecainide	Second- or third-degree AV block or right bundle branch block with associated hemiblock unless a pacemaker is in place; cardiogenic shock; known hypersensitivity to the drug; asymptomatic ventricular arrhythmias after myocardial infarction	May worsen sinus node dysfunction; increases pacing thresholds; may suppress ventricular escape rhythms; avoid concurrent administration of disopyramide or verapamil	*New or worsened ventricular tachycardia or ventricular fibrillation* in patients with sustained ventricular arrhythmias; *heart failure,* second- or third-degree AV block Dizziness; *visual disturbances;* dyspnea; hepatic dysfunction; blood dyscrasias
Propafenone	Uncontrolled congestive heart failure or cardiogenic shock; sinoatrial or AV block in the absence of an electronic pacemaker; bradycardia; bronchospastic disorders; manifest electrolyte disorders; and known hypersensitivity to the drug	Reduce dose in hepatic or renal dysfunction; may worsen arrhythmias; increases plasma digoxin or warfarin concentrations; decreases the clearance of some β blockers; quindine or cimetidine increases plasma concentrations; use cautiously with β-blockers or calcium entry blockers	New or worsened ventricular arrhythmias in patients with sustained ventricular arrhythmias; safety unknown when used to treat potentially malignant ventricular arrhythmias after myocardial infarction; aggravates asthma or chronic bronchitis; aggravates congestive heart failure; dizziness, taste disturbances, blurred vision; anorexia, nausea, and vomiting; agranulocytosis
Acebutolol	Severe sinus bradycardia; second- and third-degree AV block; overt cardiac failure; cardiogenic shock	Myocardial infarction or exacerbation of angina may occur following abrupt withdrawal; may mask symptoms of hypoglycemia or hyperthyroidism; cautious use in renal insufficiency or with concurrent α-adrenergic or catecholamine-depleting drugs	Congestive heart failure; bradycardia; hypotension; increase in AV block Fatigue; headache; dizziness; arterial insufficiency; bronchospasm; impotence
Propranolol	Cardiogenic shock; sinus bradycardia; second- or third-degree AV block; asthma; congestive heart failure	Exacerbation of angina or myocardial infarction may occur following abrupt withdrawal; may mask symptoms of hypoglycemia or hyperthyroidism; may cause severe sinus bradycardia following termination of tachycardia; may worsen hypertension in pheochromocytoma unless used with an α-adrenergic blocking drug	Congestive heart failure; bradycardia; increase in degree of AV block; hypotension Bronchospasm; arterial insufficiency; Raynaud's phenomenon; mental depression; sleep disturbances; weakness; impotence; disorientation; memory loss; blood dyscrasias
Amiodarone	Severe sinus node dysfunction; marked sinus bradycardia; second- or third-degree AV block; history of syncope due to bradycardia unless a pacemaker is in place	Raises serum digoxin concentration; potentiates the effect of oral anticoagulants; increases levels of quinidine, procainamide, phenytoin; may potentiate bradycardia or AV block when used with β blockers or calcium antagonists; may worsen arrhythmias	Sinus bradycardia *Pulmonary fibrosis;* interstitial pneumonitis; corneal microdeposits; photosensitivity; blue-gray pigmentation; hypo- or hyperthyroidism; *hepatic injury;* nausea; vomiting; anorexia; constipation; tremor; malaise; gait disturbance; *peripheral myopathy or neuropathy*
Bretylium tosylate	*Severe hypotension may occur in patients with fixed cardiac output;* may aggravate digitalis toxicity; reduce dosage in renal insufficiency	*Hypotension, especially postural hypotension;* transient hypertension and increased frequency of ventricular arrhythmias Nausea and vomiting, usually with rapid IV infusion; increases sensitivity to catecholamines	
Dilitiazem	Sick sinus syndrome; second- or third-degree AV block in absence of a ventricular pacemaker; systolic BP <90 mm Hg	Cautious use in renal or hepatic insufficiency; additive effects on AV conduction when used with digitalis or β blockers	Bradycardia; hypotension; AV block Edema; headache; nausea; dizziness; rash; abnormal hepatic enzymes
Verapamil	*Severe left ventricular dysfunction; hypotension or cardiogenic shock;* sick sinus syndrome (except with a pacemaker); second- or third-degree AV block; concurrent intravenous β blockers and intravenous verapamil; known hypersensitivity to verapamil	Reduce oral dose with hepatic dysfunction; avoid use with disopyramide; use cautiously with renal insufficiency, β blockers, quinidine, or severe hypertrophic obstructive cardiomyopathy; raises serum digoxin level; *may accelerate ventricular response in atrial flutter or fibrillation in the presence of the Wolff-Parkinson-White syndrome;* may potentiate activity of neuromuscular blocking agents	Hypotension; AV block; heart failure; bradycardia; asystole (with IV use); *severe hypotension or ventricular fibrillation when given IV to patients with ventricular tachycardia* Peripheral edema; headache; elevation of liver function tests; constipation

to those of lidocaine and has almost no effect on the ECG. Also, it is well tolerated hemodynamically.

Indications. Tocainide is indicated for the oral treatment of sustained or symptomatic unsustained ventricular arrhythmias. The drug is similar to mexiletine in its efficacy; i.e., it controls about 60 per cent of the chronic unsustained ventricular arrhythmias. There is good concordance between the effect of IV lidocaine and oral tocainide on ventricular arrhythmias.

DRUGS WITH CLASS IA ANTIARRHYTHMIC ACTION

DISOPYRAMIDE. Disopyramide has been available in the United States for the oral treatment of ventricular arrhythmias since 1978. Disopyramide suppresses normal automaticity in Purkinje fibers and depresses phase 0 of fast action potentials and slows conduction. Disopyramide appears more potent than quinidine in increasing atrial or ventricular refractoriness but seems less potent in the His-Purkinje system. Therapeutic concentrations cause little change in heart rate or PR or QT intervals and increase the QRS duration by about 25 per cent. It increases the ERP of the atrium and ventricle but not the AV node or His-Purkinje system. Disopyramide has a prominent anticholinergic action that counteracts its direct effects on the sinus and AV nodes.

Indications. Disopyramide is indicated for the treatment of symptomatic, unsustained ventricular arrhythmias. It also terminates attacks of PSVT and decreases the frequency of recurrences. It is about as effective as quinidine for preventing recurrence of atrial fibrillation after cardioversion. Disopyramide prolongs the ERP of anomalous AV connections and can control arrhythmias in the WPW syndrome.

PROCAINAMIDE. Procainamide has been used since the 1950's for the treatment of atrial and ventricular arrhythmias. The cardiac electrophysiologic effects of procainamide are similar to those of disopyramide and quinidine. It suppresses automaticity in cardiac Purkinje fibers, slows the phase 0 depolarization in fibers with fast action potentials, and delays repolarization and increases refractoriness in the atrium, His-Purkinje system, and ventricle. Procainamide produces a small increase in the PR and QT intervals in the ECG and produces a 20 to 30 per cent increase in the QRS duration at therapeutic plasma concentrations. Also, procainamide increases slightly the ERP of the atrium, has little effect on the refractoriness of the AV node, and prolongs the conduction time and ERP of the His-Purkinje system slightly in humans. Procainamide has no significant anticholinergic or α-adrenergic blocking properties.

Indications. Procainamide is indicated for the treatment of atrial fibrillation, atrial flutter, PSVT, symptomatic, unsustained ventricular arrhythmias that do not respond to β blockers, and sustained VT. It can suppress digitalis-toxic ventricular arrhythmias, but lidocaine or phenytoin is a better choice.

Pharmacokinetics. Procainamide is biotransformed in the liver to N-acetyl procainamide (NAPA), and steady-state plasma concentrations can equal or exceed those of procainamide. NAPA is qualitatively different electrophysiologically from procainamide; it has little class I action but a pronounced class III antiarrhythmic action. NAPA is eliminated by the kidney and can accumulate to toxic levels when renal or congestive heart failure is present. Procainamide's adverse effects often preclude chronic therapy.

QUINIDINE. Quinidine, an alkaloid derived from the bark of the cinchona tree, has been used for the treatment of atrial and ventricular arrhythmias since the 1920's.

Pharmacology. Quinidine has powerful direct effects on most types of cardiac cells and has significant anticholinergic and α-adrenergic blocking activity. Quinidine has little effect on normal sinus nodes, but can markedly depress abnormal ones. Quinidine substantially decreases normal automaticity in cardiac Purkinje fibers but has little effect on abnormal automaticity. Quinidine increases atrial and ventricular pacing and fibrillation thresholds. Quinidine depresses phase 0 of atrial, ventricular, and Purkinje cells. Quinidine delays repolarization and increases the effective refractory period of atrial, ventricular, and Purkinje cells. In humans, quinidine causes a small increase in heart rate and in the PR, QRS, and QT intervals in the ECG, and usually prolongs the HV interval slightly.

Indications. Quinidine is indicated for the chronic treatment of atrial flutter or fibrillation, PSVT, and symptomatic ventricular arrhythmias. For symptomatic benign or potentially malignant ventricular arrhythmias that do not respond to β blockers, quinidine can be used if the benefits outweigh the risks. Quinidine is selected for malignant arrhythmias if it renders them uninducible by programmed ventricular stimulation or if it abolishes unsustained VT from Holter recordings.

DRUGS WITH CLASS IC ANTIARRHYTHMIC ACTION

Four drugs with class IC antiarrhythmic action were approved for use in the United States: flecainide in 1986, encainide in 1987, and indecainide and propafenone in 1989. Propafenone has class II action (β blockade) as well. These four drugs have little effect on the normal sinus node but can depress abnormal sinus nodes. They decrease spontaneous phase 4 depolarization in Purkinje fibers and markedly depress phase 0 in fast-response cardiac cells. They slow conduction substantially and shorten the ERP in atrium, ventricle, and His-Purkinje system. In humans, chronic oral doses prolong the refractory periods of the atrium, ventricle, and anomalous AV connections. They increase the AH and HV intervals and the PR, QRS, and QT intervals in the ECG much more than drugs with class IA action. Encainide and propafenone have important active metabolites.

Indications. At the present time, drugs with class IC antiarrhythmic action are indicated only for the treatment of life-threatening, sustained ventricular arrhythmias when other drugs have failed. Treatment should be initiated in hospital. However, encainide and flecainide are extremely effective against PSVT in the WPW syndrome, AV nodal PSVT, and paroxysmal atrial fibrillation and have been recommended for treatment of these arrhythmias in patients without structural heart disease. Encainide and flecainide *increased* the mortality rate in the Cardiac Arrhythmia Suppression Trial, a controlled study that enrolled patients with left ventricular dysfunction and asymptomatic or minimally symptomatic ventricular arrhythmias after myocardial infarction. It is prudent to assume that other drugs with class IC action and perhaps drugs with class IA or IB antiarrhythmic action have the same effect on mortality rate.

DRUGS WITH CLASS II ANTIARRHYTHMIC ACTION

Propranolol, the first β blocker in the United States, was approved more than 20 years ago. Of the many β-adrenergic blocking drugs now available, only acebutolol and propranolol are approved for the treatment of chronic atrial or ventricular arrhythmias; atenolol and metroprolol are indicated to reduce mortality in acute myocardial infarction (when started within hours of symptom onset); and propranolol and timolol are indicated to reduce cardiovascular mortality in patients who have survived the acute phase of infarction. Timolol also reduces nonfatal reinfarction. When there are no contraindications, drugs with class II antiarrhythmic action are the preferred treatment for potentially malignant ventricular arrhythmias. There are many significant differences among the β-adrenergic blocking agents that govern the choice for an individual patient, e.g., cardioselectivity, intrinsic sympathomimetic action, electrophysiologic effects, and pharmacokinetics.

Pharmacology. Beta blockers decrease automaticity in the sinus node and His-Purkinje system when it is enhanced by sympathetic influences but have little effect when catecholamines are absent. Propranolol has little effect on phase 0 depolarization of cardiac fibers at low concentrations. At high concentrations, i.e., 1000 to 3000 ng per milliliter, phase 0 depolarization is depressed. Propranolol shortens while other β blockers can prolong action potential duration in atrial, ventricular, and particularly His-Purkinje cells; these effects are unrelated to β-blocking activity. In humans, propranolol and other β blockers increase the ERP of the AV node, a major antiarrhythmic effect, but have little effect on atrial or ventricular refractoriness.

Indications. Propranolol is indicated for supraventricular arrhythmias, particularly those induced by catecholamines and those associated with the WPW syndrome or thyrotoxicosis, for symptomatic APC's, and to control the ventricular rate in atrial flutter or fibrillation. It is also indicated for ventricular arrhythmias caused by catecholamines. Propranolol, acebutolol, or another β blocker is the first choice for the treatment of symptomatic but benign or potentially malignant VPC's.

DRUGS WITH CLASS III ANTIARRHYTHMIC ACTION

AMIODARONE. Amiodarone is a benzofuran derivative, 37 per cent iodine by weight, originally developed as a smooth muscle relaxant and coronary vasodilator to treat angina pectoris. In 1986, amiodarone was approved by the United States Food and Drug Administration as a last resort treatment for malignant ventricular arrhythmias. There have been no controlled studies of its efficacy.

Pharmacology. Amiodarone substantially prolongs action potential duration and ERP in atrium, ventricle, and Purkinje fibers (a class III action). Amiodarone slows sinus rate by a direct effect. Under laboratory conditions, amiodarone can have a substantial class I antiarrhythmic effect. In man, amiodarone slows the sinus rate and increases the PR and QT intervals in the ECG with less effect on the QRS. Also, it increases the atrial, AV nodal, and ventricular refractory periods and prolongs the HV interval (a class I action).

Indications. Amiodarone is indicated only for treatment of recurrent ventricular fibrillation or recurrent, hemodynamically unstable sustained VT that has not responded to other antiarrhythmic drugs or when other drugs cannot be tolerated. Treatment must be assessed by a method with high predictive accuracy. Endocardial electrical stimulation is the method of choice. About 20 per cent of patients with inducible VT can be rendered uninducible, and these patients do well. In another 40 to 50 per cent, the VT rate slows enough to control symptoms during sustained VT. In this group, recurrences of VT are not reduced much but usually are not fatal. Patients who have inducible symptomatic, sustained VT after being loaded with amiodarone should be considered for some alternate treatment. Because of the serious nature of the arrhythmias for which amiodarone is indicated and the unpredictable time course of effect, amiodarone should be started in a hospital setting.

BRETYLIUM TOSYLATE. Bretylium is a postganglionic adrenergic neuron blocker that was approved in the United States in 1978 for intramuscular or intravenous use as an antiarrhythmic drug.

Pharmacology. Bretylium causes marked lengthening of the action potential duration and ERP of ventricular muscle and Purkinje fibers (class III action). It is selectively taken up in peripheral adrenergic nerves and causes the acute release of norepinephrine; later, it produces chemical sympathectomy, preventing the norepinephrine release during nerve action potentials. Bretylium has no significant effect on phase 0 depolarization or conduction (i.e., it has no class I action), but it does increase the ventricular fibrillation threshold. Bretylium does not depress myocardial performance but can cause severe postural hypotension by interfering with the efferent limb of the baroreceptor reflex arc.

Indications. Bretylium is indicated for the therapy and prophylaxis of ventricular fibrillation and for the treatment of life-threatening ventricular arrhythmias, e.g., sustained VT, that have failed to respond to first-line antiarrhythmic drugs, e.g., lidocaine. Use of bretylium should be restricted to intensive care units. It is interesting that ventricular fibrillation usually responds within minutes while the full effect on unsustained VT and VPC's takes hours.

dl-SOTALOL. dl-Sotalol is an experimental drug being proposed for treatment of malignant or symptomatic, potentially malignant ventricular arrhythmias. It has class III action as well as substantial class II action. It is more effective than amiodarone at rendering sustained VT uninducible and is much safer.

DRUGS WITH CLASS IV ANTIARRHYTHMIC ACTION

VERAPAMIL. Verapamil is a papavarine derivative that has been used since 1962 as a coronary vasodilator. Later, its calcium channel blocking properties were discovered and, in 1981, it was approved for use in the United States for the treatment of angina pectoris and supraventricular arrhythmias.

Pharmacology. Verapamil slows spontaneous firing in isolated sinus node preparations; the effect is less marked in vivo because of reflex sympathetic nervous activity caused by peripheral vaso-

dilation. Verapamil decreases normal automaticity in Purkinje fibers and abolishes delayed afterdepolarizations and triggered activity in experimental digitalis toxicity. Verapamil prolongs refractoriness and conduction in the AV node by blocking Ca^{2+} channels. This action accounts for the ability of verapamil to terminate and prevent PSVT. Verapamil can abolish experimental VT due to slow potentials. Also, verapamil can delay ischemic injury and prevent arrhythmogenic electrophysiologic effects caused by transient ischemia. Verapamil also has α-adrenergic blocking properties. In humans, verapamil slows heart rate and increases the PR interval without any change in the QRS and QTc.

Indications. Intravenous verapamil is about 80 per cent effective for a rapid conversion (45 to 60 seconds) of PSVT to sinus rhythm (Table 42–11). Verapamil should not be given IV to patients with heart failure or those with wide QRS tachycardias until the rhythm is *proven* to be PSVT.

Verapamil can provide temporary control of rapid ventricular rate in atrial fibrillation. A 5- to 10-mg IV dose of verapamil slows the ventricular rate about 20 per cent for 15 to 30 minutes while a more permanent treatment is being established. Verapamil can be used orally to prevent PSVT or to help control the ventricular rate in atrial flutter or fibrillation.

Diltiazem shows promise for the acute and chronic treatment of PSVT.

DRUGS WITH MISCELLANEOUS ANTIARRHYTHMIC ACTION

ADENOSINE. Adenosine became available for use in the United States in 1990. It depresses automaticity in sinus node and conduction in the AV node; these are direct effects not blocked by atropine. A 10- to 20-mg dose of this drug terminates PSVT within 20 seconds in more than 90 per cent of cases by blocking conduction in the AV node in AV reciprocating tachycardia or in the slow antegrade AV nodal pathway in AV nodal tachycardia. It is not effective for terminating intra-atrial reentry and therefore is ineffective for atrial tachycardia, atrial flutter, or atrial fibrillation. It has less adverse hemodynamic effect than verapamil but frequently causes transient, minor adverse effects.

Bigger JT Jr, Hoffman BF: Antiarrhythmic Drugs. *In* Gilman AG, Goodman LS, Rall TW, Murad F (eds.): The Pharmacological Basis of Therapeutics, 8th ed. New York, MacMillan Publishing Company, 1990, pp 840–873. *A concise summary of the pharmacology and clinical use of antiarrhythmic drugs. Selectively referenced.*
Siddoway LA, Roden DM, Woosley RL: Clinical pharmacology of old and new antiarrhythmic drugs. Cadiovasc Clin 15:199, 1985. *A discussion of the pharmacodynamics, pharmacokinetics, drug interactions, and clinical use of antiarrhythmic drugs. Extensively referenced.*
The Physicians Desk Reference. Oradell, N.J., Medical Economics Company, Inc. *A yearly publication that gives accurate full prescribing information for all drugs.*

ELECTRICAL MODALITIES IN THE MANAGEMENT OF CARDIAC ARRHYTHMIAS

Temporary or permanent cardiac pacemakers and DC cardioversion or external defibrillation are well-established forms of electrical therapy. In 1985, an automatic implantable cardioverter/defibrillator was approved by the FDA.

Cardiac Pacemakers

Permanent pacemakers were first implanted in the 1960's, and over the ensuing 25 years the pacemaker industry has matured, providing highly sophisticated and diverse products for management of bradyarrhythmias and, to a lesser extent, tachyarrhythmias. About 100,000 pulse generators are implanted each year in the United States, about half of the world's pacemaker implants. There are approximately 500,000 patients with pacemakers living in the United States.

INDICATIONS FOR CARDIAC PACING. The joint report of the American College of Cardiology and American Heart Association divided indications into three classes: I, definitely indicated; II, possibly indicated; and III, not indicated (Table 42–12). Pacing is indicated for bradycardia with complete heart block or advanced second-degree AV block with symptoms such as transient dizziness, lightheadedness, near syncope or syncope,

TABLE 42–12. DEFINITE INDICATIONS FOR IMPLANTED PACEMAKER

A. Complete heart block, permanent or intermittent with any one of the following complications:
1. Symptomatic bradycardia
2. Congestive heart failure
3. Conditions that require treatment with drugs that suppress ventricular escape rhythms
4. Asystole ≥ 3 seconds or ventricular rate <40 per minute
5. Mental confusion that clears with temporary pacing
B. Complete heart block or advanced second-degree AV block that occurs during myocardial infarction and persists
C. Chronic bi- or trifascicular block with one of the following:
1. Intermittent complete heart block
2. Type II second-degree AV block associated with symptomatic bradycardia
D. Sinus node dysfunction with documented symptomatic bradycardia
E. Hypersensitive carotid sinus syndrome with recurrent syncope and asystole >3 seconds provoked by minimal carotid sinus pressure
F. Symptomatic supraventricular tachycardia that does not respond to medical treatment

TABLE 42–13. CODE FOR PACEMAKER MODES

Chamber Paced	Chamber Sensed	Response to Sensing
V = Ventricle	V = Ventricle	I = Inhibited
A = Atrium	A = Atrium	T = Triggered
D = Double (atrium and ventricle)	D = Double (atrium and ventricle)	D = Double (atrium triggered and ventricle inhibited)
	O = None	O = None

marked exercise intolerance, and congestive heart failure. Asymptomatic conditions that are definite indications are permanent high-grade AV block after myocardial infarction or surgical repair of congenital heart disease, or complete heart block with a ventricular rate less than 40 per minute.

LEAD PLACEMENT. More than 90 per cent of permanent pacing leads are placed via cephalic, subclavian, or external jugular veins. Most transvenous leads are stainless steel, multifilament helical coil wires insulated with polyurethane or silicone rubber. These leads are small, steerable, and fracture resistant. Leads are anchored by tines or a screw-in arrangement at their tips. Both unipolar and bipolar electrodes are commonly used. For simple ventricular pacing, one lead is placed in the right ventricular apex. For dual chamber pacing, a second lead is placed in the right atrium.

PULSE GENERATORS. Modern pacemaker generators weigh 40 to 50 grams, are powered by lithium batteries that last 7 to 10 years, and have circuitry for sensing intracardiac electrograms. Pacemakers can be interrogated to evaluate the pulse generator or reprogrammed to meet changing requirements. Multiprogrammability provides flexibility in obtaining diagnostic information and individualizing the pacemaker prescription.

MODES OF CARDIAC PACING. Pacemaker modes are expressed in the three- or five-letter notation proposed by the

Inter-Society Commission for Heart Disease Resources. Table 42–13 shows the first three letter codes. The three letters indicate the chamber paced, the chamber sensed, and the response to sensing. The fourth and fifth positions describe programmable and antitachycardia features and are used less frequently.

SELECTION OF THE PACEMAKER MODE. Selection of the appropriate pacemaker has become more complex as options have become more diverse. Table 42–14 summarizes common selections, considering the atrial rhythm and status of AV and VA conduction.

COMPLICATIONS. Transvenous implants are associated with cardiac perforation, arrhythmias, infection, thrombosis, emboli, and lead fracture or displacement. Thoracotomy carries the risk of general anesthesia, bleeding, infection, postoperative respiratory compromise, and late threshold increases. With either route of implantation, the pulse generator may erode through the skin. Pacemakers can be inhibited by intense magnetic fields such as large telephone transformers, microwave devices, diathermy, cautery, antitheft devices, and certain types of motors, e.g., electric razors. Unipolar pacemakers may be inhibited by local myopotentials. The "pacemaker syndrome" was first defined as lightheadedness or syncope related to long cycles of AV asynchrony that occurred during VOO or VVI pacing. The definition also includes (1) episodic weakness or syncope associated with alternating AV synchrony and asynchrony, (2) inadequate cardiac output associated with continued absence of AV synchrony or with fixed asynchrony (persistent VA conduction), and (3) patient awareness of beat-to-beat variation in vascular pulsation.

PACEMAKER FOLLOW-UP. Implanted pacing devices require careful follow-up. Regular transtelephonic monitoring permits early detection of battery depletion. At the present time, the principal problem in pacemaker follow-up is the diversity of pacemaker models and methods for interrogating pacemaker function.

TABLE 42–14. INDICATIONS FOR PACING MODES

	Atrial Rhythm		
AV Conduction	*Normal*	*Bradycardia*	*Bradycardia-Tachycardia*
Normal	None indicated	AAI	AAI
AV block; normal VA conduction time	VDD, DDD	DDD, DVI	DVI, VVI
AV block; prolonged VA conduction time	DVI	DVI	DVI

AAI: Fixed-rate atrial pacing occurs unless inhibited by sensed atrial complexes. This mode can be used for patients with symptomatic sinus node dysfunction and normal AV conduction.

VDD: Ventricular pulses are delivered when atrial complex is sensed and inhibited when ventricular complex is sensed. The VDD mode is used when adequate atrial rates and sensing are present, along with high-grade AV block and normal VA conduction. VDD pacing provides atrial augmentation of ventricular filling and avoids the pacemaker syndrome but is contraindicated for patients with supraventricular tachyarrhythmias.

DVI: Both chambers are paced at a preselected rate and AV interval. Pacing is inhibited by ventricular but not atrial activity. The DVI mode is used when synchronous AV contraction is needed in patients with symptomatic atrial bradycardia. The pacing rate does not increase during exercise. DVI pacing is contraindicated in patients who have supraventricular tachyarrhythmias.

DDD: Both atria and ventricles are paced and sensed. The atrial or ventricular pacemaker pulses are inhibited when either atrial or ventricular premature activity is detected. When atrial activity is sensed, a ventricular pulse is provided. This mode of pacing provides synchronous AV contraction over a wide range of heart rates. DDD pacemakers are adaptive: totally inhibited in sinus rhythm with normal AV conduction; AAI pacing during sinus bradycardia with normal AV conduction; VDD pacing during sinus rhythm with impaired AV conduction; DVI pacing during sinus bradycardia with impaired AV conduction. DDD pacemakers are contraindicated in patients with persistent or frequently occurring atrial tachyarrhythmias and those with long VA conduction times who can develop pacemaker-mediated reciprocating tachycardia.

VVI: This mode can be used for any symptomatic bradyarrhythmia. The VVI mode is contraindicated in patients who have had the pacemaker syndrome, those with congestive heart failure, and those who need rate-responsive pacing.

Rate-Responsive Pacing (VVIR): Many patients who need increased heart rate during exercise have relative contraindications for DDD pacing, e.g., inadequate sinus node function or atrial fibrillation. Rate-responsive pacing is provided by sensing the activity level and increasing the pacing rate. Heart rate can be increased by as much as 90 per minute, i.e., from 60 at rest to 150 during exercise, providing an increase in cardiac output and exercise capability.

DC Cardioversion

DC cardioversion was introduced in 1962, and has become a mainstay in the management of cardiac arrhythmias. Cardioversion depolarizes all or most of the heart, interrupts reentrant circuits, and terminates arrhythmias. It is effective for atrial fibrillation, atrial flutter, PSVT, ventricular tachycardia, or ventricular fibrillation. Drug-resistant arrhythmias, e.g., atrial flutter, may respond readily to DC cardioversion. Because of its speed, cardioversion is preferable to drug therapy for arrhythmias that adversely affect hemodynamics, such as rapid atrial arrhythmias, sustained ventricular tachycardia, or ventricular fibrillation. Elective cardioversion is indicated for atrial fibrillation of recent onset (<6 months) to control symptoms and hemodynamic abnormalities and lower the risk of systemic embolism.

LIMITATIONS AND CONTRAINDICATIONS. Chronic atrial fibrillation, i.e., greater than 6 to 12 months in duration, is so likely to recur after cardioversion that digitalis therapy may be preferred. Contributing causes (e.g., hyperthyroidism, pericardial inflammation, pulmonary thromboembolism, chronic obstructive pulmonary disease, or alcohol abuse) should be controlled before cardioversion; otherwise, atrial fibrillation is likely to recur. Sinus rhythm is difficult to maintain after cardioversion of atrial fibrillation in patients with heart failure or large left atria (>45 mm in diameter by echocardiography). In the bradycardia-tachycardia syndrome, cardioversion often produces inadequate rhythms, and atrial fibrillation usually resumes within a few hours. Cardioversion is contraindicated for arrhythmias caused by digitalis intoxication because it can precipitate ventricular fibrillation.

ANTICOAGULATION. Despite the lack of a controlled evaluation, a standard anticoagulation practice has evolved for patients with atrial fibrillation. Most patients who have been fibrillating for more than 3 weeks are anticoagulated, particularly those with (1) a history of embolization, (2) a prosthetic mitral valve, (3) an enlarged left atrium, or (4) congestive heart failure. The prothrombin time is kept at 1.5 to 2.0 times the normal value with warfarin for 3 or more weeks before and a week after cardioversion.

RESULTS. The immediate results of cardioversion are excellent (Table 42–15). The main long-term problem following cardioversion is reversion to atrial fibrillation. Class I antiarrhythmic drugs decrease the chance of recurrence of atrial fibrillation 1 year after cardioversion from about 75 to 50 per cent.

COMPLICATIONS. Few complications attend technically excellent cardioversion. Occasionally, transient SA or AV block or ventricular arrhythmias occur immediately after DC shock, especially with excessive digitalis. In the sick sinus syndrome, the sinus may fail to resume control of cardiac rhythm after cardioversion. Atropine, isoproterenol, and/or external pacing usually maintain the patient until a temporary transvenous pacemaker can be inserted. Occasionally, worsening heart failure or frank pulmonary edema occurs within a few hours after cardioversion. The cause of this syndrome is unknown. Elevation of myocardial creatine kinase after DC cardioversion is rare.

Automatic Implantable Cardioverter/Defibrillator

The first automatic implantable defibrillator (AID), a device that responded only to ventricular fibrillation, was implanted in 1980. The first automatic implantable cardioverter/defibrillator (AICD) was implanted in 1982. This unit detected and cardioverted ventricular tachycardia as well as providing defibrillation. Antitachycardia pacing was added to AICD units in the 1990's.

INDICATIONS. The AICD currently is recommended for patients who have had a documented episode of life-threatening ventricular tachyarrhythmia or cardiac arrest not associated with the acute phase of myocardial infarction. Also, patients should have inducible ventricular tachycardia or ventricular fibrillation unsuitable for drug or surgical therapy. These initial indications are being extended.

IMPLANTATION. The electrode systems are implanted via a thoracotomy. The 292-gram power unit is implanted subcutaneously in an abdominal pocket. During implantation, defibrillation thresholds and detection of ventricular tachycardia/fibrillation are tested extensively to ensure proper function. The AICD usually lasts about 5 years.

The device monitors the ECG continuously. When ventricular tachycardia or fibrillation is detected and verified, the AICD charges its capacitors and delivers a 20- to 30-joule pulse.

FOLLOW-UP. The AICD is a complex device that requires careful follow-up. Potential problems with the device include (1) depletion of the battery, (2) lead breakage or migration, (3) inappropriate discharges, (4) infection, and (5) skin erosion. After implantation, a magnet test should be performed every 2 months to evaluate the device and reform the capacitors. The rate cut-off and other features are programmable to meet changing needs during follow-up.

Between 1980 and the end of 1990 more than 10,000 AID or AICD units were implanted. Follow-up reveals a 1-year cardiovascular mortality of about 10 per cent and a sudden death rate of about 2 per cent. Although the device is complex and expensive, it is highly effective for selected patients with malignant ventricular arrhythmias.

DeSilva RA, Graboys TB, Podrid PJ, Lown B: Cardioversion and defibrillation. Am Heart J 100:881–895, 1980. *A thorough review of the history, theory, and practice of cardioversion and defibrillation.*

Frye RL, Collins JJ, DeSanctis RW, et al.: Guidelines for permanent cardiac pacemaker implantation, May 1984. J Am Coll Cardiol 4:434, 1984. *A report of a task force to review cardiac pacing. The report defines indications for cardiac pacing and makes recommendations about the selection of devices for treatment of specific clinical problems. This report is used as a standard by the medical profession, regulatory agencies, and reimbursement sources.*

Mirowski M: The automatic implantable cardioverter-defibrillator: An overview. J Am Coll Cardiol 6:461, 1985. *A review of the concepts, evolution, clinical use, and follow-up of the automatic implantable cardioverter defibrillator by the originator of the device.*

Parsonnet V, Bernstein AD: Pacing in perspective: Concepts and controversies. Circulation 73:1087, 1986. *A perspective on cardiac pacing. Provides a concise view of the history, development, practice, and future directions in cardiac pacing.*

Winkle RA, Mead RH, Ruder MA, et al: Long-term outcome with the automatic implantable cardioverter-defibrillator. J Am Coll Cardiol 13:1353–1361, 1989. *The clinical events and outcome in 270 patients with AICD implants. Provides an excellent perspective on the current use of the device.*

SURGICAL TREATMENT OF CARDIAC ARRHYTHMIAS

The objective of arrhythmia surgery may be (1) to remove the arrhythmic focus, (2) to interrupt a reentrant pathway, or (3) to prevent the ventricles from responding to supraventricular tachyarrhythmias (Table 42–16). For surgery to be seriously considered, the arrhythmia must pose significant risk to life or interfere substantially with the quality of life.

Supraventricular Arrhythmias

INTERRUPTION OF THE BUNDLE OF HIS. Atrial flutter and fibrillation can be palliated by interruption of the His bundle

TABLE 42–15. ENERGY FOR CARDIOVERSION/DEFIBRILLATION

Arrhythmia	Recommended Initial Energy* (joules)	Comments
Atrial flutter	50	100% conversion; most convert with about 25 joules.
Atrial fibrillation	200	85–95% conversion; a few patients may require 300- to 400-joule DC shocks to cardiovert.
Paroxysmal supraventricular tachycardia	100	100% conversion
Ventricular tachycardia	50	90–95% conversion; 80% convert with <10 joules; a few need 100 joules or more.
Ventricular fibrillation	300–400	90–95% defibrillation; many convert at 200 joules or below but time is of the essence in successful defibrillation.

*An energy level with a high probability of converting the arrhythmia.

TABLE 42–16. SURGERY FOR CARDIAC ARRHYTHMIAS

Arrhythmia	Operative Approach
Atrial fibrillation	Ablation of AV node and implantation of a pacemaker
	Left atrial exclusion (highly experimental)
Ectopic atrial focus	Excision of the focus after accurate mapping
PSVT (Pre-excitation)	Surgical division of anomalous AV connection
PSVT (AV nodal)	Partial catheter ablation of AV node
	Retronodal surgical resection
	Division of His bundle, implantation of pacemaker
Ventricular tachycardia (coronary heart disease)	Endocardial resection guided by mapping
Ventricular tachycardia (arrhythmogenic right ventricular dysplasia)	Simple ventriculotomy; isolation of arrhythmic site
Ventricular tachycardia (after repair of tetralogy of Fallot)	Resection of infundibulectomy scar
Multiform ventricular tachycardia (long QT syndrome)	Left stellate ganglionectomy

and implantation of a ventricular pacemaker when drug therapy cannot control ventricular rate. The need for such surgery has diminished with the advent of β-adrenergic blockers, verapamil, and catheter ablation.

Catheter Ablation. A catheter technique for His bundle ablation has been found to be safe and effective. Using fluoroscopy, a multielectrode catheter is placed so as to record the bundle of His depolarization. Then one or more large energy shocks are delivered to the electrode that records the largest His bundle depolarization. Shocks can be repeated until AV conduction is interrupted.

EXCISION OF AUTOMATIC FOCI. Rhythms originating in automatic or tiny reentrant ectopic foci can be removed or ablated. The key to removal or ablation is accurate localization by epicardial and/or endocardial activation mapping.

INTERRUPTION OF REENTRANT PATHWAYS. Surgery is very effective for PSVT that uses an anomalous AV connection as an essential portion of the circuit or for atrial fibrillation with rapid ventricular response in the WPW syndrome. Preoperative electrophysiologic studies are used to delineate the mechanism of PSVT, the site of the accessory AV connection, and the route of cardiac excitation during PSVT. During operation, the anomalous AV connection(s) is located precisely using cardiac stimulation and epi- or endocardial mapping during sinus rhythm, ventricular pacing, and PSVT. Traditionally, division of anomalous AV connections is done on cardiopulmonary bypass with the atrium open. More recently, dissection and cryoablation have been used successfully without cardiopulmonary bypass. Centers with major programs obtain cure rates greater than 85 per cent, with surgical mortalities less than 1 per cent. These results usually make surgery a better choice than drug treatment.

Sustained Ventricular Tachycardia

VENTRICULAR ANEURYSMS. The largest surgical experience has been gathered in patients with recurrent, sustained VT and coronary heart disease; most of these patients have left ventricular aneurysms, two- or three-vessel disease, and severely impaired left ventricular function. The rate of VT tends to be slow and easily induced and can be mapped during electrophysiologic studies. Accurate preoperative endocardial maps are critical because adequate endocardial maps are often impossible to obtain at surgery. At surgery, the arrhythmogenic tissue is removed or ablated with a cryoprobe. Map-guided excision, isolation, or cryoablation is about 80 per cent effective in controlling sustained VT during 1 to 3 years of follow-up. However, the perioperative mortality is about 15 to 20 per cent owing primarily to the advanced coronary disease and severity of left

ventricular dysfunction. Selection of ideal cases lowers the mortality rate to about 8 to 12 per cent.

ARRHYTHMOGENIC RIGHT VENTRICULAR DYSPLASIA. Patients who have VT due to right ventricular arrhythmogenic dysplasia usually can be cured by an incision across the dysplastic area that shows the latest activation in sinus rhythm and earliest activation during VT. Small areas of dysplasia can be excised and large areas can be isolated if simple incision is not successful.

TETRALOGY OF FALLOT. VT occurs rarely in patients who have had total repair of tetralogy of Fallot. Epicardial excitation mapping at surgery shows that VT arises in the right ventricular infundibular scar, and scar resection effects a cure.

LONG QT SYNDROME. Patients with the congenital form of the long QT syndrome can have recurrent attacks of malignant, multiform VT of the torsades de pointes type. These rhythms are associated with cardiac arrest and sudden cardiac death. Unequal sympathetic nerve traffic to the heart is part of the explanation for the heterogeneous electrophysiologic condition of the ventricles. Excision of the left stellate ganglion markedly reduces the mortality rate in high-risk patients with the congenital long QT syndrome.

Cox JL: The status of surgery for cardiac arrhythmias. Circulation 71:413–417, 1985. *A perspective on surgery for both supraventricular and ventricular arrhythmias.*

Cox JL: Patient selection criteria and results of surgery for refractory ischemic ventricular tachycardia. Circulation 79:163–177, 1989. *An update on selection of patients in the era of the automatic implantable cardioverter defibrillator.*

Cox JL, Gallagher JJ, Cain MM: Experience with 118 consecutive patients undergoing operation for the Wolff-Parkinson-White syndrome. J Thorac Cardiovasc Surg 90:490–501, 1985. *A review of a large, successful experience with surgery for anomalous AV connections.*

Guiraudon GM, Klein GJ, Sharma AD, Yee R: Surgical alternatives for supraventricular tachycardias. Am J Cardiol 64:92J–96J, 1989. *A review of the operative treatment of a wide range of supraventricular tachycardias.*

Klein GJ, Guiraudon GM: Surgical therapy of cardiac arrhythmias. Cardiol Clin 1:323–340, 1983. *A summary of concepts that form the basis for surgical treatment of cardiac arrhythmias.*

43 Sudden Cardiac Death
Douglas P. Zipes

DEFINITION AND INCIDENCE

Sudden cardiac death is unexpected natural death from cardiac causes. The cardiac cause results in a disturbance in cardiac function which produces abrupt loss of cerebral blood flow. Death occurs within 1 hour of the onset of acute symptoms. In 25 per cent of patients who die from coronary heart disease, sudden cardiac death may be the first sign of trouble. Although some patients at risk for sudden cardiac death may be symptomatic prior to the event, their complaints are often too nonspecific to be helpful. An estimated 350,000 sudden cardiac deaths occur annually in the United States, or about one every 90 seconds. This represents almost half of all cardiovascular deaths and almost one fourth of all deaths. The incidence of sudden cardiac death due to coronary heart disease is declining along with the overall decrease in coronary heart disease mortality. These decreases may relate to more frequent and effective treatment of hypertension, angina, and myocardial infarction and attention to additional risk factors.

The incidence of sudden cardiac death peaks between 0 and 6 months and between 45 and 75 years of age. Risk factors for sudden cardiac death parallel those for coronary heart disease and include male sex, cardiac enlargement, obesity, cigarette smoking, glucose intolerance, hypertension, social isolation, stress, and excess alcohol consumption. The presence of coronary heart disease and past myocardial infarction add additional risks. Following myocardial infarction, more than five to ten premature ventricular complexes (PVC's) per hour, three or more repetitive PVC's, late potentials recorded on signal-averaged electrocardiograms, and left ventricular dysfunction are variables identifying patients at increased risk of sudden cardiac death. Angiographic or hemodynamic characteristics are not significantly different between patients who have coronary artery disease and suffer sudden cardiac death and those who do not die suddenly.

Sudden cardiac death, stroke, and myocardial infarction all occur more frequently in the morning hours upon rising, from 6:00 A.M. to noon, at a time when a hypercoagulable state with increased platelet aggregability or coronary vasoconstriction exists. Autonomic mechanisms may also be important in modulating this hypercoagulable state and in triggering sudden cardiac death.

CAUSES

Substrate

Ventricular myocardial abnormalities such as hypertrophy, dilated cardiomyopathy, inflammatory changes, diseases of the heart valves, and primary electrophysiologic abnormalities (Table 43–1) are responsible for about 25 per cent of sudden cardiac deaths, with the remaining 75 per cent due to coronary artery disease. Occasionally, patients without structural heart disease suffer ventricular fibrillation. The long QT syndrome is one of several electrophysiologic abnormalities that can predispose to sudden cardiac death (Table 43–1). It may be acquired by exposure to several antiarrhythmic drugs such as quinidine, phenothiazines, and tricyclic antidepressants or may result from electrolyte disturbances such as hypokalemia or hypomagnesemia. It may also be congenital, with (Jervell-Lange-Nielsen syndrome) and without (Romano-Ward syndrome) neural deafness. Preliminary information suggests that a specific electrophysiologic mechanism is responsible, called early afterdepolarizations.

At autopsy, 90 per cent or greater narrowing of at least one coronary artery is noted in three quarters of patients dying with sudden cardiac death, and almost two thirds have three vessels with 75 per cent or more stenosis. Old myocardial infarction is

TABLE 43–1. CAUSES AND CONTRIBUTING FACTORS IN SUDDEN CARDIAC DEATH

Coronary artery abnormalities
  Coronary atherosclerosis
  Congenital abnormalities of coronary arteries
  Coronary artery embolism
  Coronary arteritis
  Miscellaneous mechanical obstructions of coronary arteries
  Functional obstruction of coronary arteries
Hypertrophy of ventricular myocardium
  Left ventricular hypertrophy associated with coronary atherosclerosis
  Hypersensitive heart disease without significant coronary atherosclerosis
  Hypertrophic myocardium secondary to valvular heart disease
  Hypertrophic cardiomyopathy
  Primary or secondary pulmonary hypertension
Myocardial diseases and heart failure
  Chronic congestive heart failure
  Acute cardiac failure
Inflammatory, infiltrative, neoplastic, and degenerative processes
Diseases of the cardiac valves
Congenital heart disease
Electrophysiologic abnormalities
  Abnormalities of the conducting system
  Prolonged QT interval syndrome
  Idiopathic ventricular fibrillation
Electrical instability related to neurohumoral and central nervous system influences
  Catecholamine-dependent lethal arrhythmias
  Central nervous system related
Sudden infant death syndrome and sudden death in children
Miscellaneous
  Sudden death during extreme physical activity
  Mechanical interference with venous return
  Dissecting aneurysm of the aorta
  Toxic/metabolic disturbances
  Mimics of sudden cardiac death

Modified from Myerburg RJ, Castellanos A: Cardiac arrest and sudden cardiac death. *In* Braunwald EB (ed.): Heart Disease: A Textbook of Cardiovascular Medicine, 3rd ed. Philadelphia, W. B. Saunders Company, 1988, pp 742–777; with permission.

found in about two thirds of autopsies. No specific high-risk coronary artery or lesion site, proximal versus distal, has been identified. Acute thrombotic occlusion is noted in 60 to 75 per cent, usually at the site of a fissured plaque, providing clues about mechanisms of sudden cardiac death. For example, in sudden cardiac death, as in unstable angina, plaque rupture with thrombus formation may result in myocardial ischemia and precipitate fatal ventricular arrhythmias. Also, platelet microthrombi from ulcerated arterial plaques may produce multiple areas of myocardial necrosis that can cause electrical instability and ventricular fibrillation. It is likely that a non–flow-limiting intimal plaque serves as a nidus for acute formation of a lumen-occluding thrombus in a significant number of patients with sudden cardiac death. Certainly coronary artery spasm or other factors that reduce myocardial blood flow without an increase in demand, as well as an increase in myocardial oxygen demand with a fixed supply, may be critical.

Prostacyclin (PGI_2), a potent inhibitor of platelet activation and a vasodilator, may be important. In dogs, PGI_2 given intravenously reduces the incidence of ventricular fibrillation after circumflex coronary artery occlusion, as do specific thromboxane synthase inhibitors. The latter presumably work by blocking conversion of prostaglandin endoperoxide PGH_2 to thromboxane A_2, causing PGH_2 accumulation, which then can be converted to prostacyclin. Prostacyclin also modulates sympathetic activity to the heart at presynaptic sites and can reduce the incidence of ventricular fibrillation by reducing sympathetic effects. Local release of serotonin in atherosclerotic vessels may also be important by reducing coronary blood flow, increasing platelet aggregation, and causing the development of an occlusive thrombus and electrical instability.

Other biochemical clues are being investigated. For example, inhibition of carnitine acyltransferase, which reduces the accumulation of long-chain acylcarnitines in the sarcolemma and the initial electrophysiologic derangements associated with hypoxia and also the accumulation of lysophosphatidylcholine, lowers the early occurrence of ventricular tachycardia or ventricular fibrillation in cats subjected to coronary artery occlusion.

Of great interest is the observation that only 20 per cent of those patients who are successfully resuscitated from ventricular fibrillation evolve an acute myocardial infarction. This means that if thrombosis of a coronary artery causes the ischemia responsible for the ventricular fibrillation, it is transient because flow must be restored to prevent infarction. Ventricular fibrillation recurs in 30 per cent within 1 year and 45 per cent by 2 years in those survivors who do not, versus only about 2 per cent in those who do, evolve a transmural myocardial infarction after resuscitation. Therefore, patients without infarction are at increased risk for another episode of sudden cardiac death.

Ischemia responsible for the biochemical changes noted above is conducive to arrhythmia development. Myocardial ischemia results in loss of membrane integrity with cellular efflux of potassium and influx of calcium, development of acidosis, reduction of transmembrane resting potentials, and enhanced automaticity in some tissues. Reperfusion causes continued influx of calcium that may result in triggered arrhythmias. The electrophysiologic changes following myocardial ischemia can create areas of slow conduction and unidirectional block, changes necessary for reentry to occur, as well as areas of abnormal automaticity and triggered activity. These factors can lead to ventricular tachycardia/fibrillation. Tissue healed after previous injury appears more susceptible to the electrical destabilizing effects of acute ischemia. The combination of a triggering event such as a premature ventricular complex and a susceptible myocardium may be the fundamental combination for development of a lethal arrhythmia. Triggering events and a susceptible myocardium may be dissociated from each other so that in the absence of a susceptible myocardium, triggering events may occur innocuously. Similarly, the presence of a susceptible myocardium without a triggering event may not give rise to arrhythmias.

Arrhythmias

More than 90 per cent of sudden cardiac deaths are due to a lethal cardiac rhythm disturbance, approximately 80 per cent to

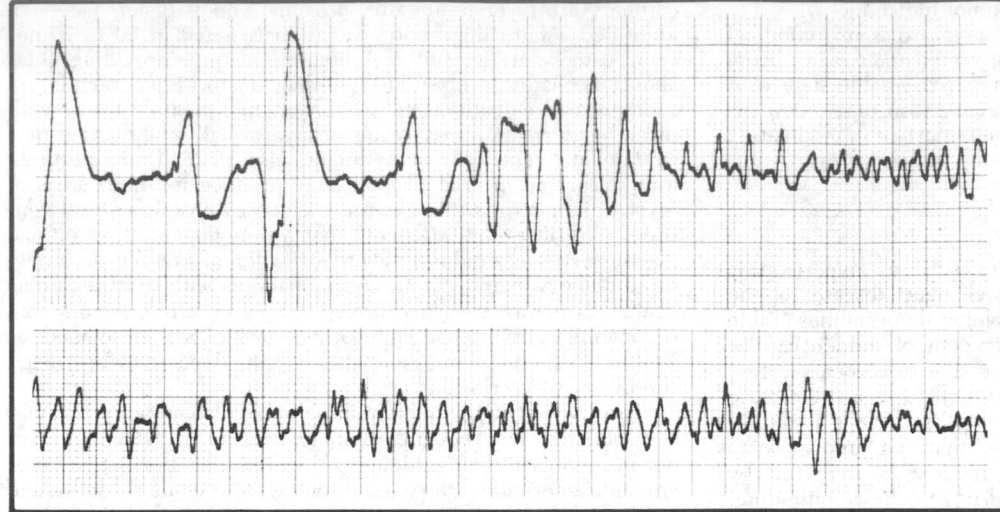

FIGURE 43–1. Ventricular tachycardia fibrillation. Several multiform premature ventricular complexes initiate a run of ventricular tachycardia that progresses to ventricular fibrillation. Monitor lead. Continuous recording.

ventricular tachycardia/fibrillation (Fig. 43–1), and 20 per cent to a severe bradyarrhythmia or ventricular asystole (Fig. 43–2). Ventricular tachycardia leading to ventricular fibrillation is often preceded by increases in sinus rate, advancing grades of ventricular ectopy, and loss of sinus arrhythmia (suggesting a decrease in vagal tone). Only a small percentage of patients have ischemic ST changes. Bradycardia and ventricular asystole occur more commonly in a severely diseased heart and may represent diffuse involvement of subendocardial Purkinje fibers by the ischemic process. Atrioventricular block occurs less often than asystole. Less frequent nonarrhythmic mechanisms of sudden cardiac death include electromechanical dissociation, ventricular rupture, cardiac tamponade, acute mechanical obstruction to flow, and acute dissection of a major blood vessel.

THERAPY AND OUTCOME

Untreated ventricular fibrillation produces irreversible brain damage within 3 to 5 minutes and death shortly thereafter. Although some patients may be resuscitated after longer periods of sustaining a ventricular tachyarrhythmia, the probability of a favorable outcome deteriorates rapidly in proportion to the duration of the unattended cardiac arrest, with older patients doing more poorly than younger. Some patients may have ventricular tachycardia with an output inadequate to maintain consciousness but sufficient to maintain brain viability, permitting a longer time interval between the onset of loss of consciousness and irreversible brain damage or death.

Therapy for a patient suffering cardiac arrest begins initially with establishing the diagnosis of the cardiac arrest, delivering a blow to the chest to attempt "thumpversion" of ventricular tachycardia, and clearing the airway. Basic life support activities including mouth-to-mouth ventilation, and chest compression should be started and continued until advanced life support activities begin. These include initially electrical cardioversion/

defibrillation for treatment of ventricular tachycardia/fibrillation, pacing for bradyarrhythmia/asystole, and drug administration. After successful resuscitation, the patient is admitted to a monitoring unit where treatment goals are to provide hemodynamic support, prevent a second cardiac arrest, and evaluate causes of the first.

Early ventricular defibrillation is the most important factor influencing survival. In the hospital, no time should be wasted in instituting electrical cardioversion or defibrillation. Out of hospital, prompt cardiopulmonary resuscitation (CPR) by bystander laypersons awaiting the arrival of emergency rescue personnel significantly improves the percentage of patients subsequently discharged alive from the hospital. Presumably this difference is due to CPR-related protection of the central nervous system.

Elements required to achieve the highest survival rates from out-of-hospital cardiac arrest include witnessed arrest, rapid telephone notification of the emergency medical service, early initiation of cardiopulmonary resuscitation, rapid arrival of emergency personnel equipped with a defibrillator, early advanced airway management, and prompt intravenous drug therapy. Significant risk factors for death after cardiopulmonary resuscitation include hypotension and pneumonia prior to arrest, time for restoration of normal rhythm exceeding 15 minutes, need for intubation, the presence of hypotension and, after resuscitation, a need for vasopressors.

The rhythm disturbance responsible for the cardiac arrest influences outcome dramatically. Patients who have ventricular tachycardia have the best prognosis but constitute the smallest group of only about 10 per cent of all cardiac arrests. It is possible that many more cardiac arrests begin as sustained ventricular tachycardia and progress to ventricular fibrillation and that patients found with ventricular tachycardia do better because their arrest is treated earlier. Forty to 60 per cent of patients who

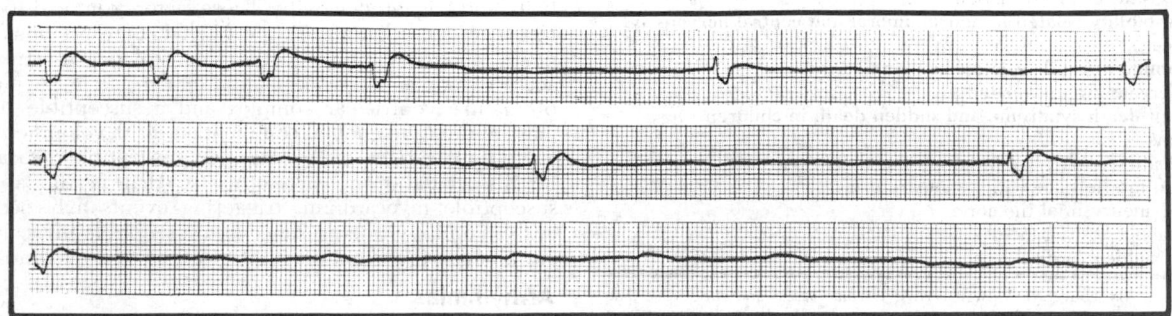

FIGURE 43–2. Sudden cardiac death due to asystole. A ventricular escape rhythm progressively slows, terminating in complete asystole. Monitor lead. Continuous recording.

have ventricular fibrillation are successfully resuscitated and admitted to the hospital alive, and about half of those are ultimately discharged alive. Patients who have bradyarrhythmia or asystole as the initiating event or at initial contact have the worst prognosis, with only about 10 per cent admitted to hospital alive and few if any subsequently surviving. Similarly, patients whose rhythm following defibrillation is a bradyarrhythmia of less than 60 beats per minute also have a poor prognosis, with 95 per cent dying prior to or during hospitalization.

Long-term therapy for prevention of ventricular tachyarrhythmias includes pharmacologic, electrical, and surgical options (see Ch. 42). In patients with ventricular tachycardia/fibrillation inducible by programmed electrical stimulation, serial electrophysiologic testing can identify drug regimens that prevent arrhythmia recurrence in approximately 20 to 40 per cent of patients. In an additional 20 per cent of patients, drugs can slow the ventricular tachycardia and reduce arrhythmia-related mortality to less than 3 per cent per year. For patients in whom ventricular tachycardia/fibrillation cannot be prevented or significantly slowed, medical antiarrhythmic therapy is generally unsuccessful and the sudden death mortality is 20 to 40 per cent per year. In these patients, surgical resection of the arrhythmogenic substrate or implantation of a pacemaker/cardioverter/defibrillator may be indicated. Both subendocardial resection and defibrillator implantation are highly effective in preventing sudden cardiac death. The choice of procedure depends on the arrhythmia diagnosis and the nature of the cardiac disease. Operative mortality is 10 to 15 per cent for surgical resection versus 3 per cent for device implantation, with left ventricular function being the most important predictor of risk. Arrhythmic mortality following device implantation is less than 2 per cent per year.

Bayes-deLuna A, Coumel P, Leclercq JF: Ambulatory sudden cardiac death: Mechanisms of production of fatal arrhythmia on the basis of data from 157 cases. Am Heart J 117:151–159, 1989. *An original study on ECG recordings of patients at the time of sudden cardiac death.*

Epstein SE, Quyyumi AA, Bonow RO: Sudden cardiac death without warning. N Engl J Med 321:320–324, 1989. *Suggestions on the coronary mechanisms responsible for sudden cardiac death.*

Kremers MS, Black WH, Wells PJ: Sudden cardiac death: Etiologies, pathogenesis and management. DM 35:381–445, 1989. *A thorough review of sudden cardiac death.*

Muller JE, Tofler GH, Stone PH: Circadian variation and triggers of onset of acute cardiovascular disease. Circulation 79:733–743, 1989. *A review of some of the triggers of sudden cardiac death.*

Winkle RA, Mead RH, Ruder MA, et al.: Long-term outcome with the automatic implantable cardioverter-defibrillator. J Am Coll Cardiol 13:1353–1361, 1989. *An original study on the largest single series of patients receiving the implantable defibrillator.*

44 Arterial Hypertension

Suzanne Oparil

Systemic hypertension is the most prevalent cardiovascular disorder in the United States, affecting over 60 million Americans. Almost 40 per cent of all black adults and more than half of the entire population over age 60 have hypertension. In spite of increasing public awareness and a rapidly expanding array of antihypertensive medications, hypertension remains one of the leading causes of cardiovascular morbidity and mortality. Efforts to prevent, diagnose, and treat hypertension remain an important concern of national health care. Advances in the diagnosis and treatment of hypertension are likely responsible for the decline in cardiovascular mortality which has occurred in the last 20 years. However, the adverse metabolic effects of some classes of antihypertensive drugs and the disappointing results of antihypertensive treatment in coronary disease prevention have raised questions that challenge traditional approaches to the management of the hypertensive patient. Antihypertensive treatment should be undertaken in the context of overall management of cardiovascular disease risk factors, and its ultimate goal should be reduction of overall cardiovascular risk.

TABLE 44–1. CLASSIFICATION OF BP IN ADULTS AGED 18 YEARS OR OLDER*

BP Range (mm Hg)	Category†
DBP	
<85	Normal BP
85–89	High-normal BP
90–104	Mild hypertension
105–114	Moderate hypertension
≥115	Severe hypertension
SBP, when DBP <90 mm Hg	
<140	Normal BP
140–159	Borderline isolated systolic hypertension
≥160	Isolated systolic hypertension

*Classification based on the average of two or more readings on two or more occasions. BP indicates blood pressure; DBP, diastolic blood pressure; and SBP, systolic blood pressure.
†A classification of borderline isolated systolic hypertension (SBP, 140 to 159 mm Hg) or isolated systolic hypertension (SBP, ≥160 mm Hg) takes precedence over high-normal BP (DBP, 85 to 89 mm Hg) when both occur in the same person. High-normal BP (DBP, 85 to 89 mm Hg) takes precedence over a classification of normal BP (SBP, <140 mm Hg) when both occur in the same person.
Reprinted with permission from The 1988 Report of the Joint National Committee on Detection, Evaluation, and Treatment of High Blood Pressure. Arch Intern Med 148:1023, 1988.

DEFINITION

Arterial hypertension is defined as elevated arterial blood pressure (BP). Since BP in the general population falls on a gaussian curve of normal distribution, it is impossible to define with precision the limits of "normal" BP. In addition, the BP of a given individual varies widely over time, depending on many variables, including sympathetic nervous system activity, posture, state of hydration, and skeletal muscle tone. Accordingly, any definition of hypertension must be arbitrary. The Joint National Committee on Detection, Evaluation and Treatment of High Blood Pressure recommends the scheme shown in Table 44–1 for the diagnosis of hypertension in individuals aged 18 years or older. The diagnosis of hypertension in adults is made when the average of two or more diastolic BP measurements on at least two subsequent visits is 90 mm Hg or higher or when the average of multiple systolic BP readings on two or more subsequent visits is consistently greater than 140 mm Hg (Table 44–2). The patient should be clearly informed that a single elevated reading does not constitute a diagnosis of hypertension but is a sign that further observation is required.

Essential, primary, or **idiopathic hypertension** is arterial hypertension of unknown cause. Over 95 per cent of all cases of arterial hypertension are in this category.

Secondary hypertension is arterial hypertension of known

TABLE 44–2. FOLLOW-UP CRITERIA FOR INITIAL BP MEASUREMENT FOR ADULTS AGED 18 YEARS OR OLDER*

BP Range (mm Hg)	Recommended Follow-up
DBP	
<85	Recheck within 2 years
85–89	Recheck within 1 year
90–104	Confirm within 2 months
105–114	Evaluate or refer promptly to source of care within 2 weeks
≥115	Evaluate or refer immediately to source of care
SBP, when DBP <90 mm Hg	
<140	Recheck within 2 years
140–199	Confirm within 2 months
≥200	Evaluate or refer promptly to source of care within 2 weeks

*BP indicates blood pressure; DBP, diastolic blood pressure; and SBP, systolic blood pressure. If recommendations for follow-up of DBP and SBP are different, the shorter recommended time for recheck and referral should take precedence.
Reprinted with permission from The 1988 Report of the Joint National Committee on Detection, Evaluation, and Treatment of High Blood Pressure. Arch Intern Med 148:1023, 1988.

cause. Fewer than 5 per cent of all cases of systemic hypertension are in this category. The importance of identifying patients with secondary hypertension is that they sometimes can be cured by surgery or can be easily controlled by specific medical treatment. Thus the morbidity and mortality of potentially ineffective empiric medical therapy can be avoided and the cumulative cost of medical treatment reduced. The most common causes of secondary hypertension are summarized in Table 44–3.

Malignant hypertension is the syndrome of markedly elevated BP (diastolic BP usually greater than 140 mm Hg) associated with papilledema. **Accelerated hypertension** is the syndrome of markedly elevated BP associated with hemorrhages and exudates (grade 3 Kimmelstiel-Wilson [K-W] retinopathy). If untreated, accelerated hypertension presumably progresses to a malignant phase. Both accelerated and malignant hypertension are associated with widespread degenerative changes in the walls of resistance vessels. These syndromes are characterized by extreme BP elevations, sudden onset, fulminant course, and evidence of severe, generalized vascular damage, including grade 3 or 4 K-W retinopathy, hypertensive encephalopathy, hematuria, and renal dysfunction. Malignant hypertension is usually fatal unless treated promptly and vigorously. If BP can be controlled, prognosis depends on the state of renal function.

Complicated hypertension is the descriptive term for arterial hypertension of any etiology in which there is evidence of cardiovascular damage related to the BP elevation. Hypertensive complications commonly include stroke, congestive heart failure, renal failure, myocardial infarction, and arterial aneurysm.

Borderline hypertension is intermittent hypertension in which some BP measurements are elevated and some are normal in the untreated patient. Patients with borderline hypertension tend to maintain pressures that are above average for the general population and are at greater risk of cardiovascular morbidity and mortality than the general population. As a group, these patients manifest increased cardiac output, more rapid heart rate, and higher left ventricular ejection rate than either the normotensive population or the population of patients with stable hypertension.

White coat or **office hypertension** refers to the elevation in BP manifested by some patients due to the stress and anxiety of an office visit. Studies using ambulatory monitoring have suggested that as many as 30 per cent of patients diagnosed as hypertensive by standard office measurements are actually normotensive. However, the true incidence and significance of this phenomenon remain controversial.

INCIDENCE AND PREVALENCE

Approximately 60 million persons in the United States have hypertension. The prevalence of hypertension increases with age in all groups: blacks, whites, men, and women (Fig. 44–1). Diastolic hypertension is roughly twice as common among 50-year-olds as among 30-year-olds, and systolic hypertension increases greatly in prevalence after age 45, probably reflecting age-regulated reductions in compliance of the large conduit vessels. Hypertension is an extremely common health problem in the geriatric population, afflicting approximately 65 per cent of the population in the 65- to 74-year-old group. Data from the 1976 to 1980 National Health and Nutrition Examination Survey (NHANES II) indicate that blacks have a higher prevalence of hypertension than whites (38 per cent versus 29 per cent). The reason for the increased prevalence of hypertension among blacks is unclear, but it has been attributed to heredity, greater salt intake, and greater environmental stress. Men have a higher overall prevalence of hypertension than women (33 per cent versus 27 per cent). Hypertension is more common in men than in women up to approximately age 50; after that time, hypertension is more common in women. The increased prevalence of hypertension in postmenopausal women is related to a combination of weight gain and hormonal alterations.

Data from NHANES II indicate that most hypertensive patients have small elevations in BP (Fig. 44–2). Approximately 50 per cent of all hypertensives in the 18- to 74-year age group, or 15 per cent of the entire adult population of the United States, have mild hypertension (see Table 44–1). These figures reflect the preponderance of white hypertensives sampled by NHANES II. Blacks tend to have more severe hypertension than whites. Five per cent of hypertensives, most of whom are elderly, have isolated systolic hypertension.

ETIOLOGY AND PATHOGENESIS OF ESSENTIAL HYPERTENSION

The cause of elevated BP cannot be identified in more than 95 per cent of cases; these individuals are said to have essential hypertension. Essential hypertension tends to cluster in families and represents a collection of genetically based diseases and/or syndromes with a number of underlying inherited biochemical abnormalities. Of the numerous pathologic features of essential hypertension, many undoubtedly represent compensatory mechanisms that offset the primary abnormality. Pathophysiologic factors that have been implicated in the genesis of essential hypertension include increased sympathetic nervous system activity, overproduction of an unidentified sodium-retaining hormone, chronic high sodium intake, inadequate dietary intakes of potassium and calcium, increased or "inappropriate" renin secretion, deficiencies of vasodilators such as prostaglandins, congenital abnormalities of the resistance vessels, diabetes mellitus, insulin resistance, obesity, increased activity of vascular growth factors, and altered cellular ion transport. The tools of molecular biology provide, for the first time, the means of defining the genetic basis of the hypertensive diseases and for designing rational preventive and therapeutic strategies. To date, no specific set of

TABLE 44–3. CAUSES OF SECONDARY HYPERTENSION

Systolic and diastolic hypertension
  Renal
    Renal parenchymal disease
      Chronic nephritis
      Polycystic disease
      Collagen vascular disease
      Diabetic nephropathy
      Hydronephrosis
      Acute glomerulonephritis
    Renal vascular disease
    Renal transplantation
    Renin-secreting tumors
  Endocrine
    Adrenal
      Primary aldosteronism
      Overproduction of 11-deoxycorticosterone (DOC), 18-OH-DOC, and other mineralocorticoids
      Congenital adrenal hyperplasia
      Cushing's syndrome
      Pheochromocytoma
    Extra-adrenal chromaffin tumors
    Hyperparathyroidism
    Acromegaly
  Pregnancy-induced hypertension
  Coarctation of the aorta
  Neurologic disorders
    Dysautonomia
    Increased intracranial pressure
    Quadriplegia
    Lead poisoning
    Guillain-Barré syndrome
  Postoperative
  Drugs and chemicals
    Cyclosporine
    Oral contraceptives
    Glucocorticoids
    Mineralocorticoids, including licorice and carbenoxolone
    Sympathomimetics
    Tyramine and MAO inhibitors
Isolated systolic hypertension
  Aging, with associated aortic rigidity
  Increased cardiac output
    Thyrotoxicosis
    Anemia
    Aortic valvular insufficiency
  Decreased peripheral vascular resistance
    Arteriovenous shunts
    Paget's disease of bone
    Beriberi

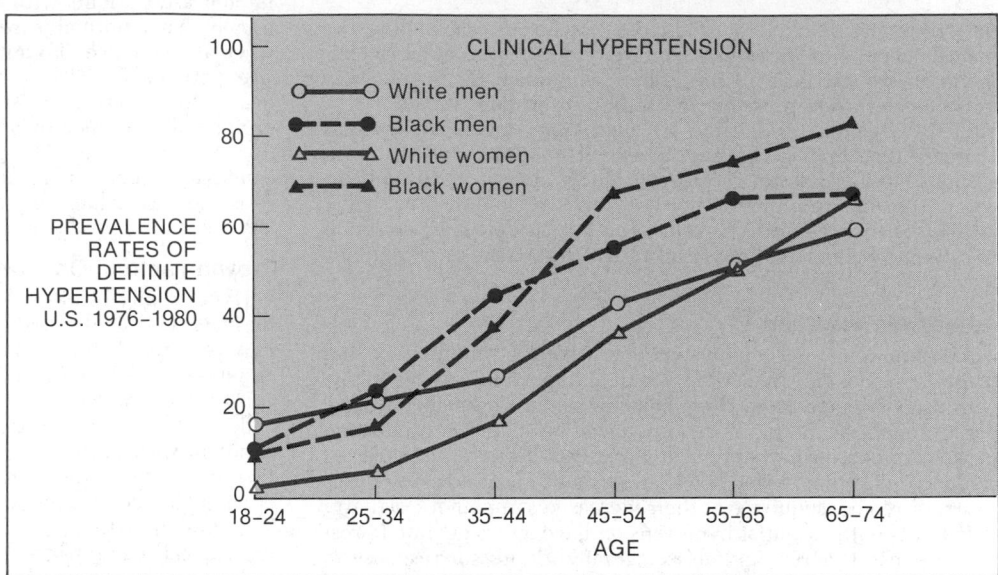

FIGURE 44–1. The prevalence of hypertension in the United States defined as the average of three blood pressure measurements of 140/90 mm Hg or higher on a single occasion or reported taking of antihypertensive medications. (Prepared using data from the 1976–1980 National Health and Nutrition Examination Survey. Modified from Hypertension Prevalence and the Status of Awareness, Treatment and Control in the United States: Final Report of the Subcommittee on Definition and Prevalence of the 1984 Joint National Committee. Hypertension 7:457–468, 1985; by permission of the American Heart Association.)

BP-regulating genes has been identified, nor have genetic markers that permit early detection of individuals at risk for developing hypertension been characterized.

Genetic Factors

The mechanisms by which BP is genetically controlled are diverse, interrelated, and incompletely understood. Studies in normotensive first-degree relatives of essential hypertensives have demonstrated differences in electrolyte excretion and circulating renin levels that may make this group susceptible to the development of hypertension. Thus, inherited abnormalities in the renin-angiotensin-aldosterone system, perhaps including alterations in sympathetic nervous drive to renin release and/or an intrinsic defect in the ability of the kidney to handle volume overload, may contribute to the pathogenesis of essential hypertension.

Specific molecular defects in cell membrane transport systems, such as pumps or cotransport, have been described in hypertensive subjects and related to the pathogenesis of hypertension. Several abnormalities in Na^+ handling, including increased passive entry of Na^+, increased maximal rate of Na^+/Li^+ exchange, and decreased apparent affinity of the Na^+-K^+ pump for internal Na^+, have been found in red blood cells of human hypertensives. An important consequence of these alterations in cellular handling of Na^+ is an increase in intracellular Na^+ concentration, which results in an increased intracellular free Ca^{2+} concentration. A positive correlation between platelet Ca^{2+} and BP has been reported. The membrane defects observed in blood cells of human essential hypertensives could be shared by other cell types, such as vascular smooth muscle cells, sympathetic neurons, and renal tubule cells, which are involved in the maintenance of vascular tone and volume homeostasis and in the pathogenesis of hypertension. Thus, the abnormalities in membrane Na^+ and Ca^{2+} handling described in human hypertensives could account for the circulatory alterations that lead to systemic hypertension. Further study is needed to determine which genes are responsible for these abnormalities and to establish more precisely the mechanisms by which their expression leads to the development of genetically mediated hypertension in humans.

Renal Sodium Handling

A defect in the excretion of salt and water may be central to the pathogenesis of hypertension. The normal kidney plays an important role in maintaining intravascular volume and BP. It responds to increments in perfusion pressure by increasing sodium and water excretion, thus reducing intravascular volume and restoring BP to normal levels. Hemodynamic, neural, and humoral factors participate in the control of volume and BP homeostasis by regulating renal sodium handling. In hypertensive subjects, this relationship is perturbed, such that higher perfusion

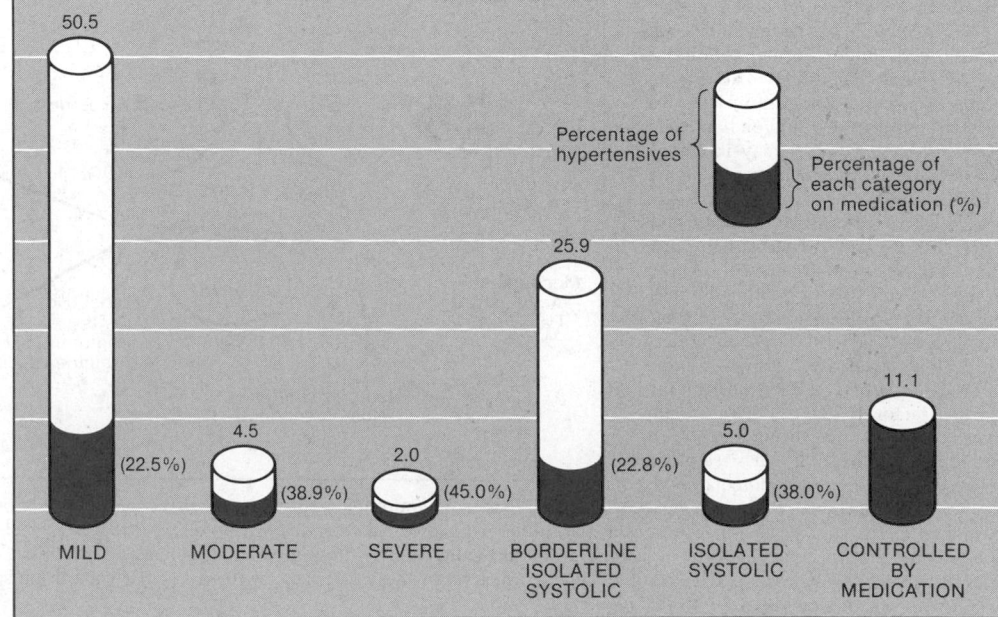

FIGURE 44–2. Percentage of civilian, noninstitutionalized population, 18 to 74 years of age, with hypertension categorized by blood pressure (BP) (*figure over column*) and percentage of each category receiving medication (*dark column*). Hypertension is defined as BP, 140/90 mm Hg or above or use of antihypertensive medication. (Prepared using data from the 1976–1980 National Health and Nutritional Examination Survey. From Hypertension Prevalence and the Status of Awareness, Treatment and Control in the United States: Final Report of the Subcommittee on Definition and Prevalence of the 1984 Joint National Committee. Hypertension 7:457–468, 1985; by permission of the American Heart Association.)

pressures are needed to produce a natriuresis, facilitating the maintenance of hypertension. A variety of neurohumoral factors, intrinsic and extrinsic to the kidney, influence the relationship between perfusion pressure and sodium excretion. In addition, a kidney subjected to elevated BP over time develops structural changes that limit its ability to excrete sodium and water in response to increases in pressure. Kidneys altered in this fashion, when transplanted into a normotensive recipient, cause that individual to become hypertensive. Thus, a defect in excretion of salt and water may be central to the pathogenesis of systemic hypertension.

Autonomic Function

The autonomic nervous system is involved in the initiation and maintenance of elevated BP in essential hypertension. In patients with early hypertension, there is evidence for diminished resting parasympathetic inhibition and enhanced sympathetic stimulation of the cardiovascular system. These patients have elevated plasma renin and norepinephrine levels and enhanced vascular responses to stress as a consequence of their increased sympathetic activity.

Patients with essential hypertension have an exaggerated pressor response to stress and an exaggerated depressor response to relaxation. Blood pressure falls during meditation and other states of relaxation and rises during isometric exercise and the stress of mental arithmetic in these patients to a greater extent than in normotensive control subjects. The impressive fall in BP that is frequently seen when a hypertensive patient is removed from his home environment and brought into the hospital suggests that environmental stress exacerbates hypertension. The increased prevalence of hypertension in urban populations compared to rural groups and the occurrence of age-related rises in BP in societies with changing value systems but not in those with a stable social structure give evidence for a psychogenic contribution to essential hypertension. Stress presumably mediates its pressor effect through the sympathetic nervous system.

Hemodynamics

Cardiac output is elevated early in the course of essential hypertension and may cause secondary increases in peripheral vascular resistance which are responsible for maintaining the hypertension. This concept of total body autoregulation has been used to explain the adaptation of resistance vessels to increases in cardiac output. According to the theory of total body autoregulation, systemic resistance vessels respond to an increased cardiac output and increased intravascular volume by constricting in order to reduce tissue blood flow to normal. Patients with essential hypertension of recent onset generally show a pattern of increased cardiac output (about 15 per cent greater than normotensive control levels), tachycardia, and venoconstriction,

with normal or even low peripheral vascular resistance at rest. In contrast, patients with longstanding established hypertension usually have normal cardiac output and increased peripheral vascular resistance. Longitudinal studies of untreated hypertensive patients have documented a fall in cardiac output, due mainly to a decrease in stroke volume, and an increase in total peripheral resistance over time. These observations are compatible with the notion that increases in cardiac output initiate essential hypertension and that changes in peripheral vascular resistance occur later and are more important in maintaining the BP elevation.

Growth Factors, Oncogenes, and Vascular Hypertrophy

Hypertrophy of blood vessels, whether primary or secondary to increases in BP and hence vessel wall tension, plays an important role in the pathogenesis of hypertension. The myogenic response to elevations in BP and flow is characterized by vasoconstriction, increased calcium influx into vascular smooth muscle cells, and, over the long term, increased myocyte growth. The resultant vascular hypertrophy tends to reduce blood flow to the tissues and to elevate intravascular pressure. Stimuli to growth of vascular smooth muscle cells are summarized in Figure 44–3. The growth factors have contractile effects on vascular smooth muscle cells and trigger many of the same cellular signaling events as are activated by vasoconstrictor agents such as norepinephrine and angiotensin II. Conversely, many of the endogenous vasoconstrictors stimulate vascular smooth muscle cell growth via receptor-mediated mechanisms. Of the endogenous vasoconstrictors, angiotensin II is a particularly important autocrine and paracrine regulator of vascular hypertrophy. Blood vessel walls contain an active renin-angiotensin system, and inhibition of vascular angiotensin II production with angiotensin-converting enzyme (ACE) inhibitors prevents or reverses vascular hypertrophy more effectively than treatment with other classes of antihypertensive agents that have equipotent blood pressure–lowering effects. Further, recent evidence suggests that captopril may prevent restenosis following angioplasty, suggesting that angiotensin II may participate in the vascular remodeling characteristic of the atherosclerotic process.

Contractile agonists and many growth factors share cellular signaling effects that are related to the vascular growth response. These agents activate phospholipase C, which hydrolyzes phosphatidylinositol bisphosphate to generate inositol trisphosphate and diacylglycerol. The former mobilizes Ca^{2+} from intracellular stores; the latter modulates Ca^{2+}-sensitive protein kinase C, which activates Na^+/H^+ exchange and alkalinizes the cell. Cellular alkalinization is associated with both vasoconstriction and growth and/or division. Alternate signaling events, including cyclic AMP production, have been described with some growth factors.

Proto-oncogenes, including c-fos, c-myc, and c-jun, that are induced in association with these signaling events render the

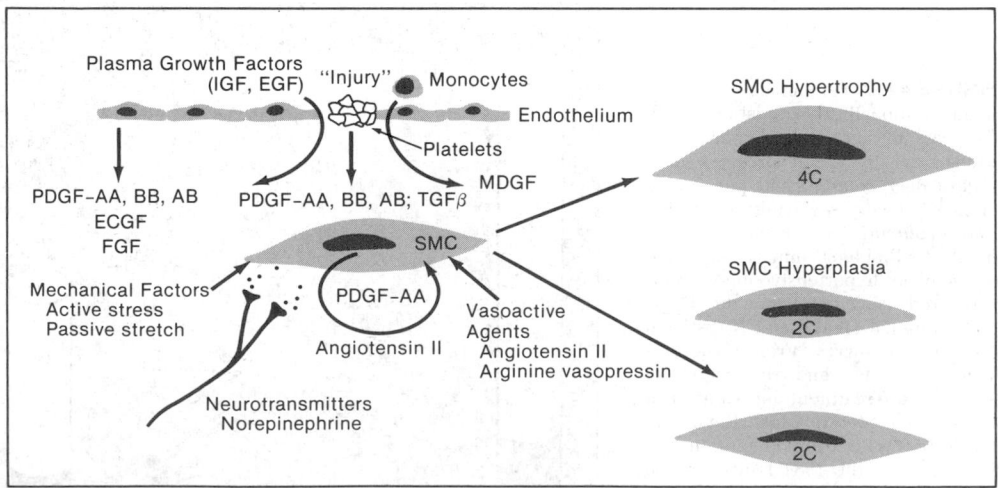

FIGURE 44–3. Factors that may play a role in growth regulation of smooth muscle cells under normal conditions and after vascular injury. The growth response of the smooth muscle cell may be hypertrophy and/or hyperplasia. Endothelial injury may influence the growth of smooth muscle cells by increased influx of plasma growth factors, such as insulin-like growth factor I (IGF), into the vessel wall through denuded vessel segments or as the result of increased endothelial macromolecular permeability; release of growth factors from platelets (e.g., platelet-derived growth factors [PDGF-AA, BB, AB]; transforming growth factor β [TGF β]) or monocytes (e.g., macrophage-derived growth factor [MDGF]) at sites of injury; or increased production of growth factors by endothelial cells (e.g., PDGF-AA, BB, and AB; endothelial-derived growth factor [ECGF]) or of smooth muscle cells themselves as a response to the injury. Other factors that may influence growth of smooth muscle cells in the absence of vessel injury include norepinephrine and other neurotransmitters, mechanical factors, and contractile agonists from circulating blood or endothelial cells or generated by smooth muscle cells themselves. (From Owens GK: Control of hypertrophic versus hyperplastic growth of vascular smooth muscle cells. Am J Physiol 257:H1755–H1765, 1989; with permission.)

cells competent to replicate their DNA in response to growth factors. Whether the protein products of these competence genes are responsible for vascular growth is uncertain. The regulation of vascular growth in hypertension is an area of active investigation and may give rise to new approaches, including gene therapy, to antihypertensive treatment.

Insulin Resistance

Peripheral resistance to insulin has been described in essential hypertension. The level of insulin resistance and the defect in whole-body glucose utilization are positively correlated with the severity of the hypertension. Insulin resistance in hypertension appears to be independent of both obesity and glucose tolerance as measured by standard glucose tolerance tests. Whole-body insulin-induced glucose uptake and nonoxidative glucose disposal (glycogen synthesis and glycolysis) are markedly reduced and plasma insulin levels are elevated, presumably as a compensatory mechanism, in insulin-resistant subjects. Several mechanisms have been hypothesized to explain the relationship between hyperinsulinemia and BP elevation (Fig. 44–4): (1) Hyperinsulinemia could elevate BP by increasing sodium reabsorption in the distal nephron and possibly in the proximal tubule as well, thus expanding plasma and extracellular fluid volume. (2) Hyperinsulinemia in the presence of normal blood glucose levels increases sympathetic nervous system activity, which can, in turn, elevate BP. (3) Insulin is a potent stimulus for receptor-mediated growth of vascular endothelial and smooth muscle cells, thus leading to increased peripheral vascular resistance and BP. (4) Insulin, by altering plasma free fatty acid levels, modulates Na^+-K^+-ATPase activity, thus altering cellular cation transport in a manner that could increase peripheral vascular tone and BP. Interventions that reduce insulin resistance, such as weight loss, diets low in carbohydrates and high in unsaturated fats, and aerobic exercise, reduce both BP and insulin resistance, supporting the concept that essential hypertension is an insulin-resistant state. Further study is needed to elucidate the relationships among hyperten-

sion, insulin resistance, and two related syndromes—obesity and diabetes mellitus.

DIAGNOSIS

Initial Evaluation

The initial evaluation of the hypertensive patient should determine baseline arterial BP, assess the degree of end-organ damage, screen for secondary causes of hypertension, identify other cardiovascular risk factors, and characterize the patient (sex, race, age, lifestyle, concomitant illnesses) to facilitate choice of therapy, drug selection in particular.

BP MEASUREMENT. The accurate and reproducible measurement of BP by the cuff technique is the most critical part of the diagnostic evaluation. On the initial visit, the BP should be taken after the patient has been seated comfortably for at least 5 minutes with his or her arm bared. Constriction of the upper arm by a rolled sleeve should be avoided, as it distorts the BP measurement. Two or three measurements should be taken at each visit, and at least 2 minutes should be allowed between readings. Proper cuff size is critical to accurate BP measurement. The cuff bladder should be long enough to encircle at least two thirds of the arm. Falsely elevated readings can be obtained when the bladder is too short, and the error is magnified if the cuff is also too narrow. Mercury manometers are preferred, but aneroid manometers can be used if they are standardized frequently against a mercury manometer.

To obtain an accurate systolic pressure, the cuff should be inflated rapidly to at least 30 mm Hg above the systolic pressure, as determined by palpation of the radial artery. This inflation is necessary to avoid underestimating the pressure because of the auscultatory gap, an unexplained disappearance of Korotkoff's sounds for some interval between systole and diastole. The systolic reading is taken as the level of pressure at which clear Korotkoff's sounds are heard with each heart beat. The diastolic reading is taken at the level when sounds become muffled (Korotkoff phase IV) and when sounds disappear (phase V). Both readings should be recorded. It is not known whether the level of muffling or of disappearance is a more accurate reflection of the intra-arterial diastolic pressure, so selection of one over the other as the clinical measurement of diastolic pressure is a matter of convenience and reproducibility. Baseline BP should be calculated from the average of two separate measurements determined at least 2 weeks apart. However, patients with diastolic BP greater than 115 mm Hg or elevated BP with evidence of ongoing end-organ damage should be started on therapy immediately.

The use of home BP recordings by either the patient or another person in the household or of 24-hour ambulatory BP recordings or both are useful, particularly in monitoring patients with labile hypertension, anxious patients whose BP readings tend to be falsely elevated in the doctor's office, and patients whose doses of antihypertensive medications need to be adjusted frequently. Home recordings should be taken at various times of day, in various positions, and during periods of both stress and relaxation in order to assess the effects of diurnal variations in hormones, posture, and emotional state on BP. Not only do home BP measurements provide additional information on the patient's true BP profile, but involving the patient in his or her care and informing him or her of therapeutic goals may provide incentive for nonpharmacologic therapies, such as weight loss, and may also enhance medication compliance. Standard sphygmomanometers and stethoscopes are appropriate for this purpose and are preferred over automated indirect BP measuring devices, which are often inaccurate. The patient's skill at BP measurement should be tested at frequent intervals by a professional.

Studies using ambulatory BP monitoring suggest that traditional office BP measurements overdiagnose hypertension by 20 to 30 per cent. In addition, these studies suggest that mean ambulatory pressures may better assess end-organ risk than do serial office measurements. These findings are controversial because of potential selection biases, uncertainty over the risks of stress-related hypertension, and the argument that office visits are no more stressful than many work and home environments. Current ambulatory monitoring systems are too cumbersome and

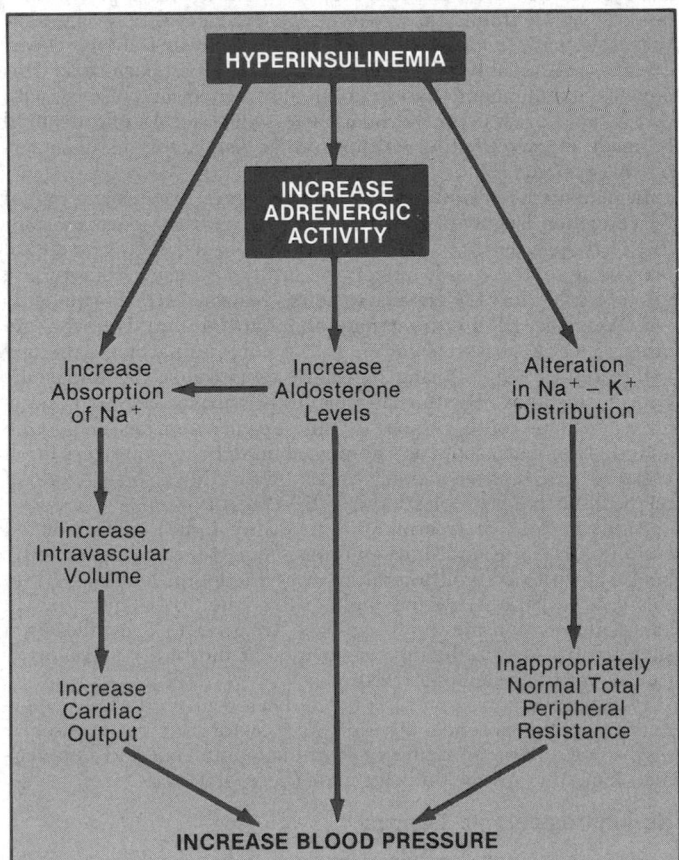

FIGURE 44–4. Physiologic mechanisms involved in insulin resistance–related hypertension. (From Reisin E: Sodium and obesity in the pathogenesis of hypertension. Am J Hypertension 3(2):164–167, 1990; with permission.)

expensive for routine assessment of BP. The controversy they have generated, however, does emphasize the value of home BP measurements made by the patient and/or the patient's family.

Accurate BP determination can be particularly difficult in elderly patients because of stiffening of arterial walls. The loss of arterial wall compliance can result in falsely elevated BP measurements by use of a standard sphygmomanometer, so-called pseudohypertension. Such an occurrence should be suspected in elderly patients diagnosed as having hypertension but lacking evidence of end-organ damage. Use of the Osler maneuver can sometimes identify this phenomenon. During the Osler maneuver, the BP cuff is inflated above the level of systolic BP. If the pulseless radial or brachial artery remains palpable, there may be sufficient stiffening of the artery to falsely elevate the BP measurement. Intra-arterial BP determinations may be necessary for the accurate diagnosis of hypertension in this setting.

Selection of Patients for Evaluation for Secondary Hypertension

Once a diagnosis of stable hypertension has been established, the need for antihypertensive treatment should be assessed, and, where indicated, diagnostic evaluation for secondary causes of hypertension should be undertaken. In view of the rarity of secondary causes of hypertension and the high cost and risk of elaborate diagnostic studies, the routine pretreatment workup should be limited to defining the severity of the hypertension and identifying its complications and associated cardiovascular risk factors. All of the secondary causes combined account for less than 5 per cent of the adult hypertensive population, but since some patients with secondary hypertension are potentially curable, diagnostic evaluation is warranted in selected patients. These include the following:

1. Those in whom routine history, physical examination, or routine laboratory data suggest a specific secondary cause
2. Those who are younger than 30 years of age, since they have the greatest prevalence of correctable secondary hypertension
3. Those in whom drug therapy is inadequate or unsatisfactory
4. Those whose hypertension has suddenly worsened
5. Older patients who develop new-onset hypertension

MEDICAL HISTORY. A careful, complete history should be obtained and a physical examination performed in all hypertensive patients before therapy is started. The medical history should include any previous history of hypertension, including prior and current antihypertensive treatment; a history of factors regarded as predisposing to hypertension, including excessive salt intake, the use of drugs that are known to elevate BP (Table 44–3), stressful occupation, and a family history of hypertension and its complications; evidence of hypertensive complications, including congestive heart failure, coronary artery disease, renal dysfunction, and stroke; and a history of other cardiovascular risk factors, including diabetes, obesity, cigarette smoking, and lipid abnormalities. Discussion of family history should include mention of familial diseases associated with secondary hypertension, including familial renal disease, polycystic kidney disease, medullary thyroid cancer, pheochromocytoma, and hyperparathyroidism. Discussion of the patient's personal habits should include exercise habits, ethanol consumption, and any unusual dietary practices. All current medications should be considered, particularly agents such as corticosteroids, nonsteroidal anti-inflammatory agents, antihistamines, sympathomimetics, appetite suppressants, phenothiazines, tricyclic antidepressants, and monoamine oxidase inhibitors that may exacerbate existing hypertension or antagonize or adversely interact with drug therapy. The physician should also begin assessing the patient's understanding of his or her illness and willingness to alter lifestyle if necessary. A history of weakness, muscle cramps, and polyuria suggests hypokalemia and the possibility of hyperaldosteronism; a history of headaches, palpitations, or hyperhidrosis suggests pheochromocytoma.

PHYSICAL EXAMINATION. The physical examination should include two or more BP measurements, at least one of which is obtained in the standing position; funduscopic examination for hypertensive retinopathy; careful examination of the cardiovascular system for evidence of congestive heart failure, cardiomegaly, myocardial dysfunction, and peripheral vascular disease; examination of the abdomen for bruits; auscultation over all scars for evidence of arteriovenous fistulas, and a careful neurologic examination for the stigmata of stroke. Since poor prognosis has been correlated with severity of retinopathy, presence of left ventricular hypertrophy, and coexisting atherosclerotic disease, physical findings related to these complications should be well documented.

LABORATORY EVALUATION. Pretreatment laboratory tests can be restricted to those generally performed as part of a routine medical checkup: hematocrit, urinalysis to exclude proteinuria and hematuria suggestive of renal disease, creatinine or blood urea nitrogen levels to assess renal function, serum potassium levels, chest film to assess heart size and rule out aortic coarctation, and electrocardiogram. Other tests that can be obtained as part of most automated blood chemistry batteries, such as the blood glucose, serum cholesterol, triglyceride, and uric acid levels, are helpful in assessing other cardiovascular risk factors and can be used as a baseline for monitoring the effects of antihypertensive treatment. Serial electrocardiograms and echocardiograms may be useful in assessing the effects of hypertension and antihypertensive treatment on the heart.

TREATMENT

The goal of antihypertensive therapy is to reduce overall cardiovascular risk. In any given patient, the decision to initiate therapy is governed by the extent of the BP elevation and the presence or absence of cardiovascular complications or additional cardiovascular risk factors, or both. Antihypertensive treatment is indicated in patients with diastolic BP measurements of 95 mm Hg or higher and in those with lesser elevations (90 to 94 mm Hg) who are at high risk of developing cardiovascular morbidity or mortality. The high-risk group includes patients with target-organ damage, diabetes mellitus, and/or other major risk factors for coronary artery disease. The initial goal of therapy is to lower diastolic BP to levels below 90 mm Hg with minimal adverse effects. Excessive BP reduction (diastolic BP below 80 mm Hg and systolic BP below 130 mm Hg) should be avoided, particularly in elderly patients and those with coronary artery disease, because it may actually increase the risk of death from ischemic heart disease, presumably secondary to coronary hypoperfusion. This J-curve phenomenon has been demonstrated in patients with and without pre-existing coronary artery disease. An effort should be made to correct other cardiovascular risk factors in all hypertensive patients.

In patients with moderate to severe hypertension, even partial BP reduction has been shown to decrease cardiovascular morbidity. Therefore, in these patients, a more limited therapeutic goal may be accepted if side effects of antihypertensive therapy are intolerable at doses necessary to achieve normal BP. For patients with diastolic BP in the range of 90 to 94 mm Hg who are otherwise at low risk, an initial trial of nonpharmacologic therapy with careful BP monitoring should be carried out. If the diastolic BP remains above 90 mm Hg despite nonpharmacologic therapy for a 3- to 6-month period, antihypertensive drugs should be added. Nonpharmacologic therapy should be encouraged in all patients with hypertension, as it may reduce the dosage of medication required for adequate BP control.

Antihypertensive treatment is probably indicated in isolated systolic hypertension, since pharmacologic therapy has recently been shown to be well tolerated and effective in lowering BP in this group. Patients with systolic BP greater than 160 mm Hg are generally considered to deserve treatment. The efficacy of such treatment in reducing cardiovascular morbidity and mortality has yet to be demonstrated.

Pharmacologic treatment is not indicated in borderline hypertension in the absence of other risk factors for cardiovascular disease or end-organ damage. Careful monitoring and nonpharmacologic therapy are indicated for these patients.

Nonpharmacologic Therapy

Since the nonpharmacologic interventions useful in hypertensive persons are not costly and are generally beneficial in promoting good health, their gradual introduction should be attempted in all hypertensive patients. Although permanent modifications in diet and lifestyle are difficult to achieve, in motivated patients, they may obviate the need for drug treatment or reduce the dosage requirements of antihypertensive drugs for adequate BP control.

WEIGHT REDUCTION. There is a clear, direct relationship between body weight and resting BP. Epidemiologic studies have consistently shown that overweight individuals have an increased risk of hypertension and increased cardiovascular risk. Weight loss is closely correlated with reduction in BP and is potentially the most efficacious of all nonpharmacologic measures in the treatment of hypertension. This effect is independent of dietary sodium restriction and is seen in both obese and nonobese hypertensive individuals. In addition to reducing BP, weight loss independently reduces cardiovascular risk and tends to improve the patient's self-image and sense of well-being. Patients should avoid appetite suppressants, which contain sympathomimetics such as phenylpropanolamine that can elevate BP. However, significant weight loss is difficult to achieve and even more difficult to maintain. Most patients regain the lost weight within 1 year. Nevertheless, all overweight hypertensive patients should be encouraged to lose weight.

ALCOHOL RESTRICTION. Alcohol consumption elevates BP, both acutely and chronically, and cross-sectional studies have demonstrated an association between increased BP and increased levels of alcohol consumption. The regular ingestion of 1 ounce of alcohol per day (two drinks) is estimated to raise systolic BP by 2 to 6 mm Hg. Therefore, abstinence or moderation of alcohol consumption (restriction of intake to 1 ounce of ethanol, corresponding to 2 ounces of 100 proof distilled liquor, 4 ounces of wine, or 24 ounces of beer daily) should be encouraged.

EXERCISE. Both cross-sectional and longitudinal studies have demonstrated a lower prevalence of hypertension in physically active people. Regular isotonic exercise, such as jogging, bicycling, or swimming, produces modest reductions in BP in persons with mild to moderate hypertension. Exercise also reduces cardiovascular risk independent of weight loss while promoting a sense of well-being. Therefore, all hypertensive patients should be encouraged to participate in regular isotonic or aerobic exercise. Current recommendations for BP reduction and reduction of overall cardiovascular risk include aerobic exercise maintaining 70 to 80 per cent of maximal heart rate (maximal heart rate calculated by subtracting age from 220) for 20 to 30 minutes three times a week. Patients should work gradually toward this goal.

DIETARY SODIUM RESTRICTION. Although dietary sodium restriction is commonly recommended by physicians to hypertensive patients, studies evaluating the antihypertensive efficacy of sodium restriction in unselected patients with essential hypertension have not demonstrated a clear benefit. A recent meta-analysis of published studies of dietary sodium restriction in hypertensive patients found only a small reduction in BP and concluded that there is little evidence that reduction of sodium intake has a beneficial effect on BP control. Further, BP increases have been observed in some hypertensive patients when dietary sodium intake is reduced. The observed heterogeneity in BP response to dietary sodium restriction has given rise to attempts to classify hypertensive patients as salt sensitive or salt resistant and to develop biochemical indices of salt sensitivity. Patients with low renin activity, frequently encountered in elderly and black patients, are more likely to respond to sodium restriction with a decrease in BP. Further, sodium restriction can minimize diuretic-induced hypokalemia and may enhance the ease of BP control with diuretic therapy and should be encouraged in patients who are receiving diuretics. Moderate sodium restriction (4 to 6 grams of salt per day) can be generally recommended to hypertensive patients, realizing that only a subset of patients will benefit. This can be effected by the simple and tolerable measures of not adding salt to food during preparation or at the table and avoiding processed foods containing salt as the preservative. Salt substitutes in which sodium is replaced with potassium are useful in hypertensive patients who do not have renal dysfunction. Patients should be instructed to avoid concomitant decreases in calcium and potassium intake.

DIETARY CALCIUM SUPPLEMENTATION. Epidemiologic studies have suggested an inverse relationship between dietary calcium intake and BP: Hypertensive persons, according to their dietary recalls, ingest less calcium than normotensive persons. Clinical studies of the BP-lowering effects of calcium supplementation have produced mixed results. Only a fraction of the hypertensive patients given oral calcium supplementation (1 gram of elemental calcium per day) show significant reductions in BP. Patients with salt-sensitive essential hypertension who are ingesting a high salt diet appear to be sensitive to the BP-lowering effects of dietary calcium, whereas patients with salt-resistant hypertension are not. This issue requires more study, but early data suggest that patients with salt-sensitive essential hypertension may benefit from oral calcium supplementation. Maintenance of oral calcium intake at levels of 1 gram per day or greater may also be beneficial for other reasons, such as the prevention of osteoporosis and gastrointestinal malignancy.

DIETARY POTASSIUM SUPPLEMENTATION. Epidemiologic studies have demonstrated an inverse relationship between dietary potassium intake and BP, and several recent controlled studies have demonstrated a small but significant reduction in BP with dietary potassium supplementation. The antihypertensive effect of potassium supplementation appears to be related to concomitant sodium intake, in that the higher the sodium intake, the more effective potassium supplementation is in reducing BP. Hypertensive patients should maintain adequate potassium intake ($\sim$ 100 mEq per day) by adequate ingestion of fresh fruits and vegetables and, if necessary, by use of potassium supplements. Potassium supplementation should be avoided or used only with extreme caution in patients with renal insufficiency, in diabetics, and in patients receiving potassium-sparing diuretics. Hypokalemia, whether due to diuretic use or to poor dietary intake, should be treated. Hypokalemia should particularly be avoided in patients receiving digoxin and in those with known coronary artery disease, as it predisposes to arrhythmia. Use of potassium-sparing diuretics should be considered in patients who are hypokalemic prior to initiation of diuretic therapy or who develop hypokalemia while receiving a nonpotassium-sparing diuretic.

SPECIAL DIETS. Dietary manipulations, such as changing to a vegetarian diet, increasing total fiber intake, decreasing total fat intake while increasing polyunsaturated fats relative to saturated fats, or increasing ingestion of fish oils, have been shown in preliminary studies to lower BP. They may, in addition, lower other cardiovascular risk factors. The mechanisms of antihypertensive action of these diets are unknown. Further studies are necessary to evaluate the role of these special diets in BP lowering, and it is premature to recommend them to patients with essential hypertension who lack other cardiovascular risk factors.

SMOKING CESSATION AND CAFFEINE RESTRICTION. Caffeine and nicotine raise BP acutely, but neither cigarette smokers nor coffee drinkers have an increased incidence of sustained hypertension, and there is no evidence that quitting smoking or caffeine products benefits BP control. Accordingly, patients should be advised to avoid cigarettes and coffee or tea immediately prior to having their BP checked. Because of the high incidence of associated malignancy and accelerated cardiovascular disease, smoking cessation should be strongly urged in all patients. Further, moderation in consumption of caffeine-containing beverages is advisable, in part because coronary disease risk may be increased in heavy coffee drinkers.

RELAXATION/STRESS REDUCTION. Relaxation and stress management produce only modest BP lowering even in highly motivated patients. Therefore, although these techniques may have beneficial side effects, including decreased anxiety and an improved sense of well-being, they have limited clinical application in the treatment of hypertension.

OVERALL RECOMMENDATIONS FOR NONPHARMACOLOGIC TREATMENT OF ESSENTIAL HYPERTENSION. Nonpharmacologic antihypertensive therapy should be used in all hypertensive patients, either as definitive treatment or as an adjunct to drug therapy. Therapy should be tailored to the individual characteristics of each patient—for example, weight reduction and exercise for the overweight patient and moderation in alcohol consumption for the heavy drinker. A reasonable generalized approach for all patients includes (1) reduction of dietary sodium and increases in dietary calcium and potassium, (2) weight loss for the overweight patient, (3) regular exercise, (4) moderation of alcohol consumption, and (5) smoking cessation. Such an approach has been shown to produce significant sustained reductions in BP while reducing overall cardiovascular risk.

Pharmacologic Therapy

THERAPEUTIC BENEFIT

Epidemiologic studies, including the Framingham Study, have clearly demonstrated that elevated BP is correlated with an increased incidence of cardiovascular disease, including stroke, renal failure, congestive heart failure, and myocardial infarction. The risk of cardiovascular complications is proportional to the degree of BP elevation. Clinical trials have shown that treatment of moderate to severe hypertension (diastolic BP > 105 mm Hg) reduces overall cardiovascular mortality. In the Veterans Administration Cooperative Study Group Trial, pharmacologic treatment of severe hypertension (diastolic BP 115 to 120 mm Hg) reduced morbidity and mortality by 90 per cent; treatment of moderate hypertension (diastolic BP 105 to 114 mm Hg) reduced overall cardiovascular complications by 50 per cent; treatment of patients with mild hypertension (diastolic BP 90 to 104 mm Hg) did not produce a significant reduction in cardiovascular morbidity and mortality overall. Only those individuals with mild hypertension who were above 50 years of age or had pre-existing cardiovascular or renal disease benefitted from therapy. Other studies, in contrast, have demonstrated clear benefits of pharmacologic treatment of patients with mild hypertension. The Hypertension Detection Follow-Up Program Study demonstrated a 20 per cent reduction in overall mortality in patients with mild hypertension (diastolic BP 90 to 104 mm Hg) who had aggressive treatment of their hypertension. Importantly, in those patients with the mildest degrees of hypertension (diastolic BP 90 to 94 mm Hg), survival was the most significantly improved. The European Working Party Trial demonstrated improved survival in elderly patients (60 to 80 years) being treated for mild hypertension. Clearly, treatment of moderate or severe hypertension significantly reduces overall cardiovascular morbidity and mortality. Although less conclusive, there is also sufficient evidence to recommend pharmacologic treatment of mild hypertension.

Most clinical trials of antihypertensive drugs have shown reductions in the incidence of congestive heart failure, renal failure, and stroke but have demonstrated less impressive reductions in morbidity and mortality from coronary artery disease. A new meta-analysis of clinical trials of antihypertensive drugs (chiefly diuretics and β blockers), in which mean reductions in diastolic BP of 5 to 6 mm Hg were achieved, showed a 42 per cent reduction in incidence of stroke and a 14 per cent reduction in coronary artery disease (Collins et al.). Diuretics and β blockers, the most commonly used medications in these large clinical trials, have metabolic side effects that increase coronary risk. Newer antihypertensive agents with fewer metabolic side effects and with neutral or even positive effects on coronary risk may reduce coronary morbidity and mortality further. Large clinical trials employing the newer agents are needed to assess their overall benefit.

GENERAL CONSIDERATIONS

The increasing number and variety of drugs available for use in hypertension, coupled with our rapidly expanding knowledge of the pathophysiology of hypertension and of the adverse effects of these drugs in individual patient groups, make it increasingly possible to individualize antihypertensive treatment. When used as monotherapy, most agents effectively control hypertension in over 50 per cent of patients with mild or moderate disease. Thus, it is possible to use a single agent to provide effective BP control with minimal side effects in many patients. Therapy should be initiated with the agent best tolerated and most likely to be effective in lowering BP in a given patient. If the initial agent is ineffective at maximal recommended doses or has undue side effects, an alternative agent from another class should be tried. When monotherapy is unsuccessful, a second agent, usually of a different class, should be added. Additional agents should be added or substituted as necessary to provide effective and well-tolerated BP control (Fig. 44–5).

Prescription of antihypertensive therapy should take into consideration the physiologic, economic, and social characteristics of each patient in order to provide effective BP control as simply and as inexpensively as possible. Expensive, complicated, and

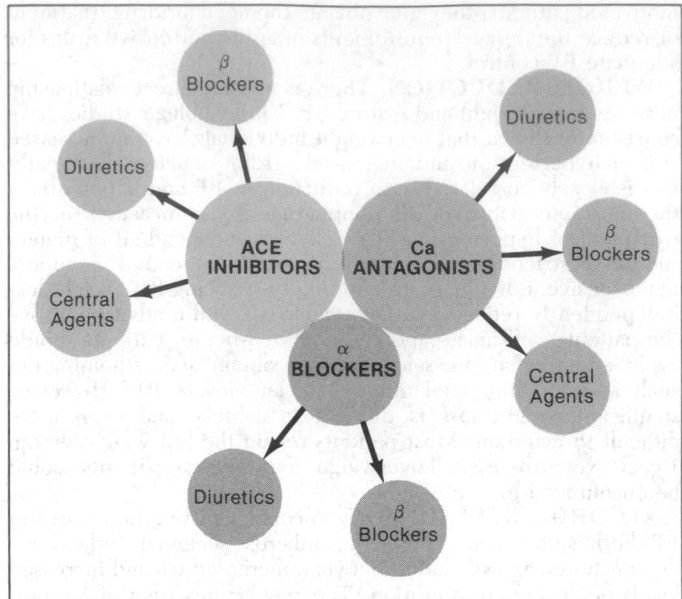

FIGURE 44–5. Proposed program for individualized antihypertensive therapy. Initial treatment should be with an angiotensin-converting enzyme (ACE) inhibitor, Ca antagonist, or α blocker. If this is unsuccessful in controlling blood pressure, an agent from another class should be substituted or a second agent should be added, as indicated in the diagram. Agents can then be added or substituted as necessary to provide effective and well-tolerated blood pressure control. (Modified from Zanchetti A: Angiotensin-converting enzyme inhibitors in essential hypertension. J Cardiovasc Pharmacol 9(Suppl 3):S2–S5, 1987; with permission.)

inconvenient regimens promote poor compliance. Patient involvement in his or her own care should be encouraged. Keeping patients informed of their illness and having patients measure and record their own BP's have been shown to improve BP control.

After initiating therapy, patients should be seen once every 1 to 4 weeks (depending on the severity of hypertension) for titration of antihypertensive drug dosage and once every 3 to 4 months once BP control is achieved. This allows for frequent assessment of treatment effectiveness and side effects and also emphasizes the physician's interest in the patient. Recommended dose ranges for individual drugs are listed with each agent in Tables 44–4 and 44–5, and for combination agents in Table 44–6. Common adverse effects are summarized in Table 44–7.

Once a patient's BP is controlled on a particular regimen, fixed combination tablets may be substituted in order to simplify the regimen and reduce medication costs (Table 44–6). However, such fixed combinations preclude individualized dosage titration, and therefore physicians may need to return to multiple tablet regimens as the patient's dose requirements change.

Step-down therapy, or withdrawal of antihypertensive medication under close monitoring, should be attempted in patients with mild or moderate hypertension whose BP has been adequately controlled for 1 year or more. Dosages should be titrated slowly downward and medications discontinued one at a time, if possible. Therapy should not be discontinued abruptly. Step-down therapy is generally most effective in patients who are also receiving nonpharmacologic treatment for their hypertension. Regular follow-up is crucial for all patients who have antihypertensive therapy discontinued, because BP can rise again to hypertensive levels, even after years of normal BP off therapy.

SPECIFIC DRUGS

DIURETICS. Thiazide diuretics were the principal agents used in most of the major trials of antihypertensive therapy that demonstrated significant reductions in overall cardiovascular morbidity and mortality, including significant reductions in congestive heart failure, stroke, and renal failure. These trials did not show significant reductions in mortality related to coronary artery disease, however. This failure to reduce the incidence of myocardial infarction, considered in conjunction with their adverse metabolic side effects, has led to growing concern about the effects of diuretics on overall cardiovascular risk, particularly in patients with mild hypertension.

Thiazide diuretics are effective in lowering BP in all patient groups, particularly in blacks and the elderly. They are inexpensive and generally well tolerated and consequently are widely used. Diuretics have been used safely in combination with all other classes of antihypertensive agents and generally provide additional BP reduction; therefore, they are a logical second agent when combination therapy is needed.

Thiazide diuretics are associated with a number of metabolic alterations, including kaliuresis, with an average fall in serum potassium of 0.6 mEq per liter, although profound hypokalemia can occur. The clinical significance of this decrease in serum potassium is controversial, but it may be arrhythmogenic in some patients. This interpretation was supported by the finding from the Multiple Risk Factor Intervention Trial (MRFIT) that patients with resting ECG abnormalities receiving thiazide diuretics had an increased incidence of sudden death. Although this finding has not been substantiated by other clinical trials, the potential arrhythmogenic effect of diuretic-induced hypokalemia remains worrisome, particularly in light of the failure of diuretics to improve coronary disease–related mortality. Hypokalemia should especially be avoided in patients at increased risk for arrhythmia, including those receiving digoxin, diabetics, and patients with known coronary artery disease.

Thiazide diuretics cause increases in total cholesterol, LDL cholesterol, and triglyceride levels. These increases tend to diminish with time, but well-controlled studies indicate that significant elevations in lipids persist with long-term thiazide treatment. Although the clinical significance of these alterations in lipid levels is not known, they may have a deleterious effect on overall cardiovascular risk.

Other metabolic side effects of thiazide diuretics include glucose intolerance, elevations in serum uric acid and calcium levels, and decreases in serum magnesium levels. These effects tend to be small but may become problematic in patients with related disorders. Therefore, thiazide diuretics should be used cautiously in diabetics and in patients with a history of gout or hypercalcemia. Other less common thiazide-induced metabolic alterations include hyponatremia and metabolic alkalosis. The most common subjective adverse effects of thiazide use are impotence, decreased libido, muscle cramps, and fatigue.

Recent studies have shown that adequate BP reduction can be achieved with much lower doses of thiazide diuretics than were traditionally used. Metabolic adverse effects tend to be minimized with the lower doses of thiazides. A starting dose of thiazide diuretic is the equivalent of 12.5 mg of hydrochlorothiazide in the general hypertensive population and 6.25 mg of hydrochlorothiazide in the elderly hypertensive patient. Because of their adverse metabolic side effects, their deleterious effects on cardiovascular risk factors, and their failure to reduce coronary morbidity and mortality, it seems prudent, when economically feasible, not to use thiazide diuretics as first-line therapy in patients with mild to moderate hypertension but to reserve them for use in combination with other classes of agents in patients with moderate to severe disease.

Loop diuretics such as furosemide and bumetanide are indicated in hypertensive patients with congestive heart failure or other edematous states or with renal insufficiency. **Potassium-sparing diuretics** are appropriate treatment for patients who are hypokalemic prior to initiation of diuretic therapy or who develop hypokalemia with the use of a non–potassium-sparing diuretic. Potassium-sparing diuretics are also magnesium sparing and may prevent the hypomagnesemia common in thiazide diuretic use. Diabetics, patients with renal insufficiency, and patients receiving ACE inhibitors, β-adrenergic blocking drugs, oral potassium

TABLE 44–4. DIURETICS FOR AMBULATORY TREATMENT OF HYPERTENSION

Generic Name	Trade Name (Manufacturer)	Adult Dosage (mg/day)	Duration (hr)	Dispensing Unit (mg)
Benzothiadiazine diuretics				
Thiazides				
Chlorothiazide	Diuril (MSD)*	250–500	6–12	250, 500
Hydrochlorothiazide	Esidrix (CIBA)	12.5–50	12–18	25
	HydroDIURIL (MSD)			50
	Oretic (Abbott)			
Bendroflumethiazide	Naturetin (Squibb)	5–20	18–36	2.5, 5.0
Benzthiazide	Aquatag (Tutag)	25–50	12–18	10
				50
	Diucen (Central)			
	Edemex (Savage)			
	Exna (Robins)			
	Lemazide (Lemmon)			
Cyclothiazide	Anhydron (Lilly)	1–2	18–24	2
Hydroflumethiazide	Saluron (Bristol)	25–50	18–24	50
Methyclothiazide	Aquatensen (Wallace)	2.5–10.0	24–48	5.0, 2.5
	Enduron (Abbott)			
Polythiazide	Renese (Pfizer)	2–4	24–48	1, 2, 4
Trichlormethiazide	Methahydrin (Merrell Dow)	2–4	24–48	2
	Naqua (Schering)			4
Indapamide	Lozol (USV Pharmaceutical)	2.5–5.0	18–24	2.5
Phthalimidines	Hygroton (USV Pharmaceutical)	12.5–50	24–72	25, 50, 100
Chlorthalidone	Chlorthalidone (Parke-Davis)			25, 50
	Thalitone (Boehringer-Ingelheim)			
Metolazone	Zaroxolyn (Pennwalt)	2.5–5.0	12–24	2.5, 5.0, 10.0
	Diulo (Searle)			2.5, 5.0, 10.0
Quinazolines	Hydromox (Lederle)	50–100	18–24	50
Quinethazone				
Loop diuretics				
Furosemide	Lasix (Hoechst-Roussel)	20–1,000	3–6	20, 40, 80
Ethacrynic acid	Edecrin (MSD)	50–400	3–6	25, 50
Bumetanide	Bumex (Roche)	0.5–2.0	1–4	0.5, 1.0
Potassium-sparing diuretics				
Spironolactone	Aldactone (Searle)	50–100	3–6	25, 50, 100
	Spironolactone (Parke-Davis)			25
Triamterene	Dyrenium (SKF)*	50–100	3–6	50, 10
Amiloride	Midamor (MSD)	5–10	24	5

*MSD = Merck Sharp & Dohme; SKF = Smith Kline & French.

supplementation, or salt substitutes high in potassium chloride are prone to hyperkalemia. Potassium-sparing diuretics should be used with caution in these patients. Dosing information for the currently available diuretics is summarized in Table 44–4.

BETA-ADRENERGIC RECEPTOR BLOCKING AGENTS. Beta-blockers are used extensively in the treatment of hypertension. They are available as nonselective agents that block β_1- and β_2-adrenergic receptors equally, cardioselective agents that have higher affinity for β_1 receptors, and agents with intrinsic sympathomimetic activity (ISA). Labetalol has both α_1-adrenergic antagonist and nonselective β antagonist activity. The antihypertensive effect of β blockers is attributed to their negative inotropic and chronotropic properties, which tend to decrease cardiac output. In addition, β blockers inhibit renin release and produce a delayed vasodilator effect of uncertain mechanism. Beta blockers have been used effectively and safely in combination with all other classes of antihypertensive agents. They must be used cautiously in combination with calcium channel blockers that have significant negative inotropic and chronotropic activity, as these effects of the two classes of agents may be additive. Beta blockers are routinely used in combination with vasodilators to blunt reflex tachycardia.

Beta blockers are more effective in lowering BP in younger patients than in the elderly and in whites than in blacks. Since β blockers are effective in the treatment of angina and in the secondary prevention of myocardial infarction, they are the drugs of choice in hypertensive patients with known coronary artery disease. Recent evidence, uncorroborated by large clinical trials, has suggested that β blockers may also be effective in the primary prevention of myocardial infarction in hypertensive patients. Beta blockers are very effective in younger patients and are the drugs of choice in hypertensive patients with sympathetic hyperactivity, as evidenced by a fast resting heart rate and a wide pulse pressure.

The most common adverse effects of β blockers are related to

TABLE 44–5. ANTIHYPERTENSIVE DRUGS IN AMBULATORY TREATMENT OF HYPERTENSION

Generic Name	Trade Name (Manufacturer)	Adult Maintenance Dose (mg/day)	Frequency of Administration (times/day)	Duration of Action (hr)
Sympatholytic agents				
Centrally acting agents				
Methyldopa	Aldomet (MSD)	250–2000	2	6–12
Clonidine	Catapres (Boehringer-Ingelheim)	0.2–0.8	2	6–12
Clonidine patch	Catapres-TTS (Boehringer-Ingelheim)	1 patch (0.1,0.2,0.3 mg)	weekly	7 days
Guanfacine	Tenex (Robins)	1–3	1	12–24
Guanabenz	Wytensin (Wyeth)	8–64	2	8–12
Reserpine and rauwolfia alkaloids	Serpasil (CIBA)	0.1–0.25	1	24
Beta-adrenergic blocking agents				
Propranolol	Inderal (Ayerst)	40–640	2	6–12
Metoprolol	Lopressor (CIBA)	100–450	2	12
Atenolol	Tenormin (ICI)	50–100	1	24
Nadolol	Corgard (Squibb)	40–320	1	24
Timolol	Blocadren (MSD)	20–60	2	6–12
Pindolol	Visken (Sandoz)	10–60	2	6–12
Acebutolol	Sectral (Wyeth)	400–1200	1 or 2	12–24
Penbutolol	Levatol (Reed & Carnrick)	20	1	24
Alpha-adrenergic blocking agents				
Prazosin	Minipress (Pfizer)	2.5–20	2 or 3	3–6
Prazosin sustained release	Minipress XL (Pfizer)	2.5–20	1	24
Terazosin	Hytrin (Abbott)	1–20	1	24
Doxazosin	Cardura (Roerig)	2–8	1	24
Mixed alpha- and beta-adrenergic blocking agent				
Labetalol	Normodyne (Schering) Trandate (Glaxo)	200–800	2	3–6
Ganglion-blocking agent				
Mecamylamine	Inversine (MSD)	2.5	2	12–24
Peripherally acting sympatholytic agent				
Guanethidine	Ismelin (CIBA)	10–300	1	24
Angiotensin-converting enzyme inhibitors				
Captopril	Capoten (Squibb)	75–450	3	4–8
Enalapril	Vasotec (MSD)	5–40	1 or 2	12–24
Lisinopril	Prinivil (MSD) Zestril (Stuart)	10–40	1	24
Quinapril*	Accupril (Parke-Davis)	5–40	1 or 2	12–24
Cilazaril*	Inhibace (Roche)	1.25–5	1	24
Calcium channel blocking agents				
Nifedipine	Procardia (Pfizer)	30–120	3 or 4	6–8
Nifedipine sustained release	Procardia XL (Pfizer)	30–90	1	24
Diltiazem	Cardizem (Marion)	90–240	3 or 4	6–8
Diltiazem sustained release	Cardizem SR (Marion)	120–240	2	12
Verapamil	Isoptin (Knoll) Calan (Searle)	240–480	3 or 4	6–8
Verapamil sustained release	Isoptin SR (Knoll) Calan SR (Searle)	120–480	1 or 2	12–24
Nicardipine	Cardene (Syntex)	30–90	3	6–8
Nitrendipine*	Baypress (Miles)	10–80	1 or 2	12–24
Isradipine*	DynaCirc (Sandoz/Glaxo)	2.5–20	2	12
Direct vasodilators				
Hydralazine	Apresoline (CIBA)	20–300	2 or 3	6
Minoxidil	Loniten (Upjohn)	5–10	1 or 2	Up to 72
Pinacidil	Pindac (Lilly)	25–50	2 or 3	3–6

*These agents have not been approved by the FDA for the treatment of hypertension.

their mechanism of action. The negative chronotropic and inotropic effects of β blockers may precipitate severe bradycardia, AV block, and congestive heart failure in susceptible patients and therefore should be avoided in patients with a history of bradycardia, cardiac conduction abnormalities, or heart failure. Beta blockers should be used with caution in patients with chronic obstructive pulmonary disease or peripheral vascular disease, since β₂ blockade may exacerbate bronchospasm, peripheral vascular constriction, and Raynaud's phenomenon. Cardioselective agents have a theoretical advantage in such patients because of their lower affinity for β₂ receptors, but this selectivity diminishes with increasing dose and is probably trivial at usual clinical doses. Central nervous system side effects such as fatigue, impotence, and decreased mental acuity can occur with β blockers, particularly in the elderly. These can be minimized with the use of less lipophilic agents, such as atenolol, acebutolol, nadolol,

TABLE 44–6. COMBINATION AGENTS FOR TREATMENT OF HYPERTENSION

Generic Name	Trade Name (Manufacturer)	Daily Dose (pills/day)	Pill Content (mg/mg)
Combination diuretics			
HCTZ/spironolactone	Aldactazide (Searle)	1–2	25/25
HCTZ/triamterene	Maxzide (Lederle)	1–2	25/75,50/75
HCTZ/triamterene	Dyazide (SKF)	1–4	25/50
HCTZ/amiloride	Modurectic (MSD)	1–2	50/15
ACE inhibitors and diuretics			
Captopril/HCTZ	Capozide (Squibb)	2–4	25/15,25/25 50/15,50/25
Enalapril/HCTZ	Vaseretic (MSD)	1–2	10/25
Beta-blocking agents and diuretics			
Propranolol/HCTZ	Inderide (Wyeth-Ayerst)	2–4	40/25,80/25
Propranolol LA/HCTZ	Inderide LA (Wyeth-Ayerst)	1	80/50 120/50 160/50
Atenolol/chlorthalidone	Tenoretic (ICI)	1	50/25 100/25
Timolol/HCTZ	Timolide (MSD)	1–2	10/25
Nadolol/bendroflumethiazide	Corzide (Princeton)	1	40/5,80/5
Labetalol/HCTZ	Normozide (Schering)	2	100/25 200/25 300/25
Vasodilators and diuretics			
Hydralazine/HCTZ	Apresazide (CIBA)	2–4	25/25,50/50 50/25
Hydralazine/HCTZ	Apresoline-Exidrix (CIBA)	2–4	25/15
Prazosin/polythiazide	Minizide (Pfizer)	2–4	1/0.5,2/0.5 3/0.5
Centrally acting agents and diuretics			
Methyldopa/chlorothiazide	Aldoclor (MSD)	2–8	250/150 250/250
Methyldopa/HCTZ	Aldoril (MSD)	2–4	250/15 250/25 500/30 500/50
Clonidine/chlorthalidone	Combipres (Boehringer-Ingelheim)	2–3	0.1/25 0.2/25 0.3/25
Reserpine/chlorothiazide	Diupres (MSD)	1–2	0.125/250 0.125/500
Reserpine/methychlothiazide	Diutensen-R (Wallace)	1–4	0.1/2.5
Reserpine/quinethazone	Hydromox (Lederele)	1–2	0.125/50
Reserpine/HCTZ	Hydropres (MSD)	1–2	0.125/25 0.125/50
Reserpine/trichlormethiazide	Naquival (Schering)	1–2	0.1/4
Reserpine/polythiazide	Renese-R (Pfizer)	0.5–2	0.25/2
Reserpine/hydroflumethiazide	Salutensin-Demi Salutensin (Bristol)	1–2	0.125/25 0.125/50
Reserpine/HCTZ	Serpasil-Esidrix (CIBA)	1–2	0.1/25 0.1/50
Reserpine/chlorthalidone	Demi-Regroton Regroton (Rorer)	1	0.25/25 0.25/50
Deserpidine/methychlothiazide	Enduronyl Enduronyl-Forte (Abbott)	0.5–2	0.25/50 0.5/5
Deserpidine/HCTZ	Oreticyl Oreticyl-Forte (Abbott)	2–4	0.125/25 0.125/50 0.250/25
Guanethidine/HCTZ	Esimil (CIBA)	1–4	10/25
Rauwolfia/bendroflumethiazide	Rauzide (Princeton)	1–4	50/4
Other combinations			
Reserpine/hydralazine	Serpasil-Apresoline (CIBA)	2–4	0.1/25 0.2/25
Reserpine/hydralazine/HCTZ	Ser-Ap-Es (CIBA)	3–6	0.1/25/15

HCTZ = Hydrochlorothiazide.

labetalol, and timolol, which are less likely to enter the brain. Beta blockers should be used with caution in insulin-dependent diabetics, as they mask symptoms and delay recovery from hypoglycemia. Beta blockers adversely effect the serum lipid profile by reducing HDL cholesterol and increasing triglycerides.

Labetalol has both α and β antagonist properties; its most prominent pharmacologic effect is α_1 adrenergic receptor antagonist activity, similar to prazosin. Labetalol is particularly effective in lowering BP in blacks and in the elderly. It has no significant effect on serum lipid levels and has been used safely in patients with chronic obstructive pulmonary disease and peripheral vascular disease. The most common side effects of labetalol include fatigue, dizziness, headache, and gastrointestinal complaints. There is a low incidence of orthostatic hypotension with labetalol.

Because of their frequent adverse effects and their negative effect on the lipid profile, traditional β-blocking agents are not recommended for initial antihypertensive therapy in the general population. They remain useful in patients with established coronary artery disease. The newer mixed adrenergic blocking agents, such as labetalol, which are generally better tolerated and have a neutral to positive effect on serum lipid levels, are recommended for initial antihypertensive therapy in the general population. Dosing information for the currently available β blockers is summarized in Table 44–5.

CALCIUM CHANNEL BLOCKERS. The calcium channel blockers inhibit vascular smooth muscle contraction by blocking the influx of calcium into the cell. Their predominant antihypertensive effect is a decrease in peripheral vascular resistance. The calcium channel blockers are effective in reducing BP in a majority of unselected hypertensive patients, but like diuretics, they are particularly efficacious in blacks and the elderly. Calcium channel blockers are useful in the treatment of angina, so they are a logical choice for the treatment of hypertension in patients with coronary artery disease. Recent evidence suggests that calcium channel blockers, like β blockers, reduce the incidence of reinfarction. The antivasospastic property of calcium channel blockers may benefit patients with Raynaud's phenomenon, esophagospasm, and irritable bowel syndrome. The calcium channel blockers have been used safely and successfully in combination with all other classes of antihypertensive agents, but they (particularly verapamil) should be used cautiously in combination with β blockers, because of common negative inotropic and chronotropic properties.

The calcium channel blockers are well tolerated and convenient now that sustained-release formulations are available. They are

TABLE 44–7. COMMON ADVERSE EFFECTS OF ANTIHYPERTENSIVE DRUGS

Drugs	Side Effects	Precautions and Special Considerations
Diuretics		
Thiazides and related sulfonamides	Hypokalemia, hyperuricemia, glucose intolerance, hypercholesterolemia, hypertriglyceridemia, sexual dysfunction	May be ineffective in renal failure; hypokalemia increases digitalis toxicity; and hyperuricemia may precipitate acute gout.
Loop diuretics	Same as for thiazides	Effective in chronic renal failure; cautions regarding hypokalemia and hyperuricemia same as above; hyponatremia may be found, especially in the elderly.
Potassium-sparing agents	Hyperkalemia	Danger of hyperkalemia in patients with renal failure or diabetes or those receiving ACE inhibitors.
Amiloride hydrochloride	Sexual dysfunction	—
Spironolactone	Gynecomastia, mastodynia, sexual dysfunction	—
Adrenergic antagonists		
Beta-adrenergic blockers	Bradycardia, fatigue, insomnia, bizarre dreams, sexual dysfunction, hypertriglyceridemia, decreased HDL cholesterol	Should not be used in patients with asthma, chronic obstructive pulmonary disease, congestive heart failure, heart block (> first degree), and sick sinus syndrome. Use with caution in patients with diabetes and peripheral vascular disease. Sudden withdrawal of these drugs may be hazardous in patients with abrupt discontinuance.
Centrally acting agents	Drowsiness, dry mouth, fatigue,	Rebound hypertension may occur with abrupt discontinuance.
Methyldopa	—	May cause liver damage and positive direct Coombs' test (rare hemolytic anemia).
Reserpine	Sexual dysfunction, nasal congestion, lethargy	Contraindicated in patients with a history of depression; use with caution in patients with a history of peptic ulcer.
Alpha₁-adrenergic blockers	"First-dose" syncope, orthostatic hypotension, weakness, palpitations, dizziness, headache, fluid retention	Use cautiously in elderly patients.
Combined α- and β-adrenergic blockers	Nausea, fatigue, dizziness, headache, orthostatic hypotension	Use with caution in patients with cardiac failure, chronic obstructive pulmonary disease, sick sinus syndrome, heart block (> first degree), diabetes.
Vasodilators		
Vasodilators	Headache, tachycardia, fluid retention	May precipitate angina in patients with coronary heart disease.
Hydralazine hydrochloride	Positive antinuclear antibody (without other changes)	Lupus syndrome may occur (rare at recommended doses).
Minoxidil	Hypertrichosis, ascites (rare)	May cause or aggravate pleural and pericardial effusions.
Angiotensin-converting enzyme inhibitors		
Angiotensin-converting enzyme inhibitors	Cough	Can cause reversible acute renal failure in patients with bilateral renal artery stenosis; neutropenia may occur in patients with autoimmune collagen disorders; proteinuria may occur (rare at recommended doses).
Calcium channel blocking agents		
Calcium channel blocking agents	Headache, hypotension, dizziness	
Verapamil hydrochloride	Constipation, bradycardia	Use with caution in patients with congestive heart failure or heart block.

free of significant metabolic adverse effects, including alterations in lipid levels. Negative inotropic effects are seen with all calcium channel blockers but are most pronounced with verapamil and can cause significant suppression of myocardial contractility. Therefore, verapamil should be avoided in patients with left ventricular dysfunction. Verapamil also has a significant negative chronotropic effect and should be used cautiously in patients with conduction abnormalities. Verapamil is indicated for the treatment for certain tachyarrhythmias and is the drug of choice in hypertensive patients who have such arrhythmias. All of the calcium channel blockers can cause constipation, but this effect is most problematic with verapamil. The most common adverse effects of the dihydropyridine derivatives (nifedipine, nitrendipine, nicardipine, isradipine) are related to their vasodilator action. These include lightheadedness, flushing, tachycardia, and periorbital and pedal edema. These adverse effects are less common with sustained-release preparations. Calcium channel blockers generally are free of central nervous system side effects, including sexual dysfunction. They are metabolized by the liver and may require dosage adjustment in patients with hepatic disease but can be used safely in patients with renal disease. All of the calcium channel blockers can increase serum digoxin levels. This is a particular problem with verapamil. Dosing information for the currently available calcium channel blockers is summarized in Table 44–5.

ANGIOTENSIN-CONVERTING ENZYME (ACE) INHIBITORS. ACE inhibitors inhibit the enzymatic conversion of angiotensin I to angiotensin II with consequent reductions in peripheral vascular resistance, sympathetic nervous system activity, and renal sodium and water retention. They effectively lower BP in all of the major subgroups of hypertensive patients, including the elderly. Blacks are generally less sensitive to the antihypertensive effects of ACE inhibition than are whites, but increasing the dose of ACE inhibitor or adding a diuretic abolishes the racial difference. ACE inhibitors reduce afterload and are the drugs of choice in patients with hypertension and congestive failure. The combination of an ACE inhibitor, diuretic, and digoxin prolongs survival in patients with severe congestive failure (New York Heart Association class IV). ACE inhibitors are particularly useful in hypertensive patients with diabetes, since they decrease proteinuria and stabilize renal function in patients with diabetic nephropathy. They are also particularly effective in the control of hypertension secondary to renal vascular disease. However, in patients with renal artery stenosis in a solitary kidney, bilateral renal artery stenosis, or transplant renal artery stenosis, ACE inhibition may precipitate acute renal failure. Renal function should be monitored closely if ACE inhibitors are used in this setting. Further, ACE inhibitors have been reported to minimize the adverse metabolic effects of diuretic therapy. Therefore, the ACE inhibitor–diuretic combination is appealing. ACE inhibitors are well tolerated and generally free of adverse effects on the CNS, sexual function, and metabolism. Specifically, they do not adversely affect lipid levels, glucose tolerance, or uric acid levels.

Class-specific adverse effects of ACE inhibitors include hypotension, hyperkalemia, acute renal failure, angioedema, and cough, which tends to be nonproductive and worse at night. Cough is the most common adverse effect of the ACE inhibitors, with an incidence that approaches 25 per cent. Hypotension is generally a first-dose phenomenon in patients who are in a high renin state, such as those on a low-salt diet or receiving diuretic therapy. It can be minimized by starting with a very low dose of ACE inhibitor and, if possible, withholding diuretics prior to initiation of ACE inhibition. Hyperkalemia rarely occurs in patients with normal renal function. However, in patients with diabetes or renal dysfunction or those receiving potassium-sparing diuretics, potassium supplements, or nonsteroidal anti-inflammatory agents, clinically significant hyperkalemia may be precipitated by ACE inhibitor therapy. Angioedema is a rare but potentially catastrophic side effect of ACE inhibitors.

Side effects of ACE inhibitors thought to be related to the sulfhydryl group (currently found in captopril only) include proteinuria, rash, taste disturbances, and bone marrow suppression. The incidence of these side effects is related to the dose of the ACE inhibitor or to the presence of renal insufficiency. When the captopril dose is limited to less than 150 mg per day in a person with normal renal function, these side effects are infre-

quent. The risk of neutropenia is highest in patients with connective tissue disease and related renal dysfunction. Rash, taste disturbances, and proteinuria tend to be self-limited and to resolve with cessation of captopril therapy. These side effects have also been reported with nonsulfhydryl-containing ACE inhibitors, but much less frequently.

Captopril should be taken prior to eating, as food may decrease its absorption. The other ACE inhibitors are well absorbed even in the presence of food. Captopril is the shortest acting of the ACE inhibitors and generally requires at least twice-daily dosing for effective BP reduction. The other ACE inhibitors have longer half-lives and are generally effective when administered once a day. All of the ACE inhibitors are excreted by the kidney and require dosage adjustment in patients with renal impairment. Dosing information for the currently available ACE inhibitors is summarized in Table 44–5.

CENTRALLY ACTING AGENTS. The traditional centrally acting antihypertensive agents—clonidine, methyldopa, and guanabenz—have been a mainstay of antihypertensive therapy for several decades. However, in recent years their use has been limited by a high incidence of side effects and the need for frequent dosing. The recent release of transdermal clonidine and long-acting guanacine, both of which allow for more convenient dosing with fewer side effects, expands the role of centrally acting agents in the treatment of hypertension.

The centrally acting agents are predominantly α_2 adrenoceptor agonists, stimulating adrenoceptors in the brain stem and hypothalamus, thereby inhibiting sympathetic outflow from the central nervous system and decreasing BP, heart rate, and peripheral vascular resistance. These agents are as effective as the other major classes of antihypertensive agents in lowering BP. They have no significant effects on glucose regulation, serum lipid levels, or renal function.

The most common side effects of the centrally acting agents are dry mouth, drowsiness, and fatigue. These occur initially in as many as 30 per cent of patients receiving the traditional centrally acting agents but tend to diminish with continued therapy. Less frequent side effects include orthostatic hypotension, sexual dysfunction, and decreased mental acuity. Transdermal clonidine and guanfacine are better tolerated and have a significantly lower incidence of side effects than the traditional agents. Abrupt discontinuation of the traditional agents, particularly clonidine, has been associated with a withdrawal syndrome characterized by headache, nausea, anxiety, vomiting, and rebound hypertension that may require emergent therapy. BP in this setting can be reduced and symptoms alleviated with reinitiation of previous therapy. The withdrawal syndrome has not been associated with transdermal clonidine or guanfacine. Approximately 10 to 20 per cent of patients receiving methyldopa develop a positive direct Coombs' reaction, but only a very small percentage (< 1 per cent develop hemolytic anemia. Drug-induced hepatitis and/or fever is rarely associated with methyldopa use. Transdermal clonidine is associated with a local rash in 10 to 15 per cent of patients. The rash is generally a mild, localized erythema, but vesicular eruptions have been reported. It disappears with discontinuation of therapy.

The centrally acting agents are effective in all the major subgroups of hypertensive patients but should be used cautiously in the elderly because of their adverse effects on baroreflex and central nervous system function. The more convenient dosing of guanfacine and transdermal clonidine makes these agents more acceptable to patients than the traditional oral centrally acting agents. Transdermal clonidine with its once-weekly dosing is well suited for patients who are forgetful, who do not like to be reminded daily of their illness, or who have their medicines administered to them by family or friends. The centrally acting agents have been used safely and successfully in combination with all of the major classes of antihypertensive agents, including diuretics. Dosing information for the currently available centrally acting agents is summarized in Table 44–5.

ALPHA-ADRENERGIC RECEPTOR BLOCKERS. The α-adrenergic antagonists lower BP by reducing peripheral vascular resistance, principally by inhibiting norepinephrine-induced vasoconstriction in vascular smooth muscle. The hypotensive effect is not accompanied by significant alterations in heart rate, cardiac output, glomerular filtration rate, or renal plasma flow. The α antagonists are effective in all major subgroups of hypertensive patients and have been used safely in combination with all of the major classes of antihypertensive agents, including diuretics and β blockers. Contrary to common clinical perception, long-term trials have not demonstrated the development of tolerance to the antihypertensive effects of the α antagonists.

The α antagonists have no significant adverse metabolic effects and, in fact, have a beneficial effect on the serum lipid profile. They decrease total cholesterol and/or LDL cholesterol and increase HDL cholesterol. Thus, the α antagonists provide a dual benefit in lowering cardiovascular risk.

The major side effects of the α antagonists include headache, dizziness, weakness, and mild fluid retention. Orthostatic hypotension, which is usually most prominent with the initial dose, can occur with all the α antagonists but is best documented with prazosin. The effect can be minimized by initiating therapy with a small dose at bedtime. The α antagonists are generally free of central nervous system–mediated side effects, such as dry mouth, fatigue, and sexual dysfunction. The development of longer-acting α antagonists with minimal side effects and positive effects on serum lipid levels expands the role of these agents as initial antihypertensive therapy, particularly in patients with underlying diseases such as chronic obstructive pulmonary disease, peripheral vascular disease, diabetes, and hyperlipidemia. Dosing information for the currently available α-adrenergic antagonists is summarized in Table 44–5.

VASODILATORS. The direct vasodilators relax arterial smooth muscle with little effect on venous capacitance vessels. BP is reduced secondary to a decrease in peripheral resistance in association with reflex-mediated increases in heart rate, stroke volume, and cardiac output, as well as expansion of the plasma and extracellular fluid volumes.

Common side effects include tachycardia, fluid retention, palpitations, headache, nasal congestion, and, in patients with underlying coronary artery disease, myocardial ischemia. It is generally necessary to administer hydralazine or minoxidil in combination with a diuretic and β blocker to minimize fluid retention and block reflex-mediated increases in heart rate and cardiac output. Long-term administration of hydralazine, particularly in doses greater than 300 mg per day, may induce systemic lupus erythematosus. The lupus reaction generally resolves following discontinuation of hydralazine therapy but occasionally may require several years for complete resolution. Side effects of minoxidil include hirsutism, which makes minoxidil unacceptable to female patients, nausea, fatigue, and skin rash. Minoxidil use has been associated with unexplained pericardial effusion, occasionally with tamponade.

The direct vasodilators are generally reserved for adjunctive therapy in patients with severe refractory hypertension. Minoxidil has been safely and effectively used in patients with severe hypertension complicated by renal insufficiency. The combination of a vasodilator and diuretic with a β blocker (triple therapy) is effective in treating patients with severe, refractory essential or renal hypertension. Dosing information for the currently available vasodilators is summarized in Table 44–5.

Special Patient Groups

THE ELDERLY. Approximately two thirds of persons between the ages of 65 and 74 years have hypertension. Both diastolic hypertension and isolated systolic hypertension in the elderly are associated with a two- to three-fold increased risk of cardiovascular mortality. Multiple clinical trials have demonstrated reduced cardiovascular morbidity and mortality with treatment of diastolic hypertension in the elderly. Whether treating isolated systolic hypertension in the elderly has a similar effect on prognosis is a topic of current study.

The drugs used in the treatment of diastolic or isolated systolic hypertension in the elderly are the same as those used in the nonelderly. Because older persons are particularly sensitive to pharmacologic intervention, antihypertensive medications should be prescribed cautiously at lower than the recommended starting dose for the general population of hypertensives and adjustments made slowly (6- to 8-week intervals). Elderly persons are more prone to orthostatic hypotension because of decreased sensitivity of their baroreceptors. Accordingly, supine and standing BP should be checked regularly in order to avoid orthostasis. Agents particularly prone to cause severe orthostatic hypotension (guanethidine, prazosin, and guanadrel) should be avoided in the elderly. All of the major classes of antihypertensive drugs have been shown to be effective in elderly patients, although the β blockers may be slightly less effective in this group.

DIABETICS. Hypertension is twice as common in diabetics as in the general population. Diabetics with hypertension have a greatly increased risk of developing cerebral vascular disease, coronary artery disease, and renal disease compared to normotensive diabetics. Nonpharmacologic approaches, including weight loss, exercise, and decreased alcohol consumption, benefit both glucose and BP control. Because of their proven effectiveness and lack of significant adverse effects, recommended first-line agents for BP control in diabetics include calcium channel blockers, ACE inhibitors, and α-adrenergic blockers. The ACE inhibitors are gaining favor in the treatment of hypertension in diabetic patients because of recent evidence that they reduce the proteinuria and slow the rate of deterioration in renal function due to diabetic nephropathy. Alpha blockers are favored as antihypertensive treatment in diabetics because of their positive effects on the serum lipid profile. Diuretics are effective in lowering BP in hypertensive diabetics, but their effects on serum potassium, lipid levels, and glucose tolerance are particularly worrisome in this group. Similarly, β blockers are effective but should be used with caution in insulin-dependent diabetics because they tend to mask the symptoms of hypoglycemia and inhibit recovery of glucose levels. Potassium supplements and potassium-sparing diuretics should be used with caution in diabetics because of the frequent occurrence of hyporeninemic hypoaldosteronism in patients with diabetic nephropathy.

BLACKS. Hypertension tends to be more common, earlier in onset, and more severe in blacks than in whites. Organ damage secondary to hypertension also occurs more frequently in blacks than in whites. However, hypertension in blacks can be treated as successfully as hypertension in whites.

Pharmacologic therapy is generally the same for blacks and whites, with only subtle differences in responsiveness to various treatment regimens. Diuretics and calcium channel blockers are very effective in the treatment of black patients. Beta blockers and ACE inhibitors provide less reduction of BP in blacks than in whites at equivalent doses, but at higher doses or in combination with diuretics, racial differences are obliterated. Centrally acting agents and vasodilators are equally effective in whites and blacks.

SECONDARY HYPERTENSION

Renal

RENOVASCULAR HYPERTENSION. Renovascular disease is the most common (1 to 2 per cent) cause of curable hypertension. Lesions of the renal vessels produce a fixed obstruction to perfusion, stimulating the intrarenal baroreceptor and perhaps the macula densa to augment renin secretion. Angiotensin and aldosterone are increased secondarily, resulting in sodium and water retention. Elevated circulating angiotensin II and aldosterone levels are primarily responsible for BP elevation early in the course of renovascular hypertension, and increased sodium and water retention and enhanced sympathetic nervous system activity play dominant roles in the chronic phase of the syndrome. Deficiencies of antihypertensive factors, such as prostaglandins and renomedullary neutral lipid, may also contribute to the pathogenesis of renovascular hypertension.

Any lesion that obstructs either large or small renal arteries can cause renovascular hypertension. The most common and clinically important of these are intrinsic lesions of the large vessels, because they can be physically removed and the hypertension either cured or ameliorated. Atherosclerotic disease is found in two thirds of patients with renovascular hypertension, fibrous or fibromuscular disease in one third. Patients with atherosclerotic renal artery lesions tend to be older and to have higher systolic BP and more frequent extrarenal arterial disease than patients with essential hypertension and are more likely to develop target-organ damage. Patients with fibromuscular disease tend to be younger and predominantly female and are less likely to develop cardiovascular complications. Prognosis is generally worse in atherosclerotic disease than in fibromuscular disease.

Patients most likely to have renovascular hypertension include those with hypertension of abrupt onset, especially in the young or in late middle age or old age; those with malignant hypertension or sudden acceleration of benign hypertension; and those who fail to respond to medical therapy. Generally, these patients have moderately severe to severe fixed diastolic hypertension. The presence of an upper abdominal bruit, particularly one that is systolic-diastolic or continuous in timing, is high pitched, and radiates laterally from the midepigastrium, is strongly suggestive of functionally significant renal artery stenosis. Such bruits have been described in one half to two thirds of patients with surgically proven renovascular hypertension. Because of the high cost of the diagnostic evaluation for renovascular hypertension, diagnostic study should be reserved for patients with one or more of the characteristics discussed above.

Screening tests for renovascular hypertension include abdominal ultrasonography, the captopril renogram, and pharmacologic screening with an ACE inhibitor. **Abdominal ultrasonography** provides an inexpensive, noninvasive means of assessing renal size and ureteral anatomy and does not require administration of radioactive isotopes. It is useful in evaluating patients in whom renal parenchymal disease and obstructive uropathy are part of the differential diagnosis. The **captopril renogram** provides an indirect index of glomerular filtration rate or estimated renal plasma flow and its dependence on intrarenal angiotensin II by measuring renal uptake of radiolabeled diethylene triamine penta-acetic acid (DTPA) or Hippuran before and after ACE inhibition with captopril. It has replaced the rapid-sequence or hypertensive intravenous pyelogram as the most commonly used screening test for renovascular hypertension. A positive captopril renogram indicates that a stenotic lesion is both hemodynamically and functionally significant and predicts a good result from renal revascularization; renal revascularization corrects the abnormalities in the captopril renogram. The sensitivity and specificity of the captopril renogram as a screening test in a large population with a low probability of disease have not yet been tested, however. **Pharmacologic screening** with an ACE inhibitor is a sensitive but not highly specific means of evaluating patients for renovascular hypertension. Administration of a single oral dose of ACE inhibitor leads to increases in plasma renin activity and decreases in BP that are exaggerated in patients with renovascular hypertension. Responses to this pharmacologic screening test reflect the angiotensin dependence of the patient's BP and thus are critically dependent on volume and sodium status. False-positive results are seen in patients who are volume depleted or are being treated with antihypertensive therapy, patients with malignant hypertension, and some patients with high- and normal-renin essential hypertension.

Diagnosis of functionally significant renal artery stenosis has traditionally been made by a combination of selective renal angiography and differential renal vein renin measurement. Renal angiography defines the anatomy of the stenotic renal artery, information needed to plan the approach to revascularization. With the advent of safe and highly effective percutaneous techniques for renal revascularization, many angiographers now elect not to perform renal vein renin determinations in patients with typical lesions but to proceed immediately to angioplasty and use the BP response as a test of the functional significance of the lesion. In some centers, the captopril renogram has replaced renal vein renin determinations as a functional test in patients with documented renal artery stenosis.

In general, the therapeutic approach to patients with renovascular hypertension is to attempt revascularization with percutaneous transluminal angioplasty at the time of diagnosis in those with anatomically favorable lesions. If angioplasty is unsuccessful or if restenosis occurs after successful dilatation, the procedure can be repeated. If repeat angioplasty is unsuccessful, surgical revascularization should be attempted in patients with favorable lesions who can tolerate the procedure, particularly if BP is uncontrolled on medical treatment or renal function is deteriorating. Only patients with anatomically unfavorable lesions and those who are not surgical candidates should receive medical treatment at the time of diagnosis without a prior attempt at revascularization. Medical therapy is used more often in older patients who have atherosclerotic renal artery disease and overt extrarenal vascular disease than in younger patients with fibromuscular disease.

ACE inhibitors, given alone or in combination with a diuretic, are generally effective in controlling BP while sparing renal function and maintaining negative sodium balance in patients with hypertension due to unilateral renal artery stenosis. These simple regimens are well tolerated and represent the medical treatment of choice in most patients with renovascular hypertension. The ACE inhibitors induce acute, reversible renal failure in a subset of patients with renovascular hypertension: those with bilateral renal artery stenosis or renal artery stenosis in a solitary kidney, whether native or allograft, or with unilateral renal artery stenosis and severe parenchymal disease in the contralateral kidney. This form of reversible renal insufficiency results from impairment in the autoregulation of glomerular filtration secondary to blockade of the intrarenal renin-angiotensin system in the presence of reduced renal artery perfusion pressure. Normal autoregulation of glomerular filtration rate, which is dependent on an intact intrarenal renin-angiotensin system, is lost when an ACE inhibitor is administered.

Renal size and function must be carefully monitored in patients being treated medically for renovascular hypertension, even if BP is satisfactorily controlled. Renal function can deteriorate and renal mass can be lost very rapidly in patients with atherosclerotic disease who are treated medically. Progressive loss of renal mass, presumably related to parenchymal ischemia due to progression of the renal artery lesion, is common in medically treated patients with renovascular hypertension and is unrelated to BP control. Significant reduction in renal length is the most sensitive index of loss of renal mass. Serial (every 3 to 6 months) estimates of renal size are important in the follow-up of patients who are receiving medical treatment for renovascular hypertension.

Adrenal

Primary aldosteronism and pheochromocytoma are relatively rare causes of hypertension which are clinically important because the associated hypertension can usually be cured with appropriate surgical or targeted drug therapy. These syndromes are discussed in detail in Ch. 217.8 and 229, respectively.

ORAL CONTRACEPTIVE–INDUCED HYPERTENSION. A small percentage of women who use oral contraceptives experience the onset of hypertension that resolves with withdrawal of oral contraceptive therapy. Genetic characteristics, such as family history of hypertension and black race, as well as environmental characteristics, such as pre-existing and occult renal disease, obesity, and middle age (> 40 years), increase susceptibility to oral contraceptive–induced hypertension. The diagnosis of oral contraceptive–induced hypertension can be made by documenting the onset of hypertension de novo during contraceptive therapy and the resolution of the hypertension on drug withdrawal. This form of hypertension usually begins during the first year of oral contraceptive administration.

Oral contraceptive–induced hypertension can, in part, be prevented by avoiding the use of these agents in women who are at high risk. Evidence of thromboembolic disease or chronic hypertension of any cause is a contraindication to use of oral contraceptive. A family history of hypertension and a personal history of pre-existing or occult renal disease or of pregnancy complicated by hypertension are relative contraindications to oral contraceptive use. Women over 35 years of age, particularly if obese, should be cautioned about the increased risk of developing hypertension while ingesting oral contraceptives. Such patients should be followed closely: BP measurement and a funduscopic examination should be performed and an interval history obtained on several occasions during the first year of treatment and at yearly intervals thereafter.

The prevalence of oral contraceptive–induced hypertension is not related to the formulation or dose of estrogen, but since the incidence of thromboembolic complications is related to the dose of estrogen in the contraceptive, it is preferable to use preparations of relatively low estrogen content.

HYPERTENSIVE CRISIS

Hypertensive crises are subclassified as hypertensive urgencies or emergencies, depending on evidence of ongoing end-organ

TABLE 44–8. ANTIHYPERTENSIVE DRUGS FOR MANAGEMENT OF HYPERTENSIVE CRISIS

Drugs	Intramuscular (mg*)	Single Dose (mg*)	Continuous Infusion (μg/kg/min)	Onset of Action	Adverse Effects
Oral agents					
Clonidine (Catapres)†	—	0.2 p.o. initially, then 0.1 at 1-hr intervals as needed up to total dose of 0.7	—	30–60 min	Hypotension, headache, nausea, dizziness
Nifedipine (Procardia)†	—	10–20 sublingually or buccally initially, then at 30-min intervals as needed × 3	—	5–10 min	Hypotension, flushing, headache, tachycardia, nausea, coronary ischemia (rare)
Parenteral agents					
Direct vasodilators					
Sodium nitroprusside (Nipride)	—	—	0.5–10	Immediate	Nausea, vomiting, muscle twitching, apprehension, sweating, thiocyanate intoxication
Diazoxide (Hyperstat)	—	50–100 at 5–10-min intervals until satisfactory BP is achieved	Rarely used	3–5 min	Tachycardia, palpitations, flushing, headache, nausea, vomiting, aggravation of angina or congestive heart failure or both, hyperglycemia, hyperuricemia, hypotension
Hydralazine (Apresoline)	10–40 at 30-min intervals until satisfactory response is achieved	10–20 at 30-min intervals until satisfactory BP is achieved	Rarely used	Intramuscularly 30 min; intravenously 5–10 min	Tachycardia, palpitations, flushing, headache, vomiting, aggravation of angina or congestive heart failure or both
Sympathetic blocking drugs					
Ganglion-blocking agent					
Trimethaphan camsylate (Arfonad)	—	—	4–90	5–10 min	Urinary retention, paralytic ileus, paralysis of pupillary reflex and accommodation of eye, dry mouth, orthostatic hypotension
Central nervous system–active agent					
Methyldopa hydrochloride (Aldomet ester)	—	250–500; may be repeated at 6-hr intervals	—	2–3 hr	Drowsiness
Alpha-adrenergic receptor blocking agents					
Phentolamine (Regitine)	5–15	5–15 (rapid injection essential)	—	Instantaneous	Tachycardia, flushing
Labetalol	—	20 initially over 2 min, then 40–80 at 10-min intervals as needed up to 300 total	2/min to a total dose of 300	Instantaneous	Postural dizziness with or without postural hypotension; paradoxical pressor responses have been reported; nausea, vomiting, scalp tingling, burning in throat and groin
Calcium channel blocking agent					
Nicardipine (Cardene)†	—	5/h initially, titrated upward by 1–2.5/h every 15 min as needed up to 15/h		1–5 min	Hypotension, flushing, headache, diaphoresis, dizziness, nausea, tachycardia

*Start with the smallest dose shown. Subsequent doses and intervals of administration should be adjusted according to the BP response.

Start infusion slowly and adjust rate according to response to BP. Constant surveillance is mandatory. Concentration of solution can be adjusted according to patient's fluid requirements.

The total dose should be contained in a volume of at least 20 ml, and the solution should be administered from a 20- or 50-ml syringe. BP should be monitored continuously during injection. Rate of injection should not exceed 0.5 ml per minute. To avoid hypotension, the injection should be stopped frequently when the BP is falling.

Diluted up to 100 ml and injected during a 30- to 60-minute period.

†Not approved by FDA for this indication.

damage. In the absence of neurologic, cardiovascular, or renal deterioration and funduscopic abnormalities, patients with severely elevated BP (> 200/120 mm Hg) require urgent treatment, but usually not hospital admission. However, in the presence of evidence of ongoing end-organ damage, patients with severely elevated BP should be treated emergently with parenteral medications in an intensive care unit. The distinction between the need for urgent versus emergent intervention is based not on the absolute BP, but instead on the effect of the BP elevation on target organs. A BP of 190/130 mm Hg may be well tolerated in a patient with chronic hypertension, whereas that BP reading in another patient may precipitate acute renal insufficiency, left ventricular failure, cerebral edema, or other vascular crisis, thereby creating a medical emergency. The triggering mechanism for the arteriolar lesion responsible for the development of accelerated or malignant hypertension is unknown but has been related to the absolute level or rate of rise of arterial pressure, the presence of disseminated intravascular clotting, or activation of the renin-angiotensin system. The syndrome is perpetuated by the deposition of fibrin in arteriolar walls, which leads to retinopathy, renal damage, and increased renin release. Usually the etiology of any particular hypertensive crisis is not known, and therapy must be generalized. However, when the etiology is known, specific treatment should be instituted whenever possible.

Symptoms of hypertensive crisis include headache, malaise, dizziness, blurred vision, chest pain, palpitations, and shortness of breath. Clinical and laboratory signs of hypertensive crisis include funduscopic changes (arteriolar narrowing, arteriovenous nicking, hemorrhages, exudates, papilledema); changes related to renal insufficiency; microangiopathic hemolytic anemia; signs of left ventricular dysfunction (gallops, jugular venous distention, cardiomegaly, tachycardia, pulmonary edema); and evidence of increased intracranial pressure (confusion, somnolence, stupor, neurologic deficits, seizures). Patients with hypertensive emergencies may present with stroke, subarachnoid hemorrhage, intracranial hemorrhage, aortic dissection, left ventricular failure, or myocardial ischemia. Importantly, however, severely elevated BP is often discovered coincidentally without any related signs or symptoms.

Evaluation of a patient with hypertensive crisis includes a pertinent history, with a special attempt to elicit symptoms relating to the etiology or consequences of the severely elevated BP. Physical examination includes determination of supine, sitting, and standing BP, neurologic evaluation, funduscopic examination, cardiac auscultation with evaluation of left ventricular size and function, and palpation of distal pulses. Chest radiography, electrocardiography, complete blood cell count with blood smear, and renal chemistries and urinalysis should be performed. If by history, physical examination, or laboratory data the patient has evidence of ongoing (new or worsening) end-organ damage, the patient should be considered to be having a medical emergency.

The goal in treating hypertensive crisis is a prompt but gradual reduction in BP to just above normotensive levels. Precipitous or excessive reductions in BP may impair the body's ability to regulate blood flow, causing end-organ hypoperfusion. Ideally, BP should be reduced to 150 to 160/100 to 110 mm Hg and maintained at that level for a few days. Then, with initiation or reinitiation of long-term therapy, BP levels can slowly be returned to the normotensive range.

Hypertensive urgencies are best treated with oral agents that allow effective titration of BP over a short period of time. Both clonidine and nifedipine are especially well suited to this purpose. Recommended dose schedules for these agents in the setting of hypertensive urgency are listed in Table 44–8. If clonidine loading successfully reduces a patient's BP, chronic clonidine therapy should be initiated. Approximately 80 per cent of the oral loading dose given daily on an every-12-hour schedule generally maintains BP adequately and serves as a good starting point for outpatient dose titration. Patients who respond acutely to nifedipine should be started on long-term calcium channel blocker therapy. All patients presenting with hypertensive urgency and treated with oral therapy should be monitored for at least 6 hours to document persistent BP reduction and should be seen in outpatient follow-up within 1 week.

Patients presenting with hypertensive emergencies require parenteral antihypertensive therapy administered in an intensive care setting. Table 44–8 lists the antihypertensive drugs most commonly used in the management of hypertensive emergencies, with recommended doses and common adverse effects. As above, the goal of therapy is to effect an immediate but gradual decline in BP to approximately 160/100 mm Hg. Most patients presenting with critically elevated BP are volume depleted, and consequently the indiscriminate administration of diuretics may exacerbate their hypertension. All patients presenting with severe hypertension should have supine and standing BP checked, and if they have orthostatic changes in BP, diuretics should be withheld. However, in patients with clinical evidence of volume overload, diuresis is indicated, both to improve left ventricular filling pressure and to reduce BP.

Calhoun DA, Oparil S: Treatment of hypertensive crisis. N Engl J Med 323:1177, 1990. *An up-to-date review of the emergency treatment of hypertension.*

Collins R, Peto R, MacMahon S, et al.: Blood pressure, stroke, and coronary heart disease. Part 2, short-term reductions in blood pressure: Overview of randomised drug trials in their epidemiological context. Lancet 335:827, 1990. *A new meta-analysis of 14 randomized trials of antihypertensive drugs, including 37,000 individuals treated for a mean of 5 years, shows significant treatment-related reduction in stroke and coronary artery disease.*

The Joint National Committee on Detection, Evaluation, and Treatment of High Blood Pressure: The 1988 Report of the Joint National Committee on Detection, Evaluation, and Treatment of High Blood Pressure. Arch Intern Med 148:1023, 1988. *Detailed recommendations for the diagnosis and pharmacologic and nonpharmacologic treatment of systemic hypertension.*

Veterans Administration Cooperative Study Group on Antihypertensive Agents: Effects of treatment on morbidity in hypertension: I. Results in patients with diastolic blood pressures averaging 115 through 129 mm Hg. JAMA 202:1028, 1967. *Demonstration that male hypertensive patients with diastolic blood pressure averaging 115 mm Hg or above represent a high-risk group in which hypertensive therapy exerts a significant beneficial effect.*

Veterans Administration Cooperative Study Group on Antihypertensive Agents: Effects of treatment on morbidity in hypertension: II. Results in patients with diastolic blood pressure averaging 90 through 114 mm Hg. JAMA 213:1143, 1970. *Demonstration that treatment of male patients with mildly elevated blood pressure is more effective in preventing congestive heart failure and stroke than in preventing the complications of coronary artery disease and that the degree of benefit of treatment is related to the level of prerandomization blood pressure.*

Working Group on Management of Patients with Hypertension and High Blood Cholesterol: National education programs working group report on the management of patients with hypertension and high blood cholesterol. Ann Intern Med 114:224, 1991. *Detailed recommendations for the management of patients with hypertension and hypercholesterolemia with or without concomitant atherosclerotic disease.*

45 Pulmonary Hypertension

Alfred P. Fishman

The normal pulmonary circulation is not prone to develop pulmonary hypertension. On the one hand, it is endowed with a large capacity, great distensibility, and low resistance to blood flow; on the other, it contains no baroregulatory mechanisms comparable to those in the systemic circulation that can go awry or overshoot. Amputation of more than half of the normal pulmonary circulation, as by pneumonectomy, or doubling of the pulmonary blood flow through normal lungs, as during exercise, elicits a barely perceptible increase in pulmonary arterial pressure. In contrast, when widespread disease or disturbed ventilation-perfusion relationships increase pulmonary vascular resistance and limit distensibility, modest increments in pulmonary blood flow generally elicit considerable increments in pulmonary arterial pressure.

Definitions

The term "pulmonary hypertension" refers to pulmonary *arterial* hypertension unless otherwise specified. Criteria for pulmonary hypertension depend on the altitude: In the resting individual at sea level, a mean pulmonary arterial pressure greater than 19 to 20 mm Hg establishes the diagnosis; the corresponding limit at altitude is higher—at about 15,000 feet, a mean pulmonary arterial pressure greater than 25 mm Hg signifies pulmonary hypertension.

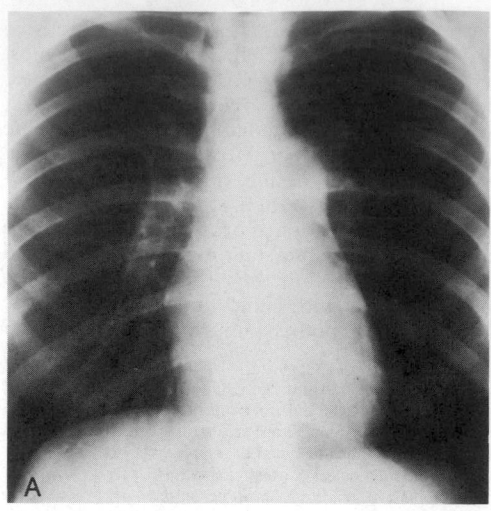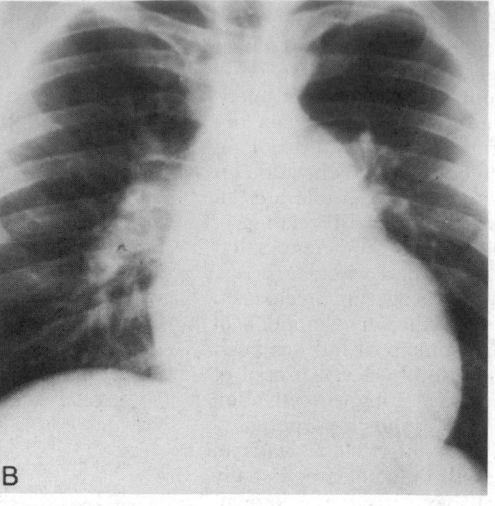

FIGURE 45–1. Pulmonary hypertension, cor pulmonale, and right ventricular failure in two patients with primary pulmonary hypertension. *A*, Pulmonary hypertension and cor pulmonale. *B*, Pulmonary hypertension, cor pulmonale, and right ventricular failure (systemic venous congestion).

Pulmonary *venous* hypertension is a different entity with respect to etiology, pathogenesis, clinical manifestations, and management. It is said to exist when pulmonary venous or left atrial pressure exceeds 12 mm Hg; this limit applies at altitude as well as at sea level. In the normal pulmonary circulation, an acute increase in pulmonary venous pressure to the range of 20 to 30 mm Hg runs the risk of causing pulmonary edema. The sample levels are less threatening when sustained chronically, as in mitral valve disease, presumably because of thickening of alveolar-capillary walls.

Cor pulmonale is a consequence of pulmonary hypertension. It is defined as enlargement of the right ventricle, i.e., hypertrophy, dilatation, or both, as a consequence of disease of the respiratory apparatus. In chronic cor pulmonale resulting from sustained pulmonary hypertension, hypertrophy usually dominates the course of the illness until the later stages when the right ventricle fails; at this juncture, dilatation generally predominates (Fig. 45–1).

THE NORMAL PULMONARY CIRCULATION

In the normal adult, the small muscular arteries and arterioles constitute the "resistance" vessels. In the adult at sea level, these vessels are thin walled and sparsely equipped with muscle; in the fetus and in the native resident at altitude, the muscle is thicker and more extensive.

Hemodynamics

Because of the low resistance and high distensibility of the pulmonary vascular bed and the pulsatile nature of pulmonary blood pressure, the large pulmonary blood flow is accomplished by only a small drop in mean pressure between the pulmonary artery and the left atrium (Table 45–1). The mean pressure difference at rest is ordinarily about 5 to 10 mm Hg.

TABLE 45–1. REPRESENTATIVE VALUES AT REST FOR THE NORMAL PULMONARY CIRCULATION AT SEA LEVEL AND AT ALTITUDE

	Sea Level	14,900 ft
Pulmonary arterial pressure (mm Hg, systolic/diastolic, mean)	20/12, 15	38/14, 25
Cardiac output (liters/min)	6.0	6.0
Cardiac index (liters min/m², body surface area)	3.1	3.1
Left atrial pressure (mm Hg)	5.0	5.0
Pulmonary vascular resistance (R units*)	0.1†	0.2

*R units express calculated resistance in terms of $\frac{mm\ Hg}{ml/sec}$. To convert to C.G.S. units (dynes · sec · cm^{-5}), the value in R units is multiplied by 1328.

†Based on the data in this table, at sea level, $R = \frac{15 - 5}{6000/60} = 0.1$ R units.

The normal pulmonary hemodynamics of adults residing at sea level and at altitude are indicated in Table 45–1. Because of the passive nature of the pulmonary vascular bed, the pulmonary arterial pressure—particularly in hypertensive states—must be assessed with respect to the pulmonary blood flow (cardiac output). At the same levels of cardiac output, the pulmonary arterial pressure is consistently higher at altitude than at sea level because of the increase in pulmonary vascular tone elicited by hypoxia.

Calculation of pulmonary vascular resistance (Table 45–1) has become a popular expedient for depicting the state of the pulmonary resistance vessels (small muscular arteries and arterioles) and for inferring whether a change in the tone of these vessels occurs after an intervention, e.g., the administration of a vasodilator agent. However, in pursuing the goal of detecting *active* change, due regard is not always paid to the possible obscuring effects of passive change. Also, for practical reasons—especially in human studies—outflow pressures (left atrium) are often ignored or assumed. In order to minimize shortcomings inherent in applying the resistance formula to a distensible system for which it was not intended, two precautions have proved useful in providing interpretable values for resistance: (1) accurate assessment should be made not only of pulmonary arterial pressure and pulmonary blood flow but also of left atrial (pulmonary wedge) pressure, and (2) if resistances before and after an intervention are to be compared, comparisons should be made at the same level of either the pressure drop across the lungs (the numerator of the resistance equation) or the pulmonary blood flow (the denominator). In this way, passive changes in the pulmonary circulation do not cloud the search for vasomotor activity. Fortunately, the second criterion becomes less stringent in states of severe pulmonary hypertension in which disease has curtailed the extent and distensibility of the pulmonary circulation.

Regulation by Local Chemical Stimuli

It was noted above that the pulmonary circulation is devoid of a baroregulatory apparatus comparable to the carotid sinus apparatus in the systemic circulation. Indeed, local stimuli dominate the control of the pulmonary circulation. Of the local stimuli, hypoxia is the most powerful. Acidosis per se is a fairly weak stimulus, except in reinforcing the pressor effect of hypoxia. Hypercapnia is also a modest pressor agent that acts, presumably, by way of the local acidosis that it generates.

SECONDARY PULMONARY HYPERTENSION

Of the two subsets of pulmonary arterial hypertension, the secondary form (Table 45–2) is by far the more prevalent. As a rule, the clinical manifestations of secondary pulmonary hypertension are dominated by signs and symptoms of the underlying disease, generally cardiac or respiratory. Pulmonary hypertension of mild to moderate degree, as in normal native residents at high altitude, is generally asymptomatic for a lifetime. In contrast,

TABLE 45–2. CLASSIFICATION OF CHRONIC PULMONARY (ARTERIAL) HYPERTENSION

Secondary
  Cardiac disease
    Acquired disorders of the left side of the heart causing
      pulmonary venous hypertension
      Left ventricular failure
      Mitral valve disease
      Left atrial myxoma
      Decrease in left ventricular compliance
    Congenital heart disease
      Pre-tricuspid
      Post-tricuspid
  Respiratory diseases
    Obstructive airways disease
    Diseases of the lung parenchyma
      Alveolar
      Interstitial
    Pulmonary vascular disease
      Collagen vascular disease
      Thromboembolic disease
    Neuromuscular disorders
      Abnormal chest bellows
      Disordered respiratory control mechanisms
Primary pulmonary (arterial) hypertension
Pulmonary veno-occlusive disease

severe pulmonary hypertension, as occurs in chronic mountain sickness or in primary pulmonary hypertension, can be accompanied by evidences of right heart failure and a tendency to easy fatiguability, syncope, arrhythmias (especially in hypoxic states), and sudden death.

The most common causes of pulmonary (arterial) hypertension are heart disease and lung disease (Table 45–2). Regardless of the root cause of the pulmonary arterial hypertension, sooner or later the resistance (precapillary) vessels of the lungs undergo anatomic change that contributes to the pulmonary hypertension. However, the initiating mechanisms are generally dissimilar in heart disease and lung disease: As a rule, pulmonary arterial hypertension secondary to acquired heart disease begins with a disorder of the left ventricle that leads to pulmonary venous hypertension followed by pulmonary arterial hypertension; rarely does an increase in pulmonary blood flow per se cause pulmonary hypertension. In contrast, an increase in pulmonary blood flow not infrequently triggers pulmonary arterial hypertension in congenital heart disease and, as during exercise, aggravates pre-existing pulmonary hypertension in both acquired and congenital heart disease.

Cardiac Disease

Acquired disorders of the left side of the heart and certain types of congenital heart disease often lead to pulmonary hypertension.

ACQUIRED DISORDERS. Left ventricular failure is the predominant cause of pulmonary hypertension and of right ventricular failure. Myocardial disorders and lesions of the mitral and aortic valves are the most common left ventricular disorders leading to pulmonary hypertension. Left ventricular disorders increase pulmonary venous pressure, which, in turn, evokes an increase in pulmonary arterial pressure that suffices to maintain antegrade flow; this automatic adjustment is presumably reflex. But, in time, three types of morphologic changes appear as a consequence of the pulmonary venous hypertension: (1) occlusive intimal and medial changes in pulmonary precapillary vessels as well as in pulmonary venules and veins; (2) perivascular interstitial edema, which not only contributes directly to the increase in resistance to blood flow but also stimulates perivascular fibrosis; under the influence of gravity, the vascular and perivascular changes are most marked in the dependent portions of the lungs; and (3) occlusion of small pulmonary vessels by emboli or thrombi; especially in states of slowed systemic blood flow, emboli are much more apt to arise from thrombi in the veins of the extremities than from the right side of the heart. Depending on the reversibility of the vascular and perivascular lesions, relief of the pulmonary venous hypertension, as by mitral valve commissurotomy or replacement for mitral valvular disease, generally reduces the pulmonary arterial pressure.

CONGENITAL HEART DISEASE. Congenital defects that produce left to right shunting of blood within the heart or between the great vessels are commonly associated with pulmonary arterial hypertension. As a rule, this shunting interferes with the normal transition from the thick-walled fetal pulmonary circulation to the thin-walled adult state. Moreover, arterial hypoxemia is often part of the congenital heart syndrome. The net effect of the interplay between the hemodynamic abnormalities, arterial hypoxemia, and the persistent fetal pulmonary circulation is to promote intimal proliferation and medial hypertrophy, which, in time, may dominate in sustaining the pulmonary hypertension and in determining its reversibility. Heart-lung transplantation has been used in small series of patients with Eisenmenger's complex. The results to date have been encouraging, i.e., about 50 per cent alive at 4 years. Deaths were due primarily to infection and, in a few instances, to bronchiolitis obliterans and cerebral embolism.

Respiratory Disease

Failure of any major component of the respiratory apparatus can lead to pulmonary hypertension. For convenience, the components can be sorted into the airways, lung parenchyma, chest bellows, and respiratory control mechanisms. In turn, pulmonary hypertension often taxes the right heart to the point of enlargement (cor pulmonale) by way of dilatation and hypertrophy.

OBSTRUCTIVE AIRWAYS DISEASE. Chronic bronchitis and emphysema (chronic obstructive lung disease, or COPD) is the most common cause of pulmonary hypertension and cor pulmonale. Even though chronic bronchitis and emphysema generally coexist, the chronic bronchitis is predominantly responsible for the alveolar hypoxia and the low Po_2, high Pco_2, and resultant low pH that lead to pulmonary hypertension. In patients with obstructive airways disease, "blue bloaters" are chronically hypoxemic and pulmonary hypertensive whereas "pink puffers" develop transient pulmonary hypertension in the course of an acute respiratory infection that leads to arterial hypoxemia. A key clinical sign of pulmonary hypertension is right ventricular enlargement (cor pulmonale). However, right ventricular enlargement may be difficult to prove in a particular patient with obstructive airways disease until right ventricular failure supervenes. The onset of right ventricular failure is often heralded by striking cyanosis, unexplained drowsiness, inappropriate behavior, systemic venous congestion, and hepatomegaly. Right ventricular gallops (S_3 and S_4) are generally present, and the murmur of tricuspid insufficiency can often be elicited. Arterial blood gas analysis reveals that the Po_2 is low ($Po_2 <$ 40 to 50 torr), the Pco_2 is high ($Pco_2 >$ 50 torr), and respiratory acidosis is present.

Electrocardiographic evidence of right ventricular enlargement is often equivocal in patients with bronchitis and emphysema because of rotation and displacement of the heart, widened distances between electrodes and the cardiac surface, and acute cardiac dilatation. As a rule, consecutive changes in the electrocardiogram are more useful than a single electrocardiogram in detecting that the right ventricle has been overloaded acutely by pulmonary hypertension: T waves in the right precordial leads (V_1 to V_3) flatten and become inverted, the mean electrical axis of the QRS complex shifts to the right, ST segments become depressed in leads II, III, and aV_F, and right bundle branch block (generally incomplete) often appears; these changes reverse as arterial hypoxemia is relieved and pulmonary blood pressures decrease.

Echocardiography is widely used as a noninvasive approach to estimating pulmonary arterial pressure. Three separate techniques are available: M-mode for determining right ventricular and atrial dimensions, two-dimensional for analysis of the motions of the right ventricular, atrial, and septal walls and of the pulmonic and tricuspid valves, and Doppler (pulse wave, continuous wave, and color flow imaging) for determining velocities of blood flow across the pulmonic and tricuspid valves. In practice, these techniques are generally applied as a package. They are costly, complex, and often inaccurate, except when pulmonary hypertension is severe enough to cause considerable tricuspid insufficiency. Consequently, cardiac catheterization is usually resorted to soon after pulmonary hypertension is suspected, with two goals in mind: (1) to determine directly the pulmonary arterial and wedge pressures and the cardiac output for the calculation of pulmonary vascular resistance; and (2) if pulmonary hypertension does exist, to assess the contribution of congenital and acquired cardiac lesions to its pathogenesis. Echocardiography can be useful in following the course of pulmonary hypertension and cor pulmonale, and the effects of pulmonary vasodilators, if it is performed serially, before and after cardiac catheterization.

Treatment of the patient with obstructive airways disease in whom pulmonary hypertension either develops or intensifies because of a bout of bronchitis or pneumonia is directed at maintaining tolerable levels of arterial oxygenation (e.g., arterial $Po_2 > 50$ mm Hg) while treating the upper respiratory infection. Because of persistent arterial hypoxemia, continuing oxygen administration may be necessary even after maximal recovery from the upper respiratory infection. This need is often met by delivering oxygen at low flow rates via a nasal cannula. It has been shown that continued, prolonged oxygen therapy can slow the progression of pulmonary hypertension and its sequelae. Pulmonary vasodilators have little role in treating pulmonary hypertension associated with obstructive airways disease if oxygen and antibiotic therapy are properly administered.

Heart-lung transplantation has been successfully applied to patients with obstructive airways disease, notably cystic fibrosis. Lung transplantation is also being tested for patients with intractable, end-stage bronchitis and emphysema (COPD), as well as for widespread pulmonary fibrosis and primary pulmonary hypertension (see below).

DISEASES OF THE LUNG PARENCHYMA. These diseases may be further subdivided into alveolar, interstitial, and vascular.

Alveolar. Pulmonary hypertension is a frequent concomitant of alveolar disorders, such as pulmonary edema and the respiratory distress syndromes. In the respiratory distress syndromes, pulmonary hypertension is quite common, occasionally in conjunction with pulmonary venous hypertension secondary to fluid overload but more often as a consequence of mechanical influences exerted by pulmonary edema and atelectasis operating in conjunction with respiratory acidosis. This concomitant disorder requires no special treatment, since it follows the course of the illness, decreasing spontaneously as the patient recovers. The pathogenesis and management of these disorders are considered elsewhere.

Interstitial. A wide variety of inflammatory processes, such as sarcoidosis, asbestosis, and "idiopathic fibrosing alveolitis," can affect the interstitium of the lungs. Early on, the major consequence is a diffusion defect in association with a restrictive ventilatory defect that is characterized by concentric reduction in lung volumes and a low diffusing capacity without evidence of airways obstruction. In time, ventilation-perfusion balances become upset and arterial hypoxemia intensifies as fibrosis progresses. At this juncture, the initial hypocapnia resulting from the reflex stimulation of intrapulmonary receptors is succeeded by eucapnia and then hypercapnia. The small muscular arteries and arterioles are caught up in the inflammatory process, and pulmonary hypertension gradually sets in as a consequence of increasing pulmonary vascular resistance due to mechanical vascular obstruction and arterial hypoxemia. The stage is then set for cor pulmonale and right heart failure.

Supplemental oxygen, especially during exercise and sleep, helps to minimize the hypoxic contribution to the pulmonary hypertension. Corticosteroids are the mainstay of therapy but are apt to be least effective when marked fibrosis and pulmonary distortion, reflected in honeycombing, dominate the condition. Lung transplantation, primarily of a single lung, has been used as a last resort in patients with widespread pulmonary fibrosis. The results reported from a few clinics in this country and abroad have been gratifying, but long-term observations are not yet available.

DISEASES OF THE PULMONARY VESSELS. In this category, the most common cause of pulmonary hypertension is thromboembolic disease. At the opposite extreme is obliterative capillary disorder of unknown etiology known as "pulmonary capillary angiomatosis." Among the more uncommon disorders is primary pulmonary hypertension (see below), which has attracted considerable attention because of its implications for the diagnosis

and treatment of other types of pulmonary hypertension. Between these extremes of incidence is a variety of pulmonary vascular diseases that cause pulmonary hypertension as part of systemic disorders, e.g., scleroderma, lupus erythematosus. The latter are often included in the category of interstitial lung disease because the interstitium as well as the vessels is often directly affected by the inflammatory process.

Collagen Vascular Disease. The incidence of pulmonary hypertension and right heart failure in systemic lupus erythematosus (SLE) is high (Fig. 45–2). The incidence of this complication of SLE is much higher in females than in males. Raynaud's phenomenon is a common occurrence in women with SLE who develop pulmonary hypertension. As a rule, the parenchyma of the lungs as well as the pulmonary blood vessels is involved in the inflammatory process leading to pulmonary hypertension.

On rare occasions, scleroderma of the lungs may affect only the microvasculature. Much more usual for progressive systemic sclerosis (scleroderma) and its variants (CREST and overlap syndromes) is for pulmonary hypertension to be a consequence of combined interstitial and vascular disease. Pulmonary hypertension is quite common in patients with progressive systemic sclerosis or the CREST syndrome but is often overlooked until manifestations of heart failure ensue.

Thromboembolic Disease. Pulmonary hypertension and cor pulmonale can occur acutely or chronically as a result of pulmonary thromboembolic disease. The acute form is caused by massive obstruction of major pulmonary arteries that generally leads to death unless the large clots either attenuate spontaneously or by thrombolytic agents or heroic surgery. Chronic pulmonary thromboembolic disease is a much more prevalent and manageable problem.

Three categories of pulmonary thromboembolic disease leading to chronic pulmonary hypertension can be identified depending on the size of the affected pulmonary arteries. This classification is useful as long as it is recognized that some degree of overlap among categories is almost inevitable. It should also be kept in mind that most instances of nonfatal pulmonary thromboembolism—a common clinical occurrence—are not associated with pulmonary hypertension because of the localized nature of the one or more embolic lesions.

Chronic pulmonary thromboembolism accompanied by pulmonary hypertension is manifested by dyspnea on exertion, easy fatiguability, and occasionally angina-like pain in the chest. Three different syndromes have been identified according to the pulmonary vessels primarily affected.

Small Pulmonary Arteries and Arterioles (Resistance Vessels). This rare syndrome can be indistinguishable in onset and progression from that of primary pulmonary hypertension (Fig. 45–3A). Indeed, not long ago, textbooks referred to it as a syndrome of "multiple pulmonary emboli." However, it now seems likely that the syndrome is caused by widespread in situ thrombi in the distal arterial tree rather than by emboli. The etiology of the widespread in situ thrombosis is speculative.

Neither angiography nor ventilation-perfusion scans are capable of identifying microvascular thrombosis as the cause of the pulmonary hypertension, but scans can exclude thromboembolic disease of larger proximal arteries. Biopsy or autopsy reveals the thrombotic nature of the occlusive vascular disease.

Treatment generally consists of long-term anticoagulation using warfarin-type agents and/or antiplatelet agents. Since the microvascular clots are organized, this antithrombotic therapy probably does more to prevent the formation of new clots than to treat the existing clots. In principle, vasodilator therapy holds as much promise in this disorder (which mimics primary pulmonary hypertension) as it does in primary pulmonary hypertension per se. However, no trials of this hypothesis are as yet available.

Intermediate Pulmonary Arteries. Moderate-sized emboli may lodge in intermediate arteries directly or after fragmentation or lysis of larger clots in major vessels. These lesions are demonstrable both by ventilation-perfusion scans and by angiography.

Once chronic pulmonary hypertension is established in patients with this type of pulmonary vascular occlusive disease, it is generally irreversible except when associated with large organized proximal clots that can be removed surgically (see next section). Attention is therefore directed at preventive measures, particularly at eliminating sources of emboli. Symptomatic relief of breathlessness, enhanced cerebration, and relief of arterial hy-

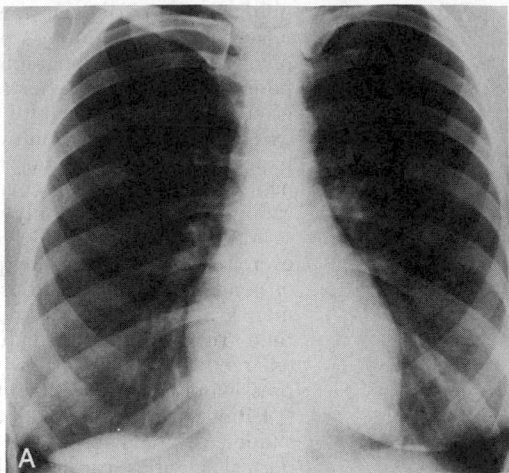
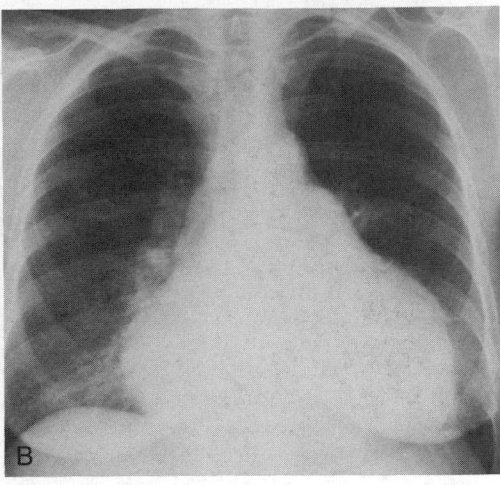

FIGURE 45–2. Pulmonary hypertension in a young woman with systemic lupus erythematosus. *A*, 1974. Pulmonary hypertension and cor pulmonale. *B*, 1981. Cor pulmonale and right ventricular failure.

poxemia can be accomplished by supplemental oxygen. Anticoagulation and/or antiplatelet therapy is routine, as described elsewhere for thromboembolic disease.

Major Pulmonary Arteries. This syndrome results from one or more large clots of long standing in the proximal pulmonary arterial tree which have been incorporated into the vessel wall and cause obstruction and pulmonary hypertension. The clot presumably originates as a large undetected embolus to the lungs. Propagation of the clot proximally and distally, followed by organization, culminates in severe pulmonary hypertension due to obstruction to pulmonary blood flow by poorly compliant proximal pulmonary vessels (Fig. 45–3*B*).

This disorder is amenable to surgery. All patients with unexplained (primary) pulmonary hypertension should be given ventilation-perfusion scans to exclude this possibility. A perfusion defect that is segmental or larger calls for selective pulmonary angiography to localize the site of the organized clot and its proximal extent.

Surgical treatment consists of thromboendarterectomy. It is indicated when clot in the proximal pulmonary arterial tree persists after prolonged anticoagulation, i.e., warfarin sodium for more than 6 months. Presurgical delineation of the extent and boundaries of the obstructive vascular lesions can be helped by combining angiography with magnetic resonance imaging and/or fiberoptic angioscopy. Surgery is formidable, entailing cardiopulmonary bypass during hypothermia punctuated by periods of circulatory arrest. Successful surgery is often followed by a bout of pulmonary edema confined to the large area of lung that was hypoperfused preoperatively. However, successful surgery is gratifying: It is followed by dramatic relief of the pulmonary hypertension and alleviation of symptoms. Lifetime anticoagulation using warfarin sodium is instituted after the surgical procedure.

NEUROMUSCULAR DISORDERS. Disorders of respiratory control mechanisms, of the chest bellows, or of a combination of the two can cause hypertension in lungs that are normal or nearly normal. These disorders, of diverse etiologies that range from kyphoscoliosis to poliomyelitis, have alveolar hypoventilation as the common denominator. Just as in the case of obstructive airways disease, the pulmonary hypertension is associated with alveolar hypoxia and arterial hypoxemia, hypercapnia, and respiratory acidosis. Because of the predominant role of alveolar hypoxia in the syndrome of alveolar hypoventilation, patients are often initially seen because of right heart failure. However, in contrast to obstructive airways disease, the abnormal alveolar and arterial blood gases are due to *global* alveolar hypoventilation rather than to ventilation-perfusion abnormalities; e.g., the alveolar-arterial P_{O_2} gradient is normal or nearly normal in the syndrome of alveolar hypoventilation, whereas it is characteristically large in obstructive airways disease.

Chest Bellows. This category includes skeletal deformity of the chest as well as muscular disorders and extreme obesity (Fig. 45–4). Severe kyphoscoliosis accompanied by dwarfing of the thorax is the prototype of chest deformities that can lead to alveolar hypoventilation. Mutilating operations on the thorax can have the same effect. The predomina mechanism is an inordinate increase in the work of breathing.

Respiratory Control Mechanisms. The Guillain-Barré syndrome or a stroke can impair the central drive to breathe sufficiently to cause alveolar hypoventilation. As indicated elsewhere, certain of the sleep apnea syndromes are also associated with alveolar hypoventilation.

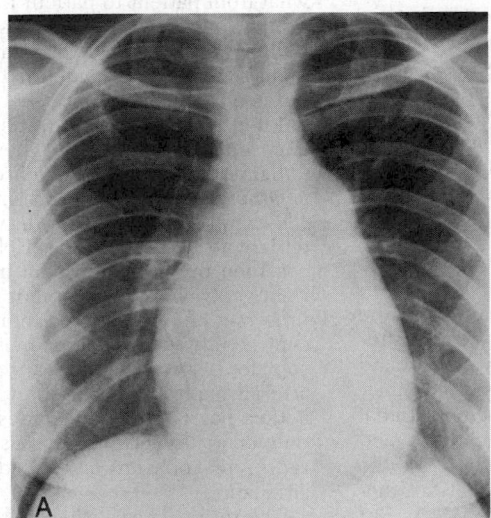
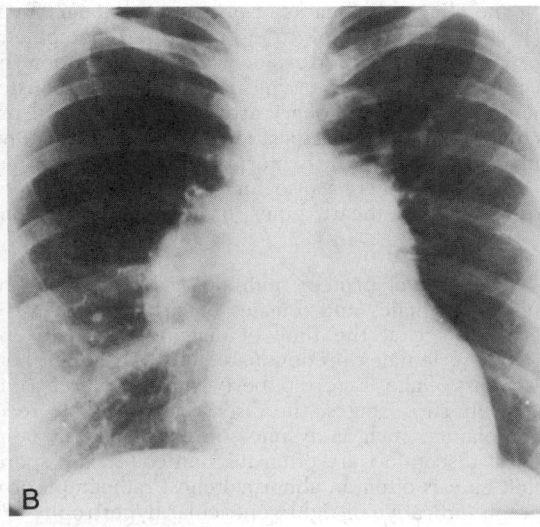

FIGURE 45–3. Pulmonary hypertension due to thromboembolic disease. *A*, A 33-year-old woman with clinical diagnosis of primary pulmonary hypertension. Autopsy showed widespread organized clots in resistance vessels (small muscular arteries and arterioles) throughout the lungs. *B*, A 35-year-old woman with organized clots in major pulmonary arteries. Note hypoperfused upper lobes. Thromboendarterectomy restored blood flow to the right upper lobe and relieved the pulmonary hypertension.

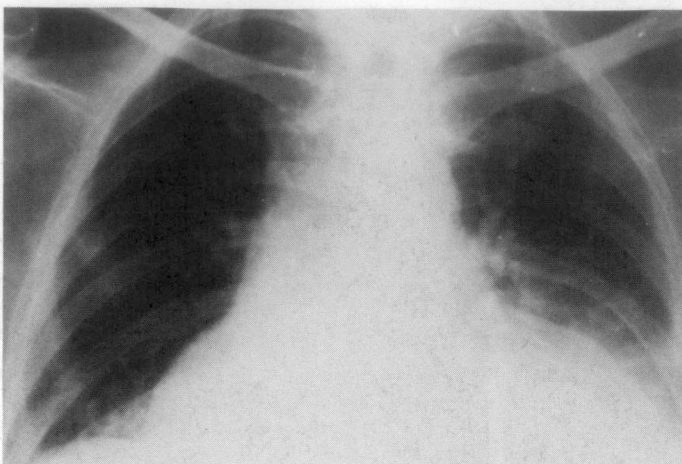

FIGURE 45–4. Cor pulmonale and severe right ventricular failure in global alveolar hypoventilation due to extreme obesity.

Chest Bellows and Respiratory Control Mechanisms. These are the true neuromuscular disorders, as exemplified by central nervous system and paralytic poliomyelitis. In these disorders, both the ventilatory drive and the respiratory muscles per se are directly affected. Alveolar hypoventilation may become manifested years after the acute infection as the ventilation finally fails to keep pace with the metabolic demand, e.g., during stress, fever, or further respiratory infection.

The treatment of alveolar hypoventilation in patients with normal lungs is ideally one of restoring ventilation toward normal or at least improving oxygenation. The practicality of these goals depends on the etiology. In kyphoscoliosis and the muscular dystrophies, ventilation can be supported at night, thereby resting the respiratory muscles, using a body cuirass. This approach is generally less feasible in extreme obesity, in which right ventricular failure that begins with alveolar hypoxia and pulmonary hypertension is accompanied by left ventricular failure due to systemic causes. When assisted ventilation is impractical, supplemental oxygen is useful in minimizing arterial hypoxemia.

PRIMARY PULMONARY HYPERTENSION

Primary pulmonary hypertension is a synonym for "unexplained" pulmonary *arterial* hypertension. The diagnosis is made by exclusion. It is an uncommon disorder that accounts for about 1 per cent of all causes of cor pulmonale encountered at autopsy. Until recently, virtually all reports of primary pulmonary hypertension dealt with sporadic cases. During the past few years, about 25 families have been identified in which the disease seems to be hereditary. Whether more painstaking family histories would show that some sporadic cases are actually familial is unknown.

The clinical hallmarks of primary pulmonary hypertension are (1) clinical, radiographic, and electrocardiographic manifestations of pulmonary hypertension; (2) demonstration by right-heart catheterization of the typical hemodynamic constellation of abnormally high pulmonary arterial pressures and pulmonary vascular resistance in association with a normal pulmonary wedge pressure and a nearly normal or low cardiac output; and (3) inability to find a cause for the pulmonary hypertension in a disorder of the heart, lungs, or systemic circulation.

Clinical Picture

Instances of primary pulmonary hypertension have been reported in males and females of virtually all ages, although the average age at the time of diagnosis is 30 to 36 years. After puberty, females predominate, most strikingly between 10 and 40 years of age. Before puberty, no sex differential is discernible.

In its early stages, the disease is difficult to recognize. Initial complaints, such as dyspnea on exertion, easy fatiguability, and chest discomfort are often discounted. In the sporadic case, the first clue is often an abnormal chest radiograph or electrocardiograph indicative of right ventricular hypertrophy (Fig. 45–5). But

these are late manifestations. In many clinics, echocardiography (all three modes) is used to buttress the clinical suspicion of pulmonary hypertension raised by the combination of otherwise unaccountable symptoms, physical examination, chest radiography, and electrocardiography. Echocardiography serves no purpose if pulmonary hypertension can be excluded on clinical grounds. Nor is it helpful in blatant pulmonary hypertension except for following noninvasively the response of pulmonary hypertension to pulmonary vasodilator therapy. Direct determination of pulmonary circulatory pressures by cardiac catheterization is currently the only way to prove the diagnosis.

When the disease is advanced, dyspnea, particularly during exercise, is common. Many patients are tachypneic and complain of nondescript chest pain as well as breathlessness. Other common symptoms are weakness, fatigue, and effort syncope. In time, right-sided heart failure develops. On rare occasion, an enlarged pulmonary artery causes hoarseness because of compression of the left recurrent laryngeal nerve.

Patients with severe pulmonary hypertension seem prone to sudden death. Thus, death has occurred unexpectedly during normal activities, cardiac catheterization, and surgical procedures and after the administration of barbiturates or anesthetic agents. The mechanisms for sudden death are not clear, although in a few instances bradycardia and atrioventricular dissociation were seen to culminate in cardiac arrest and death.

On physical examination, the jugular venous pulse usually shows a prominent "a" wave. Right ventricular hypertrophy causes a cardiac thrust along the left sternal border, and a distinct impulse is typically palpable over the region of the main pulmonary artery. The pulmonic component of the second sound is markedly accentuated, the second heart sound is narrowly split, and an ejection click is heard in the pulmonic area. Often a fourth heart sound emanating from the hypertrophied left ventricle is heard at the lower left sternal border. In some patients an ejection murmur is audible at the pulmonic area; as pulmonary arterial pressures approximate systemic arterial levels, the murmur of pulmonary valvular insufficiency (Graham-Steell) often appears.

Right ventricular failure is accompanied by jugular venous distention and an RV gallop (S_3); inspiration intensifies the gallop. The liver becomes enlarged and tender and hepatojugular reflux can be elicited; in time dilation of the failing right ventricle leads to tricuspid insufficiency manifested by a holosystolic murmur, best heard in the fourth interspace to the left of the sternum, which increases in intensity during inspiration. The liver develops expansile pulsations synchronous with the heart beat. Hydrothorax and ascites are uncommon even in the face of hepatomegaly and peripheral edema.

RADIOGRAPHY. In the early stage, the chest radiograph is generally normal. Later it shows cardiac enlargement in association with enlargement of the pulmonary trunk, while the peripheral pulmonary arterial branches are attenuated; the lung fields are free of widespread interstitial disease and may appear oligemic. Although fullness of the central pulmonary arterial trunks and peripheral "pruning" are distinctive, appearances vary somewhat from patient to patient in accord with the level and duration of the pulmonary hypertension and the age of the patient. Radiographic evidence of right ventricular enlargement (cor pulmonale) usually becomes overt only late in the course of the pulmonary hypertension (see Fig. 45–1).

Lung scans and angiography help to exclude multiple pulmonary emboli. Rarely do these procedures prove to be more enlightening than the standard chest radiograph.

Other Laboratory Tests. The electrocardiogram almost always shows some evidence of right ventricular enlargement and usually of right atrial enlargement. Echocardiography, as indicated above, can then provide additional information about the nature of the right ventricular enlargement (hypertrophy and/or dilatation), the presence of right-sided valvular insufficiencies, and myocardial contractility. Pulmonary function tests are generally normal except for a low diffusing capacity, often in association with mild arterial hypoxemia at rest. A high incidence of antinuclear antibodies has recently been described in patients with "primary" pulmonary hypertension, raising the possibility that some may represent collagen vascular disease confined to the pulmonary circulation.

The results of cardiac catheterization are consistent with diffuse

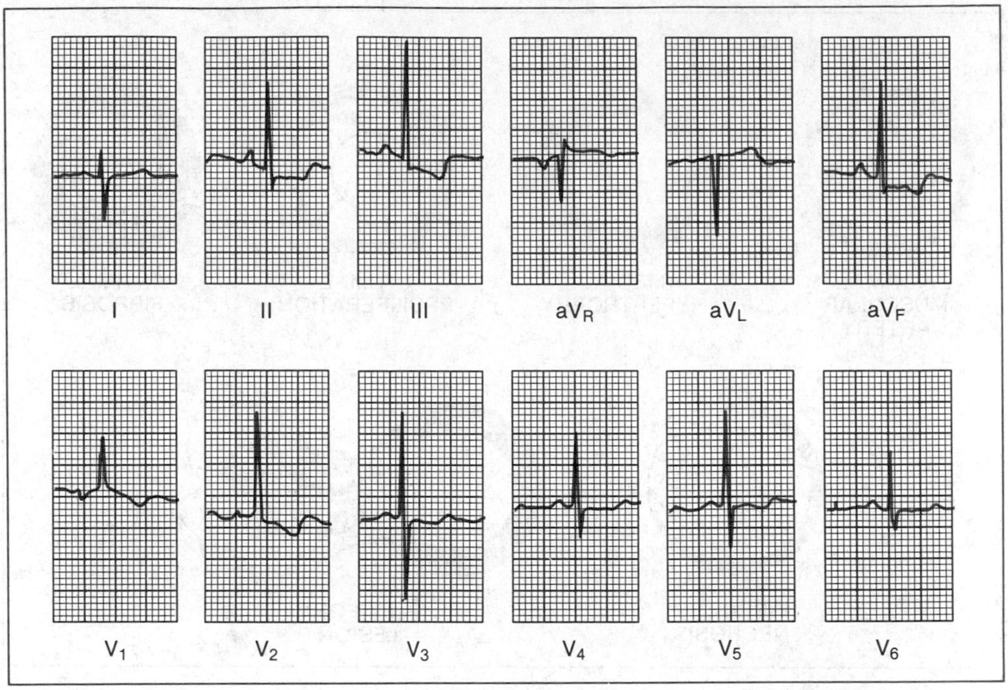

FIGURE 45–5. Unsuspected primary pulmonary hypertension. Routine electrocardiogram in an asymptomatic 32-year-old man was the first clue to the presence of primary pulmonary hypertension.

obliterative disease of the pulmonary precapillary vessels: Pulmonary arterial hypertension is associated with a normal pulmonary wedge pressure and a normal, or nearly normal, cardiac output (see Pathophysiology). Cardiac catheterization is most valuable in excluding cardiac causes of pulmonary arterial hypertension and in screening the response of the pulmonary circulation to vasodilator agents.

Pathology

With respect to corroborating the clinical diagnosis, pathology is generally most helpful in two respects: (1) excluding secondary pulmonary hypertension, and (2) demonstrating occlusive vascular disease of the small pulmonary (muscular) arteries and arterioles. For a long while, pathologists touted the "plexiform" lesion as pathognomonic of primary pulmonary hypertension. However, biopsy and autopsy have shown that the vascular lesions of primary pulmonary hypertension are quite heterogeneous (Fig. 45–6) and that plexiform lesions can also occur in instances of secondary pulmonary hypertension, e.g., Eisenmenger's complex. The heterogeneity of the pulmonary vascular lesions in primary pulmonary hypertension has been underscored by recent experience with the familial form of the disease. As things stand now, primary pulmonary hypertension seems to be the final common pathway for diverse unknown etiologies (Table 45–3), and plexiform lesions probably represent a healed pulmonary arteritis that occurred sometime in the evolution of the occlusive vascular disease.

The seat of the disease is the small pulmonary arteries (between 40 and 100 μ in diameter) and arterioles. The obliterative lesions are diverse, affecting one or more layers of the small muscular arteries and arterioles. The full-blown "classic" picture of concentric intimal fibrosis, medial hypertrophy, necrotizing arteritis, and plexiform lesions is common, but often one or more ingredients are missing. Thrombi are commonly found at autopsy in primary pulmonary hypertension but are generally assigned a subsidiary role in pathogenesis, i.e., preterminal slowing of the circulation in damaged, partially obstructed vessels, rather than a primary role.

Pulmonary capillary angiomatosis is an extraordinary cause of primary pulmonary hypertension. Proliferative lesions of the pulmonary capillary bed lead to high resistance to blood flow in a segment of the pulmonary circulation that is generally unaffected in more conventional types of primary pulmonary hypertension.

TABLE 45–3. SUGGESTED ETIOLOGIES FOR PRIMARY PULMONARY HYPERTENSION

Etiology	Comment
Autoimmune mechanisms	Especially in young women, associated with Raynaud's phenomenon and collagen diseases, such as disseminated lupus erythematosus, rheumatoid arthritis, progressive systemic sclerosis, polyarteritis nodosa, and dermatomyositis.
Persistence of fetal pulmonary vascular bed	A distinct syndrome in neonatal life that is questionably related to the adult syndrome.
Dietary pulmonary hypertension	Suggested by an outbreak of primary pulmonary hypertension related to an anorectic agent, aminorex. Only 2% of those who ingested the drug developed pulmonary hypertension, suggesting individual predisposition. Pulmonary hypertension (with different vascular lesions) also produced experimentally by ingesting seeds of leguminous plant *Crotalaria spectabilis*.
Sustained vasoconstriction	A classic suggestion that is difficult to accept as initiating mechanism; more likely a contributing factor.
Combined portal and pulmonary hypertension	Common denominator suggested by occurrence of pulmonary hypertension in some patients with hepatic cirrhosis. Also related to mechanism of dietary pulmonary hypertension.
Multiple pulmonary emboli	Once considered to be the major cause of primary pulmonary hypertension. May still be difficult to distinguish on clinical grounds but can almost always be distinguished morphologically.
Familial pulmonary hypertension	Although familial instances do occur, and individual susceptibility has been demonstrated in some instances, the connecting links between inherited defect or predisposition and clinical disease are unclear.

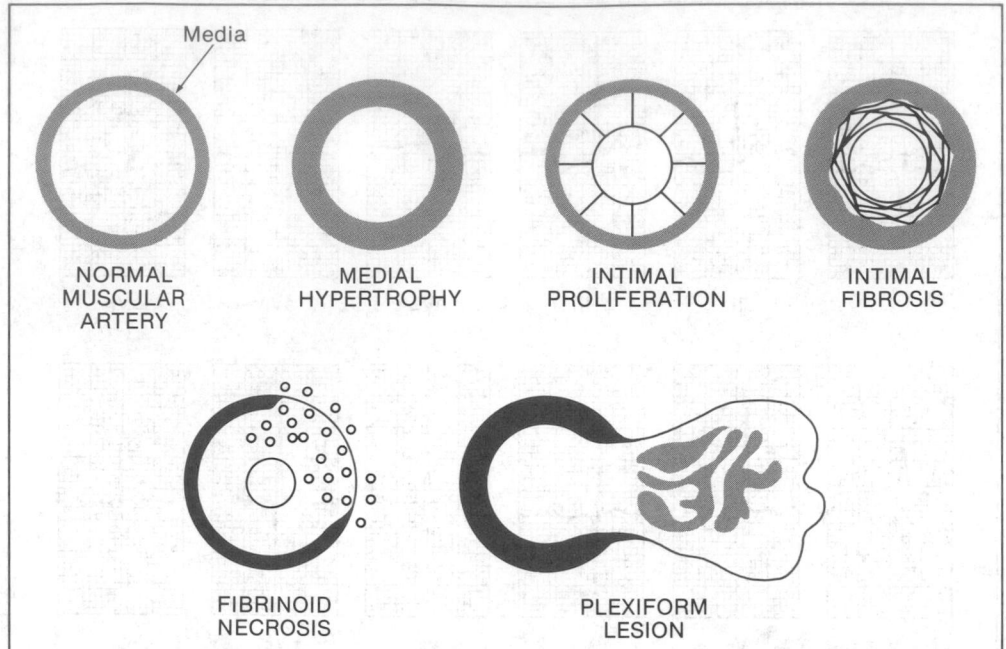

FIGURE 45–6. The heterogeneity of pulmonary vascular lesions in primary pulmonary hypertension. (Modified after Wagenvoort CN, Wagenvoort N: Pathology of Pulmonary Hypertension. Copyright © 1977. By permission of John Wiley & Sons, Inc.)

Pathophysiology

The hemodynamic hallmarks of primary pulmonary hypertension studies at rest are well known: a high pulmonary arterial pressure in association with a nearly normal cardiac output and a normal left atrial (pulmonary wedge) pressure. As a result of this constellation, calculated pulmonary vascular resistance is high, generally leading to the logical conclusion that the resistance vessels, i.e., the small muscular arteries and arterioles, are the predominant sites of vascular obstruction. During exercise, as cardiac output increases, pulmonary arterial pressures increase; the increments in pressure in the pulmonary hypertensive circuit are generally much more striking than in the normotensive pulmonary circulation.

Diagnosis

The diagnosis of primary pulmonary hypertension rests on two pillars: (1) the detection of pulmonary hypertension, and (2) exclusion of known causes of high pulmonary arterial pressure. The history is of utmost importance. For example, the occurrence of Raynaud's syndrome directs attention to the possibility of disseminated sclerosis (scleroderma). Pulmonary function tests are useful in excluding diffuse pulmonary disorders, particularly interstitial fibrosis and granuloma. Serologic testing, especially in young women, may direct attention to covert connective tissue disorders, such as lupus erythematosus. The value of cardiac catheterization in eliminating acquired or congenital heart disease has been indicated above. Even after these procedures, distinction is often not possible, particularly between primary pulmonary hypertension and pulmonary arterial hypertension secondary to pulmonary emboli. This distinction has recently come into prominence because of the increasing awareness that proximal pulmonary organized clots, i.e., in major pulmonary arteries, can be removed surgically. Evidence, as by angiography, of more recent pulmonary emboli calls for anticoagulant therapy. Finally, once the diagnosis of primary pulmonary hypertension is established, the use of vasodilators has to be weighed.

Treatment

The aim of treatment in primary pulmonary hypertension is to decrease pulmonary arterial pressure, preferably in conjunction with an increase in cardiac output. By this combination, the afterload on the right ventricle decreases and organ blood flow improves. In recent years, attempts have been made to identify pulmonary vasodilators that, by decreasing pulmonary vascular resistance, provide symptomatic relief and prolong life.

THE NATIONAL REGISTRY. To help in pursuing this goal, the National Heart, Lung, and Blood Institute has established a national registry by which experiences with the disease and with the use of pharmacologic agents can be shared. To date, about 194 patients have satisfied the criteria for inclusion in the registry and 102 have died (Dr. Carol Vreim, personal communication). Although the data have not yet been thoroughly analyzed, enough information is already on hand to underscore the difficulties in evaluating therapy: (1) The natural history of primary pulmonary hypertension is inconsistent, probably in keeping with the diverse etiologies that can elicit pulmonary hypertension. (2) Instances are being reported of long-term survival without vasodilator therapy. (3) Unless documented by morphologic studies, i.e., lung biopsy or autopsy, secondary pulmonary hypertension—notably pulmonary emboli and less often vasculitis—can masquerade clinically as primary pulmonary hypertension. (4) All vasodilators, except those destroyed during a single pulmonary circulatory transit (currently acetylcholine and prostacyclin), cannot be administered so that they act solely on the pulmonary circulation; as a corollary, all run the risk of troublesome side effects on the heart and systemic circulation. (5) For both acute and chronic administration, optimal therapeutic doses are difficult to establish. (6) Criteria for efficacy in acute studies are inconsistent; many rely almost entirely on a drop in calculated pulmonary vascular resistance even though pulmonary arterial pressure usually remains unchanged and the work of the right ventricle increases. (7) Symptomatic improvement after the acute administration of a presumed pulmonary vasodilator is most closely related to an increase in cardiac output. (8) The acute response to a pulmonary vasodilator is not a reliable predictor of the chronic response. Because of these reservations, optimism for the use of pulmonary vasodilators in primary pulmonary hypertension remains cautious. The ideal would still be prevention (as in thromboembolic disease) or treatment according to etiology (e.g., corticosteroids for interstitial granulomas due to sarcoidosis).

PULMONARY VASODILATORS. Most protocols designed to test pulmonary vasodilators acutely currently center on the response to rest and exercise. Several clinical and hemodynamic changes are sought as desirable endpoints:

1. Improvement in exercise tolerance. This increase in physical capacity is usually accompanied by an increase in cardiac output and presumably improved distribution of blood flow to peripheral organs and tissues.

2. A decrease in the level of pulmonary arterial hypertension, both at rest and during exercise.

3. A decrease in calculated pulmonary vascular resistance. Although this goal is often attained in acute experiments, its

**TABLE 45–4. SOME VASODILATOR DRUGS CURRENTLY USED
IN THE MANAGEMENT OF PRIMARY PULMONARY HYPERTENSION***

	Mechanism of Action	Acute Testing	Usual Maintenance Therapy	Major Side Effects; Comments
Nitroprusside	Directly on vascular smooth muscle; relaxes both systemic arteries and veins.	10 μg/min IV, increasing by 10 μg/min every 4 min until systemic systolic < 95 torr or PA† systolic > 10 torr over control (max 60 μg/min).	Hydralazine 10 mg every 6 h, increasing up to 50 mg every 6 h, + isosorbide dinitrate 10 mg every 6 h, increasing up to 50 mg every 6 h.	Systemic vasodilation and hypotension, cyanide toxicity at high concentrations. Half-life of a few minutes.
Hydralazine	Directly on vascular smooth muscle, presumably via prostacyclin production; greater dilator effect on arterioles than on veins; myocardial stimulant.	10 mg IV repeated once after 10 min. Resting hemodynamics followed by exercise 20 min later.	Hydralazine, start with 10 mg every 6 h, increase to 50–75 mg every 6 h.	Flushing, nasal congestion, conjunctivitis, CNS† stimulation, drug fever, muscle cramps. Lupus-like syndrome at doses of 200–400 mg/day. Side effects lessened by gradual increase in dosage. Surprisingly few side effects reported as yet in treating primary pulmonary hypertension.
Isoproterenol	Beta-adrenergic agonist; relaxes vascular smooth muscle when tone is high; increases venous return to heart; positive inotropic and chronotropic effects.	1 μg/min IV and increasing by 1 μg/min until heart rate > 120/min or PA systolic > 10 torr over control, up to maximum dose of 5 μg/min.	Isoproterenol (sublingual) 10 mg every 4 h, increasing up to 20 mg every 3 h. Terbutaline 5 mg tid.	Palpitation, tachycardia, flushing, cardiac arrhythmias exceedingly common.
Phentolamine	Alpha-adrenergic blocker; dilates both systemic arterioles and large veins; positive inotropic effect.	0.5 mg/min IV to a maximum of 10 mg.	Phentolamine 25 mg every 6 h, increasing to 50 mg every 3 h while awake. Phenoxybenzamine 10 mg daily, increasing by 10 mg every 4 days to a maximum of 40 mg daily. Prazosin 2 mg tid, increasing up to 5 mg tid.	Tachycardia, cardiac arrhythmias, angina, gastrointestinal stimulation.
Nifedipine‡§	Interferes with calcium fluxes in vascular smooth muscle.	10 mg sublingually repeated once after 15 min. Exercise 15 min later.	Nifedipine 50 mg bid.	Systemic vasodilation and hypotension; flushing, rhythm disturbances; dysesthesias, peripheral edema; currently the most popular vasodilator agent for empiric trial (without hemodynamic testing).

*Based on a table developed by a working group as part of suggested protocols for use by centers for primary pulmonary hypertension, recently established by the National Heart, Lung, and Blood Institute. Members of this working group were Drs. Edward H. Bergofsky (chairman), Michael Beaven, Alfred P. Fishman, Michael Heymann, John T. Reeves, Lynne M. Reid, and Marvin A. Sackner. (From Fishman AP [ed.]: Update: Pulmonary Diseases and Disorders. Copyright © 1982 by McGraw-Hill, Inc. Used by permission of McGraw-Hill Book Company.)

†PA = pulmonary arterial; CNS = central nervous system.

‡Some clinics prefer the calcium channel blocker diltiazem, up to 30 mg three times daily, for oral maintenance therapy.

§This use of nifedipine is not listed in the manufacturer's directive.

clinical value is doubtful unless an increase in cardiac output (with minimal increase in heart rate) occurs in conjunction with a decrease in pulmonary arterial pressure.

It should be kept in mind that agents given to relax the pulmonary vessels cause systemic vasodilation if they gain access to the systemic circulation; in turn, systemic vasodilation unloads the left ventricle. As far as the pulmonary circulation is concerned, this unloading is a passive mechanism for decreasing pulmonary arterial pressure. Instead of causing pulmonary vasodilation, pulmonary arterial pressure falls passively as blood is shifted from the pulmonary circulation to the systemic circulation. It seems likely that effective pulmonary vasodilators currently in use exert both active and passive effects.

Criteria for acute pulmonary vasodilation in response to a potential vasodilator vary from clinic to clinic. As a result, some reports using more rigid criteria, e.g., a 30 per cent drop in pulmonary vascular resistance accompanied by a drop in pulmonary arterial pressure and an increase in cardiac output, conclude that about one third of patients with primary pulmonary hypertension respond to pulmonary vasodilators. Others, using less rigid criteria, are more sanguine about the prospects for eliciting vasodilation. Clearly, because of its effects on the work of the heart, the greater the drop in pulmonary arterial pressure, the brighter the prospects for sustained clinical improvement. Evidence is accumulating that successful pulmonary vasodilation promotes long-term survival. This likelihood, plus the fact that an increase in cardiac output is almost invariably accompanied by symptomatic relief, is encouraging the search for effective pulmonary vasodilators that can be taken chronically by mouth or via the skin in dosages that do not evoke deleterious systemic side effects.

A battery of drugs was used until recently in acute testing for the capability of the hypertensive pulmonary circulation to vasodilate. These included agents that acted directly on pulmonary resistance vessels (nitroprusside and hydralazine) and others that acted on adrenergic receptors (isoproterenol, phentolamine, and the quinazoline derivative, prazosin) (Table 45–4). However,

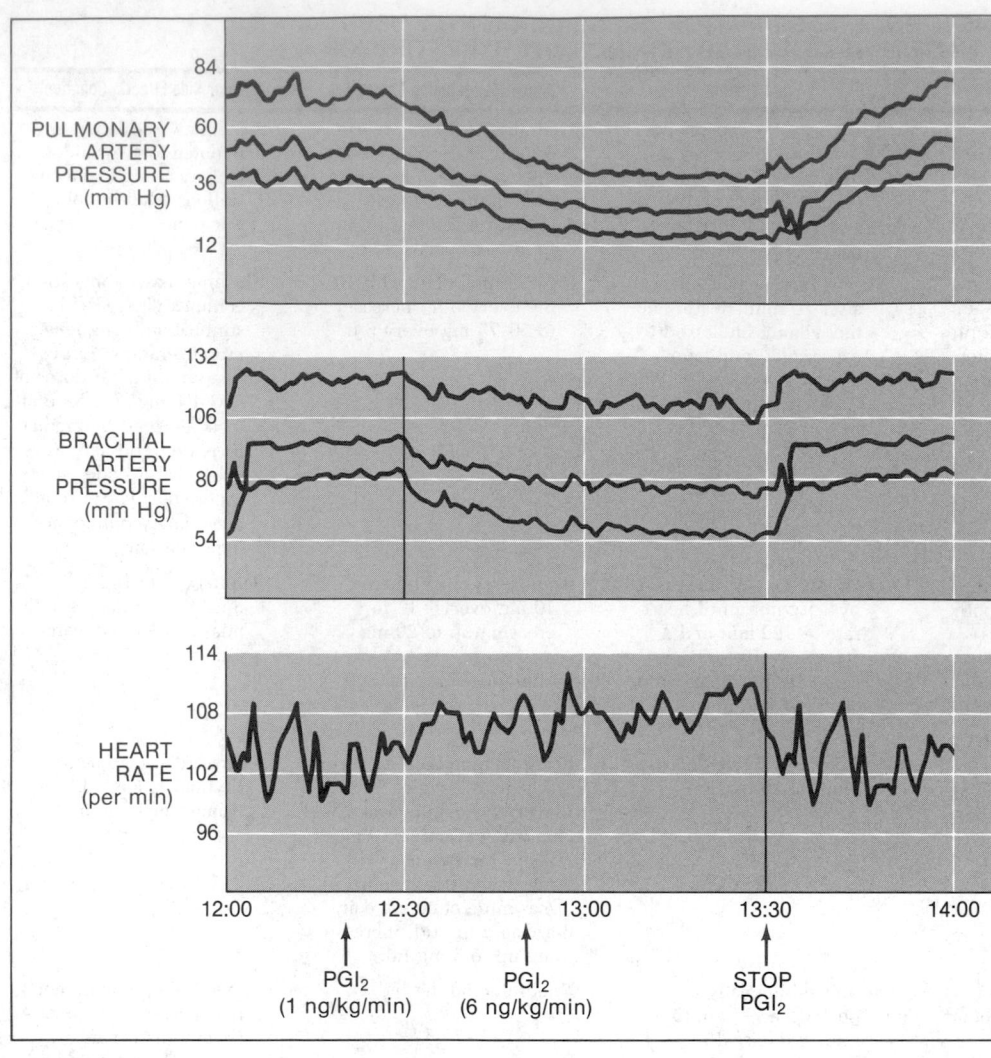

FIGURE 45–7. Prostacyclin administered intravenously to a patient with primary pulmonary hypertension. An abrupt drop in pulmonary arterial pressure occurs at the start of the infusion (with little effect on systemic arterial pressure or heart rate) (*first arrow*). Cessation of the infusion (about 1 hour later) is followed by a prompt return of pulmonary arterial pressure to high levels. (Courtesy of Dr. Harold Palevsky.)

these have been superseded during the last few years by prostacyclin and calcium channel blockers, i.e., nifedipine or diltiazem.

Prostacyclin. Enthusiasm remains high about the effectiveness of prostacyclin (PGI_2) in screening for pulmonary vasomotor responsiveness (vasodilation) in patients with primary pulmonary hypertension (Fig. 45–7). Indeed, it has come to be regarded as "the gold standard." This agent seems to have several attractive features: (1) It is a powerful relaxant of increased pulmonary vascular tone; i.e., it is a potent vasodilator; (2) it reduces pulmonary vascular resistance in a dose-dependent way so that dosage can be titrated to achieve maximal pulmonary vasodilation without undue systemic side effects, e.g., headache, nausea, flushing, and vomiting; (3) adverse effects stop when the infusion stops; and (4) it seems to indicate whether there is a vasoconstrictive element to the pulmonary hypertension that other pulmonary vasodilators might affect. Unfortunately, it is still an investigational drug available only for intravenous use.

Calcium-Blocking Agents. The designation "calcium channel blocker" or "calcium antagonist" is applied to a heterogeneous group of agents of different structural, pharmacologic, and electrophysiologic properties. The agents currently receiving the most clinical attention as potential pulmonary vasodilators are nifedipine and diltiazem. Both are administered orally for both acute testing and chronic therapy. As a rule, the agent is pushed to the limit of tolerance in attempting to achieve the optimal chronic pulmonary vasodilator effect. But severe side effects, e.g., systemic hypotension, often limit the maximum dosage. Of the two, nifedipine is the more popular. Verapamil, once used extensively, has fallen into disuse, largely because of its undesirable negative inotropic effect.

Nifedipine is a synthetic agent that is one of a large family of dihydropyridine compounds unrelated to other vasoactive or cardiotonic drugs. It is available in capsule form. The usual dose is 10 mg three or four times a day, but in some clinics higher dosages are tried until systemic side effects ensue. It is a potent systemic vasodilator used for the treatment of angina pectoris and is thought to be particularly useful when an element of coronary vasospasm is present. The latter use is not listed in the manufacturer's directive. Myocardial depressant effects are typically evident only in patients with severe ventricular dysfunction. It is now the agent of choice when acute trials using prostacyclin or nifedipine show that pulmonary vasodilation can be elicited, or it may be used empirically when preliminary hemodynamic trials of the various pulmonary vasodilators are not feasible.

HEART-LUNG TRANSPLANTATION. Technical and immunosuppressive considerations, as well as a shortage of organ donors, have exerted a large influence on the choice of transplant procedures. Currently, heart-lung transplantation is the preferred choice for primary pulmonary hypertension and certain congenital cardiac disorders affecting the heart and lungs, e.g., Eisenmenger's complex. Bilateral lung transplantation is preferred for chronic bronchitis and emphysema on the one hand and for sepsis, e.g., cystic fibrosis, on the other. Single lung transplantation is used predominantly for patients with end-stage widespread fibrosis (in whom the level of pulmonary hypertension is generally modest).

In patients with primary pulmonary hypertension, heart-lung transplantation is generally reserved for patients with limited life expectancy, e.g., 12 to 18 months, pursuing a downhill course with evident cor pulmonale, often in right ventricular failure; bouts of syncope lend urgency to surgical intervention. Many patients accepted for transplantation die while awaiting the procedure. In some patients, the prolonged infusion of prostacyclin (for 2 months to 2 years) has made it possible to sustain candidates for the operation. The results of heart-lung transplantation have been encouraging with respect to both the quality of life, e.g., improved exercise tolerance, and mortality. About 75 per cent of patients are alive after 1 year, about two thirds after the second year, and almost 50 per cent after the third year. Among the serious complications of heart-lung transplantation have been bronchiolitis obliterans and infections, both presumably related to the postoperative lifelong immunosuppression.

Prognosis

The diagnosis of primary pulmonary hypertension carries with it a poor prognosis. Although death usually occurs within a few years after the onset of symptoms, instances of long-term survival do occur. Exceptions to the rule of a short and fatal course have also been reported. Epidemics of primary pulmonary hypertension have been attributed to the ingestion of aminorex; in many patients in whom the drug was stopped, the pulmonary hypertension subsided. At present, there is no specific treatment for primary pulmonary hypertension. Pulmonary vasodilators have, in some patients, improved exercise tolerance and the quality of life but have not yet been shown to prolong life. Neither anticoagulants nor corticosteroids have been of value. The cause of death is generally right ventricular failure. In some patients, sudden death terminates the illness.

PULMONARY VENO-OCCLUSIVE DISEASE

Pulmonary venous hypertension is usually secondary to lesions of the left side of the heart (mitral valvular disease, left heart failure, left atrial myxoma) but also occurs after obstruction of large pulmonary veins (metastatic carcinoma, tuberculosis, or histoplasmosis), massively enlarged lymph nodes (sarcoidosis), or fibrosing mediastinitis of unknown cause.

However, there are also a small number of patients in whom unexplained progressive obliteration of small pulmonary veins and venules leads to pulmonary venous and then pulmonary arterial hypertension. The entity has been called pulmonary veno-occlusive disease. Despite its name, evidence of vascular injury, possibly viral, occurs not only on the pulmonary venous side but also on the pulmonary arterial side, leaving the pulmonary capillaries unaffected.

CLINICAL PICTURE. Predominantly children and young adults are affected, but the age range has been from infancy to 48 years. There seems to be no sex difference. Although hints exist of possibly related familial cardiac disorders, the patients are too few to do more than raise suspicion of a familial or common environmental cause.

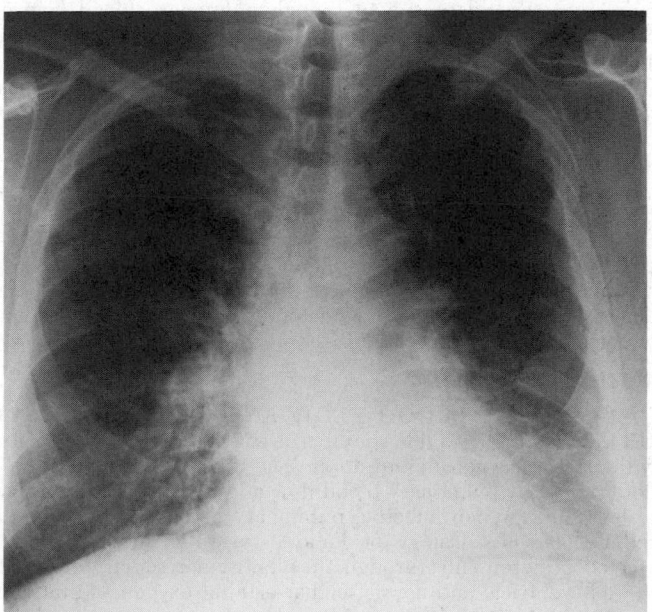

FIGURE 45–8. Pulmonary veno-occlusive disease. Severe pulmonary hypertension in association with pulmonary congestion and edema. Diagnosis was established by lung biopsy.

There is generally little clinical or hemodynamic basis for distinguishing between primary arterial pulmonary hypertension and pulmonary veno-occlusive disease. Even the pulmonary wedge pressure is usually normal in both. However, in some instances, in a patient who proves to have a normal mitral valve and left ventricle, evidence appears of pulmonary venous congestion and edema (bibasal crackles, Kerley B lines, increased vascular markings on the chest radiograph). Another clue is the occurrence of pleural effusions in a patient who otherwise seems to have primary (arterial) pulmonary hypertension. With these few exceptions, the patients are generally diagnosed as having primary (arterial) pulmonary hypertension until autopsy discloses distinctive lesions affecting primarily the small pulmonary veins and venules (see below).

LABORATORY TESTS. Cardiac catheterization discloses a high pulmonary arterial pressure, usually with a normal pulmonary wedge pressure. The low wedge pressure has been attributed to the interruption of blood flow by the occluding catheter into a venous bed in which widespread vascular occlusions preclude inflow from tributaries to the occluding catheter. In a few patients, lung biopsies have established the diagnosis during life.

PATHOLOGY. Both lungs are involved, but the venous lesions may be more marked in one region than in another (Fig. 45–8). As a rule, the pulmonary arteries as well as the pulmonary veins are affected, but the lesions are different. Most striking are the morphologic changes in the pulmonary veins and venules, which are narrowed or occluded by fibrous tissue; up to 95 per cent of the veins and venules may be affected, but complete occlusion is uncommon. Bronchial veins and bronchopulmonary anastomoses share in the occlusive process. Hypertrophy in the walls of the pulmonary arteries may also be quite striking, whereas the pulmonary capillary bed is generally unaffected. Thrombi in the pulmonary arteries are common. The lungs show congestion, edema, and focal fibrosis, which may become extensive.

Treatment has been disappointing, since the lesions are generally irreversible. Often, either anticoagulants or platelet-inhibiting agents are administered. Pulmonary vasodilators have been tried empirically with some anecdotal descriptions of effectiveness. The usual duration of life after the patient is found to have pulmonary hypertension ranges from a few weeks in infants to several years in adults, with 7 years the maximum.

Eysmann SB, Palevsky HI, Reichek N, et al.: Two-dimensional and Doppler-echocardiographic and cardiac catheterization correlates of survival in primary pulmonary hypertension. Circulation 80:353–360, 1989. *Echocardiography can be used as a guide to prognosis in primary pulmonary hypertension once the diagnosis has been made and repeat cardiac catheterization is inadvisable.*

Fishman AP: Pulmonary circulation. In Fishman AP, Fisher A (eds.): Handbook of Physiology: The Respiratory System, Vol. I. Bethesda, MD, American Physiological Society, 1986, pp 93–165. *A comprehensive survey of the regulation of the pulmonary circulation, particularly useful as a background for considering pathogenesis of clinical pulmonary hypertension. Emphasis is placed on the concept of pulmonary vascular resistance, the interpretation of pulmonary wedge pressures, and the identification of pulmonary vasomotor activity.*

Fishman AP (ed.): The Pulmonary Circulation: Normal and Abnormal. Philadelphia, University of Pennsylvania Press, 1990. *A survey of current understanding of mechanisms, management (medical and surgical), and treatment of pulmonary hypertension, including both secondary and primary. A feature of the volume is a summary of findings of the National Registry on Primary Pulmonary Hypertension, which began in 1981 and involved 35 medical centers.*

Higenbottam T, Wheeldon D, Wells F, et al.: Long-term treatment of primary pulmonary hypertension with continuous intravenous epoprostenal (prostacyclin). Lancet 1:1046, 1984. *This paper describes the first of seven patients, unmanageable by oral vasodilators, who were treated by continuous infusion of prostacyclin for months up to 2 years. After 1 year of continuous self-administration of prostacyclin intravenously, the patient remained greatly improved.*

Lloyd JE, Atkinson JB, Pietra GG, et al.: Heterogeneity of pathologic lesions in familial primary pulmonary hypertension. Am Rev Respir Dis 138:952–957, 1988. *The heterogeneity of the pulmonary vascular lesions in familial primary pulmonary hypertension argues against the idea of a unique anatomic change in pulmonary resistance vessels as the hallmark of the disease.*

Long WA, Groves BM, Rubin LJ, et al.: Acute hemodynamic effects of prostacyclin in 100 primary pulmonary hypertension patients. Ann Intern Med, in press. *A report of an interinstitutional study of prostacyclin as a vasodilator agent in primary pulmonary hypertension. This agent is now the "gold standard" for acute testing of pulmonary vasodilators.*

Loscalzo J: An overview of thrombolytic agents. Chest 97:117S–123S, 1990. *A review of the mechanisms by which thrombi develop, the pharmacologic agents to lyse thrombi, and the mechanisms of action of these agents.*

Palevsky HI, Schloo BL, Pietra GG, et al.: Primary pulmonary hypertension: Vascular structure, morphometry, and responsiveness to vasodilator agents. Circulation 80:1207–1221, 1989. *Correlation of histologic structure (obtained either by biopsy or at autopsy) with vasodilator responsiveness. An appreciably thickened intima correlated with poor pulmonary vasodilation.*

46 Congenital Heart Disease

Samuel Kaplan

Congenital diseases of the heart occur in about 8 to 10 of 1000 live births. The spectrum of severity varies widely. One fourth to one third are symptomatic in the first year of life, frequently as neonates. In others, such as in patients with a functionally normal bicuspid aortic valve, the lesion may remain silent throughout life. With the development of palliative or radical surgical treatment, another large group has evolved that was treated during infancy or childhood and has reached adult life. Accordingly, adults with congenital heart disease fall into several groups: Some have anomalies with a natural history for long survival, others have had successful palliative or "curative" surgery in childhood, and still others have had lesions that were mild in childhood but have increased in severity in adult life (e.g., aortic stenosis).

Etiology

The cause is usually unknown in individual patients. The etiology of congenital heart disease is thought to be multifactorial, primarily due to an interaction between genetic predisposition and intrauterine environmental factors. It is estimated that congenital heart disease is associated with chromosomal abnormalities in 5 per cent of cases and with single mutant genes and environmental factors in 3 per cent each. Among *chromosomal abnormalities* the prevalence of congenital heart disease is about 50 per cent in trisomy 21 (Down's syndrome), 95 per cent in trisomy 18, 90 per cent in trisomy 13, and 35 per cent in Turner's (XO) syndrome. Among *single mutant gene* disorders (autosomal dominant or recessive or X-linked phenotypes), the more frequent syndromes in which the heart is involved are hypertrophic cardiomyopathy and the syndromes of Noonan and Holt-Oram. Numerous *environmental factors* have been implicated. Women who contract rubella during the first trimester of pregnancy may give birth to infants with pulmonic stenosis (especially pulmonary artery branch stenosis), persistent patent ductus arteriosus, and less often other defects. Other viruses have also been implicated, but the evidence that they produce congenital heart disease is not so strong. These include cytomegalovirus, coxsackievirus, and herpesvirus. Among drugs implicated in congenital heart disease are the anticonvulsants, especially phenytoin and trimethadione, and lithium salts (with an apparent predilection for atrioventricular [AV] valve disease, especially Ebstein's malformation of the tricuspid valve), progesterone, warfarin, and amphetamines. The offspring of diabetic women are at greater risk for a variety of congenital heart diseases. Patent ductus arteriosus is more frequent in children born at high altitudes. It is estimated that about one half of the offspring of alcoholic mothers have congenital heart disease, usually left to right shunts.

Counseling

Parents of children with congenital heart disease are concerned about the cause and the possibility of recurrence in future pregnancies. This concern is greatest when the child is first born or the baby succumbs during the neonatal period. An explanation should be offered about the known causes of congenital heart disease and guilt feelings allayed. The prevalence of congenital heart disease in a second infant is 1 to 4 per cent. Although this figure is higher than in the general population, it is still quite low, and parents should be supported if they decide to have another child. When congenital heart disease has recurred in two siblings, the prevalence is higher in a third pregnancy (estimated to be 3 to 12 per cent). Many women with congenital heart disease who had corrective surgery during childhood have reached childbearing age. The prevalence of congenital heart disease in their children ranges from 3 to 16 per cent and is highest in left ventricular obstructive lesions. Recurrence risks are low in the offspring of fathers with congenital heart disease (1 to 3 per cent).

Circulatory Shunts

PATHOPHYSIOLOGY

MAGNITUDE AND DIRECTION. Factors that determine the magnitude and direction of intra- and extracardiac shunts are the size of the defect, pressure differences between the cardiac chambers or vessels, and resistance to ejection produced by outflow obstruction, as well as the ratio of systemic to pulmonary vascular resistance. Since normal systemic vascular pressures and resistances greatly exceed those in the pulmonary circuit, flow across small defects (such as ventricular septal defects) is from left to right but is limited in magnitude by the small opening. When the defect is large and nonrestrictive, peak systolic pressures in the ventricles are virtually identical, so that the direction and magnitude of flow are regulated by outflow resistance. If systemic vascular resistance significantly exceeds that in the pulmonary circuit with large defects (in the absence of pulmonic stenosis), torrential left to right shunts are present. The magnitude of the shunt is decreased as pulmonary vascular resistance approaches that in the systemic circuit, and it is bidirectional or right to left with continued increase of pulmonary resistance. When severe pulmonic stenosis is present, resistance to right ventricular ejection virtually equalizes peak systolic pressures in both ventricles so that flow across ventricular defects is right to left or bidirectional. A major determinant of direction and magnitude of shunting at the atrial level is the diastolic distensibility of the ventricles. Flow, frequently torrential, is from left to right, since the thin-walled right ventricle is easily filled even though atrial pressures are equal and low.

PULMONARY HYPERTENSION. This complication (see Ch. 45), common in congenital heart disease, results from increased pulmonary blood flow and/or resistance. Torrential pulmonary blood flow (as in secundum atrial septal defects) can be accommodated by the pulmonary circulation without increase in pressure. Pulmonary hypertension develops frequently in the presence of large defects at the ventricular level or communications between the aorta and pulmonary arteries. In infants and small children with these defects, "hyperkinetic" pulmonary hypertension is present. This term refers to a vasoactive pulmonary bed that undergoes vasodilation in response to oxygen or tolazoline. These agents reduce the level of pulmonary arterial pressure by pulmonary vasodilation even though pulmonary blood flow increases. Hyperkinetic pulmonary hypertension is uncommon in adults but is seen in some with secundum atrial septal defects. Generally, pulmonary vascular disease is present in adults, so that pulmonary vascular resistance is greatly increased even when pulmonary blood flow is not excessive (see Eisenmenger's Syndrome below). The status of the pulmonary vascular bed determines the clinical picture, prognosis, and feasibility of surgical treatment of intra- and extracardiac shunts. The goal of management is to prevent the development of severe pulmonary vascular changes by surgical ablation of the shunt. This implies serial measurements of pulmonary and systemic pressures and resistances, especially in infants and toddlers with large ventricular or aortopulmonary defects.

RIGHT TO LEFT SHUNTS

PULMONARY BLOOD FLOW AND SYSTEMIC DESATURATION. Right to left shunts are characteristically associated with arterial oxygen desaturation. The degree of desaturation is determined by pulmonary blood flow and the magnitude of right to left shunt. When effective pulmonary blood flow is markedly reduced (as in tetralogy of Fallot), systemic venous blood is ejected preferentially through the ventricular septal defect into the left ventricle and aorta, so that arterial oxygen saturation is severely reduced and cyanosis is obvious. On the other hand, right to left shunts may be associated with markedly increased pulmonary blood flow (as in transposition of the great arteries). In this situation pulmonary venous blood is almost fully saturated so that systemic arterial saturation is only moderately decreased. Cyanosis is not as intense in the latter group of patients, but they suffer from volume loading and failure of the left ventricle.

ARTERIAL HYPOXEMIA. *Cyanosis,* a dusky purple color of the skin but especially the mucous membranes and nail beds, is due to reduced hemoglobin in the arterial blood from right to left shunts. Clinical cyanosis may not be evident until the arterial oxygen saturation is below 85 per cent (normal is 94 to 98 per cent). *Clubbing* of fingers and toes is common, especially when arterial hypoxemia is marked. This sign may appear in childhood (beyond the age of 1 year) and is progressive. When arterial oxygen saturation returns to normal (at rest and during exercise), as occurs after surgical correction, clubbing regresses and even severe forms disappear within 2 to 3 years after operation.

When the hematocrit exceeds 65 to 70 per cent, symptoms of hyperviscosity appear and include excruciating headaches, fatigue, paresthesias, faintness, dizziness, visual disturbances, myalgias, and arthralgias. In adults these symptoms are alleviated with cautious venesection of 500 ml with immediate fluid replacement. Within 48 hours a second venesection of 500 ml can be undertaken if symptoms of hyperviscosity persist. The only indication for venesection is symptomatic hyperviscosity. A high hematocrit (65 to 75 per cent) in an asymptomatic patient is not an indication for venesection because the incidence of intravascular thrombosis (including cerebral vascular accidents) is not increased. However, repeated venesections to lower the hematocrit are not well tolerated and frequently result in iron deficiency with hypochromic and microcytic red blood cells. Furthermore, microcytosis aggravates hyperviscosity, resulting in extreme fatigue, headaches, faintness, paresthesias, dizziness, and decreased effort tolerance. These patients are treated for 1 week with small doses of oral iron (325 mg ferrous sulfate daily) because the hematocrit may rise rapidly on therapy. This treatment may be repeated for 1 to 4 weeks until iron stores are replenished and symptoms disappear. Another important cause of an elevated hematocrit is dehydration, which is treated with fluid replacement. Patients with erythrocytosis and hyperviscosity may have a bleeding diathesis due to a combination of thrombocytopenia, accelerated fibrinolysis, hypofibrinogenemia, prolonged prothrombin time, and prolonged partial thromboplastin time. These coagulation abnormalities may be improved by cautious venesection, which is used to prepare patients for elective noncardiac surgery. Patients with erythrocytosis may have hyperuricemia due to low fractional excretion (not to urate overproduction). Arthralgias are common, although acute gouty arthritis is less frequent.

BRAIN ABSCESS AND PARADOXICAL EMBOLUS. Brain abscess occurs in older children and adults. Predisposing factors include previous occlusive microcirculatory disease from thrombosis or emboli. Clinical recognition may be difficult because the onset is insidious, symptoms are vague, and fever is low grade. In others, the onset is more acute, with headache, seizures, and localized neurologic signs that are dependent on the size and site of the abscess and the presence of increased intracranial pressure. The diagnosis is established with computed tomography or magnetic resonance imaging or both. Treatment is with antibiotics, generally followed by surgical drainage. In patients with right to left shunts, venous blood bypasses the lungs so that emboli arising from systemic veins enter the systemic circulation directly to occlude an artery anywhere in the body, especially the brain. This complication is rare.

SHUNT LESIONS

Atrial Septal Defect

Atrial septal defects occur more frequently in females and are designated according to their site in the septum. The most common are in the region of the fossa ovalis (*ostium secundum defect*) and are among the most prevalent congenital cardiac anomalies in adults. A less frequent variety (*sinus venosus defect*) occupies the upper part of the atrial septum and is closely related to the entry of the superior vena cava. This structure receives one or more anomalously draining pulmonary veins, usually from the right lung. (The *ostium primum defect* is discussed under Endocardial Cushion Defect, below).

The principal factors that determine the magnitude of the left to right shunt are the size of the defect, the relative compliance

of the cardiac chambers, and the vascular resistances in the pulmonary and systemic circulations. If the defect is moderate or large (>2 cm in diameter in an adult), the greater distensibility of the right atrium and ventricle and the low pulmonary vascular resistance allow an abundant left-to-right shunt. On the other hand, in infancy the relatively thick and less compliant right ventricle limits the magnitude of left to right shunts. Large defects with torrential left to right shunts produce right atrial and ventricular enlargement, which encroaches on the left-sided chambers. Pulmonary pressures and resistances are generally normal. In the unusual instances in which they are elevated, the pulmonary circulation remains vasoactive, so that pressures and resistances return to normal after surgical ablation of the shunt. Those with severe pulmonary vascular disease are described under Eisenmenger's Syndrome.

DIAGNOSIS. Although symptoms are trivial and physical signs subtle, the diagnosis is usually made during childhood. However, many escape detection in the first decade of life and are recognized in later years only because of effort dyspnea and fatigue. Superimposed coronary artery disease or systemic hypertension can cause the left ventricle to be less distensible, favoring the development or worsening of these symptoms because of a further increase in left to right shunt and right volume overload. In some instances the presence of the defect is first appreciated when pulmonary hypertension develops with persistence of a torrential left to right shunt. The advent of atrial arrhythmias, fibrillation, flutter, or paroxysms of supraventricular tachycardia is not well tolerated. These events increase in frequency beyond the fourth decade. Some patients with an uncomplicated atrial septal defect are recognized for the first time because of an abnormal "routine" chest roentgenogram.

In children failure to gain weight is common but by no means the rule. The characteristic physical appearance is that of a thin child with nearly normal height and a gracile habitus. Generally, adults have a normal physical appearance, but again some are thin and gracile. The jugular venous pulse shows "a" and "v" waves of equal heights reflecting the normal left atrial pulse because the atria are in free communication. Dominant "a" waves suggest the presence of pulmonary hypertension, and dominant "v" waves are associated with tricuspid regurgitation. Right ventricular volume overload results in an easily palpable left parasternal lift. The importance of this sign cannot be overemphasized, and in some the dilated pulmonary artery is palpated in the second left interspace. The soft mid-systolic murmur, seldom accompanied by a thrill, is best heard at the upper left sternal edge and is produced by increased blood flow into the pulmonary artery. A loud murmur is widely transmitted to the chest anteriorly and posteriorly, especially in slightly built patients. The murmur is preceded by an accentuated first heart sound and sometimes by a pulmonic ejection sound. The auscultatory hallmark is the easily audible, widely split second heart sound. This split is virtually fixed in all phases of respiration and during the Valsalva maneuver. When the defect is large, a mid-diastolic murmur is audible at the lower left sternal edge and is produced by extravagant flow across the tricuspid valve. An early diastolic murmur of pulmonary regurgitation may accompany pulmonary hypertension, but this is rare.

The *electrocardiogram* shows right-axis deviation and right ventricular hypertrophy (generally rsR^1 in right precordial leads). This pattern is due to terminal depolarization of the hypertrophied right ventricular outflow tract. Less frequent findings include tall P waves (because of right atrial enlargement), complete right bundle branch block, a prolonged PR interval, and Wolff-Parkinson-White syndrome. Supraventricular arrhythmias may be detected in untreated adults or many years after surgical closure of the defect. These consist of atrial fibrillation or flutter, paroxysmal atrial tachycardia, and multiple premature atrial contractions. Left-axis deviation usually denotes the presence of an ostium primum atrial defect but is seen occasionally in secundum defects. Another rare finding is a normal electrocardiogram.

The *chest roentgenogram* is often distinctive, especially in adults. Varying degrees of cardiac enlargement are due to dilatation of the right atrium and ventricle, which displaces the normal or relatively small left-sided chambers posteriorly. The large pulmonary trunk contrasts with the smaller aortic knob, which is especially notable on the posteroanterior view. The primary branches of the pulmonary artery are enlarged and the vascularity is increased toward the periphery of both lung fields.

Echocardiography not only is diagnostic but also is useful in excluding other suspected anomalies. In uncomplicated secundum atrial defects the right ventricular end-diastolic dimension is increased and the ventricular septal motion is flat or paradoxical. Real-time two-dimensional echocardiograms define the location and size of the defect and also confirm the significant enlargement of the right atrium. The deformity of the ventricular septum resulting from right ventricular volume overload is recognized, and its encroachment into the left ventricular cavity is visualized. Flow disturbance across the interatrial septum can be detected by measurements based on the Doppler principle. The pulmonary and aortic flows can be estimated by two-dimensional echo and Doppler techniques, and the difference between these flows represents the shunt volume. *Mitral valve prolapse* may be associated with secundum atrial septal defects and in many instances the suspicion is raised by the echocardiogram. Since various criteria are used for the echo diagnosis of mitral valve prolapse, caution should be exercised in the diagnosis of combined atrial septal defect and mitral valve prolapse. It is probable that the association has been overestimated.

There is an ongoing debate about whether *cardiac catheterization* is indicated in all patients. Physical examination supplemented by the electrocardiogram and chest roentgenogram usually suggests the diagnosis. This can be confirmed by visualizing the site of the defect and pulmonary venous connection by echocardiography, which also estimates the pulmonary-systemic flow ratio as well as the pulmonary arterial pressure. However, cardiac catheterization should be undertaken in the adult in whom pulmonary hypertension or coexisting coronary artery disease is suspected.

NATURAL HISTORY. The vast majority of secundum atrial septal defects are recognized and treated surgically during childhood or adolescence. Spontaneous closure does occur, but this is usually prior to the age of about 3 years. Although life expectancy is shortened, adult survival is the rule and some live to an advanced age. Pregnancy is usually well tolerated, especially in women who were asymptomatic prior to pregnancy.

COMPLICATIONS. After the age of 40 years complications are frequent, and most patients who survive beyond the age of 60 years show symptoms of effort dyspnea and fatigue. Death may be unrelated to the defect, but when a relationship exists cardiac failure is the most common cause. Heart failure may be due to right ventricular failure alone or may be intensified by a dilated tricuspid valve ring with resultant incompetence. The prevalence of atrial arrhythmias increases after the fourth decade and may precipitate heart failure, especially when the ventricular response is rapid in the presence of a large shunt. Coronary artery disease or systemic hypertension may result in a less distensible left ventricle, which favors an increase in left to right shunting. Pulmonary hypertension may be due to the high pulmonary blood flow or may progress to a state in which pulmonary and systemic vascular resistances are virtually identical and the shunt is abolished or reversed (see Eisenmenger's Syndrome). Infective endocarditis is rare in isolated lesions.

TREATMENT. Treatment is surgical ablation of the shunt, especially when the pulmonary systemic flow ratio exceeds 2:1. Devices inserted through a percutaneous cardiac catheter have been developed to close secundum atrial septal defects. These devices are undergoing clinical trial and if successful would obviate the need for open heart surgery. At this time surgery is advised and is preferably accomplished between the ages of about 3 and 4 years, when the surgical risk is minimal. In these young patients the right ventricular dimension returns to normal. Surgical treatment in older children and adolescents usually improves the size of the right-sided chambers, but they may not return to normal. When the operation is performed in adults, patchy fibrosis of the chronically volume-loaded right ventricle persists, as does some degree of right ventricular dilatation. These residua may explain the blunted chronotropic response during exercise, with resultant decreased cardiac output and decreased working capacity. Nevertheless, patients in the fifth, sixth, or even seventh decade with high pulmonary blood flow and low resistance benefit

from surgical repair, which can be done with a comparatively low risk. Defects in older patients can be closed surgically despite moderate pulmonary hypertension and cardiac failure, provided there is still a significant left to right shunt. Operation is contraindicated when pulmonary vascular resistance is greatly elevated so that the shunt is abolished or reversed. Late-onset arrhythmias occur in fewer than 5 per cent, 10 to 20 years after surgery. The most common are atrial flutter, atrial fibrillation, paroxysmal supraventricular tachycardia, and frequent premature atrial contractions. Less frequent arrhythmias are sick sinus syndrome, junctional tachycardia, and complete heart block.

LUTEMBACHER'S SYNDROME

This condition consists of a secundum atrial septal defect with acquired mitral stenosis. Obstruction to left ventricular inflow aggravates the left to right shunt across the atrial septum. Atrial fibrillation is common. A prominent jugular "a" wave is visible because left atrial pressure is transmitted to the right atrium and the systemic venous return. Physical findings resemble those described under secundum atrial septal defects. Auscultatory findings of mitral stenosis are present but may not be obvious. The echocardiogram is diagnostic in that signs of mitral stenosis are superimposed on right ventricular volume overload. Patients with this condition experience great symptomatic relief after intracardiac repair.

ENDOCARDIAL CUSHION DEFECT

The embryonic endocardial cushions contribute to the development of the mitral and tricuspid valves and to the growth and convergence of the atrial and ventricular septa. Maldevelopment during this stage of cardiac morphogenesis results in varying degrees of complex malformations involving the AV valves and the atrial and ventricular septa. The *ostium primum defect* is situated in the lower portion of the atrial septum overlying both the mitral and tricuspid valves. A cleft in the anterior leaflet to the mitral valve is usual, and the tricuspid valve is frequently thickened but otherwise normal. The ventricular septum is intact functionally. *Common AV canal* (complete endocardial cushion defect) consists of a common defect of both the intra-atrial and intraventricular septa with a single AV valve. This valve, common to both ventricles, has an anterior and posterior leaflet with a lateral leaflet in each ventricle. This anomaly is relatively common in patients with Down's syndrome. *Transitional forms* are intermediate between AV canal and ostium primum defects.

OSTIUM PRIMUM DEFECTS. Ostium primum defects may be associated with recurrent lower respiratory tract infections with or without congestive heart failure during infancy and early childhood. However, the majority are asymptomatic and are recognized because of the murmur of mitral incompetence. In others, the degree of mitral regurgitation is trivial. The physical signs resemble those of ostium secundum defects with superimposed mitral regurgitation. The electrocardiogram is distinctive in that there is a superior counterclockwise frontal plane axis (left-axis deviation), varying degrees of right ventricular hypertrophy (rsR^1 is common), and sometimes voltage criteria for left ventricular hypertrophy because of mitral regurgitation. The chest radiograph simulates an ostium secundum atrial septal defect. The echocardiogram is also characteristic, showing enlargement of both right ventricle and right atrium, a low lying atrial septal defect, and a cleft in the anterior mitral leaflet. The mitral valve apparatus is displaced so that the anterior mitral leaflet encroaches upon the left ventricular outflow. Cardiac catheterization demonstrates the left to right shunt, the level of pulmonary arterial pressure, and the degree of mitral valve incompetence. Left ventriculography shows the characteristic "goose-neck" deformity produced by the abnormal position of the mitral valve. Surgical treatment is advised during infancy or childhood with the purpose of obliterating the left to right shunt and alleviating mitral valve incompetence. In adult life, many years after surgery, atrial arrhythmias may occur as described under secundum atrial septal defect. In addition, a small number of patients have progressive mitral valve incompetence that may require mitral valve replacement.

COMPLETE AV CANAL. Congestive cardiac failure, significant elevation of pulmonary artery pressures and resistances, and intercurrent pulmonary infections are common during infancy.

At that time surgical treatment is undertaken to attempt to prevent progression of these complications. Without treatment, survival of these patients to adolescence and adult life is usually associated with the development of severe pulmonary vascular disease (see Eisenmenger's Syndrome) or congenital obstruction to right ventricular outflow, which limits pulmonary blood flow.

Ventricular Septal Defect

The most common form of congenital heart disease is an isolated ventricular septal defect. Perimembranous defects are the most frequent (Fig. 46–1). The magnitude of the shunt depends on the size of the defect and status of the pulmonary vascular bed. A small defect limits the size of the left to right shunt so that cardiac chambers are normal in size and pulmonary arterial pressures and resistances remain within normal limits. Large defects are associated with a marked increase in pulmonary blood flow, as well as varying degrees of elevation of pulmonary arterial pressures and resistance. In these instances pulmonary vascular disease may be progressive, so that systemic and pulmonary vascular resistances are virtually equal (Eisenmenger's syndrome) (see Ch. 39.5).

SMALL VENTRICULAR SEPTAL DEFECTS. Spontaneous closure of the defect is frequent, especially in the first year of life, and is estimated to occur in more than one half of instances. If the defect does not close spontaneously within the first 3 years of life, the clinical condition is likely to remain unchanged. These patients are generally asymptomatic and have a normal heart size. A systolic thrill may be palpable at the lower left sternal edge and is accompanied by a harsh, loud pansystolic murmur that is widely distributed but loudest at the site of the thrill. The electrocardiogram and chest roentgenogram are normal. These defects may be visualized by two-dimensional echocardiography if they are greater than 2 mm in diameter. However, Doppler interrogation of the right ventricular septum identifies turbulence

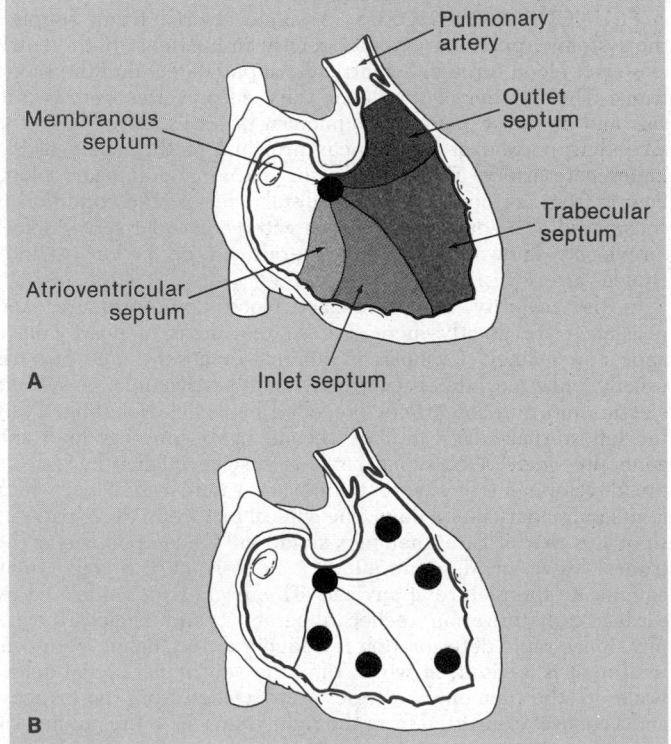

FIGURE 46–1. Diagrams of the right side of the ventricular septum. Anterior portions of the right ventricle and atrium have been removed, as has the tricuspid valve. *A,* Subdivisions of the ventricular septum. *B,* Locations of ventricular septal defects (VSD). 1. Perimembranous VSD (most common type). 2. Subpulmonic VSD (also known as infundibular, conal, or outlet VSD). 3. Atrioventricular canal VSD. 4, 5, and 6. Muscular VSD's in various parts of the septum; defects may be single or multiple. VSD's may extend to adjacent parts of the septum so that perimembranous VSD's may involve the inlet, trabecular, or outlet septum. The tricuspid valve may straddle the defect (rare in isolated VSD).

at the site of the defect, and color flow imaging confirms the site of left to right shunting. It is now believed that spontaneous closure of a small ventricular septal defect may also occur in early adult life. This notion is based on the fact that congenital ventricular septal defects are seldom found in older adults. Sometimes the development of an ejection click heralds a course that in a few years is associated with complete disappearance of all abnormal auscultatory findings when the defect is completely closed. Uncomplicated small ventricular septal defects do not require surgical closure, and the only treatment is prophylaxis against infective endocarditis.

LARGE VENTRICULAR SEPTAL DEFECTS. Large defects with unrestricted flow from the left to the right ventricle and into the pulmonary vascular bed are common in early life and rare in adults. These defects are associated with increased pulmonary vascular pressure and resistance. Furthermore, volume loading of the left heart may lead to superimposed left ventricular failure. Symptoms are present during infancy, especially between the ages of 2 and 6 months, and are produced by congestive cardiac failure, poor physical development, and recurrent pulmonary infections. These infants may respond to anticongestive measures. If this improvement is maintained, especially beyond the age of 1 year, the defect frequently decreases in size, with continuing clinical improvement. However, in a significant number, response to therapy is not maintained, physical development remains poor, and signs of pulmonary hypertension persist. In these instances surgical closure of the defect is indicated, since the mortality rate from surgery is acceptably low and soon after operation there is a growth spurt when heart failure and pulmonary hypertension regress.

Clinical improvement in some babies with a large ventricular septal defect may be due to the development of *acquired pulmonic stenosis,* which limits pulmonary blood flow. Generally, right ventricular outflow tract obstruction is due to infundibular hypertrophy and is progressive. During infancy or early childhood the clinical course changes in that signs of heart failure improve and heart size decreases because pulmonary blood flow is limited by the pulmonic stenosis. Right ventricular pressure rises to approximate that of the left ventricle, with resultant right to left shunting and cyanosis. The clinical picture resembles that of tetralogy of Fallot (see below).

VENTRICULAR SEPTAL DEFECT WITH AORTIC REGURGITATION. The ventricular septal defect is usually small or moderate in size and its presence is known from infancy. During childhood or adolescence aortic valve regurgitation occurs because of prolapse of the right or, at times, the noncoronary cusp. The clinical picture is extremely variable, from the asymptomatic child with a small left to right shunt and trivial aortic regurgitation to the symptomatic young adult with congestive cardiac failure, angina pectoris, massive cardiomegaly, and florid aortic regurgitation. The latter patient requires surgical closure of the defect and relief of aortic regurgitation; this generally requires aortic valve replacement. The asymptomatic patient with mild regurgitation needs to be observed closely. Some believe that closure of the ventricular defect prevents further prolapse of the aortic valve. Others recommend simultaneous aortic valvuloplasty prior to the development of significant valvular regurgitation and left ventricular dysfunction.

VENTRICULAR SEPTAL DEFECT WITH LEFT VENTRICULAR–RIGHT ATRIAL SHUNT. The AV septum is divided by the insertions of the tricuspid valve and the mitral valve. The insertion of the tricuspid valve is below that of the mitral. Thus, this area is common to the right atrium and left ventricle, and a defect in this area allows shunting from the left ventricle directly into the right atrium. In others the defect is below the tricuspid valve and is associated with an abnormal tricuspid septal leaflet. The physical signs simulate those of an isolated small to moderate ventricular septal defect, but color flow imaging identifies the shunt from left ventricle to right atrium. This condition should be treated surgically.

OTHER DEFECTS ASSOCIATED WITH VENTRICULAR SEPTAL DEFECTS. *Patent Ductus Arteriosus.* In some instances the murmurs of both lesions are audible, so that a continuous murmur is present at the upper left sternal edge and a holosystolic murmur is heard at the lower left sternal edge.

However, in many patients the physical findings are dominated by either the ventricular defect or the patent ductus arteriosus. Echocardiography combined with Doppler interrogation and color flow imaging is helpful in the diagnosis, disclosing shunting at the ventricular level as well as a patent ductus arteriosus.

Secundum Atrial Septal Defect. In patients with a ventricular septal defect and an ostium secundum atrial septal defect, the clinical picture is usually dominated by the ventricular defect. This combination of defects is more likely to be present during infancy and may result in torrential pulmonary blood flow, pulmonary hypertension, and congestive heart failure. The defects are recognized by echocardiography and, if uncontrolled by medical measures, are both treated surgically during the same procedure.

Coarctation of the Aorta. Signs of coarctation of the aorta usually dominate, and sometimes the signs of ventricular septal defect are erroneously attributed to the collateral circulation associated with coarctation.

Communications Between the Aorta and Pulmonary Arteries

PATENT DUCTUS ARTERIOSUS. Persistent patency of the ductus arteriosus is more frequent in females, in premature babies, in infants born at high altitude, and in infants whose first trimester of intrauterine life is complicated by maternal rubella. The aortic end of the ductus is opposite the origin of the left subclavian artery, and the vessel enters the pulmonary artery, usually at its bifurcation.

The hemodynamic effects of a patent ductus arteriosus depend on the size of the communication, the length of the ductus, and the resistance relationships between the systemic and pulmonary circulations. Generally, the flow through the ductus is small to moderate so that pulmonary arterial pressures and resistances remain normal. These patients usually are asymptomatic, and the only abnormal physical sign is a typical continuous murmur. This murmur, sometimes accompanied by a thrill, is heard best at the upper left sternal edge, rises to a peak in late systole, continues without interruption through the second sound, and wanes during the course of diastole. Larger shunts with a significant aortic runoff result in a wide pulse pressure and a "waterhammer" or bounding arterial pulse. The left atrium and ventricle enlarge to accommodate the increased pulmonary blood flow, and this is recognized by a lateral and downward displacement of the apical impulse, which is lifting in character. The typical continuous murmur is still present, but in addition an apical mid-diastolic murmur may be audible because of increased flow across the mitral valve. When pulmonary arterial pressure and resistance rise to systemic levels, flow across the ductus is limited. In patients with pulmonary hypertension, effort dyspnea is common, the wide pulse pressure disappears, and right ventricular enlargement is prominent. The auscultatory findings are dominated by those produced by pulmonary hypertension in that the typical continuous murmur disappears and is replaced by a short systolic murmur frequently preceded by an ejection click, a booming second heart sound due to loud pulmonic valve closure, and sometimes an early diastolic murmur of pulmonic valve incompetence. Occasionally the shunt through the ductus is reversed so that the descending aorta is perfused with desaturated pulmonary arterial blood. This results in cyanotic lower extremities with clubbing of the toes and normal color and shape of the fingers and fingernails.

The *electrocardiographic findings* are normal when the ductus is small. Moderate or large flows result in left ventricular hypertrophy. In the presence of severe pulmonary hypertension right ventricular hypertrophy dominates. The *chest roentgenogram* is normal if the flow is small. With larger flows the heart is enlarged because of left atrial and left ventricular prominence, the pulmonary arterial trunk and aorta are enlarged, and there is pulmonary plethora. With the development of severe pulmonary hypertension, heart size decreases, there is prominence of the right ventricle and especially the main pulmonary artery, and the size of the aorta may not be increased. In older patients the ductus may calcify. The *echocardiogram* defines and identifies the degree of chamber enlargement and visualizes the ductus.

Evidence of continuous flow is recorded using Doppler interrogation of the ductus arteriosus and the major pulmonary arteries.

Surgical correction is advisable by division of the ductus. In the adult with a large left to right shunt and normal pulmonary vascular resistance, surgery is also advised. Extensive calcification of the ductus increases the surgical risk, but surgery should still be advised if the shunt is large. Occasionally, an adult is seen with a small, hemodynamically insignificant patent ductus. The decision of surgical treatment for these patients must take into account that they are at risk for infective endocarditis, but on the other hand they may remain asymptomatic and some may experience spontaneous closure of the defect. Thus individual judgment is required in these patients. Devices inserted through a cardiac catheter have been developed to close a patent ductus arteriosus. These devices are undergoing clinical trial and if successful would obviate the need for thoracotomy.

AORTIC-PULMONARY SEPTAL DEFECT. This rare anomaly consists of a communication between the ascending aorta and the pulmonary arterial trunk. The defect is generally large and associated with a torrential pulmonary blood flow and pulmonary hypertension. Congestive cardiac failure is common during infancy and childhood. In the absence of severe pulmonary hypertension the signs are dominated by a wide pulse pressure, cardiomegaly, a systolic murmur at the left and right upper sternal edges, and occasionally a continuous murmur. The electrocardiogram generally shows biventricular hypertrophy, although isolated left or right dominance may be present. Roentgenographic examination of the chest defines the degree of cardiomegaly and shows prominence of the pulmonary artery and ascending aorta, as well as pulmonary plethora. The echocardiogram is helpful in defining the presence of two semilunar valves (which excludes the diagnosis of truncus arteriosus) and shows a normal relationship of a large aorta and pulmonary artery. The diagnosis is confirmed by aortography. The hemodynamic effects are measured at the same time by cardiac catheterization. These defects usually require surgical correction.

TRUNCUS ARTERIOSUS. A single arterial trunk supplies the systemic, pulmonary, and coronary circulations. Both ventricles eject blood through a ventricular septal defect into the single trunk. The number of semilunar valve cusps varies from two to six, and in most patients pulmonary arteries arise from the ascending portion of the truncus proximal to the origin of the innominate artery. When the major source of pulmonary blood flow is from aortopulmonary collateral arteries, the condition is considered to be pulmonary atresia with ventricular septal defect (previously known as truncus arteriosus type IV or pseudo–truncus arteriosus).

In the majority the pulmonary blood flow, pressure, and resistance are greatly increased, so that signs of heart failure appear in infancy. Cyanosis is minimal or absent. The heart is usually enlarged, the precordium is hyperdynamic, a systolic ejection murmur sometimes preceded by a click is audible along the left sternal edge, and the second heart sound is loud and generally single. Occasional patients survive infancy because of the development of severe pulmonary vascular disease, which limits pulmonary blood flow. The clinical picture in these patients simulates that of Eisenmenger's syndrome. Incompetence of the truncal valve or, less frequently, stenosis of this valve may complicate the picture at any age. The diagnosis is confirmed by cardiac catheterization, echocardiography, and angiocardiography. Since rapid deterioration is frequent during infancy, surgical treatment is advised, at which time the ventricular septal defect is closed, the pulmonary arteries are detached from the truncus, and a conduit is inserted from the right ventricle to the pulmonary arteries.

Communication Shunts Between the Aortic Root and the Right Heart

CORONARY ARTERIAL FISTULA. A fistulous branch, most frequently from the right coronary artery, enters the right atrium or right ventricle and occasionally the pulmonary trunk. The right coronary artery becomes massively dilated. Although the volume of shunt from the coronary artery to the right heart is variable, it is usually small. The diagnosis is suspected when an atypically located continuous precordial murmur is heard. The electrocardiogram and chest roentgenogram are normal. Studies using the Doppler technique demonstrate the site of entry of the fistula. The diagnosis is confirmed with an aortic root injection of contrast material that demonstrates the large, tortuous right coronary artery and its site of entry into the right heart. Surgical treatment is advised.

CONGENITAL ANEURYSMS OF THE SINUSES OF VAL-SALVA. The usual aneurysm involves the right or noncoronary sinus, which begins as a blind pouch or diverticulum. The aneurysms may remain as unruptured diverticula but usually enter the right ventricle or right atrium. Patients with these aneurysms are generally asymptomatic and the left to right shunt is small. The diagnosis is suspected because of an atypically located continuous murmur and confirmed by echocardiography and ascending aortography. Surgical treatment is advisable even in asymptomatic patients. Acute rupture of a large aneurysm in a previously healthy young adult produces a dramatic clinical picture. This is characterized by sudden onset of dyspnea, chest pain, brisk arterial pulses, and a loud continuous murmur. Cardiac failure with pulmonary edema supervenes rapidly. The electrocardiogram shows left or combined ventricular hypertrophy. The chest roentgenogram shows cardiomegaly with prominent vascular markings due to pulmonary arterial overcirculation and prominent pulmonary veins and signs of pulmonary edema. The diagnosis is confirmed by two-dimensional echocardiography and Doppler methods, supplemented by cardiac catheterization and aortography. Surgical correction is urgently indicated in acute rupture.

ANOMALOUS ORIGIN OF THE LEFT CORONARY ARTERY FROM THE PULMONARY TRUNK. The right coronary artery originates normally from the aorta, and the left coronary artery receives blood from intercoronary anastomoses so that blood flow in the left coronary artery drains *into* the pulmonary trunk. Thus left ventricular myocardial perfusion is significantly compromised. Generally symptoms are present within the first few months of life because of myocardial infarction, congestive cardiac failure, and mitral valve incompetence due to papillary muscle dysfunction. About 15 per cent of patients with this anomaly reach adult life because of exuberant intercoronary anastomoses, which may produce a continuous murmur. The electrocardiogram is important because signs of anterior and anterolateral myocardial infarction are present in a relatively young person. The chest roentgenogram shows cardiomegaly with dominance of the left ventricle. The origin of the left coronary artery from the aorta cannot be demonstrated by echocardiography. The diagnosis is confirmed by selective right coronary arteriography, which demonstrates the dilated right coronary artery, the intercoronary anastomoses, and opacification of the left coronary artery from these anastomoses as it enters the pulmonary artery. Reconstitution of normal coronary flow from the aorta to the left coronary artery is advised, although in many instances fibrosis of the left ventricle has resulted in permanent damage to ventricular function.

Pulmonary Arteriovenous Fistula

Fistulous communications between the pulmonary arteries and pulmonary veins may be multiple, small, and diffuse in both lungs or large and relatively localized. Hereditary hemorrhagic telangiectasia (Rendu-Osler-Weber syndrome) with angiomas of the buccal and nasal mucous membranes, gastrointestinal tract, and liver is present in about one half of patients or other members of their family. Desaturated pulmonary arterial blood flows through the fistula and enters the pulmonary vein without oxygenation. When total flow across the fistulous communications is significant, left atrial and left ventricular blood is desaturated, resulting in cyanosis and digital clubbing. Pulmonary arterial pressure remains normal because the flow across the fistula is at low pressure and resistance; cardiomegaly is unusual and heart failure uncommon. Hemoptysis may occur and is sometimes massive. Recurrent epistaxes and gastrointestinal bleeding are features of hereditary hemorrhagic telangiectasia. Transitory central nervous symptoms, including dizziness, vertigo, speech disturbances, visual aberrations, motor weakness, and convulsions, may result from paradoxical emboli, cerebral thromboses, or abscess. Findings on auscultation of the chest may be normal; in others soft systolic or continuous murmurs are audible anywhere

in the chest. The electrocardiogram is usually normal. Roentgenographic examination of the chest shows the presence of large fistulas only. Selective pulmonary arteriography is diagnostic and visualizes the site, extent, and distribution of the fistulas. Large localized fistulous communications are treated surgically by lobectomy or wedge resection. Smaller communications may be obliterated by embolization; these emboli are introduced selectively through a strategically placed catheter in the branch of the pulmonary artery that feeds the fistula. Successful treatment is usually followed by disappearance of symptoms, although in some there is postoperative growth of small previously unrecognized fistulas and recurrence of symptoms.

OBSTRUCTIVE LESIONS WITH OR WITHOUT SHUNTS

Tetralogy of Fallot

Fallot originally described a combination of four defects consisting of pulmonic stenosis, ventricular septal defect, overriding aorta, and right ventricular hypertrophy. The important lesions are pulmonic stenosis and ventricular septal defect. In the normally developing ventricular septum, the infundibular septum above is aligned with the muscular septum below. In Fallot's tetralogy the infundibular septum deviates anteriorly, resulting in malalignment with a ventricular septal defect at the site of malalignment. The anteriorly placed hypoplastic infundibular septum encroaches on the right ventricular outflow tract with a reciprocal increase in aortic root size so that the aorta overrides the ventricular septum. Right ventricular hypertrophy is obligatory because right ventricular pressure is systemic as a result of outflow obstruction and ejection against systemic resistance. Right ventricular outflow obstruction is usually a combination of infundibular and valvular pulmonic stenosis, but the pulmonary trunk may be small and pulmonary artery branch stenosis may be present (Fig. 46–2).

The severity of right ventricular outflow tract obstruction determines the hemodynamics and therefore the clinical picture. Severe obstruction is common, pulmonary blood flow is decreased, and blood is shunted from the right ventricle across the ventricular defect into the aorta. This right to left shunt results in systemic hypoxemia manifested as marked cyanosis, digital clubbing, and erythrocytosis. When obstruction to right ventricular outflow and a ventricular septal defect coexist without right to left shunting, the condition is known as acyanotic tetralogy of Fallot.

In severe cases, *cyanosis* is present from birth. In others, this finding develops in infancy, generally before the first birthday.

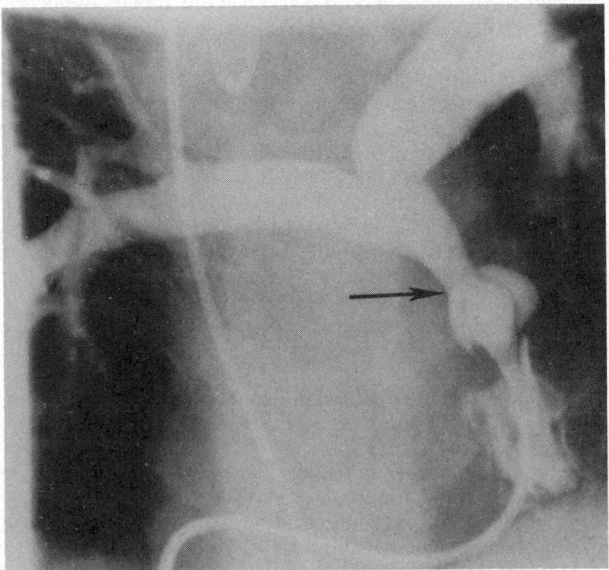

FIGURE 46–2. Cineangiograms in tetralogy of Fallot. Contrast injected in outflow of the right ventricle showing subvalvular obstruction, pulmonary valve stenosis with small annulus (*arrow*), and supravalvular stenosis with short pulmonary arterial trunk.

The absence of cyanosis in the neonatal period is related to maintenance of pulmonary blood flow via a patent ductus arteriosus, which closes spontaneously in the first few months of life. Cyanosis increases in intensity progressively during the first years and is associated with poor physical development. *Dyspnea* with exertion is usual.

Hypoxic ("blue") spells occur primarily in infants with hypoxemia. These spells consist of a sudden onset of dyspnea, restlessness, increased cyanosis, gasping respirations, and syncope. They are associated with a further decrease of arterial Po_2 and a reduction of an already compromised pulmonary blood flow. These frightening episodes are treated by placing the child in a knee-chest position and by administering oxygen and intravenous bicarbonate if acidemia develops. The frequency and severity of these episodes can be reduced by oral propranolol. However, surgical treatment is generally indicated to increase pulmonary blood flow and thus relieve the hypoxemia.

Squatting is common in children with hypoxemia, who may assume this position to relieve dyspnea associated with exertion. Physical activity is usually resumed within a few minutes. Squatting decreases the magnitude of right to left shunt by increasing systemic vascular resistance and pulmonary blood flow. Adults seldom squat because they know the limitation of their exercise tolerance and discontinue physical activity before arterial Po_2 is significantly decreased.

Physical examination confirms the presence of delayed growth and development, cyanosis, and clubbing. Characteristically, the heart size is normal but the apical impulse is tapping owing to right ventricular hypertrophy. The systolic murmur, sometimes accompanied by a thrill, is produced by the right ventricular outflow tract obstruction. Auscultatory findings are variable; the systolic murmur, which is loudest at the upper left sternal edge but is widely transmitted, may be mid- or pansystolic. The murmur is less intense when the obstruction is severe. Aortic blood flow is increased, and this may result in an early ejection click. The second heart sound is single, produced by aortic valve closure, and pulmonic valve closure is generally inaudible. In rare instances a systolic and diastolic murmur may be audible in any part of the chest, anteriorly or posteriorly, and is produced by bronchial collateral flow to the lung or rarely by a patent ductus arteriosus. This auscultatory finding is frequent with pulmonary atresia.

Roentgenographically the heart size is normal, with a rounded, elevated cardiac apex likened to a wooden shoe (coeur en sabot). There is a concavity in the region of the main pulmonary artery, and the pulmonary vasculature is diminished. The aorta is large and arches to the right in 20 per cent. The *electrocardiogram* shows right-axis deviation and right ventricular hypertrophy. Sometimes the P wave is tall and peaked. *Echocardiography* demonstrates the major intracardiac abnormalities. Echocardiographic examinations show the large ventricular septal defect, the degree of aortic override, and thick right ventricle; the right ventricular outflow tract obstruction may be visualized or inferred from Doppler turbulence in this area. The echocardiogram also helps to distinguish tetralogy of Fallot from other anomalies that may closely simulate this condition, namely, double outlet right ventricle with pulmonic stenosis, arterial transposition with pulmonic stenosis and ventricular septal defect, and a group of complex cardiac malformations consisting primarily of single ventricle and pulmonic stenosis.

These abnormalities are also excluded by *cardiac catheterization and angiocardiography*. Cardiac catheterization confirms that the peak systolic pressures in both ventricles are virtually identical and that there is a significant gradient across the right ventricular outflow. The degree and direction of shunting at the ventricular level are also demonstrated. Arterial oxygen saturation is decreased and at rest is usually between 75 and 85 per cent. Selective right ventriculography identifies the site or sites of right ventricular outflow tract obstruction, the narrowed pulmonic valve ring, the presence of abnormalities of the pulmonary arterial trunk, and any stenoses of the pulmonary arterial branches (Fig. 46–2). In patients with pulmonary atresia, the anatomy of pulmonary blood flow is complex. Although there may not be filling of the main pulmonary artery, a central confluence of left and right intrapulmonary arteries may be present. Left ventriculog-

raphy shows the position and size of the ventricular septal defect and the presence of an overriding aorta. In a few instances, a large coronary artery courses over the right ventricular outflow; preservation of this artery during surgical repair is essential. *Surgical treatment* is usually advised during infancy or childhood. The type of surgical procedure and its timing are still controversial. Infants with severe anoxemia in the first few months of life are frequently treated with a systemic to pulmonary arterial shunt to augment pulmonary arterial blood flow. Beyond the age of 1 to 2 years correction of the defect is advised, at which time any previous systemic to pulmonary shunt is taken down. Older children should have surgical correction of the anomaly because they are generally symptomatic. In all groups surgical correction is more difficult when there is severe deformity of the right ventricular outflow, including a small pulmonic valve ring. The surgical procedure consists of closure of the ventricular septal defect and relief of obstruction by infundibular resection and/or pulmonic valvotomy. Right ventricular outflow may need to be enlarged.

Ebstein's Anomaly of the Tricuspid Valve

This abnormality consists of an abnormal tricuspid valve that is displaced into the right ventricular cavity so that portions of the valve leaflet are attached to the right ventricular wall rather than to the AV ring. The portion of the right ventricle proximal to the tricuspid valve is thin, functions as an extension of the right atrium, and is known as an "atrialized right ventricle." Leaflets of the tricuspid valve are generally redundant and frequently incompetent. The right atrium is large and an atrial septal defect or patent foramen ovale may be present. Increased right atrial pressure, as from tricuspid regurgitation, results in a right to left shunt across the atrial septum and cyanosis of varying degrees. Pulmonary blood flow is decreased.

Ebstein's anomaly in adults varies considerably in severity, so that many patients have active and productive lives, but survival beyond age 50 years is unusual. Symptoms vary in intensity, and with mild anomalies the only complaint is fatigue. Cardiac arrhythmias are frequent and generally supraventricular, the most common being attacks of paroxysmal atrial tachycardia. The precordium is quiet to palpation. Auscultation reveals a systolic murmur, sometimes accompanied by a thrill over most of the anterior left chest, and third and fourth heart sounds are audible, resulting in triple or quadruple rhythms. A diastolic murmur is frequent, appears to be superficial, and may mimic a pericardial friction rub. Other auscultatory findings include multiple systolic ejection clicks and an opening snap of the tricuspid valve. The *electrocardiogram* shows right bundle branch block, tall and/or broad P waves, and a prolonged PR interval. Wolff-Parkinson-White syndrome (usually type B) is present in some. *Roentgenographic examination* shows a variable heart size; in extreme instances massive cardiomegaly is present because of great enlargement of the right atrium (Fig. 46–3). The outflow portion of the right ventricle is sometimes visible in the region usually occupied by the pulmonary artery in the posteroanterior view. The pulmonary vasculature is normal to decreased, and the aorta is small. The *echocardiogram* shows significant delay in tricuspid valve closure and an increased amplitude of motion of the tricuspid valve. The large right atrium and the displaced tricuspid valve can also be visualized. Surgical treatment should be advised in symptomatic patients, especially those with progressive cyanosis. Therapy consists of tricuspid valvuloplasty or valve replacement and ablation of the anomalous pathways between the atrium and ventricle in patients with Wolff-Parkinson-White syndrome and supraventricular tachycardia.

Tricuspid Atresia

In this condition there is no communication between the right atrium and right ventricle so that the entire systemic venous return enters the left heart through a defect in the intra-atrial septum. The left ventricle ejects blood into the normally related aorta and through a ventricular septal defect into the pulmonary arteries. If these vessels are transposed, the aorta arises from a hypoplastic right ventricle that fills from a ventricular septal defect. These patients have a marked increase in pulmonary blood flow and pressure so that heart failure and minimal cyanosis are common in infancy. Survival usually depends upon pulmonary arterial banding to limit pulmonary arterial flow. When the great arteries are normally related, the right ventricle can be minute and associated with marked pulmonic stenosis or atresia. In these patients pulmonary blood flow is derived from a patent ductus arteriosus or collateral bronchial flow. In other instances the left ventricle ejects its blood through a ventricular septal defect into a small right ventricle and then into the pulmonary artery.

Symptoms are usual during infancy and with decreased pulmonary blood flow consist of cyanosis, anoxemia, and poor physical development. Minimal cardiac enlargement is present, and the mid-systolic murmur along the left sternal edge is nonspecific. Left-axis deviation with left ventricular hypertrophy is usual, and these *electrocardiographic findings* in the presence of cyanosis suggest the diagnosis. *Roentgenograms* of the chest show pulmonary undercirculation but are otherwise nonspecific. The *echocardiogram* confirms absence of the tricuspid valve, delineates the size of the small right ventricle, confirms the presence of a large left ventricle, and identifies the presence or absence of transposition of the great arteries. Most infants with decreased pulmonary blood flow require enlargement of the intra-atrial septal defect to ensure easy communication between the two atria as well as a systemic to pulmonary shunt. In later years more radical surgery is undertaken with anastomosis of the right atrium to the pulmonary artery and closure of the intra-atrial septal defect. This procedure effectively separates pulmonary and systemic blood flows, abolishes cyanosis, and improves exercise tolerance. A similar procedure is also used in patients who had pulmonary arterial banding during infancy.

Single Ventricle

Atrial blood empties through two separate AV valves or a common valve into a single ventricle from which the aorta and pulmonary artery arise. Associated cardiac abnormalities are present, but their nature varies considerably. The most frequent ones are transposition of the great arteries, pulmonic stenosis, and aortic origin from a rudimentary outlet chamber. The clinical picture depends on the nature of the associated anomalies. If pulmonic stenosis is severe, cyanosis and anoxemia dominate. In the absence of pulmonic stenosis, pulmonary blood flow and vascular resistance are increased. The clinical picture is then dominated by congestive heart failure. Although these malformations are complex, surgical palliation is undertaken. In the presence of pulmonic stenosis the blood flow is increased with a systemic pulmonary shunt. On the other hand, high pulmonary blood flow is treated with a pulmonary arterial band. In later years, a surgical connection is established between the right atrium and pulmonary artery, and the atria are partitioned so that systemic venous return flows into the pulmonary artery and pulmonary venous return is ejected from the single ventricle into the aorta. When the aorta arises from a rudimentary chamber, systemic flow depends on an unobstructed communication between the single ventricle and the rudimentary chamber. This communication (the bulboventricular foramen) may narrow, resulting in a variable but often significant subaortic gradient. This complication may occur at any time, even postoperatively, and produces cardiomegaly and heart failure.

Inflow Obstruction to the Left Ventricle

Conditions of inflow obstruction are grouped together because they result in high pulmonary venous pressure with potential pulmonary edema. The lesions may occur anywhere from the insertion of the pulmonary veins into the left atrium to the area of the mitral valve. They are extremely rare abnormalities. *Pulmonary vein stenoses* at their site of entry into the left atrium are difficult to treat surgically or by balloon angioplasty. *Cor triatriatum* consists of a diaphragmatic partition of the left atrium. The upper portion receives the pulmonary veins, and the distal portion communicates with the mitral valve or through an atrial septal defect into the right atrium. The opening in the diaphragm is generally small so that symptoms are present in early life. The condition is surgically correctable by excision of the diaphragm and closure of associated atrial septal defects. A *supravalvular ring* above the mitral valve produces a similar clinical picture. *Congenital mitral stenosis* may be due to marked abnormality of the mitral valve apparatus, which includes fused, thickened mitral valve leaflets with short chordae, or the valve may have a parachute deformity in which the leaflets are also abnormal but the chordae converge and insert into a single papillary muscle.

Hypoplastic Left Heart Syndrome

Varying degrees of underdevelopment of the left side of the heart coexist, including marked underdevelopment of the left ventricle and atrium, and stenosis or atresia of the aortic and mitral orifices with hypoplasia of the ascending aorta. This complex malformation is a significant cause of cardiovascular death in the neonatal period. Attempts at surgical management have not been standardized.

OBSTRUCTIVE AND REGURGITANT LESIONS
Pulmonic Stenosis with Intact Ventricular Septum

Obstruction to right ventricular outflow can be valvular, subvalvular, supravalvular, or a combination of obstructions at these sites. Valvular obstruction, the most common variety, results from varying degrees of commissural fusion so that the deformed valve appears domelike. Dysplastic thick valve leaflets are less common and may accompany Noonan's syndrome. Subvalvular obstruction usually accompanies severe valvular stenosis, is due to infundibular hypertrophy, and occasionally is seen as an isolated abnormality with a normal pulmonic valve. Pulmonary arterial branch stenosis may be isolated or may occur at multiple sites and may be associated with supravalvular stenosis. These peripheral lesions are a feature of congenital rubella.

The hemodynamic consequences of valvular pulmonic stenosis are produced by the severity of obstruction. When the right ventricular outflow gradient is between 50 and 80 mm Hg the obstruction is considered to be moderate; pressures below and above that range are considered mild and severe, respectively. Pulmonary arterial pressure is normal or low. The arterial oxygen saturation is normal except when the obstruction is severe (sometimes with suprasystemic right ventricular pressure). Poor right ventricular compliance with or without an increase in right

FIGURE 46–3. Chest roentgenograms in Ebstein's anomaly of the tricuspid valve. *A,* Posteroanterior view showing globular cardiac silhouette with narrow waist simulating pericardial effusion. *B,* Left anterior oblique view showing marked cardiomegaly due to massive right atrial enlargement, which extends posteriorly (*arrows*) and also encroaches on the anterior clear space.

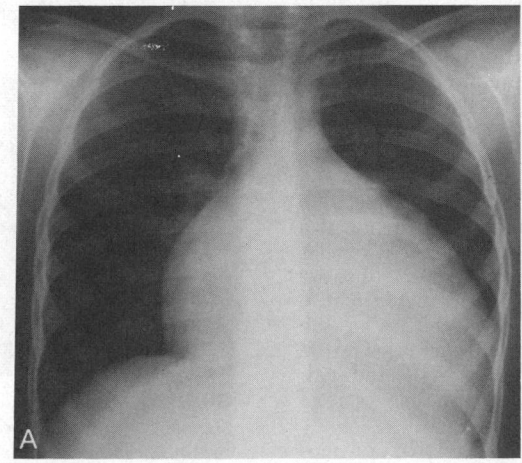
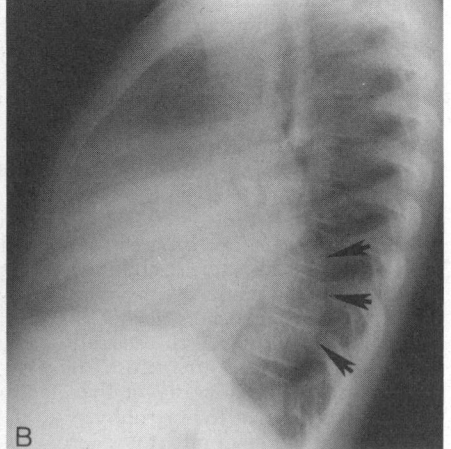

ventricular end-diastolic pressure increases right atrial pressure and may result in right to left shunting across the intra-atrial septum.

Symptoms are usually absent when the obstruction is mild or moderate, but when it is severe, effort dyspnea may be present. The physique is frequently normal, and some patients appear robust. When the stenosis is *mild*, the venous pressure is normal and the heart is not enlarged. A systolic murmur of varying intensity with mid-systolic peaking is heard best at the upper left sternal edge and is preceded by a pulmonic ejection click. The second heart sound may be normal, but the pulmonic component is frequently delayed and of normal intensity. The electrocardiogram is normal or shows signs of minimal right ventricular hypertrophy. The chest *roentgenogram* shows prominence of the pulmonary arterial trunk because of poststenotic dilatation, but the heart size and pulmonary vasculature are normal. Echocardiography shows the domed stenotic valve. When pulmonic stenosis is *moderate*, the venous pressure may be normal or slightly elevated, with a prominent "a" wave in the jugular pulse. A right ventricular parasternal lift is palpable and may be accompanied by a systolic thrill at the upper left sternal edge. The systolic murmur, frequently preceded by an ejection sound, is accentuated in late systole. The second heart sound is split with a delayed and diminished pulmonic component. Electrocardiographic evidence of right ventricular hypertrophy is usual, sometimes with a prominent spiked P wave. The chest roentgenogram shows a normal or mildly enlarged heart, prominence of the pulmonary arterial trunk, and normal pulmonary vasculature. The abnormal valve is visualized by echocardiograms.

In *severe* pulmonic stenosis cyanosis may be present, owing to a small cardiac output or a right to left shunt across the intra-atrial septum. A large presystolic "a" wave is usual in the jugular venous pulse and the increased venous pressure may be transmitted to the liver, resulting in a presystolic pulsation. The heart is moderately or greatly enlarged, with a conspicuous parasternal right ventricular lift. The systolic ejection murmur is usually loud, frequently accompanied by a thrill, and audible maximally at the upper left sternal edge, but it may radiate widely over the entire precordium and into the neck and back. The murmur is accentuated in late systole, frequently encompasses the aortic component of the second heart sound, and may be preceded by an ejection sound. The pulmonic component of the second heart sound is either inaudible or soft and very late. The electrocardiogram shows gross right ventricular hypertrophy with tall P waves attributed to right atrial enlargement. The chest roentgenogram confirms the cardiac enlargement, prominence of the right ventricle and atrium, poststenotic dilatation of the pulmonary artery, and pulmonary vasculature that is either normal or decreased. The echocardiogram demonstrates systolic doming of the stenotic leaflets into the dilated pulmonary arterial trunk. In the presence of significant obstruction, the right ventricular wall is thick, the right atrium is enlarged, and the intra-atrial septum bows toward the left. The degree of obstruction is quantified with Doppler techniques by applying a modified Bernoulli equation using peak velocity of flow ($P = 4v^2$, where P = pressure gradient and v = peak flow velocity).

Cardiac catheterization demonstrates the pressure gradient across the pulmonic valve and determines the degree of severity. Selective right ventriculography visualizes the site and nature of the obstruction. During ventricular systole contrast material is seen as a jet through the domed stenotic valve. Subvalvular hypertrophy, which may intensify the obstruction, is also demonstrated by this method.

The clinical course of patients with mild obstruction is usually good, and progression of the disease is unusual, especially in adolescence and adult life. Many with moderate obstruction also do well, although their progress needs to be evaluated at regular intervals, especially during childhood. Progression of the obstruction is detected clinically by the change in character of the murmur, which becomes accentuated in late systole. Also, the width of the splitting of the second heart sound increases as the right ventricular pressure rises. These signs are associated with an increase in the severity of the electrocardiographic signs of the right ventricular hypertrophy.

Treatment of moderate to severe obstruction is by valvulo-plasty, accomplished by a balloon catheter inserted percutaneously. Rapid inflation and deflation of the balloon placed across the valve annulus significantly increases the size of the valve orifice. This results in an immediate decrease in right ventricular pressure which is maintained for years, and recurrence of obstruction is unusual. Postvalvuloplasty pulmonary valve regurgitation is infrequent and when present is mild. The results in adults with severe obstruction may not be as good. Right ventricular dysfunction may persist despite relief of gradient, and this has been attributed to a poorly compliant ventricle because of persistent hypertrophy and fibrosis. Surgery is reserved for patients with dysplastic pulmonary valve leaflets.

Bicuspid Aortic Valve

This condition is said to occur in about 2 per cent of the population. The valve consists of two commissures and two cusps, one of which is generally larger. The bicuspid aortic valve may have normal function so that there is no systolic gradient across the valve and during diastole the valve remains competent. This normal function may continue throughout life, and the bicuspid valve may be found only incidentally at necropsy. In others, abnormality of the aortic valve can be suspected during examination of teenagers or young adults. These findings relate to minor degrees of valvular obstruction and/or incompetence. The auscultatory findings consist of short, soft systolic murmurs heard at the upper right sternal edge. An early aortic ejection click, which precedes the murmur, excludes an innocent murmur. In others, the systolic murmur may be followed by a short, high-pitched early diastolic murmur of aortic incompetence. The diagnosis may be confirmed by echocardiography, which demonstrates only two aortic leaflets (Fig. 46–4).

The natural course of bicuspid aortic valves is variable. In some, the valve may function normally for many decades and produce no abnormal clinical signs. In others the valve leaflets become thickened, fibrotic, and calcified, so that clear signs of aortic stenosis of varying severity develop during early or mid-adult life. In others, there is eversion or prolapse of one of the aortic cusps, resulting in progressive aortic regurgitation that can become severe. A bicuspid aortic valve is particularly susceptible to infective endocarditis, which may convert a benign lesion into one associated with acute severe aortic regurgitation.

Congenital Valvular Aortic Stenosis

See Ch. 49 for a discussion of this lesion.

Subvalvular Aortic Stenosis (Discrete)

Obstruction to left ventricular outflow is produced by a fibrous membrane situated just below the aortic valve. The membrane is a collar-like structure extending from the intraventricular septum and involving the anterior mitral leaflet. The high-velocity jet of blood flowing through the obstructed area during ventricular systole impinges on the aortic valve, which results in fibrous thickening and incompetence of the valve. The clinical picture simulates that of valvular aortic stenosis with important exceptions. An aortic ejection sound is usually absent, and the murmur occupies the whole of systole. This condition is frequently mistaken for a ventricular septal defect or mitral incompetence. Mild forms of obstruction may coexist with other lesions, especially a ventricular septal defect. This obstruction may be unrecognized

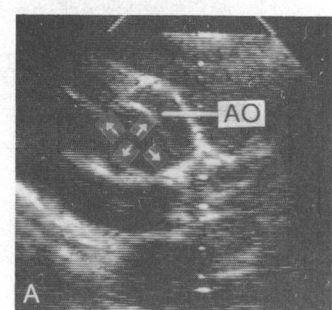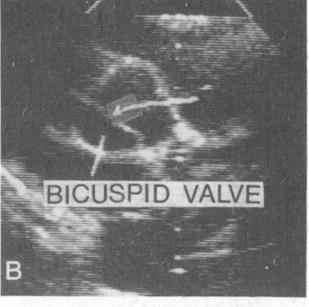

FIGURE 46–4. Short axis echocardiogram of bicuspid aortic valve (AO). *A*, Open valve orifice during systole (*arrows*). *B*, Competent bicuspid valve during diastole. Arrow points to line of apposition of valve leaflets.

at the time of surgical closure of the ventricular septal defect, and the obstruction may progress over the ensuing years. A useful differential sign is the presence of an early diastolic murmur of aortic valve incompetence, which is a common finding when the obstruction is moderate or severe. Laboratory findings simulate those described under valvular aortic stenosis. However, the echocardiogram is diagnostic in that the discrete membrane is visualized. Cardiac catheterization and angiocardiography measure the severity of obstruction and outline the membrane by left ventriculography or aortography if the aortic valve is incompetent. Indications for surgery are liberalized, since continued damage to the aortic valve should be prevented. Excision of the membrane gives immediate good results, but complications include damage to the anterior mitral leaflet with resultant regurgitation or conduction abnormalities, including complete heart block from trauma to the intraventricular septum. Furthermore, there may be recurrence of obstruction from regrowth of the membrane.

A rarer form of subaortic stenosis is a long, narrow fibromuscular channel frequently associated with hypoplasia of the aortic ring. This disease is more frequent in childhood and is difficult to treat surgically because relief of obstruction may require enlargement of the aortic valve ring. In extreme cases a valve-bearing conduit is inserted between the left ventricle and the aorta.

Hypertrophic Cardiomyopathy

See Ch. 50.

Supravalvular Aortic Stenosis

The obstruction may be localized to a segmental hourglass-shaped narrowing immediately above the aortic sinuses. Beyond the area of obstruction the aorta may be normal in diameter or show varying degrees of tubular hypoplasia, frequently involving the ascending aorta but occasionally extending for a varying length along the course of the aorta, even to its bifurcation. Aortic valve leaflets may be thickened, with resultant mild aortic regurgitation. During systole the aortic valve leaflets may impinge upon the orifices of the coronary arteries so that coronary flow is impaired; this may be further aggravated by the coronary arteries themselves, which can be enlarged and tortuous but have a narrow lumen. Supravalvular aortic stenosis is frequently associated with the *Williams syndrome*, consisting of typical facies (broad, prominent forehead, flattened bridge of the nose, epicanthal folds, and long upper lip), mild mental retardation, and low-pitched voice; children with this syndrome are particularly friendly and converse easily. In the absence of the Williams syndrome, supravalvular aortic stenosis occurs sporadically and is sometimes familial. Pulmonary arterial branch stenosis may coexist. Carotid and brachial arterial pulses may be asymmetric, with more conspicuous pulses on the right side. This finding has been attributed to preferential flow into the innominate artery. Other components of the clinical picture simulate those described under valvular aortic stenosis. Echocardiography visualizes the ascending aorta, identifies the area and severity of obstruction, and defines the degree of aortic hypoplasia. Cardiac catheterization and angiocardiography confirm the severity of the obstruction, visualize the anatomy of the aorta and the obstruction, and demonstrate severity of pulmonary arterial branch stenosis, if present. Surgical treatment to relieve the obstruction is advised when the gradient is severe. However, surgical treatment is complicated, especially when the transverse and thoracic aortae are markedly hypoplastic.

Coarctation of the Aorta

Narrowing of the aortic lumen may occur at isolated or multiple sites in the aorta. By far the most common site of discrete obstruction is just distal to the origin of the left subclavian artery. The lesion is more frequent in males and is also seen in patients with Turner's (XO) syndrome. Associated cardiac malformations are frequent, the most common being a bicuspid aortic valve, congenital aortic stenosis with or without incompetence, ventricular septal defect, and lesions of the mitral valve with or without valvular regurgitation. Extensive collateralization usually develops, especially from branches of the subclavian, internal mammary, superior intercostal, and axillary arteries. These vessels join the intercostal arteries of the descending aorta and inferior epigastric branches of the femoral arteries, which allow channels for arterial blood to bypass the area of coarctation. These collateral vessels can become enormously enlarged and tortuous by early adult life.

Children and young adults are generally asymptomatic. However, hypertension may develop in the arteries above the coarctation and may be associated with epistaxis and throbbing headaches. Other symptoms include leg fatigue, complaints of cold extremities, and occasionally intermittent claudication. Beyond the second decade coarctation may be discovered by the finding of brachial arterial hypertension during routine physical examination. The methods of presentation in adults include infective endocarditis, usually involving the aortic valve, and rupture of the aorta or dissecting aneurysm may occur, especially in the 20's and 30's. The site of rupture is either in the proximal aorta or in an aneurysm in the area of coarctation. Cerebral vascular disease with resultant cerebral hemorrhage or infarction may result from complications of hypertension or from the rupture of an aneurysm, usually of the circle of Willis. Hypertension and associated atherosclerosis of the coronary circulation may result in congestive cardiac failure, sometimes preceded by acute myocardial infarction. Pregnancy is usually well tolerated, especially if hypertension is controlled. However, the risk of aortic rupture is increased, especially toward the end of the third trimester.

Classic signs of aortic coarctation are the disparity in pulsations and blood pressures of the arms and legs. The bounding pulses of the arms and carotid vessels contrast with the weak, delayed, or absent femoral and/or distal arterial pulses in the legs. Also, the blood pressure in the arms exceeds that in the legs. This applies especially to the systolic reading, and there is a further rise of systolic blood pressure in response to exercise. If the systolic arterial pressure in the right arm exceeds that of the left arm by more than 30 mm Hg, the left subclavian artery is involved in the coarctation. Collateral arterial circulation may be visible but is usually palpable, especially in the back, at the angles of the scapulae and in the axillae. Murmurs are variable in location, quality, and intensity. The usual is a precordial midsystolic murmur heard best at the left sternal edge, but it may be loudest in the back between the scapulae. Additional systolic or sometimes continuous murmurs are audible over the anterior or posterior chest and are produced by flow through the large, tortuous collateral arteries. The *electrocardiogram* is usually normal during childhood and adolescence. In adults, varying degrees of left ventricular hypertrophy are present. *Roentgenographic* examinations during childhood may not be striking. However, prominence of the left ventricle occurs thereafter and during adult life. The heart may be moderately enlarged. Notching of the inferior border of the ribs from collateral vessels is common. This may be unilateral if one of the subclavian arteries arises below the area of coarctation. Poststenotic dilatation of the descending aorta is usual and is demonstrated by a barium esophagram, and the prominent left subclavian artery produces a shadow in the left mediastinum. *Echocardiography* visualizes the area of coarctation, the large left subclavian artery, poststenotic dilatation of the descending aorta, and associated intracardiac anomalies, especially those of the aortic valve. The site of obstruction, localized aortic aneurysms, and the aortic size are well visualized by magnetic resonance imaging. Two options are now available for therapy and consist of surgical resection or angioplasty. Successful surgical coarctectomy has been undertaken for more than four decades with a low operative mortality. Experience with angioplasty is more recent and follow-up relatively short. There is also debate as to whether angioplasty should be reserved for recoarctation, but successful angioplasty of native coarctation has also been accomplished. Long-term follow-up after surgical coarctectomy in childhood indicates that complications are frequent when patients reach adult life. These consist of recurrence of coarctation, hypertension, atherosclerotic coronary artery disease, aneurysm at the site of coarctectomy, and progressive aortic stenosis and/or regurgitation. It is therefore imperative that patients be followed regularly and treatment instituted (especially for hypertension) prior to onset of complications.

Pulmonic Valvular Regurgitation

Isolated congenital pulmonic valve regurgitation is rare and seldom produces symptoms; an early diastolic murmur at the upper left sternal edge is the only abnormal sign. However, pulmonic valvular regurgitation may accompany other conditions such as those associated with severe pulmonary hypertension or after surgical transection of the pulmonic valve ring for the treatment of severe obstruction of the right ventricular outflow.

Absence of Pulmonic Valve

Absence of the pulmonic valve is a congenital anomaly in which pulmonic valve leaflets are virtually absent. Although the lesion may be isolated it is usually associated with other defects, especially tetralogy of Fallot or isolated ventricular septal defect.

Vascular Rings and Other Aortic Arch Anomalies

The more common anomalies are double aortic arch, right aortic arch with left ligamentum arteriosum, origin of the right subclavian artery from the thoracic aorta distal to the left subclavian artery, anomalous origin of the innominate or left carotid arteries, and anomalous left pulmonary artery, which arises from the elongated pulmonary trunk and courses between the trachea and the esophagus. The clinical picture is extremely variable, and in many instances there are no symptoms. Tracheal compression, especially during infancy, produces respiratory distress with wheezing and a brassy cough. Dysphagia may occur in older patients. Surgery is advised in symptomatic patients to relieve the tracheal and esophageal compression.

THE TRANSPOSITIONS

Transposition of the Great Arteries

In this condition the aorta arises from the right ventricle and the pulmonary artery from the left ventricle. Systemic venous return is to the right atrium, and pulmonary venous return is to the left atrium. Systemic venous blood flows through the tricuspid valve into the right ventricle and is ejected into the aorta. Pulmonary venous blood flows from the left atrium through the mitral valve into the left ventricle and is ejected into the pulmonary artery. Thus, the circulations are parallel. Survival is dependent on mixture of blood through the foramen ovale, a ventricular septal defect, or patency of the ductus arteriosus. This condition is a common malformation that occurs predominantly in males, with symptoms in the neonatal period or soon thereafter.

ISOLATED "SIMPLE" TRANSPOSITION OF THE GREAT ARTERIES. In this malformation the ventricular septum is intact. Mixing of systemic and pulmonary blood occurs primarily from bidirectional shunting across the foramen ovale. This condition produces symptoms and signs of anoxemia in the neonate, is suspected in an otherwise normal neonate who is cyanotic and tachypneic, and is verified by echocardiography, which demonstrates the abnormal origin of the great arteries, as well as the fact that the aorta is usually anterior to the pulmonary artery. Emergency balloon atrial septostomy that ruptures the foramen ovale allows greater mixing at the atrial level and decompresses the left atrium. The arterial switch operation is the treatment of choice in the neonate whereby the origins of the great arteries are transected and the pulmonary artery is connected to the stump of the vessel arising from the right ventricle and the aorta to the left ventricle with implantation of the coronary arteries into the new aorta. This procedure is preferred over intra-atrial redirection of venous return because many years after the latter operation supraventricular tachy- or bradyarrhythmias or systemic (right) ventricular failure occurs.

TRANSPOSITION OF THE GREAT ARTERIES WITH VENTRICULAR SEPTAL DEFECT. When the septal defect is small, the clinical picture is similar to that of simple transposition, and many of these small defects close spontaneously. If the ventricular septal defect is large and nonrestrictive, significant mixing of blood occurs and symptoms are frequently delayed. The clinical picture is dominated by signs of congestive cardiac failure with minimal cyanosis. In the untreated state there is progressive pulmonary hypertension with severe pulmonary vascular disease. Surgical treatment is required during infancy, and the preferred procedure is the arterial switch and closure of the ventricular septal defect. Another option is pulmonary arterial banding during infancy to restrict pulmonary blood flow and prevent the onset of pulmonary vascular disease. In later years, usually during childhood, the second stage is undertaken, in which the pulmonary artery is debanded and transected, the ventricular septal defect is closed so that the left ventricle ejects blood into the aorta, and a conduit is placed from the right ventricle to the transected pulmonary artery (Rastelli procedure).

TRANSPOSITION OF THE GREAT ARTERIES WITH PULMONIC STENOSIS. The importance of this condition is that it may closely simulate the clinical picture produced by tetralogy of Fallot. The condition generally requires an aortic pulmonary shunt during infancy to increase pulmonary blood flow and relieve the symptoms of anoxemia. In later years the Rastelli procedure is undertaken.

Double Outlet Right Ventricle

In this malformation both the pulmonary artery and the aorta arise from the right ventricle, and the only outlet from the left ventricle is a ventricular septal defect. The clinical picture simulates a large, uncomplicated ventricular septal defect with pulmonary hypertension. The echocardiogram is diagnostic in that there is discontinuity between the anterior mitral leaflet and the aorta, since the latter structure arises from the right ventricle. Uncontrollable heart failure and pulmonary hypertension are frequent during infancy so that pulmonary arterial banding is usually required. In later years, generally during childhood, the Rastelli operation is advised. Another option is the arterial switch operation. Double outlet right ventricle may be complicated by pulmonic stenosis when the condition simulates that described under Tetralogy of Fallot.

Corrected Transposition (L Transposition of the Great Arteries)

This condition consists of ventricular inversion and transposition of the great arteries. Systemic venous blood enters a normal right atrium, flows through a mitral valve into the left ventricle, and is ejected into the pulmonary artery. Pulmonary venous blood flows from the left atrium through a tricuspid valve into the right ventricle and is ejected into the aorta. If the condition is uncomplicated, blood flow and hemodynamics are normal. However, associated anomalies are usual, such as ventricular septal defect, pulmonic stenosis, left AV valve (tricuspid) anomalies, including an Ebstein-like malformation of this valve, and AV conduction abnormalities—frequently complete AV block. The clinical picture is dominated by the associated lesions. The chest roentgenogram may suggest the abnormal origin of the great arteries in that the ascending aorta occupies the upper left border of the cardiac silhouette in the posteroanterior view. Since ventricular inversion is present, the electrocardiogram may show absence of q waves in leads I and V_6, initial q waves in III, aVF, and V_1, and prominent T waves in the right precordial leads. During surgical treatment the bundle of His may be injured because it is located abnormally, so that complete heart block may occur. In others, significant regurgitations via the Ebstein-like tricuspid valve requires valve replacement.

Anomalous Pulmonary Venous Connection

The anomalous pulmonary venous return may be partial or total. Partial anomalous pulmonary venous return simulates the clinical picture produced by a secundum atrial septal defect. In fact, one of these forms is the sinus venosus defect.

TOTAL ANOMALOUS PULMONARY VENOUS CONNECTION. The site of entry of the pulmonary veins may be supradiaphragmatic (into a left superior vena cava or vertical vein, coronary sinus, right superior vena cava, or right atrium) or infradiaphragmatic (portal vein, hepatic veins, or inferior vena cava). Thus, there is no connection between the pulmonary vein and the left atrium. Generally the pulmonary veins converge to form a single trunk, which then enters the systemic venous circulation. Varying degrees of pulmonary venous obstruction are present and depend on the length of the common pulmonary venous trunk before its entry into the systemic vein as well as localized areas of obstruction.

The clinical picture is variable. In some instances, especially those of infradiaphragmatic connection, pulmonary edema and cyanosis are present in the neonatal period or soon thereafter. When there is a large intra-atrial communication and obstruction to pulmonary venous return is moderate, symptoms occur in later infancy and the clinical picture is dominated by congestive cardiac failure. When pulmonary venous obstruction is absent and there is a large communication between the right and left atria, symptoms may be delayed until early childhood and very occasionally adolescence. The clinical picture of these patients simulates that produced by a large left to right shunt at the atrial level.

The *electrocardiogram* reflects the hemodynamic state so that symptomatic infants have marked right ventricular hypertrophy with prominent P waves. Chest *roentgenograms* in neonates with pulmonary venous obstruction are characterized by pulmonary edema with a normal heart size. In older infants the heart is large and pulmonary overcirculation evident. In older children with pulmonary venous connection to the left superior vena cava, the cardiac silhouette has the appearance of a snowman or figure 8. The supracardiac shadow is produced by marked dilatation of the left superior vena cava, innominate vein, and right superior vena cava. The *echocardiogram* shows signs of right volume overload, and color flow imaging identifies the site of entry of pulmonary veins. *Cardiac catheterization* demonstrates the severity of pulmonary hypertension, and pulmonary arteriograms show return of contrast material to the pulmonary veins and their anomalous site of insertion into the systemic venous circulation. Surgical treatment is indicated when the common pulmonary venous trunk is anastomosed to the left atrium, the atrial septal defect closed, and the anomalous connection to the systemic venous system obliterated. Results of surgical treatment have been good, with greatest risk in symptomatic neonates.

CARDIAC MALPOSITION

Knowledge of the position of the heart as well as the location (situs) of abdominal viscera aids in defining the nature of these anomalies. Roentgenography of the abdomen helps identify abdominal situs by localizing the position of the stomach bubble and other abdominal structures, but many viscera cannot be visualized by this method alone. Generally, atrial and visceral situs are related; if the viscera are normally located, the atria have a normal position. In abdominal situs inversus, the left atrium is usually to the right and the right atrium to the left. Location of the atria is further and more accurately assessed by evaluation of the tracheobronchial air column on chest roentgenogram. A normal tracheobronchial tree with an epiarterial bronchus on the right indicates normal atrial situs, and this finding is independent of the position of the heart.

Dextrocardia

The heart is in the right chest, and the cardiac apex points to the right. Associated abdominal situs inversus (mirror-image dextrocardia) in adults is usually associated with a normally functioning heart. However, poorly motile cilia may result in sinusitis and bronchiectasis (Kartagener's syndrome). Dextrocardia may be discovered by physical examination when the heart sounds are more clear in the right chest or accidentally on a routine chest film. The electrocardiogram demonstrates the mirror image, so that the P, QRS, and T are inverted in lead I; aV_R and aV_L are the reverse of normal, and the right precordial leads resemble those usually recorded from the left chest. *Isolated dextrocardia* with abdominal viscera in normal position (situs solitus) is invariably associated with various combinations of severe cardiac malformations, the most common being ventricular inversion, single ventricle, pulmonic stenosis, abnormalities of the AV valves, and anomalies of systemic and pulmonary venous return.

Isolated Levocardia

Isolated levocardia is accompanied by varying degrees of anomalous position of abdominal viscera (heterotaxia) so that situs inversus is partial or complete. Severe cardiac malformations are usual, including various combinations of anomalies of systemic and pulmonary venous return, common AV canal, pulmonic stenosis or atresia, defects of the atrial and ventricular septa, and single ventricle.

Mesocardia

Mesocardia is the term used when the heart is centrally located in the chest or the cardiac silhouette on roentgenogram is toward the right chest. The cardiac anatomy is normal with normal relationships of the cardiac chambers, venous return, and origin of the great arteries. Cardiac malformations are usually absent.

Asplenia Syndrome

This condition is characterized by absence of the spleen, undefinable situs of the abdominal viscera (situs ambiguus), bilateral *right-sidedness*, and complex, severe cardiac malformations. Bilateral right-sidedness is identified by bilateral trilobed lungs with bilateral epiarterial bronchi. In the majority the liver is located centrally so that the liver edge is palpable across the entire upper abdomen. The stomach is located on the right in about half the patients, and varying degrees of malrotation of the small bowel are present. Both atria have the morphologic characteristics of the right atrium. Common cardiovascular anomalies include total anomalous pulmonary venous connection, transposition of the great arteries, pulmonic stenosis or atresia, complete AV canal, single ventricle, and dextrocardia. The condition is suspected in a deeply cyanotic male infant with dextrocardia and a centrally placed liver. Howell-Jolly and Heinz bodies in the peripheral red blood cells are suggestive of asplenia, but these findings are not conclusive. Infants with asplenia are susceptible to severe intercurrent infections so that continued antibiotic prophylaxis has been suggested as a preventive measure. Aortopulmonary shunts during infancy are indicated when severe anoxemia is present owing to pulmonic stenosis, and right atrial-pulmonary shunts (Fontan) are advised in later years.

Polysplenia Syndrome

The features of this condition are multiple splenic masses (two or more), ambiguous abdominal situs, and *bilateral left-sidedness*; while cardiovascular abnormalities are frequent, they are generally not as complex as in the asplenia syndrome. The lungs are bilobed and epiarterial bronchi are absent. The liver is frequently located centrally in the upper abdomen, and the stomach is right- or left-sided. Malrotation of the bowel is common. Both atria have the morphologic features of the left atrium. The hepatic segment of the inferior vena cava is frequently absent so that systemic venous return is by way of the azygos vein. The cardiac apex points to the left in the majority. Pulmonary venous return may be normal, arterial transposition is present in only a minority, and pulmonic stenosis is unusual. The cardiac malformations are generally associated with left to right shunts at atrial or ventricular levels.

THE ADULT WITH "UNCURED" CONGENITAL HEART DISEASE

Strategies of management of symptomatic patients with congenital heart disease have changed recently so that the majority are treated during infancy or early childhood. Many adolescents and adults now exist who have trivial lesions, have remained asymptomatic, and have lived a normal lifestyle. Other patients have anomalies that are silent until adult life. Palliative surgery may have been undertaken in another group who have remained relatively well and have now approached adult life. Another cohort of patients who may not have had surgical treatment during early life develop progressive pulmonary hypertension during childhood, and in adult life their lesions are associated with severe pulmonary vascular disease. This section discusses these groups of patients.

VENTRICULAR SEPTAL DEFECTS. A significant number of patients seen in pediatric cardiac clinics have trivial shunts across a small ventricular septal defect. They remain asymptomatic throughout the growing years, and as adults the only abnormal physical sign is a long, harsh systolic murmur, which may be accompanied by a thrill and is heard best at the lower left sternal edge. It is unusual to see such patients beyond the age of 40 years so that it has been assumed that many of these defects close spontaneously. While the defect remains, these patients are at risk to develop infective endocarditis and occasionally aortic regurgitation or discrete subaortic stenosis.

VALVULAR PULMONIC STENOSIS. Generally, asymptomatic children with mild pulmonic stenosis (resting peak right ventricular pressure less than one half of systolic systemic pressure) do not require surgical treatment. There is no consensus about the course of untreated mild to moderate pulmonic stenosis. The generally held belief, however, is that progressive increase in severity is unusual, especially if the patient is beyond the age of 12 years. This optimistic view also applies to those who had a valvotomy during childhood, which relieved the obstruction. Restriction of physical activity is not required, pregnancy is well tolerated, and, although infective endocarditis of the pulmonic valve is not common, prophylaxis is advisable at the time of risk for this complication.

CONGENITAL COMPLETE HEART BLOCK. Fetal echocardiography may be prompted by the recognition of intrauterine bradycardia, and this test unmasks the presence of complete atrioventricular (AV) block. This study is especially important during pregnancy of mothers with connective tissue disease, such as systemic lupus erythematosus, since the offspring are at greater risk for complete AV block. It is suggested that antinuclear antibodies of the IgG category cross the placenta and damage the fetal conduction system. This occurs in mothers whose disease is active but also when there are no overt clinical manifestations and only positive serologic evidence is present. In about 70 per cent of children with complete AV block the lesion is isolated, and the remainder have associated complex cardiac malformations, such as ventricular inversion or single ventricle. Familial complete AV block is well recognized. Adolescents and adults with isolated congenital complete AV block are usually asymptomatic, but it is not possible to predict episodes of syncope. The pulse rate is inappropriately slow for age. The large stroke volume and vasodilatation produce jerky pulses, systolic hypertension, and cardiomegaly. Cannon waves may be visible in the jugular venous pulse. The first heart sound varies in intensity and may be followed by a nonspecific mid-systolic ejection murmur. The diagnosis is confirmed by the electrocardiogram, in which there is no constant relationship between the P waves and QRS complexes. Usually the QRS is of normal duration, which suggests that the site of the lesion is above the bundle of His. Marked ventricular slowing may be recorded by continuous, 24-hour electrocardiographic monitoring, especially during sleep. It is not known whether there is any relationship between the slow ventricular rates during sleep and the prognosis. Since patients with congenital complete AV block have been observed in late adult life, there is a generally held view that the prognosis is good. However, the lesion is not benign, in that complications may occur at any time and are not predictable. Syncope is an indication for implantation of a permanent pacemaker. Decisions about treatment in asymptomatic patients are more difficult. The demonstration of ventricular tachycardia or fibrillation during continuous electrocardiographic monitoring or graded exercise testing is an indication for pacemaker implantation. There remains a group of asymptomatic patients in whom treatment is not standardized, including those with premature ventricular contractions during and after exercise, extreme nocturnal bradycardia, and ventricular depolarization initiated from a focus low in the bundle of His.

EISENMENGER'S SYNDROME. This syndrome is associated with marked elevation of pulmonary vascular resistance with reversed or bidirectional shunt, which is intracardiac or between the aorta and pulmonary arteries. Thus, pulmonary vascular disease is the hallmark of this syndrome, and the site of the shunt is incidental. Medial hypertrophy of pulmonary arteries and arterioles is present and is associated with cellular, fibrotic, and fibroelastic intimal reactions, and in more severe forms plexiform lesions encroach into the lumen of the vessel. These changes in the pulmonary vascular bed are directly related to pulmonary arterial pressure. Extension of muscle into the peripheral arteries occurs when pulmonary hypertension is still associated with increased pulmonary blood flow. With progressive vascular disease, a reduction in the number of small arteries may precede obliterative pulmonary vascular disease.

Historically these patients are frequently symptomatic during infancy and early childhood because of congestive cardiac failure, poor physical development, and recurrent lower respiratory tract infections. As pulmonary vascular resistance rises, the left to right shunt decreases so that symptoms improve. These children may lead nearly normal lives, but their stamina is limited and mild exertional cyanosis is evident. In early adult life there is progressive anoxemia with intensification of cyanosis, digital clubbing may be extreme, and, erythrocytosis increases. Progressive decrease in effort tolerance develops over many years, culminating in congestive cardiac failure in early or mid-adult life. Other symptoms are produced by hyperviscosity, a bleeding diathesis, or hyperuricemia. Angina pectoris attributed to right ventricular ischemia, syncope, and palpitations from premature atrial or ventricular contractions may be present. Jugular venous pressure is increased, with a prominent "v" wave in the presence of complicating tricuspid valve regurgitation. Hepatomegaly and marked dependent edema with ascites are usual with heart failure. The heart size is increased to a variable extent, greatest when there are shunts at the atrial level and when there is complicating tricuspid and/or pulmonic valve incompetence. The precordium is active with a right ventricular heave along the left sternal edge. Pulmonary arterial pulsations and the second heart sound may be palpable at the upper left sternal edge. The systolic murmur varies in intensity and is frequently initiated by a pulmonic ejection click. The second heart sound is booming, single, or narrowly split in ventricular shunts, but wide, fixed splitting may be audible in isolated atrial shunts. Signs of pulmonary and/or tricuspid valve regurgitation are superimposed when there is dilatation of these valve rings secondary to pulmonary hypertension or right ventricular failure. The *electrocardiogram* shows marked right ventricular or biventricular hypertrophy with prominent P waves. Complete right bundle branch block may be present, especially when the shunt is at the atrial level. In others the electrocardiogram is influenced by the underlying anomaly (e.g., single ventricle, ventricular inversion, etc.). The *chest roentgenogram* confirms the degree of cardiomegaly. The pulmonary trunk is enlarged with prominence of the primary divisions, which diminish in caliber in the peripheral branches. The *echocardiogram* helps to identify the anatomy of the underlying intracardiac or extracardiac malformation. *Cardiac catheterization* is undertaken when the diagnosis cannot be established by clinical findings and noninvasive studies. One of the purposes of catheterization is to determine whether the pulmonary vascular bed is vasoactive, as indicated by a fall in pulmonary artery pressure and resistance during the breathing of 100 per cent oxygen. Another major indication is to exclude the presence of left ventricular inflow lesions, which result in elevation of pulmonary venous pressure and secondary pulmonary hypertension. Angiocardiography carries a small increased risk because the contrast medium may produce a fall in systemic vascular resistance and increased right to left shunting with a further fall in systemic arterial saturation.

Symptomatic *erythrocytosis* is treated with cautious venesection, and repeated phlebotomies are avoided because of the risk of iron deficiency. *Hemoptysis* occurs from coagulopathies, from rupture of pulmonary vessels, or from pulmonary arterial thrombosis or embolism. This symptom is usually limited to adult life, blood loss is not excessive, and symptomatic treatment is all that is needed. However, hemoptysis can be life threatening if associated with hypotension, an increase in the degree of hypoxemia, and the development of acidemia. Long-term anticoagulation is not indicated. *Syncope* and *sudden death* cannot be predicted, but patients with Eisenmenger's syndrome between the ages of about 20 and 40 years are at risk. The mechanism is not clear but has been attributed to arrhythmias, probably ventricular tachyarrhythmias, which result in hypotension and an increase in right to left shunting. *Pregnancy* is not well tolerated, and sudden death has been reported during the third trimester or in the postpartum period.

Treatment. Surgical treatment of the cardiac anomaly is contraindicated because these patients succumb to the effects of pulmonary vascular disease. Palliation has been successful in the presence of transposition of the great arteries, ventricular septal defect, and severe pulmonary vascular disease; the procedure involves redirection of the venous return but the ventricular defect is not closed. The experience with transplantation of the heart and lungs is still small and follow-up is short, but this therapy is being watched with interest because patients with progressive symptoms are at great risk of dying. Drugs have been used to attempt to manipulate pulmonary and systemic vascular resistance to reduce the right to left shunt; generally the results have been disappointing.

COMPLEX CARDIAC MALFORMATIONS. When pulmonic stenosis is an important part of the anomaly, surgical aortopulmonary shunting is undertaken during infancy or childhood to alleviate hypoxemia. In others with torrential pulmonary blood flow and pulmonary hypertension, pulmonary arterial banding is undertaken in infancy to prevent progressive pulmonary vascular disease. Many have now reached adolescence or adult life with normal or low pulmonary vascular resistance. These patients are candidates for operation using the Fontan principle (caval or right atrial anastomosis to the pulmonary artery).

THE ADULT WITH SURGICALLY "CURED" CONGENITAL HEART DISEASE

Surgical treatment for extracardiac anomalies has been undertaken for over four decades, and 35 years have elapsed since the introduction of surgical procedures for intracardiac congenital malformations. Immediate results after operation continue to be excellent, even dramatic, but it is now recognized that complications may develop many years after surgery.

INTRA-ATRIAL SURGERY. Many anomalies may be treated by an approach through the right atrium. These include atrial septal defects of all types, endocardial cushion defects, transposition of the great arteries, and total anomalous pulmonary venous connection. Frequently, isolated ventricular septal defects are closed surgically transatrially, and the defect (especially the more common perimembranous defect) is approached through the tricuspid valve and the shunt obliterated. Persistent *conduction disturbances* may occur immediately after operation or appear for the first time many years later. These consist of supraventricular arrhythmias (atrial flutter or fibrillation, paroxysmal supraventricular tachycardia, and junctional rhythm), sick sinus syndrome, or varying degrees of AV block. These rhythm disturbances occur even when there is complete anatomic correction of the abnormality. The treatment of these abnormalities in conduction is similar to the treatment of these arrhythmias of any cause. The *function of the right ventricle* and competence of the tricuspid valve have also been of concern, especially in transposition of the great arteries.

INTRAVENTRICULAR SURGERY. Right ventriculotomy is the approach used in most patients who require intraventricular surgery. The more common lesions treated this way include some forms of ventricular septal defect, tetralogy of Fallot with or without pulmonary atresia, and various forms of transposition of the great arteries. Some of these complications may be reduced in future years, since earlier operation is being advised, especially in some patients with tetralogy of Fallot.

Conduction Disturbances. Permanent complete heart block from intraoperative trauma to the conduction system has decreased to a point where it is no longer a major problem soon after operation. *Bifascicular block* (left anterior hemiblock with complete right bundle branch block) may occur from intraoperative trauma to the bundle of His and its branches. These patients usually remain well for many years after operation, but the conduction abnormality may progress to complete AV block. Bifascicular block does not require treatment. *Sudden unexpected cardiac arrest* may occur many years after operation. While this catastrophe may occasionally occur from complete AV block, more frequent mechanisms are ventricular tachyarrhythmias and deterioration into ventricular fibrillation. The risk of ventricular tachycardia is higher in patients who have multiple unifocal or multifocal premature ventricular contractions at rest. Bursts of ventricular tachyarrhythmia may be recorded during 24-hour electrocardiographic recording or unmasked during or immediately after graded exercise testing. While these arrhythmias may occur in patients who have had adequate relief of right ventricular outflow tract obstruction and in whom the ventricular defect is closed, there appears to be greater risk when residual defects are present, such as severe pulmonic stenosis, persistent large shunts across the ventricular septum, and right ventricular aneurysms. Significant residual defects should be treated by reoperation, and the ventricular arrhythmia may be abolished by excision of arrhythmogenic right ventricular aneurysms. Medical treatment of the ventricular tachycardia is indicated and although there is

a choice of many drugs, phenytoin (Dilantin) has been used with particular success.

Reconstruction of the Right Ventricular Outflow Tract. Treatment of extreme forms of tetralogy of Fallot, especially pulmonary atresia, and many forms of transposition of the great arteries with pulmonic stenosis or previous arterial banding requires a prosthesis to establish continuity between the right ventricle and the pulmonary artery. During the last decade the most frequently used prosthesis consisted of a Dacron tube with an aortic valve bearing a porcine heterograft. The durability of this prosthesis is unpredictable, since recurrence of obstruction may occur anywhere along its length from narrowing of the anastomotic sites or from development of an exuberant neointima that encroaches on the lumen of the Dacron tube. Because of these complications, a human valve bearing aortic or pulmonary homografts is being used with greater frequency.

Congenital Aortic Stenosis. See above.

Valvular Pulmonic Stenosis. See above.

Coarctation of the Aorta. See above.

Adams FH, Emmanouilides GC, Riemenschneider TA: Moss' Heart Disease in Infants, Children and Adolescents. 4th ed. Baltimore, Williams and Wilkins, 1989. *The standard comprehensive text on all aspects of congenital heart disease.*

Cohen M, Fuster V, Steele PM, et al.: Coarctation of the aorta. Long-term follow-up and prediction of outcome after surgical correction. Circulation 80:840, 1989.

Garson A, Nihill MR, McNamara DG, et al.: Status of the adult and adolescent after repair of tetralogy of Fallot. Circulation 59:1232, 1979. *Long-term results are evaluated with emphasis on complications in the adult.*

Girod DA, Fontan F, Deville C, et al.: Long-term results after the Fontan operation for tricuspid atresia. Circulation 75:605, 1987. *These principles are also applicable to other complex cardiac malformations with inadequate pulmonary blood flow.*

Giuliani ER, Fuster V, Brandenberg RO, et al.: Ebstein's anomaly. Mayo Clin Proc 54:163, 1979. *Clinical features and natural history are reviewed in a lucid manner.*

Kirklin JW, Barratt-Boyes BG: Cardiac Surgery. New York, John Wiley and Sons, 1986. *Comprehensive analyses of combined clinical experiences from two respected pioneers in all aspects of cardiac surgery, especially congenital heart disease.*

Kopecky SL, Gersh BJ, McGoon MD, et al.: Long-term outcome of patients undergoing surgical repair of isolated pulmonary valve stenosis. Follow-up at 20 to 30 years. Circulation 78:1150, 1988. *These long-term results set the standard against which the results of valvuloplasty will be compared.*

Mullins CE: Pediatric and congenital therapeutic cardiac catheterization. Circulation 79:1153, 1989. *A description of the present status of catheter interventional procedures for congenital heart disease.*

Perloff JK: The Clinical Recognition of Congenital Heart Disease. 3rd ed. Philadelphia, W.B. Saunders Company, 1986. *A book that focuses on the anatomic and physiologic derangements in congenital heart disease, setting the stage for an understanding of the history, physical signs, electrocardiogram, chest roentgenogram, and echocardiogram. All age groups are dealt with.*

Perloff JK, Child JS: Congenital Heart Disease in Adults. Philadelphia, W.B. Saunders Company, 1991. *All major aspects of diagnosis and management are discussed in a sophisticated and authoritative manner.*

Wernovsy G, Hougen TJ, Walsh EP, et al.: Midterm results after the arterial switch operation for transposition of the great arteries with intact ventricular septum: Clinical, hemodynamic, electrocardiographic, and electrophysiologic data. Circulation 77:1333, 1988.

47 Atherosclerosis

Russell Ross

Atherosclerosis is responsible for the majority of cases of myocardial and cerebral infarction and thus represents the principal cause of death in the United States and western Europe. Atherosclerosis is the descriptive term for thickened and hardened lesions of the medium and large muscular and elastic arteries. It is a lipid-rich lesion, in contrast with arteriosclerosis, which is the generic term used for thickened and stiffened arteries of all sizes. Other forms of arteriosclerosis include focal calcific arteriosclerosis (Mönckeberg's arteriosclerosis) and arteriolosclerosis, a disease of small vessels.

The lesions of atherosclerosis occur within the innermost layer of the artery, the intima, and are largely confined to this region of the vessel. The lesions are generally eccentric and, if they become sufficiently large, can occlude the artery and thus the vascular supply to a tissue or organ, resulting in ischemia or necrosis. If this occurs, it often leads to the characteristic clinical sequelae of myocardial infarction, cerebral infarction, gangrene of the extremities, or sudden cardiac death.

THE NORMAL ARTERY

The normal artery consists essentially of a tube lined on its luminal aspect by a continuous layer of endothelium and on its outer aspect by loose connective tissue containing fibroblasts and smooth muscle cells, which package an intermediate layer of pure smooth muscle cells that are bound together in such a manner that, by working with the elastic laminae and the collagen and proteoglycans that surround the cells, the smooth muscle cells contract and maintain the tonus of the artery wall as the blood flows through with each systole and diastole.

The lining cells of the artery, the endothelium, represent the interface with the cells of the blood. It is at this interface that different blood cell types can interact with the endothelium and, under appropriate circumstances, lead to the development of lesions of atherosclerosis. These cells are the platelet, the monocyte, and the lymphocyte. Their potential roles in atherogenesis are discussed below.

THE LESIONS OF ATHEROSCLEROSIS

The two principal forms of atherosclerosis are the early lesion, or fatty streak, and the advanced lesion, or fibrous plaque, which can become an advanced complicated lesion.

The Fatty Streak

The fatty streak is the most common and ubiquitous lesion of atherosclerosis. It occurs at all ages and in Western society is present at birth in some infants and is common in young children. The lesions of atherosclerosis are confined principally to the intima. Initially, the fatty streak appears to contain two cell types: foam cells that consist of macrophages filled with lipids (principally in the form of cholesteryl esters) and T lymphocytes (principally CD-8+ with some CD-4+ cells). The macrophages are derived from blood-borne monocytes that are chemotactically attracted into the artery wall, where they develop into foam cells. As the fatty streak enlarges, it does so by continuing attachment and migration of monocytes into the intima with their consequent development into macrophages. Subsequently, smooth muscle cells appear to migrate into the intima from the media and also begin to accumulate lipid and take on the appearance of foam cells. As the fatty streak becomes larger and more advanced, it contains varying numbers of smooth muscle cells mixed together with lymphocytes and the predominant lipid-filled macrophages. Fatty streaks can be found in young individuals at the same anatomic sites that are later occupied by advanced lesions, as well as at sites where they may either regress and disappear or remain as fatty streaks throughout life.

The Fibrous Plaque

The fibrous plaque is also located in the intima and characteristically leads to the eccentric thickening of the artery that often results in occlusion of the lumen. The fibrous plaque is typically covered at its luminal aspect by a thickened cap of dense connective tissue containing a special form of flattened, pancake-shaped smooth muscle cell that has formed the dense collagenous matrix in which it is embedded. Beneath this cap, the lesion is highly cellular and contains large numbers of smooth muscle cells, some of which may be full of lipid droplets. It also contains numerous macrophages, many of which take the form of foam cells, together with variable numbers of T lymphocytes. These collections of cells usually overlie a deeper area of necrotic foam cells and debris. This necrotic area sometimes becomes calcified and often may contain cholesterol crystals. (Figure 47–1 details the cellular composition of a fibrous plaque.)

The Complicated Lesion

The complicated lesion is a fibrous plaque that has undergone extensive degeneration and often calcification. It may contain

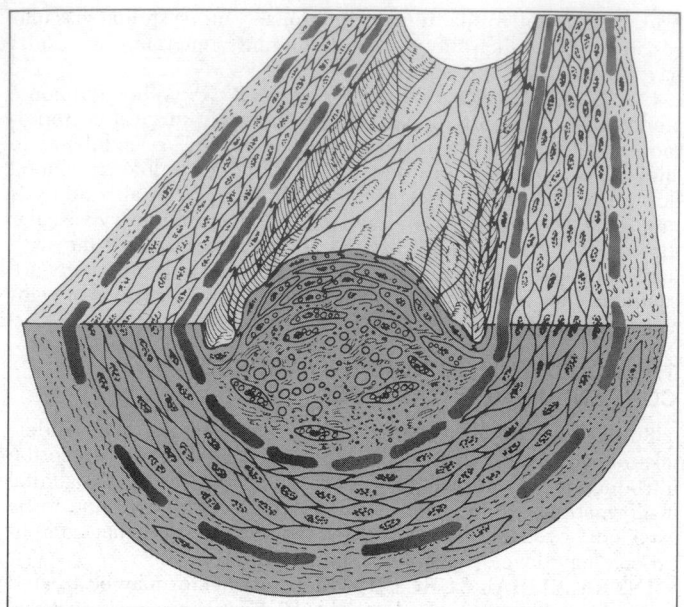

FIGURE 47–1. The *fibrous plaque*, which characteristically consists of numerous proliferated smooth muscle cells together with macrophages and variable numbers of lymphocytes. In this diagram, the fibrous plaque is covered by an intact endothelial monolayer and contains a fibrous cap of smooth muscle cells. These smooth muscle cells lie in a dense connective tissue matrix that covers a deeper collection of smooth muscle cells and macrophages, both of which may contain numerous lipid droplets and take the form of foam cells mixed together with variable numbers of lymphocytes. These collections of cells lie in a mixture of connective tissue matrix and free extracellular deposits of lipid. The fibrous plaque usually intrudes into the lumen owing to its proliferative nature. This diagram represents only in general terms the relative appearance of such a lesion.

ulcerations, cracks, and fissures, which serve as sites for platelet adherence, aggregation and thrombosis, and subsequent organization. When this occurs, thrombosis may result in sudden occlusion of the artery.

Morbid Anatomy of the Lesions

Fatty streaks are flat lesions that often appear as yellow discolorations on the surface of the artery but seldom intrude into the lumen and thus cause no clinical sequelae. The fibrous plaques and complicated lesions are raised lesions that are often pearly gray in appearance but may be discolored when associated with erythrocytes and thrombi.

Localization of the Lesions

The arteries most commonly involved with atherosclerosis are the aorta; the femoral, popliteal, and tibial arteries; the coronary arteries; the internal and external carotid arteries; and the cerebral arteries.

In the aorta, the abdominal portion is commonly involved with lesions of atherosclerosis at an earlier age, and, as in the thoracic aorta, lesions most commonly form around orifices of branches and bifurcations of the artery. There is a greater incidence of atherosclerotic lesions in the leg arteries, whereas they are relatively rare in the vessels of the upper limbs. Atherosclerosis of the smaller arteries, particularly those of the legs and the coronary arteries, is more common in cigarette smokers or in individuals who have glucose intolerance.

Coronary atherosclerosis is most prominent in the main stems of the coronary arteries, particularly in the segments closest to the ostia of the coronary vessel. The degree of luminal narrowing in the coronary arteries can be variable; however, atherosclerosis is generally present in the epicardial segment of the vessels, whereas the intramural coronary arteries are generally spared. Typically, after coronary bypass surgery, the perianastomotic site of the bypass is often (30 per cent of the time) involved in the development of a new lesion of atherosclerosis, which is probably related to mural thrombi that readily form at these sites.

The carotid and cerebral arteries generally have a patchy

distribution of the lesions of atherosclerosis, which often first appear at the base of the brain in the carotid, basilar, and vertebral arteries.

The pulmonary arteries are generally spared of lesions of atherosclerosis, except in association with pulmonary hypertension.

RISK FACTORS

The risk factor concept evolved from epidemiologic studies of the incidence of coronary artery disease conducted in the United States and in Europe. Prospective studies demonstrated a consistent association of characteristics observed in apparently healthy individuals with the subsequent incidence of coronary artery disease in the same individuals. These studies demonstrated an association between an increase in the concentration of plasma lipoproteins, principally low density lipoprotein (LDL) and thus plasma cholesterol (see Ch. 172), and the rate of occurrence of new events of coronary artery disease. Also observed was an increased incidence of the disease in relation to cigarette smoking, hypertension, clinical diabetes, age, male sex, obesity, stress and particular personality characteristics (denoted as type A), and genetic factors. Because of these associations, each of these characteristics was termed a risk factor for atherosclerosis (see Ch. 37). At least three independent predictors of risk for individuals within a population are valuable in anticipating increased incidence of atherosclerosis. These are hyperlipidemia, cigarette smoking, and hypertension.

Hyperlipidemia

There is a clear association between chronic hypercholesterolemia and increase in incidence of ischemic heart disease. The Framingham Study demonstrated this association, particularly in men between the ages of 20 and 40. When the plasma cholesterol levels are greater than 220 mg per deciliter, there is a marked increase in the relative incidence of myocardial infarction, which is most easily demonstrated in individuals with familial hypercholesterolemia. The range of normality is not entirely clear in defining cholesterol and triglyceride levels for a given population as they relate to increased risk of ischemic heart disease. However, in the United States, 200 mg per deciliter is considered to be the upper limit of normal for the plasma cholesterol level, which increases from birth through young adulthood until the age of approximately 50 in men and to somewhat older ages in women. Similarly, there is an age-related increase in plasma triglyceride levels. Triglyceride is associated with increases in very low density lipoproteins (VLDL), whereas elevation in plasma cholesterol level is generally associated with increase in LDL.

Abnormal accumulation of lipoproteins in the plasma can occur from overproduction, from deficient removal, or from a combination of these abnormalities. There are numerous forms of genetically derived hyperlipoproteinemias that are either monogenic or polygenic. Perhaps more common are forms of hyperlipoproteinemia that are secondary to other disease, such as diabetes, renal disease, alcoholism, hypothyroidism, and the dysglobulinemias, or to treatment with corticosteroids or estrogens (see Ch. 172).

HOMOZYGOUS FAMILIAL HYPERCHOLESTEROL-EMIA. Patients with homozygous familial hypercholesterolemia (FH disease) represent one of the best demonstrations of the capacity of hypercholesterolemia to induce the cellular changes that lead to atherogenesis. Although FH disease is much rarer than the secondary hyperlipoproteinemias or other forms of genetic hyperlipidemia, we know a great deal about its course in humans and in an animal model, the Watanabe heritable hyperlipidemic rabbit, as well as diet-induced hypercholesterolemia in the nonhuman primate. In the case of genetic hyperlipidemia, the plasma cholesterol and LDL levels are inordinately high owing to faulty or missing LDL receptors. When LDL is bound to its normal receptor, it suppresses the activity of the rate-limiting enzyme for cholesterol synthesis, HMG-CoA-reductase. In individuals with FH disease, the liver and peripheral cells continue to synthesize large amounts of cholesterol because absent or faulty receptors fail to generate a feedback inhibitory signal and cholesterol synthesis goes on unabated. Under these conditions, plasma cholesterol levels reach 500 to 1000 mg per deciliter or higher, and rampant atherosclerosis develops, with advanced occlusive lesions. This can occur at very young ages, and myocardial infarcts have been described in young children with this disease.

TREATMENT OF HYPERCHOLESTEROLEMIA. The Lipid Research Clinic Trials have demonstrated that it is beneficial to lower plasma levels in patients with chronic elevations of LDL. These studies showed that the decrease in plasma cholesterol levels can be correlated with a reduction in the incidence of myocardial infarction and thus atherosclerosis. Premature ischemic heart disease is usually associated with hypercholesterolemia, particularly when levels of plasma cholesterol are greater than 240 mg per deciliter. When this occurs, the incidence of atherosclerotic disease can be as high as fivefold greater than for individuals with plasma cholesterol levels below 200 mg per deciliter.

Hypertriglyceridemia is usually associated with increases in VLDL in the plasma, which may be complicated by increases in cholesterol as well. Patients with increased VLDL levels who come from families with familial combined hyperlipidemia are at increased risk for atherosclerosis, whereas those with elevated VLDL levels from families with monogenic familial hypertriglyceridemia are not at increased risk. Increased VLDL levels can increase the risk of atherosclerosis if it accompanies other risk factors, such as diabetes mellitus or cigarette smoking.

It is important to examine all patients over the age of 20 for hyperlipidemia, particularly if they have a family history of premature ischemic heart disease. This is best done by measuring the concentrations of cholesterol and triglyceride in plasma after an overnight fast. Cholesterol levels above 200 mg per deciliter or triglyceride levels above 250 mg per deciliter, or both, are indicative of hyperlipidemia, requiring attention and therapy, the first step of which should be dietary intervention. Such patients should be brought to normal weight if this is excessive and maintained on a diet low in saturated fat and cholesterol. Those with hypertriglyceridemia should limit or eliminate intake of alcohol. In general, reduction of intake of calories, cholesterol, and saturated fat is the best approach to begin with in most patients. Severe hyperlipidemia with cholesterol levels in excess of 350 mg per deciliter or triglyceride levels in excess of 400 mg per deciliter, or both, is usually representative of a genetic disorder and often first manifests with xanthomas. Such patients' families, particularly first-degree relatives, should also be examined.

If dietary approaches are unsuccessful, then regimens including bile acid–binding resins or one of the more recently developed lipid-lowering drugs should be considered (see Ch. 172). Use of such agents is dependent not only on their efficaciousness, but on their long-term effects as well. Their use before puberty and during pregnancy is currently not recommended.

High Density Lipoprotein (HDL)

In epidemiologic studies, elevations of high density lipoprotein particles in the plasma are inversely related to the incidence of atherosclerosis and its sequelae. Elevation of the HDL cholesterol level is "protective" against ischemic heart disease; conversely, the individuals with abnormally low levels of HDL are at increased risk.

HDL has been postulated to participate in transfer of cholesterol out of cells. Women generally have elevated HDL levels prior to menopause. If their HDL level is decreased in association with diabetes or obesity, they are at increased risk for ischemic heart disease. Regular strenuous exercise, decreased cigarette smoking, and diet rich in some fish oils (eicosapentaenoic acid) are associated with increased HDL levels, although the basis for the increase is poorly understood.

Cigarette Smoking

Cigarette smoking is one of the most common risk factors associated with increased incidence of atherosclerosis, and when it is reduced or eliminated, the risk of developing the disease decreases. Stroke, myocardial infarction, and intermittent claudication are common in male cigarette smokers, who, together with female smokers, show an increased incidence of symptoms associated with atherosclerosis. In addition to atherosclerosis of the large coronary arteries, cigarette smokers characteristically have occlusive disease of the leg arteries. There is a mean increase of approximately 70 per cent in the death rate and a three- to fivefold increase in the risk of ischemic heart disease in males who smoke more than one pack of cigarettes per day, compared with nonsmokers.

Sudden death is frequently associated with cigarette smoking, and of particular importance is the observation that cessation of cigarette smoking leads within a year to reduction of the risk of the sequelae of atherosclerosis to levels of that of nonsmokers. The basis for atherosclerosis in cigarette smokers is not well understood.

Glucose Intolerance and Diabetes Mellitus

Both insulin-dependent and non–insulin-dependent diabetics show at least a twofold increase in the incidence of myocardial infarction, compared with nondiabetics. Younger diabetics have a marked increase in the risk of atherosclerosis and thus of ischemic heart disease, and diabetic women appear to be even more prone than diabetic men. Gangrene of the lower extremities is one of the principal sequelae of atherosclerosis in diabetics. It is not clear what factors are responsible for the increased incidence of atherosclerosis in diabetes.

Hypertension

Elevation in blood pressure is an important risk factor associated with increased incidence of atherosclerosis and is of particular importance since this is a factor that is easily diagnosed and highly treatable. The risk of atherosclerosis and its sequelae increases progressively with increase in blood pressure, and when the blood pressure exceeds 160 mm Hg systolic and 95 mm Hg diastolic in middle-aged men the risk is five times greater than in normotensive men with blood pressure of 140 mm Hg systolic and 90 mm Hg diastolic or less. The increase in diastolic pressure may be more important than that in systolic pressure in both hypertensive men and women. After the age of 50, hypertension may be more important as a risk factor in predicting increased incidence of atherosclerosis than hypercholesterolemia. Recent intervention studies of individuals with hypertension have demonstrated that a reduction of diastolic pressure levels below 105 mm Hg can significantly reduce the incidence of symptomatic cerebrovascular disease, ischemic heart disease, and congestive heart failure in men (see Ch. 44). When multiple risk factors are present, including hypertension, it is particularly important to treat the hypertension, since it is the most easily accessible and treatable aspect of this disease process.

Obesity

When body weight is greater than 20 per cent above the norm, there is an increased risk of ischemic heart disease. Obesity may particularly accelerate atherosclerosis in individuals below the age of 50. Obesity is generally associated with hypertriglyceridemia, hypercholesterolemia, glucose intolerance, and hypertension.

Physical Activity

There are many studies related to the value of increased physical activity in reducing the incidence of ischemic heart disease. The Framingham Studies suggest that sedentary individuals are more susceptible to atherosclerosis and to sudden death than individuals who maintain an active lifestyle. It has been suggested that increased physical activity may elevate the level of HDL. Appropriately supervised physical training can improve exercise performance in patients with angina due to ischemic heart disease.

Genetic Factors

Clearly, genetic factors are critical in atherosclerosis. The best example of this is the increased incidence of atherosclerosis in individuals with homozygous familial hypercholesterolemia and familial combined hyperlipidemia. Other risk factors, such as hypertension and diabetes mellitus, can also be inherited, and it is possible that protective factors, such as increased HDL, may

also be inherited, although the latter is not well understood. As a consequence, family history must be included in assessing the risk for a given individual.

THE PATHOGENESIS OF THE LESIONS OF ATHEROSCLEROSIS

The lesions of atherosclerosis as they occur in the intima of the artery essentially consist of three biologic entities. First and foremost of these is an increase in the number of intimal smooth muscle cells, together with an accumulation of macrophages and variable numbers of lymphocytes. The increased number of smooth muscle cells is responsible for the second entity, the formation of large amounts of connective tissue matrix containing collagen, elastic fibers, and proteoglycans. The third entity, lipid, accumulates in hyperlipidemic individuals within the smooth muscle cells and the macrophages and in many instances causes them to develop into foam cells. Lipid also accumulates within the surrounding connective tissue matrix but may be absent from lesions of patients that are normocholesterolemic, subject to other risk factors. Thus the advanced lesions of atherosclerosis represent the culmination of a usually longstanding proliferative disease process in which it becomes important to understand the basis for the proliferation of smooth muscle, accumulation of macrophages, formation of new connective tissue, and accumulation of lipid.

The Response to Injury Hypothesis of Atherosclerosis

During the past 15 years, it has been possible to develop a hypothesis that takes into account most of what is known concerning risk factors, the biology of the artery wall, the cells involved, and the biologic processes that result in the lesions of atherosclerosis.

The response to injury hypothesis of atherosclerosis suggests that some form of "injury" affects the lining endothelial cells. The injury may alter the functional characteristics of the endothelium, leaving the endothelium morphologically intact. Thus endothelial injury could alter the permeability of the endothelium, its nonthrombogenic character, its ability to form vasoactive substances and growth factors, and its capacity to regenerate. At the other extreme, endothelial injury may lead to endothelial cell-cell disjunction and endothelial retraction, exposing the underlying connective tissue or accumulated foam cells, such as macrophages, that form the first and ubiquitous lesion of atherosclerosis, the fatty streak.

In hypercholesterolemic animals, including nonhuman primates, swine, rabbits, and rats, the first change that occurs in the artery wall is a chemotactic attraction of circulating monocytes and lymphocytes, which increasingly adhere to the surface of the endothelial cells in clusters located throughout the arterial tree. The adherent monocytes migrate on the surface of the endothelium, penetrate between endothelial junctions, localize subendothelially, accumulate lipid, and become intimal foam cells. The accumulation of these intimal lymphocytes and monocytes that become converted to lipid-laden macrophages represents the initial lesion of atherosclerosis, the fatty streak. These fatty streaks expand by continued attraction and accumulation of lymphocytes and monocytes in the artery. They also expand by migration of some smooth muscle cells from the underlying media into the intima, where they localize beneath the accumulated macrophages and also accumulate lipid.

With increasing time, level, and duration of hypercholesterolemia, endothelial cell-cell junctions separate and endothelial cells retract, permitting lipid-laden macrophages to enter the circulation and home to the spleen and lymph nodes. This occurs particularly at branches and bifurcations of the artery. Sometimes the exposed macrophages or connective tissue, or both, can be thrombogenic and induce platelets to adhere at these sites. Sites where mural thrombi have formed become loci of increased migration and proliferation of smooth muscle cells that accumulate and form large amounts of connective tissue matrix. Thus sites of platelet adherence and aggregation subsequently may become sites of intimal smooth muscle proliferation.

At other anatomic sites, the endothelium may remain intact, but the fatty streak expands by the continued attraction and accumulation of monocytes. Many of the macrophages in the lesions also synthesize DNA and replicate, further aggravating the proliferative component of the lesions.

Numerous investigations have attempted to determine what factors are responsible for the migration and proliferation of smooth muscle cells in the intima. Growth factors able to induce smooth muscle cell migration and proliferation can be formed and secreted by several cells. Of particular importance is the capacity of platelets to release growth factors and of activated macrophages to release the same as well as other types of growth factors. The growth factors that may play a critical role in atherogenesis include platelet-derived growth factor (PDGF), a potent growth factor for mesenchymal connective tissue cells such as fibroblasts and smooth muscle, and transforming growth factor beta (TGF-β), a factor that may act in an inhibitory fashion and can induce formation of large amounts of connective tissue.

PDGF is a potent mitogen that, at nanogram and picogram levels, can induce cells such as smooth muscle to multiply, and TGF-β can induce them to form new connective tissue. PDGF and TGF-β can be derived from platelets, from activated macrophages which are probably the principal cellular source of PDGF, and from appropriately stimulated or "injured" endothelial cells. Thus, if endothelial injury occurs, appropriate opportunities may be present for the release of mitogens such as PDGF

from all three cells. Such growth factor release may be related to increased incidence of atherogenesis in experimental animals. There is also evidence that smooth muscle cells, once they have been induced to proliferate in the artery wall, may in themselves be capable of expressing the gene for PDGF and of secreting this growth factor so that they may, in effect, stimulate themselves in an autocrine fashion to continue the proliferative response.

The response to injury hypothesis of atherogenesis suggests that the "injury" to the endothelium results in cellular changes that lead to a modified form of inflammation in which monocytes and lymphocytes enter the artery wall and the monocytes become macrophages that can secrete growth factors, act as scavenger cells, and accumulate lipid and become foam cells. The fatty streak then becomes converted into a smooth muscle proliferative lesion, or fibrous plaque, and probably does so by local release within the artery of growth factors derived from activated macrophages, injured endothelium, and/or platelets that may interact with the artery wall at sites where the protective cover of the endothelium may be altered. These changes are diagrammatically shown in Figure 47–2, which suggests how the lesions of atherosclerosis may form.

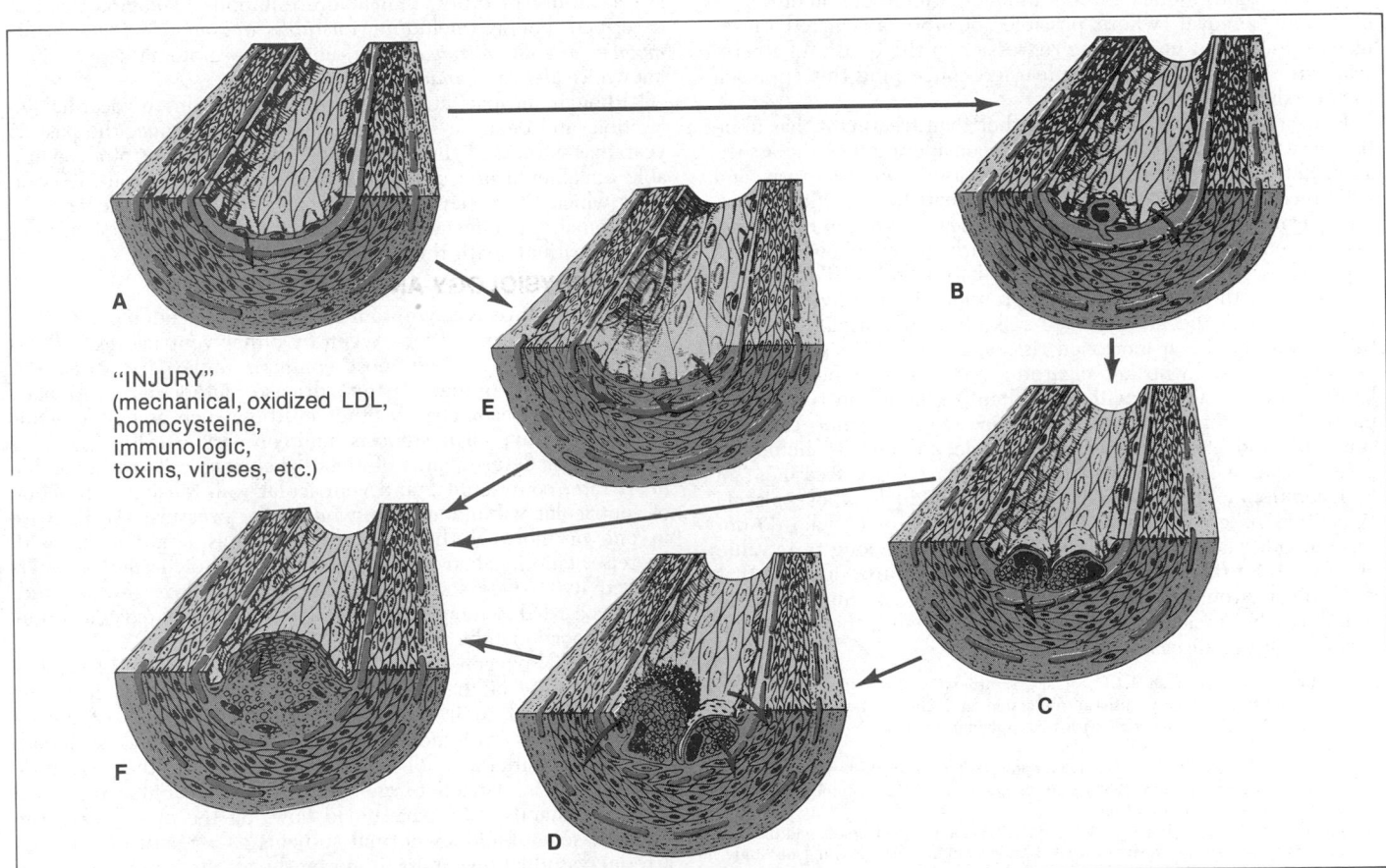

FIGURE 47–2. Endothelial injury: The response to injury hypothesis. Advanced intimal proliferative lesions of atherosclerosis may occur by at least two pathways. The pathway demonstrated by the clockwise (*long*) arrows to the right has been observed in experimentally induced hypercholesterolemia. Injury to the endothelium (*A*) may induce growth factor secretion (*short arrow*). Monocytes attach to endothelium (*B*), which may continue to secrete growth factors (*short arrow*). Subendothelial migration of monocytes (*C*) may lead to fatty streak formation and release of growth factors such as platelet-derived growth factor (PDGF) (*short arrow*). Fatty streaks may become directly converted to fibrous plaques (*long arrow* from *C* to *F*) through release of growth factors from macrophages or endothelial cells or both. Macrophages may also stimulate and/or injure the overlying endothelium. In some cases, macrophages may lose their endothelial cover and platelet attachment may occur (*D*), providing three possible sources of growth factors—platelets, macrophages, and endothelium (*short arrows*). Some of the smooth muscle cells in the proliferative lesion itself (*F*) may form and secrete growth factors such as PDGF (*short arrows*).

An alternative pathway for development of advanced lesions of atherosclerosis is shown by the arrows from *A* to *E* to *F*. In this case, the endothelium may be injured but remain intact. Increased endothelial turnover may result in growth factor formation by endothelial cells (*A*). This may stimulate migration of smooth muscle cells from the media into the intima, accompanied by endogenous production of PDGF by smooth muscle as well as growth factor secretion from the "injured" endothelial cells (*E*). These interactions could then lead to fibrous plaque formation and further lesion progression (*F*). (From Ross R: The pathogenesis of atherosclerosis—an update. N Engl J Med 314:496, 1986. Reprinted by permission of the New England Journal of Medicine.)

The response to injury hypothesis also offers an opportunity to consider means of preventing and intervening in the formation of the lesions of atherosclerosis. Clearly, alteration in lifestyle habits, including changes in dietary habits and alteration of risk factors associated with increased incidence of atherosclerosis, could be potentially important in preventing these cellular changes from occurring and possibly in inducing lesion regression.

Regression of Atherosclerosis

In experimental animals the fatty streak is clearly capable of regressing and disappearing entirely if hypercholesterolemic animals are placed on a normocholesterolemic regimen for a sufficient period of time. There is evidence to suggest that fatty streaks can also regress in humans, based upon examination of individuals who decreased their dietary intake of lipids and atherogenic foods. Fibrous plaques or complicated lesions in humans may also be partially reversible, based upon angiographic studies. It is not yet clear how far a lesion must progress before it becomes irreversible. Cessation of cigarette smoking is associated with decreased risk, and this in combination with treatment of hypertension, dietary intervention, treatment of diabetes mellitus, and removal, where possible, of other associated causes may be important in inducing regression of the lesions of atherosclerosis. More remains to be learned concerning this approach to reversing the disease process.

Prevention of atherosclerosis, rather than treatment, has to be the principal goal for all patients. In consideration of the association between hyperlipidemia and increased atherosclerosis, and with recognition of the decline in the death rate in the United States from premature ischemic heart disease, it becomes increasingly important to understand that early detection of risk and approaches toward change in dietary habits and in lifestyles are important in the prevention of atherosclerosis in individuals who may potentially be at increased risk. It is important to detect those who may be at increased risk on a familial basis, who may be hypertensive, who are cigarette smokers, or whose dietary habits could be altered with a resultant reduction in risk. Treatment of hypertension, as well as advice regarding diet, cigarette smoking, and exercise, can be valuable adjuncts to helping a patient deal with these problems. Pharmacologic treatment of hyperlipidemia should be limited to individuals whose plasma cholesterol is greater than 240 mg per deciliter or who do not respond adequately to dietary management. The long-term value of antiplatelet drugs and, potentially in the future, of drugs that may affect growth factor activity could be of importance in reducing the incidence of atherosclerosis and the long-term sequelae of this disease process.

Brown BG, Albers JJ, Fisher LD, et al.: Treatment study: A randomized trial demonstrating coronary disease regression and clinical benefit from lipid altering therapy among men with high apolipoprotein B. N Engl J Med, in press.

Brown MS, Goldstein JL: How LDL receptors influence cholesterol and atherosclerosis. Sci Am 251:158, 1984. *A discussion of how LDL receptor interactions control cholesterol metabolism.*

Gordon T, Castelli WP, Hjortland MC, et al.: Diabetes, blood lipids, and the role of obesity in coronary heart disease risk for women. The Framingham Study. Ann Intern Med 87:393, 1977.

Gordon T, Castelli WP, Hjortland MC, et al.: High density lipoprotein as a protective factor against coronary heart disease. The Framingham Study. Am J Med 62:707, 1977. *These two papers represent epidemiologic studies that relate the role of several of the principal risk factors on atherosclerosis and indicate the potential protective effect of HDL in atherosclerosis.*

Report of the Working Group on Arteriosclerosis of the National Heart, Lung, and Blood Institute. Vol. 2. Department of Health, Education and Welfare (National Institutes of Health) Publication No. 82-2035. Washington, D.C., Government Printing Office, 1981. *This represents an overview of a large number of individuals who have examined both the epidemiology and the nature of the lesions of atherosclerosis.*

Ross R: The pathogenesis of atherosclerosis—an update. N Engl J Med 314:488, 1986.

Ross R, Glomset JA: The pathogenesis of atherosclerosis. N Engl J Med 295:369, 1976. *These two papers review the anatomic structure of the artery wall, lesions of atherosclerosis, and the potential roles of the cells in atherosclerosis. They provide a hypothesis for how atherogenesis may come about.*

Steinberg D: Metabolism of lipoproteins and their role in the pathogenesis of atherosclerosis. Atherosclerosis Rev 18:1, 1988.

48 Disorders of the Coronary Arteries

48.1 ANGINA PECTORIS

William J. Rogers

Angina pectoris, a common clinical manifestation of coronary artery disease, afflicts over 3 million persons in the United States. The term "angina pectoris," derived from the Greek *ankhein* (to choke), was coined by William Heberden in 1768 to describe a clinical syndrome of exertional chest discomfort, but the cardiac origin of the syndrome was not fully appreciated until Caleb Parry proposed in 1799 that angina was due to insufficient delivery of blood to the heart muscle, particularly during exercise.

Today angina pectoris is generally defined as a discomfort within or adjacent to the chest, typically provoked by exertion or anxiety, usually lasting for several minutes, alleviated by rest, and not resulting in myocardial necrosis. Besides this common syndrome of what is often termed *classic exertional angina*, there are a variety of other clinical presentations of angina pectoris described below, including *unstable angina, variant (Prinzmetal's) angina, mixed angina,* and an asymptomatic syndrome known as *silent ischemia*.

Although incapacitating recurrent chest pain, myocardial infarction, and death are potential sequelae of angina, the past 25 years has witnessed the emergence and refinement of a remarkable armamentarium of pharmacologic and mechanical interventions which, if properly utilized, can considerably alleviate the symptomatic manifestations and extend the duration of survival of most patients with this common condition.

PATHOPHYSIOLOGY AND CLASSIFICATION

Angina pectoris is a symptom of myocardial ischemia, occurring when the requirement for oxygen by either ventricle exceeds its supply (Fig. 48–1). The most common underlying disease is atherosclerotic coronary artery disease, although occasionally angina occurs secondary to other entities, such as hypertrophic cardiomyopathy, aortic stenosis, and coronary arteritis.

The major determinants of myocardial oxygen demand include heart rate, contractility, and ventricular wall tension, a function of ventricular volume and intraventricular pressure. An increase in one or more of these determinants—as might occur with exercise, emotional stress, or other states of heightened adrenergic activity—triggers an increase in myocardial oxygen demand, and myocardial ischemia results unless myocardial oxygen supply rises proportionately.

Myocardial oxygen supply is governed by coronary blood flow and the ability of the myocardium to extract oxygen from the blood delivered to it. Unlike other organs, the heart always extracts oxygen with near maximal efficiency from the blood, even under situations of minimal demand, so there is little potential for enhanced oxygen extraction to counter increased oxygen demands. Coronary blood flow, on the other hand, can increase several-fold in normal subjects as a result of coronary arterial vasodilation, most importantly at the arteriolar level, triggered by the local build-up of lactate, adenosine, and other vasoactive substances as myocardial oxygen demands increase.

In the presence of obstructive coronary artery disease, myocardial ischemia may result when the coronary arterial stenosis prevents autoregulatory vasodilation so that coronary blood flow can no longer increase proportional to rising oxygen demands. In other situations, myocardial ischemia may occur when oxygen demands are constant but there is a *primary decrease in coronary blood flow* mediated via (1) coronary artery spasm, (2) rapid evolution of the underlying atherosclerotic plaque (plaque disruption) leading to a reduced coronary arterial lumen caliber, and/or (3) intermittent microvascular plugging by platelet aggregates.

In some patients with *exertional angina*, ischemia is primarily a manifestation of increased oxygen demands in the face of fixed coronary blood flow, whereas in patients with primary *vasospastic angina*, ischemia results when coronary artery spasm causes blood flow to diminish in the face of stable oxygen demands. However,

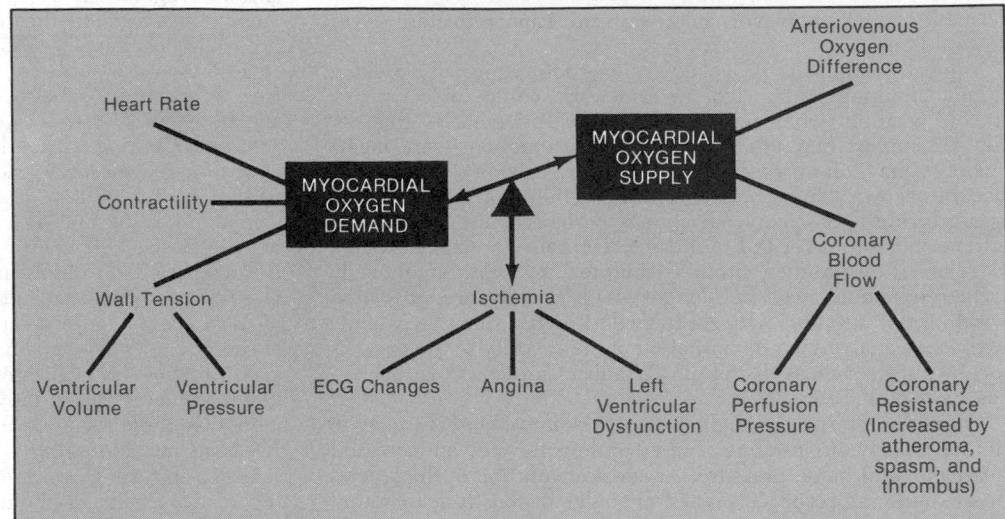

FIGURE 48–1. Ischemia occurs when oxygen demand exceeds supply.

many, if not most, patients fall between these two extremes, experiencing angina as a result of both heightened oxygen demands and diminished supply, and are said to have *mixed angina.*

As shown in Figure 48–1, angina is but one manifestation of myocardial ischemia. Ischemia typically begins in the subendocardium, where wall tension is high and compressive forces limit coronary microvascular flow, and then spreads like a wavefront toward the epicardium. The electrocardiogram often depicts ST-segment depression or T-wave inversion as manifestations of subendocardial ischemia but may show ST-segment elevation (injury current) if ischemia is prolonged and extends transmurally. These electrocardiographic changes may occur without typical anginal symptoms, a condition termed *silent ischemia.*

Segmental left ventricular contraction abnormalities occur in the region of the myocardium served by the coronary arterial branches distal to the stenosis responsible for the ischemia (the culprit lesion), and, if about 10 per cent or more of the myocardium is rendered ischemic, a reduction in global function of the left ventricle may be detectable. In addition to abnormal systolic function during ischemia, increased diastolic stiffness of the left ventricle manifests by a rising left ventricular end-diastolic pressure and rising pulmonary venous pressure. Consequently, transient clinical evidence of left ventricular failure may occur during episodic ischemia and may explain why many patients describe their angina not as pain but as a feeling of "breathlessness" or "chest tightness."

It is prognostically and clinically useful to classify anginal syndromes into stable and unstable categories. *Unstable angina* refers to angina of recent onset (within 2 months) or angina that has begun to intensify or to occur at rest or with a lower level of exertion within the previous 2 months. *Stable angina,* as the name implies, describes a relatively constant pattern of pain with regard to its severity and precipitating factors within the recent months. Some authorities classify angina of recent onset as "stable angina" if it is precipitated by moderate or severe levels of exertion and maintains a constant threshold over time, because "stable angina" has to begin at some point in time.

Of patients with unstable angina, up to 20 per cent progress to acute myocardial infarction within the next 3 months. Coronary angiography and angioscopy reveal that more than 50 per cent of patients with unstable angina have multivessel disease with eccentric, irregular, or ulcerated atherosclerotic lesions associated with endothelial disruption and adherent thrombus. Left main coronary artery disease occurs in about 10 per cent of patients with unstable angina. It is likely that unstable angina represents a point on a continuum between stable exertional angina and acute myocardial infarction.

Variant angina, originally described by Printzmetal, is characterized by rest pain accompanied by transient ST-segment changes (often ST elevation resembling acute myocardial infarction, although ST depression can also occur) and ventricular arrhythmias. Variant angina is a form of unstable angina caused by coronary arterial spasm, usually within a coronary artery narrowed by plaque, but occasionally within an angiographically normal appearing artery.

HISTORY AND PHYSICAL EXAMINATION

The diagnosis of angina pectoris often requires considerable clinical skill because there is no totally specific symptom, physical finding, or laboratory examination to confirm its presence. The history is probably the most powerful tool for diagnosing angina and provides the skilled interviewer an assessment of both the stability (or instability) of the syndrome as well as its severity (Table 48–1). The patient should be instructed to describe the chest discomfort according to its character, location, radiation, duration, precipitating and alleviating factors, accompanying symptoms, and change in pattern over the past few weeks or days.

As indicated above, the typical *history* is that of exertional chest discomfort of several minutes duration alleviated by rest. The discomfort typically involves the region of the sternum (substernal or, more properly, retrosternal location) but may instead manifest itself in any region between the jaw and epigastrium. Commonly the discomfort radiates to the shoulders or arms, especially the left, to the neck or jaw, and less commonly to the back or epigastrium. Most patients perceive angina as a deep or visceral (rather than superficial) sensation and describe it as a "tightness," "heaviness," or "choking sensation" rather than as a definite pain. The discomfort is usually of several minutes duration; discomfort of less than 1 minute's duration is rarely angina, and discomfort at full intensity exceeding 20 minutes in duration should arouse suspicion of myocardial infarction or discomfort unrelated to myocardial ischemia. The pain of

TABLE 48–1. CANADIAN CARDIOVASCULAR CLASSIFICATION OF ANGINA SEVERITY*

Class	Signs
I	"Ordinary physical activity does not cause . . . angina, such as walking and climbing stairs. Angina with strenuous or rapid or prolonged exertion at work or recreation."
II	"Slight limitation of ordinary activity. Walking or climbing stairs rapidly, walking uphill, walking or stair climbing after meals, or in cold, or in wind, or under emotional stress, or only during the few hours after awakening. Walking more than two blocks on the level and climbing more than one flight of ordinary stairs at a normal pace and in normal conditions."
III	"Marked limitation of ordinary physical activity. Walking one to two blocks on the level and climbing one flight of stairs in normal conditions and at normal pace."
IV	"Inability to carry on any physical activity without discomfort—anginal syndrome *may be* present at rest."

*From Campeau L: Grading of angina pectoris. Circulation 54:522, 1976. Reproduced by permission of the American Heart Association, Inc.

unstable angina, however, may wax and wane repeatedly over several hours.

Typically angina is provoked by exertion, especially walking uphill, climbing stairs, vigorous arm work, coitus, or exercising in cold weather (when peripheral vascular resistance is greater). The discomfort may also be provoked by emotion (fear, anger, anxiety), may follow a meal, or may occur on lying down (angina decubitus) owing to increased ventricular filling pressure, or may occur during sleep (nocturnal angina), perhaps owing to increased adrenergic output related to dreams. Typically, exertional angina is relieved promptly (within 5 minutes) by rest; emotionally triggered angina may last longer; both usually are alleviated within 3 to 5 minutes with sublingual nitroglycerin. For patients with exertional angina, quantitation of the severity of the discomfort by a scale such as that of the Canadian Cardiovascular Society can be useful (Table 48–1).

During an episode of angina, *the physical examination* may be normal or may disclose one or more of the following: an increased heart rate and blood pressure; paradoxical splitting of the second heart sound; a precordial presystolic bulge or fourth heart sound (S_4), both due to enhanced atrial contraction into a ventricle rendered stiff by ischemia; a systolic bulge due to left ventricular dyskinesis; a diastolic bulge or S_3 gallop as evidence of significant left ventricular failure; a mid- to late-systolic murmur of mitral regurgitation related to ischemia-induced mitral papillary muscle dysfunction; or transient rales or other evidence of pulmonary venous congestion.

Other conditions that should be considered in the *differential diagnosis* of angina include the following: gastrointestinal disease—especially disordered esophageal motility, gastroesophageal reflux, peptic ulcer disease, and cholecystitis; exertional bronchospasm related to asthmatic bronchitis; chest wall discomfort related to costochondritis, muscle spasm, herpes zoster, or anxiety states, the last often presenting as submammary sharp pain of a few seconds' duration; and other cardiac and vascular diseases such as pericarditis, myocardial infarction, aortic dissection, or pulmonary embolism. These should be readily distinguished from angina in most cases by a detailed history, physical examination, and appropriate laboratory tests.

LABORATORY EVALUATION

Certain laboratory studies may help to establish a diagnosis of angina pectoris by confirming the presence and extent of underlying coronary artery disease.

ELECTROCARDIOGRAM. Although often normal at baseline, the electrocardiogram (ECG) *during* an episode of spontaneous or provoked angina may demonstrate horizontal or downsloping depression of the ST segment, T-wave peaking or inversion, and, rarely, transient ST-segment elevation. Such ECG changes, when transitory and accompanied by typical anginal discomfort, make the diagnosis of myocardial ischemia with a high degree of confidence. However, taken alone, and occurring on the resting ECG, such ST and T-wave changes are regarded as nonspecific because they accompany many other conditions including hyperventilation, electrolyte abnormalities, left ventricular hypertrophy, pericarditis, myocarditis, and the administration of digitalis and other drugs.

EXERCISE ECG. The exercise ECG or graded exercise test is a widely used clinical provocative test for myocardial ischemia in which the patient is required to exercise, usually on a treadmill or bicycle, at gradually increasing workloads until ischemic electrocardiographic changes, angina, or other limiting symptoms occur. With the increasing workload of progressive exercise, heart rate and systolic blood pressure should rise. The product of heart rate and systolic blood pressure (the double product) correlates with myocardial oxygen demand and defines an anginal threshold for a given subject. During exercise a clinically positive response is the occurrence of typical anginal chest discomfort, whereas an electrocardiographically positive response is the occurrence of 0.1 mV horizontal or downsloping ST depression at 0.08 second after the J point of the ECG.

The sensitivity of the graded exercise test for diagnosing coronary artery disease ranges from 54 to 94 per cent and is greatest in patients with the most extensive coronary artery disease. The specificity (negative test when coronary disease is absent) ranges from 67 to 97 per cent. False-positive tests are *more common* when the test is utilized in patients with a low probability of coronary disease (as for example, with the screening of asymptomatic subjects), and false-positive exercise tests are *least common* in patients with a history of typical exertional angina.

Exercise testing is useful not only for diagnosing the presence of obstructive coronary artery disease, but also for following the natural course of the disease in patients with chronic stable angina, detecting high-risk coronary artery disease, and estimating prognosis. Left main or multivessel coronary artery disease is suggested by exercise-induced hypotension, by 3.0-mm or more ST-segment depression, by downsloping ST segments, and by ischemic ST depression occurring within the first 3 minutes of exercise and/or persisting 5 or more minutes after exercise. A good prognosis is suggested by a negative exercise test or one that becomes positive only after the patient has exercised for more than three stages (> 9 minutes), or to a heart rate exceeding 160 beats per minute.

Exercise testing is generally safe; experienced laboratories report a mortality of about 1 per 10,000 tests and a morbidity requiring hospitalization of 2.4 per 10,000. Exercise testing should not be performed in patients with significant aortic stenosis, hypertension, congestive heart failure, or unstable angina, and, when exercise testing is performed, resuscitative equipment should be immediately available.

RADIONUCLIDE STUDIES. Two radionuclide-enhanced accompaniments to exercise testing are commonly utilized: myocardial perfusion imaging and radionuclide ventriculography. These tests may localize the ischemic myocardial zone and are not influenced by factors that alter interpretation of the baseline ECG such as ST-T wave changes.

Exercise myocardial perfusion imaging utilizes a radionuclide (commonly, the potassium analogue, thallium-201) that, after intravenous injection during peak treadmill exercise, distributes to the myocardium via the coronary arterial circulation and is taken up rapidly by viable myocardium in proportion to coronary blood flow. Immediate imaging discloses perfusion defects (cold spots) in zones of myocardial ischemia or prior infarction (scar). Regions of myocardial perfusion deficit correlate with severe stenosis of the coronary artery supplying the region: i.e., septum—left anterior descending coronary artery; inferior wall—right coronary artery; posterolateral wall—left circumflex coronary artery. Repeat imaging 3 to 4 hours later (more reliably, 24 hours later) shows uptake of the radionuclide by previously ischemic zones, but not by zones of prior infarction, allowing differentiation of the two. For patients unable to exercise, a dipyridamole thallium examination (investigational) may be performed; patients are administered intravenous dipyridamole, which produces vasodilation of normal or minimally atherosclerotic coronary arteries, often stealing coronary blood flow from stenotic vessels and creating regional myocardial ischemia. Thallium-201 is then injected, and imaging is performed and interpreted in a manner analogous to that for exercise thallium-201 studies.

Exercise radionuclide ventriculography consists of imaging the left ventricular blood pool first at rest and then with exercise. Imaging is performed by either the "first-pass technique," in which there is injection of a large bolus of radionuclide (commonly, technetium-99m) and assessment of cardiac blood pool activity over the next few beats as the tracer is cleared, or by the multigated equilibrium technique (MUGA), in which the red blood cells are labeled with a radionuclide and composite left ventricular function is estimated from all beats occurring during the next several minutes' observation. In most normal subjects, systolic function of the left ventricle increases during exercise, and ejection fraction (ratio of stroke volume to end-diastolic volume) rises by 0.05 or greater. Myocardial ischemia is suggested if the ejection fraction with exercise fails to rise by 0.05, if it falls, or if segmental left ventricular wall motion abnormalities appear during exercise.

In general, the radionuclide enhancements to exercise testing are expensive and are not routinely required. Perfusion scintigraphy or radionuclide ventriculography can, however, be useful in interpreting the physiologic significance of angiographically proven coronary lesions, in assessing equivocal or suspected false-positive conventional exercise tests, in evaluating patients with chest pain following coronary revascularization surgery or angioplasty, in screening for residual ischemia in patients following myocardial infarction, and in assessing patients with abnormal ECG findings (e.g., left bundle branch block). Echocardiographic imaging of regional ventricular wall motion has been used in a manner analogous to radionuclide ventriculography.

CORONARY ARTERIOGRAPHY. Coronary arteriography, the selective visualization of the major epicardial coronary arteries by radiographic contrast material, is the most precise means currently available to document the presence and extent of obstructive coronary artery disease. The results of coronary arteriography coupled with assessment of left ventricular systolic function (ejection fraction) provide powerful prognostic information concerning the natural history of coronary artery disease and, along with the clinical evaluation, can suggest the need for coronary artery revascularization by angioplasty or bypass graft surgery.

Coronary arteriography is indicated in patients with angina whose symptoms are severe (class III to IV) or unstable, in patients with angina or other evidence of myocardial ischemia following myocardial infarction, and in many patients with recurrent chest pain of uncertain etiology. Coronary arteriography is also often performed in certain categories of patients in whom angina may or may not be present, for example, those over age 40 about to undergo cardiac valve replacement or other noncoronary cardiac surgery, those with refractory ventricular arrhythmias, survivors of out-of-hospital cardiac arrest, those with heart failure thought secondary to coronary artery disease, and those with convincing electrocardiographic evidence of extensive ischemia, either during exercise testing or during electrocardiographic monitoring at rest or during normal daily activities.

Coronary artery stenoses of 70 per cent or greater diameter narrowing are generally considered flow limiting and thus clinically significant; however, coronary stenoses may be considerably underestimated on arteriography. If the coronary arteriograms are normal, the smooth muscle constrictor, ergonovine maleate, may be carefully administered intravenously in an attempt to evoke angiographic and electrocardiographic evidence of localized coronary arterial spasm in patients suspected of having coronary vasospasm.

The risks of coronary arteriography are low and are related to the skill and experience of the operator and to the severity of the patient's cardiac disease; complications are increased in patients with severe left main coronary artery disease and in those with severe left ventricular dysfunction. Experienced operators report procedural mortality in 0.2 per cent, myocardial infarction in 0.25 per cent, embolization in 0.1 per cent, and severe vascular complication at the entry site in 0.7 per cent.

GENERAL MANAGEMENT

Patients diagnosed with angina pectoris should be counseled concerning the potential serious and unpredictable nature of the condition but also advised that powerful new pharmacologic and mechanical interventions are available that may ameliorate symptoms and, in many cases, extend survival. Patients with unstable angina should undergo hospital admission to rule out myocardial infarction, to receive intensive pharmacologic therapy, and, in most cases, to undergo coronary arteriography. All patients with angina should be thoroughly instructed in risk factor modification, particularly dietary management of cholesterol and saturated fat intake, smoking cessation, and blood pressure control. A search should be made for potentially correctable conditions such as aortic stenosis, severe anemia, thyrotoxicosis, and tachyarrhythmias that might be contributing to the myocardial oxygen supply/demand imbalance causing angina.

PHARMACOLOGIC THERAPY

The goals of pharmacologic therapy of angina pectoris are to restore the imbalance between myocardial oxygen demand and supply by reducing oxygen demands, increasing coronary blood flow, or both. The most important categories of antianginal drugs are the nitrates, β blockers, and calcium channel blockers. Additionally, patients with unstable angina benefit from heparin and aspirin.

NITRATES. Nitrates alleviate angina predominantly by reducing oxygen demands, but they may improve coronary blood flow as well. Nitrates reduce oxygen demands by relaxing vascular smooth muscle, producing venodilation at low dosages but arterial and arteriolar dilation as well at higher dosages. Their major effect at usual dosages is peripheral venous pooling, which diminishes systemic venous return, thus reducing left ventricular end-diastolic pressure and volume, left ventricular wall tension, and myocardial oxygen demands. To a lesser extent, the diminished peripheral arteriolar resistance lessens myocardial oxygen demands by reducing systemic blood pressure and left ventricular wall tension. Unfortunately, the fall in systemic blood pressure may trigger a slight rise in heart rate, which augments oxygen demands. Nitrates may also improve coronary blood flow by dilating coronary vessels, reversing or preventing coronary spasm, and enhancing collateral blood flow. Furthermore, the effect on lowering left ventricular end-diastolic pressure, noted above, may allow better perfusion of subendocardial tissue.

The most commonly used nitrate preparations are nitroglycerin and isosorbide dinitrate. Nitroglycerin is available in a variety of formulations: intravenous, topical, buccal, oral, sublingual, and lingual aerosol (Table 48–2), each with different onset and duration of action. For an acute anginal attack, one of the rapidly acting preparations such as sublingual nitroglycerin is preferable, whereas for chronic prophylaxis of angina a longer-acting nitroglycerin formulation such as isosorbide dinitrate is helpful. Failure to respond to long-acting nitrates may occur if inadequate doses are utilized; however, to minimize adverse reactions, these preparations should be initiated at low doses and then titrated upward until the desired clinical response or limiting side effects occur. Topical nitroglycerin paste can be an effective formulation but, for optimal absorption, it should be spread over a wide area of skin rather than concentrated beneath the applicator paper. Intravenous nitroglycerin is useful in the treatment of unstable angina in hospitalized patients. The drug is usually begun at doses of 10 to 20 μg per minute and titrated upward by dosage increments of 10 to 20 μg at intervals of 10 to 15 minutes until chest pain is controlled or until limiting side effects, such as hypotension, occur. Once pain is stabilized with intravenous nitroglycerin, substitution of one of the long-acting preparations can usually be accomplished.

Adverse reactions to nitrate administration include cutaneous flushing, headaches, postural dizziness, nausea, and vomiting. Attenuation or resolution of these side effects usually occurs with continued administration of the drug. Nitrate tolerance or hyporesponsiveness has been noted with preparations providing constant plasma levels over many hours. It is believed that nitrate tolerance can be prevented by using the smallest effective dose of nitrate, by using less frequent dosing, and by allowing a nitrate-free interval of 8 to 12 hours daily. For example, sustained release isosorbide dinitrate produces less tolerance when administered at 8:00 AM and 2:00 PM than when given at 8:00 AM and 8:00 PM; furthermore, nitroglycerin patches are more apt to retain effectiveness if there is an overnight patch-free interval.

BETA BLOCKERS. Beta-adrenergic blockers alleviate angina predominantly by reducing oxygen demand. These drugs competitively inhibit the action of catecholamines on β receptors throughout the body. By blocking the β_1 or cardiac β receptor, these agents lower heart rate, blood pressure, and myocardial contractility, three major determinants of myocardial oxygen utilization, and thus attenuate the rise in oxygen consumption normally occurring during exercise. By slowing the heart rate, β blockers also prolong diastole, allowing more time for diastolic coronary perfusion to occur, thus indirectly augmenting coronary flow.

Many β blockers are currently available (Table 48–3) in the United States, and each has the potential to diminish angina, although not all of them are currently approved for the treatment of angina. The available agents differ according to various pharmacologic properties, and these differences may favor the use of one agent over another in certain clinical situations.

For example, cardioselectivity, a feature of some β blockers, permits selective blockade of the cardiac β_1 receptor and is potentially advantageous in patients with reactive airways disease

TABLE 48–2. AVAILABLE DOSAGE FORMS OF NITROGLYCERIN AND ISOSORBIDE DINITRATE

Medication	Dosage Form	Recommended Dosage	Onset of Action (min)	Antianginal Duration
Nitroglycerin	Intravenous	Start at 10–20 μg/min	Immediate	Transient
	Aerosol spray	0.4 mg	2	10–30 min
	Sublingual	0.3–0.8 mg	2–5	10–30 min
	Transmucosal (buccal)	1–3 mg	2–5	30–300 min
	Oral sustained release	6.5–19.5 mg	15–45	2–6 h
	Topical ointment, 2%	1.2–5.0 cm	15–60	3–8 h
	Transdermal disc or patch	10–30 mg/24 h	30–60	Up to 24 h
Isosorbide dinitrate	Sublingual	2.5–10 mg	5–20	45–120 min
	Oral	20–60 mg	15–45	2–6 h
	Oral sustained release	40 mg	15–45	Up to 8 h

*Modified from Abrams J: Am J Med 74(Suppl 6B):85–94, 1983; with permission.

who are dependent upon chronic β_2 stimulation. Selectivity is lost, however, as the dose of the cardioselective β blockers is increased; furthermore, patients with true asthma rarely tolerate β blockade, regardless of the agent used. Beta blockers with longer half-life allow once-daily dosing and, theoretically, promote better patient compliance. The ultrashort-acting intravenous β blocker esmolol may be useful in patients, including those with unstable angina, in whom rapid onset of action is desired and in whom rapid reversal would be advantageous should adverse hemodynamic effects occur. Finally, agents with partial agonist activity (intrinsic sympathomimetic activity [ISA]) activate the β receptor minimally at rest, when adrenergic tone is low, but predominantly block the β receptor under situations of heightened adrenergic tone, such as exercise or anxiety. These agents are less apt to slow the resting heart rate than non-ISA β blockers, but might prove less useful in patients with unstable or rest angina because of their weak agonist activity. Unlike other β blockers, ISA β blockers have not uniformly shown potential for improving survival in patients following myocardial infarction.

For the treatment of angina, β blockers are generally administered orally in small doses and titrated upward at 1- to 2-day intervals until clinical benefit is observed, an adverse reaction occurs, or some physiologic marker of β blockade is noted, such as a slowing of the resting heart rate to 50 to 60 beats per minute. Side effects include bradycardia, hypotension, atrioventricular (AV) block, heart failure, and central nervous system complaints (fatigue, depression, nightmares). Beta blockers are, of course, contraindicated in patients already having any of those findings. Beta blockers may contribute to lack of recognition of hypoglycemia and are thus relatively contraindicated in patients with brittle diabetes. Discontinuation of β blocker therapy should be done by gradual tapering because rebound unstable angina and myocardial infarction may occur with sudden cessation.

CALCIUM CHANNEL BLOCKERS. Calcium channel blockers alleviate angina by reducing myocardial oxygen demands as well as by increasing coronary blood flow. Calcium channel blockers limit the uptake of calcium by vascular smooth muscle and cardiac muscle required for excitation-contraction coupling, and thereby produce systemic arteriolar dilation, systemic venodilation, and reduced inotropism, all of which reduce myocardial oxygen demands. Furthermore, coronary arteries are dilated and spasm is opposed, thus enhancing myocardial oxygen delivery.

The available calcium channel blockers have considerable dissimilarity in chemical structure and adverse clinical actions (Table 48–4). Two of the agents, verapamil and diltiazem, reduce sinus node automaticity, decrease AV conduction, and thus often slow the resting heart rate. Nicardipine and nifedipine, on the other hand, are potent arterial dilators, often causing mild hypotension and reflex sinus tachycardia. All of the calcium channel blockers should be used with caution in patients with significant impairment of systolic left ventricular function (ejection fraction less than 30 per cent) and discontinued if heart failure worsens. Mild peripheral edema is common with nicardipine and nifedipine, constipation is common with verapamil, and AV block may occur in response to verapamil or diltiazem, especially with concomitant β blocker use and in patients with baseline conduction abnormalities. Serum digoxin levels may also rise upon institution of a calcium channel blocker, especially verapamil.

Calcium channel blockers are of particular benefit in patients with vasospastic or mixed angina but are also effective in those having exertional angina. Therapy is generally begun with the doses shown in Table 48–4 and gradually advanced over 2- to 3-day intervals until symptoms or other evidence of ischemia improves or until a limiting adverse reaction occurs.

COMBINATION THERAPY AND CHOICE OF AGENT. The antianginal therapy preferred in a given clinical situation may be dictated by the type of anginal presentation and by concomitant medical conditions (Table 48–5). Therapy is usually begun with sublingual nitroglycerin for treatment of acute anginal attacks and a sustained release nitrate preparation for anginal prophylaxis, owing to the relatively low cost and reasonably low side effect profile of these agents. In most patients, angina is incompletely controlled with nitrates alone, necessitating the use of a second drug. For patients having exertional angina, β blockers

TABLE 48–3. BETA BLOCKERS AVAILABLE IN THE UNITED STATES*

Medication	Approved for Angina	Cardioselective	ISA	Primary Clearance	Half-Life (hrs)	Usual Dosage[1]
Acebutolol	No	Yes	Yes	Renal	3–4	400 mg qd
Atenolol	No	Yes	No	Renal	6–9	50 mg qd
Carteolol	No	No	Yes	Renal	5–6	2.5 mg qd
Esmolol	No	Yes	No	N/A	0.15	50 μg/kg/min[3]
Labetalol[2]	No	No	No	Hepatic	6–8	200 mg bid
Metoprolol	Yes	Yes	No	Hepatic	3–7	100 mg qd
Nadolol	Yes	No	No	Renal	20–24	40 mg qd
Penbutolol	No	No	Yes	Renal	5	20 mg qd
Pindolol	No	No	Yes	Both	3–4	10 mg bid
Propranolol	Yes	No	No	Hepatic	4	60 mg bid
Timolol	No	No	No	Both	4–5	10 mg bid

*Modified from The Medical Letter 31:71, 1989; with permission.
[1]Listed, except for esmolol, are the lowest maintenance doses for control of hypertension.
[2]Labetalol also has α_1 selectivity.
[3]Lowest dose for control of supraventricular tachycardia.

TABLE 48–4. CALCIUM CHANNEL BLOCKERS AVAILABLE IN THE UNITED STATES*

Medication	Initial Dosage	Resting Heart Rate	AV Block	Edema	Constipation
			Unique Adverse Reactions[2]		
Diltiazem	30 mg qid	Decreased	+ +	+	No
Sustained release	60–120 mg bid[1]				
Nicardipine	20 mg tid	Increased	No	+ + +	No
Nifedipine	10 mg tid	Increased	No	+ + +	No
Sustained release	30 mg qd				
Verapamil	80 mg tid	Decreased	+ + +	+	Yes
Sustained release	240 mg qd[1]				

*Modified from The Medical Letter 31:41–42, 1989; with permission.
[1]Initial dosage recommended for treatment of hypertension.
[2]All calcium channel blockers can cause hypotension and exacerbate heart failure.

may be combined with nitrates and often prove synergistic; i.e., β blockers prevent the nitrate-induced reflex tachycardia while the vasodilating action of nitrates reduces the tendency of β blockers to precipitate heart failure. For patients suspected of having vasospastic or mixed angina, a combination of nitrates and a calcium channel blocker is often effective. For patients having recurrent angina despite two-drug therapy, addition of the third drug (triple therapy) is often employed. For patients with persistent systems, attention should be directed toward maximizing the dose of each agent while considering the feasibility of mechanical revascularization.

ANTIPLATELET AND ANTITHROMBIN THERAPY. With the recognition that intracoronary thrombosis is often present in patients with unstable angina has come the demonstration that both aspirin and heparin may be protective against adverse events, including progression to myocardial infarction and death in patients with unstable angina. Unless there are contraindications, therefore, all patients with unstable angina should receive aspirin 325 mg daily. Hospitalized unstable angina patients should be treated with intravenous heparin with or without concomitant aspirin. The role of thrombolytic therapy for unstable angina is speculative and the subject of ongoing clinical trials. Once unstable angina stabilizes with medical therapy, angioplasty, or bypass surgery, daily aspirin therapy should be maintained for 1 year or longer.

CORONARY REVASCULARIZATION

Pharmacologic therapy, when used aggressively, can control the symptoms of angina in many patients and return them to a normal or nearly normal lifestyle. However, many physicians and patients elect to proceed with mechanical interventions for improving coronary blood flow—coronary artery bypass surgery or percutaneous transluminal coronary angioplasty. These procedures are each being performed in more than 200,000 patients annually in the United States.

TABLE 48–5. CHOICE OF ANTIANGINAL THERAPY

Situation	Choice of Therapy[1]
Type of anginal presentation	
Stable exertional angina	N, BB, CaB
Unstable angina[2]	N, CaB, BB
Vasospastic angina	N, CaB
Concomitant conditions in patient	
with angina	
Hypertension	BB, CaB
Diabetes	N, CaB
Heart failure	N, BB,[3] CaB[3]
AV block	N, nicardipine, or nifedipine
COPD, peripheral vascular disease	N, CaB, cardioselective BB[3]
Bradyarrhythmias	N, nicardipine, or nifedipine
Tachyarrhythmias	BB, diltiazem, or verapamil
Recent myocardial infarction	BB, ASA

[1]Drug of first choice for monotherapy is listed first. Combination therapy may also be used in most instances.
[2]Aspirin and intravenous heparin are also useful in unstable angina.
[3]Use with caution in this situation.
Abbreviations: BB = β blocker; CaB = calcium channel blocker; N = nitrate.

Coronary artery bypass surgery, popularized as a treatment for ischemic heart disease approximately 20 years ago, consists of anastomosing a reversed segment of saphenous vein between the ascending aorta and one or more stenotic coronary arteries. The procedure carries an operative mortality of approximately 1 to 3 per cent, higher in patients with disease of the left main coronary artery, with significant left ventricular dysfunction and with age greater than 65 years. Perioperative myocardial infarction occurs in 2.5 to 10 per cent of the patients. About 10 per cent of the grafts occlude within the first year postoperatively, 2 per cent occlude per year during the next 6 years, and 5 per cent occlude per year over the next 5 years. Owing to graft occlusion and progression of coronary artery disease in native vessels, angina recurs in 2 to 4 per cent of patients each year postoperatively. Recently, following the demonstration of lower rates of graft occlusion (1 per cent per year or less), internal mammary arteries rather than free saphenous vein grafts have been utilized as conduits, especially for left anterior descending artery revascularization.

Percutaneous transluminal coronary angioplasty was introduced by Gruentzig in 1979, primarily as a treatment for isolated, discrete, noncalcified, proximal stenoses in patients with single-vessel disease. As equipment has improved and operator experience has grown, the range of coronary artery lesions approachable by balloon angioplasty has expanded to encompass almost the entire spectrum formerly managed by bypass surgery. Currently, the only categories of patients having coronary artery disease in whom angioplasty is contraindicated are those with minimal coronary narrowing (no lesion of 60 per cent or greater diameter stenosis), left main stenoses, and severe diffuse multivessel disease. Angioplasty should not be performed unless in-hospital cardiovascular surgery backup is available.

Elective angioplasty is successful initially in approximately 90 per cent of patients; failures are due primarily to inability to cross the lesion with the balloon catheter or to abrupt reclosure of the vessel by dissection or thrombus following dilation. Procedure-related complications of elective angioplasty are as follows: death, 1 per cent; myocardial infarction, 4 to 5 per cent; emergency bypass surgery, 4 to 5 per cent. Complications are higher with emergency procedures, with multivessel disease, or when angioplasty is performed on complex (eccentric, angulated, or long) atherosclerotic lesions. A major limitation of coronary angioplasty is restenosis of the dilated artery in 25 to 30 per cent of patients, usually occurring within the first 6 months following angioplasty and usually amenable to repeat angioplasty.

Patients having balloon angioplasty have much shorter hospitalizations than those undergoing bypass surgery and are probably more likely to return to gainful employment. However, the long-term role of angioplasty compared to bypass surgery is unknown, particularly for patients having multivessel disease. The direct comparison of these two revascularization modalities in such patients is the subject of ongoing randomized clinical trials.

Revascularization with either angioplasty or bypass surgery is unequivocally indicated under two circumstances: (1) to alleviate incapacitating angina when medications have failed, and (2) to improve survival in certain patient subsets. Bypass surgery has been shown to improve longevity compared to continued medical therapy in patients with greater than 50 per cent stenosis of the left main coronary artery, in those with three-vessel coronary artery disease and abnormal ventricular function (ejection fraction between about 30 and 50 per cent), in those with multivessel disease with proximal left anterior descending artery involvement, and in those with residual ischemia (spontaneous or exercise-provoked) following myocardial infarction. Continued medical therapy rather than mechanical revascularization is recommended for patients with minimally obstructive (< 60 per cent diameter stenosis) coronary artery disease, especially if coronary artery spasm is suspected; for patients with chest pain atypical for angina and lacking confirmation of ischemia by objective testing; for patients without left main disease who have normal ejection fraction and good symptomatic response to antianginal therapy; for patients with left main coronary artery stenoses less than 50 per cent; for patients with prior bypass surgery and chest pain but without objective evidence of ischemia; for patients with severe left ventricular dysfunction (ejection fraction less than 20 per cent) whose primary limitation is heart failure rather than myocardial ischemia; and for elderly patients (>75 years) who have coronary disease but lack disabling angina.

Conti CR, Hill JA, Mayfield WR: Unstable angina pectoris: Pathogenesis and management. Curr Probl Cardiol 14:551–623, 1989. *A comprehensive summary of recent clinical experience in managing unstable angina with pharmacologic therapy, angioplasty, and bypass surgery.*

Frye RL, Fisher L, Schaff HV, et al.: Randomized trials in coronary artery bypass surgery. Prog Cardiovasc Dis 30:1, 1987. *A survey of the important randomized clinical trials comparing bypass surgery with continued medical therapy for patients with coronary artery disease.*

Hill JA, Pepine CJ: Silent myocardial ischemia. Annu Rev Med 39:213–219, 1988. *Most myocardial ischemia is asymptomatic, occurs during normal daily activities, and has prognosis, in general, similar to that of painful ischemia.*

Julian DG (ed.): Angina Pectoris. New York, Churchill Livingstone, 1985. *An exhaustive discussion of the historical background, epidemiology, prognosis, hemodynamics, clinical classification, physical examination, laboratory findings, and medical and surgical management of angina pectoris.*

Weiner DA, Frishman WH (eds.): Therapy of Angina Pectoris. A Comprehensive Guide for the Clinician. New York, Marcel Dekker, Inc., 1985. *An extensive description of the pathophysiology, clinical evaluation, and pharmacologic and mechanical therapy of angina pectoris.*

Willerson JT: Selection of patients for coronary arteriography. Circulation 72 (Suppl V):V3–V22, 1985. *A discussion of the various categories of patients commonly undergoing coronary arteriography and the rationale for each.*

48.2 ACUTE MYOCARDIAL INFARCTION

Burton E. Sobel

DEFINITIONS AND HISTORICAL CONSIDERATIONS. Literally, acute myocardial infarction is a focus of necrosis resulting from inadequate perfusion of the tissue. What is generally implied by the term, however, is the clinical syndrome resulting from such ischemia and manifested by sudden cardiac death; "typical" signs and symptoms of infarction such as crushing chest pain and diaphoresis, malignant ventricular arrhythmia, and congestive heart failure or shock; or atypical presentations that can be clinically silent or subtle with new-onset or accelerated angina, atypical chest pain mimicking "indigestion," impaired cerebral perfusion with syncope, or signs simulating those of a cerebrovascular accident or psychosis. Coronary thrombosis was recognized as a potential cause as early as 1910 in Obrastzow and Straschesko's report of coronary thrombosis with "status anginous" and respiratory embarrassment, and in 1912 by Herrick, who described clinical features typical of sudden coronary occlusion. Although diminution of perfusion has not been questioned, the contribution of thrombotic occlusion at sites of severe atherosclerosis as a primary phenomenon rather than as an epiphenomenon was resolved only recently. Its pivotal role was established unequivocally by early angiographic study of afflicted patients. Early catastrophic complications of infarction include ventricular fibrillation, rupture of the ventricular free wall, ventricular septal rupture (with shock and left to right shunting), or papillary muscle rupture (with profound mitral or tricuspid regurgitation). Later complications include ventricular mural thrombus with peripheral embolization and cerebrovascular accident, congestive heart failure with or without ventricular true

or pseudoaneurysm, ventricular dilatation and infarct expansion, and sudden cardiac death. Progression of underlying coronary artery disease in survivors of acute myocardial infarction may result in unstable angina pectoris, "silent ischemia" (with electrocardiographic [ECG] changes without symptoms), recurrent infarction, or sudden death.

INCIDENCE AND ETIOLOGY

INCIDENCE. Heart disease, the leading cause of death in the United States, accounts for more than 30 per cent of total death, most of which is attributable to acute myocardial infarction. Age-adjusted death rates for infarction have declined dramatically, however, since 1950 (from more than 300 per 100,000 population to slightly less than 200). Nevertheless, because of population growth, the total number of infarct-related deaths in the United States has not declined, and heart disease remains responsible for more years of potential life lost before age 65, regardless of gender or race, than any other illness.

Infarction accounts for 750,000 hospital admissions in the United States annually. Diagnosed coronary disease is present in as many as 7 million Americans and kills 514,000 annually. Sudden death, precluding hospitalization, occurs in more than 350,000. Even among those who die after the prehospital phase, death is most often sudden. The impressive decline in age-adjusted death rates attributable to acute myocardial infarction over the past 25 years, a decrease of as much as 47 per cent according to some estimates, probably reflects a decreased incidence and severity of coronary atherosclerosis antedating the recent intense interest in diet, fitness, and smoking cessation. It may reflect in part early and aggressive treatment of predisposing conditions such as hypertension, widespread use of β-adrenergic blockers in patients with angina, the benefits of community-based CPR and defibrillation programs, the impact of coronary care units, and consequences of aggressive revascularization.

ETIOLOGY. Although most infarcts result from thrombotic occlusion superimposed on severe coronary atherosclerosis, severe atherosclerotic disease may exist for years with no change in severity of effort-induced angina. Occurrence of angina with progressively less effort or at rest, protracted angina simulating the pain of infarction, and acceleration of angina despite intense medical management and the absence of exacerbating factors such as anemia, arrhythmia, hypertension, congestive heart failure, thyrotoxicosis, or obesity often reflect dynamic changes in obstructing plaques with consequent intermittent thrombosis. Q-wave infarcts (previously called transmural) appear to result when occlusive thrombi persist, as documented angiographically in more than 90 per cent of patients with infarction. Non–Q-wave infarcts (previously called subendocardial) result often from incomplete or spontaneously recanalized thrombotic occlusions after ischemia sufficiently persistent to elicit necrosis. Reocclusion with early recurrent infarction is common. A common denominator of all acute coronary syndromes (sudden cardiac dath, new-onset angina, unstable angina, acute myocardial infarction) appears to be instability of atherosclerotic plaques with intramural hemorrhage, fissuring, and plaque rupture, all of which may precipitate acute thrombotic occlusion.

Risk factors for infarction parallel those for atherosclerosis in general. Diabetes mellitus, hypertension, truncal obesity, smoking, increased concentrations of low density lipoprotein (LDL) cholesterol and decreased concentrations of high density lipoprotein (HDL) cholesterol in plasma, increased concentrations of lipoprotein (a), elevated plasma homocysteine, and genetic predisposition to atherosclerosis manifested by a strong family history apply to both, as discussed in Ch. 47. Changes such as hyperglycemia and elevation of triglycerides in plasma early after infarction may be inappropriately interpreted as indicative of diabetes or hyperlipidemia when in fact they reflect transiently impaired insulin release because of reduced pancreatic blood flow, augmented glycogenolysis secondary to catecholamines, increased gluconeogenesis secondary to 17-OH corticosteroids, increased concentrations of plasma free fatty acids, and augmented hepatic synthesis of triglycerides. Conversely, plasma cholesterol may be diminished because of hepatic dysfunction and may be misinterpreted as the absence of hypercholesterolemia that would otherwise be evident. The fall in HDL cholesterol is greater than that of total cholesterol and may persist for 6 to 8 weeks.

TABLE 48–6. CONDITIONS OTHER THAN CORONARY ATHEROSCLEROSIS THAT MAY CAUSE ACUTE MYOCARDIAL INFARCTION

Coronary emboli	Causes include aortic or mitral valve lesions, left atrial or ventricular thrombi, prosthetic valves, fat emboli, intracardiac neoplasms, infective endocarditis, and paradoxical emboli.
Thrombotic coronary artery disease	May occur with oral contraceptive use, sickle cell anemia and other hemoglobinopathies, polycythemia vera, thrombocytosis, thrombotic thrombocytopenic purpura, disseminated intravascular coagulation, antithrombin III deficiency and other hypercoagulable states, macroglobulinemia and other hyperviscosity states, multiple myeloma, leukemia, malaria, and fibrinolytic system shutdown secondary to impaired plasminogen activation or excessive inhibition.
Coronary vasculitis	Seen with Takayasu's disease, Kawasaki's disease, polyarteritis nodosa, lupus erythematosus, scleroderma, rheumatoid arthritis, and immune-mediated vascular degeneration in cardiac allografts.
Coronary vasospasm	May be associated with variant angina, nitrate withdrawal, cocaine or amphetamine abuse, and angina with "normal" coronary arteries.
Infiltrative and degenerative coronary vascular disease	May result from amyloidosis, connective tissue disorders such as pseudoxanthoma elasticum, lipid storage disorders and mucopolysaccharidoses, homocystinuria, diabetes mellitus, collagen vascular disease, muscular dystrophies, and Friedreich's ataxia.
Coronary ostial occlusion	Associated with aortic dissection, luetic aortitis, aortic stenosis, and ankylosing spondylitis syndromes.
Congenital coronary anomalies	Including Bland-White-Garland syndrome of anomalous origin of the left coronary artery from the pulmonary artery, left coronary artery origin from the anterior sinus of Valsalva, coronary arteriovenous fistula or aneurysms, and myocardial bridging with secondary vascular degeneration.
Trauma	Associated with and responsible for coronary dissection, laceration, or thrombosis (with endothelial cell injury secondary to trauma such as angioplasty); radiation; and cardiac contusion.
Augmented myocardial oxygen requirements exceeding oxygen delivery	Encountered with aortic stenosis, aortic insufficiency, hypertension with severe left ventricular hypertrophy, pheochromocytoma, thyrotoxicosis, methemoglobinemia, carbon monoxide poisoning, shock, and hyperviscosity syndromes.

Several causes of acute myocardial infarction (Table 48–6) other than atherosclerosis merit particular consideration. Embolization of coronary arteries secondary to infective or marantic endocarditis (associated with drug abuse or collagen vascular disease), calcium deposits or thrombi from prosthetic or calcified valves, ventricular mural thrombi, or atrial thrombi or myxomas may be responsible. Coronary thrombosis caused by trauma or by oral contraceptives in women, perhaps attributable to diminished antithrombin III or increased plasminogen activator inhibitor type 1 (PAI-1) in plasma; vasculitis; vasospasm (idiopathic or associated with cocaine or amphetamine abuse); coronary vascular degeneration (including accelerated atherosclerosis) after cardiac transplantation; or inflammatory small vessel coronary disease (0.1- to 1.0-mm diameter vessels) associated with diabetes, collagen vascular diseases, or disorders affecting extracellular matrix may be implicated.

Occasionally, acute myocardial infarction may occur in association with syndrome X (angina with "normal" coronary arteries) or variant angina. Diminished elaboration of endothelial cell–derived relaxing factor or release of vasoconstrictors such as endothelin may contribute.

PATHOLOGY AND PATHOPHYSIOLOGY

PATHOLOGY. Coronary atherosclerosis is particularly prominent at branch points of vessels. Atherosclerotic lesions appear initially as "fatty streaks"—i.e., lipid-laden cells, presumably monocytes or macrophages, adhering to the endothelial surface and ultimately penetrating the intima. More advanced fibrous plaques comprise not only lipid-laden cells but also connective tissue and proliferating smooth muscle cells. The most advanced lesions, called complicated plaques, exhibit fibrocalcific degeneration with intra- and extracellular lipid, calcium, fibrous tissue, necrotic debris, extravasated blood, and a fibrous tissue cap. Platelet-rich mural thrombi are often associated with the surface. Atherogenesis may reflect endothelial injury; permeation of atherogenic lipoproteins such as oxidized LDL; platelet and monocyte mitogens; and impaired reverse cholesterol transport attributable to low HDL. It is undoubtedly linked intimately to thrombosis. For example, platelet-derived growth factors may contribute to atherogenesis, impaired endothelial cell function caused by early atherosclerosis may predispose to platelet adhe-

sion and activation, diminished endothelial elaboration of activators of fibrinolysis or augmented release of inhibitors may predispose to thrombosis, and vasospasm in atherosclerotic vascular segments may potentiate platelet activation through augmentation of sheer forces.

The spectrum of injury manifest in myocardium depends not only on the intensity of impairment of myocardial perfusion but also on its duration. Accordingly, no conventional microscopic or gross changes may be evident in hearts of patients who die suddenly as a result of an acute coronary event. Typical infarction is manifest by coagulation necrosis followed ultimately by fibrosis. Contraction-band necrosis occurs when ischemia is followed by reperfusion or accompanied by massive adrenergic stimulation, often with myocytolysis.

In patients who succumb with a history of preceding unstable angina, morphologic manifestations of frank infarction may be lacking. However, platelet microemboli and vascular mural thrombosis of diverse ages are seen, indicative of the underlying pathophysiology involving repetitive thrombotic phenomena initiated by dynamic changes in complicated atherosclerotic plaques. In victims of infarction reflected by evolutionary ECG changes, the classic differentiation of transmural from nontransmural infarction based on ECG criteria (the presence or absence of Q waves after complete evolution of the insult) serves only as a crude generalization in view of bidirectional overlap of morphologic lesions associated with each ECG pattern.

PATHOPHYSIOLOGY. The right and left coronary arteries arise independently from individual ostia associated with right and left aortic valve cusps. The left anterior descending (LAD) and circumflex coronary arteries arise as the left main coronary artery bifurcation and supply the anterior left ventricle, the bulk of the interventricular septum, and the lateral and posterior left ventricular walls. The apex, lateral wall, and posterior wall may be supplied by the right posterior descending coronary artery, diagonals from the LAD, and the posterior left ventricular branch of the right coronary artery, respectively. When the posterior descending coronary artery that supplies the posterior interventricular septum arises from the left circumflex, the circulation is called left dominant. More often, the posterior descending artery arises from the terminal portion of the right coronary artery (right dominant circulation). The posterior left ventricular branch of the right coronary artery supplies the atrioventricular (AV) node in 90 per cent of subjects. Another branch (in 55 per cent of subjects) supplies the sinus node. The right ventricle is supplied by the right coronary artery. Although the posterior division of the left bundle branch has a dual blood supply (from both the left and right coronary arteries), the anterior fascicle of the left bundle and the right bundle are each supplied primarily by branches of the left anterior descending coronary artery.

In view of anatomic considerations it is not surprising that right coronary artery occlusion is manifested frequently by sinus bradycardia, AV block, right ventricular infarction, or left ventricular infarction of modest extent. Conversely, markedly impaired left ventricular function with pulmonary congestion or edema indicative of extensive injury and intraventricular conduction defects such as hemiblock are more typical of left coronary artery occlusion.

Acute insults are generally attributable to thrombosis initiated by hemorrhage or rupture of complicated atheromatous plaques with deprivation of blood flow to myocardium as a final common denominator. Even if recanalization is induced relatively promptly (spontaneously, mechanically, or with fibrinolytic drugs), regional myocardial perfusion may not be sustained (the "no reflow" phenomenon) because of endothelial cell swelling, platelet and leukocyte plugs, or complement-mediated microvascular inflammation. In addition to hypoxia, decreased removal of noxious metabolites, including potassium, calcium, amphiphilic lipids, and oxygen-centered free radicals, impairs ventricular performance and may evoke lethal arrhythmias. Inflammation of endocardial surfaces and stasis associated with dyskinesis can lead to ventricular mural thrombi. Epicardial inflammation may initiate the pericardial involvement seen with as many as 20 per cent of Q-wave infarcts.

Systolic Function. Even transitory deprivation of oxygen and accumulation of metabolites are manifest promptly by diminished regional systolic contractile function and wall thickening detectable by echocardiography, abnormal wall motion detectable by radionuclide ventriculography, diminished cardiac cycle–dependent variation of backscattered ultrasound detectable by tissue characterization, and, if extensive, diminished stroke volume. Restoration of perfusion may promptly restore function of depressed myocardium even after prolonged intervals ("hibernating" myocardium). Often, however, impairment of function persists even if blood flow is restored early ("stunning")—when injury is not yet irreversible. In general, hypokinesis and dyskinesis reflect the locus and extent of myocardial injury. Expansion of infarction and ventricular dilatation begin as early as 24 hours after the onset of infarction with thinning of the infarct zone and realignment of layers of tissue within and adjacent to it. Rupture, seen in 20 per cent of fatal infarcts, may result, particularly when cardiogenic shock, malignant arrhythmia, or antecedent ventricular hypertrophy is present. Rupture may occur also with small infarcts because the well-preserved ventricular function increases wall stress.

Ventricular aneurysms are seen with early cardiac imaging in as many as 20 per cent of patients with Q-wave infarction. Clinically, they may be recognized only late, manifested by congestive heart failure, recurrent ventricular arrhythmia, or recurrent emboli. They may be accompanied by persistent ST-segment elevation in electrocardiograms obtained 6 or more weeks after infarction.

Because coronary artery disease is usually generalized, ischemia "at a distance" may be evident. As left ventricular end-diastolic volume and pressure increase because of impaired regional pump function, intramural diastolic ventricular pressure increases and myocardial perfusion declines. Peripheral arterial vasoconstriction and systemic venous constriction can no longer compensate for diminished stroke volume, and blood pressure falls. With decline of cardiac output and acceleration of heart rate, coronary flow declines further. Ischemia at a distance may be manifest simply as an ECG derangement or may result in a vicious circle in which stuttering infarction ultimately leads to profound left ventricular failure and cardiogenic shock.

Normally perfused zones may initially exhibit compensatory hyperfunction with excessive wall thickening in systole. However,

as the heart dilates over 24 to 48 hours, hyperfunction regresses.

Diastolic Function. Early after the onset of infarction, distensibility of ischemic myocardium first increases and then decreases. Effective ventricular filling can be maintained only with an increase in left ventricular end-diastolic volume and pressure (LVEDP). The increased LVEDP results in elevated pulmonary venous pressure, decreased pulmonary compliance, interstitial and ultimately alveolar pulmonary edema, hypoxemia, and exacerbation of myocardial ischemic injury. As the infarct thins and shrinks and if infarct expansion does not predominate, ventricular dilatation may regress, and diastolic cardiac and pulmonary pressures may return toward normal.

Right Ventricular Function. Impaired right ventricular function was recognized initially in the extreme, when right coronary artery occlusion led to gross right ventricular infarction. However, similar manifestations can occur when inferior left ventricular infarction and right coronary or left circumflex occlusion exist in the presence of a left dominant circulation. Right ventricular dysfunction diminishes cardiac output disproportionally to left ventricular injury. High-grade bradyarrhythmias are common, including those resulting from third-degree heart block, occasional profound arterial oxygen desaturation because of augmented right atrial pressure and right to left shunting through a patent foramen ovale, and exacerbation or extension of left ventricular infarction because of hypotension and diminished cardiac output.

Compensatory Mechanisms. Reflexly augmented sympathoadrenal and vagal discharge may give rise to tachycardia, ventricular arrhythmia, and bradycardia (sinus node depression or heart block), as well as pallor, cutaneous vasoconstriction, and diaphoresis. Initially, compromised cardiac output is maintained by the combination of increased heart rate and ventricular dilatation with recruitment of the Frank-Starling mechanism. Right ventricular infarction impairs hemodynamics most dramatically early in its course. As healing progresses and the right ventricle becomes less complaint, its conduit function is restored, permitting maintenance of cardiac output at the expense of augmentation of right ventricular filling pressure.

Effects of Myocardial Infarction on Organs Other Than the Heart. Augmentation of pulmonary venous pressure may cause diminished pulmonary compliance, dyspnea, pulmonary vascular redistribution detectable radiographically, interstitial and alveolar pulmonary edema, respiratory decompensation, and hypoxemia.

Cerebral hypoperfusion may result in restlessness or, rarely, psychosis. Coupled with dyspnea in the elderly, it may be manifest only by confusion and combativeness. Increased sympathoadrenal tone reflected by markedly elevated plasma catecholamines and adrenocortical stimulation may be prominent as well. Plasma concentrations of atrial natriuretic peptide decrease initially but then increase, perhaps because of heart failure and atrial stretch. Elevated plasma concentrations of vasopressin, angiotensin (with β-adrenergic stimulation of renin release), and aldosterone contribute to fluid retention and hyponatremia. Impaired pancreatic blood flow inhibits insulin secretion.

In addition to the typical increase in erythrocyte sedimentation rate and leukocytosis, a modest increase in plasma fibrinogen and an augmentation of circulating PAI-1 occur as part of the acute phase reaction to infarction. Impairment of fibrinolysis and augmentation of platelet activation by circulating catecholamines may predispose to continuing coronary and ventricular mural thrombosis. Plasma viscosity increases because of increased fibrinogen, α_2 globulins, and hemoconcentration several days after the onset of infarction, most markedly when left ventricular failure or shock supervenes.

Determinants of Prognosis. Immediate survival depends primarily on whether or not ventricular fibrillation occurs, and if so, whether it can be treated instantly. Community-based emergency systems with defibrillation capability, the use of defibrillators by appropriately trained lay personnel, and rapid hospitalization of patients with suspected evolving infarction have improved early survival. Even among hospitalized patients, fatality is generally attributable to ventricular fibrillation, which can, of course, often be interrupted by immediate defibrillation.

Judging from ambulatory electrocardiograms and recordings obtained in coronary care units, mortality associated with acute myocardial infarction is attributable to primary ventricular fibrillation in 85 per cent or more of instances. Only rarely is electrical asystole responsible. The association between primary ventricular fibrillation and "warning arrhythmias" (high-grade ventricular ectopy and R-on-T phenomena) is not strong, although ectopy as well as fibrillation may reflect intermittent or severe ischemia with compromise of ventricular performance exacerbating ischemia, thereby predisposing to fibrillation. Ventricular premature complexes activating the ventricle during its vulnerable period can, of course, trigger fibrillation. Nevertheless, pharmacologic suppression of ventricular ectopy per se does not necessarily protect the heart against fibrillation. In fact, suppression with type IA or IC agents, β blockers, calcium channel blockers, or type III agents may increase the incidence of asystole in patients being treated with lidocaine.

In some instances mortality may result from fibrillation secondary to cardiac decompensation accompanying profound congestive heart failure, hypotension, or shock (secondary ventricular fibrillation). Accordingly, determinants of late mortality include "infarct size" measured enzymatically or by other means at the time of the index infarct (Fig. 48–2). Diminution of left ventricular ejection fraction is a powerful descriptor.

Late mortality is determined also by the likelihood of recurrent infarction and the frequency and severity of episodic ischemia. Both may reflect progression of underlying atherosclerotic coronary artery disease and thrombosis. Complex ventricular ectopy after hospital discharge predicts subsequent mortality as well. Most late cardiac death is sudden, arrhythmic death (Fig. 48–3).

The Status of the Infarct-related Artery. Coronary thrombolysis and mechanical revascularization have revolutionized primary treatment of acute myocardial infarction largely because they salvage myocardium when implemented early after the onset of ischemia. In addition, however, prognostic benefit of an open infarct-related artery is evident even when recanalization can be induced only 6 hours or more after onset of symptoms, when salvage of substantial amounts of jeopardized ischemic myocardium is no longer likely. An open infarct-related artery is reflected ultimately by improved ventricular function, improved collateral blood flow from the infarct-related artery, decreased infarct expansion, decreased ventricular aneurysm formation, improved ventricular remodeling, diminished left ventricular dilatation, decreased late arrhythmia associated with ventricular aneurysms, decreased late potentials on the signal-averaged electrocardiogram, and decreased mortality.

SIGNS AND SYMPTOMS

"Typical" Q-wave infarction is manifested by prodromal symptoms of fatigue, chest discomfort, or malaise in the days preceding the event. Onset of infarction occurs often in the early morning

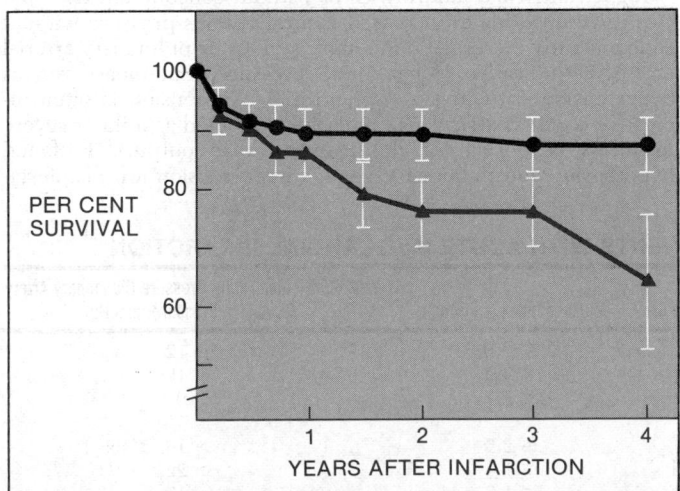

FIGURE 48–2. The influence of the extent of an initial infarct on survival. Infarct size index was estimated enzymatically and expressed as CK-g-equivalents per square meter of body surface area in 173 patients who survived for at least 24 hours. Survival was greater for those with small (< 15 CK-g-eq) (*circles*) compared with large (≥ 15 CK-g-eq) (*triangles*) infarcts. (From Geltman EM, et al.: Circulation 60:805, 1979. Reproduced by permission of the American Heart Association, Inc.)

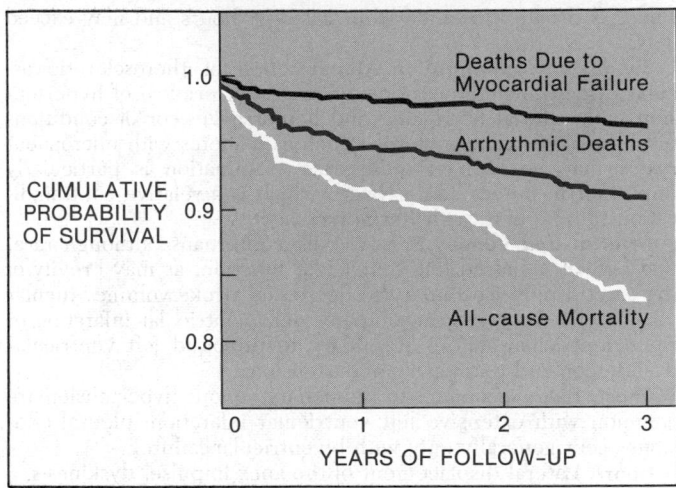

FIGURE 48–3. The large contribution of arrhythmia (sudden cardiac death) to overall mortality throughout the follow-up interval in victims of acute myocardial infarction. The ordinate shows survival from the time of hospital discharge after acute myocardial infarction. The number of patients alive and in follow-up were 0 years, 867; 1 year, 777; 2 years, 704; and 3 years, 314. (Adapted from Marcus F, et al.: Am J Cardiol 61:8, 1988; with permission.)

hours, presumably in part because of the increased catecholamine-induced platelet aggregation and diminished plasma concentrations of PAI-1 after awakening. Onset is generally not directly associated with severe exertion.

Typical pain is intense, severe, unremitting for 30 to 60 minutes, crushing or squeezing in nature, retrosternal, and often radiating down the ulnar aspect of the left arm and into the neck, teeth, or jaw. Occasionally the pain is epigastric. Diaphoresis, weakness, a sense of impending doom, profound restlessness, confusion, presyncope, hiccuping (presumably reflecting irritation of the diaphragm), nausea and vomiting, and palpitations are common. Decreased systolic ventricular performance accounts for impaired perfusion of vital organs and reflexly mediated compensatory responses to hypotension such as restlessness and impaired mentation, pallor, cutaneous vasoconstriction and sweating, tachycardia, and prerenal failure. Impaired left ventricular diastolic function leads to pulmonary vascular congestion with shortness of breath and tachypnea and pulmonary edema with orthopnea. Impaired right ventricular diastolic function leads to systemic venous hypertension, edema, hepatomegaly, and further compromise of left ventricular cardiac output.

Myocardial infarction may be clinically silent (in as many as 1 per cent of patients), with the diagnosis established only retrospectively by ECG criteria. The patient may recall only an episode of "indigestion" or nothing. Stoicism, an unusually high pain threshold, disorders impairing function of the nervous system such as diabetes mellitus, or obtundation caused by medications or impaired cerebral perfusion may prevent recognition of typical chest pain.

PHYSICAL FINDINGS TYPICAL OF ACUTE MYOCARDIAL INFARCTION. Typical clinical findings can be summarized as follows:

General Appearance. Pallor, diaphoresis, and restlessness are present.

Vital Signs. Heart rate is often increased secondary to sympathoadrenal discharge, ventricular ectopy, accelerated idioventricular rhythm, ventricular tachycardia, atrial fibrillation or flutter, or other supraventricular arrhythmias, especially when atrial infarction or heart failure is present. Bradyarrhythmias attributable to impaired sinus node function, AV nodal block, or infranodal block may be evident. The blood pressure is generally elevated initially with arterial vasoconstriction, in contrast to the case with acute pulmonary embolism, in which initial hypotension is frequent. However, with right ventricular infarction or severe left ventricular dysfunction, hypotension occurs. The respiratory rate is usually increased in response to pulmonary congestion. Coughing, wheezing, and production of frothy sputum may occur.

Fever is usually present within 24 to 48 hours and may exceed 39°C.

Funduscopic Examination. Manifestations of atherosclerotic vascular disease including copper wiring of arterioles, of hypertension with arterial narrowing and hemorrhages, or of conditions predisposing to atherosclerosis such as diabetes with microaneurysms may be seen. Funduscopic examination is particularly important to detect hemorrhage, which is a relative contraindication to treatment with fibrinolytic agents.

Arterial and Venous Pulses. Pulsus alternans, although rare, may reflect impaired left ventricular function, as may brevity of the carotid pulse secondary to decreased stroke volume. Jugular venous distention may accompany right ventricular infarction or right ventricular failure secondary to profound left ventricular dysfunction and pulmonary hypertension.

Chest. Rales secondary to pulmonary venous hypertension are common with extensive left ventricular infarction; pleural effusions occur generally only with biventricular failure.

Heart. Lateral displacement of the apex impulse, dyskinesis, a palpable S_4, and a soft S_1 may be indicative of diminished contractility of the compromised left ventricle; paradoxical splitting of S_2 may reflect left bundle branch block or prolongation of the pre-ejection period with delayed aortic valve closure despite decreased stroke volume; accentuated S_4 and S_3 may reflect diminished left ventricular compliance; a mitral regurgitation murmur indicative of either papillary muscle dysfunction or rupture or annulus dilatation may be audible even if cardiac output is diminished markedly; a pericardial friction rub may be evident. Premature ventricular beats, brief runs of ventricular tachycardia, or accelerated idioventricular rhythm are common.

Abdomen. Hepatojugular reflux may be elicited even when hepatomegaly is not marked.

Extremities. Peripheral cyanosis, edema, and pallor may indicate vasoconstriction, and diminished cardiac output may reflect right ventricular dysfunction or failure.

Neurologic Findings. Patients with acute myocardial infarction are prone to frank cerebrovascular insults as a result of ventricular mural thrombi and consequent embolization (with an incidence of approximately 1 per cent). Recrudescence of signs or symptoms of a prior cerebrovascular accident may occur secondary to diminished cerebral perfusion. In contrast, the incidence of myocardial infarction in patients with cerebrovascular accidents is substantial.

The incidence of myocardial infarction appears to be greater and its prognosis worse in patients with depression. Infarction may precipitate reactive depression whether or not β-adrenergic blocking agents or other central nervous system (CNS)–active agents are administered.

HEMODYNAMIC MANIFESTATIONS. Hemodynamic observations are of inestimable value in guiding therapy. A categorization of hemodynamic subsets of patients is shown in Table 48–7.

Patients Requiring Invasive Monitoring. Not all patients with infarction require hemodynamic monitoring with right heart catheterization and/or invasive arterial pressure monitoring.

Those who are hemodynamically stable without apparent complications such as tachycardia, refractory arrhythmia, respiratory compromise, impairment of cerebral, hepatic, or renal function, or persistent or recurrent pain indicative of recurrent or refractory ischemia, pericarditis, or incipient cardiac rupture can generally be managed without invasive hemodynamic monitoring. Effective management may be facilitated by balloon flotation right heart catheter hemodynamic monitoring in patients with pulmonary congestion indicative of pulmonary venous hypertension reflected by physical findings or chest roentgenographic abnormalities, but many patients with mild complications can be managed conservatively. Patients with peripheral hypoperfusion despite initial administration of fluids to replete or expand vascular volume and those with severe, refractory, or progressive congestive heart failure, potentially catastrophic complications of acute infarction refractory arrhythmias, persistent pain, or hemodynamic instability should be evaluated by balloon flotation right heart catheter hemodynamic monitoring.

Monitoring catheters should generally be introduced through compressible sites, particularly because of the high likelihood that thrombolytic agents will be used early in the treatment of infarction. They should remain in place for no more than 72 hours to avoid the risk of infection and can often be removed much more promptly. Sometimes ascertainment of systemic and pulmonary venous pressure, cardiac output, and peripheral vascular resistance is sufficient for subsequent management without the need for continuous monitoring. In other instances the effects of vasodilators, diuretics, agents with positive inotropic effects, and therapeutic alterations of vascular volume should be monitored over the ensuing 48 to 72 hours.

Hemodynamic Subsets. Patients are categorized with respect to cardiac output (increased, normal, or diminished), systemic arterial blood pressure (increased, normal, or diminished with or without increased or decreased systemic vascular resistance), and the presence or absence of pulmonary venous hypertension (augmented pulmonary arterial wedge pressure) (Table 48–7).

Patients without diminished systemic arterial blood pressure or pulmonary venous hypertension may have normal or hyperdynamic hemodynamics (the latter reflected by a high cardiac output with or without hypertension caused by sympathoadrenal stimulation). Systemic arterial hypotension may be attributable to relative or absolute hypovolemia or to right ventricular infarction (generally reflected by augmented systemic venous pressure). Rarely, it reflects decreased peripheral vascular resistance caused by vagotonia or sepsis. The noncompliant left ventricle requires augmented filling pressure to sustain cardiac output. Accordingly, relative hypovolemia may exist despite moderately elevated left ventricular filling pressure. Central venous pressure cannot be relied upon for assessment of vascular volume.

Right ventricular failure with or without concomitant tricuspid regurgitation leads to increased central venous pressure without concomitantly increased pulmonary venous or pulmonary arterial occlusive (indicative of left atrial) pressure. Pulmonary venous hypertension without systemic arterial hypotension is often indicative of left ventricular failure (differentiated as mild or severe in terms of normal or depressed cardiac output). Profound hypotension and pulmonary venous hypertension are manifesta-

TABLE 48–7. HEMODYNAMIC SUBSETS AMONG PATIENTS WITH ACUTE MYOCARDIAL INFARCTION

Hemodynamic Subset		Systemic Arterial Blood Pressure	Cardiac Index (L/m²/min)	Left Ventricular Filling Pressure (Pulmonary Artery Occlusive Pressure; mm Hg)
I	Normal hemodynamics	Normal	2.7 ± 0.5	≤ 12
II	Hyperdynamic state	Increased	> 3.0	< 12
III	Hypovolemia*	Decreased	≤ 2.7	≤ 9
IV	Left ventricular failure			
	A. Mild	Normal	≤ 2.5	$> 18, \leq 22$
	B. Severe	Normal or decreased	≤ 1.8	≥ 22
V	Cardiogenic shock	Decreased	≤ 1.8	≥ 18
VI	Shock attributable to right ventricular infarction†	Decreased	≤ 1.8	≤ 18

Adapted from Forrester JS, et al.: Medical therapy of acute myocardial infarction by application of hemodynamic subsets. N Engl J Med 295:1404, 1976. By permission of the New England Journal of Medicine.

*Relative hypovolemia may result in hypertension even if pulmonary artery pressure is moderately elevated (≤ 18) if left ventricular compliance is decreased associated with infarction or failure.

†Central venous (systemic venous) pressure is often markedly elevated (upper limit of normal = 6 mm Hg).

tions of cardiogenic shock. The vicious circle of cardiogenic shock—progressive infarction with declining cardiac output, further compromise of perfusion, and ultimately extensive necrosis with profound failure and shock—is generally irreversible without prompt mechanical support of the circulation and coronary revascularization with thrombolytic drugs, angioplasty, or surgery.

In general, hemodynamic status reflects the extent of left ventricular infarction. However, an infarct of modest extent superimposed on a previous infarct can profoundly compromise hemodynamics. Initial impairment of ventricular performance may exceed that attributable to irreversible injury because of myocardial stunning early after the onset of infarction. Right ventricular involvement may compromise cardiac output more than anticipated from the extent of left ventricular injury alone.

LABORATORY DETERMINATIONS

The objectives of acquiring laboratory data include determination of the presence or absence of infarction (diagnosis and differential diagnosis); characterization of the locus, nature (Q or non-Q), and extent of infarction (estimation of infarct size); detection of recurrent ischemia or infarction (extension of infarction); detection of early and late complications of infarction; and estimation of prognosis.

The complete blood count and platelet count (which may decrease after heparin) are useful not only diagnostically but in assessing suitability for treatment with thrombolytic drugs. The leukocyte count may be normal initially but generally increases within 2 hours and peaks in 2 to 4 days with predominance of polymorphonuclear leukocytes and a shift to the left. Elevations generally persist for 1 to 2 weeks. Other components of the acute phase reaction contribute to elevations of the erythrocyte sedimentation rate (ESR) within 48 hours with subsequent changes paralleling those in the leukocyte count. Because of increased pulmonary and sometimes systemic venous pressure, contraction of plasma volume is common after acute myocardial infarction, manifested not only by hemoconcentration but also by prerenal failure with elevation of plasma creatinine and blood urea nitrogen. Arterial blood gases should be assayed if necessary to evaluate hypoxemia resulting from pulmonary congestion, atelectasis, or ventilatory impairment secondary to complications of infarction or excessive sedation or analgesia. Fingertip oximetry may be adequate and can obviate the need for arterial puncture and bleeding in patients treated with thrombolytic drugs. The chest radiograph is particularly useful in determining the presence or absence of cardiomegaly (often correlated with the presence or absence of increased LVEDP or left atrial pressure, and of pulmonary venous hypertension), pulmonary edema, pleural effusions, Kerley B lines, and other criteria of congestive heart failure. A small cardiac silhouette and clear lung fields in a patient with systemic hypotension may be indicative of relative or absolute hypovolemia. A large cardiac silhouette with similar hemodynamics may reflect hemopericardium and tamponade or right ventricular infarction compromising cardiac output. Chest radiographic findings indicative of pulmonary venous hypertension may occur later and persist longer because of delay in fluid shifts between vascular, interstitial, and alveolar spaces.

Sequential ECG findings remain hallmarks of diagnosis despite the occasional occurrence of infarction without any acute changes and the nonspecific nature of some of the ECG changes that may be seen. The diagnosis can be established with certainty when typical ST elevation persists for hours and is followed by T-wave inversion within the first few days and Q waves subsequently. However, initial ST depression or T-wave inversion is difficult to differentiate from that seen with ischemia without infarction or in unrelated conditions (Table 48–8). ST-segment depression followed by T-wave inversion without evolution of Q waves can result from non–Q-wave infarction or subendocardial ischemia without infarction. Q-wave infarction cannot be differentiated from non–Q-wave infarction initially if ST elevation is lacking and Q waves have not yet developed. Infarction is often associated with nonspecific ECG changes including intraventricular conduction delays; ventricular and supraventricular arrhythmias; signs of atrial infarction, such as changes in P-wave morphology, elevation or depression of the PQ segment, atrial flutter or fibrillation, or a wandering atrial pacemaker; and signs of right ventricular infarction such as ST elevation or Q waves detectable

TABLE 48–8. CONDITIONS ASSOCIATED WITH ELECTROCARDIOGRAPHIC CHANGES THAT MAY OBSCURE OR SIMULATE THOSE INDICATIVE OF ACUTE MYOCARDIAL INFARCTION

Abnormality	Examples
Intraventricular conduction abnormalities	Left bundle branch block, left anterior superior fascicular block, infranodal arborization block, right ventricular transvenous or epicardial pacing
Electrolyte disturbances	Hypo- or hyperkalemia, hypocalcemia
Pre-excitation	Wolff-Parkinson-White syndrome
Early repolarization	
Cerebrovascular accident	
Myocarditis	Inflammatory, infiltrative, viral, collagen vascular disorders, pheochromocytoma, cardiac allograph rejection, neuromuscular disorders such as muscular dystrophy and Friedreich's ataxia
Left ventricular hypertrophy	Hypertrophic cardiomyopathy, dilated cardiomyopathy, valvular heart disease, hypertension
Right ventricular hypertrophy	Cor pulmonale, acute pulmonary embolus, pneumothorax
Cardiac tumors	
Pericarditis	

in right-sided precordial leads. The appearance of abnormalities in a large number of ECG leads is often indicative of extensive injury or concomitant pericarditis. Anterior and anterolateral infarcts tend to involve more left ventricular myocardium than inferior or true posterior infarcts.

MACROMOLECULAR MARKERS OF INFARCTION. Detection of elevated concentrations in plasma of macromolecules released from irreversibly injured myocardium has become the definitive diagnostic criterion of infarction. Enzymes, including creatine kinase (CK), aspartate serum transaminase (AST), and lactate dehydrogenase (LDH); myoglobin; and myosin light chains, among numerous other constituents, egress from irreversibly injured ischemic myocardium within several hours after the onset of the insult. Their elevated concentrations in plasma constitute sensitive diagnostic findings. Specificity is limited, however, because of their ubiquitous distribution in skeletal muscle and other tissues. Assay of activity in plasma of the MB isoenzyme of CK (MB CK) is the cornerstone of diagnosis because of the marked abundance of this isoenzyme in myocardium and virtual absence from most other tissues, and its consequent sensitivity (detection of necrosis of less than 100 mg of myocardium). Characteristic sequential changes of plasma MB CK include elevations above normal within 4 hours, a two- to 10-fold peak in 16 to 24 hours, and a return to baseline within 3 to 4 days. The magnitude and persistence of elevations are useful in estimating the extent of infarction.

Initially normal enzyme values are seen often when patients present very early after the onset of infarction. Thus, discharge from an emergency room of a patient with a history consistent with myocardial infarction should not occur without several hours of observation and repeat determinations. If infarction has occurred more than 24 hours before admission, is of very modest magnitude, or is stuttering in nature, enzyme elevations may be lacking because of the predominance of clearance over rates of release into the circulation. Assay of myosin light chains or the $LDH_1:LDH_2$ isoenzyme ratio, which remains elevated for several days after infarction because of the slow clearance of LDH, may be helpful. Late detection of infarction is sometimes facilitated by myocardial infarct scintigraphy with technetium-99m (^{99m}Tc)-pyrophosphate or radiolabeled antimyosin antibodies (investigational).

Generally, MB CK is assayed at the time of admission and at 12- to 24-hour intervals until the diagnosis is established. Determination of total CK is less specific and is redundant. Recently, assays detecting post-translational conversion of individual isoenzymes of CK to isoforms have been shown to permit even earlier diagnosis (within 2 to 3 hours of infarction). Recanalization is reflected by sudden washout of the tissue isoform into plasma. Isoform analysis is likely to become useful for monitoring interventions such as coronary thrombolysis. Determination of plasma concentrations of myoglobin, a protein with a short half-life in the circulation, offers similar promise, but results may be distorted by changes in renal function with prerenal failure.

IMAGING. Several noninvasive modalities permit detection of regional wall motion and hypokinesis or dyskinesis, as well as estimation of overall ventricular performance (Fig. 48–4). These include two-dimensional and color flow Doppler echocardiography, radionuclide ventriculography, ultrafast (cine) computed tomography, and gated magnetic resonance imaging. Because of cost considerations and convenience, only the first two are used widely. Sensitivity and specificity of abnormal wall motion as criteria of acute myocardial infarction exceed 90 per cent, particularly in patients without previous infarction. Assessment of segmental function and overall left ventricular performance has prognostic implications and is essential when infarction is extensive (elevations of MB CK exceeding 150 IU per liter) or complicated by shock or profound heart failure, in part to identify potentially surgically correctable complications and to detect ventricular true or false aneurysms and thrombi (Fig. 48–5) that can be treated with anticoagulants or fibrinolytic drugs. Imaging is useful also to detect pericardial effusion, concomitant valvular or congenital heart disease, and marked depression of ventricular function that may interdict treatment with calcium antagonists or β-adrenergic blockers. Doppler echocardiography is particularly useful in estimating the severity of mitral or tricuspid regurgitation, detecting ventricular septal defects secondary to rupture, assessing diastolic function, and monitoring cardiac output calculated from flow velocity and aortic valve area. When right ventricular infarction is suspected or when infarction is superimposed on a previous insult or associated with ECG phenomena such as left bundle branch block that obscure diagnosis, assessment of right ventricular function and delineation of regional wall motion may be particularly helpful.

Infarct-avid agents such as ^{99m}Tc-pyrophosphate and radiolabeled antimyosin antibodies (investigational) can sensitively detect infarction and define its locus. However, positive results with infarct scintigraphy cannot be obtained generally until 24

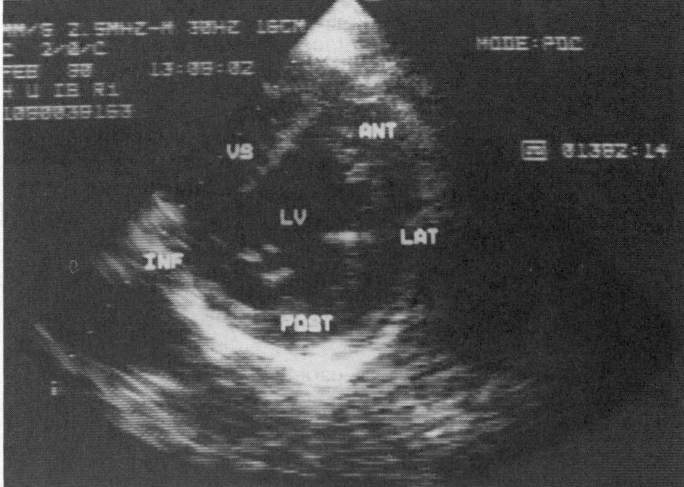

FIGURE 48–4. A still-frame short-access two-dimensional echocardiogram illustrating an inferoposterior left ventricular aneurysm after acute myocardial infarction evident as an outpocketing of the thinned left ventricular wall on the perimeter of the left ventricular cavity in the region corresponding to 6 to 9 o'clock, with the center of the clock face envisioned as central. The echo densities within the left ventricular cavity posteriorly and laterally are caused by papillary muscles. ANT = Anterior; LAT = lateral; POST = posterior; INF = inferior; VS = ventricular septum; LV = left ventricular cavity. (Courtesy of Dr. J. E. Perez, Washington University School of Medicine, St. Louis, MO.)

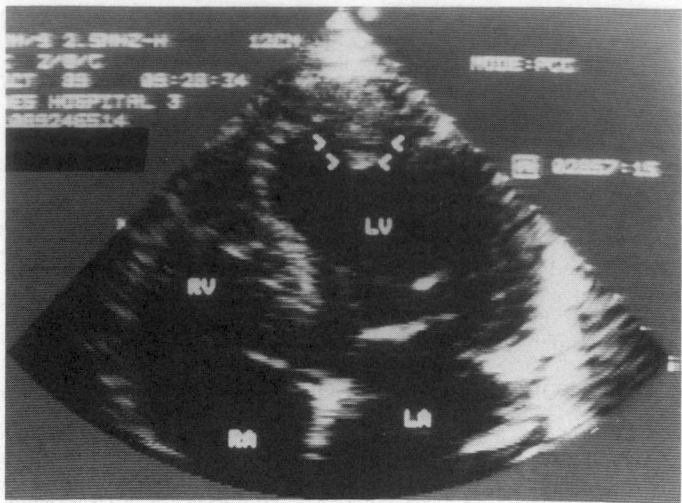

FIGURE 48–5. An apical four-chamber two-dimensional echocardiographic still frame demonstrating thrombus in the apex of the left ventricle (*arrows*) associated with acute myocardial infarction. LV = Left ventricle; RV = right ventricular; RA = right atrium; LA = left atrium. (Courtesy of Dr. J. E. Perez, Washington University School of Medicine, St. Louis, MO.)

hours or more after the onset of infarction and may be simulated by accumulation of tracer in temporally remote infarcts. Perfusion scintigraphy with tracers such as thallium-201 or ^{99m}Tc-isonitrile is sometimes useful when the diagnosis is obscure.

Positron emission tomography with tracers of intermediary metabolism (Fig. 48–6), perfusion (Fig. 48–7), or oxidative metabolism (Fig. 48–7) permits quantitative assessment of the distribution and extent of impairment of myocardial oxidative metabolism and regional myocardial perfusion (Fig. 48–8). It has been particularly useful in defining the efficacy of therapeutic interventions designed to salvage myocardium and has been used diagnostically to differentiate reversible from irreversible injury in hypoperfused zones.

DIFFERENTIAL DIAGNOSIS

When the history of acute myocardial infarction is typical, the initial electrocardiogram abnormal and followed by definitive sequential changes, and MB CK elevated in the initial or subsequent plasma samples with typical sequential changes, the diagnosis is straightforward. A presumptive diagnosis can be made when any two of these criteria are present. Unfortunately, however, the diagnosis may be obscure in patients seen very early after the onset of infarction and in those with ECG manifestations of prior ischemic or other types of heart disease, electrocardiographically silent infarcts, or atypical presentations. Differentiation from ischemia without infarction (unstable angina, aortic stenosis in the elderly, ischemia attributable to right ventricular overload, new-onset angina, or inadequate myocardial perfusion in markedly hypertrophied left ventricles or in association with marked aortic insufficiency) and from pericarditis with pain simulating that of infarction may be difficult without the aid of laboratory tests and cardiac imaging. A critical differential diagnostic consideration is aortic dissection. It should be suspected whenever pain is atypical or not associated with ECG changes typical of infarction.

Pleurodynia, pulmonary embolism or infarction, pneumothorax, pneumonitis, musculoskeletal pain associated with bursitis, the shoulder/hand syndrome, pectoral lymphadenopathy, herpes zoster before eruption of the typical vesicles, myalgia, and costochondritis may simulate infarction superficially but can usually be differentiated easily on the basis of physical findings, results of laboratory tests, and chest radiography. Pain of abdominal origin that may masquerade as infarction includes that caused by cholecystitis or cholelithiasis, pancreatitis, duodenal or gastric ulcer, gastritis, esophagitis, esophageal spasm, or esophageal reflux associated with a hiatal hernia.

CARE OF THE PATIENT

The focus of treatment differs in the prehospital, hospital (coronary care unit and step-down unit), and convalescent phases

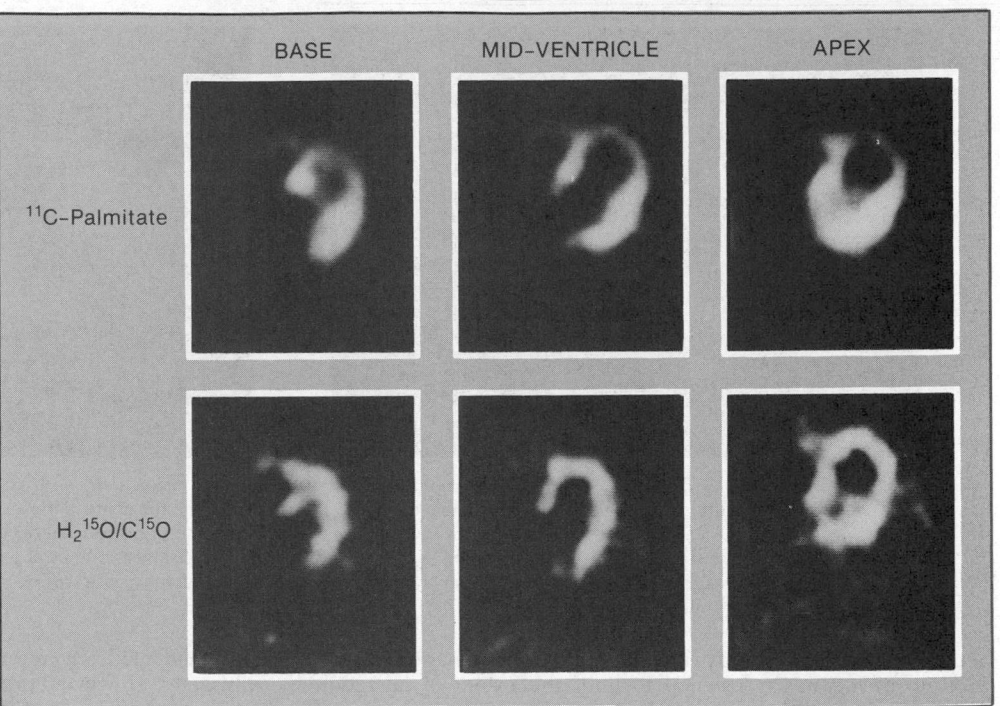

BASE   MID-VENTRICLE   APEX

^{11}C–Palmitate

$H_2^{15}O/C^{15}O$

FIGURE 48–6. Positron emission tomograms at three levels of the left ventricle obtained from a subject with myocardial infarction after late spontaneous coronary recanalization. Anterior myocardium is at the top right, the left ventricular free wall at the bottom right, and posterior myocardium at the bottom left. Reconstructions acquired after intravenous administration of ^{11}C-palmitate show the persistent anterior defect despite homogeneous myocardial perfusion imaged with $H_2^{15}O$ and blood pool subtraction with $C^{15}O$. The discontinuity posteriorly in some tomographic sections is attributable to the mitral valve apparatus. (From Bergmann SR, et al.: Prog Cardiovasc Dis 28:165, 1985; with permission.)

despite considerable overlap of objectives in each. Most death caused by infarction occurs early and is attributable to primary ventricular fibrillation. Thus, initial objectives are immediate ECG monitoring and reversal of ventricular fibrillation should it occur.

TREATMENT IN THE PREHOSPITAL PHASE. Community-based systems in Belfast, Ireland; Columbus, Ohio; Los Angeles, California; and Seattle, Washington, have conclusively documented the effectiveness of rapidly responding rescuers such as police and firefighters trained in defibrillation. Approximately 65 per cent of deaths caused by infarction occur in the first hour. More than 60 per cent (39 per cent of those who would succumb) can be saved by defibrillation initiated by a bystander or first-responding rescuer. Additional objectives of prehospital care by paramedical and emergency room personnel include adequate analgesia (generally with morphine), reduction of excessive sympathoadrenal and vagal stimulation pharmacologically, prophylaxis and treatment of malignant ventricular arrhythmias (generally with lidocaine), and support of cardiac output, systemic blood pressure, and respiration. Atropine (0.5 mg IV at 5-minute intervals to a maximum of 2 to 4 mg) is particularly useful in counteracting excessive vagal tone often underlying bradyarrhythmias and hypotension. It is indicated when heart rate is disproportionately diminished with respect to blood pressure, when hypotension (sometimes secondary to morphine) is refractory despite augmentation of left ventricular filling pressure, or when impaired AV nodal conduction with Wenckebach block is evident. If bradycardia persists, pacing may be required.

The advent of coronary thrombolysis as primary therapy for Q-wave infarction has already revolutionized management of patients in the hospital. Prehospital phase coronary thrombolysis initiated by paramedical personnel under medical supervision appears likely to become important as well because of its promise for salvaging more myocardium because of earlier interruption of ischemia.

TREATMENT IN THE HOSPITAL PHASE. Cardiac care units (CCU's) have reduced early mortality attributable to acute myocardial infarction by approximately 50 per cent, largely by immediate implementation of defibrillation. They have proven to be optimal facilities for continuous ECG monitoring, invasive

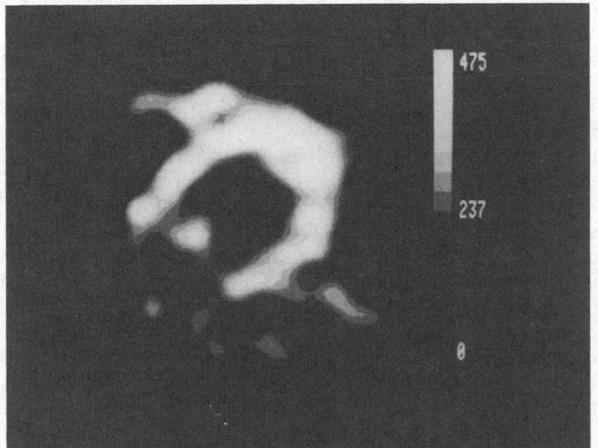

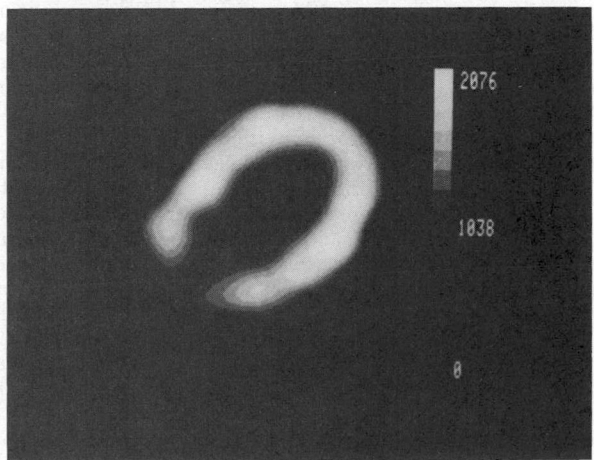

FIGURE 48–7. A single midventricular positron emission tomographic reconstruction obtained from a normal subject. Perfusion (*left*) assessed with $H_2^{15}O$ and myocardial oxidative metabolism (*right*) assessed with ^{11}C-acetate are homogeneous. The scales indicate counts per pixel. Orientation is the same as in Figure 48–6. (Courtesy of Dr. S. R. Bergmann, Washington University School of Medicine, St. Louis, MO.)

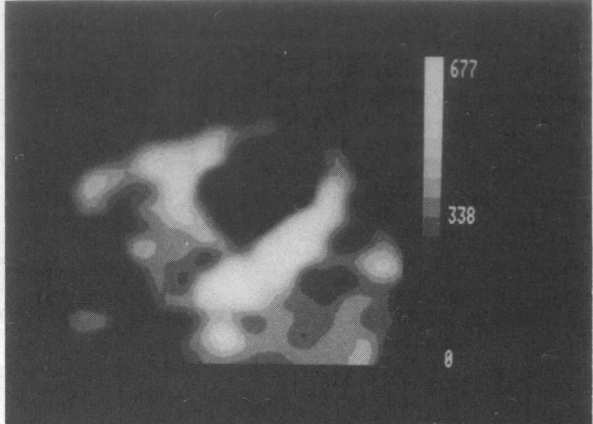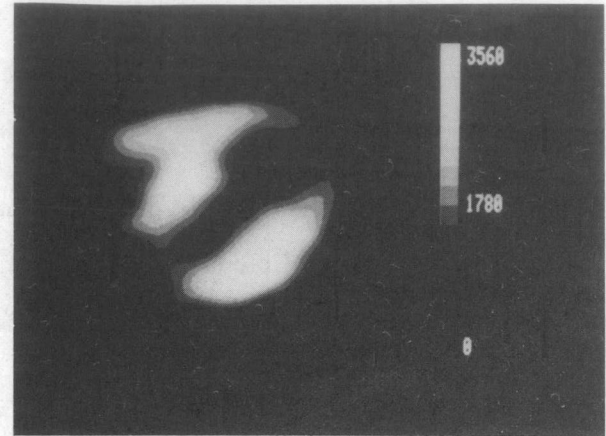

FIGURE 48–8. Midventricular tomographic reconstructions of perfusion (*left*) and oxidative metabolism (*right*) obtained after intravenous administration of $H_2^{15}O$ and ^{11}C-acetate after acute anterior myocardial infarction. A large perfusion deficit is evident anteriorly with a concordant decrease in myocardial oxygen consumption reflected by decreased ^{11}C-acetate uptake. (From Walsh MN, Geltman EM, Brown MA, et al.: Noninvasive estimation of regional myocardial oxygen consumption by positron emission tomography with carbon-11 acetate in patients with myocardial infarction. J Nucl Med 30:1798, 1989; with permission.)

hemodynamic monitoring when indicated, implementation and titration of measures designed to limit the extent of infarction and salvage jeopardized ischemic myocardium, and induction of recanalization of infarct-related arteries pharmacologically.

Care in the CCU. In addition to continuous ECG monitoring, several general measures should be implemented. Diet should include liquid only during the first 24 hours because of the risk of aspiration with the frequent nausea and vomiting, and possible cardiac arrest. Stool softeners are helpful to avoid constipation, straining, and consequent circulatory derangements. Patients with uncomplicated infarction need be confined to bed for only 1 day. Physical activity should be limited (bed-chair regimen) throughout the 2- to 3-day CCU stay, with gradual and carefully monitored resumption of ambulatory activity in the late hospital phase. Sedative, anxiolytic, and hypnotic drugs at night may be helpful but cannot replace optimal communication by compassionate physicians and nurses and the reassurance it provides. Oxygen should be given to avoid hypoxemia. High doses may be counterproductive because of vasoconstriction and lack of augmentation of myocardial oxygen delivery in normoxemic patients.

Refractory or severe pain should be treated with intravenous morphine, meperidine, or pentazocine. Repeated intravenous doses of 4 to 8 mg of morphine at intervals of 5 to 15 minutes can be given with relative impunity until the pain is relieved or toxicity is manifest by hypotension, vomiting, or depression of respiration. Prodigious quantities are sometimes required (2 to 3 mg per kilogram). Should toxicity occur, a morphine antagonist such as naloxone can reverse it. Morphine-induced hypotension in a patient without incipient or overt pulmonary edema can be minimized by maintenance of the patient in a supine position, elevation of the legs, administration of fluids, and administration of atropine if heart rate is not increased.

Continuing chest pain indicative of ischemia should be treated with agents diminishing myocardial oxygen requirements and potentiating myocardial perfusion. Intravenous nitroglycerin titrated (10 to 200 μg per minute) to avoid hypotension reduces peripheral arterial resistance and ventricular afterload. Higher doses diminish systemic venous tone, blood pressure, and ischemic zone perfusion. Favorable effects are probably mediated by diminished afterload and preload and decreased LVEDP facilitating myocardial perfusion. Although coronary vasodilation in intramural vessels is often already maximal as a result of accumulation of vasodilator metabolites locally, nitrates may dilate epicardial vessels and reduce vasospasm, thereby reducing shear forces otherwise contributing to platelet activation and potentiating propagation of coronary thrombi. Tolerance to continuously administered intravenous nitrates occurs rapidly, often within hours.

Oral calcium channel blockers such as nifedipine and diltiazem are often useful because they reduce ventricular afterload (nifed-ipine) and modestly reduce heart rate and contractility as well (diltiazem). However, prognosis appears to be affected adversely in patients with congestive heart failure or impaired left ventricular function that persists after myocardial infarction by treatment with diltiazem and possibly other calcium channel blockers as well. Oral or intravenous conventional or ultra–short-acting β-adrenergic blockers such as esmolol may ameliorate ischemia and pain by lowering heart rate and hence myocardial oxygen requirements. Theoretically, calcium antagonists and β-adrenergic blockers may exert anti-injury effects as well by diminishing inward calcium flux in cardiac myocytes.

Despite the use of effective analgesia with nitrous oxide given by inhalation in concentrations of 20 to 50 per cent combined with oxygen in Europe and elsewhere, this agent is not used widely in the United States. Its effects on ventricular afterload are favorable, and it is generally well tolerated for intervals as long as 24 to 48 hours when used intermittently.

Limitation of Infarct Size. Because the evolution of infarction is dynamic and determined in part by the imbalance between myocardial oxygen requirements and oxygen supply, early treatment focuses not only on prompt recanalization of the infarct-related artery but also on diminution of myocardial oxygen requirements without compromise of perfusion of vital organs. Myocardial protection can be enhanced with β-adrenergic blockers to reduce heart rate; arterial vasodilators such as nifedipine, nitrates, or angiotensin-converting enzyme (ACE) inhibitors to reduce ventricular afterload; and diuretics with pulmonary venous dilating properties such as furosemide and ethacrynic acid to reduce left ventricular preload. Beta-adrenergic blockers are likely to be useful in most patients without specific contraindications such as heart failure, bradycardia, or bronchial constriction. Other agents should be titrated to optimize left ventricular filling pressure (often to as high as 18 to 22 mm Hg because of decreased ventricular compliance) and cardiac output while maintaining adequate systemic arterial blood pressure (Table 48–9).

Coronary Thrombolysis. The potential value of coronary thrombolysis has been recognized for more than 30 years. Its emergence as primary therapy was delayed, however, until the pivotal role of thrombosis in causing Q-wave infarction had been established unequivocally by coronary arteriography, the impact of extensive infarction on mortality had been established, and salvage of myocardium by decreasing oxygen requirements had been found to be limited. The "modern" era of coronary thrombolysis began in the late 1970's with the demonstration that intracoronary administration of plasminogen activators recanalized occluded arteries and immediately relieved pain. Recanalization was soon documented in 70 to 75 per cent of patients given intracoronary streptokinase. However, intracoronary dosing entailed serious disadvantages including risk and delay associated with the obligatory cardiac catheterization. Intravenous administration was soon

TABLE 48–9. THERAPEUTIC INTERVENTIONS TAILORED TO SPECIFIC HEMODYNAMIC SUBSETS

Hemodynamic Subset		Intervention	Remarks
I	Normal hemodynamics	None required	
II	Hyperdynamic state	Beta-adrenergic blockade	Analgesics and anxiolytic drugs may be helpful.
III	Hypovolemia	Intravenous fluids to augment effective vascular volume	Marked increases in pulmonary artery occlusive pressure reflecting pulmonary venous hypertension and increased left ventricular filling pressure may occur if heart failure is unmasked or exacerbated; manifestations may include dyspnea, hypoxemia, bronchospasm and rales, and pulmonary congestion evident radiographically.
IV	Left ventricular failure		
	A. Mild	Systemic arterial vasodilators	Diuretics may be useful if failure is refractory.
	B. Severe	Systemic arterial vasodilators and diuretics	Cardiotonic agents may be helpful if hypotension supervenes, but their use can exacerbate the imbalance between myocardial oxygen requirements and supply; sympathomimetic and dopaminergic agents may be helpful, but their benefit on hemodynamics is usually only transitory and may exacerbate ischemic injury.
V	Cardiogenic shock	Coronary recanalization and circulatory support	
VI	Shock attributable to right ventricular infarction	Augmentation of vascular volume and cardiotonic agents	

Adapted from Forrester JS, et al.: Medical therapy of acute myocardial infarction by application of hemodynamic subsets. N Engl J Med 295:1404, 1976. By permission of the New England Journal of Medicine.

shown to be effective in recanalizing approximately 50 per cent of infarct-related arteries when streptokinase was used and 75 to 80 per cent (comparable to the optimal recanalization rates with any agent by any route of administration) when tissue-type plasminogen activator (t-PA) was used (Fig. 48–9). The superiority of intravenously administered second- compared with first-generation plasminogen activators in recanalizing coronary arteries may reflect (1) more modest plasminemia with its consequent procoagulant and platelet-activating effects counteracting thrombolysis; (2) a lack of "plasminogen steal" with consequent maintenance of high concentrations of clot-associated plasminogen available for activation to plasmin induction of lysis; and (3) the feasibility of safe administration of high concentrations of activator with less degradation of hemostatic proteins.

Induction of coronary thrombolysis with intravenously administered activators of plasminogen improves ventricular function and decreases mortality both early and late after infarction, particularly when initiated within a few hours after the onset of ischemia. Even when initiated only 6 hours or more after the onset of infarction, restoration of patency of the infarct-related artery appears to confer benefits reflected by improved collateral blood flow, improved ventricular remodeling, decreased infarct expansion, decreased late potentials manifest in signal-averaged electrocardiograms potentially indicative of arrhythmogenicity, improved late ventricular function, decreased ventricular aneurysm formation, decreased late arrhythmia associated with those aneurysms that do develop, and decreased mortality.

It is convenient and useful to consider two generations of fibrinolytic drugs. The first, typified by streptokinase, urokinase, and APSAC (acetylated plasminogen streptokinase activator complex) induces activation of free plasminogen and clot-associated plasminogen indiscriminately. First-generation drugs invariably

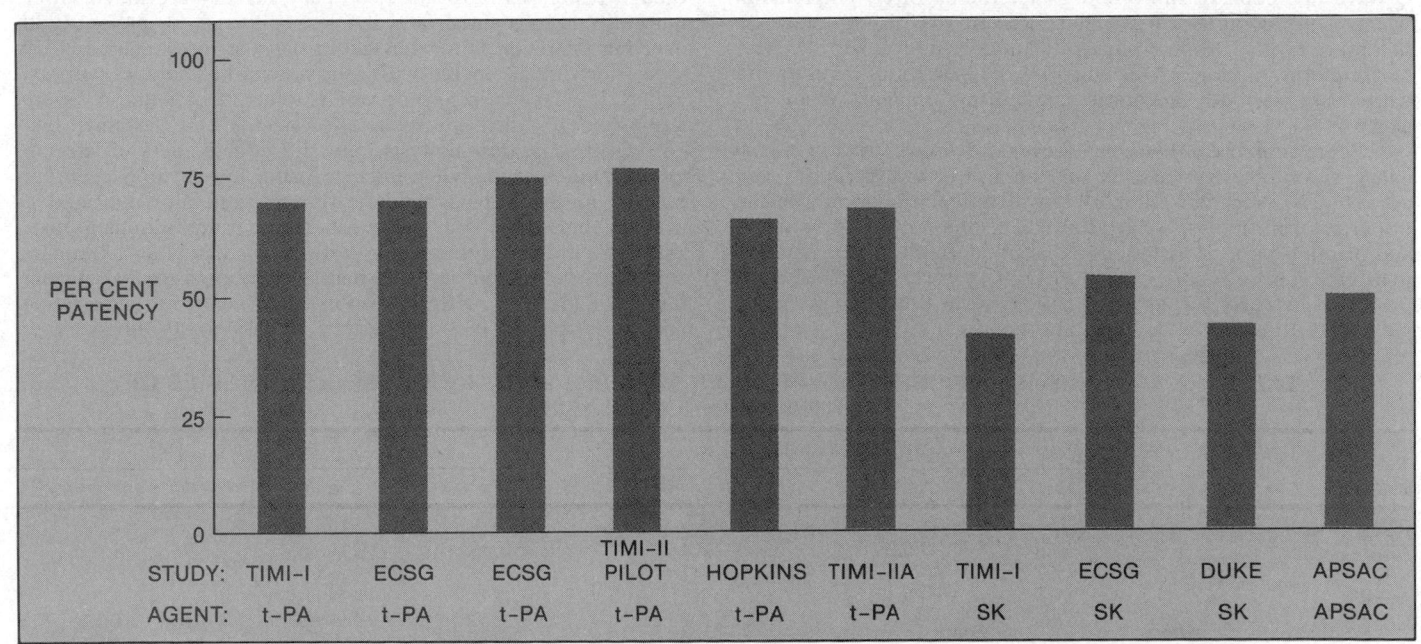

FIGURE 48–9. Angiographically defined patency of infarct-related arteries 90 minutes after treatment within 4 to 8 hours after onset of symptoms with streptokinase (SK), tissue-type plasminogen activator (t-PA), or acetylated plasminogen streptokinase activator complex (APSAC) reported in 10 large studies involving 1654 patients. TIMI = Thrombolysis in Myocardial Infarction; ECSG = European Cooperative Study Group. (From Tiefenbrunn AJ, Sobel BE: Fibrinolysis 3:1, 1988; with permission of Churchill Livingstone.)

elicit a systemic lytic state characterized by depletion of circulating fibrinogen, plasminogen, and hemostatic proteins and by marked elevation of concentrations of fibrinogen degradation products in plasma. Their lack of clot selectivity is therefore associated with an increased risk of bleeding and possible protection against early reocclusion in inadequately anticoagulated patients.

Second-generation drugs, typified by t-PA and single-chain urokinase plasminogen activator, activate plasminogen in the fibrin domain preferentially compared with free plasminogen in the circulation. Thus they exhibit relative clot selectivity. In optimal dosage they induce clot lysis without inducing a systemic lytic state. They are less prone to predispose to hemorrhage requiring transfusion.

Recanalization is more frequent and more rapid with second- than with first-generation agents, perhaps in part because of clot selectivity and lack of induction of plasminemia, which may induce procoagulant effects that attenuate fibrinolysis and plasminogen steal and diminish the intensity of fibrinolysis.

The risks of coronary thrombolysis with plasminogen activators include bleeding, most of which is confined to sites of vascular access. Marked depletion of fibrinogen indicative of a systemic lytic state may be a marker of pharmacologic effects that can lead also to bleeding. Marked prolongation of bleeding time may reflect bleeding risk somewhat more specifically. Although intracranial hemorrhage had been feared, the incidence of cerebrovascular accidents in patients treated with thrombolytic agents is no greater than that seen with conservative treatment without fibrinolytic drugs (Table 48–10). The incidence of hemorrhagic stroke is somewhat greater and that of thrombotic or embolic stroke somewhat less, but the disparity is not reflected by an increased incidence of fatal cerebrovascular accidents and is more than offset by the favorable impact of fibrinolytic agents on survival after infarction.

Plasminogen activators should not be given to patients with active internal bleeding or a bleeding diathesis, suspected aortic dissection, hemorrhagic retinopathy, recent trauma (including surgery or prolonged and traumatic cardiopulmonary resuscitation), intracranial neoplasm, or hypertensive crisis. Relative contraindications include peptic ulcer disease, remote cerebrovascular accident, and hepatic failure. Safety has not been established for pregnant women. In general, thrombolytic agents should be used in patients 75 years of age or less who present with suspected Q-wave infarction within 6 hours after the onset of symptoms in whom contraindications are not present. Treatment may be helpful in some patients first seen 6 hours or more after the onset of symptoms. Its impact on non–Q-wave infarction, infarction in patients of very advanced age, and unstable angina is not yet clear.

Adjunctive and Conjunctive Measures. Clinical efficacy of coronary thrombolysis depends on the frequency, rapidity, and persistence of recanalization, all of which depend not only on the intensity of fibrinolysis but also on the inhibition of coagulation and platelet-induced thrombosis that undoubtedly occur concomitantly. Even optimally effective coronary thrombolysis is compromised by early thrombotic reocclusion in 6 to 20 per cent of patients with initial recanalization.

Calcium antagonists have potential value as anti-injury agents in the setting of reperfusion, as antiplatelet agents, and as coronary vasodilators, effects that may minimize activation of platelets in the vicinity of lysed thrombi by reducing shear forces. Nitrates may diminish excessive coronary reactivity and hence ischemia. Reperfusion arrhythmias, if they compromise hemodynamics or threaten to degenerate into ventricular fibrillation, can often be suppressed with lidocaine. Alpha-adrenergic blocking agents are attractive theoretical alternatives. Accelerated idioventricular arrhythmia often does not require pharmacologic intervention. Perhaps of most importance are conjunctive anticoagulation with a powerful antithrombin such as heparin or hirudin (currently investigational) and conjunctive use of antiplatelet agents such as aspirin or antibodies and antagonists to the platelet glycoprotein IIb/IIIa receptor, prostacyclin and PGE_2 analogues, thromboxane receptor antagonists and synthetase inhibitors, and serotonin antagonists (all investigational at present).

Contrary to initial expectations, not all patients treated with thrombolytic drugs should be subjected to obligatory early cardiac catheterization and angioplasty. A strategy comprising arteriography and angioplasty in only those patients who exhibit recurrent or persistent symptoms and signs of ischemia appears to be safer (Table 48–11) and as effective as obligatory angiography for all patients in preserving ventricular function and reducing mortality. The value of rescue angioplasty, i.e., angioplasty performed when occlusion has proven to be refractory to recanalization with fibrinolytic drugs, has not been established.

Mechanical Revascularization. Compared with pharmacologic thrombolysis, mechanical recanalization (angioplasty or surgery) may enhance flow more markedly or more rapidly in patients who sustain infarction while in a cardiac catheterization laboratory. However, except in such rare instances or in centers dedicated to immediate angioplasty as primary therapy, it has not yet proven to be superior. Immediate angioplasty or surgery cannot be provided universally because of contention for facilities, the need for large teams of highly trained personnel on a 24-hour per day basis, and other logistic constraints. Risks of primary angioplasty exceed those of elective angioplasty for coronary artery disease with angina. Surgical facilities and personnel should be readily available in view of the 10 per cent incidence of life-threatening complications encountered. Restenosis rates after balloon angioplasty or other investigational approaches such as laser or mechanical atherectomy exceed 30 per cent within 6 months despite vigorous use of anticoagulants, antiplatelet drugs, calcium antagonists, vasodilators, and intracoronary stents. Although restenosis rates after coronary surgery are much lower, morbidity is substantial, and the mortality risk for patients with evolving infarction is not trivial. In view of the remarkably low early mortality attainable with intravenous fibrinolytics (approximately 5 per cent in appropriately selected patients in several large studies with second-generation agents), the sustained benefit of coronary thrombolysis, and the effectiveness of late mechanical intervention when indicated after initial coronary thrombolysis, mechanical revascularization is generally indicated as primary therapy only for patients with contraindications to pharmacologic thrombolysis, those with immediate life-threatening conditions such as cardiogenic shock refractory to coronary thrombolysis, and those with infarction resulting from occlusion of previously placed coronary artery bypass grafts amenable to

TABLE 48–10. INCIDENCE OF CEREBROVASCULAR ACCIDENT (CVA) IN CONTROLLED STUDIES OF CORONARY THROMBOLYSIS

Study	Thrombolytic Agent			Control Group		
	n	*Agent*	*Per Cent with CVA*	*n*	*Agent*	*Per Cent with CVA*
GISSI	5860	SK	1.1	5852	Placebo	0.9
AIMS	502	APSAC	0.4	502	Placebo	1.0
ISIS-2	8592	SK	0.7	8595	Placebo	0.8
ASSET	2516	t-PA	1.1	2495	Placebo	1.0
ECSG*	722	t-PA	1.1	366	Placebo	0.5
TOTAL	18,192		0.9	17,810		0.9

Adapted from Tiefenbrunn AJ, et al.: Coronary thrombolysis—it's worth the risk. JAMA 261:2107, 1989. Copyright 1989, American Medical Association.
*Two studies, one with placebo, one with t-PA with and without angioplasty.
GISSI = Gruppo Italiano per lo Studio della Streptochinasi nell'Infarto Miocardico; AIMS = APSAC Intervention Mortality Study; ISIS-2 = International Study of Infarct Survival; ASSET = Anglo-Scandinavian Study of Early Thrombolysis; ECSG = European Cooperative Study Group.
SK = Streptokinase; APSAC = anisoylated plasminogen streptokinase activator complex; t-PA = tissue-type plasminogen activator.

TABLE 48–11. OUTCOME AFTER INVASIVE COMPARED WITH CONSERVATIVE MANAGEMENT*

Event	Management Strategy after Thrombolysis		
	Invasive	Conservative	P Value
Death	5.2%	4.7%	0.49
Death or reinfarction	10.9%	9.7%	0.25
Coronary artery bypass grafting	11.9%	10.5%	0.18
Intracranial hemorrhage	0.9%	0.7%	0.70
Any adverse endpoint†	13.0%	10.6%	0.04

Adapted from the TIMI Group: Comparison of invasive and conservative strategies after treatment with intravenous tissue plasminogen activator in acute myocardial infarction: Results of the thrombolysis in myocardial infarction (TIMI) phase II trial. N Engl J Med 295:1404, 1976. By permission of the New England Journal of Medicine. Inclusion and exclusion criteria are delineated in the referenced article.

*The percentages of adverse clinical events during the initial 42 days of follow-up are shown in these results from a study of 3262 patients with Q-wave infarction randomized to treatment with (invasive strategy) or without (conservative strategy) obligatory angiography and angioplasty early after acute myocardial infarction treated initially with tissue-type plasminogen activator. The invasive strategy was not superior.

†Death, nonfatal reinfarction, intracranial hemorrhage, or coronary bypass grafting after angioplasty.

angioplasty. The role of salvage angioplasty for occlusions refractory to fibrinolysis remains to be established, in part because candidates are likely to have already sustained extensive irreversible injury by the time failure of thrombolysis can first be established.

PROPHYLAXIS AND TREATMENT OF ARRHYTHMIA. Continuous ECG monitoring is essential for 72 hours after the onset of infarction and optimally throughout hospitalization by telemetry to immediately detect ventricular fibrillation and numerous arrhythmias that may occur. Some degenerate into ventricular fibrillation because of augmentation of myocardial oxygen requirements, impaired ventricular performance with consequent exacerbation of ischemia, or both.

Both primary and secondary (to hemodynamic decompensation, hypoxemia, electrolyte disturbances, or progressive cardiac or pulmonary failure) ventricular fibrillation should be treated by immediate electrical countershock. Fibrillation may be confused with electrical asystole when the vector of fibrillation is perpendicular to the axis of the recording lead used for monitoring. True asystole requires confirmation with multiple leads and differentiation from fine ventricular fibrillation. If the distinction between ventricular fibrillation and asystole cannot be made with certainty, fibrillation should be assumed to be present. Other established components of cardiopulmonary resuscitation and advanced cardiac life support are invaluable, but the primacy of immediate restoration of effective cardiac rhythm cannot be overemphasized. Electrical countershock should be implemented immediately rather than deferred until after endotracheal intubation and other emergency measures. If true electrical asystole is documented, immediate external, transvenous, or transthoracic cardiac pacing is essential, although prognosis in this situation is grim.

When ventricular fibrillation accompanies acute myocardial infarction, lidocaine is the drug of choice for prevention of immediate recurrence. Prophylactic administration remains somewhat controversial because adverse effects (central nervous system depression, seizures, proarrhythmic, asystolic, and cardiodepressant effects) may offset potential benefit. Repeat bolus injections of 0.5 to 1.0 mg per kilogram body weight every 5 minutes to a total of 4 mg per kilogram, followed by maintenance infusions of 1 to 2 mg per minute are used for this purpose in younger patients without prior cardiac disease who can be treated within the first few hours after the onset of infarction when the risk of primary ventricular fibrillation is greatest. After successful resuscitation when ventricular fibrillation has occurred, lidocaine should be administered by continuous infusion (20 to 50 µg per kilogram of body weight per minute), particularly if frequent, closely coupled, multiform, or repetitive ventricular premature complexes or ventricular tachycardia occurs. Blood levels should be maintained in the range of 2 to 5 µg per milliliter. Recurrent ventricular fibrillation, refractory to lidocaine, may be suppressed after a considerable lag period by intravenous bretylium given in

5- to 10-mg per kilogram doses or by amiodarone (0.75 µg per kilogram loading dose followed by infusion of 5 to 10 µg per minute [still investigational in the United States]). Other promising antifibrillatory drugs are currently investigational in the United States.

High-grade ventricular ectopy or bursts of ventricular tachycardia should be treated with lidocaine. If they persist for more than a few hours after hospitalization, their management is similar to that applicable in other circumstances. Procainamide and quinidine are generally the drugs of choice. Torsades de pointes may respond to overdrive pacing or intravenous magnesium sulfate. Accelerated idioventricular rhythm should not be treated unless hemodynamic decompensation occurs, in which case sequential or atrial overdrive pacing or atropine may be effective.

Supraventricular Arrhythmias. Treatment of these arrhythmias is the same as when they occur under other circumstances and is indicated when they impair hemodynamics or compromise myocardial viability by augmenting oxygen requirements. Sinus tachycardia is usually secondary to excessive sympathoadrenal tone associated with extensive infarction and impaired ventricular performance, pericardial inflammation and irritation of the sinus node, relative or absolute hypovolemia, hypoxemia secondary to pulmonary venous congestion and respiratory impairment, congestive heart failure, or other potentially remediable factors. Atrial fibrillation or atrial flutter may be indicative of failure or atrial infarction. In the absence of the Wolff-Parkinson-White syndrome, these conditions should be treated with calcium channel blockers such as verapamil, digitalis glycosides, or a short-acting β-adrenergic blocker such as esmolol to control ventricular rate. Procainamide (intravenous or oral) or quinidine (oral) is often effective in restoring and maintaining sinus rhythm. When decompensation is evident, rapid atrial pacing (to terminate atrial flutter) or electrical cardioversion (to terminate either atrial fibrillation or flutter) should be used. When hemodynamics are compromised or myocardial viability is threatened, paroxysmal supraventricular tachycardias should be managed initially by augmentation of vagal tone with carotid sinus compression or the Valsalva maneuver, calcium channel blockers, intravenous adenosine, or electrical cardioversion. The safety of adenosine in patients with infarction has not yet been established unequivocally.

Bradyarrhythmias. Sinus bradycardia occurs often, particularly in patients with inferior myocardial infarction. If refractory to atropine, it may require temporary transvenous pacing. A wandering atrial pacemaker or first-degree AV block rarely requires specific treatment. Higher degrees of AV block or AV block associated with hypotension refractory to atropine may require sequential pacing to sustain adequate hemodynamics.

Long-term pacing is needed only when heart block persists throughout the hospital phase, sinus node function is markedly impaired, Mobitz II second- or third-degree block occurs intermittently, or block is associated with newly acquired bundle branch block or other criteria of conduction system impairment. It is difficult to prove that long-term pacing improves survival after myocardial infarction because mortality is so high, with the extensive infarction frequently responsible. Nevertheless, temporary transvenous pacing may stabilize hemodynamics, and long-term pacing may be justified prophylactically in patients at high risk.

TREATMENT TAILORED TO HEMODYNAMICS. Invasive hemodynamic monitoring is of inestimable value in patients with clinically complicated acute myocardial infarction. It permits rapid delineation of left ventricular filling pressure, effective vascular volume, the presence or absence of mitral regurgitation and its severity, ventricular septal rupture (with oximetry), right ventricular systolic and diastolic pressure and function, and cardiac output and peripheral vascular resistance. Selection of therapy based on hemodynamics is delineated in Table 48–9 and is predicated on the following considerations:

1. Hypertensive patients with increased cardiac output and normal pulmonary artery wedge pressure may benefit from infusions of β-adrenergic blockers such as esmolol to reduce myocardial oxygen requirements.

2. Hypotension associated with relative or absolute hypovole-

mia reflected by lack of substantial elevation (above 18 mm Hg) of left ventricular filling pressure generally responds to augmentation of vascular volume with intravenous fluids. Pulmonary artery wedge pressure should be monitored to preclude excesses leading to pulmonary edema. Hypotension with markedly elevated right ventricular diastolic, right atrial, and central venous pressures may implicate right ventricular infarction, which responds often to augmentation of vascular volume and stimulation of the heart with cardiotonic agents such as dobutamine, dopamine, or β-adrenergic agonists. Systemic arteriolar vasodilators secondarily decrease impedance of right ventricular outflow if they ameliorate left heart failure and can be used when systemic arterial diastolic pressure is adequate.

3. Sudden and profound hypotension may reflect a catastrophic insult such as pulmonary embolism (manifested by pulmonary arterial hypertension and hypoxemia) or rupture of the ventricular septum (detectable by augmented right ventricular and pulmonary artery pressure associated with an oxygen step-up in the right ventricle). Alternatively, it may reflect left ventricular papillary muscle rupture with mitral regurgitation manifested by large V waves in the pulmonary artery wedge pressure recording. When caused by free wall rupture with hemopericardium, hemodynamic manifestations of pericardial tamponade are apparent, with a diastolic pressure plateau in all four cardiac chambers, impairment of right ventricular filling, and confirmatory echocardiographic findings of pericardial fluid and diastolic right atrial and right ventricular collapse. Mechanical insults should be treated by immediate surgery if hemodynamic stability can be maintained with only pharmacologic and circulatory support. Surgery can be delayed for 1 to 2 weeks if stability can be maintained without such measures and the patient can be monitored meticulously.

4. Hypotension associated with markedly elevated pulmonary artery wedge pressure is generally indicative of severely impaired left ventricular performance and cardiogenic shock. Supportive measures and cardiotonic agents are generally ineffective unless the ischemia responsible can be relieved by coronary thrombolysis, angioplasty, or surgery. Mechanical circulatory support may be necessary to permit acquisition of definitive diagnostic information pertinent to potentially remediable insults such as septal or free wall rupture, mitral regurgitation, or coronary reocclusion. Intra-aortic balloon counterpulsation or circulatory support with a left ventricular assist device may be particularly useful as a temporizing measure or as a bridge to cardiac transplantation.

5. Pulmonary venous hypertension with normal systemic arterial pressure is indicative of relative or absolute excess of vascular volume and left heart failure that should be treated with vasodilators to reduce both ventricular preload and afterload, diminish the commonly associated mitral regurgitation accompanying left ventricular failure, and diminish left atrial and pulmonary venous hypertension. Intravenous nitroprusside, nitroglycerin, or parenteral or oral ACE inhibitors may be effective. Caution must be exercised to avoid marked changes in concentrations of electrolytes in plasma. If pulmonary congestion is severe or pulmonary edema is present but cardiac output is reasonably well maintained and associated with an adequate systemic arterial blood pressure, contraction of vascular volume by removal of fluid (phlebotomy with reinfusion of blood cell elements, slow continuous ultrafiltration, and rarely peritoneal dialysis) may be effective. If pulmonary congestion persists or if cardiac output and systemic arterial pressure are low, loop diuretics (having the advantage also of pulmonary venodilation) may be helpful. Hemodialysis is dangerous because of the risk of precipitous changes in filling pressures and cardiac performance. Cardiotonic agents (dobutamine or dopamine, digitalis, and phosphodiesterase inhibitors such as amrinone or milrinone [investigational]), previously a mainstay of therapy for congestive heart failure with diminished cardiac output and hypotension, may be necessary but entail the risk of exacerbating imbalance between myocardial oxygen supply and demand and are generally not dramatically effective alone.

6. Hypotension with or without pulmonary venous hypertension indicative of left heart failure is generally associated with increased peripheral vascular resistance in patients with infarc-

tion. In rare instances it may be decreased, in which case vasoconstrictors (such as dopamine in relatively high doses, epinephrine particularly if cardiac rate is not accelerated, and rarely, although usually fruitlessly, norepinephrine) may be indicated. The decrease of resistance is often caused by other factors, such as occult sepsis, which must of course be recognized. In patients with profound ventricular failure, circulatory support with intra-aortic balloon counterpulsation or left ventricular assist devices may permit performance of diagnostic catheterization and identification and treatment of surgically remediable lesions.

Care in the Step-down Unit. Patients with uncomplicated myocardial infarction require CCU care generally for no more than 72 hours. Subsequent care is facilitated in a step-down unit equipped with telemetry for continuous ECG monitoring. Therapeutic objectives include immediate recognition and treatment of ventricular tachycardia, ventricular fibrillation, and bradycardia caused by sinus node dysfunction or AV block; daily clinical and appropriate laboratory monitoring for prompt detection and treatment of complications, including deep venous thrombosis (sometimes manifest–by fever and Homans' sign), pulmonary emboli, post–myocardial infarction pericarditis with a friction rub, tachycardia, and fever (generally managed with aspirin to avoid impaired infarct healing that may occur with nonsteroidal antiinflammatory agents or corticosteroids), ventricular thrombi, ventricular true or false aneurysm, or catastrophic mechanical complications including cardiac rupture; treatment to minimize the risk of recurrent infarction; assessment of prognosis based on evaluation of left ventricular function, exercise tolerance, and the severity of spontaneous or inducible ischemia; and gradual and judicious progressive ambulation followed by a rehabilitation program after discharge.

In patients who have been treated with thrombolytic agents, heparin can be discontinued after 5 to 7 days, and secondary prevention of thrombosis can be continued with daily aspirin. For those with ventricular mural thrombus or extensive hypokinesis, congestive heart failure, or ventricular aneurysm predisposing to mural thrombus, anticoagulation with warfarin is appropriate for 6 months. Patients with non–Q-wave infarction without congestive heart failure should be treated with calcium channel blockers to prevent recurrence. Those with Q-wave infarction without failure or other contraindications should be treated for 6 months or more with β-adrenergic blockers devoid of intrinsic sympathomimetic activity to reduce the incidence of reinfarction and enhance survival.

Complications detected by telemetry (episodic ischemia with ST-segment deviation, arrhythmia, heart block, new-onset bundle branch block, tachycardia with minimal exertion), physical findings suggestive of congestive heart failure, markedly impaired ventricular performance documented echocardiographically or by radionuclide ventriculography, or manifestations of recurrent coronary occlusion such as recurrent pain, unexplained tachycardia, exacerbation or appearance of heart failure, hypotension, or impaired ventricular performance justify consideration of coronary arteriography before discharge from the hospital, with mechanical revascularization if indicated. In patients without such complications and particularly those treated initially with thrombolytic drugs, submaximal (7 to 10 days) or symptom-limited (predischarge) exercise testing should be performed to determine whether arteriography is indicated. Exercise-induced ischemia manifested by ST-segment depression of 1 mm or more, reversible thallium perfusion defects, a hypotensive response to modest workloads, ventricular arrhythmias, diminution of ejection fraction, or induction of wall motion abnormalities with or without angina pectoris is an indication for coronary arteriography. Marked impairment of ventricular performance (resting ejection fraction less than 40 per cent) or anticipated stringent physical occupational requirements are relative indications. Thallium scintigraphy or exercise echocardiography may be useful when baseline ECG abnormalities obscure interpretation. Dipyridamole thallium scintigraphy or dobutamine stress echocardiography (currently investigational in the United States) may substitute for exercise testing in patients unable to exercise for noncardiac reasons. Risk for development of sustained ventricular tachycardia or ventricular fibrillation can be estimated by high-resolution electrocardiography with frequency- or time-domain analysis of signal-averaged recordings, which provides criteria independent

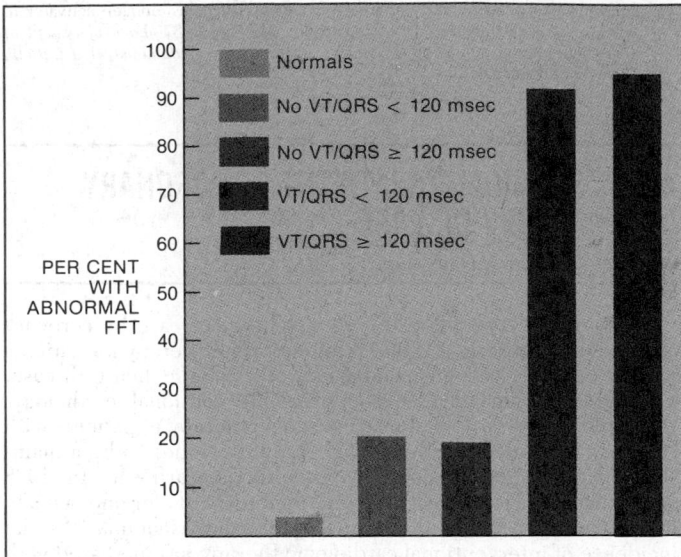

FIGURE 48–10. The predictive value for risk of sustained ventricular tachycardia (VT) of abnormalities detectable by high-resolution electrocardiography performed by fast-Fourier transform (FFT) frequency-domain analysis in 169 subjects with and without coronary artery disease and myocardial infarction categorized with respect to the presence or absence of QRS complex prolongation indicative of left bundle branch block or other intraventricular conduction delays. High-resolution ECG abnormalities correlated closely with the likelihood of occurrence of sustained VT whether or not conduction disturbances were present. (From Lindsay BD, et al.: Circulation 77:122, 1988. Reproduced by permission of the American Heart Association, Inc.)

of left ventricular dysfunction (Fig. 48–10). Ambulatory continuous ECG monitoring is often used, but the occurrence of the complex ventricular ectopy targeted for detection is generally concordant with severe left ventricular dysfunction after infarction.

CONVALESCENCE

Most patients can be discharged within 1 to 2 weeks. Complications at any time may require a longer hospital stay. Objectives of management during convalescence include (1) prevention of recurrent infarction (continued use of β-adrenergic blockers after Q-wave infarction, calcium channel blockers after non–Q-wave infarction with preserved left ventricular function, and aspirin); (2) prevention of late complications of infarction such as peripheral or cerebral embolus from ventricular mural thrombus with continued anticoagulation for 3 to 6 months in patients at high risk of harboring mural thrombi; (3) risk factor modification including

cessation of smoking, treatment of hypertension, diabetes, and hyperlipidemia, and implementation of a carefully monitored exercise rehabilitation program under supervision or for appropriately motivated patients at home; (4) prompt detection and evaluation of potential progression of underlying coronary artery disease manifested by signs or symptoms of ischemia including angina pectoris; and (5) prevention of sudden cardiac death with β-adrenergic blockers in patients without specific contraindications. Indiscriminate use of antiarrhythmic agents, particularly type I_c drugs, to suppress asymptomatic ventricular ectopy should be avoided because of the risk of increasing mortality (Fig. 48–11).

Patients with non–Q-wave infarctions require special consideration. This syndrome appears often to be a manifestation of incomplete or nonsustained thrombotic coronary occlusion. Early prognosis is good compared with prognosis for patients with Q-wave infarction. However, mortality late after infarction may exceed that after Q-wave infarction because of reocclusion, reinfarction, or sudden cardiac death reflecting recurrent ischemia. Survivors of non-Q infarction in whom ventricular function is well maintained benefit from treatment with calcium channel blockers. Beta-blockers are more likely to improve survival after Q-wave infarction; aspirin is indicated in both groups.

THE OUTLOOK

Early mortality associated with acute myocardial infarction has declined dramatically over the past three decades. Before the advent of CCU's, hospital mortality was approximately 30 per cent. Aggressive defibrillation reduced it by half. Protection of jeopardized ischemic myocardium and early pharmacologic coronary recanalization followed by mechanical revascularization when indicated have lowered mortality even further, to 5 per cent or less among patients 75 years of age or less with no contraindications to thrombolysis in whom treatment can be initiated within several hours after the onset of symptoms. Consolidation of these gains requires continued surveillance and management of patients throughout convalescence to allow recognition and prevention of recurrent ischemia; retardation of progression of coronary artery disease; prompt recognition of its occurrence; and vigorous medical, mechanical, and surgical intervention when required.

Bergmann SR: Positron emission tomography. *In* Gerson M (ed.): Cardiac Nuclear Medicine. New York, McGraw-Hill Book Company, 1990. *A comprehensive and elegant review addressing technology, instrumentation, applications in research, and utility in diagnosis.*

Braunwald E: Thirty-five years of progress in cardiovascular research. Circulation (Suppl III) 70:III-8, 1984. *Lucid and thorough articulation of the major conceptual themes and paradigms underlying treatment of acute myocardial infarction and their evolution during the modern era.*

The Cardiac Arrhythmia Suppression Trial Investigators: Preliminary report: Effect of encainide and flecainide on mortality in a randomized trial of arrhythmia suppression after myocardial infarction. N Engl J Med 321:406, 1989. *A noteworthy report of the unexpected adverse influences of type I_c antiarrhythmic agents when utilized in the treatment of ventricular ectopy in asymptomatic patients who have sustained acute myocardial infarction.*

Collen D, Topol EJ, Tiefenbrunn AJ, et al.: Coronary thrombolysis with recombinant human tissue–type plasminogen activator: A prospective, randomized, placebo-controlled trial. Circulation 70:1012, 1984. *The initial study demonstrating effective coronary thrombolysis with sparing of fibrinogen in patients with acute myocardial infarction treated with tissue-type plasminogen activator produced by recombinant DNA technology.*

Davies MJ, Woolf N, Robertson WB: Pathology of acute myocardial infarction with particular reference to occlusive coronary thrombi. Br Heart J 38:659, 1976. *A seminal study demonstrating the pathophysiologic connections between complex atherosclerotic plaques and sudden cardiac death.*

DeWood MA, Spores J, Notske R, et al.: Prevalence of total coronary occlusion during the early hours of transmural myocardial infarction. N Engl J Med 303:897, 1980. *Demonstration of the high incidence of occlusive coronary thrombi in patients studied angiographically soon after the onset of chest pain who have sustained acute Q-wave infarctions.*

Ellis AK, Little T, Masud Z, et al.: Early noninvasive detection of successful reperfusion in patients with acute myocardial infarction. Circulation 78:1352, 1988. *A recent report demonstrating the value of macromolecular markers such as myoglobin in the detection of recanalization.*

Forrester JS, Litvack F, Grundfest W, et al.: A perspective of coronary disease seen through the arteries of living man. Circulation 75:505, 1987. *Angioscopic illustrations supporting the hypothesis that acute coronary syndromes are attributable to dynamic changes in complex atherosclerotic plaques with characteristic durations of thrombosis accounting for differences between the syndromes.*

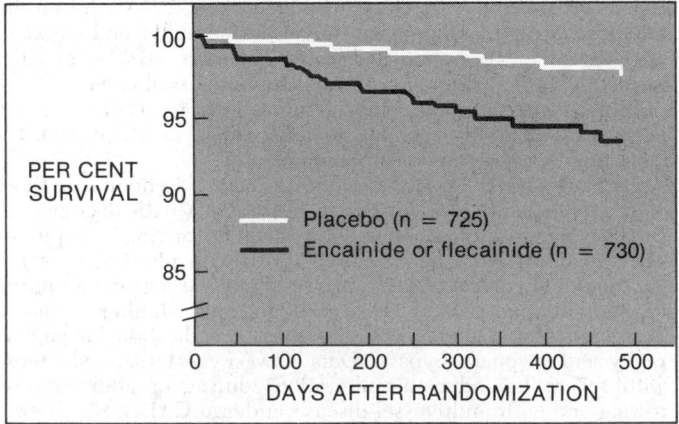

FIGURE 48–11. Survival among 1455 patients randomly assigned to treatment with encainide or flecainide compared with those assigned to placebo calculated with respect to death attributable to arrhythmia or cardiac arrest. (Adapted from Cardiac Arrhythmia Suppression Trial Investigators: N Engl J Med 321:406, 1989. By permission of the New England Journal of Medicine.)

Fry ETA, Sobel BE: Coronary thrombolysis. *In* Zipes DP, Rowlands DJ (eds.): Progress in Cardiology. Philadelphia, Lea & Febiger, 1990, pp 199–239. *A recent review of the impact of coronary thrombolysis on acute myocardial infarction with extensive reference to clinical trials performed with diverse plasminogen activators.*

Geltman EM, Ehsani AA, Campbell MK, et al.: The influence of location and extent of myocardial infarction on long-term ventricular dysrhythmia and mortality. Circulation 60:805, 1979. *An investigation establishing the association between the extent of myocardial injury sustained and long-term morbidity and mortality after acute myocardial infarction.*

Gruppo Italiano per lo Studio Della Streptochinasi nell'Infarto Miocardico (GISSI): Long-term effects of intravenous thrombolysis in acute myocardial infarction: Final report of the GISSI study. Lancet 2:871, 1987. *The pivotal report demonstrating improved survival after coronary thrombolysis in patients with acute myocardial infarction.*

Gunnar RM, Bourdillon PDV, Dixon DW, et al.: Guidelines for the early management of patients with acute myocardial infarction. A report of the American College of Cardiology/American Heart Association Task Force on Assessment of Diagnostic and Therapeutic Cardiovascular Procedures (Subcommittee to Develop Guidelines for the Early Management of Patients With Acute Myocardial Infarction). J Am Coll Cardiol 16:249, 1990. *This task force report summarizes the rationale and accepted approaches to treatment of all aspects of acute myocardial infarction based on full understanding of pertinent pathophysiologic principles.*

Jaffe AS, Serota H, Grace A, et al.: Diagnostic changes in plasma creatine kinase isoforms early after the onset of acute myocardial infarction. Circulation 74:105, 1986. *Observations indicating the value of analysis of isoforms of creatine kinase in plasma for prompt detection of acute myocardial infarction.*

Kanovsky MS, Falcone RA, Dresden CA, et al.: Identification of patients with ventricular tachycardia after myocardial infarction: Signal-averaged electrocardiogram, Holter monitoring, and cardiac catheterization. Circulation 70:264, 1984. *Delineation of the relationship between changes evident by high-resolution electrocardiography and the risk of ventricular tachycardia after acute myocardial infarction.*

Kennedy JW, Martin GV, Davis KB, et al.: The Western Washington intravenous streptokinase in acute myocardial infarction randomized trial. Circulation 77:345, 1988. *Report of a major clinical trial supporting the hypothesis that an open infarct-related coronary artery is beneficial even if recanalization cannot be induced very early after the onset of symptoms.*

Lindsay BD, Markham J, Schechtman KB, et al.: Identification of patients with sustained ventricular tachycardia by frequency analysis of signal-averaged electrocardiograms despite the presence of bundle branch block. Circulation 77:122, 1988. *Observations indicating that frequency-domain analysis of signal-averaged electrocardiograms provides information predictive of risk of sustained ventricular tachycardia even when intraventricular conduction abnormalities are present.*

Marcus FI, Cobb LA, Edwards JE, et al.: Mechanism of death and prevalence of myocardial ischemic symptoms in the terminal event after acute myocardial infarction. Am J Cardiol 61:8, 1988. *The prominence of arrhythmia as a cause of death late after acute myocardial infarction is underscored by these findings from a longitudinal study of survivors of acute myocardial infarction.*

Maroko PR, Kjekshus JK, Sobel BE, et al.: Factors influencing infarct size following experimental coronary artery occlusions. Circulation 43:67, 1971. *Laboratory observations demonstrating that myocardial infarction is a dynamic process amenable to favorable modification by reduction of myocardial oxygen requirements.*

Puleo PR, Perryman B, Bresser MA, et al.: Creatine kinase isoform analysis in the detection and assessment of thrombolysis in man. Circulation 75:1162, 1987. *The value of assay of creatine kinase isoforms in plasma for early detection of recanalization induced by fibrinolytic agents is demonstrated.*

Roberts R, Croft C, Gold HK, et al.: Effect of propranolol on myocardial infarct size in a randomized blinded multicenter trial. N Engl J Med 311:218, 1984. *Despite favorable effects in experimental animals, reduction of myocardial oxygen requirements in victims of acute myocardial infarction does not appear to reduce the extent of necrosis judging from results of this large-scale randomized multicenter study.*

Seacord LM, Abendschein DR, Nohara R, et al.: Detection of reperfusion within 1 hour after coronary recanalization by analysis of isoforms of the MM creatine kinase isoenzyme in plasma. Fibrinolysis 2:151, 1988. *A report demonstrating that serial assay of plasma creatine kinase isoforms permits very prompt detection of coronary recanalization.*

Sobel BE (ed.): Coronary thrombolysis. Review in depth. Coronary Artery Dis 1:1, 1990. *A review with components from Collen and Lijnen, Sheehan, Ohman and Califf, Guerci, and Muller and Topol addressing features of first- and second-generation fibrinolytic drugs, similarities and differences between the two, and mechanisms responsible for both.*

Tiefenbrunn AJ, Sobel BE: The impact of coronary thrombolysis on myocardial infarction. Fibrinolysis 3:1, 1989. *A review of pathophysiologic mechanisms, principles underlying treatment with plasminogen activators, and benefits resulting from early coronary thrombolysis.*

The TIMI Study Group: Comparison of invasive and conservative strategies after treatment with intravenous tissue plasminogen activator in acute myocardial infarction: Results of the thrombolysis in myocardial infarction (TIMI) phase II trial. N Engl J Med 320:618, 1989. *A definitive report from a large number of centers comparing survival after coronary thrombolysis with that following obligatory early angiography and demonstrating the advantages of a conservative strategy focusing on thrombolysis alone.*

Topol EJ, Califf RM, George BS, et al.: A randomized trial of immediate versus delayed elective angioplasty after intravenous tissue plasminogen activator in acute myocardial infarction. N Engl J Med 317:581, 1987. *Lack of benefit of immediate angioplasty after coronary thrombolysis was demonstrated initially in this important trial.*

48.3 SURGICAL TREATMENT OF CORONARY ARTERY DISEASE

Lawrence H. Cohen

The surgical treatment of coronary heart disease by coronary artery bypass grafting (CABG) is an important therapy for patients with acute and chronic syndromes of ischemic heart disease. Despite the enormous advances in interventional cardiology, thrombolytic therapy, and pharmacologic therapy of patients with coronary heart disease, surgical therapy continues to be a mainstay of direct reperfusion of ischemic myocardium. In 1988 approximately 240,000 patients underwent CABG for one of many indications of acute and chronic myocardial ischemia. As the incidence of interventional cardiologic therapy has increased with percutaneous transluminal coronary angioplasty (PTCA), the indications for CABG have changed and evolved so that the two procedures are now considered complementary to each other. PTCA is generally indicated for the less severe anatomic manifestations of obstructive coronary lesions, namely single-vessel disease, whereas CABG continues to be the treatment of choice for multivessel coronary disease.

The selection of patients for CABG has evolved strikingly since the advent of this procedure on a large scale in 1967 by the Cleveland Clinic Foundation, although a few individual cases had been done earlier by Sabiston and DeBakey. At the outset of surgical therapy, the patients who were operated upon were the younger, healthier patients with relatively few coronary lesions and good ventricular function. The patients most often considered for CABG today are those on the other end of the spectrum who tend to be older and sicker and have more advanced arterial disease, oftentimes with the ravages of coronary heart disease manifested by severe left ventricular dysfunction. In addition, there are numbers of patients with acute myocardial ischemia requiring operation who were seldom considered candidates for surgery when the operation was introduced. CABG has thus evolved into a procedure with a wide spectrum of indications requiring a considerable amount of ingenuity, new uses of conduits, better myocardial protection, and advanced techniques for life support.

INDICATIONS FOR CORONARY BYPASS SURGERY

In general, the patients selected for CABG should be those who have failed intensive medical therapy for the treatment of chronic angina or acute myocardial ischemia and who, by demonstration on coronary arteriography, have one or more significant lesions greater than 70 per cent luminal diameter. With exercise tolerance testing, radionuclear angiocardiography, and coronary arteriography, the patient's diseased coronary arteries and the impact on cardiac function can be completely evaluated.

Table 48–12 lists the clinical indications for CABG. These range from "silent" ischemia to an evolving acute myocardial infarction or massive myocardial damage.

SILENT ISCHEMIA. Patients with "silent" ischemia are those with exercise and ECG evidence of ischemia with documented coronary arterial obstruction who have no anginal symptoms. These patients often have sudden death with physical exertion. Considerable controversy has arisen about the logistics required for the identification of these patients and whether or not a positive exercise tolerance test should be indication for angiography and coronary bypass. Data now suggest that only those with severe hemodynamic alterations during or after exercise testing and with multivessel disease undergo CABG.

CHRONIC STABLE ANGINA. This is the largest group of patients who are considered for coronary bypass surgery. These patients, predominantly male and predominantly in their sixth decade of life, have effort angina or stress-related angina that is more or less controlled by medical therapy but with considerable reduction in lifestyle. These patients require β blockade, calcium

TABLE 48–12. INDICATIONS FOR CORONARY ARTERY BYPASS SURGERY

Chronic ischemia
  "Silent" ischemia
  Chronic stable angina
Acute myocardial ischemia
  Unstable angina
  Subendocardial infarction
  Postinfarction angina
  Acute evolving myocardial infarction
  Myocardial infarction with shock
With other cardiac operations
  Valve surgery
  Mechanical sequelae of myocardial infarction
    Ventricular septal defect
    Ruptured septal defect
    Left ventricular aneurysm

channel blockers, vasodilators, and antiplatelet aggregation agents, which may produce a considerable number of untoward effects. Arteriography of patients in this category shows at least two and usually three or more significant obstructions in their coronary arteries. They may have normal but often have reduced left ventricular function, especially as measured by the left ventricular ejection fraction, due to prior myocardial infarction(s). Occasionally, CABG may be considered for a patient with single-vessel disease who is symptomatic despite medical treatment, who is not a candidate for or who has failed angioplasty, and whose single diseased artery is unusually large and dominant.

UNSTABLE ANGINA. Unstable angina refers to a condition of accelerated anginal patterns not controllable by the usual medical therapy; it may manifest as rest angina, nocturnal angina, or almost continuous chest pain with ECG abnormalities indicating ischemia but not infarction, and it often requires the most intensive of therapies in the Coronary Care Unit. Patients with unstable angina should be stabilized, if possible, and treated with intravenous vasodilators such as nitroglycerin; they may occasionally even require the use of intra-aortic balloon support pump for the stabilization of hemodynamics, anginal symptoms, and ECG abnormalities. A cooperative national prospective study in the 1970's showed that stabilization of patients prior to bypass surgery is far preferable to operating on patients emergently when they are truly unstable. By decreasing left ventricular myocardial oxygen consumption, intensive β blockade and other pharmacologic agents actually decrease operative mortality when patients with this syndrome are operated upon.

SUBENDOCARDIAL INFARCTION. The patient with a subendocardial myocardial infarction has a small leak of myocardial enzymes not associated with a Q-wave type infarction pattern on ECG. Clinically, these patients are very similar in presentation to patients with unstable angina and may have severe angina. Their angiographic patterns of obstructive disease are the same as those with unstable angina, and they are considered for operation with the same degree of aggressiveness as are patients with unstable angina, provided that they are otherwise good candidates for surgery.

EVOLVING MYOCARDIAL INFARCTION. Those with evolving myocardial infarction present in the throes of a myocardial infarction, usually from occlusion of the anterior descending artery or posterior circulation, are considered for operation when they may be operated upon within approximately 6 hours of the onset of chest pain. A number of cardiac centers with excellent logistical set-ups have performed large numbers of operations in these patients with excellent results and ultimate reduction of myocardial necrosis. These large studies evolved from earlier studies which showed that patients who had sustained an acute occlusion in the cardiac catheterization laboratory, for example, could be taken to the operating room, undergo a rapid CABG procedure, generally survive, and usually abort a major myocardial infarction. These patients usually have triple-vessel coronary disease, since those with single-vessel disease are excellent candidates for thrombolytic therapy and/or PTCA. Patients with acute evolving infarction with triple-vessel disease may also be candidates for thrombolytic therapy, but if this is not successful they should be considered for expeditious operation.

POSTINFARCTION ANGINA. Postinfarction angina is an important clinical syndrome that occurs in patients who have had a myocardial infarction which was thought to be complete but is now threatening to extend either in the area of the prior infarction or in a new area of ischemia. This syndrome, left untreated, usually results in extension of the myocardial infarction and oftentimes severe mechanical sequelae of myocardial infarction. A major advance in the surgical therapy of coronary heart disease has been the aggressive treatment by CABG of this syndrome, which may occur within hours to days of the completed myocardial infarction. Untreated, it is a harbinger of further difficulty and a high mortality. Results of surgery for this syndrome are similar to those for unstable angina, provided that the patient is not in shock preoperatively.

MYOCARDIAL INFARCTION WITH SHOCK. This relatively small group of patients requiring CABG have suffered occlusion of a coronary artery which has produced massive destruction of the left ventricle, usually in excess of 40 per cent of the volume of the left ventricle. This syndrome often leads to immediate sudden death, but in some instances, by support with appropriate pharmacologic and mechanical devices, the patients are stabilized enough in the intensive care unit to be considered for emergency CABG. Careful evaluation of the residual left ventricular function in nonischemic areas and the anatomy of the distal coronary vessels is extremely critical in these patients, since patients with poor residual myocardial function or poor distal vessels are not usually candidates for conventional CABG. This treatment should be considered only in patients otherwise in good health and generally in the younger age group. Operative mortality in the best of centers averages 25 to 40 per cent.

CORONARY BYPASS WITH OTHER CARDIAC OPERATIONS. For sequelae of myocardial infarction when there is a mechanical abnormality associated with a myocardial infarction, coronary bypass is often done. These include infarction ventricular septal defect, ruptured or dysfunctional papillary muscle producing mitral regurgitation and left ventricular aneurysm, pseudoaneurysm, or left ventricular rupture. These are all sequelae of a transmural myocardial infarction and may occur from days to weeks following the original infarction and are often associated with multiple-vessel coronary disease. Coronary bypass should be done as an adjunctive procedure during simultaneous repair of these defects.

In cardiac valve disease, a very high percentage of patients in the adult population have coexistent coronary artery lesions. These patients require a concomitant coronary bypass operation if valve surgery is to be done because of the added reduction in coronary blood flow to the left ventricular myocardium imposed on the hemodynamic burden produced by the valve lesion itself. In some series of patients operated upon for valve disease, fully 30 to 40 per cent of the patients require concomitant CABG. The long-term outlook for patients with valve disease and coronary disease, despite the fact that the coronary disease may be grafted completely, is not as satisfactory as for those who have valve disease without concomitant coronary artery disease. In the workup of any adult patient for valvular heart surgery over the age of 40, coronary arteriography is generally indicated.

ANATOMIC INDICATIONS FOR CORONARY ARTERY BYPASS GRAFTING. Finally, there are some anatomic indications for CABG regardless of symptomatology. Severe occlusive lesion of the left main coronary artery of greater than 70 per cent diameter is indication for immediate surgery, regardless of the severity of the patient's clinical symptoms. Similarly, acute failure of a coronary angioplasty may often require emergency CABG, either because of failure to improve the lesion over subsequent dilations or because a failed angioplasty usually results in an acute myocardial infarction from coronary occlusion.

BASIS OF SURGICAL TREATMENT OF CORONARY ARTERY DISEASE

The basis of the surgical attack on coronary arteries is the bypass principle, one that has been in use for many years in regard to ischemic problems in many arterial beds throughout the body: the aortoiliofemoral arteries, the renal arteries, and the cerebral arteries. In a coronary bypass a conduit is sutured distal to the obstructing lesion and connected proximally to either the aorta or some other systemic artery, much as a detour in a road is used to get to a destination beyond a highway blockage. CABG utilizes autogenous conduits, since artificial grafts, which need to be sutured to coronary vessels that measure 1 to 2 mm, at the present time have poor long-term patency. A reversed saphenous vein was first used as the conduit for CABG. It is readily available and allows considerable flexibility. Other readily available conduits used since the early days of coronary surgery are the left and right internal mammary arteries. These arteries run under the chest wall bilaterally, supplying blood to the chest wall and breast, and can be dissected off the chest wall, dropped down, and used as a conduit to a coronary artery beyond the blockage. The advantages of this conduit are that it is an autogenous artery with a better size match to the coronary artery vessel and it has a natural proximal long-term patency rate better than that of the saphenous vein. The size match is better, the arterial wall is more consistent with that of coronary artery, and a number of other physiologic observations suggest that it is the bypass graft of choice for coronary arteries, particularly the left anterior descending. More recently, the gastroepiploic artery, which must be brought through the diaphragm, has also been considered for CABG.

Operations are performed on cardiopulmonary bypass with moderate systemic hypothermia and cardioplegic solutions to render the heart totally flaccid and motionless without expending energy stores and allowing for the performance of very small anastomoses. Hemodilution and the avoidance of blood transfusions are desirable and obtainable with a variety of extracorporeal perfusion techniques. Over the quarter century that CABG has been performed, complete revascularization of the patient—that is, the placement of a graft beyond every major stenosis—yields significantly better long-term survival and prevents cardiac events better than incomplete revascularization. In the average multivessel patient undergoing CABG, at least three or four bypass grafts are the rule in the modern era. The safety of the operation is unquestionably improved because of myocardial protection with various forms of cardioplegic solutions and the availability of intra-aortic balloon pumping.

The surgical mortality after coronary bypass surgery varies with the acuity of the presenting symptoms, the state of left ventricular function, and other patient risk factors. There is no statistical difference in mortality among varying numbers of grafts, but mortality is clearly dependent upon the function of the left ventricle prior to surgery. The operative mortality for coronary bypass in the multivessel younger age group with good left ventricular function is about 1 per cent. In the acutely ischemic

syndromes, operative mortality may vary from 2 to 25 per cent, depending upon whether it is postinfarction angina or acute myocardial infarction with shock. The effect of age is to perhaps double the operative mortality in patients over 70, particularly those with acute ischemic events. Increased ventilator dependency, stroke rate, etc., are also clearly more frequent in the older age group undergoing CABG.

Postoperative care consists of management of all organ subsystems, including renal, pulmonary, cerebral, and general metabolic function. Low cardiac output following cardiac surgery is treated by monitoring devices to measure cardiac output, pulmonary vascular resistance, and left and right ventricular filling pressures. Optimization of these filling pressures determines which type of pharmacologic agent or mechanical assist device to use in the management of this complication. Cardiac arrhythmias are extremely common and occur in about 30 per cent of patients, most often atrial fibrillation. Perioperative myocardial infarction (Q wave) occurs much less frequently than in previous decades, and it is now estimated to be around 2 to 5 per cent. Hypertension is often an accompanying feature and must be vigorously controlled with the use of vasodilating drugs such as nitroprusside or nitroglycerin to limit myocardial oxygen consumption in this critical postoperative period. It is of interest that unless there is severe associated hemodynamic instability, a postoperative perioperative infarction apparently has little or no effect on long-term survival and little effect on the hospital course. Mediastinitis may occur in a small percentage of cases, usually about 1 to 2 per cent in most large centers, which may be increased with the use of bilateral internal mammary arteries, particularly in diabetic patients. Postoperative management of this complication includes open drainage and irrigation and then closure with antibiotic irrigation tubes and occasionally in some instances the placement of a pectoral muscle flap to improve the healing.

Postoperative management now includes the routine use of antiplatelet therapy with daily aspirin. It has been demonstrated in randomized prospective trials that the addition of one aspirin tablet per day is effective in improving graft patency, presumably by the prevention of platelet "stickiness" in the grafts.

REOPERATIONS

Coronary bypass surgery is palliative surgery and unless the disease is totally controlled biochemically with extensive rehabilitation of patients undergoing this operation, symptoms may recur as a result of progression of disease in previously ungrafted normal vessels, or new disease may occur involving the bypass grafts themselves. Thus, reoperation is a necessity in some patients and increases with the length of time from surgery unless internal mammary artery bypass grafts are used exclusively. The indications for reoperative CABG are similar to the primary

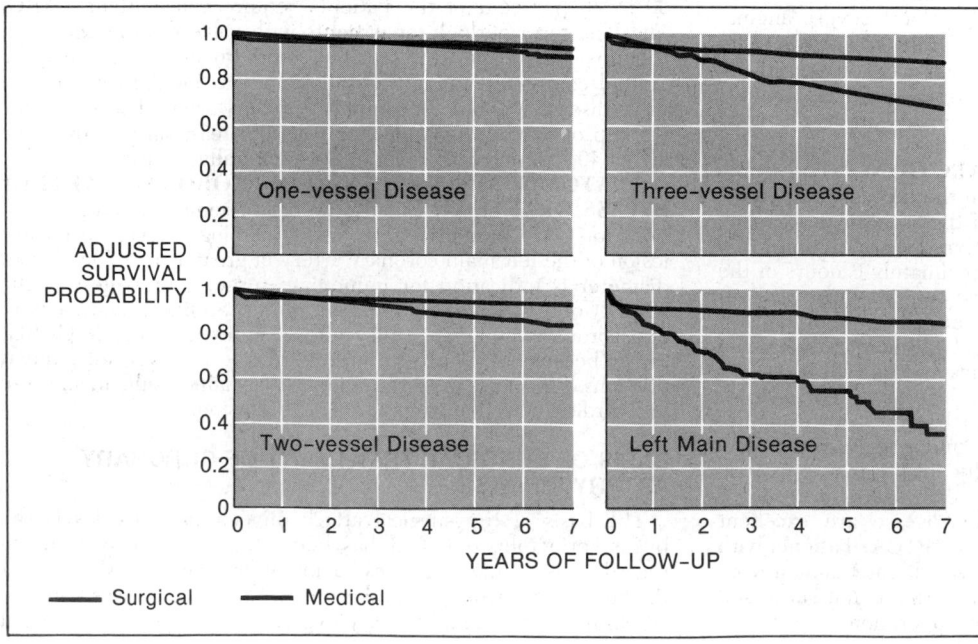

FIGURE 48–12. Survival treated medically or surgically with one-vessel, two-vessel, three-vessel, and left main coronary artery disease. (From Califf RM, et al.: JAMA 261:2077, 1989. Copyright 1989, American Medical Association.)

ADJUSTED SURVIVAL PROBABILITY

One-vessel Disease
Three-vessel Disease
Two-vessel Disease
Left Main Disease

YEARS OF FOLLOW-UP

—— Surgical   —— Medical

operation indications, but the patient must be aware that the risk is somewhat higher (5 to 10 per cent) and the benefits to be gained are somewhat lower than in the previous operation. This is because of the inherent difficulty with reoperative surgery due to the extensive adhesions around the heart, the possibility of myocardial ischemia due to manipulation of partially obstructed grafts filled with atheromatous material, and increased risk of bleeding. The risk of reoperative coronary bypass varies considerably with the experience of the team and the approach to myocardial protection.

LATE RESULTS OF CORONARY BYPASS SURGERY

The current operative mortality has stabilized at 2 to 5 per cent despite the increased number of aged patients, complexity of disease, numbers of reoperations, left ventricular dysfunction, and extension to almost all forms of acute myocardial ischemia. The probability of long-term survival and prevention of late cardiac events is related to the function of the left ventricle, complete revascularization, type of conduits used (internal mammary arteries versus saphenous veins), and patient rehabilitation. In general, the 5-year late survival of patients with multivessel disease completely revascularized is 90 to 95 per cent and the 10-year survival is 85 to 90 per cent (Figs. 48–12 and 48–13). The long-term graft patency is clearly better with an internal mammary artery than with a saphenous vein graft, 95 per cent versus 75 per cent at 5 years and 50 per cent at 10 years. It is apparent that if one considers every major clinical risk factor, the outcome with use of the internal mammary artery is statistically significantly better than that with the saphenous vein. In the long term, it is apparent that patients with left main coronary stenosis or with multivessel disease have improved survival and protection from cardiac events over similar medical patients in both prospective randomized studies and retrospective studies. Effects on ventricular function are less easy to document, but it is apparent that the ischemic or stunned myocardium may show significant improvements in left ventricular function after CABG

and that CABG may prevent further deterioration of function in the severely dysfunctional left ventricle.

Califf RM, Harrell FE, Lee KL, et al.: The evolution of medical and surgical therapy for coronary artery disease. JAMA 261:2077, 1989. *A 15-year perspective on the evolution of medical and surgical treatment, indicating that the surgical treatment, particularly in the last decade, has improved markedly so that not only the early but the late survival is improved over that with medical therapy because of newer revascularization techniques and better myocardial protection.*

Cohn LH: Surgical treatment of acute myocardial infarction. Cardiology 76:167, 1989. *This paper is a review of the various acute ischemic syndromes related to coronary occlusion and the results of both pure bypass surgery and surgery associated with the mechanical sequelae of myocardial infarction.*

Loop FD, Bruce WL, Cosgrove DM, et al.: Influence of the internal-mammary-artery graft on 10-year survival and other cardiac events. N Engl J Med 314:1, 1986. *This is a long-term follow-up of patients treated with internal mammary arteries versus those treated with only saphenous vein grafts for anterior descending coronary bypass. This large, well followed-up series (including angiography) shows conclusively that the internal mammary is the preferable conduit for coronary bypass surgery.*

Naunheim KS, Fiore AC, Wadley JF, et al.: The changing mortality of myocardial revascularization: Coronary artery bypass and angioplasty. Ann Thorac Surg 46:666, 1988. *This paper analyzes risk factors and outcomes for patients operated on in different eras and shows the marked change in the demography of patients operated upon in the late 1980's compared with the late 1970's.*

49 Valvular Heart Disease
Charles E. Rackley

The clinical manifestations of valvular heart disease result from either stenosis or incompetence of cardiac valves, or both. These mechanical disturbances lead to either pressure or volume overload on the affected chambers. The most frequently involved cardiac chamber in valvular heart disease is the left ventricle, which compensates for chronic volume or pressure overload with dilatation and hypertrophy. Myocardial oxygen requirements are related to the increased mechanical work and hypertrophy of the myocardium. In the advanced stage of valvular heart disease, myocardial decompensation, a reduction in cardiac output, and decreased coronary perfusion can impair oxygen delivery despite increased myocardial oxygen demands.

Although rheumatic heart disease remains prevalent in the temperate climates of the world, control of streptococcal infections in the United States has reduced the incidence of rheumatic fever and subsequent rheumatic heart disease. Today mitral valve prolapse is the most common valvular abnormality. A bicuspid aortic valve is the most common cause of aortic stenosis, but degeneration and calcification of the aortic valve are recognized with increasing frequency in the aging adult.

Recognition of a heart murmur on physical examination is the usual means of initially diagnosing valvular heart disease. Thus, the clinical examination remains important for detection of valvular heart disease, recognition of cardiac deterioration, and assessment of follow-up status. The noninvasive technologies of electrocardiography, chest radiography, echocardiography, radionuclide angiography, and stress testing play an important role in assessing the impact of valvular heart disease on cardiac function and determining the timing of operative intervention. Cardiac catheterization continues to be important in the accurate measurement of gradients across stenotic valves, evaluation of left ventricular function, and recognition of concomitant coronary artery disease. In recent years advances in echocardiography have resulted in more accurate assessment of valvular orifice size, and catheterization is reserved to confirm impressions and to identify underlying coronary artery disease.

GENERAL APPROACH TO THE PATIENT WITH VALVULAR HEART DISEASE

History

The patient with valvular heart disease usually recalls a history of a heart murmur, and therefore the first recognition of the

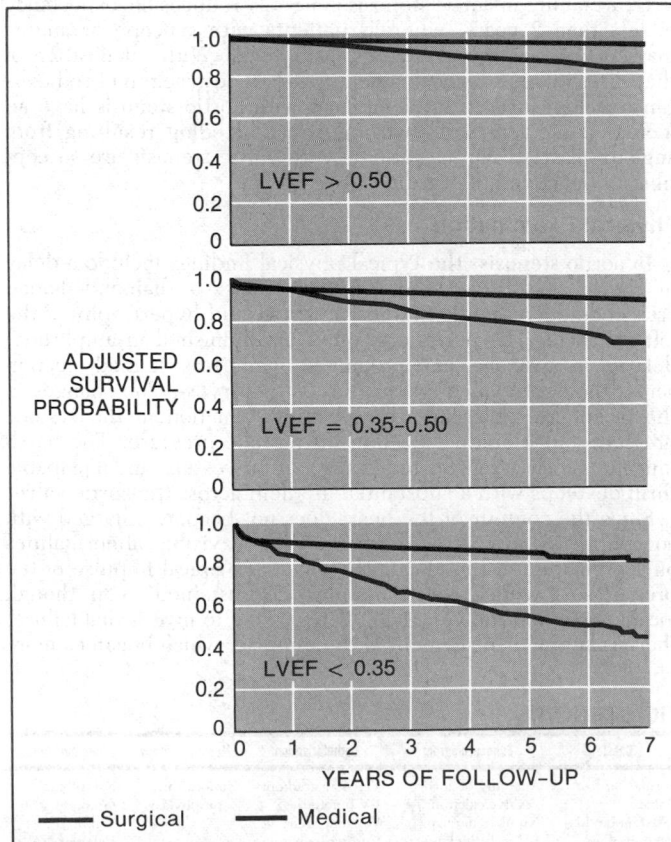

FIGURE 48–13. Projected survival of patients treated medically or surgically with a left ventricular ejection fraction (LVEF) greater than 0.50, between 0.35 and 0.50, and less than 0.35. (From Califf RM, et al.: JAMA 261:2077, 1989. Copyright 1989, American Medical Association.)

murmur may be helpful in establishing the etiology. Although cardiac murmurs are frequent in healthy, physicially active children and adolescents, congenital valvular etiologies are often recognized at birth. Detection of a heart murmur in early adulthood often suggests a congenital or rheumatic basis, whereas development of the murmur in later years is often due to the degenerative changes in valvular structure. In addition to ascertaining the earliest detection of the heart murmur, the physician should carefully assess the patient's physical activities and note the initial onset of dyspnea or fatigue. The physician's interpretation of the patient's symptoms dictates the appropriate timing of noninvasive and invasive cardiac studies as well as the decision for surgical correction.

Physical Examination

The physical examination of the patient with valvular heart disease should be performed in the standard manner. Particular attention should be paid to the vital signs. Fever should raise the possibility of infective endocarditis. Palpation of the peripheral pulse may indicate stenosis or incompetence of the aortic valve. The habitus can suggest Marfan's syndrome as well as other heritable disorders of connective tissue. Funduscopic examination can demonstrate subtleties in arterial pulsations in aortic incompetence or the characteristic hemorrhages or Roth's spots in infective endocarditis. Careful attention to the vessels in the neck can reveal abnormalities in venous pulsation, reflecting right ventricular failure or tricuspid stenosis or incompetence. Carotid arteries reveal pulsatile abnormalities and transmitted bruits from the aortic valve.

Cardiac examination must include inspection, palpation, percussion, and auscultation. These maneuvers should be performed with the patient both in the sitting and in the recumbent positions. Auscultation at the apex, left sternal border, and pulmonic and aortic areas should be performed with the patient in the sitting, recumbent, and left lateral decubitus positions as well as after mild exercise. The remainder of the examination consists of documenting fluid retention, such as hepatic enlargement, ascites, and peripheral edema.

AORTIC STENOSIS

Etiology and Pathology

Aortic stenosis (Table 49–1) can result from a congenital abnormality, rheumatic fever, or degeneration with calcification in the aging patient. A bicuspid valve is the most common congenital abnormality, and invariably there is a raphe in one of the cusps that indicates failure of the commissure to develop. Rarely, a unicuspid valve can be present at birth. Although the bicuspid valve may not be initially stenotic, fibrosis and thickening lead to eventual reduction of the orifice size with calcification. Rheumatic fever produces scarring of the leaflet margins, and there is eventual fusion of the commissures with calcification. More than 50 per cent of adults with aortic stenosis will be found to have a bicuspid valve, but fibrosis and calcification may make it difficult to determine whether the valve is bicuspid or tricuspid. In the aging patient with degenerative aortic stenosis, calcium deposits usually develop in the sinuses and annulus, whereas the margins of the leaflets remain free.

In any of the conditions producing hemodynamic stenosis of the aortic valve, the systolic hypertension in the ventricular chamber is compensated by concentric hypertrophy of the myocardial wall. As myocardial failure develops from depression of the contractile state, dilatation of the ventricle will occur. Fibrosis

of the myocardium also occurs. Myocardial oxygen consumption remains high owing to the elevation of systolic pressure within the left ventricle and the increase in left ventricular mass. Thus, significant aortic stenosis creates conditions in which high myocardial oxygen demands are inadequately supported by reduced oxygen supply, which leads to subendocardial ischemia. Eventually, with a decline in the inotropic state of the myocardium, the ventricle dilates and the ejection fraction is decreased below the normal range. Further elevation of the left ventricular end-diastolic pressure results in pulmonary venous hypertension. The increased myocardial oxygen demands in aortic stenosis with the underperfused subendocardial myocardium can produce arrhythmias, chest pain, and even sudden death. In adults there may be coexistent coronary artery disease, which further contributes to myocardial ischemia.

Clinical Features

Chest pain, syncope, and heart failure are the characteristic symptoms of aortic stenosis, even though a gradient across the valve can exist for years before the patient develops symptoms. Children with a severe gradient can suddenly develop symptoms, whereas in adults the increase in mortality occurs later in the course of the disease.

The chest discomfort is exertional and indistinguishable from that of ischemic heart disease. Approximately 50 per cent of patients with aortic stenosis above the age of 40 years have underlying coronary artery disease whether exertional chest pain is present or not. Syncope can be an initial symptom of aortic stenosis and is probably related to the same mechanism as the chest pain, that is, critical reduction in myocardial oxygen supply with increased demands. Orthostatic syncope can result from the inability of the cardiac output to increase with abrupt assumption of the upright position, whereas exertional syncope is further aggravated by peripheral vasodilatation unaccompanied by an increase in cardiac output. Arrhythmias due to myocardial ischemia can also contribute to syncope and sudden death. When aortic stenosis is found at autopsy, approximately 15 per cent of the patients will have died suddenly without previous symptoms.

Heart failure in aortic stenosis generally reduces life expectancy to less than 2 years, whereas patients with syncope or angina may survive, on the average, 2 to 5 years. With calcification of the aortic valve, hemolytic anemia due to destruction of red cells can develop; furthermore, patients with aortic stenosis have an increased incidence of gastrointestinal bleeding resulting from angiodysplasia. Finally, patients with aortic stenosis are susceptible to infective endocarditis.

Physical Examination

In aortic stenosis, the typical physical findings include a delay in the upstroke of the peripheral pulse, a diamond-shaped crescendo-decrescendo systolic murmur, and hypertrophy of the left ventricle. The peripheral pulse is diminished in amplitude, delayed in upstroke, and prolonged owing to sustained ejection across the aortic valve (pulsus tardus et parvus). The changes in the peripheral pulse are caused by a reduction in the systolic pressure and a gradual decline in diastolic pressure. The harsh murmur is often transmitted to the carotid vessels, and a palpable thrill develops with a substantial gradient across the aortic valve.

Since the contour of the heart does not become enlarged with concentric hypertrophy, there may be no visible abnormalities on examination of the chest. However, the apical impulse of the pressure-overloaded ventricle may be sustained even though localized. When the ventricle dilates owing to myocardial failure, there is lateral displacement of the impulse, which becomes more

TABLE 49–1. AORTIC STENOSIS

Etiology	Physiology	Symptoms	Physical Examination	Electrocardiogram	Chest	Echocardiogram	Catheterization	Medical Therapy	Surgical Therapy
Congenital Rheumatic Degenerative	LV* pressure overload LV hypertrophy Decreased LV compliance	Chest pain Syncope Heart failure	Delayed arterial pulse wave Aortic thrill Diamond-shaped aortic area, left sternal border and apex	LV hypertrophy	Normal cardiac size Poststenotic dilatation of ascending aorta	Anatomy of aortic valve/calcium Number of cusps LV wall thickness Echo Doppler estimate of valvular gradient Valvular area	Valvular gradient LV function Valvular area Coronary anatomy Mitral lesions	Endocarditis prophylaxis	Symptoms Gradient >50 mm Hg Valvular area <0.8 cm^2

*LV = left ventricular.

diffuse. Detection of palpable systolic vibrations over the primary aortic area, with the patient in the sitting position during full expiration, often correlates with a gradient across the aortic valve of more than 40 mm Hg. An atrial (S_4) gallop is usually audible, and an ejection click may be heard along the left sternal border. The aortic second sound becomes diminished, except in calcific stenosis of the elderly, in which the margins of the leaflets usually maintain their mobility. Fibrosis and fusion of the aortic leaflets may result in a single S_2 at the base. Mechanical or electrical prolongation of left ventricular systole can create reverse splitting of S_2. The diamond-shaped ejection murmur develops after the first sound, peaks in mid- and late systole, and disappears before the second heart sound. There is a tendency toward late peaking of the murmur with increasing severity of the stenosis. If an ejection click is present, the murmur develops immediately after the click and can sometimes be erroneously identified as a holosystolic murmur. The murmur is most intense over the aortic area and along the left sternal border, but in the elderly patient, the musical quality of the murmur can sometimes be loudest at the apex. The intensity in the apical area can be confusing and may make it difficult to distinguish this murmur from that of mitral regurgitation. A faint diastolic blow is often audible along the left sternal border, since the severely stenotic valve may have a mild degree of incompetence.

Laboratory Studies

ELECTROCARDIOGRAM. Left ventricular hypertrophy is the most common finding on the electrocardiogram, with an increase in QRS amplitude and ST-T changes of a strain pattern. Left-axis deviation can develop as well as conduction disturbances and left bundle branch block. As the left ventricle becomes noncompliant, there may be enlargement of the left atrium with a negative P wave in lead V_1. Because of myocardial fibrosis, Q waves can develop in the precordial leads, but these as well as the ST-T wave abnormalities are indistinguishable from underlying coronary artery disease.

CHEST RADIOGRAPH. Cardiac size remains unchanged in the early phase of aortic stenosis, since hypertrophy does not increase the cardiothoracic ratio. Poststenotic dilatation and prominence of the ascending aorta may be present. Calcification is often present but may require fluoroscopy for confirmation. Development of heart failure will enlarge the left ventricle and cause pulmonary congestion. Since a bicuspid aortic valve is sometimes associated with coarctation of the aorta, rib notching should always be sought on the chest film.

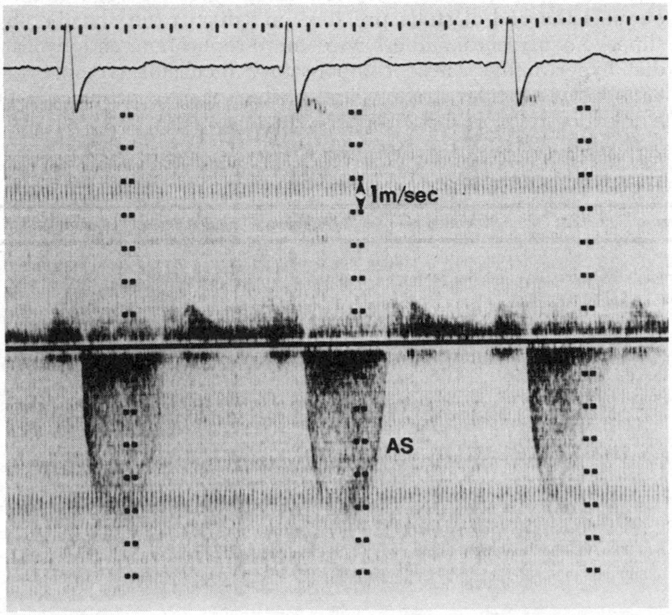

FIGURE 49-1. Continuous wave Doppler recording from the ascending aorta in a patient with severe aortic stenosis. The peak velocity is approximately 5 m/sec. Utilizing the modified Bernoulli equation, a peak instantaneous gradient across the aortic valve of 100 mm Hg can be calculated. Peak-to-peak gradient at catheterization was 80 mm Hg.

ECHOCARDIOGRAM. The echocardiogram can demonstrate thickening of the aortic leaflets, determine the number of leaflets, detect calcification of the valves, and estimate left ventricular wall thickness and function. Two-dimensional echocardiography can give an estimated size of the aortic orifice, and the Doppler technique can assess accurately the systolic pressure gradient across the valve. Thus, available echocardiographic techniques can provide accurate detection and assessment of aortic stenosis (Fig. 49-1).

CARDIAC CATHETERIZATION. The pressure gradient across the aortic valve can be accurately measured with simultaneous measurements of left ventricular and aortic pressures. A decline in cardiac output is associated with a reduced pressure gradient across the valve, and the valvular area tends to be overestimated when the cardiac output is reduced and only the pressure gradient is analyzed.

The size of the normal aortic orifice is 2.5 to 3 cm^2, and mild stenosis develops when the orifice is reduced to 0.75 to 1.5 cm^2. Moderate stenosis is present when the valvular size is less than 0.75 cm^2 and severe stenosis when the valvular area is less than 0.5 cm^2. Surgery is usually advised when the aortic valve gradient is greater than 50 mm Hg or the valve area is less than 0.8 cm^2. Left ventricular angiography is helpful in determining the presence of mitral regurgitation. With the information available from echocardiography, cardiac catheterization may be primarily indicated for coronary arteriography, since 50 per cent of patients over the age of 40 years will have underlying coronary artery disease.

Differential Diagnosis

In children, valvular aortic stenosis has to be differentiated from congenital forms of both supra- and infravalvular lesions. In hypertrophic cardiomyopathy with obstruction, the systolic ejection murmur is similar to that of valvular aortic stenosis, but the peripheral pulse is hyperdynamic with a rapid upstroke and a double-notch or bisferious contour compared with the delayed upstroke observed in valvular stenosis. With rupture of the chordae or papillary muscle, acute mitral regurgitation may produce a harsh systolic murmur. This murmur can be transmitted to the left atrial wall and aorta, resulting in a palpable and audible "aortic" murmur. However, the murmur of acute mitral regurgitation transmitted into the aortic area is holosystolic rather than midsystolic. A systolic ejection murmur accompanies significant aortic regurgitation and is generally caused by turbulence of the large stroke volume across the aortic valve.

Medical Therapy

Prophylaxis with antibiotics is indicated for dental, genitourinary, and gastrointestinal procedures in the asymptomatic patient to reduce the likelihood of infective endocarditis. Prophylaxis should be routine throughout life in a patient with a stenotic or prosthetic valve (Table 49-2). Prosthetic valves require intramuscular or intravenous antibiotics for prophylaxis. If the patient with aortic stenosis develops a supraventricular tachycardia, digitalis and an antiarrhythmic drug may be necessary to slow the ventricular response. Development of chest pain warrants catheterization to evaluate underlying coronary artery disease, but the use of nitrates should be undertaken with great caution, since arterial pressure may fall and further reduce coronary blood flow. Since life expectancy is reduced when aortic stenosis becomes symptomatic, chest pain, syncope, or heart failure warrants appropriate studies and consideration for surgery. Aysmptomatic patients with hemodynamically significant aortic stenosis are at significant risk for cardiac events within 2 years and should be followed closely.

Surgical Therapy

In children with aortic stenosis, surgery may be considered before the development of symptoms. If the pressure gradient is high, valvuloplasty can sometimes be performed before calcification has developed. The operative mortality for aortic valve replacement is 2 to 3 per cent and is less than 5 per cent if coronary bypass surgery is also performed. Even if heart failure has developed, surgery with prosthetic valve replacement can improve ventricular function. A mechanical valve will require

TABLE 49–2. ANTIBIOTIC PROPHYLAXIS IN AORTIC STENOSIS

Category	Drug	Dose and Route of Administration
Dental procedures and surgery of the upper respiratory tract		
Most patients	Penicillin	2 grams penicillin V orally 1 hour prior to procedure and 1 gram 6 hours later
Allergic to penicillin	Erythromycin	1 gram orally 1 hour prior to procedure and 500 mg 6 hours later
Prosthetic valves, not allergic to penicillin	Ampicillin and gentamicin	Ampicillin 1–2 grams plus gentamicin 1.5 mg/kg IM or IV 30 min before procedure; no repeat dose necessary
Prosthetic valves, allergic to penicillin	Vancomycin	Vancomycin 1 gram IV over 60 min, begun 60 min before procedure; no repeat dose necessary
Gastrointestinal and genitourinary tract surgery and instrumentation		
Most patients	Ampicillin and gentamicin	Ampicillin 2 grams plus gentamicin 1.5 mg/kg IM or IV 30 min before procedure; may repeat once 8 hours later
Allergic to penicillin	Vancomycin and gentamicin	Vancomycin 1 gram IV plus gentamicin 1.5 mg/kg IM or IV over 60 min before procedure; may be repeated once 8–12 hours later
Minor or repetitive procedures	Amoxicillin	Amoxicillin 3 grams orally 1 hour before procedure and 1.5 grams 6 hours later

long-term coagulation, but the porcine valve can be utilized in older patients or in those in whom anticoagulation is contraindicated. Currently, the porcine valve usually lasts 10 years or longer before deterioration in adults, but it is not recommended in children or adolescents. If indicated, coronary bypass surgery should also be performed at the time of valve replacement. The 10-year survival of combined aortic valve replacement and coronary revascularization approaches 55 per cent. Late cardiac events occur at a rate of approximately 6 per cent per year and include thromboembolic neurologic insults, myocardial infarction, congestive heart failure, endocarditis, bleeding, peripheral thromboembolism, and reoperation. Valvuloplasty is an option in severely ill or elderly patients, but the restenosis rate remains high. Octogenarians are those most likely to benefit from percutaneous valvuloplasty, since operative mortality may be as high as 30 per cent. Hospital mortality for the procedure in patients 80 years old or older has been reported at 6.5 per cent, with 1-year survival at 70 per cent. Surviving patients describe marked symptomatic improvement.

AORTIC REGURGITATION
Etiology and Pathology

Aortic regurgitation (Table 49–3) can be caused by disease conditions that render the aortic leaflets incompetent or affect the ascending aorta with dilatation of the annulus of the aortic valve. Rheumatic fever produces scarring and fibrosis of the valvular margins. Myxomatous degeneration of the aortic cusp can lead to incompetence. Hypertension, as well as arteriosclerosis, can be associated with scarring of the aortic valve and mild incompetence. Congenital lesions, such as bicuspid aortic valve, are predominantly stenotic, but scarring and calcification can result in associated incompetence as well. An aneurysm of the sinus of Valsalva may be associated with a ventricular septal defect as well as aortic regurgitation.

Conditions that affect the ascending aorta and produce valvular incompetence include syphilis, heritable disorders of connective tissue, arthritic diseases, and cystic medial necrosis of the aorta. In syphilis, the granulomatous process can result in calcification of the aorta, extreme dilatation, and ostial narrowing of the coronary arteries. Myxomatous degeneration of the aortic valve occurs in Marfan's syndrome. Ankylosing spondylitis, rheumatoid arthritis, and Reiter's syndrome are arthritic conditions that can cause aortic root dilatation and aortic cusp thickening. Cystic medial necrosis and aortic ectasia can produce extreme dilatation of the aorta with secondary aortic regurgitation. Acute aortic regurgitation can result from dissection of the aorta, perforation of the valve with infective endocarditis, rupture of a sinus of Valsalva, and mechanical complications of a prosthetic aortic valve.

Physiology

Aortic regurgitation imposes a volume overload on the left ventricle. Although the end-diastolic pressure may be normal or slightly elevated in the early phases, progressive regurgitation elevates the end-diastolic pressure and dilates the chamber by slippage of myocardial fibers, sarcomere replication, and myocardial hypertrophy. These compensatory mechanisms support a large left ventricular stroke volume, which is often achieved with an ejection fraction above 50 per cent.

TABLE 49–3. AORTIC REGURGITATION

Etiology	Physiology	Symptoms	Physical Examination	Electrocardiogram	Chest	Echocardiogram	Catheterization	Medical Therapy	Surgical Therapy
Chronic									
Rheumatic fever Connective tissue disorders Hypertension, atherosclerosis Syphilis Cystic medial necrosis Aortic ectasia Congenital heart disease	Chronic volume overload LV* dilatation LV hypertrophy	Fatigue Dyspnea Edema	Wide arterial pulse pressure Enlarged LV Diastolic aortic murmur Systolic ejection murmur Third sound Apical diastolic rumble	LV hypertrophy and strain	Enlarged LV Dilated aorta	Valvular anatomy Aortic root size Enlarged LV Mitral valve fluttering LV function	Contrast from aorta to LV LV function	Preload and afterload reduction Diuretics Digitalis	LV systolic echo dimension >55 mm Ejection fraction <50%
Acute									
Endocarditis Aortic dissection Ruptured sinus of Valsalva Prosthetic valve	Acute LV diastolic pressure and volume overload	Pulmonary edema	Loud diastolic musical murmur Right and left sternal border radiation with thrill Soft S_1 and third sound Continuous murmur if rupture into right side of heart	LV strain	Pulmonary edema Normal heart size	Valvular anatomy Aortic size and intimal flap	Contrast from aorta to LV Aortic and intimal flap	Preload and afterload reduction	Urgent surgery

*LV = left ventricle, ventricular.

The systolic ejection of a large stroke volume into the high-impedance area of the systemic circulation increases the systolic pressure. Systolic wall stress or afterload can be maintained within the normal range by hypertrophy of the myocardium, but myocardial oxygen demand is significantly increased. A progressive decline in aortic diastolic pressure due to regurgitation of blood into the left ventricle can reduce coronary blood flow and thus create conditions for subendocardial ischemia in severe chronic aortic regurgitation.

The gradual volume overload of chronic aortic regurgitation can be tolerated for years before the inotropic state of the myocardium deteriorates. Eventually, the declining ejection fraction and inotropic state, along with limits to the dilatation hypertrophy mechanism, cause marked elevation of the left ventricular filling pressure with pulmonary venous capillary congestion.

Left ventricular hemodynamics in acute aortic regurgitation, compared with those in chronic aortic regurgitation, are immediately disturbed, since the regurgitant volume may be imposed on a normal end-diastolic volume. Under such circumstances, sudden incompetence of the aortic valve can severely elevate the left ventricular filling pressure, since the acute dilatation of the left ventricle is limited. With such rapid regurgitation through the aortic valve, the mitral valve may close prematurely, and the aortic diastolic murmur may persist beyond the diminished first heart sound.

Clinical Course

Since the chronic volume overload of aortic regurgitation is well tolerated, patients may remain asymptomatic for long periods of time. The patient may be aware of prominent precordial activity as well as exaggerated pulsation of the carotid arteries. Diffuse sweating patterns and vague abdominal discomfort are less frequent symptoms. The accelerated development of angina, heart failure, or sudden death within several years has been observed in patients with a pulse pressure greater than 140/40 mm Hg and left ventricular enlargement demonstrated on electrocardiography or chest radiograph. Dyspnea, orthopnea, and paroxysmal nocturnal dyspnea result from impaired left ventricular contractility in pulmonary venous hypertension. Although tachycardia may impair ventricular function, the shortened diastolic filling period can be beneficial in reducing the duration of the aortic regurgitation. Chest pain and syncope are infrequent symptoms. Chest pain is often associated with underlying coronary artery disease, and syncope is usually attended by arrhythmias.

With acute aortic regurgitation, pulmonary edema is often the presenting manifestation. Severe chest pain suggests aortic dissection when acute aortic incompetence develops.

Physical Examination

In aortic regurgitation, the physical findings reflect the large left ventricular stroke volume into the systemic circulation and the rapid diastolic run-off into the left ventricle. The peripheral pulse is characteristically bounding, and additional manifestations of the wide pulse pressure include head bobbing, pulsation of the retinal arterioles, bounding carotid pulse, pistol shot sounds over the femoral arteries, a to-and-fro murmur elicited from the femoral artery with slight compression of the stethoscope, and capillary pulsations in the nail beds. With connective tissue and arthritic diseases that produce aortic regurgitation, there may be characteristic changes in habitus, such as the musculoskeletal type in Marfan's syndrome and kyphosis of the thoracic spine in ankylosing spondylitis.

The precordium is hyperdynamic with a laterally displaced apical impulse. The auscultatory hallmark is the high-pitched, blowing, decrescendo diastolic murmur heard best along the left sternal border while the patient is in the sitting position during full expiration. As the regurgitation becomes more severe, a diastolic rumble or Austin Flint murmur due to vibration of the anterior leaflet of the mitral valve in the regurgitant jet may be audible at the apex. If the ascending aorta is dilated, the diastolic murmur may be heard along the right sternal border as well. With extreme left ventricular dilatation, mitral regurgitation can produce an apical systolic murmur, and heart failure is attended by a ventricular gallop at the apex.

With acute aortic regurgitation due to disruption of an aortic leaflet or dissection dilating the aortic annulus, the diastolic murmur may be harsh with palpable vibrations along the left sternal border. A perforated or prolapsed aortic leaflet, as well as the detached aortic intima from dissection, can generate prominent musical qualities in the diastolic murmur.

Laboratory Studies

ELECTROCARDIOGRAM. The electrocardiogram typically reveals left ventricular hypertrophy with increased QRS voltage amplitude and ST-T wave changes of the strain pattern. With acute aortic regurgitation, the hypertrophy may be absent, and the ST-T wave changes can indicate myocardial ischemia.

CHEST RADIOGRAPHY. Significant cardiomegaly usually attends chronic aortic regurgitation, with the increase in size due to dilatation of the left ventricle. The ascending aorta is often prominent. Calcium in the aortic valve or annulus is best appreciated by fluoroscopy, but calcification of the ascending aorta caused by syphilis can be detected on the chest film. Left ventricular failure will be accompanied by pulmonary congestion and venous prominence.

ECHOCARDIOGRAM. Echocardiography has become the most useful noninvasive tool to recognize anatomic abnormalities of the aortic valve and to assess dimensions of the annulus and ascending aorta. The intensity of the regurgitant flow can be appreciated by the vibrations of the anterior mitral leaflet, and the echo Doppler and color techniques can estimate the severity of the regurgitation. Left ventricular chamber dimensions and wall thickness permit calculation of end-diastolic volume and hypertrophy. Finally, an end-systolic dimension of 55 mm has been proposed by several investigators to represent the limit of surgically reversible dilatation of the left ventricle so that aortic valve replacement should be performed before this chamber size is exceeded. Additional clinical experience has challenged the validity of the 55-mm systolic limit, since postoperative reduction in chamber size remains variable. Thus, echocardiographic studies of left ventricular dimensions and function are important in evaluation, follow-up, and timing for aortic valve replacement in aortic regurgitation.

EXERCISE TESTING. Although exercise capacity can be measured and followed periodically in patients with aortic regurgitation, exercise testing is best clinically used in combination with radionuclide angiography. A reduction in exercise ejection fraction by 5 per cent or more is considered by some an indication for surgery even in the absence of symptoms.

CARDIAC CATHETERIZATION. Cardiac catheterization can confirm the presence of aortic incompetence when contrast material injected into the aorta regurgitates into the left ventricle. The primary clinical indications for catheterization are to recognize coexisting lesions, such as mitral regurgitation, and to detect coronary artery disease. Dimensions of the aortic annulus and the ascending aorta are useful for the choice of a prosthetic device in the operative procedure.

Differential Diagnosis

In the evaluation of a diastolic murmur along the left sternal border, aortic insufficiency is far more common than pulmonic insufficiency. The pulsatile characteristics of the peripheral circulation can be helpful in differentiating an aortic from a pulmonic origin of the diastolic murmur. In systemic hypertension, accentuated tambour qualities of the second heart sound can sometimes suggest mild aortic regurgitation, but the level of the diastolic blood pressure can be helpful in distinguishing incompetence from reverberations of the second sound. Any condition that causes aortic stenosis through immobility of the valve leaflets is often accompanied by some degree of aortic regurgitation.

Medical Therapy

Antibiotic prophylaxis is indicated for the prevention of endocarditis. When symptoms of heart failure develop, vasodilating agents such as hydralazine, prazocin, or nifedipine may be beneficial, but benefits are rarely maintained. Thus, the use of digitalis, diuretics, and afterload-reducing agents is primarily of short-term benefit in aortic regurgitation.

Surgical Therapy

A major clinical decision in aortic regurgitation is the timing of aortic valve replacement before irreversible dilatation of the left ventricle has developed. The echocardiographic dimensions and evidence of reduced left ventricular function are now being utilized to advise valve replacement before symptoms of heart failure are manifested. Even after heart failure has developed, patients still improve clinically after aortic valve replacement. Valve replacement can be undertaken with a mortality of less than 3 to 5 per cent. The type of prosthetic valve will depend on the patient's age and the ability to be anticoagulated. In aortic dissection, there may also be replacement of the ascending aorta, since acute regurgitation requires intervention.

MITRAL STENOSIS

Etiology and Pathology

Rheumatic fever remains the predominant cause for mitral stenosis (Table 49–4). Calcification of the mitral valve annulus in the elderly patient can occasionally cause hemodynamic obstruction. Space-occupying lesions, such as left atrial myxoma, or thrombus formation can rarely obstruct the mitral valve. The characteristic pathologic change in rheumatic fever is fibrosis and scarring, particularly at the margins of the valve. This process can also extend into the chordae, with shortening and fusion. Eventually, fibrotic and destructive changes lead to calcification of the valve, and pulmonary venous hypertension causes thickening of the pulmonary veins and capillaries with eventual intimal and medial proliferation of the pulmonary arteries. With longstanding mitral stenosis and pulmonary hypertension, right ventricular hypertrophy and fibrosis develop.

Physiology

The hemodynamic abnormalities in mitral stenosis result from obstruction of diastolic blood flow into the left ventricle. The normal cross-sectional area of the mitral valve ranges from 4 to 6 cm^2, and turbulence of diastolic flow occurs when the valvular orifice is reduced below 2 cm^2. Increased demands for cardiac output, such as in exercise or fever, may be necessary to produce the diastolic murmur when the mitral valve orifice is reduced to 1.5 to 2 cm^2. In the second stage of progressive reduction in the mitral orifice size, a diastolic gradient develops between the left atrium and left ventricle under resting conditions when the valvular area is 1.5 to 1 cm^2. In the advanced stage, mitral orifice size is less than 1 cm^2, and left atrial and pulmonary hypertension becomes significant. The pulmonary capillary pressure often exceeds 20 to 25 mm Hg, and this leads to significant pulmonary arterial hypertension, pressure overload on the right ventricle, and compensatory hypertrophy of the right ventricle. Although the cardiac output can be maintained until the late stage of severe mitral stenosis, exercise will not produce a normal increase in cardiac output owing to impaired diastolic filling. Another hemodynamic complication in chronic mitral stenosis is atrial fibrillation due to left atrial enlargement. Atrial fibrillation and the increased ventricular response can aggravate hemodynamic abnormalities by reducing the diastolic filling period and leading to further elevation of pressure in the lungs.

Clinical Features

The average age at which rheumatic fever occurs is 10 to 12 years, and generally there is a 10-year period before the murmur of mitral stenosis can be detected. Mitral stenosis affects females more than males, and symptoms usually develop between the ages of 25 and 30 years. In temperate zones, mitral stenosis can accelerate in childhood, with severe hemodynamic impairment by the age of 10 to 12 years. Dyspnea is the most common symptom secondary to pulmonary venous hypertension and can be precipitated by any circumstance that increases cardiac output, such as exercise or febrile conditions. Paroxysmal atrial fibrillation can precipitate symptoms by increasing the ventricular rate. As the stenosis progresses, patients experience symptoms with minimal effort or at rest. With longstanding mitral stenosis and chronic pulmonary hypertension, the compensatory thickening of the pulmonary capillaries can protect the lungs from extravasation of fluid despite severe elevations of pulmonary pressure.

Systemic embolization resulting from underlying atrial fibrillation and left atrial thrombus development can also be a manifestation of mitral stenosis. Females can become symptomatic in the second trimester of pregnancy, when the blood volume increases significantly and elevates pulmonary pressures. As the blood volume diminishes late in the third trimester, the symptoms may slightly improve. With severe enlargement of the left atrium and infringement on the mainstem bronchus, persistent cough may develop. Hemoptysis can result from rupture of small vessels in the bronchi due to longstanding venous hypertension. Infective endocarditis can complicate mitral stenosis at any stage, but this generally occurs when mitral regurgitation is present as well.

Physical Examination

The classic physical findings of mitral stenosis are an accentuated first sound at the apex, an opening snap, and a diastolic rumble. If the condition is severe, the diminished peripheral pulse and blood pressure reflect a reduced left ventricular stroke volume. Patients may display typical "mitral facies" with florid congestion of the cheeks. The distended neck veins indicate right ventricular failure with secondary tricuspid regurgitation. If tricuspid stenosis coexists with mitral stenosis, a prominent *a* wave may be observed in the jugular vein.

Inspection of the precordium may reveal activity along the left sternal border, indicating right ventricular enlargement and pulmonary hypertension. On palpation, the accentuated first sound, the opening snap (OS), and the diastolic rumble can sometimes be felt at the apex. With significant right ventricular dilatation, the left ventricular apical impulse may be displaced laterally, and the right cardiac border may be percussed to the right of the sternum. The opening snap can vary from 0.04 to 0.10 second after the second sound at the apex. The higher the left atrial pressure, the closer the opening snap to the second heart sound (S_2), and thus the S_2-OS interval indicates the severity of the mitral stenosis. The opening snap is a high-pitched sound and is heard best with the patient in the left lateral decubitus position. The opening snap can sometimes be appreciated at the base of the heart but must be differentiated from a split pulmonic second sound. The diastolic rumble at the apex is a low-pitched murmur following the opening snap. If sinus rhythm is present, there will be presystolic accentuation due to atrial contraction. Since the murmur of mitral stenosis may be faint in the early stages, to complete the physical examination, the patient should exercise by performing sit-ups or hopping on one foot to increase the heart rate. With the increased flow across the mitral valve, the diastolic rumble may be more easily detected.

The diastolic murmur of pulmonic insufficiency should be sought along the left sternal border, but this can be difficult to distinguish from aortic regurgitation. A widened systemic pulse pressure favors aortic over pulmonic insufficiency with mitral stenosis. Rarely, tricuspid stenosis can simultaneously occur with

TABLE 49–4. MITRAL STENOSIS

Etiology	Physiology	Symptoms	Physical Examination	Electrocardiogram	Chest	Echocardiogram	Catheterization	Medical Therapy	Surgical Therapy
Rheumatic	Pressure overload	Dyspnea	Loud S$_1$	Broad, notched	Enlarged LA	Square wave of	Elevated PA*	Dental	Symptoms
Myxoma	LA* and	Fatigue	Opening snap	P wave in	Prominent	EF slope of	wedge	prophylaxis	Valvular area
Calcification	pulmonary	Palpitations	Diastolic rumble	lead II	pulmonary	mitral valve	pressure	Digitalis for	<1.0 cm^2
Congenital	veins	Hemoptysis	Signs of pulmonary		veins	Estimation of	and normal	atrial fibrilla-	
			hypertension:			gradient and	LV diastolic	tion	
			RVH*			orifice size	pressure	Warfarin	
			↑ P$_2$					(Coumadin)	
			Diastolic blow						

*LA = left atrium; RVH = right ventricular hypertrophy; PA = pulmonary arterial.

the mitral stenosis. The murmur of tricuspid stenosis is heard along the lower left sternal border and is greatly accentuated with inspiration. Finally, some degree of mitral incompetence often accompanies mitral stenosis and produces an apical systolic murmur of varying intensity.

Laboratory Studies

ELECTROCARDIOGRAM. The electrocardiographic changes of mitral stenosis include left atrial enlargement and right ventricular hypertrophy due to pulmonary hypertension. Characteristic notching and prolongation of the P wave are most prominent in leads II, III, and aV_F. The terminal portion of the P wave is usually negative in lead V_1. Right-axis deviation and an increased amplitude of the R wave in V_1 are evidence of right ventricular hypertrophy.

CHEST RADIOGRAPH. Radiographic evidence of mitral stenosis includes left atrial enlargement, pulmonary venous hypertension, and right ventricular prominence. The enlarged left atrium produces a double contour along the right cardiac silhouette, as well as straightening of the left cardiac border due to the large left atrial appendage. This change produces elevation of the left mainstem bronchus. The pulmonary venous hypertension redistributes the blood flow to the apices of the lungs, with a reduction in blood volume of the lower lung. Pulmonary arterial hypertension renders the hilar arteries more prominent. Kerley's B lines due to fibrosis and lymphatic engorgement appear as transverse linear densities at the lung bases above the diaphragm.

ECHOCARDIOGRAM. The echocardiogram is the most accurate noninvasive technique for detection of mitral valve stenosis (Fig. 49–2), which is recognized by the characteristic square wave motion of the E to F slope of the valve during diastole. The concordant movement of anterior and posterior mitral valve leaflets is one of the cardinal echocardiographic findings in mitral stenosis. Calcification produces additional echoes from the stenotic valve. The two-dimensional echo can accurately measure the diastolic area of the mitral valve, and the echo Doppler technique can estimate the pressure gradient across the valve, as well as left atrial and left ventricular dimensions, and provide an assessment of left ventricular function. Thrombus or a myxoma in the left atrium produces multiple echoes during diastolic filling.

EXERCISE TESTING. Treadmill or bicycle exercise testing can establish aerobic capacity and the degree of exercise impairment. These observations can be useful in following the young patient with mitral stenosis during the early stages of the disease. The response of the heart rate to exertion and early symptoms of fatigue or dyspnea can be documented with an exercise test.

CARDIAC CATHETERIZATION. Hemodynamic confirmation of mitral stenosis requires measurement of the diastolic pressure gradient across the mitral valve. Left atrial pressure can

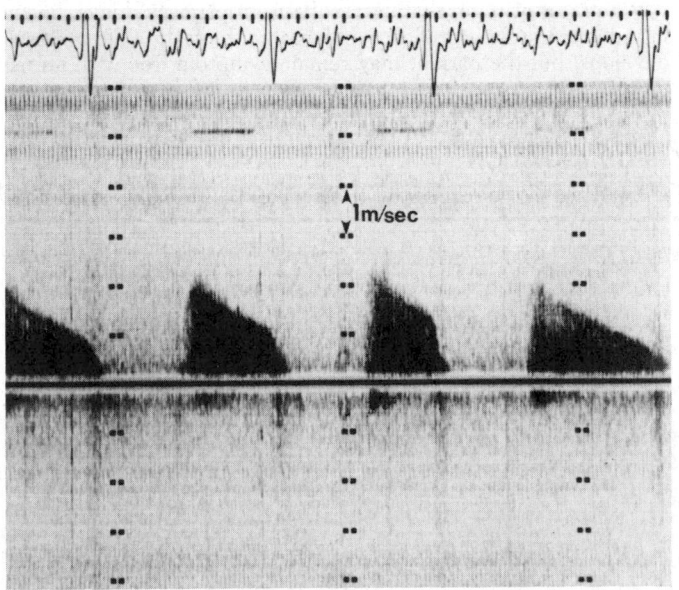

FIGURE 49–2. Continuous wave Doppler echocardiogram of mitral valve flow in a patient with mitral stenosis and atrial fibrillation.

be obtained directly through trans-septal puncture or as reflected in the pulmonary capillary wedge pressure and recorded simultaneously with the left ventricular pressure. The Gorlin formula (see Ch. 39.5) permits calculation of the mitral orifice size based on the diastolic flow derived from the forward cardiac output and the simultaneous pressure gradient across the valve. The mitral valve gradient can vary from 5 to 25 mm Hg. In an individual without symptoms, mitral valve area can range from 1.5 to 2.0 cm^2. In those exhibiting symptoms with usual activity, valvular size may be 1.5 cm^2 or less, and patients with marked limitations usually have an orifice size less than 1.0 cm^2. Sometimes, a minimal mitral valve gradient is obtained under resting circumstances, but exercise can markedly increase pulmonary pressures to the level of heart failure. At the time of catheterization, associated valve lesions should be assessed, such as mitral regurgitation, aortic stenosis, and aortic regurgitation. If the patient is above 40 years of age, coronary arteriography should also be performed.

Differential Diagnosis

Several cardiac conditions can be confused with the symptoms and physical findings of mitral stenosis. A left atrial myxoma can produce dyspnea or syncope with an opening snap and a diastolic rumble. Primary pulmonary hypertension in young women can be associated with dyspnea and an accentuated pulmonic second sound, but other auscultatory findings are lacking. An atrial septal defect can mimic mitral stenosis with an accentuated first sound, opening snap, and diastolic rumble. However, the accentuated first sound is due to tricuspid valve closure, the opening snap is a split pulmonic second sound, and the diastolic rumble is created by flow across the tricuspid valve.

Medical Therapy

Medical therapy is directed at reducing the incidence of rheumatic fever, prophylaxis for infective endocarditis, control of atrial fibrillation with a rapid ventricular response, and anticoagulation for thromboembolic phenomena. The patient should continue on rheumatic fever prophylaxis until he or she is 30 years of age.

Since atrial fibrillation can aggravate and precipitate symptoms of pulmonary congestion, digitalis should be administered to control ventricular response. Anticoagulation on a chronic basis should be considered in all patients with mitral stenosis and atrial fibrillation. If the patient develops pulmonary edema with atrial fibrillation, cardioversion should be attempted. Ideally, the patient should be anticoagulated 2 weeks prior to elective cardioversion for atrial fibrillation. Quinidine should be started 2 days before the elective procedure, and if digitalis has been administered, this may be discontinued 1 day prior to the cardioversion. If cardioversion is successful, the patient should remain on long-term anticoagulation and quinidine therapy. For thromboembolic phenomena from the left atrium, anticoagulation is indicated. For acute embolism to the extremities or abdomen, surgical embolectomy may be beneficial.

Valvuloplasty via catheter is being performed in selected patients with mitral stenosis, particularly in children, in young women desiring to become pregnant at a later date, and in the elderly at high surgical risk.

Surgical Therapy

The decision for surgery is based on the development of symptoms of pulmonary congestion during activity or at rest. In addition to pulmonary congestion, recurrent atrial fibrillation with aggravation of pulmonary congestion, thromboembolic phenomena, and hemoptysis can be indications for surgery. Mitral commissurotomy remains the procedure of choice with a pliable mitral valve without calcification or mitral regurgitation and carries an operative mortality of less than 1 per cent. This procedure should be considered particularly for the young female who has a desire for pregnancy. Sometimes commissurotomy can be performed before the development of significant symptoms. Patients may benefit for 5 to 20 years after commissurotomy, but if symptoms occur at a later time, mitral valve replacement may be required. Mitral valve replacement carries an operative mortality of 2 to 3 per cent. The type of mitral valve depends on the age of the patient as well as the circumstances for anticoagulation in a young female. The porcine valve can be inserted without the need for chronic anticoagulation but may require replacement after 10 years. If the valve is calcified or if the patient has had a previous commissurotomy, a prosthetic device is preferred. When there is a contraindication to anticoagulation, as in the aging patient, the porcine valve can be inserted.

Anticoagulation and antibiotic prophylaxis are required in patients with a prosthetic valve. Should atrial fibrillation persist with a rapid ventricular response, digitalis will still have to be administered. Long-term complications of prosthetic mitral valves, such as thrombus formation, infection, and mechanical dysfunction, are estimated to occur at a rate of 1 to 2 per cent per year. Thromboembolism occurs at a rate of 3 per cent per year with a mechanical mitral valve, whereas with the porcine valve, the incidence is 1 to 2 per cent per year.

MITRAL REGURGITATION

Etiology and Pathology

Mitral valve prolapse has now become the leading cause of mitral regurgitation (see next section), although rheumatic heart disease remains an important cause of mitral regurgitation (Table 49–5). Connective tissue disorders, coronary artery disease, annular calcification, and any condition producing left ventricular dilatation can create incompetence of the mitral valve. Several congenital cardiac conditions, such as partial atrioventricular (AV) canal, corrected transposition of the great arteries, and isolated cleft of the mitral valve seen with the ostium primum atrial septal defect, can be associated with mitral valve regurgitation.

Acute mitral regurgitation can result from sudden disruption of the normal function of the mitral valve apparatus. Ruptured mitral valve chordae from endocarditis, myxomatous degeneration of the valve, or trauma can produce sudden mitral regurgitation. Acute myocardial infarction can rupture the papillary muscle, and infective endocarditis can perforate the mitral valve leaflet or the chordae. Mechanical disturbances with a prosthetic mitral valve can lead to mitral incompetence.

Physiology

Incompetence of the mitral valve apparatus during systolic ejection permits regurgitation into the left atrium and pulmonary veins. The extent of the hemodynamic abnormalities imposed on the left ventricle and the left atrium is influenced by the chronic or acute nature of the valvular disturbance as well as the pre-existing functional state of the left ventricle. In chronic mitral regurgitation, a volume overload is imposed on the left ventricle, and the size of the regurgitant volume determines the increase in the end-diastolic volume. Systolic regurgitation into the left atrium produces a prominent v wave, which accentuates the normal filling of the left ventricle from the pulmonary venous inflow. With chronic mitral regurgitation, distensibility of the left atrium and pulmonary veins and increased compliant properties of the left ventricle permit rapid ventricular diastolic filling. As a result of the increased atrial and ventricular compliance, mean left atrial pressure and left ventricular end-diastolic pressure often remain within the normal range in chronic mitral regurgitation.

In *chronic mitral regurgitation*, the large total left ventricular stroke volume maintains the forward stroke volume despite the regurgitant volume into the left atrium. Total left ventricular output may reach six times the normal forward cardiac output. Left ventricular hypertrophy accompanies the increased left ventricular end-diastolic volume. Eventually, the contractile properties of the left ventricular myocardium decline, and the end-systolic volume is abnormally increased. The ejection fraction declines, even though the value may remain near the normal range in the early stage of left ventricular decompensation. An increase in the end-systolic volume elevates the pressure and wall stress values beyond those that can be attributed solely to changes in wall thickness or hypertrophy. This occurrence has been designated as a mismatch in afterload and preload. Even though the deterioration of the contractile state of the left ventricle may gradually elevate the left ventricular end-diastolic pressure, in rare instances the left atrium enlarges to such dimensions that ventricular end-diastolic and left atrial pressures remain normal, as encountered in the giant left atrium syndrome.

In coronary artery disease, mitral regurgitation results from abnormalities of posterior wall motion and papillary muscle function. Ischemia of the papillary muscle has been proposed as a mechanism, and disturbances in posterior wall motion are usually present with mitral regurgitation. When the residual scar after myocardial infarction exceeds 20 per cent of the total surface area of the ventricle, compensatory dilatation of the left ventricle is often attended by some degree of mitral regurgitation.

Severe dilatation of the left ventricle from either a primary volume overload or secondary myocardial decompensation eventually results in mitral regurgitation. Dilatation of the left ventricular chamber displaces the papillary muscles so that coaptation of the leaflets is impaired during systolic ejection. Conditions producing ventricular dilatation are further aggravated by depression of the contractile state, and the left ventricular hemodynamic abnormalities primarily reflect myocardial failure with an additional overload on the ventricle.

In *acute mitral regurgitation*, a sudden pressure overload is imposed on the left atrium and pulmonary veins from the left ventricular regurgitant volume. This pressure overload is intensified by the inability of the left atrium and left ventricle to dilate suddenly. The v wave in the left atrium may be as high as 60 to 70 mm Hg, resulting in acute pulmonary edema.

Clinical Features

When mitral regurgitation results from primary defects in the mitral apparatus, significant enlargement of the left ventricle develops, but the patient may remain symptom free with normal exercise tolerance. Since pulmonary venous hypertension and

TABLE 49–5. MITRAL REGURGITATION

Etiology	Physiology	Symptoms	Physical Examination	Electrocardiogram	Chest	Echocardiogram	Catheterization	Medical Therapy	Surgical Therapy
Chronic									
Prolapse	LV volume	Initially	Holosystolic apical	LV hypertrophy	Enlarged LV	Enlarged LV and	Contrast from	Afterload	Symptoms
Rheumatic	overload	asymptomatic	murmur		Enlarged LA	LA	LV to LA	reduction	LV echo
Coronary artery	LV dilatation and	Fatigue	Decreased S_1			Mitral valve	LA v wave	Diuretics	Diastolic
disease	hypertrophy	Dyspnea	Third sound			anatomy		Digitalis	dimension
Annular	LA* enlargement								>60 mm†
calcification									
Connective tissue									
disorder									
LV* dilatation									
Prosthetic valve									
Acute									
Ruptured	Pressure overload	Acute pulmonary	Harsh holosystolic	No change	Normal LV and	Abnormal mitral	Massive LA	Preload and	Surgery may be
chordae	LA and	edema	murmur radiating	Acute myocar-	LA dimen-	valve apparatus	regurgita-	afterload	urgently
Ruptured	pulmonary		into back	dial infarction	sion		tion	reduction	required
papillary	veins		Third sound		Pulmonary		Large v wave		
muscle	No change in LV				edema		Normal-sized		
Perforation of	dimension						LA		
leaflet									
Prosthetic valve									

*LV = left ventricle or ventricular; LA = left atrium or atrial.
†Proposed.

congestion are not early features of mitral regurgitation, fatigue due to reduced forward cardiac output is a more frequent symptom than dyspnea. Gradual impairment of the contractile state is attended by further enlargement of end-systolic and end-diastolic volumes and elevation of the left ventricular end-diastolic and left atrial pressures. Atrial fibrillation commonly develops when the left atrium enlarges and further aggravates heart failure.

In coronary artery disease, significant mitral regurgitation is usually accompanied by symptoms of impaired left ventricular function, such as dyspnea, fatigue, and orthopnea. This condition is sometimes designated the *ischemic cardiomyopathy syndrome.* In acute syndromes of mitral regurgitation, pulmonary edema is often the initial presentation because of the suddenly imposed pressure and volume overload on the left atrium and pulmonary venous system.

Physical Examination

The typical physical finding of mitral regurgitation is the apical holosystolic murmur, but the intensity, variation during the ejection phase, and radiation over the precordium are influenced by the underlying mechanism. The peripheral pulse can sometimes be rapid in upstroke with a short duration because of the abbreviated systolic ejection time, since a large volume of blood is regurgitated into the left atrium. The precordium may reveal a diffusely hyperdynamic impulse, and the first heart sound at the apex is diminished. The characteristic holosystolic murmur radiates into the axilla and often to the left sternal border. A protodiastolic or ventricular gallop sound is frequently audible and may be followed by an early diastolic rumble due to the large inflow of blood from the left atrium. When mitral regurgitation is caused by left ventricular dilatation and depression of the contractile state, the systolic murmur may be mid-, late, or holosystolic. Under these circumstances, the systolic murmur is usually grade II/VI or less and is accompanied by a left ventricular (S_3) gallop sound.

In acute mitral regurgitation due to rupture of the mitral valve apparatus, the murmur is harsh, grade III or IV/VI, and accompanied by a palpable thrill at the apex.

Laboratory Studies

ELECTROCARDIOGRAM. In chronic mitral regurgitation, the electrocardiogram will show evidence of left ventricular dilatation and hypertrophy with increased QRS voltage and ST-T wave changes in the lateral precordial leads. Left atrial enlargement will produce a negative P wave in lead V_1, but atrial fibrillation often develops in the late stages. When coronary artery disease is the etiology of mitral regurgitation, there is often evidence of an inferior or posterior wall myocardial infarction.

CHEST RADIOGRAPH. Left ventricular enlargement due to the volume overload can be appreciated from the standard chest film. Left atrial enlargement will cause a prominence along the right sternal border, but the pulmonary venous pattern may show no abnormalities until heart failure and venous congestion have developed.

ECHOCARDIOGRAM. The echocardiogram can define the anatomy of the mitral valve apparatus as well as left atrial and left ventricular chamber dimensions and function. Calcification of the valve leaflets and the annulus can be recognized. Depression of left ventricular ejection fraction and increases in end-diastolic and end-systolic dimensions are observed in secondary causes of mitral regurgitation with heart failure. With acute mitral regurgitation, a flail leaflet, ruptured chordae, or nidus of infection with infective endocarditis can sometimes be identified by the echocardiogram. The echo Doppler and color techniques can assess the intensity of the regurgitant jet into the left atrium. Finally, left ventricular end-diastolic and end-systolic dimensions have been used to identify the optimal time for mitral valve replacement before significant and irreversible myocardial deterioration has taken place.

EXERCISE TESTING. The standard exercise tests and radionuclide angiography can quantify functional capacity and document early deterioration in patients with mitral regurgitation.

CARDIAC CATHETERIZATION. Left ventriculography confirms mitral regurgitation by demonstrating systolic regurgitation of contrast material into the left atrium. Although the magnitude of the regurgitation can be quantified, the mechanism is not always apparent from left ventriculography. Left ventricular end-diastolic and end-systolic dimensions can be utilized to calculate ejection fraction, left ventricular mass, wall stress, and regurgitant volume per beat into the left atrium. The difference between the angiographic left ventricular stroke volume—that is, the end-diastolic volume minus the end-systolic volume on left ventriculography—and the forward stroke volume, calculated from the Fick or thermodilution methods, yields the regurgitant stroke volume per beat across the mitral valve. Coronary artery disease and the wall motion abnormalities contributing to disturbance in mitral valve function can also be confirmed at catheterization. The prominent v wave of mitral regurgitation can be recorded in the left atrium or the pulmonary capillary wedge pressure tracing. In acute mitral regurgitation, dimensions of the left ventricle and left atrium may be normal, but the regurgitant v wave can rise to 60 to 70 mm Hg. Cardiac catheterization can also detect coexistent lesions in the aortic valve. Since the left ventricular ejection fraction may be maintained in the normal range despite deterioration of the contractile state, additional assessment of the contractile state is important in all causes of mitral regurgitation. Calculation of end-systolic wall stress from pressure, volume, and wall thickness dimensions has proved useful in recognizing early deterioration of the contractile state in mitral regurgitation.

Differential Diagnosis

A holosystolic murmur identifies mitral regurgitation, even though the mechanism may not be apparent. Tricuspid regurgitation can cause a holosystolic murmur at the lower left sternal border, but inspiration accentuates the murmur more than in mitral regurgitation. If the murmur is not holosystolic, conditions such as aortic stenosis could be considered, along with papillary muscle dysfunction and mitral valve prolapse. In calcific aortic stenosis of the elderly patient, the murmur may sometimes be more prominent in the apex and may be confused with that of mitral regurgitation. A ventricular septal defect also causes a harsh holosystolic murmur at the lower left sternal border, but this generally radiates to the right of the sternum, compared with the axillary radiation of the murmur in mitral regurgitation.

Medical Therapy

In the early phase of mitral regurgitation without symptoms, only antibiotic prophylaxis is warranted. The same antibiotic program as described for mitral stenosis should be administered to these patients. When atrial fibrillation develops, digitalis is indicated to slow the ventricular response. Afterload-reducing agents, such as nitrates and antihypertensive drugs, have been found useful in maintaining the forward stroke volume in mitral regurgitation. Once heart failure develops, diuretics and inotropic agents are required, but major consideration should be given to surgery.

Surgical Therapy

The operative mortality of mitral valve replacement in mitral regurgitation has remained higher than the 2 to 3 per cent in mitral stenosis and for the symptomatic patient may range from 5 to 10 per cent. In the past, surgery has been delayed until patients develop symptoms, but the advanced symptomatic stage and depressed left ventricular function contribute to high operative mortality rates. When the ejection fraction falls below 20 per cent, operative mortality for mitral valve replacement may be as high as 25 per cent. Therefore, surgery should be considered before the patient becomes extremely symptomatic. An echocardiographic diastolic dimension greater than 60 mm has been proposed as a predictor for mitral valve replacement. In the selection of the optimal prosthetic device, the patient's age, underlying condition, and circumstances for anticoagulation must be considered. When technically feasible, valvular reconstruction is employed in order to preserve the anatomy. The mechanical prosthetic valve in the mitral position is more likely to develop thrombotic material than in other locations, so anticoagulation must be maintained. Any contraindication to anticoagulation warrants consideration of a porcine valve. Thromboembolism in patients with mechanical valves who are on anticoagulation occurs at a rate of 3 per cent per year, and for preoperative functional classes I through III, there is a yearly mortality rate of 3 per cent over a 10-year follow-up period. With a porcine valve, the rate of thromboembolism is lower but may reach 1.5 per cent per year.

MITRAL VALVE PROLAPSE

Etiology and Pathology

Although an isolated systolic click has been regarded as benign for decades, echocardiography has identified prolapse of the mitral valve in as many as 5 per cent of the adult population. A variety of synonyms include the midsystolic click–late systolic murmur, click murmur syndrome, and Barlow's syndrome. Pathologic findings include myxomatous degeneration of the valve and redundancy of the valve leaflets. These changes can also involve the chordae as well as the mitral valve. Although the underlying mechanism is still incompletely understood, these changes in the mitral valve are seen with several connective tissue diseases, including Marfan's syndrome and osteogenesis imperfecta, and sometimes with coronary artery disease. The syndrome occurs most frequently in women in early adulthood and can also be found in families.

Physiology

The abnormalities of mitral valve prolapse can affect both anterior and posterior leaflets, but the posterior leaflet is most frequently involved. With the onset of ventricular systole, normal closure of the mitral valve takes place, but redundancy of the leaflets results in further upward motion of the valve into the left atrium. Sudden cessation of the valvular motion is thought to generate the click, and the lack of proper positioning of the two leaflets results in the systolic regurgitant murmur in mid- and late systole. Occasionally, both the anterior and posterior leaflets prolapse, and in extreme conditions, there can be extensive prolapse of both leaflets in the absence of a click or murmur. In a small number of patients, progressive degenerative changes in the valve or rupture of the chordae or both can produce severe mitral regurgitation.

Clinical Features

The majority of patients with mitral valve prolapse remain asymptomatic, but a spectrum of symptoms can be encountered. Symptoms include palpitations, fatigue, chest pain, orthostatic changes, and psychological aberrations. Frequently, symptoms fail to correlate with the prominence of the physical findings and the extent of mitral regurgitation. Circulatory studies on changes in tilting, along with heart rate and blood pressure response, have led to the designation of dysautonomia in certain of these patients. In 10 to 15 per cent of affected individuals, palpitations may become frequent, and in a smaller number there may be progressive mitral regurgitation. Infective endocarditis occurs with a slightly higher incidence than in the normal population. Sudden deaths associated with this syndrome have been sporadically reported.

Physical Findings

Patients are often female, with a thin habitus and a narrow anteroposterior chest diameter. The principal findings are the early to midsystolic click and a mid- or late systolic murmur. The timing of the click as well as the characteristics of the murmur can vary widely. Often the murmur is crescendo and decrescendo, but it can be sustained in its frequency. The click or the murmur may be present alone, and not infrequently, both click and murmur are absent. The click and the murmur are influenced by the dimensions of the ventricle, and maneuvers that decrease ventricular filling, such as standing and the Valsalva maneuver, will result in movement of the click closer to the first sound, followed by early onset of the murmur. Conditions that increase filling of the ventricle, such as the squatting maneuver, can delay the onset of the click and the murmur.

Laboratory Studies

ELECTROCARDIOGRAM. The electrocardiogram may reveal a variety of T wave and ST-segment changes, along with atrial or ventricular ectopic beats. Most commonly, the T wave is slightly inverted in the inferior and lateral precordial leads, and occasionally there is associated ST-segment depression. Rarely, QT prolongation with deep coving of the T wave is seen in the precordial leads. Runs of premature beats, both from the atrium and the ventricle, can be recorded by Holter monitoring. Symptoms may not correlate with the frequency and occurrence of cardiac ectopic activity.

CHEST RADIOGRAPH. The habitus is asthenic; the chest has a narrow anteroposterior diameter, and the cardiac silhouette is elongated.

ECHOCARDIOGRAPHY. The echocardiogram is the diagnostic technique of choice for mitral valve prolapse (Fig. 49–3). In one form, late systolic prolapse of the posterior leaflet resembles an inverted question mark. In the second form, there may be prolapse of the posterior leaflet throughout the systolic ejection phase with a hammock type of configuration. The echocardiographic findings of prolapse can be recognized in the absence of the click and the murmur. At other times, the click and murmur are not attended by echocardiographically evident prolapse of the leaflet. The standard for diagnosis of mitral valve prolapse is the two-dimensional echo, which can define the plane of the mitral annulus and demonstrate extension of the mitral valve leaflets beyond the annulus into the left atrium. Color Doppler can display the amount of mitral regurgitation.

EXERCISE TESTING. Stress testing can aggravate or precipitate cardiac irritability in these patients. Furthermore, the exercise test can document the patient's fatigue and musculoskeletal symptoms, which often are at variance with the echocardiographic findings.

CARDIAC CATHETERIZATION. Although left ventriculography has been the standard invasive method for documenting redundancy and prolapse of the mitral leaflets, the precision of echocardiography has obviated the necessity of catheterization in the majority of patients with prolapse. Atypical chest discomfort sometimes requires coronary arteriography to exclude coronary artery disease. Wall motion abnormalities have been recognized on the ventriculogram, but these do not correlate with coexisting abnormalities in the coronary arteries. Prolapse of the tricuspid valve can also occur. With mitral valve prolapse in connective tissue disorders, there may be associated aortic regurgitation.

Differential Diagnosis

The mid- and late systolic murmur, as well as the crescendo-decrescendo qualities of mitral valve prolapse, can be similar to the murmur of regurgitation in papillary muscle dysfunction. In coronary artery disease or hypertrophic cardiomyopathy with

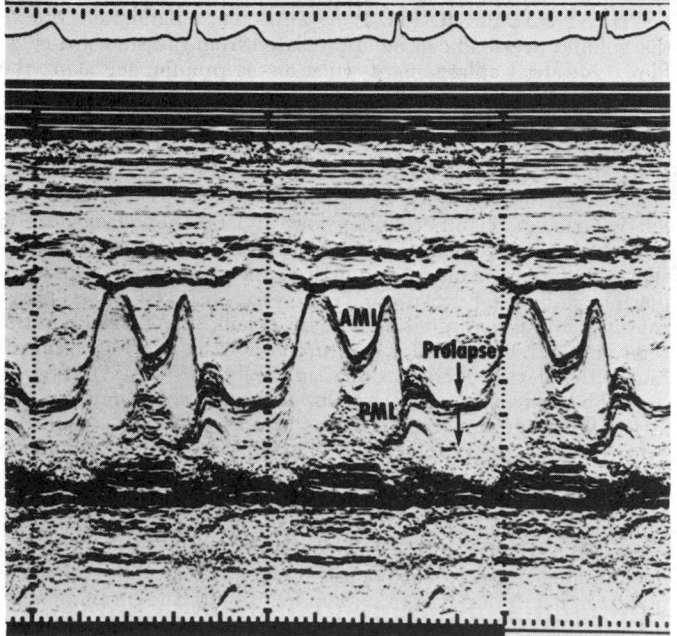

FIGURE 49–3. M-Mode echocardiogram of a patient with mitral valve prolapse. Note the systolic posterior motion of the anterior (AML) and posterior (PML) mitral valve leaflets.

obstruction, the crescendo-decrescendo murmur may be similar to that of mitral valve prolapse. However, the harsh intensity of the murmur is much louder with the hyperdynamic contraction of hypertrophic cardiomyopathy. Maneuvers that increase the murmur of mitral valve prolapse intensify the murmur of cardiomyopathy with obstruction even more. However, in the latter condition, the murmur is often holosystolic. If ventricular irritability is present, the intensity of the murmur of hypertrophic cardiomyopathy with obstruction will be much louder in the postextrasystolic beat.

Treatment

The majority of patients with mitral valve prolapse require no treatment. Ventricular ectopy and symptoms of palpitations can be effectively managed with β-blocking drugs. However, fatigue in these patients can sometimes be aggravated with β blockade. With a prolonged QT interval or syncope, treatment with an antiarrhythmic is warranted. Infrequently, control of ectopy may be difficult despite the use of standard antiarrhythmic agents.

Infective endocarditis is a potential problem in these patients. Originally, all patients were advised to have antibiotic prophylaxis. Statistical studies now suggest that only those patients with an audible click and murmur should be treated with antibiotic prophylaxis. Patients with prolapse demonstrated on echocardiography without a click or murmur may be at no greater risk than the normal population. When mitral regurgitation becomes progressive with chamber enlargement or with ruptured chordae, mitral valve replacement may be necessary. Mitral valve reconstruction and mitral valve annuloplasty are preferred by some surgeons to total valve replacement. Fortunately, for the majority of patients, reassurance and conservative follow-up constitute the best treatment.

TRICUSPID STENOSIS

The most common cause of stenosis of the tricuspid valve remains rheumatic fever, but this condition is invariably associated with involvement of left-sided valves by the same rheumatic process. Rare conditions such as carcinoid tumor, endocardial fibroelastosis, and right atrial myxoma can create stenosis or obstruction of the tricuspid valve. Tricuspid stenosis causes right atrial hypertension and elevated systemic venous pressure. Stenosis of the tricuspid valve may serve as a protective mechanism for the pulmonary vascular bed in patients with mitral stenosis. Symptoms of tricuspid stenosis are dyspnea and fatigue, but the pulmonary manifestations of mitral stenosis can diminish with the development of significant stenosis of the tricuspid valve. Pulsations in the neck veins and peripheral edema develop.

Physical examination reveals a prominent, often giant, a wave in the neck veins caused by the vigorous atrial contraction against the stenotic valve. The diastolic murmur is heard best along the left lower sternal border and is presystolic if sinus rhythm is present or midsystolic with atrial fibrillation. The murmur increases prominently with inspiration, but an opening snap is rarely heard. Since mitral stenosis is usually concurrent, the auscultatory maneuvers must specifically locate the tricuspid stenosis murmur. If tricuspid stenosis is the dominant hemodynamic lesion, pulmonary hypertension and right ventricular hypertrophy will not be detected on the physical examination.

The electrocardiographic finding is a tall, tented P wave in leads II, III, and aV$_F$ with absence of right ventricular hypertrophy. The chest radiograph should reveal a large right atrium without prominence of the pulmonary arteries. The echo Doppler technique may detect and assess the gradient across the tricuspid valve. If cardiac catheterization is performed, simultaneous catheters must be placed in the right atrium and the right ventricle for accurate detection of the pressure gradient. Respiratory variations will introduce inaccuracies in a pull-back tracing across the tricuspid valve. Treatment consists of antibiotic coverage. If surgery is performed for lesions in the left side of the heart, correction of the tricuspid lesion can also be undertaken.

TRICUSPID INSUFFICIENCY

Tricuspid insufficiency is, most commonly, secondary to right ventricular dilatation and hypertrophy. Tricuspid regurgitation can rarely result from infective endocarditis, myocardial infarction, trauma, prolapse, or congenital heart disease such as atrial septal defect or Ebstein's anomaly. Symptoms of tricuspid regurgitation are those of hepatic congestion or peripheral edema.

On physical examination, atrial fibrillation is commonly present and large cv waves can be detected in the jugular veins. The murmur is holosystolic along the left sternal border and increases with inspiration. The electrocardiogram often reveals atrial fibrillation without other significant features. The chest film demonstrates a prominent right atrium and ventricle. The echocardiogram can document prolapse of the tricuspid leaflets as well as a nidus of infection or disruption of a chorda. Contrast-echo and echo Doppler techniques can accurately detect and assess the amount of tricuspid regurgitation. Therapy usually consists of treatment of conditions leading to right ventricular failure. Should surgery be performed for left-sided lesions, the tricuspid valve can be inspected. Often the leaflets are anatomically normal, and annuloplasty is indicated rather than valve replacement. If the tricuspid valve is replaced, along with insertion of mitral and aortic prostheses, mortality remains high at 20 per cent.

PULMONIC REGURGITATION

Regurgitation of the pulmonic valve is most commonly secondary to severe pulmonary hypertension, which can be caused by mitral stenosis, chronic lung disease, or pulmonary emboli. Inflammatory diseases and endocarditis can sometimes render the pulmonic valve incompetent, and previous surgery for congenital heart disease may create pulmonic regurgitation. The murmur (Graham Steell) is typically a high-pitched diastolic blow along the left sternal border similar to that in aortic regurgitation. No characteristic electrocardiographic changes are found, but the chest radiograph often demonstrates a prominent pulmonary artery echo. The color Doppler technique easily detects regurgitation in the pulmonary outflow tract. Cardiac catheterization is useful only to exclude aortic regurgitation as a cause of the diastolic murmur. Treatment consists of management of pulmonary hypertension with medical agents or occasionally with mitral valve surgery.

PULMONIC STENOSIS

Stenotic lesions of the pulmonic valve are almost always caused by congenital malformations (see Ch. 46). Rarely, hypertrophic cardiomyopathy can involve the right side of the heart with obstruction of the right ventricular outflow tract.

Aortic Valve Disease

Letac B, Cribier A, Koning R, et al.: Aortic stenosis in elderly patients aged 80 or older: Treatment by percutaneous balloon valvuloplasty in a series of 92 cases. Circulation 80:1514, 1989. *A review by the founders of this procedure for a common valvular condition in aging patients.*
Pellikka PA, Nishimure RA, Bailey KR, et al.: The natural history of adults with asymptomatic hemodynamically significant aortic stenosis. J Am Coll Cardiol 15:1012, 1990. *Clinical guidelines for the asymptomatic patient.*

Mitral Valve Disease

Duren DR, Recker AE, Dunning AJ: Long-term follow-up of idiopathic mitral valve prolapse in 300 patients: A prospective study. J Am Coll Cardiol 11:42, 1988. *Clinical events in the most common abnormality of cardiac valves.*
Rackley CE, Edwards JE, Karp RB: Mitral valve disease. In Hurst JW (ed.): The Heart. 7th ed. New York, McGraw-Hill Book Company, 1989, p 820.
Rappaport E: Natural history of aortic and mitral valve disease. Am J Cardiol 36:221, 1975. *A 10-year follow-up of the stenotic and regurgitant lesions of the aortic and mitral valves.*

Valve Surgery

Chavez AM, Copgrove DM, Lyth BW, et al.: Applicability of mitral valvuloplasty techniques in a North American population. Am J Cardiol 62:253, 1988. *Alternatives to surgical replacement of the mitral apparatus.*
Lindblom D, Lindblom U, Quist J, et al.: Long-term survival rates after heart valve replacement. J Am Coll Cardiol 15:566, 1990. *Analysis of risk, benefits, and complications in long-term follow-up of prosthetic valves.*
Rackley CE, Katz NM, Wallace RB: Artificial valve disease. In Hurst JW (ed.): The Heart. 7th ed. New York, McGraw-Hill Book Company, 1989, p 871.

50 Diseases of the Myocardium

Joseph K. Perloff

"Cardiomyopathy" means heart (cardio) muscle disease (myopathy). The term is appropriately applied to disorders characterized by *primary* involvement of ventricular myocardium. Because these disorders of cardiac muscle are primary, they are by definition not in response to coexisting or pre-existing disease of the heart or circulation. The cardiomyopathies are best classified according to their anatomic and pathophysiologic types as dilated, hypertrophic, or restrictive (Table 50–1, Fig. 50–1). In each category, the cause or causes may or may not be known.

DILATED CARDIOMYOPATHY

DEFINITION AND GENERAL DESCRIPTION OF FINDINGS. Dilated cardiomyopathy is characterized by an increase in left ventricular or biventricular internal dimensions without a proportional increase in septal and free wall thicknesses. The principal physiologic impairment is in systolic function (depressed contractility).

Certain *general pathophysiologic principles* apply. Injured myocytes do not regenerate but are replaced by connective tissue. Hypertrophy of remaining cells does not adequately compensate for the loss of contractile elements. Ventricular volumes increase, cardiac output falls, and left ventricular filling pressure rises. Stroke volume is initially maintained despite depressed ejection fraction. This state of compensated systolic dysfunction is ultimately replaced by decompensated heart failure in which cardiac output is critically limited. The development of mitral and tricuspid regurgitation adds to the hemodynamic burden and further depresses cardiac output. Hypervolemia and peripheral vasoconstriction contribute additionally to net ventricular overload.

Three major threats confront the patient with chronic dilated cardiomyopathy, namely, progressive hemodynamic deterioration, systemic embolization, and sudden death. An insidious decrease in exercise tolerance is followed by frank exertional dyspnea, orthopnea, and paroxysmal nocturnal dyspnea. Both ventricles are usually involved, but the clinical manifestations of left ventricular failure generally predominate. The mechanisms of sudden death are diverse and include ventricular tachycardia or fibrillation, severe bradycardia, electromechanical dissociation, systemic embolization of mural thrombi from the dilated left ventricle (Fig. 50–2), and pulmonary embolization from venous thromboses.

On *physical examination*, the arterial pulse exhibits a relatively narrow pulse pressure and pulsus alternans. A "proportional pulse pressure" (calculated as the difference between systolic and diastolic blood pressures divided by the systolic pressure) of 25 per cent or less identifies approximately 90 per cent of patients with cardiac indices of 2.2 liters per minute per square meter or less. The jugular venous pulse exhibits elevated a and v waves with preserved x and y descents until tricuspid regurgitation increases the v wave and blunts the x descent. Precordial palpation identifies a displaced, hypodynamic left ventricular impulse. Auscultation detects third and fourth heart sounds. Systolic murmurs originate from mitral and tricuspid regurgitation. Occasional patients have disproportionate right ventricular failure (peripheral edema, ascites, and hepatic congestion). Im-

TABLE 50–1. PATHOPHYSIOLOGIC CLASSIFICATION OF THE CARDIOMYOPATHIES

1. Dilated
2. Hypertrophic
   a. Asymmetric (eccentric)
   b. Symmetric (concentric)
3. Restrictive (nondilated, nonhypertrophic)
   a. Increased septal/wall thickness
   b. Normal septal/wall thickness

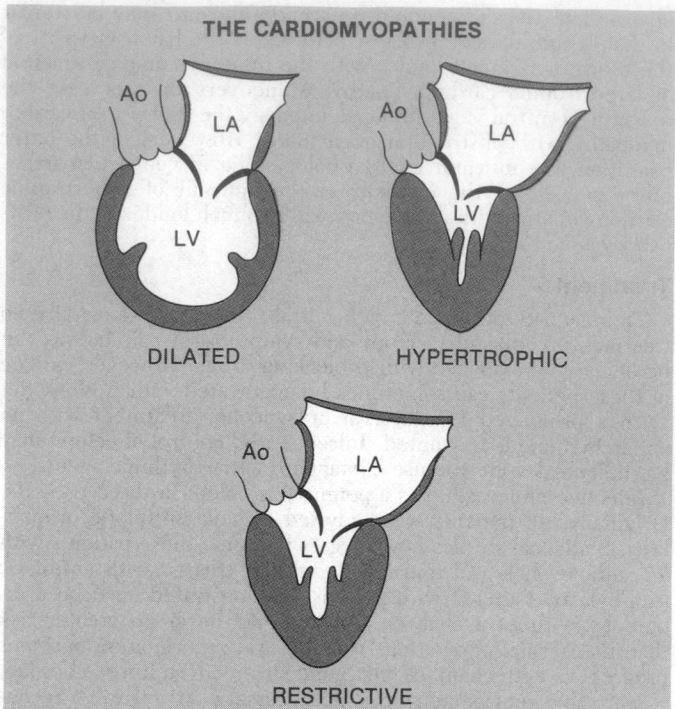

FIGURE 50–1. Schematic illustrations of dilated, hypertrophic, and restrictive cardiomyopathies. (Modified from Roberts WC, Ferrans VJ: Pathologic anatomy of the cardiomyopathies. Human Pathol 6:287, 1975. Reprinted with permission from W. B. Saunders Co.)

portantly, rales are typically absent despite elevated left ventricular filling pressure because chronic exudation of fluid is associated with an increase in lymphatic drainage so that the alveoli remain relatively dry.

The *electrocardiogram* may show nothing more than nonspecific ST-T wave abnormalities, but occasionally Q wave "infarct patterns" are present and are believed to reflect myonecrosis. Left bundle branch block is relatively frequent in chronic idiopathic dilated cardiomyopathy, but Chagas' disease is most commonly associated with right bundle branch block.

The *chest roentgenogram* reveals varying degrees of cardiomegaly. The increase in heart size principally reflects dilatation of the ventricles, although the atria are enlarged as well. Elevated left ventricular filling pressure is reflected chiefly in prominent central (hilar) pulmonary veins and in upper lobe vascular redistribution, rather than by radiologic evidence of pulmonary edema. Increased lymphatic drainage is the reason (see above).

Two-dimensional echocardiography identifies increased internal dimensions of the ventricles at end-diastole, normal or reduced septal and free wall thicknesses, and depressed ventricular function (Fig. 50–3). Although global hypokinesis is the rule, regional wall motion abnormalities occur and are believed to reflect zones of myonecrotic injury. Doppler echocardiography with color flow imaging establishes the presence and degree of atrioventricular (AV) valve regurgitation. Two-dimensional echocardiography and technetium-99m radionuclide imaging shed light on abnormal ventricular function and wall motion. Magnetic resonance imaging provides refined morphologic information and, together with two-dimensional echocardiography, serves to identify left ventricular endocardial thrombi (see Fig. 50–2).

INCIDENCE. It has been estimated that in 1989 there were approximately 140,000 patients with idiopathic dilated cardiomyopathy in the United States. Each year, approximately 20,000 new patients come to attention, and about 10,000 die.

ETIOLOGY, PATHOGENESIS, AND PATHOLOGY. The dilated cardiomyopathies are caused by myocardial injury that results in depressed systolic function and progressive ventricular dilatation. Table 50–2 lists most of the etiologic categories. Pathogenetic mechanisms—clinical and experimental—include myocarditis (infectious or noninfectious), immune or autoimmune processes, genetic factors (immune-response genes), hormonal

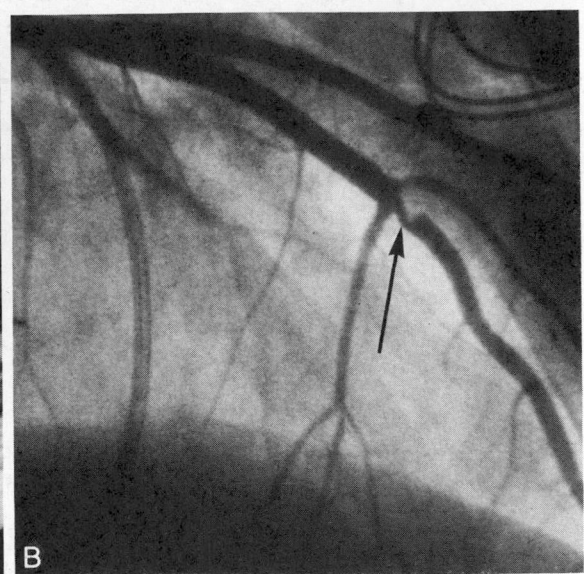

FIGURE 50–2. *A*, Two-dimensional echocardiogram showing an endocardial thrombus *(arrowheads)* in the apex of the left ventricle (LV) of a patient with dilated cardiomyopathy. *B*, Coronary arterial embolus *(arrow)* to the left anterior descending artery in another patient with idiopathic dilated cardiomyopathy.

imbalances, free radicals, calcium overload, and altered blood supply (abnormal coronary microvasculature).

The majority of cases of dilated cardiomyopathy are believed to represent sequelae of myocarditis, generally infectious. The histologic diagnosis of myocarditis is now on firmer ground because of the Dallas criteria established by a group of experienced pathologists (Fig. 50–4). Every major type of infectious agent has been implicated as causative (Table 50–2), although with widely divergent incidence. In western Europe and the United States, infectious myocarditis is most commonly due to viruses, especially enteroviruses.

The most convincingly documented cause of human myocarditis is coxsackievirus group B infection. Experimental murine coxsackievirus B3 results in an initial phase of active intramyocardial viral replication and cell necrosis during which physical exercise or immunosuppressive agents enhance replication of the virus and reinforce tissue injury. In the next phase, virus is not detectable in the myocardium. Defects in immunoregulation are believed to result in an inability to attenuate the stimulus for autoimmune responses (suppressor cell defect), ineffective viral clearance (natural killer cell deficiency), and prolonged antigenic stimulation that may trigger the immune responses. The net result is immunopathic myonecrosis. Reduction of the offending lymphocyte population appears to coincide with a decrease in late myocyte injury. Infected animals may recover, die, or progress to a late third stage in which the dilated heart contains little or no inflammation but, instead, large areas of fibrosis.

The histologic features of dilated cardiomyopathy on endomyocardial biopsy do not necessarily correspond to the symptomatic or hemodynamic status. It is likely, therefore, that many cases of primary myocarditis initially escape clinical detection. In the late phase of the natural history, active inflammatory cell infiltration is absent or nearly so. Chronic dilated cardiomyopathy is then characterized by the presence of areas of fibrosis interwoven among shrunken or hypertrophied myocytes (Fig. 50–4). At this stage, the designation *idiopathic dilated cardiomyopathy* is commonly applied because thorough clinical evaluation fails to identify a specific cause in more than 80 per cent of patients. The association in human subjects between myocardial inflammation initiated by cardiotropic viruses and the subsequent development of dilated cardiomyopathy is persuasive but not conclusive.

In South America, up to 15 per cent of the rural population have primary myocardial injury due to infection by *Trypanosoma cruzi* (Chagas' disease). Chagas' cardiomyopathy is characterized by an acute tissue invasive phase followed by a chronic phase of extensive myocardial fibrosis believed to be the result of a lymphocyte- or an antibody-mediated autoimmune reaction. Chronic chagasic injury not only affects myocytes (with a peculiar propensity to cause apical left ventricular aneurysm) but also has a predilection for specialized tissues (right bundle branch block) and for cardiac parasympathetic ganglia (denervation).

Noninfectious inflammation of the myocardium occurs with systemic diseases of connective tissues (autoimmune disorders). Systemic lupus erythematosus is an example. Of the *toxic agents* that directly injure ventricular myocardium, ethyl alcohol (ethanol) is the most common, and has been implicated in at least 10 per cent of patients with dilated cardiomyopathy. The undesirable acute myocardial effects of ethyl alcohol are masked by

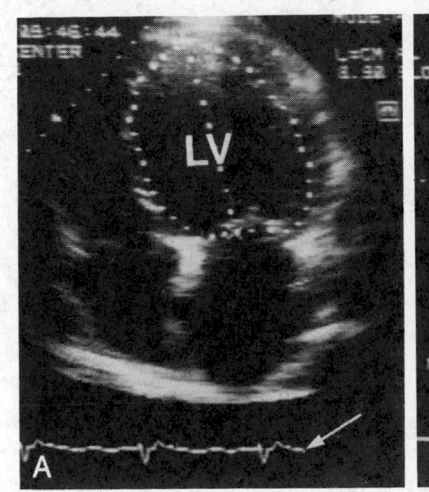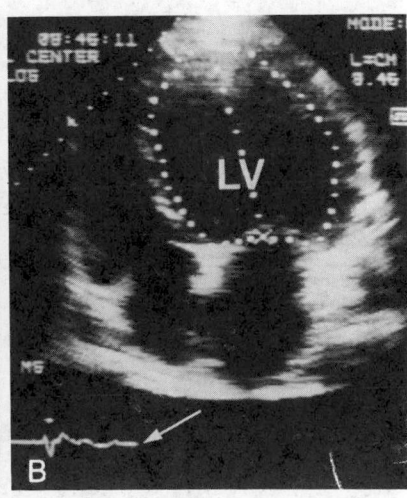

FIGURE 50–3. Two-dimensional echocardiograms with endocardial markers *(A)* during systole and *(B)* during diastole in a patient with dilated cardiomyopathy. The minimal change in dimensions indicates a markedly reduced left ventricular (LV) ejection fraction.

TABLE 50–2. ETIOLOGIC CLASSIFICATION OF THE DILATED CARDIOMYOPATHIES

I. **Idiopathic**
II. **Inflammatory**
  A. Infectious
    1. Viral
    2. Bacterial
    3. Mycobacterial
    4. Parasitic
    5. Rickettsial
    6. Spirochetal
    7. Fungal
  B. Noninfectious
    1. Autoimmune disease
    2. Peripartum
    3. Hypersensitivity reactions
    4. Transplantation rejection
III. **Toxic**
  A. Ethyl alcohol
  B. Chemotherapeutic agents
  C. Elemental compounds
  D. Catecholamines
IV. **Metabolic**
  A. Nutritional
  B. Endocrinologic
  C. Electrolyte abnormalities
V. **Familial cardiomyopathy**
  A. Neuromyopathic
    1. Progressive muscular dystrophy
    2. Myotonic muscular dystrophy
    3. Friedreich's ataxia
  B. Hereditary dilated cardiomyopathy
VI. **Abnormal coronary microvasculature**

the beneficial effects of peripheral vasodilatation and the positive inotropic response to catecholamines, but in the autonomic blockaded heart, ethanol causes a significant decrease in contractility. Both ethanol and acetaldehyde (its first metabolite) adversely affect myocardial metabolism. Alcoholic cardiomyopathy is attributed to the toxicity of ethanol and acetaldehyde on the myocardial cell. In addition to the effects of ethyl alcohol and its metabolites, constituents of the brew may also depress contractility. Cobalt added to beer to stabilize foam is a case in point. In the beriberi heart disease of chronic alcoholics, high-output heart failure of thiamine deficiency is imposed upon the depressed myocardium of alcoholic cardiomyopathy. There is a positive epidemiologic association between excessive alcohol ingestion

and systemic hypertension. An important clinical aspect of alcoholic cardiomyopathy is its reversibility, at least initially. However, pathologic studies late in the natural history reveal myocardial cell necrosis with replacement fibrosis.

A host of other toxic substances and drugs reportedly cause myocardial injury either as a result of excessive exposure or as idiosyncratic responses. Catecholamine excess may cause myonecrosis. Doxorubicin (Adriamycin) and other anthracycline chemotherapeutic agents are additional examples. The structural changes in response to anthracycline antitumor agents are dose related. Doxorubicin rarely results in acute heart failure and only occasionally produces arrhythmias or conduction disturbances. About 2 to 5 per cent of patients receiving 500 mg of the drug per square meter slowly develop overt heart failure, but over one half of patients have abnormal responses to exercise and exhibit histologic changes on endomyocardial biopsy. The microscopic pattern of doxorubicin-induced myocardial injury is characterized by the gradual appearance of vacuolar degeneration, myofibrillar loss, and juxtaposition of disrupted cells among normal cells.

The distinct clustering of *peripartum cardiomyopathy* in the last month of gestation and especially in the first 3 postpartum months supports the contention that the disorder is uniquely coupled to pregnancy. Incidence has been estimated from 1 in 3000 to 1 in 15,000 confinements. Myocardial inflammation is sufficiently frequent to warrant the designation "myocarditis," but the inflammation is not infectious. Despite diligent search, no role of cardiotropic viruses has been established. The peripartum myocardial injury is believed to result from an autoimmune mechanism triggered by release of myocyte antigens from the late-term pregnant uterus.

Metabolic derangements that adversely affect systolic function and result in dilated cardiomyopathy include endocrinopathies, trace element deficiencies, and electrolyte abnormalities. In diabetes mellitus, there is convincing evidence of a cardiopathy (myocardial injury) separate from extramural coronary artery disease. The relative roles of microvascular disease, interstitial PAS-positive material, and fibrosis remain unsettled. Dilated heart failure in hyperthyroidism principally reflects pre-existing impairment of contractile reserve made clinically overt by the hypermetabolic state. An analogy is the high-output state of beriberi (vitamin B_1 deficiency) in chronic alcoholics. In classic Asian beriberi, however, dilated heart failure is due to thiamine deficiency per se in individuals without myocardial depression from other causes. Teenagers who excessively consume processed foods deficient in thiamine may suffer from heart failure provoked by strenuous exercise. The principal initial physiologic effect of thiamine deficiency is on the peripheral circulation, but persistent deficiency may lead to dilated cardiomyopathy. Abnormal regu-

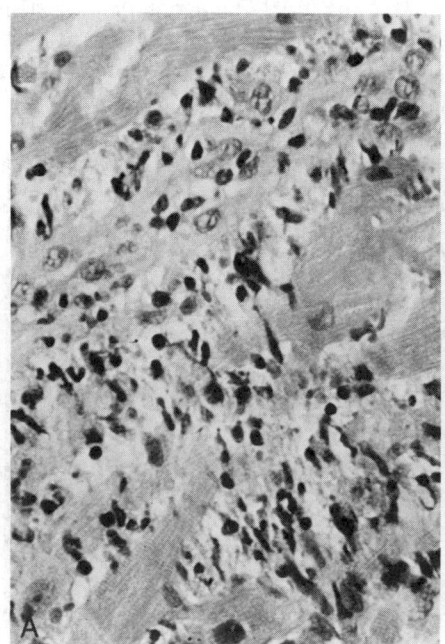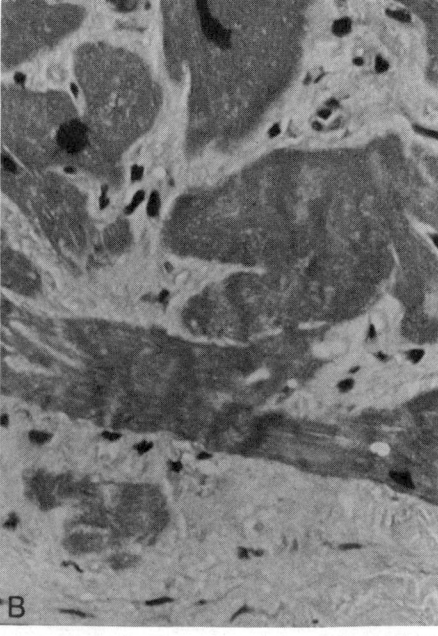

FIGURE 50–4. Endomyocardial biopsies from two patients. *A*, Early stages showing the inflammatory cells and myocyte damage of myocarditis. *B*, Late stage showing extensive replacement of myocardium by fibrous tissue.

lation of carnitine, a naturally occurring amino acid required for mitochondrial oxidation of long chain fatty acids, has also been associated with dilated heart failure.

Electrolyte disorders that adversely affect cardiac contractility include deficiencies of calcium, phosphate, magnesium, and potassium. If the availability of calcium is inadequate, ejection fraction falls, as in patients receiving large transfusions of blood preserved with citrate, which chelates calcium, or in patients with hypoparathyroidism. Hypophosphatemia leads to inadequate stores of high-energy phosphate compounds, as in alcoholism, diabetes, and hyperalimentation. Magnesium, a cofactor for thiamine-dependent reactions and for sodium-potassium adenosine triphosphatase (ATPase), may be depleted by impaired gastrointestinal absorption or increased renal excretion (diuretics).

A number of heredofamilial *neuromyopathic disorders* are associated wtih dilated cardiomyopathy. Examples include X-linked, slowly progressive muscular dystrophy (Becker dystrophy), certain patients in the late stages of Duchenne dystrophy, Friedreich's ataxia, and the childhood form (but not the adult form) of myotonic muscular dystrophy.

DIAGNOSIS. Dilated cardiomyopathy should be suspected in relatively young patients who present with cardiac enlargement, cardiac failure, systemic emboli, and ventricular arrhythmias. Chest pain indistinguishable from myocardial infarction (myonecrosis caused by the cardiotropic virus) sometimes accompanies acute myocarditis. The diagnosis of dilated cardiomyopathy hinges on firm exclusion of pre-existing or coexisting heart or vascular disease. Cardiac catheterization has given way to noninvasive diagnostic procedures, especially two-dimensional echocardiography (see Fig. 50–3), except for the exclusion of ischemic cardiomyopathy (coronary artery disease) in older patients, especially males.

If dilated cardiomyopathy presents early in its course, throat and stool cultures and viral titers should be secured and serially compared. Up to 50 per cent of patients with clinical myocarditis have evidence of recent coxsackievirus B infection, especially types 1 to 5. Myocardial inflammation has been identified by gallium-67 scintigraphy, but more specifically by endomyocardial biopsy from the right ventricular septum (Fig. 50–4). Twenty-four hour Holter monitors are used to detect ventricular arrhythmias.

TREATMENT AND PROGNOSIS. Dilated cardiomyopathy entails four major therapeutic concerns: the potential presence of ongoing myocardial injury, the hemodynamic state of the dilated heart, the threat of systemic emboli, and the risk of ventricular arrhythmias.

During the tissue-invasive stage of acute infectious myocarditis, immunosuppressive agents provoke viral replication and are therefore proscribed. The majority of patients who present with active infectious myocardial inflammation do so after the acute tissue-invasive stage. Attempts at pharmacologic suppression of persistent myocarditis require documentation of the presence of inflammation. Although immunosuppression for biopsy-proven myocarditis in human subjects remains controversial, experience with cardiac transplant patients teaches us that immunosuppressive therapy can be lifesaving. Many patients with virus-induced myocarditis improve during treatment with prednisone and azathioprine, and relapses have occurred after discontinuing immunosuppression. Whether or not immunosuppression is used, clinical status improves in up to one half of patients with biopsy-proven myocarditis. Not surprisingly, even patients who clinically improve may have persistent abnormalities of ventricular systolic function. The grim prognosis of peripartum cardiomyopathy, coupled with evidence of noninfectious myocardial inflammation, argues for treatment with immunosuppressive agents, but the relatively high incidence of spontaneous improvement is a confounding variable. Mortality rates in the acute and subacute stages of peripartum cardiomyopathy range from 30 to 60 per cent. Improvement in symptoms, heart size, and ventricular function, when it occurs, does so early, generally within 1 month of presentation. The severity of early compromise in left ventricular function does not predict long-term outcome, but if normalization of function is not achieved by 6 months, the outlook is poor. The risk of recurrences during subsequent pregnancies is related to ventricular function. Alcoholic cardiomyopathy often responds dramatically to abstention even after patients have

become significantly symptomatic. Continued ethanol consumption is associated with an inexorable deterioration and a 3-year mortality of up to 80 per cent. Abstention should be undertaken in hospital so that compliance can be assured, diet monitored, and arrhythmias controlled.

Doxorubicin (Adriamycin) cardiotoxicity is generally irreversible and is the cause of death in over 60 per cent of patients so afflicted. Careful monitoring during doxorubicin therapy minimizes the risk. Potential cardiomyopathy in response to doxorubicin can be identified by radionuclide angiography, two-dimensional echocardiography, or endomyocardial biopsy. Patients without additional cardiac risks are best studied after 450 mg per square meter of drug administration. Although a decline in ejection fraction at rest or with exercise arouses legitimate concern of myocyte damage, the frequency of false positivity mandates that damage be confirmed by endomyocardial biopsy before therapy is withdrawn. Cardiotoxicity of doxorubicin is related not only to peak levels but also to cumulative dose. Toxicity is reduced by slow infusion rates.

The treatment of dilated ventricles with depressed systolic function and elevated filling pressure requires an awareness of the complex interplay among a host of variables, including neurohormonal interactions and adaptations, and the relationship between central hemodynamics and regional blood flow. The chief pharmacologic agents employed are vasodilators (afterload reduction) and diuretics. The role, if any, of digitalis glycosides remains open to question. Vasodilator therapy and diuretics are initially employed empirically, but refined adjustments require a flotation catheter for hemodynamic monitoring in order to achieve an optimal balance between a reduction in left ventricular filling pressure and maintenance of a satisfactory cardiac output. Reductions in ventricular filling pressure and systemic vascular resistance can result in a decrease in *total* stroke volume but an increase in *forward* stroke volume, apparently due to attenuation of mitral regurgitation and a decrease in left ventricular volume.

The use of β blockade in chronic dilated cardiomyopathy is seemingly contradictory and at present controversial. There is a contrasting effect between short- and long-term administration of the β-adrenergic blocker metoprolol. Short-term administration results in acute depression of systolic function, whereas long-term administration results in improved systolic function. The following mechanisms have been proposed to account for improvement after long-term (3 to 12 months) metoprolol therapy. Chronically elevated levels of circulating catecholamines and a high local release of norepinephrine tend to worsen heart failure. There is down-regulation of β receptor density in severe heart failure. Long-term treatment with metoprolol results in moderate receptor up-regulation, which may facilitate a more normal response to sympathetic stimulation.

The risk of systemic emboli in dilated cardiomyopathy argues for the use of long-term anticoagulants, which are obligatory if a thrombus announces itself as a systemic embolus or if an endocardial thrombus is found during noninvasive imaging. Systemic emboli generally arise from a thrombus attached to the left ventricular endocardium (see Fig. 50–2). A second predisposing cause of embolization is atrial fibrillation. Pulmonary emboli are not uncommon and originate from peripheral venous thromboses rather than from right ventricular endocardium.

Sudden, unexpected cardiac arrest accounts for approximately half of all deaths in patients with dilated cardiomyopathy. The conventional wisdom attributes sudden death to ventricular tachyarrhythmias, but Holter monitoring does not reliably identify patients at risk of dying suddenly from ventricular tachycardia or fibrillation. This is so because the mechanisms of unexpected cardiac arrest in advanced heart failure are diverse. A significant majority of patients experience severe bradycardia or electromechanical dissociation at the time of arrest, with ventricular tachycardia or fibrillation occurring in the minority.

Cardiac transplantation has been a major step forward in the treatment of patients with advanced heart failure, over half of whom have primary dilated cardiomyopathy. Impressive improvements in post-transplantation survival are due chiefly to advances in immunosuppression. However, because of the substantial disparity between donor availability and patient need, every attempt should be made to stabilize candidates so that transplantation can be done electively. Patients referred for urgent transplantation cannot be considered refractory to medical therapy until vasodilators and diuretics are systematically administered during continuous hemodynamic monitoring. When that is done, oral vasodilator and diuretic therapy is possible in 80 per cent of "refractory" patients, with a 6-month actuarial survival of 75 per cent despite an initial ejection fraction of 0.15 per cent ± 0.04.

Aretz HT, Billingham ME, Edwards WD, et al.: Myocarditis: A histopathologic definition and classification. Am J Cardiovasc Pathol 1:3, 1986. *The biopsy diagnosis of myocarditis hinges on the identification of inflammatory cells and evidence of subsequent damage as defined by the Dallas criteria established in this report.*

Dec GW, Palacios IF, Fallon JT, et al.: Active myocarditis in the spectrum of acute dilated cardiomyopathies: Clinical features, histologic correlates, and clinical outcome. N Engl J Med 312:885, 1985. *A series of 27 patients with dilated cardiomyopathy of recent onset in which biopsy-proven myocarditis and subsequent improvement were frequent, whether or not immunosuppressive drugs were given.*

Luu M, Stevenson WA, Stevenson LW, et al.: Diverse mechanisms of unexpected cardiac arrest in advanced heart failure. Circulation 80:675, 1989. *This report deals with the multifactorial mechanisms of sudden death in advanced heart failure, calling attention to severe bradycardia and electromechanical dissociation in the majority of patients at the time of cardiac arrest.*

O'Connell JB, Costanzo-Nordin MR, Subramanian R, et al.: Peripartum cardiomyopathy: Clinical, hemodynamic, histologic, prognostic characteristics. J Am Coll Cardiol 8:52, 1986. *Characterization and prognosis of 14 patients who developed peripartum cardiomyopathy despite good general health and prenatal care. The relatively high incidence of myocarditis is documented and discussed.*

O'Connell JB, Mason JW: Immunosuppressive therapy in experimental and clinical myocarditis. Pathol Immunopathol Res 7:292, 1988. *This review summarizes the studies of immunosuppression in active myocarditis and describes a multicenter trial designed to resolve the issue of efficacy.*

Perloff JK (ed.): The Cardiomyopathies. Cardiology Clinics. Philadelphia. W. B. Saunders Company, 1988. *This concise volume surveys the clinical and experimental aspects of the three major categories of cardiomyopathies, covering etiology, clinical manifestations, diagnosis, and treatment.*

Regan TJ: Alcoholic cardiomyopathy. Prog Cardiovasc Dis 27:141, 1984. *A comprehensive review of the pathogenesis, preclinical course, and prognosis of alcoholic cardiomyopathy.*

THE HYPERTROPHIC CARDIOMYOPATHIES

DEFINITION. This category of cardiomyopathies is represented grossly by asymmetric (eccentric) or symmetric (concentric) hypertrophy of the left ventricle in the absence of another cardiac or systemic disease capable of producing an increase in ventricular mass (see Table 50–1). In the asymmetric variety, the septum is disproportionately thick relative to the left ventricular free wall beneath the mitral annulus (see Fig. 50–1). In the symmetric variety, the septum and left ventricular free wall are of equal thickness. Ventricular cavity size is normal or reduced in both types.

ETIOLOGY. Hypertrophic cardiomyopathy occurs in both familial and sporadic forms. Autosomal dominance is the usual mode of inheritance in the genetically transmitted form of the disease. Sporadic occurrences may represent new mutations, reduced penetrance in first-degree relatives, autosomal recessive transmission, or nongenetic occurrence. Biochemical determinants in the pathogenesis are not firmly established but have focused on two interrelated hypotheses—the proposed intrauterine links between myocyte development and norepinephrine stimulation and/or excess intracellular calcium. Studies of regional myocardial blood flow and metabolism using positron emission tomography suggest a metabolic abnormality in the disproportionately thick septum.

PATHOLOGY. Genetic hypertrophic cardiomyopathy is characterized by two gross morphologic and two histologic features. The gross morphologic features are asymmetric septal hypertrophy and a catenoid ventricular septal configuration. Asymmetric hypertrophy may involve the entire septum (base to apex, Fig. 50–5), or much less commonly the hypertrophy is principally if not exclusively apical or midventricular, at the level of the papillary muscles. The most typical histologic feature—cellular disarray—is significantly more common and quantitatively considerably more extensive in hypertrophic cardiomyopathy than in other cardiac disorders or in normal subjects. In its proper clinical and pathologic context, extensive septal cellular disarray remains an important marker of genetic hypertrophic cardiomy-

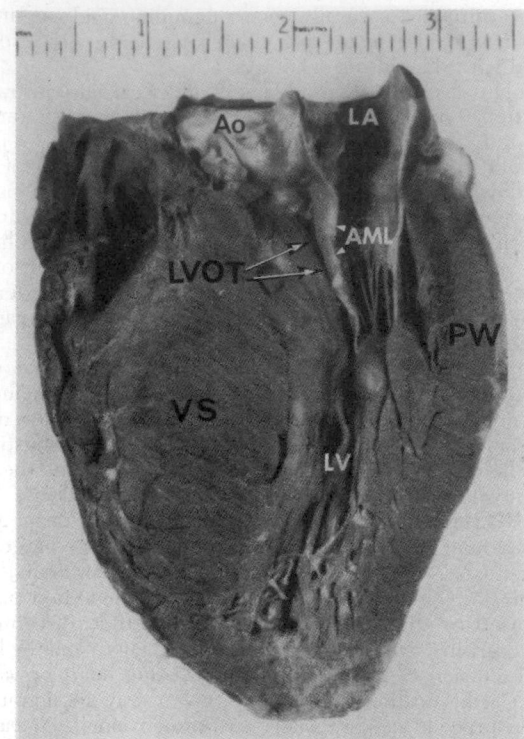

FIGURE 50–5. One of Teare's original cases of "asymmetrical hypertrophy of the heart." The ventricular septum (VS) is substantially thicker than the left ventricular posterior wall (PW). The cavity of the left ventricle (LV) is much reduced. The base of the ventricular septum bulges into the left ventricular outflow tract (LVOT) adjacent to the anterior mitral leaflet (AML). Ao = Aorta; LA = left atrium. (From Teare D: Asymmetrical hypertrophy of the heart in young adults. Br Heart J 20:1, 1958, with permission. Labels superimposed.)

opathy. The second histologic feature–thick-walled intramural coronary arteries with narrow lumens—occurs in more than three fourths of patients with genetic hypertrophic cardiomyopathy, especially in the ventricular septum. The pathogenetic and clinical significance of the thickened intramural coronary arteries is unresolved.

PHYSIOLOGY. Characterization of the physiologic derangements in genetic hypertrophic cardiomyopathy forms the basis for an understanding of the clinical manifestations, diagnosis, and treatment. The principal physiologic features include a hypercontractile left ventricular free wall (enhanced systolic function) (Fig. 50–6A), hypocontractile ventricular septum, left ventricular cavity obliteration (Fig. 50–6A), and impaired diastolic function. In the normal heart, ventricular contraction consists of an isovolumetric phase that occupies about 10 per cent of systole and an ejection phase with fiber shortening that occupies 80 to 90 per cent of systole. In genetic hypertrophic cardiomyopathy, a third phase is added. High-velocity ejection is completed in the first 60 to 80 per cent of systole, following which the cavity obliterates and the ventricle contracts isometrically. Thus, hypertrophic cardiomyopathy is characterized by enhanced systolic function, a prolonged and abnormally powerful isometric contraction phase followed by impaired relaxation and increased chamber stiffness during diastole.

Classic genetic hypertrophic cardiomyopathy is accompanied by a singular physiologic feature that continues to generate lively interest—the left ventricular to aortic dynamic pressure gradient. Entrapment of the catheter tip during cavity obliteration spuriously elevates the recorded systolic pressure within the left ventricle. However, echocardiography with Doppler interrogation and color flow imaging has provided convincing evidence of a true obstructive pressure gradient. Anterior mitral leaflet–septal contact is believed to be the cause of the gradient, and the Venturi effect is regarded as the responsible pathogenetic mechanism.

The gradient is "dynamic," a term that calls attention to its lability and its response to certain physical and pharmacologic

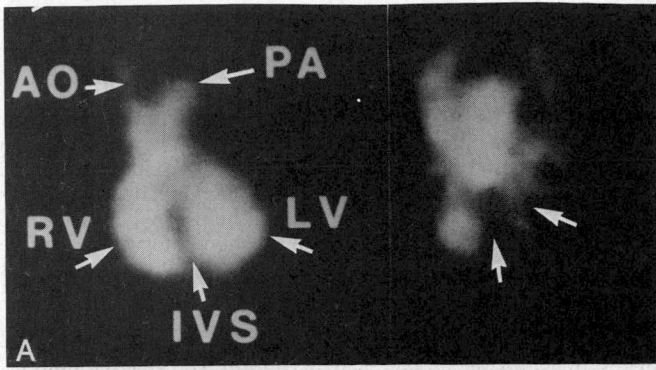

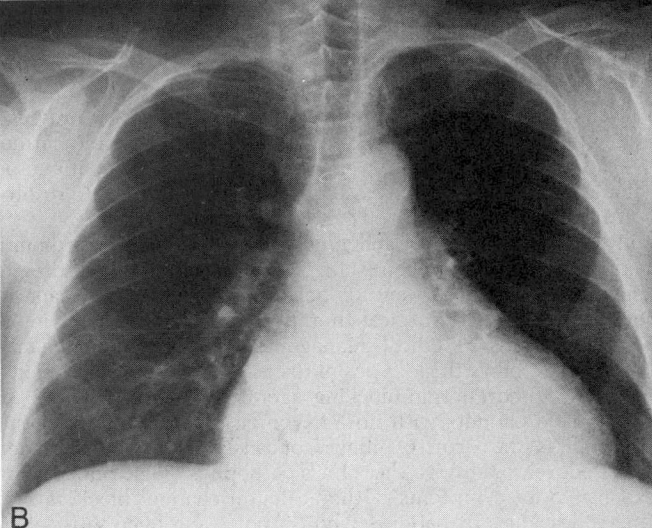

FIGURE 50–6. *A*, Technetium-99m gated radionuclide angiography in genetic hypertrophic cardiomyopathy (diastolic and systolic images). During systole, the left ventricular (LV) cavity obliterates, and the thick interventricular septum (IVS) becomes evident. RV = Right ventricle; Ao = aorta; PA = pulmonary artery. *B*, Left ventricular dilatation and failure 20 years after ventriculomyomectomy in a patient with genetic hypertrophic cardiomyopathy.

interventions. Interventions that reduce left ventricular cavity size intensify the gradient and vice versa. The gradient increases during the straining phase of the Valsalva maneuver; during prompt standing from the squatting position; following the compensatory pause initiated by a premature beat; and in response to isotonic exercise, tachycardia, digitalis, isoproterenol, amyl nitrite, and nitroglycerin. The gradient decreases during the overshoot phase of the Valsalva maneuver, during the Müller maneuver, upon squatting, in response to isometric exercise (handgrip), and in response to β-adrenergic blockade or α-adrenergic stimulation. In patients with significant gradients, administration of inotropic drugs or volume-depleting diuretics can be accompanied by sudden and serious deterioration.

CLINICAL MANIFESTATIONS. The clinical picture ranges from asymptomatic patients who are incidentally found to have hypertrophic cardiomyopathy to severely ill patients with incapacitating symptoms. The widespread use of echocardiography has allowed detection of asymptomatic patients who come to attention because of an abnormal physical examination or electrocardiogram, or because of a first-degree relative with hypertrophic cardiomyopathy. The symptomatically overt disease typically becomes manifest in relatively young adults (third to fifth decades), but it is not uncommon for patients to present after 60 years of age. In infants, the disorder presents as a murmur and marked congestive failure, with the majority of afflicted babies dying before their first birthday. In adults, it is not uncommon for the disease to declare itself dramatically as syncope or sudden death in previously healthy young persons engaged in strenuous exertion. The most common symptoms are dyspnea, fatigue, chest pain (similar to, if not identical with, angina pectoris), and syncope. The most prevalent symptom is dyspnea, which is

intensified by exertion and which is believed to be chiefly related to high end-diastolic pressures (left ventricular diastolic dysfunction). Clinical deterioration in adults is typically slow with two major exceptions—sudden death or the onset of atrial fibrillation. Loss of coordinated atrial contraction in the face of impaired left ventricular diastolic function results in acute dyspnea (sudden increase in end-diastolic and pulmonary venous pressures).

In older subjects, chest pain coupled with electrocardiographic Q waves (see later) prompts a diagnosis of atherosclerotic coronary artery disease, which may coexist. However, symptoms resembling angina pectoris occur in relatively young patients without extramural coronary artery disease, and have been attributed to small vessel (intramural) coronary disease, decreased capillary to fiber ratio of hypertrophy, and impaired diastolic function which impedes coronary blood flow. Observations based upon positron emission tomography have not detected ischemia at rest in mildly symptomatic patients.

Cerebral symptoms vary from lightheadedness to frank syncope. Patients sometimes feel pain in the upright position (promptly corrected by lying down) or in response to physical exercise. Occasional patients report such a history for years without apparent clinical deterioration. Syncope or presyncope has been attributed to disturbances in rhythm or conduction (see below), to an inability to increase cardiac output because of impaired diastolic function or obstruction to left ventricular outflow, or to stimulation of intraventricular baroreceptors that impairs peripheral vasoregulation.

The *physical examination* in asymptomatic patients without systolic gradients is unimpressive except for a relatively prominent left ventricular impulse and a fourth heart sound. The jugular venous pulse may exhibit a prominent A wave (increased force of right atrial contraction) that does not reflect pulmonary hypertension, but instead is a response to reduced distensibility of the right ventricular cavity caused by massive thickening of the ventricular septum (see Fig. 50–5). The increase in velocity of left ventricular ejection causes a brisk rate of rise of the systemic arterial pulse while the pulse pressure remains normal (small waterhammer pulse). Twin peaking of the arterial pulse coincides with a mid- to late-systolic trough, a feature better recorded than palpated. Precordial palpation sometimes detects a *triple* apical impulse composed of double systolic movement coupled with presystolic distention. A systolic thrill may be present at the apex and toward the lower left sternal edge in patients with left ventricular outflow gradients, but the thrill is related more closely to mitral regurgitation than to the outflow gradient. Auscultation detects a prominent apical fourth heart sound, a normal first sound, and at the left base a second sound that is usually normally split, sometimes narrowly split or single, and occasionally paradoxically split. Despite the increased velocity of left ventricular contraction, aortic ejection sounds are exceptional. Systolic murmurs in patients with left ventricular outflow gradients represent combinations of midsystolic murmurs caused by increased velocity of ejection and longer, if not holosystolic, apical murmurs caused by mitral regurgitation. The murmur is typically loudest at the apex, with radiation into the axilla or to the left lower sternal edge, less prominently to the base, and seldom into the neck. The systolic murmur is less important because of its presence than because of the diagnostic significance of its response to physical and pharmacologic interventions (Table 50–3). Third heart sounds occur in the presence of mitral regurgitation and are occasionally followed by brief after-

TABLE 50–3. EFFECTS OF BEDSIDE PHYSICAL INTERVENTIONS ON THE SYSTOLIC MURMUR OF HYPERTROPHIC OBSTRUCTIVE CARDIOMYOPATHY

Increased Intensity of Murmur
    Dynamic exercise
    Straining phase of Valsalva maneuver
    Prompt standing after squatting
Decreased Intensity of Murmur
    Release (overshoot) phase of Valsalva maneuver
    Squatting
    Isometric exercise (handgrip)

vibrations that create the auscultatory impression of short mid-diastolic murmurs. A high-frequency early diastolic murmur of aortic regurgitation makes the diagnosis of hypertrophic cardiomyopathy doubtful.

Electrocardiograms are normal in a minority of asymptomatic patients but are almost invariably abnormal in symptomatic patients with left ventricular outflow gradients. P-wave morphology generally shows a left atrial abnormality alone, but occasionally a right atrial configuration coexists. The PR interval is often short but only rarely associated with pre-excitation, even when the short PR interval is accompanied by initial force slurring reminiscent of a delta wave. Atrial fibrillation, the most common sustained supraventricular rhythm disturbance, is not accompanied by accelerated AV conduction. Ventricular arrhythmias are relatively common (see below). Arrhythmic syncope is ominous and heralds sudden death that is attributed to ventricular tachycardia or fibrillation. The propensity for ventricular arrhythmias has been attributed, at least in part, to electrical instability inherent in the cellular disarray (nonuniform anisotropy) and to the disparity between the duration of mechanical systole and electrical activation. The potentially malignant ventricular arrhythmias that prevail in genetic hypertrophic cardiomyopathy are essentially unknown in the hypertrophic cardiomyopathy of Friedreich's ataxia, whether asymmetric or concentric, and cellular disarray has not been found at necropsy in Friedreich's disease.

Prominent Q waves occur in upward of 50 per cent of cases. The Q waves tend to be abnormal because of their depth rather than their duration. The Q waves have been ascribed to abnormal electrophysiologic properties in areas of cellular disarray. Electrocardiographic evidence of left ventricular hypertrophy is common but not invariable and is reflected in the increased voltage and ST-segment and T-wave abnormalities. Distinctive giant T-wave inversions in mid to left precordial leads imply *apical* hypertrophic cardiomyopathy (Fig. 50–7).

In the *chest roentgenogram*, enlargement of the left atrium is relatively common, especially when significant mitral regurgitation coexists with atrial fibrillation. Left ventricular size and contour range from normal to a convex silhouette projecting to the left, inferior and posterior. The aortic root is inconspicuous.

The echocardiogram is the mainstay of the *laboratory diagnosis* of hypertrophic cardiomyopathy, providing virtually all necessary clinical diagnostic information. The cardinal echocardiographic features of genetic hypertrophic cardiomyopathy are disproportionate thickness of the ventricular septum (at least 15 mm measured at the minor axis level), with a septal/posterior wall ration of 1.5:1 or more, a small left ventricular cavity, exaggerated contractility of the left ventricular free wall, and a relatively hypocontractile ventricular septum. Two-dimensional echocardiography establishes the location and extent of disproportionate septal thickness (Fig. 50–7A) and occasionally shows a ground-glass appearance of the septum believed to be related to cellular disarray. High-velocity ejection through a left ventricular outflow tract that is narrowed by the disproportionately thick septum causes systolic anterior motion of the mitral leaflets (Venturi effect). Doppler interrogation with color flow imaging establishes the left ventricular outflow dynamics and the presence and degree of mitral regurgitation. Pulsed Doppler echocardiography (sample volume slightly on the ventricular side of the mitral annulus) has been a major step forward in characterizing the abnormalities of left ventricular diastolic function.

Technetium-99m gated radionuclide ventriculography identifies the thickness of the ventricular septum, the relative motions of septum and free wall, and the left ventricular cavity size in diastole and systole (Fig. 50–6A). Magnetic resonance imaging, with its capability of recording in multiple planes, offers refined morphologic information on the septum and free walls.

Prior to noninvasive imaging, *cardiac catheterization* provided the standards for the clinical diagnosis of hypertrophic cardiomyopathy. Catheterization is now reserved for older patients in whom coronary angiography is employed in an attempt to resolve the cause of chest pain.

TREATMENT. The management of hypertrophic cardiomyopathy includes genetic counseling, medical therapy according to hemodynamic subgroup and associated symptoms, the management of arrhythmias, surgical therapy, and prophylaxis for infective endocarditis. Medical management of the hemodynamic subgroups employs three types of drugs—calcium channel blocking agents, β-adrenergic blocking agents, and disopyramide. In symptomatic patients with no left ventricular to aortic gradient, verapamil is the drug of choice because diastolic dysfunction (impaired relaxation) is the chief pathophysiologic mechanism responsible for symptoms. Other calcium channel blockers may be as efficacious. In patients who do not experience satisfactory symptomatic improvement on verapamil alone, β blockers are added to reduce the heart rate and prolong the diastolic filling period.

Treatment of symptomatic patients with latent (provokable) left ventricular outflow gradients primarily employs β-adrenergic blockers. Calcium channel blockers might serve a useful purpose as negative inotropic agents, but drug-induced peripheral vasodilatation can augment left ventricular outflow obstruction. The negative inotropic effect of disopyramide does not run this risk (see below).

Symptomatic patients with resting left ventricular to aortic gradients are first treated with disopyramide, provided that intravenous administration appreciably reduces or abolishes the gradient. If subsequent oral administration relieves both the

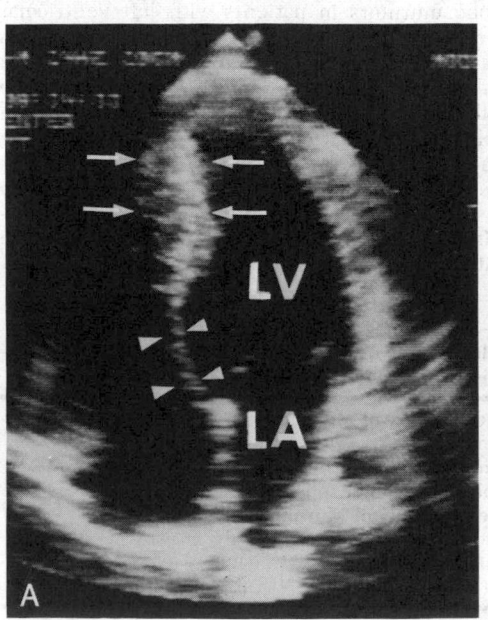

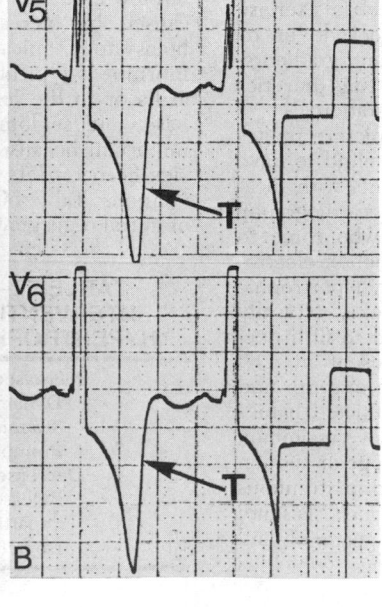

FIGURE 50–7. *A*, Two-dimensional echocardiogram showing hypertrophic cardiomyopathy involving the apical half of the ventricular septum (*arrows*). The basal septum (*arrowheads*) is not thickened. *B*, Typical electrocardiogram in apical hypertrophic cardiomyopathy showing giant T-wave negativity (*arrows*) in leads V₅ and V₆.

symptoms and the gradient, the drug is continued. If not, a β blocker can be added. Calcium channel blockers are used cautiously if at all because their vasodilating effect can appreciably augment the gradient and provoke symptoms.

The management of arrhythmias focuses on ventricular arrhythmias and atrial fibrillation. The recommended method of screening patients for ventricular arrhythmias is 48- to 72-hour ambulatory electrocardiographic monitoring. Sudden death occurs about eight times more frequently in patients with asymptomatic ventricular tachycardia recorded on this type of ambulatory monitoring than in those without ventricular tachycardia so recorded. The highest yield for asymptomatic ventricular tachycardia is in patients with resting gradients, extensive hypertrophy, syncope, or a family history of sudden death. Clinical trials have not yet shown that antiarrhythmic therapy reduces the risk of sudden death, but treatment is recommended for patients with frequent repetitive firing of three or more ventricular beats, and in the rare patient with prolonged episodes of asymptomatic ventricular tachycardia. Quinidine, procainamide, or disopyramide are initially used, with dose levels adjusted according to blood levels and according to efficacy by repeated ambulatory monitoring. Amiodarone is effective in abolishing the ventricular arrhythmias, but there are significant side effects, and recent data suggest that abolition of ventricular tachycardia on ambulatory monitoring does not prevent sudden death. The drug is best confined to high-risk patients in whom more conventional antiarrhythmic therapy has failed.

Atrial fibrillation requires treatment because of its adverse effect on diastolic filling (removal of the booster pump benefit of atrial systole and shortening of the diastolic filling period because of the increased heart rate). Every effort should be made to restore sinus rhythm. If the need is urgent, digoxin, verapamil, or a β blocker are used to slow the ventricular response while prompt cardioversion is arranged. If cardioversion is not considered urgent, the patient should be anticoagulated and treated with digoxin or β blockers, together with quinidine, procainamide, or disopyramide. If sinus rhythm is not restored, cardioversion is then required. If patients cannot be maintained in sinus rhythm, amiodarone should be considered because it may be efficacious in relatively low doses.

Surgery in hypertrophic cardiomyopathy consists of excision of a portion of the basal septum (ventriculomyomectomy). The objective is to enlarge the outflow tract, abolish the gradient, and reduce if not eliminate mitral regurgitation by reducing the Venturi effect on the mitral leaflets. Although a success rate in excess of 90 per cent has been reported in symptomatic patients with resting gradients, ventriculomyomectomy is recommended only for patients with resting gradients in whom medical therapy has failed. In patients with resting gradients and either recurrent or chronic atrial fibrillation, surgery should be considered when sinus rhythm cannot be maintained. The efficacy of successful ventriculomyomectomy in reducing the risk of sudden death remains open to question.

Susceptibility to infective endocarditis is confined to patients with resting left ventricular outflow obstruction because of the coexisting mitral regurgitation and anterior mitral leaflet/septal contact. Prophylaxis is recommended only in this subgroup.

PROGNOSIS. Except for the infant with clinically overt hypertrophic cardiomyopathy in the first year of life, the natural history is usually characterized by slow progression. The most ominous threat is sudden death, which often occurs during exercise in younger patients who were previously clinically well. Sudden death accounts for an appreciable proportion of the annual mortality, which is about 4 per cent. The advent of atrial fibrillation can rapidly and significantly accelerate clinical deterioration, and the risk of systemic embolization is relatively high. A small proportion of patients develop progressive left ventricular dilatation and failure late in the natural course of their disease or many years after ventriculomyomectomy (see Fig. 50–6B). The dilated left ventricle is extensively replaced with fibrous tissue.

Maron BJ, Nichols PF, Pickle LW, et al.: Patterns of inheritance in hypertrophic cardiomyopathy: Assessment by M-mode and two-dimensional echocardiography. Am J Cardiol 53:1087, 1984. *This important paper focuses on the mode of inheritance of hypertrophic cardiomyopathy in 367 relatives from 70 families.*
Perloff JK: Pathogenesis of hypertrophic cardiomyopathy. In Goodwin JF (ed.): Heart Muscle Disease. Lancaster, England, MTP Press Ltd., 1985, pp 7–22. *Pathogenesis is dealt with in light of anatomic, physiologic, and clinical features of hypertrophic cardiomyopathy. The catecholamine hypothesis is elaborated.*
Rosing DR, Idanpaan-Heikkila U, Maron BJ, et al.: Use of calcium channel blocking drugs in hypertrophic cardiomyopathy. Am J Cardiol 55:185B, 1985. *An important long-term drug study dealing with 227 patients treated with verapamil. A policy regarding drug administration is recommended, and the beneficial and adverse effects are reviewed.*
Sasson Z, Rakowski H, Wigle ED: Hypertrophic cardiomyopathy. In Perloff JK (ed.): The Cardiomyopathies. Philadelphia, W. B. Saunders Company, 1988. *A comprehensive critical review of all of the major aspects of hypertrophic cardiomyopathy.*
Takenaka K, Dabestani A, Gardin JM, et al.: Left ventricular filling in hypertrophic cardiomyopathy: A pulsed Doppler echocardiography study. J Am Coll Cardiol 7:1263, 1986. *Left ventricular diastolic filling characteristics were studied by pulsed Doppler echocardiography in patients with and without systolic anterior motion of the mitral leaflets.*

THE RESTRICTIVE CARDIOMYOPATHIES

DEFINITION. The restrictive cardiomyopathies, the least common of the three major categories of cardiomyopathic disorders (see Table 50–1), are characterized by a *primary* abnormality of *diastolic* function (impaired filling) with normal or nearly normal systolic function (contraction). The term "restrictive cardiomyopathy" is not appropriately applied when the primary derangement is one of systolic function that precedes and is variably associated with diastolic impairment (late-stage dilated cardiomyopathy, for example) or when impaired diastolic function is secondary to cardiac hypertrophy. The restrictive cardiomyopathies show little or no increase in end-diastolic or end-systolic dimension of either the right or left ventricle—hence the designation "nondilated, nonhypertrophic cardiomyopathy."

Ventricular filling is not a passive event in which inflow merely distends a compliant recipient chamber, but instead is a complex, active, energy-dependent process. The abnormality of diastolic filling in the restrictive cardiomyopathies results in a higher filling pressure for a given increment in volume. Ventricular filling is completed in early diastole with little or no filling in late diastole, functionally analogous to constrictive pericarditis. The differential diagnosis can be difficult, but information from echocardiography, computed tomography, and magnetic resonance imaging generally permits restrictive cardiomyopathy to be distinguished from constrictive pericarditis.

Impaired diastolic function in the restrictive cardiomyopathies can be idiopathic, i.e., in the absence of morphologically detectable myocardial or endomyocardial disease, or can occur because of interstitial deposition of abnormal substances (infiltrative), because of intracellular accumulation of abnormal substances (storage diseases), or because of endomyocardial diseases (Table 50–4).

Noninfiltrative Restrictive Cardiomyopathies

IDIOPATHIC RESTRICTIVE CARDIOMYOPATHY. This term applies to the clinical and hemodynamic findings of restric-

TABLE 50–4. CLASSIFICATION OF THE RESTRICTIVE CARDIOMYOPATHIES

Myocardial
  A. Noninfiltrative
    Idiopathic
    Scleroderma
  B. Infiltrative
    Amyloid
    Sarcoid
    Gaucher's disease
    Hurler's disease
  C. Storage diseases
    Hemochromatosis
    Fabry's disease
    Glycogen storage diseases
Endomyocardial
  Endomyocardial fibrosis
  Hypereosinophilic syndrome
  Carcinoid
  Metastatic malignancies
  Radiation
  Anthracycline toxicity

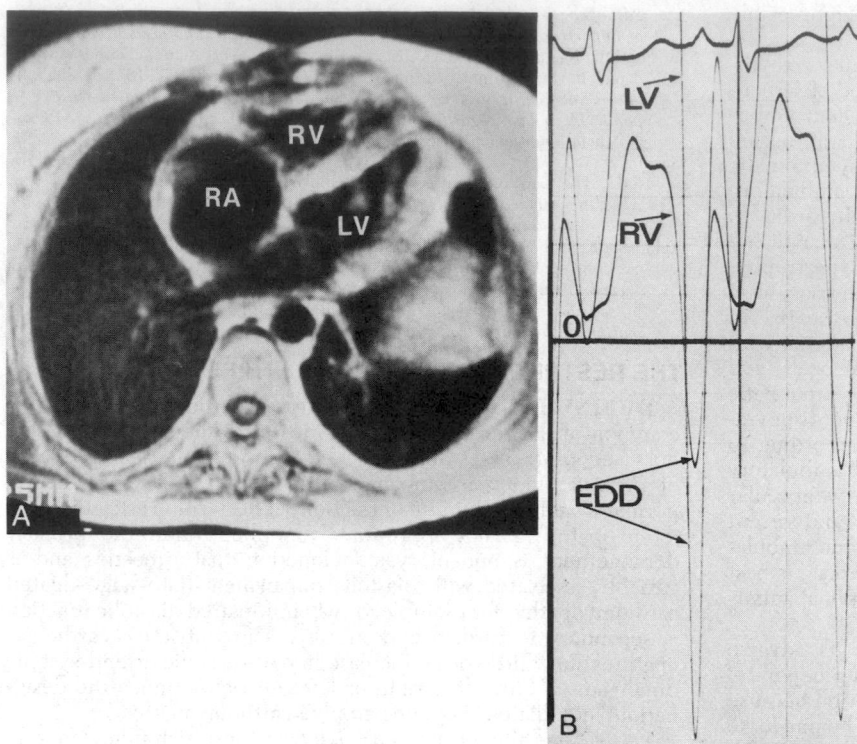

FIGURE 50–8. *A*, Magnetic resonance image in a patient with idiopathic restrictive cardiomyopathy. The right ventricle (RV) and left ventricle (LV) are normal in size, and the septum, pericardium, and ventricular free walls are of normal thicknesses. The right atrium (RA) is enlarged. The left atrium is not well shown in this view, but was also enlarged. *B*, The right ventricular (RV) and left ventricular (LV) pressure pulses show marked early diastolic dips (EDD), but the diastolic configurations differ.

tive heart disease in the absence of discernible morphologic cause. Ventricular cavity sizes and ventricular septal and free wall thicknesses are normal or nearly so. Microscopic examination including histochemical stains may show nothing more than mild interstitial fibrosis. Idiopathic restrictive cardiomyopathy is sometimes familial and is believed to be a biochemical abnormality of the energy-dependent rapid filling phase of ventricular relaxation. The decline in cytosolic calcium required for myocardial relaxation is probably mediated by sarcolemmal Na^+-Ca^{2+} exchange. The fault in idiopathic restrictive cardiomyopathy may reside in a failure of an appropriate decline in cytosolic calcium needed for relaxation.

Patients with idiopathic restrictive cardiomyopathy present with clinical signs and symptoms of high systemic and pulmonary venous pressures. The jugular venous pulse resembles that of constrictive pericarditis, and peripheral edema and ascites reinforce the impression. Atrial fibrillation is not uncommon. Auscultation detects a prominent third heart sound (right or left ventricular in origin), and murmurs of AV valve regurgitation are common. Chest roentgenograms show pulmonary venous congestion and pleural effusions. The cardiac silhouette reflects biatrial enlargement without ventricular dilatation.

Two-dimensional echocardiography with Doppler interrogation and color flow imaging discloses normal or nearly normal systolic ventricular function, impaired diastolic function, relatively normal ventricular cavity sizes, and marked biatrial dilatation in response to reduced ventricular distensibility and AV valve regurgitation. Magnetic resonance imaging is efficacious in confirming the absence of pericardial thickening (Fig. 50–8A). Intraventricular pressure pulses reveal an early diastolic dip followed by a diastolic plateau, but the configurations of the diastolic portions of the pressure pulses differ because the myocardial restriction is not uniform in the two ventricles (Fig. 50–8B).

The clinical course of idiopathic restrictive cardiomyopathy can be protracted even in the presence of chronic atrial fibrillation. High-degree heart block is relatively common and may require a permanent pacemaker. Digitalis glycosides are useful in controlling the ventricular response to atrial fibrillation but otherwise have little to offer because ventricular systolic function is normal or nearly so. The biochemical fault in idiopathic restrictive cardiomyopathy may lie in failure of the decline in cytosolic calcium required for ventricular relaxation, so calcium channel

antagonists theoretically may have a therapeutic role in improving diastolic relaxation, although their efficacy is unproven.

SCLERODERMA. Scleroderma heart disease is primarily the result of insidious fibrosis involving myocardial interstitium as well as pericardium and AV conduction. Echocardiographic studies occasionally disclose patterns of restrictive or dilated cardiomyopathy.

Infiltrative Restrictive Cardiomyopathies

AMYLOIDOSIS. Amyloid heart disease is the paradigm of the infiltrative restrictive cardiomyopathies. Amyloid causes tissue injury chiefly because interstitial deposits replace normal contractile elements of the myocardium. When amyloid fibrils consist mainly of light chains, deposition tends to involve the heart, tongue, gastrointestinal tract, nerves, and skin. When the fibrils are chiefly protein, amyloid tends to involve the liver, kidney, and spleen. The differences between these two varieties of amyloid are, however, less than categoric.

Histologically, cardiac amyloidosis is characterized by interstitial deposition in all four cardiac chambers and also in cardiac valves (especially the AV valves) in the walls of intramural coronary arteries and arterioles, in the pericardium, and in the impulse and conduction system. Deposition of amyloid in myocardial interstitium impairs diastolic ventricular function, leaving systolic function normal or nearly so, at least initially. As amyloid insidiously and progressively replaces contractile elements, systolic function suffers but may remain well preserved despite advanced amyloid infiltration.

The clinical manifestations of cardiac amyloidosis reflect the anatomic and physiologic derangements described above. Biventricular circulatory congestion is the most common feature, but right-sided congestion often dominates the clinical picture, with peripheral edema and ascites outweighing orthopnea and nocturnal dyspnea. Angina pectoris occurs in approximately one third of patients and is believed to be caused by amyloid involvement of the coronary arteries. Impairment of sinus node function and of AV conduction occurs in about 35 per cent of cases. Atrial fibrillation is a less frequent occurrence. Upwards of one third of patients experience orthostatic hypotension, lightheadedness, or frank syncope (amyloid autonomic neuropathy). Sudden death is comparatively common.

On physical examination, the arterial pulse is normal or small.

FIGURE 50–9. *A*, Two-dimensional echocardiogram in a patient with amyloid heart disease (restrictive cardiomyopathy). There is thickening of the ventricular septum (VS) and of the walls of both ventricles. The left ventricular (LV) cavity is small. There is echo dropout in the atrial septum, the inferior portion of which (*vertical arrow*) is thickened. RV = Right ventricle; RA, LA = right and left atria. *B*, Technetium-99m pyrophosphate scan (left anterior oblique view) from a patient with amyloid heart disease. The isotope accumulated in the thick ventricular septum and left ventricular free wall (*arrows*). The left ventricular (LV) cavity is small.

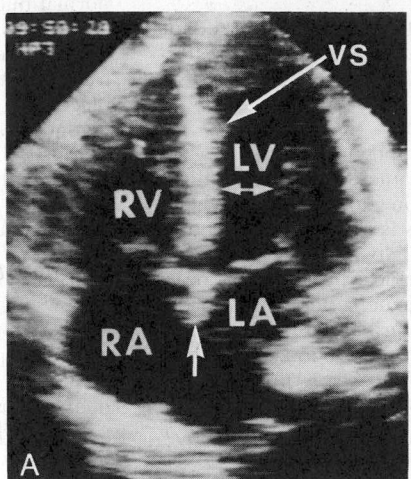
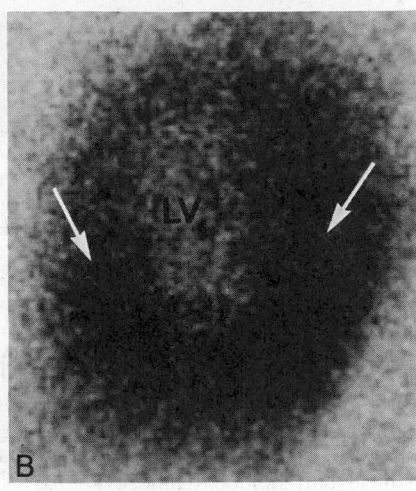

The jugular venous pulse is often visible even when the patient sits bolt upright, with wave forms that resemble those of constrictive pericarditis. Auscultation detects a soft first heart sound (PR interval prolongation), no murmur or soft systolic murmurs of AV valve regurgitation, and third heart sounds but not fourth heart sounds. Peripheral edema, hepatomegaly, and ascites are common, even in the absence of pulmonary rales and orthopnea.

The electrocardiogram shows left or right atrial P-wave abnormalities and varying degrees of AV block. QRS voltage is characteristically low. Poor R-wave progression or QS deformities in right precordial leads are believed to reflect myocardial replacement with amyloid.

Echocardiography has been a major step forward in the clinical diagnosis of cardiac amyloidosis. Two-dimensional imaging discloses a symmetric increase in thickness of the ventricular septum and left ventricular free wall, with an increase in right ventricular wall thickness, but normal to small ventricular cavity sizes (Fig. 50–9*A*). Two-dimensional imaging also serves to identify thickening of the interatrial septum (Fig. 50–9*A*), and of the AV valves. Real-time imaging often discloses a distinctive "granular/sparkling" appearance of the thickened ventricular myocardium. Rarely, the ventricular septum is thicker than the posterior wall, prompting a mistaken diagnosis of asymmetric hypertrophy. Pulsed Doppler diastolic filling patterns reflect the presence and degree of amyloid infiltration of the myocardium. Early, intermediate, and advanced stages have been identified. Advanced cardiac amyloidosis is characterized on pulsed Doppler inflow interrogation by a typical "restrictive pattern" (increased early diastolic ventricular inflow velocities with shortened deceleration times, decreased "a" velocities, and normal isovolumic relaxation time). Color flow imaging frequently reveals mitral and tricuspid regurgitation, much less commonly aortic and pulmonic regurgitation, all usually mild. Technetium-99m pyrophosphate cardiac scans are useful diagnostic adjuncts in the diagnosis of advanced cardiac amyloidosis (Fig. 50–9*B*). The mechanism of intense uptake of the tracer is unclear, but accumulation is biventricular and relates to the thickness of ventricular myocardium. Based upon the above clinical and diagnostic assessments, the diagnosis of cardiac amyloidosis can generally be made without recourse to histochemical tissue confirmation from endomyocardial biopsy.

The prognosis and clinical course of cardiac amyloidosis depend upon where in the spectrum of cardiac involvement a given patient lies. Progressive congestive heart failure and atrial fibrillation are generally reserved for patients with marked ventricular wall thicknesses, granular/sparkling tissue texture, decreased systolic function, and atrial enlargement. Amyloid involvement of major epicardial coronary arteries can cause ischemia and infarction.

Treatment of cardiac amyloidosis is supportive, usually ineffective, and occasionally inadvertently harmful. Progression cannot currently be arrested, and regression is unknown. Overzealous use of diuretics may reduce ventricular filling pressures and relieve symptoms of circulatory congestion, but at the expense of an undesirable fall in cardiac output. Digitalis glycosides are potentially proarrhythmic and have adverse effects on already depressed sinus node and AV node function. Should cardioversion be attempted for atrial fibrillation, the abnormal sinus node may fail as an effective pacemaker. An artificial ventricular pacemaker is required for high-degree heart block, but the thresholds may be abnormally high because of amyloid deposits at the site of electrode implantation. Treatment of angina pectoris with nitroglycerin may provoke hypotension owing to decreased ventricular filling and may reinforce the tendency to orthostatic hypotension.

SARCOIDOSIS. Myocardial involvement at necropsy has been identified in up to 25 per cent of patients with generalized sarcoidosis. However, only about 5 per cent of patients with proven sarcoidosis have clinically overt involvement of the heart. Physiologic derangements initially reflect interstitial infiltration that causes impaired diastolic function with normal or nearly normal systolic function. Subsequent injury to contractile elements with fibrous replacement results in impaired systolic function.

The sites most frequently involved in myocardial sarcoidosis are the left ventricular free wall, the basal aspect of the ventricular septum, the right ventricular free wall, and the walls of the atria. The basic lesion is a noncaseating granuloma, which may be accompanied by lymphocytic infiltration and patchy fibrosis. The peculiar affinity for involvement of the cephalad portion of the ventricular septum may result in complete heart block. Accordingly, cardiac sarcoidosis may dramatically announce itself as a Stokes-Adams episode or sudden death. Relevant to this discussion is the restrictive phase of sarcoid cardiomyopathy, although pulmonary hypertension, high-degree heart block, and papillary muscle dysfunction are important clinical associations.

Echocardiography and imaging with technetium-99m pyrophosphate, gallium, and thallium-201 may be useful in detecting myocardial sarcoid. Endomyocardial biopsy is seldom efficacious because the biotome is not likely to sample one of the common sites of cardiac sarcoidosis.

Prognosis is determined not only by the restrictive cardiomyopathy but also by the risks of high-degree heart block, ventricular arrhythmias, and pulmonary hypertension. Steroid treatment has been advocated for biopsy-proven myocardial sarcoidosis. Sarcoid granulomas in the heart are supposedly more responsive to steroids than granulomas in other organs. Myocardial granulomas may be replaced by connective tissue with aneurysmal thinning of the ventricular wall.

GAUCHER'S DISEASE. This is an inherited disorder of glucocerebroside metabolism. The cerebroside accumulates in the reticuloendothelial system as well as in brain and myocardium. Infiltration of the myocardium by Gaucher cells can cause decreased ventricular compliance.

HURLER'S DISEASE. This autosomal recessive disorder is the prototype of the mucopolysaccharidoses. Hurler cells laden with mucopolysaccharide moieties infiltrate the myocardial interstitium and are accompanied by increased interstitial fibrous tissue. The result is reduced diastolic distensibility (restriction). Although as many as one third of deaths in the Hurler syndrome result from congestive heart failure, it is difficult clinically to isolate myocardial involvement per se from the hemodynamic effects of infiltration of mitral and aortic valves, the ischemic effects of infiltration of coronary arteries, and the coexisting effect of systemic hypertension.

Storage Diseases

HEMOCHROMATOSIS. Primary hemochromatosis is a recessive inborn error of metabolism characterized by multiple organ parenchymal intracellular deposition (storage) of iron. Deposition of iron in reticuloendothelial cells is relatively innocuous, but parenchymal cell deposits are potentially harmful. The initial myocardial iron deposits are in the subepicardium, subendocardium, and papillary muscles, with subsequent deposition in the ventricular free walls and septum. Myocardial cell disruption is followed by fibrous replacement. The AV conduction system may be involved, but the sinus node is usually spared. Approximately one third of untreated patients with histologically proven primary hemochromatosis die of congestive heart failure. A phase of restrictive cardiomyopathy has been confirmed. Patients with clinical and hemodynamic evidence of cardiac restriction may also have decreased systolic function with normal left ventricular cavity size. Dilated heart failure is the most common ultimate sequela.

Progressive diastolic dysfunction with rising ventricular filling pressures is symptomatically expressed as effort dyspnea, but right-sided failure may dominate the clinical picture. When systolic dysfunction supervenes, the physical signs resemble those of dilated cardiomyopathy. In either case, hepatic enlargement may be due to the hemochromatosis per se rather than to passive congestion.

Symptomatic cardiac hemochromatosis is usually associated with electrocardiographic abnormalities, chiefly ST-T changes or supraventricular arrhythmias. Despite histologic involvement of ventricular muscle and atrioventricular conduction system, ventricular arrhythmias and conduction disturbances are uncommon.

Because cardiac hemochromatosis is the most common cause of death in these patients, and because phlebotomy is an effective therapy if begun early enough, accurate diagnosis is of considerable practical importance. A significant minority of patients die within a short time after the diagnosis is made. The echocardiogram initially shows a nondilated, concentrically thick left ventricle with evidence of diastolic dysfunction but normal or nearly normal ejection fraction. Suspected cardiac involvement has been confirmed by endomyocardial biopsy, although myocardial iron can be focal and variable in location. Multiple biopsy sites are necessary to minimize the chance of sampling error.

Heart failure may respond to iron depletion therapy if initiated when cardiac muscle cells are viable and before there is significant myocardial fibrosis. The corollary to this observation is that prevention of myocardial fibrosis can be achieved when early recognition of myocardial infiltration with iron is effectively treated by phlebotomy.

FABRY'S DISEASE. This is an X-linked recessive disorder of glycosphingolipid metabolism due to a specific enzyme deficiency. The result is intracellular glycolipid accumulation in vascular endothelial lysozymes as well as in heart muscle and valves (particularly mitral), skin, cornea, kidneys, gastrointestinal tract, and central nervous system. The disease is fully expressed in the male and incompletely expressed in the female (X-linked). Males usually die by the fourth or fifth decade from cardiac failure, renal failure, hypertension, or cerebrovascular disease.

Accumulation (storage) of glycolipid in cardiac muscle can result in an increase in mass and myocardial restriction. Echocardiography in the typical male with Fabry's disease reveals increased septal and free wall thicknesses (presumably a consequence of glycolipid storage) with normal left ventricular internal dimensions. Lysosomal accumulation of glycolipids in mitral leaflets does not correlate with clinical severity of disease, but left ventricular mass does.

GLYCOGEN STORAGE DISEASES. These disorders result from a deficiency of one or more of the enzymes involved in the biosynthesis and degradation of glycogen. Most cases of glycogen storage disease causing restrictive cardiomyopathy belong to type II, that is, Pompe's disease. The glycogen that is stored in cardiac muscle cells, skeletal muscle cells, and liver is biochemically normal but present in excessive amounts.

Pompe's disease is always fatal, usually within the first 2 to 3 years of life. The combination of marked cardiomegaly (increased free wall and septal thicknesses) with skeletal muscle weakness (flaccidity) in infants who appear normal at birth is diagnostically distinctive. The characteristic echocardiographic findings in Pompe's disease are dramatic thickening of ventricular septum and of right and left ventricular free walls with reduced cavity sizes. The electrocardiogram is distinctive, exhibiting a remarkable increase in QRS amplitude with a short PR interval.

Restrictive Cardiomyopathies Due to Endomyocardial Disease

ENDOMYOCARDIAL FIBROSIS. This is a common form of cardiomyopathy in tropical and subtropical Africa, is encountered less often in South America and Asia, and more recently has been reported in Western Europe and the United States in patients who have never been in the tropics. Endomyocardial fibrosis accounts for 15 to 25 per cent of deaths due to heart disease in equatorial Africa. The disease involves both the right and left ventricles in about 50 per cent of cases but is isolated to the left ventricle in approximately 40 per cent and to the right ventricle in 10 per cent. Dense endomyocardial thickening of the inflow tracts of the ventricles includes the AV valves, so that mitral and tricuspid regurgitation are important features. The ventricular outflow tracts are not involved. Functional derangements consist of impaired diastolic filling and AV valve regurgitation with relatively well-preserved systolic function. In the presence of intractable biventricular failure and AV valve regurgitation, surgical resection of the fibrous endocardium with valve replacement has been advocated as a therapeutic option.

HYPEREOSINOPHILIC SYNDROME. This syndrome is defined as (1) persistent eosinophilia of 1500 per cubic millimeter for at least 6 months, or death before 6 months; (2) lack of evidence of recognized causes of eosinophilia despite careful evaluation; and (3) signs and symptoms of organ system involvement, especially the heart and nervous system. The capability of the eosinophil and its contents to cause tissue damage (the "Gordon phenomenon") has been known for over 50 years and is held responsible for initial damage to the endocardium. Platelet thrombi form over the denuded endocardium with a morphologic evolution that ultimately results in pathologic findings indistinguishable from those described above in endomyocardial fibrosis. It has been argued persuasively that idiopathic hypereosinophilic syndrome and endomyocardial fibrosis are the same disease at different stages of development. Conversely, it has been proposed that geochemical factors (thorium excess together with magnesium deficiency) might cause tropical endomyocardial fibrosis.

Endomyocardial biopsies lend support to the hypothesis that endocardial endothelial cells and the microvasculature are the primary targets, whereas thrombosis is secondary. In any event, endocardial fibrosis and restrictive cardiomyopathy ensue. Because of the endocardial thrombi, peripheral emboli are common. Involvement of the posterior mitral leaflet and the septal and posterior tricuspid leaflets result in mitral and tricuspid regurgitation, as in endomyocardial fibrosis described above.

Echocardiography is useful in the noninvasive diagnosis. The combination of small ventricles and large atria is typical although not diagnostic, but together with apical obliteration, the diagnosis is reasonably secure.

Treatment is limited. The surgical option is as mentioned earlier for endomyocardial fibrosis.

CARCINOID ENDOCARDIAL DISEASE. The carcinoid syndrome results in cardiac involvement as a late complication in 50 per cent of cases. Endocardial abnormalities may cause a restrictive cardiomyopathy, although the principal overt cardiac manifestations reflect involvement of the pulmonic and tricuspid valves with stenosis and regurgitation. In the presence of significant pulmonic or tricuspid valve disease, detection of coexisting restriction is difficult even with current techniques of pulsed Doppler inflow interrogation.

MALIGNANT ENDOMYOCARDIAL DISEASE. Cardiac metastases are present in over 60 per cent of patients with malignant melanoma, and there is a relatively high incidence of involvement of the heart in bronchogenic carcinoma, carcinoma of the breast, lymphoma, and leukemia. Restriction of ventricular filling caused by endomyocardial infiltration is rare and is more commonly due to pericardial tumor or radiation.

RADIATION HEART DISEASE. Radiation-induced endocardial and myocardial fibrosis can cause restrictive cardiomyopathy, sometimes with disproportionate involvement of the more exposed anterior right ventricle. Functional abnormalities due to interstitial fibrosis demonstrated by echocardiography and radionuclide angiography occur up to 15 years after radiation. Importantly, the pericardium is the most frequent cardiovascular site of radiation heart disease, and the differential diagnosis between radiation-restrictive cardiomyopathy and radiation injury to pericardium is difficult.

ANTHRACYCLINE CARDIOMYOPATHY. There is convincing evidence that doxorubicin and other anthracycline antitumor agents can cause dilated cardiomyopathy as well as restrictive cardiomyopathy due to endomyocardial fibrosis. Light microscopy of biopsy specimens has disclosed fibrous thickening of the endocardium. Hemodynamic studies may record a restrictive diastolic "dip-and-plateau" in the left and/or right ventricle. The risk of myocardial injury is dose-related, although cardiotoxicity sometimes occurs at lower doses in individuals with prior mediastinal (and cardiac) radiation.

Child JS, Perloff JK: *In* Perloff JK (ed.): The Cardiomyopathies. Philadelphia, W. B. Saunders Co., 1988. *A comprehensive review of the various types of myocardial and endomyocardial restrictive cardiomyopathies.*

Cueto-Garcia L, Tajik AJ, Kyle RA, et al.: Serial echocardiographic observations in patients with primary systemic amyloidosis; Smith TJ, Kyle RA, Lie JT: Clinical significance of histopathologic patterns of cardiac amyloidosis. Mayo Clin Proc 59:547, 589, 1984. *Two comprehensive articles that deal with the pathology and serial echocardiographic diagnoses of cardiac amyloidosis.*

Dabestani A, Child JS, Henze E, et al.: Primary hemochromatosis: Anatomic and physiologic studies characteristic of the cardiac ventricles and their responses to phlebotomy. Am J Cardiol 54:153, 1984. *Clinically occult cardiac involvement was identified by echocardiography and equilibrium blood pool imaging. Therapeutic phlebotomy ameliorated or reversed the deleterious effects of cardiac iron deposition if initiated prior to irreversible connective tissue replacement.*

Fauci AS, Harley JB, Roberts WC, et al.: The hypereosinophilic syndrome. Ann Intern Med 97:78, 1982. *This comprehensive National Institutes of Health conference deals with clinical, pathophysiologic, and therapeutic considerations in the hypereosinophilic syndrome and with the relationship of the disorder to endomyocardial fibrosis.*

Siegel RJ, Shah PK, Fishbein MC: Idiopathic restrictive cardiomyopathy. Circulation 70:165, 1984. *This form of cardiomyopathy is characterized chiefly by elevated left and right ventricular filling pressures, normal global ventricular systolic function, and normal or nearly normal ventricular septal and wall thicknesses and internal dimensions in the absence of specific infiltrative disorders or of diseases of pericardium or coronary arteries.*

Stewart JR, Fajardo LF: Radiation-induced heart disease: An update. Prog Cardiovasc Dis 27:173, 1984. *An informative review of the pathology, physiology, pathogenesis, diagnosis, treatment, and prevention of radiation-induced heart disease.*

51 Diseases of the Pericardium

Ralph Shabetai

Diseases of the pericardium typically present in one or more of three clinical forms: acute pericarditis, pericardial effusion, and pericardial constriction. Pericardial involvement may progress from inflammation to effusion and then constriction, or it may present as effusion or constriction without clinical evidence of preceding inflammation.

ETIOLOGY

The pericardium may be involved in a large number and variety of diseases. The most important are listed in Table 51–1. Pericardial disease may be asymptomatic but may also cause dramatic symptoms and signs.

The clinical syndromes of pericardial disease are listed in Table 51–2.

INFECTIONS WITH LIVING AGENTS. Virus Infection. Many viruses may cause pericarditis; the common offenders are listed in Table 51–1. The number of cases of idiopathic pericarditis that are caused by preceding viral infection is unknown.

TABLE 51–1. MAJOR CAUSES OF PERICARDIAL DISEASE

1. Inflammation	
Virus	
Coxsackie (usually B)	(E)
Echo	(E)
Other	
Bacterial	
Pneumococcus	(E)
Staphylococcus	(E,C)
Meningococcus	(E,C)
Mycobacterium tuberculosis	(E,C)
Haemophilus influenzae	(C)
Other	
Fungus	
Histoplasma capsulatum	(E,C)
Other	
Other living organisms	
Parasites	(E)
Protozoa	(E)
Nonliving agents	
Trauma	(E,C)
Radiation	(E,C)
Chemical	
Chemotherapeutic agents	
2. Idiopathic	
(Many may be viral, but unproven)	(E,C)
3. Neoplastic	
Secondary to carcinoma of	
Lung	(E,C)
Breast	(E,C)
Other	
Lymphoma	(E)
Primary	
Mesothelioma	(E)
Other	
4. Metabolic	
Chronic renal disease	
Associated with dialysis	(E)
End-stage uremia	(E)
Myxedema	(E)
Chylopericardium	(E)
Hypoalbuminemia	(E)
5. Myocardial injury	
Myocardial infarction	
Acute	
Dressler's syndrome	(E)
Congestive heart failure	(E)
6. Trauma	(E,C)
Postpericardiotomy syndrome	(E)
Postoperative	(C)
7. Connective tissue disorders and hypersensitivity	
Acute rheumatic fever	
Rheumatoid arthritis	(C)
Systemic sclerosis	
Lupus erythematosus	
Drugs	
Procainamide	
Others	
8. Congenital	
Absence of left pericardium	
Partial	
Complete	
Cyst	
Other	

(E) = effusion common; (C) = constrictive pericarditis common.

Bacterial Infection. Bacterial pericarditis is still important, although the spectrum has altered. Pneumococcal pericarditis, once a frequent complication of pneumonia, is now rare, whereas infection by staphylococci, fungi, and exotic organisms is more common, especially in persons at either extreme of age and in the immunologically compromised host. Meningococcal pericarditis may be a manifestation of either direct infection or hypersensitivity.

TABLE 51–2. CLINICAL SYNDROMES OF PERICARDIAL DISEASE

Dry, fibrinous pericarditis
    Usually acute (R)
Lax pericardial effusion
    Chronic effusive
Cardiac tamponade (R)
Constrictive pericarditis
    Subacute
    Chronic
Effusive-constrictive pericarditis

(R) = Relapse or recurrence common.

Tuberculosis. Tuberculous pericarditis is less common now that tuberculosis is better controlled and treated. Pulmonary tuberculosis may be present, but often pericardial effusion may be an isolated manifestation. *Mycobacterium tuberculosis* can be recovered from only one third of effusions. Even pericardial biopsy findings are not uniformly positive. Commonly, the diagnosis is presumptive and based on circumstantial evidence, such as a positive skin test result or a history of recent contact.

Haemophilus influenzae infection is an important cause of constrictive pericarditis in children.

Fungal Infection. In an otherwise normal population fungal pericarditis is uncommon, but infection with *Histoplasma capsulatum* should be considered in patients who reside in the Ohio Valley. Similarly, coccidioidomycosis should be considered in patients who have been in the San Joaquin Valley of California.

PERICARDIAL INFLAMMATION CAUSED BY NONLIVING AGENTS. *Trauma.* Blunt and sharp trauma is an important cause of pericarditis and may lead to pericardial effusion with or without tamponade and ultimately to constrictive pericarditis. Common examples of acute trauma include gunshot and knife wounds. Impact against a steering wheel, explosions, and crushing are the major causes of blunt injuries.

Radiation. The pericardium may be exposed to considerable injury when radiotherapy is employed to treat neoplasia, for example, Hodgkin's disease and lung or breast neoplasms. The latent period between radiation and clinical pericardial disease may extend for many years.

PERICARDIAL DISEASE IN METABOLIC DISORDERS. *Renal Disease.* Pericardial disease continues to be one of the more frequent major complications of chronic dialysis and may cause cardiac tamponade. Fortunately, constrictive pericarditis is rare. The etiology is not understood: It may be a manifestation of end-stage renal disease, but the process of dialysis itself may be responsible in whole or in part.

Myxedema. Pericardial effusion may occur and accounts in part for apparent cardiomegaly on chest radiograph; it may also contribute to the low voltage and T-wave inversion that, in addition to sinus bradycardia, characterize the electrocardiogram. Pericardial effusion may contain cholesterol crystals.

CHYLOPERICARDIUM. Chylopericardium, a pericardial collection of fluid bearing a large quantity of chyle, may be idiopathic but often follows surgical or other trauma of the thoracic duct.

MYOCARDIAL INFARCTION. Acute dry, fibrinous pericarditis can be detected in about one third of patients with acute myocardial infarction. Autopsy evidence is more common. Acute pericarditis early in the course is often a contiguous inflammation over the infarction but may also represent reaction to myocardial injury. Rupture of an infarction, aneurysm, or pseudoaneurysm creates greater or lesser degrees of hemopericardium, the former usually ending fatally.

In some patients, pericarditis (often accompanied by effusion) occurs in the weeks or months following acute myocardial infarction. This syndrome (Dressler's) is thought to be a delayed autoimmune reaction and is often recurrent.

CONNECTIVE TISSUE DISORDERS. Pericardial reaction may occur in virtually all of these disorders. Acute pericarditis is a constituent of rheumatic pancarditis but does not progress to constriction. On the other hand, subacute constrictive pericarditis can occur in rheumatoid arthritis. Pericarditis is an important manifestation of lupus erythematosus, both spontaneous and induced by drugs such as procainamide, and can cause tamponade.

HEART FAILURE. In patients with fluid retention, small pericardial effusion may be seen by echocardiography.

CONGENITAL LESIONS AND CYSTS. Partial absence of the pericardium produces a striking abnormality on the chest radiograph. Pericardial cysts are more frequent. They are filled with clear fluid and most often occupy the right cardiophrenic angle, although they may occupy atypical locations. They are benign and usually produce no symptoms.

ACUTE (FIBRINOUS) VIRAL OR IDIOPATHIC PERICARDITIS

SYMPTOMS. Findings are often preceded by generalized malaise and fever. The chief symptom is chest pain, which may be either sharp or crushing. Frequently, the pain is precordial but may shift to the left side, simulating pleurisy. Characteristically, the pain is relieved by sitting up and exacerbated by deep inspiration. Thus, pericardial pain has features that may suggest either myocardial ischemia or pleural inflammation. Referral of pain to the right trapezius ridge is a specific but uncommon sign of its pericardial origin.

CLINICAL FINDINGS. *Pericardial Friction Rub: The Pathognomonic Sign of Pericardial Inflammation.* Classifically, the rub has components accompanying atrial systole, ventricular systole, and ventricular diastole (see LMSB line, Fig. 51–1). Commonly, the rub is biphasic and must be distinguished from to-and-fro murmurs. When it is monophasic, it must be differentiated from systolic murmurs. It is typically superficial and scratchy, and although it may be widely distributed over the precordium, it is usually most apparent at the left sternal edge. Appreciation is enhanced by firm pressure with the diaphragm of the stethoscope. Changes in posture and the respiratory cycle may alter the intensity. Pericardial friction rubs are often transient and should be sought frequently when pericarditis is suspected. They must be distinguished not only from cardiac murmurs but also from mediastinal crunch due to air in the mediastinum, crepitations from surgical emphysema, and artifacts produced by movement of the skin against the stethoscope.

LABORATORY FINDINGS. *Electrocardiogram.* The typical findings of pericarditis are shown in Figure 51–2. ST-segment elevation, although common, is not invariably present, depression of the ST segment being usual in leads aV_R and V_1. Depression of the PR segment, although highly specific, is less common than ST-segment elevation.

On a single tracing and without clinical information, ST-segment elevation cannot always be distinguished from the early repolarization normal variant or from the early stage of acute myocardial infarction. In the latter, evolution of the pattern in serial tracings is helpful. In acute pericarditis, the ST segment returns to baseline without inversion of the T wave (which may occur later if pericarditis becomes chronic), whereas in acute myocardial infarction, T-wave inversion typically occurs before the ST segment becomes isoelectric.

Other Laboratory Findings. The erythrocyte sedimentation rate is elevated and there is variable leukocytosis. Viral titers may confirm the origin of the illness but are seldom performed in clinical practice. Gallium radioisotope scanning may display the epicardium, but this expensive test is required only in exceptional cases. Plasma levels of cardiac enzymes may be elevated, but this determination need not be made routinely.

DIAGNOSIS. The diagnosis can usually be made reliably from symptoms and signs. When any of the conditions listed in Table 51–1 is suspected, the symptoms and signs of pericarditis should be specifically sought and the diagnosis confirmed by electrocardiography. When the pain simulates that of pleurisy, pneumonia or pulmonary infarction must be considered. When it is retrosternal and crushing, myocardial infarction must be ruled out. On occasion, other major causes of chest discomfort, such as acute pulmonary embolism or dissection of the aorta, need to be considered.

CLINICAL COURSE, PROGNOSIS, AND MANAGEMENT. Commonly, this is a self-limiting disease. However, its natural history is seldom observed, as it usually responds rapidly to treatment with nonsteroidal anti-inflammatory agents such as

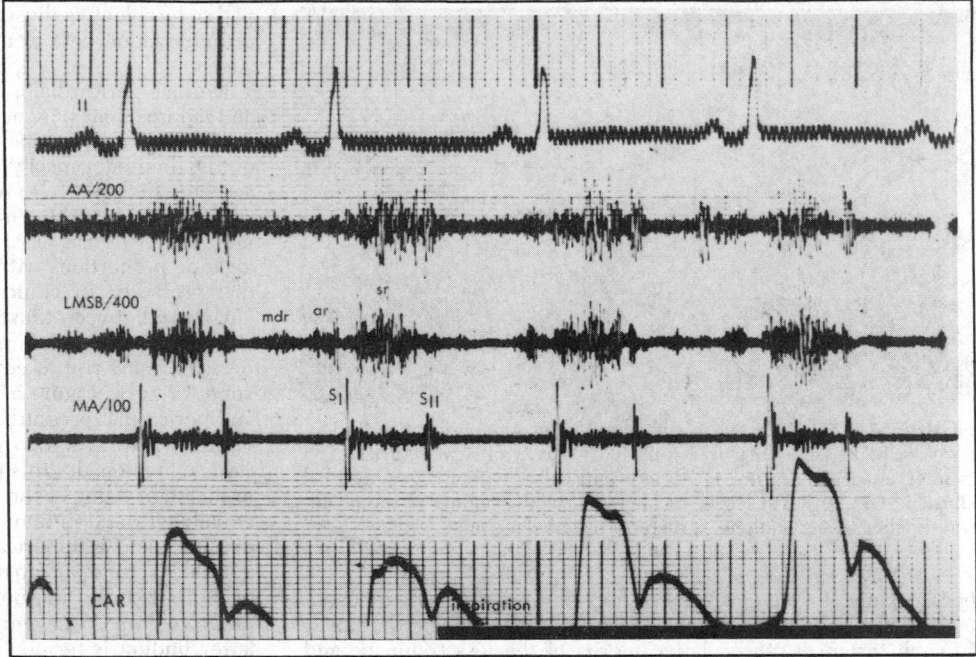

FIGURE 51–1. Phonocardiography of pericardial friction rub. AA = Aortic area; LMSB = left mid-sternal border; MA = mitral area. Note the three-component rub heard along the left mid-sternal border. Numbers refer to filter settings. (Reproduced by permission from Spodick DH: Am Heart J 81:114, 1971.)

indomethacin (25 to 50 mg three to four times a day) or ibuprofen. Even aspirin is often satisfactory. Resistant cases may require steroid treatment—for instance, prednisone, starting with 75 mg a day and rapidly tapering to the minimum dose that suppresses symptoms and signs.

Detectable pericardial effusion occurs in a small proportion of cases and may progress to cardiac tamponade. Similarly, acute pericarditis may rarely lead to chronic constrictive pericarditis.

Recurrent Pericarditis. Perhaps the most troublesome of all complications is frequent recurrence over a period of years. The patient is greatly disturbed by the frequent occurrence of disabling pain, and when steroidal agents must be used for resistant cases, their side effects may become significant.

PERICARDIAL EFFUSION

LAX PERICARDIAL EFFUSION. Pericardial effusions that do not raise intrapericardial pressure more than 3 or 4 mm Hg do not cause symptoms. The physical findings are variable and frequently do not provide valuable clinical clues. Pericardial effusion should be strongly suspected in the setting of acute pericarditis if the cardiopericardial silhouette is enlarged on the chest radiograph. A previous radiograph showing a normal-sized silhouette is particularly helpful. The diagnosis can be made with certainty by echocardiography (Fig. 51–3).

PERICARDIAL EFFUSION COMPLICATING ACUTE PERICARDITIS. When echocardiograms are performed rou-

tinely in acute pericarditis, effusion is found in a considerable proportion of cases. However, in clinical practice, echocardiography is not required if the heart size remains normal, there is no evidence of cardiac tamponade or myocarditis, and the findings subside within 48 to 72 hours after beginning treatment. Myocarditis should be suspected when depolarization changes, such as left or right bundle branch block, or conduction abnormalities develop and when a third heart sound is audible. In such cases, echocardiography is often useful in distinguishing cardiac chamber enlargement from pericardial effusion.

ETIOLOGY OF PERICARDIAL EFFUSION. The causes of pericardial effusion are indicated in Table 51–1. Pericardial effusion must always be considered in patients who have or are likely to have one of these disorders, but especially when there is or has been evidence of acute pericarditis or when there is circulatory compromise. When the patient has a possible cause of cardiac tamponade or constrictive pericarditis, pericardial disease must be ruled out before attributing circulatory abnormalities to heart disease.

PERICARDIOCENTESIS. When the venous pressure is normal, systemic arterial hypotension is absent, and the etiology of pericardial effusion has been established with reasonable certainty, pericardiocentesis is seldom needed. On the other hand, if the clinician suspects or diagnoses purulent effusion, or cardiac tamponade that is not responding satisfactorily to medical treatment, removal of pericardial fluid via a needle or open drainage

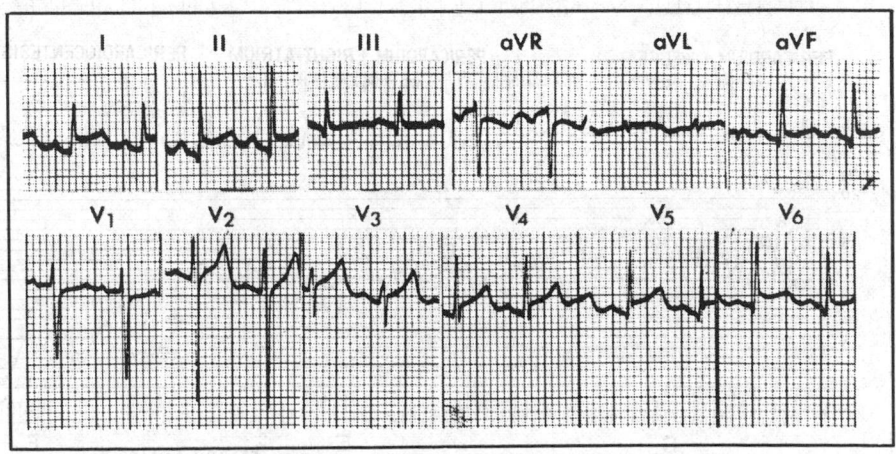

FIGURE 51–2. ECG from a case of acute pericarditis. Note the ST-segment elevation in leads I, II, aV_F and V_4 to V_6 and ST segment in leads aV_R and V_1. (From Shabetai R: The Pericardium. New York, Grune & Stratton, 1980.)

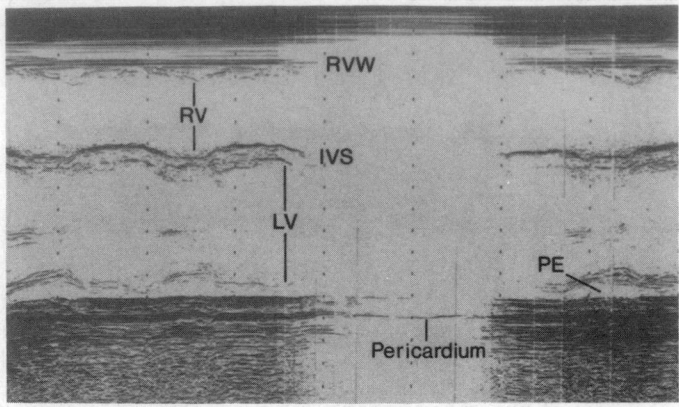

FIGURE 51–3. M-mode echocardiogram of moderate pericardial effusion. RVW = Right ventricular free wall; RV = cavity of right ventricle; IVS = interventricular septum; LV = left ventricular cavity; PE = pericardial effusion. The pericardial echo is identified in the middle of the photo, where other less echo-dense structures have been damped.

becomes necessary. In a smaller fraction of cases, pericardiocentesis is required to establish a tissue or bacteriologic diagnosis. In such instances, the relative merits of the less traumatic and less expensive pericardiocentesis, versus surgical drainage, must be weighed against local experience and preference and the relative importance of pericardial biopsy in establishing the diagnosis.

Lax pericardial effusions have minimal hemodynamic effects, but when large and chronic, as, for example, in idiopathic chronic effusive pericarditis, a number of clinicians recommend surgical drainage.

CARDIAC TAMPONADE

ETIOLOGY AND PATHOPHYSIOLOGY. Pericarditis of virtually any cause may be associated with pericardial effusion, and virtually any pericardial effusion can progress to cardiac tamponade. The important causes are indicated in Table 51–1. The pathophysiology is illustrated in Figure 51–4, taken from cardiac catheterization data from a patient with severe cardiac tamponade.

Normal pericardial pressure is subatmospheric (Fig. 51–4F) and approximates pleural pressure. When pericardial effusion rapidly accumulates, pericardial pressure rises abruptly because of the limited capacity of the parietal pericardium to stretch acutely (Fig. 51–4D). A few hundred milliliters accumulating rapidly can generate intrapericardial pressures in excess of 20 mm Hg, whereas a slowly developing effusion may assume gigantic proportions with only minimal elevation of intrapericardial pressure. In clinical practice, cases may be encountered anywhere between these two ends of the spectrum.

If effective circulation is to be maintained, systemic venous pressure must rise to equal intrapericardial pressure to maintain venous return. Figure 51–4E indicates equilibration of right atrial and pericardial pressure. Unless the pre-existing left ventricular diastolic pressure was higher than pericardial pressure during cardiac tamponade, this pressure also must rise to the same level to maintain filling of the left ventricle. Figure 51–4 A to E shows equally elevated pulmonary wedge, right atrial, right ventricular diastolic, and intrapericardial pressures. During inspiration the normal inspiratory drop of systemic venous pressure is maintained (Fig. 51–4A), but the normal systemic arterial systolic and pulse pressure drop is exaggerated during inspiration (Fig. 51–4C). The latter finding is termed pulsus paradoxus. Systemic arterial hypotension is absent (Fig. 51–4C) in mild-to-moderate cardiac tamponade. Surgical causes such as trauma or rupture of the heart or the aorta into the pericardium are usually associated with profound hypotension. In medical cases, cardiac output is often reduced to the range shown in Figure 51–4, but in surgical cases still lower cardiac outputs are often observed.

CLINICAL FINDINGS. The chief component in recognizing tamponade is thinking of it. Cardiac tamponade must be considered whenever evidence suggesting heart disease or heart failure develops in a patient who may reasonably be suspected of a disorder listed in Table 51–1. In extreme cases consciousness may be impaired, and arterial blood pressure may drop to shock

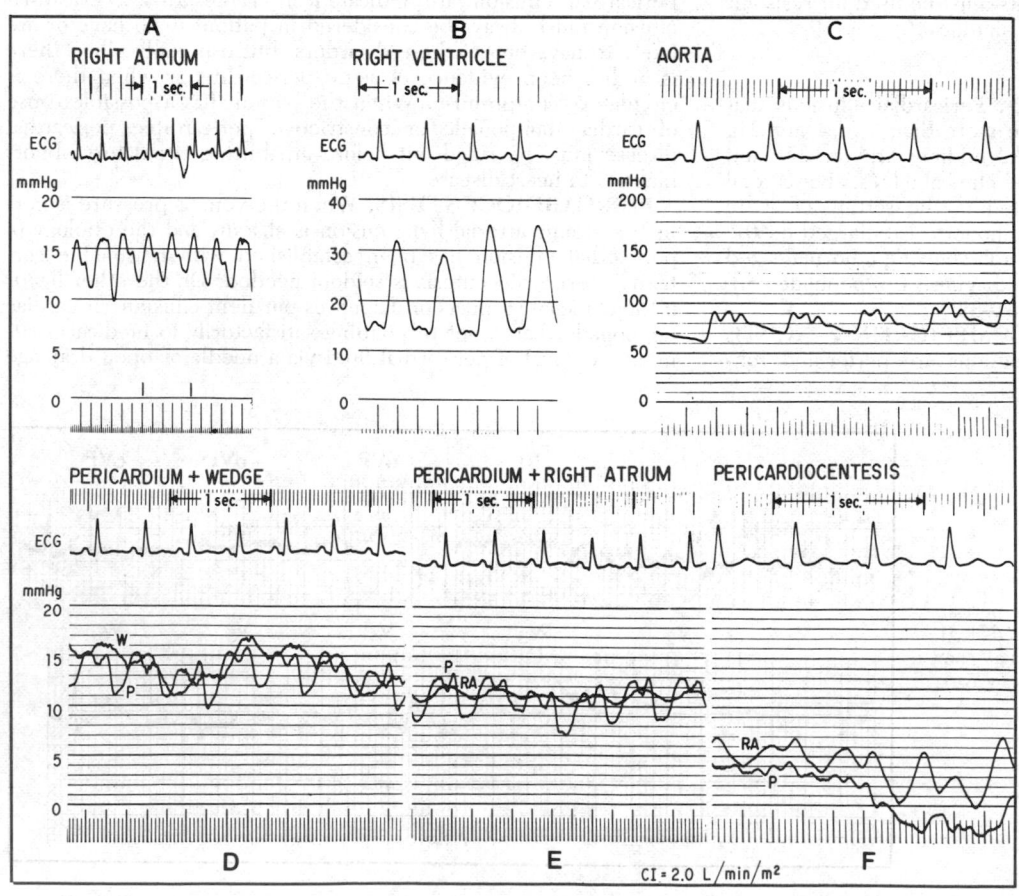

FIGURE 51–4. Hemodynamic data from a patient with cardiac tamponade. See text for discussion.

levels. Frequently there is oliguria, because cardiac tamponade, with the resulting drop in cardiac output and blood pressure, is a powerful stimulus for sodium retention by the kidney. Pericardial pain may or may not be present; often there is a sensation of fullness of the chest and sometimes frank dyspnea.

Venous Pressure. Important evidence of cardiac tamponade includes abnormal jugular venous pulses. The venous pressure is elevated, usually considerably so, unless there is concomitant acute blood loss or severe dehydration. The right atrial (and therefore the jugular) pulse is monophasic, the normal inspiratory drop is maintained, and the predominant wave is the x descent, occurring when the ventricle ejects (Fig. 51–4A). The prominent x descent is detected as a sharp inward movement of the internal jugular pulse synchronous with the carotid pulse. The y descent is reduced or abolished because of the attenuated early diastolic dip of ventricular pressure (Fig. 51–4B).

Pulsus Paradoxus. Severe pulsus paradoxus may be detectable by palpation of any arterial pulse. When extreme, the pulse disappears during inspiration; when less extreme, it diminishes but can still be palpated. In the presence of severe hypotension, pulsus paradoxus may be difficult to detect but then is usually more evident in large arteries. Pulsus paradoxus is quantified with a sphygmomanometer. As the cuff is deflated, pulsus paradoxus is estimated as the difference between pressure occurring when the first blood pressure sound can be heard only during expiration and that occurring when the sound is heard throughout the respiratory cycle. More accurate measurement requires direct monitoring of systemic arterial pressure. In clinical practice this intervention is necessary only when monitoring of arterial blood pressure is essential.

Friction Rub. In some cases of cardiac tamponade, a pericardial friction rub is present; otherwise, precordial examination tends not to be helpful.

LABORATORY FINDINGS. The echocardiogram is definitive. The chest radiograph usually shows cardiac enlargement, but in acute cases the volume of pericardial effusion may be too small to increase the cardiothoracic ratio. The electrocardiogram is often not helpful, but when pericardial effusion is large, especially in cardiac tamponade secondary to neoplasm, electrical alternans may occur. Alternation is usually confined to the QRS complex; more specific for pericardial effusion, but less common, is alternation of P, QRS, and T waves.

TREATMENT. Unless tamponade is mild or moderate and rapidly improves following medical treatment of the cause, prompt removal of pericardial fluid is mandatory. In acute cases only a small portion of the fluid need be removed, because of the steep pressure-volume curve of the pericardium. In experienced hands, pericardiocentesis has an acceptable risk. When experience is limited, tamponade is recurrent, or biopsy is needed, subxiphoid surgical drainage is preferred.

CONSTRICTIVE PERICARDITIS

DEFINITION AND ETIOLOGY. Constrictive pericarditis produces thickening, fibrosis, and often calcification of the pericardium with restriction of the diastolic filling of the ventricles. The most common causes are listed in Table 51–1. In the United States and western Europe, constrictive pericarditis most often is idiopathic, secondary to neoplasm or radiation, post-traumatic, or due to connective tissue disease. Tuberculosis and pyogenic infection are less common causes than they used to be. More subacute and fewer chronic cases are therefore seen, and heavy calcification of the pericardium is less frequent.

PATHOPHYSIOLOGY. The pathophysiology and hemodynamics are shown in Figure 51–5 from the study of a stock car driver with post-traumatic pericarditis. Panel A shows pressures recorded simultaneously from both ventricles. In early diastole there is a prominent dip of pressure, and in mid and late diastole the pressure forms a plateau. The two plateaus are elevated and equal. During early diastole, ventricular filling is faster than normal, signified by the early diastolic dip, at the end of which cardiac volume reaches the limit set by the rigid pericardium. The ventricular diastolic pressures are then elevated but do not rise through the remainder of diastole, signifying absence of further ventricular filling. Elevation of left ventricular diastolic pressure to approximately 20 mm Hg causes elevation of right ventricular systolic pressure.

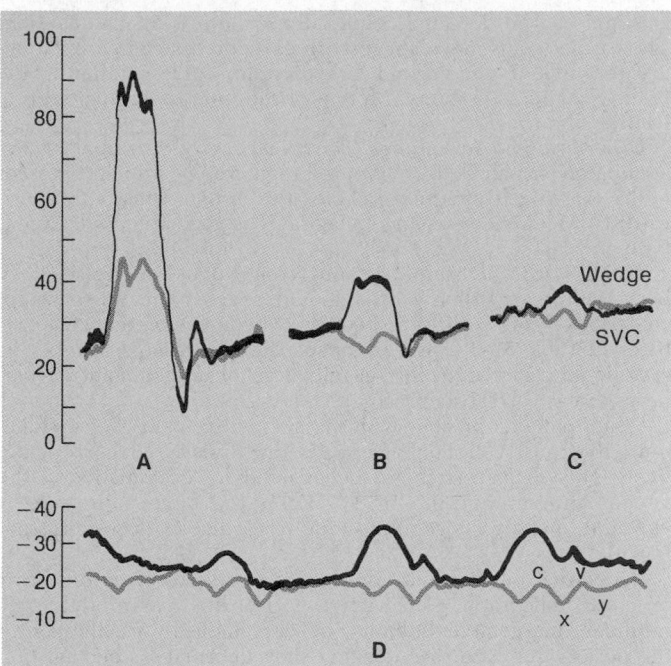

FIGURE 51–5. Hemodynamic data from a case of constrictive pericarditis. See text for details. (From Shabetai R: Profiles of constrictive pericarditis, restrictive cardiomyopathy and cardiac tamponade. *In* Grossman W [ed.]: Cardiac Catheterization and Angiography. 2nd ed. Philadelphia, Lea & Febiger, 1980.)

Panel B shows simultaneous pressure records from the right ventricle and right atrium. In contradistinction to cardiac tamponade, right atrial pressure is biphasic, showing a prominent x descent with ventricular ejection and prominent y descent coincident with the early diastolic dip of ventricular pressure. The y descent can be recognized at the bedside as a sharp inward movement of the jugular pulsation out of phase with the carotid pulse. Respiratory variation is absent. Panel C shows simultaneous pulmonary wedge and superior vena cava pressures, confirming equilibration of filling pressures on the two sides of the heart. Panel D shows pressures simultaneously recorded from the pulmonary artery and the pulmonary wedge position. In late diastole all cardiac pressures equilibrate around 20 mm Hg.

CLINICAL FINDINGS. Elevation of the filling pressure of the left side of the heart causes dyspnea and pulmonary congestion, which in severe cases is evident on the chest radiograph. Elevated filling pressure of the right side of the heart causes peripheral edema; hepatic enlargement, congestion, and dysfunction; and frequently ascites.

When ventricular filling is suddenly checked at the end of the early diastolic pressure dip, a loud third heart sound ("pericardial knock") is frequently audible. The apex beat may not be palpable, or there may be systolic retraction. Ascites is often prominent in relation to peripheral edema. The liver is usually enlarged and pulsatile. When present, palmar erythema, spider angiomas, and mild jaundice testify to severe, chronic hepatic congestion.

The abnormally small ventricular end-diastolic volume reduces stroke volume even when systolic function is well maintained, as it usually is.

LABORATORY FINDINGS. By chest radiography, the heart is normal in size to moderately enlarged. In chronic cases, particularly those associated with tuberculosis, calcification may be seen in the pericardium. The electrocardiogram usually shows T-wave inversions and frequently a wide, notched P wave due to chronic elevation of left atrial pressure. In longstanding cases, atrial fibrillation often supervenes. Liver function test results are abnormal, and hypoalbuminemia may be compounded by protein-losing enteropathy.

Echocardiography. The echocardiogram is less helpful than in pericardial effusion. Sometimes increased thickness of the pericardium can be detected, especially if there is a small effusion. The cardiac walls move abruptly in early diastole and are stationary throughout middle and late diastole, corresponding to the hemodynamic alterations. Motion of the interventricular septum is often abnormal.

Other Imaging Techniques. The thickened pericardium is more adequately visualized by computed tomography, which at present is the imaging technique of choice for chronic constrictive pericarditis. Magnetic resonance imaging is as good and, on occasion, better.

DIAGNOSIS. Systemic venous congestion not explained by heart failure or other causes should suggest the possibility of constrictive pericarditis, especially when one of the etiologies listed in Table 51–1 is present or suspected. Although nonspecific systolic murmurs are common, murmurs of predominant valvular heart disease are absent.

When patients present with massive edema and liver dysfunction, the most common erroneous diagnosis is cirrhosis of the liver. This major error can be avoided by examination of the venous pressure in the neck. When the venous pressure is elevated, anasarca is generally due to cardiac or pericardial, not hepatic, causes.

Pericardial effusion may produce a large "water-bottle" heart on chest radiograph. Constrictive pericarditis may produce only minimal enlargement but may be detectable by calcification of the pericardium. Cardiac imaging shows normal systolic function and normal cardiac valves. The ventricles are often small and fill rapidly in early diastole but not at all for the remainder of diastole. This finding, together with increased thickness of the pericardium, establishes the diagnosis.

Restrictive cardiomyopathy is a disease of heart muscle (see Ch. 50) that mimics constrictive pericarditis. Characteristically, however, left ventricular diastolic pressure exceeds that on the right. In some cases, endomyocardial biopsy and occasionally exploratory thoracotomy are needed to establish the correct diagnosis.

TREATMENT. For the vast majority of patients, the treatment of choice is pericardiectomy. The patient may be prepared by modest diuresis. With modern techniques of cardiopulmonary bypass, especially in cases that are not too far advanced, the operation yields gratifying clinical improvement; although full benefit may not be evident for about 6 months.

Engel PH: Echocardiographic findings in pericardial disease. *In* Fowler NO (ed.): The Pericardium in Health and Disease. Mt. Kisco, NY, Futura Publishing Company, 1985. *An up-to-date, well-written discussion.*

Klopfenstein HS, Schuchard G, Wann LS, et al.: The relative merits of pulsus paradoxus and right ventricular diastolic collapse in the early detection of cardiac tamponade. An experimental echocardiographic study. Circulation 71:829, 1985. *Describes the correlation between hemodynamics and echocardiographic abnormalities in cardiac tamponade.*

Shabetai R: The Pericardium. New York, Grune & Stratton, 1980. *A comprehensive monograph dealing with the normal pericardium and pericardial diseases.*

Shabetai R, Fowler NO, Fenton JC, et al.: Pulsus paradoxus. J Clin Invest 44:1882, 1965. *An experimental study of the mechanisms of pulsus paradoxus.*

Spodick DH: Pathogenesis and clinical correlations of the electrocardiographic abnormalities of pericardial disease. Cardiovasc Clin 8:201, 1977. *A well-illustrated and complete account of theory and clinical application.*

52 Miscellaneous Conditions of the Heart: Tumor, Trauma, and Systemic Disease

Bernadine P. Healy

CARDIAC TUMORS

Tumors of the heart and pericardium are uncommon, and as a cause of clinical cardiac disease they are especially rare. Consecutive autopsy studies suggest that primary tumors of the heart are seen in only 1 in 2000 postmortem examinations; tumors secondary to metastases are roughly 20 times more frequent than primary lesions. A number of factors have made cardiac tumors a more visible current medical problem. With improved medical diagnostic technology, we are more apt to recognize both primary and secondary cardiac tumors; and with better therapy, patients with metastatic neoplasms live longer, increasing the likelihood for the heart to develop secondary cancers.

In part because of their relative rarity as a cause of clinical heart disease, cardiac tumors often go unrecognized. A general awareness of the pathophysiology of the heart afflicted with tumor and the ways in which it so often mimics more common forms of heart disease is essential to diagnosis and recognition of options for therapeutic intervention.

Primary Tumors of the Heart

Primary tumors of the heart are almost always benign and are considerably less common than tumors secondary to metastatic disease. The myxoma, of endocardial origin, is overwhelmingly the most common and best known of the primary cardiac tumors. Less common is the rhabdomyoma, a benign congenital tumor of myocardium most often seen in children. The sarcoma is the predominant malignant form of primary heart tumor and includes a variety of types, such as rhabdomyosarcoma, angiosarcoma, and fibrosarcoma. Among these tumor types, the myxoma is of greatest clinical importance in terms of relative frequency, tendency to produce symptoms, and ease of diagnosis and therapy.

The cardiac myxoma has been recognized as a pathologic entity for several hundred years, occurring with an incidence of about 0.03 per cent at autopsy. Myxomas are typically solitary, smooth-surfaced, globular tumors, which vary in size from 1 to 8 cm (average 5 cm), and most are pedunculated. In about 90 per cent of cases they occur in the left atrium; most of the rest occur in the right atrium. They are attached to the interatrial septum in the region of the fossa ovalis. Clinical presentation is related to location of the tumor, as well as to the presence of a pedicle. Larger myxomas, generally over 3 cm in diameter, are more apt to be symptomatic. The presence of a pedicle, allowing the myxomas to move about in the cardiac chambers, also correlates with symptomatology.

Myxomas occur most frequently (75 per cent) in women and usually manifest with symptoms in persons between the ages of 35 and 60 years. Because myxomas are most commonly located in the left atrium, signs and symptoms of cardiac dysfunction are usually referable to left-sided cardiac disease. The most common clinical cardiac problem is congestive heart failure, present in roughly half of patients, and often the heart failure is paroxysmal and precipitated by positional change, such as lying down. Other signs include chest pain, murmurs of mitral stenosis or regurgitation or both, syncope, and arrhythmias (including atrial fibrillation, often paroxysmal in nature). Other, noncardiac manifestations of atrial myxomas include systemic or pulmonary embolism, fever, malaise, arthralgias, and hematologic abnormalities suggestive of chronic infection. With these clinical manifestations, it is not surprising that atrial myxomas often have been misdiagnosed as rheumatic mitral valve disease, infective endocarditis, fever of unknown origin, or connective tissue disease. Indeed, cardiac myxomas may be viewed as the "great simulators"; their correct clinical diagnosis is among the most challenging in internal medicine.

Some of the challenge and error in the clinical recognition of cardiac myxomas have been diminished by the advent of improved noninvasive techniques. Echocardiography, particularly two-dimensional study, readily identifies atrial tumors and has virtually eliminated the need for invasive contrast angiography. Radionuclide ventriculography (gated blood cardiac scan) will also identify a moving filling defect within the cardiac chambers and can be used in making the diagnosis of intracavitary tumor. Once the diagnosis of cardiac myxoma has been made, the only treatment is surgical excision. Undiagnosed atrial myxomas are often fatal, but when considered, are readily detected and, once detected, straightforwardly treated and virtually always cured.

Secondary Tumors of the Heart

The heart may be a target for secondary tumor invasion. Cancer has been reported to involve the heart in anywhere from 5 to 20 per cent of patients with metastatic malignant disease, with an apparent increase in reported involvement of the heart in recent years. Almost any type of primary neoplasm may involve the heart. Malignant melanomas are among the most common solid tumors that spread to the heart. Cardiac lesions occur in 40 to 50 per cent of patients with metastatic disease, and as a group, melanomas constitute approximately 3 per cent of all cardiac metastases. Leukemias frequently infiltrate the heart, with microscopic invasion evident in approximately half of patients. Other tumors that frequently metastasize to the heart include carcinomas of the lung, breast, and thyroid, the lymphomas, and the sarcomas, including Kaposi's sarcoma. Carcinomas of the lung and breast, because of their relative frequency among malignancies, together account for approximately 50 per cent of the secondary tumors of the heart.

What is most striking about cardiac invasion by metastatic tumor is that it is so often clinically silent, despite what may be extensive disease. The clinical manifestations of cardiac metastases are myriad and generally reflect the anatomic site of invasion. Congestive heart failure, cardiac arrhythmias, and signs of pericardial constriction are among the most common clinical manifestations of cardiac metastases. Myocardial ischemia and infarction may also result from coronary compression or invasion. Although most cardiac metastases are diagnosed post mortem, they may be clinically detected by a variety of means. When a malignant pericardial effusion is present, cytologic examination of pericardial fluid readily provides diagnosis. Identification of a mass in one or more cardiac chambers or of an irregularity in chamber contour or wall thickness may be accomplished by cross-sectional cardiac echocardiography, radionuclide ventriculography, or invasive contrast angiography. Pathologic examination is necessary, however, to identify tumor type. Unlike treatment for myxomas, surgery for primary or secondary malignancies of the heart is generally ineffective. The major role for cardiac surgery is to obtain tissue for pathologic diagnosis or to alleviate mechanical obstruction. Radiotherapy and chemotherapy are utilized, depending on tumor type.

CARDIAC DISEASE SECONDARY TO CANCER THERAPY. Cardiac disease or dysfunction may also occur as a consequence of chemotherapy and radiotherapy and may obscure even further the diagnosis of metastatic tumors of the heart. Many of the antineoplastic drugs, particularly doxorubicin (Adriamycin), produce a dose-dependent toxicity that leads to a dilated congestive cardiomyopathy. Doxorubicin causes a characteristic degeneration of the myocyte that can be detected by myocardial biopsy. Radiotherapy may also produce dose-dependent cardiac damage to all three layers of the heart. Pericarditis and pericardial effusions are most common, but fibrosis of the myocardium and of mural and valvular endocardium may occur. Prevention is the best therapy for radiation- and drug-induced cardiac damage, which is generally irreversible.

CARDIAC TRAUMA

Trauma is a major cause of morbidity and mortality in our society, and tragically it often affects those who are otherwise healthy. Cardiac trauma results from either a penetrating object or a nonpenetrating blunt assault on the thorax. Death may immediately occur as a result of asystole, ventricular fibrillation, or exsanguination. Those who survive long enough for transport to a hospital pose immediate diagnostic and therapeutic challenges.

Penetrating wounds of the heart are believed to be fatal in over 90 per cent of instances, with most patients never reaching medical attention. Stab and gunshot wounds may lacerate any portion of the heart. Pericardial laceration with cardiac tamponade or exsanguination is most common, usually in conjunction with rupture of some portion of the myocardium. Because of their anterior location, the right ventricle and pulmonary outflow tract are particularly susceptible. Valve lacerations leading to incompetence and coronary injuries leading to ischemia or infarction, or both, are of particular importance for survivors, who may be left with residual lesions.

The diagnosis of cardiac trauma in the setting of a penetrating wound of the thoracic cavity is not always straightforward. Patients usually present acutely with hypotension due either to cardiac tamponade or to hemorrhage. The diagnosis is assumed when profound hypotension is present in the setting of a penetrating mediastinal wound with or without an object in or near the cardiac silhouette. In this setting, emergency thoracotomy, preferably in an operating room, is virtually always necessary for both diagnosis and therapy. The wisdom of performing a diagnostic pericardiocentesis has been challenged, as false-negative readings may result from local clot formation. Pericardiocentesis may be necessary, however, to stabilize a patient with cardiac tamponade prior to emergency thoracotomy. Once the diagnosis of trauma has been made and cardiac surgical repair initiated, the survival rate may be as high as 70 per cent.

Nonpenetrating trauma to the chest cavity may also cause a similar range of cardiac injuries requiring emergency thoracotomy. Unlike penetrating wounds, however, physical evidence of trauma to the chest wall may be minimal or even absent, and the severity of chest wall trauma does not correlate with likelihood or extent of cardiac injury. Among the most common causes of cardiac trauma are steering wheel injuries to the sternum. Others include sports activities, industrial accidents, and personal assaults. The myocardium is the major site of injuries, which may range in severity from mild myocardial contusion to rupture of the ventricle or interventricular septum. Pericardial laceration, valve disruption, coronary artery thrombosis, or great vessel rupture, particularly of the ascending aorta, may also occur.

Diagnosis is difficult, since symptoms are often absent or misleading. Symptoms of chest pain similar to that associated with myocardial infarction are the most frequent. Cardiac arrhythmias and hypotension may also signal cardiac injury in the proper setting. Survivors of myocardial injury may develop false aneurysms with their usual complications. Early and late cardiac arrhythmias (atrial or ventricular) may be caused by myocardial contusions, and the electrocardiographic abnormalities may include those of myocardial infarction or acute pericarditis. Serum enzyme assays (creatine kinase, MB fraction) and echocardiography are helpful in making the diagnosis, and if coronary compromise is suggested, cardiac catheterization with coronary angiography would be appropriate. Treatment depends on the extent of cardiovascular compromise. Pain and arrhythmias alone are treated similarly to those of acute myocardial infarction, except that anticoagulants should be strictly avoided. Thoracotomy is necessary if there are signs of myocardial rupture or pericardial tamponade. Late complications, such as valvular or interventricular septal rupture or false aneurysms of the heart or aorta, require surgical correction.

CARDIAC MANIFESTATIONS OF SYSTEMIC DISEASE

The heart may be afflicted secondarily by a variety of systemic conditions and diseases. The most frequent cardiac manifestations of systemic disease are those common disorders that primarily involve the vascular system and produce cardiac dysfunction by virtue of increased volume or pressure load on the heart or interruption in blood flow to the myocardium. Systemic hypertension, whether essential, renal, or endocrine in cause, often leads to cardiac hypertrophy and heart failure. Atherosclerosis is a systemic vascular disease with the heart as a prime target. Less common are the anemias, which produce a volume load and at times hypoxic insult to the heart, leading to congestive heart failure. In addition to these widely recognized disorders, there are several systemic diseases that secondarily involve the heart in a distinctive fashion. Examples of these disorders include the connective tissue diseases (e.g., systemic lupus erythematosus [SLE], progressive systemic sclerosis, and polyarteritis nodosa); endocrine-humoral disorders (thyroid disease, pheochromocytoma, and metastatic carcinoid); and systemic infiltrative disease (amyloidosis).

CONNECTIVE TISSUE DISEASES. Although the connective tissue diseases may affect the heart only secondarily, the cardiac disorder may dominate the clinical course. In systemic lupus erythematosus, the endocardium, myocardium, and pericardium all are potential targets. A fibrinous pericarditis is a common cardiac lesion and frequently produces clinical symptoms. Fibrofibrinous thrombotic lesions may develop on the surface of the cardiac valves (a condition termed Libman-Sacks endocarditis) and are usually clinically silent. On occasion this endocarditis may lead to significant mitral or aortic valve dysfunction. Myocarditis may occur but is an infrequent result of SLE. Coronary arteritis and thromboembolism may also develop, and in patients with corticosteroid-treated lupus, in particular, there may be accelerated coronary atherosclerosis.

Progressive systemic sclerosis (PSS) or scleroderma may produce cardiac dysfunction by means of its effect on the myocardium. Focal fibrosis and necrosis of myocardium may lead to a picture of dilated congestive cardiomyopathy. Morphologic and clinical evidence now suggests that the etiology of the myocardial disease in PSS is small vessel coronary spasm, causing ischemia, i.e., a Raynaud's phenomenon of the coronary arteries. Polyarteritis nodosa may cause a focal or a diffuse coronary arteritis, with formation of coronary thrombosis or aneurysm or both. The latter may lead to myocardial ischemia or infarction and, combined with systemic hypertension, to congestive heart failure. Cardiac manifestations of the connective tissue diseases are diagnosed and treated with the standard technology and methods used for valvular, myocardial, pericardial, or coronary disease. Therapy also includes the immunosuppressive drugs used for treatment of the systemic diseases.

ENDOCRINE-HUMORAL DISORDERS. Thyroid disease has long been known to target the heart. Thyroid hormone increases oxygen consumption and metabolic rate, has a direct inotropic and chronotropic effect on the heart, and has been shown to have a direct trophic effect on the myocardium, inducing a physiologic pattern of hypertrophy. The major clinical manifestation of thyroid hormone excess is a hyperkinetic heart and circulation. Other symptoms include a variety of arrhythmias (atrial fibrillation, in particular), and, with severe disease, congestive heart failure may develop. Although less common, hypothyroidism may produce an idiopathic dilated cardiomyopathy, but its etiology is obscure. More often, hypothyroidism causes bradycardia and pericardial effusions. The latter may contain cholesterol crystals, a finding believed to be characteristic of a myxedema-associated effusion. Identification of the basis for these cardiac disorders is confirmed by abnormal serum thyroxine levels. Thyroid hormone levels should be obtained routinely in patients with idiopathic atrial fibrillation and in those with heart failure of obscure etiology.

Pheochromocytomas, which are chromaffin cell tumors, produce norepinephrine and, to a varying degree, epinephrine, which may cause systemic hypertension as well as induce direct myocardial toxicity. Autopsy studies have shown focal myocardial contraction band necrosis and fibrosis in as many as 50 per cent of patients with this tumor. Similar lesions may be produced in experimental animals with catecholamine infusions and are believed to relate to norepinephrine-induced calcium overload. Although this tumor may cause cardiomyopathy, it is exceedingly rare.

CARDIAC AMYLOIDOSIS. This disorder may be primary but occurs most often secondary to systemic conditions, including multiple myeloma, systemic amyloidosis, familial Mediterranean fever, and aging. Amyloid may infiltrate myocardium and coronary arteries, and less often the cardiac valves, and typically causes increased myocardial mass and focal fibrosis. The latter leads to decreased myocardial compliance and ultimately congestive heart failure—a picture that may simulate hypertrophic or restrictive cardiomyopathy. Cardiac amyloid deposits may also affect the conduction system of the heart, causing a variety of arrhythmias. The diagnosis of cardiac amyloid is confirmed by myocardial biopsy. Therapy for the cardiac dysfunction of amyloidosis is the standard treatment for arrhythmias or heart failure or both. A proclivity to digitalis toxicity, possibly related to conduction system infiltration by amyloid, should be considered when treating heart failure in these patients.

Doherty NE, Siegel RJ: Cardiovascular manifestations of systemic lupus erythematosus. Am Heart J 110:1257, 1985. *A review article summarizing present information on the clinical and morphologic aspects of the heart in systemic lupus erythematosus.*

Follansbee WP, Curtiss EI, Medsger TA, et al.: Physiologic abnormalities of cardiac function in progressive systemic sclerosis with diffuse scleroderma. N Engl J Med 310:142, 1984. *Description of cardiac dysfunction in patients with PSS, showing by noninvasive techniques the relationship of circulatory disturbances to ventricular dysfunction.*

Frazee RC, Mucha P Jr, Farnell MB, et al.: Objective evaluation of blunt cardiac trauma. J Trauma 26:510, 1986. *A review of the cardiovascular consequences of blunt chest trauma, describing CK-MB elevations, arrhythmias, and ven-*

tricular dysfunction as assessed by echocardiography in a wide range of cardiac injuries.

McDonnell PJ, Mann RB, Bulkley BH: Involvement of the heart by malignant lymphoma: A clinicopathologic study. Cancer 49:944, 1982. *A clinicopathologic study of the cardiovascular manifestations of lymphomatous involvement of the heart and a general review of the range of malignant tumors of the heart and how they cause cardiac dysfunction.*

Morkin E, Flink IL, Goldman S: Biochemical and physiologic effects of thyroid hormone on cardiac performance. Prog Cardiovasc Dis 25:435, 1983. *An in-depth and current review of the effect of thyroid hormone on the normal heart and its role in disease.*

Salcedo EE, Adams KV, Lever HM, et al.: Echocardiographic findings in 25 patients with left atrial myxoma. J Am Coll Cardiol 1:1162, 1983. *Describes the use of echocardiography to diagnose myxomas noninvasively.*

Schrader ML, Hochman JS, Bulkley BH: The heart in polyarteritis nodosa: A clinicopathologic study. Am Heart J 109:1353, 1985. *A clinicopathologic study of the heart in polyarteritis nodosa and a review of the literature.*

Skhvatsabaja LV: Secondary malignant lesions of the heart and pericardium in neoplastic disease. Oncology 43:103, 1986. *A review of clinical and laboratory data in 240 patients with metastatic tumors of the heart and pericardium, focusing on clinical symptoms and diagnosis.*

53 Diseases of the Aorta

Lawrence S. Cohen

The aorta is vital to the proper functioning of every organ system in the body. The coronary arteries are the first arteries to arise from the aorta, followed by vessels of the head and central nervous system and then the gastrointestinal, renal, and genitourinary arteries. Disease in any segment of the aorta, therefore, can have profound consequences upon bodily function. The aorta is susceptible to four major disease processes: *aneurysm, dissection, arteriosclerotic occlusive disease,* and *aortitis.*

At its origin the aorta is approximately 3 cm in diameter. The ascending aorta is approximately 5 cm in length, coursing in a left-to-right direction in the same ejection axis as the left ventricle. The aortic arch is also approximately 5 cm in length and takes an upward, posterior, and leftward direction, terminating along the left border of the thoracic vertebrae. The aortic arch lies entirely within the superior mediastinum. The descending thoracic aorta is contained in the posterior mediastinum. It is a bit narrower than the ascending aorta and is approximately 20 cm in length. It runs to the diaphragm at the level of the twelfth thoracic vertebra and supplies the arteries to the spinal cord. The abdominal aorta is the continuation of the thoracic aorta, ending at the level of the fourth lumbar vertebra. The average length is 15 cm, with an average diameter of 2 cm at its origin and a slightly smaller diameter at its lower end.

ANEURYSM

Definition

An aneurysm is a widening of a vessel involving the stretching of fibrous tissue within the media of the vessel. A true aneurysm is a widening of the vessel, whereas a false aneurysm represents a localized rupture of the artery with sealing over by clot or adjacent structures. The natural history of aneurysms is to enlarge. Not only does the etiologic process tend to continue and progress but also the law of Laplace is a factor. As described by Laplace, the tension in the wall of a spherical chamber enclosing a fluid under pressure is related to the pressure under which the fluid is kept and the radius of curvature of the containing vessel. As the radius increases so does wall tension. Hence, enlargement of the vessel begets more enlargement.

It is convenient to classify aneurysms according to etiology, morphology, and location. Arteriosclerosis is the most common cause of aneurysms. Other causes are cystic medial necrosis, trauma, and infection, including syphilis. Rarer causes are rheumatic aortitis, Takayasu's syndrome, temporal arteritis, and relapsing polychondritis. Marfan's syndrome is characterized by cystic medial necrosis (Ch. 187). In some forms of Ehlers-Danlos syndrome, rupture of blood vessels, including the aorta, may occur. Aneurysms can be classified into three morphologic types: (1) fusiform, in which the aneurysm encompasses the entire circumference of the aorta and assumes a spindle shape; (2)

saccular, in which only a portion of the circumference is involved and in which there is a neck and an asymmetric outpouching of the aneurysm; and (3) dissecting, in which an intimal tear permits a column of blood to dissect along the media of the vessel. This is often called a dissecting hematoma. Location is a further way to classify aneurysms. Aneurysms involve (1) the ascending aorta, including the sinuses of Valsalva; (2) the aortic arch; (3) the descending thoracic aorta, originating just distal to the left subclavian artery; and (4) the abdomen, most commonly distal to the renal arteries.

The most proximal portion of the ascending aorta comprises the sinuses of Valsalva. Aneurysms in this location are usually congenital in origin. Most involve either the right sinus or the right portion of the noncoronary sinus. Aneurysms of the sinus of Valsalva are often silent until they rupture into the right side of the heart, usually the right ventricle or right atrium. This event may occur spontaneously or may be a consequence of infective endocarditis. Other causes of aortic sinus aneurysm are Marfan's syndrome, syphilis, and infective endocarditis. Aneurysms of the ascending aorta may be arteriosclerotic, but cystic medial necrosis with or without other features of Marfan's syndrome is more common. Syphilis was once a common cause of ascending aortic aneurysm but has all but disappeared as an etiology. The more distal the aortic location of the aneurysm, the more likely it is to be arteriosclerotic.

Clinical Manifestations

Clinical manifestations of aneurysms of the thoracic aorta (other than rupture) are due to compression, distortion, or erosion of surrounding structures. Pain is the most common symptom. Pain in a gradually enlarging aneurysm is insidious and may be described as boring and deep. Increasing intensity of pain is an ominous sign and may presage impending rupture.

Aortic valve regurgitation may be associated with aneurysms of the ascending aorta. Distortion of the aortic annulus and separation of the aortic valve cusps accounts for the regurgitation. If regurgitation occurs rapidly, the clinical consequences can be dramatic, with the patient developing acute pulmonary edema. Many patients develop a murmur of aortic regurgitation gradually and may be relatively asymptomatic. Aneurysms of the transverse aortic arch are less common than are aneurysms in other sites. The consequences of such aneurysms are often formidable, since the innominate and carotid arteries arise from the transverse aortic arch. In addition, the arch is contiguous with other vital structures such as the superior vena cava, pulmonary artery, trachea, bronchi, lung, and left recurrent laryngeal nerve. Symptoms may include dyspnea, stridor, hoarseness, hemoptysis, cough, or chest pain.

The most common site of an aneurysm of the descending thoracic aorta is between the origin of the left subclavian artery and the diaphragm. Arteriosclerosis is the most common cause, with age, hypertension, and probably smoking contributing as risk factors. One factor in the pathogenesis of aneurysms of the descending aorta may be the immobility of the aorta at this site and the unique stresses imposed on the aorta immediately distal to the left subclavian artery. Distortion of the architecture in this area may result in sufficient turbulence to cause elastic tissue degeneration, accelerated arteriosclerosis, and localized dilatation.

Pain from descending thoracic aortic aneurysm is often intrascapular but can vary considerably. Hoarseness may occur from stretching of the left recurrent laryngeal nerve. Hemoptysis may occur owing to leakage into the left lung. Thoracic aortic aneurysms, like those of the abdominal aorta, threaten life by potential rupture. They are rarely complicated by thrombosis or embolism. Thoracoabdominal aneurysms involve the celiac, superior mesenteric, and renal arteries. Fortunately, they are not common, for they represent a great challenge to the vascular surgeon. Although some are caused by cystic medial necrosis, most are of arteriosclerotic origin and occur in older men.

The most common form of aneurysm is the abdominal aortic aneurysm. The prevalence of this aneurysm at autopsy is in the 1 to 3 per cent range but is even more common in men over 60. Its frequency in men outnumbers that in women by 6:1. Almost all of these aneurysms are below the renal arteries. Most are of arteriosclerotic origin, but trauma, infection (including syphilis),

and arteritis make up a small fraction. A fortunate feature of these aneurysms is their accessibility on physical examination. Rupture of an abdominal aneurysm is the greatest threat and may lead to a rapid demise because of shock and hypotension. Other less acute symptoms may also occur. Pain in the lower back is a sign of enlargement of the aneurysm and at times is a warning of impending rupture. Almost all abdominal aortic aneurysms are lined with clot or have ulcerated plaques. Embolization of atherothrombotic material may lead to a variety of symptoms, ranging from digital infarction to anuria from a shower of emboli to the kidneys.

The likelihood of rupture increases with increasing aortic aneurysm size. Sixty to 80 per cent of patients with lesions 7 cm or larger die of rupture, and 95 per cent of patients with lesions over 10 cm die of aneurysm rupture. The risk of rupture in aneurysms 5 cm or less is considerably lower. Given these data, general guidelines about surgical repair have emerged. Aneurysms associated with aortic thrombosis or distal embolic events should be repaired promptly. Aneurysms suspected of rupture or acute expansion should be treated surgically immediately. Although there are differences of opinion concerning when elective repair of asymptomatic aneurysms should be undertaken, once the aneurysm exceeds 5 cm in diameter, the prognosis on continued medical management becomes increasingly guarded.

Diagnosis

Palpation is usually the first step in diagnosing abdominal aneurysms. Ultrasound imaging is an excellent technique to confirm the diagnosis, as it is noninvasive, inexpensive, and accurate to within 2 to 3 mm of aneurysm size when compared with the findings at surgery. Computed tomographic (CT) scanning utilizing contrast material is equal in effectiveness to ultrasound in the detection and sizing of abdominal aortic aneurysms. Often lumbar spine x-ray films clearly outline the walls of an abdominal aortic aneurysm if there is calcium in the walls. Aortography, either arterial or venous with digital subtraction, may not reflect the true size of the aneurysm; an extensive laminated clot may reduce the lumen.

Joyce JW: Aneurysmal disease. *In* Spittell JA Jr (ed.): Clinical Vascular Disease. Philadelphia, F. A. Davis Company, 1983, pp 89–101. *A concise summary of aneurysmal disease, including management guidelines for aneurysms in all aortic locations.*
Spittell JA Jr: Abdominal aortic aneurysms. Hosp Pract 21:105, 1986. *This is a short, well-illustrated practical management update. Modern diagnostic tools are discussed, and management strategies are reviewed.*

DISSECTING ANEURYSM OF THE AORTA

The incidence of aortic dissections is not known exactly, but it is estimated that approximately 2000 acute cases occur in the United States each year.

Classification of aortic dissection is based upon duration and anatomic location of the dissection. Dissection is considered acute if it occurred within 2 weeks, and chronic if it occurred more than 2 weeks, prior to the institution of therapy.

Aortic dissection is more commonly classified by site of the intimal tear and extent of dissecting hematoma. In type I and type II dissections, the intimal tear is in the ascending aorta, usually within a few centimeters of the aortic valve. In type I aneurysms, the dissecting hematoma extends and involves at least the aortic arch and often the descending aorta as well. Type II aneurysms involve the ascending aorta only. Type III aneurysms are characterized by an intimal tear in the descending aorta, usually immediately distal to the left subclavian artery. The dissecting hematoma usually propagates distally but at times may extend in a retrograde manner to the aortic arch (Fig. 53–1).

Etiology

The most consistent etiologic factor in aortic disection is hypertension. Other conditions are associated with dissection in the absence of hypertension. Marfan's syndrome has been discussed. There is a peculiar association between pregnancy and dissection. It is postulated that hormonal changes during pregnancy may alter the composition of the aorta and make it more susceptible to rupture. Stresses and strains of labor may also be a factor.

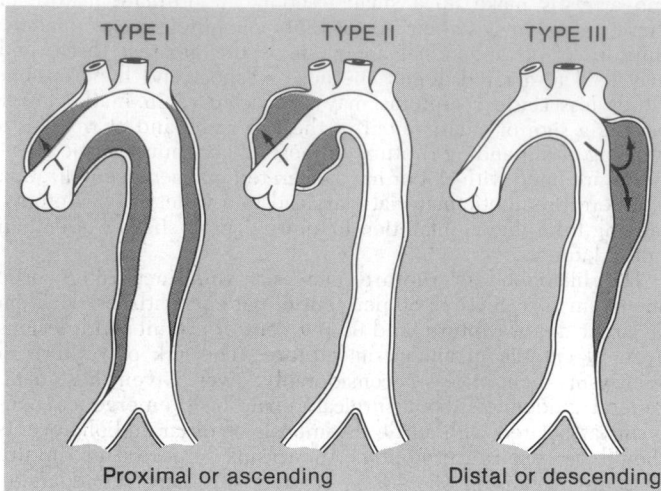

TYPE I   TYPE II   TYPE III

Proximal or ascending   Distal or descending

FIGURE 53–1. Classification of dissecting aneurysms of the aorta. (Modified from DeBakey.)

Valvular aortic stenosis, particularly that due to a bicuspid valve, is associated with dissection. Turbulence established beyond the stenotic valve increases lateral forces, thereby enhancing the likelihood of an intimal tear and development of a dissection. The association between coarctation of the aorta and dissection is well known. The years of proximal aortic hypertension prior to repair of the coarctation may establish the conditions that ultimately lead to aortic dissection. In addition, there is a high incidence of bicuspid aortic valves in patients with coarctation of the aorta. Before the advent of antimicrobial agents, syphilitic aortitis was the most common cause of aortic dissection. It is now unusual. Trauma may be a cause of dissecting aneurysm. Other unusual etiologies are the Ehlers-Danlos syndrome and relapsing polychondritis.

Pathogenesis

Aortic dissection begins most frequently in an intimal tear in the ascending aorta a short distance above the aortic valve. The primary tear is often referred to as the *entry intimal tear*. The *re-entry* or *secondary tear* occurs more distally. The basic pathologic condition resides in the underlying media, the chief supporting layer of the aorta. Most tears are transverse or circumferential, reflecting the direction of the muscular fibers of the media.

The two key ingredients of aortic dissection are arterial hypertension and medial degeneration. In any given patient, one or the other of these abnormalities may be the more important. Many patients with Marfan's syndrome or the Ehlers-Danlos syndrome develop dissecting aneurysms without ever developing hypertension. Alternatively, individuals with longstanding hypertension may develop dissection without any apparent specific weakness of the aortic medial wall. Additional factors in the pathogenesis of aortic dissections are the anatomy and motion of the heart and great vessels themselves. The heart beats an average of 70 times per minute, over 80,000 times per day, and over 35 million times per year. The heart is not absolutely fixed in place but is limited in its anterior-posterior movement by the sternum and vertebral column, respectively. Its motion is both side to side and twisting as it ejects blood into the ascending aorta. This produces a flexing stress in the ascending aorta and contributes to the frequency of ascending aortic dissections. The descending aorta becomes fixed distal to the left subclavian artery, accounting for the alternative predilection for dissection to occur at that site. Once an intimal tear occurs, the dissecting hematoma is propagated through the weakened medial wall. The forces that continue the propagation are the arterial pressure and the pulse wave properties (dp/dt) of left ventricular ejection. Some dissecting hematomas rupture back into the aortic lumen at a distal site. Rupture may also occur externally into the pericardial or pleural space.

Clinical Manifestations

Pain is often excruciating and may occur primarily in the anterior chest. It may migrate to the back as the dissecting hematoma works it way down the aorta. Patients sometimes describe an accentuation of the pain with each heart beat, suggesting the driving force of the pulse wave. Pain may occur in the neck, jaw, or teeth if the aortic arch is involved. Less common symptoms are syncope, stroke, paraplegia, or loss of pulses in any of the extremities. Rarely, a dissection may be clinically silent and be suggested only by an abnormal roentgenogram. If aortic regurgitation occurs owing to the dissection, patients may develop congestive heart failure. A diastolic murmur is usually present in these circumstances, although the duration of the murmur may be relatively short if the filling pressure in the left ventricle rises rapidly because of the acute nature of the regurgitation. Such murmurs may be heard commonly along the right sternal border.

The clinical presentation and physical findings in patients with aortic dissection are determined by the course taken by the dissecting hematoma. (1) Loss of any pulse can occur as the circulation to any major artery arising from the aorta may be compromised. (2) Aortic regurgitation may result from disruption of the supporting structures of the aortic valve. (3) Neurologic symptoms may occur if the head and neck vessels are compromised by the dissection. Paraplegia may occur owing to loss of blood supply to the spinal cord. A number of other physical findings may be seen in patients with aortic dissection. These include Horner's syndrome due to compression of the superior cervical ganglion, vocal cord paralysis and hoarseness due to pressure against the recurrent laryngeal nerve, superior vena cava syndrome, pulsating neck masses, dyspnea due to tracheal or bronchial compression, hemorrhagic pleural effusion, myocardial infarction if the hematoma dissects retrograde across a coronary ostium, and symptoms and signs of mesenteric infarction. Persistent fever has also been described.

Diagnosis

Time is often of utmost importance in management. Once the patient is stabilized, aortography should not be delayed. Routine laboratory tests do not generally add much to the diagnosis. Leukocytosis is a common but nonspecific finding. A chest roentgenogram may be normal but will often show widening of the aortic shadow (Fig. 53–2). Aortic angiography is the definitive procedure, yielding precise information necessary for proper management. The extent of the dissection, the entry and reentry

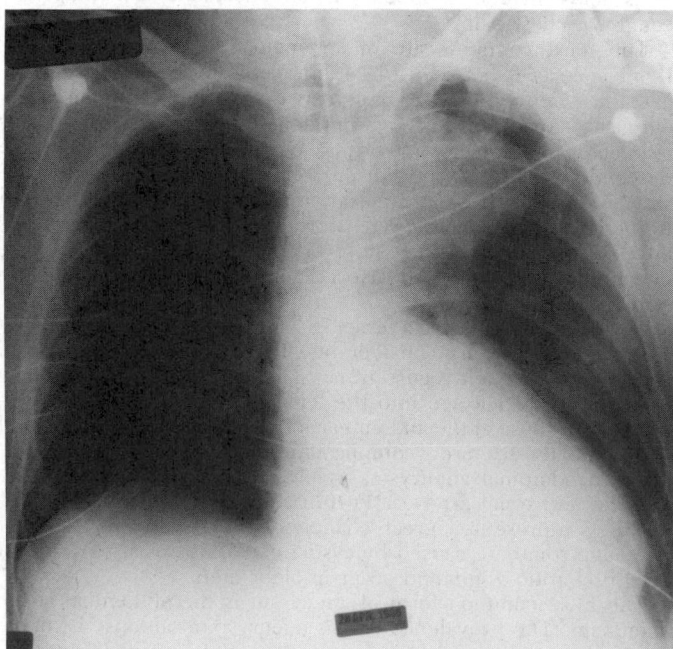

FIGURE 53–2. Chest roentgenogram of a patient with a dissecting aneurysm demonstrating marked enlargement of the aortic arch and descending aorta.

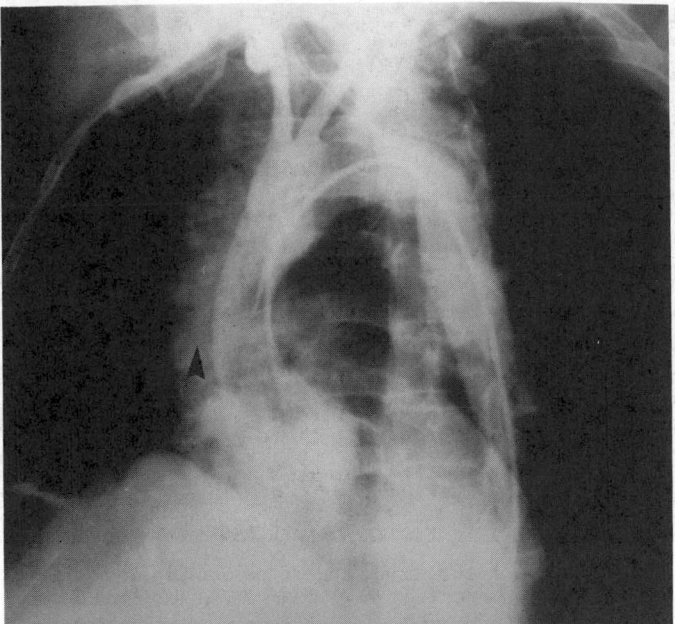

FIGURE 53–3. Aortic root angiogram in the left anterior oblique projection. The black arrowhead demonstrates the false lumen caused by the aortic dissection.

sites, the competence or degree of regurgitation of the aortic valve, and aortic branch vessel involvement can all be ascertained (Fig. 53–3).

The differential diagnosis of a patient with chest or back pain, pulmonary edema with a new murmur of aortic regurgitation, any acute neurologic syndrome, or sudden loss of pulse in an extremity should include aortic dissection.

Computed tomography with the use of contrast material is also highly accurate in demonstrating aortic dissection, although it is not always possible to perform this examination rapidly. Two-dimensional echocardiography does not necessitate the use of contrast agents or ionizing radiation and is easily performed. False-negative and false-positive diagnoses remain a problem with this procedure, but it is nevertheless useful (Fig. 53–4). Transesophageal echocardiography is a powerful new diagnostic tool, as the majority of the aorta can be imaged well from the transducer placed in the esophagus (Fig. 53–5). Magnetic resonance imaging is also capable of diagnosing aortic dissection and does not require the use of contrast agents for vascular imaging.

Prognosis

In untreated aortic dissection, the prognosis is poor. Approximately 20 per cent of patients die in 24 hours, 60 per cent in 2 weeks, and 90 per cent in 3 months. The principal cause of death is not the initial intimal tear but is related to the effects of propagation of the dissecting hematoma. Progressive aortic regurgitation may occur if the hematoma dissects in a retrograde direction. Rupture into the pericardial or pleural space is often a fatal complication.

Treatment

Prompt diagnosis and institution of therapy are critical to the success of treatment. Since the most important known factors in the propagation of the dissecting hematoma are hypertension and the rate of rise of the aortic pressure pulse (dp/dt), efforts must be undertaken to alter both of these. An intravenous drip of sodium nitroprusside is started, and the infusion is titrated to reduce the systolic blood pressure to 100 to 120 mm Hg. The infusion rate can usually be started at 1 μg per kilogram per minute. Simultaneously, propranolol should be given in intermittent intravenous boluses of 0.5 to 1.0 mg until the heart rate is in the range of 60 beats per minute. When possible, an intra-arterial line to measure blood pressure accurately and a central venous line or Swan-Ganz catheter should be utilized. Once the patient's blood pressure and other hemodynamic and clinical features are stable, aortography should be performed. Computed tomographic scanning or echocardiography may be of some diagnostic aid at this stage while awaiting aortography.

Operative intervention is usually indicated if the dissection involves the ascending aorta, as in types I and II aneurysms. These aneurysms are unstable and pose the threat of retrograde dissection, rupture, severe aortic regurgitation, or fatal pericardial tamponade. This type of acute dissection can be corrected surgically with a mortality rate in the range of 20 per cent. Type III aneurysms that involve the distal or descending aorta can generally be treated medically. If the patient's condition stabilizes, drug therapy can be continued into the chronic phase. Surgical intervention for the patient with a type III aneurysm is indicated if there is evidence of increasing size of the dissecting hematoma, impending rupture, inability to control pain, or bleeding into the pleural space.

The operative approach must be flexible and individualized. For patients with ascending aortic dissection and involvement of the annulus or root, it is often necessary to replace the entire

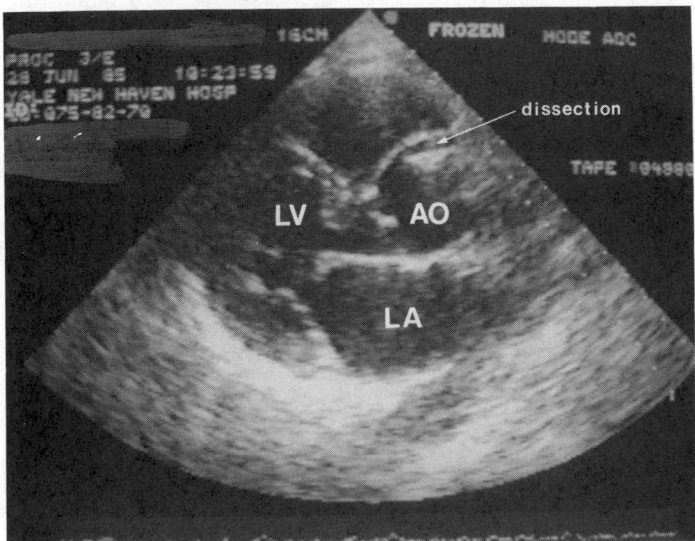

FIGURE 53–4. Echocardiogram, long-axis parasternal view of a patient with dissecting aneurysm. The dissection arises in the proximal aortic root. LV = Left ventricle; AO = aortic root; LA = left atrium.

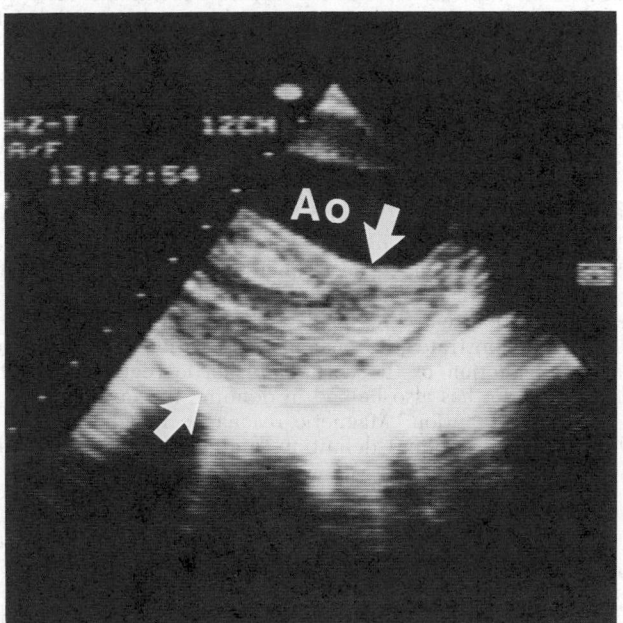

FIGURE 53–5. Transesophageal echocardiogram demonstrating an ascending aortic dissection. The top arrow points to an intraluminal clot. The bottom arrow points to the outer aortic wall.

aortic root and aortic valve with a composite conduit, which is attached proximally to the aortic annulus and distally to the aorta after obliteration of the false lumen. The coronary ostia are then reimplanted into the tubular graft. If the ascending aorta is involved but the sinuses of Valsalva are spared, operative repair consists of resection of the aneurysmal portion with replacement by a synthetic tubular graft. This same technique applies for descending aortic dissections. In all cases, the false lumen is obliterated. Management and follow-up of patients initially treated either surgically or medically is the same. Continued meticulous control of blood pressure and administration of β blockers to control dp/dt are warranted. The systolic blood pressure should be kept below 130 mm Hg at rest and the heart rate below 72 beats per minute at rest.

Cooke JP, Safford RE: Progress in the diagnosis and management of aortic dissection. Mayo Clin Proc 61:147, 1986. *This excellent short article concentrates on the available diagnostic studies in patients with aortic dissection.*

Eagle KA, Quertermous T, Kritzer GA, et al.: Spectrum of conditions initially suggesting acute aortic dissection but with negative aortograms. Am J Cardiol 57:322, 1986. *This study defines the differential diagnosis of aortic dissection, discusses the frequency of false-negative aortographic findings, and contrasts the clinical features of patients with and without dissection.*

Roberts WC: Aortic dissection: Anatomy, consequences, and causes. Am Heart J 101:195, 1981. *A well-illustrated review of aortic dissection with emphasis on pathologic findings.*

Slater EE, DeSanctis RW: The clinical recognition of dissecting aortic aneurysm. Am J Med 60:625, 1976. *The clinical, roentgenologic, and laboratory findings in 124 patients with dissecting aneurysm of the aorta are discussed. Patients with dissections of the proximal aorta were younger and had a higher incidence of Marfan's syndrome, cystic medial necrosis, anterior chest pain, pulse deficits, neurologic compromise, aortic regurgitation, and congestive heart failure. Back pain, hypertension, and atherosclerosis characterized patients with distal dissection.*

Wheat MW Jr: Acute dissecting aneurysms of the aorta: Diagnosis and treatment—1979. Am Heart J 99:373, 1980. *The author, a surgeon, presents arguments for vigorous medical therapy in order to control hypertension and rate of pressure development in the aorta.*

MARFAN'S SYNDROME

Patients with Marfan's syndrome (see Ch. 187) develop both aortic aneurysm and aortic dissection. Myxomatous degeneration of valve leaflets may also occur. The mitral valve cusps may be involved. The chordae tendineae may elongate or rupture, predisposing to mitral valve prolapse, or flail mitral valve with mitral regurgitation. Regurgitation at either the mitral or the tricuspid valve may be the most prominent finding in certain patients. However, the most commonly affected tissue is the aorta. The aorta enlarges, beginning with the sinuses of Valsalva. The enlargement most often extends to the innominate artery, although at times the entire aorta may be involved in what has been referred to as annuloaortic ectasia. Aortic dilation may begin as early as the fifth year of life or as late as the sixth decade.

Aortic regurgitation may occur secondary to participation of the aortic root in the development of an aortic aneurysm. Dissection of the aortic root may lead to acute aortic regurgitation. Dilation of the pulmonary artery is common.

Diagnosis

Dilation of the aortic root is easily measured by echocardiography. Two-dimensional echocardiography shows the classic flask-shaped dilation of the aorta extending from the aortic valve to the innominate artery (Fig. 53–6). Echocardiography may also be used to demonstrate the major complications of aortic root dilation, dissection of the aorta, and aortic regurgitation. The echocardiogram has also helped in defining the optimal time for operative intervention. Magnetic resonance imaging is also capable of giving excellent definition to abnormalities of the aorta (Fig. 53–7).

Therapy

It is now generally agreed, although not absolutely proven, that β blockade may inhibit the pace of aortic dilation. Therefore, it is appropriate to obtain serial echocardiograms in patients thought to have Marfan's syndrome. When incipient dilation of the aorta is recognized, institution of a β blocker may be warranted. By diminishing the velocity with which the left ventricle ejects blood, the forces on the weakened aortic wall may be lessened.

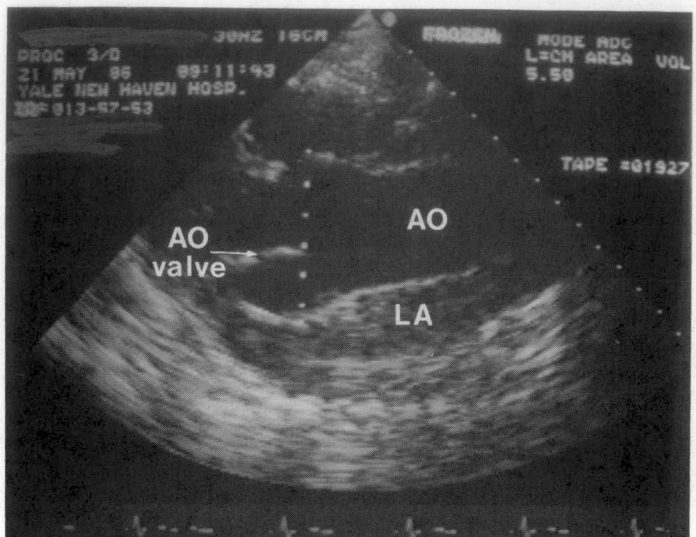

FIGURE 53–6. Echocardiogram, long-axis parasternal view of a patient with Marfan's syndrome. The sinuses of Valsalva are flared and the aortic root is dilated.

Complications of aneurysms in the ascending aorta account for more than 90 per cent of deaths from Marfan's syndrome. The likelihood of both aortic dissection and aortic regurgitation increases as the size of the aortic root increases. Operation in the face of an acute dissection is fraught with considerable hazard. Therefore, prophylactic operation is recommended if the aortic root enlarges to 6 cm on echocardiography. The operation most commonly utilized for patients with Marfan's syndrome is replacement of the ascending aortic aneurysm with a composite tube graft that includes a prosthetic valve at its proximal end. The coronaries are anastomosed to the sides of the tube graft. The aneurysm is wrapped around the tube graft to help establish hemostasis. The overall hospital mortality of the procedure is 2 per cent (Gott and colleagues). Although it may seem radical to recommend aortic replacement to a patient who may be asymptomatic, the adverse prognosis of the patient with Marfan's syndrome whose aorta dilates to greater than 6 cm in diameter probably warrants this recommendation.

Gott VL, Pyeritz RE, Magovern GJ Jr, et al.: Surgical treatment of aneurysms of the ascending aorta in the Marfan syndrome. N Engl J Med 314:1070, 1986. *The results of ascending aorta replacement with a composite graft in 50 consecutive patients with Marfan's syndrome are reported. Because of the unfavorable natural history of Marfan's syndrome, the authors recommend prophylactic repair when the aneurysm reaches a diameter of 6 cm.*

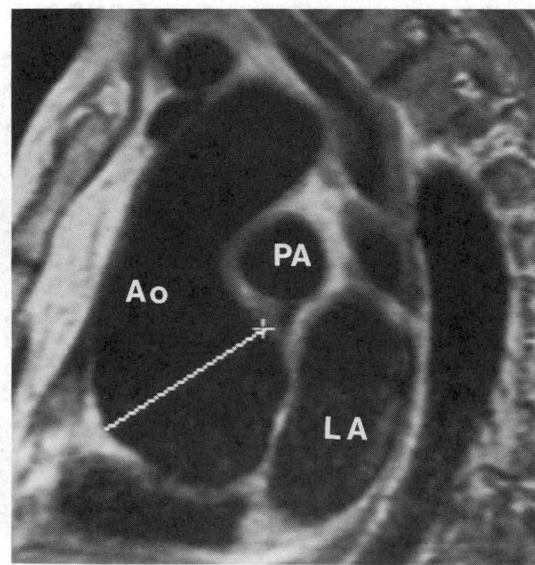

FIGURE 53–7. Magnetic resonance image, sagittal view, showing an aneurysm of the ascending aorta in a patient with Marfan's syndrome.

Halpern BL, Char F, Murdoch JL, et al.: A prospectus on the prevention of aortic rupture in the Marfan syndrome with data on survivorship without treatment. Johns Hopkins Med J 129:123, 1971. *This is one of the first articles to advocate the prophylactic use of β blockers in patients with the Marfan's syndrome in order to prevent further dilation and dissecting aneurysm.*

MISCELLANEOUS FORMS OF AORTITIS AND THE AORTIC ARCH SYNDROME

Arteritis

A number of inflammatory processes can involve the aortic arch and its major branches. Aortic arteritis, no matter what the etiology, may cause narrowing or occlusion of the major arch vessels. Blood supply to the areas supplied by the innominate artery, the left common carotid artery, and the left subclavian artery may be impaired. Symptoms may include transient ischemic attacks, syncope, disorders of vision or speech, claudication of the upper extremities or of the muscles of the jaw, decreased pulses in the neck and upper extremities, or symptoms of basilar artery insufficiency. As a group, these entities are called the aortic arch syndrome. They include aortitis due to syphilis, tuberculosis, giant cell arteritis, polyarteritis nodosa, Takayasu's syndrome, or dissecting aneurysm. Kawasaki's mucocutaneous lymph node syndrome may cause an aortitis, but the coronary arteries are the principal vessels involved. Giant cell arteritis may cause the aortic arch syndrome in addition to temporal and ophthalmic artery disease.

Takayasu's arteritis may be a more specific form of aortitis. Initially it was thought that the arteritic process was limited to the aortic arch and its branches. Subsequent studies have demonstrated that the arteritis is not confined to these areas. Three varieties are now recognized. In one type, the involvement is localized to the aortic arch and its branches. The second type involves the descending thoracic aorta and abdominal aorta without the arch. The third type contains features of both. There is a preponderance of females with "pulseless disease." Although early reports were more common in Japan, increasing numbers of patients are being recognized in the United States. The presence of hypertension with absent pulses in the upper extremities has caused this syndrome to be called reversed coarctation.

Lupi-Herrera E, Sanchez-Torres G, Marcushamer J, et al.: Takayasu's arteritis: Clinical study of 107 cases. Am Heart J 93:94, 1977. *A review of Takayasu's arteritis involving 107 patients. This entity is not limited to Asian patients. It is a nonspecific inflammatory process affecting the aorta and its main branches.*

TRAUMATIC AORTIC DISEASE

The most common form of trauma to the aorta is due to deceleration injuries, often seen in automobile accidents. Since the descending aorta is relatively immobile, deceleration injuries characteristically affect the portion of the aorta immediately distal to the left subclavian artery. Nonpenetrating aortic injury may cause internal bleeding with no external evidence of chest injury. Hypotension or shock, left hemothorax, absence of femoral pulses, and pale lower extremities round out the clinical picture. A chest roentgenogram may show mediastinal widening. Prompt surgical intervention may be life saving.

54 Vascular Diseases of the Limbs

Hermes A. Kontos

VASCULAR DISEASES OF THE LIMBS CAUSED BY ABNORMAL RESPONSES OF VASCULAR SMOOTH MUSCLE

Raynaud's Phenomenon and Disease

DEFINITION. Raynaud's phenomenon is a syndrome manifested by attacks of pallor and cyanosis of the digits in response to cold or to emotion. As the attack abates, these color changes are replaced by redness. When the disorder is primary, it is called Raynaud's disease; when it is secondary to another disease or cause, it is called Raynaud's phenomenon.

ETIOLOGY AND INCIDENCE. Raynaud's disease is the

most common cause of Raynaud's phenomenon, accounting for 60 per cent of patients with this disorder. The cause of Raynaud's disease is unknown. Although it can begin at any age, it becomes clinically manifest most commonly between the ages of 20 and 40 years. Raynaud's disease is much more common in women than in men. Two theories have been advanced to explain its occurrence. Raynaud believed that it is caused by increased sympathetic nerve activity. However, measurements of the sympathetic nerve traffic in the median nerve failed to show differences between patients with Raynaud's disease and normal individuals. Lewis discovered that attacks of Raynaud's phenomenon could be induced after interruption of the sympathetic nerves. He concluded that the cause of the disorder was a fault in the arterial wall that rendered the vessels hyperresponsive to the vasoconstrictive effects of cold. He ascribed the vasospastic attacks to spasm of the digital arteries as a result of this hypersensitivity. Little is known about the defect in the vessel wall, which renders the vessel hypersensitive to cold. The circulation of the digits of patients with Raynaud's disease is not hypersensitive to infused norepinephrine. Also, determination of the arteriovenous concentration differences of norepinephrine and epinephrine across the hand showed that there was no excessive release of catecholamines from the hands of patients with Raynaud's disease. More recently, accelerated destruction of platelets and release of agents such as serotonin or thromboxane A_2 have been proposed as causing vasoconstriction in some patients with Raynaud's phenomenon. It is not known whether platelet destruction is the cause of spasm in such patients or a consequence of it.

In a recent study, 26 per cent of patients with the variant type of angina pectoris were found to have migraine, and 24 per cent were found to have Raynaud's phenomenon. This suggested that some patients with Raynaud's phenomenon may have a generalized defect that predisposes arteries in many regions to vasospasm. An association of Raynaud's phenomenon with idiopathic pulmonary hypertension has also been reported. This association may reflect a very high level of peripheral vascular tone secondary to the severe reduction in cardiac output.

Secondary Raynaud's phenomenon is observed frequently as a manifestation of the diseases listed in Table 54–1.

In the presence of arterial obstruction, vasoconstrictive stimuli that normally do not cause clinical manifestations result in more

TABLE 54–1. CAUSES OF SECONDARY RAYNAUD'S PHENOMENON

1. Occlusive arterial disease
   a. Arteriosclerosis obliterans
   b. Buerger's disease
   c. Arterial embolism
   d. Vasculitis
   e. Arterial thrombosis
2. Connective tissue diseases
   a. Scleroderma
   b. Rheumatoid arthritis
   c. Systemic lupus erythematosus
3. Vascular injury
   a. Repetitive minor occupational trauma, as in pneumatic hammer operators, pianists, typists, or users of hand-held vibrating tools
   b. Frostbite
4. Neurogenic causes
   a. Thoracic outlet compression by cervical rib, by scalenus anticus muscle, or in hyperabduction syndrome
   b. Carpal tunnel syndrome
   c. Sympathetic causalgia
   d. Spinal cord diseases
5. Drugs or exposure to chemicals
   a. Ergotamine
   b. Ergotism
   c. Methysergide
   d. Polyvinyl chloride
   e. Beta-adrenergic receptor blockers
   f. Antimetabolite drugs (cisplatin, vinblastine, bleomycin)
6. Intravascular coagulation or aggregation
   a. Cryoglobulinemia
   b. Cold agglutinins

severe reduction in blood flow and may cause Raynaud's phenomenon.

Raynaud's phenomenon is very often associated with connective tissue diseases; it is particularly frequent in scleroderma. Almost all patients with scleroderma develop Raynaud's phenomenon at some time during the course of their illness. A distinctive syndrome consisting of calcinosis, Raynaud's phenomenon, abnormal esophageal motility, sclerodactyly, and telangiectasia (CREST syndrome) is recognized. Raynaud's phenomenon may be the presenting manifestation in connective tissue diseases and may precede the appearance of other manifestations by several years. The presence of abnormal nail fold capillaries in patients with Raynaud's phenomenon has predictive value for the future development of scleroderma. Structural changes in the vessel wall that limit flow and increase the sensitivity to vasoconstrictive influences appear to account for the frequent occurrence of Raynaud's phenomenon in these diseases. Vascular injury may also result from repetitive minor occupational trauma or from a severe exposure to cold, as in frostbite. Consequent hypersensitivity to cold causes Raynaud's phenomenon. Occupationally induced Raynaud's phenomenon is frequently secondary to exposure to a source of vibration. It is referred to as vibration white finger. It usually develops after several years of using hand-held vibrating power tools.

Neurogenic lesions cause Raynaud's phenomenon because of irritation of sympathetic nerves and consequent vasoconstriction. Intense or sustained vasoconstriction caused by drugs may also result in Raynaud's phenomenon, as in 3 to 6 per cent of patients taking β-adrenergic receptor–blocking drugs. Propranolol is the main offender. These drugs block a β-adrenergic vasodilative mechanism in the digits and may also enhance the vasoconstrictive effects of norepinephrine. A high incidence of Raynaud's phenomenon was described during administration of certain antimetabolite drugs, such as cisplatin, vinblastine, and bleomycin. Raynaud's phenomenon was associated with hypomagnesemia, which might have been responsible for vasoconstriction.

Intravascular aggregation or coagulation of blood elements may obstruct the vessels and cause ischemia and Raynaud's phenomenon.

PATHOPHYSIOLOGY. The pallor during the attack of Raynaud's phenomenon is explained by intense vasoconstriction or spasm of the digital arteries. This results in severe reduction in blood flow. In a later stage of the attack, the vasoconstriction becomes less severe, and the capillaries and veins are partially filled with blood whose hemoglobin becomes markedly deoxygenated. This accounts for the cyanosis. Upon rewarming, cyanosis is replaced by an intense red color associated with reactive hyperemia. Between attacks, blood flow to the digits is usually reduced, especially in patients who have trophic changes, but may be normal in some patients. In those patients without trophic changes, blood flow to the hand during maximum vasodilation is the same as in normal individuals, but it is severely reduced in those with trophic changes, a reflection of structural changes in the blood vessels.

PATHOLOGY. In the early stages of the disease, the digital blood vessels are histologically normal. In longstanding cases, the intima becomes thickened, and the media may be hypertrophied. In severe progressive cases, complete obstruction from thrombosis may occur, and gangrene of the tips of the digits may ensue.

CLINICAL MANIFESTATIONS. The onset of Raynaud's disease is usually gradual. The patient notices an occasional mild and short-lasting attack during winter. Over succeeding years, the severity and duration of the attacks may increase. A wide variation in severity is present. Most commonly, the attacks are provoked by exposure to cold. In some patients, attacks are also precipitated by emotion. The attacks may be terminated by rewarming, or they may abate spontaneously. Between attacks, in a warm environment, the patient is asymptomatic, and physical examination shows no abnormalities. Some patients, however, complain of chronically cold hands and feet, and they may have cold fingers with cyanosis on examination. In a typical attack of Raynaud's phenomenon, the digits become pale. Usually, all digits are affected symmetrically. The pallor is sharply demarcated at the level of the metacarpophalangeal joints, a reflection of spasm of the digital arteries. At a later stage during the attack, pallor is replaced by cyanosis. The patient may have feelings of coldness, numbness, and occasionally pain. Upon rewarming, the cyanosis is replaced by intense redness, and the patient may feel tingling or throbbing. Most commonly, only the hands are affected. Frequently, both hands and feet are affected. Rarely, the nose, cheeks, ears, and chin are affected also.

Atypical attacks are not infrequent. In these, the involvement of the digits may be asymmetric, with only one or two digits being affected. In some cases, only a portion of the digit is affected. In these instances, the most severely affected portion of the digit is the most distal one. Thus, one may see pallor of the fingertip or of the terminal phalanx of one digit. In other cases, more than one phalanx may be involved.

In severe, progressive cases, trophic changes may occur after a few years of involvement. The hair may disappear from the dorsal aspect of the digits. The nails grow more slowly and become brittle and deformed. The skin becomes atrophic, thin, and tight (sclerodactyly). Ulcerations may develop at the fingertips or around the nail bed. These heal slowly and may become infected. They are extremely painful, especially at night. When they heal, they leave characteristic small, pitted scars.

DIAGNOSIS. The diagnosis of Raynaud's phenomenon can usually be made on the basis of the history of vasospastic attacks in the digits, precipitated by cold and relieved by warming. In atypical cases or when the patient's description of the attack is not clear, provocation of an attack may be helpful. This may be done by immersing the hands in water at a temperature of 10 to 15°C. Whole-body exposure to cold is more successful in provoking attacks. A negative result does not exclude Raynaud's phenomenon.

In typical cases, Raynaud's phenomenon is easily distinguished from acrocyanosis, but when involvement is atypical, the differentiation may be more difficult. Distinguishing features include the following: The color changes in Raynaud's phenomenon are episodic, whereas in acrocyanosis they are sustained. Pallor is not a prominent feature of acrocyanosis. Cyanosis is the more typical color change, whereas in Raynaud's disease digital pallor is characteristic. In Raynaud's disease, only the digits are involved, whereas in acrocyanosis the color changes usually involve the whole hand or foot and sometimes even more proximal portions of the limbs. In Raynaud's disease the skin of the palms is usually dry, whereas in acrocyanosis it is wet and clammy with sweat. Finally, acrocyanosis rarely causes trophic changes and ulcerations.

Obstruction of major arteries from arteriosclerosis, angiitis, embolism, or thrombosis may lead to color changes in the digits that simulate Raynaud's phenomenon. The distinction is made by the demonstration of changes in arterial pulses and by the fact that the color changes in these disorders are likely to be confined to one limb rather than symmetric. Arteriography, which demonstrates the arterial lesion, is helpful. However, secondary Raynaud's phenonenon may be superimposed upon any of these diseases. In Raynaud's phenomenon, Doppler velocity studies show patent arteries and sharply peaked blood flow velocity patterns in the digits. Arteriography shows normal major arteries and diffuse spasm of the digital arteries.

The distinction of Raynaud's disease from secondary Raynaud's phenomenon is based mainly on the exclusion of disorders known to cause secondary Raynaud's phenomenon. The exclusion of obstructive arterial disease is discussed above. Connective tissue disorders, particularly scleroderma, are excluded by the absence of arthralgias or arthritis, alterations of esophageal motility, and the absence of a pulmonary oxygen diffusion defect. The presence of a normal sedimentation rate and the absence of circulating autoantibodies, such as antinuclear antibodies, provide additional reassurance. A careful occupational history is necessary to exclude Raynaud's phenomenon secondary to minor repetitive trauma. A history of drug ingestion or exposure to chemicals is helpful in identifying drug-induced Raynaud's phenomenon. Neurologic disorders can be recognized by their somatic neurologic manifestations. Thoracic outlet compression syndromes can be excluded by the appropriate maneuvers. The presence of intravascular agglutination or coagulation of the blood elements may be suspected if, in the presence of cyanosis, the blood cannot be expelled from vessels by pressure, and when there are isolated areas of redness as the attack abates during rewarming. Confirmation is obtained by demonstrating the cold agglutinins or cryoglobulins in the patient's blood.

TABLE 54–2. TREATMENT OF RAYNAUD'S PHENOMENON

Frequency and Severity of Vasospastic Attacks	Suggested Treatment
1. Rare or mild attacks	Protective measures, cessation of smoking, and no drug therapy
2. Frequent or severe attacks without trophic changes	Protective measures and calcium antagonists
3. Frequent attacks with trophic changes but no open ulcers	Protective measures plus calcium antagonists or oral reserpine plus liothyronine
4. Frequent attacks with active, painful ulcers	Intravenous PGE₁, intra-arterial reserpine followed by calcium antagonists; or reserpine plus liothyronine; or oral misoprostol

TABLE 54–3. SOME DRUGS USEFUL IN THE TREATMENT OF RAYNAUD'S PHENOMENON

1. Calcium antagonists
   a. Nifedipine*
   b. Diltiazem*
2. Alpha-adrenergic receptor blockers
   a. Phenoxybenzamine*
   b. Tolazoline
   c. Prazosin*
3. Drugs that interfere with sympathetic nerve activity
   a. Reserpine*
   b. Guanethidine*
   c. Alpha-methyldopa*
4. Vasodilators
   a. PGE₁*
   b. PGE₂*
   c. PGI₂*
   d. Iloprost
   e. Misoprostol*
5. Miscellaneous
   a. Liothyronine*

*Investigational drug for this purpose.

PROGNOSIS. The prognosis of patients with Raynaud's disease is good. There is no mortality associated with the disease and morbidity is low; it is generally limited to loss of portions of digits as a result of ulcerations. In approximately 50 per cent of patients with Raynaud's disease, the disorder improves and may disappear completely after several years. In only a fraction of 1 per cent of patients is amputation necessary. Approximately 15 per cent of patients with Raynaud's phenomenon eventually develop a connective tissue disorder, particularly scleroderma.

The prognosis in secondary Raynaud's phenomenon depends on the course of the primary disorder. In scleroderma, the prognosis is unsatisfactory, particularly when the disease has caused digital ulcerations.

TREATMENT. Management of patients with Raynaud's phenomenon must be tailored to the individual needs of the patient, taking into consideration the frequency and severity of the attacks (Table 54–2). All patients benefit from reassurance and protective measures against exposure to cold. The patients should limit the duration of exposure to cold to the greatest extent possible. They should wear heavy clothing, protecting not only the hands and feet but also the face and trunk, especially when there is a cold wind; this is important because exposure to cold of other portions of the body may reflexly induce vasoconstriction in the digits and precipitate Raynaud's phenomenon. When prolonged exposure to cold is unavoidable, the use of electrically powered or solid fuel–powered hand and foot warmers is advisable. These patients should be taught to recognize and terminate attacks by returning promptly to a warm environment, placing their hands in warm water, or using a warm-air hairblower to warm their hands rapidly. Smoking causes cutaneous vasoconstriction; therefore, tobacco smoking is contraindicated in Raynaud's phenomenon. The use of induced vasodilation by placing the hands in warm water (43°C) has been reported to raise skin temperature and minimize the severity of attacks of Raynaud's phenomenon. Biofeedback to teach patients to raise skin temperature voluntarily has been shown to limit the duration and frequency of vasospastic attacks, but its effect is nonspecific because it is also seen in control patients who received no such treatment and in those in whom biofeedback is used to teach relaxation. In patients with Raynaud's phenomenon secondary to vibration, the use of vibrating tools must cease. However, termination of exposure to vibration does not always eliminate Raynaud's phenomenon.

The simple measures outlined above usually suffice for patients with infrequent or mild attacks. When Raynaud's phenomenon is more frequent or more severe, and especially when it has resulted in trophic changes or ulcerations, these measures need to be supplemented by drugs. The aim of drug therapy is to induce vascular smooth muscle relaxation, thereby relieving spasm, raising resting blood flow, and limiting the degree of ischemia during attacks. The drugs most frequently used in treating patients with Raynaud's phenomenon are shown in Table 54–3. For most patients, the drug of choice is a calcium antagonist. Nifedipine* has been found to be effective in several well-controlled, double-blind studies. The drug is administered at a dose of 10 to 20 mg three or four times daily. Diltiazem,* at a dose of 60 mg three or four times daily, may be substituted, if nifedipine is not well tolerated or if it causes side effects. In one

study of very severely affected patients, verapamil was found not to be effective. The angiotensin-converting enzyme inhibitors enalapril and captopril are also effective in reducing the frequency and decreasing the severity of Raynaud's phenomenon. They have been less extensively studied than calcium antagonists, although they appear equally effective. Enalapril is administered by mouth in a dose of 10 to 20 mg once daily, and captopril in a dose of 25 to 50 mg two to three times daily.

Reserpine* is the best-studied drug among the group that interferes with the function of the adrenergic nervous system. It is administered by mouth in doses of 0.1 to 0.5 mg daily. In cases in which ulcerations have developed, it may be given intra-arterially in a dose of 0.5 to 1 mg, dissolved in saline and administered into the brachial or radial artery by slow infusion over several minutes. The drugs in this group may also be administered by means of tourniquet-controlled intravenous injection (Bier's block). The administration by the last two routes gives a much higher local concentration and largely avoids systemic side effects.

In controlled trials, nitroglycerin* ointment or topical prostaglandin E₂* (PGE₂) has been found effective in Raynaud's phenomenon. The topical application of these drugs is advantageous because their local relaxant action is not counteracted by reflex vasoconstriction secondary to changes in blood pressure that may occur when they are given systemically.

Prostaglandin E₁* (PGE₁) or prostacyclin* (PGI₂) administered intravenously has a beneficial effect in patients with Raynaud's phenomenon. These drugs can be given by constant intravenous infusion in a dose of 6 to 10 ng per kilogram per minute for a few hours or up to 3 days. Iloprost is an experimental stable analogue of PGI₂. It is administered intravenously in a dose of 0.5 to 2 ng per kilogram per minute for several hours. Misoprostol* is an analogue of PGE₁. It is administered by mouth in a dose of 0.2 mg three or four times daily. It is reported that the beneficial effect outlasts this therapy by several weeks. All these drugs act by inducing vasodilation and also by inhibiting platelet aggregation.

A novel but effective way of inducing vasodilation in the digits is via the iatrogenic induction of hyperthyroidism by the administration of sodium liothyronine* (triiodothyronine), 75 μg daily. The resultant hypermetabolism elicits thermoregulatory reflex cutaneous vasodilation. The combination of triiodothyronine and reserpine has been found to be most effective.

Preganglionic sympathectomy to eliminate vasoconstrictor tone may have a beneficial immediate result, but the long-term results are disappointing. The duration of benefit is limited by regeneration of the nerves. If sympathectomy is contemplated, it is advisable to try sympathetic blockade with local anesthetics to verify a beneficial result. A recently devised technique that

*Investigational drug for this purpose.

*Investigational drug for this purpose.

involves surgical stripping of the palmar and digital arteries to bring about a local sympathectomy may also be tried, but its results have not been fully evaluated.

Coffman JD, Davis WT: Vasospastic diseases: A review. Prog Cardiovasc Dis 18:123, 1975. *A comprehensive, well-referenced review of vasospastic diseases.*

Cohen RA, Coffman JD: β-Adrenergic vasodilator mechanism in the finger. Circ Res 49:1196, 1981. *Demonstration of a β-adrenergic, humorally activated, vasodilative mechanism in the arteriovenous anastomoses of the human finger. Blockade of this mechanism may explain the occurrence of Raynaud's phenomenon in patients taking β-adrenergic receptor–blocking drugs.*

Fagius J, Blumberg H: Sympathetic outflow to the hand in patients with Raynaud's phenomenon. Cardiovasc Res 19:249, 1985. *Demonstration that sympathetic nerve activity in patients with Raynaud's phenomenon under baseline conditions and during maneuvers that increase sympathetic nerve traffic does not differ from that in normal controls. The results do not support the theory that Raynaud's disease is caused by increased sympathetic nerve activity.*

Harper FE, Maricq HR, Turner RE, et al.: A prospective study of Raynaud's phenomenon and early connective tissue disease. Am J Med 72:883, 1982. *This study of capillaries of the nail fold shows that the presence of capillary abnormalities in patients with Raynaud's phenomenon may have predictive value for the future development of scleroderma.*

Janini SD, Scott JS, Coppock PAB, et al.: Enalapril in Raynaud's phenomenon. J Clin Pharmacol Ther 13:145, 1988. *Report of a prospective double-blind crossover trial showing that enalapril is effective in reducing the frequency and severity of attacks of Raynaud's phenomenon.*

Kontos HA, Wasserman AJ: Effect of reserpine in Raynaud's phenomenon. Circulation 39:259, 1969. *An analysis of the effects of reserpine given intra-arterially and orally on hand blood flow in patients with Raynaud's disease. It also contains evidence against the hypothesis that defective catecholamine metabolism may account for Raynaud's disease. Beneficial results from oral administration of reserpine are also presented.*

Miller D, Waters DD, Warnica W, et al.: Is variant angina the coronary manifestation of a generalized vasospastic disorder? N Engl J Med 304:763, 1981. *Provocative study showing high incidence of migraine and Raynaud's phenomenon in patients with variant angina, suggesting the possibility that we may be dealing with a generalized vasospastic disorder.*

Roath S: Management of Raynaud's phenomenon: Focus on newer treatments. Drugs 37:700, 1989. *Comprehensive consideration of drug therapy in Raynaud's phenomenon.*

Smith CR, Rodeheffer RJ: Treatment of Raynaud's phenomenon with calcium channel blockers. Am J Med 78 (Suppl 2B):39, 1985. *Concise consideration of the pathophysiology of Raynaud's phenomenon and review of available evidence concerning the effectiveness of treatment with calcium antagonists.*

Acrocyanosis

DEFINITION. Acrocyanosis is a rare disorder characterized by persistent cyanosis of the skin of the hands and, less commonly, of the feet associated with reduced skin temperature.

ETIOLOGY. Acrocyanosis is a primary disorder of unknown cause. It is much more common in women than in men. The onset of the disease is usually in young adults or middle-aged persons. The high incidence of the disease among patients with psychiatric disorders is of unknown significance.

PATHOPHYSIOLOGY. The smaller precapillary vessels (arterioles) are abnormally constricted, causing reduction in blood flow and accounting for cyanosis and reduced skin temperature. The veins are secondarily dilated. Constriction of the arterioles occurs under normal environmental conditions and becomes more pronounced on exposure to cold because of increased sensitivity of these vessels to the effects of cold. An important feature of acrocyanosis is the reduced venous flow. No venous obstruction is present. These features can be demonstrated by elevating the involved limb and eliminating the blue color or intensifying the blue color by placing the limb in a dependent position and overfilling the veins.

CLINICAL MANIFESTATIONS. Patients with acrocyanosis have persistent blue discoloration of the hands. Less commonly, the feet are also involved. In some cases, the blue color extends to more proximal portions of the limbs. The skin is cold, and the palms are wet and clammy from sweat. No pallor is usually present. In some cases, there may be spots of pallor surrounded by confluent cyanosis. The blue color is intensified by exposure to cold, and it is converted into purplish or red color by exposure to heat. There are few accompanying symptoms. The patient has feelings of coldness and, occasionally, numbness. Ulcerations and other trophic changes are distinctly unusual. Patients with acrocyanosis seek medical advice either because they are frightened or because the cyanosis is cosmetically unappealing.

DIAGNOSIS. The distinction between acrocyanosis and Raynaud's phenomenon is discussed above in the section on Raynaud's phenomenon. Differentiation from cyanosis secondary to arterial obstruction can be made on the basis of normal pulses, by the bilateral and symmetric occurrence of acrocyanosis, and, if necessary, by the angiographic verification of absence of obstruction. The limitation of the cyanosis to the hands and feet, the improvement in a warm environment, and the absence of reduced arterial blood saturation distinguish acrocyanosis from generalized, systemic cyanosis.

TREATMENT. Since acrocyanosis is a benign disease, no drug therapy is usually required. Reassurance and protection from cold usually suffice. In some cases, cosmetic considerations or unusually severe symptoms may necessitate drug therapy. In these cases, the same drugs that are useful in Raynaud's phenomenon may be tried.

Lewis T, Landis EM: Observations upon the vascular mechanism in acrocyanosis. Heart 15:229, 1930. *Classic description of the clinical features of acrocyanosis. Evidence is presented showing that the disease is the result of an abnormal responsiveness of the smaller blood vessels.*

Livedo Reticularis

DEFINITION. Livedo reticularis is a reticular, bluish discoloration of the skin of the extremities that produces a lacy, irregular appearance outlining central areas of normal-appearing skin. The etiology is not known. The disorder usually begins in young individuals before age 20 to 30 years. It is equally common in men and women but more often symptomatic in women.

PATHOLOGY. Proliferative lesions of the arterioles of the skin with perivascular infiltration have been described. In some cases, there may be thrombosis of arterioles leading to cutaneous infarction and ulceration. Similar changes are seen in the veins.

PATHOPHYSIOLOGY. The mechanism of livedo reticularis is presumed to be similar to that of acrocyanosis, namely, constriction of arterioles followed by stasis and dilation of capillaries and veins. The latter are filled with desaturated blood. The reticular appearance of livedo reticularis reflects the anatomic arrangement of the affected vessels. It is believed that the bluish areas represent the arborizations of peripheral capillaries from central penetrating arterioles. Blood flow is faster in the central regions closer to the penetrating arteriole, whereas the more distant areas have lower flow, with consequent stasis and cyanosis.

CLINICAL MANIFESTATIONS. Patients seek medical attention for cosmetic reasons or because they are frightened by the bluish discoloration. The lower extremities are involved more often than the upper extremities. The patient usually has no symptoms. In some cases, there may be paresthesias or a feeling of coldness. The bluish discoloration becomes more intense on exposure to cold and may disappear in a warm environment. Ulcerations occur rarely; when they do, they appear in winter and heal in summer.

TREATMENT. In most cases no treatment is required. Protection from cold and abstinence from tobacco are useful. In severe cases, drugs useful in the treatment of Raynaud's phenomenon, such as nifedipine and reserpine, may be tried.

Feldaker M, Hines EA, Kierland RR: Livedo reticularis with ulcerations. Circulation 13:196, 1956. *Report of the clinical and pathologic features of 18 patients with livedo reticularis with ulcerations. A brief review of the earlier literature is included.*

Erythromelalgia (Erythermalgia)

DEFINITION. Erythromelalgia is a disorder manifested by episodes of erythema accompanied by increased skin temperature and by pain involving the feet and, less commonly, the hands. It may be primary or secondary to other disorders. Erythromelalgia is considered further in Ch. 280.

PATHOPHYSIOLOGY. The symptoms of erythromelalgia are dependent on skin temperature. Rise in skin temperature above a certain level causes the manifestations. In each person this critical point is fairly constant. Vasodilation and consequent hyperemia are the usual causes of the rise in skin temperature. However, an increased blood flow is not essential, since once symptoms have been induced by heat, they may continue even though blood flow is reduced to zero with a cuff inflated above the systolic pressure levels. These features suggest that the cause of the disorder is abnormal sensitivity of the cutaneous pain fibers to heat or tension from the dilated blood vessels.

CLINICAL MANIFESTATIONS. The onset of the disease is

gradual. With progression, the frequency and duration of the attacks become more pronounced. Eventually, symptoms may become almost continuous and cause total disability. During an attack the patient complains of burning pain, usually in the feet and, less commonly, in the hands. The pain is usually located in the balls of the feet and in the tips of the toes and in the corresponding parts of the hands. Pain is aggravated by dependency and ameliorated by elevation of the limbs. Exposure to heat aggravates the disorder, whereas cold provides relief. Trophic changes, ulcerations, and gangrene are rare.

DIAGNOSIS. Peripheral neuropathy may cause burning pain simulating erythromelalgia. The pain may be accompanied by cutaneous vasodilation. The detection of the associated sensory and motor manifestations of peripheral neuropathy should help distinguish this condition from erythromelalgia. Arteriosclerosis obliterans or thromboangiitis obliterans may also produce localized burning pain and redness. The alterations in the arterial pulses and the absence of high skin temperature distinguish these conditions from erythromelalgia. Vascular damage from prolonged exposure to cold, as after frostbite, may simulate erythromelalgia. In these cases, the condition is more persistent, and the history of cold exposure should help make the distinction possible.

TREATMENT. Avoidance of exposure to heat, particularly dry heat, prevents attacks of erythromelalgia. Elevation of the extremity and application of cold may terminate an attack. Aspirin, 0.5 gram orally, relieves the pain in many cases. The response is sometimes so striking that it is of diagnostic value. Vasoconstrictive agents, such as methysergide or epinephrine, or β-adrenergic blocking agents, such as propranolol, have been reported to be effective in some patients. In secondary cases, treatment of the primary disorder may alleviate the attacks.

Babb RR, Alarçon-Segovia D, Fairbairn JF: Erythermalgia: Review of 51 cases. Circulation 29:136, 1964. *Description of the features of primary and secondary erythromelalgia based on a study of a large number of patients.*

Lewis T: Clinical observations and experiments relating to burning pain in the extremities, and to so-called "erythromelalgia" in particular. Clin Sci 1:175, 1933. *A classic paper with detailed clinical descriptions of the manifestations of erythromelalgia. The paper also presents clinical investigations pertinent to the pathogenesis of the disease.*

VASCULAR DISEASES OF THE LIMBS CAUSED BY DAMAGE FROM COLD

Immersion Foot (Trench Foot)

DEFINITION AND ETIOLOGY. Immersion foot is characterized by vascular damage resulting from prolonged exposure of the extremities to cold by wearing wet socks or wet footwear. Usually, the exposure is for several days at about 0°C. Dependency of limbs and immobility, as well as conditions that lead to general debility (lack of sleep and starvation), are contributory factors. The condition occurs primarily in soldiers at war.

Immersion foot has been described in survivors of shipwrecks, who were immobilized in crowded small craft for prolonged periods of time and exposed to wetness and cold. Maceration of the skin with sea water and secondary infection also contribute.

PATHOPHYSIOLOGY. This condition results from vascular injury. The initial effect of cold is to cause vasoconstriction. Loss of heat is facilitated by moisture. The resultant ischemia causes tissue and vascular injury with increased endothelial permeability. There is extensive extravasation of protein and fluid. As a result, there may be increased hematocrit, sludging, and further aggravation of ischemia.

PATHOLOGY. Little is known about the earliest pathologic change in the blood vessels in immersion foot. Most of the available information has been obtained from advanced cases with extensive vascular injury and gangrene. In these cases, the small arteries exhibit periarterial fibrosis and thickening and may be occluded. The veins show perivenous fibrosis, inflammatory reaction, and hemorrhage. The nerves may also be affected. In cases of immersion foot at relatively high temperatures, hyperhydration of the plantar stratum corneum may be the only finding.

CLINICAL MANIFESTATIONS. Three successive stages, each with distinct clinical manifestations, are recognized. During exposure to the wet, cold environment, there is vasoconstriction. The involved extremity becomes pale and cool, and the patient has paresthesias and a feeling of coldness. A second hyperemic stage follows. Patients are observed most commonly during this stage, because this is when they seek attention. The involved extremity is red, hot, and edematous. There may be pain or paresthesias. The swelling may be aggravated by heat and by placing the limb in a dependent position. Subsequently, blebs appear, filled with serous or hemorrhagic fluid. Hemorrhages may occur into the skin and subcutaneous tissue. This stage may persist for several days. In severe cases, gangrene may supervene. The condition may be complicated by lymphangitis, cellulitis, and thrombophlebitis. Mild cases or those treated early may recover after this second hyperemic phase. In other cases, a third late vasospastic phase occurs in which there is increased sensitivity to cold and typical secondary Raynaud's phenomenon, with excessive sweating, pain, and paresthesias of the lower extremities. This phase may persist for years.

TREATMENT. If the patient is seen in the initial vasoconstrictive phase, bed rest with the extremity in the horizontal position and a warm environment are necessary. During the hyperemic phase, the extremity should be placed at heart level and kept cool to diminish edema. Local care to keep the foot dry and clean should be instituted to avoid infection. Control of pain may require analgesics or narcotics. Sympathectomy may be helpful in the hyperemic stage and also in preventing the late vasospastic phenomena.

Abramson DI, Lerner D, Shumacker HB, et al.: Clinical picture and treatment of the later stage of trench foot. Am Heart J 32:52, 1946. *Clinical report based on the study of 633 patients with trench foot. Emphasis is placed on the late sequelae of the disorder.*

Frostbite

DEFINITION AND ETIOLOGY. Frostbite results from freezing of the tissues and consequent vascular injury. In most cases, frostbite occurs during prolonged exposure to temperatures below 0°C. Other environmental factors also play a role, such as high wind and humidity. Predisposing factors include vascular disease, inadequate clothing, lack of acclimatization, and general debility.

PATHOPHYSIOLOGY. Tissue damage results from cold-influenced vasoconstriction. Freezing causes water crystal formation in cells and dehydration. Endothelial damage with increased permeability to protein ensues, causes edema, and further contributes to stasis and eventual thrombosis.

PATHOLOGY. The vessels show endothelial swelling and vacuolization and proliferative changes. Subsequently, there are inflammatory reactions and atrophic changes in the skin.

CLINICAL MANIFESTATIONS. Initially, the patient notices a prickling sensation followed by numbness. The skin becomes bloodless and appears white and cold. This is followed by redness, swelling, and increased temperature. Blisters may form 24 to 48 hours after thawing. They are filled with either serous yellow or hemorrhagic fluid. There may be hemorrhages under the nail beds. Necrosis and gangrene may supervene. The subsequent course may be similar to that of sudden arterial occlusion, including ischemia and gangrene. Spontaneous amputation may require several weeks or months. After an attack of frostbite, the affected extremities may remain sensitive to cold for a period of time or permanently, and secondary Raynaud's phenomenon may occur.

TREATMENT. Frostbite should be treated with immediate rewarming. If frostbite affects deep tissues, rewarming should be done with water at 40 to 44°C. Muscular exercise of the involved limb and massage should be avoided, because they tend to increase edema and pain. If pain is severe, it should be treated with analgesics or narcotics. After the tissues have thawed, the exposed parts should remain at room temperatures. Vesicles should be left untouched, and the limb should be left exposed, without dressings. Antibiotic therapy should be used if infection is present. Sympathectomy has been reported to be beneficial in the initial stages as well as in preventing the delayed sequelae of frostbite.

Washburn B: Frostbite. N Engl J Med 266:974, 1962. *Comprehensive consideration of the clinical features, pathology, diagnosis, prevention, and treatment of frostbite.*

Chilblain (Pernio)

DEFINITION. Chilblain is an inflammatory condition of the skin of the extremities induced by cold and characterized by erythema, itching, and ulceration. The cause is unknown. It is more common in cold, damp climates, as in England, than in the United States. Women are affected more commonly than men. In most patients, the disease begins before the age of 20 years.

PATHOLOGY. In chronic cases, the lesions consist of angiitis with intimal proliferation, thickening of the arterial wall, and perivascular infiltration with lymphocytes and polymorphonuclear leukocytes. There may be necrosis of the adipose tissue and chronic inflammatory infiltrates in the subcutaneous tissue.

CLINICAL MANIFESTATIONS. Both acute and chronic forms of the disease are recognized. The typical patient is a young woman who, in the winter, notices bluish-red discoloration and edema of the skin of the lower limbs associated with burning and warmth. The lesions are persistent and are associated with itching. They generally last from 7 to 10 days and then clear up, sometimes leaving residual pigmentation of the skin. In severe cases, the lesions may become hemorrhagic, or blebs may appear. Infection may supervene.

With repeated exposure to cold, susceptible persons may develop chronic lesions. These are erythematous, ulcerative, and hemorrhagic lesions that begin as raised, red areas 0.5 to 1 cm in diameter. These lesions are then transformed into blebs and finally ulcerate. Healing occurs in the summer, leaving a permanently pigmented region.

DIAGNOSIS. Acute chilblain is distinguished from other forms of dermatitis by its characteristic distribution and by its relationship to cold. Chronic chilblain needs to be distinguished from erythema induratum and erythema nodosum. Erythema induratum of Bazin is caused by *Mycobacterium tuberculosis*. If the infection is active, the differential diagnosis may be made by the microscopic demonstration or culture of bacteria. Erythema induratum affects the upper part of the legs more frequently than the lower part. The lesions are more nodular, deeper, and infiltrative. They are also more permanent, whereas those of chronic chilblain clear up in the summer. Erythema nodosum is a more acute process, and it is usually associated with a systemic reaction, consisting of fever, malaise, and arthralgias. There is no seasonal association.

TREATMENT. In mild cases, protection from cold, local application of anti-inflammatory ointments, avoidance of scratching, and cessation of smoking are usually sufficient. In more severe cases, drugs that have been found useful in the treatment of Raynaud's phenomenon, such as reserpine or nifedipine, may be effective.

Eskell J: Reserpine in the treatment of chilblains. Practitioner 189:792, 1962. *Report of a controlled clinical trial of reserpine in patients with chilblain showing excellent benefit.*

Lynn RB: Chilblains. Surg Gynecol Obstet 99:720, 1954. *Concise description of the clinical and pathologic features of chilblain.*

Rustin MHA, Newton JA, Smith NP, et al.: The treatment of chilblain with nifedipine: The results of a pilot study, a double-blind placebo-controlled randomized study and a long-term open trial. Br J Dermatol 120:267, 1989. *Report of a controlled trial showing that nifedipine accelerated the clearance of chilblain and prevented the development of new lesions. It also caused symptomatic relief and resolution of edema and perivascular infiltration.*

VASCULAR DISEASES OF THE LIMBS CAUSED BY ORGANIC ARTERIAL OBSTRUCTION

Arteriosclerosis Obliterans

DEFINITION. Arteriosclerosis obliterans consists of segmental arteriosclerotic narrowing or obstruction of the lumen in the arteries supplying the limbs.

ETIOLOGY AND INCIDENCE. The etiology of arteriosclerosis in general is discussed in another chapter (see Ch. 47).

Arteriosclerosis obliterans is the most common cause of arterial obstructive disease of the extremities. The disease becomes clinically manifest usually between the ages of 50 and 70. It is unusual in individuals younger than 30 years of age. Men are affected more often than women. The lower limbs are involved much more frequently than the upper limbs. The most commonly affected vessel is the superficial femoral artery. The distal aorta and its bifurcation into the two iliac arteries and the popliteal artery are the next most frequent sites of involvement. The presence of diabetes mellitus influences arteriosclerosis obliterans in a number of important ways. In diabetics, arteriosclerosis

obliterans is likely to be more progressive. This is reflected in a much higher incidence of intermittent claudication in diabetics. The disease affects arterial vessels of smaller caliber and more distally located vessels more frequently than in nondiabetics. The incidence of involvement of vessels below the knee with arteriosclerosis obliterans in diabetics is considerably higher than in nondiabetics.

PATHOLOGY. The lesions of arteriosclerosis obliterans are typical atheromatous plaques involving the intima of the arteries. As a rule, there is superimposed thrombus formation. The media of the vessels shows degenerative changes. Calcification of the media is frequent and may take the form of a ringlike arrangement, as in Mönckeberg's sclerosis. Medial calcification is twice as frequent in diabetics as in nondiabetics. These arteriosclerotic lesions are segmental, and they are typically multiple. Weakening of the media may give rise to aneurysmal dilation of the involved artery. Such arteriosclerotic aneurysms are most common in the popliteal fossa or in the femoral artery below the inguinal ligament. They may be filled with thrombi.

PATHOPHYSIOLOGY. The arterial obstruction or narrowing causes reduction in blood flow during exercise or at rest. Clinical symptoms are caused by the consequent ischemia. The most important feature of the stenosis in determining ischemia is the cross-sectional area of the stenotic segment. Because the vascular bed of the extremities generally has a high resting vascular tone and, therefore, a large capacity for vasodilation, a moderate degree of stenosis can be compensated fully by downstream dilation. Stenoses that decrease the cross-sectional area of the vessel by less than 75 per cent do not usually affect resting blood flow. When the prevailing flow rates are high, as in exercise, decreases of 60 per cent or more in cross-sectional area are required before a reduction in flow occurs. Vasodilation in response to ischemia is the result of the action of local mechanisms. These include myogenic mechanisms related to reduction in intravascular pressure or metabolic mechanisms due to release of vasodilative metabolites from the ischemic tissues. These local mechanisms compete with neurogenic mechanisms that, when activated, cause vasoconstriction. Increased sympathetic activity, as from exposure to cold, may, therefore, induce ischemia in the presence of an arterial obstructing lesion.

The presence or absence of ischemia in the face of severe arterial stenosis or obstruction is frequently determined by the degree of development of collateral circulation. Some collateral vessels are present in the normal limb but are not used until obstruction takes place. They open up immediately after an acute arterial occlusion. Others take several weeks or months to become fully developed. Little is known about the responsiveness of collateral vessels. They are subject to neurogenic vasoconstriction from the action of adrenergic nerves. They dilate in response to increased blood pressure, resulting in improved collateral blood flow.

CLINICAL MANIFESTATIONS. The symptoms of arteriosclerosis obliterans are intermittent claudication, pain at rest, and trophic changes in the involved limb. Intermittent claudication denotes pain that develops in a limb on exercise and disappears when the patient rests. The pain is usually described as a cramp or a tightness or as severe fatigue of the exercising muscles. The amount of exercise necessary to induce the pain is usually constant for any given patient. The pain is usually bilateral. In some patients, the pain disappears by slowing the pace of walking without complete cessation of exercise. The location of the pain is distal to the arterial obstruction. The most frequently affected muscles are those of the calf, because of the high frequency with which the femoral artery is involved. The muscles of the lower part of the back, the buttocks, the thigh, and the foot may also be affected.

Pain at rest occurs when a pronounced reduction in resting blood flow is present. It is a sign of severe disease. The pain may be localized to one or more toes, or it may have a stocking-type distribution. The character of the pain is usually burning or gnawing. It is generally worse at night. It is improved by placing the limb in a dependent position and by cooling. There may be associated coldness and numbness, together with cyanosis or pallor of the extremity.

Examination discloses reduced or absent arterial pulses distal to the obstruction. There may be bruits audible over the aorta or its branches. These may be systolic, or they may be continuous.

In advanced cases, examination may reveal signs of ischemia. The skin temperature may be abnormally low, or there may be pallor or cyanosis. Ischemic damage may cause persistent reddish or reddish-blue discoloration. There may be trophic changes, including a dry, scaly, and shiny skin. The hair may disappear, and the toenails may become brittle, ridged, and deformed. There may be ulcerations or gangrene. The ischemic ulcers are usually at pressure points and may be inflamed and painful.

Leriche's syndrome refers to isolated aortoiliac disease, which produces a fairly characteristic clinical picture. There is intermittent claudication of the low back, buttocks, and thigh or calf muscles. There is atrophy of the limbs and pallor of the skin of the feet and legs. Impotence may also be present. Arterial pulses in the legs are absent; they may be present but weak in the femoral arteries. Systolic bruits may be audible over the femoral arteries and lower abdomen.

Arteriosclerotic aneurysms may occur, and present as pulsatile, expansible masses in the popliteal fossa or in the femoral artery below the inguinal ligament. These may cause symptoms by pressure on adjacent structures, and, occasionally, by embolism of peripheral vessels or by hemorrhage into the tissues.

DIAGNOSIS. The diagnostic approach to the patient with arteriosclerosis obliterans should be directed at establishing the site of the arterial obstruction, its severity, the degree of ischemia, and the adequacy of the collateral circulation. Palpation of the arterial pulses and auscultation of bruits usually suffice to determine the presence and site of arterial obstruction. Trophic changes and alterations in skin color and temperature indicate ischemia. The latter, as well as the adequacy of the collateral circulation, can be further ascertained by determining the blood pressure at the ankle at rest and during exercise. Several tests may be helpful. With the patient in a warm environment, so that vasoconstrictor tone is low, the leg is raised to a 45-degree angle while the patient is supine. The color of the plantar surface of the foot is observed. Pallor during this test is indicative of severe arterial insufficiency. Venous and capillary filling times can be measured when the patient shifts from the recumbent to the sitting position. Ordinarily, delay in flushing by more than 20 to 30 seconds indicates inadequate collateral circulation. The systolic blood pressure in the dorsalis pedis or posterior tibial arteries can be determined with the use of a Doppler velocitometer at rest as well as during exercise. Ordinarily, this pressure should not be lower than 90 per cent of the level of systolic pressure in the brachial artery. In the presence of severe ischemia, pressures may fall to very low levels. As a rule, pressures less than 30 mm Hg indicate ischemia of sufficient severity to cause gangrene.

The confirmation of arterial obstruction is carried out by arteriography, which is essential to establish the exact anatomy of the arterial vessels and to determine the advisability of surgery.

Arterial embolism is usually distinguishable from arteriosclerosis obliterans because of the sudden onset of the ischemic manifestations and the usually unilateral involvement. Intermittent claudication may occur in severe anemia, in venous disease, and in muscle phosphorylase deficiency (McArdle's syndrome). These conditions are distinguished from arteriosclerosis obliterans by the presence of normal pulses. Ergotamine or methysergide toxicity may cause severe vasospasm, which may affect the large arteries and diminish pulses. The history of drug ingestion may help distinguish these from arteriosclerosis obliterans. In difficult cases, angiography shows the generalized vasospasm and absence of segmental obstructions. A number of conditions of nonvascular nature, such as arthritis and lumbar disc disorders, may cause pain in the limbs and may be confused with intermittent claudication. The presence of normal pulses and other manifestations of these diseases distinguishes them from arteriosclerosis obliterans. In diabetics, ulcerations may be present as a result of diabetic neuropathy. The cause of these ulcers may be difficult to ascertain in the presence of arteriosclerosis obliterans.

TREATMENT. Patients with arteriosclerosis obliterans without evidence of ischemia should be treated medically. Limitation of physical activity, avoidance of tobacco smoking (which causes vasoconstriction), and a regular exercise program are advisable. The treatment of hyperlipidemia, if present, may prevent development of new arteriosclerotic lesions. The control of diabetes, if present, is required. Patients should maintain the skin of the affected limbs clean, dry, and soft and protect it from cold and trauma. Infections and trauma should be attended to promptly.

There is no evidence that vasodilative drugs are effective in the treatment of arteriosclerosis obliterans. In fact, they may be harmful under certain circumstances by lowering arterial blood pressure and reducing collateral blood flow or by diverting blood to proximal healthy areas, thereby reducing the perfusion pressure in the more distal portions of the limb. Pentoxifylline, 400 mg administered orally three times daily, has been shown in controlled trials to prolong the duration of exercise and the distance the patient is able to walk prior to the onset of claudication. The drug acts by increasing red cell membrane deformability, thereby reducing effective blood viscosity.

Surgical treatment is advisable when ischemia is present or if intermittent claudication seriously interferes with the patient's activities. Surgery involves either endarterectomy of the stenotic artery or a bypass operation. Bypass can be performed with either a vein graft or synthetic material. Vein grafts are preferred because of the lower incidence of thrombosis. It is essential that the presence of patent vessels below the obstruction be ascertained before the grafting procedure is carried out. Axillofemoral or femorofemoral grafts for aortoiliac disease have been successful. The larger the size of the vessels grafted, the higher the rate of successful restoration of blood flow.

Percutaneous transluminal angioplasty offers an attractive alternative to surgery in the treatment of arteriosclerosis obliterans. It is simple, has low morbidity, and is less costly than surgery. In this technique, the segmental stenosis or obstruction is dilated by suddenly inflating at the site of the lesion a balloon introduced into the artery by percutaneous catheterization. High success rates and good long-term rates of patency of the dilated vessels have been reported. Angioplasty is more successful in larger vessels, when the stenotic segment is relatively short and when the vessel is not completely occluded. Restenosis of lesions dilated by angioplasty occurs in 20 to 30 per cent of the patients within a year. It may be due to thrombosis or, more commonly, to intimal and medial proliferation.

Atherectomy is a newly introduced alternative to balloon angioplasty. In this technique, the obstructing lesion is eliminated by shaving off successive layers with a special atherectomy catheter equipped with a rotary cutting device. The technique may be advantageous when used for repeat angioplasty following restenosis.

If the anatomy of the disease makes surgery impossible and ischemic manifestations are present, bed rest is essential. The affected extremity should be kept in a slightly dependent position at 20 to 30 degrees below horizontal, and direct application of heat should be avoided. The limb is best kept warm by placing it under a cradle, under which the temperature is regulated below 38°C. Analgesics or narcotics may be required to control pain. Ulcers should be kept clean with warm saline soaks and debrided. Appropriate antibiotics should be used if infection is present. Intra-arterial administration of PGE_1,* may be beneficial in patients with gangrene or ulceration in whom surgery is not possible. Amputation may be necessary to arrest advancing gangrene. The level of amputation is chosen by the presence of warm, viable tissue having normal color.

Long-term anticoagulants are of questionable value. Fibrinolytic therapy with intravenous streptokinase is reported to be helpful in a few patients with recent onset of the disease.

Preganglionic lumbar sympathectomy may be performed as an acute intervention to treat ischemic manifestations of arteriosclerosis obliterans. Before surgery, it must be demonstrated that the interruption of sympathetic nerves is likely to cause improvement in the circulation of the limb. This is done by inducing temporary sympathetic blockade with local anesthetics. This is essential, especially in diabetics in whom peripheral neuropathy may have already produced spontaneous sympathectomy. Sympathectomy does not influence the long-term prognosis of intermittent claudication.

PROGNOSIS. Arteriosclerosis obliterans in the absence of diabetes is a slowly progressive disease. No significant deterioration may be detected for several years. In the presence of diabetes, the disease tends to progress more rapidly, and the

---

*Investigational drug for this purpose.

prognosis is less satisfactory. The location of obstructing lesions also influences the prognosis. When the lesions are in larger arteries, the probability of successful surgical intervention or percutaneous angioplasty is higher, and the prognosis is better. Frequently arteriosclerosis obliterans is only one of the manifestations of a generalized arteriosclerotic process. Mortality results from arteriosclerotic involvement of other vascular beds, such as the coronary or the cerebral circulation, with death from myocardial infarction or stroke.

Coffman JD: Intermittent claudication and rest pain. Physiologic concepts and therapeutic approaches. Prog Cardiovasc Dis 22:53, 1979. *A comprehensive, well-referenced consideration of the clinical features, diagnosis, and treatment of arteriosclerosis obliterans.*

Freiman DB, Spence R, Gatenby R, et al.: Transluminal angioplasty of the iliac and femoral arteries: Follow-up results with anticoagulation. Radiology 141:347, 1981. *Transluminal angioplasty for the treatment of obstructive disease of the iliac and femoral arteries. Excellent results are reported in 192 patients.*

Porter JM, Culter BS, Lee BY, et al.: Pentoxifylline efficacy in the treatment of intermittent claudication: Multicenter controlled double-blind trial with objective assessment of chronic occlusive arterial disease patients. Am Heart J 104:66, 1982. *A controlled trial of pentoxifylline in patients with intermittent claudication demonstrating objectively improved exercise tolerance.*

Schadt DC, Hines EA, Juergens JL, et al.: Chronic atherosclerotic occlusion of the femoral artery. JAMA 175:937, 1961. *A long-term follow-up study showing slow progression of arteriosclerosis obliterans.*

Thromboangiitis Obliterans (Buerger's Disease)

DEFINITION. Thromboangiitis obliterans is an obstructive arterial disease caused by segmental inflammatory and proliferative lesions of the medium and small arteries and veins of the limbs.

ETIOLOGY. The cause of thromboangiitis obliterans is unknown. Almost all patients with this disease are moderate or heavy smokers, particularly of cigarettes. Many show cutaneous hypersensitivity to intradermally injected tobacco products. There is a high prevalence of HLA-A9 and HLA-B5 antigens in affected persons. An autoimmune mechanism is suggested by a study of cellular and humoral immune responses of 39 patients with thromboangiitis obliterans. Lymphocytes from 77 per cent of these patients exhibited cellular sensitivity to human type I and type III collagen, both of which are constituents of the vascular wall. In addition, approximately 50 per cent had significant levels of anticollagen antibodies in their blood. By contrast, normal controls and patients with arteriosclerosis obliterans had considerably lower levels of cellular sensitivity to collagen and no circulating anticollagen antibodies.

INCIDENCE. Thromboangiitis obliterans is a disease mostly of young males. The disease begins most frequently between the ages of 20 and 40 years, and the ratio of men to women affected varies from 9:1 to as high as 75:1. There is a high prevalence of the disorder in Israel, the Orient, and in India as compared with the United States and Western Europe, suggesting the possibility of a genetic predisposition. The disease has been occasionally reported to occur in familial form.

PATHOLOGY. The disease affects small and medium-sized arteries and veins in segmental fashion. Acute lesions are manifested by proliferation of the intima and thrombosis. There is inflammatory infiltration with polymorphonuclear leukocytes, lymphocytes, and giant cells of all coats of the artery or vein, extending into the thrombus. The media remains intact. Calcium or cholesterol deposition does not occur. These lesions are distinguished from those of arteriosclerosis obliterans because of the more cellular thrombus, the preservation of the media, and the inflammatory infiltration of all coats of the vessel. Older lesions become less cellular, and eventually they may be transformed into a dense scar. Typically, in any one vessel, lesions of varying ages are seen.

CLINICAL MANIFESTATIONS. The typical patient with thromboangiitis obliterans is a young man who smokes cigarettes heavily, has manifestations of ischemia of the extremities, and has a history or evidence of superficial thrombophlebitis. Common presenting complaints are Raynaud's phenomenon with digital ulcerations or pain from ischemia. Pain in thromboangiitis obliterans may be of several types. The most frequent is pain at rest in one or more digits. This pain may be accompanied by manifestations of ischemia, such as color or temperature changes

of the skin. This type of pain may be a forerunner of ulceration or gangrene. In the presence of these trophic lesions, there may be localized pain that is aching in character and more severe at night. Another type of pain may occur along the course of the inflamed blood vessels. Ischemic neuropathy may result and cause a paroxysmal, shocklike pain, which may follow the distribution of sensory nerves. Paresthesias may accompany this type of pain. Typical intermittent claudication occurs commonly in the lower extremities. It most often occurs in the arch of the foot because of involvement of the vessels of the leg and sparing of the femoral and iliac arteries. Some patients have intermittent claudication of the forearm or hand. Sensitivity to cold with paresthesias and the development of secondary Raynaud's phenomenon are common. Migratory superficial thrombophlebitis is manifested by the development of inflamed, tender, red segments of the superficial veins, which subside over a period of several weeks.

Physical examination discloses impaired arterial pulsations in the more distal portions of the limbs, such as the radial, ulnar, dorsalis pedis, and posterior tibial arteries. The more proximal arteries are normal, a finding that contrasts with arteriosclerosis obliterans. There may be cyanosis or pallor or persistent redness in the digits, and associated changes in temperature may be noted. Postural changes in color are also common. Gangrene or ulcerations of the digits may be present in both upper and lower extremities. Edema of the foot is common. Occasional patients have involvement of visceral arteries with stenosis or occlusion of mesenteric, coronary, cerebral, or renal arteries and manifestations of ischemia of these organs.

DIAGNOSIS. The diagnosis of thromboangiitis obliterans should be entertained when there is evidence of ischemia of the extremities from arterial occlusive disease in association with migratory superficial thrombophlebitis. The age and sex of the individual and the involvement of the upper extremities are additional helpful characteristics. Arteriography may be helpful in disclosing segmental multiple occlusions of the medium-sized and small arteries associated with collateral vessel visualization. The larger arteries are generally spared, a finding that also helps distinguish the disorder from arteriosclerosis obliterans. Final confirmation may be obtained only from biopsy material of an early lesion and histologic demonstration of the characteristic inflammatory and proliferative lesion of the disease.

PROGNOSIS. Thromboangiitis obliterans is not usually life threatening except in rare individuals in whom the visceral arteries are involved. The disease, however, results in disability and amputation of the extremities in a high percentage of cases. It is generally more rapidly progressive than arteriosclerosis obliterans, especially in individuals who refuse to stop smoking.

TREATMENT. Cessation of tobacco smoking is essential. Continuation of smoking results in a progressive course. If the patient stops smoking, new lesions do not develop or they develop more rarely. The approach to the patient with thromboangiitis obliterans is generally the same as that to patients with advanced arteriosclerosis obliterans. It consists of conservative measures, including protection from cold, local care in the event of ulceration or gangrene, and eventually amputation, if these lesions occur. Sympathectomy is tried frequently and may be effective, at least temporarily, if vasospasm is a prominent feature. Vasodilative drug therapy can be tried in cases of Raynaud's phenomenon with ulcerations, but its effectiveness is questionable.

Adar R, Papa MZ, Halpern Z, et al.: Cellular sensitivity to collagen in thromboangiitis obliterans. N Engl J Med 308:1113, 1983. *An important study showing high incidence of cellular sensitivity to collagen and the presence of circulating anticollagen antibodies in patients with thromboangiitis obliterans. The results have profound implications concerning the etiology of the disease and offer possible means of differentiating it from arteriosclerosis obliterans.*

McKusick VA, Harris WS, Ottesen OE, et al.: Buerger's disease: A distinct clinical and pathologic entity. JAMA 181:5, 1962. *A concise and thoughtful consideration of the clinical features, arteriographic findings, and histopathology of 30 cases with Buerger's disease.*

Sudden Arterial Occlusion

DEFINITION. Sudden arterial occlusion may result from obstruction of an artery of the extremity by embolism or by thrombosis in situ. The clinical manifestations are the result of the consequent ischemia.

ETIOLOGY. The major cause of sudden arterial occlusion is arterial embolism. The heart is the most frequent source of emboli in this syndrome. Emboli may arise from thrombi in the left atrium in the presence of atrial fibrillation or mitral valve disease, usually mitral stenosis. Emboli may also arise from mural thrombi from a myocardial infarction or in the presence of a cardiomyopathy. Septic emboli may arise from vegetations from the mitral or aortic valves in the presence of bacterial endocarditis. Less commonly, emboli may arise from an arteriosclerotic plaque in more proximal parts of the arterial tree or from aneurysms. In rare cases, the embolus may arise from the venous side and enter the arterial tree via a patent foramen ovale (paradoxical embolism). More rarely, the embolus consists of calcium fragments from a calcified valve leaflet, cholesterol crystals from an arteriosclerotic plaque, or foreign materials such as a bullet.

Sudden arterial thrombosis occurs in about 10 per cent of the cases of arteriosclerosis obliterans. The condition is rare in thromboangiitis obliterans or in polyarteritis nodosa. Acute arterial thrombosis may occur in conditions in which the coagulability of the blood is increased in the presence of normal vessels, such as in polycythemia vera or in cryoglobulinemia. Rarely, arterial thrombosis may occur in the presence of normal vessels in infections such as septicemia, pneumonia, peritonitis, tuberculosis, ulcerative colitis, and other debilitating diseases. Trauma from penetrating wounds, as from arterial puncture or catheterization, may cause arterial occlusion.

PATHOLOGY. The structure of emboli that arise from thrombi in the heart or from aneurysms is the same as that of the parent thrombi. Emboli lodge in an artery and obstruct the vessel. There may be extension of the thrombus distally by further clotting of the blood. The fate of the embolus varies. In some cases it may become organized and finally be recanalized, and in other cases it may become fragmented and the fragments may lodge in more distal vessels.

PATHOPHYSIOLOGY. The sudden arterial occlusion causes reduction of blood flow to the more distal portions of the limb and consequent ischemia. There have been suggestions that vasoactive agents released from the emboli, such as serotonin from platelets, may cause contraction of vascular smooth muscle in more distal portions of the vascular tree and result in vasospasm that further aggravates ischemia. The severity and extent of ischemia depend on the size of the vessel occluded and on the extent of collateral circulation. The larger the occluded vessel, the more likely it is that severe ischemia would result.

CLINICAL MANIFESTATIONS. Sudden arterial occlusion causes the abrupt onset of severe pain accompanied by manifestations of ischemia in about half the patients. In the remainder, the onset is gradual with either mild pain or numbness and paresthesias. Pain is present in about 75 per cent of the cases. There may be muscular weakness or outright paralysis. A saddle embolus of the aortic bifurcation causes abdominal pain, nausea, and vomiting and may result in a shocklike state.

Examination of the patient discloses diminished or absent pulses distal to the occlusion. Evidence of ischemia is present with low skin temperature and pallor or cyanosis or a combination of the two. If the occluded artery is superficial, the site of lodgment of the embolus may be identified as a tender region. The subsequent course depends on the adequacy of the collateral circulation. If this is adequate, gradual improvement occurs. Otherwise, gangrene supervenes.

DIAGNOSIS. The diagnosis of sudden arterial occlusion is usually relatively easy in the patient who has the acute onset of pain and ischemia of an extremity. If the cause is an embolus, its source may be evident. Rarely, patients with acute thrombophlebitis of the iliac and femoral veins may have feeble or absent arterial pulses and show manifestations resembling those of ischemia from an arterial embolus. In these cases, the demonstration of the feeble pulse and the presence of distended veins and pronounced edema help make the differentiation possible.

PROGNOSIS. The outcome of acute arterial obstruction depends on the size of the vessel affected, the age of the patient, the extent of the collateral circulation, and the timing of therapeutic intervention. When a large artery is occluded, the prognosis is poor without surgical treatment. In older patients with pre-existing arterial occlusive disease, the prognosis is poor because of obstruction of multiple vessels, including collateral vessels.

TREATMENT. The goal of therapeutic intervention is the removal or dissolution of the thrombus and re-establishment of patency of the occluded artery. This goal can be achieved by surgical embolectomy or by thrombolytic therapy. Urgent embolectomy is the preferred method of treatment when a large artery is occluded, such as with a saddle embolus of the bifurcation of the aorta. When smaller vessels are occluded and the thrombus is not easily accessible or when the patient's general condition does not permit surgical intervention, intravenous or intra-arterial streptokinase or urokinase may be given, if there are no contraindications for their use. Streptokinase is given intravenously as a bolus of 250,000 IU, followed by an infusion of 100,000 IU per hour. The infusion is continued for 72 hours. Intra-arterial administration can be used instead, in a dose of about one tenth of the intravenous dose; it can be coupled with angioplasty. Thrombolytic therapy is followed by conventional anticoagulants. The success rate of thrombolytic therapy is critically dependent on how early it is administered after the onset of symptoms. It is more effective for thrombotic lesions than embolic ones. Streptokinase or urokinase cannot be safely followed by surgery because of the danger of bleeding from the arteriotomy. The choice of therapy, therefore, must be carefully considered.

If neither therapeutic approach can be used, the patient should be treated conservatively. The patient should be placed at rest. The limb should be placed in a slightly dependent position under a cradle whose temperature is controlled at 30 to 35°C. Anticoagulation with heparin should be started as soon as possible to prevent extension of the thrombus and to prevent formation of additional emboli. If vasospasm is prominent, lumbar sympathectomy may be tried to reduce vasomotor tone and improve blood flow to the limb.

When a patient is treated by conservative medical measures, he or she should be followed closely for evidence of deterioration. If this occurs, immediate surgical intervention and embolectomy should be attempted. The results of embolectomy depend, to a large extent, on the timing of intervention. Therefore, surgery should not be delayed longer than a few hours. If therapy fails, gangrene may supervene, and amputation may become necessary.

Haimovici H: Peripheral arterial embolism. Angiology 1:20, 1950. *Detailed consideration of the clinical features of the arteries of the limbs based on study of 330 cases.*

Hargrove WC, Barker CF, Berkowitz HD, et al.: Treatment of acute peripheral arterial and graft thromboses with low-dose streptokinase. Surgery 92:981, 1982. *A report of good results from the use of intra-arterial streptokinase for the treatment of acute arterial thrombosis.*

Hinton RC, Kistler JP, Fallon JT, et al.: Influence of etiology of atrial fibrillation on incidence of systemic embolism. Am J Cardiol 40:509, 1977. *A study of the pathology of arterial embolism in 333 patients with atrial fibrillation. The paper emphasizes that the risk of embolism is independent of the cause of atrial fibrillation.*

VASCULAR DISEASES OF THE LIMBS CAUSED BY ABNORMAL COMMUNICATION BETWEEN ARTERIES AND VEINS

Arteriovenous Fistula

DEFINITION. Arteriovenous fistula is an abnormal direct communication between an artery and a vein.

ETIOLOGY. Arteriovenous fistulas in the limbs may be congenital or acquired. Congenital fistulas are usually multiple; acquired ones are usually single. The most common type is iatrogenic, created to carry out renal dialysis. Acquired arteriovenous fistulas may also result from trauma caused by penetrating wounds or surgical procedures.

PATHOPHYSIOLOGY. The low resistance of the direct communication between artery and vein results in a high arterial inflow into the vein, with a resultant increase in venous pressure. The elevated venous pressure causes engorgement of the vein and distention and may lead to the production of varicose veins. In the region of the fistula, blood flow is high, whereas more distal portions are deprived of capillary blood flow and may show ischemia and trophic changes.

Large fistulas cause a reduction in systemic vascular resistance and impose a burden on the heart because of the associated increase in cardiac output. Total blood volume may be increased. Left ventricular failure may eventually result.

PATHOLOGY. In the region of the fistula the veins become thickened, whereas the artery undergoes thinning and loss of elastic and muscular fibers in the media.

CLINICAL MANIFESTATIONS. The patient may be totally asymptomatic, and the discovery of the fistula may be accidental. In other cases, there may be pain in the location of the fistula, edema, varicosities, and asymmetry in the size of the limbs. In some cases, the presenting symptoms may be those of cardiac decompensation with dyspnea on exertion, palpitations, and orthopnea. Examination of the involved limb reveals tortuous, dilated superficial veins and venous pulsation at the site of the fistula. The temperature of the skin may be high, and distal portions of the limb may show ischemic changes. A bruit or a thrill may be heard over the fistula during systole. At other times, a continuous bruit may be present. The extremity may be swollen, or the girth of the limb may be increased because of hypertrophy of the soft tissues. Temporary compression of the artery proximal to the fistula causes immediate increase in systemic vascular resistance and leads to reflex decrease in heart rate (Branham's sign), a change that may be helpful diagnostically.

DIAGNOSIS. When the fistula is superficial and large, the diagnosis can be made easily. If this is not possible from the physical examination, arteriography should be attempted for a definitive diagnosis. The oxygen saturation of the venous blood from the involved limb is higher than that of its contralateral part, and this comparison may be helpful in making the diagnosis.

TREATMENT. The treatment of choice is surgical intervention with closure of the fistula and re-establishment of the continuity of the involved artery and vein. If such restoration is not possible, ligation of the artery or vein or both may be necessary, but this may lead to arterial or venous insufficiency of the limb. In some cases, the fistula involves an anomalous artery. In this case, the ligation of the artery and the obstruction of the veins by the injection of sclerosing solutions may give a satisfactory result. It may not be practical to treat surgically patients with multiple fistulas. In these cases, conservative measures consisting of local care, relief of pain, and wearing elastic bandages may be helpful. If the fistula is inoperable and cardiac decompensation is present or threatened, amputation may be necessary.

Nickerson JL, Elkin DC, Warren JV: The effect of temporary occlusion of arteriovenous fistulas on heart rate, stroke volume, and cardiac output. J Clin Invest 30:215, 1951. *A classic study of the systemic hemodynamic effects of arteriovenous fistulas in a large number of patients.*

Rossi P, Carillo FJ, Alfidi RJ, et al.: Iatrogenic arteriovenous fistulas. Radiology 111:47, 1974. *A comprehensive review of 154 cases of iatrogenic arteriovenous fistulas. The paper provides a good review of the literature.*

Glomus Tumor (Glomangioma)

DEFINITION. Glomangioma, or glomus tumor, is a benign tumor of the glomus body.

PATHOLOGY. The glomus tumor is an encapsulated structure consisting of a hypertrophied arteriovenous anastomosis. The tumor varies in size from 0.5 to 2.5 cm in diameter. It can be found in various parts of the upper and lower extremities but is most frequently located in the nail beds.

CLINICAL MANIFESTATIONS. The most common symptom is severe burning pain in the location of the tumor. The pain may precede the appearance of the tumor. Pain may occur spontaneously, or it may be precipitated by exposure to heat or cold. Occasionally, the tumor is exquisitely sensitive to touch, and even the slightest pressure from contact with clothing may cause severe pain. Severe disability and atrophy of the limb from disuse may occur secondary to fear of pain. Examination of the involved area shows a reddish, purplish, or bluish mass that is sharply demarcated. At times, the tumor may not be easily visible or palpable. In this case, pressure with the head of a pin may help identify the location of the tumor. When it is located under the nail bed, the nail and the phalanx may be visibly deformed, thereby giving a clue to the location of the tumor. Ultrasonography or magnetic resonance imaging is useful in the diagnosis of small glomus tumors.

TREATMENT. The glomus tumor is a benign tumor. Surgical excision results in complete relief without recurrence.

Cooke SAR: Misleading features in the clinical diagnosis of the peripheral glomus tumour. Br J Surg 58:602, 1971. *The clinical manifestations of glomus tumor are described based on the study of 24 cases.*

Fornage BD: Glomus tumors in the fingers: Diagnosis with US. Radiology 167:183, 1988. *This report shows that ultrasonography is useful in the diagnosis of small glomus tumors.*

DISEASES OF THE VEINS OF THE LIMBS

Thrombophlebitis and Deep-Vein Thrombosis

DEFINITION. Thrombophlebitis refers to venous thrombosis with accompanying inflammation of the venous wall. For important practical reasons, superficial thrombophlebitis is distinguished from deep-vein thrombosis. Superficial thrombophlebitis does not cause embolic complications, but deep-vein thrombosis is a frequent cause of pulmonary embolism.

PATHOLOGY. Thrombi in veins consist mostly of red cells with a few platelets held together with fibrin. They propagate in the direction of the bloodstream by extension of the thrombotic process. They attach to the wall of the vein at one end, while the more proximal end floats freely into the lumen of the vessel. This is the portion that is commonly broken off and travels to the lungs. Varying degrees of inflammatory reaction of the venous wall may be present. Venous thrombosis may exist in the absence of inflammation, as is the case in some patients with malignancy. This is referred to as "phlebothrombosis." In most cases, however, inflammation and thrombosis coexist. The disorder may start as a pure thrombotic process, and inflammation usually occurs secondary to the presence of the thrombus.

INCIDENCE. Deep-vein thrombosis is a common disorder. It is more common in women than in men. All races seem to be affected equally, at least in developed countries. The incidence of the disease increases with advancing age. The disease is very common in hospitalized patients. Approximately one third of the patients over age 40 who have undergone major surgery or have had an acute myocardial infarction develop deep-vein thrombosis. The incidence is even higher after certain operations such as repair of hip fractures or prostatectomy. Patients with thrombotic strokes have an equally high incidence of deep-vein thrombosis. This occurs almost exclusively in the paralyzed limb.

Superficial thrombophlebitis occurs most commonly in patients with varicose veins, possibly as a result of minor trauma. It is also frequent after pregnancy. A migratory type of superficial thrombophlebitis also occurs in patients with thromboangiitis obliterans.

PATHOGENESIS. Venous stasis, injury to the venous wall, and a hypercoagulable state are the three main factors that lead to venous thrombosis. In most cases, more than one of these factors are present, and their effect may be cumulative. The combination of venous stasis and changes in the clotting mechanism of the blood accounts for the increased incidence of deep-vein thrombosis in pregnancy and during administration of oral contraceptives. Venous stasis is the major factor in the development of venous thrombosis in patients with heart disease, in paralyzed patients, in patients undergoing major surgery, in those who have varicose veins, and in healthy individuals after long trips. Increased viscosity, leading to stasis, and alterations in the clotting factors of the blood account for the high incidence of polycythemia vera. Patients with familial deficiencies of certain anticlotting factors are susceptible to recurrent thrombophlebitis. These include deficiencies of antithrombin III, protein S, protein C, and heparin cofactor II. Injury to the venous wall may result from administration of certain vasoconstrictive or chemotherapeutic agents, or it may result from infectious agents. Patients with malignancies may have migrating thrombophlebitis, which has been attributed to low-grade activation of intravascular coagulation.

CLINICAL MANIFESTATIONS. The presence of superficial thrombophlebitis is usually easily ascertained by finding the inflamed vein. This may be apparent as a red, tender cord. By contrast, deep-vein thrombosis frequently causes few distinctive clinical features; about one half of patients with deep-vein thrombosis are asymptomatic. The first manifestation of deep-vein thrombosis may be the occurrence of pulmonary embolism. Pain in the region of the thrombosed veins at rest or only during exercise and edema distal to the obstructed veins are the usual symptoms of deep-vein thrombosis. Examination of the patient may disclose several helpful manifestations. Edema or pitting of the malleolar fossa may be present and may cause loss of the normal concavity of that portion of the leg. There may be a difference between the two legs in the circumference of the calf. A difference in maximal circumference in excess of 1.4 cm in men and 1.2 cm in women is highly suspicious. The temperature of the skin may be increased as a result of the inflammatory reaction, and palpation may disclose the thrombosed veins in the calf or in the popliteal fossa. There may be tenderness to palpation. Increased resistance or pain on voluntary dorsiflexion of the foot (Homans' sign) may be present. A useful sign is the presence of tenderness on inflation of a blood pressure cuff around the calf. Most normal individuals tolerate this without pain up to pressures of 160 to 180 mm Hg.

Thrombosis of the iliac and femoral veins usually presents with a characteristic clinical picture consisting of rapidly advancing swelling of the entire limb. The thrombosed vein may be tender if it extends below the inguinal ligament. Collateral distended veins may be present in the upper thigh. In some cases, secondary ischemia may occur as a result of the very high venous pressure that impedes arterial inflow. Cyanosis of the toes and even gangrene may occur under these circumstances.

Thrombosis of the subclavian vein may result in swelling of the upper extremity, and collateral veins may be present. In axillary thrombosis, a similar clinical picture occurs; the thrombosed vein may be felt in the axilla. A history of walking on crutches or sleeping in a sitting position on a bench with the arms behind the backrest may be helpful. Thrombosis of the superior vena cava causes increased venous pressure in the neck and face with distention of the neck veins in the upper part of the chest.

In septic thrombophlebitis, there may also be systemic manifestations of infection, such as fever, chills, and leukocytosis. In cases in which septic phlebitis begins from infected needles or catheters, an inflamed, tender cord may appear at the site of the venipuncture.

DIAGNOSIS. Iliofemoral thrombophlebitis is usually easily recognized by the rapid swelling of the entire limb, engorged collateral veins in the thigh, and signs of inflammation, such as increased skin temperature.

By contrast, in the majority of cases of deep-vein thrombosis involving the calf, popliteal area, and thigh, the clinical picture is not sufficiently distinctive to allow diagnosis with a high degree of confidence. Confirmation of the diagnosis must be provided by resorting to one or more of a number of diagnostic tests. The most commonly employed tests are the following:

X-ray Venography. Venography is one of the most accurate means of making the diagnosis of deep-vein thrombosis. The test involves the injection of a contrast medium into the venous system, which has been previously emptied of blood by gravity. The test relies on finding a filling defect or a sharp cutoff, indicating the presence of occluding thrombus in the vein. The test may result in inflammatory reaction followed by thrombosis in a few cases. It is sensitive and highly specific; for these reasons, venography is considered the "gold standard" in the diagnosis of deep-vein thrombosis.

Radionuclide Venography. This test is similar to x-ray venography except that instead of contrast medium, a radioisotope, such as ^{99m}Tc-macroaggregated albumin, is injected in a foot vein. External scanning detects venous obstruction and the presence of collateral circulation. In another variation of the technique, ^{99m}Tc-labeled red cells from the patient's own blood are injected intravenously, and a blood pool scan is obtained. The sensitivity and specificity of the technique are somewhat less than those of x-ray venography. The technique is probably better in detecting venous thrombosis in the thigh than in the calf.

Radioisotope-labeled Fibrinogen. This test consists of intravenous administration of fibrinogen labeled with ^{125}I and the subsequent incorporation of the radioactive material into the thrombus. The accumulation of radioactivity is detected by external counting. This test detects an active thrombophlebitis; it may be negative in cases in which the active process has stopped but thrombi exist in the veins. The reliability of the test depends on the location of the thrombus. It is of little use in detecting pelvic thrombi because of the high background due to the bladder and iliac arteries. It is most useful in detecting thrombosis of the calf. Another disadvantage is that it requires 1 or 2 days for sufficient counts to build into the thrombosed vein for detection. This test is, therefore, most useful in longitudinal screening of high-risk populations.

Liquid Crystal Thermography. This test relies on the detection of small increases in skin temperature as a result of the venous inflammation. The test is easy to perform. It has high sensitivity but relatively low specificity. It can be a useful adjunct to ultrasonography or impedance plethysmography for monitoring patients at risk.

Ultrasonography. This test utilizes the Doppler principle to detect venous obstruction. Thus, during various maneuvers that alter venous flow, such as deep inspiration, the Valsalva maneuver, or leg compression, the ultrasonogram may detect the presence of obstructed veins. The disadvantages of the technique are that a high degree of stenosis is necessary for the test result to be abnormal and that it does not distinguish between occlusion from external pressure and occlusion by thrombus. Also, the result may be negative if an effective collateral circulation has developed. The test is most sensitive for thrombosis of the veins above the knee.

"Duplex" Ultrasonography. This technique makes use of simultaneous real-time ultrasound imaging, combined with pulsed gated Doppler evaluation of blood flow. The technique allows direct visualization of the major vascular channels together with evaluation of the blood flow. Modern instruments display the Doppler signal in the form of a colored real-time image (color-flow Doppler). This technique has excellent specificity and sensitivity for deep-vein thrombosis above the knee. It is less reliable in detecting small calf thrombi. Its reliability is so high for thrombosis in the thigh that it can be used as a substitute for venography.

Impedance Plethysmography. This test detects alterations in blood volume of the extremities by detecting changes in the electrical impedance of the tissues. The test is carried out during respiratory maneuvers or during alterations in blood flow by occluding the limb with a pneumatic pressure cuff. Like ultrasonography, this test requires significant proximal obstruction for positive results. The reported sensitivity and specificity of the last two tests are high (over 90 per cent).

Choice of Tests. The choice of tests to be performed depends to a large extent on their availability. If all are available, it is preferable to use duplex ultrasonography. Because this technique does not detect small thrombi in the calf with consistency, it is necessary to repeat the test after a few days to eliminate the possibilty of extension into the thigh of existing deep vein thrombosis in the calf. If duplex ultrasonography is not available, it is preferable to use conventional ultrasonography or impedance plethysmography and to resort to venography if the results of these tests are inconclusive. The radioactive fibrinogen test and thermography should be reserved for screening of patients at high risk.

DIFFERENTIAL DIAGNOSIS. A number of conditions that cause localized pain or edema in the lower extremities may be confused with deep-vein thrombosis. A ruptured popliteal synovial membrane or cyst (Baker's cyst) may simulate most of the manifestations of venous thrombosis. The diagnosis can be suspected if there is a history or physical findings of arthritis of the knee joint. The diagnosis may be confirmed by an arthrogram revealing the entry of dye from the joint into the calf muscles. Rupture of the calf muscles may cause pain, tenderness, and edema and may simulate thrombophlebitis. The diagnosis can be made from the history of strenuous or unusual exercise, the presence of ecchymosis from extravasated blood, and the palpation of a hematoma. Sometimes the patient reports an audible snap during the activity when the pain first occurred. The differential diagnosis is important because anticoagulants are contraindicated in this condition. A severe muscle cramp may cause pain and swelling for a considerable period of time. Other manifestations of thrombophlebitis are, however, lacking in this situation. The pain of a lumbar disc may be localized in the calf. There are no other manifestations of venous thrombosis, however, and there may be neurologic findings to identify the cause of the pain. Lymphedema is recognized by its slower and gradual onset and the absence of signs of inflammation and of collateral veins. Finally, cellulitis may be confused with superficial thrombophlebitis.

COMPLICATIONS. Pulmonary embolism is a frequent and serious complication of deep-vein thrombosis. About 80 to 90 per cent of pulmonary emboli arise in the deep veins of the lower limbs. Although deep-vein thrombosis may begin frequently in the veins of the calf, it is only when the thrombosis extends above the knee that serious pulmonary embolism occurs.

About 5 per cent of patients with deep-vein thrombosis develop venous insufficiency with stasis dermatitis (postphlebitic syndrome). This is more likely to occur in those with more proximal venous obstruction. A rare complication of iliofemoral thrombophlebitis is venous claudication, in which the patient develops pain on exercise which is relieved by rest, as in arterial occlusive disease.

PROPHYLAXIS. Prophylactic therapy against deep-vein thrombosis should be attempted in high-risk patients (Table 54–4). The exact regimen used must take into consideration the risk of deep-vein thrombosis and consequent pulmonary embolism and the potential risk of hemorrhagic complications from the prophylactic therapy. Low-dose heparin is currently the most commonly used prophylactic technique. For surgical patients, this consists of administration of 5000 units of heparin subcutaneously 2 hours before surgery and then every 8 or 12 hours until the patient is ambulatory. This method is effective in reducing the incidence of deep-vein thrombosis and pulmonary embolism in patients subjected to a variety of surgical procedures. It is also effective in reducing the incidence of deep-vein thrombosis in patients following acute myocardial infarction, but it is not known whether there is also a reduction in the incidence of pulmonary embolism. Low-dose heparin has been shown to be ineffective in patients undergoing surgery for hip fracture and hip replacement, and its effectiveness has not been established in urologic procedures. Higher dose heparin adjusted to give an activated partial thromboplastin time (APTT) in the upper limits of the therapeutic range has been reported to be more effective than low-dose heparin. In addition, the administration of dihydroergotamine mesylate, 0.5 mg subcutaneously, together with low-dose heparin, is more effective in preventing deep-vein thrombosis than heparin alone in surgical patients. Ergotamine acts by inducing venoconstriction and also by altering the coagulability of the blood. Warfarin and other similar drugs are also effective in protecting patients from thromboembolism during a variety of surgical techniques. Low molecular weight dextran given on the day of surgery and at suitable intervals thereafter has been reported in most cases to give favorable results. There is a risk of fluid overload, and, to a lesser extent, hemorrhagic complications. This method can be used in instances in which there is a high risk of bleeding from anticoagulants. Drugs that interfere with platelet aggregation, such as aspirin and other nonsteroidal anti-inflammatory agents, have not been shown convincingly to be effective as prophylactic agents. In patients in whom anticoagulation is contraindicated, such as patients with neurosurgical procedures, it is prudent to use conservative means of prophylaxis. These include early ambulation, elastic stockings, and external periodic calf compression. The external compression devices have been reported to be effective. There are no risks associated with their use; the only negative aspect is low patient acceptance during prolonged use, because they are uncomfortable or cumbersome.

TREATMENT. Anticoagulation is not necessary for the treatment of superficial thrombophlebitis. Local measures, sometimes coupled with administration of anti-inflammatory drugs, such as indomethacin, suffice to bring about healing and relief of symptoms.

Full anticoagulation is the preferred treatment for deep-vein thrombosis. Heparin is preferred for initiation of treatment because of its immediate action, whereas warfarin-type drugs may not become fully effective for a considerable period of time. Heparin inhibits coagulation by binding and activating antithrombin III, an inhibitor of activated Factor X. Heparin is best administered by constant infusion. Initially a bolus of 5000 units is given intravenously, followed by constant infusion of 750 to 1000 units per hour. The dose is adjusted by monitoring the APTT so that a level about two times the normal control is achieved. APTT is checked 4 to 6 hours after the initial bolus and once a day thereafter. An alternative method is intermittent intravenous administration of 5,000 to 10,000 units every 4 to 6 hours. If no suitable veins are found, heparin may be administered subcutaneously in a dose of 15,000 to 30,000 units every 12 hours. After 5 days of heparin therapy, oral warfarin at a dose of 10 to 15 mg daily is given until the one-stage prothrombin time (PT) is 1.2 to 1.5 times the normal level. Subsequently, a daily maintenance dose is administered to maintain the PT at the desired level. Warfarin brings about anticoagulation by decreasing the level of Factors II, VII, IX, and X. Many drugs interact with warfarin. Some of them potentiate its action and others inhibit it. If the patient requires other drug therapy while on warfarin, each drug should be carefully screened for potential interaction. If bleeding occurs in the course of heparin therapy, its effect can be counteracted by administration of 1 mg of protamine per 100 units of heparin. If bleeding develops in the course of warfarin treatment, the patient should receive vitamin K_1 intramuscularly to reduce PT to the therapeutic range (0.25 to 1.0 mg usually suffices). If bleeding is serious, blood or fresh frozen plasma may be necessary.

Thrombolysis with fibrinolytic agents, such as streptokinase or urokinase, administered intravenously in patients with deep-vein thrombosis has been shown to achieve more complete dissolution of the thrombus and better preservation of the venous architecture than conventional anticoagulants. These drugs act by causing activation of plasminogen to plasmin, thereby causing dissolution of the thrombus. Streptokinase is administered intravenously as an initial bolus of 250,000 to 500,000 IU, followed by an infusion of 100,000 IU per hour for 24 to 72 hours. The effectiveness of the drug diminishes after the first 24 hours. Urokinase is less likely to cause anaphylactic reactions, but it is more expensive. It is given in a dose of 4400 IU per kilogram as a bolus, followed by an infusion of 4400 IU per kilogram per hour for the same duration as streptokinase. Human recombinant tissue-type plasminogen activator is also capable of dissolving venous thrombi and pulmonary emboli. A controlled trial of this agent in deep-vein thrombosis is now in progress. Thrombolytic therapy is the preferred method of treatment of patients with iliofemoral or subclavian-axillary vein thrombosis. In patients with more distal deep-vein thrombosis, the high effectiveness of heparin and its lower rate of hemorrhagic complications render this the preferred method of treatment.

TABLE 54–4. PREVENTION OF VENOUS THROMBOEMBOLISM

Representative patient groups	1. Medical patients without predisposing factors on short bed rest 2. Young patients without predisposing factors undergoing brief (<1 hr) general surgical procedure	1. Medical patients with predisposing factors or on prolonged bed rest 2. Middle-aged or old patients without predisposing factors undergoing general surgical procedure longer than 1 hr	1. Patients with hip fracture 2. Patients undergoing extensive orthopedic or pelvic surgery 3. Middle-aged or old patients with predisposing factors or with previous venous thrombosis undergoing general surgical procedure longer than 1 hr
Approximate incidence of venous thrombosis	5%	20–40%	50–70%
Approximate incidence of pulmonary embolism	Almost zero	5%	10%
Suggested prophylaxis	None	Low-dose heparin or intermittent pneumatic compression	Warfarin, low-dose heparin plus either intermittent pneumatic compression or dihydroergotamine; or higher dose heparin

In patients in whom anticoagulation is contraindicated, simple measures—elevation of the extremity and local heat—should be used. When the risk of pulmonary embolism is low, as in the case of deep-vein thrombosis limited to the calf, these measures suffice. In patients with deep-vein thrombosis extending above the knee, in whom the risk of pulmonary embolism is high, implantation of an inferior vena caval filter or ligation of the inferior vena cava may also be considered. This form of therapy should also be used when anticoagulation needs to be terminated because of complications, when recurrent thromboembolism occurs in the presence of adequate anticoagulation, and when septic thromboembolic disease not controlled by antibiotics is present.

Bed rest should be continued until local signs of inflammation, including tenderness and edema, subside. After 7 to 15 days the patient is allowed to walk wearing elastic stockings. If no discomfort occurs, resumption of full activity is allowed 1 to 2 weeks later. Anticoagulation for 3 months is usually sufficient to prevent recurrence of deep-vein thrombosis.

Beisaw NE, Comerota AJ, Groth HE, et al.: Dihydroergotamine/heparin in the prevention of deep-vein thrombosis after total hip replacement. J Bone Joint Surg 70A:2, 1988. *Report of a controlled, randomized multicenter trial showing greater effectiveness of the combination of dihydroergotamine plus heparin than either drug alone in the prophylaxis of deep-vein thrombosis in patients undergoing total hip replacement.*

Grassi CJ, Goldhaber SZ: Interruption of the inferior vena cava for prevention of pulmonary embolism: Transvenous filter devices. Herz 14:182, 1989. *A consideration of the uses of inferior vena cava filters for the prevention of pulmonary embolism.*

Hirsh J, Hull RD: Treatment of venous thromboembolism. Chest 89:426S, 1986. *A thoughtful consideration of various aspects of the use of anticoagulants in the treatment of venous thromboembolism.*

Hull RD, Raskob GE, Hirsh J: Prophylaxis of venous thromboembolism: An overview. Chest 89:374S, 1986. *A concise and thoughtful analysis of the methods for preventing deep-vein thrombosis.*

Mudge M, Hughes LE: The long term sequelae of deep vein thrombosis. J Surg 65:692, 1978. *A report of long-term follow-up of patients who had evidence of venous thrombosis after surgery. The sequelae of venous thrombosis are described.*

Peterson CE, Kwaan HC: Current concepts of warfarin therapy. Arch Intern Med 146:581, 1986. *A concise consideration of the pharmacology and use of warfarin in the treatment of thrombotic disease.*

Shafer KE, Jaffe AS: Thrombolytic therapy: Current and potential uses. Drug Ther 13:95, 1983. *A concise consideration of the uses of thrombolytic agents.*

Sharma GVRK, Cella G, Parisi AF, et al.: Thrombolytic therapy. N Engl J Med 306:1268, 1982. *Detailed consideration of the use of streptokinase and urokinase in vascular thrombosis.*

White RH, McGahan JP, Daschbach MM, et al.: Diagnosis of deep-vein thrombosis using duplex ultrasound. Ann Intern Med 111:297, 1989. *A review of the use of duplex ultrasonography in the diagnosis of deep-vein thrombosis.*

Varicose Veins

DEFINITION. Varicose veins are prominent, abnormally distended, and tortuous veins.

INCIDENCE. Approximately 20 per cent of adults develop varicose veins. A familial history is present in 15 per cent of patients. They are more common in women than in men by a factor of 5 to 1. Most women date the onset of varicose veins from the time of pregnancy. The veins of the lower extremities are most frequently affected because of the effects of gravity on venous pressure.

ETIOLOGY. Congenitally absent or defective valves are a recognized cause of varicose veins in early life. Varicose veins may develop secondary to sustained elevations of venous pressure from obstruction of the veins. The cause of the obstruction may be thrombosis secondary to thrombophlebitis or external pressure, as is the case in pregnancy, ascites, and tumors. However, in most affected individuals, no clearly identifiable cause or precipitating factor can be found. The possibility of a genetically determined structural defect in the venous wall has been suggested. Individuals with varicose veins in the lower extremities have been found to have increased venous distensibility and reduced amounts of collagen and hexosamine in the wall of unaffected veins. In the face of such a generalized defect, a sustained elevation in venous pressure from the effects of gravity in the lower extremities or from other factors may lead to stretching of the walls and, finally, to incompetence of the valves and overdistention of the veins. An association of varicose veins with hemorrhoids and diverticulosis of the bowel suggests the possibility that increased intra-abdominal pressure during bowel movements may play a role in their pathogenesis.

CLINICAL MANIFESTATIONS. Most patients are asymptomatic, especially in the early stages of the disease. They may seek attention because the dilated, tortuous varicosities are cosmetically unappealing. In some cases, aching in the lower extremities and edema, especially after prolonged standing or exercise, may be present. The edema usually subsides overnight. When the communicating veins are incompetent, symptoms are more common. Prolonged venous insufficiency leads to the postphlebitic syndrome, with sustained edema, induration, and fibrosis. Eventually, trophic changes with brownish discoloration of the skin and ulceration may result. Ulcers usually occur above the medial malleolus. An incompetent communicating vein may be identified in the vicinity of the ulcer. The arterial pulses are normal, and no evidence of ischemia is present.

DIAGNOSIS. Clinical inspection suffices to make the diagnosis. The Trendelenburg test can identify the presence of defective valves and incompetent communicating veins. With the patient recumbent, the leg is elevated to empty the veins, and a tourniquet is then applied to occlude the superficial veins. The patient is instructed to resume the erect position, and the tourniquet is released. If the venous valves are incompetent, the veins immediately become distended as a result of the backflow. If two tourniquets are applied, the distention of the veins in the intervening portion of the limb identifies the presence of incompetent communicating veins. The patency of the deep venous system can be examined by venography. It is prudent to exclude other causes of edema, such as congestive heart failure and renal disease.

PROGNOSIS. The prognosis of uncomplicated superficial varicose veins is excellent. The postphlebitic syndrome, once established, is usually progressive and resistant to treatment.

TREATMENT. Simple measures usually suffice to treat uncomplicated varicose veins. These consist of frequent periods of rest with elevation of the limbs, external pressure with elastic stockings or bandages, and avoidance of obstruction of the veins by garments such as girdles. In more severe or advanced cases, ligation and stripping of the saphenous veins or injection of sclerosing solutions may become necessary to prevent the postphlebitic syndrome. An injection/compression technique in which the sclerosing solution is injected into a vein emptied of blood, followed by compression by external pressure, is simple, cheap, and effective. It is widely used in Europe. When stasis ulcers are present, local care with warm, wet dressings is necessary. If infection is present, local and systemic antibiotics may be administered. If considerable fibrosis is present, it may be necessary to excise the entire area and carry out skin grafting to eliminate ulceration.

Beresford SSA, Chant ADB, Jones HO, et al.: Varicose veins: A comparison of surgery and injection/compression sclerotherapy. Lancet 1:921, 1978. *A 5-year follow-up comparing the effects of surgery and injection/compression sclerotherapy for varicose veins.*

Hobbs JT: The Treatment of Venous Disorders: A Comprehensive Review of Current Practice in the Management of Varicose Veins and Post-thrombotic Syndrome. Philadelphia, J. B. Lippincott Company, 1977. *A well-written, comprehensive consideration of the clinical features, diagnosis, and treatment of varicose veins and post-thrombotic syndromes.*

DISEASES OF THE LYMPHATIC VESSELS OF THE LIMBS

Lymphangitis

DEFINITION. Lymphangitis is an inflammation of the lymphatic vessels. It is usually of bacterial origin.

ETIOLOGY. In most cases the responsible infective agent is the hemolytic streptococcus or *Staphylococcus aureus*, coagulase-positive. The bacteria gain access to the lymphatics via local trauma or from ulcerations. In many instances no identifiable portal of entry can be found. Infection spreads from the lymphatics to the regional lymph nodes.

PATHOLOGY. Various stages of inflammation are found in the subcutaneous tissue and regional lymph nodes.

CLINICAL MANIFESTATIONS. The local manifestation of lymphangitis consists of a red streak that appears at the site of initial entry of the infective organism and extends to the regional lymph nodes. The latter are swollen and tender. There may be a surrounding area of cellulitis. Systemic accompaniments of infection may constitute the presenting manifestations.

DIAGNOSIS. The local manifestations of lymphangitis and the accompanying systemic reaction are usually sufficient to make the diagnosis. Leukocytosis with predominance of polymorphonuclear leukocytes may be present. Confirmation is obtained by culturing the organism from the portal of entry or from the subcutaneous tissues. Acute lymphangitis may be difficult to distinguish from a generalized cellulitis or from thrombophlebitis.

PROGNOSIS. With treatment the prognosis is good when one is dealing with an initial attack in an otherwise normal limb. In the case of recurrent attacks, lymphedema may develop and residual increase in the girth of the limb may occur.

TREATMENT. This consists of systemic administration of the appropriate antibiotics. In addition, surgical drainage of the focus of infection is important. Supportive measures, including rest and elevation of the infected limb and local warm, wet dressings, are also helpful. The use of elastic support hose may be necessary for a period of several weeks to prevent lymphedema. In recurrent cases, the causes of secondary lymphedema should be sought.

Schinger A, Martin WJ, Spittell JA: Acute lymphangitis and cellulitis. Minn Med 48:191, 1965. *Concise consideration of the clinical features, diagnosis, and treatment of lymphangitis.*

Lymphedema

DEFINITION. Lymphedema refers to edema from accumulation of lymph secondary to obstruction to its flow.

ETIOLOGY AND INCIDENCE. Lymphedema can be primary or secondary. The most frequent type of primary lymphedema is simple congenital lymphedema, which is not familial and is present at birth. A congenital familial form (Milroy's disease) is inherited as an autosomal dominant trait. Another hereditary form is associated with Noonan's syndrome in about 15 per cent of cases. Lymphedema praecox becomes manifest in puberty and is associated with congenital hypoplasia of the lymphatics. A late form may become manifest in middle age.

Primary lymphedema is more common in women. Most cases are manifest at birth or become apparent before age 40. A syndrome characterized by yellow nails, recurrent pleural effusion, and lymphedema is believed to be secondary to multiple lymphatic abnormalities in the areas involved. A familial syndrome consisting of recurrent intrahepatic cholestasis and lymphedema is probably due to defective hepatic lymphatic vessels as well as those in the extremity.

Secondary lymphedema results most commonly from trauma. It commonly results from surgical removal of lymph nodes and from fibrosis secondary to radiation following surgery for cancer. Lymphoma or metastatic carcinoma involving the lymph nodes may also cause obstruction to the flow of lymph and lymphedema. Filarial infection in the tropics is a cause of secondary lymphedema.

PATHOLOGY. In cases of congenital lymphedema there is absence or hypoplasia of the lymphatic vessels. In secondary lymphedema there are numerous small, irregular lymphatics, together with tortuous and sometimes greatly enlarged varicose lymphatic vessels.

CLINICAL MANIFESTATIONS. Typically, lymphedema begins gradually with an enlargement of the involved limb without other manifestations. The swollen extremity is soft and pitting. The edema subsides at night. With time, the skin becomes thickened and cannot be raised into a fold, and the edema becomes more persistent. The lower extremities are involved most often. In about half the patients the edema is unilateral. Superimposed lymphangitis and cellulitis may occur, and in longstanding cases lymphangiosarcoma may develop.

DIAGNOSIS. The diagnosis of lymphedema may be confirmed with a radioisotope lymphogram. ^{99m}Tc-labeled rhenium sulfur colloid, ^{99m}Tc-labeled antimony trisulfide colloid, or ^{99m}Tc-labeled human serum albumin microcolloid is injected in the web spaces of the foot. The ilioinguinal region is scanned 30 and 60 minutes later. In lymphedema, the uptake of isotope by the lymph nodes is reduced, whereas in edema due to venous obstruction it is greater than normal owing to increased lymph flow. The precise diagnosis of the type of lymphedema is made by lymphangiography. Contrast medium is injected directly into a lymphatic vessel in the foot, or a water-soluble contrast agent is injected intracutaneously and taken up by the lymphatics. By this technique, a distinction can be made between absence or hypoplasia of the lymphatic vessels, on the one hand, which characterizes congenital lymphedema, and the hyperplasia and numerous small lymphatics, which characterize secondary lymphedema, on the other.

PROGNOSIS. Primary lymphedema is usually a slowly progressive disorder, not easily amenable to treatment. The prognosis of secondary lymphedema depends on the cause. In cases in which it results from infection, it can be effectively managed by treatment with antibiotics.

TREATMENT. In primary lymphedema this is aimed at keeping the limb as free of edema as possible to prevent fibrosis and secondary infection. Frequent elevation of the limb, the use of elastic stockings, and the administration of diuretics may be useful. In cases not controlled by these simple measures, benzopyrones have been reported to be useful. These drugs break down protein by activating macrophages; hence, they reduce viscosity and facilitate the flow of lymph. Surgery may be tried in advanced cases to remove subcutaneous tissue and to induce new lymph vessel formation. Anastomosis of small lymphatic vessels with veins by microsurgery has been reported to give good results in some cases.

Allen EV, Ghormley RK: Lymphedema of the extremities: Etiology, classification and treatment; report of 300 cases. Ann Intern Med 9:516, 1935. *Comprehensive consideration of the clinical features of primary and secondary lymphedema in a large series of cases.*

Browse NL: The diagnosis and management of primary lymphedema. J Vasc Surg 3:181, 1986. *A concise account of the diagnosis and management of primary lymphedema.*

Browse NL, Stewart G: Lymphoedema: Pathophysiology and classification. J Cardiovasc Surg 26:91, 1985. *An up-to-date description of the pathophysiology and classification of lymphedema.*

Gloviczki P, Calcagno D, Schirger A, et al.: Noninvasive evaluation of the swollen extremity: Experiences with 190 lymphoscintigraphic examinations. J Vasc Surg 9:683, 1989. *Report of the use of lymphoscintigraphy with ^{99m}Tc-labeled antimony trisulfide in the diagnosis of lymphedema.*

Partsch H, Wenzel-Hora BI, Urbanek A: Differential diagnosis of lymphedema after indirect lymphography with iotasul. Lymphology 16:12, 1983. *Description of the usefulness of indirect lymphangiography using a water-soluble contrast medium for the differential diagnosis of lymphedema.*

Pillar NB: Lymphoedema, macrophages and benzopyrones. Lymphology 13: 109, 1980. *Discussion of the role of macrophages in lymphedema. The effectiveness of benzopyrones in this disease is ascribed to activation of macrophages.*

Weissleder H, Weissleder R: Lymphedema: Evaluation of qualitative and quantitative lymphoscintigraphy in 238 patients. Radiology 168:729, 1988. *Report of the application of lymphoscintigraphy using ^{99m}Tc-labeled human serum albumin microcolloid in the diagnosis of lymphedema.*

55 Introduction

John F. Murray

Respiration includes all the processes that contribute to O_2 uptake and CO_2 elimination. The lungs are the major organs of gas exchange, but the nose, oropharynx, extrapulmonary airways, brain, spinal cord, nerves, thoracic cage, respiratory muscles, lymph nodes and vessels, and cardiovascular system are also involved. Thus respiratory diseases, literally interpreted, include a large variety of abnormalities arising in all the different structures concerned with gas exchange. In general, a more limited definition applies, and respiratory diseases are considered to include disturbances of the air passages, lungs, pleura, chest wall, muscles of respiration, and mediastinum (excluding the heart, systemic vessels, and esophagus).

Acute respiratory diseases are probably the most common afflictions of humankind and are responsible for more absences from school and work than any other type of illness. Chronic respiratory diseases, particularly emphysema and bronchitis, are second only to cardiovascular diseases as causes of disability payments. Cancer of the lung kills more persons each year than any other kind of malignancy. Because of the extremely high incidence of these and other respiratory diseases, it is important that all physicians, not just internists and chest specialists, be well versed in the clinical manifestations and methods of diagnosis, treatment, and prevention of the most common disorders. The material concerned with respiratory diseases here and elsewhere in the book is intended as a primer of necessary knowledge with which to recognize and to treat the major respiratory diseases; additional information is available in the references cited at the end of each chapter.

Patients with respiratory disease often seek medical attention because they have at least one of three cardinal manifestations: *cough* (including its derivative hemoptysis), *chest pain*, and *dyspnea*. These are nonspecific and sometimes trivial abnormalities, but the frequency with which they are associated with serious underlying thoracic disease means that the complaints must always be considered carefully and often become the focus of diagnostic evaluations. Because of the clinical importance of cough, chest pain, and dyspnea, the mechanisms, special features, and diagnostic approach to each symptom are briefly reviewed in the following pages. Further information can be found under the headings of the specific diseases in which these symptoms occur.

COUGH

Healthy persons seldom cough; their scant bronchial secretions, although constantly being produced, are imperceptibly carried up the tracheobronchial system by the action of cilia and, after reaching the pharynx, swallowed. Coughing is an essential defense mechanism that protects the airways from the adverse effects of inhaled noxious substances and also serves to clear them of retained secretions. Patients recognize that coughing indicates an abnormality, and this symptom is the second most common reason given for seeking medical advice.

MECHANISM. Coughing may be produced voluntarily, but more often it results from reflex stimulation. Extrathoracic cough receptors are located in the nose, oropharynx, larynx, and upper trachea. Intrathoracic rapidly adapting irritant receptors, which cause cough, are located in the epithelium of the lower trachea and large central bronchi, which are the air passages from which coughing effectively clears secretions or removes foreign material.

Depending on which cough receptors are activated, afferent stimuli travel to the brain via the trigeminal, glossopharyngeal, superior laryngeal, or vagus nerve. Efferent pathways include the recurrent laryngeal nerves, to cause closure of the glottis, and the corticospinal tract and peripheral nerves, to cause contraction of the thoracic and abdominal musculature. The cough reflex begins with a deep breath followed by glottic closure, relaxation of the diaphragm, and contraction of the expiratory muscles. Collectively, these acts generate a positive pressure of 100 to 300 mm Hg within the thorax, which is suddenly released when the glottis opens. During cough, the *volume* rate of flow out of the lungs (liters per second) is only slightly greater than or the same as it is during a forced expiratory maneuver, a fact that is not always appreciated. However, because the positive pressure in the pleural space is higher than the luminal pressure in the trachea and central bronchi, a pressure difference is created that causes the posterior membranous portion of the airway walls to fold inward and nearly to obliterate the lumen. By this means, the *linear* velocity of airflow through the narrowed channels (centimeters per second) is markedly increased, and a shearing force is created that dislodges secretions and particles from the mucosal surface.

PRODUCTIVE COUGH. The daily quantity of bronchial secretions produced by a normal person is not known, but it is sufficiently small to be removed by mucociliary action alone, and coughing and expectoration are not required. Secretions can accumulate in the tracheobronchial system in the presence of one or more of the following abnormalities: excessive production, altered physical properties, and deficient clearance. Thus, productive cough, which clears retained secretions from the airways, is an important defense mechanism and one of the hallmarks of acute and chronic inflammatory conditions of the lungs and airways. Patients who are unconscious or intubated or who, for other reasons, cannot cough must have their tracheobronchial secretions removed by suctioning to prevent the complications of atelectasis and/or bronchopulmonary infection.

NONPRODUCTIVE COUGH. In addition to the cough that serves an expectoration function, another type of cough—an irritative phenomenon—is encountered frequently. The stimulus may be mechanical, chemical, thermal, or inflammatory, including reactions from infection. There is increasing evidence that alteration of the surface epithelium of the major airways, into which the terminal filaments of irritant receptors are inserted, exposes the receptors more directly or somehow sensitizes them to the effects of stimulants; the cough reflex thus becomes hyperreactive, and coughing occurs in response to ordinarily innocuous stimuli. When the causes of chronic cough are analyzed, asthma often heads the list. Indeed, chronic nonproductive cough, especially at night, may be the sole presenting complaint of patients who subsequently prove to have bronchial asthma. An intractable, dry cough is now recognized as an important side effect of angiotensin-converting enzyme inhibitors.

COMPLICATIONS. Coughing seems to provoke more coughing. Paroxysms of coughing, as in pertussis, may terminate in vomiting, which seems to break the cycle. Paroxysmal attacks may also terminate in syncope. The mechanism of *cough syncope* is uncertain, but the effects of increased intrathoracic pressure on venous return, cardiac output, and blood flow to the brain are believed to play a role. At times, severe coughing attacks have continued to the point of utter exhaustion. The muscular force developed during coughing may be sufficient to cause occasional fractures of ribs (*cough fractures*) and even compression fractures of vertebral bodies.

DIAGNOSTIC APPROACH. It is difficult to generalize about a condition as common but as varied as coughing. Obviously, many episodes of coughing are innocent and transient. The essential first step in evaluating a patient complaining of cough is to obtain a thorough history with particular attention to the following aspects: (1) acute or chronic, (2) productive or nonproductive, (3) character, (4) time relationships, (5) type and quantity of sputum, and (6) associated features. A specific diagnosis of the cause of chronic intractable cough can be made by history alone in the majority (80 per cent) of patients.

An acute cough is usually associated with viral laryngotracheobronchitis but may signify other bronchopulmonary infections. Less commonly, acute episodes of coughing may be the chief manifestation of the inhalation of various immunologic or irritative substances. A chronic cough is the diagnostic hallmark of chronic bronchitis but also occurs in asthma, tuberculosis, bronchiectasis, and bronchogenic carcinoma. The frequency with which chronic bronchitis and bronchogenic carcinoma coexist, both being a complication of cigarette smoking, has led to the important axiom that *any change in the character or pattern of a chronic cough warrants immediate diagnostic evaluation, with special attention directed toward the detection of bronchogenic carcinoma.*

A productive cough usually implies an underlying inflammatory process, often infectious, but in many conditions in which secretions would be anticipated, the cough is described as nonproductive. The cough may be characterized as "brassy," from major airways involvement, or "barking" or "croupy," from laryngeal disease. Paroxysmal coughing with "whoops" is characteristic of pertussis. A cough that occurs mainly at night may accompany congestive cardiac failure; one occurring at meals suggests esophagogastric disease, such as hiatal hernia or diverticulum; and the cough of severe bronchitis or bronchiectasis is often worse upon awakening because of pooling of secretions during sleep. Each of these patterns tends to recur repeatedly under similar circumstances.

A description of the secretions produced in association with cough is diagnostically useful. Foul-smelling sputum indicates anaerobic infection, as in lung abscess or necrotizing pneumonia. Abundant frothy, saliva-like sputum is a well-known but rare symptom of bronchoalveolar carcinoma. Pink, foamy sputum, which is often voluminous, indicates pulmonary edema. In pneumococcal pneumonia, the classic rust-colored or "prune juice"–colored sputum may be observed. The chronic production of copious purulent sputum with intermittent blood streaking, especially on change of postures, is an important clue to bronchiectasis.

The associated features of coughing episodes are of considerable clinical importance: wheezing—a disorder with obstruction to airflow, such as asthma; stridor—involvement of the pharynx–larynx–extrathoracic trachea; fever and chills—acute infection; weakness and weight loss—tuberculosis or other chronic infection or malignancy; and recurrent pneumonias—bronchiectasis, foreign body, or obstructing tumor. In view of the importance of cigarette smoking in the pathogenesis of cough, a careful smoking history is crucial to the evaluation of cough.

Physical examination may reveal signs of pulmonary involvement that provide clues to the specific diagnosis. Regardless of the presence or absence of physical findings, evaluation of significant cough entails roentgenographic examination of the chest. When indicated, simple pulmonary function tests will demonstrate abnormalities of airflow and/or lung volumes. In patients whose routine spirometric tests are normal, bronchial provocation studies are indicated. Appropriate studies of sputum, especially culture and cytology, are often the easiest and most direct way of establishing a diagnosis. Fiberoptic bronchoscopy or other special diagnostic tests are sometimes needed.

TREATMENT. The ideal treatment of cough is elimination of its underlying cause. This is possible in most kinds of bronchopulmonary infections by suitable antimicrobial treatment of the responsible microorganism. Cessation of cigarette smoking nearly always eliminates the cough of chronic bronchitis. Disabling, irritative, nonproductive cough may be suppressed by an antitussive drug such as codeine, 15 mg every 6 hours. In contrast, productive cough should not be suppressed because retention of secretions impairs the distribution of inspired air, which worsens gas exchange, and promotes the development of atelectasis and secondary infection. Adequate hydration, not overhydration, is traditionally recommended, although its effect on pulmonary secretions is difficult to substantiate. Expectorants and ultrasonic aerosols have not been shown to be beneficial. When secretions are difficult to raise because of their physical properties and/or ineffective coughing, respiratory physical therapy with postural drainage and percussion may be helpful, and a trial is warranted.

HEMOPTYSIS

Regardless of whether the sputum is grossly bloody or merely blood streaked, the expectoration of any blood whatsoever denotes hemoptysis. Patients with chronic bronchitis may produce faintly blood-tinged sputum from time to time, but apart from this exception every patient with hemoptysis deserves a thorough diagnostic workup. A substantial proportion of all patients who expectorate bloody sputum have a serious disease, although the causes have changed in recent decades: Tuberculosis has become less common and bronchogenic carcinoma has become more common; bronchitis-bronchiectasis remains important. Other conditions that may manifest with hemoptysis include pulmonary embolism, mitral stenosis, pulmonary arteriovenous fistula, and Goodpasture's syndrome. All series include an appreciable number (5 to 15 per cent) of undiagnosed cases despite complete investigation.

Diagnostic Approach

The amount of expectorated blood may vary widely, from slight streaking of sputum to massive exsanguinating hemorrhage. The patient may not be aware of the pulmonary origin of the bleeding and often states that the blood "welled up" in his or her throat. For this reason, patients with true hemoptysis may seek the services of an otolaryngologist. Although it is always wise to examine the nasopharynx thoroughly, it is rare that hemoptysis is due to lesions in the upper respiratory tract.

Bleeding of esophageal, gastric, or duodenal origin may be confused with bleeding from the respiratory tract. Hematemesis can usually be differentiated from hemoptysis by the presence of symptoms of gastrointestinal involvement, such as nausea and vomiting, a history of peptic ulcer disease or alcoholism, or signs of cirrhosis. Prompt endoscopy will settle the issue in doubtful cases.

The history and physical examination may provide clues to the underlying cause of hemoptysis but are seldom diagnostic. Chest roentgenograms, which should be obtained in all patients complaining of hemoptysis, may reveal evidence of old or new inflammatory lesions, probable malignancies, or vascular abnormalities. At times, the underlying lesion may be obscured by the densities caused by the presence of blood itself. Once the bleeding has stopped, however, intra-alveolar blood usually clears within a week, so that delayed roentgenographic examinations are often helpful. Routine laboratory evaluation should include a complete blood count and tests to exclude a coagulopathy. It is useful to collect and measure the quantity of blood coughed up, but much may be swallowed or retained in the lungs and airways.

Virtually every patient with significant hemoptysis should undergo bronchoscopy to determine the site of bleeding and its cause, but the timing of the procedure is controversial. It is always desirable to determine from which bronchus the blood is coming; this is absolutely necessary in patients bleeding massively who are being considered for surgery, but it is also extremely difficult because the tracheobronchial system contains so much blood that it is frequently impossible to identify a bleeding point. The fiberoptic bronchoscope is often used in patients with hemoptysis, but many experts prefer the rigid scope because its larger lumen permits easier aspiration of blood and, when necessary, control of bleeding by packing.

TREATMENT. Fortunately, intrapulmonary bleeding usually stops spontaneously, and massive or life-threatening hemoptysis is unusual (fewer than 1.5 per cent of all cases). When bleeding is brisk, the patient should be hospitalized and kept with the affected lung, from which the bleeding is occurring, in the dependent position; the airways should be kept free of blood—coughing may suffice, but suction may be necessary; and strong sedatives, which abolish cough, should be avoided, but mild sedatives, to relieve anxiety, are often advisable. A thoracic surgeon should be notified about the problem, and an endotracheal tube and suction apparatus must be ready at the bedside.

If massive bleeding suddenly occurs, the tube can be inserted blindly into the right main bronchus and the balloon inflated to separate the two lungs and keep the blood confined to one of them. If circumstances permit, it is even better to put a balloon catheter, under bronchoscopic guidance, into a lobar or segmental bronchus to isolate the blood to as small a region of the lung as possible. Blood transfusions are given according to the usual clinical guidelines of quantity of blood lost, hematocrit, blood pressure, pulse rate, and urine output.

After the bleeding stops, the patient should be examined as outlined to determine the cause of the hemorrhage as well as the extent and severity of the underlying disease or diseases. Then, in consultation with a thoracic surgeon, a rational decision can be made concerning the need for and likelihood of success of an operation. Ordinarily, localized lesions (e.g., bronchial adenoma or sequestration) are resected, and generalized lesions (e.g., widespread bronchiectasis or multiple fistulas) are left alone. However, there is considerable clinical ground between these two extremes, and each patient must be considered individually.

The accepted treatment for "massive" hemoptysis has been rapid identification of the site of bleeding and, when possible, its surgical removal, usually by lobectomy but occasionally by pneumonectomy. However, the overall benefits of this approach have never been convincingly validated, and there is increasing emphasis on medical treatment followed by elective lung resection of carefully selected patients. Nonsurgical management of persistent severe hemoptysis includes bronchial artery embolism, which stops the bleeding, at least temporarily, in virtually all patients.

CHEST PAIN

Various types of chest pain are extremely common. Chest pain is one of the most frequent symptoms that cause the sufferer to seek medical attention. Because there is no clear relationship between the intensity of the discomfort and the importance of its underlying cause, all complaints of chest pain must be considered carefully. Pain that is virtually diagnostic because of its typical pattern of onset, location, and relation to effort and to respiratory movements is found in pleurisy, intercostal neuritis, costochondral disease, and disorders of the chest wall. The location and character of pain from myocardial ischemia are also characteristic but may be simulated by the pain of acute and chronic pulmonary hypertension. Occasionally, chest pain is elusive and difficult to diagnose, but it must always be taken seriously. A *meticulous history* is essential in evaluating chest pain. From the patient's story alone, a differential diagnosis can be formulated that serves as the basis for subsequent examinations.

MECHANISM. The anatomy, physiology, and biochemistry of pain in the body are reviewed in Ch. 26. Chest pain is no different from other types in that receptors and afferent pathways transmit a stimulus to the central nervous system, where that stimulus is perceived as pain. However, the capacity of various intrathoracic structures to serve as a source of pain differs. The lung parenchyma and the visceral pleura covering it are insensitive to ordinarily painful stimuli. In contrast, pain often accompanies involvement of the parietal pleura, the major airways, the chest wall, the diaphragm, or the mediastinal structures, including the heart. The mechanism of pain in myocardial ischemia is unknown, but the actuating event is clearly an imbalance between myocardial oxygen supply and demand. The pain of pericarditis may be in part related to involvement of the adjacent pleura, thus accounting for the striking respiratory component of what is primarily a cardiac disease. Pain in the esophagus is provoked by stimulation of receptors from acid reflux or muscle spasm.

PLEURAL PAIN. Pleurisy, or acute inflammation of the pleural surfaces, usually causes chest pain that has several distinctive features. The pain is restricted in distribution rather than diffuse, is nearly always on one side or the other, and tends to be distributed along the intercostal nerve zones. Pain from diaphragmatic pleurisy is often referred to the shoulder and side of the neck. The most striking and important characteristic of pleural pain is its clear relationship to respiratory movements. The pain may be variously described as "achy," "sharp," "burning," or simply a "catch," but whatever its designation, it is typically worsened by taking a deep breath, and coughing or sneezing causes intense distress. Patients with pleurisy frequently also complain of dyspnea because the aggravation of their pain during inspiration makes them conscious of every breath. Movement of the trunk, including bending, stooping, or even turning in bed, increases pleural pain, and patients usually find and remain in the position in which movements of the affected region are most restricted.

The rapidity of development of pleural pain provides a clue to its cause. An immediate onset attends pulmonary embolism or spontaneous pneumothorax; a slower but still acute onset over a few hours, especially with fever and cough, accompanies pneumonia; finally, a gradual onset over days or even weeks, often associated with features of chronic illness, such as weakness and weight loss, suggests tuberculosis or malignancy.

INTERCOSTAL NEURITIS. The distribution and superficial and knifelike quality of the pain of intercostal neuritis may resemble pleural pain and sometimes may even be mistaken for myocardial ischemia. Usually, the pain of intercostal neuritis is worsened by vigorous respiratory movements such as coughing, sneezing, and straining but, unlike pleurisy, not by ordinary breathing. A neuritic origin may be suggested by the presence of lancinating or electrical shock sensations unrelated to movements, and hyperalgesia or anesthesia over the distribution of the affected intercostal nerve provides further confirmatory evidence.

COSTOCHONDRAL DISEASE. Pain localized to the costosternal cartilaginous junctions may be confused with other, more serious causes of chest pain. The discomfort is usually described as dull with a gnawing, aching quality; there is little, if any, relationship to respiratory or other movements, although the pain may be most noticeable when the patient is lying in bed at night. The diagnostic key lies in the fact that there is tenderness to palpation that is clearly localized to one or more of the costal cartilages. Redness, swelling, and enlargement of the costal bridges (*Tietze's syndrome*) may be present, but the frequency of these is overemphasized. The most common sites of costosternal perichondritis are the second, third, and fourth cartilages, but any part of the large and complex cartilaginous shield along the central and lower portions of the anterior thoracic cage may be involved.

DISORDERS OF THE CHEST WALL. The system of joints, muscles, and fasciae involved in movements of the thoracic wall is complex. Because these structures are in constant motion throughout a person's life, it is surprising that "rheumatic" pains of the chest do not occur more frequently than they do. Fibrositis of the muscle-bone attachments may simultaneously involve the chest wall and other parts of the skeleton. Similarly, spondylitis of the thoracic spine may have its rib cage component, and many less definable skeletal disorders may produce discomfort in the chest. Localized pain in the thoracic cage may be related to unusually severe exercise or motion of the involved area. At times, the abnormality appears to be spontaneous, although even in these cases it is possible that pain was delayed in onset after either injury to the muscles of the chest wall or fractures of ribs during minor trauma or an unnoticed episode of coughing.

PULMONARY HYPERTENSION. The pain of pulmonary hypertension may simulate the pain of myocardial ischemia in its substernal location, its pattern of radiation, and its crushing or constricting quality. This type of pain may occur in patients with acute pulmonary hypertension, especially from multiple and/or massive pulmonary emboli. A similar pain has been noted in patients with chronic pulmonary hypertension from vasculitis or mitral stenosis, but the relationship is controversial. The mechanism of the pain is unknown, but it is believed to differ in the acute and chronic varieties. In the former it is related to sudden distention of the main pulmonary artery and stimulation of mechanoreceptors, and in the latter to an imbalance between the oxygen supplied to and utilized by the pressure-overloaded right ventricle. Although substernal pain related to the sudden onset of pulmonary hypertension is a well-recognized complication of pulmonary embolism, more commonly emboli cause pain in the lateral part of the chest that is typically pleuritic in character whether or not they produce pulmonary infarction.

MYOCARDIAL ISCHEMIA. Among the most important types of chest pain is that of myocardial ischemia, which is usually caused by coronary artery atherosclerosis (see Ch. 47). These attacks are provoked by an imbalance, which may be transient or permanent, between the supply of and demand for oxygen by the ventricular myocardium. Ischemic pain spans a continuum of severity from angina pectoris on the one hand to myocardial infarction on the other. Typical anginal pain is induced by exercise, heavy meals, and emotional upsets; the pain is usually described as a substernal "pressure," "constriction," or "squeezing" that, when intense, may radiate to the neck or down the ulnar aspect of one or both arms. Variant or Prinzmetal's anginal pain is similar in location and quality to typical angina pectoris but occurs in cycles at rest rather than during stressful episodes. Both typical and variant types of angina pectoris are relieved by coronary vasodilator drugs such as nitroglycerin. Typical angina also decreases with rest or removing the inciting stress. In contrast, the pain of myocardial infarction, although similar in location and character to anginal pain, is usually of greater intensity and duration, is not alleviated by rest or by nitroglycerin, may require large doses of opiates, and is often accompanied by diaphoresis, nausea, hypotension, and arrhythmias. Although patients are often short of breath during attacks of myocardial ischemia, and myocardial infarction may induce severe pulmonary edema, the pain itself is neither related to breathing nor affected by respiratory movements.

OTHER SOURCES. Pericarditis causes pain that is usually pleuritic in nature but may be steady and substernal; typically, the pain is worse while the patient is recumbent or lying on the left side. Dissecting aneurysm of the aorta is associated with severe, unremitting anterior chest pain that often radiates through to the back or into the abdomen. A deep substernal pain may result from esophageal reflux or spasm or from spontaneous mediastinal emphysema. Finally, psychogenic disorders may be associated with various forms of chest pain, the most common of which is a substernal tightness or aching sensation that may last from 30 minutes to several days. The pain may vary somewhat in intensity from time to time, and the ancillary features of myocardial infarction and a respiratory component are absent.

DIAGNOSTIC APPROACH. The approach to the general problem of the diagnosis of chest pain varies according to how seriously ill the patient is when first seen. Patients with acute chest pain who are gravely ill, as evidenced by hypotension, intense dyspnea, profuse diaphoresis, agitation, and restlessness, are usually evaluated first in the emergency room. The chief diagnostic considerations in this common clinical complex are myocardial infarction, pulmonary embolism, and dissecting aneurysm; less likely possibilities are tension pneumothorax, pericardial tamponade, and ruptured esophagus. An initial tentative diagnosis can usually be made from the results of a careful history and physical examination, supplemented by an electrocardiogram and chest roentgenograms. Except when the electrocardiogram reveals clear evidence of acute myocardial ischemia, definitive diagnosis depends on the results of later studies, such as ventilation-perfusion lung scans, pulmonary angiography, aortography, serial enzyme determinations, and coronary artery catheterization.

Patients with less severe chest pain may present during an episode of pain or afterward. Again, a detailed history of the character and behavior of the pain provides the best guide for the selection of subsequent diagnostic studies. Most patients will require an electrocardiogram, ideally taken during an episode of pain, and chest roentgenograms; then, on the basis of the results of these examinations, diagnostic evaluation proceeds as needed for the particular entities under consideration.

TREATMENT. The treatment of chest pain depends on its cause. Anginal pain responds to coronary artery vasodilator drugs, whereas myocardial infarction usually requires opiates, often in large doses. Pleural pain responds to analgesics, given as required. However, pleurisy in association with pneumonia may be alleviated by anti-inflammatory drugs such as indomethacin; in refractory cases, intercostal nerve block is needed. For costochondral and other types of chest wall pain, mild analgesia, reassurance, and time usually suffice; rapid relief can be obtained, when necessary, by injection of local anesthetic agents into the involved area.

DYSPNEA

When healthy persons undertake a steadily increasing amount of physical activity, they will eventually become aware of their breathing; the exercise required to provoke this sensation depends on their physical fitness. If they increase the level of activity even further, the awareness will increase as the sensation becomes progressively more unpleasant; if they stop exercising, the feeling will quickly disappear. The sensation experienced by normal subjects during physical exertion is aptly described as "shortness of breath" but not as dyspnea. The term dyspnea implies that the awareness is disproportionate to the stimulus and, moreover, that the sensation is abnormally uncomfortable. Many patients will describe their breathing discomfort as "breathlessness," but many others will complain only of "tightness," "choking," "inability to take a deep breath," "suffocating," and simply "can't get enough air." Thus dyspnea is difficult to define and quantify precisely, although various rating scales are in use. As with the evaluation of chest pain, a thorough history is required to explore all the vagaries of this elusive symptom.

MECHANISM. It is impossible to find a common mechanism for what appears to be the same or similar sensation of difficulty in breathing that may occur in respiratory, cardiac, erythropoietic, metabolic, and psychogenic disorders. Dyspnea in patients with respiratory diseases is believed to have a reflex origin and thus must begin with stimulation of receptors in one or more of the organs concerned with breathing. There are three types of intrapulmonary receptors (stretch, irritant, and C-fibers, which include the J- and probably other receptors), each of which has its afferent pathway to the central nervous system in the vagus nerve. There are also receptors in the muscles and tendons that participate in breathing, and chemoreceptors are situated in systemic arteries and the brain. The theory of "length-tension inappropriateness" postulates that misalignment of muscle spindles in the respiratory musculature serves as the genesis of dyspnea. An attractive explanation is that dyspnea is the subjective perception of the intensity of the stimuli that are generated by *all* the receptors activated during or in association with the act of breathing. Another theory proposes that the presence and intensity of dyspnea depend on the level of motor output to the respiratory muscles, but it is not certain how this activity is sensed.

PATTERNS. Dyspnea occurs with many underlying conditions and in several different patterns. Some of these are sufficiently characteristic to warrant separate designations. Episodes of breathlessness that wake patients from a sound sleep are called *paroxysmal nocturnal dyspnea;* these are most often observed in patients with chronic left ventricular failure but may also occur in patients with chronic pulmonary diseases because of pooling of secretions, gravity-induced decreases in lung volumes, or sleep-induced increases in airflow resistance. *Orthopnea,* or the onset or worsening of dyspnea on assuming the supine position, like paroxysmal nocturnal dyspnea, is found in patients with heart disease and occasionally in patients with chronic lung disease. The inability to assume the supine position (instant orthopnea) is particularly characteristic of the rare condition of paralysis of both hemidiaphragms. *Platypnea* denotes dyspnea that occurs in the upright position and *trepopnea* the even rarer form of dyspnea that develops in either the right or the left lateral decubitus position. Both the terms *hyperpnea,* an increase in minute volume, and *hyperventilation,* an increase in alveolar ventilation in excess of carbon dioxide production, indicate that ventilation is increased above normal. However, neither term carries any implication about the presence or absence of dyspnea.

DIAGNOSTIC APPROACH. The differential diagnosis of the dyspneic patient begins with a careful history. In patients with chronic respiratory or cardiac disease, dyspnea initially develops only during physical activity, and the amount of exertion required to provoke the symptom relates in a general way to the severity of the underlying condition. Sudden episodes of dyspnea, unrelated to physical activity, typically occur with pulmonary embolism, spontaneous pneumothorax, and anxiety; the acute attacks in each of these disorders characteristically remit, but bouts of breathlessness may recur with varying severity.

The results of the history and physical examination, routine blood tests, electrocardiography, and chest roentgenography nearly always indicate whether the dyspneic patient is suffering from a respiratory, cardiac, hematologic, renal, or hepatic abnormality. Special diagnostic studies are often then required to determine what specific kind of disease is present. Measurements of lung volumes, expiratory flow rates, and diffusing capacity, studies during exercise, and noninvasive tests of cardiac function are particularly valuable in three difficult clinical situations: (1) differentiating between dyspnea of cardiac and pulmonary origin and, if abnormalities of both systems coexist, as is often the case, estimating the severity of each; (2) identifying the presence of either pulmonary vascular obstructive disease or diffuse pulmonary infiltrative disorders in dyspneic patients whose routine studies, including chest roentgenograms, are normal; and (3) helping to establish, by ruling out significant cardiorespiratory abnormalities, that dyspnea in a given patient is psychogenic in origin (a diagnosis that is always tenuous).

TREATMENT. Unlike cough, for which there are effective antitussives, and pain, for which there are powerful analgesics, there is no category of medications for relief of dyspnea. Cure or alleviation of dyspnea depends on recognizing its origin and treating the basic abnormality. In acute reversible conditions, the dyspnea subsides along with improvement of its underlying cause. In chronic cardiac and pulmonary disorders, sufficient physical exertion will continue to provoke dyspnea, but even in these conditions rehabilitation programs can be used to enable patients to increase their physical activity up to the maximum of the limits imposed by their disease.

CONCLUSION

This introduction to the three most common and important symptoms of *all* diseases of the respiratory system is meant to supplement the material presented not only in the remainder of Part VII but also elsewhere in the book. Acute infections of the upper and lower respiratory tract caused by viruses, bacteria, fungi, protozoa, and helminths are discussed in Parts XX, XXI, and XXII. Systemic diseases in which the lungs may be involved are also discussed elsewhere: Wegener's granulomatosis (Ch. 266), eosinophilic syndromes (Ch. 150), and the "collagen diseases" (Ch. 258 to 268). Various abnormalities of the pulmonary circulation, exclusive of pulmonary embolism, and pulmonary edema, an important disorder (not disease) of the lungs, are discussed chiefly in Part VI.

Simon PM, Schwartzstein RM, Weiss JW, et al.: Distinguishable types of dyspnea in patients with shortness of breath. Am Rev Respir Dis 142:1009, 1990. *A partially successful effort to subdivide various types of dyspnea that supports the belief that different mechanisms are involved in each.*

Jones DK, Davies RJ: Massive haemoptysis. Medical management will usually arrest the bleeding. Br Med J 300:889, 1990. *Short review that supports the recent trend from surgical to medical management.*

Schneider RR, Seckler SG: Evaluation of acute chest pain. Med Clin North Am 65:53, 1981. *Comprehensive description of pain arising from different organs within the thorax; 75 references.*

Stulbarg M: Evaluating and treating intractable cough. Medical Staff Conference, University of California, San Francisco. West J Med 143:223, 1985. *Excellent review of the pathophysiology, causes, diagnosis, and management of intractable cough; 49 references.*

56 Respiratory Structure and Function

John F. Murray

Respiration can be defined as "those processes concerned with gas exchange between an organism and its environment." This definition, which emphasizes that the chief function of the respiratory system is *gas exchange*, is sufficiently comprehensive to apply to all animals, ranging from simple one-celled protozoa to infinitely more complex mammals. In human beings, the basic processes leading to gas exchange, or the uptake of O_2 and the elimination of CO_2, are usually divided into four functional subdivisions:

1. *Ventilation*—the movement of air from outside to inside the body and the distribution of air within the tracheobronchial system to the gas exchange units of the lungs.

2. *Diffusion*—the movement of O_2 and CO_2 across the alveolar-capillary membrane between the gas in alveolar spaces and the blood in pulmonary capillaries.

3. *Perfusion*—the flow of mixed venous blood through the pulmonary arterial circulation, distribution of the blood to the capillaries of the gas exchange units, and removal of the blood from the lungs through pulmonary veins.

4. *Control of breathing*—the regulation of ventilation, usually in accordance with changing metabolic demands.

VENTILATION

Air moves from outside the body into the gas exchange units of the lungs because contraction of the muscles of respiration normally generates sufficient force to expand the lungs and chest wall and to overcome the resistance and inertia in the system. This condition creates a negative pressure within the alveolar spaces that causes ambient air to flow into the lungs. The volume of gas that reaches the individual gas exchange units is determined by the mechanical properties of the lung parenchyma, airways, and chest wall, and by the force provided by the muscles of respiration (or by a mechanical ventilator).

The amount of air that enters the lung with each breath is called the *tidal volume*. When the lungs are fully expanded, the amount of gas they contain is called the *total lung capacity*. The maximal volume of gas that a person can exhale from total lung capacity is called the *vital capacity*, and the amount of gas remaining in the lungs at the end of maximal expiration is called the *residual volume*. Another important static lung volume is the *functional residual capacity*, which is the volume of gas in the lungs at the end of a normal breath. The relationships among these different lung volumes, which vary in different disorders and which will be frequently referred to, are shown in Figure 56–1.

Static Properties

Both the lungs and the chest wall are elastic structures. This means that they can be distended, and when the distending force is removed, they recoil back to their resting volumes. Although the lungs and chest wall are similar in this respect, they differ considerably in their respective resting volumes when there is no expanding force.

The elastic properties of isolated lungs are shown by the dashed line in Figure 56–1. The slope of the line, or the change in volume (ΔV) for a given change in pressure (ΔP), is known as the compliance of the lungs. This curve demonstrates that (1) the lungs collapse almost completely when there is no distending pressure; (2) the slope of the volume-pressure curve is relatively steep at low lung volumes (i.e., as the lungs are beginning to inflate, their compliance is high); and (3) at high lung volumes, the curve flattens (compliance decreases), so that little increase in volume results from a large increase in pressure. The elastic forces of the lungs originate within the tissues that are being stretched, particularly those containing elastin and collagen, and from the surface tension of the film of *surfactant* that lines the air-liquid interface of alveolar spaces. The static properties of the isolated chest wall (including the diaphragm and abdominal contents that must be displaced during breathing) are shown by the solid light red line in Figure 56–1. The chest wall is a compressible and distensible structure that contains an appreciable volume in its resting state. To decrease the volume of the thorax, a force must be applied to overcome the tendency of the chest wall to resist compression and recoil back to its resting position. Conversely, to increase the volume of the thorax, the applied force must overcome the elastic forces in the chest wall that also cause it to recoil back to its resting position.

It is useful conceptually to consider the behavior of the lungs and chest wall separately, but obviously they function together. Because their action is coupled by the pleural pressure that keeps each lung expanded against the chest wall, the lungs and chest wall ordinarily change their volumes by exactly the same amount. Thus the pressures required to change the volume of the respiratory system are obtained by simply adding the separate pressures necessary to inflate the lungs and chest wall to a given volume. The solid dark red line in Figure 56–1 indicates the pressure that must be produced by contraction of the respiratory muscles, or by a mechanical ventilator, to inflate or deflate both the lungs and the chest wall. Figure 56–1 also shows that functional residual capacity is the volume at which the inward recoil force of the lungs is equal and opposite to the outward recoil force of the chest wall; in other words, functional residual capacity is that volume at which the net force of the respiratory system is zero.

During inspiration, the force developed by the contracting muscles of inspiration meets progressively increasing (inward) recoil forces from the combined expansion of the lungs and chest wall. Furthermore, because shortening muscle fibers generate progressively less force, inspiration finally ceases at that volume (total lung capacity) at which the weakening inspiratory muscle forces can no longer overcome the increasing forces required to expand the lungs and chest wall further. Similarly, during expiration, the net force developed by the contracting muscles of expiration meets progressively increasing (outward) recoil forces from the chest wall. In children and young adults, expiration ceases at that volume (residual volume) at which the decreasing expiratory muscle forces can no longer overcome the increasing forces required to compress the chest wall further. In older persons, residual volume is governed mainly by factors that regulate the caliber and patency of peripheral airways; thus even though the expiratory muscles are capable of further compression of the thorax, emptying is prevented by airway closure and trapping of gas in the lungs.

Vital capacity, or the volume between total lung capacity and residual volume, is determined by the factors that influence maximum inspiration and expiration, i.e., the balance of forces generated by the muscles of respiration and by the mechanical properties of the lungs and chest wall combined. Changes in these variables explain the characteristic abnormalities in lung volumes that occur in patients with the respiratory disorders discussed in subsequent chapters.

Lung volumes also vary among healthy persons according to their age, sex, and physical structure (especially height). Because body build varies slightly from one ethnic group to another, it is important to have normal data that pertain to the population being studied. Measured volumes are usually expressed as both the observed value and the percentage of the predicted mean value for a normal subject of the same age, sex, and height. Measured values should not be considered abnormal unless they are clearly outside the range of values likely to be found in normal persons (100 per cent ± 20 per cent for vital capacity and 100 per cent ± 25 per cent for total lung capacity, residual volume, and functional residual capacity).

Routine tests of pulmonary function customarily include measurements by a spirometer or one of a variety of commercially available recording systems of vital capacity and of rates of expiratory airflow (see Dynamic Properties, below). These methods, however, do not measure total lung capacity, functional residual capacity, or residual volume.

To measure *all* the gas in the lungs at any of these volumes, one of two basically different methods must be used: either dilution or washout of an inert gas or whole-body plethysmography. Functional residual capacity is usually determined because it is the normal end-expiratory lung volume and thus is an easy volume for subjects to maintain during the breathing test. During the measurement of functional residual capacity, the subject exhales completely so that this volume, expiratory reserve volume, can be subtracted from the functional residual capacity to obtain the residual volume; total lung capacity is obtained by adding vital capacity to the residual volume.

Gas dilution or *washout* involves measurement of the volume and concentration of an inert gas, such as nitrogen (N_2), neon (Ne), or helium (He). These methods measure the amount of gas that communicates freely with the airways during the breathing maneuver; dilution or washout techniques do not detect gas trapped beyond closed (or very narrowed) airways and in poorly communicating regions, like bullae.

Body plethysmography involves placing the subject in the plethysmograph, a large airtight box resembling a telephone booth, and having him or her breathe through a mouthpiece in which a shutter can be closed to stop the flow of air. When the subject attempts to pant against the closed shutter, the volume of the thorax and gas in the lungs expands and contracts, which changes the pressure measured inside the mouthpiece. Movement of the thorax also changes the pressure in the box by compressing and expanding the gas surrounding the subject. From application of Boyle's law, which states that the pressure times the volume of a gas is constant if temperature remains the same, the volume of gas in the thorax can be calculated. The body plethysmograph measures all the gas present during the breathing maneuver, including that in freely communicating air spaces *and* any that may be trapped behind poorly communicating airways or in closed spaces (e.g., pneumothorax).

In normal subjects, measurements of functional residual capacity by dilution (or washout) and plethysmographic techniques are virtually identical. In contrast, in patients with airways obstruction or bullous disease, the communicating volume may be considerably less than the plethysmographic volume, and the difference is a measure of the noncommunicating (sometimes called "trapped") volume.

Dynamic Properties

To cause air to flow from outside the body into the gas exchange units, a muscular (or other mechanical) force must be exerted to overcome not only the elastic recoil properties of the lungs and chest wall but also their resistive and inertial properties. In contrast to distensibility, which is not affected by the rate of movement, the forces required to offset resistance and inertia

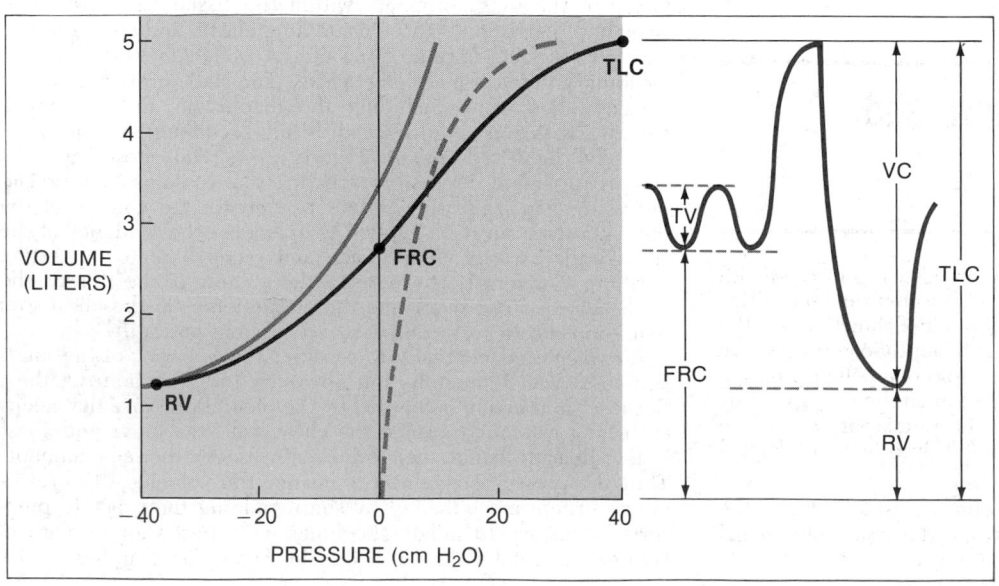

FIGURE 56–1. Schematic representation of the volume-pressure relationships of the chest wall (*solid light red line*), lungs (*dashed light red line*), and chest wall and lungs combined (*solid dark red line*). Total lung capacity (TLC) occurs when the lungs are fully expanded, and residual volume (RV) is the amount of gas remaining in the lungs at the end of a maximal expiration. Functional residual capacity (FRC) occurs at that volume at which the recoil pressures of the chest wall and lung are equal and opposite (i.e., the distending pressure = 0 cm H_2O). On the right is a spirometric tracing (volume-time) of the breathing maneuvers of the person whose pressure-volume curves are on the left. TV = tidal volume; VC = vital capacity.

are markedly influenced by the velocity of airflow. Inertial forces are ordinarily small and usually ignored, although new tests show they may be important in advanced lung diseases.

Resistance to airflow is affected chiefly by the caliber of the air passages. Although the diameter of each successive generation of airways decreases, the combined total cross-sectional area at any level increases steadily throughout the tracheobronchial tree, from the main bronchi to the peripheral airways. This means that airways resistance progressively decreases and that most of the resistance of the human tracheobronchial tree resides in large airways: Direct measurements reveal that between 50 and 80 per cent of total resistance to airflow originates in airways *greater than* 2 mm in diameter. A corollary of this observation is that substantial changes can occur in the caliber of the small peripheral airways without having much effect on total airways resistance. Hence, small airways have been called the lung's "quiet zone," and because they are frequently involved early in the evolution of clinically important lung disease, special tests have been devised to examine their functional behavior.

Changes in the cross-sectional area of airways can also result from changes in lung volume and diseases of the lung parenchyma or the airways themselves. During inflation of the lungs from functional residual capacity, airways are pulled open so that resistance to airflow decreases; during deflation, airways narrow and their resistance increases. Airway caliber changes during inflation and deflation because of the combined effects of the tethering action of the attachments between the lung parenchyma and small bronchioles and the distending effect of pleural pressure on larger airways. Elastic recoil of the lung, which governs the pull of the attachments and the magnitude of pleural pressure, affects the size of all airways, and this, in turn, affects overall resistance to airflow.

Airway narrowing may result from bronchospasm, edema of the mucosal lining, and secretions within the lumen. In addition, changes in the viscosity and density of the inspired gas affect airways resistance, and gas mixtures of different densities are sometimes used to study the dynamic properties of the tracheobronchial system.

Resistance to airflow can be measured in a body plethysmograph; however, this procedure has limited clinical usefulness. Fortunately, the important dynamic properties of the respiratory system can be assessed by several readily available tests of airways function. The simplest and most widely used of these is the forced expiratory volume in 1 second (FEV_1), expressed as a ratio of the forced vital capacity (FVC), or FEV_1/FVC (Fig. 56–2). To perform the FVC maneuver, the subject inhales fully and then exhales as rapidly and completely as possible. In normal persons, the FVC equals the vital capacity from a slow or nonexpulsive maneuver, but in patients with airways obstruction, vigorous expiration may cause airways to narrow and close prematurely, so that the FVC may be less than the vital capacity; the magnitude of the difference between the two values is an indication of the amount of air trapped behind compressed airways. The FEV_1/FVC decreases with age in normal persons after reaching adulthood and is usually higher in women than in men at all ages.

Additional measurements of airways behavior besides the FEV_1 can be obtained from the FVC maneuver (Fig. 56–2): several derivatives of time, such as the $FEV_{0.5}$ and FEV_3 (the subscript denoting the number of seconds after beginning expiration at which the expired volume is measured), the maximal expiratory flow rate (MEFR or often $MEFR_{200-1200\ ml}$, indicating that the flow rate was measured between expired volumes of 200 and 1200 ml), and the maximal mid-expiratory flow rate (MMFR or often $MMFR_{25-75\%}$, indicating, that the rate was measured between expired volumes of 25 and 75 per cent of the FVC). None of these has any particular advantage over the FEV_1 except that the MMFR is less dependent on the effort exerted by the subject than are the other variables and reflects the flow properties of small as well as large airways.

Another way of examining the events during an FVC maneuver is by recording flow against volume instead of volume against time, which provides a maximal expiratory flow-volume curve (Fig. 56–3). From these records, maximal flow rates at any given fraction of the expired vital capacity, usually 50 per cent ($\dot{V}max_{50}$) or 75 per cent ($\dot{V}max_{75}$), can be determined and reported as the percentage of the predicted values for a subject

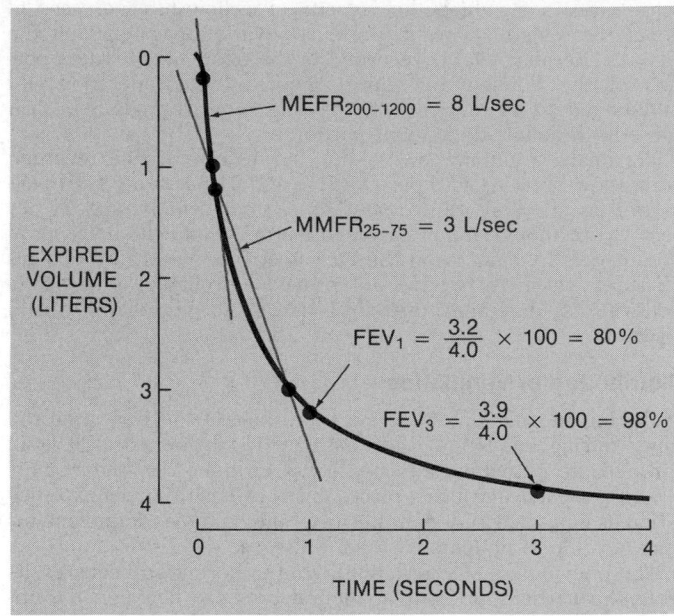

FIGURE 56–2. Schematic representation of a normal forced vital capacity (FVC) maneuver (expired volume against time, *heavy red line*) and the derivation of several variables commonly used to evaluate airways obstruction. $MEFR_{200-1200}$ = maximal expiratory flow rate, measured between expired volumes of 200 and 1200 ml; $MMER_{25-75}$ = maximal mid-expiratory flow rate, measured between 25 and 75 per cent of the total FVC; FEV_1 = forced expiratory volume in 1 second, expressed as percentage of total FVC; FEV_3 = forced expiratory volume in 3 seconds, expressed as percentage of total FVC.

of the same age, sex, and body size. The early portion of the maximal expiratory flow-volume curve, which includes peak flow, is determined by the effort exerted by the subject and is thus called the effort-*dependent* segment; the later portion is less influenced by effort and is called the effort-*independent* segment, or that part of the curve during which expiratory airflow limitation occurs. Additional effort does not increase expiratory airflow (i.e., maximal velocity is limited), because "choke points" develop in

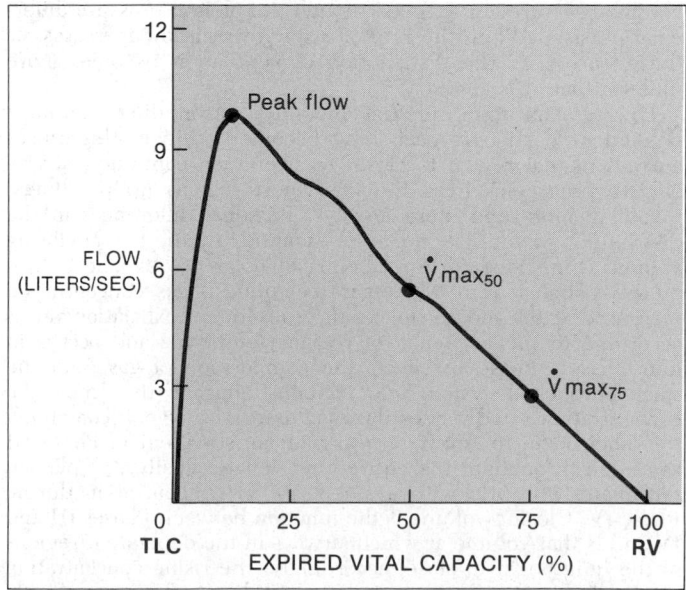

FIGURE 56–3. Typical forced expiratory flow-volume tracing of a normal adult man showing points of peak flow, maximal flow at 50 per cent expired vital capacity ($\dot{V}max_{50}$), and maximal flow at 75 per cent expired vital capacity ($\dot{V}max_{75}$). TLC = total lung capacity; RV = residual volume. (From Smith LH, Thier SO: Pathophysiology: The Biological Principles of Disease. Philadelphia, W. B. Saunders Company, 1981.)

those airways in which the velocity of airflow has increased to equal the speed at which pressures will propagate along the airways. Because events recorded in the effort-independent portion of the flow-volume curve require less cooperation and understanding by the subject, they are more reproducible than those in the effort-dependent portion.

Maximal expiratory flow-volume curves can also be recorded after a few breaths of 79 per cent He and 21 per cent O_2 (He-O_2) as well as after breathing room air (79 per cent N_2 and 21 per cent O_2). Although much has been learned about the behavior of the airways by comparing the curves obtained with the two gas mixtures, these tests have not proved as reliable as originally believed in detecting disease localized to peripheral (small) airways.

Distribution of Ventilation

During the movement of air from outside the body into the lungs during inhalation, the airstream is partitioned as it flows through the branching airways to the terminal respiratory units where gas exchange takes place. Even in healthy persons ventilation is not distributed uniformly, and marked derangements may develop in patients with lung disease.

The unevenness of ventilation found in normal subjects results from the vertical gradient of pleural pressure between the uppermost and lowermost parts of the lungs. The origins of the vertical gradient in different mammals are complex and include the weight of the lungs, their attachments at the hilum, and the shape and effects of the chest wall and abdominal contents; in humans, the weight of the lungs is the most important determinant. Because of the gradient in the pressure surrounding the lungs, alveoli are larger at the top than at the bottom, and there are regional differences in the distribution of inspired ventilation.

When breathing slowly from functional residual capacity, more inspired air is distributed to the dependent regions of the lungs than to the superior regions because the differences in pleural pressure cause the two regions to function on different segments of the same volume-pressure curve. Because the *change* in intrapleural pressure during quiet breathing is the same throughout the pleural space, the lower regions, which are operating on a steeper part of the curve and thus receive more volume for the same pressure change, inflate more than the upper regions. When inspiration continues to total lung capacity, alveoli at the top and bottom of the lungs inflate to nearly the same size because both regions are functioning on the flat portion of the volume-pressure curve, even though the pleural pressure difference persists. When the rate of inspiratory airflow increases, as during exercise, the distribution of ventilation becomes more uniform than it is at rest.

During expiration, pleural pressure surrounding the most dependent portion of each lung becomes positive; this causes airways in that region to close. As expiration continues, airway closure progresses from the lowermost regions up the lungs, involving more and more airways. Regional differences in the distribution of ventilation can be examined by the test of closing volume (Fig. 56–4). After labeling alveolar gas by one of two methods (bolus or resident gas techniques), gas concentration measured at the mouth during the subsequent exhalation varies according to the sequence of regional emptying and occurs in four phases. Phase I reflects the composition of gas from the tracheobronchial system and contains none of the label; the concentration rapidly rises during Phase II as alveoli containing the label begin to empty; a near-plateau is evident in Phase III as alveoli throughout the entire lung deflate; finally, the plateau terminates abruptly with a steep rise in concentration during Phase IV. Closing volume is the junction between Phases III and IV and is that volume at which airways in the dependent regions of the lung begin to close; accordingly, the rising concentration of the label in the subsequent expirate indicates the progressively increasing contributions from the preferentially labeled alveoli in the upper regions of the lung.

Because an increase in closing volume reflects premature closure or narrowing of airways, an increase in closing volume occurs in patients with lung disorders in which the caliber of peripheral airways is decreased from either decreased elastic

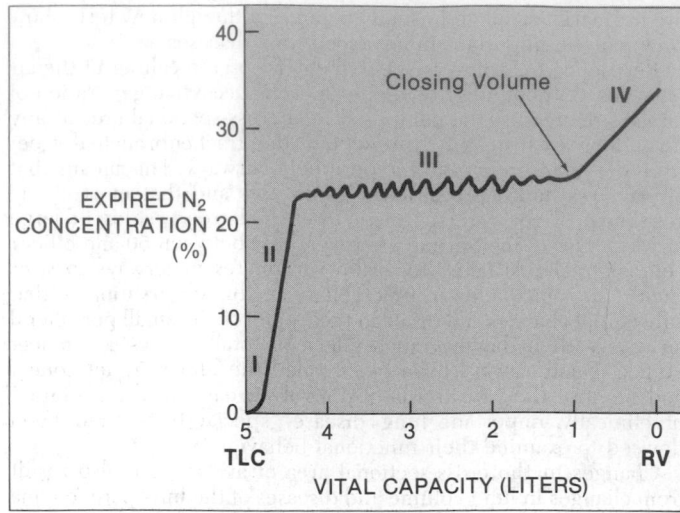

FIGURE 56–4. Representative tracing of expired nitrogen (N_2) concentration after taking a single breath of 100 per cent oxygen. An explanation of the four numbered phases (I, II, III, IV) is provided in the text. TLC = total lung capacity; RV = residual volume. (From Smith LH, Thier SO: Pathophysiology: The Biological Principles of Disease. Philadelphia, W. B. Saunders Company, 1981.)

recoil (e.g., in emphysema) or abnormalities of the airways themselves (e.g., in bronchitis or asthma). Furthermore, increases in closing volume have been detected in asymptomatic patients, usually smokers, and may be an early manifestation of lung disease. In addition, examination of the slope of Phase III is useful because it provides a sensitive measure of the adequacy of the distribution of ventilation. Well-ventilated units fill and empty more completely and rapidly than poorly ventilated units; this means that the concentration of the label will be lower in the better-ventilated regions that empty early during exhalation than in the poorly ventilated regions. Thus, the more uneven the distribution of ventilation within the lung, the steeper the slope of Phase III.

Other tests of the distribution of ventilation utilize the gamma ray–emitting properties of certain radioactive gases, chiefly ^{133}Xe, which are nontoxic and can be detected by external counters after inhalation in low concentrations. The distribution of ventilation can be assessed during a breath hold at end-inspiration after a single breath of ^{133}Xe or at intervals during its elimination by normal breathing after the lung has been labeled uniformly by rebreathing ^{133}Xe from a closed system.

Abnormalities of Ventilation

Lung diseases that cause abnormalities of ventilation are usually divided into two different categories: restrictive and obstructive ventilatory disorders. This classification is not completely satisfactory because it ignores the fact that disturbances of the distribution of ventilation are the earliest and by far the most common abnormality of ventilation and can occur in the absence of manifestations of coexisting obstructive or restrictive disorders.

DISTURBANCES OF DISTRIBUTION. Whenever a disease process involves the lung parenchyma or airways unevenly, abnormalities in the distribution of ventilation are likely to occur because more inspired gas will reach the normal regions of the lung compared with the regions distal to the sites of bronchial narrowing, or the regions in which the distensibility is impaired. Whether these functional changes can be detected depends on the extent and severity of the disease and the sensitivity of the test being used. The slope of Phase III of the closing volume maneuver is the most commonly used test for detecting early abnormalities in the distribution of ventilation. Frequency dependence of compliance is an extremely sensitive test for distribution of ventilation but is seldom used owing to its technical complexities.

RESTRICTIVE VENTILATORY DISORDERS. The term *restrictive ventilatory disorder* denotes a pattern of abnormalities in lung function. The word "restrictive" is employed to indicate a restriction of or limitation to the amount of gas within the lungs. Thus restrictive ventilatory disorders are characterized by reductions in lung volumes (Table 56–1). The hallmark of restriction is a decreased vital capacity, but because this change also occurs in obstructive ventilatory disorders, it is important to exclude the presence of airways obstruction (see Obstructive Ventilatory Disorders, below) or to demonstrate the presence of reductions in other lung volumes, particularly total lung capacity.

Many components of the lungs, chest wall, and respiratory control system determine the amount of gas that can be breathed into the lungs. Accordingly, restrictive ventilatory disorders can develop in diseases that (1) affect the chest wall or respiratory muscles (kyphoscoliosis, myasthenia gravis), (2) cause infiltrations in the lung parenchyma or air spaces (diffuse interstitial fibrosis, pulmonary edema), (3) involve the pleura (pleural thickening), (4) occupy space within the thorax (tumors, effusions, cardiac enlargement), and (5) occur after lung resection (pneumonectomy).

OBSTRUCTIVE VENTILATORY DISORDERS. The term *obstructive ventilatory disorder* denotes the constellation of abnormalities that results from limitation of expiratory airflow, regardless of its cause. Because the functional disturbances depend on the presence of increased airways resistance, obstructive ventilatory disorders are detected mainly by tests of the behavior of the respiratory system under dynamic conditions (Table 56–1). Of the available tests, the FEV_1/FVC is the most widely used, and other tests provide little additional information.

Obstructive ventilatory disorders are found in patients with asthma, bronchitis, emphysema, advanced bronchiectasis, or other diseases that cause narrowing of the tracheobronchial system. When the term "obstructive" was originally employed, it was not possible to differentiate among these various entities, so they were lumped together in the nonspecific category of chronic obstructive pulmonary disease. Now, however, it is possible by means of specialized tests of lung function to sort out the various diseases that cause airways obstruction, even when they coexist; the characteristic features of asthma, chronic bronchitis, and emphysema are described in subsequent chapters.

DIFFUSION

Diffusion can be defined as the movement of molecules from a region of higher to one of lower concentration; accordingly, diffusion tends to eliminate differences in concentration within the various regions accessible to the molecules. Diffusion is a passive process that results from the kinetic motion of the molecules, and no extra energy is required. In the lungs, O_2 moves by diffusion from alveolar gas into pulmonary capillary blood; similarly, in the peripheral tissues, O_2 moves by diffusion from capillary blood into neighboring cells. Carbon dioxide also moves by diffusion but usually in the direction opposite to that of O_2. Both O_2 and CO_2 undergo chemical reactions in the bloodstream at the start and finish of their journeys between the lungs and the peripheral tissues; O_2 reacts solely with hemoglobin, and CO_2 reacts in part with hemoglobin and in part to form bicarbonate.

Diffusing Capacity

The diffusing capacity of the lungs for any gas indicates the quantity of that gas that diffuses across the alveolar-capillary membrane per unit of time in response to the difference in mean pressures of the gas within the alveolus and pulmonary capillary. Most inert gases (e.g., N_2) diffuse across the air-blood barrier so rapidly that the amount taken up by the lungs is not detectably limited by the diffusibility of the gas and the properties of the lungs and blood but is determined solely by the solubility of the gas and the volume of tissue and blood into which it can dissolve. This phenomenon enables the use of highly soluble gases like acetylene, dimethyl ether, or nitrous oxide to measure lung tissue volume and pulmonary capillary blood flow.

The only two gases that can be used to measure the diffusing capacity of the lungs are O_2 and CO. Because of their unique ability to combine with hemoglobin, both have to diffuse across the alveolar-capillary membrane in large quantities to saturate the available hemoglobin at the gas pressure prevailing in the alveoli. Thus it may not be possible for complete equilibrium to occur before the hemoglobin-containing red blood cells leave the pulmonary capillaries and gas transfer ceases. Of the two gases, CO is much more widely used for the measurement of diffusing capacity than O_2 because of the ease and convenience of applying the various CO tests and because CO uptake is always diffusion limited. In contrast, O_2 uptake is not limited by diffusion (i.e., is not a test of diffusing capacity) in normal subjects except during heavy exercise or while breathing low concentrations of O_2.

Two general types of tests using CO are available that involve either a breath-holding maneuver (single-breath method) or continuous rebreathing (steady-state methods). These two methods yield systematically different results, largely because neither technique summarizes accurately the events taking place in the 100,000 gas exchange units of the lung, in each of which P_{CO} varies according to the ventilation and blood flow to the unit. Despite this shortcoming, measurements of pulmonary diffusing capacity have provided useful empiric information concerning the function of the lungs in healthy persons and patients with lung diseases.

The quantity of CO that will diffuse in a known period of time from alveolar gas into capillary blood and combine with hemoglobin in response to a given pressure difference between gas and blood depends on (1) the solubility and diffusibility of CO in each layer of the air-blood barrier, (2) the surface area and thickness of the barrier, and (3) the rate of the chemical reaction between CO and hemoglobin within red blood cells. Because the solubility and diffusibility of CO are physical characteristics that presumably do not change under ordinary circumstances, the two chief components of diffusing capacity are the area and thickness of the alveolar-capillary membrane available for diffusion (D_M) and the pulmonary capillary blood volume (V_C), both of which can be derived by performing several measurements of diffusing capacity (DL_{CO}) with the subject breathing gas mixtures of different concentrations of CO and O_2.

Normal values for CO-diffusing capacity depend chiefly on the person's lung volume and therefore closely correlate with body size, especially height. Less than half the total resistance to diffusion of CO from alveolar gas to capillary blood is attributable to the membrane component, and the greater fraction resides in the chemical reaction that takes place in the pulmonary capillary blood volume. Accordingly, changes in the hemoglobin concentration have a calculable effect on total CO diffusion that should be taken into account when establishing the predicted "normal" value for a patient with anemia or polycythemia.

Diffusing capacity is normally higher when a person is in the supine position than when he or she is in the erect posture because position changes the volume of blood in pulmonary capillaries, and at high compared with low lung volumes because inflation recruits alveolar-capillary surface. When blood flow to the lung increases, as in muscular exercise, capillary blood volume also increases owing to recruitment of previously nonperfused capillaries and dilation of others; these phenomena account for the progressive increase in DL_{CO} during increasingly strenuous levels of exercise. Similarly, the elevated pulmonary arterial pressures encountered in persons who live at high altitudes also recruit capillaries, increase capillary blood volume, and cause an increase in "normal" DL_{CO}. For unexplained reasons (possibly genetic), natives of high altitudes have higher DL_{CO} values than sojourners fully acclimatized to the same altitude.

TABLE 56–1. CHARACTERISTIC CHANGES IN LUNG VOLUMES AND TESTS OF AIRWAYS RESISTANCE IN PATIENTS WITH RESTRICTIVE AND OBSTRUCTIVE VENTILATORY DISORDERS*

Test	Restrictive	Obstructive
Vital capacity	Decreased	Decreased or normal
Residual volume	Decreased or normal	Increased
Total lung capacity	Decreased	Normal or increased
RV/TLC	Normal or slightly increased	Markedly increased
FEV_1/FVC	Normal or increased	Decreased
MMFR	Normal or decreased	Decreased
Slope of phase III	Normal or increased	Increased

*Abbreviations: RV/TLC = ratio of residual volume to total lung capacity; FEV_1/FVC = ratio of forced expiratory volume in 1 second to forced vital capacity; MMFR = maximum mid-expiratory flow rate.

Abnormalities of CO-Diffusing Capacity

On the basis of the physiologic principles that govern the diffusion of CO, it can be inferred that DL_{CO} may increase or decrease in patients with various cardiopulmonary disorders that affect the membrane, the capillary blood volume, or both. When tests of diffusing capacity were first used to study patients with various forms of lung disease, it was assumed that abnormalities of gas transfer would result from thickening of the air-blood barrier by a pathologic process that lengthened the pathway for diffusion of gases; this concept led to the formulation of what became widely known as the *alveolar-capillary block syndrome*. The "block" meant that the distance CO molecules had to travel from gas to blood was increased and, in turn, that extra time was required for diffusion to reach equilibrium across the air-blood barrier. Now it is known that most abnormalities of diffusion are caused by decreased capillary blood volume and that a true alveolar-capillary block is unusual.

Pulmonary vascular disorders, such as pulmonary emboli and pulmonary vasculitis, that affect (directly or indirectly) the pulmonary capillary bed decrease DL by decreasing capillary blood volume. Similarly, DL_{CO} is reduced in patients with infiltrative disorders of the interalveolar septum that obliterate or destroy capillaries. This is the usual mechanism underlying reduction of DL_{CO} in patients with sarcoidosis, diffuse interstitial fibrosis, berylliosis, or collagen diseases of the lung.

Changes in the characteristics of the membrane account for a decreased DL_{CO} in patients with diseases in which some form of intra-alveolar filling process has occurred and the air-to-blood diffusion pathway is actually lengthened: pneumonia, pulmonary edema, and alveolar proteinosis. A decrease in both membrane and blood volume components produces a low DL_{CO} in patients with disorders associated with removal or destruction of lung tissue, such as resectional surgery or emphysema.

An increase in DL_{CO} results occasionally from an increase in capillary blood volume secondary to hemodynamic changes in the pulmonary circulation: an increase in pulmonary arterial or left atrial pressures, as in congestive heart failure, or an increase in pulmonary blood flow, as in atrial septal defect. The DL_{CO} is sometimes increased in patients with bronchial asthma during an attack, but the cause of this change is not known.

PERFUSION

The pulmonary circulation delivers blood in a thin film to the gas exchange units so that O_2 uptake and CO_2 elimination can occur. The physiologic determinants of pulmonary blood flow are analogous to those of ventilation in that the total volumes of ventilation and blood flow must be adequate to meet metabolic needs, and the distribution of both must be such that proportionate amounts of inspired fresh air and incoming mixed venous blood are delivered to individual gas exchange units. Ventilatory volume is controlled by the factors that regulate breathing (see below), whereas the volume of blood flowing through the lungs is determined mainly by the extrapulmonary mechanisms that govern cardiac output.

Distribution of Pulmonary Blood Flow

Pulmonary blood flow is not distributed uniformly throughout the lungs but is normally greatest in the dependent regions, where pulmonary arterial pressure is highest, and, conversely, is least in the superior regions, where pulmonary arterial pressure is lowest. In the upright subject under resting conditions, the apices of the lungs are poorly perfused, and considerably more blood flows, even allowing for differences in the amount of lung tissue, to the basilar regions. The presence of nonuniform blood flow, which is not matched by comparable changes in ventilation, leads to important differences between regions of the lung in their defense capabilities and efficiency of gas exchange.

Regional blood flow is also governed by local factors, the most important of which is vasoconstriction secondary to alveolar hypoxia. As a consequence, blood flow is redistributed away from poorly ventilated gas exchange units, and the matching of ventilation and perfusion is preserved.

Distribution of pulmonary blood flow can readily be measured by injecting radioactive substances, such as ^{125}I-albumin aggre-gates or ^{133}Xe dissolved in saline, and then detecting their location in the lung with an external counter system. Abnormalities in the volume and distribution of pulmonary blood flow may result from diseases that involve the blood vessels themselves (emboli, vasculitis, emphysema), from compression of blood vessels (tumors, cysts), or from vasoconstriction of blood vessels (alveolar hypoxia secondary to local abnormality of ventilation).

Other Functions

The pulmonary circulation has important functions besides providing blood flow for continuous gas exchange: (1) It acts as a filter of virtually the entire venous drainage; (2) it supplies substrates for the nutrition and metabolic needs of the lung, including the synthesis of surfactant; (3) it serves as a reservoir of blood for the left ventricle; (4) it affects endocrine function by modifying the pharmacologic properties of a variety of circulating substances; and (5) it provides a large surface area for the absorption and filtration of liquids and solutes.

CONTROL OF BREATHING

The respiratory system must maintain gas exchange during periods of stress, such as exercise and other forms of increased metabolic needs. The O_2 consumption may increase more than 10-fold from rest to strenuous exercise; over this range, arterial Po_2 remains remarkably constant. The correspondence between the volume of ventilation and the demands for O_2 uptake and CO_2 elimination results from the responsiveness of three reasonably well characterized receptor systems that interact to regulate breathing in normal persons and patients with a variety of disease states: (1) receptors in the airways and lung parenchyma, (2) peripheral chemoreceptors, and (3) central chemoreceptors. Nerve impulse traffic from these receptors is integrated and modulated in the medulla with impulses arising from higher centers in the brain. The medulla can be viewed as the main headquarters for initiating, processing, and relaying messages concerning breathing to other parts of the body via nervous pathways. Some of the resulting medullary neural activity may reach the cerebral cortex and evoke conscious perception of breathing (i.e., the symptom of dyspnea); other impulses may travel through efferent pathways in the autonomic nervous system to the lungs and other organs; still other impulses may descend in the spinal cord to be processed with afferent impulses from peripheral nerves at different cord segments before finally being transmitted to the muscles of respiration and other effectors.

Abnormalities of Control of Breathing

Variations, usually increases, in the rate and depth of breathing occur in patients with many common clinical disturbances such as fever, metabolic diseases, or psychiatric disorders. Several frequently used drugs (e.g., aspirin, antidepressants, and alcohol) also affect ventilation. *Hyperventilation* occurs when ventilation increases out of proportion to CO_2 production and arterial Pco_2 decreases; *hypoventilation* is the converse. *Hyperpnea* signifies an increase in the rate and depth of breathing, such as occurs during exercise, but carries no implication concerning arterial Pco_2 values. It should be emphasized that a decrease in the O_2 pressure (Po_2) of arterial blood has several causes. In contrast, the pressure of CO_2 (Pco_2) is governed simply by the relationship between CO_2 production ($\dot{V}co_2$) and CO_2 elimination by alveolar ventilation ($Valv$):

$$Pco_2 = k\dot{V}co_2/\dot{V}alv$$

Because alveolar ventilation normally changes to keep pace with CO_2 production, for practical purposes abnormal arterial Pco_2 values can always be interpreted as indicating hyperventilation or hypoventilation.

Abnormalities of the control of breathing can result from excitation of intrapulmonary receptors (pulmonary embolism, pneumonia, asthma), depression of peripheral chemoreceptors (natives of high altitudes, sedative drugs, severe chronic bronchitis), stimulation of peripheral chemoreceptors (drugs such as doxapram), depression of central chemoreceptors (sedative drugs, obesity, myxedema, neurologic disorders), and stimulation of central chemoreceptors (drugs such as aspirin, irritative neurologic lesions). Special tests of the ventilatory response to breathing gas mixtures with increased CO_2 or decreased O_2 and a test that determines the pressure developed during the first 0.1 second of breathing against a closed mouthpiece ($P_{0.1}$) help define the physiologic derangements in these disorders.

GAS EXCHANGE

The end-product of respiration is gas exchange, which in human beings consists of maintaining the values for P_{O_2} and P_{CO_2} in arterial blood within normal limits. As stated previously, respiration consists of ventilation, including the distribution of inspired air throughout the tracheobronchial system, diffusion, blood flow, including the distribution of mixed venous blood throughout pulmonary capillaries, and the control of breathing. Each of these contributes in a unique way to gas exchange such that an impairment in one process cannot be compensated for by improvement in another.

Ambient air consists primarily of N_2 and O_2, with varying amounts of water vapor. As air is inhaled, it is warmed to body temperature and fully saturated with water vapor (P_{H_2O} 37°C = 47 mm Hg); the addition of water vapor has the effect of diluting the inspired mixture of N_2 and O_2 and reduces their respective pressures proportionately. During gas exchange in the alveoli, more O_2 is removed than CO_2 is added; this causes the volume of each respiratory unit to decrease slightly and raises the concentration and pressure of N_2 slightly. When ventilation and perfusion are each uniformly distributed to various units (Fig. 56–5), "ideal" conditions for gas exchange exist, and there is no difference between the P_{O_2} values in (mean) alveolar gas and arterial blood. The alveolar-arterial P_{O_2} difference is an important measure of the uniformity of matching of ventilation and perfusion. The difference is derived from a direct measurement of the arterial P_{O_2}, which is subtracted from alveolar P_{O_2} ($P_{A_{O_2}}$) calculated according to the following equation:

$$P_{A_{O_2}} = P_{I_{O_2}} - P_{A_{CO_2}} \left[F_{I_{O_2}} + \frac{1 - F_{I_{O_2}}}{R} \right]$$

where $P_{I_{O_2}}$ = P_{O_2} of inspired gas, $P_{A_{CO_2}}$ = alveolar P_{CO_2} (usually assumed to equal arterial P_{CO_2}), $F_{I_{O_2}}$ = fractional concentration of O_2 in inspired gas, and R = respiratory exchange ratio (often assumed to equal 0.8).

However, gas exchange in healthy lungs is not perfect because there is a small (5 to 10 mm Hg) alveolar-arterial P_{O_2} difference, which occurs because of the normal presence of a slight nonuniformity in the distribution of ventilation with respect to perfusion and a small right-to-left shunt. It is also noteworthy that the sum of the pressures of the individual gases in mixed venous blood is less than the total atmospheric pressure. Because the tissues and spaces of the body are in approximate equilibrium with venous blood, these structures are also subatmospheric. The "suction" serves to keep the lung expanded against the chest wall and to cause the reabsorption of gas from tissue spaces (e.g., a pneumothorax).

Abnormal Gas Exchange

Measurements of arterial P_{O_2} and P_{CO_2} and calculations of the alveolar-arterial P_{O_2} difference are reliable guides to the overall adequacy of respiration. In determining whether or not an abnormality is present, it must be remembered that normal values for P_{O_2}, but not P_{CO_2}, vary with age and that both P_{O_2}

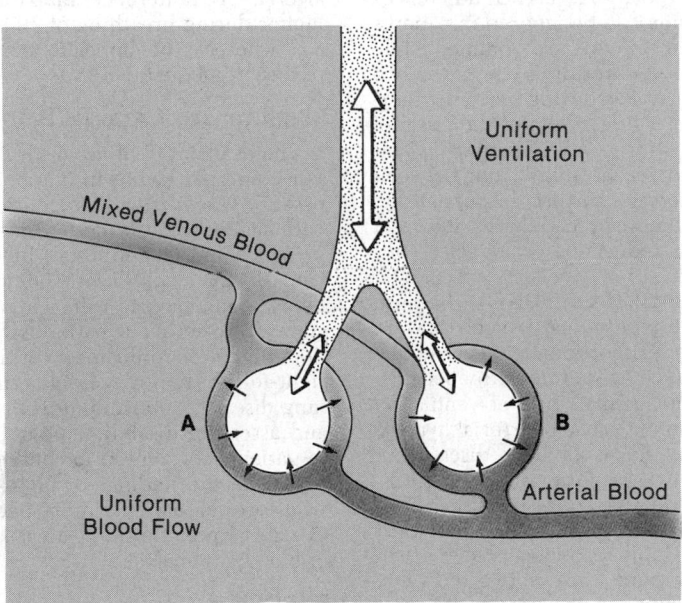

FIGURE 56–5. Schematic representation of gas exchange in an idealized two-compartment model of the lung in which there is uniform distribution of ventilation and blood flow. (Adapted with permission from Comroe JH Jr, et al.: The Lung: Clinical Physiology and Pulmonary Function Tests. 2nd ed. Chicago, Year Book Medical Publishers, 1962. Copyright © 1962, Year Book Medical Publishers, Inc.)

	A	B	A + B	Units
Alveolar ventilation	2.4	2.4	4.8	L/min
Pulmonary blood flow	3.0	3.0	6.0	L/min
Ventilation-perfusion ratio	0.8	0.8	0.8	
Mixed venous P_{O_2}	40	40	40	mm Hg
Mixed venous S_{O_2}	75	75	75	per cent
Mixed venous P_{CO_2}	46	46	46	mm Hg
Alveolar P_{O_2}	101	101	101	mm Hg
Arterial P_{O_2}	101	101	101	mm Hg
Arterial S_{O_2}	97.5	97.5	97.5	per cent
Arterial P_{CO_2}	40	40	40	mm Hg
Alveolar-arterial P_{O_2} difference	0	0	0	mm Hg

and P_{CO_2} are influenced by the altitude at which the subject is living. There are five physiologic mechanisms known to cause arterial hypoxia, defined as a decrease below normal of arterial P_{O_2}: (1) hypoventilation, (2) decreased diffusion, (3) ventilation-perfusion imbalance, (4) right-to-left shunting of blood, and (5) breathing air (or a gas mixture) with a low P_{O_2}. Except for a few uncommon clinical examples, such as breathing air with its P_{O_2} reduced by combustion of O_2 and addition of smoke or suffocation, item 5 can be ignored. Items 1 to 4 can be distinguished, at least for practical clinical purposes, by analyzing the values from a given blood specimen and a few easy tests.

HYPOVENTILATION. The simplest disturbance of gas exchange occurs when not enough fresh air is breathed into alveolar spaces to raise pulmonary capillary P_{O_2} to normal levels and to allow CO_2 to leave the bloodsteam. Although arterial P_{CO_2} may theoretically increase in patients with other disturbances of gas exchange (ventilation-perfusion abnormalities and right-to-left shunts), for clinical purposes an elevated value should be interpreted as indicating alveolar hypoventilation.

Pure hypoventilation is a relatively uncommon clinical event. When it is found, depression of the central nervous system resulting from anesthetic agents or other sedative drugs is the usual cause. More commonly, hypoventilation occurs in association with other disturbances of oxygenation. When these coexist, they can be recognized by the fact that the decrease in arterial P_{O_2} is more than can be accounted for by the increase in arterial P_{CO_2}.

IMPAIRED DIFFUSION. Decreased diffusion, from either loss of pulmonary capillaries or thickening of the air-blood barrier, does not usually cause important alveolar-arterial P_{O_2} differences *at rest*. Thus abnormalities of diffusion can be ignored in patients with arterial hypoxia whose blood specimens are obtained while they are resting. In contrast, impaired diffusion is one of the two major causes of severely worsening hypoxia during exercise (right-to-left shunting of blood is the other). Regardless of the cause of the diffusing impairment, under resting conditions there is sufficient time to allow gas transfer to reach equilibrium between gas and blood. However, during exercise, cardiac output and the velocity of blood flow through pulmonary capillaries increase; thus the time for gas transfer is reduced and alveolar–end-capillary P_{O_2} differences may occur.

VENTILATION-PERFUSION MISMATCHING. Because the distributions of inspired air and pulmonary blood flow in normal lungs are neither uniform nor proportionate to each other, a slight ventilation-perfusion imbalance exists in healthy persons. Moreover, increased (above normal) mismatching of ventilation and perfusion is by far the most common cause of arterial hypoxia encountered clinically. Virtually all forms of lung disease are associated with a detectable ventilation-perfusion abnormality.

When a unit is underventilated relative to its perfusion (i.e., has a low ventilation-perfusion ratio), O_2 uptake by that unit must decrease so that the P_{O_2} of its end-capillary blood is lower than normal; P_{CO_2} tends to increase but cannot rise above the value in mixed venous blood (Fig. 56–5). Thus the process affects values for P_{O_2} more than P_{CO_2}. Furthermore, in those units that are overventilated owing to a redistribution of inspired air, the high ventilation-perfusion ratio causes P_{O_2} to increase and P_{CO_2} to decrease. But there is an important difference in the effects of these changes in pressures on the actual quantities (contents) of O_2 and CO_2 in the capillary blood leaving units with high ventilation-perfusion ratios. Given the shapes of the respective dissociation curves, O_2 content is not appreciably increased but CO_2 content is decreased. Thus increasing ventilation with respect to perfusion in some regions corrects the tendency to CO_2 retention that would otherwise exist but does not correct the hypoxia caused by low ventilation-perfusion relationships in other units. Another invariable consequence of a ventilation-perfusion abnormality is an increase in the alveolar-arterial P_{O_2} difference.

RIGHT-TO-LEFT SHUNTING. A small right-to-left shunt of blood is found in normal persons, and shunts of considerable magnitude may occur in patients with pulmonary disease. A right-to-left shunt may be visualized as a pathway (or pathways) through which mixed venous blood flows from the right to the left side of the heart without having perfused functioning gas exchange units along the way. Thus there is a continuous admix-

ture of venous blood that has flowed through the abnormal pathway with arterialized blood from normal pathways in the lungs. Arterial hypoxia and an increased alveolar-arterial P_{O_2} difference occur that vary in severity with the magnitude of the shunt and its O_2 content. Right-to-left shunts may occur through intracardiac communications in patients with congenital heart disease. In patients with lung disease, although shunts may be extremely large, they seldom occur through abnormal vascular channels such as pulmonary arteriovenous fistulas; instead, they are caused by blood perfusing normal vessels in regions of the lung that are atelectatic or in which alveoli are filled with edema fluid, pus, or blood; in either case, because gas transfer is impossible, a shunt occurs.

The consequences of a right-to-left shunt are similar to those of a ventilation-perfusion imbalance owing to basic similarities between the two disturbances. A shunt can be viewed as an extreme ventilation-perfusion abnormality in which there is perfusion but *no* ventilation at all. It is impossible to differentiate between a ventilation-perfusion disturbance and a right-to-left shunt while the subject is breathing ambient air; therefore the effects of both are combined and designated venous admixture or a "shuntlike" effect. The two causes of hypoxia can be differentiated by giving the patient 100 per cent O_2 to breathe and measuring arterial P_{O_2} after all the N_2 has been washed out of the lungs. When a ventilation-perfusion abnormality exists, the N_2 is replaced by O_2 and all the blood perfusing the lungs equilibrates at a high P_{O_2} (approximately 600 mm Hg); in this way 100 per cent O_2 is said to "correct" a ventilation-perfusion disturbance. In contrast, in the presence of a right-to-left shunt, the admixture of mixed venous blood continues despite breathing 100 per cent O_2, and arterial hypoxia persists. In fact, the alveolar-arterial P_{O_2} difference in patients with a right-to-left shunt is higher during breathing of 100 per cent O_2 compared with room air, whereas the opposite occurs in patients with ventilation-perfusion inequalities.

Significance of Arterial Blood Gas Values

The availability of accurate rapid analyzers for measuring P_{O_2}, P_{CO_2}, and pH has been one of the major clinical advances of the past 25 years. Virtually the entire therapeutic approach to patients with acute and chronic respiratory failure is dictated by the presence and magnitude of blood gas and pH abnormalities (see Ch. 70). Every physician should know the mechanisms of arterial hypoxia and how to differentiate them, because it is important clinically whether a patient's hypoxia results from hypoventilation, impaired diffusion, ventilation-perfusion mismatching, or right-to-left shunting. Evaluating the course and prognosis of the lung disease, determining the need for and outcome of therapy, and assessing disability, operability, and the limits of resection in patients considered for pulmonary surgery all depend to some extent on the findings of blood gas analysis. Thus all physicians who care for patients must become familiar with the technique of arterial puncture and must know how to interpret the results of blood gas analysis.

EXERCISE

Tests of pulmonary function are customarily performed with the subject seated at rest. The results of these studies provide useful information about the functional abnormalities that characterize common and important pulmonary diseases. Occasionally, the results of routine tests are perfectly normal in symptomatic patients, usually those with exertional dyspnea. In these circumstances, tests during exercise may reveal severe functional disturbances that lead to further evaluation and a diagnosis of either pulmonary vascular or parenchymal infiltrative diseases. Exercise tests are also essential to document the presence of and mechanisms underlying disability.

Chang HK, Paiva M (eds.): Respiratory Physiology. New York, Marcel Dekker, Inc., 1989. *Detailed and authoritative review for advanced students.*

Murray JF: The Normal Lung: The Basis for Diagnosis and Treatment of Pulmonary Disease. 2nd ed. Philadelphia, W. B. Saunders Company, 1986. *Review of normal anatomy, pulmonary physiology, and structure-function correlations.*

Roussos C, Macklem PT (eds.): The Thorax, Parts A and B. New York, Marcel Dekker, Inc., 1983. *Extremely thorough, authoritative discussion of the interrelationships among the thorax, lungs, and respiratory muscles in health and disease.*

Taylor AE, Rehder K, Hyatt RE, et al.: Clinical Respiratory Physiology. Philadelphia, W.B. Saunders Company, 1989. *Useful introduction to pulmonary physiology and its many clinical applications.*

Wagner PD, Rodriguez-Roisin R: State of the art. Clinical advances in pulmonary gas exchange. Am Rev Respir Dis 14:883, 1991. *A summary of the pathophysiologic insights gained from studies of pulmonary gas exchange in various common clinical diseases.*

Wasserman K, Hansen JE, Sue DY, et al.: Principles of Exercise Testing and Interpretation. Philadelphia, Lea and Febiger, 1987. *An instructive and practical book for all persons interested in exercise physiology.*

Wilson AF (ed.): Pulmonary Function Testing: Indications and Interpretations. Orlando, Fla., Grune & Stratton, 1985. *Good summary of pulmonary function testing; well referenced.*

57 Asthma

Jeffrey M. Drazen

DEFINITION

Asthma is a clinical syndrome characterized by recurrent episodes of airway obstruction that resolve spontaneously or as a result of treatment. The etiology of asthma remains unknown. The resolution of the airway obstruction in asthma is a critical feature that distinguishes it from forms of chronic obstructive lung disease. Asthma is also associated with hyperresponsiveness of the airways to a variety of inhaled stimuli; this condition is manifested as an exaggerated bronchoconstrictor response to stimuli that have little or no effect in normal subjects. Current evidence, outlined in Pathogenesis and Pathology below, suggests that asthma may comprise a number of distinct disease entities.

EPIDEMIOLOGY AND STATISTICS

Asthma is an extremely common disorder affecting men and women equally; approximately 4 per cent of the population of the United States has signs and symptoms consistent with a diagnosis of asthma. Although most cases of asthma begin before the age of 25, asthma may begin anytime throughout life. Asthma is a common reason to seek medical treatment. In the United States in 1988, there were 15 million outpatient visits to physicians for asthma and nearly 2 million inpatient hospital days of treatment. More than 4 billion dollars per year are spent on asthma care.

PATHOGENESIS AND PATHOLOGY

Despite the high prevalence of asthma, its cause remains unknown. It is established that the episodic airway narrowing that constitutes an asthma attack results from obstruction of the airway lumen to airflow. Three distinct pathobiologic processes account for this obstruction: (1) constriction of airway smooth muscle, (2) thickening of the airway epithelium, and (3) the presence of liquids within the confines of the airway lumen. Among these mechanisms, the first has received the greatest attention. In this regard, constriction of airway smooth muscle due to the local release of bioactive mediators or neurotransmitters is the most widely accepted reason for airway obstruction in asthma. The sources and mechanisms of release of such molecules in human asthma are still speculative, but potential sources have been identified from experimental studies in lower animals and in isolated human tissues. The cellular sources and mediators thought to be of importance in asthma are summarized below.

HISTAMINE. Histamine, or beta-imidazolylethylamine, was identified as a potent endogenous bronchoactive agent more than 80 years ago. Mast cells, which are prominent in airway tissues, constitute the major pulmonary source of histamine. Recent studies with novel potent antihistamines indicate a role for histamine as one of the mediators of bronchospasm in asthma.

ACETYLCHOLINE. Acetylcholine released from intrapulmonary motor nerves that are branches of the vagi effects constriction of airway smooth muscle through direct stimulation of muscarinic receptors. In the airways these receptors are predominantly of the M_3 subtype. The utility of atropine (and its congeners) in the treatment of asthma provides the major evidence for the importance of acetylcholine in the pathogenesis of asthma.

KININS. Bradykinin and related molecules are cleaved from plasma precursors by the actions of enzymes known as kallikreins. Although there are many sources of kallikreins, at least one type is released from mast cells after appropriate activation. Although no bradykinin synthesis inhibitors or receptor antagonists are in clinical study or use, the potential importance of bradykinin derives from its potency and from the release of kinin-forming enzymes from a cell of potential importance in asthma, the mast cell.

ADENOSINE. Adenosine is a purine nucleoside that is formed during the rapid extracellular metabolism of adenosine triphosphate (ATP). A possible role of adenosine in asthma was first suggested based on the observation that theophylline at therapeutic levels effectively antagonizes the activity of adenosine at the receptor level. Both oral and inhaled forms of theophylline have also been shown to inhibit the adenosine-induced bronchoconstriction in human asthmatics. This evidence for the importance of adenosine in asthma lost some of its strength when enprofylline, a xanthine with a poor adenosine-antagonist effect, was documented to be a more potent antiasthmatic drug than theophylline.

LEUKOTRIENES. The sulfidopeptide leukotrienes—LTC_4, LTD_4, and LTE_4—constitute the material previously known as slow-reacting substances of anaphylaxis, or SRS-A. These molecules and LTB_4 are derived by the sequential lipoxygenation of arachidonic acid, which is released from cell membrane phospholipids during cellular activation. Mast cells, eosinophils, and alveolar macrophages have the enzymatic capability required to produce sulfidopeptide leukotrienes from membrane phospholipids. Two enzyme systems, 5-lipoxygenase and LTC_4 synthase, and a cytosolic protein known as 5-lipoxygenase-activating protein are required to produce the sulfidopeptide leukotriene LTC_4. This molecule is transported out of the cell where it is synthesized and processed extracellularly to LTD_4 and LTE_4. LTC_4 and LTD_4 are about 3000 times more potent than histamine as contractile agonists, while LTE_4 is about 300 times more potent than histamine. Preliminary clinical studies with leukotriene receptor antagonists or synthesis inhibitors have shown efficacy in the treatment of asthma.

PLATELET-ACTIVATING FACTOR (PAF). PAF is a phospholipid with an ether rather than an ester link to a long-chain (C_{16}–C_{20}) fatty acid in the sn−1 position, an acetyl moiety in the sn−2 position, and phosphatidylcholine in the sn−3 position. It is derived from lyso-PAF by the action of specific acetyltransferases and is produced by a variety of inflammatory cells, including mast cells and eosinophils. PAF, through action at specific receptors, is a moderately potent airway contractile agonist, but since the receptors mediating this constriction are rapidly tachyphylactic, it is unlikely that PAF has a major direct role in asthmatic bronchoconstriction. PAF has the ability to induce a state of prolonged airway hyperresponsiveness (see below), which is characteristic of the asthmatic condition.

TACHYKININS. Tachykinins are a series of small peptides, on the order of 10 residues in length, which share a common carboxy terminal sequence—Phe-X-Gly-Leu-Met-NH$_2$. Three tachykinins—substance P, neurokinin A (substance K), and neurokinin B—are found in the terminal axon dendrites of certain sensory nerves. When these nerves are stimulated by appropriate sensory stimuli, the peptides are released into the airway microenvironment, where they can induce airway smooth muscle constriction as well as mucus secretion through action at specific receptors. As these sensory signals pass the terminal ramifications of the axon on their way to the central nervous system, antidromic conduction occurs. Conduction of the antidromic signal to the sensory nerve endings is accompanied by further local release of tachykinins. This process has been termed as "axon reflex." Ordinarily, the peptides released from the nerves are rapidly degraded by specific peptidases located at or near the site of their action or release; inhibition of the function of these peptidases enhances the biologic effects of released peptides. These small peptides have been implicated in asthmatic responses because many stimuli known to cause their release in lower animals have been shown to induce asthma attacks in humans.

Each of these putative mediators of asthma has the potential to effect airway obstruction; their action in concert may induce severe bronchospasm. It is not unreasonable to speculate that there are a variety of asthmatic diatheses that differ in the profile of mediators released, elaborated, or left unchecked at or near their site of action on airway smooth muscle. Elucidation of these pathways may fragment the syndrome we now know as asthma into many diseases.

Pathology of the Asthmatic Response

The pathology of mild asthma, as derived from bronchoscopic and biopsy studies, is characterized by edema and hyperemia of the mucosa and by infiltration of the mucosa with mast cells, eosinophils, and lymphocytes bearing the CD4 phenotype. The lamina propria is thickened, with deposition of types III and V collagen (Fig. 57–1). In cases of more severe asthma, there is thickening of the airway wall due to hypertrophy and hyperplasia of the airway glands and secretory cells, hyperplasia of airway smooth muscle, as well as further deposition of submucosal collagen. Airway epithelium may be shed, leading to a denuded airway. These changes occur in a patchy fashion in mild asthma and become more widespread as the disease becomes more severe. Morphometric studies of airways from asthmatic subjects have demonstrated airway wall thickening of sufficient magnitude to increase airflow resistance and enhance airway responsiveness. In severe asthma, the airway wall is thickened markedly, and there is patchy airway occlusion by a mixture of hyperviscous mucus and shed airway epithelium.

Physiologic Changes in Asthma

The consequence of the airway obstruction induced by smooth muscle constriction, thickening of the mucosa, or free liquid within the airway lumen is an increased resistance to airflow. This condition is manifested by increased airway resistance (R_{aw}) and decreased flow rates throughout the vital capacity. At the onset of an asthma attack, obstruction occurs at all airway levels; during the resolution of the attack, changes reverse first in the large airways (i.e., mainstem, lobar, segmental, and subsegmental bronchi) and then in the more peripheral airways. This anatomic sequence of onset and reversal is reflected in the physiologic changes monitored during an asthmatic episode (Fig. 57–2). As an asthma attack resolves, flow rates first normalize high in the vital capacity, and only later do they resolve low in the vital capacity. Because asthma is an airway disease, there are no primary changes in the static pressure-volume curve of the lungs. However, during an acute attack of asthma, airway narrowing may be so severe as to result in airway closure. Individual lung units tend to close at a volume that is near their maximal volume; this tendency produces a change in the pressure-volume curve such that for a given contained gas volume within the thorax there will be decreased elastic recoil. The decreased elastic recoil at a given overall lung volume further depresses expiratory airflow rates.

Additional factors influence the mechanical behavior of the lungs in the course of an acute attack of asthma. During inspiration, the pleural pressure drops far below the 4 to 6 cm H_2O below atmospheric pressure usually required for tidal airflow. The expiratory phase of respiration also becomes active as the patient tries to force air from the lungs. As a consequence, peak pleural pressures during expiration, which normally are only a few centimeters of water above atmospheric pressure, may be as high as 20 to 30 cm H_2O. The low pleural pressures during inspiration tend to dilate airways, while the high pleural pressures during expiration tend to narrow airways. During an asthma attack, the net effect is to increase airflow resistance during expiration much more than during inspiration.

The respiratory rate is usually rapid during an acute asthma attack. The tachypnea is not driven by abnormalities in arterial blood gas composition, but rather by stimulation of intrapulmonary receptors, with subsequent effects on the respiratory centers. A consequence of airway narrowing combined with the rapid airflow rates is that there is a heightened mechanical load on the ventilatory pump. During a severe asthma attack, the load can increase the work of breathing by a factor of 10 or more and can predispose to fatigue of the ventilatory muscles.

The patchy nature of the asthmatic airway narrowing results in a maldistribution of ventilation (V) relative to pulmonary perfusion(Q). There is a shift from the normal situation, in which V/Q units with a ratio of near unity are preponderant, to a distribution involving a large number of alveolar-capillary units with a V/Q ratio less than unity. The net effect is to induce arterial hypoxemia. In addition, the hyperpnea of asthma is reflected as hyperventilation with a low arterial P_{CO_2}.

CLINICAL PRESENTATION

History

During an asthma attack, patients seek medical attention for shortness of breath accompanied by cough, wheezing, and anxiety. The degree of breathlessness experienced by the patient is not closely related to the degree of airflow obstruction but is often influenced by the acuteness of the attack. Dyspnea may occur only with exercise, so-called *exercise-induced asthma;* may occur after exposure to a specific known allergen, referred to as *extrinsic asthma;* or may occur for no identifiable reason, so-called *intrinsic asthma.* There are variants of asthma in which cough, hoarseness, or inability to sleep throughout the night are the only symptoms. Identification, through careful questioning, of a provoking stimulus both helps to establish the diagnosis of asthma and may help in therapy if the stimulus can be avoided. Most patients with asthma will complain of shortness of breath when exposed to rapid changes in the temperature and humidity of inspired air. For example, in less temperate climates during the winter months, this commonly occurs when the patient leaves a heated house. Airway narrowing induced by breathing cold, dry air forms the basis of one of the diagnostic tests for asthma (see below).

Physical Examination

VITAL SIGNS. A rapid respiratory rate, often 25 to 40 breaths per minute, is common during an acute asthma attack. Tachycardia is also common, as is the presence of pulsus paradoxus, an

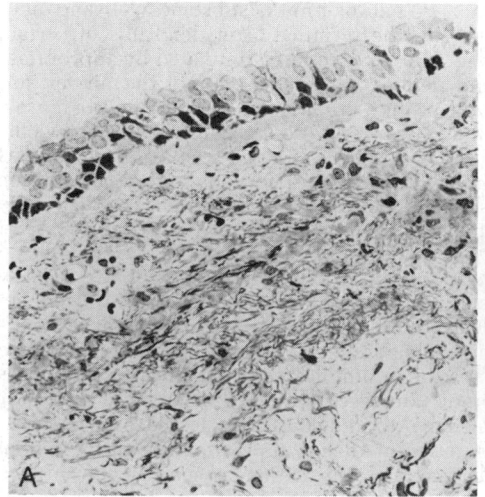
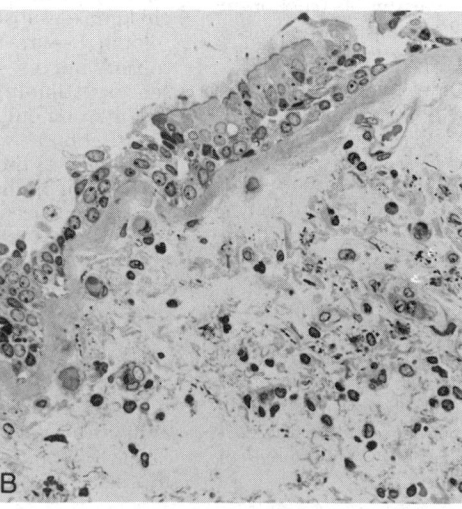

FIGURE 57–1. Photomicrographs of endobronchial biopsy specimens from a normal (*A*) and a mildly allergic asthmatic subject (*B*). The airway biopsy from the asthmatic individual demonstrates the characteristic subepithelial fibrosis, edema, and inflammatory cell infiltration not seen in the normal subject. (Photomicrograph courtesy of W.R. Roche, University of Southampton, United Kingdom.)

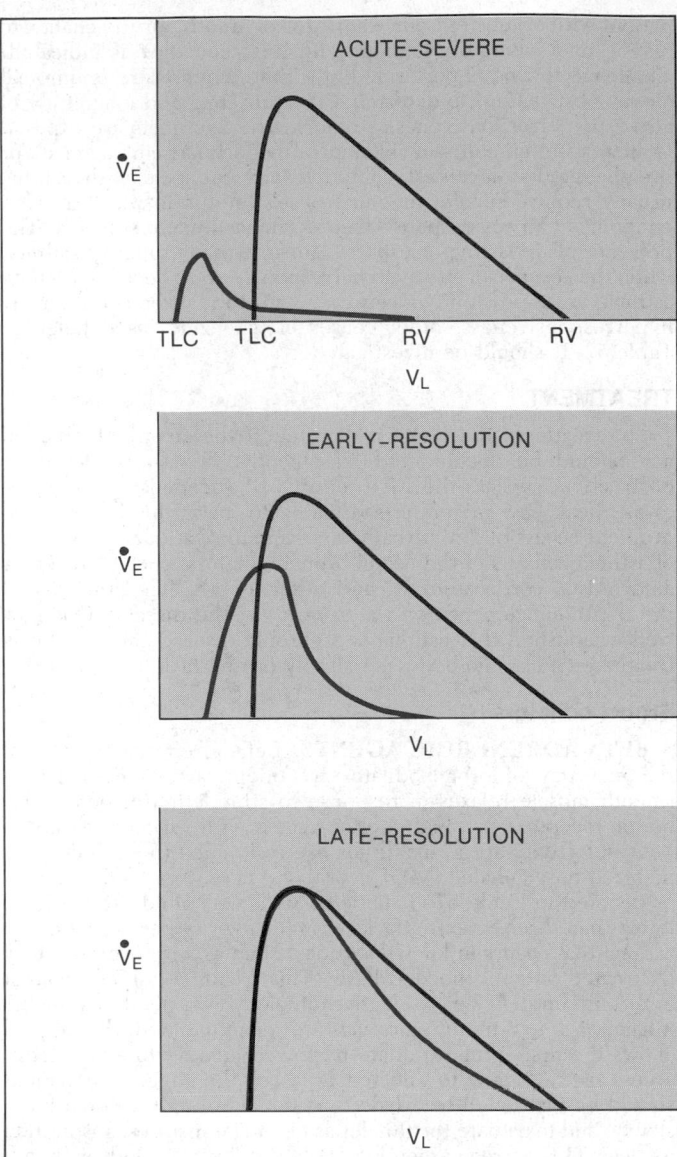

FIGURE 57–2. Schematic flow-volume curves in various stages of asthma; in each figure the colored line depicts the normal flow-volume curve. Predicted and observed total lung capacity (TLC) and residual volume (RV) are shown in the top panel. Note that TLC and RV decrease as flow rates increase with attack resolution. $\dot{V}_E$ = expiratory flow rate; V_L = lung volume.

exaggerated inspiratory fall in the systolic pressure. The magnitude of the pulsus paradoxus is related to the severity of the attack.

THORACIC EXAMINATION. Inspection will reveal that the patient is using the accessory muscles during inspiration; the skin over the thorax may be retracted into the intercostal spaces during inspiration. The chest is usually hyperinflated, and the expiratory phase is prolonged relative to the inspiratory phase. Percussion of the thorax demonstrates hyperresonance with loss of the normal variation in dullness due to diaphragmatic movement. Auscultation reveals wheezing, the cardinal physical finding in asthma; the presence of wheezing does not, however, establish asthma as the diagnosis (Table 57–1). Wheezing is commonly heard during both inspiration and expiration, although it is louder during the latter phase of respiration. The wheezing is characterized as polyphonic in that more than one pitch may be heard at a given time. There may be other accompanying adventitious sounds, including rhonchi, suggestive of free secretions in the airway lumen, or rales, indicative of localized infection or cardiac failure. The loss of intensity or absence of breath sounds in a patient with asthma is an indication of severe airflow obstruction.

TABLE 57–1. DIFFERENTIAL DIAGNOSIS OF WHEEZING OTHER THAN ASTHMA

Common
Acute bronchiolitis (infectious, chemical)
Aspiration (foreign body)
Bronchial stenosis
Cardiac failure
Chronic bronchitis
Cystic fibrosis
Eosinophilic pneumonia

Uncommon
Airway obstruction due to masses
   External compression
      Central thoracic tumors, superior vena cava (SVC) syndrome, substernal thyroid
   Intrinsic airway
      Primary lung cancer, metastatic breast cancer
Carcinoid syndrome
Endobronchial sarcoid
Pulmonary emboli
Systemic mastocytosis
Systemic vasculitis (polyarteritis nodosa)

Laboratory Findings

PULMONARY FUNCTION FINDINGS. A decrease in airflow rates throughout the vital capacity is the cardinal pulmonary function abnormality in asthma. Although essential for the diagnosis of asthma, it is not specific, as other obstructive diseases share this feature. The peak expiratory flow rate (PEFR), forced expiratory volume in the first second (FEV_1), and maximal midexpiratory flow rate (MMEFR) are all decreased in asthma. In very severe asthma, the dyspnea may be so severe as to prevent the patient from performing a complete spirogram. In this case, if 1 second of forced expiration can be recorded, useful values for the PEFR and FEV_1 can be obtained. Gradation of attack severity *must* be assessed by objective measures of airflow; there are no other methods that can do this in an accurate and reproducible fashion. Table 57–2 relates the severity of the attack to the relative depressions of airflow rates. As the attack resolves, PEFR and FEV_1 increase in concert while the MMEFR remains substantially depressed. Further resolution of obstruction is indicated by a normalization of both the FEV_1 and the PEFR while the MMEFR remains depressed. Even when the attack is resolved clinically, it is not uncommon to observe residual depression of the MMEFR, which may resolve over a prolonged course of treatment. Representative schematic flow-volume curves during an asthma attack are shown in Figure 57–2. If the patient is able to cooperate fully, measurements of lung volumes will show increases in total lung capacity (TLC) and residual volume (RV) during the acute attack that resolve with treatment.

ARTERIAL BLOOD GASES. Blood gas analysis need not be done in individuals with mild asthma. If, however, the asthma is of sufficient severity to merit prolonged observation, blood gas analysis is indicated; in such cases, hypoxemia and hypocarbia are the rule. With the subject breathing room air, the Pa_{O_2} is usually between 55 and 70 torr, and the Pa_{CO_2} is usually between 25 and 35 torr. At the onset of the attack, there will be an appropriate pure respiratory alkalemia, while with attacks of prolonged duration, the pH will normalize owing to compensatory metabolic acidemia. The presence of a normal Pa_{CO_2} in a patient with moderate to severe airflow obstruction is reason for concern, as it may indicate that the mechanical load on the respiratory system is greater than what can be sustained by the ventilatory muscles and that respiratory failure is imminent. When the Pa_{CO_2} rises in such settings, the pH will fall quickly because the bicarbonate stores will have been depleted as a result of renal compensation for the prolonged preceding respiratory alkalemia. Since this chain of events can occur rapidly, close observation is indicated for asthmatics with "normal" P_{CO_2} levels and moderate to severe airflow obstruction.

OTHER BLOOD FINDINGS. Asthmatic subjects are commonly atopic; thus blood eosinophilia is common. In addition, elevated serum immunoglobulin E (IgE) levels are common;

TABLE 57–2. RELATIVE SEVERITY OF AN ASTHMATIC ATTACK AS INDICATED BY PEFR, FEV₁, AND MMEFR

Test	Per Cent of Predicted	Asthma Severity
PEFR	80% or greater	
FEV$_1$	80% or greater	No spirometric abnormalities
MMEFR	80% or greater	
PEFR	80% or greater	
FEV$_1$	70% or greater	Mild asthma
MMEFR	55%–75%	
PEFR	60% or greater	
FEV$_1$	45%–70%	Moderate asthma
MMEFR	30%–50%	
PEFR	Less than 50%	
FEV$_1$	Less than 50%	Severe asthma
MMEFR	10%–30%	

PEFR = peak expiratory flow rate; MMEFR = maximal mid-expiratory flow rate; FEV$_1$ = forced expiratory volume in the first second.

epidemiologic studies indicate that asthma is unusual in subjects with low IgE levels. If indicated by the patient's history, specific radioallergosorbent (RAST) assays for IgE directed against likely offending antigens can be obtained. Although unusual, asthma alone can result in elevated levels of serum transaminases, lactate dehydrogenases, muscle creatine phosphokinase, ornithine transcarbamylase, and antidiuretic hormone.

RADIOGRAPHIC FINDINGS. The chest radiograph is often normal in subjects with asthma. Severe asthma is associated with hyperinflation, as indicated by depression of the diaphragm and abnormally lucent lung fields. Complications of severe asthma, including pneumomediastinum or pneumothorax, may be detected radiographically. In mild to moderate cases of asthma without adventitious sounds other than wheezing, a chest radiograph need not be obtained; if the asthma is of sufficient severity to merit hospital admission, a chest radiograph is advised.

ELECTROCARDIOGRAPHIC FINDINGS. The electrocardiogram is usually normal, save for a sinus tachycardia, in acute asthma. However, right-axis deviation, right bundle branch block, "P pulmonale," or even ST segment and T wave abnormalities may arise from severe asthma and resolve as the attack subsides.

SPUTUM FINDINGS. The sputum of the asthmatic patient may be clear or opaque with a green or yellow tinge. The presence of color does not invariably indicate infection, and examination of a Gram-stained and Wright-stained sputum smear is necessary. Often the sputum will contain eosinophils, Charcot-Leyden crystals (crystallized eosinophil proteins), Curschmann's spirals (bronchiolar casts composed of mucus and cells), or Creola's bodies (clusters of airway epithelial cells with identifiable cilia).

Differential Diagnosis

Asthma is easy to recognize in a younger patient without comorbid medical conditions who has exacerbating and remitting airway obstruction accompanied by blood eosinophilia. The rapid response to bronchodilator treatment (see below) is usually all that is needed to establish the diagnosis firmly. However, in the patient with cryptic episodic shortness of breath, airway challenge testing by a laboratory familiar with this procedure is indicated. Challenge testing is performed at a time when there is minimal airway obstruction, to determine the presence and magnitude of airway hyperresponsiveness. In such tests, subjects are exposed to increasing amounts of inhaled bronchoconstrictor agonists or breathe graded levels of cold, dry air. Subjects with asthma usually require smaller amounts of a stimulus to reach a given endpoint in airway response than do nonasthmatic subjects. The presence of airway hyperresponsiveness strongly suggests asthma, while the absence of airway hyperresponsiveness does not exclude asthma as a possibility. However, in the absence of airway hyperresponsiveness, other causes of wheezing, as detailed in Table 57–1, should be investigated.

TREATMENT

The treatment of asthma is directed at the airway obstruction and should be documented by objective measures of airflow obstruction, such as the FEV$_1$ or PEFR. Inexpensive and easy-to-use peak flow meters are available to make this latter measurement accessible to virtually all asthmatic patients. Treatment of asthma consists of the use of bronchodilators, specific receptor antagonists, corticosteroids, and other agents. The intensity of the treatment depends on the severity of the disease. It is now well established that asthma is a chronic disease and should be treated on a chronic basis, not simply from attack to attack.

Bronchodilators

BETA-ADRENERGIC AGENTS. Beta-adrenergic agents are the mainstay of bronchodilator treatment. Constricted airway smooth muscle relaxes in response to stimulation of beta$_2$-adrenergic receptors. Beta-adrenergic agents with varying degrees of beta$_2$ selectivity are available for use in inhaled (by nebulizer or metered-dose inhaler [MDI]), oral, or parenteral preparations, as detailed in Table 57–3. Patients with very mild asthma (i.e., fewer than three or four attacks of mild severity per year) or with asthma that occurs in known settings, such as with exercise, may be treated on an as-needed basis. This treatment should consist of a long-duration beta$_2$-selective inhaler. Two "puffs" from the inhaler at 3- to 5-minute intervals are recommended; the interval allows the first "puff" to dilate narrowed airways to allow better access of the agent to affected areas of the lung. The patient should be instructed to exhale to residual volume, to breathe in slowly, and to actuate the inhaler as he or she inspires. Inspiration to near TLC is recommended, followed by a period of breath holding on the order of 5 seconds, to allow smaller aerosol particles to deposit in more peripheral airways. Aerosol "spacers" are available from many manufacturers for the patient who has difficulty coordinating inspiration and inhaler actuation. Patients with mild to moderate disease should use their inhalers on a regular, daily basis (at 6- to 8-hour intervals) rather than only when they become symptomatic. Depending on the specific type of inhaled beta agent employed, use of the inhaler is possible between scheduled intervals if symptoms of airflow obstruction occur. Patients with moderate to severe asthma may benefit from the addition of an oral beta$_2$ agent used as indicated by the manufacturer.

The routine use of parenteral beta agonists in adults is not encouraged, as careful studies have shown that inhaled agents

TABLE 57–3. BETA AGONISTS FOR ASTHMA TREATMENT*

Drug	Beta$_2$ Selective	Inhaled	Oral	Parenteral	Comments
Albuterol	Yes	Yes	Yes	No	Available as an MDI or for nebulization
Ethylnorepinephrine	No	No	No	Yes	Fewer central nervous system effects than with epinephrine
Epinephrine	No	Yes	No	Yes	MDI available without prescription
Isoetharine	Yes	Yes	No	No	Available as an MDI or for nebulization
Isoproterenol	No	Yes	No	Yes	Parenteral form is for intravenous use only
Metaproterenol	Yes	Yes	Yes	No	Available as an MDI or for nebulization
Perbuterol	Yes	Yes	No	No	Available as an MDI
Terbutaline	Yes	Yes	Yes	Yes	Although beta$_2$ is selective in animals, clinical studies do not show selectivity when given subcutaneously

The "Form Available for Administration" heading spans the Inhaled, Oral, and Parenteral columns.

*Based on market drugs in the United States as of February 1, 1990.
MDI = metered-dose inhaler.

have equal efficacy, without the systemic side effects that accompany the use of parenteral agents.

THEOPHYLLINE. Theophylline and aminophylline are bronchodilators of moderate potency used in both inpatient and outpatient management of asthma. The mechanism of action of their effect is not established with certainty but likely is related either to the inhibition of the breakdown of cyclic adenosine monophosphate (AMP) by phosphodiesterase or to the inhibition of adenosine receptors. The utility of theophylline is limited by its toxicity and by the wide variations in the rate of its metabolism both in a single individual over time and among individuals in a population. As a result of this wide variability, monitoring of plasma theophylline levels is indicated to be sure that patients are appropriately treated. Acceptable plasma levels for therapeutic effects are between 10 and 20 μg per milliliter; higher levels are associated with gastrointestinal, cardiac, and central nervous system toxicity, including anxiety, headache, nausea, vomiting, diarrhea, cardiac arrhythmias, and seizures. The last two, catastrophic complications of toxicity may occur when plasma levels exceed 20 μg per milliliter without antecedent mild side effects. Because of these potentially life-threatening complications from treatment, plasma levels need to be monitored with great frequency in hospitalized patients receiving intravenous aminophylline and with less frequency in stable patients receiving, on an outpatient basis, one of the long-acting theophylline preparations. The use of theophylline preparations in patients with mild to moderate asthma managed with other medications has been recently questioned.

Receptor Antagonists

ANTIHISTAMINES. When antihistamines were first developed in the 1940's and 1950's, they were used in asthmatic subjects with unremarkable effect and major soporific side effects. In the past decade, newer, more potent H_1 receptor antagonists, such as terfenadine and astemizole, have emerged, with fewer central nervous system side effects. Although these compounds have not yet come into widespread use for the treatment of asthma, data from clinical trials indicate that they produce bronchodilation and alleviate asthmatic symptoms. It is likely that H_1 receptor antagonists will soon be used more frequently in asthma.

ANTICHOLINERGICS. Atropine has been known to be beneficial in the treatment of asthma for more than a century. Its mechanism of action is thought to be inhibition of the effects of acetylcholine released from intrapulmonary motor nerves that run in the vagus and innervate airway smooth muscle. The central nervous system side effects of atropine, which limited its utility, have been overcome with the development of ipratropium bromide, which is available as a metered-dose inhaler. Although ipratropium bromide has a salutary effect on cough in asthma and is useful in conjunction with a beta$_2$ inhaler in chronic stable asthma, it is not effective treatment for acute bronchospasm.

OTHER RECEPTOR ANTAGONISTS. Antagonists active at the putative receptors for LTD_4 and PAF are being clinically tested for use in the treatment of asthma. Initial trials in both laboratory-induced and spontaneously occurring asthma have shown efficacy, but there are currently no marketed drugs with this mechanism of action available for use in treating asthma.

Anti-inflammatory Agents

SYSTEMIC CORTICOSTEROIDS. Corticosteroids are a widely used and effective treatment for patients with moderate to severe asthma. Their mechanism of action in asthma is not established with certainty but has been linked to the diminished phlogistic potential of the cells resident within the airway as well as a reduction in the number of inflammatory cells within the airway. There is no consensus on the specific type, dose, or duration of dose of corticosteroid to be used in the treatment of asthma. In nonhospitalized patients refractory to standard antiasthma therapy, initial dosages on the order of 40 to 60 mg of prednisone per day tapered over 7 to 14 days are recommended. It has been clearly shown that in patients who cannot stop taking steroids without recurrent uncontrolled bronchospasm, the use of alternate-day oral steroids is preferable to daily treatment. In the patient who requires hospital treatment of his or her asthma, but who is not considered to have life-threatening asthma, an initial intravenous bolus of 2 mg per kilogram of hydrocortisone, followed by continuous infusion of 0.5 mg per kilogram per hour, has been shown to be effective therapy, with beneficial effects observable within 12 hours of starting treatment. In attacks of asthma that are considered life threatening, the use of intravenous methylprednisolone, 125 mg every 6 hours, has been advocated. In each case as the patient improves, oral steroids are substituted for intravenous steroids, and the dose is tapered over 1 to 3 weeks; as outlined below, the addition of inhaled steroids to tapering oral steroids is recommended.

INHALED CORTICOSTEROIDS. Inhaled corticosteroids, which have minimal systemic and side effects, have been shown to be an effective adjunctive therapy to bronchodilators for moderate to severe asthma. Their mechanism of action is presumed to be secondary to the reduction of intraluminal and airway mucosal inflammation. A number of studies have shown that at the recommended doses it is possible to withdraw oral steroids from steroid-dependent asthmatic patients; recent studies have suggested that the use of two to four times the recommended dose of inhaled steroid (i.e., four to six inhalations four to six times per day) results in further improvement in indices of airflow obstruction and asthmatic symptoms. The addition of inhaled steroids to the regimen of any asthmatic who has required a course of oral steroids is strongly advised. The major side effect from inhaled steroids is oral thrush; the risk and severity of this complication can be reduced through the use of aerosol spacers and good oropharyngeal hygiene.

OTHER ANTI-INFLAMMATORY DRUGS. The use of systemic gold (as is used in rheumatoid arthritis) or oral methotrexate has been suggested as adjunctive treatment for patients with severe chronic asthma who cannot be removed from high-dose corticosteroid treatment. These treatments are experimental, and their routine use is not advocated.

Disodium Cromoglycate

Disodium Cromoglycate is a mast cell membrane–stabilizing agent that is of value in the prophylactic treatment of asthma. It is most useful in patients with identifiable stimuli eliciting an asthmatic response, such as exercise or allergen exposure.

Specific Treatment Scenarios

ASTHMA IN THE EMERGENCY ROOM. When a patient with asthma presents for acute emergency care, objective measures of the severity of the attack, including quantification of pulsus paradoxus and measurement of airflow rates (PEFR or FEV_1), should be obtained in addition to the usual vital signs. If the PEFR or FEV_1 is less than 40 per cent of the predicted value, but the attack does not appear to be clinically life threatening, inhaled beta$_2$ agents and intravenous aminophylline (dose to be determined by the patient's previous treatment status) should be given. If the attack is prolonged and has failed to respond to treatment with bronchodilators, intravenous steroids (40 to 60 mg of methylprednisolone) should be administered. Inhaled treatments should be repeated at 20- to 30-minute intervals until the PEFR or FEV_1 improves to greater than 40 per cent of the predicted value. If this improvement fails to occur within 2 hours, admission to the hospital for further treatment is strongly advocated. In the patient whose PEFR and FEV_1 are greater than 60 per cent of predicted values on admission to the emergency room, treatment with inhaled beta$_2$ agonists alone is likely to result in an objective improvement in airflow rates. If a significant improvement occurs, such patients can usually be treated on an outpatient basis with the use of inhaled beta$_2$ agonists; the addition of oral theophylline or of oral or inhaled corticosteroids may be of value, depending on the severity of the attack and the rapidity of its response to treatment. For the patients whose PEFR and FEV_1 are between 40 and 60 per cent of predicted values at the time they are initially evaluated in the emergency care setting, a treatment plan varying in intensity between the two cited above is indicated. It is important to realize that failure to achieve an objective response to treatment, as recorded by measurements of PEFR or FEV_1, is an indication for more intense therapy.

STATUS ASTHMATICUS. The asthmatic subject in whom

the PEFR or FEV₁ does not increase above 40 per cent of the predicted value with treatment, who develops an increasing Pa_{CO_2} without an improvement in the indices of airflow obstruction, or who develops major complications, such as pneumothorax or pneumomediastinum, should be admitted to the hospital in a care environment where he or she can be closely monitored. Frequent treatments with inhaled beta agonists, intravenous aminophylline to achieve maximal plasma levels, and high-dose intravenous steroids are indicated. Oxygen should be administered by face mask or nasal cannula. If there is objective evidence of infection, it should be treated. If the patient's condition fails to improve with treatment and respiratory failure appears imminent, bronchodilator treatment should be intensified to the maximum tolerated by the patient. If indicated, intubation of the trachea and mechanical ventilation can be instituted; in this case the goal should be to provide ventilation just adequate to sustain life and *not to normalize* arterial blood gases. For example, a Pa_{CO_2} of 50 to 60 torr is acceptable for a patient in status asthmaticus.

THE PREGNANT ASTHMATIC. Asthma may be exacerbated, remain unchanged, or remit during pregnancy. There need not be substantial departures from the ordinary management of an asthmatic during pregnancy; however, unnecessary medications should be avoided. Systemic steroids should be used sparingly to avoid fetal complications, and certain drugs should be avoided. These include tetracycline as a treatment for intercurrent infection; atropine and atropine-like drugs, since they may cause fetal tachycardia; terbutaline during active labor because of its tocolytic effects; and iodine-containing mucolytics, such as saturated solution of potassium iodine (SSKI). The use of prostaglandin $F_{2\alpha}$ as an abortifacient should be avoided in asthmatics.

Barnes PJ: A new approach to the treatment of asthma. N Engl J Med 321:1517, 1989. *A good summary of current approaches to the treatment of asthma.*

Beasley R, Roche WR, Roberts JA, et al.: Cellular events in the bronchi in mild asthma and after bronchial provocation. Am Rev Respir Dis 139:806, 1989. *A review of the cellular physiology involved in bronchospastic responses.*

Jeffrey PK, Wardlaw AJ, Nelson FC, et al.: Bronchial biopsies in asthma. An ultrastructural, quantitative study and correlation with hyperreactivity. Am Rev Respir Dis 140:1745, 1989. *A good discussion of the pathology and tissue changes in asthma.*

Rossing TH: Methylxanthines in 1989. Ann Intern Med 110:502, 1989. *A good discussion of the pharmacology of methylxanthine.*

58 Chronic Airways Diseases

Richard A. Matthay

CHRONIC BRONCHITIS AND EMPHYSEMA

Chronic generalized airway disorders that are not the direct result of a "specific" bronchopulmonary disease are discussed in this chapter. Common to most of these diseases is chronic airways obstruction, caused most frequently by a diffuse involvement of peripheral (small) airways or, more rarely, by localized obstruction of central (large) airways. The designation *chronic obstructive pulmonary disease* (COPD) is an imperfect, although widely utilized, term, since it includes several specific disorders with different clinical manifestations, pathologic findings, therapy requirements, and prognoses.

Four *diffuse* airway disorders are examined in this chapter: simple chronic bronchitis, asthmatic bronchitis, chronic obstructive bronchitis, and emphysema. Some classifications include all of these entities in the broad term COPD. Moreover, various combinations of these disorders coexist; for instance, patients often have chronic obstructive bronchitis as well as emphysema. Localized airways obstruction, above and below the tracheal bifurcation, is discussed in a separate section of this chapter.

DEFINITIONS OF TERMS. Unfortunately, *chronic bronchitis* has been used variably to refer to a simple smoker's cough or, as in the British literature, to severe COPD. To reduce ambiguity, in this discussion, chronic bronchitis is considered "simple," "obstructive," or "asthmatic," and thus these three terms are applied. It is useful clinically to differentiate between the extremely common simple chronic bronchitis and the less common but often devastating form, chronic obstructive bronchitis. These two entities are therefore described in separate sections.

Simple chronic bronchitis, a syndrome characterized primarily by a chronic productive cough, is the result of low-grade exposure to bronchial irritants in an individual without hyperreactive airways. This syndrome is associated with enhanced mucus secretion, reduced ciliary activity, and impaired resistance to bronchial infection. Simple chronic bronchitis is defined in clinical terms: (1) excessive production of mucus; (2) presence of symptoms, largely cough, on most days for at least 3 months annually during 2 or more successive years; and (3) exclusion of bronchiectasis, tuberculosis, or other causes of these symptoms. The term does not describe the underlying process, which may vary widely. The patient population ranges from those who are asymptomatic except for a morning "cigarette cough" productive of mucus in small amounts (*simple chronic bronchitis*) to patients with a severe, disabling condition manifested by increased resistance to airflow, hypoxia, and often hypercapnia (*chronic obstructive bronchitis*). Chronic obstructive bronchitis, which develops in a relatively small proportion of individuals with simple chronic bronchitis, results in irreversible narrowing of airways. Because the obstruction is in bronchioles and bronchi 2 mm or less in diameter, the term *small airways disease* has been used.

Exposure to bronchial irritants in individuals with hyperreactive, or "twitchy," airways can lead to bronchospasm (i.e., bronchial smooth muscle constriction), frequently accompanied by excessive mucus production and edema of bronchial walls. Recurrent episodes of symptomatic bronchospasm are called *asthma* (discussed in Ch. 57). The present discussion must consider bronchospasm, since a degree of reversible airways obstruction often accompanies other reactions to inhaled noxious agents. In fact, episodic airways obstruction is common in individuals with chronic bronchitis. This combination, called *asthmatic bronchitis*, may closely resemble classic asthma. The term *chronic asthmatic bronchitis* is applied in patients with persistent airways obstruction, a chronic productive cough, and a major problem of episodic bronchospasm.

Emphysema, another lung response to noxious stimuli, is characterized by abnormal, permanent enlargement of air spaces distal to the terminal bronchioles, accompanied by destruction of their walls, and without obvious fibrosis. The alterations in emphysema cause reduction in lung elastic recoil, which permits excessive airway collapse upon expiration and leads to irreversible airflow obstruction.

These definitions are not mutually exclusive; there is considerable crossover between the emphysematous (type A) and bronchial (type B) findings listed in Table 58–1. For example, most individuals with emphysema also have a chronic productive cough. It may be difficult to determine the relative importance of emphysema and chronic obstructive bronchitis, with obliteration of small airways. Accordingly, general terms such as *chronic obstructive pulmonary disease (COPD)* have been used to describe this clinical syndrome.

PATHOPHYSIOLOGY OF AIRWAYS OBSTRUCTION. Airways obstruction denotes slowing of forced expiration. As outlined in Ch. 56, the speed of forced expiration is determined primarily by three factors: intrinsic resistance of the airways, compressibility of the airways, and lung elastic recoil. Reduced maximal expiratory flow (V̇max) results from high airways resistance, reduced lung recoil, and/or excessive airways collapsibility.

In general, a low FEV₁/FVC* ratio is indicative of airflow obstruction; the amount of reduction in FEV₁ itself establishes the severity of the obstruction (Fig. 58–1). Some prefer to use $FEF_{25-75\%}$, the average flow over the middle half of a forced expiration.

Actual V̇max values have been measured, commonly at 50 per cent or 75 per cent of the forced expired volume (V̇max₅₀% or

---

*Fev₁ = forced expiratory volume in 1 second; FVC = forced vital capacity; FEF = forced expiratory flow.

TABLE 58-1. FEATURES OF THE EMPHYSEMATOUS AND BRONCHIAL TYPES OF COPD

	Emphysematous (Type A)	Bronchial (Type B)
Clinical features		
Dyspnea	Insidious onset, slowly progressive	Often noted first only during chest infections
Sputum	Usually scant and mucoid	Often copious and purulent
Weight loss	Often marked	Usually slight or absent
Chronic cor pulmonale with heart failure	Infrequent until terminal stages of the disease	Common
Chest examination	Quiet chest (except slight wheeze at end expiration), marked hyperinflation	Noisy chest, slight hyperinflation
Chest radiograph	Hyperlucent, overinflated lung; often regional attenuation of vessels	Often evidence of old inflammatory disease
Physiologic tests		
Total lung capacity	Increased	Normal or slightly decreased
Residual volume	Markedly increased	Moderately increased
Lung compliance, static	Increased	Near normal
Lung compliance, dynamic	Normal or slightly low	Very low
Lung recoil	Markedly reduced	Variable
Inspiratory airways resistance	Normal	Increased
Diffusing capacity	Markedly reduced	Variable
Arterial P_{O_2}	Slight reduction at rest; usually falls with exertion	Often very low at rest; variable change with exertion
Arterial P_{CO_2}	Usually normal or low	Often chronically elevated
Resting pulmonary artery pressure	Normal or slightly elevated at rest; increases with exertion	Often markedly elevated at rest
Cardiac output	Often low	Usually near normal

$\dot{V}max_{75\%}$, respectively*). $\dot{V}max_{75\%}$ has become popular in epidemiologic studies because it appears to be more sensitive than the FEV_1.

In clinical practice, FEV_1 is used more widely because it is easy to measure, is quite reproducible, has a relatively narrow normal range, and tends to reflect the clinical severity of disease.

A variety of physiologic abnormalities are associated with obstructive airways disorders (also discussed in Ch. 56). Increased venous admixture and hypoxemia develop owing to ventilation-perfusion mismatching. Unless there is an increase in overall ventilation, this mismatching may also lead to increased physiologic dead space and hypercapnia. Carbon dioxide retention is likely when airways obstruction is severe, respiratory muscle fatigue occurs, and the drive to breathe is depressed. Air trapping and an increase in residual volume develop because obstructed airways tend to close prematurely during a maximal exhalation. In emphysema, total lung capacity may be enhanced as well. The pulmonary diffusing capacity measurement is usually reduced in emphysema owing to loss of functioning alveolar-capillary membrane surface area.

Because of the large total cross-sectional diameter of the small airways, marked alterations are required to produce discernible changes in the FEV_1 values. Several potentially more sensitive tests have been proposed to detect mild abnormalities of the small airways: closing volume, helium response of the maximal expiratory flow volume (MEFV) curve, and frequency dependence of compliance. Although these tests are not used routinely, they may prove useful in research studies for detecting subclinical disease.

Burrows B: Airways obstructive diseases: Pathogenetic mechanisms and natural histories of the disorders. An overview of obstructive lung disease. Med Clin North Am 74:547, 1990. *This is the lead article of an 18-chapter symposium on obstructive lung diseases. The entire symposium is recommended reading and an excellent source of original references.*

Fishman AP: The spectrum of chronic obstructive disease of the airways. *In* Fishman AP (ed.): Pulmonary Diseases and Disorders. 2nd ed. New York, McGraw-Hill Book Company, 1988, p 1159. *A concise, clearly written description of the different types of airways obstructive disorders and how they overlap.*

Snider GL, Kleinerman J, Thurlbeck WM, et al.: The definition of emphysema. Am Rev Respir Dis 132:182, 1985. *Succinct statement of the definition, anatomic subtypes, and clinical diagnosis of emphysema.*

Thurlbeck WM: Pathophysiology of chronic obstructive pulmonary disease. Clin

Chest Med 11:389, 1990. *Overview of pathophysiology associated with airways obstruction.*

Simple Chronic Bronchitis and Asthmatic Bronchitis

PREVALENCE AND PATHOGENESIS. "Simple chronic bronchitis" refers to a productive cough for at least 3 months of the year for 2 consecutive years. It affects 10 to 25 per cent of the adult population. Cough with sputum production is more common in men than in women and more common in persons over the age of 40 than in younger individuals. All forms of chronic bronchitis are strongly linked to cigarette smoking. Thus, a large proportion of cigarette smokers, particularly those over age 45, fit the diagnostic criteria for simple chronic bronchitis. Some occupations (e.g., those involving dust, handling grain, and mining) are associated with an abnormally high incidence of chronic bronchitis, even after statistics are corrected for smoking habits. Few individuals with simple chronic bronchitis consult a physician, and then the visit is usually prompted by acute or recurrent respiratory tract infections or wheezing in addition to chronic cough. *Chronic asthmatic bronchitis* tends to develop in elderly individuals; most commonly, they are smokers.

Three direct effects of inhaling bronchial irritants cause chronic bronchitis: (1) stimulation of mucus secretion in the airways, (2) impaired mucus clearance due in part to interference with ciliary activity, and (3) lowered resistance to bronchopulmonary infection because of disturbed alveolar macrophage function. Cough develops owing to accumulation of secretions. As a result of bacterial colonization by organisms usually found in the nasopharynx, normally sterile bronchi now harbor organisms.

Although cigarette smoking is the most important of the identifiable causal factors, not all smokers experience mucus hypersecretion, and no more than 15 to 20 per cent develop airflow obstruction. Little is known about the reasons for the variable susceptibility to hypersecretion and airflow obstruction in smokers or why reversible airways obstruction develops in many patients with chronic bronchitis. Retention of secretions may be a major factor in some instances. Immunologic factors and other mediators of bronchoconstriction may play a role, since some patients have subacute or chronic bronchospasm resembling classic asthma.

PATHOLOGY. Enlargement of mucous glands in the large airways, the most characteristic abnormality, is primarily due to increased numbers of their constituent cells (hyperplasia) rather than to enlargement of cells (hypertrophy). Retained bronchial secretions and variable degrees of inflammatory changes in the bronchial walls are also identified. Narrowing or obliteration of some small airways, increased mucus in these airways, and

---

*Because use of these symbols has caused confusion, it has been suggested that $\dot{V}max_{50\%}$ and $\dot{V}max_{75\%}$ be expressed as $FEF_{50\%}$ and $FEF_{75\%}$, respectively. Moreover, $\dot{V}max_{75\%}$ as defined herein has sometimes been reported as $\dot{V}max_{25\%}$, the 25% referring to the portion of the FVC remaining when the flow measurement is made.

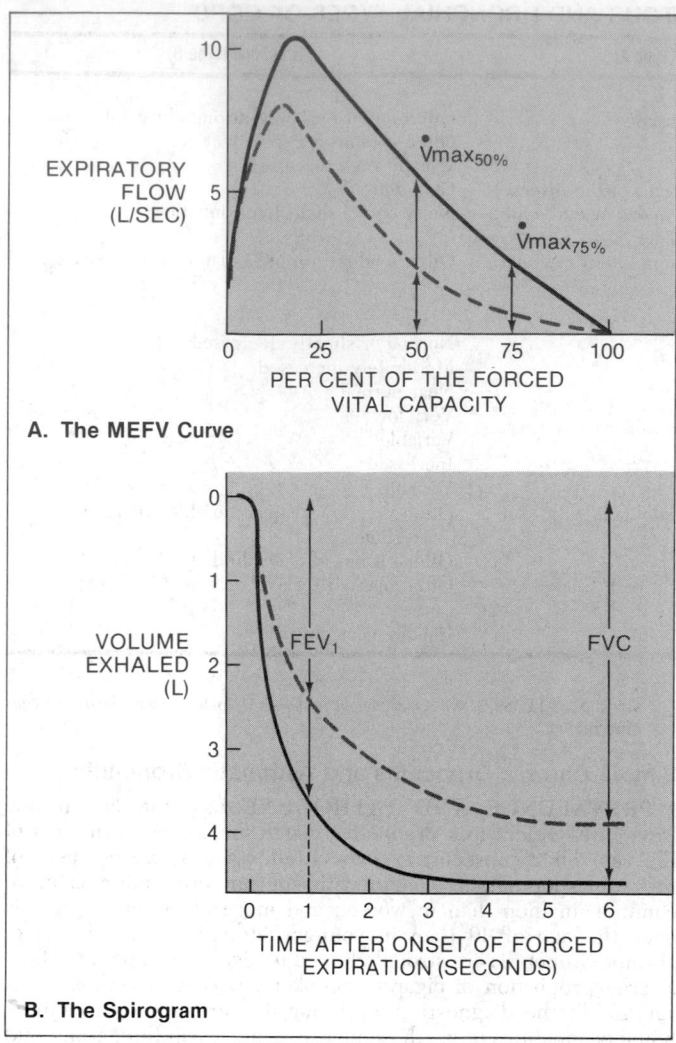

A. The MEFV Curve

B. The Spirogram

FIGURE 58–1. Solid lines are used to show a normal maximal expiratory flow-volume (MEFV) in *A* and a normal spirogram in *B*. Broken lines indicate typical curves for a patient with mild airways obstruction. Measurements of the forced vital capacity (FVC), the forced expiratory volume at 1 second (FEV$_1$), and forced flow rates at 50 per cent and 75 per cent of the FVC ($\dot{V}max_{50\%}$ and $\dot{V}max_{75\%}$) are depicted as vertical lines. (Adapted from Burrows B: Chronic airways disease. *In* Wyngaarden JM, Smith LH Jr (eds.): Cecil Textbook of Medicine. 17th ed. Philadelphia, W. B. Saunders Company, 1988, p 412).

scattered centrilobular emphysema may be found, even though clinically significant obstruction is absent. Since asymptomatic smokers may have similar small airways and emphysematous changes, it is unclear whether these alterations are related to simple chronic bronchitis, except through a common association with cigarette smoking.

CLINICAL MANIFESTATIONS. When the disease is mild, *cough* occurs when the patient arises or usually after he or she smokes the first cigarette of the day. The cough is productive of a small amount of mucoid sputum and occurs most regularly in the winter months. As the severity increases, the patient coughs throughout the day, symptoms are present throughout the year, sputum volume increases, and episodes of severe coughing develop. Near the end of a severe paroxysm of coughing, wheezing may occur, probably owing to cough-induced bronchospasm. Lying down may induce wheezing, which is probably caused by retained secretions, for cough often provides relief.

Symptoms associated with purulent sputum, suggesting overgrowth of bacteria, may reappear after a viral respiratory infection. *Hemophilus influenzae* and *Streptococcus pneumoniae* may be present, but sputum cultures usually show normal nasopharyngeal flora.

Bacterial organisms probably represent secondary pathogens

rather than being the primary cause of these exacerbations of symptoms. During exacerbations, various degrees of bronchospasm may also develop, blurring the distinction between such episodes and asthma. Whereas *blood-streaked sputum* is noted occasionally, severe or repeated hemoptysis may indicate a more serious entity, such as a pulmonary neoplasm.

The sputum may become chronically purulent as the disorder progresses, and the term *mucopurulent bronchitis* may be applied at this stage of the disease. Rarely, drug-resistant organisms (e.g., *Pseudomonas aeruginosa*) are identified on sputum cultures, especially if the patient has received multiple antibiotics.

In mild disease, the physical examination may be normal. As the disease advances, variable coarse crackles, which may clear or change location with coughing, and scattered wheezes are heard. A forced expiratory maneuver often induces a wheeze or a paroxysm of coughing.

If reversible airways obstruction is present, the patient may resemble the typical asthmatic person, with wheezing and slowing of forced expiration as prominent features.

LABORATORY FINDINGS. The chest radiograph, blood counts, and the differential smear are all normal in the uncomplicated case. Leukocytes and a mixed flora of organisms are noted on sputum examination. Although spirometry often shows some slowing of forced expiration, flow rates may be normal in simple bronchitis. Individuals with *chronic asthmatic bronchitis* may have severe airways obstruction even between acute attacks. During episodes of bronchospasm in patients with asthmatic bronchitis, functional abnormalities are more severe, and both blood and sputum eosinophilia may be present.

COURSE AND PROGNOSIS. In patients with simple chronic bronchitis, symptoms may fluctuate widely. Increased cigarette use, inclement weather, and acute respiratory infections all tend to enhance cough and sputum production. Cessation of smoking in mild cases usually leads to disappearance of symptoms. A slight reduction in ventilatory function is common in simple chronic bronchitis, but progressive respiratory insufficiency does not necessarily develop.

The long-term outcome of patients with asthmatic bronchitis has not been studied extensively. Some patients may become asymptomatic for years after an initial excellent response to therapy, while others require progressively more medication to control bronchospasm. Progress to irreversible airways obstruction occurs in at least a few patients despite good medical management.

DIFFERENTIAL DIAGNOSIS. A persistent, productive cough not attributable to an upper respiratory tract disorder, an allergic reaction of the airways, a specific endobronchial disease, or parenchymal lung disease justifies the diagnosis of chronic bronchitis. Exclusion of a parenchymal lesion requires a chest radiograph. Moreover, a careful upper airway examination should be done, and physical findings, such as a persistent, localized wheeze, must be sought to identify a localized airways disorder. Cystic fibrosis must be excluded in children and in young adults who have severe symptoms of chronic bronchitis (see Ch. 64). In addition, in individuals with one of the immotile cilia syndromes, symptoms of chronic bronchitis may be noted (see Ch. 64).

When there is no identifiable source of chronic bronchial irritation, the diagnosis of simple chronic bronchitis should be made with caution. Sputum and blood eosinophilia should be sought in a nonsmoking patient whose symptoms are associated with exposure to allergens or in a patient with episodes of combined wheezing and dyspnea. Asthmatic bronchitis, which may respond to bronchodilators or corticosteroids, is suggested by high eosinophil levels.

Bronchoscopy and even bronchography or a computed tomography (CT) scan of the chest may be indicated to rule out an endobronchial lesion or localized bronchiectasis in patients with severe or repeated hemoptysis or with physical findings suggesting localized disease. In the routine case, these procedures are not indicated.

Severe mucopurulent bronchitis may be difficult to distinguish from bronchiectasis. In fact, in persons with severe bronchitis, the bronchi may show mild, diffuse, cylindrical dilatation. Saccular bronchiectasis is suggested by (1) repeated pneumonias in the same lung zone, (2) honeycombed areas on the chest radiograph, and (3) recurrent hemoptysis. Bronchography provides an accurate diagnosis, but this invasive procedure is usually indicated only if resection of the bronchiectatic area or areas is considered. Otherwise there is little difference between the therapy for mucopurulent bronchitis and that for bronchiectasis. CT of the chest has been used successfully to diagnose localized and diffuse bronchiectasis.

TREATMENT. Cigarette smoking should stop, and any other bronchial irritants should be removed initially, since this step alone may relieve the symptoms. If the symptoms persist after the maximal effort to avoid provoking factors, the following measures are applied.

Antibiotic Therapy. Infection is considered present when the patient is producing a noneosinophilic, purulent sputum. A 7- to 10-day course of tetracycline or ampicillin (1 gram daily in divided doses) or double-strength sulfamethoxazole-trimethoprim (one tablet twice daily) should be administered. Failure of this antibiotic therapy to clear the sputum warrants a sputum culture and sensitivity test. Successive doses of different antibiotics should be avoided, since this may lead to resistant flora. Therapeutic failure generally is due to inadequate drainage of the airways more often than to an improper choice of antibacterial drugs.

The antibiotic may have to be changed on the basis of drug susceptibility studies when resistant organisms are cultured from the sputum. (For severe, purulent exacerbations, penicillin has proved to be inadequate therapy.)

Bronchodilators. The bronchodilator agents are the mainstays for managing bronchospasm associated with simple chronic bronchitis and for control of any reversible component of COPD. They are also useful in conjunction with bronchial hygiene therapy, described below. Both of the main classes of bronchodilators, the methylxanthines and the beta-adrenergic agonists, help to relieve bronchospasm and to prevent recurrent attacks. The inhaled route of administering beta-adrenergic drugs is usually more effective and rapid in relieving bronchospasm than the oral route. Patients must be carefully instructed, however, in the proper technique for utilizing inhalers. Inhaled atropine may exhibit a combined beneficial effect of reducing copious amounts of sputum and partially relieving bronchospasm in the person with severe bronchitis. The principles and details for therapeutic application of these agents are described in Ch. 57.

Corticosteroids. When significant airways obstruction persists or recurs in the patient with asthmatic bronchitis in spite of maximal therapy with bronchodilators, corticosteroids are indicated. If the patient is ambulatory, modest dosages (e.g., 20 to 40 mg of prednisone per day) are administered for several days and then tapered to the lowest dose that will sustain improvement. Often, improvement is rapid, and the drug can be discontinued in 7 to 10 days. Thereafter, a short "burst" of corticosteroids is used to treat occasional relapses. In some patients, tapering corticosteroids leads to recurrence of symptoms. In these individuals, the dose should be maintained as low as possible to relieve bronchospasm and to prevent recurrent attacks. Alternate-day single-dose corticosteroids should be used for maintenance if possible.

Once bronchospasm has been relieved and a maintenance dose of corticosteroid achieved, an inhaled, poorly absorbed preparation such as beclomethasone should be added. This medication is inhaled from a pressurized container, two to four puffs (100 to 200 g) two to four times daily, depending upon the preparation. The inhaled agent may permit reduction in the maintenance dose of corticosteroid without recurrence of bronchospasm. When significant bronchospasm is present, inhaled corticosteroid agents should be avoided, since this medication may aggravate bronchoconstriction and fail to reach the distal airways. For some patients, premedication with an inhaled bronchodilator (e.g., a beta-adrenergic agent) may relieve airway irritation and permit successful use of inhaled corticosteroids. In general, inhaled corticosteroids replace 7.5 to 10 mg per day of oral prednisone.

After the addition of an inhaled agent, the dose of oral prednisone should be reduced slowly (over several months) to avoid adrenal insufficiency in a corticosteroid-dependent patient who has received months or years of systemic medication. In up to 30 per cent of patients, oropharyngeal candidiasis occurs because of inhaled corticosteroids. This condition responds, however, to specific therapy and rarely requires discontinuation of the inhaled preparation. Nasal symptoms, previously controlled by oral prednisone, may recur, requiring reinstitution of oral agents.

Bronchial Hygiene. These measures are designed to clear retained bronchial secretions. Deep breathing followed by deliberate coughing is the most important maneuver. Sputum production may be more effective if the most involved lung regions are in the superior position (postural drainage) and chest percussion and vibration are applied.

Bronchial hygiene measures may be better tolerated and more effective if the patient is premedicated with an inhaled bronchodilator and then inhales a bland mist to loosen secretions. Although some patients are convinced of its efficacy, objective benefits of bland mist therapy have been difficult to establish. Because patients' reactions to this therapy vary, only measures that prove effective should be continued, since the full program is uncomfortable and time consuming.

To avoid inspissation of secretions, patients should be encouraged to keep well hydrated. Intravenous fluids may be required for acute exacerbations. Although the efficacy of expectorant medications has not been established, some authorities recommend 10 to 12 drops of a saturated solution of potassium iodide three times daily. This program is associated with a high rate of side effects, some severe; yet it does seem beneficial in some patients. Cough syrups and lozenges have little effect on the viscosity of bronchial secretions, but they may relieve a "tickle" in the throat of many persons with bronchitis. Cough sedatives should be used only for acute episodes of a severe, nonproductive cough and are otherwise contraindicated.

Treatment of Severe Exacerbations. Severe exacerbations of asthmatic bronchitis can be life threatening, particularly when associated with severe airways obstruction. The approach to status asthmaticus outlined in Ch. 57 is appropriate, although the patient with asthmatic bronchitis may require more attention to bronchial hygiene measures to clear secretions than does the person with asthma.

Anthonisen NR, Manfreda J, Warren CPW, et al.: Antibiotic therapy in exacerbations of chronic obstructive pulmonary disease. Ann Intern Med 106:196, 1987. *Double-blind placebo controlled trial that reports significant benefit from antimicrobial therapy during exacerbations of chronic bronchitis.*
Burrows B: Irreversible airways obstruction and asthma. Pract Cardiol 8:69, 1982. *This article presents in more detail views concerning the overlap of reversible and irreversible airways obstructive diseases.*
Burrows B, Lebowitz MD, Barbee RA, et al.: Interactions of smoking and immunological factors in relationship to airways obstruction. Chest 84:657, 1983. *This paper presents evidence that chronic asthmatic bronchitis may result from an interaction of the irritant effects of smoking and immunologic factors.*
Iafrate RP, Massey KL, Hendeles L: Current concepts in clinical therapeutics: Asthma. Clin Pharm 5:206, 1986. *A quality review of the use of bronchodilators and corticosteroids in reversible airways diseases.*
IPPB Trial Group: Intermittent positive pressure breathing therapy of chronic obstructive pulmonary disease. Ann Intern Med 99:612, 1983. *This study establishes that there is no significant benefit in positive-pressure breathing over other modalities of delivering bronchodilators.*
Sachs FL: Chronic bronchitis. In Pennington JE (ed.): Respiratory Infections: Diagnosis and Management. New York, Raven Press, 1983, p 113. *Comprehensive review of the etiologic role and need for treatment of respiratory infection during exacerbations of chronic bronchitis.*
Stoller JK, Wiedemann HP: Chronic obstructive lung diseases: Asthma, emphysema, chronic bronchitis, bronchiectasis, and related conditions. In George RB, Light RW, Matthay MA, Matthay RA (eds.): Chest Medicine. 2nd ed. Baltimore, Williams and Wilkins, 1990. *Comprehensive discussion of the various obstructive lung diseases and their management.*

Chronic Obstructive Bronchitis and Emphysema

PREVALENCE AND PATHOGENESIS. As a major cause of chronic disability in older individuals, chronic obstructive bronchitis and emphysema (COPD) rank behind only heart disease and schizophrenia in the United States. Trends over the past two decades suggest a 60 per cent increase in the prevalence of COPD. This disease is the fifth leading cause of death in the United States, and there has been a 22 per cent increase in the death rate from this condition over the past 20 years. Approximately 75,000 individuals per year die of COPD in the United States, one-half the number of persons dying annually of lung cancer.

Emphysema is common and increases with age. It is present at autopsy in approximately 65 per cent of adult men and 15 per cent of adult women. The prevalence of emphysema is strongly related to cigarette smoking.

Chronic obstructive pulmonary disease is usually diagnosed in those between the ages of 55 and 65. The greater incidence in men than in women most likely reflects the lower incidence of smoking in women in earlier decades. Recent trends, however, show that more teenage girls than boys are starting to smoke. Thus, in several decades COPD may be as common, or more common, in women.

Smoking. Patients with COPD have some combination of chronic obstructive bronchitis and pulmonary emphysema, both of which are closely associated with cigarette smoking. Longitudinal studies confirm a dose-response relationship between cigarette smoking and the rate of pulmonary function decline in patients with COPD. The chronic, progressive destruction of the alveolar structures characteristic of emphysema is thought to occur because of an imbalance between the proteases (proteolytic enzymes) and antiproteases in the lower respiratory tract. According to this concept, proteases, particularly polymorphonuclear neutrophil (PMN) elastase and possibly elastases in pulmonary alveolar macrophages (PAM's), work unimpeded to destroy alveolar structures and their elastin network. Cigarette smokers have increased numbers of PAM's, and PMN's are recruited into their lungs, so that increased numbers of both cell types are recoverable on bronchoalveolar lavage. Recruitment of PMN's into the lungs may occur as a result of the elaboration of chemotactic factors by PAM's stimulated by cigarette smoke. Moreover, smoke components can cause elastase to be released by PMN's by inducing cytotoxic reactions and by stimulating secretion from viable cells. Macrophages exposed to cigarette smoke in vitro or in vivo increase secretion of an elastase-like enzyme. This potential for a greatly increased protease (primarily elastase) burden must be counteracted by the antiprotease defense system of the lungs.

The protease-antiprotease theory of the pathogenesis of emphysema has received further support from the recognition that patients with severe (homozygous phenotype) alpha$_1$-antitrypsin deficiency have markedly reduced levels of serum alpha$_1$-antitrypsin and progressive panacinar emphysema. As might be expected, when studied by bronchoalveolar lavage, patients with severe alpha$_1$-antitrypsin deficiency have little or no alpha$_1$-antitrypsin in their lower respiratory tracts. Nor do they have alternate antiprotease protection against neutrophil elastase.

Compared with nonsmokers, cigarette smokers without alpha$_1$-antitrypsin deficiency also show reduced elastase inhibitory capacity because of inactivation of alpha$_1$-proteinase inhibitor (alpha$_1$-PI). Chemical oxidation of alpha$_1$-PI by material in cigarette smoke is postulated as a major cause of the observed decrease in elastase inhibitory capacity. Smoking may interfere with elastin repair mechanisms, as documented by studies both in vivo and in vitro.

Severe genetic deficiency of serum alpha$_1$-antitrypsin occurs in 0.5 to 2 per cent of patients with COPD. Typically, in such individuals, emphysema is likely to develop by age 40 in smokers and by age 60 in nonsmokers. Presumably, prolonged exposure to irritants, primarily cigarette smoke, further reduces lung antiprotease defenses and induces low-grade inflammation and destructive changes in the parenchyma of the lungs.

The protease-antiprotease hypothesis of the pathogenesis of emphysema does not readily explain all of the observations in experimental and human emphysema. For instance, experimental enzyme-induced emphysema is panacinar rather than centrilobular, the more common type in humans with chronic airflow obstruction. Further, it does not explain the predominant localization of centrilobular emphysema to the upper lung zones or of panacinar emphysema to the lung bases or of paraseptal emphysema to the regions beneath the pleura and adjacent to fibrous septa. There is a close relationship between slowing of forced exhalation and cigarette smoking. The average heavy smoker has a 40- to 45-ml per year decline in FEV$_1$, whereas the average nonsmoking adult shows a decline of only 20 to 25 ml per year. Nonsmokers with alpha$_1$-antitrypsin deficiency have approximately an 80-ml per year decline in FEV$_1$; cigarette smokers with this deficiency have approximately a 150-ml per year decline. When individuals with alpha$_1$-antitrypsin deficiency stop smoking, this excess rate of decline in FEV$_1$ ceases. Nevertheless, the average effect of cigarette smoking alone does not explain the more severe reduction in FEV$_1$ noted in patients with COPD.

Moreover, why is it that only a minority of smokers develop clinically significant COPD? Some individuals may be particularly susceptible for various reasons: respiratory disorders in childhood, intercurrent respiratory infections, and genetic factors, for example.

Can COPD be detected early by screening lung function in young to middle-aged adults? Longitudinal studies are attempting to identify susceptible cigarette-smoking individuals with an excessive rate of decline in pulmonary function throughout adult life. The hypothesis is that the individual who will develop COPD later in life should be identifiable by age 40 because he or she will show at least a mild ventilatory abnormality by then. There is no direct evidence yet, however, that any physiologic test applied early in life detects the individual who will develop disabling COPD.

Alpha$_1$-Antitrypsin Deficiency. A deficiency in serum antiproteolytic activity associated with a susceptibility to COPD has been noted in several families. The protease inhibitor, or "Pi," phenotype of the subject determines the serum's trypsin inhibitory capacity. Two M genes (Pi MM phenotype) are present in normal individuals. When only Z genes are present (Pi ZZ phenotype), serum alpha$_1$-antitrypsin levels are severely reduced (<50 mg per deciliter), and the alpha$_1$-antitrypsin that is present in plasma is less effective in inhibiting neutrophil elastase than the alpha$_1$-antitrypsin in individuals with the Pi MM phenotype. Deficiency of alpha$_1$-antitrypsin is transmitted as an autosomal recessive trait. This antiproteolytic deficiency, present in approximately 1 in 4000 of the population, is associated with hepatitis in infancy and the development of emphysema in the third, fourth, and fifth decades. Present in 3 to 5 per cent of the population, the heterozygotic state (Pi MZ phenotype) is associated with a moderately reduced serum antiproteolytic activity, but no predilection for developing an excess of respiratory disorders. Several other Pi genes have been identified (of which S is the most common), but only the Z gene clearly leads to COPD. In Ch. 121 the hepatic manifestations of alpha$_1$-antitrypsin deficiency are discussed.

PATHOLOGY. Alveolar wall destruction with a nonuniform pattern of air space enlargement is the basic abnormality in emphysema. The orderly appearance of the acinus and its components is disturbed and may be lost, as air spaces are fewer in number but enlarged. In centrilobular emphysema, the process is most severe in the central portion of the lobule, whereas in panacinar emphysema, the defect occurs uniformly throughout the acinus. Both centrilobular and panacinar emphysema may be noted in the same lung. In severe centrilobular emphysema, the entire acinus may ultimately become involved. Centrilobular emphysema generally is the most common form of emphysema in patients with chronic airflow obstruction.

In large airways, inflammation is noted in and around air passages, with narrowing of the lumina, impaction of mucus, and obliterative changes. Abnormalities of the small airways are usually not obvious on cursory examination and require careful morphometric studies.

CLINICAL MANIFESTATIONS. Dyspnea is usually the predominant complaint, but some patients consult a physician initially because of cough, wheezing, recurrent respiratory infections, or, occasionally, weakness or weight loss. Patients may date the onset of chronic symptoms to an acute respiratory infection. In some, shortness of breath is present only during acute exacerbations.

A productive cough is usually present, associated with a thick or "sticky" sputum varying widely in quantity. Copious amounts of purulent sputum, coupled with a severe cough, are noted by some patients.

The physical examination may yield normal findings relatively early in the illness (FEV$_1$ > 1.0 liter). Auscultation of the chest may reveal rhonchi, or the chest may be quiet, particularly in patients with extensive emphysema. Wheezing, which may be absent on quiet breathing, can often be heard on forced exhalation. As the disease progresses, marked hyperinflation with low diaphragm and a reduced area of cardiac dullness are common. Labored breathing, at times through pursed lips, may be noted after minimal exertion or even at rest. Patients tend to lean forward on their elbows when sitting, assuming a stooped posture, while using accessory muscles of respiration. Cyanosis and dependent edema may be noted.

Occasionally, patients first seek medical attention when signs of right ventricular failure due to cor pulmonale appear. In such cases, the FEV_1 is likely to be below 1 liter and the arterial Po_2 below 45 mm Hg. The pulmonary hypertension in these patients with COPD and cor pulmonale is most closely related to the severity of hypoxemia.

Table 58–1 shows features of relatively distinctive COPD clinical syndromes and their associated underlying pathologic conditions. These two clinical types of COPD, emphysematous (type A) and bronchial (type B), represent extremes of presentation; most individuals, if followed chronically, develop a mixture of findings from the type A and type B groups. Type A patients, described as "pink puffers," often hyperventilate, maintaining normal or nearly normal arterial O_2 and CO_2 tensions. In contrast, type B patients, "blue bloaters," often have a low arterial O_2 tension, high CO_2 tension, cyanosis, and right-sided congestive heart failure. The "blue bloater" syndrome may also result from disordered breathing during sleep, a common problem in patients with COPD.

LABORATORY FINDINGS. The routine blood count and differential study are normal except for erythrocytosis in some COPD patients with hypoxemia. When eosinophilia is found, a reversible (asthmatic-bronchitic) component of the disease should be suspected.

Early in the disease, the chest radiograph may be normal; however, in severe emphysema, lung hyperinflation and an increased retrosternal air space, with flattening of the diaphragm and regional attenuation of blood vessels, are usually noted. Frank bullae outlined by hairline margins are present in some cases. The chest radiograph should not be the sole basis for the diagnosis of COPD, for individuals with perfectly normal lung function may have radiographic findings typical of the disease. Chest CT has frequently been used to determine with accuracy the presence of emphysema and to quantify its severity.

Persistent reduction in FEF rates is the most typical finding in COPD. Two lung volume measurements, the residual volume and the ratio of residual volume to total lung capacity, are elevated. Ventilation-perfusion mismatch and nonuniformity of ventilation are also typical findings, whereas arterial hypoxemia and physiologic shunting vary among patients. When the diffusing capacity is very depressed and the total lung capacity is clearly increased, emphysema is likely to be extensive.

Ventilation-perfusion lung scans should be interpreted cautiously when pulmonary emboli are suspected. These scans reveal the uneven ventilation and perfusion typical of COPD. Areas of diminished perfusion may be mistaken for pulmonary emboli. Accordingly, when pulmonary embolism is suspected in a patient with COPD, a pulmonary angiogram is often required for definitive diagnosis.

The electrocardiogram tends to be normal, particularly early in the course of the disease. Later, the axis is shifted to the right, and there are early R waves in the precordial leads V_1 and V_2 and net negative electrical forces in leads V_5 and V_6. Especially during exacerbations, peaked P waves ("P pulmonale") are present. Unfortunately, these changes do not correlate well with pulmonary artery hypertension and cor pulmonale. The presence of R waves over the right precordium is the most reliable indication of cor pulmonale.

COURSE AND PROGNOSIS. Initially, the response to bronchodilator therapy is variable, dependent upon the degree of bronchospasm. Thereafter, the disease progresses slowly, with an annual average decrement in FEV_1 of 50 to 75 ml. Because the variability in FEV_1 may be greater than the true annual decline, a follow-up of several years is required to determine the rate of loss of lung function. If the patient stops smoking, cough and sputum production may cease. However, most other symptoms progress gradually.

In terms of absolute FEV_1, patients are dyspneic upon moderate exertion when the value is 1.2 to 1.5 liters; they are forced to be relatively sedentary at 1.0 liter; and they are often invalids when the FEV_1 is 500 ml or less. As the FEV_1 drops below 1 liter, severe arterial hypoxemia, hypercapnia, and cor pulmonale are often evident.

Median survival varies considerably. Despite initially very low FEV_1 values, some individuals live 12 to 15 years. Generally, however, when the FEV_1 is more than 1.2 liters, patients survive about 10 years; when the FEV_1 is 1.0 liter, survival is approxi-

mately 5 years; and when the FEV_1 is less than 700 ml, survival is about 2 years. Signs of a poor prognosis include a resting tachycardia, severe arterial hypoxemia or hypercapnia or both, and evidence of cor pulmonale. If a patient resides at altitudes higher than 3500 feet, longevity is reduced.

Increased cough and dyspnea are hallmarks of periodic worsening of the disease. Symptoms characteristically occur after an acute respiratory infection and may be accompanied by bronchospasm. Such exacerbations in patients with severe COPD may be life threatening and may lead to acute respiratory failure as well as right ventricular failure. The latter occurs secondary to pronounced increases in pulmonary artery pressure and pulmonary vascular resistance, which, in turn, are due primarily to hypoxic pulmonary vasoconstriction.

DIFFERENTIAL DIAGNOSIS. Three criteria are required to diagnose COPD: (1) The FEV_1 must be reduced, and this reduction must be proportionately more than any lowering in the FVC (i.e., both the predicted percentage of FEV_1 and the $FEV_1/$FVC ratio must be depressed); (2) in spite of intensive, prolonged medical treatment, this slowing of forced expiration must persist; and (3) other bronchopulmonary disease that might explain the observed physiologic abnormalities must be excluded. Sufficient evidence for the last criterion generally includes absence of extensive parenchymal abnormalities on the chest radiograph and absence of any signs of upper airways obstruction, such as neck mass, stridor, or narrowing of the upper airway seen on the chest radiograph. Irreversibility of the obstructive ventilatory defect may be more difficult to establish. This factor is discussed further in the treatment section.

Assessing the relative contribution of emphysema and intrinsic airway changes can also be difficult. Emphysema is usually severe when the diffusing capacity is very depressed and the chest radiograph shows hyperlucent lungs with attenuation of the vascular markings. In contrast, if the diffusing capacity is normal or nearly normal, extensive emphysema is unlikely. Esophageal balloon measurements, which are required to assess lung elastic recoil (the best guide to the severity of emphysema), are seldom justified as part of the clinical evaluation.

If there is a family history of emphysema or emphysema-type COPD develops at an early age, a homozygous alpha$_1$-antitrypsin deficiency should be considered. Suspicion is heightened when the patient is a nonsmoker or a woman or when the chest radiograph shows a bibasilar distribution of emphysematous changes. Laboratory confirmation is provided by almost complete absence of alpha$_1$ globulin, by a markedly reduced serum trypsin inhibitory capacity, and, most specifically, by demonstration of a pattern of a pure Z phenotype on crossed immunoelectrophoresis of the serum.

TREATMENT. The following are therapeutic goals in patients with COPD: (1) to relieve the portion of airway obstruction that is reversible; (2) to control cough and sputum production; (3) to eliminate and prevent airway infections; (4) to increase exercise tolerance to the maximum allowable at the individual's level of physiologic deficit; (5) to control remedial disease complications, such as arterial hypoxemia and cardiovascular problems; (6) to avoid smoking and other airway irritants, narcotics and sedatives, and noncritical surgery, all of which aggravate the disease; and (7) to relieve the anxiety and depression that are often present in the patient with COPD.

In spite of treatment, most patients with severe COPD show progressive ventilatory deterioration; yet therapy should not be withheld. A comprehensive therapeutic program can reduce symptoms, decrease the frequency of hospital admissions, prevent premature death, and permit patients to lead a more active and satisfying life.

A formal rehabilitation program using a team approach is effective. Nevertheless, good results can also be obtained by a dedicated individual physician, assisted, perhaps, by an office nurse who can help patients with physical therapy and bronchial hygiene measures.

Initial Treatment. During the initial visit, it is impossible to predict with certainty the degree of reversibility of airways obstruction in a patient with COPD. Therefore, all patients should be considered as having potentially reversible disease. Bronchodilators should be administered according to tolerance, as outlined in the therapy for asthmatic bronchitis and asthma. Smoking should be discontinued and other bronchial irritants avoided. As mentioned in the therapy for simple chronic bronchitis, bronchial hygiene measures and, when indicated by purulent mucus production, antibiotics should be used. Diuretics should be given when heart failure is present. In addition, the Pneumovax vaccine and yearly administration of the influenza vaccine are indicated.

The effects of this initial therapy both on symptoms and on pulmonary function test results should be determined and adjustments made in medication to minimize side effects. Apparently ineffective measures (e.g., postural drainage that leads to no symptom relief or sputum production) should be discontinued. Next, if further reversibility of the disease is considered possible, a 3- to 4-week trial of corticosteroids can be initiated. If the acute inhalation of bronchodilator produces a 20 per cent improvement in FEV_1 or if there is a similar increase in FEV_1 several days or weeks after intensive bronchodilator therapy, corticosteroids are likely to be beneficial. Several other findings suggest that corticosteroids may help: (1) a noisy chest or wheeze upon auscultation, (2) sputum or blood eosinophilia, (3) evidence of atopy (e.g., history of hay fever, an elevated serum immunoglobulin E [IgE] level, positive results of allergy skin tests), or (4) associated nasal polyps or vasomotor rhinitis.

Generally, 20 to 40 mg of prednisone daily is given for 3 to 4 weeks, and spirometry tests are used to assess the efficacy of this medication. Other bronchodilators are continued at full doses. When improvement is noted, the corticosteroid dose should be tapered to the lowest maintenance dose possible, as outlined for asthmatic bronchitis. If there is no significant improvement in FEV_1 (e.g., >20 per cent), corticosteroids should be tapered slowly and discontinued.

Maintenance Therapy. Frequently, objective improvement (i.e., increase in FEV_1) cannot be demonstrated with bronchodilator therapy. Yet oral theophylline, combined with an inhaled beta-adrenergic agent, is recommended to prevent superimposed bronchospasm. In COPD, theophylline can (1) enhance respiratory muscle function, in both the fatigued and the nonfatigued state; (2) augment right and left ventricular systolic pump function while decreasing pulmonary artery pressures and pulmonary vascular resistance (potentially helpful in patients with cor pulmonale); and (3) in some patients, reduce dyspnea. The beta-adrenergic agents also improve biventricular systolic pump performance and decrease pulmonary vascular resistance. Whether any of these potentially salutary effects are additive or synergistic when oral theophylline is administered in conjunction with beta-adrenergic agents has not been established.

Aerosolized adrenergic agents are also used (1) to relieve acute attacks of dyspnea; (2) prior to exposure to known bronchial irritants, such as cold air; or (3) as a regular part of a bronchial hygiene program.

If a patient with COPD shows improvement in airflow rates (particularly FEV_1) with bronchodilators or adrenocortical hormones, these agents should be maintained, as in asthmatic bronchitis. Those with a productive cough, retained secretions, or repeated episodes of bronchopulmonary infection should be treated with the same measures as described for simple chronic bronchitis. In addition, some other forms of treatment are uniquely applicable to patients with COPD.

Physical Therapy. Exercise has not been shown to improve lung function, but it may enhance cardiovascular fitness and train skeletal muscles to function more efficiently, thus increasing exercise tolerance. Accordingly, unless contraindicated by an underlying cardiac abnormality, progressively increasing exercise (usually walking) should be prescribed. In most cases, the program can be recommended directly by the physician, but if the patient is severely disabled, a trained physical therapist can initiate an appropriate exercise program. Arterial blood gas levels should be obtained when the patient is at rest and after exercise, prior to instituting a vigorous exercise program, particularly if the FEV_1 is less than 1 liter. Supplemental oxygen should be used during exercise if the patient becomes severely hypoxemic.

Although breathing exercises probably do not alter the usual breathing pattern of COPD, occasionally they are recommended to encourage diaphragmatic breathing. Perhaps it is more useful and more realistic to teach patients slow, deep breathing as a quicker, more effective method for relieving dyspnea than rapid, shallow "panic" breathing. Breath holding should be avoided during exertion. Many authorities now recommend inspiratory muscle training by breathing against a graded resistor, but mechanical devices, intermediate positive-pressure breathing (IPPB) machines, and emphysema belts are of unproven value.

Oxygen Therapy. In some individuals with COPD, there are clear indications for home oxygen therapy. One indication is development of severe exertional hypoxemia (PaO_2 < 40 mm Hg) in patients who respond to supplemental oxygen therapy with an increase in exercise tolerance. A second indication is found in patients with severe, persistent arterial hypoxemia at rest (PaO_2 < 55 mm Hg), accompanied by secondary signs of hypoxemia, after all other therapeutic measures have been exhausted and the patient has completely recovered from exacerbation of the disease. Both continuous oxygen therapy and that spanning 12 to 15 hours per day prolong survival, but continuous therapy (i.e., 10 to 24 hours per day) is associated with longer survival. To raise the PaO_2 to the necessary 60 to 80 mm Hg usually requires 1 to 3 liters of oxygen per minute via nasal prongs.

Since patients may become habituated to this therapy and thus increase their invalidism, oxygen should not be prescribed solely for episodes of dyspnea.

Environmental Control. All patients with severe COPD should be cautioned to avoid high altitudes, and supplemental oxygen may be required for those with severe hypoxemia when they travel by air. Moreover, COPD patients with severe hypoxemia should reside at altitudes below 4000 feet. A change in residence may be indicated in patients who live in areas with heavy air pollution.

Cold winter climates are avoided by some patients who find relief in either warm desert climates or warm, humid regions. No specific climate has been shown to alter the overall course of the disease. Accordingly, the economic and social hardships of a move should be weighed carefully against the potential symptomatic benefit provided by relocation to a more agreeable climate. Before moving, the patient should spend a trial period in the new climate to assess symptomatic benefit.

Treatment of Edema and Cor Pulmonale. Even in the absence of frank right-sided congestive heart failure, pedal edema is common, and control is usually obtained with small doses of diuretics. Ankle edema associated with cor pulmonale is more difficult to control, but oxygen combined with diuretics often suffices. Digitalis is useful for enhancing right ventricular function only if there is concomitant left ventricular failure; accordingly, digitalis should be reserved for combined right and left ventricular failure. Phlebotomy is not required in most oxygen-treated patients but may transiently relieve central nervous system symptoms, especially when the hematocrit is above 60 per cent.

Treatment of Hypercapnia. Chronic hypercapnia is common in late stages of COPD, but it requires no therapy. However, during exacerbations, blood gases must be monitored closely for severe respiratory acidosis, and all narcotics, sedatives, and tranquilizers should be avoided. In patients with stable chronic hypercapnia, mechanically assisted ventilation and respiratory stimulants are unnecessary.

Surgical Therapy. In the absence of significant emphysema (e.g., that manifested by a moderate to severe reduction in diffusing capacity), bullectomy may benefit patients with large bullae compressing normal or nearly normal lung. Careful, detailed preoperative evaluation is required to select suitable candidates for operation.

Supportive Measures. Careful, detailed education of the patient regarding the nature of the disease is essential. The significance of symptoms such as purulent sputum production, potential side effects of medication, and therapeutic goals should be explained. A prompt, prearranged treatment plan for intercurrent exacerbations should be discussed with the patient.

Above all, within the limits of respiratory impairment and within the constraints of therapy, these patients should be encouraged to have an active lifestyle with daily exercise. Some patients benefit from vocational rehabilitation and occupational therapy.

Replacement Therapy in Severe Alpha$_1$-Antitrypsin Deficiency Emphysema. Chronic, weekly replacement or monthly therapy with intravenous alpha$_1$-antitrypsin concentrate of normal plasma has been undertaken at the National Heart, Lung and Blood Institute in individuals with severe alpha$_1$-antitrypsin deficiency. Serum alpha$_1$-antitrypsin was elevated to levels that are probably required for effective antielastase protection of the lungs (average posttherapy level achieved, 130 mg per deciliter; average pretherapy level, 31 mg per deciliter). Alpha$_1$-antitrypsin levels after bronchoalveolar lavage increased in these individuals to about 60 per cent of normal, associated with an equivalent restoration of functional antineutrophil elastase activity. Moreover, the incidence of adverse reactions was limited to a transient postinfusion fever in fewer than 1 per cent of the patients.

Recently, recombinant DNA methodology has been used to produce alpha$_1$-antitrypsin molecules. The future may bring widespread clinical application of this potentially less expensive material administered by intravenous infusion or by inhalation to patients with the PiZZ phenotype. When only mild airways disease is present, this therapy will re-establish the lung antineutrophil elastase defenses and protect the alveolar walls from elastolytic attack.

Treatment of Exacerbations. Antibiotics, increased bronchodilator medications, and even corticosteroids are often indicated for acute exacerbations. Immediate hospitalization is required for severe hypoxemia, increasing carbon dioxide tension, or congestive heart failure. Ch. 40 and 70 outline the management of decompensated cor pulmonale and acute respiratory failure, respectively. The same management utilized in patients with status asthmaticus is indicated in COPD patients with superimposed refractory bronchospasm.

Anthonisen NR: Hypoxemia and O$_2$ therapy. Am Rev Respir Dis 126:729, 1982. *A succinct review of the British and American studies establishing that oxygen therapy prolongs life in patients with hypoxemic COPD.*

De Marco FJ Jr, Wynne JW, Block AJ, et al.: Oxygen desaturation during sleep as a determinant of the "blue and bloated" syndrome. Chest 79:621, 1981. *One of several papers by this group of investigators proposing that sleep-related breathing disorders are important in COPD patients.*

Gadek JE (ed.): Alpha–1-antitrypsin deficiency. Am J Med 84 (suppl 6A):1, 1988. *Extensive monograph detailing the pathogenesis and potential treatment modalities for lung disease associated with alpha$_1$-antitrypsin deficiency.*

Higgins MW, Keller JB: Estimating your patients' risk of COPD. J Respir Dis 4:97, 1983. *This paper discusses the use of routine spirometric testing to detect subjects who are at high risk of developing clinically significant airways obstructive disease.*

Hubbard RC, Brantly ML, Sellers S, et al.: Anti-neutrophil-elastase defenses of the lower respiratory tract in alpha$_1$-antitrypsin deficiency directly augmented with an aerosol of alpha$_1$-antitrypsin. Ann Intern Med 111:206, 1989. *Establishes that inhaled alpha$_1$-antitrypsin restores epithelial lining fluid levels of alpha$_1$-antitrypsin and antineutrophil-elastase activity in patients with severe alpha$_1$-antitrypsin deficiency.*

Janoff A: Elastases and emphysema. Current assessment of the protease-antiprotease hypothesis. Am Rev Respir Dis 132:417, 1985. *Reviews 10 years of progress in elucidating the pathogenesis of emphysema.*

Petty TL (ed.): Chronic obstructive pulmonary disease. 2nd ed. New York, Marcel Dekker, 1985. *Comprehensive text on all aspects of COPD.*

Snider GL: Pulmonary disease in alpha$_1$-antitrypsin deficiency. Ann Intern Med 111:957, 1989. *Succinct, up-to-date statement on the pathogenesis and therapy of lung disease in patients with alpha$_1$-antitrypsin deficiency.*

LOCALIZED AIRWAYS OBSTRUCTION

Extrinsic compression of airways, intraluminal obstruction, and diseases of the airways themselves all can cause localized airways obstruction. Signs and symptoms depend upon the location of the obstruction and upon whether it is partial or complete, variable or fixed. The discussion of localized lesions is divided into obstructions above and below the bifurcation of the trachea.

Obstruction Above the Tracheal Bifurcation

PARTIAL OBSTRUCTION. Stridor, frequently accompanied by inspiratory retraction of the intercostal spaces, is the principal finding in partial obstruction above the main (tracheal) carina. On both forced inspiration and forced expiration, airflow rates are reduced, and there may be a characteristic appearance to the MEFV curve. As shown in Figure 58–2, the site and nature of the obstruction determine the findings on spirometry. When the obstruction is severe, hypoxemia and hypercapnia may result owing to reduced overall ventilation.

Among the intrinsic airways diseases that can cause partial airways obstruction are (1) tonsil and adenoid enlargement, especially in young children; (2) stenosing lesions secondary to trauma; (3) neoplams or granulomatous processes (e.g., sarcoidosis, fungi) involving the hypopharynx, larynx, vocal cords, or

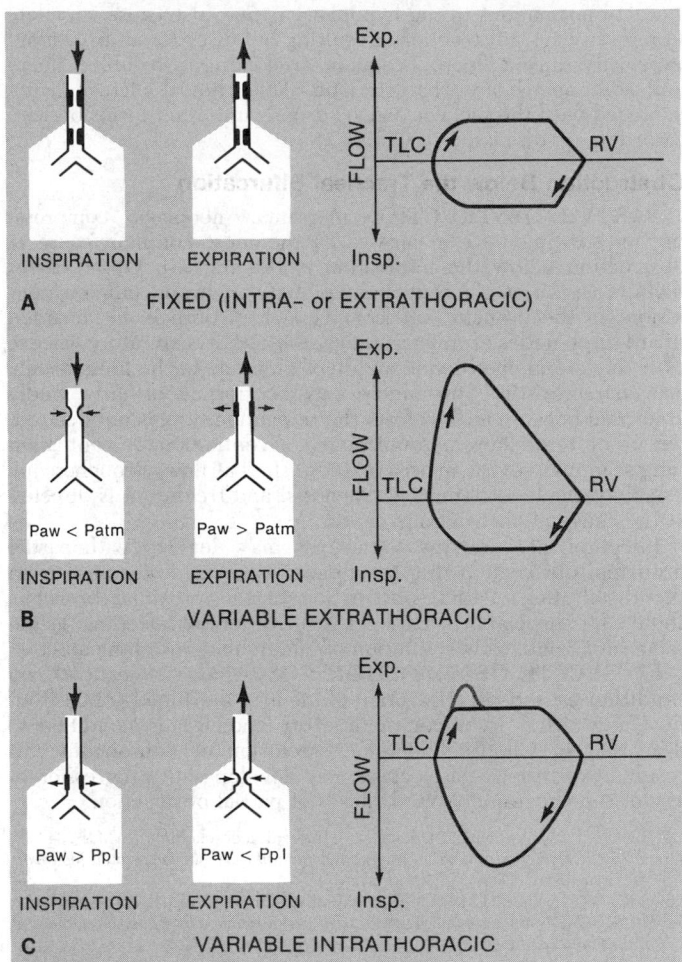

FIGURE 58–2. Airways obstruction above the carina may produce characteristic flow-volume abnormalities, depending on the type and site of obstruction. *A,* If the obstruction is fixed, both inspiratory and expiratory flows will be decreased whether the obstruction is intrathoracic or extrathoracic (for purposes of illustration, obstruction is shown in both locations). Note that this pattern is usually seen when the obstruction is at the level of the thoracic inlet. *B,* When a variable obstruction is extrathoracic in location, the airway narrows during inspiration when airway pressure (P$_{aw}$) is less than atmospheric pressure (P$_{atm}$) and inspiratory flow is diminished. Expiratory flows are often limited, but to a lesser extent. *C,* When a variable obstruction is intrathoracic in location, airway pressure is less than pleural pressure (Ppl) during expiration, and expiratory flow is diminished. Inspiratory flows are often limited, but to a much lesser extent. (Reproduced with permission from Burrows B, et al: Respiratory Disorders—A Pathophysiologic Approach. 2nd ed. Copyright © 1983 by Year Book Medical Publishers, Inc., Chicago.)

trachea; (4) bilateral paralysis of the vocal cords; (5) spasm or edema of the larynx; or (6) inflammation in several locations—the pharynx (e.g., peritonsillar abscess), the larynx (e.g., croup), or the trachea (e.g., diphtheria). An enlarged thyroid, a paratracheal neoplasm, or a mediastinal infection can cause extrinsic compression of the airways. An artificial airway, tracheostomy, or surgical repair is indicated when the primary cause of the obstruction cannot be eliminated.

COMPLETE OBSTRUCTION. Rapid asphyxiation results unless complete obstruction above the main carina is relieved promptly. There is a pathognomonic presentation, with absent airflow at the mouth in spite of both inspiratory efforts and inspiratory retraction of the intercostal muscles. Aspiration of poorly chewed food (so-called "café coronary") is the most common cause of acute obstruction. If a sharp blow to the back fails to dislodge the obstructing material, forced pressure is applied to the epigastrium—the *Heimlich maneuver.*

When the glossopharyngeal structures fall back in some obese individuals, complete obstruction of the upper airway occurs.

Local abnormalities in the hypopharynx may also cause complete upper airways obstruction, resulting in disordered breathing, especially during sleep. Frequent awakening, a troubled sleep, and somnolence are characteristic. This clinical picture, often confused with the pickwickian syndrome and other forms of sleep disorders, is discussed in Ch. 203.

Obstruction Below the Tracheal Bifurcation

PARTIAL OBSTRUCTION. A primary neoplasm, compressing or growing into an airway, is the most common cause of obstruction below the bifurcation of the trachea. Other causes include aspiration of foreign bodies, acute or chronic inflammatory lesions of the bronchi, and compression of bronchi by enlarged hilar lymph nodes or mucous plugs. A localized expiratory wheeze over the site of obstruction and hyperinflation of the lung distally are characteristic. Spirometry may be normal or only mildly abnormal because airflow from the remaining lung is unimpaired; yet other tests show nonuniformity of ventilation. A ventilation lung scan may reveal an area of diminished airflow. Bronchoscopy usually provides a definitive diagnosis, and treatment is directed at the cause of obstruction.

Infection and perhaps an abscess may develop with partial bronchial obstruction due to impaired secretion clearance from the distal lung. Partial obstruction of the proximal bronchus should be suspected in patients with recurrent infections in the same lung zone, slow resolution of pneumonia, or a lung abscess.

COMPLETE OBSTRUCTION. "Obstructive atelectasis" is a condition caused by absorption of air into the bloodstream from the lung distal to a complete obstruction. This condition is discussed in Ch. 59. Complete occlusion of a bronchus and resultant obstructive atelectasis may develop with progression of any of the above-mentioned causes of partial obstruction.

Heimlich HJ: A life-saving maneuver to prevent food-choking. JAMA 234:398, 1975. *The original report on a standard method to remove aspirated food from the airways.*

Loughlin GM, Taussig LM: Upper airway obstruction. Semin Respir Med 1:131, 1979. *This is an excellent review of upper airways obstructive disorders in infants and children.*

Miller RD: Obstructing lesions of the larynx and trachea: Clinical and pathophysiologic aspects. *In* Fishman AP (ed.): Pulmonary Diseases and Disorders. 2nd ed. New York, McGraw-Hill Book Company, 1988, p 1173. *An excellent review of the causes, consequences, and treatment of tracheolaryngeal obstruction.*

59 Abnormalities of Lung Aeration

Richard A. Matthay

LOCALIZED HYPOAERATION (ATELECTASIS)

Atelectasis, or reduced aeration of the lung, is present in many bronchopulmonary disorders and assumes a variety of forms. A total loss of ventilation to a lung region (i.e., with total airway collapse) leads to a shunt wherein blood traversing this region fails to participate in gas exchange and behaves as if it were moving directly from the right to the left side of the heart. Accordingly, total atelectasis causes an "absolute" shunt. In contrast to the shuntlike effect of increased venous admixture present in most bronchopulmonary diseases, the absolute shunt is not fully corrected by inhalation of 100 per cent oxygen.

TYPES OF ATELECTASIS AND THEIR PATHOGENESIS. *Obstructive atelectasis* is a condition of alveolar collapse that develops within a few hours after obstruction of an airway distal to the tracheal bifurcation. The collapse occurs because gas in the lung behind the obstruction is slowly absorbed into the bloodstream. If the lung is filled with oxygen-rich gas rather than ambient air, the alveoli collapse more rapidly. Nitrogen in ambient air is poorly soluble, whereas oxygen is rapidly absorbed into the bloodstream. As a result, high inspired oxygen tensions encourage the development of atelectasis behind obstructing mucous plugs.

Contraction atelectasis occurs when fibrotic changes in a local area of the lung increase its recoil. Contraction, or shrinkage, of the involved lung, rather than complete airlessness, results.

Patchy atelectasis develops throughout the lung owing to alveolar instability in adult and infant (newborn) respiratory distress syndromes.

A large pneumothorax, pleural effusion, or other space-occupying lesion in the thorax can increase intrapleural pressure, causing a portion of the lung to decrease in volume. This *compression atelectasis* is more appropriately called *relaxation atelectasis* because the atelectasis results from the tendency of the lung to recoil when the distending forces are relaxed. As small airways close in the affected region because of marked relaxation atelectasis, any air remaining distally is absorbed into the bloodstream.

Although its pathologic significance is unclear, *platelike atelectasis* may be visible on the chest radiograph. This condition is characterized by horizontal radiopaque streaks, usually in the lung bases. Commonly associated with poor lung aeration, these streaks are seen when the patient has been unable to breathe deeply for a sustained period or when the diaphragm is elevated, such as after intra-abdominal surgery.

CLINICAL MANIFESTATIONS. The chronicity and extent of the process determine the physiologic and clinical consequences of atelectasis. When the obstruction evolves slowly, typical of bronchial neoplasms, usually few or no symptoms develop and hypoxemia is minimal. In contrast, profound dyspnea and severe hypoxemia often develop after the acute collapse of a large section of the lung. As blood flow through the nonventilated lung diminishes over several hours, symptoms and hypoxemia lessen. The acute situation typically involves obstructive atelectasis due to aspiration of a foreign body or to retention of secretions (which may develop in the postoperative period).

The type of atelectasis determines the physical findings. In obstructive or contraction atelectasis, the physical findings depend upon the amount of lung involved. In major atelectasis, the trachea and mediastinum shift to the affected side, the diaphragm is elevated, and the involved hemithorax is smaller and shows less respiratory motion than does the unaffected side. Patchy atelectasis is associated with findings like those of the respiratory distress syndrome reviewed in Ch. 70. The underlying condition (e.g., pleural effusion, pneumothorax, space-occupying lesion) determines the findings in relaxation atelectasis. Platelike atelectasis is primarily diagnosed on the basis of a chest radiograph and presents no distinctive abnormalities on physical examination.

DIAGNOSIS, TREATMENT, AND OUTCOME. The chest radiograph confirms the presence of atelectasis. When obstructive atelectasis is suspected, bronchoscopy is required to establish the cause; it may be possible to remove the occluding material through the bronchoscope. However, a bronchogenic neoplasm should always be considered when obstructive atelectasis is present and the patient is not severely ill.

Treatment is directed at the underlying disorder in nonobstructive forms of atelectasis.

When relaxation atelectasis is relieved (e.g., by insertion of a chest tube for a large pneumothorax), the lung usually returns to normal. However, obstructive atelectasis often is accompanied by secondary complications, such as infection, which lead to abscess formation, localized bronchiectasis, and fibrosis. Moreover, after prolonged collapse, the affected lung may fail to reexpand after the obstruction is removed. The *middle lobe syndrome* exhibits a typical sequence of events. In this syndrome, the middle lobe bronchus in the right lung has usually been compressed by large hilar lymph nodes in tuberculosis or other granulomatous lung diseases. Even after the lymph nodes finally decrease in size, the affected lung fails to expand fully, there are often bronchiectatic changes, and the lobe may be a site of recurrent or chronic infection. Although less common, the same sequence of events may occur in other lung regions. The involved lung may have to be resected if recurrent pneumonia, chronic suppuration, or repeated episodes of hemoptysis develop.

LOCALIZED HYPERAERATION

BLEBS AND BULLAE. Blebs are small collections of gas that are entirely enclosed within the visceral pleura. The gas resides between the multiple leaves of the visceral pleura rather than within the lung itself. Blebs are the uncommon result of dissection of air from the lung interstitium into the lung septa and thence into and between the layers of visceral pleura. Blebs are not clinically important except on the rare occasions that they rupture and cause a spontaneous pneumothorax. Sometimes blebs are visible on the plain chest radiograph, particularly in the lung apex; they are more easily seen when there is a pneumothorax and partial collapse of normal surrounding lung.

Bullae are larger air spaces in the parenchyma of the lung (> than 1 cm in diameter) that are associated with destruction. A bulla denotes severe, localized emphysema causing the formation of a large air space. Bullae may occur with several different types of emphysema and are common in patients with chronic obstructive bronchitis and emphysema. Individuals without any generalized obstructive airways disorder and without diffuse emphysema may also develop bullae.

Bullae are commonly located in the apices of the lungs and are often multiple. A lack of an endothelial lining distinguishes bullae from cysts. Moreover, on the chest radiograph, bullae have "hairline" (thin) margins and, unlike cysts, are usually irregularly shaped, are frequently trabeculated, and rarely contain fluid.

When they become large enough to compromise the function of the remaining normal lung and cause shortness of breath, bullae are clinically important. However, like blebs, when small, they are of little significance, unless they rupture and lead to a pneumothorax.

A difficult clinical problem may be to ascertain whether dyspnea is secondary to diffuse emphysema of the lungs or to bullae (observed on the chest radiograph). Surgery may be indicated in the latter case, but it is contraindicated in the former. Ventilation-perfusion radionuclide lung scans, computed tomography (CT) scans, and pulmonary angiograms may be necessary to make this distinction and to evaluate the state of the remaining lung. As a rule, unless associated generalized obstructive airways disease is present, bullae that occupy less than half a hemithorax do not cause severe dyspnea and significant functional impairment. Moreover, when diffuse disease is present, severe slowing of expiratory airflow is unusual, even with very large bullae. An ideal surgical candidate has moderate to severe dyspnea, bullae that fill most of a hemithorax, only mild slowing of flow rates on forced expiration, good perfusion of normal remaining lung on lung scan and pulmonary angiogram, and no evidence of significant emphysema (e.g., the diffusing capacity measurement is normal or only moderately reduced, and lung compliance studies are normal).

The diagnosis is usually made on the basis of the chest radiograph; however, on physical examination, a tympanitic percussion sound and reduced breath sounds may be noted over very large bullae. The radiolucency of a very large bulla on the chest film may be mistaken for a pneumothorax.

BRONCHOGENIC CYSTS. Bronchogenic cysts may occur in the mediastinum or within the lung parenchyma. These congenital malformations can be differentiated from bullae by their epithelial lining. On the chest radiograph, mediastinal cysts are seen as masses in the hilar, the paraesophageal or paratracheal, and, most commonly, the subcarinal region. In the parenchyma, these cysts are most often found in the lower lobes and are usually filled with a proteinaceous material, unless they become infected and communicate with the bronchial tree. They may have thin, even paper-thin, walls. During early development, acquired lung cysts often have relatively thick walls; later even those resulting from lung abscesses may have very thin walls that simulate those of bullae.

Large cysts may cause respiratory symptoms in young children, but adults with these large lesions are usually asymptomatic, and the abnormality tends to be an incidental finding on the chest radiograph. In the differential diagnosis, mediastinal cysts must be distinguished from other mediastinal masses. Lung cysts must be differentiated from acute lung abscesses, cavitated carcinomas, and cystic bronchiectasis. Frequently, thoracotomy and resection of the lesion are required to obtain a specific diagnosis, although chest CT combined with needle aspiration has been useful for diagnosis and drainage.

Only when they have a bronchial connection (communication) do bronchogenic cysts manifest as abnormalities in lung aeration. Although often partially filled with fluid, they may appear as air spaces when there is a bronchial communication. Infection in

fluid-filled cysts is unusual, but if it occurs and does not resolve after a course of antibiotics, the cysts may have to be removed surgically. Cysts containing air can often be distinguished from bullae by their regular outline, lack of trabeculation, and the presence of a fluid level. Distinguishing bronchogenic cysts in the lung from thin-walled cavities secondary to granulomatous infections, prior abscesses, previous pulmonary infarcts, and squamous cell carcinomas may be more difficult.

BRONCHOPULMONARY SEQUESTRATION. In *bronchopulmonary sequestrations* of the intralobular type, cystic lesions may be identified. This sequestration is caused by abnormal budding in the tracheobronchial tree of the early embryo. The involved area is found most often in the bases of the lungs posteriorly, and the affected lung region is nonfunctional. On the chest radiograph, involved areas are opaque.

Only when there is a bronchial communication do air-containing cysts develop, and in such situations secondary infection is the prime concern. These lesions are asymptomatic and are incidental findings on the chest radiograph unless infection develops. An aortogram that shows an abnormal vascular supply distinguishes a sequestration from a simple cyst. The arterial supply to some sequestrations arises at least partially from below the diaphragm. Surgical excision is the only treatment.

THE UNILATERAL HYPERLUCENT LUNG. Swyer-James (also called Macleod's) syndrome, a rare disorder, is generally discovered on the chest radiograph. Increased translucency of one hemithorax is noted because of diminished vascular markings in the lung on that side. On the inspiration chest radiograph, the affected lung is usually not hyperinflated. However, air trapping has been described, and an expiration chest radiograph may show hyperinflation of the affected lung relative to the other uninvolved lung and shift of the mediastinum to the unaffected side. Extensive bronchitis and bronchiolitis are usually noted on biopsy. These abnormalities likely date from childhood. In fact, in some children the condition develops 6 months to 5 years after viral bronchiolitis, and there is a history of some such occurrence in more than half of the patients. Dyspnea, a productive cough, and occasionally hemoptysis may occur.

At bronchoscopy, no obstruction of the main bronchi can be observed. But bronchography shows irregular dilatation of the bronchi to the fifth order, with failure to fill the peripheral airways, and an appearance characteristic of bronchiolar obliteration. Patency of the pulmonary artery on the angiogram differentiates Swyer-James syndrome from pulmonary artery stenosis or atresia. On the affected side, the lung scan shows reduced ventilation and perfusion. Pulmonary function test findings are variable and usually include some evidence of airways obstruction and an increase in residual volume, suggesting air trapping. Severe expiratory obstruction of airflow is uncommon.

Resection is not indicated, and treatment is usually limited to managing infection.

Allison RS, Chirnside AM: Pulmonary sequestration: A review of 12 cases. NZ Med J 596:381, 1983. *Well-written, complete coverage of the types, presentation, and management of pulmonary sequestration.*

Fraser RG, Paré JAP, Paré PD, et al.: Bullous disease of the lung. *In* Diagnosis of Diseases of the Chest. Vol. III. 3rd ed. Philadelphia, W. B. Saunders Company, 1990, p 2166. *In-depth review of blebs, bullae, and cysts, as well as the unilateral hyperlucent lung.*

Fraser RG, Paré JAP, Paré PD, et al.: Roentgenologic signs in the diagnosis of chest disease. *In* Diagnosis of Diseases of the Chest. Vol. I. 3rd ed. Philadelphia, W. B. Saunders Company, 1988, p 472. *Excellent overview of atelectasis.*

Murphy DMF, Fishman AP: Bullous disease of the lung. *In* Fishman AP (ed.): Pulmonary Diseases and Disorders. Vol. 2. 2nd ed. New York, McGraw-Hill Book Company, 1988, p 1219. *Detailed review of blebs, bullae, and cysts of the lung.*

Primrose WR: Spontaneous pneumothorax: A retrospective review of etiology, pathogenesis, and management. Scott Med J 29:15, 1984. *Succinct, up-to-date review of spontaneous pneumothorax.*

Proto AV, Tocino I.: Radiographic manifestations of lobar collapse. Semin Roentgenol 15:117, 1980. *A comprehensive, superb review of chest radiographic features of lobar collapse.*

Rodgers BM, Harman PK, Johnson AM: Bronchopulmonary foregut malformations—the spectrum of anomalies. Ann Surg 203:517, 1986. *A review of the various foregut malformations, including both bronchogenic cysts and sequestration, complete with ultrasound and CT images and a quality bibliography.*

Wagner RB, Johnston MR: Middle lobe syndrome. Ann Thorac Surg 35:679, 1983. *The etiology, pathophysiology, and therapy of this syndrome are up to date.*

60 Interstitial Lung Disease

Ronald G. Crystal

General Description

The interstitial lung diseases (ILD) are a heterogeneous group of diffuse inflammatory disorders of the lower respiratory tract. The term "interstitial lung disease" refers to the fact that the interstitium of the alveolar walls is thickened, usually by fibrosis. While this is true, the ILD are also characterized by derangements of the epithelial and endothelial cells of the alveolar walls and, in many cases, of the small airways and/or blood vessels of the lung parenchyma.

There are many disorders associated with ILD. In some, the ILD is the only manifestation; in others it is a part of a systemic disorder. The natural history of many of the ILD is one of slowly progressive loss of the functional alveolar-capillary units, often eventuating in respiratory insufficiency and death. Because of their insidious nature and the nonspecificity of the accompanying symptoms, such as dyspnea on exertion or a nonproductive cough, the ILD may go undiagnosed and untreated until large numbers of alveolar-capillary units become scarred and irrevocably lost.

These disorders are inflammatory diseases; the bulk of the damage to the lung parenchyma is caused by activated inflammatory cells that have accumulated in the alveolar structures. The diagnosis, staging, and treatment of the ILD require defining the character and intensity of the inflammation in the lung and the derangements of the alveolar structures caused by the inflammation.

Anatomy

The lower respiratory tract is composed of alveoli, grapelike units branching off the terminal bronchioles, and the vascular network of pulmonary arterioles, capillaries, and venules that bring blood to and from the lung (Fig. 60–1). The walls of the alveoli are lined by a single layer of epithelial cells resting on a thin, continuous basement membrane. Ninety-five per cent of the alveolar surface is covered by type I epithelial cells, with the remainder by type II epithelial cells, the cell that produces surfactant, the material that prevents alveolar collapse. Underneath the epithelial basement membrane is the alveolar interstitium, a region containing mesenchymal cells and supporting connective tissue matrix composed of collagen, elastic fibers, proteoglycans, and various glycoproteins. The pulmonary capillaries form a branching network of tubes lined by a single layer of endothelial cells resting on their own basement membrane. The capillaries weave through the interstitium in such a way that the capillary basement membrane often abuts the epithelial basement membrane beneath the type I epithelial cells. It is at these sites that air and blood are in closest approximation and where gas exchange takes place.

The normal alveolar wall is thin (5 to 10 μm wide) compared with the space occupied by air (200 to 300 μm). In the ILD, the walls are thickened several-fold and the space for air is correspondingly less. The derangements that accompany the thickening of the alveolar walls in the ILD can be conceptualized in two groups (Fig. 60–2). In the distortion form of derangement, typified by sarcoidosis and the early phases of hypersensitivity pneumonitis, the alveolar walls are deformed by the accumulation of inflammatory cells in the interstitium, altering the normal architecture. Because there is little injury to the normal structures, this form of derangement is often reversible if the process causing the distortion is eliminated. In the fibrosis form of derangement, typified by idiopathic pulmonary fibrosis and the inorganic dust disorders, the epithelial surface is often altered: Type I epithelial cells are lost, and the surface is repopulated with cuboidal cells derived from proliferating type II cells and bronchiolar cells migrating down from the terminal airways. Alveolar capillary endothelial cells are injured and lost. The interstitium is thickened with edema and proliferation of mesenchymal cells and accumulation of connective tissue products secreted by these cells, particularly collagen. The interstitium is scarred and fibrotic—hence the term "fibrotic lung disease" is also used to refer to these ILD. In the more aggressive forms of fibrosis-type derangements, there are breaks in the epithelial basement membrane through which the interstitial contents protrude; this condition often expands into intra-alveolar fibrotic masses called "intra-alveolar buds" that are eventually incorporated into the alveolar wall, expanding its mass. As the fibrotic form of ILD progresses, the alveolar-capillary units become less distinguishable, and the lung parenchyma takes on the appearance of "end-stage lung" characterized by masses of fibrotic tissue interspaced with cystic areas representing the remnants of alveoli and dilated terminal bronchioles.

Epidemiology

The epidemiology for most of the ILD is not carefully defined, but it is estimated that in the United States their prevalence is approximately 20 to 40 per 100,000 of the population. Conven-

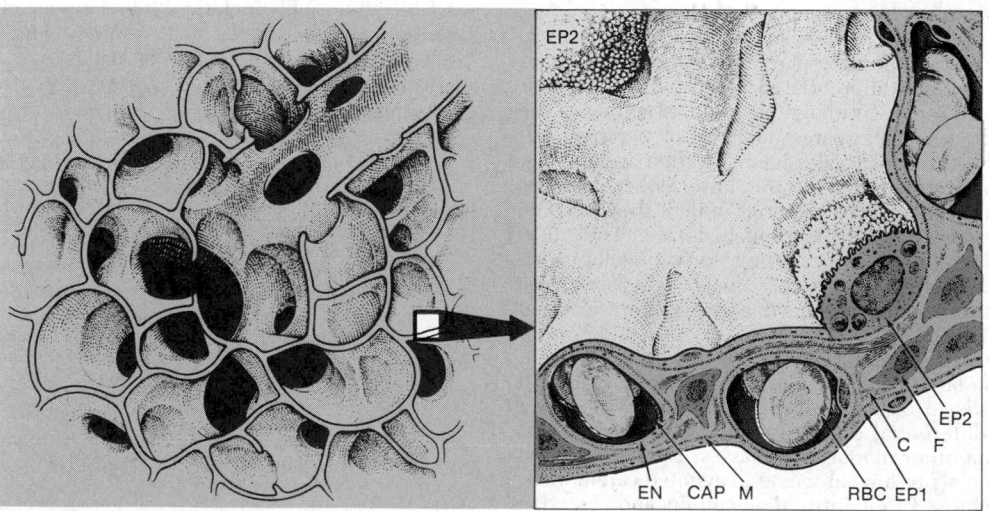

FIGURE 60–1. Structure of the normal lower respiratory tract. *Left,* Representation of a low-power view of the distal lung; the terminal bronchiole is shown but the pulmonary artery and vein are omitted. *Right,* Representation of a high-power view of an alveolus; the cut surface demonstrates the type I (EP1) and type II (EP2) epithelial cells, endothelial cells (EN), basement membranes (M), red blood cells (RBC) in the capillaries (CAP), fibroblasts (F; the most common form of mesenchymal cell in the interstitium), and connective tissue (C). Inflammatory cells are not shown. (From Crystal RG, Bitterman PB, Rennard SI, et al.: Interstitial lung diseases of unknown cause: Disorders characterized by chronic inflammation of the lower respiratory tract. N Engl J Med 310:154, 1984. Reprinted with permission of the New England Journal of Medicine.)

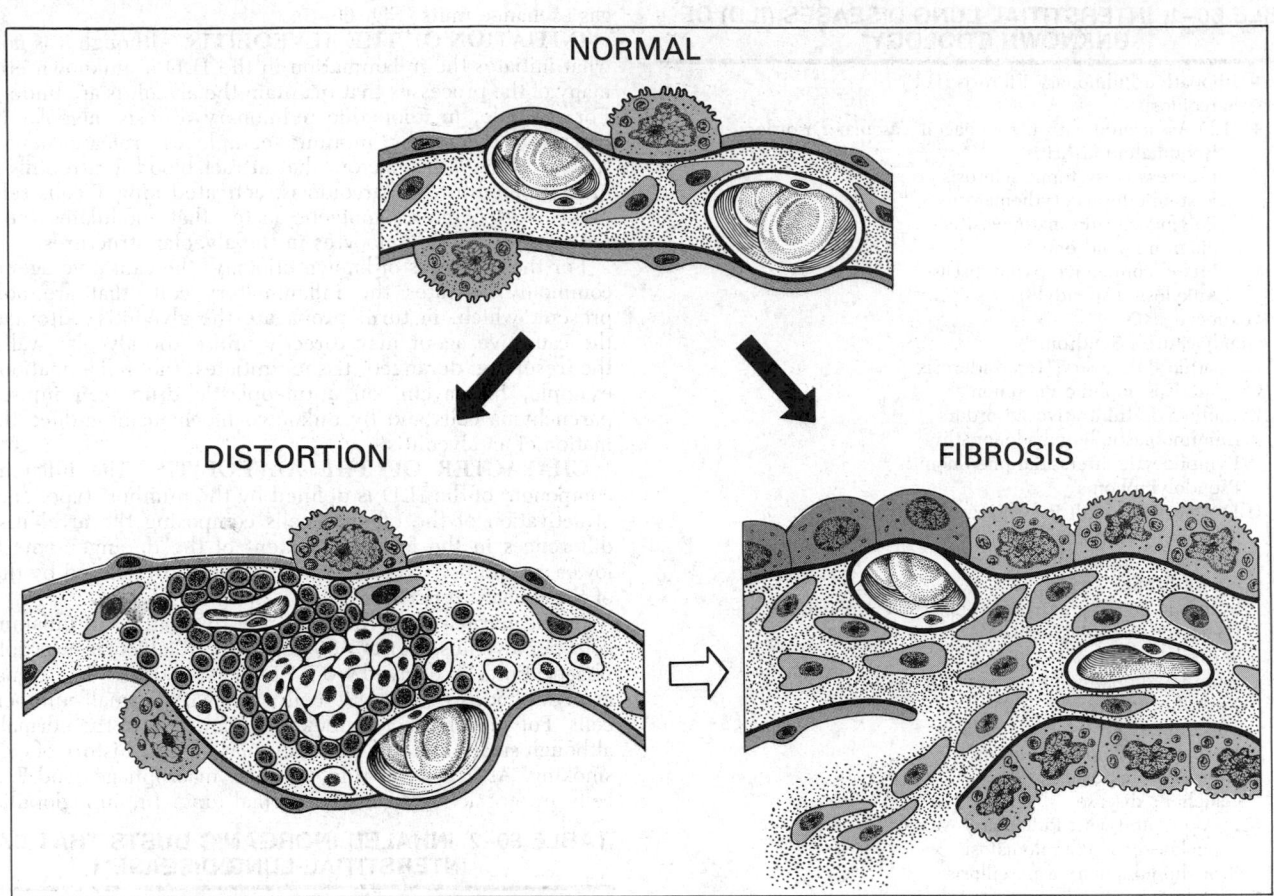

FIGURE 60–2. Typical forms of derangement of alveolar structures in the interstitial lung disorders. *Top*, Schematic of a cut surface of the normal alveolar wall. Shown are the type I and II epithelial cells, endothelial cells lining the capillaries, basement membranes, mesenchymal cells, and interstitial connective tissue. The few inflammatory cells normally present are not shown. *Lower left*, Schematic of a similar view of the alveolar wall deranged by the distortion caused by the accumulations of inflammatory cells. The example used is that of sarcoidosis, in which T cells (primarily CD4+ cells) (pale red) macrophages (white), and granulomas (massed accumulation of macrophages) distort the normal alveolar walls. *Lower right*, Schematic of a similar view of the alveolar wall deranged by fibrosis. The example used is that of idiopathic pulmonary fibrosis. In contrast to the distortion type of derangement, in which there is little damage and change in the lung parenchyma, in the fibrotic form of derangement the type I cells are injured, leaving denuded basement membrane. In some areas, the interstitial contents protrude into the air space, causing intra-alveolar fibrosis. Note that some of the injured type I cells have been replaced by the type II cells and bronchiolar cells that have migrated down from the airways. Capillaries are injured; the basement membranes are thickened; there are expanded numbers of mesenchymal cells; and the density of connective tissue is increased. In the fibrotic type of derangement, there are also large numbers of inflammatory cells distorting the alveolar wall (not shown). In some cases of the distortion kind of derangement, there is sufficient damage to the parenchymal components that the derangements shift into a more fibrotic-type situation.

tionally, the ILD are categorized as those of unknown and known etiology. ILD of known etiology have more subcategories than do ILD of unknown etiology; however, in terms of total numbers of patients, the ILD of unknown etiology predominate. The most common ILD of unknown etiology (Table 60–1) are idiopathic pulmonary fibrosis (IPF), chronic ILD associated with the collagen vascular disorders, and sarcoidosis. Much less common are histiocytosis X, Goodpasture's syndrome, chronic eosinophilic pneumonia, idiopathic pulmonary hemosiderosis, and the ILD associated with the pulmonary vasculitides. The other ILD of unknown etiology are very rare, with fewer than 1000 cases of each reported in the world literature.

The ILD of known etiology are most commonly due to the inhalation of inorganic dusts, particularly crystalline silica, asbestos, and coal dust (Table 60–2), the hypersensitivity pneumonitides (diseases caused by the repeated inhalation of organic dust; Table 60–3), and the drug-induced ILD (Table 60–4). Much less frequent are the ILD resulting from paraquat, radiation, the sequelae of known infectious agents, and the inhalation of gases, aerosols, chemical dusts, fumes, and vapors (Table 60–5). Occasionally, however, large populations develop ILD when exposed

to a single agent at one time, such as occurred in Bhopal, India, in 1984 when methyl isocyanate was released into a crowded urban area.

Differential Diagnosis

The initial problem in assessing ILD is to differentiate it from other disorders that may also present with symptoms of respiratory deficiency and diffuse infiltrates on the chest radiograph (Table 60–6). In general, pulmonary edema, high-flow states, hemorrhage, and aspiration pneumonitis can be easily differentiated from the ILD by history and physical examination. The major problem is in ensuring that the patient does not have an infection or malignancy, diagnoses that require an appropriate evaluation of specimens from the lower respiratory tract for the presence of infectious agents or malignant cells, respectively. In some cases, such as opportunistic organisms associated with human immunodeficiency virus (HIV) infection or with filarial infestation, serologic studies are also necessary.

The diagnosis of a specific ILD is made by a combination of historical, physical examination, blood, urine, roentgenographic, physiologic, scintigraphic, and bronchoscopic criteria. In addi-

TABLE 60–1. INTERSTITIAL LUNG DISEASES (ILD) OF UNKNOWN ETIOLOGY*

- Idiopathic Pulmonary Fibrosis (IPF)
- Sarcoidosis
- ILD Associated with the Collagen Vascular Disorders
  Rheumatoid arthritis
  Progressive systemic sclerosis
  Systemic lupus erythematosus
  Polymyositis/dermatomyositis
  Sjögren's syndrome
  Mixed connective tissue disease
  Ankylosing spondylitis
Histiocytosis X
Goodpasture's Syndrome
Idiopathic Pulmonary Hemosiderosis
Chronic Eosinophilic Pneumonia
Lymphocytic Infiltrative Disorders
  Immunoblastic lymphadenopathy
  Lymphocytic interstitial pneumonitis
  Pseudolymphoma
ILD Associated with Pulmonary Vasculitides
  Wegener's granulomatosis
  Lymphomatoid granulomatosis
  Churg-Strauss syndrome
  Systemic necrotizing vasculitides ("overlap" vasculitides)
  Hypersensitivity vasculitis
Inherited Disorders
  Familial idiopathic pulmonary fibrosis
  Neurofibromatosis
  Tuberous sclerosis
  Hermansky-Pudlak syndrome
  Niemann-Pick disease
  Gaucher's disease
ILD Associated with Pulmonary Airway Disease
  Bronchocentric granulomatosis
  Bronchopulmonary aspergillosis
Lymphangioleiomyomatosis
Alveolar Proteinosis
ILD Associated with Liver Disease
  Chronic active hepatitis
  Primary biliary cirrhosis
ILD Associated with Bowel Disease
  Whipple's disease
  Ulcerative colitis
  Crohn's disease
Weber-Christian Disease
Amyloidosis
Hypereosinophilic Syndrome
Pulmonary Veno-occlusive Disease
ILD Caused by Failure of Other Organs
  Chronic left ventricular failure
  Chronic left-to-right intracardiac shunt
  Chronic renal disease with uremia
Graft-vs.-Host Disease
Recovery Phase of Adult Respiratory
  Distress Syndrome

*Disorders indicated with "●" are the most common ILD of unknown etiology.

tion, unless an agent of known etiology is apparent (e.g., long-term asbestos exposure), it is mandatory to evaluate the disease by morphologic means, usually by open lung biopsy. The only exception to this rule is when the ILD is in clear association with a systemic disorder (e.g., a collagen vascular disease, Goodpasture's syndrome) in which the diagnosis can be made by evaluation of organs other than the lung.

Pathogenesis

The ILD are inflammatory disorders in which most of the derangements of the alveolar walls, including the fibrosis, are mediated by inflammatory/immune cells that have accumulated in the lung parenchyma. The inflammation, usually referred to as the "alveolitis" of the disease, not only involves the alveoli but often involves the walls of small airways and sometimes the pulmonary blood vessels. The critical importance of the alveolitis is simply stated: Although dysfunction of the alveolar-capillary units causes the symptoms and impairment of the patient, it is the alveolitis that causes the derangements of the alveolar-capillary units, resulting in their dysfunction and eventual loss as gas exchange units (Fig. 60–3).

INITIATION OF THE ALVEOLITIS. Although it is not clear what initiates the inflammation in the ILD of unknown etiology, many of the processes that maintain the alveolitis are understood. For example, in idiopathic pulmonary fibrosis, alveolar macrophages, activated by immune complexes, release neutrophil-specific chemotactic factors that attract blood neutrophils to the lung. In contrast, in sarcoidosis, activated lung T cells release a monocyte-specific chemotactic factor that modulates the accumulation of blood monocytes in the alveolar structures.

For the disorders of known etiology, the causative agent most commonly activates the inflammatory cells that are normally present, which, in turn, propagate the alveolitis. Alternatively, the causative agent may directly injure the alveolar walls, and the resulting deranged tissue initiates the inflammation. For example, bleomycin, an antineoplastic drug, can injure lung parenchyma cells and by unknown mechanisms induce the formation of an alveolitis.

CHARACTER OF THE ALVEOLITIS. The inflammatory component of the ILD is defined by the number, type, and state of activation of the effector cells composing the alveolitis. The differences in the form and extent of the derangements to the lower respiratory tract in these disorders are defined by the sum of these characteristics.

In the normal lung there are approximately 80 inflammatory cells per alveolus. Most (>80 per cent) are alveolar macrophages, phagocytic cells derived from blood monocytes. The remainder are lymphocytes, mostly T cells, but with a small number of B cells. Polymorphonuclear leukocytes are rare in the normal lung, although small numbers do accumulate with a history of cigarette smoking. As a general rule, alveolar macrophages and T and B cells are not activated in the normal lung. Immunoglobulins are

TABLE 60–2. INHALED INORGANIC DUSTS THAT CAUSE INTERSTITIAL LUNG DISEASE*†

Silica (variants of SiO_2)
- Crystalline silica ("silicosis")
  Amorphous
Silicates
- Asbestos ("asbestosis")
  Talc (hydrated Mg silicates; "talcosis")
  Kaolin (china clay, hydrated aluminum silicate)
  Diatomaceous earth (Fuller's earth, aluminum silicate with Fe and Mg)
  Nepheline (hard rock containing mixed silicates)
  Aluminum silicates (sericite, sillimanite, zeolite)
  Portland cement
  Mica (principally K and Mg aluminum silicates)
Carbon (with or without crystalline silica)
- Coal dust ("coal worker's pneumoconiosis")
  Graphite ("carbon pneumoconiosis")
Metals
  Beryllium ("berylliosis" or "chronic beryllium disease")
  Aluminum ("aluminosis")
    Powdered aluminum ("aluminum lung")
    Bauxite (aluminum oxide; "Shaver's disease")
  Barium (powder of baryte or $BaSO_4$; "baritosis")
  Iron ("siderosis")
  Tin ("stannosis")
  Antimony (oxides and alloys)
  Mixed dusts
    Hematite (mixed dusts of iron oxide, silica, and silicates; "siderosilicosis")
    Mixed dusts of silver and iron oxide ("argyrosiderosis")
  Hard metals
    Titanium oxide
    Tungsten, titanium, hafnium, niobium, cobalt, and vanadium carbides
    Cadmium
Rare earths (cerium, scandium, yttrium, lanthanum)
$CuSO_4$ neutralized with hydrated lime (Bordeaux mixture; "vineyard sprayer's lung")

*The most common inorganic dust–induced interstitial lung diseases are indicated with "●."

†Disorders given a specific name are indicated in quotes in parentheses; others are referred as "(name of the dust) pneumoconiosis."

TABLE 60–3. INHALED ORGANIC DUSTS THAT CAUSE INTERSTITIAL LUNG DISEASE*

Disorder	Causative Agent†
● Farmer's lung	M. faeni, T. vulgaris, A. fumigatus, T. candidus
● Humidifier lung, air conditioner lung	T. vulgaris, T. candidus, thermotolerant bacteria, protozoa, Penicillium species, Naegleria gruberi
● Bird breeder's disease‡	Avian proteins, feathers
Maple bark stripper's lung	Cryptostroma corticale
Cheese worker's lung	A. clavatus, Penicillium caseii
Malt worker's lung	A. clavatus, A. fumigatus
Sequoiosis	Aureobasidium pullulans, Graphium species
Paprika splitter's lung	Mucor stolonifer
Wheat weevil disease	Sitophilus granarius
Suberosis	Penicillium frequentans
Bagassosis	T. sacchari
Mushroom worker's lung	M. faeni, T. vulgaris
Pituitary snuff lung	Porcine and bovine proteins
Wood-pulp worker's disease	Alternaria species
Sauna-taker's disease	Aureobasidium species
Detergent worker's lung	Bacillus subtilis
Lycoperdonosis	Lycoperdon bovista
Rodent handler's disease	Serum and urine constituents
Dry rot disease	Merulius lacrymans
Wood-dust worker's lung	Unknown
Furrier's lung	Unknown
New Guinea lung	Saccharomonospora irridis
Coptic disease (mummy unwrapper's disease)	Antigens associated with mummy wrappings
"Summer-type" disease	Cryptococcus neoformans Cephalosporium species§ Streptomyces albus§ Bacillus subtilis§

*The most common interstitial lung disorders caused by inhaled organic antigens are indicated with "●."

†M. = Micropolyspora; T. = Thermoactinomyces; A. = Aspergillus.

‡Includes pigeons, parakeets, budgerigars, turkeys, chickens, and ducks.

§Hypersensitivity pneumonitis has been described in association with these agents, in circumstances in which no common name has been given to the disorder.

present in the normal lower respiratory tract (IgG > IgA >> IgM), as are some complement components. Macromolecules that defend against inflammatory injury, including antiproteases and antioxidants, are also present.

Active, untreated ILD are generally characterized by a marked increase in the number of inflammatory cells in the alveolar walls and on the alveolar epithelial surface. Commonly, this increase in numbers of effector cells is also characterized by a shift in

TABLE 60–4. DRUGS THAT CAUSE INTERSTITIAL LUNG DISEASE

Antineoplastic Agents	Cardiovascular Drugs	Anti-Inflammatory Agents
Azathioprine	Hydralazine	Gold salts
Bleomycin	Procainamide	Phenylbutazone
Cyclophosphamide	Beta blockers (pro-	Beclomethasone
Methotrexate	pranolol, practolol,	Naproxen
Nitrosoureas	pindolol, acebutolol)	
Carmustine (BCNU)	Tocainide	**Oral Hypoglycemic Agents**
Lomustine (CCNU)	Amiodarone	Chlorpropamide
Semustine (methyl-CCNU)	Reserpine	Tolbutamide
Chlorozotocin (DCNU)	**Central Nervous System Drugs**	Tolazamide
Melphalan	Phenytoin	**Miscellaneous**
Busulfan	Carbamazepine	Penicillamine
Chlorambucil	Chlorpromazine	Allopurinol
6-Mercaptopurine	Imipramine	Cromolyn sodium
6-Thioguanine	Amitriptyline	Hydrochlorothiazide
Mitomycin C	Methylphenidate	Mineral oil
Procarbazine	Dantrolene	Intravenous drugs con-
Uracil mustard	Mephenesin	taining particulate
Zinostatin		material
	Ganglionic Blocking Agents	Silicone used for tissue
Antibiotics	Mecamylamine	augmentation
Nitrofurantoin	Hexamethonium	
Penicillins	Pentolinium	
Sulfonamides		
Erythromycin		
Tetracycline		
Isoniazid		
para-Aminosalicylic acid		
Niridazole		

TABLE 60–5. OTHER AGENTS KNOWN TO CAUSE INTERSTITIAL LUNG DISEASE

Paraquat
Radiation
Sequelae of Known Infectious Agents
  Bacteria — *Mycoplasma*
  Mycobacteria — *Legionella pneumophila*
  Fungi — Parasites
  Viruses
Inhaled Agents Other Than Inorganic or Organic Dusts
  Gases
    Oxygen — Sulfur dioxide
    Oxides of nitrogen — Methyl isocyanate
    Chlorine gas
  Aerosols
    Aspiration pneumonia — Pyrethrum (a natural insecticide)
    Fats
    Oils — Toluene diisocyanate
  Chemical dusts
    Synthetic fibers (Orlon, polyesters, nylon, acrylic)
    Bakelite
    Vinyl chloride, polyvinyl chloride powder
  Fumes
    Oxides of Zn, Cu, Mn, Cd, Fe, Mg, Ni, Se, Sn, Sb, V, and brass
    Diphenylmethane diisocyanate
    Trimellitic anhydride
  Vapors
    Hydrocarbons
    Mercury
    Thermosetting resins

their relative proportions. Different patterns of alveolitis are generally referred to by the cell types that are most abundant. For example, when the inflammation is dominated by neutrophils and macrophages, it is referred to as a neutrophil-macrophage alveolitis. The alveolitis patterns most frequently observed in ILD are a macrophage-dominant alveolitis, a lymphocyte-macrophage alveolitis, and a neutrophil-macrophage alveolitis. Eosinophils play a role in the alveolitis of many ILD but rarely dominate it. Subcategories of the common alveolitis patterns have also been described. For example, the granulomatous lung disorders, sarcoidosis and berylliosis, are characterized by a CD4 + T-helper cell–macrophage alveolitis, while chronic hypersensitivity pneumonitis is usually characterized by a CD8 + T-suppressor/cytotoxic cell–macrophage alveolitis, sometimes including neutrophils.

In addition to the numbers and types of inflammatory cells

TABLE 60–6. DISORDERS INVOLVING THE LOWER RESPIRATORY TRACT THAT CAN BE CONFUSED WITH INTERSTITIAL LUNG DISEASE*

Pulmonary Edema
Neoplasms
  ● Leukemic infiltration
  ● Lymphoma
  ● Lymphangitic spread of carcinoma
    Multiple metastases
    Primary pulmonary malignancy
Infections
  ● Viruses†
    Fungi
    Bacteria‡
  ● Mycobacteria
  ● Parasites§
  ● *Mycoplasma*
    Psittacosis
    Q fever
  ● *Pneumocystis carinii*
Pulmonary Hemorrhage
Aspiration

*Disorders frequently confused with the ILD are indicated with "●."

†Of the viruses known to involve the lung—influenza, cytomegalovirus (CMV), varicella zoster, measles, and HIV are most commonly confused with ILD.

‡Particularly *Legionella*.

§*Pneumocystis* and filarial disease are commonly mistaken for ILD.

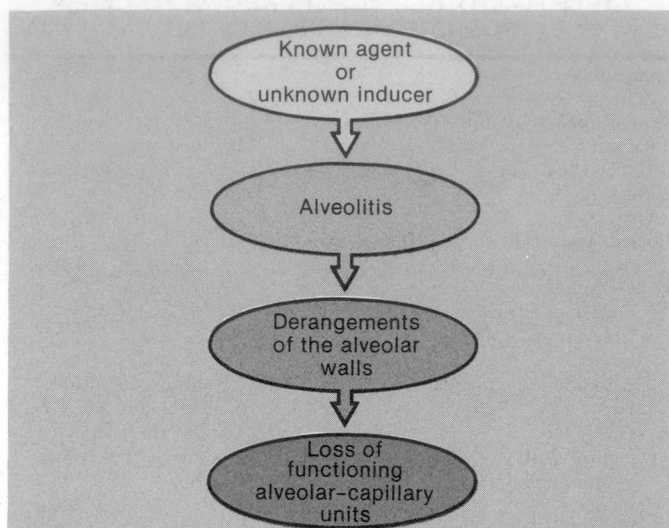

FIGURE 60–3. Pathogenesis of the interstitial lung diseases of unknown and known etiology. In both groups, the inflammation (alveolitis) is responsible for the bulk of the derangements of the alveolar walls. In some disorders, the deranged wall components may accelerate the alveolitis by recruiting additional inflammatory cells. In the disorders of known etiology, the causative agent may directly damage the alveolar structures, which, in turn, initiates and/or accelerates the alveolitis.

present, the consequences of the alveolitis critically depend on the state of activation of these cells. The simple presence of the inflammatory cells in the alveolar structures distorts the alveolar walls but usually is not damaging. When activated, however, some inflammatory cells can injure the alveolar walls, particularly sensitive type I epithelial cells and capillary endothelial cells. If the alveolitis is self-limiting, or if it is suppressed by therapy before the injury becomes too severe, the architecture of the lower respiratory tract can be re-established and normal lung function restored. If, however, the injury is extensive, with mesenchymal cell proliferation and collagen deposition, the normal architecture of the affected alveolar-capillary units can never be fully re-established. Therapeutic success in treating ILD means suppression of the alveolitis and thus prevention of further loss of alveolar-capillary units.

DISTORTION AND FIBROSIS. Whether the derangements of the alveolar walls take the form of distortion and/or fibrosis is dictated by the characteristics of the alveolitis. It is important to recognize that while the distortion type of derangement is usually reversible if the inflammation is suppressed, the consequences of the fibrosis form of derangement are commonly sufficient to prevent a return to the normal architecture.

Accumulation of sufficient numbers of any type of inflammatory cells results in some distortion of the tissue. However, this form of derangement is most significant when the inflammation involves lymphocytes and macrophages, such as when there is an accumulation of activated CD4+ T-helper cells that direct the formation of granuloma. Together, the T cells and masses of macrophages distort the normal architecture but usually do not cause permanent damage.

The fibrosis form of derangement is characterized by injury to parenchymal components, together with the accumulation of mesenchymal cells and their secreted connective tissue products. The neutrophil is the most damaging of all inflammatory cells by virtue of its highly reactive oxygen metabolites that are toxic to the parenchymal cells and its connective tissue–specific proteases that can damage the interstitial collagens and basement membranes. Injury to the epithelial basement membrane has profound consequences because the epithelial cells no longer have a surface upon which to migrate, making it impossible to reconstruct a normal alveolar surface. The eosinophil can also injure lung parenchymal cells and connective tissue, but on a per cell basis it is less potent than the neutrophil. Activated human alveolar macrophages release toxic oxidants and thus can be cytotoxic to

normal lung parenchymal cells. The macrophage also mediates the accumulation of mesenchymal cells and the connective tissue that characterizes the fibrosis type of derangement of the alveolar walls. The fundamental problem is the accumulation of mesenchymal cells in the alveolar walls. Since mesenchymal cells are major producers of collagen, the consequence of an increase in mesenchymal cell numbers is an accumulation of collagen in the alveolar interstitium. As a result, the alveolar wall is thickened and scarred and has decreased compliance. The macrophage mediates the accumulation of mesenchymal cells by releasing exaggerated amounts of at least three mediators, platelet-derived growth factor, fibronectin, and a form of insulin-like growth factor 1 (also called "alveolar macrophage–derived growth factor"). Platelet-derived growth factor, a product of the *c-sis* oncogene, attracts mesenchymal cells and is a potent stimulus for mesenchymal cells to begin traversing the cell cycle. Fibronectin, a 440,000-dalton glycoprotein, attracts mesenchymal cells, attaches them to the extracellular matrix, and stimulates them to enter the cell cycle. The alveolar macrophage form of insulin-like growth factor 1, an 18,000-dalton protein, induces the platelet-derived growth factor or fibronectin-primed mesenchymal cells to continue through the cell cycle and proliferate.

Clinical Features

HISTORY. Occasional patients are detected as having ILD because a routine chest radiograph is noted to be abnormal, but most come to medical attention because of symptoms related to the chest. All ILD are characterized by abnormalities in the transfer of oxygen from air to blood secondary to slowly progressive derangement of the lower respiratory tract. The initial symptoms are those of insufficient oxygen transfer, such as *fatigue* and *breathlessness with exertion*. These symptoms are often initially denied by the patient or are attributed to being "out of shape" or "overweight" or to a prior chest infection, usually a viral syndrome. As the disease progresses, the dyspnea becomes more apparent and eventually is felt when the patient is at rest. In contrast to cardiac-induced dyspnea, paroxysmal nocturnal dyspnea and orthopnea are rare, as are platypnea and trepopnea. Nonproductive cough, pleuritic pain, and hemoptysis are less common presenting complaints. Early in the disease, chest pain is rare, although later, when pulmonary hypertension develops, substernal discomfort may be noted.

The history also plays an important role in the diagnosis of the type of interstitial disease. Since a large number of agents cause ILD, a careful exposure history is essential to determine not only the agents to which the patient has been exposed but also the circumstances, intensity, and duration of exposure. Exposure to agents that cause ILD may be found in nonclassic situations. For example, silicosis has been described in workers involved in the manufacture of pencils, furniture, and tombstones; talcosis in the manufacture of rubber condoms; and hypersensitivity pneumonitis in office buildings where the offending organic antigen was located in the air conditioning system.

The lack of a history of exposure to a known agent that causes interstitial disease is very important in diagnosing the ILD of unknown etiology. For example, pulmonary sarcoidosis is very difficult to distinguish from berylliosis unless there is a negative history of beryllium exposure. Similarly, idiopathic pulmonary fibrosis is difficult to diagnose if an exposure history is unavailable or if there is a clear history of sufficient exposure to one or more agents that cause ILD. Some ILD of unknown etiology are associated with diseases that often involve other organs, such as the collagen vascular disorders, primary biliary cirrhosis, and Wegener's granulomatosis, which may be suspected from the history.

PHYSICAL EXAMINATION. The chest expansion is typically reduced, reflecting the reduced total lung capacity of individuals with ILD. Most have fine, crackling inspiratory and expiratory rales, heard best at the posterior lung bases. These rales have a characteristic sound, described as "Velcro-like" (i.e., the sound of unwrapping a blood pressure cuff) or like the sound of rubbing hair together. Coarse rales, wheezing, and rhonchi are occasionally heard. As the disease progresses, these patients may be tachypneic at rest, but unlike individuals with emphysema, they do not use the accessory muscles of respiration and do not assume the posture of placing their hands on their thighs to "fix" the upper body to assist in respiration.

Early in the disease, examination of the heart is normal. Later, an accentuated P₂ reflects mild pulmonary hypertension. Eventually, obvious evidence of pulmonary hypertension is noted, including a right ventricular heave. Patients with ILD rarely develop frank right-sided failure with liver enlargement and peripheral edema, presumably because they die of the complications of insufficient oxygen delivery before the right ventricle deteriorates.

Clubbing of the fingers and sometimes the toes is common in ILD, particularly in idiopathic pulmonary fibrosis and asbestosis. Cyanosis occurs, but usually very late in the disease. Other physical findings in ILD are those associated with problems with oxygen transport (e.g., left ventricular failure, central nervous system signs) and those characteristic of associated diseases (e.g., the rash of systemic lupus erythematosus, the skin changes of scleroderma).

LABORATORY STUDIES. No blood test is diagnostic for one ILD, and the intensity and character of the alveolitis are not reflected in the blood. The hemoglobin and hematocrit are usually normal despite associated hypoxemia, and the white blood cell count and differential usually bear no relationship to the alveolitis. In most ILD, the sedimentation rate is elevated.

A patient with suspected ILD should have routine blood screening tests for hematologic, liver, renal, and muscle abnormalities and collagen vascular disorders. Screening for HIV infection is mandatory, as some opportunistic infections associated with the HIV-positive state can mimic ILD, and the pulmonary inflammation associated with HIV infection can cause ILD. Other blood tests directed toward specific diseases may be ordered as the workup proceeds and the specific disease is suspected. For example, serologic tests for antibodies against organic antigens are ordered only in the context of suspected hypersensitivity pneumonitis and anti–basement membrane antibodies only when Goodpasture's syndrome is suspected.

Rheumatoid factor and antinuclear antibodies are occasionally present in low titer and do not necessarily indicate the presence of an underlying collagen vascular disorder. Plasma immunoglobulins may be elevated, but this finding is usually nonspecific. Except in those circumstances in which the disease is systemic (e.g., sarcoidosis, a collagen vascular disorder), other screening blood studies are generally normal.

The electrocardiogram (ECG) is usually normal in ILD except for evidence of pulmonary hypertension. As the loss of alveolar-capillary units progresses, the ECG demonstrates a pattern of right atrial and ventricular strain. The hypoxemia of ILD may exacerbate coexisting coronary heart disease, evoking arrhythmias and evidence of coronary insufficiency, particularly with exercise.

RADIOGRAPHIC STUDIES. The posteroanterior and lateral chest films have a major role in establishing the diagnosis of ILD, although 5 to 10 per cent of patients with biopsy-proven disease have a normal chest film. A ground-glass pattern may be seen early in the disease. More typically, the chest radiograph demonstrates a diffuse, finely nodular, reticular, or reticulonodular pattern usually more prominent at the bases (Fig. 60–4). As the disease evolves, the pattern becomes coarser, with cystic areas appearing and, finally, a honeycomb pattern. Initially the pulmonary arteries appear normal, but in the later stages of ILD, evidence of pulmonary hypertension may be present.

A definitive diagnosis of a specific ILD can never be made by the chest radiograph alone. However, certain radiographic patterns are typical of specific diseases or groups of diseases and thus are very helpful in establishing a diagnosis. For example, some ILD are also characterized by hilar and/or paratracheal lymph node enlargement, while others manifest pleural disease.

Except for rare circumstances, radiographic studies other than the routine chest film have little use in the evaluation of ILD. Oblique films, tomography, bronchography, and angiography are occasionally used to evaluate localized lesions on a background of ILD but usually are difficult to interpret. Computed tomographic (CT) scans of the chest are routinely used in the evaluation of those patients in whom questionable hilar or pleural lesions are being evaluated. CT scans are being evaluated for use in assessing the extent of parenchymal changes, but standard criteria for abnormalities are not yet established.

PULMONARY FUNCTION TESTS. The classic physiologic alterations in ILD include reduced lung volumes (vital capacity, total lung capacity), reduced diffusing capacity, and a normal or

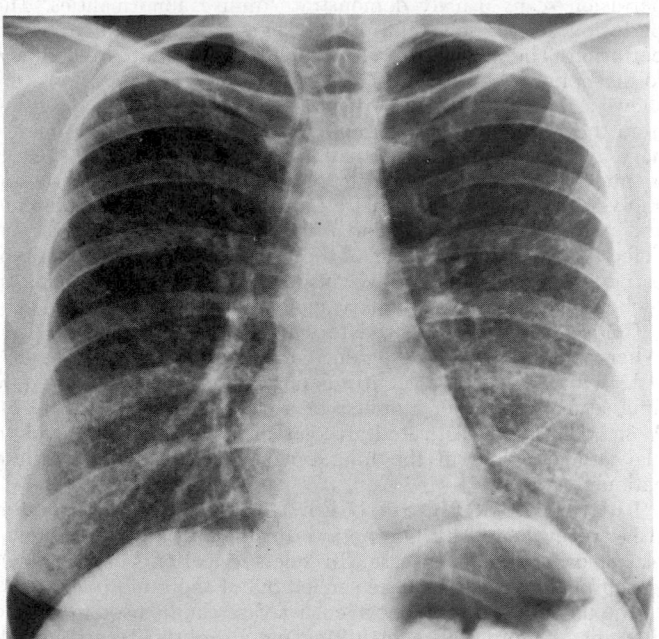

FIGURE 60–4. Chest radiograph of a patient with idiopathic pulmonary fibrosis, typical of the radiographic findings of many interstitial lung diseases. There is a diffuse reticulonodular infiltrate throughout the lung fields, most prominent at the bases. The heart and pleura are normal.

supranormal ratio of forced expiratory volume in 1 second to forced vital capacity. In some ILD, sensitive tests such as flow-volume curves and maximal flow-static recoil curves can detect mild limitation of airflow. Measurement of static lung compliance demonstrates decreased lung volumes for a given transpulmonary pressure, and an increased maximal transpulmonary pressure, i.e., very high negative pressures (relative to the atmosphere), must be generated to open the fibrotic alveoli.

Arterial blood gases typically show mild hypoxemia; carbon dioxide retention is rare, even late in the course of the disease. Patients with ILD tend to hyperventilate and have a reduced PCO₂ and compensated respiratory alkalosis, mostly as a result of an increase in respiratory rate. The drive to hyperventilate is not due to hypoxemia or abnormalities in acid-base status but rather to the subjective sense of dyspnea or to an increased stimulation of the respiratory center from neural signals arising in the deranged lung parenchyma. With exercise, the arterial PO₂ drops, while the PCO₂ remains constant. The loss of alveolar-capillary bed in ILD and hence the limitation of cardiac output seriously impair oxygen delivery and thereby markedly limit the exercise tolerance of these patients. This leads to their propensity to suffer hypoxic damage to vital organs. The arterial pH is usually normal in ILD, but it can fall with exercise as a consequence of oxygen deprivation of muscles, which then resort to anaerobic metabolism.

At rest, the hypoxemia of ILD results from abnormal matching of pulmonary ventilation and perfusion. With exercise, however, an apparent "diffusion block" also contributes. It was originally thought that this block resulted from a limited oxygen diffusion through the thickened alveolar walls, but it is now recognized to be due to red blood cells passing through the functioning pulmonary capillaries too rapidly to permit full saturation of hemoglobin. In rare instances, some of the hypoxemia of ILD results from shunts, either in the lung parenchyma or through a patent foramen ovale in the setting of pulmonary hypertension.

The loss of pulmonary capillary bed in ILD is associated with pulmonary hypertension, first with exercise only and later at rest. The pulmonary hypertension is thought to result from mechanical reasons (e.g., the loss of pulmonary capillary bed) and not from hypoxia-induced vasoconstriction or from local mediators. Right ventricular end-diastolic pressure rises late in the disease, but this rarely leads to frank right-sided failure.

SCINTIGRAPHIC STUDIES. Conventional ventilation and

perfusion scans usually demonstrate diffuse abnormalities. The perfusion scans show multiple subsegmental areas of impaired perfusion. The normal, upright individual has limited blood flow to the upper lobes at rest. The perfusion scan in ILD, however, shows a redistribution of perfusion to the upper lobes, resulting from the loss of pulmonary capillary bed and developing pulmonary hypertension. The ventilation scan shows multiple subsegmental areas of reduced ventilation. Comparison of the perfusion and ventilation scans demonstrates numerous areas of ventilation and perfusion mismatch. The presence of numerous perfusion defects limits the usefulness of these techniques in evaluation of patients with ILD who have suspected pulmonary emboli. In such circumstances, pulmonary angiography is mandatory.

Gallium-67 scans are used to evaluate the alveolitis of ILD. Whereas the normal lung parenchyma takes up little gallium-67, ILD with an active alveolitis demonstrate positive gallium-67 lung scans with either a diffuse or a patchy pattern (Fig. 60–5). A high density of activated alveolar macrophages is thought to play a major role in the lung uptake of gallium-67 in these patients.

BRONCHOSCOPIC STUDIES. Most patients with suspected ILD are evaluated by fiberoptic bronchoscopy to rule out neoplastic or infectious disease. In selected patients (see below), transbronchial biopsy can be carried out at the same time.

The technique of bronchoalveolar lavage can be used to sample the inflammatory cells constituting the alveolitis. To accomplish this, the bronchoscope is wedged into a distal bronchus, and aliquots of sterile saline are used to recover the inflammatory cells and epithelial lining fluid of the lower respiratory tract. In normal individuals, 80 per cent or more of the recovered cells demonstrate alveolar macrophages, with the remainder being lymphocytes (almost all T cells). Polymorphonuclear leukocytes are normally rare. In patients with ILD, the pattern of alveolitis is reflected by the cells recovered by lavage. For example, in pulmonary sarcoidosis, the proportions of T cells may be 30 to 60 per cent, while in idiopathic pulmonary fibrosis, the proportion of neutrophils is often greater than 10 per cent. The diagnostic usefulness of bronchoalveolar lavage has not been established, but it can help to orient the clinician to the category of alveolitis that is present. Furthermore, because alveolar macrophages are phagocytic and ingest foreign materials present in the lung parenchyma, bronchoalveolar lavage can also be used to help diagnose specific agents that cause ILD, including inorganic dust diseases.

BIOPSY. The diagnosis of many ILD depends upon pathologic studies of lung parenchyma. The method of choice is the open lung biopsy, usually performed in the right middle lobe or lingula in an area of "average" disease as judged by the chest film. Transbronchial biopsy through the fiberoptic bronchoscope is useful for diagnosing sarcoidosis, but for most other ILD the samples are too small for a definitive diagnosis to be made.

Staging and Therapy

A patient with ILD should be evaluated to assess the contribution of the disease to functional impairment. The activity of the disease process should be independently assessed. Once both are known, rational decisions can be made concerning prognosis and therapy.

ASSESSMENT OF IMPAIRMENT. The consequences of ILD are assessed by history, chest radiograph, and lung function testing. A careful history of the patient's sensation of breathlessness, combined with an estimate of exercise tolerance, allows a rough estimate of lung derangement. The chest radiograph is somewhat more objective, and comparison with prior films helps to determine if the disease has become more extensive. Pulmonary function tests are the most accurate means to assess impairment. Of the tests routinely available, vital capacity, total lung capacity, diffusing capacity, and arterial Po_2 most accurately gauge the loss of functioning alveolar-capillary units. Measurements of the changes in Po_2 with exercise and of static compliance are more sensitive indicators of the extent of the impairment, but these tests are more difficult to perform and are not widely available.

ASSESSMENT OF ACTIVITY. Alveolitis is confined to the lower respiratory tract, so that its character or extent is difficult to measure directly. Circulating immune complexes and angiotensin-converting enzyme have been suggested as measures of the alveolitis in idiopathic pulmonary fibrosis and sarcoidosis, respectively, but neither test is very sensitive or specific. Similarly, attempts to correlate the chest radiograph or lung function tests with morphologic evidence of the alveolitis have been disappointing, and thus neither can be used to evaluate the alveolitis accurately.

Open lung biopsy, bronchoalveolar lavage, and *gallium-67 scanning* are the best present methods to stage alveolitis. Open biopsy is the most accurate method but is very rarely performed more than once in the course of the disease. Bronchoalveolar lavage and gallium-67 scanning are both sensitive to and specific for the alveolitis, but neither has been fully validated for routine clinical use. At this time, bronchoalveolar lavage is most useful for evaluating the intensity of the neutrophil, eosinophil, and lymphocyte components of the alveolitis and gallium-67 scanning for the macrophage component.

THERAPY. The principal aim of therapy in ILD is to suppress the alveolitis. For the ILD of unknown etiology, the conventional approach is to treat with oral corticosteroids, usually prednisone. Relatively high doses are used (1 mg per kilogram daily) for 1 to 2 months, followed by tapering doses over 2 to 3 months to maintenance levels (0.25 mg per kilogram per day), which are continued for varying periods. The corticosteroids are generally given once daily; it is not known if alternate-day regimens are equally effective. There has never been a large controlled trial of corticosteroids in any ILD, but some patients with ILD respond to corticosteroids in a fashion that cannot be explained by spontaneous remission. "Successful" therapy does not necessarily

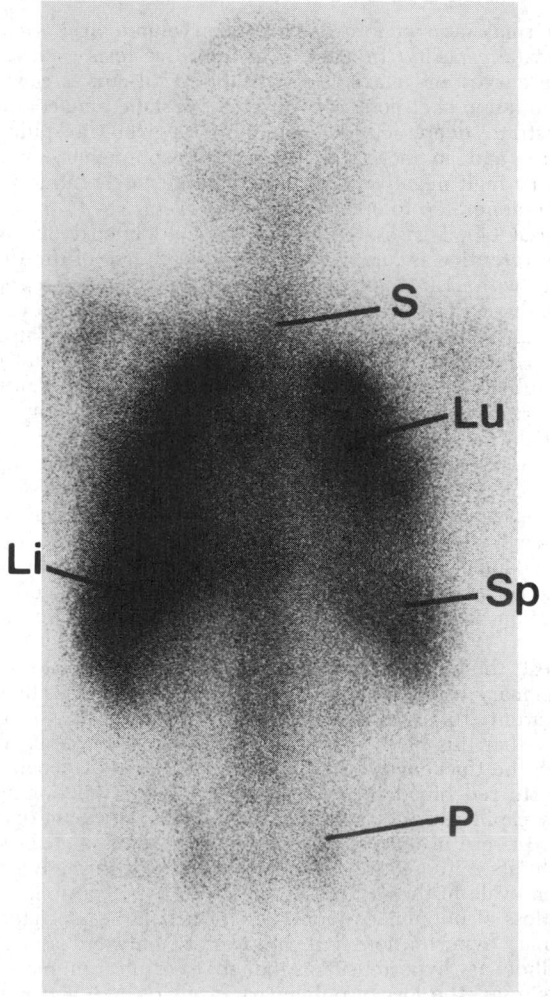

FIGURE 60–5. Gallium-67 scan of a patient with sarcoidosis. There is diffuse uptake of the isotope throughout the lung parenchyma (Lu). Structures that normally take up gallium-67 are also seen, including the spine (S), liver (Li), spleen (Sp), and pelvis (P).

mean improvement in pulmonary function, chest radiograph, or subjective symptoms, since severely damaged alveoli are lost forever. In this context, successful suppression of the alveolitis usually means no further loss of alveoli. If improvement does occur, it likely results from suppression of the contribution of the inflammation itself to the derangements of the alveolar structures.

If the disease stabilizes, the corticosteroids are usually tapered. If the deterioration begins again after a period of quiescence, corticosteroids are often restarted, but their efficacy under these circumstances is limited. A variety of cytotoxic and other anti-inflammatory drugs have also been used in the treatment of the ILD of unknown etiology, but there has been no controlled series to demonstrate their efficacy.

For the ILD of known etiology, the initial treatment is to remove exposure to the causative agent. If the inflammation persists for months after removal from the known agent, patients are usually treated in a fashion similar to that used for ILD of unknown etiology. The exception to this rule is most of the pneumoconioses, for which no therapy is used.

In all ILD, attention should be given to prompt treatment of lung infections. Bronchodilators are sometimes used in mid to late course in these diseases to help mobilize secretions. Oxygen therapy, particularly with exercise, is often used as the patient reaches the late stage of ILD, but its efficacy in increasing the lifespan of these patients is unproved.

INTERSTITIAL LUNG DISEASES OF UNKNOWN ETIOLOGY

The ILD of unknown etiology represent the majority of all cases of ILD. Although of unknown etiology, each represents a specific entity with distinct features (see Table 60–1). The best understood ILD of unknown etiology are idiopathic pulmonary fibrosis and sarcoidosis.

Idiopathic Pulmonary Fibrosis (IPF)

CLINICAL MANIFESTATIONS. IPF, the "classic" fibrotic lung disease, is characterized by a neutrophil–alveolar macrophage alveolitis and progressive scarring of alveolar-capillary units. In the past IPF was sometimes called the Hamman-Rich syndrome, but this designation is not generally used now. Typically, IPF first manifests in middle age, but all age groups can be affected. The sex distribution is equal. Patients present with dyspnea on exertion and/or a dry cough, often following a viral illness. Fever is rare. Physical examination demonstrates dry, bibasilar rales, often associated with clubbing of the fingers and sometimes of the toes. The chest radiograph typically shows a diffuse reticulonodular infiltrate most prominent at the bases without hilar or pleural abnormalities. Some patients have various "autoimmune" abnormalities that likely represent nonspecific epiphenomena. Circulating immune complexes are common. Pulmonary function tests yield typical findings for ILD, i.e., reduced volumes and diffusing capacity. Routine tests of airflow are normal, but sensitive tests reveal mild airflow limitation, an observation that correlates with morphologic evidence of narrowing of small airways. Patients with IPF have mild resting hypoxemia that drops significantly with physical activity. Typically, a resting Po_2 of 80 torr will fall to 50 torr with the exercise equivalent to walking up one flight of stairs. Ventilation and perfusion studies reveal diffuse, patchy abnormalities with mismatching of air and blood. The gallium-67 scan usually shows a diffuse uptake of isotope throughout the lung parenchyma, and bronchoalveolar lavage reveals an alveolitis pattern dominated by neutrophils and macrophages, with fewer numbers of lymphocytes and eosinophils. The epithelial lining fluid of the lower respiratory tract contains elevated levels of immunoglobulin G (IgG), immune complexes, and neutrophil products, including collagenase and myeloperoxidase. Open lung biopsy shows a diffuse alveolitis that is patchy in its intensity. There is marked derangement of the alveolar walls with a fibrosis-type pattern, including denudation of the epithelial basement membranes; replacement of the type I epithelial cells by type II epithelial cells and bronchiolar cells; loss of capillaries; and expansion of the interstitium with edema, increased numbers of mesenchymal cells, and masses of deranged collagen fibers. The epithelial basement membranes have holes through which the interstitial fibrosis extends into the air spaces.

The clinical course of IPF is characterized by progressive loss of alveolar-capillary units, with eventual respiratory failure and death occurring an average of 5 years after the onset of symptoms. Occasional patients have a rapidly progressive course; others may live for 10 or more years. IPF is associated with a higher than expected incidence of myocardial infarction and pulmonary embolism and, in association with cigarette smoking, a high incidence of lung carcinoma.

DIFFERENTIAL DIAGNOSIS. Although the term "IPF" suggests that the diagnosis is one of exclusion, its features are so characteristic that the diagnosis is usually not difficult. Most confusion arises in distinguishing IPF from ILD associated with the collagen vascular disorders; however, the latter are systemic diseases, whereas IPF is compartmentalized to the lung. To exclude the ILD of known etiology that can mimic IPF, it is mandatory to take a careful history of past exposures to agents that can cause ILD. An open lung biopsy is necessary for diagnosis, but IPF cannot be diagnosed using morphologic criteria alone. While the biopsy features of IPF fit the morphologic categories of "usual interstitial pneumonitis (UIP)," "desquamative interstitial pneumonitis (DIP)," or, more commonly, a mixture of UIP and DIP, these features are not specific for IPF and can be found in other ILD of both known and unknown etiology.

PATHOGENESIS. IPF likely results from uncontrolled inflammatory processes that ensue after any of a variety of insults to the lower respiratory tract of susceptible individuals. The susceptibility to this disease is probably inherited but links to a specific gene locus have not been made. The neutrophil-macrophage–dominated alveolitis, the first known manifestation of IPF, may be driven by immune complexes of unknown origin formed within the lower respiratory tract. The immune complexes are probably associated with enhanced lung B cell immunoglobin production, with at least some of the immunoglobulins directed against local self-antigens. These immune complexes activate alveolar macrophages to release neutrophil-specific chemotactic factors that recruit neutrophils to the alveolar structures. The neutrophils damage the alveolar walls by releasing toxic oxygen radicals and proteases. IPF macrophages spontaneously release exaggerated amounts of platelet-derived growth factor, fibronectin, and the alveolar macrophage form of insulin-like growth factor 1 and thus expand the numbers of mesenchymal cells, resulting in fibrosis of the alveolar walls.

STAGING AND THERAPY. The degree of lung damage in IPF is determined by history, chest radiograph, and pulmonary function testing. The intensity of the alveolitis of IPF can be gauged by gallium-67 scanning and bronchoalveolar lavage, with particular emphasis placed on the intensity of the neutrophil component of the alveolitis. The use of corticosteroids, usually lifelong, is the conventional therapy. Approximately 10 to 20 per cent of patients with IPF improve with corticosteroids, particularly if the disease is detected early, before the alveolitis causes significant abnormalities. The second line of therapy is either the addition of massive doses of methylprednisolone sodium succinate (Solu-Medrol) (2 grams given intravenously [IV] once weekly) or oral cyclophosphamide (1.5 mg per kilogram per day). Either approach helps suppress the alveolitis, but the long-term efficacy is unknown.

Sarcoidosis

Sarcoidosis (Ch. 67) is a multisystem granulomatous disease of unknown etiology characterized in affected organs by a CD4+ T-helper cell–mononuclear phagocyte inflammatory process, noncaseating granulomas, and derangement of normal tissue architecture. While most organs can be affected by sarcoidosis, the lower respiratory tract is the site that most commonly causes morbidity and mortality. Pulmonary sarcoidosis is characterized by sharply circumscribed granulomas in the alveolar, bronchial, and vascular walls, composed of tightly packed cells derived from the mononuclear phagocyte system. In some cases, the alveolar walls are deranged in a fashion similar to that seen in IPF, but much less so. Significant interstitial fibrosis occurs in 20 to 25 per cent of patients. Sarcoidosis is described in detail in Ch. 67 and will not be discussed further here.

ILD Associated with the Collagen Vascular Disorders

All collagen vascular disorders are associated with ILD. In most cases the collagen vascular disorder is apparent before lung involvement is noted, but occasionally the ILD develops first and the other characteristic systemic signs and symptoms appear later. In either case, these disorders are frequently confused with IPF.

RHEUMATOID ARTHRITIS (Ch. 258). The ILD associated with rheumatoid arthritis include (1) an IPF-like disorder, (2) Caplan's syndrome (rheumatoid arthritis associated with coal worker's pneumoconiosis), (3) pulmonary parenchymal rheumatoid nodules, (4) pulmonary arteritis, and (5) apical fibrobullous disease. A few patients with rheumatoid arthritis have been described with dyspnea, severe irreversible airway obstruction with hyperinflation, and morphologic evidence of obliterative bronchiolitis. While some of this terminal airway disease may be related to penicillamine therapy, it may represent another manifestation of rheumatoid arthritis in the lung parenchyma.

The IPF-like disorder is by far the most common pulmonary manifestation of rheumatoid arthritis. Approximately 25 per cent of chest radiographs of patients with rheumatoid arthritis show interstitial changes, and the diffusing capacity is reduced in 50 per cent of all patients. In most cases the lung disease is much milder than IPF. The pathogenesis of the ILD is unknown but assumed to be the consequence of the same processes that affect the joints. The alveolitis is similar to IPF, but the neutrophil component is much less evident. There is no relationship between the extent of disease and the titer of the rheumatoid factor. Most cases of ILD associated with rheumatoid arthritis do not need to be treated. If treatment is instituted, guidelines similar to those for IPF are used. Gold salts, a common therapy for rheumatoid arthritis, can also induce ILD. There is no way to distinguish between gold salt- and rheumatoid arthritis–induced ILD, except that the gold-induced disease may reverse when the drug is discontinued.

PROGRESSIVE SYSTEMIC SCLEROSIS (PSS) (Ch. 262). The most common form of ILD associated with PSS is similar to IPF. The incidence of ILD among patients with PSS is very high; at autopsy, morphologic changes are found in 90 per cent and radiographic evidence of ILD is found in 30 to 40 per cent of patients. PSS patients with the CREST syndrome (calcinosis, Raynaud's phenomenon, esophageal involvement, sclerodactyly, and telangiectasia) rarely develop ILD. The ILD associated with PSS is generally indolent, but if it becomes symptomatic, the 4-year survival rate is about 50 per cent. Although PSS is considered a connective tissue disorder with fibrosis as its main feature, patients with the ILD associated with PSS have an alveolitis, albeit milder than that of IPF. Gallium-67 scans are often positive. For most patients, the alveolitis is dominated by macrophages, but neutrophils and sometimes lymphocytes play a role. The ILD linked with PSS is associated with a higher than normal incidence of bronchogenic carcinoma, particularly bronchoalveolar cell carcinoma.

Occasional patients with PSS develop an ILD characterized by pulmonary hypertension, with relatively less disease of the alveolar-capillary units. Morphologically, there is thickening of the pulmonary arteries with fibrosis and some inflammation. Many of these patients develop rapidly progressive respiratory failure.

The pathogenesis of the ILD associated with PSS is unknown. The therapeutic guidelines are unclear, although patients with progressive disease usually are treated in a similar fashion to those with IPF. Penicillamine has been suggested as an alternative therapy, but its efficacy is unproved.

SYSTEMIC LUPUS ERYTHEMATOSUS (SLE) (Ch. 261). The common manifestations of SLE in the lung include pleurisy with or without effusion, atelectasis, and acute pneumonitis. Less frequently, SLE manifests as uremic pulmonary edema, diaphragmatic dysfunction, parenchymal hemorrhage, or chronic ILD. Most cases of chronic ILD have pulmonary features similar to those of IPF, together with the systemic findings of SLE. Rarely, ILD associated with SLE can also manifest with a lymphocytic alveolitis similar to Sjögren's syndrome, a disorder similar to idiopathic pulmonary hemosiderosis, or a hypersensitivity vasculitis–like condition. Together, the incidence of acute and chronic pulmonary involvement in SLE is fewer than 20 per cent of all cases of SLE, and chronic ILD occurs in fewer than 5 per cent. Chronic ILD can appear insidiously or follow the acute pneumonitis of SLE, a severe illness characterized by fever, tachypnea, radiographic evidence of patchy or diffuse infiltrates, and hypoxemia. The pathogenesis of the ILD associated with SLE is thought to result from the deposition of circulating immune complexes in the alveolar walls. Therapy is usually with corticosteroids, but specific treatment guidelines have not been established. SLE can be associated with pulmonary infection, and this must be distinguished from ILD before corticosteroid therapy is started.

POLYMYOSITIS/DERMATOMYOSITIS (Ch. 268). The incidence of ILD in polymyositis/dermatomyositis is 5 to 10 per cent. The proportion of patients who develop ILD before the extrapulmonary manifestations is higher in polymyositis/dermatomyositis than in any other collagen vascular disorder. The ILD is similar to IPF, but its pathogenesis is unclear. Patients are usually treated with corticosteroids, but methotrexate has been suggested as alternative therapy.

SJÖGREN'S SYNDROME (Ch. 263). Approximately 3 per cent of patients with Sjögren's syndrome develop ILD that manifests as either a mild IPF-like disease or, more commonly, a disorder with a lymphocyte-dominant alveolitis, similar to the lymphocytic infiltration of other organs in these patients. This lymphocytic form of ILD can be mild to severe and can undergo transformation to a lymphocytic malignancy, an event that is invariably fatal. Therapy of either ILD associated with Sjögren's syndrome is controversial; corticosteroids, immunosuppressive agents, and no therapy have all been advocated.

MIXED CONNECTIVE TISSUE DISEASE (Ch. 262). Up to 80 per cent of patients with this systemic disorder have ILD. The lung disease is usually like IPF. Pulmonary hypertension is common and can occur without significant parenchymal involvement. Therapy is usually with corticosteroids, with or without cytotoxic agents.

ANKYLOSING SPONDYLITIS (Ch. 259). Lung disease, manifested as chest wall restriction and upper lobe fibrobullous disease, occurs in about 1 per cent of patients with ankylosing spondylitis. Most patients are asymptomatic, but colonization with organisms such as *Aspergillus* or atypical mycobacteria is common, and hemoptysis and pneumothorax occur in the late stages of the disease. While HLA-B27 (HLA = human leukocyte antigen) is strongly associated with ankylosing spondylitis, it is not common in those patients with the associated ILD. The morphology of the ILD is like that of IPF, together with localized destruction of alveolar walls and bullae. There is no known therapy.

Histiocytosis X

Histiocytosis X (HX) (Ch. 149), also called "pulmonary Langerhans' cell granulomatosis," "primary pulmonary histiocytosis," and "eosinophilic granuloma," is a fibrotic-destructive disorder of the lower respiratory tract associated with an intense mononuclear phagocyte–dominant alveolitis. HX is grouped with the other proliferative disorders of the mononuclear phagocyte system, such as Letterer-Siwe and Hand-Schüller-Christian disease. In adults, HX is primarily a lung disease, although bone, skin, and central nervous system manifestations do occur. At least 50 per cent of all patients have chronic symptoms, and the disease can be fatal. More than 1000 cases have been reported; most new patients are 20 to 40 years of age, and there is an equal sex distribution. Almost all patients with HX have been cigarette smokers.

The patient with HX presents with a nonproductive cough, dyspnea on exertion, or chest pain. Spontaneous pneumothorax occurs in 10 per cent of cases; fever, weight loss, hemoptysis, and wheezing are occasionally noted. Bone involvement is present in a minority of patients. Posterior pituitary involvement with diabetes insipidus is unusual, as are skin lesions. Physical examination commonly reveals decreased breath sounds and rales. The chest radiograph shows upper and midzone small, irregular nodules superimposed on a delicate cystic pattern. The costophrenic angles are usually clear, and the pleura and hila are normal. Pulmonary function tests show a mixed restrictive-obstructive pattern with reduced lung volumes, reduced diffusing capacity, airflow limitation, and hypoxemia that worsens with exercise.

Definitive diagnosis is made by open lung biopsy. The disease is focal but poorly demarcated. There are sites of intense alveolitis dominated by alveolar macrophages and Langerhans' cells. Gallium-67 scans are negative or only mildly positive. Bronchoalveolar lavage reveals a macrophage-dominant alveolitis, and Langerhans' cells can be detected in lavage by ultrastructure and the T6 monoclonal antibody. The pathogenesis of this rare entity is discussed in Ch. 149. The lung disease in adults is considered untreatable.

Goodpasture's Syndrome

Goodpasture's syndrome (Ch. 79) is characterized by diffuse pulmonary hemorrhage, ILD, glomerulonephritis, and circulating anti–glomerular basement membrane (anti-GBM) and anti–alveolar basement membrane (anti-ABM) antibodies. It is assumed that the anti-GBM and anti-ABM antibodies are identical and cross-react with identical components in the kidney and lung basement membranes. Goodpasture's syndrome can be mimicked by SLE, Wegener's granulomatosis, and the systemic necrotizing vasculitides. In the appropriate clinical setting, the diagnosis of Goodpasture's syndrome is straightforward but does require (1) demonstration of the circulating antibodies, (2) characteristic linear deposits of immunoglobulin along the glomerular basement membrane, and (3) demonstration that the antibodies (either those circulating or those eluted from the kidney) are specific. It is usually not necessary to obtain lung tissue to make the diagnosis, but the diagnosis can be confirmed by histologic and immunofluorescence study of lung tissue obtained by transbronchial biopsy.

Almost all of the anti–basement membrane antibodies in Goodpasture's syndrome are IgG, but immunoglobulin A (IgA) anti-GBM and anti-ABM antibodies have been described in the setting of pulmonary hemorrhage and glomerulonephritis. The basement membrane antigen (or antigens) against which the antibodies are directed is thought to be a portion of type IV (basement membrane) collagen that is somehow unmasked in the kidney and lung.

Goodpasture's syndrome occurs mostly in young men. In most cases, evidence of alveolar hemorrhage precedes the clinical evidence of renal disease. Hemoptysis occurs in almost all cases, tends to be recurrent, and occasionally is massive and life threatening. In such cases, death is from asphyxiation. Anemia is almost always present. The chest radiograph reveals interstitial and alveolar infiltrates. The patchy infiltrates due to the hemorrhage often clear, but the interstitial markings, reflecting chronic ILD, often remain. Histologic findings include alveolar hemorrhage, hemosiderin-laden macrophages, focal areas of alveolitis, and interstitial fibrosis. Linear deposits of IgG can be detected in the alveolar walls.

Spontaneous remissions of Goodpasture's syndrome can occur but are rare. Therapy generally consists of corticosteroids, cytotoxic agents, and plasmapheresis.

Idiopathic Pulmonary Hemosiderosis (IPH)

IPH is a rare disorder of unknown cause characterized by alveolar hemorrhage, iron deficiency anemia, transient parenchymal infiltrates on the chest radiograph, and ILD. The disease is most common in individuals less than 20 years of age, but adult cases are seen. The disease is occasionally found in families, but a genetic basis has not been proved. IPH is compartmentalized in the lung and must be distinguished from Goodpasture's syndrome, Wegener's granulomatosis, SLE, and the vasculitides.

The patient with IPH presents with repetitive acute episodes of dyspnea, cough with hemoptysis, and fever. Iron deficiency anemia is common. The chest radiographs associated with these acute episodes reveal transient infiltrates, a miliary pattern, or massive confluent shadows. On this background of intermittent episodes, a chronic ILD develops, with increasing dyspnea, rales, clubbing, and pulmonary hypertension. While the childhood form of the disease is aggressive, with a mean survival of about 3 years, adult IPH tends to be more insidious. Lung function tests are typical for ILD, but the diffusing capacity may be falsely high owing to increased uptake of the carbon monoxide (used as the test gas) by free hemoglobin in the lung parenchyma. Hemosiderin-laden macrophages in sputum or lavage fluid suggest prior parenchymal hemorrhage. In the appropriate clinical setting, when there are no detectable anti-GBM antibodies, a definitive diagnosis of IPH can be made with an open lung biopsy revealing

focal hemorrhage, a macrophage-dominant alveolitis with siderin-positive macrophages, and typical findings of ILD. The pathogenesis of this disorder is unknown. Corticosteroids are generally used to treat the acute episodes and the chronic ILD, but there is no evidence regarding their efficacy.

Chronic Eosinophilic Pneumonia (CEP)

CEP is a chronic ILD characterized by cough, dyspnea, malaise, fever, night sweats, weight loss, variable degrees of blood eosinophilia, and a chest film revealing peripheral, nonsegmental, nonmigratory infiltrates. Rarely, acute cases can result in the rapid development of respiratory failure. Hilar adenopathy rarely occurs. Asthma accompanies CEP in 50 to 60 per cent of cases. High proportions of eosinophils are sometimes recovered in sputum or by lavage. A very high sedimentation rate is common, and elevated levels of immunoglobulin E (IgE) during acute episodes have been described. The histologic findings of CEP include a diffuse alveolitis dominated by eosinophils and macrophages with fewer numbers of neutrophils and lymphocytes. Eosinophilic abscesses, multinucleated giant cells, angiitis of small pulmonary vessels, and interstitial fibrosis are common.

Although the stimulus to the accumulation of the eosinophils in the lung is unknown, the eosinophil can damage the cells and matrix of the alveolar walls through its release of toxic oxygen radicals, collagenase, and major basic protein, a highly charged polypeptide associated with the eosinophil granules.

An open lung biopsy is required to make a definitive diagnosis. However, because CEP usually responds dramatically to corticosteroids, a tentative diagnosis is often made on clinical grounds only, without biopsy confirmation, and corticosteroid therapy is instituted. In some patients, the disease is only partly suppressed by corticosteroids, and long-term treatment is required.

Lymphocytic Infiltrative Disorders

This is a group of rare, diffuse ILD characterized by infiltration of the alveolar structures by cells of the lymphocyte series. Most patients present with cough and dyspnea, occasionally with fever. All of the lymphocyte infiltrative disorders of lung can progress to frank lymphoma.

Immunoblastic lymphadenopathy (also called angioimmunoblastic lymphadenopathy) is a systemic disorder, usually of elderly individuals, characterized by generalized lymphadenopathy, hepatosplenomegaly, and variable amounts of ILD. The disease has no known etiology, but associations with drugs have been reported, including antibiotics and phenytoin. A skin rash is observed in one third of cases; there may be a coexistent collagen vascular disorder or hemolytic anemia. There are polyclonal increases in serum immunoglobulins. The alveolar structures exhibit a pleomorphic alveolitis representing all levels of lymphocyte differentiation. Diagnosis is usually made by lymph node biopsy. The disease can remit spontaneously, but patients die of progressive respiratory failure, infection, or malignancy. The response to therapy with corticosteroids and/or cytotoxic agents is variable.

Lymphocytic interstitial pneumonitis is limited to the lung. The signs and symptoms are typical for an insidious, slowly progressive ILD. It is most common in women in their 40's, but it is observed in males and all age groups. The chest radiograph characteristically shows diffuse reticulonodular infiltrates. Most patients have dysproteinemias. Some cases, particularly in the pediatric population, are associated with HIV infection. Hypergammaglobulinemia and hypogammaglobulinemia have been described, and an association with Sjögren's syndrome is common. The diagnosis is made by an open lung biopsy revealing diffuse parenchymal infiltration with mature lymphocytes, plasma cells, and immunoblasts. Granulomas are sometimes observed. Because the infiltrating cells may form germinal centers, the disease is sometimes called "pseudolymphoma." The prognosis of lymphocytic interstitial pneumonitis is variable, and some patients progress to end-stage lung disease or lymphoma. Treatment is with corticosteroids and/or immunosuppressive agents.

ILD Associated with Pulmonary Vasculitis

Many of the systemic vasculitides result in ILD as a consequence of a pulmonary vasculitis causing a secondary alveolitis and derangements of the alveolar structures.

Wegener's granulomatosis is a granulomatous vasculitis of the upper and lower respiratory tracts and kidney (Ch. 266). There is a limited form of the disease without clinically apparent renal disease. All patients have pulmonary involvement, but only one third have symptoms related to the lungs. Airway involvement is common. The parenchymal lung disease can appear as discrete nodules and/or diffuse ILD; either can undergo necrosis and cavity formation. Hemoptysis, cough, sputum production, dyspnea, and pleuritic pain are common. Lung function tests reveal a mixed restrictive-obstructive pattern. Diagnosis is usually made by open lung biopsy. Untreated disease is usually fatal, but with cyclophosphamide therapy long-term survival is the rule.

Lymphomatoid granulomatosis is a systemic vasculitis involving the lung, skin, central nervous system, and kidneys. The lung is always affected, but involvement of other organs is variable. In the lung, the walls of the blood vessels are infiltrated with typical and atypical lymphocytes, together with some granulomas, and there is associated ILD. A mild form of lymphomatoid granulomatosis has been described ("benign lymphocytic angiitis and granulomatosis"). The disease is most common in middle age. Multiple, fleeting nodular densities are seen on the chest film; occasionally there are diffuse infiltrates. Death is usually due to parenchymal destruction with sepsis and occasionally to massive hemoptysis. The diagnosis is usually established by biopsy of the lung or skin. The lung disease often responds to corticosteroids and cyclophosphamide, but the central nervous system lesions do not. Lymphoma occurs in about 10 per cent of cases.

The *Churg-Strauss syndrome* (allergic angiitis and granulomatosis) (Ch. 264) is a form of systemic necrotizing vasculitis that almost always involves the lung, unlike classic polyarteritis nodosa, which rarely does. The pulmonary manifestations, consisting of asthma and diffuse infiltrates, often precede systemic involvement by 1 or 2 years. A history of allergy is common. An elevated sedimentation rate and total eosinophil count are common. The systemic vasculitis involves skin, heart, and gastrointestinal tract. Diagnosis is made by open lung biopsy, which shows a granulomatous vasculitis with eosinophilic infiltration, a secondary diffuse alveolitis, interstitial granulomas, and fibrosis. Treatment is the same as for the other pulmonary vasculitides.

Hypersensitivity vasculitis represents a heterogeneous group of vasculitides whose development is thought to be related to sensitization to antigens such as drugs or serum proteins. Skin involvement is most common; most cases do not involve the lung. When they do, there is a small-vessel polymorphonuclear leukocyte vasculitis with fibrinoid necrosis and secondary ILD. Diagnosis is usually made by skin biopsy, and the disorder is often self-limiting. A similar disorder can occur in association with mixed cryoglobulinemia or Henoch-Schönlein purpura.

Inherited Disorders

There is a small group of rare ILD that are clearly inherited. Almost all are autosomal dominant disorders, although the autosomal recessive disorders Hermansky-Pudlak syndrome, Niemann-Pick disease, and Gaucher's disease may rarely be associated with ILD.

FAMILIAL IDIOPATHIC PULMONARY FIBROSIS. This is a chronic, usually fatal autosomal dominant disorder identical to IPF. Symptoms usually begin in the fifth or sixth decade, but the disease can be manifested earlier. Some of the asymptomatic children of affected family members have evidence of a mild alveolitis yet with normal lung function, suggesting that the disease begins with an alveolitis.

NEUROFIBROMATOSIS (Ch. 467). Von Recklinghausen's disease is an autosomal dominant disorder characterized by pigmented skin lesions and neurofibromas of the peripheral and central nervous systems. In 10 to 20 per cent of adult cases there is a coexisting ILD and/or bullous lung disease. The ILD has histologic features similar to those of IPF, but it is not known whether it responds to similar therapies.

TUBEROUS SCLEROSIS (Ch. 467). This is a hamartomatous autosomal dominant disorder involving the central nervous system, skin, kidneys, eyes, bones, heart, and, in 1 per cent of patients, the lungs. Although the hamartomatous "tumors" are composed of various cell types in most affected organs, in the

lung they are composed only of smooth muscle cells. The accumulation of smooth muscle cells in the alveolar interstitium causes ILD, together with parenchymal destruction. Unlike most ILD, there is little alveolitis. The chest radiograph shows diffuse infiltrates and honeycombing, and lung function tests show a mixed pattern with a dominant obstructive pattern. Pneumothorax is common. There is no known therapy.

ILD Associated with Pulmonary Airway Disease

This term refers to disorders in which the ILD is likely secondary to a primary airway disease. It is unclear if there are many such diseases or only one. The characteristic lesions are necrotic granulomas in the bronchial walls, with the bronchiolar lumina filled with palisading epithelioid cells, cellular debris, and polymorphonuclear leukocytes. A diffuse alveolitis and nongranulomatous fibrosis-type derangements of the alveolar walls are usually present. Approximately one third of patients have asthma, blood eosinophilia, mucus plugging, fungal hyphae identifiable in the airways, and positive sputum cultures for *Aspergillus* organisms. These patients are usually referred to as having *bronchopulmonary aspergillosis* (see Ch. 406). It is unclear, however, whether the fungus is a primary cause of the disease or represents a secondary process.

The remaining two thirds of patients, referred to as having *bronchocentric granulomatosis*, do not have asthma, microscopic evidence of fungi, or blood eosinophilia. The disease can present in an insidious manner or as an acute febrile illness. The chest film usually shows nodular or mass lesions; diffuse infiltrates are seen in about 20 per cent of cases. Lung function tests demonstrate a mixed obstructive-restrictive pattern. Corticosteroids are usually the therapy of choice.

Lymphangioleiomyomatosis

This is a rare disease of women, almost always of childbearing age, characterized by the proliferation of benign but atypical smooth muscle cells in walls of the lymphatics of the lower respiratory tract, pleura, mediastinum, and retroperitoneum. Although it is an ILD characterized by thickening and derangements of the alveolar walls, very little inflammation is present. Eventual destruction of the alveolar walls is common. The clinical findings include dyspnea, recurrent unilateral or bilateral chylous pleural effusions, pneumothorax, hemoptysis, and occasionally peritoneal chylous effusions. The chest radiograph has a characteristic reticulonodular pattern on a background of diffuse cystic changes, similar to that seen in HX. Lung function tests reveal a mixed obstructive-restrictive pattern. An open lung biopsy is required to make the diagnosis. It has been theorized that the disease results from an abnormal response to estrogens, and thus oophorectomy, progesterone, and tamoxifen therapy have all been tried in these patients. There is no proven efficacy of such therapies, and the disease is almost always fatal, usually within 10 years of diagnosis.

Alveolar Proteinosis

In this disorder the alveoli are filled with a periodic acid–Schiff (PAS)–positive lipid and protein-rich granular material. There may be an accompanying mononuclear cell alveolitis and fibrosis-type derangements of the alveolar walls. Although of unknown etiology, alveolar proteinosis can be associated with silicosis, hematologic malignancies, bronchogenic cyst, and mycobacterial and fungal diseases of the lung. Why this material accumulates in the alveoli is unknown but is speculated to result from the breakdown of cells in the lower respiratory tract, from the overproduction of substances normally secreted into the alveolar spaces (e.g., surfactant), from increased transudation of plasma proteins, or from decreased alveolar clearance mechanisms.

The disease usually begins insidiously with dyspnea as the initial symptom. The chest radiograph has a characteristic diffuse, finely nodular alveolar filling pattern. Lung function tests show decreased lung volumes and diffusing capacity. There is usually hypoxemia secondary to pulmonary blood shunting by filled alveoli. Open lung biopsy is ordinarily required for the diagnosis. However, in the appropriate clinical setting, bronchoalveolar lavage recovery of the typical material, together with transbronchial biopsy evidence of alveoli filled with PAS-positive material, is usually diagnostic. Alveolar proteinosis can be fatal but can also spontaneously resolve. The recommended therapy is massive whole-lung lavage with the patient under general anesthesia. Corticosteroid therapy has no proven use and may lead to the development of opportunistic infections.

Miscellaneous Other ILD of Unknown Etiology

There are several ILD of unknown etiology that are reasonably well defined but so rare that there is little information available concerning their pathogenesis and no apparent guidelines relating to their staging and therapy. These are included by list in Table 60–1 but will not be discussed individually here.

INTERSTITIAL LUNG DISEASE OF KNOWN ETIOLOGY

Approximately 135 agents are known to cause ILD, but together they are responsible for only one third of all cases of ILD. In terms of numbers of patients that come to medical attention, the most important agents are crystalline silica, asbestos, coal dust, organic dusts of the *Micropolyspora* and *Thermoactinomyces* genera and those derived from avian proteins, some antineoplastic drugs, nitrofurantoin, and hyperoxia.

Inhaled Inorganic Dusts

ILD resulting from the chronic inhalation of an inorganic dust is called a "pneumoconiosis" (see Table 60–2). The most common are silicosis, asbestosis, and coal worker's pneumoconiosis. The common pneumoconioses are all characterized by fibrosis-type derangements of the lower respiratory tract.

There are several important principles relevant to understanding the pneumoconioses. (1) The dusts themselves cause little damage to the lung parenchyma; it is the inflammatory response to the dusts that causes the loss of functional alveolar-capillary units. (2) A number of defense mechanisms prevent such dusts from reaching the alveoli, and others remove most dusts that might reach the lower respiratory tract. Just because an individual has been exposed to an inorganic dust does not mean that the dust has necessarily caused ILD. (3) Abnormalities on a chest radiograph consistent with exposure to an inorganic dust do not prove that the individual has a functionally significant ILD. (4) These chronic disorders result from the inhalation of high concentrations of inorganic dusts over many years; i.e., history of a brief exposure sometime in the past is not sufficient evidence to implicate a particular dust. (5) No known therapy has proven efficacy for any pneumoconiosis; current "treatment" for all pneumoconioses is permanent removal from inhalation of the causative agent. (6) Many individuals exposed to inorganic dusts also have a history of chronic cigarette smoking; this must be taken into account when evaluating these patients. (7) Physical evidence of the inorganic dust in the lung is useful but not critical in making the diagnosis of a common pneumoconiosis (silicosis, asbestosis, coal worker's pneumoconiosis) as long as the chronic exposure history is very clear and unambiguous. For the other inorganic dusts, however, biopsy evidence is required to make a definitive diagnosis. (8) While the miners and millers who work around these inorganic dusts represent the "classic" exposure situations, inorganic dust materials are widely used in manufacturing. A careful occupational history is required, or the exposure history may be missed. *Coal worker's pneumoconiosis, silicosis, asbestosis,* and *berylliosis* are described in Ch. 527, Occupational Pulmonary Disorders.

Inhaled Organic Dusts

The repeated inhalation of certain organic dusts (see also Ch. 527) causes a granulomatous ILD called *hypersensitivity pneumonitis* or *extrinsic allergic alveolitis.* The term "hypersensitivity pneumonitis" is reserved for those ILD caused by organic dusts derived from living sources. A large number of organic dusts have been implicated (see Table 60–3), but the most common are the thermophilic organisms of the *Micropolyspora* and *Thermoactinomyces* groups and those derived from avian proteins.

The nomenclature relating to hypersensitivity pneumonitis is confusing because the name of the disease usually refers to the situation of exposure (e.g., "maple bark stripper's disease," "humidifier lung"), even though the organic dusts causing different diseases may be identical. For example, *Thermoactinomyces vulgaris* can cause "farmer's lung," "humidifier lung," and "mushroom worker's lung." The most common exposure situations are farmers exposed to moldy hay, individuals exposed to organic antigens growing in humidifiers and air conditioners, and bird breeders, particularly those raising pigeons. The other exposure situations are varied, and the list is ever expanding (see Table 60–3).

Classically, 4 to 6 hours after inhalation of the antigen, a sensitized individual develops acute symptoms of hypersensitivity pneumonitis, including fever, cough, dyspnea, and malaise. The chest film at this time shows diffuse parenchymal infiltrates, and lung function tests demonstrate decreased lung volumes, decreased diffusing capacity, mild airflow limitation, and hypoxemia. If the individual is removed from the antigen exposure, there is gradual improvement in symptoms, the chest film, and lung function tests over a 24-hour period. If the exposures are few, there are few sequelae other than the acute episodes. However, in some individuals, for unknown reasons, repetitive exposure leads to a chronic ILD characterized by lymphocyte-macrophage alveolitis occasionally mixed with neutrophils. Initially, the derangements are of the distortion type, with lymphocytes and granulomas in the alveolar walls. Later, however, there are fibrotic changes, including intra-alveolar fibrosis. Rarely, the chronic form develops in an insidious manner without the acute episodes.

The diagnosis of hypersensitivity pneumonitis is made in the context of a history of exposure to a known causative antigen, the presence of ILD, the presence of antigen-specific antibodies in the blood, and an open lung biopsy demonstrating the characteristic morphology. The gallium-67 scan is usually positive, and bronchoalveolar lavage shows a lymphocyte-macrophage alveolitis, mixed with neutrophils when the exposure has been recent. When the history is typical, a biopsy is not necessary to make the diagnosis, but there must be a clear demonstration of the acute symptoms 4 to 6 hours after inhalation of the antigen.

The mechanisms by which sensitization to these organic dusts causes either the acute or the chronic disease are unknown. T cells, the majority of which have suppressor/cytotoxic (CD8+) surface markers, dominate the alveolitis. The T cells in the lung and blood are sensitized to the offending antigen. Besides the circulating antigen-specific immunoglobulins, levels of IgG and immunoglobulin M (IgM) are increased in the lower respiratory tract. However, there is no evidence that the immunoglobulins play a role in the pathogenesis of the disease, and immune complexes have not been convincingly demonstrated in the lower respiratory tract. One of the confusing aspects of this disease is that although many exposed individuals become sensitized to the organic antigen (as manifested by the presence of antigen-specific antibodies in the blood), only a very small proportion will develop either the acute or the chronic symptoms of hypersensitivity pneumonitis.

The prognosis of chronic hypersensitivity pneumonitis is not clear. In those with farmer's lung, there is a 10 per cent mortality over 6 years, with an additional 30 per cent having significant functional impairment. Management of hypersensitivity pneumonitis is directed toward removing the patient from the source of the antigen and suppressing the alveolitis, usually with corticosteroids.

Drug-Induced ILD

Drug-induced ILD are disorders in which the lower respiratory tract is structurally and/or functionally deranged as a result of a pharmacologic agent. The list of drugs reported to cause ILD is large (see Table 60–4) and includes those producing acute, subacute, and chronic ILD. Drug-induced ILD can be serious and sometimes fatal, but they are usually effectively treated simply by recognizing the disorder and discontinuing the responsible drug.

It is generally assumed that many of the drug-induced ILD are "hypersensitivity" reactions, but proof of an immune basis for these diseases is circumstantial at best. In many cases, it is thought that the drug injures the lung parenchyma in some fashion to initiate an alveolitis that propagates the injury.

Typically, the acute and subacute forms of drug-induced ILD present with respiratory decompensation following a prodrome of fever and cough. At this time there are usually increased heart and respiratory rates, dry rales, and, occasionally, cyanosis. The chest radiograph shows a patchy or diffuse reticulonodular infiltrate that can be confused with pulmonary edema. Pleural effusions are common. Blood studies often show eosinophilia and arterial hypoxemia and hypocarbia. Lung function tests are typical for ILD, and the gallium-67 scan is often positive. Open lung biopsy demonstrates parenchymal cell injury, edema of the alveolar wall, fibrin in the air spaces, and a patchy lymphocyte-macrophage alveolitis, sometimes mixed with neutrophils and/or eosinophils. In some cases, the course is rapidly downhill, requiring mechanical ventilation and oxygen administration. The disease is usually reversible if the drug is discontinued but can be fatal if this is not done early in the course.

One major area of confusion in conceptualizing and categorizing the drug-induced ILD disorders has resulted from the use of the term "pulmonary infiltration with eosinophilia (PIE) syndrome" to describe patients receiving drugs who develop an acute or subacute disorder characterized by blood eosinophilia and parenchymal infiltrates on the chest film. However, the PIE syndrome is far from diagnostic as a drug-induced ILD. Many non–drug-associated ILD of both known (e.g., acute beryllium-induced disease) and unknown etiology (e.g., IPF, sarcoidosis) can be associated with blood eosinophilia, and tropical pulmonary eosinophilia caused by filarial infestation presents in an identical manner. In addition, there is no evidence that the blood eosinophilia has any relevance to the pathogenesis of the disease in the lung. Thus, most clinicians have abandoned the concept of the PIE syndrome and simply think of these disorders as part of the spectrum of ILD in which the presence of blood eosinophilia is a helpful, but not definitive, clue to the diagnosis.

The chronic form of drug-induced ILD is much more insidious and difficult to associate with a drug as the etiologic agent. Fever is less common, and patients usually present with typical ILD. Occasionally there is blood eosinophilia. Because of the insidious nature of the chronic form of drug-induced ILD, many clinicians use lung function tests, particularly the diffusing capacity, to follow patients on drugs commonly associated with the development of ILD. The gallium-67 scan is usually positive. Open lung biopsy usually shows a lymphocyte-macrophage alveolitis with mixed numbers of polymorphonuclear leukocytes. The derangements are of the fibrosis type, often with intra-alveolar fibrosis. Unlike the acute and subacute forms of the drug-induced ILD, the chronic form often persists after the drug is discontinued. The reasons why this occurs are not clear, but it is likely that the injury to the parenchyma has been sufficient to establish a chronic alveolitis that propagates the disorder in the absence of the initial stimulus. In such cases, therapeutic strategies are directed toward suppressing the alveolitis, usually with corticosteroids.

ANTINEOPLASTIC AGENTS. *Bleomycin*-induced disease is common; up to 10 per cent of patients receiving bleomycin develop some ILD, and 1 per cent die of the ILD. Toxicity from this agent occurs in both acute and chronic forms and is potentiated by concomitant therapy with oxygen or irradiation. *Busulfan* lung disease occurs in 2 to 3 per cent of those receiving the drug. The disease is chronic, usually takes at least 1 year of therapy before it appears, and usually does not respond to withdrawal of the drug or to corticosteroids. *Methotrexate*-induced ILD can appear in acute or chronic form. Leucovorin or corticosteroids are not protective, but recovery is common once the drug is stopped. There are increasing numbers of reports of ILD induced by the *nitrosoureas*. The incidence of toxicity is about 1 per cent and occurs 2 months to 3 years after initiation of therapy. *Procarbazine* causes an acute ILD with pleural effusions, peripheral eosinophilia, and an eosinophilic alveolitis. Although *cyclophosphamide* is used to treat many ILD of unknown etiology, it can rarely cause acute or chronic ILD. Several other antineoplastic agents are reported to cause ILD, but very rarely.

ANTIBIOTICS. ILD induced by *nitrofurantoin* is a common adverse drug reaction, occurring in both acute and chronic forms. The acute form, 5 to 10 times more frequent than the chronic form, occurs in sensitized individuals within 1 month of reinstituting treatment. The disease almost always clears when the drug is discontinued. The chronic disease occurs following 6 to 12 months of therapy. Approximately 60 per cent have positive antinuclear antibodies. The prognosis is good once the drug is stopped, but permanent loss of lung function is common, and approximately 10 per cent die of the disease. The ILD caused by other antibiotics are also mostly acute disorders and are very rare.

CARDIOVASCULAR DRUGS. *Hydralazine* and *procainamide* induce an acute ILD similar to that associated with SLE. In contrast to spontaneously occurring SLE, which is common in blacks and women, the ILD produced by both of these drugs occurs more commonly in whites and affects a significant number of men. Most affected individuals have serum antinuclear antibodies. The disease usually disappears when the drug is stopped. Other drugs that can cause a similar syndrome include isoniazid, phenytoin, and allopurinol. Increasingly, ILD has been observed in association with amiodarone, a useful antiarrhythmic agent. The ILD is usually dose dependent and self-limiting but can be chronic even after the drug has been discontinued. The beta blockers can cause chronic ILD, but rarely. The disease is insidious and like IPF but is often associated with fibrosis elsewhere in the body.

OTHER DRUGS. *Gold salts* can induce ILD after 1 to 6 months of therapy; this form of ILD can be difficult to distinguish from the ILD associated with rheumatoid arthritis. The disease is thought to represent a hypersensitivity reaction. *Mineral oil*–induced ILD, sometimes called "lipoid pneumonia," results from the aspiration of mineral oil used as nose drops or ingested as a laxative. The open lung biopsy demonstrates a typical picture of lymphoid cells, lipid-laden macrophages, and fibrosis. With an appropriate history, however, the diagnosis can be made by recovering lipid-laden macrophages by bronchoalveolar lavage. The intravenous use of drugs meant for oral use can cause ILD by virtue of the presence of particulate material in the drugs, including talc, starch, maltose, or quinine. The disease is usually chronic and characterized by foreign body granulomatous reactions affecting pulmonary capillaries.

Many other drugs are known to cause acute and/or chronic ILD, and the list is ever expanding. Because these disorders are all potentially curable if the drug is stopped, it is critical to have a high index of suspicion of drug-induced disease whenever confronted by a patient with ILD.

Other Agents Known to Cause ILD

Beyond inorganic dusts, organic dusts, and drugs, the most important known causes of ILD are paraquat, radiation, the sequelae of prior infectious processes, hyperoxia, and chronic aspiration pneumonia. The others are very rare and mostly represent anecdotal case reports (see Table 60–5).

PARAQUAT. Poisoning with the herbicide paraquat can occur with oral, parenteral, aerosol, or dermal exposure. Paraquat is available in granules, aerosols, and liquid concentrates; ingestion of the liquid either by accident or by suicidal intent is the most common means of paraquat poisoning. Paraquat is an extremely potent cause of parenchymal derangement and fibrosis and consequent respiratory insufficiency. As little as 1 teaspoon of the concentrate can be fatal. The disease is usually acute, but chronic cases have been described. In acute cases, dyspnea, fever, fatigue, and gastrointestinal complaints occur 1 to 5 days after poisoning. Mouth, pharyngeal, and esophageal ulcerations are common following oral ingestion. Diffuse radiographic changes of ILD are quickly followed by rapidly progressive respiratory failure, usually requiring ventilatory support. Open lung biopsy reveals a neutrophil-macrophage alveolitis and alveolar wall derangements typical of ILD, but very severe. In addition to interstitial fibrosis, intra-alveolar fibrosis is common. In these acute cases, there is a rough correlation between plasma levels of paraquat and survival. If the plasma paraquat concentration 8 hours after ingestion is greater than 1200 μg per liter, death is inevitable. In addition to these acute cases, intermittent low-dose skin exposure may be hazardous and may lead to a chronic ILD.

Paraquat causes ILD by virtue of its propensity to be taken up by parenchymal cells of the lower respiratory tract, where it generates toxic oxygen radicals sufficient to damage the normal parenchymal components severely. There is a secondary alveolitis that further injures the parenchyma and mediates the development of fibrosis-type derangements. Treatment of paraquat poisoning is mostly supportive. Attempts should be made to remove the paraquat (gastric lavage with bentonite, Fuller's earth, or charcoal, followed by charcoal hemoperfusion). Since hyperoxia accelerates paraquat-induced injury, oxygen concentrations should be kept as low as possible. Antioxidant therapy (e.g., vitamin E) has been suggested, but its efficacy is unknown. In chronic cases, corticosteroids are usually used to suppress the alveolitis.

RADIATION. ILD resulting from thoracic irradiation is a common sequela of radiotherapy of breast, lung, or esophageal carcinoma and lymphoma and is potentiated by the concomitant use of antineoplastic drugs known to cause ILD. Radiation-induced lung disease is described in Ch. 530.

SEQUELAE OF KNOWN INFECTIOUS AGENTS. All types of infections of the lower respiratory tract may occasionally result in significant injury and fibrosis. Usually, the ILD remains localized to the site of infection and does not progress after eradication of the infectious agent. A typical example is the localized upper lobe scars left by mycobacterial infection. ILD has been described following *Mycoplasma* infection as well as *Legionella* pneumonia, and there are scattered reports of viral infections causing a progressive ILD. A significant number of individuals with HIV infection develop mild ILD. In some cases, this results from the inflammation associated with opportunistic infections, but in others, it is likely that the inflammation with resulting ILD is secondary to the local HIV infection. Tropical pulmonary eosinophilia due to chronic microfilarial infestation is a subacute ILD (see Ch. 437.3) and can evolve into a chronic ILD.

INHALED AGENTS OTHER THAN INORGANIC OR ORGANIC DUSTS. These agents include gases, aerosols, chemical dusts, fumes, and vapors. Most are rare causes of ILD, and there is little information available concerning pathogenesis, clinical course, staging, or therapy. Most are acute disorders that reverse when the agent is removed unless significant injury to the parenchyma has occurred.

The most common gas causing ILD is *oxygen*. The inhalation of high concentrations of oxygen over several days often causes parenchymal lung damage, particularly in the setting of acute respiratory failure in the intensive care situation (see Ch. 70). Oxygen toxicity can also be chronic. In contrast, the inhalation of gases such as the oxides of nitrogen, chlorine gas, and sulfur dioxide almost always cause only acute injury; if the patient survives the initial insult and respiratory failure, there are rarely any sequelae. In contrast, many of the survivors of methyl isocyanate exposure develop chronic fibrosis-type ILD.

Aerosols are particles of liquid suspended in a gas. The most common examples of ILD due to aerosol inhalation are the acute and chronic ILD resulting from aspiration of gastric contents (see Ch. 528) and the aspiration of mineral oil. Exposure to aerosols of cooking oils, pyrethrum (a neutral insecticide used in commercial and household products), and toluene diisocyanate has also been implicated as a cause of ILD.

ILD due to the inhalation of chemical dusts such as synthetic fibers, Bakelite, and vinyl chloride and polyvinyl chloride powder are probably hypersensitivity-type disorders similar to those associated with the repeated inhalation of organic dusts from living sources. Little is known about the clinical course of these disorders. ILD have also followed the inhalation of various fumes and vapors (see Table 60–5).

Cooper JAD, Jr (ed.): Drug-induced pulmonary disease. Clin Chest Med 2:1, 1990. *Details the pathogenesis and clinical findings in all of the drug-induced interstitial lung disorders.*

Crystal RG, Ferrans VJ: Reactions of the interstitial space to injury. *In* Fishman AP: Pulmonary Diseases and Disorders. New York, McGraw-Hill, 1988, pp 711–738. *General concepts of the processes that derange the alveolar walls.*

Crystal RG, Bitterman PB, Rennard SI, et al.: Interstitial lung diseases of unknown cause: Disorders characterized by chronic inflammation of the lower respiratory tract. N Engl J Med 310:154, 235, 1984. *A general review of the interstitial lung disorders of unknown etiology.*

Crystal RG, Ferrans VJ, Basset F: Biologic basis of pulmonary fibrosis. *In* Crystal RG, West JB (eds.): The Lung. Scientific Foundations. New York, Raven Press, 1991, pp 2031–2046. *Overview of the concepts underlying the development of fibrosis in the interstitial lung disorders.*

Crystal RG, Gadek JE, Ferrans VJ, et al.: Interstitial lung disease: Current concepts of pathogenesis, staging, and therapy. Am J Med 70:542, 1981. *Overviews the concepts of the pathogenesis of the interstitial lung disorders and emphasizes the approaches to staging and therapy.*

Davis WB, Crystal RG: Chronic interstitial lung disease. *In* Simmons DH (ed.):

Current Pulmonology. Vol. V. New York, John Wiley and Sons, 1984, pp 347–473. *Reviews each of the interstitial lung disorders.*

DuBois R, Saltini C, Holroyd K, et al.: Granulomatous processes. *In* Crystal RG, West JB (eds.): The Lung. Scientific Foundations. New York, Raven Press, 1991, pp 1925–1938. *General concepts of granulomatous disorders of the lung.*

Keogh BA, Crystal RG: Alveolitis: The key to the interstitial lung disorders. Thorax 37:1, 1982. *Summarizes the importance of alveolitis in the interstitial disorders.*

Morgan WKC, Seaton A: Occupational Lung Diseases. 2nd ed. Philadelphia, W. B. Saunders Company, 1984. *Overall summary of the interstitial lung disorders resulting from the inhalation of inorganic dusts.*

Rom R, Crystal RG: Consequences of chronic particulate exposure. *In* Crystal RG, West JB (eds.): The Lung. Scientific Foundations. New York, Raven Press, 1991, pp 1885–1898. *Recent review of the pathogenesis of the common pneumoconioses.*

Schwarz MI, King TE (eds.): Interstitial Lung Disease. Toronto, B. C. Decker, 1988. *General review of interstitial lung disease.*

61 Introduction to Pneumonia

Waldemar G. Johanson, Jr.

Pneumonia is a term used to indicate inflammation of the distal lung—terminal airways, alveolar spaces, and interstitium. To improve the precision of communication, the term "pneumonia" is usually further qualified with words that imply an etiology, mechanism, anatomic site, or clinical course. Thus, descriptors such as "viral bronchopneumonia," "aspiration pneumonia," "chronic interstitial pneumonia," or "acute bacterial pneumonia" serve to identify patients with clinical illnesses characterized by signs and symptoms of lung inflammation in a variety of clinical situations. This chapter will provide the background for the chapters that deal with specific forms of bacterial pneumonia (see Part XIX).

PATHOPHYSIOLOGY. Bacterial pneumonia can be simply defined as a condition that results when host defense mechanisms are insufficient to meet a bacterial challenge presented to the lungs. This definition emphasizes the two key aspects of bacterial pneumonia—host defenses and the type and route of bacterial challenge.

Bacterial Challenges to the Lungs. Bacteria may be introduced into the lungs by any of four routes (Table 61–1). The most common routes are aspiration of contaminated oropharyngeal secretions and inhalation of airborne bacteria. Organisms arriving in the lungs via the bloodstream may produce pneumonia, but the originating site of infection and the severe systemic effects of sepsis usually outweigh the importance of the resulting pneumonia. Direct extension from a focus of infection adjacent to the lungs is uncommon, and the initial site of infection is always more important.

Aspiration of contaminated oropharyngeal secretions is by far the most common route of lung inoculation leading to pneumonia. Organisms transmitted from person to person are usually deposited in the nose or mouth by one means or another, including the inhalation of large droplets generated by cough, sneeze, or even talking. These organisms initially establish themselves in the nasopharynx or oropharynx, where they join the plethora of organisms already present and multiply to achieve high local concentrations. They gain entry into the lungs in a bolus of secretions in the company of other organisms. Aspiration of large amounts of oropharyngeal secretions occurs regularly in individuals with impaired levels of consciousness, but aspiration of small volumes of secretions occurs regularly, at least during sleep, in normal people as well. The concentration of aerobic bacteria in upper respiratory tract secretions is about 10^8 organisms per

TABLE 61–1. ROUTES OF BACTERIAL INOCULATION OF THE LUNGS

Aspiration of contaminated oropharyngeal secretions
Inhalation of airborne bacteria
Bacteremia
Direct extension into the lungs

milliliter, while that of anaerobic organisms is about 10 times greater. Thus, aspiration of even small quantities of oropharyngeal secretions causes inoculation of the lung with an enormous bacterial challenge.

The number of bacteria present in ambient air is small, although some are available for inhalation with each breath. The organisms present are highly selected by environmental conditions, as they must have survived aerosolization, drying, temperature changes, and ultraviolet irradiation. Further, since only a few bacteria will be inhaled with each breath, those that arrive in the lungs must be capable of causing infection with a very small inoculum; this is not true for most pathogenic bacteria. In fact, the inability of investigators in the early twentieth century to produce pneumonia in experimental animals by exposing them to massive numbers of aerosolized bacteria nearly halted research on the airborne transmission of disease. Subsequently it was learned that a few organisms meet all of the criteria listed above and are often transmitted by the airborne route. *Mycobacterium tuberculosis* was one of the first to be identified. The infective dose may be as low as a single organism, most often resulting in only a positive skin test as the evidence of infection. Many viruses are transmitted by this route as well. However, the list of bacteria capable of transmission by this route is short and includes only organisms that are unusually invasive, such as the plague bacillus, and organisms particularly adapted to certain environments, such as *Legionella*, so that they are present in large numbers in the air in confined spaces, such as buildings served by contaminated air conditioning systems. Organisms capable of airborne transmission often produce outbreaks of infection when groups of susceptible people are exposed, a striking characteristic of *Legionella* infections, for example.

Host Defenses. A variety of mechanisms defend the host against bacterial invasion of the respiratory tract. Some of them should be evident from the discussion above. The anatomy of the upper air passages is an important aspect of defense against inhaled particulates, including bacteria. Droplets that exceed 10 μ in diameter are deposited by inertial impaction in the upper airways, a process that is promoted by the angulations of these structures. About 90 per cent of particles 5 to 10 μ in diameter are deposited along the tracheobronchial tree, while only those particles that are 0.5 to 3 μ in diameter tend to be deposited in the alveoli. Smaller particles tend to behave like gas molecules and are exhaled to a large extent. "Droplet nuclei" is the term applied to particles about 1 to 3 μ in diameter containing a single bacterium, the likely infecting unit for organisms transmitted by the airborne route.

Organisms that are deposited in the upper air passages are immediately exposed to local secretions. The antibacterial capacity of normal respiratory secretions has been investigated for many years without a firm conclusion. There is little doubt that an antibacterial effect can be demonstrated under various experimental conditions or in vitro. These effects have been attributed to a variety of factors, including lysozyme, complement, immunoglobulins, and products of resident bacteria. The biologic significance of these factors remains uncertain, however. Of much greater significance is the process of physical removal effected by the movement of secretions toward the esophagus and ultimate swallowing.

To avoid physical removal, newly arrived bacteria must persist in the upper air passages. This is facilitated by adherence of bacteria to the regional epithelium. Normal mucosal cells of the upper respiratory tract contain cell-surface receptors for a variety of bacteria. The chemical nature of receptors for different species of bacteria is highly variable, and the site of the receptor may be either an integral part of the cell surface or contained in proteins attached to the cell. For example, *Streptococcus pyogenes* binds to fibronectin, a protein that is not an integral constituent of the cell membrane but is acquired normally by respiratory mucosal cells following exposure to respiratory secretions. By contrast, gram-negative bacilli such as *Escherichia coli* or *Pseudomonas aeruginosa* adhere in large numbers to respiratory cells only after the surface fibronectin is removed. While many details of bacteria–host cell adherence remain to be defined, it is clear that this phenomenon is a major determinant of the composition of the normal bacterial flora of the oropharynx and that changes in

adherence are important in promoting or inhibiting colonization of this region by exogenous bacteria.

Under ideal conditions aspiration of oropharyngeal secretions is prevented by the normal swallowing mechanisms and the presence of reflexes that close the vocal cords when foreign materials enter the larynx. The latter are highly effective in preventing the aspiration of large volumes of fluid in normal persons but apparently do not prevent the aspiration of small volumes, at least during sleep. In view of the high concentration of bacteria in oropharyngeal secretions, aspiration of even 0.0001 ml may be important in initiating pneumonia, depending upon the nature of the bacteria aspirated and the state of lung defenses. Aspiration of such volumes may be an everyday occurrence in normal people and the infrequence of pneumonia may be due principally to lung defenses.

The first line of defense against bacteria that have gained entry into the lungs is physical removal from the airways. This is accomplished by the mucociliary escalator, an integrated multifaceted system consisting of the ciliated cells lining the airways, the secretory cells (goblet cells and submucosal glands), and the secretions. Propulsion of secretions toward the mouth is provided by cilia beating at the incredible rate of 1200 times per minute. However, the effectiveness of this activity depends on the perpendicular depth and the viscosity of secretions. The perpendicular depth of secretions within the airways appears to be relatively constant. This is somewhat puzzling when one considers the total cross-sectional area of the airways, which becomes markedly smaller as the numerous peripheral airways converge on the fewer central bronchi and ultimately on the trachea alone. Mucus moves twice as rapidly in the trachea as in small bronchi, but the difference in area is much greater, a finding that has led to speculation that fluid in secretions must be resorbed in proximal airways to maintain the perpendicular depth of the mucous layer in a range compatible with the length of the cilia. Obviously, processes that impair ciliary movement, cause excessive secretion of respiratory mucus, or change the viscosity of secretions may each hinder the effectiveness of this transport system.

Bacteria that penetrate to the distal airways or alveoli are killed in situ prior to physical transport out of the lung. The principal mechanism of bacterial killing is ingestion and killing by phagocytic cells. The quantitative aspects of this phenomenon have been extensively investigated in experimental animals, using a variety of bacterial species. The initial experiments were performed with relatively nonpathogenic staphylococci, and the results indicated that the antibacterial capacity of the lung is enormous and that phagocytosis and killing are accomplished almost solely by resident alveolar macrophages. This finding fits nicely with the concept that the lung is normally sterile and that polymorphonuclear leukocytes constitute a very small proportion of the total phagocytic cells on the alveolar surface. Further, these experiments indicated that neither antibody nor other humoral components are required for phagocytosis of bacteria on the alveolar surface. Subsequent experiments with more highly pathogenic bacteria showed that the situation is more complicated; some species cause a prompt recruitment of neutrophils, and in fact, bacterial killing appears to depend much more upon the availability of neutrophils than on the presence of alveolar macrophages. Further, clearance of viable bacteria from the lung is enhanced by the presence of specific antibody and is delayed in the absence of complement, findings that indicate an important role for circulating factors.

In general, bacterial killing is more efficient following aerosol deposition than following deposition of a fluid bolus containing equal numbers of bacteria. The reasons for this difference are not entirely clear but probably have to do with the local concentration of bacteria; changes induced in the organisms by the process of aerosolization, e.g., loss of capsular material; and the antiphagocytic effects of the fluid bolus in which the bacteria are suspended.

If bacteria on the alveolar surface are not promptly engulfed and killed, an inflammatory response swiftly develops that is characterized by interstitial and alveolar edema and an influx of neutrophils from the vascular space. The chemoattractants responsible for the latter may include bacterial products, activation of complement proteins that are present in small concentration in alveolar lining fluid, and the elaboration of neutrophil chemotactic factors by alveolar macrophages. In any case, once alveolar edema and inflammation are initiated, the process of bacterial ingestion and killing is remarkably retarded. As neutrophils and bacteria accumulate, the local milieu becomes acidic and hypoxic, since ventilation is impaired by alveolar filling. These conditions further impair phagocyte function, so that a population of viable organisms persists, albeit with a reduced rate of multiplication.

In the preantibiotic era, patients with pneumonia often improved dramatically on about the seventh day of illness with a sudden loss of fever, a process that was termed the "crisis" or "breaking of the fever." This event correlated with the development of antibody, which interrupted the standoff between bacteria and phagocytes in the consolidated regions of lung. This clinical phenomenon rarely occurs with antibiotic treatment because the drugs assist in bacterial killing. However, many antibiotics penetrate lung tissue poorly, and treatment must be relatively prolonged.

Community-acquired pneumonias are usually due to a single organism, an observation that appears to contradict the aspiration mechanism that necessarily includes multiple species. The susceptibility of individual bacterial species to lung defenses varies widely. While mucociliary transport is presumably equally effective for all bacteria, phagocytosis by the resident alveolar macrophages clearly is not. Further, previous exposure or immunization may have led to the development of antibody against some species, a factor that promotes phagocytosis and killing by neutrophils. The result of these differences is that the lung's defenses select the organism (or organisms) that will go on to cause pneumonia—the species most capable of evading phagocytosis and killing.

A number of conditions are clinically associated with an increased risk of bacterial pneumonia. Many of these have been confirmed in studies of experimental animals in attempts to relate susceptibility to pneumonia to specific defects in one or another of the lung's defenses (Table 61–2).

CLINICAL MANIFESTATIONS. The signs and symptoms associated with bacterial pneumonia vary widely, depending on several factors, most importantly the nature of the offending pathogen and the state of the host. Extremes in presentation can be easily described, although most patients will fall somewhere between. At one extreme is the previously healthy person with pneumococcal pneumonia. Such patients complain of a brief prodromal upper respiratory illness followed by fever, a single shaking chill, pleuritic chest pain, and a cough productive of purulent or "rusty" sputum. Physical examination reveals signs of consolidation, which are readily confirmed by chest radiography. Gram's stain of the sputum reveals numerous neutrophils and abundant pneumococci. In such a patient there is no doubt that a lower respiratory tract infection is present, and the stain of the sputum strongly suggests the etiology. At the other extreme might be an elderly, confused patient who presents only with deterioration in mental function. Physical examination reveals only rhonchi without signs of consolidation, and the chest radiograph shows only bilateral lower lobe interstitial infiltrates that might represent acute or chronic changes. Gram's stain of the sputum (obtained with difficulty) shows many squamous epithelial cells, a few neutrophils, and a pleomorphic bacterial flora that includes both gram-positive and gram-negative organisms. In such patients it may not be clear whether or not the patient has pneumonia, and the information at hand offers few clues regarding etiology.

The history-taker should explore the presence of risk factors, including chronic illnesses, recent acute illnesses, illness in family members, use of alcohol or other drugs, and possible exposures to infectious agents. A thorough physical examination, posteroanterior and lateral chest radiographs, and blood leukocyte count with differential should be performed. On the basis of the data available from these steps, it is usually possible to conclude that pneumonia is present. The remaining task is to determine its etiology.

Controversy exists over the proper microbiologic evaluation of the patient with pneumonia because of questions of sensitivity, specificity, cost, and benefit. These problems are created basically by the presence of abundant organisms in the upper tract and the resultant contamination of expectorated specimens. Further, since most patients with pneumonia respond satisfactorily to simple, relatively nontoxic antibiotic regimens, the need to document the etiology of the process is uncertain. It is impossible to define rules that apply to all patients, and knowledgeable physicians will differ in their approach to an individual patient.

There is little disagreement that sputum should be examined microscopically. The portion chosen should be purulent and contain fewer than 10 squamous cells and more than 25 leukocytes per low-power field. A well-done Gram stain will disclose whether or not one species of organism predominates. Often, such specimens contain a vast preponderance of a single species, and if these are encapsulated gram-positive diplococci (pneumococci), clumps of large gram-positive cocci (staphylococci), or small pleomorphic gram-negative coccobacilli (*Haemophilus*), a presumptive diagnosis can be made. Problems arise when a predominant organism is less apparent, when enteric gram-negative bacilli are present, or when an adequate specimen cannot be obtained. Special stains for acid-fast organisms, fungi, *Legionella*, *Pneumocystis carinii*, and others should be used selectively when the clinical situation suggests infection with one of these organisms.

Aerobic culture of expectorated sputum suffers from a lack of sensitivity (organisms causing pneumonia are not detected) and specificity (organisms are present that are not the cause of pneumonia); both have been estimated to occur in up to 50 per cent of cases. The results may be improved by microscopic screening of the specimen prior to culture. Other approaches have included washing the specimen repeatedly to remove contamination by oral secretions and using quantitative culture techniques on the assumption that the organism causing pneumonia will be present in the greatest concentration. While both of these techniques have merit, the time and effort required to perform them preclude their use as a routine part of the evaluation of a sputum specimen.

Contamination of sputum by oral secretions may be avoided by collecting the specimen proximal to the mouth. The most direct approach involves puncture of the trachea with a large-bore needle and insertion of a plastic cannula into the trachea, a technique called transtracheal aspiration. If secretions cannot be harvested by suction, a small amount of sterile saline is injected through the cannula and suction is reapplied. In the hands of experienced operators, this technique provides better results than sputum examination in some situations. It is most useful in documenting the absence of bacteria in the secretions of individuals with nonbacterial (e.g., viral, mycoplasmal, and so on) pneumonias, but these pneumonias can usually be strongly suspected on clinical grounds alone. In patients in whom an accurate bacteriologic diagnosis is urgently required, such as elderly or immunocompromised patients, contamination of tracheal secretions by aspirated oropharyngeal secretions renders the technique of less value. Absolute contraindications to transtracheal aspiration include abnormal bleeding or clotting values and an uncooperative patient. The major complications are bleeding and the occurrence of barotrauma, usually manifested as subcutaneous emphysema in the neck only. Because of the risk of bleeding, the procedure should not be performed in patients with a small trachea (children) or in those with a markedly impaired cough who may not be able to expectorate blood effectively. Transtracheal aspiration remains an excellent method for identifying anaerobic bacteria as responsible for pleuropulmonary infections, if this diagnosis cannot be made by other means.

Another method for bypassing the mouth in the collection of

TABLE 61–2. CONDITIONS ASSOCIATED WITH INCREASED RISK OF BACTERIAL PNEUMONIA

Condition	Impaired Defense Mechanism
Chronic airway obstruction	Reduced mucociliary transport Alveolar hypoxia
Pulmonary edema	Reduced phagocyte function
Unconsciousness	Increased aspiration
Immunoglobulin deficiency	Impaired phagocytosis
Neutropenia	Impaired phagocytosis
Viral infection	Altered mucosal adherence Reduced mucociliary transport Impaired phagocytosis

specimens is to aspirate directly from the area of lung consolidation, using either physical findings or fluoroscopy to guide the approach. This technique, called transthoracic lung aspiration, has proved to be an excellent technique in children with complicated pneumonias, since sputum samples may be impossible to obtain. In adults, especially those with underlying lung disease, the rate of complications, particularly pneumothorax and bleeding, limits its usefulness. This direct approach is further compromised by the fact that the false-negative rate may be as high as 30 per cent.

Fiberoptic bronchoscopy provides a relatively safe way to collect specimens from the periphery of the lung. Specially designed protected brushes are available that permit the operator to obtain endobronchial specimens that have not been contaminated by proximal airway secretions, even though the instrument has traversed the upper airways. Complications of the procedure are infrequent, and the major limiting factors are expense and time. In addition to the small specimens collected by brushing of the peripheral airways, sterile fluid can be instilled and aspirated to obtain material from a larger area of the lung (bronchoalveolar lavage).

Immunologic techniques, such as immunofluorescence, enzyme-linked immunoassay, and DNA hybridization, hold great promise for determining the cause of pneumonia. However, compared with conventional cultures, these techniques are expensive and relatively insensitive. They detect the presence of only a narrow spectrum of related organisms. Because of this specificity, they have a limited role in the evaluation of patients with pneumonia and should be considered only when specific organisms are strongly suspected on clinical grounds.

Last, it must be remembered that cultures of the blood and pleural fluid, if positive, provide results that are highly specific. However, only about 30 per cent of patients with bacterial pneumonia are bacteremic. About the same percentage of pleural fluid aspirates are positive in the absence of antibiotic therapy, but since only 10 to 15 per cent of patients with pneumonia have a pleural effusion, the applicability of this approach is limited. Nevertheless, blood cultures should be obtained in patients with serious illness due to pneumonia, and a diagnostic thoracentesis should be performed in patients with effusions large enough to be aspirated safely.

Proper utilization of these techniques must be individually determined for each patient with pneumonia. In many patients, the history, physical examination, radiographic studies, and evaluation of the sputum by Gram's stain provide all the data that might be reasonably required. Additional procedures should be reserved for those patients in whom a delay in making an accurate diagnosis will have serious consequences or those in whom the diagnosis cannot be reasonably suspected on the basis of simpler approaches.

RADIOGRAPHIC PATTERNS. Careful examination of posteroanterior (PA) and lateral chest radiographs is an invaluable adjunct in the diagnosis of pneumonia and should be part of the evaluation of every patient in whom significant respiratory infection is suspected. While a specific microbiologic diagnosis is seldom, if ever, possible on the basis of radiographic data alone, important clues to the etiology of pneumonia and its distribution and severity may be gained by this technique. Pathogens frequently associated with particular radiographic patterns are summarized in Table 61–3.

The presence of shadows corresponding to pulmonary lobes or segments (lobar or segmental infiltrates) should strongly suggest a bacterial etiology for pneumonia. Such lobar pneumonia is most commonly caused by one of the aerobic pathogens, such as *Streptococcus pneumoniae, H. influenzae,* or *Klebsiella pneumoniae.* These infections may be confined to a single lobe or segment or may involve multiple areas of the lung. Radiographically, the infiltrates are usually dense and homogeneous, frequently with obscuration of the borders between adjacent structures (e.g., heart borders or diaphragm). This obliteration of mutual radiographic borders is often termed the "silhouette sign" and is very useful in the localization of densities within the lung parenchyma.

Less well defined and inhomogeneous radiographic densities, often described as "patchy" or "streaky" infiltrates, are commonly observed in bronchopneumonia, a pattern of infection involving

TABLE 61–3. COMMON RADIOGRAPHIC PATTERNS OF PNEUMONIA AND ASSOCIATED PATHOGENS

Pattern	Pathogen
Lobar or segmental infiltrates	*Streptococcus pneumoniae, Haemophilus influenzae, Klebsiella pneumoniae, Escherichia coli, Legionella* species
Inhomogeneous infiltrates (patchy or streaky opacities)	*Mycoplasma pneumoniae,* viruses, mixed aerobic/anaerobic organisms (e.g., aspiration), *Legionella* species
Diffuse homogeneous infiltrates	*Legionella* species, viruses, *Pneumocystis carinii*
Nodular opacities	Mycobacterial species, *Aspergillus, Candida,* organisms involved in hematogenous spread of infection
Cavitary infiltrates	*Staphylococcus aureus,* gram-negative organisms, anaerobes, *Mycobacterium tuberculosis, Aspergillus*

airways rather than lobes and segments. This radiographic pattern may be seen in infections caused by a wide variety of organisms, including bacteria and viruses, and may occur in virtually any clinical setting, including aspiration of oropharyngeal contents by debilitated individuals and the relatively mild pneumonia caused by *Mycoplasma pneumoniae* in otherwise healthy, ambulatory adults.

Diffuse pulmonary infiltrates are less commonly caused by the typical aerobic or anaerobic pathogens associated with lobar pneumonia or bronchopneumonia. This pattern may be indicative of infection with viruses (such as cytomegalovirus or influenza), *Legionella pneumophila,* or opportunistic pathogens such as *P. carinii.* In addition to infection, diffuse homogeneous infiltrates may also be due to pulmonary edema, lung hemorrhage, interstitial lung disease, or the lung injury associated with the adult respiratory distress syndrome (ARDS), making the differential diagnosis of this radiographic pattern particularly complicated. For this reason, the detection of infection superimposed on other forms of lung pathology may be especially difficult and often requires the use of specialized diagnostic techniques, such as bronchoscopy or open lung biopsy.

Important information can be derived not only from the size and shape of the radiographic density but also from its character. In this regard, cavitary shadows generally suggest the presence of a necrotizing infection, with associated destruction of lung tissue. Organisms that frequently produce this radiographic picture include *Staphylococcus aureus,* gram-negative bacteria, mixed anaerobic organisms (such as those associated with aspiration of oropharyngeal contents), *Aspergillus* species, and *Mycobacterium tuberculosis.* Less commonly, nonnecrotizing infection occurring in an area of lung containing cysts or bullae may have a cavitary appearance on the radiograph in the absence of frank lung destruction.

Pulmonary infection may be associated with the appearance of nodular lesions on the chest radiograph. These nodular shadows can range widely in size, from the miliary (<2 mm) lesions of tuberculosis to the large cavitating lesions of septic embolization to the lung. In general, however, disseminated nodular lesions suggest the presence of infection borne to the lung from another source via the bloodstream. Consideration must be given to primary sites of infection, such as endocarditis of the valves of the right side of the heart and septic thrombophlebitis. In patients with unexplained fever despite prolonged courses of antibiotics, fungal infection (e.g., *Candida albicans*) should be considered.

The chest radiograph may also yield valuable information about infectious involvement of structures outside the parenchyma of the lung, including the pleural surface and thoracic lymph nodes. Pleural effusions occur in a wide variety of respiratory infections, including bacterial, viral, fungal, and mycobacterial illnesses. Lateral decubitus radiographs are helpful in documenting the presence of free pleural fluid, and thoracentesis is frequently necessary to distinguish transudative and uncomplicated parapneumonic effusions from complicated parapneumonic effusions or empyema, which may require drainage (see Ch. 62 and 69). Needle pleural biopsy may be useful in the diagnosis of granulomatous infections involving the pleura.

Enlargement of mediastinal and hilar lymph nodes is uncommon in acute bacterial infection of the lung. When present in association with pneumonia, this finding should suggest infection by fungal pathogens or mycobacteria, or an underlying malignancy.

Loss of volume of a pulmonary segment or lobe (partial or complete atelectasis) should raise suspicion regarding an endobronchial lesion obstructing a large airway, with associated infection in the obstructed segment. Such lesions may include bronchogenic carcinoma, foreign body, or mucous plug.

Green GM, Jakab GJ, Low RB, et al.: Defense mechanisms of the respiratory membrane. Am Rev Respir Dis 115:479, 1977. *Still the best, most comprehensive review of lung defense mechanisms.*

Onofrio JM, Toews GB, Lipscomb MF, et al.: Granulocyte-alveolar-macrophage interaction in the pulmonary clearance of *Staphylococcus aureus*. Am Rev Respir Dis 127:335, 1983. *Illustrates how the lung defenses vary in response to differing bacterial challenges.*

Palmer DL, Jones CC: Diagnosis of pneumococcal pneumonia. Semin Respir Infect 3:131, 1988. *A thoughtful review of the usefulness of immunologic studies in diagnosing pneumococcal infections.*

Van Uffelen R, van Saene HKF, Fidler V, et al.: Oropharyngeal flora as a source of bacteria colonizing the lower airways in patients on artificial ventilation. Intensive Care Med 10:233, 1984. *Demonstrates the progression from oropharyngeal colonization to colonization of distal airways to bacterial pneumonia.*

Wanner A: Clinical aspects of mucociliary transport. Am Rev Respir Dis 116:78, 1977. *An excellent, complete review of the mucociliary system.*

62 Lung Abscess

John G. Bartlett

DEFINITION. Lung abscess literally means a collection of pus within a destroyed portion of the lung; thus there are numerous possible causes of such a lesion (Table 62–1). As used clinically, however, the term "lung abscess" refers to a pulmonary infection with parenchymal necrosis, generally caused by bacteria other than mycobacteria. Lung abscesses are usually solitary, but occasionally multiple discrete lesions are observed. Numerous small abscesses confined to a given region of the lung are sometimes referred to as "necrotizing pneumonia." Because they share a common pathogenesis, there is considerable overlap among aspiration pneumonia, lung abscess, and necrotizing pneumonia, and each of these may lead to and coexist with an empyema (a collection of pus within the pleural space).

ETIOLOGY. As indicated in Table 62–1, many different underlying processes can lead to the formation of a lung abscess. By far the most important are necrotizing pulmonary infections, and, of these, anaerobic bacteria are responsible for the majority.

TABLE 62–1. DIFFERENTIAL DIAGNOSIS OF A CAVITARY LESION IN THE LUNG

Necrotizing infections
  Bacteria: Anaerobic bacteria, *Staphylococcus aureus*, enteric gram-negative bacteria, *Pseudomonas aeruginosa*, *Legionella*, *Streptococcus pyogenes*, *Hemophilus influenzae*, *Pseudomonas pseudomallei*, *Actinomyces*, *Nocardia*, *Streptococcus pneumoniae* (?)
  Mycobacteria: *Mycobacterium tuberculosis*, *M. kansasii*, *M. avium-intracellulare*
  Fungi: *Coccidioides immitis*, *Histoplasma capsulatum*, *Blastomyces hominis*, *Cryptococcus neoformans*, *Aspergillus*, *Phycomycetes* (*Mucor*)
  Parasites: *Entamoeba histolytica*, *Paragonimus westermani*
  Septic embolism: *S. aureus*, anaerobes, and so on

Cavitary infarction
  Bland infarction (with or without superimposed infection)
  Vasculitis: Wegener's granulomatosis, periarteritis

Neoplasms
  Bronchogenic carcinoma, metastatic carcinoma, lymphoma (with or without superimposed infection)

Miscellaneous lesions
  Cysts or bullae with fluid collections, sequestration

These organisms account for essentially all "putrid" lung abscesses and nearly all that have been classified as "nonspecific" or "primary." Most of these infections involve multiple bacterial species, which may include aerobic organisms. The dominant bacteria are *Fusobacterium nucleatum*, *Bacteroides melaninogenicus*, *B. intermedius*, peptostreptococcus, aerobic streptococci, and microaerophilic streptococci.

Pneumonia, particularly cases caused by *Staphylococcus aureus* and *Klebsiella pneumoniae*, may also be complicated by abscess formation. Less frequent but well-documented agents of lung abscess include *Streptococcus pyogenes* (group A beta-hemolytic streptococci), *Streptococcus pneumoniae* (especially type 3), *Streptococcus milleri*, *Haemophilus influenzae* (type B), *Pseudomonas aeruginosa*, *Pseudomonas pseudomallei* (melioidosis), *Actinomyces* (actinomycosis), *Legionella*, *Nocardia*, *Paragonimus westermani* (lung fluke), and *Entamoeba histolytica* (amebiasis). Enteric gram-negative bacilli other than *K. pneumoniae* may cause lung abscess, but this occurs almost exclusively in debilitated patients with severe associated medical-surgical conditions. Necrotizing alveolitis is a separate entity diagnosed by microscopic examination and usually caused by *P. aeruginosa;* sometimes these microabscesses coalesce to form radiographically detectable cavities.

INCIDENCE AND PREVALENCE. The incidence of primary lung abscess has decreased substantially since the prechemotherapeutic era. Nevertheless, most large academic centers encounter 10 to 30 cases annually.

EPIDEMIOLOGY. Most lung abscesses, and nearly all involving anaerobic bacteria, involve the normal flora of the oropharynx. Abscesses involving *S. aureus* or gram-negative bacilli are more likely to be nosocomial in origin. Amebic lung abscess results from the direct extension of an hepatic abscess through the diaphragm into the lung. *Nocardia* causes lung abscess almost exclusively in immunocompromised hosts, especially in recipients of corticosteroids. Septic pulmonary emboli commonly lead to multiple solitary abscesses in noncontiguous sites and are usually caused by *S. aureus*, anaerobic bacteria, or *P. aeruginosa;* hematogenous abscesses are most often found in intravenous drug abusers with tricuspid valve endocarditis and patients with septic thrombophlebitis. Lung abscesses due to *P. westermani* and melioidosis are usually acquired in the Far East or Indonesia.

PATHOGENESIS. The formation of an anaerobic lung abscess nearly always involves two coexisting abnormalities: (1) periodontal infection, such as gingivitis or pyorrhea, which provides the inoculum; and (2) aspiration, which provides access to the lung parenchyma. The usual causes for aspiration are those that compromise consciousness and the gag reflex, such as alcoholism, drug addiction, general anesthesia, seizure disorder, sedative use, or neurologic disorders. Other factors predisposing to aspiration include dysphagia resulting from esophageal disorders or neurologic deficits; disruption of the usual mechanical barriers, as with nasogastric intubation, tracheostomy, or nasogastric feeding tubes; or pharyngeal anesthesia, as seen with dental procedures or surgery involving the upper airway. Most healthy persons periodically aspirate small inocula from the upper airways, but these are readily cleared by the normal cough reflex and other pulmonary defense mechanisms without deleterious consequences. Patients who develop aspiration pneumonia and lung abscesses presumably do so because of the relatively large inocula of bacteria and failure of the usual protective mechanisms.

The initial lesion is pneumonitis, or "aspiration pneumonia," which typically involves dependent pulmonary segments, e.g., those favored by gravitational flow. The dependent pulmonary segments in patients who aspirate in the recumbent position are the superior segments of the lower lobes or posterior segments of the upper lobes. Aspiration in the upright or semi-upright position favors involvement of the basilar segments of the lower lobes. Patients who have a defined period of known or probable aspiration demonstrate with sequential radiographs that 7 to 14 days are usually required for the appearance of a typical air-fluid level on chest radiograph.

CLINICAL MANIFESTATIONS. Patients with anaerobic abscesses tend to have indolent symptomatology with medical complaints dating for 2 or more weeks before presentation. The usual symptoms are fever, malaise, cough, sputum production, and pleuritic pain. The frequent observation of weight loss and anemia provides testimony to the chronicity of the infection. There may be "chilliness," but frank rigors are rare, and their presence suggests organisms other than anaerobes. The cough often becomes more productive at the time of cavitation, and it is at this time that the patient is most likely to note the onset of putrid sputum, which is considered diagnostic of anaerobic infection. Putrid sputum is found in 60 per cent of patients with a confirmed anaerobic etiology. Many patients will also note that the sputum has an unusually noxious taste. Most patients have a history of compromised consciousness or other risk factors for aspiration, and many have periodontal infection. Nevertheless, about 10 per cent of patients with anaerobic lung abscesses have no identifiable predisposing condition. Occasional patients with anaerobic lung abscesses are edentulous; the incidence of underlying bronchogenic neoplasms seems particularly high in this group. Patients with lung abscesses due to *S. aureus*, gram-negative bacilli, and amebae usually have a more fulminant course, with the precipitous onset of symptoms. Other features that may be noted in this group include chills, the lack of putrid discharge, and the absence of the usual associated findings. The physical findings in the early phases of disease are those of pneumonia, with or without a pleural effusion. At a later stage there may be amphoric or cavernous breath sounds, pleural effusions are common, and approximately 25 per cent of patients have an associated empyema.

DIAGNOSIS. The diagnosis of lung abscess is usually established on the basis of a chest radiograph showing a parenchymal infiltrate with a cavity containing an air-fluid level (Fig. 62–1). The differential diagnosis of this roentgenographic finding is included in Table 62–1. Certain roentgenographic features may provide clues to the presence of an infected cyst, bulla, or sequestration. Massive pulmonary fibrosis with necrosis from occupational exposure is usually distinctive. A loculated empyema with an air-fluid level may be differentiated from lung abscess with computed tomography.

Studies for an etiologic agent are often hampered by the limitations of bacteriologic analysis of expectorated sputum. These specimens are useful in detecting mycobacteria, pathogenic fungi, and parasites, and they may be used for cytologic studies. However, routine aerobic cultures often give erroneous results, and they are not valid for meaningful anaerobic culture owing to the universal presence in oral secretions of anaerobes that con-taminate the specimen during passage through the upper airways. Blood cultures are useful, primarily for patients with infections involving *S. aureus* or gram-negative bacilli, but most patients with anaerobic abscesses do not have bacteremia. Pleural fluid is a valuable culture source for both aerobic and anaerobic bacteria in any patient with an empyema, so that thoracentesis should be performed before treatment is begun. For most patients with anaerobic pulmonary infections restricted to the pulmonary parenchyma, the preferred specimen source is from a transtracheal aspiration, from a transthoracic needle aspirate, or from a fiber-optic bronchoscopy utilizing a double-lumen catheter with a distal occluding plug, combined with quantitative cultures. Specimen collection prior to institution of antibiotic therapy is preferred. In most cases of anaerobic abscesses, the etiologic agents will not be defined, and the therapeutic regimen will be selected empirically. Bronchoscopy, which used to be performed routinely in patients with lung abscesses, is now usually restricted to patients who fail to respond to antibiotic treatment or who have an atypical clinical presentation. Major concerns are a cavitating neoplasm, an obstructing tumor, or a foreign body.

TREATMENT. The most important facets of the treatment are the administration of appropriate antibiotics and adequate drainage of any associated empyema. Physiotherapy with postural drainage should be utilized when possible; however, this must be done with considerable caution in patients with large lung abscesses because of the possibility of spillage of purulent contents, with extensive involvement of other lobes.

The drugs of choice for the treatment of abscesses caused by aerobic pyogenic microorganisms, *Mycobacterium tuberculosis*, fungi, and *Entamoeba histolytica* are reviewed in detail elsewhere in this volume. For aspiration-related lung abscess involving anaerobic bacteria, the three antimicrobial regimens recommended are penicillin, clindamycin, or penicillin plus metronidazole. Penicillin has traditionally been regarded as the favored drug on the basis of its long, well-established track record. There is considerable variation in the dosage recommendations, but most authorities recommend doses of 10 to 20 million units given intravenously per day. This is continued until the patient is afebrile and clinically improved, at which time treatment is changed to intramuscular or oral penicillin using penicillin G, penicillin V, ampicillin, or amoxicillin in doses of 500 to 750 mg three or four times daily. Some authorities suggest an arbitrarily selected total duration of treatment of 3 to 6 weeks, whereas others continue treatment until the chest radiograph changes have cleared or there is only a small, stable residual lesion. The

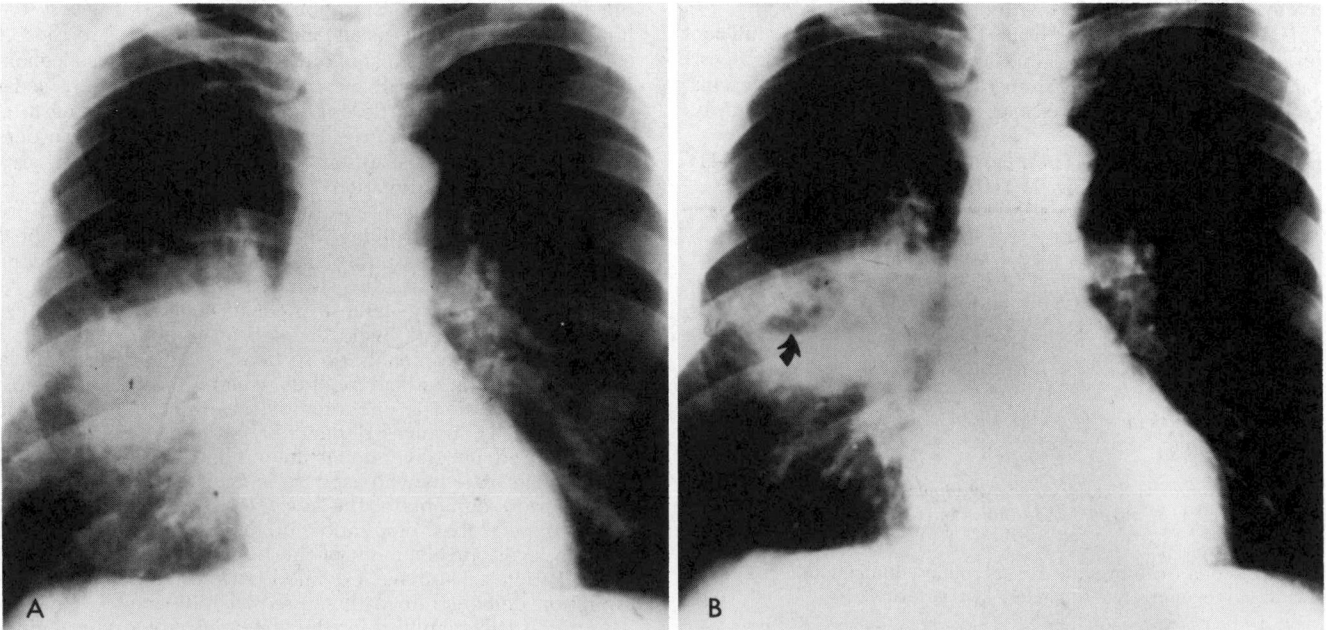

FIGURE 62–1. Chest radiographs of a 55-year-old alcoholic man. The first film (*A*) shows pneumonitis involving the superior segment of the right lower lobe, a common segment for aspiration pneumonia. The second radiograph (*B*), taken 1 week later, shows cavitation with an air-fluid level as indicated by the arrow. A transtracheal aspirate yielded *F. nucleatum*, *B. melaninogenicus*, and anaerobic streptococci. The final diagnosis was aspiration pneumonia with progression to lung abscess due to anaerobic bacteria.

latter criterion commonly requires 2 to 4 months or longer but may be necessary to prevent relapses.

Clindamycin is active against most penicillin-resistant anaerobes that are found in 20 to 25 per cent of cases, including many or most strains of *B. melaninogenicus*, *B. fragilis*, *B. ruminicola*, and *B. ureolyticus*. Some regard clindamycin as the preferred agent for all lung abscesses due to anaerobic bacteria; others advocate it only for patients who fail to respond to penicillin, have a contraindication to penicillin, or have a serious infection with a fulminant course. The usual regimen is 600 mg given intravenously every 6 to 8 hours until the patient is afebrile and clinically improved, followed by 300 mg orally four times daily. An alternative regimen is penicillin G (above doses) combined with metronidazole (2 gm orally per day in two to four divided doses). Metronidazole is active against nearly all clinically important anaerobes, but penicillin must be added owing to the probable importance of aerobic and microaerophilic streptococci.

The necessity to treat the aerobic components of mixed aerobic-anaerobic infections is controversial, but this is generally advocated for patients who are seriously ill or fail to respond to clindamycin. In such cases, most penicillins are considered equally effective against oral anaerobes, including penicillin G, penicillin V, ampicillin, amoxicillin, ticarcillin, and piperacillin. However, antistaphylococcal penicillins, such as nafcillin or oxacillin, are considered inferior and unacceptable. Cephalosporins are considered nearly equivalent to penicillins in terms of in vitro activity, although the clinical experience is limited. Imipenem and any combination of a betalactam–betalactamase inhibitor are considered almost universally active against clinically important anaerobes. The activity of tetracyclines and erythromycin is variable. Quinolones and trimethoprim-sulfamethoxazole are unacceptable for infections caused by anaerobic bacteria.

Patients with lung abscesses involving *S. aureus* should be treated with a penicillinase-resistant penicillin or a first-generation cephalosporin. Vancomycin is the preferred agent for methicillin-resistant strains of *S. aureus*. This agent or clindamycin may be used for patients with a contraindication to beta-lactam antibiotics. Penicillin G is the preferred agent for infections involving group A beta-hemolytic streptococcal infection. Antibiotic selection for infections involving gram-negative bacilli requires in vitro sensitivity data. This usually consists of an aminoglycoside combined with an expanded-spectrum penicillin, such as ticarcillin for *P. aeruginosa* or a cephalosporin for Enterobacteriaccae. Sulfonamides are preferred agents for *Nocardia* infections.

The expected response to antimicrobial agents is subjective improvement with decreased fever within 3 to 7 days and elimination of fever within 7 to 14 days. The putrid odor of the sputum, when initially present, usually resolves in 3 to 10 days. Delayed response may indicate large cavity size, poor host status, obstruction, erroneous antimicrobial selection, a wrong diagnosis, drug fever, a complicating empyema requiring drainage, or an abscess that requires drainage by physiotherapy, bronchoscopy, or surgery. Radiographic response is delayed; in fact, there is often extension of the infiltrate and increased cavity size or new cavity formation during the first week. Chest radiographs should be followed at 2- to 3-week intervals with the expectation that infiltrates will clear or there will be a small residual scar or a thin-walled cyst.

Bronchoscopy is indicated in patients with an atypical presentation and in those who fail to respond to recommended antimicrobial regimens. The major purpose of the procedure is to differentiate cavitating neoplasms and to detect underlying lesions, such as bronchogenic neoplasms, bronchostenosis, or a foreign body. It may also be used to facilitate drainage.

The major indications for surgery are an uncontrollable or life-threatening hemorrhage, a bronchogenic neoplasm, a bronchial obstruction, or a lung abscess that proves absolutely refractory to medical treatment. Medical failures are rare but are most common in patients with an obstructed bronchus, those with extremely large abscesses, those with abscesses that have been present for an extended period before the institution of treatment, and those with infections involving certain bacteria such as gram-negative bacilli. The usual surgical procedure is lobectomy. Patients with prohibitive operative risks may benefit from percutaneous drainage, but care must be taken to avoid contamination of the pleural space.

PROGNOSIS. The natural course of lung abscesses was best studied in the prechemotherapeutic era. Treatment at that time was nearly equally divided between conservative management using postural drainage and supportive care, and surgery. The mortality rate was about 33 per cent in both groups, and another third of patients developed a chronic debilitating disease or suffered recurrent symptoms. The availability of the Jackson bronchoscope to facilitate drainage had no important bearing on outcome. The technique of resectional surgery was developed at about the time penicillin became available, and the relative merits of these two approaches as the primary therapeutic modality were widely debated. During the past two decades, however, the majority of patients have been treated with antibiotics alone, including those with "delayed closure" (i.e., the persistence of a cavity demonstrated by a chest radiograph at 4 to 6 weeks after the initiation of antibiotic therapy), because most of these cavities eventually resolve if the antibiotics are continued long enough. The mortality rate for aspiration-related lung abscess is currently reported at 5 to 6 per cent. Findings that herald a relatively poor prognosis include (1) large cavity size, particularly cavities greater than 6 cm in diameter; (2) prolonged symptoms prior to presentation, especially symptoms for more than 6 weeks; (3) necrotizing pneumonia characterized by multiple small abscesses in contiguous segments; (4) patients who are elderly, debilitated, or immunologically compromised; (5) abscesses associated with bronchial obstruction; and (6) abscess due to aerobic bacteria, including *S. aureus* and gram-negative bacilli.

PREVENTION. The major preventive measures are factors used to reduce the incidence or magnitude of aspiration, appropriate care of periodontal disease, early treatment of pneumonia, and adequate courses of antimicrobials to prevent relapses.

Bartlett JG: Anaerobic bacterial infections of the lung. Chest 91:6, 1987. *A review of anaerobic pleuropulmonary infections, including 83 cases of lung abscesses with bacteriology, clinical features, and management guidelines.*

Hagan JL, Hardy LD: Lung abscess revisited. A survey of 184 cases. Ann Surg 197:755, 1983. *Update on the surgical point of view concerning lung abscess; 11 per cent were operated on.*

Landay MJ, Christensen EE, Bynum LJ, et al.: Anaerobic pleural and pulmonary infections. AJR 134:233, 1980. *The authors review the roentgenographic features of anaerobic pleuropulmonary infections, including response to antibiotic treatment.*

Levison ME, Mangura CT, Lorber B, et al.: Clindamycin compared to penicillin for the treatment of anaerobic lung abscess. Ann Intern Med 98:466, 1983. *The authors show the superiority of clindamycin versus intravenous penicillin in terms of response rates, relapse rates, and time to defervescence.*

Snow N, Lucas A, Horrigan TP: Utility of pneumonotomy in the treatment of cavitary lung disease. Chest 87:731, 1985. *A description of the procedure and results with percutaneous drainage.*

63 Bronchiectasis

Roger Bone

DEFINITION

The definition of bronchiectasis is primarily an anatomic one, expressed as the *irreversible* dilation of one or more proximal and medium-sized bronchi due to destruction of the muscular and elastic supporting tissues of the bronchial walls. Destruction is generally the result of recurrent or chronic inflammation and intermittent healing with fibrosis. Chronic cough and copious sputum production are nearly universal; dyspnea and orthopnea occur in severe cases.

HISTORICAL PERSPECTIVE AND CURRENT ETIOLOGIES

Before the advent of antibiotics and vaccines, bronchiectasis was a much more significant contributor to patient morbidity and mortality than it is today. Measles, pertussis, tuberculosis, and a variety of childhood respiratory infections commonly set the stage for the development of bronchiectasis. Immunization and aggressive antibiotic therapies have rendered these diseases much less significant precursors to bronchiectasis in the United States; in the developing countries, however, these diseases remain common antecedents.

With immunization and antibiotics also comes the declining absolute incidence of bronchiectasis. Although infection remains a major component in the disease, those cases that do occur are often in patients with one or more predisposing conditions (Table 63–1).

Bronchial Obstruction

Aspiration of foreign bodies (most notably in children), tumors, and occasionally mucus impaction can lead to infection, dilation of bronchi, and subsequent destructive changes. These are generally focal rather than diffuse processes. Bronchiectasis may develop years after aspiration of foreign bodies or inhalational injury. Obstruction, per se, does not appear to cause bronchiectasis but facilitates the condition by interfering with bronchial clearance and thereby encouraging infection.

Congenital or Hereditary Conditions

The cilia of individuals with the immotile cilia syndrome exhibit structural alterations (dynein arms are absent or aberrant) that render them immotile or dyskinetic. The syndrome is probably transmitted as an autosomal recessive trait. Lack of ciliary motility is apparent in several body systems. Men with the condition are infertile, owing to immotile sperm; women have decreased fertility as well. Such patients are prone to the recurrent infections characteristic of bronchiectasis because cilia of the respiratory tract are unable to beat or because they have functional alterations. Mucociliary clearance of bacteria and phagocytic debris is inhibited; chronic sinusitis and bronchiectasis may result.

Patients with Kartagener's syndrome, a subset of the immotile cilia syndrome, may, in addition to bronchiectasis and sinusitis, exhibit situs inversus. It is presumed that situs inversus represents the chance result of embryonic migration of viscera, rather than the normally cilia-dependent placement of internal organs.

Bronchiectasis in patients with cystic fibrosis is a reflection of defects in exocrine gland secretion. In this country, nearly half of the cases of bronchiectasis in children or young adults are attributable to cystic fibrosis. Copious amounts of thickened

TABLE 63–1. PREDISPOSING FACTORS FOR BRONCHIECTASIS

Bronchopulmonary infections	Pertussis, measles; *Staphylococcus aureus*, *Klebsiella*, *Mycobacterium tuberculosis*, *Haemophilus influenzae*; adenovirus, influenza, herpes simplex; viral bronchiolitis; mycotic (histoplasmosis) or mycoplasmal (?) infection
Bronchial obstruction	Foreign body aspiration; neoplasm; hilar adenopathy (tuberculosis, sarcoidosis); mucoid impaction; chronic obstructive pulmonary disease (COPD; chronic bronchitis, asthma); acquired tracheobronchial disease; amyloidosis
Congenital anatomic defects	Bronchomalacia, bronchial cysts, cartilage deficiency, tracheobronchomegaly, ectopic bronchus, endobronchial teratoma, tracheoesophageal fistula; pulmonary sequestration, pulmonary artery aneurysm; yellow-nail syndrome
Immunodeficiency states	Congenital agammaglobulinemia; acquired immune globulin deficiency; chronic granulomatous disease
Hereditary defects	Ciliary defects (immotile cilia syndrome, ciliary dyskinesia, Kartagener's syndrome); alpha$_1$-antitrypsin deficiency; cystic fibrosis
Miscellaneous	Young's syndrome; recurrent aspiration pneumonias (alcoholism, neurologic disorders, lipoid pneumonia); irritant inhalation (ammonia, nitrogen dioxide, smoke, talc, silicates, detergents); after heart/lung transplantation (associated with obliterative bronchiolitis)

Adapted from Swartz MN: Bronchiectasis. *In* Fishman AP (ed.): Pulmonary Diseases and Disorders. 2nd ed. New York, McGraw-Hill Book Company, 1988, p 1559; with permission of McGraw-Hill, Inc.

secretions promote the development of infection (for more information, see Ch. 64).

Intralobar sequestration of the lung is a congenital malformation that consists of a detached segment of pulmonary tissue that has a systemic arterial blood supply and that is attached to normal lung and covered by the same pleura. In adults, pneumonia in the sequestered segment may occur. In general, the detached segment has no bronchial attachment to the rest of the lung and, therefore, is not filled with air. With infection, however, connections may become established, allowing progression to bronchiectasis.

Bronchiectasis is also associated with immunodeficiency states; defects in humoral immunity more frequently lead to the disorder than do defects in cellular immunity. Panhypogammaglobulinemia, especially, may lead to bronchiectasis. Such patients have a greatly increased susceptibility to repeated bacterial infections and therefore are at increased risk.

Other Causes

Although no longer common in the United States, bronchiectasis can follow necrotizing pneumonias caused by the tubercle bacillus or staphylococci. Previously, necrotizing pneumonia was not uncommon secondary to measles, pertussis, and influenza. In addition, one third to two thirds of patients with Young's syndrome, a combination of obstructive azospermia and chronic sinopulmonary infections, will develop bronchiectasis. Central bronchiectasis is a finding associated with allergic bronchopulmonary aspergillosis. Brief mention should also be made of the very rare "yellow-nail syndrome"—a combination of lymphedema of the lower extremities, recurrent pneumonia, bronchiectasis, and yellow discoloration of the nails.

PATHOGENESIS AND PATHOLOGY

It is likely that infection and at least some degree of obstruction are necessary for the development of bronchiectasis. Bronchiectatic changes may become irreversible if obstruction persists or if infection produces further bronchial inflammation, destruction, and dilation.

Current views on the pathogenesis of bronchiectasis describe the following scenario. An inhalational or parenteral injury occurs (e.g., corrosive chemical, infectious agent, particulate agent). If the precipitating event is a respiratory infection, it is not necessarily a serious one. Obstruction and stasis occur because secretions, epithelial injury, or a relatively minor obstruction inhibit drainage and clearance and allow infection to continue. The process may be exacerbated in a vulnerable host (one with immunodeficiency, ciliary dysfunction, or reactive airways). Often, the initial insult is unknown; it may be that in the susceptible host repeated cycles of bacterial infection with increasing airway obstruction and destruction develop.

Bronchial dilation predominantly involves medium-sized bronchi but may extend to more distal regions. Bronchi may be dilated to greater than four times their normal size and are often filled with purulent secretions. Peripheral airways in involved regions are often obstructed. In addition, viscous secretions slow mucociliary clearance, and the proteolytic activity of polymorphonuclear leukocytes (of the inflammatory process) contributes to tissue destruction. There is also evidence that purulent secretions themselves are rich in proteases (elastase, collagenase, and cathepsin G) and may be at least partially contributory. The mucosal surface is swollen, inflamed, frequently ulcerated, and sometimes necrotic. Formation of granulation tissue may lead to alterations in the bronchial epithelial lining. This condition is often described as being "polypoid" in appearance—ciliated columnar epithelium is replaced by cuboidal cells or fibrous tissue.

The lower lobes are most frequently involved, the left much more often than the right, presumably because of anatomic differences in drainage attributable to the angle and diameter of more proximal segments. In left lower lobe bronchiectasis, the posterior basal segment is almost always involved, and the apical segment is usually spared.

The radiologic appearance of bronchiectasis can be classified into three types, increasing in severity. In *cylindrical* or *fusiform* bronchiectasis, bronchi are relatively straight and not greatly increased in diameter. Bronchi in *varicose* bronchiectasis are typically dilated and irregular and exhibit bulbous, distorted terminations. The bronchial lumen may be totally obliterated by fibrous tissue; distal portions may become epithelium lined and fluid filled. *Saccular* or *cystic* bronchiectatic segments are dilated, ballooning into pus-filled cavities called saccules as they approach the periphery. These saccules represent totally destroyed and fibrosed segments of the bronchial tree. Larger, more proximal segments may remain relatively unchanged, except for marked inflammation in the bronchial walls and polyposis of bronchial epithelium. The morphology of saccular bronchiectasis is probably attributable to extension of the inflammatory process of the bronchial walls to supporting structures and surrounding lung parenchymal tissue, which are destroyed or fibrosed. Polyposis of bronchial mucosa partially obstructs bronchi proximal to saccular regions, preventing drainage. As a result, these more proximal regions become distended with pus. Squamous metaplasia is common in saccular bronchiectasis but is uncommon in the other types.

Clinical Manifestations and Clinical Course

Today, most clinically significant bronchiectasis originates in early childhood but may not become apparent until much later. Predisposing factors, such as cystic fibrosis, the immotile cilia syndrome, or immunodeficiency states, are usually present.

Cough (sometimes paroxysmal) and sputum production (frequently purulent)—often more severe upon awakening—are observed in 90 per cent of patients. In the preantibiotic era, sputum volumes of as much as 600 ml per day were seen in those with advanced, untreated disease. Fetid sputum and foul breath were also common. Today, these extreme presentations are unlikely; antibiotics and postural drainage have greatly reduced the volume of sputum and have prevented the development of secondary growth of anaerobic bacteria that contributes to such purulence.

Recurrent episodes of infection exacerbate established bronchiectasis. Intercurrent infections may be accompanied by fever, cough, sputum production, and dyspnea. Anorexia and weight loss are associated with multiple bronchiectatic episodes, as is wheezing. Hemoptysis was very common in the past but is not as common today, since the infectious aspect of the disease can be treated. Sinusitis sometimes accompanies bronchiectasis, especially in patients with ciliary defects and immunodeficiency states.

Bronchiectatic patients usually show abnormalities on physical examination. Persistent, medium to coarse, "moist crackles" over involved lobes are most significant. The crackles begin early in inspiration, continue to mid-inspiration, and then fade by the end of inspiration. Diffuse rhonchi and prolonged expiratory phases may also be evident. In patients with extensive disease, dullness and decreased breath sounds may be heard over involved regions. Respiratory expansion may be either increased or decreased. Patients with advanced disease or disease complicated by emphysema may show hyperexpansion, but hyperexpansion is more common in children.

In the preantibiotic era, clubbing and cyanosis were common as the disease progressed (40 per cent of cases). Metastatic abscesses, especially in the brain, were well known. At present, these are all unusual. The incidence of cor pulmonale has also declined dramatically in these patients, except in those with cystic fibrosis and considerable lung destruction. Secondary amyloidosis is rare.

DIAGNOSIS

Since the definition of bronchiectasis is an anatomic one, diagnosis of the disease is based upon demonstration of morphologic alterations in the bronchial tree. Generally, radiologic techniques are used. Patients should also be evaluated for the presence of one of the familial causes of bronchiectasis (Table 63–2)—unless there has been an obvious precipitating event. Bronchiectasis should be suspected in any patient presenting with chronic productive cough (especially if sputum is purulent or there is intermittent blood streaking).

Chest Radiographs

Chest radiographs are crucial for documenting regions of increased markings, cavities, and atelectasis. However, routine chest radiographs may appear normal, especially in the early phases of bronchiectasis (7 to 10 per cent of patients). Often, all that may be seen are nonspecific markings in localized segments of lung. Tubular shadows (tram tracks, tram lines), mucoid impactions, or gloved finger shadows are more significant. Tubular shadows reflect the thickening of bronchial walls, peribronchial fibrosis, and alveolar collapse. Mucoid impactions or gloved finger shadows appear when secretions and pus fill airways with radiodense material.

Compensatory hyperinflation of uninvolved lung regions is common, especially in patients with cystic fibrosis.

Bronchography

Bronchography used to be considered the best method of confirming bronchiectasis and evaluating the extent of its progress. However, it is rarely done, since severely compromised patients or those with bronchospasm may have adverse reactions. In addition, bronchographic studies should not be performed in patients with active disease. Bronchography is rarely indicated today and should not be obtained unless the results will be important to a treatment decision. One example would be to document localized bronchiectasis that might be amenable to surgery. If they are needed, bronchograms should be obtained after several months, when reversible damage to airways has had time to resolve.

Computed Tomography (CT)

In almost all instances, CT replaces the need for bronchography. Adequate visualization of bronchiectatic segments is usually possible, and the problems noted above do not occur with this technique.

Bronchoscopy

Though not of use in diagnosing bronchiectasis, bronchoscopy is useful in identifying obstructions or sources of hemoptysis and in removing secretions. Biopsy of bronchial (or nasal) mucosa for

TABLE 63–2. DIAGNOSTIC FEATURES OF FAMILIAL BRONCHIECTASIS

Disorder	Clinical Findings	Laboratory Tests
Cystic fibrosis (see Ch. 64)	Pancreatic insufficiency, mucoid *Pseudomonas* strain, obstructive azoospermia, infertility	Sweat chloride
Immotile cilia syndrome	Infertility, sinusitis, otitis media, Kartagener's syndrome (with or without dextrocardia)	Electron microscopy of cilia, absent mucociliary clearance, immotility in living cells (nasal, sperm)
Alpha$_1$-antitrypsin deficiency	Emphysema, cirrhosis	Serum alpha$_1$-antitrypsin, Pi typing
Immunoglobulin G (IgG) deficiency	Recurrent infections	Quantitative Ig, IgG subclass
Immunoglobulin A (IgA) deficiency	Autoimmune phenomena, atopy	Quantitative Ig
Williams-Campbell syndrome	Disease restricted to chest	On bronchography, expiratory collapse of proximal bronchi
Neutrophil deficiencies	Recurrent infections (with or without thrombocytopenia, with or without pancreatic disease)	Blood smear, differential leukocyte count, nitroblue tetrazolium dye test
Complement deficiencies	Recurrent infections	C3 levels, CH50 determination

From Newth CJL: Bronchiectasis. *In* Wyngaarden JB, Smith LH Jr (eds.): Cecil Textbook of Medicine. 18th ed. Philadelphia, W. B. Saunders Company, 1988, p 439; with permission.

electron microscopic evaluation may be used to confirm ciliary dyskinesia.

Sinus Radiographs

Radiographic evaluation may be helpful in identifying patients in whom sinusitis accompanies bronchiectasis (e.g., immotile cilia syndrome, Young's syndrome).

Pulmonary Function

Patients with extensive bronchiectasis have impairments similar to those seen in chronic bronchitis or emphysema. Cough in patients with saccular or varicose bronchiectasis produces premature collapse of large bronchi, leading to obstruction of expiratory airflow and to air trapping. This collapse is probably due to the inflammatory destruction of proximal bronchial walls. Ineffective cough leads to retention of secretions, predisposing patients to further infection.

Disturbances in respiratory function are dependent upon the anatomic type of bronchiectasis and the degree of lung compromise. Pulmonary function tests in patients with diffuse involvement usually reveal airway obstruction. Forced vital capacity (FVC), forced expiratory volume in 1 second (FEV_1), FEV_1/FVC, and forced expiratory flow ($FEF_{25-75\%}$) are all decreased, and residual volume is increased. Decreased ventilation, perfusion, and ventilation-perfusion ratios are found in involved regions. Nitrogen washout studies may show evidence of maldistribution of inspired air. Hypoxemia may occur in severe bronchiectasis; but carbon dioxide retention tends to occur only in those patients with concomitant severe bronchitis or advanced emphysema. Persistent or progressive hypercapnea is an ominous finding, one that reflects advanced disease and cor pulmonale.

Additional Studies

Sputum cultures may yield evidence of *Haemophilus influenzae*, *Streptococcus pneumoniae*, *Streptococcus pyogenes*, *Pseudomonas aeruginosa*, *Pseudomonas cepacia*, *Staphylococcus aureus*, or *Aspergillus*, as well as a number of other organisms. Accurate determination of infective organisms has obvious implications for antibiotic therapies.

White blood cell counts and differentials may help to confirm active infection and to distinguish bronchiectasis from lymphoproliferative disorders. Arterial blood gas levels aid in the assessment of severe respiratory compromise. Sweat chloride tests in patients with bronchiectasis may detect previously undiscovered cystic fibrosis. Quantitative immunoglobulin determinations should be obtained if immunodeficiency is suspected. Nasal or bronchial biopsy is indicated when the immotile cilia syndrome is suspected.

Differential Diagnosis

Bronchiectasis represents permanent lung destruction and needs to be distinguished from reversible changes caused by such entities as pneumonia, bronchitis, and atelectasis, as well as from foreign body aspiration, tuberculosis, and lung abscess. In addition, the presence of any of the numerous predisposing conditions needs to be determined.

COMPLICATIONS

Severe complications are relatively uncommon; hemoptysis does occur. An early onset of disease, especially in those with cystic fibrosis or immunodeficiencies, is associated with decreased lifespan. Such complications as lung abscesses, pneumonia, progression of infection through the pleura to produce bronchopleural fistulas, or empyema are more common in this population than in those who acquire bronchiectasis later in adult life.

TREATMENT AND PROGNOSIS

Since anatomic destruction is irreversible, efforts are directed at medical therapies to prevent disease progression and to control symptoms. Antibiotics to combat (or occasionally prevent) infections, postural drainage, chest physical therapy, hydration, discontinuation of smoking, bronchodilators (in patients with bronchospasm), oxygen (for hypoxic patients during acute exacerbations or for those with chronic respiratory insufficiency), and

treatment for sinusitis are used as appropriate. Patients with bronchiectasis should also receive annual influenza vaccines.

The choice of antibiotics should be guided by the results of the sputum culture. However, these cultures often grow "normal flora," so ampicillin is generally chosen for empiric use. Trimethoprim-sulfamethoxazole or tetracycline is appropriate for patients for whom penicillins are contraindicated. One to 3 weeks of antibiotic therapy may be required to achieve the desired therapeutic effects. Long-term antibiotic therapy and courses of inhaled antibiotics have not proved effective.

Progression within involved bronchial segments is common, but extension to normal regions is unusual. Underlying diseases such as cystic fibrosis, asthma, and the immotile cilia syndrome may render the entire bronchial system vulnerable. Appropriate use of antibiotics is effective in controlling symptoms and minimizing dysfunction and disease progression.

Resection may be curative in that small subset of patients with severe localized disease. Patients with advanced bilateral disease are not surgical candidates and may do well with medical therapies alone. Rarely, surgery is indicated for a patient with massive hemoptysis resulting from vascular deformity within a bronchiectatic segment. If the patient is unable to tolerate surgical resection, bronchial artery embolization may be warranted.

Barker AF, Bardana EJ Jr: Bronchiectasis: Update of an orphan disease. Am Rev Respir Dis 137:969, 1988. *A concise review with 214 references, outlining pathology, etiology, host-insult pathogenesis, prognosis, and suggested evaluation.*

Le Roux BT, Mohlala ML, Odell JA, Whitton ID: Suppurative Diseases of the Lung and Pleural Space. Part II: Bronchiectasis. Chicago, Year Book Medical Publishers, 1986, pp 95–159. *Review with exhaustive bibliography and excellent section on historical perspective; focuses primarily on surgical management of bronchiectasis.*

Slutzker AD, Kinn R, Said SI: Bronchiectasis and progressive respiratory failure following smoke inhalation. Chest 95:1349, 1989. *Case presentation of patient who developed bronchiectasis after inhalational injury.*

Swartz MN: Bronchiectasis. *In* Fishman AP (ed.): Pulmonary Diseases and Disorders. 2nd ed. New York, McGraw-Hill Book Company, 1988, pp 1553–1579. *Comprehensive, well-referenced, and well-illustrated examination of the subject.*

64 Cystic Fibrosis
Roger Bone

DEFINITION

Cystic fibrosis (CF) is a heritable disease that follows an autosomal recessive pattern of transmittance. A child born to two heterozygous carriers has a 1:4 risk of having the disease, a 1:2 chance of being a carrier, and a 1:4 chance of neither being a carrier nor having the disease. CF is the most common lethal genetic disease in the United States; the approximate frequency in Caucasians is 1 in 2000. On the basis of this figure, it is estimated that 1 in 20 is a carrier of the defective gene. Blacks and Asians are seldom affected. CF is characterized by abnormal eccrine and exocrine gland function; mucous glands produce viscous secretions, which lead to chronic pulmonary disease, insufficient pancreatic and digestive function, and abnormally concentrated sweat.

HISTORICAL PERSPECTIVE

Although there are numerous historical associations between salty skin and early death, CF was first described as a distinct clinical entity in the late 1930's. It was initially referred to as "cystic fibrosis of the pancreas," to describe the histologic appearance of that organ late in the course of the disease. Only later was it recognized that all exocrine glands were involved.

PATHOLOGY AND PATHOGENESIS

There have been several diverse lines of research into the basic etiology of CF. The more prominent theories included searches for alterations in the physicochemical properties of exocrine secretions (e.g., defective macromolecular secretion), the regulation of exocrine gland secretions, electrolyte transport, and abnormalities in serum.

Though it has been known for the past few years that the gene for CF is located on the long arm of chromosome 7, the gene has only recently been isolated. The encoded protein contains 1480 amino acids, is very similar to other membrane proteins, and may, in fact, be an ion channel. A deletion of three base pairs in the genetic code results in loss of a phenylalanine residue at position 508. It is believed that the defective protein may be at least partially responsible for alterations in cyclic adenosine monophosphate (cAMP)–mediated chloride secretion.

With the isolation, in late 1989, of the genetic defect that presumably leads to CF, a unifying hypothesis is beginning to emerge. In normal individuals, chloride channels are located on the luminal membranes of epithelial cells. When these channels are open, chloride ions move into the airway lumen, producing an osmotic gradient that draws water into the lumen (Fig. 64–1). Abnormalities in sweat electrolytes of CF patients are probably due to chloride impermeability of the sweat duct epithelium. Anomalous mucus of the lungs and other organs may result from inadequate amounts of water on the luminal side of epithelial membranes, secondary to excessive sodium reabsorption or failure to secrete chloride, either of which would favor water movement from secretions into tissues. There is evidence to suggest that several CF mucous secretions contain inadequate amounts of water and that physical properties of mucous secretions are highly dependent on water content. If altered regulatory mechanisms are the source of these water and electrolyte transport abnormalities, it is possible that the secretion of macromolecules by exocrine cells is not properly controlled and that excessive amounts of mucous glycoproteins and other elements are secreted, which would further diminish clearance of secretions. It is now hoped that research in these directions will have a bearing on new therapies or potential cures for CF. Further efforts will most likely focus on epithelial cell regulatory mechanisms.

CLINICAL MANIFESTATIONS AND CLINICAL COURSE

Cystic fibrosis manifests in any number of ways and can mimic other clinical entities (Fig. 64–2). Early gastrointestinal involvement (i.e., meconium ileus, failure to thrive) leads to the diagnosis of more than 10 per cent of CF patients at birth or during infancy. More typical presentations, however, include early onset of respiratory symptoms such as cough and recurrent respiratory infections later in life.

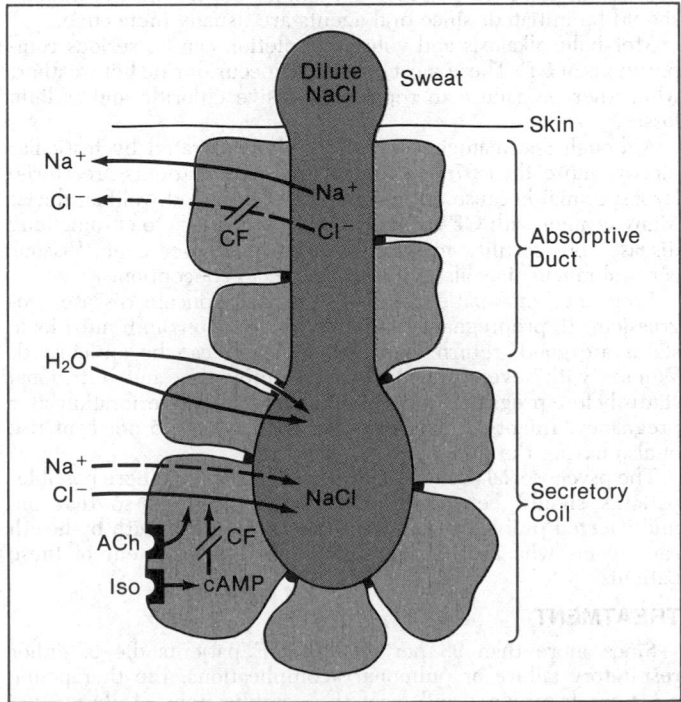

FIGURE 64–1. Electrolyte transport by sweat glands. (From Welsh MJ, Fick RB: Cystic fibrosis. J Clin Invest 80:1523, 1987. Reproduced from *The Journal of Clinical Investigation* by copyright permission of the American Society for Clinical Investigation.)

In many patients, intermittent episodes of acute respiratory infections persist longer than would be expected. Coughing increases and becomes worse at night and upon the patient's awakening. Sputum is viscous and purulent. Disease progression is often marked by a gradual decline in pulmonary function and is punctuated by acute exacerbations. The clinical course of CF is known to change suddenly with the onset of a number of complications. Poor nutritional status (or malnutrition, if present) often correlates with the severity of the pulmonary disease.

DIAGNOSIS

Radiology

Hyperinflation is noted early in the course of CF. As the disease progresses, hyperinflation and evidence of bronchitis increase, and there may be indications of peripheral cuffing, mucus impaction, or bronchiectasis.

Pulmonary Function

It is thought that newborns with CF have normal lung function, but within a short time many children show evidence of decreasing pulmonary function. There is usually demonstrable obstruction of small airways (e.g., decreased maximal mid-expiratory flow rates, reduced expiratory flow rates at low lung volumes, increased residual volume/total lung capacity [RV/TLC] ratios). Spirometry, lung volume measurements, and oxygenation levels are most frequently used to monitor pulmonary function and disease progression. Oxygenation gradually worsens throughout life; when arterial P_{O_2} values remain below 55 mm Hg, pulmonary hypertension is often present. Significant arterial P_{CO_2} elevations or forced expiratory volume in 1 second (FEV_1) values less than 30 per cent of those predicted portend end-stage disease; survival then averages 29 months.

Patients with CF often display airway hyperreactivity, which can be demonstrated by exercise testing, histamine challenge, or response to bronchodilators.

Sputum Culture

Although *Staphylococcus aureus*, *Pseudomonas aeruginosa*, and *Pseudomonas cepacia* are sometimes found in sputum cultures from patients with pulmonary diseases other than CF, their association with this disease is so consistent that attempts to obtain sputum cultures have become an integral part of evaluating any patient suspected of having CF. Sputum cultures may also be useful during exacerbations of the disease.

Pancreatic Function

Ninety to 95 per cent of patients with CF exhibit some degree of exocrine pancreatic dysfunction. Enzyme deficiency leads to maldigestion of protein and fat, which produces bulky, foul-smelling stools. If untreated, these patients fail to gain weight, and growth is inhibited. Poor growth can also be the result of increased energy expenditures associated with the work of breathing in those with severe respiratory symptoms.

Sweat

The discovery that an excessive loss of salt occurs in the sweat of CF patients has been used as the most important diagnostic criterion. Although the sweat glands of patients with CF are histologically normal, they function abnormally—producing secretions that are nearly isotonic, rather than the hypotonic solutions excreted by normal individuals.

Quantitative pilocarpine iontophoresis, performed in laboratories with established expertise, remains the standard for diagnosis of CF. A minimum of 100 mg of sweat needs to be collected, and results should be confirmed by a second test. In children, sodium and chloride concentrations exceeding 60 mEq/per liter are considered diagnostic of CF; in adults the level is 70 mEq per liter.

COMPLICATIONS

Respiratory

The major source of morbidity in patients with CF is pulmonary disease. Atelectasis is not uncommon, and it is usually associated with few symptoms. Evidence of bronchiectasis is common in CF

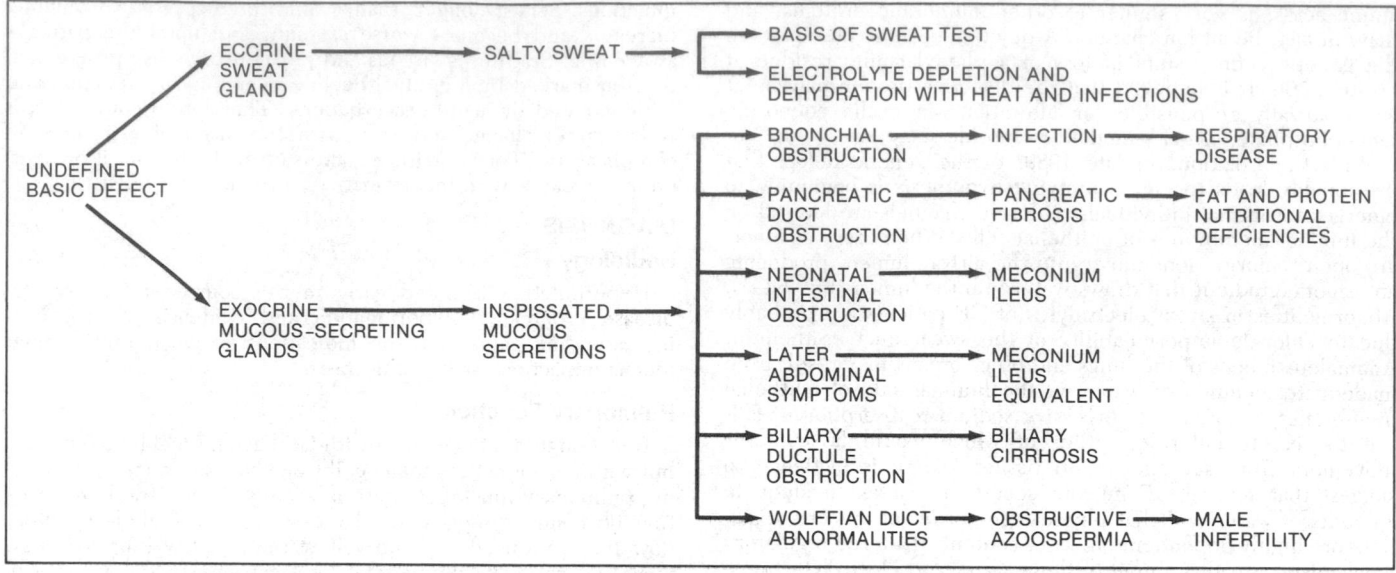

FIGURE 64–2. Clinical manifestations of cystic fibrosis. (From Newth CJL: Cystic fibrosis. *In* Wyngaarden JB, Smith LH Jr (eds.): Cecil Textbook of Medicine. 18th ed. Philadelphia, W. B. Saunders Company, 1988, p 440; with permission.)

patients by 5 to 10 years of age. Chest physiotherapy and antibiotics are often successful in re-expanding atelectatic regions. Surgical resection is only rarely considered, since the bronchiectasis is diffuse.

Pneumothorax is a common complication of CF. Up to one third of older patients experience recurrent episodes of pneumothorax. Because of this high rate, after an initial pneumothorax, attempts are often made to obliterate the pleural space by instillation of sclerosing agents, such as tetracycline. Insertion of a chest tube is usually considered only when the pneumothorax involves more than 10 per cent of a hemithorax.

Hemoptysis may occur if there is an erosion of pulmonary tissue that impinges on a bronchial blood vessel. Small amounts of blood-streaked sputum are common, but expectoration of more significant volumes of blood (>30 ml) often requires hospitalization. Massive hemoptysis is relatively uncommon in patients with CF, but when it occurs, it is life threatening. Bronchoscopy or surgery may be necessary, but radiographically guided bronchial artery embolization is becoming a more frequent treatment maneuver.

Respiratory failure (hypoxemia, hypercarbia) in a patient with CF becomes increasingly difficult to manage. Since CF patients tend to respond poorly to, and experience more complications from, mechanical ventilation than do patients in respiratory failure secondary to other conditions, mechanical ventilation is generally instituted only in the event of acute precipitating events, such as infectious pneumonia or other reversible complications. With disease progression, hypoxemia increases, and pulmonary hypertension and cor pulmonale develop in virtually all CF patients.

Although as many as 50 per cent of patients with CF exhibit antibodies to *Aspergillus fumigatus* in their serum, only a small number develop allergic aspergillosis. Expectoration of rusty brown plugs of sputum is suggestive of this condition.

Digital clubbing occurs in nearly every patient with CF and is often present early in the course of the pulmonary manifestations of this disease. Severity seems to correlate with the degree of pulmonary dysfunction. Hypertrophic pulmonary osteoarthropathy occurs in up to 15 per cent of adolescent and adult CF patients and is often characterized by pain in the joints on ambulation. Symptoms tend to subside when pulmonary symptoms improve.

Other

Intestinal obstruction (caused by meconium ileus or meconium ileus equivalent) can usually be treated medically; intussusception or rectal prolapse usually requires surgical intervention. Patients with CF are often prone to episodes of acute or chronic, crampy,

lower right quadrant abdominal pain, reflecting partial intestinal obstruction. These episodes can usually be treated with oral mineral oil and N-acetylcysteine used in conjunction with hyperosmolar enemas that contain agents such as diatrizoate methylglucamine.

Symptomatic biliary cirrhosis occurs in 2 to 5 per cent of CF patients. Patients present with hyperbilirubinemia, ascites, and peripheral edema. Although bleeding esophageal varices are an infrequent complication of CF, they are seen in some patients secondary to hepatic cirrhosis and portal hypertension. Endoscopy is generally used to sclerose the affected vessels.

As fibrosis of the exocrine pancreas continues, hyperglycemia may be encountered in patients with CF, especially in the second and third decades. Diabetes mellitus occurs in approximately 10 per cent of adult CF patients. If diabetes occurs, insulin therapy should be initiated, since oral agents are usually ineffective.

Metabolic alkalosis and volume depletion can be serious complications of CF. These most commonly occur during hot weather, when there is failure to replace excessive chloride and sodium losses.

Although spermatogenesis can be demonstrated by testicular biopsy, more than 97 per cent of male CF patients are sterile (azoospermia) because of incompletely developed wolffian ducts. Many women with CF are anovulatory secondary to chronic lung disease, but fertility may be as high as 20 per cent. Viscous cervical mucus may also prove a barrier to conception.

Pregnancy in a patient with CF can complicate disease progression. If prepregnancy pulmonary function and nutritional status are good, return to pregravid levels can be anticipated. Women with severely compromised pulmonary and nutritional status before pregnancy often show accelerated deterioration after pregnancy. Infants of mothers with CF have a 2.5 per cent risk of also having the disease.

The psychosocial aspects of CF are formidable. Where possible, patients should be cared for in special centers so that the multifaceted problems of the disease can be dealt with by health care teams who are experienced in the management of these patients.

TREATMENT

Since more than 98 per cent of CF patients die of either respiratory failure or pulmonary complications, the therapeutic goals are to prevent and treat the complications of obstruction and infection in the airways, enhance mucus clearance, and improve nutrition. Antibiotics are the key element to increasing survival in this population of patients. Frequent courses of antibiotic therapy are usually necessary; some patients may require them nearly continuously. Antibiotic selection should be guided by sputum culture.

Several species demonstrate great affinity for the respiratory tracts of patients with CF—*Staphylococcus aureus, Pseudomonas aeruginosa,* and, more recently, *Pseudomonas cepacia.* Indeed, their presence is suggestive of CF. Patients with demonstrable infection by *S. aureus* are most often treated with dicloxacillin, cephalexin, the newer cephalosporins, or chloramphenicol. Ciprofloxacin is also being increasingly used but is recommended only for patients older than 10 years of age. Early in the course of the disease, *Pseudomonas* organisms may be sensitive to tetracycline, trimethoprim-sulfamethoxazole, or chloramphenicol, but infection by these organisms is most often treated by using a combination of an intravenously given aminoglycoside and a semisynthetic penicillin (more popular combinations include gentamicin-carbenicillin and tobramycin-ticarcillin). Once found in the sputum, however, *P. aeruginosa* rarely, if ever, is eradicated. Therapeutic benefit therefore seems to be derived from reduction in the microbial load, rather than elimination of the infecting organism. Of late, *P. cepacia* is emerging as a serious problem for CF patients. This species tends to develop resistance to multiple antibiotics and has been associated with severe, frequently fatal pneumonia. *Haemophilus influenzae* infection is most often treated with ampicillin, trimethoprim-sulfamethoxazole, or chloramphenicol.

Chest Physiotherapy

Percussion and postural drainage are mainstays in the treatment of CF. Clearance of pulmonary secretions to prevent the complications that result from plugging of the airways with viscous mucous secretions and the infections that may arise distal to obstruction constitutes a crucial component of therapy.

Bronchodilators

Although positive effects can be demonstrated in the laboratory, long-term benefit from the use of bronchodilators for CF patients has not been established.

Nutrition

Most patients can be maintained on normal diets with pancreatic enzyme supplementation (usually enteric-coated capsules taken with meals). Because defective fat metabolism may lead to deficiencies in the fat-soluble vitamins (i.e., A, D, E, K), supplementation with these is often necessary. Many patients with CF also have higher than normal caloric needs—presumably resulting from the increased workload of breathing and maldigestion.

Exercise and Rehabilitation

Exercise tolerance in patients with CF correlates with the severity of pulmonary obstruction. Although exercise does not improve pulmonary function, it does improve cardiorespiratory fitness, and a program of physical conditioning is recommended. Long-term oxygen therapy can be used for chronic hypoxemia.

PROGNOSIS

Over the past three decades, there can be no question that comprehensive treatment programs have increased the overall survival of patients with CF. In the 1950's, patients lived only a few years; at present, the median survival is to age 24, and significant numbers of patients survive well beyond that. Clinical complexity and individual variability, however, make predictions in any given patient difficult. As mentioned previously, numerous factors are associated with unfavorable prognoses. CF patients who initially present with respiratory symptoms seem to have poorer prognoses. Once lung disease is established, colonization by *Pseudomonas* may indicate a poor prognosis. Males, those who maintain weight, and those in whom pancreatic exocrine function is relatively well preserved seem to do much better than those with severe insufficiency. The most significant determinant of the clinical course is the severity of the pulmonary disease and the rate at which it progresses.

To date, using marker techniques, it has been possible to screen only for carriers of the genetic defect within families of living CF patients. Recent advances in identification of the defective gene promise to have profound effects on our ability to detect heterozygotes, thereby allowing prevention of this devastating disease.

Boat TF: Cystic fibrosis. *In* Murray JF, Nadel JA (eds.): Textbook of Respiratory Medicine. Philadelphia, W. B. Saunders Company, 1988, pp 1126–1152. *Outstanding overview; especially clear review of the clinical manifestations of CF; 207 references.*

Fick RB, Stillwell PC: Controversies in the management of pulmonary disease due to cystic fibrosis. Chest 95:1319, 1989. *Addresses the questions of antibiotic administration (ambulatory, nebulized), corticosteroid use, nutritional support, exercise as a substitute for postural drainage, and surgical resection in this patient population.*

Halley DJJ, Bijman J, deJonge HR, et al.: The cystic fibrosis defect approached from different angles—new perspectives on the gene, the chloride channel, diagnosis and therapy. Eur J Pediatr 149:670, 1990.

O'Loughlin EV: Cystic fibrosis: An inborn error of cellular electrolyte transport? J Paediatr Child Health 26:126, 1990.

Michel BC: Antibacterial therapy in cystic fibrosis: A review of the literature published between 1980 and February 1987. Chest 94(Suppl 2):129S, 1988. *Numerous comparative tables compiled over a 7-year period; 67 references.*

Rubio TT: Infection in patients with cystic fibrosis. Am J Med 81(Suppl 1A):73, 1986. *Compilation and comparison of data from antimicrobial therapy studies over the past 16 years; 40 references.*

Scanlin TF: Cystic fibrosis. *In* Fishman AF (ed.): Pulmonary Diseases and Disorders. 2nd ed. New York, McGraw-Hill, 1988, pp 1273–1294. *An excellent overview, especially regarding the genetics, pathology, evaluation, treatment, natural history, and complications of CF.*

Thomassen MJ, Demko CA, Doershuk CF: Cystic fibrosis: A review of pulmonary infections and interventions. Pediatr Pulmonol 3:334, 1987. *A state-of-the-art review of the topic as of August 1986; 184 references.*

65 Pulmonary Embolism

Robert M. Senior

DEFINITION

Pulmonary embolism is the impaction of material into branches of the pulmonary arterial bed. Although they may completely prevent blood flow, most pulmonary emboli do not produce necrosis of lung parenchyma ("pulmonary infarction") because (1) a dual circulation (bronchial and pulmonary) supports lung parenchymal tissue and (2) exchange of oxygen and carbon dioxide can occur directly between the tissue and alveolar gas. Most pulmonary emboli are blood clots ("thromboemboli"); much more rarely, neoplastic cells, fat droplets (Ch. 66), air bubbles, exogenous materials (such as talc and cornstarch particles in intravenous drug abusers), or pieces of intravenous catheters and catheter introducers occlude pulmonary vessels. The ensuing discussion deals with pulmonary thromboembolism.

PATHOGENESIS

Pulmonary embolism is a complication of venous thrombosis; that is, emboli come from thrombi in peripheral veins, principally the deep veins of the lower extremities and pelvis (Ch. 54), and "travel" through the circulation to the pulmonary artery. In fact, in 70 per cent of patients with pulmonary thromboembolism, coexisting thrombi can be found in the deep veins of the thighs or pelvis. In the remaining cases, it is presumed that the emboli either come from other sites that escape detection or represent the entire thrombus that originated in the lower extremities. Thrombosis of superficial veins of the lower extremities does not lead to pulmonary thromboemboli, and thrombosis confined to deep veins in the leg distal to the popliteal vein infrequently leads to pulmonary thromboemboli. The renal veins can be a source of thromboemboli, particularly in patients with the nephrotic syndrome, but thromboemboli in nephrotic patients do not necessarily arise only from the renal veins. Pulmonary thromboemboli seldom originate in veins of the upper extremities, head, or neck, but they may arise from mural thrombi in the right side of the heart. Venous thromboemboli may be trapped in the right atrium or ventricle, from which they embolize to the lungs intact or fragment in the heart and shower the lungs with emboli at one time or at different times.

Venous thrombosis can be attributed to one or more of the

TABLE 65–1. CLINICAL RISK FACTORS FOR VENOUS THROMBOSIS AND PULMONARY THROMBOEMBOLISM

Common	Uncommon
Surgical and nonsurgical trauma, including burns	Acquired
Congestive heart failure	Lupus anticoagulant
Immobilization (bed rest, stroke, prolonged travel, and so forth)	Nephrotic syndrome
	Inflammatory bowel disease
	Persistent thrombocytosis
Malignancy	Polycythemia vera
Previous deep venous thrombosis	Paroxysmal nocturnal hemoglobinuria
Pregnancy, particularly in the puerperium and after cesarean section	Inherited
	Antithrombin III deficiency
Estrogen therapy	Protein C deficiency
Age over 50	Protein S deficiency
Obesity (?)	Plasminogen activator deficiency
	Elevated plasminogen activator inhibitor
	Homocystinuria

following: stasis of blood, increased tendency for blood to coagulate, and endothelial injury. Many clinical situations have been associated with the risk of proximal deep venous thrombosis (Table 65–1), but practically speaking, most are associated with decreased blood flow in lower extremity veins due to immobilization, elevated systemic venous pressure, extrinsic pressure on pelvic and lower extremity veins, intraluminal venous blockage from previous venous thrombosis, or decreased venous tone.

Pulmonary embolism occurs in 1 to 2 per cent of patients over age 40 following general surgery. The incidence is higher (5 to 10 per cent) with orthopedic surgery of the hip or knee. The risk associated with surgery is increased by advanced age, obesity, a lengthy operative period, underlying malignancy, pre-existent venous disease, prolonged bed rest after surgery, and postoperative infection. Venous stasis due to immobilization is probably a major reason for venous thrombosis associated with surgery, but other factors come into play: increased blood coagulability associated with release of tissue thromboplastin and exposure of subendothelium, postoperative decreased blood fibrinolytic activity, and vessel damage, particularly in surgery of the lower extremities or pelvis.

Cancers of the lung, breast, and abdominal viscera have a strong association with venous thromboembolism, and the thromboembolism may antedate clinical recognition of the malignancy. Factors released from tumors may increase blood coagulability, decrease fibrinolytic activity, and alter endothelial surfaces. Malignancies also predispose to deep venous thrombosis by leading to venous stasis through immobilization and surgical interventions. Some evidence in women with breast cancer points to a thrombogenic effect of anticancer drug therapy. Prolonged bed rest from any cause and paralysis resulting from stroke are also associated with a high incidence of venous thrombosis. Pulmonary embolism is commonly found at autopsy in patients who die of congestive heart failure.

In pregnancy, multiple factors predispose to venous thrombosis: (1) venous stasis induced by compression on pelvic veins, increased intra-abdominal pressure, and hormonal relaxation of vascular smooth muscle; (2) altered blood rheologic properties; and (3) increased concentrations of factors in the coagulation cascade (fibrinogen, Factors VII, VIII, IX, and XII), with concomitant reductions in antithrombin III and fibrinolytic activity. There may be a greater risk of thromboembolism during pregnancy, but there is clearly an increased risk in the puerperal period, particularly after cesarean section. Estrogen therapy has been linked with a higher incidence of venous thrombosis, and the risk appears related to the dose, but the precise degree of increased risk and the mechanisms involved are not certain. Multiple possibilities have been considered, including reduction in antithrombin III concentration, decreased plasminogen activator level, increased platelet aggregability, increased blood viscosity, and increased distensibility of peripheral veins leading to venous stasis.

When pulmonary embolism occurs without an obvious predisposing factor, and particularly when there is a family history of venous thrombosis, one should consider the possibility of a hereditary decrease in an anticoagulant factor (antithrombin III, proteins C and S, or tissue plasminogen activator) or a hereditary increase in plasminogen activator inhibitor (Ch. 155).

INCIDENCE

Pulmonary embolism is a major cause of morbidity and death. The annual incidence in the United States has been estimated at approximately 600,000. About one third of the episodes are fatal, with nearly all of the fatalities either sudden (within 1 hour of onset) or undiagnosed during life. In approximately half of the people who die, there is serious underlying disease apart from venous thrombosis. Autopsy studies have reported pulmonary embolism as a major cause of death (10 to 20 per cent of all deaths occurring in hospitals and 15 per cent of postoperative deaths). The incidence of fatal pulmonary embolism in hospitalized patients may be declining. In one medical center, the incidence of autopsy-documented fatal pulmonary embolism fell from 9.3 per cent to 3.8 per cent over a recent 10-year period. It is interesting that during the same years, there was a concomitant increase, from 4 per cent to approximately 12 per cent, in the percentage of adult patients given anticoagulant therapy.

PATHOPHYSIOLOGY

Pulmonary emboli produce respiratory and hemodynamic responses that reflect the extent of pulmonary vascular obstruction, the time elapsed since embolization, and the presence or absence of pre-existent heart or lung disease.

HYPERPNEA AND ALVEOLAR HYPERVENTILATION. Acute pulmonary embolism stimulates ventilation. The increase in minute ventilation, manifested clinically by increased respiratory rate, usually offsets the increased physiologic dead space produced by obstruction of the pulmonary vascular bed, so that the arterial P_{CO_2} (Pa_{CO_2}) does not rise. On the contrary, the Pa_{CO_2} typically falls below 35 mm Hg, indicating that hyperpnea does not occur solely to preserve a normal Pa_{CO_2}. Similarly, alveolar hyperventilation is not due to hypoxemia, as it occurs even when arterial oxygenation is normal, and it cannot be abolished with supplemental inspired oxygen. The stimulus for alveolar hyperventilation is unknown but presumably involves reflexes initiated from the pulmonary parenchyma in the area of the obstructed vessel. A reduction of Pa_{CO_2} below baseline may occur even among those with chronic hypercapnia. Although a lower than normal Pa_{CO_2} is usual, the Pa_{CO_2} rises in individuals who cannot increase their minute ventilation adequately to compensate for the increased physiologic dead space—for example, in those with neuromuscular disease, those receiving controlled mechanical ventilation, or those with severe pleuritic pain. The Pa_{CO_2} may also rise when there is massive embolization that confines pulmonary blood flow to a severely reduced portion of the pulmonary vascular bed.

HYPOXEMIA. A decrease in arterial oxygen tension (Pa_{CO_2}) is common in acute pulmonary embolism. The mechanisms are complex. Ventilation-perfusion ($\dot{V}a/\dot{Q}$) inequality seems to be the predominant mechanism early in the course of pulmonary embolization, with intrapulmonary shunting as the dominant cause after 48 hours. Regional bronchoconstriction, atelectasis, and pulmonary edema are postulated as the anatomic basis for these physiologic defects. If cardiac output fails to keep up with metabolic demands, as is common with massive pulmonary embolism, mixed venous oxygen saturation falls and accentuates the effects of abnormal $\dot{V}a/\dot{Q}$ and intrapulmonary shunting. If pulmonary hypertension develops and a patent foramen ovale is present, blood may be shunted from the right to left within the heart, another factor causing arterial hypoxemia.

PULMONARY HYPERTENSION AND ACUTE COR PULMONALE. Pulmonary thromboembolism is the most common cause of acute pulmonary hypertension. The rise in pulmonary arterial pressure results primarily from mechanical blockage of the pulmonary vascular bed. Vasoconstrictive reflexes and mediators may also contribute. The rise in mean pulmonary arterial pressure tends to match the extent of blockage of the pulmonary arterial tree, but in patients without pre-existing cardiac or pulmonary disease, mean pulmonary arterial pressure is usually below 20 mm Hg unless pulmonary vascular obstruction exceeds 50 per cent. Pressures of 20 to 40 mm Hg occur only with 50 per cent to 75 per cent obstruction. The pressure seldom rises above 40 mm Hg because the normal right ventricle is incapable of generating higher pressures. A mean pulmonary arterial pressure above 40 mm Hg indicates chronic right ventricular hypertrophy secondary to recurrent pulmonary emboli or other diseases. When a sudden and marked increase in pulmonary vascular resistance causes the mean pulmonary arterial pressure to approach 40 mm Hg, several events occur. Right ventricular diastolic pressure, right atrial pressure, and systemic venous pressure all increase. The cardiac index falls below 2.5 liters per minute per square meter, and systemic hypotension and other clinical signs of hemodynamic distress appear.

PATHOLOGY

Most episodes of acute pulmonary embolism involve multiple emboli. Both lungs are affected about two thirds of the time. Lower lobe vessels are involved more often than upper lobe vessels, and the right lung is affected more often than the left. Emboli in the main branches of the right or left pulmonary arteries are seen in only a small percentage of patients. A large embolus obstructing the main pulmonary artery or straddling the pulmonary artery bifurcation (so-called "saddle embolus") is uncommon even in fatal acute pulmonary embolism. When a thromboembolus is poorly organized, it is apt to fragment in passage through the heart and is thus more likely to impact in smaller vessels than are organized thromboemboli.

The likelihood that emboli will cause pulmonary infarction is determined by the size of the vessels involved, by the extent of obstruction, by the potential for delivery of bronchial arterial blood flow, and by the adequacy of ventilation to the lung tissue supplied by the blocked pulmonary arteries. Occlusions of segmental arterial vessels or smaller branches are more apt to lead to infarction than are emboli lodged in larger vessels. Infarction is also more likely in the setting of elevated pulmonary capillary pressure from any cause—hence the frequency of infarction in patients with congestive heart failure—but otherwise healthy individuals can develop infarcts. Histologically, pulmonary infarction is characterized by intra-alveolar hemorrhage and necrosis of alveolar walls, but little inflammation. Cavitation rarely develops without coexisting pulmonary infection or an infected thrombus.

CLINICAL MANIFESTATIONS

The clinical features of pulmonary embolism can be diverse and confusing and range from no symptoms to sudden death. Occasionally, the principal manifestations are fever, arrhythmias, or refractory congestive heart failure. Usually, however, the presentations are not obscure. Three clinical patterns predominate: (1) sudden dyspnea with no physical findings but tachypnea; (2) sudden pleuritic chest pain and dyspnea accompanied by findings consistent with pleural effusion and pulmonary consolidation; and (3) sudden apprehension, chest discomfort, and dyspnea, with findings of acute cor pulmonale (accentuated pulmonic closure sound in the second left interspace, right ventricular lift, jugular venous distention) and systemic hypotension. It is this last pattern that may culminate in death within a few minutes.

The type of pattern that develops depends upon the extent of pulmonary arterial tree blockage, whether there is pre-existent cardiopulmonary disease, and whether pulmonary infarction occurs. Severe disturbances in pulmonary and systemic hemodynamics seldom occur unless extensive vascular obstruction or pre-existent heart or lung disease is present. Pleuritic pain and signs of pulmonary consolidation and pleural effusion indicate that embolization involves one or more peripheral pulmonary arterial branches. Large discrepancies may exist between the severity of embolization and symptoms. Some patients with massive embolization may appear remarkably comfortable, whereas others with minimal embolization may show great distress.

The most common symptoms of pulmonary embolism are dyspnea and chest pain, each occurring in more than 80 per cent of patients (Table 65–2). Tachypnea is the most common sign. Hemoptysis, on the other hand, often considered typical, is not

TABLE 65–2. SYMPTOMS AND SIGNS IN 327 PATIENTS WITH PULMONARY EMBOLI

Symptoms	Per Cent	Signs	Per Cent
Chest pain	88	Respirations above 16/min	92
Pleuritic	74	Rales	58
Nonpleuritic	14	S₂P* increased	53
Dyspnea	84	Pulse above 100/min	44
Apprehension	59	Temperature above 37.8°C	43
Cough	53	Phlebitis	32
Hemoptysis	30	Gallop	34
Sweats	27	Diaphoresis	36
Syncope	13	Edema	24
		Murmur	23
		Cyanosis	19

*S_2P = intensity of the pulmonic component of the second heart sound.

Apprehension, syncope, increased pulmonic component of the second heart sound, gallop, diaphoresis, murmur, and cyanosis occurred more often with massive emboli (angiographically, at least two lobar arteries obstructed), whereas hemoptysis and pleuritic pain were more often present with submassive emboli.

From Bell WR, Simon TL, DeMets DL: The clinical features of submassive and massive pulmonary emboli. Am J Med 62:355, 1977; with permission.

a usual finding. Its absence, therefore, is not evidence against pulmonary embolism. Similarly, deep venous thrombosis of the lower extremities is seldom clinically apparent. A recent prospective study of adults presenting to the emergency room with pleuritic chest pain found, by pulmonary arteriography, that 21 per cent had pulmonary emboli. Emboli were not found in those under age 40 without risk factors for venous thrombosis; however, among the subjects over 40 without risk factors, 18 per cent had abnormal pulmonary arteriograms.

DIAGNOSIS

Although the history and physical examination may suggest the pulmonary embolism, a diagnosis that rests on clinical grounds alone is often incorrect. The differential diagnosis of pulmonary embolism can encompass many disorders, but principally those leading to acute shortness of breath, substernal or pleuritic chest pain, hemoptysis, and hemodynamic collapse. Thus, at times the possibility of pulmonary embolism must be distinguished from asthma, the hyperventilation syndrome, pneumothorax, pulmonary edema, a fractured rib, herpes zoster before the appearance of vesicles, pleurodynia, pleuritis due to collagen vascular diseases, pneumonia, empyema, bronchiectasis, bronchogenic carcinoma, acute myocardial infarction, pericarditis, dissecting aortic aneurysm, esophageal rupture, and upper abdominal processes such as acute cholecystitis. Several features discount the diagnosis of pulmonary embolism: (1) the absence of a precipitating factor for deep venous thrombosis, (2) recurrent chest pain in the same location, (3) pleuritic chest pain of more than 1 week's duration that is increasing in severity, (4) pleuritic chest pain with normal findings on the chest radiograph, (5) hemoptysis of greater than 5 ml with normal findings on the chest radiograph, (6) pericardial friction rub, (7) purulent sputum, and (8) spiking fever in excess of 39°C lasting more than 1 week.

DIAGNOSTIC STUDIES. When pulmonary embolism is suspected, confirmation of the diagnosis depends upon establishing that there is intravascular obstruction to pulmonary arterial blood flow. The definitive means of making the diagnosis is by pulmonary arteriography; however, a high degree of certainty can also be achieved with ventilation-perfusion scanning. Other approaches to visualizing the pulmonary circulation, such as computed tomography and magnetic resonance imaging, as well as methods of visualizing intrapulmonary thrombi using radioisotopically labeled platelets or monoclonal antibodies to platelet antigens and fibrin, are under development.

Arterial blood gas measurement, the electrocardiogram, the chest radiograph, and thoracentesis may help in the evaluation of patients suspected of having pulmonary embolism, either by favoring or by discounting diagnoses with which pulmonary embolism can be confused, but these studies lack specificity and therefore cannot be used in place of imaging the pulmonary circulation. Many efforts have been made to develop blood tests with specificity for the diagnosis of pulmonary embolism. None has been found useful.

Arterial Blood Gases. Typically in pulmonary embolism, there is a reduction in Pa_{O_2} and a concomitant reduction in Pa_{CO_2}. In patients with arteriographically proven acute pulmonary embolism who do not have previous cardiopulmonary disease, Pa_{O_2} values are less than 50 mm Hg in 13 per cent, 50 to 59 mm Hg in 19 per cent, between 60 and 80 mm Hg in 55 per cent, and greater than 80 mm Hg in 13 per cent. In those with a normal Pa_{O_2}, there is usually an increased alveolar-arterial oxygen difference, reflecting reduced efficiency of alveolar gas exchange, but even a normal alveolar-arterial oxygen difference does not exclude the diagnosis. A Pa_{O_2} less than 50 mm Hg is confined to those with greater than 50 per cent occlusion of major pulmonary arterial branches; however, in individuals with underlying cardiopulmonary disease, less severe degrees of pulmonary vascular obstruction can be associated with severe hypoxemia. Arterial blood gas abnormalities have no specificity for pulmonary embolism (similar abnormalities occur in conditions with which pulmonary embolism is confused).

Electrocardiogram. The main value of the electrocardiogram is to help exclude acute myocardial infarction. The most common finding in pulmonary embolism is sinus tachycardia. With emboli that provoke a substantial rise in pulmonary arterial and right-sided cardiac pressures, patterns of S_1, Q_3, T_3, inverted T waves in leads V_{1-3}, right ventricular strain, right-axis deviation, right bundle branch block, and atrial arrhythmias may occur. These changes, when they occur, are apt to be transient, lasting a few minutes or hours, disappearing as the pulmonary arterial pressure returns toward normal.

Chest Radiograph. A normal chest radiograph is uncommon in acute pulmonary embolism, but the usual radiographic findings are nonspecific: elevation of one of the hemidiaphragms with basilar atelectasis, infiltrates, and unilateral pleural effusion. Cardiac dilatation, dilatation of the main branches of the pulmonary artery, and zones of oligemia may occur with massive embolization. Besides lacking specificity, the chest radiograph shows a poor correlation with pulmonary arteriographic findings. Parenchymal densities tend to be in the lower lung fields, pleural based, and triangular and are ordinarily associated with pleural effusions. These densities usually represent extravascular blood rather than infarcted tissue. In summary, the principal value of the chest radiograph is to help exclude other possible diagnoses.

Thoracentesis. Pleural effusions, usually unilateral, are common with pulmonary embolism. The fluid is most often an exudate and is often hemorrhagic (but has a low hematocrit).

Ventilation-Perfusion Lung Scans. Isotopic scans of pulmonary perfusion ($\dot{Q}$ scans) provide a sensitive, safe means of assessing regional pulmonary blood flow and therefore have proved to be of great value in the diagnosis of pulmonary embolism. They can be performed alone or in combination with isotopic scans of ventilation ($\dot{V}$ scan). The combination of scans ($\dot{V}/\dot{Q}$ scans) is more specific than the $\dot{Q}$ scan alone. $\dot{V}/\dot{Q}$ lung scanning has become the accepted means of initially assessing the patient suspected of having pulmonary embolism. The strategy of using these scans is summarized in Figure 65–1.

A $\dot{Q}$ scan requires intravenous administration, with the patient supine, of technetium-99m–labeled particles of macroaggregated albumin, followed by scanning of the thorax with a gamma counter in a minimum of six views (anterior, posterior, right and left lateral, and right and left posterior oblique). The particles, which are slightly larger in diameter than the cross-section of the precapillary vessels of the pulmonary circulation, are injected into a peripheral vein, flow through the peripheral and central venous circulation, the right side of the heart, and the main pulmonary arteries, and finally lodge in precapillary vessels, where they remain for hours. The standard dose of particles blocks less than 0.2 per cent of the pulmonary precapillary vessels in the normal pulmonary vascular bed. For a $\dot{V}$ scan, the patient usually inhales and then rebreathes air containing radioactive gas, most often xenon-133, or aerosolized radiolabeled particles. Images of the initial breath, equilibration, and washout of the tracer are obtained. Typically, the xenon $\dot{V}$ scan is performed before the $\dot{Q}$ scan in the posterior projection with oblique views during washout. The patient is upright if possible. Besides xenon-

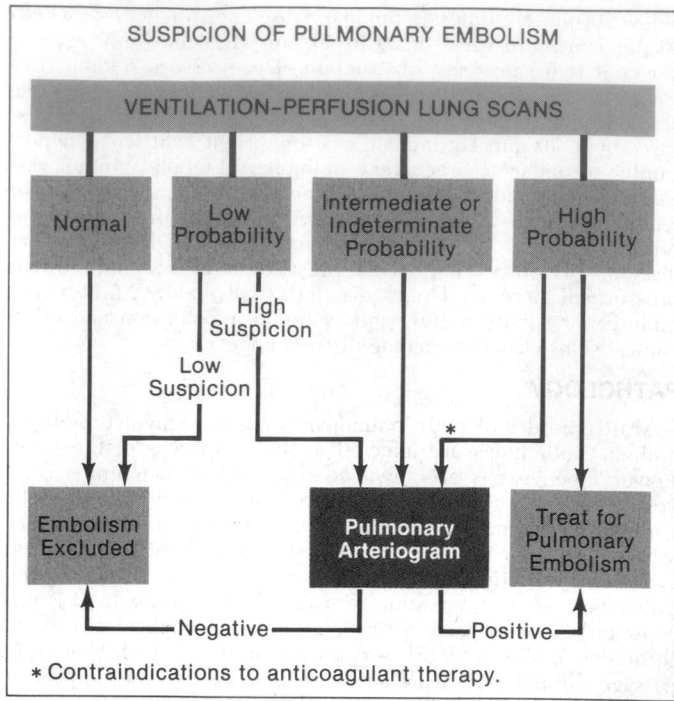

FIGURE 65–1. Ventilation-perfusion lung scanning in the evaluation of the patient suspected of having pulmonary embolism.

133, two other isotopes that are increasingly used for $\dot{V}$ scanning are krypton-81m– and technetium-99m–labeled particles in aerosols, which have the advantage over xenon-133 of enabling scans to be obtained in the same views as the $\dot{Q}$ scan with minimal radiation exposure.

A normal $\dot{Q}$ scan eliminates the diagnosis of pulmonary embolism. A normal scan reveals a homogeneous distribution of activity with an image that conforms to the lungs. In the presence of a pulmonary embolus, the radiolabeled particles are prevented from reaching vessels distal to the embolus, and the scan shows one or more perfusion defects in the image. The sensitivity of the $\dot{Q}$ lung scan to pulmonary arterial obstruction is excellent, as obstruction of vessels 3 mm in diameter or more leads to defects. Perfusion defects generally show some resolution within 4 to 5 days, but substantial abnormalities commonly persist for several weeks and may be present even a year later.

Defects on $\dot{Q}$ lung scans are interpreted in conjunction with the chest radiograph. Defects that do not have a corresponding abnormality on the chest radiograph are scored by number and size for the probability of pulmonary embolism. Single defects smaller than segments carry low probability for pulmonary embolism, whereas multiple defects that are segmental or larger carry a substantially higher probability for pulmonary embolism. Perfusion defects that have corresponding abnormalities on the chest radiograph are called "indeterminate," although some evidence indicates that a perfusion defect can be assigned a probability of embolus score based upon its size relative to the radiographic abnormality.

The limitation of the $\dot{Q}$ scan is nonspecificity. Besides emboli, perfusion defects can be caused by lesions that compress pulmonary vessels, by increased pulmonary vascular resistance, by regional alveolar hypoxia, and by regional loss of pulmonary parenchyma, as in pulmonary emphysema. In practice, obstructive lung disease is the most common clinical condition causing perfusion defects that are not due to pulmonary embolism.

The $\dot{V}$ lung scans increase the specificity of the $\dot{Q}$ scans for diagnosing pulmonary emboli because pulmonary emboli do not usually disrupt regional ventilation as much as regional blood flow, unlike other causes of perfusion defects, especially obstructive lung disease (Table 65–3). $\dot{V}$ scans may indicate the preservation of ventilation when there are perfusion defects ("$\dot{V}/\dot{Q}$ mismatches"), the loss of ventilation when there are perfusion defects ("$\dot{V}/\dot{Q}$ matches"), and delays of washin or washout indicative of obstructive lung disease. $\dot{V}/\dot{Q}$ mismatches establish a higher probability of pulmonary emboli than do perfusion defects alone. With some patterns of V̇/Q̇ mismatch, the diagnosis of pulmonary embolism can be made with virtual certainty (Fig. 65–2). Matched V̇/Q̇ defects are less likely to represent pulmonary embolism, but pulmonary embolism is not excluded.

A multicenter study to evaluate the sensitivity and specificity of V̇/Q̇ scanning in the diagnosis of pulmonary embolism has been completed recently in the United States. This prospective investigation of pulmonary embolism diagnosis (referred to as the PIOPED Study) employed V̇/Q̇ scanning and pulmonary arteriography in a large, randomly selected sample of individuals suspected of having acute pulmonary embolism. The results support the findings of earlier studies (Table 65–3): (1) High-probability scans were confirmed with definitive arteriographic findings of emboli in most cases; (2) normal scans were seldom associated with arteriographic findings of emboli; (3) among low-probability scans the occurrence of embolism was small, particularly when the clinical suspicion for embolism was low; and (4) intermediate or indeterminate scans were of little help in predicting the results of arteriography. Notably, in the majority of instances in which arteriograms were abnormal, scans were abnormal but did not indicate a high probability of embolism.

Pulmonary Arteriography. Pulmonary arteriography is the definitive test for the diagnosis of pulmonary embolism. It involves insertion of a catheter into the pulmonary artery, usually by a percutaneous approach through one of the femoral veins. After the catheter is advanced at least as far as the right or left mainstem branch of the pulmonary artery, or more selectively into lobar or segmental branches, the contrast medium is injected and films are taken in rapid sequence. Radiographic images—anterior, oblique, or lateral views—are examined for filling defects (Fig. 65–3) in branches of the pulmonary artery; these establish the diagnosis of pulmonary embolism. Abrupt terminations ("cutoffs") of pulmonary arterial branches also indicate that diagnosis, although less definitely. The filling defects or cutoffs should be present in vessels of at least 2 to 3 mm in diameter. Other types of abnormalities, including delayed filling and a diminished number of small vessels, are not diagnostic. A normal study has rarely been proved wrong. Arteriography should be done promptly after the onset of symptoms, but it is doubtful that there will be major changes within a few days in most cases.

Pulmonary arteriography is indicated when scans demonstrate an intermediate probability of pulmonary embolism. It is also warranted in the following circumstances: (1) when V̇/Q̇ scans suggest a high probability of pulmonary embolism but there are concerns about using anticoagulation therapy; (2) before using thrombolytic agents; (3) when there are clear-cut contraindications to anticoagulation therapy, so that other forms of treatment will be needed; and (4) when anticoagulation therapy has apparently failed and surgical treatment is being contemplated.

When V̇/Q̇ scans are interpreted as indicating a low probability of pulmonary embolism, it has been considered reasonable to be guided by clinical suspicion about the need for arteriography (see Fig. 65–1). Since approximately 10 per cent of these patients will have an abnormal arteriogram, some clinicians contend that

pulmonary arteriography should be done routinely in this situation, irrespective of the level of clinical suspicion. Recent studies, however, cast doubt on whether pulmonary arteriography is necessary in any patients having low-probability scans because long-term follow-up of such individuals indicates that they are unlikely to have clinically apparent pulmonary emboli over the subsequent year without anticoagulant therapy. Assessing the proximal deep veins of the lower extremities may be important in this setting. In a large prospective series, Hull and associates found that an abnormal V̇/Q̇ scan, but not one of high probability, combined with normal results on serial noninvasive tests for thrombosis of proximal veins, carried a very good prognosis without anticoagulant therapy.

Many experts in this field believe that pulmonary arteriography is underutilized because physicians have unwarranted concerns about the safety of the procedure. Pulmonary arteriography for the diagnosis of pulmonary embolism has proved to be very safe. In large series, the risk of a serious complication is 1 to 2 per cent and of death, about 0.25 per cent. The deaths have occurred almost exclusively in people with severe pulmonary hypertension who were given large amounts of contrast media.

THERAPY

Nearly all patients with acute pulmonary embolism who survive long enough to have the diagnosis confirmed will survive the acute episode. Accordingly, the primary goal of therapy is to prevent a recurrence that might be fatal. Additional goals are to reduce the morbidity of the acute episode and to prevent chronic pulmonary hypertension.

The overall therapeutic approach is summarized in Figure 65–4. The cornerstone of therapy is the use of anticoagulant drugs, since most patients with acute pulmonary embolism are hemodynamically stable and do not have a contraindication to anticoagulants. Patients who are treated with therapeutic doses of anticoagulants for an appropriate period seldom have a recurrence of pulmonary embolism, and fatal recurrences are rare indeed. Thrombolytic therapy accelerates restoration of pulmonary blood flow and normal pulmonary hemodynamics and therefore is the initial therapy for massive pulmonary embolism that has produced hemodynamic instability. When anticoagulants and thrombolytic agents are contraindicated or prove ineffective, therapy consists of interruption of the inferior vena cava, combined with pulmonary embolectomy in patients with hemodynamic instability.

Supportive measures can reduce the morbidity of the acute episode and, on occasion, are essential to sustain the patient through a period of hemodynamic crisis. These measures include supplemental oxygen to correct hypoxemia, analgesics for pleuritic pain, and hemodynamic and ventilatory support.

ANTICOAGULANT THERAPY. Anticoagulant therapy guards against future embolization by preventing the formation of new deep venous thrombi and the propagation of residual thrombi in the deep venous system. During anticoagulant ther-

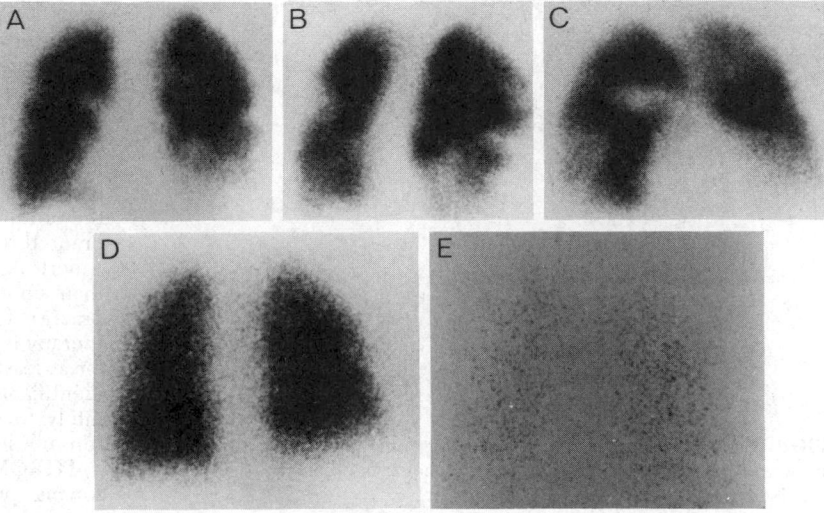

FIGURE 65–2. Selected views of ventilation-perfusion lung scans in a 60-year-old man who experienced sudden, severe shortness of breath 14 days after a suprapubic prostatectomy. The perfusion scans—(*A*) posterior, (*B*) right posterior oblique, and (*C*) left posterior oblique—show multiple segmental defects; the ventilation scans are normal—(*D*) at equilibrium and (*E*) at 1 minute of washout. This combination of scan findings indicates a high probability of pulmonary embolism and with the clinical setting is sufficient to make the diagnosis of pulmonary embolism. (Courtesy of Dr. Keith C. Fischer.)

TABLE 65–3. INTERPRETATION OF VENTILATION-PERFUSION (V̇/Q̇) SCINTIGRAMS

Category	Pattern	Approximate Frequency of Pulmonary Embolism Detected by Pulmonary Arteriogram (%)
Normal	No perfusion defects	0
Low probability	Small V̇/Q̇ mismatches	10
	V̇/Q̇ matches without corresponding roentgenographic changes	
	Perfusion defect substantially smaller than roentgenographic density	
Intermediate probability	Severe, diffuse obstructive pulmonary disease with perfusion defects	30
	Perfusion defect of same size as roentgenographic change	
	Single segmental mismatch*	
High probability	Two or more segmental mismatches	90
	Perfusion defect substantially larger than roentgenographic density	

*Controversy exists regarding the important categorization of a single segmental mismatch. This has been considered either of high or intermediate probability. The more conservative interpretation, that is, intermediate probability, has been used in this table.

Adapted from Biello DR: Radiological (scintigraphic) evaluation of patients with suspected pulmonary thromboembolism. JAMA 257:3257, 1987; with permission. Copyright 1987, American Medical Association.

apy, pulmonary emboli and residual deep venous thrombi either organize or undergo dissolution or both. Anticoagulation does not, however, hasten resolution of the thromboemboli within the lungs.

Table 65–4 presents a regimen of anticoagulant agents. Heparin is the initial therapy because its effect is immediate. It may also be a more effective antithrombotic agent than warfarin. Heparin, an acidic glycosaminoglycan obtained from pig intestinal mucosa or beef lung, accelerates the inhibitory effect of antithrombin III upon the coagulation enzymes, thrombin, and Factors IXa, Xa, XIa, and XIIa. In patients who are suspected of having pulmonary embolism, an intravenous bolus of heparin (5000 to 10,000 units) should be given while diagnostic studies are under way, unless there is intracranial bleeding, intracranial lesions predisposed to bleed, or active internal bleeding, all of which are absolute contraindications to heparin.

Heparin is usually administered intravenously by continuous infusion. Intermittent intravenous injection and subcutaneous injection are alternative means of administration, but a higher incidence of bleeding complications may occur with intermittent injection, and it is difficult to establish the correct dose with the subcutaneous route. The risk of recurrent venous thromboembolism is low if the activated partial thromboplastin time is maintained 1.5 to 2 times the control (about 25 seconds beyond the control) at all times. Accordingly, this is the goal of therapy. The usual daily dose is 25,000 to 50,000 units. Heparin therapy should be monitored particularly closely during the first few days

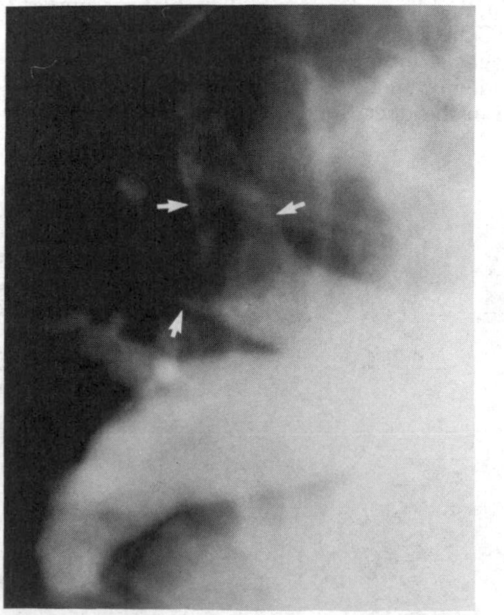

after the thromboembolic event, as the heparin requirements are greatest then.

The most common and most serious complication of heparin therapy is bleeding. The risk of bleeding may be more closely related to risk factors, such as trauma, recent surgery, recent invasive procedures, and the inhibition by heparin of platelet function, than to the absolute anticoagulant effect produced by the drug. Thrombocytopenia may also complicate therapy and cause bleeding. Approximately 10 per cent of patients exhibit platelet counts less than 100,000 per cubic millimeter during heparin therapy; there seems to be no correlation between this complication and the type of heparin used. The thrombocytopenia, which appears to have an immunologic basis, seldom occurs until after several days of therapy. A rare complication of heparin-induced thrombocytopenia is thrombosis, mainly of arteries. With long-term administration, heparin can cause accelerated osteoporosis.

After 1 to 2 days of heparin therapy, oral anticoagulation with warfarin is begun. Both agents are continued together for 4 to 5 days, after which the heparin is discontinued. Warfarin acts in the liver to inhibit the gamma-carboxylation of specific glutamic acid residues in several vitamin K–dependent coagulation factors: Factors II, VII, IX, and X (Ch. 155). These gamma-carboxyglutamic acids are required for calcium binding and the expression of functional activity. Since these coagulation cofactors have different half-lives in the circulation, the rates at which they diminish in activity are variable after the start of therapy. The prothrombin time is most sensitive to Factor VII, which has the shortest half-life (4 to 6 hours).

The rationale for overlapping heparin therapy with the first period of warfarin therapy is to ensure a full anticoagulant effect during the time required for depression of the level of all four coagulation cofactors affected by warfarin. It is also done to reduce the risk of thrombosis during the induction of warfarin, since warfarin lowers the concentration of protein C, a vitamin K–dependent protein that has anticoagulant properties because of its capacity to degrade Factors Va and VIIIa proteolytically. Warfarin is not used during pregnancy, since it is teratogenic. In pregnancy, only heparin is used for anticoagulant therapy, and its use has been found safe for the fetus and protective for the mother without producing an incidence of bleeding greater than that expected for the nonpregnant individual.

The dose of warfarin needed for prophylaxis against venous thromboembolism should be adjusted to achieve an increase in the prothrombin time to 1.3 to 1.5 times the control (using rabbit brain thromboplastin for the assay, as is customary in North America). This range is therapeutic and produces less bleeding than amounts aiming for 1.5 to 2 times the control, as was the practice for many years. The optimal duration of anticoagulant therapy is not known. It is generally advised to continue therapy for at least 3 months in all patients, to extend therapy as long as identifiable risk factors are resolving, and to give therapy indefinitely to patients in whom an increased risk for deep venous thrombosis is permanent.

FIGURE 65–3. Pulmonary arteriogram showing filling defects in branches of the pulmonary artery, indicative of pulmonary embolism. (Courtesy of Dr. Noah Susman.)

THROMBOLYTIC THERAPY. Thrombolytic agents, by dissolving pulmonary emboli and thrombi in the deep venous

TABLE 65–4. GUIDELINES FOR ANTICOAGULANT THERAPY WITH HEPARIN AND WARFARIN IN PULMONARY EMBOLISM

Embolism Suspected	Embolism Confirmed
Obtain baseline APTT,* PT, and platelet count and give heparin bolus (5000–10,000 units) IV	Give loading dose of heparin (5000 units) and start constant IV infusion at approximately 1000 units/hr
Order diagnostic test: ventilation-perfusion lung scan or pulmonary arteriogram	Monitor APTT at 6 hr and thereafter until the APTT is stabilized between 1.5 and 2.0 times control value
	Monitor platelet count every 3–4 days while administering heparin
	Start warfarin on day 1 or 2 by instituting the estimated daily maintenance dose (usually 4–10 mg)
	After at least 5 days of heparin therapy and 4–5 days of joint therapy, stop heparin and check PT 4 hr later
	Maintain PT off heparin at 1.3 to 1.5 times control or pretreatment value (using rabbit brain thromboplastin)
	Maintain full-dose anticoagulation for at least 3 mo in patients without continuing risk factors, longer in other patients

*APTT = activated partial thromboplastin time; PT = one-stage prothrombin time (1.3 times control performed with rabbit brain thromboplastin is roughly equal to 2.0 times control with human brain thromboplastin); IV = intravenous.

Adapted from Hyers TM, Hull RD, Weg JG: Antithrombotic therapy for venous thromboembolic disease. Chest 95:37S, 1989; with permission.

system, can alleviate the hemodynamic disturbances caused by pulmonary emboli, eliminate the source of further emboli, and perhaps diminish postphlebitic complications in the lower extremities. Two thrombolytic agents, streptokinase and urokinase, have been used for a number of years. A third, tissue-type plasminogen activator (TPA), generated by recombinant DNA methods, has been used in limited trials, but it is not yet approved by the Food and Drug Administration for the treatment of pulmonary embolism.

Streptokinase and urokinase convert circulating endogenous plasminogen to plasmin, a potent serine protease that dissolves fibrin. Urokinase cleaves plasminogen to plasmin directly, whereas streptokinase forms a complex with plasminogen, allowing expression of plasminogen's normally hidden active site, which then cleaves other plasminogen molecules to plasmin. At equivalent dosage, streptokinase is considerably cheaper than urokinase, but, unlike urokinase, it can produce febrile and allergic reactions. Plasmin formed by either agent lyses the fibrin clot in pulmonary emboli, but unfortunately it also cleaves other molecules in the circulation, including fibrinogen and Factors V and VIII, and it leads to consumption of circulating plasmin inhibitors, in particular, alpha$_2$-antiplasmin. Thus, besides solubilizing pulmonary emboli and deep venous thrombi, these agents can solubilize hemostatic plugs where they are important, such as at incisional sites, and can reduce hemostatic competence generally.

Thrombolytic agents can restore pulmonary arterial pressure and pulmonary parenchymal perfusion toward normal faster than does heparin, but this effect does not appear to result in improved survival rates or pulmonary perfusion when patients are studied a few weeks after the acute episode. Moreover, concerning the rate of recurrence of pulmonary embolism, there is no difference between thrombolytic agents and anticoagulants. With thrombolytic agents, pulmonary capillary blood flow after a year may be more normalized than if only heparin were used, but this is of questionable clinical importance, since pulmonary impairment is rare following pulmonary emboli in either case. One setting in which thrombolytic therapy may offer a clear advantage over heparin is that of angiographically proven massive pulmonary embolism that has produced hemodynamic instability. In this case, the rapid reduction in vascular occlusion that may be achieved with thrombolytic therapy may prove life-saving. Some preliminary evidence has suggested a greater speed of clot resolution with TPA than with other thrombolytic agents, but the studies showing such an effect have not used comparable doses, so these data are difficult to interpret.

The typical thrombolytic regimen involves a loading dose of streptokinase or urokinase, followed by a continuous intravenous infusion for 12 to 24 hours. Other regimens that have been proved effective include single large-bolus infusions of thrombolytic agent into the right atrium over a few minutes and continuous infusions of low-dose thrombolytic agent directly into the

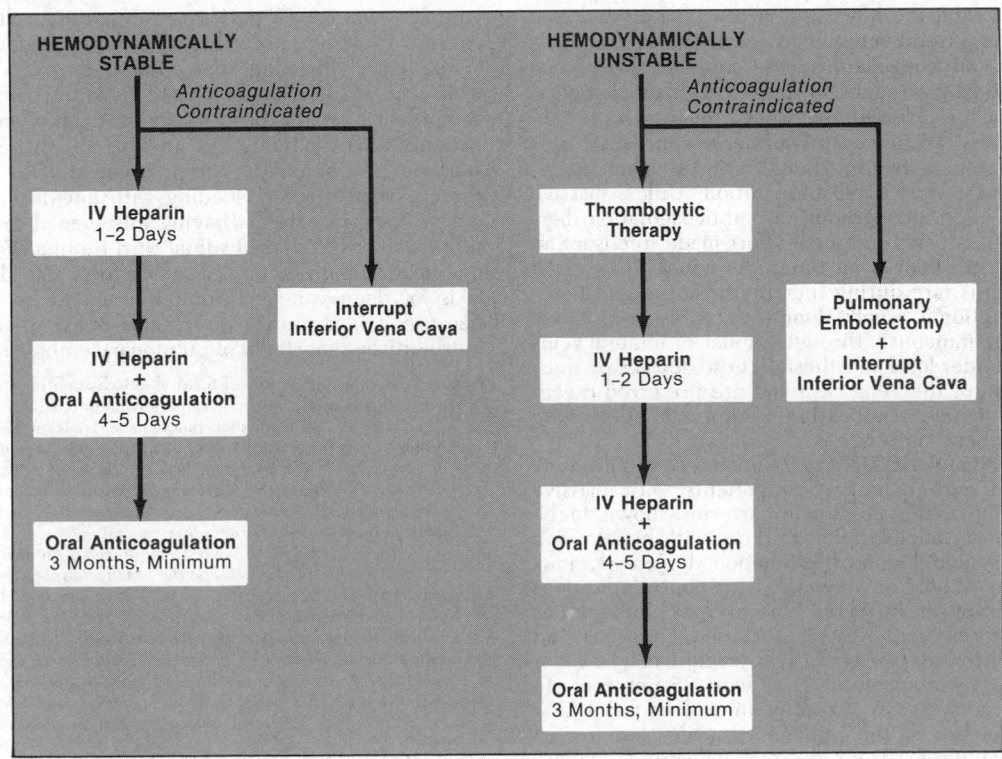

FIGURE 65–4. The therapy of pulmonary embolism.

pulmonary artery at the site of the clot, in combination with systemic heparinization. Whatever thrombolytic regimen is used, it should be followed by anticoagulant therapy (Fig. 65–4).

There is no ideal test for monitoring patients given thrombolytic agents. The usual approach is to document either an anticoagulant effect (lengthening of the prothrombin time, partial thromboplastin time, or thrombin time) or evidence of fibrinogen or fibrin degradation (decreased fibrinogen concentration or increased titers of fibrin degradation products) or both. Because these agents digest substrates besides fibrin in pulmonary emboli, proof that a thrombolytic agent has exerted some effect according to these tests does not, however, prove that it has had an effect upon pulmonary emboli. Nor is it possible to use results from these tests to titrate the dose. On the other hand, clinical effectiveness is usually apparent from improvement in the patient's cardiopulmonary status.

Because thrombolytic agents may start or aggravate bleeding, they are absolutely contraindicated when active internal bleeding is present or within a few months of stroke, neurologic or ophthalmic surgery, or head injury. They are relatively contraindicated within 10 days of major surgical procedures or biopsies of internal organs or arteriographic studies, during pregnancy and the first 10 days post partum, and in a variety of medical states associated with increased risk of bleeding, such as severe hypertension. In the patient who is critically ill from pulmonary emboli, however, the danger of bleeding must be weighed against the potential benefits and the risks of alternate forms of therapy.

VENA CAVAL INTERRUPTION. The principal reasons for interruption of the inferior vena cava are (1) absolute contraindications to anticoagulant therapy (active internal bleeding and recent central nervous system lesions that are bleeding or are predisposed to bleeding), (2) severe internal bleeding that develops during therapeutic anticoagulation, and (3) recurrent emboli despite adequate anticoagulation. Infrequently, vena caval interruption is necessary for septic embolism, after pulmonary embolectomy, or after massive embolization of such severity that further embolization might well be fatal. In the last-noted situation, anticoagulation therapy is used as well.

Like anticoagulation therapy, interruption of the vena cava is only preventive against future emboli. It does not promote resolution of emboli already in the lungs, and it does not correct the hemodynamic effects of emboli. In addition, it may not provide permanent protection against pulmonary embolism, since collateral veins bypassing the interruption can enlarge and provide other routes for thromboemboli to reach the lungs. Since most bleeding during anticoagulant therapy is not life threatening and can be controlled by a reduction in anticoagulant dosage, a conservative approach is advised regarding the interruption of the vena cava. Similarly, recurrence of pulmonary embolism after anticoagulation therapy is begun should not be taken as an automatic indication for vena caval interruption. Unless massive embolism is documented angiographically, anticoagulation therapy should be continued, with maximal effort made to ensure an adequate anticoagulant effect at all times. As noted above, fatal pulmonary embolism is rare during therapeutic anticoagulation.

Vena caval interruption is usually done with umbrellas or filters that are inserted percutaneously through jugular or femoral veins while the patient is under local anesthesia. These devices produce only partial occlusion of the vena cava and are preferred except for septic emboli, in which case ligation or clipping is done with the patient under general anesthesia.

PULMONARY EMBOLECTOMY. Pulmonary embolectomy is rarely performed and is limited to patients with massive pulmonary emboli involving pulmonary arteries shown to be accessible on pulmonary angiography, to those with hypotension and end-organ (brain and kidney) dysfunction despite maximal medical support, and to those in whom there are contraindications to thrombolytic therapy or in whom thrombolytic therapy has proved ineffective. Few patients meet these conditions and survive long enough to have surgery. The surgical mortality for emergency pulmonary embolectomy is at least 25 per cent. In contrast, elective surgery for symptomatic, unresolved pulmonary emboli in large branches of the pulmonary artery has proved effective and reasonably safe. The procedure for chronic emboli, which amounts to an endarterectomy for removal of organized

thromboemboli, can improve functional status, reduce pulmonary arterial pressure, and normalize pulmonary arterial perfusion and arterial oxygenation.

PROGNOSIS

The majority of deaths from pulmonary embolism occur either too quickly for therapy to be given or because the condition is not recognized. If pulmonary embolism goes untreated, survival is only 70 per cent, with death occurring as a result of recurrent thromboembolism within a few weeks of the first episode. In contrast, among those individuals in whom a diagnosis is made and therapy begun, 92 per cent survive and do so without sequelae. Among those few individuals who do not survive despite therapy, two thirds of the deaths are due to associated critical diseases. In those in whom death is caused by pulmonary embolism, systemic hypotension is usually present at the onset of the episode, and pulmonary vascular obstruction is usually greater than 75 per cent. Even when hypotension and acute cor pulmonale are present at the onset of acute pulmonary embolism, however, it does not necessarily mean a fatal outcome. Clinical signs of massive embolization can subside quickly, presumably because vascular obstruction decreases as a result of fragmentation or remodeling of the emboli or because pulmonary vasoconstrictive reflexes and mediators dissipate. The presence of pulmonary infarction has no effect on survival.

In fewer than 1 per cent of those who survive acute pulmonary thromboembolization, the emboli persist and result in a chronic syndrome of exertional dyspnea, pulmonary hypertension, right ventricular enlargement, and right ventricular failure. Individuals presenting with this syndrome usually have a history that contains clues to recurrent episodes of pulmonary embolism and to conditions predisposing to venous thromboembolic disease.

PREVENTION

Several therapeutic regimens reduce the risk of deep venous thrombosis and by doing so decrease the risk of pulmonary thromboembolism. These regimens—which include early ambulation after surgery, low-dose subcutaneous heparin, low-dose warfarin, dextran, external pneumatic calf compression, and gradient elastic stockings—are easy to use, have minimal complications, and require essentially no laboratory monitoring. The most thoroughly proven regimen, low-dose subcutaneous heparin (5000 units twice daily), is effective for (1) general surgery patients with high-risk features (over age 40, obese, previous deep venous thrombosis or pulmonary embolism, current malignancy, and complex surgery), (2) patients undergoing urologic or gynecologic surgery (excluding procedures for gynecologic malignancies), and (3) patients with congestive heart failure and those recovering from acute myocardial infarction. Low-dose subcutaneous heparin is not effective for prophylaxis of deep venous thrombosis in patients with traumatic hip fracture. In that situation, low-dose warfarin or pneumatic compression should be used. Because there is some risk of bleeding with low-dose heparin, it should not be used in patients having intracranial or eye surgery or in those who have suffered spinal cord trauma. For these situations, pneumatic compression is a satisfactory, safe alternative. Prophylaxis for deep venous thrombosis should be used more widely because it is the only way that a substantial reduction in the morbidity and mortality of pulmonary embolism will be achieved.

Collins R, Scrimgeour A, Yusuf S, et al.: Reduction in fatal pulmonary embolism and venous thrombosis by perioperative administration of subcutaneous heparin: Overview of results of randomized trials in general, orthopedic, and urologic surgery. N Engl J Med 318:1162, 1988. *Analysis of randomized trials of prophylactic subcutaneous heparin therapy in various types of surgery indicates that this therapy greatly decreases pulmonary emboli, deep venous thromboses, and deaths due to pulmonary emboli, without causing a concomitant increase in deaths from other causes.*

Dalen JE, Hirsh J (eds.): 2nd ACCP Conference on Antithrombotic Therapy. Chest 95:1S, 1989. *Detailed articles on the practical aspects of anticoagulant therapy.*

Hull RD, Raskob GE, Carter CJ, et al.: Pulmonary embolism in outpatients with pleuritic chest pain. Arch Intern Med 148:838, 1988. *Prospective study of individuals presenting to an emergency room with pleuritic pain showing a substantial occurrence of pulmonary embolism in those over age 40 and in those with predisposing factors for venous thrombosis.*

Hull RD, Raskob GE, Coates G, et al.: A new noninvasive management strategy for patients with suspected pulmonary embolism. Arch Intern Med 149:2549, 1989. *A prospective study with long-term follow-up showing an excellent prognosis without anticoagulant therapy in individuals suspected of having acute pulmonary embolism whose lung scan is not of high probability and* whose lower extremity proximal veins do not show thrombosis on serial impedance plethysmography.

Levine M, Hirsch J, Weitz J, et al.: A randomized trial of a single bolus dosage regimen of recombinant tissue plasminogen activator in patients with acute pulmonary embolism. Chest 98:1473, 1990. *A prospective study of recombinant tissue plasminogen activator (rt-PA) therapy in patients with acute symptomatic pulmonary embolism who were receiving heparin. Patients given a 2-minute infusion of rt-PA at 0.6 mg per kilogram had more resolution of perfusion defects on lung scans 24 hours later than patients given a saline palcebo, but at 7 days the resolution of scans was the same in both groups.*

Mitchell JP, Trulock EP: Tissue-plasminogen activator for pulmonary embolism resulting in shock: Two case reports and discussion of the literature. Am J Med 90:260, 1991. *Two patients with relative contraindications to thrombolytic therapy received 100 mg of recombinant tissue plasminogen activator over 2 to 3 hours for pulmonary emboli causing shock. In both patients, there was almost complete restoration of normal hemodynamics within a few hours.*

Moser KM: Venous thromboembolism. Am Rev Respir Dis 141:235, 1990. *Review of deep venous thrombosis and pulmonary thromboembolism, with particular emphasis on the importance of prevention.*

The PIOPED Investigators: Value of the ventilation/perfusion scan in acute pulmonary embolism: Results of the Prospective Investigation of Pulmonary Embolism Diagnosis (PIOPED), JAMA 263:2753, 1990. *A multicenter, prospective study that used pulmonary arteriography to assess the sensitivity and specificity of lung scans in the diagnosis of pulmonary embolism.*

66 Fat Embolism Syndrome

Robert M. Senior

DEFINITION

Fat embolism syndrome refers to the constellation of clinical manifestations that may develop when fat droplets become impacted in the pulmonary microvasculature and other microvascular beds, especially in the brain. The principal clinical features of fat embolism syndrome are respiratory failure, cerebral dysfunction, and petechiae.

CLINICAL SETTING

Fat embolism syndrome occurs almost exclusively as an early complication of traumatic fractures of the pelvis and of long bones, particularly the shaft of the femur. Delays in stabilization of fractures and periods of systemic hypoperfusion after trauma increase the risk of the syndrome. The syndrome develops in 2 to 25 per cent of persons with fresh long bone fractures, depending on criteria for the diagnosis and selection of patients at risk. In contrast, it rarely follows elective orthopedic surgery on long bones, even though fat droplets can be found routinely in the venous blood draining the operative sites. Other forms of trauma that rarely result in fat embolism include massive soft tissue injury, severe burns, and liposuction. Nontraumatic settings occasionally lead to fat embolism. These include conditions associated with fatty liver, prolonged corticosteroid therapy, acute pancreatitis, osteomyelitis, and conditions causing bone infarcts, such as sickle cell hemoglobinopathy.

DIAGNOSIS

There are no laboratory tests that are diagnostic of fat embolism syndrome. Looking for fat droplets in the blood, urine, and sputum is not helpful in making the diagnosis, as droplets may not be present in patients who clearly have fat embolism syndrome but may be found after traumatic fractures in patients without evidence of the syndrome. It is possible, however, that bronchoalveolar lavage and staining the lavage cells with oil red 0 may be helpful. In a recent study, large fat droplets were found in the lavage cells of patients with definite fat embolism syndrome and of patients with possible fat embolism syndrome that was later proved, whereas fat droplets were rare in the lavage cells from normal persons and patients with other causes of respiratory distress. The diagnosis is based on the presence of at least one of the following features within the first 72 hours after traumatic fracture: (1) otherwise unexplained dyspnea, tachypnea, arterial hypoxemia, and diffuse alveolar infiltrates on the chest radiograph; (2) otherwise unexplained confusion or other signs of cerebral dysfunction; and (3) petechiae over the upper half of the body, including the axillae, conjunctivae, and oral mucosa. The diagnosis is definite if all three criteria are present. Further support for the diagnosis is provided by fluffy retinal exudates and hemorrhages and unexplained fever. The diagnosis is unlikely if the signs and symptoms first begin more than 72 hours after the injury. In these situations, more probable causes of respiratory distress are pulmonary edema from massive fluid replacement, aspiration, sepsis, pneumonia, or venous thromboembolism.

PATHOGENESIS

The cellular mechanisms leading to fat embolism syndrome are not fully understood, but it is clear that the syndrome is not simply a consequence of mechanical obstruction of small vessels by fat droplets. An important aspect of the pathogenesis appears to be endothelial injury caused by fatty acids released from impacted fat droplets by lipoprotein lipase, with ensuing increased microvascular permeability and fluid leakage into interstitial spaces.

The fat droplets found in small vessels are from the trauma site. As the first microvascular bed encountered by fat droplets in the venous circulation, the lungs bear the brunt of fat embolization. Presumably, fat emboli in other organs, especially the brain, reach those sites by passing through the pulmonary microvasculature or through right-to-left shunts in the heart.

Although the effects of fatty acids upon endothelium appear to be important in the mechanism of lung injury, the pathogenesis of respiratory failure may be more complex in some cases. Other tissue components besides fat may be liberated from fracture sites, and these as well as the injured pulmonary endothelium may activate the clotting, complement, and contact systems. Thus, the pathogenesis of lung injury may be multifactorial, as in other forms of the adult respiratory distress syndrome, involving thrombi, mediators of inflammation, and products of inflammatory cells.

Hypoxemia explains brain dysfunction in many cases, but not all. In some fatal cases, cerebral symptoms reflect direct brain injury with many fat emboli and associated hemorrhage and necrosis. Moreover, patients with comparable hypoxemia from causes other than fat embolism syndrome seldom have brain dysfunction, and occasional patients with fat embolism syndrome have neurologic features that precede hypoxemia or are disproportionate to the degree of hypoxemia.

The reason for the petechiae is not known, although in some patients thrombocytopenia and disseminated intravascular coagulation may be present. There is also no explanation for the striking localization of the petechiae to the pectoral regions and conjunctivae.

THERAPY

Management of fat embolism syndrome is supportive and consists primarily of ensuring good arterial oxygenation. Supplemental oxygen is given to maintain the arterial oxygen tension in the normal range, 75 to 90 mm Hg. If endotracheal intubation and ventilatory support are necessary, positive end-expiratory pressure may reduce the need for high concentrations of inspired oxygen. Restricting fluid intake and even giving diuretics, if systemic perfusion can be maintained, may minimize fluid accumulation in the lungs. The role of corticosteroids is controversial; there is no clear-cut evidence that they are helpful.

In patients with acute long bone fractures, the risk of fat embolism syndrome is reduced by prompt surgical stabilization of the fractures and by correcting or preventing decreased systemic perfusion. In addition, administration of corticosteroids for a short period (for example, 1.5 mg per kilogram of methylprednisolone intravenously at 8-hour intervals for 2 days) seems to prevent development of the syndrome.

PROGNOSIS

The mortality from fat embolism syndrome is 10 per cent or less and thus is clearly much lower than the 50 per cent or greater mortality for most causes of the adult respiratory distress syndrome. Even severe respiratory failure associated with fat embolism seldom leads to death. In one report of 54 cases, there was not a single fatality from the syndrome, although severe hypoxemia was common during the acute stages.

Chastre J, Fagon J-Y, Soler P, et al.: Bronchoalveolar lavage for rapid diagnosis of the fat embolism syndrome in trauma patients. Ann Intern Med 113:583, 1990. *A report indicating that looking for fat droplets in alveolar macrophages and neutrophils recovered by bronchoalveolar lavage is helpful in making the diagnosis of the fat embolism syndrome.*

Eddy AC, Rice CL, Carrico CJ: Fat embolism syndrome: Monitoring and management. J Crit Ill 2:24, 1987. *Reviews many aspects of posttraumatic fat embolism syndrome.*

Guardia SN, Bilbao JM, Murray D, et al.: Fat embolism in acute pancreatitis. Arch Pathol Lab Med 113:503, 1989. *Describes a patient with fatal fat embolism syndrome that occurred without trauma.*

Peltier LF: Fat embolism: A perspective. Clin Orthop Rel Res 232:263, 1988. *Reviews the progress in understanding the pathogenesis of fat embolism syndrome and its management since the first diagnosis in 1873.*

67   Sarcoidosis

Barry L. Fanburg

DEFINITION

Sarcoidosis, a multisystem granulomatous disease, begins most frequently in people between 20 and 40 years old. The etiology is unknown, but alterations in the immune system are clearly involved in its pathogenesis. Organ involvement is usually asymptomatic, and the disease most frequently regresses spontaneously, but it may progress to a more chronic state of fibrosis with severe functional impairment of various organs. No natural animal models of sarcoidosis have been discovered.

EPIDEMIOLOGY AND GENETICS

Sarcoidosis occurs with similar manifestations world wide, but its incidence differs strikingly, from 0.04 per 100,000 in Spain, for example, to 64 per 100,000 in Sweden. The reported numbers are susceptible to considerable error based upon procedures for evaluation, but large unexplained differences in prevalence clearly exist. The occurrence in blacks has been reported to be more frequent than that in whites. The majority of cases occur during adulthood, but sarcoidosis is also present in the pediatric population.

The disease has been reported to be transmissible in experimental animals, but this work still has not been rigorously tested for confirmation. Sarcoidosis is not contagious in humans.

Familial occurrences have been reported in approximately 200 instances, but no specific patterns of parent-child or sibling relationships have emerged. Sarcoidosis has been reported in twins, with a preponderance of monozygotic over dizygotic twins. The disease seems not to be linked with specific human leukocyte antigen (HLA) types.

IMMUNOLOGY

A postulated schema for the immunopathology of sarcoidosis is presented in Figure 67–1. The macrophage most likely initiates the cellular response of sarcoidosis, possibly in response to some unknown presenting antigen. Various factors released by the macrophage, such as interleukin 1, cause accumulation and proliferation of helper T lymphocytes. Factors secreted by the lymphocytes attract and immobilize other inflammatory cells. In addition, B lymphocytes are stimulated to produce increased amounts of immunoglobulins, and fibroblasts are stimulated to proliferate. As the response becomes less active, the number of T lymphocytes decreases, and suppressor T lymphocytes predominate.

As a result of these various immunologic interactions, (1) inflammatory cells proliferate in the affected organ (forming the granuloma), (2) cutaneous delayed hypersensitivity responses to common antigens are depressed, and (3) immune globulins are synthesized and circulate in excess. In addition, circulating immune complexes may be present; high levels of serum antibodies to common environmental antigens such as *Mycoplasma pneumoniae* and various viruses frequently occur; antibody responses to immunization may be exaggerated; and circulating rheumatoid factor, antinuclear antibody, and autoantibodies to T lymphocytes may be present.

Intradermally injected extracts of homogenized tissue of involved organs from patients with sarcoidosis are capable of producing a delayed inflammatory reaction in patients with sarcoidosis. This antigen that causes the so-called *Kveim-Siltzbach reaction* has not been purified, and the basis for its response has not been defined. The reaction differs from a cutaneous delayed hypersensitivity reaction in that it takes 4 to 6 weeks to develop and then persists for several months.

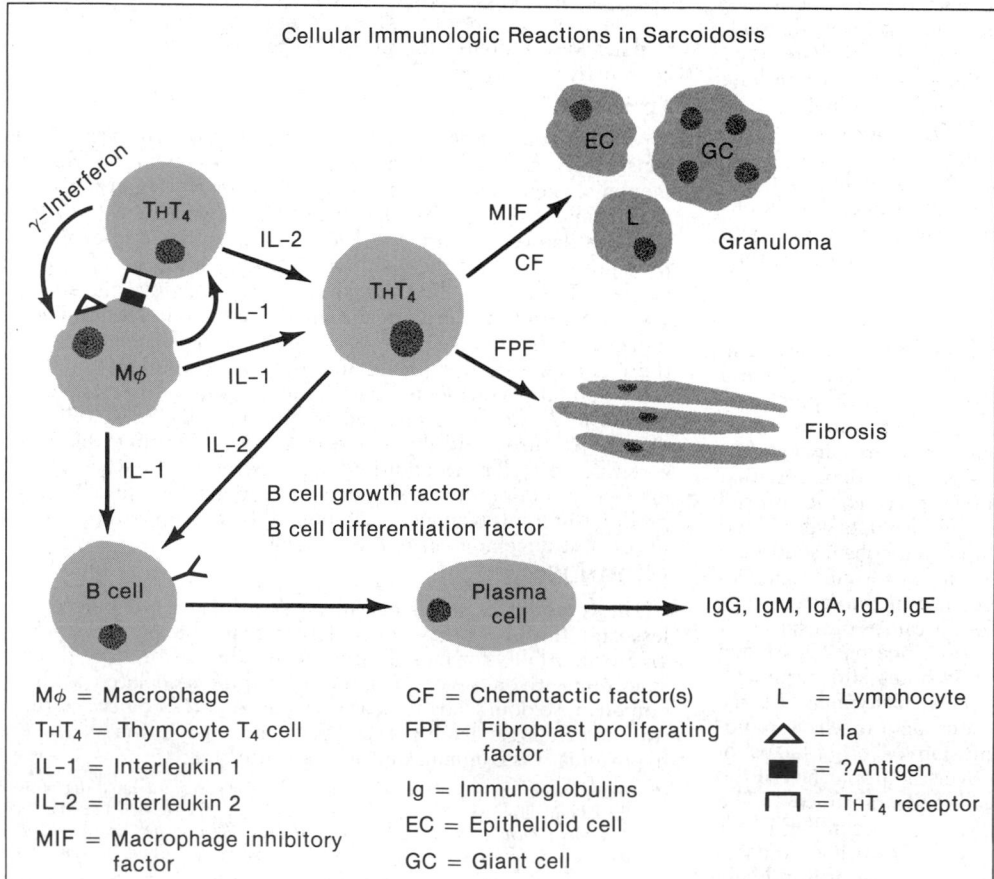

FIGURE 67–1. Immunologic abnormalities associated with sarcoidosis.

CLINICAL PRESENTATION

Sarcoid lesions may develop in almost any organ system, so that the clinical presentation is quite varied (Fig. 67–2). In fact, "silent" granulomas are frequently present in multiple organs. Most characteristically, the patient is asymptomatic, but the disease is detected by an abnormal chest radiograph, usually showing bilateral symmetric hilar adenopathy often associated with paratracheal adenopathy (Fig. 67–3) and/or reticulonodular parenchymal infiltrates. Patients with sarcoidosis may also present with hilar and paratracheal adenopathy in association with some combination of acute peripheral arthritis, uveitis, and erythema nodosum (the so-called "acute sarcoidosis," or Loeffgren's syndrome). Except for Loeffgren's syndrome, significant constitutional symptoms other than those of fatigue are unusual in sarcoidosis. When anorexia, weight loss, and fever are present, other diseases should be strongly considered.

Lungs

The lungs are the most frequently involved organ, and pulmonary symptoms, when present, include dyspnea on exertion, nonproductive cough, and wheezing. Dyspnea is usually caused by fibrotic or granulomatous pulmonary parenchymal disease, but it may also result from granulomatous obstruction of the upper airways. Granulomas in the nose may cause nasal congestion and in the larynx may result in hoarseness. Hemoptysis is rare in sarcoidosis but may occur from an associated mycetoma in advanced cavitary sarcoidosis. Acute dyspnea secondary to a pneumothorax also occasionally develops in patients with more advanced fibrotic pulmonary disease. Pleural involvement has been reported but is unusual.

Skin

Erythema nodosum may be associated with sarcoidosis as a secondary vasculitic reaction. Sarcoid granulomas also occur directly in the skin to produce a variety of small, asymptomatic macular and papular lesions that are present either superficially or more deeply in the dermis. *Lupus pernio*, consisting of violaceous plaques over the nose, cheeks, and ears, is the most commonly described skin lesion. It may be disfiguring. Granulomas may also occur in scar tissue.

Eyes

Ophthalmologic lesions most commonly consist of inflammation of the uveal tract, but the conjunctiva, retina, and lacrimal glands may also be involved. These lesions may produce nonspecific ocular symptoms of visual impairment and discomfort; chronic lesions may progress to blindness. Anterior uveitis in combination with parotitis and facial nerve palsy has been referred to as *Heerfordt's syndrome.*

Nervous System

Almost any portion of the neurologic system may be affected by sarcoidosis, and the diagnosis may prove difficult. The most common cranial nerve to be involved is the facial nerve, but any cranial nerve may be affected. Disease of the optic nerve may result in papilledema. Palsies of the ninth and tenth cranial nerves manifest as dysphagia, absent gag reflex, and vocal cord paralysis, and disease of the eighth cranial nerve occurs as deafness, tinnitus, and vertigo. Mononeuropathy or polyneuropathy of peripheral nerves causes sensory loss, paresthesias, or motor weakness. Meningitis produced by sarcoidosis is usually insidious in presentation and chronic in its course. Diabetes insipidus results from involvement of the hypothalamus or posterior pituitary gland. Granulomas of the brain may produce a space-occupying lesion and cause headaches, seizures, or focal symptoms. Rarely, personality changes have been observed, and the total constellation of findings resulting from multiple areas of involvement of the nervous system by sarcoidosis may bewilder the diagnostician.

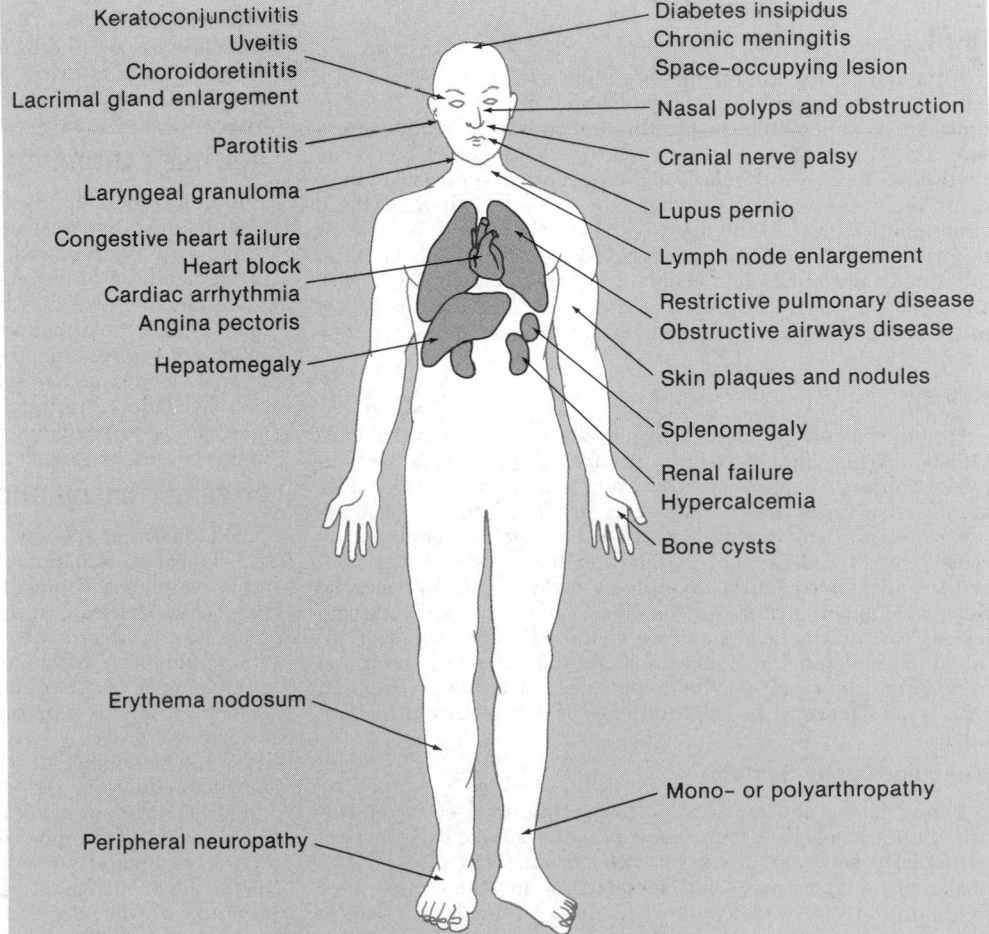

FIGURE 67–2. Organ abnormalities associated with sarcoidosis.

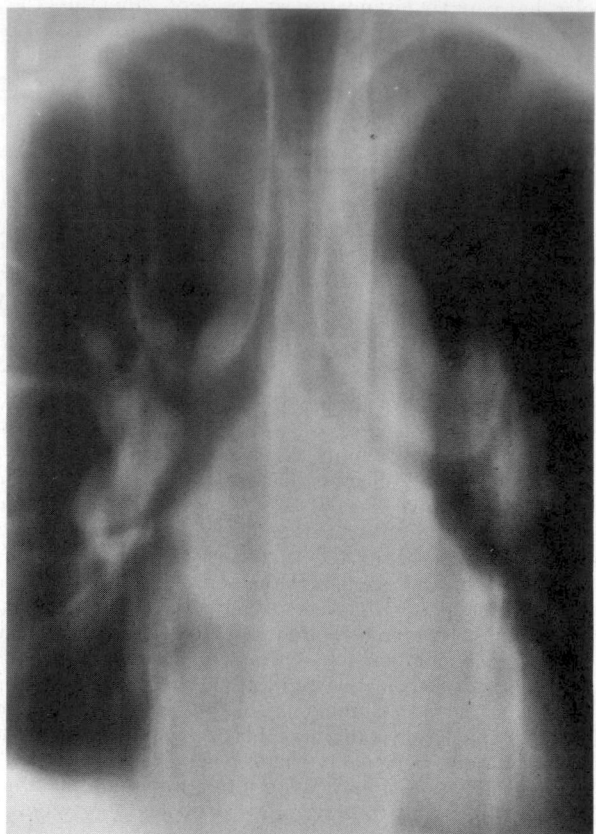

FIGURE 67–3. Tomogram of chest showing hilar and paratracheal adenopathy. (From Murray JF, Nadel J: Textbook of Respiratory Medicine. Philadelphia, W. B. Saunders Company, 1987.)

Heart

Although cardiac granulomas are often present on autopsies of patients with sarcoidosis, symptomatic cardiac involvement is unusual. Granulomatous or fibrotic cardiac lesions resulting from sarcoidosis may cause congestive heart failure, heart block, arrhythmias (often ventricular), angina pectoris, ventricular aneurysm, recurrent pericardial effusion, or sudden death. Since these abnormalities may also be due to other causes, it may be difficult to prove a relationship to sarcoidosis. Cor pulmonale is an infrequent presentation, occurring usually in association with advanced pulmonary fibrosis, but there has been the rare report of pulmonary hypertension without severe restrictive lung disease.

Kidneys

Granulomas of the kidneys are usually infrequent and asymptomatic. When kidney failure occurs, other lesions such as pyelonephritis, nephrocalcinosis, and hyalinization of various kidney structures are usually present. The kidneys may be severely and irreversibly damaged by calcium nephropathy caused by altered calcium metabolism that produces hypercalcemia and hypercalciuria. Symptoms of kidney failure may be the predominant feature of sarcoidosis in these cases. Sarcoid lesions can enzymatically activate vitamin D precursors to 1,25-dihydroxycholecalciferol, thereby increasing intestinal absorption of calcium. The result may be hypercalcemia and hypercalciuria, with renal damage from nephrocalcinosis and recurrent nephrolithiasis.

Musculoskeletal System

Bones, joints, and muscles are frequently involved in sarcoidosis. Bone changes are found most often in chronic cases and are particularly common in blacks with chronic skin disease. The phalanges, metacarpals, and metatarsals are the bones most frequently involved. Osteoporosis, cystic or reticulated changes, and external manifestations of digital deformation and dystrophic

nails may be present. Joints are usually spared destructive changes except in the vicinity of bone lesions.

Arthritic changes may also manifest acutely by monoarthralgias or polyarthralgias or arthritis of the larger joints, such as the ankles, knees, wrists, or elbows. The associated symptoms may be migratory and usually recede with no residual deformities. Although, like the liver, muscles frequently contain asymptomatic granulomas, acute myositis and chronic myopathy with associated muscular enzyme abnormalities are uncommon findings in sarcoidosis. Gout may complicate sarcoidosis, presumably owing to overproduction of purines in widespread granulomas.

Miscellaneous

Although diffuse granulomas may be present, clinical manifestations of liver, gastrointestinal, or pancreatic disease are very unusual. Similarly, clinical evidence for involvement of the endocrine and reproductive systems is rare. As noted earlier, posterior pituitary and hypothalamic involvement may result in diabetes insipidus. Hypopituitarism from anterior pituitary disease occurs very rarely. Alteration in fertility by sarcoidosis has not been described. Peripheral lymph nodes, in contrast to hilar nodes, are seldom more than moderately enlarged and usually go unnoticed by the patient. Although the spleen is moderately enlarged in 5 to 10 per cent of patients, gross enlargement that causes discomfort and predisposes to rupture occurs rarely. Thrombocytopenia is occasionally present and may be associated with hypersplenism. Hypercalcemia may produce nonspecific anorexia and vomiting.

PHYSICAL FINDINGS

Physical findings in the chest in sarcoidosis are often normal despite radiographic abnormalities that may be extensive. Fever is absent, except with Loeffgren's syndrome. Other physical findings usually relate to granulomatous or fibrotic involvement of a specific organ system. Skin lesions may be readily apparent or found only with careful examination. Subcutaneous or muscle nodules may be identified. Slit-lamp examination may be necessary to demonstrate ocular lesions. Lymph nodes are often palpable but usually only moderately enlarged. As noted above, hepatosplenomegaly may be present. Digits may be deformed by bone lesions, and the nails may be dystrophic in cases of chronic disease. Acute arthritic changes may be apparent, in particular in association with erythema nodosum, and must be differentiated from associated gout.

ROUTINE LABORATORY STUDIES

Routine laboratory evaluation may reveal lymphopenia, hyperglobulinemia, hypercalcemia, and/or hypercalciuria. The platelet count is rarely decreased. It is unusual for the sedimentation rate to be significantly elevated, except with Loeffgren's syndrome. Liver function tests may be moderately abnormal, and, in particular, alkaline phosphatase levels may be elevated. With complications of the disease, the expected but nonspecific changes in arterial blood gases and serum chemistries accompany respiratory or renal failure, respectively. Cerebrospinal fluid examination may show nonspecific pleocytosis and increased protein in meningitis caused by sarcoidosis.

DIFFERENTIAL DIAGNOSIS

The differential diagnosis of sarcoidosis depends largely upon the clinical presentation of the patient. With hilar lymphadenopathy, lymphoma is most frequently considered; with pulmonary parenchymal disease, a wide variety of diffuse interstitial diseases must be considered (Ch. 61). Tuberculosis and other granulomatous pulmonary infections must always be ruled out. Eosinophilic granuloma is another diagnostic possibility, particularly when diabetes insipidus is present. Exposure to beryllium may produce disease very similar to sarcoidosis. Pulmonary sarcoid nodules raise the possibility of primary or metastatic tumor. Similarly, sarcoid nodules in the breast or brain may be thought to be tumor. Conglomerate lesions with hilar retraction or eggshell calcification of lymph nodes may be confused with silicosis. Hypercalcemia in sarcoidosis raises the question of a number of metabolic or malignant disorders, especially primary hyperparathyroidism (Ch. 235). Arthritis or arthralgia associated with sarcoidosis may be confused with acute rheumatic fever or gout.

The isolated finding of granulomas on biopsy of various tissues raises the possibilities of foreign body reactions, fungal or tubercular infections, and malignancy associated with granulomatous reactions. Granulomas occurring only in the liver may result in confusion between granulomatous hepatitis and sarcoidosis. The presence of granulomas in the intestinal wall may suggest Crohn's disease. Finally, renal and hepatic impairment or cardiac abnormalities occurring in sarcoidosis may be caused by more common coexisting diseases rather than by sarcoidosis itself.

RADIOLOGIC EVALUATION

Radiologic evaluation of the chest is particularly useful in sarcoidosis, since the disease is so often asymptomatic and so often involves the thorax. Radiologic abnormalities that occur in sarcoidosis have been arbitrarily classified as follows: grade 0—absence of abnormal radiographic findings; grade 1—lymph node enlargement without pulmonary parenchymal abnormalities; grade 2A—combination of lymph node and diffuse pulmonary parenchymal disease; grade 2B—diffuse parenchymal disease without lymph node enlargement; and grade 3—radiographic changes indicating more chronic disease with pulmonary fibrosis ("honeycombing" or hilar retraction). The most frequent parenchymal abnormality is reticulonodularity, consisting of fine linear densities and small, irregular nodules measuring 3 to 5 mm in diameter (Fig. 67–4). Large, conglomerate lesions may be present in association with hilar retraction (Fig. 67–5). Parenchymal infiltrates are at times "fluffy" and have an alveolar pattern. Single or multiple large nodules may occur and may be confused with tumor. Small nodules may cause a miliary pattern suggestive of tuberculosis.

A large variety of other changes may be present on the radiograph. Pleural effusion occurs rarely in sarcoidosis. Mediastinal or hilar lymph nodes may show eggshell calcification. In addition to bullous changes, true cavities may be present that, at times, contain mycetomas. Lobar atelectasis may be caused by intrabronchial granulomas, and postobstructive bronchiectasis may be present. In addition to the more common locations in the short tubular bones of the hands and feet, lytic or sclerotic bone lesions may occur in the ribs.

Computed tomographic (CT) scans can demonstrate lymphadenopathy more clearly and, in particular, can detect anterior mediastinal and subcarinal lymph nodes that have gone undetected on conventional films of the chest (Fig. 67–6). This examination, however, is needed in only a limited number of patients with sarcoidosis.

PHYSIOLOGIC CHANGES

The most common pulmonary physiologic changes occurring in sarcoidosis are decreases in vital capacity and diffusing capacity.

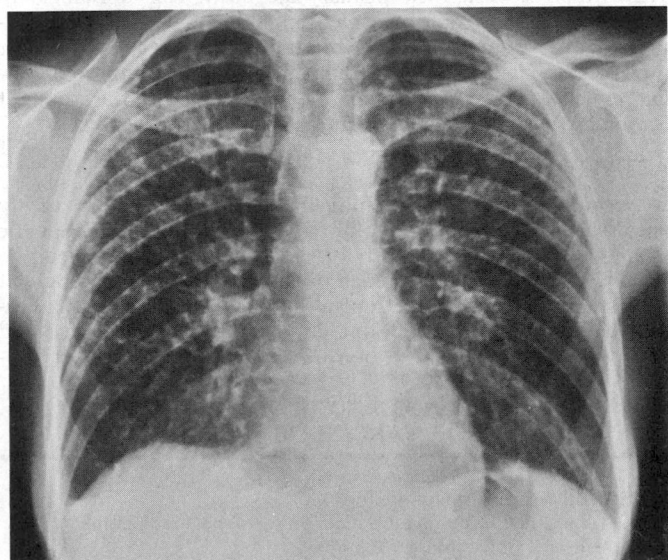

FIGURE 67–4. Chest radiograph showing typical reticulonodular appearance of parenchymal sarcoidosis. (From Murray JF, Nadel J: Textbook of Respiratory Medicine. Philadelphia, W. B. Saunders Company, 1987.)

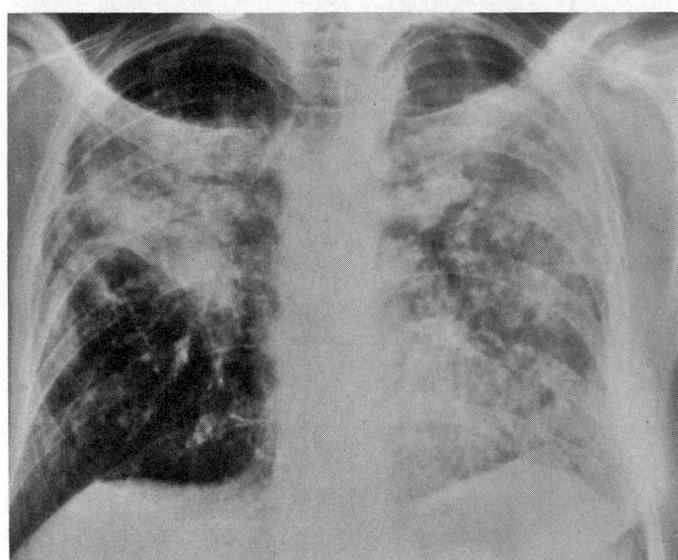

FIGURE 67–5. Chest radiograph showing large conglomerate lesions associated with hilar retraction. (From Murray JF, Nadel J: Textbook of Respiratory Medicine. Philadelphia, W. B. Saunders Company, 1987.)

Although useful in determining the extent of functional impairment at the onset and in following the course of the disease, physiologic changes do not correlate well with symptoms or radiologic abnormalities. At times pulmonary function studies are totally normal despite radiologic evidence of pulmonary disease. Conversely, functional abnormalities, especially of diffusing capacity, may be present when the lung parenchyma appears normal radiographically. Evidence of airway obstruction may also be present, and, at times, this is the predominant feature of sarcoidosis, causing confusion with asthma. An elevation in arterial PCO_2 is unusual, but moderate arterial hypoxemia may be present. As with other interstitial diseases, arterial hypoxemia often worsens with exercise.

APPROACH TO DIAGNOSIS

With a very typical presentation (i.e., bilateral symmetric hilar and paratracheal lymphadenopathy in an asymptomatic patient 20 to 40 years of age or in one with erythema nodosum, uveitis, and arthralgias), the clinical diagnosis of sarcoidosis can be made with a high degree of certainty by physicians familiar with this disease (Table 67–1). In all other cases in which the diagnosis is less clear, further support must be obtained by examination of biopsy material.

Diagnosis by Biopsy

Typical sarcoid granulomas consist of whorls of epithelioid cells surrounding multinucleated giant cells, which may or may not contain inclusion bodies (Fig. 67–7). Mononuclear cells are present at the periphery of the granulomas, and various amounts of fibrosis and/or hyalinization are present throughout the tissue. True caseation is unusual. The histologic appearance, even when typical, is always nonspecific. To strengthen the diagnosis of sarcoidosis, infectious agents and foreign bodies must be excluded by special stains, cultures, and examination under polarized light.

What tissue should be examined by biopsy? In the absence of specific skin lesions, transbronchial biopsy of the lung is usually most specific, since rarely, if ever, will nonspecific granulomas be found (in contrast to liver or lymph nodes). Approximately 60 per cent of patients with sarcoidosis show granulomas on transbronchial lung biopsy even if their chest radiographs are normal; this number increases to 85 to 90 per cent when there is a parenchymal abnormality on chest radiograph. If the transbronchial biopsy yields negative findings but a high suspicion of sarcoidosis exists and there is obvious parenchymal disease on the chest radiograph, a repeat transbronchial biopsy may be justified. Other reasonable approaches at this juncture of evaluation include mediastinoscopy or, at times, open lung biopsy.

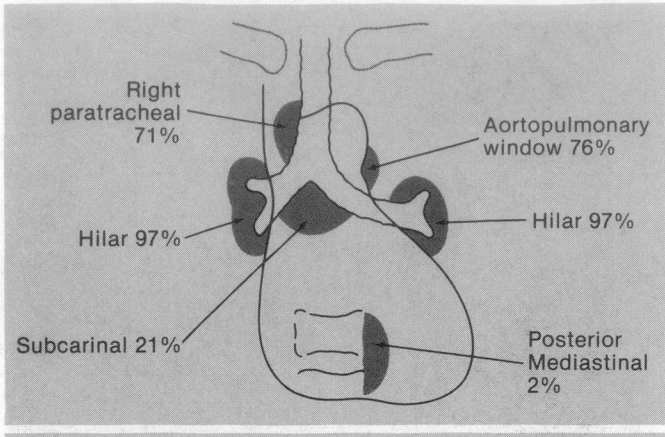

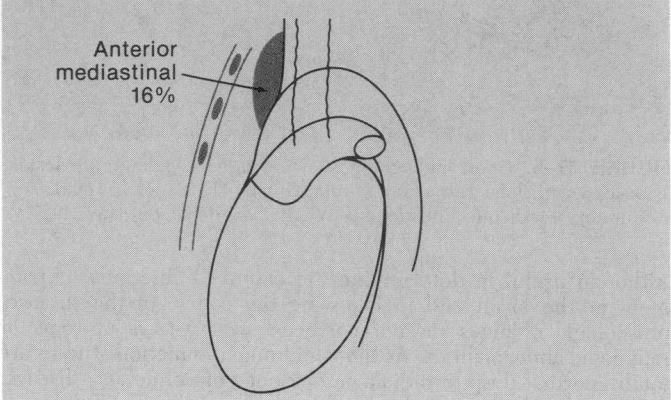

FIGURE 67–6. Schematic representation of CT detection of thoracic lymphadenopathy in sarcoidosis. (Reprinted from Rodan BA, Putman CE: Radiologic alterations in sarcoidosis. *In* Fanburg BL [ed.]: Sarcoidosis and Other Granulomatous Diseases of the Lung. New York, Marcel Dekker, 1983. By courtesy of Marcel Dekker, Inc.)

Blind conjunctival, lacrimal gland, or gingival biopsies are frequently not rewarding in the absence of overt disease at these locations. When these tissues are involved, however, the yield is high. Biopsies of skin lesions are particularly useful, since they may show granuloma and, in association with other findings, may provide an easy diagnosis if foreign body granuloma can be excluded. Biopsy of idenfiable subcutaneous or muscle lesions may also be diagnostic. Biopsy of lesions of erythema nodosum shows a nonspecific panniculitis or vasculitis and therefore is not diagnostic. Other localized lesions, such as those of the pharynx or larynx, require direct biopsy for diagnosis. Diagnosis by biopsy sometimes becomes problematic for neurologic disease caused by sarcoidosis when other tissues do not provide a positive diagnosis, since the involved tissue is often not easily accessible.

Other Available Tests

The Kveim-Siltzbach test lacks precision, and the required antigen is not readily available. It is therefore rarely used. Anergy

TABLE 67–1. FEATURES CONSIDERED IN THE DIAGNOSIS OF SARCOIDOSIS

Primary
1. Clinical and radiologic presentation
2. Biopsy material showing granuloma, but no mycobacterial, fungi, or refractile material

Secondary
1. Anergy to skin tests
2. Positive Kveim-Siltzbach reaction (infrequently performed)
3. Significant elevation of serum angiotensin I–converting enzyme with exclusion of other obvious diseases associated with elevation (e.g., Gaucher's disease, leprosy)

Current Research Modalities
1. Evaluation of cells obtained by bronchial lavage
2. Gallium-67 scanning

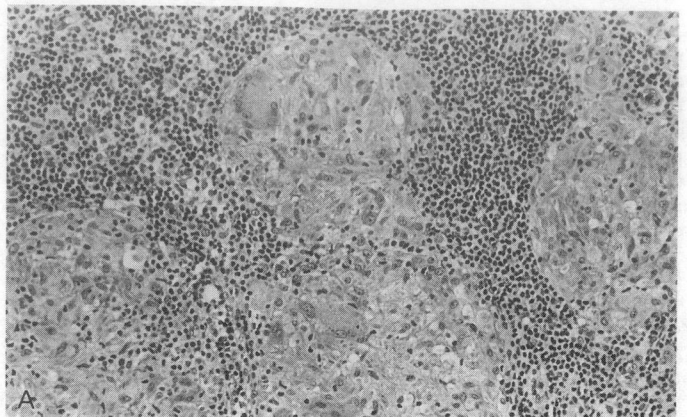

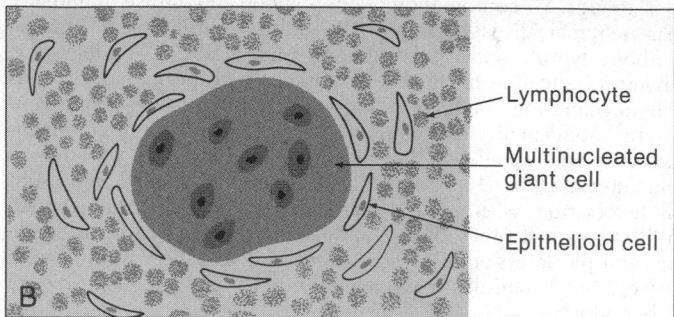

FIGURE 67–7. Typical histologic appearance of the granuloma of sarcoidosis with accompanying schematic representation.

to delayed hypersensitivity skin test antigens is a frequent finding but is obviously not diagnostic of sarcoidosis. Similarly, characterization of cells obtained by bronchial lavage and the use of gallium–67 scanning of the lungs are not in themselves diagnostic of sarcoidosis, although abnormalities consistent with that diagnosis may be found. For this reason, and because of cost and radiation exposure, these last two tests are not routinely justified currently for diagnosis in clinical practice. However, gallium–67 scanning may be useful in detecting unsuspected organ involvement by sarcoidosis, such as that of parotid glands. This observation may support the diagnosis.

Serum angiotensin I–converting enzyme activity is often elevated in sarcoidosis, but a number of other diseases may be similarly associated with its increased activity (e.g., miliary tuberculosis, leprosy, Gaucher's disease). If these diseases can be readily excluded, measurement of this enzyme may be useful. This is the case when the primary diagnostic considerations are lymphoma and sarcoidosis, since angiotensin I–converting enzyme activity is not increased in lymphoma. Elevations of other proteolytic enzymes in serum, such as lysozyme and thermolysin-like metalloendopeptidase, have been evaluated but are not yet commonly used for diagnostic purposes.

ACTIVITY OF DISEASE

Sarcoidosis may remit spontaneously; the concept of "activity of disease" is therefore useful when considering therapeutic strategies (Table 67–2). Activity of disease is very difficult to define, since occult granulomatous lesions may exist throughout many tissues of the body. Clinical findings provide some indication of activity of disease, but often in a nonquantitative and imprecise way, especially when the patient is relatively asymp-

TABLE 67–2. INDICATORS OF "ACTIVITY" OF SARCOIDOSIS

1. Clinical features
2. Worsening of symptoms
3. Worsening of pulmonary function tests/chest radiograph
4. Elevation of serum calcium level
5. Elevation of serum angiotensin I–converting enzyme level
6. Gallium scanning positivity
7. Evidence of alveolitis on bronchial lavage

tomatic. Radiologic and pulmonary function study changes may also be helpful in assessing activity of disease. Bronchoalveolar lavage to measure the percentage of lymphocytes as a reflection of parenchymal inflammation has been advocated. A high percentage of lymphocytes has been referred to as high-intensity alveolitis, denoting a poorer prognosis, but this approach has not gained wide acceptance. Gallium–67 scanning of the lung, which is also thought to reflect inflammation, has been proposed as an indirect method to monitor the intensity of alveolitis; the utility of this assessment of disease activity, similar to that of bronchoalveolar lavage, will need to be determined by more extensive prospective testing. Since elevated activity of serum angiotensin I–converting enzyme in sarcoidosis may be derived from epithelioid cells or granulomas, it has been suggested, without convincing evidence, that serum levels of this enzyme may reflect the granuloma "load" of the body. On the basis of this premise, its measurement is sometimes used to follow disease activity, but there is no assuredly accurate independent assessment of its validity as a guide to therapy or prognosis.

THERAPY

Many patients with sarcoidosis show spontaneous total remission of disease in a period up to 3 years. As many as 80 to 90 per cent of those with hilar and mediastinal lymphadenopathy or Loeffgren's syndrome alone may have remission; fewer patients with parenchymal involvement experience remission spontaneously. Other patients show arrest of the disease with moderate fibrosis, and a small percentage of patients develop progressive fibrosis and organ impairment. Once the disease remits spontaneously, only rarely does it recur. Treatment with corticosteroids causes granulomas to regress but does not appear to affect the natural course of the disease, since granulomas may recur if therapy is stopped. Since the disease may remit spontaneously and since steroids may cause significant side effects, treatment is usually started only if there is an indication of interference with the function of a vital organ (lungs, kidneys, eyes, heart, or central nervous system) or if hypercalcemia is present. All patients with sarcoidosis should be followed carefully so that therapy can be started as soon as deterioration of organ function has been detected.

Prednisone is usually the drug of choice for the treatment of sarcoidosis. The usual starting dosage is 30 to 40 mg per day, but at times a schedule of 50 to 60 mg every other day is used for initial therapy. A response in terms of symptoms or radiologic findings should be seen within 2 to 4 weeks. The steroid dose should be tapered after several weeks, and the eventual maintenance dose should be the lowest one that is effective in maintaining the response that is being followed (see below). Often 10 to 15 mg of prednisone every other day, a dosage that has a low risk of side effects, will suffice. Attempts to stop therapy may be tried after several months, but evidence of disease activity (symptoms, chest radiographic abnormalities, or worsening of pulmonary function) may recur, and prednisone may have to be restarted.

What are the best parameters to follow as indicators of disease activity? As noted earlier, measurements of disease activity are imprecise. Certainly, clinical symptoms should be assessed carefully, and chest radiographic and pulmonary function changes often give indication of disease activity. However, both radiographic abnormalities and pulmonary function changes correlate poorly with clinical parameters. Serum angiotensin I–converting enzyme levels are easily obtained and may provide clues to activity, but tests such as bronchial lavage and gallium–67 scanning are still largely experimental. Failure of response may indicate irreversible fibrosis, a situation in which steroid therapy causes more potential risk than benefit.

All of the usual side effects associated with steroid therapy may occur in patients treated for sarcoidosis (Ch. 27). The dose can usually be reduced sufficiently, however, so that infection with opportunistic organisms occurs rarely. Cosmetic problems of weight gain and fluid accumulation are often the most bothersome side effects. More difficult decisions about steroid therapy arise when there are associated disorders, such as diabetes mellitus, that may be exacerbated by these agents. Since tuberculin skin tests will become positive in patients with sarcoidosis who contract tuberculosis, appropriate prophylaxis or treatment should

be given when the tuberculin skin test is positive or converts to positivity.

Topical steroids have been used for dermatologic and ophthalmologic lesions, and chloroquine and methotrexate have been used for sarcoidosis of the skin. Indomethacin and other nonsteroidal anti-inflammatory agents may be useful for arthritis occurring in Loeffgren's syndrome. Aerosolized steroids approved for use in the United States have not been effective for pulmonary sarcoidosis, but other aerosolized preparations are being tried in Europe. Sarcoidosis that manifests with bronchoconstriction does not respond well to conventional bronchodilator therapy other than steroids. It remains to be determined whether avoidance of sunlight will significantly influence calcium metabolism in sarcoidosis. Dietary calcium restriction may be considered when hypercalcemia is present.

Bascom R, Johns CJ: The natural history and management of sarcoidosis. Adv Intern Med 31:213, 1986. *This is an excellent general review of this controversial area, with 138 references.*

Fanburg BL: Sarcoidosis and Other Granulomatous Diseases of the Lung. New York, Marcel Dekker, 1983. *A comprehensive textbook covering both clinical and experimental aspects of sarcoidosis.*

James DG, Williams WJ: Sarcoidosis and Other Granulomatous Disorders. Philadelphia, W.B. Saunders Company, 1982. *Another good monograph with an extensive review of all phase of sarcoidosis. Excellent clinical descriptions and comprehensive references.*

Roberts WC, McAllister HA Jr, Ferrans VJ: Sarcoidosis of the heart: A clinicopathologic study of 35 necropsy patients (Group I) and review of 78 previously described necropsy patients (Group II). Am J Med 63:86, 1977. *A good compilation of cases of sarcoidosis of the heart.*

Rockoff SD, Ronatagi PK: Unusual manifestations of thoracic sarcoidosis. Am J Radiol 144:513, 1985. *A comprehensive coverage of radiologic features of sarcoidois.*

Stern BJ, Krumholz A, Johns C, et al.: Sarcoidosis and its neurological manifestations. Arch Neurol 42:909, 1985. *A superb review of neurologic manifestations of sarcoidosis.*

Thomas PD, Hunninghake GW: Current concepts of the pathogenesis of sarcoidosis. Am Rev Respir Dis 135:747, 1987. *A current review with emphasis on immunologic features in sarcoidosis.*

Venet A, Hance AJ, Saltini C, et al.: Enhanced alveolar macrophage–mediated antigen-induced T-lymphocyte proliferation in sarcoidosis. J Clin Invest 75:293, 1985. *Further information about immunologic abnormalities in sarcoidosis.*

68 Pulmonary Neoplasms

Charles H. Scoggin

The lung can be affected by a variety of neoplasms (Table 68–1). Bronchogenic carcinoma accounts for more than 90 per cent of all lung tumors. The major management questions of lung cancer are the following: Is the tumor resectable? Is the tumor small cell lung cancer? Other tumors may metastasize to the lung. Benign tumors of the lung are infrequent compared with malignant tumors.

BRONCHOGENIC CARCINOMA

Lung cancer, a primary neoplasm arising within the airways, is a frequent and important neoplasm. In the United States, it is the leading fatal neoplasm of men and women. In 1990, it is estimated that approximately 142,000 will die of lung cancer in the United States. This figure represents 28 per cent of all cancer deaths in the United States. Lung cancer is strongly associated with the use of tobacco products, particularly with cigarettes. Although surgery or radiation therapy may lead to eradication of tumors in a small number of patients, the majority of people with lung cancer will have advanced disease at the time of diagnosis and will die of the disorder within 1 year of its detection. Determining the cell type and the stage of the disease is important in the clinical management of lung cancer, since these factors will affect treatment and prognosis. Four types of tumors account for 95 per cent of all lung malignancies: squamous cell (epidermoid), adenocarcinoma (including alveolar cell), large cell (also known as large cell anaplastic), and small cell lung cancer. Small

TABLE 68–1. WORLD HEALTH ORGANIZATION CLASSIFICATION OF LUNG TUMORS

I. Epithelial tumors
  A. Benign
    1. Papillomas (squamous cell and "transitional")
    2. Adenomas (includes pleomorphic and monomorphic)
  B. Dysplasia, carcinoma in situ
  C. Malignant
    1. Squamous cell carcinoma (epidermoid carcinoma)
    2. Small cell carcinoma
    3. Adenocarcinoma (includes acinar, papillary, bronchiolar, alveolar, and solid with mucus formation)
    4. Large cell carcinoma (giant cell and clear cell)
    5. Adenosquamous carcinoma
    6. Carcinoid tumor
    7. Bronchial gland carcinomas (includes adenoid cystic and mucoepidermoid carcinoma)
    8. Others
II. Soft tissue tumors
III. Mesothelial tumors
  A. Benign mesothelioma
  B. Malignant mesothelioma
IV. Miscellaneous tumors
  A. Benign
  B. Malignant
    1. Carcinosarcoma
    2. Pulmonary blastoma
    3. Malignant melanoma
    4. Malignant lymphoma
    5. Others
V. Secondary tumors
VI. Unclassified tumors
VII. Tumor-like lesions
  A. Hamartoma
  B. Lymphoproliferative lesions
  C. Tumorlet
  D. Eosinophilic granuloma
  E. "Sclerosing hemangioma"
  F. Inflammatory pseudotumor
  G. Others

cell lung cancer is distinguished from other types of lung cancer because it often shows a clinical response to chemotherapy.

Incidence and Prevalence

No population group is exempt from lung cancer. Lung cancer is the leading cause of cancer-related death of men in 28 developed countries of the world. In 1986, lung cancer surpassed breast cancer as the leading cause of death from cancer in women in the United States. The worldwide incidence of lung cancer is anticipated to continue to increase owing to the spread of the use of cigarettes, particularly in the Third World.

Lung cancer, as a major health problem, is a phenomenon of the twentieth century. In 1912, only 374 cases of primary lung neoplasms had been reported in the world's medical literature. There is little doubt that the exposure to cigarette smoke and other carcinogens accounts for the rapid increase in the occurrence of lung cancer.

The exact incidence of each type of lung cancer is difficult to determine. Squamous cell carcinoma is thought to be the most frequent form of the tumor (30 to 35 per cent of all cases), followed by adenocarcinoma, large cell carcinoma, and small cell carcinoma. Adenocarcinoma may be the most frequent lung cancer of women currently, but there is evidence that small cell lung cancer may soon surpass it.

Lung cancer occurs principally in those between the ages of 45 and 75 years. All histologic types of lung cancer in men peak at approximately 70 to 74 years of age. In women, adenocarcinoma peaks at an earlier age than in men (50 to 59 years).

Epidemiology

CIGARETTE SMOKING. About 80 to 90 per cent of all cases of lung cancer are caused by smoking cigarettes (see also Ch. 10 and 158). Cigarette smoking causes cancer in humans and experimental animals in a dose-dependent manner. Consumption of cigarettes is commonly quantitated as number of packs smoked per day and number of years smoked ("pack years"). A person who has smoked 2 packs per day for 20 years (40 pack years) has a 60- to 70-fold increased risk of developing lung cancer compared with a person who has never smoked. Because the duration of smoking is strongly associated with risk of lung cancer, the incidence and death rate from lung cancer are highest in the older age groups. Other factors that are important are depth of inhalation and tar and nicotine content of cigarettes.

Decreased smoking of cigarettes is associated epidemiologically with a declining incidence of lung cancer. A reduction in the prevalence of smoking among men in Sweden, Australia, Canada, and the United States has resulted in a reduction or slowing of deaths from lung cancer in men. A lag phase of about 20 years exists between an increase in cigarette smoking in a particular population and a rise in deaths from lung cancer. This lag is reflected in the current rise in deaths from lung cancer among women of the United States, among whom there was an increase in cigarette consumption in the 1950's. A similar phenomenon is thought to account for the increasing occurrence of lung cancer among Japanese men.

Passive inhalation of cigarette smoke may also be a risk factor for lung cancer. Passive smoke inhalation may cause both lung cancer and breast cancer in women. Sidestream smoke has a higher concentration than mainstream smoke of carcinogens such as nitrosamines, naphthalene, and benzopyrene.

OCCUPATIONAL ASSOCIATIONS. Occupational exposures also increase the incidence of lung cancer: uranium (in miners), haloethers (such as dichloromethyl ether and chloromethyl methyl ether), arsenical fumes, isopropyl oil, nickel, metallic iron, iron oxide, and beryllium. Asbestos exposure in nonsmokers is associated with a four- to fivefold increased incidence of lung cancer. Asbestos and radon gas act as cocarcinogens with cigarette smoke. Smoking increases the risk of bronchogenic cancer 80- to 90-fold in persons also exposed to asbestos. Radon gas exposure may also occur as an environmental pollutant in heavily insulated homes. As many as 12 per cent of homes in the United States may contain unhealthy levels of radon gas. Chronic inflammation of the lung, such as from interstitial fibrosis and areas of scarring, is associated with the occurrence of adenocarcinoma. Certain genetic determinants, such as levels of aryl hydrocarbon hydroxylase, may also be important.

Pathogenesis

CELL OF ORIGIN. The development of lung cancer is a multistep process. The pulmonary endodermal cell seems to be the common stem cell of origin of all lung cancer cell types. Because it demonstrates certain amine precursor uptake and decarboxylation (APUD) properties, small cell lung cancer has been hypothesized to arise from Kulchitsky's cell. There is no direct evidence to support this hypothesis, however.

CIGARETTE SMOKE. Cigarette smoke contains many carcinogens in both the gaseous and the particulate phases. Nitrosamines and other compounds are thought to be important in the gaseous phase. Carcinogens in the particulate phase include benzopyrene and related polycyclic aromatic hydrocarbons, nitrosonornicotine, polonium, and arsenic. Reduction in particulate factors correlates with a decreased incidence of lung cancer.

CELLULAR CHANGES. In the natural history of bronchogenic cancer, bronchial epithelial cells first become cytologically abnormal. At this stage, they are not malignant, not are they invariably predictive of the eventual development of malignancy. The next step is carcinoma in situ, i.e., carcinomatous changes localized above the basement membrane and productive of no symptoms. The next change is epidermal invasion by tumor cells, followed by metastasis of the tumor. In situ tumors are indolent and slow growing. As malignancy progresses, so too does the rapidity of tumor spread.

CELLULAR EVENTS. Three aspects of the cellular events that attend the transformation of normal bronchial epithelial cells to malignant cells are important: (1) damage to cellular DNA; (2) alteration in cellular oncogene expression; and (3) tumor-derived factors that stimulate cellular division.

Cigarette smoke, ionizing radiation, and chemical carcinogens damage cellular DNA, in part through inducing chromosomal deletions and rearrangements and point mutations. The most

TABLE 68–2. CLINICAL MANIFESTATIONS OF LUNG CARCINOMA

1. Due to primary lesions
   Cough   Wheezing
   Dyspnea   Weight loss
   Hemoptysis   Fever
   Sputum   Pneumonia
2. Due to local extension
   Chest pain   Dysphagia
   Hoarseness   Pericardial effusion
   Superior vena cava syndrome   Pleural effusion
   Pancoast's syndrome   Diaphragm paralysis
   Horner's syndrome
3. Extrapulmonary manifestations

widely recognized chromosomal abnormality seen in lung cancer is a deletion of genetic material in the 3p14 to 23 region in the malignant, but not the normal, cells of patients with small cell lung cancer. Activation of oncogenes appears to be a common event in bronchogenic carcinoma (Ch. 157). Expression of members of both the *ras* and the *myc* oncogene families has been found in lung tumor cells, in contrast to normal lung cells. Another important factor is the production of so-called "autocrine growth factors" by lung cancer cells. Cultured small cell lung cancer cells secrete growth factors into their media. This feature is thought to account for their decreased requirement for serum growth factors. One such factor is bombesin/gastrin-related peptide. These growth factors stimulate cell division constantly. They may be of future clinical importance in that monoclonal antibodies to bombesin/gastrin-related peptide inhibit tumor growth of cells in culture and in experimental animals.

Clinical Manifestations

SYMPTOMS OF LUNG CANCER (Table 68–2). Most patients with lung cancer have some symptoms that cause them to seek medical attention. A typical patient will present with pulmonary complaints such as cough, hemoptysis, and weight loss. Only 5 to 15 per cent of patients are asymptomatic when discovered to have bronchogenic carcinoma.

Some Characteristics of Specific Tumors. *Squamous cell*, or *epidermoid*, *carcinoma* usually begins as a central lesion that tends to invade locally. The patient often presents with symptoms referable to the airways, such as cough, dyspnea, or hemoptysis. It may also invade the chest wall, diaphragm, or mediastinum. Unlike other primary lung neoplasms, squamous cell tumors may cavitate.

Adenocarcinoma usually begins as a peripheral lesion. It is more aggressive than squamous cell carcinoma. Symptoms at the time of diagnosis often reflect invasion of lymph nodes, pleura, or the other lung or metastasis to other organs, such as the central nervous system or adrenal glands. *Bronchioloalveolar carcinoma*, a special subtype of adenocarcinoma, usually accounts for no more than 1 to 5 per cent of primary lung neoplasms. Bronchioloalveolar carcinoma often manifests as a solitary pulmonary nodule (approximately 60 per cent) but may also appear as a localized infiltrate or area of lobar consolidation mimicking infection. *Large cell carcinoma* usually manifests as a bulky peripheral mass.

Small cell lung cancer should be carefully distinguished from non–small cell lung cancer, from which it differs both in biologic features and in clinical manifestations (Table 68–3). Small cell lung cancer commonly begins as a central tumor, but 70 to 90 per cent of patients have disease outside the original hemithorax at the time of detection. Because of its propensity to metastasize and to produce paraneoplastic syndromes, small cell lung cancer is usually symptomatic for 3 months or less before diagnosis. In contrast, symptoms associated with squamous cell carcinoma appear, on the average, 8 months before the diagnosis is made, and up to 25 per cent of patients with adenocarcinoma are asymptomatic at presentation. The severity of symptoms is also an important prognostic factor, particularly in small cell lung cancer. The more severe the tumor symptoms, the worse the prognosis.

Symptoms Referable to the Chest. Most patients with bronchogenic carcinomas present with symptoms referable to the chest, sometimes reflecting the area of lung involved. Central or endobronchial tumors can manifest as dyspnea, cough, hemoptysis, wheezing, or pneumonitis with fever and purulent sputum. Even small tumors may cause a disproportionately high degree of dyspnea. Hemoptysis, a common complaint, is more frequent in non–small cell lung cancer, since small cell lung cancer is often submucosal in location, without ulceration into the airway itself. Peripheral tumors may manifest as chest pain due to pleural or chest wall involvement.

Spread to thoracic lymph nodes is common in lung cancer, especially in small cell lung cancer. Regional spread to hilar and mediastinal nodes may cause dysphagia due to esophageal compression, hoarseness because of recurrent laryngeal nerve compression, Horner's syndrome due to sympathetic nerve involvement, and elevation of the hemidiaphragm from phrenic nerve compression. Superior sulcus, or Pancoast's, tumor may involve the brachial plexus, resulting in a C7–T2 neuropathy with pain, numbness, and weakness of the arm.

Cardiac involvement is seen at autopsy in 20 to 25 per cent of patients with small cell lung cancer, but less frequently in those with non–small cell lung cancer. Clinical findings of cardiac involvement are arrhythmias, cardiomegaly, and pericardial effusion with pericardial friction rub. Cardiac tamponade may occur.

Systemic Symptoms. Constitutional symptoms of anorexia, weight loss, and generalized weakness are common in lung cancer. Patients may also have fever without obvious infection.

Tumors that obstruct the superior vena cava cause the superior vena cava syndrome: swelling of the head and neck, breast enlargement, and prominence of the superficial veins of the thorax. Bronchogenic carcinoma, particularly small cell lung cancer, may demonstrate extrathoracic spread to other organ systems. Metastasis to the spinal cord causes spinal cord pain and symptoms of cord compression. Pain may precede weakness and sensory changes by days. Metastasis to the liver may cause pain, chemical dysfunction of the liver, and biliary obstruction. Metastasis to the bone may result in pain or bone marrow invasion.

Paraneoplastic Syndromes. Paraneoplastic syndromes are remote effects of tumor. They are described in detail in Ch. 161

TABLE 68–3. COMPARISON BETWEEN NON–SMALL CELL LUNG CANCER AND SMALL CELL LUNG CANCER

	Small Cell Lung Cancer	Non–Small Cell Lung Cancer
Cytopathology	Scant cytoplasm; indistinct nucleoli	Large amount of cytoplasm; prominent nucleoli
Cytogenetics	Deletion of 3p14 → 23	No known specific chromosomal alteration
Biochemistry and hormone production	Multiple enzymes and hormones (neuron-specific enolase, creatinine kinase BB, L-dopa decarboxylase, ACTH, bombesin, ADH, somatostatin, MSH)	Ectopic hormone production rare; paraneoplastic syndromes less common than in small cell lung cancer
Clinical presentation	Hemoptysis rare; most patients symptomatic at presentation; usually metastatic at presentation	Hemoptysis common, symptoms less frequent at time of presentation; dissemination at presentation less common than in small cell carcinoma
Treatment		
Surgery	Seldom, if ever, indicated	Primary hope for cure
Radiation	Limited role; palliation and perhaps prophylaxis of CNS metastasis	Palliation, possible cure
Chemotherapy	Main treatment (up to 80 per cent response)	Effect on survival undetermined

ACTH = adrenocorticotropic hormone; ADH = antidiuretic hormone; MSH = melanocyte-stimulating hormone; CNS = central nervous system.

and 162, to which the reader is referred. They lead to metabolic and neuromuscular disturbances unrelated to the primary tumor, metastases, or treatment. Paraneoplastic syndromes may be the first sign of the tumor or of tumor recurrence. They do not necessarily indicate that a tumor has spread. Paraneoplastic syndromes often respond to treatment of the primary tumor. Osteoarthropathy associated with lung cancer is seen in up to 30 per cent of patients with lung cancer but is rare in patients with small cell lung cancer. Manifestations include digital clubbing and painful periosteal inflammation. Periosteal elevation usually involves the long bones. It may be confused with certain forms of arthritis, including rheumatoid arthritis. Endocrinologic manifestations are well recognized in bronchogenic carcinoma. Up to 10 per cent of epidermoid tumors secrete humoral factors, resulting in hypercalcemia and hypophosphatemia. Metastasis to the adrenal glands may rarely result in adrenal insufficiency. Other endocrinologic manifestations, most common with small cell lung cancer, include Cushing's syndrome due to production of adrenocorticotropic hormone (ACTH), hyperpigmentation from production of melanocyte-stimulating hormone (MSH), and rarely the "somatostatinoma syndrome," which consists of vomiting, abdominal pain, diarrhea, mild diabetes, and cholelithiasis. Patients with lung cancer develop the syndrome of inappropriate antidiuretic hormone secretion (SIADH) in 10 to 15 per cent of cases (Ch. 161). Neuromyopathic manifestations of lung cancer are rare (<5 per cent) but may dominate the clinical picture when they occur (Ch. 162). Such manifestations include the Eaton-Lambert syndrome (seen in small cell lung cancer), polymyositis, subacute cerebellar degeneration, spinocerebellar degeneration, and peripheral neuropathies. Nonbacterial (marantic) endocarditis, migratory thrombophlebitis (Trousseau's syndrome), and disseminated intravascular coagulation as complications of malignancy are described in Ch. 159.

CLINICAL FINDINGS OF LUNG CANCER. Physical examination often does not reflect either the presence of lung cancer or the state of the disease. Digital clubbing may be found in up to 12 per cent of patients and gynecomastia in 5 to 7 per cent of patients (the latter most frequently associated with large cell anaplastic cancer). Acanthosis nigricans may be found with adenocarcinoma, and hyperpigmentation of the palms and soles may be seen with squamous cell carcinoma (Ch. 163). Obstruction of the superior vena cava may cause superior vena cava syndrome. Examination of the head may disclose the presence of Horner's syndrome, i.e., a unilaterally constricted pupil, enophthalmos, narrowed palpebral fissure, and loss of sweating on the same side of the face. Endobronchial obstruction may result in a localized wheeze detected during physical examination of the chest. Lobar collapse may result in an area of decreased breath sounds and dullness to percussion. Decreased movement of a hemidiaphragm may occur as a consequence of phrenic nerve compression. Liver metastasis may cause hepatic enlargement or nodularity. Weakness, altered reflexes, and decreased sensation may be found in patients with tumors metastatic to the central nervous system.

Diagnosis of Bronchogenic Carcinoma

The diagnosis of lung cancer requires detecting the tumor, establishing its cell type, and defining the stage of the malignancy. Determining cell type is important because it guides the approach both to staging and to treatment.

THE CHEST RADIOGRAPH. The presence of lung cancer is usually suggested by abnormalities on the chest radiograph. The most frequent finding is a mass in the lung field. Lesions usually cannot be detected if they are less than 5 to 6 mm. Tumors occur in the right lung more than in the left (3:2) and in the upper lobes more than in the lower lobes. Secondary manifestations seen on the chest radiograph include lobar collapse, pleural effusion, pneumonitis, elevation of the hemidiaphragm, hilar and mediastinal adenopathy, and erosion of ribs or vertebrae due to metastases. Alveolar cell cancer can manifest as a localized infiltrate mimicking pneumonia.

HISTOLOGIC DIAGNOSIS. When lung cancer is suspected, the next step in evaluation after the chest radiograph should be that of obtaining tissue specimens for histologic examination. The diagnostic yield of sputum cytologic evaluation will depend upon the adequacy of the specimen, the expertise of the cytologist, the type of tumor, and the number of specimens examined (three or four specimens are considered adequate). Sputum cytologic study is more likely to be negative in patients with small cell lung cancer than in those with non–small cell lung cancer. A negative sputum study should never be regarded as conclusive evidence for absence of carcinoma.

Bronchoscopy is important both for determining if a tumor is present and for obtaining tissue for histologic diagnosis. The combination of bronchial brushing and forceps biopsy is positive 90 to 93 per cent of the time with tumors located in proximal airways. Bronchial washings are less successful (approximately 80 per cent positive). For lesions that are not proximal enough in the airways for direct visualization, transbronchial biopsy with fluoroscopic guidance may be utilized. Yield of histologic diagnosis is 25 per cent for tumors less than 2 cm in diameter and 65 per cent for larger lesions. Transbronchial needle aspiration can also be employed. Peripheral lesions can be aspirated using a transthoracic needle with guidance by multiplane fluoroscopy or chest computed tomography (CT). Success rates as high as 95 per cent have been reported. Pneumothorax is the major complication. Contraindications to pulmonary biopsy include pulmonary hypertension, hypoxemia with carbon dioxide retention, and a bleeding diathesis.

If a diagnosis is not established by cytologic study of the sputum, bronchoscopy, or needle biopsy, thoracotomy may be necessary. The decision to undertake thoracotomy should be a reasoned one, weighing the importance to the patient of making the diagnosis against other factors such as age or other complicating illness.

In some circumstances, a histologic diagnosis can be made by biopsy of metastatic sites, such as liver, lymph nodes, bone, or bone marrow. When tumor involves the pleural space, combined thoracentesis and pleural biopsy will provide a diagnostic yield of up to 90 per cent.

SCREENING STUDIES. Screening studies for early stages of lung cancer, using chest radiographs alone or in combination with sputum cytology, have been proposed for cigarette smokers who are 45 years of age or older; however, recent trials examining the outcome of screening have failed to demonstrate a benefit. Carcinoembryonic antigen (CEA), neural peptides, and neurogenic enzymes are not currently useful in detecting lung tumor, its metastases, or its recurrence.

Staging of Lung Cancer

Lung cancers are staged first for location (anatomic staging) and then for the patient's ability to withstand various treatments aimed at curing the tumor or increasing life expectancy (physiologic staging). Staging for non–small cell lung cancer differs from that for small cell lung cancer.

NON–SMALL CELL LUNG CANCER. For non–small cell lung cancer, the first and most important decision is whether or not the tumor is operable. Routine staging to exclude inoperable patients has increased the survival of patients undergoing surgical resection of lung cancer. Table 68–4 lists a widely used tumor, node, and metastasis (TNM) system for classifying lung cancer.

Patients with stages I and II are considered candidates for surgical resection. Certain patients with stage III cancer may be candidates for surgery with postoperative irradiation of the mediastinum. Surgical resection of N2 disease is controversial. Detection of mediastinal lymph node involvement with cancer is best determined by mediastinoscopy for tumors in the right hemithorax. Tumor assessment of the left hemithorax requires an anterior exploration (a Chamberlain procedure). Transbronchial and percutaneous needle aspiration is sometimes used to evaluate hilar lymph nodes. Size alone cannot be used to judge whether or not mediastinal lymph nodes are involved with metastatic cancer; however, enlarged nodes in the presence of known bronchogenic carcinoma argue strongly for metastatic disease. CT scanning of the chest is useful in excluding the presence of other tumors in the chest. In addition, scanning of the adrenal glands can be useful in determining if adrenal enlargement, possibly due to metastases, is present. Routine bone scan, CT scanning, liver scan, and bone radiographs are not recommended unless the physical examination or history suggests that these organs are involved. Magnetic resonance imaging (MRI) may be helpful in

TABLE 68–4. TNM CLASSIFICATION OF LUNG CANCER

Primary Tumor (T)

TX: Tumor present as determined by presence of malignant cells in bronchopulmonary secretions, but not radiographically or bronchoscopically visible; no evidence of primary tumor

T0: No evidence of primary tumor

T1S: Carcinoma in situ

T1: Tumor 3 cm or less surrounded by lung or visceral pleura, but without evidence of invasion proximal to lobar bronchus at bronchoscopy

T2: Tumor more than 3 cm or tumor invading visceral pleura or associated with obstructive pneumonitis or atelectasis; involving less than entire lung; at bronchoscopy, proximal extent of visible tumor must be within a lobar bronchus or at least 2 cm distal to carina

T3: Tumor of any size with direct extension into chest wall, diaphragm, or mediastinal pleura or pericardium without involving heart, great vessels, trachea, esophagus, or vertebral body; also includes superior sulcus tumors and tumor in main bronchus within 2 cm of carcina but not involving carina

T4: Tumor of any size invading mediastinum or involving heart, great vessels, trachea, esophagus, vertebral body, or carina or presence of malignant pleural effusion

Nodal Involvement

N0: No demonstrable metastasis to regional lymph nodes

N1: Metastasis to peribronchial or the ipsilateral, or both, hilar lymph nodes, including direct extension

N2: Metastasis to ipsilateral mediastinal lymph nodes and subcarinal lymph nodes

N3: Metastasis to contralateral mediastinal lymph nodes, contralateral hilar lymph nodes, ipsilateral or contralateral scalene or supraclavicular lymph nodes

Distant Metastasis (M)

M0: No (known) distant metastasis

M1: Distant metastasis present—specify site(s)

Stage Grouping

Occult carcinoma	TX	N0	M0
Stage 0	T1S	Carcinoma in situ	
Stage I	T1	N0	M0
	T2	N1	M0
Stage II	T1	N1	M0
	T2	N1	M0
Stage IIIa	T3	N0	M0
	T3	N1	M0
	T1–3	N2	M0
Stage IIIb	Any T	N3	M0
	T4	Any N	M0
Stage IV	Any T	Any N	M1

examining adrenal glands, defining hilar masses, and demonstrating chest wall invasion.

SMALL CELL LUNG CANCER. Small cell lung cancer has often metastasized at the time of diagnosis; the TNM system has not proved to be useful. Small cell lung cancer is defined as either limited or extensive (Table 68–5). Limited disease is confined to one hemithorax, with or without involvement of mediastinal lymph nodes. Spread of disease beyond this point is extensive. In addition, performance status is also an important prognostic factor. Survival correlates with degree of symptoms and functional impairment.

Treatment of Bronchogenic Carcinoma

NON–SMALL CELL LUNG CANCER. Both surgery and radiation therapy may benefit patients with non–small cell lung

TABLE 68–5. TWO-STAGE CLASSIFICATION OF SMALL CELL LUNG CANCER

Limited disease (30%)
1. Primary tumor confined to hemithorax
2. Ipsilateral hilar lymph nodes
3. Ipsilateral and contralateral supraclavicular lymph nodes
4. Ipsilateral and contralateral mediastinal lymph nodes
5. Pleural effusion

Extensive disease (70%): more advanced than limited
1. Metastasis in the contralateral lung
2. Distant metastasis (brain, bone, liver, and so on)

cancer, but chemotherapy remains experimental. Newer modalities, such as laser bronchoscopy, may lead to symptomatic improvement by relieving endobronchial obstruction and may have a role in the treatment of carcinoma in situ.

Surgery. Surgical resectability of lung cancer is determined in large measure by the extent of lymph node metastasis. Patients with stage I and stage II non–small cell lung cancer (Table 68–5) should be treated with surgical resection aimed at cure. Patients with stage III disease characterized by ipsilateral intranodal mediastinal lymph node involvement may benefit from surgical resection of the primary and involved lymph nodes. Intranodal disease is defined as tumor completely confined within the capsule of the mediastinal lymph nodes. These patients should also receive postoperative mediastinal irradiation. Patients with superior sulcus tumors that have not metastasized to mediastinal lymph nodes or systemically should be treated with preoperative irradiation and en bloc resection. Irradiation is usually given as 3000 rads in 10 treatments, followed in 3 to 6 weeks by surgical resection. En bloc surgical resection of tumors that have invaded the chest wall, but have not metastasized systemically or to the mediastinal lymph nodes, may benefit. Surgical resection of both superior sulcus and chest wall tumors is associated with increased surgical mortality, compared with other less extensive surgical resections of lung cancer.

Limited resection of tumors yields results comparable to those obtained with more extensive surgical procedures. In general, lobectomy is recommended. Even less extensive procedures, such as lobar segment and wedge resection, are usually reserved for patients with peripheral lesions or limited pulmonary function.

Approximately 40 per cent of patients with non–small cell lung cancer undergo thoracotomy, with an overall 5-year survival from 10 to 35 per cent. At the time of thoracotomy, 75 per cent of patients undergo tumor resection with the aim at cure. The overall survival of patients resected for cure varies according to histopathologic type of tumor: squamous cell carcinoma, 37 per cent; adenocarcinoma, 27 per cent; large cell undifferentiated carcinoma, 27 per cent; and bronchoalveolar carcinoma, 56 per cent. Stage of the tumor is also an important determinant of surgical survival: stage I, 54 per cent; stage II, 35 per cent; and stage III without systemic or mediastinal lymph node metastasis, 19 per cent.

Pulmonary function is another very important factor in the evaluation of patients for surgery. Forced vital capacity greater than 2 liters and a forced expiratory volume in the first second (FEV_1) of greater than 50 per cent of the forced vital capacity predict that a patient can tolerate the consequences of pneumonectomy. Radionuclide scanning has generally replaced differential spirometry as a method of assessing the lung to be resected for its contribution to overall respiration.

Elderly patients should not be excluded from consideration for resection of tumor. The most limiting factor of survival in this age group is not age, but the tumor. Bronchogenic carcinoma is a highly aggressive tumor in the elderly. The average life expectancy of patients with untreated tumor is 8 months. This compares with an average life expectancy in the United States of 11.1 and 14.8 years, respectively, for men and women aged 70 years. Elderly patients carefully selected for surgery have a 5-year survival of 35 to 42 per cent.

Radiation Therapy. Most non–small cell lung cancers are responsive to radiation treatment. Radiation therapy is indicated in patients with stage III disease without metastases or in stage I or stage II patients who refuse surgical treatment. A consistently small but reproducible group of patients with disease in the chest alone benefit from radiation treatment aimed at cure. Patients with operable lung cancer may have a 5-year survival rate with radiation therapy alone of up to 21 per cent. Treatment is generally 5500 to 6000 rads by either split course or continuous fraction irradiation. Acute esophagitis is a common complication. Patients receiving irradiation of a lung for cure of cancer may develop radiation pneumonitis; therefore, patients must have pulmonary function equivalent to that necessary to tolerate pneumonectomy.

Most tumors will respond to irradiation by decreasing in sizes; however, radiation treatment of patients with nonresectable non–small cell lung cancer has been disappointing in prolonging survival.

Postoperative mediastinal irradiation is recommended in patients who have undergone resection and who have intranodal lymph node involvement, but preoperative and postoperative adjuvant radiotherapy for T2 and T3 tumors has not been shown to be beneficial and may even be detrimental. The single exception appears to be superior sulcus, or Pancoast's, tumor.

TREATMENT OF PATIENTS WITH DISSEMINATED NON–SMALL CELL LUNG CARCINOMA. Seventy per cent of patients with non–small cell lung cancer have unresectable disease at the time of diagnosis or thoracotomy. In such patients, irradiation and other forms of palliative treatment are very important.

Radiation Therapy. Irradiation effectively decreases tumor size to reduce endobronchial obstruction and to re-expand the atelectatic lung. Important intrathoracic complications may respond to irradiation: the superior vena cava syndrome, 80 to 90 per cent; hemoptysis, 84 per cent cough, 60 per cent; and atelectasis, 23 per cent. Radiation therapy may also palliate bone pain and cerebral metastases.

Chemotherapy. A response rate of 30 to 40 per cent in non–small cell lung cancer has been achieved with cisplatin regimens, especially in combination with etoposide (VP–16) and/or mitomycin C. This should not be regarded as routine therapy. Substantive improvement in symptoms and survival remains to be proved. Potential benefit to the patient must be weighed against chemotherapy-induced side effects. Peripheral neuropathy, not severe myelosuppression, is usually the main dose-limiting factor. The effectiveness of combined modalities such as chemotherapy plus radiotherapy or chemotherapy plus surgery is still unproved.

SMALL CELL LUNG CANCER. The median survival of patients with untreated small cell lung cancer from the time of diagnosis is 2.8 months. Fewer than 1 per cent of untreated patients will survive 5 years. The treatments of choice for small cell lung cancer are chemotherapy and radiation. Surgical resection has little, if any, role, because at the time of detection the tumor has usually spread beyond the limits of surgical removal. For example, the mean survival with radiation therapy alone (284 days) is statistically greater than the mean survival with surgical treatment (199 days), although it remains very low.

Chemotherapy. Small cell lung cancer is highly responsive to chemotherapy. Moderately intensive therapy with three agents is usually given initially in an attempt to eradicate the tumor. The use of additional drugs beyond three is associated with a disproportionate increase in side effects compared with benefit. Examples of currently employed regimens are cyclophosphamide, methotrexate, and lomustine (CCNU); cyclophosphamide, doxorubicin, and vincristine; and cyclophosphamide, doxorubicin, and etoposide (VP–16). These regimens appear to be approximately equal in producing responses and long-term survival. Objective responses usually occur within 6 to 12 weeks after initiation of treatment. The effective length of treatment is yet to be established. Most protocols involve treatment for 12 months or less. Alternating non–cross-resistant combinations of drugs and using intensive therapy with autologous bone marrow transplantation have not been shown to increase survival. Combined modalities of irradiation and chemotherapy may be of use in limited disease, although this has yet to be conclusively proved.

Most chemotherapy regimens produce a greater than 80 per cent response rate in all patients. Complete response, defined as the absence of any evidence of residual tumor, is seen in greater than 50 per cent of patients with limited disease and in 20 per cent of patients with extensive disease. This results in a median survival of about 14 months in patients with limited disease and 7 months in patients with extensive disease. Twelve to 15 per cent of patients with limited disease will survive 6 to 11 years.

Aggressive chemotherapy produces complications and symptoms in all patients. All experience anemia and leukopenia. Opportunistic infection is an important complication. Approximately 60 per cent of neutropenic patients experience febrile episodes. Herpes zoster occurs in 8 to 12 per cent of patients with small cell lung cancer treated with chemotherapy. Other complications include nausea, vomiting, alopecia, hemorrhagic cystitis, mucositis, electrolyte imbalance, possible cardiotoxicity, and peripheral neuropathy. A long-term complication of chemotherapy for small cell lung cancer is a secondary malignancy: leukemia, lymphoma, and other neoplasms. Risk appears to increase with intensity of drug dosage and the number of drugs utilized. Finally, patients successfully treated for small cell carcinoma are still at risk for non–small cell carcinoma.

Radiation Therapy. Radiation therapy is of proven benefit in controlling bone pain, spinal cord compression, superior vena cava syndrome, and bronchial obstruction. More than 90 per cent of patients have been reported to have palliation of symptoms due to brain metastases. The use of radiation therapy in combination with chemotherapy is controversial and should be reserved for experimental studies.

Prophylactic Cranial Irradiation. Although chemotherapy has increased the survival of patients with small cell lung cancer, this survival has been accompanied by an increased risk of relapse in the central nervous system. The cumulative risk of central nervous system metastases at 2 years may be as high as 80 per cent. This risk is reduced to about 3 to 12 per cent with the use of prophylactic cranial irradiation. Unfortunately, this decreased rate of brain metastasis is not associated with increased survival. Prophylactic cranial irradiation is generally reserved for patients who have achieved a complete response in chemotherapy, but even in these patients, the benefit in terms of increased survival is slight. In all other patients, cranial irradiation should be used when central nervous system metastases are diagnosed. Most patients who survive long term exhibit memory loss, confusion, ataxia, loss of vision, and dysphonia. This encephalopathy is probably a complication of cranial irradiation with a possible contribution by chemotherapy as well.

OTHER CONSIDERATIONS IN THE TREATMENT OF LUNG CANCER

Bone Metastasis. The metastasis of lung cancer to bone most frequently causes pain, but pathologic fracture may also occur. Bone involvement is best detected by bone scan, although large lesions will be visible radiographically. Pain can usually be palliated by radiation to the involved areas.

Hypercalcemia. Hypercalcemia is one of the most important complications of lung cancer. Serum calcium values in excess of 12 mg per deciliter are considered life threatening. Treatment is aimed at lowering the serum calcium level. Treatment of hypercalcemia is discussed in detail in Ch. 235.

Central Nervous System Metastasis. Metastases from lung cancer to the central nervous system usually cause symptoms in proportion to their size and location. Corticosteroids are effective in relieving acute symptoms of increased intracranial pressure in about 75 per cent of patients. Doses of 8 to 12 mg of dexamethasone should be administered on an acute basis. Osmotic agents given to reduce intracranial pressure, such as a 20 per cent solution of mannitol administered intravenously, may be useful in treating cerebral herniation. Acute control of increased pressure should be followed by radiation therapy.

Pleural Effusion. Malignant pleural effusion frequently complicates bronchogenic carcinoma. It is exudative in nature. The diagnosis is made by cytologic examination of the fluid and by pleural biopsy. Effusions complicated by dyspnea or pain should be drained. If the fluid recurs, obliteration of the potential pleural space should be accomplished by introducing a sclerosing agent. This is best performed by insertion of a chest tube to drain the effusion completely, followed by the instillation of 1 gram of tetracycline dissolved in 100 ml of normal saline and 50 ml of 1 per cent lidocaine (Xylocaine) into the chest through the tube. The tube should then be clamped and the patient turned into different positions to distribute the sclerosing fluid along the pleural surface. The tube is then allowed to drain until the amount of fluid over a 12- to 14-hour period is 100 ml or less. Malignant pleural effusions with pH less than 7.0 are associated with a very poor prognosis.

Weakness and Weight Loss. Weight loss, muscle weakness, and difficulty in eating are frequent and distressing manifestations of lung cancer. The pathophysiology of weight loss in lung cancer is poorly understood but can be partially explained by altered carbohydrate and protein metabolism and the release of toxic factors into the circulation. The use of aggressive nutritional support in lung cancer patients in whom traditional forms of treatment have been ineffective is of limited value and may even be adverse.

Cough and Dyspnea. Reversible causes of cough and dyspnea, such as bronchospasm, bronchitis, and pneumonitis, should be excluded. The mainstays of cough control are narcotic cough suppressants. Narcotics and tranquilizers used in low dosage may produce remarkable relief of severe dyspnea. When clearance of large airway secretions becomes difficult, patients may "rattle" when they breathe (so-called "death rattle"). This is particularly distressing to family members. In patients who are terminally ill, scopolamine, 0.4 to 0.6 mg given subcutaneously every 4 hours as necessary, will tend to dry up secretions and relax the smooth muscle of the airways. It is preferred to atropine, since the former is a central nervous system depressant, in contrast to atropine, which is a stimulant.

Pain. The therapeutic goal of managing pain, the most common symptom of advanced lung cancer, should be not only its relief but also its prevention. Narcotics should be taken every 4 hours around the clock to prevent the patient from awakening with pain. There is no single optimal dosage schedule for narcotics. Most patients have their pain controlled with 30 mg of morphine, or its equivalent, given orally on a 4-hour basis. Patients, families, and those caring for the patient should be counseled that tolerance and addiction do not present real clinical problems in patients with advanced lung cancer. The most common adverse side effects of narcotic treatment are constipation and nausea, which must preferably be prevented, but treated aggressively if they appear.

Patients who have been treated for lung cancer with apparent success continue at risk for a second primary lung cancer, or "metachronous" tumor. Such tumors can have a histologic pattern identical with or different from the first primary tumor. Metachronous tumors occur in 1 to 3 per cent of patients with lung cancer. Treatment is determined by the same factors that affect other primary lung tumors; however, the physiologic impact of treatment of the first primary cancer may limit surgical resection or radiation dosage.

Bunn PA (ed.): Lung cancer. Issue dedicated to Mary Jean O'Leary Matthews. Semin Oncol 15:197, 1988. *Very comprehensive review of non–small cell and small cell lung cancer, including biology, pathology, molecular genetics, diagnostic techniques, staging, and treatment.*

Carney DN: The biology of lung cancer. Acta Oncol 28.1, 1989. *Concise review of biology of lung cancer with emphasis on tumor markers.*

Eddy DM: Screening for lung cancer. Ann Intern Med 111:232, 1989. *Excellent review of all recent trials examining screening for lung cancer with lung roentgenography and sputum cytology. Concludes routine screening not recommended because of cost, lack of benefit, and potential harm.*

Filderman AE, Shaw C, Matthay RA: Lung cancer part 1: Etiology, pathology, natural manifestations, and diagnostic techniques. Invest Radiol 21:80, 1986. *Particularly good for summarization of roentgenographic manifestations of primary pulmonary malignancies.*

Horton AW: Indoor tobacco smoke pollution. A major risk factor for both breast and lung cancer? Cancer 62:6, 1988. *Reviews risk of involuntary smoke inhalation and risk of breast and lung cancer.*

Iannuzzi MJ, Scoggin CH: Small cell lung cancer: State of the art. Am Rev Respir Dis 134:593, 1986. *Focuses on clinical and investigational aspects of small cell lung cancer.*

Rapp E: Chemotherapy can prolong survival in patients with advanced non–small cell lung cancer—report of a Canadian multicenter randomized trial. J Clin Oncol 6:633, 1988. *Reports on 18-center study sponsored by National Cancer Institute of Canada. In 251 patients studied, survival increased by 7 weeks in treated patients, but with significant toxicity.*

Webb WR: The role of magnetic resonance imaging in the assessment of patients with lung cancer: A comparison with computed tomography. J Thorac Imaging 4:65, 1989. *Reviews role of CT, but also presents the advantages and disadvantages of MRI. MRI has superior ability to discriminate certain tissues and is helpful in demonstrating chest wall invasion, defining mediastinal masses, detecting hilar masses, and distinguishing recurrent tumors from fibrosis in patients with prior irradiation.*

Whang-Peng J, Bun PA, Kao-Shan CS, et al: A nonrandom chromosomal abnormality, del3p(14–23), in human small cell lung cancer (SCLC). Cancer Genet Cytogenet 6:119, 1982. *Description of a chromosomal abnormality found in small cell lung cancer.*

OTHER MALIGNANCIES OF THE LUNG

Carcinoid Tumors

These tumors, sometimes termed "bronchial adenomas," are in fact distinct entities with different clinical courses and histologic manifestations. Three types are recognized: bronchial carcinoids, cylindromas, and mucoepidermoid tumors. Tumors may manifest with endobronchial obstruction or hemoptysis. Carcinoid tumors, including bronchial carcinoids, are considered in Ch. 230.

Scheithauer BW, Carpenter PC, Block B, et al.: Ectopic secretion of a growth hormone–releasing factor: Report of a case of acromegaly with bronchial carcinoid tumor. Am J Med 76:605, 1984. *Reviews different extrapulmonary manifestations of bronchial carcinoid tumors.*

Primary Lymphoma of the Lung

Hodgkin's disease and non-Hodgkin's lymphoma are discussed in Ch. 147 and 148. Such lymphoma may arise in the lymph nodes of the chest or within the lung itself. Patients with tumor involving the lung may present with weight loss, fever, cough, or pleuritic chest pain. Pleural effusion may be an initial or complicating manifestation.

Non-Hodgkin's tumors arising within the parenchyma of the lung are often discrete masses with or without hilar and mediastinal lymph node enlargement. An intrathoracic Hodgkin's tumor mass may cavitate or compress the bronchial tree to cause atelectasis or postobstructive pneumonitis. A common differential diagnosis of hilar adenopathy is that between lymphoma and sarcoidosis (Ch. 67). Enlargement of anterior mediastinal lymph nodes suggests lymphoma, as this is an unusual region of lymphadenopathy in sarcoidosis.

Other lymphoproliferative disorders that involve the lung are pseudolymphoma and lymphocytic interstitial pneumonitis. Pseudolymphoma appears as a nodular lesion, whereas lymphocytic interstitial pneumonitis manifests as a diffuse infiltrate. The diagnosis is made by histologic examination of lung biopsy specimen. Distinguishing between benign disease and true pulmonary lymphoma may be difficult. Some patients who initially present with an apparently benign lymphoproliferative disorder later develop malignant lymphoma. The development of hilar or mediastinal lymphadenopathy suggests the presence of malignancy.

The diagnosis of lymphoproliferative disorders of the lung depends upon histologic examination of tissue obtained by bronchoscopy, transbronchial biopsy, mediastinoscopy, or thoracotomy.

The treatment of Hodgkin's and non-Hodgkin's lymphomas of the lung involves the use of radiation or chemotherapy as would be employed for nonpulmonary lymphoma (Ch. 147 and 148). Pseudolymphoma can be removed by surgical resection. No established treatment for lymphocytic interstitial pneumonitis exists, although chemotherapy has been attempted.

Colby TV, Carrington CB: Pulmonary lymphomas: Current concepts. Pathol Annu 14:884, 1983. *Presents criteria for and classification of pulmonary lymphoid lesions.*

Uncommon Primary Lung Malignancies

Cylindromas are the second most common tumors of the trachea and bronchi. (The most common tumors are bronchogenic carcinomas.) The tumors arise from the mucous glands of the bronchial epithelium. The most common symptoms are airway obstruction and cough. Men and women are equally affected, and the age of occurrence ranges from 30 to 65 years. The diagnosis is made by bronchoscopy and biopsy. Treatment is by surgical resection, although cure may be difficult owing to the tumor's propensity to metastasize.

Mucoepidermoid tumors also arise from the bronchial mucous glands and usually manifest in persons between the ages of 40 and 55. The diagnosis is made by the bronchoscopic finding of a polypoid endobronchial mass, followed by biopsy. Treatment is by surgical resection; the prognosis is better than that with cylindroma. *Carcinosarcoma,* an unusual tumor, contains both malignant epithelial elements and sarcomatous changes. It may occur as a peripheral mass or as an endobronchial lesion; it is treated by surgical resection. *Pulmonary blastomas,* which usually occur in the periphery of the lung, are thought to arise from mesoderm. Surgical resection is the indicated treatment, but the prognosis is poor.

Primary sarcomas of the lung, which are very rare, include fibrosarcomas, leiomyosarcomas, hemangiopericytomas, and osteosarcomas. Treatment is by surgical resection. More recently, Kaposi's sarcoma has been recognized as a cause of pulmonary disease in patients with the acquired immunodeficiency syndrome (AIDS). It may be difficult to distinguish from infection. The diagnosis requires lung biopsy.

Olnibene FP, Steis RG, Macher AM, et al.: Kaposi's sarcoma causing pulmonary infiltrates and respiratory failure in the acquired immunodeficiency syndrome. Ann Intern Med 102:471, 1985. *Description of 66 patients with acquired immunodeficiency syndrome and 30 episodes of pulmonary Kaposi's sarcoma.*

Tumors Metastatic to the Lung

Both hematogenous and lymphatic spread of carcinomas and sarcomas may involve the lung. Patients are often asymptomatic; however, metastatic lesions may cause dyspnea, cough, and chest pain. Diffuse hematogenous tumor spread may cause vascular obstruction, manifested by cor pulmonale with hilar enlargement and clear lung parenchyma.

The radiographic appearance of pulmonary metastases may give some clue to the primary tumor. Solitary nodules are usually associated with cancers from breast, colon, kidney, rectum, cervix, and melanoma. These tumors may also diffusely involve the lung, leading to multiple large nodules or micronodules. In addition, a micronodular pattern is also seen with tumors from the thyroid, trophoblastic tissue, or bone sarcomas. Large, well-defined pulmonary nodules, sometimes with associated hilar enlargement, occur with testicular germinal cell tumors.

Tumors that spread lymphatically include carcinomas from the stomach, pancreas, thyroid, larynx, and lung. These tumors may spread to lung lymphatics through hilar lymph nodes or from parenchymal lymphatics that have been invaded by hematogenous metastases. Enlargement of lung lymphatics is radiographically visible as linear shadows similar to Kerley's lines.

Pleural involvement may appear as a pleural-based mass or as pleural effusion. Metastatic lesions, particularly synovial cell tumors and other bone tumors, may lead to pneumothorax. Certain metastatic lesions may cavitate: metastatic sarcomas, carcinomas of the colon, and epidermoid carcinomas of the head, neck, and the female reproductive system. Osteogenic sarcomas or chondrosarcomas display calcification in metastatic lesions.

The diagnosis of metastatic lesion is confirmed by the histologic examination of tissue obtained by sputum cytology, fiberoptic bronchoscopy, or occasionally thoracotomy. Cytologic findings are positive in as many as 50 per cent of patients. Bronchoscopy and needle biopsy have similar success rates. Decisions on how aggressive to be in seeking confirmation by tissue study of suspected metastatic lesions must be made thoughtfully. The risk to the patient must be weighed against the question of how the confirmation of metastasis will alter the management of the patient.

Treatment of metastases will usually be based upon management of the primary neoplasm. Certain metastatic lesions should be considered for surgical resection, especially those arising from osteogenic sarcomas. On occasion, resection of a solitary metastasis from other primary sources has been reported to be associated with increased survival, but usually without any controlled study. In considering surgical resection of a metastasis, the following criteria should be met: (1) absence of other metastatic lesions within the lung on CT, (2) no evidence of metastasis involving other organs, and (3) sufficient physiologic reserve to tolerate a more extensive resection if simple wedge resection is deemed inadequate.

In general, this means the criteria used for determining tolerance of surgical resection of primary lung cancer should be applied when contemplating resection of metastatic lesions.

In summary, surgical resection of pulmonary metastasis should be considered when the primary tumor is under control, the patient is a good surgical risk, other approaches to treatment are unsatisfactory, and all of the tumor can be resected.

Beattie EJ: Surgical treatment of pulmonary metastases. Cancer 54:2729, 1984. *Brief review of metastatic lesions to the lung that may be appropriate for multiple surgical resections.*

Mountain CF, McMurtrey MJ, Hermes KE: Surgery for pulmonary metastasis: A 20-year experience. Ann Thorac Surg 38:323, 1984. *Report of results of the M.D. Anderson Hospital and Tumor Institute with surgical resection in 443 patients with various tumors metastatic to the lung.*

BENIGN NEOPLASMS OF THE LUNG

Benign neoplasms of the lung are uncommon. They may occur as solitary nodules within lung parenchyma or as endobronchial lesions. Symptoms are nonspecific and include cough, dyspnea, chest pain, and pneumonia.

HAMARTOMAS. Hamartomas, the most common benign tumors of the lung, are usually diagnosed in adults. The tumors consist of unorganized elements, such as fat, fibrous tissue, epithelial tissue, cartilage, and calcification. Calcification leads to the "popcorn" radiographic appearance of the tumor. The majority of hamartomas occur as solitary nodules within lung parenchyma, but about 10 per cent are endobronchial. Hamartomas should be removed because of the potential complications of hemorrhage and bronchial obstruction resulting in atelectasis and pneumonia.

PAPILLOMAS. Papillomas, which arise from the trachea and bronchi, are most commonly found in children. They may be diffuse, leading to repeated pneumonias, bronchiectasis, atelectasis, and chronic infection. Because of diffuse involvement, management may be difficult, and repeated bronchoscopy may be required in an attempt to remove these tumors. Malignant changes may also occur.

OTHER TUMORS. Uncommon benign tumors of the lung include granular cell myoblastomas, lipomas, fibromas, leiomyomas, chondromas, and hemangiomas. They usually first appear as masses radiographically. Complications are similar to those of other benign neoplasms. Surgical removal is the usual treatment.

Arrignoni MG, Woolner LB, Bernatz PE, et al.: Benign tumors of the lung: A ten-year surgical experience. J Thorac Cardiovasc Surg 60:589, 1970. *Excellent review of 130 patients with benign tumors of the lung. Includes clinical, radiographic, and pathologic features.*

SOLITARY PULMONARY NODULE

A solitary pulmonary nodule is a single lesion, regardless of size, surrounded by lung parenchyma on at least two thirds of its circumference, not touching the hilum or mediastinum, and without associated atelectasis or pleural effusion. Important etiologies of solitary pulmonary nodules include neoplasia, infection, and collagen vascular disease. Because of the wide variety of cause and differing treatments, determining the etiology is very important (Table 68–6).

Etiology

Both benign and malignant tumors may manifest as a solitary pulmonary nodule. Approximately 40 per cent of solitary pulmonary nodules are malignant, and of these, 85 to 90 per cent are bronchogenic carcinoma. Bronchogenic carcinomas that are detected as solitary nodules have a much more favorable prognosis (24 per cent 5-year survival) than do those with more complicated presentations (5 to 8 per cent 5-year survival). Patients detected with solitary nodules at stage I of bronchogenic carcinoma have been reported to have almost a 50 per cent 5-year survival. Most benign hamartomas appear as solitary pulmonary nodules. Three to 10 per cent of solitary pulmonary nodules are due to malignancies metastatic to the lung from other organs, especially from renal cell carcinoma, Wilms' tumor, Ewing's sarcoma, choriocarcinoma, bladder carcinoma, rhabdomyosarcoma, osteosarcoma, melanoma, and carcinomas of the breast, colon, testis, head, and neck.

The most common infection that manifests as solitary nodules is that caused by *Coccidioides immitis*. Echinococcal cysts may also appear as a single nodule, as may the lesions of *Histoplasma*

TABLE 68–6. ETIOLOGIES OF SOLITARY PULMONARY NODULES

1. Primary lung malignancies
2. Metastatic malignancies to the lung
3. Benign tumors or tumor-like conditions

Hamartoma	Pseudolymphoma
Herniation of omentum	Herniation of liver
Hemangioma	

4. Pulmonary infections

Fungal	Mycobacterial
Bacterial	Hydatid cyst

5. Foreign body pneumonitis

Lipid pneumonia	Amyloidosis
Pneumoconiosis	Aspiration pneumonia
Talc granulomas	

6. Pulmonary vascular disorders

Pulmonary infarct	Pulmonary hemosiderosis
Pulmonary hemorrhage	

capsulatum and *Blastomyces dermatitidis*. Tuberculosis rarely manifests as a solitary pulmonary nodule.

Certain collagen vascular disorders may present as pulmonary nodules, especially rheumatoid arthritis and Wegener's granulomatosis. Although usually multiple lesions occur, occasionally only a single nodule may be seen. Unusual causes of solitary nodules are pulmonary infarcts and vascular malformations.

Evaluation

The sequence of the approach to a patient with a solitary pulmonary nodule is outlined in Figure 68–1. Evaluation of patients with solitary pulmonary nodules begins with a thorough history and physical examination. Travel to an area endemic for fungal disease such as coccidioidomycosis suggests, but does not prove, this etiology. Weight loss and other constitutional symptoms are consistent with malignancy, although early stages may be asymptomatic. Joint changes may suggest rheumatoid nodules. Age is also an important consideration. Primary lung cancer is uncommon in patients who have never smoked and who are below the age of 30 years. Patients over the age of 50 years with new solitary nodules, particularly if they have smoked, have an increased incidence of malignancy. Geography is also important. Fungal disease is a more common etiology in persons who reside in or have recently visited the American Southwest, whereas malignancy is a more common cause of solitary nodules in individuals living in areas nonendemic for fungal infections such as coccidioidomycosis.

An important step in the evaluation of a solitary pulmonary nodule is a comparison of its radiographic appearance with that of a previous film. A benign etiology is suggested by a lesion that has not enlarged in 2 or more years. On the other hand, if the nodule is new or if there has been progressive enlargement, malignancy or infection is much more likely. Most malignant solitary nodules have a volume doubling time of 60 to 150 days, with a mean of 120 days. In spherical lesions, an increase in diameter of 26 per cent equates to one doubling in volume. Calcification within the node is usually a sign of a benign lesion. Patterns of calcification seen with benign lesions are a dense central nidus of calcium, a concentric or laminated pattern, a diffuse pattern, or a clustered or "popcorn" pattern. Small amounts of calcium may be seen within 1 to 3 per cent of bronchogenic carcinomas or osteosarcomas metastatic to the lung. CT has two important roles in evaluating solitary pulmonary nodules. First, imaging and densitometry can be helpful in detecting calcification. Tomograms of the lung may also serve this purpose. Second, other nodules not seen with standard anteroposterior and lateral chest radiographs may be detected on CT. The use of CT densitometry to identify malignancy by low-density numbers remains experimental.

If a previous radiograph is not available, or if an enlarging lesion is suspected, the ultimate determination of etiology of a solitary nodule is dependent upon either culture confirmation of infection or histologic examination. A lesion can be considered benign only if a specific diagnosis is obtained. Sputum for tuberculosis should be obtained only if tuberculosis is highly suspected. Cytologic findings in sputum are positive in only 10 per cent or fewer of patients with endobronchially invisible bronchogenic carcinomas and 20 per cent of patients with malignancies metastatic to the lungs.

Once the etiology of a solitary nodule is ascertained, treatment will depend upon cause. When a lesion is not obviously benign, percutaneous transthoracic needle aspiration, fiberoptic bronchoscopy, or thoracotomy is indicated. Needle aspiration biopsy yields a specific diagnosis in 85 to 90 per cent of cases. It is helpful to establish a diagnosis of malignancy in patients in whom surgery is not contemplated but in whom a specific diagnosis will help guide management. Fiberoptic bronchoscopy with transbronchial biopsy and bronchial brushing has the advantage over needle aspiration because it is useful in staging lung cancer and has a lower complication rate. Success in obtaining a diagnosis is dependent upon the size of the nodule. Solitary pulmonary nodules less than 2 cm in size or within 2 cm of the hilum are difficult to diagnose with bronchoscopy. Thoracotomy is the most direct means of establishing a diagnosis; however, transthoracic needle biopsy may be used as an alternative to thoracotomy in lesions less than 2 cm in diameter. It also offers the best chance for cure of lung cancer. The possibility of small cell lung cancer is not necessarily a reason for avoiding thoracotomy. Surgical resection of small cell lung cancer presenting as a solitary pulmonary nodule may have a 5-year survival comparable to that with other forms of nodular bronchogenic carcinoma treated with surgical resection (approximately 24 per cent). Indications for thoracotomy include suspicion that the lesion is malignant and resectable and the absence of major surgical risk factors. Contraindications are severe underlying lung disease or heat disease. Mediastinoscopy is indicated only if the chest radiograph shows mediastinal widening, if the solitary nodule is greater than 3 cm in diameter, or if the nodule is centrally located near the hilum of the lung.

Stauffer JL: What to do when you detect a solitary pulmonary nodule. J Respir Dis 7:17, 1986. *Excellent summary of management of solitary pulmonary nodule based upon etiologic consideration and the yield of particular diagnostic approaches. Practical and rational.*

Swensen SJ, Jett JR, Payne WS, et al.: An integrated approach to evaluation of the solitary pulmonary nodule. Mayo Clin Proc 65:173, 1990. *Focuses on integrated approach for detection and evaluation of solitary nodule, particularly using CT and transthoracic needle biopsy.*

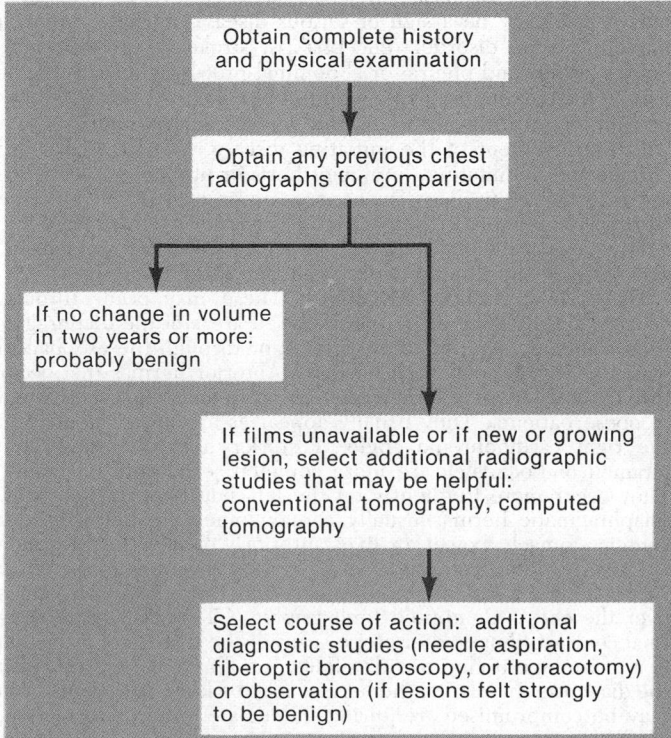

FIGURE 68–1. Approach to the patient with a solitary pulmonary nodule.

(Flowchart contents:)

Obtain complete history and physical examination

Obtain any previous chest radiographs for comparison

If no change in volume in two years or more: probably benign

If films unavailable or if new or growing lesion, select additional radiographic studies that may be helpful: conventional tomography, computed tomography

Select course of action: additional diagnostic studies (needle aspiration, fiberoptic bronchoscopy, or thoracotomy) or observation (if lesions felt strongly to be benign)

---

69 Diseases of the Diaphragm, Chest Wall, Pleura, and Mediastinum

Bartolome R. Celli

THE DIAPHRAGM

The diaphragm is the most important muscle of respiration. Shaped like a thin dome, it separates the thoracic and abdominal cavities. It has two components: the central noncontractile tendon and the muscle fibers that arise from it and radiate down and outward to insert distally into the circumferential caudal limits of the ribcage. There is a hiatus for each of the structures that pass from the thorax to the abdomen. The diaphragm is neurologically controlled via the phrenic nerve, the motoneurons of which arise in the cervical spinal cord at levels C3–C5. The anatomic arrangement of the diaphragm and its coupling to the ribcage-abdomen account for its mechanical action. Diaphragmatic contraction acts to displace the abdominal contents downward and to raise the ribs up and outward. This action results in the creation of the negative intrapleural pressure of inspiration. Like the heart, the diaphragm, and, to a lesser degree, the other respiratory muscles, must intermittently contract throughout a person's life. Unlike the heart, it has no intrinsic contractile mechanism, and the respiratory cycle is regulated by a complex set of centrally organized neurons and several peripheral feedback mechanisms that synchronizes the diaphragm with many other muscles. This arrangement must be so, since the diaphragm serves other, nonrespiratory functions, such as speech, defecation, and parturition. The blood supply to the diaphragm is very rich and is arranged in such a way as to minimize interruption during contraction. Nevertheless, the muscle itself is highly oxygen dependent.

Disorders of the Diaphragm

DYSFUNCTION AND FATIGUE. The most frequent cause of diaphragmatic dysfunction is lung hyperinflation, either acute, like in asthma, or chronic, like in chronic obstructive pulmonary disease (COPD). Hyperinflation shortens the diaphragmatic fibers and changes the shape of the diaphragm to a flatter state in which the more horizontal fibers do not generate the normally lifting and expanding action of the ribcage but rather produce an inward deforming change in the lower ribcage (Hoover's sign in COPD). These changes, coupled with the increased ventilatory loads secondary to airways resistance and with changes in lung and chest wall compliance, result in greater work by the diaphragm. If the increased demand of energy to perform this work outstrips the energy supply, the diaphragm will fatigue, and ventilation may fail. Diaphragmatic fatigue can be determined by the use of pressure measurements across the diaphragm (transdiaphragmatic pressure, or Pdi) or by the more elaborate power-spectrum analysis of electromyographic signals. Fortunately, both correlate well with simpler clinical signs, such as increased respiratory rate with progressively shallower breathing. As fatigue increases, ventilation is maintained by intermittent expansions of the ribcage and abdomen (respiratory alternans) and then by paradoxical inward motion of the abdomen during inspiration (abdominal paradox). The strategies available to improve diaphragmatic muscle function in patients with impending fatigue are listed in Table 69–1. If the fatigue has resulted in hypercapnia and acidosis, mechanical ventilation must be instituted so that the respiratory muscles can rest. When ventilation is assisted, it should be done for at least 1 to several days, since muscle fatigue of the kind causing ventilatory failure may take that long to abate.

DISORDERS OF DIAPHRAGMATIC MOTION. Diaphragmatic paralysis may be unilateral, which is usually secondary to phrenic nerve involvement by a tumor (bronchogenic carcinoma

TABLE 69–1. THERAPEUTIC MODALITIES TO IMPROVE DIAPHRAGMATIC FUNCTION

Reduce mechanical load
1. Decrease airways resistance (bronchodilators, treat infection, decrease inflammation)
2. Reduce hyperinflation
3. Decrease ventilatory requirements (administer oxygen, control fever, avoid caloric loads)

Improve respiratory muscle contractility and endurance
1. Oxygen therapy
2. Improve nutrition
3. Improve cardiovascular performance
4. Correct electrolytes (sodium, potassium, calcium, phosphorus)
5. Administer drugs that improve contractility (theophylline, β_2 agonist, caffeine)
6. Check for hypothyroidism or drugs that impair contractility (aminoglycosides)
7. Ventilatory muscle training

Improve respiratory muscle coordination and energy conservation
Rehabilitation
Respiratory muscle resting

being the most frequent). It may result as a complication of neurologic diseases, such as myelitis, encephalitis, poliomyelitis, and herpes zoster. It may result from trauma to the thorax or cervical spine or from compression by benign processes, such as a substernal thyroid, an aortic aneurysm, and infectious collections. With the advent of extensive cardiac surgery, paralysis secondary to cooling of the phrenic nerve has been increasingly noted. Occasionally, the paralysis may be idiopathic. In patients with normal lungs, unilateral paralysis is usually asymptomatic and rarely requires treatment. The diagnosis is suspected when, in the chest roentgenogram, the diaphragmatic leaflet is elevated and is confirmed fluoroscopically by observing paradoxical diaphragmatic motion on sniff and cough. Bilateral paralysis usually results from high cervical trauma (C3–C5) or from myopathies. The myopathy may be generalized (muscular dystrophy, polymyositis, hypothyroidism) or may be limited or may primarily affect the diaphragm (acid maltase deficiency, collagen vascular disorders). In many cases, the etiology remains unknown. The patients may become symptomatic early. The dyspnea is characteristically worsened when the patient assumes the supine position, since abdominal contents displace the diaphragm into the thorax. This situation also results in a significant drop in the vital capacity (>500 ml) and in oxygen saturation. Fluoroscopic observation of diaphragmatic excursions is less reliable in this condition, since the flaccid diaphragm may lag behind the ribcage expansion when accessory muscles contract, thus giving the impression of diaphragmatic contraction. The diagnosis can be suspected by the presence of abdominal paradoxical retraction with inspiration. It can be confirmed by measurement of transdiaphragmatic pressure with and without electromyographic recording. Phrenic nerve conduction time helps establish the diagnosis of neuropathy. The treatment of ventilatory failure secondary to bilateral paralysis consists of intermittent ventilation that has been achieved with different methods (external negative ventilation, nasal positive-pressure ventilation, and rocking beds). In some cases, such as after cardiac surgery, the paralysis will resolve with time, and the ventilation may be discontinued. When used on a permanent basis, but in those with intact muscle function (e.g., in high quadriplegics), diaphragmatic pacing has been life saving.

HICCUP. Hiccup, or singultus, is a common disorder produced by spasm of the diaphragm that is followed by sudden closure of the glottis during an inspiratory effort. Hiccups are usually self-limited but may persist for days or weeks and become very disturbing. In most patients, a cause is never found, but it may occasionally be a sign of serious disease, such as a central nervous system disorder (encephalitis, stroke, tumor), uremia, herpes zoster, and pleural or abdominal processes that invade or irritate the diaphragm. Prolonged hiccups are sometimes psychogenic in origin. In general, hiccups will subside spontaneously or with improvement of the initiating disease. When hiccups are chronic and debilitating, local anesthesia or phrenic nerve crushing may be required (permanent paralysis may occur with the latter). Diaphragmatic flutter is a rare disorder in which rhythmic contractions of the diaphragm occur at a rate of 1 to 8 per second. The etiology and treatment are similar to those of hiccups.

DIAPHRAGMATIC HERNIAS. These may occur through congenitally weak or incompletely fused areas of the diaphragm, from traumatic rupture of the muscle or through the esophageal hiatus (>70 per cent of all hernias). Anterior hernias that occur through the foramina of Morgagni are rare and tend to be found in obese patients. They usually appear as a rounded density in the right cardiophrenic angle. Posterior hernias through the foramen of Bochdalek are more common, especially in infants. They occur more frequently on the left side than on the right. Diaphragmatic hernias usually contain omentum but may also contain stomach, bowel, or liver anteriorly or kidney and spleen posteriorly. The diagnosis is suspected on the basis of the chest roentgenogram and in some cases when there is borborygmus over the chest. Computed tomographic (CT) scans, gastrointestinal contrast films, radioisotope scans of the liver, and induction of a pneumoperitoneum with a follow-up film may help establish the diagnosis. In infants, the hernias may be large, and ventilation may be compromised, requiring immediate surgical correction. In the asymptomatic adult with previous evidence of a hernia, observation is indicated. Surgery may be needed for diagnosis or to relieve strangulation of sac contents. Traumatic diaphragmatic hernias may result from direct penetrating injuries or from abdominal compression. The severity of symptoms depends upon the extension of abdominal contents into the thorax and the presence of strangulation. In other cases, several years may elapse before respiratory and abdominal symptoms recur. The treatment in these cases is surgical. Eventration may resemble a hernia but instead consists of a localized elevation of the diaphragm resulting from impaired muscle development or weakness. It is more frequent in the right anteromedial portion and tends to occur in middle-aged, obese persons. Once differentiated from neoplasm, it rarely requires surgical treatment.

Celi BR: Clinical and physiologic evaluation of respiratory muscle function. Clin Chest Med 10:199, 1989. *Comprehensive, up-to-date review covering the clinical aspects and practical application of respiratory muscle function.*

Newsom-Davis J, Goldman M, Loh L, et al.: Diaphragm function and alveolar hyperventilation. Q J Med 45:87, 1976. *It establishes the role of diaphragmatic dysfunction in generating ventilatory failure. It also introduces intermittent external ventialtion as a therapeutic modality.*

Rochester DF: The diaphragm: Contractile properties and fatigue. J Clin Invest 75:1397, 1985. *Excellent review of the anatomy and physiology of the diaphragm. It covers our understanding of dysfunction and fatigue.*

THE CHEST WALL

The chest wall is an integral part of the pump that moves air in and out of the lungs. It consists of the bony thoracic cage (ribs, sternum, and vertebrae) and the various muscles of respiration. Besides the diaphragm, the intercostal and scalenus muscles are active even during quiet breathing in normal persons. Other muscles, such as the sternocleidomastoid, pectoralis minor and major, serratus anterior, latissimus dorsi, and trapezius, may participate in respiration in cases of increased ventilatory demand. Even the abdominal muscles can take part in ventilation; by contracting in exhalation, they lengthen the inspiratory muscles and place them in an advantageous position for the next inspiratory contraction. The thoracic cage system is a major determinant of ventilation and of static and dynamic lung volumes. Diseases that disrupt the system will alter ventilation and the ventilation-perfusion relationship, thus causing hypoxemia or hypercapnia. Primary disorders of the chest wall may occur from impairments of the neuromuscular apparatus or of the bony thoracic cage. Since alterations in the neuromuscular apparatus are dealt with in different parts of the text, this section discusses primary alterations of the bony thoracic cage.

Disorders of the Chest Wall

The most important diseases of the bony thoracic cage are listed in Table 69–2. They are all linked by a similar pathophysiologic process: (1) alveolar hypoventilation, (2) changes in chest wall compliance, (3) variable lung compression, (4) ventilation-perfusion imbalance, and (5) pulmonary hypertension and cor pulmonale. Clinical symptoms include dyspnea without significant cough, sputum, or pain. The physical examination usually establishes the diagnosis and helps determine the presence of cor pulmonale.

KYPHOSCOLIOSIS. Deformities of the dorsolumbar spine are by far the most common causes of symptomatic derangements of the chest wall. Scoliosis consists of lateral angulation and rotation of the spine and can be categorized as right (most frequent) or left, according to the direction of the convexity of the primary curvature. Kyphosis is less important and consists of anteroposterior angulations of the spine. The severity of scoliosis is quantified by measuring the angle (Cobb's angle) between the upper and lower portions of the spinal curve on a roentgenogram. Only when this angle exceeds 70 degrees is any abnormality of respiratory function detectable. When the angle is greater than

TABLE 69–2. MOST IMPORTANT RIBCAGE DERANGEMENTS

Spine
    Scoliosis (idiopathic, congenital, paralytic)
    Kyphosis
    Ankylosing spondylitis

Sternum, Ribs, or Pleura
    Pectus excavatum
    Thoracoplasty
    Fibrothorax

120 degrees, dyspnea and early respiratory failure are expected. The ribs over the convex side of the deformity are separated and rotated posteriorly, giving rise to the kyphoscoliotic hump. On the concave side, the ribs are crowded and displaced anteriorly. This, combined with decreased thoracic height, results in forward bulging of the anterior wall. Kyphoscoliosis usually begins in childhood and has no specific etiology in most cases. Primary muscle diseases and congenital disorders account for a very small fraction of the total. The patients who have angles greater than 70 degrees may begin to develop symptoms upon exerting effort, and as the angulation increases, respiratory failure and cor pulmonale gradually develop. This situation may result in death in the fourth to sixth decade. If the scoliosis is not severe and does not progress, life expectancy may be normal. Static lung volumes are decreased in relation to the severity of the scoliosis. Chest wall and, to a lesser degree, lung compliance are also decreased. The determination of regional lung function shows ventilation-perfusion shifts that result in hypoxemia. When the mechanical load, caused by progressive scoliosis or superimposed infection, is such that the muscles fail, the hypoxemia may be associated with hypercapnia. Hypoventilation and hypoxemia may become worse during sleep, which accounts for the frequent worsening of some patients with otherwise stable kyphoscoliosis.

Several therapeutic approaches are used in kyphoscoliosis and thoracic disorders in general. Surgical correction includes traction, plasters, and attempts to straighten the scoliosis by the use of rods. The effects appear mostly cosmetic (it prevents prgression of the curvature), and the improvement in function is minimal. In patients who are hypoxemic, the addition of oxygen is beneficial. Kyphoscoliosis is one of the few diseases in which the administration of intermittent positive-pressure ventilation results in increases in tidal volume with temporary improvement in lung compliance and lung volumes. In patients with chronic ventilatory failure from scoliosis, nighttime ventilatory assistance either with external devices or with tracheostomy results in reversal of the failure. Efforts must be made to prevent airways disease and to induce the patient to stop smoking. Bronchospasms and respiratory infections must be treated aggressively. If obese, the patient should lose weight.

ANKYLOSING SPONDYLITIS. This inflammatory disease results in the fusion of costotransverse and vertebral joints but also involve sternomanubrial and clavicular joints. With relative fixation of the ribcage in an inspiratory position, most of the ventilatory movement is performed by the diaphragm-abdomen, which is already placed at a mechanical disadvantage, as shown by a normal or greater than normal functional residual capacity. In contrast to kyphoscoliosis, cor pulmonale and ventilatory failure are the exception. Some patients with ankylosing spondylitis may develop upper lobe fibrosis with minimal alterations in gas exchange.

PECTUS EXCAVATUM. This condition is a congenital deformity of the lower portion of the sternum with symmetric bowing of the anterior ribs. In infants it tends to occur with multiple abnormalities and is associated with high mortality. It may also be associated with mitral valve prolapse. When the deformity is severe, the heart and mediastinal structures are laterally displaced. Although some patients may fail to increase cardiac output during exercise in a normal fashion, functional impairment for the most part is limited. Surgical correction is mainly done for cosmetic reasons.

SEQUELAE OF THORACOPLASTY. Thoracoplasty is the general term applied to a series of surgical procedures employed from 1940 to 1950 for the treatment of tuberculosis. The procedures included resection of several ribs with collapse of the lung underneath the resected area. This situation results in paradoxical retraction of that portion of the chest wall. Although it was originally thought to have minimal physiologic consequences, there has been a significant increase in the development of cardiorespiratory failure with cor pulmonale in those patients.

FIBROTHORAX. Fibrothorax resulting from pleural diseases such as intense hemothorax or asbestosis is also considered a primary disease of the chest wall, since the lung itself may not be affected. The disorder may occasionally result in ventilatory and cardiac failure. The treatment of both conditions is similar to that of patients with kyphoscoliosis. Occasional pleurectomy may help patients with fibrothorax secondary to pleural fibrosis.

FLAIL CHEST. This condition is produced by double fractures of three or more adjacent ribs or by combined sternal and rib fractures. The flail segment will paradoxically move inward during inspiration and outward during expiration. The inefficient ventilation increases the work of breathing, which may be even more inefficient if (as is often the case) there is concomitant neuromuscular impairment. Flail chest occurs most frequently with accidental chest trauma, but it also can occur after cardiopulmonary resuscitation. Hypoxemia is very often present as a result of ventilation-perfusion inequality from the flail segment and the frequent underlying lung contusion. It is clear that in most cases artificial ventilation for internal fixation of the flail segment is not necessary. It should be reserved for patients with ventilatory failure. Supportive care with attention to maintaining adequate oxygenation, clear airways, and prevention of infections is the preferred therapy for most patients. When the flail segment is large, operative chest wall fixation may be considered.

Bergofsky EH: Respiratory failure in disorders of the thoracic cage. Am Rev Respir Dis 119:643, 1979. *Still the most comprehensive work on this topic. Easy to read, excellent review.*

Holppner VH, Cockcroft DW, Dosman JH, et al.: Nighttime ventilation improves respiratory failure in secondary kyphoscoliosis. Am Rev Respir Dis 129:240, 1984. *Reviews the use of nighttime ventilation and its effectiveness in reverting ventilatory failure in cases of "pump fatigue."*

Todd TR, Shamji F: Pathophysiology of chest trauma. Thorax 33:979, 1985. *Excellent review of the pathophysiologic changes in respiratory function secondary to chest trauma. Reviews the controversies in treatment.*

THE PLEURA

Anatomy and Physiology

The pleura consists of a layer of variable-sized mesothelial cells and normally has a smooth, glistening, and semitransparent appearance. It is supported by a network of connective and fibroelastic tissue, lymphatics, and vessels. The mesothelial cells are rich in microvilli, and their most important function is to deliver glycoproteins rich in hyaluronic acid, which helps decrease friction between the lung and chest wall. The pleura is defined as "parietal" where it covers the surface of the chest wall, diaphragm, and mediastinum. The parietal pleura is supplied with blood from the systemic circulation, contains sensory nerves, and has cells that are very rich in microvilli. The visceral pleura is that layer covering the entire surface of the lungs, including the interlobar fissures. Its blood supply arises from the low-pressure pulmonary circulation, it has no sensory nerves, and its cells have a lower number of microvilli. Both pleural layers are separated by a cavity and are lubricated by 5 to 10 ml of fluid. This arrangement allows the lung to expand, retract, and deform with ease. It also helps maintain the lung in an inflated state by coupling it with the chest wall. Both functions decrease the work of breathing.

The pleural fluid has a low protein concentration (< 2 grams per deciliter) with a pH and glucose level similar to those of blood. Pleural fluid is formed primarily from the parietal pleura, and part of its turnover is dependent on the same Starling forces that govern vascular and interstitial fluid exchange elsewhere. The parietal pleura has a hydrostatic pressure similar to that of the systemic circulation (30 cm H_2O), while that of the visceral pleura depends on the pulmonary circulation (10 cm H_2O). Oncotic pressure is similar in both (25 cm H_2O), but the pressure within the pleural cavity is affected by the gravity gradient. Thus the pleural space is heterogeneous with a nondependent portion where Starling forces favor outpouring of fluid to the cavity and into parenchymal capillaries. Recent evidence reveals that stomas are present over the parietal surface of the low mediastinum, low chest wall, and diaphragm. These stomas and "lacunae" empty into lymphatics. The current thought is that these subpleural parietal lymphatics represent the major pathway for liquid and solute drainage of the pleural space. Alterations in any of the components of this formation-resorption mechanism frequently lead to the accumulation of pleural fluid. Excessive increases in hydrostatic forces or decreases in oncotic pressures result in low-protein "transudates." Increased outpouring by the capillaries or cells or blocking of lymphatics results in high-protein "exudates." The mechanisms that lead to the accumulation of pleural fluid are shown in Table 69–3.

TABLE 69–3. MECHANISMS THAT LEAD TO ACCUMULATION OF PLEURAL FLUID

1. Increased hydrostatic pressure in microvascular circulation (e.g., congestive heart failure)
2. Decreased oncotic pressure in microvascular circulation (e.g., severe hypoalbuminemia)
3. Decreased pressure in the pleural space (e.g., complete lung collapse)
4. Increased permeability of the microvascular circulation (e.g., pneumonia)
5. Impaired lymphatic drainage from the pleural space (e.g., malignant effusion)
6. Movement of fluid from the peritoneal space (e.g., ascites)

Diagnostic Procedures

HISTORY AND PHYSICAL EXAMINATION. Although a patient's history may suggest pleural disease, it is neither sensitive nor specific. The most frequent symptoms are chest pain, dyspnea, and cough. They may be absent in some large effusions and in critically ill patients. When present, the pain is usually unilateral and sharp and worsens with inspiration, cough, or ribcage movements. It may radiate to shoulder, neck, or abdomen. Dyspnea may result from the compression of lung tissue secondary to the accumulation of fluid, thus creating a ventilation-perfusion mismatch. It may also result from mechanical alterations in diaphragmatic and other respiratory muscles as the amounts of fluid change their length-tension relationship. The degree of dyspnea relates to the volume of fluid, to the intrathoracic pressure it generates, and to its effect on mechanics and gas exchange. Finally, pleural effusions that accumulate in patients with minimal lung compromise are well tolerated, whereas similar effusions in patients with underlying severe lung disease may cause ventilatory failure. The physical examination varies, depending on the severity of the effusion and the underlying lung or systemic disease. Patients breathe shallowly and rapidly, they may have decreased excursions in the affected hemithorax (splinting), and breath sounds are decreased in the affected area. Percussion shows dullness with absent tactile fremitus over the area. Frequently, there are E to A changes (egobronchophony) at the upper border of the fluid.

RADIOLOGIC EXAMINATION. An effusion can be suspected when blunting and medial displacement of the sharp costophrenic angle are present. Accumulation of fluid between the base of the lung and the diaphragm (subpulmonic effusion) is suspected when there is apparent elevation of the hemidiaphragm or widening of the shadow between the gas-containing stomach and the lower margin of the left lung. Up to 300 ml of fluid may fail to be seen in a posteroanterior chest roentgenogram, whereas as little as 150 ml may be seen in a lateral decubitus film. A supine film (frequent in patients in intensive care units) may obscure the diagnosis as the fluid layers posteriorly. A pseudotumor occurs when fluid loculates in an interlobar fissure, most commonly in the minor fissure, and gives the radiologic appearance of a tumor. A clue to the diagnosis is the presence of pleural fluid elsewhere and a biconvex lenticular configuration of the mass. When an effusion is suspected, an upright or a lateral decubitus film is usually confirmatory. A collection of pleural air and fluid (hydro-, pyo-, hemopneumothorax) usually produces horizontal and not concave margins. A pneumothorax is identified by noting the contrast between the water density of the visceral pleura centrally and the gas lucency without vascular markings laterally. Small pneumothoraces may be harder to diagnose, but an expiratory film may help outline it. Pleural plaques may be seen when calcified, and if not calcified, they may be detected when the plaques are viewed tangentially but not en face. Other tumors and loculated effusions may be difficult to define. Ultrasonography and CT may provide better definition of pleural and, in many cases, parenchymal abnormalities.

THORACENTESIS AND PLEURAL FLUID ANALYSIS. Thoracentesis may be performed for diagnostic or therapeutic purposes. A thoracentesis is diagnostic in approximately 75 per cent of patients, and even when not diagnostic it helps exclude other important diagnoses, such as empyema. Diagnostic thoracentesis requires a relatively small amount of material (30 to 50 ml), usually obtained with a small-gauge needle. As a rule, newly

TABLE 69–4. CHARACTERISTICS OF PLEURAL FLUID TRANSUDATES

	Absolute Value	Pleural Fluid/ Serum Value
Protein	<3 grams/dl	<0.5
Lactate dehydrogenase (LDH)	<200 units/L	<0.6
Glucose	<60 mg/dl	1.0
White blood cell count	<1000	—

discovered effusions should be tapped. Although there are no absolute contraindications to a diagnostic thoracentesis, relative contraindications include a bleeding diathesis, anticoagulation, a small volume, mechanical ventilation, and low risk-benefit ratio. Therapeutic thoracentesis involves removing larger amounts of fluid. No more than 1000 to 1500 ml should be removed at one time, since pulmonary edema may occur in the re-expanded underlying lung, especially in those cases of tension effusions.

Although the classification of pleural fluid into *transudate* or *exudate* is not absolute, it has proved helpful in directing the clinician to the most useful studies and in suggesting possible diagnoses. To differentiate transudates and exudates, it is cost effective to obtain the following tests on the fluid obtained: total protein, lactate dehydrogenase (LDH), white blood cell count (WBC) with differential, and either glucose level or pH. Table 69–4 shows the characteristics of transudates. Transudates are due to imbalances in hydrostatic and oncotic pressures, such as those seen in congestive heart failure or hypoalbuminemia. They may also result from the peritoneum to the pleural space.

Exudates are defined by the presence of at least one of the following criteria: (1) a pleural fluid/serum protein ratio greater than 0.5; (2) a pleural fluid/serum LDH ratio greater than 0.6; and (3) a pleural fluid LDH greater than two-thirds that of serum. The results obtained from the analysis of exudative effusions suggest some diseases, as shown in Table 69–5. The diagnoses that can be established by thoracentesis include malignancy (malignant cells), empyema (pus), tuberculosis (positive acid-fast bacillus for smear or cultures), fungal infection (positive KOH or culture), lupus pleuritis (LE cells), chylothorax (high triglyceride levels or presence of chylomicrons), urinothorax (a pleural fluid/serum creatinine ratio of >1), and esophageal rupture (an increased pleural fluid amylase level and pH around 6.0). Since many diagnoses may produce exudative pleural fluid with overlapping values, acid-fast and Gram's stains, aerobic and anaerobic cultures, cell count and differential, and cytologic analysis should be included in the study of these effusions. A predominance of polymorphonuclear leukocytes is most compatible with bacterial infection, while lymphocytes (particularly with a paucity of mesothelial cells) suggest tuberculosis. Lymphocytes are also seen in lymphoma and leukemic effusions. Abundant eosinophils are usually nonspecific and suggest longstanding fluid. When not due to trauma, a bloody effusion is most likely the result of malignancy or pulmonary infarction. A white effusion suggests chyle, choles-

TABLE 69–5. CORRELATION OF PLEURAL FLUID EXUDATE FINDINGS AND CAUSATIVE DISEASE

Tests	Diseases
pH < 7.2	Empyema, malignancy, esophageal rupture, rheumatoid, lupus and tuberculous, pleuritis
Glucose (<60 mg/dl)	Infection, rheumatoid pleurisy, tuberculous and lupus effusions, esophageal rupture
Amylase (>200 units/dl)	Pancreatic disease, esophageal rupture, malignancy, ruptured ectopic pregnancy
Rheumatoid factor, ANA, LE cells	Collagen vascular diseases
Complement (decreased)	Lupus erythematosus, rheumatoid arthritis
Red blood cells (>5000/ml)	Trauma, malignancy, pulmonary embolus
Chylous effusion (triglycerides > 110 mg/dl)	Violation of thoracic duct (trauma, malignancy)
Biopsy (+)	Malignancy, tuberculosis

terol, or lymphoma. A black fluid suggests *Aspergillus* pleural involvement. A yellow-green color may be seen in rheumatoid pleurisy. A putrid odor is diagnostic of anaerobic empyema, while an ammonia odor suggests urinothorax. The value of other diagnostic markers, such as adenosine deaminase (ADA), beta$_2$-microglobulin, and lysozyme, remains to be determined. The complications of thoracentesis include pain, bleeding (local, pleural, or abdominal), pneumothorax, infection, and spleen or liver puncture. With therapeutic thoracentesis, up to 50 per cent of patients experience a temporary fall in PaO$_2$ of as much as 20 mm Hg.

PERCUTANEOUS PLEURAL BIOPSY. This biopsy is indicated in the evaluation of the patient with undiagnosed exudative effusion (particularly those with lymphocytic predominance), since the most frequently diagnosed diseases are malignancy and tuberculosis. The procedure is performed with the patient under local anesthesia, using a hook-type needle (Cope or Abrams). The contraindications are as follows: a small or loculated pleural effusion; an uncooperative patient; and anticoagulation or bleeding diathesis, including azotemia with abnormal bleeding time. Since pleural seeding may not be uniform, multiple samples are needed. The overall diagnostic yield is around 60 per cent for malignancy and 75 per cent for tuberculosis.

EXPLORATION OF THE PLEURA. In most of the 5 to 10 per cent of cases of patients with pleural effusion in whom a diagnosis cannot be established, the effusion will disappear spontaneously or the cause will become evident. In those patients in whom a diagnosis is considered necessary, a biopsy can be directly obtained through thoracoscopy (introduction of a rigid scope with a cold light source). Besides its high yield, thoracoscopy is useful because it may be performed with the use of local anesthesia and sedatives. In some other cases, it is necessary to perform an open pleural biopsy with the patient under general anesthesia. The main advantage is the possibility of obtaining larger specimens and concomitant lung tissue.

Disorders of the Pleura

TRANSUDATIVE EFFUSIONS

Congestive heart failure is the most common cause of transudative effusions. The evidence indicates that effusions result from biventricular failure with venous hypertension. They are more often bilateral, usually larger on the right, and on the chest roentgenogram, they are associated with vascular congestion and cardiomegaly. In chronic heart failure (months), the total protein level may be greater than 3 grams per deciliter. Thoracentesis is indicated if the patient is febrile, the effusion is very large and unilateral, and there is pleuritic pain or hypoxemia that is disproportionate to the degree of failure. Transudates may also occur in 5 to 10 per cent of patients with cirrhosis of the liver, usually with ascites. This transudate is secondary to movement of ascitic fluid through diaphragmatic defects or lymphatic channels. The effusion is more frequent on the right (70 per cent). If the diagnosis is in doubt, injection of radioactive tracer in the ascitic fluid will show up in the chest within hours of administration. The pleural effusion very often improves as the ascites improves. Occasionally, chemical pleurodesis has been effective in relieving symptomatic recurrent effusions. The transudative effusion seen in up to 20 per cent of patients with the nephrotic syndrome is due to decreased oncotic pressure (hypoalbuminemia) and increased hydrostatic forces. It is frequently bilateral and improves with correction of the protein-losing nephropathy. Peritoneal dialysis and atelectasis may also cause transudative effusions. A rare form of transudate is that seen in obstructions of the urinary system. The effusion (urinothorax) is usually ipsilateral with the obstruction and has the characteristic odor of urine. Relief of the obstruction results in prompt resolution of the effusion.

EXUDATIVE EFFUSIONS

INFECTIONS. Parapneumonic effusion (pleural fluid associated with pneumonias or lung abscess) is the most common cause of exudates. The effusions can be divided into two types: uncomplicated, which resolve spontaneously with antibiotics, or complicated, which require drainage to resolve fully. Complicated effusions are usually rich in white cells (empyema) and/or have a positive Gram stain or cultures. Uncomplicated effusions are usually small, contain moderate amounts of polymorphonuclear neutrophils (PMN's), a glucose level similar to that of blood, a pH higher than 7.3, and an LDH less than 500 units per liter. In contrast, complicated effusions have a large number of PMN's many times over 100,000 per cubic millimeter, a pH less than 7.2, a glucose level lower than 40 grams per deciliter, and an LDH greater than 1000 units per liter. If the effusion is also purulent and contains bacteria, immediate draining is necessary. The more of these features the effusion has, the more likely it is that drainage is needed. Drainage itself is best achieved with a standard chest tube placed in the most dependent portion of the pleural space. If the fever persists over 48 to 72 hours, the pleural space drainage is inadequate (such as when fluid becomes loculated), the antibiotic is inappropriate, or the diagnosis is wrong. If drainage is not effective because of loculation, insertion of an additional tube or instillation of intrapleural streptokinase has been effective. Poorly treated empyemas may result in communications with the bronchial tree (bronchopleural fistulas) or skin (bronchopleurocutaneous fistulas). These require surgical therapy (open drainage with rib resection, decortication, and extensive reconstruction). In some patients whose main problem is uncontrolled pleural sepsis, a thoracotomy with drainage and decortication may be life saving. Pleural involvement by nonbacterial, nontuberculous infection is uncommon and, when present, is usually small. Fungal diseases rarely affect the pleura except for coccidioidomycosis, which may cause a hypersensitivity pleuritis.

OTHER INFECTIVE-INFLAMMATORY DISORDERS. Exudative and frequently infected pleural effusions may result from subdiaphragmatic processes such as upper abdominal abscess, of which a subphrenic site is the most common location. Very frequently postoperative in origin, they may result from hepatic diseases and gastrointestinal perforations. The patients are usually febrile and dyspneic and manifest an elevated hemidiaphragm with ipsilateral decreased motion. Abscesses may also develop in the liver or spleen. Antibiotics alone may not be sufficient, and drainage may be necessary. Pancreatitis and pancreatic pseudocyst can cause pleural effusions, more often on the left side or bilaterally. These exudates may be blood tinged. The amylase level is higher than that in the serum. It tends to normalize as the pancreatic problem improves. Esophageal rupture is an urgent cause of pleural effusion. Close to one half of cases are secondary to endoscopy or esophageal dilatation. It may also be secondary to a foreign body or trauma or may occur spontaneously (Boerhaave's syndrome). Patients complain of chest pain, dyspnea, and dysphagia. Fever is universal, and half will have subcutaneous emphysema. The roentgenogram may confirm the subcutaneous emphysema and may show pneumothorax more frequently on the left side. Pleural effusion occurs in 75 per cent of cases. The fluid findings depend on the time of thoracentesis. Early on, the exudate contains abundant PMN's, to be followed by high concentrations of salivary amylase. Later, anaerobic organisms from the mouth will seed the space, and the pH will rapidly fall and approach a value of 6.0. The diagnosis is established by using barium sulfate or water-soluble water compounds with the patient in the appropriate lateral decubitus position. Early diagnosis and prompt surgical correction result in a greater than 90 per cent survival. If surgical closure is delayed, antibiotics for anaerobes, parenteral nutrition, and mediastinal and pleural drainage are necessary.

TUBERCULOSIS. Pleural effusion occurs in most cases of pulmonary tuberculosis but is frequently inapparent. The effusion may accompany the primary infection, in which case it is serous and results from a hypersensitivity phenomenon. These patients, who are usually febrile, may recover without treatment, but close to two thirds of them will develop active tuberculosis in the following 5 years. A second form occurs when a subpleural focus of *Mycobacterium tuberculosis* ruptures into the pleural space. The immunologic reaction between proteins or the bacterium itself and lymphocytes results in alterations in vascular permeability and an accumulation of cells that characterizes the tuberculous effusion. It is usually rich in protein (>4 grams per deciliter), with a leukocyte count around 5000 cells, of which 90 to 95 per cent are lymphocytes. A predominance of PMNs may occur the first few days after penetration of the bacillus to the pleural space. The glucose level may be low, but rarely lower than 20 mg per deciliter. The pH ranges between 7.0 and 7.3, with a pH over 7.4 virtually excluding tuberculosis. The fluid is characteristically free of mesothelial cells. Recently, the presence of ADA and lysozyme has been found to correlate with tuberculosis. The use of enzyme-linked immunosorbent assay (ELISA) for demonstration of mycobacterial antigen is gaining acceptability. Acid-fast bacilli in a smear are seen in fewer than 10 per cent of cases. Multiple-sample closed pleural biopsy is positive in 50 per cent to 80 per cent of cases, while a culture is positive in 30 per cent to 70 per cent. With all three methods combined, the yield is close to 95 per cent. The clinical presentation may vary, from simulation of an acute pneumonia (60 per cent of cases), with fever, nonproductive cough (80 per cent), and chest pain (75 per cent), to a subacute or more chronic form, with fever being the predominant symptom. The chest roentgenogram shows a normal heart size and small to moderate effusions (4 per cent are actually large). Parenchymal disease is seen in one third of cases. Intermediate-strength purified protein derivative (PPD) is positive in 70 per cent of patients, and if repeated after 6 to 8 weeks, it may become positive in those with a prior negative test. Standard treatment for pulmonary tuberculosis, including isoniazid and rifampin, results in resolution of the fever within 2 weeks, although occasionally the fever may persist for 6 to 3 weeks. The effusion resolves by 6 weeks but may persist for 3 to 4 months. Very ill patients may be helped by short-term corticosteroids. Rarely, surgical drainage of tuberculous empyema or decortication may be necessary.

OTHER INFECTIOUS EFFUSIONS. Actinomycosis, caused by the anaerobic organism *Actinomyces israelii*, may produce purulent pleural effusions. The effusions may bulge the thoracic wall and drain through the chest. Sulfur granules (whitish-yellow or brown interwoven filaments) can be identified in the fluid. Pleural effusions are also common in *Nocardia* infection of the lungs. The effusion is usually purulent with abundant PMN's. Sulfonamides are the treatment of choice. Aspergillosis of the pleura is uncommon, but an inflammatory, thickened pleura is frequently seen in progressive invasive aspergillosis. Pleural effusions due to parasitic diseases are still uncommon but are increasing in frequency, especially among Third World immigrants. Paragonimiasis causes pleural thickening or effusion in up to 48 per cent of patients. This effusion has a triad of characteristic findings: low glucose (<10 grams per deciliter), high LDH (>1000 units per liter), and low pH (<7.1). Complement fixation antibodies higher than 1:64 are diagnostic. Amebiasis and echinococcosis are rare diseases only occasionally seen in most U.S. hospitals.

HEMOTHORAX. Frank blood in the pleural space (hematocrit >20 per cent) is usually the result of trauma, hemothorax, hematologic disorders, or pleural malignancies. Left-sided pneumothorax, particularly with an associated widened mediastinum may indicate rupture or dissection of the aorta. Pleural blood often does not clot and can be readily removed by lymphatics if small. Larger effusions require tube drainage. Persistent bleeding requires surgical correction.

CHYLOTHORAX. Leakage of the lymph from the thoracic duct (chyle) most commonly results from malignancy involving the mediastinum (50 per cent), lymphoma being the most frequent. It may also result from thoracic surgery (20 per cent) or trauma (5 per cent). Since chyle collects within the posterior mediastinum, the chylothorax may not appear for days, until the mediastinal pleura ruptures. The usual milky appearance of the effusion may be confused with a cholesterol effusion or an effusion with many leukocytes. The best diagnostic criterion is the presence of a triglyceride concentration greater than 110 mg per deciliter, with rare instances of values between 50 and 110 mg per deciliter. The major complications of chylothorax are malnutrition and immunologic compromise, as fat, protein, and lymphocytes are depleted with repeated thoracentesis or chest tube drainage. Treatment should include drainage of the pleural space, a decrease in chyle formation by intravenous hyperalimentation, and a decrease in oral intake, with the possible addition of medium-chain triglycerides, which are directly absorbed into the portal circulation. In those cases in which drainage persists, thoracic duct ligation should be considered if the cause is traumatic. If the chylothorax is secondary to tumor, the treatment should address the primary cause. The triad of slow-growing yellow nails, lymphedema, and pleural effusions is termed the "yellow nail syndrome." It is due to either hypoplastic or dilated lymphatics.

IMMUNOLOGIC CAUSES OF PLEURAL EFFUSIONS. Clinical rheumatoid pleurisy occurs in close to 5 per cent of patients with rheumatoid disease, even though autopsy studies suggest up to 50 per cent involvement. It has a striking male predominance, and the effusion appears within 5 years after the onset of the disease; nevertheless, effusions have been known to occur up to 20 years before the onset of articular disease. The fluid is an exudate with a low glucose level (<30 mg per deciliter) and pH and a high LDH level. The complement level in the fluid is usually low, with high titers of rheumatoid factors. The patients may complain of pleuritic chest pain or dyspnea. Fever is not common, in contrast with lupus pleuritis. The effusion does not resolve quickly, but rather over several months; occasionally, it persists for years. The major complication is fibrosis with lung trapping, so that anti-inflammatory agents and careful administration of corticosteroids may be tried. Pleuritic pain or effusion can be the presenting manifestation in 5 per cent of patients with systemic lupus erythematosus (SLE) and can occur at some point in the course of the disease in close to 50 per cent of patients. Pain (86 per cent), cough (64 per cent), dyspnea (50 per cent), pleural friction rub (71 per cent), and fever (57 per cent) are commonly seen. The effusions are exudates, which, in the majority of cases, have normal pH and glucose. The hemolytic complement (especially C–3 and C–4 components) is low, and classic LE cells may be present in the pleural fluid. LE pleuritis is likely if the antinuclear antibody (ANA) titer in the fluid is 1:160. Spontaneous resolution of LE pleuritis is uncommon, but the response to corticosteroids is usually dramatic, with disappearance of the pleuritis within 2 weeks. Sarcoidosis, Wegener's granulomatosis, Sjögren's syndrome, and immunoblastic lymphadenopathy are rare causes of pleural effusions that may involve an immunologic mechanism for their formation.

OTHER CONDITIONS AFFECTING THE PLEURA

ASBESTOSIS. This condition is frequently associated with pleural disease. It may be an effusion, often unilateral, small, and serosanguineous. The cell count is lower than 6000 cells per milliliter with a predominance of either PMN's or mononuclear cells. Eosinophilia of up to 50 per cent of cells has been described. The diagnosis is suspected with known asbestos exposure of variable duration and intensity. The exclusion of malignant mesothelioma when pleural plaques coexist may be difficult and requires follow-up of 2 to 3 years. The effusion tends to resolve in 1 month to a year. When it resolves, it leaves a blunted angle in more than 90 per cent of patients, with 50 per cent showing diffuse pleural thickening. Calcification of the plaques occurs late (20 to 40 years after exposure). Close to 5 per cent of patients may have underlying pulmonary parenchymal asbestosis.

MEIG'S SYNDROME. This syndrome consists of the following triad of features: benign fibroma or other ovarian tumors, ascites, and large effusions (usually on the right side). Most commonly seen shortly after menopause, the symptoms are those of chronic illness, chest pain, and increased abdominal girth. Fluid moves from the abdomen to the thorax through small diaphragmatic defects or lymphatics. The fluid is usually an exudate with a paucity of mononuclear cells. When the condition is suspected, an abdominal CT scan can be done in addition to the pelvic examination and will document the ovarian tumors. Their removal results in resolution of the effusion within 2 to 3 weeks.

UREMIA. Different from the urinothorax and hydrothorax of the nephrotic syndrome, the effusion of uremia accompanies a polyserositis. It is usually an exudate with varying amounts of blood. The effusions will resolve with treatment of the uremia, but repeated thoracentesis may be needed if the patient is very symptomatic (dyspnea, cough, chest pain).

MISCELLANEOUS CAUSES OF INFLAMMATORY EFFUSIONS. Other causes of effusions with an inflammatory component include radiation therapy, esophageal sclerotherapy, enteral feeding misplacement, drug-induced pleural disease (nitrofurantoin, dantrolene, methysergide, methotrexate, procar-bazine, amiodarone, practolol, mitomycin, bleomycin, and minoxidil). Pleuritis in a lupus-like syndrome has been associated with procainamide, hydralazine, isoniazid, and quinidine. It usually resolves after discontinuation of the medicine and may occasionally require corticosteroids.

MALIGNANCY. Malignant effusions probably are the most common cause of exudate in patients over the age of 60. Direct invasion by carcinoma of the lung is the most frequent cancer, while tertiary spread from liver metastasis or chest wall lymphatic invasion is the most frequent mechanism in breast cancer. Ovarian and gastric cancers represent close to 5 per cent of cases, while 7 per cent of patients may have an unknown primary malignancy at the time of initial diagnosis. The patients may be asymptomatic or may develop cough, pain, and dyspnea; the last-named seems related to changes in chest wall compliance and improves after thoracentesis. The effusion is an exudate with abundant red blood cells (30,000 to 50,000 per milliliter) and mononuclear cells (lymphocytes >50 per cent). Occasionally (5 per cent to 10 per cent), they are transudative, and close to one third may have a pH lower than 7.3 or a glucose level less than 60 mg per deciliter. Pleural fluid cytology is positive in close to 60 per cent of cases, and the biopsy increases the yield only to 70 per cent. Thoracentesis should be repeated if the diagnosis is still suspected. Malignant pleural effusion carries a very poor prognosis, with the exception of breast and small cell carcinoma of the lung, both of which may respond temporarily to therapy. The best method short of pleurectomy or pleural abrasion for control of recurrent malignant effusion is the intrapleural instillation of tetracycline after drainage through a chest tube.

Lymphomas. These may cause exudative effusions, which are frequently diagnostic in the case of non-Hodgkin's lymphoma. Mediastinal invasion with lymphatic blockage and effusion on this basis is suggestive of Hodgkin's lymphoma. Although the prognosis for patients with lymphomatous pleural effusion is poor, they often respond to chemotherapy.

Malignant Mesothelioma. This tumor is related to asbestos exposure in 80 per cent to 90 per cent of cases. Patients usually present with symptoms of dyspnea, cough, weight loss, and pain. Smoking is not a factor. The tumors are diffuse and often encase the underlying lung. The effusion may be massive and often bloody and, in 70 per cent cases, may have a pH lower than 7.3. Cytology is controversial because even when positive it may be difficult to differentiate from metastatic carcinoma. Elevated levels of hyaluronic acid have been documented, and special stains and electron microscopy of biopsy tissue may help in the diagnosis. The prognosis is dismal, with a median survival of 6 to 12 months after diagnosis. Malignant mesotheliomas may be confused with benign mesotheliomas, which have the histologic features of a fibroma. Benign mesotheliomas may reach a large size and may be pedunculated (migrating with position changes). They are often associated with hypertrophic pulmonary osteoarthropathy and clubbing. Treatment involves surgical removal of the mass.

PNEUMOTHORAX. Pneumothorax is defined as an accumulation of gas in the pleural space. It may be caused by (1) perforation of the visceral pleura and entry of gas from the lung; (2) penetration of the chest wall, diaphragm, mediastinum, or esophagus; or (3) gas generated by microorganisms in an empyema. In cases in which gas originates in the lung, the rupture may occur in the absence of known disease (simple pneumothorax) or as a result of parenchymal disease (secondary pneumothorax).

Simple, spontaneous pneumothorax occurs most commonly in previously healthy men 20 to 40 years of age and is due to spontaneous rupture of subpleural blebs at the apex of the lungs. The right lung is more frequently involved than the left, and recurrence is frequent (30 per cent ipsilateral, 10 per cent contralateral). The patients usually present with an acute onset of pain, dyspnea (related to size of pneumothorax), and cough. Physical examination reveals decreased breath sounds and tactile fremitus with increased resonance on the side of the pneumothorax. The chest roentgenogram classically shows the visceral pleural line. As stated before, a small pneumothorax may become evident only with an expiratory or lateral decubitus film. Small amounts of fluid (sometimes blood) are present in 25 per cent of patients. Tension pneumothorax (caused by increased positive pressure through a "ball-value" air leak) can cause mediastinal shift and compromise circulation. Observation may suffice for a small pneumothorax (<20 per cent of the hemithorax) in an asymptomatic patient, since it reabsorbs in 7 to 14 days. Larger pneumothoraces can be treated with air aspiration. In patients with pneumothorax that occupies more than 50 per cent of the hemithorax, in those with tension pneumotherapy, or in those who are very symptomatic, a chest tube should be placed. The tube can be connected to suction or placed under a water seal. The tube should be left 2 to 4 days until the leak seals. After recurrent episodes, chemical pleurodesis or surgical correction is necessary.

Secondary or complicated pneumothorax occurs as a result of trauma or other pulmonary diseases. Widespread emphysema is the most common process causing secondary pneumothorax. It may be caused by rupture of an infected abscess, with spillage of the material into the pleural space (pyopneumothorax). Also seen, but less frequently, are asthma; certain interstitial lung diseases (idiopathic fibrosis, eosinophilic granulomatosis, sarcoidosis, tuberous sclerosis); neoplasms (sarcoma, bronchogenic carcinoma); some rare diseases, such as Marfan's and Ehlers-Danlos syndromes; and endometriosis (catamenial pneumothorax). Iatrogenic injuries (e.g.,) insertion of central lines) and barotrauma are frequently seen in the intensive care unit. The treatment of pneumothorax in patients with underlying lung disease should be aggressive. The patient should be hospitalized and a chest tube inserted, since spontaneous expansion is rare, and because of the decreased pulmonary reserve, even small or moderate pneumothorax may cause significant ventilatory compromise. Surgery must not be regarded lightly since the rate of complications is high, but it may be life saving in some patients. In patients on ventilatory support, a pneumothorax will always be under tension and requires immediate insertion of a chest tube. If a bronchopleural fistula persists, a portion of the minute ventilation will exit through it; hence it is necessary to increase ventilation to compensate for this loss. For severe leak, high-frequency low-pressure ventilation or synchronized chest tube occlusion may be helpful. Frequent complications of chest tube insertion include re-expansion pulmonary edema, lung trauma or infarction, subcutaneous emphysema, bleeding, and infection of a previously sterile pleural space.

Light RW, MacGregor MI, Luchsinger PC, et al.: Pleural effusions: The diagnostic separation of transudates and exudates. Ann Intern Med 77:507, 1972. *Classic paper that divides effusions into transudative or exudative types on the basis of pleural fluid/serum ratios of LDH and protein.*

O'Rourke JP, Yee E. Civilian spontaneous pneumothorax: Treatment options and long-term results. Chest 96:1302, 1989. *Retrospective review of a large number of patients (130) with discussion of therapeutic options.*

Pistolesi M, Miniati M, Giuntini C: Pleural liquid and solute exchange. Am Rev Respir Dis 140:825, 1989. *Reviews the physiology and pathophysiology of pleural liquid. It summarizes the new concepts that have increased the importance of lymphatic drainage for fluid and solute exchange.*

Sahn SA. The pleura: State of the art. Am Rev Respir Dis 138:184, 1988. *Extensive in-depth review of pleural effusions: cause, presentation, and differential diagnosis. With 594 references, the most complete review.*

Wied U, Halkier E, Holier-Madson K, et al.: Tetracycline versus silver nitrate pleurodesis in spontaneous pneumothorax. J Thorac Cardiovasc Surg 86:591, 1983. *Controlled trial that determined the superiority of tetracycline over silver nitrate.*

THE MEDIASTINUM

The mediastinum is the anatomic space that lies in the mid-thorax and separates the two pleural cavities. It is limited by the diaphragm below and the suprasternal thoracic outlet above. The mediastinum contains several vital structures in a small space. Thus, regardless of the cause, mediastinal abnormalities can produce major symptoms. For clinical purposes, it is convenient to divide the mediastinum into anterior, middle, and posterior compartments (Fig. 69–1). The anterior compartment is bounded posteriorly by the pericardium, ascending aorta, and brachial cephalic vessels and anteriorly by the sternum. It contains the thymus, substernal extensions of the thyroid and parathyroid glands, blood vessels, pericardium, and lymph nodes. The middle compartment extends from the posterior limit of the anterior compartment to the posterior pericardial line. It contains the heart, great vessels, trachea, main bronchi, lymph nodes, and

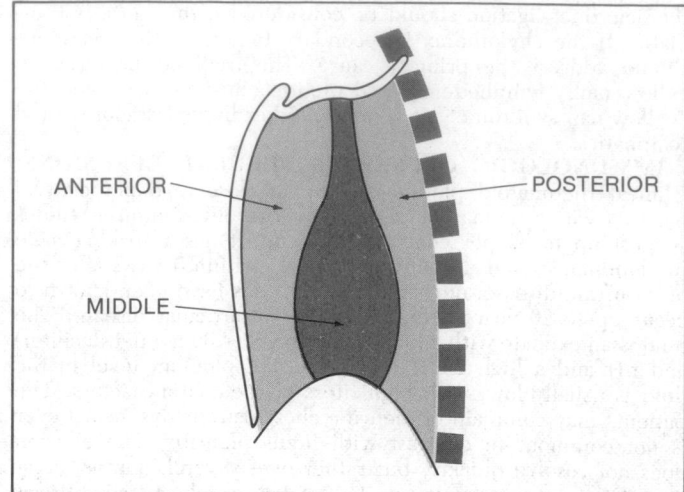

FIGURE 69–1. Anatomic compartments of the mediastinum.

phrenic and vagus nerves. The posterior compartment extends from the posterior pericardial line to the dorsal chest wall. It contains the vertebrae, descending aorta, esophagus, thoracic duct, the azygos and hemiazygos veins, the lower portion of the vagus, the sympathetic chains, and the posterior mediastinal nodes.

Signs and Symptoms of Mediastinal Masses

Most patients with mediastinal masses are asymptomatic, and the finding is incidental on a chest roentgenogram obtained for another reason. The most common symptoms are chest pain, cough, hoarseness, and dyspnea, while stridor, dysphagia, and Horner's syndrome are less frequent. Occasionally, some syndromes are associated with a primary mediastinal lesion. Myasthenia gravis is seen in nearly half of patients with thymoma. Hypoglycemia has been observed in patients with mesotheliomas, fibrosarcomas, and teratomas. Parathyroid tumors may induce hypercalcemia, and neurogenic tumors may press upon the spinal cord, causing neurologic symptoms. The signs on the physical examination are usually minimal and nonspecific. The mass may produce superior vena caval obstruction with typical signs of facial edema, dilated neck veins, and upper extremity edema. The masses may erode the trachea, esophagus, and great vessels, with life-threatening consequences.

Diagnosis of Mediastinal Masses

Most mediastinal masses are detected on a plain chest roentgenogram (Figs. 69–2 and 69–3). CT of the chest should be the initial procedure for evaluating most patients (Fig. 69–4), since it provides good visualization and definition of mediastinal struc-

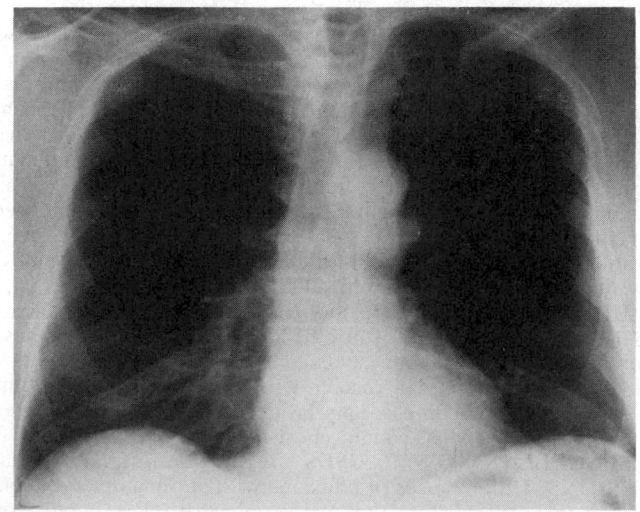

FIGURE 69–2. Posteroanterior roentgenogram of a patient with a mass in the superior portion of the anterior mediastinum.

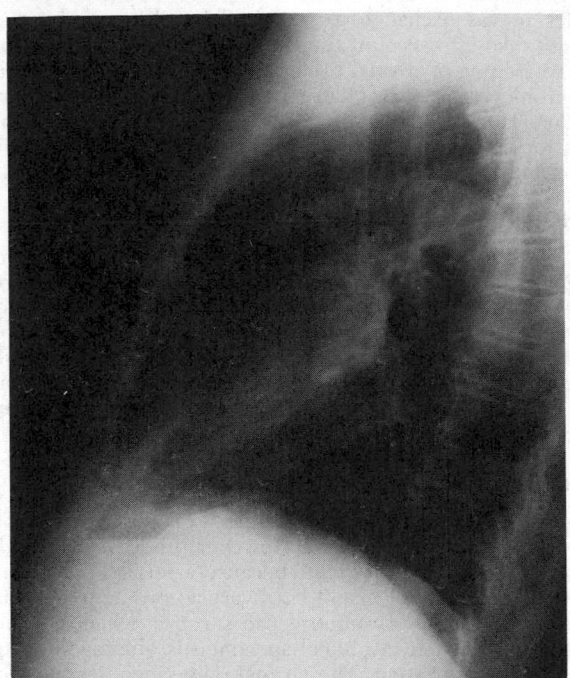

FIGURE 69-3. Lateral chest radiograph of same patient as in Figure 69–2.

TABLE 69–6. MOST FREQUENT CAUSES OF MASSES IN THE MEDIASTINUM

Anterior	Middle	Posterior
Thymoma	Lymphoma	Neurogenic tumors
Lymphoma	Cancer	Enteric cysts
Teratogenic tumors	Cysts	Esophageal lesions
Thyroid	Aneurysms	Aneurysms
Parathyroid	Hernia (foramen of	Diaphragmatic hernias
Aneurysms	Morgagni)	(foramen of Bochdalek)

Neurogenic Tumors. These are the most common primary mediastinal tumors (20 per cent). They are located in the posterior mediastinum. Nonspecific chest pain and nonproductive cough with occasional compression of intercostal nerves and trachea and bronchi are the most frequent symptoms. Most tumors are benign, originating in the nerve sheath (neurilemoma, neurofibroma) or sympathetic ganglion cells (ganglioneuroma). Neuroblastomas (malignant tumors of sympathetic ganglion cell) have a better prognosis than the same tumors occurring as primary malignancies in the adrenals. Neurofibromas may occur in association with von Recklinghausen's disease. Ganglioneuromas and neuroblastomas may secrete hormones that cause flushing, diarrhea, and hypertension. Pheochromocytomas may occasionally arise in the mediastinum. Neurogenic tumors should be resected and postoperative radiation therapy given to neuroblastomas.

Lymphoreticular Tumors. Thymomas account for 20 per cent of mediastinal tumors and are located in the superior portion of the anterior mediastinum. Two thirds of them are malignant. Myasthenia gravis is seen in 40 per cent of cases, and other paraneoplastic syndromes, such as Cushing's syndrome, refractory anemia, and hypogammaglobulinemia, have been reported. All thymomas should be regarded as malignant, and surgical resection should be done, followed by radiation. Lymphatic tumors (17 per cent) also arise in the anterior mediastinum. Hodgkin's lymphoma is the most frequent and carries the best prognosis. Non-Hodgkin's lymphoma, plasmacytomas, and angiomatous lymphoid hamartomas with a similar clinical presentation carry a worse prognosis. Teratomatous tumors constitute 10 per cent of mediastinal tumors. One third of them are malignant at diagnosis. Also located in the anterior compartment, they are embryologically and histologically linked to the thymus. Cystic teratomas are more frequent and may contain squamous cells, hair follicles, sweat glands, cartilage, and linear calcifications. *Intrathoracic goiter* (10 per cent) is usually a benign nodular or follicular enlargement of the thyroid gland. Three quarters of patients present with stridor, cough, and dyspnea. Most frequently located in the anterior mediastinum, it occasionally causes the superior vena cava (SVC) syndrome. Benign cysts are usually asymptomatic and occur as an incidental roentgenographic finding. Bronchogenic cysts develop around the paratracheal area or carina and are seen in the middle and posterior compartments. They are filled with liquid and are lined with respiratory epithelium and cartilage but do not communicate with the tracheobronchial tree. Pericardial cysts occur in the anterior compartment and cardiophrenic angle. They contain clear liquid and are lined by flattened endothelial or mesothelial lining with a bland, fibrous wall. Enteric cysts are located in the posterior mediastinum and are lined by gastric or intestinal epithelium. All developmental cysts are potentially hazardous in that they may become infected, bleed, or rupture into the mediastinum or pleural cavity.

Vascular Tumors. These tumors may have a primary origin in the mediastinum. Vascular hamartoma, lymphangioma, and hemangioma are benign tumors, whereas hemangiopericytoma is malignant. Mesenchymal benign (lipoma) or malignant (liposarcoma, mesothelioma, rhabdomyosarcoma, and mesenchymoma) tumors are rare causes of mediastinal masses.

HERNIAS. Hernias through the diaphragm may also manifest as mediastinal masses. They may be retrosternal through the foramen of Morgagni, posterolateral through the foramen of Bochdalek, or, most commonly, through the esophageal hiatus. When gas is contained in the herniated organ, the presumptive diagnosis is easily made.

PNEUMOMEDIASTINUM. This condition may occur second-

tures. If the patient is asymptomatic and if noninvasive information obtained by CT with and without contrast suggests a benign process, conservative management with careful follow-up is justified. The radiologic evaluation may include angiography and barium esophagogram. The role of magnetic resonance imaging (MRI) is currently being investigated, specifically in the evaluation of vessels and blood flow, in which no contrast solution is needed. In patients in whom a specific diagnosis cannot be established by radiologic methods, it may be necessary to obtain tissue for histologic diagnosis. Classically, anterior and middle compartment lesions are reached through mediastinoscopy or mediastinotomy. Thoracotomy may be needed for middle and posterior compartment lesions or when surgery is the treatment of choice for the suspected lesion. Direct sampling, using fluoroscopy or CT-guided needle aspiration, has proved useful, especially in patients whose underlying conditions made thoracotomy or mediastinoscopy a risky procedure.

Disorders of the Mediastinum

TUMORS. The most common cause of a mediastinal mass in older patients is a metastatic carcinoma (most commonly, bronchogenic carcinoma). In young adults, primary mediastinal pathology is more frequent. The common origin of tumors by location is shown in Table 69–6.

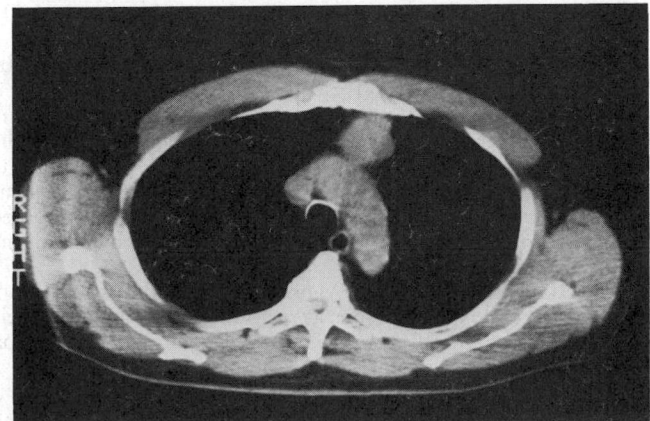

FIGURE 69–4. CT of same patient as in Figures 69–2 and 69–3. The mass proved to be a thymoma. (Courtesy of Elon Gale, M.D., Department of Radiology, Boston Veterans Administration Medical Center.)

ary to a tear in the esophagus or tracheobronchial tree or from the dissection of air from ruptured alveoli. Tears in the esophagus and tracheobronchial tree commonly have a traumatic origin, whereas an alveolar rupture may occur spontaneously or as a complication of artificial ventilation. Air may track to the neck and rest of the body, producing subcutaneous emphysema, or into the pleural space and cause pneumothorax. Patients complain of retrosternal pain and dyspnea. There may be subcutaneous emphysema with the classic crepitus. Auscultation may reveal a crunching sound synchronous with the heartbeat (Hamman's sign). Rarely, cardiac function is compromised. A lateral chest roentgenogram is usually diagnostic. Simple, spontaneous pneumomomediastinum usually resolves without treatment. When it is severe or results from organ rupture, surgical drainage and repair are required.

SUPERIOR VENA CAVA (SVC) SYNDROME. The SVC syndrome results from the obstruction of blood flow through the superior vena cava. Besides dilatation of the collateral veins of the upper thorax and neck and edema and congestion of the face, patients may have headache, dyspnea, dysphagia, and wheezes. Malignancy is the most frequent cause of SVC syndrome, with bronchogenic carcinoma responsible for more than 70 per cent of cases and lymphoma a distant second. Fibrosing mediastinitis can also occur after granulomatous diseases such as histoplasmosis or in association with the ingestion of methysergide. Aortic aneurysm and retrosternal thyroid are relatively benign causes of SVC syndrome. Because of vessel dilatation, invasive procedures are contraindicated. An effort must be made to obtain tissue elsewhere, and irradiation or chemotherapy must be begun before attempts are made to obtain mediastinal tissue.

Benjamin SP, McCormack LJ, Effler DB, et al.: Primary tumors of the mediastinum. Chest 67:297, 1972. *Excellent experience with 215 patients with mediastinal tumors managed by two surgeons. It establishes the prevalence and localization of primary mediastinal masses.*

Putgatch RD, Faling LJ, Robbins AH, et al.: CT diagnosis of benign mediastinal abnormalities. A J R 135:685, 1980. *Examines the evidence that supports the concept that CT scan of the thorax should be the initial procedure used to evaluate mediastinal masses.*

Weisbrod GL: Percutaneous fine needle aspiration biopsy of the mediastinum. Clin Chest Med 8:27, 1987. *It reviews the experience with fluoroscopy and CT-guided needle aspiration. It reiterates that experience and good cytopathologic interpretation are important to the success of the procedure.*

70 Respiratory Failure

John F. Murray

Adequate respiration consists of the uptake of sufficient amounts of O_2 and the elimination of sufficient amounts of CO_2 to maintain P_{O_2} and P_{CO_2} in arterial blood at their respective normal values. It follows that *respiratory failure* is associated with disturbances in the exchange of O_2 and CO_2 between gas in alveoli and blood in pulmonary capillaries and that these abnormalities must be reflected by changes in the P_{O_2} and P_{CO_2} in arterial blood. Thus respiratory failure is defined as a condition in which arterial P_{O_2} is below the normal range (excluding hypoxemia from intracardiac right-to-left shunting of blood) or arterial P_{CO_2} is above the normal range (excluding respiratory compensation for metabolic alkalosis). This definition, which is physiologically precise as well as clinically applicable, implies that the diagnosis of respiratory failure depends chiefly on laboratory analysis of arterial blood and not on clinical findings.

Respiratory failure is not a disease but a disorder of function that can be caused by a variety of conditions that affect the lungs; in some instances, the lungs are completely normal (e.g., overdose of sedative drugs). Respiratory failure is analogous to heart failure and renal failure, both of which represent the consequences of impaired normal function resulting from numerous disparate diseases.

Respiratory failure is traditionally divided into acute and chronic varieties, depending on the time it takes for the abnormalities in gas exchange to occur. This arbitrary classification does not take into account the common clinical occurrence of an acute worsening of arterial P_{O_2} and P_{CO_2} in a patient who already has chronic respiratory failure as a result of some underlying disorder. However, the distinction between acute and chronic respiratory failure has important etiologic and therapeutic implications and will be referred to subsequently.

PATHOPHYSIOLOGY OF RESPIRATORY FAILURE

In human beings, respiration has been subdivided into four functional processes: *ventilation, diffusion, perfusion,* and *control of breathing.* Each of these contributes uniquely to the maintenance of normal values of P_{O_2} and P_{CO_2} in arterial blood. Therefore, abnormalities in any one of the four processes, if sufficiently severe, will cause respiratory failure; furthermore, in many common respiratory disorders, multiple abnormalities coexist.

Normal Gas Exchange

The physiology of normal gas exchange is described in Ch. 56 and will not be reviewed here. However, understanding what is meant by normal is important, because arterial P_{O_2} varies with age, and both arterial P_{O_2} and P_{CO_2} vary according to the altitude (i.e., the prevailing barometric pressure) at which the person happens to be when the blood specimen is obtained and to the extent of acclimatization. The normal range includes the biologic variabilities among individuals and the analytic variations inherent in the measurements. Because the diagnosis of respiratory failure should be made in the laboratory and not at the bedside, the physician's ability to establish the diagnosis depends on the accuracy of the laboratory tests used to measure P_{O_2} and P_{CO_2}. Normal mean arterial P_{O_2} (Pa_{O_2}) values in subjects 20 years of age or older can be calculated from the regression equation $Pa_{O_2} = 100.1 - 0.323$ (age in years). The normal range of variation is $\pm$ 5 mm Hg from the mean value. Arterial P_{CO_2} does not vary with age and is normally within the range of 40 ± 5 mm Hg in healthy persons at sea level. Values of P_{O_2} *below* or P_{CO_2} *above* normal limits indicate the presence of respiratory failure.

Abnormal Gas Exchange

The pathophysiology of abnormal gas exchange is also discussed in Ch. 56 and 71. Hypoventilation, impaired diffusion, ventilation-perfusion mismatching, right-to-left shunting of blood, and breathing air with a low P_{O_2} all cause arterial hypoxia (a decrease below normal of P_{O_2}); in contrast, for practical purposes, only hypoventilation causes arterial hypercapnia (an increase above normal of P_{CO_2}). In view of the therapeutic importance of recognizing the abnormal mechanism (or mechanisms) leading to a patient's respiratory failure, each will be reviewed briefly.

HYPOVENTILATION. Alveolar hypoventilation is present when the arterial P_{CO_2} is increased. Furthermore, as arterial P_{CO_2} increases, P_{O_2} decreases *except* when the patient is breathing gas with an enriched concentration of O_2. Because arterial P_{O_2} and P_{CO_2} change in opposite directions by nearly the same amount during hypoventilation, the contribution of hypoventilation to the patient's arterial hypoxia can be readily assessed. (In a 60-year-old person, for example, if $P_{O_2} = 50$ mm Hg and $P_{CO_2} = 70$ mm Hg, both have changed from their normal values by the same amount [30 mm Hg] and "pure" hypoventilation is present; in contrast, if $P_{O_2} = 30$ mm Hg and $P_{CO_2} = 70$ mm Hg, the change from normal of P_{CO_2} does not account for the entire change in P_{O_2}; therefore, some other cause in addition to hypoxia from hypoventilation must be present.) Arterial hypoxia from alveolar hypoventilation is not associated with an increased alveolar-arterial P_{O_2} difference and is "corrected" by breathing 100 per cent O_2.

IMPAIRED DIFFUSION. Abnormalities of diffusion do not cause arterial hypoxia in persons at rest unless they are extremely severe. Although these occur in occasional patients with respiratory failure, for practical purposes the possible contributions of an abnormality of diffusion to a given patient's arterial hypoxia can be ignored except during exercise or at high altitude. This practice is permissible because diffusion disturbances, even when marked, cause only relatively small increases in the patient's alveolar-arterial P_{O_2} difference, and this abnormality, if it exists, is readily corrected by adding small amounts of O_2 to the inspired air.

VENTILATION-PERFUSION IMBALANCE. When gas exchange units receive more blood flow than ventilation, arterial hypoxia results. Mismatching of ventilation and perfusion is by far the most common cause of arterial hypoxia and can be recognized by giving the patient 100 per cent O_2 to breathe; this causes the alveolar-arterial Po_2 difference from pure mismatching that is present while the patient breathes room air to decrease and arterial Po_2 to increase to normal values (>550 mm Hg). It is important, when performing this test, to use 100 per cent O_2 and to allow enough time for N_2 to be eliminated from the lungs; otherwise, the results are unreliable. Although a "pure" ventilation-perfusion inequality can lead to CO_2 retention, this is an uncommon cause of hypercapnia because as arterial Pco_2 tends to increase, it stimulates peripheral and central chemoreceptors and increases ventilation; this, in turn, reduces Pco_2 back to normal values but, owing to the shape of the oxyhemoglobin dissociation curve, does not correct the hypoxia.

RIGHT-TO-LEFT SHUNTS. Shunts of blood from right to left may occur through abnormal anatomic communications in the lung (e.g., pulmonary arteriovenous fistula) but much more frequently by perfusion of lung units that are completely unventilated because they are either collapsed (atelectasis) or filled with fluid (pulmonary edema, pneumonia, intra-alveolar hemorrhage). Regardless of the cause, an alveolar-arterial Po_2 difference results that increases when the patient breathes 100 per cent O_2 compared with when the patient breathes room air. For reasons similar to those occurring in patients with ventilation-perfusion imbalances, CO_2 retention seldom occurs in patients with right-to-left shunts.

DECREASED INSPIRED Po_2. Expected values of arterial Po_2 are corrected for the influence of decreasing barometric pressure; strictly speaking, therefore, the effects of high altitude on inspired Po_2 and the resulting decreased arterial Po_2 are not an abnormal cause of hypoxia, even though the hypoxia may be severe and dangerous. Occasionally, pathologic hypoxia occurs when ambient Po_2 is reduced because of combustion of O_2 or because of dilution by some other gas, both of which may occur in fires. However, this phenomenon is not of importance when interpreting the results of analysis of arterial blood specimens obtained in the hospital or clinic.

HYPERCAPNIA. In contrast to arterial hypoxia, which may result from five different pathophysiologic derangements, arterial hypercapnia can always be interpreted as signifying alveolar hypoventilation. This is true because arterial Pco_2 (Pa_{CO_2}) is governed by the relationship between CO_2 production ($\dot{V}co_2$) and alveolar ventilation ($\dot{V}A$): $Pa_{CO_2} = k\dot{V}co_2/\dot{V}A$. Normally, however, even when CO_2 production increases markedly, alveolar ventilation increases proportionally and arterial Pco_2 is maintained within fairly narrow limits. Thus an increase in arterial Pco_2 can always be viewed as respiratory failure in the sense that alveolar ventilation is inadequate to eliminate all the CO_2 being produced at that time. Severe ventilation-perfusion imbalances and right-to-left shunts can produce hypercapnia, but this is uncommon because, as already emphasized, alveolar ventilation usually increases and restores CO_2 to normal values.

An increase or decrease in Pco_2 in the blood has a direct effect on the amount of carbonic acid in the blood and a reciprocal effect on pH. Acute changes in Pco_2 have a more profound effect on pH than chronic changes owing to differences in plasma bicarbonate concentrations. With acute increases or decreases in Pco_2, there is little change in bicarbonate level and a considerable change in pH; after 3 to 5 days of a sustained change in Pco_2, renal compensation has increased plasma bicarbonate in hypercapnia and decreased it in hypocapnia, both tending to restore pH toward normal. Many patients with respiratory failure have mixed respiratory and nonrespiratory acid-base disturbances, which are difficult to define without knowledge of their time course and the level of plasma bicarbonate.

Right-Sided Heart Failure

Acute respiratory failure can cause acute right-sided heart failure (acute cor pulmonale). The normal right ventricle is not a good pressure generator and cannot sustain sudden pressure loads over 40 to 50 mm Hg. Thus acute right-sided heart failure may develop in any condition in which pulmonary vascular resistance increases abruptly; this happens most commonly in patients with massive pulmonary emboli with obstruction of much of the pulmonary vascular bed (usually >60 per cent). At times, acute cor pulmonale complicates the course of patients with severe bronchial asthma or other forms of marked airways obstruction.

Acute right-sided heart failure may also occur in patients with chronic lung disease during an episode of acute respiratory failure. Most of these patients have right ventricular hypertrophy (chronic cor pulmonale) to begin with, and a subclinical or stable condition is aggravated by the added effects of the superimposed acute lung disease (usually bronchitis or pneumonia). In these patients, right ventricular function is worsened for several reasons: (1) Alveolar hypoxia and acidemia cause pulmonary arterial vasoconstriction; (2) certain lung diseases reduce the cross-sectional area available for perfusion; (3) hyperinflation of the lung increases pulmonary vascular resistance; and (4) arterial hypoxia may depress myocardial contractility. These factors are important to recognize because they are reversible and usually respond well to appropriate treatment of the intercurrent acute disorder.

CAUSES OF RESPIRATORY FAILURE

Because respiratory failure is defined as the presence of arterial hypoxia with or without hypercapnia, two physiologically different types are recognized: failure of ventilation, which is characterized by abnormalities of both O_2 and CO_2, and failure of oxygenation, in which only O_2 is abnormal. For convenience, the multiple causes of respiratory failure can be classified according to which component of the respiratory system is involved, and whether they are either acute or chronic in onset.

Diseases Causing Airways Obstruction

ACUTE. Obstruction may result from acute diseases that involve any portion of the upper and lower airways. The presence of respiratory failure depends on the magnitude and extent of the narrowing. Obstruction of the *extra*thoracic airway (nasopharynx, larynx, extrathoracic portion of the trachea) usually causes stridor, a characteristic alteration of breathing that is associated with harsh, high-pitched respiratory noises that are louder and more pronounced during inspiration than expiration. In contrast, obstruction of the *intra*thoracic airways causes wheezing, an abnormality of breathing in which expiration is louder and longer than inspiration.

Obstruction of the upper airways can result from (1) inflammation-induced swelling of the mucosa secondary to infections, allergic reactions, and, less commonly, thermal or mechanical injuries and (2) impaction of foreign bodies or, occasionally, tumors. Acute obstruction of the upper airways is particularly likely to develop in infants and young children, who have smaller and hence more vulnerable upper passages than do older children and adults.

Acute obstruction of the lower airways is usually caused by swelling of the mucosa, secretions in the lumen, or bronchospasm. Accordingly, bronchial asthma, infections, bronchiolitis, and the inhalation of chemicals (such as nitrogen dioxide in silo-filler's disease) are important causes of acute respiratory failure.

CHRONIC. Diffuse obstruction may result from disorders originating in bronchi (bronchiectasis), bronchioles (bronchiolitis), or the lung parenchyma (emphysema). These abnormalities characteristically progress gradually and lead to chronic respiratory failure. Of considerable importance are the intercurrent episodes of acute disease, usually pneumonia or bronchitis, that complicate the underlying disorder and often worsen the severity of existing respiratory failure.

Diseases Causing Parenchymal Infiltration

ACUTE. The most common cause of acute infiltration of the parenchyma is pneumonia, which usually has an infectious origin but occasionally is caused by inhalation or aspiration of a toxic chemical. Whether acute respiratory failure develops depends on the extent and severity of the disease. Immunologic reactions from drugs, migrating parasites, or leukoagglutinins are uncommon causes of acute respiratory failure but are important because of their special therapeutic requirements.

CHRONIC. More than 100 different conditions can cause chronic diffuse parenchymal infiltration. When severe, any of these can cause chronic respiratory failure. As in patients with chronic airways obstruction, patients with chronic infiltrative diseases may have intercurrent episodes of bronchopulmonary infection that cause acute worsening of their underlying respiratory status.

Diseases Causing Pulmonary Edema

CARDIOGENIC. Pulmonary edema in patients with heart disease may be acute or chronic in onset; both varieties are caused by an increase in the hydrostatic pressure within pulmonary capillaries. Pulmonary edema may follow an acute myocardial infarction or acute left ventricular failure of any cause (hypertensive crises, arrhythmias), or it may be precipitated in patients with valvular or other forms of chronic heart disease by sudden changes in their cardiorespiratory status (from arrhythmias, hypoxemia, or increased systemic blood pressure). Chronic pulmonary edema is found in patients with chronic, usually refractory, heart failure, but even in these patients the amount of edema increases and decreases according to changing hemodynamics and therapy.

INCREASED PERMEABILITY. Acute pulmonary edema can accompany certain conditions that do not involve the heart. The basic pathophysiologic abnormality in most of these disorders appears to be an increased permeability of the pulmonary capillary endothelium and overlying alveolar epithelium. Generalized pulmonary edema with accompanying severe hypoxemia from right-to-left shunting of blood, diffuse infiltrations on chest radiographs, and decreased pulmonary compliance constitute what is known as the *adult respiratory distress syndrome (ARDS)*. This syndrome (not disease) includes the composite manifestations of diffuse injury to the lung parenchyma, which may occur in association with certain usually identifiable clinical disorders (Table 70–1); of these, the sepsis syndrome (infection with systemic complications, such as hypotension and/or metabolic acidosis) is by far the most common. Histologic examination early in the evolution of ARDS reveals prominent injury to the type I alveolar epithelial cells, less severe damage to the capillary endothelium, hyaline membranes, proteinaceous pulmonary edema, and intra-alveolar hemorrhage. Later, the injury may clear or may evolve into a proliferative pattern, with hyperplasia of type II epithelial cells, infiltration by connective tissue cells, and deposition of collagen. Unless the underlying cause of ARDS is rapidly reversible (heroin, air embolism, near-drowning), the clinical course is apt to be prolonged and complicated and is associated with a high mortality (60 to 70 per cent). However, death is much more likely to result from multiple organ failure (see Ch. 71) than from intractable respiratory failure.

TABLE 70–1. PARTIAL LIST OF CONDITIONS THAT HAVE BEEN ASSOCIATED WITH THE ADULT RESPIRATORY DISTRESS SYNDROME

Infections	Inhaled toxins
Sepsis syndrome	O_2 (high concentrations)
Pneumonia (any cause)	Smoke
Trauma	Corrosive chemicals (NO_2, Cl_2,
Fat emboli	NH_3, phosgene, cadmium)
Lung contusion	Hematologic disorders
Nonthoracic trauma (including	Intravascular coagulation
head injury)	Massive blood transfusion
Liquid aspiration	Metabolic disorders
Gastric juice	Pancreatitis
Fresh and salt water (drowning)	Uremia
Hydrocarbon fluids	Paraquat ingestion
Drug overdose	Miscellaneous
Heroin and other opiates	Increased intracranial pressure
Salicylates	(including seizures)
Propoxyphene	Eclampsia
Barbiturates	Post cardioversion
	Radiation pneumonitis
	Post cardiopulmonary bypass

Pulmonary Vascular Diseases

ACUTE. Pulmonary embolism is usually accompanied by a decreased arterial Po_2 and Pco_2, the former from ventilation-perfusion mismatching and the latter reflecting the hyperventilation that nearly always occurs. Pulmonary embolism is also an important cause of worsening respiratory failure in patients with underlying chronic lung disease. Fat emboli and emboli from platelet-fibrin aggregates during disseminated intravascular coagulation are recognized causes of ARDS.

CHRONIC. Pulmonary vasculitis and recurrent thromboembolism are not common conditions and, when present, usually do not cause respiratory failure until the late stages of the disease. Recurrent thromboembolism occurs in intravenous drug abusers and in patients with chronic peripheral venous thrombi, sickle cell anemia, and schistosomiasis. Pulmonary vasculitis occurs in patients with scleroderma, other collagen diseases, and primary pulmonary hypertension.

Diseases of the Chest Wall and Pleura

ACUTE. The most important cause of sudden respiratory failure from acute disorders involving the thoracic cage is injury to the chest wall. Segmental fractures of several ribs or fractures of ribs on both sides of the sternum can result in a flail chest. Besides the impairment of ventilatory function that results from the unstable chest wall, gas exchange abnormalities are often compounded by contusion of the lung underneath the site of injury. Spontaneous or traumatic pneumothorax is an important cause of acute respiratory failure, which may be severe and which often afflicts otherwise healthy persons.

CHRONIC. Severe idiopathic or acquired kyphoscoliosis can cause chronic respiratory failure, which is often associated with cor pulmonale. Patients with massive pleural effusion (or effusions) or with thickened, constrictive pleural layer (or layers) may also have chronic respiratory failure.

Disorders of the Neuromuscular System

Disorders of the neuromuscular system are classified according to which part of the effector system is involved, i.e., the brain, neuronal pathways, or muscles of respiration, rather than into acute and chronic varieties. Patients with these disorders often have perfectly normal lungs; respiratory failure occurs from inability to ventilate normally.

BRAIN DISORDERS. Probably the most common cause of respiratory failure from impaired function of the central nervous system is the use of sedative drugs or anesthetic agents. Suppression of ventilatory drive from opiates, barbiturates, psychic depressants, alcohol, and a variety of sedative drugs results in hypoxia and hypercapnia that may be life threatening. Ventilatory stimuli can also be depressed by many diseases of the central nervous system, including vascular diseases, tumors, and infections.

SPINAL CORD AND PERIPHERAL NERVE DISORDERS. Injuries to the cervical or high thoracic spinal cord may produce immediate respiratory failure from paralysis of the muscles of respiration. Loss of anterior horn cell function in patients with poliomyelitis was an important cause of acute and chronic respiratory failure but is seldom encountered now because of the widespread use of vaccination. Polyneuritis, whether postinfectious (Guillain-Barré syndrome) or toxic, is an uncommon but important cause of respiratory failure in view of its inherent reversibility.

MUSCULAR DISORDERS. The final effectors in the system that controls breathing are the skeletal muscles of respiration. When these muscles are involved by generalized myopathies, such as muscular dystrophy or myasthenia gravis, respiratory failure results. Respiratory failure in patients with myasthenia gravis occurs during myasthenic or cholinergic crises. In contrast, respiratory failure in patients with muscular dystrophy is nearly always chronic and related to an advanced stage in the progression of the disease.

SLEEP APNEA. Brief periods of apnea occur in normal persons during deep sleep. Much more prolonged episodes associated with severe hypoxia have been documented in patients with massive obesity, chronic mountain sickness, enlarged tonsils, and many other disorders. Apnea results from either failure of ventilatory drive or obstruction of the upper airway. Severe sleep apnea can cause chronic respiratory failure, cor pulmonale, psychosis, and pathologic daytime sleepiness, a condition occasionally called the pickwickian syndrome, with somewhat dubious literary authenticity. Sleep apnea is discussed at greater length in Ch. 447.

CLINICAL MANIFESTATIONS

Given the great variety of disorders that can cause respiratory failure, it is obvious that the clinical manifestations in a given patient depend in large part on which underlying disease he or she has; these are dealt with elsewhere in this text. When respiratory failure ensues and if the blood gas disturbances are sufficiently severe, the signs and symptoms of hypoxia, and possibly hypercapnia, become superimposed upon the signs and symptoms of the underlying disease. The clinical manifestations of hypoxia and hypercapnia are nonspecific and usually occur late in the evolution of the clinical problem. This statement underscores the earlier axiom that the diagnosis of respiratory failure is made in the laboratory by blood gas analysis and not at the bedside by clinical examination.

Hypoxia

The signs and symptoms of acute hypoxia are chiefly caused by abnormalities in central nervous system and cardiovascular function. Characteristic features are impaired judgment and motor instability, a clinical picture closely resembling that of acute alcoholism. As hypoxia worsens, the brain stem is affected, and death results from depression of the medullary respiratory centers. The initial cardiovascular effects of acute hypoxia are tachycardia and increased blood pressure; when hypoxia is very severe, bradycardia, myocardial depression, and shock ensue. Recognizable cyanosis of the lips, mucous membranes, and nail beds usually occurs when the concentration of reduced hemoglobin in the capillaries is greater than 5 grams per deciliter. Accordingly, cyanosis can result from decreases in either arterial P_{O_2} or blood flow. In patients with lung disease, cyanosis cannot be detected by most physicians until arterial P_{O_2} is less than 50 mm Hg; some observers cannot recognize cyanosis unless arterial P_{O_2} is less than 40 mm Hg!

In patients with chronic hypoxia, the central nervous system manifestations are drowsiness, inattentiveness, apathy, fatigue, and delayed reaction time. The chronic cardiovascular effects are often minimal, but pulmonary hypertension or even cor pulmonale with signs of right-sided heart failure may be detected on clinical examination. One of the hallmarks of chronic hypoxia is erythrocytosis, which may cause noticeable plethora and changes in the hemoglobin concentration, hematocrit ratio, or red blood cell count.

Hypercapnia

The physiologic consequences of hypercapnia depend not only on the amount of excess CO_2 in the body but also on the rate at which retention develops. Increases in P_{CO_2} from acute respiratory failure lead to a constellation of progressive disturbances of central nervous system function: apprehension, confusion, drowsiness, coma, and death. The vascular responses represent a mixture of vasoconstriction, from generalized sympathetic activity, and vasodilation, from local accumulation of CO_2; thus the cardiovascular abnormalities are variable and depend on whether vasoconstrictor or vasodilator influences predominate. Tachycardia and sweating are usually present, but blood pressure may be high, low, or normal.

In contrast, if P_{CO_2} increases slowly, compensation takes place and the clinical consequences may be minimal at values of arterial P_{CO_2} that would cause death if reached suddenly. There are numerous patients with arterial P_{CO_2} values over 100 mm Hg who are ambulatory and at times living active lives, although most breathe supplementary O_2 to prevent life-threatening hypoxia. Patients with hypercapnia from chronic respiratory failure frequently complain of headaches and drowsiness; these symptoms are probably attributable to the potent cerebral vasodilating effect of excess CO_2. In addition, patients with chronic hypercapnia may have papilledema, muscular twitching, coarse myoclonic jerky motions, and asterixis. At times, the neurologic findings simulate those of a brain tumor.

TREATMENT OF ACUTE RESPIRATORY FAILURE

The time course of worsening abnormalities varies in patients with acute respiratory failure from almost instantaneous (flail chest, pulmonary embolism) to a gradual crescendo during a period of several hours or even days (respiratory tract infections, bronchial asthma). The demands for treatment and the speed with which it must be provided obviously differ from one patient to another. It is difficult to generalize about such an extremely variable clinical condition, but the principles of treatment of acute respiratory failure are as follows: *first*, establish an airway, administer O_2, and maintain adequate alveolar ventilation; *second*, identify and treat the underlying condition and monitor the patient's progress carefully.

Establish an Airway

The upper airway tends to be occluded in unconscious patients because of relaxation of the oropharyngeal muscles and tongue and the presence of saliva, vomitus, and other secretions. When respiratory arrest occurs away from medical facilities, all material should be cleared from the oropharynx, and the victim should be placed on his or her back with the head tilted backward as far as possible and the jaw extended forward. Sometimes these simple maneuvers are all that is required to enable breathing to resume spontaneously. Further details about the treatment of cardiorespiratory arrest are provided in Ch. 71.

An airway can be established by three different methods: an oropharyngeal tube, an endotracheal tube passed via the nose or mouth, and a tracheostomy. Selection of the procedure depends on available facilities and personnel and on the site and severity of the obstruction.

OROPHARYNGEAL AIRWAY. An oropharyngeal airway is valuable in unconscious patients who are breathing spontaneously (e.g., during recovery from general anesthesia, after a cerebrovascular accident). An oropharyngeal airway is also useful in patients who are apneic during emergency resuscitation but who are receiving some form of assisted ventilation (mouth-to-mouth respiration, bag-mask system). Although an oropharyngeal tube is commonly used in these clinical circumstances, its role must be viewed as temporary, either while the patient is waking up or until an endotracheal tube can be inserted.

ENDOTRACHEAL TUBE. The preferred method of establishing an airway in most emergencies is with an endotracheal tube. Once inserted, the tube is used to remove secretions and to provide ventilation. Endotracheal tubes can usually be passed quickly through the nose or, at times, through the mouth into the trachea by an experienced person; the airway is then sealed by inflating a balloon near the tip of the tube. Endotracheal tubes should be used in nearly all patients with acute respiratory failure severe enough to require control of their airways.

TRACHEOSTOMY. Emergency tracheostomy was formerly the only way of quickly establishing an airway in patients with acute respiratory failure. Now, emergency tracheostomy is contraindicated except in one clinical situation: acute obstruction of upper airways (e.g., from foreign bodies, trauma, or inflammation). Otherwise, intubation with an endotracheal tube is the treatment of choice for control of the airway. Tracheostomy, if needed, can be performed electively at a later time in the operating room under ideal conditions. There is virtually no mortality and very little morbidity with an elective tracheostomy, in contrast to the high incidence of complications associated with emergency tracheostomy performed at the bedside.

The decision to convert a satisfactory endotracheal intubation to a tracheostomy is not an easy one and must be individualized in each case. The availability of tubes of inert plastic with low-pressure cuffs permits endotracheal tubes to be used for weeks rather than days without prohibitive injury; the main mechanical difference between endotracheal and tracheostomy tubes is the trauma to the vocal cords from the former and problems related to the stoma in the latter. The usual reasons for performing a tracheostomy in a patient with a satisfactory endotracheal tube are (1) failure to control secretions (sometimes it is difficult to suction the lungs adequately, especially the left side, through a long endotracheal tube) and (2) the need for prolonged (i.e., several weeks) intubation for assisted ventilation and/or removal of secretions (these circumstances are uncommon but occur particularly in patients with neuromuscular disease and chest wall injuries).

The presence of a tube and its cuff in the airways can cause necrosis of the mucosa of the trachea; at times the entire airway wall may be eroded with penetration of the esophagus (tracheo-esophageal fistula) or a neighboring blood vessel (innominate artery), causing severe hemorrhage. Delayed complications after extubation are caused by damage to the trachea or larynx from the tube or cuff; injury to the vocal cords merely impairs phonation, but serious and life-threatening obstruction to airflow can result from stenosis or malacia of the tracheal wall. These complications should be considered and evaluated in any patient who complains of persisting hoarseness or who develops breathlessness or stridor at any time after endotracheal intubation.

HUMIDIFICATION. Insertion of an endotracheal or tracheostomy tube bypasses the normal source of humidification of the inspired air. When this occurs and unhumidified air or gas mixture is breathed, the result is drying of the mucosa and impairment of mucociliary clearance. Thus as long as the upper airway is bypassed, patients must receive air or a mixture of O_2 that is fully saturated with water vapor at their body temperature. This is easily accomplished if the patient is being ventilated, because most commercial ventilators have heated humidifiers in the circuit. If the patient is breathing spontaneously, humidified gas can be delivered through a T-piece connected to the endotracheal or tracheostomy tube. When proper humidification is carried out, remember that there is *no* insensible water loss through the respiratory tract when evaluating the patient's daily fluid balance.

Administer Oxygen

Acute respiratory failure, by definition, includes decreased arterial Po_2. When respiratory failure is severe, death results from the central nervous system or cardiovascular consequences of hypoxia. During emergencies, supplementary O_2 is given without worrying about the concentration being used; in general, the higher the concentration of O_2, the better. After the patient's emergency condition has stabilized, attention is directed to administering O_2 in the lowest possible concentration required to correct the hypoxia. Any more O_2 than required to raise arterial Po_2 to a safe level exposes the patient to the direct toxicity of O_2 on the lung parenchyma and other undesirable effects: suppression of alveolar macrophage function and mucociliary clearance. In patients with chronic obstructive pulmonary disease, especially those with chronic hypercapnia, the administration of O_2 is likely to worsen the CO_2 retention. The further increase in Pco_2 can be explained in part by suppression of preexisting hypoxic ventilatory drive; the remaining increase can be accounted for through the effects of O_2 on the breathing pattern and matching of ventilation-perfusion. In general, the higher the inspired O_2 concentration, the greater the CO_2 retention; this observation underlies the use of "low-flow" O_2 for these patients, as described below under Treatment of Chronic Respiratory Failure.

The usual goal of O_2 therapy in acute respiratory failure is to raise arterial Po_2 to between 60 and 80 mm Hg. Because these values lie on the flat portion of the oxyhemoglobin dissociation curve, most of the available hemoglobin is saturated with O_2; raising arterial Po_2 values even higher adds very little additional O_2 to the blood and may require increases in alveolar Po_2 concentrations to toxic levels. At times, especially when the mechanism of arterial hypoxia is right-to-left shunting of blood, arterial Po_2 may be considerably less than 60 mm Hg even with the patient breathing 100 per cent O_2. When this occurs, other maneuvers, such as addition of end-expiratory pressure, are required to raise arterial Po_2 and to allow a reduction in inspired O_2 concentration.

There are several ways of giving supplementary O_2 to a patient. Which method is chosen depends on the cause and severity of the arterial hypoxia and convenience to the patient. It is important to emphasize that no method can be relied upon to produce a certain increase in arterial Po_2; the response depends on which physiologic mechanism (or mechanisms) is responsible for the

hypoxia. Thus it is always advisable to monitor the effects of O_2 administration by serial analyses of arterial blood.

NASAL CANNULAS OR PRONGS. Nasal cannulas, catheters, or prongs can be used to administer enriched concentrations of O_2. These devices work well even when patients breathe through their mouths. However, because of the drying effects of unhumidified O_2 on the nasal mucous membranes, if more than 5 to 6 liters per minute is needed to achieve satisfactory arterial oxygenation, other methods of administration, such as face masks, are advisable.

RESERVOIR MASKS. When high concentrations of O_2 (40 to 80 per cent) are needed in patients who are not intubated, reservoir masks are used. To ensure optimal efficiency of operation, the masks must be tight fitting to avoid leaks; because this often causes discomfort, it is difficult to deliver high concentrations of O_2 by reservoir masks for long periods.

OTHER METHODS. Virtually all mechanical ventilators have regulators that can be set to deliver an inspired O_2 concentration that ranges from 21 to 100 per cent. The most reliable way of ensuring that patients actually receive high concentrations of O_2 (60 to 100 per cent) when they need it is to use a mechanical ventilator connected to an endotracheal or tracheostomy tube.

Maintain Alveolar Ventilation

Emergency resuscitation after respiratory arrest requires ventilation by mouth-to-mouth respiration or a bag and mask device. As soon as possible thereafter, if the patient does not resume spontaneous breathing, intubation and ventilation by a mechanical ventilator are indicated. Similar considerations apply to patients with acute respiratory failure whose breathing is insufficient to maintain adequate gas exchange. The main indications for mechanical ventilation are ventilatory failure, shown by an elevated or rising Pco_2, or severe refractory hypoxia, shown by a low Po_2 that cannot be corrected without high concentrations of O_2 and often end-expiratory pressure. Special indications include the need to produce alkalosis, as in head injuries and certain drug overdoses; to stabilize the thorax, as in traumatic injuries that result in flail chest; or to aspirate secretions, as in bronchopulmonary infections and failure to cough.

MECHANICAL VENTILATION. The different types of ventilators and modes of ventilation are described in Ch. 71. In general, the settings that are chosen depend on whether or not the patient can initiate each breath and what the underlying disorder is. Patients who cannot synchronize their breathing with the machine frequently become agitated, and their gas exchange deteriorates further. This problem can often be solved by alternate settings of the ventilator; if not, the patient must be sedated or at times paralyzed.

END-EXPIRATORY PRESSURE. Mechanical ventilators ordinarily raise airway pressure during inspiration and allow it to fall to zero (atmospheric) pressure during expiration; this pattern of assisted ventilation is known as intermittent positive-pressure ventilation, or IPPV. At times, it is desirable to add positive pressure to the airway during expiration as well as inspiration to hold the lung at a higher end-expiratory lung volume (functional residual capacity) than it would reach at zero end-expiratory pressure; this pattern of assisted ventilation is known as continuous positive-pressure ventilation, or CPPV. Keeping the lung at a high end-expiratory lung volume prevents closure of alveoli and airways during expiration, redistributes pulmonary edema fluid out of alveoli, and often improves arterial Po_2 considerably. Positive end-expiratory pressure (or PEEP) is particularly useful in patients with the conditions that cause the adult respiratory distress syndrome (Table 70–1).

Although end-expiratory pressure usually results in an improvement in arterial Po_2 and O_2 content, it may also decrease cardiac output by impairing venous return. Accordingly, the actual delivery of O_2 to the tissues of the body may decrease. Thus it is important to monitor both the respiratory and the circulatory responses to end-expiratory pressure to determine the optimal amount of pressure and the need for additional therapeutic interventions. Another common and serious hazard of end-expiratory pressure is its tendency to cause spontaneous pneumothorax and pneumomediastinum.

Identify and Treat the Underlying Condition

Acute respiratory failure always has a precipitating cause. Consequently, the cause of the condition should be identified as soon as possible after emergency measures have been started and the patient's condition has stabilized. Usually, the diagnosis can be established easily by a thorough history and physical examination, analysis of the blood and urine, and chest roentgenogram. Helpful auxiliary tests include those that evaluate central nervous system or cardiac function, those that determine the presence of drugs or poisons in the body, and bacteriologic study of secretions and blood.

Treatment obviously depends on the underlying cause, and the reader is referred to the appropriate chapters of this book for information about therapy for specific pulmonary and other disorders that lead to acute respiratory failure. In all patients with acute respiratory failure, careful attention should be paid to fluid balance. Overhydration is a frequent and serious complication that can usually be avoided by careful attention to fluid replacement and, when needed, monitoring of pulmonary capillary (wedge) pressure.

Many patients cared for in intensive care units are nutritionally depleted at the time of admission or become so soon afterward. Because morbidity and mortality are closely linked to nutritional status, it is important that this be assessed and, when necessary, treated by appropriate enteral or parenteral supplementation.

Monitor the Patient's Progress

The need for monitoring varies from patient to patient according to the response to initial treatment. If the disorder is readily reversible (e.g., bronchial asthma), the patient may respond sufficiently to go home shortly after being seen and treated. Other less rapidly responding conditions causing acute respiratory failure often require hospital care, and seriously ill patients are best treated in special acute care facilities (intensive care units) when available. Intensive care units provide an institutional focus of trained personnel and special equipment for the care of critically ill patients.

All seriously ill patients should have frequent measurements of blood pressure, constant monitoring of heart rate, careful recording of fluid intake and output, and determination of weight daily. Arterial blood gas analysis should be performed as often as needed but usually at least once daily. Special studies include measurement of cardiac output and placement of a Swan-Ganz catheter in the pulmonary artery for determination of pulmonary arterial and wedge pressures and sampling of mixed venous blood; this information is very helpful in guiding fluid replacement and ventilator adjustments, including levels of end-expiratory pressure. In general, wedge pressure values should be maintained in the normal range (5 to 10 mm Hg) and not allowed to increase above 15 mm Hg, especially in patients with ARDS. Less reliance is being placed now, compared with previous years, on values of mixed venous Po_2 as a guide to O_2 delivery, especially in disorders such as sepsis and ARDS. Attention is currently directed at improving O_2 delivery by increasing cardiac output through pharmacologic means or by increasing O_2 content through transfusions of packed red blood cells.

TREATMENT OF CHRONIC RESPIRATORY FAILURE

Patients with chronic lung disease often have sufficient alterations in their daily arterial Po_2 and Pco_2 values that they are said to be in chronic respiratory failure. Therapeutic regimens for these patients, whose disease is relatively stable, are delivered mainly on an outpatient basis and are designed to meet two objectives: (1) preventing or minimizing the number and severity of the intercurrent complications that would otherwise occur and (2) treating maximally all reversible elements of the underlying disorder. Many of the specific remedies are used for both purposes, and the approaches to preventive and maintenance therapy for patients with the most common chronic lung diseases—asthma, bronchitis, and emphysema—are discussed in Ch. 57 and 58.

Despite emphasis on preventing intercurrent complications, these attacks continue to plague the lives of patients with chronic lung disease. Acute episodes of bronchopulmonary infection, pneumothorax, pulmonary embolism, surgical procedures, and misuse of sedatives all add their effects to those of the underlying lung disease and frequently produce serious disturbances of blood gases. These episodes are potentially life threatening, are usually associated with prolonged morbidity, and frequently require hospitalization. The principles of therapy are to maintain oxygen-

ation while treating all new, presumably reversible, elements of the disease in an effort to restore the patient to his or her former level of function.

Oxygen

Patients with chronic obstructive lung disease and superimposed episodes of acute respiratory failure nearly always have severe hypoxia from a combination of hypoventilation and ventilation-perfusion mismatching. Typical arterial blood values are a Po_2 of approximately 30 mm Hg, a Pco_2 of 70 mm Hg, and a pH of 7.30. Neither the hypercapnia nor the acidemia is life threatening, but the hypoxia is potentially fatal. Thus treatment is directed mainly at alleviating the disturbance in oxygenation; the changes in Pco_2 and pH will return to the baseline values for that patient as the acute condition improves. In view of the possibility that O_2 therapy may depress ventilation and cause the Pco_2 to increase further, O_2 is given initially in low concentrations (1 to 3 liters per minute). The goal is to raise Po_2 to satisfactory levels (50 to 60 mm Hg) without depressing ventilation to the extent that unacceptable increases in Pco_2 and decreases in pH (particularly) occur.

The O_2 is usually started at 2 liters per minute, and an arterial blood specimen is analyzed 15 to 30 minutes later to determine the patient's response. Depending on the Po_2 value, the flow of O_2 can be adjusted. If hypoventilation and acidemia result from too much O_2 (e.g., a Po_2 of 80 mm Hg, a Pco_2 of 80 mm Hg, and a pH of 7.25), the supplementary O_2 should *not* be discontinued, but the flow rate should be decreased. This is necessary because the Po_2 decreases much faster than the stimulus to breathe returns, and cardiac arrest or other serious complications of hypoxia may result.

Intubation-Assisted Ventilation

Low-flow O_2 given in the manner described provides satisfactory relief of hypoxia in most patients with respiratory failure from chronic lung disease. Although the goal of low-flow O_2 is an arterial Po_2 of 50 to 60 mm Hg, at times one has to be satisfied with 40 to 50 mm Hg. When oxygenation cannot be achieved without intolerable hypercapnia and acidemia, the decision whether to intubate and ventilate the patient must be made. Experience with intubation and mechanical ventilation in this group of patients has not been rewarding, particularly because of the prolonged need for assisted ventilation once intubation is performed and the poor prognosis for lengthy survival and return to useful life after recovery from the acute episode. There are no firm guidelines to intubation and assisted ventilation in patients with chronic obstructive pulmonary disease who develop superimposed acute respiratory failure, and it is helpful to have ascertained the wishes of the patient before the event occurs.

Bronchodilators

Most intercurrent episodes of acute respiratory failure in patients with chronic obstructive pulmonary disease are associated with increased airways resistance from the presence of secretions, edema of the mucosa, and bronchospasm. Because it is impossible to discriminate among these, bronchodilator drugs are always included in the treatment regimen to take advantage of the reversibility of whatever element of bronchospasm is present.

When patients seek medical attention for intercurrent attacks, they frequently have already tried—and failed to respond to—oral and aerosolized bronchodilators. In this circumstance, the mainstays of treatment are aerosolized beta$_2$-sympathomimetic drugs, administered at 1- or 2-hour intervals for the first 12 to 24 hours, and intravenous corticosteroids, either methylprednisolone, 60 mg, or hydrocortisone, 100 mg, given intravenously every 6 hours. Much higher doses of corticosteroids (e.g., methylprednisolone, 15 mg per kilogram of body weight per day in divided doses) have been proposed, but there is no evidence to suggest that these are more efficacious in this clinical setting than the lower doses recommended above. Intravenous theophylline, although less popular now than before, and aerosolized anticholinergic drugs are often used as supplementary therapy in patients who are sick enough to warrant hospitalization.

Antimicrobials

Infections are the most frequent and important cause of acute respiratory failure in patients with chronic underlying lung disease. Intercurrent attacks usually begin as a typical cold, with rhinitis, pharyngitis, and headaches. Shortly afterward, lower respiratory involvement appears with increasing cough, sputum production, purulence, wheezing, and breathlessness. These episodes occur several times a year in most patients with chronic obstructive pulmonary disease. (It should be noted that fever, leukocytosis, and new roentgenographic infiltrations are uncommon in this syndrome.) When airway infection is present, the sputum not only is purulent but usually contains numerous microorganisms detectable by Gram's stain of the secretions. Sputum cultures, however, often fail to reveal pathogenic bacteria, although at times *Streptococcus pneumoniae* and/or *Haemophilus influenzae*, may be grown. Regardless of the presence or absence of identifiable pathogens, oral treatment with ampicillin (250 to 500 mg every 6 hours), a combined preparation of trimethoprim-sulfamethoxazole (160 mg and 800 mg, respectively, every 12 hours), or tetracycline (250 to 500 mg every 6 hours) frequently results in decreased volume of sputum, thinning of the secretions, change in sputum appearance from purulent to mucoid, and improvement in blood gases. If parenteral therapy is indicated, second-generation cephalosporins are useful.

When pneumonia is present, signified by the presence of new infiltrations on the chest roentgenogram, Gram's stain of the sputum is likely to show one bacterial species predominating, and the initial selection of antimicrobials should cover this organism. Therapy can be revised, if necessary, when the results of the sputum cultures are available.

Control of Secretions

Many patients complain of thick, tenacious sputum that is troublesome to clear. Although it seems desirable to attempt to alter the character of these secretions to facilitate their removal, there is no clear evidence that it is possible to do so by pharmacologic means. Iodides, enzymes, detergents, and acetylcysteine, administered orally or by aerosol, have been tried extensively, but none has been shown convincingly to be effective. Moreover, each has potential toxic side effects. Similarly, mist tents and ultrasonic nebulizers, once widely used, are seldom employed today. The best way to control secretions is to treat infection with antimicrobials and to ensure adequate (but not excessive) hydration by the administration of intravenous fluids.

Patients with troublesome sputum retention may require intermittent nasotracheal suction to control the volume of secretions. Manual or mechanical percussion serves to loosen secretions and enhances their removal in patients who have retained sputum in their airways. Respiratory physical therapy, especially when carried out by a skilled therapist, may result in an increase in arterial Po_2 related to the improvement in the distribution of ventilation from clearance of sputum.

Treatment of Heart Failure

Cor pulmonale is an inevitable complication of severe chronic lung disease. Right ventricular hypertrophy followed by heart failure occurs secondary to the increased work load imposed on the ventricle by the changes in the pulmonary circulation from the effects of lung disease. Resistance to blood flow through the lungs increases when pulmonary blood vessels are destroyed (as in emphysema), obstructed (as in pulmonary thromboembolism), narrowed (from vasoconstriction), or compressed (breathing at high lung volumes), or when the blood is unusually viscous (polycythemia). Patients whose cor pulmonale is well compensated or even inapparent while their chronic lung disease is stable often develop acute right-sided heart failure during intercurrent attacks of acute respiratory failure. Peripheral edema, increased venous pressure, and an enlarged, painful liver are important clues to the presence of acute cardiac decompensation.

Most patients with right-sided heart failure from cor pulmonale, even if severe, have a satisfactory diuresis when they are put to bed, given O_2, and treated appropriately for their underlying lung disease. Diuretics may make patients feel more comfortable by diminishing peripheral edema and hepatic and gastrointestinal congestion faster than spontaneous diuresis; but if used, the drugs should be administered orally in low doses. Intravenous ethacrynic acid or furosemide can cause excessive renal loss of Cl^- that worsens existing acid-base disturbances and depletes intravascular volume sufficiently to decrease cardiac output and blood pressure. A particularly dangerous situation occurs in patients who already have coexisting nonrespiratory (metabolic) alkalosis, often from Cl^--losing diuretics, in addition to their hypercapnia from chronic respiratory failure; when the measures designed to improve ventilation lower arterial Pco_2, the metabolic alkalosis becomes "unmasked," and arterial pH becomes markedly alkaline. When this occurs, the patients can develop cardiac arrhythmias, become comatose, or manifest convulsive seizures or other focal neurologic abnormalities.

If an element of pulmonary edema or pulmonary vascular congestion is present from left-sided heart failure, this may also respond to diuretics. Whether left-sided heart failure can occur secondary to purely right-sided disease is controversial. Of greater importance are coexisting causes of left-sided involvement (e.g., valvular disease, coronary atherosclerosis); furthermore, chronic hypoxia and severe polycythemia may impair left ventricular as well as right ventricular function.

Present evidence indicates that digitalis preparations are not beneficial in patients with cor pulmonale. Also, the use of digitalis is hazardous in patients with chronic respiratory failure owing to the sudden shifts in acid-base balance and electrolyte concentrations that may occur in these patients. Therefore, digitalis drugs should be used only in patients with digitalis-responsive arrhythmias or coexisting left-sided heart failure.

Respiratory Stimulants

With few exceptions, respiratory stimulants are obsolete. Nikethamide, picrotoxin, and ethamivan have been replaced by other less hazardous and more efficient methods of maintaining ventilation. Doxapram, a drug that works by stimulating carotid chemoreceptors rather than neurons in the brain, appears to be much safer than centrally acting stimulants. The chief use of doxapram is to minimize or prevent the depression of ventilation, with consequent increase in Pco_2 and decrease in pH, that occurs in some hypoxic patients with hypercapnia who are given O_2 to breathe. Almitrine, another drug that stimulates the carotid chemoreceptors but that can be administered orally, is widely used in Europe to improve arterial Po_2 in outpatients with chronic respiratory failure. This drug has not been approved by the Food and Drug Administration for use in the United States.

Sedation

All sedative drugs should be avoided in patients with chronic lung disease and intercurrent acute respiratory failure, including diazepam (Valium) and chlordiazepoxide (Librium), which can suppress ventilation. Exceptions to this cardinal rule are made from time to time, but usually only when the patient is being mechanically ventilated and sedation is required to enable breathing synchronous with the machine.

Postoperative Complications

Patients with chronic respiratory failure are high-risk operative candidates. Moreover, the closer the surgical incision to the thorax, the higher the incidence of postoperative complications. Despite this caveat, it is safe to say that virtually *all* patients who have respiratory failure can safely undergo *non*thoracic surgery or *nonresectional* thoracic surgery. Postoperative complications can be anticipated and often prevented by attention to the general principles of care outlined in this chapter. Close observation and monitoring are usually required, and these can best be carried out in an intensive care unit.

Derene J-P, Fleury B, Pariente R: Acute respiratory failure of chronic obstructive pulmonary disease. Am Rev Respir Dis 138:1006, 1988. *Recent state-of-the-art review of this common and important complication.*

Johanson WG, Peters JI: Respiratory failure: Pathophysiology and treatment. *In* Murray JF, Nadel JA (eds.): Textbook of Respiratory Medicine. Philadelphia, W.B. Saunders Company, 1988, p 2017. *Detailed discussion of the physiologic abnormalities and therapy directed to improve them.*

Murray JF, Matthay MA, Luce JM, Flick MR. An expanded definition of the adult respiratory distress syndrome. Am Rev Respir Dis 138:720, 1988. *A synthesis of 20 years of studies of this elusive syndrome.*

Pingleton SK: Complications of acute respiratory failure. Am Rev Respir Dis 137:1463, 1988. *A useful compendium of the subject with 420 references.*

PART VIII

CRITICAL CARE MEDICINE

71 Critical Care Medicine

John M. Luce
and Philip C. Hopewell

CHARACTERISTICS OF CRITICAL CARE MEDICINE

Critical care medicine is a body of knowledge that is applied to the management of severely ill patients in critical care units. Many kinds of patients require critical care, but most have dysfunction or failure of one or more organ systems. Circulatory and respiratory failures are the most common kinds of organ system failure dealt with in critical care units. This chapter focuses on their pathophysiology, monitoring, and management.

Critical care medicine is practiced for the most part by internists, anesthesiologists, surgeons, and pediatricians. The parent boards of these disciplines recognize that critical care medicine may become a specialty and now provide certification of special competence in critical care medicine. The American Board of Internal Medicine gave its first critical care certifying examination in 1987. This and subsequent examinations have been taken primarily by pulmonologists, cardiologists, and general internists. These physicians are expected to be familiar with all areas of internal medicine that are relevant to severely ill patients, in addition to ethical issues in critical care.

Consistent with this broad approach, the interdependence of organ systems must be kept in sharp focus in critical care practice. Limited attention to one component of an illness, even if it is predominant, will frequently yield a therapeutic approach that is detrimental to the patient as a whole. For example, treatment directed toward reducing intravascular volume in a patient with the adult respiratory distress syndrome (ARDS) may adversely affect renal and central nervous system function. Conversely, an increase in intravascular volume given to raise cardiac output in a patient with left ventricular infarction may result in noncardiogenic pulmonary edema if parenchymal lung injury pre-exists. Physicians caring for severely ill patients must synthesize an overall management strategy that supports several organ systems and often incorporates the view of numerous consultants. This is one of the major challenges of critical care.

ATTRIBUTES OF CRITICAL CARE UNITS

Critical care units were first developed in the 1950's for patients who required mechanical ventilation because they had poliomyelitis or were recovering from anesthesia. Currently, various kinds of critical care units are found in almost all acute care hospitals in the United States containing more than 200 beds. These units are defined by their ability to provide the environment, facilities, and personnel for the care of severely ill patients. The important features of critical care units are listed in Table 71–1.

Critical care units may have a general orientation, treating all kinds of severely ill patients, or be more specialized, accepting only specific categories of patients as defined by the kind of

TABLE 71–1. FEATURES OF CRITICAL CARE UNITS

High nurse-patient ratio
Ready accessibility of physicians
Ability to provide invasive cardiovascular and respiratory monitoring
Availability of respiratory support techniques
Ability to provide supervised continuous infusion of pharmacologic
    agents

illness (for example, burn units), organ system involved (coronary and acute neurologic units), specialty service designation (medical and surgical units), or the patient's age (neonatal and pediatric units). In addition to having the basic attributes listed in Table 71–1, specialized units provide medical personnel specifically skilled in the area of care provided by the units and have available particular forms of technology with applications generally limited to the category of patients accepted by them.

Critical care units need administrative policies and procedures that differ from those of other hospital areas. Because of the severity of the illness of their patients, critical care units require clear delineation of administrative and medical lines of authority and responsibility. Critical care units must also have general guidelines for admission and discharge of patients, specifically described roles for nurses and respiratory therapists, standing orders, and programs of continuing staff education and quality assurance. The existence of such policies reduces the apparent ambiguity often inherent in the difficult environment of a critical care unit and enables prompt decision making by health care professionals.

MONITORING OF CARDIOVASCULAR AND RESPIRATORY FUNCTION

The term monitoring refers to the repeated or continuous assessment of patients and their physiologic functions. Critical care units are designed to provide such assessment, particularly as it pertains to specific organ systems. Thus, vital signs, mental status, and urinary output are regularly measured. In addition, a variety of noninvasive and invasive procedures may be performed to measure the cardiovascular and respiratory variables listed in Table 71–2.

Cardiovascular Monitoring

The adequacy of cardiac output ($\dot{Q}T$) and tissue perfusion can be inferred from the strength of peripheral pulses, the warmth and color of the hands or feet, and the time required to refill superficial capillaries after they have been blanched; normally, 2 to 3 seconds is required. Most critical care units also have the capacity to monitor and record heart rate (HR) and heart rhythm electrocardiographically. Manually or mechanically inflatable sphygmomanometers may be used to measure systemic arterial pressure (P_{SA}).

MONITORING OF SYSTEMIC ARTERIAL PRESSURE. Heart rate and P_{SA} may be determined in an on-line fashion with indwelling systemic arterial catheters, which may also be used to obtain samples for systemic arterial blood gas analysis. These catheters are usually placed in the radial or femoral artery. Complications such as local hematoma formation, ischemia distal to the site of insertion, and local infection may be minimized by using pressure dressings, devices that continually flush the catheters with dilute solutions containing heparin, and sterile catheter insertion and maintenance techniques, respectively.

Although HR is easy to measure, stroke volume (SV) is difficult to estimate and requires radionuclide or ultrasonographic studies that cannot routinely be performed at the bedside. Because of this, clinicians commonly must infer SV by estimating preload, one of its three determinants. Preload cannot be measured directly in patients, but it is equivalent to ventricular end-diastolic volume, which itself is similar to—but not always the same as—ventricular end-diastolic pressure.

MONITORING OF CENTRAL VENOUS PRESSURE. Right ventricular end-diastolic pressure may be obtained by passing a catheter into the superior vena cava and measuring mean right atrial pressure ($P_{\overline{RA}}$) when the tricuspid valve is open. Central venous pressure (CVP) monitoring carries the risk of perforating a major vein or the right atrium and providing a nidus for infection, especially if the catheter is inserted in an unsterile fashion or left in place too long. Nevertheless, the pressure measurement provides an approximation of right ventricular preload, if ventricular compliance is normal.

Central venous pressure measurement may also be used to estimate left ventricular end-diastolic pressure and volume if one assumes that right and left ventricular pressures are similar in diastole. The $\overline{P_{RA}}$ is particularly helpful when it is less than its normal level of approximately 5 mm Hg, inasmuch as pressure in the right ventricle is seldom much higher than that in the left. However, the $\overline{P_{RA}}$ may be increased owing to elevated pressure in the pulmonary circulation when left ventricular pressure is normal, just as left ventricular pressure may be elevated when right ventricular pressure is normal. Because of this, it may be preferable to assess left ventricular pressure more directly.

MONITORING OF PULMONARY ARTERY PRESSURE. Left ventricular end-diastolic pressure may be estimated by passing a balloon-tipped catheter into the central venous circulation. With the balloon inflated, the catheter travels with venous blood through the right atrium, right ventricle, and main pulmonary artery; the pressure tracings obtained as the catheter passes through these structures are depicted in Figure 71–1. The catheter then floats into a branch of the pulmonary artery and "wedges" there. Blood flow distal to the balloon ceases, and the "wedge" or pulmonary artery occlusion pressure (P_{PAO}) measured at the catheter tip just distal to the balloon reflects the downstream pressure. This pressure usually is equal to left atrial pressure (P_{LA}), which is the same as left ventricular end-diastolic pressure when the mitral valve is open, assuming that pulmonary venous pressure is not higher. The left ventricular end-diastolic pressure is assumed to be an approximation of left ventricular end-diastolic volume, that is, preload.

In addition to estimating preload, the pulmonary artery catheter with a thermistor incorporated may be used to measure $\dot{Q}_T$. This measurement is done using the indicator dilution technique, in which a bolus of cold liquid, usually dextrose in water, is injected through the proximal port of the catheter that is located in the right ventricle when the distal port is in the pulmonary artery. The cold liquid mixes with venous blood as it flows from the ventricle into the artery, where the temperature decrease is detected by the thermistor. The change in temperature then is used to calculate $\dot{Q}_T$. Although the $\dot{Q}_T$ of the right ventricle is measured, it is assumed to be equivalent to that of the left ventricle.

The indications for pulmonary artery catheterization are listed in Table 71–3. The contraindications include lack of vascular access, untreatable bleeding disorders, and instability of the patient that does not allow time for the procedure. The complications of pulmonary artery catheterization include vascular laceration during insertion and infection, as with central venous catheterization. In addition, because the catheter is passed through the heart, it may cause arrhythmias and heart block. For this reason, pulmonary artery catheterization should be performed under the guidance of electrocardiographic monitoring, with resuscitation equipment and intravenous lidocaine available. A temporary transvenous pacemaker should also be available for patients with pre-existing left bundle branch block, because additional right bundle branch block may develop as the catheter is inserted. The catheter should be passed quickly through the ventricle and should be removed if significant ventricular arrhythmias develop.

Once the catheter is in the pulmonary artery, it may cause vessel rupture or infarction if it migrates into a distal vessel. These complications may be avoided by determining the position of the catheter tip on chest radiographs, monitoring the P_{PA} waveform to be certain that the P_{PAO} tracing is not present when the balloon is deflated, and making sure that a P_{PAO} tracing can be obtained only by inflating the balloon with at least 1 ml of air.

Proper interpretation of measurements made with central venous and pulmonary artery catheters requires that intravascular pressures be referenced to the extravascular pressures around them. Thus, the P_{PAO} will actually be lower than the true ventricular filling pressure if it is measured in a spontaneously breathing patient during inspiration, when pleural pressure may be greatly negative. On the other hand, the P_{PAO} will be higher than the true filling pressure if it is measured in a mechanically

TABLE 71–2. NORMAL VALUES FOR SELECTED CARDIOVASCULAR AND RESPIRATORY VARIABLES

Variables	Symbol	Mean	Range
Heart rate	HR	70 beats/min	60–80 beats/min
Stroke volume	SV	70 ml/beat	60–80 ml/beat
Cardiac output	$\dot{Q}_T$	5 L/min	4–6 L/min
Mean pulmonary artery pressure	$\overline{P_{PA}}$	15 mm Hg	9–18 mm Hg
Mean left atrial (pulmonary arterial occlusion) pressure	$\overline{P_{LA}}$ ($\overline{P_{PAO}}$)	10 mm Hg	2–14 mm Hg
Pulmonary vascular resistance	PVR	80 dyne • sec • cm^{-5}	70–90 dyne • sec • cm^{-5}
Mean systemic arterial pressure	$\overline{P_{SA}}$	85 mm Hg	70–105 mm Hg
Mean right atrial (central venous) pressure	$\overline{P_{RA}}$ (CVP)	5 mm Hg	0–8 mm Hg
Systemic vascular resistance	SVR	1240 dyne • sec • cm^{-5}	950–1350 dyne • sec • cm^{-5}
Systemic arterial carbon dioxide tension	Pa_{CO_2}	40 mm Hg	35–45 mm Hg
Fraction of inspired oxygen	FI_{O_2}	0.21	
Systemic arterial oxygen tension	Pa_{O_2}	95 mm Hg	90–100 mm Hg
Carbon dioxide production	$\dot{V}_{CO_2}$	200 ml/min	180–220 ml/min
Oxygen consumption	$\dot{V}_{O_2}$	250 ml/min	225–275 ml/min
Minute ventilation	$\dot{V}_E$	6 L/min	5–7 L/min
Dead space ventilation (per breath)	V_D	150 ml	125–175 ml
Tidal volume	V_T	450 ml	400–500 ml
Dead space to tidal volume ratio (per breath)	V_D/V_T	0.32	0.30–0.35
Respiratory rate	F	17/min	12–22/min
pH	pH	7.40	7.38–7.42
Bicarbonate concentration	$[HCO_3^-]$	24 mEq/dl	22–26 mEq/dl
Hemoglobin	Hb	15 grams/ml	14–16 grams/ml
Systemic arterial oxygen saturation	Sa_{O_2}	98%	96%–100%
Systemic arterial oxygen content	Ca_{O_2}	20 ml/dl	19–21 ml/dl
Mixed venous oxygen tension	$P\bar{v}_{O_2}$	40 mm Hg	38–42 mm Hg
Mixed venous oxygen saturation	$S\bar{v}_{O_2}$	75%	72%–78%
Mixed venous oxygen content	$C\bar{v}_{O_2}$	15 ml/dl	14–16 ml/dl
Arterial–mixed venous oxygen content difference	$C(a - \bar{v})_{O_2}$	5 ml/dl	4–6 ml/dl
Shunt fraction	$\dot{Q}_S/\dot{Q}_T$	<7%	
Maximum inspiratory pressure	MIP	-70 cm H_2O	-60 to -80 cm H_2O
Vital capacity	VC	50 ml/kg	40–60 ml/kg
Forced expiratory volume in 1 second	FEV_1	75% of VC	70%–80% of VC

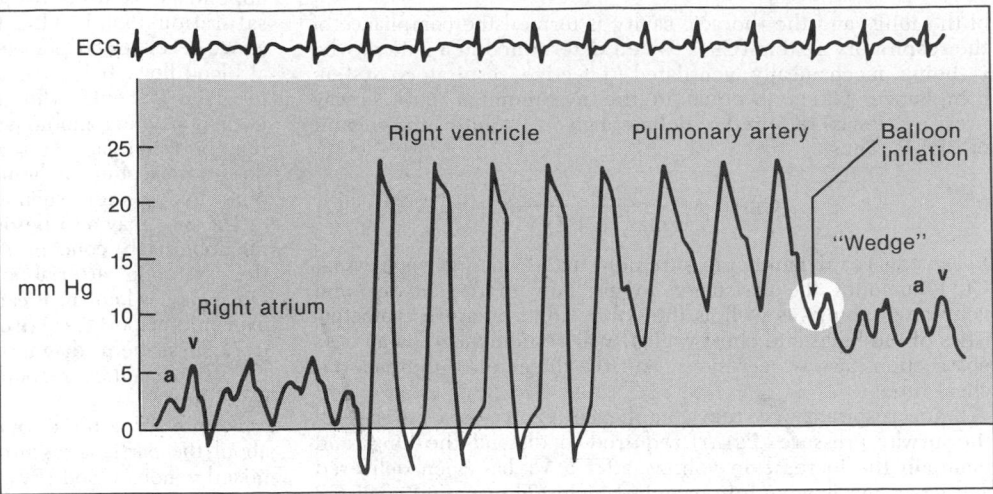

FIGURE 71–1. Tracing of pressures during passage of a pulmonary artery catheter from the internal jugular vein into the pulmonary artery. Pressures and waveform are normal. (From Matthay MA: Invasive hemodynamic monitoring in critically ill patients. Clin Chest Med 4:233, 1983.)

ventilated patient during an inspiration with positive pressure. To avoid erroneous interpretation, the PPAO should be measured in end-expiration. If patients are receiving positive end-expiratory pressure (PEEP) at levels above 10 cm H_2O from the ventilator, approximately one quarter of the PEEP should be subtracted from the measured PPAO to approximate the true PPAO. It is less important to subtract an exact amount than it is to recognize that the PPAO is at best an approximation of left ventricular end-diastolic pressure, which itself is only an approximation of left ventricular end-diastolic volume.

The combination of systemic and pulmonary artery catheterization also facilitates measurement of the pressure across the systemic ($\overline{PSA}$ minus $\overline{PRA}$) and pulmonary (mean pulmonary artery pressure [$\overline{PPA}$] minus $\overline{PLA}$ or $\overline{PPAO}$) circulations. In concert with QT, these data allow determination of the systemic and pulmonary vascular resistances (SVR, PVR). Pulmonary artery catheterization also provides information about mixed venous blood gas values, as discussed in the next section. Characteristic patterns of cardiovascular and respiratory dysfunction that may be identified by combined systemic and pulmonary artery catheterization are listed in Table 71–4 and are discussed in greater detail later in this chapter.

Respiratory Monitoring

Physical examination may be very helpful in assessing respiratory function. For example, intercostal muscle retraction may reflect respiratory distress. Inward movement of the abdominal wall during inspiration, a sign called abdominal paradox, signifies that the diaphragm is not contracting normally and frequently presages ventilatory failure. In addition, hypoxemia may be suspected if cyanosis of the lips and palate is detected. Nevertheless, cyanosis is an insensitive finding, and respiratory failure can be diagnosed only through systemic arterial blood gas analysis.

ASSESSMENT OF VENTILATION. Samples of systemic arterial blood for measurement of the partial pressures of carbon dioxide (Pa_{CO_2}) and oxygen (Pa_{O_2}), pH, and the bicarbonate concentration ($[HCO_3^-]$) may be obtained from either repeated percutaneous arterial punctures or indwelling arterial catheters. The Pa_{CO_2} is used to assess the adequacy of ventilation and to diagnose hypercapnic respiratory failure, also called ventilatory failure. Similarly, the pH and $[HCO_3^-]$ measurements can be used to determine whether hypercapnia is acute or chronic.

TABLE 71–3. INDICATIONS FOR PULMONARY ARTERIAL PRESSURE MONITORING

To help distinguish cardiogenic from noncardiogenic pulmonary edema
To provide information in the differential diagnosis of shock
To assist in determining the cause of hypoxemia
To characterize the patterns of abnormal cardiovascular function after myocardial infarction
To monitor the effects of various cardiovascular and respiratory therapies

An approximation of Pa_{CO_2} may be made by measuring the end-tidal carbon dioxide tension (PET_{CO_2}) in expired gas. This is most conveniently measured in mechanically ventilated patients. If the PET_{CO_2} is to substitute for the Pa_{CO_2}, the two values should be correlated, using several paired measurements. The PET_{CO_2} usually is slightly less than the Pa_{CO_2}.

Ventilatory variables such as respiratory rate (F) and tidal volume (VT) and their product, the minute ventilation (VE), may be accurately measured by a technique called respiratory inductance plethysmography, which uses wire coils embedded in bands that fit around the chest and abdomen to detect movements of these areas. These variables may also be measured by a pneumotachograph or other types of spirometers in patients who are breathing through endotracheal tubes. Neither alveolar ventilation (VA) nor dead space ventilation (VD) can be directly measured, although the value of VA may be inferred if VE and VD are known. The ratio of VD to VT per breath can be calculated in patients whose Pa_{CO_2} and PET_{CO_2} are known, using the modified Bohr equation:

$$VD/VT = \frac{Pa_{CO_2} - PET_{CO_2}}{Pa_{CO_2}} \quad (1)$$

The VD/VT is usually 0.30 to 0.35 in healthy persons breathing spontaneously. In patients with normal lungs being mechanically ventilated, the VD/VT is approximately 0.50.

Carbon dioxide production ($\dot{V}CO_2$) may be measured by closed systems in patients breathing spontaneously or receiving mechanical ventilation. Once $\dot{V}CO_2$ is measured, VD/VT is calculated from Equation 1, and VA is inferred, one can determine which abnormality in the alveolar ventilation relationship (Equations 5 and 6) is responsible for ventilatory failure.

Three other variables that reflect ventilatory capability are the maximum inspiratory pressure (MIP), the vital capacity (VC), and the ratio of the forced expiratory volume in 1 second (FEV_1) to the forced VC. In the MIP maneuver, a manometer is used to measure the negative pressure that patients can generate when inspiring from a low lung volume. An MIP that is less negative than -20 cm H_2O suggests the need for ventilatory support, whereas an MIP that is more negative than -20 cm H_2O correlates with successful weaning from mechanical ventilation.

The VC, the greatest amount of gas that can be inhaled or exhaled in a single breath, can be measured with any of a variety of spirometers. The normal VC is approximately 50 ml per kilogram of body weight. A VC of less than 10 ml per kilogram usually indicates the need for institution or continuation of mechanical ventilation. The FEV_1 can also be measured by spirometry. Normally, the FEV_1 is approximately 75 to 80 per cent of the forced VC; reductions in this ratio may occur in patients with airways obstruction due to asthma or chronic obstructive pulmonary disease (COPD).

ASSESSMENT OF RESPIRATORY SYSTEM COMPLIANCE. The amount of pressure required to increase the volume of the lungs and the thoracic cavity is termed the compliance of the respiratory system (CRS). When determined in a patient who is being mechanically ventilated, effective respiratory system compliance (CEFF) is equal to the maximum or peak airway pressure (Pmax) required to deliver a given VT minus the amount of PEEP. Thus,

$$C_{EFF} = \frac{V_T}{P_{max} - PEEP} \quad (2)$$

Because it is a dynamic measurement made when gas is flowing, CEFF includes the resistance to gas flow in the airways and ventilator tubing, as well as the volume and pressure characteristics of the lungs and chest wall. It will be influenced by airways obstruction, airway secretions, and the diameter of the endotracheal tube.

Static respiratory system compliance (CSTAT) is a measure of the airway pressure (PSTAT) required to distend the lungs and maintain the increase in volume after a VT has been delivered and gas is not flowing into or out of lungs. The amount of PEEP should be subtracted in determining this pressure. Thus,

$$C_{STAT} = \frac{V_T}{P_{STAT} - PEEP} \quad (3)$$

Because it is a static measurement, CSTAT reflects only the compliance of the lungs and chest wall and is not affected by resistance to gas flow. It will be decreased (normal level is 50 to 60 ml per centimeter of water) by conditions, such as ARDS, that decrease lung volume. Weaning from mechanical ventilation is difficult if CSTAT is less than 25 ml per centimeter of water.

ASSESSMENT OF AUTO-PEEP. Another measurement that may be made on mechanically ventilated patients is intrinsic or auto-PEEP. Auto-PEEP occurs in patients with airways obstruction and other disorders who fail to complete expiration either during spontaneous breathing or before they receive the next breath from a mechanical ventilator. This results in air trapping that produces positive pressure at end-expiration. The auto-PEEP effect can reduce cardiac filling pressures and $\dot{Q}_T$ and elevate PPAO readings unless it, like intentionally administered PEEP, is accounted for. Auto-PEEP can be measured in mechanically ventilated patients by stopping airflow at end-expiration just before the next breath, allowing the pressure in the airways and the ventilator tubing to equilibrate, and reading the pressure from the ventilator manometer.

ASSESSMENT OF ARTERIAL OXYGENATION. Just as measurement of Pa_{CO_2} is the means by which ventilatory failure is diagnosed, failure of arterial oxygenation can be diagnosed only by determining the Pa_{O_2}. Introducing the values for Pa_{CO_2} and the partial pressure of oxygen in inspired gas (PI_{O_2}) into the alveolar gas equation (Equation 7) enables determination of the alveolar-arterial oxygen pressure difference, $P(A - a)_{O_2}$, as will be discussed. This information in turn provides insight into the probable cause of hypoxemia in a given patient.

Because systemic arterial blood sampling may be associated with complications, a less invasive approximation of the state of arterial oxygenation often is desirable. This may be accomplished through pulse oximetry, in which the differential absorption of

certain wavelengths of light passed through a finger or other appendage is used to calculate the systemic arterial oxygen saturation (Sa_{O_2}). This technique accurately measures Sa_{O_2} above levels of 80 per cent in patients with adequate peripheral blood flow. It is particularly helpful as a continuous measurement in patients who are relatively stable and in whom a normal oxyhemoglobin saturation curve enables good correlation between Sa_{O_2} and Pa_{O_2}. The Sa_{O_2} measured by oximetry does not account for hemoglobin that is saturated by substances other than oxygen, such as carbon monoxide.

The Sa_{O_2} may also be derived from the Pa_{O_2}. The Sa_{O_2}, the hemoglobin (Hb) concentration, and Pa_{O_2} are the determinants of the systemic arterial oxygen content (Ca_{O_2}). (Equation 9). Once Ca_{O_2} is known, it can be multiplied by the $\dot{Q}_T$ to determine oxygen transport ($\dot{T}o_2$) (Equation 8). Thus, systemic arterial blood gas analysis helps diagnose failure of oxygen transport, determine the abnormalities responsible for such failure, and assess its severity.

Pulmonary arterial blood gas analysis provides information about the partial pressure, saturation, and content of oxygen in mixed venous blood ($P\bar{v}_{O_2}$, $S\bar{v}_{O_2}$, $C\bar{v}_{O_2}$). In addition, $S\bar{v}_{O_2}$ may be measured continuously with oximetric pulmonary artery catheters. In combination with values for $\dot{Q}_T$ and Ca_{O_2} obtained by systemic arterial blood gas analysis, the $C\bar{v}_{O_2}$ may be inserted into Equation 10 to calculate the oxygen consumption ($\dot{V}o_2$). Alternatively, $\dot{V}o_2$ may be determined directly by measuring concentrations of oxygen in inspired and expired gas and the inspired and expired volumes. Even if $\dot{V}o_2$ is not calculated or precisely known, the decrease in $P\bar{v}_{O_2}$, $S\bar{v}_{O_2}$, and $C\bar{v}_{O_2}$ and the increase in the arterial–mixed venous content difference, $C(a - \bar{v})_{O_2}$, that characterize inadequate oxygen transport can be assessed by analysis of systemic and pulmonary artery blood gas samples, as can the increase in $P\bar{v}_{O_2}$, $S\bar{v}_{O_2}$, and $C\bar{v}_{O_2}$ and the decrease in $C(a - \bar{v})_{O_2}$ that characterize inadequate oxygen extraction.

MEASUREMENT OF SHUNT FRACTION. Finally, combined systemic and pulmonary artery blood gas analysis may be used to quantitate the contribution to hypoxemia of right-to-left intrapulmonary shunting of blood. This analysis may be performed in patients receiving 100 per cent oxygen, using the following shunt equation:

$$\frac{\dot{Q}_S}{\dot{Q}_T} = \frac{Cc'_{O_2} - Ca_{O_2}}{Cc'_{O_2} - C\bar{v}_{O_2}} \quad (4)$$

where $\dot{Q}_S$ is the volume of shunted blood and Cc'_{O_2} is an approximation of end-capillary blood oxygen content, assuming Pc'_{O_2} to be the same as PA_{O_2}, and calculating Cc'_{O_2} on the basis of that assumption. The shunt equation is based on the Fick equation (Equation 10), which will be discussed. A simpler but less precise way of estimating intrapulmonary shunt, which is also based on the Fick equation and assumes a normal $C(a - \bar{v})_{O_2}$ of 5 ml per deciliter of blood, is to divide the $P(A - a)_{O_2}$ by 15 to 20. The normal $\dot{Q}_S$ is 7 per cent or less of $\dot{Q}_T$.

ASSESSMENT OF TISSUE OXYGENATION. As suggested by the previous discussion, the data obtained from combined systemic and pulmonary artery blood gas analysis may be very helpful in managing critically ill patients. Nevertheless, not all

TABLE 71–4. HEMODYNAMIC PATTERNS IN CARDIOVASCULAR AND RESPIRATORY DISORDERS

Situation	PSA	PRA	PPA	PPAO	$C(a - \bar{v})_{O_2}$	$\dot{Q}_T$	PVR	SVR	$P\bar{v}_{O_2}$
Airways obstruction	→↓	→↑	↑	→	→	→↓	↑	→	→
Hypovolemic shock	↓	↓	↓	↓	↑	↓	↑	↑	↓
Pulmonary thromboembolism	↓	↑	↑	→↓	↑	↓	↑	↑	↓
Cardiac tamponade	↓	↑	↑	↑	↑	↓	→	↑	↓
Cardiogenic shock	↓	↑	↑	↑	↑	↓	↑	↑	↓
Right ventricular infarction	↓	↑	→	→	↑	↓	→	→↑	↓
Distributive shock	↓	↓	↓	↓	↓	↑	↓	↓	↑

PSA = systemic arterial pressure; PRA = right atrial or central venous pressure; PPA = pulmonary arterial pressure; PPAO = pulmonary arterial occlusion pressure; $C(a - \bar{v})_{O_2}$ = arterial–mixed venous oxygen content difference; $\dot{Q}_T$ = cardiac output; PVR = pulmonary vascular resistance; SVR = systemic vascular resistance; $P\bar{v}_{O_2}$ = mixed venous oxygen tension.

such patients require such sophisticated monitoring techniques, and the techniques still cannot provide an ideal assessment of oxygenation of a tissue level. The same can be said for serial measurement of serum lactate levels, which some physicians use as a monitoring tool. Despite these and other technologic advances in critical care monitoring, assessment of tissue oxygenation probably is best performed by analyzing individual organ system function by simple biochemical tests, such as renal and hepatic indices, measurement of urine output, and observation of mental status.

PATHOPHYSIOLOGY OF CIRCULATORY AND RESPIRATORY FAILURE

Aerobic metabolism in humans is made possible by four processes that involve the cardiovascular and respiratory systems: (1) *ventilation*, in which oxygen is inhaled from the atmosphere and carbon dioxide is excreted into it; (2) *arterial oxygenation*, in which oxygen is transferred from the alveoli into mixed venous blood in the pulmonary capillaries in exchange for carbon dioxide; (3) *oxygen transport*, in which oxygen is carried in systemic arterial blood to the tissues; and (4) *oxygen extraction and utilization*, in which the tissues take up oxygen from the blood and give up carbon dioxide, which is transported in mixed venous blood to the lungs.

Impairments in any or all of these four processes commonly occur in critically ill patients. As a result, much of critical care monitoring and management involves preventing or correcting the various impairments. In the following section, the four processes are discussed in greater detail, and examples of disorders that cause disturbances in the processes are given (Table 71–5).

Ventilation

The adequacy of ventilation is determined by measurement of the Pa_{CO_2} in systemic arterial blood. At sea level, the normal Pa_{CO_2} is approximately 40 mm Hg. Hypoventilation and hypercapnia exist when the Pa_{CO_2} exceeds this level, and hypercapnic respiratory failure is diagnosed when the Pa_{CO_2} is 50 mm Hg or

TABLE 71–5. KINDS OF CIRCULATORY AND RESPIRATORY FAILURE

Failure	Definition	Abnormality	Examples
Ventilatory failure	Inadequate alveolar ventilation	High Pa_{CO_2}	Narcotic or sedative drug overdose Asthma Chronic obstructive pulmonary disease Neuromuscular diseases
Failure of arterial oxygenation	Inadequate oxygenation of systemic arterial blood	Low Pa_{O_2}	Pneumonia Asthma Chronic obstructive pulmonary disease
Failure of oxygen transport	Inadequate supply of oxygenated blood to tissues	Low Ca_{O_2} or $\dot{Q}T$ or both Low $P\bar{v}_{O_2}$, $S\bar{v}_{O_2}$, $C\bar{v}_{O_2}$ Increased $C(a - \bar{v})_{O_2}$ Lactic acidosis	Anemia Carbon monoxide poisoning Hypovolemic shock Obstructive shock Cardiogenic shock Cardiorespiratory arrest
Failure of oxygen extraction	Inadequate tissue oxygen uptake	Low $\dot{V}_{O_2}$ High $P\bar{v}_{O_2}$, $S\bar{v}_{O_2}$, $C\bar{v}_{O_2}$ Decreased $C(a - \bar{v})_{O_2}$ Lactic acidosis	Cyanide poisoning Distributive shock Adult respiratory distress syndrome Multiple organ system failure

Pa_{CO_2} = systemic arterial carbon dioxide tension; Pa_{O_2} = systemic arterial oxygen tension; Ca_{O_2} = systemic arterial oxygen content; $\dot{Q}T$ = cardiac output; $P\bar{v}_{O_2}$ = mixed venous oxygen tension; $S\bar{v}_{O_2}$ = mixed venous oxygen saturation; $C\bar{v}_{O_2}$ = mixed venous oxygen content; $C(a - \bar{v})_{O_2}$ = arterial–mixed venous oxygen content difference; $\dot{V}_{O_2}$ = oxygen consumption.

greater at sea level, unless this is a compensation for metabolic alkalosis. Hypercapnic respiratory failure is also called ventilatory failure.

The pathophysiology of ventilatory failure is explained by examining the factors that determine the Pa_{CO_2}. The Pa_{CO_2} is directly related to the body's carbon dioxide production per minute ($\dot{V}_{CO_2}$) and inversely proportional to $\dot{V}A$. Thus,

$$Pa_{CO_2} \simeq \frac{\dot{V}_{CO_2}}{\dot{V}_A} \qquad (5)$$

The normal $\dot{V}_{CO_2}$ of a healthy young person is approximately 200 ml per minute; the $\dot{V}_A$ is approximately 5 liters.

Alveolar ventilation is equal to the $\dot{V}E$, which is the amount of gas that enters the upper respiratory tract each minute, minus the $\dot{V}D$, which is the inhaled gas that does not participate in gas exchange, either because it remains in the upper airways or because it enters areas of the lung where blood flow is insufficient for the matching of ventilation and perfusion. The minute ventilation is the product of $\dot{V}T$ (normally 450 ml) and F (normally 12 to 22 per minute). Thus,

$$Pa_{CO_2} \simeq \frac{\dot{V}_{CO_2}}{(\dot{V}_T \times F) - \dot{V}_D} \qquad (6)$$

From Equations 5 and 6 it follows that hypercapnia can occur (1) if $\dot{V}_{CO_2}$ increases and $\dot{V}_A$ does not, (2) if $\dot{V}_A$ decreases and $\dot{V}_{CO_2}$ does not, or (3) if $\dot{V}_D$ increases out of proportion to $\dot{V}E$. An example of the first situation might be a patient who becomes febrile owing to sepsis syndrome and thereby increases $\dot{V}_{CO_2}$ but cannot increase $\dot{V}_A$ because of respiratory muscle weakness. Patients with severe asthma and COPD may have ventilatory failure because $\dot{V}_A$ is reduced owing to airways obstruction, especially when $\dot{V}_{CO_2}$ is increased. A primary reduction in $\dot{V}_A$ also is seen in narcotic or sedative drug overdose. Diseases such as ARDS, in which $\dot{V}_D$ may increase owing to vascular obstruction, can cause ventilatory failure if patients cannot increase $\dot{V}E$ because of, for example, oversedation.

The physiologic consequences of hypercapnia depend largely on the rate of increase in Pa_{CO_2} and the level it reaches. An increased Pa_{CO_2} dilates cerebral blood vessels, increases cerebral blood flow, and may cause headaches and eventually obtundation. More important, every 1 mm Hg rise in Pa_{CO_2} causes the pH in systemic arterial blood to fall by 0.0075 unit. The acute respiratory acidosis that results may depress the function of the heart and other organs until the plasma $[HCO_3^-]$ rises and buffers the fall in pH. Thus, gradual increases in Pa_{CO_2} are compensated for by an increasing $[HCO_3^-]$. Chronic metabolic alkalosis of this sort is of little physiologic consequence. However, as discussed in the next section, an increase in Pa_{CO_2} will result in a reduction of the partial pressure of oxygen in alveolar gas and thus a decrease in the partial pressure of oxygen in systemic arterial blood unless supplemental oxygen is administered.

Arterial Oxygenation

The adequacy of arterial oxygenation is determined by the Pa_{O_2}, which in healthy young persons is approximately 95 mm Hg at sea level. Hypoxemia exists when the Pa_{O_2} is below this value, and hypoxemic respiratory failure is diagnosed if the Pa_{O_2} is less than 50 to 60 mm Hg at sea level. Hypoxemic respiratory failure is also called failure of arterial oxygenation.

The alveolar gas equation states that the partial pressure of oxygen in alveolar gas (PA_{O_2}) is equal to the partial pressure of oxygen in inspired air (PI_{O_2}) minus the partial pressure of carbon dioxide in alveolar gas (PA_{CO_2}), divided by the respiratory quotient (RQ). Thus,

$$PA_{O_2} = PI_{O_2} - \frac{PA_{CO_2}}{RQ} \qquad (7)$$

The PI_{O_2} is equal to the fraction of inspired oxygen (FI_{O_2} normally = 0.21) times the barometric pressure corrected for water vapor ($PB - 47$ mm Hg) and is approximately 150 mm Hg at sea level.

The PA_{CO_2} is equal to the Pa_{CO_2} and therefore normally is 40 mm Hg. The RQ is the ratio of $\dot{V}CO_2$ to $\dot{V}O_2$ and usually is assumed to be 0.8. Substituting these values in Equation 7, the PA_{O_2} should equal approximately 100 mm Hg in healthy young persons breathing ambient air at sea level. Normally, with an FI_{O_2} of 0.21, the difference between PA_{O_2} and Pa_{O_2}, the $P(A - a)_{O_2}$, is less than 10 mm Hg.

From Equation 7 and the normal value for $P(A - a)_{O_2}$ just derived, it follows that a fall in the Pa_{O_2} to below 50 to 60 mm Hg can occur if PI_{O_2} decreases, if Pa_{CO_2} increases, or if $P(A - a)_{O_2}$ increases. A marked decrease in PI_{O_2} might occur while breathing air at high altitude where PB is reduced or in a fire that consumes oxygen; in the latter case, FI_{O_2} will be less than 0.21. An increase in Pa_{CO_2} above 40 mm Hg is ventilatory failure by definition; thus, ventilatory failure may cause failure of arterial oxygenation unless the PI_{O_2} is increased by the administration of supplemental oxygen to offset the fall in PA_{O_2}. An increased $P(A - a)_{O_2}$ is primarily the result of two processes: ventilation-perfusion mismatching and shunting of mixed venous blood either within the heart or past unventilated areas of the lung, the most extreme form of ventilation-perfusion mismatching. The hypoxemia associated with asthma and COPD is largely attributable to ventilation-perfusion mismatching, whereas the hypoxemia associated with ARDS is attributable to intrapulmonary shunting.

The physiologic consequences of hypoxemia depend on the rate of decline of Pa_{O_2} and its severity and duration. Some persons who are born at high altitude or who have congenital cyanotic heart disease live normally with a Pa_{O_2} less than 50 mm Hg. However, failure of arterial oxygenation usually leads to some mental impairment and reduced exercise performance regardless of its chronicity, and it is likely to be catastrophic in depressing organ function in patients unaccustomed to hypoxemia.

Oxygen Transport

The amount of oxygen transported to the tissues is the product of the cardiac output $\dot{Q}T$ and the Ca_{O_2}. Thus,

$$\dot{T}O_2 = (\dot{Q}T)(Ca_{O_2}) \tag{8}$$

The Ca_{O_2} is the oxygen that is bound to Hb plus the small amount that is dissolved in plasma. This is described by the following equation:

$$Ca_{O_2} = (1.39)(Hb)(Sa_{O_2}) + (0.003)(Pa_{O_2}) \tag{9}$$

where 1.39 is the oxygen-carrying capacity of Hb in milliliters per gram and 0.003 is the solubility of oxygen in plasma at 37°C in milliliters of oxygen per milliliter of blood. If arterial blood has an Hb concentration of 15 grams per milliliter and the Hb is 98 per cent saturated, the Hb carries 19.7 ml of oxygen per deciliter of blood. The amount of oxygen in solution at a Pa_{O_2} of 95 mm Hg is 0.3 ml per deciliter of blood. Thus, the Ca_{O_2} normally is 20 ml of oxygen per deciliter of blood, or 200 ml of oxygen per liter. Multiplying by the normal $\dot{Q}T$ of 5 liters per minute, $\dot{T}O_2$ is approximately 1 liter per minute.

The relationship between Pa_{O_2}, Sa_{O_2}, and Ca_{O_2} is described by the oxyhemoglobin dissociation curve (Fig. 71–2). Some laboratories use an idealized version of this curve to calculate the Sa_{O_2} and Ca_{O_2} from the measured Pa_{O_2}. However, the idealized curve assumes that Hb and metabolic status are normal. In patients the oxyhemoglobin dissociation curve frequently is shifted to the left owing to alkalosis, Hb with a high affinity for oxygen, or carbon monoxide poisoning (in which Hb also binds carbon monoxide more avidly than oxygen, causing a functional anemia). As a result of this left shift, the Sa_{O_2} is higher at a given Pa_{O_2}, so less oxygen is extracted by the tissues. By contrast, the curve is shifted to the right by acidosis, Hb with a weak affinity for oxygen, and 2,3-diphosphoglycerate, which is produced in increased amounts in response to hypoxia. This right shift results in a lower Sa_{O_2} for a given Pa_{O_2}, so that more oxygen is extracted by the tissues. The true Sa_{O_2} can be known only by oximetric analysis of arterial blood, a fact that is of particular relevance in evaluating patients with carbon monoxide poisoning.

Inspection of the oxyhemoglobin dissociation curve reveals other important aspects of $\dot{T}O_2$. One is that with a normal Hb concentration the Ca_{O_2} remains near 20 ml per deciliter of blood above a Pa_{O_2} of 60 mm Hg and Sa_{O_2} of 90 per cent, but the Ca_{O_2} diminishes rapidly below these levels. Because of this, the physiologic consequences of hypoxemia usually begin to occur at a Pa_{O_2} of approximately 60 mm Hg and can be avoided if the Pa_{O_2} is raised above this level. Note also that the Ca_{O_2} can be increased only slightly by raising the Pa_{O_2} above the normal level of 95 mm Hg. This is because the Hb is fully saturated at this level and only a little more oxygen can be dissolved in blood.

The oxyhemoglobin dissociation curve also gives information regarding the $P\bar{v}_{O_2}$, $S\bar{v}_{O_2}$, and $C\bar{v}_{O_2}$. The relationship between these values and their counterparts in systemic arterial blood is described by the Fick equation, which holds that the oxygen extracted by the tissues, the $\dot{V}O_2$, is the difference between the oxygen transported to the tissues, the $\dot{T}O_2$, and the oxygen returned from the tissues in mixed venous blood to the right side of the heart, which is the product of $\dot{Q}T$ and the $C\bar{v}_{O_2}$. By combining terms, the Fick equation can be expressed as follows:

$$\dot{V}O_2 = \dot{Q}T (C[a - \bar{v}]_{O_2}) \tag{10}$$

Figure 71–2 shows that the $P\bar{v}_{O_2}$ normally is approximately 40 mm Hg, the $S\bar{v}_{O_2}$ is 75 mm Hg, the $C\bar{v}_{O_2}$ is 15 ml per deciliter of blood, and the $C(a - \bar{v})_{O_2}$ is 5 ml per deciliter blood; given a $\dot{Q}T$ of 5 liters per minute, $\dot{V}O_2$ is approximately 250 ml of oxygen per minute. These values indicate that normally only 25 per cent of the oxygen in systemic arterial blood is extracted by the tissues, leaving a large oxygen reserve. Patients characteristically call upon this reserve when $\dot{V}O_2$ increases or when $\dot{T}O_2$ decreases owing to a fall in $\dot{Q}T$, Ca_{O_2}, or both. This in turn causes a decrease in the $P\bar{v}_{O_2}$, $S\bar{v}_{O_2}$, and $C\bar{v}_{O_2}$ and an increase in the $C(a - \bar{v})_{O_2}$.

A shift from aerobic to anaerobic metabolism and an increased production of lactic acid may be observed in conditions such as severe anemia; carbon monoxide poisoning; hypovolemic, obstructive, and cardiogenic shock; and cardiorespiratory arrest. These findings are associated with decreases in the $P\bar{v}_{O_2}$ below 30 mm Hg, in the $S\bar{v}_{O_2}$ below 60 per cent, and in the $C\bar{v}_{O_2}$ below 10 ml of oxygen per deciliter of blood, and an increase in the $C(a - \bar{v})_{O_2}$ above 10 ml per deciliter. Such values are indicative of failure of oxygen transport.

From Equation 8, it can be seen that inadequate oxygen transport can result from a decrease either in Ca_{O_2} or in $\dot{Q}T$. Cardiac output itself is the product of HR and SV. Thus,

$$\dot{Q}T = (HR)(SV) \tag{11}$$

Heart rate, which normally averages about 70 beats per minute, is determined by autonomic influences on the intrinsic cardiac pacemakers. Stroke volume, which averages 70 ml per beat, is determined by three factors: (1) preload, the length of cardiac muscle fibers at the start of contraction, which is equal to ventricular end-diastolic volume and is approximated as end-diastolic pressure; (2) afterload, the tension the heart muscle develops during systole, which usually is equated with the blood pressure or the vascular resistance that the ventricle must overcome to pump blood into either the pulmonary or the systemic circulation; and (3) contractility, the inotropic state of the muscle, which may be expressed as the velocity of muscle shortening.

Cardiac output also is equal to the perfusion pressure (Pcirc) across the circulation into which the ventricle is pumping, which is the difference between arterial inflow and venous outflow pressures, divided by the resistance of that circulation (Rcirc). Thus,

$$Rcirc = Pcirc/\dot{Q}T \tag{12}$$

Pulmonary vascular resistance is equal to $\overline{P}PA$ minus $\overline{P}LA$ divided by $\dot{Q}T$. Normally, $\overline{P}PA$ = approximately 15 mm Hg, $\overline{P}LA$ = 10 mm Hg, and $\dot{Q}T$ = 5 liters per minute, so PVR = 1 mm Hg per liter per minute; this usually is multipled by 80 and expressed as 80 dyne • sec • cm^{-5}. On the other hand, SVR is equal to $\overline{P}SA$ minus $\overline{P}RA$, divided by the $\dot{Q}T$. Normally, $\overline{P}SA$ = approximately 85 mm Hg, $\overline{P}RA$ = 5 mm Hg, and $\dot{Q}T$ = 5 liters per minute, so SVR = 16 mm Hg per liter per minute, or 1280 dyne • sec • cm^{-5}.

Oxygen Extraction

Some critically ill patients shift from aerobic to anaerobic metabolism and develop lactic acidosis despite what appears to be a normal or even increased $\dot{Q}T$ and Ca_{O_2}. Such patients have what may be called failure of oxygen extraction. They characteristically have a $P\bar{v}_{O_2}$ of greater than 60 mm Hg, a $S\bar{v}_{O_2}$ of greater than 80 per cent, a $C\bar{v}_{O_2}$ of greater than 18 ml of oxygen per milliliter, and a $C(a - \bar{v})_{O_2}$ of less than 5 ml of oxygen per milliliter of blood. In keeping with Equation 10, failure of oxygen extraction is characterized by a reduction in $\dot{V}_{O_2}$. Such a reduction occurs in cyanide poisoning, in which the cyanide ion interrupts intracellular mitochondrial oxygen transport. More common examples are distributive shock, ARDS, and the syndrome of multiple organ system failure (MOSF).

GENERAL MANAGEMENT OF CIRCULATORY AND RESPIRATORY FAILURE

Abnormalities in ventilation, arterial oxygenation, oxygen transport, and oxygen extraction may exist separately or coexist in critically ill patients As a result, management of such patients may require therapy to improve these processes either independently or at the same time. The following section provides a general approach to improving ventilation, arterial oxygenation, oxygen transport, and oxygen extraction.

Therapy to Improve Ventilation

The Pa_{CO_2} may be improved by manipulating the variables that affect it: $\dot{V}_{CO_2}$ and $\dot{V}A$ ($\dot{V}A$ is equal to $\dot{V}E - \dot{V}D$). Manipulation of $\dot{V}A$ may involve any or all components of the respiratory system. These include the respiratory control centers in the brain stem that regulate $\dot{V}A$, the nerves that transmit messages from the control centers to the respiratory muscles, the muscles themselves, the chest wall to which the muscles are attached, the pleura that lines the lungs, the lung parenchyma, and the upper and lower airways.

Ventilation may be improved in patients who have overdosed on narcotics by the administration of intravenous naloxone in 0.4-mg doses as required. Antagonists to benzodiazepines and other sedatives are not yet generally available in the United States, although the excretion of some of the drugs that depress ventilation may be enhanced by hemodialysis or charcoal hemoperfusion. At the very least, narcotics and sedatives should be administered cautiously to patients at risk of ventilatory failure. Intravenous doxapram in a bolus of 140 mg and a continuous infusion of 2 mg per minute has been used to overcome drug-induced ventilatory depression and to forestall mechanical ventilation in a variety of patients whose ventilatory failure is thought to be reversible, such as those recovering from anesthesia or having exacerbations of COPD. However, neither this agent nor other ventilatory stimulants can forestall mechanical ventilation indefinitely.

Disorders of the chest wall, such as in massive obesity and kyphoscoliosis, are not usually amenable to specific treatment. This is not true, however, of neuromuscular diseases that cause respiratory muscle weakness or paralysis, as will be discussed. Beyond therapies for neuromuscular diseases, there are few measures that improve respiratory muscle weakness. Theophylline increases ventilatory capacity in some, but not all, patients with COPD. Nutrition also improves respiratory muscle function to a limited extent, but it also increases $\dot{V}_{CO_2}$, which may offset any increase in $\dot{V}E$.

Pleural and parenchymal diseases limit $\dot{V}A$ by restricting lung expansion and by increasing $\dot{V}D$. These disorders also increase the work of breathing, which increases $\dot{V}_{CO_2}$ and may fatigue the respiratory muscles. Evacuation of the pleural space, usually by means of tube thoracostomy, is called for in patients compromised by pneumothorax, hemothorax, or pleural empyema.

Anatomic obstruction of the upper airways should be removed or bypassed when it causes or could cause hypercapnia; this rule applies to excessive soft tissues as well as to aspirated material. Inspissated secretions frequently cause or contribute to ventilatory failure in a variety of patients, including those with neuromuscular diseases, asthma and COPD, and ARDS. Removal of secretions may be facilitated by chest physiotherapy or gentle endotracheal suctioning. In a recent study, iodinated glycerol facilitated secretion clearance in outpatients with COPD, although the effects of this oral mucolytic agent on $\dot{V}A$ and Pa_{CO_2} were not determined.

The $\dot{V}_{CO_2}$ may be reduced by lowering the metabolic rate and thereby the need for increased ventilation. For example, seizures may respond to phenytoin administration (50 mg per minute given intravenously, up to a loading dose of 1000 mg, followed by 300 mg per day). Shivering may be prevented by chlorpromazine (25 to 75 mg given intramuscularly). Fever may be reduced by the administration of antipyretics, such as aspirin or acetaminophen, which are more effective than cooling blankets or sponge baths in decreasing core temperature.

Unfortunately, the increase in $\dot{V}D$ caused by obliteration of the pulmonary vasculature due to disorders such as ARDS is rarely amenable to medical measures. Increases in the $\dot{V}D$ caused by pulmonary thromboembolism may be treated with thrombolytic agents, such as streptokinase.

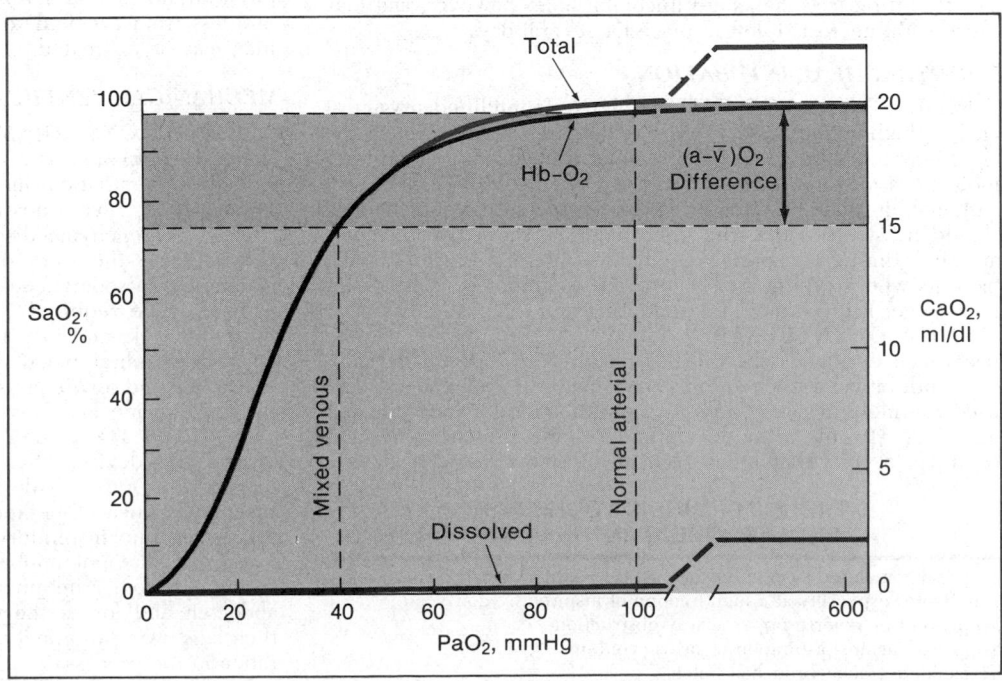

FIGURE 71–2. The oxyhemoglobin dissociation curve, relating the partial pressure of oxygen in systemic arterial blood (Pa_{O_2}), in millimeters of mercury, to systemic arterial oxygen saturation (Sa_{O_2}), in per cent, and to the oxygen content of systemic arterial blood (Ca_{O_2}), in milliliters per deciliter of blood. A normal hemoglobin (Hb) concentration of 15 grams per deciliter of blood is assumed, as is an unshifted dissociation curve. Note that the curve descends steeply below Pa_{O_2} values of 50 to 60 mm Hg, indicating severely reduced oxygen-carrying capacity of Hb below this Pa_{O_2}. The lower line represents oxygen bound to Hb plus oxygen dissolved. Note that dissolved oxygen contributes little to Ca_{O_2} at a Pa_{O_2} in the normal range. (From Luce JM, Tyler ML, Pierson DJ: Intensive Respiratory Care. Philadelphia, W.B. Saunders Company, 1984.)

Therapy to Improve Arterial Oxygenation

The Pa_{O_2} may be improved by manipulating the variables that affect it: Pa_{CO_2}, P_{IO_2}, and $P(A - a)_{O_2}$. Thus, if hypoventilation is the sole cause of hypoxemia, as might be the case in a narcotic overdose, the Pa_{O_2} increases as the Pa_{CO_2} decreases in response to naloxone. Similarly, if the P_{IO_2} is reduced by the combustion of oxygen in a fire or by residence at high altitude, the Pa_{O_2} should improve if the patient breathes atmospheric air with an F_{IO_2} at the same P_B as at sea level. Patients whose $P(A - a)_{O_2}$ is increased require therapy for the underlying cause of their hypoxemia as well as supplemental oxygen.

POSITIONING. Alveolar collapse, also called atelectasis, commonly occurs in dependent regions of the lung. Atelectasis is particularly problematic in supine patients whose lung expansion is limited by obesity, pain on deep breathing, or the presence of restricting bandages over the abdomen or chest. Positioning such patients upright from time to time and relieving their pain with narcotics may greatly improve the Pa_{O_2}.

Adults with unilateral parenchymal lung disorders, such as pneumonia, may become more hypoxemic when their diseased lung is dependent. The Pa_{O_2} of these patients may improve when they lie on the side of the nondiseased lung. Pulmonary edema fluid tends to collect in dependent lung regions because the intravascular hydrostatic pressure is greatest there. For this reason, the Pa_{O_2} of patients with pulmonary edema may improve, at least temporarily, if they are moved from the supine to the prone position. Unfortunately, such positioning may complicate nursing care.

OXYGEN DELIVERY SYSTEMS. Hypoxemia usually responds to increasing the F_{IO_2} and thereby the P_{IO_2}. The hypoxemia associated with disorders such as asthma and COPD that are characterized by ventilation-perfusion mismatching but not by intrapulmonary shunt usually is relieved by supplemental oxygen at a low F_{IO_2}. An F_{IO_2} of 0.24 to 0.35 can usually be achieved by delivering oxygen through nasal prongs at flow rates of 5 to 6 liters per minute; higher flow rates dry the nasal mucosa and do not further increase the F_{IO_2} because patients dilute the oxygen with ambient air. Open face masks provide a higher flow of humidified, premixed air and oxygen at an F_{IO_2} of up to 0.5. Such masks can be combined with a Venturi device that allows precise setting of the F_{IO_2} to avoid ventilatory depression in patients who have chronic carbon dioxide retention.

Tightly fitting face masks with a nonrebreathing valve and reservoir bag can be used to provide even higher concentrations of oxygen in patients whose hypoxemia is caused by shunting associated with disorders such as severe pneumonia and ARDS. Tightly fitting face masks are uncomfortable, however, and may cause nasal necrosis if left in place for several days.

ENDOTRACHEAL INTUBATION

INDICATIONS FOR INTUBATION. Humidified oxygen at an F_{IO_2} higher than 0.50 is most reliably delivered through the closed system provided by an endotracheal tube. The other indications for endotracheal intubation are listed in Table 71–6. Although intubation often precedes mechanical ventilation, it should be stressed that the indications for these two therapies and their timing are not necessarily the same. For example, some patients who are intubated to prevent aspiration of gastric contents never require mechanical ventilation.

KINDS OF INTUBATION. Endotracheal intubation may be performed either via the translaryngeal route through the nose or mouth or via a tracheostomy. Tracheostomy tubes once were used routinely in patients requiring intubation for longer than 1 or 2 days. However, the development of low-pressure and high-compliance cuffs that limit tracheal damage from nasal or oral

TABLE 71–6. INDICATIONS FOR ENDOTRACHEAL INTUBATION

To provide a closed system for mechanical ventilation or oxygen
  delivery, especially at a high fraction of inspired oxygen
To prevent or reverse upper airway obstruction
To protect against aspiration of gastric contents
To facilitate tracheobronchial toilet

tubes, the demonstration that such tubes can be left in place for weeks and even months without severe sequelae, and the documentation of complications after tracheostomy have led to a preference for orotracheal or nasotracheal intubation over tracheostomy in all but a few patients. Such patients include those with laryngeal fractures and those who will require intubation for longer than a month or so. Tracheostomy tubes generally are more comfortable than translaryngeal tubes. Tracheostomy tubes also are easier to suction through, and talking may be made possible by fitting the tubes with a device that directs a stream of air retrograde through the larynx above the cuff site.

Nasal intubation provides good support for the endotracheal tube and often allows patients to swallow their secretions better than when the tube passes orally. Oral intubation may allow passage of a tube with a larger diameter (8 mm or more) than that which the nostril will accommodate and usually is the preferred route during emergency intubations. Whichever route is chosen, the tube diameter should be sufficient to seal the trachea without cuff pressures in excess of 20 to 25 mm Hg. These pressures should be monitored regularly. Tube position should be determined by chest radiograph immediately following insertion and on a regular basis thereafter. Intubation of the right mainstem bronchus, which extends from the trachea at less of an angle than the left mainstem bronchus, should be sought in particular.

COMPLICATIONS OF INTUBATION. In one study, more than half of all patients receiving endotracheal intubation suffered adverse consequences. Excessive cuff pressure requirements (>20 mm Hg), self-extubation, and inability to seal the airway were the most common complications with nasotracheal and orotracheal tubes, occurring in 62 per cent of all endotracheal intubations. Problems associated with tracheostomy, which occurred in 66 per cent of intubations, included stomal hemorrhage, excessive cuff pressure requirements, and subcutaneous emphysema. Follow-up studies of patients receiving intubation and mechanical ventilation revealed a higher incidence of tracheal stenosis after tracheostomy (65 per cent) compared with translaryngeal intubation (19 per cent), although laryngeal complications were more common with nasal and oral tubes.

EXTUBATION. In general, endotracheal tubes may be removed when the original indications for their insertion are no longer present. For example, extubation frequently follows the return of consciousness and an adequate gag reflex in previously comatose patients or the restoration of adequate ventilation and arterial oxygenation in patients with respiratory failure. If an endotracheal tube has been in place only briefly, it may be removed after secretions have been suctioned from above the cuff site and the patient has been seated upright. Depending on physical and mental status, a patient with a tracheostomy may progress from a cuffed to a noncuffed or fenestrated tube and then may be extubated.

MECHANICAL VENTILATION

INDICATIONS FOR MECHANICAL VENTILATION. Mechanical ventilation may be necessary in patients who have inadequate ventilation, inadequate arterial oxygenation, or both. Furthermore, severe airway obstruction caused by asthma and COPD or parenchymal disease caused by disorders such as ARDS may increase the work of breathing to levels that cannot be maintained in spontaneous breathing. Finally, mechanical ventilation may be required in clinically unstable patients, such as those in shock, and in patients who require hyperventilation to decrease cerebral blood flow and intracranial pressure. These indications and severe physiologic abnormalities that may indicate the need for mechanical ventilation are listed in Table 71–7.

DEVICES TO ASSIST VENTILATION. Ventilation can be assisted by devices that substitute for the functions of the diaphragm. One such device is the rocking bed, which swings the patient in a 60-degree arc, forcing the weak or paralyzed diaphragm into inspiratory and expiratory positions by gravity. Another is the pneumobelt, which is used by patients in the sitting position. The pneumobelt intermittently squeezes the abdomen and forces the diaphragm cephalad. The diaphragm then falls owing to gravity, creating a marginally effective inspiration in the process.

NEGATIVE-PRESSURE VENTILATION. Ventilation can

**TABLE 71–7. INDICATIONS FOR
MECHANICAL VENTILATION**

Acute hypercapnia
Minute ventilation greater than 10 L/min
Vital capacity less than 10–15 ml/kg body weight
Maximum inspiratory pressure more positive than −20 cm H_2O
Dead space to tidal volume fraction 0.60 or more
Acute hypoxemia (Pa_{O_2} less than 50–60 mm Hg, especially if inspired
  oxygen fraction is 0.4 or more, or $P(A − a)_{O_2}$ greater than 300 mm Hg
  on inspired FI_{O_2} of 1.0)
Clinical instability
Need for hyperventilation therapy

Pa_{CO_2} = systemic arterial carbon dioxide tension; Pa_{O_2} = systemic arterial oxygen
tension; $P(A − a)_{O_2}$ = systemic alveolar-arterial oxygen pressure difference;
FI_{O_2} = fraction of inspired oxygen.

also be supported by devices that generate a negative pressure around the chest during inspiration to substitute for the negative pleural and airway pressures normally created by contraction of the respiratory muscles. Negative-pressure ventilation can be achieved by enclosing the entire body, except the head and neck, in an "iron lung," by encompassing the thorax in a garment wrap, or by fitting a cuirass to the anterior chest. Like machines that substitute for the diaphragm, negative-pressure ventilators are best suited to stable patients with neuromuscular diseases whose lungs are normal and who do not require endotracheal intubation for delivery of oxygen at a high FI_{O_2}.

POSITIVE-PRESSURE VENTILATION. Because of the limitations of the aforementioned devices, positive-pressure ventilation (PPV) is the kind of mechanical ventilation most widely used today. With PPV, gas is delivered under positive pressure, usually through an endotracheal tube, into the airways and the lungs. In contrast to negative-pressure ventilation, PPV produces a positive airway pressure during inspiration. This pressure inflates the alveoli, providing both ventilation and arterial oxygenation while reducing the work of breathing.

Most positive-pressure ventilators may be used to deliver gas up to either a preset pressure or volume. The first approach allows limits to be established on the Pmax used for lung inflation but allows VT and hence V̇E to vary, depending on CRS. Alternatively, the ventilators may deliver a preset VT at whatever Pmax is required for lung inflation, which guarantees V̇E but may increase Pmax and pressure in the alveoli. Cycling of standard ventilators occurs whenever a certain pressure or volume is reached or at preset time intervals. Time-cycled ventilation is used primarily in infants or in adults who are ventilated at a high F that precludes pressure or volume cycling.

Modes of Positive-Pressure Ventilation. Perhaps the simplest mode of PPV is *controlled mechanical ventilation* (CMV), in which the ventilator delivers gas at a preset F and either a preset Pmax or VT (Table 71–8). Volume-cycled CMV most often is used in patients who are unconscious owing to illness or drugs, who are being intentionally hyperventilated, or who are recovering from anesthesia. Patients whose ventilatory drives are intact must often be hyperventilated or given sedatives to diminish their tendency to breathe asynchronously with the ventilator while receiving CMV. As with most other modes of PPV, an inspiratory to expiratory (I/E) ratio of 1:3 or less generally is used with CMV to allow adequate time for expiration and thereby avoid auto-PEEP. Because patients receiving CMV cannot increase their V̇E voluntarily, their ventilatory status must be followed closely. Thus, the advantage of CMV—complete control of ventilatory function—is also its major limitation.

Assisted mechanical ventilation (AMV) is a PPV mode in which the patient triggers the ventilator to deliver a preset VT. Triggering is accomplished by generating an airway pressure less than that in the ventilator and tubing; if the ventilator is sensitive to this pressure, it will increase F and V̇E in response to the demands of the patient. The machine will not trigger if it is insensitive, however, and if unduly sensitive it will trigger in response to small fluctuations in airway pressure in addition to attempts to breathe. The latter problem may be circumvented by establishing a proper sensitivity or, if this is not possible, by sedating the patient. Because sedation or neurologic changes may prevent patients from adjusting V̇E, an obligatory backup (or CMV) rate that will provide to the minimum allowable V̇E should

be used with AMV. The combination of AMV and CMV, which is called the assist/control mode, offers the great advantage of responding to changes in the patient's status without the close monitoring required of CMV. Traditionally, AMV and CMV have been referred to as intermittent positive-pressure ventilation (IPPV).

A third mode of PPV is *intermittent mandatory ventilation* (IMV), in which the ventilation delivers a preset VT at specific intervals while also providing a flow of gas for spontaneous breathing. The form of IMV most often used today is synchronized IMV (SIMV), in which ventilator breaths are delivered only after the end of a spontaneous expiration, so the patient's lungs are not hyperinflated by receiving spontaneous and machine-delivered inspirations simultaneously. With SIMV, the ventilator F may be set high enough to provide most, if not all, of the patient's V̇E initially; F then may be lowered as the patient improves. The potential benefits of SIMV include less asynchronous breathing and fewer sedation requirements, reducing mean airway pressure by combining spontaneous and machine breaths, and improving respiratory muscle function by allowing patients to breathe spontaneously. Disadvantages include the lack of a backup to guarantee V̇E in unstable patients and the possibility of causing respiratory muscle fatigue in patients who receive SIMV at a low ventilator F.

Another PPV mode is *high-frequency ventilation* (HFV), in which gas is delivered to the lungs using either a conventional ventilator with very high internal compressibility, high-pressure jet sources, or an oscillator that entrains ambient air. The ventilator F with HFV is greater than 60 per minute, the I/E ratio is very small, and the VT is either greater than the patient's anatomic VD (convective flow HFV) or less than the VD (nonconvective flow HFV). Although adequate ventilation with a VD/VT in excess of 1.0 would seem to be physiologically impossible, nonconvective flow HFV can achieve adequate carbon dioxide elimination in some patients, probably by enhanced diffusion in the lung. Both convective and nonconvective flow HFV usually produce a Pmax that is less than that with other modes of PPV, although the small I/E ratio usually produces auto-PEEP. The

**TABLE 71–8. MODES OF
POSITIVE-PRESSURE VENTILATION**

Mode	Description	Advantages/Disadvantages
Controlled mechanical ventilation (CMV)	Ventilator F, VT (and thus V̇E) preset	May be used with sedation or paralysis; ventilator cannot respond to ventilatory needs
Assisted mechanical ventilation (AMV) or assist/control	Ventilator VT preset, but patient can increase F (and thus V̇E)	Ventilator may respond to ventilatory needs; ventilator may undertrigger or overtrigger, depending on sensitivity
Intermittent mandatory ventilation (IMV)	Ventilator delivers preset VT and F, but patient may also breathe spontaneously	May decrease asynchronous breathing and sedation requirements; ventilator cannot respond to ventilatory needs
Synchronized intermittent mandatory ventilation (SIMV)	Same as IMV, but ventilator breaths delivered only after patient exhales	Same as IMV, plus patient's lungs not overinflated by receiving spontaneous and ventilator breaths at same time
High-frequency ventilation (HFV)	Ventilator F is increased and VT may be smaller than VD	May reduce peak airway pressure; may cause auto-PEEP
Pressure support ventilation (PSV)	Patient breathes at own F; VT determined by inspiratory pressure and respiratory system compliance	Increased comfort and decreased work of breathing; ventilator cannot respond to ventilatory needs
Pressure control ventilation (PCV)	Ventilator peak pressure, F, and inspiratory time preset	Peak inspiratory pressures may be decreased; hypoventilation may occur
Inverse ratio ventilation (IRV)	Inspiratory time exceeds expiratory time	May improve gas exchange by increasing time spent in inspiration; may cause auto-PEEP

F = rate; VT = tidal volume; VD = dead space; V̇E = minute ventilation; PEEP = positive end-expiratory pressure.

lower Pmax supports the use of HPV in treating patients with bronchopleural fistulas and conditions such as ARDS. However, ventilation and arterial oxygenation may be inadequate with HFV.

Pressure support ventilation (PSV), a fifth mode of PPV, augments spontaneous ventilatory efforts with a level of positive airway pressure that is preset to achieve a desired VT. This mode of ventilation allows patients to set their own F and timing of breaths, which may be more comfortable than other modes of PPV. Pressure support ventilation also is useful in overcoming the work of breathing through an endotracheal tube. Inasmuch as patients must initiate breaths with PSV, it should not be used in unstable patients and is most applicable during weaning.

A sixth PPV mode is *pressure control ventilation* (PCV). With this mode, gas is not delivered at a constant VT. Instead, it is delivered until a preset Pmax is reached, and the patient's VE is determined by the preset Pmax, ventilator F, and inspiratory time. In contrast to the square wave gas flow pattern used with CMV and AMV, inspiratory flow with PCV decelerates when the Pmax is reached. Advocates of this mode state that complications are reduced with PCV because Pmax is limited. In addition, the decelerating waveform is thought to provide ventilation of more alveoli. This feature might be particularly helpful in patients with ARDS, although PCV may not provide a VE that is sufficient to prevent hypoventilation.

Inverse ratio ventilation (IRV) is the final mode of PPV discussed in this chapter. With IRV, the I/E ratio is increased above the normal level of 1:3 or less to 1:1 or more. The rationale for this approach is that the longer duration of inspiratory positive pressure will open stiff or fluid-filled alveoli and the shorter expiratory time will not allow these alveoli to collapse. Peak airway pressure may also be lower than with other modes of PPV, although the increase in I/E time probably increases auto-PEEP. One drawback to IRV is that this mode often is uncomfortable and requires sedation or paralysis of the patient.

Complications of Positive-Pressure Ventilation. One possible result of PPV is that inflation at high pressure may damage the lung. Such damage has been described traditionally as barotrauma, implying that it is the consequence of pressure changes. However, because alveolar distention occurs as a result of changes in pressure, "volutrauma" may be an equally accurate term. Pneumothorax is a common kind of barotrauma, but subcutaneous and mediastinal emphysema, parenchymal lung cysts, and systemic air embolism may also occur. Some investigators believe that PPV at high pressures and volumes also causes bronchopulmonary dysplasia and diffuse alveolar damage identical to what is found in ARDS and may either cause or perpetuate the syndrome.

In addition to these respiratory effects, PPV may also compromise the cardiovascular system. This is because the positive airway pressure during inspiration reduces venous return to the chest and may depress QT. This effect may be increased if auto-PEEP is produced by PPV. On the other hand, it may be decreased if adequate time is allowed for airway and alveolar pressure to return to ambient levels during exhalation.

An early study reported pneumothorax in 4 per cent of patients receiving PPV in the form of CMV and AMV. Other complications included hyperventilation (11 per cent), hypoventilation (10 per cent), atelectasis (5 per cent), pneumonia (4 per cent), and massive gastric distention with air (1 per cent). Proponents of newer modes of PPV, such as PCV and IRV, claim that complications are limited with their use, but no data support this claim.

Weaning from Positive-Pressure Ventilation. Mechanical ventilatory support generally can be withdrawn when the reasons for its initiation no longer are present. This usually means complete or near-complete resolution of the patient's disease process, whether or not it involves the lungs. Such resolution should be reflected in clinical stability, a return of VE to below 10 l per minute, spontaneous VT to between 10 and 15 ml per kilogram, MIP to more negative than -20 cm H_2O, VD/VT to below 0.6, Pa_{O_2} to above 50 to 60 to 100 mm Hg on an FI_{O_2} of 0.4, and $P(A - a)_{O_2}$ to less than 300 mm Hg on an FI_{O_2} of 1.0.

Weaning from AMV and other modes of PPV may be accomplished by connecting the endotracheal tube to a piece of tubing, called a T-piece, that is connected to a source of oxygen that is diluted with air to create the desired FI_{O_2}. The patients then may breathe spontaneously through the T-piece at their own F and

TABLE 71–9. INDICATIONS FOR POSITIVE END-EXPIRATORY PRESSURE

To prevent or reverse atelectasis
To facilitate weaning from mechanical ventilation
To improve arterial oxygenation at a low inspired oxygen fraction

VT until they meet some or all of the weaning criteria just described. Otherwise healthy persons recovering from anesthesia or drug overdoses may be put on a T-piece when they wake up and may be extubated after a brief (15 to 30 minutes) period. Chronically ventilated patients may be put on a T-piece for a few minutes each hour or a few hours each day. When their respiratory muscles are less fatigued and they can tolerate longer periods on a T-piece, discontinuation of the ventilator may be appropriate.

Weaning from SIMV may be accomplished by progressively reducing the ventilator F until the patient can maintain an adequate VE by breathing spontaneously. Patients initially receiving AMV or other PPV modes can be weaned with SIMV without ever using a T-piece. Finally, SIMV and PSV may be combined to facilitate weaning. The PSV level is reduced as long as the patient's VT remains adequate; SIMV is begun at an intermediate rate and reduced to an F of 2 or so to inflate the lungs periodically and limit atelectasis.

POSITIVE END-EXPIRATORY PRESSURE

Positive end-expiratory pressure improves arterial oxygenation by increasing lung volume. This has the effect of preventing or reversing atelectasis and redistributing intra-alveolar edema fluid either into a thinner meniscus within the alveoli or out into the interstitium of the lung. The end result is recruitment of alveoli for better oxygen exchange. It should be noted that PEEP does not improve ventilation; in fact, the Pa_{CO_2} may increase because PEEP increases VD/VT by distending the airways and alveoli.

INDICATIONS FOR POSITIVE END-EXPIRATORY PRESSURE. One indication for PEEP is to prevent or reverse atelectasis (Table 71–9). For example, low levels of PEEP, such as 5 cm H_2O, are commonly administered to intubated patients who are supine in bed. Some investigators believe that low levels of PEEP facilitate weaning from mechanical ventilation by maintaining higher lung volumes while patients breathe through an endotracheal tube. They therefore continue PEEP during T-piece trials and when patients are receiving SIMV at a low ventilator F, with or without PSV.

The other major indication for PEEP is to improve arterial oxygenation in patients with diffuse parenchymal lung disorders, such as ARDS. Because their hypoxemia is primarily due to

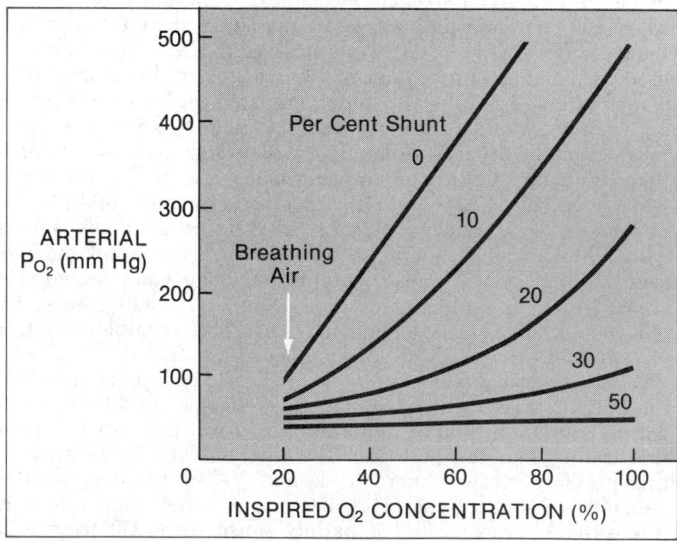

FIGURE 71–3. The relationship of the partial pressure of oxygen in systemic arterial blood (Pa_{O_2}) to the fraction of inspired oxygen (FI_{O_2}) with increasing amounts of shunt. Note that with 30 per cent of the cardiac output being shunted, there is only a slight increase in Pa_{O_2}. (From West JR: Pulmonary Pathophysiology: The Essentials. © 1977, The Williams & Wilkins Co., Baltimore.)

intrapulmonary shunt, such patients often cannot be oxygenated adequately even at an $F_{I_{O_2}}$ of 1.0, as illustrated in Figure 71–3. Administered in levels in excess of 5 cm H_2O, PEEP usually improves the Pa_{O_2} of these patients. It also allows the $F_{I_{O_2}}$ to be reduced to levels of 0.6 or less, thereby minimizing the risk of oxygen toxicity.

MODES OF POSITIVE END-EXPIRATORY PRESSURE. Positive end-expiratory pressure can be administered to spontaneously breathing patients through either a tightly fitting face mask or an endotracheal tube, in which case it is called continuous positive airway pressure (CPAP). It may also be combined with IPPV to create what is called continuous positive-pressure ventilation (CPPV). The improvement in oxygenation that may be produced by these two modes of PEEP depends primarily on the increase in lung volume they achieve, which in turn depends on the increase in airway pressure. As illustrated in Figure 71–4, the increase in airway pressure generally is greater with CPPV than with CPAP. Because of this, patients who merely have atelectasis may often be managed solely with CPAP. However, because they also have edema and because their ventilatory needs are greater, patients with diffuse parenchymal lung disease generally receive CPPV.

COMPLICATIONS OF POSITIVE END-EXPIRATORY PRESSURE. Like its benefits, the complications of PEEP are related to lung volume and airway pressure. The delivery of gas at high pressure to achieve an increase in lung volume throughout the ventilatory cycle is more likely to cause barotrauma (or "volutrauma") than is the delivery of pressurized gas solely during inspiration. It is also more likely to decrease venous return to the chest and thereby depress P_{SA} and $\dot{Q}T$. Although the incidence of complications due to PEEP has not been well studied, it appears to be significant if high levels are used.

WEANING FROM POSITIVE END-EXPIRATORY PRESSURE. Patients who are receiving low levels of PEEP for atelectasis can usually be weaned from PEEP without difficulty. Premature withdrawal or reduction of PEEP in patients with diffuse parenchymal lung disorders can worsen oxygenation, however, and cause clinical deterioration that requires hours or days of therapy to reverse. For this reason, PEEP should be withdrawn slowly, in small (2 to 5 cm H_2O) decrements, with close monitoring of Pa_{O_2} or Sa_{O_2} in such patients. Premature

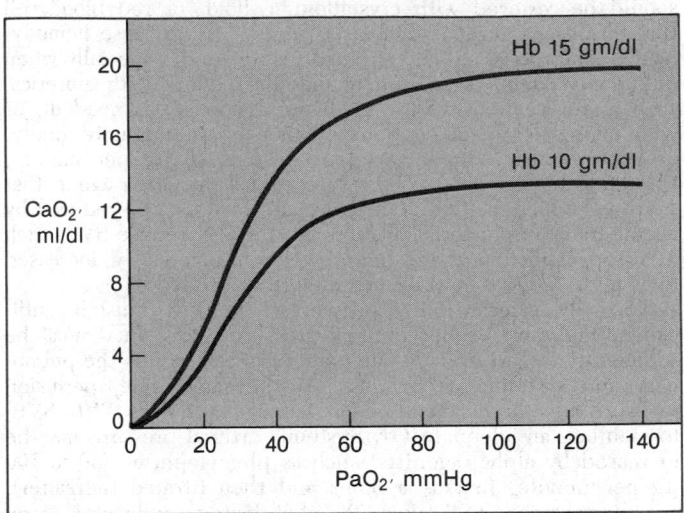

FIGURE 71–5. Importance of blood hemoglobin (Hb) concentration in oxygen transport. At a Pa_{O_2} of 80 mm Hg, arterial blood oxygen content (Ca_{O_2}) can be increased by 50 per cent by raising Hb from 10 to 15 grams per deciliter in an anemic patient. (From Luce JM, Tyler ML, Pierson DJ: Intensive Respiratory Care. Philadelphia, W. B. Saunders Company, 1984.)

reduction of PEEP can be avoided if the disease process for which PEEP was initiated has resolved or is substantially improved, if the Pa_{O_2} is 80 mm Hg or greater on an $F_{I_{O_2}}$ of 0.4 or less, and if these conditions have been present for several hours.

Therapy to Improve Oxygen Transport

Oxygen transport may be improved by manipulating the variables that affect it: Ca_{O_2} and $\dot{Q}T$. The major determinants of Ca_{O_2} are the Hb concentration and Sa_{O_2}. Most physicians are familiar with the need to optimize Sa_{O_2} by the methods discussed earlier, but many forget that $\dot{T}o_2$ can often be improved by restoring the Hb concentration to normal, as depicted in Figure 71–5.

Carbon monoxide poisoning causes a functional anemia that may impair $\dot{T}o_2$. The oxyhemoglobin dissociation curve is also shifted to the left in patients with carbon monoxide poisoning, which results in less oxygen being available to the tissues. Because the Pa_{O_2} is normal, the possibility of carbon moxide poisoning may be overlooked unless the Sa_{O_2} or the Ca_{O_2} is measured directly. Carbon monoxide poisoning is treated with supplemental oxygen at an $F_{I_{O_2}}$ of 1.0 and occasionally with hyperbaric oxygenation. Both of these maneuvers improve $\dot{T}o_2$ by dissolving oxygen in plasma and displacing carbon monoxide from Hb.

Manipulation of $\dot{Q}T$ in patients with failure of oxygen transport often involves administration of drugs to alter HR, SV, and vascular pressures and resistances (Table 71–10). Alteration of HR includes measures to reverse bradyarrhythmias or tachyarrhythmias if they are present. In general, sinus bradycardia severe enough to compromise $\dot{Q}T$ and P_{SA} may be treated with parasympatholytic drugs, such as atropine (0.5 to 1.0 mg intravenously); with beta$_1$- and beta$_2$-adrenergic agonists, such as isoproterenol (1 to 2 mg in 500 ml of dextrose and water given at 2 to 20 μg per minute); or with cardiac pacing. Sinus tachycardia may be treated by correcting its underlying causes, which include hypovolemia, pain, and hyperthyroidism.

Supraventricular tachycardia may respond to vagal maneuvers, such as carotid sinus massage; beta$_1$ and beta$_2$ antagonists, such as esmolol (5 grams in 500 ml of dextrose and water given as a loading dose of 500 μg per kilogram over 1 minute, followed by an infusion of 50 μg per minute for 4 minutes); and calcium channel blockers, such as verapamil (5 to 10 mg given intravenously as needed). Ventricular tachycardia is treated with lidocaine or bretylium; ventricular fibrillation is treated with electrical defibrillation. The use of these therapies in cardiopulmonary resuscitation is discussed later.

Manipulation of SV requires alterations of its three determinants: preload, afterload, and contractility. For example, preload

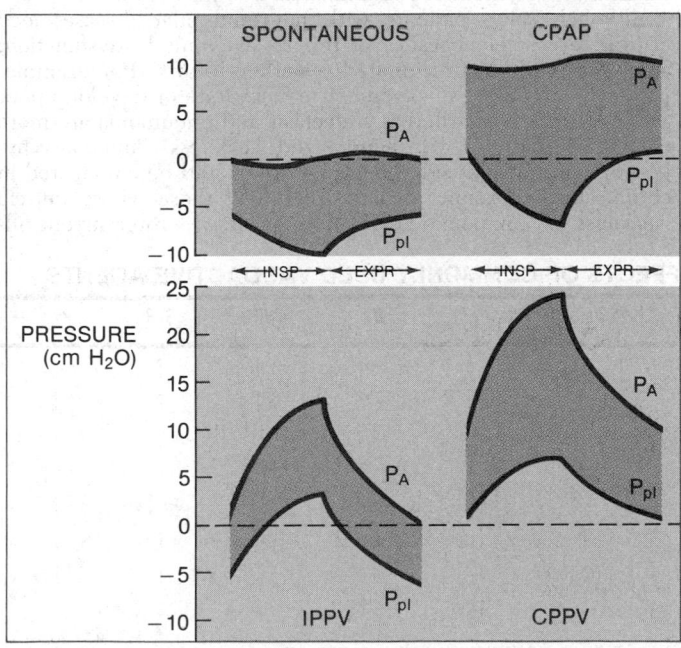

FIGURE 71–4. Schematic representations of airway (P_A) and pleural (P_{pl}) pressures with spontaneous respiration, spontaneous respiration with continuous positive airway pressure (CPAP), intermittent positive-pressure ventilation (IPPV), and continuous positive-pressure ventilation (CPPV). Note that with CPAP and CPPV, the pressure gradient between the airway and the pleural space is increased compared with spontaneous respiration and IPPV, respectively. (From Hinshaw HC, Murray JF [eds.]: Diseases of the Chest. Philadelphia, W.B. Saunders Company, 1980.)

should be restored with crystalloid, colloid, or red blood cell transfusions, when it is decreased sufficiently to cause hemodynamic compromise. When preload is increased, especially when pulmonary edema is present, it may be reduced with diuretics, such as furosemide (40 mg given intravenously as needed), or with nitroglycerin (given transcutaneously, sublingually, orally, or intravenously; the intravenous dose is 10 μg per minute, titrated as high as 200 to 300 μg per minute) or other agents that cause venodilation. Left ventricular afterload may be reduced by agents that cause arterial dilation and thereby reduce SVR, such as nitroprusside (10 μg per minute given intravenously, increased to as high as 300 to 400 μg per minute as needed).

Normally, arterial inflow pressures ($\overline{P_{PA}}$, $\overline{P_{SA}}$) must be sufficiently high and venous outflow pressures ($\overline{P_{LA}}$, $\overline{P_{RA}}$) must be sufficiently low to provide adequate perfusion across the pulmonary and systemic circulations. At the same time, perfusion pressure must be balanced by circulatory resistances (PVR, SVR) to maintain an adequate $\dot{Q}_T$. Systemic arterial pressure may be increased by alpha$_1$ agonists, such as phenylephrine (50 to 100 μg per minute, first as a bolus and then titrated thereafter), norepinephrine (4 to 8 mg in 500 ml of dextrose and water, given at 4 to 12 μg per minute), or high-dose dopamine. Left atrial pressure and P_{RA} may be reduced by nitrates and other agents that decrease preload. Similarly, SVR may be increased by alpha$_1$ agonists and decreased by drugs such as nitroprusside.

The drugs most commonly used to improve $\dot{Q}_T$ in critically ill patients are dopamine and dobutamine. Dopamine may be given in low doses (usually 2.0 to 5.0 μg per minute) to enhance renal and mesenteric perfusion through its dopaminergic effects. Intermediate-dose (5.0 to 10.0 μg per minute) dopamine improves $\dot{Q}_T$ through its beta$_1$ effects, whereas high-dose (>10.0 μg per minute) dopamine increases P_{SA} through its alpha$_1$ properties. The pharmacologic effects of dopamine are not always predictable in all patients, and the drug must be carefully titrated to achieve its desired effects.

Unlike dopamine, dobutamine does not selectively enhance renal and mesenteric perfusion because it lacks dopaminergic properties. It also does not generally increase P_{SA} or P_{AO} because its alpha$_1$ properties are balanced by its beta$_1$ properties; in fact, dobutamine may reduce P_{SA} and P_{AO} in some labile patients when its beta$_2$ properties predominate. However, dobutamine improves $\dot{Q}_T$ through its beta$_1$ properties. If P_{SA} is reduced, dobutamine may be combined with high-dose dopamine or other alpha$_1$ agonists. The usual dose of dobutamine is 2.5 to 10 μg per minute, up to a maximum dose of 30 μg per minute.

Therapy to Improve Oxygen Extraction

Oxygen extraction may be improved by increasing $\dot{V}_{O_2}$. In patients with cyanide poisoning, this has traditionally involved administering amyl nitrate by inhalation and sodium nitrite intravenously; these drugs produce methemoglobin, which binds free cyanide ions. Intravenous sodium thiosulfate then is given to enhance conversion of cyanide to thiosulfate, which is less toxic and is readily excreted. Vitamin B$_{12}$A will soon be available for treating cyanide poisoning in the United States.

Unfortunately, no simple antidote exists for the disturbances in oxygen extraction associated with distributive shock, ARDS, and MOSF. The general approach to these conditions is to improve T_{O_2}, as is discussed further on.

PATHOPHYSIOLOGY, MONITORING, AND MANAGEMENT OF COMMON CAUSES OF CIRCULATORY AND RESPIRATORY FAILURE

Neuromuscular Diseases Causing Respiratory Failure

A wide variety of neuromuscular diseases cause weakness or paralysis that may lead to hypercapnic respiratory failure. These disorders may involve the upper motor neurons (e.g., traumatic quadriplegia), lower motor neurons (e.g., amyotrophic lateral sclerosis), peripheral nerves (e.g., Guillain-Barré syndrome), myoneural junction (e.g., myasthenia gravis, botulism), or the muscles themselves (e.g., muscular dystrophies). The overall approach to patients with these conditions is to diagnose and treat specific neuromuscular disease, if possible, to ascertain precipitating factors prompting critical care unit admission, to evaluate the need for respiratory support, to provide such support on an acute basis, and to consider chronic support when required.

Once weakness or paralysis is appreciated, most neuromuscular diseases causing these symptoms can be differentiated by means of clinical characteristics, cerebrospinal fluid analysis, provocative tests such as the administration of cholinergic drugs, nerve conduction studies and electromyography, and occasionally muscle biopsy. In terms of specific therapy, plasmapheresis is used for patients with the Guillain-Barré syndrome (Ch. 497). Myasthenia gravis is treated with relatively long-acting anticholinesterase agents, such as pyridostigmine, and with plasmapheresis, corticosteroids, and thymectomy (Ch. 509). Specific therapy for botulism involves elimination of malabsorbed neurotoxin from the gut by means of enemas and gastric lavage, administration of trivalent antitoxin, administration of high-dose penicillin, and surgical debridement of contaminated wounds (Ch. 309).

Although some patients with neuromuscular disease need critical care solely because of progressive muscle dysfunction, admission often is precipitated by other factors. For example, patients with bulbar involvement may aspirate or develop upper airway obstruction, whereas atelectasis and pneumonia are more common in patients with generalized weakness. Pulmonary hypertension and right-sided heart failure should be anticipated in chronically hypoxemic patients, including those whose muscle weakness is compounded by kyphoscoliosis. Intercurrent ill-

TABLE 71–10. CARDIOVASCULAR AND RESPIRATORY EFFECTS OF COMMONLY USED VASOACTIVE AGENTS

Agent	HR	$\overline{P_{SA}}$	$\overline{P_{RA}}$	$\overline{P_{PA}}$	$\overline{P_{PAO}}$	$C(a-\bar{v})_{O_2}$	$\dot{Q}_T$	PVR	SVR	$P\bar{v}_{O_2}$
Phenylephrine	→	↑	↑	→↑		→↓	→	→↑	↑	→↓
Norepinephrine	↑	↑	↑	↑	↑	↓	→↑	→↑	↑	↑
Epinephrine	↑	↑	↑	→↑	↑	↓	↑	→	↑	↑
Dopamine, low dose	→	→	→	→		→↓	→↑	→	→	→↑
Dopamine, intermediate dose	↑	→	→	→	→↓	↓	↑	→	→↓	↑
Dopamine, high dose	→↑	↑	↑	→		↓	↓	↑	↑	↓
Dobutamine	↑	↓	↓	→↓	↓	↓	↑	→↓	↓	↑
Isoproterenol	↑	↓	↓	→↓	↓	↓	↑	→↑	↓	↓
Metaproterenol/albuterol	→↑	→↑	→	→↓	→	→	→↑	→	→	→
Nitroglycerin	→↑	↓	↓	→↓	↓	↓	↓	↓	↓	↓
Nitroprusside	↑	↓	↓	↓	→↓	↓	↑	→↓	↓	↑
Esmolol	↓	→↓	→	→	→↑	↑	↓	↓	→	↓
Morphine	→↑	↓	→	↓	→	↑	↓	→	↓	↓

HR = heart rate; $\overline{P_{SA}}$ = mean systemic arterial pressure; $\overline{P_{RA}}$ = mean right atrial or central venous pressure; $\overline{P_{PA}}$ = mean pulmonary arterial pressure; $\overline{P_{PAO}}$ = mean pulmonary arterial occlusion pressure; $C(a-\bar{v})_{O_2}$ = arterial–mixed venous oxygen content difference; $\dot{Q}_T$ = cardiac output; PVR = pulmonary vascular resistance; SVR = systemic vascular resistance; $P\bar{v}_{O_2}$ = mixed venous oxygen tension.

nesses, such as urinary tract infection and pulmonary thromboembolism, may also occur.

The need for respiratory support in patients with neuromuscular disease can be assessed by the MIP and VC maneuvers. As noted earlier, intubation and mechanical ventilation generally are required if the MIP is less negative than -20 cm H_2O and the VC is approximately 10 ml per kilogram. It should be noted that impaired clearance of secretions may occur at a VC that is less than 30 ml per kilogram and may require intubation but not mechanical ventilation.

Hypoxemic respiratory failure in patients with neuromuscular disease can usually be treated adequately with supplemental oxygen delivered through nasal prongs or a face mask, coupled with frequent repositioning and the delivery of CPAP via a tightly fitting face mask to treat atelectasis. Intubation and mechanical ventilation are usually called for, however, if muscle strength and lung volumes have declined to the level mentioned previously and always are necessary if hypercapnia is acute and severe. Patients with rapidly reversible muscle weakness or paralysis should be intubated by the translaryngeal route in most instances, but tracheostomy is indicated if patients require intubation for longer than a month or so.

No particular kind of ventilatory support has been demonstrated to be superior in patients with neuromuscular disease, although PPV is preferred to negative-pressure ventilation in the critical care unit, especially if admission has been prompted by pneumonia or some other intermittent illness that requires supplemental oxygen at a high FI_{O_2}. The value of various modes of PPV is also open to debate. Nevertheless, because SIMV can be used only in those patients who can generate substantial inspiratory pressures, patients with severe weakness or paralysis are ventilated at least initially with CMV or AMV. In patients who are improving, SIMV may be used if it does not cause fatigue. Weaning by SIMV, T-piece, or PSV should be attempted only when patients demonstrate improvement in the MIP and VC.

Oxygen transport usually is adequate in patients with neuromuscular disease who are not hypoxemic or anemic and who do not have concurrent cardiac disease. Nevertheless, autonomic dysfunction in patients with Guillain-Barré syndrome and other disorders may take the form of either overactivity or underactivity of the sympathetic nervous system. Hypertension, diaphoresis, and tachycardia may be treated with titratable agents, such as esmolol, to prevent overswings in HR and PsA. The hypotension that often accompanies spinal cord injury and other conditions may be treated with intravenous fluids or alpha$_1$ agonists, such as phenylephrine or high-dose dopamine. Bradycardia is treated with atropine. Patients with profound vagal tone in whom bradycardia progresses to asystole may be candidates for cardiac pacing.

Patients with neuromuscular disease also require emotional support. These patients frequently regress psychologically, owing occasionally to central nervous system involvement by their disease and more commonly to their complete dependence on the people caring for them. They and their families usually need frequent reminders that their needs will be met by nurses, physicians, respiratory therapists, and other health care professionals. If their neuromuscular disease can be corrected with time or treatment, they should also be told that their recovery can be expected, in months if not in days.

The difficult question remains of how to help patients who are not expected to recover neuromuscular function. Some patients whose phrenic nerve nuclei are damaged but whose phrenic nerves and diaphragm are intact may be candidates for electrophrenic ventilation, in which the nerves are repetitively stimulated in the lower neck or upper thorax. Others who maintain nearly normal arterial blood gas values only while awake may be ventilated during sleep with rocking beds, pneumobelts, chest cuirasses, and other negative-pressure devices, or by PPV delivered through the mouth or the nose or via a tracheostomy. Unfortunately, however, most patients with chronic severe neuromuscular disease must receive negative- or positive-pressure ventilation around the clock at home or in the hospital. This situation may be unacceptable to the patients and their families.

Asthma and Chronic Obstructive Pulmonary Disease

The primary pathophysiologic abnormalities in asthma and COPD are (1) an increased resistance in airflow resulting from

narrowing of the airways by bronchospasm, inflammation, and mucus and (2) loss of airway tethering forces by parenchymal lung destruction. The airflow resistance causes air trapping and an abnormal increase in lung volume. Patients also have hypoxemia caused by mismatching of ventilation and perfusion and hypercapnia caused by the airways obstruction itself plus fatigue of the respiratory muscles.

In patients with asthma and COPD, Pa_{CO_2} usually begins to increase when the FEV_1 is reduced to approximately 750 ml or 25 per cent of the predicted value. This reduction may result from gradually progressive disease but more often occurs in the setting of acute exacerbations of obstruction due, for example, to acute bronchitis. An increase in Pa_{CO_2} without a deterioration in FEV_1 may be the result of decreased ventilatory drive due to narcotic or sedative drugs or the inhalation of oxygen at a high FI_{O_2}. Alternatively, it may result from increased V_{CO_2} in a patient with a limited ability to increase V_A. As previously described, the distinction between acute and chronic respiratory acidosis can be determined by analyzing the relationships between Pa_{CO_2}, pH, and $[HCO_3^-]$. Acute hypoventilation obviously dictates a more prompt response than chronic partially compensated respiratory acidosis, as is also true in patients with neuromuscular disease.

Metabolic acidosis is a more ominous finding than pure respiratory acidosis in the setting of airways obstruction. It implies a failure of oxygen transport to meet the demands imposed by the increased work of breathing. This failure may result from a decrease in Ca_{O_2} due to processes such as hypoxemia or anemia or a decrease in $\dot{Q}T$ due to concurrent ischemic heart disease, inadequate intravascular volume, or auto-PEEP caused by air trapping. Unless patients with inadequate oxygen transport improve, their condition will rapidly deteriorate.

Patients with asthma and COPD may be treated with beta$_2$-adrenergic agonists, theophylline, anticholinergic agents, and corticosteroids (Ch. 57 and 58). Beta$_2$ agonists, such as metaproterenol and albuterol, relax bronchial smooth muscle through their action on beta$_2$ receptors in the airways and have little effect on beta$_1$ receptors in skeletal muscles, systemic vessels, and the heart. They, therefore, are preferred to agents such as epinephrine and isoproterenol that have mixed beta$_1$ and beta$_2$ properties. The usually mild tachycardia, tremulousness, and other cardiovascular side effects of beta$_2$ agonists can be minimized if the drugs are taken in aerosol form. Average doses of aerosolized metaproterenol and albuterol are 15 mg and 2.5 mg, respectively, given every 2 to 4 hours.

Theophylline has fallen into disfavor because of its limited bronchodilating properties and its potential for toxicity. Theophylline may be administered as aminophylline in a loading dose of 5 to 6 mg per kilogram given intravenously, followed by an infusion of 0.4 to 0.9 mg per kilogram per hour to achieve a mean serum level of approximately 10.0 μg per milliliter. Serum levels should be followed regularly in patients receiving intravenous theophylline.

Aerosolized anticholinergic agents such as ipratropium bromide, which may be given via an inhaler at a dose of 0.04 mg every 2 to 4 hours, are both effective and safe owing to their lack of systemic side effects. Corticosteroids suppress inflammation and increase responsiveness to beta$_2$ stimulation. These agents are available in aerosol, oral, or intravenous forms. In patients critically ill with asthma and COPD, intravenous methylprednisolone is commonly administered in the range of 0.5 to 1.0 mg per kilogram four times per day.

Although hypoxemia invariably is present in patients with severe airways obstruction, the degree of reduction in Pa_{O_2} is generally not sufficient to require respiratory support other than supplemental oxygen delivered with external devices. Hypoxemia should usually be corrected only to a Pa_{O_2} of approximately 60 mm Hg, using as low an FI_{O_2} as possible to avoid ventilatory depression. If a high FI_{O_2} must be used in patients with intercurrent illnesses such as pneumonia, endotracheal intubation and mechanical ventilation may be required.

One cannot definitely state what the criteria are for intubating and ventilating patients with severe airways obstruction. Arterial blood gas and pH values at a single point in time showing marked acute respiratory acidosis with or without metabolic acidosis may be sufficient information on which to base the decision to provide mechanical ventilation. More commonly, however, it is necessary to evaluate the patient during a period while drugs are being administered and to assess the response to therapy. If blood gas values are worsening or not improving in spite of maximal treatment, mechanical ventilation is the next logical step. In addition to the objective evaluation provided by arterial blood gas and pH measurements, subjective assessments are also of value. Patients who are confused, somnolent, or uncooperative may require ventilatory support because their mental status may indicate inadequate oxygen transport and because they cannot cooperate with conservative management.

Severe airways obstruction presents a difficult situation in which to apply PPV. There is need to allow adequate expiratory time to avoid auto-PEEP, but also slow inspiratory flows are desirable to optimize the distribution of ventilation and to minimize the airway pressure required to deliver a preset V_T. To accomplish these goals, at least early in the course of mechanical ventilation, it often is necessary to sedate the patient receiving CMV or AMV in order to provide a slow ventilator F, which allows a small I/E ratio to be used. Some patients will benefit from SIMV in this situation. The V_T should be between 7 and 10 ml per kilogram, and the $F_{I_{O_2}}$ should be adjusted to provide an adequate Pa_{O_2}. The Pa_{CO_2} may rise owing to the relatively low F and V_T, but the pH will not fall precipitously if the rise is gradual. If the Pa_{CO_2} remains elevated, or if the patient already has chronic hypoventilation, it is important not to reduce the Pa_{CO_2} rapidly because doing so will result in uncompensated metabolic alkalosis.

Positive end-expiratory pressure would appear to be contraindicated in patients with asthma and COPD whose lung volumes already are increased above normal. Certainly, high levels of PEEP are potentially dangerous; they also are unnecessary because these patients do not have failure of arterial oxygenation due to diffuse parenchymal lung disease. Nevertheless, PEEP in levels of approximately 5 cm H_2O does not commonly cause hyperinflation in patients with airways obstruction. Indeed, low levels of PEEP may reduce the work or breathing of some obstructed patients by preventing airway collapse during expiration.

The adequacy of oxygen transport in patients with asthma and COPD can generally be assessed by physical examination, measurement of urine output, and monitoring of Psa. Central venous and pulmonary artery catheterization is rarely required but may be helpful in evaluating patients whose Qt is known or suspected to be depressed and in evaluating their response to fluids and agents such as dopamine or dobutamine. The elevation of $Ppao$ by auto-PEEP should be taken into account when estimating intravascular volume. Serial measurements of $Ceff$ in ventilated patients may be useful in assessing the severity of airways obstruction and the response to therapy.

In patients with airways obstruction, weaning from mechanical ventilation may also present difficulties. Patients with asthma may usually be weaned and extubated quickly after they have responded to treatment. Patients with COPD may at best have marginal lung function, however, with persistent retention of carbon dioxide. In general, the arterial blood gas pattern that exists when the patient is "well" should be approximated while mechanical ventilation is still being used. Ideally, weaning with SIMV or a simple T-piece with or without PSV and small amounts of PEEP then can proceed, using previously described criteria.

In some instances, patients with COPD never meet the objective criteria for weaning and extubation. When this occurs, the decisions regarding weaning and extubation are based on subjective criteria, such as level of alertness, cooperation of the patient, and prognosis. These factors obviously cannot be quantitated. Once the patient has demonstrated the ability to maintain a desired V_E spontaneously for 30 to 60 minutes, the endotracheal tube should be removed.

It is important to determine which patients with COPD have a component of reversible respiratory dysfunction and which patients have simply reached the end stage of their disease, as is true of patients with neuromuscular disorders. Although chronic negative- or positive-pressure ventilation may be used to maintain life in a patient with end-stage airways obstruction, the decision to pursue this course should be carefully considered by the patient and the family, preferably before mechanical ventilation is begun.

Adult Respiratory Distress Syndrome and Multiple Organ System Failure

A constellation of clinical, radiographic, and pathophysiologic findings that result from diffuse injury to the lung parenchyma defines ARDS. The characteristics of this syndrome are (1) severe hypoxemia due to intrapulmonary shunting of blood, (2) decreased Crs due to decreased compliance of the lung, and (3) the presence of diffuse infiltration on the chest radiograph. The common abnormality that accounts for these features is an increase in the permeability of the endothelium of the pulmonary capillary and the epithelium of the alveolar wall. This increased permeability allows fluid to leak from the capillary into the alveolus, even though the hydrostatic pressure within the capillary is normal; hence, noncardiogenic pulmonary edema results.

The adult respiratory distress syndrome is associated with a variety of clinical conditions, the most common of which is sepsis syndrome. A partial list of these conditions is found in Table 71–11. The injury to the lung that occurs in these conditions may be delivered either via the airways or via the circulation. In many instances (e.g., gastric aspiration or diffuse pneumonia), lung injury would appear to be direct. In others (e.g., sepsis syndrome or pancreatitis), the injury presumably is indirect and is mediated by circulating substances.

Regardless of the type or mechanism of injury, the damage to the lungs of patients with ARDS is diffuse, compared with the damage in diseases such as unilateral pneumonia. The damage is nonhomogeneous, however, and some areas of lung parenchyma may be spared. In damaged areas, the lung is atelectatic, edematous, and hemorrhagic. Microscopic examination reveals intraalveolar collections of proteinaceous fluid, red blood cells, and inflammatory cells. Microthrombi or white cell aggregates may be seen in small vessels. After 24 to 48 hours, hyaline membranes formed by fibrin that has escaped through the capillaries line the alveoli. Subsequently, as repair of the injury occurs, fibrosis may ensue.

Reduction in lung volume is characteristic of ARDS and is caused by a combination of atelectasis, edema fluid, and inflammation and perhaps fibrosis replacing alveolar air. This decrease in lung volume contrasts with the increase in lung volume of patients with airways obstruction. It is largely responsible for the decrease in Crs associated with ARDS, which traditionally has been attributed primarily to lung stiffness. The work of breathing increases considerably because of the decreased Crs.

The major and most frequent gas exchange abnormality in ARDS is hypoxemia caused by the loss of functional alveoli. In severe forms of ARDS, as the process evolves from injury to repair, gas exchange abnormalities also evolve. Lung fibrosis may result in obliteration of capillaries and coalescence of alveoli to produce an increased VD/VT. Unless VE can be increased, which may be difficult, hypercapnia will result.

Some, but not all, patients with ARDS develop dysfunction or failure of one or more organ systems sequentially or simultaneously. By contrast, other patients develop the syndrome of MOSF without having ARDS, although they may have less severe degrees of parenchymal lung injury. Multiple organ system failure is associated with the same clinical conditions as ARDS. Furthermore, as with ARDS, it most commonly is associated with sepsis syndrome. This observation suggests that ARDS is a respiratory manifestation of MOSF, just as distributive shock is

TABLE 71–11. CONDITIONS ASSOCIATED WITH THE ADULT RESPIRATORY DISTRESS SYNDROME AND MULTIPLE ORGAN SYSTEM FAILURE

Sepsis syndrome
Severe trauma
Diffuse pneumonia
Burns and smoke inhalation
Multiple transfusions
Pancreatitis
Anaphylaxis
Drug overdose
Cardiorespiratory arrest

a cardiovascular manifestation. Alternatively, ARDS and MSOF may be aspects of sepsis syndrome. Indeed, some investigators have broadened the use of the term sepsis syndrome to include any generalized inflammatory process that may cause or contribute to widespread organ dysfunction.

This generalized inflammatory process may be mediated by a variety of circulating substances with vasoactive, inflammatory, and tissue-damaging properties. These substances, which may include endotoxin, histamine, arachidonic acid metabolites, complement, myocardial depressant factor, and tumor necrosis factor, may cause systemic vasodilation, microvascular vasoconstriction, altered myocardial contractility, capillary microembolization, and endothelial cell disruption. The end result is increased capillary permeability with intravascular fluid loss, interstitial fluid accumulation, impaired microcirculatory blood flow, and inadequate tissue oxygenation in the lungs and other organs. Patients may die of refractory hypotension, hypoxemia attributable to ARDS, or other manifestations of MOSF, such as disseminated intravascular coagulation.

The diagnoses of ARDS and MOSF are made clinically because there are no reliable markers for the disorders. The diagnoses are supported by documenting the presence of the associated conditions just discussed. Pulmonary artery catheterization, which may aid in management, also suggests the diagnosis of ARDS and MOSF if the characteristic patterns of distributive shock and inadequate oxygen extraction are observed.

It is not clear whether the term sepsis syndrome should be applied to patients with ARDS and MOSF who are not truly infected. Nevertheless, such patients probably should be assumed to be infected unless there is another explanation for their condition. If bacterial infection is suspected or known to exist, broad-spectrum antibiotics, such as ampicillin, metronidazole, and gentamicin, should be given intravenously to cover gram-positive and gram-negative pathogens, and the choice of agent then tailored to culture results. Suspected or documented infections with other organisms should be treated appropriately. In addition, abscesses should be sought by computed tomography (CT) and other techniques when appropriate. If detected, they should be drained percutaneously or at surgery.

The unusual patient with MOSF who does not have severe parenchymal lung disease may benefit from endotracheal intubation and mechanical ventilation merely because he or she is hemodynamically unstable. Vital organ perfusion may also be enhanced if the work of breathing is reduced by mechanical ventilation. Patients with ARDS, however, invariably require both PPV and PEEP to improve arterial oxygenation. The need for such support may be evaluated by monitoring the Pa_{O_2} and $P(A - a)_{O_2}$. Respiratory or metabolic acidosis is ominous in this setting. Because patients with ARDS, MOSF, or both may deteriorate rapidly, it generally is better to provide intubation and mechanical ventilation earlier rather than later.

The use of PPV in patients with ARDS and MOSF varies. Most physicians probably administer CMV, AMV, or IMV with a VT of 10 to 15 ml/kg, an I/E ratio of 1:3 or greater, and a Pmax as required to deliver a VT in the aforementioned range. Positive end-expiratory pressure is used at levels necessary to reduce the FI_{O_2} to 0.6 or less. Increasing concern over the possible effects of high alveolar pressures and volumes in causing barotrauma has led some investigators to advocate the use of HFV, PCV, and IRV despite the fact that these newer modes of PPV have not been shown to be superior to older ones. When older modes of PPV are employed, it is argued, VT should be as low as 5 to 7 ml per kilogram, ventilators should be pressure cycled, and high levels of PEEP should be avoided if possible, even if the FI_{O_2} exceeds 0.6 in the process.

It is not clear that the current concepts of the pathogenesis of lung injury and therapies based upon them will prove superior to concepts and therapies accepted earlier. Nevertheless, it does appear prudent to use all modes of PPV and PEEP carefully. Most patients with ARDS and MOSF probably can be adequately ventilated and oxygenated by CMV, AMV, and IMV at a relatively low VT and a Pmax of less than 50 cm H_2O. If Pmax exceeds this amount, PCV may be added with or without IRV. Positive end-expiratory pressure should be used at the lowest possible level to achieve an FI_{O_2} of 0.6 or less.

Because barotrauma is such a concern, CSTAT should be monitored frequently in patients receiving PPV and PEEP. In addition, the amount of auto-PEEP should be measured by the method cited previously. Although the auto-PEEP often caused by PCV and IRV has been considered undesirable, auto-PEEP may be just as potentially useful as intentionally administered PEEP in recruiting alveoli. The important point is to include the amount of auto-PEEP in the overall measurement of PEEP so that its effects can be anticipated.

Appropriate use of intravenous fluid is an essential component of the management of ARDS and MOSF. Because pulmonary capillary permeability is increased, administration of fluid, which raises the capillary hydrostatic pressure, tends to increase the amount of lung water. The relationship between capillary hydrostatic pressure and extravascular lung water is shown schematically in Figure 71–6.

On the other hand, adequate pulmonary perfusion may be important in preventing or ameliorating lung damage, and systemic perfusion clearly is essential in maintaining renal, cardiac, and central nervous system function. Thus, the effects of crystalloid, colloid, or red blood cell administration should be carefully monitored with clear endpoints in mind. In addition to measuring PSA and other variables, indices of end-organ perfusion, such as urine output and mental status, should be followed.

Pulmonary artery catheterization may be extremely helpful in assessing hemodynamic status, at least early in the course of ARDS and MOSF. Although the correlation between PPAO and the outcome of these disorders has not been determined, it appears reasonable to maintain the PPAO at a normal or slightly lower than normal level as long as perfusion of vital organs is maintained. If perfusion is inadequate or if QT is depressed by the patient's underlying disease or its treatment, the circulation can be supported with dopamine or dobutamine.

Ideally, the combination of specific therapy for associated conditions, such as sepsis syndrome, and appropriate cardiovascular and respiratory system support should improve T_{O_2} in patients with ARDS and MOSF. It is important to keep this goal in mind for at least three reasons. First, T_{O_2} and its components (Ca_{O_2} and QT) can be quantified, and therapies that increase one component at the expense of the other may be modified. Second, because there is no specific antidote for the inadequate oxygen extraction that so often characterizes ARDS and MOSF, therapies to improve T_{O_2} are the only ones available.

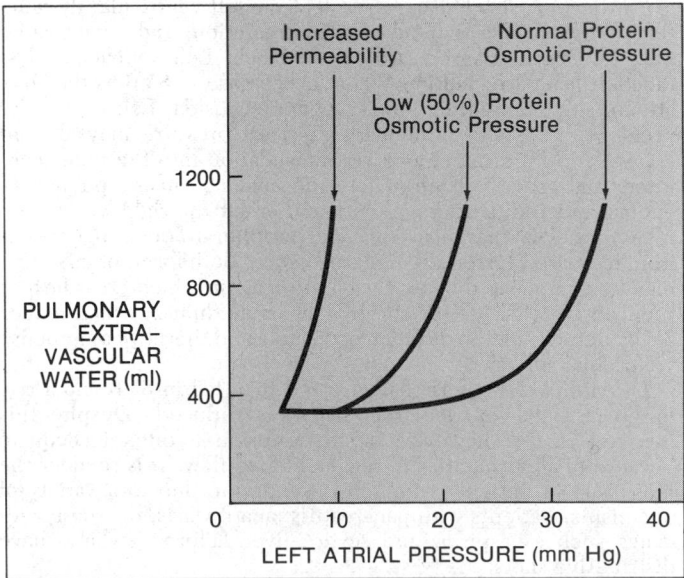

FIGURE 71–6. Schematic representation of the relationship between pulmonary extravascular water volume and left atrial or pulmonary artery occlusion pressure. Right curve represents the relationships when both microvascular permeability and plasma protein osmotic pressures are normal; middle curve represents normal permeability but a reduction in plasma protein osmotic pressure of 50 per cent; left curve shows relationship when permeability of the capillaries is increased. (From Hopewell PC, Murray JF: Adult respiratory distress syndrome. *In* Moser KM, Spragg RG [eds.]: Respiratory Emergencies. 2nd ed. St. Louis, The C.V. Mosby Company, 1982; with permission.)

A third reason to improve $\dot{T}_{O_2}$ is that the apparent failure of oxygen extraction in patients with ARDS and MOSF may actually be a complicated form of failure of oxygen transport. This is supported by the demonstration that $\dot{V}_{O_2}$ appears to be dependent upon $\dot{T}_{O_2}$ at some critical level of $\dot{T}_{O_2}$ in these conditions. It is also supported by the finding that some patients with ARDS and MOSF increase $\dot{V}_{O_2}$ and resolve their lactic acidosis with increases in $\dot{T}_{O_2}$. Given this finding, some investigators advocate fluid loading, hypertransfusion with red blood cells, or the administration of dobutamine to patients with ARDS and MOSF to increase Ca_{O_2} and $\dot{Q}_T$ to arbitrarily high levels. The general benefit of this approach has not been determined, however, and it cannot be recommended at the present time.

Large doses of corticosteroids, such as methylprednisolone, have also been given to patients with sepsis syndrome, ARDS, and MOSF and to those at risk of these disorders. These agents have not been shown to improve outcome from the sepsis syndrome, to prevent or ameliorate ARDS, or to influence the development of MOSF, however. Prostaglandin E_1, a pulmonary vasodilator with anti-inflammatory properties, also does not improve survival despite its salutary effect on $\dot{Q}_T$. Broad-spectrum nonabsorbable antibiotics have been given to some patients in the hope that selective decontamination of the gut may reduce a potential source of bacteria and endotoxin, but few data support this strategy. Studies of antiendotoxin antibodies currently are being performed in the hope that these agents will affect the underlying pathogenesis of these conditions. Other experimental therapies designed to neutralize other mediators and cytokines that may be responsible cannot be recommended until they are proved effective in large clinical trials.

Shock (also see Ch. 41)

The concepts contained in Equations 11 and 12 help to explain the various kinds of shock that produce inadequate oxygen transport and oxygen extraction. For example, hypovolemic shock, in which $\dot{Q}_T$ is depressed because SV is inadequate, is associated with either hemorrhage or other intravascular fluid losses. Obstructive shock may result from pulmonary thromboembolism, in which right ventricular output falls because PPA and PVR increase, or from cardiac tamponade, in which an accumulation of pericardial fluid interferes with ventricular filling and SV.

Cardiogenic shock usually results from left ventricular dysfunction following massive myocardial infarction; right ventricular infarction rarely causes cardiogenic shock. Left ventricular dysfunction leads to a fall in SV and an increase in SVR as the body attempts to maintain PSA and coronary perfusion. Left ventricular pressure, PLA, and pulmonary capillary pressure may also increase, and fluid may move via transudation into the pulmonary interstitial space and ultimately the alveoli, causing pulmonary edema and reducing Pa_{O_2}. With either left or right ventricular infarction, PRA may increase, and peripheral edema may result from increased systemic venous pressure. Both forms of infarction may be complicated by bradyarrhythmias, in which $\dot{Q}_T$ is further reduced by a fall in HR, and by tachyarrhythmias, which reduce SV by decreasing the duration of diastole and thereby compromise ventricular filling.

Distributive shock is characterized by a fall in SVR and a rise in $\dot{Q}_T$ as left ventricular afterload is reduced. Despite this increase in $\dot{Q}_T$, however, organ perfusion is often inadequate because of abnormalities in regional blood flow. It is seen for the most part in patients with sepsis syndrome due to a variety of organisms. Patients with pancreatitis, anaphylaxis, overdose with drugs such as aspirin, and severe liver failure may also have distributive shock.

The monitoring of patients with all kinds of shock should involve repeated measurement of vital signs and urine output. Because most patients with shock are hypotensive, they may require systemic arterial catheterization for continuous measurement of PSA. The combination of systemic and pulmonary artery catheterization may also aid in their evaluation and management.

Treatment of the various kinds of shock is based on their underlying pathophysiology. For example, hypovolemic shock is best treated with intravascular fluids, including blood, that restore preload. Alpha$_1$ agonists, such as phenylephrine or high-dose

dopamine, that increase Pcirc and Rcirc should be used only temporarily to support PSA because they do not affect the underlying volume loss. Similarly, obstructive shock should be treated with measures that relieve the obstruction. Thus, the abnormal rise in PPA and PVR that accompanies pulmonary thromboembolism may be ameliorated by thrombolytic agents. Oxygen should also be administered to prevent increases in PVR caused by alveolar hypoxia. At the same time, SV may be restored in patients with cardiac tamponade by removing pericardial fluid. The circulation can be supported in patients with these conditions with volume infusion and dobutamine to increase $\dot{Q}_T$, given in concert with alpha$_1$ agonists, if necessary, to maintain PSA and perfusion of the coronary circulation.

The treatment of cardiogenic shock following left ventricular infarction depends on the patient's PLA, as approximated by PPAO. If the PPAO is decreased, $\dot{Q}_T$ may be increased by improving preload. Conversely, if PPAO is increased, it may be decreased by agents that reduce preload, left ventricular afterload, or both variables. Morphine (1 to 10 mg or more given intravenously) is a potent venodilator that reduces preload; this agent also relieves pain and thereby reduces the liberation of endogenous catecholamines that increase SVR during infarction. Nitroglycerin also reduces preload by its effects on the venous circulation and limits ischemia through coronary vasodilation. Nitroprusside is preferred in reducing afterload because its effects are more pronounced on the arterial circulation. It should be noted that decreasing PPAO by reducing preload or afterload will in turn reduce pulmonary capillary pressure and edema formation and also PRA. If right ventricular infarction has occurred, the output of that ventricle may be improved either by volume infusion or by dobutamine. In patients with infarction of either ventricle, PSA may be supported with alpha$_1$ agonists, if necessary, to ensure adequate coronary perfusion.

The general approach to patients with distributive shock is to ensure adequate preload, to add alpha$_1$ agonists to increase PSA and SVR if necessary, and to administer dopamine in low doses to maintain renal and mesenteric blood flow. Dopamine may also be used in beta$_1$- and alpha$_1$-range doses in patients with sepsis syndrome, pancreatitis, and severe liver failure. Epinephrine, which also has alpha$_1$ and both beta$_1$ and beta$_2$ properties, traditionally has been given to patients with anaphylaxis at doses of 0.5 to 1.0 mg (5 to 10 ml of a 1:10,000 solution). Although dobutamine may be useful in increasing $\dot{Q}_T$ in patients with distributive shock, it may cause hypotension and require the simultaneous administration of alpha$_1$ agonists. Isoproterenol probably should be avoided because it is a beta$_1$ and beta$_2$ agonist without alpha$_1$ effects and therefore has unopposed vasodilating properties.

Finally, many patients in shock require mechanical ventilation because of lung disease or to decrease respiratory work. If patients with shock are allowed to breathe spontaneously, a greater portion of the $\dot{Q}_T$ must be diverted to the respiratory muscles. Perfusion of the heart and brain is aided when PPV is provided to experimental animals in shock.

Cardiorespiratory Arrest

Cardiorespiratory arrest is the most profound form of cardiogenic shock and also the most extreme example of failure of oxygen transport. Cessation of effective $\dot{Q}_T$ may be the culmination of a variety of shock states but most commonly is the result of ventricular fibrillation, occurring either primarily or in the course of left ventricular infarction. As $\dot{Q}_T$ abruptly falls, release of catecholamines results in peripheral vasoconstriction in an attempt to preserve blood flow to the brain, heart, and respiratory muscles at the expense of other organs, just as occurs in less severe shock. Lactic acid production increases unless $\dot{Q}_T$ is restored, and the effectiveness of catecholamines is diminished. This in turn results in generalized vasodilation that reduces the distribution of blood flow to vital organs.

Oxygen consumption by the brain is normally about 5 ml of oxygen per minute per 100 grams of brain tissue, and cerebral blood flow averages 50 ml per minute per 100 grams of tissue. Cerebrovascular resistance is minimal during cardiorespiratory arrest because the cerebral circulation cannot autoregulate, so cerebral blood flow is totally dependent on cerebral perfusion pressure, determined by the $\overline{P_{SA}}$ minus intracranial pressure

(ICP), the effective venous outflow pressure of the brain. Central nervous system injury develops when cerebral blood flow is less than approximately 18 ml per minute per 100 grams of tissue. Anaerobic cerebral metabolism is stimulated, but the subsequent increase in lactic acid further induces neuronal damage. Because oxygen utilization is nonuniform within the brain, some areas, such as the frontal and temporal lobes, are more susceptible to ischemia than are areas of lower metabolic activity.

Myocardial $\dot{V}o_2$ is approximately 10 ml of oxygen per minute per 100 grams of tissue in the normally beating heart and 5 ml of oxygen per minute per 100 grams of tissue during ventricular fibrillation. Assuming a normal Ca_{O_2} and an oxygen extraction of 75 per cent, a myocardial blood flow of 60 ml per minute per 100 grams of tissue would be required to meet normal metabolic needs; with ventricular fibrillation this figure would be 25 ml per minute per 100 grams of tissue. Coronary vascular resistance is also likely to be minimal during cardiorespiratory arrest unless coronary vascular disease is present, so myocardial blood flow will be dependent on coronary perfusion pressure, which is the difference between Psa and Pra during diastole. As Psa falls during arrest, myocardial blood flow will fall below the vital levels given earlier, and ischemic injury will result. Myocardial injury will be particularly severe in the presence of coronary artery disease unless metabolic needs are reduced as blood flow is restored.

Cardiorespiratory arrest is treated with cardiopulmonary resuscitation (CPR). This technique is based on the goal of augmenting both Ca_{O_2} and $\dot{Q}T$ by a series of basic life support maneuvers until advanced cardiac life support can be applied (Table 71–12). An important determinant of success in CPR is the provision of adequate $\dot{V}A$ to normalize Pa_{CO_2} and pH. When cardiac arrest occurs in nonintubated patients, the first step is to open the airway and ensure its patency. The most common cause of obstruction is the tongue. This situation may be corrected simply by tilting the head backward and lifting the chin or lower jaw forward. Mouth-to-mouth ventilation then has to be applied unless a foreign body is obstructing the airway. Two quick breaths sufficient to make the chest wall rise should be given in single-rescuer CPR.

A resuscitator's exhaled air may provide an FI_{O_2} of approximately 0.17 during mouth-to-mouth ventilation, and carbon dioxide will be eliminated because of passive lung deflation. This should alleviate the need for HCO_3^-, which is no longer recommended to reverse metabolic acidosis because it adds carbon dioxide to the body and may cause respiratory acidosis. Commonly, however, oxygen exchange within the lungs is not normal, and significant hypoxemia develops. For this reason, supplemental oxygen should be administered as soon as it is available. Both oxygenation and ventilation can be accomplished via a tightly fitting face mask and ventilation bag, preferably one capable of delivering an FI_{O_2} of 1.0. Endotracheal intubation provides the most reliable closed system for oxygenation and ventilation and also protects the airway against the aspiration of gastric contents.

Closed-chest compression should be administered to patients who do not have a palpable pulse. The patient should be supine and on a firm surface. Sufficient pressure should be applied to the lower half of the sternum to depress it 4 to 5 cm in most adults and 2 cm in children in order to increase Psa. The pressure should be relaxed after each compression, allowing the sternum to return to its relaxed position, which will reduce Pra and enhance coronary perfusion. The recommended compression-relaxation ratio is 1:1, and the rate of compressions should be between 80 and 100 per minute. The adequacy of closed-chest compression should be determined by attempting to palpate a carotid or femoral pulse produced by the compression.

The mechanism by which closed-chest compression causes

TABLE 71–12. BASIC LIFE SUPPORT

Establish unresponsiveness
Call for help
Position victim
Open airway
Check for foreign body in airway
Institute mouth-to-mouth breathing
Check for pulse
Initiate closed-chest compression

blood to circulate is not clear. The original "cardiac pump" theory held that by compressing the chest the heart was squeezed between the sternum and the vertebral column, producing a mechanical systole in which right and left ventricular pressures exceed pulmonary artery and aortic pressures, respectively, causing forward blood flow. Release of the pressure caused diastolic filling of the ventricles because of the gradient between the peripheral venous system and the intrathoracic structures. More recent data suggest that it is the total intrathoracic pressure that causes forward blood flow rather than cardiac compression ("thoracic pump" theory). For example, cough in itself has sustained cardiac output and consciousness in patients with ventricular fibrillation. A variety of experimental studies are consistent with this contention, but "new CPR" based on this model has not proved to be more effective than conventional CPR.

The arrival of persons with additional training or equipment marks the start of advanced cardiac life support. Electrocardiographic monitoring enables proper application of direct-current countershock for defibrillation or conversion of ventricular tachycardia. A current of 200 to 360 joules should be used for ventricular fibrillation. The current given should be increased if there is no response to the initial shock. In patients with ventricular fibrillation, epinephrine should be administered, routinely in doses of 1 mg, or 10 ml of a 1:10,000 dilution, either intravenously (preferably via a central venous catheter) or via an endotracheal tube before countershock is applied. Epinephrine constricts peripheral vessels through its $alpha_1$ effects and enhances myocardial contractility through its $beta_1$ effects; this combination improves cerebral and cardiac perfusion. Intravenous lidocaine in a bolus of 1 mg per kilogram, followed by additional boluses and a continuous infusion of 1 to 4 mg per minute, may also be helpful in treating ventricular ectopy, as may bretylium (initial intravenous bolus of 5 to 10 mg per kilogram, followed by an infusion of 1 to 2 mg per minute). Calcium chloride is no longer recommended in the treatment of cardiorespiratory arrest because it has not been shown to be effective and because it may contribute to ischemic injury.

All patients who have been resuscitated successfully should be transferred as quickly as possible to a critical care unit if they are not there already. At a minimum, electrocardiographic monitoring should be provided. The need for pulmonary artery catheterization depends on the causes and consequences of the cardiorespiratory arrest. Often, at least transiently, it is necessary to provide mechanical ventilation to allow rest and functional recovery of the respiratory muscles and to minimize their oxygen needs.

The major determinant of return of brain function is the adequacy of cerebral perfusion during the period of cardiac arrest. Subsequently, after recovery of cardiac function, all factors that influence oxygen delivery to the brain should be evaluated and made normal when possible. Measures to prevent possible elevations in ICP, such as head elevation, controlling arterial pH and Pa_{CO_2}, and treating seizures and agitation, should be undertaken. Barbiturate loading has not been demonstrated to minimize brain damage; calcium channel blocking agents are being studied at the present time.

ETHICAL ISSUES IN CRITICAL CARE MEDICINE

Critical care units have been utilized in more or less their present form for approximately 25 years, yet their contribution to health care has not been quantified. Studies of patients suspected of having a myocardial infarction have suggested that if there are no early (initial 2 hours in one study, at 24 hours in another) indications of complications, management in a coronary care unit does not offer any advantage over management in a hospital room or at home. Similarly, the outcome of patients with bacteremic pneumococcal pneumonia has not been found to be improved by critical care.

Other diseases commonly encountered in the critical care setting continue to have a poor outcome. One study demonstrated that the in-hospital mortality rate for patients with ARDS who required mechanical ventilation with an FI_{O_2} of 0.5 or greater for more than 24 hours was 66 per cent; patients who required an FI_{O_2} of 1.0 with a PEEP level of 5 cm H_2O or more for 2 hours, or an FI_{O_2} of 0.6 and a PEEP level of 5 cm H_2O or more for 12 hours, had a mortality rate of 92 per cent. The mortality rates of patients with cardiogenic and distributive shock remain between 50 and 75 per cent despite the introduction of pulmonary artery catheterization, a finding that has led to questions regarding the value of this monitoring technique. Cardiopulmonary resuscitation, when performed on hospitalized patients or persons older than 70 years of age out of the hospital, may be successful less than 10 per cent of the time. The survival rate of patients with three or more organ failures after 5 days in a critical care unit approached zero in one large investigation.

Data such as these imply that critical care is of little or no value in several categories of illness. Yet patients in the postoperative period and patients with cardiac arrhythmias, narcotic and sedative drug overdose, reversible neuromuscular diseases, hypovolemic and obstructive shock, and asthma and COPD clearly benefit from critical care. Furthermore, most clinicians treating severely ill patients have hope that the patients will survive, and they thus request that critical care be provided, almost regardless of the published prognosis. One reason for this is that prognostication is difficult in individual patients despite data derived from groups. Another is that patients and their families usually desire critical care if it will prolong life, assuming that self-awareness and social interaction are maintained. A third reason is that physicians may respond to what has been called the technologic imperative: the desire to do everything possible despite the ratio of benefit to cost.

Critical care is extraordinarily expensive. The issue of who should be admitted to critical care units and how aggressively they should be treated is a social, as well as medical, concern. Until this issue is resolved, physicians should base decisions regarding critical care primarily on the wishes of well-informed, mentally capable patients or their surrogates. Patients and surrogates who request critical care should receive it if they can benefit and if space permits. On the other hand, the wishes of mentally capable patients who choose against therapies such as endotracheal intubation and mechanical ventilation should be respected. If the mental capacity to make decisions is not clear, hospital ethics committees may become involved.

Orders not to initiate CPR, which are also called "do not resuscitate," or "DNR," orders, may be written at the request of patients, as just discussed, or may be initiated by physicians, when to the best of their knowledge CPR will not be successful in the broad sense of restoring meaningful life. In most instances, such decisions should be discussed with the patient and, when appropriate, with his or her family. The order should then be written in standard fashion in the order sheet, and a note describing the basis for the order and the decisions that took place should be included in the chart. Such orders clarify the ambiguity that surrounds the decisions concerning critical care for patients with irreversible illnesses and relieve nurses or uninvolved physicians from the responsibility of deciding not to initiate CPR.

Some patients with pre-existing DNR orders may still benefit from critical care. Treating airways obstruction, metabolic abnormalities, or arrhythmias may at least temporarily improve the patient's condition, making the existence of DNR orders a moot point. Nevertheless, DNR orders, when written in a critical care unit, usually represent the start of withholding or withdrawal of life support. Life-sustaining care was withheld or withdrawn from only 5 per cent of the patients in a recent study, but such withdrawal or withholding precipitated about half of the deaths occurring in critical care units. The reason for limiting care was a poor prognosis, including brain death, the complete and irreversible loss of the functions of the cerebral hemisphere and brain stem. Most of the patients from whom life support was withheld or withdrawn were not brain dead, but they nonetheless were not mentally capable of participating in the decision-making process. Only a few had previously expressed their wishes regarding critical care in a "living will" or other format. As a result, family members or other patient surrogates usually had to make decisions limiting treatment on the basis of the physician's recommendations. Developing the prognostic knowledge to make such recommendations on a more rational basis and managing the death of severely ill patients are among the major responsibilities of those who participate in critical care medicine.

Bihari D, Smithies M, Gimson A, et al.: The effects of vasodilation with prostacyclin on oxygen delivery and uptake in critically ill patients. N Engl J Med 317:397, 1987. *Describes the presence of an "oxygen debt" in patients with the adult respiratory distress syndrome and how the "debt" can be repaid with maximization of oxygen transport.*

Danek SJ, Lynch JP, Weg JG, et al.: The dependence of oxygen uptake on oxygen delivery in the adult respiratory distress syndrome. Am Rev Respir Dis 122:387, 1980. *The first clinical study of oxygen supply dependence in patients with the adult respiratory distress syndrome.*

Danis M, Patrick DL, Southerland LI, et al.: Patients' and families' preferences for medical intensive care. JAMA 260:797, 1988. *Through interviews with survivors of critical care and relatives of nonsurvivors, the authors conclude that most patients welcome such care if it prolongs meaningful life.*

Darioli R, Perret C: Mechanical controlled hypoventilation in status asthmaticus. Am Rev Respir Dis 129:385, 1984. *Intentional underventilation of asthmatics to reduce the risk of barotrauma is described.*

Dorinsky PM, Gadek JE: Mechanisms of multiple nonpulmonary organ failure in ARDS. Chest 96:885, 1989. *A recent review of organs other than the lungs that fail in patients with the adult respiratory distress syndrome. Explanations for this phenomenon are offered.*

Gilbert EM, Haupt MT, Mandanas RY, et al.: The effect of fluid loading, blood transfusion, and catecholamine infusion on oxygen delivery and consumption in patients with sepsis. Am Rev Respir Dis 134:873, 1986. *Administering fluids, blood, or catecholamines increased oxygen consumption in patients with septic shock and lactic acidosis.*

Hook EW III, Horton CA, Schaberg DR: Failure of intensive care unit support to influence mortality from pneumococcal bacteremia. JAMA 249:1055, 1983. *This study illustrates that critical care has had no major impact on the outcome of bacteremic pneumococcal pneumonia.*

Kelly MA: Critical care medicine—a new specialty? N Engl J Med 313:24, 1988. *Traces the evolution of critical care medicine.*

Knaus WA, Draper EA, Wagner DP, et al.: An evaluation of outcome from intensive care in major medical centers. Ann Intern Med 104:3, 1986. *Patient outcome was related primarily to the interaction and coordination of critical care unit staff.*

Krischer JP, Fine EG, Weisfeldt ML, et al.: Comparison of prehospital conventional and simultaneous compression-ventilation cardiopulmonary resuscitation. Crit Care Med 17:1263, 1989. *Describes a recent trial of "new" versus conventional CPR; the "new" form was not superior.*

Lain DC, DiBenedetto R, Morris SL, et al.: Pressure control inverse ratio ventilation as a method to reduce peak inspiratory pressure and provide adequate ventilation and oxygenation. Chest 95:1081, 1989. *A clinical study of the effectiveness of pressure control and inverse ratio ventilation as compared with assisted mechanical ventilation.*

Luce JM: Ethical principles in critical care. JAMA 263:696, 1990. *A recent review of the application of ethical principles, such as beneficence, in the critical care unit.*

MacIntyre NR: Respiratory function during pressure support ventilation. Chest 89:677, 1986. *A small trial of pressure support ventilation during weaning.*

Montgomery AB, Stager MA, Cerrico CJ, et al.: Causes of mortality in patients with the adult respiratory distress syndrome. Am Rev Respir Dis 132:485, 1985. *This study demonstrates that most patients with the adult respiratory distress syndrome die of septic complications, including MOSF.*

Norcini JJ, Shea JA, Langdon LO, et al.: First American Board of Internal Medicine critical care examination: Process and results. Crit Care Med 17:7, 1989. *Describes the physicians who took the first ABIM critical care examination and what was expected of them.*

O'Quin RJ, Marini JJ: Pulmonary artery occlusion pressure: Clinical physiology, measurement, and interpretation. Am Rev Respir Dis 128:319, 1983. *A guide to using and interpreting flow-directed pulmonary artery catheters.*

Parillo JE, Burch C, Sheshamer JH, et al.: A circulating myocardial depressant substance in humans with septic shock: Septic shock patients with a reduced ejection fraction have a circulating factor that depresses myocardial cell performance. J Clin Invest 76:1539, 1985. *This investigation provides the best evidence yet for circulating myocardial depressant factor.*

Pepe PE, Marini JJ: Occult positive end-expiratory pressure in mechanically ventilated patients: The auto-PEEP effect. Am Rev Respir Dis 126:166, 1982. *Describes the effects of auto-PEEP and how to measure this parameter in ventilated patients.*

Sahn SA, Lakshiminarayan S, Petty JL: Weaning from mechanical ventilation. JAMA 235:2208, 1976. *Reviews the best overall approach to the task of weaning, although it does not include newer ventilatory modes.*

Shoemaker WC, Kram HB, Appel PL: Therapy of shock based on pathophysiology, monitoring, and outcome prediction. Crit Care Med 18:S19, 1990. *Argues in favor of increasing oxygen transport in patients in shock.*

Smedira NG, Evans BH, Grais LS, et al.: Withholding and withdrawal of life support from the critically ill. N Engl J Med 322:309, 1990. *This recent study documents why, how, and under what circumstances life support was withheld or withdrawn from patients in two critical care units.*

Stauffer JL, Olson DE, Petty TL: Complications and consequences of endotracheal intubation and tracheotomy. Am J Med 70:65, 1981. *The best prospective study of the complications of endotracheal intubation by the translaryngeal route or via tracheostomy.*

Wanzer SH, Federman DD, Adelstein SJ, et al.: The physician's responsibility toward hopelessly ill patients. N Engl J Med 320:844, 1989. *A consensus of ethicists and clinicians reviews how to deal with hopelessly ill patients in critical care units.*

Zwillich WC, Pierson DJ, Creagh CE, et al.: Complications of assisted ventilation: A prospective study of 354 consecutive episodes. Am J Med 57:161, 1974. *A study of complications in patients receiving assisted mechanical ventilation.*

PART IX
RENAL DISEASES

72 Approach to the Patient with Renal Disease

Thomas E. Andreoli

This chapter provides an overview of the cardinal manifestations of diseases of the kidney or urinary tract, together with a relatively simple classification of these disorders. There are four sections. The first section contains a brief consideration of the cardinal functions of the kidney. A more detailed analysis of renal physiology is presented in Ch. 73. The second section enumerates briefly the approach to patients affected with the more common syndromes involving the kidneys and urinary tract. The third section describes the consequences of complete or nearly complete failure of renal function, that is, the uremic syndrome. Finally, the last section considers the relationship between the adaptive response to a reduction in nephron mass and the potential contribution of one of these adaptive responses, renal hyperfiltration, to the pathogenesis of progressive renal disease.

CARDINAL ELEMENTS OF RENAL FUNCTION

URINE FORMATION. The kidneys maintain constancy of the volume and composition of body fluids by forming urine, whose composition is ultimately determined by the dietary intake of solute and water and by the rate and kind of metabolic transformation of endogenous and exogenous carbohydrates, proteins, lipids, and nucleic acids. The kidneys also serve as the major route for the excretion of a large number of drugs. The formation of urine serves two purposes: a *regulatory* function, that is, the maintenance of a constant volume and composition of body fluids; and an *excretory* function, that is, elimination of endogenous and exogenous metabolic end-products.

Urine is formed by a sequence of five events:

1. The glomerulus filters approximately 180 liters of extracellular fluid daily across glomerular capillaries and the visceral epithelium of Bowman's capsule, using as a driving force the mean arterial pressure. The glomerular capillary endothelium and basement membrane and the visceral epithelium of Bowman's capsule are freely permeable to water and solutes of relatively low molecular weight (that is, under 6000 to 8000), moderately permeable to large molecular weight species such as myoglobin (molecular weight, approximately 16,000), and virtually impermeable to macromolecules such as albumin. Filtration is also influenced by molecular charge as well as size. The result is an isotonic, virtually protein-free filtrate whose daily volume is more than 10-fold greater than the volume of extracellular fluid (ECF).

2. The proximal tubule isotonically reabsorbs approximately two thirds of the glomerular filtrate. In the process, certain alterations in the composition of tubular fluid are produced by specialized transport mechanisms: the preferential absorption of sodium with bicarbonate rather than chloride; the virtually complete absorption of organic solutes such as glucose and amino acids; and the absorption of organic acids such as uric acid and other nonamino acids in early segments of the proximal nephron, followed by secretion of these acids into tubular fluid in the late proximal nephron. Thus the volume of tubular fluid delivered to the loop of Henle is approximately one third of the volume of glomerular filtrate, has a sodium concentration equal to that of plasma and a bicarbonate concentration about 10 per cent of that in plasma, and contains little or no glucose or amino acids.

3. The loop of Henle dissociates the absorption of sodium and water. The descending limb of Henle passively abstracts water into the hypertonic medullary interstitium, concentrating the tubular fluid. Conversely, the essentially water-impermeable thick ascending limb of Henle actively absorbs approximately 25 per cent of filtered sodium chloride but little water. As a result, about 18 liters of tubular fluid enter the distal convoluted tubule daily. This fluid, which is approximately 10 per cent of the initial glomerular filtrate, is also maximally dilute, having an osmolality of approximately 50 mOsm per kilogram of H_2O.

4. The distal convoluted tubule primarily absorbs sodium under the influence of aldosterone and secretes protons, ammonia, and potassium.

5. The collecting duct system regulates the osmolality of urine. When antidiuretic hormone (ADH) is present, water is absorbed across the collecting duct and tubular fluid equilibrates osmotically with the hypertonic medullary interstitium; when ADH is absent, the water permeability of collecting ducts is at a minimum and a dilute urine is excreted.

THE KIDNEY AS AN ENDOCRINE RECEPTOR. Among many hormones that regulate renal function, three are of particular importance: parathyroid hormone (PTH), aldosterone, and ADH. PTH enhances the absorption of calcium and magnesium and inhibits the absorption of phosphate and bicarbonate in the proximal tubule by increasing intracellular cyclic $3',5'$-adenosine monophosphate (cAMP). PTH also stimulates the renal conversion of 25-hydroxycholecalciferol, the major metabolite of vitamin D_3, to 1,25-dihydroxycholecalciferol, which is the major biologically active form of vitamin D_3 (Ch. 233).

Aldosterone and other mineralocorticoids stimulate the rate of sodium absorption in the distal nephron. Aldosterone also increases the rate of net potassium secretion and net proton secretion (and consequently the rate of bicarbonate regeneration) by the distal nephron.

ADH promotes the formation of a hypertonic urine both by increasing the rate of salt absorption in the thick ascending limb of Henle and by increasing the water permeability of the collecting duct system. Both actions are mediated by ADH-dependent increases in cytosolic cAMP in those renal tubular segments.

THE KIDNEY AS AN ENDOCRINE ORGAN. The kidney plays a major role in prostaglandin production, in the operation of the kallikrein-kinin system, and in the degradation of low molecular weight proteins. The kidney is also the major site for the synthesis of erythropoietin and of renin. Erythropoietin is a glycoprotein produced by renal enzymatic action on a circulating precursor of hepatic origin. The principal action of erythropoietin is to stimulate the rate of red blood cell production by the bone marrow. Synthetic human erythropoietin, produced using recombinant technology, is now available for use in patients with chronic renal failure who are undergoing chronic dialysis.

Renin is secreted by the granular cells of the juxtaglomerular apparatus in response to reductions in renal perfusion pressure or in effective circulating volume. Renin increases the rate of conversion of angiotensinogen to angiotensin I, which in turn is a precursor of angiotensin II. In turn, angiotensin II is a potent vasoconstrictor agent and a strong stimulus to thirst and to aldosterone production. Thus, the kidney, by way of renin production, plays a central role in the volume repletion reaction.

EVALUATION OF PATIENTS WITH RENAL DISEASE

Renal diseases may be intrinsic or may occur as manifestations of systemic disease. Thus the initial history and physical examination are often quite variable in different diseases. The same considerations apply to routine urinalysis, to initial blood chemistry measurements, and to more specialized renal imaging tests, such as renal ultrasonography or intravenous pyelography. Consequently, these findings are considered in the context of the various cardinal renal syndromes.

THE MAJOR RENAL SYNDROMES

Renal disorders are often nonspecific in their manifestations—as hematuria, azotemia, hypertension, or metabolic acidosis, for example. The interpretation of a group of findings obtained by history, physical examination, and routine laboratory studies, however, may be used to describe some of the more common syndromes and disorders affecting the kidneys and urinary tract, which are briefly described below.

THE UNDERPERFUSION SYNDROMES. Table 72–1 lists the major groups of diseases characterized by renal hypoperfusion: (1) renal hypoperfusion secondary to a reduction in effective circulating volume, (2) renal ischemia because of occlusive disease in one or both renal arteries, and (3) reversible renal vasoconstriction secondary to acute transplant rejection or certain drugs.

All three classes of disorders reduce effective renal perfusion and thus are characterized by certain common features. These include (1) a reduced fractional excretion of sodium, (2) hyperreninemia and secondary hyperaldosteronism, and (3) nuclear renal scintiscans indicative of renal underperfusion. When renal underperfusion is severe, oliguria and azotemia also ensue. However, the clinical manifestations of the three groups of disorders differ significantly.

Renal hypoperfusion secondary to a *reduction in effective circulating volume* may occur in association with true volume contraction; an increase in vascular capacitance, as in sepsis; sequestration of fluid in interstitial compartments, as in ascites and the hepatorenal syndrome; or an inability to transfer fluid from the venous to the arterial limbs of the circulation, as in severe congestive heart failure, constrictive pericarditis, or pericardial tamponade. When the effective circulating volume is sufficiently reduced, the kidneys are hypoperfused, the glomerular filtration rate is reduced, and renin is released. This results in oliguria, an elevation in serum blood urea nitrogen (BUN) and creatinine concentrations, and a reduced fractional excretion rate for sodium (that is, generally less than 1 per cent). Although plasma renin levels are elevated, the patients are ordinarily normotensive, presumably because the effective circulating volume is decreased.

Renal ischemia produced by *occlusive disease* of the renal arteries results in renin release from the ischemic kidney without a reduction in effective circulating volume and consequently is manifested primarily as hypertension, since pressor activity is elevated while filling of the arterial tree is normal or only slightly reduced. If the renal arterial occlusive disease is limited to one kidney and the contralateral kidney retains normal function, azotemia is absent. However, if the hypertension results in injury to the unaffected kidney, azotemia may ensue. When both renal arteries are involved, azotemia occurs when renal ischemia is sufficiently severe that renal autoregulatory mechanisms are inadequate to maintain an adequate glomerular filtration rate.

Reversible vasoconstriction of renal microcirculation is a third mechanism for producing renal hypoperfusion, renal salt avidity, and azotemia. This phenomenon occurs in acute renal transplant rejection and in response to certain nephrotoxic agents, particularly cyclosporine and amphotericin B. Restoration of renal perfusion and improvement in renal function generally occur if the

TABLE 72–1. THE UNDERPERFUSION SYNDROMES

Class	Examples
Reduced effective circulating volume	Circulatory collapse
	Congestive heart failure
	Cirrhosis with ascites
Occlusive renal artery disease	Renal artery atherosclerosis
	Fibromuscular hyperplasia
Vasoconstriction of renal micro-vasculature	Acute transplant rejection
	Cyclosporine nephrotoxicity
	Amphotericin B nephrotoxicity

acute rejection episode is treated successfully or when the offending nephrotoxic agent is discontinued.

THE RENAL PARENCHYMAL SYNDROMES. *Acute Glomerular Disorders.* **Glomerulonephritis and the Nephrotic Syndrome** (Ch. 79). Two major types of disorders affect the glomerulus: (1) the *acute nephritic syndrome*, characterized mainly by inflammatory and/or necrotizing lesions within glomeruli, and (2) the *nephrotic syndrome*, a predominantly noninflammatory derangement of the glomeruli characterized by an abnormal "leakiness" of the glomeruli to albumin and other macromolecules.

The etiologic, histologic, and clinical characteristics of the glomerulonephritic and nephrotic syndromes overlap to a considerable degree: (1) A given disease process—for example, systemic lupus erythematosus (SLE)—may produce a mild, focal glomerulonephritis with hematuria, mild proteinuria, but no azotemia; a diffuse proliferative glomerulonephritis with hematuria, proteinuria, and severe renal failure; or membranous nephropathy characterized by a relatively pure nephrotic syndrome. (2) Glomerular lesions may evolve; for example, Goodpasture's syndrome can begin as a mild, focal nephritis and progress to a diffuse, necrotic glomerulonephritis. (3) The extent of glomerular injury, as viewed on renal biopsy, correlates generally but inexactly with the severity of the clinical picture. (4) A given pathogenic mechanism—for example, immune complex disease—may in some instances result in acute glomerulonephritis and in other cases in a pure nephrotic syndrome. (5) In certain disorders such as membranoproliferative nephritis, both a nephritic picture and a nephrotic picture may coexist. (6) The same histologic picture—for example, in nil disease—may occur either as a primary renal disorder or in association with a systemic disorder such as Hodgkin's disease.

These diverse glomerular disorders can be somewhat arbitrarily classified by four major patterns that may be defined by the initial presentation of the patient (Table 72–2). Table 72–3, in turn, lists the most common diseases that present as nephritic, nephrotic, and mixed syndromes. As indicated in Table 72–3, the acute glomerular syndromes may occur as primary renal disorders—for example, postinfectious glomerulonephritis—or in association with a systemic disease—for example, SLE. Accordingly, the clinical findings vary considerably. In primary renal disorders, the antecedent history may reveal nothing except a prior, recent infection and a recent history of hematuria. In Goodpasture's syndrome, pulmonary symptoms may also be present. The physical findings are generally limited to edema and/or hypertension. In glomerular disorders associated with systemic diseases such as vasculitis, gammopathies, or diabetes, the history and physical examination may reveal findings typical of those disorders. Alternatively, a glomerular disorder may commonly be the first manifestation of a systemic disease, as in, for example, SLE.

The Mild Acute Glomerulonephritis Syndromes. In this class of glomerular inflammation, glomerular blood flow is sufficient to

TABLE 72–2. CLASSIFICATION OF MAJOR ACUTE GLOMERULAR SYNDROMES

Class of Disorder	Major Derangement	Major Findings
1. Mild acute glomerulonephritis	Mild glomerular inflammation	Hematuria, proteinuria Absent or mild azotemia Absent or mild edema
2. Severe acute glomerulonephritis	Extensive glomerular inflammation Renal ischemia Primary tubular sodium acquisitiveness	Hematuria, proteinuria Azotemia Plasma volume expansion Hypertension Edema Circulatory overload (if severe)
3. Pure nephrotic syndrome	Glomerular protein leak	Massive proteinuria Reduced plasma oncotic pressure Anasarca Normotensive Sensitive to diuretics
4. Mixed disorders	1 plus 3 or 2 plus 3	Hematuria Massive proteinuria Azotemia (variable) Hypertension (variable) Edema

TABLE 72–3. MAJOR ACUTE GLOMERULAR SYNDROMES

Common Presentation	Primary Renal Disorders	Systemic Disorders
Nephritic syndrome	Postinfectious glomerulo-nephritis Idiopathic rapidly progressive (crescentic) glomerulonephritis Goodpasture's syndrome Hemolytic-uremic syndrome Hereditary nephritis	Vasculitis: SLE Polyarteritis nodosa Wegener's granulomatosis Henoch-Schönlein purpura
Nephrotic syndrome	Idiopathic nil disease Membranous nephropathy Focal sclerosis	Nil disease in Hodgkin's disease Membranous nephropathy in neoplasia, SLE, and drug toxicity Focal sclerosis in heroin abuse, vesicoureteral reflux, and AIDS Essential cryoglobulinemia Gammopathies Diabetic nephropathy
Nephritic/nephrotic syndrome	Membranoproliferative glomerulonephritis type I type II (dense deposit disease) Mesangioproliferative glomerulonephritis (IgA/IgG nephropathy)	Vasculitides, particularly SLE Diabetic nephropathy

SLE = systemic lupus erythematosus; AIDS = acquired immunodeficiency syndrome; IgA = immunoglobulin A; IgG = immunoglobulin G.

maintain the glomerular filtration at a normal or nearly normal rate. Mild acute glomerulonephritis is characterized by hematuria, red cell casts, modest proteinuria, minimal azotemia, and mild or no edema. Because renal perfusion is not severely compromised, hypertension or salt retention or both are generally absent.

The Diffuse Acute Glomerulonephritis Syndromes. These glomerulonephritic syndromes are usually characterized by diffuse glomerular inflammation and/or necrosis sufficiently severe that hematuria and proteinuria are accompanied by a reduction in filtation rate and, consequently, azotemia of varying degrees. Simultaneously, for reasons that are not well understood, sodium acquisitiveness in acute glomerulonephritis is considerably greater than that expected solely from the reduction in glomerular filtration rate. Plasma albumin is generally normal, so that a significant fraction of retained sodium remains in the vascular compartment and may result in hypertension, plasma volume dilution, circulatory overload, congestive heart failure, and a suppression of plasma renin activity.

Nephrotic Syndrome. In the pure nephrotic syndrome, the glomerular filtration barrier is abnormally permeable to macromolecules, so that massive proteinuria occurs even though the filtration rate may be normal. This large urinary loss of protein contributes to the characteristic hypoalbuminemia in such patients. Hypercholesterolemia also occurs and correlates closely with the degree of hypoalbuminemia.

Nephrotic patients are usually salt acquisitive and edematous. In the nephrotic syndromes the reduced plasma oncotic pressure leads to translocation of fluid to the interstitium, a reduced effective circulating volume, and a secondary sodium acquisitiveness and edema. Patients with the pure nephrotic syndrome often are normotensive, rarely develop circulatory overload, and frequently have elevated plasma renin activities. As further evidence for a reduced effective circulating volume, severely nephrotic patients may have postural hypotension even in the presence of anasarca and may have hemoconcentration and renal hypoperfusion with attendant azotemia following excessive diuretic use.

The Interstitial Nephritis Syndromes (Ch. 80). In the interstitial nephritis syndromes, the primary abnormality is damage to the tubulointerstitial system of the kidney, with secondary glomerular damage. Thus renal tubular function tends to be deranged disproportionately to reductions in glomerular filtration rate.

Generalized tubulointerstitial disorders often damage the juxtaglomerular apparatus and therefore tend to impair renin pro-

duction. As a consequence of hyporeninemia, aldosterone production is curtailed. This combination generally results in hyporeninemia, hypoaldosteronism, modest degrees of salt wasting, hyperkalemia, and hyperchloremic metabolic acidosis. These abnormalities occur even when the glomerular filtration rate is only modestly reduced.

Urinary abnormalities such as hematuria and proteinuria are usually, but not always, relatively modest in patients with tubulointerstitial disease. Three general classes of tubulointerstitial diseases can be defined:

1. *Chronic tubulointerstitial disease* may occur as a consequence of any of a large number of diseases that produce chronic damage to the renal interstitium: chronic hypertension, with progressive ischemia to the renal interstitium; diabetes mellitus, in which microvascular disease within the kidney effects the same end result; occlusive disease of smaller renal vessels, as in sickle cell disease; chronic pyelonephritis; and gout; other causes include exogenous toxins, notably illicit alcohol containing lead, and analgesic abuse, particularly the combination of phenacetin and aspirin. Chronic interstitial disease is generally detected in individuals who have modest degrees of sodium wasting, hyperkalemia, metabolic acidosis, and an acidic urine. These abnormalities may occur even when only mild degrees of azotemia exist. The plasma renin activity is generally reduced, as are rates of aldosterone secretion. Hematuria and massive proteinuria are not common in chronic interstitial disease.

2. *Acute allergic interstitial disease* occurs when patients are treated with antibiotics, notably penicillin and related drugs, or with nonsteroidal anti-inflammatory agents. In addition to producing electrolyte abnormalities similar to those described above for chronic interstitial nephritis, acute allergic interstitial nephritis may severely reduce glomerular filtration and may be associated with marked hematuria and proteinuria and with oliguria.

Oliguria and azotemia associated with acute allergic interstitial nephritis may be difficult to differentiate from those of acute tubular necrosis. In this setting an electrolyte pattern of hyperkalemic, hyperchloremic metabolic acidosis, a reduced plasma renin activity and rates of aldosterone secretion, an elevated fractional excretion rate for sodium, eosinophilia, and the presence of eosinophils in the urine would strongly suggest acute allergic interstitial nephritis.

3. *Acute pyelonephritis*, a form of acute interstitial nephritis due to bacterial invasion of the kidney, usually produces a septic picture with fever, flank pain, leukocytosis, and dysuria (Ch. 84). Factors that predispose to acute pyelonephritis are often present, such as diabetes mellitus, obstructive uropathy, prior instrumentation of the urinary tract, or bacterial endocarditis with septic renal emboli. The most useful clues to the presence of acute pyelonephritis include findings of sepsis, costovertebral angle tenderness, pyuria, leukocyte casts, the presence of bacteria in unspun samples of urine, and positive urine cultures.

Isolated Tubular Defects (Ch. 82). In addition to tubular derangements secondary to diffuse tubulointerstitial disease, there are a number of specific defects of tubular function.

Proximal Tubular Defects. *Renal glycosuria* occurs when the glucose threshold of the proximal nephron is reduced. *Renal phosphate wasting* results when the rate of proximal absorption of phosphate is reduced. Similarly, *aminoaciduria* may result from tubular defects that are either generalized or specific. Finally, the rate of bicarbonate absorption by the proximal nephron may be reduced, resulting in profound bicarbonate wasting, a syndrome entitled *proximal renal tubular acidosis* (Ch. 82).

Renal phosphate wasting, renal glycosuria, renal aminoaciduria, and proximal renal tubular acidosis occurring simultaneously constitute Fanconi's syndrome (Ch. 82). These proximal tubular defects may be congenital or may be found in association with heavy metal poisoning of the proximal nephron, notably by copper in Wilson's disease, following exposure to toxic agents such as maleic acid, and in the gammopathies.

Possible Loop of Henle Defect. The pathogenesis of *Bartter's syndrome* has not been elucidated (Ch. 82). Yet it appears that many of the findings of Bartter's syndrome, including profound salt wasting, potassium wasting, and compensatory hypertrophy of the juxtaglomerular apparatus with hyperreninemia, may be the result of a salt-absorptive defect in the thick ascending limb. A clinical syndrome resembling Bartter's syndrome commonly occurs because of surreptitious ingestion of furosemide or furosemide-like diuretics.

Distal Tubular Defects. *Distal, gradient-limited renal tubular acidosis* represents a specific defect of the distal nephron (Ch. 82). In this disorder the distal nephron is abnormally permeable to protons and cannot therefore maintain an adequately acid urine. In contrast to patients who have tubulointerstitial disease, the classic electrolyte abnormalities in distal, gradient-limited renal tubular acidosis include a tendency to salt wasting, hyperchloremic metabolic acidosis, a urine that is relatively alkaline with respect to arterial pH, and profound hypokalemia. The hypokalemia of distal, gradient-limited renal tubular acidosis is probably a consequence of aldosterone release in response to salt depletion. In contrast to proximal renal tubular acidosis or to the hyperkalemic, hyperchloremic renal tubular acidosis of diffuse tubulointerstitial disease, gradient-limited distal renal tubular acidosis is frequently associated with severe nephrocalcinosis, renal calculi, renal infection, and progressive destruction of renal mass.

Distal, gradient-limited renal tubular acidosis may occur congenitally. The disorder may also occur as a consequence of exposure to exogenous agents, notably amphotericin B and lithium, and in association with the gammopathies.

Collecting Duct Defects. The unique tubular defect of the collecting duct is nephrogenic diabetes insipidus (NDI), in which the collecting duct is refractory to the action of ADH (Ch. 214). Patients with NDI are consistently polyuric, even when large amounts of ADH are administered. The disorder may occur congenitally; in association with certain systemic disorders, such as Sjögren's syndrome and sarcoidosis; and as a result of lithium intoxication or exposure to the antibiotic demethylchlortetracycline.

The Renal Calculus Syndrome. The origin and composition of renal calculi are described in Ch. 88; most renal calculi contain magnesium-ammonium-phosphate, calcium oxalate, uric acid, a combination of calcium oxalate and uric acid, or cystine as their main crystalloids. Of these, all but uric acid stones are radiopaque.

Renal calculi may be asymptomatic and detected only on routine radiographic examination of the kidney, especially isolated calculi that do not move down the urinary tract and staghorn calculi lodged within the renal pelvis. Calculi may obstruct urine flow and consequently lead to pyelonephritis. Therefore, in any patient in whom pyelonephritis is suspected, a careful radiographic and urologic examination for renal calculi is mandatory. *Renal colic* refers to the passage of a renal calculus from the renal pelvis into the ureter characterized by exquisite pain, generally beginning in the flank and radiating into the groin. Patients almost always describe renal colic as the worst pain they have ever experienced. Renal colic is almost invariably accompanied by hematuria, unless the calculus is lodged within a ureter and produces complete unilateral obstruction to urine flow. Under these circumstances, the urine voided by the patient represents red cell–free urine from the unaffected kidney.

Kidney stones are among the more common renal disorders. It is generally prudent, particularly in patients with multiple renal calculi or with a family history of renal calculi, to look for potential underlying causes for stone formation (for example, gout, absorptive hypercalciuria, cystinuria, distal, gradient-limited renal tubular acidosis, or primary hyperparathyroidism). The presence of nephrocalcinosis should alert the physician to the possibility of distal, gradient-limited renal tubular acidosis or to primary hyperparathyroidism.

The patient with renal colic also warrants an evaluation for obstructive uropathy on the affected side and for urinary tract infection. These approaches generally involve culture of the urine, plain films of the abdomen, and, when indicated, ultrasonography of the kidneys, excretory urography, evaluation of parathyroid function, and evaluation for an absorptive hypercalciuric state.

Renal Cystic Disease (Ch. 89). There are three major forms of renal cystic disease: single or multiple cysts, polycystic kidney disease, and microcystic disease of the renal medulla. The clinical characteristics, significance, and clinical presentations of these three kinds of renal cysts vary significantly. There is no evidence that true simple cysts, multiple simple cysts, or polycystic kidney disease progresses to renal neoplasia. However, in more than 30 per cent of patients undergoing chronic hemodialysis therapy for more than 5 years, multiple single cysts develop. These are sometimes termed acquired polycystic kidney disease. About 10 per cent of these cystic transformations subsequently undergo malignant transformation.

Isolated simple cysts, either single or multiple, form sporadically for unknown reasons within the renal parenchyma, generally within the renal cortex. Single cysts in particular usually cause no symptoms; they are generally detected in one of two circumstances: episodes of renal trauma that provoke cyst rupture and hematuria, or on routine excretory urography. The true single, simple cyst (in contrast to the cystic neoplasm; see below) is innocuous and needs no therapy. *Multiple simple cysts* probably represent an extension of the process described above and are also similarly innocuous unless they encroach on renal parenchyma. Multiple simple cysts should be distinguished from polycystic kidney disease, a disorder with a more ominous prognosis. These two forms of multicystic disease can be distinguished by excretory urography; in individuals with multiple simple cysts, the overall size of the kidney is normal and the calyceal system is not elongated and only minimally distorted.

Adult polycystic kidney disease is a form of nephropathy that is generally inherited by autosomal dominance with incomplete penetrance. If a parent has polycystic kidney disease, approximately one half of the progeny will ultimately develop the disorder, although the time at which polycystic kidney disease becomes manifest is highly variable.

Polycystic kidney disease may present with recurrent bouts of hematuria, renal colic, hypertension, or urinary tract infection because of intrarenal obstruction due to cysts. Many patients with polycystic kidney disease develop renal failure, although the rate and extent of development of renal failure depend on the degree of penetrance of the autosomal dominant trait.

Three factors distinguish between patients with polycystic kidney disease and those with multiple simple cysts: (1) a positive family history consistent with an autosomal dominant trait; (2) enlargement of the kidneys, generally detected as a pole-to-pole diameter in excess of 15 to 17 cm and a cortical thickness in excess of 3 cm; and (3) elongation and deformation of the caliceal structure from the progressive enlargement of the parenchymal cysts.

Microcystic kidney disease of the renal medulla, a disorder of children generally inherited as a recessive trait, is characterized by progressive disruption and destruction of the renal medullary architecture by multiple cysts. The disease is generally detected when young children complain of fatigue and are noted to have mild degrees of proteinuria, anemia, and azotemia. The clinical course is characterized by an inordinately high requirement for salt intake in order to maintain blood pressure and an adequate filtration rate and by stunted growth due to chronic illness, to uremia, and to excessive urinary calcium losses. Nephrons are gradually destroyed, usually with progression to end-stage renal disease before the age of 30.

Renal Neoplasia (Ch. 91). Two major classes of renal tumors occur in adults: *renal cell carcinomas* (sometimes called hypernephromas), which originate in the renal cortex, and *transitional cell tumors* of the renal pelvis. Hypernephromas are versatile tumors and are often difficult to diagnose. Many patients present simply with painless hematuria. However, hypernephromas also produce a number of unusual syndromes, including polycythemias, presumably due to excessive erythropoietin production; hypertension, presumably because the neoplasm acts as the equivalent of an arteriovenous fistula and results in renin release by the affected kidney; fever of unknown origin; and hypercalcemia (see Table 91–3).

Transitional cell tumors of the renal pelvis commonly present as hematuria, which may be painless or accompanied by renal colic from the clots that are passed. The systemic manifestations described for hypernephroma are uncommonly found in transitional cell tumors. Examination of urine cytology by a Wright's stain of the urinary sediment may provide a useful diagnostic clue to the presence of these tumors.

Acute Renal Failure (Ch. 76). Acute renal failure refers either to the sudden cessation of urine flow or to sudden oliguria. Acute renal failure caused by acute glomerular disorders is generally evident from the findings described above for the acute glomerulonephritic syndromes. The general approach to the differential diagnosis of acute renal failure, particularly in hospitalized patients, involves the distinction between three major classes of disorders: (1) the underperfusion syndromes indicated in Table 72–1; (2) intrarenal syndromes, especially acute tubular necrosis and acute allergic interstitial nephritis; and (3) postrenal syndromes, that is, oligoanuria resulting from urinary tract obstruction.

The general approach to these patients involves the following cardinal maneuvers: (1) an assessment of circulatory dynamics; (2) a careful history to assess possible antecedent hypotension or exposure to nephrotoxic agents, coupled with a measurement of the fractional excretion of sodium; and (3) renal ultrasonography to exclude the possibility of obstruction of both kidneys, or obstruction of a solitary kidney, as in an individual with renal agenesis or with renal transplantation. These maneuvers are generally helpful in distinguishing between prerenal, intrarenal, and postrenal causes of oliguria. Invasive hemodynamic monitoring, coupled with a fluid challenge, may still be required to exclude rigorously the possibility of oliguria due to a reduced effective circulating volume. A percutaneous renal biopsy may be needed to distinguish between acute tubular necrosis and acute allergic interstitial nephritis. Renal ultrasonography has reduced strikingly the need for retrograde ureteral catheterization as a means for excluding obstructive uropathy.

THE POSTRENAL SYNDROMES (Ch. 81). The postrenal syndromes result from obstruction of urine flow at various loci in the urinary tract from the renal papillae to the urethral meatus. Azotemia and oliguria occur in urinary tract obstruction only when the urinary tract is obstructed bilaterally or when obstruction exists in a sole functioning kidney. The degree of azotemia depends upon the extent of the obstruction; partial obstruction may produce only moderate degrees of azotemia, while complete obstruction of the urinary tract obviously produces anuria. Obstruction of urine flow can irreversibly damage the kidneys. If the obstruction is partial or nearly complete, renal function may be preserved for as long as 4 to 5 weeks following the onset of obstruction. Obstructive uropathy also carries with it the possible complication of urinary tract infection.

Bilateral ureteral obstruction most frequently occurs at three major sites: (1) the *ureteropelvic junction*, where the obstruction is generally due to scar formation or, less commonly, to renal vessels crossing the ureter; (2) the site where the ureters cross the *pelvic brim*—neoplasms are the primary cause of such obstruction, particularly extensive carcinoma of the cervix; and (3) the *ureterovesical junction*, because of either neoplasm or scar formation. Less commonly, other disorders such as *retroperitoneal fibrosis* or disseminated retroperitoneal lymphoma may cause bilateral ureteral obstruction between the ureterovesical junction and where the ureters cross the pelvic brim. The probability of renal calculi causing bilateral ureteral obstruction is small unless one kidney is already nonfunctional and a stone obstructs the outflow of urine from the other kidney. Prostatic enlargement is a common cause of partial or complete obstruction to urine outflow. In contrast to the case in ureteral obstruction, the urinary bladder distends and often results in overflow urinary incontinence. The patient may therefore present with azotemia secondary to a profound reduction in glomerular filtration and yet have significant volumes of urine flow.

Urinary tract obstruction represents a potentially remediable cause of renal failure; every attempt should be made to exclude obstructive uropathy in individuals who are oliguric or anuric. Renal ultrasonography has simplified this task greatly, since it noninvasively detects whether or not the renal calyces are dilated and the ureters are narrowed, as occurs in ureteropelvic junction obstruction; or whether the ureters and renal calyces are both dilated, as occurs in ureterovesical obstruction or urethral obstruction.

RENAL FAILURE: THE UREMIC SYNDROME

The uremic syndrome (Ch. 77) occurs when the functional renal mass is reduced sufficiently that the kidney is no longer able to carry out excretory functions, functions relating to the regulation of the volume and composition of body fluids, functions as an endocrine receptor, and functions as an endocrine organ. The manifestations of *acute* uremia may differ from those of

chronic uremia, but these differences relate more to the rate of development of renal failure than to fundamental differences in pathophysiology.

Uremia is in part a syndrome of "autointoxication." While the chemical agents responsible for this autointoxication have not been clearly identified, uremic syndromes may be ameliorated by dialysis (which generally removes molecules having molecular weights less than 1000 to 2000), and severe protein restriction may minimize the rate of development of the uremic symptoms. Thus it is plausible to presume that the retention of the end-products of protein metabolism, reflected primarily by the BUN and serum creatinine levels as well as by other factors such as acidosis, is responsible for many of the manifestations of the uremic syndrome.

In early stages, chronic uremia is manifested by relatively nonspecific systemic symptoms, including anorexia, a metallic taste, systemic weakness, and easy fatigability. Hypertension is commonly present, but signs of circulatory volume overload may be absent if dietary solute intake has been curtailed because of anorexia. As uremia progresses, these findings increase in severity and are often accompanied by vomiting, progressively increasing pruritus, marked pallor, and central nervous system symptoms such as lethargy and confusion. In advanced uremia, frank coma and seizure, as well as pericarditis, are common findings. However, advanced central nervous system manifestations of uremia, such as pericarditis or peripheral neuropathy, are relatively infrequent in modern clinical practice because of early intervention with dialysis therapy.

In uremia the major electrolyte alterations include hypocalcemia, presumably due to the inability to form 1,25-dihydroxycholecalciferol as renal mass is reduced and to hyperphosphatemia; hyperphosphatemia, resulting from a reduction in glomerular filtration rate; and metabolic acidosis, which results from a reduction in the renal excretion of "fixed" acids (that is, incompletely combusted organic acids; and sulfate and phosphate, which represent the end-products of protein and nucleic acid metabolism, respectively).

The occurrence of hyperkalemia among uremic individuals is variable and depends on a number of factors, including the rate of potassium intake, the rate of tissue catabolism, and the rate at which renal failure has evolved. In general, patients in whom the uremic syndrome evolves acutely do not develop adaptive mechanisms (either renal or extrarenal) for potassium elimination and are therefore more prone to develop hyperkalemia. In contrast, individuals who approach end-stage renal disease gradually may often be normokalemic even when the glomerular filtration rate is less than 5 per cent of normal. Two factors may account for this phenomenon: (1) The development of renal disease is accompanied by asthenia and anorexia, so that dietary intake of potassium may be minimized; and (2) both renal and extrarenal mechanisms for more efficient potassium excretion are gradually developed.

Uremia, whether acute or chronic, is a catabolic disorder. In individuals with acute renal failure, even extensive hyperalimentation fails to prevent the loss of approximately 0.5 to 1.0 pound daily. In chronic renal failure, weight loss is more gradual and less easily perceived by patients. But in both acute and chronic renal failure, asthenia and loss of lean body mass are inevitable sequelae.

As the functional renal mass is diminished, erythropoietin production is also reduced. Thus within 2 to 3 weeks of the onset of acute renal failure, the combination of diminished erythrocyte production and an accelerated rate of red cell destruction invariably reduces the hematocrit level to the range of 20 to 25 per cent. Similar hematocrits are found in patients with chronic renal failure, particularly prior to dialysis therapy. Polycystic kidney disease represents an exception in that profound reductions of glomerular filtration rate may occur coincident with the maintenance of a hematocrit well in excess of 30 per cent. Presumably, the large renal mass of polycystic kidney disease produces sufficient erythropoietin to maintain an adequate hematocrit.

Individuals with acute renal failure do not develop significant bone disease. In contrast, individuals with chronic, severe reductions in glomerular filtration rate and in functional renal mass often have significant bone disease, termed renal osteodystrophy

(Ch. 237). At least four factors may contribute to the complex bone disorders in uremia: (1) The synthesis of 1,25-hydroxycholecalciferol in the kidney is reduced, with consequent diminished calcium absorption from the gut. (2) The calcium malabsorption leads to secondary hyperparathyroidism, which mobilizes calcium from bone in an attempt to maintain a normal level of serum ionized calcium and in the process produces osteitis fibrosa (Ch. 235). (3) Bone calcium is exchanged for retained protons in buffering the metabolic acidosis of chronic renal failure with partial maintenance of acid-base homeostasis, but at the expense of progressive dissolution of bone. (4) The uremic state impairs protein synthesis in bone and with this the formation of osteoid.

In short, the uremic syndrome results from varying impairment in the ability of the kidney to meet all of its normal metabolic and physiologic obligations: to regulate the volume and composition of body fluids, to excrete the end-products of metabolism, to serve as an endocrine receptor, and to serve as an endocrine organ. Within that framework the particular manifestations of uremia in any given patient will depend largely on the rate at which kidney failure has occurred, the severity of the renal failure (that is, the extent to which residual nephron mass is able to maintain homeostasis), and the homeostatic stresses to which the individual is subjected.

ADAPTATION TO RENAL INJURY AND THE PATHOGENESIS OF PROGRESSIVE RENAL FAILURE

Two additional characteristics of nearly all forms of chronic renal disease warrant particular consideration. First, nephron loss may be accompanied by *adaptive functional changes* in residual nephrons, which tend to minimize the effects of reducing the functional nephron mass on the chemical composition of blood. This argument, generally termed the *intact nephron hypothesis*, considers that in chronic renal disease the function of residual nephrons may be normal or supranormal. Among the cardinal adaptive characteristics described by the intact nephron hypothesis have been an increased glomerular filtration rate per nephron with elevated serum BUN concentrations or increased rates of protein feeding, and an increase in the rate of phosphate excretion per nephron mediated through secondary hyperparathyroidism, such that, in chronic renal failure, serum phosphate levels do not rise until the glomerular filtration rate is reduced to about 30 per cent of normal.

Second, these adaptive responses may ultimately be harmful to the kidney: For example, the maintenance of relatively normal serum calcium and phosphate concentrations in a setting of modest reductions in glomerular filtration rate (that is, to 30 to 40 per cent of normal) by secondary hyperparathyroidism is achieved at the expense of bone dissolution. Likewise, recent observations have provided evidence that increases in protein intake lead to glomerular hyperperfusion and that the elevated glomerular filtration rate produced by this hyperperfusion can result in progressive glomerulosclerosis. Thus, in principle, glomerular hyperperfusion produced by a protein intake that is large in relation to the residual nephron mass could contribute to the progression of chronic renal disease. A corollary to this hypothesis is the possibility that dietary protein restriction early in the course of chronic renal failure might slow the rate of progression of renal disease. A federally sponsored trial assessing the potential benefits of low-protein diets in preserving renal function in various stages of chronic renal failure is currently in progress.

Glassock RJ, Ward H, Adler S: The primary and secondary glomerular diseases. Curr Nephrol 13:1–47, 1990. *A helpful classification of primary glomerular disorders and those secondary to systemic diseases.*

Hricak H: Radiologic assessment of the kidney. *In* Brenner BM, Rector FC (eds.): The Kidney. Philadelphia, W.B. Saunders Company, 1991, pp 969–992. *A discussion of renal imaging studies.*

Klahr S, Schreiner G, Ichikawa I: The progression of renal disease. N Engl J Med 318:1657, 1988. *A detailed analysis of the factors contributing to progressive chronic renal failure.*

Levey AS, Madaio MP, Perrone RD: Laboratory assessment of renal disease: Clearance, urinalysis, and renal biopsy. *In* Brenner BM, Rector FC (eds.): The Kidney. Philadelphia, W.B. Saunders Company, 1991, pp 968–969. *A concise approach to the laboratory evaluation of patients with renal disease.*

Levine E, Grantham JJ, Slusker SL, et al.: A computed tomographic study of acquired cystic disease and renal tumors in long-term dialysis patients. AJR 142:125, 1984.

73 Structure and Function of the Kidneys

*Saulo Klahr**

This chapter reviews the structure and function of the normal mammalian kidney as a framework for understanding the derangements that occur with kidney disease.

RENAL STRUCTURE

The kidneys are located retroperitoneally with their upper and lower poles opposite the twelfth thoracic and third lumbar vertebrae, respectively. Because of the presence of the liver, the right kidney is generally lower than the left. Each adult kidney weighs 130 to 170 grams and measures about 12 by 6 by 3 cm. Through the hilus of the kidney pass a renal artery and vein, lymphatics, a nerve plexus, and the *renal pelvis*, which subdivides into the *three major calices* and subsequently into eight or more *minor calices*. A coronal section of the kidney reveals two distinct regions: the medulla and the cortex. The *renal medulla* is composed generally of 12 to 18 conical masses, the *pyramids*. The base of each pyramid is located on the corticomedullary boundary, and the apex extends toward the renal pelvis, forming the *papilla*, which projects into the minor calix. Each papilla is perforated by the distal end of 15 or more *terminal collecting ducts* (of Bellini). The *renal cortex*, about 1 cm in thickness, covers the base of the pyramids and extends medially between the individual pyramids to form the renal columns (of Bertin).

BLOOD SUPPLY

Each kidney is usually supplied by a single artery originating from the aorta at the level of the first lumbar vertebra. This artery generally divides into two branches (anterior and posterior) which enter the renal sinus and give rise to upper, middle, and lower branches *(lobar arteries)*. As these arteries enter the renal parenchyma they form the *interlobar arteries* that course toward the cortex along the lateral borders of the medullary pyramids and then form the *arcuate arteries* at the base of the renal medulla. The *intralobular arteries*, branching at right angles from the arcuate vessels, course through the cortex to the periphery. They give rise to *afferent arterioles*, each of which ends in a fine capillary bed known as a glomerulus. Thus, the glomerulus is supplied by a single afferent arteriole and drained, in turn, by an *efferent arteriole*, which emerges at the glomerular vascular pole and immediately ramifies into numerous peritubular capillaries that surround the tubular segments of the cortex. The *vasa recta*, which extend medially into the medulla, are the capillaries that originate from efferent arterioles of juxtamedullary glomeruli.

The venous system follows the same pattern as the arterial system, with the capillaries forming venules that unite into intralobular, arcuate, lobular, and ultimately renal veins. Each renal vein drains into the inferior vena cava.

THE NEPHRON

The nephron is the functional unit of the kidney. There are approximately 1,200,000 nephrons in each human kidney. Each is composed of a malpighian corpuscle (the *glomerulus* and *Bowman's capsule*) and its attached *tubule*. The tubule contains several distinct anatomic and functional segments: proximal tubule, loop of Henle, distal convoluted tubule, and collecting tubule. The junction of collecting tubules forms the collecting ducts, which traverse the medulla and terminate at the tip of the papilla. There are two distinct populations of nephrons in the human kidney: those with glomeruli located in the outer cortex *(superficial nephrons)* and those with glomeruli situated near the

*The author wishes to thank Dr. David Warnock for assistance in the revision of this chapter.

corticomedullary junction (*juxtamedullary nephrons*). The superficial nephrons, which constitute about 85 per cent of the total nephron population, have short loops of Henle that frequently do not penetrate the medulla. The juxtamedullary nephrons have long loops of Henle that extend into the inner medulla and are in close apposition to the vasa recta.

GLOMERULUS. The glomerulus (Fig. 73–1) is a network of capillaries originating from the afferent arteriole. After dividing into four to eight lobules to form the glomerular tuft, the capillaries rejoin to form the efferent arteriole, which leaves the glomerulus at the vascular pole. The glomerular tuft is surrounded by *Bowman's capsule*, which is an extension of the basement membrane and connective tissue of the proximal tubule. The *urinary* or *Bowman's space* separates the capsule from the glomerular tuft. Bowman's capsule contains a single layer of squamous cells (*parietal epithelial cells*), which undergo an abrupt transition to taller columnar cells typical of the proximal tubule at the urinary pole of the glomerulus. In the glomerular tuft there are three distinct cell types (endothleial, mesangial, and epithelial), a capillary wall (basement membrane), and an interstitial or supporting region (mesangium).

Capillary Wall. The capillary wall contains endothelial cells, a basement membrane, and epithelial cells (see Fig. 73–1). The *endothelial cells* line the capillary lumen. Fenestrae or pores (approximate diameter of 700 Å) covered by thin diaphragms are present in the attenuated endothelium. The *basement membrane*, a structure with an average thickness in the adult of 3200 Å, contains three distinct areas: a central electron-dense *lamina densa* and, on either side, a *lamina rara externa* and *lamina rara interna* (see Fig. 73–1). The major constituents of the basement membrane are collagen and glycoprotein. Thickening of this structure is seen in a number of glomerular diseases. The *visceral epithelial cells*, or *podocytes*, are the largest of the glomerular cells. Extending from the body of the podocyte are primary processes, from which individual *foot processes*, or *pedicels*, project to come into contact with the lamina rara externa of the basement membrane. Between the foot processes is a space (*filtration slit* or *slit pore*) 250 to 400 Å wide, which is covered by a thin membrane, the *filtration slit diaphragm*, which is located approximately 600 Å from the basement membrane. This slit diaphragm is a zipper-like structure composed of rectangular

pores (40 to 140 Å in a cross-section). The estimated total area of these pores is approximately 3 per cent of the total surface area of the glomerular capillaries. In renal diseases characterized by proteinuria the pedicels of the podocytes are replaced by a continuous band of cytoplasm adjacent to the lamina rara externa (fusion of foot processes).

The Mesangium. The mesangium, the interstitial portion of the glomerular lobules, is composed of *mesangial cells* (axial or intercapillary) and *mesangial matrix*. The latter is a homogeneous fibrillary material containing mucopolysaccharides and glycoprotein. The mesangial cells, which have phagocytic properties, resemble smooth muscle cells, contain myosin, and usually do not communicate directly with the vascular space. The mesangium is unique in that entry of a substance into the space does not require passage through a capillary basement membrane. In human glomerulonephritis, immune deposits are found in the mesangium, often exclusively.

THE TUBULE. The renal tubule is composed of distinct anatomic and functional segments: the *proximal convoluted tubule*, the *pars recta* or *straight portion* of the proximal tubule, the *thin descending* and *ascending limbs of Henle's loop*, the *thick ascending limb of Henle's loop*, the *distal convoluted tubule*, the *cortical collecting tubule*, and the *medullary collecting duct*. These segments differ in their location, length, diameter, characteristics of the lining epithelium, including number and size of mitochondria, appearance of intercellular channels, presence of luminal microvilli (brush border), and complexity of basal infoldings. The functional differences among nephron segments are described below.

JUXTAGLOMERULAR APPARATUS. The juxtaglomerular apparatus is a region near the glomerular vascular pole in which the transition occurs between the *thick ascending limb* and the *distal convoluted tubule* and the *afferent* and *efferent arterioles* come into juxtaposition. Here, the cells of the distal tubule become taller and more numerous (*macula densa*), and cells derived from the afferent arteriole (*juxtaglomerular cells*) are present between the distal tubule and the vascular pole (Fig. 73–1). These cells may be granular (containing renin) or agranular. Adrenergic nerve endings have been demonstrated in the juxta-

FIGURE 73–1. Schematic representation of the glomerulus, illustrating the three major types of cells (endothelial, epithelial, and mesangial) and the close relationship of the macula densa to afferent and efferent arterioles ("juxtaglomerular apparatus"). Notice that there is no basement membrane interposed between the mesangium and the lumen of the capillaries. The inset shows a magnified view of the capillary wall, illustrating the gaps between the endothelial cells (fenestrae), the three layers of the basement membrane, and the foot processes of the epithelial cells. For more details see text.

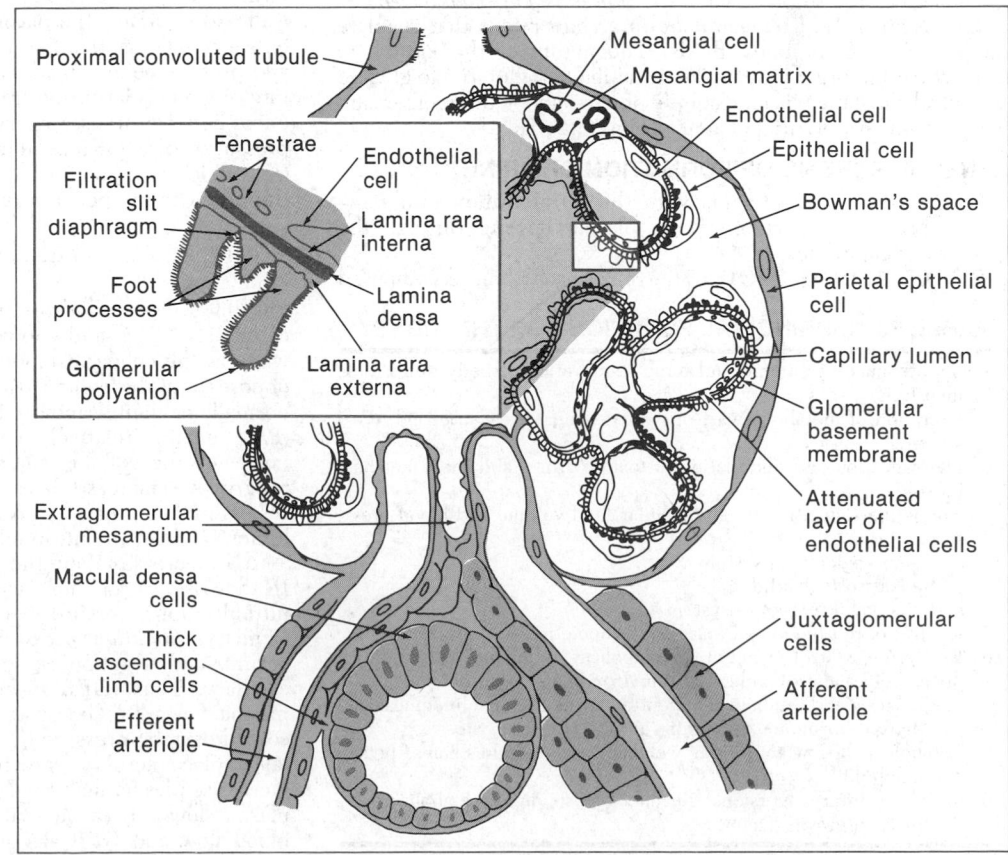

glomerular region. Signals originating from the macula densa can affect glomerular filtration rate (tubuloglomerular feedback).

INTERSTITIUM

The interstitial connective tissue of the kidney is scant and consists primarily of *reticular fibers* and *interstitial cells*. It is more prominent in the medulla than in the cortex. In addition to capillaries, the interstitium contains *lymphatics* and *motor* and *sensory nerves*. This region may be infiltrated by white blood cells and contain increased amounts of connective tissue in a variety of renal diseases.

NORMAL RENAL FUNCTION

The principal functions of the kidney are summarized in Table 73–1. The kidneys play a central role in the *maintenance of volume and ionic composition of body fluids* (homeostasis) by regulating the rate of excretion of water and/or ions. The large changes in urine volume and composition, which occur in response to alterations in the diet, reflect the adaptability of the kidney to the requirements of homeostasis. There is no fixed normal volume or composition of the urine. Normal homeostatic renal function is defined by the capacity of the organ to vary the volume and composition of the urine over a wide range.

The kidney is the main route of excretion of fixed (nonvolatile) metabolic waste products. These substances usually serve no biologic function, and some of them are potentially toxic. Examples include urea (end-product of protein metabolism), uric acid (end-product of nucleic acid metabolism), and creatinine (end-product of creatine metabolism). The kidney also *eliminates exogenous chemicals (drugs, toxins)* and their metabolites.

The kidney participates in endocrine functions as well. In addition to its capacity to *metabolize and excrete certain hormones*, the kidney is the site of *production* of *renin, erythropoietin, prostaglandins, 1,25-dihydroxycholecalciferol*, and *kinins*. It is the target organ for several hormones (e.g., parathyroid hormone, atrial peptide, antidiuretic hormone, angiotensin, aldosterone).

The kidney is also involved in the *catabolism of small molecular weight proteins* and in *metabolic interconversions* that regulate the composition of body fluids. The ability of the kidney to convert certain organic acids (lactic, alpha-ketoglutaric) to glucose (a neutral substance) is an example of a metabolic interconversion that minimizes potential changes in plasma pH.

GENERAL SCHEME OF FORMATION OF URINE

Formation of urine begins with the ultrafiltration into Bowman's space of a portion of the plasma flowing through the glomerular capillaries.

RENAL BLOOD FLOW. The renal circulation is composed

TABLE 73–1. PRINCIPAL FUNCTIONS OF THE KIDNEY

1. Maintenance of volume and ionic composition of body fluids (homeostasis)
2. Excretion of metabolic waste products—e.g., urea, uric acid, creatinine
3. Detoxification and elimination of toxins, drugs, and their metabolites
4. Endocrine regulation of extracellular fluid volume and blood pressure
   a. Renin-angiotensin system
   b. Renal prostaglandins
   c. Renal kallikrein-kinin system
5. Control of red blood cell mass: erythropoietin
6. Endocrine control of mineral metabolism: formation of 1,25-dihydroxycholecalciferol and 24,25-dihydroxycholecalciferol
7. Degradation and catabolism of peptide hormones: insulin, glucagon, parathyroid hormone, calcitonin, growth hormone, etc.
8. Catabolism of low molecular weight proteins: light chains, beta$_2$-microglobulin
9. Metabolic interconversions: gluconeogenesis, lipid metabolism
10. Synthesis of growth factors

of two capillary beds in series: the glomerular and the peritubular capillaries. The glomerulus has a high intracapillary hydrostatic pressure because it is interposed between two arterioles, i.e., resistance vessels. Therefore, filtration is favored. The second capillary system (peritubular capillaries in the cortex, vasa recta in the medulla) is a high-flow, low-pressure system that acts as a reservoir for tubular reabsorption and secretion.

The kidneys receive 25 per cent of the cardiac output, or approximately 1.1 liters of blood per minute. In subjects with a physiologic hematocrit of 45 per cent, total renal plasma flow is about 600 ml per minute. Cortical blood flow is about 75 per cent and medullary blood flow 25 per cent of total renal blood flow. Only 1 per cent of the renal blood flow reaches the papilla. As blood flows through the glomerular capillaries, hydrostatic forces drive filtration of 20 per cent of the plasma volume (120 ml per minute) across the capillary wall into Bowman's space (glomerular filtration). The ratio of glomerular filtration rate (GFR) to renal plasma flow is called the *filtration fraction*.

Renal blood flow is maintained relatively constant (*autoregulation*) even in the face of wide variations (80 to 180 mm Hg) in renal arterial perfusion pressure by changes in renal vascular resistance proportional to changes in perfusion pressure. Since the afferent and efferent arterioles determine renal vascular resistance, changes in arteriolar resistance alter renal blood flow. Recent evidence suggests that endothelium-derived relaxing factor (EDRF) and endothelins are major regulators of renal blood flow and vascular resistances. Autoregulation of renal blood flow maintains a constant GFR despite alterations in arterial perfusion pressure. Although the kidneys are innervated by adrenergic nerve fibers, renal sympathetic tone probably does not play a significant role in regulating renal blood flow under basal conditions. Thus, denervation or alpha- or beta-adrenergic blockers does not alter renal blood flow. However, augmented sympathetic activity (e.g., fright, pain, exercise, norepinephrine, congestive heart failure) increases renal vascular resistance and reduces renal blood flow. Both afferent and efferent arterioles contract, but GFR falls less than renal blood flow, suggesting that catecholamines have their major effect at the efferent arteriole. Renal blood flow is increased in infections or by substances inducing fever (pyrogenic reaction), presumably as a consequence of nitric oxide release by macrophages.

GLOMERULAR FILTRATION RATE. The initial step in the formation of urine (ultrafiltration) occurs across the glomerular wall and separates the plasma water and its nonprotein constituents (crystalloids) that enter Bowman's space from the blood cells and protein (colloids), which remain in the capillary lumen. The rate of glomerular ultrafiltration (GFR) is governed by the differences between transcapillary hydrostatic (ΔP) and colloid osmotic pressures ($\Delta \Pi$). GFR is influenced also by the filtration coefficient (K_f), which is a function of both total capillary surface area and the permeability per unit of surface area. Thus:

$$GFR = K_f(\Delta P - \Delta \Pi) \text{ or } GFR = K_f[(P_{GC} - P_{BS}) - \Pi_{GC}]$$

The difference in hydrostatic pressure (ΔP) between glomerular capillaries (P_{GC}) and Bowman's space (P_{BS}) favors filtration, whereas the colloid osmotic pressure inside the capillaries (Π_{GC}) opposes it. (The colloid osmotic pressure in Bowman's space is normally negligible and can be disregarded.) Hydrostatic pressure (P_{GC}) remains relatively constant along glomerular capillaries; however, the colloid osmotic pressure (Π_{GC}) undergoes a large progressive increase because filtration of "protein-free fluid" results in an increase of protein concentration along the capillary lumen. Hence, the mean effective pressure for ultrafiltration ($\Delta P - \Delta \Pi$) decreases along the glomerular capillary as $\Delta \Pi$ increases. If the rise in glomerular capillary Π is such that effective ultrafiltration pressure becomes zero before the end of the capillary, *filtration pressure equilibrium* ($P_{GC} = \Pi_{GC} + P_{BS}$) occurs, and filtration ceases before the end of the glomerular capillary. Thus, GFR is highly dependent on the glomerular plasma flow rate, because at high flow rates, a slower rise in colloid osmotic pressure (Π_{GC}) occurs. Thus, glomerular filtration takes place across a greater length of the capillary. Hence, increased plasma flow tends to elevate GFR, whereas decreased plasma flow may cause a fall in GFR. As noted previously, renal blood flow and GFR are autoregulated within a wide range of renal arterial pressure. When perfusion pressure falls, the resistance of the afferent arteriole decreases. Thus, glomerular plasma flow and GFR are maintained. Below 80 to 90 mm Hg, renal plasma flow and GFR vary directly with arterial pressure, and the GFR ceases when the pressure falls below 50 mm Hg.

At a physiologic GFR of 120 ml per minute, the filtration rate per nephron (assuming 2,400,000 nephrons in both kidneys) would be 50 nanoliters per minute. However, just as superficial and juxtamedullary nephrons differ anatomically, they also appear to differ functionally. The larger juxtamedullary glomeruli have filtration rates that are about twice as high as the superficial ones. The physiologic implications of this extensive heterogeneity are not clear, although it has been suggested that redistribution of intrarenal blood flow toward deeper nephrons is associated with salt retention and may contribute to edema in hepatic disease and congestive heart failure.

Alterations by disease states of any of the primary determinants discussed above may modify GFR. Thus, GFR can fall as a result of (1) decreased hydrostatic pressure in glomerular capillaries (marked hypotension); (2) increased hydrostatic pressure in Bowman's space (intratubular or urinary tract obstruction); (3) elevated glomerular plasma oncotic pressure as a consequence of increased concentration of proteins in the systemic circulation (dehydration: vomiting, diarrhea); (4) decreased renal plasma flow, which may lead to filtration equilibrium at a more proximal region along the glomerular capillary and hence may decrease the total surface area of capillary available for filtration (e.g., congestive heart failure, hepatic disease); or (5) a decrease in the filtration coefficient (K_f) due to a fall in permeability or to a reduction in total surface area available for filtration (intrinsic renal disease: certain nephrotoxins, acute or chronic glomerulonephritis).

Permselectivity of the Glomerular Capillary Wall. The glomerular capillary wall is highly permeable to small solutes and water. Molecules the size of inulin (molecular weight 5200) or smaller are present in the glomerular filtrate at the same concentration as in plasma water. Constituents with increasing *molecular size* exhibit progressively decreasing concentration in the filtrate.

In addition to molecular size, *molecular configuration, deformability*, and *net electrical charge* influence the filtration of macromolecules across the glomerular capillary wall. Negatively charged dextrans, of comparable size to albumin (a polyanion), have a clearance similar to that of albumin (less than 1 per cent that of inulin). By contrast, uncharged (neutral) dextran molecules of the same size as albumin are filtered at a much greater rate (20 per cent the rate of inulin), and filtration of cationic (positively charged) dextrans is even greater. Therefore, at constant molecular size, negative charge of the solute restricts and positive charge accelerates its filtration, suggesting that, phenomenologically, glomerular filtration occurs through pores with negative charges. A negatively charged glycoprotein ("*glomerular polyanion*"), predominantly found lining the foot processes of the epithelial cells, has been identified. Loss of these negative charges, in certain glomerular diseases, may lead to increased filtration of albumin.

HOMEOSTATIC AND EXCRETORY FUNCTIONS OF THE KIDNEY

The formation of urine begins with the elaboration of a protein-free plasma ultrafiltrate across the glomerular capillaries (*glomerular filtration*). As this ultrafiltrate flows through the renal tubule, solutes and water are reabsorbed from lumen to blood (*reabsorption*). Other solutes are secreted into the tubular lumen from the blood (*secretion*). In some cases, both processes (reabsorption and secretion) affect a given substance, permitting flexible regulation of its excretion. Quantitatively, about 170 liters of fluid are ultrafiltered daily, of which less than 1 liter to more than 10 liters may be excreted as urine, depending on the water balance of the individual. Large amounts of filtered sodium, chloride, calcium, magnesium, and phosphate are reabsorbed, with the quantity remaining in the final urine varying according to the dietary intake of each one of these solutes. Substances such as glucose, amino acids, and bicarbonate are almost completely reabsorbed and, under physiologic conditions, do not appear in the urine. The contribution of tubular transport to homeostasis is discussed in more detail below.

TUBULAR TRANSPORT. The renal tubule can be divided functionally into three major segments: (1) the proximal tubule, (2) the loop of Henle, and (3) the distal nephron. Although there are physiologic and morphologic subdivisions of these segments, it is possible to ascribe a general function to each. The proximal tubule reabsorbs, rather nonselectively, a large fraction (two thirds) of the glomerular filtrate. The loop of Henle has unique water and solute transport properties and serves to establish a hyperosmolar medullary interstitium that influences the ultimate concentration or dilution of the urine. The distal nephron is the site of fine regulation of water and electrolyte excretion and appears to be the main target of hormones that control these processes. Since the tubule segments are arranged in series, the function of any segment depends not only on its own intrinsic transport characteristics but also on the volume and composition of the fluid delivered to it from the previous segment.

Proximal Tubule. The proximal tubule reabsorbs sodium, several other solutes, and water at a high rate. Active sodium reabsorption and hydrogen ion secretion are the essential processes to which transport of chloride, several organic solutes, and water is coupled by a variety of mechanisms. Fluid transport is isosmotic, so that concentration gradients of solute across the wall are small. Functionally, the proximal tubule can be divided into three segments:

Initial Portion of the Proximal Tubule. Sodium reabsorption in this portion occurs through cells and intercellular spaces. Transcellular reabsorption of sodium is active, generating a small transtubular electrical potential (1 to 5 mV, lumen negative) (Fig. 73–2). It requires entry of sodium across luminal (brush border) membranes and extrusion of sodium across basolateral membranes. Entry of sodium across luminal membranes is passive and occurs (1) by diffusion, (2) coupled to the transport of other solutes (e.g., glucose, amino acids, phosphate), and (3) in exchange with H^+ secreted from cell to lumen. Sodium extrusion from cells into the intercellular spaces and across the basolateral membrane is an active (energy-requiring) process that is accomplished by the sodium-potassium pump (Na^+-K^+-ATPase). These processes transport solutes out of the lumen and generate slight osmotic gradients which drive water absorption across the permeable proximal tubule.

Preferential reabsorption of bicarbonate from H^+ secretion occurs in this segment, with bicarbonate concentration falling and chloride concentration increasing to an equivalent degree along this segment of the tubule. The reabsorption of glucose and amino acids is active, is coupled to sodium transport, and is nearly complete in this segment. Some permeant solutes, such as urea, are partially reabsorbed by a passive mechanism because of the increase in their luminal concentration as water is absorbed.

Distal Two Thirds of the Proximal Tubule. The luminal fluid of the last two thirds of the proximal tubule is characterized by a low concentration of bicarbonate and by the absence of glucose and amino acids. The tubular fluid remains isosmotic with plasma and has the same concentration of sodium as does the filtrate. The concentration of chloride in the lumen, however, exceeds the concentration of chloride in the peritubular capillary. This concentration gradient for chloride favors its diffusion out of the lumen, generating a lumen-positive potential (which is on the order of 1 to 3 mV). In experiments in vitro in which luminal and peritubular fluids have identical compositions, active sodium transport occurs. Therefore, sodium chloride reabsorption in this segment primarily occurs by active transcellular transport, with a smaller passive flow due to the positive luminal potential and solvent drag.

This segment is the main site of secretion of organic acids (penicillin, uric acid) and other substances such as creatinine. Its rate of sodium and fluid transport is slower, and its capacity for glucose and amino acid reabsorption is modest compared with that of the early segments of the proximal tubule.

Modulation of Reabsorption by the Proximal Tubule. Proximal reabsorption conserves most of the filtered fluid and all of a number of essential solutes. Several factors modulate the transport rate at the proximal tubule and therefore influence the performance of subsequent segments by altering their load.

Transtubular Physical Factors. The hydrostatic pressure (P) in the peritubular capillaries is markedly decreased compared with that in the glomerular capillaries. The colloid osmotic pressure

(II) is increased owing to filtration of a "protein-free fluid" at the glomeruli. These "Starling forces" thus favor the uptake of fluid by the peritubular capillaries. When II falls or P rises, the uptake of fluid by peritubular capillaries decreases. This leads to fluid accumulation in the interstitium, increased hydrostatic pressure in this space, and a decrease in net fluid reabsorption.

Glomerular tubular balance refers to a direct relationship between GFR and the prevailing rates of proximal tubular reabsorption and has been ascribed to changes in II in the peritubular circulation that result from changes in GFR (increases in GFR and hence in filtration fraction lead to a greater protein concentration and increases in II in the efferent arterioles and peritubular capillaries; a decrease in GFR has the opposite effect). Thus, when GFR increases, a greater amount of fluid is delivered to the proximal tubule; however, the resulting rise in peritubular II leads to a proportional increase in the reabsorption of fluid in this segment so that the percentage of the filtrate reabsorbed in the proximal tubule remains constant. An alternative mechanism accounting for glomerular tubular balance is a link between fluid reabsorption in the proximal tubule and flow rates of tubular fluid. Increases in GFR, and hence in proximal tubular flow, augment reabsorption; decreases in GFR and in flow decrease reabsorption.

Effects of Hormones on Sodium Reabsorption by the Proximal Tubule. Parathyroid hormone acutely reduces sodium and fluid reabsorption in the proximal tubule; catecholamines may stimulate fluid reabsorption in this segment. Locally generated angiotensin II stimulates sodium reabsorption across the apical membrane of the proximal tubule. Atrial natriuretic peptide antagonizes this effect of angiotensin II on sodium reabsorption.

Loop of Henle. The loop of Henle, which is interposed between the proximal and distal tubules, is a hairpin-shaped structure extending into the renal medulla (Fig. 73–2). Under physiologic conditions it reabsorbs about 25 per cent of the filtered sodium and chloride and 15 per cent of the filtered water. In consequence, the isotonic fluid entering Henle's loop becomes hypotonic to plasma before entering the distal tubule.

The maintenance of water balance requires the excretion of urine of varied tonicity. The formation of a dilute (hypotonic to plasma) or concentrated (hypertonic to plasma) urine takes place by means of a *countercurrent system* that involves not only the loops of Henle but also the distal tubule, the collecting ducts,

and the blood vessels supplying these segments. The excretion of a hypertonic urine involves two basic steps: (1) creation of a hypertonic medullary interstitium and (2) osmotic equilibration of the fluid that enters the medullary collecting duct with the hypertonic interstitium. Antidiuretic hormone (ADH) is required in this latter process. Hypotonic urine is excreted when the fluid that enters the medullary collecting duct does not equilibrate with the hypertonic interstitium owing to low levels or absence of ADH.

In normal human subjects the maximal osmolality of urine that can be achieved is around 1200 mOsm per kilogram. Since the tubular fluid reaches this osmolality by equilibration with the medullary interstitium, it follows that the interstitium must have a similar osmolality. *Countercurrent multiplication* is the process by which the interstitial osmolality is increased from 285 mOsm in the cortex (the same osmolality as plasma) to 1200 mOsm in the papilla. The thin descending and ascending limbs of juxtamedullary nephrons lie in close proximity to each other in the medulla. Flow through them is countercurrent. Fluid obtained from thin ascending limbs has a lower osmolality than fluid obtained from thin descending limbs at comparable levels in the papilla. This is due to functional differences. Whereas the descending limb is highly permeable to water, slightly permeable to urea, and highly impermeable to sodium, the ascending limb is highly permeable to sodium, moderately permeable to urea, and impermeable to water. In normal mammals, the medullary interstitium is hyperosmotic owing to the accumulation of high concentrations of both urea and sodium chloride. The isotonic fluid delivered from the proximal tubule becomes progressively hypertonic as it traverses the thin descending limb owing to net water flow from lumen to interstitium. The highest osmolality of the luminal fluid is achieved at the tip of the loop. This hyperosmolar fluid becomes diluted progressively as it flows up the thin ascending limb, owing to the movement of sodium without water from the lumen to the interstitium. Urea present in the interstitium diffuses inward. However, since the permeability of this segment to sodium chloride is greater than to urea, the net effect is a greater exit of sodium chloride than urea entry, resulting in net addition of solute to the interstitial fluid, and since the thin ascending limb is impermeable to water, the fluid becomes hypotonic with respect to the interstitial fluid at the same level.

The thick ascending limb of the loop actively reabsorbs sodium chloride. The luminal transport step is a furosemide-inhibitable $Na^+/K^+/2Cl^-$ cotransporter. This segment is essentially imperme-

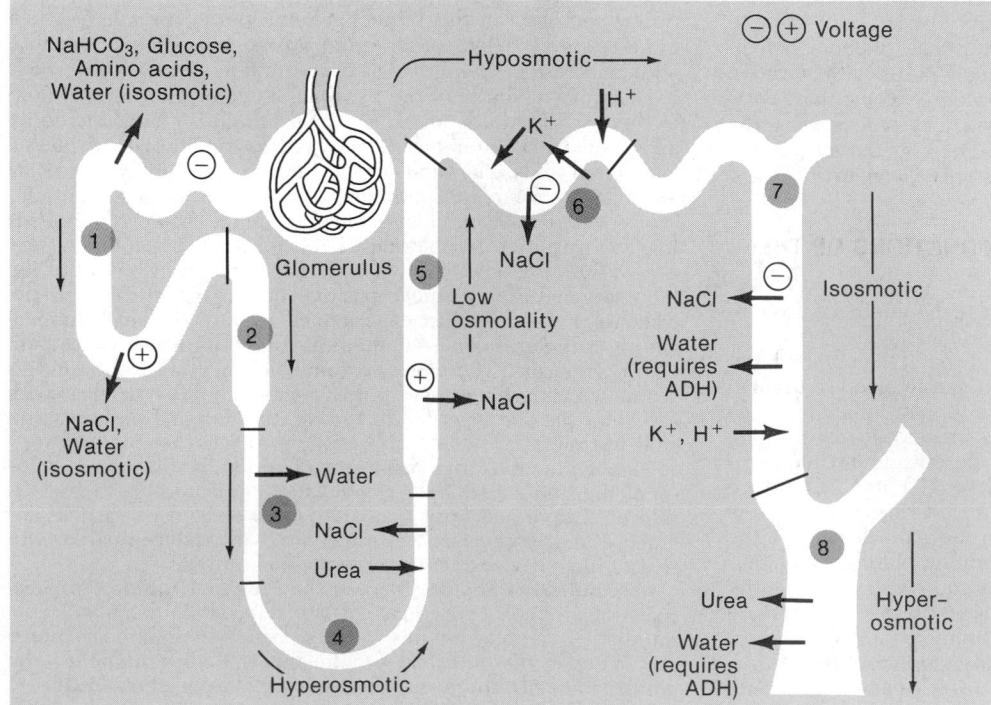

FIGURE 73–2. Schematic representation of the principal processes of transport in the nephron. In the early portion of the proximal tubule (1) salt and water are reabsorbed at high rates, in isotonic proportions. Bulk reabsorption of most of the filtrate (65 to 70 per cent) and virtually complete reabsorption of glucose, amino acids, and bicarbonate take place in this segment. In the pars recta (2) organic acids and bases are secreted and continuous reabsorption of sodium chloride takes place. The loop of Henle comprises three segments; the thin descending (3) and ascending (4) limbs and the thick ascending limb (5). The fluid becomes hyperosmotic, because of water abstraction, as it flows toward the bend of the loop and hyposmotic, because of sodium chloride reabsorption, as it flows toward the distal convoluted tubule (6). Active sodium reabsorption occurs in the distal convoluted tubule and in the cortical collecting tubule (7). This latter segment is water impermeable in the absence of ADH, and the reabsorption of sodium in this segment is increased by aldosterone. The collecting duct (8) allows equilibration of water with the

hyperosmotic interstitium when ADH is present. In the absence of ADH, a large volume of dilute urine is excreted. (Adapted from figure by A Iselin, from Burg MB: Hosp Pract 13:99, 1978. Reproduced with permission.)

able to water, even when ADH is present; therefore, salt transport from lumen to interstitial fluid further decreases the osmolality of the luminal fluid and increases the osmolality of the interstitium, accounting for the countercurrent multiplication that occurs in the renal medulla. The amount of urea present in the fluid of the thick ascending limb is higher than in the fluid entering the thin descending limb. This is due to water abstraction, in excess of urea, out of the latter segment and net urea entry (recycled from the collecting duct) into the thin ascending and descending limbs of Henle's loop.

The fluid emerging from the loop of Henle is virtually always hyposmotic (about 150 mOsm per kilogram) compared with plasma, regardless of the final urine osmolality. With low or absent ADH, the luminal fluid in the collecting system does not equilibrate with the interstitium. Hence, the volume of fluid delivered to the tip of the collecting duct is increased and its osmolality decreased compared with plasma. The osmolality of this fluid can be further decreased to as low as 30 mOsm per kilogram by the reabsorption of solute in excess of water in distal tubule and cortical and medullary collecting ducts.

Since the maximal urine osmolality cannot exceed that in the interstitium, the ability to conserve water by excreting a highly concentrated urine is reduced when the hypertonicity of the medullary interstitium is decreased. This may occur when papillary urea accumulation is reduced, as occurs in protein malnutrition, as a consequence of decreased urea production, or due to reduced interstitial sodium chloride accumulation (use of loop diuretics, hypercalcemia). Reduced levels or absence of ADH (diabetes insipidus) or unresponsiveness of the collecting duct to the action of ADH (nephrogenic diabetes insipidus) may prevent equilibration of the fluid in the collecting duct with the hypertonic interstitium, leading to an impairment in water conservation.

Distal Nephron (Distal Convoluted Tubule, Cortical Collecting Tubule, and Medullary Collecting Duct). The distal nephron accomplishes the final and delicate adjustments in the reabsorption of water, sodium, chloride, phosphate, and calcium in response to aldosterone, ADH, and parathyroid hormone.

The *distal convoluted tubule* is defined anatomically as the segment that extends from the macula densa to the site of transition from homogeneous cells to a mixture of dark and light cells (typical of the collecting duct). The distal convoluted tubule is essentially impermeable to water and unresponsive to ADH. Sodium chloride is reabsorbed at a slower rate than in the proximal tubule or in the loop, but against large concentration gradients. The rate of reabsorption is proportional to the load. The transtubular electrical potential, lumen negative, is related to the reabsorption of sodium and varies from −10 in the initial portion to −45 mV in the distal portion. Most of the reabsorption of sodium chloride occurs transcellularly. Potassium is secreted in this segment from peritubular capillary into the lumen, and there appears to be an active H⁺ transport mechanism located at the luminal membrane, especially at the transition of distal convoluted tubule to cortical collecting tubule.

The *cortical collecting tubule* extends from the end of the distal tubule to the corticomedullary junction. Under basal conditions, water permeability is negligible in this segment. It is increased markedly by ADH. Sodium chloride is actively reabsorbed at this level; therefore, in the absence of ADH the luminal fluid osmolality falls further. When ADH is present the luminal fluid equilibrates with the cortical interstitial fluid and becomes isosmotic with plasma; at the same time, luminal urea concentrations rise (see above). The transtubular electrical potential is about 35 mV, lumen negative; it is related to active reabsorption of sodium and is highly dependent on the levels of mineralocorticoids, which increase sodium reabsorption. Potassium and hydrogen are secreted in this segment. Aldosterone increases sodium reabsorption as well as potassium and H⁺ secretion in this portion of the nephron (Fig. 73–2).

The *medullary collecting duct* starts at the corticomedullary junction and ends on the surface of the papilla. Water and urea permeabilities are low in the absence of ADH. Continuous sodium chloride reabsorption at this level, in the absence of ADH, results in a further drop in urine osmolality. ADH increases water and urea permeability and allows the equilibration of the luminal osmolality with that of the hypertonic interstitium.

To recapitulate, in the proximal tubule salt and water are transported at high rates, in isotonic proportions. Bulk reabsorp-

tion of most of the filtrate (65 to 70 per cent) and virtually complete reabsorption of "metabolically useful" solutes (glucose, amino acids, bicarbonate) take place in this segment. The *loop of Henle* comprises three segments with strikingly different properties of active transport and permeability of water and solute. Because of these properties, the medullary interstitium is made hyperosmolar and acts as the driving force for final water reabsorption. The loop reabsorbs additional sodium chloride (about 25 per cent of that filtered) and water (about 15 per cent of the filtrate) and leaves about 10 per cent of the sodium and 15 per cent of the water to be reabsorbed in the last segments of the tubule.

The distal convoluted tubule and the collecting tubule can establish large sodium gradients between fluid in the lumen and in the peritubular capillary. The collecting ducts, water impermeable in the absence of ADH, become permeable to water in response to the hormone. It is in these segments that the final volume and osmolality of the urine are determined. Salt transport occurs at a slower rate than in the preceding segments but against large concentration gradients. The final regulation of salt excretion takes place in these segments, under the influence of aldosterone. Potassium and H⁺ excretion are regulated also in these segments.

ROLE OF THE KIDNEY IN SODIUM CHLORIDE HOMEOSTASIS. Normally the kidney regulates sodium balance (and hence extracellular fluid volume) in a very efficient manner. The daily intake of sodium varies considerably. In the Western world the average diet contains about 170 mEq per 24 hours. About 98 per cent of this amount is excreted in the urine. However, this represents less than 1 per cent of the amount of sodium filtered (140 mEq per liter × 170 liters = 23,800 mEq) each day. Thus, maintenance of sodium homeostasis is primarily a function of the renal tubule and reabsorption of filtered sodium; changes in GFR appear to be quantitatively less important. Thus, (1) sizable increases in GFR, not accompanied by extracellular fluid (ECF) volume expansion, do not result in a marked natriuresis because of glomerular tubular balance (see above), and (2) the natriuresis of ECF volume expansion occurs under experimental conditions in which GFR is maintained constant or even decreased experimentally. When a normal subject increases the intake of salt, urine sodium excretion increases progressively and reaches a steady-state level equal to intake. During the interval of adjustment, positive sodium balance occurs, with an accompanying retention of water and consequent gain in body weight. When salt intake is suddenly reduced, the opposite effects are observed. Sodium excretion decreases, reaching a level equal to intake within 3 to 5 days with a reduction in total body water and body weight.

Several physiologic mechanisms ordinarily control sodium reabsorption by the kidney to maintain the sodium content of ECF. Changes in sodium mass are not sensed as such, but secondarily as changes in ECF volume. Total ECF volume changes are sensed through their effects on circulatory dynamics ("effective arterial blood volume"). The determinants of effective arterial blood volume are (1) the degree of filling of the arterial tree, which depends in large part on cardiac output, and (2) peripheral vascular resistance, which depends on the compliance of the peripheral vessels and the magnitude of the arterial runoff. Decreases in effective volume (dehydration, hemorrhage, venodilation, venous pooling) lead to renal retention of salt. Increases in effective volume (saline administration, excessive salt intake) lead to a rise in salt excretion by the kidney.

Factors That Influence the Tubular Reabsorption of Sodium. Alterations in effective arterial volume affect handling of sodium by the kidney through the renin-angiotensin-aldosterone system, the sympathetic nervous system, and other less well-defined factors. The last category probably includes changes in intrarenal hydrostatic and oncotic pressures (so-called physical factors), natriuretic (or salt-losing) hormones such as atrial natriuretic peptides, and possibly the distribution of blood flow within the kidneys.

Role of Physical Factors in the Reabsorption of Sodium. A fall in effective arterial blood volume (dehydration, hemorrhage) and the consequent decline in blood pressure decrease renal perfusion. In response to reductions in renal perfusion pressure, glomerular plasma flow decreases more than does glomerular capillary hydrostatic pressure, resulting in a fall in GFR that is proportionally less than the decline in renal plasma flow. This disparity is due to a greater vasoconstriction of efferent compared with afferent arterioles in response to increased levels of catecholamines and angiotensin II. The lesser fall in GFR compared with renal plasma flow increases filtration fraction and hence the concentration of protein in the efferent arterioles and peritubular capillaries. In addition, vasoconstriction of the efferent arteriole results in a fall in hydrostatic pressure (P) in the peritubular capillaries. The increase in Π and the decrease in P in the peritubular capillaries augment sodium and water reabsorption along the proximal segments of the nephron. Thus, in response to contraction of effective arterial volume, the glomerular and peritubular microcirculations act in concert to minimize fluid losses by both lowering GFR and augmenting salt and water reabsorption by the tubules.

Expansion of the ECF volume elicits opposite effects. The increase in renal perfusion pressure leads to not only a rise in GFR but also a proportionally greater rise in renal plasma flow; consequently filtration fraction falls. The net effect is a decrease in peritubular protein concentration and hence in Π, with a decrease in reabsorption of fluid by peritubular capillaries. The importance of such physical factors in the normal control of sodium and water reabsorption is not exactly clear. Since alterations in Π and P in the peritubular capillaries influence fluid reabsorption mainly, if not exclusively, in the proximal tubule, it is likely that changes in physical factors are important only when fluid balance deficits or gains are very large (as, for example, with severe hemorrhage or marked expansion of the ECF volume). Whether significant changes in proximal reabsorption occur in response to more modest alterations in fluid balance (as might result, for example, in response to a diet very low or very high in sodium chloride) remains uncertain.

Redistribution of Blood Flow. Another mechanism potentially altering sodium excretion is redistribution of blood flow. It has been suggested that nephrons with superficially placed glomeruli have less capacity to reabsorb sodium than others. If so, at any given total GFR, the relative amounts of fluid filtered by the two different nephron populations would be an important determinant of sodium excretion. Redistribution of GFR toward the "high reabsorption nephrons" (juxtamedullary nephrons) would be associated with decreased sodium excretion because of the greater capacity of these nephrons to reabsorb sodium. Despite the attractiveness of this theory, evidence favoring it is scant.

Renin-Angiotensin-Aldosterone. Sodium balance is controlled also by *mineralocorticoid hormones, mainly aldosterone.* Only a small but significant fraction (some 2 per cent) of the filtered sodium is under hormonal control. Yet loss or gain of an amount of sodium equivalent to 2 per cent of the filtered load (about 500 mEq per day) has profound effects on sodium balance. Aldosterone increases sodium reabsorption in the distal tubule and collecting duct. Lack of aldosterone leads to loss of sodium in the urine. The factors controlling aldosterone secretion include (1) angiotensin, (2) plasma concentration of potassium, (3) adrenocorticotropic hormone (ACTH), and (4) plasma Na+ concentration. Circulating levels of angiotensin are increased by hemorrhage, dietary salt restriction, changes in distribution of blood and fluids (venous pooling and edema-forming states), and other states of increased secretion of renin. *Renin* is a proteolytic enzyme secreted by the granular cells of the juxtaglomerular apparatus. The mechanisms controlling its release seem to depend on (1) changes in renal perfusion pressure, (2) factors reflecting the rate of delivery of sodium chloride to the macula densa, and (3) activity of the renal sympathetic nerves. When perfusion pressure or the delivery of sodium falls, or the activity of the sympathetic nerves increases, the release of renin is enhanced. Renin acts on a substrate in plasma, *angiotensinogen,* to form *angiotensin I* (a decapeptide). *Converting enzyme* splits two amino acids from angiotensin I to form *angiotensin II* (an octapeptide). The latter is a potent hormone, central to the regulation of salt and water balance. It produces vasoconstriction and stimulates the secretion of aldosterone, thirst, and the renal reabsorption of sodium. Another split product of angiotensin, *angiotensin III* (a heptapeptide), also increases aldosterone secretion from the zona glomerulosa of the adrenal.

Natriuretic Hormones. A 28-amino acid peptide produced in the cardiac atria (atrial peptide), which has both natriuretic and vasodilating properties, participates in the regulation of extracellular fluid volume and electrolyte balance. Recently an "atrial-like" natriuretic peptide has been shown to be produced in the kidney. Its role is unknown. In addition, a natriuretic substance of hypothalamic origin that inhibits Na+-K+-ATPase activity, displaces ouabain that is bound to cellular membranes, and cross-reacts with digoxin antibodies has been described. The roles of these natriuretic substances in the regulation of renal sodium excretion have not been fully defined, but are most apparent during volume expansion.

Other Hormonal Agents. Cortisol, estrogen, growth hormone, and insulin all can enhance sodium reabsorption. Glucagon, progesterone, and parathyroid hormone can decrease it. It is almost certain that when circulating levels of these hormones are elevated (as, for example, estrogen during pregnancy), significant influences occur on sodium reabsorption and thereby excretion. However, there is no evidence that any of them, unlike the factors described previously, are controlled specifically as part of the homeostatic regulation of sodium balance. Of great interest is the possible role played by intrarenally produced substances such as *prostaglandins* and *kinins*. These agents are potent vasodilators and may reduce sodium reabsorption, by altering regional intrarenal vascular resistance or by direct actions on the tubular cells. Their levels change with alterations of sodium balance, but it is not yet clear how extensively they participate in the renal regulation of sodium excretion. In addition, locally generated vasoconstrictors (thromboxanes, endothelins) may affect renal blood flow and tubule function.

Renal Nerves. The renal sympathetic nerves play a prominent role in sodium homeostasis by modulating (1) secretion of aldosterone via the renin-angiotensin system, (2) intrarenal physical factors, (3) the reabsorptive activity of the tubular cells themselves, and (4) GFR. Yet, because of the many other known (and potential) factors involved, a transplanted and, therefore, denervated kidney maintains sodium homeostasis quite well.

RENAL REGULATION OF WATER EXCRETION. The capacity to regulate renal excretion of water, independent of solute excretion, maintains the osmolality of body fluids within narrow limits despite wide variations in intake of water. Roughly 170 liters of water are filtered daily. Of this amount, less than 2 liters, or about 1 per cent of the amount filtered, are excreted. Except for setting an upper limit for the amount of water that can be excreted per unit time, GFR is not involved in the regulation of water excretion. This upper limit assumes importance only when GFR is profoundly reduced as in acute renal failure or advanced chronic renal disease.

The tubule is the major site for renal regulation of water excretion. Net absorption of water occurs all along the nephron and is due to passive diffusion of water down its concentration gradient into a region of higher osmolality. In the proximal tubule, this gradient is established by the active transcellular transport of sodium chloride and other solutes. About two thirds of the filtered water is reabsorbed isosmotically in the proximal tubule. Reabsorption of water in this segment is intimately related to the reabsorption of sodium. Since water reabsorption in the remaining segments of the nephron is to a large extent independent of the reabsorption of solute, the process is referred to frequently as the reabsorption of solute-free water, or simply *free water.*

The reabsorption of free water is dependent largely on interrelationships among four factors: (1) the concentration of solute in the interstitium through which the renal tubule passes, (2) the concentration of solute in the tubular fluid, (3) the permeability of the renal tubule to water and solute, and (4) the circulating levels of ADH. About 15 per cent of the filtered water enters the distal tubule. A variable fraction of this water is reabsorbed by the distal tubules and collecting ducts. Absorption of this final fraction is controlled by antidiuretic hormone (ADH), which serves as the main regulator of the osmolality of body fluids. ADH is synthesized by nerve cells in the hypothalamus and liberated from their terminals in the posterior lobe and pituitary stalk. The major stimulus for the secretion of ADH into the circulation is an increase in plasma osmolality, mediated by osmoreceptors, which are exquisitely sensitive to changes in osmolality. The feedback system they provide helps to maintain the tonicity of plasma within a standard deviation of ±2 mOsm (a change of less than 1 per cent). Although changes in osmolality are the most sensitive and therefore the primary regulators of ADH release, alterations in ECF volume can modulate ADH release through a baroreceptor pathway, and override the effects of tonicity. However, secretion of ADH is not increased unless volume loss is greater than 10 per cent. Baroreceptor stimulation appears to mediate the increase in ADH secretion resulting from volume contraction. This effect is potentiated by elevated levels of circulating catecholamines, which act directly on these receptors. Angiotensin II, prostaglandins, and nicotine may also affect ADH release through activation of arterial baroreceptors. When a surfeit of body water develops, ADH release is inhibited and a dilute urine is excreted; when a water deficit is present, free water is reabsorbed and the urine becomes concentrated with respect to plasma.

The human kidney can dilute urine 10-fold with respect to plasma (to about 30 mOsm per kilogram) but can concentrate it to a maximum of only fourfold with respect to plasma (to about 1200 mOsm per kilogram). The daily volume of urine depends on the intake of fluid and can be varied from 600 ml to over 24 liters. When a large load of water is ingested, the following events occur: (1) The osmolar concentration (osmolality) of plasma falls; (2) over the next 15 to 20 minutes ADH levels fall, and as a consequence the flow rate of urine increases, reaching a maximum in 45 to 60 minutes. The maximal increase in urine flow occurs when free water excretion is about 15 per cent of GFR.

ROLE OF THE KIDNEY IN THE PRESERVATION OF POTASSIUM BALANCE. The daily intake of potassium ranges from 50 to 150 mEq. Most of the potassium ingested is absorbed (less than 10 mEq is excreted in the stool); thus, maintenance of balance requires the daily excretion of an amount of potassium identical to that absorbed from the gut. Under physiologic conditions, approximately 70 per cent of the potassium filtered is reabsorbed in the proximal tubule. The loop of Henle reabsorbs the remaining 20 to 30 per cent. Distal segments of the nephron can both reabsorb and secrete potassium. The balance between distal reabsorption and secretion determines the net urinary excretion of this cation. On a normal diet (100 mEq per day) the kidneys excrete approximately 90 mEq of potassium per day. The secretion of potassium is influenced by the potassium concentration in renal distal tubular cells, by the magnitude of the electrochemical gradient between cell interior and tubular lumen, and by the luminal flow rate. The factors that regulate potassium excretion in the urine are summarized in Table 73–2. If potassium intake is increased acutely, renal excretion of potassium can rise

TABLE 73–2. FACTORS THAT REGULATE POTASSIUM EXCRETION IN THE URINE

Condition		Effect on K⁺ Excretion
Dietary K⁺	High	Increase
	Low	Decrease
Serum levels of K⁺	High	Increase
	Low	Decrease
Levels of mineralo- or glucocorticoid hormones	High	Increase
	Low	Decrease
Tubular fluid or urine flow rate	Fast	Increase
	Slow	Decrease
Sodium excretion in the urine	High	Increase
	Low	Decrease
Most diuretics		Increase
K⁺-sparing diuretics (spironolactone, triamterene, amiloride)		Decrease
Inhibitors of renin release or angiotensin II formation (NSAID's, beta blockers, ACE inhibitors)		Decrease
Metabolic alkalosis		Increase
Metabolic acidosis		Decrease
Augmented urine excretion of impermeant anions (sulfate, carbenicillin)		Increase

more than 10-fold. About 50 per cent of the amount administered appears in the urine within 12 hours. The renal response to potassium deprivation is sluggish. Excretion falls to levels of 10 to 15 mEq per 24 hours only after 7 to 14 days of a potassium-free diet. During this interval a deficit of as much as 200 mEq of potassium may be incurred. In adults with increased catabolism (infections, surgery), the renal excretion of potassium may exceed the amount ingested.

Urinary excretion of potassium (Table 73–2) depends on its rate of secretion by the distal tubule. Increased net secretory rates of potassium in this segment could be due to (1) increased active uptake by the peritubular membrane leading to increased cell potassium concentration and increased passive leak across the luminal membrane, (2) increased permeability of the luminal membrane to potassium, (3) decreased active reabsorption of potassium by the luminal membrane, (4) increased lumen-negative electrical potential difference, or (5) increased luminal flow rate.

A high concentration of potassium in distal tubular cells is maintained through the action of a Na⁺-K⁺-ATPase located in the peritubular membrane. Potassium uptake via this pump is stimulated by high plasma levels of potassium, alkalosis, aldosterone, and increased sodium reabsorption. All factors that raise cell potassium (increased peritubular pump activity, dehydration) favor its diffusion into the lumen. If the cellular potassium concentration falls (potassium deprivation, acidosis, dilution of body fluids), the rate of potassium translocation into the lumen falls and may be less than the potassium uptake across the luminal membrane. Under these conditions, net reabsorption of potassium may replace net potassium secretion.

The difference in electrical potential across the entire distal tubular cell is established by the active reabsorption of sodium and is about 50 mV (lumen negative to peritubular fluid). The cell interior is negative (−70 mV) in relation to the peritubular capillary. Thus, the luminal membrane potential difference is about 20 mV (cell negative to lumen). This electrical profile favors a greater leak of potassium across the luminal membrane than across the peritubular membrane. Thus, potassium is pumped into distal tubular cells and then leaks across the luminal membrane into the tubular lumen. Such passive translocation of potassium from the cell into the lumen depends not only on the electrical potential difference across the luminal membrane but also on the chemical concentration gradient. An increased lumen-negative electrical potential or factors that increase cellular potassium or lower luminal potassium have been shown to augment potassium secretion.

Augmented sodium reabsorption in the distal tubule increases lumen electro-negativity, which favors potassium secretion from the cell interior into the tubular fluid. Hence, increased distal sodium reabsorption favors potassium excretion. For example, diuretic administration increases sodium delivery distally, which, in turn, increases potassium excretion, particularly in patients with secondary aldosteronism. Hyperkalemia increases potassium excretion by two mechanisms: It stimulates aldosterone secretion directly, and it also enhances renal secretion, presumably via increased cell content of potassium. Alkalosis enhances and acidosis depresses potassium secretion, probably by inducing corresponding changes in renal cell potassium. The rates of *distal tubular flow* also influence potassium excretion, presumably because of the rapid dissipation of the concentration of potassium in the tubular lumen at higher flow rates.

ROLE OF THE KIDNEY IN ACID-BASE BALANCE. The kidney maintains plasma pH in a physiologic range by regulating the concentration of plasma bicarbonate. This is accomplished by the reabsorption of filtered bicarbonate, and the excretion in the urine of 50 to 100 mEq of H⁺ in the form of ammonium (NH₄⁺) and titratable acid (the amount of alkali required to titrate the urine to the pH of plasma). Disodium phosphate (Na₂HPO₄) present in the filtrate is converted to NaH₂PO₄, which accounts for most of the titratable acid excreted in the urine. Net excretion of acid (titratable acid + ammonium excretion − bicarbonate excretion) equals the daily production of nonvolatile acids under physiologic conditions. Both the *reclamation* of filtered bicarbonate and the *regeneration* of bicarbonate depend on the secretion of H⁺ from the tubular cells into the lumen. The secreted H⁺ is generated within the tubular cells by the *carbonic anhydrase*-catalyzed hydration of CO_2 to H_2CO_3, which immediately dissociates into H^+ and HCO_3^-. The H^+ is secreted into the tubular fluid, and the bicarbonate, concomitantly produced intracellularly, enters the peritubular capillary. Thus, H^+ secretion results in addition of bicarbonate to plasma. When the H^+ secreted into the lumen combines with filtered bicarbonate, it forms H_2CO_3, which quickly dissociates to CO_2 and H_2O. As a consequence, a bicarbonate disappears from the lumen, and the net effect is bicarbonate reabsorption (reclamation).

At a physiologic GFR of 170 liters per day and a plasma bicarbonate level of 24 mEq per liter, the reabsorption of over 4000 mEq of bicarbonate requires the secretion of an equivalent amount of H^+, whereas the excretion of net acid requires the secretion of 50 to 100 mEq of H^+ daily (Table 73–3). The process of bicarbonate reclamation operates to reabsorb all the filtered bicarbonate below a critical serum concentration, the *bicarbonate threshold concentration*, which in adult humans is normally about 24 mEq per liter, essentially identical to the concentration of bicarbonate in plasma. When plasma bicarbonate concentration rises and/or GFR is increased, the filtered load of bicarbonate is increased and renal reclamation is incomplete. The excess bicarbonate escapes into the urine, enabling the plasma bicarbonate concentration to return to the threshold level. Under physiologic conditions the virtually complete reabsorption of bicarbonate serves to preserve bicarbonate stores but does not replace the bicarbonate consumed in the buffering of nonvolatile acids. If the secreted H^+ combines with buffers, such as HPO_4^- or NH_3, a new bicarbonate ion (de novo synthesis) is added to the peritubular capillary blood. This results in replacement of the bicarbonate consumed in buffering the daily acid load (Table 73–3).

At times, net acid excretion is absent or has a negative value. This occurs after ingestion of an alkaline load (bicarbonate or substances that can be metabolized to bicarbonate). Ammonium excretion accounts for two thirds and titratable acid for one third of the urinary excretion of acid. When the daily H^+ load increases (e.g., increased catabolism, infection), the rise in acid excretion by the kidney is usually due to increased ammonium excretion. Ammonia (NH_3), produced within the renal proximal tubular cells from glutamine, diffuses into the peritublar capillary or lumen down its concentration gradient. In the lumen it combines with H^+ to form NH_4^+. As noted, each mole of NH_4^+ excreted results in the de novo generation of 1 mole of bicarbonate. Thus, when metabolic acidosis develops and the need for regenerating bicarbonate increases, synthesis of ammonia and NH_4^+ excretion usually increase.

Hydrogen secretion occurs in both proximal and distal segments of the nephron. As the concentration of bicarbonate in the lumen decreases, the concentration of H^+ increases, and as a result a limitation is imposed on the net rate of H^+ secretion. The maximal H^+ gradient achievable between cell and collecting duct lumen is about 800:1 (luminal fluid pH of 4.5).

Factors That Regulate the Renal Secretion of Hydrogen Ions. The major factors that influence the renal secretion of H^+ are (1) *effective circulating volume*, (2) *arterial pH and P_{CO_2}*, (3) *plasma concentration of potassium*, and (4) *mineralocorticoids (aldosterone)*.

Effective Circulating Volume. Hydrogen ion secretion is increased during volume depletion (increased sodium reabsorption) and diminished during ECF volume expansion. Hydrogen secretion is stimulated also when significant amounts of nonreabsorbable anions, i.e., sulfate ions, are present in the distal nephron and when sodium reabsorption is enhanced by any mechanism. Thus, the effective circulating volume of the ECF and the amounts of nonreabsorbable anion accompanying sodium through the distal nephron are important determinants of renal H^+ secretion.

Arterial pH and P_{CO_2}. Net acid excretion is increased with acidosis and decreased with alkalosis. Acidosis, resulting from a decrease in the plasma concentration of bicarbonate (metabolic acidosis) or induced by an elevation in P_{CO_2} (respiratory acidosis), augments H^+ excretion and increases the renal synthesis of bicarbonate. Metabolic alkalosis (increased plasma bicarbonate) or respiratory alkalosis (decreased P_{CO_2}) has the opposite effects. The effects of arterial pH on net acid excretion are most likely mediated by changes in renal tubular cell pH. Elevations in arterial P_{CO_2} increase bicarbonate reabsorption, and a fall in arterial P_{CO_2} reduces bicarbonate reabsorption.

Plasma Potassium Concentration. Hypokalemia increases and hyperkalemia decreases H^+ excretion. These effects are due to changes in intracellular H^+ concentration induced by cation shifts between the ICF and the ECF. In hypokalemia, potassium leaves the cell and is replaced by H^+ and sodium. The increase in intracellular H^+ concentration (intracellular acidosis) leads to the enhanced H^+ secretion and bicarbonate reabsorption associated with potassium depletion. In addition, hypokalemia stimulates renal ammonia production. The opposite occurs with hyperkalemia.

Aldosterone. Aldosterone stimulates secretion of both potassium and hydrogen in the distal nephron. Excess of aldosterone may cause metabolic alkalosis, and its deficiency may lead to hyperchloremic metabolic acidosis and hyperkalemia by decreasing H^+ and K^+ excretion.

ROLE OF THE KIDNEY IN MINERAL HOMEOSTASIS. The kidney regulates the homeostasis of minerals not only by modifying the excretion of phosphate, calcium, and magnesium (see below) but also by influencing the metabolism of vitamin D. Vitamin D_3 (cholecalciferol) is metabolized to 25(OH) cholecalciferol in the liver and subsequently to $1,25(OH)_2D_3$ and $24,25(OH)_2D_3$ in the kidney. The $1,25(OH)_2D_3$ is the calcemic hormone produced in the renal cortex in response to hypophosphatemia or elevated levels of parathyroid hormone (when hypocalcemia occurs), and $24,25(OH)_2D_3$ is produced preferentially when the mineral balance is normal. The $1,25(OH)_2D_3$ increases absorption of calcium and phosphate from the gut as well as mineral mobilization from bone. The role of $24,25(OH)_2D_3$ is less well defined; it seems to promote bone mineralization and suppress parathyroid hormone release.

REGULATION OF PHOSPHORUS METABOLISM. The kidneys play a major role in maintaining the serum phosphorus concentration within narrow limits, about 3.0 to 4.5 mg per deciliter in adults. On an average diet, 1 gram of phosphorus is ingested daily, of which 700 mg is absorbed and the rest is excreted in the stool. The kidneys filter about 7 grams of phosphorus daily, of which 6.3 grams (90 per cent) is reabsorbed and 700 mg is excreted in the urine. As serum phosphorus and filtered load of phosphorus rise, the capacity to reabsorb phosphorus increases until a transport maximum (Tm) for phosphorus reabsorption is reached when serum phosphorus concentrations are between 6 and 9 mg per deciliter. Under physiologic conditions, about 70 per cent of the filtered phosphorus is reabsorbed in the proximal tubule and 10 to 15 per cent in the distal tubule and collecting ducts; thus, 5 to 20 per cent of the filtered phosphorus is excreted in the urine. In other words, the tubular reabsorption of phosphate (TRP) ranges normally from 80 to 95 per cent.

Numerous factors (the major ones being dietary phosphorus load and the serum levels of parathyroid hormone) affect the reabsorption of phosphorus. Phosphorus reabsorption approaches 100 per cent in patients fed a very low-phosphorus diet. In contrast, patients ingesting 2 to 3 grams of phosphorus daily can excrete 60 to 70 per cent of this amount in the urine. Changes in phosphorus intake affect phosphorus excretion directly and also by altering the levels of ionized calcium that modify the release of parathyroid hormone. Parathyroid hormone decreases phosphorus reabsorption in both proximal and distal segments of the nephron. An excess of parathyroid hormone may increase fractional excretion of phosphorus from a basal value of 10 per cent to 30 per cent or more. In the absence of parathyroid hormone the tubular capacity to reabsorb phosphorus is increased. Additional factors affect phosphorus reabsorption by the

TABLE 73–3. ROLE OF THE KIDNEY IN ACID-BASE BALANCE

Function	mEq/24 hr
1. Reabsorption of filtered bicarbonate ("reclamation")	$\cong 4000$
2. Generation of new bicarbonate (net excretion of acid)	50–100
a. Ammonium excretion	35–65
b. Titratable acid excretion	15–35

kidney. Volume expansion of the ECF, calcitonin, glucocorticoids, metabolic acidosis or alkalosis, and glycosuria increase urinary phosphorus excretion. On the other hand, growth hormone, insulin, and respiratory acidosis decrease phosphorus excretion. Vitamin D and its metabolites increase phosphorus reabsorption by the kidney.

RENAL REGULATION OF CALCIUM METABOLISM. Serum calcium concentrations in humans are maintained between 9 and 10 mg per deciliter despite wide variations in dietary calcium intake. Total serum calcium consists of ultrafilterable calcium (approximately 60 per cent of the total) and calcium bound to protein, primarily albumin. The ultrafilterable fraction includes both the ionized calcium (50 per cent of the total) and calcium complexed to citrate, bicarbonate, and phosphate, which represents 10 per cent of total serum calcium. Serum calcium levels are maintained relatively constant through modification of calcium absorption from the gastrointestinal tract, changes in renal calcium excretion, and mobilization of calcium from bone.

Approximately 1000 mg of calcium is ingested daily in the diet. About 800 mg appears in the stool (from unabsorbed dietary calcium and intestinal secretion) and 200 mg in the urine. The percentage of dietary calcium absorbed from the intestine increases when calcium intake is low and decreases when it is high. Parathyroid hormone and vitamin D participate in these adaptations. Thus, in patients fed a low-calcium diet, the development of mild and transient hypocalcemia increases the release of parathyroid hormone, which augments the renal conversion of $25(OH)D_3$ to $1,25(OH)_2D_3$. This latter compound increases intestinal calcium absorption and mobilizes calcium from bone, synergistically with parathyroid hormone. Thus, serum calcium returns toward normal. On the other hand, in patients fed a high-calcium diet, the mild hypercalcemia that may occur suppresses the release of parathyroid hormone, leading to decreased activity of the renal 1-hydroxylase enzyme and reduced production of $1,25(OH)_2D_3$.

The kidneys filter approximately 10 grams of calcium per day, but usually less than 200 mg appear in the urine. Thus over 98 per cent of the filtered load is reabsorbed. Approximately 55 per cent of the filtered calcium is reabsorbed in the proximal tubule, 20 to 30 per cent in the loop of Henle, 10 to 15 per cent in the distal tubule, and 2 to 8 per cent in the terminal nephron, including the collecting duct. Most maneuvers that decrease sodium and fluid reabsorption in the proximal tubule (infusion of saline, administration of acetazolamide, or mild to moderate hypercalcemia) decrease calcium reabsorption in this segment as well. The reabsorption of calcium in the loop of Henle also parallels sodium reabsorption. It is only distal to the loop of Henle that calcium and sodium are influenced separately and independently.

Parathyroid hormone stimulates the renal absorption of calcium and decreases urinary calcium excretion. Acute parathyroidectomy increases calcium excretion despite a fall in total serum calcium and hence in the filtered load of calcium. However, the degree of calciuria declines when the plasma concentration of calcium falls below 7 mg per deciliter. Pharmacologic doses of vitamin D usually increase intestinal absorption of calcium and bone resorption, leading to increases in serum calcium, the filtered load of calcium, and urinary calcium excretion. Metabolic acidosis or phosphate depletion produces hypercalciuria. Both furosemide and ethacrynic acid inhibit sodium and calcium transport in the thick ascending limb of Henle's loop and increase calcium excretion. Chronic administration of thiazides results in natriuresis and hypocalciuria. This effect may be due to contraction of ECF volume and increased calcium reabsorption in the proximal segments. In addition, thiazides may directly stimulate calcium reabsorption in the distal segment.

RENAL REGULATION OF MAGNESIUM METABOLISM. Total body magnesium is approximately 2000 mEq (or 25 grams). About 60 per cent of total body magnesium is found in bone. Another 20 per cent is present in muscle. Only a small fraction (about 1 per cent) is present in the ECF. The normal plasma concentration of magnesium in humans is 1.7 to 2.2 mg per deciliter, of which 80 per cent is ultrafilterable and the remainder protein bound. Most of the ultrafilterable magnesium is ionized. Roughly 300 mg or 25 mEq of magnesium is ingested daily in the diet. About two thirds of this amount appears in the stool and one third is eliminated in the urine. The kidney filters about 2 grams of magnesium daily, and approximately 100 mg (5 per cent) appears in the urine; thus, 95 per cent of the filtered magnesium is reabsorbed. Renal excretion of magnesium can be reduced to less than 0.5 per cent of the filtered load during magnesium deprivation. On the other hand, during infusion of magnesium or among patients with advanced chronic renal insufficiency the kidney can excrete 40 to 70 per cent of the filtered magnesium. The proximal tubules reabsorb about 20 to 30 per cent of the filtered magnesium, with 50 to 60 per cent being reabsorbed in the loop of Henle. Expansion of the ECF volume, produced by infusion of saline or chronic administration of mineralocorticoids, reduces the reabsorption of magnesium. A diet deficient in magnesium or the administration of parathyroid hormone enhances the reabsorption of magnesium in the thick ascending limb of Henle's loop. Infusions of calcium, ingestion of alcohol, administration of glucose, diets containing large amounts of magnesium, and diuretics such as furosemide or ethacrynic acid increase the urinary excretion of magnesium. Nephrotoxins, most notably cisplatin and aminoglycosides can cause severe renal Mg^{2+} wasting.

OTHER NONEXCRETORY FUNCTIONS OF THE KIDNEY

In addition to its role in the secretion of renin and the metabolism of vitamin D already discussed, the kidney has several other nonexcretory functions.

REGULATION OF THE RED BLOOD CELL MASS. *Erythropoietin* promotes the differentiation, proliferation, and maturation of red blood cell precursors in the bone marrow. Erythropoietin is produced by interstitial cells and by endothelial cells lining the peritubular capillaries of the cortex and outer medulla of the kidney. The stimulus to increased erythropoietin production by the kidney appears to be decreased renal oxygen tension or decreased renal perfusion (anemia, hypoxia, renal ischemia) or circulatory alterations induced by vasoconstrictors such as norepinephrine, angiotensin, or vasopressin. Increased erythropoietin levels may be seen in association with renal artery stenosis, renal cysts, renal cell carcinoma, and hydronephrosis and after renal transplantation. Production of erythropoietin decreases with hyperoxia, an excess red blood cell volume, and reduced functional renal mass.

RENAL METABOLISM OF PLASMA PROTEINS AND PEPTIDE HORMONES. The kidney is an important catabolic site for low molecular weight proteins (less than 50,000) but not for proteins with a molecular weight exceeding 68,000 (e.g., albumin, immunoglobulins).

Low molecular weight proteins are filterable. In the absence of tubular reabsorption they would be excreted quantitatively in the urine. Reabsorption of proteins or their catabolic products by the kidney prevents their loss in the urine, thereby conserving nutritionally important components. The proteins catabolized by the kidney are broken down to amino acids or polypeptides prior to return into the renal venous blood. The kidney, therefore, contributes to the regulation of their concentrations in plasma and precludes extensive loss of protein components in the urine.

In some patients with abnormalities of renal tubular function, low molecular weight proteins may appear in the urine in the absence of albumin owing to decreased tubular reabsorption. Conversely, in patients with reduced GFR the fractional catabolic rate of low molecular weight proteins (lysozyme, ribonuclease, beta_2-microglobulins, insulin, proinsulin, gastrin, glucagon, parathyroid hormone, Bence Jones protein, retinol binding protein, and growth hormone) is decreased and their levels in plasma are elevated.

Insulin, parathyroid hormone, and glucagon are catabolized by the kidney by filtration and subsequent tubular reabsorption as well as by peritubular uptake.

The catabolism of albumin, immunoglobulins, and larger plasma proteins is relatively low, with the kidney accounting for less than 5 per cent of their fractional catabolic rate, unless the nephrotic syndrome is present, in which case albumin catabolism could be significantly increased owing to both urinary losses and increased tubular degradation.

SYNTHESIS OF GROWTH FACTORS. Insulin-like growth factor I (IGF-I) is synthesized in the kidney. IGF-I is localized throughout the collecting ducts in both cortex and medulla. The steady-state levels of IGF-I mRNA in the collecting duct are influenced by the levels of circulating growth hormone. Receptors for IGF-I are present in proximal tubular basolateral membranes but not in membranes from the collecting duct, suggesting that IGF-I produced in the latter site exerts its biologic effect in the proximal tubule (paracrine action). Renal IGF-I is very likely involved in kidney growth or hypertrophy. A role for IGF-I in the regeneration of proximal tubule cells following ischemic injury has also been proposed.

THE KALLIKREIN-KININ SYSTEM. Kallikrein is a peptidase produced in various tissues, including the kidney, which acts on a specific substrate (kininogen) to split off a peptide, kinin. The kinin is destroyed by plasma and tissue peptidases (kininases). Kinins are potent vasodilators. The renal kallikrein-kinin system may constitute a local hormonal mechanism involved in the regulation of renal blood flow and sodium excretion. Renal kallikrein is probably produced by the cortex and excreted into the urine. It acts on a kininogen substrate to produce the potent vasodilator decapeptide (kallidin). Kallikrein excretion is augmented by reduced sodium intake. In contrast, high sodium intake decreases it. Administration of mineralocorticoids increases the excretion of kallikrein, and the increased kallikrein excretion of a low-salt diet is blocked by aldosterone antagonists (spironolactones). However, the role of the renal kallikrein system in sodium homeostasis is not yet established.

RENAL PROSTAGLANDINS. The prostaglandins are 20-carbon unsaturated fatty acids. Both vasodilator prostaglandins (PGE_2, prostacyclin, or PGI_2) and vasoconstrictor substances (thromboxanes) are synthesized in renal cortex (by arteries and glomeruli) and medulla (by interstitial and collecting duct cells) from free arachidonic acid, released from phospholipids. Renal prostaglandins may play a role in control of blood flow and GFR and in sodium and water excretion. They affect renin secretion as well. Prostaglandins may also modulate phosphorus transport and regulate renal ammonia synthesis. Their synthesis is stimulated by bradykinin, angiotensin II, ADH, and catecholamines. The last substances are vasoconstrictors that tend to diminish renal plasma flow. Therefore when constrictor stimuli are operative, renal prostaglandin production may increase, resulting in maintenance of renal blood flow.

Two other pathways of arachidonic acid metabolism have been described in the kidney: (1) an NADPH-dependent mono-oxygenase pathway that leads to the formation of 19- and 20-hydroxyeicosatetranoic acid (19-HETE and 20-HETE), 19-ketoarachidonic acid, and 1,20-dicarboxylic acid; and (2) a calcium-dependent lipoxygenase pathway with synthesis of 15-HETE, 12-HETE, and leukotrienes. The physiologic or pathophysiologic importance of these pathways is unknown, but it should be remembered that the HETE's are potent chemotactic compounds and, therefore, may play a role in inflammatory glomerular disease. Leukotrienes are known to contract vascular and nonvascular smooth muscle and enhance vascular permeability. Thus, they may play a role in the control of renal blood flow and GFR.

Cogan MG: Renal effects of atrial natriuretic factor. Ann Rev Physiol 52:699–708, 1990. *Comprehensive description of the role of atrial natriuretic peptides on glomerular filtration rate and tubular function.*

DuBose TD Jr. (ed.): Acidification mechanisms. Semin Nephrol 10(2):91–180, 1990. *Several contributions in this issue cover different aspects of proton secretion and bicarbonate reabsorption in the nephron.*

Hammerman MR: The growth hormone–insulin-like growth factor axis in kidney. Am J Physiol 257:F503–F514, 1989. *An authoritative editorial on the role of insulin-like growth factors in the kidney.*

Khraibi AA, Knox FG: Renal hemodynamics and sodium chloride excretion. *In* Klahr S, Massry SG (eds.): Contemporary Nephrology. Vol. V. New York, Plenum Publishing Company, 1989, pp 35–79. *A lucid update written by major contributors in the field of renal physiology.*

Norris SH: Renal eicosanoids. Semin Nephrol 10:64–88, 1990. *A detailed review of the role of arachidonic acid metabolites in health and disease.*

Tisher CC, Madsen KM: Anatomy of the kidney. *In* Brenner BM, Rector JC (eds.): The Kidney. 3rd ed. Philadelphia, W. B. Saunders Company, 1986, pp 3–60. *An excellent and clearly written review of kidney structure.*

Vane JR, Angaard EE, Botting RM: Regulatory functions of the vascular endothelium. N Engl J Med 323:27–36, 1990. *An excellent review of the role of vasoconstrictors and vasodilators produced by the vascular endothelium.*

74 Investigations of Renal Function

Vincent W. Dennis

Methods are available to assess the functional integrity of the glomerular ultrafiltration barrier; the presence of urogenital inflammation; the overall rate of glomerular filtration; the ability to dilute, concentrate, or acidify urine; and the ability to conserve or to excrete specific solutes. Measurements of certain values in blood and urine detect abnormalities in renal function and may occasionally point to specific etiologies, but a final diagnosis usually requires direct or indirect visualization of the kidneys and urogenital system or morphologic examination of renal tissue.

PROTEINURIA. Increased urinary excretion of protein is one of the most common and most easily detected signs of renal disease. The normal excretion rate of urinary protein is less than 150 mg per 24 hours for adults, but values as high as 300 mg per 24 hours may occur in apparently healthy adolescents. The normal composition of urinary protein includes about 40 per cent albumin, 40 per cent tissue proteins originating from renal and other urogenital tissues, 15 per cent immunoglobulins and their fragments, and 5 per cent other plasma proteins. Abnormalities may occur in both the quantity and the composition of urinary proteins.

Urinary protein is usually detected by a colorimetric test ("dipstick test"), which depends on the ability of proteins, especially albumin, to alter the color reaction of a pH-sensitive dye. Such qualitative tests may detect protein concentrations as low as 15 mg per deciliter and give a positive test result if a normal amount of protein is present in a concentrated volume of urine. Conversely, abnormal rates of protein excretion may remain undetected in large volumes of dilute urine. It is therefore important to have some estimate of the degree of urine concentration when interpreting a qualitative test for protein. A positive qualitative result for urinary protein usually warrants quantification of the absolute protein excretion rate per 24 hours. Alternatively, the protein-creatinine ratio of a random daytime urine sample correlates well with values from 24-hour collections. Proteinuria usually results from (1) elevated plasma concentration of normal or abnormal proteins, (2) increased glomerular permeability, (3) decreased tubular reabsorption of normally filtered proteins, and (4) alterations in renal hemodynamics (Table 74–1).

Overflow Proteinuria. Changes in plasma protein concentrations may alter the rates of protein excretion by both the normal and the abnormal kidney. This type of proteinuria may occur from the presence in plasma of increased concentrations of proteins not normally present in significant amounts. Examples include light-chain immunoglobulin fragments such as Bence Jones protein associated with plasma cell disorders (see Ch. 151) or myoglobin associated with rhabdomyolysis. The presence of abnormal proteins in either plasma or urine may be confirmed by electrophoresis. Changes in the concentration of normal plasma proteins may also influence passage across the *abnormal* glomerular capillary wall. For example, increases or decreases in the plasma concentration of albumin may increase or decrease its rate of urinary excretion without necessarily indicating improvement or worsening of the renal conditions that led to proteinuria.

Increased Glomerular Permeability. The glomerular capillary wall consists of capillary endothelium, basement membrane, visceral epithelium, and mesangium. Each of these four anatomic components contributes directly or indirectly to the formation and maintenance of the functional ultrafiltration barrier that limits the passage of proteins into the urinary space. The glomerular capillary wall restricts the passage of plasma proteins according to their size (steric hindrance) and surface charge (electrostatic hindrance). At any given molecular size, negative charges on the glomerular capillary basement membrane hinder the passage of negatively charged molecules more than positively charged molecules.

A number of systemic and primary renal diseases may affect one or more glomerular structures and thereby increase the effective permeability of the glomerular capillary wall to proteins. The degree of proteinuria may range from 0.2 to greater than 20 grams per 24 hours. Proteinuria that exceeds about 3 to 5 grams of normal plasma protein per 24 hours provides direct evidence of increased effective permeability of the glomerular capillary wall, since these amounts exceed those that may be filtered by the normal glomerulus and reabsorbed by the renal tubules. Such massive losses of plasma proteins may be responsible for changes in plasma oncotic pressure and thereby set in motion the events that are manifest clinically as the nephrotic syndrome (see Ch. 79).

Because of its low molecular weight and its dominance among plasma proteins, albumin is typically the major urinary protein in this type of proteinuria. However, the relative proportion of albumin in the urine, even if corrected for changes in its proportion in plasma, is lower in some forms of renal diseases than in others. *Selective proteinuria* refers to the ability of the glomerulus to retain higher molecular weight proteins despite increased filtration of low molecular weight proteins. A highly selective proteinuria therefore consists almost exclusively of increased excretion of albumin, whereas a poorly selective proteinuria contains proportionately greater amounts of higher molecular weight proteins and is generally associated with severe disruption of the glomerular capillary wall. This selectivity may be attributed to the glomerulus only if the composition of urinary proteins is not affected significantly by downstream events such as tubular reabsorption. This requirement is presumably met with levels of proteinuria that exceed 3 to 5 grams per 24 hours, but the selectivity pattern of lesser amounts of proteinuria may be significantly influenced by tubular reabsorption. To define glomerular selectivity requires measurements of the relative clearances of specific proteins with increasing molecular weights, such as albumin (69,000), transferrin (90,000), gamma globulin (150,000), and alpha$_2$-glycoprotein (820,000). Although attractive in theory and potentially useful as an index of the severity of glomerular damage, the techniques required to characterize the selectivity of proteinuria are generally too laborious and too imprecise to have achieved widespread clinical applicability. Nevertheless, heavy proteinuria characterized by the dominance of albumin and the absence of higher molecular weight globulins is typical of minimal change or nil lesion (see Ch. 79), whereas the detection of a nonselective pattern is highly suggestive of the presence of some other form of otherwise undefined glomerular disease.

Microalbuminuria refers to increases in albumin excretion that are detectable by sensitive immunoassay but not by current standard clinical techniques. The presence of microalbuminuria in diabetics may predict the development of diabetic nephropathy, whereas its absence may forecast a more favorable prognosis.

Tubular Proteinuria. Many polypeptides and low molecular weight proteins normally present in plasma are filtered freely at the glomerulus and are reabsorbed by the tubules. Examples include polypeptide hormones such as insulin, glucagon, and parathyroid hormone and plasma proteins with a molecular weight smaller than 20,000. Once filtered, these proteins are absorbed by specific endocytic processes that bind and engulf the filtered proteins. The presence of tubular disorders, especially injuries that result from various antibiotics or heavy metals (see Ch. 80), may be associated with increased urinary excretion of low molecular weight proteins and relatively slight increases in the excretion of albumin (*tubular proteinuria*). This pattern is in marked contrast to the predominance of albumin in the urine of patients with glomerular disorders. Patients characterized clinically as having tubulointerstitial rather than glomerular diseases have increased urinary protein excretion (generally less than 2 grams per 24 hours) and increased renal clearance of beta$_2$-microglobu-

lin, especially relative to albumin. Beta$_2$-microglobulinuria is less likely to occur in those disease processes such as diabetes mellitus that cause proteinuria via effects on glomerular permeability. The clinical significance of tubular proteinuria is unclear at this time because there is still insufficient documentation of correlations between tubular proteinuria and detailed functional, biochemical, and morphologic descriptions of the underlying diseases in which it has been observed.

Proteinuria from Altered Renal Hemodynamics. Changes in protein excretion rate may also occur in response to changes in renal hemodynamics. Exercise, major motor seizures, change to the standing position, fever, and vasoactive agents such as renin, angiotensin, and norepinephrine increase urinary protein excretion by mechanisms that seem related to reductions in renal blood flow. Changes in renal blood flow may alter urinary protein excretion in normal subjects as well as in those with abnormal rates of protein excretion. Possible mechanisms include local increases in protein concentration within the glomerular capillary, increased effective permeability of the glomerular capillary wall, increased transglomerular hydrostatic pressure, and increased effective filtration area. Hemodynamic increases in urinary protein excretion are generally transient or additive to other causes of proteinuria.

LEUKOCYTURIA. The urinary leukocyte excretion rate in apparently healthy individuals ranges between 0 and 300,000 leukocytes per hour; rates greater than 400,000 per hour are generally regarded as abnormal. If appropriate cleansing precautions are used, there is no difference in leukocyte excretion rates between apparently healthy males and females or between urine samples obtained from suprapubic puncture and midstream urine.

In practice, leukocyte excretion rates are estimated indirectly by microscopic examination of urinary sediment resuspended after centrifugation of approximately 10 ml of urine. Abnormal leukocyturia probably exists when more than 5 white blood cells occur per high-power field. However, about 20 per cent of urine specimens from patients excreting more than 400,000 white blood cells per hour may demonstrate fewer than 5 leukocytes per high-power field. The indirect method thus underestimates the prevalence of abnormal leukocyturia, although increased numbers of white blood cells per high-power field appear to correspond well to increased rates of leukocyte excretion. Leukocyturia results frequently from urinary tract infection (see Ch. 84) but may also indicate other causes of inflammation, such as tubulointerstitial diseases (see Ch. 80).

HEMATURIA. The detection of hematuria is aided by the widespread use of the multifunctional "dipstick," which includes a section impregnated with orthotolidine. The test is sufficiently sensitive to detect the equivalent of greater than 10,000 red blood cells per milliliter of urine but is negative in normal individuals despite the wide range of red blood cell excretion rates. A positive orthotolidine test occurs in the presence of free hemoglobin or myoglobin in urine. Free hemoglobin in the urine generally results from the lysis of red blood cells in the urine but may also reflect free hemoglobin in the plasma. When indicated, this question can be resolved by direct measurements of plasma hemoglobin and haptoglobin concentrations. Myoglobin in the urine is detected by the differential precipitation of hemoglobin with ammonium sulfate, by spectrophotometry of the ferricyanide derivatives of hemoglobin and myoglobin, by the co-migration on paper electrophoresis of myoglobin with hemoglobin C, or, preferably, by direct immunoassay of myoglobin in plasma or

TABLE 74–1. TYPES OF PROTEINURIA*

Type	Mechanism	Quantity	Molecular Weight	Examples
Overflow	Increased filtration of abnormal plasma proteins across normal glomeruli	Variable (0.2 to >10 grams)	Low (<40,000)	Bence Jones proteinuria, myoglobinuria
Glomerular	Defective glomerular retention of normal plasma proteins	>3–5 grams	High (>68,000)	Glomerulonephritis, nephrotic syndrome
Tubular	Defective reabsorption of normally filtered plasma proteins	<2 grams	Low (<40,000)	Interstitial nephritis, antibiotic injury, heavy metals
Hemodynamic	Increased filtration and possibly decreased reabsorption	<2 grams	Variable (20,000–68,000)	Transient proteinuria, congestive heart failure, fever, seizures, exercise

*Values >150 mg per 24 hours.

urine. Myoglobinuria is usually accompanied by marked increases in plasma concentrations of creatine phosphokinase (CPK).

As with leukocytes, the presence of red blood cells in urine is quantified in terms of red blood cells per high-power field and is normally 0 to 1 in males but may be slightly higher in females. The persistent presence in males or females of even small numbers of red blood cells in urine is cause for concern and may indicate the presence of a coagulopathy, hemoglobinopathy, renal parenchymal disease, tumor, trauma, or inflammation anywhere along the renal and urinary tract (Table 74–2). Hematuria accompanied by proteinuria generally indicates renal parenchymal disease.

GLOMERULAR FILTRATION RATE. Measurements of glomerular filtration rate are used clinically largely as estimates of the mass of functional renal tissue or of the number of functioning nephrons. To be useful in the measure of glomerular filtration rate, a substance should be filtered freely at the glomerulus and not secreted, reabsorbed, catabolized, or synthesized by the kidney. The substance should be harmless, inexpensive, and easy to administer and measure accurately. A number of exogenous substances fulfill some of these requirements, but there is no ideal material of endogenous origin. Overall, however, the most useful indicators of glomerular filtration rate are measurements of the plasma creatinine concentration and creatinine clearance. Creatinine is an end-product of creatine metabolism. Its endogenous production averages about 15 mg per kilogram of body weight per day, correlates with muscle mass, and tends to be constant for a given individual. Creatinine is filtered freely at the glomerulus and is secreted by the proximal tubule to an extent that may increase with elevated plasma concentration. The excretion rate of creatinine thus reflects the combined effects of filtration and secretion, and normally the clearance of creatinine exceeds the glomerular filtration rate. The secretion of creatinine is inhibited by certain drugs, such as cimetidine and trimethoprim, which may increase the plasma creatinine concentration without affecting glomerular filtration rate. Ketonemia may cause spurious increases in measurements of plasma creatinine because acetoacetate interferes with certain automated analytic techniques (Table 74–3).

Figure 74–1 shows the theoretic relationship between plasma creatinine concentration and creatinine clearance and the relationship between creatinine clearance and other measures of glomerular filtration rate, such as inulin clearance. The relationship between plasma creatinine and creatinine clearance is described by a rectangular hyperbola. This reflects the mathematical reality that values on the horizontal axis are determined by the reciprocals of values on the vertical axis, since the formula for creatinine clearance includes the serum creatinine concentration in the denominator. To the extent that creatinine clearance and glomerular filtration rate are equivalent, the same ideal relationship should apply between observed glomerular filtration rate and plasma creatinine concentration, but deviations from this ideal occur.

In the normal range, measurements of plasma creatinine concentration include a significant and variable component of noncreatinine chromogen that is not excreted in the urine. This overestimate offsets in part the error introduced by the renal secretion of creatinine, so that in this range creatinine clearances correlate well with other measures of glomerular filtration rate.

TABLE 74–2. CAUSES OF HEMATURIA ISOLATED FROM OTHER URINE ABNORMALITIES

Urologic
  Urogenital tumor
  Renal cyst or solid tumor
  Nephrolithiasis or urolithiasis (usually painful)
Hematologic
  Coagulopathies, inherited or acquired
  Hemoglobinopathies, especially sickle trait
Nephrologic
  Glomerulopathies, especially immunoglobulin A (IgA) nephropathy
  Benign essential hematuria (attenuated glomerular basement membrane)
Menstruation

TABLE 74–3. FACTORS THAT AFFECT PLASMA CREATININE CONCENTRATION WITHOUT CHANGES IN GLOMERULAR FILTRATION RATE

Increase	
Ketonemia	Spurious increase in automated measurements by acetoacetate
Cimetidine, trimethoprim	Inhibition of tubular secretion
Decrease	
Muscle wasting	Reduced creatinine production
Low protein diet	Reduced creatinine ingestion and production

In the presence of renal failure, plasma creatinine concentration rises much more so than that of noncreatinine chromogens, and thus measurements of plasma creatinine concentration approach the true creatinine concentration. Moreover, in the presence of moderate degrees of renal failure, the secretory component of creatinine excretion may increase until the glomerular filtration rate falls below about 10 ml per minute. For these reasons, in the presence of moderate renal failure the clearance of creatinine tends to overestimate the glomerular filtration rate. In advanced renal failure (glomerular filtration rate less than 10 ml per minute), creatinine clearance again approximates the glomerular filtration rate (Fig. 74–1). Despite these shortcomings, measurement of the plasma creatinine concentration is the most useful estimate of filtration rate largely because of the ease with which repeated measurements may be made in individual patients along the course of their disease. In view of the insensitivity in detecting reductions in the glomerular filtration rate to the 50 to 80 ml per minute range, values in the upper range of normal need to be interpreted with special caution and correlated with other clinical data. Patients with chronic renal disease should have at least one and perhaps annual measurements of their 24-hour creatinine excretion to monitor possible changes in creatinine production. Measurements of urinary creatinine are less useful in acute renal failure, since values do not generally reflect a steady state. In the acute setting, about 3 days are required for plasma creatinine concentrations to achieve a steady state, and thus clinically detectable changes may lag behind the time of injury.

The most accurate measures of glomerular filtration rate in humans are obtained with the use of a number of exogenous

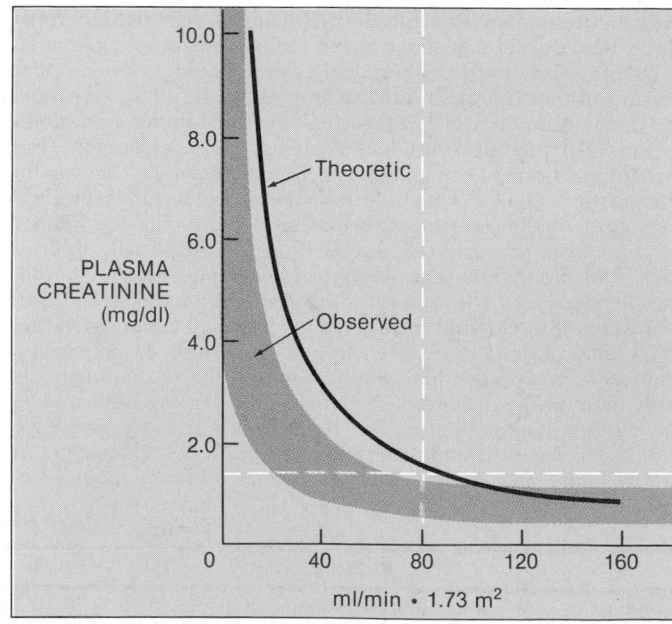

FIGURE 74–1. Relationship between plasma creatinine concentrations and various measures of glomerular filtration rate. The solid line depicts the theoretical relationship between plasma creatinine concentration and creatinine clearance. The color-screened area represents the relationship between plasma creatinine and noncreatinine measures of glomerular filtration rate. The dashed lines denote the limits of normal values. Note the extent to which normal plasma creatinine values may occur in spite of reduced filtration rates.

substances, such as insulin, or a variety of radioisotopically labeled compounds, such as ^{125}I-iothalamate. Standard clearance techniques for these measurements require injection of the compound to a steady-state plasma concentration and then the timed collection of urine.

The blood urea nitrogen (BUN) concentration is an imperfect quantitative indicator of renal filtration despite its frequent use for this purpose. Urea is synthesized by the liver from ammonia derived from the catabolism of proteins and amino acids. Urea production is therefore variable and is influenced by hepatic as well as dietary conditions. At the kidneys, urea is filtered, reabsorbed, and secreted. Reabsorption dominates, but the rate of reabsorption varies with the degree of hydration. Those conditions, such as dehydration, that tend to increase the renal reabsorption of volume also increase the reabsorption of urea. Accordingly, blood urea nitrogen concentration may increase without any abnormality in renal function. Conversely, in the presence of renal excretory failure and reduced filtration rate, the BUN concentration may be influenced significantly by the degree of dietary protein intake. For these reasons, measurement of plasma creatinine concentration provides a more reliable index of renal filtration rate than the BUN. The BUN is used mainly to quantify the balance between the accumulation and excretion of nitrogenous metabolites (i.e., the degree of uremia), especially in the presence of more than moderate reductions in glomerular filtration rate.

RENAL CONCENTRATING AND DILUTING ABILITY. The total solute concentration of urine is generally assessed clinically by measurement of urinary specific gravity, which relates the weight of a unit volume of urine to an equal volume of water. Because of its simplicity, this technique has persisted despite well-recognized deficiencies. Errors of technique relate primarily to poor calibration of the hygrometer, but even in the absence of faulty technique the specific gravity of urine provides only a rough indication of urinary osmolality. For example, urines that contain high concentrations of urea have lower specific gravities than expected for their osmolality, and urines that contain higher density solutes, such as glucose, iodinated contrast material, or protein, have higher specific gravities relative to their osmolalities. Within these limitations, however, there is a useful correlation between the specific gravity and osmolality of urine such that urinary osmolality in milliosmoles per kilogram of water may be estimated as 40 times the increase in specific gravity of urine above the value of water, which is 1.000. Thus, urine with a specific gravity of 1.007 would have an estimated osmolality of 280 mOsm, similar to that of plasma, and urine with a specific gravity of 1.020 would be distinctly concentrated, with an estimated osmolality of 800 mOsm. Nonetheless, measurements of urinary specific gravity represent only crude estimates of osmolality, and, when indicated, accurate measures of urinary

osmolality may be made easily by measurement of freezing point depression in a cryoscopic osmometer.

Maximal urinary concentrating ability is measured by restricting fluid intake until the patient loses a minimum of 3 per cent or a maximum of 5 per cent of body weight, or until three consecutive urine specimens show no further increase in osmolality. These results are usually achieved within 16 hours of fluid restriction but may occur much earlier in patients with severe inability to conserve water. Once either one of these endpoints is achieved, additional information may be obtained by the subcutaneous administration of 5 units of aqueous vasopressin to determine if any further increase in urinary osmolality can be achieved. Normal subjects achieve maximal urinary osmolality of 1000 ± 200 (SD) mOsm without further change after vasopressin. Patients who have complete or incomplete defects in antidiuretic hormone secretion (ADH), nephrogenic diabetes insipidus, or psychogenic polydipsia will have abnormal and distinctive patterns of response (Fig. 74–2).

Maximal diluting capacity of the kidney is assessed by the rapid administration of 1200 ml of water by mouth to a fasting subject. The osmolality of three hourly urine specimens is measured and should achieve values lower than 80 mOsm or a specific gravity of 1.002. Measurements of the rate or extent of excretion of the administered water are quite variable and are not generally useful. Both maximal diluting and maximal concentrating ability of the kidney may be impaired by diuretics, especially potent loop diuretics such as furosemide and ethacrynic acid, and by diuretic states such as glucosuria.

ACIDIFICATION CAPACITY. The urine is normally more acidic than body fluids because of the endogenous production and renal excretion of nonvolatile acids derived primarily from sulfate and phosphate contained in dietary protein. Even at low pH, however, the amount of acid excreted as free hydrogen ion is negligible (pH 5.0 equals 0.01 mEq H^+ per liter). Most hydrogen ion is excreted in the form of ammonium or titratable acids. For these reasons, the pH of a random specimen of urine provides only limited information about renal function and essentially no reliable information about the systemic acid-base status.

Assessment of the renal acidification capacity is accomplished by the *ammonium chloride tolerance test*. The basis of this test is to induce mild metabolic acidosis by the administration of ammonium chloride by mouth and to measure the maximal depression in urinary pH, the maximal excretion rate of ammonium and titratable acid, and the percentage of excretion of the administered hydrogen ion equivalent. Because the purpose of the ammonium chloride is to induce metabolic acidosis, its administration is not necessary if acidosis is present spontaneously. Indications for the ammonium chloride test are generally

FIGURE 74–2. Patterns of changes in urine osmolality in response to prolonged water deprivation. DI = diabetes insipidus.

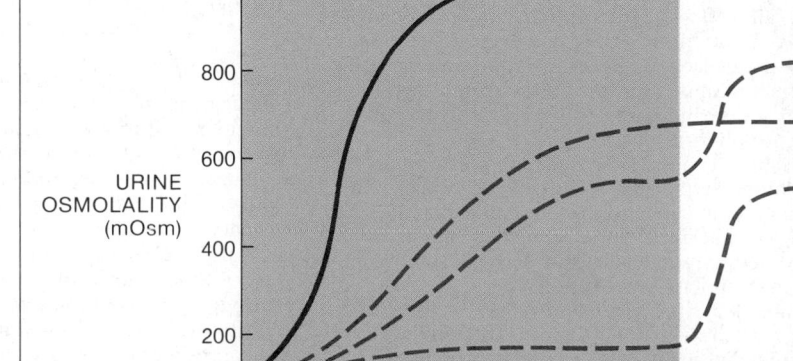

restricted to those conditions, usually suspected abnormalities in distal tubular function, that are associated with only mild reductions in glomerular filtration rate. Ammonium chloride, 0.1 gram per kilogram, is administered by mouth, and urine is collected hourly for 6 to 8 hours. A normal response is to achieve a urinary pH of 5.4 or less and to excrete at least 30 per cent of the administered hydrogen ion equivalent. An abnormal response consists of failure to acidify the urine below pH 5.4 despite a measured reduction in arterial pH. This defines a distal renal tubular acidosis and indicates a defect in maximal acidification capacity. The ammonium chloride tolerance test is not generally performed in patients with renal insufficiency, but, if performed, these patients usually achieve reduction in the urinary pH below 5.4, although there is reduced excretion of ammonium and titratable acid.

URINARY ELECTROLYTES. Measurements of urinary sodium, potassium, and chloride may provide important information but only in a limited set of clinical circumstances. Two types of measurements are made. The absolute daily excretion of sodium, potassium, or chloride (milliequivalents per day) is derived from the electrolyte concentration of a 24-hour collection of urine. Such measurements provide quantification of the daily intake of these electrolytes, provided that two requirements are met. First, total body weight must be constant to indicate balance between intake and output. Second, electrolyte excretion must be limited to the urine, and losses via the gastrointestinal tract or skin must be negligible. Under these conditions, the daily excretion of sodium, potassium, or chloride will reflect the dietary intake, but this information has only limited clinical value.

Measurement of the *concentration* of sodium, potassium, or chloride in a random urine sample may provide information of importance in certain circumstances, such as the evaluation of hyponatremia, acute oliguria, volume depletion, hypokalemia, and metabolic alkalosis. In the evaluation of hyponatremia, a urinary sodium concentration less than 10 mEq per liter indicates the presence of reduced effective extracellular volume with an appropriate increase in mineralocorticoid and ADH activity that leads to the renal retention of sodium and solute-free water. Higher urinary sodium concentrations indicate significant renal losses of sodium such as might occur from diuretics or, less commonly, from mineralocorticoid or glucocorticoid insufficiency or with volume expansion from the inappropriate secretion of ADH. Similarly, in the evaluation of patients with reduced extracellular volume, urinary sodium concentrations greater than 10 to 20 mEq per liter indicate that the kidney is participating in the loss of sodium and volume, perhaps because of diuretics or renal or adrenal insufficiency, whereas urinary sodium concentrations less than 5 to 10 mEq per liter indicate that losses of sodium and volume are occurring via extrarenal routes.

In the setting of acute oliguria, urinary sodium concentration greater than 20 to 40 mEq per liter occurs frequently with acute renal failure or incomplete obstruction, whereas urinary sodium concentrations are generally less than 20 mEq per liter in the presence of severe volume depletion (prerenal azotemia), acute glomerulonephritis, congestive heart failure, coexistent liver disease, or acute renal failure from radiocontrast material or acute rejection (Ch. 76). As is often the case, however, these values may be modified by many factors, including the administration of diuretics, and urinary sodium concentrations are not generally regarded as sufficiently discriminatory to be useful in the differential diagnosis of acute oliguria.

The urinary potassium concentration may be useful in the evaluation of unexplained hypokalemia. In the presence of hypokalemia, urinary potassium concentrations greater than 20 mEq per liter indicate significant renal losses, such as might occur from diuretics, increased mineralocorticoid activity, or magnesium deficiency. Urinary potassium concentrations less than 10 mEq per liter indicate that the hypokalemia may be related to gastrointestinal losses, such as may occur from the surreptitious use of laxatives or may indicate changes in plasma potassium concentration without potassium deficits, such as may occur with hypokalemic periodic paralysis (see Ch. 507).

Urinary chloride concentrations provide important information in the evaluation of metabolic alkalosis. Persistent metabolic alkalosis results most often from the depletion of chloride via the gastrointestinal tract or urine. In the presence of metabolic alkalosis, urinary chloride concentrations greater than 10 mEq per liter suggest the presence of diuretic-induced increases in chloride excretion, severe depletion of potassium, Bartter's syndrome, or increased adrenocortical hormone activity. On the other hand, urinary chloride concentrations less than 10 mEq per liter point to losses of chloride via extrarenal routes, usually vomiting, and indicate further that the metabolic alkalosis is likely to respond to replacement of volume with normal saline.

IMAGING OF THE KIDNEYS AND UROGENITAL TRACT

Imaging techniques of importance in the evaluation of renal abnormalities include roentgenography, ultrasonography, radionuclide studies, and magnetic resonance imaging (MRI). These techniques are used (1) to visualize the number, size, and location of the kidneys; (2) to identify the presence and site of obstruction; (3) to detect and to characterize mass lesions; (4) to visualize renal arteries and veins; and (5) to guide percutaneous diagnostic and therapeutic interventions, such as biopsy and nephrostomy. The choice of a technique is based on its relative simplicity, its safety, its potential to yield results that for a particular suspected disorder are neither falsely positive (lack of specificity) nor falsely negative (lack of sensitivity), and its potential to provide additional information not already available from previous studies.

ROENTGENOGRAPHIC STUDIES. The most simple radiologic study of the kidneys and urogenital system is the plain roentgenogram of the kidneys, ureter, and bladder (KUB), which will often reveal abnormal calcifications and may reveal renal size if the kidneys are not obscured by overlying bowel. If indicated, tomography may be necessary to determine the renal outlines.

Excretory Urogram. The excretory urogram, also known as the intravenous pyelogram, or IVP, is the classic radiologic method to detect anatomic abnormalities of the kidneys and ureters and to evaluate patients with renal abnormalities. The basic excretory urogram is performed by the intravenous injection of iodinated contrast material, which is filtered at the glomerulus and concentrated within the tubular lumina and collecting system by the renal reabsorption of volume. Visualization of the contrast material within the renal parenchyma yields a *nephrogram*, and visualization within the major collecting system yields a *pyelogram*. Each of these phases is dependent on the amount of radiocontrast material that is delivered to the kidneys and filtered and also on the degree of extraction of volume that concentrates the dye within the parenchyma and collecting system. Modern radiocontrast materials are not secreted. Patients with renal insufficiency (e.g., those with plasma creatinine values >3 to 4 mg per deciliter) may not have adequate filtration and concentration of radiocontrast to allow detailed visualization, especially relative to their increased risk for adverse reactions.

A nephrogram normally appears within 1 to 3 minutes after injection of the contrast material. The nephrogram provides an opportunity to determine the number of kidneys, their size and configuration, and the possible presence of inhomogeneous areas or filling defects. In addition, the symmetric and timely appearance of nephrograms bilaterally provides qualitative information on the relative blood flow and filtration rate of each kidney. The pyelogram phase occurs within 5 minutes after the injection of dye as the nephrogram fades. This phase allows visualization of the caliceal system, ureters, and bladder and provides opportunities to detect abnormalities in shape, size, or drainage that might result from intrinsic defects or from extrinsic compression. Vascular or outflow obstructions may result in marked delays in the onset of both the nephrogram and the pyelogram phases.

Retrograde Pyelography. Retrograde pyelography is the direct injection of radiocontrast material into the ureter and upper urinary tract. The approach to this area is achieved via insertion of a ureteral catheter under direct visualization through cystoscopy. Some form of anesthesia may be required. Although retrograde pyelography was used frequently to assess renal size and to evaluate the possibility of ureteral obstruction in patients who presented with advanced renal failure, these questions are now resolved more readily with ultrasonography. Retrograde pyelography does provide more direct and improved visualization of the ureters and calices, and this visualization is useful in the localization and diagnosis of tumors and obstructions.

Percutaneous Pyeloureteral Techniques. The combination of

visualizing techniques such as roentgenographic fluoroscopy or ultrasonography and the availability of percutaneous catheters allows placement of a catheter in the renal pelvis, calices, or perirenal space if these spaces are distended by abnormal collections of fluid. Percutaneous catheter placement allows drainage and irrigation of pyonephrosis, abscesses, and obstructions, as well as placement of temporary nephrostomy catheters.

Renal Arteriography and Venography. The renal vasculature is visualized with radiocontrast material injected via a catheter introduced usually through the femoral vessels. Renal arteriography is performed most often to evaluate possible renal arterial stenosis as a cause or aggravating factor in systemic hypertension and to evaluate renal mass lesions. In general, cystic mass lesions are devoid of vasculature and may stretch and distort normal renal vessels and calices. Solid tumors are frequently vascular with irregular and erratic vessels that fill early as a blush of contrast material.

Renal venography is limited largely to searches for renal vein thrombosis and venous extension of renal cell carcinoma. Because renal venography requires the injection of dye against usually heavy renal venous outflow, turbulence may on occasion distort the distribution of dye and give the appearance of an intravascular filling defect. For this reason, renal venography is sometimes performed with intra-arterial infusion of epinephrine to reduce renal blood flow.

Digital Subtraction Angiography. Digital subtraction angiography uses high-quality image intensifiers and video camera recordings to visualize major arterial vessels following the rapid intravenous injection of radiocontrast material. Standard x-ray sources are used to produce sequential images at rates of about one per second, beginning at the time of injection of radiocontrast material into a central or peripheral artery or vein. Images are intensified electronically, displayed on a video camera, digitized, and stored on magnetic tape in a memory system. Images obtained prior to the arrival of radiocontrast material at a particular vascular region are subtracted electronically from the subsequent images to enhance the contrast between vessels and other tissues. With regard to the detection of renovascular diseases, digital subtraction venous angiography has an overall accuracy of about 70 to 80 per cent, compared with conventional arteriography. Technically successful studies are generally sensitive enough to detect significant renovascular lesions, but false-positive results may be as frequent as 20 to 30 per cent. Because venous angiography does not require an arteriotomy, it can be performed without hospitalization at considerably less cost than direct arteriography.

Computed Tomography. Computed tomography (CT) represents a sophisticated extension of roentgenography and may be performed with or without contrast material. Its usefulness in the evaluation of renal abnormalities consists primarily in its application as a tertiary mode after excretory urograms and ultrasonography to detect and localize mass lesions. Computed tomography may detect cystic masses as small as 0.5 cm in diameter, but the sensitivity is less for noncalcific solid masses (Fig. 74–3). Computed tomography is also useful in detecting and evaluating obstruction and dilatation of the major collecting system in patients allergic to iodinated contrast material or for whom ultrasonography is inconclusive for technical reasons, such as interference by bone, calcifications, or gas.

Adverse Effects of Urography. Two types of adverse effects should be considered in relation to the performance of excretory urograms, angiograms, or CT with intravenous contrast material. First, any exposure to radiation is associated with a finite, statistical risk of permanent alteration in DNA. Depending on the question being asked, alternative modes of visualization, such as ultrasonography, might be considered in certain circumstances, especially those that involve pregnancy or repeated examinations over time.

The second type of adverse effect of excretory urography relates to toxic reactions to the iodinated contrast material. The overall incidence of adverse reactions to intravenous contrast is about 5 per cent for the general population and about 10 per cent for those with any allergies. The most common reactions involve nausea or urticaria; about 10 per cent of reactions will involve life-threatening events, such as hypotension, laryngeal edema, or cardiac arrhythmias.

Radiocontrast urography is a remarkably safe procedure, es-

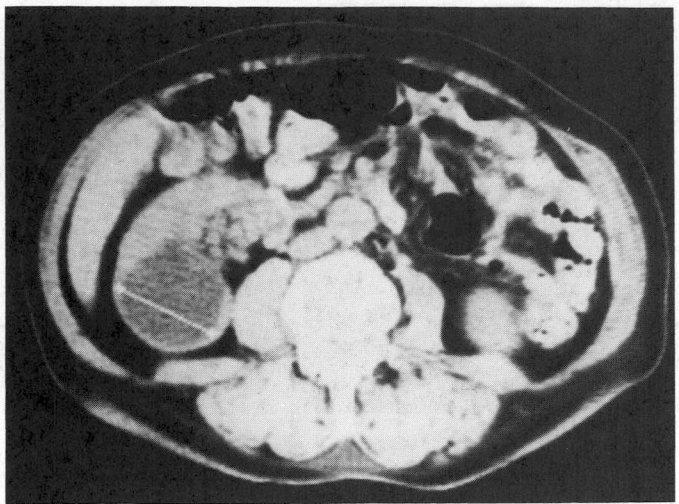

FIGURE 74–3. Computed tomography (CT) of the abdomen. The orientation is looking upward from toes to head. The right kidney is visualized at this level, but only a small portion of the left kidney is shown. There is a large, well-demarcated, homogeneous mass (white diagonal) in the right kidney that has the density of water rather than tissue. This is characteristic of a renal cyst.

pecially when performed in essentially healthy individuals. Not unexpectedly, radiocontrast materials are less safe in individuals who are less healthy. The single most important risk factor for radiocontrast-induced renal injury is the presence of pre-existent renal disease, such as that likely to be present in patients with diabetes mellitus, multiple myeloma, and generalized atherosclerotic disease. Renal function may also deteriorate more frequently following administration of intravenous radiocontrast in patients with advanced age, marked dehydration, hyperuricemia, or proteinuria. Appropriate precautions are indicated: consideration of alternative modes of visualization, attention to optimal hydration, and use of the minimal amount of contrast material consistent with an adequate examination.

ULTRASONOGRAPHY. Ultrasonography represents a major advance in the noninvasive visualization of the kidneys and genitourinary system. The acoustic impedance of a tissue to ultrasonic waves is the product of its density and the velocity of sound in that tissue. Significant differences in acoustic impedance occur among tissues that differ in their content of water, fat, collagen, minerals, and other solids, and interfaces between these tissues will reflect portions of the sound energy back to the transmitting transducer. These reflections are recorded as electrical signals and may be visualized by various display modes. The brightness modulation, or B-mode, displays echoes as bright dots plotted along the vertical and horizontal axes of an oscilloscope at positions corresponding to their point of origin in the area being scanned and in degrees of brightness that correspond to their amplitude. So-called "real-time" imaging, or sonofluoroscopy, produces repetitive scans that give the impression of a continuous image.

Sonography can usually allow delineation of the renal outlines and measurement of the longitudinal and transverse dimensions (Fig. 74–4). Difficulties may arise from overlying ribs that may obscure the upper poles or from similarities in the acoustic impedance of perirenal fat and renal cortex such that the renal margins are poorly defined. The structures within the renal parenchyma are sufficiently similar that few intrarenal echoes are produced except by the vascular and caliceal structures of the renal pelvis. Advanced gray-scale examination of the kidney may permit identification of the cortex, medulla, arcuate vessels, and renal pyramids. The ureters are not normally visualized unless distended.

B-mode ultrasonography has been combined with pulsed Doppler and color Doppler systems to form duplex imaging systems that also provide estimates of the velocity of blood flow in regions or vessels localized precisely by sonography. Doppler techniques depend on the observation that sound waves emanating or

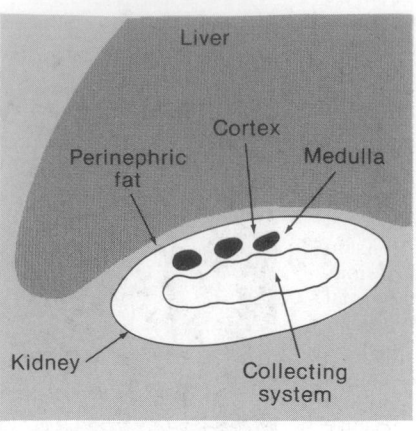

FIGURE 74–4. Ultrasonography *(left)* and schematic *(right)* of a normal right kidney. This was obtained anteriorly by transmission through the liver.

reflected from objects in motion shift their frequency ("Doppler shift") and that the intensity of the Doppler shift is directly proportional to the velocity of the objects in motion, which in the clinical context are red blood cells. Duplex ultrasonography is highly dependent on the skills of the operator but has emerging applications in suspected diseases of the major renal arteries or veins and in acute failure of the transplanted kidney.

The primary applications of ultrasonography to the evaluation of renal abnormalities include assessment of renal size, especially in the presence of severe renal failure, evaluation of mass lesions detected by excretory urography, examination of the perinephric area, and detection and grading of hydronephrosis. Renal ultrasonography may serve as the primary imaging procedure for patients with unexplained acute renal failure, for diabetics and other individuals at higher risk for adverse reactions to contrast material, in the presence of pregnancy, and to diagnose suspected polycystic kidney disease.

Evaluation of Renal Mass Lesions. Ultrasonography is used widely and effectively in the evaluation of renal mass lesions detected by excretory urography. Fluid-filled cysts as small as 1 to 2 cm in diameter may be detected, but reliable detection and evaluation of consistency generally require lesions greater than 2.5 to 3.0 cm. The primary application of ultrasonography is to describe the ultrasonographic characteristics of mass lesions ac-

cording to three patterns: cystic, solid, or complex. Cystic lesions are free of internal echoes, have smooth, sharply defined margins, and cause accentuation of echoes from their far wall. Solid lesions have less distinct margins because of attenuation of the signal by solid tissue and also demonstrate internal echoes related to vessels, connective tissue, or hemorrhage. Complex lesions represent features of both patterns. Because of the inherent limitations of the technique, ultrasonographically defined lesions should be described simply as having the *characteristics* of cysts or solids. Physically solid lesions that may appear on ultrasonography as cysts include melanomas, lymphomas, and certain metastases. Localized areas of hydronephrosis may also appear as cysts.

Renal ultrasonography is most nearly diagnostic in adult polycystic kidney disease and severe hydronephrosis. In other instances, ultrasonography should be regarded as informative rather than diagnostic. In the evaluation of renal mass lesions, combinations of ultrasonography, CT (Fig. 74–3), and arteriography may distinguish between benign cysts and potentially malignant solid tumors with remarkable accuracy. Clinical judgment will still be needed to decide whether even a 90 to 95 per cent level of accuracy is sufficient in an individual instance or whether surgery is indicated to obtain a definite diagnosis.

RADIONUCLIDE SCINTILLATION IMAGING. Radionuclide imaging has not achieved a major role in the evaluation of the kidneys and urinary tract. Two advantages of these techniques, however, make them useful in special circumstances. First, radionuclide imaging does not require the injection of radiocontrast material. Second, radionuclide studies are relatively simple and rapid and may be performed repeatedly at intervals of 24 to 48 hours. For these reasons, radionuclide imaging has perhaps its greatest application in the evaluation of patients at high risk for adverse reaction to radiocontrast material and in the evaluation of patients in the period immediately after renal transplantation. Otherwise, these techniques have few advantages over more direct radiologic and ultrasonographic methods.

With regard to the kidneys, radionuclide imaging techniques involve the intravenous injection of an agent labeled with a radionuclide that emits gamma radiation. Use of a scintillation camera allows the performance of dynamic studies that monitor the passage of a radiopharmaceutical agent through the vascular, renal parenchymal, and urinary tract compartments. Static studies examine the local accumulation of radionuclide activity. At present, radiopharmaceuticals of value in studies of the kidney contain either ^{131}I or ^{99m}Tc (technetium).

Static Imaging. Static imaging of the kidney consists of the administration of a radiopharmaceutical agent, usually ^{99m}Tc-glucoheptonate, that accumulates within the renal parenchyma and persists for several hours. Static imaging provides information on the location, size, and contour of functional renal tissue and may reveal areas of inhomogeneity or filling defects.

Dynamic Imaging. Dynamic scintillation imaging consists of the intravenous injection of a radiopharmaceutical agent and the visualization of its course through the vascular, renal parenchymal, and urinary collecting system by external monitoring of regional radioactivity with a scintillation camera. The time course of the appearance and disappearance of radioactivity is recorded

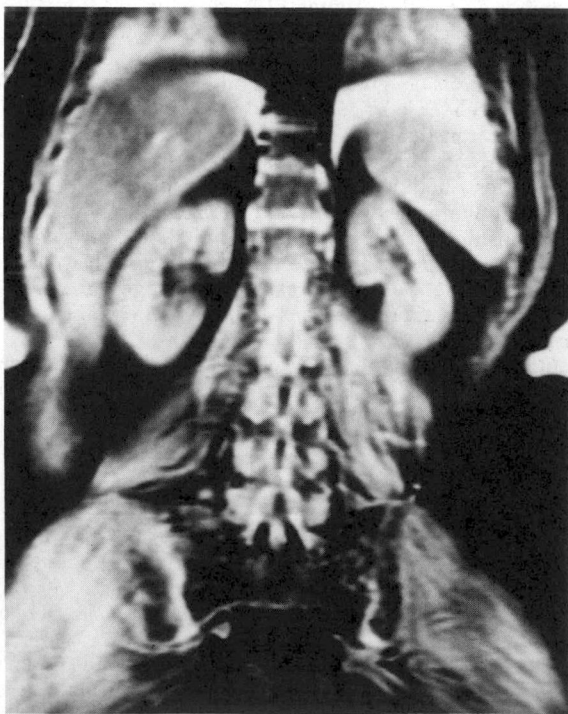

FIGURE 74–5. Magnetic resonance image (MRI) of two normal kidneys in an elderly woman.

in intervals as brief as 1 second. The radiopharmaceuticals used most frequently include ^{131}I-orthoiodohippurate, which is excreted by secretion with only a small component of filtration, and ^{99m}Tc-diethylenetriamine pentacetic acid (DTPA), which is excreted by filtration only.

The time-activity data observed for the passage of either radionuclide generally delineate three discrete phases. The vascular phase is the first 15 to 60 seconds after injection and consists of a rapid increase in radioactivity in the region viewed by the scintillation camera. The second phase occurs over the next 3 to 5 minutes and consists of slower accumulation of regional radioactivity. The third, or excretory, phase refers to the decrease in activity that occurs as the radionuclide is excreted from the region of interest. Unilateral or bilateral disturbances in renal blood flow, renal filtration, renal tubular function, or excretion cause disturbances in the various phases of this renogram. Although some efforts have been made to provide quantification of the various phases, interpretation of renograms still depends for the most part on the recognition of patterns in the scintillation displays. Dynamic imaging is especially useful for comparing excretory function between the right and left kidneys when renal dysfunction is asymmetric, such as may occur with congenital, vascular, or urologic disorders.

MAGNETIC RESONANCE IMAGING. Magnetic resonance imaging represents a new and emerging diagnostic technology that uses high magnetic fields and radiofrequencies to construct images. The method avoids the use of ionizing radiation or the administration of contrast material. Imaging depends instead on the water content and the chemical behavior of hydrogen compounds in the tissues themselves. Magnetic resonance imaging provides images in a tomographic format similar to CT (Fig. 74–5). The technique is very sensitive to blood flow and represents an excellent method for evaluating major vascular structures for patency or tumor involvement.

RENAL BIOPSY

Biopsy of the renal parenchyma by either the percutaneous or the open technique is useful (1) to define the morphologic expression of primary renal diseases, (2) to determine the type and extent of renal involvement by systemic diseases, and (3) to diagnose systemic diseases. The performance of renal biopsy is seldom necessary to *diagnose* systemic diseases. Systemic lupus erythematosus, diabetes mellitus, thrombotic thrombocytopenic purpura, multiple myeloma, Wegener's granulomatosis, and amyloidosis may on occasion display pathognomonic features on renal biopsy, but of these diseases only amyloidosis is likely to require renal biopsy for diagnosis. The others are diagnosed more readily by other means.

Renal biopsy is performed most frequently via the percutaneous technique. The indications for percutaneous biopsy are listed in Table 74–4; the contraindications are the presence of a single kidney, bleeding disorders, and uncontrolled hypertension. In experienced hands, percutaneous renal biopsy is a safe and effective technique that should provide sufficient tissue in more than 90 per cent of the attempts. Complications occur in 5 to 10 per cent of the attempts, and the most frequent complication is gross hematuria that usually resolves uneventfully in 24 to 48 hours. The formation of a perirenal hematoma may on occasion

TABLE 74–4. INDICATIONS FOR RENAL BIOPSY

Presumptive presence of glomerular disease
    Heavy proteinuria (>3 to 5 grams/24 hr)
    Nephrotic syndrome
    Acute nephritic syndrome
Proteinuria with hematuria
Renal involvement by systemic disease
    Connective tissue disease
    Vasculitis
    Amyloidosis
    Suspected Goodpasture's disease
Unexplained acute renal failure
Persistent acute renal failure (beyond 2 to 4 weeks)
Renal transplantation
    Acute rejection
    Chronic rejection
    Recurrence of original disease

require surgical evacuation. Microscopic hematuria occurs very frequently and is not generally considered a complication. Complications that occur less frequently include persistent bleeding, formation of arteriovenous fistula, aggravation of hypertension, and inadvertent biopsy of nonrenal tissue, such as muscle, liver, pancreas, spleen, or small bowel. Although fluoroscopy and ultrasonography may on occasion be useful or even necessary to localize the kidney for biopsy, it is not clear that these added maneuvers diminish the occurrence of complications or notably improve the rate of success. Complications of percutaneous renal biopsy occur more often in younger patients and in those with hypertension or small, diseased kidneys. Because hemorrhagic complications of percutaneous renal biopsy are the most common, the patient should be advised to refrain from strenuous exercises, especially lifting, and from contact sports for at least 2 weeks after biopsy.

The information obtained from a renal biopsy depends on the quality of tissue examination. Tissue should be examined by light microscopy, immunofluorescence microscopy, and, on occasion, electron microscopy. Accurate morphologic definition of possible primary renal disease or of the type and extent of renal involvement by systemic disease is often essential prior to making therapeutic decisions that might involve the use of life-threatening immunosuppressive therapy and to informing the physician and patient about the expected natural history of any renal abnormality. Moreover, for those renal disorders that may be treated ultimately by renal transplantation, knowledge of the nature of the original renal disease is important to predictions of whether that disease is likely to recur in the transplanted kidney.

Dennis V. W., Robinson R. R.: Clinical proteinuria. *In* Stollerman G. H., Harrington W. J., Lamont J. T., et al. (eds.): Advances in Internal Medicine. Chicago, Year Book Medical Publishers, 1986, pp 243–263. *This article provides more detail on the mechanisms and clinical classifications of proteinuria isolated from other renal abnormalities.*

Hertzberg B. S., Carroll B. A.: Ultrasonography of the vascular system. *In* Taveras J. M., Ferrucci J. T. (eds.): Radiology Diagnosis-Imaging-Intervention. Vol 2. Philadelphia, J. B. Lippincott Company, 1990, pp 1–19. *Readable background information on the theory and applications of Doppler imaging.*

Schwab S. J., Hlatky M. A., Pieper K. S., et al.: Contrast nephrotoxicity: A randomized controlled trial of a nonionic and an ionic radiographic contrast agent. N Engl J Med 320:149, 1989. *A recent and extensive study of some of the variables in radiocontrast injury in a general population undergoing angiographic study.*

Walser M.: Progression of chronic renal failure in man. Kidney Int 37:1195, 1990. *A scholarly examination of the methods and results of studies contending that chronic renal failure progresses inexorably and that selected interventions alter that course.*

75 Disorders of Fluid Volume, Electrolyte, and Acid-Base Balance

Thomas E. Andreoli

INTRODUCTION

Electrolyte abnormalities often occur as manifestations of underlying illnesses. In turn, fluid and electrolyte abnormalities, of themselves, produce systemic derangements. This chapter considers four major derangements of fluid and electrolyte balance, namely, volume disturbances, osmolality derangements, abnormalities of potassium balance, and acid-base disorders.

In health, the functional capacities of the mechanisms regulating water and electrolyte balance are so large that one can vary the intake of solutes and water over a wide range without developing perceptible metabolic disturbances. But the limits between which solute and water intake can be varied become narrower as the degree of functional impairment progresses. For example, salt intake in normal individuals can vary from approximately 10 mEq per day to several hundred milliequivalents per day without affecting volume homeostasis. In the presence of chronic renal disease, the minimal requirement rises and the maximal tolerance decreases, so that dietary salt intake must be kept within a much narrower range if volume depletion or volume overload is to be avoided.

75.1 VOLUME DISORDERS

PHYSIOLOGIC CONSIDERATIONS

Protection of extracellular fluid volume is the most fundamental characteristic of fluid and electrolyte homeostasis. It is helpful to use the term *effective circulating volume (ECV)*. The latter cannot be defined in an absolute sense, nor can it be measured explicitly. In operational terms, effective circulating volume may be viewed as adequate filling of the arterial tree, that is, an arterial flow rate sufficient to maintain adequate perfusion of body tissues. The mechanisms regulating volume balance respond primarily to changes in the ECV.

The Body Fluid Compartments

In healthy adults, body water comprises approximately 60 per cent of body weight and exists in two compartments: The intracellular compartment (ICF) contains two thirds of body water, or 40 per cent of body weight; the extracellular compartment (ECF) contains the remaining one third of total body water; and total blood volume, that is, plasma plus formed elements, constitutes one third of the total ECF volume. This "rule of thirds" for the body fluid compartments is useful in the assessment of most clinically encountered fluid and electrolyte disorders. Thus in a healthy 70-kg man, total body water comprises about 40 liters, of which 25 liters is intracellular. The functional extracellular fluid volume is 15 liters, 5 liters of which is blood; and since the normal hematocrit is 40 to 45 per cent, total plasma volume is approximately 2.75 to 3.0 liters.

More than 95 per cent of total body sodium is extracellular, and sodium and its associated anions, primarily chloride and bicarbonate, constitute the principal solutes of the ECF. Albumin and other macromolecules present in plasma are restricted to the vascular bed and constitute 5 per cent of plasma volume, so that plasma is about 95 per cent water. Since capillaries are freely permeable to water and small solutes, interstitial fluid is a protein-poor, but not entirely protein-free, ultrafiltrate of plasma.

Potassium is the principal cation of intracellular fluid, and nearly 98 per cent of total body potassium is intracellular. The principal anions of intracellular fluid vary among different cells. In muscle cells, they include phosphate, sulfate, and negatively charged macromolecules; and in red blood cells, they include the latter anions as well as chloride and bicarbonate.

Regulation of Fluid Transfer Among Compartments

The transfer of fluid between vascular and interstitial compartments occurs at the capillary level and is governed by the balance between hydrostatic pressure gradients and plasma oncotic pressure gradients. This relation may be stated by the familiar Starling equation:

$$J_v = K_f (\Delta P - \Delta \pi)$$

where J_v is rate of fluid transfer between vascular and interstitial compartments, K_f is the water permeability of the capillary bed, ΔP is the hydrostatic pressure difference between capillary and interstitium, and $\Delta \pi$ is the oncotic pressure difference between capillary and interstitial fluids. Under normal circumstances, interstitial tissue pressure is low and the ΔP term in the Starling equation represents the integrated hydrostatic pressure gradient from arteriolar to venular ends of a capillary. Since interstitial fluid is protein poor, the $\Delta \pi$ term in the Starling equation represents the oncotic pressure of plasma proteins, principally albumin; 5 grams of albumin per deciliter of plasma exerts an oncotic pressure of about 15 mm Hg.

Protection of Fluid Balance

As noted earlier, protection of the ECV is the single most fundamental characteristic of body fluid homeostasis. This pri-

TABLE 75–1. THE INTEGRATED VOLUME RESPONSE

	Systemic Hemodynamic Changes	External Salt and Water Balance
Response	Tachycardia ↑ Peripheral resistance ↓ Venous capacitance	Thirst Renal Na$^+$, water retention
Onset	Minutes	Hours
Major activators	Catecholamines ADH Angiotensin II Endothelin 1 Prostaglandin H$_2$ Thromboxane A$_2$	Catecholamines Aldosterone ADH
Major inactivators	Prostaglandin E$_2$ Atriopeptin Nitric acid	Prostaglandin E$_2$ Atriopeptin

ADH = antidiuretic hormone.

macy is underscored by the fact that, in circumstances in which multiple physiologic variables are threatened simultaneously, the homeostatic response invariably protects ECF volume even at the expense of aggravating another electrolyte disorder. For example, a volume-contracted patient who is replenished with water, and not sodium, will retain water and become hyponatremic in an attempt to avoid circulatory collapse. Likewise, the maintenance of metabolic alkalosis in a patient who has vomited and is not repleted with salt depends, in part, on an elevated renal absorptive capacity for sodium bicarbonate. The latter maintains fluid balance at the expense of pH homeostasis.

Two cardinal mechanisms protect extracellular fluid volume: alterations in systemic hemodynamic variables and alterations in external sodium and water balance. Both mechanisms maintain filling of the arterial tree and consequently are activated by external fluid losses; by inability to transfer fluid from the interstitium to the venous system, for example, in ascites; or by impaired fluid transfer from venous to arterial systems, for example, in congestive heart failure, pericardial tamponade, or constrictive pericarditis.

The combination of alterations in systemic hemodynamic variables and alterations in external water and solute balance can be termed the "integrated volume response" (Table 75–1). Increases in pulse rate and blood pressure are modulated not only by ADH, catecholamines, and angiotensin II but also by a series of factors derived from vascular endothelial cells. These factors include endothelin 1, a 21-residue peptide with potent vasoconstrictor properties, and thromboxane A$_2$ and prostaglandin H$_2$, both derived from the cyclo-oxygenase pathway in vascular endothelial cells. The major inactivators of these systemic hemodynamic changes include prostaglandin E$_2$ and atriopeptin, both of which are discussed below, and nitric oxide, an endogenous vasodilator released by vascular endothelial cells.

There are differences in the two response systems, indicated in Table 75–1. Tachycardia, peripheral arteriolar vasoconstriction, and peripheral venoconstriction occur within minutes of external fluid losses, whereas renal salt and water conservation lag behind by 12 to 24 hours. The sensitivities of the two limbs also differ. For example, a 2 to 3 per cent decrease in extracellular fluid volume, which amounts to the loss of 40 to 60 mEq of sodium, results in virtual elimination of sodium from the urine but produces negligible changes in systemic hemodynamic factors, such as heart rate, blood pressure, or systemic vascular resistance. Since there is 2500 to 3000 mEq of exchangeable sodium in the ECF, the system for conserving renal sodium is remarkably sensitive.

Renal Volume Regulation

Figure 75–1 provides a schematic summary of the renal factors regulating volume homeostasis. In general, the system is characterized by a positive limb, activated by volume contraction, and by negative feedback, activated by volume repletion. The separate details of this mechanism are as follows.

SENSING AND EFFECTOR ELEMENTS. Changes in effective ECF volume that exceed acceptable physiologic limits are sensed by baroreceptors located in both the high- and the low-pressure regions of the circulation. The low-pressure barorecep-

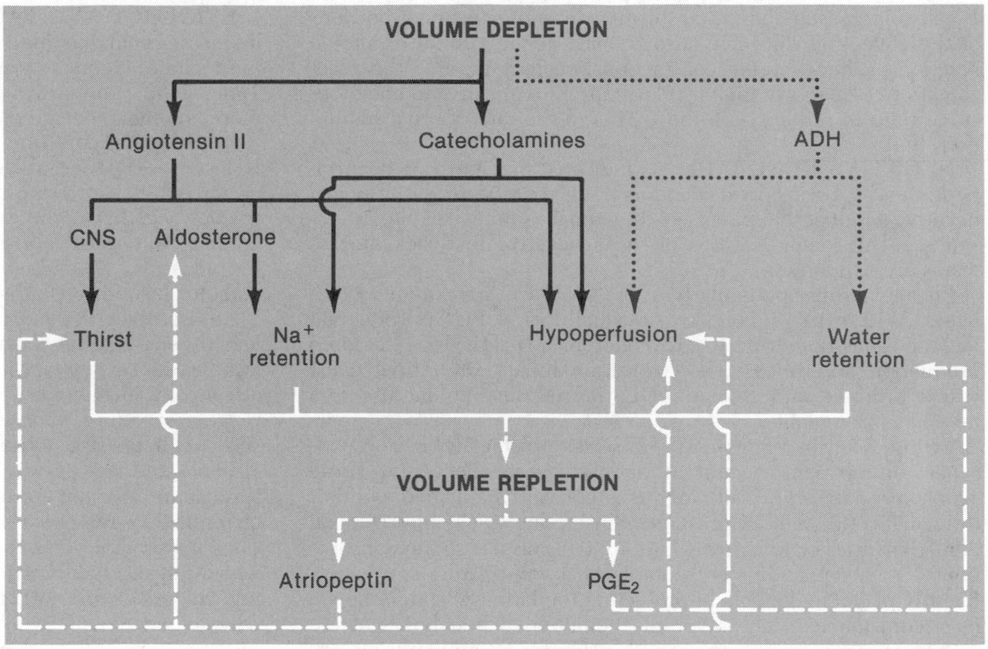

VOLUME DEPLETION

FIGURE 75–1. The volume repletion reaction. The solid and dotted lines originating from "volume depletion" indicate positive mechanisms activated when volume depletion is modest and severe, respectively. The dashed lines originating with "volume repletion" indicate negative feedback mechanisms.

tors are located primarily in the left atrium and in major thoracic veins, whereas the arterial high-pressure baroreceptors are located in the sinus body and aortic arch. Both sets of baroreceptors respond to pressure and stretch stimuli associated with changes in ECV. Activation of these extrarenal baroreceptors by relatively slight reductions in effective circulating volume results in increased sympathetic nerve activity and in rises in plasma catecholamine activity.

This catecholamine response raises blood pressure by increasing arteriolar resistance and heart rate, while simultaneously decreasing venous capacitance. Increases in arteriolar resistance also reduce capillary hydrostatic pressure and therefore promote fluid transfer from interstitial fluid to the vascular compartment. Within the kidney this increase in arteriolar resistance results in renal hypoperfusion. Moreover, adrenergic nerve terminals are in direct contact with proximal renal tubular epithelial cells, and direct stimulation of renal sympathetic nerves increases proximal tubular sodium absorption.

A second effector mechanism activated by stimulation of extrarenal baroreceptors is release of antidiuretic hormone (ADH). When blood volume is isotonically contracted by more than 8 to 10 per cent, afferent stimuli carried by the ninth and tenth cranial nerves result in nonosmotic ADH release by the neurohypophysis. In turn, ADH enhances renal water conservation and, because the hormone also has potent vasoconstrictor activity, reduces renal perfusion.

In addition to these extrarenal baroreceptors, the renal juxtaglomerular apparatus serves as an intrarenal baroreceptor system. Sympathetic nerve stimulation, reductions in afferent arteriolar blood pressure, or reductions in the rates of distal tubular sodium delivery enhance renin release by the juxtaglomerular apparatus. Renal renin release into plasma accelerates the formation of angiotensin II according to the following general scheme:

Renin Substrate
↓ renin
Angiotensin I
↓ pulmonary converting enzyme
Angiotensin II
↓ circulating angiotensinase
Angiotensin III

The octapeptide angiotensin II has three major effects on volume conservation: (1) It is a potent pressor agent; on a molar basis, angiotensin II is a more potent vasoconstrictor than norepinephrine. (2) Angiotensin II is the major stimulus to aldosterone secretion and consequently is a key factor modulating renal sodium conservation. (3) The angiotensin II formed in the central

nervous system is a potent stimulus to thirst. The heptapeptide angiotensin III is also a potent vasoconstrictor but is not as potent a stimulator of aldosterone secretion as is angiotensin II; angiotensin III also stimulates thirst.

Finally, as indicated in Table 75–1, factors produced and released by vascular endothelial cells also play a major role in modulating systemic hemodynamics. The vasoconstricting factors include the potent vasoconstrictor peptide endothelin 1. Moreover, endothelin 1 is also released from the posterior pituitary and may play a role in modulating ADH release. The vasoconstrictor agents derived from the cyclo-oxygenase pathway in vascular endothelial cells include thromboxane A_2 and prostaglandin H_2. Nitric oxide produced by vascular endothelial cells is the major endogenous nitrovasodilator.

RENAL ELEMENTS. The kidneys respond to slight reductions in ECV by increasing the rate of proximal tubular sodium absorption without disturbing either the glomerular filtration rate (GFR) or osmoregulatory mechanisms. In normal circumstances, approximately 70 per cent of filtered sodium is absorbed by the proximal nephron. As long as euvolemia persists, the fractional rate of proximal sodium absorption remains constant when the GRF is varied; this constant relation is referred to as *glomerulotubular balance.*

A number of factors modulate glomerulotubular balance in association with changes in ECV. In empiric terms, this modulation includes a downsetting of glomerulotubular balance in volume-expanded states and an increase in the rate of fractional proximal sodium absorption when filling of the arterial tree is impaired. Among these factors, the hemodynamic regulation of oncotic pressure in peritubular capillaries seems to have a dominant role. At relatively low concentrations, angiotensin II has a vasoconstricting effect on efferent, but not afferent, glomerular arterioles. Therefore this agent, by increasing the glomerular filtration fraction, can increase peritubular capillary oncotic pressure and thereby enhance proximal tubular rates of sodium absorption. At high concentrations, angiotensin II, like norepinephrine, produces afferent glomerular arteriolar constriction, which results in reductions in GFR and in renal ischemia.

The kidney responds to modest sodium depletion by increasing the rate of tubular sodium absorption without altering the GFR. Glomerulotubular balance is reset upward, so that a greater fraction of glomerular filtrate is absorbed in the proximal nephron; both direct stimulation of renal nerves and the effect of angiotensin II on efferent glomerular arterioles contribute in part to this resetting of glomerulotubular balance. Angiotensin II also provides a second mechanism for renal sodium conservation by increasing the rate of aldosterone secretion, which enhances sodium absorption in the terminal regions of the distal tubule.

Finally, increased sodium absorption by more terminal portions of the collecting duct may also be part of the volume repletion reaction. When volume contraction becomes severe, the vasoconstrictive effects of high levels of norepinephrine and angiotensin II tend to reduce both the GFR and the rate of renal sodium excretion.

NEGATIVE FEEDBACK. As indicated in Figure 75–1, atriopeptin and E series prostaglandins (PGE) constitute the principal negative feedback elements of the renal volume regulatory response. The major features of these negative feedback mechanisms are as follows.

Prostaglandins, particularly of the E series, are potent vasodilators. Within the kidney, two cardinal loci of PGE_2 production include renal glomeruli, where angiotensin II activates eicosanoid production and release, and renal medullary interstitial cells, which produce and release PGE_2 in response to increases in medullary osmolality.

As indicated in Figure 75–1, E series prostaglandins suppress renal volume conservation by at least three effects: (1) These agents are natriuretic, although it is not yet established whether the natriuretic effect of prostaglandins is due to changes in renal hemodynamics or to a direct inhibition of tubular sodium absorption. (2) Prostaglandins are potent renal vasodilators and consequently play a major role in protecting the kidneys from ischemia in circumstances such as volume depletion, when levels of the vasoconstrictor agents angiotensin II and norepinephrine are increased. (3) PGE_2 is a direct antagonist of the renal tubular effects of ADH and thus impairs renal water conservation.

An important therapeutic principle follows from a consideration of the renal vasodilatory effects of prostaglandins. Specifically, the use of aspirin and other nonsteroidal anti-inflammatory agents should be avoided in circumstances characterized by a high degree of sodium avidity, that is, by a reduction in ECV. These agents inhibit prostaglandin synthesis and thus reduce the rate of prostaglandin production. Consequently, in sodium-avid states, the use of aspirin or other nonsteroidal anti-inflammatory agents increases the rate of development of renal ischemia and hence azotemia.

Atriopeptin, or atrial natriuretic peptide, is the second negative feedback element in the renal volume regulatory response. This hormone is released from cardiac atrial storage granules in response to atrial distention; immunoreactive atriopeptin has also been identified within the central nervous system. Atriopeptin is discussed in detail in Ch. 211. In the present context, three actions of atriopeptin have particular pertinence: (1) Centrally released atriopeptin suppresses pituitary ADH release and angiotensin II–mediated thirst. (2) Atriopeptin of cardiac origin inhibits aldosterone secretion and hence renal Na^+ conservation; atriopeptin may also block terminal nephron Na^+ absorption directly. (3) Atriopeptin is a potent vasodilator that increases renal blood flow strikingly. The last-named effect also accounts in part for the natriuretic effects of this peptide.

SUMMARY. When considered in an overall context, two features of the volume repletion reaction illustrated in Figure 75–1 are noteworthy. First, redundant mechanisms protect ECV. Thus, angiotensin II release, catecholamine release, and ADH release all produce overlapping results.

Second, the magnitude of the volume repletion reaction varies, depending on the degree of volume contraction. In modestly volume-contracted states, peripheral vasoconstriction and renal sodium conservation occur, but renal blood flow, GFR, and osmoregulation are unaffected. When volume contraction becomes advanced, nonosmotic ADH release, angiotensin II–mediated thirst, and reductions in the rate of salt delivery to the loop of Henle act in concert to produce hyponatremia. Finally, when catecholamine release and angiotensin II release become sufficiently great that renal blood flow is compromised beyond autoregulatory limits, prerenal azotemia ensues.

VOLUME DEPLETION

DEFINITION. A true hypovolemic state is one in which there is a reduction in total body water, functional ECF volume, and ICF volume; it occurs when the rate of salt and water intake is less than the combined rates of renal plus extrarenal volume losses. In chronic volume-contracted states, input and output may be equal.

ETIOLOGY AND PATHOGENESIS. Three major groups of diseases, occurring individually or in combination, account for most clinically encountered states of true volume contraction. Table 75–2 summarizes these three sets of disorders and the more common specific diseases in each group.

Hormone Deficit. Volume contraction can occur whenever there is loss of ADH or aldosterone. Untreated *diabetes insipidus*, either pituitary or nephrogenic, produces profound volume contraction and hypertonic encephalopathy in patients denied free access to water. The obligatory loss of solute-free water in diabetes insipidus may be as high as 10 to 18 liters daily. Both forms of diabetes insipidus are discussed in Ch. 214.

Addison's disease may impair aldosterone production and hence lead to renal sodium wasting. A second major cause of aldosterone lack occurs in *hyporeninemic hypoaldosteronism*, which may accompany interstitial renal disease. Disorders that damage the renal interstitium, such as hypertension, diabetes mellitus, gout, sickle cell disease, chronic ingestion of lead-containing illicit alcohol, and analgesic abuse, can suppress the ability of the juxtaglomerular apparatus to produce renin. In turn, the low rate of renin secretion results in low rates of aldosterone secretion. Thus hyporeninemic hypoaldosteronism represents a disorder in which impaired aldosterone production results in renal salt wasting, hyperkalemia, and metabolic acidosis. It is not yet known why hyperkalemia, which is a potent stimulus to aldosterone secretion, fails to enhance rates of aldosterone secretion in patients with hyporeninemic hypoaldosteronism.

Renal Deficits. A number of disorders impairing renal tubular sodium or water conservation can lead to volume contraction. For convenience, these derangements may be grouped into three classes.

First, various tubular nephropathies are characterized by specific deficits in salt or water absorption. As mentioned above, nephrogenic diabetes insipidus and interstitial renal disease may produce water and sodium wasting, respectively. Because interstitial renal disease often results in hyperchloremic, hyperkalemic metabolic acidosis, the term "renal tubular acidosis, type IV" is often applied to this disorder. However, the general term "renal tubular acidosis" also includes other sodium-wasting disorders accompanied by hyperchloremic acidosis, such as proximal tubular acidosis, a specific proximal defect in bicarbonate reabsorption, and gradient-limited distal renal tubular acidosis, a specific defect in distal tubular sodium bicarbonate regeneration (Ch. 82).

Alternatively, Bartter's syndrome is a specific tubular nephropathy that results in failure of sodium chloride absorption by distal regions of the nephron; the disorder is accompanied by excessive production of prostaglandins by the renal medullary interstitium and is characterized by sodium chloride wasting, juxtaglomerular hyperplasia, high renin levels, and secondary hyperaldosteronism; the last-named results in hypokalemic metabolic alkalosis.

TABLE 75–2. MAJOR CAUSES OF VOLUME DEPLETION

Renal Losses	Extrarenal Losses
Hormonal Deficit	**Hemorrhage**
Pituitary diabetes insipidus	**Cutaneous Losses**
Aldosterone insufficiency	Sweating
Addison's disease	Burns
Hyporeninemic hypoaldosteronism	
Interstitial nephritis	
Renal Deficits	**Gastrointestinal Losses**
Specific tubular nephropathies:	Vomiting
Renal tubular acidosis	Diarrheal disorders
Proximal	Gastrointestinal fistulas
Distal, gradient-limited	Tube drainage
Bartter's syndrome	
Nephrogenic diabetes insipidus	
Diuretic abuse	
Postobstructive diuresis	
Excessive filtration of	
nonelectrolytes:	
Osmotic diuresis	
Generalized renal disease:	
Chronic renal failure	

Inhibition of tubular sodium absorptive processes due to *chronic diuretic abuse* may also lead to salt wasting, volume contraction, and specific metabolic acid-base abnormalities. These abnormalities are discussed below in connection with Table 75–5 (see below). Diuretics such as furosemide and thiazides produce serum electrolyte changes indistinguishable from those of Bartter's syndrome.

Profound but reversible defects in tubular salt and water absorption may occur during *postobstructive diuresis*, that is, shortly after relief of partial or complete urinary tract obstruction. Salt and water losses may also occur in the *diuretic phase* of acute tubular necrosis. However, profound salt and water losses associated with the diuretic phase of acute tubular necrosis are seen uncommonly if extracellular fluid volume is carefully controlled during oliguric acute tubular necrosis.

Third, glomerular filtration of large amounts of nonelectrolytes may produce volume deficits by overwhelming renal tubular reabsorptive capacity for salt and water; in this instance, water losses predominate, so that hypernatremia generally occurs. This phenomenon, termed *osmotic diuresis* or *solute diuresis*, occurs in diabetic ketoacidosis, hyperglycemic hyperosmolar coma, or hyperalimentation with large glucose loads in chronically debilitated patients; in patients with burns, in whom there are abnormally high rates of urea production; and during mannitol or glycerol administration to patients with central nervous system disorders requiring reductions of intracranial pressure.

Finally, in *chronic renal failure* of any cause, there is an obligatory loss of sodium. The extent of obligatory sodium loss in chronic renal failure is most pronounced in cystic renal diseases, notably medullary cystic disease and polycystic kidney disease (Ch. 89).

Extrarenal Losses. In addition to hemorrhage, two other classes of extrarenal losses account for volume contraction. Simple dehydration may result from increased insensible water loss in *excessive sweating* due to high ambient temperatures or to fever. Because sweat usually contains less than 50 mEq per liter of sodium, the ICF and the ECF share the water loss, and body water osmolality rises while ECF volume loss is modest. *Burns* allow the loss of large amounts of plasma and interstitial fluid through affected areas and therefore can lead rapidly to profound ECF losses.

Finally, gastrointestinal volume losses occur when portions of the 8 to 10 liters of normal gastrointestinal secretions are lost, particularly in secretory diarrheas. Volume depletion is most commonly the consequence of vomiting, gastric drainage, or diarrhea but may occur with any type of bowel fistula. Loss of hydrochloric acid from the stomach may produce metabolic alkalosis, whereas loss of sodium bicarbonate from pancreatic secretions lost through the lower gastrointestinal tract, as in diarrhea, may produce metabolic acidosis.

CLINICAL MANIFESTATIONS. The clinical findings in states of true volume contraction are due both to underfilling of the arterial tree and to the renal and hemodynamic responses to this underfilling. In mild or partially compensated volume contraction, particularly when the latter has occurred gradually, the patient may exhibit nothing more than mild postural giddiness, postural tachycardia, and weakness. In more advanced stages of volume depletion, particularly those occurring acutely, there may be hypotension when the patient is recumbent, tachycardia, and a reduced urine volume. Finally, when volume contraction is severe, the combination of profound fluid loss and increased sympathetic activity produces circulatory collapse characterized by oliguria, a nondetectable blood pressure (except by Doppler studies), tachycardia when the patient is recumbent, and cold extremities. In short, the clinical manifestations of mild to severe volume contraction may range from minimal symptoms to life-threatening circulatory collapse.

The lack of physical findings does not exclude the presence of mild to moderate volume contraction in a given patient. In the postoperative period, 7 to 10 per cent blood volume losses in patients are often accompanied by normal vital signs and by only slight decreases in the central venous pressure or the pulmonary capillary wedge pressure.

Skin turgor and the moistness of mucous membranes are valuable indices to the volume of body water in infants but are unreliable in adults. In young adults, reductions in skin turgor do not occur unless profound volume contraction is present, and

normal loss of skin elasticity makes skin turgor difficult to assess in older patients. Similarly, mouth breathing and other factors affect the oral mucosa independently of external volume balances.

The signs and symptoms of volume contraction, regardless of cause, are referable to a reduction in ECV. Consequently, the clinical findings in volume contraction depend primarily on the interplay among four major factors: the magnitude of the volume loss; the rate of volume loss; the nature of the fluid loss, that is, whether the fluid loss is primarily water, a combined sodium plus water loss, or a blood loss; and finally, the responsiveness of the vasculature to volume reduction. Some simple considerations illustrate these relations.

The clinical manifestations of volume contraction are obviously related intimately to the volume and rate of fluid loss. For example, an acute gastrointestinal hemorrhage of 1 liter of blood can easily result in oliguria, coupled with the signs and symptoms of circulatory collapse, while the hematocrit remains constant. In other words, the hemorrhage is sufficiently acute that fluid flux from the interstitial to the vascular bed makes a negligible contribution to expanding the vascular bed. However, the same amount of gastrointestinal blood loss occurring more slowly—for example, over a 1-day period—permits a partial transfer of fluid from the interstitium to the vascular bed and consequently produces a fall in hematocrit; but since the ECV is at least partially restored by this fluid shift, the volume of urine flow and the hemodynamic response to volume contraction may be minimally affected.

Second, the kind of fluid loss significantly affects the clinical findings in volume contraction. Consider, for example, a 1-liter loss of different kinds of body fluids in a 70-kg man having a total body water of 40 liters and a hematocrit of 45 per cent. The acute loss of 1 liter of predominantly solute-free water, as in diabetes insipidus, produces a 2.5 per cent reduction in blood volume; urine flow and systemic hemodynamics are minimally affected. The acute loss of 1 liter of predominantly extracellular fluid produces a 6.6 per cent reduction in blood volume, since sodium is confined to the ECF; in this circumstance, modest oliguria and tachycardia while the patient is recumbent ensue. Last, the acute loss of 1 liter of blood by hemorrhage reduces blood volume by 20 per cent, thus resulting in profound oliguria and near circulatory collapse.

Finally, peripheral vasoconstriction and tachycardia represent important physiologic responses to volume losses. Consequently, the signs and symptoms of volume contraction, even of modest degree, are amplified appreciably in patients with diminished myocardial reserve or reduced sympathetic nervous system function. The former occurs commonly in cardiomyopathies of any cause or in pericardial tamponade or pericardial constriction. The latter occurs commonly in patients subjected to prolonged bed rest, in diabetic patients with autonomic neuropathy, and as a consequence of therapy with certain antihypertensive drugs.

DIAGNOSIS. The pulse, blood pressure, and changes of these variables with position, together with a clinical estimate of the venous pressure and skin temperature, provide an initial assessment of circulatory dynamics. Because these findings may be inconclusive in moderate degrees of volume contraction, a fluid challenge is useful in the evaluation of critically ill patients in whom a volume deficit is thought to be a contributory factor to a reduced cardiac output. A convenient way of achieving this goal is to administer 500 ml of normal saline over 1 to 3 hours.

In patients with a normal cardiac reserve, the effect of a fluid challenge may be monitored safely by evaluating the pulse, blood pressure, and urine flow. In patients with impaired cardiac function, the use of a flow-directed Swan-Ganz catheter for measurement of the pulmonary capillary wedge pressure or cardiac output, as estimated by thermal dilution, provides more precise indicators to early volume overload secondary to a fluid challenge. Because volume contraction is associated with vasoconstriction, both in the venous and the arterial circuits, transient changes in the pulmonary capillary wedge pressure may not accurately reflect the volume status of the patient. During volume expansion, the wedge pressure rises and subsequently falls. The initial pressure elevation is due to fluid infusion into a vasoconstricted, low-capacity vascular bed and should not be misinterpreted to indicate adequacy of volume repletion. The subsequent reduction in wedge pressure coincides with decreases in arterial resistance coupled to increases in venous capacitance. Finally, central venous pressure measurements provide unreliable estimates of pulmonary vascular volume.

The cardinal laboratory findings associated with volume contraction follow directly from the volume repletion mechanism summarized in Figure 75–1. The kidney initially responds to a decrease in effective circulating blood volume by reducing urine volume and sodium excretion. Severe degrees of volume contraction also reduce filtration rate and result in prerenal azotemia.

The urinary sodium concentration and the fraction of filtered sodium excreted in the urine, denoted as Fe_{Na}, are clinically useful indices of renal sodium avidity. The Fe_{Na} is calculated as the urine to plasma sodium concentration ratio divided by the urine to plasma creatinine concentration ratio. In the volume-contracted state, the urinary sodium concentration is generally less than 10 mEq per liter and the Fe_{Na} is less than 1 per cent, whereas in acute tubular necrosis, the urinary sodium concentration is greater than 40 mEq per liter and the Fe_{Na} is greater than 1 per cent. These indices are useful in the differential diagnosis between acute oliguric tubular necrosis and volume contraction associated with prerenal azotemia, with certain notable exceptions.

The urinary sodium indices are not reliable determinants of volume contraction when there is obligatory renal sodium wasting, as in interstitial nephritis. When volume contraction is due to the renal losses listed in Table 75–2 (except for diabetes insipidus), the urinary sodium concentration and the Fe_{Na} may both be elevated even when volume losses are large enough to produce azotemia. The urinary sodium excretion may also be elevated in volume contraction due to upper gastrointestinal losses associated with vomiting or gastric drainage. This occurs during early metabolic alkalosis if the filtered load of bicarbonate exceeds the renal tubular reabsorptive capacity for bicarbonate. During this interval, the urinary chloride concentration is a more reliable index of renal salt avidity. Finally, antecedent diuretic therapy may invalidate Fe_{Na} measurements.

TREATMENT. The major goal of the treatment of volume contraction is to expand the ECV by replacing fluid deficits. The type of fluid, the route and rate of fluid administration, and the total amount of fluid to be given will vary with the particular circumstance. For example, a mild, nonpersisting upper gastrointestinal hemorrhage may be treated appropriately by infusion of normal saline, whereas a major, persisting upper gastrointestinal hemorrhage will generally require replacement with whole blood.

The degree to which a given volume of crystalloid solution expands the ECV depends on solution composition. If glucose metabolism is normal, the infusion of 5 per cent dextrose in water (D_5W) is equivalent to administering solute-free water, which distributes uniformly in total body water. Since less than 10 per cent of total body water is in the intravascular compartment, infusion of 1 liter of D_5W expands the intravascular volume by 75 to 100 ml, that is, by about 2 per cent.

Sodium-free solutions, such as D_5W, are used principally in hypertonic volume-contracted states, such as diabetes insipidus or excessive sweating. If large volumes of glucose-containing solutions are given rapidly, the urine must be monitored for glycosuria, since the osmotic diuresis produced by the latter will cause urinary losses of both sodium and water.

Solutions containing sodium as the principal solute preferentially expand the extracellular fluid volume. Infusion of 1 liter of a normal saline solution increases blood volume by about 300 ml, or about 6 per cent; the remaining portion is distributed in the interstitial compartment. Hypotonic sodium-containing salt solutions expand intravascular volume in a manner intermediate between that of D_5W and normal saline. Sodium-containing crystalloid solutions are indicated primarily in volume-contracted states secondary to renal or gastrointestinal sodium losses (Table 75–2). They are also useful adjuncts to therapy in burns and in hemorrhage.

Colloid-containing solutions, such as iso-oncotic albumin solutions and plasma, preferentially expand the intravascular compartment, since large molecules like albumin are mainly restricted to the intravascular space. This kind of fluid replacement is most helpful in burns, in which cutaneous protein losses are appreciable, and in circulatory collapse, in which rapid intravascular expansion is critical. In most other instances of volume contraction, the use of colloid-containing solutions is difficult to justify, since the half-life of infused albumin in ill patients is relatively short, only 4 to 6 hours, and the cost of colloid solutions such as iso-oncotic albumin is more than 50 times greater than that of an equal volume of crystalloid solution.

Finally, blood, which contains formed elements, is the most potent expander of the intravascular space. A unit of packed red blood cells will remain entirely in the vascular bed. In most hemorrhagic situations, the combination of packed red blood cells with either normal saline solutions or colloid solutions is adequate for volume replacement. There are few circumstances in modern practice, with the possible exception of massive hemorrhagic shock, in which whole-blood therapy for volume expansion is utilized.

CIRCULATORY COMPROMISE WITHOUT TRUE VOLUME CONTRACTION

DEFINITION. In the previous section, we considered those disorders characterized by inadequate filling of the arterial tree that occur because of fluid losses between the patient and the external environment. Clearly, the cardinal signs and symptoms of these disorders are referable to responses accompanying the integrated volume repletion reaction (Fig. 75–1). There are also disorders in which inadequate arterial filling occurs in the absence of external fluid losses. The signs and symptoms of these disorders mimic closely those that characterize true volume contraction.

ETIOLOGY AND PATHOGENESIS. Table 75–3 lists three commonly encountered classes of derangements that may manifest clinically with tachycardia, acute hypotension, oliguria, azotemia, and a reduced Fe_{Na}. These disorders can be termed "non–volume-contracted circulatory compromise," with the understanding that the term "non–volume-contracted" refers to the absence of body fluid losses between the patient and the external world.

Impaired Cardiac Output. A profound collapse of cardiac output, due to acute myocardial infarction with pump failure (cardiogenic shock) or to acute pericardial tamponade, may clearly result in circulatory collapse. In this instance, failure to fill the arterial tree and to maintain an ECV occurs because the heart fails to translocate blood adequately from venous to arterial beds.

Increased Vascular Capacitance. Circulatory collapse with its attendant signs and symptoms occurs when there is a sudden increase in the capacitance of the vascular bed, most notably in the venous part of the circulation. This kind of increase in ratio of vascular capacitance to vascular volume occurs most commonly in sepsis but may also be seen in circumstances in which peripheral vasodilators, particularly those having a postarteriolar locus of action, are administered injudiciously.

Vascular-Interstitial Fluid Shifts. Profound hypotension, tachycardia, progressive oliguria, and azotemia are also encountered when there is a rapid translocation of fluid from vascular to interstitial compartments, presumably because of a sudden, profound increase in the permeability characteristics of peripheral capillaries. Some common derangements of this type include infarction of the small or large intestine, extensive tissue trauma, acute pancreatitis, and rhabdomyolysis. An analogous mechanism—namely, a marked increase in the permeability of pulmonary capillaries—is also presumed to account for the formation of noncardiogenic pulmonary edema in the adult respiratory distress syndrome.

DIAGNOSIS AND THERAPY. The diagnosis and therapy of

TABLE 75–3. CIRCULATORY COMPROMISE WITHOUT EXTERNAL FLUID LOSSES

I. **Impaired Cardiac Output**
  Acute myocardial infarction
  Pericardial tamponade
II. **Increased Vascular Capacitance**
  Septic shock
III. **Vascular → Interstitial Fluid Shifts**
  Acute pancreatitis
  Bowel infarction
  Rhabdomyolysis
  Noncardiogenic pulmonary edema

acute myocardial infarction with circulatory collapse and of acute pericardial tamponade are considered in detail in Part VI of this book. It is, however, worth citing certain factors particularly germane to the management of fluid therapy in such patients. In individuals affected either by right ventricular infarction or by pericardial tamponade, maintenance of adequate filling of the systemic arterial tree depends critically on providing a relatively high venous preload to the right side of the heart. Attempts at volume contraction in patients with right ventricular infarcts or pericardial tamponade may exacerbate systemic hypotension. Thus treatment of these disorders generally requires concomitant hemodynamic monitoring with a flow-directed Swan-Ganz catheter to avoid excessive preload to the left side of the heart.

In patients with left ventricular infarction and systemic hypotension, particular attention should be directed to excluding the possibility that antecedent true volume depletion—for example, with prolonged diuretic therapy and salt restriction prior to the myocardial infarction—may be a significant contributor to what otherwise might be mistaken for true cardiogenic shock. The findings of acute left ventricular infarction, systemic arterial hypotension, the absence of pulmonary edema on the chest radiograph, a reduced pulmonary capillary wedge pressure, and an antecedent history of prolonged diuretic therapy, when taken together, indicate that improved systemic hemodynamics may be achieved by cautious attempts at volume expansion carried out in combination with serial measurements of the cardiac output and the pulmonary capillary wedge pressure.

The distinction between hypotension due to true volume contraction and that due to an increase in the capacitance-volume ratio of the vascular bed, as occurs in sepsis, is often difficult. This distinction is particularly difficult in individuals who have been in intensive care units for prolonged periods of time and in those at high risk for developing sepsis, such as cancer patients treated with potent chemotherapeutic agents. A useful clue to the presence of septic circulatory collapse is the occurrence of warm extremities coupled with hypotension and oliguria, since true hypovolemia, particularly when advanced, is ordinarily accompanied by profound peripheral vasoconstriction and hence cool and often cyanotic extremities.

True hypovolemia and sepsis may also coexist. In such a circumstance, invasive hemodynamic monitoring may be helpful. Both in true hypovolemia and in sepsis, the pulmonary capillary wedge pressure is reduced; but in septic circulatory collapse, the calculated systemic vascular resistance falls, because of peripheral vasodilation, whereas in true hypovolemia, peripheral vasoconstriction ordinarily raises the systemic vascular resistance. The diagnosis of disorders producing rapid transfer of fluids from the vascular bed to the interstitium, such as trauma, acute pancreatitis, or rhabdomyolysis, is generally evident from clinical appraisal.

The treatment of patients with sepsis and an increased vascular capacitance-volume ratio, as well as those individuals with rapid vascular to interstitial fluid shifts, has as a mainstay the administration of sufficient sodium-containing fluids, generally isotonic saline, to permit adequate filling of the arterial tree. This therapy necessarily expands total body water, particularly in the vascular and interstitial compartments. Consequently, during recovery from the underlying disorder, care must be taken to avoid unnecessary expansion of the vascular bed and consequently the risk of volume-mediated cardiac decompensation.

VOLUME EXCESS

DEFINITION. Volume-expanded states are characterized by an increase in total body water, which is accompanied, in most but not all circumstances, by an increase in total body sodium. Total body salt and water may be increased while the ECV is decreased. In other words, certain volume-expanded states are characterized by dissociation between total body salt and water and the ECV.

ETIOLOGY AND PATHOGENESIS. Volume expansion occurs whenever the rate of salt or water intake exceeds the rate of renal plus extrarenal losses; in chronic volume expansion, the external salt and water balance may be normal. A convenient way of considering volume-expanded states is to view them in the context of three different classes of physiologic explanations (Table 75–4).

TABLE 75–4. DISORDERS OF VOLUME EXCESS

I. Disturbed Starling Forces (Reduced effective circulating volume; edema formation) Systemic venous pressure increases: Right heart failure Constrictive pericarditis Local venous pressure increases: Left heart failure Vena cava obstruction Portal vein obstruction Reduced oncotic pressure: Nephrotic syndrome Combined disorders: Cirrhosis	**II. Primary Hormone Excess** (Increased effective circulating volume) Primary aldosteronism Cushing's syndrome SIADH **III. Primary Renal Sodium Retention** (Increased effective circulating volume) Acute glomerulonephritis

SIADH = syndrome of inappropriate antidiuretic hormone production.

Disturbances in Starling Forces. The most common diseases encountered in which both volume expansion and edema occur are those in which derangements in the Starling forces regulating fluid transfer between capillaries and interstitium tend to promote expansion of the interstitial compartment at the expense of the ECV. Consequently, renal sodium retention and edema occur. By definition, this group of disorders is characterized by increases in capillary hydrostatic pressure, by decreases in capillary oncotic pressure, or by a combination of these two factors.

Four groups include most edematous states characterized by abnormal Starling forces (Table 75–4). First, the systemic venous pressure may be increased because of primary cardiac disorders, such as right-sided heart failure or constrictive pericarditis. Second, local elevations in pulmonary or systemic venous pressure may occur, as in left-sided heart failure, vena caval obstruction, or portal vein obstruction. Third, a reduction in plasma oncotic pressure, and consequently a net increase in the tendency for fluid to transude from capillaries to interstitium, accounts plausibly for edema formation in the nephrotic syndrome. Finally, a combination of these factors may be responsible for edema formation. For example, both hypoalbuminemia and portal hypertension are major contributory factors to the development of ascites in hepatic cirrhosis.

Plasma renin activity and aldosterone concentrations in these disorders tend to be elevated, although the results also tend to be variable. In advanced cases of disorders characterized by increases in local or systemic venous pressure, most notably in severe congestive heart failure and in cirrhosis, hyponatremia may occur; this finding represents an ominous prognostic sign. Finally, edema formation due to such derangements of Starling forces may result in the "third space" phenomenon, namely, the sequestration of large volumes of interstitial fluid in regions such as the pleural or peritoneal cavities.

Primary Hormonal Excess. These disorders include those disturbances in which there is unregulated production of mineralocorticoids or ADH. The volume expansion that occurs in states of mineralocorticoid excess, such as primary hyperaldosteronism, is due to sodium retention and is accompanied by a primary, preferential expansion of the ECF and consequently by hypertension. The serum sodium level is generally normal. In the syndrome of inappropriate ADH production (SIADH), primary water retention occurs. Consequently, the volume expansion involves both the ICF and ECF; dilutional hyponatremia is the hallmark of SIADH, whereas hypertension is uncommon. Edema is not characteristic in either of these two disorders. Instead, patients with primary aldosteronism or SIADH reach a volume-expanded steady state in which output equals input.

Primary Renal Sodium Retention. The kidneys may also retain sodium abnormally when the ECV is normal and there is no effector excess. For example, in acute glomerulonephritis unidentified renal mechanisms are primarily responsible for edema formation. Patients with acute glomerulonephritis retain salt and water and become hypertensive without reductions in the GFR or in ECV. Furthermore, sodium retention and edema develop when plasma renin activity and aldosterone concentration are normal or reduced and when the serum albumin concentration is normal. Thus, the renal tubule may be abnormally avid for sodium in acute glomerulonephritis. Congestive heart failure may occur as a secondary consequence of the volume expansion.

DIAGNOSIS AND TREATMENT. The recognition and management of volume-expanded states depend on proper identification and treatment of the underlying disorder. Clearly, the cornerstones of therapy in volume-expanded states characterized by sodium excess include salt restriction and diuretics. Table 75–5 provides a summary of some of the major diuretics used commonly and certain of their properties. For convenience, these drugs have been classified according to their sites of action in the nephron.

Proximal Diuretics. The cardinal example of a proximal tubular diuretic is acetazolamide, a carbonic anhydrase inhibitor that blocks proximal reabsorption of sodium bicarbonate. Consequently, prolonged use of acetazolamide may lead to hyperchloremic acidosis, in contrast to all other diuretics, which act at loci prior to the late distal nephron. Metolazone, a congener of the thiazide class of diuretics, blocks sodium chloride absorption in two nephron sites by unknown mechanisms. Specifically, in addition to an action on the early distal tubule, metolazone also inhibits proximal tubular sodium chloride absorption. Since the major locus for phosphate absorption is in the proximal nephron, the phosphaturia accompanying metolazone administration exceeds considerably that observed with other thiazide class diuretics.

Proximal diuretics are rarely used as primary diuretic therapy in modern practice. More commonly, these diuretics, particularly metolazone, are used as supplements to loop diuretics in instances in which loop diuretics alone are ineffective in producing diuresis.

Loop Diuretics. Loop diuretics, such as ethacrynic acid and furosemide, produce diuresis by inhibiting the coupled entry of Na^+, Cl^-, and K^+ across apical plasma membranes in the thick ascending limb of Henle. The latter is responsible for the reabsorption of approximately 25 per cent of filtered sodium. The natriuretic dose-response characteristics of these diuretic agents are considerably more linear than those of all other currently used diuretics. Consequently, the loop diuretics are, for practical purposes, the most potent diuretics currently available; therefore these drugs are commonly referred to as "high-ceiling" diuretics.

Furosemide is the most commonly used loop diuretic. The drug may be administered orally, generally at dosages of 20 to 60 mg every 6 to 8 hours. The onset of action occurs within 1 to 2 hours and is dissipated at 6 hours. Intravenous furosemide, generally in dosages of 20 to 80 mg at 6-hour intervals, is useful in circumstances in which acute diuresis is required, as, for example, in acute pulmonary edema. The onset of action occurs within 10 to 20 minutes, and the effect is dissipated at 3 to 4 hours. Although the dose-response curve with furosemide is more linear than with diuretics of the thiazide class, there is little justification for using intravenous furosemide dosages in excess of 120 to 160 mg. Rather, it is more prudent, in instances of

diuretic resistance, to employ combined diuretic therapy—for example, using metolazone together with furosemide.

Early Distal Tubule Diuretics. Early distal tubule diuretics, such as thiazide and metolazone, interfere primarily with sodium chloride absorption in the earliest segments of the distal convoluted tubule. The thiazide diuretics appear to exert their effect by blocking sodium entry from tubular fluid across apical plasma membranes into distal tubular cells.

With the exception of acetazolamide (which impairs bicarbonate absorption), hypokalemia and metabolic alkalosis may complicate the administration of proximal diuretics, loop diuretics, and early distal tubular diuretics. This occurs because the rate of sodium delivery to terminal distal tubular regions, where a significant fraction of potassium and proton secretion occurs, is a major factor promoting these two processes. Consequently, an increased delivery of salt to the late distal nephron, occasioned by inhibition of sodium reabsorption in the proximal tubule, the ascending limb of Henle, or the early distal tubule, leads to accelerated rates of proton and potassium secretion and consequently to hypokalemia and metabolic alkalosis.

In general, early distal tubular diuretics are utilized for the same circumstances as loop diuretics. The major exception to this statement occurs in disorders of calcium metabolism. Loop diuretics are calciuric and therefore are a valuable adjunct to the management of acute hypercalcemia. In contrast, thiazide diuretics promote hypocalciuria and calcium retention and are therefore useful in managing hypercalciuric states, but not hypercalcemia.

Late Distal Nephron Diuretics. Finally, a group of agents inhibit sodium absorption in terminal regions of the distal tubule and concomitantly suppress indirectly potassium secretion and proton secretion. Spironolactone competes with aldosterone; the primary use of this agent is restricted to conditions of aldosterone excess, either primary or secondary. Alternatively, both triamterene and amiloride operate independently of aldosterone. These agents directly block sodium uptake by late distal tubular cells and concomitantly suppress indirectly both potassium and proton secretion. Accordingly, hyperkalemic, hyperchloremic metabolic acidosis may complicate the injudicious use of spironolactone, triamterene, or amiloride. These diuretics are useful especially in managing disorders characterized by secondary hyperaldosteronism, such as cirrhosis with ascites, and in promoting diuresis in hypokalemic patients.

One factor common to the treatment of disorders with reduced ECV's and expanded ECF volumes merits particular consideration. A major factor in edema formation is an increase in the Starling forces promoting fluid translocation from the vascular to interstitial spaces. When potent diuretics are administered to patients with portal hypertension or with hypoalbuminemia, urinary sodium excretion may exceed the rate at which salt and water are transferred from the interstitium to the vascular bed. As a result, vigorous diuretic therapy may result in volume contraction, reduced salt delivery to diluting segments, nonosmotic ADH release, and consequently hyponatremia. In advanced cases of diuretic abuse, hypotension, hemoconcentration, and azotemia also occur.

A like effect occurs in volume-expanded patients, particularly

TABLE 75–5. CHARACTERISTICS OF COMMONLY USED DIURETICS

Diuretic	Primary Effect	Secondary Effect	Complications
I. Proximal Diuretics			
Acetazolamide	↓ Na^+/H^+ exchange	↑ K^+ loss, ↑ HCO_3^- loss	Hypokalemic, hyperchloremic acidosis
Metolazone	↓ Na^+ absorption	↑ K^+ loss, ↑ Cl^- loss	Hypokalemic alkalosis
II. Loop Diuretics			
Furosemide	} ↓ Na^+:K^+:$2Cl^-$ absorption	↑ K^+ loss, ↑ H^+ secretion	Hypokalemic alkalosis
Ethacrynic acid			
III. Early Distal Diuretics			
Thiazide	} ↓ Na^+ absorption	↑ K^+ loss, ↑ H^+ secretion	Hypokalemic alkalosis
Metolazone			
IV. Late Distal Diuretics			
Aldosterone antagonists			
Spironolactone			
Nonaldosterone antagonists	} ↓ Na^+ absorption	↓ K^+ loss, ↓ H^+ secretion	Hyperkalemic acidosis
Triamterene			
Amiloride			

those exhibiting a third space effect and having significant hypo-albuminemia, if relatively large volumes of ascitic fluid are removed by paracentesis. In this circumstance, the transudation of fluid from the vascular space to the interstitial space may result in circulatory collapse.

Johnston CI, Hodsman PG, Kohzuki M, et al.: Interaction between atrial natriuretic peptide and the renin, angiotensin, aldosterone system. Am J Med 87(Suppl 6B):24S, 1989. *A review of the renin-angiotensin system and the interaction with atriopeptin.*

King AJ, Brenner BM, Anderson SH: Endothelin: A potent renal and systemic vasoconstrictor peptide. Am J Physiol 256:F1051, 1989. *A description of the physiology of endothelin.*

Palkovits M, Geiger H, Bahner U, et al.: Atrial natriuretic factor in central nervous system regulatory mechanisms: Effect of experimental alterations in water and salt homeostasis and blood pressure. Miner Electrolyte Metab 16:42, 1990. *A summary of current information about atriopeptin.*

Stein JH, Kunau RT (eds.): Diuretics II: Clinical uses. Semin Nephrol 8:317, 1988. *A complete issue of this journal devoted to the clinical application of diuretics.*

Weinman EJ, Andreoli TE (eds.): Diuretics I: Physiology, biochemistry and pharmacology. Semin Nephrol 8:197–314, 1988. *A complete issue of this journal devoted to the physiology of diuretics.*

75.2 OSMOLALITY DISTURBANCES

PHYSIOLOGIC CONSIDERATIONS

In normal individuals, the serum osmolality is virtually constant from day to day, and the serum sodium concentration is an accurate index of body water osmolality. In fact, the normal ranges for serum sodium concentrations or for serum osmolalities in populations of healthy individuals reflect small differences in body water osmolality among individuals, rather than on variations in body water osmolality in a given individual.

It is useful to define "effective ECF osmolality," since the osmoregulatory mechanisms that adjust water balance in normal individuals are determined primarily by changes in cell volume that result from variations in effective ECF osmolality. In dilutional states, the measured and effective ECF osmolalities are approximately equal, since ECF dilution also produces ICF dilution and, at least acutely, cell swelling. Osmoregulatory mechanisms are activated when ECF hypertonicity is due to a solute that is excluded from cells and therefore produces, at least acutely, cell shrinkage; in this case, the measured and effective ECF osmolalities are approximately equal. If the ECF osmolality is increased by solutes such as urea, which penetrate cell membranes readily, acute cell shrinkage does not occur and osmoregulatory mechanisms are not activated. In this case, the measured ECF osmolality is greater than the effective ECF osmolality.

The serum osmolality can be approximated from the following formula:

$$\text{Osmolality} = 2[\text{Na}^+] + \frac{[\text{glucose}]}{18} + \frac{[\text{BUN}]}{2.8}$$

where the glucose and blood urea nitrogen (BUN) concentrations are expressed as milligrams per deciliter and the serum sodium concentration is expressed as milliequivalents per liter. In normal circumstances, glucose contributes 5.5 mOsm per kilogram of H_2O to the serum osmolality. When hyperglycemia occurs, the effective ECF osmolality rises because glucose entry into cells is limited. When azotemia occurs, the effective ECF osmolality does not rise because urea enters cells readily.

Cell Volume Regulation

Starling forces regulate fluid transfer between the ICF and the ECF. Because plasma membranes cannot tolerate even small hydrostatic gradients, the operational Starling forces between ICF and ECF are almost entirely osmotic. Significant changes in cell volume, particularly in the central nervous system, are by themselves potentially lethal. Thus the goals of fluid transport between the ECF and ICF are to maintain constancy of cell volume and to maintain a negligible hydrostatic pressure gradient between cells and the ECF. Since cell membranes are freely permeable to water, these two goals are achieved when the ECF osmolality is normal and intracellular and extracellular osmolalities are identical.

Since cell membranes are partially permeable to sodium and potassium, there is a tendency for sodium to leak into cells and for potassium to leak out of cells. Because impermeant macromolecules account for a large fraction of intracellular anions, passive sodium and potassium movements tend toward a Donnan distribution, in which total intracellular cations would exceed total interstitial cations, in precise analogy to the way in which total plasma water cations exceed total interstitial cations. If these passive cation movements across cell membranes were unopposed, osmotic water movement into cells would tend to produce cell lysis. Consequently, active transport mechanisms are required to balance intracellular and interstitial cation concentrations.

Specifically, both sodium leakage from the ECF into cells and potassium leakage out of cells into the ECF are counterbalanced exactly by active outward sodium transport coupled to active inward potassium transport. These active transport events maintain the intracellular cation (and therefore osmolar) content equal to that of extracellular fluid and also maintain the predominant extracellular and intracellular distributions of sodium and potassium, respectively. Thus because cellular cation pumps balance cellular cation leaks, cells are *operationally* impermeable to sodium and to potassium. Active sodium efflux coupled to active potassium influx is mediated by membrane-bound $(\text{Na}^+ + \text{K}^+)$–adenosine triphosphatase (ATPase), and the activity of these cellular cation pumps accounts for more than 50 per cent of the basal caloric consumption.

Cation transport mediated by $(\text{Na}^+ + \text{K}^+)$-ATPase is the major factor regulating cell volume when the effective ECF osmolality is normal. When the effective ECF osmolality is increased or decreased, additional processes are required to maintain the constancy of cell volume. These auxiliary mechanisms are of particular importance in minimizing potentially lethal changes in brain volume because of osmotic water shifts into or out of brain cells.

In chronic hypotonic disorders, cell swelling is offset by the loss of potassium chloride from cells. This potassium chloride efflux mechanism appears to be activated by small increases in cell volume produced by ECF dilution. In chronic hypernatremia, brain shrinkage is minimized by the accumulation of additional solutes within brain cells. These latter solutes, often called "idiogenic osmoles," include amino acids and other solutes, including myoinositol, betaine, and urea. As will be discussed in the section on treatment, these auxiliary transport processes affect significantly the therapeutic approach to patients with osmoregulatory failure.

Water Balance

The key elements regulating water balance are summarized in Figure 75–2. The osmoreceptors, both for ADH release and for thirst, respond to small changes in effective ECF osmolality, while baroreceptors respond to changes in ECV. As little as a 2 per cent increase in effective ECF osmolality causes shrinkage of osmoreceptor cells and stimulation of both ADH release from the posterior pituitary and thirst. A second way of stimulating both ADH release and thirst involves volume-mediated stimuli that can operate independently of changes in plasma osmolality. When the ECV volume is reduced by approximately 10 per cent, these volume-dependent mechanisms stimulate ADH release.

Until recently, it was commonly thought that increases in plasma osmolality and in plasma volume directly suppressed water repletion. It now seems likely, however, that suppression of thirst and of ADH release depends on at least two factors, namely, the oropharyngeal reflex (OPR) and release of atrial natriuretic peptide, the latter occurring, in all likelihood, both systemically and in the central nervous system.

SENSORS AND EFFECTORS. Three kinds of *sensor* elements adjust water balance. Two of these, osmoreceptors and the thirst center, respond to small changes in effective ECF osmolality, whereas baroreceptors respond to changes in ECV. The osmoreceptors are situated in the supraoptic and paraventricular nuclei of the hypothalamus, whereas the thirst center is in the organum vasculosum of the anterior hypothalamus. As little as a 2 per cent increase in effective ECF osmolality produced by solutes such as sodium chloride, but not urea, causes shrinkage

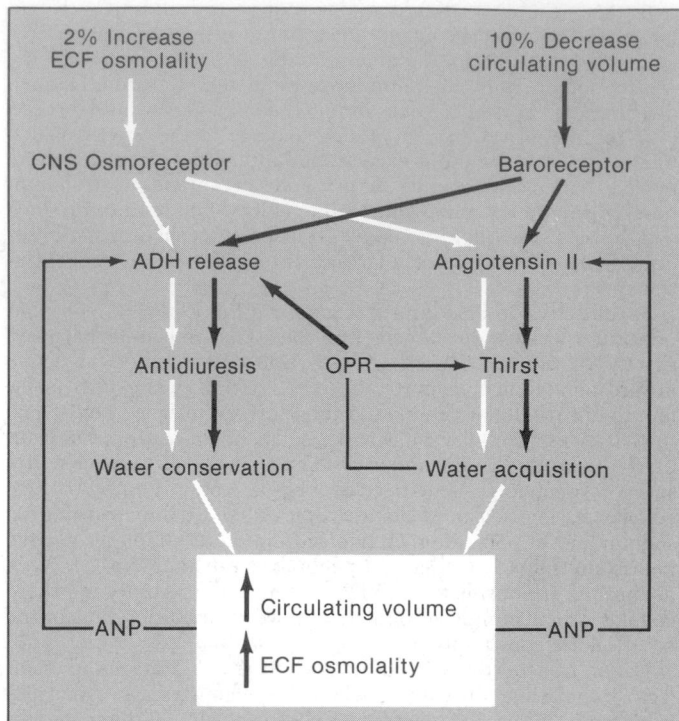

FIGURE 75–2. The water repletion reaction. The white arrows are positive water conservation processes activated by osmolality. The red arrows are water conservation processes that are volume activated. The black arrows indicate negative feedback. (From Reeves WB, Andreoli TE: The posterior pituitary and water metabolism. *In* Wilson JD, Foster DW [eds.]: Williams Textbook of Endocrinology. 8th ed. Philadelphia, W. B. Saunders Company, 1992.)

of osmoreceptor cells and thirst center cells. The osmoreceptors stimulate the release of the *effector* hormone ADH from storage sites in the posterior pituitary gland. The stimulation of thirst by the thirst centers depends on centrally produced angiotensin II.

Endothelin 1 is also released from the posterior pituitary in response to water deprivation. Moreover, administered endothelin 1 increases plasma ADH levels. Thus, endothelin 1 may have a central role in modulating ADH release.

When the ECV is reduced by more than 10 per cent, volume-dependent blood volume produces afferent signals, carried by the ninth and tenth cranial nerves, which result in nonosmotic ADH release. Volume contraction also acts as a potent stimulus to thirst via angiotensin II.

THE ANTIDIURETIC RESPONSE. The cardinal characteristics of the antidiuretic response depend primarily on the integrated activity of two regions of the nephron: the medullary thick ascending limb of Henle, referred to as the diluting segment; and the collecting duct, which may be termed the concentrating segment.

The medullary thick ascending limb absorbs a large amount, possibly as much as 25 per cent, of the filtered load of sodium. Some of this reabsorbed sodium is trapped in the renal medullary interstitium, thus accounting in large part for the hypertonicity of the renal medullary interstitium. However, the medullary thick limb of Henle is also impermeable to water. Consequently, salt abstraction from the thick limb of Henle accounts simultaneously for the development of medullary hypertonicity, thus permitting, in the presence of ADH, maximal antidiuresis, and for the appearance of maximally dilute urine in early distal convolutions, thus permitting, in the absence of ADH, maximal water diuresis.

In normal individuals, approximately 18 liters daily of tubular fluid reaches the early distal tubule; the osmolality of this fluid is quite dilute, approximately 50 mOsm per kilogram of H_2O. Thus in the total absence of ADH and volume contraction, maximal rates of water diuresis include a urinary volume of 18 liters per day having an osmolality of 50 mOsm per kilogram of

H_2O. During antidiuresis, ADH increases the water permeability of collecting ducts (Ch. 214). Tubular fluid equilibrates osmotically with the hypertonic medullary interstitium, reducing urinary volume, concentrating the urine, and conserving body water. When ADH is absent, the water permeability of collecting ducts is low, and absorption of tubular fluid is reduced, so that it escapes unchanged as hypotonic urine.

Finally, since collecting ducts are partially permeable to water in the absence of ADH, a reduced volume of hypotonic fluid reaching collecting ducts equilibrates partially with the medullary interstitium, thereby limiting the ability to dilute urine maximally. In some experimental circumstances, sufficiently significant reductions in the rate of solute excretion result in formation of a hypertonic urine when ADH is absent.

NEGATIVE FEEDBACK. Water repletion activates a negative feedback of water conservation by at least two systems, atriopeptin and OPR (Fig. 75–2). Immunoreactive atriopeptin is released both within the central nervous system and by secretory granules in cardiac atria. The centrally released atriopeptin can suppress ADH release and thirst. Oropharyngeal stimulation by water suppresses ADH release and thirst prior to absorption of water or a fall in plasma osmolality. This mechanism, termed the oropharyngeal reflex, probably depends on neural traffic between the oropharynx and the central nervous system.

Finally, intrarenal PGE_2 suppresses the effects of ADH on nephron segments. PGE_2 is produced by renal interstitial cells in response to increases in medullary osmolality. In turn, PGE_2 impairs water conservation by inhibiting the actions of ADH on nephron segments involved in the antidiuretic response, namely, the medullary thick ascending limb and the collecting duct.

HYPOTONIC DISORDERS

DEFINITION. A hypotonic disorder is one in which the ratio of solutes to water in body fluids is reduced, and the serum osmolality and serum sodium are both reduced in parallel. True hypotonicity must be distinguished from disorders in which the *measured* serum sodium is low while the measured serum osmolality is either normal or increased.

The distinction among these disorders is presented in Table 75–6. The measured serum sodium can be reduced either because there is an increased concentration of small, nonsodium solutes restricted to the ECF or because of a laboratory artifact. In hyperglycemia or excessive mannitol administration, these solutes, which are restricted to the ECF, draw water from the cellular compartment. The serum sodium level is therefore reduced, even though the serum osmolality may be increased. When a small, nonsodium solute is distributed in total body water, as in ethanol intoxication or in azotemia, the serum osmolality rises but the serum sodium concentration remains normal, resulting in an "osmolar gap." The latter is a useful diagnostic aid in intoxication with the different alcohols shown in Table 75–6.

Instances of spurious hyponatremia due to hyperlipemia or hyperproteinemia are becoming less common as more laboratories adopt the use of ion-selective electrodes to measure the serum sodium concentration.

TABLE 75–6. DISTINCTION BETWEEN APPARENT AND REAL HYPOTONICITY

Condition	Measured Serum [Na⁺]	Measured Serum Osmolality
True hypotonicity	↓	↓
Increased nonsodium ECF solutes		
Hyperglycemia	↓	↑
Mannitol administration	↓	↑
Increased nonsodium ECF and ICF solutes		
Ethanol	Normal	↑
Ethylene glycol	Normal	↑
Methanol	Normal	↑
Isopropyl alcohol	Normal	↑
Laboratory artifact		
Hyperlipemia	↓	Normal
Hyperproteinemia	↓	Normal

ETIOLOGY AND PATHOGENESIS. Hyponatremia and simultaneous body water hypotonicity develop whenever water intake exceeds the sum of renal plus extrarenal water losses; in chronic hyponatremia, the net water intake and net water output may be equal. Thus hyponatremia and body fluid hypotonicity occur when there is a primary increase in water ingestion, when the ability of the kidney to dilute urine maximally is limited, or when a combination of these factors is operative.

Dilutional hyponatremia may be the consequence of an absolute increase in water intake that exceeds the ability of a normal kidney to excrete free water, as in *primary polydipsia*, occasionally referred to as psychogenic polydipsia. Patients with this disorder ingest unusually large volumes of water, often in excess of 10 to 15 liters per day, and generally develop mild, clinically asymptomatic hyponatremia.

However, polydipsia may contribute to rather severe hyponatremia in individuals with underlying psychiatric illness. Episodic polydipsia and hyponatremia occur in 3 to 5 per cent of patients in mental hospitals, and polyuria occurs in more than 60 per cent of patients in mental hospitals. This disorder is sometimes described by the acronym PIP syndrome (psychosis, intermittent hyponatremia, and polydipsia). The cause of this syndrome is uncertain. Most patients have, in addition to polydipsia, excessive vasopressin secretion. Carbamazepine, sometimes used to control agitation in psychotic patients, may also contribute to hyponatremia.

More commonly, hyponatremia occurs because the ability of the kidney to excrete a maximally dilute urine is reduced. This inability to dilute urine maximally occurs because of (1) reductions in the rate of salt absorption by the diluting segment, that is, the thick ascending limb of Henle; (2) sustained nonosmotic release of ADH; or (3) a combination of these factors. Table 75–7 summarizes these disorders.

Reduced Sodium Delivery to Diluting Segments. These disorders occur when a reduced sodium intake, without significant sodium depletion or ECF volume contraction, decreases the rate of sodium delivery to the diluting segment and consequently impairs the maximal rate of dilute urine formation, the minimal urinary osmolality, or both. Beer potomania, although an uncommon disorder, illustrates this mechanism for hyponatremia nicely.

Patients with beer potomania derive a substantial part of their caloric intake from the ingestion of large volumes of beer, which contains little salt or protein. Because sodium and urea are the major urinary solutes, dietary restriction of these solutes, particularly sodium, increases the fractional rate of proximal sodium absorption, diminishes the rate of salt delivery to diluting segments, and in turn limits the daily rate of formation of dilute urine. For example, the minimal urinary osmolality is approximately 50 mOsm per kilogram of H_2O; consequently, the excretion of 15 liters of highly dilute urine requires the excretion of 750 mOsm of solute. If the daily urinary solute excretion falls, the maximal amount of dilute urine formed daily is also reduced. Moreover, partial equilibration of reduced volumes of collecting duct fluid with the renal medullary interstitium impairs even further the daily excretion of dilute urine.

Hyponatremia due to reduced solute intake is not restricted to individuals with beer potomania but may occur during starvation,

TABLE 75–7. HYPONATREMIA REFERABLE TO IMPAIRED RENAL EXCRETION OF WATER

I. Reduced Sodium Delivery to the Diluting Segment	III. Mixed Disorders
Starvation	Volume contraction (Addison's disease)
Beer potomania	Edema with deranged
? Myxedema	Starling forces
II. Primary Excess of ADH	(congestive heart failure,
SIADH	constrictive pericarditis,
Drug-induced ADH production	and cirrhosis)
Drug potentiation of ADH action	
Trauma	
Potassium depletion	
? Myxedema	
? Acute intermittent porphyria	

TABLE 75–8. MAJOR CAUSES OF SIADH

Malignant Neoplasia
Carcinoma: bronchogenic, pancreatic, ureteral, prostatic, bladder
Lymphoma and leukemia
Thymoma and mesothelioma
Central Nervous System (CNS) Disorders
Trauma
Infection
Tumors
Porphyria
Pulmonary Disorders
Tuberculosis
Pneumonia
Ventilators with positive pressure

when intake may be dramatically reduced without parallel reductions in water intake. This form of hyponatremia occurs with increasing frequency in elderly patients in nursing homes who are inadequately supervised.

Patients with beer potomania or starvation are to be distinguished from individuals in whom a reduced ECV accompanied by an increase in total body water or by a reduction in GFR reduces the rate of salt delivery to diluting segments and collecting ducts (see below). In short, beer potomania and starvation are classic examples in which a reduced rate of delivery to the diluting segment, in the absence of ADH release, blunts significantly urinary diluting power in the absence of profound gains or excesses in total body water.

Primary Effector ADH Excess. The Syndrome of Inappropriate ADH Production (SIADH). In SIADH, hyponatremia occurs as a result of sustained endogenous production and release of ADH or ADH-like substances; the ECV is normal or increased, and there are no other physiologic or pharmacologic stimuli to ADH release. Table 75–8 lists the major causes of SIADH. A similar process may account in part for the hyponatremia seen in myxedema.

Antidiuretic hormone, or a peptide having comparable biologic activity, is produced by tumors. Increased ADH levels, estimated by either bioassay or radioimmunoassay, have also been noted in patients with cranial disorders such as skull fractures, subdural hematomas, subarachnoid hemorrhage, and brain tumors; in acute intermittent porphyria; and possibly in myxedema. Four different patterns of plasma ADH concentrations have been described in patients with SIADH. Figure 75–3 illustrates three of these patterns; the shaded area in Figure 75–3 illustrates the normal relation between plasma ADH levels and serum osmolality. The pattern denoted "erratic ADH release" in Figure 75–3 accounts for about 37 per cent of patients with SIADH; the hormone is released completely independently of osmotic control. About one third of patients with SIADH have a "reset osmostat"; there is an abnormally low threshold for ADH secretion, but if sufficiently hyponatremic, these patients with SIADH can produce a maximally dilute urine. About 16 per cent of patients with SIADH exhibit the "ADH leak" pattern, namely, sustained ADH production below the osmotic threshold, and normal increases in serum ADH levels with osmotic challenge (Fig. 75–3). Finally, about 14 per cent of patients with SIADH have no detectable abnormality in ADH levels; they fail, for reasons not yet understood, to dilute urine maximally.

The typical features of SIADH are listed in Table 75–9. The cardinal results of the sustained water conservation in SIADH are twofold: hyponatremia and volume expansion. In fact, patients with SIADH who are allowed free access to water generally gain about 3 kg in water weight, or, in other words, nearly 10 per cent of body water. In that respect, patients with SIADH differ from those with hyponatremia secondary to salt depletion, Addison's disease, or diuretic excess, since patients with the latter disorders are volume contracted. However, patients with SIADH, although volume expanded, do not develop edema and thus differ in that respect from patients with congestive heart failure or cirrhosis.

When total body water is expanded by about 10 per cent by water conservation in SIADH, a natriuresis occurs even in the face of hyponatremia. Thus the patient with SIADH reaches a

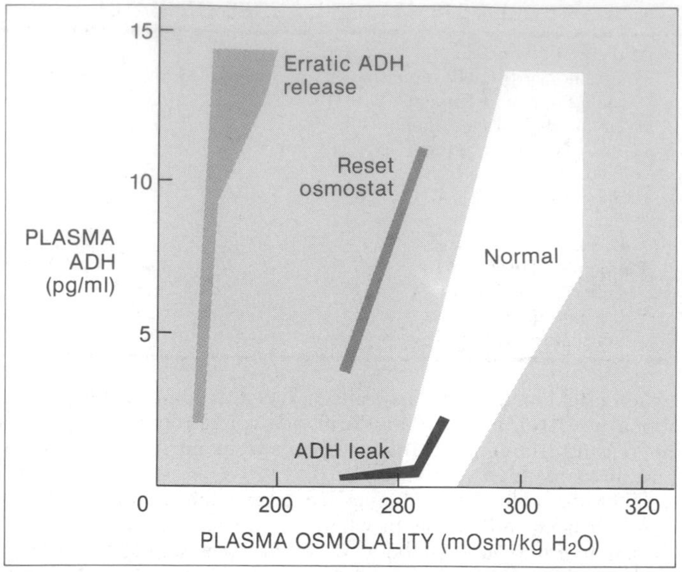

FIGURE 75–3. The patterns of serum ADH abnormalities in SIADH. The shaded areas indicate the normal relation between increases in effective ECF osmolality and ADH levels; the normal osmotic threshold is lower than the normal serum osmolality. The three shaded areas indicate ADH patterns in SIADH. (Adapted from Zerbe R, Strope L, Robertson G: Vasopressin function in the syndrome of inappropriate diuresis. Annu Rev Med 31:315, 1980. With permission from the Annual Review of Medicine, Vol. 31, © 1980 by Annual Reviews, Inc.)

steady state in which body water is expanded by water retention and in which natriuresis, even in the face of hyponatremia, prevents edema formation.

The causes for the natriuresis that is characteristic of SIADH are multiple. First, volume expansion will result in enhanced release of atriopeptin, which enhances urinary sodium wasting both by enhancing glomerular filtration and probably by suppressing tubular sodium absorption. Second, the volume expansion of SIADH also reduces the rate of proximal tubular sodium absorption, as well as the rate of proximal uric acid absorption.

In short, SIADH is a disorder in which hormone-stimulated water conservation results in hyponatremia, volume expansion, and consequently an increased GFR, tubular sodium wasting, and reduced net tubular absorption of creatinine and uric acid, but no edema formation. These characteristics are summarized in Table 75–9. Finally, as indicated in connection with Figure 75–3, the urinary osmolality in patients with SIADH may be either inappropriately high for the level of serum osmolality or maximally dilute.

Other Causes of Excessive ADH Production and/or Release. Table 75–7 lists other circumstances in which an increased level of ADH is the primary factor responsible for hyponatremia. A number of commonly used drugs stimulate ADH release: vincristine, cyclophosphamide, carbamazepine, phenothiazines, morphine, barbiturates, chlorpropamide, amitriptyline, thiothixene, and clofibrate. Chlorpropamide also potentiates the effect of ADH on the water permeability of collecting ducts. The posterior pituitary peptide oxytocin (Pitocin) also has an antidiuretic action, although oxytocin is a much less potent antidiuretic agent than is vasopressin. Thus the administration of intravenous hypotonic solutions containing oxytocin for the purpose of inducing labor may result in profound hyponatremia. Trauma or surgical stress also stimulates ADH release.

Ordinarily, diuretic-induced hyponatremia is related to volume contraction; this kind of body fluid dilution will be discussed below. Chronic severe potassium depletion induced by diuretics can also result in ADH release, although the mechanisms by which potassium depletion stimulates ADH release are unknown.

Mixed Disorders. Hyponatremia occurs commonly in true volume contraction and in edematous states in which filling of the arterial tree is impaired. The former disorders include patients in whom both ECF and total body water are reduced; the latter group comprises those patients with deranged Starling forces,

notably local or systemic increases in venous pressure, which result in inadequate filling of the arterial tree. In both sets of disorders, two factors contribute, individually or in unison, to the pathogenesis of hyponatremia: nonosmotic, volume-mediated ADH release and reductions in the rate of sodium delivery to the diluting segment.

Volume contraction is a potent nonosmotic stimulus to ADH release. Figure 75–4 shows the relations between osmotic and nonosmotic, volume-mediated stimuli and plasma ADH levels in experimental animals; entirely comparable responses occur in humans. Increases in plasma osmolality are related linearly to increases in plasma ADH levels. The relation between blood volume depletion and plasma ADH levels is nonlinear. However, with depletion of more than 7 to 10 per cent blood volume, plasma ADH levels rise sharply and produce an antidiuretic effect even when the plasma osmolality is reduced below normal. In other words, volume-mediated, nonosmotic ADH release occurs primarily when circulatory dynamics are moderately to severely advanced; in that circumstance, volume-mediated stimuli override osmotically mediated ADH release, and hyponatremia ensues.

A second factor that accounts for hyponatremia in volume-contracted states is an inability to dilute urine maximally because the rate of sodium delivery to diluting segments in the thick ascending limb is reduced. This situation occurs because increased rates of proximal tubular sodium absorption are stimulated by reduced sodium intake or by inadequate filling of the arterial tree in conditions with combined ECF volume expansion and reduced arterial tree filling. The significance of volume contraction as a pathogenic factor in this type of hyponatremia can be gauged by noting that hyponatremia occurs during volume contraction in experimental animals with pituitary diabetes insipidus.

Hyponatremia is a common feature of untreated Addison's disease and occurs because of a combination of circumstances. In mineralocorticoid deficiency, the major factors responsible for an inability to handle water loads appear to be ECF volume contraction, glomerular filtration reduction, enhanced proximal tubular salt absorption, and volume-mediated, nonosmotic ADH release. Glucocorticoid deficiency also impairs the ability to handle water loads. One of the factors responsible for water retention in Addison's disease is nonosmotic ADH release, which results from impaired cardiac function.

Hyponatremia occurs commonly in advanced stages of disorders characterized by edema formation and a reduced ECV (Table 75–7), particularly in intractable heart failure and advanced hepatic cirrhosis with ascites. Reduced rates of salt delivery to diluting segments of the renal tubule clearly contribute to the impairment in water excretion in these disorders. In patients with heart failure or severe ascites, the plasma concentrations of ADH tend to be inappropriately high with respect to plasma osmolality, so that nonosmotic ADH release may contribute to the development of hyponatremia in these disorders. Furthermore, since nonosmotic ADH release occurs only with profound reductions in blood volume (Fig. 75–4), the occurrence of hyponatremia in congestive heart failure or cirrhosis indicates profound arterial underfilling. This observation correlates well with the ominous prognosis of hyponatremia in these disorders.

CLINICAL MANIFESTATIONS. The clinical features of hyponatremia are produced by the brain swelling that accompanies acute dilution of total body water and generally become manifest when the serum sodium concentration falls to 120 mEq per liter or less. The early symptoms include lethargy, weakness, and somnolence, which proceed rapidly to seizures, coma, and death as hyponatremia worsens. Untreated acute water intoxication is nearly uniformly fatal and represents a medical emergency. In chronic hyponatremia, central nervous system manifestations are

TABLE 75–9. MAJOR CHARACTERISTICS OF SIADH

Hyponatremia
Volume expansion without edema
Natriuresis
Hypouricemia
Normal or reduced serum creatinine level
Normal thyroid and adrenal function

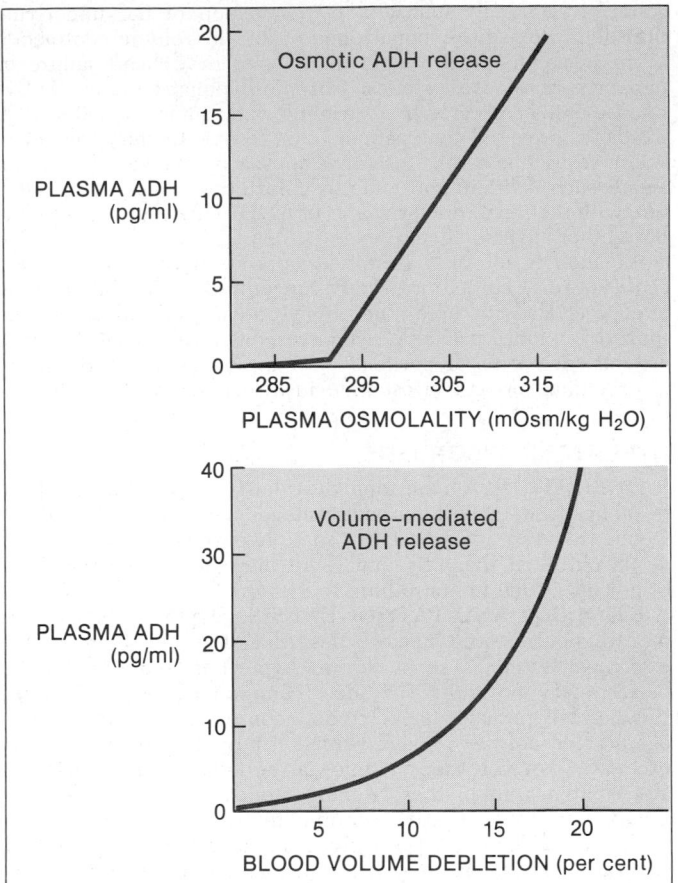

FIGURE 75–4. Relation between plasma ADH concentrations and either effective ECF osmolality (*upper plot*) or the per cent of blood volume depletion (*lower plot*). (Adapted from Dunn FL, Brennan TJ, Nelson AE, et al.: The role of blood osmolality and volume in regulating vasopressin secretion in the rat. J Clin Invest 52:3212, 1973. By copyright permission of the American Society for Clinical Investigation.)

far less common, even when the serum sodium concentration is as low as 100 mEq per liter, because the loss of brain solutes, principally potassium chloride, minimizes brain cell swelling for a given reduction in body water osmolality.

DIAGNOSIS. Hyponatremia should be considered whenever there is a sudden deterioration in central nervous system function, particularly in circumstances such as intractable heart failure, hepatic cirrhosis with ascites, or the administration of large volumes of intravenous fluids. The hyponatremic patient should be evaluated to determine the underlying condition that produced body fluid dilution. This evaluation should include a careful history and physical examination; measurement of the serum creatinine, BUN, and electrolytes; measurement of the urinary sodium concentration, or the Fe_{Na}; measurement of serum and urinary osmolalities; and, when appropriate, evaluation of thyroid and adrenal function.

The history and physical examination are generally adequate for recognizing disorders such as beer potomania or compulsive water ingestion or for noting the ingestion of drugs that stimulate ADH release or enhance ADH action. The presence of edema is characteristic of individuals in whom hyponatremia occurs because of a reduced ECV coupled to ECF volume expansion. In myxedema or Addison's disease, the typical clinical or laboratory findings of these disorders are generally present (Ch. 216 and 217).

The most difficult differential diagnosis among hyponatremic disorders involves the distinction between patients who are modestly volume contracted and those who have SIADH. In both circumstances, the serum sodium and the serum osmolality are reduced, whereas the urinary osmolality is inappropriately high with respect to the reduced serum osmolality. Nonosmotic water conservation in SIADH and in volume contraction is recognized by the presence of a urinary osmolality greater than 120 to 150

mOsm per kilogram of H_2O in association with a reduced serum osmolality. The distinction between the two disorders therefore depends on a clinical and laboratory assessment of ECV.

Patients who are volume contracted may provide a history of volume losses or of diuretic ingestion and may exhibit the signs of ECF volume contraction discussed previously in the section on volume depletion. When the volume losses are due to extrarenal causes, the urinary sodium concentration is less than 10 to 15 mEq per liter and the Fe_{Na} is generally less than 1 per cent. The presence of hyperuricemia may also be a useful clue to the possibility of ECF volume contraction. Prerenal azotemia may occur if the volume contraction is severe. Patients with SIADH are generally normovolemic or slightly volume expanded and therefore exhibit none of the signs of volume contraction. The serum BUN and creatinine levels are normal, and the serum uric acid level is generally reduced. The urinary sodium concentration usually exceeds 30 mEq per liter, and the Fe_{Na} is greater than 1 per cent. Tests of adrenal function yield normal results.

The above studies usually discriminate between SIADH and extrarenal volume contraction. When ECF volume contraction is due to renal salt wasting, urinary sodium losses generally persist unless volume contraction is profound. Moreover, as noted previously (see Volume Depletion), the blood pressure and pulse may be normal in states of modest volume contraction. A useful diagnostic and therapeutic maneuver in this situation is to observe the results of water restriction. When water intake is restricted to 600 to 800 ml daily, patients with SIADH exhibit a highly characteristic response: A 2- to 3-kg weight loss is accompanied by correction of hyponatremia and cessation of salt wasting, usually over a period of 2 to 3 days. If weight loss fails to correct both hyponatremia and urinary sodium wasting simultaneously, the diagnosis of SIADH is doubtful. Rather, renal sodium wasting with ECF volume contraction, due to Addison's disease or the other renal salt-losing disorders listed in Table 75–2, is the more probable diagnosis.

TREATMENT. The goal of treatment in hyponatremia is to correct body water osmolality and therefore restore cell volume to normal by raising the ratio of sodium to water in extracellular fluid. The increase in ECF osmolality draws water from cells and therefore reduces their volume. The choice of therapeutic approach, and whether or not net sodium and water balance is adjusted to be positive or negative during therapy, depends on the serum sodium concentration, the rate at which hyponatremia has developed, the clinical status of the patient, and the underlying disorder.

Acute Hyponatremia. Acute hyponatremia associated with a serum sodium concentration below 120 mEq per liter and with central nervous system manifestations requires immediate therapy. In volume-contracted states, the treatment of choice is to raise the serum sodium level to 125 to 130 mEq per liter over a 6-hour interval by administering hypertonic 3 to 5 per cent saline. As is discussed below, the rapid elevation of serum sodium to values greater than 125 mEq per liter may be hazardous. Since the desired effect is to correct body water osmolality, the amount of sodium administered must be sufficient to raise total body water osmolality to approximately 250 mOsm per kilogram of H_2O, that is, to approximately twice the desired serum sodium concentration. A convenient formula for calculating this sodium requirement is as follows:

$$[125 - \text{measured serum Na}^+] \times 0.6 \text{ body weight} = \text{required mEq of Na}^+$$

The serum sodium level is in milliequivalents per liter, and the body weight is in kilograms. Since 60 per cent of body weight is water, the formula allows an estimate of the amount of sodium required to raise body water osmolality to 250 mOsm per kilogram of H_2O.

The administration of hypertonic saline solutions is hazardous in volume-expanded, salt-retaining states such as congestive heart failure. Furthermore, in SIADH associated with volume expansion and sodium wasting, hypertonic saline alone is ineffective in correcting hyponatremia because the administered salt is excreted promptly in a relatively concentrated urine.

A preferable alternative is to use normal saline in combination with furosemide administration. The diuretic induces urinary salt loss and therefore reduces the risk of ECF volume expansion. Moreover, the diuresis induced by furosemide is characterized by the excretion of urine having a sodium concentration that is appreciably lower than that in plasma. Consequently, the combination of intravenously administered normal saline with a furosemide-induced diuresis of urine that is dilute with respect to plasma provides an effective way of raising the serum sodium level in SIADH or other volume-expanded states. By adjusting the rates of salt administration to be less than urinary salt losses, reductions in ECF volume can be produced simultaneously.

Rate and Magnitude of Correction of Acute Hyponatremia. Since loss of brain solute is a compensatory mechanism for preserving brain cell volume in dilutional states, a serum sodium level of 140 mEq per liter is relatively hypertonic to brain cells that have become partially depleted of solute as a result of hyponatremia. Consequently, raising the serum sodium rapidly to levels greater than 120 to 125 mEq per liter can result in central nervous system damage, such as central pontine myelinolysis. Furthermore, raising the serum sodium concentration to greater than 120 mEq per liter is probably unnecessary.

The major, and still unresolved, controversy surrounding the treatment of hyponatremia concerns the rate at which hyponatremia should be corrected. Mortality rates for severe hyponatremia of 33 to 86 per cent have been cited in support of prompt correction of hyponatremia. These estimates, however, derive largely from single case reports and small series of patients. Thus, these data may overestimate the mortality from hyponatremia. For example, a recent retrospective analysis of all patients with severe hyponatremia (less than 110 mEq per liter) at two university-affiliated hospitals found a mortality rate of only 8 per cent, with most deaths attributed to underlying diseases. Slow or delayed correction of hyponatremia was not associated with higher mortality or with neurologic complications. But the risk of developing neurologic complications was greatest in patients whose serum sodium concentrations were corrected at a rate greater than 0.6 mEq per liter per hour (14 mEq per day).

It has been suggested that rapid correction of hyponatremia may lead to central pontine myelinolysis. This is a demyelinating lesion of the pons, with destruction of myelin sheaths but sparing of the axis cylinders and nerve cells. The majority of patients in whom it has been described have had some form of debilitating disease, such as malnutrition or alcoholism. The clinical characteristics include flaccid quadriplegia or paraplegia, facial weakness, dysphagia, dysarthria, and coma. The possible role of the rate of correction of hyponatremia in the development of central pontine myelinolysis remains uncertain. For example, the incidence of central pontine myelinolysis in hyponatremia is very low, and the rate of correction in patients who develop this condition is no faster than in those who do not. Furthermore, central pontine myelinolysis generally occurs in settings in which additional risk factors, such as alcoholism or malnutrition, could be responsible for the lesion. In experimental animals, the rapid correction of severe hyponatremia to normal sodium levels results in diffuse necrotic brain lesions, whereas rapid correction of mildly hyponatremic levels does not. Thus, the extent of correction and the rate of correction are important factors in the development of neurologic complications.

Given these considerations, it is prudent to correct the serum sodium concentration at a rate of 0.5 mEq per liter per hour until it reaches 120 to 125 mEq per liter. However, young women with acute symptomatic hyponatremia are at greater risk than men for suffering respiratory arrest, severe neurologic sequelae, and death. Thus, it is reasonable to treat these patients with hypertonic saline in an attempt to raise the serum sodium concentration to 125 mEq per liter at a rate of 1.0 to 1.5 mEq per liter per hour. At this point, the patient should be asymptomatic, and the serum sodium level can be gradually returned to normal over several days with water restriction. Overcorrection of the serum sodium concentration (to greater than 130 mEq per liter) is unnecessary and potentially harmful. Even in acutely developing hyponatremia, symptoms and central nervous system signs are uncommon until the serum sodium concentration falls below 120 mEq per liter.

Chronic Hyponatremia. Mild, asymptomatic chronic hyponatremia is generally managed by correction of the underlying disorder, when the hyponatremia occurs in volume contraction or in salt-retaining states, such as congestive heart failure or hepatic cirrhosis with ascites. Chronic hyponatremia in SIADH may be easily corrected by restricting water intake to 800 to 1000 ml daily, provided that patients can adhere to the program of water restriction. An alternative approach involves the use of agents such as lithium or demethylchlortetracycline, which interfere with the renal tubular effects of ADH. However, both agents have other adverse effects.

As another alternative, some workers have recommended reducing renal ability for urinary concentration by administering large oral loads of urea, thereby producing a modest osmotic diuresis. A more palatable maneuver, effective in patients who are not edematous, hypertensive, or in congestive heart failure, is to administer oral furosemide in association with a high-salt diet.

HYPERTONIC DISORDERS

DEFINITION. A hypertonic disorder is one in which the ratio of solutes to water in total body water is increased. All hypernatremic states are hypertonic. In some hypertonic disorders, such as uncontrolled hyperglycemia, the increase in effective ECF osmolality is due to nonsodium solutes.

ETIOLOGY AND PATHOGENESIS. Hypernatremia develops whenever water intake is less than the sum of renal and extrarenal water losses; in chronic hypertonic states, net water balance may be zero. The most common causes of clinically significant hypernatremia occur as a consequence of three pathogenic mechanisms: impaired thirst; solute or osmotic diuresis; excessive losses of water, either via the kidneys or extrarenally; and combinations of these derangements. These disorders are grouped in Table 75–10 according to the primary pathogenic mechanism. There is also a group of miscellaneous disorders, such as hypokalemia, hypercalcemia, and interstitial renal disease, as well as chronic renal failure, which either partially impair renal urinary concentrating ability or partially blunt the responsiveness of collecting ducts to ADH. These disorders rarely cause significant hypernatremia and are not discussed further.

Inadequate Intake of Water. This problem occurs in patients who are comatose or who are otherwise unable to communicate thirst. Because of the exquisite sensitivity of thirst mechanisms to changes in effective body water osmolality, hypernatremia due to inadequate water intake is rare in conscious patients allowed free access to water. Rarely, patients will have a primary thirst deficiency. Patients with Cushing's syndrome or primary hyperaldosteronism commonly have slight elevations in the serum sodium level for unknown reasons.

Finally, "essential hypernatremia" is characterized by a slightly elevated serum sodium level that occurs in the conscious state. The defect in patients with essential hypernatremia appears to be an insensitivity of thirst centers and osmoreceptors to osmotic stimuli. However, both thirst and antidiuresis occur when these patients are volume contracted. Consequently, it has been inferred that volume-mediated stimuli to thirst and ADH release are intact in patients with essential hypernatremia. This disorder may be either congenital or acquired, sometimes in association with histiocytic infiltration of the central nervous system.

Osmotic Diuresis. This is another mechanism for producing renal water losses in excess of sodium losses and therefore

TABLE 75–10. MAJOR CAUSES OF HYPERNATREMIA

I. Impaired Thirst
    Coma
    Essential hypernatremia
II. Solute Diuresis
    Osmotic diuresis: diabetic ketoacidosis, nonketotic hyperosmolar coma, mannitol administration
III. Excessive Water Losses
    Renal
        Pituitary diabetes insipidus
        Nephrogenic diabetes insipidus
    Extrarenal
        Sweating
IV. Combined Disorders
    Coma plus hypertonic nasogastric feeding

hypertonicity. Osmotic diuresis occurs commonly in uncontrolled glycosuria and may occur during mannitol administration for the treatment of increased intracranial pressure. Since these solutes are restricted to the ECF, the serum sodium level is generally reduced in the early stages of osmotic diuresis, and the effective ECF osmolality is increased primarily by the impermeant nonsodium solute. In prolonged osmotic diuresis, net water losses may be sufficiently great that hypernatremia develops. In this circumstance, the increase in effective ECF osmolality is due to the combined effects of hypernatremia and the nonsodium solute. Hypernatremia due to an osmotic urea diuresis can occur if large amounts of protein and amino acids are administered by nasogastric tube, or if tissue catabolism is great, as in burns. In this circumstance, hypernatremia is entirely responsible for the increased effective ECF osmolality.

Hypernatremia may also occur when large amounts of hypertonic sodium solutions are administered, particularly in patients whose renal function is compromised. Two common examples of this condition include the rapid intravenous administration of multiple ampules of sodium bicarbonate during cardiopulmonary resuscitation and the administration of large amounts of sodium bicarbonate to patients with lactic acidosis.

Hypernatremia may also complicate the administration of normal saline solutions when the endogenous osmolar solute load is high and renal concentrating ability is limited. Patients with diabetic ketoacidosis, who are generally young, have sufficient urinary concentrating ability that hypernatremia does not occur when normal saline solutions are used in the treatment of ketoacidosis. In contrast, the nonketotic hyperglycemic syndrome generally occurs in elderly patients, who can have partial impairment of urinary concentrating power. In this setting, hypernatremia can occur during therapy with normal saline solutions. This complication can be avoided by treating with half-normal saline and thus providing sufficient solute-free water for urinary elimination of the osmolar glucose load.

Excessive Water Losses. Impairment of ADH production, release, or action, as in pituitary or nephrogenic diabetes insipidus, can lead to profound water deficits and to hypernatremia. In such circumstances, the urine volumes are large, the urinary osmolality is low, and the net rate of solute excretion is low, in contrast to individuals undergoing osmotic diuresis, in whom rates of urinary solute excretion are elevated. The diabetes insipidus syndromes arc considered in detail in Ch. 214.

Striking water losses may also occur with excessive sweating, particularly during rigorous physical activity by untrained individuals exercising in high humidity. This phenomenon plays a major role in the evolution of heat stroke.

Combined Disorders. Finally, hypertonic dehydration may occur as a combination of these events. A common example in modern clinical practice involves the injudicious administration of large amounts of carbohydrate or amino acids by nasogastric tube, coupled with limited amounts of water, to stroke patients unable to communicate thirst.

CLINICAL MANIFESTATIONS AND DIAGNOSIS. Since two thirds of body water is intracellular, primary water losses tend to have modest effects on circulating volume unless fluid losses are profound. Rather, the clinical manifestations are produced by brain shrinkage that results from increases in effective ECF osmolality. Thus the symptoms of hypertonicity produced either by hypernatremia or by impermeant nonsodium solutes such as glucose are referable to the central nervous system and range from somnolence and confusion to coma, respiratory paralysis, and death. The degree of symptomatology varies with the degree of hypertonicity and with the rate at which hypertonicity develops. In acute hypertonicity, symptoms generally appear when the effective ECF osmolality exceeds 320 to 330 mOsm per kilogram of H_2O, and coma and respiratory arrest may occur when the ECF osmolality exceeds 360 to 380 mOsm per kilogram of H_2O. Chronic hypertonicity generally produces fewer central nervous system manifestations, because brain cells accumulate idiogenic osmoles, which minimize the tendency for brain shrnkage.

TREATMENT. The treatment of acute hypernatremia requires the administration of isotonic dilute saline solutions, generally by an intravenous route. The following factors should be borne in mind when treating acute hypernatremia.

In the highly volume-contracted patient with severe hyperna-

tremia, the administration of isotonic saline solutions has two advantages. It provides fluid resuscitation in impending cardiovascular collapse. Moreover, the isotonic salt solution, which is hypotonic with respect to the hypertonic patient, avoids an unnecessary rapid fall in the serum sodium level.

Rapid correction of hypertonicity to a normal serum osmolality is hazardous. Since accumulation of idiogenic osmoles by brain cells is a compensatory mechanism for preserving brain volume in hypertonic disorders, a normal serum osmolality may be relatively hypotonic to brain cells that have accumulated idiogenic solutes. Hence if the serum osmolality is reduced rapidly, central nervous system damage due to brain swelling may occur. A useful guide to circumventing this difficulty is to reduce the serum sodium level by no more than 1 mEq per liter during every 2 hours of the first 2 days of treatment.

Finally, if solutions of D_5W are administered at a rapid rate, hyperglycemia and osmotic diuresis may occur and hence aggravate the hypertonic state. In this circumstance, the use of a 2.5 per cent dextrose solution in one-quarter normal saline is advisable. This solution has been particularly useful in treating hypernatremia associated with volume contraction in children with pituitary or nephrogenic diabetes insipidus.

Ayus JC, Krothapalli RK, Arieff AI: Treatment of symptomatic hyponatremia and its relation to brain damage: A prospective study. N Engl J Med 317:1190, 1987. *A prospective study showing little relation between the rate of correction of hyponatremia and the occurrence of central pontine myelinolysis.*

Berl T: Treating hyponatremia: Damned if we do and damned if we don't. Kidney Int 37:1006, 1990. *A discussion of the relative merits of rapid versus slow correction of hyponatremia.*

Buckalew VM Jr: Hyponatremia: Pathogenesis and management. Hosp Pract 21:49, 1986. *An excellent description of the treatment of hyponatremia.*

Goldman MB, Luchins DJ, Robertson GL: Mechanisms of altered water metabolism in psychotic patients with polydipsia and hyponatremia. N Engl J Med 318:397, 1988. *An account of factors causing hyponatremia in hospitalized patients with affective disorders.*

Reeves WB, Andreoli TE: The posterior pituitary and water metabolism. *In* Wilson JD, Foster DW (eds.): Williams Textbook of Endocrinology. 8th ed. Philadelphia, W. B. Saunders Company, 1992. *A complete analysis of the physiology of water metabolism and osmotic derangements.*

Sterns RH: Severe symptomatic hyponatremia: Treatment and outcome. Ann Intern Med 107:656, 1987. *An extensive retrospective analysis of acute symptomatic hyponatremia that argues that rapid correction of hyponatremia is hazardous.*

Thompson CS, Andreoli TE: Hyponatremia and hypernatremia. *In* Callaham ML (ed.): Decision Making in Emergency Medicine. Philadelphia, B.C. Decker, 1990, pp 172–175. *A practical guide to the diagnosis and treatment of hyponatremia and hypernatremia.*

Zerbe R, Strope L, Robertson G: Vasopressin function in the syndrome of inappropriate diuresis. Annu Rev Med 31:315, 1980. *The patterns of ADH response in SIADH.*

75.3 DISTURBANCES IN POTASSIUM BALANCE

PHYSIOLOGIC CONSIDERATIONS

The body contains approximately 3500 mEq of potassium, of which only 60 mEq, or about 2 per cent, is extracellular. In normal circumstances external potassium balance depends mainly on dietary potassium intake and renal potassium excretion; fecal potassium losses are only about 10 mEq per day unless diarrhea is present. Since 98 per cent of potassium is located intracellularly, primarily in skeletal muscle, regulation of the serum potassium concentration depends not only on external potassium balance but also on potassium exchanges between the intracellular and extracellular compartments.

Transfer Between ICF and ECF

The intracellular compartment acts as a large potassium reservoir in series with the small ECF potassium pool. In potassium-depleted states, a 1 mEq per liter fall in the serum potassium level requires the loss of about 100 to 200 mEq of potassium; hence the bulk of external potassium loss comes from the cellular compartment. Conversely, if large amounts of potassium are administered acutely, the rise in serum potassium level is less than would be expected if the administered potassium were distributed solely in the ECF. In this situation, cellular uptake of potassium obviously occurs and prevents greater increases in the serum potassium concentration. This ability of cells to accumulate potassium can be enhanced strikingly by chronic administration of high-potassium diets.

A number of *effector* mechanisms regulate the partition of potassium between the ICF and ECF. These include active and passive ionic transcellular transport processes.

ACTIVE TRANSPORT PROCESSES. The cardinal transport process regulating K^+ distribution between ICF and ECF is cell membrane–bound $(Na^+ + K^+)$-ATPase, which actively transports potassium into cells and therefore counterbalances the passive leak of potassium from cells into interstitial fluid. Insulin is a second effector that promotes potassium transfer from ECF to ICF. This hormone promotes cellular uptake of potassium independently of cellular glucose uptake by increasing $(Na^+ + K^+)$-ATPase activity. Insulin also reduces sodium permeability; the resultant cellular hyperpolarization of cells produces a passive driving force for potassium accumulation within cells. Furthermore, hyperkalemia augments insulin release. Thus hyperkalemia may be the sensor that stimulates release of insulin, which then serves as an effector for potassium entry into cells. Beta-adrenergic agents, particularly beta$_2$ agonists such as terbutaline, also promote cellular potassium uptake by enhancing $(Na^+ + K^+)$-ATPase activity; it is not yet known whether hyperkalemia can provoke beta agonist release, as it does for insulin release. Finally, mineralocorticoids such as aldosterone, in addition to enhancing renal potassium excretion (see below), also enhance cellular potassium uptake; the mode of aldosterone action in the latter instance is not understood.

PASSIVE TRANSPORT PROCESSES. A number of passive effector mechanisms also regulate the partition of potassium between the ICF and the ECF. First, alterations in the pH of ECF reproducibly shift potassium between the ICF and the ECF: Systemic acidosis, whether metabolic or respiratory, promotes potassium efflux from cells, whereas systemic alkalosis, either metabolic or respiratory, promotes cellular potassium uptake. As a general rule, a reduction in plasma pH of 0.1 unit raises the serum potassium level by 0.6 mEq per liter, whereas a plasma pH increase of 0.1 unit produces a similar reduction in serum potassium. The mechanisms for these pH-induced potassium shifts between ICF and ECF are not understood.

Second, cellular shrinkage produced by increases in effective ECF osmolality raises the intracellular potassium concentration and thereby increases the driving force for passive potassium leakage from the ICF to the ECF. This leakage may result in hyperkalemia when large glucose loads are administered to insulin-deficient diabetic patients who also have hyporeninemic hypoaldosteronism; the insulin lack limits cellular reentry of potassium, and the aldosterone deficiency limits renal potassium excretion. Increases in cellular potassium concentrations produced by cellular shrinkage also contribute significantly to the hyperkalemia of diabetic ketoacidosis, because hyperglycemia raises cellular potassium levels by cell shrinkage and insulin lack prevents accelerated potassium reentry into cells.

Finally, brain cells and renal tubular cells lose potassium when exposed to chronic ECF hypotonicity. However, muscle cells, which are the largest component of ICF potassium, do not appear to participate in this process. Consequently, hypotonic disorders, by themselves, have little effect on the serum potassium level or on external potassium balance.

Renal Handling of Potassium

The kidneys process potassium strikingly differently from the way in which they process sodium. Sodium excretion involves filtration, partial tubular absorption, and appearance of nonabsorbed sodium as urinary sodium excretion. When dietary sodium intake is varied, there is a prompt adjustment in urinary sodium excretion, either in the upward direction, when sodium intake is increased, or in the downward direction, when sodium intake is curtailed.

In contrast, virtually all dietary potassium, ordinarily about 50 to 200 mEq per day, appears in the urine because of tubular secretion of potassium by terminal nephron segments, particularly the late distal convoluted tubule and the cortical collecting duct. These regions of the nephron can increase rates of potassium secretion significantly if dietary potassium intake is augmented; and they carry out net absorption of potassium in kaliopenic states. In other words, these terminal nephron segments regulate external potassium balance by adjusting *renal output* to balance *intake*.

A convenient way of considering distal nephron handling of potassium, and the ways in which effector mechanisms modulate this process, is shown in Figure 75–5. The dashed lines indicate passive processes, and the solid lines denote active transport processes. Basolateral membranes of all terminal nephron segments, including the thick limb of Henle, the distal tubule, and the collecting duct, share two common characteristics: a passive leakage pathway for K^+ efflux and an active $(Na^+ + K^+)$-ATPase for cellular K^+ uptake. The apical membranes of these nephron segments also contain passive potassium leakage pathways, which can be blocked by barium. In the thick ascending limb of Henle, apical membranes contain a furosemide-sensitive coupled entry step that involves electroneutral $Na^+{:}K^+{:}2Cl^-$ co-transport, driven by the electrochemical sodium gradient between lumen and cells. In distal tubular and collecting ducts, Na^+ entry into cells involves sodium-specific channels that are blocked by amiloride. Thus in the ascending limb, coupled electroneutral sodium entry into cells does not result in luminal electronegativity (in fact, the lumen in the thick ascending limb is electropositive), whereas in the distal tubule and collecting duct, amiloride-sensitive ionic sodium entry produces luminal electronegativity.

The majority of net K^+ secretion occurs in these latter two segments and is driven indirectly by the rate of sodium entry into cells, which increases luminal electronegativity and increases the activity of basolateral $(Na^+ + K^+)$-ATPase, thus raising cell potassium concentrations. In the loop of Henle, little net potassium secretion occurs, because the lumen is electropositive and because coupled $Na^+{:}K^+{:}2Cl^-$ transport from lumen to cells recycles secreted potassium back into cells.

The major elements of the *effector systems* that regulate distal nephron potassium excretion include the rate of distal tubular sodium delivery, dietary potassium intake, plasma pH, aldosterone, impermeant anions, and tubular flow rates. When distal sodium delivery rates are increased, increased sodium entry into cells across apical membranes is accompanied by increased activity of pump $(Na^+ + K^+)$-ATPase, which tends to raise intracellular potassium concentrations. Second, either an increase in

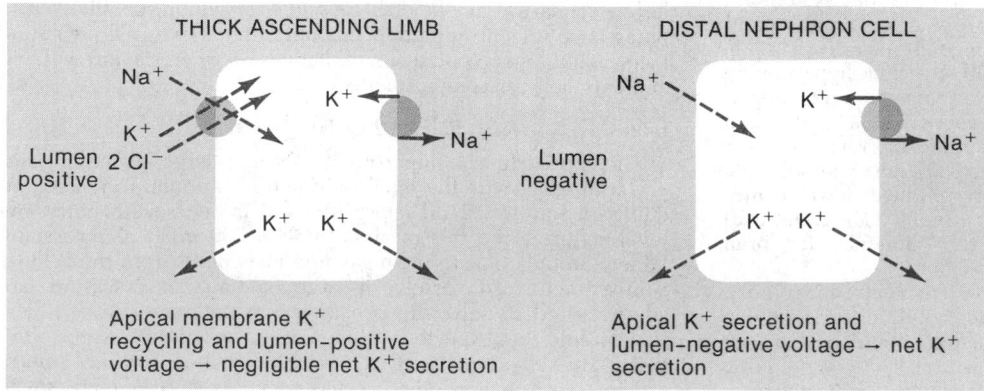

FIGURE 75–5. Handling of potassium in late nephron segments, including the thick ascending limb and the distal nephron. The dashed arrows represent passive transport processes, and the solid arrows represent active transport processes. In the thick ascending limb, K^+ recycling into cells by $Na^+{:}K^+{:}2\,Cl^-$ co-transport and the lumen-positive voltage reduce the rate of net K^+ secretion. Most urinary K^+ comes from net K^+ secretion by terminal nephron segments, particularly the late distal convoluted tubule and the cortical collecting tubule.

THICK ASCENDING LIMB

DISTAL NEPHRON CELL

Na$^+$
K$^+$
Lumen positive
2 Cl$^-$
K$^+$
Na$^+$
K$^+$ K$^+$

Apical membrane K$^+$ recycling and lumen–positive voltage → negligible net K$^+$ secretion

Na$^+$
Lumen negative
K$^+$
Na$^+$
K$^+$ K$^+$

Apical K$^+$ secretion and lumen–negative voltage → net K$^+$ secretion

dietary potassium intake or an increase in plasma pH tends, as indicated above, to raise cellular potassium content. Third, urinary excretion of impermeant anions such as sulfate, carbenicillin, or penicillin produces greater luminal electronegativity. Fourth, aldosterone and mineralocorticoids, whose kaliuretic effects may be dissociated from their sodium-sparing effects, increase the permeability of luminal membranes to potassium. These hormones may also augment distal tubular ($Na^+ + K^+$)-ATPase activity. Among these factors, the rate of aldosterone secretion and the rate of distal salt delivery to terminal nephron segments are the cardinal variables.

Each of the above factors modulates one or another portion of a generalized mechanism, namely, an electrochemical gradient favorable to the passive movement of potassium from tubular cells to urine and consequently for net potassium secretion. Conversely, reductions in sodium delivery, potassium restriction, reductions in plasma pH, and mineralocorticoid lack all reduce the magnitude of passive potassium movement from cells to tubular fluid and therefore tend to decrease net potassium secretion. Finally, increases in tubular flow rates, as in osmotic diuresis, also promote potassium secretion, whereas reductions in tubular flow rates decrease potassium secretion. The mechanism responsible for this effect is unknown.

The net rate of urinary potassium excretion in any given circumstance therefore depends on the interplay of these multiple factors in modulating the common effector mechanism for potassium secretion. For example, mineralocorticoid excess in primary aldosteronism commonly leads to severe potassium wasting. This kaliuresis can be curtailed by dietary sodium restriction and accentuated by dietary sodium loading. Conversely, in hyporeninemic hypoaldosteronism, hyperkalemia may be prevented by ensuring a liberal intake of sodium.

The renal adaptation to excess potassium loads occurs over a 24- to 36-hour period. Consequently, hyperkalemia from the ingestion of large oral potassium loads is uncommon in normal individuals. But the renal response to dietary potassium restriction is more sluggish and requires 7 to 10 days for full development. Even under the latter circumstances, urinary potassium losses are rarely less than 20 mEq per day.

Excitable Tissues and the ICF/ECF Potassium Ratio

The clinical consequences of hypokalemia and hyperkalemia are generally due to changes in the excitable characteristics of heart, skeletal muscle, and smooth muscle. Excitable tissues, such as nerve, heart, and skeletal muscle, share certain common properties. At rest excitable tissues are far more permeable to potassium than to sodium. The cell interior is electronegative with respect to extracellular fluid, and this voltage is largely determined by the logarithm of the ratio of intracellular (K_i) to extracellular (K_o) potassium concentrations. When excitable tissues are suddenly depolarized to their threshold voltage, sodium permeability increases profoundly with an accompanying increase in the sodium to potassium permeability ratio. This sodium entry into the cells of excitable tissues occurs through sodium-specific

channels having electronegative sites that are activated by sudden depolarization. During depolarization, rapid sodium entry produces the initial spike of the action potential, and the cell interior becomes electropositive.

This voltage-dependent increase in sodium permeability during depolarization to threshold is the most fundamental characteristic of excitable tissues (except in tissues such as the atrioventricular node, where Ca^{2+} influx into cells is responsible for the action potential). If an excitable cell is partially depolarized in the resting state, the rate of rise of action potentials is reduced; the prolonged resting depolarization, by undefined mechanisms, reduces the increase in sodium permeability that accompanies the action potential. This effect of resting depolarization on reducing sodium permeability during action potentials is referred to as inactivation.

Repolarization of excitable cells occurs more slowly than depolarization. During repolarization, potassium permeability rises with respect to sodium permeability, and there is passive potassium efflux from the cell to the ECF. This potassium efflux restores the electronegativity of the cell interior. In nerve and skeletal muscle, potassium efflux occurs almost immediately after the initial spike of the action potential. In cardiac muscle, potassium efflux follows the absolute refractory period and coincides with the relative refractory period (phase 3) of the cardiac action potential.

Hyperkalemia reduces the K_i/K_o ratio and consequently partially depolarizes electrical tissues at rest. Hyperkalemia also increases the potassium permeability of excitable cells. The results of these changes on cardiac excitation are illustrated in the left-hand panel of Figure 75–6. Because partial resting depolarization decreases the rate of sodium entry into cells during excitation, the rate of phase zero depolarization is slower and the peak of phase zero depolarization is markedly reduced. The increased potassium permeability accelerates repolarization and shortens the plateau phase. The net effect of progressive hyperkalemia is therefore to make the heart progressively refractory to excitation.

The effects of hypokalemia on excitable tissues are more complex. Because the K_i/K_o ratio rises in hypokalemia, excitable cells at rest should be hyperpolarized. This occurs initially, but resting depolarization eventually follows, because the high K_i/K_o ratio, by itself, reduces the potassium permeability of excitable cells. The effects of hypokalemia on cardiac muscle fibers are shown in the right-hand panel of Figure 75–6. At rest the cell is partially depolarized because the reduced potassium permeability allows the high extracellular to intracellular sodium ratio to make the cell interior less negative. The initial spike of the action potential is less affected than in hyperkalemia because the reduced potassium permeability offsets the reduced sodium permeability during phase zero depolarization. Since potassium efflux determines the rate of repolarization, the reduced potassium permeability prolongs the relative refractory period. The net effect of these changes in cardiac tissue is to increase the

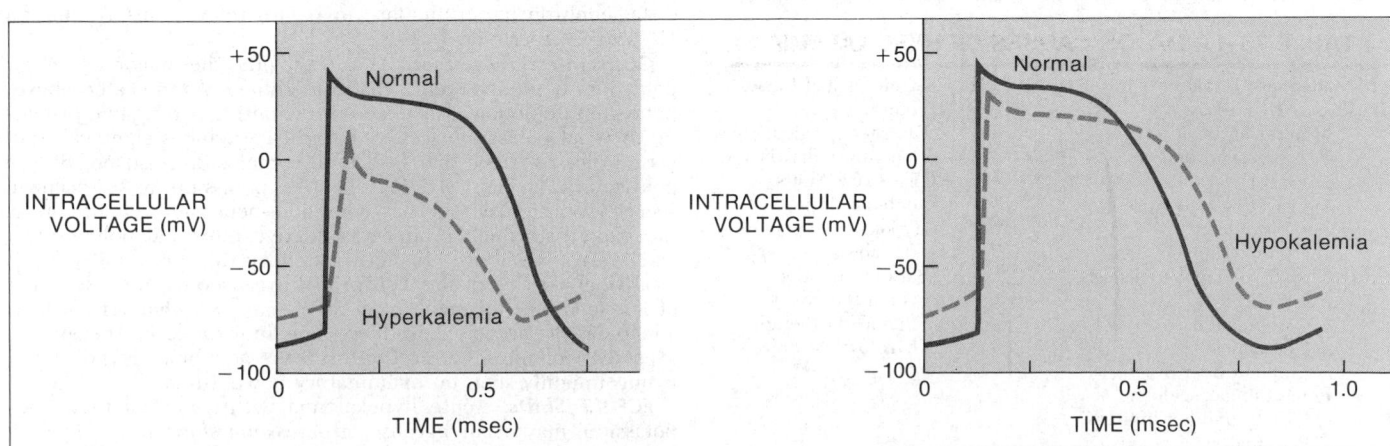

FIGURE 75–6. The effect of increases or decreases in serum potassium on the cardiac action potential. The solid lines represent the normal cardiac action potential; the dashed lines represent the cardiac action potential with either hyperkalemia (*left*) or hypokalemia (*right*).

likelihood of sinus bradycardia and, because of a prolonged relative refractory period, the risk of arrhythmia formation. In skeletal muscle the reduction in membrane permeability to potassium produced by hypokalemia leads, in severe hypokalemia, to generalized paralysis.

HYPOKALEMIA AND POTASSIUM DEPLETION

DEFINITION. Chronic hypokalemia generally reflects a reduction in total body potassium. A 1-mEq reduction in serum potassium level generally implies the net loss of 100 to 200 mEq of potassium from the body. In extreme body potassium depletion, the serum potassium level may be as low as 1.5 to 2.0 mEq per liter. Acute reductions in serum potassium level without parallel reductions in total body potassium occur when potassium is shifted from the ECF to the ICF.

ETIOLOGY AND PATHOGENESIS. Hypokalemia and simultaneous potassium depletion occur whenever renal plus extrarenal potassium losses exceed potassium intake. In advanced body potassium depletion, intake and output of potassium may be equal. The four major causes for hypokalemia are given in Table 75–11.

Inadequate Intake. Reduced potassium intake may result in potassium depletion and hypokalemia because maximal renal conservation of potassium requires, as indicated above, 7 to 10 days. During this interval, the net renal potassium loss may be as much as 150 to 200 mEq.

Excessive Renal Losses. Many of the causes for renal potassium wasting can be analyzed in terms of factors that modulate the common effector system for potassium secretion. *Mineralocorticoid excess* accelerates distal tubular potassium secretion (Fig. 75–5). Consequently, hypokalemia occurs regularly in primary hyperaldosteronism, in Cushing's syndrome, and in secondary hyperaldosteronism. *Chronic licorice ingestion* produces a syndrome that mimics primary hyperaldosteronism, because glycyrrhizinic acid, a component of licorice extract, has physiologic properties similar to those of aldosterone.

In *Bartter's syndrome* sodium chloride wasting and secondary aldosteronism may contribute to potassium depletion (Ch. 82). However, potassium depletion in Bartter's syndrome may also occur either when aldosterone secretion rates are normal or following bilateral adrenalectomy. Consequently, it is believed that a tubular defect in potassium handling also contributes to the hypokalemia of Bartter's syndrome.

Most diuretics having a locus of action prior to the late distal tubule (Table 75–5) increase urinary potassium losses. Enhanced sodium delivery to distal nephron segments is the major factor responsible for the kaliuresis produced by these diuretics, and sodium restriction or volume depletion tends to minimize diuretic-induced potassium losses. Carbonic anhydrase inhibitors such as acetazolamide inhibit proximal bicarbonate absorption and thereby accentuate potassium losses. Distal tubular segments are relatively impermeable to bicarbonate; consequently, increased delivery of bicarbonate to distal nephron regions has an impermeant anion effect that increases luminal electronegativity in these nephron regions.

Osmotic diuresis is commonly associated with increased renal potassium losses, because increased tubular flow rates enhance net potassium secretion. In diabetic ketoacidosis renal potassium losses are common. Yet patients with diabetic ketoacidosis and a reduced total body potassium commonly present with hyperkalemia, because metabolic acidosis tends to promote potassium shifts from the ICF to the ECF. Consequently, profound hypokalemia may develop if body potassium is not replenished concomitantly with insulin therapy and ECF volume expansion (Ch. 218).

Potassium depletion is seen frequently in *chronic metabolic alkalosis*. When the alkalosis is associated with volume contraction, secondary hyperaldosteronism results in renal potassium losses. Potassium depletion in chronic metabolic alkalosis is also enhanced if bicarbonaturia is present, because of the impermeant anion effect produced by bicarbonate delivery to terminal nephron segments. In fact, the hypokalemia associated with upper gastrointestinal fluid losses, as in vomiting or nasogastric suction, is primarily the result of the renal potassium losses produced by secondary hyperaldosteronism or bicarbonaturia or both. The potassium losses from the upper gastrointestinal tract are small, since upper gastrointestinal tract fluid contains only about 10 mEq of potassium per liter.

Hypokalemia may develop during therapy with certain *antibiotics*. Carbenicillin or other penicillin-like antibiotics exist as sodium or potassium salts of impermeant anions and promote kaliuresis because they increase net sodium excretion and because of an impermeant anion effect. Amphotericin B increases the permeability of luminal membranes to potassium and therefore promotes potassium secretion. Gentamicin produces potassium losses by unknown mechanisms.

Hypokalemia and potassium depletion are common findings in *distal, gradient-limited renal tubular acidosis* (Ch. 82). Increased distal sodium delivery and the impermeant anion effect produced by bicarbonate wasting account for most of the potassium losses seen in proximal renal tubular acidosis. Consequently, salt restriction, which enhances the rate of proximal sodium bicarbonate absorption in this disorder, also tends to correct potassium depletion. In gradient-limited distal renal tubular acidosis, hypokalemia may be accentuated by volume losses and secondary hyperaldosteronism. Other factors, not yet understood, also contribute to hypokalemia in this disorder. Hyperkalemia, rather than hypokalemia, commonly accompanies the hyperchloremic acidosis of interstitial disease (type IV acidosis) or of voltage-dependent renal tubular acidosis (see below).

Liddle's syndrome is a rare tubular disorder characterized by hypokalemia, metabolic alkalosis, hypertension, and normal aldosterone secretion rates. Therapy with triamterene, but not with aldosterone antagonists such as spironolactone, ameliorates the disorder. These findings suggest that terminal nephron sodium avidity and potassium secretion independent of aldosterone are major factors in the pathogenesis of Liddle's syndrome. Thus in operational terms, Liddle's syndrome may be described as distal nephron hyperfunction, in regard to Na^+ absorption and H^+ and K^+ secretion.

Gastrointestinal Losses. These provide the major route for potassium depletion, other than the kidney. As indicated above, potassium depletion associated with vomiting is referable primarily to renal potassium losses. Diarrhea produces significant potassium losses, since diarrheal fluid contains 30 mEq per liter of potassium. The most striking diarrheal potassium losses occur in secretory diarrheas, such as with non–beta islet cell tumors of the pancreas, which produce vasoactive intestinal polypeptide, and in laxative abuse. In both secretory diarrheas and chronic laxative abuse, hypokalemia is probably caused by increased rates of K^+ secretion through apical membrane K^+ channels. Villous adenomas of the colon produce potassium depletion because of excessive colonic K^+ secretion from the adenoma. Hypokalemia is uncommonly seen in inflammatory bowel disease.

ECF-ICF Shifts. Acute hypokalemia with a normal total body potassium may occur because of *potassium shifts* from the ECF to the ICF. In *hypokalemic periodic paralysis*, acute shifts of potassium from the ECF to the ICF produce limb and trunk paralysis. The periodic attacks are often precipitated by high-carbohydrate meals. Patients with the disorder can often abort

TABLE 75–11. MAJOR CAUSES OF HYPOKALEMIA

I. **Inadequate Intake**	III. **Gastrointestinal Losses**
II. **Excess Renal Loss**	Vomiting
Mineralocorticoid excess	Diarrhea, particularly
Bartter's syndrome	secretory diarrheas
Diuresis	IV. **ECF → ICF Shifts**
Diuretics with a pre–late	Acute alkalosis
distal locus	Hypokalemic periodic
Osmotic diuresis	paralysis
Chronic metabolic alkalosis	Barium ingestion
Antibiotics	Insulin therapy
Carbenicillin	Vitamin B_{12} therapy
Gentamicin	Thyrotoxicosis (rarely)
Amphotericin B	
Renal tubular acidosis	
Distal, gradient-limited	
Proximal	
Liddle's syndrome	
Acute leukemia	
Ureterosigmoidostomy	

attacks by exercising affected muscles. The chronic use of acetazolamide can prevent attacks. A condition resembling hypokalemic periodic paralysis occurs with the ingestion of *barium salts* and is endemic in China, where the disorder is referred to as "Pa-Ping." Barium appears to produce hypokalemia by blocking K^+ channels in skeletal muscle and thus blocking efflux of potassium from the ICF to the ECF. *Insulin* therapy and *vitamin B_{12}* therapy also promote potassium shifts from the ECF to the ICF. Hypokalemia can also result rarely from thyrotoxicosis, especially in Asian males, for reasons that are unclear.

CLINICAL MANIFESTATIONS. The clinical effects of potassium deficiency are manifest in one or more organ systems, including skeletal muscle, heart, kidneys, and the gastrointestinal tract. The most serious disturbances are those affecting the neuromuscular system. At serum potassium concentrations in the range of 2.0 to 2.5 mEq per liter, muscular weakness is likely to occur; with more severe hypokalemia, the patient may develop areflexic paralysis, in which case respiratory insufficiency is an immediate threat to survival. The severity of the neuromuscular disturbance tends to be proportional to the speed with which the potassium level has declined.

Losses of large amounts of potassium from skeletal muscle may be accompanied by rhabdomyolysis and myoglobinuria. Hence, rhabdomyolysis sometimes occurs in military recruits subject to severe exercise, sweating, and ECF volume contraction. The secondary hyperaldosteronism that follows excessive salt loss produces urinary potassium wasting and consequently potassium depletion. Potassium depletion secondary to malnutrition and vomiting is also one of the pathogenic mechanisms in alcoholic rhabdomyolysis.

The electrocardiographic abnormalities of potassium depletion, shown in Figure 75–7, affect primarily repolarization segments of the electrocardiogram, in keeping with the effects of hypokalemia on the action potential. The common electrocardiographic manifestations of hypokalemia include sagging of the ST segment, depression of the T wave, and elevation of the U wave. With

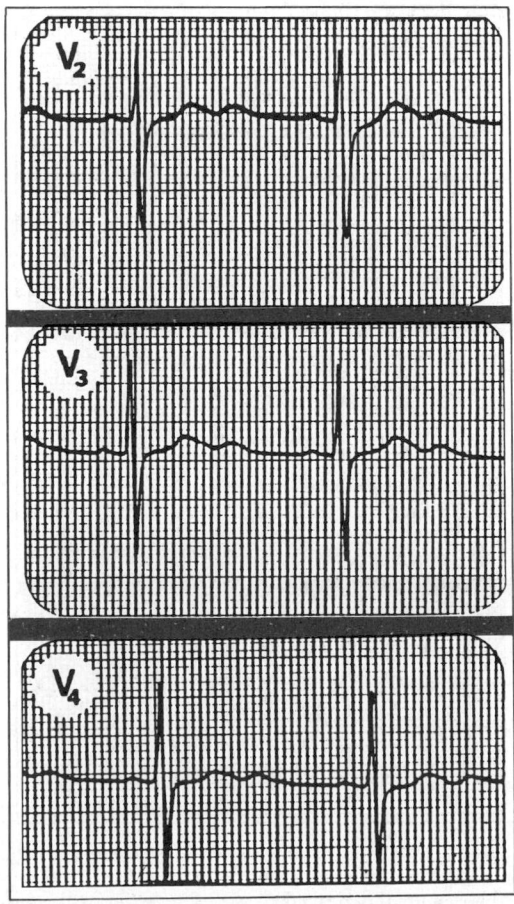

FIGURE 75–7. The electrocardiographic manifestations of hypokalemia. The serum potassium was 2.2 mEq per liter. Note that the ST segment is prolonged, primarily because of a V wave following the T wave, and that the T wave is flattened.

marked hypokalemia, the T wave becomes progressively smaller and the U waves show increasing amplitude. In some cases the merging of a flat or positive T wave with a positive U wave may erroneously be interpreted as a prolonged QT interval. Ordinarily, there are no serious clinical consequences from the abnormalities in cardiac excitation. In patients treated with digitalis, hypokalemia may precipitate serious arrhythmias.

Longstanding potassium depletion may produce renal tubular damage, referred to as hypokalemic nephropathy. Potassium deficiency also affects smooth muscle of the gastrointestinal tract and can result in paralytic ileus.

TREATMENT. The treatment of hypokalemia involves replacement therapy with potassium salts and attempts to correct the underlying disorder. Since diuretic abuse is probably the most common cause for hypokalemia in routine clinical practice, every attempt should be made to identify diuretic ingestion.

Except in extreme circumstances, oral rather than parenteral potassium replacement is prudent. However, when gastrointestinal function is impaired, or when neuromuscular manifestations of hypokalemia are present, parenteral therapy with potassium may be advisable. Since potassium deficits involve both the ICF and the ECF, their correction requires the transfer of administered potassium from the ECF into the ICF. The major problem in parenteral therapy is to avoid intravenous administration of potassium at rates sufficiently great to produce hyperkalemia. A prudent protocol to follow is to add potassium chloride to intravenous solutions at a final concentration of 40 to 60 mEq per liter and to administer no more than 10 to 20 mEq of potassium per hour. Except in unusual circumstances, the total amount of potassium administered daily should not exceed 200 mEq. The serum potassium level should be monitored at appropriate intervals; the frequency of monitoring should be determined by the patient's clinical condition, by the initial serum potassium, by the rate at which the serum potassium changes in a given patient, and by the patient's renal function. Because the electrocardiographic manifestations of hypokalemia are subtle, the electrocardiogram should not be used as a guide to replacement therapy.

Although potassium chloride is the salt of choice for intravenous potassium replacement, oral potassium chloride solutions are not well tolerated because of gastrointestinal irritation. Enteric-coated potassium chloride tablets are to be avoided, because they produce small bowel ulcerations. Oral potassium is administered most conveniently in the form of organic salts such as gluconate or citrate. This form of therapy is, however, not effective in hypokalemic metabolic alkalosis with hypochloremia. In this circumstance, chloride supplementation is required together with potassium replacement and is most easily achieved by administering sodium chloride supplementation.

HYPERKALEMIA AND POTASSIUM EXCESS

DEFINITION. Chronic hyperkalemia can occur with little or no increase in total body potassium. However, acute increases in serum potassium concentrations, produced by potassium shifts from the ICF to the ECF, can occur even when total body potassium is normal or reduced.

ETIOLOGY AND PATHOGENESIS. Hyperkalemia develops whenever the rate of potassium intake or the rate of potassium efflux from cellular to extracellular fluids exceeds the sum of renal plus extrarenal potassium losses. The renal mechanisms for potassium excretion adapt efficiently to increases in the rate of potassium influx to extracellular fluid, particularly from dietary sources. Hence acute or chronic hyperkalemia due to exogenous potassium intake is uncommon, unless renal mechanisms for potassium excretion are compromised. In the latter setting injudicious potassium administration may result in hyperkalemia. This occurs most commonly when intravenous potassium chloride is administered too rapidly; when potassium salts of antibiotics such as penicillin are administered; when transfusions are given with blood that has been stored for long periods; or when salt substitutes containing potassium are used. The occurrence of hyperkalemia in these settings usually requires that renal potassium excretion be impaired.

Acute or chronic hyperkalemia occurs most commonly either

TABLE 75–12. MAJOR CAUSES OF HYPERKALEMIA

I. Diminished Renal Excretion	II. Transcellular Shifts
Reduced GFR	Acidosis
Acute oliguric renal failure	Cell destruction
	Trauma, burns
Chronic renal failure	Rhabdomyolysis
Reduced tubular secretion	Hemolysis
Addison's disease	Tumor lysis
Hyporeninemic hypoaldosteronism	Hyperkalemic periodic paralysis
Potassium-sparing diuretics	Diabetic hyperglycemia
	Insulin dependence plus aldosterone lack
Voltage-dependent renal tubular acidosis	Depolarizing muscle paralysis
	Succinylcholine

GFR = glomerular filtration rate.

because of diminished *renal excretion* or because there is a sudden *transcellular shift* of potassium from the ICF to the ECF. The major causes for hyperkalemia listed in Table 75–12 follow this format.

Diminished Renal Excretion. Hyperkalemia may occur in *acute oliguric renal failure* of any cause. In *chronic renal failure*, hyperkalemia generally does not occur until the GFR has reached markedly low levels. Hyperkalemia may be precipitated in chronic renal failure, however, either by the development of acidosis or, as indicated above, by the injudicious administration of potassium salts. Hyperkalemia also occurs with little or modest reduction in the GFR, if there is impairment of potassium secretion by terminal nephron regions. This occurs in *Addison's disease*, in *hyporeninemic hypoaldosteronism*, and with the injudicious administration of *potassium-sparing diuretics*, such as triamterene or spironolactone. Hyperkalemia in Addison's disease and hyporeninemic hypoaldosteronism may also be exacerbated by the administration of beta-blocking agents or converting enzyme inhibitors.

Hyperkalemia is also a characteristic feature of *voltage-dependent renal tubular acidosis*. The latter is a specific defect in sodium transport of distal nephron segments. This blockade of distal sodium absorption reduces luminal electronegativity and consequently impairs both proton secretion and potassium secretion. Thus, voltage-dependent renal tubular acidosis, like hyporeninemic hypoaldosteronism, is characterized by sodium wasting and hyperkalemia. In hyporeninemic hypoaldosteronism, the urine is acidic, and plasma levels of aldosterone are reduced even during volume contraction, whereas in voltage-dependent renal tubular acidosis, there is impaired urinary acidification but a normal plasma aldosterone response to volume contraction.

Finally, in each of the disorders characterized by diminished renal potassium excretion, hyperkalemia can be aggravated by ECF volume contraction, which reduces sodium delivery to terminal nephron segments, or by acidosis, which promotes cellular potassium efflux.

Transcellular Shifts. The second class of disorders causing acute hyperkalemia includes situations in which there is an abrupt shift of potassium from the ICF to the ECF. This shift occurs in acidosis or in circumstances that result in *cell destruction;* the latter occurs commonly with tissue trauma, burns, rhabdomyolysis, or hemolysis, as well as with lysis of large masses of tumor cells. As indicated previously, hypokalemia predisposes to rhabdomyolysis. Thus the sudden occurrence of hyperkalemia in potassium-depleted patients is a diagnostic clue to the development of rhabdomyolysis.

Hyperkalemic periodic paralysis is an autosomal dominant disorder in which sudden increases in the serum potassium level result in muscle paralysis. The hyperkalemia is often provoked by dietary potassium intake or by exercise. Myotonia occurs commonly in the disorder and appears either between attacks or immediately preceding attacks. The pathogenesis of the disorder is not understood. The acute paralytic attack can be treated by intravenous administration of calcium gluconate or glucose and insulin. Chronic treatment with diuretics such as acetazolamide minimizes the frequency of attacks.

Paradoxical hyperkalemia occurs when *sudden hyperglycemia*

develops in insulin-dependent diabetics who also have interstitial renal disease and associated hyporeninemic hypoaldosteronism. The sudden increase in ECF osmolality draws water from cells, raises intracellular potassium concentrations, and therefore promotes passive potassium efflux from cells. The insulin lack minimizes cellular reentry of potassium, and the aldosterone deficiency blunts renal potassium excretion. Insulin therapy promptly corrects the hyperkalemia. Finally, anesthetic agents or other drugs that cause a *depolarizing muscle paralysis*, such as succinylcholine, promote potassium efflux from muscle cells. The loss of cell electronegativity in this situation increases passive potassium efflux from muscle cells.

Pseudohyperkalemia may occur in thrombocytosis or leukocytosis, because clotting of blood promotes potassium release from these cells and may be identified by noting that the *serum* potassium level is elevated while the *plasma* potassium level is normal. This kind of artifact occurs most commonly in patients with myeloproliferative disorders.

CLINICAL MANIFESTATIONS. The most important clinical manifestations of hyperkalemia relate to alterations in cardiac excitability. For this reason the electrocardiogram is the single most important guide in appraising the threat posed by hyperkalemia and in determining how aggressive a therapeutic approach is necessary.

The electrocardiographic manifestations of hyperkalemia, shown in Figure 75–8, follow directly from the effects of hyperkalemia on cardiac action potentials (see Fig. 75–6). The earliest manifestation of hyperkalemia is the development of peaked T waves, which become evident when the serum potassium level exceeds 6.5 mEq per liter. This peaking of the T waves is a manifestation of the accelerated repolarization of the cardiac action potential produced by hyperkalemia. When the potassium concentration exceeds 7 to 8 mEq per liter, diminished cardiac

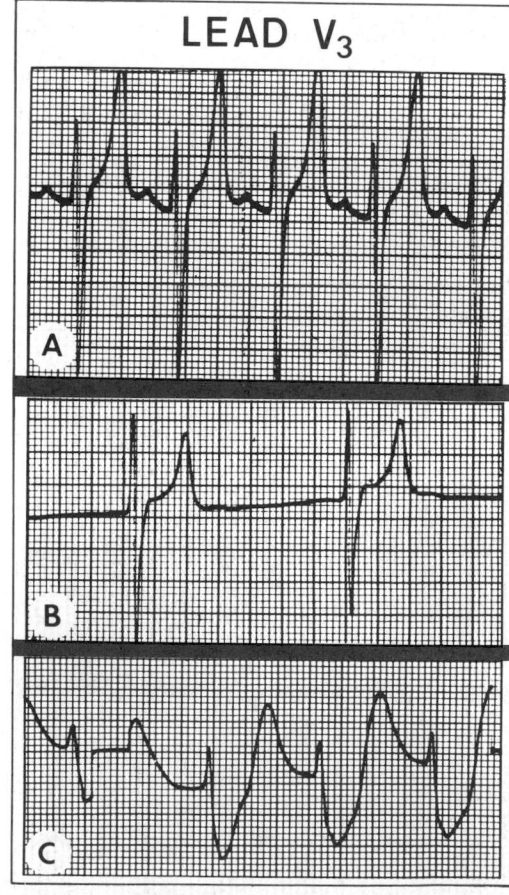

LEAD V₃

FIGURE 75–8. The effects of progressive hyperkalemia on the electrocardiogram. All of the illustrations are from lead V_3. *A*, Serum K^+ = 6.8 mEq per liter; note the peaked T waves together with normal sinus rhythm. *B*, Serum K^+ = 7.7 mEq per liter; note the peaked T waves and absent P waves. *C*, Serum K^+ = 8.9 mEq per liter; note the classic sine wave with absent P waves, marked prolongation of the QRS complex, and peaked T waves.

excitability results in prolongation of the PR interval, followed by a loss of P waves and widening of the QRS complex. These changes indicate progressive inexcitability of cardiac muscle and are referable to hyperkalemia-induced inactivation of sodium permeability during the initial spike of the action potential. When the serum potassium level exceeds 8 to 10 mEq per liter, the electrocardiogram may develop a sine wave pattern and cardiac standstill can occur.

The correlation between serum potassium concentrations and electrocardiographic abnormalities is approximate at best; in a given patient, progression from peaked T waves to a sine wave pattern may occur rapidly, particularly if the serum potassium concentration rises rapidly. Therefore the development of peaked T waves in conjunction with hyperkalemia should be viewed as a serious disorder; more advanced electrocardiographic manifestations of hyperkalemia should be treated as life-threatening medical emergencies.

TREATMENT. Three kinds of maneuvers are used in the treatment of hyperkalemia: agents such as glucose plus insulin, sodium bicarbonate, or beta agonists, which promote the transfer of potassium from the ECF to the ICF; maneuvers that enhance potassium elimination from the body, such as administration of diuretics or exchange resins or dialysis; and the use of calcium, which does not alter serum potassium concentrations but counteracts the effects of hyperkalemia on cardiac excitability.

Both insulin and sodium bicarbonate promote potassium entry into cells. The administration of 25 grams of glucose, together with 10 units of regular insulin, is an effective way of reducing the serum potassium level rapidly. The glucose may be administered over 30 minutes as a 20 per cent solution, or it may be given as a 50 per cent glucose solution. Insulin promotes potassium entry into cells, and glucose is administered to prevent hypoglycemia. In insulin-dependent diabetic patients in whom sudden hyperglycemia has precipitated the hyperkalemia, insulin administration alone suffices to reduce the serum potassium concentration.

Administering 40 to 150 mEq of sodium bicarbonate intravenously over a 30- to 60-minute interval also promotes potassium entry into cells, particularly if acidosis is also present. This maneuver should be used with caution in patients with compromised renal function because of the risks of hypernatremia and of ECF volume overload.

Potassium shifts from extracellular to intracellular fluids may also be enhanced by the use of aerosolized specific beta$_2$ agonists; albuterol is a commonly used agent of this kind. Agents such as albuterol are most helpful in the management of mild hyperkalemia in chronic disorders such as chronic renal failure and hyperkalemic periodic paralysis.

None of the maneuvers described above removes potassium from the body. Gastrointestinal potassium losses may be produced by the use of cation exchange resins in the sodium cycle, such as sodium polystyrene sulfonate (Kayexalate). Each gram of the resin contains approximately 1 mEq of sodium and exchanges for about 1 mEq of potassium. This stoichiometry is not precise, since the sodium form of the resin also exchanges for other cations in gastrointestinal secretions, including calcium. In chronic hyperkalemia, 20 grams of Kayexalate may be given three or four times a day in a 70 per cent solution of sorbitol. The sorbitol creates an osmotic diarrhea and enhances resin passage through the gastrointestinal tract. In acute circumstances, Kayexalate may also be administered by enema, generally as 100 grams of resin suspended in 200 ml of 20 per cent sorbitol. The use of chronic Kayexalate therapy in patients with chronic renal failure carries with it the risk of sodium overload.

In settings of extreme hyperkalemic cardiotoxicity, when P waves are absent and the QRS complexes are widened, the administration of calcium gluconate, 10 to 30 ml of a 10 per cent solution over a 10- to 20-minute interval, may be life saving. This approach should be undertaken with constant electrocardiographic monitoring and should be used with extreme caution in patients who have received digitalis. In the latter circumstances, calcium administration may unmask digitalis intoxication, especially if other agents are used simultaneously to reduce the serum potassium level. Calcium salts should not be added to bottles of intravenous fluids containing bicarbonate, because water-insoluble calcium salts will form.

The influence of calcium salts in minimizing the cardiotoxic

effects of hyperkalemia may be understood by noting, as described under Physiologic Considerations, that depolarization of excitable tissues by elevating serum K$^+$ concentrations inactivates sodium channels and that the extracellular sides of these sodium channels are electronegative. Divalent cations such as calcium provide a remarkably effective way of screening these electronegative sites. Thus calcium salts raise the voltage gradient across sodium channels by screening electronegative surface charges of these channels on their extracellular fluid sides and consequently restoring the voltage-dependent excitability of these channels.

Finally, acute hemodialysis or peritoneal dialysis provides another mechanism for potassium removal from the body. This approach is particularly advantageous in acute renal failure; when patients are volume expanded and sodium administration may produce congestive heart failure; or when there is a continued efflux of large amounts of potassium from the ICF to the ECF, as in burns or rhabdomyolysis.

Brem AS: Disorders of potassium homeostasis. Pediatr Clin North Am 37:419, 1990. *A concise clinical guide to disorders of potassium balance.*

Brown RS: Extrarenal potassium homeostasis. Kidney Int 30:116, 1986. *An account of extrarenal factors regulating potassium homeostasis.*

Castellino P, Bia M, DeFronzo RA: Adrenergic modulation of potassium metabolism in uremia. Kidney Int 27:793, 1990. *The role of beta-adrenergic agents in regulating potassium homeostasis in uremia.*

Clausen T, Everts ME: Regulation of the Na, K-pump in skeletal muscle. Kidney Int 35:1, 1989. *A description of the (Na$^+$ + K$^+$)-ATPase in skeletal muscle and its regulation by insulin and beta agonists.*

Kurtzman NA, Gonzalez J, DeFronzo R, et al.: A patient with hyperkalemia and metabolic acidosis. Am J Kidney Dis 15:333, 1990. *A concise account of the renal tubular disorders causing hyperkalemia.*

Montoliu J, Almirall J, Ponz E, et al.: Treatment of hyperkalemia with salbutamol inhalation. J Intern Med 228:35, 1990. *A description of the use of beta agonist nebulization in hyperkalemia.*

Tsien RW, Hess P: Excitable tissue—the heart. In Andreoli TE, Hoffman JF, Fanestil DD, et al. (eds.): Physiology of Membrane Disorders. New York, Plenum, 1986, pp 469–490. *A meticulous description of the ionic basis for the cardiac action potential.*

75.4 DISTURBANCES IN ACID-BASE BALANCE

PHYSIOLOGIC CONSIDERATIONS

The pH of arterial blood and interstitial fluid normally ranges between 7.38 and 7.42 despite wide variations in dietary intake of acids or alkali. The arterial pH range over which cardiac function, metabolic activity, and central nervous system function can be maintained is narrow; the widest range of pH values compatible with life is from 6.8 to 7.8, or an interval of one pH unit.

The major buffer system in extracellular fluid is the bicarbonate–carbonic acid pair. The relation between pH, bicarbonate, and carbonic acid concentrations in ECF may be expressed according to the familiar Henderson-Hasselbalch equation.

$$pH = pK + \log \frac{HCO_3^-}{H_2CO_3}$$

where pK is the carbonic acid dissociation constant, HCO_3^- is the plasma bicarbonate concentration, and H_2CO_3 is the plasma carbonic acid concentration. The H_2CO_3 concentration is given by αPa_{CO_2}, where α is the Co_2 solubility constant, and has a value of 0.03, and Pa_{CO_2} is the arterial carbon dioxide tension. Therefore, with a Pa_{CO_2} of 40 mm Hg, the Henderson-Hasselbalch equation becomes the following:

$$7.4 = 6.1 + \log \frac{24 \text{ mM/L}}{1.2 \text{ mM/L}}$$

The arterial pH provides a qualitative, but not quantitative, index to total body water acid-base status because, at any given time, about two thirds of an acid or alkali load is buffered by proton shifts into or out of the ICF, respectively. For this reason, some prefer to use the term "acidemia" for acidosis and "alkalemia" for alkalosis to connote that plasma pH measurements provide quantitative information about the pH status of plasma and interstitial fluid and only qualitative information about total body acid-base balance.

A convenient way to consider the total body buffering capacity is as follows. Bicarbonate is predominantly an extracellular anion, and the total ECF bicarbonate content in a 70-kg man having 15 liters of ECF is (24 mEq per liter $\times$ 15 liters), or 360 mEq HCO_3^-. However, about two thirds of a given acid or alkali load is buffered within cells. Consequently, the total body buffering capacity, often referred to as the "bicarbonate space," is calculated as:

$$(\text{Arterial } HCO_3^- \times 0.6 \text{ body weight})$$

that is, using total body water as an index to total buffering capacity. The bicarbonate space is also an index to net acid excess or net base excess. If the arterial HCO_3^- concentration in a 70-kg man is reduced to 15 mEq per liter while the Pa_{CO_2} remains constant, the net acid excess (or net base deficit) is $(24 - 15)$ mEq per liter $\times$ 42 liters = 378 mEq. Conversely, if the arterial HCO_3^- concentration rises to 33 mEq per liter while the Pa_{CO_2} remains constant, the net base excess (or acid deficit) is 378 mEq.

Proton shifts between the ECF and ICF stabilize the plasma pH against acute fluctuations. But the ultimate maintenance of pH balance requires that input of acid or base into the body be matched by output of acid or base, so that the HCO_3^-/H_2CO_3 ratio and the total bicarbonate content in the ECF remain constant. The cardinal systems involved in these external processes are the kidneys, for bicarbonate balance, and the lungs, for carbon dioxide balance.

Carbon Dioxide Production and Elimination

VOLATILE ACID INPUT. The largest source of endogenous acid production is from combustion of glucose and fatty acids to carbon dioxide and water or, in other words, to a volatile acid. During aerobic glycolysis, that is, cellular respiration, glucose oxidation involves oxygen utilization and carbon dioxide production according to the following reaction:

$$C_6H_{12}O_6 + 6O_2 \rightarrow 6CO_2 + 6H_2O$$

Since red blood cells contain carbonic anhydrase (c.a.), carbon dioxide hydration in erythrocytes yields the following:

$$CO_2 + H_2O \xrightleftharpoons{\text{c.a.}} H_2CO_3 \rightleftharpoons H^+ + HCO_3^-$$

The protons formed from carbonic acid dissociation are buffered by hemoglobin, whereas bicarbonate leaves red blood cells in exchange for chloride (the familiar chloride shift). In other words, carbon dioxide generation is equivalent to carbonic acid formation, and the bulk of hydrogen ion formed is buffered intracellularly.

A simple way of calculating the daily rate of nonvolatile acid production is to note, from the above reactions, that the production of 1 mole of metabolic water and 1 mole of carbon dioxide represents, through dissociation of carbonic acid, the formation of 1 mole of hydrogen ions.

Since the molecular weight of water is 18, 1 liter of water contains about 55 moles of water. Consequently, the average rate of metabolic water production, about 400 ml daily, yields 22,000 mmol of water and an equal number of carbon dioxide molecules. Thus the rate of volatile acid production amounts to about 22,000 mEq of hydrogen ion daily. The cellular combustion of carbohydrates and fatty acids to carbon dioxide and water is remarkably efficient. Under normal circumstances, organic anions such as lactate and keto acids, which derive from incomplete combustion of carbohydrates and fatty acids, have plasma concentrations of approximately 5 mEq per liter.

VOLATILE ACID OUTPUT. Pulmonary ventilation excretes the carbon dioxide formed by cellular respiration. During blood transit through the lungs, bicarbonate reenters red blood cells and combines with protons to form carbonic acid, which dissociates to carbon dioxide and water. The carbon dioxide so formed diffuses freely through red blood cells and alveolar epithelium, so that the rate of carbon dioxide excretion is governed primarily by the rate of minute ventilation.

MODULATION OF RESPIRATION. The prime factors normally regulating alterations in the rate of minute ventilation are subtle changes in cerebrospinal fluid (CSF) pH or arterial pH. Sensor chemoreceptors in central medullary centers or in the carotid body are activated by small reductions in CSF pH or arterial pH, respectively; the pH reduction can result either from carbon dioxide accumulation or from nonvolatile acid accumulation, which reduces the plasma bicarbonate concentration. In most circumstances, central medullary chemoreceptors provide the major impetus to altering ventilatory response, and the carotid body chemoreceptors serve as relatively minor stimuli to ventilation. The medullary respiratory centers therefore serve as the major *effector* mechanism for regulating carbon dioxide output by increasing ventilation rate.

The ventilatory response for carbon dioxide removal involves an increase in both tidal volume and respiratory rate. On an average, for every 1 mEq per liter reduction in plasma bicarbonate produced by metabolic acidosis, increased minute ventilation will produce a 1.0 to 1.2 mm Hg fall in the Pa_{CO_2}. In most circumstances, the maximum reduction in Pa_{CO_2} produced by the hyperventilatory response to severe metabolic acidosis is to a Pa_{CO_2} of 12 to 15 mm Hg; hyperventilation to Pa_{CO_2} values less than 10 mm Hg in metabolic acidosis almost never occurs. Conversely, an increase in arterial pH reduces the rate of minute ventilation and therefore results in carbon dioxide retention. For increases in plasma bicarbonate concentrations to 35 mEq per liter, the Pa_{CO_2} usually remains less than 50 mm Hg. When profound metabolic alkalosis occurs, the Pa_{CO_2} may rise further but virtually never exceeds 65 mm Hg.

Renal Bicarbonate Processing

In addition to volatile acid production due to carbon dioxide formation, cellular metabolism also results in the formation of a number of nonvolatile acids. The major source for nonvolatile acid production is the metabolism of sulfur-containing amino acids, such as cysteine and methionine, which results in sulfuric acid formation. Consequently, the daily rate of nonvolatile acid production is closely related to dietary protein intake and to the rate of endogenous protein catabolism. Nonvolatile acids also derive from oxidation of phosphoproteins and phospholipids, which results in phosphoric acid formation; nucleoprotein degradation, which yields uric acid; and incomplete combustion of carbohydrates and fatty acids, which produces lactic acid and the keto acids.

The daily rate of nonvolatile acid production under normal conditions is about 1 mEq per kilogram of body weight. Thus daily nonvolatile acid production would consume the total body fluid buffering capacity in about 2 weeks, were it not for the fact that the kidneys excrete nonvolatile acids and, in so doing, regenerate bicarbonate. Since the minimal urinary pH ordinarily attainable is 5.0 and the amount of nonvolatile acid to be excreted is about 70 mEq per day, renal hydrogen ion excretion, which is equivalent to renal bicarbonate regeneration, occurs mainly as protons trapped in an undissociated form by urinary buffers.

The kidneys also filter large quantities of bicarbonate daily: For a normal plasma bicarbonate concentration of 24 mEq per liter and a glomerular filtration of 180 liters per day, the net amount of bicarbonate filtered daily is approximately 4300 mEq, or about four times the total body buffering capacity. Thus, in addition to generating new bicarbonate, the renal tubules must also absorb filtered bicarbonate.

BICARBONATE REABSORPTION. Virtually all filtered bicarbonate is absorbed, together with sodium, by the proximal tubule. Within renal tubular cells, CO_2 is hydrated to H_2CO_3. Apical membrane Na^+ exchange permits H^+ secretion into urine and Na^+ entry into cells, with subsequent absorption of sodium bicarbonate into blood.

The rate of proximal bicarbonate reabsorption is modulated by the same *effectors* that regulate proximal sodium absorption. Among these, the ECV exerts a central effect. Volume expansion, which resets glomerulotubular balance downward, reduces the fractional rate of proximal bicarbonate reabsorption. Conversely, volume contraction raises the bicarbonate threshold by increasing the fractional rate of proximal tubular sodium bicarbonate reabsorption.

Two other *effectors* regulate, in operational terms, the rate of bicarbonate reabsorption. One of these is the arterial Pa_{CO_2}: High

Pa_{CO_2} values raise the apparent bicarbonate threshold, whereas low Pa_{CO_2} values reduce the rate of bicarbonate reabsorption. This factor accounts for the compensatory increase in plasma bicarbonate concentrations in respiratory acidosis. Second, hypokalemia also increases the rate of bicarbonate reabsorption, presumably by raising the intracellular hydrogen ion concentration. This factor accounts for the fact that in hypokalemic, hypochloremic metabolic alkalosis associated with volume contraction, alkalosis can persist after volume deficits are restored. In this circumstance, correction of potassium deficits is required for correction of the alkalosis.

BICARBONATE REGENERATION. The excretion of nonvolatile acids and the simultaneous renal regeneration of bicarbonate occur principally in distal nephron segments. Distal renal tubular cells hydrate carbon dioxide to carbonic acid, which dissociates to protons, which are secreted into urine, and bicarbonate anions, which are absorbed into blood. The major mode of proton secretion in terminal nephron segments, particularly collecting tubules, involves an apical membrane proton-ATPase.

The secreted protons titrate urinary buffers, principally phosphate, while sodium is absorbed. Thus the overall reaction is as follows:

$$Na_2HPO_4 + H^+ + HCO_3^- \longrightarrow NaH_2PO_4 + NaHCO_3$$
$$\textit{(filtered)} \qquad\qquad\qquad \textit{(excreted)} \quad \textit{(absorbed)}$$

Titratable acid formation normally accounts for about one third of renal acid excretion. The remaining two thirds of acid excretion is accounted for by ammonia (NH_3) secretion by the following sequence:

$$NaR + NH_3 + H^+ + HCO_3^- \longrightarrow NaHCO_3 + NH_4R$$
$$\textit{(filtered)} \qquad\qquad\qquad\qquad \textit{(reabsorbed)} \quad \textit{(excreted)}$$

where NaR is the filtered sodium salt of a nonvolatile acid, NH_3 is ammonia produced by renal tubular cells, and the protons and bicarbonate come from carbon dioxide hydration by tubular cells.

Distal acid excretion and bicarbonate absorption are accompanied by sodium absorption. Consequently, *effector* systems that enhance distal sodium absorption, such as aldosterone or increased rates of sodium delivery to terminal nephron segments, also promote terminal nephron hydrogen ion excretion. Three other *effector* mechanisms also increase the rate of hydrogen ion excretion: (1) Delivery of sodium to terminal nephron segments in association with impermeant anions such as sulfate favors proton movement from tubular cells to lumen. (2) Hypokalemia enhances hydrogen ion excretion, particularly in sodium-acquisitive states, presumably because hypokalemia is accompanied by a fall in intracellular pH. (3) Acidosis stimulates ammoniagenesis by renal tubular cells; consequently, in metabolic acidosis, increases in the rate of renal acid excretion are referable primarily to increased rates of ammonium excretion. In other words, these last-named three effector systems enhance renal acid excretion by creating a favorable situation for proton transfer from tubular cells to urine. Conversely, aldosterone deficiency, alkalosis, or reduced rates of salt delivery to terminal nephron segments reduce renal capacity for acid excretion.

pH Disequilibria Between Plasma and CSF

Central rather than arterial chemoreceptors are the prime sensors for pH-mediated changes in respiration. The ventilatory responses to pH changes mediated by respiratory processes and by metabolic processes therefore differ. The blood-brain barrier is freely permeable to carbon dioxide. Consequently, pH changes produced exclusively by hyperventilation or hypoventilation occur almost simultaneously in arterial plasma and in the CSF, and the respiratory response to primary increases or decreases in Pa_{CO_2} occurs almost instantaneously. The blood-brain barrier imposes a lag, however, in the rate at which arterial bicarbonate equilibrates with the CSF. Thus in metabolic acidosis, the arterial pH and bicarbonate concentration fall more rapidly than they do in the CSF; and in metabolic alkalosis, the CSF pH and bicarbonate concentration rise more slowly than they do in arterial plasma. Consequently, in the early stages of acute metabolic acidosis, there may be a 1- to 3-hour delay in the development of a maximal hyperventilatory response. Conversely, when metabolic acidosis is corrected rapidly, hyperventilation may persist for a few hours because of a delay in the rise of cerebrospinal fluid pH.

An unusual situation relating to this effect occurs in diabetic ketoacidosis and in certain other metabolic acidoses associated with impaired central nervous system function. In these situations, carotid body chemoreceptors, rather than central medullary chemoreceptors, provide the major stimulus to respiration driven by a reduced arterial pH. The rapid correction of ECF acidosis by bicarbonate administration reduces the rate at which carotid body chemoreceptors drive ventilation. When this occurs, Pa_{CO_2} levels in plasma and in the CSF rise almost simultaneously; but because of a lag in the rate of bicarbonate entry into the CSF, the CSF bicarbonate/carbonic acid ratio tends to fall. In severe diabetic ketoacidosis, this situation can result in an actual fall in CSF pH simultaneously with a rise in arterial pH produced by intravenous bicarbonate administration.

DEFINITION OF ACID-BASE ABNORMALITIES

The arterial pH is determined by the ratio of the bicarbonate–carbonic acid buffer system, as expressed in the Henderson-Hasselbalch equation. These data also provide an index of total body acid-base balance, because, as indicated in the preceding section, the majority of body buffering occurs within cells. Acid-base disturbance can therefore occur either by altering the serum bicarbonate concentration, referred to as a "metabolic" disorder, or by altering arterial carbon dioxide tension, referred to as a "respiratory" disorder. A convenient way for considering these disturbances is illustrated in Figure 75–9, which illustrates pH isobars (for pH 7.0, 7.4, and 7.8) calculated according to the Henderson-Hasselbalch equation for the bicarbonate concentrations and Pa_{CO_2} values listed on the ordinate and abscissa, respectively.

TYPES OF ACID-BASE ABNORMALITIES. The left-hand panel in Figure 75–9 shows the directional changes in Pa_{CO_2} and bicarbonate concentrations that *initiate* the four basic types of acid-base abnormalities. *Respiratory acidosis* results from hypoventilation and reduces pH by raising the Pa_{CO_2}. *Respiratory alkalosis* results from hyperventilation and raises pH by reducing the Pa_{CO_2}. *Metabolic alkalosis* occurs when increases in the plasma bicarbonate concentration raise pH, and *metabolic acidosis* occurs when reductions in plasma bicarbonate decrease pH.

Any of these initial acid-base disturbances activates *compensatory responses*, illustrated in the right-hand panel of Figure 75–9, that tend to minimize the pH changes produced by the initial acid-base abnormality. By comparing the directional arrows in the left- and right-hand panels of Figure 75–9, it becomes evident that the initial disturbance in any of these four acid-base abnormalities tends to displace the arterial pH away from the pH 7.4 isobar and that the compensatory response partially restores arterial pH values toward the pH 7.4 isobar. The arterial pH, Pa_{CO_2}, and plasma bicarbonate concentrations illustrated in the right-hand panel of Figure 75–9 are the values usually observed clinically in the four primary acid-base disturbances.

The Compensatory Responses. As indicated in Figure 75–9, a compensatory response blunts the effect of the initial insult on pH homeostasis. In *primary respiratory disorders*, the renal response is to change the proximal tubular bicarbonate threshold and consequently the plasma bicarbonate concentration. A good rule of thumb is that for every 1 mm Hg rise or fall in the arterial Pa_{CO_2}, the plasma bicarbonate concentration rises or falls, respectively, by approximately 0.3 to 0.5 mEq per liter. This renal adaptive response is relatively slow, however, and requires 24 to 48 hours for complete expression. Consequently, the renal response to a respiratory acid-base disorder affords relatively little pH compensation in the first 12 to 18 hours in acute respiratory acidosis or alkalosis.

In chronic respiratory acidosis, as, for example, in chronic obstructive pulmonary disease, renal bicarbonate retention provides adequate but not complete compensation for CO_2 retention. Chronic respiratory alkalosis is relatively uncommon in clinical settings. The renal response to chronic respiratory alkalosis is discussed below.

The pulmonary response to primary *metabolic acid-base disorders* involves an alteration in the rate of minute ventilation. In

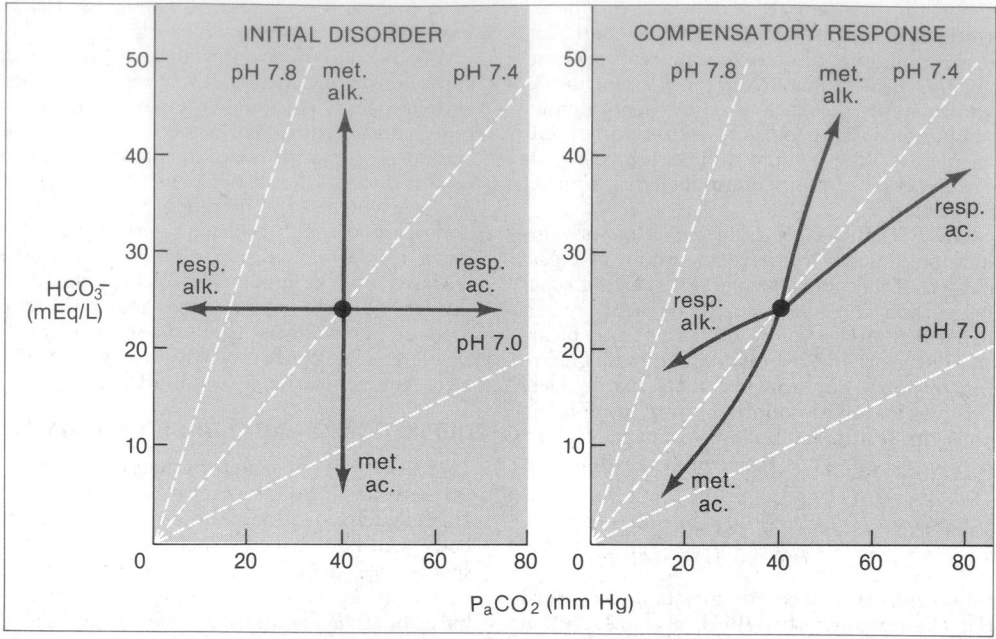

FIGURE 75–9. Schematic frame of reference for considering acid-base disturbances. The dotted lines are the pH isobars for pH values of 7.8, 7.4, and 7.0 computed from the Henderson-Hasselbalch equation for given combinations of arterial bicarbonate values (vertical axes) and arterial carbon dioxide tensions (horizontal axes). The graph on the left shows the initial derangement in HCO_3^- concentrations in metabolic acidosis and metabolic alkalosis and the initial $PaCO_2$ derangement in respiratory acidosis and respiratory alkalosis. Note that each of the four changes in either HCO_3^- or $PaCO_2$ tends to displace the arterial pH from the pH 7.4 isobar. The graph on the right, labeled "Compensatory Response," indicates the general trend of pH, HCO_3^-, and $PaCO_2$ changes actually observed in the four primary acid-base disturbances: respiratory acidosis, respiratory alkalosis, metabolic acidosis, and metabolic alkalosis. Respiratory acidosis and alkalosis are accompanied by compensatory renal bicarbonate retention and loss, respectively. Metabolic acidosis and alkalosis are accompanied by compensatory hyperventilation and hypoventilation, respectively. Note that the compensatory response in each of the four acid-base disorders tends to restore arterial pH values toward the pH 7.4 isobar.

general, a 1 mEq per liter decrease or increase in the plasma bicarbonate concentration produces a 1.0 to 1.2 mm Hg decrease or increase in the arterial Pa_{CO_2}, respectively. This ventilatory response begins within minutes of the onset of the metabolic abnormality. The full expression of the ventilatory response may be delayed for 1 to 3 hours if, as noted above, a pH disequilibrium exists between plasma and CSF.

Three other characteristics of these compensatory responses should be noted. The compensatory responses do not, in general, provide complete compensation for the initial abnormality. Moreover, the magnitude of the compensatory response may vary in individual patients and may be affected by pre-existing conditions. For example, the ventilatory response to sepsis with lactic acidosis is considerably less in patients with chronic obstructive pulmonary disease than in normal individuals. Finally, a near-normal arterial pH may also be due to offsetting metabolic derangements rather than to physiologic compensatory processes. For example, in diabetic ketoacidosis, a fall in arterial pH may be offset by a metabolic alkalosis secondary to vomiting rather than by Kussmaul's ventilation (see below).

THE SERUM ANION GAP. Sodium is the principal cation in extracellular fluids. The sum of plasma chloride plus bicarbonate concentrations is less than the serum sodium concentration; the remaining anions required for electroneutrality, generally not reported with routine serum electrolyte measurements, are referred to as unmeasured anions, or as the serum anion gap. A convenient formula for calculating the serum anion gap is the following:

$$\text{Serum anion gap} = Na^+ - (Cl^- + HCO_3^-)$$

where Na^+, Cl^-, and HCO_3^- are the serum sodium, chloride, and bicarbonate concentrations, respectively. The serum anion gap includes primarily phosphates and sulfates derived from tissue metabolism; lactate and keto acids arising from incomplete combustion of carbohydrates and fatty acids; and negatively charged protein molecules, principally albumin. The normal value for

unmeasured anions, or the serum anion gap, is 10 to 12 mEq per liter; albumin and other proteins normally account for about half of the anion gap.

An *increased* serum anion gap generally indicates the presence of metabolic acidosis. The factors responsible for this kind of metabolic acidosis are discussed in the next section.

A *reduced* serum anion gap provides a clue to the presence of certain other disorders. The anion gap will be reduced if the sodium concentration falls while the chloride plus bicarbonate concentrations are unchanged or, in other words, when the concentration of another cation in serum is increased while the serum osmolality remains normal. This may occur in multiple myeloma of the immunoglobulin G (IgG) variety if the myeloma proteins are cationic at pH 7.4. Hyperviscosity syndromes may also result in a reduced anion gap because of a laboratory artifact: When serum is excessively viscous, automatic pumps deliver decreased volumes of serum to a flame photometer, producing artifactual reductions in sodium concentrations. Rarely, lithium intoxication, hypermagnesemia, and hypercalcemia raise nonsodium cation concentrations sufficiently high to reduce the anion gap.

The serum anion gap will also be decreased if the serum sodium concentration remains normal while the serum chloride plus bicarbonate concentrations are increased. This situation occurs most commonly in hypoalbuminemia. A low serum anion gap also occurs in bromide intoxication, since colorimetric techniques for serum chloride determinations give spuriously high values for chloride plus bromide when bromide is present in relatively high concentrations in serum.

THE URINARY ANION GAP. The urinary anion gap, defined as

$$\text{Urinary anion gap} = (Na^+ + K^+) - Cl^-$$

is a useful measurement in evaluating patients with hyperchloremic acidosis. The test provides an approximate index of urinary NH_4 excretion, as measured by a negative urinary anion gap, that

TABLE 75–13. CHARACTERISTICS OF DISTAL RENAL TUBULAR ACIDOSIS (RTA) SYNDROMES

Condition	Urinary pH	Serum K+	Urinary Anion Gap	Response to Furosemide		Aldosterone Secretion
				Urinary pH	*Urinary K+*	
Gradient-limited RTA	>5.5	↓	Positive	Unchanged	↑	Normal
Hyporeninemic hypoaldosteronism	<5.5	↑	Positive	↓	↑	Reduced
Voltage-dependent RTA	>5.5	↑	Positive	Unchanged	Unchanged	Normal

is, urinary $(Na^+ + K^+)$ is less than urinary Cl^-. Thus, in hyperchloremic metabolic acidosis, a normal renal response would be a negative urinary anion gap, generally in the range of 30 to 50 mEq per liter. In such an instance, it is likely that the hyperchloremic acidosis is due to gastrointestinal losses rather than a renal lesion. In contrast, a positive urinary anion gap implies a renal tubular disorder, as is discussed below.

URINARY RESPONSE TO ORAL FUROSEMIDE. The urinary response to oral furosemide loading is another useful test for evaluating tubular acidifying capability. The rationale for the test is that in normal individuals blockade of sodium absorption in diluting segments by furosemide increases sodium delivery to distal nephron segments where potassium and protons are secreted (see above) and increases the rate of excretion of the latter two moieties. Consequently, the oral administration of 40 to 80 mg of furosemide should be followed, in a subsequent 4- to 6-hour urinary collection, by an increase in urinary sodium excretion and fractional sodium excretion, an increase in urinary potassium excretion and fractional potassium excretion, and a reduction in urinary pH. In some renal tubular acidosis syndromes, proton and/or potassium excretion is impaired (Table 75–13).

METABOLIC ACIDOSIS

ETIOLOGY AND PATHOGENESIS. A convenient way to consider the metabolic acidoses is to divide them into two groups: normal anion gap and increased anion gap metabolic acidoses (Table 75–14). The pathogeneses of these two groups differ appreciably.

NORMAL ANION GAP METABOLIC ACIDOSIS. The metabolic acidoses having a *normal anion gap* result whenever there are abnormally high net bicarbonate losses. This situation may occur because the kidneys fail to reabsorb or regenerate bicarbonate; because there are extrarenal losses of bicarbonate; or because excessive amounts of substances yielding hydrochloric acid have been administered.

Bicarbonate Losses. Bicarbonate losses occur either when the proximal tubule fails to absorb virtually all filtered bicarbonate, that is, when the apparent bicarbonate threshold is reduced, or when there are losses of bicarbonate from the gastrointestinal tract.

Renal bicarbonate wasting occurs in *proximal renal tubular acidosis*, either alone or as part of Fanconi's syndrome (Ch. 82). The apparent threshold for bicarbonate in this disorder is set below the normal value of 26 mEq of bicarbonate per deciliter of glomerular filtrate and may be as low as 15 to 20 mEq of bicarbonate per deciliter of glomerular filtrate. Consequently, bicarbonate wasting occurs whenever the plasma bicarbonate level is raised above the apparent renal threshold for bicarbonate.

Attempts to correct the acidosis of proximal renal tubular acidosis by bicarbonate administration are generally unrewarding, because increases in the plasma bicarbonate level produced by administering bicarbonate salts are accompanied by corresponding increases in bicarbonaturia. A promising approach to this disorder involves reducing the ECV by sodium restriction. This maneuver exploits the fact that ECF contraction resets glomerulotubular balance upward and consequently increases the fractional rate of sodium, and hence bicarbonate, reabsorption by the proximal tubule.

A converse of this situation is sometimes referred to as *dilutional acidosis*. Individuals who are volume expanded reduce the fractional rate of sodium bicarbonate absorption by the proximal tubule and consequently develop mild reductions in plasma bicarbonate concentrations. *Carbonic anhydrase inhibitors* such

as acetazolamide inhibit proximal sodium bicarbonate absorption, resulting in metabolic acidosis. *Primary hyperparathyroidism* also reduces the apparent bicarbonate threshold in the proximal tubule; mild degrees of hyperchloremic acidosis are commonly noted in patients with this disorder.

Gastrointestinal bicarbonate wasting can occur in several circumstances. Both pancreatic and small bowel secretions are rich in bicarbonate; pancreatic fluid, for example, has a pH of approximately 8.0. Hence *diarrheal states* and *ileal drainage* can result in significant bicarbonate losses. *Ureterosigmoidostomy* results in metabolic acidosis because the colon can secrete bicarbonate in exchange for chloride. Thus in patients with this surgical procedure, urine reaching the colon is alkalinized by bicarbonate exchange for chloride, thereby producing a net bicarbonate loss.

Failure of Bicarbonate Regeneration. The second major group of disorders producing hyperchloremic acidosis includes those disorders in which the ability of the distal nephron to regenerate bicarbonate is impaired. Three different tubular disorders account for the majority of cases of renal hyperchloremia encountered clinically. *Classic gradient-limited renal tubular acidosis* is a tubular disorder in which proton secretion may be normal, but because the distal tubule is unable to maintain a steep urine to blood proton concentration gradient, secreted protons are recycled back to blood. The administration of large quantities of phosphate salts permits the excretion of large amounts of titratable acid in this disorder, because the pH of the phosphate buffer system is 6.8, that is, relatively high. Potassium wasting and hypokalemia are common in distal gradient-limited renal tubular acidosis, owing at least in part to secondary hyperaldosteronism stimulated by sodium wasting.

In *hyporeninemic hypoaldosteronism*, which generally occurs in association with interstitial disease, the distal tubular derangements include diminished rates of sodium absorption and diminished rates of proton and potassium secretion. Aldosterone secretion is impaired. Consequently, sodium wasting and hyperkalemic, hyperchloremic acidosis are the hallmarks of this disorder. Diuretics such as *triamterene, spironolactone,* and

TABLE 75–14. MAJOR CAUSES OF METABOLIC ACIDOSIS

Normal Anion Gap	Increased Anion Gap
I. **Bicarbonate Loss**	I. **Reduced Excretion of Inorganic Acids**
Proximal renal tubular acidosis	Renal failure
Dilutional acidosis	II. **Accumulation of Organic Acids**
Carbonic anhydrase inhibitors	
Primary hyperparathyroidism	Lactic acidosis
Diarrheal states	Ketoacidosis: alcoholic
Small bowel drainage	diabetic
Ureterosigmoidostomy	starvation
II. **Failure of Bicarbonate Regeneration**	Ingestion: salicylates
Distal, gradient-limited renal tubular acidosis	paraldehyde
Hyporeninemic hypoaldosteronism	methanol
Diuretics: triamterene, spironolactone	ethylene glycol
III. **Acidifying Salts**	
Ammonium chloride	
Lysine hydrochloride	
Arginine hydrochloride	
Parenteral hyperalimentation	

amiloride, which interfere with distal tubular sodium absorption, proton secretion, and potassium secretion, also result in hyperkalemic, hyperchloremic metabolic acidosis (Table 75–5).

Finally, *voltage-dependent renal tubular acidosis*, also known as hyperkalemic tubular acidosis, is a disorder characterized by an impaired ability of the distal nephron to absorb sodium and by an inability to secrete either potassium or protons. The latter two secretory deficits appear to be secondary to the defect in sodium absorption, which diminishes the magnitude of the lumen-negative transepithelial voltage in those nephron segments. Aldosterone secretion is normal.

Table 75–13 provides a summary of the distinguishing features of the three renal tubular acidosis syndromes. It should be noted that when hyporeninemic hypoaldosteronism is associated with extensive interstitial disease, the ability to increase urinary potassium excretion or decrease urinary pH in response to furosemide may be blunted.

Acidifying Salts. The third major group of conditions producing hyperchloremic acidosis includes the administration of *acidifying salts*, such as ammonium hydrochloride, lysine hydrochloride, or arginine hydrochloride. In each instance, metabolism of the ammonium or of the amino acids leads to hydrochloric acid formation. *Parenteral hyperalimentation* without the administration of adequate amounts of bicarbonate or bicarbonate-yielding solutes (such as lactate or acetate) can also produce hyperchloremic metabolic acidosis. The acidosis occurs because the synthetic amino acids used in hyperalimentation mixtures contain positively charged amino acids, such as arginine, lysine, and histidine, which yield proton equivalents when metabolized.

INCREASED ANION GAP METABOLIC ACIDOSIS. Metabolic acidoses characterized by an increased anion gap occur either because the kidneys fail to excrete inorganic acids, such as phosphate or sulfate, or because there is net accumulation of organic acids.

Reduced Acid Excretion. Renal failure, either acute or chronic, results in metabolic acidosis with an increased anion gap due to retention of sulfates and phosphates. In chronic renal failure metabolic acidosis occurs because the net amount of ammonium excreted daily falls as functional renal mass diminishes. The plasma bicarbonate concentration in most patients with chronic renal failure ranges between 16 and 20 mEq per liter. Although this degree of acidosis appears relatively modest, the daily acid load is buffered by bone salts; this buffering may contribute to the osteopenia of chronic renal failure (Ch. 237). In acute tubular necrosis, acidosis occurs because of generalized tubular dysfunction, including impaired net acid excretion. The plasma bicarbonate level generally remains above 16 mEq per liter unless sepsis, profound hypoxia, or extensive tissue necrosis complicates the disorder.

Organic Acid Accumulation. Accumulation of organic acids represents the second major cause for metabolic acidosis with an increased anion gap and is the most common cause for acute metabolic acidosis. Normally, the complete combustion of carbohydrates and fatty acids to carbon dioxide and water is highly efficient and results in the production of approximately 22,000 mEq of hydrogen ion per day. Thus, the lungs eliminate, as expired carbon dioxide, more than 300 times as much acid as the 70 mEq of fixed acid excreted daily by the kidneys as titratable acid plus ammonia. Processes that impair cellular respiration, and therefore result in nonvolatile rather than volatile acid production, lead to profound metabolic acidosis. In these circumstances, the interplay of four cardinal factors determines the magnitude of the anion gap acidosis.

The first two of these factors are insulin and glucagon, and the interplay between these two hormones. In disorders such as diabetic ketoacidosis or starvation, insulin lack accelerates lipolysis while aerobic glycolysis is impaired. Concomitantly, glucagon increases augment ketogenesis by the liver.

The third variable is the rate of cellular respiration, which in practical terms is determined by the rate of tissue perfusion with oxygen and the functional state of mitochondria. Lactic acidosis due to hypoperfusion or phenformin therefore is an anion gap acidosis caused by impaired cellular respiration.

The last factor determining the magnitude of the anion gap for such conditions is the extent of renal perfusion, which in turn regulates the proximal renal tubular threshold for organic acid excretion. Thus in diabetic ketoacidosis, volume expansion with normal saline can convert a large anion gap acidosis to a normal anion gap acidosis, not by correcting the underlying metabolic derangement, which requires insulin, but simply by increasing the rate of renal organic acid excretion.

The syndrome of *lactic acidosis* results from impaired cellular respiration. Lactic acid is produced in muscle, red blood cells, and other tissues as a consequence of anaerobic glycolysis. Lactic acid oxidation involves reduction of nicotine adenine dinucleotide (NAD) by lactic acid dehydrogenase (LDH) according to the following reaction:

$$\text{Lactate} + \text{NAD} \underset{\text{LDH}}{\overset{}{\rightleftharpoons}} \text{pyruvate} + \text{NADH}$$

Cellular respiration involves mitochondrial oxidation of pyruvate and NADH to carbon dioxide and water. When lactic acidosis occurs because of impaired cellular respiration, the lactate to pyruvate ratio (L/P) rises, as does the NADH/NAD ratio. Thus glycolysis in a setting of impaired cellular respiration results in increased production of nonvolatile lactic acid. Lactic acidosis should not be confused with states in which serum lactate levels are elevated with normal L/P and NADH/NAD ratios, as, for example, in vigorous exercise. Lactic acidosis is also characterized by negative serum nitroprusside (Acetest) reactions, since Acetest tablets react with acetoacetic acid and acetone, but not with lactic acid or beta-hydroxybutyric acid. In lactic acidosis the beta-hydroxybutyric acid/acetoacetic acid ratio is elevated in parallel with the increased NADH/NAD ratio.

Lactic acidosis occurs most commonly in disorders characterized by inadequate oxygen delivery to tissues, such as shock, septicemia, and profound hypoxemia. Drug-induced lactic acidosis may occur with phenformin therapy and isoniazid toxicity; in both circumstances, oxygen utilization by tissues is thought to be impaired. Lactic acidosis also occurs in association with leukemia and diabetes mellitus. A negative serum Acetest reaction in patients with diabetes acidosis is a valuable clue to the coexistence of diabetic ketoacidosis and lactic acidosis. There is also a spontaneous, idiopathic form of lactic acidosis in debilitated patients, which is almost uniformly fatal.

A second group of disorders characterized by an anion gap metabolic acidosis includes those disorders in which cellular respiration may not be impaired, but accelerated rates of organic acid production, particularly from lipolysis, result in an increased anion gap. *Alcoholic ketoacidosis* occurs in patients with chronic alcoholism and a recent history of binge drinking, little or no food intake, and recurrent vomiting. Hypoglycemia may be present. The major pathogenic mechanism for alcoholic ketoacidosis is accelerated lipolysis and hepatic ketoacid production because of relative decreases and increases in the secretion rates for insulin and glucagon, respectively. The Acetest reaction is variably positive, and the beta-hydroxybutyrate/acetoacetate ratio is elevated. Lactate utilization is diminished in this disorder. Patients with alcoholic ketoacidosis have beta-hydroxybutyric acid, rather than lactic acid, as the principal nonvolatile acid. *Diabetic ketoacidosis* is the most common cause of metabolic acidosis with an increased anion gap and occurs because of increased rates of ketogenesis due to insulin lack and inadequate carbohydrate combustion. *Starvation* produces metabolic acidosis by essentially the same mechanism: increased hepatic ketogenesis with reduced caloric intake. Thus in a general sense, alcoholic ketoacidosis, diabetic ketoacidosis, and starvation share at least one common feature: accelerated lipolysis and ketogenesis due to a relative insulin lack coupled with a relative glucagon excess.

Finally, a number of ingested substances result in severe metabolic acidosis with a large anion gap. *Salicylism* produces a complex set of acid-base abnormalities. Salicylates stimulate ventilation through central mechanisms; the decrease in Pa_{CO_2} then results in reductions in plasma bicarbonate concentrations. Since salicylate is a relatively strong acid, the ingestion of large quantities of salicylate can, by itself, contribute to metabolic acidosis and an increased anion gap. Salicylates also interfere with mitochondrial function. As a consequence, a number of as yet unidentified organic acids accumulate in serum and are the major factors responsible for the anion gap acidosis of salicylism.

A number of other agents, including *paraldehyde, methanol,* and *ethylene glycol,* also produce severe metabolic acidosis with organic acid accumulation. In methanol poisoning, formic acid (an end-product of methanol metabolism) accounts in large part for the reduction in serum bicarbonate concentration. In ethylene glycol intoxication, glycolic and lactic acid accumulation accounts for the majority of the reduction in plasma bicarbonate level; however, oxalate deposition in tissues is clearly a major factor in ethylene glycol toxicity. The organic acids responsible for an increased anion gap in paraldehyde intoxication have not been identified.

DIAGNOSIS AND TREATMENT. The diagnosis of metabolic acidosis requires analysis of serum electrolytes and, when indicated, measurement of arterial pH and Pa_{CO_2}. A cardinal clinical manifestation of metabolic acidosis is hyperventilation, which, when severe, is manifest as Kussmaul's respiration. In patients with chronic metabolic acidosis, however, hyperventilation may be difficult to detect clinically.

Severe metabolic acidosis exerts a negative inotropic effect on the heart, which depends, at least in part, on the fact that acidosis diminishes tissue responsiveness to catecholamines. Thus in lactic acidosis, negative inotropy sets the stage for a potentially lethal chain of events: poor tissue perfusion → lactic acidosis → decreased cardiac function → further reduction in tissue perfusion.

Acidosis also affects the delivery of oxygen to tissues. In acidosis, the Bohr effect shifts the oxyhemoglobin dissociation curve to the right. This compensatory mechanism permits the delivery of oxygen to inadequately perfused tissues. However, the protective characteristics of the Bohr effect may be offset by the effect of pH variation on red blood cell 2,3-diphosphoglycerate (2,3-DPG). Increases in red cell 2,3-DPG also shift the oxyhemoglobin dissociation curve to the right. However, acidosis tends to reduce red blood cell 2,3-DPG; this may offset partially the compensatory Bohr effect and therefore aggravate inadequate tissue oxygenation in acidosis.

Since metabolic acidosis is a manifestation of a variety of different diseases, the treatment of metabolic acidosis varies, depending on the underlying process and on the acuteness and severity of the acidosis. Certain general principles serve as useful guidelines for therapy. Those disorders characterized by *failure of bicarbonate regeneration* or *reduced excretion of inorganic acids* represent acidoses in which the kidneys fail to excrete a normal load of nonvolatile acid or, in other words, fail to regenerate approximately 70 mEq of bicarbonate daily. Thus the treatment of these metabolic acidoses requires removal of the offending agent, if patients are receiving triamterene or spironolactone, and the administration of relatively modest amounts of bicarbonate. In chronic renal failure, alkali therapy is generally not required unless the plasma bicarbonate level falls below 16 to 18 mEq per liter. If the acidosis is more severe, bicarbonate supplementation in the form of Shohl's solution (see below) may be instituted. Caution should be exercised to avoid sodium overload or the appearance of tetany, if overalkalinization occurs.

In distal, gradient-limited renal tubular acidosis, the administration of 30 to 60 mEq of bicarbonate daily, either as sodium bicarbonate tablets or as Shohl's solution, usually corrects the acidosis. A 650-mg sodium bicarbonate tablet provides 7.7 mEq of bicarbonate. Shohl's solution is a mixture of sodium citrate and citric acid; 1 ml of Shohl's solution yields the equivalent of 1 mmol of sodium bicarbonate. The cost of sodium bicarbonate, either as tablets or as common baking soda, is considerably less than that of Shohl's solution.

Potassium supplementation is also required in treatment of the disorder. In children with distal renal tubular acidosis, greater quantities of bicarbonate, in the range of 5 to 14 mEq of alkali per kilogram per day, are usually required to avoid growth retardation.

The therapy of patients with metabolic acidosis due to *external bicarbonate loss* varies with the nature of the disorder. As indicated above, sodium restriction, and an attendant rise in the apparent bicarbonate threshold, may be helpful in treating proximal renal tubular acidosis. In acute metabolic acidosis due to gastrointestinal losses, the net bicarbonate deficit may be roughly calculated, as indicated previously, from the reduction in "bicarbonate space," or total body buffering capacity, as follows:

$$(24 \text{ mEq/L} - \text{measured plasma } HCO_3^-) \times 0.6 \text{ body weight (kg)}$$

Bicarbonate therapy should be instituted when the arterial pH falls below 7.1. It is prudent to administer sufficient sodium bicarbonate intravenously to raise the plasma bicarbonate concentration to 16 mEq per liter over a 12- to 24-hour interval, rather than to repair the entire bicarbonate deficit. Calculation of the bicarbonate deficit in this manner is valid only if there are no further bicarbonate losses. If the latter persist, as in cholera or other types of secretory diarrhea, the daily amount of bicarbonate given to maintain the plasma bicarbonate concentration in the range of 16 mEq per liter may actually exceed the calculated bicarbonate space.

The treatment of acidoses due to *accumulation of organic acids* varies with the disorder. In *lactic acidosis,* therapy should be directed toward improving tissue perfusion. Because the disorder results from a failure of conversion of lactic acid and other organic acids to carbon dioxide and water, large amounts of sodium bicarbonate, sometimes in excess of 1000 mEq per 24-hour period, have been used in attempts to avoid lethal acidosis.

The treatment is complicated by the fact that the response to alkali therapy is not predictable. In experimental lactic acidosis, dichloroacetate can raise arterial pH by suppressing endogenous lactic acid production, but bicarbonate therapy worsens the disorder by increasing the rate of splanchnic bed lactate production. Moreover, large amounts of sodium bicarbonate (in the form of ampules containing 44.5 mmol of sodium bicarbonate per 50 ml) can produce cellular shrinkage due to hypertonicity and circulatory overload due to ECF volume expansion. Finally, in controlled clinical trials in patients with lactic acidosis, sodium bicarbonate therapy has failed to improve circulatory dynamics when compared with equimolar sodium chloride therapy.

The treatment of *alcoholic ketoacidosis* generally requires only the administration of saline solutions and glucose. Alkali therapy should not be used unless the metabolic acidosis is in the lethal range. The same considerations apply to starvation ketosis. The insulin release provoked by glucose administration suppresses lipolysis and consequently the overproduction of keto acids.

In *diabetic ketoacidosis,* insulin therapy promotes glucose utilization and, consequently, complete oxidation of keto acids; simultaneously, ketogenesis is reduced. Therefore alkali therapy is ordinarily not required in the disorder. Furthermore, because the hyperventilatory response to acidosis in some diabetic patients is governed by arterial rather than central medullary chemoreceptors, intravenous sodium bicarbonate administration may result in arterial alkalinization, a reduction in the rate of minute ventilation, and a potentially lethal fall in CSF pH. Sodium bicarbonate therapy in diabetic ketoacidosis should therefore be reserved for initial therapy of the disorder when the arterial pH is below 7.0 to 7.1 and cardiac contractility is impaired. Finally, because *salicylates, methanol,* and *ethylene glycol* are by themselves tissue toxins, appropriate therapy for ingestion of these toxins includes not only alkalinization but also hemodialysis for removal of the offending agent. Ethanol can be administered to slow the rate of metabolism of methanol to formic acid.

METABOLIC ALKALOSIS

ETIOLOGY AND PATHOGENESIS. The maintenance of the plasma bicarbonate concentration depends on renal bicarbonate reabsorption and renal bicarbonate regeneration (that is, net acid excretion). Consequently, although metabolic alkalosis may be *initiated* by the loss of hydrogen ion from the body—for example, during gastric drainage—the *maintenance* of a sustained metabolic alkalosis requires that the net rate of renal bicarbonate reabsorption or renal bicarbonate generation, or both, be greater than normal. In other words, a steady-state elevation of plasma bicarbonate concentrations to levels greater than 24 mEq per liter requires increased activity of one or more of the effector mechanisms regulating bicarbonate handling by renal tubules. In normal individuals it is therefore difficult to produce metabolic alkalosis by simple alkali loading.

Table 75–15 lists the major clinical causes of metabolic alkalosis. The table includes two disorders in which the apparent threshold for proximal bicarbonate reabsorption is increased, namely, volume contraction and potassium depletion, and disorders that increase net bicarbonate regeneration, including increased rates

TABLE 75–15. MAJOR MECHANISMS FOR METABOLIC ALKALOSIS

ECF volume concentration
Potassium depletion
Increased distal salt delivery
Mineralocorticoid excess
Liddle's syndrome
Bicarbonate loading (posthypercapnic alkalosis)
Delayed conversion of administered organic acids

of distal salt delivery and mineralocorticoid excess, either primary or as a consequence of volume contraction. Table 75–15 also lists Liddle's syndrome, in which the pathogenesis of alkalosis is obscure.

Volume contraction can sustain metabolic alkalosis because of an increase in the apparent rate of bicarbonate reabsorption by the proximal tubule. The most common cause for initiating this kind of alkalosis is hydrochloric acid loss caused by vomiting or gastric suction. In the early stages of gastric fluid losses, there is a modest sodium bicarbonate diuresis, but urinary sodium chloride excretion is reduced. As volume contraction becomes increasingly severe, sodium conservation occurs and potassium bicarbonate is excreted in an attempt to maintain pH homeostasis. Finally, when potassium depletion becomes severe, urinary sodium plus potassium excretion is sharply reduced and paradoxical aciduria occurs: The urine is acidic while the plasma bicarbonate level and pH are both elevated. *Contraction alkalosis* is a frequently misunderstood term; the designation should be reserved for those patients in whom metabolic alkalosis has developed and volume contraction maintains the alkalosis by increasing the apparent proximal tubular threshold for bicarbonate reabsorption. Thus contraction alkalosis is a mirror image of the dilutional acidosis listed in Table 75–14.

Potassium depletion from any cause, when sufficiently severe, can sustain metabolic alkalosis initiated by acid loss, for example, during gastric drainage. Presumably, potassium loss from cells is accompanied by increased hydrogen ion concentrations within cells, including renal tubular cells. Thus potassium depletion, when sufficiently severe, can raise the rate of renal tubular bicarbonate reabsorption and hence maintain a metabolic alkalosis. Consequently, when serum potassium concentrations are reduced to about 2 mEq per liter, metabolic alkalosis due to gastric fluid loss becomes saline resistant but responsive to potassium chloride administration.

Situations in which there occurs *enhanced delivery of sodium chloride* to terminal nephron segments enhance renal acid excretion and therefore lead to metabolic alkalosis by increasing the rate of renal bicarbonate generation. This effect occurs with loop diuretics (Table 75–5), such as furosemide or ethacrynic acid, and with the proximal tubular diuretic metolazone. These diuretics also contribute to the maintenance of metabolic alkalosis by contracting ECF volume and by promoting potassium depletion. Salt wasting is common in *Bartter's syndrome;* metabolic alkalosis due to renal bicarbonate generation is therefore a common feature of the disorder. The administration of large amounts of *impermeant anions* such as carbenicillin also favors distal hydrogen ion secretion. Thus carbenicillin therapy is one of the few circumstances in which an increased anion gap and metabolic alkalosis can be produced simultaneously by the same agent.

Mineralocorticoid excess, either primary or secondary, can also result in metabolic alkalosis because of renal bicarbonate generation. The disorder can occur in volume-expanded patients, as, for example, in primary hyperaldosteronism, in which the alkalosis is unresponsive to sodium chloride loading; and in patients with a reduced ECV and secondary hyperaldosteronism. The alkalosis of mineralocorticoid excess occurs primarily because of increased generation of bicarbonate by terminal nephron segments (or, in other words, by increased renal acid excretion) and is clearly accentuated by potassium depletion. *Liddle's syndrome* is a disorder of unknown cause in which metabolic alkalosis, hypokalemia, and hypertension occur because of an increase in sodium avidity by terminal nephron segments, which can be blocked by triamterene therapy.

When viewed in this context, the disorders listed in Table 75–15, with the exception of posthypercapnic alkalosis, result in metabolic alkalosis by two general kinds of mechanisms. First, metabolic alkalosis may be initiated by a loss of acid from nonrenal sources, for example, gastric fluid loss; and the kidney maintains the metabolic alkalosis by raising the rate of proximal tubular bicarbonate reabsorption. This is the primary mechanism responsible for the alkalosis associated with ECF volume contraction or potassium depletion. Second, the generation of metabolic alkalosis may occur intrarenally, because of increased rates of renal bicarbonate generation (or net acid excretion). This appears to be the major factor responsible for the alkalosis accompanying increased rates of salt delivery to the terminal nephron, mineralocorticoid excess, and Liddle's syndrome. Obviously, there may be considerable degrees of overlap. For example, loop diuretics increase rates of salt delivery to terminal nephron segments and therefore enhance bicarbonate generation. However, these agents also produce hypokalemia and ECF volume contraction and as a consequence raise the apparent threshold for bicarbonate reabsorption. Similarly, in primary aldosteronism, increased distal nephron bicarbonate generation as a cause for alkalosis is accentuated by the effects of hypokalemia on bicarbonate reabsorption.

In normal circumstances it is nearly impossible to produce metabolic alkalosis by increasing dietary alkali intake. In certain situations, however, *bicarbonate loading* can produce either a transient or a steady-state alkalosis. One such circumstance is *posthypercapnic alkalosis.* Patients with chronic hypercapnia develop compensatory increases in plasma bicarbonate concentrations: On an average, chronic hypoventilation results in a 0.3 to 0.5 mEq per liter rise in serum bicarbonate level for each 1.0 mm Hg increase in excess of a Pa_{CO_2} of 40 mm Hg. If ventilatory status is improved acutely, the Pa_{CO_2} will fall quickly but the plasma bicarbonate level will remain elevated, particularly if the patient is salt acquisitive because of congestive heart failure or ECF volume contraction. A common way to accentuate posthypercapnic alkalosis is to maintain patients on ventilators having high positive end-expiratory pressures (PEEP), which causes a central tourniquet effect that reduces cardiac output.

Delayed conversion of *accumulated organic acids* is a second mechanism for producing transient metabolic alkalosis. This may occur after insulin therapy for diabetic ketoacidosis, during the recovery phase of lactic acidosis, and following high-efficiency hemodialysis. In the last-named circumstance, acetate in the dialysis bath is taken up rapidly during dialysis. The accumulated acetate, which represents "potential bicarbonate," is then converted to bicarbonate after dialysis has been completed. Prolonged metabolic alkalosis because of alkali loading is a common feature of the *milk-alkali syndrome.* The alkalosis occurs because of prolonged ingestion of absorbable alkali in patients with impaired renal function due to hypercalcemic nephropathy. Frequent vomiting and attendant ECF volume contraction may also contribute to alkalosis in this disorder.

CLINICAL FEATURES AND DIAGNOSIS. There are no specific signs or symptoms of metabolic alkalosis. Relatively severe metabolic alkalosis can result in cardiac arrhythmias. Severe metabolic alkalosis can also result in severe hypoventilation, especially in patients with reduced renal function. Tetany and increased neuromuscular irritability, which are quite common in acute respiratory alkalosis, are very rare in chronic metabolic alkalosis. Rather, since hypokalemia generally accompanies metabolic alkalosis, muscular weakness and hyporeflexia are often seen in chronic metabolic alkalosis.

The diagnosis is inferred in most cases by routine measurements of serum electrolytes and can be confirmed by arterial blood gas analysis. Hypokalemia is generally present. The finding of an unexplained hypokalemic metabolic alkalosis is suggestive of the presence of Cushing's syndrome due to an extrarenal neoplasm.

The urinary chloride concentration is a useful index for distinguishing metabolic alkalosis due to volume contraction from that due to primary mineralocorticoid excess. In volume-contracted states, the urinary chloride concentration is generally less than 10 mEq per liter. Volume-contracted patients with Bartter's syndrome or volume-contracted patients taking diuretics generally have elevated urinary chloride concentrations. The combination of postural hypotension, hypokalemic metabolic alkalosis, and a urinary chloride concentration greater than 20 mEq per liter is therefore suggestive of diuretic abuse or Bartter's syndrome.

TREATMENT. In metabolic alkalosis associated with hypokalemia and volume contraction, appropriate therapy consists of volume expansion with saline solutions and of potassium replacement (see Disturbances in Potassium Balance). If the metabolic alkalosis is sufficiently severe that significant hypoventilation is present ($Pa_{CO_2} > 60$ mm Hg), the administration of dilute hydrochloric acid or other acidifying salts, such as lysine hydrochloride or arginine hydrochloride, may be required. The use of these amino acid salts carries with it the risk of hyperkalemia that is in excess of that expected simply from the change in arterial pH, presumably because these agents promote potassium efflux from cells. Ammonium chloride, lysine hydrochloride, or arginine hydrochloride should not be used in patients with significant liver disease.

If diuretic abuse can be identified, use of these agents should be discontinued. Indomethacin may partially correct the abnormalities of Bartter's syndrome, although potassium supplementation is almost invariably required. Triamterene is effective in preventing potassium wasting in Liddle's syndrome.

Hypokalemia and metabolic alkalosis due to primary hyperaldosteronism are best treated by potassium chloride supplementation, which tends to correct the metabolic alkalosis partially. Dietary sodium restriction in this disorder also tends to reduce renal potassium wasting. Of course, neither of these maneuvers provides definitive therapy for primary hyperaldosteronism.

MIXED METABOLIC DISORDERS

Mixed metabolic derangements occur commonly. Consequently, the evaluation of metabolic acid-base abnormalities depends on a simultaneous assessment of the anion gap, serum electrolytes, and, when appropriate, arterial blood gases. Electroneutrality requires that the sum of the principal anions in serum (Cl^- + HCO_3^- + anion gap) equals the serum sodium level. Thus unless the serum sodium level changes, a change in the serum concentration of one or more of these principal anions necessitates a reciprocal change in the remaining anions.

Table 75–16 indicates the pattern of serum anion concentrations in single and mixed acid-base disorders. In the single acid-base disturbances, the change in the concentration of one anion is usually balanced by a reciprocal change in one other anion. For example, in hyperchloremic acidosis, the increase in chloride concentration equals the decrease in bicarbonate concentration.

In mixed disorders, the anion patterns are more complex. In a mixed metabolic alkalosis combined with an anion gap acidosis (e.g., diabetic ketoacidosis complicated by vomiting), the identifying pattern is an increased anion gap offset partially or entirely by a reduction in chloride; the serum bicarbonate level is variable. In an anion gap plus hyperchloremic acidosis, the reduction in bicarbonate is offset by increases in both chloride and the anion gap. Finally, in metabolic acidosis combined with hyperchloremic acidosis (e.g., vomiting combined with interstitial nephritis), offsetting changes in serum bicarbonate and chloride concentrations may result in normal anion concentrations.

TABLE 75–16. ANION PATTERNS IN METABOLIC ACID-BASE DISORDERS

Condition	Serum Anion Concentrations		
	HCO_3^-	Cl^-	Anion Gap
Simple Disorders			
Hyperchloremic acidosis	↓	↑	nl
Anion gap acidosis	↓	nl	↑
Metabolic alkalosis	↑	↓	nl
Mixed Disorders			
Metabolic alkalosis + anion gap acidosis	nl, ↑, or ↓	↓	↑
Anion gap acidosis + hyperchloremic acidosis	↓	↑	↑
Metabolic alkalosis + hyperchloremic acidosis	nl	nl	nl

nl = normal.

RESPIRATORY ACIDOSIS

ETIOLOGY AND PATHOGENESIS. Respiratory acidosis occurs whenever there is impairment in the rate of alveolar ventilation. Carbon dioxide elimination involves the following sequence: transfer of carbon dioxide from tissues to the lungs in the form of venous bicarbonate; formation of carbon dioxide within red blood cells by a reversal of the chloride shift, described previously in connection with tissue buffering mechanisms; perfusion of the lungs with systemic venous blood; diffusion of carbon dioxide from pulmonary capillaries to alveoli; and alveolar ventilation. Under normal circumstances, the rate of carbon dioxide hydration within red blood cells and the rate of carbon dioxide diffusion from pulmonary capillaries into alveoli are sufficiently rapid that carbon dioxide accumulation is virtually synonymous with hypoventilation.

Acute respiratory acidosis occurs when there is a sudden depression of the medullary respiratory center, as in narcotic overdose or anesthesia; when there is paralysis of the respiratory muscles, as in profound hypokalemia, neuromuscular disorders (myasthenia gravis), or the administration of agents that impair neuromuscular transmission (aminoglycoside antibiotics); when there is airway obstruction, as in foreign body aspiration or profound bronchospasm; when trauma, such as flail chest, impedes ventilation; and when an acute insult is imposed on a chronic hypercapnic state.

Chronic respiratory acidosis generally occurs in individuals with chronic bronchitis, emphysema, and bullous lung disease; in patients with extreme kyphoscoliosis; and in individuals with extreme obesity (pickwickian syndrome).

The arterial pH and plasma bicarbonate concentrations differ in acute and chronic respiratory acidosis. The compensatory response to carbon dioxide retention is to increase the apparent renal threshold for bicarbonate reabsorption. In general, the plasma bicarbonate concentration rises by approximately 0.3 to 0.5 mEq per liter for every millimeter of Hg increase in the Pa_{CO_2} over 40 mm Hg, until the Pa_{CO_2} reaches 80 mm Hg. This compensatory increase in plasma bicarbonate concentration requires 2 to 3 days for complete expression. Conversely, when chronic hypercapnia is relieved suddenly, there is a 2- to 3-day lag in renal bicarbonate excretion, resulting in posthypercapnic alkalosis.

These concepts are also useful in evaluating the possibility of mixed acid-base disorders occurring in association with respiratory acidosis. For example, since the rate of compensatory bicarbonate retention is delayed in acute respiratory acidosis, the presence of an elevated plasma bicarbonate concentration in a setting of acute carbon dioxide retention should be a clue to the simultaneous occurrence of acute respiratory acidosis and metabolic alkalosis. Similarly, because renal bicarbonate reabsorption is an effective compensatory mechanism for chronic carbon dioxide retention, plasma bicarbonate concentrations below 28 to 30 mEq per liter in patients having chronic Pa_{CO_2} values in excess of 50 mm Hg should alert one to the possible coexistence of acute metabolic acidosis and chronic respiratory acidosis.

Since hypercapnia is synonymous with alveolar hypoventilation, patients with carbon dioxide retention are invariably hypoxemic. A compensatory polycythemia occurs commonly in chronic hypercapnic states.

CLINICAL MANIFESTATIONS. The clinical manifestations of respiratory acidosis vary, depending on the severity of the disorder and on the rate at which carbon dioxide retention has occurred. Acute increases in Pa_{CO_2} values result in somnolence, in confusion, and ultimately in *carbon dioxide narcosis*. Asterixis may also be present. Because carbon dioxide is a cerebral vasodilator, the blood vessels in the optic fundi are often dilated, engorged, and tortuous; in severe hypercapnic states, frank papilledema may occur.

TREATMENT. The only practical treatment for acute respiratory acidosis involves treatment of the underlying disorder and ventilatory support. The possibility of drug abuse should always be considered in otherwise healthy patients who suddenly develop acute respiratory depression; consequently, naloxone (Narcan) therapy should be considered in all comatose patients seen in the emergency room in whom no apparent cause for respiratory depression can be identified.

In patients with chronic hypercapnia who develop sudden increases in Pa_{CO_2} values, attention should be directed toward identifying factors such as pneumonia or pulmonary embolism, which may have aggravated the underlying disorder. It should be emphasized again that oxygen therapy in patients with chronic hypercapnia should be instituted with extreme caution, since hypoxemia may be the primary stimulus to respiration in this setting. Consequently, in such patients, sudden increases in the arterial Pa_{CO_2} produced by oxygen administration may result in cessation of respiration. The administration of alkalinizing salts has no place in the management of chronic respiratory acidosis.

RESPIRATORY ALKALOSIS

ETIOLOGY AND PATHOGENESIS. Respiratory alkalosis occurs when hyperventilation reduces the arterial Pa_{CO_2} and consequently increases arterial pH. Acute respiratory alkalosis is most commonly the result of the hyperventilation syndrome in anxiety. Acute hyperventilation may also occur because of damage to the respiratory centers; in acute salicylism; in fever and septic states; and in association with pneumonia, pulmonary emboli, or congestive heart failure. The disorder may also be produced iatrogenically by injudicious mechanical ventilatory support. Chronic hyperventilation occurs in the acclimation response to exposure to high altitudes (a low ambient oxygen tension), in advanced hepatic insufficiency, and in pregnancy.

During acute hyperventilation, plasma bicarbonate concentrations fall by approximately 3 mEq per liter when the Pa_{CO_2} falls to about 25 mm Hg. This fall in plasma bicarbonate level is due largely to proton shifts from the ICF to the ECF and tends to minimize acute changes in arterial pH. In chronic hyperventilation, renal bicarbonate loss provides the compensatory response to the reduction in Pa_{CO_2}. In experimental studies with dogs, approximately 2 to 4 days are required for a maximal renal compensatory response, which involves approximately a 0.4 mEq per liter reduction in plasma bicarbonate concentrations for every 1 mm Hg fall in Pa_{CO_2}.

Hyperventilation and respiratory alkalosis may also occur, as mentioned previously, following the correction of metabolic acidosis and particularly in diabetic ketoacidosis. In all likelihood, hyperventilation persists in this setting because of the lag in the rate at which plasma bicarbonate concentrations rise with respect to ECF bicarbonate concentrations during correction of metabolic acidosis.

CLINICAL MANIFESTATIONS AND TREATMENT. Chronic hyperventilation may be asymptomatic. The acute hyperventilation syndrome is characterized by light-headedness, paresthesias, circumoral numbness, and tingling of the extremities. Tetany occurs in severe cases. Both the acute metabolic alkalosis and the reduction in ionized calcium contribute to the increased neuromuscular excitability.

The treatment of acute respiratory alkalosis involves correction of the underlying disorder. When severe anxiety provokes the hyperventilation syndrome, air rebreathing with a paper bag generally terminates the acute attack. If this maneuver fails, sedation may also be required. If an individual is to be exposed to high altitude, 2 days of pretreatment with acetazolamide, 500 mg daily, will produce a mild metabolic acidosis that will offset the initial respiratory alkalosis on exposure to high altitude and thus minimize symptoms due to hyperventilation on initial exposure to high altitude.

Androgué HJ, Rashad MN, Gorin AB, et al.: Assessing acid-base status in circulatory failure. Differences between arterial and central venous blood. N Engl J Med 320:1312, 1989. *A comparison of arterial blood gases with central venous blood measurements.*
Batlle DC, Hizon M, Cohen E, et al.: The use of the urinary anion gap in the diagnosis of hyperchloremic metabolic acidosis. N Engl J Med 318:594, 1988. *An account of the urinary anion gap in renal tubular disorders. The data in Table 75–13 are adapted in part from this paper.*
Cooper DJ, Walley KR, Wiggs BR, et al.: Bicarbonate does not improve hemodynamics in critically ill patients who have lactic acidosis. Ann Intern Med 112:492, 1990. *This paper compares the effects of sodium chloride and those of sodium bicarbonate on pH balance and hemodynamics in critically ill patients with lactic acidosis.*
Feinstein EI (ed.): Severe metabolic acidosis in an intoxicated patient. Am J Nephrol 8:323, 1988. *An account of the metabolic acid-base derangements in licit and illicit alcohol ingestion.*
Kitabchi AE, Murphy MB: Diabetic ketoacidosis and hyperosmolar hyperglycemic nonketotic coma. Med Clin North Am 72:1545, 1988. *A clinical summary of these two disorders.*
Kurtzman NA, Gonzalez J, DeFronzo R, et al.: A patient with hyperkalemia and metabolic acidosis. Am J Kidney Dis 15:333, 1990. *A concise account of the renal tubular disorders causing hyperkalemia and the diagnostic approach to these disorders.*
Madias NE: Lactic acidosis. Kidney Int 29:752, 1986. *A superb discussion of lactic acidosis.*
Norris SH, Kurtzman NA: Does chloride play an independent role in the pathogenesis of metabolic alkalosis? Semin Nephrol 8:101, 1988. *An analysis of the pathophysiology of metabolic alkalosis.*
Stacpoole PW, Lorenz AC, Thomas RG, et al.: Dichloroacetate in the treatment of lactic acidosis. Ann Intern Med 108:58, 1988. *The use of dichloroacetate in the treatment of lactic acidosis.*
Winter SD, Pearson JR, Gabow PA, et al.: The fall of the serum anion gap. Arch Intern Med 150:311, 1990. *A good summary of anion gap acidosis.*

76 Acute Renal Failure

Jared J. Grantham

DEFINITION

Acute renal failure is a syndrome characterized by a relatively rapid decline in renal function that leads to the accumulation of water, crystalloid solutes, and nitrogenous metabolites in the body. Clinically significant acute renal failure is usually associated with a daily increase in the serum creatinine and urea nitrogen levels (azotemia) greater than 0.5 and 10 mg per deciliter, respectively. *Oliguria*, a rate of urine flow less than 400 ml per day, may be observed, but in some cases the urine output may exceed this limit (*nonoliguric* acute renal failure). Complete cessation of urine flow, *anuria*, is relatively uncommon.

ETIOLOGY

Acute renal failure may be seen in a wide variety of clinical settings (Table 76–1). A systematic approach to the causes of acute renal failure facilitates diagnosis in the individual patient. It is important to remember that acute renal failure is a bilateral process, except in patients with only one functioning kidney.

Prerenal

Prerenal causes lead to renal failure by decreasing the effective perfusion of kidney parenchyma. An absolute decrease in blood volume (hypovolemia), the most common prerenal disorder, may be caused by skin, gastrointestinal, and renal losses of water and electrolytes, hemorrhage, and sequestration of fluids in body cavities. In some conditions the kidneys respond as though the blood volume were decreased, when in fact the measured volume is normal or even increased. These oliguric states include congestive heart failure (which may be precipitated by myocardial infarction or dysrhythmia), sepsis, anaphylaxis, and liver failure. Bilateral renal artery occlusion can occur spontaneously owing to emboli from the heart or from an atheromatous aorta. Embolism of atheroma may occur in the course of difficult surgical procedures involving the abdominal aorta.

Postrenal

Although quite rare, *bilateral ureteral obstruction* may be due to calculi, shed papillae in analgesic nephropathy, thrombus, neoplasms, and iatrogenic causes. Commonly in bilateral obstruction one kidney is blocked for several days or weeks before obstruction of the contralateral kidney causes acute renal failure. Acute ureteral obstruction of a solitary kidney is seen occasionally. Acute renal failure can be caused by *urethral obstruction* due to prostatic hypertrophy, prostatitis, bladder and prostate tumors, bladder rupture, calculi, and iatrogenic causes. In hospitalized patients with indwelling urinary catheters, the patency and correct placement of the catheter should always be checked in the evaluation of acute renal failure.

Bilateral renal venous occlusion is rare but may be seen in hypercoagulable states, with intra-abdominal neoplasms, or secondary to surgical procedures.

TABLE 76–1. CAUSES OF ACUTE RENAL FAILURE SYNDROME

Location of Primary Disorder	Clinical Examples
Prerenal	
Absolute decrease in effective blood volume	Hemorrhage, skin losses (burns, sweating), gastrointestinal losses (diarrhea, vomiting), renal losses (diuretics, glycosuria), fluid pooling (peritonitis, burns)
Relative decrease in blood volume (ineffective arterial volume)	Congestive heart failure, dysrhythmias, sepsis, anaphylaxis, liver failure
Arterial occlusion	Bilateral thromboembolism, thromboembolism of solitary kidney, aortic or renal artery aneurysm
Postrenal	
Ureteral obstruction	Bilateral or solitary kidney (calculi, neoplasm, clot, retroperitoneal fibrosis, iatrogenic)
Urethral obstruction	Prostatitis
Venous occlusion	Bilateral or solitary kidney (renal vein thrombosis, neoplasm, iatrogenic)
Intrarenal	
Vascular	Vasculitis, malignant hypertension, vasopressors, eclampsia, microangiopathy, hyperviscosity states, nonsteroidal anti-inflammatory drugs, hypercalcemia, iodinated radiocontrast agents
Glomerulus	Acute glomerulonephritis
Tubular injury	
Ischemia	Profound hypotension, postrenal transplant, vasopressors, microvascular constriction
Intratubular pigments	Hemoglobinuria, myoglobinuria
Intratubular proteins	Myeloma
Intratubular crystals	Uric acid, oxalate, sulfonamides, phenazopyridine hydrochloride
Tubulointerstitial	Interstitial nephritis due to drugs, infection, radiation
Nephrotoxins	Antibiotics (gentamicin, kanamycin, neomycin, amikacin, tobramycin, streptomycin, cephaloridine, amphotericin B); metals (mercury, bismuth, uranium, arsenic, silver, cadmium, iron, antimony); solvents (carbon tetrachloride, glycol, tetrachlorethylene); iodinated contrast agents; streptozotocin, cisplatin

Intrarenal

The renal arterial and arteriolar *blood vessels* may be involved in vasculitis, malignant hypertension, eclampsia, and microangiopathies. Pronounced vasospasm leading to acute renal failure may be seen in scleroderma, during systemic infusions of norepinephrine, secondary to the use of nonsteroidal anti-inflammatory compounds, iodinated radiocontrast agents, or diet pills, or in hypercalcemic states.

Glomerular inflammation (acute glomerulonephritis, Ch. 79) may cause acute renal failure by sharply reducing renal blood flow. *Renal tubules* are susceptible to a number of insults. *Ischemic* injury, sometimes progressing to frank necrosis, may be seen secondary to profound hypotension, especially in elderly persons. The term *acute tubular necrosis* (ATN) is frequently used to describe a clinical syndrome in which there is a simultaneous and progressive deterioration of glomerular and tubular function in the absence of documented glomerular or interstitial nephritis, vascular disease, or obstruction of the collecting system. In the vast majority of patients with ATN, the initiating event is either a decrease in renal plasma flow or exposure to a nephrotoxic agent. In spite of its wide usage, however, the term ATN is not a valid histologic description of the renal injury. In general, the term *acute renal failure* is to be preferred. Rarely, ischemia may be severe enough to cause irreversible necrosis of renal parenchyma. Kidneys transplanted from cadaver sources often undergo oliguric renal failure. The intravenous administration of powerful vasoconstrictors, such as norepinephrine, may cause acute ischemic tubular injury in certain susceptible patients. Renal tubules are susceptible to injury by high levels of urinary pigments (hemoglobinuria, myoglobinuria), especially in the setting of renal hypoperfusion and ischemia. Several serum proteins are potentially nephrotoxic, including kappa and lambda light chains, which may be abundantly excreted in patients with multiple myeloma. Renal tubules may be occluded by uric acid, oxalate, sulfonamide, or pyridium crystals, leading to acute renal failure.

A wide variety of chemicals are potential tubular toxins. Antibiotics of the aminoglycoside class (one of the most common iatrogenic nephrotoxins), streptomycin, cephaloridine, and amphotericin all injure renal tubules when given in excessive doses. These agents are apparently nephrotoxic even at low therapeutic doses in patients who are oliguric or hypotensive or who have underlying renal disorders. The combined effects of aminoglycosides and certain cephalothin drugs appear to be additive in causing acute renal failure. Heavy metal poisoning is seen rarely but may cause acute tubular necrosis and renal failure. Iodinated radiocontrast agents may directly injure renal tubules in patients with underlying disorders such as diabetes mellitus, systemic lupus erythematosus, and chronic renal insufficiency from nearly any cause. Chemotherapeutic agents such as streptozotocin and cisplatin almost routinely cause acute renal injury that may progress to acute renal failure. Phencyclidine, a psychotropic agent, has caused acute renal failure in a few patients.

INCIDENCE

Acute renal failure is a relatively common syndrome. The incidence in the general outpatient population is not known; in one study about 5 per cent of patients on medical and surgical units in a general hospital experienced an episode of acute renal failure. Approximately 60 per cent of cases are related to surgery or trauma; the remainder have medical or obstetric causes. Overall, about one half of cases of acute renal failure in hospitalized patients may be iatrogenic.

PATHOGENESIS

Ischemia and nephrotoxins are the most common causes of acute renal failure listed in Table 76–1. There are at least three important phases in the acute renal failure syndrome due to ischemia or nephrotoxins. In the first, or *initiation*, phase the kidneys are subjected to an insult that produces parenchymal injury (e.g., temporary cessation of renal blood flow; nephrotoxins or pigments; see Table 76–1 and Fig. 76–1). In some patients who are hypovolemic, the initiation phase can be overridden by plasma volume expansion and the acute renal failure syndrome aborted. More commonly, however, the initiation phase causes profound renal vasoconstriction and an initial decrease in renal blood flow. The initiation phase is followed by the *maintenance* phase, during which renal vasoconstriction may persist, thereby decreasing the formation of glomerular filtrate. The hydraulic permeability of the glomeruli is usually decreased, diminishing further the ability of glomeruli to form filtrate. In addition to factors operating within the glomeruli, injury to renal tubules causes the cells to slough from the basement membranes to form casts that can obstruct urine flow. Moreover, the damaged epithelium of the tubules allows the small amount of glomerular filtrate that is formed to leak back into the peritubular capillaries. These four factors—vasoconstriction, decreased glomerular permeability, intratubular obstruction, and tubular back leak of filtrate (Figs. 76–1 and 76–2)—operate in concert to depress the effective glomerular filtration rate (GFR) in the ischemic and nephrotoxic types of acute renal failure listed in Table 76–1.

In some cases the renal blood flow may return to relatively normal levels 24 to 48 hours after the initiation phase. Despite this, the GFR remains very low owing to the decreased glomerular hydraulic permeability, tubular obstruction, or tubular back leak of filtrate.

The third stage in the pathogenetic sequence is the *recovery* phase. Healing of renal parenchyma and recovery of function may be expected in most types of acute renal failure.

CLINICAL MANIFESTATIONS

The onset of acute renal failure usually follows the initiating event by an interval varying from a few hours to as long as several

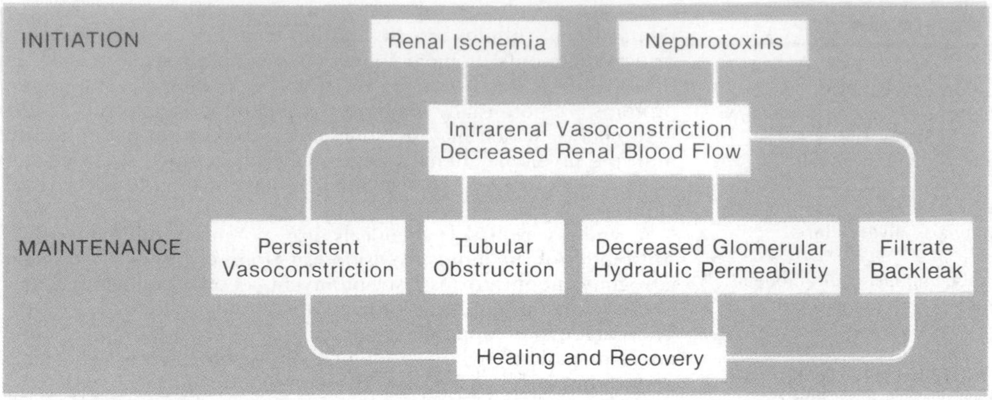

INITIATION	Renal Ischemia	Nephrotoxins

Intrarenal Vasoconstriction
Decreased Renal Blood Flow

| MAINTENANCE | Persistent Vasoconstriction | Tubular Obstruction | Decreased Glomerular Hydraulic Permeability | Filtrate Backleak |

Healing and Recovery

FIGURE 76–1. Pathogenesis of acute renal failure.

days. Patients and physicians usually first notice a reduction in urinary volume in the oliguric types of acute renal failure. Facial edema, tight-fitting rings, and weight gain reflect the retention of water. Rarely, pulmonary edema may be an initial manifestation. Renal pain is uncommon except in association with acute infection, urolithiasis, and tumors. Hematuria is seen in nephritic syndromes and vascular occlusive states but is uncommon in nephrotoxic and transient ischemic states.

The serum creatinine and urea levels rise steadily. In severely oliguric persons of average size, the serum creatinine level rises about 1.5 to 2.0 mg per deciliter per day. When the measured increase in serum creatinine exceeds this range, one should consider hypercatabolic factors; when the measured increase is less, renal clearance of creatinine may be greater than the rate of urine volume flow would suggest. The serum urea nitrogen level usually rises in concert with the creatinine level. However, urea production is altered by food intake, by tissue catabolism, and by blood within the intestines; consequently, the urea levels do not reflect the performance of the kidneys as well as do creatinine levels.

Hyperkalemia due to inadequate renal excretion of potassium may be life threatening early in the course of acute renal failure. Metabolic acidosis due to inadequate renal excretion of hydrogen ions is seen later on. Hyponatremia may be seen in patients who drink unlimited amounts of water or other fluids. Hypocalcemia, hyperphosphatemia, hyperuricemia, and anemia usually develop after several days unless there are mitigating factors, such as rhabdomyolysis and hemolysis. Serum amylase levels may be twice normal in the absence of pancreatitis.

The uremic syndrome develops gradually and, in addition to the features mentioned above, is characterized by the progressive development of anorexia, nausea, vomiting, nervous irritability, hyperreflexia, asterixis, seizures, and coma. Hemorrhagic signs include ecchymoses, gastric and colonic hemorrhage, and pericarditis.

DIAGNOSIS

When renal failure is recognized, it is important to determine the probable cause and remediable factors underlying kidney dysfunction. Table 76–2 lists several key components in the diagnostic approach to renal failure.

The initial objective is to determine whether the renal failure is acute or chronic. The diagnostic evaluation starts at the patient's bedside. With conversant ambulatory patients, the onset of renal dysfunction can usually be determined based on historical changes in urine output (oliguria, polyuria, nocturia), abnormal urine color, and changes in body weight. Chronic renal failure is further indicated by anemia, osteodystrophy, lipiduria, bilateral small kidneys, neuropathy, and a modestly elevated serum level of uric acid.

In the differential diagnosis of acute renal failure, it is important to distinguish among *prerenal, postrenal,* and *intrarenal* factors.

Prerenal Failure

Prerenal failure is suggested by a history of rapid weight loss, flu-like illness, lack of fluid ingestion, bleeding, nasogastric aspiration, diuretic therapy, or orthostatic dizziness. In prerenal failure due to *extracelluar fluid volume contraction,* the physical examination may reveal orthostatic hypotension and tachycardia, poor venous filling and a "thready" pulse, and peripheral vasoconstriction with cool extremities and dry mucous membranes. When prerenal failure occurs in *euvolemic* or *hypervolemic* patients, one usually finds signs of congestive heart failure or liver failure, including distended veins, a third heart sound, pulmonary rales and wheezes, ascites, jaundice, and peripheral edema.

Urinary indices (Table 76–3) show concentrated urine (relatively high specific gravity and osmolality), low fractional excretions of sodium and chloride, and a high urine to plasma creatinine ratio. Diuretics can diminish the diagnostic usefulness of urinary indices and should not be used prior to collecting urine for

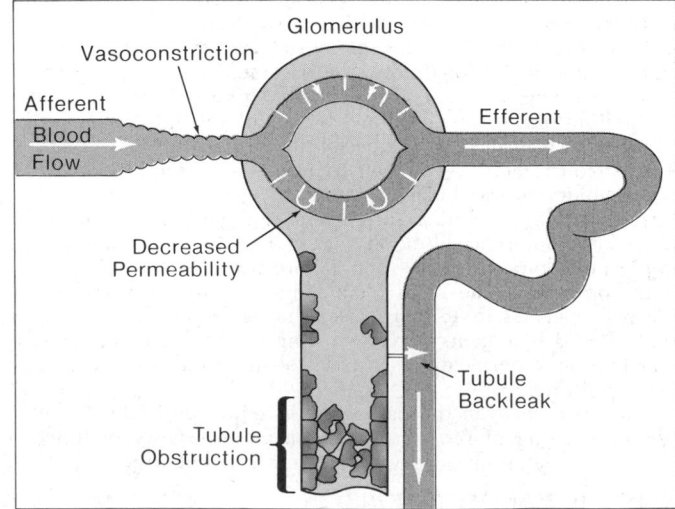

FIGURE 76–2. Possible mechanisms contributing to oliguria in acute renal failure.

TABLE 76–2. DIAGNOSTIC APPROACH TO RENAL FAILURE

1. Review of medical history, clinical setting, medications
2. Physical examination, including evaluation of hemodynamic status
3. Urinalysis, including careful sediment examination
4. Simultaneous chemical analysis of blood and urine. Osmolality, urea, creatinine, sodium, chloride, potassium, uric acid
5. Bladder catheterization
6. Fluid-diuretic challenge
7. Radiologic studies
    Ultrasonography
    Radioisotope scans (pertechnetate ^{99m}Tc, ^{131}I-hippurate)
    CT scan
    Pyeloureterography
        Intravenous pyelography
        Retrograde pyelography
        Antegrade (percutaneous) pyelography
8. Renal biopsy

TABLE 76–3. URINARY INDICES IN ACUTE RENAL FAILURE

Index	Prerenal	Acute Tubular Injury
Urinary osmolality, mOsm/kg H_2O	> 500	< 350
Urinary sodium, mEq/liter	< 20	> 40
Urinary/plasma creatinine	> 40	< 20
Fractional sodium excretion*	< 1	> 1

$$* \frac{\text{Urine/Serum [Na]}}{\text{Urine/Serum [creatinine]}} \times 100$$

analysis. Urinalysis and urinary sediment examination are usually unremarkable except for hyaline casts.

When the physical and chemical findings point to prerenal acute azotemia due to a *decrease in extracellular fluid volume*, a fluid challenge of 500 to 1000 ml of isotonic saline may stimulate urine formation in the average adult. In the author's opinion, mannitol and diuretics are contraindicated in volume-depleted patients with prerenal azotemia. In prerenal azotemia associated with an *expanded extracellular fluid volume*, diuretics may be indicated as part of the general plan to improve cardiac function.

Prerenal azotemia due to occlusion of renal arteries is revealed by radioisotope screening tests and arteriography. Urine output generally is scanty. Urinalysis may show hematuria and proteinuria, and urinary indices show an inability to concentrate urinary solutes (Table 76–3).

Postrenal Failure

Obstruction to the flow of urine may be acute or chronic (see Ch. 81). In most cases of acute obstruction of the *upper tract*, the patient notices pain in the flank or lower abdominal regions and fluctuating urine output. *Urethral* obstruction usually causes urinary frequency, dribbling, and lower abdominal fullness. In urinary tract obstruction, infected urine is commonly observed.

The onset of renal failure due to obstruction of the urinary drainage system can be difficult to determine. To cause renal failure, the urinary drainage from both kidneys must be compromised; alternatively, the patient may have only one kidney. Chronic progressive processes, such as retroperitoneal neoplasia, can obstruct the drainage of one ureter weeks or months before the contralateral ureter is obstructed. Obstructive uropathy should be suspected in patients with adenopathy, abdominal scars, palpable bladder, flank tenderness, prostatic enlargement, or pelvic masses with induration.

Urinary findings are nonspecific. The sediment contains leukocytes and erythrocytes in infected patients. The urinary indices are variable. In acute obstruction the indices are identical to those seen in prerenal failure; in obstructions more than 2 days in duration the indices are similar to those seen in intrarenal tubular injury (Tables 76–2 and 76–3).

Bladder catheterization may be diagnostic. With upper tract obstruction, ultrasonography in the hands of an experienced radiologist is the most useful diagnostic test. Rarely, acute obstruction of the urinary tract may occur without dilation of the renal pelvis and cannot be detected by sonography. The ^{131}I-hippurate scan is a noninvasive test that is useful for determining the number and placement of the kidneys and the potential for return of renal function in obstructive uropathy. Bilateral upper tract obstruction is usually nonsynchronous. In such cases the hippurate scan shows asymmetric accumulation of the isotope. The kidney showing the most intense uptake of hippurate is the best candidate for return of function after relief of obstruction. Intravenous pyelography is useful to localize the site of obstruction, but adequate renal function is needed to concentrate the contrast material in the urinary tract. Retrograde pyelography should be reserved for those cases in which the noninvasive methods are not available or those in which equivocal results have been obtained. In some cases the computed tomographic (CT) scan may provide anatomic confirmation of obstruction.

Occlusion of the renal veins is suggested by a history of a hypercoagulable state, pulmonary emboli, hematuria, or proteinuria. Urinary indices are not diagnostic. Radioisotope studies of renal perfusion may be suggestive, but definitive diagnosis depends on renal arteriography or venography.

Intrarenal Failure

Renal failure due to intrinsic dysfunction is suggested by a history of multisystem disease (e.g., systemic lupus erythematosus, vasculitis), fever, malaise, skin rash, hypertension, gross hematuria, hypotensive episode, or exposure to nephrotoxins.

The urinalysis is an invaluable guide in the diagnosis of intrarenal failure. Acute glomerulonephritis is characterized by hematuria, proteinuria, erythrocyte casts, and granular casts. Lipid bodies and broad waxy casts suggest a chronic process. Pus casts indicate acute or chronic interstitial inflammation. Urinary eosinophils are seen in allergic interstitial nephritis. Crystalluria is observed in urate and oxalate disorders. Physicians should be able to recognize these formed elements in the urine and should personally examine a freshly prepared urinary sediment. Acute inflammation of the preglomerular arterioles may or may not be associated with alterations in glomerular capillaries. In the absence of glomerular capillary inflammation, the urinalysis reflects ischemic tubular injury due to reduced renal blood flow. Acute tubular injury does not give specific urinary sediment findings, but celluluria, epithelial cell casts, and coarse granular casts should raise the index of suspicion.

Urinary indices (Table 76–3) are very helpful in differentiating between conditions that cause injury to preglomerular arterioles and glomeruli and those that cause acute tubular injury. In the former the indices show a prerenal pattern, whereas in acute tubular injury the fractional excretion of sodium is increased and the urinary osmolality approaches that of plasma. The conditions that may exhibit low or normal fractional sodium excretion at some point in the course of the acute renal failure syndrome are listed in Table 76–4.

Radiologic tests are relatively nonspecific in the evaluation of intrarenal failure. The ^{131}I-hippurate scan shows accumulation of isotope in both kidneys if some renal perfusion is preserved and viable tubules remain. Renal arteriography may show microaneurysm formation in polyarteritis nodosa. Renal biopsy is usually indicated in the evaluation of glomerulonephritis, vasculitis, or interstitial nephritis but is not commonly used when pyelonephritis or acute tubular injury is suspected.

TREATMENT

There are at least four major objectives in the treatment of acute renal failure: (a) correct the reversible causes, (b) prevent additional injury, (c) convert oliguric to nonoliguric renal failure, and (d) provide general metabolic support during the maintenance and recovery phases of the syndrome.

Correct Reversible Causes

Prerenal and postrenal factors contributing to renal function should be corrected insofar as is possible. Drugs that interfere with renal perfusion or that are directly nephrotoxic should be stopped. In hypotensive patients the blood pressure should be restored by discontinuing antihypertensive drugs and administering isotonic volume-expanding solutions. In elderly patients with longstanding hypertension, a "normal" blood pressure of 110/70 may in fact be inadequate to generate glomerular filtrate. If there is doubt about the status of the plasma volume, an intravenous challenge of isotonic saline (500 to 1000 ml) is warranted. Accident victims with crushed extremities may re-

TABLE 76–4. CONDITIONS ASSOCIATED WITH FRACTIONAL SODIUM EXCRETION LESS THAN 1 PER CENT IN ACUTE RENAL FAILURE SYNDROME

Intense Intrarenal Vasoconstriction
1. Iodinated radiocontrast
2. Acute bilateral ureteral obstruction
3. Severe burns
4. Sepsis
5. Pigment excretion (myoglobin, hemoglobin)
6. Nonsteroidal anti-inflammatory drugs
7. Amphotericin B
8. Norepinephrine, dopamine
9. Liver disease
10. Cardiopulmonary bypass

Vascular Inflammation
1. Acute glomerulonephritis
2. Acute vasculitis
3. Renal transplant rejection

quire several liters of isotonic saline when they are freed from entrapment. In the states listed in Table 76–4 associated with a low fractional sodium excretion due to intrarenal vasoconstriction, a volume challenge combined with 40 to 80 mg of intravenous furosemide may reverse the oliguric state and, in some cases, prevent the maintenance phase of acute renal failure.

Prevention of Additional Injury

Radiocontrast agents are potentially harmful to patients in the maintenance phase of acute renal failure, and alternative diagnostic methods should be used whenever possible. CT scans are often done with contrast enhancement, and physicians are not always aware of this "hidden" source of iodinated radiocontrast material. Nonsteroidal anti-inflammatory drugs and nephrotoxic antibiotics should be avoided if possible. Drug dosages should be adjusted according to guidelines for renal failure, and plasma drug levels should be monitored when possible.

Convert Oliguria to Nonoliguria

Oliguria in and of itself is not harmful, and a normal urinary flow rate does not accelerate the healing process in the acute renal failure syndrome. Nonetheless, the management of patients with acute renal failure is simplified, and the survival rate may be improved by converting oliguria to nonoliguria with diuretics and fluid administration. A trial of furosemide (2 to 10 mg per kilogram given intravenously) is warranted. If urine output exceeding 40 ml per hour is achieved, additional doses of diuretic may be given periodically.

General Support

Conservative management without dialysis may be adequate in many cases. Indwelling urinary catheters should be avoided in uncomplicated cases. Intermittent catheterization using careful sterile technique is usually sufficient in oliguric obtunded patients. In all patients careful attention to fluid status is crucial to successful management. Daily weight measured by a competent assistant or physician is essential in the evaluation of changes in fluid balance. Catabolic patients may be expected to lose about 0.5 kg per day. As a rule of thumb, patients can be allowed to drink a volume of fluid (water, tea, coffee) equal to 500 ml plus the amount of the preceding 24-hour urine output. In febrile patients this fluid limit can be increased. In anorectic patients the fluids are given intravenously.

Sodium, potassium, and chloride are not given to patients in the maintenance phase of acute renal failure, except coincidentally in the food they eat. This may amount to about 1 mEq per kilogram of Na, K, and Cl daily. Protein intake is restricted to 0.7 to 1.0 gram per kilogram of body weight per day and is principally composed of foods high in essential amino acid content. Carbohydrates and fats are given to ensure an adequate caloric intake. In patients who cannot eat, intravenous infusion of essential amino acids and glucose may be necessary, but this regimen contributes a considerable fluid load.

In addition to measurements of daily weight, fluid intake and fluid output, serial determinations of blood pressure (supine and upright), serum electrolytes, creatinine, urea nitrogen, and blood hematocrit are essential for patient management. Hyperkalemia exceeding 6 mEq per liter is a potentially serious complication that can be handled temporarily by ingestion of polystyrene sulfonate exchange resin (25 to 50 grams) in a solution containing sorbitol. Electrocardiographic changes showing widened QRS complexes or atrioventricular (AV) dissociation demand immediate treatment with intravenous sodium bicarbonate (88 mmole), glucose and insulin (25 units regular insulin per liter of 10 per cent glucose), and calcium gluconate (10 per cent solution, 10 to 30 ml). These measures will generally control the serum potassium level until dialysis can be initiated. (See Ch. 75 for a discussion of hyperkalemia.)

Dialysis may be necessary in certain patients in the maintenance phase of acute renal failure. The indications for dialysis include severe hyperkalemia (serum $K^+ > 6.5$ mEq per liter after treatment), severe metabolic acidosis (serum bicarbonate < 10 mEq per liter after bicarbonate therapy), pulmonary edema due to fluid overload, progressive azotemia (urea nitrogen > 100, creatinine > 10 mg per deciliter), encephalopathy, seizures, bleeding diathesis, pericarditis, and uremic enteropathy.

In uncomplicated cases, peritoneal dialysis may be the most suitable method of treatment. This procedure avoids the wide shifts in blood volume and blood solute composition encountered in hemodialysis, and anticoagulants are not used. Peritoneal dialysis can be used for prolonged treatment if recovery of renal function is slow.

In many cases, one must remove solutes and water from the blood faster than can be achieved by peritoneal dialysis. Also, patients with acute renal failure frequently have pre-existing abdominal injuries. In such cases hemodialysis is the preferred dialytic method. One has rapid access to the circulation by percutaneous catheterization of femoral or subclavian veins. In hemorrhagic states, systemic heparinization is not feasible, and regional anticoagulation with citrate or prostacyclin may be necessary.

PROGNOSIS

The prognosis for recovery must be viewed from at least two perspectives: (1) patient survival and (2) recovery of renal function.

Patient Survival

With the advent of modern dialysis techniques, few if any patients with the acute renal failure syndrome die of uremia. Death is usually a consequence of the underlying disease that caused the acute renal failure or is secondary to trauma and/or sepsis. The mortality rate in traumatized septic patients with acute renal failure is disturbingly high (40 to 80 per cent).

Recovery of Renal Function

The prognosis for recovery of renal function depends on the nature of the underlying disorder that initiated the renal dysfunction. All acute renal failure due to prerenal causes is potentially reversible. In postrenal failure, renal function may be expected to stabilize or improve significantly if the obstruction is relieved.

Acute renal failure due to intrarenal causes has a variable outcome. Glomerulonephritis and vasculitis may respond to immunosuppressive therapy, with complete recovery of renal function. Acute renal failure due to renal tubular injury is usually reversible, provided that the cause of ischemia is removed or nephrotoxins are avoided. Recovery of renal function to near-normal levels is more likely in nonoliguric than in oliguric patients, and in subjects who have strong images on the ^{131}I-hippurate renal scan. The duration of the period of poor renal function is highly variable. Recovery of renal function takes longer in elderly patients than in young persons. Recovery is also prolonged in patients who develop acute renal failure in addition to a chronic renal disorder that compromises baseline function.

The major improvements in renal function usually appear in the first and second weeks after the beginning of the recovery phase. Some mild defects in renal function may persist for months or years after a bout of acute tubular injury.

PREVENTION

The opportunity for major prevention of acute renal failure is in the hands of physicians and surgeons. A few simple measures will diminish the incidence of acute renal failure acquired in the hospital: (1) Patients should be adequately hydrated before receiving iodinated radiocontrast material. (2) Adequate hydration is necessary before certain surgical procedures, specifically repair of abdominal aortic aneurysm and renal transplantation. (3) Adequate hydration is essential before and during chemotherapy using cisplatin and streptozotocin. (4) Pretreatment with allopurinol before chemotherapy of massive tumors will diminish uric acid excretion. (5) Nonsteroidal anti-inflammatory drugs should be avoided in patients with renal diseases. (6) Nephrotoxic antibiotics should be avoided or carefully monitored.

Better, OS, Stein JH: Early Management of shock and prophylaxis of acute renal failure in traumatic rhabdomyolysis. N Engl J Med 322:825, 1990. *Seismic catastrophes entrap victims, leading to rhabdomyolysis and acute renal failure. The critical role of fluid therapy is emphasized in this timely article.*

Brezis M, Rosen S, Epstein FH: Acute renal failure. In Brenner BM, Rector FC Jr (eds.): The Kidney. 3rd ed. Philadelphia, W. B. Saunders Company, 1986, pp 735–799. *This is an exhaustive compendium with 1003 references.*

Harwood TH, Hiesterman DR, Robinson RG, et al.: Prognosis for recovery of function in acute renal failure. Arch Intern Med 136:916, 1976. *A simple noninvasive radioisotope test (^{131}I-hippurate) is shown to be useful in judging the prognosis for recovery of renal function.*

Hou SH, Bushinsky DA, Wish JB, et al.: Hospital-acquired renal insufficiency: A prospective study. Am J Med 74:243, 1983. *A disturbing study that establishes in one hospital the risk for developing acute renal failure.*

Myers BD, Morna SM: Hemodynamically mediated acute renal failure. N Engl J Med 314:97, 1986. *The clinical patterns of acute renal failure are examined systematically in this excellent paper.*

77 Chronic Renal Failure

David G. Warnock

Chronic renal failure (CRF) is a functional diagnosis characterized by a progressive and generally irreversible decline in glomerular filtration rate (GFR). It is caused by a large number of diseases. Nearly 158,000 Americans were treated for end-stage renal disease (ESRD) during 1987. The prevalence in 1977 was only 45,000 patients, so it is apparent that the ESRD programs are expanding. Approximately 12 per cent of the U.S. population was black in 1987, while nearly 28 per cent of the patients in the Medicare ESRD program were black; it is clear that renal failure is much more likely in blacks than in whites. Figure 77–1 summarizes the incidence of CRF for 1987 according to causes (U.S. Renal Data System Report). Diabetes and hypertension are now recognized as the leading causes of CRF in the United States.

This chapter considers the pathophysiology and clinical manifestations of CRF, an approach to the patient with CRF, and principles of management.

PATHOPHYSIOLOGY AND CLINICAL MANIFESTATIONS

The clinical constellation of signs and symptoms of end-stage renal failure is known as the "uremic syndrome" (Table 77–1). In the initial phases of advancing renal failure, most organs function normally, so that the patient often seeks medical attention only when his or her disease has progressed to the uremic stage.

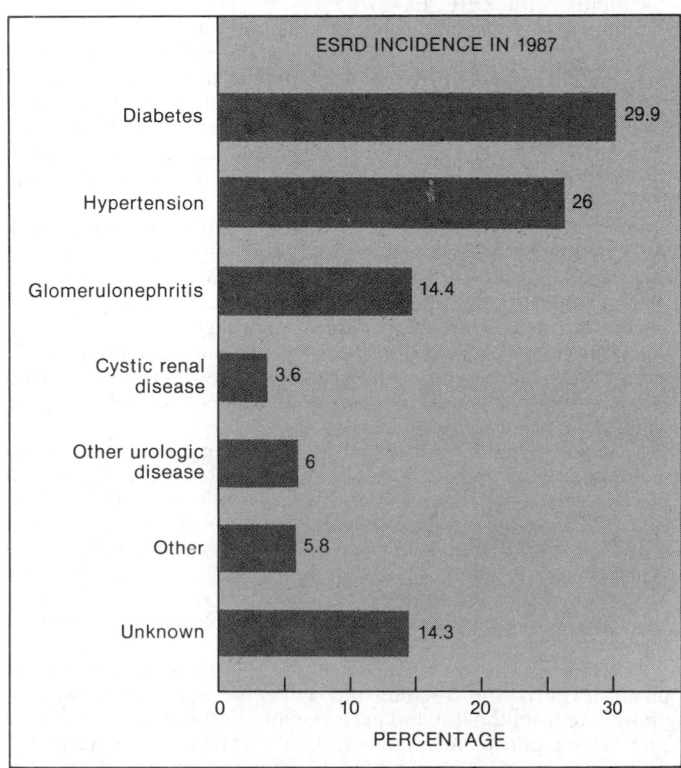

FIGURE 77–1. Histogram of primary renal diseases leading to end-stage renal disease. (Data based on U.S. Renal Data System, 1988.)

TABLE 77–1. THE UREMIC SYNDROME

1. Electrolyte disorders
   a. Potassium: hyperkalemia, total body depletion
   b. Sodium: salt-losing nephropathy, sodium retention
   c. Acidosis: metabolic acidosis with high "anion gap," type IV renal tubular acidosis (hyporeninemic hypoaldosteronism)
   d. Calcium (see Table 237–1): tendency toward hypocalcemia—phosphate retention and secondary hyperparathyroidism, with vitamin D deficiency
   e. Phosphate: hyperphosphatemia contributes to disorders of calcium metabolism
   f. Magnesium: accumulation due to excessive intake
   g. Aluminum: accumulation due to excessive intake
2. Cardiovascular abnormalities
   a. Accelerated atherosclerosis
   b. Hypertension
   c. Pericarditis
   d. Myocardial dysfunction
3. Hematologic abnormalities
   a. Anemia: erythropoietin deficiency, iron deficiency
   b. Leukocyte dysfunction: infection
   c. Hemorrhagic diathesis: defective platelet function
4. Gastrointestinal disorders
   a. Anorexia, nausea, vomiting, gastroparesis
   b. Gastrointestinal bleeding
   c. Disorders of taste
5. Renal osteodystrophy (see Table 237–1)
   a. Osteomalacia
   b. Osteitis fibrosa (secondary hyperparathyroidism)
   c. Osteosclerosis
   d. Osteoporosis
6. Neurologic abnormalities
   a. Central nervous system: insomnia, fatigue, psychological symptoms, asterixis
   b. Peripheral neuropathy: stocking-glove sensory neuropathy
7. Myopathy: especially of proximal muscles
8. Impaired carbohydrate tolerance: peripheral resistance to insulin, hypoglycemia
9. Endocrine and metabolic disorders
   a. Glucose intolerance: insulin resistance, insulin degradation, hypoglycemia
   b. Other endocrine disorders: fertility, sterility
   c. Hypothermia
10. Hyperuricemia: clinical gout is rare; pseudogout occurs
11. Pruritus, soft tissue calcification, uremic frost

Normally, the adult patient is unaware of advancing renal failure until the GFR has decreased to less than 15 ml per minute. When conservative medical management is no longer adequate, alternative approaches, such as dialysis or transplantation (see Ch. 78), must be considered.

The uremic syndrome results from functional derangements of many organ systems, although the prominence of specific symptoms may vary from patient to patient (Table 77–1). In this chapter, the pathophysiology and clinical manifestations of uremia are discussed by components, even though this is arbitrary and not all of them may be present in the same patient. Azotemia refers to the retention of nitrogenous waste products as renal insufficiency develops. Uremia refers to the final stages of progressive renal insufficiency when the complex, multiorgan system derangements become clinically manifest. A variety of metabolites of proteins and amino acids have been considered possible uremic toxins, but the clinical symptoms of uremia correlate to their blood levels rather poorly. Uremia, in the general sense, results from the accumulation of such metabolites and from the progressive failure of renal catabolic, metabolic, and endocrinologic processes.

WATER, ELECTROLYTE, AND ACID-BASE METABOLISM IN UREMIA. Renal and extrarenal compensatory mechanisms maintain electrolyte and water metabolism in a nearly normal state until the late stages of renal failure. However, characteristic changes develop as renal function declines.

Potassium. The normal human dietary intake of potassium is 1 mEq per kilogram of body weight per day, more than 90 per cent of which is excreted by the kidneys. The potassium excreted in the urine has been largely secreted by distal nephron segments beyond the macula densa. The intracellular concentration of potassium is important in net potassium secretion. The accumulation of potassium in the distal tubular cells is related to the activity of Na-K-ATPase (adenosine triphosphatase) in the basolateral membranes of these cells. The activity of the cell Na-K-ATPase is controlled by diet and mineralocorticoid status. Both normal and uremic subjects adapt to high-potassium diets by increasing potassium excretion per nephron. In addition, the gut can increase its ability to secrete potassium and serves as an important adjunct for potassium adaptation in CRF.

In spite of these adaptive processes, potassium homeostasis in patients with CRF is not normal. In advanced CRF, the serum potassium concentration tends to be higher than normal, even though body stores of potassium may be reduced. Hyperkalemia can be accentuated by trauma, surgery, anesthesia, blood transfusion, acidosis, or increased dietary intake. It can produce serious cardiac abnormalities, but many patients are asymptomatic until cardiac arrest occurs. Occasional patients complain of muscle weakness or paresthesias. The major warning signs are those detected by electrocardiography and include peaked T waves and prolongation of the PR interval and QRS complex.

Sodium. The kidney has a remarkable ability to maintain total body sodium within normal limits until the very end stages of CRF. As renal disease progresses, the remaining nephrons must excrete a proportionately greater quantity of dietary sodium to maintain total body sodium balance. This observation has led to a search for humoral factors that might be responsible for the increased natriuresis per nephron observed in CRF.

Sodium Wasting. Some patients with CRF have salt-losing nephropathy and may lose sodium chloride to the point of extracellular volume contraction and hypotension. These patients will require dietary salt supplementation to prevent their hypotensive symptoms. A variety of renal diseases may be associated with salt wasting, including pyelonephritis, medullary cystic disease, hydronephrosis, interstitial nephritis, and milk-alkali syndrome. The collecting ducts are damaged in these conditions and cannot regulate the final urinary excretion of sodium chloride.

Sodium Retention. Many patients with CRF are unable to increase sodium chloride excretion to appropriate levels with increases in dietary intake. Most come to a new steady state with increased total body weight. When these patients receive an extra salt load, they excrete it promptly and maintain their state of volume expansion. These patients often have the physical findings of expanded extracellular fluid volume: hypertension, peripheral edema, pulmonary vascular congestion, and cardiomegaly. The clinical picture often suggests heart failure, and valvular heart disease or cardiomyopathy may be suspected. Some patients with normal cardiac output may develop relentless sodium retention and require hemofiltration for volume control. These patients tend to be diabetic or have other causes of severe nephrotic syndrome. Volume overload worsens hypertension and thus accelerate all forms of CRF.

Acid-Base Balance. The kidney normally regulates blood pH within narrow limits by reabsorption (proximal tubule) and regeneration (distal tubule) of bicarbonate by secretion of protons into the urinary fluid. When diets high in alkali content are ingested, the kidney excretes less acid, whereas with acid ash diets and endogenous acid production, the kidney reabsorbs and regenerates bicarbonate and secretes hydrogen ion in amounts sufficient to maintain systemic acid-base balance. A maximally acidic urine in the human has a pH of 4.5 to 5.0. The total quantity of acid that can be excreted is a function of the amount of buffer that is excreted and the net rate of proton secretion. The excreted buffers may be filtered or generated; the most important filtered buffer is phosphate, and the most important buffer generated within the kidney is ammonia.

In chronic renal disease, there is a progressive reduction in net ammonia secretion. While the urinary pH may be maximally acid in CRF, the total amount of acid secretion is reduced owing to the limitation on buffer delivery to the distal tubule. In disease processes that disproportionately affect the medulla, the ability to form maximally acidic urine may also be compromised. Metabolic acidosis develops when exogenous intake and endogenous production of acid exceed renal net acid excretion. In chronic metabolic acidosis, extrarenal buffering mechanisms become involved, including bone salts and intracellular buffers. These buffering mechanisms allow for maintenance of relatively stable, but reduced, blood bicarbonate concentrations when the urinary net acid excretion rate cannot keep up with endogenous production of acid. Loss of bone buffer stores contributes to the development of osteomalacia and renal osteodystrophy. As the GFR falls below 10 ml per minute, there is retention of various organic anions and a progressive rise in the "anion gap" $[Na - (Cl + HCO_3)]$ to around 20 to 24 mEq per liter, with a reciprocal fall in plasma bicarbonate concentration ("uremic acidosis"). The serum bicarbonate concentration does not usually fall below 12 to 15 mEq per liter. This chronic metabolic acidosis is well tolerated by most patients with CRF, probably reflecting its slow development and respiratory compensation. The overall buffer reserve is limited, however, so that acute acid-base challenges (ketoacidosis, sepsis) can cause severe worsening of the metabolic acidosis.

Another form of renal acidosis, distinct from the uremic acidosis described above, is type IV renal tubular acidosis (RTA), or hyporeninemic hypoaldosteronism with hyperkalemia and hyperchloremic acidosis. This condition can occur in the early stages of CRF when the GFR is only moderately depressed. At this stage the kidney still has the capacity to excrete various organic acids, and therefore patients with type IV RTA, in contrast to those with uremic acidosis, have normal anion gaps. There is a reciprocal fall in plasma bicarbonate levels as chloride concentration increases. Type IV RTA is often seen in all forms of CRF but is most characteristically seen in diabetic patients with progressing renal disease or those with predominantly tubulointerstitial disease. It is described further and compared with other types of RTA in Chapter 82. Potassium retention and overt hyperkalemia are the most significant manifestations of hyporeninemic hypoaldosteronism in CRF.

Calcium. The total serum calcium concentration in patients with CRF is significantly lower than normal, although usually above 7.5 mg per deciliter. Great variability exists, and occasionally the calcium level is very low. Patients with CRF tolerate the hypocalcemia quite well, and rarely is a patient symptomatic from the decreased calcium concentration. Tetany is surprisingly uncommon. It is occasionally precipitated by the infusion of sodium bicarbonate, but the usual muscle twitching and cramping of CRF are primary neuromuscular disorders unrelated to hypocalcemia.

Patients with CRF have decreased intestinal absorption of calcium, and consequently fecal calcium loss exceeds that of normal subjects. Jejunal and ileal malabsorption of calcium in CRF can be corrected by oral administration of active vitamin D analogues. In addition, patients with either acute renal failure or CRF are resistant to the normal calcemic action of parathyroid hormone (PTH). The mechanism of resistance may be secondary to a decreased permissive effect of $1,25\text{-}(OH)_2D_3$ on the bone action of PTH.

Phosphate retention develops as renal insufficiency progresses. With increases in serum phosphate level, there is deposition of calcium phosphate into soft tissues and a fall in serum calcium concentration (both total and ionized). The decrease in serum calcium levels is a potent stimulus to PTH secretion and leads to functional hyperplasia of the parathyroid glands. In addition, the kidney is a major site for catabolism of PTH, so CRF is invariably associated with secondary hyperparathyroidism and elevated circulating levels of PTH.

A subgroup of CRF patients develops hypercalcemia after some months on hemodialysis, usually owing to persistent secretion of PTH from glands that have previously undergone hyperplasia. Occasionally, these patients become symptomatic with bone pain or exhibit signs of metastatic calcification. Parathyroidectomy may be indicated if other causes of hypercalcemia are ruled out. Measurements of serum levels of intact PTH and ultrasonographic localization of hyperplastic glands in the neck are very helpful in this setting.

Phosphate. The most important determinant of serum phosphate level is the relationship between net reabsorption of phosphate from the gut and excretion of phosphate by the kidney. The serum phosphate concentration is higher than normal in patients with a GFR below 20 ml per minute, but actual retention of phosphate can be documented with even less severe declines in GFR.

The retained phosphate is of major pathogenetic importance in the development of secondary hyperparathyroidism in CRF. It is postulated that there are periodic decreases in phosphate excretion as nephrons progressively drop out. The resultant increases in plasma phosphate concentration lead to reciprocal decreases in serum calcium concentration, increased secretion of PTH, and decreased tubular reabsorption of phosphate. This adaptive mechanism will maintain a normal serum phosphate concentration until GFR has fallen to approximately 20 per cent of normal. However, if dietary phosphorus intake is not reduced in patients with advancing renal disease, these adaptive mechanisms cannot compensate fully and hyperphosphatemia ensues. If hyperphosphatemia can be prevented, the expected rise in serum parathyroid hormone will be blunted. In addition to dietary restriction, intestinal absorption of phosphate can be reduced by the use of compounds that bind phosphate in the gut in nonabsorbable form. It appears that calcium carbonate is an effective phosphate binder when taken with meals. Calcium carbonate enhances gut calcium absorption, provides a base equivalent for the treatment of metabolic acidosis, and also effectively binds dietary phosphate. This approach avoids the potentially toxic effects of aluminum (dementia, anemia, bone disease) that can result from the use of aluminum-containing antacids and phosphate binders in patients with CRF.

Magnesium. Patients with CRF tend to have modest elevations in serum magnesium concentration when the GFR has fallen below 20 ml per minute. The urinary excretion of magnesium is diminished, and intestinal magnesium absorption continues normally. Most CRF patients with hypermagnesemia have no associated symptoms or findings. Nevertheless, it is prudent to discontinue magnesium-containing antacids and cathartics in patients with a GFR below 20 ml per minute.

CARDIOVASCULAR ABNORMALITIES. Cardiovascular complications are common in patients with CRF and can be classified into three main categories: atherosclerosis and hyperlipidemia, hypertension, and pericarditis. There may also be a primary myocardial dysfunction in uremia that responds to acute dialysis.

Atherosclerosis. Accelerated atherosclerosis is one of the major factors limiting the longevity of patients with CRF. The most characteristic lipid abnormality is elevated triglyceride concentrations with normal or slightly elevated plasma cholesterol levels (type IV). The incidence of elevated triglyceride concentrations is higher in patients maintained on chronic hemodialysis than in nondialyzed patients. There appears to be a positive relationship between the elevation of plasma triglyceride levels and the increased incidence of occlusive coronary disease. The cause of hypertriglyceridemia in CRF is unknown, but current evidence favors a defect in triglyceride removal rather than an increase in triglyceride production.

Hypertension. Hypertension is common in chronic renal disease, being present in the majority of patients at the onset of maintenance dialysis. At least two factors contribute to its high incidence in CRF: (1) The tendency toward sodium retention and volume expansion is perhaps the most important. Expansion of the extracellular volume is accompanied by an initial rise of cardiac output followed by a rise in peripheral resistance. Patients with volume-sensitive hypertension may have increasing problems with blood pressure control as they progress into renal failure. (2) Alterations of the renin-angiotensin axis are also important contributors to the pathogenesis of hypertension. Angiotensin-converting enzyme inhibitors effectively control hypertension in CRF and can be used as long as hyperkalemia is avoided. A small number of patients with hypertension can be controlled only by bilateral nephrectomy. The vast majority of patients with CRF will have much better control of their hypertension once fluid volume is controlled by dialysis.

Brenner and colleagues have focused their attention on glomerular capillary hypertension rather than systemic arterial pressure. It is known that reduction in renal mass causes functional and structural hypertrophy of the remaining intact nephrons. Increases in glomerular capillary pressures and blood flow may be a central factor in this adaptive hypertrophy. The role of adaptive glomerular hyperfiltration in the progression of chronic renal disease must be viewed as somewhat controversial. This hypothetical framework has provided a therapeutic approach that emphasizes the potential contribution of protein restriction and the use of antihypertensive agents that are effective at the level of the glomerular capillary in the treatment of progressive renal insufficiency

Pericarditis. "Uremic pericarditis" is a term that refers to pericarditis of unknown etiology occurring in association with uremia. Conventionally, pericarditis is classified as "uremic" or "dialysis associated." However, since the pathophysiologic characteristics are similar in both settings, the division into two distinct subtypes appears arbitrary, and therefore the continued use of the term "uremic pericarditis" seems justified. Uremic pericarditis was originally described in nondialyzed patients, whereas currently it is most common in patients who are not dialyzed adequately. Characteristically, the pericardial fluid is hemorrhagic. The onset of pericarditis is usually signaled by pain, often on the left side of the chest with respiratory accentuation. Pain is often severe and frequently associated with a friction rub. The friction rub can be loud, generalized, and even palpable but may also be evanescent. Tamponade can occur with signs of falling blood and pulse pressures, raised jugular venous pressure, and poorly perfused extremities. The hemorrhage is thought to originate from sheared pericardial capillaries that have developed in response to uremic inflammation of the pericardium. It is recognized that in previously nondialyzed patients uremic pericarditis responds to dialysis more rapidly than in patients who develop pericarditis during dialysis. However, the pericarditis in this latter group usually responds to intensification of hemodialysis. Pericarditis should be viewed as potentially lethal, and it may require surgical intervention if tamponade becomes evident. Two-dimensional echocardiography can be very helpful in documenting the magnitude of the pericardial effusion and assessing its functional significance. If "diastolic collapse" can be demonstrated with this technique, then emergent surgical drainage is indicated.

HEMATOLOGIC ABNORMALITIES. Hematologic abnormalities are among the most consistent manifestations of uremia. These abnormalities include anemia, bleeding, and granulocyte and platelet dysfunction.

Anemia. Many patients with CRF have severely reduced hematocrits. Hematocrits in the 15 to 20 per cent range are not uncommon. The manifestations of anemia include pallor, tachycardia, a wide pulse pressure with accentuation by exercise, a systolic ejection murmur best heard over the pulmonary area, and the precipitation of angina pectoris in patients with underlying coronary artery disease.

The primary cause of anemia in CRF is a deficiency of erythropoietin, which is a glycoprotein normally produced in the kidney in response to hypoxia. It is responsible for normal red blood cell differentiation from stem cells. Decreased erythropoietin production results primarily from destruction of renal parenchyma and causes normochromic, normocytic anemia. Circulating inhibitors and protein deprivation that in turn decreases erythropoietin production may also contribute to erythropoietin deficiency.

Other factors may contribute to anemia. Many patients on maintenance hemodialysis are iron deficient. Inadequate iron intake is very common in CRF, and iron deficiency may develop in dialyzed patients because of frequent blood sampling and accidental losses during the course of dialysis. Red blood cell survival is shortened in uremia, probably owing to mechanical factors and changes in the red blood cell membrane composition. In addition, patients with CRF may have additional factors that contribute to anemia, including microangiopathic hemolysis as a result of hypersplenism, and folate and iron deficiency. Erythropoietin therapy has greatly improved the sense of well-being of patients on chronic dialysis. Although difficulties may arise because of iron deficiency, exacerbation of previous hypertension, and seizure disorders, the overall response is gratifying. Although now widely prescribed for the majority of patients on chronic dialysis, the optimal dosing regimens and target hematocrits are still open to debate. The role of erythropoietin therapy in patients with CRF who have not yet become dialysis dependent is being actively investigated. Very careful dose titration is required, since any worsening of hypertension may accelerate the onset of overt renal failure.

Leukocyte Dysfunction. Although the granulocyte count is usually normal, some patients have a tendency toward granulocytopenia or lymphopenia. Moreover, the chemotactic response of granulocytes is subnormal. These factors contribute to impairments in acute inflammatory responses and delayed hypersensitivity and may account for an enhanced susceptibility to infection in CRF.

Hemorrhagic Diathesis. A hemorrhagic tendency, manifested by epistaxis, menorrhagia, or excessive bleeding or bruising after trauma, is common in CRF. Whole-blood clotting time and prothrombin time are usually normal. Bleeding time may be prolonged, perhaps related to the associated abnormalities of platelet function. Platelets are often decreased in number owing to increased peripheral destruction. In addition, there are functional defects, such as decreased adhesiveness and aggregation. These abnormalities are often rapidly corrected by hemodialysis and may be secondary to a dialyzable uremic toxin (e.g., guanidinosuccinic acid). The abnormal bleeding time is not rapidly corrected by dialysis and, as such, may not be a reliable prospective guide to the risk of bleeding complications.

INFECTIONS. Most patients with CRF develop serious infections during the course of their disease. The increased susceptibility to infection could be due to deranged or deficient humoral or cellular immunity, impaired inflammatory reaction, or increased exposure to pathogenic bacteria and viruses. Humoral immunity is, in general, intact. Most patients have normal humoral responses to vaccines, but there may be a requirement for more aggressive immunization, as demonstrated by the difficulty in achieving full responses to hepatitis B vaccine in patients with CRF. Cellular defense mechanisms are often deficient, with impairment of delayed hypersensitivity. Patients with CRF may have low lymphocyte counts, and their lymphocytes do not respond normally to mitogenic stimulation. The neutrophil count is usually normal in CRF, and it rises appropriately in response to infection. However, leukocytes of uremic subjects have a decreased phagocytic function. The chemotactic response of polymorphonuclear leukocytes is also depressed; this function improves with hemodialysis. In addition, patients on hemodialysis are often exposed to bacterial and viral infections. Staphylococcal sepsis is commonly due to cutaneous contamination through the arteriovenous hemodialysis access. Gram-negative sepsis also occurs with greater frequency. Often an infected urinary tract can be implicated as the cause. There is an increase in the frequency of hepatitis in dialysis patients that is related to multiple blood transfusions. The disease is usually asymptomatic, but it can be severe. A significant fraction of patients with CRF who contract hepatitis become chronic carriers. The incidence of hepatitis has been diminished with erythropoietin therapy, effective hepatitis screening, and vaccinations.

GASTROINTESTINAL DISORDERS. Gastrointestinal disorders are common in patients with uremia. Their symptoms have varying presentations and may be quite distressing. The most common early symptom is loss of appetite. Many uremic patients then develop nausea and vomiting, sometimes severe enough to cause loss of salt and water, leading to volume depletion and negative caloric balance, which results in weight loss. The specific cause of these symptoms has not been identified, but they quickly resolve with the institution of dialysis.

Gastrointestinal bleeding is also common in uremic patients. Often it is of minor magnitude and is detected by positive stool guaiac test results, but it can be severe as well. The gastrointestinal bleeding may be the result of scattered petechiae, ulceration, or angiodysplasia. There is also an increased incidence of peptic ulcer disease in CRF. The platelet defects contribute to the increased frequency of gastrointestinal bleeding characteristic of uremic patients, but structural abnormalities must not be overlooked.

OSTEODYSTROPHY. "Renal osteodystrophy" is an all-inclusive term for the skeletal changes in uremia, which include, in decreasing order of frequency, osteitis fibrosa, osteomalacia, osteoporosis, and osteosclerosis (see Ch. 237). Osteitis fibrosa is almost universal in advanced renal failure, the exceptions being those patients with rapidly progressive disease and a short duration of uremia. A number of patients exhibit abnormal radiographs, and some complain of actual bone tenderness or muscle weakness. Renal osteodystrophy becomes a major limi-

tation for patients on long-term dialysis. Spontaneous fractures and bone pain, due to osteitis fibrosa and osteomalacia, can have severe functional consequences. Although vitamin D deficiency plays a major role in osteomalacia, there is a growing realization that aluminum-induced bone disease and iron overload may also contribute to the development and progression of renal osteodystrophy.

NEUROPATHY. Many patients with CRF have abnormalities in central and peripheral nervous system function. Tiredness, insomnia, and psychological symptoms, including agitation, irritability, depression, regression, and rebellion, are common. Patients with secondary hyperparathyroidism have abnormal electroencephalograms (EEG's) characterized by increased frequency of slow wave activity. Patients with secondary hyperparathyroidism caused by CRF may show improvement in their EEG's and psychological symptoms after parathyroidectomy. The mechanism by which PTH exerts these effects on the central nervous system is not known, but a variety of mechanisms may be involved, including changes in brain calcium content, abnormal neuroendocrinologic responses, and alterations in ion transport systems involved in normal neurotransmission.

Peripheral neuropathy is also common in CRF. Clinical manifestations include painful paresthesias of extremities, twitchings, "restless leg syndrome," loss of deep tendon reflexes, muscular weakness, and occasional sensory deficits. Lower extremities are involved much more frequently than upper extremities. Diminished deep tendon reflexes and vibratory sense may be found, but the most common presentation is sensory loss in a stocking-glove distribution. Peripheral neuropathy can be drug induced, but its pathophysiology in most patients is unknown. Diabetic patients can develop peripheral neuropathy as part of their underlying disease processes, which only worsens as their CRF progresses.

MYOPATHY. Muscular weakness and wasting develop slowly but are common in patients with end-stage renal failure. Proximal muscles are affected more than distal muscles. There are no distinct histologic features of uremic myopathy, and the precise cause has not been defined. Nutritional factors obviously play a central role in the development and treatment of uremic myopathy. The resting transmembrane potential difference of skeletal muscle cells is abnormally low, and the average mean duration of the action potential is significantly shortened in uremic individuals. The reflexes and results of the sensory examination are normal, and there is no evidence of myositis. In inadequately dialyzed uremic patients, intracellular sodium and chloride contents are elevated, whereas potassium content is reduced. These findings are consistent with either increased permeability of the muscle membrane to these ions or decreased active efflux of sodium. These abnormalities can be corrected by dialysis and have been used as an index of the adequacy of hemodialysis. Polymyositis syndromes with elevated creatinine phosphokinase levels have been observed in patients with CRF, especially in conjunction with various drugs, including colchicine, clofibrate, and lovastatin.

ENDOCRINE AND METABOLIC DISORDERS. Carbohydrate Metabolism. Carbohydrate metabolism is often abnormal in patients with CRF. Fasting blood glucose values are normal or slightly elevated, but glucose tolerance may be abnormal. This state of impaired glucose tolerance is often termed *uremic pseudodiabetes mellitus*. Severe hyperglycemia does not occur unless the patient receives a large load of glucose, e.g., during peritoneal dialysis with hypertonic glucose solutions. Nevertheless, the requirement for exogenous insulin decreases in insulin-dependent diabetics as renal failure progresses. At least two different mechanisms are responsible for the simultaneous coexistence of abnormal glucose tolerance and a decreased requirement for exogenous insulin: (1) enhanced peripheral resistance to insulin and (2) a decreased renal clearance of insulin.

A number of possibilities may explain the insulin resistance in uremia. First, some uremic substances may interfere with the action of insulin, since aggressive hemodialysis decreases exogenous requirements for insulin. Second, potassium deficiency may alter the nature of insulin released from the pancreas. Indeed, proinsulin-insulin ratios rise in nonuremic patients who are potassium deficient. Third, there is decreased binding of insulin to peripheral receptors in CRF. Whatever the reason (or reasons), patients with CRF clearly have some degree of peripheral resistance to insulin.

Insulin is filtered and metabolized by the kidney. With progressing CRF, blood insulin concentrations rise owing to decreased extraction of insulin by renal proximal tubular cells. These observations explain the decrease in insulin requirements of diabetics with progressing CRF, but it is also necessary to postulate a degree of peripheral resistance to insulin to explain the carbohydrate intolerance ("uremic pseudodiabetes") of nondiabetic subjects with CRF. A small number of patients with CRF will not manifest insulin resistance and may in fact develop severe, life-threatening hypoglycemia.

Other Endocrine Disturbances. Pituitary, thyroid, and adrenal function is relatively normal in CRF, although some compromise may be observed in response to stress, infections, and so on. Sexual function is often compromised in CRF, with amenorrhea and infertility occurring in women and impotence and oligospermia occurring in men. Reduced estrogen and testosterone levels can often be observed, and prolactin excess may be of pathogenetic importance.

Hypothermia. Patients with CRF often have reduced basal metabolic rates and abnormalities in temperature regulation. The deficiency or reduced activity of the ubiquitous Na-K-ATPase may play a central role in the reduced rate of metabolism. Overt hypothermia is very common in CRF, with a resetting of the normal temperature from 37°C to as low as 35.5°C. This observation is of practical importance in assessing fever in patients with CRF; a temperature of 37.5°C may denote a serious, acute infection that requires appropriate antibiotic coverage.

Elevation of Uric Acid Level. Approximately two thirds of the total uric acid excretory load is normally removed each day by the kidney. With progression of CRF, hyperuricemia is a consistent finding once GFR has decreased to 20 per cent of normal. However, the correlation between the rise of the serum uric acid level and the severity of CRF is poor. Only rarely does the serum uric acid concentration rise above 10 mg per deciliter unless dehydration is superimposed. Whether or not the elevated serum uric acid levels hasten the development of ESRD is not known. Symptomatic gout does occur in patients with CRF, as well as other forms of arthritis, including "pseudogout" due to crystalline deposits other than uric acid, and deposition of amyloid and beta$_2$-microglobulin.

Pruritus. Generalized pruritus is a frequent symptom of CRF and is occasionally severe and intractable. Usually, there are no dermatologic findings. To date, no single causative factor has been identified. Implicated factors include some dialyzable product of uremia, a high calcium-phosphorus product in extracellular fluid with deposition of calcium salts in the dermal structures, and abnormalities in nerve end-plates. Symptomatic relief has been reported with more frequent dialysis, parathyroidectomy, dietary protein restriction, and exposure to ultraviolet light. Other dermatologic conditions include a sallow, yellow discoloration due to deposition of "urochromes," bronze discoloration due to hemochromatosis, uremic frost due to deposition of urea crystals on the skin surface, and metastatic calcifications.

APPROACH TO THE PATIENT WITH UREMIA

The principles of approach to the uremic patient are based on the general precepts of internal medicine. A detailed clinical history is imperative, with special emphasis on urinary tract symptoms, such as nocturia, hematuria, dysuria, polydipsia, and polyuria. Also of special importance is a complete history of systemic diseases, of exposure to toxins and infections, and of renal diseases in the family. The medical history will often be of diagnostic significance. The physical examination should emphasize the blood pressure, retina, cardiovascular system, renal examination with auscultation for bruits and palpation of size, rectal examination for size of prostate in men, gynecologic examination for pelvic masses in women, extremity examination for edema and nail bed findings, and neuroskeletal examination for evidence of myopathy, neuropathy, and osteodystrophy. Laboratory tests should include a complete blood count and urinalysis.

Additional studies should determine whether a patient has acute reversible renal failure, acute worsening of CRF resulting from aggravating factors, or a chronic progressive disease. Again, the history is important. It is unlikely that a patient with acute renal disease is asymptomatic with elevations of serum creatinine and blood urea nitrogen (BUN) above 10 and 100 mg per deciliter,

respectively. On the other hand, patients with slowly progressing CRF are often asymptomatic with much higher elevations of serum creatinine and BUN. In CRF, the hematocrit tends to be lower, the phosphate concentration is higher, and the urinary sediment is usually benign. However, none of these tests is specific enough to differentiate with certainty between acute renal failure and CRF.

Determination of the kidney size can be helpful in establishing the chronicity of renal disease. Renal sonograms can be used to estimate renal size and identify hydronephrosis or cystic masses. If the kidneys are significantly reduced in size, this almost always indicates chronicity and irreversibility. Normal kidney size tends to favor an acute process, although exceptions exist. Chronic renal processes in which kidney size may be normal or larger than normal include polycystic kidney disease, amyloidosis, scleroderma, and diabetes mellitus. Thus normal renal size does not rule out a chronic process. The sonogram may reveal asymmetric renal size, which may be due to unilateral renal agenesis, or renal arterial disease processes, which would suggest a need for arteriography to assess the renal arteries directly.

It is also important to differentiate between renal and extrarenal causes of azotemia. Extrarenal causes of progressive azotemia may be either prerenal or postrenal. Prerenal causes are those disease processes that decrease the blood flow to the kidneys. This decrease may result from true extracellular fluid volume depletion or from effective volume depletion, as seen with cardiac and liver failure. It is also imperative to rule out postrenal causes of azotemia, including lower or upper urinary tract obstruction. Lower urinary tract obstruction may be diagnosed by having the patient void completely and then measuring the residual urine volume in the bladder via catheterization. By far the most common cause in men is an enlarged prostate. Any time a uremic patient with anuria is seen, it is imperative that lower urinary tract obstruction be ruled out, especially if accompanied by symptoms such as hesitancy in initiating the urinary stream, slow urinary stream, and incontinence. Upper urinary tract obstruction can be established by ruling out residual urine in the bladder and demonstrating dilated renal calices, pelvis, and ureters above the obstruction with sonography. The most common causes of upper urinary tract obstruction include renal stones, congenital obstruction, and bladder cancer. Superimposed volume depletion can limit the usefulness of sonography in diagnosing upper urinary tract obstruction.

Once it has been determined that uremia is secondary to renal parenchymal disease and not due to prerenal or postrenal causes, the physician must ascertain whether a treatable form of parenchymal disease is present. The most common forms of treatable renal disease are listed in Table 77–2. Renal biopsy and arteriography may be helpful and are often considered. In general, although renal arteriography produces excellent visualization of the kidney, it is of limited diagnostic value in patients with uremia. It may be helpful in patients suspected of having polyarteritis nodosa, tumors (although uremia is an uncommon association), and renal disease secondary to severe hypertension. Asymmetry in renal size in the setting of severe hypertension suggests renal artery stenosis and should be evaluated by arteriography.

Renal biopsy may give a definitive histologic diagnosis, provided it is performed before the disease has progressed to such

TABLE 77–2. TREATABLE TYPES OF PARENCHYMAL RENAL DISEASE

Acute hypertensive nephropathy
Analgesic nephropathy
Hemolytic-uremic syndrome
Hypercalcemic nephropathy
Interstitial nephritis
Lupus nephritis
Multiple myeloma
Oxalate nephropathy
Pyelonephritis
Rapidly progressing glomerulonephritis with crescents
Renal vein thrombosis
Wegener's granulomatosis

a degree that the only possible morphologic interpretation is ESRD. Renal biopsy can be performed by a percutaneous route with local anesthesia or as an open biopsy with the patient under general anesthesia. The associated morbidity and mortality are low, but the possibility of complications nevertheless exists. For these reasons, renal biopsy is probably indicated in only a small number of patients with uremia; on the other hand, an argument can be made for an aggressive approach to renal biopsy in those patients who have not yet progressed to end-stage renal failure. Although a consensus does not exist among nephrologists, biopsy should not be done unless the physician has strong feelings that the information to be gained will influence management. In that light, serious consideration of any of the treatable renal diseases listed in Table 77–2 should be pursued with renal biopsy. Contraindications to renal biopsy include uncorrectable bleeding tendencies, severe hypertension, bacteriuria, suspicion of perinephric abscess, hydronephrosis, and extreme obesity. Biopsy is often most useful in patients with normal-sized kidneys and progressive renal disease if they have (or are suspected of having) nephrotic syndrome, collagen vascular disease (especially systemic lupus erythematosus), tubulointerstitial disease, or rapidly progressive glomerular disease.

MANAGEMENT

The management of patients with CRF can be divided conveniently into three separate categories: treatment of aggravating factors, treatment of specific complications of uremia, and consideration of optimal diet and general principles in the long-term follow-up of patients with CRF. We will consider those principles of management that are common to all forms of CRF regardless of etiology.

Aggravating Factors

Patients with CRF are highly susceptible to factors that may cause a deterioration of renal function. These must be sought meticulously and treated immediately so that the underlying renal failure will not be worsened permanently. Table 77–3 lists factors that may rapidly worsen renal function in a patient with previously stable CRF.

VOLUME DEPLETION. One of the most common causes of worsening renal function in a patient with CRF is vascular volume depletion. Vascular volume depletion can be the result of either absolute volume depletion or contraction of the effective arterial blood volume. Common causes of volume depletion include the aggressive use of diuretics coupled with salt and water restriction, and gastrointestinal loss of fluid from either vomiting or diarrhea. Vascular volume depletion can also be "effective" and associated with decreases in renal blood flow. Therefore, aggravating factors that cause decreases in renal blood flow can produce rapid rises in serum creatinine concentrations (Table 77–3). Physical signs of volume depletion should thus be sought. In addition, urinary electrolyte measurements often suggest volume depletion. Patients with CRF may rapidly and irreversibly decrease their GFR with volume depletion, so it is imperative for treatment, either oral or intravenous fluid replacement, to be started as soon as feasible. Patients with CRF who are not on chronic dialysis should be hospitalized if there is any doubt that adequate volume repletion can be carried out on an outpatient basis.

DRUGS. Patients with CRF are often treated with a variety of drugs, many of which are nephrotoxic. Table 77–4 lists the nephrotoxic drugs. Of these, the aminoglycoside antibiotics are a common cause of worsening renal failure. In addition, prostaglandin synthesis inhibitors can decrease the creatinine clearance in patients with CRF, especially in a setting of volume depletion. It is prudent to obtain a detailed drug ingestion history whenever a CRF patient with an accelerating rate of renal failure is seen. In addition, drug dosing appropriate to the level of renal function is important to avoid superimposed nephrotoxicity (Table 77–4).

OBSTRUCTION. Acute (less than a day) or subacute (less than a few weeks) obstruction of the urinary tract can occur from multiple causes in patients with CRF. Urinary tract obstruction is conveniently divided into that from tubular causes and that from posttubular causes. The more common etiologies for tubular obstruction include uric acid crystal deposition (as observed with malignancies) and Bence Jones protein deposition (in association with multiple myeloma). More common causes of posttubular obstruction include prostatic hypertrophy and/or prostatism; necrotic papillae, especially in patients with diabetes; and ureteral stones. When the clinical symptoms suggest urinary tract obstruction, it is important that prompt diagnostic and therapeutic measures are undertaken. Rapid in-and-out catheterization rules out bladder obstruction, whereas ultrasonography is useful in ruling out ureteral obstruction. If any doubt persists, then retrograde pyelography should be performed. These measures are simple and safe, and appropriate intervention often prevents progression of azotemia.

INFECTION. Urinary tract infections are significantly worsened when obstruction is present. The rate of infection rises especially after repeated catheterization. Although infection limited to the urinary tract rarely causes progression of renal failure, specific attention should be directed toward evaluating proteinuria, pyuria, and bacteriuria. Increased proteinuria and exaggerated pyuria suggest urinary tract infection. A culture of clean-catch urine should be done under these circumstances. If infection is documented, specific antibiotics are indicated. Care must be exercised to adjust the drug dosage for the degree of renal failure. Uremic patients are also more prone to other infections, such as pneumonia and sepsis, on a de novo basis. These systemic infections, if present, in turn may compromise renal blood flow and result in worsening uremia. The index of suspicion should be high for sepsis in hypotensive CRF patients with urinary tract infection in whom the serum creatinine level is rising.

TOXINS. The list of potential nephrotoxins is long. Therefore, it is important to obtain a good exposure history in patients with CRF. In a hospitalized patient with CRF, when the serum creatinine level starts to rise rapidly, one must consider exposure to radiocontrast materials, nephrotoxic antibiotics, and vasodilators. Volume-depleted patients with CRF, especially diabetics and individuals with multiple myeloma, may experience worsening renal disease because of volume depletion. Fortunately, the prognosis is quite good if the patients are adequately hydrated; it appears that the incidence and severity of contrast dye nephrotoxicity have been reduced with this approach.

HYPERTENSIVE CRISIS. Many patients with CRF are hypertensive. Indeed, hypertension is one of the significant risk factors that may accelerate the rate of progression of renal disease. Thus, strict attention must be paid to adequate control of blood pressure in patients with CRF. Occasionally, patients with CRF develop malignant hypertension with rapidly deteriorating renal function. It is imperative that the blood pressure is quickly controlled in these patients. Even so, the restoration of renal blood flow may be delayed if there are significant vascular abnormalities secondary to accelerated hypertension. This recovery phase can take months, with gradual improvement in the renal function.

METABOLIC FACTORS. Of the metabolic abnormalities that worsen the progression of renal disease, the rises in calcium-phosphorus products are among the most common. The rise in the calcium-phosphorus product not only causes soft tissue calcification but also may be a precipitating factor in the progression of renal disease. This is especially true in patients with multiple

TABLE 77–3. AGGRAVATING FACTORS FOR PROGRESSION OF RENAL DISEASE

1. Vascular volume depletion
   a. Absolute: aggressive use of diuretics, gastrointestinal fluid losses, dehydration
   b. Effective: low cardiac output, renal hypoperfusion with atheroembolic disease, ascites with liver disease, nephrotic syndrome
2. Drugs: aminoglycosides, prostaglandin synthesis inhibitors in a setting of renal hypoperfusion, diuretics in dosage to cause volume depletion
3. Obstruction
   a. Tubular: uric acid, Bence Jones protein
   b. Posttubular: prostatic hypertrophy, necrotic papillae, ureteral stones
4. Infections: sepsis with hypotension, urinary tract infections
5. Toxins: radiographic contrast material
6. Hypertensive crises
7. Metabolic: hypercalcemia, hyperphosphatemia

TABLE 77–4. ANTIBIOTIC DOSAGE IN CRF

Major Reduction in Dosage	Moderate Reduction in Dosage	Minor or No Reduction in Dosage	Agents That Should Not Be Used
Flucytosine	Ampicillin	Amphotericin B	Bacitracin
Gentamicin	Carbenicillin	Cefotaxime	Chlortetracycline
Kanamycin	Cefazolin	Cefoperazone	Nitrofurantoin
Oxytetracycline*	Cephaloridine	Chloramphenicol	
Streptomycin	Cephalothin	Clindamycin	
Tetracycline*	Cloxacillin	Doxycycline	
Tobramycin	Co-trimoxazole	Erythromycin	
Vancomycin	(trimethoprim-sulfamethoxazole)	Isoniazid	
	Methicillin	Lincomycin	
	Moxalactam	Nafcillin	
	Oxacillin		
	Penicillin G		
	Ticarcillin		

*Although tetracyclines are not significantly nephrotoxic per se, their dosage should be reduced in CRF because of their hepatotoxicity with increased blood levels (especially with chlortetracycline) and because their antianabolic actions cause an increase in blood urea nitrogen disproportionate to the degree of renal failure. If tetracyclines are indicated in renal failure, doxycycline is the drug of choice because it is cleared by hepatic routes.

myeloma. Vitamin D supplementation and the use of calcium carbonate as a phosphate binder provide reasonable control of the calcium-phosphorus product. Careful monitoring of the serum calcium level and dietary phosphate restriction are also important adjuncts to the care of patients with CRF.

Complications of Uremia

WATER AND ELECTROLYTE ABNORMALITIES. Hyperkalemia. The mean serum potassium concentration is higher than normal, whereas the total body potassium content is lower than normal in CRF. Serum potassium concentrations up to 6 mEq per liter are well tolerated in patients with CRF. However, patients with CRF have difficulty in excreting an acute potassium load. Therefore, potassium concentrations above 6 mEq per liter require treatment. One should initially determine whether the hyperkalemia is a result of some aggravating factor, such as volume depletion, tissue breakdown, transient worsening of acidosis, drugs (spironolactone, amiloride, triamterene, continued oral potassium supplements, converting enzyme inhibitors, nonsteroidal anti-inflammatory agents, beta blockers), fever, or high intake of potassium. If hyperkalemia is of modest degree and due to some aggravating factor, the therapy should be directed toward correcting the source of hyperkalemia. Discontinuation of oral potassium supplements and dietary potassium restriction are rational first steps. However, if hyperkalemia is severe, skeletal muscle weakness and electrocardiographic changes may be present. This situation represents a medical emergency and requires immediate intracellular transfer of potassium and rapid removal of potassium from the body. The treatment of hyperkalemia is described in detail in Ch. 75.

Abnormalities of Sodium Balance. Total body sodium content dictates total extracellular fluid volume. Although the fractional excretion of sodium per nephron increases as renal disease progresses, patients with CRF are nevertheless susceptible to both volume contraction and volume expansion. Since even mild volume depletion may adversely affect renal function in patients with CRF, it is prudent to maintain these patients in a somewhat volume-expanded state. Volume-sensitive hypertension and pulmonary edema are limiting factors, but it is even more hazardous to keep a patient completely free of edema. If a patient should develop orthostatic hypotensive symptoms, salt intake should be liberalized. Ideally, dietary salt intake should be decreased in proportion to the decrease in GFR. Some of the sodium may be given as sodium bicarbonate to correct metabolic acidosis. If the patient is poorly compliant and becomes volume expanded, the use of diuretics, such as furosemide alone or in combination with a thiazide, is indicated, assuming that underlying kidney function is sufficient to permit a satisfactory clinical response to these drugs. If volume expansion causes severe symptoms and does not respond to conventional techniques, acute peritoneal dialysis or hemodialysis is indicated. Hyponatremia and hypernatremia are treated with the same general principles of water restriction or free water administration as in any other patient. Neurologically symptomatic, life-threatening hyponatremia may require the ad-

ministration of hypertonic sodium chloride, but the resultant volume expansion may then require acute dialysis.

CARDIOVASCULAR ABNORMALITIES. It is important to control the cardiovascular complications of patients with CRF to improve their potential longevity. Hypertriglyceridemia and hypertension are the primary risk factors leading to accelerated atherosclerosis and high cardiovascular mortality. It is not clear whether the course of atherosclerotic vascular disease in patients with CRF can be altered. Even patients who have undergone successful renal transplantation seem to have an increased incidence of cardiovascular deaths. Nevertheless, it seems advisable to adhere to the same dietary principles in patients with hypertriglyceridemia and CRF as in patients without CRF (see Ch. 172). If clofibrate or cholesterol synthesis inhibitors are used, the dose should be decreased proportionately to the degree of renal failure to prevent adverse side effects.

Hypertension is the result of numerous interrelated factors in patients with CRF. It is most commonly volume dependent and volume sensitive. Thus, one of the primary objectives is to decrease intravascular volume, an approach that is sufficient to control hypertension in most patients. If the patient has an adequate urinary volume, the judicious use of diuretics together with a decrease in the dietary intake of salt and water is indicated. Of the available diuretics, furosemide and bumetanide are preferred because of their effectiveness. Excess fluid can also be removed in patients on dialysis by ultrafiltration during the procedure. If volume contraction is not sufficient, then the same general principles apply to the treatment of hypertension as in any other patient (see Ch. 44). Additional drugs, such as clonidine, calcium channel blockers, and beta blockers, may be required. Oral inhibitors of angiotensin-converting enzyme have been shown to be particularly useful in some patients. Minoxidil, a direct smooth muscle vasodilator, has also been advocated in patients with otherwise refractory hypertension. There still exists an extremely small number of patients with malignant hypertension that cannot be controlled by any medical regimen. These patients may respond to bilateral nephrectomy.

The diagnosis of uremic pericarditis requires hospitalization and treatment for fear of impending cardiac tamponade. The best initial therapy is daily dialysis for approximately a week. Indomethacin is not effective in uremic pericarditis. If pericarditis remains refractory to increased frequency of dialysis, intrapericardial injection of nonabsorbable steroids may prove therapeutic. Some patients will require partial pericardiectomy if they develop circulatory impairment that does not respond to medical management.

HEMATOLOGIC ABNORMALITIES. The anemia of CRF often improves with maintenance hemodialysis. The rise in hematocrit is not due to stimulation of erythropoietin production but rather to the removal of some circulating factor (or factors) that inhibits the normal response to erythropoietin.

Besides achievement of the best possible metabolic status of the patient with either hemodialysis or transplantation, two general considerations exist for the treatment of anemia: long-term medical management and transfusion. The general aim of medical treatment is to increase the hematocrit to reasonable levels without secondary side effects. Because patients with CRF, especially those on maintenance hemodialysis, are iron deficient, supplemental iron should be given. Iron can be given daily as a ferrous salt or on a periodic basis as intravenous iron dextran. Oral iron supplementation is inexpensive and is associated with very few side effects. Unfortunately, some patients do not absorb iron normally in spite of hemodialysis and require periodic intravenous iron dextran. No consensus on the frequency or dosage exists, and there is the potential for iron overload with hemosiderosis and occasional anaphylactoid reaction to intravenous iron dextran. Most patients with CRF do not have folate deficiency unless they are receiving maintenance dialysis treatment; routine folate supplementation is advisable.

Clinical trials have been recently carried out with recombinant human erythropoietin for the treatment of uncomplicated anemia in patients with ESRD. Gratifying and dose-dependent rises in the hematocrit occurred in response to intravenous erythropoietin administration. The phase III trial confirms that recombinant erythropoietin represents a major breakthrough in treating the anemia of ESRD.

The above findings with erythropoietin have changed the indications for transfusions and androgen therapy in CRF. Many patients with CRF tolerate extraordinarily low hematocrits surprisingly well. This tolerance may be due to increased release of oxygen from hemoglobin during chronic anemia. Substantial increases in overall well-being are observed when the hematocrit is maintained between 25 and 30 per cent. Higher levels are associated with side effects, including hypertension, headaches, and occasionally seizures.

INFECTIONS. Infections are more common in uremic than nonuremic patients. The general approach to the use of antibiotics should be the same in both groups of patients. Ideally, the antibiotic dose should be adjusted by monitoring the serum concentration of the antibiotic. However, this often is not feasible, and therefore after an initial normal loading dose, dosage levels must be adjusted for the degree of renal failure if the antibiotic is excreted by the kidney (Table 77–4). Some antibiotics are more nephrotoxic than others, and nephrotoxicity is potentiated in CRF. If drug sensitivities allow a choice in the treatment of a given infection, the physician should chose the least nephrotoxic antibiotic that is therapeutic.

RENAL OSTEODYSTROPHY. Hyperparathyroidism, decreased amounts of active vitamin D metabolites, and chronic metabolic acidosis all contribute to the development of renal osteodystrophy, as noted above. The goals of treatment are to normalize these abnormalities to the greatest extent possible.

NEUROPATHY. No specific treatment exists for either central or peripheral neuropathy. However, both objective and subjective improvement may occur by prolonging the periods of dialysis and by using dialyzers with a larger surface area. A gratifying improvement in peripheral neuropathy has been noted following successful renal transplantation, even in patients who were well dialyzed before transplantation.

MYOPATHY. No specific therapy exists for myopathy. Patients may improve dramatically with adequate dialysis. Some patients have shown improvement of myopathy following treatment with active vitamin D analogues and aggressive nutritional supplementation. Erythropoietin has a generalized anabolic effect, which may be very useful in this setting. Some patients with secondary hyperparathyroidism may benefit from parathyroidectomy.

CARBOHYDRATE METABOLISM. Abnormalities of carbohydrate metabolism in the nondiabetic patient are of no or minimal clinical significance. In the diabetic patient, insulin dosages must be adjusted to maintain serum glucose values at normal levels. Often, smaller insulin doses will be adequate as CRF progresses. Overt hypoglycemia may develop in a small number of patients with CRF.

URIC ACID. Although uric acid levels are consistently elevated in CRF, they are rarely much above 10 mg per deciliter. There is little evidence to suggest that asymptomatic hyperuricemia should be treated. Elevated uric acid levels in uremic patients should be treated only when there are tophaceous deposits or symptomatic gout. If treatment is elected, allopurinol is the drug of choice, since patients with CRF do not respond to uricosuric agents. Because of potential toxic side effects, the allopurinol dose should be decreased to no more than 100 mg per day in patients with chronic uremia.

PRURITUS. No specific therapy has withstood the test of time in the treatment of pruritus. A few patients get relief following topical application of emulsified oils or the use of oral antihistamine agents. Some patients have benefited from lowering the serum phosphate concentration by more effective dialysis and phosphate restriction. Parathyroidectomy has sometimes relieved intractable pruritus.

Diet

An appropriate diet can be critically important in the management of patients in CRF, for it may provide symptomatic improvement and may also slow the rate of loss of residual renal function. Although nutritional and caloric intake should be individualized for obese and malnourished patients, some general principles are applicable to all patients. In general, the higher the amount of protein in the diet, the higher the serum urea concentration. This occurs because amino acids are metabolized to form urea in addition to all other nitrogenous waste products that have been implicated by factors causing the uremic syndrome. Reducing the amount of protein in the diet lowers the BUN and reduces symptoms. Moreover, the difficulties in controlling serum phosphorus and acidosis are overcome, since a high protein intake is always associated with a high intake of phosphates as well as other inorganic ions. However, if dietary protein intake is too low, protein malnutrition will occur, with loss of strength, body weight, and muscle mass. This condition can be avoided if the protein requirements are met by providing 0.6 gram of protein per kilogram of body weight per day, of which at least 60 per cent contains proteins rich in essential amino acids, e.g., eggs, lean meat, and milk. A high-calorie intake can improve nitrogen utilization at very low nitrogen intakes, so that a diet of adequate calories manifests a protein-sparing (anticatabolic) effect. Providing about 30 kcal per day generally suffices, although this figure may be lowered for obese patients or raised for patients weighing less than their ideal body weight. Accumulated waste products can be reduced even further by lowering the daily protein intake to approximately 20 grams of protein per day, but only if the diet is supplemented with essential amino acids or a mixture of essential amino acids and their alpha-ketoanalogues. Such a regimen will maintain adequate protein nutrition for prolonged periods in patients with advanced renal failure. Alpha-ketoanalogues of essential amino acids are aminated in the body to form essential amino acids and hence body protein. Nitrogen, which otherwise would have accumulated as waste products, is therefore used to build body proteins. Unfortunately, this approach is extremely expensive. Low-protein diets in which daily minimum requirements are met and the very low protein diet supplemented with mixtures of amino acids may slow the rate of loss of residual renal function and possibly postpone the time when therapy with chronic hemodialysis becomes necessary. Compliance in this setting is probably the rate-limiting factor.

Diets should be supplemented with the water-soluble B vitamins plus vitamin C and folic acid; there is no need to supply additional vitamin A or E. Vitamin D should be reserved for treatment of severe renal osteodystrophy. In general, dietary sodium does not need to be severely restricted unless hypertension or edema is present. Most patients with CRF can readily excrete sodium until renal function is markedly impaired (creatinine clearance less than 10 ml per minute), but they cannot rapidly reduce salt excretion when dietary sodium is markedly restricted. For most patients, the diet should contain at least 1.5 to 2.0 grams of sodium per day. As long as the amount of urine excreted is greater than 1 liter per day, it is unusual to have to restrict potassium in the diet. Renal potassium excretion is promoted by increasing the dietary salt content. With use of these guidelines, uremic symptoms and the consequences of renal insufficiency can be controlled for most patients. Once chronic hemodialysis becomes necessary, the diet should be altered to meet the added requirements related to dialysis therapy.

Patients with CRF should be seen at regular intervals to monitor the progress of their disease. The frequency of these visits will depend upon the presence of other diseases, e.g., hypertension and heart failure, and on how rapidly residual renal function is being lost. All patients should be seen at least every 3 months, at which time a medical history is taken and a physical examination is performed. In addition, laboratory values, including hematocrit, white blood cell count, serum urea nitrogen and creatinine concentrations, and electrolyte values, should be obtained. Monitoring the progress of renal insufficiency is generally accomplished by measuring the serum creatinine concentration as an indirect index of the GFR. Alternatively, 24-hour urine collections can be obtained to measure creatinine and urea clearances, as an approximation of the GFR and a general indication of dietary protein intake. For most patients, the loss of residual renal function proceeds at a constant rate; this rate is different for each patient, although generally patients with polycystic kidney disease have a slower rate of loss of renal function than do those with diabetic nephropathy. When the reciprocal of serum creatinine concentration reaches 0.1 or less (a creatinine concentration of 10 mg per deciliter), the patient is close to the time when dialysis becomes necessary. It must be emphasized that the serum creatinine level is a reflection of muscle mass, which decreases as CRF progresses. In addition, creatinine secretion may be relatively well maintained as the GFR falls, so that creatinine clearance and serum creatinine will progressively overestimate the "true" GFR. Therefore, wide variations exist between individual patients with CRF when serum creatinine values are compared with the GFR. These considerations eliminate any absolute relationship between the serum creatinine level and the need for dialysis. Nevertheless, in the individual patient, the serum creatinine concentration provides the most immediately available marker for following the progression of renal insufficiency.

Dubach UC, Rosner B, Sturmer T: An epidemiologic study of abuse of analgesic drugs: Effects of phenacetin and salicylate on mortality and cardiovascular morbidity (1968–1987). N Engl J Med 324:159, 1991. *The authoritative 20-year follow-up on Dr. Dubach's group of 623 Swiss women who were exposed to phenacetin. A classic of epidemiologic research and clinical investigation.*

Eschbach JW, Abdulhadi MH, Browne JK, et al.: Recombinant human erythropoietin in anemic patients with end stage renal disease: Results of a phase III multicenter clinical trial. Ann Intern Med 111:992, 1989. *This is an important report of results from the phase III clinical trial using recombinant human erythropoietin to treat uncomplicated anemia in patients with end-stage renal failure undergoing hemodialysis. The authors demonstrate a remarkable dose-dependent rise in hematocrit in response to intravenous erythropoietin, which eliminates transfusions, reduces iron overload, and improves quality of life.*

Ihle BU, Becker GJ, Whitworth JA, et al.: The effect of protein restriction on the progression of renal insufficiency. N Engl J Med 321:1773, 1989. *A prospective, randomized study of 64 patients with CRF. There was a fourfold increase in ESRD in those patients who ate a regular diet, compared with those on a protein-restricted diet.*

Klahr S, Schreiner G, Ichikawa I: The progression of renal disease. N Engl J Med 318:1657, 1988. *A scholarly review of the physical, hormonal, and metabolic factors that may be involved in the progression of renal disease.*

Kopple JD, Jahn H, Massry SG, et al.: Kidney Int 36(Suppl 27):S1, 1989. *This supplement represents contributions from more than 100 leading interdisciplinary specialists on various aspects of uremia. Clinical symptoms, pathogenesis, and treatment of uremia and its complications are discussed in great detail.*

Meyer TW, Anderson S, Rennke HG, et al.: Reversing glomerular hypertension stabilizes established glomerular injury. Kidney Int 31:752, 1987. *These studies support the view that glomerular hypertension is an essential hemodynamic derangement that is responsible for progressive renal injury in the rat. Reduction of glomerular capillary pressure with converting enzyme inhibition or dietary protein restriction can arrest the progression of renal injury in the remnant rat model even if therapy is delayed until glomerular injury is established.*

Rostand SG, Brown G, Kirk K, et al.: Renal insufficiency in treated essential hypertension. N Engl J Med 320:684, 1989. *Despite acceptable blood pressure control, renal function may continue to deteriorate in approximately 15 per cent of treated patients. Black patients were twice as likely as white patients to have elevations in serum creatinine concentrations, even though diastolic blood pressure was maintained at 90 mm Hg.*

Salusky IB, Foley FN, Nelson P, et al.: Aluminum accumulation during treatment with aluminum hydroxide and dialysis on children and young adults with chronic renal disease. N Engl J Med 324:527, 1991. *A very provocative report that suggests that aluminum accumulation is a serious problem with serious sequelae in ESRD, even at previously accepted "safe" doses.*

Slatopolsky E, Weerts C, Norwood K, et al.: Long-term effects of calcium carbonate and 2.5 mEq/liter calcium dialysate on mineral metabolism. Kidney Int 36:897, 1989. *Calcium carbonate was shown to be an effective phosphate binder in large doses (10.5 grams per day). Hypercalcemia was prevented by lowering dialysate calcium concentration, thus obviating phosphate binders that contain aluminum.*

US Renal Data System: USRDS 1989 Annual Report. The National Institutes of Health, National Institute of Diabetes and Digestive and Kidney Diseases, Bethesda, Md., August 1989.

Warnock, DG: Uremic acidosis. Kidney Int 34:278, 1988. *A review of the renal responses to chronic acidosis, with an emphasis on the adaptations that develop during chronic renal insufficiency. The importance of chronic metabolic acidosis in the development of renal osteodystrophy is emphasized.*

Wollam GL, Tarazi RC, Bravo EL, et al.: Diuretic potency of combined hydrochlorothiazide and furosemide therapy in patients with azotemia. Am J Med 72:929, 1982. *A crossover study that demonstrates the importance of plasma volume expansion in chronic renal disease patients with hypertension. Hydrochlorothiazide caused a diuresis in patients who were resistant to furosemide.*

78 Treatment of Irreversible Renal Failure

78.1 DIALYSIS

Robert G. Luke

Each year approximately 1.3 in 10,000 of the United States population develop end-stage renal disease (ESRD) and require one of the various forms of renal replacement therapy: chronic hemodialysis in a center or at home; continuous ambulatory or cycling peritoneal dialysis (CAPD or CCPD); or transplantation from a live-related or cadaveric donor. For almost all of the United States population, most of the costs of such treatment are covered by the Renal Medicare Program, and by the early 1990's approximately 130,000 patients are expected to participate. The number of patients with ESRD continues to increase about 10 per cent per year, but most rapidly in the age group over 65 years. Diabetic glomerulosclerosis and hypertensive nephrosclerosis now contribute equally to cause 60 per cent of all ESRD, with chronic glomerulonephritis (5 per cent), polycystic kidney disease (7 per cent) and chronic interstitial kidney disease (5 per cent) accounting for most of the rest. Overall the program is a success, since it provides ready access to renal replacement therapy for virtually all U.S. residents with ESRD. Cost per patient (approximately $32,000 per year) has fallen, when inflation is considered.

The overall incidence of ESRD is four times greater in blacks than in whites, and all except congenital causes are increased in blacks.

Choice of renal replacement therapy is dictated by the availability of a live-related donor (best results), the age of the patient (transplantation is less frequently performed over the age of 65 years), and the presence of important systemic extrarenal disease (which may preclude surgery or immunosuppression). Preliminary hemodialysis is usually necessary before cadaveric transplantation. Home hemodialysis requires the support of a partner, an adequate home, self-motivation by the patient, and reasonably stable medical circumstances. Such patients have better rehabilitation and survival rates than those on in-center hemodialysis, but this may relate to patient selection factors. The cost of home dialysis is less than that of in-center dialysis. In general, patients are best served when all modalities of treatment for ESRD are readily available and well integrated.

TECHNICAL ASPECTS

As renal excretory function becomes progressively impaired, solutes accumulate in the body and eventually contribute to the uremic syndrome (see Ch. 77) and, ultimately, to death. These solutes, especially those of low molecular weight such as urea, can be removed efficiently from the blood by the process of diffusion across a semipermeable membrane down a chemical concentration gradient (dialysis). Substances higher in concentration in the dialysate than in the plasma, such as bicarbonate, will diffuse into the plasma. The membrane must be nontoxic and compatible with red blood cells, white blood cells, platelets, and plasma proteins. A synthetic membrane is used in extracorporeal hemodialysis; the lining membrane of the peritoneal cavity is used in peritoneal dialysis.

Hemodialysis

Membranes of varying hydraulic conductivity and solute permeability can be used in dialyzers of varying surface area and extracorporeal blood volume (100 to 250 ml in adults) to accommodate patients of different sizes, including infants. To remove accumulated sodium chloride and water, ultrafiltration across artificial membranes is induced by a transmembrane hydrostatic pressure, either positive on the blood side or negative on the dialysate side. The removal of over 1 liter of fluid per hour is feasible and predictable based on the ultrafiltration coefficient of the dialyzer. The essential components of a dialysate delivery and monitoring system of an artificial kidney apparatus are shown in Figure 78–1. Blood flow rates of 200 to 300 ml per minute are usual. Heparin is given intermittently or infused continuously (1000 to 10,000 units in total) to prevent clotting of blood in the dialyzer during the 3- to 6-hour procedure; dosage is controlled by the whole-blood or activated clotting time.

Dialysate contains normal serum levels of sodium and chloride, a variable potassium concentration (0 to 4 mEq per liter) depending on the patient's need for removal of potassium, and acetate (normally metabolized to bicarbonate) or bicarbonate (35 mEq per liter) to correct the metabolic acidosis. Bicarbonate may be preferable to acetate in some patients, either because acetate is not metabolized normally (in which case the normally transient increase in "anion gap" in the plasma will persist) or because it may contribute to hypotension during the hemodialysis procedure. A slight respiratory alkalosis is common during dialysis because of loss of CO_2 across the dialyzer. It persists transiently at the end of the hemodialysis procedure because, although the extracellular base deficit has been corrected, the respiratory center continues to respond transiently to intracellular acidosis. Calcium levels in the dialysate—3.5 mEq per liter—are higher than ionized calcium levels in blood to allow a calcium influx

from the dialysate, since most patients with chronic renal failure are in negative calcium balance. Dialysate flow rates are usually 500 ml per minute and thus the patient's blood "sees" 120 liters of fluid during a standard 4-hour dialysis.

High-flux dialysis now allows selected patients shorter dialysis times (2 to 3 hours) because of newer, more permeable membranes with higher clearances and dialyzers that allow more precise control of the rate of ultrafiltration. Patients must have a vascular access that permits blood flow rates of 300 ml per minute and must avoid high interdialytic intake of sodium chloride and water because of the limited time for fluid removal. Bicarbonate is required in the dialysate.

Peritoneal Dialysis: CAPD and CCPD

In peritoneal dialysis clearances of low molecular weight substances are less than those for hemodialysis (for example, a urea clearance of 20 to 25 ml per minute versus 150 ml per minute for hemodialysis), but clearance of some larger, perhaps also toxic, substances is greater because of the greater permeability of the peritoneal membrane to these larger molecules and the longer duration of treatment. When required, fluid removal is carried out by means of osmotic movement of water using high concentrations of glucose (1500 to 4500 mg per deciliter) in the dialysate. Exchange volumes during peritoneal dialysis are commonly 1 to 3 liters each hour. Several types of automated machines are available that deliver set volumes of fluid into the abdomen and then allow drainage after a set "dwell" time. The most common type now in use is the cycler, which is relatively simple, uses commercially prepared dialysate in bags, and automatically cycles up to 16 liters of dialysate in and out of the abdomen during a period of 8 hours (often overnight). Heparin (no systemic effect) and antibiotics are usually added during treatment of peritonitis, the most common complication of the procedure.

CAPD makes use of the fact that small molecular weight solutes reach complete equilibration with peritoneal fluid in 4 to 6 hours. Thus the patient exchanges 1.5 to 3.0 liters of sterile dialysate containing hypertonic glucose (1.5, 2.5, or 4.25 per cent) and physiologic electrolytes three to five times a day through a Tenckhoff peritoneal dialysis catheter and is able to maintain adequate removal of solutes and water. Since insulin-dependent diabetics have more complications of vascular access because of their vasculopathy and since regular insulin can be given in the dialysate with excellent control of the blood sugar, CAPD offers advantages to patients with diabetic glomerulosclerosis. In infants and children, the higher peritoneal surface area relative to body size also facilitates CAPD. In contrast to poorer dialysis of small molecular weight solutes compared with hemodialysis, dialysis of larger molecules (molecular weight >500) is increased. Many patients have been managed successfully by CAPD for 5 to 10 years, but long-term technique failure rates remain higher than for chronic hemodialysis, mainly because of problems with the peritoneal catheter or recurrent peritonitis.

CCPD is increasingly popular because the number of daily "connects" is reduced from four to two by employing the cycler during sleep and a single prolonged CAPD-type daytime exchange. This method is convenient for working patients or for blind or disabled patients who require helpers with their connections. When patients on CAPD or CCPD are admitted to the hospital and cannot perform exchanges, the cycler is usually employed. Rapid, hourly exchanges with the cycler are also useful for treating peritonitis.

Permanent vascular access is usually obtained by creation of an end-to-side arteriovenous fistula in the forearm or insertion of a prosthetic arteriovenous graft when the vessels themselves are inadequate. The fistula functions longer and, if feasible, is preferable. The permanent indwelling peritoneal catheter is made of radiopaque Silastic, is 25 cm long, and includes an intra-abdominal (located in the pelvis), subcutaneous (with a Dacron felt cuff barrier to bacteria at each end), and external segment.

SELECTION OF TREATMENT MODALITY

There is general agreement that successful renal transplantation offers the best rehabilitation, especially if a compatible related live donor is available (see Ch. 78.2). Unfortunately, the rate of renal transplantation in the United States appears to have reached

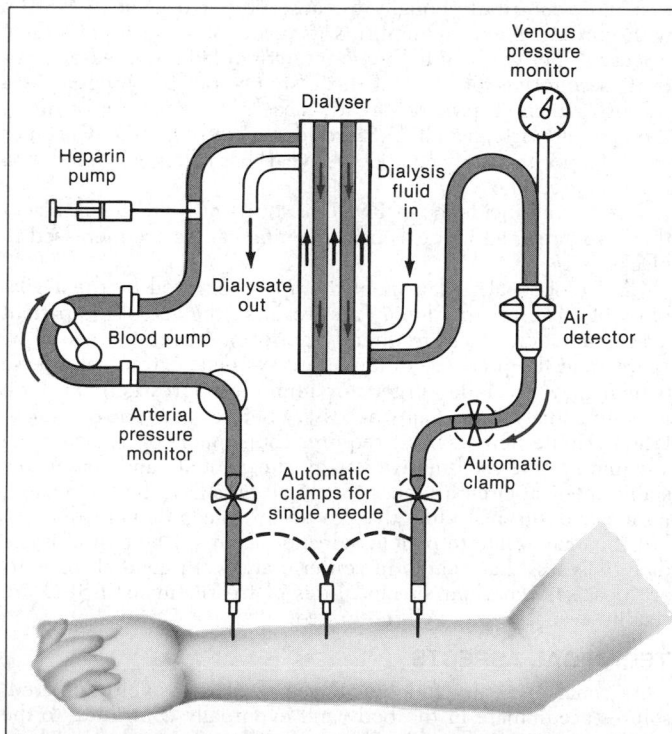

FIGURE 78–1. Essential components of a dialysis delivery system, which, together with the dialyzer, make up an "artificial kidney." In isolated ultrafiltration, no dialysis fluid is used (bypass mode). Also shown is the apparatus for using a single needle for inflow and outflow of blood from the patient. (From Keshaviah PR, Shaldon S: In Drukker W, Parsons FM, Maher JF [eds.]: Replacement of Renal Function by Dialysis. 3rd ed. Boston, Martinus Nijhoff Publishers, 1988.)

a plateau at about 10,000 per year, because of the continued high refusal rates by families of potential cadaveric donors. This means that the vast majority of ESRD patients must continue to rely on some form of dialysis therapy. This situation is influenced by age: Under 25 years of age, 50 per cent of patients with ESRD have a functioning transplant, but over 60 years of age, only 2 per cent have one. Many patients utilize all forms of renal replacement therapy at some stage of their treatment—for example, after loss of function of an allograft or after failure of vascular or peritoneal access.

All patients should have a thorough explanation of, and exposure to, all of the various renal replacement therapies, unless a specific absolute contraindication to one modality exists (e.g., human immunodeficiency virus [HIV] seropositivity for renal transplantation). Relative indications and contraindications are common (Table 78–1). The intermittent nature of clearance in hemodialysis contrasts with its continuity in CCPD or CAPD.

Initiation of Dialysis

Before initiating chronic dialysis, careful discussion with the patient and family should address the issue of whether such treatment is in the patient's best interest. For example, if there is extensive irremediable extrarenal disease, such as severe cerebrovascular disease or a painful malignancy, it may be wiser to continue conservative treatment only. Uniformly brief survival in patients with acquired immunodeficiency syndrome (AIDS) and ESRD has in general discouraged chronic dialysis in such patients. This is not true for patients who are HIV seropositive only.

Dialysis should be initiated when conservative management of chronic renal failure is beginning to be inadequate but before the development of uremic symptoms. In general, dialysis becomes necessary at a creatinine clearance of 4 to 8 ml per minute or a serum creatinine of about 10 mg per deciliter. However, the patient's general clinical state is more important than the level of blood urea nitrogen (BUN) or creatinine. It is especially important to institute therapy before the onset of pericarditis, peripheral neuropathy, or an impaired nutritional state secondary to anorexia or other uremic gastrointestinal symptoms, as subsequent recovery is then quite prolonged and mortality rate increased. A vascular access site should be prepared, if feasible, a few months before dialysis to allow it to mature adequately. If uremia develops abruptly, acute vascular access can be maintained for up to several months by an indwelling subclavian vein catheter or intermittently via the femoral vein. Permanent peritoneal access is prepared 1 to 2 weeks prior to use to prevent fluid leaks, which predispose to peritoneal and subcutaneous infections.

In *diabetic nephropathy* renal failure may accelerate or compound microangiopathic complications—especially retinopathy, gastropathy, and peripheral neuropathy—and many nephrologists therefore prefer to initiate replacement therapy earlier in such patients, perhaps when the serum creatinine level approximates 4 to 8 mg per deciliter. The progression of diabetic glomerulosclerosis to ESRD at that stage tends to be quite rapid.

Hypertension is an important complication in most patients who reach ESRD. Patients surviving for 20 years or more on chronic dialysis uniformly demonstrate good control of blood pressure. Antihypertensive medications can usually be tapered after initiation of dialysis, and blood pressure can be controlled by adjustment of plasma and extracellular fluid volume by ultrafiltration during dialysis and by dietary salt and water restriction. Sympatholytic drugs or drugs that cause postural hypotension are best avoided, since they interfere with the ability to remove fluid adequately by ultrafiltration. A reduction in urinary volume commonly accompanies the onset of dialysis because of lessening of solute osmotic diuresis. The concept of "dry weight" is a clinically important one in a patient on chronic dialysis, regardless of modality of therapy. This is the postdialysis weight at which the patient has an acceptable blood pressure and a plasma volume adequate for avoiding symptoms of diminished cardiac output or of pulmonary congestion. Short-term changes in weight are always due to salt and water deficits or excesses, but careful supervision is required to detect changes in body mass in either direction over longer periods. Interdialytic weight gains should not exceed 2 to 3 kg but unfortunately often do so in patients who are not compliant with dietary salt and fluid restrictions.

Most dialysis patients thus have "volume-dependent" hypertension and require antihypertensive medications only if they are noncompliant with salt and water intake. In perhaps 10 per cent of patients, however, blood pressure is "renin dependent," and hemodialysis is accompanied by persistent rebound hypertension due to rising circulating levels of angiotensin II resulting from ultrafiltration of plasma. Previously bilateral nephrectomy was sometimes employed to control blood pressure in such patients, but the advent of such potent drugs as captopril and minoxidil has virtually eliminated the need for this procedure. Furthermore, it is especially important to avoid bilateral nephrectomy when some recovery of renal function may occur in time, as after an episode of primary or secondary malignant hypertension or after rapidly progressive glomerulonephritis.

Dialysis disequilibrium describes a syndrome in which confusion, headache, and focal neurologic signs develop owing to more rapid dialysis of solutes from the plasma than from the intracellular compartment, especially from the brain. Thus an osmotic gradient can be set up between brain cells and extracellular fluid and lead to cerebral edema. This complication usually occurs in patients with acute or chronic renal failure and uremic symptoms and/or a very high BUN. Short dialysis with a low blood flow usually prevents this problem, which does not occur in patients maintained on chronic dialysis and is extremely rare during initiation of any of the forms of peritoneal dialysis because of their lesser efficiency.

Hepatitis B (Hb$_x$Ag) is carried in the plasma of some patients

TABLE 78–1. SELECTION OF TREATMENT*

Clinical Factor	Preferred Modality	Comment
Insulin-dependent diabetes mellitus	PD	See text
Obesity	HD	Glucose load, hyperlipidemia with PD
Noncompliance	HD	Peritonitis with self-connects, missing exchanges
Work requires travel	PD	Freedom from machine
Severe peripheral vascular disease	PD	Avoids vascular access, ischemia, steal syndromes
Severe angina, congestive heart failure	PD	Less cardiovascular stress and hypotension and smoother control of extracellular fluid and vascular volume
Hernia	HD	PD may exacerbate or cause; repair before PD
Back pain	HD	PD may exacerbate
Ostomy	HD	Infection
Extensive intra-abdominal adhesions	HD	Difficulty with catheter placement, low clearance
Large, muscular build	HD	Better clearance
Small build or child	PD	Relatively good PD clearance
Transplant planned	PD/HD	HHD requires 6 weeks to train vs. 1 week for PD
Transplant not possible or unacceptable in younger patient	HHD	Longer survival of treatment modality than PD; independence
Hypoalbuminemia	HD	Loss of 12 grams/day of protein in PD fluid

*Transplant is not considered here but, if feasible, is generally preferred.
PD = CAPD or CCPD; HD = hemodialysis; HHD = home hemodialysis.

TABLE 78-2. RELATIVE INDICATIONS FOR PERITONEAL DIALYSIS (PD) OR HEMODIALYSIS (HD) FOR MANAGEMENT OF ACUTE RENAL FAILURE

Clinical Circumstance	Comment
1. Recent cerebral surgery, vascular accident or trauma	PD preferred; risk of hemorrhage with heparin and of fluid shifts in brain during HD
2. Hypercatabolic states (e.g., multiple injuries)	HD preferred; PD may not provide adequate clearance of urea, and so on
3. Recent cardiac surgery or myocardial infarction	PD preferred; increased risks of hypotension and arrhythmias with HD
4. Recent abdominal surgery	HD preferred; loss of fluid via incisions during PD; ileus requires surgical placement of PD catheter
5. Acute hemorrhage or severe coagulopathy	PD preferred; but in certain circumstances HD without heparin feasible
6. Complicating severe lung disease	HD preferred; PD may cause atelectasis and impair vital capacity by interfering with movement of diaphragm

with chronic renal failure, who therefore constitute a serious risk to dialysis staff and other patients, since there is repeated exposure to the patient's blood. Separate dialysis facilities and staff are needed for such patients if home dialysis or transplantation is not feasible. Routine monitoring for Hb$_s$Ag is now performed in patients initially testing negative for the antigen, and active immunization is available and indicated for patients and staff. Non-A, non-B hepatitis also remains an epidemiologic problem. Universal precautions (gloves, gown and mask, and special arrangements for disposal of needles) are now routine in dialysis units and offer adequate protection against the less infective HIV. Routine testing of patients and staff and isolation of HIV-seropositive patients are not required.

The Achilles heel of CAPD and CCPD is peritonitis, most often due to gram-positive skin organisms. Fortunately, most episodes can be managed in an outpatient setting with intraperitoneal antibiotics. Fungal peritonitis usually requires catheter removal; recurrent or multiple gram-negative organisms suggest primary intra-abdominal pathology, such as diverticulitis.

Hemodialysis and acute peritoneal dialysis are also employed in the treatment of acute renal failure, the most frequent cause of which is acute tubular necrosis (see Ch. 76). These patients are often quite ill, and survival is aided by frequent "prophylactic" dialysis to maintain a BUN of less than 100 mg per deciliter. The relative merits of hemodialysis and peritoneal dialysis for acute renal failure are outlined in Table 78-2.

Continuous Arteriovenous Hemofiltration

The technique of continuous arteriovenous hemofiltration can be uniquely valuable, especially in patients with acute cardiorenal failure and a low cardiac output. This procedure employs a membrane with a very high ultrafiltration coefficient, which allows fluid and solute removal at low blood perfusion pressures and flow rates. No blood pump or complex monitoring devices are required, and the procedure can be readily performed in an intensive care setting with femoral artery and vein cannulation in very ill, often fluid-overloaded patients in whom hemodialysis or peritoneal dialysis would be very difficult or impossible. Intravenous administration of electrolyte replacement solutions may be necessary with intravenous nutrition if indicated. Heparin is needed.

ROUTINE MANAGEMENT

Patients on chronic hemodialysis usually require a slightly reduced protein intake (0.8 to 1.0 gram per kilogram), but a more stringent control of salt and potassium intake, to maintain satisfactory levels of blood urea nitrogen, potassium, and blood pressure. CAPD patients are encouraged to ingest 1.0 to 1.2

grams per kilogram because of dialysate protein losses. Depending on peritoneal ultrafiltration rates, they may also tolerate a higher intake of salt and water. Hyperkalemia remains a significant cause of death in patients on chronic dialysis, usually due to dietary indiscretion. Monitoring of adequacy of dialysis requires assessment both of clinical well-being, including nutritional state, and of BUN and serum electrolytes, including calcium and phosphorus. The BUN reflects urea production rates and is dependent on protein intake and endogenous protein catabolism as well as on adequacy of urea removal by dialysis. Provided nutrition and protein intake are adequate, a BUN less than 90 mg per deciliter immediately prior to dialysis is usually acceptable. Plasma chemistries are checked monthly in the absence of clinical problems. Because of controlled prospective studies on the amount of dialysis necessary to prevent uremic complications, the increased use of high-flux, shorter time dialysis, and the use of lower dialysis plasma flows (higher hematocrits secondary to erythropoietin treatment), prescription of dialysis treatment is now being more closely individualized in terms of the patient's size and protein intake, duration of dialysis, type of dialyzer, and required clearance and dialysis blood flow rates.

In most patients, supplemental oral base (sodium bicarbonate) is not required; the serum HCO$_3$ should be kept above 20 mEq per liter in the predialysis blood. Dialysis is almost always inadequate to maintain serum phosphorus in an acceptable range (3.5 to 5.0 mg per deciliter) and, as in the conservative management of renal failure, oral phosphate binders are necessary. Aluminum hydroxide contributes to aluminum toxicity (see below), and its use is avoided or minimized by substituting calcium carbonate or acetate, by the prudent use of magnesium-containing antacids, and by avoidance of high-phosphate foods. Because of loss of water-soluble vitamins, including folic acid, from the blood during dialysis, routine administration of supplements of these substances is necessary. Oral iron is also given because there is a chronic small loss of blood that cannot be returned to the patient at the end of each dialysis. Use of recombinant human erythropoietin is now routine for treatment of renal anemia and constitutes the major therapeutic advance since the start of chronic dialysis in the 1960's. The replacement hormone is given intravenously during each dialysis or is administered subcutaneously. Hematocrit is maintained at about 35 per cent; lack of response usually indicates iron deficiency or malignant or chronic inflammatory disease. Hypertension sometimes develops as the hematocrit increases, but it usually responds to reduction of extracellular fluid volume.

COMPLICATIONS OF CHRONIC DIALYSIS

The major clinical complications experienced by patients on chronic dialysis are renal osteodystrophy, vascular access infections and thromboses, pericarditis and ascites, beta$_2$-microglobulin amyloidosis, and acquired renal cystic disease. (Table 78-3). The major cause of death remains cardiovascular disease, but the high incidence of coronary atherosclerosis probably reflects the risk factors of hypertension, smoking, and hyperlipidemia (and perhaps of a high calcium-phosphate product) rather than any specific effects of chronic dialysis per se. Dialysis does cause some cardiovascular stress during the procedure owing to ultra-

TABLE 78-3. COMPLICATIONS IN PATIENTS ON CHRONIC DIALYSIS

Accelerated cardiovascular disease	During dialysis
Hypertension	Hypotension
Renal osteodystrophy	Cramps
Serositis	Bleeding
Pericarditis	Leukopenia with pulmonary
"Dialysis ascites"	sequestration of WBC's
Pleural effusion	Hypoxia
Access infections and thrombosis	Electrolyte disturbances
Dialysis dementia	Dialysis disequilibrium
Pseudogout, tenosynovitis	CAPD
Pruritus	Exacerbation of symptoms of
Poor nutrition	abdominal hernia or back
Hepatitis B (Hb$_s$Ag) carrier state	pain
A$_2$ amyloid	Peritonitis
Acquired renal cystic disease	

WBC's = white blood cells.

filtration and reduction of plasma volume and to a modest reduction of arterial oxygen levels (by 10 to 20 mm Hg). This latter is due to hypocarbia secondary to loss of CO_2 across the dialyzer or to sequestration of blood leukocytes in alveolar capillaries after the activation of complement by the dialyzer membrane; a transient leukopenia is usual during the first hour of dialysis. Episodes of hypotension and hypoxia secondary to those dialysis effects frequently provoke angina in patients with coronary vascular disease.

Renal osteodystrophy is discussed elsewhere from the standpoint of both pathogenesis and treatment (see Ch. 237). Normal serum levels of calcium, phosphate, bicarbonate, and parathormone should be maintained. Calcium supplements, phosphate binders, and 1,25-$(OH)_2$ cholecalciferol (given orally or given intravenously during hemodialysis) may be needed. Rarely, soft tissue calcification, hypercalcemia, and progressive osteitis fibrosa cystica may necessitate subtotal parathyroidectomy. Osteomalacia usually responds to 1,25-$(OH)_2$ cholecalciferol, but one resistant type, in which an excess of aluminum is found on bone biopsy, appears to respond only to diminishing bone aluminum by chelating agents, such as desoxyferamine.

Serositis, manifested by pleural effusion, ascites, or pericarditis, may complicate chronic dialysis. The pathogenesis is not established, although onset often accompanies infection, stress, or protein catabolism. The diagnosis is dependent on elimination of other causes. In general, the abnormal fluid has the characteristics of an exudate and, especially in the case of the pericardial sac, may be hemorrhagic. Patients with pericardial effusion may develop pericardial tamponade, especially during dialysis, when intravascular volume and pressure in the right side of the heart are being reduced. Atrial arrhythmias are also common. If pericardial effusion occurs, dialysis should be carried out daily with very careful control of anticoagulation. If hemodynamic, radiologic, or ultrasonic assessment shows no improvement, surgical treatment by pericardial stripping or medical treatment by pericardiocentesis and insertion of a locally long-acting steroid, such as triamcinolone, is indicated. "Dialysis ascites" can be an intractable management problem. Poor nutrition and fluid overload often contribute, and insertion of a LeVeen shunt (one-way valve with bacterial filter between peritoneum and vena cava) may be necessary. Tuberculosis is an important differential cause of these complications, and diagnosis is dependent on histologic findings and culture, since anergy is common. Pleural effusion is less common and less troublesome than pericarditis and ascites.

Access infections are commonly due to *Staphylococcus aureus* infection, may be associated with bacteremia or septicemia or even bacterial endocarditis, and may require excision of the graft. Nafcillin and vancomycin are commonly used; the latter is convenient, since the absence of renal excretion often permits maintenance of adequate blood levels by weekly intravenous dosage during hemodialysis. Access problems are the most frequent cause of admission to hospital in the dialysis population. These include thrombosis, aneurysms, and infection of the graft. Arteriovenous fistulas last, on the average, longer than synthetic grafts, but each may function for several, even many, years. Steal syndromes may develop with pain in the hand during dialysis, especially in patients with diabetic vascular disease. Very high blood flows through fistulas may contribute to congestive heart failure, but this is quite unusual.

Dialysis dementia is a progressive fatal disease of the central nervous system associated with speech and motor defects, dementia, and seizures. It is now rare because of improved procedures for preparation of dialysate from tap water and reduction in its aluminum content. Past and present use of oral aluminum-containing phosphate-binding agents, however, continues to be associated with aluminum toxicity manifested as microcytic anemia (unresponsive to iron), muscle weakness, and a bone syndrome of pain and pathologic fractures unresponsive to 1, 25-$(OH)_2$ cholecalciferol or parathyroidectomy—indeed, it is made worse by the latter. Diagnosis is by special staining for aluminum of a nondecalcified bone biopsy. Serum aluminum levels, even after desoxyferamine infusion, are not reliable for diagnosis. Treatment involves infusion of desoxyferamine during dialysis, supplemented, as necessary, by a specific cartridge in the dialysis circuit to increase clearance of the aluminum-desoxyferamine complex.

Pseudogout and *tenosynovitis* occur quite frequently in dialysis patients and respond well to drugs such as indomethacin. *Pruritus* is a troublesome symptom and is sometimes attributable to a high blood calcium-phosphate solubility product or to hyperparathyroidism. In some cases, pruritus, despite correction of the above factors, remains resistant to treatment.

The *dialysis procedure* itself may be complicated by hypotension and muscle cramps; both are related to rates of ultrafiltration and usually respond to injections of small amounts of hypertonic fluids, such as 0.3 M NaCl or 20 per cent mannitol. Contributory causes of hypotension are autonomic insufficiency, diminished cardiac function, and hypotensive drugs. In patients who are prone to ventricular ectopy, it is important to avoid hypoxia by use of supplemental oxygen and rapid changes in serum potassium by modifying dialysate potassium concentration. This is especially true in patients on cardiac glycosides. Other complications of the dialysis procedure are air embolism, bleeding secondary to heparin, loss of blood due to clotting of the dialyzer, and electrolyte disturbances due to errors in the dialysate. Fortunately, these are all now quite unusual. Indeed, death or serious morbidity due to complications of the hemodialysis procedure itself in properly trained or supervised patients is now exceedingly rare.

Two important new syndromes are recognized as complications after 5 or more years of dialysis: beta$_2$-microglobulin (A$_2$) amyloidosis and acquired renal cystic disease. A$_2$ amyloidosis results from retention of beta$_2$-microglobulin (molecular weight of 11,800; component of human leukocyte antigen [HLA] proteins on most cell membranes), which accumulates, after polymerization, in bone, joints, and tendons; carpal tunnel syndrome, bone pain, and arthritis are common. There is no specific treatment; prevention may be possible by use of more permeable dialyzer membranes. Intrarenal cysts also develop in patients on dialysis, but not after renal transplantation. Because some of these progress into renal adenocarcinoma, intermittent ultrasound examinations are probably indicated in patients on long-term dialysis.

LIMITATIONS OF DIALYSIS

For chronic dialysis, hemodialysis remains the "gold" standard, and many patients continue to do well even after 10 to 15 years of treatment. The 5-year survival rate for American patients is 40 per cent and ranges from 90 per cent in children to 20 per cent in adults over 64 years. This form of treatment is inherently limited, however, because of low clearances and because the endocrine and regulatory functions of the native kidney are not replaced by the "artificial kidney," (except for erythropoietin and 1, 25-$(OH)_2$-cholecalciferol.) Indeed, life saving though dialysis is, the patient with an endogenous creatinine clearance of even 20 ml per minute is usually better off than one on maintenance chronic dialysis or CAPD.

Especially in elderly patients with multisystem disease who may not improve on chronic dialysis, a "trial of dialysis" for a defined period of a few weeks may be indicated. Withdrawal from chronic dialysis in such circumstances by an informed patient is ethical.

Drukker W, Parsons FM, Maher JF: Replacement of Renal Function by Dialysis. 2nd ed. Boston, Martinus Nijhoff Publishers, 1988. *This is a complete reference work for all technical and clinical aspects of dialysis.*

Fisher JW, Bommer J, Heidelberg JE, et al.: Statement on the clinical use of recombinant erythropoietin in anemia of end-stage renal disease. Am J Kidney Dis 14:163, 1989. *A full discussion of current indications and methods for use of erythropoietin in patients with ESRD.*

Kleinman KS, Coburn W: Amyloid syndromes associated with hemodialysis. Kidney Int 35:567, 1989. *A complete and thoughtful review of the new amyloidosis related to beta$_2$-microglobulin.*

Salusky IB, Foley J, Nelson P, et al.: Aluminum accumulation during treatment with aluminum hydroxide and dialysis in children and young adults with chronic renal disease. N Engl J Med 324:527, 1991. *Aluminum hydroxide is less effective than calcium carbonate as a phosphate-binding agent for the control of hyperphosphatemia and is associated with aluminum retention in patients who are receiving chronic dialysis therapy.*

Sherrard DJ, Andress DL: Aluminum-related osteodystrophy. Ann Intern Med 39:307, 1989. *A concise review of aluminum toxicity and its primary manifestations.*

Twardowski ZJ, Nolph KD, Khanna R: Peritoneal dialysis: New concepts and applications. *In* Stein JH (ed.): Contemporary Issues in Nephrology. Vol 22. New York, Churchill-Livingstone, 1990. *A comprehensive and up-to-date account of clinical status of all aspects of CAPD and CCPD treatment and complications of therapy.*

78.2 RENAL TRANSPLANTATION

John J. Curtis

In the 1920's, Alexis Carrel developed the technique of vascular anastomoses. This momentous surgical breakthrough made possible David Hume's and Joseph Murray's human allograft attempts in the early 1950's. Similarly, Willem Kolff fashioned dialysis techniques and machinery that set the stage for George Thorn's group at Harvard Medical School to advance clinical dialysis to a viable and familiar therapy. Both accomplishments were eventually joined, with synergistic results, to effect truly dramatic changes in the management of chronic renal disease.

Those involved in other forms of organ transplantation envy the advantages produced by the combination of dialysis techniques and allograft transplantation. Because of the combination of these two effective renal replacement therapies, the volume of kidney transplant operations is vastly greater than that of other transplantation procedures. Patients can freely move back and forth between dialysis and transplantation, so that life does not depend on only one form of treatment. Kidney transplantation leads the field of organ replacement therapies by a large and growing margin.

Other advances in knowledge flow from these milestone developments. Peter Medawar's description of second set reactions and his insights into cellular immunology were preeminent advances in thinking. Both ideas are still actively advancing our understanding of human life. The close collaboration of pharmaceutical companies such as Burroughs-Wellcome and clinical researchers such as Roy Calne resulted in the development of azathioprine. Azathioprine made kidney transplantation possible in nonrelated individuals.

Today, several pharmaceutical companies are in the forefront of advancing transplantation. In few areas of endeavor are the accomplishments of academic centers, clinicians, industry, government, and patients themselves so truly beneficial to all concerned. The advance in kidney transplantation is one of medicine's success stories of the 1980's.

IMMUNOLOGIC ASPECTS OF KIDNEY TRANSPLANTATION

In kidney transplantation, the translation of understanding of the human immune system into clear-cut clinical advances is dramatic. Small lymphocytes are central to the problem of kidney allograft rejection. Both T and B lymphocytes are important players in kidney allograft rejection. B lymphocytes make circulating antibodies. The T lymphocyte, however, is critical: Acute rejection is dependent on the presence of T lymphocytes.

T lymphocytes constitute a heterogeneous group: Helper, suppressor, cytotoxic, and natural killer (NK) T lymphocytes are recognized by the presence of characteristic antigens on their cell membranes. The helper T lymphocyte is required for the rejection process. It participates in initial recognition of foreign antigen on transplanted tissue. Foreign antigens stimulate the T helper lymphocyte to release lymphokines that produce both growth and differentiation of other T and B lymphocytes.

Newly developed immunosuppressive agents target T lymphocytes and the lymphokines they produce. These new agents may be both more potent and more specific than those used in the past. Further understanding of the methods by which foreign antigens are presented to lymphocytes and the lymphokine communication network (in which the T helper cell is central) will yield more specific immunosuppression.

In the late 1960's, Daussett advanced the science of immunology with the description of the human lymphocyte antigen (HLA) system. The major histocompatibility complex (MHC), which in humans is on chromosome 6, codes for two classes of antigens (class I [A, B, and C] and class II [D, DR, DQ, DP, and DO]) on both cell membranes. Inheritance of these cell antigen markers is co-dominant. Each parent transmits one set of HLA antigens (haplotype) to his or her child. Nearly all cells, except red blood cells, express class I antigens, while B lymphocytes, monocytes, and endothelial cells express class II antigens. These antigens are pivotal in the rejection process.

Transplantation usually succeeds if all known class I and class II antigens between donor and recipient are identical. Unfortunately, from a matching prospective, the MHC is the most polymorphic coding system known in human biology. Most donors and recipients cannot be perfectly matched for MHC coded antigens unless the organ comes from a close family member. Figure 78–2 shows that siblings of a given patient with ESRD may be either two-haplotype matches (25 per cent likelihood), one-haplotype matches (50 per cent likelihood) or zero-haplotype matches (25 per cent likelihood). True parents are usually a one-haplotype match. As noted in the figure, ABO blood groups must also be compatible to ensure successful transplantation.

In animal and human recipients of kidney allografts, matching for both class I and class II antigens correlates with successful graft outcomes. The source of most human kidney transplants, however, is a cadaveric donor (a donor who has died but whose kidneys are still viable). Finding a good HLA match is more difficult from cadavers than from blood relatives. Although retrospective analysis of cadaveric transplantation data shows the benefit of class I and class II matching, the benefit is not as dramatic as for kidneys from relatives.

Transplantation centers in the United States currently follow a policy of mandatory sharing of six-antigen (both class I and class II) matches for cadaveric kidneys. Organ banks consider other factors besides HLA match (e.g., the patient's age and length of time on a waiting list) in the distribution of cadaveric kidneys.

Unquestionably important for both living-related transplantation and cadaveric transplantation is the "crossmatch" test. Tissue typing laboratories perform this test before all kidney transplant operations. Technicians incubate leukocytes from the potential donor (living-related or cadaveric) with serum from the potential recipient and serum complement. If the serum of the recipient destroys the membranes of the leukocyte of the potential donor, the laboratory reports the test as positive.

The surgeon usually cancels the transplant operation if the crossmatch is positive. Such a result signifies circulating antibodies against the HLA antigens. A positive crossmatch predicts nearly immediate and severe ("hyperacute") allograft rejection if the transplant is done. Investigators are testing modifications of the crossmatching procedure to find a more sensitive, yet more specific, test. The current tests, however, have all but eliminated hyperacute rejections. More sensitive tests could decrease other types of early rejection ("accelerated rejections").

Currently, many patients on waiting lists for kidney transplants have developed broad anti-HLA sensitization. Exposure to blood transfusions, failed previous transplants, or pregnancy causes such sensitization to HLA antigens. Nearly one third of patients awaiting transplantation fall into this "highly sensitized," difficult-to-transplant category. Such patients benefit from receiving the best HLA antigen match possible.

Physicians have tried other strategies, such as plasmapheresis and extracorporeal immunoadsorption, to find a suitable method of overcoming the problem of circulating preformed antibodies. These trials offer promise but are not yet established practice. The more common use of erythropoietin in patients awaiting transplantation will reduce the exposure to blood transfusions. The introduction of this new therapy to dialysis promises to decrease the rate of development and degree of circulating antibodies in patients with ESRD.

INDICATIONS FOR KIDNEY TRANSPLANTATION

The most common diseases that result in referral of patients for transplantation are (1) diabetes mellitus with renal failure, (2) hypertensive renal disease, and (3) glomerulonephritis. These three causes of ESRD account for nearly 75 per cent of candidates.

No specific cause of intrinsic and irreversible renal failure is considered a contraindication to kidney transplantation. Nonetheless, all patients should have reversible causes of renal dysfunction excluded (e.g., incomplete obstruction) prior to consideration of renal replacement therapy. Most patients undergo a period of chronic dialysis prior to receiving an allograft. Listed in Table 78–4 are selected diseases that can cause renal failure and need special consideration before renal transplantation is

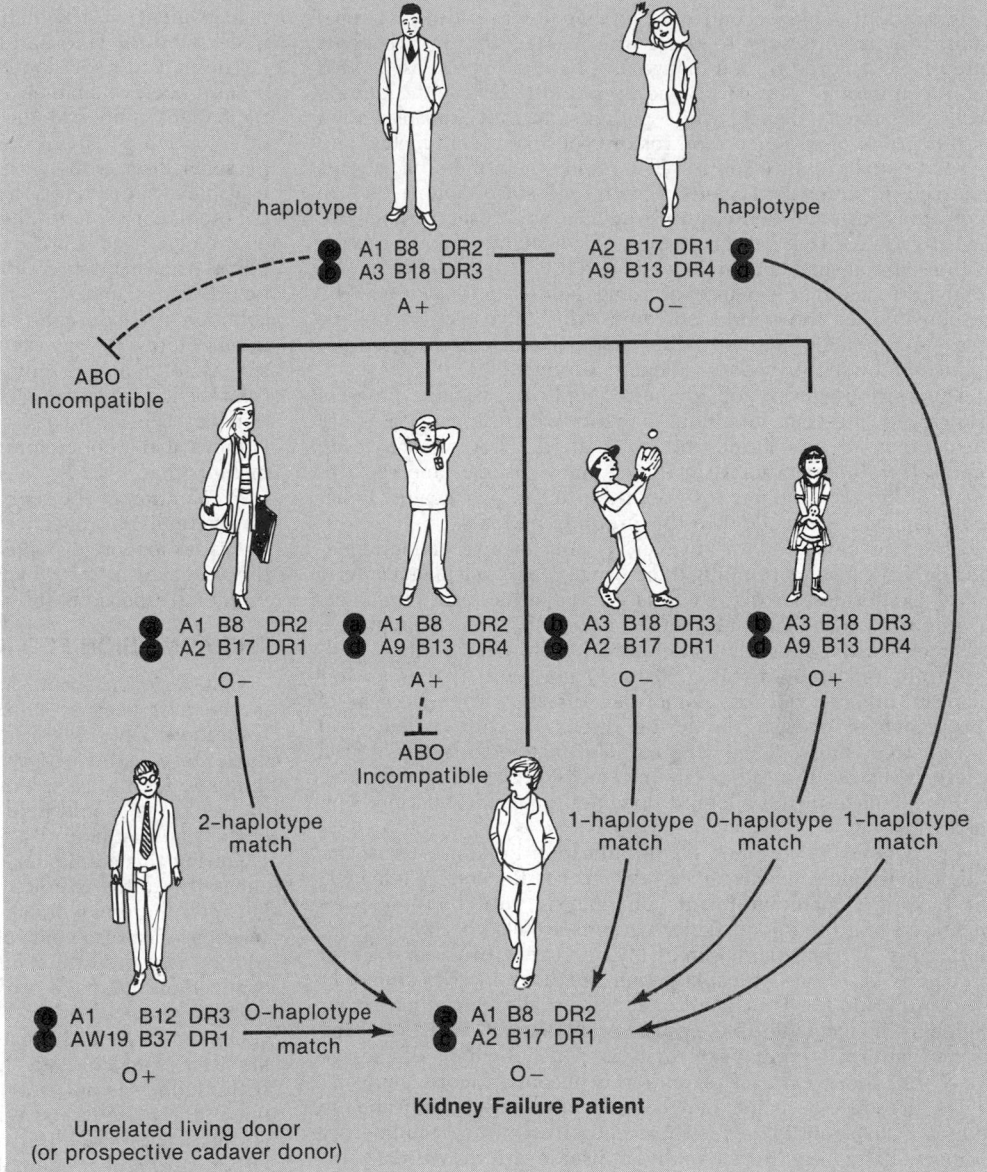

FIGURE 78–2. Family tree of HLA genotypes and unrelated HLA genotype.

chosen as therapy. The listed diseases are not contraindications to transplantation, yet the outcome may be less satisfactory for patients with these diseases compared with other renal diseases.

Patients with renal failure induced by diabetes (Kimmelstiel-Wilson disease) make up the greatest population of patients currently referred for transplantation. A decade ago, such patients were not routinely considered for kidney transplantation, but today many nephrologists consider this the treatment of choice for diabetic patients. The change in medical practice for this condition has resulted in a major extension of life expectancy of patients whose kidneys fail from diabetes.

The long-term outcome for patients with diabetes is less likely to result in full rehabilitation than for patients with forms of renal disease that do not have other organ involvement. Although allograft replacement restores normal renal function to such patients, kidney transplantation does not correct the diabetes. Long-term complications of diabetes do not reverse, and new complications develop. Eventually, other organ involvement with diabetic disease limits both survival and rehabilitation in diabetic recipients of renal allografts.

Today, living-related transplantation offers patients with diabetic renal failure the highest likelihood of prolonged survival. Most centers perform transplantations earlier in diabetic patients than in those referred with other forms of renal disease. If diabetic patients can undergo transplantation before extensive damage occurs in other organs, such as the eye and heart, rehabilitation will be more satisfactory. Late referral of diabetic patients is not in their best interest. Such patients may develop severe neurologic and cardiovascular disease to a degree that excludes them from transplantation.

Hypertension is better treated than in the past, yet the

TABLE 78–4. FACTORS LIMITING SUCCESS OF RENAL TRANSPLANTATION IN CERTAIN DISEASES

Disease	Comment
Hemolytic uremic syndrome	Disease can recur and cause graft failure rapidly; cyclosporine may increase the risk of recurrence.
Sickle cell disease	Improved hematocrit can result in increased incidence of sickle crises.
Scleroderma	Long-term vascular and gastrointestinal problems of scleroderma can limit rehabilitation.
Oxalosis	Recurrence of stone disease can be severe.
Cystinosis and Fabry's disease	Disease activity continues.
Focal glomerulosclerosis	Graft loss from recurrence is common.

incidence of end-stage renal failure due to hypertension has not decreased. It ranks second only to diabetes as a cause of renal failure in patients sent to renal transplant units. Such patients often have suffered from a malignant phase of hypertension. It is more common for elevated blood pressure to destroy the kidneys of black patients than of white patients. Kidney transplantation in this group of patients often restores normal renal function and normal blood pressure control. The reason the number of patients referred to transplant centers with end-stage failure due to hypertension is not decreasing is unclear and deserves intensive investigation. Black patients tend to have slightly poorer success with renal transplants than do white patients. The high prevalence of hypertension as a cause of renal failure in blacks may be responsible for the poorer outcome. Most investigators believe that immunologic factors, rather than original disease, are responsible for slightly poorer allograft survival.

The various forms of glomerulonephritis usually progress (slowly) to end-stage function. Patients with these diseases are ideal candidates for kidney transplantation. They often have no medical problems other than their kidney disease, and replacement of kidney function restores them to normal health. Rehabilitation can be excellent in this group of patients.

Listed in Table 78–4, however, is one form of glomerulonephritis that causes continuing difficulty in renal transplant centers. Focal glomerulosclerosis (FGS) is an idiopathic form of glomerulonephritis that (like many other forms of glomerulonephritis) can recur in the allograft. Patients with FGS have a rate of graft loss from recurrent disease (20 to 30 per cent) that is greater than in other forms of glomerular disease. The problem of recurrence of disease should be discussed with patients and prospective family kidney donors. The histologic lesion of focal sclerosis can occur in other circumstances (e.g., reflux nephritis), and recurrence in the allograft does not appear to be a problem in such cases.

Age is never an absolute contraindication to kidney transplantation. Although infants have had successful transplantations, most centers maintain infants on dialysis until body size has increased to 10 to 20 kg. Older patients are also becoming more numerous in transplant clinics. Older age (>60 years) never precludes successful transplantation but does increase the risks of complications. Transplant centers usually encourage older patients who have multiple medical problems (rather than isolated kidney failure) to remain on dialysis. On both ends of the age spectrum, however, transplantation is becoming more common.

The presence of malignancy is considered a contraindication to kidney transplantation, as is severe atherosclerotic or pulmonary disease. Patients with active liver disease are also usually excluded. Infection with the HIV virus is a relative contraindication. Anecdotal case reports suggest that such patients may progress more rapidly from carrier status to clinical AIDS when given immunosuppressive therapy. Social circumstances (inability to take medications or arrange follow-up) can also make kidney transplantation an impossibility.

EVALUATION OF THE DONOR AND RECIPIENT OF THE KIDNEY TRANSPLANT

The transplant team that will perform the surgery and follow-up should evaluate the donor (living-related) and potential recipient of the transplant. This evaluation is best done at the center where the transplantation will be done, before the actual transplantation date. The evaluation team usually includes a transplant surgeon, nephrologist, urologist, social worker, and psychiatrist.

Evaluation of the living donor focuses on three issues. Physicians must document that the patient does not have any significant medical problems that would increase the risk of surgery. The donor's motives should be appraised to ensure that the donation is altruistic. Finally, the renal function and the anatomy of the donor's renal arteries need to be defined, usually with a renal arteriogram. This evaluation is best performed in the hospital.

Evaluation of the recipient also has three goals. The physicians should assess the patient's overall medical status, aware that the recipient may face both major surgery and potent immunosuppression in the future. Emphasis should be placed on the recipient's cardiovascular risks and urologic status. The recipient's

original disease often is uncertain, and the transplant center should attempt to define this for the record. Knowledge of the original kidney disease is often important in the posttransplant management of the patient. Finally, the recipient needs to understand the risks and benefits of transplantation surgery.

The patient's social circumstance and ability to arrange follow-up also need evaluation. A discussion that explores the degree of the patient's understanding of the disease process and the planned intervention is part of the evaluation. Both audiovisual aids and personal discussions with nurses, physicians, and other kidney transplant patients are key to the patient's preparation.

Potential recipients found to have correctable cardiovascular or urologic lesions are encouraged to have repair of the lesions before transplantation. Bilateral nephrectomy of native kidneys before transplantation is rarely done. In the past, this was a more common procedure for the control of severe hypertension. A nephrectomy is suggested if the native kidneys are infected in such a fashion that only their removal will protect the patient from serious infections after transplantation. Occasionally, patients excrete such large amounts of protein from diseased native kidneys that nephrectomy is recommended because of protein malnutrition.

Preparation of the recipient with deliberate blood transfusions was a common procedure before the routine use of cyclosporine but is no longer so popular as in the past. An understanding of the mechanism by which such blood transfusions altered the immune response is still a matter of investigation.

THE ADMISSION FOR KIDNEY TRANSPLANTATION

Cadaveric transplant operations can be better "planned" than in the past because improved allograft harvesting and storage techniques have removed some of the urgency from the procedure. It is not elective surgery, however, and is still highly dramatic for the recipient. The pretransplantation evaluation of the recipient should help prepare the patient for the actual day of the transplantation.

During this admission, the transplant surgeon places a kidney allograft into the recipient's iliac fossa. An anastomosis is created between the donor renal artery and the hypogastric artery. The surgeon must also connect the donor renal vein to the iliac vein and implant the ureter into the recipient's bladder. These three connections all have variations, and all need skillful surgical technique.

On return from the operating room, the transplant recipient's first transplant admission has begun. Three issues face the patient. If the kidney is not working immediately ("immediate nonfunction"), the reason (or reasons) need to be identified. If the kidney is working, careful observation for possible rejection is begun. In either case, a new immunosuppressive regimen starts.

Immediate nonfunction of the allograft is becoming less common with improvement of techniques for procurement and storage. It is due, most often, to an acute tubular necrosis (ATN)–like syndrome in which there is reversible ischemic damage to the allograft that will heal, given time. Recent evidence strongly suggests that this phenomenon, while similar to classic ATN, differs in that the immune system plays a major role.

Obstruction, vascular thrombosis, and ureteral compression from hematoma should be considered in cases of primary nonfunction. Renal scans and ultrasound tests, as well as the patience of the managing physician, are indicated. Occasionally, an immediate return to the operating room is required. Most patients with immediate nonfunction, however, have reversible renal impairment that does not require surgical intervention.

Allografts that work immediately after the release of the vascular clamps engender immediate optimism. Observation is key in the postoperative management. It is usually in the first 3 months after transplantation that reversible acute rejections commonly occur. Many of these rejections occur during the initial hospital stay. All patients should have daily assessment of renal function, and when physicians notice impairment, a rapid diagnosis of cause (rejection versus other causes) is in order. Despite pressures to cut costs, early discharge is not in the best interest of the kidney transplant patient, although most feel well within a few days after the transplant operation. The more frequently that patients are observed in the months after transplantation, the better their care and the greater the likelihood that rejections will be reversed. The transplant physician should encourage close observation as a more important goal than early discharge.

During the first hospital stay, patients are given potent immunosuppressive agents. Immunosuppressive regimens remained stable from the 1960's through the early 1980's. Azathioprine and prednisone were the two drugs employed. Physicians became experienced with these two agents and with their predictable complications and eventually settled on the proper dose and schedule.

The Food and Drug Administration (FDA) approved cyclosporine in 1983 for general use in transplantation. Since then, the transplant community has developed a frenzy for new and different immunosuppressive protocols. Transplant centers often change to new protocols before research groups test the older protocols with randomized controlled trials. Nonetheless, as transplant groups have experimented with new and different immunosuppressive agents, results have improved markedly over the results seen with "conventional therapy" (azathioprine and prednisone).

Currently, many centers in the United States use sequential, or "induction," therapy. Four drugs are used. Initially, either antilymphocyte globulin (ATG) or monoclonal antibody (OKT3) is given as the primary immunosuppressive agent. These anti–T lymphocyte agents are continued until the allograft functions well. Then, cyclosporine, azathioprine, and prednisone are added, and ATG or OKT3 is discontinued shortly thereafter. Other groups begin with a regimen of cyclosporine, azathioprine, and prednisone immediately preceding the transplant operation ("triple drug therapy"). Some groups believe that a combination of cyclosporine and prednisone, or cyclosporine alone, is adequate therapy.

Many groups treat recipients of living-related allografts with a different immunosuppressive regimen than that used for recipients of cadaveric kidneys. Living-related donor recipients generally require less immunosuppression. These patients are usually given lower doses of fewer different immunosuppressive agents.

The addition of cyclosporine and the routine use of anti–T lymphocyte agents, while credited with improved allograft success rates, make management more complex. Cyclosporine can cause impairment of renal function that is difficult to distinguish from rejection. OKT3 and ATG can cause febrile reactions and may result in renal dysfunction.

Cyclosporine has revolutionized organ transplantation. Transplant groups have achieved a 10 to 15 per cent improvement in initial and long-term allograft survival rates with cyclosporine. Some investigators believe that the added immunosuppression of this agent overcomes the risks of rejection with poorly matched allografts. Others suggest that preparation of recipients with pretransplant blood transfusions is no longer necessary. Both of the above benefits of cyclosporine remain controversial. Most agree, however, that cyclosporine has improved allograft success rates while allowing a decrease in other immunosuppressive agents. Fewer fungal or bacterial infections occur in transplant recipients despite the decreased use of other immunosuppressants.

Cyclosporine does not affect the immunorecognition or priming of T lymphocytes to express surface receptors. Its mechanism of action is inhibition of synthesis of interleukin 2 and gamma-interferon. This is a more specific and more easily reversed action than that associated with glucocorticoids and antimetabolites. Increasing specificity of immunosuppressive agents is leading to both improved allograft survival and greater safety.

Unfortunately, one of cyclosporine's major side effects is nephrotoxicity. Investigators have shown acute, "reversible," and chronic kidney damage. Cyclosporine also markedly slows recovery from ATN and potentiates nephrotoxicity due to other substances. Cyclosporine is difficult to monitor, and clinical toxicity is common even in experienced hands. Besides nephrotoxicity, cyclosporine commonly causes tremor, palmar and plantar paresthesia, hyperglycemia, hepatotoxicity, hypertrichosis, gingival hypertrophy, and hyperkalemia.

As of this writing, OKT3 is the only monoclonal antibody commercially available. The antibody is directed against the T lymphocyte receptor for antigen and is thus a "pan" T lymphocyte agent. More specific monoclonal antibodies remain in investigational status.

OKT3 is effective in the treatment of acute rejection. Most patients who do not respond to the more traditional acute rejection therapy (bolus methylprednisolone) respond well to OKT3. This antibody is also used as prophylactic immunosuppression in the immediate posttransplant period as part of some sequential protocols. It is one of the most potent agents available for reversal and prevention of T lymphocyte–mediated rejection.

Like cyclosporine, however, OKT3 has several drawbacks. Humans develop antibodies against this murine antibody that eventually limit its effectiveness. After a single course of treatment, many patients do not respond to further therapy. Unfortunately, the reversed rejection episodes sometimes flare or recur. OKT3 that is given intravenously usually produces a "first-dose reaction" that results from cytokine release.

This first-dose reaction varies markedly among patients, from mild to life threatening. Fever, chills, dyspnea, wheezing, tachycardia, hypotension, nausea, and vomiting are common. The fever is of special concern because febrile patients with renal transplant may also be infected and OKT3-induced temperature elevation may mimic fever from other critical causes.

OUTPATIENT FOLLOW-UP

If the transplant admission goes without complication, it is possible for patients to be discharged as early as a week after surgery. Unless arrangements can be made for daily outpatient visits after discharge, however, most centers keep patients in the hospital for longer periods. Complications can lengthen this first admission to months. Geography, financial resources of the patient, facilities of the center, and clinical judgment of the physicians involved result in initial hospital stays that vary markedly in length. The author's opinion is that longer initial in-hospital stays are to the benefit of the patient. Nonetheless, whether patients are in the hospital or are outpatients, the two major problems faced by them in the initial period are infection and rejection.

Two forms of rejection have already been alluded to previously: hyperacute rejection and accelerated rejection. Both, by definition, occur before the end of the first week. Hyperacute rejection is rare with current crossmatch techniques. Accelerated rejections are less well understood and more common. Accelerated rejections often do not respond to therapy and some investigators believe that such rejection episodes also suggest the presence of circulating antibodies. It is possible that more sensitive crossmatch techniques will decrease the frequency of accelerated rejections.

Acute and chronic rejections are more common. Acute rejection episodes occur in most kidney transplant recipients. These episodes usually occur after the first week and can occur at any time, even years after the transplant. Mediated by T lymphocytes, such rejections are often associated with marked cellular infiltration of the allograft with edema. Vascular lesions also occur and suggest a poor prognosis.

Most acute rejection episodes, if diagnosed early, will respond to increased dosages of immunosuppressive agents. Diagnosis is usually made when a sudden impairment in the function of the allograft is noted. Other causes of impaired function must be ruled out. Confirmation of acute rejection can be obtained with renal scans and allograft biopsies. The most common other reason for impaired allograft function is toxicity from cyclosporine.

Chronic rejection is a phenomenon less well understood than acute rejection. Most cadaveric allografts eventually show histologic changes of rejection. These changes are mostly vascular and are similar to the histology of nephrosclerosis. Eventually, the allograft develops fibrosis and glomerular lesions that appear secondary to ischemia. There is neither a good understanding of chronic rejection nor an accepted effective therapy.

Serial "flow sheet" measurements of serum creatinine concentration reveal a gradual trend for slow but progressive impairment of allograft function. The renal scan reveals a more marked loss of renal blood flow than of glomerular filtration rate (GFR), and renal biopsy reveals fibrosis and vascular narrowing. Patients are generally asymptomatic. Recurrence of original kidney disease and cyclosporine toxicity are two other causes of allograft impairment that can mimic chronic rejection.

Despite the fact that the serum creatinine concentration is a somewhat gross measurement of renal function, it is the most commonly used test for clinical follow-up. Other tests are regularly promised in the literature to diagnose rejection earlier and more definitively. None of these laboratory tests, however, has yet replaced the serum creatinine level. Blood urea nitrogen and urinalysis are routinely obtained. It is the sequential measurement of serum creatinine concentration, however, that proves most useful clinically.

Renal scans and isotope measurements of renal blood flow (^{131}I-orthoiodohippurate) and GFR (^{99m}Tc-diethylenetriamine) are employed frequently to provide additional functional assessment of renal function. Ultrasound has proved useful for visualizing the structure of the allograft and to rule out obstruction. It has almost replaced the use of intravenous pyelography (IVP). Arteriography of the transplant renal artery is useful in making the diagnosis of stenosis. Although an invasive procedure, an arteriogram of the allograft can also provide information about the small vessels of the allograft in a more global fashion than renal biopsy. Biopsy of the allograft is also an invasive procedure. Transplant physicians believe that it gives the most useful assessment of the allograft and aids in differentiating the causes of allograft dysfunction. When other clinical assessment leaves considerable doubt in the mind of the managing physician concerning the cause of impaired function, a biopsy is indicated. More recently, the technique of fine-needle biopsy has gained popularity. This technique is considerably safer than the percutaneous core biopsy, yet its sensitivity and specificity remain controversial.

Infections during the first few weeks after transplantation cause fever and can cause impairment of allograft function. They may be confused with rejection. Wound, intravenous line, and catheter-related infections are common and are not usually due to opportunistic organisms when they occur within a few weeks of transplantation.

Opportunistic infections usually occur a month or more after the transplant operation. While *Aspergillus*, *Nocardia*, and *Toxoplasma* were once somewhat common, newer immunosuppressive protocols have resulted in a change in the spectrum of opportunistic infections. Viral infections, especially cytomegalovirus, have become dominant. Many investigators believe this is a result of the use of more specific anti–T lymphocyte preparations, such as OKT3. Infection with cytomegalovirus can be asymptomatic. It also can be so severe as to cause coma and death. Fortunately, most of these infections after transplantation, characterized by spiking fevers, leukopenia, and general malaise, last only 1 to 2 weeks and then resolve without sequelae.

Immunosuppressed kidney transplant patients believed to be infected should be hospitalized and aggressively managed. Infections in this group are the leading early cause of mortality, and aggressive management can usually reverse the process without need of sacrificing the allograft.

LONG-TERM FOLLOW-UP

Long-term immunosuppression is surprisingly well tolerated by most kidney transplant recipients. Nonetheless, it is this therapy that accounts for most of the posttransplant morbidity and mortality. Vascular disease, infections, malignancy, and chronic liver disease pose the most serious problems for recipients of kidney transplants. Immunosuppressive agents either cause or aggravate these four medical problems. Table 78–5 lists some of the more common medical problems encountered in kidney transplant clinics.

Like the general population, kidney transplant patients are most likely to die of atherosclerotic vascular disease. Kidney transplant patients, however, die of myocardial infarctions and cerebrovascular accidents at an earlier age. The reason for this precocious onset of vascular disease is not entirely understood.

Kidney transplant patients experience a high incidence of hypertension. The hypertension is multifactorial in nature. Some immunosuppressive drugs (cyclosporine and prednisone) can cause hypertension, as does kidney disease. Even if the allograft is normal, the diseased native kidneys can maintain elevated blood pressure. Stenosis of the artery of the transplanted kidney may also be a factor.

TABLE 78–5. MEDICAL COMPLICATIONS AFTER KIDNEY TRANSPLANTATION

Cardiovascular Events
  Myocardial infarction
  Cerebrovascular accident

Hypertension
  Stenosis of transplant renal artery
  Native kidney induced
  Drug induced
  Renal impairment of the allograft

Malignancies
  Skin carcinomas
  Lymphomas

Erythrocytosis
  Induced by native kidneys (?)
  Thromboembolic disease

Bone Disease
  Osteoporosis
  Aseptic necrosis
  Persistent hyperparathyroidism

Infections
  Listeria monocytogenes
  Pneumocystis carinii
  Cryptococcus
  Aspergillus
  Nocardia
  Toxoplasma
  Mycobacteria
  Legionella pneumophila
  Cytomegalovirus (CMV)
  Herpes simplex virus (HSV)
  Varicella zoster virus (VZV)
  Hepatitis viruses
  Papovaviruses
  Human immunodeficiency virus (HIV)
  Epstein-Barr virus (EBV)

Gastrointestinal Problems
  Peptic ulcer
  Pancreatitis
  Diverticulitis
  Hepatitis

Glucocorticoid-Induced Complications
  Obesity
  Cataracts
  Hyperglycemia
  Myopathy

Endocrine and Metabolic Disorders
  Secondary hyperparathyroidism
  Proximal and distal types of renal tubular acidosis
  Asymptomatic hyperuricemia and gout
  Mild hyperkalemia
  Glycosuria without an increased serum glucose concentration
  Hypophosphatemia

Miscellaneous
  Idiopathic polyarthritides
  Hirsutism
  Lymphocele
  Warts
  Psychiatric affective disorders

Kidney transplant patients have abnormal lipid profiles that physicians consider a risk factor for atherosclerotic death. These abnormal lipid patterns are believed to be an effect of the immunosuppressive drugs. Some patients continue to have proteinuria in the nephrotic range after transplantation, which may contribute to the abnormal lipid profile.

Besides hypertension and abnormal lipid profiles, there is convincing evidence that renal transplant patients usually have vascular disease even before the transplant. This vascular disease may relate to their time on dialysis and the hypertension associated with their chronic renal failure.

Most successful recipients of renal transplants enjoy a quality of life that is superior to that achieved on dialysis. Women frequently give birth after transplantation, and men can father children. It is unusual for patients with successful transplants not to return to full-time employment. Many return to a lifestyle similar to that preceding the onset of kidney disease. On the other hand, the experience of chronic disease, frequent hospitalizations, disability financing, and fear of allograft failure with long-term complications of transplant immunosuppression limit full rehabilitation for some patients.

In the United States in 1987, the average 1-year allograft survival rate was 77 per cent for recipients of cadaveric kidneys. It was 90 per cent for recipients of allografts from relatives. This is a remarkable advance compared with survival rates of 50 per cent for cadaveric kidneys just a few years ago. Some individual centers now experience cadaveric allograft survival rates of nearly 90 per cent. Mortality and morbidity continue to decrease as allograft survival rates increase. It seems likely that even these rates of success will improve in the near future.

The long-term use of immunosuppressive agents causes or aggravates most of the complications listed in Table 78–5. Investigators are directing considerable efforts at making such therapy unnecessary. Soon patients may be able to tolerate foreign antigens of the donor kidney but react normally to other foreign antigens. Limited tolerance has been achieved in animal models. If similar types of tolerance can be created in humans, graft survival will improve, and the morbidity and mortality of kidney transplantation will be drastically reduced.

Success can create problems. The number of patients on waiting lists for kidney transplantation is growing faster than the number of transplant operations. In 1988, there were only 4083 cadaveric donors in the United States. About 2000 living-related donor transplants are performed each year, and this number has been relatively stable for the past 5 years. The shortage of donor kidneys is the most consequential limitation of kidney transplantation as we enter the 1990's.

Alexander JW: The cutting edge: A look to the future of transplantation. Transplantation 49:237, 1990. *A review of the growth of kidney transplantation and predictions about future growth.*

1989 Annual Data Report of the United States Renal Data System. Washington, D.C., National Institutes of Health, pp 1–41. *Most recent statistics concerning ESRD treatment in the United States.*

Claas FHJ, van Rood JJ: The hyperimmunized patient: From sensitization toward treatment. Transplant Int 1:53, 1988. *The reasons that patients develop antibodies against HLA antigens and current strategies for dealing with this problem are reviewed.*

Combined Report on Regular Dialysis and Transplantation in Europe, XIX, 1988. Nephrol Dialysis Trans 4 (Suppl 4):5, 1989. *A review of recent trends in immunosuppressive regimens in Europe.*

Kahan BD: Cyclosporine. N Engl J Med 321:1725, 1989. *A detailed description of cyclosporine from pharmacology to future prospects.*

Shapiro ME, Reed MH, Strom TB, et al.: The role of a primate model of renal transplantation in the development of new monoclonal antibodies. Am J Kidney Dis 14 (Suppl 2):58, 1989. *A brief description of testing of new monoclonal antibodies.*

79 Glomerular Disorders
William G. Couser

About 120,000 patients in the United States require hemodialysis or transplantation for chronic renal failure at an annual cost in excess of 2 billion dollars. Two thirds of these have some glomerular disease.

In this chapter, glomerular diseases are classified on a clinical basis into three groups: (1) primary renal diseases that usually present with the abrupt onset of hematuria, red cell casts, proteinuria, and decreased glomerular filtration rate (GFR) (acute nephritic syndrome or glomerulonephritis [GN]); (2) primary renal diseases that usually present with the insidious onset of heavy proteinuria and relatively normal GFR (nephrotic syndrome); and (3) secondary glomerular diseases resulting from renal involvement by a variety of systemic illnesses, which may be either nephritic or nephrotic. This approach has the virtue of simplicity, but it is useful only if its limitations are fully appreciated. Distinguishing between primary and secondary renal diseases is sometimes difficult and arbitrary. For example, im-

munoglobulin A (IgA) nephropathy is recognized as a primary renal disease, and Henoch-Schönlein purpura is classified as a secondary one, although they probably represent only differing clinical manifestations of the same process and often overlap. Most of the diseases that present as acute GN may cause the nephrotic syndrome, although they do so uncommonly, and some nephrotic glomerular diseases may occasionally exhibit nephritic features.

IMMUNE MECHANISMS AND THE GLOMERULAR RESPONSE TO INJURY

Two immunologic mechanisms of glomerular disease are generally accepted: (1) Rare patients develop GN due to deposition of antibody to glomerular basement membrane (GBM) antigens, which results in a typical uninterrupted linear staining pattern along all glomerular capillary walls when viewed by immunofluorescence microscopy (see Fig. 79–7). (2) Much more commonly, GN is associated with discontinuous, or granular, deposits of immunoglobulin and complement (see Figs. 79–2B, 79–3B, and 79–8). These deposits may occur at three sites: (1) within the glomerular mesangium, as in IgA nephropathy, Henoch-Schönlein purpura, and early lupus nephritis; (2) along the subendothelial surface of the capillary wall between endothelial cells and GBM, as seen in more severe forms of lupus nephritis and type I membranoproliferative glomerulonephritis (MPGN); and (3) on the outer, subepithelial surface of the capillary wall, as in membranous nephropathy and the so-called subepithelial "humps" in poststreptococcal glomerulonephritis (PSGN). Granular, or immune complex, deposits at mesangial and subendothelial sites either can result from the passive glomerular trapping of preformed immune complexes from the circulation or may form in situ owing to initial glomerular localization of free antigens followed by antibody binding to them. Subepithelial immune complex deposits appear to form only on a local basis. Figure 79–1 illustrates schematically how immune deposits at each of these sites are related to normal glomerular structures and some of the morphologic lesions that result.

Several glomerular diseases that are believed to be immunologically mediated do not have immune deposit formation in glomeruli. For example, minimal change nephrotic syndrome (MCNS) exhibits a marked increase in capillary wall permeability without immune deposits or histologic changes; and idiopathic rapidly progressive glomerulonephritis (RPGN) is characterized

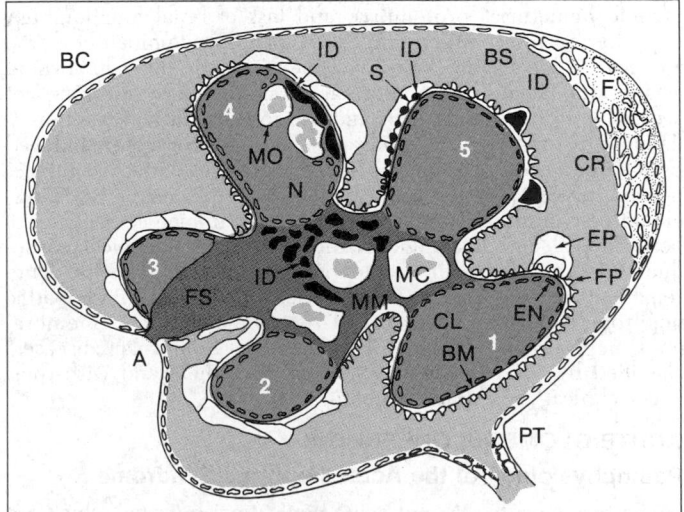

FIGURE 79–1. A highly schematized illustration of a cross-section of a single glomerulus showing normal glomerular architecture and some of the characteristic changes seen in glomerular diseases. One lobule with five capillary loops is illustrated within Bowman's capsule (BC). The capillary loops are supported by the intercapillary mesangium, containing mesangial cells (MC) and mesangial matrix (MM). Note that the normal glomerular capillary wall (loop 1) is composed of three layers: Endothelial cells (EN), basement membrane (BM), and epithelial cells (EP) with epithelial cell foot processes (FP).

TABLE 79-1. SUMMARY OF PRIMARY RENAL DISEASES THAT PRESENT AS ACUTE GLOMERULONEPHRITIS

Diseases	Poststreptococcal Glomerulonephritis (PSGN)	IgA Nephropathy	Goodpasture's Syndrome	Idiopathic Rapidly Progressive Glomerulonephritis (RPGN)
Clinical Manifestations				
Age and sex	All ages, mean 7, 2:1 male	15–35, 2:1 male	15–30, 6:1 male	Mean 58, 2:1 male
Acute nephritic syndrome	90%	50%	90%	90%
Asymptomatic hematuria	Occasionally	50%	Rare	Rare
Nephrotic syndrome	10–20%	Rare	Rare	10–20%
Hypertension	70%	30–50%	Rare	25%
Acute renal failure	50% (transient)	Very rare	50%	60%
Other	Latent period of 1–3 weeks	Follows viral syndromes	Pulmonary hemorrhage; iron deficiency anemia	None
Laboratory Findings	↑ ASO titers (70%) Positive streptozyme (95%) ↓ C3–C9 Normal C1, C4	↑ Serum IgA (50%) IgA in dermal capillaries	Positive anti-GBM antibody	Positive ANCA
Immunogenetics	HLA-B12, D "EN" (9)*	HLA-Bw 35, DR4 (4)*	HLA-DR2 (16)*	None established
Renal Pathology				
Light microscopy	Diffuse proliferation	Focal proliferation	Focal→diffuse proliferation with crescents	Crescentic GN
Immunofluorescence	Granular IgG, C3	Diffuse mesangial IgA	Linear IgG, C3	No immune deposits
Electron microscopy	Subepithelial humps	Mesangial deposits	No deposits	No deposits
Prognosis	95% resolve spontaneously 5% RPGN or slowly progressive	Slow progression in 25–50%	75% stabilize or improve if treated early	75% stabilize or improve if treated early
Treatment	Supportive	None established	Plasma exchange, steroids, cyclophosphamide	Steroid pulse therapy

*Relative risk

by severe glomerular inflammatory changes with crescent formation without detectable immune deposits.

The type and severity of histologic and functional glomerular disease induced by immune deposits in glomeruli depend on many factors, including the quantity, composition, and site of the deposits. Most glomerular antibody deposits contain predominantly immunoglobulin G (IgG), which activates complement via the classic complement pathway. When deposits are in mesangial and subendothelial sites, they are accessible to circulating inflammatory cells. Chemotactic and immune adherence mechanisms recruit participation of neutrophils, macrophages, and platelets and these effector cells cause damage to glomeruli by release of proteolytic enzymes and toxic oxygen metabolites. An inflammatory glomerular lesion results, with clinical manifestations that include hematuria, proteinuria, and loss of renal function. IgA deposits activate complement less well and predominantly by the alternate complement pathway. When immune deposits form at a subepithelial site, as in membranous nephropathy, they are not accessible to circulating cells and the resulting lesion is a noninflammatory one, with the nephrotic syndrome apparently induced by a direct effect of the C5b–9, or membrane attack complex, portion of complement on capillary wall permeability. Thus, glomerular immune complex deposits may induce a spectrum of both clinical and histologic manifestations. The clinical consequences range from the acute nephritic syndrome with acute renal failure, as seen in some cases of PSGN, to idiopathic nephrotic syndrome with normal renal function, as in membranous nephropathy. Table 79–1 lists the glomerular diseases, classified by the mechanisms that produce them and with their major clinical presentations noted.

ACUTE GLOMERULONEPHRITIS

Pathophysiology of the Acute Nephritic Syndrome

The terms *acute GN* and *acute nephritic syndrome*, which are synonymous, refer to the abrupt onset of hematuria and proteinuria, usually associated with some impairment in renal function and often with retention of salt and water, leading to hypertension and edema. Virtually all of these abnormalities are present in patients with PSGN but are less frequently found with other causes of the acute nephritic syndrome. The most common primary renal diseases that produce the acute nephritic syndrome are summarized in Table 79–2, where their major distinguishing clinical and pathologic features are compared. The syndrome may

also result from MPGN, which is discussed under diseases that cause the nephrotic syndrome, and from glomerular involvement in several of the systemic diseases to be discussed subsequently.

HEMATURIA. Hematuria is the hallmark of the acute nephritic syndrome. When hematuria is associated with proteinuria and red blood cell (RBC) casts, it usually reflects an acute glomerular inflammatory process that has the potential for rapid loss of renal function. RBC's probably reach the urine through breaks or "gaps" in the capillary wall and form casts as they become embedded in concentrated tubular fluid with an increased protein concentration. Hematuria and RBC casts may occasionally be seen in other diseases in which capillary wall

TABLE 79-2. CLASSIFICATION OF RAPIDLY PROGRESSIVE (CRESCENTIC) GLOMERULONEPHRITIS

Type of RPGN	Frequency
Anti-GBM Antibody–Mediated RPGN	20%
Goodpasture's syndrome	
Idiopathic anti-GBM nephritis	
Membranous nephropathy with crescents	
RPGN Associated with Granular Immune Deposits	40%
Postinfectious	
Poststreptococcal glomerulonephritis	
Bacterial endocarditis	
"Shunt" nephritis	
Visceral abscesses, other nonstreptococcal infections	
Noninfectious	
Systemic lupus erythematosus	
Henoch-Schönlein syndrome	
Mixed cryoglobulinemia	
Solid tumors	
Primary Renal Disease	
Membranoproliferative glomerulonephritis	
IgA nephropathy	
Idiopathic "immune complex" nephritis	
RPGN Without Glomerular Immune Deposits	40%
Vasculitis	
Polyarteritis	
Hypersensitivity vasculitis	
Wegener's granulomatosis	
Idiopathic RPGN	

PROTEINURIA. In acute GN, proteinuria invariably accompanies hematuria but rarely exceeds 3.5 grams per day and is therefore in the "nonnephrotic" range. Proteinuria in acute GN reflects an increased urinary content of serum proteins due to some combination of three factors: (1) a generalized increase in the permeability characteristics of the glomerular capillary wall itself, (2) altered glomerular hemodynamics, and (3) mechanical disruptions in capillary wall structure. Thus, proteinuria in acute GN is "nonselective" and contains serum globulins as well as albumin. The pathophysiology of glomerular protein excretion is discussed in more detail below under Nephrotic Syndrome.

IMPAIRED RENAL FUNCTION. When glomerular inflammation is severe enough to cause hematuria and proteinuria, the GFR is usually reduced. This may range from a minimal reduction in GFR with normal serum creatinine values to oliguria or anuria requiring dialysis. Multiple factors account for the reduced GFR, including the effects of acute immune injury on glomerular pathophysiology and the development of glomerular intracapillary thromboses, acute tubular necrosis secondary to glomerular ischemia, tubular obstruction by casts, and compression of the glomerular tuft by proliferating epithelial cells forming crescents. The return of renal function to normal depends not only on cessation of the process that initiated the injury but also on the extent of irreversible structural changes that have occurred, such as necrosis, sclerosis, and fibrosis.

HYPERTENSION. Hypertension is a common manifestation of the acute nephritic syndrome in PSGN and may be a presenting sign in older patients. It is largely volume dependent, reflecting impaired renal excretion of sodium and water, with reduced levels of plasma renin and aldosterone. Hypertension can generally be controlled by strict adherence to sodium restriction.

EDEMA. Edema in the acute nephritic syndrome, like hypertension, reflects extracellular fluid volume expansion due to renal retention of salt and water. The mechanisms of renal sodium retention in acute GN are poorly understood but include a reduced filtered sodium load as well as enhanced sodium reabsorption in either the distal nephron or deep juxtamedullary nephrons. Edema and fluid retention are seen in more than 90 per cent of patients with acute PSGN but are less common in other diseases causing the acute nephritic syndrome. Unlike nephrotic edema, in the nephritic syndrome, edema is often present in nondependent areas, such as eyelids, face, and hands. The key to management is effective sodium restriction, since diuretics may not be effective in the acute stage of GN.

Couser WG: Mediation of immune glomerular injury. J Am Soc Nephrol 1:13, 1990. *An in-depth review of the pathogenetic mechanisms that underlie immune glomerular disease.*

Madaio MP, Harrington JT: Medical intelligence. Current concepts: The diagnosis of acute glomerulonephritis. N Engl J Med 309:1299, 1983. *This short review provides a useful outline of the diagnosis and classification of acute glomerulonephritis, emphasizing the distinctive clinical and laboratory features of each of the diseases that cause the acute nephritic syndrome.*

Whitley K, Keane WF, Vernier RL: Acute glomerulonephritis: A clinical overview. Med Clin North Am 68:259, 1984. *This article reviews the pathogenetic mechanisms, clinical presentations, laboratory features, and renal biopsy findings in each of the major disease entities that cause acute glomerulonephritis.*

Isolated Hematuria

The presence of persistent abnormal hematuria (more than five RBC's per high-power field in more than one fresh-voided urine specimen), without systemic disease, RBC casts, significant proteinuria, or impaired renal function, is a common medical problem that may or may not reflect renal parenchymal disease. It is more common in children and adolescents than in adults. A careful medical and urologic evaluation must be performed with appropriate laboratory, radiologic, and urologic procedures to exclude nonglomerular lesions of the urinary tract, such as infection, prostatism, papillary necrosis, polycystic and medullary sponge kidney, renal or urinary tract tumors, arteriovenous malformations, renal stones, blood dyscrasias, and hemoglobinopathies. The presence of dysmorphic RBC's in the urine by phase microscopy suggests a glomerular origin for hematuria. The "loin pain–hematuria syndrome" is a disorder usually seen in young women taking oral contraceptives who develop recurrent episodes of gross hematuria accompanied by loin pain and mild

hypertension in the absence of proteinuria or reduced renal function. The condition appears to be benign and is reversible when oral contraceptives are discontinued.

If no cause of hematuria can be found and no evidence of systemic or renal disease is present, isolated hematuria appears to be a benign entity, and only careful follow-up is indicated. Renal biopsy is performed in such patients only if evidence of progressive renal disease develops or if the patient requires further evaluation for other purposes such as insurance or employment. When such patients do undergo renal biopsy, the results usually reveal a mild, nonprogressive form of glomerular disease, often focal GN with or without mesangial IgA deposits.

Bauer DC: Evaluation of hematuria in adults. West J Med 152:305, 1990. *A concise review of the causes of hematuria in adults and the approach to diagnosis as it should be pursued by a primary care physician.*

Trachtman H, Weiss RA, Bennett B, et al.: Isolated hematuria in children: Indications for a renal biopsy. Kidney Int 25:94, 1984. *This paper reviews the findings in 76 children and adolescents who had biopsies for isolated hematuria and identifies a family history of hematuria and episodes of gross hematuria as the best predictors of significant renal pathology.*

Isolated Proteinuria

A more detailed discussion of proteinuria is given in Ch. 74. Like isolated hematuria, proteinuria in the nonnephrotic range *without* hematuria or decreased renal function may indicate a significant glomerular disease but usually does not. When increased urinary protein excretion is suggested by qualitative analyses such as the dipstick test, it must be confirmed by an accurate measurement of 24-hour protein excretion. Values in excess of 150 mg per day in adults, and 140 mg per square meter per day in children, are regarded as abnormal if an accurate 24-hour urine collection has been obtained. Reliable estimates of proteinuria can also be obtained by measuring protein-creatinine ratios in random daytime urine specimens. Values in excess of 0.2 are abnormal and above 3.5 suggest nephrotic range proteinuria. Abnormal protein excretion may be intermittent or persistent (fixed).

INTERMITTENT PROTEINURIA. The most common causes of intermittent proteinuria are *exercise*, assumption of the *upright position* (postural proteinuria), and *fever*. Up to 10 per cent of patients admitted on a routine medical basis may exhibit transient proteinuria. The basis for proteinuria in most of these conditions is probably hemodynamic, although subtle alterations in glomerular architecture have not been excluded. Total protein excretion is usually less than 2.0 grams per day, renal function is normal, and 20-year follow-up studies have shown resolution of the proteinuria in a majority of cases with no evidence of progressive renal disease.

PERSISTENT PROTEINURIA. Persistent or fixed proteinuria can also occur without glomerular disease. *"Overflow" proteinuria* occurs when excess production of filterable, low molecular weight proteins exceeds the tubular reabsorptive capacity, as occurs with the production of lysozyme (molecular weight 14,000) in myelomonocytic leukemia or L-chains in plasma cell dyscrasias such as multiple myeloma. In some cases up to 5.0 grams of L-chains may be excreted daily. Another nonglomerular cause of proteinuria is renal tubular disease in which normal quantities of proteins such as lysozyme or beta$_2$-microglobulin are filtered but not reabsorbed. This situation can result in urinary excretion of up to 2.0 grams of such proteins daily in a variety of interstitial nephropathies and disorders of tubular function.

Isolated, fixed, nonnephrotic proteinuria of glomerular origin is associated with an increased incidence of hypertension and a somewhat decreased life expectancy in long-term follow-up studies, but progressive renal disease is rare. Renal biopsy in such patients usually reveals some glomerular abnormality. The spectrum of lesions in isolated proteinuria is wide and similar to that discussed above in isolated hematuria. In patients with fixed proteinuria of less than 2.0 grams per day without hematuria, systemic disease, or impaired renal function, renal biopsy is usually not performed unless a change in clinical status occurs or the patient requests a biopsy for other purposes.

Abuelo JG: Proteinuria: Diagnostic principles and procedures. Ann Intern Med 98:186, 1983. *A well-written summary of the different types of proteinuria, their causes and prognosis, with emphasis on the approach to evaluation of patients with mild proteinuria and normal renal function.*

SPECIFIC RENAL DISEASES THAT PRESENT AS ACUTE GLOMERULONEPHRITIS (GN) (see Table 79–1)

The prototype of acute postinfectious GN is PSGN, but glomerular disease may follow infection with a variety of other bacterial and nonbacterial agents: both gram-positive and gram-negative bacteria, viruses, mycoplasma, fungi, protozoa, helminths, and spirochetes. Many of these associations have been noted only in patients with endocarditis or infected ventriculoatrial shunts. It is important to distinguish between specific postinfectious glomerular diseases, such as PSGN, and the nonspecific role of many infections, particularly viral illnesses, in producing "exacerbations" of underlying glomerular disease. These exacerbations are usually characterized by a transient increase in proteinuria and hematuria associated with the infection, usually without an intervening latent period.

Poststreptococcal Glomerulonephritis (PSGN)

Etiology, Incidence, and Epidemiology. GN occurs only following infection with a group A (beta-hemolytic) streptococcus of nephritogenic M type, usually type 12 in the United States. Streptococcal pharyngitis is the most common antecedent event in the North, and PSGN occurs with a frequency of less than 5 per cent after a latent period of 6 to 20 days (average of 10). The disease is often sporadic, occurs in the winter and spring, is more common in males, and is accompanied by serologic evidence of recent streptococcal infection in more than 80 per cent of cases. In the South, streptococcal pyoderma or impetigo is more common, the attack rate is higher (25 to 50 per cent), the latent period is longer (14 to 21 days, average of 20), and the disease affects males and females equally, often occurring in epidemic form in more temperate climates in the summer and fall.

Pathogenesis. Granular immune complex deposits in glomeruli cause the clinical and histologic features of PSGN. The presence of these deposits, hypocomplementemia, and the latent period between infection and the onset of GN suggest that the disease is similar to experimental acute serum sickness, in which acute GN is mediated by formation of glomerular deposits containing antigen and antibody to it 8 to 10 days following a single injection of antigen. The deposits are thought to reflect glomerular trapping of circulating immune complexes, but they may also form on a local basis. Streptococcal antigens have been identified in glomerular deposits early in PSGN in some patients. The presence of C3 in the deposits and the prominent infiltrate of neutrophils and mononuclear cells in the acute stage suggest a lesion that is mediated by complement, neutrophils, and macrophages.

Pathology. Figure 79–2 illustrates the typical findings in acute PSGN by light microscopy, IF, and EM. The histologic lesion in PSGN is a diffuse (all glomeruli involved) proliferative GN with a marked hypercellularity involving glomerular endothelial and mesangial cells, as well as neutrophils and mononuclear cells with narrowing or occlusion of capillary loops (Fig. 79–2A). Proliferation of epithelial cells in Bowman's space results in formation of glomerular "crescents" in severe disease. Extensive crescent formation is seen in about 5 per cent of patients and correlates with a more severe initial disease and reduced likelihood of complete recovery. Coarsely granular deposits of IgG and C3 occur along the glomerular capillary walls and in the mesangium (Fig. 79–2B). By electron microscopy there are discrete electron-dense subepithelial nodules or "humps" (Fig. 79–2C) that persist for about 8 weeks. Subepithelial humps are a highly characteristic feature of PSGN, although they may occasionally be seen in other types of bacterial postinfectious GN and type I MPGN.

Clinical Findings. PSGN is the prototype of the acute nephritic syndrome and causes all of the findings discussed above under Pathophysiology of the Acute Nephritic Syndrome. The disease is most common in children between 3 and 12 years of age, with a mean age of about 7, and is rare in infancy and in adults over 50. The typical presentation of PSGN is the abrupt onset of hematuria (90 per cent), which is usually evident as dark or *"smoky" urine*, accompanied by *malaise* and sometimes gastrointestinal symptoms, such as abdominal pain, nausea, and vomiting. Central nervous system manifestations may include headaches

and occasionally seizures. *Edema* is an early and frequent sign, often in a periorbital distribution most evident on arising and sometimes progressing to peripheral edema and anasarca. *Hypertension* is present in 60 to 70 per cent of patients and reflects renal retention of salt and water with volume overload. Proteinuria is usually present as well. About 20 per cent of hospitalized patients develop nephrotic range proteinuria, usually transiently and during the recovery phase. Renal function is impaired in about 50 per cent of patients.

Prognosis. Three clinical courses can be defined in PSGN: complete recovery, no recovery, or partial recovery with progressive disease. In more than 90 per cent of cases, complete recovery occurs with spontaneous diuresis in an average of 4 to 7 days. Even patients who require dialysis during the acute phase usually recover spontaneously without specific therapy. Abnormal hematuria and proteinuria may persist for up to 2 years. Progressive renal disease is a very uncommon consequence of PSGN, however, if renal function returns to normal and proteinuria is less than 500 mg per day.

Fewer than 5 per cent of patients with PSGN have oliguria lasting more than 9 days; the prognosis in these patients is worse. Although spontaneous complete recovery has been reported with oliguria or anuria for up to 25 days, this is unusual. Many patients with prolonged oliguria have a crescentic glomerular lesion. About half of these will still recover spontaneously. In the remainder, the disease behaves like RPGN, with no recovery at all or with only partial recovery of renal function, which may be followed by persistent proteinuria and progressive renal disease, leading to renal failure in months to years. Patients with PSGN who have oliguric renal failure lasting more than 1 week, particularly adults, should undergo a renal biopsy. If extensive crescent formation is found, they should be considered for therapy as outlined below under Treatment.

Laboratory Features. Laboratory findings consist of an abnormal urinalysis, elevated antibodies against streptococcal exoenzymes, and reduced serum complement levels. The urinalysis usually reveals signs of glomerular inflammation with proteinuria, RBC's, white blood cells (WBC's), and casts. RBC casts are present in 60 to 85 per cent of cases when a freshly voided urine is examined. The urine is often concentrated and exhibits biochemical characteristics of prerenal azotemia, including a low urinary sodium concentration, indicating severe glomerular disease with good preservation of tubular function.

Beta-hemolytic streptococci are detected by culture in only 25 per cent of untreated patients, but serologic tests generally confirm recent streptococcal infection. The anti–streptolysin O (ASO) titer exceeds 200 Todd units within 1 to 3 weeks and may remain elevated for months. An increase in ASO titer may not be seen if penicillin therapy is initiated early or if the antecedent infection was in the skin. Antibodies to other streptococcal enzymes are usually elevated as well. The streptozyme test utilizes five of these antigens in a single assay and is quite sensitive and specific. More than 90 per cent of patients with PSGN have a reduced level of total hemolytic complement or C3 during the first 2 weeks of illness, with most returning to normal within 8 weeks. The pattern of complement component depression suggests alternate pathway activation, with levels of C1q and C4 usually normal.

Diagnosis. The differential diagnosis of acute GN with hypocomplementemia includes other forms of postinfectious GN, such as subacute bacterial endocarditis (SBE) or shunt nephritis, systemic lupus erythematosus (SLE), and type I MPGN. Only MPGN is difficult to exclude by clinical and laboratory criteria. A similar pattern of alternate complement pathway activation is seen in MPGN, a disease that may also occasionally follow streptococcal infection, and MPGN must be considered when nephrotic range proteinuria and hypocomplementemia persist for longer than 2 months. The diagnosis of PSGN can usually be made by the presence of typical clinical features of the acute nephritic syndrome following a streptococcal infection by an appropriate latent period, and by hypocomplementemia and serologic evidence of recent streptococcal infection. Because patients with PSGN usually recover spontaneously and no specific therapy is indicated, the diagnosis is often made clinically without a renal biopsy. Biopsy is indicated, however, if atypical features are present, such as prolonged oliguria, anuria, persistent hypocomplementemia, the nephrotic syndrome, or clinical or serologic evidence of systemic disease.

Treatment. In most patients with PSGN, there is no need for specific therapy, since spontaneous recovery can be anticipated. Antibiotics should be given if cultures are positive for group A streptococci, but penicillin therapy does not alter the incidence or severity of PSGN. Manifestations of sodium retention, such as hypertension, edema, and congestive heart failure, can usually be managed with careful sodium restriction, but diuretics and antihypertensive agents may be employed if necessary. Dialysis may be required temporarily in some patients, most of whom will still recover normal renal function spontaneously.

There are no data on which to base a recommendation for therapy in patients with prolonged oliguria and a crescentic glomerular lesion on biopsy. Although up to 50 per cent of such patients may recover spontaneously, the prognosis is sufficiently guarded to warrant considering therapy with pulse steroids or plasma exchange, as outlined below under RPGN.

Nissenson AR, moderator: Post-streptococcal acute glomerulonephritis: Fact and controversy. Ann Intern Med 91:76, 1979. *An excellent overview of the microbiology, epidemiology, clinical manifestations, laboratory features, pathogenesis, and sequelae of PSGN, with 128 references.*

Rodriguez-Iturbe B: Epidemic poststreptococcal glomerulonephritis. Kidney Int 25:129, 1984. *An excellent review of the pathogenesis, laboratory findings, clinical features, and long-term prognosis in acute poststreptococcal nephritis, with 65 references.*

Glomerulonephritis in Subacute Bacterial Endocarditis (SBE)

Glomerular disease in SBE ranges in severity from the proteinuria and hematuria seen in 70 per cent of patients, usually with normal renal function, to occasional cases of crescentic GN with acute renal failure. It is more common in chronic cases with right-sided cardiac involvement and negative blood cultures, as may occur in patients who abuse drugs. A wide variety of organisms have been implicated, most commonly *Staphylococcus aureus* and *Streptococcus viridans*. A similar syndrome may be seen in patients with infected ventriculoatrial shunts for hydrocephalus (shunt nephritis), often due to *Staphylococcus albus*. Serologic abnormalities are often present, including hypocomplementemia with activation of both the classic and the alternate complement pathways, cryoglobulinemia, and positive rheumatoid factor. Renal biopsy usually demonstrates a focal proliferative GN, often with necrosis and intracapillary thrombi. Granular deposits of IgG, IgM, and C3 occur in mesangial and subendothelial areas, implicating an immune complex rather than an embolic mechanism in the pathogenesis of the lesion. Renal function usually returns to normal following appropriate antibiotic

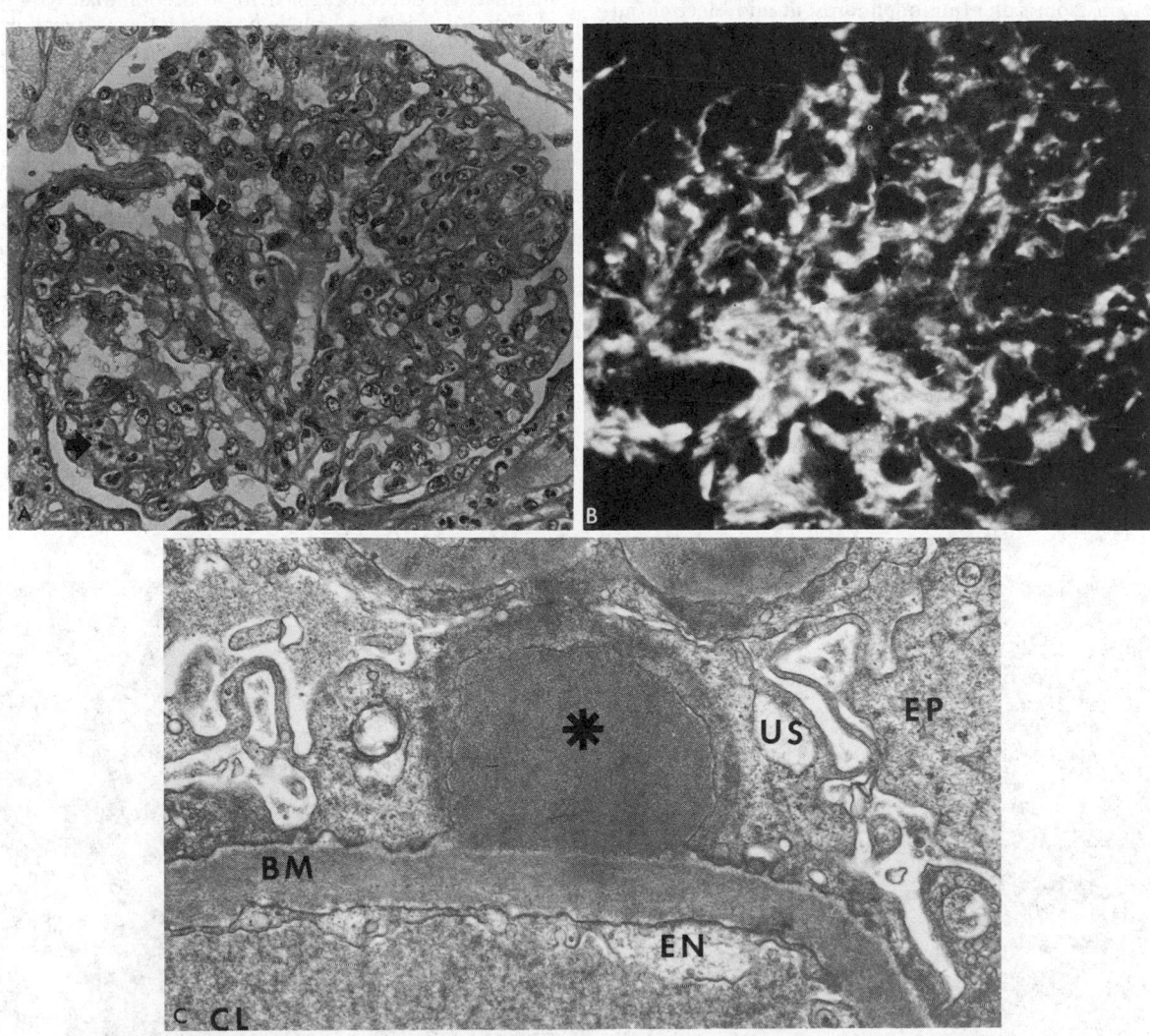

FIGURE 79–2. The renal lesion of poststreptococcal glomerulonephritis (PSGN). *A,* Light microscopic section of a renal biopsy from a patient with acute PSGN showing a marked increase in glomerular cells and infiltration by polymorphonuclear leukocytes (*arrows*) (periodic acid–Schiff stain; ×300). *B,* Immunofluorescent staining for IgG from the same biopsy reveals a coarse, granular pattern of deposits on the capillary walls and in the mesangium (×350). *C,* Electron microscopy in acute PSGN reveals a characteristic electron-dense "hump" on the subepithelial surface (*) with effacement of epithelial foot processes around the deposit. BM = Basement membrane; CL = capillary lumen; EN = endothelial cell; EP = epithelial cell; US = urinary space (×14,400). (Reproduced with permission from Couser WG, Salant DJ, Stilmant MM. *In* Flamenbaum W, Hamburger RJ [eds.]: Nephrology. Philadelphia, J.B. Lippincott Company, 1982, pp 265–301.)

therapy and eradication of the infection. However, recovery may be slow if the lesion is severe or crescents are present.

Feinstein EI, Eknoyan G, Lister BJ, et al.: Renal complications of bacterial endocarditis. Am J Nephrol 5:457, 1985. *This discussion, with 69 references, of endocarditis and glomerulonephritis in a patient who is an intravenous drug abuser presents a comprehensive review of glomerular disease associated with both endocarditis and drug abuse.*

Neugarten J, Gallo GR, Baldwin DS: Glomerulonephritis in bacterial endocarditis. Am J Kidney Dis 3:371, 1984. *This paper reviews 107 patients with endocarditis and notes that 22 per cent had glomerulonephritis with a spectrum of renal lesions and that Staphylococcus aureus was the predominant organism. The relationship among renal lesion, therapy, and prognosis is discussed.*

Glomerulonephritis with Visceral Abscesses

The abrupt onset of acute renal failure associated with proteinuria, hematuria, and red cell casts may occur in patients with a pyogenic visceral abscess. Abscesses are most frequently located in the respiratory tract but have been reported at numerous other sites, including the abdomen and uterus. Endocarditis may be present but usually is not, and blood cultures are commonly negative. In contrast to PSGN, SBE, and shunt nephritis, serologic studies, including complement levels, are usually normal. A variety of bacteria have been implicated. The glomerular lesion is usually a proliferative GN with crescents, and monocytes may be prominent in glomeruli. Immunofluoresent and electron microscopic studies do not usually reveal immune deposits, so that the pathogenesis of this lesion is unclear. Recovery of renal function has occurred in about half of the patients reported with acute renal failure who were successfully treated to eradicate the infection, but the overall mortality is quite high.

Beaufils M: Glomerular disease complicating abdominal sepsis. Kidney Int 19:609, 1981. *A detailed review of nonstreptococcal postinfectious glomerulonephritis, including SBE- as well as abscess-related lesions. The frequency with which renal biopsies reveal glomerular disease as a cause of acute renal failure in patients with sepsis is striking, since most such patients would not be so extensively studied in the United States.*

Glomerular Disease in Acquired Immunodeficiency Syndrome (AIDS)

Up to 50 per cent of patients with AIDS have abnormal proteinuria, and 10 per cent develop nephrotic syndrome. A variety of glomerular, tubular, and interstitial lesions have also been noted, presumably induced by infections, drug exposure, and other factors. However, a majority of patients with nephrotic syndrome have focal glomerulosclerosis. A rapid loss of renal function may occur in this subset of patients.

Bourgoignie JJ, Meneses R, Ortiz C, et al.: The clinical spectrum of renal disease associated with human immunodeficiency virus. Am J Kidney Dis 12:131, 1988. *A review of 100 cases of AIDS with renal manifestations that emphasizes the frequency of nephrotic syndrome and focal glomerulosclerosis as well as the poor prognosis of this type of renal lesion.*

Glassock RJ, moderator: Human immunodeficiency virus (HIV) infection and the kidney. Ann Intern Med 112:35, 1990. *This authoritative review covers all aspects of renal involvement in AIDS, including fluid and electrolyte disturbances, AIDS nephropathy, and HIV infection in patients on dialysis or undergoing renal transplantation.*

IgA Nephropathy (Berger's Disease)

Overview and Incidence. IgA nephropathy is the most common cause of primary glomerular disease in Europe, Australia, and the United States. The disease is now regarded as a monosymptomatic form of *Henoch-Schönlein purpura* (HSP), but clinical manifestations are milder than in HSP and are usually confined to the kidney. HSP is discussed later in this chapter and also in Ch. 154.

Pathogenesis. The pathogenesis of the renal lesion in IgA nephropathy and HSP is not known. It appears to be a consequence of mesangial formation of immune deposits composed predominantly of IgA (see Fig. 79–3B). The IgA may represent the antibody component of an immune complex containing a nonrenal antigen. A similar glomerular lesion may develop in liver disease associated with elevated portal pressure. The glomerular IgA deposits appear to be predominantly polymeric and of mucosal origin, which may reflect the association of disease activity with viral infections of the upper respiratory and gastrointestinal tracts.

Pathology. The typical lesion of IgA nephropathy has a focal distribution, meaning that some glomeruli are involved while others are spared, and is also segmental, with lesions in some glomerular tufts but not others (Fig. 79–3A). Mesangial expansion and hypercellularity are common, but the characteristic lesion is focal and segmental proliferative GN. When crescents are present, they are usually small and rarely involve more than 30 per cent of glomeruli. Immune deposits are present diffusely in the mesangium of all glomeruli and contain IgA as the predominant immunoglobulin, accompanied by C3 in 60 per cent and IgG in 30 per cent of cases (Fig. 79–3B). C1q and C4 are usually absent, suggesting alternate complement pathway activation. Some patients have deposits along the subendothelial aspect of the capillary wall or in the subepithelial space and generally have more severe disease and more proteinuria.

Clinical and Laboratory Findings and Diagnosis. IgA nephropathy is two to three times more common in males than in females, and most patients present before the age of 35. The classic

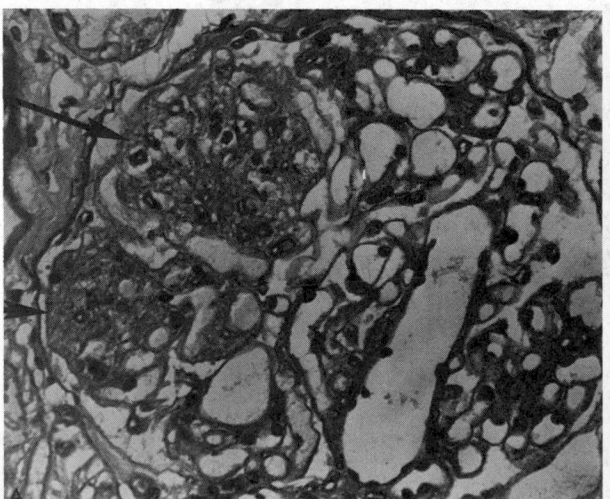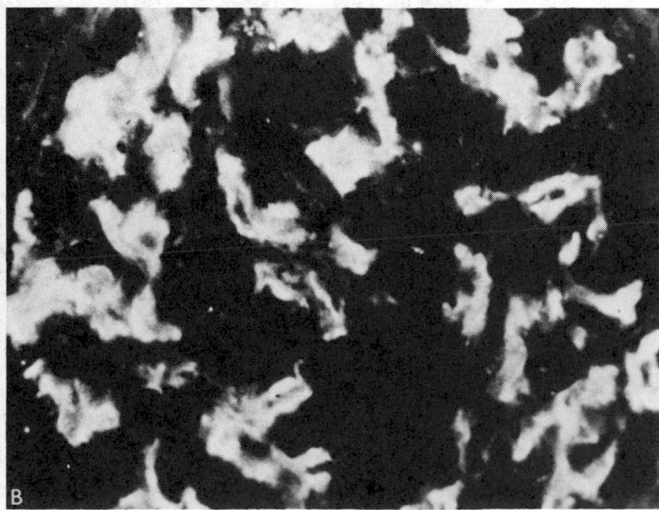

FIGURE 79–3. The renal lesion of IgA nephropathy. *A*, Light microscopic section from a patient with gross hematuria and focal glomerulonephritis due to IgA nephropathy. There is segmental involvement of the glomerulus, which shows mesangial matrix increase and hypercellularity in two lobules (*arrows*). Adjacent lobules are essentially normal (periodic acid–Schiff stain, ×350). *B*, Immunofluorescence microscopy on the same biopsy reveals bright, diffuse staining for IgA in all mesangial areas. No significant capillary wall staining is present. IgG and C3 may be found in a similar pattern but with less intensity (×450). (Reproduced with permission from Couser WG, Salant DJ, Stilmant MM. *In* Flamenbaum W, Hamburger RJ [eds.]: Nephrology. Philadelphia, J.B. Lippincott Company, 1982, pp 265–301.)

presentation is *gross hematuria* that occurs coincident with, or immediately following (24 to 48 hours), a viral upper respiratory infection (50 per cent), flu-like illness (15 per cent), a gastrointestinal syndrome (10 per cent), or other infectious prodrome. Associated findings often include mild fever, malaise, myalgias, dysuria, and loin pain. The remainder of cases are identified during medical evaluation for persistent, asymptomatic hematuria or proteinuria. The absence of a latent period, as well as normal levels of complement and antistreptococcal antibodies, distinguishes this disease clinically from PSGN. Moreover, other features of the acute nephritic syndrome, including edema and hypertension, are seen in fewer than half of the patients. Only about 25 per cent of patients have impaired renal function during active disease, and the serum creatinine level rarely exceeds 3 mg per deciliter. Proteinuria is usually less than 1 gram per day. A subset of patients with steroid-sensitive nephrotic syndrome may have mesangial IgA deposits but are believed to have primary MCNS.

Gross hematuria usually lasts only 2 to 6 days, but microscopic hematuria often persists between attacks. Fifty per cent of patients will have only a single episode of gross hematuria. The remainder have recurring episodes for many years, often preceded by viral infections.

There are no laboratory findings diagnostic of IgA nephropathy. About half of all patients have elevated serum levels of IgA that do not correlate with disease activity. Circulating immune complexes containing IgA are present intermittently, and deposits of IgA, C3, and fibrin may be present in the dermal capillaries of normal skin. The incidence of this disease is greater in persons with HLA-Bw 35 and HLA-DR4 (HLA, human leukocyte antigen) phenotypes.

Course and Prognosis. Progression to renal failure occurs in 15 to 20 per cent of patients within 6 months, and a 50 per cent death or dialysis rate is projected over 20 years. While there are no clinical or pathologic features that permit accurate prediction of progression, patients who tend to do worse are male, have a prolonged clinical course, develop hypertension or proteinuria exceeding 3 grams per day, or have extensive glomerulosclerosis present on biopsy.

Treatment. No specific form of therapy has been shown to alter the long-term clinical course of this disease. Rigorous control of hypertension is important. Mesangial deposits of IgA occur with a high frequency in renal allografts but rarely compromise graft function.

Clarkson AR, Woodroffe AJ, Aarons I, et al.: IgA nephropathy. Ann Rev Med 38:157, 1987. *A very current and detailed summary of IgA nephropathy that includes comments on clinical manifestations, pathology, natural history, and pathogenesis.*
D'Amico G: The commonest glomerulonephritis in the world: IgA nephropathy. Q J Med 64:709, 1987. *An in-depth review of IgA nephropathy with an excellent summary of the rationale for designing treatment options.*
Julian BA, Waldo FB, Rifai A, et al.: IgA nephropathy, the most common glomerulonephritis worldwide. Am J Med 84:129, 1988. *A concise but complete review of the epidemiology, clinical features, immunopathogenesis, and approach to therapy of IgA nephropathy from an experienced clinical center.*

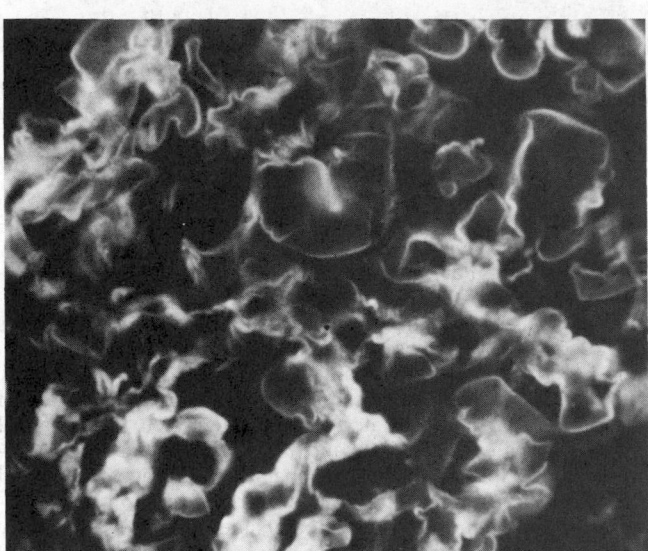

FIGURE 79–5. Immunofluorescence microscopy on a renal biopsy from a patient with Goodpasture's syndrome reveals continuous, uninterrupted, linear deposition of IgG along all capillary walls. This pattern is characteristic of anti-GBM disease ($\times 450$). (Reproduced with permission from Couser WG, Salant DJ, Stilmant MM. *In* Flamenbaum W, Hamburger RJ [eds.]: Nephrology. Philadelphia, J.B. Lippincott Company, 1982, pp 265–301.)

Rapidly Progressive Glomerulonephritis (RPGN)

Overview. The term RPGN is applied to any glomerular disease in which rapid loss of renal function occurs in association with extensive crescent formation in many glomeruli, usually more than 50 per cent (Fig. 79–4). RPGN may occur in severe cases of a wide variety of glomerular diseases, which are listed in Table 79–2, or it may occur alone as a primary renal disease. The classification system used here is based on pathogenetic mechanisms. Accurate prognosis and selection of appropriate therapy require that the underlying mechanisms be defined. About 20 per cent of cases of RPGN are mediated by anti-GBM antibody deposition and 40 per cent by glomerular immune complex formation (usually in association with some systemic disease process such as PSGN or SLE), and 40 per cent are primary renal lesions with no significant glomerular immune deposits, which are classified here as idiopathic RPGN (Table 79–2).

RPGN DUE TO ANTI-GBM ANTIBODY. Although much is known of the mediation of immune glomerular injury from studies of experimental anti-GBM nephritis, this mechanism accounts for fewer than 5 per cent of cases of GN seen clinically. Anti-GBM GN is characterized by the abrupt onset of a proliferative GN, usually with crescents, and a characteristic linear deposition of IgG seen along the GBM by immunofluorescence (Fig. 79–5). In about two thirds of cases, pulmonary hemorrhage accompanies GN, and the disease is termed Goodpasture's syndrome. The remaining one third of patients have anti-GBM nephritis without pulmonary involvement.

Goodpasture's Syndrome. Pathogenesis. The events that initiate anti-GBM antibody production are not known. Antibody reactive with GBM and alveolar basement membrane mediates the glomerular disease in anti-GBM nephritis with and without pulmonary hemorrhage. The development of lung hemorrhage appears to require the presence of prior lung damage to allow antibody deposition. Genetic factors are clearly important in this disease. There is a strong association with HLA-DRw2 (relative risk of 15 to 34 times normal). Anti-GBM antibody production is a self-limited event usually lasting several months. Exacerbations

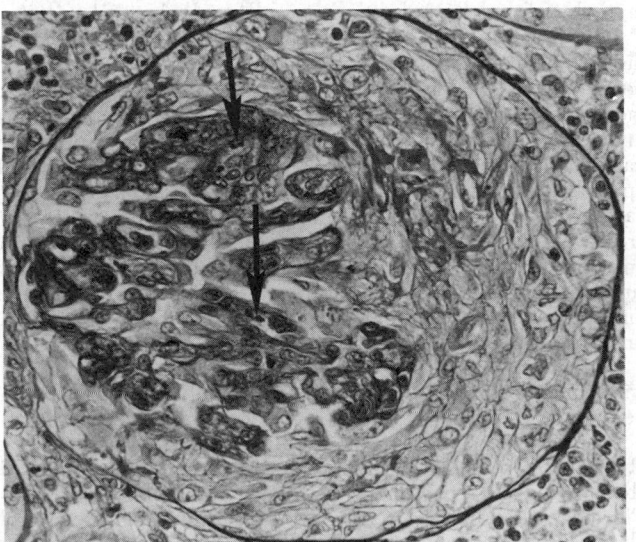

FIGURE 79–4. Light microscopy from a patient with idiopathic RPGN reveals the presence of a large cellular crescent in Bowman's space surrounding and compressing the glomerular capillary. A few polymorphonuclear leukocytes are seen in the glomerulus (*arrows*) (periodic acid–Schiff stain, $\times 275$). (Reproduced with permission from Couser WG, Salant DJ, Stilmant MM. *In* Flamenbaum W, Hamburger RJ [eds.]: Nephrology. Philadelphia, J.B. Lippincott Company, 1982, pp 265–301.)

of disease associated with increased antibody levels may be triggered by infectious complications. Antibody binding to GBM mediates glomerular injury by mechanisms that involve complement activation and participation of both neutrophils and macrophages. Fibrin deposition in Bowman's space is believed to initiate glomerular crescent formation.

Pathology. The early histologic lesion in Goodpasture's syndrome is a focal proliferative and necrotizing GN that progresses to diffuse involvement with crescent formation. Extensive interstitial infiltrates may also be present, perhaps owing to antibody deposition on tubular basement membranes. There is a characteristic, continuous, linear pattern of IgG deposition along the capillary wall, accompanied by C3 in about 70 per cent of cases (Fig. 79–5). Tubular basement membrane deposits may also occur. Electron microscopy is not diagnostic.

Clinical Features. Goodpasture's syndrome is a disease of young males (6:1 male-female ratio) characterized by a triad of *pulmonary hemorrhage, GN,* and *anti-GBM antibody production.* It usually begins with pulmonary hemorrhage manifested as hemoptysis, pulmonary alveolar infiltrates seen on the radiograph, dyspnea, and iron deficiency anemia. The pulmonary symptoms are followed within days to weeks by the development of hematuria, proteinuria, and rapid loss of renal function. Over half of patients with Goodpasture's syndrome are azotemic when first seen. Hypertension and fluid retention are uncommon. Preceding flu-like illness or exposure to other pulmonary toxins, such as volatile hydrocarbon solvents and cigarettes, is common. Until recently, 80 per cent of cases required treatment for end-stage renal disease within 1 year, although some patients with mild disease recover spontaneously. Up to 30 per cent of patients may die as a consequence of the pulmonary hemorrhage.

Laboratory Findings and Diagnosis. The only laboratory finding specific for anti-GBM nephritis is the demonstration of antibody to GBM in the serum or as linear deposits of IgG in glomeruli. The antibody can be detected quickly in serum by indirect immunofluorescence using normal human kidney substrate in a test that is similar to the fluorescent antinuclear antibody test. The indirect immunofluorescence assay is positive in 80 to 90 per cent of patients with Goodpasture's syndrome. More sensitive enzyme-linked immunosorbent assays (ELISA) are also available and are positive in more than 95 per cent of patients. It is urgent to make a diagnosis and to initiate therapy early in RPGN of all types. An anti-GBM assay, as well as a renal biopsy, should therefore be obtained as soon as possible after the diagnosis of RPGN is suspected. The demonstration of anti-GBM antibody is critical, since a variety of other diseases may result in similar pulmonary and renal manifestations, including SLE, polyarteritis nodosa, Wegener's granulomatosis, and other forms of systemic necrotizing vasculitis.

Treatment. As in all forms of RPGN, the success of treatment is critically dependent upon how quickly it is initiated. The overall survival rate in Goodpasture's syndrome has risen from less than 10 per cent 15 years ago to over 50 per cent today owing to earlier diagnosis and detection of milder cases, better general medical care, and probably some improvements in specific therapy for the disease. There is little evidence that oral steroids or immunosuppressive agents alone significantly alter the course of the renal lesion. The pulmonary hemorrhage commonly responds either to high-dose oral prednisone therapy or to intravenous "pulse" methylprednisolone (see treatment of idiopathic RPGN below). However, steroid pulse therapy does not appear to benefit the renal lesion. Most centers now treat anti-GBM disease with vigorous plasma exchange therapy combined with prednisone, 1 mg per kilogram per day, and cyclophosphamide, 2 to 3 mg per kilogram per day. Plasma exchanges of up to 4 liters per day are performed on a daily or alternate-day basis until anti-GBM antibody is no longer detectable in the circulation and disease progression has halted. Therapy may require several weeks. Replacement is with albumin or, when pulmonary hemorrhage is active, with fresh frozen plasma. Overall survival in anti-GBM nephritis appears to be improved by plasma exchange therapy. However, the response rate in patients who are oliguric on presentation or who have serum creatinine levels exceeding 6 mg per deciliter is very low, again emphasizing the need for early diagnosis. In patients with end-stage renal disease due to anti-GBM nephritis, renal transplantation appears to be safe if delayed until anti-GBM antibody is no longer detectable in the serum.

Anti-GBM Glomerulonephritis Without Pulmonary Hemorrhage. Some patients have the same anti-GBM antibody–mediated renal disease as seen in Goodpasture's syndrome, but antibody localization does not occur in lungs and pulmonary hemorrhage is therefore absent. The patients are generally older than those with Goodpasture's syndrome (mean age about 50), and males and females are equally affected. In all other respects, the clinical and pathologic findings, course, and treatment are the same as those discussed above for Goodpasture's syndrome. Because such patients present with an idiopathic form of acute RPGN without pulmonary hemorrhage and may respond to plasma exchange therapy, it is important that the possibility of anti-GBM nephritis be considered in all patients who present in this fashion and that circulating anti-GBM antibody studies and renal biopsy be performed early.

Savage COS, Pusey CD, Bowman C, et al.: Antiglomerular basement membrane antibody mediated disease in the British Isles 1980–4. Br Med J 292:301, 1986. *Experience with 71 patients in a single center is reviewed, disclosing two patterns of disease: young women in their twenties with Goodpasture's syndrome and women in their sixties with glomerulonephritis alone. The poor response to plasma exchange in patients with serum creatinine levels exceeding 6 mg per deciliter or in those requiring dialysis is emphasized.*

Walker RG, Scheinkestel C, Becker GJ, et al.: Clinical and morphological aspects of the management of crescentic anti–glomerular basement membrane antibody (anti-GBM) nephritis/Goodpasture's syndrome. Q J Med 543:75, 1985. *This review of 22 patients with anti-GBM nephritis details the clinical features of this disease. Anuria and greater than 80 per cent crescents are identified as poor prognostic signs, and a beneficial effect of plasma exchange is suggested.*

RPGN DUE TO GLOMERULAR IMMUNE COMPLEX FORMATION. Patients with RPGN associated with granular deposits of immunoglobulin and complement in glomeruli account for about 40 per cent of all patients seen with crescentic GN. In most cases the glomerular disease is a manifestation of some well-defined systemic illness, such as SLE, Henoch-Schönlein purpura, or other forms of vasculitis, or of another well-defined primary renal disease, such as PSGN, MPGN, or, rarely, IGA nephropathy. In all of these disorders, the correct diagnosis can usually be made from the associated clinical, laboratory, and pathologic findings. Prognosis depends considerably on the underlying disease. For example, about 50 per cent of patients with RPGN secondary to streptococcal infection will recover spontaneously without specific therapy, while in RPGN due to SLE spontaneous recovery virtually never occurs. Therapy for the glomerular disease per se is the same as that outlined below under treatment for idiopathic RPGN and includes the use of methylprednisolone pulse therapy and/or plasma exchange.

IDIOPATHIC RPGN. *Pathogenesis.* RPGN as a primary renal disease is usually not associated with significant glomerular deposits of anti-GBM antibody or immune complexes. The disease mechanism in such patients is undefined but probably immune in nature. Whatever the mechanism leading to capillary wall damage, leakage of fibrin into Bowman's space apparently initiates epithelial cell proliferation and crescent formation. Some of the vague prodromal clinical manifestations, the development of crescentic GN without immune deposits, and the frequent presence of anti-neutrophil cytoplasmic antibody (ANCA) are quite similar to findings in several of the vasculitides. This disease is a form of vasculitis, although inflammatory changes are confined primarily to the glomerular capillaries.

Pathology. There is extensive glomerular crescent formation with circumferential cellular crescents usually involving 50 to 100 per cent of glomeruli (see Fig. 79–4). There is a rough correlation between the percentage of glomeruli with crescents, the severity of clinical disease, and the prognosis. Prominent proliferative changes suggest a postinfectious etiology and a better prognosis. Fibrinogen and fibrin polymers are present in the crescents. The glomeruli at most show only focal granular deposits of IgM and C3, which are nonspecific. Electron microscopy may show "gaps" or rupture of the capillary wall but usually does not show immune deposits.

Clinical Manifestations and Diagnosis. Idiopathic RPGN is a disease of older patients (mean age of 58). There is a slight male predominance. Many patients have a prodrome that resembles a viral illness with myalgias; arthralgias; loin, back, and abdominal pain; fever; and malaise. Minor hemoptysis is common, and fleeting pulmonary infiltrates may be seen on the radiograph. No specific inciting events have been identified. RPGN presents as an acute nephritic syndrome, including *hematuria, proteinuria, and rapidly decreasing renal function,* often without hypertension or edema. As in anti-GBM nephritis, the progression of renal disease is usually very rapid, with up to 50 per cent of patients oliguric at the time of presentation and half of these sufficiently uremic to require immediate dialysis. The remaining patients may require dialysis within 1 to 3 weeks. At the time of presentation, the disease is often relatively acute and potentially reversible.

The laboratory features of idiopathic RPGN are entirely non-specific. ASO titers, antinuclear and anti-GBM antibodies, circulating immune complexes, and complement levels are normal or negative. The diagnosis is made by renal biopsy in a patient with deteriorating renal function, evidence of glomerular disease in the urinary sediment, absence of anti-GBM antibody, and lack of clinical or serologic evidence of other systemic diseases, such as SLE.

Treatment and Prognosis. Treatment with oral steroids and/or cytotoxic agents has been of little apparent benefit, and a death or dialysis rate of about 75 per cent in 2 years is reported. Favorable prognostic factors include a young age at the time of onset, a history of a preceding infectious episode, absence of oliguria and hypertension, a serum creatinine level below 6 mg per deciliter at presentation, and fewer than 50 per cent crescents in the renal biopsy. Success rates approaching 75 per cent have been reported in patients treated with either methylprednisolone pulse therapy or plasma exchange. Methylprednisolone, 30 mg per kilogram to a maximum of 3 grams, is given intravenously over 20 minutes on a daily or alternate-day basis three times, followed by oral prednisone, 2 mg per kilogram, which is tapered over several months. About 75 per cent of patients, including some who were oliguric and on dialysis, have shown a dramatic response, with a return of renal function to normal or nearly normal levels. Responses have generally been evident within 5 to 10 days and have continued over 4 to 6 weeks. About 25 per cent will progress to renal failure despite an impressive initial response. Very similar results have been reported in patients treated with intensive plasma exchange (plus prednisone and cyclophosphamide). Neither form of therapy has yet been shown in a prospective, controlled study to improve long-term patient or kidney survival over what might be achieved with more conservative measures. Until such data are available, the author's feeling is that both pulse therapy and plasma exchange probably represent significant advances in the treatment of idiopathic RPGN. Steroid pulse therapy is safer and cheaper and appears to be as effective as plasma exchange. There are no data on the efficacy of cytotoxic drugs in this disease. However, if there is evidence of segmental necrotizing glomerular lesions, ANCA, or systemic manifestations consistent with vasculitis, cyclophosphamide should probably be given concurrently with steroids.

Idiopathic RPGN appears to recur rarely in allografted kidneys.

Couser WG: Rapidly progressive glomerulonephritis: Classification, pathogenetic mechanisms, and therapy (in-depth review). Am J Kidney Dis 11:449, 1988. *A very current and complete review of RPGN with emphasis on pathogenetic mechanisms and therapy, including 195 references.*

Falk RJ, Jennette JC: Anti-neutrophil cytoplasmic autoantibodies with specificity for myeloperoxidase in patients with systemic vasculitis and idiopathic necrotizing and crescentic glomerulonephritis. N Engl J Med 318:1651, 1988. *This paper emphasizes the utility of determining ANCA levels in patients with idiopathic crescentic glomerulonephritis and the overlap between this disease and small vessel vasculitis, including Wegener's granulomatosis.*

Glassock RJ: Natural history and treatment of primary proliferative glomerulonephritis: A review. Kidney Int 28:S136, 1985. *In this review of treatment of several forms of glomerulonephritis, the section on crescentic glomerulonephritis provides a thoughtful and comprehensive review of the literature on treatment of RPGN, with useful guidelines and recommendations.*

NEPHROTIC SYNDROME

The nephrotic syndrome is not a disease; it is a group of signs and symptoms commonly seen in patients with glomerular diseases that are characterized by a marked increase in capillary wall permeability to serum proteins rather than (or sometimes in addition to) glomerular inflammatory changes. The primary abnormality in nephrotic syndrome is the excretion of large amounts (greater than 3.5 grams per day) of protein in the urine. Other manifestations that may occur secondary to *proteinuria* include *hypoalbuminemia, edema, hyperlipidemia,* and *lipiduria.* In contrast to the acute nephritic syndrome, the onset of the nephrotic syndrome is usually insidious, gross hematuria and red cell casts are infrequent, and renal function is often normal at the time of presentation.

The list of diseases that may cause the nephrotic syndrome is extensive and includes virtually every disorder that may affect the glomerulus. About one third of adults and one tenth of children have the nephrotic syndrome as a manifestation of some systemic disease, usually diabetes, SLE, or amyloidosis. In two thirds of adults and most children, the nephrotic syndrome is idiopathic and a manifestation of one of three types of primary glomerular disease: MCNS or its variants, membranous nephropathy, or MPGN. The relative frequencies of these diseases and their identifying characteristics are presented for comparison in Table 79–3. It is important to note that the occurrence of the nephrotic syndrome in patients over 45 may be associated with occult malignancy. The association of Hodgkin's disease with MCNS and of solid tumors of the lung, breast, and gastrointestinal tract with membranous nephropathy is discussed below. All of the diseases discussed in the section on acute GN can also cause the nephrotic syndrome, although they do not commonly do so.

Pathophysiology of the Nephrotic Syndrome

PROTEINURIA. Glomeruli are normally perfused with plasma containing more than 60,000 grams of protein per day, but less than 150 mg of protein is excreted in the final urine. The filtration barrier, which includes the endothelial cells, basement membrane, epithelial cells, and slit diaphragms, restricts the transcapillary passage of proteins on the basis of their size, shape, and electrical charge. The size barrier is primarily at the level of the endothelial cells and GBM. The glomerular filtration barrier is discussed in Ch. 73.

Glomerular hemodynamic factors also alter protein filtration. Thus, in situations of reduced renal perfusion, renal blood flow (RBF) may be reduced while GFR is maintained by adaptive changes in other determinants of GFR, such as intracapillary hydraulic pressure. Under these circumstances the filtration fraction (GFR/RBF) is increased, resulting in a higher than normal protein concentration at the efferent end of the glomerular capillary. This may produce an increased diffusion of protein across the capillary wall, resulting in proteinuria in the absence of glomerular disease in conditions such as congestive heart failure and other states of reduced renal perfusion (see Isolated Proteinuria, above).

Proteinuria, the hallmark of the nephrotic syndrome, exceeds 3.5 grams per day in adults or 40 mg per square meter per hour in children. Fixed nephrotic range proteinuria with the nephrotic syndrome generally occurs only in the presence of diffuse glomerular disease. The immune mechanisms that cause an increase in the permselective properties of the glomerular capillary wall may induce a loss of net negative charge on the capillary wall, as appears to occur in MCNS, leading to a marked increase in urinary albumin excretion without significant change in the excretion of other serum proteins (*selective proteinuria*). Other diseases with extensive capillary wall immune deposits, such as membranous nephropathy, or disorders of basement membrane biochemistry or structure, such as those found in diabetes or hereditary nephritis, are associated with apparent structural defects and increased filtration of all serum proteins (*nonselective proteinuria*). More than 40 grams of protein may be excreted in the urine each day in some patients. It is this loss of protein that leads to the other clinical and biochemical manifestations of the nephrotic syndrome.

HYPOALBUMINEMIA. Serum albumin concentration decreases to less than 3.0 grams per deciliter when the rate of urinary protein loss and renal catabolism of filtered albumin (which may exceed 10 grams per day in the nephrotic syndrome) exceeds the rate of hepatic synthesis. Hepatic albumin synthesis is normally 12 to 14 grams per day in adults and may increase in the nephrotic syndrome but can be limited by various factors, including age, poor nutritional status, and liver disease. Thus, some patients may exhibit significant hypoalbuminemia with proteinuria of less than 10 grams per day, while others excreting larger amounts of protein are better able to maintain serum albumin levels.

EDEMA. Edema in the nephrotic syndrome results in part from a reduction in plasma oncotic pressure such that capillary hydraulic pressure exceeds oncotic pressure in peripheral capillaries and fluid leaves the capillaries. Although the reduction in effective circulating volume that occurs may result in increased renal retention of salt and water through normal compensatory mechanisms, more than 50 per cent of patients with the nephrotic syndrome have normal or increased plasma volume and normal or low levels of plasma renin during sodium retention, suggesting a primary renal contribution to salt retention in the nephrotic syndrome through mechanisms that remain poorly defined.

HYPERLIPIDEMIA. Hyperlipidemia is common in the nephrotic syndrome and is inversely proportional to the serum albumin concentration. Hypercholesterolemia and elevated phospholipids are the most constant abnormalities observed, but increased levels of low and very low density lipoproteins, triglycerides, and chylomicrons are also seen. The primary mechanism appears to be increased hepatic synthesis of cholesterol, triglycerides, and lipoproteins, but reduced catabolism of these compounds has also been demonstrated.

LIPIDURIA. In a nephrotic urinary sediment, lipids are seen as free fat, oval fat bodies (degenerated renal tubular epithelial cells containing cholesterol esters), and fatty casts, all of which exhibit a Maltese cross pattern under polarizing light. Lipiduria parallels the level of urine protein excretion rather than the serum lipid levels.

Complications of the Nephrotic Syndrome

The most clinically important metabolic complications of the nephrotic syndrome are severe protein malnutrition, which may require appropriate nutritional supplementation, hypercoagulability with a tendency to form thrombi in both renal and peripheral veins leading to thromboembolic complications, and acute renal failure.

Hypercoagulability is thought to be a consequence of altered clotting factor levels in the nephrotic syndrome, including reduced levels of factors IX, XI, and XII; elevated levels of factors V and VIII, fibrinogen, beta-thromboglobulin, and platelets; a reduction in levels of antithrombin III and antiplasmin; and increased susceptibility of platelets to aggregation. There is a high incidence (10 to 40 per cent) of thrombus formation in renal, pulmonary, and peripheral veins, and occasionally in arteries, with frequent thromboembolic phenomena. The incidence of renal vein thrombosis appears to be particularly high in patients with the nephrotic syndrome due to membranous nephropathy. Routine anticoagulation is not indicated unless emboli occur.

Acute renal failure in the nephrotic syndrome very rarely occurs owing to rapid progression of the underlying renal disease, since most diseases that cause the nephrotic syndrome progress very slowly. However, acute renal failure does occur as a consequence of several potentially treatable disorders superimposed on nephrotic glomerular disease. These include (1) reduced renal perfusion due to low plasma volume, which can result in acute tubular necrosis, particularly following a surgical procedure or biopsy; (2) interstitial renal edema in patients with MCNS and significant peripheral edema, who may develop intrarenal swelling sufficient to produce increased intrarenal pressure, cessation of filtration, and acute renal failure (this may be reversible with diuretic therapy); (3) drug-induced allergic interstitial nephritis, particularly in patients receiving diuretic therapy; (4) bilateral acute renal vein thrombosis; and (5) reduced glomerular perfusion due to nonsteroidal anti-inflammatory drugs, which inhibit synthesis of vasodilatory prostaglandins and reduce glomerular plasma flow in states of volume contraction or diffuse glomerular disease. Nonsteroidal anti-inflammatory agents may also cause acute allergic interstitial nephritis, which may be accompanied by a reversible nephrotic syndrome with a glomerular lesion like that in MCNS.

Other complications that may also be associated with the nephrotic syndrome include reduced levels of IgG (which may dispose to bacterial infection); proximal tubular dysfunction with signs of Fanconi's syndrome; deficiencies of trace metals such as iron, copper, and zinc; and loss of vitamin D with development of osteomalacia and secondary hyperparathyroidism. Measurements of thyroid function, such as thyroxine (T_4) radioimmunoassay and triiodothyronine (T_3) resin uptake, may falsely suggest reduced function, but free T_4 and thyroid-stimulating hormone (TSH) levels are generally normal.

Bernard DB: Extrarenal complications of the nephrotic syndrome (nephrology forum). Kidney Int 33:1184, 1988. *A detailed and comprehensive review of the pathophysiology and treatment of systemic complications of nephrotic syndrome presented in a lucid and comprehensive fashion, with 153 references.*

TABLE 79–3. SUMMARY OF PRIMARY RENAL DISEASES THAT PRESENT AS IDIOPATHIC NEPHROTIC SYNDROME

	Minimal Change Nephrotic Syndrome (MCNS)	Focal Glomerular Sclerosis (FGS)	Membranous Nephropathy	Membranoproliferative Glomerulonephritis (MPGN)	
				Type I	Type II
Frequency*					
Children	75%	10%	<5%	10%	
Adults	15%	15%	50%	10%	
Clinical Manifestations					
Age	2–6, some adults	2–6, some adults	40–50	5–15	
Sex	2:1 male	1.3:1 male	2:1 male	male-female	
Nephrotic syndrome	100%	90%	80%	60%	
Asymptomatic proteinuria	0	10%	20%	40%	
Hematuria	20%	60–80%	60%	80%	
Hypertension	10%	20% early	Infrequent	35%	
Rate of progression	Does not progress	10 years	50% in 10–20 years	10–20 years	5–15 years
Associated conditions	Allergy, Hodgkin's disease	None	Renal vein thrombosis, cancer, SLE	None	Partial lipodystrophy
Laboratory Findings	Manifestations of nephrotic syndrome	Manifestations of nephrotic syndrome	Manifestations of nephrotic syndrome	Low C1, C4, C3–C9	Normal C1, C4, low C3–C9 C3 nephritic factor
Immunogenetics	HLA-B8, B12 (3.5)†	Not established	HLA-DRW3 (12–32)†	Not established	
Renal Pathology					
Light microscopy	Normal	Focal sclerotic lesions	Thickened GBM, spikes	Thickened GBM, proliferation, lobulation	
Immunofluorescence	Negative	IgM, C3 in lesions	Fine granular IgG, C3	Granular IgG, C3	C3 only
Electron microscopy	Foot process fusion	Foot process fusion	Subepithelial deposits	Mesangial and subendothelial deposits	Dense deposits
Response to Steroids	90%	15–20%	May be slow progression	Not established	

*Approximate frequency as a cause of idiopathic nephrotic syndrome. About 10 per cent of adult nephrotic syndrome is due to various diseases that usually present with acute glomerulonephritis (Table 79–1).

†Relative risk.

Cameron JS: The nephrotic syndrome and its complications. Am J Kidney Dis 10:157, 1987. *A stimulating and provocative analysis of what is known of the pathophysiology of fluid retention in nephrotic syndrome and including an analysis of the causes and treatment of some of the underlying disorders by an experienced clinician and student of these diseases.*

Kaysen GA, Myers BD, Couser WG, et al.: Biology of disease: Mechanisms and consequences of proteinuria. Lab Invest 54:479, 1986. *An in-depth review that correlates the pathophysiology of glomerular protein filtration with observations in patients with nephrotic syndrome and discusses the mechanisms and the consequences of massive urinary protein loss.*

Primary Renal Diseases That Present as the Nephrotic Syndrome

MINIMAL CHANGE NEPHROTIC SYNDROME (MCNS)

As indicated in Table 79–3, MCNS accounts for about 75 per cent of cases of idiopathic nephrotic syndrome in children and up to 20 per cent of adults. Synonyms include minimal change disease, nephropathy or glomerulopathy, lipoid nephrosis, and nil disease.

Pathogenesis. The pathogenesis of MCNS is not known. The disease is characterized by a loss of net negative charge on the capillary wall and can recur promptly in the transplanted kidney, suggesting the presence of a circulating factor that neutralizes glomerular polyanion, resulting in loss of the charge barrier and a selective type of proteinuria. The association of MCNS with Hodgkin's disease, its responsiveness to steroids and alkylating agents, and the tendency for remission to follow some viral infections, particularly measles, have focused attention on the possibility of an abnormality in T lymphocytes, perhaps involving production of a lymphokine with properties that induce increased glomerular capillary permeability.

Pathology. By definition, the diagnosis of MCNS requires the absence of abnormalities on light microscopy and of immune deposits on immunofluorescence. Diffuse epithelial cell foot process effacement, or "fusion," is the abnormality usually seen on electron microscopy, but some morphologic abnormalities may occur in MCNS, including mild to moderate focal or diffuse proliferation of mesangial cells; mesangial deposits of IgM, IgA, or C3 seen on immunofluorescence; and the presence of focal glomerulosclerosis (FGS) by light microscopy. In the presence of FGS, response to steroids is poor, and progressive loss of renal function is commonly seen. This observation has led several authors to consider FGS a separate disease (see below). However, in some patients the FGS lesion appears to develop late in the course of MCNS and may simply be a histologic marker of a more severe and less responsive form of MCNS mediated by a similar mechanism.

Mesangial proliferation and mesangial IgM deposits may occur together or separately and usually predict a poor (or delayed) response to steroids and an increased possibility of progression. As with FGS, there have been attempts to classify such disorders into separate disease categories (mesangial-proliferative GN, IgM nephropathy). When progression occurs in patients with MCNS and mesangial proliferation and/or IgM deposits, glomeruli develop changes typical of FGS.

Clinical Features. The peak incidence of MCNS is in children 2 to 6 years of age, in whom it virtually always presents as a full-blown nephrotic syndrome. In childhood, boys are affected twice as often as girls. One third of patients have a preceding upper respiratory tract infection or other identifiable antecedent event. In the absence of volume contraction, renal function and blood pressure are normal, but up to one third of patients, when first seen, may have a reduced GFR due to hypovolemia and reduced renal perfusion. Urinary protein excretion may exceed 40 grams per day in severe cases, and the serum albumin level is less than 2.0 grams per deciliter in more than 90 per cent of children. The complications of this disease are discussed above under complications of the nephrotic syndrome in general. In addition, there is an association between MCNS and Hodgkin's disease in which the nephrotic syndrome may be the presenting sign of an occult lymphoma. Allergic reactions to nonsteroidal anti-inflammatory agents may produce nephrotic syndrome and MCNS on biopsy, usually associated with interstitial nephritis and reduced renal function.

Laboratory Findings. The laboratory findings in MCNS are those of the nephrotic syndrome of any etiology. Proteinuria is "selective" (greater than 90 per cent albumin) in about 85 per cent of cases. Complement levels are usually normal. A consistent finding is a marked reduction in ASO titers (less than 100 Todd units).

Course and Treatment. Before steroids and modern antibiotics were available, the spontaneous remission rate in MCNS was estimated at 25 to 40 per cent. During that era, the mortality rate in children exceeded 50 per cent in 5 years owing to infections or thromboembolic complications. The mortality rate now is about 7 to 12 per cent in nephrotic children and less than 2 per cent in those who respond to steroids. Some of this improvement reflects the development of effective antibiotics and better general medical care. Steroid therapy has never been shown in a controlled study to improve survival in patients with MCNS. However, the usual dramatic resolution of the nephrotic syndrome following steroid administration, as well as the fact that survival has improved since the presteroid era, has led to the widespread belief that such treatment is beneficial.

Conventional doses of oral prednisone are 60 mg per square meter per day in children and 2 mg per kilogram per day in adults, given daily for 4 weeks, followed by alternate-day therapy for 4 more weeks and then a tapering course over 4 to 6 months. Within 4 weeks, 90 per cent of children will have responded, and 90 per cent of adults will respond within about 8 weeks. There is little value in continuing steroid therapy beyond 8 weeks if abnormal levels of proteinuria persist. The 10 per cent of patients who fail to respond generally have FGS (see below).

Of the steroid responders, roughly 50 per cent will remain free of proteinuria or develop infrequent relapses that respond to steroids, eventually entering permanent remission. The remainder will become either "frequent relapsers" (more than twice a year) or steroid dependent, often with a high incidence of steroid side effects. Some can be managed conservatively with salt restriction, diuretics, and a high-protein diet. In children, the clinical manifestations of the nephrotic syndrome are usually more severe, and steroid toxicity may require the use of an additional drug. Both cyclophosphamide, 2 to 3 mg per kilogram per day (75 mg per square meter per day in children), and chlorambucil, 0.2 to 0.3 mg per kilogram per day, given for 8 to 12 weeks, have been shown to increase the frequency and duration of remission in steroid-sensitive MCNS. However, because of their gonadal toxicity, teratogenic potential, and other side effects, these agents should be used only when both the nephrotic syndrome and steroid side effects are severe. About half of such patients treated with a second drug are reported to be in remission 4 years later, suggesting that complete remission can be achieved with drug therapy in almost 90 per cent of patients with MCNS.

Meyrier A, Simon P: Treatment of corticoresistant idiopathic nephrotic syndrome in the adult: Minimal change disease and focal segmental glomerulosclerosis. Adv Nephrol 17:127, 1988. *A comprehensive analysis of therapeutic approaches and responses to therapy as well as prognosis in adult patients with MCNS and FSG. This paper is unique in separating adults from children and emphasizes the indications and complications of cytotoxic drug therapy.*

Nolasco F, Cameron JS, Heywood EF, et al.: Adult-onset minimal change nephrotic syndrome: A long-term follow-up. Kidney Int 29:1215, 1986. *This paper reviews the clinical course and response to therapy in 89 adults with MCNS and documents a higher incidence of complications and slower response to therapy compared with children with this disease.*

FOCAL GLOMERULOSCLEROSIS (FGS)

Overview. FGS is a histologic lesion found in some patients with otherwise typical MCNS, and it correlates well with steroid resistance and progressive renal failure. Controversy exists regarding whether it should be classified as a separate glomerular disease or should be viewed as one end of a spectrum that ranges from pure steroid-responsive MCNS with no morphologic abnormalities to typical FGS. The author favors the views that mesangial proliferation, mesangial IgM deposits, and FGS are part of the MCNS spectrum. However, the clinical features of patients with idiopathic nephrotic syndrome and FGS in early biopsies are sufficiently different from those who do not have these lesions to warrant separate consideration.

Pathogenesis. The etiology and pathogenesis of the lesion of FGS are unknown. Presumably, the basic mechanism underlying the generalized increase in capillary wall permeability may be the same as that in MCNS, and the structural lesion may be the consequence of either the greater severity of this process in such patients or the presence of some additional, as-yet-unidentified factor (or factors). Experimentally, FGS has been attributed to glomerular hypertension and hypertrophy.

Pathology. The diagnosis of FGS is made by renal biopsy in which sclerotic lesions are seen only in some glomeruli (focal) and within an affected glomerulus are present only in some capillary loops (segmental). The presence of sclerosis involving occasional entire glomeruli (global sclerosis) is a common finding that increases with age in all patients and does not have prognostic significance. The FGS lesion itself is an expansion of the mesangial matrix, with wrinkling and collapse of adjacent capillary loops, development of periodic acid–Schiff (PAS)–positive intracapillary hyaline deposits, adhesions to Bowman's capsule, and often foamy cells and focal epithelial cell proliferation (Fig. 79–6). Glomeruli that do not contain the lesion of FGS exhibit changes identical to those of MCNS, indicating that the increase in capillary permeability is a diffuse one not confined to the areas of sclerotic lesions. Interstitial infiltrates and tubular atrophy usually accompany lesions of FGS. IgM and C3 are frequently deposited nonspecifically in sclerotic lesions and may occasionally be seen more diffusely in the mesangium.

Clinical Features. FGS is present in 5 to 15 per cent of patients with idiopathic nephrotic syndrome and is associated with a higher frequency of hematuria (65 per cent), hypertension (10 per cent), and renal insufficiency (10 per cent) on presentation than is seen in MCNS (Table 79–3). Sterile pyuria is also common. Proteinuria is nonselective, presumably reflecting the focal areas of structural damage to the capillary wall associated with lesions of FGS. While most patients have the nephrotic syndrome, a significant minority are detected with asymptomatic proteinuria, a finding that is rarely seen in MCNS. When all of these features accompany the finding of FGS in an early biopsy, only about 20 per cent of such patients will respond to steroid therapy and many of these do not remain steroid responsive. The presence of the nephrotic syndrome, hematuria, hypertension, decreased renal function, and mesangial hypercellularity on biopsy tends to indicate a poor prognosis.

A smaller group of patients appears to have clinically typical MCNS without hematuria or hypertension but shows early lesions of FGS on biopsy. Often such biopsies are obtained later in the course of the disease after several episodes of steroid-responsive nephrotic syndrome, and such patients may remain steroid responsive for many years and progress very slowly or not at all. When all patients with FGS on initial biopsy are studied, only about 40 per cent are in renal failure at the end of 10 years.

Laboratory Features. There are no distinctive laboratory abnormalities, except for the increased incidence of hematuria and presence of nonselective proteinuria, that differentiate patients with FGS from those with pure MCNS.

Course and Treatment. Patients with FGS on initial biopsy, especially if hematuria, hypertension, and nephrotic syndrome are present, are often resistant to steroids and may progress to renal failure in an average of about 10 years. The level of proteinuria is clearly related to prognosis, and 80 per cent of all patients with nonnephrotic proteinuria retain normal renal function for more than 10 years. About 15 to 20 per cent of all patients with FGS and the nephrotic syndrome will show a response to steroids, sometimes months to years after therapy, a phenomenon that justifies a trial of steroid therapy as outlined above for MCNS in such patients. A remission can be induced in up to 40 per cent of adults with combined steroid and cytotoxic drug therapy. If a remission is achieved, the prognosis is considerably better, and such patients may behave like those with MCNS. Alkylating agents such as cyclophosphamide and chlorambucil have been shown to increase the frequency and duration of steroid-induced remission in FGS, as they have in MCNS.

Patients with FGS who progress to renal failure have a high incidence of recurrent disease in renal transplants. Factors that have been correlated with recurrence include mesangial hypercellularity, a rapidly progressive course (less than 3 years), and receipt of a well-matched living-related donor transplant. In four-antigen matches, the recurrence rate may be as high as 80 per cent, although it is less than 50 per cent for all patients with end-stage renal disease due to FGS. With recurrence, patients develop the nephrotic syndrome within a few hours to 1 week, accompanied by lesions of FGS in the transplant and usually a shortened graft survival.

Korbet SM, Schwartz MM, Lewis EJ: The prognosis of focal segmental glomerulosclerosis of adulthood. Medicine 66:304, 1986. *This detailed analysis of 46 patients with idiopathic nephrotic syndrome and focal glomerulosclerosis emphasizes clinical features, prognosis, and therapy.*

Meyrier A, Simon P: Treatment of corticoresistant idiopathic nephrotic syndrome in the adult: Minimal change disease and focal segmental glomerulosclerosis. Adv Nephrol 17:127, 1988. *A comprehensive analysis of therapeutic approaches and responses to therapy as well as prognosis in adult patients with MCNS and FSG. This paper is unique in separating adults from children and emphasizes the indications and complications of cytotoxic drug therapy.*

Pei Y, Cattran D, Delmore T, et al.: Evidence suggesting under-treatment in adults with idiopathic focal segmental glomerulosclerosis. Am J Med 82:938, 1987. *This analysis of 103 cases of FGS from Canada emphasizes the remission rate of up to 40 per cent with appropriate steroid and cytotoxic drug therapy and points out the markedly improved prognosis in adult patients who experience a remission.*

HEROIN NEPHROPATHY. In some centers, up to 25 per cent of new cases of FGS and 10 per cent of all cases of end-stage renal disease occur in young adults with a history of parenteral drug abuse, usually including heroin. Other renal lesions such as GN secondary to bacterial endocarditis, hepatitis B–associated membranous nephropathy, large vessel vasculitis, amyloidosis, and interstitial nephritis related to embolized foreign material are also seen in addicts. However, the entity of nephrotic syndrome with FGS, hypertension, and rapidly progressive renal disease appears to be the most common drug-related lesion. A similar lesion may cause nephrotic syndrome in patients with AIDS (see above), with or without a history of drug abuse. Discontinuation of drug use has resulted in stabilization or improvement in renal function in some patients, but no other form of therapy has proved beneficial. The role of the injected drugs or other foreign substances in the pathogenesis of this lesion is not known.

Dubrow A, Mittman N, Ghali V, et al.: The changing spectrum of heroin-associated nephropathy. Am J Kidney Dis 5:36, 1985. *This study of 35 heroin abusers with nephrotic syndrome confirms the presence of FGS as a common underlying lesion but emphasizes the increasing frequency with which amyloid is seen as the cause of nephrotic syndrome.*

Membranous Nephropathy

Overview. Membranous nephropathy is an uncommon disease in childhood but is the most common cause of idiopathic nephrotic

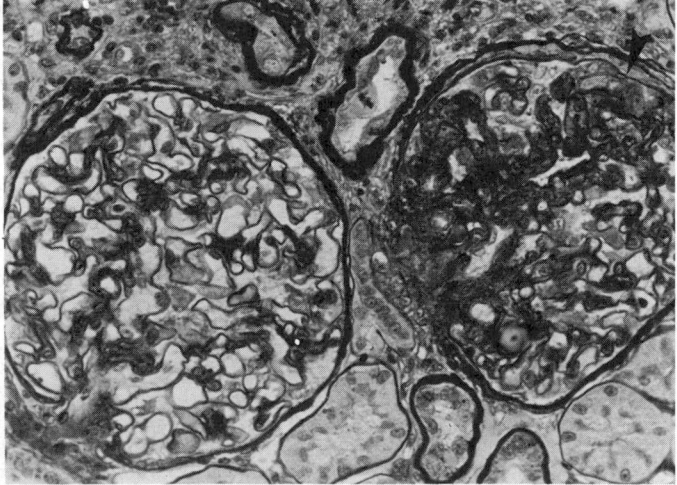

FIGURE 79–6. Renal biopsy from a patient with nephrotic syndrome, FGS, and decreased renal function. By light microscopy the glomerulus on the left appears almost normal with only slight mesangial matrix increase, while the glomerulus on the right is partially sclerotic with an adhesion to Bowman's capsule at one o'clock (*arrowhead*). Two atrophic tubules with thickened basement membranes in the upper part of the field are surrounded by fibrosis and mononuclear cells. (Periodic acid–Schiff stain, ×350.) (Reproduced with permission from Couser WG, Salant DJ, Adler S, et al. *In* Brenner BM, Lazarus JM [eds.]: Acute Renal Failure. Philadelphia, W.B. Saunders Company, 1983, p 403.)

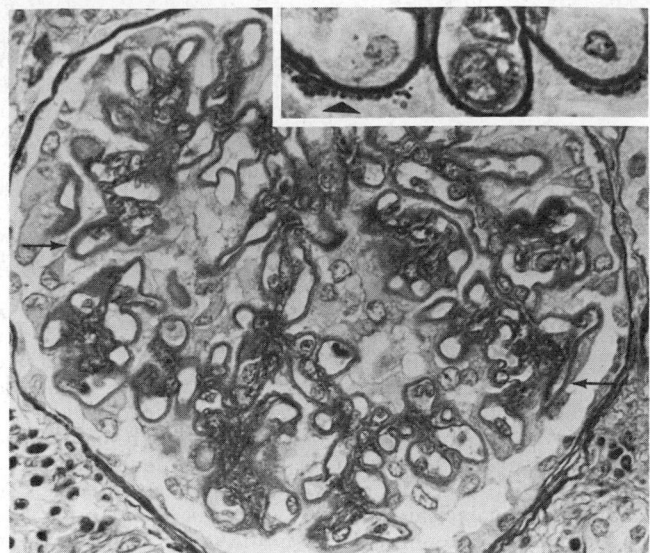

FIGURE 79–7. Light microscopy in early membranous nephropathy shows minimal thickening of the glomerular capillary walls (*arrows*) without any increase in cells or mesangial matrix. In the inset, three capillary loops stained with silver methenamine demonstrate the "spike" of basement membrane between deposits (*arrowheads*) (periodic acid–Schiff stain, ×350; inset: silver methenamine stain, ×900). (Reproduced with permission from Couser WG, Salant DJ, Stilmant MM. *In* Flamenbaum W, Hamburger RJ [eds.]: Nephrology. Philadelphia, J.B. Lippincott Company, 1982, pp 265–301.)

syndrome in adults, in whom it accounts for about 50 per cent of all cases (Table 79–3). As with all other causes of idiopathic nephrotic syndrome, the diagnosis can be made only by renal biopsy.

Pathogenesis. Experimentally, subepithelial immune deposits may result from the binding of antibody to an epithelial cell membrane antigen or to exogenous antigens that become localized at this site, usually on the basis of charge-charge interactions with glomerular anionic structures. In humans, the idiopathic form of membranous nephropathy appears to be an autoimmune disease. Subepithelial immune deposits induce proteinuria by a mechanism that probably involves the C5b–9, or membrane attack, portion of the complement system.

The role played by inciting agents, such as drugs or hepatitis

virus, in initiating this process is unknown. A strong association exists between idiopathic membranous nephropathy and HLA-DRw3 (a relative risk of about 4), an association also noted in patients who develop membranous nephropathy while taking drugs. Although most cases are idiopathic, some develop in association with a variety of other conditions, including *drugs* (penicillamine, gold, captopril), *infectious agents* (hepatitis B, various parasitic infestations), *SLE*, and *malignancy,* particularly solid tumors of the lung, breast, and gastrointestinal tract. The nephrotic syndrome may be the presenting sign of an otherwise occult neoplasm, and older patients with idiopathic membranous nephropathy should be carefully evaluated for malignancy. An identical lesion occurs in about 15 per cent of patients with SLE and may be the presenting sign of this disease when other systemic and serologic manifestations are absent. Young females who present with what appears to be idiopathic membranous nephropathy must be carefully followed for later development of SLE. Other associations, such as those with Sjögren's syndrome, mixed connective tissue disease, diabetes, thyroiditis, syphilis, sarcoidosis, and sickle cell disease, are documented but rare.

Pathology. On light microscopy, glomeruli may appear entirely normal early, but as the disease progresses, a diffuse thickening of capillary walls occurs without any increase in glomerular cellularity (Fig. 79–7). A silver methenamine stain usually demonstrates the spikelike extensions of basement membrane between areas of subepithelial deposits, and the subepithelial deposits themselves may be seen with a PAS stain. A diffuse, very finely granular pattern of immune deposits of IgG and C3 is found along the subepithelial surface of all capillary loops (Fig. 79–8). Electron microscopy demonstrates electron-dense deposits in an exclusively subepithelial distribution with effacement of overlying foot processes (Fig. 79–9).

Clinical Manifestations. The mean age of onset of idiopathic membranous nephropathy in the United States is 40 to 50, and males predominate about 2 to 1. However, the disease has been reported in patients as young as 2 and as old as over 70. More than 80 per cent of patients present with the nephrotic syndrome, but 20 per cent may be seen first with asymptomatic proteinuria. Microscopic hematuria is present in about 60 per cent of cases in adults, but red cell casts are rare. Hypertension is uncommon and renal function is usually normal at the time of presentation. The association of membranous nephropathy with other disease processes has been discussed above under Pathogenesis.

Two complications of this disease are important: (1) Patients may develop a *superimposed anti-GBM nephritis* with crescent formation and a clinical course similar to that of RPGN. This

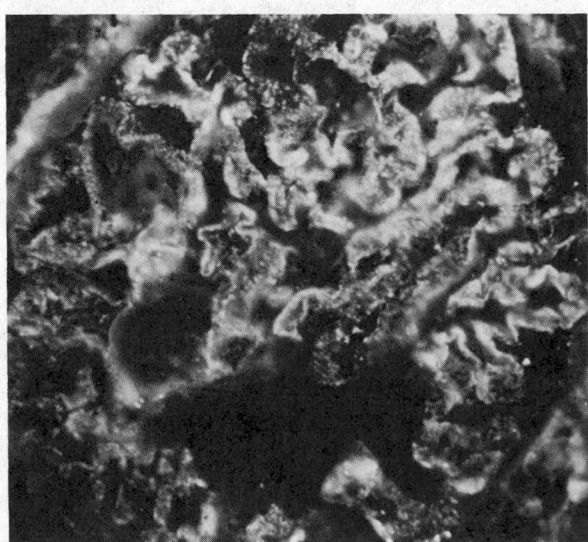

FIGURE 79–8. Immunofluorescence microscopy in membranous nephropathy demonstrates diffuse, finely granular staining of IgG (and C3) on all capillary walls, usually without mesangial deposits (×400). (Reproduced with permission from Couser WG, Salant DJ, Stilmant MM. *In* Flamenbaum W, Hamburger RJ [eds.]: Nephrology. Philadelphia, J.B. Lippincott Company, 1982, pp 265–301.)

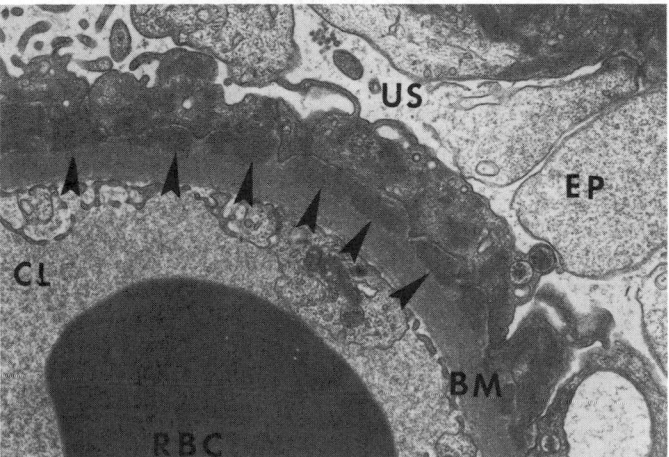

FIGURE 79–9. Electron micrograph of a glomerulus in membranous nephropathy showing many electron-dense subepithelial deposits (*arrowheads*) between the basement membrane and effaced epithelial cell foot processes. A red blood cell is present in the capillary lumen (×15,000). BM = Basement membrane; CL = capillary lumen; EP = epithelial cell; RBC = red blood cell. (Reproduced with permission from Couser WG, Salant DJ, Adler S, et al. *In* Brenner BM, Lazarus JM [eds]: Acute Renal Failure. Philadelphia, W.B. Saunders Company, 1983, p 406.)

possibility must be considered in otherwise stable patients who experience a rapid deterioration in renal function accompanied by a nephritic urine sediment. (2) An incidence of *renal vein thrombosis* as high as 50 per cent has been reported in membranous nephropathy. Any patient in whom a thromboembolism is suspected should be studied for renal vein thrombosis and treated with long-term anticoagulation to reduce thromboembolic complications if a venous thrombosis is demonstrated.

Laboratory Studies. There are no laboratory abnormalities specific for idiopathic membranous nephropathy. Because of the frequency of various associated conditions, the laboratory workup should include determinations of antinuclear and anti-DNA antibody, serum complement levels, rheumatoid factor, cryoglobulins, hepatitis B antigen, VDRL, and tests to exclude diabetes. In older patients, a careful clinical and radiologic search for occult malignancy is justified. If the patient has unusual flank pain, hematuria, or a reason to suspect pulmonary emboli, the renal veins should be studied by venography.

Course and Treatment. The disease has a widely variable clinical course, with substantial fluctuations in proteinuria and an uncertain prognosis. The spontaneous remission rate is about 25 per cent in adults. Another 25 per cent of patients have persistent nephrotic range proteinuria for many years but retain normal renal function. The remaining 50 per cent of adults, and 10 to 15 per cent of children, experience a slowly progressive deterioration of renal function that results in end-stage renal disease in an average of about 15 years, although more rapid progression may be seen. No clinical or pathologic criteria have been identified that will predict the future clinical course in an individual patient.

The variable clinical course in idiopathic membranous nephropathy makes any assessment of benefits from therapy difficult, since large numbers of patients must be followed in a prospective controlled fashion to obtain meaningful data. The results of steroid therapy have been inconsistent and generally not clearly beneficial. Concomitant administration of cyclophosphamide appears to have a definite beneficial effect in reducing proteinuria and slowing disease progression. Since fewer than 50 per cent of patients will develop progressive disease, the author recommends cytotoxic drugs only in males with proteinuria in excess of 10 grams per day and in patients with evidence of progressive loss of renal function.

Recurrent membranous nephropathy in a renal transplant is rare but has been reported in several patients who have progressed to end-stage renal disease in a period of 4 years or less. Recurrence usually has not adversely affected graft survival. Significantly more cases of de novo membranous nephropathy have been reported in renal allografts than cases of recurrence, and the disease is a relatively common cause of the nephrotic syndrome in transplant patients.

Couser WG, Abrass CK: Pathogenesis of membranous nephropathy. Ann Rev Med 39:517, 1988. *A current review of the present understanding of the pathogenetic mechanisms in membranous nephropathy as they relate to treatment and prognosis; with 81 references.*

Ponticelli C, Zucchelli P, Passerini P, et al.: A randomized trial of methylprednisolone and chlorambucil in idiopathic membranous nephropathy. N Engl J Med 320:8, 1989. *The latest results of a large controlled study of therapy in membranous nephropathy comparing steroids and cytotoxic drugs with no treatment document impressive benefits of this therapeutic approach in inducing a remission of nephrotic syndrome and preserving renal function. While the specific agents and protocols used here may be arbitrary, the efficacy of steroid and cytotoxic drug therapy in membranous nephropathy is well established by this study.*

MEMBRANOPROLIFERATIVE GLOMERULONEPHRITIS (MPGN)

Overview. The term membranoproliferative glomerulonephritis refers to a clinicopathologic entity found primarily in young adults and characterized by idiopathic nephrotic syndrome, hypocomplementemia, and a histologic lesion having the lobular appearance of glomeruli with both thickening of the basement membrane and cellular proliferation. These histologic and clinical features are probably common to at least two separate and perhaps unrelated diseases, which are now referred to as type I MPGN (that with subendothelial immune deposits) and type II MPGN (dense deposit disease). Type I MPGN is about twice as common as type II, and the two diseases cause about 10 per cent of cases

of idiopathic nephrotic syndrome in both children and adults (Table 79–3). However, unlike the other glomerular diseases that cause idiopathic nephrotic syndrome, about 20 per cent of patients present with an acute nephritic syndrome, and nephritic features are common in both of these diseases.

Pathogenesis. Type I MPGN. Several features of type I MPGN suggest that it is a chronic immune complex GN: (1) the granular deposits of IgG and C3 in a subendothelial and mesangial distribution, (2) the activation of the classic complement pathway, (3) the frequent presence of cryoglobulins and circulating immune complexes, (4) the presence of similar lesions in patients with some forms of postinfectious GN, including shunt nephritis and nephritis associated with chronic hepatitis B antigenemia, and (5) the production of similar lesions in animals immunized chronically with a foreign serum protein. However, the etiology of the disease, the nature of the antigen (or antigens) involved, and the reasons for the chronicity of the process remain unknown.

Type II MPGN. This disease does not appear to be an immune deposit disease, and the nature of the dense deposits remains unclear. Despite much study of the unique abnormalities in complement metabolism associated with this disease, and the identification of C3 nephritic factor in the serum, the role of the complement abnormalities, if any, in the pathogenesis of the disease remains undefined. There is no animal model of dense deposit disease, and similar lesions have not been described in other renal diseases.

Pathology. Type I MPGN. Light microscopy reveals a diffuse proliferative GN with thickening of the glomerular capillary walls, increase in mesangial cells and matrix, and a lobulated appearance of the glomerulus (Fig. 79–10). The thickened capillary walls are due to subendothelial immune deposits and interposition of mesangial matrix between GBM and endothelium, resulting in a double contour, splitting, or "tram track" appearance of the capillary walls on silver stain. Crescents are present in fewer than 10 per cent of cases. Coarsely granular deposits of C3, and often of IgG, IgM, C4, properdin, and fibrin, occur in the mesangium and in peripheral capillary loops in a pattern much like that seen in diffuse proliferative, or class IV, SLE. By electron microscopy, there are dense subendothelial and mesangial deposits present as well as mesangial matrix interposition with capillary wall thickening and narrowing of the capillary lumen.

Type II MPGN. The histologic findings in type II MPGN are very similar to those in type I disease except that crescents are present in up to 30 per cent of patients and correlate with a worse prognosis. The dense deposits may be seen as PAS-positive, ribbon-like deposits within the capillary wall as well as along

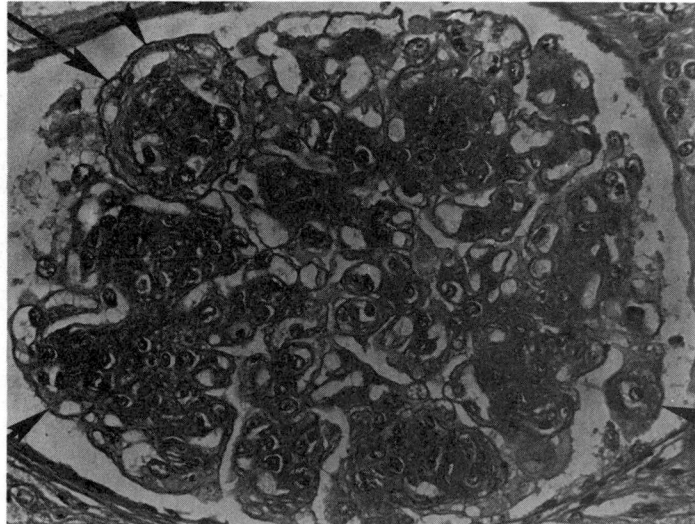

FIGURE 79–10. Light microscopy in membranoproliferative glomerulonephritis shows glomerular hypercellularity, segmental thickening of the basement membrane (*arrowheads*), and lobulation of glomerulus (*arrows*). (Periodic acid–Schiff, ×350.) (Reproduced with permission from Couser WG, Salant DJ, Stilmant MM. *In* Flamenbaum W, Hamburger RJ [eds.]: Nephrology. Philadelphia, J.B. Lippincott Company, 1982, pp 265–301.)

Bowman's capsule and tubular basement membrane. C3 is present along the margins of these deposits. Granular immune deposits of IgG are much less common than in type I disease. Electron microscopy reveals extensive replacement of the lamina densa with homogeneous, dark-staining material that may also be seen in the mesangium, Bowman's capsule, and tubular basement membrane.

Clinical Features. There are only minor differences in the clinical manifestations of types I and II MPGN. What follows is a description of patients with the more common type I disease. The differences observed in type II disease are commented on below. MPGN is a disease of children and young adults, rarely seen before age 5 and relatively uncommon after age 30. Males and females are affected approximately equally. The nephrotic syndrome is the presenting sign in about 50 per cent of patients and develops during the course of the disease in more than 80 per cent. Up to 20 per cent may present with an acute nephritic syndrome (which is more common in type II), and the remainder are detected with asymptomatic hematuria or proteinuria or both. Preceding upper respiratory tract infections have occurred in about half of patients with type I MPGN and may have been streptococcal. Hematuria is a common feature of the disease. Hypertension is present in one third, and 25 per cent have a reduced GRF on initial presentation.

The clinical course is quite variable. One third of patients develop end-stage renal disease within 6 to 10 years, one third have persistent nephrotic syndrome with relatively stable renal function, and one third have persistent nonnephrotic proteinuria or hematuria. Fewer than 5 per cent experience spontaneous remissions. In the long term, at least 50 per cent of patients with type I will reach end-stage renal disease in 15 to 20 years, while type II progresses somewhat more rapidly (6 to 10 years). Poor prognostic signs include a reduced GFR at onset, the presence of the nephrotic syndrome, early hypertension, gross hematuria, and the presence of either crescents or sclerosis on a renal biopsy.

Type I MPGN recurs in about 25 per cent of patients who receive renal transplants but rarely interferes with graft function.

The clinical features of type II disease that differ from those of type I include a higher frequency of both the nephrotic syndrome and acute nephritic episodes, a lower frequency of asymptomatic hematuria and proteinuria, more rapid progression to renal failure (probably due to the greater frequency of nephritic episodes), more frequent and persistent hypocomplementemia (see below), and a higher frequency of recurrence in transplants. Type II disease is also associated with partial lipodystrophy in some patients.

Laboratory Abnormalities. Type I MPGN is characterized by fluctuating levels of complement with depression of both classic (C1q, C4) and alternate pathway components at some time in most patients. In type II disease, hypocomplementemia is more frequent and persistent, and only alternate pathway activation is usually seen with a reduction in C3 and other alternate pathway proteins such as properdin and factor B, while classic pathway components are usually normal. Most type II patients have a circulating IgG autoantibody (C3 nephritic factor, or C3 Nef) directed against the C3 convertase of the alternate complement pathway. The definitive diagnosis of either type I or type II MPGN can be made only by renal biopsy with complete immunofluorescence and electron microscopic studies.

Treatment. Improvement or stabilization in renal function in MPGN has been reported with 2-year courses of alternate-day steroid therapy and with a "cocktail" of drugs including steroids, cytotoxic agents, anticoagulants, and antiplatelet agents. However, side effects of such treatments are significant. There is currently no therapeutic regimen of established safety and efficacy in these diseases.

Bennett WM, Fassett RG, Walker RG, et al.: Mesangiocapillary glomerulonephritis type II (dense-deposit disease): Clinical features of progressive disease. Am J Kidney Dis 13:469, 1989. *This paper reviews 27 patients with dense deposit disease and documents the clinical features as well as the clinical and morphologic correlates of a poor prognosis.*

Cameron JS, Turner DR, Heaton J, et al.: Idiopathic mesangiocapillary glomerulonephritis. Comparison of types I and II in children and adults and long-term prognosis. Am J Med 74:175, 1983. *An excellent clinical review of 104 well-studied patients that discusses the clinical and laboratory findings in types I and II MPGN, the differences between children and adults, and the long-term prognosis and prognostic features.*

GLOMERULAR INVOLVEMENT IN SYSTEMIC DISEASES

The most common systemic diseases resulting in glomerular involvement are the various forms of vasculitis. With the group of diseases referred to as systemic necrotizing vasculitis, a distinction is made between necrotizing vasculitis involving medium-sized and larger vessels (the polyarteritis nodosa group, including classic PAN, allergic granulomatosis, and "overlap" syndromes), and necrotizing vasculitis involving small vessels and capillaries (hypersensitivity vasculitis or microscopic PAN plus several well-defined clinical syndromes, including SLE, HSP, and mixed essential cryoglobulinemia). The only other common vasculitic syndrome with significant renal involvement is Wegener's granulomatosis.

Polyarteritis Nodosa (PAN)

Classic PAN, a disease of older adults sometimes associated with drug abuse (particularly amphetamines) and hepatitis B antigenemia, is described in detail in Ch. 265. Renal involvement, which occurs in 90 per cent of cases, is usually manifest first as hematuria with an active urinary sediment and mild proteinuria. In 70 per cent of cases, the renal lesion is primarily an ischemic one caused by vasculitic involvement of arcuate and interlobular arteries. This involvement is best demonstrated by abdominal angiography and is generally not seen on renal biopsy. Aneurysmal dilatation is present in renal, hepatic, and mesenteric vessels. In 30 per cent of patients, a focal necrotizing GN with crescents may be seen. Both types of glomerular involvement may sometimes occur in the same patient. Immune deposits are generally not found in the glomerulus, and the pathogenesis of the renal disease is uncertain. Renal failure is a major cause of death and may either be a slowly progressive process or develop acutely in association with accelerated hypertension. In patients with PAN who develop hypertension and acute renal failure, renal cortical necrosis is common, and there is little reversibility. More often, the disease is a slowly progressive one in which vigorous control of hypertension, use of oral steroids, and addition of cytotoxic agents, such as cyclophosphamide, have achieved 5-year survival rates of more than 80 per cent of patients in uncontrolled studies.

Milder renal lesions may occur in the other two subgroups of this category. In allergic granulomatosis, allergic symptoms, asthma, pulmonary involvement, and eosinophilia are prominent features of the disease. In the overlap syndromes, both allergic manifestations and small vessel involvement may occur in the presence of the classic large vessel involvement seen in PAN.

Balow JE: Renal vasculitis. Kidney Int 27:954, 1985. *A comprehensive review of the classification, pathogenesis, and clinical features of the various forms of systemic necrotizing vasculitis involving the kidney. The utility of angiography in the diagnosis of PAN and the indications for cytotoxic drug therapy are stressed.*

Wegener's Granulomatosis

Wegener's granulomatosis is a granulomatous and necrotizing vasculitis but also involves large vessels, usually of the upper and lower respiratory tract and kidney (see Ch. 266). The disease presents most frequently in the fourth or fifth decade of life and affects more men than women. Presenting signs usually are respiratory and include purulent rhinorrhea, painful sinusitis, otitis, keratoconjunctivitis, oral ulcerations, and multiple bilateral nodular pulmonary infiltrates. Renal involvement eventually develops in more than 80 per cent of patients and, if left untreated, may result in the death of up to 30 per cent. Early renal involvement is manifest by hematuria, proteinuria, and mild renal impairment with a focal and necrotizing proliferative GN, usually without immune deposits. However, severe diffuse necrotizing and crescentic GN may develop rapidly. Necrotizing granulomatous vasculitis may be seen in biopsies of the respiratory tract but is often not evident in renal biopsies. The presence of granulomas may be the only pathologic finding that distinguishes Wegener's granulomatosis from PAN. Spontaneous improvements in renal disease have not been reported. Antineutrophil cytoplasmic antibody levels are usually elevated in Wegener's granulomatoses and may parallel disease activity. Although the diagnosis can usually be made on clinical grounds, a renal biopsy is generally performed early in the disease to identify potentially severe renal involvement that may be clinically silent and to distinguish Wegener's granulomatosis from other diseases with pulmonary and renal manifestations, such as Goodpasture's syndrome, which would be treated differently. Prognosis and therapy are discussed in Ch. 266.

Sack KE: Wegener's granulomatosis (medical staff conference). West J Med 150:329, 1989. *A current review of the clinical manifestations, diagnosis, approach to cytotoxic drug therapy, and complications of treatment of Wegener's granulomatosis.*

Hypersensitivity Vasculitis (Microscopic PAN, Allergic Vasculitis, Leukocytoclastic Angiitis)

Hypersensitivity vasculitis is a form of systemic necrotizing vasculitis of small vessels in which the clinical manifestations do not fall into a well-recognized syndrome, such as SLE, HSP, or essential mixed cryoglobulinemia (see Ch. 264). The disease is believed to be a manifestation of immune complex formation in small vessels and frequently follows exposure to some offending antigen, such as an infectious agent, drug, or foreign protein, by about a 7- to 10-day latent period. However, about half of patients will not have an identifiable antecedent event. The skin is most commonly involved, with palpable purpura. Other frequent manifestations include microangiopathic hemolytic anemia and pulmonary infiltrates with hemoptysis.

Clinical renal involvement is present in about 50 per cent of cases and is usually manifest initially as asymptomatic proteinuria associated with a segmental necrotizing GN on biopsy. Impairment in renal function is present in 20 to 40 per cent of cases, and up to 10 per cent may develop acute oliguric renal failure. Antineutrophil cytoplasmic antibodies are often positive in these patients. On biopsy, these patients generally have extensive necrotizing glomerular lesions with abundant crescent formation and negative immunofluorescence studies. Treatment considerations are similar to those outlined above for idiopathic RPGN, including high-dose steroid pulse therapy and possibly plasma exchange. There is good evidence to support the use of additional cytotoxic agents, such as cyclophosphamide, in the treatment of RPGN due to vasculitis.

Serra A, Cameron JS, Turner DR, et al.: Vasculitis affecting the kidney: Presentation, histopathology, and long-term outcome. Q J Med 210:181, 1984. *Fifty-three patients with vasculitis involving the kidney are reviewed. The finding of a segmental necrotizing glomerular lesion accompanied by systemic symptoms, such as fever, malaise, or weight loss, was considered diagnostic of a small vessel vasculitis. Clinical features in such patients were identical to those in patients who had histologic evidence outside the kidney. The paper is an excellent review of the wide spectrum of clinical manifestations of vasculitis and the frequency of crescentic glomerulonephritis in such patients as well as the relatively poor prognosis.*

Wilkowski MJ, Velosa JA, Holley KE, et al.: Risk factors in idiopathic renal vasculitis and glomerulonephritis. Kidney Int 36:1133, 1989. *This review from the Mayo Clinic of 170 patients with renal vasculitis and glomerulonephritis provides useful data on clinical manifestations and prognostic features in this disorder.*

Systemic Lupus Erythematosus (SLE)

The current diagnostic criteria and clinical manifestations of SLE are considered in more detail in Ch. 261. This section discusses only renal involvement. About 70 per cent of patients have clinical manifestations of renal disease, ranging from microscopic hematuria and proteinuria to an acute nephritic syndrome with acute renal failure and typical nephrotic syndrome. Renal biopsies reveal some abnormalities in most patients.

CLASSIFICATION. The most common classification system used for renal involvement in SLE is the World Health Organization (WHO) classification based on histopathologic criteria (Table 79–4).

Class I (Normal Kidneys). Only very rarely do patients with diagnostic criteria for SLE have entirely normal kidneys by light microscopy, immunofluorescence, and electron microscopy, and they do not have clinical manifestations of glomerular disease.

Class II (Minimal or Mesangial Lupus Nephritis). This is the earliest and mildest form of renal involvement in SLE and is characterized by mesangial deposits of immunoglobulin and C3 with (class IIB) or without (class IIA) focal proliferative changes seen on light microscopy. Clinical manifestations of proteinuria and hematuria are present in most patients, but the nephrotic syndrome and renal insufficiency are very uncommon and do not develop unless progression to a more severe lesion occurs, as happens in about 20 per cent of patients. Five-year survival is higher than 90 per cent, and no specific therapy is indicated for the renal lesion.

Class III (Focal Proliferative Lupus Nephritis). This is a stage in a continuum between mesangial lesions alone and diffuse proliferative lupus nephritis. Focal proliferative changes are present in fewer than 50 per cent of glomeruli, but all glomeruli contain immune deposits of IgG, IgA, C3, and usually IgM and fibrin-related antigens. Deposits are predominantly mesangial, but occasional subendothelial deposits may be seen. All patients have proteinuria, but the nephrotic syndrome and renal insufficiency occur in fewer than 20 per cent and may remit following steroid therapy. Serologic abnormalities, including hypocomplementemia, are more severe than in class II disease. Long-term prognosis with this lesion is also good (90 per cent 5-year survival). However, there is a relatively high incidence of transformation to class IV disease, resulting in a reduction in 5-year survival to about 70 per cent, with almost half of the deaths occurring from renal failure. The most reliable predictor of progression is probably the presence of subendothelial deposits on electron microscopy.

Class IV (Diffuse Proliferative Lupus Nephritis). This is the severest of the glomerular lesions in lupus, with proliferation seen in more than 50 per cent of glomeruli, frequently with crescent formation and necrosis. Extensive mesangial and subendothelial deposits contain all immunoglobulins, C3, and fibrin. Mesangial and subendothelial deposits are present on electron microscopy, often with subepithelial deposits as well. Proteinuria is seen in all patients, and nephrotic range proteinuria is present in 50 per cent at onset and 90 per cent some time during the course of the disease. Renal function is decreased in 75 per cent at the time of presentation, and serologic evidence of disease activity, including hypocomplementemia, elevated levels of anti-DNA antibody, and circulating immune complexes, is present in most patients. The long-term prognosis for this lesion has improved considerably over the years, with most centers now achieving survival rates of about 75 per cent at 5 years. The best prognosis is in those patients in whom a remission of the nephrotic syndrome and normalization of serologic parameters are achieved within 1 year of starting therapy.

Class V (Membranous Lupus Nephritis). About 15 per cent of patients with SLE develop a glomerular lesion that may be indistinguishable from idiopathic membranous nephropathy, with extensive subepithelial deposits of all immunoglobulins and C3. The nephrotic syndrome and a slowly progressive renal disease are common (see Table 79–3). Patients may have undetectable levels of antinuclear antibody at the time of presentation. The

TABLE 79–4. HISTOLOGIC CLASS, CLINICAL PRESENTATION, AND PROGNOSIS IN SLE NEPHRITIS

Histologic Type	WHO Class	Frequency (%)*	Proteinuria (%)	Nephrotic Syndrome† (%)	Azotemia‡ (%)	Death (%)	Uremic Death (%)
Normal	I	<5					
Mesangial	II	15	68	0	12	18	0
Focal proliferative	III	20	100	15	18	30	11
Diffuse proliferative	IV	50	100	87	75	58	36
Membranous	V	15	100	88	20	38	6

*Per cent of patients with SLE who show this lesion on biopsy.
†Proteinuria exceeding 3.0 grams per 24 hours.
‡Serum creatinine exceeding 1.2 mg per deciliter or BUN exceeding 25 mg per deciliter.

incidence of systemic manifestations of SLE and serologic abnormalities in general is also lower in patients with a membranous lesion. The long-term prognosis for patients with this lesion does not differ significantly from those with class II disease. As in idiopathic membranous nephropathy, there appears to be an increased incidence of renal vein thrombosis. Therapy as discussed under idiopathic membranous nephropathy is usually recommended.

TREATMENT OF LUPUS NEPHRITIS. In patients with active renal disease and a class III or IV lesion, steroids have a beneficial effect in lupus nephritis. High-dose steroid therapy is given for a period of 4 to 6 weeks and subsequently tapered and adjusted according to responses in renal function, serologic parameters, and extrarenal disease. In the presence of crescents and deteriorating renal function, steroid pulse therapy, as discussed above under idiopathic RPGN, may result in more rapid return to maximal renal function. The addition of a cytotoxic agent, such as cyclophosphamide, to oral steroid therapy may result in better preservation of renal function in a subset of patients with evidence of active class III or IV disease and mild chronic changes by biopsy. Thus a renal biopsy appears to be useful as a basis for selecting therapy in patients with active lupus nephritis. Administration of cyclophosphamide as a monthly intravenous pulse provides a therapeutic effect equivalent to a daily oral dose, with fewer side effects.

With development of renal failure, disease activity in SLE usually subsides. Renal transplantation has been carried out in a large number of patients without significant problems.

Balow JE: Lupus as a renal disease. Hosp Pract 23:129, 1988. *An excellent overview of the immune basis for lupus nephritis, the clinical and pathologic features, the classification and approach to therapy, which emphasizes the extensive National Institutes of Health (NIH) experience, and results with steroids and pulse cyclophosphamide.*

Balow JE, moderator: Lupus nephritis. Ann Intern Med 106:79, 1987. *This review from a group with extensive experience in the classification and treatment of lupus nephritis summarizes current understanding of the pathogenesis and treatment of renal disease in SLE.*

Henoch-Schönlein Purpura (HSP)

Henoch-Schönlein syndrome, or anaphylactoid purpura, is another systemic necrotizing vasculitis of small vessels in which systemic manifestations include palpable purpura (100 per cent) on the lower extremities and buttocks due to a leukocytoclastic vasculitis of dermal vessels; arthralgias of large joints, usually the knees and ankles (70 per cent); gastrointestinal involvement with colic and bleeding (25 per cent); and renal involvement, usually with a focal necrotizing GN (see Ch. 154). About 30 per cent of patients have clinical evidence of renal disease in the form of hematuria or acute nephritic syndrome. Except for the systemic manifestations, the disease is very similar in its morphologic and clinical characteristics to IgA nephropathy but is of somewhat greater severity. Typically, the disease presents with an acute nephritic syndrome, usually without edema or hypertension, developing within 3 months of the onset of other systemic manifestations of HSP. Many patients have an infectious episode prior to the onset of renal disease. Up to 25 per cent of adults may develop a severe crescentic lesion with RPGN. The nephrotic syndrome has been reported to develop in over 50 per cent, and progressive renal failure occurs in at least 25 per cent of patients. The renal involvement is much less severe in children. Predictors of progressive disease include presentation with an acute nephritic syndrome, nephrotic syndrome, crescents, and subepithelial deposits or subendothelial "lead-shot" lesions by EM. Most patients have self-limited episodes of renal involvement, usually lasting 1 week or less. However, recurrences are common.

The pathogenesis of HSP is unknown but is presumed to be immunologic and similar to that of IgA nephropathy. Similar immunogenetic associations in the two diseases, as well as the clinical, histologic, and immunopathologic similarities, strongly suggest that a common underlying disease mechanism is involved.

No treatment has been shown to be of benefit in the nephritis of HSP. Short courses of steroids may be useful in controlling systemic manifestations but do not appear to benefit the renal lesion. Patients who develop crescents and a clinical picture of RPGN should be considered for treatment as outlined above under idiopathic RPGN.

Fogazzi GB, Pasquali S, Moriggi M, et al.: Long-term outcome of Schönlein-Henoch nephritis in the adult. Clin Nephrol 31:60, 1989. *This paper describes 16 adult patients with HSP and reviews the literature. The clinical manifestations are well reviewed and the poor prognosis in adults emphasized.*

Meadow AR, Glasgow EF, White RHR, et al.: Schönlein-Henoch nephritis. Q J Med 41:241, 1972. *This older article provides an excellent review of the clinical features in a large series of adult patients with HSP.*

Essential Mixed Cryoglobulinemia (EMC)

Low concentrations of mixed cryoglobulins, usually type III with polyclonal IgG and IgM with rheumatoid factor activity, are seen in a variety of immune glomerular disorders, autoimmune diseases, vasculitides, and neoplastic syndromes, in which they rarely produce symptoms (Ch. 264). Type II mixed cryoglobulins, composed of monoclonal IgM rheumatoid factor and polyclonal IgG, are characteristic of a disorder called essential mixed cryoglobulinemia (EMC), in which dependent vascular purpura, Raynaud's phenomenon, arthralgias, weakness, and GN are the principal clinical manifestations. Cryoprecipitates from these patients often contain hepatitis B antigen. The disease is one of middle age and affects women somewhat more often than men.

Renal involvement is present in about 40 per cent of cases and is usually preceded by purpura and arthralgias. The severity of renal disease ranges from microscopic hematuria and proteinuria to an acute nephritic syndrome with acute renal failure. In contrast to most of the other vasculitic syndromes, the nephrotic syndrome is a rather frequent occurrence, and severe hypertension is common. Laboratory abnormalities include a markedly elevated sedimentation rate, cryoglobulins, rheumatoid factor activity, and sometimes an artifactual decrease in levels of early complement components, with C3 and later components often normal. The glomerular lesion is a diffuse proliferative and exudative GN, sometimes accompanied by vasculitis, with large PAS-positive proteinaceous deposits present in many capillaries. The subendothelial capillary deposits are composed predominantly of IgG and IgM, with lesser amounts of C3 and fibrin. In patients with acute nephritic syndrome and renal failure, the prognosis is poor. However, in all patients with renal disease more than 50 per cent may recover with or without therapy, and the survival rate at 10 years is about 75 per cent. Although steroids and cytotoxic agents alone have not been shown to be of consistent benefit in the renal lesion, plasma exchange therapy may improve the prognosis in patients with severe renal disease.

D'Amico G, Colasanti G, Ferrario F, et al.: Renal involvement in essential mixed cryoglobulinemia: A peculiar type of immune-mediated renal disease. Adv Nephrol 17:219, 1988. *This is an excellent and detailed analysis of the renal disease in essential mixed cryoglobulinemia, with a description of clinical features, pathology, natural history, and response to therapy, including over 50 references.*

Thrombotic Microangiopathy (Hemolytic Uremic Syndrome and Thrombotic Thrombocytopenic Purpura)

Hemolytic uremic syndrome (HUS) and thrombotic thrombocytopenic purpura (TTP) are referred to collectively by some authors as thrombotic microangiopathy. The two disorders can be clinically indistinguishable, may have a common, although poorly understood, pathogenesis, and respond to similar therapy.

HEMOLYTIC UREMIC SYNDROME (HUS). HUS is a syndrome of microangiopathic hemolytic anemia, thrombocytopenia, and renal impairment, which usually occurs abruptly in children about 3 to 10 days following episodes of gastroenteritis or viral upper respiratory tract infection. Gastroenteritis is often associated with verotoxin producing *Escherichia coli* infections. A similar syndrome occurs less commonly in adults, often associated with complications of pregnancy or during the postpartum period (postpartum acute renal failure) or associated with the use of oral contraceptives. HUS also occurs in adults following treatment with a variety of antineoplastic agents. Acute renal failure develops in up to 60 per cent of children but usually resolves spontaneously within about 2 weeks with only supportive therapy. Chronic renal failure occurs in only 10 per cent of patients, usually those who suffer loss of renal function in a gradual, progressive manner, who have oliguria lasting longer than 2 weeks, or who have total anuria. Laboratory features of the disease include microangiopathic hemolytic anemia, thrombocytopenia, increased numbers of reticulocytes, elevated bilirubin levels, reduced haptoglobin levels, and elevated levels of fibrin split products, usually with only minimal laboratory evidence of disseminated intravascular coagulation. In TTP (see below) levels of fibrin split products are less commonly elevated. The glomerular lesion is one of intimal hyperplasia of arterioles and intracapillary fibrin thrombi, sometimes with areas of focal necrosis. The anemia and thrombocytopenia are presumably due to trapping of platelets and destruction of red cells in the areas of capillary thrombosis. The pathogenesis of the syndrome is unknown but probably involves glomerular endothelial cell injury by some as yet unidentified circulating factor, with subsequent fibrin deposition and thrombosis.

In typical HUS in children, only supportive therapy, including early dialysis, is required, since the rate of spontaneous recovery is very high. In adults, the prognosis is considerably worse because renal involvement is more severe and development of bilateral cortical necrosis more common. This is particularly true in cases associated with pregnancy and oral contraceptives. No form of therapy has been determined to be effective in HUS, although aspirin, antiplatelet agents, heparin, fresh frozen plasma infusions, and plasma exchange have all been advocated by some authors. In adults with severe disease, treatment with plasma exchange as described below for TTP, in addition to steroids, antiplatelet agents, and aspirin, is probably indicated.

THROMBOTIC THROMBOCYTOPENIC PURPURA (TTP). TTP is clinically and pathologically very similar to HUS (see Ch. 154). The differences that distinguish this end of the spectrum of thrombotic microangiopathy are (1) a more common occurrence in young adults, (2) fever as a frequent manifestation of the disease, (3) neurologic abnormalities that tend to predominate and cause death, and (4) a lesser degree of renal involvement, with acute renal failure in only about 10 per cent of cases. Hematuria is the most common manifestation of renal disease. Proteinuria, generally less than 5 grams per day, and a serum creatinine level in excess of 2 mg per deciliter occur in about 50 per cent of cases. Histologically, the renal lesion is the same as that in HUS. TTP has a considerably worse prognosis than HUS, with about a 75 per cent mortality within 3 months, and spontaneous recovery is rare.

A wide variety of therapeutic regimens have been employed in TTP. The most promising results have been obtained with plasma exchange, often in combination with fresh plasma, antiplatelet agents, and steroids, a regimen that has produced rather dramatic clinical remissions in several patients with apparently severe and advanced disease. In refractory cases, splenectomy may confer an additional benefit.

Kaplan BS, Proesmans W: The hemolytic uremic syndrome of childhood and its variants. Semin Hematol 24:148, 1987. *This scholarly review by pediatric nephrologists emphasizes the multiple etiologies of HUS and provides an excellent overview of management.*

Remuzzi G: HUS and TTP: Variable expression of a single entity (nephrology forum). Kidney Int 32:292, 1987. *This nephrology forum by an experienced clinical investigator is a lucid review of the classification, clinical features, pathology, pathogenesis, and treatment of HUS/TTP. The review emphasizes the similar features of these two overlapping syndromes, with 191 references.*

80 Tubulointerstitial Diseases and Toxic Nephropathies

T. Dwight McKinney

COMMON FEATURES OF TUBULOINTERSTITIAL DISEASES

Tubulointerstitial disease (tubulointerstitial nephritis or nephropathy, interstitial nephritis) refers to a diverse group of acute and chronic disorders that primarily affect the renal tubules and interstitium. In contrast, in other primary renal diseases, most notably glomerulonephritis, the tubules and interstitium are only secondarily involved. Approximately 30 per cent of all cases of

chronic renal insufficiency in the United States result from tubulointerstitial diseases. Usually the cause of tubulointerstitial disease can be identified. Renal function may improve or stabilize with appropriate therapy.

CLINICAL MANIFESTATIONS

In tubulointerstitial diseases, functional renal tubular defects, which are present to some degree in advanced renal insufficiency of any cause, are frequently out of proportion to the degree of renal insufficiency as measured by reduction in glomerular filtration rate (GFR). In fact, the finding of such a disproportional loss of tubular compared with glomerular function should lead one to suspect the diagnosis of tubulointerstitial disease (Table 80–1). Urinary concentration in response to water deprivation or exogenous antidiuretic hormone may be reduced, particularly in chronic interstitial nephritis. This may result in decreased maximal urinary osmolarity, polyuria (generally <3 liters per day), and nocturia. Concentration defect, an acquired form of nephrogenic diabetes insipidus, may result from interference with the action of antidiuretic hormone on the collecting ducts or anatomic damage or disruption of the medullary structures involved in the urinary concentrating mechanism (Ch. 214). Damage to the proximal tubules may result in excessive urinary excretion of substances normally reabsorbed in this location. Bicarbonaturia (proximal renal tubular acidosis), phosphaturia, aminoaciduria, uricosuria, glycosuria, kaliuresis, and low molecular weight proteinuria may occur. These losses may cause low plasma levels of some of these substances, particularly phosphate, bicarbonate, and urate. The presence of multiple proximal tubular defects is referred to as Fanconi's syndrome (Ch. 82). In addition to proximal renal tubular acidosis, failure of the distal nephron to acidify the tubular fluid maximally results in classic distal renal tubular acidosis. Hyperkalemic (type 4) distal renal tubular acidosis may also occur. All of these cause a hyperchloremic (normal anion gap) metabolic acidosis (Ch. 75). Hyperkalemia may result from a primary failure of potassium secretion by the distal nephron but more commonly results from decreased renal production of renin and subsequent secondary hypoaldosteronism. Patients with tubulointerstitial disease may also fail to conserve sodium normally. In some, this is due to the hyporeninemic hypoaldosteronism noted above. Renal sodium wasting may result in signs of extracellular fluid volume depletion when sodium intake is restricted and may cause worsening of renal function. With acute and, to a lesser extent, chronic interstitial nephritis, these tubular defects may be accompanied or, indeed, overshadowed by other signs, symptoms, and laboratory abnormalities of renal failure (Ch. 76 and 77).

DIAGNOSIS

A specific diagnosis of tubulointerstitial renal disease can often be made or inferred from historical information, physical examination, or laboratory tests. Renal biopsy is the most definitive

TABLE 80–1. MANIFESTATIONS OF RENAL TUBULOINTERSTITIAL DISEASES

1. Tubular dysfunction disproportionate to reduction in GFR
2. Tubular abnormalities
   a. Reduced maximal urinary concentrating ability (polyuria, nocturia)
   b. Renal tubular acidosis (hyperchloremic metabolic acidosis)
   c. Partial or complete Fanconi's syndrome
      Phosphaturia   Uricosuria
      Bicarbonaturia   Glycosuria
      Aminoaciduria
   d. Sodium wasting
   e. Hyperkalemia
3. Renal endocrine deficiencies
   a. Hyporeninemic hypoaldosteronism (hyperkalemia, metabolic acidosis)
   b. Calcitriol deficiency (renal osteodystrophy)
   c. Erythropoietin deficiency (anemia)
4. Urinalysis
   a. May be normal but usually contains cellular elements
   b. Proteinuria is usually modest (<3.5 grams per day) and consists largely of low molecular weight "tubular" proteins, such as lysozyme and beta$_2$-microglobulin

method of diagnosis, but this is not always necessary. Pathologic features are discussed below. Radiographic, ultrasonographic, and radionuclide examinations generally show only evidence of acute or chronic renal insufficiency but may provide a specific diagnosis, such as urinary tract obstruction or polycystic kidney disease.

PROGNOSIS AND TREATMENT

The prognosis usually depends on the specific cause of tubulointerstitial renal disease, as discussed below. General supportive therapy, such as treatment of electrolyte disorders, and management of acute and chronic renal failure are discussed in Ch. 76 and 77.

COMMON FEATURES OF TOXIC NEPHROPATHIES

The term toxic nephropathy refers to those renal disorders resulting directly or indirectly from exposure of the kidneys to exogenous chemicals and physical factors, including both drugs and environmental agents, and abnormal concentrations of substances normally present in the body fluids, such as calcium and uric acid. Drug-related renal disease is the most important cause of toxic nephropathy. Toxic nephropathy often results in tubulointerstitial disease, but it is not synonymous with it.

Several factors predispose the kidneys to toxic injury: (1) The kidneys receive approximately 20 per cent of the resting cardiac output and, therefore, are exposed to more blood-borne materials than any other organ except the lungs. (2) The high metabolic rate of the renal tubules required for active transport processes makes them particularly vulnerable to toxic insults. (3) The large glomerular capillary surface area is a major site for trapping immune complexes or for antigen-antibody reactions in situ. (4) Some substances (e.g., aminoglycosides) are selectively concentrated in the renal cortex because of specific transport processes located in the proximal tubules, whereas others (e.g., phenacetin) are concentrated in the medulla owing to the renal countercurrent system. This selective concentration accounts, in part, for the anatomic distribution of damage by some nephrotoxins. (5) Certain substances are converted to less soluble forms with resultant precipitation (e.g., urate to uric acid) consequent to acidification of tubular fluid in the distal nephron. This may lead to tubular obstruction.

Nephrotoxins injure the kidneys in a variety of ways, both direct and indirect (Fig. 80–1). Indirect injury, for example, may result from immunologic reactions or from secondary effects, such as drug-induced hypotension or hemolysis. These mechanisms, alone or in concert, may cause an array of renal disorders, ranging from isolated functional tubular defects to reversible acute renal failure to progressive end-stage renal disease.

ACUTE INTERSTITIAL NEPHRITIS

PATHOLOGY AND PATHOGENESIS

Characteristically, in acute interstitial nephritis (AISN) mononuclear cells infiltrate the interstitium, particularly in the cortex. Eosinophils, especially in cases of drug-related AISN, and occasionally small numbers of polymorphonuclear leukocytes may also be present. Inflammatory cells may invade the tubule walls and, in severe cases, may be associated with areas of tubular necrosis. The infiltrate may be diffuse or patchy; the extent of the infiltrate corresponds in general to the degree of renal functional impairment. In addition to the cellular infiltrate, the renal tubules are separated by interstitial edema, but no fibrosis is present. With prolonged AISN, interstitial fibrosis may develop, and the pathologic picture may merge into that of chronic interstitial nephritis. In primary AISN the glomeruli are generally normal, although there may be some mesangial prominence. The predominant mononuclear inflammatory cells in infiltrates are T cells. Both helper/inducer and suppressor/cytotoxic T cells are present. These observations suggest that both T cell–mediated delayed hypersensitivity reactions and cytotoxic T cell injury may be involved in AISN. In some cases immunoglobulins and complement components are demonstrable in the interstitium and/or tubular basement membrane by immunofluorescence. Rarely, electron microscopy may reveal electron-dense deposits in these areas, suggestive of immune complexes. Finally, in occasional cases there may be linear deposition of immunoglobulins and complement in the tubular basement membrane, indicative of anti–tubular basement membrane antibodies. There is, therefore, considerable evidence for immune injury mediated by cellular and humoral mechanisms as the cause of AISN. Usually, however,

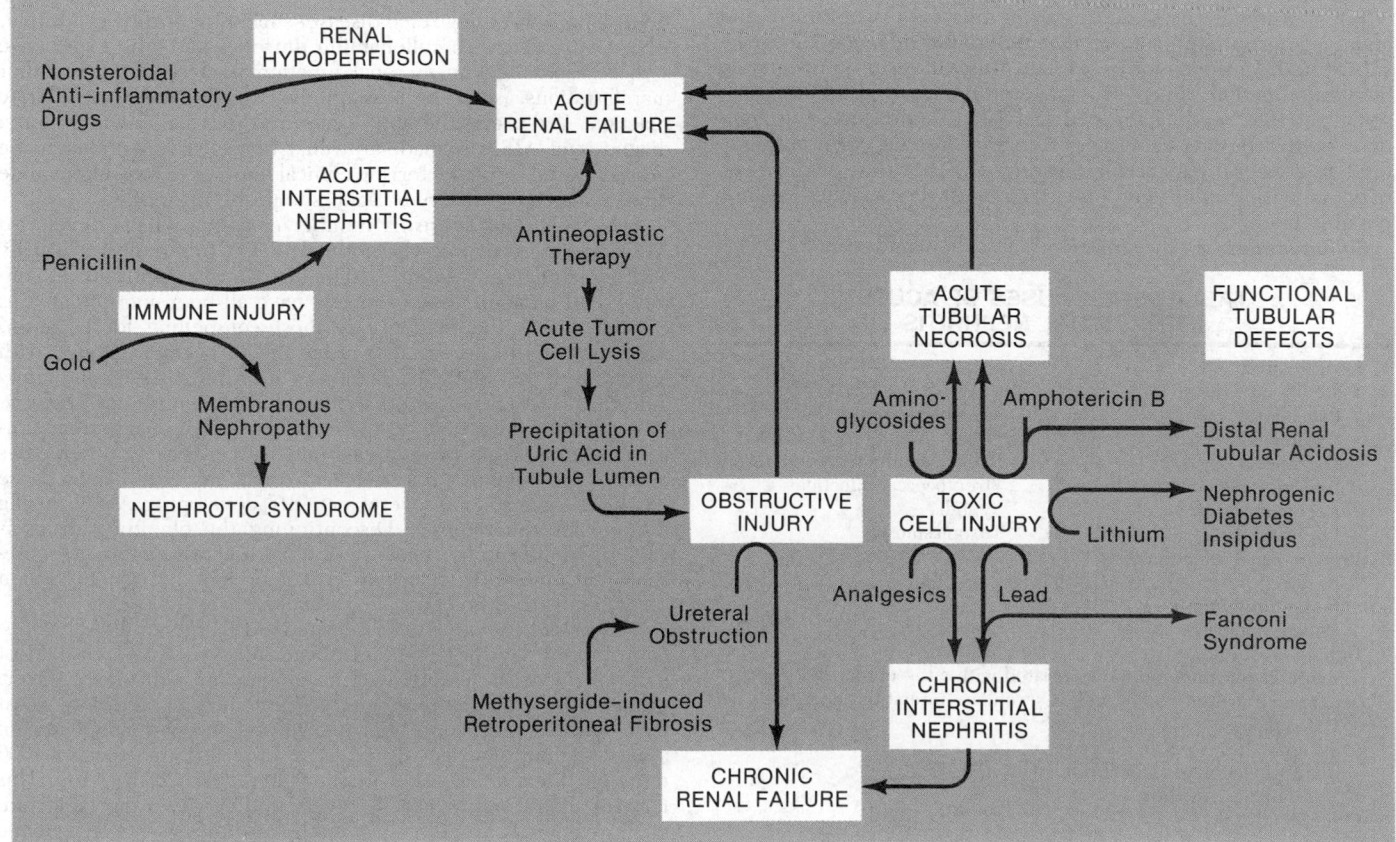

FIGURE 80–1. Types of toxin-induced renal disease.

the immunopathogenetic mechanisms involved in a given case of AISN remain unknown.

ETIOLOGY

Acute interstitial nephritis may result from a variety of causes (Table 80–2). Drug-related AISN is becoming more frequently recognized as an important cause of acute renal insufficiency, probably because of (1) the more widespread use of renal biopsy, (2) the increasing number of drugs being used, and (3) the characteristic clinical presentation.

DRUG-INDUCED ACUTE INTERSTITIAL NEPHRITIS. The list of drugs that have been implicated as etiologic in AISN continues to expand (Table 80–3). AISN is a rare complication of drug therapy, but because of the frequency with which these agents are used, drugs account for a substantial portion of all cases of acute renal failure.

Penicillins. Several penicillin congeners may cause AISN, including amoxicillin, ampicillin, carbenicillin, methicillin, mezlocillin, nafcillin, oxacillin, and penicillin G. Methicillin has been responsible for most reported cases, but the clinical syndrome is similar for the other penicillins. It is reasonable to presume that AISN may occur with any penicillin. Typically, penicillins have been taken for about 2 weeks prior to the onset of signs and symptoms of AISN, but this time interval has varied from 2 days to several weeks. The disorder appears to be more frequent in men and children. There is no correlation between the dosage of the drug administered and subsequent development of AISN. The most frequent manifestations are hematuria (which may be gross and associated rarely with red cell casts in the urinary sediment), proteinuria (usually less than nephrotic range), pyuria (eosinophiluria is frequently present and strongly suggests the diagnosis of AISN), fever eosinophilia (this may be evanescent), azotemia (often associated with oliguria), and skin rash. Serum immunoglobulin E (IgE) levels may be elevated. Renal sodium wasting and hyperchloremic metabolic acidosis with hyperkalemia (hyperkalemic distal renal tubular acidosis) may also occur. The pathogenesis of the disorder is uncertain. Binding of penicillin haptens to renal tubule basement membranes may result in formation of anti–tubular basement membrane antibodies, but evidence for this mechanism is not convincing in most patients.

For treatment, the offending drug must be discontinued, and another appropriate drug for the underlying infection should be substituted. In the majority of cases, this will result in restoration of renal function. Recovery may require several weeks, with some patients needing interval dialysis. A short course of high-dose corticosteroids (1 mg per kilogram per day of prednisone for 1 to 2 weeks) may accelerate recovery, but the added risk in patients with underlying infections must be weighed against possible benefits.

Sulfonamides. Both antimicrobial sulfonamides and sulfon-

TABLE 80–2. CAUSES OF ACUTE INTERSTITIAL NEPHRITIS

1. Drug-related (Table 80–3)
2. Systemic infections

Brucellosis	Mycoplasmal pneumonia
Cytomegalovirus	Polyomavirus
Diphtheria	Rocky Mountain spotted fever
Infectious mononucleosis	Streptococcal infections
Legionnaires' disease	Syphilis
Leptospirosis	Toxoplasmosis

3. Primary renal infections
    Bacterial pyelonephritis (Ch. 84)
    Renal tuberculosis
    Fungal nephritis
4. Immune disorders
    Acute glomerulonephritis associated with anti–tubular basement
      membrane antibodies and/or secondary interstitial nephritis
      (Ch. 79)
    Systemic lupus erythematosus
    Acute rejection of a renal transplant (Ch. 78.2)
    Necrotizing vasculitis
5. Other conditions
6. Idiopathic

TABLE 80–3. DRUGS ASSOCIATED WITH ACUTE INTERSTITIAL NEPHRITIS

Antimicrobial Drugs

Cephalosporins	Para-aminosalicylic acid
Chloramphenicol	Penicillins*
Ciprofloxacin	Polymyxin B
Erythromycin	Rifampin*
Ethambutol	Sulfonamides*
Isoniazid	Tetracyclines
	Vancomycin

Nonsteroidal Anti-inflammatory Drugs*

Miscellaneous

Allopurinol*	Methyldopa
Antipyrene	Phenindione
Azathioprine	Phenylpropanolamine
Bismuth	Phenytoin
Captopril	Probenecid
Carbamazepine	Sulfinpyrazone
Cimetidine	Sulfonamide diuretics*
Clofibrate	Triamterene
Gold	

*Most frequent or clinically important.

amide diuretics (thiazides, furosemide, chlorthalidone, acetazolamide) have been implicated in AISN. Although frequently these are prescribed in combination with other drugs (e.g., sulfamethoxazole plus trimethoprim as antimicrobials and hydrochlorothiazide plus triamterene as diuretics), it is most likely that the sulfonamide moiety of these combinations is responsible for AISN. Typically, evidence for AISN develops several days after therapy is begun, but rechallenge of a patient with a past history of sulfonamide-induced AISN may result in signs and symptoms within hours of exposure. The clinical presentation is in many ways similar to that described for the penicillins. Pyuria, hematuria, eosinophilia, and azotemia are frequent. A skin rash is present in a minority of patients. Renal failure may be severe and may require temporary dialysis, but recovery is the rule when the offending drug is discontinued. A brief course of corticosteroids may hasten recovery if no contraindication to their use is present.

Drug-induced AISN should be particularly considered in patients with underlying renal disease, such as nephrotic syndrome, who are treated with sulfonamide diuretics and who experience a more rapid decline in renal function than expected or other manifestations, such as eosinophilia, that suggest an allergic reaction. If diuretic therapy is required in a patient in whom a diagnosis of AISN is made by renal biopsy or presumed to be present based on characteristic clinical findings, a nonsulfonamide diuretic, such as ethacrynic acid, should be prescribed.

Antituberculous Drugs. A number of patients have developed AISN while receiving chemotherapy for tuberculosis, usually with more than one agent. Although rifampin, isoniazid, ethambutol, and para-aminosalicylic acid have all been incriminated as causing AISN, the evidence is most compelling for rifampin. AISN appears to occur more often and to be more severe with intermittent therapy with rifampin or after reinstitution of therapy following a drug-free interval than during continuous therapy. Fever, chills, flank pain, and anuria may develop after readministration of a single dose of rifampin. In contrast to other types of acute renal failure, transient hypercalcemia of unknown cause has been reported in several patients developing AISN during therapy for tuberculosis. Discontinuing the offending drugs is generally followed by recovery of renal function, although sometimes rather slowly. Corticosteroids do not appear to hasten recovery of renal function.

Allopurinol. Allopurinol-associated AISN generally develops after several days of treatment (mean interval of 3 weeks). Most patients have an exfoliative maculopapular skin rash, fever, eosinophilia, and decreased renal function. In addition, most have evidence of acute hepatic injury. Elevations of serum aspartate aminotransferase, sometimes to values in excess of 1000 units per liter, are present in about two thirds of patients. This form of allopurinol toxicity is severe and carries a mortality rate of approximately 20 per cent. Deaths result from severe systemic reactions, sepsis, gastrointestinal bleeding, or acute hepatic or renal failure. The cause of allopurinol toxicity is uncertain. Clinical and laboratory manifestations suggest a severe systemic hypersensitivity reaction. Most reported patients have been treated with conventional doses of the drug (200 to 400 mg per day), but most have had underlying renal insufficiency prior to development of allopurinol toxicity. Serum concentrations of the major metabolite of allopurinol, oxipurinol, are elevated in renal insufficiency. Hypersensitivity to this or another metabolite may be responsible for the syndrome. In addition, about one half of the reported patients were receiving concomitant diuretic therapy. Whether this represents a causal relationship or merely coincidence is uncertain, as allopurinol is commonly prescribed to treat hyperuricemia that develops with diuretic therapy. Treatment of allopurinol toxicity consists of discontinuing the drug and instituting supportive measures, including dialysis, when indicated. Although corticosteroids have been given to many patients, their efficacy is unproved. The incidence of allopurinol toxicity can be reduced by prescribing the drug only for clearly documented indications, such as recurrent gouty arthritis or uric acid nephrolithiasis, and not for asymptomatic hyperuricemia per se (including diuretic-induced hyperuricemia). The dose should be reduced in patients with underlying renal insufficiency.

Other Drugs Associated with AISN. Of the numerous other drugs reported to cause AISN, perhaps the most important are the nonsteroidal anti-inflammatory drugs (see Ch. 29). For the remainder of the agents listed in Table 80–3, AISN appears to be a very rare complication. Nevertheless, when manifestations characteristic of AISN occur in patients receiving these drugs (or other drugs not listed), the diagnosis of AISN should be entertained. In this setting it may be simplest to discontinue the suspected drug and replace it with an alternative agent. On the other hand, in patients for whom no suitable alternative exists, it may be necessary to confirm or exclude the diagnosis of AISN by renal biopsy.

AISN ASSOCIATED WITH INFECTION. Systemic bacterial, viral, rickettsial, mycoplasmal, and parasitic infections have been associated with AISN. Infections with group A beta-hemolytic streptococci are, perhaps, the most frequent, especially in children. The pathogenesis of AISN related to systemic infection is uncertain. Possibly, renal deposition of antigens related to the infectious agent elicits humoral and cell-mediated immune reactions that result in renal injury, as discussed earlier. Many patients with AISN associated with systemic infections have received antibiotic therapy and may have drug-induced AISN (see above). Therapy consists of treatment of the underlying infection and supportive measures. The prognosis for recovery of renal function is usually quite favorable.

Acute bacterial pyelonephritis is a common cause of AISN. The clinical presentation with fever, chills, flank pain, and bacteriuria is characteristic (Ch. 84). Similarly, renal parenchymal fungal and mycobacterial infections may cause acute renal interstitial inflammation. All of these can result in renal scarring but only rarely cause acute renal failure.

AISN ASSOCIATED WITH IMMUNE DISORDERS. Varying degrees of acute and chronic interstitial nephritis may accompany numerous renal or systemic diseases of presumed immune origin. Several types of glomerulonephritis are associated with interstitial inflammation that may be out of proportion to the degree of glomerular injury (Ch. 79). In some, there may be antibodies to the tubular basement membranes. Although glomerulonephritis is generally the primary renal lesion in systemic lupus erythematosus, interstitial nephritis is the predominant finding in some patients (Ch. 79 and 261). Acute and chronic interstitial inflammation is the hallmark of renal transplant rejection (Ch. 78.2). Renal involvement with necrotizing vasculitis is generally manifest as a focal segmental glomerulonephritis, but in some patients, particularly those with Wegener's granulomatosis, there may be prominent interstitial involvement.

OTHER CONDITIONS ASSOCIATED WITH AISN. Sarcoidosis (Ch. 67), may involve the kidneys in a number of ways, including acute (granulomatous) interstitial nephritis, chronic interstitial nephritis (often associated with hypercalcemia and hypercalciuria), and primary glomerulonephritis. Rarely, AISN may cause acute renal failure in sarcoidosis. There have been isolated case reports of AISN following therapy with recombinant leukocyte interferon.

IDIOPATHIC AISN. In occasional patients with AISN, a specific cause cannot be identified. Some of these have evidence, such as eosinophilia, suggesting a hypersensitivity reaction to an unknown antigen. In addition to acute interstitial inflammation, renal biopsies sometimes demonstrate evidence for anti–tubular basement membrane antibodies. Others have granulomatous interstitial nephritis in the absence of an obvious etiology. The course of idiopathic AISN is variable, with some patients recovering spontaneously or in response to corticosteroid therapy and others progressing to renal insufficiency.

CLINICAL MANIFESTATIONS

In AISN the GFR may decline abruptly, often with oliguria. The urinary sediment typically contains numerous leukocytes. In cases of drug-induced AISN, eosinophils are frequently present as well. Hematuria is ordinarily present, and red blood cell casts, although rare, may be observed. Proteinuria is usually present but modest (<3.5 grams per day), except in AISN due to nonsteroidal anti-inflammatory drugs (see below). The fractional excretion of sodium tends to be high, as it is in most cases of acute tubular necrosis (see Ch. 76). A spectrum of renal tubular defects may be present (Table 80–1). In cases of drug-induced AISN (see above), other manifestations of drug allergy, such as fever, skin rash, and eosinophilia, are frequent. In AISN occurring as part of a systemic process, such as systemic lupus erythematosus, clinical and laboratory manifestations of the primary disease may dominate the clinical presentation. The diagnosis of AISN is established by examination of renal tissue obtained by biopsy (or autopsy). In drug-induced AISN, the diagnosis is often inferred from characteristic clinical and laboratory findings. The outcome of AISN depends on the underlying disease process. In drug-induced disease, renal function generally improves once the offending drug is stopped. Corticosteroid therapy may be beneficial, as discussed above. With prolonged and severe AISN, variable degrees of chronic renal insufficiency may result.

CHRONIC INTERSTITIAL NEPHRITIS

PATHOLOGY

Chronic interstitial nephritis (CISN) is characterized pathologically by interstitial fibrosis with atrophy and loss of renal tubules. The glomeruli may be normal but frequently are contracted. There is generally a patchy interstitial infiltrate of chronic inflammatory cells. The renal vasculature may show evidence of associated hypertension. In addition to these general findings, there may be others that suggest a specific disease, such as casts typical of multiple myeloma.

ETIOLOGY (Table 80–4)

CISN may result from persistence or progression of many of the acute forms of interstitial nephritis (Table 80–2) or may evolve without an obvious preceding phase of acute injury. Many of the specific causes of CISN are discussed subsequently; some of the remainder are commented on briefly below.

Urinary tract obstruction (including vesicoureteral reflux), the single most important cause of CISN, is discussed in Ch. 81. Perhaps the second most important group of disorders comprises those caused by nephrotoxins, most of which are discussed later as toxic nephropathies. In addition to exogenous toxins, certain endogenous chemical abnormalities may result in CISN. The major renal complication of *chronic hypokalemia* is nephrogenic (vasopressin-resistant) diabetes insipidus, which results in mild polyuria, but chronic interstitial nephritis with modest renal insufficiency may rarely occur as well. *Hypercalcemia* also produces mild polyuria due to nephrogenic diabetes insipidus. Acute hypercalcemia also acts on the glomeruli and renal vasculature to reduce GFR in a manner largely reversible with correction of hypercalcemia. Chronic hypercalcemia results in nephrocalcinosis and chronic interstitial nephritis with reduced GFR that may be only slowly and incompletely reversible. In addition, nephrocalcinosis may cause distal renal tubular acidosis (Ch. 82). In the absence of urinary tract obstruction, *chronic bacterial pyelonephritis* rarely causes severe renal failure. Renal *tuberculosis* can

TABLE 80–4. CAUSES OF CHRONIC INTERSTITIAL NEPHRITIS

1. Persistence or progression of acute interstitial nephritis (Table 80–2)
2. Chronic urinary tract obstruction (Ch. 81)
3. Nephrotoxins
   Drugs: analgesics, nitrosoureas
   Endogenous substances: hypercalcemia, hypokalemia, oxalate, uric acid
   Metals: cisplatin, copper, lead, lithium, mercury
   Radiation
4. Chronic bacterial pyelonephritis (Ch. 84) or renal tuberculosis (Ch. 332)
5. Immune disorders
   Chronic glomerulonephritis with interstitial nephritis (Ch. 79)
   Chronic rejection of a renal transplant (Ch. 78.2)
   Systemic lupus erythematosus (Ch. 261)
   Sjögren's syndrome (Ch. 263)
6. Associated with neoplasia or paraproteinemias
   Leukemia   Waldenström's macroglobulinemia
   Lymphoma   (Ch. 151)
   Amyloidosis (Ch. 197)   Cryoglobulinemia (Ch. 79)
                             Multiple myeloma (Ch. 151)
7. Cystic diseases
   Medullary cystic disease
   Polycystic kidney disease (Ch. 89)
8. Miscellaneous
   Diabetes mellitus   Advanced renal failure
   Sickle cell   Idiopathic
     hemoglobinopathies
   Vascular diseases

result in acute and chronic tubulointerstitial disease. Tuberculous ureteral strictures may cause hydronephrosis.

A variety of *immune disorders* may be associated with both acute and chronic interstitial nephritis, including several types of glomerulonephritis (Ch. 79), chronic renal transplant rejection (Ch. 78.2), and systemic lupus erythematosus (Ch. 261). Renal involvement in *Sjögren's syndrome* is usually in the form of CISN. The most common functional abnormalities are distal renal tubular acidosis and urinary concentrating defects (Ch. 263).

Neoplastic and *paraproteinemic* disorders may be associated with CISN. In patients with lymphomas and leukemias, particularly acute lymphoblastic leukemia, neoplastic cells may infiltrate the renal interstitium and cause renal enlargement. Adjacent renal tubules may be compressed and destroyed, but renal function is rarely compromised. Renal disease in patients with *amyloidosis* (Ch. 197), *Waldenström's macroglobulinemia* (Ch. 151), and *mixed cryoglobulinemia* (Ch. 79) usually involves the glomeruli, but, rarely, there may be prominent tubulointerstitial involvement. Renal failure is a common cause of death in patients with *multiple myeloma*, especially in those with Bence Jones proteinuria (monoclonal immunoglobulin light chain paraproteins). CISN, often associated with cast nephropathy, is the most important cause of renal failure in multiple myeloma. Large, dense eosinophilic casts occur within the tubule lumina, surrounded by a chronic interstitial infiltrate. Renal failure appears to result both from obstruction of the renal tubules by these casts and/or from direct toxic effects of the Bence Jones proteins. In addition to renal insufficiency, multiple myeloma may cause proximal and distal renal tubular acidosis, Fanconi's syndrome, urinary concentrating defects, and the nephrotic syndrome. The last is usually associated with renal amyloidosis. Recovery from renal failure due to CISN with cast nephropathy is rare in contrast to that occurring from other abnormalities in these individuals, particularly hypercalcemia.

MISCELLANEOUS FACTORS

In *diabetes mellitus* and *sickle cell hemoglobinopathies*, CISN may be accompanied by papillary necrosis. Hyperkalemia and hyperkalemic distal renal tubular acidosis may occur in both. In diabetic patients this is generally due to hyporeninemic hypoaldosteronism. Urinary concentrating defects are particularly common in sickling disorders. Chronic reduction in renal blood flow from a variety of *renovascular disorders* causes atrophy of both

the renal tubules and the glomeruli, along with interstitial fibrosis. *Advanced renal disease* of any etiology results in interstitial fibrosis with mild interstitial inflammation, tubular atrophy, and glomerulosclerosis characteristic of the "end-stage" kidney. Cysts of varying size may also be present. In many cases, these changes are so severe that it is not possible to determine whether the underlying cause of renal failure was tubulointerstitial, glomerular, or vascular in origin. In occasional cases of CISN, sometimes accompanied by granulomas, no recognized cause can be identified.

CLINICAL AND LABORATORY MANIFESTATIONS

The clinical manifestations may be primarily those of renal tubular functional defects (Table 80–1) or may primarily reflect those of advanced renal failure. Sterile pyuria may be seen, but, in contrast to AISN, eosinophilia and eosinophiluria are not. Historical and laboratory findings may suggest a specific diagnosis, e.g., flank pain, and radiographic or ultrasonographic evidence of hydronephrosis suggesting obstructive nephropathy. Clinical presentations unique to certain entities are discussed elsewhere.

TOXIC NEPHROPATHIES (Table 80–5)

Drug-induced acute interstitial nephritis, an important type of nephrotoxic renal injury, is discussed in the preceding section with other causes of acute interstitial nephritis. Other important toxic nephropathies are discussed below.

Analgesic Nephropathy

Chronic interstitial nephritis leading to chronic renal failure may result from excessive consumption of certain analgesic agents. In the United States, 2 to 10 per cent of all cases of end-stage renal disease are thought to be due to analgesic nephropathy (AN). In other countries, AN is an even more important cause of chronic renal failure. For example, about 20 per cent of all cases of end-stage renal disease in Australia result from AN. The drugs most commonly associated with AN are phenacetin or acetaminophen (phenacetin is largely converted to acetaminophen soon after ingestion), usually in combination with aspirin. Generally, the offending agents are taken in the form of proprietary drugs, but sometimes they are obtained by prescriptions from physicians. In many countries the availability of phenacetin in proprietary drugs is now greatly restricted. Acute acetaminophen poisoning may cause acute renal failure due to acute tubular necrosis (Ch. 76).

PATHOGENESIS AND PATHOLOGY

Although phenacetin, acetaminophen, and aspirin may be nephrotoxic when consumed in large quantities over extended periods, there is some debate about which of these may be the most noxious to the kidney. The combination of acetaminophen or phenacetin with aspirin appears to be more nephrotoxic than either drug alone. Prospective epidemiologic studies show a convincing correlation between the amount of phenacetin or acetaminophen consumed and the development of renal disease.

TABLE 80–5. PROMINENT OR COMMON NEPHROTOXINS

Anticonvulsants: paramethadione, phenytoin, trimethadone
Antihypertensive drugs: angiotensin-converting enzyme inhibitors
Antimicrobials: aminoglycosides, amphotericin B, cephalosporins, ethambutol, isoniazid, para-aminosalicylic acid, penicillins, rifampin, sulfonamides, tetracyclines, pentamidine, acyclovir
Antineoplastic agents: cisplatin, methotrexate, mitomycin C, nitrosoureas, radiation
Sulfonamide diuretics: acetazolamide, chlorthalidone, furosemide, thiazides
Endogenous compounds: Bence Jones proteins, calcium, hemoglobin, myoglobin, oxalate, uric acid
Halogenated alkanes, hydrocarbons, and solvents: carbon tetrachloride, ethylene glycol, paraquat, toluene
Iodinated radiographic contrast media
Metals: arsenic, bismuth, cadmium, copper, gold, lead, lithium, mercury
Nonsteroidal anti-inflammatory drugs
Miscellaneous compounds: acetaminophen, allopurinol, amphetamines, azathioprine, cimetidine, cyclosporine, heroin, methoxyflurane, methysergide, D-penicillamine, phenacetin, phenindione, silicon

The generally accepted requirement for the presumptive diagnosis of AN is a cumulative ingestion of 3 kg or more of the above drugs or daily consumption of 1 gram per day for 3 or more years. In most reported cases of AN, consumption has far exceeded these amounts.

The pathogenesis of AN is still uncertain. Both aspirin and acetaminophen are concentrated within the kidney, and for acetaminophen, and perhaps aspirin, a concentration gradient exists within the kidney from the renal cortex to the medulla. Phenacetin and acetaminophen are metabolized to reactive species that covalently bind to proteins and result in oxidative tissue damage by depleting reducing equivalents such as glutathione. Aspirin may exacerbate this toxicity by inhibiting glutathione production. In addition, aspirin is a potent inhibitor of prostaglandin synthesis. This latter action may lead to a reduction in renal medullary blood flow and result in ischemic damage. In addition to aspirin, other nonsteroidal anti-inflammatory drugs that also inhibit prostaglandin synthesis have been associated with papillary necrosis. The ultimate importance of these other drugs as a cause of chronic interstitial nephritis will require long-term observations, as many of them have been only recently used on a wide scale.

In the initial stages of AN, there is patchy necrosis of interstitial cells, loops of Henle, and capillaries in the inner medulla, with calcium deposition and lipid accumulation in the involved areas. With continued exposure to these drugs, the process progressively involves the outer medulla and often results in total papillary necrosis. In advanced stages, the renal cortex is thin, and the renal tubules are atrophic. There is interstitial fibrosis accompanied by a round cell infiltrate. The glomeruli are initially spared, but later they and the arterioles become sclerotic. If AN is complicated by bacterial infection, focal collections of acute inflammatory cells are evident. The necrotic papillae may remain in situ, often with cavities in them, or they may totally detach from the medulla and slough into the renal pelvis.

CLINICAL AND LABORATORY MANIFESTATIONS

AN is usually associated with a characteristic group of signs, symptoms, and laboratory findings. The diagnosis of AN is often overlooked because patients frequently do not admit to taking analgesics or, if they do, will not provide a true estimate of the amount consumed. When the diagnosis is suspected, therefore, the possibility of AN should be vigorously pursued by discussions with family members or physicians who have cared for the patient previously. AN occurs more frequently in women (usually middle age) with a female-male ratio of 3:1 to 6:1. Although patients may consume analgesics for a variety of complaints, especially headaches, more often than not there is no disease that warrants taking large amounts of analgesics. In many patients there is a large psychological component to their clinical presentation. In some patients there is a family history of heavy analgesic use. Anemia is present in most patients and is frequently more severe than can be attributed to their degree of renal insufficiency. In addition to renal insufficiency, anemia may result from hemolysis or gastrointestinal blood loss due to peptic ulcer disease or gastritis, which also occur commonly. Hypertension is present in about one half of patients but generally appears after renal disease is obvious. Malignant hypertension occasionally develops.

Urinalysis frequently reveals pyuria. Urinary tract infections are present in approximately one half of patients at some point and may be associated with leukocyte casts in the urinary sediment. Sloughing of a necrotic papilla into the urinary tract may be associated with gross hematuria, flank pain (ureteral colic), passage of tissue in the urine, and an abrupt decline in renal function. Proteinuria is generally modest (< 2 grams per day), but as the disease progresses, occasional patients develop focal sclerosing glomerulopathy with heavy proteinuria. Generally, progression to end-stage renal failure occurs over a period of several years. Renal tubular abnormalities may be reflected by hyperchloremic metabolic acidosis due to decreased renal acidification, mild polyuria with an inability to concentrate the urine above the osmolality of blood due to nephrogenic diabetes insipidus, and an inability to reduce appropriately urinary sodium excretion with sodium deprivation (renal salt wasting).

Early in the course of the disease, the kidneys may be of normal size and contour when evaluated radiographically or by ultrasonography. In the late stages, the kidneys are small with a thin cortex and an irregular surface. A variety of findings on intravenous urography or retrograde pyelography—including caliceal clubbing, papillary cavities, and caliceal filling defects due to the presence of a sloughed papilla (ring sign)—may suggest papillary necrosis. Demonstration of papillary necrosis in the absence of its more common causes (e.g., diabetes mellitus, urinary tract obstruction, often with infection, or sickle cell disease) should suggest AN. Finally, patients with AN are at increased risk for development of transitional cell carcinoma of the urinary tract, particularly of the renal pelvis. The appearance of hematuria should lead to prompt evaluation to exclude a uroepithelial neoplasm. This evaluation should generally include examination of the urine for neoplastic cells, cystoscopy, and retrograde pyelograms.

PREVENTION AND THERAPY

Obviously, avoidance of drugs implicated as causes of AN will prevent the disorder. Public education about the dangers of excessive analgesic consumption is important. In Canada removal of phenacetin from proprietary analgesic mixtures has been associated with a decline in the incidence of AN. This has not been the case in Australia, however.

The most important factor in treatment of established AN is cessation of analgesic use. For individuals who habitually abuse analgesics, this requires a great deal of education and encouragement. Often psychological counseling is needed. For patients with diseases requiring analgesics—e.g., rheumatoid arthritis—alternative forms of therapy are indicated. With cessation of analgesic use, renal function will generally stabilize or improve. If renal disease is clearly established and drug use continues, renal function inexorably declines, often to the point of end-stage renal disease, over a period of several years. Urinary tract infections, ureteral obstruction from sloughed papillae, hypertension, and dehydration are conditions that may cause a more rapid decline in renal function, and all should be treated promptly.

Nonsteroidal Anti-inflammatory Drugs

During the last decade, several drugs that inhibit production of the various prostaglandins have been marketed. These agents are referred to collectively as nonsteroidal anti-inflammatory drugs (NSAID's) (see Ch. 29). With more widespread use of these drugs, several renal and electrolyte complications have been recognized.

The functions of renal prostaglandins have yet to be completely elucidated. Vasodilator prostaglandins (PGE_2, PGI_2) are important in maintaining renal blood flow in states of sodium depletion or when "effective" arterial blood volume is low. These states are generally associated with elevated levels of circulating angiotensin II and catecholamines. By causing renal vasodilation, prostaglandins preserve renal blood flow while allowing angiotensin II and catecholamines to maintain systemic blood pressure by increasing systemic vascular resistance. Prostaglandins also cause a natriuresis, stimulate renin release, and antagonize the effect of antidiuretic hormone. Many of the renal and electrolyte complications of prostaglandin inhibition by NSAID's (Table 80–6) are predictable, based on these recognized functions of the prostaglandins.

TABLE 80–6. RENAL AND ELECTROLYTE COMPLICATIONS OF NONSTEROIDAL ANTI-INFLAMMATORY DRUGS

1. Renal failure
   a. Hemodynamic (major risk factors are sodium depletion and low "effective" arterial blood volume)
   b. Acute interstitial nephritis with or without the nephrotic syndrome
   c. Glomerulonephritis associated with diffuse vasculitis
   d. Papillary necrosis with chronic interstitial nephritis
2. Sodium and fluid retention
3. Hyperkalemia, metabolic acidosis (occurs more often in patients with renal insufficiency, sodium depletion, or other factors predisposing to hyperkalemia)

HEMODYNAMICALLY MEDIATED ACUTE RENAL FAILURE. This has been reported in several patients receiving NSAID's, most notably indomethacin. This type of renal failure appears to result from renal hypoperfusion and occurs shortly after drug therapy is instituted. Patients at risk are those with sodium depletion (e.g., from diuretic therapy) or low "effective" arterial blood volumes (e.g., nephrotic syndrome, congestive heart failure, and hepatic cirrhosis with ascites), older individuals, and patients with underlying renal disease. Individuals receiving triamterene may be especially at risk. This type of acute renal failure is usually associated with oliguria and low fractional excretion of sodium and thus resembles prerenal azotemia (see Ch. 76). The urinary sediment is generally unremarkable. Renal biopsies have shown evidence of acute tubular necrosis. Azotemia generally resolves promptly after discontinuation of the offending drug. Occasional patients, however, require temporary dialysis.

ACUTE INTERSTITIAL NEPHRITIS (AISN). AISN resulting in acute renal failure has been described in several patients in association with NSAID's, particularly fenoprofen. Heavy proteinuria, often in the nephrotic range, is peculiar to this form of drug-induced AISN. In addition to copious proteinuria, there are other features of AISN due to NSAID's that differ from those associated with other drugs. For example, eosinophilia, eosinophiluria, and skin rashes are uncommon. As with other types of drug-induced AISN, however, urinalysis frequently reveals microscopic hematuria and pyuria. In addition to histopathologic changes of AISN (described earlier), electron microscopy of the glomeruli reveals fusion of podocyte foot processes. Unlike hemodynamically mediated acute renal failure, AISN usually appears only after the offending drug has been administered for several days to several months. The disorder usually resolves with discontinuation of the drug, but recovery may not occur until several months later, and interval dialysis may be required. Corticosteroid therapy is believed by many to hasten recovery, and in the absence of contraindications, it is reasonable to prescribe a short course of high-dose corticosteroids (1 mg per kilogram per day of prednisone) if renal failure is severe and spontaneous recovery does not occur within several days of stopping the drug.

OTHER RENAL COMPLICATIONS OF NSAID's. In addition to the above causes of acute renal insufficiency, *systemic vasculitis* with *glomerulitis* and *papillary necrosis* with chronic interstitial nephritis may occur rarely in association with NSAID's.

RETENTION OF SODIUM (AND FLUID). This is perhaps the most common renal side effect of NSAID's. Although this retention may not present a problem in persons with normal cardiovascular and renal function, it may result in worsening of pre-existing congestive heart failure or hypertension. Finally, inhibition of prostaglandin synthesis may result in *hyperkalemia* and *metabolic acidosis* due to inhibition of renin secretion and secondary hypoaldosteronism. Underlying renal insufficiency, sodium depletion, or concomitant administration of other drugs that predispose to hyperkalemia (e.g., potassium-sparing diuretics) increases the risk for developing the latter electrolyte abnormalities.

Antimicrobial Drugs

Renal damage from penicillin, sulfonamide, and antituberculous antimicrobials usually results from AISN, described earlier. Additional antibiotics may cause renal disease manifested in other ways.

AMINOGLYCOSIDES. The aminoglycosides, excreted primarily by glomerular filtration, accumulate in the renal cortex to levels higher than those in serum. They may cause several renal tubular functional abnormalities, the most clinically relevant of which are potassium and magnesium wasting, which may result in hypokalemia and hypomagnesemia. The most important manifestation of aminoglycoside renal toxicity, however, is acute renal failure. This results from both a direct effect of these drugs on glomerular filtration and tubular toxicity causing acute tubular necrosis. Up to 10 per cent of patients receiving aminoglycosides develop some degree of acute renal failure, accounting for 10 to 15 per cent of all cases of this disorder in the United States. Generally, this failure is manifested by a rise in the serum creatinine level after several days of therapy with one of the aminoglycosides. At times, renal failure may become evident only after the drug has been discontinued. Acute renal failure is usually mild and of the nonoliguric variety. However, oliguria and severe renal failure requiring dialysis may be seen.

The most nephrotoxic aminoglycoside is neomycin, which is, therefore, not administered parenterally. It may rarely cause acute renal failure when given orally or by enema to decrease the bowel flora. The least nephrotoxic is streptomycin. Tobramycin and netilmicin are, perhaps, less nephrotoxic than gentamicin and amikacin. Risk factors for development of aminoglycoside toxicity include the dose of drug administered; the length of therapy; simultaneous administration of other potential nephrotoxins, particularly cephalosporins; renal insufficiency; advanced age; extracellular fluid volume depletion; liver disease; and, possibly, potassium depletion. In older individuals the GFR normally declines, although this is unaccompanied by an elevated serum creatinine level. Failure to consider this variable when calculating the maintenance dose of aminoglycosides is a major (and preventable) factor in production of acute renal failure.

Management of acute renal failure following aminoglycoside administration consists of discontinuing the drug and substituting another appropriate antibiotic if continued treatment is necessary. When no alternative antibiotic can be found, aminoglycosides may be continued in appropriately reduced doses. In this setting, serum aminoglycoside levels should be monitored. Supportive measures are similar to those indicated with acute renal failure of other causes (Ch. 76). The prognosis for recovery of renal function after several days is excellent.

CEPHALOSPORINS. Renal failure due to acute tubular necrosis and acute interstitial nephritis may rarely accompany treatment with the cephalosporins. The combination of a cephalosporin and an aminoglycoside carries a risk higher than for either drug alone, requiring close monitoring of renal function when this combination of agents is used.

TETRACYCLINES. Tetracyclines inhibit protein synthesis and, therefore, shunt amino acids into urea. The enhanced synthesis of urea elevates the blood urea nitrogen (BUN) without a concomitant elevation of serum creatinine or a reduction in GFR. In normal individuals this is of little consequence. In patients with underlying insufficiency, however, the increase in BUN may be dramatic. With the exception of doxycycline and minocycline, which do not accumulate in renal failure and which require only minor dosage adjustments, tetracyclines should be avoided in individuals with significant renal insufficiency. Demeclocycline causes a dose-related nephrogenic diabetes insipidus. This property has been used to treat some hyponatremic patients, particularly those with the syndrome of inappropriate secretion of antidiuretic hormone (Ch. 75). Demeclocycline has been reported to cause acute renal failure, however, when used to treat hyponatremic patients with hepatic cirrhosis. Although the renal failure is reversible, demeclocycline (and other tetracyclines) should be avoided in these patients. Outdated tetracyclines can cause Fanconi's syndrome.

AMPHOTERICIN B. Most patients receiving more than 2 grams of this antifungal agent develop one or more renal abnormalities. Defects in distal nephron function are the first to appear: distal renal tubular acidosis, nephrogenic diabetes insipidus, and renal potassium wasting. These alterations may occur without a reduction in GFR and are generally reversible with discontinuation of the drug. Metabolic acidosis and hypokalemia should be treated with supplemental alkali and potassium salts. Acute renal insufficiency, which may be progressive and incompletely reversible, is a major side effect of amphotericin B. This side effect is dose related and appears to result both from direct renal tubular toxicity and from ischemia due to renal vasoconstriction. Acute renal failure is more likely to occur in patients who are sodium depleted from whatever cause: diuretics, vomiting, and so on, and in patients with underlying renal insufficiency. Sodium repletion may protect against amphotericin B nephrotoxicity. Once moderate azotemia is present (BUN > 50 mg per deciliter), consideration should be given to prescribing the drug on alternate days or to temporarily discontinuing therapy until renal function improves. The risk of renal insufficiency has to be weighed, of course, against the severity of the underlying infection and whether alternative antifungal therapy is available.

Acute renal failure resulting from acute tubular necrosis is an uncommon, but important, complication of iodinated radiographic contrast agents used, for example, in intravenous urography, arteriography, or contrast-enhanced computed tomography. The incidence of acute renal failure associated with these agents has varied in large series from 0 to 13 per cent but is much higher in certain groups of patients. Risk factors include underlying renal insufficiency, diabetes mellitus, older age, dehydration, history of prior acute renal failure following use of contrast agents, multiple contrast procedures in a short period, concomitant exposure to other nephrotoxins, and, perhaps, multiple myeloma. In addition, acute renal failure is more likely after administration of larger doses of these agents. Clearly, individuals at highest risk are diabetic patients with renal insufficiency. The incidence of acute renal failure following exposure to these agents in this population of patients may be as high as 75 per cent. In the absence of other risk factors, diabetes per se does not appear to pose a major risk.

Pathogenetic factors in radiocontrast-induced acute renal failure may include ischemia resulting from renal arteriolar vasoconstriction due to the hypertonicity of these agents, tubular obstruction due to precipitation of proteins, and direct tubular toxicity. In addition, as with any drug, anaphylaxis with hypotension is a rare cause of acute renal failure. Patients who develop acute renal failure generally have an elevation in serum creatinine level within 24 hours of exposure to radiocontrast agents. The peak in creatinine elevation typically occurs within 7 days. Renal insufficiency is usually moderate and resolves in a few days, but it may be severe and necessitate temporary dialysis. With advanced underlying renal disease, the acute insufficiency may be irreversible. In patients at risk, the serum creatinine concentration should be measured the day after exposure to these agents to determine if nephrotoxicity has occurred. A persistent nephrogram at this time also suggests renal injury.

Prevention of renal failure in patients at high risk includes avoidance of dehydration, minimizing the amount of contrast administered (no more than 0.88 mg of iodine per kilogram of body weight), and using alternative diagnostic methods such as ultrasonography, if possible. Non-ionic agents do not appear to be any less nephrotoxic than ionic ones. Hypertonic mannitol (25 to 50 grams given over 1 hour) immediately following exposure to radiographic contrast agents may reduce the incidence of acute renal failure in high-risk patients. Treatment of acute renal failure due to contrast agents is similar to that resulting from other etiologies (Ch. 76).

Nephropathies Resulting from Antineoplastic Therapy

Several drugs used in the treatment of neoplasia may produce renal toxicity. Some of these may cause isolated abnormalities in renal tubular function, whereas others may produce acute or chronic renal insufficiency. For some of these compounds, renal damage represents the dose-limiting toxicity.

CISPLATIN. Cisplatin and its metabolites are eliminated primarily by urinary excretion. Acute tubular necrosis, which may occur after intravenous administration of the drug, is dose related, being uncommon with single doses less than 50 mg per square meter but occurring in most patients with doses above 100 mg per square meter. The cause of cisplatin toxicity is uncertain, but it appears similar to that produced by other heavy metals (see below). Concomitant administration of cisplatin and other nephrotoxins, such as aminoglycosides, increases the risk of acute renal failure. Generally, azotemia appears a few days after administration of the drug and is usually reversible over a period of 2 to 4 weeks. With severe acute renal failure and/or repeated administration of cisplatin, chronic renal insufficiency due to chronic interstitial nephritis may develop. The incidence of acute renal failure due to cisplatin can be reduced by ensuring adequate hydration and establishing a saline diuresis prior to and during administration of the drug and by continuously infusing the drug slowly over several hours or a few days. Hypomagnesemia due to renal magnesium wasting may occur in as many as 50 per cent of patients treated with cisplatin. Hypomagnesemia may be severe, may develop in the absence of renal insufficiency, and may persist for several weeks following cisplatin therapy. Other renal tubular abnormalities, such as potassium wasting, decreased urinary concentrating ability, and low molecular weight proteinuria, may also be observed but are generally of little clinical importance.

METHOTREXATE. This folic acid antagonist is eliminated principally by urinary excretion. Nephrotoxicity is rare with low doses (5 to 60 mg per square meter). With high-dose therapy (500 to 7500 mg per square meter), the drug precipitates in the renal tubule lumina and causes acute renal failure from tubular obstruction. Direct tubular toxicity may also play a role. Nephrotoxicity may be reduced by vigorous (intravenous) hydration to maintain a urine flow of greater than 100 ml per hour for several days following high-dose therapy. In addition, the urine pH should be kept above 7 by alkali administration, since methotrexate is more soluble in alkaline solutions. Development of renal insufficiency prolongs the half-life of methotrexate and increases the likelihood of systemic toxicity.

NITROSOUREAS. A number of nitrosoureas used in cancer chemotherapy, including streptozocin, carmustine (BCNU), lomustine (CCNU), and methyl CCNU, may produce several types of renal toxicity. Streptozocin may cause proteinuria, sometimes resulting in nephrotic syndrome, due to glomerular injury; acute tubular necrosis leading to acute renal failure; and a variety of renal tubular abnormalities, including proximal renal tubular acidosis, glycosuria, phosphaturia, and aminoaciduria. Proteinuria is generally the first manifestation of renal toxicity. Should this occur, therapy should be withheld and only cautiously restarted if this resolves. Azotemia developing after streptozocin should lead to permanent discontinuation of the drug. The other nitrosoureas given in multiple courses over several weeks have been associated with a very high incidence of chronic renal insufficiency. In one series the majority of patients receiving at least six courses of therapy developed insidious chronic renal insufficiency, sometimes resulting in uremia, without an antecedent episode of acute renal failure and without abnormalities in the urinary sediment. The principal pathologic findings are chronic interstitial nephritis and glomerulosclerosis. Any nitrosoureas should generally be discontinued at the first sign of an otherwise unexplained decrease in renal function.

MITOMYCIN C. There is a 5 to 40 per cent incidence of nephrotoxicity following mitomycin C therapy. Toxicity is dose related and generally appears after repeated courses and/or a cumulative dose of 60 mg per square meter. Renal injury is manifested by proteinuria (usually mild) and azotemia. Renal insufficiency may develop gradually or abruptly. In the latter instance, the clinical features are similar to those of the hemolytic uremic syndrome (Ch. 79) and include thrombocytopenia, microangiopathic hemolytic anemia, and acute renal failure. Renal pathologic findings consist of glomerular alterations (mesangial fragmentation, capillary thrombi, and hemorrhage) and thrombosis and fibrinoid necrosis of the arterioles. There is no established therapy except for supportive measures for renal failure developing after administration of mitomycin C. Renal function should be monitored closely in patients receiving this drug, and therapy should probably be discontinued if otherwise unexplained azotemia occurs.

MISCELLANEOUS ANTINEOPLASTIC AGENTS. Nephrotoxicity has occasionally been reported with other cancer chemotherapeutic agents, including 5-azacytidine, daunorubicin, doxorubicin, mithramycin, dacarbazine, and recombinant leukocyte A interferon. Administration of recombinant interleukin 2 to patients with advanced cancer is commonly associated with acute renal insufficiency, probably resulting from severe prerenal azotemia. Finally, therapy resulting in massive acute killing of neoplastic cells may cause the tumor lysis syndrome (see below).

RADIATION NEPHRITIS (Also see Ch. 530). Exposure of the kidneys during abdominal irradiation for cancer may subsequently result in damage of varying degree. Manifestations range from mild proteinuria, urinary concentrating defects, and benign hypertension with a reduced GFR to malignant hypertension with end-stage renal failure. Evidence for renal damage occurs several months to years after renal irradiation, and the severity bears a general relationship to the amount of irradiation received. Clinically evident renal injury is uncommon with less than 1000 to 2000 cGy but develops in approximately 50 per cent of patients receiving doses higher than this. In the early stage of radiation nephritis, tubular necrosis, medial and intimal thickening of the small renal arteries, and damage to the glomerular endothelium are present. Later, glomerulosclerosis, collagenous thickening of the small renal arteries, and interstitial fibrosis are prominent. The incidence of radiation nephritis can be minimized by limiting the total dose of abdominal irradiation in a single course to 2000 cGy over 2 weeks and by shielding the kidneys as much as possible. Malignant hypertension resulting from unilateral radiation nephritis can be cured by nephrectomy.

URIC ACID AND THE TUMOR LYSIS SYNDROME. Patients with certain hematologic malignancies, particularly acute lymphoblastic leukemia and poorly differentiated lymphomas, may rarely develop spontaneous acute renal failure from obstruction of the renal tubules by uric acid. More frequently, this complication follows aggressive chemotherapy or radiation therapy, which kills cells and releases massive amounts of purine uric acid precursors. The resulting hyperuricemia greatly increases the filtered load of urate. Its solubility is exceeded in acidified tubular urine, and uric acid precipitation occurs in the renal tubules, often resulting in acute obstructive renal failure. A ratio of urinary uric acid/creatinine concentrations greater than 1:1 suggests the diagnosis of acute uric acid nephropathy. During massive cell lysis, phosphate is also released in large amounts, and hyperphosphaturia with intrarenal precipitation of calcium phosphate may contribute to the renal failure. Hyperkalemia due to release of intracellular potassium may also be observed. Prevention of acute renal failure secondary to massive tumor cell killing includes establishing a urinary output of 3 or more liters per 24 hours and treatment with high-dose allopurinol (300 to 400 mg per square meter per day) prior to institution of cytotoxic therapy. The role of urinary alkalinization is uncertain. Although this will increase the solubility of uric acid, a high urinary pH will favor precipitation of phosphate salts in the renal tubules. If renal failure occurs despite the foregoing precautions, hemodialysis is indicated for supportive therapy and for removing uric acid and other cellular products. This practice allows renal function to recover, generally in a few days. Chronic interstitial nephritis (gouty nephropathy), a complication of chronic hyperuricemia and gout, is discussed in Ch. 183.

Metal Nephropathies

The diagnosis and treatment of intoxication with trace metals are discussed in detail in Ch. 533. Only certain aspects of this subject related to the kidney are discussed below. Acute intoxication with some metals may cause both acute renal injury with a reduction in GFR and renal tubular dysfunction. With chronic intoxication, the most common form of injury is chronic interstitial nephritis manifested by renal tubular abnormalities with or without reduction in GFR. In certain instances glomerular injury may also occur. Metal intoxication is often treated by chelation therapy. Unfortunately, some of the drugs used for this purpose, e.g., penicillamine, may also be nephrotoxic, as discussed below.

LITHIUM. Lithium carbonate, used in the treatment of affective disorders, causes a variety of renal abnormalities. The most frequent is a form of vasopressin-resistant nephrogenic diabetes insipidus. This is of little consequence in most patients. Polyuria (urine volumes > 3000 ml per day) may result but usually abates when lithium therapy is stopped. The diuretic amiloride may significantly reduce the polyuria associated with lithium. Incomplete distal renal tubular acidosis and mild renal sodium wasting may also result from lithium therapy. Chronic interstitial nephritis occurs in some lithium-treated patients. However, since CISN is more frequent in individuals with affective disorders than in the general population, the importance of lithium is debated. However, a history of acute lithium intoxication may predispose to development of chronic renal insufficiency.

LEAD. Lead poisoning may result from acute exposure, such as from ingestion of lead-containing paint, but more often from chronic exposure, such as in foundry and battery workers or from consumption of illicit alcoholic beverages ("moonshine"). Acute intoxication, more common in children, is manifested primarily by abdominal colic, hemolytic anemia, and encephalopathy. Acute interstitial nephritis with eosinophilic inclusions in the proximal tubular cells, tubular necrosis with a reduction in GFR,

and Fanconi's syndrome may also occur. Whether acute lead intoxication without further exposure results in chronic renal disease in later years is unclear. Chronic lead intoxication causes interstitial nephritis with variable reductions in GFR and renal tubular dysfunction. Some patients develop gout and hypertension as a result of chronic lead intoxication ("saturnine gout"). Chronic lead intoxication should be considered in individuals with the triad of gout, hypertension, and chronic renal insufficiency. A history of exposure to lead should be sought and a $CaNa_2$–ethylenediaminetetra-acetic acid (EDTA) infusion carried out to evaluate lead stores (Ch. 533). Treatment of acute lead intoxication consists of preventing further exposure to the metal, supportive care, and chelation with dimercaptopropanol (BAL) or $CaNa_2$-EDTA. Chronic renal insufficiency resulting from lead may sometimes improve during chelation therapy but may also progress despite this therapy.

MERCURY. Acute intoxication with mercurial salts may cause tubular necrosis and severe renal failure. The strong affinity of mercury for sulfhydryl groups, along with the hypotension that frequently accompanies acute intoxication, probably accounts for the acute renal injury. Acute exposure may occur rarely in industrial settings or with intentional ingestion of mercurial salts. Treatment of acute poisoning from mercurial salts consists of chelation therapy with dimercaptopropanol or penicillamine and supportive care (Ch. 533). Chronic exposure to organomercurials may result in subtle renal damage manifested by increased urinary excretion of low molecular weight proteins and renal tubular enzymes (tubular proteinuria). Chelation therapy is ineffective in removing organomercurials. Chronic exposure to mercurial compounds may also cause the nephrotic syndrome as a result of glomerular damage, most commonly from membranous nephropathy. The pathogenesis of this disorder is uncertain, as mercury is not demonstrable in the glomeruli.

GOLD. Proteinuria may complicate the treatment of rheumatoid arthritis with gold salts, more frequently with parenteral than with oral administration. Proteinuria may develop at any time, but usually after several months of therapy. Rarely, it may be severe enough to result in the nephrotic syndrome associated with membranous nephropathy. It is unlikely that gold per se is directly responsible for the glomerular injury, since the metal can be demonstrated in the renal tubules, but not in the glomeruli. Gold may in some way modify an intrinsic protein so that it becomes antigenic and elicits the immune reactions that produce membranous nephropathy. Membranous nephropathy may also occur in patients with rheumatoid arthritis who have not been treated with gold. The appearance of proteinuria in a patient receiving gold should prompt discontinuation of the drug. This practice generally results in disappearance of the proteinuria, but this disappearance may occur only several months later.

ARSENIC. Arsenic is used in a number of industrial applications and is present in several commercial products, such as insecticides. In addition, illicit alcohol may be contaminated with the metal. Gastrointestinal symptoms and peripheral neuropathy are the most prominent manifestations of acute arsenic poisoning but acute tubular necrosis may also occur. Like mercury, arsenic has a high affinity for sulfhydryl groups of proteins. Cellular damage resulting from this interaction and from hypotension are the most likely causes of acute renal damage. Treatment of arsenic poisoning includes supportive measures and chelation therapy with dimercaptopropanol. Arsine gas may cause acute renal failure secondary to hemoglobinuria from acute hemolysis and from hypotension.

CADMIUM. With chronic low-level exposure—for example, in alkaline battery workers—cadmium accumulates in the renal cortex. This may result in mild proteinuria, of both glomerular and tubular origin, and in early renal insufficiency. The incidence of proteinuria increases with the length of exposure.

MISCELLANEOUS METALS. *Bismuth* has been reported to cause both acute tubular necrosis and the nephrotic syndrome. Acute *copper* poisoning may produce acute tubular necrosis, most likely resulting from hemolysis with hemoglobinuria and from hypotension. Chronic copper accumulation in Wilson's disease (Ch. 192) may be associated with proximal renal tubular acidosis and other components of Fanconi's syndrome and mild renal insufficiency. In rare instances, renal injury has been reported with *antimony, thallium,* and *uranium* intoxication. *Platinum* nephrotoxicity is discussed under cisplatin.

Oxalate

End-stage renal failure from chronic interstitial nephritis and from recurrent nephrolithiasis is the major complication of primary hyperoxaluria and may rarely occur in enteric hyperoxaluria as well (Ch. 171).

Acute intoxication with ethylene glycol is the major cause of acute renal failure due to oxalate. Ethylene glycol is the principal component of antifreeze and is usually ingested by desperate alcoholics, by children accidentally, or in a suicide attempt. Ethylene glycol is metabolized to several toxic substances, one of which is oxalic acid. Intoxication with ethylene glycol causes acute renal failure, profound metabolic acidosis of the anion gap variety (Ch. 75), and acute central nervous system and pulmonary dysfunction. Renal failure results from massive deposition of oxalate within the renal tubules. This is usually accompanied by large numbers of calcium oxalate crystals in the urinary sediment. Ethylene glycol intoxication is managed by (1) administration of ethyl alcohol to slow the metabolism of ethylene glycol by competing for alcohol dehydrogenase; (2) hemodialysis to remove the parent compound, to allow treatment with sodium bicarbonate therapy, which may be required in amounts that would otherwise result in pulmonary edema and hypernatremia, and to treat acute renal failure; and (3) administration of pyridoxine and thiamine to help shunt ethylene glycol into other metabolic pathways that result in less toxic metabolites. If patients survive acute intoxication, chances for recovery of renal function are good, but many will require temporary dialysis for several days prior to functional renal recovery.

Angiotensin-Converting Enzyme (ACE) Inhibitors

Acute renal failure has been reported in patients with bilateral renal artery stenosis or stenosis of the renal artery supplying a solitary kidney following treatment with ACE inhibitors. Usually, ACE inhibitor–associated acute renal failure is thought to be hemodynamic in origin, resulting from loss of autoregulation of renal blood flow and GFR. Sometimes, however, acute renal failure following captopril therapy has been accompanied by skin rash, eosinophilia, and eosinophiluria, a constellation of findings strongly suggesting allergic interstitial nephritis. Acute renal failure in both the above settings generally resolves with discontinuation of the ACE inhibitor but may recur upon rechallenge with the drug. Membranous nephropathy with the nephrotic syndrome may also occur in association with captopril therapy. This complication may resolve slowly after discontinuation of the drug. Membranous nephropathy occurring during therapy with captopril and penicillamine (see below) may possibly be related to the active sulfhydryl group that they contain.

D-Penicillamine

Therapy with this drug for metal chelation, rheumatoid arthritis, scleroderma, or cystinuria is complicated by proteinuria in 4 to 7 per cent of patients, often sufficiently severe to result in the nephrotic syndrome. Proteinuria, which may be associated with mild azotemia, usually results from membranous nephropathy (Ch. 79). Rarely, rapidly progressive glomerulonephritis accompanied by pulmonary hemorrhage occurs. Proteinuria generally resolves or decreases when D-penicillamine therapy is discontinued, but usually only after several months.

Methoxyflurane

This fluorinated anesthetic agent may cause a dose-related postoperative nephrogenic diabetes insipidus and acute renal failure. Similar complications have rarely been reported with enflurane. The initial polyuric acute renal failure may progress to oliguria in severe cases. Renal function may recover after several days, but persistent renal failure, which has required long-term dialysis, may develop. The pathogenesis of methoxyflurane-induced acute renal failure is uncertain. The drug is metabolized to fluoride and oxalate. Although oxalate is nephrotoxic (see above), it is believed that the major toxic product is fluoride, since nephrotoxicity correlates with blood levels of this ion and fluoride produces nephrotoxicity in experimental animals. Volume depletion due to the urinary concentrating defect may also contribute to acute renal failure.

Miscellaneous Nephrotoxins

Exposure to *hydrocarbons*, frequently in the form of paint or glue sniffing, has been associated with a variety of (generally) reversible abnormalities, including azotemia, renal tubular acidosis, Fanconi's syndrome, proteinuria, hematuria, and pyuria. Similar findings may result from exposure to halogenated alkane solvents, such as *carbon tetrachloride*, and insecticides, such as *paraquat*. *Silicon* exposure—for example, in sandblasters—has been implicated in a connective tissue–like disease with multiple serologic abnormalities and progressive renal failure associated with both glomerular and renal tubular pathologic changes that appear to be immune mediated.

Heroin abuse is associated with a variety of glomerular lesions, including amyloidosis, and glomerulonephritis due to bacterial endocarditis or hepatitis B infection. In some patients, however, these etiologies cannot be implicated. Most commonly, focal sclerosing glomerulopathy is found, often resulting in the nephrotic syndrome. Recently, it has been found that many of these patients have human immunodeficiency virus (HIV) infections with or without full-blown acquired immunodeficiency syndrome (AIDS) (Part XXI). Heroin-associated nephropathy generally results in progressive renal failure unless abuse of the drug is stopped.

The nephrotic syndrome may occur as a rare complication of *trimethadione* and *methimazole*. *Sulfonamides* and intravenous *amphetamines* may cause systemic vasculitis that results in renal damage from segmental renal infarction or glomerulonephritis (Ch. 79 and 264). Acute renal insufficiency is a major complication of *cyclosporine A* therapy of organ transplantation (Ch. 78.2). Administration of cyclosporine A for several months may be associated with occlusion of renal arterioles, CISN, and a reduced GFR. The antiviral drug acyclovir may cause acute renal failure because of precipitation of the agent in the tubular lumina with resultant intrarenal obstruction. A similar process may occur in patients treated with high-dose sulfadiazine. Pentamidine used to treat *Pneumocystis carinii* and other protozoal diseases results in acute renal insufficiency in approximately 25 per cent of cases. *Nifedipine*, like many other drugs, may cause prerenal azotemia because of hypotension but, in addition, may also rarely cause reversible acute renal failure in the absence of a fall in blood pressure and without abnormalities in the urinary sediment.

Retroperitoneal fibrosis as a complication of long-term treatment of migraine headaches with *methysergide* may obstruct the ureters. *Anticoagulant therapy* may cause ureteral obstruction from intraluminal blood clots or from ureteral compression by a retroperitoneal hematoma.

Acute and Chronic Interstitial Nephritis

Adler SG, Cohen AH, Border WA: Hypersensitivity phenomena and the kidney: Role of drugs and environmental agents. Am J Kidney Dis 5:75, 1985. *An excellent review of the various types of immune-mediated renal injury that may result from numerous pharmacologic agents.*

Benabe JE, Martinez-Maldonado M: Tubulo-interstitial nephritis associated with systemic disease and electrolyte abnormalities. Semin Nephrol 8:29, 1988. *This paper provides a concise review of interstitial diseases associated with hypokalemia, hypercalcemia, hyperuricemia, multiple myeloma, sarcoidosis, Sjögren's syndrome, systemic lupus erythematosus, and tuberculosis (136 references).*

Boucher A, Droz D, Adafer E, et al.: Characterization of mononuclear cell subsets in renal cellular interstitial infiltrates. Kidney Int 29:1043, 1986. *Using monoclonal antibodies, the authors found that the predominant mononuclear cells in interstitial cellular infiltrates of 33 renal biopsies, including 11 with AISN or CISN, were T cells. However, the relative proportions of the different T cells subsets varied among the biopsies.*

Cameron JS: Allergic interstitial nephritis: Clinical features and pathogenesis. Q J Med 66:97, 1988. *A very good review of this topic, with an emphasis on drug-induced AISN and pathogenetic factors (165 references).*

Cotran RS, Rubin RH, Tolkoff-Rubin NE: Tubulo-interstitial diseases. *In* Brenner BM, Rector FC Jr (eds.): The Kidney. 3rd ed. Philadelphia, W. B. Saunders Company, 1986. *An excellent review of this topic (353 references).*

Eknoyan G: Chronic tubulointerstitial nephropathies. *In* Schrier RW, Gottschalk CW (eds.): Diseases of the Kidney. 4th ed. Boston, Little, Brown and Company, 1988. *A detailed review of this topic (337 references).*

Hande KR, Noone RM, Stone WJ: Severe allopurinol toxicity. Am J Med 76:47, 1984. *This report describes 7 patients with allopurinol toxicity treated by the authors and reviews another 78 cases from the literature. Dosage guidelines for allopurinol for patients with varying degrees of renal insufficiency are proposed.*

Hostetter TH, Hostetter MK: Infection-related chronic interstitial nephropathy.

Semin Nephrol 8:11, 1988. *This paper provides an excellent discussion of the pathogenetic factors responsible for the renal damage that may accompany renal infections.*

Toto RD: Review: Acute tubulointerstitial nephritis. Am J Med Sci 299:392, 1990. *A recent review of the pathogenesis, pathophysiology, differential diagnosis, and treatment of this disorder (114 references).*

Toxic Nephropathy (General References)

Humes HD, Weinberg JM: Toxic nephropathies. *In* Brenner BM, Rector FC Jr (eds.): The Kidney. 3rd ed. Philadelphia, W. B. Saunders Company, 1986. *An extensive, and well-written review with 579 references.*

Roxe DM, Krumlovsky FA: Toxic interstitial nephropathy from metals, metabolites and radiation. Semin Nephrol 8:72, 1988. *This paper contains a succinct review of nephrotoxicity resulting from cadmium, mercury, uranium, lead, oxalate, and radiation (102 references).*

Walker RJ, Duggin GG: Drug nephrotoxicity. Ann Rev Pharmacol Toxicol 28:331, 1988. *A concise review of the pathophysiologic mechanisms involved in aminoglycoside, amphotericin B, cephalosporin, acetaminophen, and cyclosporine A nephrotoxicity (74 references).*

Weinberg JM: The cellular basis of nephrotoxicity. *In* Schrier RW, Gottschalk CW (eds.): Diseases of the Kidney. 4th ed. Boston, Little, Brown and Company, 1988. *This chapter provides an exhaustive review of the pathophysiology of nephrotoxic renal injury (581 references).*

Analgesic Nephropathy

Buckalew VM Jr, Schey HM: Renal disease from habitual antipyretic analgesic consumption: An assessment of the epidemiologic evidence. Medicine 65:291, 1986. *This paper reviews the worldwide evidence that indicates that habitual analgesic use is an important cause of renal diseases (74 references).*

Eknoyan G, Qunibi WY, Grissom RT, et al.: Renal papillary necrosis: An update. Medicine 61:55, 1982. *A comprehensive review of the various causes of papillary necrosis, including analgesic nephropathy.*

Kincaid-Smith P, Nanra RS: Lithium-induced and analgesia-induced renal diseases. *In* Schrier RW, Gottschalk CW (eds.): Diseases of the Kidney. 4th ed. Boston, Little, Brown and Company, 1988. *This recent chapter contains a thorough review of these disorders (298 references).*

Sandler DP, Smith JC, Weinberg CR, et al.: Analgesic use and chronic renal disease. N Engl J Med 320:1238, 1989. *This paper describes the results of a multicenter case-control study of 554 adults with recently diagnosed kidney disease. The risk of developing renal disease was markedly increased in individuals who used phenacetin or its major metabolite acetaminophen on a daily basis.*

Nonsteroidal Anti-inflammatory Drugs

Dunn MJ, Patrono C (eds.): Renal effects of nonsteroidal anti-inflammatory drugs. Am J Med 81(Suppl 2B):1, 1986. *The several papers from the proceedings of this symposium deal with most aspects of this topic (1068 references).*

Henrich WL: Nephrotoxicity of nonsteroidal antiinflammatory agents. *In* Schrier RW, Gottschalk CW (eds.): Diseases of the Kidney. 4th ed. Boston, Little, Brown and Company, 1988. *This chapter contains a thorough discussion of the renal, fluid, and electrolyte complications of NSAID's (159 references).*

Porile JL, Bakris GL, Garella S: Acute interstitial nephritis with glomerulopathy due to nonsteroidal anti-inflammatory agents: A review of its clinical spectrum and effects of steroid therapy. J Clin Pharmacol 30:468, 1990. *This paper reviews 43 reported cases of acute renal failure and/or nephrotic range proteinuria occurring after treatment with NSAID's. The disorder was more frequent in women and the elderly and had a good prognosis for resolution with discontinuation of the NSAID. The authors believe the evidence suggests that steroids do not alter the course of this disorder.*

Antimicrobial Drugs

Branch RA: Prevention of amphotericin B–induced renal impairment: A review on the use of sodium supplementation. Arch Intern Med 148:2389, 1988. *This paper reviews the evidence that suggests that sodium loading may ameliorate amphotericin B nephrotoxicity.*

Fisher MA, Talbot GH, Maislin G, et al.: Risk factors for amphotericin B nephrotoxicity. Am J Med 87:547, 1989. *This report indicates that risk factors for amphotericin B nephrotoxicity include drug dose, diuretic use, and abnormal baseline renal function.*

Humes HD, O'Connor RP Jr: Aminoglycoside nephrotoxicity. *In* Schrier RW, Gottschalk CW (eds): Diseases of the Kidney. 4th ed. Boston, Little, Brown and Company, 1988. *An up-to-date comprehensive review of this disorder (265 references).*

Perez-Ayuso RM, Arroyo V, Camps J, et al.: Effect of demeclocycline on renal function and urinary prostaglandin E_2 and kallikrein in hyponatremic cirrhotics. Nephron 36:30, 1984. *In this report, five of eight hyponatremic cirrhotic patients given demeclocycline developed acute reversible renal insufficiency with a reduction in GFR from an average of 72 to 31 ml per minute.*

Sawyer MH, Webb DE, Balow JE, et al.: Acyclovir-induced renal failure. Am J Med 84:1067, 1988. *This report describes four patients with intrarenal obstruction and crystalluria resulting from acyclovir.*

Radiographic Contrast–Induced Nephrotoxicity

Berkseth RO, Kjellstrand CM: Radiologic contrast–induced nephropathy. Med Clin North Am 68:1, 1984. *A comprehensive review of this topic (101 references).*

Cronin RE: Southwestern Internal Medicine Conference: Renal failure following

radiologic procedures. Am J Med Sci 298:342, 1989. *A recent and excellent review of this topic (148 references).*

Schwabe SJ, Hlathy MA, Pieper KS, et al.: Contrast nephropathy: A randomized controlled trial of a nonionic and an ionic radiographic contrast agent. N Engl J Med 320:149, 1989. *In this study, 443 patients were randomized to undergo cardiac catheterization with either an ionic or a nonionic contrast agent. There was no difference in the nephrotoxicity of the two agents in patients at low or high risk of developing acute renal failure.*

Nephrotoxicity Associated with Antineoplastic Therapy

Belldegrun A, Webb DE, Austin HA III, et al.: Renal toxicity of interleukin-2 administration in patients with metastatic renal cell cancer: Effect of pretherapy nephrectomy. J Urol 141:499, 1989. *In this study of 135 patients with advanced cancer, including 52 with renal cell carcinoma, posttherapy depression of renal function was more severe in patients whose pretherapy serum creatinine concentration was elevated to 1.5 mg per deciliter or higher.*

Narins RG, Carley M, Bloom EJ, et al.: The nephrotoxicity of chemotherapeutic agents. Semin Nephrol 10:556, 1990. *This paper provides succinct reviews of the nephrotoxicity associated with several contemporary chemotherapeutic agents (89 references).*

Hainsworth JD, Johnson DH, Porter LL: Nephrotoxicity associated with antineoplastic therapy. *In* McKinney TD (ed.): Renal Complications of Neoplasia. New York, Praeger, 1986. *A thorough review of this topic with a particularly extensive discussion of cisplatin nephrotoxicity (174 references).*

Hande KR: Hyperuricemia, uric acid nephropathy and the tumor lysis syndrome. *In* McKinney TD (ed.): Renal Complications of Neoplasia. New York, Praeger, 1986. *A comprehensive review of this topic (86 references).*

Jorkasky DK, Singer I: Drug-induced tubulo-interstitial nephritis: Special cases. Semin Nephrol 8:62, 1988. *This paper provides a concise review of the nephrotoxicity associated with several drugs, including methotrexate, cisplatin, and the nitrosoureas (118 references).*

Rieselbach RE, Garnick MB: Renal diseases induced by antineoplastic agents. *In* Schrier RW, Gottschalk CW (eds.): Diseases of the Kidney. 4th ed. Boston, Little, Brown and Company, 1988. *This chapter provides a thorough review of this topic (179 references).*

Metal Nephropathies

Cullen MR, Robins JM, Eskenazi B: Adult inorganic lead intoxication: Presentation of 31 new cases and a review of recent advances in the literature. Medicine 62:221, 1983. *This article describes clinical characteristics in 31 patients with lead intoxication resulting from industrial exposure, along with a review of the topic (207 references).*

Falck FY Jr, Keren DF, Fine LJ, et al.: Protein excretion patterns in cadmium exposed individuals. High resolution electrophoresis. Arch Environ Health 39:69, 1984. *In this study, 7 of 39 men chronically exposed to industrial sources of cadmium had mild proteinuria, and 5 had mild elevations of serum creatinine concentrations.*

Katz WA, Blodgett RC Jr, Pietrusko RG: Proteinuria in gold-treated rheumatoid arthritis. Ann Intern Med 101:176, 1984. *In this report, 41 of 1283 (3 per cent) patients receiving oral gold treatments for rheumatoid arthritis developed proteinuria. In 9 this was in the nephrotic range. The results suggest that oral gold is less nephrotoxic than parenteral gold therapy.*

Tubbs RR, Gephardt GN, McMahon JT, et al.: Membranous glomerulonephritis associated with industrial mercury exposure. Am J Clin Pathol 77:409, 1982. *This report describes two patients with industrial exposure to mercury who developed biopsy-proven membranous nephropathy with heavy proteinuria. In one case proteinuria resolved after cessation of exposure to mercury, and this correlated with a decline in urinary mercury excretion from high to normal values.*

Wedeen RP: Heavy metals. *In* Schrier RW, Gottschalk CW (eds.): Diseases of the Kidney. 4th ed. Boston, Little, Brown and Company, 1988. *This chapter reviews the renal complications that may accompany intoxication with several heavy metals (161 references).*

Toxic Nephropathy (Miscellaneous References)

Baldwin DS, Gallo GR, Neugarten J: Drug abuse with narcotics, amphetamines and other agents. *In* Schrier RW, Gottschalk CW (eds.): Diseases of the Kidney. 4th ed. Boston, Little, Brown and Company, 1988. *This chapter provides a good discussion of the several renal complications that may result from drug abuse, along with representative photographs of histopathologic findings (118 references).*

Diamond JC, Cheung JY, Fang LST: Nifedipine-induced renal dysfunction. Am J Med 77:905, 1984. *This paper describes four patients with underlying renal insufficiency who had reversible acute declines in renal function during nifedipine therapy in the absence of hypotension.*

Gabow PA, Clay K, Sullivan JB, et al.: Organic acids in ethylene glycol intoxication. Ann Intern Med 105:16, 1986. *This paper describes three patients with ethylene glycol intoxication, acute renal failure, and metabolic acidosis successfully treated by a combination of ethanol infusion and hemodialysis.*

Hricik DE, Dunn MJ: Angiotensin-converting enzyme inhibitor induced renal failure: Causes, consequences, and diagnostic uses. J Am Soc Nephrol 1:845, 1990. *This is a comprehensive review of this topic. Emphasis is placed both on the renal failure that may accompany administration of this class of drugs in individuals with renovascular disease and the potential use of these agents for diagnosing renovascular disease.*

Krochak RJ, Baker DG: Radiation nephritis: Clinical manifestations and pathophysiologic mechanisms. Urology 27:389, 1986. *A succinct review of this topic.*

Myers BD, Sibley R, Newton L, et al.: The long-term course of cyclosporine-associated chronic nephropathy. Kidney Int 33:590, 1988. *This paper describes the progressive decrease in renal function and the histologic changes occurring in a group of 37 cardiac transplant recipients treated with cyclosporine A. Compared with a group of 24 other patients with other types of immunosuppression treated for the same length of time (24 months), patients treated with cyclosporine A had a higher incidence of hypertension and proteinuria and a lower GFR.*

Ntoso KA, Tomaszewski JE, Jimenez SA, et al.: Penicillamine-induced rapidly progressive glomerulonephritis in patients with progressive systemic sclerosis: Successful treatment of two patients and a review of the literature. Am J Kidney Dis 8:159, 1986. *Two cases of crescentic glomerulonephritis due to penicillamine are described along with a brief review of types of renal disorders that may complicate therapy with this drug.*

Streicher HZ, Gabow PA, Moss AH, et al.: Syndromes of toluene sniffing in adults. Ann Intern Med 94:758, 1981. *Clinical features of 25 cases of toluene sniffing are reported. The most prominent renal-electrolyte manifestation was hyperchloremic metabolic acidosis.*

81 Obstructive Uropathy

Saulo Klahr

Obstructive uropathy refers to the structural or functional changes in the urinary tract that impede the normal flow of urine. It occurs in a wide variety of settings and is a relatively common cause of impaired renal function (obstructive nephropathy). Obstructive uropathy may also cause dilatation of the urinary tract (hydronephrosis). Since the consequences of obstructive uropathy are potentially reversible, prompt diagnosis and appropriate treatment are important to prevent permanent loss of renal function, which is directly related to the degree and duration of the obstruction.

INCIDENCE

Obstructive uropathy, a relatively common disorder, is seen in all age groups. Hydronephrosis has been found at autopsy in 3.5 to 3.8 per cent of adults and in 2 per cent of children, mostly as a consequence of congenital abnormalities of the urinary tract. Urolithiasis occurs predominantly in young adults (ages 25 to 45) and is three times more common in men than in women. In patients older than 60 years, obstructive uropathy is seen more frequently in men than in women owing to benign prostatic hyperplasia and prostatic carcinoma. In 1985, approximately 166 patients per 100,000 population were hospitalized with a presumptive diagnosis of obstruction, and 387 patient visits per 100,000 population were related to obstructive uropathy. Approximately 450,000 surgical procedures for benign prostatic hyperplasia are performed annually in the United States.

ETIOLOGY

Obstruction can occur anywhere in the urinary tract from the renal tubules (uric acid nephropathy) to the urethral meatus (phimosis) (Table 81–1). Clinically, it is helpful to divide the causes of obstruction into *upper urinary tract* (lesions located above the ureterovesical junction) and *lower urinary tract* (below the ureterovesical junction) factors. The causes of upper urinary tract obstruction can be divided into *intrinsic* (intraluminal or intramural) and *extrinsic* (Table 81–1). Intraluminal obstruction is due to stones, clots, or sloughed papillary tissue. Intramural causes are either anatomic (tumors, strictures) or functional (defects in peristalsis: pyeloureteral or vesicoureteral junctions). Extrinsic causes of obstruction can be classified based on the system of origin of the obstructing lesion (Table 81–1).

Clinically, the age and sex of the patient are helpful in narrowing the differential diagnosis. In children, congenital causes of obstructive uropathy are common (stenosis at the ureteropelvic or ureterovesical junction, urethral valves, and so on). In the middle-aged woman, cervical cancer is a common cause of extrinsic ureteral or ureterovesical junction obstruction. In elderly men, benign prostatic hyperplasia and prostatic carcinoma are frequent causes of obstruction.

PATHOLOGY AND PATHOPHYSIOLOGY

The effects of urinary tract obstruction on renal function are due to several factors with complex interactions. Following the

TABLE 81–1. CAUSES OF URINARY TRACT OBSTRUCTION

Upper Urinary Tract	Lower Urinary Tract

A. Intrinsic Causes
 1. Intraluminal
   a. Intratubular deposition of crystals (uric acid, acyclovir)
   b. Ureter: stones, clots, renal papillae
 2. Intramural
   a. Ureteropelvic or ureterovesical junction dysfunction
   b. Ureteral valve, polyp, stricture, or tumor
 B. Extrinsic Causes
 1. Vascular system
   a. Aneurysm: abdominal aorta, iliac vessels
   b. Aberrant vessels: ureteropelvic junction
   c. Venous: retrocaval ureter
 2. Reproductive system
   a. Uterus: pregnancy, prolapse, tumors, endometriosis
   b. Ovary: abscess, tumors, ovarian remnants
   c. Gartner's duct cyst, tubo-ovarian abscess
 3. Gastrointestinal tract: Crohn's disease, diverticulitis, appendiceal abscess, tumors, pancreatic tumor, abscess, or cyst
 4. Retroperitoneal disease:
   a. Retroperitoneal fibrosis (idiopathic, radiation, drugs)
   b. Inflammatory: tuberculosis, sarcoidosis
   c. Hematomas
   d. Primary tumors (lymphoma, sarcoma, and so on)
   e. Metastatic tumors: cervix, bladder, colon, prostate, and so on)
   f. Lymphocele
   g. Pelvic lipomatosis
	1. Phimosis, meatal stenosis, paraphimosis
	 2. Urethra: strictures, stones, diverticulum, posterior or anterior urethral valves, periurethral abscess, urethral surgery
	 3. Prostate: benign hyperplasia, abscess, carcinoma
	 4. Bladder
	   a. Neurogenic bladder: spinal cord defect or trauma, diabetes, multiple sclerosis, cerebrovascular accidents, Parkinson's disease
	   b. Bladder neck dysfunction
	   c. Bladder calculus
	   d. Bladder cancer
	 5. Trauma
	   a. Straddle injury
	   b. Pelvic fracture
	 6. Drugs: spinal anesthesia, anticholinergics, smooth muscle depressants

onset of obstruction, pressures in the renal pelvis and tubules increase, resulting in dilatation of these structures and flattening of the renal papilla. Renal damage is probably initiated by high intraureteral and high intratubular pressures. Decreases in renal blood flow cause ischemia, cellular atrophy, and necrosis. In addition, parenchymal infiltration by macrophages and T lymphocytes may cause scarring of the kidney. Superimposed infection may accelerate the destruction of the kidney in this setting.

Normal urine flow from the renal pelvis to the bladder depends on ureteral peristalsis and a progressive decrease in hydrostatic pressure from Bowman's space to the renal pelvis. Ureteral peristalsis generates high intraluminal pressures, which propel the bolus of urine along the ureter. Contraction of circular muscle fibers in the ureter prevents transmission of this pressure to the kidney. Impaired urine flow in the urinary tract leads to a rise in the pressure and volume of urine proximal to the obstruction. In this setting, contraction of the circular muscle fibers may be lost, and high intraureteral pressures are transmitted to the kidney. This situation results in increased intratubular pressure. The rise in intratubular pressure without a similar rise in intraglomerular pressure decreases the net hydrostatic filtration pressure across glomerular capillaries, resulting in a fall in the glomerular filtration rate (GFR) (Fig. 81–1).

After the onset of complete obstruction, there is an initial period of renal vasodilatation lasting 1 to 3 hours, which is followed by progressive vasoconstriction of the renal circulation. This renal vasoconstriction leads to a decrease in renal blood flow, a decrease in intraglomerular pressure, and a decrease in the GFR (Fig. 81–1). The vasoconstriction is mediated by angiotensin II and thromboxane A_2. These two compounds, through their effects on mesangial cell contraction, may also decrease the glomerular surface area available for filtration. The decrement in glomerular surface area may explain the greater decrease in the GFR than in renal plasma flow observed in obstruction.

As a consequence of increased intrarenal levels of angiotensin II, there is an increase in the synthesis of prostaglandin E_2 (PGE_2) and prostacyclin. These eicosanoids are vasodilatory substances that also antagonize the effects of angiotensin II on mesangial cell contraction. Hence, in the setting of obstruction, the increased synthesis of both PGE_2 and prostacyclin tends to prevent the GFR and renal blood flow from decreasing further. After the release of obstruction in experimental animals, the administration of inhibitors of prostaglandin synthesis, such as nonsteroidal anti-inflammatory agents, decreases the GFR and renal blood flow.

Partial obstruction of the urinary tract may also decrease renal blood flow and the GFR. In addition, functional tubular defects are prominent. There is an inability to concentrate the urine and a decreased excretion of hydrogen ion and potassium. The concentrating defect is due in part to decreased osmolality of the renal medulla, probably related to decreased sodium reabsorption in the thick ascending limb of Henle's loop, and to the removal of medullary solutes (sodium, urea) as a consequence of the initial increase in medullary blood flow seen in obstruction. A decrease in the hydro-osmotic response of the cortical collecting duct to vasopressin also contributes to the concentrating defect. The decreased hydrogen ion and potassium excretion is due to impaired secretion of these ions in distal segments of the nephron, presumably as a consequence of a diminished response to the action of aldosterone. Secondary to increased tubular pressure and dilatation, there is also disruption of intercellular tight junctions, resulting in increased tubular permeability to solutes and in inhibition of sodium reabsorption.

CLINICAL MANIFESTATIONS

The clinical manifestations of urinary tract obstruction depend on the location (upper or lower urinary tract), degree (complete or partial), and duration (acute or chronic) of the obstruction (Table 81–2).

The symptoms of upper and lower urinary tract obstruction differ. Patients with acute complete obstruction may present with acute renal failure. Patients with chronic partial obstruction (chronic hydronephrosis) may be asymptomatic, may have intermittent pain, or may present with symptoms and laboratory findings of impaired renal function, including inability to concentrate the urine, manifested as nocturia and/or polyuria, with or without elevated levels of blood urea nitrogen (BUN) and serum creatinine.

Pain and Renal Colic

Pain, due to distention of the bladder or to stretching of the collecting system or the renal capsule, is a common presenting symptom in obstructive uropathy, particularly in patients with ureteral calculi. Classic "renal colic" is a steady crescendo, severe pain located in the flank (in the case of stones lodged in the upper third of the ureter) or radiating to the labia, testicles, or groin (stones in the lower two thirds of the ureter) and may be associated with sweating and vomiting. The acute attack may last less than 30 minutes or as long as a day. Pain radiating into the flank during micturition is said to be pathognomonic of vesico-ureteral reflux. Chronic partial obstruction may cause intermittent flank pain. Pain may be elicited in some of these patients by administration of diuretics and/or excessive fluid intake. Physical examination may be normal or may reveal flank tenderness in patients with acute upper urinary tract obstruction. In patients with lower urinary tract obstruction, a distended, palpable, and occasionally painful bladder may be found. Careful rectal examination in men or pelvic examination in women should be performed, since it may reveal prostatic enlargement or pelvic masses.

Changes in Urinary Output

Anuria and acute renal failure occur in patients with complete bilateral ureteral obstruction, with complete lower urinary tract obstruction, or with unilateral ureteral obstruction when there is a solitary kidney. In patients with partial or incomplete obstruction of the urinary tract, the urinary output may be normal or increased (polyuria). Occasionally, such patients may develop marked polyuria and increased thirst (a diabetes insipidus–like syndrome). This condition may cause hypernatremia. A pattern of oliguria or anuria alternating with polyuria or the acute onset of anuria strongly suggests the presence of obstructive uropathy.

Hematuria

Gross hematuria may be seen in obstruction, particularly when it is due to stones. In the presence of gross hematuria, clots may cause ureteral obstruction.

Palpable Masses

Longstanding obstructive uropathy may increase kidney size. Such patients may have increased abdominal girth or a palpable flank mass. Hydronephrosis is a common cause of a palpable

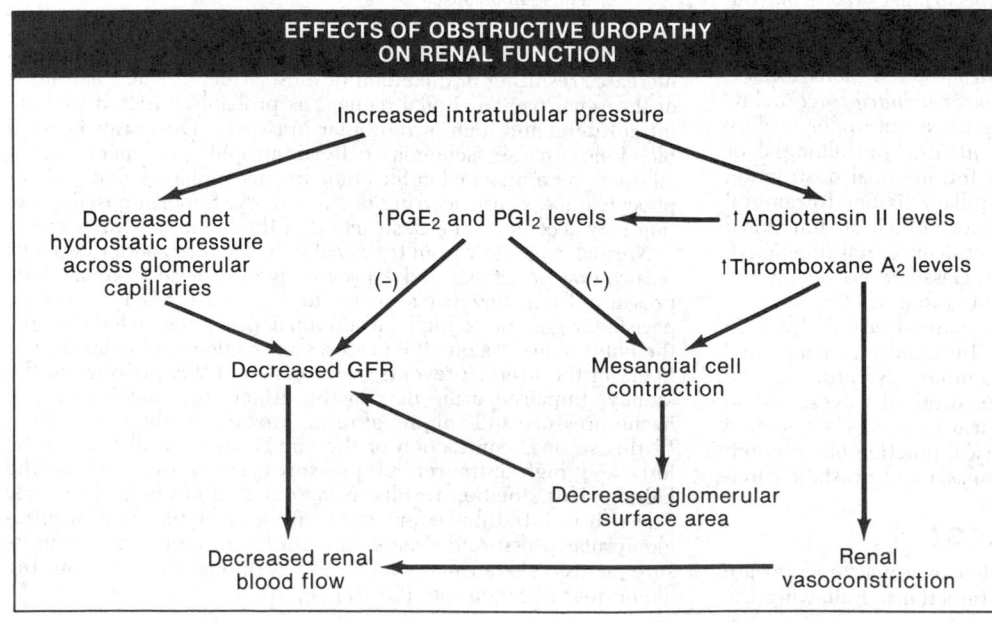

EFFECTS OF OBSTRUCTIVE UROPATHY ON RENAL FUNCTION

Increased intratubular pressure

Decreased net hydrostatic pressure across glomerular capillaries

↑PGE₂ and PGI₂ levels ← ↑Angiotensin II levels

↑Thromboxane A₂ levels

(−) (−)

Decreased GFR

Mesangial cell contraction

Decreased glomerular surface area

Decreased renal blood flow ← Renal vasoconstriction

FIGURE 81–1. Increased levels of prostaglandin E_2 (PGE_2) and prostacyclin (PGI_2) tend to antagonize (−) the effects of angiotensin II and thromboxane A_2 on mesangial cell contraction and renal vasoconstriction. Hence, they tend to prevent GFR from decreasing further.

TABLE 81–2. CLINICAL MANIFESTATIONS AND LABORATORY FINDINGS IN URINARY TRACT OBSTRUCTION

1. No symptoms (chronic hydronephrosis)
2. Intermittent pain (chronic hydronephrosis)
3. Elevated levels of BUN and serum creatinine with no other symptoms (chronic hydronephrosis)
4. Renal colic (usually due to ureteral stones or papillary necrosis)
5. Changes in urinary output
   a. Anuria or oliguria (acute renal failure)
   b. Polyuria (incomplete or partial obstruction)
   c. Fluctuating urinary output
6. Hematuria
7. Palpable masses
   a. Flank (hydronephrotic kidney; usually in infants)
   b. Suprapubic (distended bladder)
8. Hypertension
   a. Volume dependent (usually due to chronic bilateral obstruction)
   b. Renin dependent (usually due to acute unilateral obstruction)
9. Repeated urinary tract infections or infection that is refractory to treatment
10. Hyperkalemic, hyperchloremic acidosis (usually due to defective tubular secretion of hydrogen and potassium)
11. Hypernatremia (seen in infants with partial obstruction and polyuria)
12. Polycythemia (increased renal production of erythropoietin)
13. Lower urinary tract symptoms: hesitancy, urgency, incontinence, postvoid dribbling, decreased force and caliber of urinary stream, nocturia

abdominal mass in children. In patients with lower urinary tract obstruction, particularly that due to benign prostatic hyperplasia, a suprapubic mass may be caused by a distended bladder. This part of the physical examination should not be neglected in patients with anuria and suspected obstructive uropathy. This type of obstruction is readily reversed by the placement of a catheter in the bladder.

Hypertension

Hypertension is commonly associated with renal disease regardless of its etiology. Patients with urinary tract obstruction may have hypertension due to (1) fluid retention and expansion of the extracellular fluid volume, (2) increased renin secretion, and (3) possibly decreased synthesis of medullary vasodepressor substances. In some patients with obstructive uropathy, the hypertension may be coincidental. Hypertension may occur in about one third of patients with acute unilateral obstruction and is usually, but not always, renin dependent. Release of acute obstruction should ameliorate the hypertension when the two are causally related.

In patients with chronic bilateral obstruction, the hypertension is usually due to impaired sodium excretion and expansion of the extracellular fluid volume (volume-dependent hypertension). In such patients, the circulating levels of renin are usually suppressed.

Urinary Tract Infections or Infection That Is Refractory to Treatment

Repeated urinary tract infections without apparent cause are suggestive of obstruction. Infection is more common in patients with lower urinary tract obstruction. This may be due to decreased bacterial "washout" and increased bacterial adherence to the mucosa of the bladder. Moreover, in the presence of obstruction, eradication of the infection is difficult. In noninstrumented patients, the finding of unusual organisms (*Proteus, Pseudomonas*) in urine cultures should suggest the presence of underlying obstruction. Thus, in patients with repeated urinary tract infections or persistent infection refractory to treatment, the possibility of underlying urinary tract obstruction should be considered.

Increased Levels of Blood Urea Nitrogen and Serum Creatinine

Obstructive uropathy is a potential cause of impaired renal function and end-stage renal disease and should be considered in the differential diagnosis, particularly in patients with a normal urinary sediment and no previous history of renal disease. Ob-

struction of the urinary tract may occur in patients with established renal parenchymal disease and cause an acceleration in the rate of progression.

Hyperkalemic Hyperchloremic Metabolic Acidosis

A hyperkalemic, hyperchloremic (non–anion gap) metabolic acidosis may be present in patients with urinary tract obstruction. It is seen more frequently in elderly individuals. The abnormality is due to decreased hydrogen ion and potassium secretion by distal segments of the nephron and may be caused by a decrease in aldosterone production and/or refractoriness of the distal tubule to the actions of this mineralocorticoid. Hyperchloremic metabolic acidosis may occur in the absence of hyperkalemia and results from a selective defect in hydrogen ion secretion.

Polycythemia

Polycythemia that subsides after relief of obstruction is a rare manifestation of urinary tract obstruction. Increased renal production of erythropoietin, presumably due to ischemia, may account for the development of polycythemia.

Lower Urinary Tract Symptoms

Patients with obstruction of the lower urinary tract may develop symptoms such as decreased force and caliber of the urine stream, intermittency, incontinence, postvoid dribbling, hesitancy, and urgency. Alterations in the process of micturition due to neurogenic bladder disease may also result in urgency, frequent urination, and urinary incontinence (overflow incontinence).

DIAGNOSTIC APPROACH

The presence of obstructive uropathy may not be obvious. Definitive tests are needed to exclude this diagnosis in suspected cases. Early diagnosis and prompt treatment are essential, since the degree of renal impairment resulting from obstructive uropathy is related to its severity and duration. The diagnostic approach to obstructive uropathy depends on the symptoms and the clinical findings of patients presenting with asymptomatic renal insufficiency, renal colic, or acute renal failure and anuria (Fig. 81–2).

When obstruction is suspected, the history may be of value: previous urinary tract infections, drugs ingested, and the presence of lower urinary tract symptoms (see above). In the hospital setting, the pattern of urinary output can be ascertained from input and output records. The physical examination may yield some clues: tenderness in the costovertebral angle, a mass in the flank area, and muscle rigidity over the kidney area. Abdominal distention and diminished peristalsis accompany acute renal colic. A suprapubic mass may be due to bladder outlet obstruction. The urinalysis may yield important clues: Is there hematuria, bacteriuria, or a urinary pH greater than 7.5 to indicate stones and/or infection with urea-splitting organisms? The urinary sediment should be carefully examined for the presence of crystals (uric acid, cystine, and so forth). Laboratory studies should include an assessment of renal function (BUN, serum creatinine).

The tests utilized to diagnose obstructive uropathy are summarized in Table 81–3. *Ultrasound* is a noninvasive diagnostic test used as the initial procedure in suspected obstruction. The main finding detected by ultrasound is dilatation of the urinary tract. In a few instances, the ultrasound may give false-negative results because dilatation does not occur as a consequence of dehydration or too recent an onset of obstruction (Fig. 81–2). *Plain films of the abdomen (kidneys, ureter, bladder [KUB])* are particularly useful in patients with renal colic because ureteral calculi may be visualized (Fig. 81–2). They also provide information on renal and bladder morphology, such as size differences between the two kidneys or an enlarged bladder suggestive of outlet obstruction. The *intravenous pyelogram (IVP)* is used to investigate acute renal colic (Fig. 81–2). The excretion of contrast media may be delayed in patients with a low GFR because of a decrease in the filtered load of the dye. In such patients, the procedure should be extended until the collecting system and the site of obstruction are identified. This identification may require obtaining delayed films. The IVP is not useful in patients with compromised renal function, particularly those with serum

TABLE 81–3. DIAGNOSTIC TESTS UTILIZED IN OBSTRUCTIVE UROPATHY

Upper Urinary Tract Obstruction
Sonography (ultrasound)
Plain films of the abdomen (KUB)
Excretory or intravenous pyelography (IVP)
Retrograde pyelography
Isotopic renography
Computed tomography
Magnetic resonance imaging
Pressure flow studies (the Whitaker test)
Lower Urinary Tract Obstruction
Some of the tests listed above
Cystoscopy
Voiding cystourethrogram
Retrograde urethrogram
Urodynamic tests
    Debimetry
    Cystometrography
    Electromyography
    Urethral pressure profile

Reproduced by permission from Klahr S: Obstructive uropathy. *In* Jacobson HR, Striker GE, Klahr S (eds.): The Principles and Practice of Nephrology. Philadelphia, B.C. Decker, 1991, pp 432–441.

creatinine levels greater than 3 to 4 mg per deciliter. It also has the risk of potential nephrotoxicity. *Retrograde pyelography* requires the retrograde injection of radiocontrast and is used to visualize the ureter and collecting system when the IVP cannot be done or is not justified because of a history of allergic reaction to contrast material or other contraindications. This procedure can identify both the site and the cause of the obstruction. *Isotopic renography* can be used to diagnose upper urinary tract obstruction. It requires the intravenous injection of a radionuclide and subsequent imaging with a gamma scintillation camera. This imaging can be combined with intravenous furosemide administered 20 to 30 minutes after injection of the isotope. Other diagnostic procedures for obstructive uropathy include *computed tomography* and *magnetic resonance imaging*. Computed tomography is particularly useful in the diagnosis of causes of obstruction. Occasionally, obstruction of the upper urinary tract is difficult to diagnose using the techniques described above, and *pressure flow studies* (the Whitaker test) may be required. This test consists of measuring pressure differences between the renal pelvis and the bladder during the infusion, at a known rate, of fluid into the renal pelvis.

A number of diagnostic tests are useful in the diagnosis of lower urinary tract obstruction. These include a *voiding cystourethrogram*, which is utilized to investigate the presence of vesicoureteral reflux as a cause of dilatation of the urinary tract. *Cystoscopy* allows visual inspection of the entire urethra and bladder during the same procedure. However, this procedure requires the use of anesthesia in children and young adults. The anterior urethra can be assessed by *retrograde urethrogram*, which is performed by occluding the urethral meatus using a syringe or a catheter and injecting contrast medium. However, a retrograde urethrogram is not adequate to evaluate the posterior urethra. This anatomic area is best examined by an *excretory or retrograde cystogram*. The two tests combined usually provide a complete study of the urethra. *Urodynamic* tests with measurements of urine flow rate per unit time are useful to evaluate bladder outlet obstruction. Measurement of *urine flow rate* (*debimetry*) is a noninvasive test that examines the interplay between the expulsive force of the detrusor muscle and urethral resistance. *Cystometrography* can be used to assess the force of the detrusor muscle in the bladder, and it quantifies the pressure-volume relationships of this organ. Dyssynergy of the bladder sphincter refers to the inability of the sphincter to relax during contraction of the detrusor muscle and is seen in patients with neurologic disorders. This type of resistance is better analyzed by *electromyography* and *urethral pressure profiles*. About 25 per cent of children with spina bifida have detrusor sphincter dyssynergia at birth.

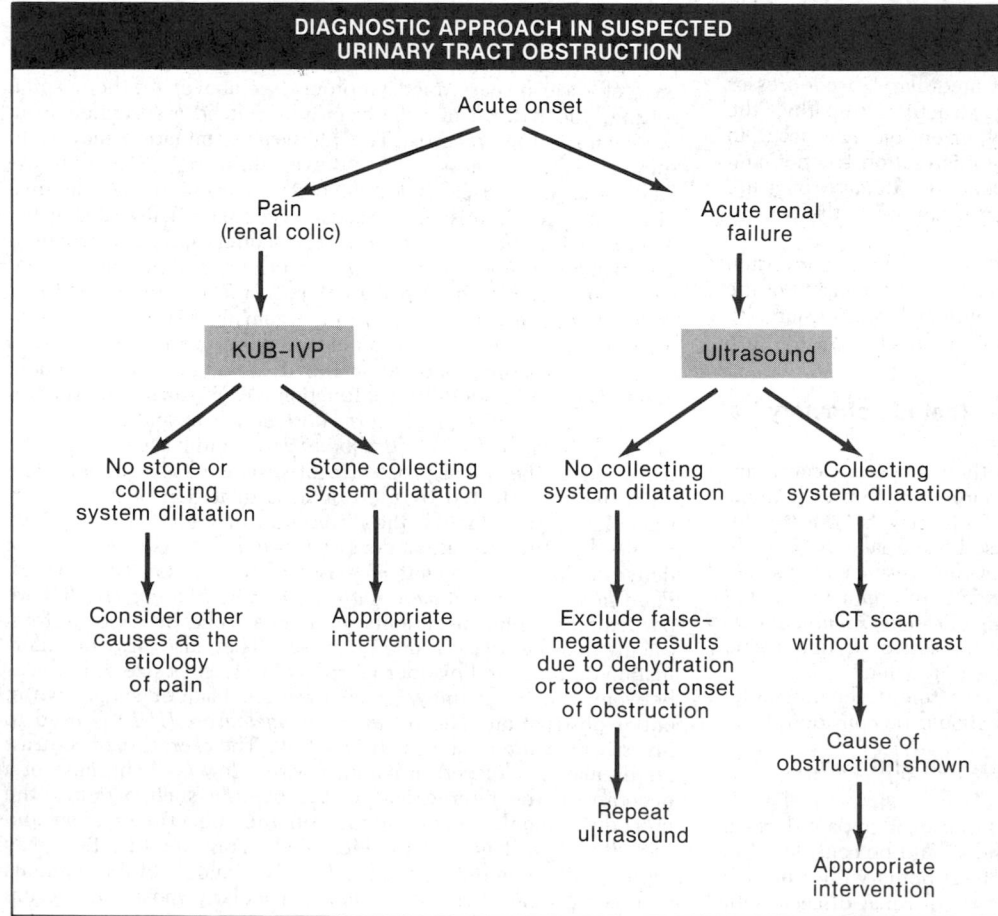

FIGURE 81–2. Scheme of diagnostic approach to urinary tract obstruction. KUB (kidney, ureter, bladder) = a flat film of the abdomen without contrast material; IVP = intravenous pyelography; CT = computed tomography.

TREATMENT

After the diagnosis of obstructive uropathy is established, it is necessary to decide whether or not surgery or instrumentation is required. The goals of therapy are (1) restoration and/or preservation of renal function, (2) relief of pain and/or other symptoms of obstruction, and (3) prevention or eradication of infection.

Acute Obstruction (Complete)

Complete bilateral ureteral obstruction presenting as acute renal failure requires prompt intervention. The site of obstruction determines the approach in these patients. If the obstruction is distal to the bladder, the placement of a urethral catheter may suffice. In some cases a suprapubic cystostomy is required. If the obstruction is located in the upper urinary tract, placement of percutaneous nephrostomy tubes or passage of a retrograde ureteral catheter may be necessary. Nephrostomy tubes not only provide drainage of the urine but also can be used for the local infusion of pharmacologic agents to treat infection, calculi, and so on. In patients with urinary tract infection and generalized sepsis, prompt relief of the obstruction is necessary, and appropriate antibiotic therapy is indicated. Sometimes dialysis may be required prior to instrumentation or surgery in patients with obstruction and acute renal failure.

Acute Obstruction (Partial)

Calculi are the most common cause of ureteral obstruction. Their treatment includes relief of pain, elimination of obstruction, and treatment of infection. Pain can be relieved by intramuscular injection of a narcotic analgesic. Stones less than 5 mm in diameter do not usually require surgical intervention or instrumentation. About 90 per cent of these stones are passed spontaneously. If the stones are 5 to 7 mm, however, only about half will pass, and stones larger than 7 mm usually are not passed spontaneously. High fluid intake to increase the urinary volume to at least 2 liters per day may help to mobilize the stone. The urine must be strained through a gauze sponge to recover the calculi for analysis. If the stone completely occludes the ureter and does not move, surgical treatment is necessary. Endourology refers to the closed controlled manipulation of the entire urinary tract. Endourologic methods can be used in the successful treatment of stones obstructing the ureter in about 98 per cent of patients. In addition, this approach shortens the hospital stay to 3 to 4 days and the convalescence period to only 4 to 7 days. Extracorporeal shock wave or ultrasound lithotripsy involves the focusing of electrohydraulic or ultrasonically generated shock waves to disintegrate the stone. The method is effective for ureteral calculi of 7 to 15 mm that lie above the pelvic brim. The stone is disintegrated in 90 per cent of patients, and all particulate matter passes within a 3-month period. Morbidity is low. However, all patients should be followed up for stone recurrence and should be given preventive therapy. In addition, there is a question of posttreatment hypertension, which requires follow-up. In selected individuals, the procedure can be done on an outpatient basis. Most patients are back at work 2 to 3 days after shock wave therapy. Calculi located distal to the pelvic brim can be approached from below. Antibiotics are useful when infections complicate renal calculi. The choice of antibiotic depends on appropriate urine cultures and sensitivity studies.

Chronic Partial Obstruction

Surgical intervention can be delayed sometimes for weeks or even months in patients with low-grade obstruction or partial chronic obstruction. However, prompt relief of partial obstruction is indicated when (1) there are repeated episodes of urinary tract infection, (2) the patient has significant symptoms (dysuria, voiding dysfunction, flank pain), (3) there is urinary retention, or (4) there is evidence of recurrent or progressive renal damage.

Lower Urinary Tract Obstruction

Urethral and bladder neck obstruction requires surgery in patients with recurrent infections who are ambulatory, particularly when reflux, renal parenchymal damage, marked urinary retention, repeated bleeding, or other symptoms are present. Obstruction secondary to benign prostatic hyperplasia is not always progressive. Therefore, a patient with minimal symptoms, no infection, and a normal upper urinary tract may be followed safely until he or she and the physician agree that surgery is desirable. Urethral strictures in men can be treated by dilatation or direct visual internal urethrotomy. The incidence of bladder neck and urethral obstruction in women is low. Hence, urethral dilatation, internal urethrotomy, meatotomy, and revision of the bladder neck in women are seldom indicated.

When obstruction is the result of neuropathic bladder function, dynamic studies are essential to determine therapy. The main goals of therapy should be (1) to establish the bladder as a urine storage organ without causing renal injury and (2) to provide a mechanism for bladder emptying that is acceptable to the patient. Patients fall into two categories, those with atonic bladders secondary to lower motor neuron injury and those with unstable bladder function due to upper motor neuron disease. The neurogenic bladder seen in diabetes mellitus is usually the result of lower motor neuron disease. Requesting these patients to void at regular intervals achieves satisfactory emptying of the bladder. Occasionally, these individuals respond to cholinergic agents, such as bethanechol chloride (Urecholine). Alpha-adrenergic blockers relax urethral sphincter tone but have only limited success because of side effects. The best treatment for patients with significant residual urine and recurrent urosepsis is the establishment of clean, intermittent self-catheterization at regular intervals. The goal is to catheterize four or five times per day so that the amount of urine drained from the bladder does not exceed 400 ml. This technique may be successful but requires the patient's acceptance and adequate training. In patients with a hypertonic bladder, the major goal is to improve its storage function. The use of anticholinergic agents may be indicated. Occasionally, chronic, clean, intermittent self-catheterization is necessary. In all patients with neurogenic bladders, chronic indwelling catheters should be avoided if possible, owing to risk of infection and other complications.

POSTOBSTRUCTIVE DIURESIS

Postobstructive diuresis refers to the marked natriuresis and diuresis that occasionally follow the relief of obstruction. This diuresis is characterized by excretion of large amounts of sodium, potassium, magnesium, and other solutes. Although usually self-limited, the losses of solutes and water may result in hypokalemia, hyponatremia or hypernatremia, hypomagnesemia, and marked volume depletion. In many patients, a brisk diuresis after relief of obstruction may represent a physiologic response to expansion of the extracellular fluid volume occurring during the period of obstruction. This postobstructive diuresis is appropriate and does not compromise the volume status of the patient. Postobstructive diuresis in this setting can be prolonged by overzealous replacement of salt and water after relief of obstruction.

Fluid replacement is justified only when excessive losses of sodium and water occur that are inappropriate for the volume status of the patient and are presumably due to an intrinsic tubular defect in sodium and water reabsorption. Fluid replacement in these patients is guided in large part by what is excreted. Intravenous fluid administration may be necessary, but urinary losses should be replaced only to the extent necessary to prevent extracellular fluid volume contraction or electrolyte imbalance.

PROGNOSIS

The return of renal function after relief of obstruction is variable and is influenced by the severity and duration of obstruction. Other events that condition the degree of recovery of renal function include the presence of infection, stones, pre-existing renal disease, and/or the underlying cause of the obstruction. Renal cortical thickness is a prognostic indicator of residual renal function in patients with chronic hydronephrosis. Patients with a very thin cortex have lost considerable renal function.

In experimental animals, the GFR reached 70 per cent of normal 2 years after relief of ureteral obstruction of 1 week's duration, 50 per cent of normal after 2 weeks of obstruction, and 20 per cent of normal after 4 weeks of obstruction. In rats with unilateral ureteral obstruction of 24 hours' duration, 15 per cent of nephrons were nonfunctional 2 months after relief of obstruction. The normalization of the GFR in these animals was due to hyperfiltration in the remaining functional nephrons. If similar changes occur in humans, short-term obstruction may result in loss of functional nephrons, which may go undetected because the GFR returns to normal owing to hyperfiltration in the remaining nephrons.

Klahr S, Bander SJ: Obstructive nephropathy. *In* Massry SG, Glassock RJ (eds.): Textbook of Nephrology. Vol I. 2nd ed. Orlando, Fla., The Williams and Wilkins Company, 1989, pp 889–909. *A recent and detailed discussion of clinical, pathologic, and diagnostic issues in obstructive nephropathy.*

Klahr S, Clayman RV, Bahnson RR: Obstructive uropathy. *In* Glassock RJ (ed.) Current Therapy in Nephrology and Hypertension. Vol 2. Toronto, B.C. Decker Publishers, 1987, pp 67–72. *Discusses the therapeutic approach to the patient with urinary tract obstruction or postobstructive diuresis.*

Klahr S, Harris K, Purkerson ML: Effects of obstructive uropathy on renal functions. Pediatr Nephrol 2:34, 1988. *A recent review on the pathophysiology of obstructive nephropathy with numerous references.*

82 Specific Renal Tubular Disorders

Martin G. Cogan

The diverse reabsorptive functions of the kidney are generally segregated so that specific nephron segments are responsible for specific transport functions. As described in Ch. 73, the proximal nephron is responsible for the reabsorption of most of the filtered bicarbonate, glucose, amino acids, uric acid, phosphate, and low molecular weight proteins. The loop of Henle reabsorbs over half the filtered sodium chloride as well as divalent cations. The distal nephron (including the cortical and medullary collecting ducts), under the influence of aldosterone, reabsorbs the final quantity of sodium and secretes hydrogen and potassium ions. The terminal collecting ducts can be induced by antidiuretic hormone to permit water reabsorption and thereby cause urinary concentration.

Genetic and acquired conditions can affect one or more of the reabsorptive or secretory transport processes within each of these nephron segments, as illustrated in Table 82–1. Depending on the transport sites affected, these diseases lead to abnormal wastage or retention of specific solutes. For instance, within a given nephron segment, there may be a selective transport defect for a single solute (e.g., bicarbonate in proximal renal tubular acidosis or glucose in renal glycosuria) or for a class of solutes (e.g., dibasic amino acids in cystinuria). Alternatively, those solutes whose transport is modulated by a specific hormone may be affected by a hormone-deficient or -resistant state (e.g., in hypoaldosteronism or diabetes insipidus). Finally, there are diseases that affect all solutes normally transported by a given nephron segment (e.g., all proximal transported solutes in Fanconi's syndrome). Luminal, cellular, or peritubular components of the overall transport process can be responsible for each of these situations. The following sections, and other chapters as identified in Table 82–1, describe some of the more common transport defects of the individual nephron segments.

DISORDERS OF PROXIMAL NEPHRON FUNCTION

The proximal nephron is responsible for reabsorbing 80 to 99 per cent of several filtered solutes, including glucose, amino acids, and bicarbonate. Detection of one or more of these solutes in the urine at normal filtered loads implies a disorder of proximal transport.

Renal Glycosurias

The renal glycosurias are caused by inherited or acquired defects in proximal tubule glucose reabsorption such that glycosuria occurs in the absence of hyperglycemia.

PATHOPHYSIOLOGY. Glucose is reabsorbed across the luminal membrane of the proximal tubule by a stereospecific carrier that requires sodium. The amount of glucose reabsorbed changes in proportion to filtered glucose load until a maximal reabsorptive capacity, or "Tm," is reached, as shown in Figure 82–1. Some-

what before saturation is attained, glucose reabsorption is incomplete, representing the "splay" in the response. The initial point of the splay represents that filtered glucose concentration or load, called the "threshold," at which reabsorption no longer equals filtration and glucose appears in the urine. The normal threshold concentration is 200 to 240 mg per deciliter, well above the normal plasma glucose concentration, so little glucose (< 125 mg per day) appears in the urine of a normal individual. The kinetics of glucose reabsorption have been compared with the behavior of an enzyme system: The Tm is equivalent to the Vmax, whereas the Km is related to the degree of splay. In the two major types of renal glycosurias, either the capacity (type A, Vmax or Tm mutation) or the affinity (type B, Km, or degree of splay mutation) of glucose reabsorption is altered (Fig. 82–1). In either case, the threshold is reduced, so that glucose is spilled into the urine at a normal plasma glucose concentration. The glycosuria is markedly exaggerated when filtered glucose concentration is elevated by intravenous hypertonic glucose infusion.

SYMPTOMS AND ETIOLOGIES. Renal glycosurias (Table 82–1) are relatively unusual, with a prevalence (depending on the stringency of diagnostic criteria) of about 0.2 to 0.6 per cent. They are usually inherited in an autosomal recessive manner. Homozygotes have more severe glycosuria than heterozygotes. Usually, but not invariably, Vmax and Km variants of the syndrome are inherited separately. On renal biopsy, there are no consistent distinguishing pathologic features. In contrast to the aminoacidurias, there is no coexisting intestinal transport defect for glucose. Renal glycosuria is completely asymptomatic (i.e., affected individuals do not have polydipsia or polyuria).

Intermittent glycosuria is not unusual during pregnancy (second and third trimesters) and during the terminal phases of chronic renal insufficiency. In both cases, an increase in tubular flow rate, due to an increase in total or in single-nephron glomerular filtration rate (GFR), is probably the primary cause of the functional alteration in glucose transport kinetics. In a rare syndrome in children, malabsorption of two sugars, glucose and galactose, in both the jejunum and the kidney, causes diarrhea and mellituria.

DIAGNOSIS AND TREATMENT. Diagnosis should be based on finding a urinary glucose excretion of greater than 500 mg per 24 hours (on a diet containing 30 kcal per kilogram, of which 50 per cent is carbohydrate) in the absence of hyperglycemia (plasma glucose < 140 mg per deciliter). The glucose oxidase method should be used to confirm that the excreted sugar is glucose in order to exclude other mellituric conditions (pentosuria, fructosuria, sucrosuria, maltosuria, galactosuria, and lactosuria). Appropriate tests should be performed to rule out coexistent tubular transport defects (of amino acids, bicarbonate, phosphate, and uric acid) typical of the Fanconi syndrome, and diabetes mellitus must be excluded, using standard clinical and laboratory evidence. If desired, differentiation of the Vmax or Km variants can be accomplished by glucose loading.

The condition is completely benign with respect to symptoms and to renal functional deterioration. Treatment is unnecessary. Prolonged fasting should be avoided to prevent the unusual complication of hypoglycemia and ketosis.

Renal Aminoacidurias

The renal aminoacidurias are inherited disorders in which one or a group of amino acids are excreted by the kidney (in the absence of hyperaminoacidemia) and are usually also malabsorbed by the intestine (Table 82–1).

GENERAL CONSIDERATIONS. Amino acids are avidly reabsorbed in the proximal nephron, so that only about 2 per cent of the filtered amino acid load is excreted in the urine (except for glycine, 5 per cent, and histidine, 8 per cent). In general, most amino acids are transported by a stereospecific carrier across the luminal membrane of the proximal nephron, accompanied by sodium and driven by the lumen-to-cell sodium concentration gradient. Under some circumstances, amino acids can also be secreted. Reabsorptive kinetics are similar to those of glucose (Fig. 82–1). Five major luminal membrane carriers for reabsorption exist, each of which transports a specific group of amino acids: basic amino acids (cystine, lysine, arginine, and ornithine); acidic amino acids (glutamic and aspartic acids); neutral amino acids (alanine, serine, threonine, valine, leucine, isoleucine, phenylalanine, tyrosine, tryptophan, and histidine); imino-glycine amino acids (proline, hydroxyproline, and glycine); and

TABLE 82–1. CLINICAL SYNDROMES ASSOCIATED WITH NEPHRON TRANSPORT DEFECTS

Proximal Nephron

I. *Selective transport defects*
  A. Renal glycosurias
    1. Primary
    2. Combined:
      a. Glucose/galactose malabsorption
      b. Glucoglycinuria
  B. Renal aminoacidurias
    1. Basic aminoacidurias
      a. General: cystinuria (cystine, lysine, arginine, ornithine)
      b. Specific: hypercystinuria, dibasic aminoaciduria (lysine, arginine, ornithine), lysinuria
    2. Neutral aminoacidurias
      a. General: Hartnup disease
      b. Specific: methioninuria, tryptophanuria, histidinuria
    3. Iminoglycinuria
      a. General (proline, hydroxyproline, glycine)
      b. Specific: glycinuria
    4. Dicarboxylic aminoaciduria
      a. General (glutamic, aspartic acids)
  C. Proximal renal tubular acidosis
    1. Primary: idiopathic or genetic
    2. Transient (infants)
    3. Carbonic anhydrase deficiency, inhibition, alteration
      a. Drugs: acetazolamide, sulfanilamide, mafenide acetate
      b. Idiopathic?
  D. Renal uric acid disorders (see Ch. 183, 184)
  E. Phosphate and calcium disorders (see Ch. 234, 235)
II. *Nonselective transport defects: Fanconi's syndrome*
  A. Primary: idiopathic or genetic
  B. Genetically transmitted systemic diseases
    1. Cystinosis
    2. Lowe's syndrome
    3. Wilson's disease
    4. Tyrosinemia
    5. Hereditary fructose intolerance
    6. Pyruvate carboxylase deficiency
  C. Dysproteinemic states
    1. Multiple myeloma
    2. Monoclonal gammopathy
  D. Secondary hyperparathyroidism with chronic hypocalcemia
    1. Vitamin D deficiency or resistance
    2. Vitamin D dependency
  E. Drugs and toxins
    1. Outdated tetracycline
    2. Methyl-3-chromone
    3. Streptozotocin
    4. Glue
    5. Gentamicin
  F. Heavy metals
    1. Lead
    2. Cadmium
    3. Mercury
  G. Tubulointerstitial diseases
    1. Sjögren's syndrome
    2. Medullary cystic disease
    3. Renal transplantation
  H. Other diseases
    1. Nephrotic syndrome
    2. Amyloidosis
    3. Osteopetrosis
    4. Paroxysmal nocturnal hemoglobinuria

Loop of Henle

I. *Bartter's syndrome*
II. *Drugs*
  A. Furosemide
  B. Bumetanide
  C. Ethacrynic acid

Distal Nephron

I. *Selective transport defects*
  A. Classic distal RTA
    1. Primary: genetic or idiopathic
    2. Genetically transmitted systemic diseases
      a. Ehlers-Danlos syndrome
      b. Hematologic disorders: hereditary elliptocytosis, sickle cell anemia, carbonic anhydrase I deficiency or alteration
      c. Medullary cystic disease
      d. With nerve deafness
      e. Glycogenosis type III
    3. Autoimmune diseases
      a. Hypergammaglobulinemia: hyperglobulinemic purpura, cryoglobulinemia, familial
      b. Sjögren's syndrome
      c. Thyroiditis
      d. Pulmonary fibrosis
      e. Chronic active hepatitis
      f. Primary biliary cirrhosis
      g. Systemic lupus erythematosus
    4. Diseases associated with nephrocalcinosis
      a. Primary hyperparathyroidism
      b. Vitamin D intoxication
      c. Hyperthyroidism
      d. Hypercalciuria: idiopathic or genetic
      e. Hereditary fructose intolerance
      f. Medullary sponge kidney
      g. Fabry's disease
      h. Wilson's disease
    5. Drug or toxic nephropathies
      a. Amphotericin B
      b. Toluene
      c. Glue
      d. Analgesics
      e. Cyclamate
    6. Tubulointerstitial diseases
      a. Chronic pyelonephritis secondary to urolithiasis
      b. Obstructive uropathy
      c. Renal transplantation
      d. Leprosy
      e. Hyperoxaluria
    7. Miscellaneous
  B. RTA of glomerular insufficiency
  C. Hypermineralocorticoid and other potassium secretory disorders (see Ch. 217)
II. *Nonselective transport defects: generalized distal RTA, hyperkalemia, and renal salt wasting*
  A. Primary mineralocorticoid deficiency (see Ch. 217)
  B. Hypoangiotensinemia
    1. Converting enzyme inhibitors: captopril, enalapril
    2. Angiotensin receptor blockers
  C. Hyporeninemic hypoaldosteronism
    1. Diabetic nephropathy
    2. Tubulointerstitial nephropathies
    3. Nephrosclerosis
    4. Nonsteroidal anti-inflammatory agents
    5. Acquired immunodeficiency syndrome (AIDS)
  D. Mineralocorticoid-resistant hyperkalemia
    1. Without salt wasting: genetic
    2. With salt wasting
      a. Childhood forms
      b. Tubulointerstitial nephropathies: methicillin, obstructive nephropathy, transplantation, sickle cell disease, cyclosporine
      c. Drugs: spironolactone, amiloride, triamterene

Loop and Medullary Collecting Ducts

I. *Diabetes insipidus* (see Ch. 214)
II. *SIADH* (see Ch. 214)
III. *Other concentrating and diluting disorders*

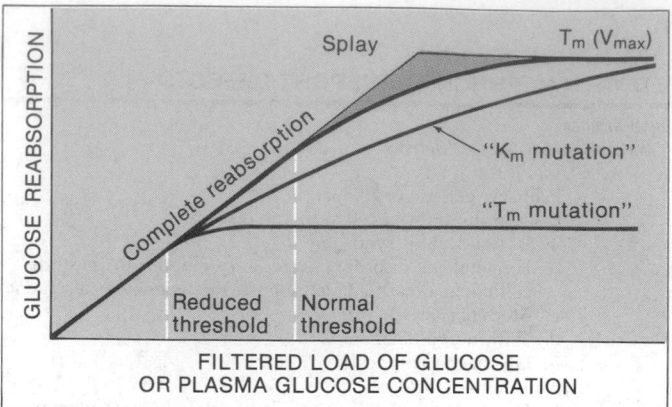

FIGURE 82–1. Kinetics of renal glucose reabsorption and the two variants of renal glycosuria. (Modified from Cogan MG: Disorders of proximal nephron function. Am J Med 72:278, 1982; with permission.)

beta-amino acids (beta-aminoisobutyric acid, beta-alanine, and taurine). Inherited dysfunction of a carrier results in urinary loss of the entire amino acid group: cystinuria (basic aminoaciduria); dicarboxylic aminoaciduria; Hartnup disease (neutral aminoaciduria); and iminoglycinuria. There is no clinical disorder yet described of beta-amino acid transport. There are also other carriers (>25 are estimated to exist) that selectively transport only one or several members of a given amino acid group. Disorders of these carriers cause even more selective aminoaciduria: hypercystinuria, histidinuria, and lysinuria.

Many of the amino acid carriers in the proximal nephron are also expressed on the luminal membrane of gastrointestinal epithelial cells. Defective gastrointestinal absorption therefore occurs conjointly with increased renal excretion of the amino acid or acids in question. Amino acid dimers can be normally absorbed by the gut, however, so that nutritional problems arising from amino acid malabsorption are unusual. Furthermore, gut absorption is not so constrained by time as that in the renal tubule, i.e., does not require such rapid response.

For diagnosis of a renal aminoaciduria, a high plasma level of the amino acid must first be excluded. Excessive filtration of an amino acid can overwhelm the tubular transport carrier for it and other members of its amino acid family and result in one or more aminoacidurias. These "overflow" aminoacidurias are discussed in Ch. 176 to 181. By contrast, the renal aminoacidurias are associated with low or normal levels of plasma amino acid concentrations because the aminoaciduria is due to defective proximal tubular transport.

CYSTINURIA. One of the most common aminoacidurias is *cystinuria* (basic aminoaciduria), an autosomal recessive disease estimated to affect about 1:7000 individuals (between 1:1000 and 1:20,000, depending on the population studied). Urinary spillage of lysine, arginine, and ornithine is asymptomatic. Cystine, however, is the least soluble of naturally occurring amino acids, and it therefore tends to precipitate to form cystine urolithiasis. Cystinuria accounts for about 1 to 2 per cent of all urinary calculi. Stone formation usually becomes manifest during the second and third decades of life, though presentation may occur from infancy to the ninth decade, and males are more severely affected. Cystine stones are yellow-brown and have a granular appearance. Such stones are radiopaque, can create staghorn calculi, and frequently form a nidus for calcium oxalate stone formation. Symptoms include renal colic, which may be associated with obstruction or infection or both. Evidence associating cystinuria with central nervous system disorders has been tenuous. A more general discussion of nephrolithiasis is found in Ch. 88.

The diagnosis of cystinuria should be considered in any patient with a renal calculus, even if the stone is composed primarily of calcium oxalate (since cystine might have been the formation nidus). The typical hexagonal crystals may be recognized on urinalysis, especially in a concentrated, acidic, early morning specimen. A useful screening test is the cyanide-nitroprusside test, which detects a cystine concentration of about 75 to 125 mg

per liter. Because of false-positive results, a definitive diagnosis requires thin-layer or ion-exchange chromatography or high-voltage electrophoresis. Excretion ratios in an adult of greater than 18 mg of cystine per gram of creatinine confirm the diagnosis. The dibasic amino acids will also be increased in excretion per gram of creatinine: lysine >130 mg; arginine >16 mg; and ornithine >22 mg. Persons with homozygous cystinuria routinely excrete more than 250 mg of cystine per gram of creatinine, usually about 0.5 to 1.0 gram per day. Cystinuria has three allelic variants, classified according to whether coexisting intestinal and renal basic amino acid transport is completely absent (types I and II) or variably reduced (type III) and whether heterozygotes have normal (type I) or supernormal (types II and III) urinary cystine and basic aminoaciduria.

Medical therapy of cystinuria is aimed at decreasing the urinary concentration below the solubility limit of 300 mg of cystine per liter. The most practical approach is to increase fluid intake to about 3 to 4 liters per day. The polyuria must be maintained at all times, including nighttime, when the urine otherwise tends to become concentrated and acidic. Cystine solubility can also be increased by alkalinizing urinary pH, but a urinary pH of greater than 7.5 is necessary to achieve a salutary effect. Avoidance of excessive intake of methionine, the metabolic precursor of cystine, is a reasonable adjunctive therapy but is ineffective as a sole therapy. When conservative measures fail, D-penicillamine is recommended, usually in a dose of 1 to 2 grams per day. This drug forms a mixed disulfide of penicillamine-cysteine, which is much more soluble than cystine alone. Free cystine excretion then falls to an acceptable level. Unfortunately, penicillamine causes fever and a rash in as many as 50 per cent of patients, and sometimes arthralgias and severe hypersensitivity reactions. In some cases the drug can be readministered at a lower dose following an adverse reaction. Pyridoxine should be given as a supplement, since penicillamine can deplete this cofactor. Other investigational agents, such as N-acetyl-D-penicillamine, mercaptopropionylglycine, glutamine, and chlordiazepoxide, have also been found to reduce cystine excretion.

HARTNUP DISEASE. Hartnup disease, a neutral aminoaciduria, is a rare autosomal recessive disorder (1:16,000 births) in which the clinical presentation is dominated by nicotinamide deficiency. Since up to 50 per cent of nicotinamide is normally supplied by metabolism of tryptophan, malabsorption and renal loss of tryptophan contribute to nicotinamide deficiency, especially when dietary nicotinamide is insufficient. Thus, this disorder exemplifies the importance of both the intestinal and the renal transport defects. Clinical signs of nicotinamide deficiency are intermittent and usually worse in children and include pellagra in sun-exposed areas, cerebellar ataxia, and sometimes psychiatric disturbance.

Hartnup disease should be suspected in a patient with pellagra or cerebellar symptoms who does not have a history of niacin deficiency. The diagnosis can be confirmed by chromatography of the urine. Sibs of an affected individual should be examined for heterozygosity. Supplemental nicotinamide (40 to 250 mg per day) suffices to prevent pellagra and neurologic problems.

OTHER AMINOACIDURIAS. Less common aminoacidurias lacking clinical manifestations include iminoglycinuria, isolated hypercystinuria (without hyperexcretion of other basic amino acids), isolated glycinuria, and dicarboxylic aminoaciduria. Mental retardation predominates in the rare disorders of hyperdibasic aminoaciduria, isolated lysinuria, histidinuria, and methioninuria.

Proximal Renal Tubular Acidosis (RTA)

Proximal RTA is a hyperchloremic, hypokalemic metabolic acidosis caused by a selective defect in proximal acidification, which is characterized by a normally acidic urine during acidosis but marked bicarbonate wasting when plasma bicarbonate concentration is normalized.

PATHOPHYSIOLOGY. The proximal nephron reabsorbs 85 to 90 per cent of the filtered bicarbonate, predominantly by Na^+/H^+ exchange and the enzymatic degradation of H_2CO_3 to CO_2 and H_2O by carbonic anhydrase (Fig. 82–2). Interference with the normal operation of Na^+/H^+ exchange or of carbonic anhydrase activity therefore results in excess delivery of bicarbonate to the distal nephron and, because of the limited distal bicarbonate reabsorption capacity, into the urine. Thus, the

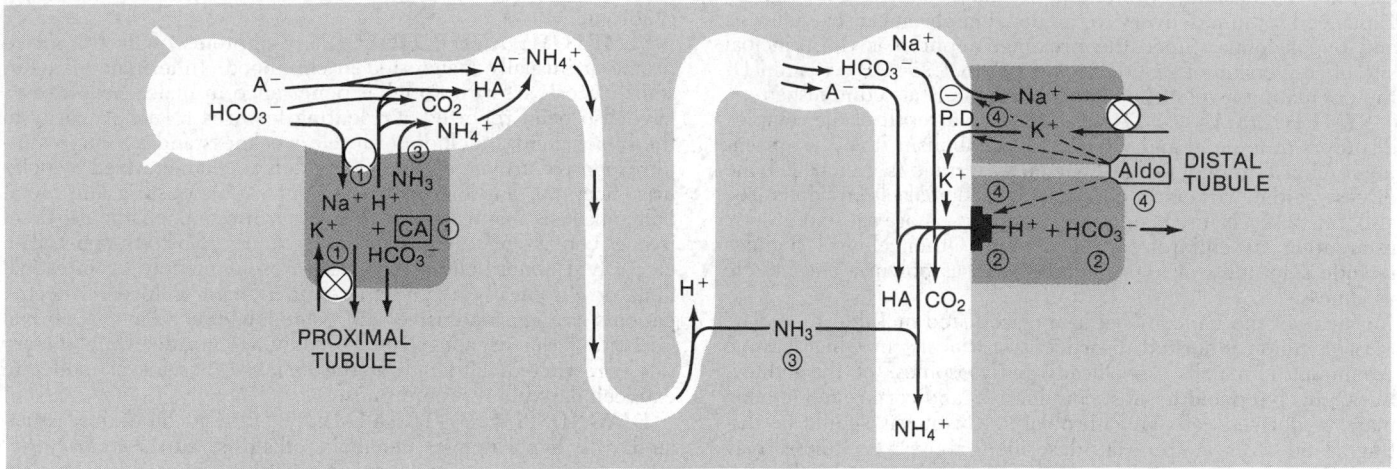

FIGURE 82–2. Sites of impaired renal acidification (RTA). The proximal tubule reabsorbs most of the filtered bicarbonate by hydrogen ion secretion. Proximal acidification is dependent on sodium and carbonic anhydrase and is energetically driven by the lumen-to-cell sodium gradient. Disorders of proximal acidification, proximal RTA, may result from defects (labeled 1) in the Na^+/H^+ exchanger, carbonic anhydrase activity, or the activity of the basolateral Na^+-K^+ ATPase. The distal nephron is regulated by aldosterone to reabsorb sodium and secrete hydrogen ions. Distal acidification is responsible for titrating both remaining filtered buffer (labeled A^-) to form titratable acids (HA) and proximally produced ammonia (NH_3) to form ammonium (NH_4^+). Disorders of distal acidification include defects of the proton pump or basolateral bicarbonate exit step (labeled 2) in classic distal RTA, in ammonia production or delivery (labeled 3) in the RTA of glomerular insufficiency, or in aldosterone levels or target sites (labeled 4) in generalized distal RTA.

urinary wastage of 15 per cent or more of the filtered bicarbonate load at a normal blood bicarbonate concentration is pathognomonic of proximal renal tubular acidosis (RTA). The excess delivery of the relatively impermeant bicarbonate to the distal nephron also results in accelerated potassium secretion and hypokalemia. As the plasma bicarbonate concentration and filtered load fall owing to defective proximal bicarbonate reabsorption and subsequent urinary bicarbonate wastage, absolute bicarbonate delivery to the distal nephron progressively decreases. At a certain point, usually when the plasma bicarbonate concentration is 15 to 18 mM, the distal nephron can cope with the delivery from the proximal tubule. At this stage, bicarbonaturia disappears, urinary pH can be lowered normally, and net acid excretion is equivalent to endogenous acid production. Acid-base homeostasis is re-established at the expense of metabolic acidosis.

SYMPTOMS AND ETIOLOGIES. Manifestations of proximal RTA are attributable to acidemia (growth retardation, anorexia and malnutrition, volume depletion), potassium depletion (muscular weakness, polyuria, nocturia, polydipsia), and disordered calcium/phosphate/parathormone/vitamin D metabolism (osteomalacia and other bone diseases). Proximal RTA is a rare disorder, usually found when carbonic anhydrase is defective or is inhibited, or in conjunction with the full Fanconi syndrome (Table 82–1).

DIAGNOSIS AND TREATMENT. Laboratory findings of proximal RTA are those of a hyperchloremic, hypokalemic metabolic acidosis. When the patient is acidemic, the urine is acidic and net acid excretion equals endogenous acid load (Table 82–2). When bicarbonate is infused to normalize the plasma bicarbonate concentration, massive bicarbonaturia results (≥15 per cent of the filtered load). Proximal RTA is usually not isolated but rather associated with the full Fanconi syndrome.

Therapy of the underlying disease should be undertaken if possible (e.g., multiple myeloma) or offending drugs or toxins discontinued (e.g., heavy metals). When this is not possible, proximal RTA is treated with large amounts of sodium and potassium bicarbonate. As the plasma bicarbonate concentration rises with treatment, distal bicarbonate delivery increases, causing more potassium wasting and the need for further potassium supplementation. Because of the inability to correct the disorder fully with bicarbonate alone, volume contraction utilizing diuretics, especially thiazides, is also used to stimulate fractional proximal bicarbonate reabsorption. Therapy with vitamin D is indicated when signs of vitamin D deficiency exist.

Nonselective Proximal Nephron Dysfunction: The Fanconi Syndrome

In the Fanconi syndrome, the entire array of proximal transport functions is impaired, resulting in glycosuria, generalized aminoaciduria, proximal RTA, phosphaturia, and uricaciduria.

PATHOPHYSIOLOGY. The lumen-to-cell sodium gradient provides the driving force in the proximal tubule for the absorption of glucose, amino acids, phosphate, and organic acids and for secretion of hydrogen ions needed to reabsorb bicarbonate. Disruption of this common driving force serves as an attractive hypothesis to explain the global functional impairment of reabsorption of solutes in the proximal tubule observed in the Fanconi syndrome. Collapse of the sodium gradient could arise by several mechanisms: a primary disturbance of the Na^+-K^+ adenosinetriphosphatase (ATPase), increased permeability of the cell to sodium, or reduced metabolic energy due to an abnormality in the redox potential or in intracellular phosphate supply.

In addition to the solutes described above, there is disordered reabsorption, and sometimes depressed serum concentrations, of

TABLE 82–2. RENAL TUBULAR ACIDOSES

Type	Renal Defect	GFR	Plasma [K⁺]	Proximal Acidification: HCO_3^- Reabsorption (During HCO_3^- Loading)	Distal Acidification: Minimal Urinary pH (During Acidosis)	UAG ≈ − Urine [NH_4^+] (During Acidosis)
Proximal	↓ Proximal acidification	N	↓	↓	< 5.5	0 or +
Classic distal	↓ Distal pH gradient	N	↓	N	> 5.5	0 or +
Glomerular insufficiency	↓ NH_3 production	↓	N	N	< 5.5	0 or +
Generalized distal	↓ Aldosterone action	↓	↑	N	< 5.5	0 or +

N = normal; UAG = urinary anion gap = [Na] + [K] − [Cl] ≈ − [NH_4]; GFR = glomerular filtration rate.

calcium, magnesium, citrate, and low molecular weight proteins. Enhanced sodium delivery to the distal nephron causes kaliuresis and hypokalemia. Since the proximal nephron is the principal site of conversion of 25-OH vitamin D to 1,25-$(OH)_2$ vitamin D, the circulating level of this latter hormone is also diminished.

SYMPTOMS AND ETIOLOGIES. As a result of the complex disorders of mineral and vitamin D metabolism, the most prominent clinical finding of the Fanconi syndrome is metabolic bone disease, either rickets in children or osteomalacia in adults (see also Ch. 234). Nausea, episodic vomiting, anorexia, and growth retardation in children are frequent. Other clinical findings include symptoms of hypokalemia, such as polyuria and muscle weakness.

Causes of the Fanconi syndrome are listed in Table 82–1. The most common inherited disorder is *cystinosis*, in which cystine accumulates in cells, specifically in lysosomes, of the kidney, liver, gut, lymphoid tissues, conjunctiva, and cornea and in bone marrow–derived cells and fibroblasts. Cystinosis should be distinguished from cystinuria, described above. Cystinosis may present as the Fanconi syndrome, followed by renal failure, in the first 2 years of life (infantile nephropathic form) or in the adolescent years. It is usually relatively benign if it first appears in adulthood, causing only asymptomatic cystine deposits in the conjunctiva, cornea, and bone marrow. An interesting inducible form of the Fanconi syndrome is *hereditary fructose intolerance* (HFI), caused by a deficiency of aldolase B activity. Ingestion of fructose in affected individuals causes acute symptoms, including nausea, vomiting, abdominal pain, and neurologic dysfunction (Ch. 170).

In adults, acquired Fanconi's syndrome is most often caused by dysproteinemias, heavy metal (especially chronic cadmium or acute lead) exposure, or immunologic diseases (Table 82–1). An older adult presenting with the Fanconi syndrome should be assumed to have multiple myeloma until proved otherwise.

DIAGNOSIS AND TREATMENT. Diagnosis of the Fanconi syndrome is established by finding consequences of the full array of proximal nephron dysfunction: glycosuria, generalized aminoaciduria, proximal RTA, phosphaturia, hypouricemia, hypovitaminosis D, and secondary hypokalemia. Underlying causes of the Fanconi syndrome (Table 82–1) should be sought. Serum and urine electrophoresis should be obtained in adults to rule out multiple myeloma.

Treatment of the Fanconi syndrome requires supplements of bicarbonate (up to 15 to 20 mEq per kilogram of body weight per day), potassium, phosphate, magnesium, and vitamin D. Treatment of the underlying disease, of course, varies widely. Effective results have been reported in the treatment of cystinosis with cysteamine, of Wilson's disease with penicillamine, of hereditary fructose intolerance with fructose restriction, and of heavy metal intoxication with removal from metal exposure or chelation (for lead).

DISORDERS OF FUNCTION OF THE ASCENDING LIMB OF THE LOOP OF HENLE

The thick ascending limb of the loop of Henle reabsorbs sodium chloride by means of a luminal Na-K-2Cl system. A lumen-positive potential difference and parallel transport systems effect potassium, calcium, and magnesium reabsorption. Defective reabsorption by the thick ascending limb of Henle occurs during diuretic treatment or in Bartter's syndrome.

Bartter's Syndrome

Bartter's syndrome consists of a constellation of findings, including hypokalemia and metabolic alkalosis with hyperreninemic hyperaldosteronism. Hypertension and edema are absent.

PATHOPHYSIOLOGY. Evidence that dysfunction of the thick ascending limb of Henle is the proximate cause of Bartter's syndrome comes primarily from free-water clearance studies. Mild extracellular volume depletion causes hyperreninemic hyperaldosteronism and the juxtaglomerular hyperplasia found on renal biopsy. Enhanced sodium chloride delivery to the collecting duct stimulates potassium secretion (exacerbated by concurrent hyperaldosteronism) leading to hypokalemia, as well as hydrogen ion secretion resulting in metabolic alkalosis. Accelerated kinin

and prostaglandin (especially PGE_2 and prostacyclin) production occurs and may account for the vascular unresponsiveness to pressors and various other phenomena known to occur in Bartter's syndrome.

SYMPTOMS AND ETIOLOGY. Symptoms of Bartter's syndrome are usually manifested in childhood. Inheritance is autosomal recessive, with a higher penetrance in males. Adult cases have also been reported. Presenting features relate primarily to the hypokalemia, including muscle weakness and a vasopressin-unresponsive urinary concentrating defect, characterized by polyuria, nocturia, and enuresis. Divalent cation wasting and metabolic alkalosis may conspire to cause symptoms characteristic of hypocalcemia, including Trousseau's and Chvostek's signs. The electrolyte abnormalities can also present acutely as intestinal ileus or chronically as growth retardation in children. Affected patients are normotensive and nonedematous, have a normal GFR, and can usually conserve sodium chloride when dietary salt is restricted, although at the expense of signs of moderate extracellular volume compromise.

DIAGNOSIS AND TREATMENT. Other conditions associated with hypokalemia, metabolic alkalosis, and secondary hyperreninemic hyperaldosteronism must be excluded before making a diagnosis of Bartter's syndrome. Surreptitious vomiting, chronic diarrheal states, or surreptitious diuretic or laxative administration can cause symptoms indistinguishable from those of Bartter's syndrome. These disorders are associated with extracellular volume depletion, and therefore the urinary chloride level is less than 20 mEq per liter, unless diuretics are being actively consumed. Thus, the diagnosis of Bartter's syndrome must be preceded by confirmation that urinary chloride concentration is more than 20 mEq per liter and by negative screening test results for diuretics in the urine and for laxatives in the stool (phenolphthalein test). States of primary hyperreninism or hypermineralocorticoidism can be readily excluded, since they are usually associated with hypertension.

Therapy of Bartter's syndrome is primarily aimed at ameliorating the kypokalemia by disrupting the renin-angiotensin-aldosterone and kinin-prostaglandin axes. Potassium supplementation, magnesium repletion, propranolol, spironolactone, prostaglandin inhibition, and captopril have all been used, but each has usually been met with incomplete success.

DISORDERS OF DISTAL NEPHRON FUNCTION

The distal nephron, including the distal convoluted tubule and the collecting ducts, is responsible for reabsorbing the final quantity of sodium in the tubular fluid and for secreting potassium and hydrogen ions. Inherited and acquired defects exist for selective or combined disorders of sodium, potassium, and acid-base regulation.

Classic Distal Renal Tubular Acidosis (RTA)

Classic distal RTA is a hypokalemic, hyperchloremic metabolic acidosis owing to a selective defect in distal acidification. It is characterized by an inability to lower the urinary pH normally and therefore by subnormal urinary net acid excretion.

PATHOPHYSIOLOGY. The distal nephron (especially the cortical and medullary collecting ducts) is normally capable of lowering the urinary pH fully 2 to 3 pH units below that of blood to titrate filtered buffers (principally phosphate) to form titratable acids and endogenously produced ammonia to form ammonium (Fig. 82–2). If the distal nephron is incapable of lowering the luminal pH below 5.5 when challenged by metabolic acidosis, a classic distal RTA is present. Because of the inappropriately high urinary pH, net acid excretion (titratable acid plus ammonium minus bicarbonate) is subnormal, less than acid production by the body. Accelerated potassium secretion occurs, presumably because there is reduced competition by proton secretion for the electrochemical driving forces in the distal nephron. The acidification defect may result from an insufficient number of proton-secreting pumps in the distal nephron. Alternatively, there may be backleak of acid across the luminal membrane, so that establishment of a pH gradient is prevented even when proton secretion is normal.

SYMPTOMS AND ETIOLOGIES. Distal RTA is found in infants, children, and adults. Symptoms may be those of acidosis or hypokalemia, as described above. Nephrocalcinosis and nephrolithiasis are common, either as a cause or as a result of classic distal RTA. However, bone disease is not as frequent as in proximal RTA. Classic distal RTA may also be genetic (most frequently autosomal dominant) or due to autoimmune diseases, drugs and toxins, and various tubulointerstitial diseases (Table 82–1).

DIAGNOSIS AND TREATMENT. The findings of hyperchloremic, hypokalemic metabolic acidosis with an inappropriately high urinary pH (>5.5) and diminished net acid excretion confirm the diagnosis (Table 82–2). Laboratory features of classic distal RTA sometimes resemble those of diarrhea, since both are associated with hyperchloremic, hypokalemic metabolic acidosis with a urinary pH greater than 5.5. If differentiation cannot be made on clinical grounds, it can be facilitated by measuring the urinary anion gap, defined as urinary $[Na] + [K] - [Cl]$, which is proportionate to the negative value of urinary $[NH_4]$. Diarrhea has a large, negative urinary anion gap, and thus a high urinary ammonium concentration (accounting for the high urinary pH), while classic distal RTA has a zero or positive urinary anion gap and a low urinary ammonium concentration (because of impaired acidification). In individuals with a normal plasma bicarbonate concentration, the failure to lower urinary pH below 5.5 following an acute acid challenge with NH_4Cl defines the syndrome of incomplete classic distal RTA (see Ch. 75 for details of the NH_4Cl test). Treatment with alkali is generally very effective. The daily dose of alkali in adults is 1 to 3 mEq per kilogram, to compensate for the normal acid production by the body plus a small amount of urinary bicarbonate wastage. In contrast to proximal RTA, urinary potassium wasting is ameliorated with alkali therapy. Children require more alkali than adults, about 5 to 14 mEq per kilogram per day. Prognosis with respect to stabilization of GFR in adults or growth in children is excellent with provision of adequate alkali therapy.

RTA of Glomerular Insufficiency

This disorder is a normokalemic, hyperchloremic metabolic acidosis associated with moderate renal insufficiency (GFR of 20 to 30 ml per minute). It results from deficient ammonia delivery and is characterized by an appropriately low urinary pH but subnormal urinary net acid (ammonium) excretion.

PATHOPHYSIOLOGY. When the GFR falls to about 20 to 30 ml per minute owing to any intrinsic glomerular or tubulointerstitial disease, a normokalemic metabolic acidosis is frequently found. The cause of this acidosis is thought to be either deficient ammonia production or impairment in the urinary trapping of ammonia as ammonium (Fig. 82–2). In either case, proximal bicarbonate reclamation and the ability to lower the urinary pH to less than 5.5 are intact, but the failure to generate sufficient acid excretion to equal intake results in systemic acidosis.

SYMPTOMS AND ETIOLOGY. The degree of metabolic acidosis is generally mild, and plasma bicarbonate concentration is usually greater than 15 mEq per liter. Acidemia exacerbates the osteodystrophy of progressive renal disease. Although tubulointerstitial diseases are thought to produce this form of RTA more commonly than glomerular diseases, this distinction has been difficult to verify. This hyperchloremic metabolic acidosis should be distinguished from the high anion gap (normochloremic) uremic metabolic acidosis secondary to retained organic acids that usually occurs when glomerular insufficiency is more severe (GFR <20 ml per minute). The two acidoses may coexist.

DIAGNOSIS AND TREATMENT. A hyperchloremic, normokalemic metabolic acidosis that occurs when the GFR falls to about 20 to 30 ml per minute is typical of the RTA of glomerular insufficiency. Although net acid, specifically ammonium, excretion is subnormal (reflected by a zero or positive urinary anion gap) the urinary pH is appropriately acidic (Table 82–2). Mineralocorticoid levels are not diminished. Treatment consists of 1 to 3 mEq per kilogram per day of alkali therapy to compensate for daily acid ingestion and production.

Nonselective Distal Nephron Dysfunction: Generalized Distal RTA, Hyperkalemia, and Renal Salt Wasting

These disorders arise from global dysfunction of the distal nephron due to aldosterone deficiency or antagonism and are characterized by hyperkalemic, hyperchloremic metabolic acidosis caused by subnormal net acid excretion and frequently by renal salt wasting.

PATHOPHYSIOLOGY. When sodium is reabsorbed in the distal nephron under the influence of aldosterone, luminal sodium concentration can be reduced to very low levels, less than 10 mEq per liter (sometimes ≤1 mEq per liter). Sodium reabsorption creates a lumen-negative potential difference, favoring secretion of potassium and hydrogen ions (Fig. 82–2). Disruption of sodium reabsorption and of potassium and hydrogen secretion may therefore be ascribable to a defect in the integrity of the distal nephron cell, deficient aldosterone production or action, diminished sodium reabsorption, or blunting of the lumen-negative potential by enhanced chloride reabsorption. Any of these processes lead to diminished total hydrogen ion and potassium excretion and therefore metabolic acidosis with hyperkalemia. The hyperkalemia also serves to depress renal ammoniagenesis independently, which exacerbates the defect in renal acidification. The ability to lower the urinary pH normally (a qualitative distal nephron function at low buffer strength) remains intact (Table 82–2).

SYMPTOMS AND ETIOLOGIES. The symptoms of generalized distal RTA in children or adults usually relate to the acidosis itself or occasionally to the neuromuscular consequences of hyperkalemia. Renal salt wasting can cause extracellular volume depletion and hypotension when sodium chloride intake is reduced. The most common forms of generalized distal RTA result from a reduction in aldosterone level or prevention of its action (Table 82–1). The adrenal synthesis of aldosterone may be directly impaired, as in Addison's disease or in inherited enzymatic defects, such as 18- or 21-hydroxylase deficiencies. More commonly, primary hyporeninemia caused by diabetic nephropathy, hypertensive nephrosclerosis, or tubulointerstitial diseases can also reduce aldosterone levels. Finally, end-organ unresponsiveness to mineralocorticoid with high circulating levels of aldosterone occurs in various tubulointerstitial diseases, especially those that have a predilection for the medulla and papilla of the kidney (e.g., analgesic abuse, sickle cell disease, and obstructive nephropathies).

DIAGNOSIS AND TREATMENT: HYPERKALEMIC, GENERALIZED DISTAL RTA. Generalized distal RTA is unique among the hyperchloremic metabolic acidoses in being a hyperkalemic disorder (Table 82–2). Glomerular filtration rate is invariably reduced in the forms associated with hyporeninemia or tubulointerstitial nephropathy but may be at levels (≥30 ml per minute) above those typically found in the RTA of glomerular insufficiency.

Treatment of the hyperkalemia and generalized distal RTA is effected with 9-α-fludrocortisone, 0.1 mg per day, when mineralocorticoid is deficient. When hyporeninemia is the cause, high doses of the synthetic mineralocorticoid are required (up to 0.5 mg per day) because of associated mineralocorticoid resistance. Hypertension can be precipitated with this treatment. A loop diuretic (furosemide or ethacrynic acid) is also useful, especially when hypertension precludes administration of mineralocorticoid, because it enhances urinary potassium excretion even when endogenous aldosterone is low. Useful adjuncts to diuretic therapy include dietary potassium restriction (≤50 mEq per day), alkali therapy to compensate for daily acid generation (sodium bicarbonate, 1 to 3 mEq per kilogram per day), and sometimes short-term use of cation exchange resin.

DIAGNOSIS AND TREATMENT: RENAL SALT WASTING. Renal salt wasting becomes apparent when dietary sodium chloride intake becomes less than the minimal threshold for sodium chloride excretion. Renal salt wasting is diagnosed when, in response to acute reduction of sodium intake (10 mEq per day), urinary sodium excretion remains inappropriately elevated, typically greater than 50 mEq per day, and weight loss is significant (>3 kg). Progressively severe extracellular volume depletion occurs with development of hypotension and renal insufficiency. This diagnostic maneuver is not without hazard, since symptomatic hypovolemia or hyperkalemia can be precipitated and should be performed only under close supervision.

Therapy for renal salt wasting secondary to aldosterone deficiency or partial resistance requires physiologic or supraphysiologic mineralocorticoid replacement, as described above. In all other cases, sodium chloride supplementation is indicated to prevent volume depletion in the event sodium intake is curtailed. The dose of sodium chloride prescribed, in the diet and salt tablets, should exceed that amount of sodium chloride spilled into the urine by the patient when dietary salt was restricted.

General

Cogan MG: Disorders of proximal nephron function. Am J Med 72:275, 1982. *This paper presents an overview of the physiology, pathophysiologic mechanisms, and clinical disorders of proximal nephron function.*

Sebastian A, Hulter HN, Kurtz I, et al.: Disorders of distal nephron function. Am J Med 72:289, 1982. *This article is a thoughtful, pathophysiologically oriented overview of the various clinical dysfunctions of potassium and hydrogen ion secretion.*

Renal Glycosurias

Wen S-F: Glycosurias. *In* Gonick HC, Buckalew VM Jr (eds.): Renal Tubular Disorders. New York, Marcel Dekker, 1985, pp 159–199. *This chapter presents an excellent discussion of the physiology of glucose transport and the pathophysiology and clinical spectrum of the renal glycosurias.*

Renal Aminoacidurias

Foreman JW, Segal S: Aminoacidurias. *In* Gonick HC, Buckalew VM Jr (eds.): Renal Tubular Disorders. New York, Marcel Dekker, 1985, pp 131–157. *This chapter presents an excellent overview of the physiology of amino acid transport and the clinical spectra of the aminoacidurias.*

Segal S, Thier SO: Cystinurias. *In* Scriver CR, Beaudet AL, Sly WS, et al. (eds.): The Metabolic Basis of Inherited Disease. 6th ed. New York, McGraw-Hill Book Company, 1989, pp 2479–2496. *This is an authoritative review of the most common of the aminoacidurias.*

Fanconi's Syndrome

Brewer ED: The Fanconi syndrome: Clinical disorders. *In* Gonick HC, Buckalew VM Jr (eds.): Renal Tubular Disorders. New York, Marcel Dekker, 1985, pp 475–544. *This is a superb, exhaustive review of the pathophysiology, clinical presentations, and principles of treatment of the multiple causes of the Fanconi syndrome.*

Roth KS, Foreman JW, Segal S: The Fanconi syndrome and mechanisms of tubular transport dysfunction. Kidney Int 20:705, 1981. *An excellent review of the pathogenetic mechanisms of this syndrome.*

Bartter's Syndrome

Gill JR, Bartter FC: Evidence for a prostaglandin-independent defect in chloride reabsorption in the loop of Henle as a proximal cause of Bartter's syndrome. Am J Med 65:766, 1978. *This paper describes in vivo studies pinpointing the tubular site of the reabsorptive defect in Bartter's syndrome.*

Stein JH: The pathogenetic spectrum of Bartter's syndrome. Kidney Int 28:85, 1985. *This article reviews the variety of clinical presentations and current concepts of pathogenesis of this heterogeneous syndrome.*

Renal Tubular Acidosis

Batlle DC, Hizon M, Cohen E, et al.: The use of the urinary anion gap in the diagnosis of hyperchloremic metabolic acidosis. N Engl J Med 318:594, 1988. *The use of the urinary anion gap to distinguish hyperchloremic acidosis of diarrhea from classic distal RTA is clearly explained.*

Cogan MG, Arieff AI: Sodium wasting, acidosis and hyperkalemia induced by methicillin interstitial nephritis. Evidence for selective distal tubular dysfunction. Am J Med 64:500, 1978. *This article describes the standard evaluation and treatment of a patient with marked renal salt wasting.*

Cogan MG, Rector FC Jr: Acid-base disorders. *In* Brenner BM, Rector FC Jr (eds.): The Kidney. 4th ed. Philadelphia, W. B. Saunders Company, 1991. *This chapter is a comprehensive review of acid-base homeostasis, including the RTA's.*

Harrington JT, Cohen JJ: Metabolic acidosis. *In* Cohen JJ, Kassirer JP (eds.): Acid-Base. Boston, Little, Brown and Company, 1982, pp 121–126. *This chapter describes the pathophysiology and clinical manifestations of metabolic acidoses.*

Schambelan M, Sebastian A, Biglieri EG: Prevalence, pathogenesis and functional significance of aldosterone deficiency in hyperkalemic patients with chronic renal insufficiency. Kidney Int 17:89, 1980. *This paper provides one of the most comprehensive reviews of the heterogeneous causes of generalized distal (type IV) RTA.*

83 Diabetes and the Kidney

Bryan D. Myers

INCIDENCE AND PREVALENCE

Among the 15,000 patients entering chronic dialysis and kidney transplantation programs in the United States each year, the development of end-stage renal failure can be attributed to diabetes mellitus in approximately 25 per cent. Diabetic glomerulopathy, a complex disorder associated with a diffuse expansion of collagenous components of the glomerulus, is the predominant cause of the renal failure. The diabetic patient is also prone to other renal diseases, such as pyelonephritis, papillary necrosis, and obstructive nephropathy, that occasionally cause or exacerbate renal failure (Ch. 81 and 84). Diabetic patients with glomerulopathy are more susceptible to these associated renal disorders than are those who do not have glomerulopathy. Most victims of end-stage diabetic renal disease have longstanding type I diabetes, defined here as juvenile-onset and insulin-dependent diabetes (see Ch. 218). Patients with type II diabetes, characterized by a more advanced age of onset and not requiring insulin for control of hyperglycemia, are not spared from diabetic glomerulopathy but constitute a substantial minority among diabetic patients in end-stage renal failure programs.

CLINICAL AND LABORATORY FEATURES OF DIABETIC GLOMERULOPATHY

The natural history of diabetic glomerulopathy has been best documented in type I patients. Early abnormalities of glomerular function and structure appear to be invariable in all type I diabetics, but only 30 to 50 per cent will develop a progressive, proteinuric form of diabetic glomerulopathy. The evolution of the glomerulopathy in this subset of type I diabetics may be thought of as a continuum of glomerular injury divisible into three stages (Fig. 83–1). The first stage of occult glomerulopathy cannot be diagnosed by conventional laboratory techniques and lasts for approximately 10 years. It is followed by two clinically evident stages of increasingly severe glomerular injury. Both are identified by the presence of proteinuria, while the milder, intermediate second stage merges with the advanced third stage with the development of azotemia. The clinical and laboratory features of this prolonged and progressive glomerular disease are reviewed by each stage separately.

Stage 1—Occult Diabetic Glomerulopathy

During this stage, the type I diabetic patient is devoid of clinical symptoms and signs of glomerulopathy. The most striking laboratory finding is a 20 to 40 per cent *elevation of the glomerular filtration rate* (GFR) above that found in age-matched normal control subjects. Such hyperfiltration could be partly attributable to a generalized hypertrophy of glomeruli, with an ensuing increase in the glomerular capillary filtration surface area. However, striking elevations of GFR in poorly controlled diabetic patients can be lowered within a matter of hours following restoration of normoglycemia, though not fully corrected. A parallel *increase in renal plasma flow*, measured by the clearance of *p*-aminohippurate, and also reversible by lowering blood glucose levels, points to a contribution by hemodynamic factors to the hyperfiltration. Notwithstanding the responsiveness of vasomotor regulation in the kidney to alterations in the metabolic milieu, GFR tends to remain elevated even with good metabolic control of the diabetic state. Not until proteinuria ushers in the intermediate second stage of the glomerulopathy does the GFR fall into the normal range.

The stage 1 glomerular hyperfiltration is sometimes accompanied by transient increases in the urinary albumin excretion rate that are measurable only by sensitive, immunochemical techniques. Healthy adolescents and young adults excrete albumin in their urine at rates of up to 15 μg per minute. Some patients with type I diabetes of short duration excrete albumin at rates in excess of 15 μg per minute but less than 100 μg per minute, which is roughly the threshold detectable by conventional techniques. This *microalbuminuria* is inferred to represent an increase in the transglomerular filtration of albumin rather than a decrease in tubular reabsorption of a normal, filtered albumin load. Microalbuminuria tends to be associated with the most striking degrees of hyperfiltration observed among type I diabetics, suggesting that it may also have a hemodynamic basis. It is exaggerated by exercise, which causes an increase in the intraluminal hydraulic pressure of the glomerular capillaries, and is blunted, although not abolished, by restoration of normoglycemia.

Early in the course of type I diabetes, hypertrophy of nephrons results in a consistent increase in kidney size. Hyperfiltration, renal hyperemia and enlargement, and intermittent microalbuminuria are all characteristic of this early occult stage, but hypertension, an important complication of diabetic glomerulopathy, is not prevalent. The incidence of hypertension in large diabetic populations without proteinuria is no different from that in nondiabetic populations.

Stage 2—Intermediate Diabetic Glomerulopathy

Stage 2, intermediate diabetic glomerulopathy, is characterized by *increasing proteinuria, declining GFR,* and the development of *hypertension* and *edema.* This stage is heralded by the development of sustained microalbuminuria, which increases over 2 or more years into a range (>250 µg per minute) that is easily measurable by dipstick. Once overt proteinuria has become manifest, its magnitude tends to reflect the rate of deterioration of glomerular capillary wall function that typifies the second stage of diabetic glomerulopathy. As indicated in Figure 83–1, proteinuria tends to increase exponentially with time and to be related inversely to GFR.

The onset of proteinuria is also accompanied by an increasing prevalence of hypertension and by the development of edema. Edema becomes clearly evident long before urinary protein losses reach nephrotic proportions (>3.5 grams per 24 hours). It worsens and often becomes refractory to diuretic therapy once proteinuria is sufficient to cause hypoproteinemia, however.

The proteinuria of stage 2 diabetic glomerulopathy has no pathognomonic characteristics, but several features distinguish it from other glomerular diseases: (1) From the onset of the second stage, immunoglobulins and other large plasma proteins are excreted in the urine in large quantities along with albumin, signifying an early loss of barrier size-selectivity in this disorder. (2) Persistent and even heavy urinary losses of plasma proteins in stage 2 diabetic glomerulopathy are often not accompanied by hypoproteinemia. Inasmuch as the conventional definition of the nephrotic syndrome requires hypoproteinemia in addition to heavy proteinuria and edema, stage 2 diabetic glomerulopathy does not always exemplify the nephrotic syndrome. An important role in edema formation is ascribed to reduction of plasma oncotic pressure in patients with the nephrotic syndrome as classically defined; the absence of hypoproteinemia, and hence the maintenance of normal plasma oncotic pressure, in much of stage 2 diabetic glomerulopathy implicates alternate mechanisms of edema formation. (3) Neither edema formation nor, for that matter, hypertension can be related unambiguously to a stimulated renin-angiotensin-aldosterone system. Rather, diabetic glomerulopathy is usually associated with normal or low circulating levels of active renin. In contrast, the circulating level of prorenin is frequently enhanced. Since prorenin is an inactive prohormone, the biologic significance of this finding is uncertain. The plasma concentration and urinary excretion rate of aldosterone tend, like active renin, also to be normal or depressed, despite the presence of edema. In fact, proteinuric diabetic glomerulopathy probably constitutes the most common example of hyporeninemic hypoaldosteronism, and such patients not infrequently exhibit the syndrome of generalized distal type IV renal tubular acidosis (see Ch. 82). Thus, both the mechanism by which edema is formed and the basis for the widespread prevalence of hypertension in stage 2 diabetic glomerulopathy remain obscure.

Stage 3—Advanced Diabetic Glomerulopathy

The third, advanced stage represents the terminal 2 or 3 years of what is typically a 20- to 25-year process. Its onset is delineated by the development of *azotemia.* Retention of urea, creatinine, and other nitrogenous compounds generally becomes apparent once the GFR has declined to less than one third of normal levels. As with the intermediate stage that precedes it, GFR in the third and terminal stage of diabetic glomerulopathy has been observed to decline at rates that are rather predictable for a given patient. Whereas the actual rate of GFR decline varies widely among individuals, it averages 1 ml per minute per month when hypertension is poorly controlled and can be halved by efficacious lowering of blood pressure. The prototypical case in Figure 83–1 is illustrative of a patient with poorly controlled hypertension, in whom GFR is predicted to decline from a normal value approximating 120 ml per minute at the onset of stage 2 to zero at the end of stage 3 over a period of 10 years. Not only does GFR decline irrevocably, resulting in progressive azotemia, but also *edema* and *hypertension* tend to worsen in the third and final stage of the disease. Similarly, *proteinuria* continues to be massive and *hypoproteinemia* finally results. Although reduced plasma protein concentration and the lowered GFR serve to lower the filtered protein load, urinary protein excretion rate is maintained at massive levels, reflecting increasing leakiness of the glomerular capillary wall to large plasma proteins.

By the time the third, advanced stage of diabetic glomerulopathy is reached, *widespread microangiopathy* involving the retinae and peripheral nerves is invariable. Although its extent varies among patients, retinopathy is frequently associated with

FIGURE 83–1. The glomerular filtration rate (*black line*) and albumin excretion rate (*red line*) have been plotted against time to chart a hypothetical course typical of diabetic glomerulopathy. The course of the disease has been divided into three stages, which are described in the text.

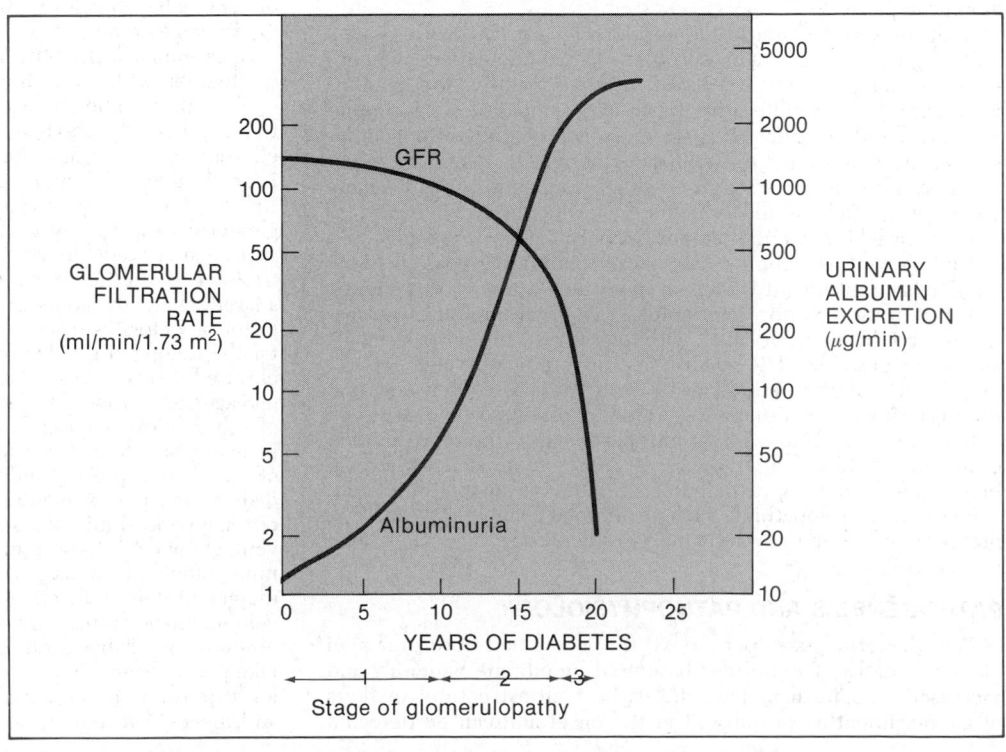

visual impairment sufficient to result in functional blindness. The effects of peripheral and more particularly of autonomic neuropathy may be equally devastating. This is particularly true when autonomic neuropathy results in partial paresis of the bladder. Progressive urinary retention may exacerbate renal insufficiency in stage 3 glomerulopathy by resulting in a superimposed obstructive nephropathy. Obstructive nephropathy in turn may predispose the already vulnerable patient to ascending pyelonephritis and/or ischemic papillary necrosis, thereby compromising renal function even further. (For more detailed discussion of obstructive nephropathy, see Ch. 81.)

Given the prolonged duration of diabetes mellitus, by the time stage 3 glomerulopathy is reached, many patients will be 40 years of age or more, an age group in which exuberant atherosclerosis is accelerated in part by the presence of longstanding hypertension and in part by lipid abnormalities that attend the diabetic state. Coronary artery disease, cerebrovascular disease and stroke, and peripheral vascular disease are all common in the third stage of diabetic glomerulopathy and account collectively for the majority of fatalities. The eventual need for substitution therapy in end-stage renal failure programs occurs in a setting, therefore, in which serious extrarenal complications are prevalent and impair the effectiveness of rehabilitation generally achieved by such therapy.

DIAGNOSIS

Proteinuria due to diabetic glomerulopathy is accompanied by typical changes of glomerular histopathology. These include a striking accumulation of extracellular matrix, which results in an expansion of the mesangium and a widening of the glomerular capillary wall caused by a thickened glomerular basement membrane. The acellular expansion of the mesangium tends to affect all glomeruli in a global fashion; thus, the histopathologic term used for this variety of diabetic glomerular disease is diffuse intercapillary glomerulosclerosis. Not infrequently, mesangial matrix accumulation occurs in a segmental fashion, however, resulting in the formation of acellular spherical nodules at the center of single or multiple peripheral glomerular lobules (Fig. 83–2) and termed nodular glomerulosclerosis. A nodular accumulation of mesangial matrix material, indistinguishable from that observed in diabetic subjects, has been associated with dysproteinemia, notably that associated with a monoclonal proliferation of B lymphocytes or plasma cells. Provided that the latter entity is excluded, however, the finding of diffuse or nodular glomerulosclerosis in a proteinuric diabetic subject is diagnostic of diabetic glomerulopathy.

A diagnosis of diabetic glomerulopathy can be made with a high degree of certainty in a proteinuric diabetic patient, without resort to biopsy, which carries a finite risk for the patient. Background and proliferative types of retinopathy, for example, are correlated strongly with the presence of diffuse or nodular glomerulosclerosis in a proteinuric diabetic. The diagnostic probability can be further strengthened by using noninvasive imaging techniques, such as ultrasonography or nephrotomography, to demonstrate kidney enlargement. Nephrotoxic acute renal failure caused by contrast agents occurs more commonly in patients with diabetic glomerulopathy than in any other category of patients. For this reason nephrotomography (or other radiologic procedures) should be performed without the use of contrast agents whenever possible. The coexistence of retinopathy and nephromegaly in diabetic patients with proteinuria is so constant that the performance of a diagnostic renal biopsy need be considered only when these factors are absent, particularly when the duration of diabetes is less than 10 years. In these circumstances, a renal biopsy has frequently revealed other, and presumably unrelated, primary glomerulopathies, such as minimal change nephropathy, membranous glomerulopathy, and proliferative glomerulonephritis (Ch. 79).

PATHOGENESIS AND PATHOPHYSIOLOGY

The diabetic state per se is the presumed forerunner of glomerulopathy. Glomerular basement membrane widening and increased mesangial matrix, the earliest ultrastructural markers of glomerulopathy, are absent at the onset and can be detected

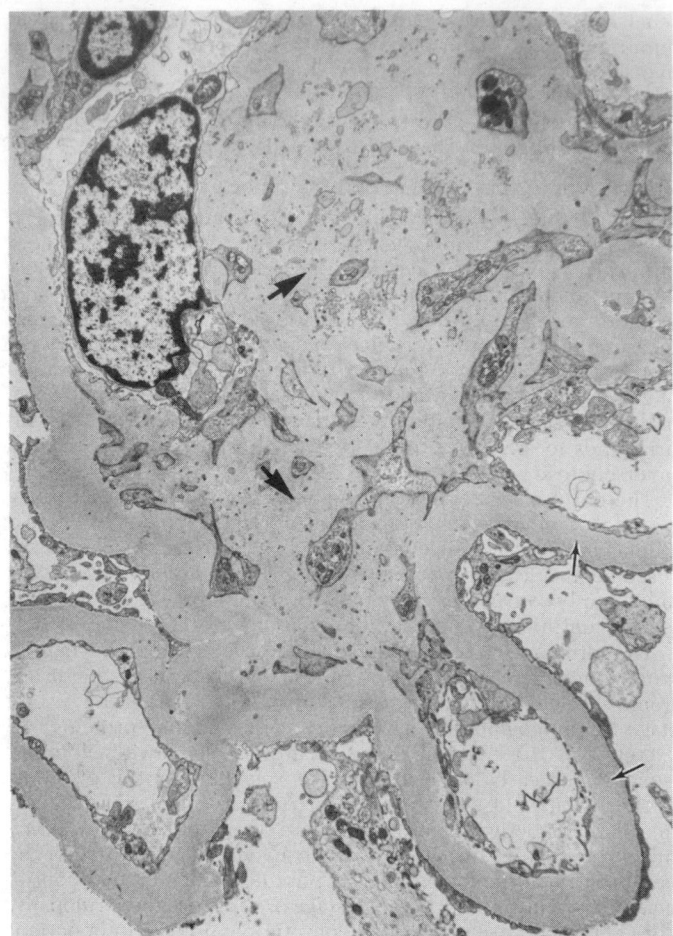

FIGURE 83–2. Electron photomicrograph of a portion of a glomerulus from a patient with proteinuric, diabetic glomerulopathy (magnification ×5000). A striking increase in collagenous components has resulted in (1) widening of the basement membrane of peripheral capillary loops (*small arrows*), and (2) expansion of the matrix of the glomerular mesangium (*large arrows*). The latter alteration is responsible for compressing and ultimately obliterating the glomerular capillary network.

only after some years of type I diabetes. An identical sequence has been observed in experimental diabetes induced in a variety of mammalian species with the use of pancreatic beta cell toxins or pancreatectomy.

As in humans, the GFR is substantially elevated in the insulin-treated rat with experimental diabetes of short duration. The early hyperfiltration is a consequence of altered vasomotion in the major resistance vessels of the renal cortex. Dilatation of the efferent and especially the afferent glomerular arterioles results in an elevation of glomerular capillary perfusion rate and pressure. By contrast, those determinants of GFR that are intrinsic to the glomerular capillary wall, namely, hydraulic conductivity and the surface area available for filtration, are unaltered. Thus hyperfiltration early in the course of diabetes in rodents appears to have a largely hemodynamic basis. It remains to be determined which factor or factors associated with the diabetic state are responsible for the deranged renal vasoregulation. Hyperglycemia per se, or elevated levels of vasodilator glucoregulatory hormones, such as glucagon and growth hormone, may be implicated. Abnormalities of other hormonal regulators of glomerular perfusion rate and pressure have also been identified. Thus, increased production of vasodilator prostaglandins by glomerular cells isolated from diabetic rats points to an imbalance in favor of local vasodilatation of renal cortical microvessels. Experimental maneuvers that prevent glomerular hyperemia and hypertension—such as the administration of an angiotensin-converting enzyme inhibitor or dietary protein restriction—largely prevent the subsequent development of proteinuria as well as the histopathologic damage observed in diabetic rats not so protected. These findings are taken to indicate that hemodynamic factors serve as a stimulus for an ensuing accumulation of extracellular matrix components and, hence, subsequent glomerulosclerosis.

Whether or not glomerular capillary hypertension and hyperperfusion are unique causes of an accumulation of extracellular matrix components, there seems little doubt that this lesion is responsible for the progressive reduction of GFR that typifies the second and third stages of clinical diabetic glomerulopathy. As shown in Figure 83–2, expansion of the mesangial matrix occurs at the expense of the surrounding glomerular capillary loops, with progressive reduction of the surface area available for filtration. By the time the end of the third stage of diabetic glomerulopathy has been reached, the mesangium will have encroached upon most glomerular capillary loops to the point that they have become almost totally obliterated.

The process by which the glomerular basement membrane becomes widened has been presumed to be responsible for the alteration in the glomerular capillary wall, causing it to become permeable to large plasma proteins. Surprisingly, however, no correlation whatsoever exists between glomerular basement membrane width and proteinuria. While the structural basis of proteinuria remains obscure, the functional nature of the disturbance in glomerular permselectivity has been elucidated by the use of physiologic techniques in vivo in which the clearance of probe filtration markers of graded size has been used to define the size-selective properties of the glomerular filter. One such study has revealed that proteinuria in diabetic glomerulopathy can be accounted for by the development within the glomerular capillary wall of a subpopulation of enlarged, protein-permeable pores. In contradistinction to the diffuse widening of the basement membrane seen by electron microscopy (Fig. 83–2), the enlarged pores can be estimated to be few in number and to behave as isolated defects in the glomerular capillary wall.

PROGNOSIS AND TREATMENT

The profound loss of filtering surface area and the disruption of glomerular membrane pore structure that underlie stage 2 and 3 glomerulopathy in diabetics are unlikely to be reversible. Attempts to maintain blood glucose in such patients in a normal range have failed to prevent or attenuate the progression of renal insufficiency. Meticulous control of hypertension, however, may slow the rate of decline of the GFR. Together with antihypertensive therapy, attention to and correction of coexistent cardiac failure, obstructive nephropathy, pyelonephritis, and other events that may lower the GFR independently of the glomerulopathy represent the mainstay of therapy of proteinuric glomerulopathy.

On the basis of our current understanding of the pathophysiology and pathogenesis of diabetic glomerulopathy, a strong case can be made for identifying early stage 2 disease by the detection of sustained microalbuminuria, particularly when it is associated with ophthalmoscopic evidence of diabetic retinopathy. The institution of measures that are likely to lower glomerular perfusion rate and pressure are regarded also to be likely to attenuate the rate of progressive glomerular injury. Such protective measures include dietary protein restriction and lowering of blood pressure, even within the so-called normal range established by the World Health Organization (<169/95 mm Hg). A growing body of evidence suggests that converting enzyme inhibitors have a more marked antiproteinuric effect than other antihypertensive agents, and studies are currently under way to determine whether they are also uniquely or disproportionately GFR sparing. Notwithstanding the absence of evidence for increased activity of the circulating (endocrine) renin-angiotensin system, it could be that a local (paracrine) system is implicated in the genesis of progressive glomerular injury in diabetic subjects. Inhibition of this local system provides a possible basis for a specific renoprotective effect of converting enzyme inhibitors. It should be emphasized, however, that the rationale for protective therapy with converting enzyme inhibitors is at the moment based on purely theoretical considerations. Prolonged and carefully controlled trials with this class of agents have yet to be conducted to confirm that it indeed has a GFR-sparing effect.

Once end-stage renal failure has supervened, the diabetic patient should be referred for treatment to a dialysis and/or transplantation center (Ch. 77 and 78). Many diabetic patients respond favorably to and enjoy a good quality of life with these modalities of treatment. With special attention to the unique problems of the diabetic patient with renal failure, the survival rates achieved with dialysis, particularly chronic ambulatory peritoneal dialysis, or following renal transplantation, are today approaching those achieved for nondiabetic patients.

Hostetter TH, Rennke HG, Brenner BM: The case for intrarenal hypertension in the initiation and progression of diabetic and other glomerulopathies. Am J Med 72:375, 1982. *A lucid review of the pathophysiology of diabetic glomerulopathy, citing virtually every important reference to this subject.*

Hostetter TH, Troy JL, Brenner BM: Glomerular hemodynamics in experimental diabetes mellitus. Kidney Int 19:410, 1981. *An elegant micropuncture study demonstrating the hemodynamic basis for glomerular hyperfiltration in early experimental rat diabetes.*

Luetscher JA, Kraemer FB, Wilson DM: Increased plasma inactive renin in diabetes mellitus. N Engl J Med 312:1412, 1985. *The abnormalities in the renin-angiotensin system in diabetic glomerulopathy are clearly delineated.*

Mauer SM, Steffes MW, Ellis EN, et al.: Structural-functional relationships in diabetic nephropathy. J Clin Invest 74:1143, 1984. *A review of the authors' use of electron microscopy and elegant morphometric techniques to chart the evolution and progression of diabetic glomerulopathy.*

Morelli E, Loon N, Meyer TW, et al.: Effects of converting enzyme inhibition on barrier function in diabetic glomerulopathy. Diabetes 39:76, 1990. *The sieving behavior of glomeruli was analyzed in 16 glomerulopathic patients in whom a 12-week course of enalapril lowered the urinary protein excretion rate. A theoretical analysis of dextran sieving profiles revealed that enalapril shifted the glomerular pore size distribution to pores of smaller radius. The improved barrier size-selectivity was unaccompanied by changes in glomerular hemodynamics, suggesting that inhibition of converting enzyme may modulate the intrinsic membrane properties of the glomerular barrier.*

Myers BD, Winetz JA, Chui F, et al.: Mechanisms of proteinuria in diabetic nephropathy: A study of glomerular barrier function. Kidney Int 21:96, 1982. *Modern physiologic techniques and mathematical modeling are used to describe the glomerular capillary wall as an ultrafiltration membrane; the defect in the glomerular filter of proteinuric diabetics is elucidated.*

Omachi R: The pathogenesis and prevention of diabetic nephropathy. West J Med 145:222, 1986. *This summary of a recent medical grand rounds offers a review of the topic with 57 references.*

Parving HH, Hommel E, Smidt UM: Protection of kidney function and decrease in albuminuria by captopril in insulin-dependent diabetics with nephropathy. Br Med J 297:1086, 1988. *A demonstration that chronic inhibition of converting enzyme with captopril lowers albuminuria and halves the rate at which GFR declines over a 24-month interval.*

Viberti GC, Bilous RW, Mackintosh D, et al.: Monitoring glomerular function in diabetic nephropathy. Am J Med 74:256, 1983. *A careful prospective study of the effects of metabolic control on proteinuric glomerulopathy. Its message is pessimistic.*

Zatz R, Meyer TW, Rennke HG, et al.: Predominance of hemodynamic rather than metabolic factors in the pathogenesis of diabetic glomerulopathy. Proc Natl Acad Sci USA 82:5963, 1985. *The protective effect of lowering glomerular pressures and flows on sclerosing diabetic glomerulopathy is well documented.*

84 Urinary Tract Infections and Pyelonephritis

Vincent T. Andriole

DEFINITION

Urinary tract infection refers to both microbial colonization of the urine and tissue invasion of any structure of the urinary tract. Bacteria are most commonly responsible, although yeast, fungi, and viruses may produce urinary infection. Urinary tract infections may be relatively mild, such as the "honeymoon cystitis" syndrome, or catastrophic, such as a perinephric abscess in a diabetic. Urinary tract infections are often categorized by the site of infection, which is convenient for the purpose of discussion. However, it is often not possible to diagnose the various types of infections on clinical grounds alone.

Significant bacteriuria refers to sufficient numbers of bacteria in the urine to denote active infection rather than contamination. A bacteria count over 100,000 organisms per milliliter in a fresh "clean-catch" midstream specimen is a reliable indicator of active urinary tract infection but does not indicate whether the infection is cystitis or pyelonephritis. In addition, women with acute cystitis may have more than 10^3 but less than 10^5 bacteria per milliliter in midstream urine cultures.

Asymptomatic bacteriuria refers to large numbers of bacteria in the urine without producing symptoms. Dysuria and frequency in the absence of significant bacteriuria are common problems among young women. This entity has been called the *acute urethral syndrome* and in 25 per cent of patients is caused by *Chlamydia trachomatis*.

Cystitis and *acute pyelonephritis* are symptomatic infections of the bladder and kidney, respectively. *Perinephric and renal abscesses*, uncommon complications of urinary infections, usually occur in (1) urinary tract obstruction; (2) bacteremia, particularly staphylococcal or candidal bacteremia; and (3) immunocompromised individuals, particularly diabetics.

Complicated infections refer to bacteriuria in association with structural or neurologic defects in the voiding mechanism (vesicoureteral reflux, neurogenic bladder), foreign bodies (stones or indwelling catheter), or intrinsic renal disease (diabetic nephropathy or polycystic kidney disease).

Chronic pyelonephritis refers to the pathologic and radiologic findings of chronic cortical scarring, tubulointerstitial damage, and deformity of the underlying calix. Chronic bacterial pyelonephritis can be *active*, which occurs in patients with persistent *complicated* infection, or *inactive*, which consists of focal sterile scars of a past infection. Recurrent infection can result in multiple scars combined with active foci of infection. In the absence of obstruction, reflux, foreign bodies, or an immunocompromised host (notably the diabetic patient), urinary tract infections rarely cause the shrunken, scarred kidneys of end-stage chronic pyelonephritis.

Other disease states can produce renal lesions that mimic "chronic pyelonephritis." Identical characteristics can be observed, in the absence of infection, in patients who suffered from severe vesicoureteral reflux in childhood. This entity, *reflux nephropathy*, refers to the radiographic triad of intrarenal reflux and vesicoureteral reflux, scarring, and loss of parenchymal mass in the absence of other obstructive lesions and can ultimately lead to end-stage renal failure with scarred, shrunken kidneys. "Reflux nephropathy" may result from "autoimmune" renal damage rather than bacterial infection of the kidney. Nevertheless, the combination of recurrent infection and reflux nephropathy can also result in chronic pyelonephritis. *Analgesic nephropathy* may produce papillary necrosis and may also mimic bacterial pyelonephritis on radiography.

PATHOGENESIS

The normal urinary tract is free of bacteria except for some organisms normally present near the external meatus and some staphylococci and diphtheroids normally found in the distal urethra. Urine, as a culture medium, generally supports bacterial multiplication. However, high concentrations of urea and hyperosmolality (which are present in the renal medulla), an acid pH, and urinary organic acid are generally unfavorable to bacterial growth. In addition, the dynamics of the urinary flow (washout) and antibacterial properties of the lining membrane of the urinary tract and of the vaginal and periurethral epithelial cells appear to be important defense mechanisms.

Urinary tract infections result most commonly from ascending transurethral invasion of the bladder by pathogenic gram-negative aerobic bacilli normally present in the large bowel and perineum, particularly of women. Sequentially, bacteria migrate from the anus to the periurethral area and along the urethra into the bladder, where infections occur if the organisms become established. This pathogenic mechanism helps explain the higher rate of urinary tract infection in women, whose urethras are shorter than those of men, and the marked frequency of the urinary tract infection associated with instrumentation of the urethra and the bladder. In addition, the increased vaginal fluid pH and altered vaginal microflora present in bacterial vaginosis are associated with *Escherichia coli* introital colonization and acute symptomatic urinary tract infection in young women who use diaphragms.

Other pathways from the large bowel to the urinary passages and kidneys include the hematogenous and lymphatic routes. The hematogenous route, a less common mechanism for renal infection, generally, but not always, requires antecedent structural damage to the kidney. Staphylococcal bacteremia can produce multiple microabscesses in the kidney (*renal carbuncle*). Disseminated *Candida albicans* infections in the immunocom-

promised host can involve the kidney. Finally, septic emboli, particularly in the setting of bacterial endocarditis, represent a classic mode for hematogenously disseminated infection of the kidney.

The renal medulla, because of its unique hypertonicity, is much more susceptible to infection than is the cortex. In experimental pyelonephritis, as few as 10 to 100 *E. coli* organisms may produce infection in the medulla, whereas 100,000 are required to infect the cortex. The increased susceptibility of the medulla is thought to be due to impaired leukocyte mobilization and phagocytosis in the hypertonic environment.

Microbial virulence factors are also important in the pathogenesis of symptomatic urinary infections. *E. coli* strains isolated from patients with pyelonephritis are more likely to (1) possess large amounts of K (capsular) antigen, (2) adhere in larger numbers to human urinary epithelial cells, and (3) possess surface pili, than are strains found in asymptomatic bacteriuria. The virulence of *Proteus* species may be related to their urease content and ammonia production.

CLINICAL MANIFESTATIONS

The symptoms of acute urinary tract infections are varied and include frequency, dysuria, burning pain on urination, suprapubic discomfort, passage of cloudy and occasionally blood-tinged urine, fever, costovertebral angle tenderness or flank pain, and rigors. Urinary tract symptoms, particularly dysuria, occur in 20 per cent of women each year, although only half seek medical attention. Approximately equal numbers of these women have the acute urethral syndrome (urethritis), bladder bacteriuria (cystitis), or renal infection.

In general, clinical grounds form an uncertain basis for separating patients with the acute urethral syndrome from those with either bladder or renal bacteriuria because frequency, burning, and suprapubic pain are found approximately equally in all three groups of patients. Costovertebral angle tenderness and fever may be present as frequently in patients with the acute urethral syndrome as in those with renal bacteriuria. Rigors occur almost equally (15 per cent) in patients with the acute urethral syndrome and those with cystitis. Similarly, tenderness in the region of one or both kidneys occurs not infrequently in lower urinary tract infections. However, sudden fever to 38.9° to 40.6°C, shaking chills, aching costovertebral or flank pain, and symptoms of sepsis are more characteristic of acute pyelonephritis than of cystitis or urethritis.

Laboratory tests show a polymorphonuclear leukocytosis in both cystitis and pyelonephritis. Pyuria is seen in urethritis, cystitis, and pyelonephritis, but white blood cell casts are more typical of pyelonephritis. Stain of the sediment and urine cultures reveal numerous bacteria, usually gram-negative bacilli. Cultures of blood may also be positive in some cases of pyelonephritis. A simple but convenient way of identifying infection of the urinary tract is by examining the urine (see below): The microscopic presence of bacteria in the urine generally indicates more than 100,000 colonies per milliliter of urine. However, the microscopic absence of bacteria does not exclude the diagnosis of urinary infection.

Impaired renal function or acute hypertension is rarely seen in acute pyelonephritis, but renal concentrating ability may be impaired. Also, subclinical forms of acute pyelonephritis may occur because tests that differentiate "upper" (kidney) from "lower" (bladder) infection may indicate the presence of renal infection in the absence of flank pain or fever. However, the only reliable tests, ureteral catheterization and bladder washout, are considered to be research maneuvers. A search for antibody-coated bacteria in the urine as a marker of renal bacteriuria may be performed, but the sensitivity and specificity of this test are not optimal. Pyelonephritis at times presents with symptoms that do not point to the urinary tract. Some patients may have only backache without demonstrable renal tenderness. Others have upper or lower abdominal pain, together with symptoms of disturbed gastrointestinal function. Some complain only of general fatigue.

In the absence of obstructive lesions of the urinary tract or host immunocompromise, as in diabetics, upper or lower urinary tract infections are generally self-limited, lasting 10 to 14 days. When obstruction or host immunocompromise is present, pyelonephritis may be complicated by papillary necrosis, perinephric abscess, or renal carbuncle. These complications should be suspected when persistent flank pain, fever, and leukocytosis are unresponsive to otherwise adequate chemotherapy (see below).

Acute urinary tract infection complicated by pyelonephritis may occur in patients subjected to urethral instrumentation, particularly long-term indwelling catheters. Sepsis from pyelonephritis is a major cause of death in individuals having neurologic disorders requiring long-term indwelling catheters.

DIAGNOSIS

Microscopic Methods

Rapid diagnostic methods are available either (1) by preparation of a Gram's stain of either centrifuged or uncentrifuged urine and examination with an oil immersion lens or (2) by study of either centrifuged or uncentrifuged urine, employing the high-dry objective under reduced light, with or without methylene blue stain. The presence of any bacteria on Gram's stain of centrifuged urine correlates best (97 per cent) with quantitative culture (100,000 bacteria per milliliter of urine). Examination of the unstained sediment for the presence of any bacteria is also very helpful and can be done during routine examination for formed elements. Pyuria, arbitrarily defined as 10 or more leukocytes per high-power field in the centrifuged specimen, can also be detected by the leukocyte esterase dipstick test. The presence of pyuria in a midstream urine sample suggests the likelihood of a urinary tract infection. Some erythrocytes may be seen in the urine, and gross hematuria may occur when inflammation in the bladder is intense. Proteinuria is not common in urinary tract infections, but in fulminant pyelonephritis, as in other severe acute interstitial nephritides, significant degrees of proteinuria may occur transiently.

Significant Bacteriuria

The concept of "significant bacteriuria" was introduced to distinguish between those bacteria that actually multiply in the urine and bacteria that are contaminants. This distinction can be made by knowledge of the site and manner in which the urine is collected from the patient and by enumeration of the number of organisms present in the sample. The criterion of 100,000 or more organisms per milliliter of urine for the diagnosis of significant bacteriuria is an excellent operational definition when the clear-voided method is used, in both males and females, to collect specimens that are processed promptly. However, bacterial counts lower than 100,000 colonies per milliliter may occur in patients with true bacteriuria. Specifically, some women with acute bacterial cystitis, who present with dysuria and frequency (the acute urethral syndrome), may have as few as 100 bacteria per milliliter of urine. Isolation of multiple species from the urine usually indicates contamination, especially in the asymptomatic person.

Urine collected by suprapubic aspiration or bladder catheterization is less likely to be contaminated. In this instance, bacterial counts of fewer than 100,000 organisms per milliliter are likely to be significant.

Bacteriologic Findings

The species of bacteria most likely to be recovered from individuals with bacteriuria depends upon prior history of infection, prior antimicrobial therapy, hospitalization, and instrumentation of the urinary tract. Enterobacteriaceae are the most common organisms identified. *E. coli* accounts for more than 80 per cent of all species recovered in uncomplicated cases, whereas *Proteus, Klebsiella, Enterobacter, Pseudomonas,* enterococci, and staphylococci are more often found in patients who have had previous infection or instrumentation. Occasionally, *Serratia marcescens, Acinetobacter, Candida albicans,* and *Cryptococcus neoformans* may produce infection of the urinary tract in diabetics and in immunosuppressed or corticosteroid-treated patients. Coliforms are also the most common organisms responsible for the acute urethral syndrome in women who have fewer than 10^5 bacteria per milliliter of urine, although *Staphylococcus saprophyticus* and *Chlamydia trachomatis* are responsible for some cases. Patients with the acute urethral syndrome caused by *Chlamydia trachomatis* have pyuria but sterile bladder urine when cultured with standard bacteriologic media.

Anaerobes are commonly present in the distal urethra and the vagina and are abundant in the gut, but they rarely produce urinary tract infection. Suprapubic aspiration of urine or examination of tissues is needed to prove anaerobic infections. When responsible, anaerobes are usually associated with complicated, longstanding infections.

Radiology

Radiographic evaluation of the urinary tract is undertaken to detect correctable lesions that may contribute to the severity or recurrence of urinary tract infections. Evaluation is indicated in men with any type of urinary tract infection or in instances of documented bacteremia. In women, urography is not indicated unless a complication, such as papillary necrosis, perinephric abscess, renal carbuncle, or tumor, is suspected because the patient is unresponsive to otherwise adequate chemotherapy.

EPIDEMIOLOGY AND NATURAL HISTORY

Bacteriuria in the newborn population has been difficult to study because of problems inherent in urine collection. Cultures of urine obtained by bladder puncture suggest an incidence of 1 to 2 per cent. Infection of the urinary tract in this age group may be part of a generalized, life-threatening gram-negative sepsis and is more common in boys than girls. Symptomatic urinary tract infections are more prevalent among girls in preschool years and are often associated with obstructive or neurogenic lesions. Urologic investigation is valuable in this age group. *Urologic evaluation is mandatory in males of any age because of the high frequency of structural abnormalities found* (valves, malformation, and obstructive and neurogenic lesions).

The incidence of bacteriuria among school girls is 1 to 2 per cent; it is only 0.03 per cent in boys of the same age. The incidence of bacteriuria in females rises about 1 per cent per decade.

Urinary tract infection is common after marriage. The pathogenesis of the "honeymoon cystitis" syndrome remains unclear. Physical factors associated with sexual activity in previously sexually nonactive women may play a prominent role. Many patients with "honeymoon cystitis" (up to 50 per cent) have dysuria due to local irritation rather than infection, and this should be clearly differentiated by culture.

Bacteriuria of pregnancy varies from 2 to 6 per cent, depending upon age, parity, and socioeconomic group. Acute symptomatic pyelonephritis develops later in pregnancy in approximately 20 per cent of these women. However, there is no evidence that isolated episodes of pyelonephritis in pregnant women lead to chronic urinary tract infections after these women cease childbearing activities. Early detection and treatment of bacteriuria in pregnancy prevent the emergence of symptomatic infection.

Elderly women may have frequencies of bacteriuria as high as 10 per cent; this rate may increase in hospitalized patients, particularly diabetics. Bacteriuria in men begins to appear in "prostate years" and is often initiated by instrumentation.

Role of Instrumentation

Bacteriuria persists in 1 to 2 per cent of relatively healthy individuals following a single catheterization; the risk is higher in the debilitated patient and in men with prostatic obstruction. With open indwelling catheter drainage, bacterial colonization exceeds 90 per cent within 3 to 4 days. This may lead to life-threatening pyelonephritis and gram-negative sepsis. Fortunately, it is largely preventable by (1) careful criteria for catheterization and (2) use of aseptic closed drainage. The catheter should be removed as soon as it is no longer needed.

Intermittent self-catheterization coupled with abdominal pressure may be of benefit in patients with neurogenic bladders and may result in minimal urinary tract infections.

TREATMENT

The goal of treatment is to eradicate bacteria from the urinary tract in order to relieve symptoms, prevent renal damage, and diminish the likelihood of spread of infections to other sites. Prophylaxis is used to prevent recurrent symptomatic infection. Suppression, although rarely effective, is used to diminish the number of bacteria in the urine or tissue. Indications for therapy depend on the potential of infection to give rise to symptoms or damage to the urinary tract and the likelihood that treatment will be effective (Fig. 84–1).

Asymptomatic Bacteriuria

Asymptomatic bacteriuria should probably not be treated except in those patients who are at high risk of developing symptomatic infections. Thus, treatment of asymptomatic bacteriuria is indicated in pregnant patients to prevent symptomatic illness in the third trimester; in patients who may have major predisposing factors to renal disease, such as diabetic or polycystic kidneys, or who have anatomic or neurologic abnormalities; and in patients who are immunocompromised or who will undergo urologic manipulation. If the treatment fails to eradicate asymptomatic infections in such individuals, further treatment should be reserved for acute symptomatic episodes. In contrast, asymptomatic bacteriuria in females should not be treated in the absence of underlying structural or neurologic lesions, since the likelihood that renal damage will occur is slight. Furthermore, short courses of therapy, when effective, are commonly followed by reinfection. In addition, asymptomatic bacteriuria in patients with indwelling catheter and in the very elderly or nonambulatory patients should not be treated, because the toxicity and expense of therapy may outweigh the risk of disease.

Symptomatic Urinary Tract Infection

Acute uncomplicated episodes of symptomatic bacteriuria localized to the lower urinary tract (bladder or urethra) can be treated effectively with oral single-dose therapy: amoxicillin–clavulanic acid (Augmentin), 3 grams (given as one 500-mg Augmentin tablet plus 2.5 grams of amoxicillin); co-trimoxazole (trimethoprim, 0.32 gram, plus sulfamethoxazole, 1.6 grams), two double-strength tablets; or the newer quinolones—ciprofloxacin (100 mg or 250 mg) or norfloxacin (800 mg). Single-dose therapy usually fails to eradicate either renal bacteriuria or complicated infections. In addition, single-dose therapy is more effective in suburban then in inner-city women with cystitis and in women less than 25 years of age than in women more than 40 years of age. Higher cure rates may be achieved in inner-city or older women with trimethoprim, 0.16 gram, plus sulfamethoxazole, 0.8 gram, or ciprofloxacin, 250 mg, or norfloxacin, 400 mg, twice daily for 3 days. Symptomatic urethritis caused by *Chlamydia trachomatis* should respond to oral doxycycline (100 mg twice daily) or tetracycline (500 mg four times per day) for 7 days.

Pyelonephritis requires a 7- to 14-day or longer course of therapy. Acute uncomplicated pyelonephritis can be treated orally with co-trimoxazole for 14 days on an outpatient basis. Complicated infections in which obstruction or a foreign body is not removed may not respond to such a course. Hematogenous pyelonephritis requires specific therapy directed at the invading organism.

The choice of an oral or parenteral agent depends upon the severity of the infection and the patient's ability to take the oral agent. Drugs are selected on the basis of cost, side effects, and antibacterial spectrum. Antimicrobial susceptibility tests should be used to guide therapy of recurrent episodes. Effective oral agents include sulfonamides, tetracyclines, ampicillin, amoxicillin, cinoxacin, ciprofloxacin, norfloxacin, cephalosporins, co-trimoxazole, trimethoprim, and nitrofurantoin. The last three drugs are useful in recurrent infections, because emergence of resistant strains occurs infrequently.

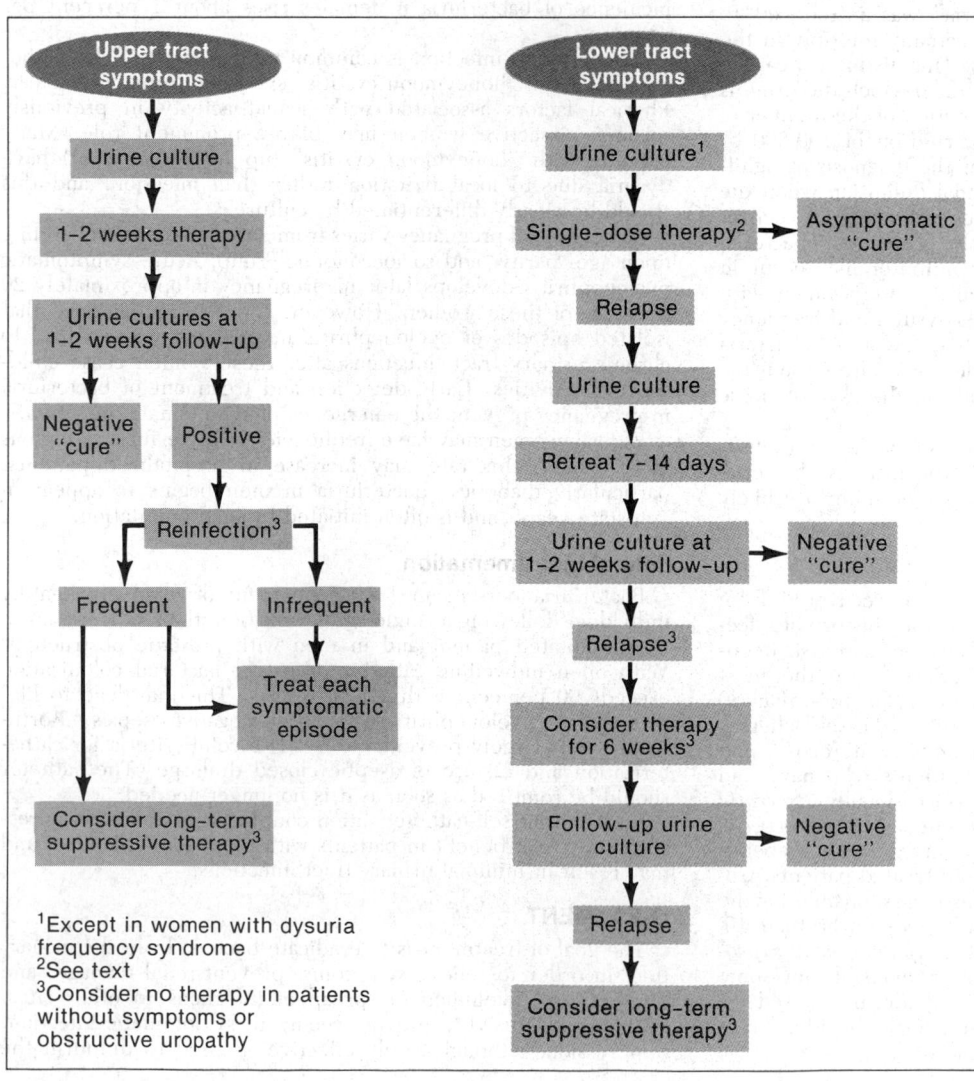

FIGURE 84–1. Management of urinary tract infections.

The initial attack of urinary tract infection is usually due to *E. coli*, which is sensitive to most antimicrobial agents and therefore may be treated "blindly" with the agents described above, with equal success. However, the widespread use of these agents for other infections has decreased their previous reliability. For example, approximately 40 per cent of *E. coli*, including those that are community acquired, are now resistant to ampicillin and amoxicillin.

Microscopic examination of urine and urine cultures have been the mainstay for accurate diagnosis of urinary tract infections. Pretreatment urine cultures are probably not essential, however, and are not cost effective in selected young women with acute dysuria and pyuria, in whom the probability of uncomplicated bacterial cystitis is high. These patients respond to short-course empiric therapy. Urine cultures can be reserved for those in whom therapy has failed. In contrast, pretreatment urine cultures should be obtained in symptomatic infants, children, men, and the elderly; patients with suspected pyelonephritis or complicated infection; patients with relapsing infections; those with *symptomatic* catheter- or instrument-associated nosocomial infection; and pregnant women to detect covert bacteriuria of pregnancy.

When therapy is successful, bacteriuria should disappear within 24 hours even if pyuria and symptoms continue. A repeat urine culture should be obtained after 72 hours of treatment in those patients who have had a pretreatment culture. A positive culture at this time denotes treatment failure. It is important to recognize bacteriologic failure early and to change to another drug. Parenteral agents, such as ampicillin, a cephalosporin, or an aminoglycoside, may be required in some instances or when the patient is too ill to receive an oral agent. A follow-up culture 1 week after the completion of antimicrobial therapy is recommended to document a cure.

Some authors recommend routine follow-up cultures several times over the ensuing year to detect recurrent bacteriuria, but this practice is prohibitively expensive and difficult to justify on medical grounds in asymptomatic patients.

Recurrent Infections

Recurrence of infection in the few weeks after treatment is usually due to persistence of the same focus, whereas later recurrence, particularly in women, is more often a result of reinfection. Frequent recurrent infections may be managed either by close follow-up and treatment of each episode or by prophylaxis with nitrofurantoin, trimethoprim, or co-trimoxazole as a single bedtime dose.

Urinary antiseptics, such as methenamine mandelate or hippurate, require an acidic urine, preferably at pH 5.5, and are of little value unless their use is accompanied by agents that consistently lower urinary pH, such as high-dose ascorbic acid (1000 mg daily). Methenamine, however, is an effective "suppressant" agent and is best used after infection is eradicated by a more effective drug.

Prophylaxis, when given for 3 to 6 months, is effective for recurrent infections of the reinfection type in women. Cessation of prophylaxis, however, results in a significant incidence of recurrence in individuals having structural abnormalities of the urinary tract or intrinsic renal structural defects. In those circumstances, prophylaxis should be reinstituted. Generally, the therapeutic agent should be changed if bacteriuria persists during treatment. This latter circumstance usually means an organism resistant to the agent is now colonizing the urine. Prophylaxis is ineffective in patients with indwelling catheters and will only lead to emergence of resistant bacteria.

The patient should be instructed to drink fluids generously and void frequently. Double voiding in patients with vesicoureteral reflux is recommended. Voiding after sexual intercourse is felt by some to decrease the chance of recurrent infection, but postcoital use of prophylactic agents is probably more effective.

Complicated Infections

Complex urinary infections, i.e., those in the presence of obstructive uropathy, neurogenic bladders, or catheters, are exceedingly difficult to eradicate. They are often best left untreated except for management of acute episodes. Suppressive therapy should be considered ineffective if bacterial populations in the urine are not reduced to less than 1000 per milliliter. The key to management is relief of obstruction or the removal of foreign bodies. Intermittent catheterization has benefited some patients with neurogenic bladders.

COMPLICATIONS

While most urinary tract infections, including pyelonephritis, are self-limited and easily treated, there are three severe complications of pyelonephritis with which the clinician must be familiar: *renal papillary necrosis, renal abscess* (renal carbuncle), and *perinephric abscess*. These complications are uncommon and occur most often in patients with underlying structural renal abnormalities or host immunocompromise (particularly diabetes).

Renal Papillary Necrosis

Renal papillary necrosis, an ischemic necrosis of the renal papilla and adjacent portions of the renal medulla, may be seen in association with severe pyelonephritis, diabetes mellitus, sickle cell anemia, obstructive uropathy, and analgesic abuse. Although infection appears to be the most important factor in the pathogenesis of this lesion, the peculiarities of blood supply of the medulla must also be a factor. This helps explain the frequent occurrence of the lesion in patients with diabetes and generalized vascular disease, as well as the role of obstruction, which must impair blood supply to this area. The zone of necrosis may occur from the extreme tip of the pyramid as far proximal as the corticomedullary junction. Eventually this may slough, with migration of chunks of necrotic tissue down the urinary passages.

The clinical manifestations of renal papillary necrosis are intensification of symptoms of pre-existing pyelonephritis. There may be pain in the lumbar region, colicky pain along the ureteral radiation, hematuria, and high fever. Manifestations of gram-negative bacteremia may supervene. This lesion should be considered in elderly patients with diabetes who show rapid deterioration in clinical status with signs of active pyelonephritis and increasing renal decompensation.

The diagnosis can sometimes be made by finding pieces of renal medullary tissue in the urinary sediment. Pyelography may demonstrate cavities and sinuses in the region of the papillae. The classic ring-shadow pattern results from detachment of a papilla and its outline within the contrast-filled cavity.

Therapy should be directed toward control of infection and measures employed to improve the status of patients who have diabetes mellitus or who are habitual abusers of analgesic agents.

Renal Abscess

Renal abscesses usually occur as a result of extension of a pyelonephritis process. Up to one half of the cases, however, arise from hematogenous spread, by virulent organisms such as *Staphylococcus aureus*, from a distant focus.

A renal abscess may be identified by intravenous pyelography, ultrasonography, computed tomography, or magnetic resonance imaging. It should be suspected whenever a urinary tract infection fails to respond to an adequate course of appropriate antibiotics. Blood and urine cultures may be negative, so empiric antibiotic regimens may be needed to cover gram-negative rods and staphylococci. Surgical drainage is usually required in addition to parenteral antibiotics, although early diagnosis may eliminate the need for surgery in some patients.

Perinephric Abscess

Perinephric abscesses are notoriously difficult to diagnose. They have an insidious onset, with symptoms usually present for over 2 weeks at the time of presentation. Fever and unilateral flank pain are common presenting symptoms. The diagnosis should be considered in the evaluation of any patient with a fever of unknown origin. A recent history of urinary tract infection should alert one to the possibility of a perinephric abscess, although this piece of history is often absent. More than two thirds of patients with perinephric abscesses have either diabetes or kidney stone disease.

Perinephric abscesses occur almost exclusively from the rupture of an intrarenal abscess. Diagnosis can be established by ultrasonography, computed tomography, or magnetic resonance imaging. Surgical drainage is mandatory.

Andriole VT: Current concepts of urinary tract infections. *In* Weinstein L, Fields BN (eds.): Seminars in Infectious Disease. Vol III. New York, Thieme-Stratton, 1980, pp 89–130. *The author's review of practical diagnostic methods, microbiologic concepts, host defenses, clinical syndromes, and treatment of urinary tract infections.*

Andriole VT: Renal and perirenal abscesses. *In* Schrier RW, Gottschalk CW (eds.): Diseases of the Kidney. 4th ed. Boston, Little, Brown and Company, 1987, pp 1049–1064. *A detailed review of the pathogenesis, diagnosis (including the value of diagnostic radiology), and treatment of infections in and around the kidney.*

Andriole VT: Urinary tract infections. Infect Dis Clin North Am 1:713, 1987. *A multiauthored text on all aspects of urinary tract infections in adults and children.*

Andriole VT: Urinary tract infections: Recent developments. J Infect Dis 156:865, 1987. *An update on current theories on the pathogenesis of urinary tract infections.*

Jenkins RD, Fenn JP, Matsen JM: Review of urine microscopy for bacteriuria. JAMA 255:3397, 1986. *An update on the value of urine microscopy.*

Johnson JR, Stamm WE: Urinary tract infections in women: Diagnosis and treatment. Ann Intern Med 111:906, 1989. *A current guide for antimicrobial therapy in urinary tract infections.*

Kunin CM: Detection, Prevention and Treatment of Urinary Tract Infections. 4th ed. Philadelphia, Lea & Febiger, 1986. *An excellent text that describes the pathogenesis, management, and prevention of urinary tract infections.*

Mayrer AR, Miniter P, Andriole VT: Immunopathogenesis of chronic pyelonephritis. Am J Med 75 (Suppl 1B):59, 1983. *Recent studies describing immunologic mechanisms of renal injury and scarring, which produce a histopathologic picture of chronic pyelonephritis.*

Stamm WE, Hooten TM, Johnson JR, et al.: Urinary tract infections: From pathogenesis to treatment. J Infect Dis 159:400, 1989. *A review of our understanding of the pathogenesis of urinary tract infections.*

85 Vascular Disorders of the Kidney

Jordan J. Cohen

RENAL ARTERY OCCLUSION

Partial occlusion (stenosis) of the main renal artery, or one or more of its branches, is common and typically results in hypertension. The clinical features of renovascular hypertension are discussed in Ch. 44. This section considers total or nearly total occlusion of the arterial supply to all or a portion of the kidney.

CAUSES (Table 85–1). Thrombosis in situ rarely occurs in the absence of a severely diseased or damaged vessel. Macroemboli of the renal circulation are far more common as a cause of complete occlusion than are in situ thrombi. (Atheroemboli are

TABLE 85–1. CAUSES OF RENAL ARTERY OCCLUSION

Thrombosis, in situ
    Progressive atherosclerosis
    Blunt trauma
    Inflammation (e.g., polyarteritis, thromboangiitis obliterans)
    Aortic or renal artery aneurysm
    Aortic or renal artery dissection
    Angiographic catheter
    No obvious cause ("spontaneous")

Macroemboli
    Atrial fibrillation
    Mitral stenosis
    Mural thrombus
    Atrial myxoma
    Infective endocarditis
    Prosthetic valve
    Paradoxical emboli (patent foramen ovale)

Atheroemboli
    Abdominal aorta surgery
    Blunt trauma
    Angiographic catheters
    Anticoagulation (?)
    No obvious cause ("spontaneous")

considered in the following section.) Approximately 90 per cent of renal artery emboli originate in the heart. Of these, most arise from the left atrium and are a consequence of atrial fibrillation due to arteriosclerotic heart disease. Although 20 per cent of the cardiac output normally goes to the kidney, only 2 to 3 per cent of the systemic emboli derived from the heart lodge in the renal circulation. The number, the size, and the consistency of individual embolic particles vary with the nature of the underlying process and determine the extent of renal involvement. Large emboli can occlude the main renal artery, but, more frequently, embolic material reaches primary or secondary branches of the vessel. Thus, total infarction of the kidney is much less common than is ischemia or segmental infarction. The presence of one or more accessory renal arteries in 20 to 30 per cent of people and of a generally rich capsular circulation also reduces the likelihood of extensive infarction. In most instances, the embolic event involves only one kidney; bilateral emboli and emboli to a solitary kidney do occur and are associated with greater morbidity.

CLINICAL MANIFESTATIONS. Sudden occlusion of a renal artery, whether from embolus or thrombosis, results in a wide spectrum of clinical manifestations in accordance with the caliber of the vessel or vessels involved and with the pre-existing status of the renal circulation. Occlusion of a primary or secondary branch of the renal artery in a patient with well-established collateral circulation due to chronic, high-grade stenosis may produce little or no infarction and, hence, few or no signs or symptoms; conversely, occlusion of the main renal artery in an otherwise normal kidney may result in immediate infarction of most of the organ and in a dramatic clinical presentation. Renal infarction typically results in the acute onset of vague, nonspecific flank pain that is described as dull and aching in character. The pain may, however, resemble that due to renal colic, cholecystitis, or pancreatitis. Nausea and vomiting are frequent; gross hematuria is *not* common. The symptoms usually subside within 3 to 4 days.

Fever is an infrequent finding at onset but often appears within 1 to 2 days. Hypertension is often present. The white blood cell count is usually elevated, and a leftward shift in the differential count is characteristic. Microscopic hematuria is common but may be absent. Striking elevations of serum lactate dehydrogenase (LDH) levels and lesser elevations of serum glutamic-oxaloacetic transaminase (SGOT) are characteristic. The blood urea nitrogen (BUN) and serum creatinine levels typically rise transiently in unilateral infarction; more severe and protracted degrees of renal functional impairment, including acute oliguric renal failure, may follow bilateral renal infarction or infarction of a solitary kidney.

DIAGNOSIS. The diagnosis of renal artery occlusion and infarction is often difficult because the clinical findings are frequently meager and nonspecific. As a result, fewer than 1 per cent of autopsy-proven cases may be diagnosed ante mortem. The intravenous pyelogram typically reveals reduced or absent function in the involved kidney or kidneys; retrograde pyelography usually reveals no abnormality. Indeed, a normal retrograde study in a kidney that makes no urine and fails to visualize on intravenous pyelography is virtually diagnostic of arterial occlusion. Radionuclide scanning of the kidney may show segmental perfusion defects or complete absence of perfusion. Definitive diagnosis of renal artery occlusion, however, requires renal angiography. In addition, angiography can often distinguish between embolic and thrombotic occlusion. Angiography should be reserved for those patients in whom the diagnostic information is crucial for making management decisions because the risk of the procedure in this setting is appreciable.

TREATMENT. The choice of therapy for acute renal artery occlusion varies widely with individual circumstances (Table 85–2). As a rule, unilateral renal artery occlusion should be treated conservatively, especially if a branch vessel or vessels are in-

TABLE 85–2. TREATMENT OPTIONS FOR RENAL ARTERY OCCLUSION

Observation
Anticoagulation
Thrombolytic therapy followed by anticoagulation
Percutaneous transluminal angioplasty
Surgical embolectomy or endarterectomy
Partial or total nephrectomy

volved; observation alone or coupled with anticoagulation often results in recanalization and avoids the high risk of surgery. Patients with bilateral occlusion or occlusion in a solitary kidney generally fare better with operative intervention. Mortality rates as high as 35 per cent have been reported in patients undergoing acute revascularization procedures. Fibrinolytic therapy followed by anticoagulation can be considered an alternative to surgery in selected cases. Recovery of renal function is a complex function of the duration and magnitude of the occlusion, the extent of collaterals, the degree of associated cardiovascular disease, and the skill and experience of the operative team. Hemodialysis can be used as a temporizing maneuver if the degree of renal functional impairment warrants. Recovery of renal function has been reported to occur after as long as 1 month of oliguric renal failure due to renal artery occlusion. Given that irreversible renal damage occurs within 60 minutes of total renal ischemia induced experimentally, such occurrences of recovery after lengthy delay underscore the important role of renal collaterals.

Percutaneous transluminal angioplasty has proved successful as an alternative to surgery for stenotic lesions of the renal artery and for occlusive lesions as well. Nephrectomy should not be considered unless unequivocal evidence of total infarction is present or hypertension is uncontrollable.

RENAL ARTERY ATHEROEMBOLI

CAUSES. Renal artery atheroembolization is a complication of severe erosive (ulcerative) atheromatosis of the abdominal aorta. Atheroemboli may occur with great frequency in patients with this condition, but, fortunately, in only a small fraction does the process culminate in significant clinical abnormalities. Events that can trigger the release of cholesterol-laden embolic material from ulcerative plaques are listed in Table 85–1.

CLINICAL MANIFESTATIONS. Atheroemboli characteristically lodge in vessels smaller than the interlobular arteries. As a consequence, macroscopic renal infarction does not usually occur, and the clinical picture is usually bland. The insidious development of renal insufficiency is the mode of presentation in most instances of severe atheroemboli. Hypertension is frequently present and may be severe. Distal embolization in the lower extremities, occasionally associated with livedo reticularis, is frequent. Acute pancreatitis and gastrointestinal bleeding can occur and indicate more widespread embolization. Laboratory findings are nonspecific and give evidence of steady or episodic decline in renal function over a period of days, weeks, or even months. Eosinophilia is common, but its cause is unknown. Urinalysis reveals nothing characteristic and is frequently normal. Kidney size is usually normal or only slightly reduced.

DIAGNOSIS. The diagnosis frequently goes undetected, and a high index of suspicion is warranted in the appropriate clinical setting. Diagnosis is made by renal biopsy. Cholesterol crystals contained in the embolic material are dissolved during routine preparation of the histologic sections, leaving pathognomonic biconvex, cleftlike structures in the occluded vessels. Skin and muscle biopsies of the lower extremities, especially from clinically affected sites, may contain similar lesions.

TREATMENT. No effective therapy is available for this condition. Anticoagulants are *not* helpful and may in fact foster atheroemboli by delaying healing of the atheromatous ulcers in the aorta. Unfortunately, once renal manifestations are evident, the process often progresses unrelentingly to renal failure.

RENAL VEIN THROMBOSIS

CAUSES (Table 85–3). Renal vein thrombosis in infants is typically an acute catastrophic event triggered by a volume-depleting illness, such as profuse diarrhea. The consequences are sudden cessation of renal function, engorgement and enlargement of the kidneys, and ultimate renal infarction and atrophy if venous obstruction is not relieved. Fortunately, acute renal vein thrombosis of such magnitude is rare in older children and adults.

TABLE 85–3. CAUSES OF RENAL VEIN THROMBOSIS

Reduced renal blood flow (especially in infants)
Nephrotic syndrome (especially in membranous glomerulopathy)
Renal cell carcinoma
Inferior vena caval thrombosis
External compression (e.g., retroperitoneal fibrosis, tumor)

Renal vein thrombosis in adults is typically of insidious onset and is almost always superimposed on an established disease. It occurs most frequently in association with idiopathic nephrotic syndrome, especially that due to membranous glomerulopathy. Predisposing factors may include reduced antithrombin III levels, reduced intravascular blood volume (often aggravated by diuretic therapy), thrombocytosis, and elevated liver-derived clotting factors. Patients with renal cell carcinoma often develop renal vein thrombosis consequent to tumor invasion of the renal vein.

CLINICAL MANIFESTATIONS. In the typical circumstance in which gradual occlusion of the renal vein occurs, the process may progress without any outward sign. Mild abdominal or back pain may be present, but severe pain is uncommon. Pulmonary emboli occur during the course of approximately half of all patients with chronic renal vein thrombosis and are frequently the initial manifestation of the condition. Renal vein thrombosis can also cause unexplained deterioration in renal function in patients with the nephrotic syndrome. Chronic renal vein thrombosis itself results in no characteristic findings on physical examination or laboratory testing. Heavy proteinuria occurs frequently in patients with this condition but reflects the presence of pre-existing nephrotic syndrome; it is not the result of renal vein thrombosis itself.

DIAGNOSIS. The index of suspicion may be heightened greatly by the clinical setting (e.g., recurrent pulmonary emboli in a patient with nephrotic syndrome) or by findings on intravenous pyelography (e.g., large kidneys with splayed calices due to interstitial edema, notching of the upper ureters due to collaterals). Definitive diagnosis, however, requires visualization of the renal vein. Selective renal venography is generally relied upon for unequivocal visualization of the vessel and its branches, but adequate visualization of the main vein can often be obtained with ultrasound, computed tomography, or magnetic resonance imaging.

TREATMENT. Long-term anticoagulation remains the treatment of choice in chronic, subtotal renal vein thrombosis. Fibrinolytic therapy for a few days prior to instituting anticoagulation should be considered in patients with more serious manifestations of renal vein thrombosis (e.g., acute flank pain coupled with a rising serum creatinine level, rapidly recurring pulmonary emboli).

Harrington JT, Kassirer JP: Renal vein thrombosis. Ann Rev Med 33:255, 1982. *An excellent, clinically relevant review.*

Keating MA, Althausen AF: The clinical spectrum of renal vein thrombosis. J Urol 133:938, 1985. *A well-referenced review of historical and modern concepts of the etiology and management of renal vein thrombosis.*

Lessman RK, Johnson SF, Coburn JW, et al.: Renal artery embolism: Clinical features and long-term follow-up of 17 cases. Ann Intern Med 89:477, 1978. *An excellent detailed review and follow-up of one of the larger series of patients with renal artery embolism; emphasizes the nonoperative management.*

Llach F: Hypercoagulability, renal vein thrombosis, and other thrombotic complications of nephrotic syndrome. Kidney Int 28:429, 1985. *An editorial review of the coagulation abnormalities and clinical features of renal vein thrombosis in patients with the nephrotic syndrome.*

Ouriel K, Andrus CH, Ricotta JJ, et al.: Acute renal artery occlusion: When is revascularization justified? J Vasc Surg 5:348, 1987. *Retrospective analysis of a single medical center's 20-year experience with the management of acute renal artery occlusion.*

Stanley JC, Whithouse WMJ: Occlusive and aneurysmal disease of the renal arterial circulation. DM 30:7, 1984. *A readable review emphasizing the diagnosis and therapy of common afflictions of the renal arteries.*

86 Renal Disease in Pregnancy

John P. Hayslett

The detection and clinical management of renal disease in the gravid woman are complicated by concern for fetal development and survival, as well as for the health of the patient. In addition, clinical evaluation requires knowledge of the physiologic changes in volume status and renal function that accompany pregnancy.

RENAL FUNCTION IN PREGNANCY. Pregnancy is characterized by a gradual, cumulative retention of 500 to 900 mEq of sodium and 6 to 8 liters of water, which are distributed between maternal extracellular fluid and the fetus. Despite an expansion in plasma volume of 30 to 45 per cent, mean blood pressure falls approximately 15 per cent owing to a reduction in peripheral vascular resistance. The glomerular filtration rate (GFR) and plasma flow increase by 30 to 50 per cent by the twelfth week of gestation, an elevation that is sustained until term (Fig. 86–1). Evaluation of GFR, therefore, should take into account expected levels during gestation and should not compare measured values with normal levels in the nonpregnant population. Since renal hemodynamics may be affected by position, a convenient way of measuring GFR in later pregnancy is with a timed (e.g., 4 hours) water-loaded creatinine clearance with the woman lying on her side, a position associated with the highest values.

Because of the increase in GFR, the levels of creatinine and blood urea nitrogen (BUN) fall to approximately 0.5 mg per deciliter and 9 mg per deciliter, respectively. Plasma concentrations above 0.8 mg per deciliter of creatinine and 13 mg per deciliter of urea nitrogen should alert the physician to the possibility of renal insufficiency. Plasma osmolality falls from approximately 280 mOsm • kg H_2O to 270, owing to a resetting of the osmostat; the plasma uric acid level falls to 3 to 4 mg per deciliter and plasma bicarbonate to approximately 20 mEq per liter (because of mild respiratory alkalosis). Glucosuria and aminoaciduria may occur during pregnancy owing, in part, both to increases in filtered load and to a transient reduction in the renal threshold of absorption. The ureters dilate during pregnancy and may remain dilated for as long as 12 weeks post partum with no implication of outflow obstruction.

PREECLAMPSIA (PREGNANCY-INDUCED HYPERTENSION)

DEFINITION. Preeclampsia, unique to human pregnancy, is characterized by hypertension in late pregnancy, usually accompanied by edema, and by proteinuria. It may rapidly progress to a convulsive phase, called eclampsia. Onset is usually insidious after the thirty-second week of pregnancy, but it may occur as early as the twenty-fourth week. In women with a hydatidiform mole, preeclampsia has been reported to occur in the first two trimesters. The usual sequence is edema and hypertension, followed by proteinuria, although proteinuria may occasionally precede hypertension. The disease usually subsides rapidly after delivery. Clinical criteria for diagnosis vary, depending on changes in blood pressure considered to be abnormal in preg-

nancy. In general, hypertension in the third trimester is defined by a blood pressure measurement of 140/85 mm Hg or greater if sustained for 4 to 6 hours, or an increase of 30 mm Hg or more in systolic blood pressure and 15 mm Hg or more in diastolic pressure above values measured during the early stages of pregnancy. The major differential diagnosis involves a distinction among preeclampsia, essential hypertension, and primary renal disease, although preeclampsia can be superimposed on the other two clinical entities.

INCIDENCE. Preeclampsia occurs worldwide with an incidence that varies between 2 per cent and 25 per cent in different populations. In the United States, the quoted incidence is 6 to 7 per cent. Individuals with a poor socioeconomic status may be at higher risk for developing the syndrome; the incidence is reduced by adequate prenatal care, with special attention to weight gain and monitoring of blood pressure. The syndrome occurs predominantly in primigravidas and especially at the extremes of reproductive age.

CLINICAL MANIFESTATIONS. Clinical symptoms of severe disease may include headache, epigastric pain, apprehension, and visual disturbances. While diastolic hypertension may be prominent, systolic blood pressure seldom exceeds 160 mm Hg, except when associated with underlying essential hypertension. Funduscopic examination may reveal segmental arteriolar narrowing and a generalized glistening fundus indicative of retinal edema. The ocular changes reflect vasoconstriction. Signs of central nervous system hyperexcitability are regarded as ominous, since they often precede convulsions, which account for most of the fetal and maternal morbidity and mortality associated with the disease. Laboratory findings include a rate of protein excretion exceeding 300 mg per day but most often below 2 grams per day, although occasionally reaching nephrotic levels of greater than 3 grams per day. There is a reduction in GFR and renal plasma flow to about 30 to 35 per cent of that in pregnancy control subjects. Owing to elevated levels of the GFR in normal pregnancy, however, BUN and serum creatinine levels may not appear to be elevated in toxemic patients, especially if compared with nonpregnant control values. Plasma uric acid levels rise in preeclampsia to about 5.0 mg per deciliter in mild toxemia and to over 7.0 mg per deciliter in severe states, because of a fall in its renal clearance. Some women with preeclampsia manifest coagulation abnormalities, thrombocytopenia, and/or liver function abnormalities.

PATHOGENESIS AND PATHOLOGY. The cause of preeclampsia is not understood. Plasma levels of aldosterone and renin are lower than in normal pregnant individuals but still may be inappropriately high in relation to salt intake and volume status. Many primigravidas who eventually develop toxemia exhibit increased sensitivity to the pressure effects of infused

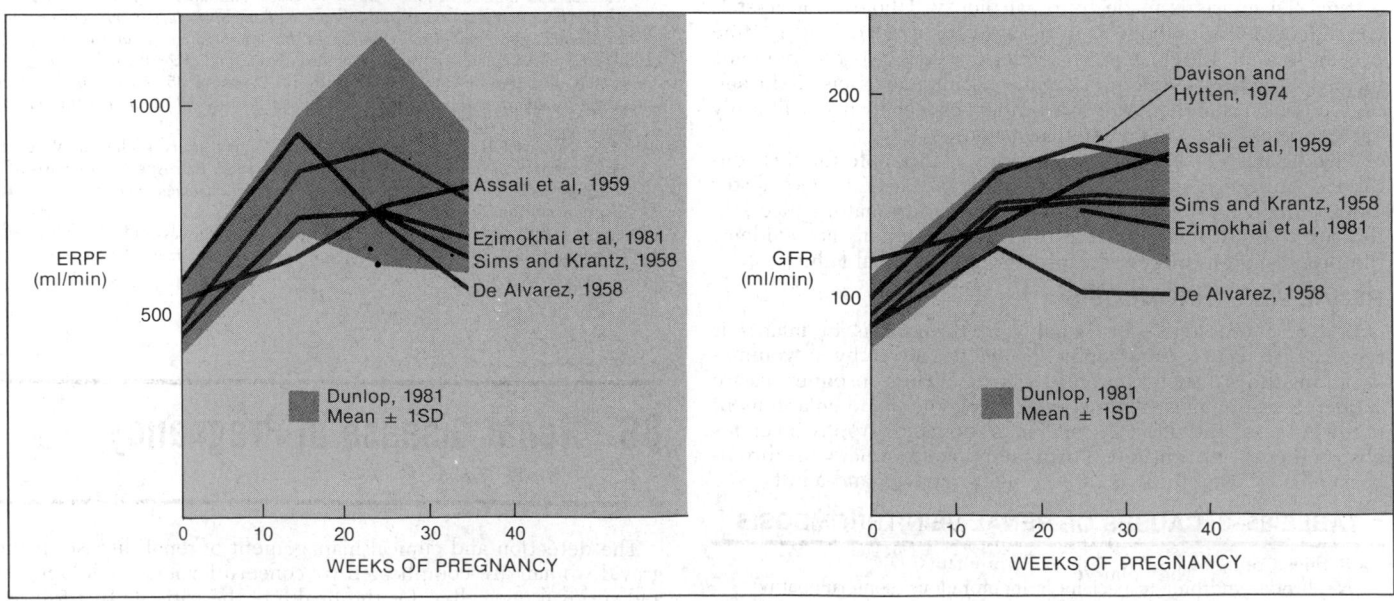

FIGURE 86–1. Changes in effective renal plasma flow (ERPF) and glomerular filtration rate (GFR) during the course of normal pregnancy. (From Davison JM, Dunlop W: Changes in renal hemodynamics and tubular functions enclosed by normal human pregnancy. Semin Nephrol 4:198, 1989; with permission.)

angiotensin many weeks before they become hypertensive. Most recently, evidence has suggested that abnormalities in eicosanoid metabolism may play a role in the pathogenesis of preeclampsia, reflecting an imbalance between production of vasodilating prostacyclin and the vasoconstrictor effects of thromboxane.

The histopathologic renal changes in toxemia, primarily confined to the glomerulus, are termed *glomerular capillary endotheliosis*. The glomeruli are large and swollen, with encroachment on capillary lumina by swollen and vacuolated endothelial and mesangial cells. Occasionally, small subendothelial deposits and fibrin deposits may be seen, but immunofluorescence studies are often negative for deposition of immunoglobulins. The characteristic lesion of endotheliosis seems to be invariably present, even when preeclampsia is mild, resolving a few weeks or months after delivery.

TREATMENT AND PROGNOSIS. All patients suspected of having preeclampsia should be hospitalized. The majority of patients with mild preeclampsia respond to bed rest and sedation. If the fetus is mature, delivery is induced. When gestational age is less than 34 weeks and disease is mild, one may temporize. In patients with diastolic blood pressure levels higher than 95 to 100 mm Hg, antihypertensive agents are administered, usually in the form of alpha-methyldopa, which can be combined with vasodilators or beta-blocking agents. In general, diuretic agents are avoided in the treatment of hypertension in pregnancy because of the risks of reducing placental blood flow. The definitive treatment for toxemia is delivery, which is indicated as soon as fetal maturity is achieved. Hyperreflexia or convulsions require immediate efforts to reduce the level of hypertension and depress central nervous system hyperexcitability. Most obstetric units employ parenteral magnesium sulfate to achieve these aims, along with monitoring of plasma magnesium levels to ensure that therapeutic levels of approximately 6 to 8 mEq per liter are maintained.

RENAL PARENCHYMAL DISEASES

Pregnancy occurs in women with pre-existing renal disease, and pregnant women are susceptible to the same kinds of disease that exist in the nongravid state. Three important clinical questions concerning these patients warrant further discussion: (1) What are the criteria that help to distinguish preeclampsia from other causes of renal dysfunction? (2) Does pregnancy adversely influence the course of the underlying renal or systemic disease? (3) Does the presence of renal insufficiency or nephrotic syndrome significantly reduce the likelihood for a successful fetal outcome?

DIFFERENTIAL DIAGNOSIS OF RENAL DISEASE IN PREGNANCY. Since the clinical hallmarks of preeclampsia— e.g., hypertension, proteinuria, and edema—are also manifested by most other types of renal parenchymal disease, a diagnostic evaluation cannot be based on these clinical features alone. Preeclampsia does not occur before the twentieth week of gestation, except in hydatidiform mole or multiple-gestation pregnancies. The differential diagnosis is therefore simplified if clinical signs of renal disease are known to exist prior to conception or in the early stages of pregnancy. In patients who are not observed until the last trimester of pregnancy, however, identification of the cause of renal dysfunction is often difficult. Multisystem involvement resulting in abnormal liver function tests and coagulation studies suggests preeclampsia. Renal biopsy, which could demonstrate the pathognomonic changes of preeclampsia, provides the only absolute method of confirming the diagnosis of preeclampsia, but few investigators advocate this procedure during gestation. When there is urgency about establishing the nature of the renal injury lesion because of treatment strategies, renal biopsy should be performed during the week immediately following delivery. During pregnancy, therefore, management in most cases must rely on a presumed clinical diagnosis. Since the clinical manifestations of preeclampsia usually resolve spontaneously within 4 to 6 weeks post partum, persistence of hypertension, proteinuria, or renal insufficiency strongly suggests a primary renal disease.

Information on the relative incidence of the various causes of hypertension and proteinuria during gestation has been reported in a large series of patients in whom the diagnosis was confirmed by renal biopsy performed within 6 days of delivery. These studies highlight the difficulty in establishing the correct diagnosis by clinical criteria. In most of these patients, a presumed diagnosis of preeclampsia was made during pregnancy. Among primigravidas, the incidence of preeclampsia, primary renal disease, and hypertensive glomerulosclerosis was 83 per cent, 12 per cent, and 5 per cent, respectively. In multiparous patients, in contrast, preeclampsia occurred in only 38 per cent of patients, while renal disease accounted for 26 per cent of cases and hypertensive renal disease for 24 per cent.

INFLUENCE OF PREGNANCY ON UNDERLYING RENAL DISEASE. Pregnancy does not significantly alter the course of pre-existing primary renal disease due to either glomerular or tubulointerstitial injury in patients with normal or nearly normal renal function. The effect of pregnancy on underlying disease, when renal insufficiency is more severe, (serum creatinine > 1.5 mg per deciliter) is less certain because of insufficient data. Although increased proteinuria, often to nephrotic levels, occurs in nearly one half of patients with a glomerulonephropathy, there is no constant relationship between pregnancy and long-term changes in the GFR. In general, the course of renal disease in these patients follows the expected course defined by the underlying pattern of injury.

There is less information on the effect of pregnancy on renal disease associated with systemic disorders. Pregnancy in diabetic patients does not appear to accelerate the onset of diabetic glomerulosclerosis or alter the natural course of renal disease in subjects with signs of renal disease before conception. In contrast, pregnancy may adversely influence systemic lupus erythematosus (SLE), as reflected in relapses and exacerbations of this disease in patients with an established diagnosis and a relatively high incidence of de novo onset of SLE during pregnancy and in the immediate postpartum period. In patients with established SLE but no clinical signs of active SLE for 6 to 12 months before conception, the clinical course during pregnancy is relatively mild and the live birth rate is approximately 90 per cent. In contrast, about half of all patients with clinical evidence of active SLE at the time of conception have subsequent exacerbations, which are often severe and associated with increased fetal loss.

An increase in urinary protein excretion in subjects with glomerulonephropathies is common during pregnancy and frequently results in the clinical manifestations of nephrotic syndrome. Sodium retention usually tends to become more severe in the last trimester. In most cases, proteinuria spontaneously returns to pregestational levels after delivery. An increase in the rate of edema formation should be anticipated during the later stages of pregnancy in patients with moderate or severe proteinuria and can be blunted by the introduction of a diet with low sodium content. The use of diuretics in pregnancy is controversial because of the possible induction of reduced placental blood flow. Conservative measures to control edema formation, including dietary measures and bed rest, are preferred. The judicious use of natriuretic agents, however, may be useful in patients with severe edema who fail to respond to conservative measures.

INFLUENCE OF RENAL DISEASE ON FETAL OUTCOME. Numerous studies have shown a live birth rate of 90 to 95 per cent in pregnancies associated with primary renal disease with normal or nearly normal renal function (serum creatinine < 1.4 mg per deciliter) and an absence of severe hypertension. These pregnancies, however, are characterized by high rates of preterm deliveries and fetal growth retardation. Analysis has shown an inverse correlation between the severity of blood pressure elevation and rates of fetal survival and birth weight. In patients with moderate or severe renal insufficiency (serum creatinine ≥ 1.5 mg per deciliter), live birth rates are reduced by 20 to 40 per cent, with proportional changes in morbidity. Fetal outcome in pregnancies associated with diabetic nephropathy is affected by the same factors found in primary renal disease and by complications present in all diabetic pregnancies, which include increased rates of macrosomia, major congenital defects, and neonatal complications.

ACUTE RENAL FAILURE IN PREGNANCY

Acute renal failure during pregnancy results from severe injury to tubular epithelial cells because of renal ischemia or the action of nephrotoxic agents. The cell injury may be reversible, with an eventual complete restoration of renal function; or it may be irreversible and lead to renal cortical necrosis. Renal cortical necrosis is characterized by the development of fibrosis within the cortex in a diffuse or patchy pattern, with relative sparing of the medullary portions of the kidney. Cortical necrosis is uncommon in nonpregnant individuals but occurs more often in pregnancy, especially in patients more than 30 years of age with third trimester abruptio placentae. It has been suggested that increased reactivity of the renal vasculature to vasoactive amines in pregnancy and local activation of coagulation may play an important role in the induction of tissue injury leading to cell death.

In addition to the usual causes of acute renal failure, some types of renal insults are unique to pregnancy. Septic abortion and hyperemesis gravidarum may cause renal failure in early pregnancy, while severe preeclampsia, placenta previa, and abruptio placentae are causative factors in the later stages of pregnancy. Clinical management of acute renal failure in pregnancy is comparable to that in nonpregnant patients. There is a high incidence of fetal loss associated with acute renal failure, but outlook has improved because of advances in dialytic therapy during pregnancy.

Barron WM, Murphy MB, Lindheimer MD: Management of hypertension during pregnancy. In Laragh JH, Brenner BM (eds.): Hypertension: Pathophysiology, Diagnosis and Management. New York, Raven Press, 1990, pp 1809–1827. *This chapter reviews blood pressure in normal pregnancy, the classification of hypertension in pregnancy, the pathogenesis and management of preeclampsia, and treatment of hypertension in pregnancy.*

Katz AI, Davison JM, Hayslett JP, et al.: Pregnancy in women with kidney disease. Kidney Int 18:192, 1980. *An analysis of a large series of pregnancies associated with primary renal disease. An excellent source for references.*

Reece EA, Coustan DR, Hayslett JP, et al.: Diabetic nephropathy: Pregnancy performance and feto-maternal outcome. Am J Obstet Gynecol 159:56, 1988. *An analysis of a large series of patients with diabetic nephropathy that compares risk factors associated with primary and diabetic renal disease.*

87 Hereditary Chronic Nephropathies

Wadi N. Suki

Several genetically transmitted renal disorders of unknown pathogenesis may fall under this heading. This chapter will discuss two of these disorders, Alport's syndrome and the nail-patella syndrome. Some hereditary disorders of renal tubular function are described in Ch. 82. Other genetic disorders that may be associated with renal disease are listed in Table 87–1 and discussed in the section on Metabolic Diseases (Part XIV).

ALPORT'S SYNDROME

DEFINITION. Also known as "chronic hereditary nephritis," this syndrome is characterized by the familial occurrence in successive generations of a progressive nephritis, more severe in males, manifested invariably by hematuria and frequently associated with a sensorineural hearing deficit.

GENETICS. The mode of transmission in most kindreds is consistent with X-linked dominant inheritance, and the gene has been localized to the middle of the long arm of the X-chromosome. Autosomal recessive and autosomal dominant inheritances have also been described in certain kindreds, suggesting that this disorder may be genetically heterogeneous.

INCIDENCE AND PREVALENCE. Several hundred kindreds of all races and geographic origins have been described. Alport's syndrome accounts for nearly 5 per cent of patients with end-stage renal disease.

PATHOLOGY AND PATHOGENESIS. Early in the disease, the kidneys may be normal or large in size, but they shrink with progression of the disease. Under light microscopy, the glomeruli may be normal or show some hypertrophy of epithelial cells and increase in mesangial matrix. Later changes consist of mesangial cell proliferation, thickening and splitting of glomerular and tubular basement membranes, thickening of Bowman's capsule, tubular cell atrophy, interstitial fibrosis, and the presence of foam

TABLE 87–1. INHERITED RENAL DISEASES*

Disorders of Tubular Function
  Proximal tubule
    Cerebro-oculorenal syndrome of Lowe
    Cystinosis (Fanconi's syndrome)
    Cystinuria
    Galactosemia
    Glycogen storage (von Gierke's) disease
    Glycinuria
    Hartnup disease
    Hepatolenticular degeneration (Wilson's disease)
    Hereditary fructose intolerance
    Hypophosphatemic vitamin D–resistant rickets
    Iminoaciduria
    Proximal renal tubular acidosis
    Pseudohypoparathyroidism
    Renal glucosuria
  Distal/collecting tubule
    Distal renal tubular acidosis
    Nephrogenic diabetes insipidus
Disorders of Renal Structure
  Agenesis
  Cystic disorders
    Hepatocerebrorenal syndrome of Zellweger
    Medullary sponge kidney
    Medullary cystic disease
    Polycystic kidney disease, adult type
    Polycystic kidney disease, infantile type
    Renal retinal dysplasia
  Duplication
  Renal malformations with extrarenal anomalies
Biochemical Disorders
  Alkaptonuria
  Cystinosis
  Diabetes mellitus
  Glycosphingolipidosis (Fabry's disease)
  Hepatolenticular degeneration (Wilson's disease)
  Hyperuricemia
  Primary hyperoxaluria (oxalosis)
  Xanthine oxidase deficiency
Systemic Disorders
  Amyloidosis
  Asphyxiating thoracic dystrophy (Jeune's disease)
  Charcot-Marie-Tooth disease
  Laurence-Moon-Biedl syndrome
  Osteo-onychodysplasia (nail-patella syndrome)
Hereditary Chronic Nephropathies
  Benign recurrent hematuria
  Hereditary chronic nephritis
  Hereditary chronic nephritis with hyperprolinemia
  Hereditary chronic nephritis with thrombocytopathy
  Hereditary immune nephritis
  Infantile nephrosis

*Includes diseases that affect the kidney secondarily.

cells. Electron microscopy characteristically reveals both thinning and irregular thickening of the glomerular and tubular basement membranes, with splitting of the lamina densa into several lamellae separated by lucent zones containing electron-dense round granulations.

The etiology of Alport's syndrome appears to be the absence of a 28-kilodalton peptide component of the noncollagenous domain of the alpha$_1$ chain of type IV collagen in basement membrane. This peptide has been labeled the Goodpasture antigen (see below).

CLINICAL MANIFESTATIONS. The disease is discovered in 70 per cent of patients by the age of 6 years, the rest of the cases being discovered at any age thereafter up to and well into adulthood. Persistent or intermittent microscopic hematuria is universally present. Gross hematuria, especially after exercise or respiratory infections, may occur in 60 per cent of affected children but rarely in adults. Proteinuria is present in 70 per cent of patients. It is usually mild but reaches the nephrotic range in 30 to 40 per cent of patients. Sensorineural hearing loss in the high-frequency (4000 to 8000 Hz) range is observed in 40 to 60 per cent of patients, predominantly in males. Its detection may require audiometric testing, but it may progress to clinical deafness. Ocular disorders, especially anterior and posterior lenticonus and spherophakia, are seen in 15 per cent of patients. The renal disease may be mild and nonprogressive, especially in women, or may progress with the development of azotemia and hypertension, culminating in chronic renal failure and uremia. Progression occurs predominantly in males, with a predilection to those with massive proteinuria, deafness, and lenticonus. Renal failure may occur in childhood or in adulthood, and in affected males usually before age 40 years. Affected females may experience decline of renal function during pregnancy.

In several kindreds, patients with classic Alport's syndrome have been reported to have thrombocytopenia with giant platelets manifested clinically by bruising, epistaxis, and gastrointestinal bleeding and in the laboratory by prolonged bleeding time. A few cases have also been associated with hyperprolinemia (Ch. 172), leiomyomatosis, and a variety of other disorders.

DIAGNOSIS. The presence of progressive renal disease in one family member younger than age 50, other than the proband, and the presence of neural hearing loss in the patient or a relative form the basis for the diagnosis of Alport's syndrome in a patient with hematuria with or without proteinuria, azotemia, or hypertension. Differential diagnosis includes benign familial hematuria, a nonprogressive disorder characterized by a uniformly thin glomerular capillary basement membrane, and IgA nephropathy (Berger's disease), a glomerulonephritis with distinctive findings on light, electron, and especially immunofluorescent microscopic examination of the renal glomerulus. The audiometric findings, ocular manifestations, and family history, coupled with the changes in the glomerular and tubular basement membranes, usually should distinguish Alport's syndrome from other renal disorders.

TREATMENT. There is no specific treatment for Alport's syndrome, and no therapy is known to alter its course. Only conventional management of progressive renal disease is available. Peritoneal dialysis or hemodialysis and related or cadaveric donor kidney transplantation have been utilized with degrees of success at least matching those in other renal disorders. In fact, improvement of hearing deficit has been reported after renal transplantation. Recurrence of the renal lesion has not been observed following transplantation, but several patients have developed Goodpasture's syndrome in the renal graft caused by an antibody directed against the basement membrane antigen, which is absent in Alport's syndrome.

NAIL-PATELLA SYNDROME

An autosomal dominant trait also known as osteo-onychodysplasia, this disorder of mesenchymal tissue is characterized by atrophic or absent fingernails, hypoplasia or aplasia of the patella, accessory conical iliac horns, thickening of the scapula, and subluxation of the radial heads at the elbow. In 40 per cent of patients, the kidneys may be involved, as manifested by mild proteinuria and, rarely, hematuria. Occasionally, the nephrotic syndrome and progression to renal failure (27 per cent) may be observed. Light microscopy shows glomerular cellular proliferation, mesangial sclerosis, and basement membrane thickening. Electron microscopy reveals areas of rarefaction in the lamina densa of the glomerular basement membrane filled with bundles of curvilinear fibrils having the typical periodicity of collagen. No specific therapy exists for this disorder. Renal transplantation has been carried out without evidence of recurrence of the disease in the transplanted organ.

Bennett WM, Musgrave ME, Campbell RA, et al.: The nephropathy of the nail-patella syndrome. Am J Med 54:304, 1973. *A good description of the renal disorder in the nail-patella syndrome.*

Kashtan CE, Michael AF: Hereditary nephritis. Semin Nephrol 9:135, 1989. *An excellent review of the biochemical defect in, and the genetic transmission of, Alport's syndrome.*

88 Renal Calculi
Charles Y.C. Pak

DEFINITION

Renal calculi (kidney stones, nephrolithiasis) are abnormal concretions occurring in the kidneys, consisting of crystalline components and an organic matrix. They are typically located within the calices or pelvis and may become lodged in the ureter or bladder as they are passed. Nephrolithiasis should be differentiated from nephrocalcinosis, which is calcification of renal parenchyma. Stones originating in the bladder (bladder stones) are rare in industrialized countries, although they were common in antiquity and are still frequent in certain countries in Southeast Asia.

Nephrolithiasis affects 1 to 5 per cent of the population, with a recurrence rate in afflicted individuals of 50 to 80 per cent and an annual incidence rate of 0.1 to 0.3 per cent. Calcareous (calcium-containing) renal stones account for 80 to 95 per cent of stones and are principally composed of calcium oxalate and calcium phosphate, usually occurring as mixtures. The remaining stones are composed of uric acid, cystine, magnesium ammonium phosphate (struvite), and, rarely, xanthine, 2,8-dihydroxyadenine, triamterene, or silicate (Table 88–1).

ETIOLOGY AND PATHOGENESIS

Renal stones form by an initial crystallization of a nidus (termed nucleation) from a supersaturated urine with subsequent crystal growth and aggregation of the nidus into a macroscopic stone. Kidney stones are not simply masses of crystals. They usually have an organic matrix that gives form, cohesiveness, and sometimes a remarkably regular structure to the stone. At the present time, abnormalities in the amount or composition of stone matrix have not been demonstrated to be important in stone pathogenesis. It is impossible to dissolve the amounts of calcium, oxalate, and phosphate present in normal urine in 1 or 2 liters of distilled water. Obviously, therefore, there are substances present in normal urine that impede crystallization and sustain supersaturation. These normal inhibitors are not fully characterized but seem to include pyrophosphate, citrate, magnesium, and certain organic macromolecules (such as glycosaminoglycans and glycoproteins).

All patients with stones are presumed to have some physiologic derangements that make them susceptible to stone formation, although no cause can be demonstrated by current techniques in 3 per cent of patients. These derangements alter urinary concentration of stone-forming constituents and of inhibitors to cause supersaturation and facilitate crystallization (Table 88–2).

Crystallization involves three steps: *nucleation* (formation of nidus), *crystal growth* (enlargement of crystal size), and *crystal agglomeration* (clumping of crystals that are formed to attain a large size). It requires supersaturation of urine and reduced urinary content of inhibitors.

Supersaturation can result from (1) too little urine output (a concentrated urine), (2) an absolute increase in the amount of a stone constituent excreted over a period of time, such as calcium, oxalate, or uric acid, or (3) an alteration in urine pH. Low urinary pH (< 5.5) increases urinary saturation of uric acid, whereas high urinary pH raises that of calcium phosphate and magnesium ammonium phosphate.

Reduction in the concentration of inhibitors of crystallization in the urine may be of great importance in stone pathogenesis, by facilitating crystallization. Some inhibitors (such as citrate) may be directly measured in urine, providing diagnostic utility. Other inhibitors (such as glycoproteins) that are difficult to analyze

TABLE 88–1. COMPOSITION OF RENAL STONES*

Type	Percentage
Calcium oxalate	70
Calcium phosphate	10
Hydroxyapatite	
Brushite	
Tricalcium phosphate	
Carbonate apatite	
Magnesium ammonium phosphate	5–10
Uric acid	< 5
Cystine	1
Xanthine and other	< 1

*Some stones occur as mixtures. Percentages are calculated for the predominant stone types.

can sometimes be assessed indirectly from the overall inhibitor activity against crystallization of stone-forming salts.

Other factors may be important in stone formation. (1) *Stasis*: Most embryonic stones are probably harmlessly washed out in the urine. Stasis allows time for nascent stone to grow. (2) *Heterogeneous nucleation*: Crystallization may begin in a supersaturated solution that is seeded with a crystal of a different (heterogeneous) composition but one that has an analogous surface topography. This process of one crystal growing on the surface of another is known as epitaxy. Many stones are mixed in composition and perhaps represent epitaxial growth.

HYPERCALCIURIA. As noted, calcium is a constituent of 80 to 95 per cent of kidney stones. Hypercalciuria is the single most frequent abnormality found in patients with stone diathesis. Hypercalciuria is often statistically defined and varies with body size and diet. In general, the normal upper limit for urinary calcium is 300 mg per day on a diet containing 1000 mg of calcium per day (some authorities use a figure of 4 mg per kilogram per day) and 200 mg per day on a diet with a daily composition of 400 mg of calcium and 100 mEq of sodium (urinary calcium tends to parallel urinary sodium so that dietary sodium should ideally be controlled). Hypercalciuria can result from (1) enhanced absorption from dietary sources, (2) primary renal wastage with secondary enhanced absorption, (3) excessive resorption from storage in bone, or (4) a combination of the above (Fig. 88–1). These different forms will be discussed briefly.

Absorptive hypercalciuria, the most common abnormality, is encountered in 30 to 40 per cent of patients with kidney stones. Increased absorption of dietary calcium may rarely occur from excessive ingestion of milk and other dairy products, from vitamin D excess (Ch. 233), or from the altered vitamin D metabolism associated with sarcoidosis (Ch. 67). Absorptive hypercalciuria usually refers, however, to a primary idiopathic increase in intestinal absorption of calcium. The consequent rise in serum calcium concentration tends to suppress parathyroid function (PTH ↓). Hypercalciuria ensues from the increased renal filtered load of calcium and the reduced renal tubular reabsorption of calcium associated with suppression of the secretion of parathyroid hormone (PTH). Serum calcium is typically maintained within the normal range because of compensatory hypercalciuria. In its usual presentation, the disorder tends to be familial and is believed to occur independently of hypophosphatemia or altered vitamin D metabolism. There is some evidence that it represents a jejunal disease characterized by a selective intestinal hyperabsorption of calcium in this intestinal segment.

Renal hypercalciuria, as a form of "idiopathic hypercalciuria,"

occurs less commonly than absorptive hypercalciuria and originates from an impaired renal tubular reabsorption (renal leak) of calcium. The ensuing decline in serum calcium causes secondary hyperparathyroidism, which in turn stimulates the renal synthesis of 1,25-dihydroxyvitamin D (Fig. 88–1). Thus, the skeletal mobilization and intestinal absorption of calcium may be secondarily increased, effects that restore serum calcium concentration to normal and further contribute to the hypercalciuria. The possibility that there may be a more generalized disturbance in proximal tubular function is shown by an exaggerated natriuretic response to thiazide and calciuric response to a carbohydrate load.

Resorptive hypercalciuria results from excessive bone resorption, most commonly from the hypersecretion of PTH. Three to 5 per cent of all kidney stones are caused by primary hyperparathyroidism (Table 88–2); conversely, 10 to 30 per cent of patients with primary hyperparathyroidism present with renal stones. The hypercalcemia of hyperparathyroidism causes hypercalciuria by augmenting the renal filtered load of calcium. The intestinal calcium absorption may also be increased secondarily, consequent to parathyroid hormone-dependent stimulation of the synthesis of 1,25-dihydroxyvitamin D; this increased calcium absorption further contributes to the hypercalciuria. Hypercalciuria secondary to net bone resorption is also seen in thyrotoxicosis, multiple myeloma, pseudohyperparathyroidism of malignancy, metastatic disease of bone, and immobilization (acute osteoporosis) and with spontaneous or iatrogenic Cushing's syndrome.

Fasting hypercalciuria with normal levels of serum PTH is neither absorptive hypercalciuria (because of the presence of apparent renal calcium leak) nor renal hypercalciuria (since parathyroid stimulation is lacking). This picture may result from several disturbances. (1) *Enhanced 1,25-dihydroxyvitamin D synthesis*: It may cause parathyroid suppression and an acquired renal calcium leak. (2) *Renal phosphate leak*: It may produce hypophosphatemia and increased synthesis of 1,25-dihydroxyvitamin D. (3) *Combined renal proximal tubular defect*: Renal calcium leak may coexist with high 1,25-dihydroxyvitamin D production occurring primarily or secondarily from renal phosphate leak.

HYPEROXALURIA. Oxalate is the second most common constituent of kidney stones, after calcium (Table 88–1), but the great majority of patients with calcium oxalate stones have no abnormality of oxalate metabolism. Sustained hyperoxaluria, which may be defined as the excretion of greater than 60 mg of oxalate per 1.73 square meters per 24 hours, occurs only (1) in primary hyperoxaluria, a rare genetic disorder described in Ch. 171, (2) in pyridoxine deficiency, (3) rarely with excessive ingestion of ascorbic acid, and (4) from enhanced absorption of dietary oxalate, termed enteric hyperoxaluria.

TABLE 88–2. PATHOGENESIS OF NEPHROLITHIASIS

Cause	Percentage of Patients with Stones	Sex Predominance	Stone Composition
Hypercalciuria			
Absorptive hypercalciuria	20–40	Male	Ca oxalate, Ca phosphate
Renal hypercalciuria	5–8	Equivalent	Ca oxalate, Ca phosphate
Fasting hypercalciuria with normal PTH*	15–25	Male	Ca oxalate, Ca phosphate
Primary hyperparathyroidism	3–5	Female	Ca phosphate, Ca oxalate
Hyperoxaluria			
Primary	Rare	Equivalent	Ca oxalate
Enteric	<2	Equivalent	Ca oxalate
Dietary	2–15	Male	Ca oxalate
Hyperuricosuric calcium nephrolithiasis	10–40	Male	Ca oxalate, Ca phosphate
Hypocitraturic calcium nephrolithiasis			
Renal tubular acidosis	1–10	Equivalent	Ca phosphate, Ca oxalate
Other	9–40	Male	Ca oxalate, Ca phosphate
Uric acid stone diathesis	15–30	Male	Uric acid, Ca oxalate, Ca phosphate
Hypomagnesiuric calcium nephrolithiasis	5–10	Equivalent	Ca oxalate
Cystinuria	<1	Equivalent	Cystine
Infection lithiasis	1–5	Female	Struvite, carbonate apatite
Low urine volume	10–50	Female	Ca oxalate
No physiologic disturbance	< 5	Female	Ca oxalate

*PTH = parathyroid hormone.

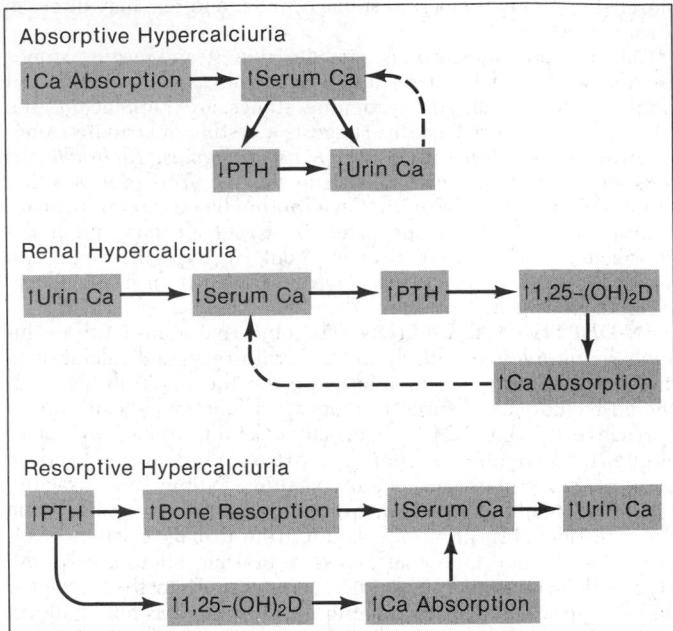

Absorptive Hypercalciuria

↑Ca Absorption → ↑Serum Ca

↓PTH → ↑Urin Ca

Renal Hypercalciuria

↑Urin Ca → ↓Serum Ca → ↑PTH → ↑1,25-(OH)₂D

↑Ca Absorption

Resorptive Hypercalciuria

↑PTH → ↑Bone Resorption → ↑Serum Ca → ↑Urin Ca

↑1,25-(OH)₂D → ↑Ca Absorption

FIGURE 88–1. Pathophysiologic schemes for hypercalciuria. (After Pak CYC: Kidney stones. *In* Foster DW, Wilson JE [eds.]: Williams Textbook of Endocrinology. Philadelphia, W. B. Saunders Company, 1985, pp 1256–1273.)

Enteric hyperoxaluria, which is encountered in approximately 2 per cent of patients with stones, occurs typically in patients with ileal disease (ileal resection, jejunoileal bypass surgery, inflammatory disease of the small bowel). In ileal disease in which there is malabsorption of fat, the intraluminal content of divalent cations, particularly calcium, may be reduced by being bound to unabsorbed fatty acids. Thus, calcium is not normally available to bind and limit oxalate absorption. The resulting enlarged free intestinal oxalate pool increases absorption and renal excretion of oxalate. Oxalate absorption may be stimulated primarily as well, especially in the colon, since patients with ileostomies do not have hyperoxaluria. Low urine volume (from an excessive intestinal loss of fluid) and defective urinary inhibitor activity (from an impaired renal excretion of citrate and magnesium) probably contribute to calcium stone formation in ileal disease. Low urinary pH (from intestinal alkali loss) may cause formation of uric acid stones.

In hypercalciuria associated with increased calcium absorption (e.g., absorptive hypercalciuria), a mild increase in oxalate excretion may be found (up to 50 mg per day). The total amount of oxalate absorbed from the gut may be high because more calcium is absorbed and less calcium is available intraluminally to bind oxalate.

HYPERURICOSURIC CALCIUM OXALATE STONE DIATHESIS. Hyperuricosuria may be the only discernible biochemical abnormality associated with calcium oxalate stones (10 per cent), although it often coexists with hypercalciuria or hypocitraturia (40 per cent). Most patients with hyperuricosuric calcium oxalate nephrolithiasis do not suffer from clinical gout. The hyperuricosuria is usually dietary in origin, since a history of high purine intake may often be disclosed and normal urinary uric acid excretion values may be restored by purine restriction. Less commonly, hyperuricosuria results from a primary overproduction of uric acid. The urinary pH typically exceeds 5.5, so that dissociated urate rather than uric acid predominates. It is believed that urates facilitate crystallization of calcium oxalate, either directly by inducing heterogeneous nucleation or indirectly by removing macromolecular inhibitors through adsorption.

HYPOCITRATURIA. Citrate reduces urinary saturation of calcium salts by complexing calcium, as well as inhibits the crystallization of these salts. Crystal agglomeration of calcium oxalate is particularly retarded by citrate. Thus, hypocitraturia would be expected to increase the tendency toward the formation of calcium-containing kidney stones. Hypocitraturia is encountered in any acidotic condition, such as renal tubular acidosis,

chronic diarrheal states, thiazide-induced hypokalemia (which causes intracellular acidosis), ingestion of excessive animal protein (which has a high acid-ash content), and strenuous physical exercise (which produces lactic acidosis). Distal (type I) renal tubular acidosis, often in an incomplete form, may first manifest with nephrolithiasis. The cause for stone formation is multifactorial and probably includes hypercalciuria (from induced renal leak of calcium by acidosis), enhanced dissociation of phosphate, an increased saturation of calcium phosphate (from high urinary pH), as well as an impaired inhibitor activity (from defective excretion of citrates). Renal tubular acidosis is described in greater detail in Ch. 82. Hypocitraturia of excessive intestinal alkali loss has been found not only in ileal disease (enteric hyperoxaluria) but also in postgastrectomy states and ulcerative colitis. Hypocitraturia should be suspected in patients with hypercalciuric nephrolithiasis who continue to form stones while on thiazide therapy. Another cause of hypocitraturia is urinary tract infection (probably from bacterial degradation of citrate). The cause for hypocitraturia often remains unknown. Hypocitraturia may occur as a sole abnormality (10 per cent) but is usually associated with other causes of nephrolithiasis (50 per cent).

URIC ACID STONES. Approximately two thirds to three fourths of the uric acid synthesized in the body is excreted in the urine. The rest is excreted in the intestine and largely destroyed by bacterial degradation. Uric acid excretion varies widely with diet. Urinary values greater than 600 mg per 1.73 square meters per 24 hours after 3 days of a diet moderately restricted in purine probably represent endogenous overproduction. In the study of patients with kidney stones, it is more important to measure uric acid excretion on the patient's usual diet. In this case, an excretion of more than 750 mg for women and more than 800 mg for men would be considered abnormally high.

Uric acid stones usually form in urines with a pH of less than the dissociation constant for uric acid (5.5), especially when there are absolute increases in uric acid (hyperuricosuria). Thus, the amount of urinary free uric acid is increased. Uric acid stones often occur in primary gout, which may be accompanied by low urinary pH and hyperuricosuria (Ch. 183), or in secondary causes of purine overproduction, such as myeloproliferative states, glycogen storage disease, and malignancy. Chronic diarrheal syndromes (ulcerative colitis, regional enteritis, jejunoileal bypass surgery) may cause uric acid stones by inducing net alkali deficit (thereby reducing urinary pH) and lowering urine volume (thereby augmenting urinary concentration of uric acid).

Most patients with uric acid stones do not have clinical gout, secondary purine overproduction, or diarrheal syndromes. Urinary pH is invariably low without dietary excess of animal proteins. Some of them may have asymptomatic hyperuricemia or family history of gouty arthritis and may also form calcium-containing stones. The term *gouty diathesis* has been used to describe this condition.

CYSTINURIA. A cystine kidney stone forms only in a patient with the genetic disorder cystinuria (Ch. 82). Other forms of aminoaciduria are not associated with the excretion of enough cystine to form stones. Cystinuria is characterized by a disturbance in renal and intestinal handling of lysine, arginine, ornithine, and cystine. Stone formation, occurring in a minority of patients with cystinuria, is the result of an excessive renal excretion of cystine and its low solubility in urine. Cystine solubility is pH dependent; at pH 5, 170 to 300 mg of cystine may be dissolved in each liter of urine, whereas at pH 7.5, 220 to 500 mg of cystine may go into the solution. Many patients with homozygous cystinuria who are prone to cystine stone formation excrete more than 250 mg of cystine per day.

INFECTION. Urinary tract infections with urea-splitting organisms may be associated with renal stones of struvite (magnesium ammonium phosphate) and varying amounts of calcium phosphate. Ammonia formed by enzymatic degradation of urea by bacterial urease undergoes hydration to form ammonium and hydroxyl ions. The resulting alkalinity of urine augments dissociation of phosphate to form more triphosphate ions and reduces the solubility of struvite. Thus, the urinary environment becomes supersaturated with respect to struvite. Although struvite stones may form de novo from infection alone, they may sometimes occur as a complication of other causes of renal calculi, such as hypercalciuria. The presence of a struvite stone is presumptive evidence for concurrent or previous urinary tract infection.

MISCELLANEOUS. A minority of patients (10 per cent) present with low urine volume (< 1 liter per day) without any of the previously mentioned causes. Habitual decreased drinking of fluids may have contributed to stone formation. It has been reported that oxalate exchange in peripheral red blood cells is significantly increased in patients with "idiopathic" calcium oxalate nephrolithiasis and that this disturbance may be corrected by treatment with thiazide or amiloride. The significance of this finding is uncertain, since intestinal absorption and renal excretion of oxalate (given without calcium) are normal, and urinary oxalate is not affected by thiazide in patients with absorptive or renal hypercalciuria.

RENAL STRUCTURAL ABNORMALITIES. Nephrolithiasis may also be found in association with *renal structural abnormalities*, such as ectopic kidney, polycystic kidney, and horseshoe kidney. In this situation, it is generally believed that stones, usually composed of struvite or calcium phosphate, form secondarily to urinary tract infection. Medullary sponge disease is often associated with calcareous renal calculi. There is no convincing evidence that the structural abnormality causes stone formation, since metabolic abnormalities (such as the three forms of hypercalciuria) are usually found in medullary sponge disease, in similar distribution to that of patients without this disease.

IDIOPATHIC STONE DIATHESIS. In less than 5 per cent of patients, no physiologic abnormality can be discerned. The cause for stone formation remains unknown.

CLINICAL MANIFESTATIONS

Patients with renal stones may be asymptomatic; may pass small, sandlike concretions with relatively little pain; or may experience severe symptoms from ureteral obstruction, localized trauma, or infection. Renal colic is the manifestation of ureteral spasm produced by the irritation of a stone and accompanying obstruction. Microscopic hematuria is almost invariably present; gross hematuria, even clots, may sometimes accompany renal colic. Pain may begin in the costovertebral angle or the flank and may migrate toward the groin; sometimes pain moves into, and may be most severe in, the testis or penis in the male. Pain may subside after the stone or clot has passed, but the process may take several hours, even days, if the stone is impacted or if ureteral swelling impedes migration. Women frequently report that the pain of renal colic is more severe than that of labor. Infection arising from stones may lead to fever, flank tenderness, dysuria, and frequency of urination.

DIAGNOSIS

INITIAL SCREEN. The first step in the diagnosis of the cause of a kidney stone is to secure the stone for analysis, if at all possible. The analysis should preferably be carried out by a crystallographic technique, which can sometimes reveal the sequence of stone formation from the central nidus to the periphery.

All patients with renal stones should have a carefully taken history, abdominal roentgenographic examination, urinalysis and culture, and a routine blood screen.

A positive family history of renal calculi suggests absorptive hypercalciuria or, more rarely, cystinuria, primary hyperoxaluria, or type I renal tubular acidosis. Absorptive hypercalciuria should be suspected in middle-aged white men who have a history of recurrent calcium-containing stones and a family history of renal stones. Renal hypercalciuria may be present in patients with a history of recurrent urinary tract infection, especially if the infection preceded the onset of the stone disease. A high-calcium diet may aggravate the stone disease in those with an intestinal hyperabsorption of calcium. Patients with gout may form stones of either uric acid or calcium oxalate. A history of chronic diarrhea, ileal disease, or intestinal surgery should arouse the suspicion of uric acid or calcium oxalate stones (enteric hyperoxaluria or hypocitraturic calcium nephrolithiasis). A high purine intake may cause hyperuricosuria and contribute to stone formation in hyperuricosuric calcium oxalate nephrolithiasis. Acetazolamide may impair renal acidification and cause formation of calcium phosphate stones. Excessive ingestion of vitamin D and

of oxalate-rich foods (such as spinach, nuts, and tea) may increase oxalate excretion.

Calcium-containing stones, struvite stones, and cystine stones are radiopaque. Uric acid stones and the rarely encountered xanthine and 2,8-dihydroxyadenine stones are radiolucent (see Ch. 184). A staghorn calculus suggests a cystine or struvite stone. Positive urine culture for *Proteus, Pseudomonas, Klebsiella,* or *Staphylococcus* in association with an alkaline urine indicates that the stone is probably struvite. On a routine blood screen, primary hyperparathyroidism is suggested by hypercalcemia and hypophosphatemia (Ch. 235); primary gout by hyperuricemia; and defective acidification by the electrolyte picture of hyperchloremic metabolic acidosis.

IN-DEPTH EVALUATION. The objective of in-depth evaluation, applicable particularly to those with recurrent calculi, is to discern the specific metabolic cause for the nephrolithiasis. It should include a measure of parathyroid function (serum immunoreactive PTH) and 24-hour urinary calcium, oxalate, uric acid, citrate, total volume, sodium, and pH (on random diets and on diets restricted with respect to calcium, sodium, and oxalate). Ideally, it should include a measure of renal tubular reabsorption and intestinal absorption of calcium (from urinary calcium levels during fasting and following excessive oral ingestion of calcium). Hypercalciuria should be defined with respect to the particular diet during which urinary calcium is determined as noted above. If the stone is not known to contain calcium, a qualitative test for urine cystine is indicated.

The nature of parathyroid function distinguishes the three forms of *hypercalciuria*. Primary hyperparathyroidism is suggested by parathyroid stimulation in the setting of hypercalcemia, absorptive hypercalciuria by normal or suppressed parathyroid function with normocalcemia and hypercalciuria, and renal hypercalciuria by parathyroid stimulation with normocalcemia and hypercalciuria. The fasting urinary calcium level is invariably increased in renal hypercalciuria and is frequently elevated in primary hyperparathyroidism, whereas it is typically normal in absorptive hypercalciuria. Intestinal calcium absorption is always increased in absorptive hypercalciuria and is often high in renal and resorptive hypercalciurias. Fasting hypercalciuria with normal parathyroid function is suggested by high fasting urinary calcium levels in the setting of normal levels of serum calcium and PTH.

In *enteric hyperoxaluria*, the urinary calcium level is typically low (< 100 mg per day) and the urinary oxalate level is high (often > 80 mg per day). Serum calcium and magnesium levels may be low, parathyroid function may be stimulated, metabolic acidosis may be present, and the urinary citrate level is low (< 320 mg per day). Hypocitraturia is also found in hypocitraturic calcium nephrolithiasis.

Urinary uric acid consistently exceeds 600 mg per day (and often > 750 to 800 mg per day), and pH is greater than 5.5 in *hyperuricosuric calcium oxalate nephrolithiasis.* Urinary pH is usually low (< 5.5) *in uric acid lithiasis* and high (> 7.5) in *struvite lithiasis.* Urine pH is high (> 6.9) in complete type I *renal tubular acidosis* and high normal or high (> 6) in the incomplete form.

TREATMENT

Kidney stones are heterogeneous in pathogenesis and not infrequently are manifestations of a generalized multisystem disorder. By and large, kidney stones cannot be treated medically in the sense of causing their dissolution. The goal of medical treatment is to stop growth or new formation of stones by correcting the specific underlying physicochemical and physiologic derangements. Stone prophylaxis often entails a prolonged program. It is particularly important, therefore, to ensure patient compliance, few complications, and reasonable costs.

GENERAL TREATMENT. The initial treatment program, applicable to all patients with renal calculi, consists of a high fluid intake to ensure a minimum urine volume of 2 liters per day. At least 3 liters of fluids should be drunk each day, distributed throughout the day. In general, any fluid (with the exception of milk and oxalate-rich tea in certain disorders to be enumerated) may be consumed. In patients with intestinal hyperabsorption of calcium, intake of dairy products and certain calcium-rich foods should be limited. Oxalate intake should be restricted in patients with calcium oxalate stones. An excessive dietary intake of sodium should be discouraged, since this may enhance calcium excretion. Urinary tract infection should be vigorously treated.

Activity of Stone Diathesis. As noted, as many as 5 per cent of the population may have a kidney stone at some time. Some patients, usually men, have a single calcium oxalate stone in middle life and are not subsequently affected. Clearly, it would not be wise to begin a lifetime program of pharmacologic intervention without some knowledge of the prognosis of the stone diathesis in the individual patient. In the absence of remediable disorders, such as primary hyperparathyroidism, it is often wise following a first stone episode to institute the general measures noted above and then to follow patients carefully to document whether new stones are forming or old stones are enlarging before more vigorous measures are instituted.

SPECIFIC MEDICAL TREATMENT. Specific programs may be required when the aforementioned conservative measures are ineffective in controlling stone formation and there is continued activity of stone diathesis.

Treatment of Hypercalciuria. The surgical removal of abnormal parathyroid tissue is clearly the treatment of choice for kidney stones secondary to the hypercalciuria of primary hyperparathyroidism. Following parathyroidectomy, serum 1,25-dihydroxyvitamin D levels, intestinal calcium absorption, and urinary calcium levels decline toward normal. Parathyroidectomy may also ameliorate the extrarenal manifestations of primary hyperparathyroidism, such as bone disease and peptic ulcer disease (Ch. 235). Similarly, the hypercalciuria of vitamin D excess, sarcoidosis, thyrotoxicosis, multiple myeloma, and malignancies may respond to specific therapies directed toward those systemic entities. The main problem is in the management of remaining forms of hypercalciuria. Several agents that have proved to be useful will be individually discussed.

Thiazides (and related compounds such as chlorthalidone) are unique among diuretics in their ability to augment the renal tubular reabsorption of calcium and therefore to reduce urinary calcium. At a dosage of hydrochlorothiazide of 50 mg once or twice a day, or an equivalent amount of related drugs, thiazides represent the treatment of choice for renal hypercalciuria. Thiazides correct the renal leak of calcium and thereby reverse the sequence of parathyroid hyperactivity, increased synthesis of 1,25-dihydroxyvitamin D, and enhanced absorption of intestinal calcium. The urinary saturations of calcium oxalate and calcium phosphate are reduced. Thiazides may be equally effective in the control of absorptive hypercalciuria, at least during the first 2 years of therapy. However, some patients may show an attenuation of the hypocalciuric response with chronic treatment. Moreover, thiazide therapy may cause hypokalemia and hypocitraturia. To overcome these problems, urinary calcium levels should be monitored, and potassium supplement (preferably as potassium citrate) should be provided.

Sodium cellulose phosphate (Calcibind) should be used only in patients with normophosphatemic absorptive hypercalciuria without bone disease in whom hypercalciuria cannot be controlled by dietary calcium restriction or by thiazide. When given orally, it forms a nonabsorbable complex with calcium that is then excreted in the feces. About 2.5 to 5 grams of this resin with each meal is sufficient to limit the amount of luminal calcium available for absorption and to restore normal urinary calcium levels. This reduces urinary saturation of calcium salts, particularly that of calcium phosphate, without overly stimulating parathyroid function or causing bone disease. Urinary oxalate may increase, because less calcium may be available intraluminally to complex oxalate, so that a moderate dietary restriction of oxalate is recommended. Oral magnesium supplementation should be provided, since this drug also binds magnesium. Sodium cellulose phosphate is contraindicated in primary hyperparathyroidism, in other states of excessive skeletal calcium mobilization, in renal hypercalciuria, in growing children or postmenopausal women, and in states of normal intestinal calcium absorption because it tends to stimulate parathyroid function and thereby produces or aggravates bone disease.

Orthophosphates, as neutral or alkaline soluble salts of sodium or potassium or both, are potentially absorbable from the intestinal tract, unlike sodium cellulose phosphate. When given orally (at a dosage of 1.5 to 2.0 grams of phosphorus per day in divided doses), they decrease urinary calcium and increase urinary phosphate levels. They reduce urinary saturation of calcium oxalate, although they may increase that of calcium phosphate. Moreover, urinary inhibitor activity may be increased, probably consequent to the increased renal excretion of inhibitors, such as pyrophosphate and citrate. Orthophosphates are optimally indicated in the management of renal phosphate leak because of the possibility that they may restore normal levels of serum 1,25-dihydroxyvitamin D and calcium absorption. Orthophosphates are contraindicated in moderate or severe hypercalcemia and in renal failure because of the danger of metastatic calcification and in urinary tract infection because of the danger of struvite or calcium phosphate stone formation.

Treatment of Enteric Hyperoxaluria. A limitation of dietary oxalate intake and potassium citrate therapy (to be discussed) may be helpful in lowering oxalate and increasing pH and citrate levels in urine, respectively. A high fluid intake is essential to overcome intestinal fluid loss. Oral administration of large amounts of calcium or magnesium has been recommended for the control of nephrolithiasis of enteric hyperoxaluria. Although urinary oxalate levels may decrease, the concurrent rise in urinary calcium may obviate the beneficial effect of this therapy in some patients. Cholestyramine does not generally cause a sustained reduction in oxalate excretion.

Treatment of Hyperuricosuric Calcium Nephrolithiasis. This form of hyperuricosuria usually results from a diet high in purine precursors of uric acid. It should therefore be subject to effective dietary therapy. Unfortunately, many patients cannot or do not choose to maintain this dietary restraint. Allopurinol, 300 mg per day orally, will produce normal or subnormal levels of urinary uric acid and thereby may inhibit urate-induced crystallization of calcium oxalate.

Treatment of Hypocitraturic Calcium Nephrolithiasis. In renal tubular acidosis (distal), sodium citrate or potassium citrate (60 to 120 mEq per day in divided doses) may augment citrate excretion (see Ch. 82 for details). In the absence of renal insufficiency, potassium citrate is preferable because it could reduce urinary calcium and correct potassium deficiency. In *chronic diarrheal states*, potassium citrate in a liquid form is recommended to allow for rapid absorption (60 to 120 mEq per day). Hypocitraturia is sometimes very severe and recalcitrant to alkali therapy. In *thiazide-induced hypocitraturia*, potassium citrate (30 to 40 mEq per day in two divided doses in a slow-release tablet form) is generally sufficient to correct both hypokalemia and hypocitraturia. In other causes of hypocitraturia, a sufficient dose of potassium citrate may be provided to restore normal urinary citrate levels. The efficacy of potassium citrate is shown in Figure 88–2.

Treatment of Uric Acid Stones. In uric acid diathesis, administration of potassium citrate may increase urinary pH and create an environment in which uric acid is more soluble. Moderate amounts of alkali (30 to 60 mEq of potassium citrate per day in divided doses), sufficient to raise urinary pH to a range of 6 to 6.5, may be effective in preventing formation of both uric acid and calcium stones. Sodium alkali, especially in high dosages, may cause formation of calcium stones. If hydration and alkali therapy are ineffective, allopurinol should be used to decrease uric acid stone formation. See the discussion in Ch. 183 on gout for more details.

Treatment of Cystinuria (see Ch. 82). If a high fluid intake and alkali therapy are ineffective in reducing cystine concentration below saturation of cystine, D-*penicillamine* (1 to 2 grams per day in divided doses) may be required. This compound reduces urinary cystine content by forming a more soluble mixed disulfide with cysteine. Unfortunately, penicillamine treatment may be complicated by serious side effects, including nephrotic syndrome, dermatitis, and pancytopenia. Alpha-mercaptopropionylglycine, which lowers urinary cystine by a similar mechanism, may be advantageous because of its apparent reduced toxicity.

Treatment of Struvite (Magnesium Ammonium Phosphate) Stones. If a longstanding effective control of infection with urea-splitting organisms can be achieved, there is some evidence that new struvite stone formation can be averted or some dissolution of existing stones may be achieved. Unfortunately, such a control is difficult to obtain with antibiotic therapy alone. It is difficult

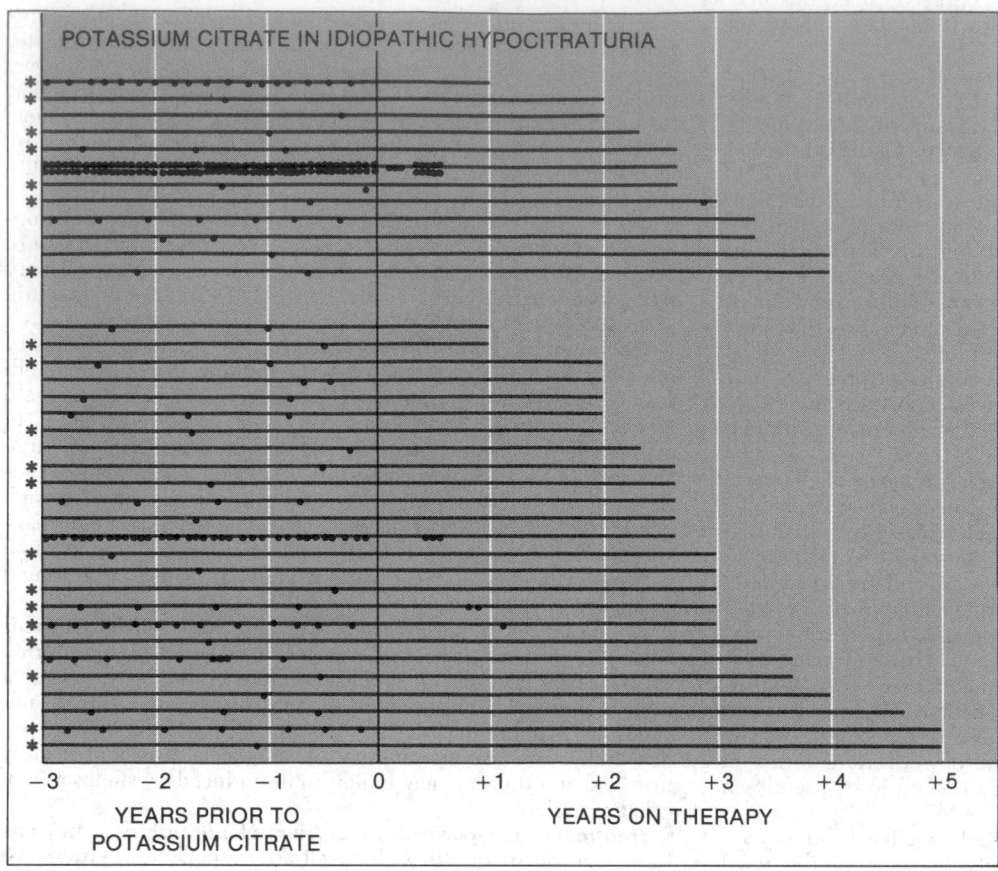

FIGURE 88–2. Effect of potassium citrate therapy on new stone formation. Each line represents one patient. An asterisk before the line indicates the presence of pre-existing stone(s). Each point shows new stone formation.

to eliminate the infection completely from an existing struvite stone because the stone often harbors the organisms within its interstices. Even if sterilization of urine is achieved by antibiotic therapy, reinfection often occurs from harbored organisms. Addition of acetohydroxamic acid, a urease inhibitor, at a dosage of 250 mg three times per day, may be more effective in controlling struvite stone formation. If not, surgical removal of stones should be considered.

Surgical Treatment

The goal of surgical treatment is removal of existing stones, whereas that of medical treatment is prevention of recurrent stone formation.

Removal of stones may become mandatory when nephrolithiasis is complicated by obstruction, infection, gross hematuria, or intractable pain. Dramatic progress has been made in techniques for stone removal. Certain stones may now be removed less invasively via percutaneous nephroscopy and by extracorporeal shock wave lithotripsy. The latter procedure, now widely introduced in the United States, utilizes focused, electrically generated shock waves to fragment stones within a human kidney without incision. Single stones of moderate size (≤ 1 cm in diameter) located in the renal pelvis are particularly amenable to this treatment. The risk of obstruction, pain, and retained fragments is higher for multiple stones and larger stones. Not all stones are amenable to shock wave lithotripsy alone (e.g., staghorn calculi and stones in lower ureter). The criteria for the choice of different methods are undergoing rapid refinement as further experience is gained with new approaches.

Coe FL: Nephrolithiasis: Pathogenesis and Treatment. Chicago, Year Book Medical Publishers, 1979. *A detailed review of current concepts of cause and treatment of calcareous as well as noncalcareous stones.*

Drach GW, Dretler S, Fair W, et al.: Report of the United States cooperative study of extracorporeal shock wave lithotripsy. J Urol 135:1127, 1986. *A review of results of extracorporeal shock wave lithotripsy among 2501 patients undergoing this procedure in the United States.*

Millman S, Strauss AL, Parks JH, et al.: Pathogenesis and clinical course of mixed calcium oxalate and uric acid nephrolithiasis. Kidney Int 22:366, 1982. *A useful review of the intriguing and important interactions of uric acid and oxalate in stone pathogenesis.*

Pak CYC: Ch. 1, 3–7, 9–12. *In* Resnick MI, Pak CYC (eds.): Nephrolithiasis. Philadelphia, W. B. Saunders Company, 1990. *A comprehensive discussion of the pathogenesis and treatment of renal calculi.*

Pak CYC: Citrate and renal calculi. Miner Electrolyte Metab 13:257, 1986. *A review of the utility of the use of potassium citrate in the management of renal calculi.*

Pak CYC, Britton F, Peterson R, et al.: Ambulatory evaluation of nephrolithiasis: Classification, clinical presentation and diagnostic criteria. Am J Med 69:19, 1980. *A detailed description of the outpatient protocol that provides diagnostic criteria for different causes of nephrolithiasis.*

89 Cystic Disease of the Kidney

Patricia A. Gabow

Renal cystic diseases are characterized by epithelium-lined cavities filled with fluid or semisolid debris within the kidneys. The cysts may be single or multiple, inherited or acquired, occurring in infancy or old age, clinically silent or symptomatic, producing renal insufficiency. This discussion focuses on simple cysts, polycystic kidney disease, acquired cystic disease, and medullary cystic disorders.

Certain clinical settings suggest specific cystic disorders (Fig. 89–1 and Table 89–1). An abdominal mass in a neonate or infant should raise the consideration of either autosomal dominant (ADPKD) or recessive polycystic kidney disease (ARPKD). Renal failure in adolescence suggests ARPKD or medullary cystic disease. The finding of a solitary cyst in a 50-year-old person is most compatible with a simple cyst. A history of renal disease in a family raises the possibility of ADPKD, ARPKD, or medullary cystic disease. Recurrent renal stones can occur in ADPKD or medullary sponge kidneys. The onset of gross hematuria in a patient undergoing chronic hemodialysis raises the possibility of acquired cystic disease.

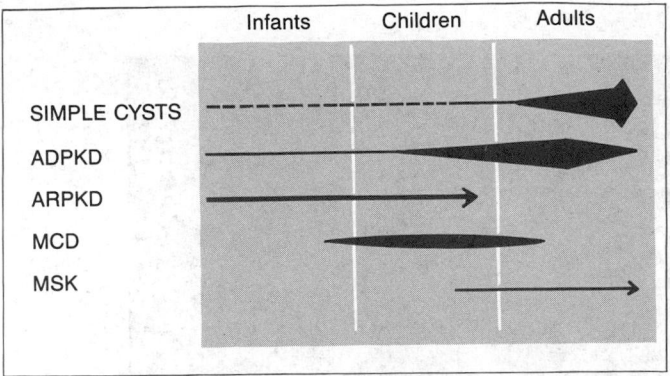

FIGURE 89–1. Ages of renal cystic disease patients.

SIMPLE CYSTS

Simple renal cysts, the most common and clinically least significant of all the cystic disorders, increase in frequency with age from 0.1 to 4 per cent in children to 50 per cent of the population over 50 years of age. Often simple cysts are asymptomatic and an incidental finding during abdominal imaging studies. Occasionally, patients with simple cysts present with hematuria or flank pain, thereby raising the question of malignancy within the cyst. With renal ultrasonography, a simple cyst demonstrates smooth walls, good sound transmission, and no intracystic debris. If the ultrasonographic pattern differs from this, computed tomography (CT) should be performed. Information from the two modalities should permit accurate differentiation of benign from malignant lesions in almost all cases. The CT scan has obviated cyst puncture for diagnosis. Occasionally, simple cysts with benign characteristics cause pain or are associated with renin-dependent hypertension. Such cysts can be punctured with ultrasonographic guidance, drained, and sclerosed with instillation of alcohol into the cyst. For another discussion of renal masses, see also Ch. 91.

Bosniak M: The current radiological approach to renal cysts. Radiology 158:1, 1986. *A comprehensive review of the subject.*

Ozgur S, Cetin S, Ilker Y: Percutaneous renal cyst aspiration and treatment with alcohol. Int Urol Nephrol 20:481, 1988. *A discussion of the role of sclerotherapy of simple cysts.*

POLYCYSTIC KIDNEY DISEASE

Polycystic kidney disease includes ADPKD and ARPKD, which were previously labeled adult polycystic kidney disease and infantile or childhood polycystic kidney disease, respectively.

Since ADPKD can be detected in childhood or even in infancy or in utero, the pattern of inheritance rather than age of onset distinguishes these disorders.

Autosomal Dominant Polycystic Kidney Disease (ADPKD)

ADPKD has a worldwide prevalence of 1 in 200 to 1 in 1000. It is the most common hereditary disease in the United States, affecting 500,000 people. The clinical disorder can be caused by at least two different genes. The most common type, ADPKD1, is carried on chromosome 16. The location of the other gene has not been determined. Complete penetrance of the gene is estimated to occur by 90 years of age. The gene defect produces a systemic disease with cysts in the kidneys and other organs, most commonly in the liver, and occasionally in the pancreas and ovaries and with frequent structural abnormalities in the gastrointestinal tract, the vascular tree, and the cardiac valves.

PATHOGENESIS AND PATHOLOGY. The pathogenesis of ADPKD has not been established. However, altered epithelial cell growth, secretion, and extracellular matrix have all been shown to occur in ADPKD. These abnormalities could, in fact, contribute to cyst development and extrarenal manifestations. Cells are not simply stretched to permit a tubular outpouching to become a cyst; cell numbers must increase. With electron microscopy, polypoid lesions have been noted throughout the cyst walls in both experimental cystic disease and human ADPKD.

The hyperplasia, exemplified by the polyps, illustrates the altered growth that is present in ADPKD. Fluid secretion must also be altered to form a cyst; altered growth without secretion would result in adenomas rather than cysts. The basement membrane also appears abnormal in cell culture systems of human ADPKD renal cyst epithelium. In fact, a primary or secondary disorder of extracellular matrix formation—e.g., basement membrane and other collagen types—offers the best current pathogenetic explanation for the extrarenal manifestations. Thus, studies of cyst epithelium suggest that the genetic defect either directly or indirectly alters cell growth, secretion, and/or matrix formation.

CLINICAL MANIFESTATIONS. Patients usually present either for screening because of a family history of the disease or for evaluation of symptoms. Pain and hematuria are the most common clinical manifestations. Flank pain and back pain are common and can be constant or intermittent, mild or severe and disabling. Both microscopic hematuria and gross hematuria occur. One third of patients have microscopic hematuria on a random

TABLE 89–1. CHARACTERISTICS OF RENAL CYSTIC DISORDERS

Feature	Simple Cysts	ADPKD	ARPKD	ACKD	MCD	MSK
Inheritance pattern	None	Autosomal dominant	Autosomal recessive	None	Often present, variable pattern	None
Incidence or prevalence	Common, increasing with age	1/200 to 1/1000	Rare	40% in dialysis patients	Rare	Common
Age of onset	Adult	Usually adults	Neonates, children	Older adults	Adolescents, young adults	Adults
Presenting symptom	Incidental finding, hematuria	Pain, hematuria, infection, family screening	Abdominal mass, renal failure, failure to thrive	Hematuria	Polyuria, polydipsia, enuresis, renal failure, failure to thrive	Incidental, urinary tract infections, hematuria, renal calculi
Hematuria	Occurs	Common	Occurs	Occurs	Rare	Common
Recurrent infections	Rare	Common	Occurs	No	Rare	Common
Renal calculi	No	Common	No	No	No	Common
Hypertension	Rare	Common	Common	Present from underlying disease	Rare	No
Method of diagnosis	Ultrasound	Ultrasound, gene linkage analysis	Ultrasound	CT scan	None reliable	Excretory urogram
Renal size	Normal	Normal to very large	Large initially	Small to normal, occasionally large	Small	Normal

ADPKD = autosomal dominant polycystic kidney disease; ARPKD = autosomal recessive polycystic kidney disease; ACKD = acquired cystic kidney disease; MCD = medullary cystic disease; MSK = medullary sponge kidney.

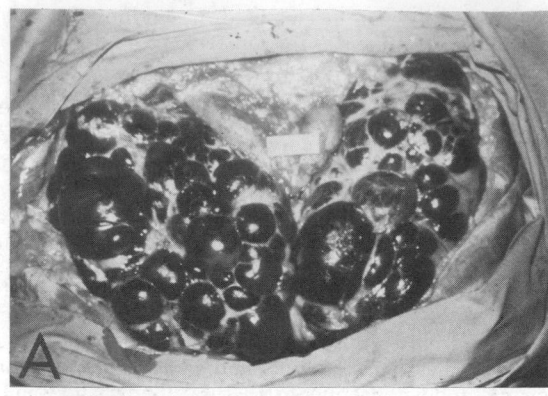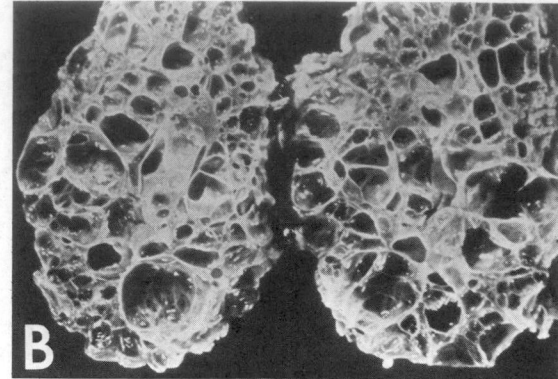

FIGURE 89–2. Autosomal dominant polycystic kidney disease (ADPKD) in situ *(A)* and on cut section *(B)*. Note diffuse, bilateral distribution of cysts. (Courtesy of F. E. Cuppage, Kansas City, Kan.; from Brenner BM, Rector FC Jr [eds.]: The Kidney. 3rd ed. Philadelphia, W. B. Saunders Company, 1986, p 1346.)

urinalysis, and a similar percentage have at least one episode of gross hematuria. Some patients present with complications, such as urinary tract infections, renal calculi, or retroperitoneal bleeding. Early in the course of ADPKD, the kidneys can be normal in size with only a few cysts. Ultimately, the kidneys enlarge and may attain the size of a football, weighing as much as 8 kg. The end-stage kidney appears to be virtually replaced by cysts throughout the renal parenchyma (Figs. 89–2 and 89–3).

The extrarenal manifestations of ADPKD are detailed in Table 89–2. The most common is hepatic cysts, which occur in 40 to 60 per cent of patients. Like renal cysts, hepatic cysts increase in number and/or size over time; however, unlike renal cysts,

hepatic cysts rarely occur before puberty, appear to increase in size and number from pregnancy, and very rarely produce functional impairment. Hepatic cysts can also become infected. Colonic diverticulosis appears to be another clinically important gastrointestinal manifestation and may be complicated by perforation and intra-abdominal abscess.

Hypertension, the most common cardiovascular manifestation of ADPKD, occurs in 60 per cent of patients before the onset of renal insufficiency. The hypertension appears to be related to the renin-angiotensin system. Intracranial aneurysms occur in 10 to 40 per cent of patients with ADPKD. Rarely, a subarachnoid hemorrhage is the presenting manifestation of ADPKD. Cardiac valve abnormalities are common; 26 per cent of all patients with ADPKD have mitral valve prolapse, often accompanied by palpitations and atypical chest pain. Myxomatous degeneration occurs in some patients and may require valve replacement.

As might be expected in a disorder with altered cell growth, renal adenomas are common, but it is not certain whether renal cell carcinoma is more common in ADPKD than in the general population. However, malignancy may present with asymmetric renal enlargement, increasing frequency or amount of hematuria, and weight loss; the frequency of these symptoms, as well as the underlying structural abnormalities in the kidney, often make the diagnosis of renal malignancy difficult in patients with ADPKD.

The natural history of renal functional impairment with ADPKD is variable. Renal failure may occur as early as the first decade of life, or renal function may be well maintained into the eighth decade. End-stage renal disease rarely occurs before 40 years of age. Approximately 50 per cent of patients have well-preserved renal function at 70 years of age. Renal function is less well maintained in ADPKD patients with hypertension. Other factors that influence long-term prognosis are less well defined.

DIAGNOSIS. The method of diagnosing ADPKD depends upon the level of certainty needed, the patient's symptoms, and the need for anatomic information (Table 89–3). A screening algorithm utilizing blood pressure, serum creatinine concentra-

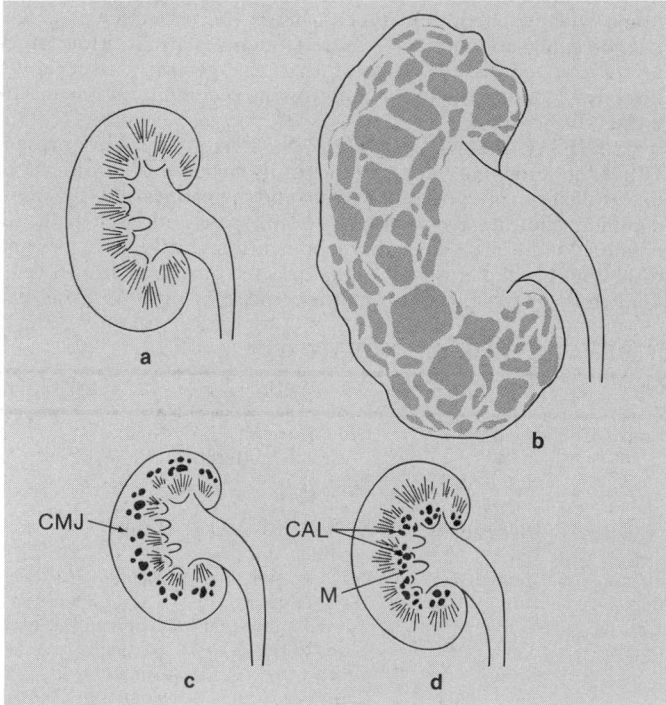

FIGURE 89–3. Schematic drawing of a cut section of *(a)* a normal kidney, measuring 12 cm with normal papilla, cortex, medulla, and corticomedullary junction, and *(b)* a kidney from a patient with ADPKD. The kidney is large, measuring 29 cm, and contains cysts throughout the cortex and medulla, which vary in size from 1 mm to 5 cm. *c,* A kidney from a patient with medullary cystic disease. The kidney is small, measuring 8 cm with a scarred surface. The cysts are at the corticomedullary junction (CMJ) and are small, measuring 1 to 5 mm across. *d,* A kidney from a patient with medullary sponge kidney; these are multiple ductal dilations measuring 1 to 5 mm in diameter, giving the medulla (M) a porous appearance. Some dilations contain calculi (CAL). (*c* and *d* from Spence HM, Singleton R: What is sponge kidney disease and where does it fit in the spectrum of cystic disorders? J Urol 107:176, © by Williams & Wilkins, 1972.)

TABLE 89–2. SYSTEMIC INVOLVEMENT IN AUTOSOMAL DOMINANT POLYCYSTIC KIDNEY DISEASE (ADPKD)

I. **Genitourinary**
    Polycystic kidney
    Renal adenoma/hypernephroma
    Renal calculi
    Ovarian cysts
II. **Gastrointestinal**
    Hepatic cysts
    Pancreatic cysts
    Diverticula
III. **Cardiovascular**
    Hypertension
    Cardiac valvular abnormalities
    Intracranial aneurysms
IV. **Musculoskeletal**
    Hernia formation

TABLE 89–3. METHODS OF DIAGNOSIS IN ADPKD

Method	Limitation
Renal concentrating ability in algorithm	Untested in children No anatomic information
Ultrasonography	May miss 2–6% of patients with cysts Highly operator and reader dependent Will not identify precystic gene carriers May miss rare patient with small cysts
CT scan	Radiation and contrast exposure Difficult to perform in children Expense Will not identify precystic gene carriers
Gene linkage analysis	Requires other family members to participate Requires that physician understand interpretation of results Expense Provides no anatomic information on organs involved

From Gabow PA: Autosomal dominant polycystic kidney disease—more than a renal disease. Am J Kidney Dis 16:403–413, 1990.

tion, and renal concentrating ability is inexpensive and easy but is the least reliable method. Imaging studies depend upon detectable cysts. The demonstration of the characteristic bilateral renal cystic involvement is best accomplished by renal ultrasonography. Occasionally, in children or young adults screening studies demonstrate only a few cysts in one or both kidneys. In adults, CT scan with contrast medium occasionally reveals more cystic involvement than is apparent by ultrasonography. Nonetheless, imaging studies that reveal only a few cysts require differentiation of early ADPKD from multiple simple cysts (Table 89–4). The patient's age and the presence of extrarenal involvement are helpful in this instance (Fig. 89–1). Since simple cysts are uncommon in children, the finding of any cysts in a child in an ADPKD family strongly suggests the disorder. However, in an individual over age 50 with similar ultrasonographic findings, the diagnosis is much less certain. The presence of extrarenal involvement, particularly hepatic cysts, lends support to the diagnosis of ADPKD. The information on gene location now permits identification of presymptomatic carriers of ADPKD1 through gene linkage analysis. If there is a need for definitive diagnosis, this technique can be utilized in many families and can predict gene status with 99:1 likelihood. As gene linkage is expensive, requires the cooperation of other family members, and supplies no anatomic information, it is probably best reserved for patients with nondiagnostic imaging studies.

It is not necessary to establish the presence of extrarenal involvement in all patients with ADPKD. Currently, total abdominal ultrasonography for detection of extrarenal cysts, echocardiography for diagnosis of cardiac valve lesions, carotid angiography, and CT scan of the head in search of intracranial aneurysm are not recommended in ADPKD patients without specific clinical indications.

TREATMENT. The treatment for patients with ADPKD is aimed at preventing complications of the disease and preserving renal function. Patients and family members should be educated about the inheritance and manifestations of the disease. Episodes of gross hematuria should be managed conservatively with bed rest, analgesics, and hydration. Urinary tract instrumentation, including Foley catheter placement, should be avoided because of the increased risk of serious urinary tract and renal cyst infections. Patients suspected of having a urinary tract infection should have urine and blood cultures. Selection of antibiotic therapy depends upon the presumed site of infection. Bladder and renal parenchymal infections can be treated as they are in other patients. Failure to respond to appropriate antibiotic treatment suggests cyst infections. In this instance, the antibiotic must be one that enters cyst fluid. These agents include chloramphenicol, trimethoprim-sulfamethoxazole, and ciprofloxacin.

Hypertension should be aggressively treated. The role of phosphorus and/or protein restriction or of cyst decompression in the preservation of renal function has not yet been established in ADPKD. Repeat imaging studies need not be performed unless new clinical symptoms occur. CT scan is the method of choice for establishing the diagnosis of complications, such as intracystic or retroperitoneal hemorrhage, renal calculi, or renal

malignancy. A serum creatinine analysis should be performed yearly prior to the development of renal insufficiency and at least every 6 months thereafter. Patients with ADPKD and renal failure respond as well as patients with other renal disease to renal replacement therapy. A more general discussion of the treatment of renal failure is found in Ch. 78.

Chapman AB, Johnson A, Gabow PA, et al.: The renin-angiotensin-aldosterone system and autosomal dominant polycystic kidney disease. N Engl J Med 323:1091, 1990. *A study of mechanisms of hypertension in ADPKD.*

Gabow PA: ADPKD—more than a renal disease, Am J Kidney Dis 16:403, 1990. *A review of both renal and extrarenal manifestations of ADPKD.*

Gabow PA, Johnson AM, Kaehny WD, et al.: Risk factors for the development of hepatic cysts in autosomal dominant polycystic kidney disease. Hepatology 11:1033, 1990. *A comprehensive study of the correlates of hepatic cysts in ADPKD.*

Gardner KD, Bernstein J (eds.): The Cystic Kidney. Dordrecht, Kluaer Academic Publishers, 1990. *This comprehensive book addresses the genetic, clinical, and pathogenetic aspects of all types of cystic disease.*

Reeders ST, Germino GG, Gillespie GAJ: Recent advances in the genetics of renal cystic disease. Mol Biol Med 6:81, 1989. *A review of human genetic data in ADPKD and experimental genetic data as they relate to pathophysiology of disease.*

Autosomal Recessive Polycystic Kidney Disease (ARPKD)

ARPKD is a rare disorder that has been classified as perinatal, neonatal, infantile, and juvenile types based on age of onset. The presenting manifestations include abdominal masses, failure to thrive, or urinary tract infections. The pathogenic mechanism is not understood. The kidneys are large early in life and may diminish in size with time. The cut surface of the kidney reveals radially oriented fusiform cysts. As in ADPKD, ultrasonography is the diagnostic method of choice. Examination of the parents and in some instances liver biopsy of the affected child are necessary to distinguish ARPKD from the childhood presentation of ADPKD. Normal renal ultrasonography in the parents strongly suggests ARPKD. In addition, children with ARPKD, particularly the juvenile form, often have hepatic fibrosis, frequently resulting in portal hypertension. As with other forms of renal disease, aggressive early treatment of hypertension may be important in the preservation of renal function. Children with ARPKD usually progress to end-stage renal disease before adolescence; in the perinatal form, this occurs within the first few weeks of life. Treatment of the chronic renal failure of ADPKD is similar to that for other childhood renal diseases.

Kaariainen H: Polycystic kidney disease in children: A genetic and epidemiological study of 82 Finnish patients. J Med Genet 24:474, 1987. *A review of presentation of both ADPKD and ARPKD in a population.*

TABLE 89–4. COMPARISON OF MULTIPLE SIMPLE CYSTS AND EARLY ADPKD

Feature	Multiple Simple Cysts	ADPKD
Family history	No	60%
Ultrasonographically demonstrable cysts in other family member(s)	No	90%
Sex distribution	M > F	M = F
Renal size	Normal	Normal to mildly enlarged
Kidneys involved	Usually unilateral, may be bilateral	Usually bilateral, may be unilateral early
Cyst distribution	Cortical	Cortical and medullary
Cyst size	Usually <2 cm, occasionally larger	<2 cm early
Blood in cysts	Rare	Common
Hepatic cysts	No	40–60%; likelihood increases with age
Intracranial aneurysm	No	10–40%
Mitral valve prolapse	No	26%
Hypertension	Rare	60%
Gene linkage analysis for chromosome 16	No	Likely

ACQUIRED CYSTIC KIDNEY DISEASE (ACKD)

Acquired cystic disease refers to the development of cysts in previously noncystic kidneys in patients with end-stage renal disease, almost exclusively in those undergoing dialysis. Reported frequencies range from 40 to almost 100 per cent, increasing with the years of dialysis. Although most patients have no symptoms from the cysts, others develop bleeding, which can be retroperitoneal, intrarenal, or into the pelvocaliceal system with resulting hematuria. Renal tumors, most commonly adenomas, but occasionally carcinomas, complicate this disorder. Although the diagnosis can be established with ultrasonography, CT scan is the diagnostic method of choice in ACKD because the kidneys and cysts are often small. Episodes of hematuria can be treated as in ADPKD. Severe, recurrent hematuria can be treated with renal arterial embolization, as it is not critical to preserve renal parenchyma in patients on dialysis. Renal tumors less than 3 cm in diameter can be followed with a yearly CT scan; larger tumors require surgery because of their greater propensity for malignancy.

Matson MA, Cohen EP: Acquired cystic kidney disease: Occurrence, prevalence, and renal carriers. Medicine 69:217, 1990. *A comprehensive review of the subject.*

MEDULLARY CYSTIC DISORDERS

Medullary cystic disease and medullary sponge kidney are the most common of the medullary cystic disorders. Medullary cystic disease has also been labeled nephronophthisis, cystic medullary complex, and renal-retinal dysplasia (because of the coincidence of retinitis pigmentosa in some families). Medullary cystic disease is uncommon; only about 300 cases have been reported. A familial pattern appears to be present in a majority of cases. Both the autosomal recessive and dominant forms of inheritance occur. Recessive transmission appears more common in the childhood presentation, and dominant inheritance is more frequent with the adult presentation.

PATHOGENESIS AND PATHOLOGY. No pathogenetic theory has been defined. The kidneys are small and generally display some cysts at the corticomedullary junction and in the medulla (Fig. 89–3). An acystic form of the disorder appears to occur. The glomeruli are hyalinized, and the tubules vary in appearance, from atrophic to tortuous. The tubular basement membrane is often irregular, with some areas thickened and others thinned and split; in addition, the composition of the tubular basement membrane appears abnormal. The interstitium reveals fibrosis and mononuclear cell infiltrate. This interstitial involvement suggests some as yet undefined relationship with other immune and nonimmune tubulointerstitial disease. It has been postulated that medullary cystic disease may be the end stage of other tubulointerstitial disease.

CLINICAL MANIFESTATIONS AND DIAGNOSIS. A majority of patients present in childhood or early adolescence with polydipsia, polyuria, and enuresis; this constellation presumably reflects a defect in urinary concentrating ability and secondary polydipsia. Often the children demonstrate growth retardation and anemia.

It has been suggested that renal salt wasting occurs in the disorder in excess of the impaired sodium conservation that accompanies any end-stage renal disease. The possibility of salt wasting should be considered prior to sodium restriction.

Diagnosis of the disorder is often difficult. The urinalysis is frequently unremarkable, and proteinuria is generally minimal. Imaging studies reveal only small end-stage kidneys. The disease in some patients is simply labeled "chronic renal failure" or "chronic pyelonephritis." The disorder should be considered in children or young adults who present with renal insufficiency, small kidneys, and a family history of renal disease. No specific treatment exists. Management is that appropriate for any child with renal insufficiency, with attention to growth, to bone disease, and in particular to sodium balance. The possibility of retinal abnormality must also be considered in the initial evaluation.

Cohen AH, Hoyer JR: Nephronophthisis: A primary tubular basement membrane defect. Lab Invest 55:564, 1986. *Data supporting abnormal basement membrane composition are presented.*

Helczyski L, Landing BH: Tubulointerstitial renal diseases of children: Pathologic

features and pathogenetic mechanisms of Fanconi's familial nephronophthisis, antitubular basement membrane antibody disease, and medullary cyst disease. Pediatr Pathol 2:1, 1984.

Chapman AB, Johnson A, Gabow PA, et al.: The renin-angiotensin-aldosterone system and autosomal dominant polycystic kidney disease. N Engl J Med 323:1091, 1990. *A review of both renal and extrarenal manifestations of ADPKD.*

MEDULLARY SPONGE KIDNEY

Medullary sponge kidney is a relatively common disorder, affecting between 1 in 5000 and 1 in 20,000 individuals. There is no known pathogenetic mechanism. Tubular dilatations occur within the medullary collecting ducts (Fig. 89–3). Patients present with recurrent hematuria, urinary tract infections, or renal calculi. The diagnosis is established with excretory urography, which reveals normal-sized kidneys with medullary ductal ectasia. The appearance on excretory urogram has been described as a "bouquet of flowers" or a "paintbrush." Often a plain film of the abdomen reveals renal calculi or calcification in the cystic areas. For this reason, other causes of nephrolithiasis and nephrocalcinosis need to be considered. Coincident hyperparathyroidism is common in medullary sponge kidney, and therefore both serum calcium and 24-hour urinary calcium determinations should be obtained and, if indicated, a serum parathyroid hormone level (Ch. 235). Conversely, as many as 20 per cent of patients presenting with nephrolithiasis may have medullary sponge kidney. Other clinical manifestations of medullary sponge kidney reflect the structural alterations in the renal papillae, with a consequent decreased renal concentrating ability, impaired acidification with an incomplete renal tubular acidosis, and an impairment in renal potassium excretion in response to acute potassium loading. Despite these defects, serum electrolyte concentrations are almost always normal. Treatment includes appropriate management of renal infections and renal calculus disease (Ch. 88). Urinary tract obstruction must be considered during acute episodes of renal colic. In the absence of obstruction, renal function remains normal.

Green J, Szylman P, Sznajder II, et al.: Renal tubular handling of potassium in patients with medullary sponge kidney. Arch Intern Med 144:2201, 1984. *Presentation of renal tubular defects in medullary sponge kidney.*

Morris RC, Yamaughi H, Palubinskas AJ, et al.: Medullary sponge kidney. Am J Med 38:883, 1965. *Twenty patients with medullary sponge kidney and some related abnormalities are discussed.*

Parks JH, Coe FL, Strauss AL: Calcium nephrolithiasis and medullary sponge kidney in women. N Engl J Med 306:1088, 1982.

Zawada ET Jr, Sica DA: Differential diagnosis of medullary sponge kidney. South Med J 77:686, 1984. *Differential diagnosis—a case report with excretory urography.*

90 Anomalies of the Urinary Tract

Richard D. Williams

Congenital aberrations of the urinary tract occur in more than 10 per cent of the population. They vary in severity from lesions incompatible with life to those that are insignificant and detected only incidentally during studies prompted by unrelated causes. Often the anomalies, although not intrinsically detrimental, predispose to infection, lithiasis, and chronic renal failure, which lead to their recognition.

KIDNEY

ANOMALIES OF NUMBER. *Bilateral renal agenesis* is rare (1 in 4800 births), more frequent in males (3:1 ratio), and typically accompanied by oligohydramnios, Potter's facies, and pulmonary hypoplasia; this complex results in death within a few days of birth. *Unilateral renal agenesis* is more common (1 in 1100 births), generally involves the left kidney, and is seen more often in males (ratio 1.8:1). Renal absence is considered secondary to lack of a ureteral bud. Occasionally, a presumptive diagnosis of unilateral renal absence may be made in males when an ipsilateral vas deferens is absent on palpation. In only 10 per cent of renal agenesis cases is the adrenal absent. Extrarenal tissue or *supernumerary kidneys* are extremely rare (no more than 66 cases have been described); they are distinct from ureteral and caliceal duplication, to be described further on.

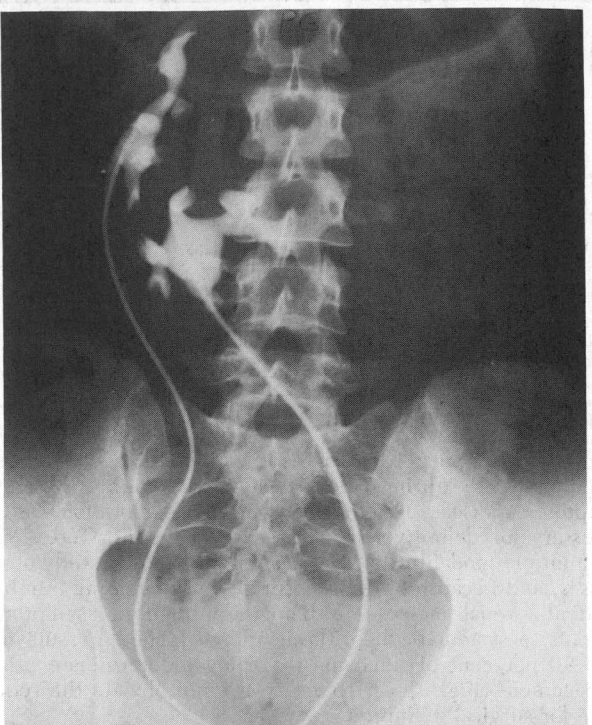

FIGURE 90–1. Bilateral retrograde ureteropyelogram of crossed renal ectopia.

ANOMALIES OF POSITION (ECTOPIA). These are due to abnormal renal ascent: They include lumbar and pelvic and the less common thoracic or crossed ectopic varieties (Fig. 90–1). As a group they occur in 1 in 900 cases and reach clinical significance only when they are mistaken for tumor during exploratory surgery or because of associated genital anomalies. Anomalies of fusion fall into this same category, since the abnormality leads to lack of ascent; *fused pelvic kidneys* or *horseshoe kidneys* (typically fused at their lower poles) are prevented from normal ascent by the inferior mesenteric artery (Fig. 90–2). These latter two anomalies are associated with recurrent infection and calculi in 10 to 20 per cent of patients and with a 30 per cent incidence of ureteropelvic junction obstruction. *Nephroptosis* is the descent toward the pelvis of a normally ascended kidney when the upright posture is assumed; it is seen in adults and is perhaps due to poor renal fixation in the retroperitoneum. This condition, which is not an anomaly per se, is usually asymptomatic and does not require surgical correction. Anomalies of rotation, commonly termed *malrotation*, are due to incomplete ventromedial rotation during ascent and are rarely related to any functional abnormality.

ANOMALIES OF THE RENAL PARENCHYMA. There is a heterogeneous group of cystic and dysplastic lesions of the kidney. The most important group of disorders comprises those that produce cystic abnormalities, described in detail in Ch. 89. *Renal dysplasia* occurs in several forms: (1) *Multicystic kidneys* are malformed, nonfunctioning, generally unilateral, and invariably associated with ipsilateral ureteral atresia. When both kidneys are involved, the manifestations and prognosis are similar to those in patients with bilateral renal agenesis. (2) *Segmental dysplasia* or *hypoplasia* is rare; it is not usually associated with significant renal complications, except in the bilateral and generalized form. (3) *Total renal dysplasia* is associated with lower urinary tract obstruction, such as *posterior urethral valves* or functional bladder outlet obstruction, as in the "*prune-belly*" syndrome.

RENAL VASCULATURE

Multiple renal arteries occur in 15 to 20 per cent of the population. They are of little significance, except when they are inadvertently injured during an operation or (rarely) when they cause caliceal infundibular obstruction or (more often) *ureteropelvic junction obstruction*. *Congenital renal artery aneurysms* are infrequent; they are differentiated from acquired lesions by their location at the bifurcation of the main renal artery or at a distal branch point. The lesions require surgical treatment only if resulting hypertension is uncontrolled or if they are calcified and/or have a diameter of more than 2.5 cm. *Congenital arteriovenous fistulas* are rare but may result in hematuria, hypertension, and/or cardiac failure (if large), necessitating surgical intervention.

COLLECTING STRUCTURES AND URETER

Caliceal anomalies include *diverticuli, hydrocalycosis, megacalycosis,* and *infundibular stenosis.* They are clinically important only when urinary stasis results in recurrent infection and/or stone formation. *Ureteropelvic junction obstruction* is one of the more frequent causes of hydronephrosis in childhood. Bilaterality is not unusual, and the condition is often asymptomatic; however, flank pain (particularly following diuresis), urinary infection, and gross hematuria (following minor trauma) are frequent findings on presentation. Relief of symptoms as a rule follows surgical repair (pyeloplasty), although normalization of the radiologic abnormality is infrequent.

Ureteral duplication is the most common ureteral anomaly; it may be incomplete, with the duplicated ureters combining to form only one entrance per side into the bladder, or complete, with two or more ureters coursing toward the bladder on one or both sides (Fig. 90–3). Most often, completely duplicated ureters enter the bladder. The ureter from the upper pole is always placed inferior in the bladder to that of the lower pole ureter and often drains in an ectopic site, such as the bladder neck, prostate, or seminal vesicle in the male or mid-urethra in the female, resulting in obstruction and hydroureteronephrosis. The ureter from the lower pole often obtains poor implantation within the bladder, which may result in vesicoureteral reflux and possibly recurrent infection and hydroureteronephrosis. Ureteral ectopia can also occur in the absence of duplication but results in similar sequelae.

Ureteral reflux can be unrelated to duplication but may instead be due to an abnormal implantation of the ureter into the bladder, with a resulting poorly developed trigone and deficient lower ureteral muscle. This condition can cause recurrent urinary infection in children; however, surgical reimplantation is necessary only in severe cases, while newer transurethral injection methods may be sufficient in milder forms. Other ureteral anomalies include *ureterocele,* a congenital distal ureteral meatal stenosis; *megaloureter,* an abnormality of the ureteral musculature allowing massive ureteral dilatation, often without caliceal distortion; *ureteral valves; ureteral diverticuli;* and *retrocaval ureter,* an anomaly of the formation of the vena cava causing the ureter to course behind the cava.

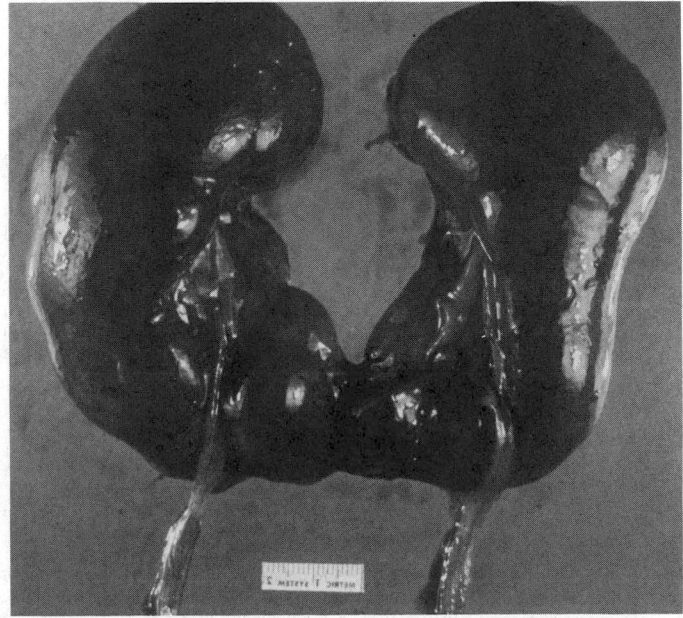

FIGURE 90–2. Gross pathologic specimen of horseshoe kidneys.

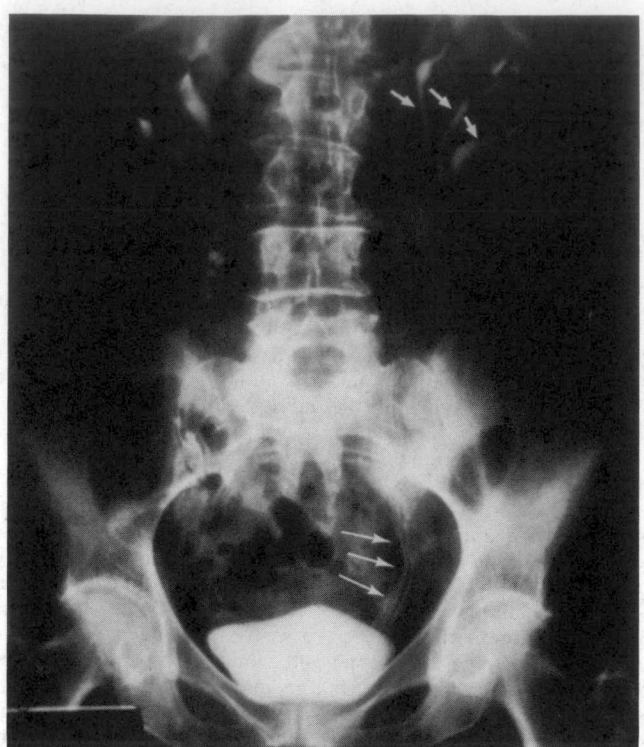

FIGURE 90-3. Intravenous urogram showing right ureteral triplication *(arrows)*. (Courtesy of John Dyhrberg, M.D., Portland, Maine.)

BLADDER

Anomalies of the bladder are very infrequent and include (1) *complete absence* (agenesis), which results in a persistent cloaca; (2) *duplication*, which may be complete with separate ureteral openings drained by separate urethras, or incomplete with a septum or hour-glass deformity; (3) *urachal* anomalies, which may appear as a patent connection to the umbilicus, a *diverticulum* at the dome of the bladder, or a *urachal cyst* along the course of the partially obliterated urachus; and (4) *exstrophy*, which is the most common severe anomaly of the bladder. Exstrophy represents a midline defect in closure of the bladder wall, lower abdominal muscles, pubic bones, and anterior urethra *(epispadias)*. The *"prune-belly" syndrome* is a complex anomaly in which absence of the abdominal muscles is associated with bilateral cryptorchidism, ureteral dilatation and reflux, and an irregular, capacious bladder with a dilated proximal urethra.

URETHRA

Hypospadias is the most common urethral anomaly in males (1 in 300 live births). The lesion results from failure of ventral fusion of the urogenital folds. It may present as a ventrally displaced meatus on the distal penile shaft or, in more severe forms, with the meatus opening more proximal on the shaft or in the perineum. These latter forms are often associated with a ventral penile chordee. Isolated *epispadias* (failure of dorsal closure of the urethra) occurs in males or females and is usually associated with incontinence. Congenital *urethral strictures* are infrequent. Although *meatal stenosis* is common, it is thought to be acquired, inasmuch as it generally is seen only in circumcised boys. Congenital *urethral diverticuli* are not rare, yet they generally are small and of no consequence. Finally, *megalo-urethra*, a markedly dilated anterior urethra, often associated with poor development of the erectile corpora, is rarely seen.

Arey LB: Developmental Anatomy. 7th ed. Philadelphia, W. B. Saunders Company, 1974. *The most complete text describing the derivation of congenital anomalies.*

Caldamone AA: Anomalies of the bladder and cloaca. *In* Gillenwater JY, et al. (eds.): Adult and Pediatric Urology. Chicago, Year Book Medical Publishers, 1987, p 1809. *An excellent discussion of the subject in a comprehensive textbook.*

Perlmutter AD, Retik AA, Bauer SB: Anomalies of the upper urinary tract. *In* Walsh PC, et al. (eds.): Campbell's Urology. 5th ed. Philadelphia, W. B. Saunders Company, 1986, p 1665. *A complete and well-referenced treatise on the subject.*

91 Tumors of the Kidney, Ureter, and Bladder

Richard D. Williams

Benign and malignant renal tumors are either primary in the kidney and its surrounding connective tissue or collecting structures, or secondary (involving the kidney from adjacent organs or distant sites of origin). By definition, any mass within the kidney is a "renal tumor," but only solid masses are considered in this chapter. Cystic lesions of the kidney are discussed in Ch. 89. A classification of renal tumors is presented in Table 91-1.

APPROACH TO THE PATIENT WITH A RENAL MASS

In the past, most renal masses were detected on excretory urograms (IVP) during an evaluation prompted by signs or symptoms of disease (Table 91-2). Surgical exploration was often necessary for definitive diagnosis and treatment. Today, there are multiple modalities for the accurate diagnostic study of renal masses, and because of their sensitivity an increasing number of incidental renal masses are being identified in asymptomatic patients. A systematic algorithmic approach should result in less than 10 per cent of renal masses being indeterminate prior to management (Fig. 91-1). Its use will often obviate the requirement for surgical definition.

The IVP with nephrotomography is still the study of first choice and can accurately define 75 per cent of renal masses. A demonstrated renal mass will require renal ultrasonography (US) to determine more accurately whether the mass is cystic or solid (Fig. 91-2). If the mass fulfills all US criteria for a simple cyst (65 per cent of renal masses) there is no need for further workup, inasmuch as US is over 95 per cent accurate (Ch. 89). In the symptomatic patient, however, initial workup by computed tomographic (CT) scan, bypassing US, is appropriate. When a mass is suspected on IVP but not confirmed on US (15 per cent of cases), either an isotopic scan of the renal cortex with ^{99m}Tc dimercaptosuccinic acid (DMSA) or renal CT is required, particularly in symptomatic patients.

If the mass on US is solid or complex (20 per cent of cases), a renal CT scan (both with and without intravenous injection of iodine contrast) has replaced renal arteriography as the next diagnostic step. CT is as accurate as, and obviates the potential morbidity of, angiography in defining renal masses. Contrast enhancement of the usually highly vascular renal cancer on a CT study leaves little doubt as to the nature of a solid mass. In addition, CT can usually give sufficient local staging information to allow definitive surgical management. When contrast enhancement on CT is coupled with areas of a negative CT number (relative tissue density in Hounsfield units) typical of fat, a diagnosis of angiomyolipoma is appropriate and no further workup is required. In indeterminate cases, arteriography or needle aspiration cytology or both may be needed to define the diagnosis

TABLE 91-1. CLASSIFICATION OF RENAL TUMORS

Benign Tumors
 Adenoma
 Oncocytoma
 Mesoblastic nephroma
 Hamartoma-angiomyolipoma
 Leiomyoma
 Hemangioma
Primary Malignant Tumors
 Renal cell carcinoma (adenocarcinoma)
 Nephroblastoma (Wilms' tumor)
 Urothelial carcinoma (renal collecting system and pelvis)
 Sarcoma
Secondary Malignant Tumors (Direct Extension or Metastatic)
 Adrenal carcinoma
 Retroperitoneal sarcoma, pancreas, colon
 Lung, stomach, breast
 Reticuloendothelial—lymphoma and Hodgkin's disease, and
  hematologic—leukemia and multiple myeloma

TABLE 91–2. PRESENTING SYMPTOMS, LABORATORY FEATURES, OR PHYSICAL FINDINGS IN PATIENTS WITH RENAL CELL CARCINOMA

Finding	Occurrence (%)
Hematuria	50–60
Elevated erythrocyte sedimentation rate (ESR)	50–60
Abdominal mass	24–45
Anemia	21–41
Flank pain	35–40
Hypertension	22–38
Weight loss	28–36
Pyrexia	7–17
Hepatic dysfunction	10–15
Classic triad (gross hematuria, flank pain, and palpable abdominal mass)	7–10
Hypercalcemia	3–6
Erythrocytosis	3–4
Acute varicocele	2–3

Data from Skinner DG, et al.: Diagnosis and management of renal cell cancer. Cancer 28:1165, 1971; Chisholm GD: Nephrogenic ridge tumors and their syndromes. Ann NY Acad Sci 230:402, 1974; Fallon B: Renal parenchymal tumors. *In* Culp DA, Loening SA (eds.): Genitourinary Oncology. Philadelphia, Lea & Febiger, p 202, 1985.

further; however, in these unusual cases, final definition will likely require surgery.

In general, the nature of primary renal parenchymal masses in adults is readily defined via this algorithm. While MRI is equal to CT in diagnosing renal masses and is better in local tumor staging, other than defining the presence and cephalad extent of intravascular tumor thrombi, this information does not obviate or change the surgical approach. Thus, the less expensive CT is favored.

Cronan JJ, Zeman RK: Renal mass imaging: The internist's role. Am J Med 81:1026, 1986. *A succinct discussion of the imaging modalities available for renal mass evaluation, including cost and efficacy considerations.*

Cronan JJ, Zeman RK, Rosenfeld AT: Comparison of computerized tomography, ultrasound and angiography in staging renal cell cancer. J Urol 127:712, 1982. *A definitive study showing CT to be the most accurate modality for staging renal cell carcinoma (RCC).*

Hricak H, Thaeii RF, Carroll PR, et al.: Detection and staging of renal neoplasms: A reassessment of MRI. Radiology 166:643, 1988. *A definitive discussion of the role of MRI in defining solid renal masses.*

Richie JP, Garnick MD, Seltzer D, et al.: CT scan for diagnosis and staging of renal cell cancer. J Urol 129:1114, 1983. *A substantial series of patients studied by CT with surgical correlation of results.*

BENIGN RENAL TUMORS

Renal adenoma is the most common benign solid parenchymal lesion. Those under 3 cm in size have been designated as "benign," yet they tend to occur in circumstances similar to lesions larger than 3 cm (which are considered cancerous), i.e., in patients above 40 years of age, with a male to female ratio of 2 or 3 to 1. Small "renal adenomas" (<3 cm) are virtually indistinguishable histologically from renal adenocarcinomas and a few have in fact metastasized. Since the biology of these small tumors cannot be predicted preoperatively, most urologic oncologists consider them to be malignant and recommend radical nephrectomy. In highly selected lesions (solitary kidney, bilateral tumors, renal insufficiency, von Hippel–Lindau syndrome) subtotal nephrectomy is appropriate, however.

Renal oncocytoma, a subtype of adenoma accounting for 3 to 5 per cent of renal tumors, has a characteristic pale brown gross appearance and contains cells with an acidophilic cytoplasm that are thought to arise from the intercalated cells of the collecting ducts. These tumors, although sometimes several centimeters in size, are generally asymptomatic. The typical spoke-wheel pattern on angiography is not sufficiently specific to exclude a malignant lesion preoperatively, and therefore treatment continues to be radical nephrectomy.

Acquired renal cystic disease has been described in up to 45 per cent of patients with end-stage renal disease with an increas-

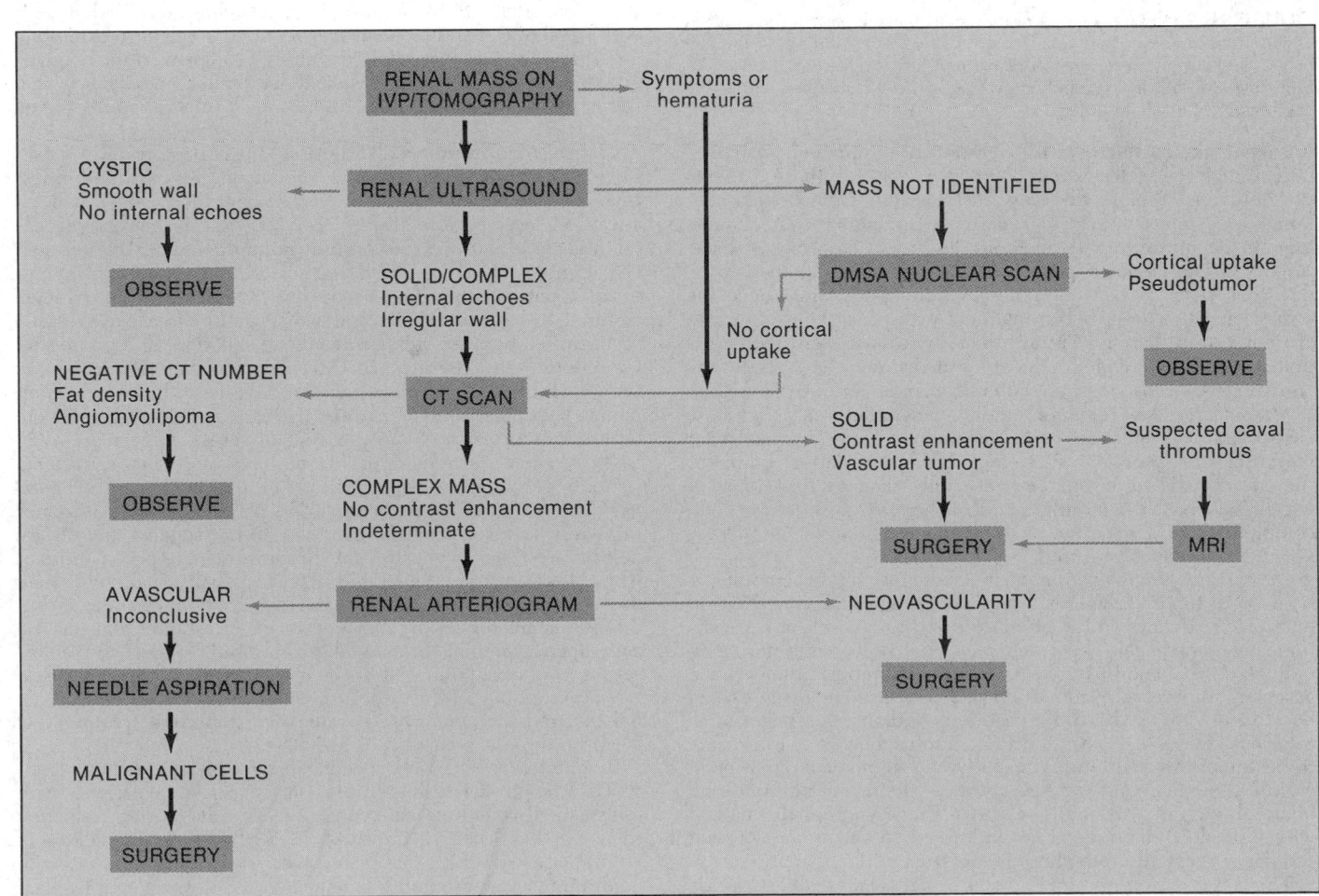

FIGURE 91–1. Algorithm for the workup of a renal mass.

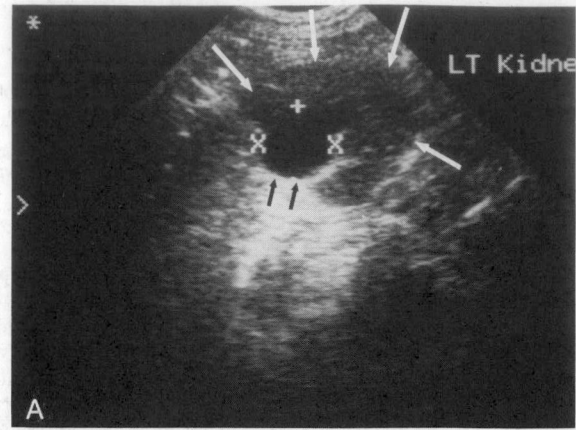

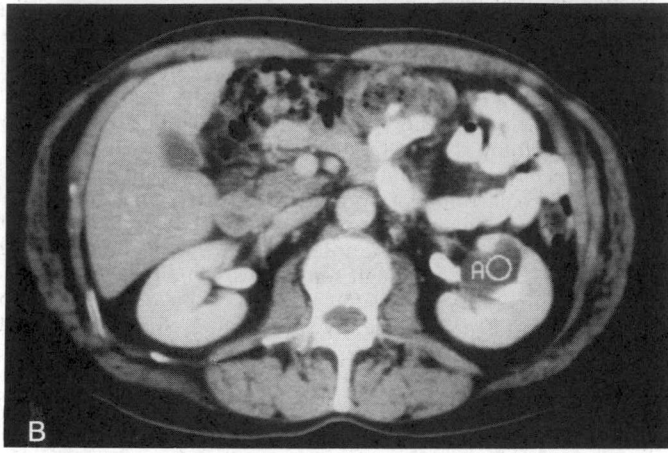

FIGURE 91–2. *A*, Left renal ultrasonogram showing normal renal parenchyma *(long arrows)*, parapelvic cyst (× and +) exhibiting no internal echoes and strong posterior wall *(short arrows)*. *B*, Transaxial CT of the same patient showing parapelvic cyst (A). The CT number within the cyst was 10 Hounsfield units.

ing incidence correlated with duration of either hemo- or peritoneal dialysis. Approximately 10 per cent of these patients develop renal tumors that vary histologically from benign adenomas and oncocytomas to renal cell carcinomas. The tumors tend to be multiple and bilateral. The metastatic rate of these tumors is only about 6 per cent. The etiology is thought to be due to a poorly excreted, nondialyzable metabolite, since the entity has been described in patients with renal failure but who are not yet on dialysis. These tumors tend to present with gross hematuria. It is recommended that all patients be screened by annual renal ultrasonography after 3 years of chronic dialysis.

Mesoblastic nephroma, a benign congenital renal tumor of early childhood, must be distinguished from the highly malignant nephroblastoma, or Wilms' tumor. Unlike the latter, however, the mesoblastic nephroma is commonly diagnosed at birth or within the first few months of life. The prognosis is excellent; complete surgical resection is curative, and neither chemotherapy nor radiotherapy is required.

Hamartoma-angiomyolipoma is seen most often in adult patients with tuberous sclerosis (adenoma sebaceum, epilepsy, and mental retardation) and is often detected as a result of retroperitoneal hemorrhage. The tumors may be quite large and commonly multiple and bilateral. As their name implies, they contain vascular, adipose, and smooth muscle elments. The diagnosis can be difficult to establish for patients without the stigmata of tuberous sclerosis. Computed tomography, however, can define these tumors by exhibiting a negative CT number in areas of fat within the mass and can in addition delineate multiple and bilateral tumors with more clarity. The asymptomatic patient with typical CT findings of fat within a < 5 cm tumor does not require surgery; the prognosis is excellent without treatment.

There is a variety of *other benign renal tumors* which include *fibroma,* a renal medullary fibrous mass most commonly found

in females; *lipoma,* adipose deposition within or around the kidney, often perihilar or within the renal sinus; *leiomyoma,* a not uncommon retroperitoneal tumor that may arise from the renal capsule or renal vessels; and *hemangioma,* occasionally accounting for hematuria with an elusive cause. Because these and other less common benign tumors are not frequently seen, it is often quite difficult to establish a diagnosis. When these tumors are accompanied by symptoms or produce a renal mass with caliceal distortion, the final diagnosis is generally made by the pathologist after the kidney is removed.

Fallon B, Williams RD: Renal cancer associated with acquired cystic disease of the kidney and chronic renal failure. Semin Urol 4:228, 1989. *A complete review of the literature and discussion of the probable causes of ARCD.*

Oesterling JE, Fishman EK, Goldman SM, et al.: The management of renal angiomyolipoma. J Urol 135:1121, 1986. *An excellent discussion of presenting findings and conditions for conservative management.*

Storkel S, et al.: The human chromophobe cell renal carcinoma: Its probable relationship to intercalated cells of the collecting duct. Virchows Arch 56:237, 1989. *Early data suggesting that oncocytomas may originate from collecting tubules.*

PRIMARY MALIGNANT TUMORS

RENAL CELL CARCINOMA. Renal cell carcinoma is the most common renal malignancy in adults, accounting for 3 per cent of all malignancies and approximately 9000 deaths per year in the United States. The tumor is also called renal adenocarcinoma, Grawitz' tumor, hypernephroma, and nephrocarcinoma, although renal cell carcinoma (RCC) has become a universally accepted designation. RCC appears to arise from cells of the proximal convoluted tubule. Risk factors include cigarette smoking and maleness (ratio of 2 or 3 to 1). Persons with HLA antigen types BW44 and DR8 may be more prone to develop renal cancer, and evidence suggests that oncogenes localized to the short arm of chromosome 3 may have etiologic implications. RCC is occasionally familial and is more common in patients with von Hippel–Lindau disease, horseshoe kidneys, adult polycystic kidney disease, and acquired renal cystic disease from renal failure. Histologically, RCC is of three varieties: the classic "clear cell" type characterized by uniformly large, cholesterol-laden cells with small nuclei and rare mitoses; a granular cell type exhibiting a darker staining cytoplasm containing numerous mitochondria, and more numerous mitoses; and an uncommon spindle cell (sarcomatoid) variety that has fusiform cells and variability in cell size.

Clinical Manifestations. The classic presenting triad of *hematuria, flank pain,* and a *palpable abdominal mass* is found in less than 10 per cent of patients and among those only with far advanced local tumors (Table 91–2). Gross or microscopic hematuria alone, however, is present in approximately 60 per cent of patients with RCC. The detection of renal tumors in asymptomatic patients has increased, but 30 per cent of patients continue to have local extension or metastatic disease at the time of diagnosis. Because of its protean manifestations and propensity for curious metastatic sites, RCC has been dubbed the "internist's tumor" (Table 91–3). Indeed, paraneoplastic syndromes are common in patients with RCC: *pyrexia* (fever as a presenting symptom occurs in approximately 15 per cent of cases), *hypertension* (20 to 40 per cent), *erythrocytosis* (3 to 4 per cent), *hypercalcemia* (3 to 6 per cent), *anemia* (20 to 40 per cent), and *hepatic dysfunction* (10 to 15 per cent). The paraneoplastic syndromes may raise suspicion of RCC but they do not suggest metastases; neither are they prognostic, since removal of the primary tumor when there is no demonstrated metastasis will usually eliminate the associated syndrome. Hepatic dysfunction (Stauffer's syndrome), characterized by elevated levels of alkaline phosphatase and alpha$_2$-globulin, prolonged prothrombin time, and a low serum level of albumin, all in the absence of hepatic metastases, is an exception to this rule, since in such cases there is an unexplained high recurrence rate after definitive treatment of localized disease.

Diagnosis. There is no specific diagnostic laboratory test for RCC. The physician must often suspect RCC in patients with unexplained constitutional symptoms. The diagnostic evaluation relies on the algorithm previously described for investigation of renal mass (see Fig. 91–1). A mass suspected on IVP with nephrotomograms should be confirmed by ultrasonography. If it is solid on US, an abdominal CT scan (Fig. 91–3) will, in

TABLE 91-3. SOME UNUSUAL OR SYSTEMIC MANIFESTATIONS OF RENAL CELL CARCINOMA

Fever
Weight loss, inanition
Anemia
Erythrocytosis
Leukemoid reaction, eosinophilia
Thrombocytosis
Hypercalcemia
Hypertension (with or without renin ↑)
Cushing's syndrome (ACTH)
Stauffer's syndrome (hepatopathy)
Galactorrhea (prolactin)
Amyloidosis
Congestive heart failure (AV fistula)
Thrombophlebitis
Inferior vena cava obstruction
Left varicocele
Budd-Chiari syndrome
von Hippel–Lindau disease

Adapted from Cronin RE, et al.: Renal cell carcinoma: Unusual systemic manifestations. Medicine 55:191, 1976. © 1976, The Williams & Wilkins Company, Baltimore. ACTH = adrenocorticotropic hormone; AV = arteriovenous.

approximately 95 per cent of cases, be sufficient to establish the diagnosis. MRI can also establish the diagnosis and be useful for staging. A renal vein or caval thrombus is common and may change the surgical approach to treatment, so the presence of a thrombus should be determined by US or MRI. In equivocal cases a venacavogram may be necessary for definition and/or determination of the cephalad extent of the thrombus before operation. The CT scan is sufficient for determining local extension and/or local lymph node involvement, although if nodal findings would obviate surgical management, needle biopsy confirmation is recommended.

Staging and Treatment. It is important to determine the presence of metastases before determining therapy. No benefit has been ascribed to removal of the primary tumor in patients with known metastases unless the patient is symptomatic, the metastasis is solitary and amenable to resection, or a promising medical therapeutic protocol is planned (see below). Spontaneous regression of metastases following surgical removal of the primary tumor is calculated at 0.5 per cent, whereas the surgical mortality is nearly 2 per cent in these patients. The common primary metastatic sites beyond the ipsilateral adrenal and local lymph nodes are lung and long bones. A chest roentgenogram and CT and a radionuclide bone scan are routine staging modalities.

Therapy of RCC depends entirely on the staging system summarized in Table 91–4. In patients with Stages I (T_1–T_2), II (T_{3a}), and IIIa (T_{3b}, T_{3c}, T_{4b}), treatment consists of a radical nephrectomy, which includes removal of the kidney and ipsilateral adrenal intact within its surrounding fascia, as well as removal of a possible intracaval thrombus. The local hilar lymph nodes are included, but a formal para-aortic node dissection is not warranted. The prognosis for patients so treated approximates a

50 to 70 per cent 5-year survival (Table 91–4). Patients with lymph node involvement (Stage IIIb, c [T_{1-3} N_{1-4}]) have a 15 to 35 per cent 5-year survival despite surgical treatment, and those with distant metastases (Stage IV [T_{1-4} N_{1-4} M_+]) generally have less than a 5 per cent 5-year survival no matter what treatment is employed.

Treatment of metastatic disease has included radiotherapy, chemotherapy, and immunotherapy, with none of these modalities emerging as clearly beneficial in effecting long-term survival. Hormonal therapy with medroxyprogesterone has less than a 5 per cent response rate. A variety of other hormonal agents, including testosterone, tamoxifen, nafoxidine, and estramustine, have similarly shown few responses. Approximately 20 per cent of patients with metastatic RCC were reported to respond to vinblastine. Immunotherapy with bacille Calmette-Guérin (BCG), *Corynebacterium parvum*, and xenogeneic immune ribonucleic acid (RNA) has been tried with limited success. Recent trials of recombinant alpha-interferon show up to a 20 per cent response rate with an occasional complete remission. Adoptive immunotherapy entails production of augmented autologous lymphocytes (LAK cells) by incubation with interleukin-2 in vitro. LAK cells are then reinfused into the patient. Early results showed a 33 per cent response rate in patients with pulmonary metastases, but confirmatory studies showed only a 16 per cent response rate and the toxicity of the treatment was great, and the duration of remissions was brief. Isolation of lymphocytes from the tumor incubated in IL-2 (TIL cells) was hoped to be more efficacious, although, to date, specificity of the cells produced toward autologous tumor cells is low; attempts to enhance specificity are in progress. Recent data suggest that alpha-interferon and IL-2 combined have an objective response rate of 30 per cent, but long-term data are not yet available. Although radiation therapy is not important in primary treatment, it can provide short-term control of symptomatic bone metastases.

Crusinberry R, Williams RD: Immunotherapy of renal cell carcinoma. Semin Surg Oncol (in press). *A review of the current treatment modalities and results.*
DeKernion JB: Treatment of advanced renal cell cancer—traditional methods and innovative approaches. J Urol 130:2, 1983. *A superb and inclusive review of the treatment of disseminated RCC.*
Fisher BI, Coltman CA, Doroshow JH, et al.: Metastatic renal cancer treated with interleukin-2 and lymphokine-activated killer cells: A phase II clinical trial. Ann Intern Med 108:518, 1988. *Adoptive immunotherapy data in perspective.*
Garnick MB, Richie JP: Renal neoplasia. *In* Brenner BM, Rector FC Jr. (eds.): The Kidney. 3rd ed. Philadelphia, W. B. Saunders Company, 1986, pp 1533–1550. *An excellent general review of renal cell carcinoma, sarcomas of renal origin, and Wilms' tumor, with 141 references.*
Holland JM: Cancer of the kidney—natural history and staging. Cancer 32:1030, 1973. *The classic article on RCC containing a complete description of the staging system.*
Krown SE: Interferon treatment of renal cell carcinoma. Cancer 59:64, 1986. *An exhaustive and authoritative review of interferon therapy for renal cancer.*
Williams RD: Renal, perirenal, and ureteral neoplasms. *In* Gillenwater JY, et al. (eds.): Adult and Pediatric Urology. Chicago, Year Book Medical Publishers, 1987, p 513. *A treatise on all aspects of upper urinary tract tumors.*

NEPHROBLASTOMA. Nephroblastoma (Wilms' tumor) is the most common malignant neoplasm of the urinary tract in childhood. It is diagnosed in one third of cases when the child is under the age of 2 and in two thirds of cases when the child is under the age of 4.

Clinical Manifestations and Diagnosis. The tumor is palpable in as many as 80 per cent of cases, often noted by a parent. Pain is initially present in 50 per cent of cases, hematuria (usually microscopic) in 10 to 20 per cent, and hypertension due to high renin levels in up to 60 per cent. The diagnosis is established first by IVP, which commonly shows caliceal distortion. Calcification within the mass occurs in 10 to 15 per cent of cases. Abdominal US or CT scans are useful to determine tumor extension and the possibility of bilaterality (this occurs in approximately 10 per cent of patients). Arteriography is necessary only in bilateral cases.

If there still is doubt about the differential diagnosis (after the studies just described are done), measurement of urine vanillylmandelic acid should help rule out neuroblastoma. The metastatic workup should be directed to the lungs, liver, and opposite kidney. A chest roentgenogram and CT and an abdominal CT are sufficient. Nephroblastoma, as is the case with RCC, often

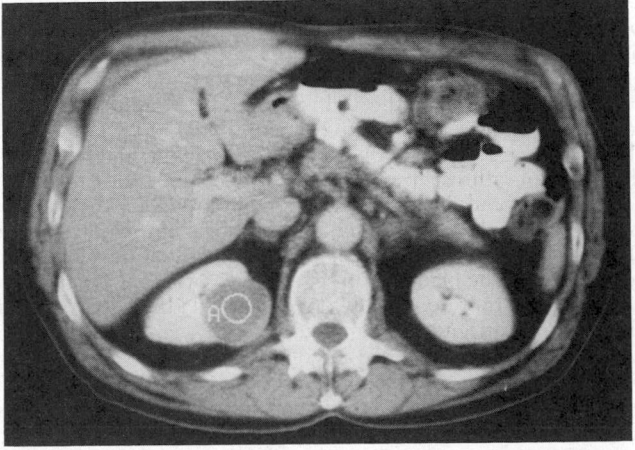

FIGURE 91–3. Transaxial CT showing enhanced solid renal cancer in left kidney (A). The CT number within the mass was 59 Hounsfield units.

TABLE 91–4. STAGING SYSTEMS AND PROGNOSIS FOR RENAL CARCINOMA

Conventional Stage		TNM Stage		5-Year Survival (%)
I. Tumor confined to renal parenchyma	T_1 (small tumor with minimal calyceal distortion) T_2 (large tumor with calyceal deformity)			60–70
II. Tumor extension to perirenal fat or ipsilateral adrenal, but confined within Gerota's fascia	T_{3a}			50–65
IIIa. Tumor thrombus in renal vein or vena cava	T_{3b} (renal vein involvement) T_{3c} (renal vein and caval involvement below the diaphragm) T_{4b} (caval involvement above the diaphragm)	N_0 (nodes negative)	M_0 (lack of distant metastases)	50–60 (renal vein) 25–35 (vena cava)
IIIb. Regional nodal involvement	T_{1-3}	N_1 (single homolateral regional node involved) N_2 (multiple regional, contralateral, or bilateral nodes involved) N_3 (fixed regional nodes involved) N_4 (juxtaregional nodes involved)		15–35
IIIc. Combination of IIIa and IIIb	T_{3-4}	N_{1-4}		15–35
IVa. Spread to contiguous organs except ipsilateral adrenal	T_{4a}	N_{0-4}		0–5
IVb. Distant metastases	T_{1-4}	N_{0-4}	M_1	0–5

Data from Robson CJ, Churchill BM, Anderson W: The results of radical nephrectomy for renal cell carcinoma. J Urol 101:297, 1969; Skinner DG, Colvin RB, Vermillion CD, et al.: Diagnosis and management of renal cell carcinoma. Cancer 28:1165, 1971; Johnson DE, Swanson DA, Von Eschenbach AC: Tumors of the genitourinary tract. In Smith DR (ed.): General Urology. Los Altos, Calif., Lange Medical Publications, 1984.

produces a tumor thrombus in the inferior vena cava, which may have to be delineated by venacavography. Abdominal US or MRI is also a reasonable alternative to establish this possibility.

Treatment. The development of successful treatment of nephroblastoma is rightfully heralded as one of the most significant advances in cancer therapy of the past few years. The prognosis has improved from a 25 per cent survival in the 1960's to a current rate of over 85 per cent disease-free survival, if there is no distant dissemination or unfavorable histology.

The initial treatment of nephroblastoma is complete surgical removal of the primary tumor and kidney, even when there are metastases. A transabdominal approach will allow the safest access and the necessary visibility of the liver, para-aortic nodes, and contralateral kidney for complete staging. Occasionally radiotherapy or chemotherapy may be required preoperatively to decrease the bulk of massive tumors. Needle biopsy is necessary to establish the diagnosis first, however. Combined therapy is indicated postoperatively in all patients but is dependent upon accurate staging, completeness of surgical extirpation, and tumor histology. A tumor confined to the kidney or Gerota's fascia requires only postoperative administration of actinomycin D and vincristine, whereas for all others the best results are obtained with radiation therapy to the tumor bed plus administration of actinomycin D, vincristine, and doxorubicin. Additional areas of current investigation include radiation therapy with triple drug versus quadruple drug (addition of cyclophosphamide) for cases with unfavorable histology (anaplasia or sarcomatous elements). Wilms' tumor may occasionally be seen in adults; similarly, RCC occurs but rarely in children.

D'Angio GJ, et al.: Treatment of Wilms' tumor: Results of the third National Wilms' Tumor Study. Cancer 64:349, 1989. *The most current study results and description of ongoing protocols.*

Pizzo PA, et al.: Solid tumors of childhood. In DeVita VT Jr, Hellman S, Rosenberg SA (eds.): Cancer Principles and the Practice of Oncology. Philadelphia, J. B. Lippincott, 1989. *An excellent discussion of pediatric solid tumors in the definitive cancer textbook.*

UROTHELIAL TUMORS. Malignant tumors of the urothelial lining of the urinary tract include those involving the collecting structures of the kidney (renal pelvis and calices), ureter, and bladder. These tumors are transitional cell cancers (TCC) in over 90 per cent of cases, with an occasional squamous cell carcinoma (often in association with chronic inflammation due to stone formation in the upper tracts and with *Schistosoma haematobium* infestation in the bladder) and rarely adenocarcinoma (commonly associated with embryologic hindgut remnants such as a persistent urachus in the dome of the bladder). TCC tends to be multifocal, occurring bilaterally in the upper tracts in a few cases but with an increasing frequency of simultaneous occurrence or recurrences in the ureter and particularly in the bladder. In each location there is a strong association of TCC with cigarette smoking, exposure to certain industrial chemicals (particularly aromatic amines), and chronic abuse of phenacetin-containing analgesics.

TCC of the Renal Pelvis and Calices. **Clinical Manifestations and Diagnosis.** The presenting finding is gross or microscopic hematuria in more than 60 per cent of cases. In contrast to RCC, constitutional symptoms and paraneoplastic syndromes are few. Generally the diagnosis is made by the finding of a filling defect in a calix, infundibulum, or renal pelvis on IVP. US can be utilized to eliminate the possibility of a nonopaque calculus. Examination of the urine by an experienced cytologist can be diagnostic of TCC, although the site will be undetermined. Cystoscopy with retrograde pyelography, including ureteral wash or brush cytology, may be required to establish the diagnosis. Ureteroscopy may be useful in equivocal cases. CT scanning may be useful in determining local extent of tumor. Arteriography is not diagnostically useful. The tumors tend to metastasize to lung and bone, and therefore a chest roentgenogram and CT and a bone scan are often indicated. Since these tumors tend to be multifocal, careful preoperative scrutiny of the opposite side of the urinary tract (on IVP) and of the bladder and urethra by direct cystourethroscopy is recommended.

Treatment and Prognosis. Treatment of renal urothelial cancer is radical nephroureterectomy, with removal of the entire ureter. Because 40 to 50 per cent of patients have or develop similar tumors within the bladder, direct cystourethroscopy is a necessary postoperative routine, usually done quarterly the first year, twice the second year, and then annually.

Most of these tumors are low grade and noninvasive, and the 5-year tumor-free survival rate after complete removal of the ipsilateral upper tract is more than 90 per cent. Patients with high-grade and/or invasive lesions, however, have a poor prognosis (<15 per cent 5-year survival). Chemotherapeutic combinations, which have begun to show activity in TCC of the bladder,

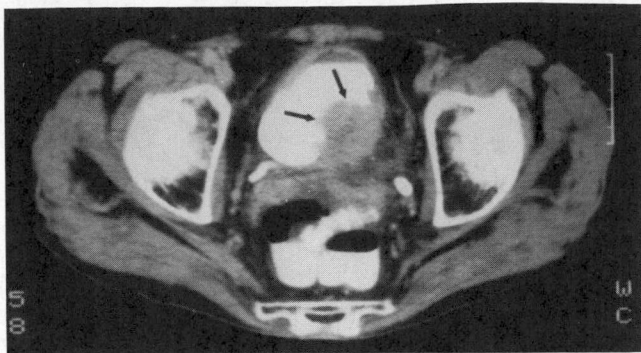

FIGURE 91–4. Transaxial CT of large bladder cancer invasive into perivesical fat (*arrows*).

are also efficacious in metastatic TCC from the upper tracts (see below).

***TCC of the Ureter.* Clinical Manifestations and Diagnosis.** These tumors are most often detected secondary to gross or microscopic hematuria, but occasionally present with renal colic due to obstructing blood clots. Diagnosis is commonly made by the finding of a ureteral filling defect on IVP. If the ureter is totally obstructed with a resultant lack of contrast excretion, cystoscopy with retrograde ureterography or ureteroscopy is required to demonstrate the lesion. As in renal pelvis TCC, ureteral urine or brush cytology can be diagnostic. Abdominal CT scans can aid in local staging, as can chest roentgenograms, and CT and bone scanning assist in detecting distant metastases.

Treatment and Prognosis. Prognosis is determined by the histologic grade of the lesion and the depth of invasion. Selected low-grade lesions may be successfully treated by segmental resection, particularly in patients with renal insufficiency or a solitary kidney, but the definitive approach remains nephroureterectomy, as in renal pelvis TCC. Prognosis of low-grade noninvasive lesions is greater than 70 to 80 per cent 5-year survival, but for the higher grade, usually invasive lesions the prognosis is dismal. Treatment of metastatic disease is rarely successful; however, as with TCC of the renal pelvis, the newer combinations of chemotherapy are promising (see below).

TCC of the Bladder. Bladder cancer affects over 20,000 people and accounts for nearly 10,000 deaths annually in the United States. Men are affected at least twice as often as women.

Clinical Manifestations and Diagnosis. Hematuria occurs at presentation in 68 per cent of patients and classically is total (throughout the stream) whether microscopic (as tested by a three-glass test) or gross. The degree of hematuria does not parallel the size of the lesion. Bladder irritability (frequency and dysuria) in the absence of infection is also a common (25 per cent) presenting complaint, particularly in males.

Intravenous pyelography is not sufficiently sensitive to detect small bladder tumors, but it is helpful in detecting upper tract TCC in the 10 per cent of patients with simultaneous lesions and in predicting bladder wall invasion in patients with concomitant unilateral ureteral obstruction. Urine cytology may establish the diagnosis of TCC but not the site. Definitive diagnosis requires cystoscopy and transurethral bladder biopsy under anesthesia, at which time a bimanual examination can predict whether the tumor has extended beyond the bladder wall. Metastases are local into adjacent pelvic structures and lymph nodes and distant to lungs and bones, and therefore staging of deeply invasive tumors is by chest roentgenograms, CT of the chest and abdomen (Fig. 91–4), and bone scanning.

Treatment and Prognosis. Nearly 80 per cent of bladder TCC's are low grade and noninvasive (stage 0, T_a) or invade only into the lamina propria (stage A, T_1). Patients with such lesions have an 85 per cent 5-year survival rate when treated by complete transurethral resection of the tumor(s). The lesions tend toward multiple recurrences in more than 50 per cent of patients, and

therefore cystoscopic surveillance is a mandatory postoperative routine. Intravesical chemotherapy with thiotepa, doxorubicin, mitomycin-C, BCG, or more recently alpha interferon has been used successfully for prophylaxis in patients with multiple or recurrent superficial low-grade tumors, resulting in 50 to 70 per cent reduction in recurrences. Importantly, only about 20 per cent of patients presenting with superficial bladder TCC subsequently develop high-grade and/or invasive disease.

Unfortunately, 80 per cent of patients with invasive bladder TCC are found so at initial presentation. In patients with deeply invasive disease, stage B_1 (T_2) refers to superficial muscle invasion, stage B_2 (T_{3a}) to deep muscle invasion, and stage C (T_{3b}) to full-thickness bladder wall invasion. In the absence of metastases current best efforts at cure of invasive disease require pelvic lymphadenectomy and radical cystectomy (complete removal of the bladder and prostate in males and the bladder, urethra, and uterus in females). This approach affords a 50 to 60 per cent 5-year survival rate in patients with stage B_1, B_2 or C disease. Patients with pelvic lymph node (stage D_1, T_{2-4} N_+) or distant metastases (stage D_2, T_{2-4} N_+ M_+) have less than a 15 per cent 5-year survival rate. Recent advances in therapy include potency-sparing bladder removal and continent urinary diversion to the abdominal skin (external) or to the urethra (internal), obviating the necessity of wearing a stomal appliance.

Metastatic disease is difficult to treat, but combination chemotherapy with vinblastine, methotrexate, and cisplatin with or without doxorubicin is showing a durable 30 to 50 per cent complete remission rate. This significant advance, if consistent, may alter the surgical approach to bladder TCC in the future. Indeed, research protocols, including precystectomy chemotherapy or combined radiation and chemotherapy in the hope of bladder salvage, are in progress. As yet, evidence is not available to suggest that either is better than cystectomy alone.

SARCOMAS. Renal sarcomas are rare; they include rhabdomyosarcoma, liposarcoma, fibrosarcoma, osteogenic sarcoma, and, most commonly, leiomyosarcoma (60 per cent). In general, sarcomas are quite malignant and usually detected at a late stage, and thus have a poor prognosis. The diagnostic approach is similar to that for RCC. Treatment is surgical with wide local excision; however, local recurrence and subsequent distant metastases are the rule.

Catalona WJ: Bladder cancer. *In* Gillenwater JY, et al. (eds.): Adult and Pediatric Urology. Chicago, Year Book Medical Publishers, 1987, p 1000. *A superb discussion of all aspects of bladder cancer in the definitive urology textbook.*

Droller MJ: Transitional cell cancer: Upper tracts and bladder. *In* Walsh PC, Gittes RF, Perlmutter AD (eds.): Campbell's Urology. Philadelphia, W. B. Saunders Company, 1986, pp 1343–1440. *A detailed and complete discussion of uroepithelial cancer diagnosis and treatment.*

Wahle S, et al.: CMV chemotherapy for extensive urothelial carcinoma. World J Urol 6:158, 1988. *A comprehensive review of the newer and more effective chemotherapeutic regimens for urothelial cancer.*

SECONDARY MALIGNANT TUMORS

Tumors of the lung, stomach, and breast most commonly metastasize to the kidney, but the metastases are usually clinically silent except for microscopic hematuria. More than 50 per cent of patients with primary lung cancer have renal metastases at autopsy. Routine use of staging abdominal CT in a variety of primary malignancies is expected to increase the premorbid diagnosis of secondary renal tumors. Adjacent tumors of the adrenal, colon, and pancreas, and sarcomas may spread contiguously into the kidney. Reticuloendothelial tumors, such as lymphoma and Hodgkin's disease, and hematologic malignancies, such as leukemia and multiple myeloma, may infiltrate the kidney, but this type of renal involvement is almost never primary or symptomatic. Other forms of renal involvement in multiple myeloma are described in Ch. 151.

Mayer RJ: Infiltrative and metastatic disease of the kidney. *In* Riesselback RE, Garnick MB (eds.): Cancer and the Kidney. Philadelphia, Lea and Febiger, 1982, p 707. *A complete review of secondary cancers in the kidney.*

PART X
GASTROINTESTINAL DISEASES

92 Introduction to Gastrointestinal Diseases

Robert K. Ockner

In gastroenterology, as in most fields of medicine, the decade of the 1980's witnessed remarkable advances in understanding of the etiology, pathogenesis, diagnosis, and treatment of disease. For example, three distinct hepatitis viruses were newly characterized, liver transplantation became an established form of treatment for advanced liver disease, neuropeptides and the enteric nervous system became more fully defined as key elements in the control of gastrointestinal function, and potent new inhibitors of gastric acid secretion became firmly established in the management of acid-peptic disease.

Despite these and other notable examples of progress, however, new challenges have appeared, and previously recognized ones have continued to resist the advance of science and technology. Thus, the newly recognized and characterized agents of hepatitis C and D and the acquired immunodeficiency syndrome remain unresolved scientific and clinical issues, while more familiar diseases pose new challenges as their respective natural histories and epidemiologies are more fully appreciated. For example, genetic hemochromatosis is far more common than had been recognized (Ch. 193), and the major problem in the management of peptic ulcer disease appears to be prevention of recurrence rather than induction of initial healing (Ch. 98).

These fundamentally scientific issues, albeit of profound impact, have arisen in the context of equally profound changes in the socioeconomic, cultural, and political milieu. Increasing awareness of the limitation of fiscal and other resources, coupled with a massive increase in new information, has forced major changes in medical research, training, practice, and financing, and these seem likely to continue unabated into the next century. Clearly the solution to many of today's most important health problems will depend upon international efforts and cooperation that, in some respects, are only beginning.

The cornerstone of medicine will remain, however, the thoughtful, compassionate, and efficient care of the patient. This, in turn, continues to depend on a careful and thorough history and physical examination in order that an appropriate differential diagnosis be formulated and that the proper diagnostic and therapeutic options be selected.

HISTORY

A carefully obtained history usually provides information important to an understanding of the basis for the patient's symptoms and for the planning of indicated diagnostic studies. Systemic symptoms, such as anorexia, weight loss, fatigue, fever, and emotional changes, are nonspecific but may be prominent. When caused by digestive disorders, these symptoms are usually associated with other evidence, such as abdominal pain, diarrhea, or jaundice, that more directly links them to digestive disease. Occasionally, however, systemic symptoms may be the only clinical manifestations of such diseases as inflammatory bowel disease, abdominal lymphoma, or pancreatic cancer. Similarly, systemic diseases that secondarily involve the digestive organs,

such as sarcoidosis and vasculitis, may be manifested only by general and constitutional symptoms. In these settings, special diagnostic studies, such as liver "function" tests, liver biopsy, or abdominal angiography, may be needed to document digestive system involvement. When symptoms more directly suggest digestive disease, their clinical and diagnostic significance requires a careful and systematic approach.

Abdominal pain, one of the most important and frequent presenting symptoms, must be carefully explored for location, quality, and temporal characteristics. Thus, epigastric pain typically arises from the stomach, proximal duodenum, or pancreas, whereas that in the right upper quadrant may reflect liver or biliary tract disease. Periumbilical pain is suggestive of small intestinal origin, the right lower quadrant of the cecum or appendix, and the lower mid-abdomen of the colon and rectum. The quality of the pain is also significant and reflects the dual nature of pain fibers and pathways that serve the intra-abdominal structures, as noted later. Intermittency of abdominal pain is often characteristic and warrants an exploration of factors that precipitate or alleviate it, such as its relationship to eating, bowel pattern, sleep, or emotional state. For example, duodenal ulcer pain is not usually present in the morning on arising but typically begins 30 minutes to 1 hour after meals or during the night, when it may awaken the patient and elicit the desire for food or antacid. Atypical manifestations of digestive disorders are not uncommon, especially among older patients and those taking certain medications such as corticosteroids. In both of these settings, for example, acute cholecystitis may be painless.

Mood and emotional stress may aggravate or even seem to produce many digestive symptoms. Because of the substantial role that emotions may play, digestive complaints are often more difficult to interpret than are symptoms referable to other organ systems. While emotional factors within the range of "normal" may influence many gastrointestinal functions and symptoms, certain eating disorders, such as anorexia nervosa and bulimia (Ch. 202) and some cases of morbid obesity (Ch. 203), are usually associated with clinically significant psychopathology. A patient's psychological profile may sometimes provide significant positive evidence pointing toward the diagnosis of irritable bowel syndrome, for example, which otherwise depends entirely on the exclusion of demonstrable "organic" pathology. Notably, disorders of swallowing, unlike other complaints such as abdominal discomfort or change in bowel habit, are almost always attributable to demonstrable organic disease. Although emotional factors may profoundly influence digestive function and the management of digestive diseases, there is no evidence that they alone account for the etiology or pathogenesis of diseases that in the past have been so represented, such as peptic ulcer disease or ulcerative colitis. Nor is there convincing evidence that certain personality types are predisposed to these disorders.

Other symptoms that must be specifically addressed include dysphagia (difficulty in swallowing), odynophagia (painful swallowing), heartburn, nausea, vomiting, hematemesis, melena, diarrhea, and constipation. For all symptoms, it is necessary to be as quantitative as possible (e.g., with respect to frequency, duration, or severity of a symptom, volume of stool or vomitus, or interval between aggravating or mitigating factors and the onset of their effects).

The background upon which a symptom occurs is also quite important. Thus, abdominal pain or melena in a patient with a documented history of peptic ulcer suggests ulcer recurrence.

Pain, bilious vomiting, or diarrhea in a patient with previous ulcer surgery, on the other hand, may be evidence of a complication of the surgery itself. And jaundice in a patient with chronic ulcerative colitis could be consistent with any of several possible explanations, including medication-induced hemolysis or liver injury, viral hepatitis transmitted by blood transfusion, or primary sclerosing cholangitis. Finally, a history of alcohol ingestion or abuse may provide the critical information to account for any of several manifestations of digestive disease, including jaundice, gastrointestinal hemorrhage, or severe abdominal pain caused by acute pancreatitis.

In the initial evaluation of the patient who presents with manifestations of digestive disease, the medical history must not be limited to matters directly related to gastroenterology. Thus, epigastric pain or gastrointestinal hemorrhage in a patient taking nonsteroidal anti-inflammatory agents suggests the presence of gastric erosions induced by the medication. And sudden onset of severe abdominal pain in a patient with known systemic vasculitis or advanced atherosclerosis immediately raises the possibility of intestinal ischemia.

In many instances, the patient and those close to him or her are unable to provide sufficient detail or documentation. In such cases, diagnosis and management may depend critically on access to medical records, including previous clinical and laboratory findings, biopsy and imaging studies, diagnoses, and treatments.

PHYSICAL EXAMINATION

A thorough physical examination is also an essential part of the initial evaluation of the patient with apparent digestive disease. It may provide crucial information about the patient's general health, for example, to determine if a patient is a suitable candidate for urgent surgery. It may also provide clues to a systemic explanation for abdominal complaints; for example, intestinal pseudo-obstruction may develop in a patient with progressive systemic sclerosis. Significant weight loss may reflect anorexia, dysphagia, malabsorption, or the catabolic effects of inflammatory or neoplastic disease. Finally, it may provide clues to the extent or severity of newly recognized digestive disease, such as cutaneous spider angiomata or asterixis in a patient with liver disease or uveitis or erythema nodosum in a patient with inflammatory bowel disease.

Examination of the abdomen may disclose distention caused by ileus, intestinal obstruction, ascites, or mass or may demonstrate the abdominal venous collaterals associated with portal hypertension or inferior vena cava obstruction. On palpation, the patient may intentionally tense the muscles of the abdominal wall in order to mitigate the actual or feared discomfort resulting from pressure of the examiner's hand on a tender organ or mass ("voluntary guarding"), or the musculature may be reflexly in spasm or rigid because of peritonitis-induced irritation of nerve endings in the parietal peritoneum. Midline tenderness in the epigastrium is typical of peptic ulcer disease or pancreatitis, whereas right upper quadrant tenderness suggests disease of the liver or biliary tract. If the tenderness is well localized to the region of the mid-clavicular line below the right costal margin, inflammation of the gallbladder is suggested, whereas tenderness just below and along much of the costal margin, especially if associated with the liver edge, suggests hepatic inflammation or a distended liver capsule. Tenderness of the right lower quadrant, possibly associated with guarding or spasm, is consistent with acute appendicitis, whereas a tender mass in this area suggests Crohn's disease or other chronic inflammatory or neoplastic process involving the ileocecal area, such as tuberculosis or lymphoma. Similar findings in the left lower quadrant, on the other hand (i.e., suggestive of a "left-sided appendicitis") are consistent with sigmoid diverticulitis. Examination of the liver should include not only an attempt to identify its lower edge, but also to characterize it with regard to form (i.e., sharp and nontender as in normal individuals, or rounded and possibly irregular as in cirrhosis) and consistency (firm as in cirrhosis or hard as in cancer), to determine whether it is tender, and to measure its cephalad-caudad span by defining its upper and lower borders. The clinical detection of ascites is often possible by demonstrating flank dullness, shifting dullness, or fluid wave, but if the volume of ascites is small, the relative nonspecificity of these signs makes their interpretation uncertain, in which case

sonography may be necessary. Auscultation may detect an hepatic friction rub, suggesting malignancy. Abdominal bruits indicate turbulent vascular flow, usually in the mesenteric vessels or the splenic or renal arteries, but their correlation with intestinal ischemia is poor. Abdominal aortic aneurysms can be detected by deep palpation in the epigastrium. Their size and the presence or absence of symptoms are important determinants of their prognosis with respect to the probability of rupture and the possible need for elective resection. An abdominal mass may be found in association with pancreatic pseudocyst, Crohn's disease, abdominal aortic aneurysm, abscess, or malignancy.

LABORATORY EVALUATION AND SPECIAL TESTS

Certain tests, such as the complete blood count and tests for fecal occult blood, are sufficiently informative and inexpensive that they may be considered routine in the evaluation of virtually all patients with digestive disease. Other studies, including those to assess intestinal absorption or the status of the liver, are employed as indicated (laboratory tests for the liver are discussed in Ch. 116). Endoscopy and the various methods for imaging play an essential role in the diagnosis of certain disorders, and therapeutic endoscopy and interventional radiology are increasingly contributing to treatment of some conditions, replacing more conventional surgical approaches (Ch. 93 and 94). Rapid scientific and technologic progress in these areas will require continuing evolution of clinical decision-making with respect to their use. Various biopsy and fine-needle aspiration techniques are available for the histopathologic characterization of known or suspected disease, and esophageal manometry may be useful in the diagnosis of certain esophageal diseases (Ch. 96). The decision to employ these options may be straightforward or complex. Without exception, such decisions need to take into consideration available alternatives, accuracy, safety, cost, and their possible impact on management.

MAJOR SYMPTOMS OF DIGESTIVE DISEASE

The symptoms discussed in the following section may occur in many digestive diseases. For a discussion of malabsorption syndromes and the causes of jaundice, the reader is referred to Ch. 102 and 115, respectively.

Disorders of Appetite and Feeding Behavior

The control of feeding behavior is complex and is often disturbed as an early manifestation of digestive disease. Subjectively, several sensations are involved. **Appetite** is the desire to ingest food, whether or not there is a physiologic need for nutrient. **Hunger,** in contrast, is the perceived need for nutrient replacement and is usually associated with a particular epigastric sensation of food craving ("hunger pangs"). **Satiety** is the diminished sensation of appetite and of hunger produced by feeding, whereas **anorexia** is the absence of appetite and hunger, usually because of illness, physiologic or pharmacologic factors, or emotion. "Feeding" and "satiety" centers in the hypothalamus play an important role in the regulation of feeding behavior. These centers appear to respond to changes in plasma levels of glucose and free fatty acids, as well as, directly or indirectly, to concentrations of humoral or paracrine mediators, including insulin, glucagon, α_2 agonist sympathomimetic amines, opioids, growth hormone–releasing factor, pancreatic polypeptide, and other neuropeptides. Cholecystokinin, released from enterocytes in the proximal intestine by the action of luminal fatty acids and amino acids, is thought to influence the sensation of satiety via its effect in the hypothalamus.

The pathophysiologic basis for the appetite-suppressant effects of many illnesses, and of digestive diseases in particular, is not well understood, although presumably the regulatory factors noted above and possible other factors as well are involved. Anorexia nervosa, bulimia, and hyperphagia seem to represent instances of a predominantly emotional basis for abnormal feeding behavior, but the pathophysiology of these illnesses is not known. Rarely, hyperphagia may reflect hypothalamic disease.

Nausea and Vomiting

The unpleasant triad of nausea, retching, and vomiting serves teleologically as a method to eliminate potentially injurious substances from the upper gastrointestinal tract. The process can also occur as the result of various chemical, humoral, or physical influences or disease states. **Nausea,** an undefinable and unmistakable sensation mediated via unknown neural pathways, is associated with hypersalivation, diminished gastric tone and peristalsis, increased duodenal tone, and duodenal-gastric reflux. **Retching** is characterized by spasmodic respiratory movements against a closed glottis with contractions of the abdominal musculature, during which the pyloric sphincter is closed and the lower esophageal sphincter relaxed (Fig. 92–1). Repeated herniations of the abdominal esophagus and gastric cardia during this phase may account for the occasional occurrence of Mallory-Weiss tears or the Boerhaave syndrome (Ch. 96). During **vomiting** itself, a sustained contraction of the abdominal musculature associated with the status of the gastric sphincters noted above results in a forceful expulsion of gastric contents. Other physiologic phenomena may accompany the process, including changes in cardiac rhythm and in intestinal and colonic motility.

The initiation and coordination of these events depend on two specialized areas of the brain, i.e., the vomiting center in the lateral reticular formation and the chemoreceptor trigger zone (CTZ) in the area postrema in the floor of the fourth ventricle. The vomiting center, which is directly excited by visceral afferent fibers from the gastrointestinal tract, serves to coordinate other medullary centers in producing the patterned response to the wide variety of noxious stimuli and disease processes that affect the digestive tract, mesentery, peritoneum, and ureters and that are associated with vomiting. An intact vomiting center is also required for the CTZ to cause vomiting. Because the CTZ is in a region in which the blood-brain barrier is poorly developed, it is influenced by a wide variety of endogenous and exogenous substances in plasma, including various chemical agents and transmitters. It also mediates radiation sickness and, in some species, motion sickness.

The timing of vomiting and the characteristics of the vomitus should be noted. For example, psychogenic vomiting typically occurs during or soon after a meal and rarely if ever is delayed as long as 12 hours. Conversely, vomiting due to gastric outlet obstruction or impaired motility tends to be somewhat delayed and usually occurs more than an hour after a meal. Vomiting that

TABLE 92–1. MAJOR CAUSES OF VOMITING

Psychogenic (including anorexia nervosa and bulimia)
Pain
Intracranial disease
Drugs and toxins
Pregnancy
Metabolic disorders
Cyclic vomiting of childhood
Gastric retention (including gastric dysmotility and pyloric obstruction)
High small intestinal obstruction
Visceral inflammation, ischemia, or perforation
Peritonitis

occurs in the morning before breakfast is typical of pregnancy and may also be associated with alcohol ingestion, uremia, or increased intracranial pressure. The presence of old food suggests impaired gastric emptying, whereas undigested food may possibly have come from an esophageal or Zenker's diverticulum. The presence of bile in vomitus excludes obstruction at the gastric pylorus or in the proximal duodenum. A feculent odor suggests prominent bacterial overgrowth, as may occur in intestinal obstruction, gastrocolic fistula, or longstanding intestinal stasis syndrome.

The causes of vomiting are many and not limited to the digestive system or the abdomen (Table 92–1). Psychogenic vomiting is often associated with anorexia nervosa or bulimia. Intracranial diseases, especially those associated with increased pressure, are typically associated with projectile vomiting, but more ordinary emesis also occurs. Many drugs and toxins cause vomiting, either through a direct effect on the CTZ or indirectly through their effects on the digestive tract, for example the gastric mucosa. Vomiting is frequently a problem confined to the first trimester of pregnancy but in severe cases (hyperemesis gravidarum) may persist through the third trimester. The mechanism for cyclic vomiting of childhood is unknown. Certain metabolic diseases, including disorders of fatty acid and amino acid metabolism, may be associated with episodic vomiting and possibly stupor or coma. The intra-abdominal causes of vomiting include inflammation, obstruction, ischemia, and perforation involving virtually any portion of the digestive tract, as well as peritonitis.

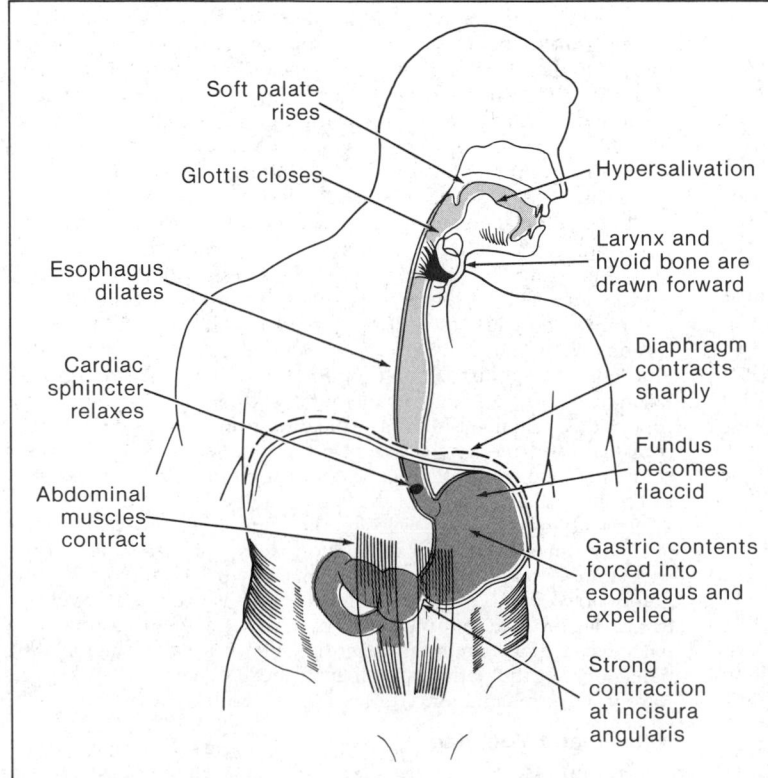

FIGURE 92–1. A diagrammatic summary of the act of vomiting in man. (From Feldman M: Nausea and vomiting. *In* Sleisenger M, Fordtran J [eds.]: Gastrointestinal Disease: Pathophysiology, Diagnosis, Management. 4th ed. Philadelphia, W. B. Saunders Company, 1989.)

Although it occasionally serves to eject noxious material from the stomach, vomiting usually accomplishes little of evident value. Moreover, it may be associated with both mechanical and metabolic complications. During vomiting, the gastroesophageal junction and the esophagus itself are subjected to substantial pressures and shearing forces. Occasionally, these mechanical forces produce the Mallory-Weiss or, rarely, the Boerhaave syndrome, which are associated with upper gastrointestinal bleeding and esophageal perforation, respectively (Ch. 96).

The metabolic complications of vomiting result from sustained losses of water and electrolytes in the vomitus, leading to hypokalemic metabolic alkalosis (Fig. 92–2). Hypokalemia reflects the combined effects of K^+ losses in vomitus, lack of K^+ intake, and K^+ loss in urine as the result of exchange of K^+ for Na^+ in the renal tubule (Ch. 75). The latter process is in turn a result of depletion of volume and Na^+, leading to extracellular fluid volume contraction and activation of the renin-angiotensin-aldosterone system. Alkalosis reflects loss of H^+ in vomitus, together with a K^+ depletion–induced shift of H^+ into cells in exchange for K^+ and into the urine in response to the aldosterone effect in the presence of K^+ depletion. The clinical manifestations of these changes are described in Ch. 75.

Heartburn and Dysphagia

Heartburn is a retrosternal burning sensation that may be accompanied by excessive salivation ("waterbrash"). It results usually from acid-peptic irritation of the esophageal mucosa, which may or may not be associated with histopathologic evidence of esophagitis. Thus, it is most commonly a manifestation of hiatal hernia or disorders that result in diminished lower esophageal sphincter pressure, so that it fails to prevent flow (reflux) of gastric contents down the hydrostatic pressure gradient from stomach to intrathoracic esophagus. It may be aggravated by bending over or by recumbency, especially after a meal.

Dysphagia (difficult or impaired swallowing) and **odynophagia** (painful swallowing) virtually always reflect organic disease in-

volving the esophagus, proximal stomach, gastroesophageal junction, or pharynx. Disease processes that can produce these symptoms include mucosal inflammation (e.g., esophagitis), mechanical obstruction (e.g., stricture or tumor), or motility disorder (e.g., achalasia or systemic sclerosis). In dysphagia, the patient complains of the sensation of food "sticking," "stopping," or "hanging up," usually felt above or at the level of the abnormality.

Chest pain may also be an important and confusing symptom of esophageal disease, usually reflecting spasm or severe inflammation. Because of its retrosternal location, radiation, and often squeezing or constricting quality, it may be very difficult to distinguish clinically from pain of cardiac origin and may even be associated with electrocardiographic abnormalities. Many individuals with so-called noncardiac chest pain are found to have motility disorders of the esophagus, including "nutcracker esophagus," or diffuse esophageal spasm (Ch. 96). Patients with long-standing esophageal disease may develop respiratory complications, such as bronchospasm, resulting from chronic, recurrent, and often subclinical aspiration.

Abdominal Pain

Abdominal pain, or a variant of it, such as indigestion, is one of the most important symptoms of digestive disease, often providing to the patient the first hint that something is amiss and providing to the physician information that is often helpful in diagnosis. Many aspects of abdominal pain have been discussed previously under the topic of the medical history. Abdominal pain varies widely in severity, quality, and location. Because it is, by definition, "subjective," the significance of pain in relation to other symptoms and to underlying disease processes can be evaluated only by thoughtful and systematic discussions with the patient.

Abdominal pain is diverse in type, reflecting the dual sensory innervation of the abdominal structures and the characteristics of each of the fiber types and pathways involved: (1) *Visceral fibers,*

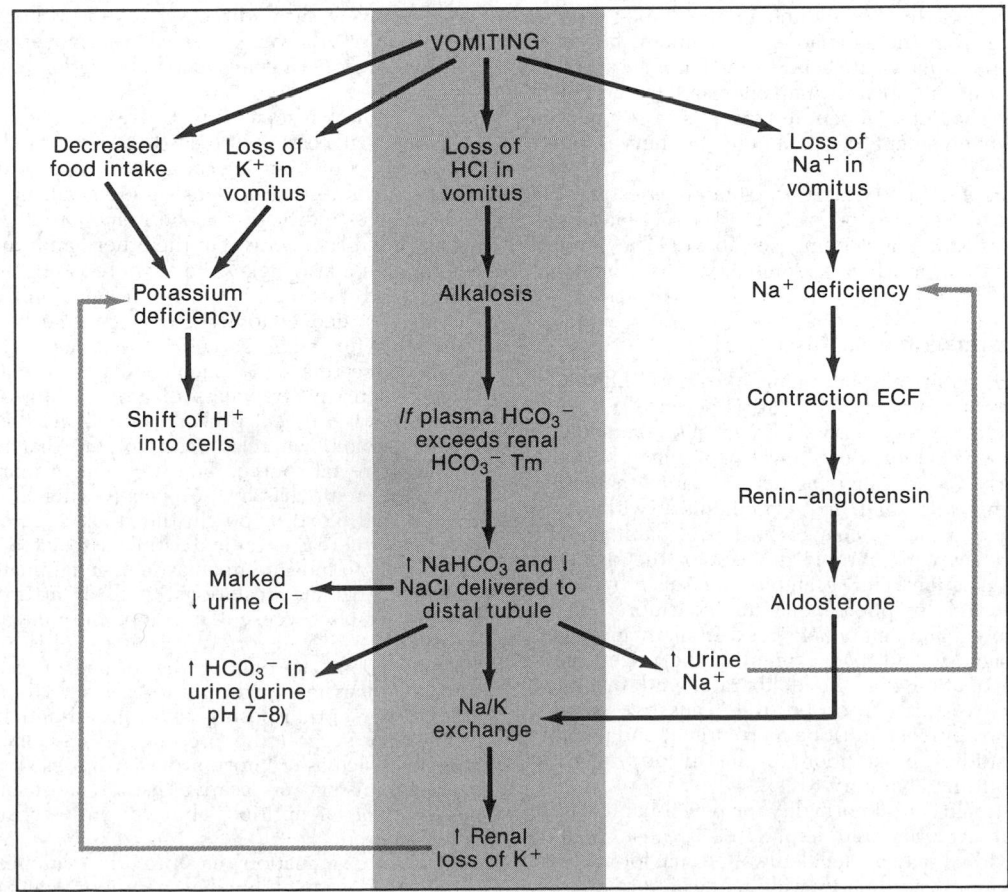

FIGURE 92–2. Metabolic consequences of vomiting. (From Feldman M: Nausea and vomiting. *In* Sleisenger M, Fordtran J [eds.]: Gastrointestinal Disease: Pathophysiology, Diagnosis, Management. 4th ed. Philadelphia, W. B. Saunders Company, 1989.)

largely type C, are present in the muscular walls of the hollow viscera and in the capsule of the solid organs and conduct afferent impulses from these sources via the vagus nerve. Innervation is usually bilateral. Pain conducted by these fibers is often perceived as midline in location, poorly localized but generally dull, cramping, or burning in quality, gradual in onset, prolonged in duration, and associated with autonomic manifestations such as nausea, vomiting, and diaphoresis. (2) *Somatic fibers*, largely type A-delta present in skin and muscle, innervate principally the parietal peritoneum and enter the spinal cord via the intercostal nerves. Pain conducted by these fibers tends to be sharper, more intense, more sudden in onset, and far more precisely localized than visceral pain. For example, the pain associated with intestinal obstruction, early acute cholecystitis, or uncomplicated peptic ulcer is typically visceral, whereas that associated with an acute peritonitis resulting from ulcer perforation is usually somatic.

Abdominal pain can be caused by (1) tension, stretching, or forceful contraction of the musculature of a hollow viscus, such as the intestine or gallbladder, (2) ischemia, presumably mediated by the local accumulation of metabolites and chemical mediators of inflammation, (3) local or generalized inflammation of the parietal peritoneum, (4) neoplastic or fibrotic involvement of nerve fibers, or (5) extra-abdominal causes, such as certain metabolic disorders (e.g., acute intermittent porphyria) or extra-abdominal pain referred to an intra-abdominal location.

Beyond the explanations that can be derived from these basic principles, certain empiric observations have related specific pain patterns to a particular organ or other site of origin. Esophageal pain, such as occurs in spasm or esophagitis, is located retrosternally, usually at or above the level of disease. If the pain is severe, it may be felt in the back. Pain arising from the stomach or duodenum is also midline and usually perceived in the epigastrium; if severe, it too may be felt in the back, a phenomenon that does not necessarily imply perforation of an ulcer. Small intestinal pain, as occurs with obstruction or ischemia, is usually periumbilical and, if severe, may also be felt in the back. Colonic pain is localized to the midline in the hypogastrium, whereas pain arising from the gallbladder or common bile duct is felt in the right upper quadrant. Pancreatic pain is localized to the mid- to left side of the epigastrium, but may also be felt in the back or the left shoulder, depending on its severity and on whether there is involvement of diaphragmatic nerves, e.g., during acute pancreatitis.

Significant information may be derived from an assessment of the temporal characteristics of the pain and its relationship to certain events such as eating or sleeping (see above). The physical examination of the patient in whom abdominal pain is a dominant symptom is described in Ch. 112.

Diarrhea and Constipation (Ch. 101 and 109)

Changes in bowel habit may be among the most difficult of gastrointestinal symptoms to evaluate. This is because the range of what is considered to be normal is very broad among individuals and because in any given individual bowel habits may be influenced by a similarly broad range of determinants that differ greatly in their significance and in the immediacy with which they must be addressed. Thus, changes in bowel habit may be caused not only by acute or chronic diseases of the digestive system and by medications, for example, but also by extra-abdominal diseases and by phenomena not considered to be "organic," such as mood and emotional stress. In many instances, the approach to diagnosis and management of the recent onset of diarrhea or constipation may be deliberate, and involve a gradual, stepwise investigation of possible causative factors; whereas in others the approach must be more urgent and possibly requires invasive studies in addition to the history, physical examination, and routine laboratory tests.

Definitions of normality or abnormality for bowel habits are of necessity somewhat arbitrary and imprecise, because what is normal for one individual may be decidedly abnormal for another. Stool frequency has an extraordinarily wide range of normal, from perhaps two or three per day to only one per week or longer, averaging one to two per day. Stool weight, accounted for mostly by water, is normally 50 to 200 grams per day but is not well correlated with stool frequency, because the extent to which the fecal mass is dehydrated during its passage through the colon varies considerably. Diarrhea can be defined as a stool weight of more than 200 grams or as more than three bowel movements per day (Ch. 101). Constipation is more difficult to define, as it involves not only stool frequency but also stool dehydration in the colon, i.e., its hardness. This and other characteristics, such as the ease or discomfort of stool passage or the sensation of a need to pass stool, are more difficult to quantify and therefore not very helpful. Perhaps the most reliable indicator of possibly disturbed physiology is the perception by the patient that an established pattern has changed, either to a degree or for a duration that seems beyond the range of variation which he or she considers normal. Such a change can reflect a change in either the amount of water excreted in the stool or the motility of the colon, or both.

Approximately 9 liters of water enter the gastrointestinal tract from exogenous and endogenous sources each day. Stool frequency and weight are therefore directly influenced by the extent to which water is absorbed from or secreted into the lumen of the small and large intestines. Essentially all water movement into and out of the intestinal lumen is passive. It is driven by osmotically active solutes that have been secreted, absorbed, or generated within the lumen through the breakdown of larger molecules by digestive enzymes or intestinal flora. Thus, abnormalities of fecal water excretion (i.e., diarrhea, or, to a lesser extent, constipation) reflect corresponding abnormalities in the digestion, absorption, or secretion of solutes. On this basis, diarrhea can be classified according to the source of these solutes. For example, the maldigestion or malabsorption of ingested nutrient solutes may occur in the malabsorption syndrome or in disaccharidase deficiency (so-called osmotic diarrhea). Or diarrhea may result from excessive secretion of inorganic ions such as Cl^- (so-called secretory diarrhea), as may occur in tumors that produce hormonal secretagogues, (e.g., "pancreatic cholera") or through the effects of bacterial enterotoxins, and the effects of nonabsorbed fatty acids and bile acids on the colonic mucosa. Changes in motility alone tend to influence stool frequency but have relatively little direct effect on volume. Suppression of bowel motility, however, retards the movement of luminal contents and may permit increased absorption of solutes and thus of water.

The medical history may provide useful clues to diagnosis. Diarrhea that ceases with fasting suggests that a nonabsorbed component of diet may be causative, either directly via an osmotic effect (e.g., intestinal malabsorption syndrome or disaccharidase deficiency) or indirectly via the induction of colonic secretion by nonabsorbed fatty acids. On the other hand, diarrhea that continues through a fast suggests that there is ongoing active secretion of ions, and thus water, into the lumen. This could be mediated either by an endogenous secretagogue, such as a tumor-derived humoral factor (e.g., vasoactive intestinal polypeptide), or by an exogenous secretagogue, such as a bacterial enterotoxin produced in cholera or in "traveler's diarrhea." Stools that are large in volume tend to reflect processes involving the small intestine or proximal colon, whereas small volume diarrhea suggests a left colonic or rectal source. The duration of diarrhea is often very important. Acute diarrhea, especially when associated with fever, cramps, and blood or pus in the stool, suggests invasive enteric infection, whereas chronic diarrhea associated with weight loss is more likely to indicate neoplastic or inflammatory bowel disease. Extraintestinal manifestations, such as arthritis or skin or eye lesions, are often present in idiopathic inflammatory bowel disease (Ch. 103). A history of recent travel is especially important and may point to one of the organisms associated with the traveler's diarrhea syndrome (Ch. 101). Homosexual contact or other factors predisposing to acquired immunodeficiency syndrome may suggest the presence of an opportunistic intestinal infection, such as cryptosporidiosis. In obscure cases of diarrhea, a careful history of laxative use is most important, and the possibility of surreptitious abuse of these substances must always be considered.

Physical examination may provide evidence of extraintestinal manifestations, an abdominal mass, perianal pathology associated with inflammatory bowel disease, or a neuropathy or other evidence of vitamin deficiency, reflecting a malabsorption syndrome. Laboratory evaluation of clinically significant diarrhea should routinely include examination of the stool for occult blood, leukocytes, enteric pathogens, and ova and parasites. Sigmoidoscopy with biopsy or swab and culture of rectal lesions may be indicated in selected cases, such as those in which symptoms are especially severe or protracted.

Sleisenger M, Fordtran J (eds.): Gastrointestinal Disease: Pathophysiology, Diagnosis, Management. 4th ed. Philadelphia, W. B. Saunders Company, 1989.

Zakim D, Boyer T (eds.): Diseases of the Liver. 2nd ed. Philadelphia, W. B. Saunders Company, 1990. *Two recent, authoritative, and extensively referenced texts.*

93 Diagnostic Imaging Procedures in Gastroenterology

Susan D. Wall

With the development of increasingly complex diagnostic imaging procedures in gastroenterology, the importance of direct communication with the consulting radiologist has increased. Clinical information regarding each diagnostic question is essential to tailoring the studies; none is "routine." In addition to conventional plain films of the abdomen and barium examination of the gastrointestinal tract, radiographic procedures of interest to the gastroenterologist include computed tomography, ultrasonography, endoscopic retrograde cholangiopancreatography, percutaneous transhepatic cholangiography, enteroclysis, radionuclide scanning, and magnetic resonance imaging.

COMPUTED TOMOGRAPHY

The faster scan time (2 to 3 seconds) and higher spatial resolution available with current computed tomography (CT) have improved greatly the images of the alimentary tract as well as of the pancreas (Fig. 93–1), liver, and gallbladder. Computed tomography continues to be an important modality for the investigation of possible hepatic tumor, pancreatic carcinoma, and retroperitoneal adenopathy. Less recognized is its contribution to the evaluation of the acute abdomen. When the diagnosis is unclear, CT is helpful in diagnosing possible pancreatitis (Fig. 93–2), perforated viscus, and subdiaphragmatic abscess, and in assessing the extent of Crohn's disease or bowel ischemia. It can detect extraluminal abscess associated with appendicitis and

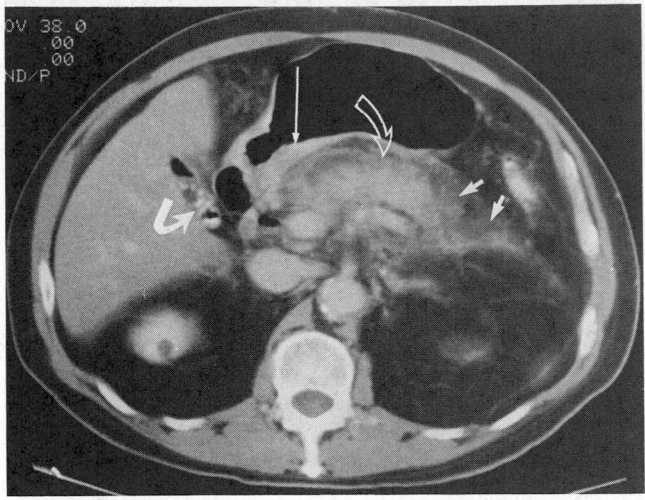

FIGURE 93–2. Computed tomography of acute pancreatitis. Abnormally dense fat surrounds the swollen pancreas *(open curved arrow)*. Free pancreatic fluid *(short arrows)* is present in the left anterior pararenal space, and the air-distended stomach has a thickened antral wall *(straight arrow)*. Note cholelithiasis *(closed curved arrow)*.

diverticulitis (Fig. 93–4) and can sometimes help in the decision regarding surgical versus nonsurgical management. Computed tomography also can detect free intra- or retroperitoneal air and small amounts of contrast material that have extravasated from the gastrointestinal tract (Fig. 93–3); it provides excellent visualization of the mesentery. It is the modality of choice for evaluation of suspected complications of pancreatitis, such as necrosis, abscess, pseudocyst, and colonic or mesenteric inflammation (Ch. 106).

Percutaneous fine needle aspiration (PFNA) with CT guidance can diagnose pancreatic carcinoma, primary and metastatic tumor of the liver, and sometimes tumor involvement of enlarged lymph nodes. False-negative results occur, but this procedure often obviates the need for diagnostic laparotomy. Furthermore, PFNA can diagnose a suspected abscess (Fig. 93–3), which can be variable and nonspecific in its radiographic appearance. Percutaneous drainage of an intra-abdominal or pelvic abscess with CT guidance is a nonsurgical treatment option for selected patients; it can palliate others until surgery is performed.

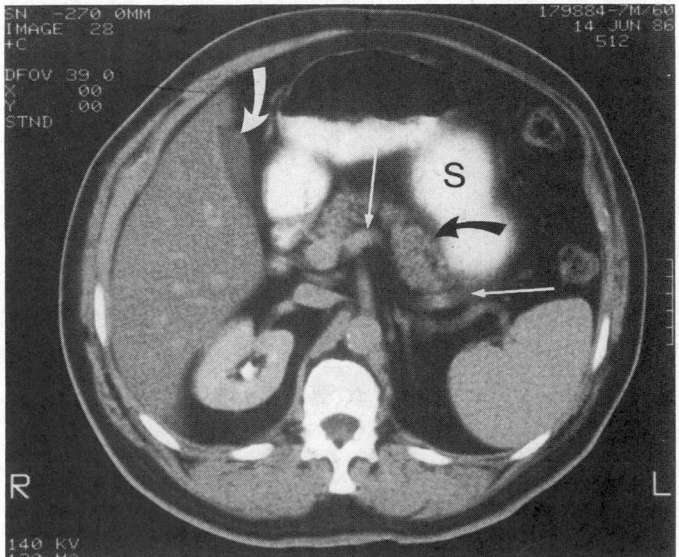

FIGURE 93–1. Normal computed tomogram. One cm thick transverse image (supine, patient's right to reader's left) is at the level of the pancreas *(black arrow)*, which is behind the contrast-filled stomach (S). The splenic artery is posterior to the splenic vein *(straight white arrows)*, which abuts the posterior margin of the tail and neck of the pancreas. The density of the right kidney is enhanced because of intravenous contrast material. *Curved white arrow* points to gallbladder.

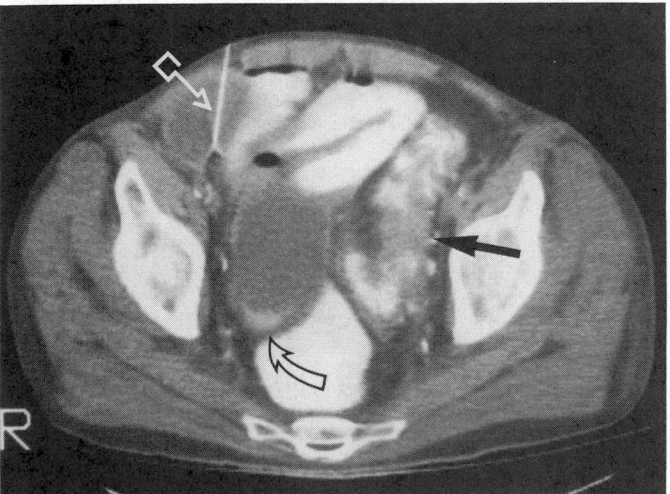

FIGURE 93–3. Computed tomography of diverticular abscess. Percutaneous fine-needle aspiration *(boxed white arrow)* of pelvic fluid collection diagnosed abscess in this patient with thickening of the wall of the sigmoid colon *(straight black arrow)* and diverticulitis. Note second fluid collection with small amount of contrast material *(curved black arrow)* extravasated from the diseased colon. Abscesses were drained percutaneously until the patient was well enough for surgery.

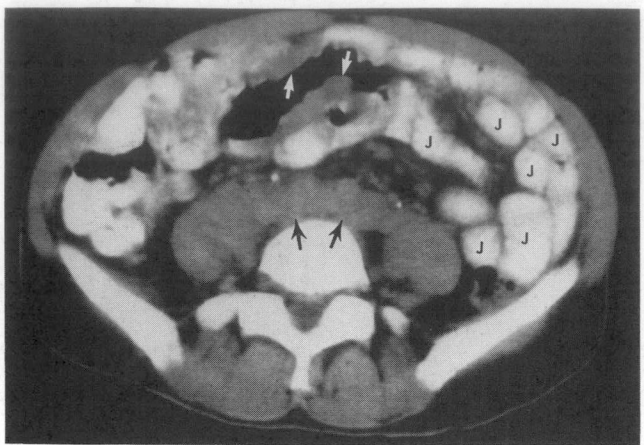

FIGURE 93–4. Small bowel Kaposi's sarcoma. Focal thickening *(arrows)* of a single segment of small bowel is due to Kaposi's sarcoma in this patient with acquired immunodeficiency syndrome. Note the normal jejunum (J) proximal to the tumor and the retroperitoneal lymphadenopathy *(black arrows)* anterior to the spine.

Computed tomography sometimes replaces barium contrast examination as the initial study of the gastrointestinal tract. Barium examination, which provides mucosal detail and delineation of the intraluminal contour, cannot demonstrate thickening of the wall, and the barium causes severe artifacts on CT images, precluding the possibility of a diagnostic study. Moreover, even unsuspected disease in the gastrointestinal tract, both primary and secondary, often is detected initially with CT. Assessment of thickening of the esophageal, gastric, and bowel wall is possible with current CT (Fig. 93–4), and surrounding organs may also be evaluated, especially regarding inflammatory processes, such as diverticulitis, appendicitis, Crohn's disease, pancreatitis, and possible perforated ulcer. Computed tomography has limited value in the regional staging of gastrointestinal malignancies because of its limited accuracy in determining tumor invasion into adjacent tissues. Indications for preoperative evaluation of patients with rectosigmoid colon carcinoma, for example, include suspected extensive disease or complications such as perforation. Computed tomography is more helpful in determining recurrence postoperatively. A baseline study is performed 2 to 4 months after resection, with follow-up comparison studies every 6 months for 2 years. New or enlarging masses in the pelvis suggest recurrent tumor; CT-guided biopsy can be performed for tissue diagnosis.

Balthazar EJ, Robinson DL, Megibow AJ, et al: Acute pancreatitis: Value of CT in establishing prognosis. Radiology 174:331, 1990. *A prospective study of 88 patients demonstrating radiographic findings predictive of serious complications.*

Moss AA: Imaging of colorectal carcinoma. Radiology 170:308, 1989. *Editorial overview of both preoperative staging and detection of postoperative recurrence.*

Sugarbaker PH: Surgical decision making for large bowel cancer metastatic to the liver. Radiology 174:621, 1990. *A superb summary of the current radiologic, laboratory, and medical considerations regarding this issue.*

Welch TJ, Sheedy PF II, Johnson CD, et al: CT-guided biopsy: Prospective analysis of 1,000 procedures. Radiology 171:493, 1989. *A valuable report documenting the high sensitivity, specificity, and predictive value of this safe alternative to more invasive diagnostic procedures such as laparotomy.*

ULTRASONOGRAPHY

Abdominal pelvic ultrasonography (US) is noninvasive, requires no ionizing radiation, and can be performed with a portable unit. Ultrasonography is superior to other modalities in differentiating cystic from solid lesions and is highly sensitive in detecting ascites. Because of the superb ability to demonstrate gallstones (Fig. 93–5), US has replaced oral cholecystography for the diagnosis of cholelithiasis. Interest in oral cholecystography has been renewed, however, with the development of extracorporeal shock wave lithotripsy and the attending need to determine the number and size of gallstones. Ultrasound is an effective and efficient first examination of suspected liver tumors (Ch. 124). It is the primary screening examination for hepatobiliary disease

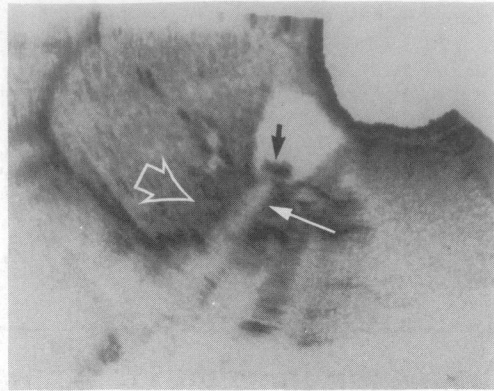

FIGURE 93–5. Ultrasound of cholelithiasis. Sagittal image (patient's head to reader's left) demonstrates a single gallstone *(black arrow).* The sound waves easily pass through the fluid (bile) in the gallbladder—hence the "posterior acoustical enhancement" *(open arrow)* characteristic of a cystic structure. The echogenic stone impedes the sound waves—hence the "posterior shadowing" *(straight white arrow)* characteristic of a gallstone. This "static" ultrasound image produces black echoes on white background.

and often is the only study needed. Dilatation of the intra- and extrahepatic biliary system can be detected (Fig. 93–6), but the distal common bile duct often is not seen adequately with US. Similarly, the tail or body of the pancreas or both are well visualized less often than the head, principally because of interference by the overlying gas-filled bowel. Ultrasonography, which plays a complementary role with CT in many diseases, often is the preferred modality when follow-up examination is needed, as in pancreatic pseudocyst, abdominal aortic aneurysm, and drained fluid collections. Percutaneous fine needle aspiration and drainage procedures can be performed with ultrasonographic guidance with greater ease and less cost than with CT.

Recent advances in ultrasound involve the application of a transducer to an exposed organ at surgery or through an endoscope. Ultrasonography has facilitated the intraoperative search for pancreatic islet cell tumor and occasionally demonstrates unsuspected multiple tumors. Endosonography requires an end-viewing fiberoptic gastroscope, which is modified to incorporate a transducer. This new imaging procedure can demonstrate the wall thickness of the esophagus, stomach, and duodenum and identify both diffuse and focal intramural lesions. It may also be valuable for the diagnosis of early pancreatic lesions. Preoperative assessment of rectal carcinoma with a high-frequency, 7.5 to 10 MHz endorectal transducer is reported to be at least as accurate as CT and magnetic resonance imaging in local staging of tumor.

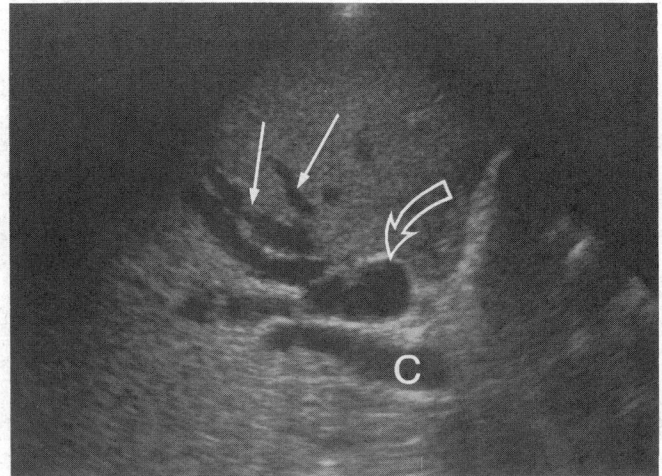

FIGURE 93–6. Ultrasound of dilated bile ducts. Dilatation of the intrahepatic *(straight arrows)* and extrahepatic *(curved arrow)* bile ducts is well demonstrated on the sagittal ultrasound image of a patient with distal biliary obstruction. (C indicates the inferior vena cava.) This real-time ultrasound image produces white echoes on black background.

Carroll BA: US of the gastrointestinal tract. Radiology 172:605, 1989. *An excellent review of the state of the art.*

Rifkin MD, Erlich MS, Marks G: Staging of rectal carcinoma: Prospective comparison of endorectal US and CT. Radiology 170:319, 1989. *Comparison of 102 consecutive patients demonstrated US to be as accurate as CT, or more so, in the preoperative staging of rectal cancer.*

ENDOSCOPIC RETROGRADE CHOLANGIOPANCREATOGRAPHY

Endoscopic retrograde cholangiopancreatography (ERCP) is performed with the fluoroscopic guidance of the radiologist. The papilla of Vater is visualized through a fiberoptic endoscope, and the common bile duct or the pancreatic duct or both are cannulated. Water-soluble iodinated contrast material is injected, and images are taken of the opacified biliary tree or pancreatic duct (Fig. 93–7). ERCP is performed specifically to evaluate the pancreatic duct or follows US or CT in demonstrating distal biliary obstruction. When a constricting or obstructing lesion is seen in the distal common bile duct, biopsy or papillotomy can be performed. A further discussion of ERCP is contained in Ch. 106.

TRANSHEPATIC CHOLANGIOGRAPHY

Percutaneous transhepatic cholangiography is used to visualize the intra- and extrahepatic biliary tree following CT, US, or ERCP that has demonstrated proximal obstruction of the common hepatic or common bile duct. It is performed by injecting water-soluble iodinated contrast material through a flexible 23-gauge

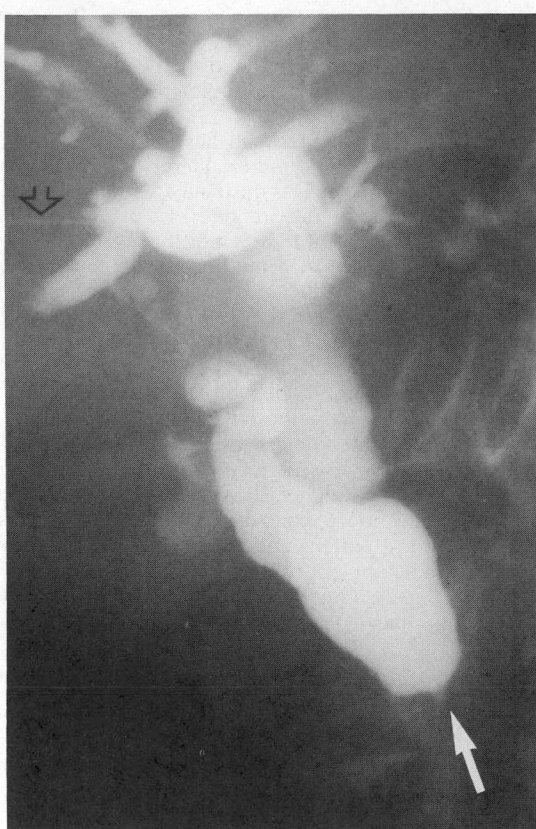

FIGURE 93–8. Percutaneous transhepatic cholangiogram. Dilatation of the biliary tree is demonstrated after percutaneous puncture and opacification of a dilated intrahepatic duct with a long 23-gauge needle *(open black arrow)*. The distal common bile duct is abruptly narrowed and obstructed *(white arrow)* owing to cholangiocarcinoma.

needle introduced percutaneously into the intrahepatic biliary tree under fluoroscopic guidance. After the biliary tree is opacified, multiple radiographs are taken in order to characterize the suspected site of blockage or narrowing (Fig. 93–8). This study provides the surgeon with the best demonstration of possible anastomotic sites of the biliary tree in the porta hepatis. Serious complications such as bile peritonitis or intraperitoneal hemorrhage occur in less than 2 per cent of cases. Biliary obstruction can be treated in patients who are poor surgical risks by several interventional procedures, including percutaneous stricture dilatation, percutaneous drainage, or insertion of a biliary endoprosthesis. The last procedure can be performed percutaneously or via an ERCP in conjunction with a percutaneous transhepatic technique.

McLean GK, Burke DR: Role of endoprostheses in the management of malignant biliary obstruction. Radiology 170:961, 1989. *State-of-the-art review of endoscopic versus percutaneous approaches to biliary drainage.*

Steinberg HV, Torres WE, Nelson RC: Gallbladder lithotripsy. Radiology 172:7, 1989. *Approach to extracorporeal shock wave lithotripsy (ESWL) described by experts in the field.*

ENTEROCLYSIS

Procedures used to study the small bowel include the "dedicated" small bowel follow-through, single- and double-contrast enteroclysis, and the peroral pneumocolon. Examination of the small bowel should not accompany most studies of the esophagus, stomach, and/or duodenum because the high-density barium used for the latter interferes with visualization of detail of the small bowel, especially the jejunum. Consequently, lesions that are present may be seen poorly or may be missed, and often it is nearly impossible to exclude abnormality. Hence, the traditional "upper gastrointestinal series with small bowel follow-through" is no longer the examination for small intestinal disease. An exception to this is the patient in whom the terminal ileum is the only suspected site of involvement. In this case, the peroral

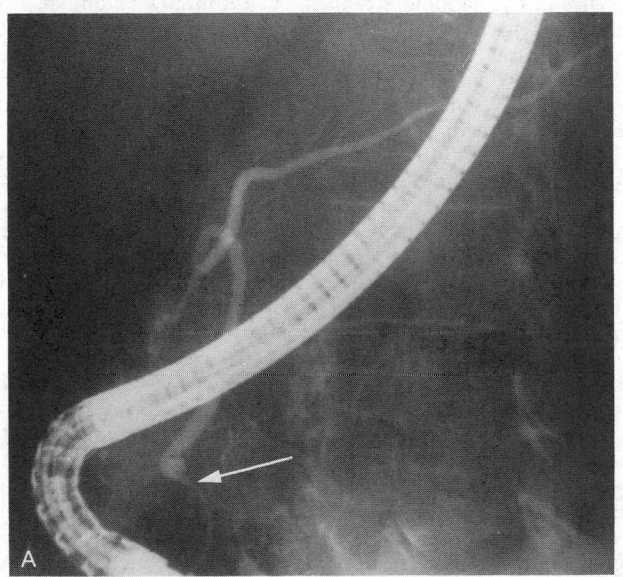

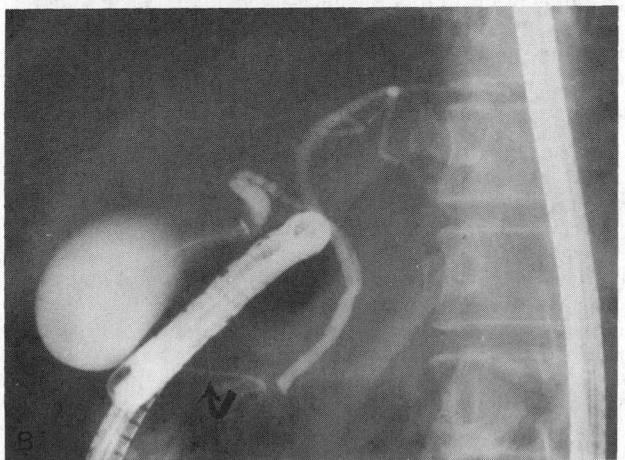

FIGURE 93–7. Normal endoscopic retrograde cholangiopancreatogram. *A,* Normal pancreatogram. The cannula *(arrow)* at the tip of the fiberoptic endoscope has been inserted into the papilla of Vater under direct visualization and the pancreatic duct opacified. *B,* Normal cholangiogram. The gallbladder, cystic duct, common hepatic duct, and common bile duct are visible. *Arrow* indicates cannula in the papilla of Vater.

pneumocolon may be the most precise approach. It is performed with introduction of insufflated air per rectum when orally administered thin barium has reached the cecum. With reflux of air across the ileocecal valve, double-contrast images of the terminal ileum are obtained.

Enteroclysis, also known as small bowel enema, refers to the direct introduction of contrast material after peroral intubation of the first loop of jejunum or, less optimally, the distal duodenum. It allows for a controlled rate of delivery of contrast material independent of gastric emptying and thus optimizes luminal distention. The double-contrast method uses air or methylcellulose to provide fine detail to the folds of the small bowel. Enteroclysis has been advocated as the most accurate method for the detection of focal lesions in the small bowel. However, it is comparable to a dedicated (tubeless) small bowel study for the detection of lesions due to Crohn's disease and tumor and is only slightly more sensitive for adhesions. A dedicated small bowel study does not immediately follow examination of the esophagus, stomach, or duodenum; it is performed with frequent, intermittent spot films by the radiologist. Enteroclysis, which is more lengthy and requires more expertise by the radiologist, is tolerated less well by the patient and, most importantly, involves a much greater radiation exposure. Preparation requires colon cleansing as well as 24 hours of clear liquid diet in order to clear the small bowel of particulate matter.

Dehn TCB, Nolan DJ: Enteroclysis: The diagnosis of intestinal obstruction in the early postoperative period. Gastrointest Radiol 14:15, 1989. *Demonstrates the efficacy of enteroclysis regarding this clinical problem.*

RADIONUCLIDE IMAGING

Acute cholecystitis is usually due to obstruction of the cystic duct by a calculus. Scanning with technetium-labeled iminodiacetic acid (^{99m}Tc HIDA), which is excreted by the hepatobiliary system, is valuable when such a diagnosis is in question. Visualization of the liver, bile ducts, gallbladder, and bowel occurs within 60 minutes of injection in normal, fasting patients (Fig. 93–9). Visualization of the gallbladder excludes the diagnosis of obstruction of the cystic duct. Nonvisualization of the gallbladder with normal visualization of the common bile duct and bowel indicates cystic duct obstruction (Fig. 93–10). Nonvisualization of both the gallbladder and the bowel can occur in conditions involving cholestasis without cystic duct obstruction, such as hepatocellular disease, total parenteral nutrition, and obstruction of the distal common bile duct. Ultrasonography is more sensitive regarding the detection of cholelithiasis but is less accurate in the diagnosis of acute cholecystitis.

Gastric mucosa secretes ^{99m}Tc pertechnetate. It can be used to detect ectopic gastric mucosa, especially in Meckel's diverticulum and sometimes in Barrett's esophagus. Ectopic gastric mucosa is present in most symptomatic Meckel's diverticula and in nearly all that bleed, but only half of the bleeding Meckel's diverticula in adults are detected by this study. False-positive results are common. This method of detecting Meckel's diverticulum is far more useful in children.

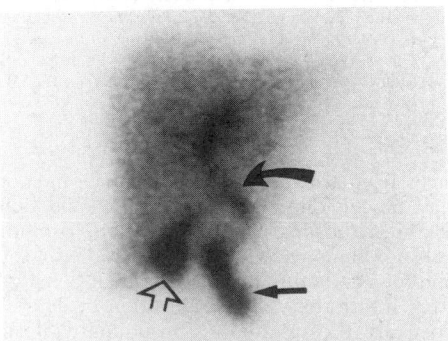

FIGURE 93–9. Normal Tc HIDA scan. Technetium-99m labeled iminodiacetic acid (HIDA) has been excreted by the liver in this normal, fasting patient. Within 60 minutes of intravenous injection, there is visualization of the common bile duct (*curved arrow*), gallbladder (*open arrow*), and duodenum (*straight arrow*).

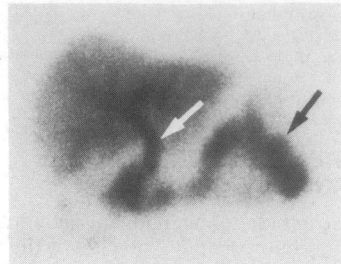

FIGURE 93–10. Tc HIDA of acute cholecystitis. Visualization of the common bile duct (*white arrow*) and small bowel (*black arrow*) without visualization of the gallbladder indicated obstruction of the cystic duct in this fasting patient with acute cholecystitis.

There are two nuclear medicine procedures available for the detection of acute and chronic gastrointestinal bleeding sites, both of which rely upon the extravasation of the radionuclide into the intestinal lumen. Injected ^{99m}Tc sulfur colloid remains in the circulation only briefly, and therefore its use requires active bleeding (approximately 2 ml per minute) at the time of the study. This disadvantage, which is shared with angiography, does not apply to ^{99m}Tc-labeled autologous erythrocytes because they remain in circulation. With the latter procedure, intermittent bleeding of 10 to 20 ml per hour may be detected on delayed views. The reliability of both procedures is greater for the colon and small bowel than for the esophagus, stomach, and duodenum because of overlapping structures in the upper abdomen. *Angiography* for gastrointestinal hemorrhage is used when the site of bleeding cannot be identified by endoscopy or radionuclide imaging or when transcatheter infusion or embolization therapy is indicated. Visceral angiography of most abdominal pathologic conditions has been replaced by other diagnostic procedures, but it is indicated still in the evaluation of vascular occlusive disease, in polysystemic vasculitis, and preoperatively for hepatic tumors.

Disorders of gastric motility are not well evaluated by barium radiographic techniques because these techniques are not quantitative, are relatively insensitive, and are not physiologic. Procedures using radiolabeled food with continuous gastric monitoring may yield quantitative data, such as gastric half-emptying time. Furthermore, with radionuclide imaging gastric emptying of solids versus liquids can be assessed simultaneously.

Liver scanning with ^{99m}Tc sulfur colloid is used for the assessment of size, shape, and position; identification of space-occupying lesions such as tumor, abscess, or hematoma; and evaluation of hepatocellular disease. Sensitivity for the detection of primary and metastatic tumor is comparable to that of CT (which is slightly more accurate) and that of US (which is slightly less sensitive). The newer technique of liver scanning with SPECT (single photon emission computed tomography) imaging produces three-dimensional cross-sectional tomographic images and eliminates the overlapping influences of the surrounding radioactivity. Thus, the sensitivity for small (2 cm) space-occupying lesions is increased.

McAtee JG, Kopecky RT, Frymoyer PA: Nuclear medicine comes of age: Its present and future roles in diagnosis. Radiology 174:609, 1990. *An overview of current uses of radionuclide imaging with an up-to-date list of references.*

MAGNETIC RESONANCE IMAGING

A very brief and simplified summary of the physics of magnetic resonance (MR) imaging is presented here as a background. Hydrogen nuclei (protons) have a dipole moment and therefore behave as would a magnetic compass. In MR scanning, the protons align with the strong magnetic field but are easily disturbed by a brief radiofrequency (rf) pulse of very low energy and then are altered in their alignment. As the protons return to their orientation with the magnetic field, they release energy of a rf that is strongly influenced by the biochemical environment. T_1 and T_2 relaxation times are a description of the released energy, which is detected, mathematically analyzed, and displayed as a two-dimensional proton-density map according to the "signal intensity" of each tissue. Because the water molecule contains two hydrogen nuclei, changes in distribution of water in tissue, as well as its overall concentration, strongly influence the "intensity" of the MR signal. Hence, MR can provide superior

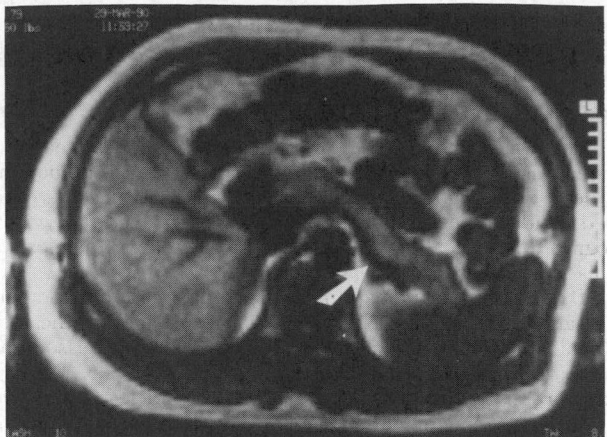

FIGURE 93–11. Normal abdominal magnetic resonance. TurboFlash (Seimens, Magnetom Imager, 1.5 Tesla) (TR = 507 msec, TE = 4 msec) transaxial image of the upper abdomen was acquired in less than 1 second. The tail of the pancreas abuts the splenic hilum and the body is seen anterior to the splenic vein *(arrow)*. Multiple segments of small bowel are seen posterior to the transverse colon.

contrast differentiation of tissues with varying amounts of water compared with conventional radiographic modalities, which depend only upon the attenuation of the roentgenographic beam. In addition, fat emits a strong signal because of the abundance of lipid protons. Other advantages of MR include its noninvasiveness, lack of ionizing radiation, and ability to image directly in transaxial, sagittal, coronal, and nonorthogonal planes. Its disadvantages include cost, limited availability, slow scanning time, and problems associated with the powerful magnetic field. The last-named precludes imaging patients with a cardiac pacemaker or metallic clips on intracranial blood vessels. Moreover, critically ill patients cannot easily be monitored because of limited access to the patient during the study and because the strong magnetic field prohibits the presence of resuscitative equipment made of metal.

Physiologic motion limits the diagnostic capability of MR in the abdomen. With current imaging times of minutes for most scanners (as opposed to a few seconds for CT), respiration and peristalsis cause blurring and artifact, especially of pancreatic and bowel images. Several recently developed techniques have decreased the scan time to seconds and sometimes milliseconds. This makes it possible to image the pancreas (Fig. 93–11) and the mesenteric alimentary tract with MR in addition to the fixed segments as in the rectum (Fig. 93–12) and distal esophagus. Magnetic resonance imaging may have a greater sensitivity to primary and metastatic liver tumors compared with CT, US, and nuclear medicine; but whether it has greater specificity has not been established. The very long T_2 value of most cavernous hemangiomas makes it possible to noninvasively differentiate this common, incidentally noted, benign liver tumor from hepatic malignancy, either primary or metastatic. Magnetic resonance can also image blood vessels noninvasively, and as such may be useful to evaluate the patency of surgical shunts for portal hypertension. The effect of the presence of a paramagnetic substance, such as ferric iron, on the T_1 and T_2 relaxation times alters the MR signal intensity of involved tissue. Hence, MR can detect hemosiderosis and hemochromatosis (Ch. 193) and intravenously introduced ferric iron can enhance the detection of hepatic and splenic metastases. Similarly, paramagnetic substances such as gadolinium-DTPA can be used as contrast-enhancing agents. Magnetic resonance can image the gallbladder,

FIGURE 93–12. Magnetic resonance of rectal tumor. *A,* Transverse T_1 weighted image (TR = 0.5 sec, TE = 30 msec) demonstrates thickening of the rectum (r) due to cloacogenic carcinoma, which is isointense with the surrounding uninvolved muscle. Normal structures demonstrated include the gluteus muscle *(curved black arrow),* which is emitting a low-intensity signal, subcutaneous fat *(white arrows),* which is emitting a high-intensity signal, the right ischium *(open arrow)* and the right femoral head *(curved white arrow). B,* T_2 weighted image of the same area demonstrates a relative increase in the signal intensity of the tumor *(straight arrow)* because of prolongation of its T_2 relaxation time. It now can be differentiated from the adjacent, noninvolved muscle *(curved arrow),* which has retained a normal low-intensity signal.

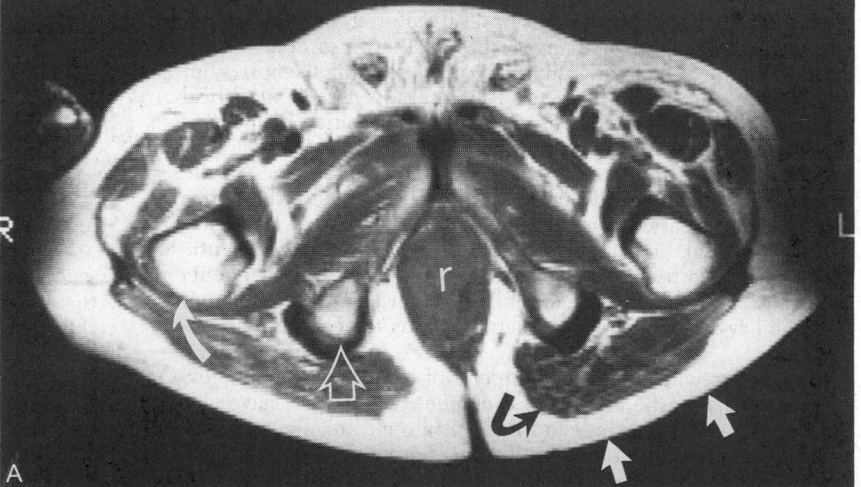

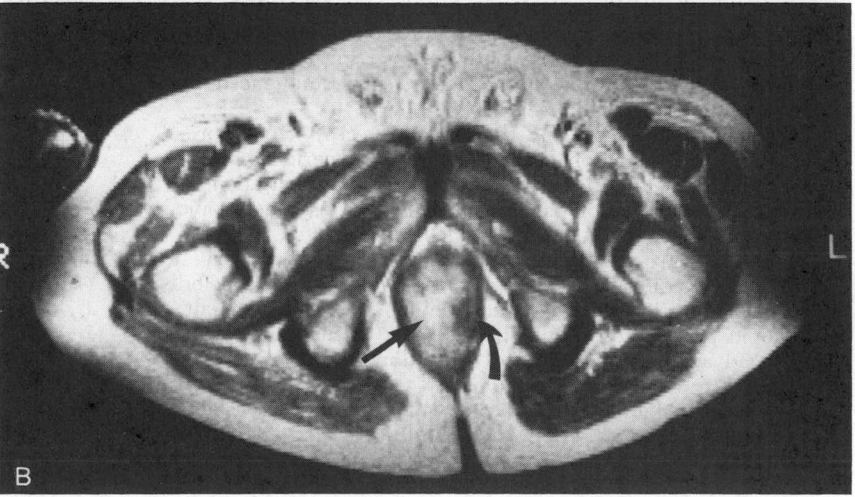

detect cholelithiasis, and differentiate concentrated from nonconcentrated bile. With further development, it may become the procedure of choice for assessing not only morphology but also function of the gallbladder and for diagnosing acute cholecystitis.

Magnetic resonance spectroscopy (MRS) of tissue specifically localized by imaging techniques is a new procedure that is still in the research stage of development. It has not yet achieved clinical applicability in the abdomen, but early work indicates some promise of diagnostic value in the study of high-energy phosphate metabolism (^{31}P) and in imaging sodium (^{23}Na), fluorine (^{19}F), and carbon (^{13}C). Such a procedure, which would facilitate the in vivo study of the biochemistry of normal and diseased organs, is technically more demanding than proton imaging. Because of great potential clinical impact, research is progressing rapidly.

deLange EE, Fechner RE, Wanebo HJ: Suspected recurrent rectosigmoid carcinoma after abdominoperineal resection: MR imaging and histopathologic findings. Radiology 170:323, 1989. *Early work demonstrates limitations, especially regarding specificity.*

Hahn PF, Stark DD, Weissleder R, et al: Clinical application of superparamagnetic iron oxide to MR imaging of tissue perfusion in vascular liver tumors. Radiology 174:361, 1990. *Demonstrates improved diagnostic accuracy in the detection and characterization of focal liver lesions.*

Pykett IL: NMR imaging in medicine. Sci Am 246:78, 1982. *An excellent, understandable review of the physical principles of MRI.*

94 Gastrointestinal Endoscopy

Jack A. Vennes

Remarkable progress in optical engineering and in fiberoptics during the past two decades has basically altered the understanding and management of many gastrointestinal disorders. Fiberoptic techniques were initially used primarily for diagnosis, but increasingly they have been used for therapy. Excellent optical resolution and tip control permit direct visualization of mucosal abnormalities, with photographic record as desired. End-viewing instruments are adapted to visualize all mucosal surfaces of the esophagus, stomach, and duodenum or, alternatively, the entire colon. An internal channel permits routine aspiration, air insufflation, mucosal biopsy, or cytologic examination. Therapeutic devices can also be precisely directed. Side-viewing instruments are used for visualizing the ampulla of Vater and for cannulation of the biliary and pancreatic ductal systems for contrast visualization.

Coincident with the development of fiberoptic techniques, other new diagnostic and often therapeutic modalities have also been developed using radiographic, ultrasound, or nuclear scanning. The problem is often to decide, therefore, which of these diagnostic and therapeutic alternatives is best and most cost effective for patients. Proper sequencing of radiologic, ultrasonic, nuclear, and endoscopic techniques requires an understanding of relative procedural strengths by both the referring physician and the consultant. Procedural choices may also be influenced by factors of cost and available skill.

The diagnostic accuracy and therapeutic success of most procedures are dependent on operator skill and experience. Inexperience not infrequently results in increased complications—including the complication of an erroneous diagnosis. Endoscopic training programs are generally available, integrated with the disciplines of gastroenterology or colorectal or general surgery.

Endoscopy is contraindicated if a perforated viscus is suspected or if the diagnostic results are unlikely to affect management. Endoscopic procedures should be carefully discussed with patients in advance for reassurance. Procedures done by trained personnel are generally well tolerated after light parenteral sedation and analgesia. Topical pharyngeal anesthesia usually improves acceptance of upper tract endoscopy and indeed is often the only medication required for safe, minimally uncomfortable examinations with modern small-caliber endoscopes.

Discussions in this chapter focus on the clinical attributes and capacities of endoscopic procedures and only secondarily on the diseases being investigated. Disease and discovery are intertwined as usual.

ESOPHAGOGASTRODUODENOSCOPY

Endoscopic examination of the entire esophagus, stomach, and duodenum (EGD) is accomplished with routine examination to the deep descending duodenum. All mucosal surfaces are visualized, and photographic records are often made of visually recognized abnormalities. Histologic and cytologic diagnosis can be made as indicated.

INDICATIONS. Indications for diagnostic and therapeutic EGD are listed in Table 94–1. EGD is most often indicated in the evaluation or discovery of possible acid-peptic disease, malignancy, or gastrointestinal bleeding (see Color Plate 1). Endoscopy used "just in case" disease is found leads to overutilization, but management of a presumed disease without diagnostic confirmation often turns out to be underutilization. Both extremes are frequently cost *ineffective*. Therapeutic use of endoscopic techniques is briefly discussed with each procedure in this chapter.

Patients frequently seek medical help for upper abdominal discomfort and associated dyspeptic symptoms of relatively recent onset. If other findings indicative of serious disease are absent, a trial of therapy may be indicated as a first diagnostic test. Most respond to a trial of therapy directed toward their presumed acid-peptic problem. EGD is therefore indicated for the perhaps 30 per cent of all patients with dyspeptic symptoms because symptoms continue despite 14 days of therapy.

Irritable bowel syndrome does not usually require endoscopy, but there are occasional exceptions. Other problems that usually do not require endoscopy include intermittent dyspepsia, heartburn responding to medical therapy, and asymptomatic or uncomplicated hiatal hernia. Uncomplicated duodenal bulb ulcer seen on radiograph that responds to therapy does not usually require endoscopy unless symptoms recur quickly.

Acid-Peptic Disease

Acid-peptic disease, i.e., reflux esophagitis, gastric ulcer, or duodenal ulcer, can be strongly suspected on the basis of the history, but one cannot confidently predict the specific site or pathologic condition. Symptoms of reflux esophagitis are quite specific, but other gastroduodenal lesions frequently coexist (Ch. 96). The presence of esophageal reflux symptoms correlates

TABLE 94–1. INDICATIONS FOR ESOPHAGOGASTRODUODENOSCOPY (EGD)

A. Upper abdominal distress that persists despite an appropriate trial of therapy
B. Upper abdominal distress associated with signs suggesting serious organic disease (e.g., anorexia and weight loss)
C. Dysphagia or odynophagia
D. Esophageal reflux symptoms that are persistent or progressive despite appropriate therapy
E. Persistent vomiting of unknown cause
F. Other system disease in which the presence of upper gastrointestinal pathologic conditions might modify other planned management; examples include patients with a history of gastrointestinal bleeding who are scheduled for renal transplantation, long-term anticoagulation, and chronic nonsteroidal therapy for arthritis
G. Radiographic findings of:
  1. A neoplastic lesion, for confirmation and specific histologic diagnosis
  2. Gastric or esophageal ulcer
  3. Evidence of upper tract stricture or obstruction
  4. Mass
H. Gastrointestinal bleeding:
  1. As the first procedure in most actively bleeding patients
  2. When surgical therapy is contemplated
  3. When rebleeding occurs after acute, self-limited blood loss
  4. When portal hypertension or aortoenteric fistula is suspected
  5. For endoscopic therapy of upper gastrointestinal bleeding
  6. For presumed chronic blood loss and iron deficiency anemia when colonoscopy findings are negative

Modified from Appropriate Use of Gastrointestinal Endoscopy. American Society for Gastrointestinal Endoscopy, 1989.

well with the presence of endoscopic findings and less well with histologic findings. Local symptoms in the mid or lower esophagus are usually predictive of disease location, whereas high substernal symptoms may be due to disease anywhere in the esophagus. Gastric or duodenal ulcers are usually symptomatic, but in patients with previous gastric or duodenal ulcer, asymptomatic recurrences are discovered in 5 per cent or more of patients who have had endoscopy in long-term studies.

EGD is more sensitive and specific than radiographic studies in evaluating disease of the upper gastrointestinal tract, although neither is infallible. Radiographic studies are least sensitive in evaluating lesions without apparent depth, such as flat stomal postgastrectomy ulcers, giant duodenal ulcers involving an entire wall of the duodenal bulb, or erosive esophagitis.

Cancer

Malignant lesions of the upper gastrointestinal tract are generally evident as exophytic masses protruding into the lumen (Ch. 99). Flat, infiltrative lesions do occur occasionally, however. In the esophagus, such lesions may resemble a benign stricture, and in the stomach (linitis plastica), the primary features are stiffness and poor distensibility. Malignancy may occasionally present as ulceration; accurate evaluation of all esophageal and gastric ulcers is therefore mandatory and challenging. At least 75 per cent of malignant ulcers are correctly identified by endoscopic visual criteria, as asymmetric folds or nodules that randomly form the crater rim and extend irregularly into surrounding mucosa. Malignant tissue is often seen as multihued. Benign ulcers are typically smoother with more crater depth and with more symmetry and less randomness, and a zone of erythema is present at the junction of the crater and rim.

Histologic and cytologic data should be added to the endoscopic evaluation of all suspicious lesions and most gastric ulcers. This results in a sensitivity (positive when disease is present) and specificity (negative when disease is absent) of 95 per cent. Brush or lavage cytology is a particularly important adjunct in evaluating the smooth, infiltrative esophageal stricture or the linitis plastica gastric lesion or the occasional superficial, spreading, flat gastric cancer. Primary gastric lymphoma may present as an ulcer, ulcerated mass, or large, asymmetric folds. Specific histologic features are frequently present only in submucosal tissue.

Mucosal polyps are rare in the stomach and rarer still in the duodenum and esophagus. Submucosal or intramucosal polypoid defects overlain with normal mucosa are usually pancreatic rests or leiomyomas and can be left in place. Adenomatous polyps have premalignant potential, which increases with size. All polypoid lesions should be endoscopically visualized, with biopsy or removal with snare cautery. Multiple small, hyperplastic polyps are not premalignant and need not all be removed, and no surveillance is indicated. Adenomas should be excised endoscopically when feasible. Very large lesions may require surgical removal. Surveillance is indicated after removal of gastric adenomatous polyps.

Other upper gastrointestinal malignancies originating in the pancreas or biliary tree do not usually extend into gastric or duodenal mucosa, and they require other diagnostic studies (see below). Ampullary carcinoma is usually visible *if* the papilla of Vater is adequately seen via a conventional end-viewing endoscope or a side-viewing instrument (see below).

Upper Gastrointestinal Bleeding (see Ch. 111)

EGD is the most informative procedure when further information is indicated for management of the acutely bleeding patient, particularly if done within 12 hours of admission. Information obtained includes (1) location and identity of the bleeding source; (2) whether bleeding is continuing; (3) whether bleeding is arterial; (4) which of multiple lesions is bleeding; and (5) whether a visible vessel is present in an ulcer base. These endoscopic observations are available in 85 per cent of patients with acute bleeding and influence prognosis and management decisions. There is no evidence that endoscopy initiates further bleeding. A precise diagnosis of the status and source of gastrointestinal bleeding is requisite for successful management. Endoscopic methods for controlling active bleeding are often effective. When indications for these techniques become clearer, more early endoscopy of acute bleeding will likely be indicated (see below).

The source of chronic gastrointestinal blood loss or iron deficiency anemia in men is usually discovered in the colon. EGD may be indicated by history suggesting upper tract sources or after negative findings on colonoscopy in patients with chronic blood loss.

Therapeutic Applications of Esophagogastroduodenoscopy

Therapeutic endoscopic procedures commonly carried out in the upper gastrointestinal tract include removal of foreign bodies, dilation of benign or malignant esophageal strictures, sclerotherapy of bleeding esophageal varices, placement of percutaneous gastrostomies, and electrocoagulation of focal bleeding lesions. Foreign bodies in the esophagus or stomach can usually be removed by techniques that employ snares or forceps as grasping devices. Protective overtubes may be used to prevent soft tissue injury or aspiration. Impaction of food may occur because of an underlying esophageal abnormality, and careful esophagoscopy after removal of food may reveal a benign or malignant stricture or may suggest a motility disorder.

Esophageal strictures found to be benign on careful evaluation can be successfully dilated. If the course of the esophagus is tortuous, if the stricture is tight and does not admit the endoscope, or if epiphrenic diverticula are present, dilation is safely done over a guide wire passed under fluoroscopic control. Tapered bougies, metal olives, or inflatable balloons of progressively increasing diameter may be passed over the wire. Following this, endoscopy and biopsy are done to assess whether there is a malignant lesion. Less complex strictures that only partially occlude the lumen may, after endoscopy, be safely dilated with tapered bougies without wire guidance and without further endoscopy. A maintenance dilation schedule with individualized intervals is important. Dilation intervals can often be lengthened as stricture inflammation subsides.

Management of malignant esophageal strictures is directed to the goal of reducing tumor mass and allowing the unobstructed passage of food, liquids, and oral secretions. The options available include surgery, radiation therapy, or such endoscopic procedures as repeated esophageal dilation, dilation and endoscopic placement of a stent across the malignant narrowing (or across a tracheoesophageal fistula), or use of laser energy to restore the lumen by tumor destruction. All of these latter procedures have good reported results; all require skill for success and safety; and all can be done without prolonged hospitalization. Local skills are often valid determinants. Quality survival time is usually brief, but 85 to 90 per cent of patients can be helped, with a complication rate of about 5 per cent.

Several endoscopic measures have proved effective in controlling upper gastrointestinal bleeding. Endoscopic variceal sclerosis by intravariceal and perivariceal injection of various sclerosants controls the acute variceal hemorrhage of portal hypertension in 90 per cent of patients. Prophylactic sclerosis may also prevent future hemorrhage. Endoscopic variceal sclerosis reduces the risk of rebleeding, with fewer hospital days and transfusions, but survival is not significantly prolonged.

Focal nonvariceal bleeding can often be controlled using electrocoagulation with monopolar or bipolar current delivery or combined electrocoagulation and thermal heater probe techniques or laser photocoagulation. Neodymium yttrium aluminum garnet (YAG) laser energy is carried through the endoscope via a flexible wave guide and converted to thermal energy when precisely directed to an absorptive (bleeding) area. Bleeding is controlled in up to 90 per cent of lesions, including those with brisk arterial bleeding, but rebleeding rates are significant with all methods. Laser equipment is expensive and not portable. Perforation, although of low risk, is a definite hazard with all techniques.

Diagnostic endoscopy is urgently indicated if one or more of several clinical risk factors are present: a large volume bleed as evidenced by orthostasis, copious hematemesis, and need for transfusions. Urgent endoscopy is also indicated if portal hypertension and variceal bleeding are suspected with an active rebleed in the hospital or if there is a history of previous aortic aneurysm repair. Endoscopic observations include the site of bleeding and whether bleeding persists.

Eighty-five per cent or more of upper gastrointestinal bleeding episodes stop spontaneously; how then do we select those patients who need endoscopic control of bleeding? A pigmented, elevated visible vessel in the ulcer base, a fresh adherent clot, or continuing active bleeding are all observable risk factors for further bleeding and are indications for endoscopic therapy, most frequently with electrocoagulation or heater probe techniques. Surgery or angiographic occlusion of bleeding vessels is required for some whose bleeding is unusually brisk.

Percutaneous endoscopic gastrostomy (PEG) is a useful method for providing selected patients with long-term enteral feeding. Candidates are those with a functioning gut and chronically inadequate oral intake. Some may have recurrent aspiration secondary to upper esophageal dysfunction. Specific indications include neurologic disorders that affect the swallowing mechanism or that result in diminished food intake secondary to a decreased sensorium, or cancer of the pharynx or upper esophagus that does not totally obstruct (so that an endoscope can be passed). Percutaneous endoscopic gastrostomy is not indicated in postgastrectomy patients or in those with midline abdominal scar, severe, uncorrectable coagulopathy, or respirator dependency. The decision to initiate chronic enteral feeding can be a difficult one, involving the wishes of patient and family and the gravity of the underlying disease. Once the decision is made, however, PEG is a simple and safe method.

COMPLICATIONS. Complications from EGD are rare with modern small-caliber, flexible instruments but do occur. A morbidity of 0.13 per cent and a mortality of 0.0004 per cent have been reported. During or following endoscopic examination, perforation has occurred in the upper esophagus near the cricopharyngeus, through Zenker's diverticula, and through areas of tumor. Use of sedative or analgesic drugs may transiently suppress respiration, especially in elderly patients or those with severe obstructive pulmonary disease. Aspiration during endoscopy is very unlikely unless there is vomiting due to massive bleeding or gastric outlet obstruction. Cardiovascular complications, sepsis, prolonged bleeding, or thrombophlebitis from intravenous medications occur rarely.

COLONOSCOPY AND FLEXIBLE SIGMOIDOSCOPY

The entire colon is now routinely accessible to high-resolution viewing with biopsy, brush cytology, polypectomy, and photography of observed lesions. Much has been learned of the polypcancer progression, and significant control of colon cancer is within cost-effective reach of the trained endoscopist.

INDICATIONS. The indications for colonoscopy are listed in Table 94–2. As with EGD, colonoscopic examination is primarily used to evaluate possible cancer, inflammation, and bleeding. The procedure is contraindicated in the presence of fulminant colitis; acute, severe diverticulitis; or probable perforated viscus. Colonoscopy is generally not indicated for stable irritable bowel syndrome, acute diarrhea, upper gastrointestinal bleeding, or rectal bleeding with an anorectal source on anoscopy or sigmoidoscopy. Other nonindications include routine follow-up of inflammatory bowel disease (except as noted in Table 94–2) and routine preoperative examination of patients undergoing elective abdominal surgery for noncolonic disease.

Flexible fiberoptic sigmoidoscopy (FFS) is usually carried out with 60-cm instrumentation, although a 35-cm endoscope is available. Training requirements are less rigorous than those for colonoscopy. Indications for FFS are listed in Table 94–3. At least 60 per cent of colon cancers and potential colon cancers (neoplastic polyps) are located in the rectosigmoid and lower descending colon and thus are in reach of the "screening" FFS. FFS has the same contraindications as colonoscopy and is generally not indicated when colonoscopy is indicated (see Table 94–3). FFS is specifically not indicated for polypectomy because colonoscopy is needed, and full colonic preparation is necessary to prevent possible explosions during electrocautery. Preparation for FFS is simple, using two enemas, whereas preparation for colonoscopy requires a two-day liquid diet preparation or total

TABLE 94–2. INDICATIONS FOR COLONOSCOPY

A. Evaluation of an abnormality on barium enema that is likely to be clinically significant, such as a filling defect or stricture
B. For discovery and excision of colonic polyps:
  1. When polyps are seen on barium enema radiograph
  2. When neoplastic polyps are detected by proctosigmoidoscopy
C. Evaluation of unexplained gastrointestinal bleeding:
  1. Clinically significant hematochezia
  2. Melena with a negative upper gastrointestinal workup
  3. Presence of unexplained fecal occult blood
D. Unexplained iron deficiency anemia
E. Surveillance for colonic neoplasia
  1. Examination to "clear" entire colon of synchronous cancer or neoplastic polyps in a patient with a treatable cancer or neoplastic polyp
  2. Follow-up examination at two- to three-year intervals after resection of a colorectal cancer or neoplastic polyp and an adequate initial "clearing" colonoscopy
  3. Patients with a strongly positive family history of colonic cancer
  4. In patients with chronic ulcerative colitis: colonoscopy every one to two years with multiple biopsies for detection of cancer and dysplasia in patients with:
    a. Pancolitis of greater than seven years' duration
    b. Left-sided colitis of over 15 years' duration (no surveillance needed for disease limited to rectosigmoid)
F. Chronic inflammatory bowel disease of the colon if more precise diagnosis or determination of the extent of activity of disease will influence immediate management
G. Therapeutic colonoscopy, as control of bleeding or colonic decompression

Modified from Appropriate Use of Gastrointestinal Endoscopy. American Society for Gastrointestinal Endoscopy, 1989.

gut lavage with large volumes of an isotonic solution. The place for FFS is assured as a more comfortable, more informative replacement for rigid proctosigmoidoscopy at nearly equivalent cost.

Polyps and Cancer of the Colon (see Ch. 105)

Colonoscopy to evaluate the possibility of colon cancer or its precursor polyps is usually indicated after an abnormality is detected by barium enema or proctosigmoidoscopy or if there is unexplained lower gastrointestinal bleeding. If occult blood is detected in the interior of a passed stool, colonoscopy will identify an age-related 20 to 30 per cent incidence of adenomatous polyps and 8 to 15 per cent incidence of cancers. During active bleeding, colonoscopy may present technical difficulties in accurately locating the bleeding source. Repeat colonoscopy may be necessary after cessation of bleeding for accurate colonic assessment.

After endoscopic removal of neoplastic polyps or after resection of colon cancer, continued surveillance is indicated, since the patient is now identified as being at risk for later colon cancer. A "clearing" examination may be optionally done once within 12 months to be certain no polyps or cancers were missed at the first examination. Thereafter, follow-up examination every 3 years will detect new lesions before they become infiltrating carcinomas, since the process from polyp inception to infiltrating cancer appears to take up to 7 years. The only way to rule out cancer within a polyp is to remove it completely for histologic examination. Other conditions associated with increased risk for cancer also require surveillance (Table 94–2).

Most colonic polyps are hyperplastic and are not premalignant. In neoplastic polyps, cancer risk increases with increasing dysplasia and villoglandular transformation and also with size. Pedunculated polyps with an uninvolved stalk and with cancer confined to the mucosa can be cured by snare cautery removal.

TABLE 94–3. INDICATIONS FOR FLEXIBLE FIBEROPTIC SIGMOIDOSCOPY (FFS)

A. Screening of asymptomatic patients at risk for colonic neoplasia
B. Evaluation of suspected distal colonic disease when there is no indication for colonoscopy
C. Evaluation of the entire colon in conjunction with barium enema radiographs

Modified from Appropriate Use of Gastrointestinal Endoscopy. American Society for Gastrointestinal Endoscopy, 1989.

Most colonoscopists remove all polyps greater than 5 mm in diameter. Polyps less than 5 mm may be neoplastic; coagulation or a coagulation biopsy technique during colonoscopy is used to remove them.

Inflammatory Bowel Disease (see Ch. 103)

Most patients with inflammatory bowel disease do not require colonoscopy for diagnosis. At times, however, colonoscopy may provide unique and important information. Differentiation between granulomatous colitis (Crohn's disease) and ulcerative colitis is usually possible with colonoscopy and multiple biopsies. The anatomic extent of disease can be determined. The presence or absence of inflammatory bowel disease can be determined more accurately when clinically suspected despite absence of radiographic or sigmoidoscopic findings.

Diagnostic colonoscopy in ulcerative colitis is at times necessary to evaluate a stricture or a mass seen on barium enema. Occasionally, strictures are malignant with submucosal tumor spread. Pseudopolyps are not premalignant and need not be histologically examined. Polyps may be neoplastic or malignant, however, and those that are larger than 1 cm in diameter and are friable and irregular in color or configuration should be biopsied. In surveillance examinations of patients with ulcerative colitis, multiple biopsies are obtained throughout the involved colon. When moderate to severe dysplasia is consistently found, colectomy is usually recommended.

Polypectomy is the main therapeutic use of colonoscopy. Endoscopic control of bleeding is not usually feasible. Electrocautery of angiodysplastic lesions in the cecum and ascending colon has been successful, but new lesions may appear within months. Dilation of anastomotic strictures by balloons passed over a guide wire or through the endoscope is occasionally useful.

COMPLICATIONS. Diagnostic colonoscopy has a complication rate of 0.5 per cent, which rises to 1 per cent when polypectomy is added, with hemorrhage and perforation being the principal complications.

ENDOSCOPIC RETROGRADE CHOLANGIOPANCREATOGRAPHY (ERCP)

The side-viewing endoscope and the technique for identifying and cannulating the ampulla of Vater result in diagnostic quality radiographic study of both the common bile duct and the pancreatic duct in 90 per cent of attempts (Fig. 93–7). Failure may result from anatomic distortions due to prior surgery, tumor infiltration, or the duodenal edema of acute pancreatitis.

INDICATIONS. Indications for ERCP are listed in Table 94–4. Endoscopic retrograde cholangiopancreatography is generally not helpful in evaluating abdominal pain of obscure origin in the absence of objective findings suggesting pancreatic or biliary disease. Known or suspected gallbladder disease is not an indication for ERCP in the absence of evidence for bile duct involvement. Study of patients with acute pancreatitis is usually deferred until a second episode has established its recurrent nature, unless there is evidence to suggest gallstone disease.

TABLE 94–4. INDICATIONS FOR ENDOSCOPIC RETROGRADE CHOLANGIOPANCREATOGRAPHY (ERCP)

A. Evaluation of the jaundiced patient suspected of having treatable biliary obstruction

B. Evaluation of the patient without jaundice (with or without prior cholecystectomy) whose clinical presentation suggests bile duct disease

C. Therapeutic pancreatic or biliary endoscopy, e.g., endoscopic sphincterotomy, balloon dilatation of strictures, stent placement across strictures; these procedures frequently require follow-up endoscopy

D. Evaluation of signs or symptoms suggesting pancreatic malignancy when results of ultrasound (US) and/or computed tomography (CT) are equivocal or normal

E. Evaluation of recurrent or persistent pancreatitis of unknown etiology

F. Preoperative evaluation of the patient with chronic pancreatitis

G. Evaluation of possible pancreatic pseudocyst undetected by CT or US and for known pseudocyst prior to planned surgical therapy

Modified from Appropriate Use of Gastrointestinal Endoscopy. American Society for Gastrointestinal Endoscopy, 1989.

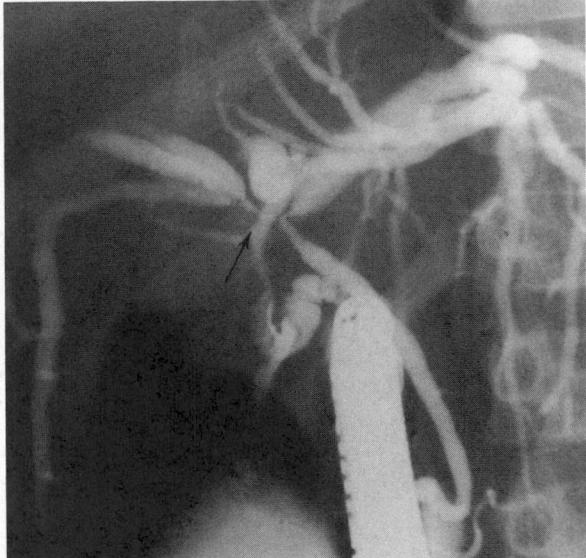

FIGURE 94–1. Retrograde cholangiogram: bile duct cancer. Multiple strictures at the bifurcation of the common hepatic duct (*arrow*) are due to a primary bile duct cancer (Klatskin tumor). Intrahepatic ducts are dilated and partially obstructed. The extrahepatic ductal system distal to the tumor is of normal caliber, here seen coursing medial to the endoscope.

Pancreatic malignancy clearly demonstrated on CT or ultrasonography need not be further evaluated with ERCP except for stent placement.

Other tests besides ERCP provide diagnostic evidence of pancreatic and biliary disease: percutaneous transhepatic cholangiography (PTC), computed tomography (CT), and ultrasonography (US). Transabdominal fine-needle aspiration cytology with CT, US, or ERCP guidance is also helpful, as malignant cells are found by this means in 85 per cent of patients with pancreatic cancer.

In evaluating suspected biliary obstruction, a cholangiogram is usually obtained prior to therapy (Fig. 94–1). When the patient has fever, pain, and icterus, choledocholithiasis is suspected with high clinical accuracy. One may then proceed directly to cholangiography by PTC or preferably by ERCP if endoscopic sphincterotomy is planned. Ultrasonography is usually performed to assess ductal dilatation, but this is of limited value, as calculi often reside in undilated ducts.

When the presence of extrahepatic obstruction and its etiology are less certain, US as the initial study provides useful information at reasonable cost. For example, a normal gallbladder without calculi makes choledocholithiasis unlikely. Masses in the pancreas, bile duct, or porta hepatis, diffuse pancreatic enlargement, or grossly dilated bile ducts direct an appropriate specific disease evaluation.

Ultrasonography and CT have improved greatly in their ability to detect pancreatic malignancy (Ch. 107). Equivocal results at times require confirmation by ERCP. Cut-off or stenosis of pancreatic duct and often of bile duct (double-duct sign) is a reliable ERCP finding of carcinoma (Fig. 94–2). Patients with chronic pain and suspected chronic pancreatitis who are surgical candidates should have preoperative pancreatography and cholangiography to assess patency of the main pancreatic duct and to assess possible stricture of the intrapancreatic bile duct. Differentiating chronic pancreatitis from pancreatic cancer may be impossible, as the pancreatic duct is often dilated and tortuous with dilated, stubby lateral branches in both diseases (Fig. 94–3). Downstream ductal stricturing in the pancreatic head is the hallmark of malignancy, however.

Therapeutic Applications of Endoscopic Retrograde Cholangiopancreatography

In endoscopic retrograde sphincterotomy (ERS), soft tissues and sphincter fibers of the papilla and intraduodenal portion of

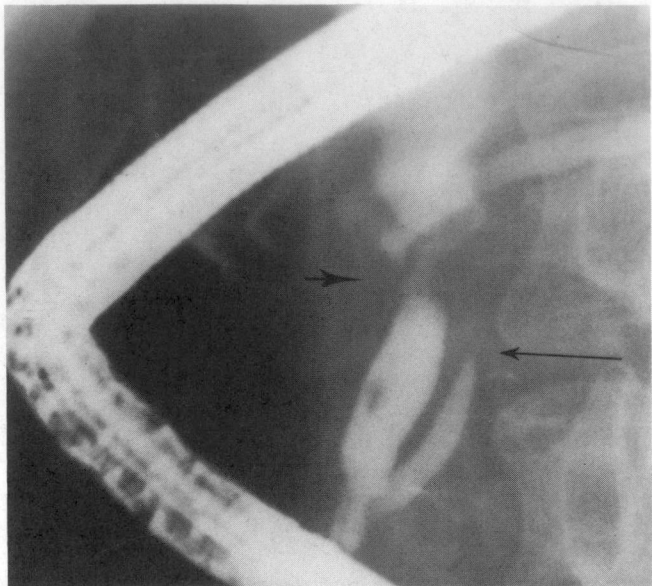

FIGURE 94–2. Pancreatogram and cholangiogram: pancreatic cancer. Both ducts are outlined by retrograde instillation of contrast at the bottom of the picture. Both the common bile duct (*large arrow*) and the pancreatic duct (*small arrow*) are strictured in the classic "double duct sign" of pancreatic cancer.

the common bile duct are divided with electrocautery to relieve ductal obstruction due to common duct stones or papillary stenosis. Endoscopic retrograde sphincterotomy has assumed a major role in the management of choledocholithiasis and offers a relatively safe and simple alternative to surgical management.

Biliary calculus obstruction is relieved by ERS in 85 to 90 per cent of attempts. Complications of hemorrhage, pancreatitis, perforation, and cholangitis occur in 3 to 8 per cent of cases with a mortality rate of 0.4 per cent. Late complications of re-stenosis or re-formed stones occur in 1 to 8 per cent of patients.

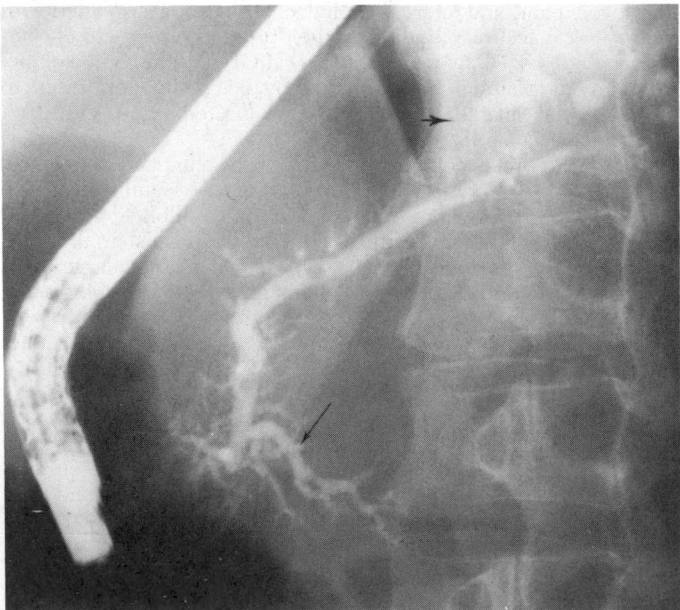

FIGURE 94–3. Pancreatogram: chronic pancreatitis. The main pancreatic duct is moderately dilated and unobstructed. The lateral branches are dilated, tortuous, and stubby. The duct from the uncinate process is prominent (*small arrow*). A small pseudocyst (*large arrow*) is barely visible overlying the spine in this oblique view. Filling defects in the main pancreatic duct may be calculi or air bubble artifact. With progression of the disease the main pancreatic duct may become more tortuous and dilated.

Endoscopic retrograde sphincterotomy is now widely considered the therapy of choice for patients with symptomatic stones in the common bile duct. The procedure is often carried out immediately following ERCP as soon as the presence of stones in the duct is confirmed. It is clearly safer and cheaper than surgery in these generally elderly patients and more successful than percutaneous transhepatic extraction. Cholangitis and gallstone pancreatitis usually respond dramatically to decompression. About 40 per cent of patients with symptomatic choledocholithiasis have never had cholecystitis, and therefore their gallbladders are intact. Almost all contain calculi. After removing duct calculi with ERS, should the gallbladder be electively removed to preclude further cholecystitis or migration of stones into the now open biliary tree? Or may the gallbladder be left in place and removed only as future symptoms dictate? Experience with patients at high surgical risk suggests the safety and success of waiting, as the probability of cholecystitis does not exceed 5 per cent per year in these generally elderly patients.

Papillary stenosis is a poorly defined disorder or group of disorders in which recurrent biliary colic or occasionally pancreatitis is thought to result from papillary fibrosis or sphincter dysfunction. Diagnostic criteria include a dilated bile duct, slow ductal drainage, cholestasis following painful episodes, and elevated basal sphincter of Oddi pressure during manometry. The problem arises most commonly in women who have had a cholecystectomy either for cholelithiasis or for biliary colic-like pain without stones. Endoscopic retrograde sphincterotomy is often curative for carefully selected patients with papillary stenosis.

Placement of plastic stents across biliary strictures is the second major therapeutic extension of ERCP. Most strictures are caused by inoperable pancreatic or bile duct carcinoma, and other treatment options are surgical or transhepatic decompression. A catheter containing a guide wire is introduced via the endoscope through the stricture, and a stent is passed over the catheter. The distal end is left in the duodenum, bile drainage is restored, and barbed flaps prevent dislodgment of the stent. The procedure is successful in 90 per cent of attempts. Present-day stents remain patent for 5 months or more and can be rather easily replaced.

COMPLICATIONS. In 1 per cent of patients, acute pancreatitis follows ERCP, usually beginning within 2 hours of the procedure as a clinically mild complication. Biliary sepsis occurs less commonly but is more serious and even life threatening. Introduction of even a few bacteria into a semiclosed space—bile duct, gallbladder, pancreatic pseudocyst—may occasionally have serious septic consequences. Organisms may be introduced from the unsterile gastrointestinal tract or from instruments. Stringent cleaning and disinfection techniques are mandatory, including periodic cultures of equipment. Sepsis is prevented by prompt surgical, endoscopic, or transhepatic decompression of discovered obstruction within 24 hours of ERCP, plus judicious use of appropriate parenteral antibiotics.

LAPAROSCOPY

Laparoscopy permits direct inspection of much of the anterior abdominal space. A pneumoperitoneum is created and a rigid or flexible laparoscope is introduced through a puncture in the abdominal wall, with the patient under local anesthesia and mild sedation. The procedure is well tolerated; complications of bleeding or bowel perforation occur in only 0.1 to 0.2 per cent. When it is clinically important to assess focal or diffuse liver disease, laparoscopy, by combining assessment of gross appearance and guided biopsy, is 90 per cent accurate, substantially better than percutaneous blind liver biopsy. This is true whether the disease is diffuse (cirrhosis) or focal (metastatic nodules). More than two thirds of the liver and variable parts of the gallbladder, spleen, peritoneum, and diaphragm can usually be visualized. The colon and small bowel are variably open to inspection.

The major indications for laparoscopy are (1) inspection and guided biopsy of the liver in suspected diffuse or focal disease, when the information will affect therapy and (2) evaluation of exudative ascites (malignancy versus inflammation). Determination of the presence or absence of abdominal metastases may be important in assessing operability. The procedure is contraindicated in the presence of acute peritonitis, intestinal obstruction, severe coagulopathy, infection of the abdominal wall, or severe

PLATE 1   GASTROINTESTINAL DISEASES

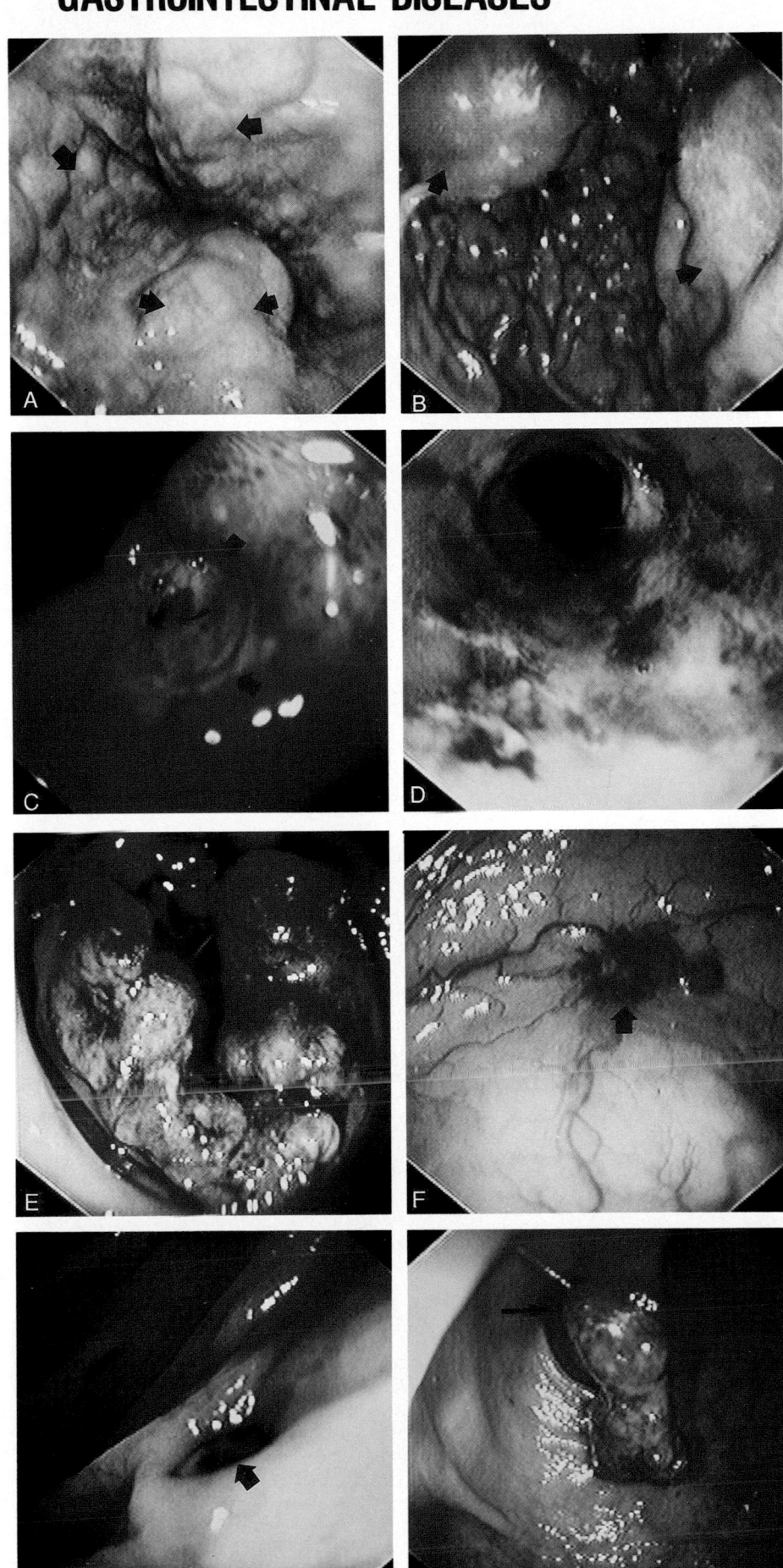

Endoscopy and colonoscopy in gastrointestinal hemorrhage.

A, Esophageal varices. Large serpiginous dilated submucosal veins (arrows) are noted coursing longitudinally down the distal esophagus.

B, Gastric varices. The endoscope has been turned around on itself to examine the gastric cardia, where large submucosal masses are seen projecting into the lumen (arrows).

C, Duodenal bulbar ulcer. A white excavated base is noted just inside the pylorus (large arrows) containing a dark red central artery oozing blood (small arrow).

D, Esophagitis. The normal pink esophageal mucosa is replaced by white exudate overlying extensive superficial erosions in a patient with reflux esophagitis.

E, Colonic cancer. Nearly all the lumen is obstructed by a fungating, bleeding colonic malignancy.

F, Vascular ectasia of the cecum. The normal delicate branching mucosal vessels are altered by a "coral reef" (arrow) telangiectatic lesion in an elderly patient with recurrent bouts of hematochezia.

G, Diverticulum of colon. Clotted blood can be seen within an outpouching of the colonic wall (arrow) in a patient with massive hematochezia.

H, Colonic polyp. An irregular fleshy mass on a pedicle (arrow) is noted projecting into the bowel lumen. Polypectomy subsequently removed and retrieved an adenomatous polyp.

PLATE 2   GASTROINTESTINAL DISEASES

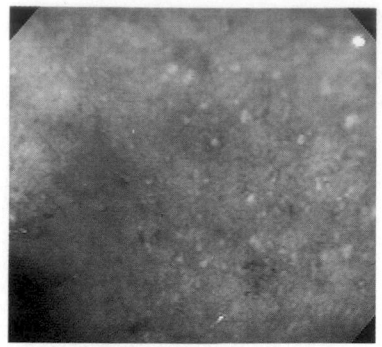

A, Mild ulcerative colitis seen on endoscopy. Granular-appearing mucosa with friability and pinpoint ulceration.

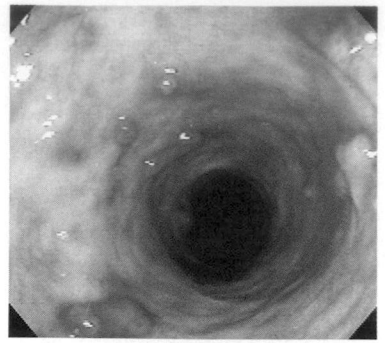

B, Quiescent ulcerative colitis seen on endoscopy. Distorted vascular pattern with residual "pseudopolyps."

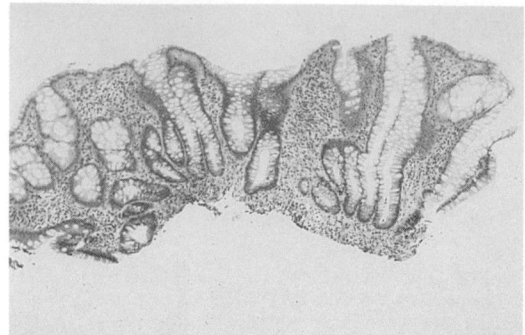

C, Mucosal biopsy of quiescent ulcerative colitis. Distorted, branching glands with reduced goblet cell mucus and minimal chronic inflammation.

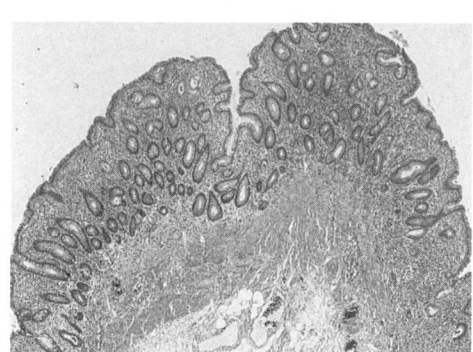

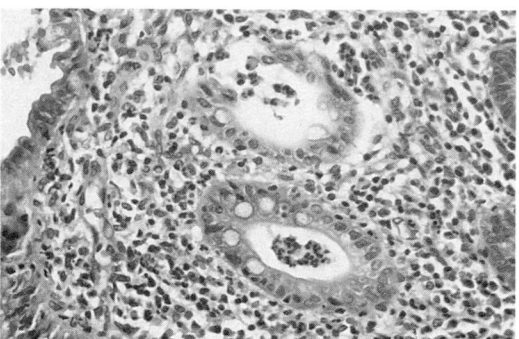

D, Mucosal biopsy of active ulcerative colitis. *Left,* Low power. Acute and chronic inflammation. *Right,* High power. Crypt abscess.

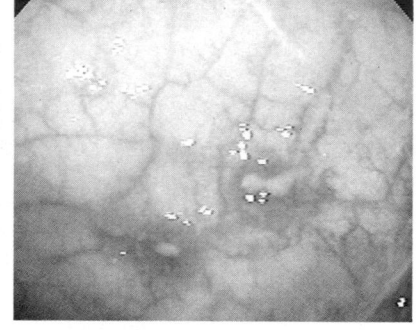

E, Aphthoid ulcer of Crohn's disease. Note normal surrounding mucosa.

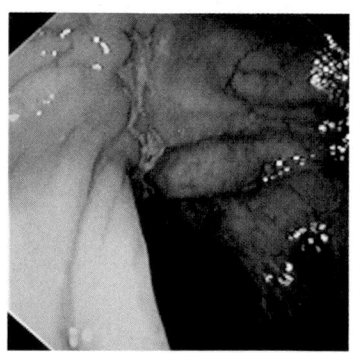

F, Crohn's disease. Linear ulceration.

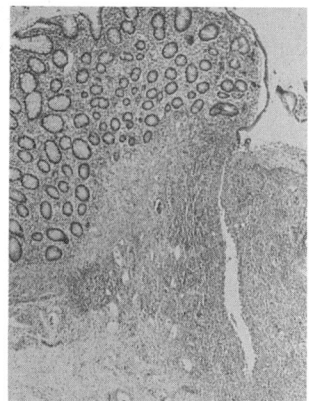

G, Mucosal biopsy of Crohn's disease. Focal inflammation with fissuring ulceration.

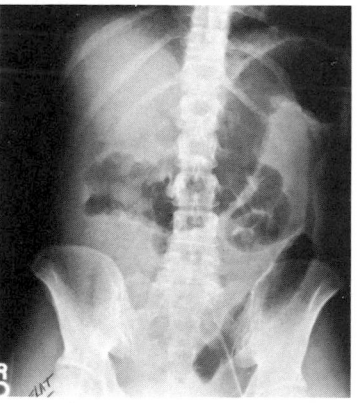

H, Abdominal flat-plate demonstrating toxic megacolon with dilated, ahaustral colon.

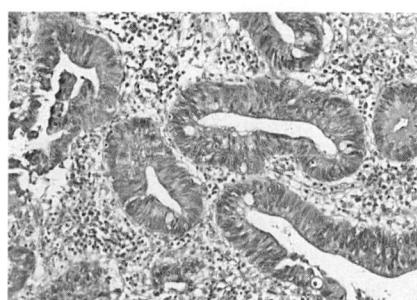

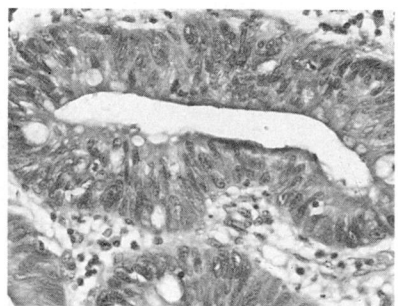

I, Low-power *(left)* and high-power *(right)* views of mucosal dysplasia with hyperchromatic epithelial cells and mucus depletion with stratification and loss of polarity.

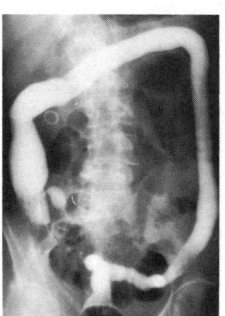

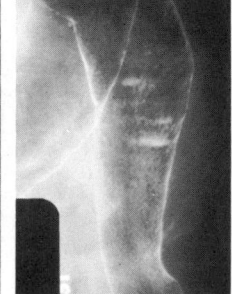

J, Left and *right,* Air-contrast barium enema of ulcerative colitis with contiguous loss of haustration and sandpaper-like granularity.

PLATE 3   GASTROINTESTINAL DISEASES

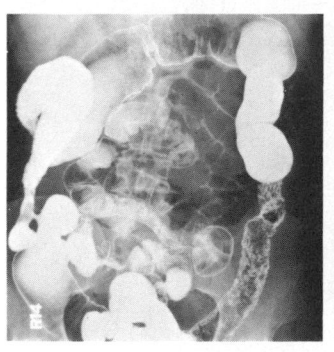 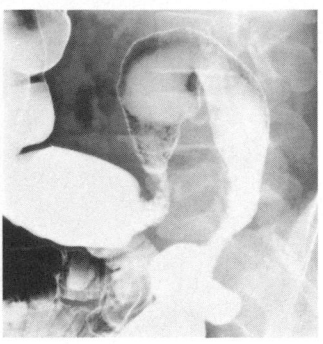

A, Left and *right,* Air-contrast barium enema of Crohn's disease of the colon with asymmetric linear ulceration, cobblestone mucosa, and rectal sparing.

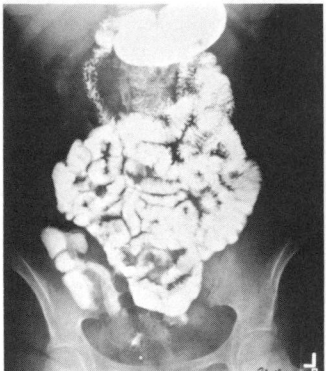 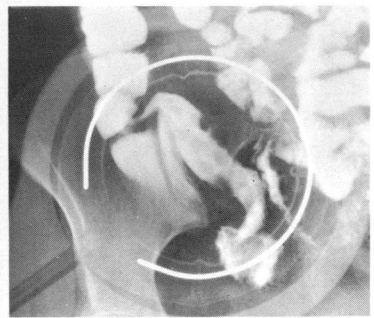

B, Left and *right,* Small bowel follow-through of ileal Crohn's disease, showing separation of loops of distal ileum and cobblestone appearance.

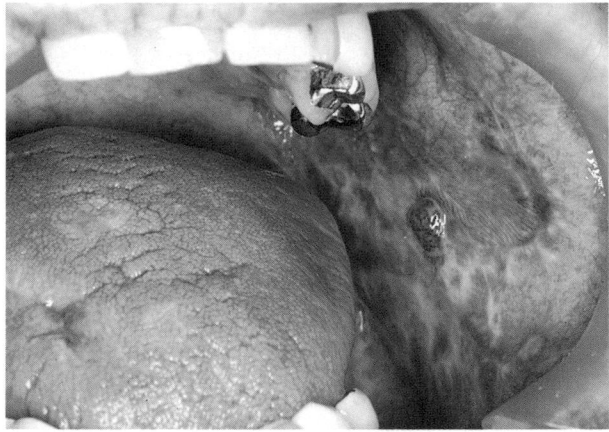

C, Erosive lichen planus in a 62-year-old woman. Note the white striae and central ulceration. Similar lesions were present on the opposite buccal mucosa.

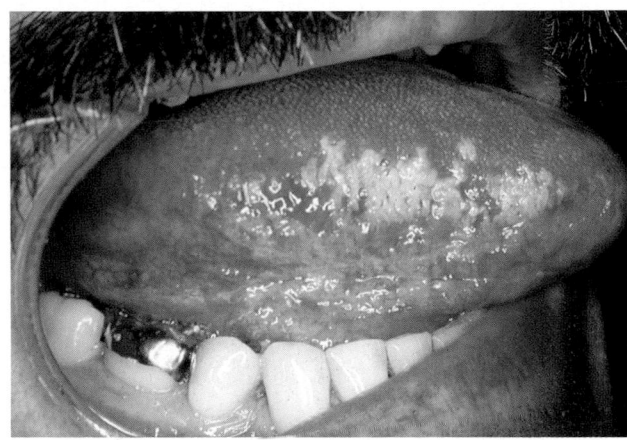

D, Hairy leukoplakia in a 38-year-old man. This was the first sign of HIV infection. One year later he developed *Pneumocystis carinii* pneumonia. (Courtesy of Dr. D. Greenspan.)

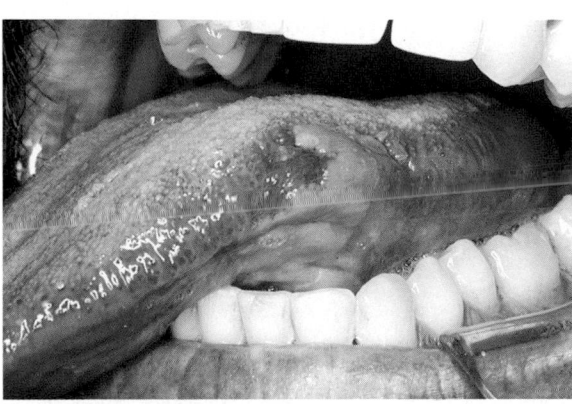

E, Erythroplakia anterior to leukoplakia in a 40-year-old man with a history of frequent cigarette smoking for many years. Histologically, the white area showed epithelial thickening and hyperkeratosis, whereas the red area showed moderately severe dysplasia.

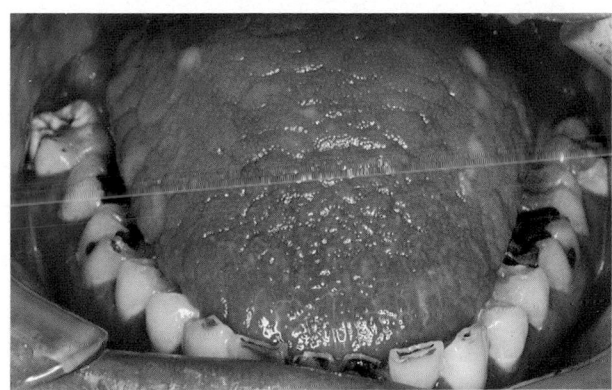

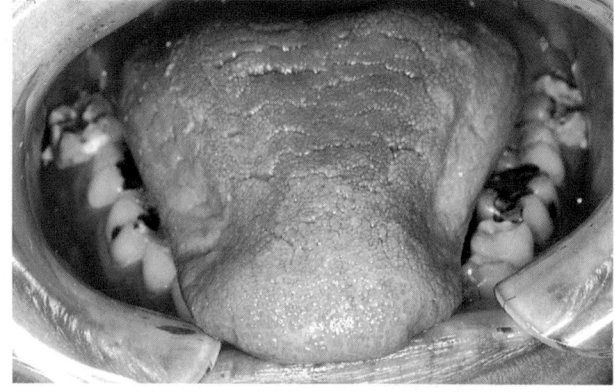

F, Chronic erythematous candidiasis in a 28-year-old woman with severe xerostomia from primary Sjögren's syndrome. *Top,* Dorsal tongue before treatment, showing erythema, atrophy of filiform papillae, and fissuring. Note caries in incisors. *Bottom,* Resolution of most of these changes after 4 months of intermittent topical antifungal therapy.

PLATE 4 CARDIOLOGY AND RHEUMATOLOGY

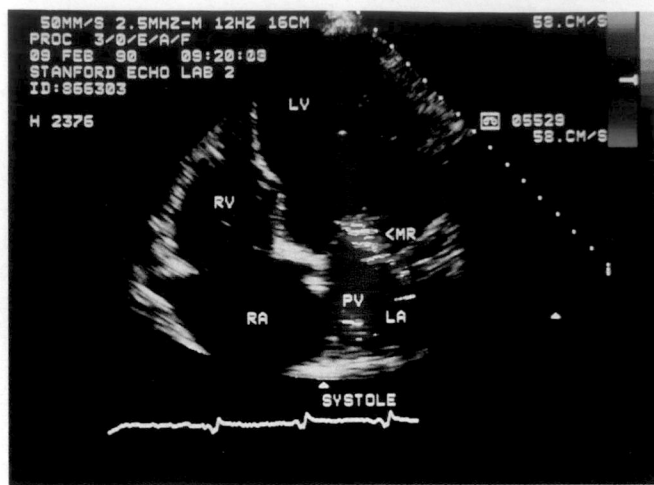

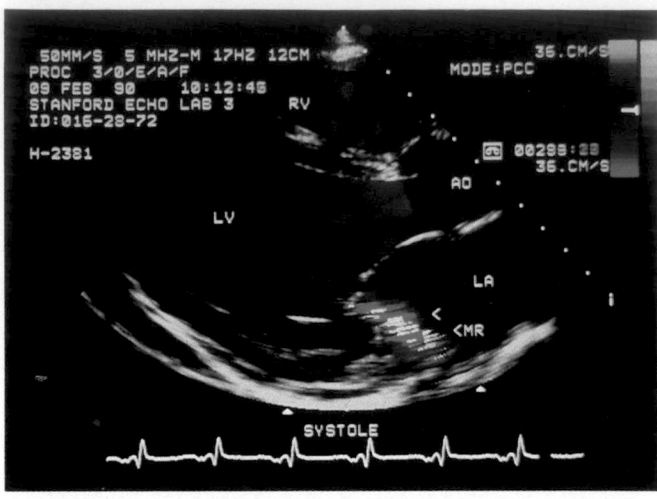

A, A two-dimensional echocardiographic image with Doppler color flow mapping superimposed to indicate blood flow. A portion of the image contains color-coded information regarding the direction and velocity of flow. Shades of orange represent flow toward the transducer, and shades of blue represent flow away from the transducer. Pulmonary venous (PV) flow into the left atrium is noted in orange during systole, while mitral regurgitation (MR) is indicated by the eccentric color at the lateral left atrial wall, extending from the area of the mitral valve. The mitral regurgitation signal contains blue, orange, and white, giving a mosaic pattern that is typical of high-velocity turbulent flow. LA = Left atrium; LV = left ventricle; RA = right atrium; RV = right ventricle.

B, A two-dimensional echocardiogram with Doppler flow mapping superimposed on a portion of the image. The color information is represented in the sector of the imaging plane extending from the apex of the triangular plane to the two small arrows at the bottom of the image plane. Mitral regurgitation (MR) is indicated *(open arrows),* extending from the mitral valve leaflets toward the posterior aspect of the left atrium (LA) during systole. The mosaic of colors representing the mitral regurgitant signal is typical of high-velocity turbulent flow. The low-intensity orange-brown signal represents flow directed away from the transducer on the chest wall, and the blue shades represent blood in the left ventricular outflow tract moving toward the transducer. AO = Aorta; LV = left ventricle; RV = right ventricle.

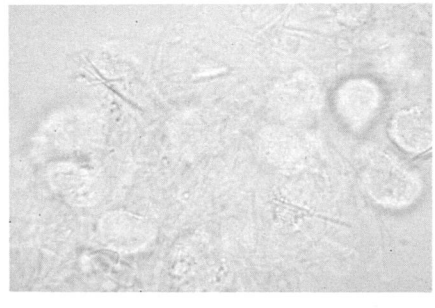
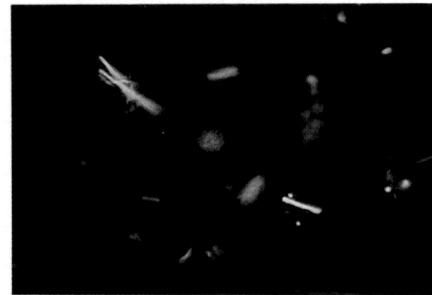
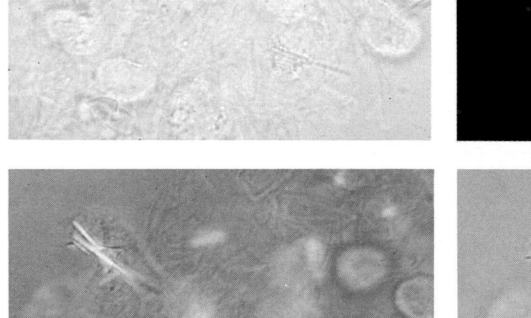
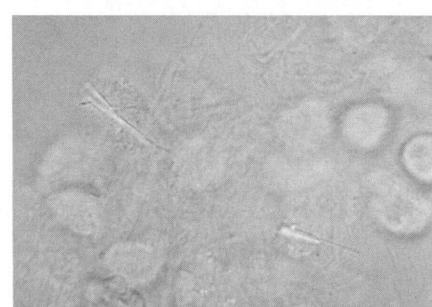

C, Monosodium urate crystals in synovial fluid aspirate. *Top left,* Plain light microscopy. *Top right,* Polarized light. *Bottom left,* First-order red compensator with axis of vibration perpendicular to crystals (2 o'clock to 7 o'clock). *Bottom right,* First-order red compensator with axis of vibration parallel to crystals (11 o'clock to 4 o'clock).

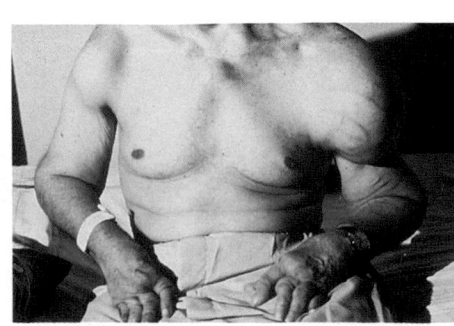
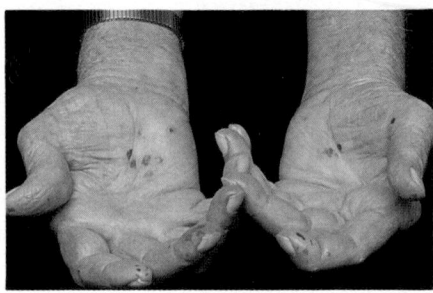
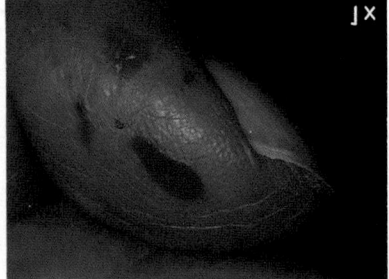

D, Large synovial cysts of the shoulders, especially on the left, in a patient with chronic deforming rheumatoid arthritis.

E, Left and *right,* Rheumatoid vasculitis with small brown infarcts of palms and fingers in chronic rheumatoid arthritis. (Courtesy of Dr. Martin Lidsky, Houston, Texas.)

ascites in patients with portal hypertension. Peritoneal adhesions as a result of peritonitis are absolute contraindications. The relative risks of postoperative adhesions and surgical scar must be weighed against the diagnostic importance.

FUTURE OF ENDOSCOPY

Endoscopic instrumentation is approaching optimal size and optical resolution, in both fiberoptic and emerging electronic video endoscopy equipment. The number of skilled endoscopists has increased so that precise diagnostic studies are generally available to most patients.

Endoscopy is contributing enormously to management of gastrointestinal disease and will continue to do so. A clearer understanding of the colonic polyp-cancer progression will likely be available in the next few years. Colonoscopic polypectomy will play a key role in altering the course of this major malignancy. It is likely that nearly all cases of common duct stones will be treated endoscopically in the near future. Removal of the gallbladder via a laparoscopic approach is attracting wide interest. Measures for successful control of gastrointestinal bleeding are greatly improving. Their influence on mortality should soon become clear.

Optimal management of patients with benign or malignant biliary obstruction is not clearly dependent on a single technique. Endoscopists, radiologists, and surgeons working together will likely evolve an integrated approach with indications for each of several options.

Fleischer DE, Goldberg SB, Brunning TH, et al.: Detection and surveillance of colorectal cancer. JAMA 261:580, 1989. *A current discussion of a topic slowly coming into focus.*

Infante-Riward C, Esnaola S, Villeneuve J-P: Role of endoscopic variceal sclerotherapy in the long-term management of variceal bleeding: A meta-analysis. Gastroenterology 96:1087, 1989. *The final role of endoscopic variceal sclerosis is not yet clear.*

Proceeding of the consensus conference on therapeutic endoscopy in bleeding ulcers. Gastrointest Endosc Suppl 36, 1990. *An important position statement on the current role of endoscopy.*

Ranshohoff DF, Lang CA, Kuo HS: Colonoscopic surveillance after polypectomy: Considerations of cost effectiveness. Ann Intern Med 114:177, 1991. *Useful analysis of the effectiveness of routine follow-up colonoscopy.*

Soll AH: Pathogenesis of peptic ulcer and implication for therapy. N Engl J Med 322:909, 1990. *Our understanding of acid-peptic disease is finally providing a rational basis for effective therapy.*

Vaira D, Ainley C, Williams S, et al.: Endoscopic sphincterotomy in 1000 consecutive patients. Lancet 2:431, 1990. *A broad review of experience with endoscopic sphincterotomy for choledocholithiasis.*

Van Stielmann G, Pearman NW, Goff JS, et al.: Endoscopic cholangiography and stone removal prior to cholecystectomy. Arch Surg 124:787, 1989. *Endoscopic retrograde sphincterotomy for bile duct stone removal poses a question—what to do with the often silent remaining gallbladder.*

95 Diseases of the Mouth and Salivary Glands

Troy E. Daniels

At least 200 primary lesions or diseases occur in the oral mucosa, gingiva, teeth, jaws, and minor or major salivary glands. In addition, many systemic diseases or drugs can cause secondary abnormalities of the oral mucosa or salivary glands. This chapter briefly discusses only the most common and important of the mucosal and salivary gland diseases, to provide a basis for developing a differential diagnosis and guiding treatment and referral. More complete coverage of these topics can be found in specialized texts cited at the end of the chapter.

ORAL MUCOSAL DISEASES

Acute Ulcerations

Painful short-term ulcerations, the most common oral mucosal lesions, are usually caused by mechanical trauma, immunologic mechanisms, and bacterial or viral infections (Table 95–1). Soon after formation, ulcers in the mouth become covered by a white to gray pseudomembrane, analogous to the scab that forms on

TABLE 95–1. COMMON AND SIGNIFICANT ORAL MUCOSAL LESIONS

Ulcers
  Acute (many are self-limiting)
    Mechanical trauma
    Recurrent aphthous ulcers/Behçet's syndrome
    Viral (herpes simplex,* varicella-zoster,* hand-foot-and-mouth disease,* herpangina,* rubeola*)
    Erythema multiforme/Stevens-Johnson syndrome
    Drug reaction
    Primary syphilis (chancre)
    Gonorrhea
  Chronic
    Squamous cell carcinoma
    Mucocutaneous diseases (pemphigus,* pemphigoid,* erythema multiforme, lichen planus,† lupus erythematosus†)
    Microbial infections (tuberculosis, leprosy, actinomycosis, noma, various fungi)
White lesions
  Squamous cell carcinoma (early)
  Leukoplakia
  Frictional keratosis
  Smokeless tobacco–associated lesions
  Nicotine stomatitis (palate)
  Lichen planus (reticular and plaque types)
  Pseudomembranous candidiasis (thrush)
  Hyperplastic candidiasis (candidal leukoplakia)
  Hairy leukoplakia (HIV-associated) (usually on lateral tongue)
  Geographic tongue
  Pseudomembrane-covered ulcers (see above)
  Mucous patch or condyloma latum of secondary syphilis
Red lesions
  Squamous cell carcinoma (early)
  Erythroplakia (epithelial dysplasia)
  Erythematous (atrophic) candidiasis
  Median rhomboid glossitis
  Mucocutaneous diseases (see above)
  Angular cheilitis
  Telangiectasias and purpuras
  Kaposi's sarcoma (blue to purple color)

*Vesicles present in early lesion formation
†Ulcers usually associated with white-red lesions

dry epidermis. Pseudomembrane-covered ulcers are usually distinguished from the white hyperkeratotic lesions described below by their clinical features of pain, a flat surface, and an erythematous periphery. Traumatic ulcers are characterized by their location on the tongue or inside of the cheeks or lips, their proximity to the chewing surfaces of the teeth, and the irregularity of their borders.

APHTHOUS ULCERS. These idiopathic recurrent ulcers, which afflict at least 90 per cent of the population, occur on all areas of the oral mucosa except the hard palate, gingiva, and vermilion. They are well-defined circles and may be single or multiple. There are three clinical forms: (1) minor, which are flat, less than 1 cm in diameter, and last only 5 to 10 days; (2) major, which have raised borders, are larger than 1 cm, and often last for weeks or months; and (3) herpetiform, which are usually clusters of very small ulcers that resemble recurrent herpetic lesions but are not preceded by vesicles and do not contain detectable viruses. Lesions clinically identical to minor aphthous ulcers occur in Behçet's syndrome (Ch. 269). Aphthous ulcers are occasionally associated with macrocytic anemias or gluten-sensitive enteropathy and may become more frequent and severe in association with human immunodeficiency virus (HIV) infection (Table 95–2).

Minor or herpetiform aphthous ulcers may not require treatment. Topical steroids, such as fluocinonide ointment in Orabase, can reduce the severity and duration of the lesions only if used with prodromal symptoms or early signs. Major aphthae usually require treatment by topical or systemic corticosteroids and occasionally are biopsied to rule out neoplasia.

VIRAL ULCERS. Several types of virus (most commonly herpes simplex) may cause oral mucosal vesicles that, after lasting a few days at most, quickly become shallow ulcers. In the initial infection by herpes simplex virus, usually in children, numerous

TABLE 95–2. ORAL LESIONS ASSOCIATED WITH HIV INFECTION

Kaposi's sarcoma
Candidiasis
  Pseudomembranous
  Hyperplastic
  Erythematous
Other opportunistic fungal infections (e.g., histoplasmosis or
  coccidioidomycosis)
Epithelial lesions
  Aphthous ulcers (increased frequency, duration, or size)
  Virus-associated epithelial hyperplasias
    Hairy leukoplakia
    Oral wart
    Focal epithelial hyperplasia (Heck's disease)
    Condyloma acuminatum
  Herpes zoster
Exaggerated forms of gingivitis and inflammatory periodontal disease
Decreased salivary gland function
Parotid gland enlargement (benign lymphoepithelial lesion)
Non-Hodgkin's lymphoma

vesicles may appear on any oral mucosal site (primary herpetic gingivostomatitis), accompanied by malaise, headache, fever, and cervical lymphadenopathy. Many patients previously exposed to this virus develop recurrent lesions, most commonly as clusters of small vesicles on the lips (herpes labialis); only a few develop intraoral recurrent herpes, as clusters of vesicles on the keratinized mucosa of the gingiva or hard palate. Such lesions tend to recur at the same site, but the frequency decreases with age.

Oral mucosal vesicles/ulcers may also accompany the initial infection by the varicella-zoster virus in children with chickenpox (Ch. 374), and unilateral lesions may occur with herpes zoster (Ch. 476), affecting branches of the trigeminal nerve. Uncommonly, oral mucosal lesions may be caused by different types of coxsackievirus (Ch. 377), appearing on any oral site in hand-foot-and-mouth disease (Ch. 380) or on the soft palate or pharynx in herpangina. After infection by the measles (rubeola) virus, small ulcers (Koplik's spots) form on the inside of the cheeks 1 to 2 days before development of the skin rash (Ch. 367).

ERYTHEMA MULTIFORME. In this mucocutaneous disease, painful oral mucosal ulcerations develop rapidly in as many as half of the patients. The lesions may be confined to the mouth, with no skin involvement. The affected patients, usually young adults with minimal or no systemic symptoms, present with irregularly shaped ulcers that can be small and few in number or involve large areas of the mucosa, most commonly the lower labial mucosa. These lesions may be distinguished from those of primary herpes by the absence of oral vesicles and systemic symptoms or the presence of characteristic skin lesions (Ch. 293). A major variant of this disease is the Stevens-Johnson syndrome.

VENEREAL INFECTIONS. Primary syphilis may present as a solitary, indurated, painless ulcer on the oral mucosa which resolves spontaneously in 4 to 6 weeks (Ch. 340). Uncommonly, *Neisseria gonorrhoeae* may cause oral ulcers, usually in the pharynx, that may be confused with oral ulcers of other causes.

Oral Squamous Cell Carcinoma

Approximately 4 per cent of all cancers occur in the mouth, largely squamous cell carcinomas of the mucosal epithelium. Oral carcinoma occurs usually in the fifth decade or beyond, in men twice as frequently as in women, and with long-term use of tobacco (more than 80 per cent of cases). The tongue is the most common site, followed by the lip, oropharynx, and mouth floor.

Oral carcinoma usually presents as a chronic, indurated, cratered ulcer, but early lesions of squamous cell carcinoma may appear as white or red macules (see Table 95–1). Most oral carcinomas develop on normal-appearing mucosa, but about 15 per cent arise within a pre-existing oral mucosal leukoplakia or erythroplakia (described below). The overall 5-year survival is approximately 50 per cent, but early treatment of small, localized lesions can lead to survival rates as high as 90 per cent.

Other Chronic Ulcerations

Chronic multifocal oral mucosal lesions composed of ill-defined areas of erythema and ulceration may be caused by several of the

mucocutaneous diseases. They are among the most difficult oral mucosal lesions to diagnose and are discussed below with the red lesions (see Table 95–1). Several microbial infections can lead to indurated, chronic oral mucosal ulcerations with moderate symptoms—e.g., ulcers overlying granulomas associated with tuberculosis, leprosy, actinomycosis, histoplasmosis, or coccidioidomycosis.

White Lesions

White plaques are commonly found in the mouth but, like ulcerations, have a wide variety of causes and outcomes. The term "leukoplakia" applies to a white plaque that does not rub off and whose appearance is not indicative of another disease. Leukoplakia can occur in any area of the mouth and usually exhibits benign hyperkeratosis on biopsy. On long-term follow-up, between 2 and 6 per cent of these lesions will have undergone malignant transformation into squamous cell carcinoma. Areas of leukoplakia with a corrugated surface or mixed with areas of erythema are often found in the lower labial or buccal vestibule of those who use smokeless tobacco.

Frictional keratoses are often found posterior to the lower third molar teeth as irregular white plaques and on the buccal mucosa as white lines adjacent to the dental occlusion. Unlike leukoplakia, these lesions rarely become malignant.

LICHEN PLANUS. Oral lesions of lichen planus occur in about 1 per cent of the population, usually as a bilateral reticular network of linear white plaques, with or without adjacent areas of erythema (atrophy or erosion) or ulcers (see Color Plate 3C). The presence of mucosal atrophy, erosion, or ulceration usually causes pain or sensitivity to certain foods. Most lesions can be adequately controlled by topical application of fluocinonide ointment mixed with an equal weight of Orabase for periods of several weeks to several months, although recurrence is common.

ORAL CANDIDIASIS. This fungal disease has three clinical forms: pseudomembranous (thrush), erythematous (atrophic), and hyperplastic (candidal leukoplakia). Pseudomembranous candidiasis, usually of relatively short duration, occurs on any site and consists of white plaques that can be rubbed off, leaving a red or bleeding base. The lesion of hyperplastic candidiasis has fungal hyphae within the surface layers of hyperkeratotic epithelium; it does not rub off and is most frequently located on the anterior buccal mucosa or on the tongue. All forms of oral candidiasis represent overgrowth of *Candida* species from the oral flora, induced by a variety of causes. These include suppression of bacterial flora by systemic antibiotics, chronic xerostomia, uncontrolled diabetes mellitus or anemia, and immunosuppression (especially in HIV-infected patients) (Table 95–2). Treatment of erythematous candidiasis is discussed below with the red lesions.

HAIRY LEUKOPLAKIA. This recently identified lesion is a white plaque occurring most frequently on the lateral surfaces of the tongue, mainly in HIV-infected persons (see Color Plate 3D). *Candida* may be present in the surface layers, but the lesion is not eliminated by effective antifungal therapy and contains large quantities of Epstein-Barr virus. Its diagnosis should be followed by determination of whether HIV antibody is present in the patient's serum.

GEOGRAPHIC TONGUE. Also called "benign migratory glossitis," this is a benign idiopathic condition affecting the dorsal tongue of about 2 per cent of the population. It is characterized by well-defined circular areas of relatively atrophied filiform papillae bordered by arcs of normal or hyperplastic filiform papillae; the lesions change in location, or "migrate," over time. Treatment is usually not necessary.

SECONDARY SYPHILIS. Secondary syphilis may present well-defined white plaques on the labial or palatal mucosa, called "condyloma latum" (or "split papule," because of their lobulated periphery).

Red Lesions

Solitary red macules or plaques ("erythroplakia") are less common in the mouth than white lesions but should be viewed with concern because many may exhibit microscopic dysplasia or carcinoma in situ (see Table 95–1). They are often associated with areas of leukoplakia (see Color Plate 3E). However, a red macule occurring in the midline of the posterior dorsal tongue, classified as median rhomboid glossitis, is an idiopathic but uniformly benign condition that is often associated with localized overgrowth of *Candida* species.

ERYTHEMATOUS (ATROPHIC) ORAL CANDIDIASIS. This chronic condition is characterized by diffuse mucosal erythema and atrophy of the filiform papillae on the dorsal tongue (see Color Plate 3F) or by ill-defined red macules on the palate, tongue, or buccal mucosa. Symptoms of oral mucosal burning and sensitivity to certain foods accompany the condition, which is frequently associated with xerostomia. In patients wearing removable dentures, there may be mucosal erythema confined to the denture-bearing area.

These lesions can be resolved with topical nystatin or clotrimazole-containing preparations or with systemic ketoconazole; these are usually administered for several months. In patients with xerostomia who have remaining natural teeth, topical antifungal preparations containing sucrose or glucose must be avoided to prevent caries. Oral use of vaginal tablets is safe and effective. Systemic ketoconazole may not be effective in patients with severe xerostomia. Effective treatment leads to significant improvement in oral symptoms, regardless of the cause of the candidiasis. Treatment of denture-associated candidiasis also requires appropriate treatment of the denture to remove the organisms; failure to do so leads to recurrence.

ANGULAR CHEILITIS. Erythema or crusting of the labial angles is usually caused by *Candida*. It is usually associated with intraoral candidiasis and in such cases topical treatment of the angular cheilitis should be accompanied by intraoral or systemic antifungal treatment.

MUCOCUTANEOUS DISEASES. Some mucocutaneous diseases involving immunologic abnormalities affect the oral mucosa—e.g., pemphigus vulgaris, mucous membrane pemphigoid, atrophic or erosive lichen planus, and lupus erythematosus. The appearance of oral lesions caused by these diseases is frequently similar. The diagnosis requires examination of a biopsy specimen by routine histopathology and usually also by direct immunofluorescence examination to identify characteristic depositions of immunoglobulins and complement components in the basement membrane zone with pemphigoid, lupus, or lichen planus or in the inter–epithelial cell spaces with pemphigus.

Pemphigus vulgaris usually presents as oral mucosal vesicles that rapidly rupture, leaving painful erosions or ulcerations. These are followed by development of skin lesions (Ch. 525). Rarely, the lesions remain confined to the mouth.

Lesions of mucous membrane pemphigoid are usually confined to the oral mucosa or conjunctivae and occur in patients over 50 years of age. They begin as vesicles that quickly rupture, leaving ulcers and areas of atrophic epithelium that are chronic but only moderately symptomatic. Use of topical fluocinonide for several months, as described above for lichen planus, is sometimes sufficient treatment of the oral lesions, but some patients need systemic treatment (Ch. 525).

Some cases of atrophic or erosive lichen planus do not show the characteristic reticular keratotic lesions described above and may be clinically indistinguishable from mucous membrane pemphigoid. In those cases, direct immunofluorescence examination of a biopsy specimen of intact mucosa is required for diagnosis.

Oral mucosal lesions of lupus may occur in patients who have systemic lupus erythematosus (SLE), in patients who do not have SLE but later develop that disease, or in patients who do not develop SLE. In this latter group, the lesions of mucosal lupus may be analogous to the skin lesions of chronic discoid lupus. Lesions of oral lupus are characterized by reticular hyperkeratotic figures associated with erythema and may resemble atrophic lichen planus. The lesions may be controlled by topical fluocinonide or intralesional triamcinolone.

Lesions of Kaposi's sarcoma associated with HIV infection frequently appear first on the oral mucosa, especially the palate. They begin as macules with a blue or purple color, at which time they need to be distinguished from purpura. Later, they spread radially and expand vertically (Table 95–2).

Pigmentations

Brown or gray-black macules on the oral mucosa are relatively common and may be caused by localized increase in melanin production, proliferation of melanin-producing cells, or deposition of local or systemically distributed pigmented substances

TABLE 95–3. PIGMENTATIONS OF THE ORAL MUCOSA (BROWN OR GRAY-BLACK IN COLOR)

Increased melanin production (flat lesions)
  Oral melanotic macule
  Ephelis (lip)
  Systemic diseases: Addison's disease, von Recklinghausen's disease of skin, Albright's syndrome, Peutz-Jeghers syndrome
Proliferation of melanin-producing cells (flat or raised lesions)
  Pigmented cellular nevi (benign and premalignant types)
  Atypical melanocytic hyperplasia
  Malignant melanoma
Nonmelanin pigmentation
  Amalgam tattoo
  Focal deposition of systemically distributed heavy metal (lead, bismuth, mercury, others) at sites of chronic inflammation
  Systemically administered drugs (chloroquine, minocycline, cyclophosphamide)

(Table 95–3). Mucosal pigmentation may occur after long-term administration of chloroquine, minocycline, or cyclophosphamide. Malignant melanoma can occur at any oral mucosal site but develops most frequently on the mucosa or gingiva covering the maxilla. Diagnosis of any of these is usually established by biopsy and knowledge of relevant underlying conditions.

ORAL SOFT TISSUE TUMORS

Connective Tissue Hyperplasias

The most common oral soft tissue tumors are small, pedunculated masses of hyperplastic fibrous connective tissue covered by normal-appearing mucosa (Table 95–4). These lesions are usually found on the inside of the cheeks or lips, in areas where they are subject to frequent irritation by the teeth. Similar lesions may be present at the border of an ill-fitting denture or may occur in clusters on the hard palate under an ill-fitting denture ("palatal papillomatosis").

Generalized enlargement of the gingiva may be caused by chronic administration of phenytoin, cyclosporine, or nifedipine. It can also be associated with a hereditary defect or be caused by an infiltration of white blood cells in some types of leukemia, especially acute monocytic. The drug-associated cases apparently represent an exaggerated response in susceptible patients to commonly occurring local irritants, such as dental plaque and calculus. The cause of this susceptibility is unknown.

TABLE 95–4. ORAL SOFT TISSUE TUMORS

Connective tissue hyperplasia (normal-appearing overlying mucosa)
  Irritation fibroma
  Denture associated hyperplasia
  Palatal papillomatosis
  Generalized gingival hyperplasia
    Drug-induced (phenytoin, nifedipine, cyclosporine)
    Hereditary
Reactive hyperplasia (erythematous overlying mucosa)
  Pyogenic granuloma/pregnancy tumor
  Peripheral giant cell granuloma
  Inflammatory gingival hyperplasia
  Hyperplastic lingual tonsil
Epithelial masses (usually irregular white surface)
  Papilloma/oral wart
  Squamous cell carcinoma
  Verrucous carcinoma
  Focal epithelial hyperplasia (Heck's disease)
  Condyloma acuminatum (venereal wart)
  Keratoacanthoma (on lips)
Salivary duct obstruction (minor salivary glands)
  Mucocele/ranula (usually fluctuant)
  Salivary stone (sialolith)
Underlying connective tissue or salivary gland neoplasms
Other malignant diseases
  Metastatic lesions
  Local or generalized leukemic infiltrates in the gingiva (esp. with acute monocytic leukemia)

Reactive Hyperplasias

Small masses with surfaces that are ulcerated or only partially covered by normal-appearing mucosa usually represent reactive lesions in the form of pyogenic granulomas (whose frequency increases during pregnancy), peripheral giant cell granulomas, or lymphoid hyperplasia of the lingual or other tonsillar tissue. The granulomas are most often located on the gingiva. Rarely, such lesions may represent a metastatic neoplasm.

Epithelial Tumors

Small, white, wartlike epithelial masses are common and can occur in any area of the oral mucosa. They are occasionally classified as epithelial neoplasms, but most do not continue to grow. Human papillomavirus types 2, 6, 11, and 13 have been identified in some but not all of these wartlike lesions. Usually, these lesions are classified generically as papillomas but require identification of virus or further clinical evidence to confirm the diagnosis of a viral disease. A large wartlike lesion on the oral mucosa should raise the suspicion of verrucous carcinoma.

Salivary Duct Obstruction

Mucoceles are small, fluctuant, frequently recurring nodules that occur commonly on the inside of the cheeks and lips, the posterior palate, and the mouth floor. They are caused by injury and blockage of the excretory duct of one of the numerous minor salivary glands. Sialoliths may be apparent as hard nodules covered by normal-appearing mucosa in the submandibular or sublingual ducts of the mouth floor or, uncommonly, in areas of minor salivary glands. Both types of lesions require conservative surgical excision.

SALIVARY GLAND DISEASES

Primary Diseases of Salivary Glands

Patients with enlargement of a major or minor salivary gland usually bring the clinician a diagnostic challenge (Table 95–5). More than 20 types of benign or malignant salivary gland neoplasms may present as unilateral enlargement of a major gland that is firm and nontender to palpation. Most of these tumors can also arise in minor glands as a firm submucosal nodule on the palate or the labial or buccal mucosa. Uncommonly, unilateral major gland enlargement may be caused by an inflammatory lesion, such as benign lymphoepithelial lesion or other chronic sialadenitis. Observation of any of these lesions should be followed by appropriate imaging and biopsy.

Major salivary gland enlargement that is markedly painful and tender to palpation suggests bacterial sialadenitis and usually requires administration of systemic antibiotics, initially oral penicillin.

Bilateral Salivary Gland Enlargement and Decreased Salivary Secretion Associated with Systemic Diseases

The best-known cause of bilateral salivary gland enlargement is infection by the mumps virus in children (Table 95–5). The incidence of mumps has decreased in the United States by more than 90 per cent since the introduction of an effective vaccine in 1967, but the number of cases began to rise again in the late 1980's, apparently as a result of reduced use of the vaccine (Ch. 16). Uncommonly, a less acute, mumpslike illness may occur in adults in association with cytomegalovirus, influenza, or coxsackie A virus infection.

Sjögren's syndrome is characterized in about one third of patients by the development of firm, nontender or only slightly tender enlargement of major salivary glands (Ch. 263). The enlargement is bilateral but often asymmetric and may slowly wax and wane. Salivary secretion usually decreases gradually, and the resulting xerostomia can impair speech and swallowing and be associated with rapidly progressive dental caries, symptomatic oral candidiasis, and difficulty in wearing dentures. In severe cases, the oral mucosa may appear dry and sticky and saliva will not be expressible from the major ducts. Signs of erythematous candidiasis (see above) are seen in about one third of patients with Sjögren's syndrome.

The salivary component of Sjögren's syndrome is most reliably diagnosed in a labial salivary gland biopsy specimen of at least

TABLE 95–5. CAUSES OF SALIVARY GLAND ENLARGEMENT

Usually unilateral
  Benign or malignant salivary gland neoplasms (more than 20 different histopathologic types)
  Bacterial infection
  Chronic sialadenitis (single gland)
Usually bilateral, often asymmetric (associated with decreased salivary secretion)
  Viral infection (mumps, cytomegalovirus, influenza, coxsackie A)
  Sjögren's syndrome (benign lymphoepithelial lesion)
  Chronic granulomatous diseases (sarcoidosis, tuberculosis, leprosy, syphilis)
  Recurrent parotitis of childhood
  Human immunodeficiency virus infection
Bilaterally symmetric, soft, nontender, parotid only
  Sialadenosis (asymptomatic parotid enlargement), idiopathic or associated with:
    Diabetes mellitus
    Hyperlipoproteinemia
    Hepatic cirrhosis
    Anorexia/bulimia
    Chronic pancreatitis
    Acromegaly
    Gonadal hypofunction
    Phenylbutazone use

five glands. Examination must show focal lymphocytic sialadenitis in most or all of the specimen and exclude nonspecific chronic sialadenitis or pathology indicative of another disease, such as noncaseating granuloma. A patient's symptoms of oral dryness are important, but, being subjective and nonspecific (Table 95–6), they are not diagnostic. Results from functional studies or imaging of salivary glands are not specific to Sjögren's syndrome.

Several chronic granulomatous diseases, such as sarcoidosis, tuberculosis, leprosy, and syphilis, can cause bilateral enlargement and decreased function of salivary glands. The clinical and serologic features of sarcoidosis may closely mimic those of Sjögren's syndrome, and the distinction must be made by salivary gland biopsy.

Some patients with HIV infection develop major salivary gland enlargement and reduced salivary secretion associated with lymphocytic infiltration of a different type than in Sjögren's syndrome. Solitary benign lymphoepithelial lesions may occur in parotid glands of intravenous drug–abusing patients (see Table 95–2).

Recurrent parotitis of childhood includes episodes of unilateral or bilateral parotid enlargement. Salivary secretion may be reduced during flares of this illness, but usually without prominent secondary symptoms or signs. This condition, of unknown cause, usually subsides after puberty. Some serologic evidence suggests an association with Epstein-Barr virus infection.

TABLE 95–6. CAUSES OF DECREASED SALIVARY SECRETION (XEROSTOMIA)

Temporary
  Effects of short-term drug use (e.g., antihistamines)
  Virus infections (esp. mumps)
  Dehydration
  Fear
Chronic
  Effects of chronically administered drugs (especially antidepressants, MAO inhibitors, neuroleptics, parasympatholytics, some combinations of drugs for treating hypertension)
  Chronic diseases (with gland enlargement in some patients)
    Sjögren's syndrome
    Granulomatous diseases (sarcoidosis, tuberculosis, leprosy, syphilis)
    Amyloidosis
    Human immunodeficiency virus infection
  Graft-versus-host disease
  Therapeutic radiation to the head and neck
  Depression
  Absent or malformed glands (rare)

Asymptomatic Parotid Enlargement (Sialadenosis)

Parotid glands can develop bilateral, symmetric enlargement that is soft and nontender to palpation and not associated with xerostomia (see Table 95–5). Usually, results of sialography and salivary scintigraphy are within normal limits. Histopathologic examination reveals only serous acinar cell hypertrophy with vacuolation and loss of granulation in the secretory cell cytoplasm, but biopsy of the affected glands is not indicated for diagnosis. Diagnosis is established by the clinical presentation and (if necessary to rule out Sjögren's syndrome or sarcoidosis) a normal labial salivary gland biopsy.

This chronic, noninflammatory, and non-neoplastic condition may occur alone or may be associated with a variety of systemic diseases, including diabetes mellitus, hyperlipoproteinemia, hepatic cirrhosis, anorexia/bulimia, chronic pancreatitis, acromegaly, and gonadal hypofunction. It can also result from use of phenylbutazone or be a reaction to iodine-containing contrast media.

Impaired Salivary Secretion (Xerostomia) Without Gland Enlargement

The very common symptom of dry mouth is most often a side effect of chronically administered drugs. Many classes of drugs reduce unstimulated salivary secretion through anticholinergic or other mechanisms (Table 95–6). At least initially, most of these drugs do not interfere with stimulated salivary production in response to gustatory, olfactory, or masticatory stimuli. This means that patients experience the symptoms soon after beginning to use the drug, but produce sufficient amounts of saliva during a meal for normal chewing and swallowing. The effects are dose-dependent and are frequently seen in those patients using several of the tricyclic antidepressants, most neuroleptics, monoamine oxidase inhibitors, and all parasympatholytics. A combination of drugs for treatment of hypertension may cause symptoms of dry mouth, but usually not to the extent of the drugs listed above.

Several systemic diseases affect salivary secretion. As noted above, most patients with Sjögren's syndrome, some with sarcoidosis, and a few patients with HIV infection experience symptoms of dry mouth of various degrees of severity, with or without salivary gland enlargement (see Table 95–2). In addition, patients who have primary or secondary amyloidosis with salivary gland deposition may develop impaired secretion. Depressed patients not receiving drug treatment for their depression are thought by some to have decreased resting salivary secretion and to complain more frequently of symptoms of dry mouth.

Radiation to the head and neck region for treatment of a malignant tumor usually produces profound xerostomia before therapy is completed, with only a slight recovery of secretory capacity in the months following treatment. Graft-versus-host disease following bone marrow transplantation can also produce xerostomia, but it is usually less severe than that following radiation therapy to the head and neck. Secretory capacity usually recovers when the reaction resolves.

Clinical Management of Patients with Chronic Xerostomia

Severe chronic xerostomia from any cause produces a risk for dental caries in approximate proportion to the impairment of salivary secretion. This secondary caries can largely be prevented if appropriate measures are taken as soon as the xerostomia begins. Remaining teeth should be protected by an adequate dental caries prevention program, monitored by a dentist, that includes daily application of an appropriate topical fluoride and removal of dental plaque, counseling on control of dietary carbohydrates that can cause caries, and placement of dental restorations as necessary.

Chronic erythematous oral candidiasis is a frequent sequela of chronic xerostomia, and its treatment and retreatment, as noted above, improve the patient's oral symptoms.

Symptomatic treatment of mild to moderately severe chronic xerostomia can include sialogogues such as sugarless hard candies or chewing gum, frequent sips of water, and use of saliva substitutes at night. Severe xerostomia, especially that following radiation, can be improved by systemic pilocarpine, 10 to 15 mg three times a day, if not contraindicated.

Ellis GL, Auclair PL, Gnepp DR (eds.): Pathology of the Salivary Glands. Philadelphia, W. B. Saunders Company, 1991. *This current text includes comprehensive discussion of neoplastic, infectious, reactive, and autoimmune salivary gland diseases.*

Genco RJ, Goldman HM, Cohen DW (eds.): Contemporary Periodontics. St Louis, C. V. Mosby Company, 1990. *This text provides thorough and current coverage of the etiology and treatment of localized periodontal diseases and devotes a large section to the effect of systemic conditions on the periodontium.*

Jones JH, Mason DK (eds.): Oral Manifestations of Systemic Diseases. 2nd ed. London, Bailliere Tindall, 1990. *This international reference text provides comprehensive coverage of essentially all oral manifestations of systemic diseases.*

Newbrun E: Cariology. 3rd ed. Chicago, Quintessence Books, 1989. *A concise and readable monograph on the causes, prevention, and management of dental caries.*

Regezi JA, Sciubba JJ: Oral Pathology: Clinical-pathologic Correlations. Philadelphia, W. B. Saunders Company, 1989. *This useful and comprehensive text discusses and illustrates the clinical features, differential diagnosis, pathogenesis, and pathology of most diseases affecting the mouth and salivary glands.*

96 Diseases of the Esophagus

Sidney Cohen

The esophagus, a relatively simple organ, is responsible for the transport of materials from the mouth to the stomach and for the prevention of retrograde flow of gastric contents. Antegrade flow is achieved by the act of swallowing with the initiation of primary peristalsis. Gastroesophageal reflux is prevented by the physiologic lower esophageal sphincter.

Disorders of the esophagus occur when one or both of the major esophageal functions become impaired. Abnormalities in esophageal transport may be due to disruption of peristalsis by a neuromuscular disorder or by an organic obstructing lesion. The physiologic lower esophageal sphincter may contribute to transport disorders when relaxation of its tonically elevated pressure is impaired. Disorders of peristaltic function such as achalasia occur together with abnormalities in sphincter relaxation. When the lower esophageal sphincter fails to function as an effective barrier to reflux, the patient develops gastroesophageal reflux with the associated complications of mucosal inflammation (peptic esophagitis).

The symptoms of esophageal disease relate closely to the abnormality in function. Disorders in transport lead to difficulty in swallowing or dysphagia. Abnormal esophageal contraction may cause chest pain. Gastroesophageal reflux leads to heartburn and postural regurgitation of food into the mouth.

The esophagus and its sphincters function through complex neural, humoral, and myogenic mechanisms. The upper esophageal sphincter, pharynx, and upper one third of the esophagus are composed of skeletal muscle. The lower two thirds of the esophagus and the lower esophageal sphincter are smooth muscle. Disorders of skeletal muscle such as polymyositis affect the upper portions of the swallowing mechanism. Disorders of smooth muscles such as scleroderma affect the distal esophagus and the lower esophageal sphincter.

The neurohumoral control of the esophagus is incompletely understood. The initiation of peristalsis by swallowing involves both cholinergic and noncholinergic pathways as well as myogenic mechanisms. The relaxation of the lower esophageal sphincter during swallowing is initiated by nonadrenergic inhibitory nerves in the vagus. These nerves may release vasoactive intestinal peptide (VIP). The sphincter responds to many peptides including gastrin, secretin, substance P, and glucagon. The role of these peptides in the physiologic control of the sphincter is not clear, but they may cause the wide fluctuations in sphincter pressure that follow a meal.

DYSPHAGIA. Consciousness of bolus arrest during swallowing, even if transient, indicates esophageal dysfunction. The patient usually uses the term "sticks," "hesitates," "pauses," or "hangs up" and often indicates the site of arrest with a finger.

Bolus arrest closely associated with the act of swallowing is dysphagia. The sensation of a substernal lump (globus hystericus) present one-half hour after eating is not dysphagia. Most patients consider mild dysphagia a normal phenomenon. "I just swallowed something that was too big." Thus, often they do not spontaneously mention the presence of dysphagia unless questioned closely.

A specialized type of dysphagia occurs when the bolus cannot be propelled from the mouth or hypopharynx into the esophagus, so-called "transfer dysphagia." This type of dysphagia is most commonly related to neurologic disease or to pharyngeal muscle weakness.

The sensation of dysphagia is localized to the suprasternal notch or substernal region. The exact location of the sensation is of little use in pinpointing the site of bolus arrest. Dysphagia for a liquid bolus usually indicates an esophageal motor disorder. Dysphagia for solids can be seen either with an organic obstruction (stricture or cancer) or secondary to esophageal motor disorders.

The patient's response to dysphagia can also provide useful information about the cause of dysphagia. If the bolus must be regurgitated, and if an attempt to force the bolus down with water is met by a sudden return of the fluid, then an organic obstruction should be suspected. If the patient is able to force the bolus down by posturing, by performing a Valsalva's maneuver, by repeated swallowing, or by ingesting fluid, then a motor disorder is more likely. Inexorable progression of dysphagia over months usually signals the presence of organic narrowing, either a lumen-obliterating carcinoma or a stricture caused by active peptic esophagitis.

Dysphagia is never an expression of a purely psychiatric disorder; it is not a manifestation of hysteria. Some patients with well-established esophageal disease such as achalasia report that their dysphagia is often worse at a time of severe emotional tension. Such observations have led many patients (and unfortunately some physicians) to believe that dysphagia is a matter for the psychiatrist rather than the gastroenterologist. Such an opinion can lead to subsequent embarrassment or tragedy, especially if an esophageal carcinoma is overlooked.

ODYNOPHAGIA. Pain upon swallowing, odynophagia, is another cardinal symptom of esophageal disease. Bolus arrest producing dysphagia can sometimes progress to a sensation of pain as esophageal obstruction continues. However, odynophagia usually occurs during the transit of the bolus and disappears once the swallowed material has left the esophagus. It may be mild in intensity so that the patient is merely aware of the location of the swallowed bolus. This is most commonly seen in patients with reflux disease. It can be of such intensity that the patient refuses to swallow any solids or liquids and expectorates saliva. Odynophagia can be seen after involvement of the mucosa by *reflux*, by *radiation*, or by *viral* or *fungal infections*. Odynophagia can be an uncommon manifestation of carcinoma or of a localized ulcer caused by a lodged tablet. Odynophagia thus localizes a process to the esophagus but gives no clue to pathogenesis.

HEARTBURN (PYROSIS). Heartburn or pyrosis is the most common manifestation of esophageal disease, so much so that it is difficult to recruit "normal" subjects, if strict histories are taken to eliminate any who have ever had heartburn. The term "burning" rather than "pain" is usually used, although heartburn can increase in intensity until it is perceived as pain. Patients commonly illustrate heartburn with a movement of the open hand up and down the sternum. This is in contrast to the stationary tightly clenched fist of angina pectoris. Heartburn is usually relieved, even if only temporarily, by taking antacids. A constant burning, unrelieved by antacids, may well be of esophageal origin, but it does not represent heartburn. Heartburn is often worse after recumbency or lifting and may follow overeating or alcoholic indiscretion.

REGURGITATION. Regurgitation of fluid contents into the mouth often accompanies heartburn. Sometimes such regurgitation is associated with eructation; often it accompanies bending over, lifting, or lying down at night. The bitter regurgitated fluid is often described as yellow-brown or green. Regurgitation at night may lead to stridor or to wheezing, a hoarse voice, and other respiratory symptoms from unrecognized reflux. Less commonly, regurgitated fluid is not from the stomach or duodenum, but from fluid retained in an *achalasic esophagus* or in a large

pharyngeal diverticulum. An uncommon but fascinating process that can be confused with regurgitation is *rumination*. In this condition, recently eaten food is propelled back into the mouth from the stomach by a strong contraction of the abdominal wall musculature. The food commonly is rechewed, reswallowed, and again returned to the mouth (Ch. 202).

ESOPHAGEAL COLIC (SPONTANEOUS ESOPHAGEAL PAIN). In addition to the discomfort from severe reflux, which can advance from heartburn into pain, abnormal motor activity of the esophageal muscle can cause severe pain clinically indistinguishable from angina pectoris in terms of intensity, radiation, relationship to exercise, and even response to nitroglycerin. Chest pain of esophageal origin can radiate directly through to the back and is often found in patients who also notice dysphagia. Esophageal colic can last from 5 to 10 seconds to hours.

HEMATEMESIS. Although vomiting blood is less specific for esophageal disease than are many of the symptoms listed above, hematemesis can signal the presence of esophageal varices, of mucosal ulceration resulting from esophageal reflux, of a rent of the mucosa of the lower esophagus, or, uncommonly, of an ulcerating carcinoma or leiomyoma of the esophagus. Although bleeding from the esophagus may be life threatening, more often it is a slow ooze, usually caused by esophageal reflux disease, which presents clinically as an iron deficiency anemia.

Berk JE (ed.): Bockus' Gastroenterology. 4th ed. Philadelphia, W. B. Saunders Company, 1985, pp 666–850. *Reference textbook chapters on esophagus. Good source for recent references.*

Pope CE II: Chapters on the esophagus. *In* Sleisenger MH, Fordtran JS (eds.): Gastrointestinal Disease. 4th ed. Philadelphia, W. B. Saunders Company, 1989. *Reference textbook on esophageal disease.*

GASTROESOPHAGEAL REFLUX DISEASE

DEFINITION. Gastroesophageal reflux disease (GERD) refers to the varied clinical manifestations of reflux of stomach and duodenal contents into the esophagus. It is preferable to the term "reflux esophagitis" because the latter expression tends to mean different things to the clinician, the endoscopist, and the pathologist. Although it may be associated with a sliding hiatus hernia, "symptomatic hiatus hernia" is a term that tends to put the emphasis on the wrong anatomic entity and pathophysiology. Gastroesophageal reflux disease can be characterized by any combination of symptoms and radiologic, endoscopic, or pathologic changes. In its milder manifestations, it is a common disease; its most florid state is uncommon but may be life threatening.

PATHOGENESIS. Several factors must work in concert to produce clinical effects of esophageal reflux. All persons will demonstrate short bursts of reflux if monitored with an intraesophageal pH probe over 24 hours. This reflux is seen postprandially and usually in the upright position. Those in whom reflux has produced symptoms or pathologic changes will demonstrate more prolonged episodes of reflux, which tend to occur at night. The factor or factors that cause this difference are not known. However, important differences between persons with and without reflux might help explain these findings.

The *lower esophageal sphincter* (LES) is a specialized bundle of circular muscle at the lower end of the esophagus with different physical and pharmacologic characteristics when compared with the circular muscle above and below it. There is a tendency for mean LES pressure to be significantly lower in subjects with GERD compared with normal persons, but LES pressures are not very useful in predicting whether reflux is present in an individual patient unless the pressure is very low. The most common event associated with reflux appears to be an *inappropriate relaxation of the lower esophageal sphincter*, i.e., LES relaxation unassociated with either swallowing or the distention of the esophageal body by refluxed fluid. Thus, two abnormalities of LES may be associated with reflux: a sphincter with very low tone, as measured by lower esophageal sphincter pressure, or inappropriate relaxation of a normally competent sphincter.

Several factors are important in removing refluxed material. The upright position facilitates esophageal emptying by gravity. Peristaltic waves initiated by swallowing or by esophageal distention help remove the refluxed material. Acid placed within the esophagus is cleared less well by patients with GERD than by normal subjects, even though the manometric tracings seen in both groups seem identical. Clearing occurs in two phases. The bulk of the fluid is returned to the stomach by a peristaltic contraction; the remainder of the acid film clinging to the esophageal wall is neutralized by swallowed saliva.

The composition and perhaps the quantity of the refluxed material also play a role in the production of GERD. Gastric acid and pepsin seem clearly important in the pathogenesis of GERD. Bile salts and possibly pancreatic enzymes may be responsible in those patients in whom acid is absent. The combination of bile salts plus acid is more injurious to the esophagus than either agent alone. Other less well-studied factors such as altered or abnormal esophageal mucus, swallowed saliva of high bicarbonate content, and diminished resistance of the esophageal mucosa to digestion may be important in determining the amount of mucosal damage in GERD.

Esophageal squamous epithelium reacts to reflux by an increase in the basal cell or germinative layer. The dermal pegs are increased in height and may become more vascular. If the process becomes more severe, the epithelial layer is destroyed, with the appearance of microulcers and classic signs of inflammation in the lamina propria, such as infiltration with polymorphonuclear leukocytes and edema. Even deeper lesions cause first submucosal, then muscular inflammation and fibrosis, resulting in an esophageal stricture. Why reflux is so common, yet inflammation and stricture formation so relatively uncommon, is not known.

Other conditions can be associated with the pathogenesis of reflux. Reflux during pregnancy, once thought to be due to the increased abdominal pressure from the fetus, may be due mainly to diminished LES strength caused by extra estrogen and progesterone. Weight gain also tends to aggravate reflux through an unknown mechanism. As expected, resection of the lower esophageal area for cancer or myotomy for achalasia can lead to severe postoperative reflux (see below). Gastroesophageal reflux with stricture formation is especially severe in patients with progressive systemic sclerosis.

ROLE OF HIATUS HERNIA. The presence of a hiatus hernia is now considered to be much less of a factor in GERD than previously thought. Some radiologists find hiatus hernias in a large percentage of patients, no matter what the reason for the examination. Others rarely demonstrate a hiatus hernia. It is not appropriate to spend a great deal of time trying to define whether a hiatus hernia is present or absent in dealing with most patients with GERD. The important entity to investigate is reflux, not hiatus hernia.

SYMPTOMS OF GASTROESOPHAGEAL REFLUX DISEASE. *Heartburn* is the most common manifestation of GERD. It can vary from an occasional mild burning after overeating to an ever-present, severe discomfort that severely limits a patient's lifestyle. It may be accompanied by *regurgitation* of gastric contents either into the mouth or into the respiratory tree. This latter group of patients may complain of nocturnal wheezing, hoarseness, a need to clear the throat repeatedly, and a sensation of deep pressure at the base of the neck. This group of symptoms may be the primary clinical presentation and more prominent than the classic symptoms of GERD.

Dysphagia is often present in those with significant GERD. Although dysphagia may be severe and even mark the onset of stricture formation, it usually is mild and must be carefully sought. Dysphagia of GERD is for solids, and the dysphagia is usually overcome by swallowing repeatedly or by washing down the bolus with some water. Dysphagia without anatomic strictures has been noted in about three fourths of patients scheduled for antireflux surgery. Many patients with GERD do not complain of bolus arrest, but rather of being aware of the location of each solid morsel as it travels down the esophagus.

Blood loss may result from esophageal erosion and shallow ulcers. Rarely producing life-threatening hemorrhage, the erosions are much more likely to weep quietly over a prolonged period of time, producing iron deficiency anemia. Some of these patients have very few other clinical manifestations of GERD, and the condition is discovered by endoscopy during an evaluation of occult gastrointestinal bleeding. Patients who vigorously and repeatedly abuse alcohol seem prone to develop severe erosive esophagitis with bleeding; this lesion heals with abstinence from alcohol without other major antireflux therapy.

DIAGNOSIS. The history and clinical manifestations of GERD are the most important aids in the establishment of the diagnosis; objective testing is used to quantify the extent and severity of the process. In the evaluation of an individual, questions to be answered dictate the appropriate test.

Does reflux exist and, if so, to what degree? This question might arise either if another condition such as pulmonary disease is present and a causal relationship is being sought, or if some idea of the frequency and extent of reflux is important. Reflux during a barium swallow in adults is uncommon unless vigorous provocative maneuvers are employed. When spontaneous reflux of barium is seen, it usually denotes free reflux. Children reflux barium more easily than do adults. The pH probe can be used either for short-term studies of 15 to 30 minutes or for more prolonged periods (24 hours). If repeated bursts of reflux are demonstrated during a 15-minute period, then severe reflux is present. At the same time, the ability of the esophagus to clear itself of refluxed acid can be evaluated. Usually a manometric catheter is attached to the pH probe in order to locate it in the esophagus; this catheter can also estimate the LES pressure. Very low values of LES pressure such as 1 to 2 mm Hg (normal, about 20 mm Hg) are of prognostic value.

Twenty-four-hour pH monitoring can be performed with a portable unit, which allows the patient to follow an almost normal lifestyle. During the prolonged monitoring period, the relationship between symptoms (heartburn, pain, wheezing) and episodes of reflux can be ascertained, and calculations can be made of the number of episodes of reflux and the amount of time the esophagus is acidified.

Reflux can be measured noninvasively by scanning of the esophageal area with a gamma camera after placing a solution of ^{99m}Tc sulfur colloid in the stomach. An abdominal binder is used to stress the gastroesophageal junction if free reflux is not seen. This technique seems to be of most value in infants and children, who tolerate esophageal tubes very poorly.

Could reflux be responsible for the patient's symptoms? This question might be asked if pain is the predominant symptom rather than more classic heartburn. This question can be answered with the same catheter assembly used to measure LES pressure and acid reflux. After a 5-minute period of dripping normal saline through one of the pressure catheters whose opening has been localized to the upper esophagus, this infusion is changed to 0.1 N hydrochloric acid without the patient's knowledge. Reproduction of the symptoms within 30 minutes of acid infusion (usually 4 to 5 minutes into the infusion) and rapid disappearance of the symptom with a switch back to saline infusion suggests an esophageal cause of the discomfort.

As another approach, the patient is asked to signal the time of discomfort during prolonged pH monitoring of the esophagus. If the patient signals discomfort at the same time that reflux is demonstrated by the pH probe, then a causal relationship is made more likely. Prolonged pH monitoring has shown good correlation between periods of reflux and heartburn as well as other unexplained chest pain syndromes.

What has reflux done to the esophageal mucosa? A barium swallow detects gross changes such as stricture formation or a deep esophageal ulcer but misses the much more common shallow ulcerations and erosions. These are detected by direct inspection with the endoscope. Only discrete lesions such as erosions and ulcerations should be taken as proof of esophageal damage; such endoscopic findings as erythema, edema, or friability are subject to wide interobserver variation. If the mucosa appears absolutely normal, as it is in approximately one third of patients with moderate to severe symptoms of GERD, a biopsy can demonstrate the changes of reflux.

A logic tree of how these tests might be used is shown in Table 96–1. A patient whose symptoms are severe enough to seek medical attention might be screened with a barium swallow. Uncommonly, reflux is demonstrated, a stricture found, or a deep ulcer seen. This might lead to immediate endoscopy for more complete evaluation. If a patient presents with hematemesis and reflux symptoms, endoscopy might appropriately be used as the first step. After first evaluation, it is appropriate to begin therapy (see Treatment, below). Only if there is a poor response to therapy should an acid perfusion test be used to confirm the diagnosis. At the same time, the presence of reflux can be checked, an estimate of LES pressure and acid clearance obtained, and the presence or absence of peristaltic waves determined.

More intensive therapy should be instituted at this point. If it

TABLE 96–1. DIAGNOSIS OF REFLUX

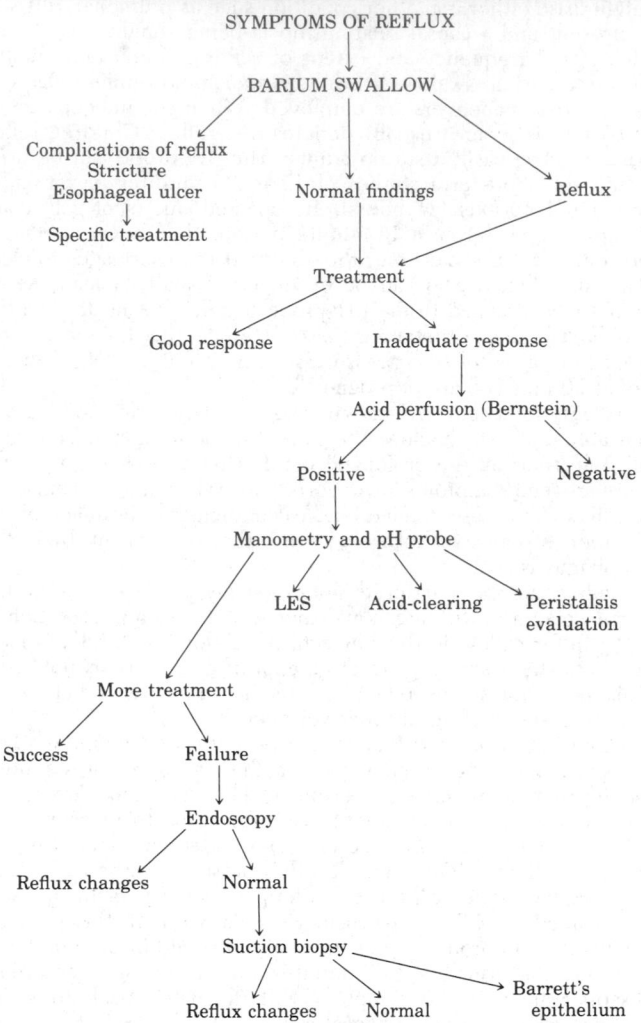

SYMPTOMS OF REFLUX

BARIUM SWALLOW

Complications of reflux
Stricture
Esophageal ulcer → Normal findings → Reflux

Specific treatment

Treatment

Good response → Inadequate response

Acid perfusion (Bernstein)

Positive → Negative

Manometry and pH probe

LES → Acid-clearing → Peristalsis evaluation

More treatment

Success → Failure

Endoscopy

Reflux changes → Normal

Suction biopsy

Reflux changes → Normal → Barrett's epithelium

---

fails and the patient is still symptomatic, endoscopy can be employed to see if gross disease is still present in the face of maximal therapy. If the appearance of the mucosa is normal grossly in the presence of overwhelming symptoms, biopsies can be obtained to search for objective evidence of reflux damage. This scheme will restrict extensive testing to those who have failed medical therapy and who are presumably candidates for surgical treatment. This algorithm can be modified if the patient has blood loss or severe dysphagia. Endoscopy is now being more widely used as the initial diagnostic study because of its overall sensitivity and specificity.

COMPLICATIONS OF GASTROESOPHAGEAL REFLUX DISEASE. Esophageal Stricture. Of the many who complain of symptoms of GERD, only a few develop esophageal strictures. Usually beginning at the lower end of the esophagus, strictures may migrate over years to the midesophagus or higher. Columnar epithelium is found below the stricture. Presumably those who develop strictures have had deep circumferential ulceration of the esophageal mucosa due to reflux damage. Instead of healing with only minimal submucosal and muscular fibrosis, these patients develop esophageal obstruction with a narrowed esophageal lumen. If reflux can be controlled, these strictures disappear.

Dysphagia is the clinical hallmark of esophageal stricture formation. Unlike the relatively mild dysphagia seen in uncomplicated GERD, the dysphagia in patients with strictures tends to be constant and slowly progressive, causing the patient to alter the type of food taken. If a bolus becomes arrested in the stricture, it is usually necessary for the bolus to be regurgitated back into the mouth before further intake of food or fluids is possible.

Strictures are most easily evaluated by barium swallow. Sometimes the extent of the strictured area is overestimated unless the esophagus below the stricture can be fully distended by barium. For mild strictures, the ingestion of a bread or marshmallow bolus can draw attention to slight luminal narrowing when the bolus impacts there. Once demonstrated, endoscopy with biopsy and/or brush cytology is in order to make certain that the stricture is benign.

Esophageal Ulcer. In addition to the more common shallow ulcerations, deep esophageal ulcers may complicate severe GERD. These ulcers, which retain barium and usually project outside the wall of the esophagus, characteristically produce severe and unrelenting pain, often with radiation of the pain through to the back. Brisk hemorrhage is another manifestation, from erosion either through to an esophageal artery or, more catastrophically, into the nearby aorta. The presence of an ulcer can be suspected on a barium swallow and confirmed endoscopically. The ulcer is usually found to reside in columnar (Barrett's) epithelium.

Columnar Epithelium. In some patients who have suffered severe esophageal ulceration as a result of GERD, the healing epithelium is replaced not with squamous epithelium but with a specialized columnar epithelium. The junctional zone between squamous and columnar epithelium can progress orad over years. Columnar epithelium is found at and below midesophageal strictures and around deep esophageal ulcers, although it can be found on routine biopsy of patients with severe GERD. Its major clinical importance is not only as a marker of severe reflux but also as a precursor for adenocarcinoma of the esophagus (see under Esophageal Tumors).

Pulmonary Aspiration. If refluxed material breaches the upper esophageal sphincter, it may easily spill into the larynx and tracheobronchial tree. Some patients react to such a spill with intense respiratory stridor. Others seem to tolerate the presence of refluxed contents in the larynx and tracheobronchial tree with milder laryngeal or respiratory symptoms. It is even possible that the gastric contents do not have to reach the larynx; instillation of acid in the esophagus of susceptible individuals while they are in the upright posture can be shown to cause closing of small bronchial airways by a vagal reflex.

None of the clinical features of pulmonary aspiration (Table 96–2) is pathognomonic. Taken together they point toward reflux and aspiration as a possible etiology. Diagnostic proof of the relationship is difficult with current techniques. Radioisotopes placed in the stomach have been demonstrated the next morning to be in the lungs by gamma camera scanning, but this cannot be demonstrated in the majority of patients. Only correction of reflux with subsequent disappearance of pulmonary symptoms can prove the relationship.

TREATMENT OF GASTROESOPHAGEAL REFLUX DISEASE AND ITS COMPLICATIONS. Medical Management. Most mildly symptomatic patients with reflux and some moderately afflicted individuals can be helped by manipulations designed to alter the frequency or type of esophageal reflux. Many patients respond to the simple measures outlined in Table 96–3. Elevation of the head of the bed by 6 to 8 inches is the simplest and most effective form of therapy. Twenty-four-hour pH monitoring has shown that this simple measure decreases the frequency and length of reflux episodes. The use of pillows to elevate the thorax does not work well, as patients tend to roll off the pillows during the night. A foam rubber wedge can be used if the bed frame cannot be moved. Avoiding food and fluid for at least 3 hours before retiring decreases the amount of material available for reflux at night. Avoidance of food that the patient finds distressing, such as fatty foods, chocolate, and onions, makes sense but has never been subjected to clinical trial.

TABLE 96–2. CLINICAL FEATURES OF PULMONARY ASPIRATION

1. Onset of "asthma" in patients over 30 years of age without a family history of asthma or industrial exposure
2. Nocturnal or early morning cough
3. Nocturnal wheezing
4. Hoarseness, especially on arising
5. The need to clear the throat repeatedly
6. A feeling of constant pressure deep in the neck

TABLE 96–3. TREATMENT OF GASTROESOPHAGEAL REFLUX DISEASE

Simple measures
1. Elevation of head of the bed
2. Avoidance of food and fluid intake before bedtime
3. Reduction of fat in diet
4. Liquid antacid (aluminum hydroxide, magnesium hydroxide) 1 and 3 hours after meals and at bedtime
5. Avoidance of cigarettes and alcohol
6. Weight loss

Measures for resistant cases
1. Alginic acid–antacid (Gaviscon), 15 ml four times a day
2. Bethanechol (Urecholine),* 10 or 25 mg four times a day
3. Metoclopramide (Reglan),* 10 mg three times a day
4. Cimetidine,* 300 mg four times a day
5. Ranitidine,* 150 mg twice a day
6. Famotidine,* 20 mg twice a day
7. Omeprazole,* 20 mg every day
8. Fundoplication

*Higher doses of an H_2 antagonist or omeprazole may be required in some cases.

Neutralization of acid is approached by taking 30 ml of aluminum hydroxide-magnesium hydroxide antacid 1 and 3 hours after meals and at bedtime. In recalcitrant cases, hourly antacids may be tried, with substitution of pure aluminum hydroxide gel to control diarrhea produced by the magnesium ion. Most patients do not tolerate such a regimen for long.

An attempt should be made to have the patient stop smoking, drinking alcohol, and overeating. Most patients, however, apparently prefer to suffer with reflux symptoms rather than to give up these mainstays of life.

If these simple measures are not effective, more vigorous treatment is indicated. Alginic acid-antacid, 15 ml after each meal and at bedtime, is more effective than placebo and as effective as antacids. It is worth trying but often does not control symptoms of severe reflux. Bethanechol, a parasympathomimetic agent, can be used in doses of 10 or 25 mg four times a day. Metoclopramide, 10 mg three times a day, can be helpful, but central nervous system side effects limit its usefulness.

The H_2 antagonists in the usual dosage range for duodenal ulcer improve symptoms of heartburn better than a placebo. Higher dosage regimens, cimetidine 800 mg, ranitidine 300 mg, or famotidine 40 mg, each twice per day, have been more effective for control of symptoms and healing of peptic esophagitis. Healing of esophageal erosions with H_2 antagonists usually takes 12 to 16 weeks.

The potassium-hydrogen ATPase inhibitor, omeprazole, 20 mg once per day, can sometimes give dramatic symptom relief and healing of esophagitis in 4 to 8 weeks.

Once healing has been achieved with either an H_2 antagonist or omeprazole, recurrence rates exceed 80 per cent if no maintenance therapy is utilized. Maintenance therapy for esophagitis generally requires full dosage, in contrast to the reduced maintenance dose used for duodenal ulcer.

Surgical Management. In a patient in whom adequate trial of medical management as outlined above has not brought good results in a 6-month period, and in whom there is good objective evidence of reflux, surgical correction of reflux should be considered. Current surgical therapy, regardless of exact techniques, attempts to restore sphincter competence by surrounding the lower end of the esophagus with a cuff of gastric fundal muscle. This is done either completely, as in the Nissen fundoplication, or partially (Hill repair, Belsey repair).

A well-done fundoplication can restore a competent lower esophageal sphincter, reduce gastroesophageal reflux, heal peptic esophagitis, and even lead to reversal of peptic stricture. Barrett's epithelium may regress in a limited number of cases, but usually the columnar epithelium does not disappear. The Nissen fundoplication seems to provide the most satisfactory long-term improvement.

A surgeon experienced in the techniques of antireflux surgery is necessary for good postoperative results. Technique is all important. Although some individual surgeons have enviable postoperative results, antireflux surgery has a relatively poor reputation in many medical communities. Currently, a conservative approach toward antireflux surgery seems indicated.

Treatment of Complications. Esophageal strictures, if only mildly symptomatic, can be handled by careful attention to dietary intake, improvement of dentition, and institution of medical therapy. Techniques of dilation have proliferated in recent years, but they still require an experienced operator. Short, simple strictures can be dilated with weighted rubber or Teflon dilators (Hurst, Maloney). Tortuous or angulated strictures are more easily approached over a previously placed guide wire. This, in turn, can be passed through an endoscope or under radiographic control. Graded steel olives (Eder-Peustow), a dilator with graded increases of size (Celestin), or a balloon with a fixed maximal diameter (Cooke) can be passed over the previously placed wire. Alternatively, a balloon of fixed maximal diameter can be passed through the large channel of an endoscope during diagnostic endoscopy, and dilation can be done under direct vision. Once the lumen is restored to a diameter of 13 to 15 mm, most patients swallow without difficulty. If the stricture is stable and requires dilation only every 4 to 6 months, nothing else is necessary.

Some patients do not tolerate dilation or require vigorous dilation every 3 to 4 weeks. This is an indication for definitive antireflux operation, following which the stricture may regress. Unfortunately, many strictures persist after attempts at antireflux surgery. Esophageal replacement by colon, jejunum, or stomach is a surgical maneuver of last resort; such procedures have relatively high morbidity and mortality. Those afflicted by strictures may have significant lung and cardiovascular disease that makes them unsuitable operative candidates. The use of high-dose H_2 antagonists or preferably omeprazole along with dilation of the stricture has led to healing of the mucosa and lower requirements for repeated stricture dilation.

Esophageal ulcers also represent a major therapeutic problem. Although cimetidine therapy may heal an ulcer, antireflux surgery, if tolerated, is a more reliable mode of treatment. If not, gastric radiation can be employed as in esophageal stricture.

Columnar epithelium may be premalignant. There is no way short of esophageal resection to make certain that the epithelium can be removed. Adequate antireflux therapy causes regression of columnar epithelium in a rare patient, but further study is necessary before antireflux surgery can be recommended as a treatment for columnar epithelium. The effect of omeprazole therapy on the columnar epithelium is not known. Currently, columnar epithelium is followed closely with periodic endoscopic biopsies to look for dysplasia and early changes of adenocarcinoma. Dysplasia can be graded using specific criteria. The persistence of confirmed high-grade dysplasia is an indication for esophagectomy.

Treatment of the pulmonary complications of reflux depends on the age of the patient. Infants who present with recurrent bronchitis can be treated by postural methods and by thickening the formula. In adults, attention to posture at night is most important (see above). Since diagnostic methods that establish a direct causal relationship between reflux and lung disease are lacking, caution is advised in offering surgery to those who present with primary pulmonary problems and in whom reflux is demonstrated.

Castell DO, Wu WC, Ott DS: Gastroesophageal Reflux Disease. Mt. Kisco, NY, Futura Publishing Company, 1985, pp 1–324. *Monograph with good literature review.*

Spechler SJ, Goyal RK: Barrett's esophagus. N Engl J Med 315:362, 1986. *Up-to-date review of columnar epithelium.*

MOTOR DISORDERS OF THE ESOPHAGUS

DEFINITION AND PATHOGENESIS. The muscular tube of the esophagus is guarded at both ends by specialized bundles of muscle, the upper and lower esophageal sphincters (UES, LES). Material from the oropharynx is injected at a high velocity (in the case of liquids), and precise coordination is required to link the muscles of the oropharynx, UES, body of the esophagus, and LES into a functional unit. Failure of any or all of these components results in an esophageal motor disorder.

Failure of the oropharyngeal and UES units can be caused either by primary muscle disease such as *myotonia dystrophica* or *dermatomyositis* or by neurologic lesions involving the innervation of these muscle groups. *Brain stem infarcts, multiple sclerosis*, and *amyotrophic lateral sclerosis* serve as examples for the latter process.

The pathogenesis of motor abnormality of the esophageal body is less well understood. The striated muscle that constitutes the upper one quarter to one third of the body can be affected by primary muscle disease, such as *myotonia dystrophica*, or by metabolic disease affecting muscle function, such as *hypothyroidism*. The smooth muscle seems more resistant to muscular disease, but the intrinsic nervous network can be involved in *Chagas' disease* and *achalasia*. In the latter disease, there is infiltration of Auerbach's plexus with lymphocytes or actual disappearance of the neuron cell bodies in the plexus.

The motor disorders of the body of the esophagus have historically been classified as *achalasia* or *diffuse spasm*. In achalasia, dysphagia and esophageal retention predominate; the radiograph shows a dilated esophagus with a distal beak, and manometry reveals a high pressure in the LES with no or incomplete relaxation as well as only simultaneous low-amplitude contractions in response to a swallow. Diffuse spasm has been characterized as a clinical syndrome of esophageal colic or dysphagia or both; segmental contractions seen by radiograph; and a manometric picture of some peristaltic waves interspersed with periods of slight simultaneous elevation of the baseline pressure in several leads surmounted by simultaneous contractions. Another common manometric abnormality is high-amplitude, long-duration waves that are peristaltic and can be associated with either esophageal colic or dysphagia or both (nutcracker esophagus). There are many variations of these "classic" diseases, and progression from diffuse spasm to achalasia has been documented in the same individual. Many nonspecific motor disorders of the esophagus do not fit these syndromes. The pathophysiology of these nonspecific disorders has not been described. It seems best at the present state of knowledge to be descriptive of the features of a motor disorder without being too precise about an actual name of the disorder.

SYMPTOMS. The type of symptom produced is a function of the level and extent of the problem. *Weakness of the oropharyngeal musculature* may cause *transfer dysphagia*—the inability to propel a solid or liquid bolus from the pharynx to the esophagus. Patients are aware usually that they cannot begin the act of deglutition. Solids are usually more troublesome than liquids. Palatal weakness may lead to *nasal regurgitation* of fluids or to *laryngeal aspiration* because of muscular failure to seal off the larynx. Such weakness may be signaled by a nasal quality of the voice.

Incoordination of UES relaxation has been suggested as a cause of transfer dysphagia and for the production of Zenker's diverticulum, but current high-fidelity methods fail to show such incoordination. Transfer dysphagia accompanied by a prominent cricopharyngeal impression on a barium swallow ("cricopharyngeal achalasia") similarly shows no defect in relaxing or in timing when studied by modern manometric methods.

Motor disorders in the body of the esophagus produce either *dysphagia* or *pain*, or both. The dysphagia may be intermittent or continuous. It may be manifest both for solids and for liquids. It is rare for the arrested material to be regurgitated; often posturing (throwing the shoulders back and extending the neck) or a Valsalva maneuver helps the material pass into the stomach.

Pain or esophageal colic is the other major clinical presentation of motor disorders. The pain is usually substernal, described as a feeling of pressure or aching, radiating to the back as well as to the neck, jaw, and arms. It can range in intensity from a transient discomfort to an overwhelming, agonizing pain similar to that of a major myocardial infarction or dissecting aortic aneurysm. The pain may last for only 5 to 10 seconds or may be present for hours. The differentiation between angina pectoris and esophageal colic may be impossible on clinical grounds; both may be related to exercise, have the same intensity and distribution, and respond to sublingual nitroglycerin.

Failure of the lower esophageal sphincter may present with two separate symptom complexes. If the sphincter fails to relax on deglutition (as occurs in achalasia), dysphagia and retention of contents in the body of the esophagus occur. This failure, coupled with loss of peristalsis (achalasia), leads to marked esophageal

retention, regurgitation, and overflow of esophageal contents into the tracheobronchial tree. If there is primary muscle failure of the sphincter, as occurs in *scleroderma*, massive reflux and the consequences of GERD follow.

DIAGNOSIS. A careful history is essential in choosing the correct diagnostic tools for evaluating esophageal motor disorders. If the difficulty is thought to be in the oropharynx and upper esophageal sphincter, a cineradiograph would offer the most information. The cine film allows for frame-by-frame analysis of this rapidly moving portion of the gastrointestinal tract. Incoordination of tongue and palate, unilateral pharyngeal weakness, and aspiration of small amounts of barium into the trachea on swallowing can be shown. Air double-contrast examinations of the pharynx can elucidate an unsuspected hypopharyngeal carcinoma. A diverticulum or prominence of the cricopharyngeal muscle can also be seen. Manometric examination of the hypopharynx and upper esophageal sphincter has not been helpful.

Radiology offers the best chance of diagnosis when the motor disorders have relatively static changes. In achalasia the body of the esophagus commonly dilates with retention of food, secretions, and barium (Fig. 96–1). Special attention can be paid to the terminal end of the esophagus. In achalasia, there is a smooth, tapering beak. Any irregularity of this beak should lead to a vigorous search for an infiltrating neoplasm of the cardia, which can exactly mimic achalasia clinically and radiologically.

If the esophageal muscle is atonic, as is seen in far-advanced scleroderma, barium and even air are retained for long periods of time in the supine position. Assumption of the upright position rapidly clears the barium from the esophagus and leaves a double-contrast view of a dilated esophagus.

The radiologist has more difficulty when the motor abnormality is more intermittent (Fig. 96–2). Such a radiologic appearance is not always evidence for a clinically important motor disorder; elderly patients often show similar radiologic findings and yet are totally asymptomatic.

Manometric examination allows more prolonged evaluation of esophageal motor function and is the only method that allows lower esophageal sphincter function to be directly determined. Normally, a swallow causes a peristaltic wave to be detected sequentially by pressure detectors spaced along the esophagus.

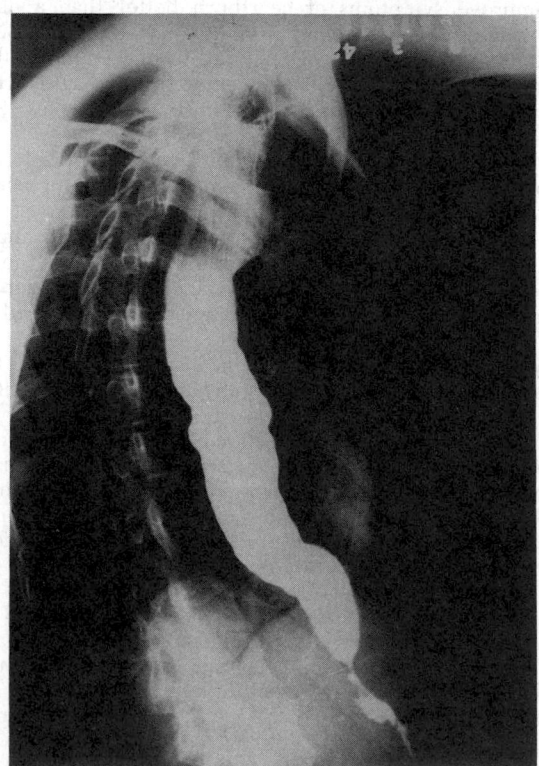

FIGURE 96–1. Radiologic appearance of achalasia. The esophageal body is dilated and terminates in a narrowed segment. (Courtesy of Dr. FE Templeton. From Pope CE II: *In* Sleisenger MH, Fordtran JS [eds.]: Gastrointestinal Disease. 3rd ed. Philadelphia, W. B. Saunders Company, 1983.)

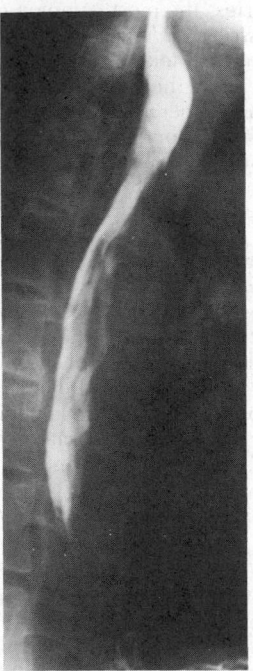
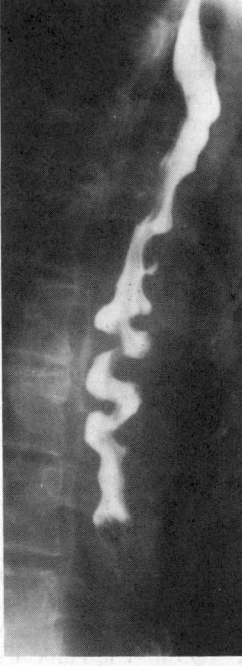

FIGURE 96–2. Radiologic appearance of diffuse spasm. Two spot films were taken within 10 seconds of each other. A fairly normal appearance on the left changes rapidly to an appearance of numerous contractions. (Courtesy of Dr. CA Rohrmann. From Pope CE II: *In* Sleisenger MH, Fordtran JS [eds.]: Gastrointestinal Disease. 3rd ed. Philadelphia, W. B. Saunders Company, 1983.)

Aperistalsis (no response to a swallow), simultaneous single or multiple contractions, prolonged contractions of high amplitude and low velocity, and spontaneous activity not related to swallowing can be recorded. Some of the "classic" patterns associated with diseases are shown in Figure 96–3. Many subjects present with dysphagia and/or chest pain in different patterns. It is best to describe the radiologic and manometric findings in the individual patient and then try to relate them to the classic syndrome most closely resembled. Also, one syndrome (diffuse spasm) may progress over time to another (achalasia).

Manometric examination can be of special benefit in the evaluation of chest pain if the patient happens to have an attack

of chest pain during the examination. If the chest pain is accompanied by motor activity that allows the manometrist to predict onset, intensity, and disappearance of the chest pain by watching the manometric tracing, the diagnosis of an esophageal origin of chest pain is firmly established. Similarly, if pH is being simultaneously monitored and the episodes of chest pain correlate closely with drops in intraesophageal pH, an esophageal origin of pain is likely. Conversely, if typical chest pain occurs but there is no change in motor activity or pH over control values, an esophageal cause of pain is unlikely. Unfortunately, such definitive statements can be made only in about 20 per cent of the patients examined.

Pharmacologic stimulation of the esophagus has been employed for diagnostic purposes using such agents as mecholyl, pentagastrin, bethanechol, and edrophonium. Edrophonium (Tensilon) is the most widely used provocative agent for inducing chest pain along with simultaneous esophageal spasm. The cholinesterase inhibitor is short acting and extremely safe in clinical usage. Provocative testing has been helpful in delineating the cause of chest pain in patients with normal baseline esophageal manometry.

Endoscopy is useful in the evaluation of motor disorders, for inspection of the cardia with a retroflexed view from the stomach to rule out an infiltrating carcinoma, and for excluding inflammatory disorders.

TREATMENT. Of the various motor disorders of the esophagus, *achalasia* seems most amenable to relief. Since the problem in achalasia is one of obstruction of the lower end of the esophagus by a sphincter that does not relax, all forms of therapy are directed at relief of this obstruction. Short-term improvement in clinical symptoms and in scintigraphic esophageal emptying may occur with isosorbide dinitrate, a long-acting nitrate, or with nifedipine, a calcium channel blocker. The place of long-term pharmacologic management of achalasia has not been established. Dilation with a large Hurst bougie may give temporary relief; a few patients have been maintained for long periods of time with weekly self-dilations, but this treatment is no longer recommended. Much more effective is dilation with a pneumatic bag under radiographic control. This should be performed by an expert, since perforation even in good hands may occur in about 5 per cent of patients. Pneumatic dilation is preferable initially for all patients.

Surgery is reserved for those in whom bag dilation fails or those who do not wish to be exposed to the risk of perforation. Direct section of the lower esophageal sphincter muscle (my-

FIGURE 96–3. Idealized manometric patterns. *A*, The normal swallow consists of a progressive wave with a wave of short duration and rapid rise time in the striated upper esophagus. The lower esophageal sphincter shows a fall in pressure coincident with swallowing. *B*, In achalasia the striated muscle sometimes, but not always, produces a typical wave. The smooth muscle portion of the esophagus has a simultaneous low-amplitude contraction that follows the striated muscle contraction. The elevated pressure in the LES shows either incomplete or no relaxation. *C*, Diffuse spasm shows an elevation of the baseline after swallowing, on top of which are superimposed repetitive simultaneous contractions. LES pressure may be high and relaxation may terminate prematurely. *D*, High-amplitude, long-duration waves (nutcracker esophagus). The wave is peristaltic but of high amplitude. Duration is increased and velocity of propagation may be decreased. *E*, Scleroderma. Striated muscle contraction is normal, but the amplitude of contraction in the smooth muscle is reduced or may be absent. Sphincter pressure is low.

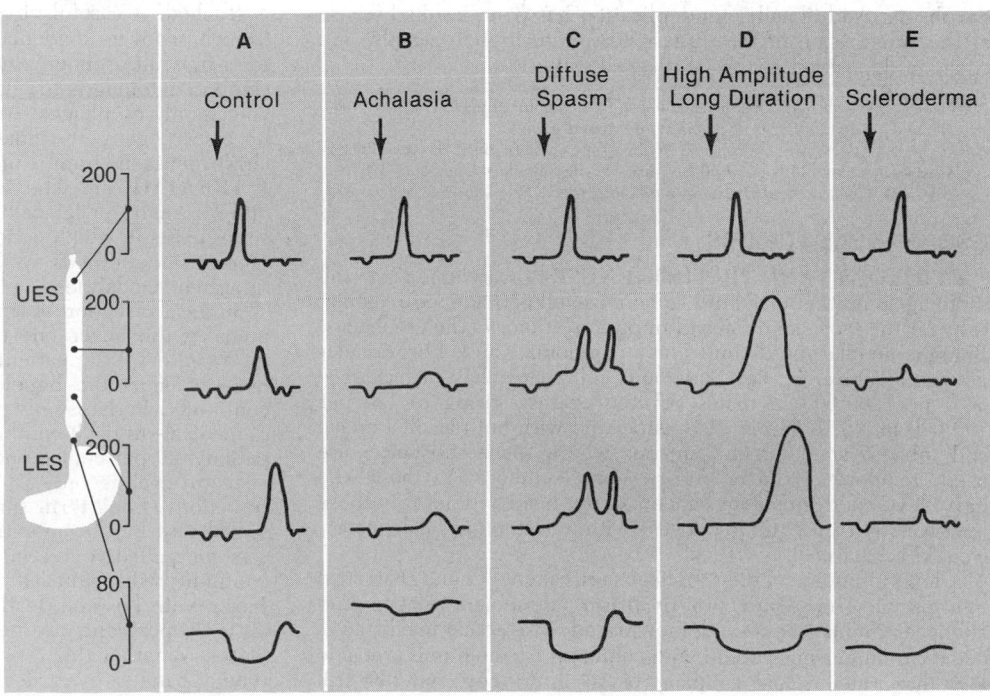

otomy) is carried out, sparing some gastric muscle fibers to prevent postoperative reflux (Heller procedure). Amazingly, after both bag dilation and myotomy, manometry reveals return of normal peristalsis in 10 per cent of those with achalasia. Many surgeons currently combine a "loose" fundoplication along with the Heller myotomy. Postoperative gastroesophageal reflux with esophagitis and peptic stricture of the esophagus may occur in patients if the myotomy abolishes all lower esophageal sphincter pressure and if no fundoplication is performed. This observation is difficult to explain in view of the degeneration of Auerbach's plexus in the intramural nervous network, thought to explain the pathogenesis of this disease.

Treatment of most other motor disorders is much more difficult. Patients with diffuse spasm can be given nitroglycerin, anticholinergics, or calcium channel antagonists. Balloon dilation has also been suggested to be of benefit in diffuse spasm and has been helpful in those patients with abnormal lower esophageal function, high basal tone with impaired relaxation. Division of all the circular muscle with a long myotomy has been tried, but the long-term results of this procedure are not always favorable.

Treatment of other nonspecific motor disorders associated with chest pain can be equally frustrating. Prescribing sublingual nitroglycerin is justifiable. If it is ineffective, long-acting nitrate therapy will probably not work. Anticholinergic drugs benefit only a few. Calcium channel antagonists reduce the force of the esophageal contractions and relieve pain. Meperidine (Demerol) has been uniformly useful. Obviously this medication is not a good long-term solution to the problem. Long myotomies have been tried in selected patients; occasional good long-term results have been obtained. It would seem wise not to subject any patient to myotomy until that patient has been observed manometrically during an attack and an esophageal origin of pain has been firmly established. Recently, a form of microvascular coronary artery disease has been suggested as a cause of chest pain in patients with "nutcracker" esophagus. The description of this new cardiac disease has further confused this field and has emphasized the reluctance to perform long esophageal myotomies in patients with esophageal chest pain.

The treatment of scleroderma and other conditions marked by aperistalsis revolves mostly around the associated reflux. If there is no obstruction at the lower end of the esophagus, either by a malfunctioning sphincter or by an organic narrowing, aperistalsis is amazingly well tolerated, usually with only mild dysphagia for solids. Caution should be employed in offering antireflux surgery to patients with scleroderma, as a tight fundoplication without any peristalsis in the body of the esophagus leads to severe dysphagia. Additionally, fundoplication has poor results because of the progression of the disease to severe muscle atrophy and collagen deposition in the esophageal wall.

Blackwell JN, Castell DO: Oesophageal chest pain: A point of view. Gut 25:1, 1984. *Review of the esophagus as a source of anginal pain.*

Ouyang A, Cohen S: Motor disorders of the esophagus. *In* Berk JE (ed.): Bockus' Gastroenterology. 4th ed. Philadelphia, W. B. Saunders Company, 1985, pp 690–704. *Good current review of motor disorders.*

ESOPHAGEAL TUMORS

ETIOLOGY AND PATHOGENESIS. Carcinoma of the esophageal epithelium, both squamous cell and adenocarcinoma, is by far the most common and important tumor of the esophagus. Benign neoplasms (leiomyoma, papilloma, and fibrovascular polyps) are rarer by far. Squamous cell cancer has an incidence of 4 per 100,000 in males (United States), rising to 130 per 100,000 in North China. It is associated with both alcohol intake and tobacco smoking in countries where these substances are used. Esophageal cancer occurs more commonly in those who have developed squamous cancers of the head and neck, in those with lye strictures, and in patients with untreated or inadequately treated achalasia.

Adenocarcinoma of the esophagus arises in columnar (Barrett's) epithelium. The sequence of dysplasia, adenoma formation, and adenocarcinoma has been demonstrated. The actual incidence of adenocarcinoma in a patient with columnar epithelium is probably less than the original estimate of 10 to 15 per cent but still represents a significant problem.

SYMPTOMS. In Western countries, the most common clinical symptom of carcinoma is *progressive dysphagia* over a 6- to 8-month period until only liquids can be taken. The obstruction reflects circumferential involvement of the esophageal wall by tumor and does not occur until the cancer is biologically rather far advanced. The dysphagia may be accompanied by a *steady, boring pain*, which signals mediastinal involvement and inoperability. In the Orient but not in the United States, pain is often a relatively early sign of a localized and thus resectable tumor. Unexplained persistent chest pain should always be investigated by a careful double-contrast radiographic view of the esophagus or by endoscopy.

More advanced lesions manifest themselves with *halitosis, weight loss*, and *coughing after drinking fluid*. The last-named symptom is caused either by nearly complete esophageal lumen obstruction with overspill into the larynx or by the development of a tracheoesophageal fistula. Hoarseness from involvement of the recurrent laryngeal nerve by tumor and hematemesis are unusual symptoms. Nail bed clubbing can be seen with both benign and malignant tumors.

Since dysphagia is the most common presenting symptom of neoplasm of the esophagus, the physician is responsible for making absolutely certain that cancer is not the cause of dysphagia. Early diagnosis affords the only chance for cure. Early diagnosis allows the patient, family, and physician to plan better all aspects of the patient's future.

DIAGNOSIS. The clinical suspicion of a cancer of the esophagus should lead immediately to an esophagogram, possibly with double-contrast techniques. Any irregularity, especially if it narrows the lumen, mandates further evaluation. If dysphagia is present, the radiologist should give a bolus of barium-soaked bread or a large marshmallow to discover any possible sites of arrest.

In the presence of symptoms but a normal barium swallow, endoscopy with biopsy and brushing of any suspicious lesion for examination of tissue and of exfoliated cells is indicated. The endoscopist should always obtain a good retroflexed view of the cardia from below to make certain that an adenocarcinoma of the gastroesophageal junction has not been overlooked.

If narrowing has been seen by barium swallow, endoscopy with biopsy and cytologic brushings of the involved area must be done. With the fiberoptic endoscope, numerous blind biopsies from as deep in the lesion as possible will be most helpful. Biopsy of visible tissue will often reveal only inflammatory tissue. Sometimes as many as eight or nine biopsies must be obtained before tumor is recovered.

Once a tumor is identified, certain procedures in addition to chest films are essential for staging before a therapeutic decision is reached. A careful physical examination for nodal metastases, bronchoscopy for evidence of tracheal involvement, liver function tests plus ultrasonography for evidence of liver metastases, and computed tomographic (CT) scanning for mediastinal nodal involvement, esophageal wall thickness, and liver metastases are necessary before the final therapeutic plan is decided upon. A chest roentgenogram is mandatory.

TREATMENT. The ideal treatment of esophageal cancer, either for cure or for palliation, has not yet been developed. No series exists in which patients were carefully staged with the best noninvasive methods available and then randomized to different treatment modalities.

Surgical resection of squamous cell carcinoma and adenocarcinoma of the lower one third of the esophagus is preferred in most centers if the patient does not have widespread metastases. Surgery offers the benefit of rapidly restoring esophagogastric continuity. Perhaps only one quarter of all patients presenting to a medical-surgical center have a resectable tumor; of these patients 20 per cent do not survive the operative period, and 5-year survival is only 5 to 10 per cent, even with extensive resections. Long-term survival cannot be predicted in the individual case by the operative findings. There is growing enthusiasm for palliative resection with restoration of gastrointestinal continuity with stomach or colon. Surgical results in China and Japan, with hospital deaths of 5 per cent and 5-year survivals of 20 to 30 per cent, are better than those quoted for the United States. Whether this represents better technical skill, a different type of patient, or earlier diagnosis is not certain.

Radiotherapy is employed in lesions of the upper one third of the esophagus and often in middle third tumors as well. This form of therapy has little hospital mortality, although it carries some short-term and long-term morbidity. With ideal home situations, radiotherapy can be carried out on an outpatient basis. Approximately 40 per cent of tumors cannot be destroyed with conventional 6000-rad therapy. Combination of pre- and postoperative radiation with resective therapy has been employed, but there is no good evidence that such combined therapy is better. Adenocarcinomas occasionally respond to radiotherapy but are not as radiosensitive as squamous cell carcinomas.

When obvious extraesophageal spread is present, palliation with bougienage to restore and maintain an adequate esophageal lumen may be done. If performed with a guide wire under fluoroscopic guidance, such therapy is not hazardous in skilled hands. If dilation does not offer lasting relief, then a Silastic tube can be placed perorally for relief of esophageal obstruction. Such tubes are also of great benefit in the treatment of a malignant tracheoesophageal fistula. Another useful approach is the destruction of intraluminal tumor and restoration of an adequate lumen by laser therapy or an intraluminal heatcoagulating probe.

Choice of therapy will depend on the location and size of the lesion, presence or absence of spread, cell type, and the skills of the medical community. Until an adequate randomized trial after adequate staging is carried out, choice of treatment modality will continue to be a matter of preference.

Earlam R, Cunha-Melo JR: Oesophageal squamous cell carcinoma. Br J Surg 67:381, 457, 1980. *Two articles present exhaustive literature reviews of surgical and radiotherapy of esophageal carcinoma.*

Livstone EM: General considerations of tumors of the esophagus. *In* Berk JE (ed.): Bockus' Gastroenterology. 4th ed. Philadelphia, W. B. Saunders Company, 1985, pp 818–840. *Review of diagnostic and therapeutic considerations in esophageal carcinoma.*

OTHER CONDITIONS

RINGS AND WEBS. During early development, the lumen of the esophagus becomes completely obliterated and then is recanalized to form the adult hollow viscus. A failure of this process leads to atresia or a residual web. Such webs usually occur in the upper esophagus, often with eccentric openings; occasionally they are multiple. A much more common web or ring is located in the terminal esophagus, has a symmetric opening, and is usually at the junction between squamous and the normal transitional or columnar epithelium of the stomach (Fig. 96–4). This latter ring (Schatzki's ring) can be demonstrated in many individuals if cine studies of the lower esophageal zone are used. It produces symptoms infrequently but in a character-

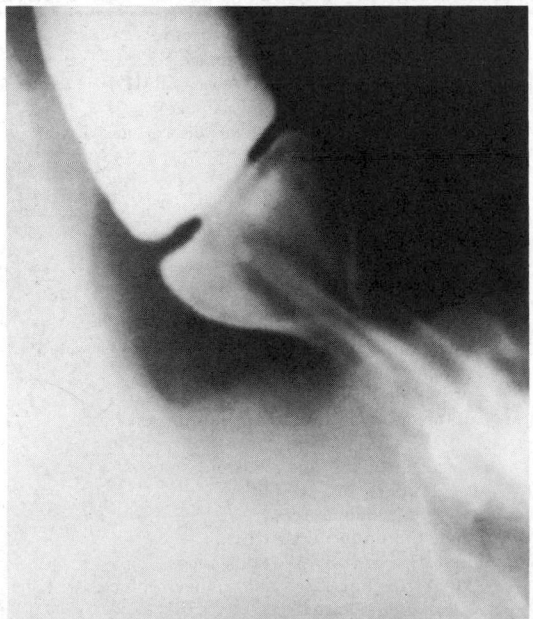

FIGURE 96–4. Lower esophageal ring (Schatzki's ring). This ring consists of a symmetric thin web located in the terminal esophagus. (From Pope CE II: *In* Sleisenger MH, Fordtran JS [eds.]: Gastrointestinal Disease. 3rd ed. Philadelphia, W. B. Saunders Company, 1983.)

istic manner. An acquired web located in the postcricoid area is sometimes associated with iron deficiency anemia (Plummer-Vinson syndrome).

All these types of webs or rings cause dysphagia for solids, and the impacted bolus usually has to be regurgitated. The lower esophageal ring (Schatzki's ring) has a characteristic clinical presentation that allows the diagnosis to be made by history. Every 3 to 4 months, after a bolus of meat or bread, the patient complains of dysphagia and total inability to swallow solids or liquids. The bolus is regurgitated, and then the patient can continue to eat normally. If the patient comes to the emergency room with an impacted bolus of meat, nothing is seen after the impacted bolus is removed with the operating endoscope, and the disorder is labeled "hysterical dysphagia." The lower esophageal ring is not well seen with the rigid endoscope. Lower esophageal rings may be dilated using a through-the-endoscope balloon or a bougie. Rings of less than 12.0 mm across their narrowest diameter cause symptoms and require rupture.

Treatment of all webs involves mechanical disruption either with a dilator or with the endoscope. Treatment of iron deficiency anemia causes the postcricoid webs to disappear. Only very rarely is a surgical approach to a web or ring necessary.

DIVERTICULA OF THE ESOPHAGUS. Zenker's diverticulum of the pharynx is not anatomically an esophageal diverticulum, as its neck is above the upper esophageal sphincter muscle, but custom has dictated its inclusion in description of esophageal diverticula. An epiphrenic diverticulum usually occurs on the right side of the esophagus just above the lower esophageal sphincter. Other diverticula are at the level of the carina and are known as traction diverticula, although traction by scar tissue is rarely demonstrated. Scleroderma is occasionally associated with numerous wide-mouthed diverticula scattered along the length of the esophagus. Large-amplitude motor waves have been associated with midbody diverticula and either achalasia or motor incoordination with epiphrenic diverticula.

Symptoms vary widely; many diverticula are found by accident during barium examination of the esophagus. If a patient with dysphagia is found to have a diverticulum, it is difficult to tell whether the diverticulum or the associated motor disorder is the cause. Zenker's diverticulum often has a classic symptom complex, particularly when it becomes large. It retains saliva and food particles, which may either be aspirated or cause repeated postprandial throat clearing with production of liquid and food particles. Patients with this type of diverticulum can often press on the neck and empty the diverticulum. The pouch can become so large that it can compress the esophagus anteriorly and obstruct it. In the presence of diverticula great caution must be exercised in passing tubes into the esophagus or stomach. Zenker's diverticulum is a special problem, since tubes naturally enter it rather than the esophageal opening, and the risk of perforation into the mediastinum is great. Traction and epiphrenic diverticula do not require treatment. Zenker's diverticulum, if large, may require diverticulectomy or diverticulopexy with coincident section of the cricopharyngeus muscle. Most techniques for diverticulectomy automatically accomplish cricopharyngeal section at the same time. If the diverticulum is small, it may regress after section of the cricopharyngeus.

INFECTIONS OF THE ESOPHAGUS. Two major infections involve the esophagus: *Candida* and *herpesvirus* infections. Although both are most common in immunocompromised hosts, such as those on steroids undergoing cancer chemotherapy or those afflicted with AIDS, either or both can invade apparently healthy hosts. Both can be found incidentally at autopsy or during endoscopy for other indications. Most commonly, infection of the mucosa leads to odynophagia of rather marked degree. Dysphagia for both solids and liquids usually accompanies the odynophagia and can be of such intensity that weight loss is rapid. Herpes esophagitis may present with hematemesis.

Although the radiograph occasionally reveals a shaggy mucosa in the case of monilial involvement, and occasionally even a stricture, endoscopy is the best method of detecting and confirming infectious involvement. *Candida* can present as isolated white plaques, which can be confused with glycogenic acanthosis, or progress to form confluent ulcerations with an overlying membrane. Herpesvirus tends to produce isolated ulcers, but extensive involvement can produce confluent ulcerations. Biopsy of the ulcerated area usually shows either invasive hyphae of *Candida* or characteristic nuclear changes of the squamous cells when herpesvirus is present. Cytologic washings occasionally demonstrate the same change.

Treatment depends on correct identification of the etiologic agent. For *Candida* infection, an assessment of the degree of severity is needed. For mild noninvasive disease, topical therapy with 250,000 units of nystatin (Mycostatin) every 2 hours suffices. For more serious infections, low-dose intravenous amphotericin therapy has been successful, the dose being individualized on the basis of weight and renal status. Treatment with miconazole and ketoconazole appears promising. For severe esophageal infections, ketoconazole should be given in doses of 200 mg to 400 mg per day for 8 to 10 days. Herpesvirus infection is treated with acyclovir.

ESOPHAGEAL INJURIES. Caustic Ingestion. Caustic burns of the esophagus occur in children by accident; adults usually suffer such burns because of suicide attempts. Lye crystals, and especially liquid lye preparations for drain cleaning, are the most common cause. The speed of lye injury is so great that attempts to neutralize the caustic are futile. Detergents and Clorox also find their way into the esophageal lumens of both children and adults. The history is all important, but the degree of esophageal injury still must be assessed endoscopically as an emergency. Significant esophageal damage has been seen even without oral burns; conversely, oral burns do not necessarily mean that the material has reached the esophagus. If there is no esophageal reaction after apparent caustic ingestion, further care directed toward the esophagus will not be necessary.

The accepted therapy of a definite lye or caustic burn remains unsupported by clinical trials. For burns with solid lye or other solid agents, steroids have been recommended, at an initial dose of 80 mg per day, tapering to 20 mg per day until esophageal healing. Most clinicians also use broad-spectrum antibiotics. If liquid lye has been the damaging agent, serious consideration of emergency esophagogastrectomy is in order, as lesser measures have met with unacceptably high mortality.

Damage by Medication. A new form of iatrogenic illness of the esophagus has recently become evident. Ingested pills tend to lodge in the esophagus and damage the mucosa in a localized area. Tetracycline, doxycycline, ascorbic acid, and quinidine have all been indicted, and the list will undoubtedly grow. Normal individuals can retain small capsules in the esophagus, even when swallowing in the upright position. The clinical syndrome consists of steady burning or chest pain, accompanied by local odynophagia, all occurring 4 to 6 hours after ingestion of one of the offending capsules or tablets. Endoscopy usually shows a localized mucosal ulcer, which heals without a scar or may lead to a stricture requiring dilation. Symptomatic therapy is adequate, but prophylaxis seems to be a more practical idea. Pills of the offending class should be taken in the upright position with several swallows of water.

Esophageal Trauma. The esophagus is well protected by the thoracic cage but can be involved either by blunt trauma (automobile accidents) or by penetrating missiles (gunshots, knives). Often the surgeon's attention is directed toward more life-threatening damage to heart, lungs, or major blood vessels, and it is understandable that a rent in the esophagus may thus be overlooked. This unfortunate oversight, however, is followed by mediastinitis, which may worsen an already grave situation. Iatrogenic perforation with endoscope, dilator, or, very rarely, nasogastric tube leads to a similar complication.

Vomiting itself can cause esophageal injury, either mucosal (*Mallory-Weiss*) or through-and-through rupture (*Boerhaave's syndrome*). The mucosal lesion first described by Mallory and Weiss has been recognized much more frequently since the advent of rapid emergency endoscopy with fiberoptic endoscopes. Classically, the patient has repeated attacks of retching, productive at first of gastric contents and later of bright red blood. One quarter of patients shown to have a Mallory-Weiss tear have no prior history of vomiting. The tear is usually in the gastric mucosa just below the gastroesophageal junction, although it can extend through the junction and up into the esophageal mucosa. Diagnosis of this condition is almost always made at endoscopy; the

rent is usually seen as the endoscope is being withdrawn from the stomach into the esophagus. The majority of such lesions heal with conservative therapy. Angiographic or surgical therapy is necessary in less than 5 per cent. Bleeding has been stopped by direct application of electrocoagulation through the endoscope.

Vomiting can also cause a complete tear in the esophageal wall. Unlike the Mallory-Weiss lesion, the tear in Boerhaave's syndrome is located above the gastroesophageal junction on the left side. It usually follows vomiting, but other marked increases in intra-abdominal pressure such as lifting a heavy weight or straining at stool have been associated with a tear. The clinical diagnosis can be extremely difficult; often patients with esophageal rupture are thought to have a myocardial infarct, pneumothorax, a perforated viscus, or pancreatitis. Air in the mediastinum or the rapid appearance of a hydrothorax on the left usually leads to the correct diagnosis.

The diagnosis of esophageal perforation can usually be established by a cautious radiographic examination with water-soluble material. Barium may be used only if a rent is not demonstrated by the water-soluble agent. Immediate surgical repair is the accepted method of treatment of esophageal perforation. In those too ill for surgery, treatment consists of nasogastric suction, antibiotics, and subsequent mediastinal drainage if necessary.

Pope CE II, McDonald GB: Rings and webs; Diverticula; Involvement of the esophagus by infections, systemic illnesses, and physical agents. *In* Sleisenger MH, Fordtran JS (eds.): Gastrointestinal Disease. 4th ed. Philadelphia, W. B. Saunders Company, 1989. *Textbook review of these various conditions.*

97 Gastritis

Andrew H. Soll

Gastritis can be defined by gross appearance, histopathology or clinical presentation, thus defying simple categorization (Table 97–1). The term "gastritis," which implies inflammation, is a misnomer, for some of the entities considered lack appreciable inflammatory change—e.g., erosions due to aspirin or other nonsteroidal anti-inflammatory drugs (NSAID's). The terms "acute" and "chronic" have not been used here to segregate gastritis because these distinctions are rarely useful. The normal gastric mucosa has a remarkable ability to resist acid-peptic injury;

TABLE 97–1. CLASSIFICATION OF "GASTRITIS"

Erosive/hemorrhagic gastric disease
 NSAID-induced gastric damage
 Stress-related mucosal disease (SRMD)
 Alcohol-induced mucosal damage
 Chronic erosive (diffuse varioliform) gastritis
Nonerosive gastritis
 Fundal gland gastritis
  Atrophic gastritis
  Pernicious anemia
 Antral gland gastritis
 Gastritis and *Helicobacter pylori*
 Postoperative alkaline gastritis
Unusual or specific forms of gastritis
 Infectious gastritis
  Phlegmonous gastritis
  Syphilis, tuberculosis, anisakiasis
  Infections in immunocompromised host
   Viral (CMV, herpes)
   Fungal (*Candida*, histoplasmosis)
   Tuberculosis, syphilis
 Gastric ischemia
 Radiation-induced gastritis
 Ingestion of corrosive substances
 Ménétrier's disease (giant hypertrophic gastritis)
 Eosinophilic gastritis
 Granulomatous gastritis
 Vascular ectasia
  Watermelon stomach (antral vascular ectasia)
  Other vascular anomalies

TABLE 97–2. MECHANISMS IN MUCOSAL DEFENSE

97 GASTRITIS / 649

Pre-epithelial mechanisms
  Mucus secretion/layer
  Bicarbonate output
Cellular mechanisms
  Apical membrane barrier to acid backdiffusion
  Cellular disposal of acid load
  Cellular defense against injury
  Restitution (resealing of injury areas of epithelium)
  Cellular replication
Post-epithelial mechanisms
  Blood flow
  Mesenchymal and inflammatory cells

The mucous layer creates a physical barrier to pepsin diffusion and stabilizes a pH gradient generated by bicarbonate output. The apical surface of mucosal cells resists acid backdiffusion, and cells are capable of disposing of an acid load. Intrinsic cellular mechanisms resist some forms of injury, but are poorly understood. Epithelial cells rapidly move across intact basement membrane to seal defects in the epithelium. Epithelial cells rapidly regenerate to replenish sloughed daughter cells. Blood flow is critical to maintaining mucosal integrity, proving nutrients and removing backdiffused acid. Lastly, mesenchymal cells and macrophages contribute to the critical wound-healing process.

several components mediate its defense (Table 97–2 and see Fig. 98–4). Efforts to establish the key element have not been successful, probably because the mechanisms are multiple, thus providing important redundant lines of defense.

CLINICAL PERSPECTIVES. Gastritis is often blamed for chronic abdominal pain, but the link between symptoms and gastritis is poorly established. For example, NSAID's produce both gastric damage and symptoms, yet neither is predictive of the other. In patients who have dyspeptic symptoms not linked to macroscopic ulcers, i.e., "nonulcer dyspepsia," it is helpful to distinguish those patients with postprandial indigestion, fullness, belching, bloating, nausea, early satiety, epigastric pain, and fatty food intolerance. This symptom complex is often indicative of *gastroparesis*, a diagnosis that can be confirmed with a nuclide gastric emptying study. This entity is frequently idiopathic but may be associated with diabetes, drug ingestion, or connective tissue diseases. An association between nonerosive gastritis and gastroparesis has been hypothesized, although not firmly established. Chronic abdominal pain is occasionally associated with back, chest, and abdominal wall musculoskeletal symptoms and can be reproduced by pressure on a paraspinous trigger point. This suggests the presence of a "back-gut" syndrome; an exhaustive workup can often be avoided, particularly if symptoms are relieved with a trial of local therapy (trigger point injection with lidocaine or physical therapy). Caution is necessary, since visceral pathology may trigger secondary musculoskeletal symptoms.

DIAGNOSIS. The diagnosis of gastritis may be suspected by a careful history, e.g., the prior ingestion of NSAID's or alcohol. Although barium radiographs may be suggestive, endoscopy coupled with the history is much more likely to establish a diagnosis by providing characteristic macroscopic or biopsy findings.

EROSIVE/HEMORRHAGIC GASTRIC DISEASE

NSAID-INDUCED GASTRIC DAMAGE. NSAID use is associated with petechiae, erosions, and ulcers in the gastric mucosa. In contrast to non-NSAID ulcers, however, only about half of NSAID-associated gastric ulcers occur in a surrounding area of diffuse gastritis. In these latter individuals, *Helicobacter pylori*, a putative factor in nonerosive gastritis, is also found, leaving no reason to implicate NSAID's as a causative factor for the gastritis. Thus, neither acute nor chronic inflammation is a major part of the spectrum of NSAID-induced gastroduodenal damage. Petechiae due to bleeding into the mucosa are frequent but of little clinical significance. Erosions, unlike ulcers, are superficial breaks that do not extend deeper than the mucosa itself and therefore do not cause perforation or severe bleeding. Superficial gastric lesions from NSAID ingestion may occasionally lead to iron deficiency anemia from chronic blood loss or to an acute upper gastrointestinal hemorrhage from a severe erosive process. Gastric erosions are often blamed for occult blood in the stool of patients taking NSAID's, but a thorough workup is appropriate. The incidence of other lesions (e.g., colonic polyps)

is the same in such patients as in those with occult blood in their stool who are not taking NSAID's.

STRESS-RELATED MUCOSAL DISEASE (SRMD). SRMD occurs during severe illness, most frequently in the intensive care unit setting, as a function of the severity of the underlying acute medical or surgical illness (e.g., respiratory or renal failure, sepsis, hypotension, trauma, or the postsurgical state). Mucosal lesions also occur in patients with severe burns (Curling's ulcers) and with central nervous system disease, trauma, or surgery (Cushing's ulcers). The etiology is multifactorial, resulting from a compromise in mucosal blood flow or in other elements of mucosal defense in the presence of acid/peptic activity in gastric juice (Table 97–2). The lesions are diffuse, superficial breaks in the acid-secreting mucosa. Bleeding, generally a slow ooze, may become severe because of the widespread mucosal involvement. Cushing's ulcers tend to be deeper and occasionally perforate, possibly reflecting the acid hypersecretion that can occur with central nervous system lesions. Lesions begin rapidly; for example, erosive changes can be found in the majority of patients examined endoscopically immediately after completion of open heart surgery. About 10 to 20 per cent of ICU patients develop gastric bleeding; the risk increases with severity of the underlying illness. Once bleeding has started, the mortality rate of the underlying condition doubles or triples.

Diagnosis. Gastrointestinal bleeding in the ICU setting requires accurate diagnosis; the initial step entails determining if bleeding is from an upper gastrointestinal source (Ch. 111). Melena may occur with right-sided colonic bleeding and hematochezia may occur with brisk upper gastrointestinal bleeding. Blood may be absent from the nasogastric aspirate if bleeding is intermittent or from a duodenal source. The consistent finding of bile without blood in the nasogastric aspirate argues for a bleeding site distal to the ligament of Treitz. If the nasogastric aspirate is bloody, it is worth determining how rapidly this blood clears with lavage and gravity drainage (suction aspiration may induce artifacts endoscopically indistinguishable from acute erosions). The only practical method for diagnosis is endoscopy. In the decision to do endoscopy the potential benefits of making a specific diagnosis must be weighed against the risks of endoscopy (premedication, respiratory and circulatory compromise, and possible bleeding or perforation). Any patient who has begun to bleed deserves aggressive medical management (see below), with endoscopy reserved for those patients in whom bleeding is brisk enough to warrant consideration of additional measures. Endoscopy can reveal a discrete ulcer or a focal lesion other than SRMD, which may respond to specific therapy.

Treatment and Prevention. Medical, endoscopic, and surgical treatment of bleeding due to SRMD all yield discouraging results, so prevention is of particular importance. Patients sick enough to be at risk deserve prophylaxis. Since gastric ischemia is a likely causative factor in SRMD, efforts to improve volume status, cardiac output, and respiratory function are critical to both treatment and prevention. The incidence of bleeding is generally decreased if the gastric pH is maintained above 3.5, a pH level above which pepsin activity is markedly reduced. An antacid drip or hourly antacids (15 to 30 ml) via a nasogastric tube can neutralize the gastric lumen. H_2 blockers are approved for intravenous use; slow bolus infusion is effective in increasing gastric pH (cimetidine 300 mg every 8 hours; ranitidine 50 mg every 12 hours; famotidine 20 mg every 12 hours). Continuous infusion may provide smoother control of pH; for example, an infusion of cimetidine (300 mg priming dose, 37.5 mg per hour) produces effective gastric neutralization. Omeprazole, the H^+-K^+-ATPase inhibitor, is likely to be effective for preventing SRMD, but it is not yet approved by the Food and Drug Administration for parenteral use, nor has efficacy for this indication been established. Sucralfate is also effective in reducing bleeding due to SRMD; nasogastric administration is required (1 gram every 6 hours).

ALCOHOL AND MUCOSAL DAMAGE. Characteristic subepithelial hemorrhages, with the endoscopic appearance of "blood under a plastic wrap," are commonly found in individuals abusing alcohol. Although termed "hemorrhagic gastritis," these lesions are composed of hemorrhage and edema in the interstitial space under the surface epithelium, without inflammation. Usually the bleeding is mild. If more severe bleeding is found, associated lesions, such as portal hypertension, peptic ulcer, or a Mallory-Weiss tear, should be sought (Ch. 98).

CHRONIC EROSIVE (DIFFUSE VARIOLIFORM) GASTRITIS. This entity, of unknown pathogenesis, which consists of erosive changes usually involving the antrum, can be diagnosed only in the absence of the use or abuse of NSAID and/or alcohol. Symptoms are nonspecific and include abdominal pain, nausea, vomiting, anorexia, weight loss, and sometimes bleeding. Occasionally isolated antral erosions are found without symptoms or progression to other entities.

NONEROSIVE GASTRITIS

CLASSIFICATION. Nonerosive gastritis refers to inflammatory change in a mucosa that is often grossly normal, and lacks, as the name implies, erosive changes. Nonerosive gastritis can be classified by whether the fundus (type A) or antrum (type B) is primarily involved and by whether the inflammation is superficial (involving the foveolar or gastric pit region and upper portion of the lamina propria), deep (involving the gastric glands that contain parietal and chief cells), or atrophic (with decreased or absent glandular elements and mucosal thinning). The term "active" reflects infiltration by polymorphonuclear leukocytes. Once glandular atrophy develops, the inflammatory infiltrate may be minimal. Other important features are intestinal and pseudopyloric metaplasia and dysplastic epithelial changes. With intestinal metaplasia, gastric mucosal cells may be replaced by typical goblet cells and absorptive cells; rudimentary intestinal villi may form. With pseudopyloric metaplasia the parietal and chief cells of fundic glands are replaced by mucous glands indistinguishable from normal antral glands. Fundal and antral gland gastritis constitute two distinct forms of nonerosive gastritis.

With *fundal or type A gastritis*, the inflammatory changes are usually maximal along the greater curvature in the fundus and body. Characteristic parietal cell antibodies occur in most patients, and pernicious anemia may develop (Ch. 132). Inflammatory change is usually much less marked in the antrum than in the fundus. Hyposecretion of acid occurs as a function of fundal glandular atrophy; the relative absence of glandular atrophy in the antrum accounts for the ability of many of these patients to develop marked hypergastrinemia as the feedback inhibition of acid on gastrin release is lost. Fundal gastritis and a decrease in maximal acid secretion may be a normal concomitant of aging, but only a small proportion of affected individuals go on to develop pernicious anemia.

Antral or type B gastritis has several features distinguishing it from fundal gastritis, including the predominance of antral inflammatory change, a lack of progression to atrophic gastritis, and an association with both peptic ulcer and *H. pylori.*

ETIOLOGY AND ASSOCIATIONS. The cause(s) of chronic gastritis remains unknown. Factors hypothesized to cause or exacerbate gastritis include chronic trauma, gastric bacteria, toxins, and thermal insult. A role for reflux of duodenal juice, containing bile and pancreatic enzymes, has been postulated but without supporting data. Lysolecithin, formed by the action of the pancreatic enzyme phospholipase A on biliary lecithin, can be refluxed from the duodenum. The detergent action of lysolecithin may disrupt the surface epithelial barrier to acid backdiffusion, thus creating a chronic insult that could provoke an inflammatory response. Chronic infection with *H. pylori,* as discussed below, is a leading candidate for causing nonerosive antral gastritis; the association with fundal gastritis is less well founded. Multiple factors probably interact in the pathogenesis of nonerosive gastritis; for example, the inflammatory infiltrate induced by *H. pylori* may disrupt normal mucosal architecture, thus interfering with mucosal resistance to acid/peptic injury and to refluxed bile. End-stage gastric atrophy may be accompanied by an intact surface epithelium and little inflammatory infiltrate, possibly because with achlorhydria the acid-peptic exacerbation of the inflammatory response is removed.

Pernicious anemia (Ch. 132) is on the end of the spectrum of fundal gastritis, although fundal gastritis may not reflect only a single disease mechanism. Despite histamine-fast achlorhydria, some patchy nests of parietal and chief cells may still be found.

Hypergastrinemia is present in about three fourths of patients with pernicious anemia. The absence of hypergastrinemia in achlorhydric patients suggests extensive antral gastritis.

Immunologic mechanisms appear to be operative in fundal, but not antral, gastritis. About 90 per cent of patients with pernicious anemia (fundal gastritis) have antibodies against parietal cells, which appear to react with the parietal cell H^+-K^+-ATPase. Antibodies reacting with intrinsic factor also occur, and such antibodies may block the vitamin B_{12} binding site. Whether these antibodies mediate immunologic damage or simply reflect a secondary reaction is unclear. Sera from patients with pernicious anemia contain an antibody reported to be cytotoxic to canine gastric mucosal cells. Pernicious anemia is also associated with other diseases in which immunologic mechanisms appear operative, such as Hashimoto's thyroiditis, hypothyroidism, hyperthyroidism, insulin-dependent diabetes mellitus, and vitiligo.

Genetic factors are important in pernicious anemia; family members of patients have an increased incidence of atrophic gastritis, achlorhydria, vitamin B_{12} malabsorption, and antibodies to parietal cells and intrinsic factor. There are no data regarding genetic factors in gastritis without pernicious anemia.

CLINICAL PRESENTATION. Nonerosive gastritis is frequently found in asymptomatic individuals; blaming this entity for dyspeptic symptoms is not justified. Despite this disclaimer, it has been hypothesized that altered motility resulting in symptomatic gastroparesis may be associated with nonerosive gastritis. An association between reflux esophagitis and altered esophageal motility (esophageal spasm) is well recognized. If symptoms suggestive of gastroparesis are elicited, a gastric emptying study should be performed. If gastric emptying is delayed, endoscopy is necessary to exclude a mechanical gastric outlet obstruction. Patients with pernicious anemia may develop symptoms secondary to vitamin B_{12} deficiency (Ch. 132). Macroscopic endoscopic findings (erythema, petechiae, nodularity, pallor, and atrophy) are generally nonspecific. Diagnosis requires biopsy, and multiple biopsies may be required, since the histopathology may be patchy. The ratio of pepsinogen I (present in fundic chief cells) to pepsinogen II (present in both chief cells and surface epithelial cells) falls with the degree of glandular atrophy.

NATURAL HISTORY OF GASTRITIS. About half of "normal" subjects over 50 years of age are thought to have superficial gastritis, which can progress to an atrophic pattern over the subsequent 10 to 20 years.

Enterochromaffin-like cells may undergo hyperplasia in atrophic gastritis, as in the Zollinger-Ellison syndrome (Ch. 98). It is probable that the severe and sustained hypergastrinemia found in these conditions has a trophic effect on enterochromaffin-like (ECL) cells, a population of endocrine cells identified by characteristic granules and silver staining properties. Carcinoid tumors composed of ECL cells have been described in atrophic gastritis and in the Zollinger-Ellison syndrome, the latter primarily in association with multiple endocrine neoplasia (MEN) type I. ECL cells do not contain serotonin, and thus these tumors do not produce the carcinoid syndrome found with tumors composed of serotonin-containing enterochromaffin (EC) cells (Ch. 230). Gastric carcinoids occurring without hypergastrinemia are solitary, aggressive tumors, whereas carcinoids associated with hypergastrinemia and ECL cell hyperplasia are generally indolent and multifocal. Antrectomy coupled with local excision deserves consideration as an alternative to total gastrectomy in atrophic gastritis with carcinoid tumor formation, since achlorhydria-induced hypergastrinemia exerts a trophic effect on these ECL tumors. This situation provides a logical indication for a gastrin receptor antagonist, when one becomes available for clinical use.

Gastric adenocarcinomas have been reported to occur with increased frequency with atrophic gastritis, but the assessment of increased risk is variable, ranging from nil to threefold in different series (Ch. 99).

TREATMENT. No specific therapy exists for fundal gastritis. Replacement of vitamin B_{12} is, of course, indicated in pernicious anemia. Delayed gastric emptying can be treated with the prokinetic agent metoclopramide (5 to 20 mg, 1 hour before meals and at bedtime). The liquid preparation (5 mg per milliliter) is generally more effective, since gastric emptying of tablets is also delayed. Parenteral administration may also be of benefit, particularly during the first few days of therapy. Metoclopramide has a high incidence of central nervous system side effects. Its use should be restricted to instances in which therapy is clearly warranted and effective and patients should be monitored closely for these side effects.

It is reasonable to evaluate family members of patients with pernicious anemia for gastritis and vitamin B_{12} deficiency. Some advocate performing endoscopy at the time of an initial diagnosis of pernicious anemia, obtaining sufficient antral and fundal biopsies to assess the severity of intestinal metaplasia and epithelial dysplasia. Although imperfect, these findings are the best indicators of the cancer risk. Using this approach, only those patients with severe dysplasia would warrant close follow-up and/or surgical intervention.

GASTRITIS AND *Helicobacter pylori*. *H. pylori*, a gramnegative microaerophilic organism, may be the most common worldwide human infective agent. No reservoir other than the human stomach has been identified and the epidemiology is unknown. The organism is fastidious but can be cultured with careful technique. *H. pylori* can be identified as a bent or spiral rod on specific silver stains (Warthin-Starry or Giemsa) or by careful examination of routine hematoxylin and eosin–stained sections. Serology sensitively detects antibodies to *H. pylori*. The organism has a very high urease activity, which allows identification in biopsies by a rapid test or in vivo by using a breath test for $^{13}CO_2$ following an oral ^{13}C-urea load. *H. pylori* is found embedded in the mucous layer and tends to cluster over intracellular junctions. *H. pylori* is found in nearly all biopsies showing active antral gastritis with polymorphonuclear infiltration, whereas the organism is unusual in the histologically normal stomach (Table 97–3). Since it is unethical to experimentally administer an organism that may cause disease and may be difficult to eradicate, studies of causality must be indirect. Two investigators have self-administered *H. pylori*, however, with subsequent development of acute superficial gastritis associated with epigastric pain, nausea, and vomiting. Thus, it appears that *H. pylori* can induce a form of acute, superficial gastritis. Additional evidence that *H. pylori* causes active gastritis is that eradication of the organism reduces active inflammation, which remains unchanged following similar treatment without its eradication. It is possible, of course, that the gastritis comes first, creating an environment suited for colonization with *H. pylori*. Although *H. pylori* and antral gastritis are clearly associated, no such association has been shown between *H. pylori* and fundal gastritis, gastric atrophy, or gastric cancer.

Although *H. pylori* is clearly associated with antral gastritis, no clinical benefit has been established to result from eradication of this organism. The organism is difficult to treat; delayed recurrences with the same strain are frequent, and thus multiple antibiotic regimens, usually including colloidal bismuth and metronidazole, have been evaluated. Since there are other effective modalities for ulcer healing, therapy directed at the eradication of *H. pylori* should await demonstration of beneficial effects on the natural history of gastritis or peptic ulcer disease.

Two "epidemics" of acute, superficial gastritis, have been reported. Despite the absence of glandular gastritis and the presence of histologically robust parietal cells, acid secretion was markedly reduced, suggesting release of a factor inhibiting acid secretion. These epidemics occurred before recognition of *H. pylori*, but retrospective analysis revealed histology and serology consistent with *H. pylori* infection.

GASTRITIS ASSOCIATED WITH PEPTIC ULCER. Antral

TABLE 97–3. ANTRAL GASTRITIS AND *H. PYLORI*

		Antral Gastritis	
		+	−
H. pylori Status	+	233	5
	−	2	87

Normal subjects and individuals with duodenal and gastric ulcer or with ulcer-negative dyspepsia underwent endoscopic biopsy, which was then graded for active antral gastritis. *H. pylori* status was also ascertained using culture. Note the very tight association between the presence of *H. pylori* and antral gastritis. (Data from Rauws EAJ, Lagenberg W, Houthoff HJ, et al.: *Campylobacter pyloridis*–associated chronic active gastritis. A prospective study of its prevalence and the effects of antibacterial and antiulcer treatment. Gastroenterology 94:33, 1988.)

gastritis has been associated with both gastric and duodenal ulcer. Some of the differences between gastric and duodenal ulcer may be explained by the patterns of the associated gastritis. In patients with ulcers, antral gastritis is not age-related, in contrast to normal subjects. The fundic mucosa in patients with duodenal ulcer is usually robust and "juvenile" (they generally secrete more acid than normals) and lacks the development of the fundal gastritis that is often seen with aging. Patients with gastric ulcer, in contrast to duodenal ulcer, tend to have more severe antral gastritis. Mild to moderate superficial fundal gland gastritis is also more common with gastric than with duodenal ulcer. There is a close association between antral gastritis, peptic ulcer, and *H. pylori*; the causal nature of these interactions will remain controversial until properly designed, controlled trials firmly establish that the presence or absence of the bacterium alters that natural history of the gastritis and ulcer disease.

POSTOPERATIVE ALKALINE GASTRITIS. Macroscopic gastritis with a dramatic red color may rapidly develop after gastric resection or pyloroplasty, but this endoscopic appearance does not correlate with symptoms, bile reflux, or histologic inflammation. The occurrence of this difficult-to-treat complication of surgery for peptic ulcer is another indication to do the least physiologically disruptive operation (i.e., highly selective vagotomy), when possible.

UNUSUAL OR SPECIFIC FORMS OF GASTRITIS

PHLEGMONOUS GASTRITIS. This is a rarely encountered, purulent process involving the gastric submucosa and wall. Streptococci, but also staphylococci, *E. coli*, and *Proteus*, have been implicated. The course is fulminant and medical management is ineffective, leaving surgery as a drastic, but unavoidable, last resort.

OTHER INFECTIONS. As with infections in all other sites, the spectrum of gastric infections is expanded and altered in the immunocompromised host. Gastric tuberculosis, diagnosed by finding caseating granulomas and positive cultures, occurs in AIDS. Secondary syphilis may involve the stomach with thickened folds and erosions. Despite the frequency of esophageal candidiasis, gastric ulcers appear to be only colonized by these organisms. Mycelia may occur at the ulcer margin, but antifungal therapy does not alter ulcer healing, suggesting a lack of clinical importance. Cytomegalovirus can involve the stomach in the immunocompromized host. The ascaris-like larva, *Anisakis*, present in raw fish, may infect the normal gastric mucosa, producing pain and dyspepsia. *Strongyloides stercoralis* involves the small intestine much more frequently than the stomach and can cause dyspepsia. The diagnosis is made by examining duodenal aspirates or stool specimens.

GASTRIC ISCHEMIA. Ischemic gastric injury is rarely recognized, although erosive changes have been reported with vasculitis and atheromatous embolization. Whether chronic gastric ulcers have an ischemic component remains speculative.

MÉNÉTRIER'S DISEASE. Ménétrier's disease (giant hypertrophic gastritis) is a specific entity of unknown etiology characterized by the triad of giant folds, in the fundus and body of the stomach, hypoalbuminemia secondary to a protein-losing gastropathy, and the histologic features of foveolar (gastric pit region) hyperplasia with gland atrophy, cystic dilation, and increased mucosal thickness. Tortuous gastric folds may resemble the cerebral cortex. Hypochlorhydria is generally present, but a hypersecretory variant has been described. Symptoms are variable and may include abdominal pain, nausea, vomiting, weight loss, and edema. The disease is more common in men than in women, generally presenting after age 50, although a childhood form exists. Large folds, especially involving the greater curvature of the gastric body, are found on radiography. Typical biopsies can confirm the diagnosis, but variant patterns warrant the less specific diagnosis of idiopathic hypertrophic gastropathy. The differential diagnosis includes gastrinoma syndrome, infiltrating carcinoma, lymphoma, and amyloidosis. Large gastric folds are found without any associated pathology and also have been reported associated with *H. pylori* infection; the relevance of this organism to hypertrophic gastritis remains unclear. Usually no therapy is indicated, but anticholinergics and H_2 blockers may reduce gastric protein loss. Accompanying ulcers and erosions usually respond to standard antiulcer therapy (Ch. 98). No increased risk of cancer has been established.

EOSINOPHILIC GASTRITIS. Eosinophils may infiltrate the gastrointestinal mucosa and muscular layers, especially with antral involvement, in association with peripheral eosinophilia as an idiopathic syndrome. Thickening of gastric mucosal folds and wall rigidity are common. Antral motility may be altered, leading to gastric retention. Patients may present with eosinophilia, nausea, vomiting, or pain. Rarely, serosal involvement results in ascites. Milk-sensitive enteropathy of infancy, connective tissue disorders, and parasitic infections should be ruled out. Glucocorticoid therapy may be useful, and surgery may be needed if mechanical outlet obstruction occurs.

GRANULOMATOUS GASTRITIS. Granulomas in the gastric mucosa may occur in association with generalized diseases such as sarcoidosis, Crohn's disease, or infections. Crohn's disease may involve the duodenum, pylorus, antrum, and gastric body (in that order) in association with disease in the small intestine or colon. Mucosal granulomas may also be incidental findings or occur in eosinophilic granulomas or in isolated, idiopathic granulomatous gastritis. Involved portions of the stomach may be rigid or narrow or have thickened folds on radiographic examination, findings that must be distinguished from malignancy. The antrum is most often involved, and granulomas may occur in all layers of the stomach. Ulcerated lesions may perforate. Patients are often operated upon because of the difficulties in differentiating this entity from malignancy. Once the diagnosis is made, it is important to exclude potentially curable diseases (e.g., tuberculosis, histoplasmosis, syphilis) or treatable processes (e.g., sarcoidosis, Crohn's disease). With malignancy and associated diseases excluded, the patient can be followed, since spontaneous resolution has been reported.

WATERMELON STOMACH. This entity, also known as gastric antral vascular ectasia, represents another nongastric condition. At endoscopy, the antrum has erythematous folds or linear angioid streaks; the convergence of the latter at the pylorus in a pattern reminiscent of a watermelon prompted the naming of this entity. Biopsy can be diagnostic, demonstrating dilated antral vasculature with intravascular fibrin thrombi and fibromuscular hyperplasia. This uncommon lesion can present with either acute gastrointestinal bleeding or with chronic iron deficiency anemia. Corticosteroid therapy has been tried with uncertain success. Antrectomy is effective in eliminating bleeding; however, success has also been reported with repeated coagulation using endoscopic laser or heater probes.

Dooley CP, Cohen H: The clinical significance of *Campylobacter pylori*. Ann Intern Med 108:70, 1988. *Basic review of Helicobacter pylori in relationship to gastrointestinal disease. This field is rapidly changing, so conclusions will be different when new studies are available.*

Laine L, Weinstein WM: Histology of alcoholic hemorrhagic "gastritis": A prospective evaluation. Gastroenterology 94:1254, 1988. *Critical assessment of histopathology of alcohol-related gastric damage.*

Petrini JL Jr., Johnston JH: Heat probe treatment for antral vascular ectasia. Gastrointest Endosc 35:324, 1989. *Description of heat probe therapy for this entity. Provides references for description of the lesion.*

Robert A, Kauffman GL Jr.: Stress ulcers, erosions, and gastric mucosal injury. *In* Sleisenger MH, Fordtran JS (eds.): Gastrointestinal Disease. 4th ed. Philadelphia, W. B. Saunders Company, 1989, pp 772–791. *Good overview of the pathophysiology and therapy of gastric mucosal injury and stress related mucosal damage.*

Soll AH, Kurata JH, Walsh JH: Ulcer epidemiology conference. Gastroenterology 96:561, 1989. *Compendium of articles summarizing the consequences of NSAID-associated ulcers.*

Weinstein WM: Gastritis. *In* Sleisenger MH, Fordtran JS (eds.): Gastrointestinal Disease. 4th ed. Philadelphia, W. B. Saunders Company, 1989, pp 792–813. *Comprehensive summary of the various forms of gastritis.*

98 Peptic Ulcer

98.1 PATHOGENESIS

Charles T. Richardson

DEFINITION

Ulcers are defects in the gastrointestinal mucosa that penetrate the muscularis mucosa. This distinguishes them from superficial erosions, which do not extend through the muscularis mucosa. Peptic ulcers usually occur in the stomach, pylorus, or duodenal bulb but also can develop in the esophagus and the postbulbar duodenum. In patients with markedly increased acid secretion (as in Zollinger-Ellison syndrome) ulcers sometimes develop in the distal duodenum and jejunum. Peptic ulcers occasionally occur in the ileum in or near Meckel's diverticula.

Originally, all ulcers in the upper gastrointestinal tract were believed to be caused by the aggressive action of hydrochloric acid and pepsin on the mucosa. Thus they became known as "peptic ulcers." Although acid and pepsin are secreted by most patients with benign ulcers, they are not the only causes of ulcers. Thus, the term "peptic ulcer" may be a misnomer. Ulcers probably result from several different pathogenetic mechanisms. In general, ulcers occur when luminal aggressive factors overcome opposing mucosal defenses. Mechanisms believed important in the pathogenesis of ulcer disease are discussed in greater detail below.

NORMAL PHYSIOLOGY

STRUCTURE. The stomach is divided into four anatomic regions: the cardia, fundus, body, and antrum (Fig. 98–1). *Parietal cells*, which secrete hydrochloric acid, and *chief cells*, which secrete pepsinogen, are located primarily in the fundus and body, although a few are found in the antrum. *Gastrin (G) cells* are located in the antrum.

Gastric mucosa is made up of a series of pits and glands (Fig. 98–2). The pits contain surface epithelial cells, whereas the glands contain mucous, parietal, endocrine, and chief cells. Normal gastric juice is a mixture of parietal secretion (acid and intrinsic factor) and nonparietal secretions (mucus, bicarbonate, sodium, potassium, and pepsinogen). Pepsinogen is converted to pepsin in the presence of hydrochloric acid.

CONTROL OF GASTRIC SECRETION. Three endogenous chemicals (acetylcholine, gastrin, and histamine) stimulate acid secretion (Fig. 98–3): (1) *Acetylcholine*, believed to be a neural transmitter, is released by vagal efferent neurons. Vagal stimulation of acid secretion occurs when humans see, smell, taste, chew, or think about appetizing food. (2) *Gastrin* is a hormone responsible for acid secretion. Protein in food is the most potent stimulant of gastrin release, but vagal stimulation, calcium, other cations such as magnesium and aluminum, and alkalinization of the antrum also release gastrin. Gastrin release is inhibited by acid within the lumen of the antrum. (3) *Histamine* stimulates acid secretion via a paracrine mechanism. Mastlike cells that contain histamine are located in the lamina propria of the stomach in close proximity to parietal cells. When histamine is liberated from mast cells, it diffuses through intercellular spaces to reach parietal cells. Acetylcholine, gastrin, and histamine are believed to act on receptors on parietal cell membranes to cause acid secretion (see Ch. 98.3, on medical therapy of peptic ulcer disease).

Mechanisms within parietal cells that lead to acid secretion are not well defined. It is believed that cyclic adenosine monophosphate (AMP) is important in the mediation of histamine-stimulated acid secretion, while calcium entry into parietal cells is believed to play a role in gastrin- and acetylcholine-stimulated secretion. A hydrogen/potassium adenosine triphosphatase (ATPase) enzyme is located on the luminal surface of parietal cells (Ch. 98.3). This enzyme serves as a proton pump, which is the final step in secretion of hydrogen ions.

PRODUCTS OF GASTRIC SECRETION. In the pathogenesis of peptic ulcer the two most important products of gastric secretion are hydrochloric acid and pepsin.

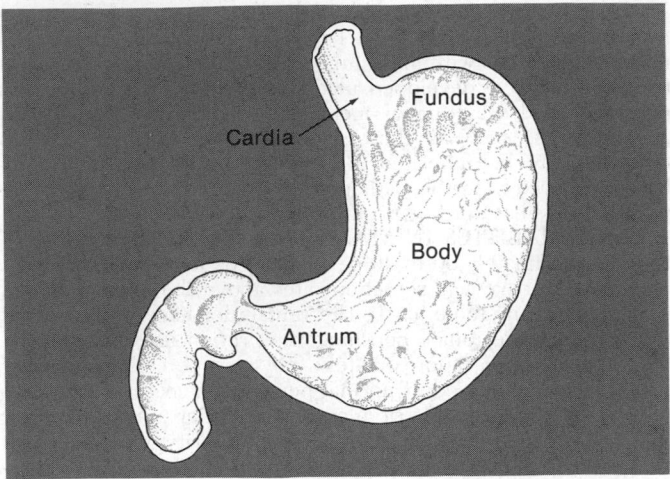

FIGURE 98–1. Anatomic divisions of the stomach.

Secretion of Acid. Basal acid output (BAO) is the amount of acid secreted under fasting or unstimulated conditions. Peak acid output (PAO) or maximum acid output (MAO) is acid secreted in response to an injection of either pentagastrin or histamine, the maximal amount of acid that a normal subject or patient with ulcer disease can secrete. MAO reflects the number of parietal cells in an individual, and the ratio of BAO to MAO represents the fraction of parietal cell mass functioning under basal conditions. Thus, if a patient has an increased amount of gastrin, acetylcholine, or histamine near parietal cells or if there is increased sensitivity of parietal cells to normal amounts of these stimulants, BAO will be increased, as will the BAO/MAO ratio. Such a patient is said to have a basal acid hypersecretory state, such as the Zollinger-Ellison syndrome (see below).

Upper and lower limits of normal acid secretion are shown in Table 98–1. Men usually secrete more acid than do women. This can be explained, in part, by differences in body size, but men secrete more acid than do women even when corrections are made for weight and lean body mass.

Secretion of Pepsin. Pepsin is secreted into the lumen as an inactive precursor, pepsinogen. Pepsinogen secretion usually accompanies acid secretion. Although mechanisms controlling pepsinogen secretion are less well understood, cholinergic stimulation is believed to be a major mediator. Once pepsinogen is secreted into the gastric lumen, it is converted by acid to pepsin,

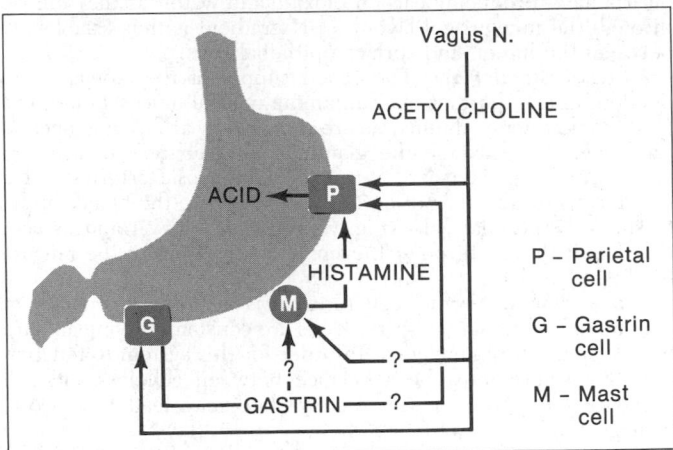

FIGURE 98–3. Model illustrating the chemical stimulants of acid secretion. Acetylcholine originates in the vagus nerves; gastrin is released from gastrin cells in the antrum; and histamine is liberated from mast cells in the lamina propria of the gastric mucosa.

the active enzyme. The optimal pH for conversion of pepsinogen to pepsin ranges between 1.8 and 3.5.

MAINTENANCE OF NORMAL MUCOSAL INTEGRITY. Several mechanisms are believed important in protecting gastric and duodenal mucosa from damage by acid, pepsin, bile, pancreatic enzymes, and other possible aggressive factors. These defensive mechanisms include mucus, bicarbonate, mucosal blood flow, and cell renewal after injury. Endogenous prostaglandins currently are the most likely candidates as mediators to control these defensive mechanisms.

Mucus. This secretory product is a gel that forms a thin, protective coat over superficial mucosal cells (Fig. 98–4). Mucus has several functions: (1) to protect underlying cells from mechanical forces of digestion; (2) to lubricate the mucosa, assisting movement of food over mucosal surfaces; (3) to retain water within the mucous gel and thereby provide an aqueous environment for underlying cells; and (4) to form an unstirred layer impeding, but not blocking, diffusion of hydrogen ions from the lumen to the apical membrane of epithelial cells. Under normal conditions, mucus is constantly being produced but also is being removed continuously by mechanical forces during mixing and grinding of food and by pepsin, which degrades mucus into soluble glycoprotein subunits. However, secretion and degradation of mucus remain in equilibrium under normal conditions.

Bicarbonate. This is secreted by surface epithelial cells in the stomach and duodenum and also by Brunner's glands in the duodenum. Although some bicarbonate reaches the lumen, much of the secreted bicarbonate remains below or within the mucous layer (Fig. 98–4). Thus, the mucosal surface is in contact with fluid that contains a high pH relative to the lumen of the stomach. Under normal conditions, hydrogen ions are neutralized by

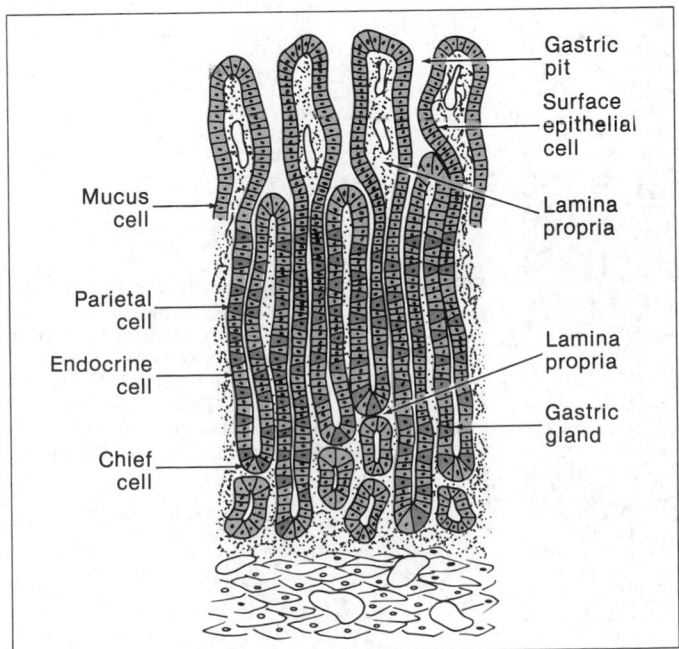

FIGURE 98–2. Diagram demonstrating the cell types lining the pits and glands of the gastric mucosa.

TABLE 98–1. UPPER (ULN) AND LOWER (LLN) LIMITS OF NORMAL ACID SECRETION IN HEALTHY MEN AND WOMEN

	Acid Output (mmol/hr)*			
	Basal	Peak	Maximum	Basal/Maximum
Men (N = 172)				
ULN	10.5	60.6	47.7	0.31
LLN	0	11.6	9.3	0
Women (N = 76)				
ULN	5.6	40.1	31.2	0.29
LLN	0	8.0	5.6	0

*Acid output (volume of gastric juice times concentration of acid) is measured in 15-minute intervals and is expressed in mmol/hr. Basal acid output is the sum of acid secreted during four 15-minute periods. Peak acid output is the sum of the highest two 15-minute periods after pentagastrin or histamine stimulation multiplied by two. Maximum acid output is the sum of four 15-minute intervals after pentagastrin or histamine stimulation.

bicarbonate (producing carbon dioxide and water) as they diffuse through the mucous gel layer. A pH gradient is thus established between the lumen and surface epithelial cells.

Mucosal Blood Flow. The blood supply of the stomach and duodenum is important in maintaining normal mucosal integrity. Gastric and duodenal mucosae are supplied by arborizing mucosal capillaries that traverse the glandular area of the stomach and duodenum. An extensive system of submucosal arteries and a submucous plexus of arteries and veins regulate the blood supply to surface epithelial cells (Fig. 98–4). Blood flow removes acid that might diffuse through the mucosa, especially if the mucosa has been damaged.

Cell Renewal. Normal cell renewal is an important factor in maintaining mucosal integrity. Cells are constantly dying and are being replaced by new cells. In order for this system to function normally, there must be a balance between cell loss and cell renewal. Disruption of this steady state may lead to mucosal damage.

Endogenous Prostaglandins. Prostaglandins of the E, F, and I types are found in the gastric and duodenal mucosa. When administered exogenously, prostaglandins stimulate secretion of mucus and bicarbonate, increase mucosal blood flow, and enhance mucosal regeneration after injury. Prostaglandins also may have a trophic effect on the mucosa. Duodenal mucosal prostaglandins appear to stimulate basal duodenal bicarbonate secretion. Exogenously administered prostaglandins protect the mucosa of animals against a variety of noxious agents, including boiling water, ethanol, bile acids, and aspirin, a property termed "cytoprotection." On the basis of such studies of exogenously administered prostaglandins, it is presumed that endogenous prostaglandins also possess cytoprotective properties and that they may help regulate the defensive mechanisms described above.

ABNORMALITIES IN PATIENTS WITH DUODENAL OR GASTRIC ULCERS

GENETIC PREDISPOSITION. Heredity has been postulated to play a role in the pathogenesis of ulcer disease in some patients. Several rare genetic syndromes are associated with peptic ulcer disease. Multiple endocrine neoplasia I syndrome is the most common example (Ch. 228). Additionally, several pathophysiologic abnormalities believed to be associated with increased acid and pepsin secretion or increased gastric emptying have been discovered, and several of these have been found in "ulcer families." For example, in several families an increased level of serum pepsinogen I was inherited as an autosomal dominant trait. Since serum pepsinogen I concentrations reflect chief cell mass and correlate with maximum acid output, members of these families may have developed ulcers because of either increased pepsin or acid secretion or increased secretion of both. Other abnormalities, such as those leading to diminished mucosal defense, may be inherited also. The importance, if any, of hereditary factors in the pathogenesis of peptic ulcer disease in most patients has not been established.

ABNORMALITIES IN SECRETION OF ACID AND PEPSIN. Approximately 30 to 40 per cent of patients with duodenal ulcer disease have acid secretion rates above the upper limits of normal shown in Table 98–1. The remainder have values within the normal range. Since pepsinogen secretion usually accompanies acid secretion, approximately the same percentage of ulcer patients have increased or normal pepsinogen secretion.

Most patients with gastric ulcers have either normal or lower than normal acid secretion rates. Only a minority of patients with gastric ulcer disease (for example, a few patients with Zollinger-Ellison syndrome) have secretion rates above the normal range. The fact that most gastric ulcer patients have normal or lower than normal acid secretory rates does not exclude acid and pepsin as the cause of gastric ulcer disease in an individual patient but suggests that other factors may be involved (see below). This same concept applies to patients with duodenal ulcers who have normal rates of acid secretion. In fact, the role that acid or pepsin or both play in the pathogenesis of either gastric or duodenal ulcers is not known. It is assumed that acid is involved in the pathogenesis of ulcer disease in patients with higher than normal rates of acid secretion (see below). It is also assumed that pepsin is an essential factor in acid-mediated ulcer disease.

Three mechanisms for increased basal acid secretion are known: (1) increased stimulation by *gastrin* (Zollinger-Ellison syndrome, retained antrum syndrome, and antral gastrin [G] cell hyperplasia or hyperfunction); (2) increased stimulation by *acetylcholine* (vagal hyperfunction); and (3) increased *histamine* stimulation (systemic mastocytosis or basophilic leukemia). Other causes of basal hypersecretion may exist, but so far they have not been described. Ulcers presumably occur in patients with these disorders because of increased levels of acid and pepsin. All of the currently recognized syndromes causing increased basal acid secretion are rare. Of the group Zollinger-Ellison syndrome is the most common and will be discussed separately (see Ch. 98.6).

REFLUX OF BILE AND PANCREATIC JUICE. Bile acids, lysolecithin, and pancreatic enzymes are believed to be aggressive factors that lead to ulceration in some patients, especially some

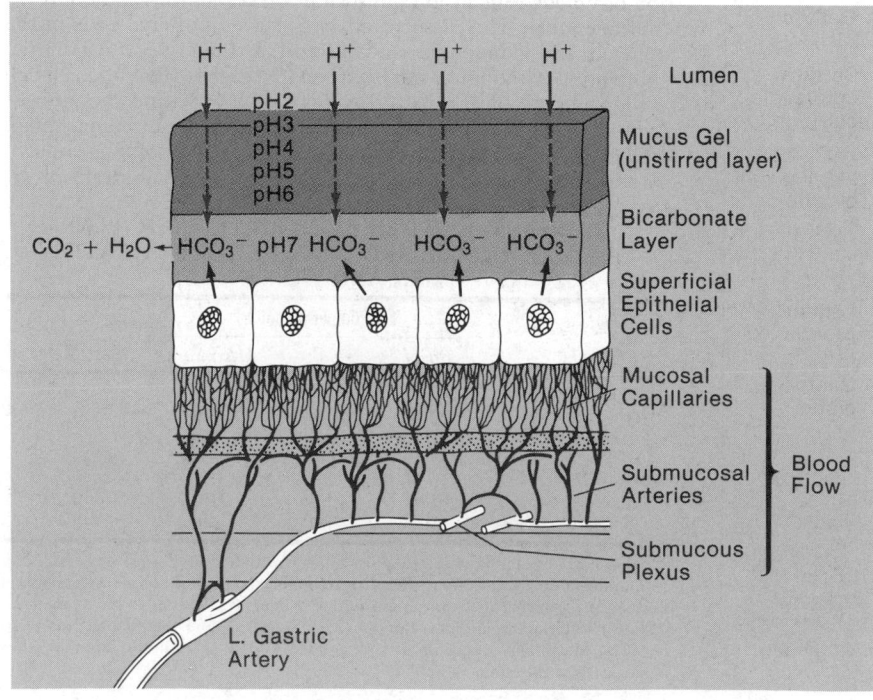

FIGURE 98–4. Model illustrating mechanisms maintaining mucosal integrity. Superficial epithelial cells secrete mucus and bicarbonate, which aid in maintaining a pH gradient between lumen and mucosa and protect the underlying epithelial cells from damage by acid and pepsin. Epithelial cell renewal and mucosal blood flow also are believed to be important mechanisms in maintaining mucosal integrity.

of those with gastric ulcers. It has been postulated that duodenal contents reflux into the stomach causing gastritis that, in turn, predisposes to gastric ulceration. Some patients with gastric ulcers may have an incompetent pyloric sphincter that allows reflux of bile or pancreatic enzymes or both into the stomach.

Two mechanisms have been proposed whereby bile and pancreatic juice may damage gastric mucosa: first, alteration of mucus overlying surface epithelial cells, reducing its protective effect; and second, damage to the so-called gastric mucosal barrier (the ability of the stomach to maintain electrical and hydrogen ion concentration gradients between lumen and blood). When these protective mechanisms are disrupted, the mucosa becomes more permeable to the damaging effects of acid and pepsin. Although bile and pancreatic juice have been postulated as the cause of gastric ulcers in some patients, a cause-and-effect relationship has not been clearly established.

ABNORMALITIES OF MUCOSAL DEFENSE. Little is known at the present time about how disruptions in mucosal integrity may lead to ulceration, although there are several theoretic ways in which this might occur. For example, some patients may secrete *reduced amounts of mucus* or *structurally abnormal mucus*. Both could lead to a weaker mucous gel layer.

Diminished blood flow may lead to cell injury and ulceration in some patients. Gastric mucosal ischemia is believed to be a factor in the pathogenesis of acute mucosal injury, as occurs in patients with severe medical or surgical illnesses (stress ulceration). Whether similar reductions in blood flow contribute to the development of chronic gastric or duodenal ulcers is not known. There are fewer collateral blood vessels on the lesser curvature of the stomach compared with the greater curvature. Whether this anatomic difference in blood supply leads to reduced blood flow to the lesser curvature with subsequent ulceration in some patients is not known, but most gastric ulcers do occur on the lesser curvature.

Decreased bicarbonate secretion is a possible cause for diminished mucosal defense. Gastric bicarbonate secretion has been measured in patients with duodenal ulcer disease and found not to be significantly different from that in normal subjects. However, bicarbonate secretion from the duodenum is decreased in some duodenal ulcer patients. Reduced pancreatic bicarbonate secretion into the lumen of the duodenum could theoretically lead to increased acidity in the duodenal bulb with subsequent duodenal ulceration, but patients with pancreatic insufficiency seem not to have a higher incidence of duodenal ulcers. The role of possible *abnormalities in cell renewal* in the pathogenesis of peptic ulcer is entirely speculative at the present time.

Prostaglandin content in gastric or duodenal mucosa might be diminished, leading to abnormalities of mucosal defense (see above) and ulceration. Studies have led to conflicting reports, however, so that it is impossible at this time to evaluate adequately the possible role of endogenous prostaglandins in the pathogenesis of gastric or duodenal ulcers.

EMOTIONAL STRESS. The mechanism or mechanisms by which emotional stress might contribute to ulcer disease in some patients are unclear. Certain emotions such as hostility, resentment, guilt, and frustration are associated with increased gastric acidity. Furthermore, basal acid secretion has been reported to increase during stressful interviews and prior to surgery in ulcer patients or before difficult school examinations in healthy subjects. Patients have been described who developed acid hypersecretion and gastric ulcer disease during periods of severe emotional stress. With alleviation of stress, acid secretion diminished and symptoms and ulcerations disappeared. Thus, certain emotions can cause increased acid secretion that in turn may lead to ulceration in certain patients. Emotional stress may alter factors that maintain mucosal integrity and thereby result in ulcers because of decreased mucosal defense. Although controlled studies suggest a relationship between emotional stress and ulcer disease in some patients, its exact role is uncertain.

DELAYED GASTRIC EMPTYING. Delayed gastric emptying has been postulated to have a role in the pathogenesis of gastric ulcer disease, possibly through retention of food in the stomach, which, in turn, might increase gastrin release and acid secretion. Prolonged gastric emptying, perhaps due to antral hypomotility, has also been thought to cause stasis and delayed clearing of duodenal contents (bile and pancreatic enzymes) that had refluxed into the stomach. This in turn could damage gastric mucosa,

cause gastritis, and lead to ulceration. Currently, delayed emptying is believed to be related to ulceration in only a minority of patients.

EXOGENOUS FACTORS. The most important exogenous factors that have been associated with peptic ulcer disease are cigarette smoking and the use of nonsteroidal anti-inflammatory drugs. Interest has increased during the past several years in the possible relationship between *Helicobacter pylori* and peptic ulcer disease. The possible association with adrenocorticosteroid therapy, alcohol, or caffeine is more tenuous.

Cigarette Smoking. Whether cigarette smoking is related to the pathogenesis of ulcer disease is unclear, although epidemiologic data suggest an association between the two: (1) Smoking is more common among patients with ulcers than among control subjects. (2) There is a positive correlation between the quantity of cigarettes smoked and the prevalence of ulcer disease. (3) Death due to peptic ulcer disease is more likely among patients who smoke than among those who do not. (4) Duodenal ulcers are less likely to heal in cigarette smokers than in nonsmokers. (5) Duodenal ulcers recur more frequently in smokers than in nonsmokers. Whether this applies also to patients with gastric ulcers is not known.

Nonsteroidal Anti-inflammatory Drugs (NSAID's). These medications inhibit prostaglandin synthesis and cause decreased mucus and bicarbonate secretion, diminished mucosal blood flow, and perhaps reduced cell renewal. Aspirin and other NSAID's cause superficial mucosal erosions in the stomach, presumably by reducing the factors believed important in maintaining mucosal integrity and likely cause chronic gastric or duodenal ulcers. NSAID's are an important cause of upper gastrointestinal bleeding from gastric and duodenal erosions and ulcers. Bleeding secondary to these drugs appears to be more common in elderly patients.

Adrenocorticosteroid Therapy. An association between treatment with glucocorticoids (especially prednisone) and peptic ulcer disease has been both supported and denied in conflicting studies. There appears to be a higher incidence of ulcer disease in patients taking large doses of glucocorticoids for long periods of time.

Infectious Agents. Cytomegalovirus (CMV) has been isolated from gastric ulcers in a few patients receiving immunosuppressive drugs and in patients with post-transfusion CMV mononucleosis. *Candida albicans* also has been found in gastric ulcers in several patients. Whether these organisms caused the ulcers or whether the organisms were there secondarily is not known. Herpesviruses have never been isolated from gastric or duodenal ulcers, but one study indicated that antibodies to Herpesvirus type I occurred more frequently and in higher titers in patients with duodenal ulcers than in control subjects.

Helicobacter pylori has been associated with gastric antral gastritis. There is circumstantial evidence that this organism may be related to the pathogenesis of peptic ulcer disease. How the organism might cause ulcers is unclear. It could disturb the normal defense mechanisms described above and this, in turn, lead to ulceration. The organism might produce a toxin that disrupts normal mucosal integrity which, in turn, would predispose to ulceration. More studies are needed before *H. pylori* can be established as an important cause of gastric or duodenal ulcers.

Alcohol or Caffeine-Containing Beverages. Even though both of these substances stimulate acid secretion, there is no evidence that either causes gastric or duodenal ulcers.

Peterson WL: Current concepts: *Helicobacter pylori* and peptic ulcer disease. N Engl J Med 324:1043, 1991. *This is a succinct summary of this topic of great current interest concerning the possible role of infection in gastritis and peptic ulcer.*

Richardson CT: Gastric ulcer. In Sleisenger MH, Fordtran JS (eds.): Gastrointestinal Disease. 4th ed. Philadelphia, W. B. Saunders Company, 1989. *The factors involved in the pathogenesis and therapy of gastric ulcer are discussed.*

Soll AH: Duodenal ulcer diseases. In Sleisenger MH, Fordtran JS (eds.): Gastrointestinal Disease. 4th ed. Philadelphia, W. B. Saunders Company, 1989. *The pathophysiologic abnormalities found in various groups of duodenal ulcer patients are discussed as well as the therapy of duodenal ulcer.*

Soll AH: Pathogenesis of peptic ulcer and implications for therapy. N Engl J Med 322:909, 1990. *This is an excellent, current review of factors believed important in the pathogenesis of peptic ulcer diseases.*

98.2 EPIDEMIOLOGY, CLINICAL MANIFESTATIONS, AND DIAGNOSIS

Lawrence R. Schiller

EPIDEMIOLOGY

Peptic ulcer disease is a common disorder; 5 to 10 per cent of all individuals develop peptic ulcer in their lifetime. Although ulcer disease is a common cause of morbidity, it is a relatively rare cause of death. The annual prevalence of symptomatic peptic ulcer disease in the United States is approximately 18 per 1000 adults, but the current mortality rate is only 2.5 per 100,000. Approximately 350,000 new cases of ulcer present each year in the United States.

Ulcer incidence varies by site, sex, and age. Symptomatic duodenal ulcer is more common than symptomatic gastric ulcer in both men (5.5 to 1) and women (2.8 to 1). Men are twice as likely as women to develop a duodenal ulcer but equally likely to develop a gastric ulcer; sex differences may be narrowing, however. Duodenal ulcer usually first produces symptoms between the ages of 25 and 55 years (peak occurrence at age 40) and gastric ulcer most commonly between 40 and 70 years of age (peak occurrence at age 50).

Hospitalization and mortality rates for duodenal ulcer disease seem to be declining in the United States, suggesting that the prevalence of duodenal ulcer may be declining. It is unclear whether this reflects an actual change in the prevalence of duodenal ulcer, a change in the criteria for hospitalization, or a change in the way mortality data are recorded. Hospitalization and mortality rates for gastric ulcer seem to be stable or increasing slightly, especially among the elderly. This has been attributed to increasingly widespread use of nonsteroidal anti-inflammatory drugs by these patients. Substantial differences in ulcer prevalence from country to country remain unexplained at present.

Epidemiologic studies have suggested strong associations between the occurrence of peptic ulcer and (1) cigarette smoking, (2) genetic factors, such as blood group O, (3) personality profiles, and (4) infection with *Helicobacter pylori*. Both gastric and duodenal ulcer are associated with active infection by *Helicobacter* in the gastric antrum, but the issue of cause and effect is not yet settled. There is no convincing evidence that alcohol ingestion or diet is associated with the development of peptic ulcer. Peptic ulcer is more prevalent than normal in patients with chronic obstructive pulmonary disease, cirrhosis, renal failure or transplantation, and renal stone (even when hyperparathyroidism is not present). Less firm associations have been suggested with coronary heart disease and polycythemia vera.

SYMPTOMS

DYSPEPSIA. Peptic ulcer usually presents as a painful upper abdominal disorder with the constellation of symptoms known as *dyspepsia*. Dyspepsia is poorly defined by both patients and physicians and often includes such symptoms as nausea, vomiting, anorexia, and fullness and bloating in addition to pain or discomfort. Most patients thought to have ulcers because of "typical dyspepsia" are not found to have peptic ulcer by radiography or endoscopy but instead have other diseases or are classified as having "non-ulcer" (functional) dyspepsia. The opposite can also be true; patients with symptoms such as heartburn, which might suggest gastroesophageal reflux, may actually have peptic ulcer. Thus it is impossible to differentiate ulcer reliably from any other condition causing dyspepsia on the basis of history alone.

PAIN. The clinical diagnosis of ulcer disease has usually been based on the location of pain, its character, and the factors aggravating or alleviating it. For example, ulcer pain is classically described as being located in the epigastrium and as burning or gnawing in character. Pain in this location also occurs in a majority of patients with "non-ulcer" dyspepsia, however, and pain of this character actually occurs in a minority of patients with either gastric or duodenal ulcer. Some patients describe ulcer pain as a cramping sensation not unlike hunger pangs, but descriptions of the character of pain are often hard to obtain in an unbiased way

and are difficult to assess. Typical ulcer pain is said to be relieved by ingestion of food or antacids, but this is also quite variable. A better predictor of the presence of peptic ulcer (especially duodenal ulcer) is an episodic pattern of pain. Individual episodes of pain usually are short lived, lasting for minutes rather than hours. Episodes of pain usually occur in clusters lasting from days to weeks, interspersed with long symptom-free periods. Recurrence is typical for peptic ulcer; some patients with ulcer report annual recurrences of pain during particular seasons such as spring or fall. Changes in the character of ulcer pain may herald ulcer complications, such as penetration or perforation (see Ch. 98.5).

The cause of ulcer pain remains unknown. Ulcer pain is usually attributed to increased acidity at the ulcer site and the relief of pain to a decrease in luminal acidity. This theory is consistent with the classic onset of pain several hours after a meal, when gastric emptying has reduced the buffering capacity of gastric contents and intraluminal acidity rises. Attempts to induce pain by perfusing the ulcer site with acid have not uniformly produced pain, however. In several studies ingestion of placebo with no buffering capacity was as effective as ingestion of active antacid in relieving ulcer pain. In addition, ingestion of food sometimes worsens pain. Alternative mechanisms for the production of ulcer pain have been proposed, such as abnormal gastric or duodenal motor function, but are similarly unproved.

COMPLICATIONS. Peptic ulcers frequently fail to produce dyspepsia or pain (perhaps as often as one third of the time) and therefore may present de novo as a complication, such as bleeding, obstruction, or perforation. These are discussed in Ch. 98.5.

PHYSICAL EXAMINATION

The physical examination is usually not helpful in uncomplicated peptic ulcer disease. Epigastric tenderness is an insensitive and nonspecific finding and correlates poorly with the presence of an active ulcer crater. When ulcer disease is complicated by obstruction, perforation, penetration, or bleeding, important physical findings may be present (see Ch. 98.5).

Rarely, peptic ulcer is associated with multisystem syndromes that may produce physical findings. For instance, systemic mastocytosis, stiff skin syndrome, pachydermoperiostosis, and multiple lentigines-ulcer syndrome may have cutaneous findings. Ulcer-tremor-nystagmus syndrome and amyloidosis may produce both peptic ulcer and neurologic findings.

DIAGNOSTIC VISUALIZATION

The definitive diagnosis of ulcer depends on visualizing the ulcer crater by radiography or endoscopy. Radiography is well tolerated (even in patients in fragile condition), readily available, and comparatively inexpensive, making it an excellent screening test. However, radiography may miss as many as 20 per cent of peptic ulcers. Endoscopy is more accurate and allows directed biopsy and cytologic study of suspicious lesions but cannot always be done safely in uncooperative patients or those whose condition is unstable. In the United States, where endoscopy currently costs from three to five times as much as radiography, upper gastrointestinal radiographs, preferably with both single-contrast and double-contrast techniques, are often the initial diagnostic test. In symptomatic patients with no radiographic abnormalities or with equivocal evidence of ulcer, endoscopy can establish or exclude the diagnosis of active ulcer disease. In situations in which there is little difference in cost between endoscopy and radiography, endoscopy is preferable in the investigation of patients with dyspepsia because of its greater sensitivity in diagnosis. Endoscopy is also preferable in patients with acute gastrointestinal bleeding because the risk of rebleeding can be assessed better and therapy can be delivered, if necessary.

DUODENAL ULCER. If a duodenal ulcer is demonstrated radiographically (Fig. 98–5), no further diagnostic evaluation is necessary and treatment can be started. Since duodenal ulcers are rarely malignant, endoscopic biopsy is not necessary. Follow-up examinations to assess healing of a duodenal ulcer need not be done routinely. However, if symptoms fail to subside with therapy, endoscopy should be done to prove the diagnosis of ulcer before considering surgery (see Ch. 98.4).

GASTRIC ULCER. If a gastric ulcer is found on the radiograph (Fig. 98–6), malignancy should be rigorously excluded, particularly if there is any suspicion by the radiologist that the ulcer

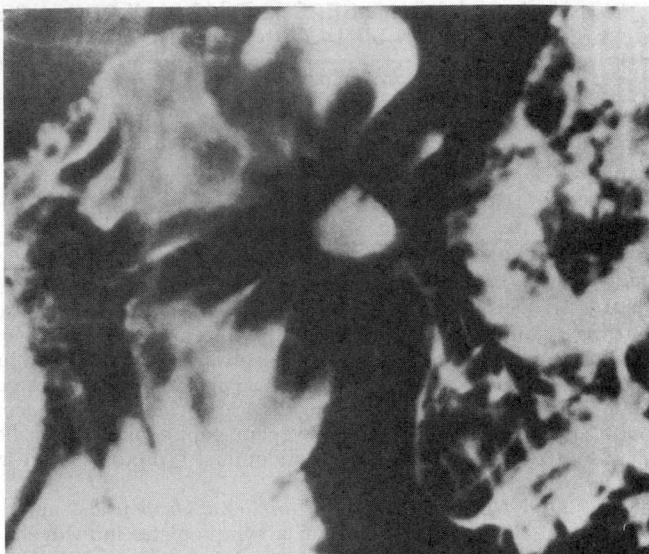

FIGURE 98–5. Duodenal ulcers are recognized when barium is retained within an ulcer niche. In this example barium has collected in an ulcer at the base of the duodenal bulb along the posterior wall. Folds radiate to the margin of this ulcer. (From Goldberg HI: *In* Sleisenger MH, Fordtran JS [eds.]: Gastrointestinal Disease. 2nd ed. Philadelphia, W. B. Saunders Company, 1978.)

may be malignant. Malignancy should be suspected if (1) the ulcer is located completely within the gastric wall or in an intraluminal mass, (2) there is nodularity of the ulcer base or of adjacent gastric mucosa, (3) there are no folds radiating to the ulcer margin, or (4) the ulcer is large. Malignancy can best be excluded by direct endoscopic visualization of the gastric ulcer to obtain brush cytologic specimens and to obtain a minimum of six

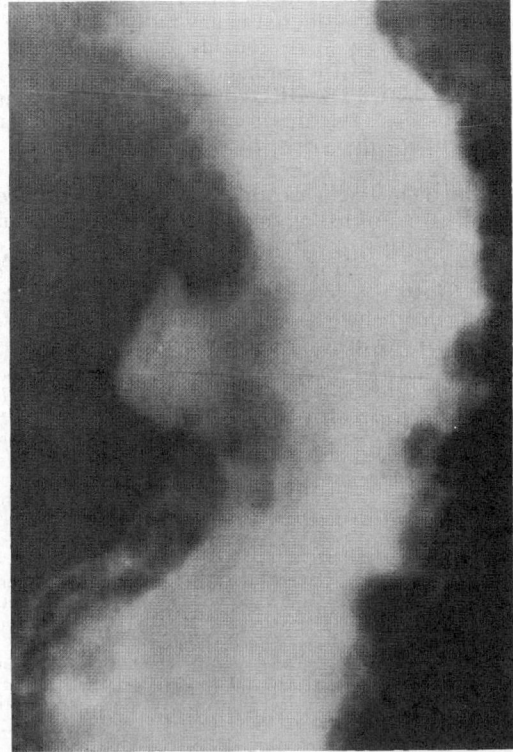

FIGURE 98–6. This ulcer of the lesser curve of the stomach demonstrates several features typical of benign gastric ulcers: The ulcer crater projects beyond the contour of the gastric wall, the margin of the ulcer crater is sharply defined and smooth, the ulcer is surrounded by a broad lucent band—an ulcer collar—resulting from edema at the ulcer orifice, and mucosal folds radiate from the ulcer collar. (From Goldberg HI: *In* Sleisenger MH, Fordtran JS [eds.]: Gastrointestinal Disease. 2nd ed. Philadelphia, W. B. Saunders Company, 1978.)

to eight pinch biopsy specimens for careful pathologic examination. This approach will lead to an accurate diagnosis in more than 95 per cent of cases. Some investigators recommend that patients with radiographically benign-appearing gastric ulcers not have endoscopy initially but that malignancy be excluded by repeating a radiographic study or by endoscopy after a period of therapy to prove that the ulcer has healed completely. Whether initially endoscoped and found benign or not, all gastric ulcers should be followed to healing to exclude malignancy. This can be done best by endoscopy after treatment for 8 to 12 weeks to allow healing to occur. Surgery may be needed to exclude malignancy in nonhealing gastric ulcer even if multiple endoscopic biopsies yield negative results (Ch. 98.4).

LABORATORY STUDIES

SERUM GASTRIN LEVELS. Radioimmunoassay of gastrin is useful in screening patients with known ulcer disease for Zollinger-Ellison syndrome (Ch. 98.6) and other rare hypersecretory states. The reasons for identifying these patients are (1) they may have a more severe course marked by excessive complications such as bleeding, obstruction, or perforation; (2) therapy is different, particularly surgical therapy (see Ch. 98.4); (3) associated but undiagnosed diseases of other organs, such as multiple endocrine neoplasia type I, may cause morbidity; and (4) gastrinomas associated with Zollinger-Ellison syndrome may be malignant and cause death from metastasis. Early recognition of Zollinger-Ellison syndrome makes possible effective control of symptoms and sometimes allows resection of tumor and cure of the disease (Ch. 98.6).

Measurement of serum gastrin concentrations in all patients with peptic ulcer disease is not cost effective because the incidence of Zollinger-Ellison syndrome is low (less than 1 per cent of patients with peptic ulcer disease). Table 98–2 lists the selective clinical situations in which obtaining a fasting serum gastrin level may be useful, although even with this selectivity the likelihood of identifying a patient as having Zollinger-Ellison syndrome is low.

If fasting serum gastrin concentrations are elevated (> 200 pg per milliliter) in patients not taking medications that alter intragastric pH such as high-dose antacids, H_2-receptor antagonists, or omeprazole, gastric acid secretion should be measured in order to prove that gastrin levels are not elevated in response to hypochlorhydria or achlorhydria, such as that due to pernicious anemia, atrophic gastritis, gastric cancer, or vagotomy. A finding of high serum gastrin levels and increased basal acid output limits the differential diagnosis to only a few entities (Table 98–3). If both fasting gastrin levels and basal acid secretion are very high (> 1000 pg per milliliter and > 15 mmol per hour, respectively), a diagnosis of Zollinger-Ellison syndrome is likely.

When fasting gastrin levels or basal acid outputs or both are less markedly elevated and the diagnosis of Zollinger-Ellison syndrome is unclear, the response of serum gastrin concentration to an intravenous injection of secretin may be helpful. In individuals with Zollinger-Ellison syndrome, intravenous injection of pure Secretin-Kabi, 2 U per kilogram of body weight, results in a prompt and pathognomonic rise of gastrin of greater than 200 pg per milliliter within 2 to 10 minutes. Patients with other hypergastrinemic conditions (Table 98–3) and normal individuals do not

TABLE 98–2. CLINICAL SITUATIONS IN WHICH MEASUREMENT OF SERUM GASTRIN LEVELS IS INDICATED

Family history of peptic ulcer
Ulcer associated with hypercalcemia or other manifestations
   of multiple endocrine neoplasia type I
Multifocal peptic ulcer
Peptic ulceration of postbulbar duodenum or jejunum
Peptic ulceration associated with diarrhea*
Chronic unexplained diarrhea*
Enlarged gastric folds on upper GI radiograph
Before surgery for "intractable" ulcer
Recurrent ulcer after ulcer surgery

*Not due to antacid ingestion.
GI = Gastrointestinal.

show this elevation. Gastrin secretion rises with calcium infusion also, but this rise is less reliable diagnostically than that following injection of secretin.

Differentiation of other rare hypergastrinemic syndromes (Table 98–3) can be made on the basis of (1) history of ulcer surgery (retained antrum syndrome, discussed in Ch. 98.4) or small bowel resection, (2) demonstration of gastric outlet obstruction by radiography or endoscopy, (3) laboratory evidence of renal failure, or (4) response of serum gastrin levels to a meal. Patients with antral G cell hyperplasia or hyperfunction more than double their already elevated fasting gastrin levels after ingestion of a protein meal. Patients with Zollinger-Ellison syndrome do not usually have this exuberant response to a meal.

ACID SECRETORY TESTING. Gastric acid secretion is measured by placing a vented nasogastric tube in the gastric antrum under fluoroscopic guidance and aspirating gastric juice with a suction pump. By measuring the volume and acid concentration (determined either by titration to pH 7.0 or indirectly from pH measurements), the quantity of acid secreted by the stomach can be calculated. Basal acid output (BAO) is defined as the amount of acid produced during four consecutive 15-minute periods. Vmax for acid secretion is estimated by injecting a maximally effective dose of gastric secretagogue. Pentagastrin (6 µg per kilogram), the biologically active carboxyl-terminal fragment of gastrin, is preferred for this purpose. Histamine or betazole (Histalog) can also be used. Stimulated secretion is expressed as peak acid output (PAO, the sum of the two highest consecutive 15-minute periods after injection multiplied by 2) or as maximal acid output (MAO, the sum of four consecutive 15-minute periods after injection). Values for acid secretion in healthy subjects and ulcer patients are shown in Table 98–1. In the absence of hypergastrinemia, measurement of gastric acid secretion is usually unnecessary in patients with peptic ulcer. Basal and peak acid output are increased in duodenal ulcer patients as a group (see Ch. 98.1), but knowledge of the level of acid secretion has no therapeutic implications for the individual patient at present. Measurement of acid secretion rates is sometimes useful preoperatively so that postoperative values can be compared and the effect of the operation on acid secretion can be assessed (see Ch. 98.4). When ulcer disease occurs in the presence of achlorhydria, malignancy should be suspected.

OTHER LABORATORY TESTS. The interest in *H. pylori* as a possible etiologic factor in peptic ulcer has spawned a number of tests for the presence of this organism. These include biopsy of antral mucosa with special stains, bacterial culture, immunologic tests, and tests based on bacterial metabolism, such as the ^{13}C-urea breath test. The clinical indications for any of these tests are unclear at present, since the implications of a positive test for subsequent management have not yet been defined.

In patients with recurrent gastric ulcer, blood salicylate levels may be helpful in detecting surreptitious aspirin ingestion.

Measurement of serum pepsinogen concentrations has been proposed as a surrogate test for direct measurement of gastric acid secretion. While the correlation of the two tests is good in large groups, individual values show too much variation to be useful for most clinical purposes.

DIFFERENTIAL DIAGNOSIS

Peptic ulcer can usually be distinguished from painful intestinal disorders that customarily produce discomfort in the periumbilical or lower quadrants of the abdomen (e.g., appendicitis or diverticulitis). Disorders affecting the viscera of the upper abdomen or chest are more difficult to differentiate from peptic ulcer

TABLE 98–3. CAUSES OF INCREASED FASTING SERUM GASTRIN CONCENTRATIONS AND INCREASED BASAL ACID OUTPUT

Zollinger-Ellison syndrome
Retained antrum syndrome
Massive small bowel resection (?)
Chronic gastric outlet obstruction (?)
Renal failure
Antral G cell hyperplasia or hyperfunction

TABLE 98–4. COMMON DISEASES THAT MAY PRODUCE EPIGASTRIC PAIN SIMULATING PEPTIC ULCER

Myocardial infarction
Pleurisy
Pericarditis
Esophagitis
Cholecystitis
Pancreatitis
Irritable bowel syndrome

disease (Table 98–4). Differentiation of these disorders can often be made by considering the acuteness of pain, lack of response to eating or antacids, changes of pain with changes in position, radiation of pain, and the presence of physical findings such as rebound tenderness, all of which are atypical in uncomplicated peptic ulcer disease. Because ulcer disease is common and ulcer symptoms are often variable, however, peptic ulcer must be considered as a possible cause of abdominal symptoms even in patients with atypical symptoms.

FUNCTIONAL DYSPEPSIA. *Functional dyspepsia* ("nonulcer" dyspepsia) is diagnosed when a symptomatic individual is not found to have an ulcer or other structural disease, such as cholelithiasis. The causes of this syndrome are unknown. It is likely that several different problems can lead to dyspepsia. It has been estimated that 20 to 30 per cent of patients with this diagnosis eventually develop peptic ulcer; therefore, some of these patients may really have evanescent ulcers that evade diagnosis. Some of these patients have a disruption of normal gastric motor function. Gastrokinetic agents such as metoclopramide or domperidone reverse both symptoms and motor dysfunction in some of these patients. Longer clinical trials are needed before such therapy can be generally recommended for patients with functional dyspepsia.

GASTRIC CANCER. Many patients with gastric cancer present with dyspepsia (Ch. 99). This diagnosis should be considered in particular when dyspepsia is associated with weight loss or evidence of occult gastrointestinal blood loss in an elderly individual or when radiographic or endoscopic appearances of gastric ulcer are suspicious for malignancy. However, a diagnosis of cancer should also be considered in any individual with a benign-appearing gastric ulcer, since roughly 2 to 5 per cent of such ulcers contain foci of gastric carcinoma.

MISCELLANEOUS DISORDERS. A variety of other diseases can produce dyspepsia that may mimic that of peptic ulcer. These conditions include *infiltrative diseases* of the stomach such as hypertrophic gastritis, tuberculosis, syphilis, Crohn's disease, and other granulomatous gastritides (see Ch. 97); *duodenal obstruction* by polyps, webs, or an annular pancreas; and *intestinal parasitosis* by *Giardia* or *Strongyloides*. More common diseases causing dyspeptic symptoms include *biliary tract disease* and *pancreatitis*. These can often be suspected by history, but tests such as sonography, cholecystography, and serum amylase determinations are usually necessary to confirm their diagnosis.

Graham DY: *Campylobacter pylori* and peptic ulcer disease. Gastroenterology 96:615, 1989. *Detailed review of possible relationships of infection by* Helicobacter pylori *and peptic ulcer disease.*
Kurata JH: Ulcer epidemiology: An overview and proposed research framework. Gastroenterology 96:569, 1989. *Introductory review and critique of epidemiologic techniques in ulcer disease.*
Richardson CT: Gastric ulcer. *In* Sleisenger MH, Fordtran JS (eds.): Gastrointestinal Disease: Pathophysiology, Diagnosis, Management. 4th Ed. Philadelphia, W. B. Saunders Company, 1989, pp 879–909. *Excellent review of clinical aspects of gastric ulcer disease.*
Soll AH: Duodenal ulcer and drug therapy. *In* Sleisenger MH, Fordtran JS (eds.): Gastrointestinal Disease: Pathophysiology, Diagnosis, Management. 4th Ed. Philadelphia, W. B. Saunders Company, 1989, pp 814–879. *Encyclopedic review of current knowledge about duodenal ulcer.*
Talley NJ, McNeil D, Piper DW: Discriminant value of dyspeptic symptoms: A study of the clinical presentation of 221 patients with dyspepsia of unknown cause, peptic ulceration, and cholelithiasis. Gut 28:40, 1987. *Analysis of symptoms in dyspepsia.*

98.3 MEDICAL THERAPY

Walter L. Peterson

In the healthy human stomach and duodenum, the potential for acid and pepsin to damage epithelium is effectively balanced by mucosal defense factors that act to prevent such damage.

Peptic ulcers occur when mucosal defense is disrupted in the presence of acid and pepsin. Potential mechanisms for this disruption include, but are not limited to, depletion of endogenous prostaglandins and *Helicobacter pylori* gastritis. Once formed, an ulcer remains as long as acid and pepsin overwhelm attempts at cellular regeneration. The goal of therapy is to shift the balance in favor of cell regeneration to effect healing of the ulcer, the clinical benefits of which are (a) relief of ulcer pain and (b) prevention of complications. Once an ulcer has healed, these early objectives may be extended by therapy designed to prevent recurrence.

Therapeutic agents used to accomplish these goals include antisecretory agents, antacids, sucralfate, and bismuth.

ANTISECRETORY AGENTS

Acid secretion may be reduced either by blocking the interaction of histamine or acetylcholine with their receptors on parietal cells (histamine H_2-*receptor antagonists* or *antimuscarinic drugs*) or by interfering with the intracellular machinery of the parietal cell (*prostaglandins* or *substituted benzimidazoles*) (Fig. 98–7).

H_2-RECEPTOR ANTAGONISTS. The effects of histamine are mediated through H_1 and H_2 receptors. H_1 receptors are located in the smooth muscle of the bronchus and small bowel, and H_2 receptors are located on parietal cells and the uterus. H_1 receptors are blocked by classic antihistamines such as diphenhydramine (Benadryl); H_2 receptors are blocked by specific H_2-receptor antagonists, which effectively lower both fasting and food-stimulated gastric acid secretion. There are four commercially available H_2-receptor antagonists for the acute treatment of duodenal or gastric ulcers. *Cimetidine* (Tagamet) is highly effective in the treatment of peptic ulcers in doses of 300 mg four times a day, 400 mg twice a day, or 800 mg at bedtime. *Ranitidine* (Zantac), used as 150 mg twice a day or 300 mg at bedtime, *famotidine* (Pepcid), used as 20 mg twice a day or 40 mg at bedtime, and *nizatidine* (Axid), used as 150 mg twice a day or 300 mg at bedtime, have subsequently become available. These agents are equal to cimetidine in effectiveness, with no clinical advantage of any one over the other three. Ulcers heal in over 80 per cent of patients after 6 to 8 weeks of therapy. Maintenance therapy with half-doses at bedtime also reduces the incidence of recurrent ulceration. These agents are remarkably safe, although side effects have been reported. Most reports deal with cimetidine and ranitidine, since the other two agents have not been in use long enough for a confident assessment of side effects. Central nervous system side effects (e.g., headache, mental confusion) are rare, reversible, and seen more often in patients with liver and renal failure. Gynecomastia and impotence have been reported, but in general the incidence is not significantly different from that of control groups. A number of drug interactions have been reported, predominantly with cimetidine, whereby concomitant administration with the H_2-receptor antagonist leads to increased levels of the agent in question. While there is potential for problems with drugs that have low therapeutic-to-toxic ratios (e.g., theophylline, warfarin, and phenytoin), the impact on patient management is minimal.

ANTIMUSCARINIC DRUGS. The classic antimuscarinic drugs reduce fasting and food-stimulated acid secretion by about 50 per cent and 30 per cent, respectively. However, these drugs also block other muscarinic receptors and produce unwanted side effects such as drowsiness, blurred vision, and urinary hesitancy. Therefore, these drugs (as well as the centrally active tricyclic antidepressant drugs trimipramine and doxepin, which possess antimuscarinic properties) have no role as first-line therapy for peptic ulcers.

PROSTAGLANDINS. Several methylated analogues of prostaglandin E_1 and E_2 have been developed which, when given in high doses, reduce gastric acid secretion by interfering with the generation of cyclic adenosine monophosphate (cAMP) in the parietal cell (Figure 98–7). Results of ulcer healing with these agents have been unimpressive, however, when compared to H_2-receptor antagonists. In addition, there has been a substantial incidence of diarrhea as well as the potential for abortion. Unfortunately, when lower doses (i.e., "cytoprotective" doses) of prostaglandin analogues are used, there is no effect on ulcer healing. Thus, most companies have abandoned their agents.

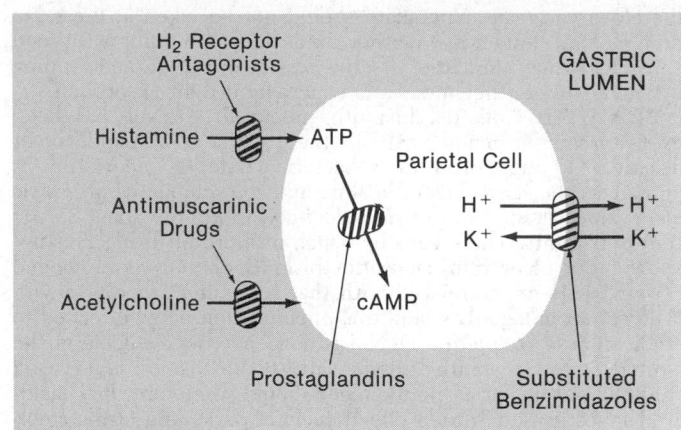

FIGURE 98–7. Sites of action of four drugs employed to inhibit acid secretion.

Only misoprostol (Cytotec) is commercially available and it is approved in doses of 200 µg four times a day only for the prevention of NSAID-induced gastric ulcers in patients at high risk of ulcer complications. The prostaglandin story is one of unfulfilled promises.

SUBSTITUTED BENZIMIDAZOLES. Drugs of this class, the prototype of which is omeprazole, are extremely potent inhibitors of gastric acid secretion. These drugs inhibit H^+-K^+–adenosine triphosphatase (ATPase), an enzyme found at the acid secretory surface of parietal cells that mediates final transport of hydrogen ions (via exchange with potassium ions) into the gastric lumen (Fig. 98–7). There is a prolonged duration of action, even when blood levels of drug are undetectable.

Omeprazole (Losec) in doses of 20 mg once daily produces ulcer healing modestly better than do H_2-receptor antagonists when the latter are given in standard doses. Because the cost of omeprazole is $0.50 to $1.00 higher per day than standard regimens of H_2-receptor antagonists, its major role should be in patients who might require larger than usual doses of H_2-receptor antagonists (e.g., patients with refractory ulcer, Zollinger-Ellison syndrome, severe esophagitis). The sustained hypochlorhydria produced by omeprazole results in hypergastrinemia, which, in rats, has led to the development of enterochromaffin-like cell hyperplasia and carcinoid tumors. The hypergastrinemia is reversible, however, and no such drug-related tumors have been documented in humans. Nevertheless, this drug should be used judiciously until more experience has been gained.

ANTACIDS. Antacids react with hydrochloric acid to form a salt and water, thereby reducing gastric acidity. Large doses (1000 mmol per day neutralizing capacity) of aluminum and magnesium hydroxide antacids are highly effective in healing gastric and duodenal ulcer, as effective as H_2-receptor antagonists. Such large doses often result in diarrhea, however. This property of antacids, as well as the advent of more convenient H_2-receptor antagonists, has relegated antacids to a position as supplemental rather than primary therapy for peptic ulcer. Interestingly, more recent studies from outside the United States suggest that low-dose antacids (e.g., one tablet, 25 mmol neutralizing capacity, four times daily) are as effective as large dose regimens. No such studies have been performed in this country.

SUCRALFATE

Sucralfate (Carafate) is the aluminum hydroxide salt of a sulfated disaccharide, sucrose octasulfate. Its mechanisms of action are uncertain. It has been suggested that sucralfate (1) forms a viscous shield over an ulcer crater, preventing acid from reaching regenerating ulcer tissue, (2) adsorbs bile acids or pepsin or both in the lumen, (3) stimulates the generation of local prostaglandins, (4) binds epidermal growth factor to the ulcer, or (5) acts as a scavenger of toxic free radicals. However it acts, sucralfate is effective for the acute therapy of duodenal ulcer in doses of 1 gram four times a day or 2 grams twice a day and as maintenance therapy in a dose of 1 gram twice a day. Results with gastric ulcer are less well studied. The drug is not absorbed and is therefore very safe. Sucralfate should not be taken at the same time as food, antacids, or other medications. Binding with food or antacids may limit the effectiveness of the drug, and binding by sucralfate of other medications may limit their absorption.

BISMUTH. Colloidal bismuth subcitrate (DeNol) has been used abroad for many years in the treatment of peptic ulcer disease. Although bismuth is bactericidal to *H. pylori*, this is unlikely to be its means of healing an active duodenal or gastric ulcer, since eradication of *H. pylori* occurs in only about 25 per cent of patients. The means by which bismuth heals ulcers is not known, but ulcer remission after bismuth therapy is prolonged in some patients compared with that seen after treatment with H_2-receptor antagonists, and this phenomenon may be related to eradication of *H. pylori*. DeNol is not currently available in the United States. Bismuth subsalicylate (Pepto-Bismol) is less well studied, and its use in peptic ulcer should, therefore, be considered investigational. Side effects include darkening of the stool, and, because of the potential for bismuth encephalopathy, long-term administration of bismuth is to be avoided.

If *H. pylori* is proven to have a role in the pathogenesis of peptic ulcers, its eradication may become a goal of treatment. Accomplishment of this goal, however, will likely require therapy with both a bismuth compound and at least one antibiotic.

TREATMENT OF PATIENTS WITH PEPTIC ULCER

At this writing, drugs available in the United States as therapy for patients with peptic ulcers include the H_2-receptor antagonists and sucralfate. Antimuscarinic agents, omeprazole, misoprostol, and antacids are also marketed but, for the reasons detailed above, are not recommended for first-line therapy. A physician should also be aware of several factors that at one time or another have been considered important in ulcer therapy.

COMPLEMENTARY FACTORS IN PEPTIC ULCER THERAPY. Factors to consider in this category include diet, smoking, alcohol or analgesic use, sedatives, and the need for hospitalization.

Diet. Diet therapy was once the standard treatment of peptic ulcer disease. Now, it is clear that no specific diet is of proven benefit in ulcer therapy. Patients should avoid whatever foods cause them discomfort but otherwise eat whatever they like. Because food, especially milk, stimulates acid secretion, between meal or bedtime snacks should be taken in moderation.

Smoking. There are many important reasons (other than the presence of a peptic ulcer) to encourage patients to stop smoking. Patients who do not smoke heal ulcers more often and more rapidly than those who smoke. The mechanism of this adverse effect on peptic ulcers is not known, although components of cigarettes may reduce endogenous generation of prostaglandins.

Alcohol. There is no evidence that alcohol ingestion retards ulcer healing. Nevertheless, because alcohol damages gastric mucosa, patients with ulcers who choose to drink should be advised to drink in moderation.

Analgesics. Drugs that inhibit prostaglandin synthesis (aspirin, nonsteroidal anti-inflammatory drugs [NSAID's]) are not only ulcerogenic but may predispose an ulcer to bleed. Therefore, patients with documented ulcer disease should be advised to discontinue the agent if at all possible. Patients with nonhealing ulcers should be queried regarding NSAID or aspirin use, and patients with documented ulcer who must continue taking NSAID's should be given prophylactic therapy with misoprostol (gastric ulcer) or an H_2-receptor antagonist (duodenal ulcer).

Sedatives. Although emotional stress may play a role in the pathogenesis of peptic ulcers in some patients, routine use of sedative drugs is of no proven benefit in ulcer therapy.

Hospitalization. Hospitalization should be reserved for patients with complications of ulcer disease (bleeding, perforation, penetration, obstruction) (see Ch. 98.5) or patients with ulcer pain refractory to routine medical management. In other situations, hospitalization is not warranted and has not been shown to lead to more rapid healing.

INITIAL MANAGEMENT OF PEPTIC ULCER. Patients should be treated initially with a single-drug, full-dose regimen of an H_2-receptor antagonist or sucralfate for duodenal ulcer and

an H_2-receptor antagonist for gastric ulcer. Duodenal ulcers are usually treated for 4 to 6 weeks; if at that time the patient is symptom-free, therapy is stopped with no further evaluation by radiography or endoscopy. Gastric ulcers are treated for 8 weeks, at which time assessment of healing is made, preferably with endoscopy or barium radiography. Follow-up evaluation to document ulcer healing is done to ensure that the ulcer is benign. Biopsies are taken any time an unhealed gastric ulcer is noted.

MANAGEMENT OF PATIENTS WITH UNHEALED ULCER. If a symptomatic duodenal ulcer or any gastric ulcer remains unhealed after initial therapy, the first steps are to ensure that the diagnosis of benign peptic ulcer is correct, to redouble efforts to have the smoking patient cease, and to inquire regarding aspirin or NSAID use. For duodenal ulcer, one will wish to increase the dose of H_2-receptor antagonist (if that was initial therapy) or change to omeprazole. Since medical therapy today can reduce gastric acidity as well as or better than can surgery, surgical therapy is almost never indicated for nonhealing duodenal ulcer. Of course, development of complications (e.g., bleeding) on medical therapy or noncompliance may mandate surgery. For patients with unhealed gastric ulcer, the first step is to treat longer with the same regimen, since gastric ulcers are usually larger than duodenal ulcers and, of necessity, take longer to heal. If healing still does not occur, the dose of H_2-receptor antagonist may be increased or therapy changed to omeprazole. If at any time the fear of cancer is overriding or if intensive therapy still fails to heal the ulcer, surgery should be considered. For patients who are not operative candidates, misoprostol has been reported to produce healing where H_2-receptor antagonists had not.

LONG-TERM MAINTENANCE THERAPY. Once an ulcer has healed with full-course therapy, long-term treatment with any of the H_2-receptor antagonists or sucralfate significantly reduces the high incidence of recurrent ulcer (as high as 70 to 80 per cent in 1 year). Not every patient requires such therapy, however. Patients who have bled from an ulcer should receive maintenance therapy with H_2-receptor antagonists in the hope that rebleeding will not occur and that surgery will not be necessary. Maintenance therapy is also given to those patients with frequent or especially severe recurrences for whom surgery might otherwise be considered. Unless a patient is a poor operative candidate, surgery is recommended if the ulcer recurs during maintenance therapy.

TREATMENT OF PATIENTS WITH ZOLLINGER-ELLISON SYNDROME. Patients with Zollinger-Ellison syndrome (ZES) pose a special problem. Because of constant gastrin-induced hypersecretion of acid, they are always at risk of ulceration and ulcer complications. The treatment is discussed in Ch. 98.6.

Feldman M, Burton ME: Drug therapy: Histamine$_2$-receptor antagonists—standard therapy for acid-peptic disease. N Engl J Med 323:1672, 1749, 1990. *Excellent recent review.*

Graham DY: Prevention of gastroduodenal injury induced by chronic nonsteroidal anti-inflammatory drug therapy. Gastroenterology 96:675, 1989. *Concise review of a controversial area.*

Lipsy RJ, Fennerty B, Fagan TC: Clinical review of histamine$_2$ receptor antagonists. Arch Intern Med 150:745, 1990. *Concise review of available H$_2$-receptor antagonists with long list of references.*

Maton PN: Omeprazole. N Engl J Med 324:965, 1991. *This is an excellent recent article in the* Drug Therapy *review series; with 181 references. It is the best starting point for reading about this new class of inhibitors of gastric acid secretion.*

Richardson CT: Gastric ulcer. *In* Sleisenger MH, Fordtran JS (eds.): Gastrointestinal Disease. 4th ed. Philadelphia, W. B. Saunders Company, 1989, pp 879–909. *Includes a detailed discussion of clinical results with therapeutic agents for gastric ulcer.*

Soll AH: Duodenal ulcer. *In* Sleisenger MH, Fordtran JS (eds): Gastrointestinal Disease. 4th ed. Philadelphia, W. B. Saunders Company, 1989, pp 814–879. *Excellent, detailed discussion of all aspects of duodenal ulcer disease.*

Wagstaff AJ, Benfield P, Monk JP: Colloidal bismuth subcitrate. A review of its pharmacodynamic and pharmacokinetic properties, and its therapeutic use in peptic ulcer disease. Drugs 36:132, 1988. *Encyclopedic review of bismuth subcitrate, a drug that may gain increased prominence in ulcer therapy if the H. pylori story holds up.*

Walan A, Bader J-P, Classen M, et al.: Effect of omeprazole and ranitidine on ulcer healing and relapse rates in patients with benign gastric ulcer. N Engl J Med 320:69, 1989. *Documents the results with omeprazole, 40 mg daily, in benign gastric ulcer. Also suggests a role for omeprazole in healing gastric ulcer in patients receiving concurrent NSAID therapy.*

98.4 SURGICAL THERAPY

Richard C. Thirlby

INDICATIONS

Peptic ulcers can be managed medically in most patients. Surgery may be required, however, to treat patients with complications of ulcers (hemorrhage, perforation, or obstruction) or patients with intractable ulcer disease. The decision to operate for intractability is difficult and is made primarily on subjective criteria. The physician and the patient must decide when pain and multiple ulcer recurrences become intolerable or intractable. Failure of medical therapy occurs when an ulcer does not heal on medication, when ulcers recur during maintenance medical treatment, or after multiple ulcer recurrences. Pain, interruption of livelihood or lifestyle, and history of major complications all influence the decision to refer patients for surgery. Pain per se is not an indication. Endoscopy should be performed before elective surgery to document the presence of an active ulcer in a patient with intractable pain, because the pain may arise from another cause. Although the frequency of elective operations for peptic ulcers continues to decline, the frequency of emergency operations for complications of peptic ulcers (e.g., bleeding, perforation) remains nearly constant.

SURGICAL PROCEDURES

SUBTOTAL GASTRECTOMY. Subtotal gastrectomy (65 to 75 per cent gastrectomy) was the standard operation for duodenal ulcer disease for many years. This procedure was effective in preventing ulcer recurrence in 90 to 95 per cent of cases, but the incidence of long-term postoperative complications was excessive (Table 98–5). This procedure is no longer recommended for treating patients with duodenal ulcers but is occasionally necessary in treating patients with gastric ulcers (see below).

TRUNCAL VAGOTOMY AND PYLOROPLASTY. Vagotomy eliminates cephalic (vagal) stimulation of acid secretion and reduces basal acid output by 80 to 90 per cent and maximal (peak) acid output by 50 to 60 per cent. Truncal vagotomy also denervates the antral pump mechanism, leading to delayed gastric emptying. This can be overcome by adding a drainage (gastric emptying) procedure to vagotomy either as a pyloroplasty (Fig. 98–8) or a gastrojejunostomy.

Operative mortality with vagotomy and pyloroplasty is less than 1 per cent (Table 98–5). Even when this procedure is performed as an emergency, operative mortality is relatively low in contrast to an operative mortality of 9 to 15 per cent after emergency vagotomy and antrectomy (see below). Vagotomy and pyloroplasty is the surgical treatment of choice for most patients with bleeding ulcers and is also used by some surgeons to treat patients with intractable ulcer disease.

TRUNCAL VAGOTOMY AND ANTRECTOMY. Resection of the gastric antrum, or antrectomy, removes gastrin-containing mucosa and diminishes the gastric phase of food-stimulated acid secretion. Antrectomy alone reduces acid secretion, and the combination of an antrectomy with a vagotomy leads to an even greater reduction of acid output (reducing basal acid output by 90 per cent and peak acid output by 70 to 80 per cent).

The combination of truncal vagotomy and antrectomy (Fig. 98–8) is frequently considered the standard elective operation for duodenal ulcer disease because ulcers recur rarely after this procedure. However, operative mortality is approximately 1 per cent, and long-term postoperative complications occur frequently

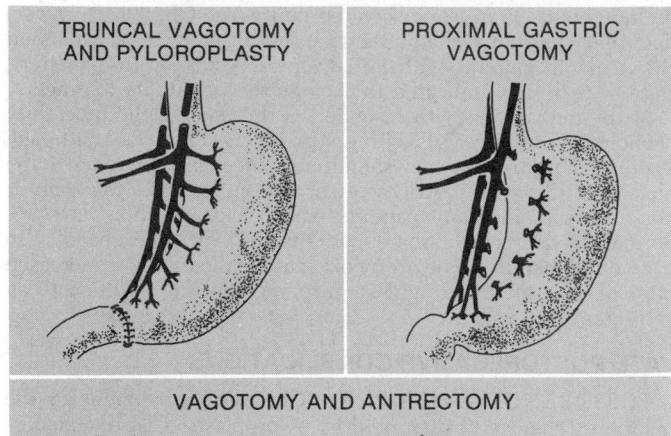

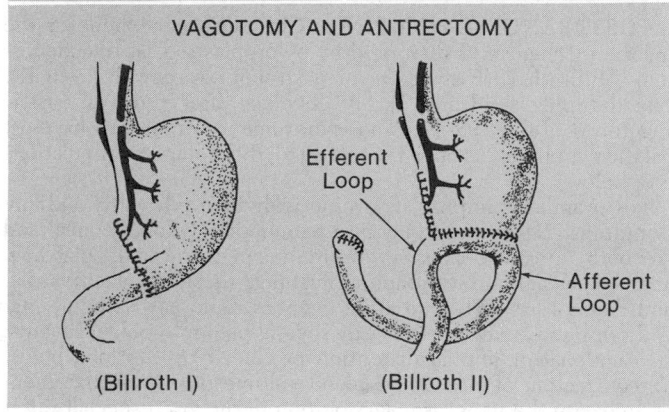

FIGURE 98–8. Model illustrating surgical procedures for peptic ulcer disease.

(Table 98–5). Therefore, proximal gastric vagotomy is gaining favor in some centers.

PROXIMAL GASTRIC VAGOTOMY. The parietal cell mass can be selectively denervated (proximal gastric vagotomy) (Fig. 98–8) while antral innervation and motor function remain intact. This operation reduces acid secretion while maintaining normal gastric emptying. Since many of the late sequelae of other acid-reducing procedures (e.g., dumping, diarrhea) are secondary to abnormal gastric emptying, the theoretic advantage of proximal gastric vagotomy is to reduce acid secretion with minimal mortality and long-term postoperative morbidity (Table 98–5).

Proximal gastric vagotomy is not indicated in patients with gastric outlet obstruction, active pyloric channel ulcers, prepyloric ulcers, or most patients with actively bleeding ulcers. Complicated peptic ulcer disease (history of bleeding or perforation) or high acid outputs do not contraindicate this procedure. Proximal gastric vagotomy is the operation of choice in many hospitals for patients undergoing elective operations for duodenal ulcers.

SPECIAL CONSIDERATIONS IN PATIENTS WITH GASTRIC ULCERS

The indications for operation and the surgical management of gastric ulcers are the same as for duodenal ulcers except that gastric cancer is a concern in patients with nonhealing gastric ulcers. If endoscopy with multiple biopsies and brush cytology specimens indicates that a gastric ulcer is benign, cancer is

TABLE 98–5. SURGICAL PROCEDURES FOR TREATMENT OF PEPTIC ULCER DISEASE

| | Operative Mortality | | Late Postoperative Complications | | | | | |
| | | | Dumping | | Diarrhea | | | |
	Elective	*Emergency*	MILD*	SEVERE	MILD*	SEVERE	*Weight Loss*	Incidence of Recurrent Ulcers
Subtotal gastrectomy	1%	10%	60%	5%	15%	0%	50%	5–10%
Truncal vagotomy and pyloroplasty	<1%	<7%	20%	2%	20%	2%	5–39%	7–10%
Truncal vagotomy and antrectomy	1%	9–15%	30%	2–5%	20–30%	2%	10–42%	1%
Proximal gastric vagotomy	0.1%	1%	0.5%	0%	1–2%	0%	0–5%	10%

*Nearly all patients have some change in bowel habits. Numbers are averages of many series and reflect clinically important symptoms.

excluded with 95 to 98 per cent certainty (see Ch. 99). However, if an ulcer has not healed after 12 weeks of medical management (15 weeks in patients with initial ulcers > 2.5 cm in diameter), surgery is usually indicated to exclude the possibility of cancer.

Antrectomy alone with resection of the ulcer is the procedure of choice in most patients with gastric ulcers (Fig. 98–8), although a subtotal gastrectomy is sometimes necessary to remove the ulcer and all of the gastric ulcer-prone epithelium. Vagotomy is not necessary in many patients, since acid secretion rates are normal or decreased. Some patients, on the other hand, also have duodenal ulcers or prepyloric gastric ulcers, have increased rates of acid secretion, and require vagotomy in addition to an antrectomy.

LATE POSTOPERATIVE COMPLICATIONS

POSTPRANDIAL DUMPING. This can occur whenever the pyloric mechanism is disrupted by pyloroplasty, gastroduodenostomy (Billroth I) (Fig. 98–8), or gastrojejunostomy (Billroth II). The dumping syndrome rarely develops after proximal gastric vagotomy (Table 98–5). The syndrome is transient in most patients and can usually be managed by dietary manipulations (see below).

Postprandial dumping syndrome is divided into early and late symptoms. *Early* symptoms occur immediately after a meal and are both intestinal (nausea, vomiting, epigastric pain, diarrhea, and dyspepsia) and vasomotor (flushing, dizziness, tachycardia, and diaphoresis). The initiating event is rapid gastric emptying, and symptoms may be caused by several pathophysiologic events: (1) duodenal or jejunal distention produced by the food bolus, (2) contraction of circulating blood volume due to displacement of fluid into the hyperosmolar solution in the gut (especially after consumption of refined carbohydrates), and (3) release of vasoactive hormones (serotonin, bradykinin, vasoactive intestinal peptide).

Late postprandial dumping symptoms occur 1 to 3 hours after a meal and are believed to result from hypoglycemia. The mechanism is presumed to be a rapid rise in blood glucose after ingestion of a large carbohydrate meal. This leads to an exaggerated insulin response followed by reactive hypoglycemia.

Treatment of the dumping syndrome is largely dietary (Table 98–6). Medications such as serotonin antagonists or antimuscarinic drugs are ineffective in most patients, although somatostatin analogues may prove efficacious. Reconstructive surgery aimed at slowing the transit of food through the small intestine using reversed intestinal segments or Roux-en-Y jejunal interpositions is indicated in the 2 to 5 per cent of patients who are severely disabled (Fig. 98–9).

POSTVAGOTOMY DIARRHEA. Diarrhea is common following gastric surgery, especially when vagotomy is included. In 20 to 30 per cent of patients, diarrhea is clinically important and in 2 per cent it is incapacitating (see Table 98–5). The pathogenesis is unclear, and diagnosis of postvagotomy diarrhea should not be made without excluding *inflammatory bowel disease*, *lactose deficiency*, *celiac sprue*, or other causes of diarrhea, because gastric surgery may unmask previously silent diseases.

Treatment of postvagotomy diarrhea is largely dietary (Table 98–6). Medications (antidiarrheal agents, opiates, cholestyramine, and aluminum hydroxide–containing antacids) may be helpful in some patients. Approximately 2 per cent of patients require reoperation (using reversed intestinal segments) to control disabling diarrhea.

WEIGHT LOSS. Weight loss occurs frequently after antrectomy (see Table 98–5). In general, it develops in proportion to the extent of gastric resection and occurs most commonly after a Billroth II gastrojejunostomy (see Fig. 98–8). Weight loss after gastric surgery most commonly results from inadequate caloric intake. Early satiety resulting from a small gastric remnant may cause patients to limit meal size. Fear of eating because of postprandial symptoms or diarrhea may also prevent patients from consuming adequate calories. Other causes of weight loss include bacterial overgrowth that can occur in the afferent limb (blind loop) of a Billroth II anastomosis (see Fig. 98–8), delayed and reduced mixing of pancreatic secretions with meals, and in rare cases celiac sprue. Bacterial overgrowth leads to hydrolysis

TABLE 98–6. DIETARY TREATMENT OF DUMPING SYNDROMES AND POSTVAGOTOMY DIARRHEA

1. Follow low-carbohydrate, high-protein, high-fat diet.
2. Avoid refined carbohydrates and concentrated carbohydrates such as sugar, jelly, cake, pie, pudding, candy; substitute complex carbohydrates such as starch.
3. Eat six small meals a day.
4. Drink fluids between meals rather than immediately before or during meals.
5. Eat slowly.

of conjugated bile salts and also damage to small intestinal absorptive cells. In turn, this causes malabsorption of fat, fat-soluble vitamins, and other nutrients. Malabsorption of calcium and vitamin D may combine to produce osteomalacia and osteoporosis. Bacteria also utilize vitamin B_{12}; this may lead to B_{12} deficiency.

Antibiotics (metronidazole, 250 mg three times a day) or surgical conversion of a Billroth II to a Billroth I anastomosis reduces bacterial overgrowth and may restore vitamin B_{12}, fat, and fat-soluble vitamin absorption toward normal. Weight loss and malabsorption may be helped also by dietary manipulations (Table 98–6), calcium and vitamin supplementation, antidiarrheal drugs, pancreatic enzymes, or a gluten-free diet in patients with celiac sprue.

ANEMIA. Anemia after surgery for ulcer disease can be caused by deficiency of iron, vitamin B_{12}, or folate. Iron deficiency is frequent after gastric resection. Malabsorption of iron and bleeding from recurrent ulcers or peristomal gastritis contribute to iron deficiency. Vitamin B_{12} deficiency may occur either because of atrophic gastritis (loss of parietal cells that secrete intrinsic factor) or because of bacterial overgrowth in the afferent loop of a Billroth II anastomosis (see Fig. 98–8). Folate deficiency is uncommon and presumably is caused by malabsorption of folate from food and by decreased ingestion of dietary folate.

Evaluation of anemic patients after surgery for peptic ulcer requires measurements of serum iron, vitamin B_{12}, and folate and assessment of stool for occult blood. Parenteral administration of vitamin B_{12} (1000 μg per month intramuscularly) and oral or intravenous iron (Imferon) may be required if deficiencies are documented. If bacterial overgrowth is suspected in patients with a Billroth II anastomosis, antibiotics (e.g., metronidazole, 250 mg three times a day) may be helpful.

ALKALINE REFLUX GASTRITIS AND ESOPHAGITIS. Reflux of duodenal contents, particularly bile, into the gastric remnant is believed to cause gastritis and esophagitis (see Ch. 97). Symptoms include continuous, burning abdominal pain,

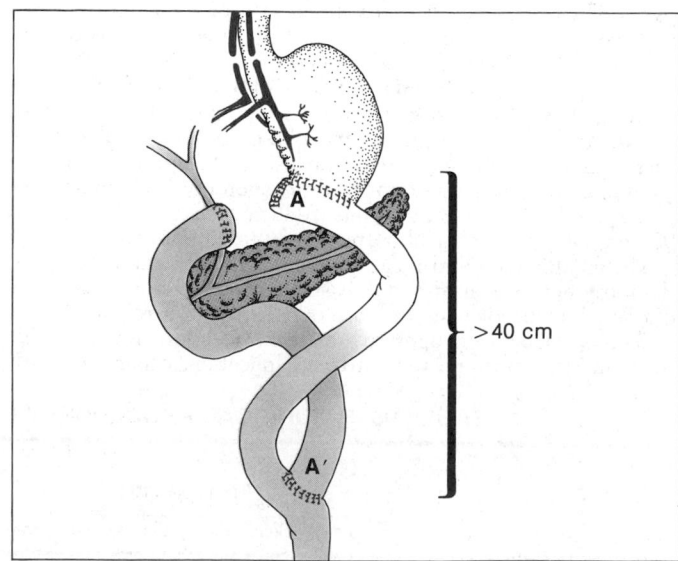

FIGURE 98–9. Model illustrating truncal vagotomy, antrectomy, and Roux-en-Y gastrojejunostomy (see text). Jejunum is divided at A-A′ with distal end (A) anastomosed to stomach. Pancreaticobiliary secretions are thus diverted from the stomach by at least 40 cm of interposed intestine (pancreaticobiliary secretions shown in red).

nausea, and vomiting of bile-containing material. Establishing reflux and inflammation as the cause of pain is difficult, since many asymptomatic postgastrectomy patients have similar endoscopic or histologic findings. No test definitively confirms that pain is caused by reflux.

Results of medical treatment with drugs that bind bile salts (cholestyramine or aluminum hydroxide–containing antacids) are poor. Roux-en-Y jejunal interposition prevents reflux of duodenal contents into the gastric remnant and esophagus and relieves symptoms in most patients (Fig. 98–9). However, many patients with alkaline reflux gastritis have slow gastric emptying and do poorly after Roux-en-Y diversion, developing a syndrome of nausea, vomiting, and abdominal pain.

AFFERENT LOOP SYNDROME. This can occur in patients who have a Billroth II–type gastroenterostomy (Fig. 98–8). Symptoms occur when pancreatic and biliary secretions collect in a partially obstructed afferent loop, causing distention and pain. Eventually, the fluid bypasses the partial obstruction, rushes into the stomach, and provokes vomiting. Thus, the symptom complex is characterized by postprandial cramping epigastric pain followed by projectile vomiting. Pain is relieved after vomiting. The vomitus is voluminous, contains bile, and does not contain food because food has left the stomach and passed through the efferent loop. Management of severe symptoms requires operative revision of the gastrojejunal anastomosis.

POSTOPERATIVE RECURRENT PEPTIC ULCER

Postoperative ulcers can develop in the stomach, the duodenum, or the jejunum in patients with a Billroth II gastrojejunostomy (marginal ulcer) (Fig. 98–8). The incidence varies for the different operations (Table 98–5). The clinical presentation is characterized by pain in only one half of patients, and complications, especially bleeding, are frequent. Diagnosis of postoperative recurrent ulcer is best made by endoscopy because upper gastrointestinal barium studies are poor at identifying postoperative ulcers.

Incomplete vagotomy is responsible for postoperative recurrent ulcers in the majority of patients. Other uncommon causes include *Zollinger-Ellison syndrome, retained antrum syndrome, ulcerogenic drugs* (aspirin or other nonsteroidal anti-inflammatory drugs), *silk surgical sutures* at the anastomosis, or *antral G cell hyperplasia*. Serum gastrin concentrations should be measured in all patients with recurrent ulcers to rule out Zollinger-Ellison syndrome (see Ch. 98.6) or retained antrum syndrome.

Sham feeding is the best test for diagnosis of incomplete vagotomy (see Ch. 98.1). An appetizing meal is presented to a patient, and the meal is chewed but not swallowed. Acid output is measured during the test by aspirating gastric secretions through a nasogastric tube. Acid output induced by sham feeding greater than 10 per cent of pentagastrin-stimulated peak acid output implies intact vagal innervation of the stomach.

The use of histamine H_2-receptor antagonists is the first choice for the treatment of postoperative recurrent ulcers caused by incomplete vagotomy. Postoperative recurrent ulcers heal with standard doses of histamine H_2-receptor antagonists in 60 to 90 per cent of patients, and reoperation may not be necessary. Lifetime maintenance therapy (e.g., ranitidine, 150 mg, at bedtime) is required in all patients to prevent further recurrence and complications. The indications for reoperation in patients with recurrent ulcer secondary to incomplete vagotomy are (1) failure to heal with H_2-receptor antagonists, (2) recurrence on maintenance therapy with H_2-receptor antagonists, (3) a complication (bleeding, obstruction, or perforation) associated with recurrent ulcer, or (4) noncompliance with long-term medical therapy. The choice of reoperation should be individualized. If sham feeding confirms incomplete vagotomy, and if the patient has had an emptying procedure such as a pyloroplasty or a gastroenterostomy at the initial operation, transthoracic revagotomy usually should be performed. Antrectomy (or re-resection) is indicated in patients who have a complete vagotomy as judged by sham feeding.

Jordan PH Jr.: Indications for parietal cell vagotomy without drainage in gastrointestinal surgery. Ann Surg 210:29, 1989. *Review of a single institution's experience with 658 parietal cell (proximal gastric) vagotomies. Overall results were excellent in patients with intractable, perforated, and even bleeding duodenal ulcers.*

Jordan PH Jr.: Operations for peptic ulcer disease and their early postoperative complications. *In* Sleisenger MH, Fordtran JS (eds.): Gastrointestinal Disease. 4th ed. Philadelphia, W. B. Saunders Company, 1989. *A general review of the surgical treatment of peptic ulcer disease, including indications for surgery and a description of the operations.*

McConnell DB, Baba GC, Deveney CW: Changes in surgical treatment of peptic ulcer disease within a Veterans Hospital in the 1970s and the 1980s. Arch Surg 124:1164, 1989. *Current status of trends in rates of elective and emergency operations for peptic ulcers.*

Meyer JA: Chronic morbidity after ulcer surgery. *In* Sleisenger MH, Fordtran JS (eds.): Gastrointestinal Disease. 4th ed. Philadelphia, W. B. Saunders Company, 1989. *Detailed review of pathophysiology and treatment of postgastrectomy syndromes.*

Schirmer BD: Current status of proximal gastric vagotomy. Ann Surg 209:131, 1989. *Excellent review of historical, physiological, clinical, and technical aspects of proximal gastric vagotomy.*

98.5 COMPLICATIONS

Mark Feldman

Approximately one of three patients with peptic ulcer disease experiences *bleeding, perforation,* or *obstruction* at some point in the course of his or her disease. Patients with a peptic ulcer in the pyloric channel or postbulbar duodenum, with combined duodenal and gastric ulcer, and with Zollinger-Ellison syndrome are especially likely to experience complications. The incidence of complications has not changed since introduction of histamine (H_2) blockers. Complications may cause death before the patient can be brought to a hospital or before definitive treatment can be carried out.

BLEEDING

Bleeding is the most common complication of peptic ulcer disease, occurring in 15 to 20 per cent of patients with duodenal ulcer and 10 to 15 per cent of patients with gastric ulcer. Risk of bleeding is unrelated to duration of ulcer disease; one of three to one of four patients have no history of ulcer disease when he or she presents with bleeding. The mortality rate for a single bleeding episode (5 to 10 per cent) has not changed in the past several decades.

Hemorrhage results from erosion of the ulcer into a blood vessel. The most common sign of acute bleeding is melena, with or without hematemesis. Although these symptoms usually indicate major blood loss (> 1000 ml), melena may occur with loss of as little as 50 to 75 ml of blood. In some patients with major hemorrhage, gastrointestinal transit of blood may be so rapid that the stool is bright red or maroon. Moreover, a nasogastric aspirate may not contain blood if active bleeding from a duodenal ulcer does not reflux into the stomach. Thus, the combination of hematochezia and a bloodless nasogastric aspirate can occur in patients with bleeding peptic ulcer. The hemoglobin and hematocrit on admission may not reflect the severity of bleeding if sufficient time has not elapsed to allow for compensatory hemodilution. Therefore, the severity of acute bleeding is better assessed by the blood pressure and pulse rate. A systolic blood pressure of less than 100 mm Hg and a pulse rate of more than 100 beats per minute, both taken with the patient supine, suggest major blood loss, as do a fall in blood pressure of greater than 10 mm Hg and an increase in pulse of more than 20 beats per minute after the patient assumes an upright position.

Peptic ulcer is the most common source of acute upper gastrointestinal bleeding (accounting for 40 to 50 per cent of cases). The differential diagnosis, however, includes esophagogastric varices, erosive and hemorrhagic gastritis, and Mallory-Weiss laceration. Less common causes include benign and malignant gastric neoplasm, esophagitis, duodenitis, vascular anomaly (e.g., angiodysplasia and arteriovenous malformation), and aortoenteric fistula, usually in patients with a prosthetic aortic graft. Peptic ulcers may also cause chronic or intermittent bleeding, resulting in iron deficiency anemia. In such instances, it is mandatory to exclude other causes of chronic blood loss, such as colonic cancer, before attributing the bleeding to a peptic ulcer (Ch. 105).

Certain factors may, if present, adversely affect clinical outcome in patients with bleeding peptic ulcers: (1) severe, continuing hemorrhage; (2) early rebleeding, usually occurring within 3 to 5 days of initial stabilization; (3) age greater than 60 years; (4) associated diseases, especially involving the cardiovascular system, lungs, and liver; (5) history of ingestion of nonsteroidal anti-inflammatory drugs; and (6) endoscopic visualization of a blood vessel in the base of the ulcer.

Various therapeutic measures have been employed in patients with bleeding ulcers, including nasogastric suction, antacid therapy, and inhibition of gastric acid-pepsin secretion with histamine H_2-receptor antagonist drugs or with somatostatin. None of these measures, alone or in combination, has been proved to stop active bleeding, to prevent rebleeding, to decrease need for surgery, or to reduce mortality.

Ulcers that are actively bleeding or that have a visible vessel are sometimes treated endoscopically using electrodes (monopolar, multipolar, heater probes), laser (argon, neodymium: yttrium aluminum garnet), or by injecting alcohol, epinephrine, or other agents into the ulcer base. While all of these modalities can usually stop active bleeding, it is not yet clear which is most effective in preventing rebleeding, reducing transfusion requirements, and reducing the need for emergency surgery. It is also uncertain whether any of these newer modalities will reduce mortality rates.

Continuous bleeding from an ulcer or major bleeding that recurs in the hospital commonly is an indication for surgery. Urgent surgery in patients with bleeding peptic ulcers carries a mortality rate two- to threefold higher than elective surgery. Emergency surgical therapy for bleeding duodenal ulcer consists of suture ligation of the bleeding vessel, along with truncal vagotomy and pyloroplasty, parietal cell vagotomy, or truncal vagotomy and antrectomy. Vagotomy without gastric resection has a higher in-hospital rebleeding rate than truncal vagotomy and antrectomy but a lower operative mortality rate. For bleeding gastric ulcer, the distal stomach, including the ulcer, is usually resected. If the ulcer is quite proximal in the stomach, the ulcer is usually biopsied and oversewn, followed by distal gastrectomy. Emergency surgery stops bleeding in 90 to 95 per cent of cases. In poor surgical candidates, angiography with arterial embolization using Gelfoam or autologous clot may stop bleeding.

Following discharge from the hospital, patients should receive an H_2 blocker by mouth for 4–8 weeks to facilitate ulcer healing. Once medical therapy is stopped, a patient has a 30 to 50 per cent chance of bleeding again from an ulcer. The severity of the initial bleeding event is not correlated with the severity of subsequent bleeding. Late rebleeding may be partly preventable by prolonged, nocturnal therapy with an H_2 blocker (e.g., 150 mg ranitidine), but more studies are needed.

Armstrong CP, Blower AL: Non-steroidal anti-inflammatory drugs and life threatening complications of peptic ulceration. Gut 28:527, 1987. *One of several case-controlled studies from the United Kingdom linking NSAID use and life-threatening ulcer complications (bleeding, perforation).*

Christensen A, Bousfield R, Christiansen J: Incidence of perforated and bleeding peptic ulcers before and after the introduction of H_2-receptor antagonists. Ann Surg 207:4, 1988. *Study shows nearly constant annual incidences of ulcer bleeding (5 to 10 per 100,000) and perforation (4 to 10 per 100,000) from 1974 to 1984 in Denmark, despite introduction of H_2 blockers in 1977.*

Christensen J, Ottenjann R, Arx FV: Placebo-controlled trial with the somatostatin analogue SMS 201-995 in peptic ulcer bleeding. Gastroenterology 97:568, 1989. *Demonstrates no benefit of a 5-day intravenous course followed by subcutaneous somatostatin analogue (octreotide) in stopping ulcer bleeding or preventing rebleeding.*

Laine L: Multipolar electrocoagulation in the treatment of active upper gastrointestinal tract hemorrhage. A prospective controlled trial. N Engl J Med 316:1613, 1987. Multipolar electrocoagulation in the treatment of peptic ulcers with nonbleeding visible vessels. A prospective, controlled trial. Ann Intern Med 110:510, 1989. *Two controlled trials showing benefit of multipolar electrocoagulation of actively bleeding ulcers or ulcers with a visible vessel.*

Murray WR, Laferla G, Cooper G, et al.: Duodenal ulcer healing after presentation with haemorrhage. Gut 27:1387, 1986. *Controlled study showing 4-week healing rate of 80 per cent with ranitidine (150 mg twice a day) compared to 25 per cent with placebo after a duodenal ulcer hemorrhage.*

Therapeutic endoscopy and bleeding ulcers. JAMA 262:1369, 1989. *NIH consensus development conference which reviews different endoscopic techniques available for control of bleeding ulcers.*

PERFORATION

An ulcer may penetrate the wall of the duodenum or stomach, resulting in (1) *free perforation*—rupture into the peritoneal cavity with spillage of duodenal or gastric contents; (2) *penetration*—erosion into and confinement by a solid organ, such as pancreas, liver, or spleen; or (3) *fistula formation*—extension into a hollow viscus, such as the common bile duct, pancreatic duct, gallbladder, or intestine.

Free perforation occurs in 6 to 11 per cent of patients with duodenal ulcer and in 2 to 5 per cent of patients with gastric ulcer, during the course of known peptic ulcer disease or as the initial manifestation. Free perforation occurs more commonly in men, in elderly patients, and in patients who ingest nonsteroidal anti-inflammatory agents. Ulcers on the anterior duodenal wall are more likely to perforate, while ulcers on the posterior wall are more likely to bleed. A posterior duodenal ulcer may occasionally perforate into the lesser sac and cause back pain rather than signs of generalized peritonitis. Most perforated gastric ulcers arise from the lesser curvature. In approximately 10 per cent of cases, peptic ulcer perforation is complicated by significant bleeding.

Free perforation characteristically causes sudden, severe, constant abdominal pain that reaches maximal intensity rapidly. The pain is initially present in the upper abdomen but quickly becomes generalized. Movement exacerbates the pain so that the patient prefers to lie on his or her back without moving. Marked abdominal tenderness to palpation and diffuse, boardlike rigidity of the abdominal wall musculature are present. Hypotension and tachycardia usually occur owing to intraperitoneal fluid losses. Hemoconcentration and leukocytosis are usually present, whereas fever often is absent. The serum amylase level is mildly elevated in one of six patients. Upright abdominal or chest radiographs show free air (pneumoperitoneum) in approximately 75 per cent of cases. If pneumoperitoneum is not evident and there is clinical suspicion of perforation, it may be helpful to insufflate 400 to 500 ml of air into the stomach through a nasogastric tube and then to obtain upright radiographs of the chest and abdomen (pneumogastrography) or to administer a contrast agent such as meglumine diatrizoate (Gastrografin) through the tube or by mouth. Free air can also be diagnosed by sonography. However, definite diagnosis of perforated peptic ulcer often is not established until surgery is performed, and radiologic studies should be done expeditiously to avoid delays in therapy. The differential diagnosis of perforated ulcer is discussed in Ch. 98.2.

The presentation of free perforation may be atypical: (1) A perforation may close rapidly with only minimal contamination of the peritoneal cavity and with rapid, spontaneous clinical improvement. (2) Abdominal pain and physical findings may be less impressive in elderly patients and in patients with neurologic or psychiatric problems or both. Such patients may present with unexplained shock. (3) Fluid may leak into the peritoneal cavity slowly and collect in the right paracolic gutter, resulting in a clinical presentation simulating that of acute appendicitis.

Treatment of free perforation is usually surgical. In most cases, surgery is carried out to establish the diagnosis and to patch the perforation with a piece of omentum (Graham's closure). Whether definitive ulcer surgery should be carried out also at the time of patching a perforation is controversial. Many physicians will perform parietal cell vagotomy, truncal vagotomy and pyloroplasty, or truncal vagotomy and antrectomy for perforated duodenal ulcer (or distal gastrectomy for perforated gastric ulcer) if there has been a long history of ulcer disease or previous ulcer complications. If perforation occurred more than 8 to 12 hours earlier, definitive surgery is usually not performed because of extensive peritoneal soiling. If a perforated gastric ulcer is not resected, the ulcer should be biopsied because 10 per cent of perforated gastric ulcers are malignant. Medical therapy of free perforation, usually reserved for high-risk patients, consists of nasogastric suction and intravenous fluids and broad-spectrum antibiotics. In a recent study, about two thirds of patients could be treated medically, while one third required surgery. Whether perforation is treated surgically or medically, H_2 blockers should be prescribed orally for 4 to 8 weeks to facilitate ulcer healing.

Mortality from free perforation is approximately 5 to 15 per cent for duodenal ulcer and somewhat higher for gastric ulcer, especially if the gastric ulcer is near the cardia. Factors associated with a poor outcome in perforated duodenal ulcer are longstanding (> 48 hours) perforation prior to surgery; preoperative shock; serious concurrent illnesses; and old age.

Penetration into solid organs such as the pancreas occurs with unknown frequency, since penetration can be diagnosed with certainty only at surgery or autopsy. These patients almost always have a long history of ulcer disease and usually present with intractable ulcer pain. Serum amylase and lipase levels may be elevated with posterior penetrating ulcers.

A *fistula*, an uncommon form of perforation, from a duodenal ulcer usually extends into the common bile duct; one from a gastric ulcer usually extends into the colon or duodenum. Patients with duodenocholedochal fistula may be asymptomatic but have air in the biliary tree, or they may present with cholangitis and abnormal liver function tests. The fistula is usually demonstrated by an upper gastrointestinal series, in which case barium refluxes from the duodenal bulb into the biliary tree. The fistula may close during medical treatment, although surgery may be required in some cases. Gastrocolic or gastrojejunocolic fistula caused by perforated gastric ulcer is often associated with ingestion of nonsteroidal anti-inflammatory drugs. These patients may present with diarrhea and malabsorption. The usual treatment is surgical. A gastric ulcer in the antrum may also perforate into the duodenal bulb, resulting in two or even three channels from the stomach to the duodenum.

Chang-Chien C, Lin H, Yen C, et al.: Sonographic demonstration of free air in perforated peptic ulcers: Comparison of sonography with radiography. J Clin Ultrasound 17:95, 1989. *Since many patients with abdominal pain now receive abdominal sonography, the ability to detect free air with this method is important to recognize.*
Crofts TJ, Park KGM, Steele RJC, et al.: A randomized trial of nonoperative treatment for perforated peptic ulcer. N Engl J Med 320:970, 1989. *Controlled study which suggests that an initial period of careful observation and medical therapy is often safe, except in patients above age 70.*
Simpson CJ, Lamont G, Macdonald I, et al.: Effect of cimetidine on prognosis after simple closure of perforated duodenal ulcer. Br J Surg 74:104, 1987. *Controlled trial showing that cimetidine is superior to placebo in relieving symptoms and preventing morbidity after simple closure of perforated duodenal ulcer.*
Svanes C, Salvesen H, Larssen TB, et al.: Trends in and value and consequences of radiologic imaging of perforated gastroduodenal ulcer. A 50-year experience. Scand J Gastroenterol 25:257, 1990. *Compares plain film and use of water-soluble contrast agents in diagnosis of ulcer perforation and emphasizes that these procedures delay treatment by at least 2 hours.*

OBSTRUCTION

Gastric outlet obstruction occurs in approximately 5 per cent of patients with duodenal or gastric ulcer and is especially common if the ulcer is located in the pyloric channel. Obstruction is caused by edema, smooth muscle spasm, fibrosis, or a combination of these processes. Obstruction usually occurs after ulcer disease of many years duration but may occasionally occur as the initial manifestation. Mortality rates from obstruction in peptic ulcer disease are 7 to 26 per cent, depending on the age of the patient and the presence or absence of associated diseases.

Obstruction delays gastric emptying and commonly causes nausea, vomiting, epigastric fullness or bloating, anorexia, early satiety, and a fear of eating (sitophobia). Significant weight loss may result. Epigastric pain is frequent and may be relieved temporarily by vomiting. Symptoms have usually been present for weeks or months. Vomiting, which may be delayed an hour or more after eating, is often copious and may contain undigested food but usually no bile. Physical examination may reveal volume depletion (hypotension, tachycardia, and dry skin and mucous membranes), visible peristalsis in the epigastrium, or a succussion splash over the stomach.

Any of the following objective measurements support the diagnosis of gastric retention: (1) aspiration of more than 300 ml of gastric fluid 4 or more hours after a meal (a large-bore tube may be necessary for measuring this); (2) aspiration of more than 200 ml of gastric fluid the morning after an overnight fast; or (3) removal of more than 400 ml of gastric fluid 30 minutes after instilling 750 ml of isotonic saline into the empty stomach (*saline load test*). Gastric retention may be appreciated on a plain abdominal radiograph (large, dilated stomach containing solid debris) and documented by an upper gastrointestinal series or radionuclide scintigraphy. Gastric retention is not always caused by gastric outlet obstruction. It may result from gastric atony, as in diabetic gastroparesis, from vagotomy, or as a side effect of medications. Gastric outlet obstruction, which is caused by peptic ulcer disease in 80 to 90 per cent of cases, can usually best be established by endoscopy. The other common cause is carcinoma of the antrum. Less common causes include gastric lymphoma,

pancreatic carcinoma, pancreatitis, hypertrophic pyloric stenosis, eosinophilic gastritis, Crohn's disease, antral caustic stricture, antral polyp, and annular pancreas.

Laboratory studies usually reflect intravascular volume depletion (hemoconcentration, prerenal azotemia) and a hypokalemic, hypochloremic metabolic alkalosis due to vomiting. If extensive weight loss has occurred, hypoalbuminemia, cutaneous anergy, and a low serum transferrin concentration may be present. The urine is usually concentrated and contains less than 10 mEq of chloride per liter, but the urinary sodium concentration and pH are variable, depending on the renal tubular threshold for bicarbonate reabsorption.

Therapy of gastric outlet obstruction has three goals: gastric decompression and resolution of obstruction; replacement of fluids and electrolytes; and nutritional support. Gastric decompression is accomplished by continuous nasogastric suction for at least 72 hours. With prolonged obstruction, gradual gastric dilation occurs, and this interferes with the contractile function of gastric smooth muscle. Electrolyte disturbances such as hypokalemia can also contribute to gastric motor dysfunction. Saline load tests, performed serially, may have prognostic value. For example, a return of more than 300 ml after 24 hours of nasogastric suction suggests that obstruction will not resolve and that surgery may be required. After 72 hours, a return of less than 200 ml is a favorable sign and usually indicates that the tube can be removed and the patient can be fed liquids. Intravenous fluids and electrolytes are given to replace pre-existing and current losses. Isotonic saline containing 10 to 20 mEq of potassium chloride per liter is satisfactory in most cases. Losses of gastric acid from continuous gastric aspiration can be curtailed by administering H_2-receptor antagonists (cimetidine, ranitidine, or famotidine) intravenously. If suction is carried out for only a few days, 5 per cent dextrose solution administered intravenously, along with soluble vitamins, may suffice. If prolonged suction proves necessary, parenteral intravenous hyperalimentation should be instituted. This is especially valuable if the patient has lost significant lean body mass.

Approximately 50 per cent of patients with obstruction improve with medical management. If obstruction does not resolve in 3 to 7 days, surgery may be necessary. There is controversy over which operation is best: truncal vagotomy and antrectomy, truncal vagotomy and drainage (pyloroplasty or gastrojejunostomy), or subtotal gastrectomy. Some surgeons are reluctant to perform truncal vagotomy for fear of postoperative gastric atony, although this complication is uncommon. Gastrojejunostomy (without gastric resection or truncal vagotomy) is associated with a high rate (30 to 40 per cent) of recurrences of ulcer. Nonsurgical dilation of the obstructed pylorus using balloons passed through an endoscope is a newly introduced therapy that has not yet been compared with surgery in a controlled study. Nevertheless, approximately 80 per cent of patients can be successfully treated by dilation followed by oral H_2 blockers. Follow-up of patients receiving dilation is short, however (<2 years), and thus the long-term effectiveness remains to be established.

Graham D: Complications of peptic ulcer disease and indications for surgery. In Sleisenger MH, Fordtran JS (eds.): Gastrointestinal Disease. 4th ed. Philadelphia, W. B. Saunders Company, 1989, p 925. *Comprehensive review with extensive references.*
Griffin SM, Chung SCS, Leung JWC, et al.: Peptic pyloric stenosis treated by endoscopic balloon dilatation. Br J Surg 76:1147, 1989. *Uncontrolled study of 25 patients with gastric outlet obstruction dilated endoscopically with 9 months of median follow-up. Excellent results in 20 patients.*

98.6 ZOLLINGER-ELLISON SYNDROME
Charles T. Richardson

DEFINITION

The Zollinger-Ellison syndrome is defined by both chemical and clinical criteria: (1) an increased serum gastrin concentration, (2) an increased basal acid output, (3) an increased ratio of basal to peak (pentagastrin-stimulated) acid output, (4) the presence of peptic ulcer disease or diarrhea or both, and (5) a gastrin-producing tumor. Not all patients with an elevated serum gastrin concentration and hypersecretion of acid have tumors that can be identified at surgery or by noninvasive tests such as sonography or computed tomography. Presumably, such patients have tumors that are too small to be identified, or they have hyperplasia of the islets of Langerhans, a condition known as microadenomatosis.

CLINICAL MANIFESTATIONS

Zollinger-Ellison syndrome occurs most frequently between ages 35 and 65 years and more commonly in men than in women.

Abdominal pain resulting from an ulcer is the most common clinical finding. Ulcers usually occur in the duodenal bulb but also may develop in the postbulbar duodenum, jejunum, stomach, or esophagus. Complications of ulcer disease, such as bleeding or perforation, occur in 40 to 50 per cent of patients at some time during their course and may be the presenting manifestation. Forty-five per cent of patients have esophageal symptoms consisting of heartburn, dysphagia, or both. *Diarrhea* is a frequent complaint and may precede ulceration in some patients or occur without ulcers in others (5 to 10 per cent). *Fat malabsorption* (steatorrhea) is occasionally noted.

About 20 to 30 per cent of patients with Zollinger-Ellison syndrome have multiple endocrine neoplasia (MEN I) syndrome and thus have a hereditary form of peptic ulcer disease (Ch. 228). These patients may have parathyroid or pituitary tumors and clinical findings such as hypercalcemia, renal stones, or increased prolactin levels. It is unlikely that peptic ulcer disease occurs with increased frequency in association with parathyroid adenomas except in patients who also have MEN I syndrome.

In some patients, Cushing's syndrome can develop as a result of either pituitary disease or ectopic adrenocorticotropic hormone (ACTH) production by gastrinomas. Patients with ectopic ACTH production frequently have metastatic gastrinoma, for example, in the liver.

PATHOPHYSIOLOGY

Peptic ulcers in patients with Zollinger-Ellison syndrome presumably result from increased secretion of acid and pepsin driven by excessive amounts of circulating gastrin. Gastrin also has a trophic effect on parietal (acid-secreting) cells that leads to an increased parietal cell mass.

Diarrhea results almost exclusively from the large volumes of fluid secreted by the stomach and is relieved in most patients by aspirating gastric juice via a nasogastric tube or more conveniently by treating patients with H_2-receptor antagonists or omeprazole (see below).

Steatorrhea may occur for several reasons: (1) excess acid damages small bowel epithelial cells, causing a mucosal defect that limits transport of fat and perhaps other nutrients across the mucosa; (2) pancreatic lipase is inactivated by acid, which impairs hydrolysis of triglycerides and contributes to fat malabsorption; (3) acid may decrease the amount of conjugated bile acids in the duodenum and upper jejunum, resulting in inadequate formation of micelles for fat absorption (Ch. 102).

DIAGNOSIS

Zollinger-Ellison syndrome should be suspected in patients who have (1) ulcers in unusual locations, such as the postbulbar duodenum or jejunum, (2) ulcers that persist despite medical treatment, (3) ulcers and diarrhea, (4) abnormally large gastric folds or thickened duodenal and/or jejunal folds, (5) ulcers and manifestations of other endocrine tumors such as renal stones, (6) a family history of ulcer disease, and (7) recurrent ulcers after ulcer surgery.

These criteria call for measurement of the serum gastrin concentration (see Table 98–2). If the level is abnormally high, a gastric analysis should be performed. Zollinger-Ellison syndrome is a likely diagnosis if the serum gastrin level is elevated, basal acid output is increased (>10.6 mmol per hour in men and 5.6 mmol per hour in women), and the ratio of basal to peak acid output (pentagastrin stimulated) is greater than 0.40:1.0. The diagnosis can be confirmed by performing a secretin stimulation test (see Ch. 98.2). This test is especially helpful in patients with serum gastrin concentrations or basal acid outputs that are only slightly increased. A positive secretin test, along with an increased serum gastrin concentration and basal acid output, establishes the diagnosis of Zollinger-Ellison syndrome in over 95 per cent of patients.

Tumors are found at surgery in 40 to 70 per cent of patients with Zollinger-Ellison syndrome and are usually located in the pancreas. Tumors have also been found in the duodenum, stomach, greater omentum, transverse mesocolon, and other areas of the peritoneal cavity. Computed tomography (CT) is useful in detecting gastrinomas and therefore should be performed in patients suspected of having the Zollinger-Ellison syndrome. A positive CT scan is almost always correct, whereas a negative CT scan is less reliable. Angiography and sonography are helpful adjuncts to CT. Since some gastrinomas have been found in the stomach or duodenum, upper endoscopy also should be performed to look for tumors. Techniques such as intraoperative sonography or transhepatic venous sampling to measure gastrin from tributaries draining the pancreas or duodenum have been helpful in localizing tumors.

THERAPY

For many years total gastrectomy was the treatment of choice for patients with Zollinger-Ellison syndrome. All of the acid-secreting mucosa as well as the antrum is removed, with subsequent cure of peptic ulcers and diarrhea. However, many of the late postoperative complications that occur in patients with ordinary peptic ulcer disease develop after total gastrectomy (see Ch. 98.4). Furthermore, in some centers mortality is higher with total gastrectomy than with other surgical procedures for ulcer disease.

With the advent of H_2-receptor antagonists and omeprazole, it has become possible to treat patients medically. Reducing acid secretion with an H_2-receptor antagonist or omeprazole effectively treats symptoms related to the disease in most patients. However, larger than normally prescribed doses, as well as more frequent administration, are often required. For example, 600 mg of cimetidine every 4 hours or 300 mg of ranitidine every 8 hours may be necessary to reduce acid secretion adequately.* A few patients have required even larger and more frequent doses of H_2-receptor antagonist. For example, a few patients have required as much as 5 to 10 grams of cimetidine daily. The dose of H_2-receptor antagonist may be reduced by treating patients concomitantly with an antimuscarinic drug such as glycopyrrolate or isopropamide (see Fig. 98–7), since antimuscarinic drugs have been shown to enhance the inhibitory effect on acid secretion of H_2-receptor antagonists. Many patients can be treated with once-daily doses of omeprazole (see Ch. 98.3). Even when using this more potent inhibitor of acid secretion, higher than normal doses must be prescribed in many patients. For example, doses as high as 60 to 120 mg have been required in some patients and doses of 60 mg twice daily have been needed in a few patients to reduce acid secretion effectively.

Medical treatment alone with H_2-receptor antagonists or omeprazole is not ideal for two reasons: First, complications of ulcer disease have occurred in some patients, and second, medical therapy does not provide an opportunity to search for resectable tumors, more than half of which are believed to be malignant. Because of this, a reasonable approach to treating patients with Zollinger-Ellison syndrome is laparotomy to search for resectable tumors present in about 20 to 30 per cent of patients, followed by medical therapy with H_2-receptor antagonists or omeprazole. At laparotomy a careful search for resectable tumors should be carried out. This includes intraoperative endoscopy with transillumination of the stomach and duodenum and intraoperative sonography.

Vagotomy may be combined with medical therapy in some patients to reduce acid secretion and to add to the inhibitory effect of medication. Treatment with a drug is still necessary, although the dose of H_2-receptor antagonist or omeprazole can sometimes be reduced. Regardless of the therapy used (tumor search followed by medical therapy alone or medical therapy combined with vagotomy), close follow-up to ensure compliance with the regimen is mandatory.

---

*May exceed maximum recommended daily dose.

Jensen RT, Doppman JL, Gardner JD: Gastrinoma. *In* Brooks F, Dimagno E, Gardner JD, et al.: The Exocrine Pancreas: Biology, Pathology and Disease. New York, Raven Press, 1986, pp 727–745. *An excellent review of the clinical manifestations, diagnosis, and treatment of patients with Zollinger-Ellison syndrome.*

McGuigan JE: The Zollinger-Ellison Syndrome. *In* Sleisenger MH, Fordtran JS (eds.): Gastrointestinal Disease. 4th ed. Philadelphia, W. B. Saunders Company, 1989.

Wolfe MM, Jensen RT: Zollinger-Ellison syndrome: Current concepts in diagnosis and management. N Engl J Med. 317:1200, 1987. *Both of the last two references review the pathophysiology, diagnosis, and treatment of Zollinger-Ellison syndrome and give extensive references to the recent literature for this disorder.*

99 Neoplasms of the Stomach

Sidney J. Winawer

The majority of gastric neoplasms are malignant, in contrast to the colon, where the reverse is true. Although gastric carcinoma is steadily decreasing in the United States, it still represents a major public health problem throughout the world. In some countries it is the most frequent cancer and the leading cause of death from cancer. In the United States gastric carcinoma is responsible for 90 to 95 per cent of malignant disease of the stomach. Approximately 5 per cent of all primary gastric malignancy is Hodgkin's disease (HD) and non-Hodgkin's lymphoma, particularly the latter, since HD rarely involves the stomach as a primary site. The sarcomas, including leiomyosarcoma, liposarcoma, neurogenic sarcoma, and fibrosarcoma, are all relatively rare malignant tumors that may involve the stomach. Leiomyosarcoma of the stomach represents about 1 per cent of gastric cancers.

CARCINOMA OF THE STOMACH

EPIDEMIOLOGY. The incidence of gastric cancer varies markedly in different areas of the world. It is extremely common in Japan, Latin America west of the Andes, some parts of the Caribbean, and Eastern Europe; moderately common in Finland, Austria, and Czechoslovakia; and uncommon in the United States, Australia, New Zealand, and other Anglo-Saxon countries. Colorectal cancer tends to be rare where gastric cancer is common and vice versa. The low incidence in the United States is a recent development (Fig. 99–1), since gastric cancer was the most common known cancer in the United States 40 to 50 years ago. Other countries that previously had a high incidence have also begun to show a decrease. The reasons for this are unknown. Environmental factors are considered important in the etiology of gastric cancer, as evidenced by populations migrating to areas of either low or high risk and taking on the risk of the area of migration. Japanese moving to Hawaii have a decreased incidence of gastric cancer in subsequent generations, and there is a further reduction with migration to the mainland. The incidence of colonic cancer increases with this migration.

ETIOLOGY. *Dietary influences* are thought to be important, but without direct proof. Consumption of barbecued meals, smoked or pickled fish and sauces, and alcohol and deficiencies of magnesium and vitamin A have all been postulated but unproved as causes of gastric cancer (Table 99–1).

Nitrosamines are powerful carcinogens for animals. They can be formed easily from common, secondary, tertiary, and quaternary amines by combining these with nitrite (the nitrosation reaction). This reaction can take place under varying conditions of pH and temperature, so that nitrosamines may be formed in the soil, under conditions of food storage, during food preparation such as frying bacon, or in the body. Bacteria may play a role by catalyzing the amine nitrite union or by reducing nitrate to nitrite. Thus the achlorhydric stomach is considered a favorable site for nitrosamine synthesis. The necessary amines can be found in many foods and medications, whereas nitrate and nitrites are found naturally in food and water and are present in food preservatives. Ascorbic acid (vitamin C) blocks the nitrosation reaction in the test tube. The increased intake of vitamin C and refrigeration have been postulated to be responsible for the

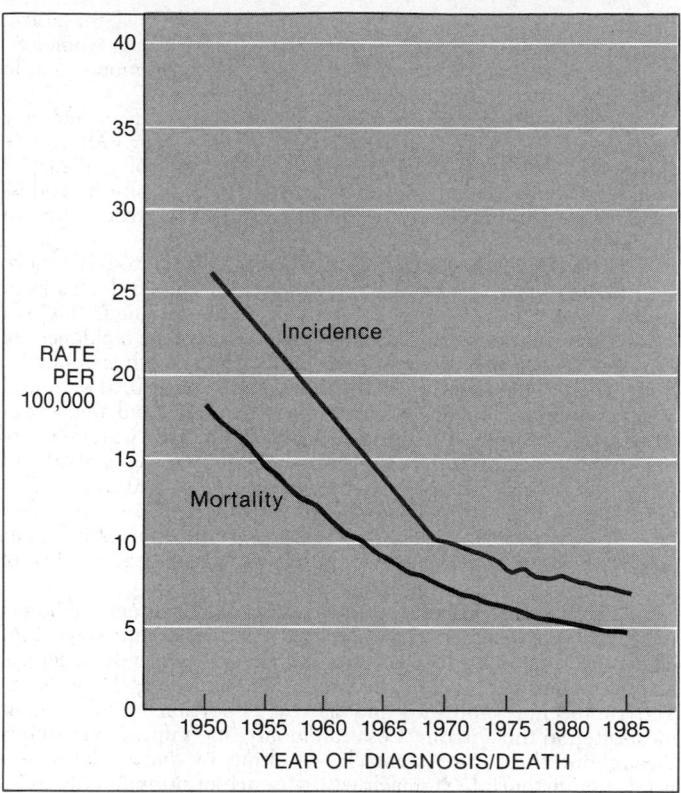

FIGURE 99–1. Incidence and mortality of gastric adenocarcinoma in the United States. (Data obtained and modified from the NCI Annual Cancer Statistics Review including Cancer Trends: 1950–1985 and is representative of the United States population.)

decrease in gastric cancer in the United States over the last few decades, but the nitrite hypothesis itself remains to be validated.

Blood group A is associated with a higher incidence of gastric cancer even in areas of the world where gastric cancer is rare. This fact and the threefold increase in gastric cancer among first-degree relatives, (parents, siblings, children) of gastric cancer patients has raised the possibility of an inherited or familial component.

Pernicious anemia had been considered a premalignant condition, but the prior high incidence of gastric cancer seen in this disease is no longer seen. This may be a reflection of the progressively decreasing incidence of gastric cancer being observed worldwide. Although atrophic gastritis is usually seen in association with gastric cancer, this disorder is extremely common, and the vast majority of such patients never develop cancer.

Adenomatous polyps of the stomach, especially those larger than 2 cm, may occasionally give rise to carcinoma. Most stomach polyps, however, are hyperplastic and do not become malignant.

Subtotal resection for benign disease results in chronic atrophic gastritis from either bile reflux or removal of the gastrin trophic factor. This has been shown to produce gastric cancer in animals. It has also been shown to result in gastric cancer after a 10-year

TABLE 99–1. DIETARY FINDINGS FROM CASE CONTROL STUDIES OF GASTRIC CANCER*

Positive Association	Negative Association
Salted fish	Vegetables
Pickled vegetables	Fruit
Salty foods	Milk
Smoked fish	Meat
Starchy foods	Squash
Cabbage, potatoes	Eggplant
Cooked cereals	Lettuce
Bacon	Celery
	Animal fat

*United States (including Hawaii), Japan, Norway, England, and Israel.

interval in persons living in countries at increased risk for gastric cancer, especially in men, who are at higher risk than women.

Immunologic deficiencies, particularly the common variable type, may cause a predisposition to gastric cancer.

Gastric ulcer does not transform into cancer. Cancer foci may be present in association with an ulcer, however. All gastric ulcers must be suspected of having small areas of malignancy even when the ulcer appears benign by radiography or endoscopy. Biopsy and cytologic examination reveal the true nature of the lesion.

INCIDENCE AND PREVALENCE. It is estimated that there were 20,000 new cases of gastric cancer and 14,000 deaths from gastric cancer in the United States in 1990. Although this is a substantial number, a dramatic decline in the incidence of stomach cancer has occurred here and in many other countries (Fig. 99–1). The magnitude of the decline varies. In the United States the age-adjusted mortality rate for males and females of all races decreased 25 per cent from 1973 to 1985. Carcinoma of the stomach occurs most frequently between the ages of 50 and 70 years and is rare in patients younger than 30 years. The incidence and mortality rise steeply with age. Rates are higher in males than females by 2 to 1. Risk of gastric cancer is higher among those of low socioeconomic status. The 5-year survival of 16 per cent has not changed in recent years.

PATHOLOGY. Carcinoma of the stomach is adenocarcinoma that usually is manifested pathologically in one of four ways (Fig. 99–2): (1) Most often it appears as a bulky mass with deep central ulceration projecting into the lumen and invading the wall. (2) The tumor may infiltrate and narrow a portion of the lumen, most often in the antrum. Less commonly, the infiltration extends throughout the entire stomach, resulting in *linitis plastica*—a fixed, nondistensible stomach with absence of normal folds and a narrowed lumen. (3) Polypoid or exophytic carcinoma with or without a stalk may occur and be difficult to distinguish from a benign polyp on radiograph. (4) More rarely, carcinoma of the stomach may occur as a superficially spreading tumor involving only the mucosal surface and producing a granular appearance. This is unlike linitis plastica, which extends through the entire thickness of the wall. *Early gastric cancer* is a term used to characterize very superficial cancer that is detected by screening radiography or endoscopy primarily in asymptomatic people. This has the same anatomic and male-female distribution as the more advanced stage. Prognosis is excellent even with lymph node involvement. It is commonly seen in Japan and rarely in the United States.

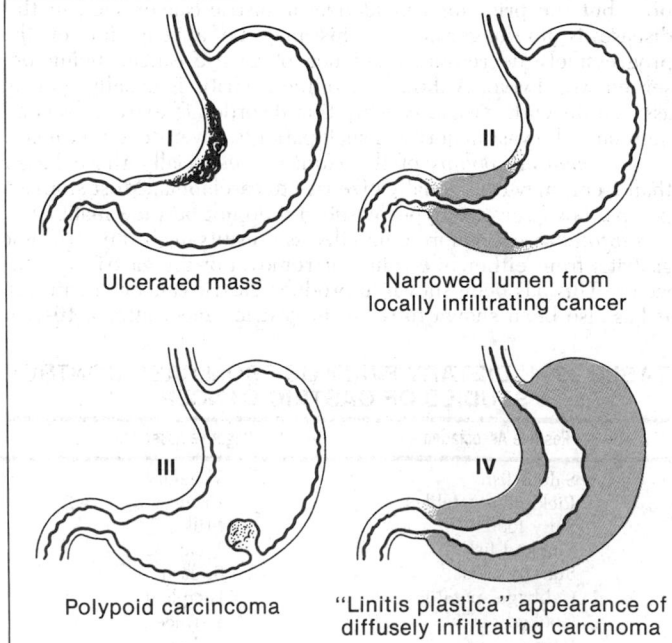

FIGURE 99–2. Diagrammatic representation of various presentations of gastric carcinoma.

(Figure labels:)
I — Ulcerated mass
II — Narrowed lumen from locally infiltrating cancer
III — Polypoid carcincoma
IV — "Linitis plastica" appearance of diffusely infiltrating carcinoma

TABLE 99–2. STAGING OF GASTRIC CANCER*

Stage		Tumor, Nodes, Metastasis
0	(T_{is}, N_0, M_0)	T_{is}—Limited to mucosa
I	(T_1, N_0, M_0)	T_1—Limited to mucosa and submucosa
II	$(T_{2,3}; N_0, M_0)$	T_2—To but not through serosa
		T_3—Through serosa but not adjacent structures
III	$(T_{4a}, N_0, M_0; T_{1-4}, N_{1-2}, M_0)$	T_{4a}—Through serosa and involves adjacent structures
		N_1—Perigastric nodes within 3 cm of tumor
		N_2—Perigastric nodes more than 3 cm from tumor (within celiac group)
IV	$(T_{4b}, N_{0-3}, M_0; T_{1-3}, N_3, M_0;$ Any T, Any N, $M_1)$	T_{4b}—Involves liver, diaphragm, pancreas, abdominal wall, retroperitoneum, small bowel, or duodenum via serosa
		N_3—Other intra-abdominal nodes (retroperitoneal, mesenteric, etc.)
		M_1—Distant metastasis

*From American Joint Committee on Cancer: Manual for Staging of Cancer. Philadelphia, J.B. Lippincott Company, 1983

Gastric carcinomas may be well-differentiated adenocarcinomas or may be so anaplastic as to resemble diffuse histiocytic lymphoma or sarcoma. A true carcinoma in situ is rarely found and is confined entirely to the glands (Table 99–2). This is more commonly seen at the surface of large adenomatous polyps of the stomach.

In about 75 per cent of patients with carcinoma of the stomach the tumors are found in the distal third. The lymphatic flow from such tumors is in the direction of the subpyloric nodes and porta hepatis and along both curvatures. The tumor very rarely spreads to the pancreaticolineal nodes, in contrast to proximal and mid-stomach lesions. Celiac and pancreatic nodal involvement occurs from lesions in all areas. In addition to invasion of lymph nodes, gastric carcinoma invades local structures: the lower end of the esophagus by submucosal spread, the pancreas, the transverse colon, the peritoneum, and, rarely, the duodenum. Hematogenous spread results in pulmonary, pleural, liver, brain, and bone metastases.

CLINICAL MANIFESTATIONS (Table 99–3). Early carcinoma of the stomach is frequently asymptomatic. *Anorexia* and *weight loss* are nonspecific symptoms and not well correlated with the size of the tumor. *Early satiety,* particularly with linitis plastica; *bloating; dysphagia; epigastric distress;* or more severe epigastric boring pain may be later symptoms. *Vomiting* is commonly a later symptom that may be caused by pyloric obstruction but may occur with other levels of obstruction. Vomiting also occurs without obstruction and may be secondary to the motility disturbance that a fixed mass in the wall produces. The pain is similar to that of peptic ulcer in about one fourth of patients, particularly when the tumor has ulcerated. In most patients, however, the pain usually occurs after eating and is not relieved by foods or antacids. Boring pain radiating to the back may indicate penetration of the tumor into the pancreas.

Dysphagia may occur with more proximal lesions, particularly

TABLE 99–3. ADENOCARCINOMA OF THE STOMACH

Associated With	Clinical Manifestations
Environment—geographical differences	Anorexia, early satiety, weight loss
Diet—? nitrosamines	Dysphagia, vomiting, weakness
Blood group A—genetic	Epigastric distress to severe, boring pain
Atrophic gastritis	Anemia, occult blood in stools
Adenomatous polyps (>2 cm)	Epigastric mass, signs of metastases
Subtotal resection for benign ulcer disease in high-risk countries	Rare—Virchow's node, Blumer's shelf, Trousseau's syndrome, acanthosis nigricans

when they have invaded the area around the cardioesophageal junction or spread submucosally to the esophagus, which is common in fundal lesions. Weakness and fatigue from *anemia* caused by chronic occult blood loss are common, although acute massive bleeding and hematemesis are unusual. Angina pectoris, congestive heart failure, and rarely cerebral ischemia may occur because of the anemia. Perforation occurs in a very small percentage of patients and can simulate peptic ulcer. When the tumor metastasizes, additional symptoms may include jaundice or right upper quadrant pain from liver metastases, cough from lung metastases, hiccups, and vague abdominal discomfort and bloating from peritoneal seeding and ascites.

Physical examination during the early stages of gastric carcinoma may be completely unremarkable. Later there may be signs of weight loss and anemia. When the tumor has disseminated, hepatomegaly from metastases, jaundice, or ascites may be present. Splenomegaly may occur if the portal or splenic vein is invaded. A palpable *epigastric mass* is present in less than one half of patients and usually, but not always, indicates extensive involvement. Rarely, left supraclavicular adenopathy (Virchow's node), a nodular perirectal wall (Blumer's shelf), or umbilical nodules give evidence of metastatic spread.

Several extragastric signs may precede the detection of an underlying malignancy. These include recurrent thrombophlebitis (Trousseau's syndrome); acanthosis nigricans, a verrucous, hyperpigmented, elevated skin lesion involving primarily the flexor spaces of the body; neuromyopathy characterized by localized sensory and/or motor disturbances; and profound central nervous system involvement with abrupt onset of confusion, memory defects, hostility, or ataxia. More detailed descriptions of the paraneoplastic syndromes are contained in specific chapters in Part XIII.

Laboratory studies usually disclose iron deficiency, or megaloblastic anemia if the tumor is associated with untreated pernicious anemia. *Occult blood in the stool* is present in less than half of the patients. Most patients have gastric acid present but in reduced amounts. A few have achlorhydria after maximal stimulation with pentagastrin. A few have hypersecretion, especially with antral tumors. Therefore the presence of acid does not ensure that carcinoma is not present. Abnormalities in liver function, particularly a markedly elevated alkaline phosphatase and 5'nucleotidase level, suggest liver metastases. Microangiopathic hemolytic anemia has been reported in several patients with gastric cancer. Rarely, protein-losing enteropathy occurs with ulcerated carcinomas of the stomach. Elevation of carcinoembryonic antigen is a late finding, usually in the presence of metastatic disease.

DIAGNOSIS. Roentgenologic Diagnosis. Most gastric cancers will be suspected on roentgenologic examination. The standard upper gastrointestinal series has been refined to include barium contrast studies capable of detecting very small lesions. With the gastric mucosa covered by a thin layer of barium and distended with air or gas, multiple projections are taken, which outline almost the entire stomach surface. Refinement of technique can be accomplished by using high-density barium, CO_2, simethicone for gas dispersion, and glucagon to induce gastroparesis. With such methods films showing fine detail may be produced and small mucosal lesions visualized.

The radiologist is usually able to define the characteristics of a benign versus malignant lesion and suggest a histologic diagnosis. For example, lymphoma of the stomach may be suspected by the extensive involvement, multiple shallow ulcerations, and giant rugal hypertrophy caused by infiltrative disease, and by the fact that the duodenum may be involved in the neoplastic process. A gastric ulcer often gives difficulty, but radiologic accuracy is in the range of 80 per cent. Characteristic radiographic signs that suggest a malignant lesion are the presence of an ulcer in a mass, irregular folds stopping short of the ulcer crater, and an irregular ulcer base. It is essential, however, to determine the nature of the ulcer by endoscopy with biopsy and cytology. Generally the location of an ulcer is not important in determining malignancy. Ulcers on the greater and lesser curvatures have about equal frequency of malignancy. Rigidity, loss of distensibility, unchanging contour, and irregular peristalsis are characteristic of a malignant lesion; when extensive infiltration from linitis plastica is present, a "leather bottle" appearance may result.

Endoscopy with Biopsy and Cytology. Fiberoptic endoscopy has increased the diagnostic yield over radiology alone. When combined with biopsy and brush cytology, the diagnostic accuracy is in the range of 95 to 99 per cent in various series. About one half of early gastric cancers present as small ulcerations; some have slight elevation or depression of the adjacent mucosa. The next most common type is a small polyp. Appearance at endoscopy may be misleading. Directed tissue sampling techniques, such as biopsy or brush cytology, should be used on any suspicious area, whether it is raised, depressed, or ulcerated. With more advanced carcinoma a specific tissue diagnosis can also be achieved with high accuracy by directed biopsy and cytology. Endoscopy is now being used also to stage and treat gastric cancer. Endoscopic ultrasonographic probes are highly accurate in evaluating depth of penetration of the cancer through the wall and extension to lymph nodes. This information can complement CT scans or standard ultrasonography in defining the extent of the tumor. The use of endoscopy to diagnose malignancies of the stomach is described in greater detail in Ch. 94.

TREATMENT. At present *surgery* provides the only satisfactory curative treatment for gastric cancer. The high frequency of regional node metastases plays a major role in the choice of the surgical procedure and the results of various therapeutic efforts. When the tumor is localized in the distal portion of the stomach, the omentum as well as nodes in the region of the porta hepatis and the pancreatic head are dissected, and a generous subtotal gastrectomy is performed. For tumors in the pars media and the proximal stomach, total gastrectomy may be indicated to obtain an adequate margin and for dissection of the predictable lymphatic spread in all directions. Distal pancreatectomy and splenectomy are usually necessary. There is little doubt that operative mortality is greater after total gastrectomy than after subtotal resection, and the procedure should be avoided whenever possible.

With extensive bleeding or obstruction, a palliative limited subtotal gastric resection can be done even in the presence of residual cancer. Palliative total gastrectomy should almost never be done. Resection of recurrent cancer in the gastric remnant may be of palliative value even when a cure is not obtained.

Chemotherapy is often suggested for unresectable gastric adenocarcinoma in an effort to decrease symptoms and prolong survival. The most widely used drug has been 5-fluorouracil (5FU), with an overall partial response rate of 15 to 20 per cent. Other agents such as mitomycin-C, doxorubicin (Adriamycin), and the various nitrosoureas have also been used as single agents with varying response. Combined use of several agents such as 5FU, doxorubicin, and mitomycin-C has resulted in some studies in a better response rate but has not improved survival.

Adjuvant chemotherapy following apparently curative surgery is an attractive concept for gastric carcinoma because of its high recurrence rate. Micrometastases are undoubtedly frequently present after surgery, and it has been postulated that chemotherapy might be most effective against such minimal disease. However, multiple trials with single agents have not shown success. Several trials using adjuvant chemotherapy with combinations of agents are in progress and may provide an answer to this very important question, although to date no effective adjuvant program has been demonstrated.

Radiation therapy is generally unsatisfactory, since gastric carcinomas are not very radiosensitive. Occasionally palliation may be obtained for persistent bleeding, obstruction, or pain. An occasional patient with inoperable gastric carcinoma has had prolonged survival with radiation therapy. Combining 5FU with radiation can provide a synergistic response.

Patients with gastrointestinal cancer frequently have complications associated with their disease or its treatment that require vigorous supportive treatment. Many aspects of the patients' general condition require consideration and treatment, including the management of infection; anemia; gastrointestinal bleeding; fluid and electrolyte loss secondary to vomiting, diarrhea, or fistula formation; disabling ascites; pain; and poor nutrition. Endoscopic laser treatment is also being evaluated as a palliative approach to keeping the lumen open in unoperated upon or recurrent cancer in order to maintain nutrition. Total parenteral nutrition is being utilized more frequently to supply the daily caloric requirement of patients with gastric cancer. Preoperative and postoperative use of this modality enables patients to withstand the rigors of surgery and to tolerate more effectively the postoperative period, including the use of chemotherapy.

PROGNOSIS. The 5-year survival rate depends upon whether or not adjacent lymph nodes contain cancer. The presence of perigastric lymph node metastases indicates a less than 15 per cent chance for survival. Early diagnosis plays a role in prognosis because a long period of time between the onset of cancer and its diagnosis favors lymphatic spread. In the Japanese studies, resection of gastric cancer limited to the mucosa and submucosa had a more than 80 per cent cure rate; when disease was limited to the mucosa, cure rate was 90 to 95 per cent. Linitis plastica and infiltrating lesions have a very poor prognosis compared with polypoid or exophytic disease.

PREVENTION. Until we learn more of the etiologic factors in gastric carcinoma we cannot practice primary prevention. We can only practice a limited degree of secondary prevention, i.e., detect the disease at an earlier stage in minimally symptomatic people in order to prevent its devastating consequences. The mass survey approach utilized in Japan is not practical in the United States because of the relatively low incidence of gastric cancer.

LYMPHOMA OF THE STOMACH (Ch. 147 and 148)

Primary lymphoma represents about 5 per cent of all primary malignant tumors of the stomach, and non-Hodgkin's lymphoma accounts for most of these. It is extremely rare for Hodgkin's disease (HD) to involve the stomach as a primary lesion. Patients with lymphoma are generally about a decade younger than those with carcinoma of the stomach, and males are affected more frequently. Pain is the most frequent symptom, and mild anemia is common, owing to gastrointestinal bleeding (which on occasion can be massive). A palpable mass is the most common presenting physical finding. Studies of maximal stimulation of gastric acid secretion have not been done in a large group of patients, but achlorhydria seems to be unusual. Secondary lymphoma involving the stomach is common in the course of disseminated lymphoma but is difficult to diagnose.

Lymphoma of the stomach frequently presents radiographically as a bulky mass and less frequently as a diffusely infiltrating tumor—the most common form of secondary lymphoma—giving the appearance of large folds on upper gastrointestinal series, frequently associated with multiple nodular defects and ulcerations. Lymphoma of the stomach often resembles superficially spreading carcinoma, linitis plastica, or solitary adenocarcinoma. Gastroscopy with directed biopsy and brush cytology gives a higher yield than was previously appreciated. Exophytic lesions provide a diagnosis in about 88 per cent of cases; the infiltrative type does not yield as high an accuracy.

Pseudolymphoma is a gastric lesion that may be confusing. This diffuse or discrete lesion is an atypical inflammatory response in the region of benign gastric ulcers. It is frequently difficult for the pathologist to differentiate pseudolymphoma from a true lymphoma.

In patients with lymphoma of the stomach there is a significant incidence of nontumorous lesions such as stress ulcer, hemorrhagic gastritis, and monilial gastritis. Therefore in such patients with upper gastrointestinal bleeding or other symptoms referable to the stomach, it is important that a careful diagnostic approach be undertaken to determine the possible nontumor cause of the sign or symptom.

Treatment of primary lymphoma of the stomach is usually surgical resection followed by 3600 to 4000 rads of radiotherapy, particularly if lymph nodes are involved. Some have advocated radiotherapy alone because of the marked sensitivity of lymphoma to radiation. If lymphoma involves the stomach secondarily, radiotherapy or chemotherapy or both are indicated. The 5-year survival following surgery for primary lymphoma of the stomach is in the range of 50 per cent for non-Hodgkin's lymphoma and less for HD, suggesting that HD is already disseminated when initially found in the stomach. The best prognosis for primary tumors occurs with small lesions confined to the stomach, differentiated into tumor follicles without lymph node involvement and with only superficial infiltration of the wall.

OTHER MALIGNANT TUMORS OF THE STOMACH

Leiomyosarcoma of the stomach represents about 1 per cent of gastric cancers and may present with a large intramural mass with central ulceration. Systemic symptoms are minimal, but massive bleeding or a palpable mass of which the patient is aware may be the presenting complaints. The tumor may be slow growing; 5-year survival following resection is in the range of 50 per cent. Metastases to the liver and nodes are common, but these patients have a better prognosis than those with other metastatic tumors. Liposarcoma, fibrosarcoma, myxosarcoma, and neurogenic sarcoma are extremely rare and present with symptoms similar to those of leiomyosarcoma. Neurogenic sarcoma can be associated with von Recklinghausen's disease.

Metastatic disease to the stomach from other sites is not common but may simulate primary gastric cancer. Malignant melanoma and breast and lung carcinomas are the most frequent offenders. In breast cancer the metastatic lesions may be ulcerative, of linitis plastica type, or polypoid.

LEIOMYOMAS AND BENIGN TUMORS

Leiomyomas are commonly found at postmortem examination but are rarely of clinical significance. They occur equally in men and women, and are usually found in the midportion and antrum of the stomach. They may grow toward the mucosa, encroach on the lumen, and cause mucosal effacement and secondary ulceration. They may grow in the direction of the serosa, producing a mass that is predominantly extrinsic. Simultaneous inward and outward growth results in a dumbbell shape. These features are also characteristic of leiomyosarcomas, and differentiation on radiography or gastroscopy is difficult. Bleeding is common and epigastric pain may simulate peptic ulcer disease. On roentgen examination the findings are usually an intramural filling defect with or without secondary ulceration. Gastroscopic examination reveals effaced but normal mucosa overlying the mass. Central ulceration may be seen.

Asymptomatic leiomyomas need not be removed while symptomatic lesions are excised locally.

Neurofibroma occasionally associated with von Recklinghausen's disease, neuroma, lymphangioma, ganglioneuroma, lipoma, carcinoid, and hamartoma associated with Peutz-Jeghers syndrome all may involve the stomach. About 10 per cent of hamartomas of the stomach and duodenum in Peutz-Jeghers syndrome become malignant.

ADENOMAS

Adenomas of the stomach are relatively rare lesions. Most polyps of the stomach are hyperplastic, not neoplastic, and do not become malignant. Adenomatous polyps are the usual neoplastic type of polyp. These are more frequent in men than in women and are generally seen in patients over 50. Patients with familial adenomatous polyposis or Gardner's syndrome (Ch. 105) have a 30 per cent probability of having polyps in the upper gastrointestinal tract. These are usually hyperplastic in the stomach and adenomatous in the duodenum. Patients with Peutz-Jeghers syndrome occasionally have similar findings. Bleeding, dyspepsia, and nausea are the most common symptoms, but most patients are asymptomatic. The diagnosis may be strongly suspected when a rounded smooth defect in the stomach on upper gastrointestinal series or a mass covered by mucosa with or without a stalk is detected by radiograph or endoscopy.

The size of polyps strongly influences management. It is rare for a polyp under 2 cm to show malignant change. In view of their potential for malignancy (present and future), polyps larger than 2 cm or polyps of any size causing significant symptoms should be removed. Pedunculated polyps can now be safely removed by cautery-snare technique through the fiberoptic endoscope. For sessile polyps more than 2 cm in diameter, a segmental gastric resection may be necessary. If carcinoma is diagnosed histologically at the time of surgery, subtotal gastric resection should be done. Multiple gastric polyps are usually hyperplastic and of no significance.

TUMORS OF THE DUODENUM

Adenocarcinoma of the duodenum is rare but is more common than lymphoma, which, in turn, arises more commonly in the jejunum and ileum. The second and third portions of the duodenum are the usual sites of adenocarcinoma except when associated with Crohn's disease, in which it is in the ileum. Cancer in the duodenal bulb is exceedingly rare. Adenocarcinoma of the duodenum more frequently affects men and develops at a younger age than carcinoma of the stomach or colon. The tumor tends to grow into the lumen or to invade the wall of the duodenum. Cramping abdominal pain, anorexia, weight loss, vomiting, and melena are common. Jaundice or fever may result from obstruction of the ampulla of Vater or the common bile duct when the carcinoma involves the second portion of the duodenum. The tumor may simulate benign postbulbar ulceration. The diagnosis is usually made by radiologic examination and confirmed by endoscopy. Pancreaticoduodenectomy is necessary. Five-year survival ranges between 4 and 15 per cent.

Lymphoma, leiomyosarcoma, carcinoid, metastatic cancer, and benign tumors may involve the duodenum, and these are discussed in more detail in Ch. 105. In general, these lesions are manifested as an intramural and submucosal mass with the exception of lymphoma and metastatic cancer, which frequently are exophytic and ulcerate. Any tumor, benign or malignant, may occur in a diverticulum at the descending portion of the duodenum. Aberrant pancreatic tissue may produce a submucosal filling defect in the duodenum, which may resemble a neoplastic lesion. Also, hyperplasia or adenoma of Brunner's glands may produce multiple polypoid defects in the duodenal bulb and is frequently associated with hypersecretion, duodenal ulcer and, rarely, Zollinger-Ellison syndrome. A prominent ampulla of Vater may resemble a neoplastic lesion radiographically. Endoscopy may be necessary to clarify the situation.

Brooks JJ, Enterline HT: Primary gastric lymphomas. A clinicopathologic study of 58 cases with long-term follow-up and literature review. Cancer 51:701, 1983. *A large series of primary gastric lymphomas with long-term follow-up (average 12.8 years). Five- and 10-year survival rates were 57 and 46 per cent, respectively. Statistically significant prognostic variables were smaller tumor size, superficial mural invasion (submucosal only), and pathologic stage 1 disease.*

Fleischer D, Sivak MV: Endoscopic Nd:YAG laser therapy as palliative treatment for advanced adenocarcinoma of the gastric cardia. Gastroenterology 87:815, 1984. *Endoscopy has taken on therapeutic potential for palliative treatment of gastric cancer with lasers, especially in the relief of obstruction at the gastroesophageal junction.*

Kurtz RC, Lightdale CJ, Winawer SJ, et al.: Endoscopy and gastrointestinal neoplasm: Diagnosis and management. Curr Probl Cancer 5:4, 1980. *This monograph describes the techniques and applications of endoscopy in patients with cancer of the gastrointestinal tract, including the stomach.*

Lawrence W Jr.: Gastric cancer. CA 36:5, 1986. *This monograph reviews the status of epidemiology, etiology, staging, pathology, and prognosis from a clinician's point of view.*

Le Chevalier T, Smith FP, Harter WK, et al.: Chemotherapy and combined modality therapy for locally advanced and metastatic gastric carcinoma. Semin Oncol 12:46, 1985. *An overview of therapeutic results. Response rates are still disappointing, and combination protocols have not as yet been dramatically better.*

Lightdale CJ, Botet JF, Kelsen DP, et al.: Diagnosis of recurrent upper gastrointestinal cancer at the surgical anastomosis by endoscopic ultrasound. Gastrointest Endosc 35:407, 1989. *The fiberoptic endoscope has advanced from solely a diagnostic instrument to one that has the capability of staging. Incorporation of an ultrasonographic probe into the scope now permits the endoscopist to see beyond the mucosal surface.*

Nomura A: Stomach. In Schottenfeld D, Fraumeni Jr. (eds.): Cancer Epidemiology and Prevention. Philadelphia, W. B. Saunders Company, 1982, pp 624–637. *A comprehensive dissertation on all aspects of gastric cancer from a worldwide epidemiologic point of view.*

O'Brien MJ, Burakoff R, Robbins EA, et al.: Early gastric cancer, clinicopathologic study. Am J Med 78:195, 1985. *Early gastric cancer as seen in United States patients is discussed. The disease is not seen often in the United States because of late diagnosis but is the same disease as early gastric cancer seen in Japan.*

Schafer LW, Larson DE, Melton LJ, et al.: Risk of development of gastric carcinoma in patients with pernicious anemia: A population-based study in Rochester, Minnesota. Mayo Clin Proc 60:444, 1985. *This study demonstrates the present lack of significant risk of gastric cancer in patients with pernicious anemia. The prior association was probably related to the higher incidence of gastric cancer worldwide. The risk for gastric cancer is no longer being expressed in this population.*

Shiu MH, Karas M, Nisce LZ, et al.: Management of primary gastric lymphoma. Ann Surg 195:196, 1982. *The surgical management of primary gastric lymphoma is presented in this paper and put into clinical perspective.*

Shiu MH, Moore E, Sanders M, et al.: Influence of the extent of resection on survival after curative treatment of gastric carcinoma. Arch Surg 122:1347, 1987. *Surgery varies with the size and location of the gastric cancer. This paper presents data and concepts underlying a rational operative approach to patients.*

Sonenberg A: Endoscopic screening for gastric stump cancer—would it be beneficial? Gastroenterology 87:489, 1984. *This paper provides a good perspective as well as a useful review of literature. Gastric stump cancer is a real entity but*

is expressed primarily in individuals living in countries at high risk for gastric cancer.

Winawer SJ, Posner G, Lightdale CJ, et al.: Endoscopic diagnosis of advanced gastric cancer. Factors influencing yield. Gastroenterology 69:1183, 1975. *Diagnostic yield was higher for exophytic lesions than for infiltrative tumor, and directed brush cytology alone was more productive than directed biopsy alone. Combination of infiltrative character and location in antrum or cardia often resulted in nondiagnostic biopsy and cytology specimens.*

100 Disorders of Gastrointestinal Motility

William J. Snape, Jr.

NORMAL MOTILITY IN STOMACH, SMALL INTESTINE, AND COLON

Motility of the gastrointestinal tract regulates the orderly movement of ingested material through the gut to ensure adequate absorption of nutrients, electrolytes, and fluid. Transit of intraluminal contents through the stomach, small intestine, and colon depends on the coordination of regional control of intraluminal pressure. Sphincters, interposed at several discrete areas along the length of the bowel, not only regulate the forward movement of intraluminal contents but impede the retrograde flow of intestinal contents. Unlike in the esophagus, external physical forces such as gravity have little impact on the movement of gastrointestinal intraluminal contents. Coordinated gastrointestinal motility depends on neural and hormonal control of sphincter, longitudinal, and circular smooth muscle contraction and relaxation.

SMOOTH MUSCLE. Changes in tension of the smooth muscle wall control regional intraluminal pressures, which in return regulate movement of intraluminal contents through the bowel. Movement of luminal contents from the stomach to the distal colon requires coordination between phasic and tonic contractions and relaxation of the intrinsic smooth muscle tone (peristaltic reflex), since luminal contents move from a high-pressure zone to a lower one. Differences in the physiologic control of contraction or relaxation of the muscle in each region determine the local pressure gradients. Myoelectric activity, including slow waves and spike potentials, coordinates regional intestinal smooth muscle contractions by controlling their frequency and by electrically linking neighboring smooth muscle cells (Fig. 100–1). The slow wave is a cyclic change in membrane potential that

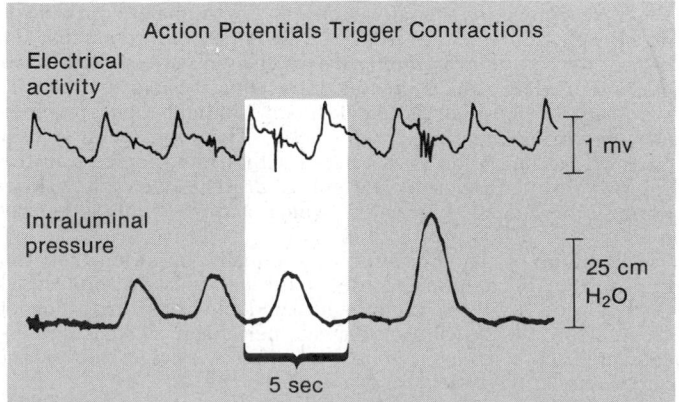

FIGURE 100–1. Simultaneous electrical and mechanical activity in the canine jejunum. The electrical signal was recorded from an extracellular electrode in the tunica muscularis; it shows a regular cycle of depolarization-repolarization at 12 to 14 cycles per minute. Superimposed on some of these cycles (basic electrical rhythm, slow wave, or pace-setter potential) are more rapid oscillations (fast waves, spikes). When spiking occurs, the smooth muscle contracts, causing intraluminal pressure to rise (lower tracing).

occurs in smooth muscle from the stomach, small bowel, and colon. The slow wave frequency of a smooth muscle cell is intrinsic to the cell, but it can be modified by the activity in neighboring cells. A pacemaker region sets the dominant frequency of each region of the gastrointestinal tract. Calcium influx during spike potentials, superimposed upon the slow waves, results in smooth muscle cell contraction.

Tight electrical coupling of gastric smooth muscle cells is responsible for progressive propagation of the slow waves, oral to caudal, along the proximal to distal slow wave gradient. Therefore, without a change in the slow wave frequency, contractions also propagate in an oral to caudal direction. In the small intestine and colon, in addition to tight intercellular coupling, regional differences in slow wave and contraction frequency maintain the forward movement of intraluminal contents. A higher contraction frequency elevates mean pressure, stimulating movement of intraluminal contents distally into the lower pressure area. Higher intraluminal pressure in the descending colon creates a pressure gradient that regulates the movement of intraluminal contents back to the transverse colon and forward to the sigmoid colon. Therefore, a pressure amplitude gradient, rather than a frequency gradient, determines colonic transit. In the colon the dominance of contractions in the proximal descending colon and splenic flexure mixes the intraluminal contents and is responsible for a storage area in the transverse colon. Another motility pattern, the propagating contraction, is under neural control and propagates the fecal content distally from the transverse colon for further storage in the sigmoid colon.

Circular and longitudinal muscles have different functions. Throughout the gut, circular contractions segment the lumen, mixing the contents to expose the mucosa to continually different contents. The longitudinal muscle shortens the bowel, moving intraluminal contents forward.

Sphincters are high-pressure zones interposed through the gastrointestinal tract. The upper esophageal and external anal sphincters are localized bands of skeletal muscle. The lower esophageal sphincter is not an anatomically distinct structure; in contrast, the pylorus is a localized collection of smooth muscle. The ileocecal valve, a valvelike structure separating the colon and the ileum, responds like a sphincter. The internal anal sphincter is a localized collection of circular smooth muscle surrounded by the external anal sphincter. Contraction or relaxation of the sphincters is controlled by enteric neurotransmitters or by circulating peptide hormones, in response to changes in pressure in the surrounding bowel or physiologic stimuli, such as eating or emotional stress. In general, proximal distention relaxes all sphincters; distal distention contracts sphincters.

Contraction of gastrointestinal smooth muscle requires an increase in the intracellular calcium concentration. Regulation of intracellular calcium begins at the smooth muscle cell membrane. When receptors are activated, inositol triphosphate is produced, which releases calcium from the sarcoplasmic reticulum, or voltage- or receptor-operated calcium channels are opened. Each of these mechanisms increases intracellular calcium, which is necessary for phosphorylation of the myosin light chain, required for cross-bridge formation with actin. The rapid actin-myosin cross-bridge formation is associated with a rapid increase in the velocity of smooth muscle shortening. Cross-bridge cycling slows during a prolonged contraction, which conserves muscle energy use.

Relaxation of smooth muscle is equally important for the transport of intraluminal contents through the gastrointestinal tract. Cyclic AMP production, initiated by ligand activation of receptors on the smooth muscle cell membrane, decreases intracellular calcium concentration by initiating calcium movement into sarcoplasmic reticulum or out of the cell.

Enteric Nervous System. Enteric neurons contain many different excitatory and inhibitory neurotransmitters (Table 100–1). Many nerve cells release more than one neurotransmitter upon stimulation. The complex interaction among inhibitory and excitatory neurotransmitters coordinates bowel activity. Although some neurotransmitters are generally stimulating (e.g., acetylcholine) and others inhibitory (e.g., vasoactive inhibitory polypeptide [VIP]), some neurotransmitters may control the motility pattern through different effects on nerve and muscle (opiates

TABLE 100–1. ENTERIC NEUROTRANSMITTERS AFFECTING GASTROINTESTINAL MOTILITY

Excitatory	Inhibitory
Acetylcholine	Vasoactive intestinal polypeptide (VIP)
Neurokinins	Calcitonin gene-related peptide
Gastrin-releasing peptide	Adenosine triphosphate
Neurotensin	Neurotensin
Enkephalin	Enkephalin
Cholecystokinin	Somatostatin
5-Hydroxytryptamine	Neuropeptide Y

stimulate muscle and inhibit acetylcholine release) or by different regional effects (neurotensin relaxes gastric muscle and stimulates small intestinal and colonic muscles). In addition to the efferent neurons, afferent neurons provide important signals for control of the motility through relaying sensations from one region of the gut to other regions or to the central nervous system (CNS).

The intrinsic enteric neurons of the gastrointestinal tract have numerous interconnections (Fig. 100–2). Input comes from the CNS, internuncial neurons, and interaction with afferent neurons via the prevertebral ganglia. Sympathetic and cholinergic fibers, which originate in the CNS and travel in the vagus, splanchnic, lumbar colonic, or sacral nerves, regulate the output of neurotransmitters from the myenteric plexus. Control of the myenteric plexus is mediated by intestinal afferent neurons and CNS neurons, interacting in the celiac, superior mesenteric, and inferior mesenteric ganglia. The interaction of interneurons within the myenteric plexus controls neural output to the gut. Each site of neural interconnection may be a potential target for future therapeutic intervention.

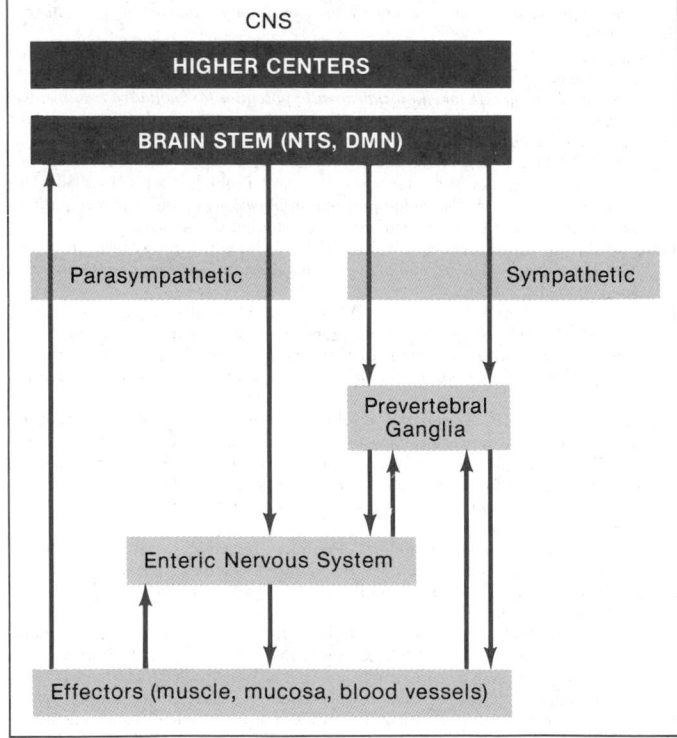

FIGURE 100–2. Schematic diagram showing control levels for neural regulation of gastrointestinal effector function. The enteric nervous system integrates information from the periphery and the central nervous system and modulates effector function. In prevertebral ganglia, afferent inputs from the gut and descending inputs through the sympathetic branch of the autonomic nervous system are integrated into output that has primarily inhibitory effects on gut motility. Autonomic nuclei of sympathetic and parasympathetic nerves located in the brain stem integrate inputs from the periphery and the cortex. Output reaches the gut via the parasympathetic and sympathetic nerves. NTS = Nucleus tractus solitarius; DMN = dorsal motor nucleus. (Adapted from Mayer EA, Raybould H: Role of neural control in gastrointestinal motility and visceral pain. *In* Snape WJ Jr. [ed.]: Pathogenesis of Functional Bowel Disease. New York, Plenum Medical Book Company, 1989, pp 13–35.)

Enteric Peptide Hormones. Peptides, released from the gastrointestinal mucosa into the blood after eating, act as hormones and affect gastric, small intestinal, and colonic smooth muscle contractions. As in the enteric nervous system, a counterbalance between stimulating peptides (gastrin, cholecystokinin, and motilin) and inhibitory peptides (enteroglucagon and peptide yy) controls motility. Further flexibility is gained in the peptide hormone modulation of motility by regional variation in response to a peptide (e.g., cholecystokinin stimulates gallbladder emptying and inhibits gastric emptying). Blood levels of the enteric hormonal peptides reach their maximum approximately 30 to 60 minutes after eating. In contrast to the enteric neurotransmitters, which affect motility soon after the stimulus does, the hormones may mediate a delayed gastrointestinal response to eating.

In summary, the neurohumoral control of gastrointestinal smooth muscle involves interactions among the CNS, local neural reflexes, and circulating hormones. This control mechanism modulates smooth muscle contraction and regulates the coordinated movement of intraluminal contents through the entire gastrointestinal tract.

Gastrointestinal Transit. Regulated smooth muscle contractions result in coordinated changes in gut intraluminal pressure, which controls the transit of chyme through the gastrointestinal tract. Each of the major sections of the gastrointestinal tract has a specific function that requires a different transit pattern. Different transit patterns exist during fasting and after eating. Eating ends the fasting motility pattern and initiates a postprandial transit pattern in each segment of the alimentary tract. Emotional stress and physical exercise modulate these patterns but are not the primary controls.

Stomach. As an initial response to eating, the proximal stomach relaxes to accommodate the volume of a meal. The distal stomach grinds the masticated chunks of food to less than 1-mm diameter and regulates the delivery of the processed gastric contents to the intestine synchronous with the release of digestive enzymes. Gastric emptying adjusts to the different physical and chemical characteristics of the food. Emptying of liquids is faster ($T_{1/2}$ = 6 to 12 min) than that of solids ($T_{1/2}$ = 45 to 70 min). Specific chemoreceptors regulate gastric emptying of different substances. Gastric emptying of glucose solutions is regulated so that approximately 2 kcal of glucose is emptied per minute; an equiosmolar solution of saline empties more rapidly. The gastric fundal tone regulates liquid emptying, whereas antral contractions control the rate of solid food emptying. Therefore, the stomach prepares as well as transports the gastric contents.

Small Intestine. The small intestine slowly moves the chyme distally, which allows mixing of the contents with digestive enzymes and absorption of the nutrients, electrolytes, and water. The transit time for material to move through the small intestine and appear in the cecum is approximately 40 to 180 minutes. In addition to controlling the distal transit of nutrients, the small intestine must clear the extruded dead cells and bacteria. The migrating motor complex (MMC) (Fig. 100–3), which occurs during fasting, removes these indigestible luminal contents. The MMC consists of three different phases: Phase 1 is a period of inactivity; phase 2 is a period of intermittent phasic contractions similar to the postprandial pattern; and phase 3 is a continuous period of contractions, which are at the slow wave frequency indigenous for that region of the bowel. The entire complex migrates from the stomach to the ileum. Phase 3 propels the intestinal contents that remain during fasting.

Colon. Regulation of colonic transit allows the colon to absorb additional water and electrolytes and to store the fecal waste for elimination. Eating stimulates aborad and orad movement of luminal contents. This back and forth shuttling mixes the luminal contents and allows greater time for absorption by the colonic mucosa. The transverse and rectosigmoid colons are separate sites of storage. Propagating contractions transport the luminal contents distally and appear necessary for normal bowel movements. The transit time is approximately 40 to 80 hours for excretion of one-half of the colonic content.

CLINICAL ASSESSMENT OF GASTROINTESTINAL MOTILITY

HISTORY AND CLINICAL EXAMINATION. Although symptoms can originate from disturbances of any part of the gastrointestinal tract, particular symptoms may suggest dysfunction of a specific site. In motility disturbances of each of the distinct organs (stomach, small intestine, colon), cramping abdominal pain occurs frequently, often after eating. The location of the pain can indicate the most likely source—epigastric for stomach, periumbilical or generalized for small intestine, or lower quadrants for the colon. In fact, pain referred from the anatomic location of the colon may occur in any of the abdominal quadrants. Colonic pain resolves after a bowel movement or passing flatus.

Early satiety or postprandial vomiting occurs in patients with delayed transit through the stomach and upper small bowel. Both symptoms can also result from organic nonmotility disorders (e.g., gastritis), which are not discussed in this chapter. Because receptive relaxation of the stomach is usually intact, postprandial vomiting secondary to obstruction of the gastric outlet is characteristically voluminous and may not occur until after eating several meals. When disturbed motility causes either symptom, the pathophysiologic defect may be secondary to reduced receptive relaxation, a low threshold for sensory nerve recognition of gastric distention, or uncoordinated antroduodenal contractions. Rapid gastric emptying causes symptoms of the "dumping syndrome," which include sweating, weakness, occasional orthostasis, tachycardia, and diarrhea (Ch. 98.5).

If massive gastric retention (>750 ml) is present, findings include a soft mass in the left upper quadrant. In a fasting patient, recovery of more than 150 ml of gastric contents via nasogastric tube, especially if old food is present, suggests gastric retention. An abdominal radiograph shows a large fluid-filled viscus in the left upper quadrant. If the patient is vomiting acutely, nasogastric suction should be initiated for therapy, and the hypovolemia and metabolic alkalosis should be treated.

Intestinal pseudo-obstruction may present with symptoms that are difficult to differentiate from those of true obstruction. Abdominal distention and pain occur in both anatomic and functional disorders of the gastrointestinal tract. Distention is an objective physical sign in patients with pseudo-obstruction, but in patients with the irritable bowel syndrome, the sensation of bloating may be secondary to a defect in sensory recognition. Tightly fitting clothes are uncomfortable to these patients. There is no increase in bowel gas in patients with the irritable bowel syndrome complaining of abdominal bloating.

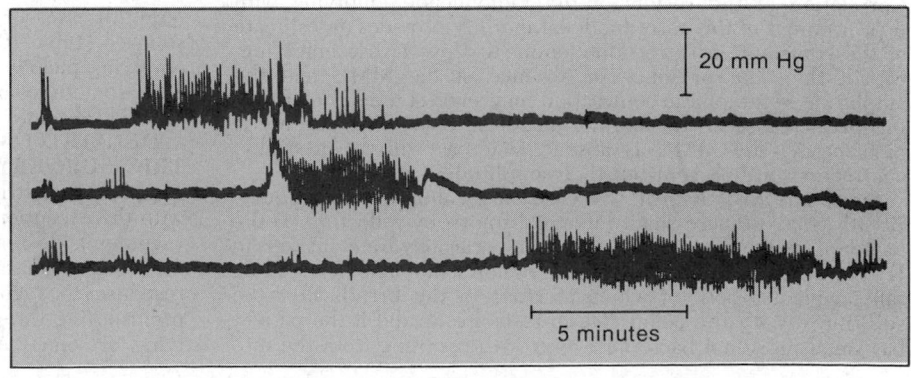

FIGURE 100–3. The activity front of the interdigestive motor complex is characterized on manometric tracings by a burst of rhythmic contraction waves that progress down the intestine. The top tracing is in the distal duodenum. The pressure ports are 25 cm apart. (From VanTrappen G, Janssen SJ, Hellmans J, et al.: The interdigestive motor complex of normal subjects and patients with bacterial overgrowth of the small intestine. J Clin Invest 59:1158, 1977, by copyright permission of the American Society for Clinical Investigation.)

20 mm Hg

5 minutes

Bowel sounds are loud with high-pitched rushes in patients with obstruction. If the obstruction has been present a long time, the bowel sounds are quieter or absent. In acute ileus or pseudo-obstruction the bowel sounds are quiet but usually present. If the ileus is associated with a severe abdominal insult, such as peritonitis or surgery, the bowel sounds are absent.

Vomiting is a common symptom of intestinal pseudo-obstruction, acute ileus, and a high anatomic obstruction. If the obstruction is in the distal small intestine, distention is a more prominent complaint than vomiting. In distal obstructions the vomitus, when present, has a feculent odor. An abdominal radiograph usually shows a cut-off between dilated and nondilated bowel in a true obstruction. In acute ileus or pseudo-obstruction the bowel is dilated throughout, with air visible in the rectum.

Alterations in bowel habit (diarrhea or constipation) are the cardinal symptoms of motor disorders of the gastrointestinal tract, but they do not specifically identify the pattern of motility. In the absence of a defect in mucosal absorption, diarrhea results from more rapid transit of intestinal contents through either the small intestine or the colon (Ch. 101). The mechanism of rapid transit through the small intestine is unclear, but diarrhea due to altered colonic motility is associated with an increased frequency of propagating contractions. Constipation generally results from slow colonic transit due to either colonic inertia or increased segmenting contractions, which impede the forward movement of the intraluminal contents. Propagating contractions are markedly decreased or absent in patients with constipation.

The frequency, character, and volume of bowel movements should be carefully defined in each patient. More than three bowel movements a day defines excessive frequency. Stool volume is increased in small bowel–mediated diarrhea, whereas low-volume stools result from disordered colonic motility. Stools may vary in consistency from liquid to merely soft. Constipation is defined as fewer than three bowel movements each week. The constipated stool generally has a lower volume (weight) and is firmer than normal stools, since more water has been absorbed. These strict definitions may exclude the patient complaining of constipation who has stools of normal size and consistency but who strains to defecate. The patient who has only increased straining may have a functional anal outlet obstruction.

MOTILITY TESTS. Regional differences in anatomy and physiologic controls in the gastrointestinal tract require distinct procedures to measure motility and transit. In addition to identifying the motility disturbance responsible for the patient's symptoms, standardized motility tests allow objective assessment of response to treatment.

Gastric emptying of liquids and solids must be measured independently to provide a full description of the organ's function. Gastric emptying is best assessed using standardized measurements of the respective emptying rates of liquids and solids. These measurements can be performed simultaneously using different radionuclides to tag the liquid and the solid phases. The bedside assessment of the gastric transit of a bolus of isotonic saline may be a useful and inexpensive screening test. After a period of 30 minutes, the residual should be less than 40 per cent of an oral volume of 750 ml administered. Estimation of gastric emptying from an upper gastrointestinal barium study often does not provide useful information. Changes in gastric fundic pressure can be measured by placing a large balloon in the fundus and measuring the tone before and after a meal. Correlation of the results of the radionuclide emptying with measurement of the antroduodenal motility provides an estimate of the contribution of the duodenum to slow gastric emptying. In addition, the presence or absence of the MMC and the amplitude of the phasic contraction may suggest a neuropathic or myopathic cause of the motility disorder. Thus, with an enteric neuropathy, the MMC is absent, whereas with a myopathy, contractions are present but their amplitude is decreased.

Small intestinal transit is measured by different techniques. Breath tests estimate small intestinal transit by reflecting (1) the bacterial metabolism of nonabsorbable carbohydrate marker to H_2, or (2) the bacterial release of a radionuclide label from a bile salt conjugate, both of which increase in the breath after the substrates reach the colon. These tests are invalid if the patient has small intestinal bacterial overgrowth resulting from the mo-

tility dysfunction or a blind loop of intestine, since the bacteria release the marker proximal to the ileocecal valve. The appearance in the right lower quadrant (cecum) of a radionuclide-labeled nonabsorbable marker ingested with a meal also provides an estimate of small intestinal transit. Measurement of intraluminal pressures in the small intestine may document abnormalities in the fasting MMC and the postprandial motility response. As in the stomach, concomitant use of transit and manometric studies allows the contribution of the enteric nerves and smooth muscle to the motility disorder to be estimated objectively.

Global colonic transit can be easily measured by orally administering radiopaque markers and measuring the distribution of the markers throughout the colon 5 days later. If no markers are then present within the colon, the patient probably is not constipated. In the constipated patient the localization of the markers to the rectosigmoid region suggests that the patient has a rectoanal outlet dysfunction. If the markers are distributed throughout the colon, there is a colonic motility disturbance. Regional emptying times can be calculated from this test. Once the motility defect has been localized to the colon, more specific transit and motility tests, measuring increases in intraluminal pressure and segment transit times with radionuclide markers, are available in specialized centers. The absence of a postprandial increase in segmenting contractions suggests a neural lesion, whereas low amplitude postprandial contraction suggests a disturbed smooth muscle function. Anorectal manometry shows whether the anal sphincter contributes to outlet dysfunction. The internal anal sphincter relaxes and the external anal sphincter contracts after the rectum is distended. If this spinal reflex is absent, an abnormality of the enteric neurons controlling the internal anal sphincter is suggested.

Cohen S, Snape WJ Jr.: Movement of the small and large intestine. *In* Sleisenger MH, Fordtran JS (eds.): Gastrointestinal Disease: Pathophysiology, Diagnosis, Management. 4th ed. Philadelphia, W. B. Saunders Company, 1989, pp 1088–1105. *Complete review of associations between alteration in physiology and presentation of small intestinal and colonic disease.*

Meyer JH: Motility of the stomach and gastroduodenal junction. *In* Johnson LR (ed.): Physiology of the Gastrointestinal Tract. 2nd ed. New York, Raven Press, 1987, pp 613–630. *Comprehensive review of physiology of the region; contains all major references and basic mechanism.*

Sarna SK, Otterson MF: Small intestinal physiology and pathophysiology. Gastroenterol Clin North Am 18:375, 1989. *Excellent review of pathophysiology of intestinal motility disorders.*

Szurszewski JH: Electrophysiological basis of gastrointestinal motility. *In* Johnson LR (ed.): Physiology of the Gastrointestinal Tract. 2nd ed. New York, Raven Press, 1987, pp 383–422. *Comprehensive review of physiology of the region; contains all major references and basic mechanism.*

DISORDERS OF GASTRODUODENAL MOTILITY

Delayed Gastric Emptying

Delayed gastric emptying is a more frequent source of symptoms than is excessively rapid emptying. The only significant cause of excessively rapid emptying, resulting in the "dumping syndrome," is partial gastric resection, the incidence of which is decreasing as the indications for gastric surgery diminish (Ch. 98.5). Chronic delayed gastric emptying (gastroparesis) is caused most often by an intrinsic disturbance in gastric or upper gastrointestinal motility and requires specific therapy of the underlying neuromuscular disorder. Acute gastroparesis, which is most frequently associated with an electrolyte disturbance, ketoacidosis, systemic infection, or an acute abdominal insult, is managed by treating the underlying disease, not the gastric motility disorder.

Delayed gastric emptying may be associated with other systemic diseases or may be due to a primary dysfunction of the stomach (Table 100–2). The typical symptoms of delayed gastric emptying include early satiety, nausea, and vomiting. Phytobezoars sometimes occur in these patients as well, especially if the MMC is absent.

DELAYED GASTRIC EMPTYING COMPLICATING GASTRIC SURGERY. Delayed gastric emptying not infrequently complicates gastric surgery for peptic ulcer disease. Vagotomy, with the exception of the highly selective vagotomy (parietal cell vagotomy), decreases fundic relaxation, antral contractions, and coordinated relaxation of the pylorus. The expected physiologic response to vagotomy is rapid emptying of liquids, possibly predisposing the patient to dumping syndrome, and slow emptying of solids. Although most often patients have no gastric

Delayed gastric emptying
Postvagotomy
Diabetes mellitus
Viral infections
Reflux esophagitis
Brain stem lesions
Anorexia nervosa
Tachygastria

Rapid gastric emptying
Dumping syndrome
Pancreatic insufficiency
Celiac sprue
Zollinger-Ellison syndrome
Duodenal ulcer

symptoms following abdominal vagotomy, approximately 5 to 10 per cent have delayed gastric emptying. This complication is more likely to occur if the patient had gastric outlet obstruction due to his or her primary disease. Antral contractions are poorly coordinated owing to irregular antral slow wave activity. Gastric MMC activity is often absent, although intestinal MMC remains normal.

Metoclopramide, a putative dopamine receptor antagonist, improves symptoms in many patients with delayed gastric emptying after a vagotomy. The usual dose of metoclopramide (10 mg orally, four times a day) causes anxiety, fatigue, or sedation in about 15 per cent of patients. Domperidone, also a dopamine antagonist, does not cross the blood-brain barrier and has fewer CNS side effects. Cisapride, which releases acetylcholine from the enteric neurons, may be useful, but this agent is currently approved only for investigational use in the United States.

Roux-en-Y anastomoses after gastric resection occasionally cause poor gastric emptying, especially of solids (Ch. 98.4). The MMC and the postprandial motor response are abnormal in the roux limb. Delayed gastric emptying of solids is the major functional disturbance; liquid gastric emptying may be normal. Patients with severe vomiting can be treated with subcutaneous bethanechol, further gastric resection, or elimination of the roux loop. The patient's symptoms may be recalcitrant to other prokinetic agents, such as metoclopramide or cisapride. Leuprolide may reduce symptoms in some patients.

DIABETIC GASTROPARESIS. Delayed gastric emptying complicating diabetic ketoacidosis resolves as the patient improves, but the stomach is sometimes massively distended, exhibits mucosal bleeding, and may require decompression by nasogastric tube. Chronic delayed gastric emptying, associated with longstanding insulin-dependent diabetes mellitus, is a greater clinical problem. Such patients have frequent episodes of nausea and vomiting, which affect food intake and complicate insulin requirements. Retinopathy, nephropathy, peripheral neuropathy, and other complications are commonly present. Absence of the gastric MMC, necessary for the emptying of nondigestible material larger than 1 mm, predisposes the diabetic patient to the development of bezoars, causing abdominal discomfort, early satiety, and vomiting. Vagal neuropathy is thought to be the pathogenesis of gastric stasis in diabetes mellitus, although a demonstrable autonomic neuropathy is not always present. Early in the patient's course gastric emptying of liquids may be rapid, although in many patients emptying of liquids is slow from the initiation of symptoms. Gastric emptying of solids is slow throughout the course of the disease.

Metoclopramide improves the symptoms of gastric stasis in patients with diabetes mellitus both by increasing gastric emptying and by decreasing the CNS recognition of nausea and distention. Gastric emptying is rarely normalized after treatment with metoclopramide, even though symptoms may be completely alleviated. Bethanechol also stimulates an increase in gastric motility and improves symptoms in patients with diabetic gastric stasis. Cisapride, which has no demonstrated CNS effect, improves both symptoms and gastric emptying. Cisapride also improves the emptying of nondigestible solids and may prevent the occurrence of bezoars. Erythromycin improves gastric emptying by increasing MMC activity in recent studies.

ANOREXIA NERVOSA. This psychiatric disorder, which oc-

curs predominantly in young women, is characterized by excessive weight loss (Ch. 202). The gastric emptying of solids, but not of liquids, is slowed in patients with anorexia nervosa, but not in patients with bulimia nervosa. The delayed gastric emptying is associated with antral dysrhythmia, fundal hypotonia, decreased postprandial plasma concentrations of norepinephrine and neurotensin, and impaired autonomic function (decreased resting diastolic blood pressure and skin conductance). The mechanism causing delayed gastric emptying is unclear. Patients with equal weight loss but without the psychiatric disorder do not have delayed gastric emptying. Interestingly, gastric emptying in obese patients is more rapid than in healthy subjects.

Repletion of the patient's calories improves gastric emptying in the absence of prokinetic medicine. Bethanechol, metoclopramide, and cisapride increase the emptying of solids by stimulating antral motility. The ultimate success of prokinetic drugs for anorexia nervosa is unclear, since they treat only the peripheral symptom of gastric emptying. Reversal of the underlying psychiatric disturbance appears necessary for complete resolution of symptoms.

MISCELLANEOUS CAUSES. *Tachygastria* is a condition of unknown etiology which presents as intractable vomiting that causes failure to thrive in infants and as vomiting in young adults. Tachygastria is caused by rapid slow wave activity in the antral smooth muscle segment, which becomes the dominant pacemaker initiating orad propagating contractions. Parvovirus-like agents (Norwalk or Hawaii viruses) can slow gastric emptying. The decreased gastric emptying associated with an acute viral infection usually resolves quickly. Up to 25 per cent of patients with reflux esophagitis, associated with an incompetent lower esophageal sphincter, have delayed gastric emptying, which must be corrected in order to treat the reflux esophagitis adequately. Lesions such as tumors, infarction, or viral encephalitis that affect the vagal complex in the medulla can delay gastric emptying.

Rapid Gastric Emptying

Rapid gastric emptying occurs in some patients with duodenal ulcer disease and Zollinger-Ellison syndrome as a result of duodenal insensitivity to an acid load. Rapid liquid emptying occurs in patients with pancreatic insufficiency and possibly with celiac sprue because of poor feedback inhibition of gastric motility by fat due to a maldigestion or malabsorption. The dumping syndrome is discussed in Ch. 98.5.

McCallum RW: Motor function of the stomach in health and disease. *In* Sleisenger MH, Fordtran JJ (eds.): Gastrointestinal Disease. 4th ed. Philadelphia, W. B. Saunders Company, 1989, pp 675–712. *Comprehensive review of pathophysiology of gastroduodenal motility disorder; complete bibliography.*

DISORDERS OF SMALL INTESTINAL MOTILITY

Motility disorders of the small intestine can most usefully be categorized by their respective motility patterns, although some symptom complexes (e.g., postprandial bloating) foil simple categorization. Small intestinal motility may be hypoactive, hyperactive, or uncoordinated. Decreased intestinal motility reflects either absent or fewer MMC's during fasting or a minimal increase in postprandial motility in the different regions of the small bowel. Conversely, increased motility is reflected in increased numbers of fasting MMC's or an augmented intraluminal pressure response to eating. Uncoordinated intestinal motility can be caused by retrograde MMC's and clustered contractions. For rational therapy it is important to determine if the decreased intestinal motility is due to a neuropathy or a myopathy. In general, increased or uncoordinated motility is secondary to neural dysfunction. A disease may affect both the enteric nerves and smooth muscle and may present with different abnormalities in motility during its course (e.g., progressive systemic sclerosis). Table 100–3 lists the conditions associated with chronic disordered small intestinal motility.

In patients with motility disorders, qualitatively similar transit patterns may result in different symptoms. For example, patients with the irritable bowel syndrome may have delayed small intestinal transit that results in constipation. In contrast, a patient with pseudo-obstruction may have a greater delay in intestinal transit that results in diarrhea due to bacterial overgrowth.

TABLE 100–3. SMALL INTESTINAL MOTILITY DISORDERS

Decreased motility
Hollow visceral myopathy (primary intestinal
pseudo-obstruction)
Progressive systemic sclerosis (late)
Amyloidosis
Muscular dystrophy
Duchenne's
Myotonic
Hypothyroidism
Jejeunal diverticulosis
Jejeunoileal bypass

Increased or uncoordinated motility
Primary visceral neuropathy
Carcinoma-associated visceral neuropathy
Progressive systemic sclerosis (early)
Irritable bowel syndrome
Diabetes mellitus
Infectious diarrhea
Mass lesion of brain stem
Amyloidosis
Hyperthyroidism
Carcinoid syndrome
Shy-Drager syndrome

Therefore, symptoms may not be helpful in determining the etiology of a disease process.

Patients with slow intestinal transit tend to complain of nausea, vomiting, abdominal distention, and periumbilical abdominal cramps. Although constipation can occur with delayed intestinal transit, diarrhea is more common. The MMC, which propels bacteria and sloughed, dead epithelial cells from the small intestine into the colon, is often absent or severely deranged by an enteric neuropathy. Bacterial overgrowth due to a diminished number of MMC's deconjugates bile salts, causing steatorrhea and diarrhea. The absence of postprandial motility impedes the normal transit through the small intestine.

Diarrhea is generally the result of rapid intestinal transit because of decreased time of contact of the luminal contents with the mucosa. The patients also may have maldigestion and malabsorption due to poor mixing of the dietary material with the digestive enzymes and bile salts. Borborygmi may also disturb the patient.

Decreased Intestinal Motility

HOLLOW VISCERAL MYOPATHY (INTESTINAL PSEUDO-OBSTRUCTION). This disorder is the prototype for myopathic diseases of the small intestine. The disease generally displays vacuolization or degeneration of the smooth muscle in the circular or longitudinal layers, separately or together, without affecting the enteric nerves. In some cases the muscle is not histologically altered. Defective slow wave generation or actin-myosin cross-bridge formation may cause the myopathy. The contractions are decreased in amplitude and number, but usually the MMC is present because the nerves are unaffected (Fig. 100–4). The MMC may function poorly, however, because of the low-amplitude contractions. The motility pattern differs from that associated with a partial small bowel obstruction in which 3 to 10 clustered contractions occur regularly, separated by 1-minute intervals of quiescence.

Patients usually present with symptoms and signs of small intestinal stasis without evidence of an anatomic obstruction or of a secondary cause for pseudo-obstruction (Table 100–3). Hollow visceral myopathy is familial, but random, nonfamilial cases are probably more common. With familial primary intestinal pseudo-obstruction, parts of the urinary system (bladder, renal pelvis) may also be dilated as a result of abnormal smooth muscle contraction. Familial visceral myopathy is also associated with a high incidence of intestinal malrotation.

Anatomic bowel obstruction or acute ileus must be excluded before making the diagnosis of pseudo-obstruction. Acute adynamic ileus occurs most frequently after abdominal surgery, peritonitis, intra-abdominal vascular accidents, or a severe electrolyte imbalance. Ileus or obstruction can cause hypovolemia or third-space accumulation of fluid. The signs and symptoms of acute ileus are similar to those of chronic disorders of decreased intestinal motility, but in contrast treatment of the initiating cause results in resolution of the symptoms. Acute ileus or obstruction is treated by decompression via a nasogastric tube, replacement of fluid volume, and correction of electrolyte and acid-base imbalances.

The therapy of hollow visceral myopathy is generally highly unsatisfactory. Metoclopramide has little efficacy in treating patients with pseudo-obstruction, but the newer prokinetic agent cisapride shows promise in the therapy of severe small intestinal motility disorders, especially in those patients with postprandial hypomotility with a normal fasting pattern. Intestinal bypass surgery should be avoided in patients with pseudo-obstruction. Occasionally antibiotics may be of help if a blind loop syndrome with bacterial overgrowth is present.

PROGRESSIVE SYSTEMIC SCLEROSIS (Ch. 262). This is the most common "collagen vascular disease" to cause disordered intestinal motility, although polymyositis and systemic lupus erythematosus may rarely do so. Approximately 40 per cent of patients with progressive systemic sclerosis have intestinal in-

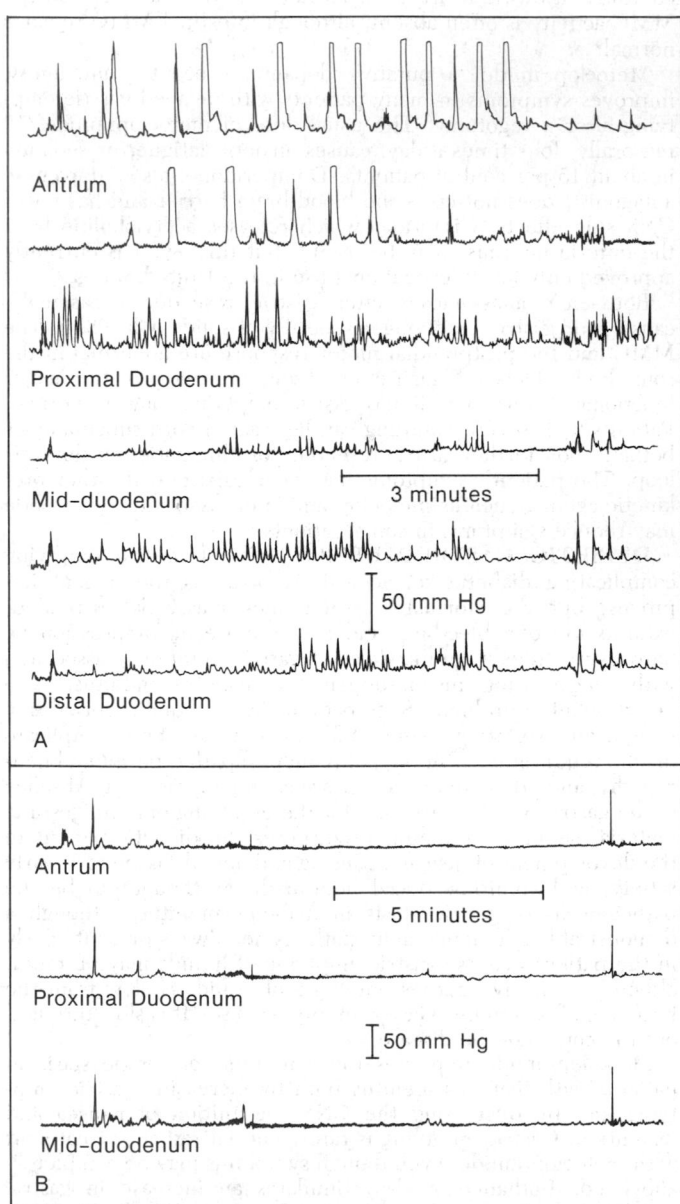

FIGURE 100–4. Postprandial gastroduodenal manometry recordings from a healthy subject (*A*) and a patient with myopathic pseudo-obstruction (*B*). The postprandial response is decreased in the patient with pseudo-obstruction. (From Hyman PE: Absent postprandial duodenal motility in a child with cystic fibrosis: Correction of the symptoms and manometric abnormality with cisapride. Gastroenterology 90:1274, 1986.)

volvement consisting of defects in both neural and smooth muscle. Early in the course of the disease, signs of a neuropathy predominate, whereas collagen later replaces smooth muscle and a myopathy becomes the major component of the disease. In symptomatic patients, characteristically postprandial motility is markedly reduced. Since a neuropathy is often present, the MMC's are absent. In general, patients become symptomatic only after extensive replacement of the smooth muscle with collagen. In contrast to hollow visceral myopathy, muscle cells in progressive systemic sclerosis are decreased in number but morphologically normal. Since the number of functional smooth muscle cells is decreased, pharmacologic stimulation with prokinetic drugs is generally unsuccessful.

OTHER CONDITIONS. *Amyloidosis* of the small intestine may cause either a myopathy or a neuropathy, depending on its distribution. Several of the *muscular dystrophy* syndromes may affect the intestinal smooth muscle in addition to skeletal and cardiac muscle. *Hypothyroidism* decreases the slow wave frequency and amplitude of contraction of the intestine, which may result in atony. *Jejunal diverticulosis* is secondary to pseudo-obstruction, which predominantly involves the small intestine. The histologic pattern is similar to that of progressive systemic sclerosis in most patients, although some patients have a neuropathy.

Increased or Uncoordinated Motility

VISCERAL NEUROPATHY. Intestinal motility can be increased, as well as uncoordinated, in patients with visceral neuropathy because of a decrease in neural inhibition. The hallmark of visceral neuropathy is a patchy loss of nerve tracts, a decreased number of neurons, or fragmentation and dropout of axons. Specialized silver stains are needed for the accurate histologic diagnosis of an enteric neuropathy.

Primary visceral neuropathy can be familial or random. Familial cases may be associated with other neural lesions, including mild autonomic insufficiency, mental retardation, altered sensory recognition of position, and absent deep tendon reflexes. Random cases may be secondary to injury from a viral infection or an environmental toxin or to carcinomatous neuropathy (Ch. 162). The motility patterns associated with visceral neuropathy are variable, probably because different disease complexes have not been separated at this time. In general, during fasting a neuropathy disrupts either the propagation or configuration of the MMC. In some patients the MMC may be absent. Eating may initiate no contractions or uncoordinated contractions or may fail to inhibit MMC's in patients with neuropathy.

IRRITABLE BOWEL SYNDROME. In this common disorder, to be discussed more fully under colonic disorders, symptoms of abdominal pain and an altered bowel habit consistent with the irritable bowel syndrome may be associated with abnormal motility in the small intestine as well as in the colon. Balloon distention of the small intestine provokes characteristic abdominal pain in some patients. Two patterns of contractions, "discrete clustered contractions" and "prolonged propagated contractions," are associated with abdominal pain more frequently in patients with the irritable bowel syndrome than in healthy control subjects.

DIABETES MELLITUS. The diarrhea associated with diabetes mellitus is most likely due to small intestinal motility disturbances. Abnormal manometric patterns in diabetics, who also have gastroparesis, include decreased motility or uncoordinated bursts of small intestinal contractions. The MMC's can be present, deranged, or absent in diabetic patients. Patients with a central autonomic nervous system disturbance, Shy-Drager syndrome, have similar findings to patients with diabetes (Ch. 452). Diabetic diarrhea may respond to treatment with the α_2-adrenergic agent clonidine.

OTHER DISORDERS. *Infectious diarrhea* (e.g., due to enterotoxigenic *E. coli* or *Shigella*) initiates a significant motility disorder, characterized experimentally by powerful aborad migrating contractions. *Brain stem mass lesions* can either slow the small intestinal MMC or initiate an activity front simultaneously at different levels of the small intestine, through an effect on the vagal motor complex and the autonomic nuclei in the medullary reticular formation. *Amyloid* can affect the enteric nerves of the small intestine as well as replace smooth muscle. *Hyperthyroid-ism* increases the slow wave frequency of the bowel, which is a possible cause of the frequently associated diarrhea. *Carcinoid syndrome* with increased 5-hydroxytryptamine production increases the migration velocity of the MMC and increases the cycling frequency.

Malagelada J-R, Camilleri M, Stanghellini V: Manometric Diagnosis of Gastrointestinal Motility Disorders. New York, Thieme-Stratton, 1986. *A monograph on the diagnosis of motility disorders but dealing also with normal physiology and the pathophysiology of the common and uncommon disorders of motility. The bibliography is extensive and will guide the reader into any area.*
Kellow JE, Phillips SF: Functional disorders of the small intestine. *In* Snape WJ Jr. (ed.): Pathogenesis of Functional Bowel Disease. New York, Plenum Medical Book Company, 1989, pp 171–198. *Extensive discussion of pathophysiology of small intestinal motility disturbance; extensive bibliography.*

DISORDERS OF COLON MOTILITY

Orderly transit of contents through the colon "fine tunes" the absorption of salt and water. If the transit is too slow, the mucosa can extract too much water and the stool becomes hard, resulting in constipation. Rapid transit causes frequent, soft stools. Diarrhea caused by colonic motility disorders is low in volume (less than 400 ml per day), since most intestinal fluid is absorbed in the small intestine (Ch. 101). Table 100–4 lists the diseases or syndromes that cause disordered colonic motility. Many of the systemic diseases that affect gastric and small intestinal motility also alter colonic motility.

Either increased or decreased segmenting contractions can slow transit through the colon. A functional partial obstruction results from increased segmenting contractions, since the movement of the colonic contents is impeded by the segmentation. The colonic contents also move slowly if colonic segmenting activity is decreased (colonic inertia). Propagating contractions are invariably absent in patients with slow colonic transit and constipation, suggesting that these contractions are necessary for net forward movement of feces into the distal rectosigmoid.

Patients with diarrhea and rapid colonic transit have decreased colonic segmenting contractions and increased numbers of contractions propagating into the rectum. As a result, intraluminal contents are rapidly transported distally. When these powerful contractions carry the colonic contents into the rectum, the patient experiences urgency.

Cramping abdominal pain referable to the colon occurs predominantly in the lower abdominal quadrants, but it can be felt anywhere over the anatomic distribution of the colon. This pain is characteristically relieved by flatus or a bowel movement. Although the patients feel bloated, ascribed to increased gastrointestinal gas, they actually have normal amounts of bowel gas. Tenesmus, a feeling of incomplete evacuation, is associated with rectosigmoid spasm.

Slow Transit with Increased Segmenting Contractions

PRIMARY CONSTIPATION. Most people experience brief periods of constipation during their lives; treatment is usually not

TABLE 100–4. PATHOGENESIS OF COLONIC MOTILITY DISORDERS

Slow transit
  Increased segmenting contraction
    Primary constipation
    Irritable bowel syndrome (spastic)
    Diverticular disease
    Anal outlet obstruction
      Congenital—Hirschsprung's disease
      Acquired
  Decreased segmenting contractions
    Irritable bowel syndrome (inertia)
    Primary colonic pseudo-obstruction
    Ogilvie's syndrome
    Diabetes mellitus
    Progressive systemic sclerosis
    Spinal cord injury
Rapid transit
    Functional diarrhea
    Bile salt diarrhea
    Surreptitious abuse of laxatives

necessary unless the symptoms last for several months. Infrequent bowel movements (less than every other day) result in hard fecal pellets, which require straining to eliminate, because of slow colonic transit and the ensuing desiccation of the stool. Patients do not complain of abdominal pain but rather have nonspecific symptoms of bloating, increased flatus, and mild malaise. Fecal impactions, which rarely occur except in elderly or sedentary patients, may cause overflow diarrhea or bleeding from stercoral rectal ulcers.

Although the pathophysiology of primary constipation is poorly understood, most patients respond quickly to increasing fiber in their diet. The chronic use of osmotic laxatives, dioctyl sodium sulfosuccinate, or stimulant laxatives has the potential to damage the myenteric plexus, causing an unresponsive "cathartic colon."

IRRITABLE BOWEL SYNDROME (SPASTIC). Symptoms of the irritable bowel syndrome occur in up to 25 per cent of otherwise healthy individuals. Although most common in women in early adulthood, the irritable bowel syndrome can begin after the age of 45 years. In such older patients, however, it is extremely important to exclude other disease, including carcinoma of the colon or colonic diverticular disease.

Cramping abdominal pain of colonic origin and an altered bowel habit are the hallmarks of the irritable bowel syndrome. The symptoms are intermittent with variable periods of remission. Eating, especially a large meal with a high fat content, or episodes of emotional stress increase the pain. Constipation alternating with an increased frequency of low-volume stools is the "classic" bowel pattern, although patients may have more frequent looser stools at the onset of an attack of the irritable bowel or may complain only of constipation. A perception of uncomfortable abdominal distention and increased fecal mucus are common adjunctive symptoms.

Patients with constipation-predominant irritable bowel syndrome have an increased prevalence of colonic slow waves at a frequency of 3 cycles per minute compared with normal individuals. In approximately 60 per cent of patients with constipation-predominant irritable bowel syndrome, segmenting contractions are increased after eating a meal, whereas in the remainder no increase in motility and little mixing movement of the fecal contents in the colon occur. The increased segmenting contractions shuttle the colonic contents back and forth in the transverse and descending colon. When present, the normal increase in postprandial motility is delayed. There are subtle differences in symptoms in the two groups of patients; nausea and vomiting are more prominent symptoms in patients with little postprandial motility (colonic inertia). Propagating contractions are absent in both groups of patients.

Balloon distention of the rectum or other regions of the colon causes abdominal pain at a lower threshold in patients with the irritable bowel syndrome than in healthy people. This is not a generalized increase in pain perception because the patients generally feel less somatic pain. The abnormal pathophysiology in visceral sensory nerves and in colonic motility combines to cause the classic symptoms of the irritable bowel syndrome.

The diagnosis of the irritable bowel syndrome requires exclusion of other diseases. Functional diarrhea, variably lumped into the irritable bowel syndrome, is discussed in detail later in reference to rapid transit. The rigor used to exclude the diagnosis of other diseases depends on the age and clinical presentation of the patient. The major differential diagnoses include carcinoma of the colon, diverticulitis, and inflammatory bowel disease. After a careful history and physical examination, the stool should be examined for occult blood. Patients over the age of 40 years definitely should have colonoscopy or barium enema to exclude anatomic colonic disease. If the symptoms persist, especially that of diarrhea, the terminal ileum should be visualized to exclude inflammatory bowel disease (Ch. 103).

Once organic disease is excluded, the irritable bowel syndrome is best treated by reassuring the patient, explaining the cause of symptoms, and instituting some alterations of the diet. Decreasing dietary fat reduces colonic intraluminal pressure. An increase in soluble and insoluble dietary fiber decreases water net absorption and intraluminal pressure, respectively. Pharmacologic agents should be used only if counseling and dietary changes have no effect on symptoms. Anticholinergics, the next line of

therapy, decrease the colonic contractions and may relieve symptoms. Combined therapy with dietary fiber supplements and anticholinergics has enhanced efficacy. Diarrhea and fecal continence may improve following a dietary fiber supplement owing to increased bulk. Anxiolytics or antidepressants should be used only after documenting a psychoneurosis.

ACQUIRED DIVERTICULAR DISEASE OF THE COLON. Diverticular disease, mucosal outpouchings through the colonic wall that occur as the patient ages, results in a spectrum of abnormalities extending from no symptoms to diverticulitis. Diverticular disease may occur more often in patients who had the irritable bowel syndrome in their youth.

Acquired diverticula, which occur most frequently in the left colon, result from increased intraluminal pressure pushing sleeves of mucosa through perivascular weaknesses in the wall of the colon juxtaposed to the taeniae coli. The predilection for the left colon results from the decreased colonic diameter there leading to increased pressures, as predicted by Laplace's law: Intraluminal pressure is directly correlated with wall tension and inversely correlated with bowel diameter. Decreased dietary fiber and distal colonic smooth muscle hypertrophy contribute to elevation in distal colonic intraluminal pressure.

The symptoms of *painful colonic diverticular disease* are similar to those of irritable bowel syndrome but are more likely to be localized in the left lower quadrant. When *diverticulitis* occurs as a complication, the patient may have similar symptoms with the addition of fever, left lower quadrant mass, leukocytosis, and occult blood in the stool (Ch. 112). Gross hematochezia is more frequent in asymptomatic patients with diverticula (Ch. 112). Diverticula can be diagnosed by barium enema or colonoscopy. Muscular hypertrophy gives a saw-tooth pattern visible on barium enema. Narrowing due to diverticular inflammation can be difficult to differentiate from carcinoma of the colon.

Painful diverticular disease of the colon is best treated by decreasing the intraluminal pressure, similar to the therapy in the irritable bowel syndrome. Narcotics, especially morphine, should be avoided because of an exaggerated increase in smooth muscle contraction.

ANAL OUTLET OBSTRUCTION. Constipation may result from a disturbance in the elimination of stool through the anal sphincter. Elimination normally begins by the involuntary relaxation of the internal anal sphincter after distention of the rectum. The patient uses voluntary control to open the rectoanal angle and relax the external anal sphincter. A disturbance of any component of this mechanism leads to constipation.

Hirschsprung's disease is the congenital absence of enteric neurons in the submucosal and myenteric plexuses, due to an arrest of the embryonic caudad migration of the enteric neurons along the gut. The aganglionic segment remains contracted, causing dilatation of the proximal normal bowel. The severity of symptoms and the age at diagnosis are related to the length of the aganglionic segment. Involvement of the rectum or additional parts of the colon results in constipation or obstipation in infancy, requiring emergent resection of the aganglionic bowel and a pull-through anastomosis to the anus.

Abnormalities in anal physiology are a significant cause of constipation; impaired anal sphincter relaxation occurs relatively frequently in adults. The absent rectoanal reflex may be secondary to a short aganglionic segment (short-segment Hirschsprung's disease), to chronic distention with a fecal impaction, or to an insufficient distention stimulus due to an enlarged rectal vault. In acquired megacolon, relaxation of the internal anal sphincter may be impaired if a large volume is not used to distend the rectum. Some patients have subtle histologic abnormalities in the myenteric plexus, suggesting that an acquired neuropathy may also account for the abnormal sphincter response. In the spastic pelvic floor syndrome (animus) the external anal sphincter and the puborectalis relax poorly or the levator ani contracts poorly, leading to impaired opening of the rectoanal angle. This acquired condition, which occurs more often in multiparous women, can prevent the patient from normal stool evacuation. Anal outlet dysfunction can be diagnosed as a cause of constipation by observing the accumulation of the fecal markers in the rectum and by abnormal anal manometry.

Impaired internal anal sphincter relaxation in an adult patient may respond to a posterior anal sphincter myomectomy. Patients who have difficulty in opening the rectoanal angle or who have animus may sometimes respond to biofeedback training.

Slow Transit with Decreased Segmenting Contractions

Patients with decreased segmenting contractions have symptoms similar to those in patients with increased contractions. The colonic inertia form of the irritable bowel syndrome and primary colonic pseudo-obstruction may be the same pathophysiologic disturbance. Postprandial increases in colonic motility are absent in both, but the colon is dilated in primary intestinal pseudo-obstruction, explaining the increased incidence of abdominal distention. Constipation is a major symptom in both conditions. Ogilvie's syndrome is the primary colonic pseudo-obstruction, usually paraneoplastic.

Constipation is present in many patients with longstanding, insulin-requiring diabetes mellitus, progressive systemic sclerosis, or thoracic spinal cord lesions. Colonic motility is not increased postprandially in these patients. In the patients with diabetes or spinal cord lesions, colonic smooth muscle can be stimulated with exogenous drugs, suggesting a neural lesion, not a myopathy. In progressive systemic sclerosis the colon cannot increase intraluminal pressure after drug stimulation, as expected in a neuropathy.

It is difficult to treat patients with decreased colonic motility. In patients with neuropathy and normal smooth muscle function, prokinetic drugs have had some success. In patients with a myopathy it is unlikely that pharmacologic stimulation will have much effect.

Rapid Transit

FUNCTIONAL DIARRHEA. Some patients have functional, painless diarrhea with fecal urgency but with no associated anatomic or histologic abnormality of the gastrointestinal tract. These patients present with small frequent stools, consistent with a large bowel abnormality, and fecal incontinence is relatively frequent because their anal sphincters cannot retard evacuation of a liquid stool. Lactose intolerance must be excluded either by history or by a lactose tolerance test. The diarrhea is greater than that in the spastic irritable colon syndrome, and abdominal pain may be absent.

Segmenting postprandial contractile activity is decreased in functional diarrhea. Propagating contractions are increased and propagate into the rectum, possibly accounting for the increased urgency and fecal incontinence that occur in these patients. The lack of segmenting contractions to impede forward movement or transit may exacerbate the urgency. Specific foods may stimulate an increase in prostaglandin E_2 production by the colon, which could initiate the diarrhea. Increased concentrations of fecal bile salts, which occur in some patients, may contribute to the functional diarrhea also. Bile salts irritate colonic sensory nerves and thereby stimulate frequent propagating contractions in the colon through irritation of sensory nerves.

Microscopic or collagenous colitis presents as functional diarrhea without obvious anatomic abnormalities. The diagnoses can be made by histologic examination of the rectal biopsy.

In the treatment of functional diarrhea, antidiarrheal agents such as the opioid analogues, loperamide, or diphenoxylate are used to decrease symptoms. Fecal continence improves as the stool consistency becomes firmer. Some patients may require biofeedback training to maintain continence. If excess bile salts contribute to the diarrhea, low doses of cholestyramine may decrease the diarrhea. Microscopic and collagenous colitis may respond to 5-aminosalicylic compounds.

Surreptitious Laxative Abuse. Surreptitious laxative abuse is a common cause of functional diarrhea (Ch. 101). Oxyphenisatin and bisacodyl stimulate increased numbers of propagating contractions and diarrhea. Patients may take these or other laxatives as a manifestation of a psychiatric disorder. It is a challenge to the physician to make the correct diagnosis.

Ulcerative Colitis. There is rapid transit of colonic contents through the colon, in addition to increased mucosal secretion, in patients with active ulcerative colitis. As in the other colonic causes of diarrhea, propagating contractions are increased in number and propagate into the rectum, accounting for the significant incidence of fecal incontinence. The rapid transit improves as the mucosal inflammation decreases after therapy for the underlying inflammation (Ch. 103).

Devroede GJ: Constipation: Mechanism and management. *In* Sleisenger MH, Fordtran JS (eds.): Gastrointestinal Disease. 4th ed. Philadelphia, W. B. Saunders Company, 1989, pp 331–368. *This is a complete examination of the pathophysiology and treatment of constipation.*

Snape WJ Jr.: Irritable bowel syndrome. *In* Snape WJ Jr. (ed.): Pathogenesis of Functional Bowel Disease. New York, Plenum Medical Book Company, 1989. *This summarizes the field, providing 150 references for further study.*

DRUGS THAT AFFECT GASTROINTESTINAL MOTILITY

As understanding of the pathophysiology of gastrointestinal motility disorders grows, the number and the diversity of the drugs that are available for therapy increase (Table 100–5). Drugs that stimulate motility may indiscriminately increase smooth muscle contractions or increase a specific motility function, such as MMC initiation. Many of the drugs on the list, used for treatment of other systemic diseases, may precipitate gastrointestinal symptoms as a side effect.

Excitatory Agents

Drugs that excite the gastrointestinal tract should be used to treat decreased motility when the smooth muscle can functionally contract. In general, patients who benefit from these agents have an enteric neuropathy with decreased release of endogenous stimulatory neurotransmitters or an increased release of inhibitory neurotransmitters. When the smooth muscle is absent or severely damaged, the prokinetic drugs are rarely helpful. Acetylcholine analogues, such as bethanechol, stimulate both longitudinal and circular gastrointestinal smooth muscle by directly binding to the M_2 muscarinic receptor to release inositol triphosphate or to open

TABLE 100–5. EFFECTS OF DRUGS ON SMALL AND LARGE INTESTINAL CONTRACTILITY

Drug	Effect on Stomach	Effect on Small Intestine	Effect on Colon	Mechanism of Action
Acetylcholine analogues	Excitatory	Excitatory	Excitatory	Agonist of muscarinic receptors on muscle cells
Neostigmine	Excitatory	Excitatory	Excitatory	Acetylcholine esterase inhibitor
Metoclopramide	Excitatory	Excitatory	Excitatory	Dopamine antagonist (central, peripheral)
Domperidone	Excitatory	Excitatory	No effect	Dopamine antagonist (peripheral)
Cisapride	Excitatory	Excitatory	Excitatory	Unknown
Macrolide antibiotic	Excitatory	Excitatory	?	Binds to motilin receptor
Leuprolide acetate	?	Excitatory	?	Reduces progesterone and relaxin
Atropine	Inhibitory	Inhibitory	Inhibitory	Antagonist of muscarinic receptor
Secoverine	?	Inhibitory	Inhibitory	Antagonist of M_2 muscarinic receptors on muscle cells
Papaverine	?	?	Inhibitory	Unknown
Calcium channel blockers	Inhibitory	Inhibitory	Inhibitory	Blocks voltage-operated calcium channels
Nitrate compounds	?	Inhibitory	Inhibitory	Blockade of receptor-operated calcium channels; Increase of intracellular cGMP
Peppermint oil	?	Inhibitory	Inhibitory	Unknown
Cholecystokinin antagonists	?	?	?	Blocks CCK receptors

receptor-operated or voltage-dependent calcium channels. Drugs that block acetylcholinesterase increase endogenous acetylcholine concentration at the myoneural junction. These drugs have a theoretical advantage in regulating as well as in increasing motility, since the distribution of acetylcholine release is predetermined by the autonomic nervous system.

Dopamine antagonists can variably increase motility throughout the gastrointestinal tract. Metoclopramide, a centrally and peripherally acting dopamine antagonist, increases gastric emptying and transit through the small intestine and the colon. Metoclopramide is useful in diabetic gastroparesis, in the placement of small intestinal tubes in patients with ileus, and in diabetic constipation. It has little therapeutic value in symptomatic patients with progressive systemic sclerosis or in many patients with pseudo-obstruction. Domperidone, a peripherally acting dopamine antagonist, mainly increases gastric emptying and has little therapeutic effect in small intestinal or colonic motility disorders.

Cisapride may stimulate motility through antagonism of a serotonin (5-hydroxytryptamine) receptor in the bowel. Cisapride stimulates gastric emptying, increases small intestinal transit, and stimulates colonic contractility. Cisapride may improve symptoms in patients with decreased gastric emptying, small intestinal pseudo-obstruction, or colonic inertia. This drug is not currently available in the United States.

Erythromycin, one of the macrolide antibiotics, stimulates MMC activity by binding at the motilin receptor on the small intestinal smooth muscle cell. Normal MMC activity is absent in many patients with neuropathic pseudo-obstruction. The clinical usefulness of this agent remains to be established.

Leuprolide acetate may improve symptoms secondary to functional disturbances of small intestinal motility. This drug is believed to work by decreasing the concentrations of the smooth muscle inhibitory hormones progesterone and relaxin.

Inhibitory Agents

Inhibitory drugs should be most useful for treating patients whose symptoms result from increased motility, which causes uncoordinated movement of the intestinal contents. The inhibitory drugs may block the receptors for excitatory neurotransmitters or block the increase in intracellular calcium necessary for normal smooth muscle contraction.

Anticholinergic drugs, which inhibit muscarinic receptor stimulation, are sometimes effective in the treatment of the small intestinal or colonic variants of the irritable bowel syndrome. The anticholinergics must be used with care in patients who may develop urinary retention (e.g., prostatism) or glaucoma.

Calcium channel blockers inhibit the increase in intracellular calcium that is necessary for smooth muscle contraction. Several classes of calcium channel blockers, including verapamil and the dihydropyridines, are available. The dihydropyridine, nifedipine, decreases smooth muscle contraction and may be used in some patients with increased small intestinal or colonic motility.

Nitrate compounds inhibit smooth muscle contraction, probably through an increase in the intracellular concentration of cyclic guanosine monophosphate and a decrease in calcium influx into the smooth muscle cell.

Peppermint oil is a relaxant of smooth muscle, which improves symptoms in some patients with the irritable bowel syndrome. In the future, a new class of agents, cholecystokinin antagonists, may prove useful in the treatment of multiple gastrointestinal motility disorders.

Burks TF: Actions of drugs on gastrointestinal motility. *In* Johnson LR (ed.): Physiology of the Gastrointestinal Tract. 2nd ed. New York, Raven Press, 1987, pp 723–744. *Extensive references are provided for the background of drug action.*

Camilleri M, Malageladn JR, Abell TL, et al.: Effect of six weeks of treatment with Cisapride in gastroparesis and intestinal pseudo-obstruction. Gastroenterology 96:704, 1989. *Report of efficacy for the new class of prokinetic drugs.*

Corazziari E, Ricci R, Biliodtti D, et al.: Oral administration of loxiglumids (CCK antagonist) inhibits postprandial gallbladder contraction without affecting gastric emptying. Dig Dis Sci 35:50, 1990. *Interesting study showing the potential of the new medication.*

101 Diarrhea

Guenter J. Krejs

Diarrhea is defined as the presence of stool liquidity (instead of formed or soft stool) and an increase in daily stool weight, the upper normal limit of which is 200 grams in industrialized societies. Diarrhea is usually associated with increased stool frequency (more than three bowel movements per day) and is often accompanied by urgency, perianal discomfort, and incontinence. Some patients may have increased frequency and liquidity of stools, however, when their daily stool weights are less than 200 grams. Since diarrhea results from a disturbance in the normal flow and transport of gut fluids, the normal physiology of absorption in the digestive tract is first considered.

NORMAL PHYSIOLOGY

DELIVERY, FLOW, AND ABSORPTION RATES. During fasting, the intestine contains very little fluid, but when three normal meals per day are eaten, about 9 liters of fluid are delivered to the proximal duodenum. Approximately 2 liters of this fluid are from ingested food and liquids, the rest being digestive secretions.

The volume of chyme that passes through different segments of the small bowel depends on the type of food that has been eaten. For example, meals containing high concentrations of sugar are hypertonic, and when such meals are ingested, the volume of material passing through the jejunum is even greater than the volume that enters the proximal duodenum. On the other hand, after isotonic or hypotonic meals (such as a meal of steak, potatoes, and tea), the volume of fluid traversing the jejunum is much less than that which was delivered to the duodenum. (These considerations are especially important in patients who have had gastric surgery or intestinal resection.) In either case, the osmolality of chyme is adjusted toward that of plasma as fluid travels through the duodenum and upper jejunum, and by the time chyme reaches the ileum, most of the dietary sugars, amino acids, and fats have been absorbed. Fluid arriving at the ileum is mainly an isotonic salt solution and therefore similar in its ionic composition to plasma. The ileum absorbs much, but not all, of this salt solution. About 1 liter per day of this isotonic unabsorbed ileal fluid enters the colon. Although ileal fluid resembles plasma with regard to its sodium and potassium concentrations, the concentrations of chloride and bicarbonate are quite different, being approximately 70 and 60 mEq per liter, respectively.

The colon can absorb 2 to 4 liters of isotonic salt solution per day (even more in patients with secondary hyperaldosteronism associated with salt depletion). The presence of nonabsorbable and osmotically active solutes from the diet and from bacterial action, a relatively slow rate of absorption from the rectosigmoid, and timely bowel movements prevent complete fluid absorption and desiccation of the fecal mass. About 100 ml of fluid is excreted in the feces; its sodium and chloride concentrations are about 50 mEq per liter, while the potassium concentration is about 90 mEq per liter. This fluid also contains a high concentration of volatile fatty acids (from bacterial action on nondigestible carbohydrates), which dissipate most of the unabsorbed or secreted bicarbonate ions and which often cause stool fluid to be hypertonic to plasma. Since the gastrointestinal tract does not have a diluting mechanism, the osmolality of fecal fluid is never less than the osmolality of plasma.

To summarize, daily volumes of fluid traversing the duodenum are 9 liters, traversing the ileocecal valve area are 1 liter, and traversing the anal sphincter are 0.1 liter. Stated in another way, the small bowel absorbs 8 liters of fluid per day and empties 1 liter into the colon, and the colon absorbs 0.9 liter. Theoretically 2 to 4 liters of fluid would have to be delivered to the colon per day before diarrhea would ensue, provided that delivery rates were steady, the fluid contained no abnormal solutes, and colon function was normal. Unfortunately, the latter qualifications do not apply in many gastrointestinal diseases.

TRANSPORT PHYSIOLOGY. The mechanisms responsible for fluid absorption differ in different regions of the gut and in different species. According to the model for the ileum shown in Figure 101–1, the brush border membrane contains a carrier that facilitates the simultaneous entry of Na^+ and glucose into the cells; Na^+ cannot enter without glucose. A separate pair of exchange carriers works together to facilitate the simultaneous and electrically neutral entry of Na^+ and Cl^-. Na^+ enters in exchange for H^+, and Cl^- enters in exchange for HCO_3^-. If these two exchange carriers operate at the same rate, Na^+ and Cl^- are absorbed in equal amounts, and H^+ and HCO_3^- are secreted in equal amounts and react in the lumen to form CO_2 and water. However, the anion carrier usually operates more rapidly than the cation carrier, and there is a net secretion of HCO_3^-. (This accounts for the high concentration of HCO_3^- and the low concentration of Cl^- in fluid that the ileum delivers to the colon.) Once inside the cell (via either the Na^+-H^+ exchange or the Na^+-glucose carrier), Na^+ is pumped out of the cell across the basolateral membrane by a pump that is probably an Na^+-K^+ adenosine triphosphatase (ATPase). Chloride and glucose exit the basolateral membrane by facilitated or passive diffusion.

Sodium pumping at the basolateral membrane causes a potential difference (PD) across the mucosa (serosal side positive). However, the tight junctions between small bowel mucosal cells (the "shunt pathway") are "leaky," and passive diffusion of anions (in the absorptive direction from lumen to plasma) or cations (in the secretory direction) readily dissipates the PD. Therefore, the residual PD across small bowel mucosa is only 2 to 4 mV.

Colonic cells and colonic transport are somewhat different. The brush border membrane apparently has a carrier for Na^+ that is not influenced by glucose or other actively absorbed nonelectro-

lytes (glucose is not absorbed in the colon). There is no convincing evidence for Na^+-H^+ exchange, but the brush border membrane appears to have an anion exchange carrier that facilitates chloride absorption and bicarbonate secretion. The tight junctions are "tight," so the electrical gradient generated by the basolateral membrane pump is sustained. The PD is, therefore, about 30 mV (serosal side positive).

Potassium movement in all regions of the gut is passive, in response to electrochemical gradients. Thus, passive potassium absorption in the colon is retarded (owing to the high lumen-negative PD), and the potassium concentration in fecal fluid is much higher than in plasma (up to 100 mEq per liter). Water movement throughout the gut is passive, secondary to osmotic pressure gradients generated by active solute transport.

NORMAL SMALL BOWEL SECRETION. Small intestinal cells normally secrete as well as absorb electrolytes and water, with the secretory rate normally being of less magnitude than the absorptive rate, so that the net effect of small bowel transport processes is absorption of fluid. (Although it is possible that the same cell might both absorb and secrete, the putative small bowel secretion probably originates in crypt cells, whereas absorption takes place from villous cells.) This is an extremely important concept, because it means that a hormone or toxin might reduce net absorption rate in either of two ways: (1) by stimulating secretion, or (2) by inhibiting absorption. In either case, the observed effect is reduced absorption. Similarly, a hormone or a toxin might cause small bowel secretion by stimulating active secretion, so that it overwhelms the normal absorptive process; or a hormone or a toxin could cause secretion by inhibiting absorption, so that the normal small bowel secretion is unmasked. In fact, many toxins and hormones appear capable of both stimulating secretion and inhibiting normal absorption (see below). In patients with diarrhea caused by toxins or hormones, it is difficult to ascertain which of these factors is predominant.

In the colon, absorption takes place from the surface epithelial cells. There is no evidence for or against a normal colonic secretion.

PATHOPHYSIOLOGY OF DIARRHEA

Diarrhea may result from one or more of the following four mechanisms. There is, in addition, a miscellaneous group for which a single mechanism cannot currently be identified:

1. Poorly absorbable, osmotically active solutes in the intestinal lumen.
2. Active ion secretion.
3. Deranged intestinal motility.
4. Altered mucosal morphology or loss of absorptive surface.
5. Miscellaneous (several mechanisms or pathophysiology not clearly understood).

Osmotic Diarrhea

Osmotic diarrhea is caused by the accumulation of nonabsorbed solutes in the gut lumen. There are three main subtypes: (1) ingestion of poorly absorbable solutes, such as saline purgatives; (2) maldigestion of ingested food, such as in lactase deficiency; and (3) failure of a mucosal transport mechanism, such as in glucose-galactose malabsorption (Table 101–1). Being osmotically active, these solutes cause water and salts to be retained within the intestinal lumen, resulting in diarrhea.

Osmotic diarrhea stops when the patient fasts (or stops ingesting the poorly absorbable solute). Furthermore, the fecal fluid has a large solute gap; i.e., normal electrolytes do not account for much of the fecal fluid osmolality (fecal solute gap = [osmolality] − 2[(Na^+) + (K^+)]; the factor of 2 is to account for anions in stool water). An exception is congenital chloridorrhea, in which unabsorbed chloride prevents water absorption. In chloridorrhea the chloride concentration in fecal fluids exceeds the sum of the concentration of sodium and potassium. Such fecal fluid analysis is performed on supernatant stool water following centrifugation of a stool sample in a test tube (30 minutes at 2000 g). In most instances, electrolytes and osmolality will provide meaningful information only if the stools are liquid enough that at the end of centrifugation the supernatant stool water constitutes at least one third of the total sample. In osmotic diarrhea resulting from

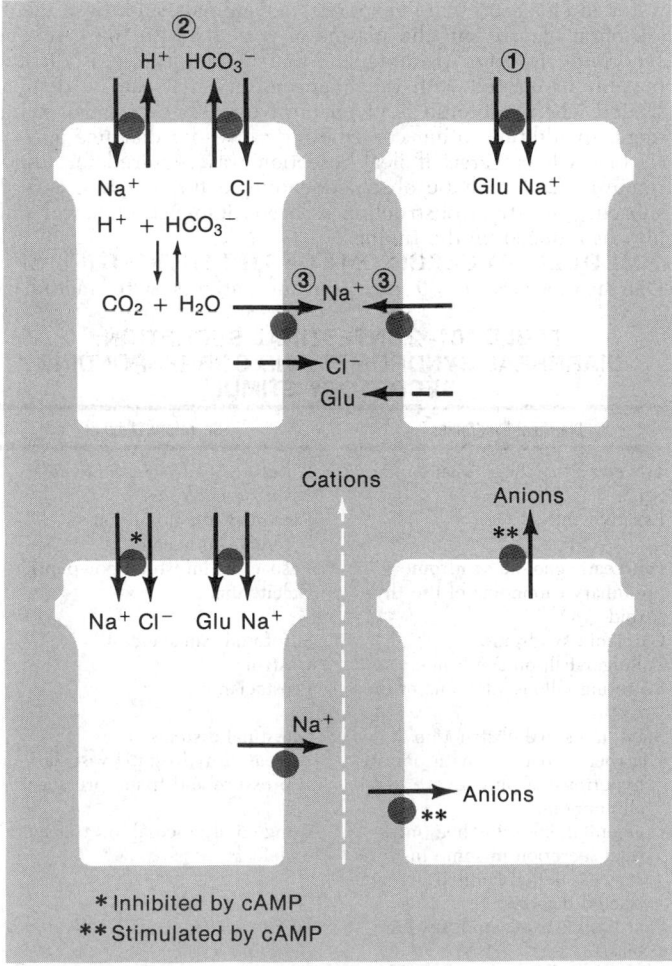

FIGURE 101–1. *Top,* Active transport mechanisms in the human ileum. *1,* Brush border glucose-sodium carrier. *2,* Double exchange carriers for neutral NaCl entry. *3,* Basolateral membrane sodium pump. *Bottom,* Model of cyclic AMP–mediated change in intestinal transport. Active anion secretion is stimulated (**), and there is inhibition of neutral NaCl entry across the brush border membrane (*). The glucose-sodium entry carrier and the basolateral membrane sodium pump are intact. Cations are secreted passively via the tight junction pathway.

*Inhibited by cAMP
**Stimulated by cAMP

TABLE 101–1. CAUSES OF OSMOTIC DIARRHEA

Ingestion of poorly absorbable solutes
  Magnesium sulfate, sodium sulfate, citrate-containing laxatives
  Some antacids—$Mg(OH)_2$
  Mannitol, sorbitol (chewing gum, diet candy)
Maldigestion
  Disaccharidase deficiencies (lactose, sucrose-isomaltose,
    trehalose intolerance)
  Gastrocolic fistula, jejunoileal bypass, short bowel syndrome
  Postgastrectomy, postvagotomy state
  Chronic intestinal ischemia
  Lactulose therapy
Mucosal transport defects
  Glucose-galactose malabsorption
  Chloridorrhea
  Congenital sodium diarrhea
  General malabsorption in diffuse disease of small bowel mucosa

carbohydrate malabsorption, the concentration in stool of short-chain fatty acids is high, and thus the pH is low (pH 4.0 to 6.0). In some instances it is necessary to measure magnesium (normal less than 12 mM), sulfate (normal less than 5 mM), and phosphate (normal less than 12 mM) in stool water to identify the cause of osmotic diarrhea, especially in surreptitious laxative abuse.

Normal fecal fluid, which can be isolated from stool by dialysis methods, often has a modest solute gap (mainly because of unabsorbed carbohydrates and their bacterial products). Therefore, the presence of a solute gap is suggestive of osmotic diarrhea only if stool volume losses are substantially higher than normal. For example, a modest osmotic gap with a stool weight of only 200 grams per 24 hours would not by itself be suggestive of osmotic diarrhea.

Secretory Diarrhea

The net effect of a secretory stimulus on intestinal mucosa can be either inhibition of absorption or a net luminal gain (secretion) of water and electrolytes. This sequence of net movement changes may follow a dose-response curve, with a low secretagogue dose (e.g., circulating vasoactive intestinal polypeptide [VIP] concentration) inhibiting intestinal water and ion absorption and a high dose causing net secretion. On a cellular level, both processes can occur at the same time, with inhibition of villus absorption and enhancement of crypt secretion in the small bowel.

Secretory diarrhea is recognized clinically by certain features: Stools are large in volume and watery (more than 1 liter per day), and diarrhea persists with fasting. The stool osmolality can be totally accounted for by normal ionic constituents: $([Na^+] + [K^+]) \times 2$ equals stool osmolality, which is close to the osmolality of plasma. Table 101–2 gives the major causes of secretory diarrhea. A few examples are discussed in detail.

ENTEROTOXIN-INDUCED SECRETION. The classic disease in this category is Asiatic cholera (Ch. 317). Intestinal secretion is caused by cholera toxin; the morphologic appearance of intestinal mucosa, however, remains normal. An increase in intracellular cyclic adenosine monophosphate (cAMP) in cholera mediates active ion secretion by the enterocytes (Fig. 101–1B). Patients may lose 10 to 20 liters of watery stool per day. Mortality was high prior to the introduction of oral rehydration solutions. This therapy is successful because glucose-stimulated sodium absorption remains normal despite ongoing secretion.

Enterotoxigenic *Escherichia coli* strains can produce one or more of at least three types of toxins (one heat-labile and two heat-stable toxins). Intestinal secretion caused by these toxins is responsible for many episodes of acute diarrhea, including traveler's diarrhea (Ch. 319). Enterotoxin is produced by a large number of other bacteria, some of which are also capable of tissue invasion (*Campylobacter jejuni, Yersinia enterocolitica, Salmonella, Shigella, Clostridium difficile, Staphylococcus aureus, Klebsiella pneumoniae, Aeromonas, Plesiomonas*).

PANCREATIC CHOLERA SYNDROME (Ch. 220). High circulating levels of VIP cause intestinal water and electrolyte secretion that results in large-volume diarrhea. In adults, VIP production usually comes from tumors originating in pancreatic islet cells, whereas in children these tumors are often gangli-

oneuromas or ganglioneuroblastomas. The disease can be mimicked by prolonged intravenous VIP infusion in healthy subjects. This syndrome is also known as Verner-Morrison syndrome, VIPoma syndrome, or watery diarrhea-hypokalemia-hypochlorhydria (WDHH) syndrome. Diarrhea disappears when plasma VIP levels return to normal following tumor resection. Fifty per cent of patients have metastatic disease at diagnosis, however, so that resection is not possible.

In one study of patients with pancreatic cholera, mean daily stool weights averaged 4224 grams during a regular diet and 1817 grams during fasting. Hypokalemia and metabolic acidosis due to large fecal potassium and bicarbonate losses are prominent features, whereas hypochlorhydria is variable. Cosecretion of calcitonin, pancreatic polypeptide, PHM (peptide histidine methionine), or helodermin by these tumors has been found in a number of patients.

IDIOPATHIC SECRETORY DIARRHEA. Patients with this syndrome present with the large-volume secretory diarrhea and other clinical features of pancreatic cholera, but no evidence of tumor or of an abnormally elevated concentration of a circulating secretagogue can be found. These patients undergo extensive negative investigations that often include exploratory laparotomy. Autopsy examination may also be unrevealing, and the etiology remains unknown. Both the severity of this syndrome and the prognosis vary widely. Spontaneous resolution of the diarrhea may occur after several months. A few patients respond to opiates.

CARCINOID SYNDROME (Ch. 230). Diarrhea is a common manifestation of the carcinoid syndrome, occurring in about 70 to 80 per cent of patients. In most patients, intestinal secretion can be demonstrated. Serotonin and substance P elicit intestinal water and ion secretion in experimental animals, and these agents are often elevated in the plasma of patients with the carcinoid syndrome. In other patients, the diarrhea appears episodic and possibly associated with the hypermotility that can be demonstrated when serotonin is given intravenously to normal volunteers. In addition, other contributing causes for diarrhea may be (1) bile salt catharsis if ileal resection was required for tumor removal, (2) lymphatic obstruction due to tumor mass, and (3) subacute intestinal obstruction as a consequence of bowel wall fibrosis induced by the tumor.

MEDULLARY CARCINOMA OF THE THYROID (Ch. 216). Diarrhea occurs in 30 per cent of patients with medullary

TABLE 101–2. INTESTINAL SECRETION: DIARRHEAL SYNDROMES AND CORRESPONDING SECRETORY STIMULI

Diarrheal Syndromes	Secretory Stimulus
Traveler's diarrhea, Asiatic cholera	Enterotoxins (*Escherichia coli, Vibrio cholerae*)
Laxative abuse	Laxatives (phenolphthalein, senna, bisacodyl)
Pancreatic cholera syndrome	Vasoactive intestinal polypeptide
Medullary carcinoma of the thyroid	Calcitonin
Carcinoid syndrome	Serotonin, substance P
Zollinger-Ellison syndrome	Gastrin
Secreting villous adenoma of the rectum	Prostaglandins
Small intestinal obstruction	Intestinal distention
Diarrhea in patients with portal hypertension plus severe hypoalbuminemia	Increased hydrostatic vascular pressure and tissue pressure
Congenital chloridorrhea (intestinal secretion in some instances); lethal familial protracted diarrhea	Congenital mucosal ion transport defects
Giardiasis, strongyloidosis, amebiasis	Unknown mechanism activated by protozoa
Idiopathic chronic secretory diarrhea (pseudopancreatic cholera syndrome)	Unknown
Collagen vascular diseases (scleroderma, systemic lupus erythematosus, mixed connective tissue disease)	Unknown
Intestinal lymphoma	Unknown

carcinoma of the thyroid and may precede the presence of a palpable thyroid mass. Circulating calcitonin is the major mediator of intestinal secretion in this syndrome. Since this tumor may be part of multiple endocrine neoplasia syndromes (Ch. 228), first-degree relatives need to be investigated by measuring basal and postprovocation (intravenous pentagastrin) plasma calcitonin concentrations. Other than in medullary carcinoma of the thyroid, calcitonin is also found in high concentrations in the plasma and tumor tissue of a number of patients with endocrine pancreatic tumors (VIPoma, somatostatinoma), but usually it is not the predominant peptide.

ZOLLINGER-ELLISON SYNDROME (Ch. 98.6). The secretory diarrhea that occurs in gastrinoma (Zollinger-Ellison syndrome) has a unique pathophysiology. Owing to the gastric hypersecretion caused by high concentrations of circulating gastrin, an excessive load of acidic fluid enters the small bowel and overwhelms the intestinal absorptive capacity. In such patients, daily delivery of up to 24 liters of acidic fluid to the jejunum can occur in the fasting state. Although the percentage of decrease in luminal flow rates in the intestine is similar to that in healthy subjects, the remaining fecal volume is often still in excess of 1 liter per day. Other factors that may play a role in causing diarrhea in gastrinoma are the functional or morphologic impairment of the mucosal brush border by the abnormal acid milieu, the direct effect of excessive gastrin on the small bowel mucosa (reducing absorption), and inactivation of pancreatic lipase by the acidic fluid, causing a mild degree of steatorrhea. Low intraluminal pH may also cause some of the primary bile acids to become insoluble, leading to a reduction of micelle formation and a mild degree of steatorrhea.

BILE ACID DIARRHEA. Watery diarrhea in cholerrheic enteropathy results from the secretory effect of malabsorbed bile acids on colonic mucosa. Interruption of the normal enterohepatic circulation of bile acids can be caused by three types of bile acid malabsorption. Type I is due to ileal disease or resection. Type II, which is less common, consists of a selective ileal transport defect for bile acids. Type III is bile acid malabsorption in the postcholecystectomy and postvagotomy state. Cholestyramine is the treatment of choice for type I and type II bile acid diarrhea. Patients with type III are rarely found to have secretory concentrations of fecal bile acids and rarely respond to cholestyramine.

Deranged Intestinal Motility

On a priori grounds, three major derangements might cause diarrhea: (1) Abnormally reduced peristalsis may allow bacterial overgrowth in the small bowel. (2) "Intestinal hurry" may reduce contact time between the small bowel mucosa and its contents and thus result in delivery of abnormally large and qualitatively abnormal fluid loads to the colon. This occurs in spite of the fact that absorption in the small bowel is normal per unit of time. (3) Premature emptying of the colon caused by an abnormality of its contents, or by intrinsic colonic "irritability" or inflammation, results in a reduced contact between luminal contents and colonic mucosa and therefore increased volume and liquidity of the stools.

Some diarrheal diseases due, at least in part, to deranged motility are irritable bowel syndrome, malignant carcinoid syndrome, postvagotomy diarrhea, diarrhea resulting from diabetic neuropathy, diarrhea resulting from thyrotoxicosis, and the diarrhea associated with postgastrectomy dumping syndrome. Abnormal motility may also contribute to acute diarrhea caused by infections. Stool analysis in diarrhea due to a motility disturbance may be consistent with that in osmotic diarrhea if nutrient absorption is impaired in the small bowel or may resemble that in secretory diarrhea, if, following nutrient absorption, the ileocecal transit volume remains largely unabsorbed. Alternatively, a mixed pattern can exist, with electrolytes accounting for an osmolality equal to that of plasma and an additional component making stool water hyperosmolar, owing mainly to bacterial metabolism of malabsorbed carbohydrates in the collection unit following passage of the stool. Irritable bowel syndrome and fecal incontinence are discussed in more detail.

IRRITABLE BOWEL SYNDROME. In the United States, up to 50 per cent of all patients seen by primary care physicians for digestive tract problems have irritable bowel syndrome. Diarrhea is usually referred to as functional diarrhea, since no obvious cause can be found on extensive routine clinical testing. On special investigations, altered myoelectric activity in the large bowel and a significant acceleration in small bowel transit have been demonstrated in patients with irritable bowel syndrome and diarrhea. At the present time, however, it is unclear what clinical relevance these findings may have in the diagnostic and therapeutic management of such patients.

Although functional diarrhea as part of the irritable bowel syndrome is generally considered a diagnosis by exclusion, this does not mean that extensive testing is necessary when one is initially confronted with such a patient. Rather, a positive diagnosis can often be made at the first interview. This is based mainly on a typical history: abdominal pain of long duration (often for several years), discomfort and pain in different areas of the abdomen, bloating associated with various so-called food intolerances, and alternating diarrhea and constipation. Functional diarrhea may show a temporal relation to meal intake, and nocturnal diarrhea is typically absent. Furthermore, signs of systemic disease, such as weight loss, are usually absent. Classically, patients are female and in their 20's and 30's, and a history of emotional conflict, stress, or anxiety is common.

In functional diarrhea, stool weight rarely exceeds 500 grams per day (normal less than 200 grams). In a patient who complains of an increased frequency of defecation, a normal or nearly normal 24-hour stool weight may be the first clue to fecal incontinence, a diagnosis often confused with functional diarrhea.

INCONTINENCE. Most patients whose major disability is due to fecal incontinence present to their physician with "diarrhea." Either they are embarrassed to mention the incontinence, or they interpret it as a manifestation of severe diarrhea. If patients do mention incontinence, the physician also usually attributes it to voluminous diarrhea. In most instances, however, these patients are suffering primarily from a defect in the continence mechanisms rather than from severe diarrhea. As a matter of fact, quantitative stool collections usually reveal rather small fecal volumes, even though stools are soft to liquid in consistency. In any case, the major problem in most such patients is in the anal continence mechanisms. The most frequent causes for sphincter dysfunction are previous anal surgery for fissures, fistulas, or hemorrhoids; episiotomy or tear during childbirth; anal Crohn's disease; and diabetic neuropathy.

Anal sphincter training may improve sphincter function and reduce the frequency of incontinent episodes. It is also important to establish the cause of diarrhea if possible, since effective therapy of the diarrhea usually prevents further incontinence. Symptomatic therapy with opiate drugs is helpful in some patients. There is recent interest in surgical treatment for incontinence, but no good prospective studies have been done. No therapy for incontinence in patients with diarrhea, whether involving drugs, biofeedback, or surgery, has included objective data that convincingly establish its benefit.

Morphologic Alterations

Efficient intestinal absorption requires that the intestinal mucosa be intact with a well-functioning blood supply and intact neural connections. A large number of diseases can cause diarrhea by disrupting the normal anatomy of the intestine (Table 101–3).

VIRAL GASTROENTERITIS. It is estimated that every year 5 million children less than 2 years of age die in developing countries as a consequence of acute diarrhea. Rotavirus is responsible for at least 50 per cent of these infections. The pathogenesis of viral diarrhea is thought to be as follows. The virus enters the absorptive epithelial cells on the tip of the villus, and these cells are sloughed off. Crypt cells then move quickly to replace the lost enterocytes. These cells, however, are immature and cannot absorb effectively. Their sucrase and lactase activities are low, whereas adenylate cyclase activity and cAMP content are normal (in contrast to cholera, in which sucrase and lactase activities are normal and adenylate cyclase activity and cAMP content are increased). There is no enhanced water and electrolyte secretion in viral gastroenteritis; however, sodium-stimulated glucose absorption is markedly diminished. Malabsorption of water, electrolytes, and nutrients results until the infection subsides and mature enterocytes again coat the surface of the villus.

TABLE 101–3. DIARRHEA DUE TO DISRUPTION OF STRUCTURAL INTEGRITY OF THE INTESTINE

Viral gastroenteritis
Bacterial infection with tissue invasion
Sprue (tropical, nontropical, collagenous)
Whipple's disease
Radiation enteritis
Drugs (e.g., chemotherapeutic agents)
Amyloidosis
Collagen vascular diseases (systemic lupus erythematosus, scleroderma, mixed connective tissue disease)
Inflammatory bowel disease (Crohn's disease, ulcerative colitis, microscopic and collagenous colitis)
Eosinophilic gastroenteritis
Intestinal lymphoma
Ileocecal tuberculosis
Intestinal ischemia, mesenteric vasculitis
Diverticulitis
Pelvic inflammatory disease
Acquired immunodeficiency syndrome (AIDS)

SPRUE (Ch. 102). The changes associated with sprue involve villous atrophy and a marked diminution in the effective absorptive surface of the bowel. When studied with intestinal perfusion techniques, such patients demonstrate jejunal secretion. This can be expected from the observation that the mucosa in total villous atrophy consists only of crypts, and crypts normally secrete fluid and electrolytes. Diarrhea is a result of fat and carbohydrate malabsorption. Typically, there is no diarrhea when these patients fast, suggesting that the colon reabsorbs the small bowel secretions. In rare cases patients with sprue have severe secretory diarrhea; a stool output as high as 5 liters a day has been observed.

RADIATION ENTERITIS. Acute radiation enteritis usually occurs within the initial weeks of radiation exposure and is characterized by abdominal cramping, diarrhea, nausea, and vomiting. With the passage of time, symptoms abate, and a quiescent period ensues. The average onset of further symptoms is 1 year, but symptoms may occur at any time. Malabsorption of varying degree for bile acids, fat, carbohydrate, and vitamin B_{12} is observed. Interference with absorption occurs owing to infiltration of the mucosa by inflammatory cells and luminal narrowing of the submucosal arterioles with fibrin plugs. Disturbances in motility due to the effects of radiation on the muscularis propria can also contribute to the diarrhea. Late-appearing structural changes with intermittent obstruction, mucosal ulceration, and fistula formation may also lead to diarrhea. Medical therapy with antidiarrheal agents, broad-spectrum antibiotics for bacterial overgrowth, and prednisone rarely provides total control of symptoms. Ultimately, 15 per cent of patients require surgical intervention, such as segmental resection or fistula closure.

LOSS OF ABSORPTIVE SURFACE. The diarrhea that results from intestinal resection may be on the basis of the region removed (e.g., ileum, with its special transport sites for active bile acid absorption) or of the length of bowel resected. At least 50 per cent of the small bowel is required in order to avoid diarrhea and malnutrition associated with the short bowel syndrome.

AIDS (ACQUIRED IMMUNODEFICIENCY SYNDROME) (Part XXI). Small intestinal morphologic alterations and consequent malabsorption and diarrhea are common among patients with AIDS. Infectious agents (*Giardia, Salmonella, Cryptosporidium,* and *Stronglyoides*) and Kaposi's sarcoma can cause gastrointestinal disturbances in AIDS. There remains a group of patients, however, who do not have identifiable infectious or parasitic agents or Kaposi's sarcoma but who still manifest diarrhea, malabsorption, and weight loss. Such patients have abnormal D-xylose and fat absorption. Duodenal biopsies reveal blunting of the villi and an inflammatory infiltrate in the lamina propria. This condition is referred to as AIDS enteropathy. Other patients with AIDS may demonstrate a histiocytic infiltrate (pseudo-Whipple's disease) containing numerous acid-fast organisms. *Mycobacterium avium-intracellulare* has been isolated in these patients.

MICROSCOPIC COLITIS. Some patients with chronic diar-

rhea demonstrate inflammation of colonic mucosa despite a normal appearance of the colon on barium enema and colonoscopy. The histologic changes consist of excess neutrophils and round cells in the lamina propria, cryptitis, and reactive changes of surface epithelial cells. When colonic absorption is measured in these patients by perfusion techniques, water and electrolyte absorption is either abolished or abnormally low. Thus, the normal ileocecal transit volume (1 liter per day) remains largely unabsorbed, and stool weights are typically in the range of 400 to 800 grams per day.

Miscellaneous Causes of Diarrhea

Table 101–4 gives a list of diseases in which several of the discussed mechanisms may cause diarrhea or in which the pathophysiology is not clearly understood.

DIAGNOSIS

Although the cause of diarrhea is obvious in many clinical situations, in many others it is not. Here we are concerned with a diagnostic approach to the patient with diarrhea in whom the cause is unknown.

History and Physical Examination

When the stools are consistently large in volume, the underlying cause of diarrhea is likely to be located in the small bowel or in the proximal colon. By contrast, in small-volume diarrhea, in which the patient has frequent urges to defecate but passes only small amounts of feces or mucus, the disorder is usually in the left portion of the colon and rectum. Passage of blood mixed in with the diarrheal stool usually indicates inflammation of the mucosa, less often a neoplasm. Passage of nonbloody mucus suggests irritable bowel syndrome, as does a history of small-volume diarrhea alternating with constipation. Frothy stools and excessive flatus suggest fermentation of unabsorbed carbohydrates. Excessively foul stools suggest putrefaction of unabsorbed amino acids. Visible oil or fat indicates severe steatorrhea. Fecal soiling (incontinence) suggests an anal sphincter defect. Diarrhea in a patient with features of anorexia nervosa suggests laxative abuse.

There are, of course, many other pertinent facts obtainable from the history, including previous surgery, drug intake (Table 101–4), symptoms of systemic illness, travel, and related illnesses in family members. In chronic and recurrent diarrhea, an association of exacerbation of diarrhea with emotional stress should be sought, an association that may suggest irritable bowel syndrome. The patient's sexual history should be discussed, as male homosexuals have a high incidence of shigellosis, giardiasis, other intestinal infections, and the usually recognized venereal diseases. Diarrhea may be the presenting manifestation of AIDS.

The physical examination may provide clues to the cause of diarrhea. Some physical findings, as well as other clinical associations that may assist in the diagnosis of diarrhea, are listed in Table 101–5.

Diagnostic Tests

ROUTINE EXAMINATION OF STOOL. Unless the diagnosis is readily apparent from the history and physical examination, certain relatively simple studies on the stool should routinely be

TABLE 101–4. MISCELLANEOUS CAUSES OF DIARRHEA

Drugs
    Diuretics, cardiac glycosides, propranolol, quinidine, colchicine, antibiotics, methotrexate, 6-mercaptopurine, 5-fluorouracil, guanethidine, ethanol
Endocrine disorders
    Addison's disease, hypoparathyroidism
Neurologic diseases
    Tabes dorsalis, multiple sclerosis, myelitis, encephalitis, heat stroke, Charcot-Marie-Tooth disease, myotonia dystrophica, orthostatic hypotension
Toxicologic disorders
    Lead poisoning
Immunoglobulin deficiency
Allergy
Systemic mastocytosis

TABLE 101–5. CLUES TO DIAGNOSIS OF DIARRHEA FROM OTHER SYMPTOMS, SIGNS, AND LABORATORY TESTS

Symptom or Sign Associated with Diarrhea	Diagnoses To Be Considered
Arthritis	Ulcerative colitis, Crohn's disease, Whipple's disease
Liver disease	Ulcerative colitis, Crohn's disease, bowel malignancy with metastasis to liver
Fever	Ulcerative colitis, Crohn's disease, amebiasis, lymphoma, tuberculosis
Marked weight loss	Malabsorption, inflammatory bowel disease, cancer, thyrotoxicosis
Eosinophilia	Eosinophilic gastroenteritis, parasitic disease
Lymphadenopathy	Lymphoma, Whipple's disease, AIDS
Neuropathy	Diabetic diarrhea, amyloidosis
Postural hypotension	Diabetic diarrhea, Addison's disease, idiopathic orthostatic hypotension
Flushing, large liver	Malignant carcinoid syndrome
Proteinuria	Amyloidosis
Perianal disease or right lower quadrant abdominal mass	Crohn's disease
Purpura	Celiac disease
Peptic ulcer	Zollinger-Ellison syndrome, antacid therapy, gastrocolic fistula
Following cholecystectomy	Bile acid malabsorption
Frequent infections	Immunoglobulin deficiency, AIDS
Immunodeficiency	Giardiasis, nodular lymphoid hyperplasia, celiac sprue
Hyperpigmentation	Whipple's disease, celiac disease, Addison's disease
Good response to corticosteroids	Ulcerative colitis, Crohn's disease, Whipple's disease, Addison's disease, pancreatic cholera, eosinophilic enteritis
Good response to antibiotics	Bacterial overgrowth in small intestine, tropical sprue, Whipple's disease, celiac disease

performed. Regardless of the clinical classification, the information obtained usually narrows the diagnostic possibilities.

Stain for Pus. The presence or absence of intestinal inflammation can often be ascertained by examination of a stained stool specimen. Wright's or methylene blue stains are satisfactory. The presence of large numbers of white blood cells is diagnostic of inflammation. The presence of rare, scattered white cells is within normal limits.

In patients with acute or traveler's diarrhea, pus in the stool suggests invasion of the mucosa by *Shigella, E. coli, Entamoeba histolytica, Salmonella, Campylobacter,* gonococci, or other invasive organisms. In general, shigellosis and invasive *E. coli* infections cause more pus than do *Salmonella* and *E. histolytica* infections. Antibiotic-related colitis may or may not be associated with pus. Diarrhea caused by noninvasive organisms that produce enterotoxins (toxigenic *E. coli,* for example), viruses, and *Giardia* is not associated with pus in the stool.

In patients with chronic and recurrent diarrhea or diarrhea of unknown etiology, pus suggests colitis of some type—idiopathic ulcerative colitis, Crohn's colitis, antibiotic-associated colitis, amebic colitis, ischemic colitis, or tuberculous colitis. Pus is especially abundant in idiopathic ulcerative colitis and tends to be less so in amebic colitis. It is usually absent in microscopic colitis. Absence of pus on a single examination does not, of course, absolutely rule out any of these entities. Radiation-induced disease of the large or small bowel or Crohn's disease limited to the small intestine may or may not be associated with pus in the stool. Pus is not present in the stools of patients with irritable bowel syndrome, most causes of malabsorption syndrome, laxative abuse, viral gastroenteritis, and giardiasis.

Occult Blood. Occult (or gross) blood in association with diarrhea usually indicates inflammation and therefore usually has the same significance as pus in the stools (see above). When blood is present in diarrheal stools that do not contain pus, one should consider neoplasms of the colon, heavy metal poisoning, and acute ischemic damage to the gut.

Sudan Stain for Fat. If excess fat is evident on Sudan stain, steatorrhea is probably present, and the various causes of malabsorption syndromes should be considered (see Ch. 102). Most such patients have chronic and recurrent diarrhea; steatorrhea in a patient with acute or traveler's diarrhea suggests giardiasis.

Alkalinization. A pink color following alkalinization of a stool or urine sample indicates phenolphthalein ingestion as the cause of diarrhea. The test is so easily and quickly done, and the significance of a positive result is so great, that it should be carried out routinely in female patients with chronic diarrhea. Surreptitious laxative ingestion is rarely seen in males.

OTHER TESTS. Evidence of systemic illness has obvious implications in the etiology of diarrhea (Table 101–5). For instance, a history of flushing and diarrhea leads to determination of urinary 5-hydroxyindoleacetic acid (Ch. 230). The order in which tests are carried out, assuming that further tests are necessary, varies according to the physician's intuition regarding a particular patient. Certain of the diagnostic tests deserve brief discussion here.

Search for Infectious and Parasitic Organisms. It is important to complete the examination for parasites and to have adequate bacterial cultures in progress prior to examination of the patient with radiologic contrast media because barium interferes with successful demonstration of pathogens. Failure to find *Giardia* in stool samples is not strong evidence against giardiasis; sometimes it is necessary to examine duodenal fluid in order to demonstrate this organism. *Cryptosporidium* can be revealed by acid-fast stain of feces subjected to a flotation technique for concentration. Special culture methods are required if the presence of infection by *Gonococcus, Campylobacter,* or *Yersinia* is to be established. A microimmunofluorescent test with monoclonal antibodies can be used on a rectal mucosal smear to assess for chlamydial proctitis. Serologic tests for amebae and lymphogranuloma venereum may assist in the diagnosis in some patients. Finally, tests for clostridial toxin in fecal fluid help in the diagnosis of pseudomembranous colitis.

Proctosigmoidoscopy. Proctosigmoidoscopy is helpful in establishing the presence or absence of mucosal inflammation. In antibiotic-associated diarrhea, it may reveal pseudomembranes. Proctosigmoidoscopy is often essential in patients with chronic and recurrent diarrhea and in patients with diarrhea of unknown etiology. The findings are especially apt to be abnormal in those whose stools contain pus or blood or both; they are usually normal in patients with diarrhea caused by the various malabsorption syndromes.

Proctosigmoidoscopy to investigate diarrhea should be done without enemas, laxatives, or suppositories. Such preparation may wash away exudate, distort the mucosa, induce trauma, and possibly obscure evidence of disease or create the false impression of disease. In almost all instances, fecal matter can easily be aspirated or pushed aside, and since most abnormalities are diffuse, fecal matter does not interfere greatly with a satisfactory examination. The presence of solid stool in the rectum of a patient who supposedly has diarrhea is also revealing, suggesting that an acute diarrhea is subsiding, that the patient may have irritable bowel syndrome, that the diarrhea is an illusion, or that the diarrhea is secondary to fecal impaction.

Since proctitis may not be evident grossly, even to the experienced eye, mucosal smears should always be obtained and stained for pus. The mucosa should be carefully examined for melanosis coli, although melanosis may be present microscopically even if it is not present grossly.

Rectal Biopsy. Biopsy can often be helpful in the evaluation of patients with diarrhea. The main disorders that might be detected by biopsy, but not by smears and stool examination, are amyloidosis, Whipple's disease, microscopic colitis, granulomatous inflammation, melanosis coli, intestinal spirochetosis (other than that caused by *Treponema pallidum*), and schistosomiasis. Biopsy is indicated in patients with diarrhea of unknown origin, especially in a search for melanosis coli and unsuspected colitis that may not have been evident grossly. It is the opinion of this author that irritable bowel syndrome should not be diagnosed until after a rectal mucosal smear has shown that pus is not present and a rectal biopsy is found to reveal no abnormality. The biopsy should be taken from the posterior wall of the rectum on a valve.

Although the risk is uncertain, some clinicians believe that a rectal biopsy with large forceps predisposes to a colonic perforation if a barium enema is done within 10 days of the biopsy.

Quantitative Fecal Fat. Collected stools (usually for 72 hours) should be quantitatively analyzed for fat content (1) when malabsorption is suggested by the history and physical examination, (2) when the qualitative test for fecal fat is positive, or (3) routinely in patients with diarrhea of unknown origin. If steatorrhea is present, the differential diagnosis of malabsorption syndrome can be pursued (see Ch. 102). Of course, the results of this test must be interpreted with knowledge of the approximate intake of dietary fat. Stool weight in grams (which is equivalent to stool volume in milliliters) should also be noted and recorded (see below).

Twenty-four-hour Stool Volume. For reasons indicated under History and Physical Examination above, knowledge of stool volume helps localize the region of the intestine that is most likely responsible for diarrhea, and in several instances specific information on stool volume is of great diagnostic help. For example, stool volumes greater than 500 ml per day are rarely seen in patients with irritable bowel syndrome, and stool volumes of less than 1000 ml per day provide evidence against pancreatic cholera syndrome. In addition, very large measured stool volumes will alert the physician to the need for vigorous fluid replacement therapy.

Collection of 24-hour stool specimens is easy to do in the initial phases of a diarrhea workup, prior to barium radiographs, enemas, or other preparations. With a little effort, it can be accurately done on an outpatient basis. If a record of stool frequency is kept, the average volume of each stool can be calculated, and the results may give useful insight.

In special instances, e.g., in diarrhea of unknown origin, it is useful to measure stool electrolytes and osmolality and to determine whether or not the diarrhea persists during a 48-hour fast (while the patient is given glucose and salt solutions intravenously). These results help establish whether the diarrhea is secretory or osmotic in type (see Pathophysiology, above). If the osmolality of stool water is less than 250 mOsm per kilogram, water has been added to the stool to simulate diarrhea. A sodium concentration in fecal water that is higher than that of plasma indicates contamination by urine.

Vasoactive Intestinal Polypeptide (VIP) and Other Circulating Agents. The pancreatic cholera syndrome should be considered if diarrhea of unknown origin has lasted longer than 4 weeks, is secretory in type, and is severe (more than 1 liter per day and/or associated with hypokalemia and salt and water depletion), and if surreptitious laxative abuse and organic disease of the gastrointestinal tract have been excluded. The incidence of this syndrome is 1 in 10 million population per year. Only in this rare subgroup of patients is serum assay for VIP, PHM, and calcitonin likely to be helpful. Other gastrointestinal hormones such as pancreatic polypeptide (PP) may be elevated in plasma and serve as markers of endocrine pancreatic malignancy. In the United States, Dr. O'Dorisio's laboratory (Columbus, Ohio) and, in England, Dr. Bloom's laboratory (London) offer a gastrointestinal hormone profile that can be obtained from a single plasma sample. Blood needs to be drawn in iced tubes containing ethylenediamine tetra-acetic acid (EDTA) with aprotinin added to inhibit serum peptidases (aprotinin [Trasylol], 0.5 ml [5000 Kallikrein Inactivator Units] per 10 ml of blood). After immediate centrifugation in a refrigerated centrifuge, plasma is stored at $-25°C$ or lower until sent in a frozen state on Dry Ice to the appropriate laboratory.

Therapeutic Trials. In some instances therapeutic trials are indicated as diagnostic tests. (Obviously, in most instances, the results must be considered suggestive rather than conclusive.) These trials may include pancreatic enzymes, antibiotics (also as part of the Schilling test), metronidazole or quinacrine (for giardiasis), cholestyramine (for bile acid malabsorption), indomethacin (for prostaglandin synthetase inhibition), and various diets (lactose free, carbohydrate free, low fat, and avoidance of any specific food to evaluate the unlikely possibility of food allergy).

THERAPY

The most satisfactory therapy is to cure the underlying disease. When this is not possible, certain drugs may ameliorate the disease and thus reduce the severity of diarrhea (prednisone for inflammatory bowel disease is an example). In a few instances, the disease cannot be ameliorated, but there is fairly specific therapy for the diarrhea, such as cholestyramine for bile acid malabsorption.

At present, unfortunately, in many patients the disease process responsible for diarrhea cannot be satisfactorily suppressed, and specific therapy is lacking. Supportive and symptomatic therapy is required in such instances.

Fluid Replacement

The most important aspect of therapy in acute and traveler's diarrhea, and in some patients with chronic diarrhea, is prevention or correction of salt and water depletion. This can be done by oral ingestion of liquids and salty foods, oral glucose-saline solutions, or intravenous fluid therapy, as dictated by the clinical situation. Two points deserve emphasis. First, soft drinks, tea, and citrus juices contain little, if any, sodium chloride (even Gatorade contains only 23 mEq per liter of sodium chloride). Second, oral glucose-saline solutions or liquids plus salty foods will actually worsen the diarrhea (in terms of stool volume) as they help correct fluid depletion. The oral rehydration solution recommended by the World Health Organization contains the following in millimoles (grams) per liter: glucose, 111 (20); NaCl, 60 (4); KCl, 20 (2); NaHCO₃, 30 (2); and osmolality is 331 mOsm per kilogram. In some patients, particularly those with short bowel syndrome, a high sodium concentration is needed in the oral rehydration solution to achieve a positive sodium and fluid balance. To prevent hypertonicity of such a solution, glucose is best given as a polymer. Glucose polymer consists of linear chains of mostly five to nine glucose units and is obtained from hydrolysis of starch. Glucose polymer is available as Polycose (Ross Laboratories, Columbus, Ohio) or Moducal (Mead Johnson, Evansville, Indiana) and in England as Caloreen (Roussel Ltd., Wembly Park, England). Glucose polymer is readily hydrolyzed in the gut lumen, providing glucose to the sodium-glucose carrier in the brush border. The solution contains the following in millimoles (grams) per liter: glucose polymer, 20 (20); NaCl, 120 (7); KCl, 10 (1); and osmolality is 280 mOsm per kilogram. Various flavoring substances can be added to this solution (e.g., Kool Aid).

Avoidance or Treatment of Perianal Discomfort

Helpful therapy consists of the following: (1) avoidance of soap, toilet paper, washcloths, and towels; (2) gentle washing with warm water on absorbent cotton after each bowel movement, followed by gentle, thorough drying with absorbent cotton; (3) if seepage is present, absorbent cotton retained next to the anal orifice and held in place by snug underwear; (4) sitz baths for 10 minutes two or three times a day; and (5) hydrocortisone creams (1 per cent). In addition to these measures, patients may obtain relief by additional gentle cleaning with soft pads containing witch hazel (Tucks). Locally applied anesthetic ointments may be transiently helpful, but ointments restrict perspiration and anesthetics may irritate the perianal skin, so these agents should be used only for short periods of time. It is important to recognize specific treatable conditions, such as perianal moniliasis.

Opiates

Codeine, diphenoxylate with atropine (Lomotil), and loperamide reduce urgency, bowel movement frequency, and stool volume in a wide variety of acute or chronic diarrheal illnesses. This is not to say that they have a beneficial effect in every patient; but they do in most, so that when groups of patients are studied, both stool frequency and stool volume are reduced to a statistically significant extent. Of the three drugs, loperamide and codeine are usually somewhat superior to diphenoxylate; loperamide may have less tendency than codeine to cause addiction. Codeine, however, is much less expensive. In chronic diarrhea, the drugs may be given once a day in a maximally tolerated dose or several times daily in smaller doses.

Opiate drugs are generally thought to reduce diarrhea through reducing the propulsive activity of the gut and thereby reducing stool frequency. This mechanism might also enhance contact time between intestinal mucosa and luminal contents. Assuming that at least part of the gut mucosa is in an absorbing and not a secretory state, this would allow greater absorption of fluid and thereby reduce stool volume. In vitro opiates have also been reported to stimulate sodium chloride absorption and to have antisecretory action against several secretagogues. These effects cannot be demonstrated in clinical situations using therapeutic doses of opiate drugs.

Opiates should not be used in patients with severe ulcerative colitis with impending toxic megacolon, and there is evidence suggesting that they may prolong the diarrhea in shigellosis and perhaps in diarrheal diseases caused by other invasive bacteria and in antibiotic-associated diarrhea. These reservations notwithstanding, opiates are often of benefit in the symptomatic relief of diarrhea in patients with less severe ulcerative colitis and with many acute infectious diarrheal illnesses. Obviously, they should be prescribed only when diarrhea is causing significant disability.

There are rare case reports suggesting that opiate drugs can be a cause of paradoxical diarrhea.

Bismuth Subsalicylate

Bismuth subsalicylate may prevent infection with enterotoxin-producing *E. coli* organisms. In addition, this agent brings mild symptomatic relief in patients with acute infectious diarrhea, whether bacterial or viral in origin. The mechanism of the effect is unknown. The dose is 30 to 60 ml every 30 minutes for eight doses. Patients should be warned that this medication may turn their stools black. If the patient is on other medications, possible drug interaction should be considered.

Antibiotics in Acute and Traveler's Disease (Ch. 319)

For at least two reasons, antibiotics should not usually be used. First, in most patients they do not shorten the duration of illness. Second, their use risks the development of antibiotic-associated diarrhea or colitis, superimposed on whatever was causing the diarrhea initially. This greatly confuses the problem if the diarrhea becomes chronic.

In mild disease (small-volume diarrhea, no chills or fever, no blood or pus in the stool), antibiotics should not be prescribed unless a specific indication emerges from the bacteriology and parasitology laboratory. In patients who are severely ill, especially if they have blood or pus in the stool, antibiotic therapy aimed at shigellosis is reasonable, pending the result of stool culture.

Antisecretory Drugs

A specific and potent inhibitor of intestinal secretion is not available. On the basis of in vitro observations and individual case reports, a number of agents can be tried on an empiric basis. Phenothiazines inhibit secretion caused by cholera toxin and *E. coli* enterotoxins; aspirin, indomethacin, and other non-steroidal anti-inflammatory agents reduce secretion mediated by prostaglandins (inhibition of prostaglandin synthesis); glucocorticoids decrease mucosal inflammation and enhance NaCl absorption (increase in Na-K-ATPase activity); nicotinic acid, clonidine, lidamidine,* and lithium carbonate may increase intestinal NaCl absorption (inhibition of adenylate cyclase); and cromoglycate may inhibit release of mediators of allergic reaction in the intestine. When diarrhea is due to circulating agents (VIPoma, carcinoid), a somatostatin analogue given subcutaneously may abolish diarrhea by decreasing secretagogue release from tumor tissue.

Bo-Linn GW, Vendrell DD, Lee E, et al.: An evaluation of the significance of microscopic colitis in patients with chronic diarrhea. J Clin Invest 75:1559, 1986. *First description of microscopic colitis as a separate disease entity. Patients reveal abolished water and electrolyte absorption during colonic perfusion studies.*

Field M, Fordtran JS, Schultz SG (eds.): Secretory Diarrhea. Bethesda, Md., American Physiological Society, 1980. *Sixteen chapters by different experts on various aspects of the pathophysiology of secretory diarrhea. The emphasis is on basic research, although there is a highly original chapter on the pharmacology of antidiarrheal drugs.*

Fine KD, Krejs GJ, Fordtran JS: Diarrhea. *In* Sleisenger MH, Fordtran JS (eds.): Gastrointestinal Disease. 4th ed. Philadelphia, W. B. Saunders Company, 1989, pp 290–315. *A detailed description of the physiology of the human intestinal tract with regard to water and electrolyte movement and the pathophysiology of chronic diarrhea.*

*Investigational agent.

Krejs GJ (ed.): Diarrhoea. Clin Gastroenterol 15, No 3, 1986. *Thirteen chapters on the pathophysiology and clinical investigation of diarrhea. Contains re-evaluation of criteria for defining secretory diarrhea and extensive description of diarrhée motrice (diarrhea due to motility derangement).*

Krejs GJ: VIPoma syndrome. Am J Med (in print). *An extensive description of pancreatic cholera syndrome, the most prominent example of secretory diarrhea caused by a circulating agent.*

Lambert HP (ed.): Infections of the GI tract. Clin Gastroenterol 8, No 3, 1979. *Twelve excellent chapters by different experts dealing with the pathophysiology of diarrhea, viral infections, pathogenic mechanisms in bacterial diarrhea, E. coli, Shigella, food poisoning, typhoid and paratyphoid fever, Campylobacter enteritis, traveler's diarrhea, antibiotic-associated colitis, antibiotic resistance, and antimicrobial agents. The book contains much practical and clinically useful information.*

Read NW, Krejs GJ, Read MG, et al.: Chronic diarrhea of unknown origin. Gastroenterology 78:264, 1980. *A detailed account of the clinical problems encountered in patients with intractable and difficult-to-diagnose chronic diarrhea.*

Santangelo WC, Krejs GJ: Gastrointestinal manifestations of the acquired immunodeficiency syndrome. Am J Med Sci 292:328, 1986. *Complete review of enteric infections, parasitic infestations, enteropathy, gastrointestinal bleeding, and neoplasms in patients with AIDS.*

102 Malabsorption
Phillip P. Toskes

The malabsorption syndrome refers to a clinical condition in which a number of nutrients and minerals are not normally absorbed; almost always, however, lipids fail to be normally absorbed. At times the absorption of a single nutrient may be selectively impaired. A sound knowledge of normal absorptive processes allows the physician to pursue a logical approach to the diagnosis and treatment of the patient with malabsorption.

NORMAL ABSORPTION OF NUTRIENTS

Absorption is the integration of those processes whereby the products of digestion pass from the lumen of the intestine through the small intestinal enterocyte to appear in the general circulation via the lymphatics or the portal vein. Although the digestive process is initiated by acid and pepsin within the stomach, the exocrine pancreas has the major role in digesting fat, carbohydrate, and protein by its secretion of lipase, amylase, and proteases. Fat is eventually broken down to monoglycerides and fatty acids; carbohydrate, to disaccharides and monosaccharides; and proteins, to peptides and amino acids. These forms of nutrients are absorbed through the intestinal enterocyte. The villi and microvilli of the small intestine provide an enormous area for absorption. The motility of the intestine and the contraction of the microvilli allow molecules to pass through an "unstirred layer" adjacent to the microvilli.

Nutrients pass through the enterocyte by several processes: active transport, passive diffusion, facilitated diffusion, and endocytosis. Active transport and passive diffusion are the main mechanisms whereby nutrients pass through membranes. *Active transport* moves nutrients against a chemical or electrical gradient, requires energy, is carrier mediated, and is subject to competitive inhibition. *Passive diffusion* does not require energy and allows nutrients to pass through a membrane according to chemical concentration and electrical gradients. Passive diffusion, best typified by water absorption, is not carrier mediated and does not demonstrate competitive inhibition. *Facilitated diffusion* is similar to passive diffusion but may be carrier mediated and may be subject to competitive inhibition. *Endocytosis* is a process whereby nutrients are engulfed by parts of the cell membrane. Although endocytosis may be most important in the neonatal period, this absorptive mechanism may also occur to some extent in the adult and may be involved in the absorption of antigens.

Absorption of nutrients may be regionalized (Table 102–1). Although many nutrients can be absorbed throughout the small intestine, each nutrient has a major site of absorption. When areas of the intestine are damaged or resected, the remaining intestine usually adapts effectively to absorb the nutrients that

TABLE 102–1. REGIONALIZATION OF NUTRIENT ABSORPTION

Nutrient	Major Site of Absorption
Fat	Proximal small intestine
Protein	Mid small intestine
Carbohydrate	Proximal and mid small intestine
Iron	Proximal small intestine
Calcium	Proximal small intestine
Folic acid	Proximal and mid small intestine
Cobalamin (vitamin B_{12})	Distal small intestine (ileum)
Other water-soluble vitamins	Proximal and mid small intestine
Bile salts	Distal small intestine (ileum)
Water and electrolytes	Small intestine and colon (especially cecum)

would normally have been absorbed by those areas. Two noteworthy exceptions to this adaptation process are cobalamin (vitamin B_{12}) and bile salts. If the distal ileum has been resected, the subject can *never* actively absorb these two nutrients again. This has important clinical implications, especially for cobalamin. Patients who have had their distal ileum resected must receive monthly parenteral cobalamin or they will develop macrocytic anemia and neuropathy secondary to cobalamin deficiency (Ch. 132).

Fat Absorption

Dietary fat is ingested largely as long-chain triglycerides, the absorption of which is a complex process involving the pancreas, liver, small intestine, and lymphatics (Fig. 102–1). Nevertheless, the process is very efficient; the coefficient of fat absorption is greater than 93 per cent, i.e., less than 7 per cent of ingested fat escapes absorption and appears in the stool per day. A breakdown in any one of these steps (Fig. 102–1) leads to malabsorption of fat (steatorrhea). A thorough knowledge of this physiologic process allows a logical approach to be pursued in the evaluation of the patient with steatorrhea.

Some triglyceride digestion begins in the stomach by lingual and gastric lipases. Triglyceride is emulsified in the stomach, and fat is slowly emptied into the duodenum, where its entry, and that of acid, release cholecystokinin-pancreozymin and secretin. As a result, the pancreas secretes enzymes and bicarbonate, and the gallbladder contracts to release bile salts. Bicarbonate maintains the pH of the intestinal lumen above 4, allowing pancreatic lipase to be effective in hydrolysis of triglycerides to yield free fatty acids and monoglycerides. Another pancreatic protein, colipase, facilitates the interaction between lipase and triglyceride for effective lipolysis. Fatty acids and monoglyceride interact with conjugated bile salts to form molecular aggregates or micelles (Fig. 102–1). A critical concentration of bile salts for micelle formation (5 to 15 μmol per milliliter) is maintained by a very efficient enterohepatic circulation of bile salts. Although the total

bile salt pool is only 2 to 4 grams, 95 per cent of bile salts is actively absorbed in the ileum and returned to the liver by the portal venous system. Each day 20 to 30 grams of bile salts recirculate in this enterohepatic circulation. Only about 200 to 600 mg of bile salts is excreted in the feces per day and must be replaced by hepatic biosynthesis from cholesterol.

Micellar fat passes through the "unstirred" water layer covering the surface of the enterocyte. Because of their solubility in the lipid-rich surface membrane, the fatty acids and monoglycerides are released and diffuse into the enterocyte. Fatty acid–binding protein (low molecular weight cytosolic protein) avidly binds long-chain fatty acids in the enterocyte and transports them to the smooth endoplasmic reticulum, where they are re-esterified with monoglyceride to form triglyceride. Absorbed cholesterol is also largely esterified with fatty acids for optimal transport. The intestine must also synthesize phospholipids and specific proteins (apoproteins) in order to incorporate these nonpolar lipids into lipoproteins, the major transport vehicles for fat transport in lymph and plasma (Ch. 172). These polar components are added to the surface of the lipid droplet, producing lipoproteins called chylomicrons. Chylomicrons are concentrated in the Golgi apparatus and then discharged through the lateral basal portion of the cell to the interstitium and mesenteric lymph to be delivered via the thoracic duct to the vena cava.

Medium-chain triglycerides (C-6 to C-12 fatty acids) are absorbed quite differently and more effectively than are long-chain triglycerides (C-16 to C-18 fatty acids) described above. Medium-chain triglycerides (MCT) (1) are more completely hydrolyzed by pancreatic lipase, (2) do not require bile salts for absorption, (3) can be directly taken up into the enterocyte and hydrolyzed by a mucosal lipase to fatty acids, (4) do not need to be re-esterified, (5) are not incorporated into lipoproteins, and (6) can pass directly into the portal venous system, transported as fatty acids bound to albumin. These characteristics of MCT allow its therapeutic use to improve fat absorption in a number of diseases in which dietary triglyceride absorption is impaired.

Fat-soluble vitamins (A, D, E, K) are absorbed after micellar solubilization and are transported into lymph with chylomicrons. In the case of vitamin A, the free vitamin is esterified within the enterocyte with palmitic acid, transported via chylomicrons in the lymph and stored as retinol palmitate in the liver. Vitamin metabolism is described more fully in Ch. 204.

Carbohydrate Absorption

Carbohydrate is ingested in the form of starch, sucrose, and lactose. Salivary and pancreatic amylases hydrolyze starch to oligosaccharides and disaccharides. All carbohydrate must be digested to a final monosaccharide product before it can be absorbed. Disaccharides are split by membrane-bound disaccharidases located on the microvilli of the enterocyte. Lactose is digested by lactase to glucose and galactose; sucrose, by sucrase to glucose and fructose; and maltose by maltase to two molecules of glucose. These monosaccharides are then transported through the enterocyte to the portal blood. Glucose and galactose are

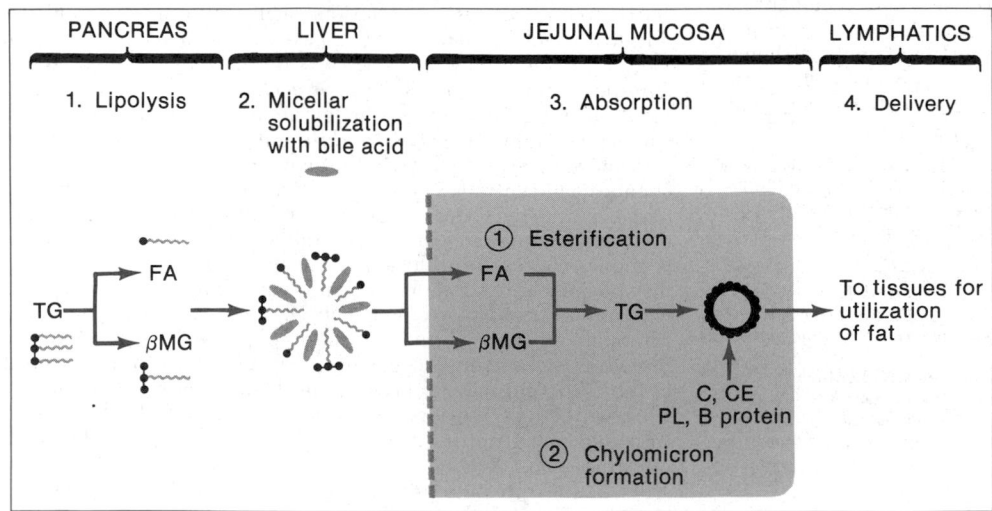

PANCREAS	LIVER	JEJUNAL MUCOSA	LYMPHATICS
1. Lipolysis	2. Micellar solubilization with bile acid	3. Absorption	4. Delivery

① Esterification

② Chylomicron formation

C, CE PL, B protein

To tissues for utilization of fat

FIGURE 102–1. Schematic of intestinal absorption, showing the participation of the pancreas, liver, and intestinal mucosal cell in fat absorption. (From Wilson FA, Dietschy JM: Gastroenterology 61:911, 1971. Copyright 1971, The Williams & Wilkins Company, Baltimore.)

absorbed by active transport requiring sodium. Fructose is transported by facilitated diffusion. Glucose is transported into the enterocyte, probably bound along with sodium to a protein carrier. These monosaccharides are transported out of the cell by active sodium extrusion across the basolateral aspect of the enterocyte via a sodium pump.

Protein and Amino Acid Absorption

The digestion of dietary protein is initiated in the stomach by acid and pepsin but is largely completed by pancreatic proteases, both endopeptidases (trypsin, chymotrypsin, elastase) and exopeptidases (carboxypeptidase). Pancreatic proteases secreted in inactive forms (zymogens) must be activated. Enterokinase from the small intestinal mucosa activates trypsin from trypsinogen, and trypsin then activates all of the other protease precursors. The digestive products of pancreatic proteases are peptides containing two to six amino acids as well as single amino acids. Peptidases on the microvillus membrane or in the cytosol of the enterocyte further hydrolyze oligopeptides to free amino acids, which are directly absorbed in the portal vein.

The L forms of amino acids are actively transported in the enterocyte by specific energy-requiring, sodium-dependent processes. There are several specific transport systems for amino acids: (1) the dibasic amino acid system, which is often abnormal in cystinuria; (2) the neutral amino acid system, which is abnormal in Hartnup disease; (3) the iminoglycine system; and (4) the dicarboxylic acid system. Intact di- and tripeptides are also actively transported across the enterocyte membrane without hydrolysis by peptidases on the microvillus membrane. These peptides are hydrolyzed in the cytosol of the enterocyte to amino acids, which are then released into the circulation.

Water and Electrolyte Absorption

Over 7 liters of water (both ingested and reabsorbed from intestinal secretion) is absorbed by the small intestine per day through the process of passive diffusion. Absorption of water often follows that of glucose and electrolytes in order to maintain isotonicity of intraluminal contents.

Sodium is actively transported linked to an exchange with H^+ in the jejunum and ileum and with Cl^- and HCO_3^- in the ileum. Na^+ transport is enhanced by glucose absorption in the jejunum (via the glucose-Na^+ carrier on the microvillus membrane) and by solvent (water) drag. Some Na^+ also moves down a gradient across the mucosa, i.e., by passive diffusion. Changes in the concentration of sodium in the lumen depend on relative rates of exchange of both sodium and water between blood and lumen. Potassium passively diffuses from the lumen of the proximal small intestine and into the lumen of the distal small intestine.

Calcium Absorption

Calcium is actively absorbed in the duodenum largely regulated by the active form of vitamin D_3–1,25-dihydroxycholecalciferol (calcitriol). Vitamin D_3 from the diet is metabolized first by the liver (25-hydroxylation) and then by the kidney (1-hydroxylation) to form 1,25-dihydroxycholecalciferol (1,25[OH]$_2$D$_3$) (Ch. 233). This process is influenced by parathyroid hormone levels, which are regulated by plasma levels of ionized calcium. Calcitriol stimulates the synthesis of calcium-binding protein, alkaline phosphatase, and a calcium-activated ATPase—all involved in active calcium transport. Absorption of vitamin D, a fat-soluble vitamin, is often impaired in the malabsorptive syndromes such that calcium absorption is diminished. Fatty acids within the lumen of the intestine may also directly impair absorption by binding calcium. In turn, the unavailability of ionized calcium in the lumen leads to excessive absorption of oxalate and a resulting propensity to form calcium oxalate kidney stones.

Iron Absorption (Ch. 131)

The average intake of iron from dietary sources is 15 to 25 mg per day, of which 0.5 to 2.0 mg is normally absorbed. Iron is absorbed as inorganic iron (cereals, vegetables) or as heme iron (meat). For optimal absorption, inorganic iron must be released from dietary components to soluble iron complexes in the intestinal lumen. Gastric acid enhances the absorption of inorganic iron (both Fe^{3+} and Fe^{2+}) by facilitating its chelation with sugars, amino acids, bile, and ascorbic acid. Such iron complexes remain in solution at the alkaline pH of the duodenum—the major site of iron absorption. Inorganic iron is absorbed from the intestinal lumen by the mucosa and then transported to the blood by mechanisms that are still not clear. A mucosal regulatory system keeps much of the iron trapped within the enterocyte, to be excreted into the feces depending on the need for iron, as determined by body stores of iron or by the rate of erythropoiesis. Organic iron (heme iron) is absorbed more efficiently than is inorganic iron. Heme is split from globin and absorbed as an intact metalloporphyrin at an alkaline pH. Iron is released from heme by heme oxygenase intracellularly. In plasma, iron is transported bound to transferrin, a specific globulin, to various tissues for use or storage.

Iron absorption is increased in iron deficiency, pregnancy, idiopathic hemochromatosis, and any conditions in which there is active erythropoiesis. Absorption is decreased in chronic infection and after the ingestion of large amounts of iron. Diffuse disease of the duodenum such as nontropical sprue may impair iron absorption and lead to iron deficiency.

Folic Acid Absorption

Dietary folic acid is conjugated with glutamyl peptides; prior to its absorption, these polyglutamates must be deconjugated to monoglutamates by folic deconjugase, an enzyme found on the microvillus membrane. Folate monoglutamates are absorbed by active transport at low concentrations of folate and by passive diffusion at high concentrations of folate. Folic acid undergoes an enterohepatic circulation. Since its body stores are limited, the major cause of folate deficiency is poor dietary intake of fresh fruits and vegetables. Folic acid deficiency may also occur if there is extensive damage to the proximal small intestine (e.g., nontropical sprue) or secondary to the use of a number of medications (sulfasalazine, phenytoin, trimethoprim) that inhibit its absorption. Other causes of folate deficiency are listed in Table 132–1.

Cobalamin (Vitamin B₁₂) Absorption (Ch. 132)

The current concept of cobalamin absorption and transport is depicted in Figure 102–2. Cobalamin, found in animal protein, is released from protein in the stomach by the synergistic action of both acid and pepsin. Cobalamin initially binds to a cobalamin-binding protein (R binder or cobalophilin), also secreted by the stomach. The cobalophilin-cobalamin complex is degraded by pancreatic proteases within the duodenal lumen, with release of cobalamin to bind with gastric intrinsic factor (a glycoprotein secreted by the parietal cells). After intrinsic factor binds cobalamin, the intrinsic factor–cobalamin complex passes down the small intestine until it reaches the distal 60 cm of the ileum, where it binds to a specific receptor of the brush border. In the absence of the terminal ileum, intrinsic factor–mediated cobalamin absorption ceases, although large doses of cobalamin (milligram in contrast to microgram amounts) may lead to adequate absorption by passive diffusion throughout the gastrointestinal tract.

Intrinsic factor does not enter the ileal cell and is not absorbed. Transcobalamin II (TCII), the most important transport protein for cobalamin, picks up cobalamin in the ileal mucosa and promotes its uptake by tissues throughout the body. The TCII-cobalamin complex enters tissues via endocytosis, with cobalamin being released by lysosomal proteolysis.

At equilibrium, the majority of circulating cobalamin is attached to cobalophilin, which is also found in saliva, gastric secretions, intestinal secretions, semen, and tears. It also moves continuously in an enterohepatic circulation. The function of the ubiquitous cobalophilins is unclear, but they may prevent or retard the absorption and dissemination of a variety of cobalamin analogues, either produced by bacteria or even found within multivitamin supplements.

CLASSIFICATION AND CLINICAL MANIFESTATIONS OF MALABSORPTION

Causes of Malabsorption

Table 102–2 divides the causes of the malabsorption syndrome into nine categories, based upon its pathophysiology (see Fig. 102–1). Some conditions have multiple reasons for malabsorption

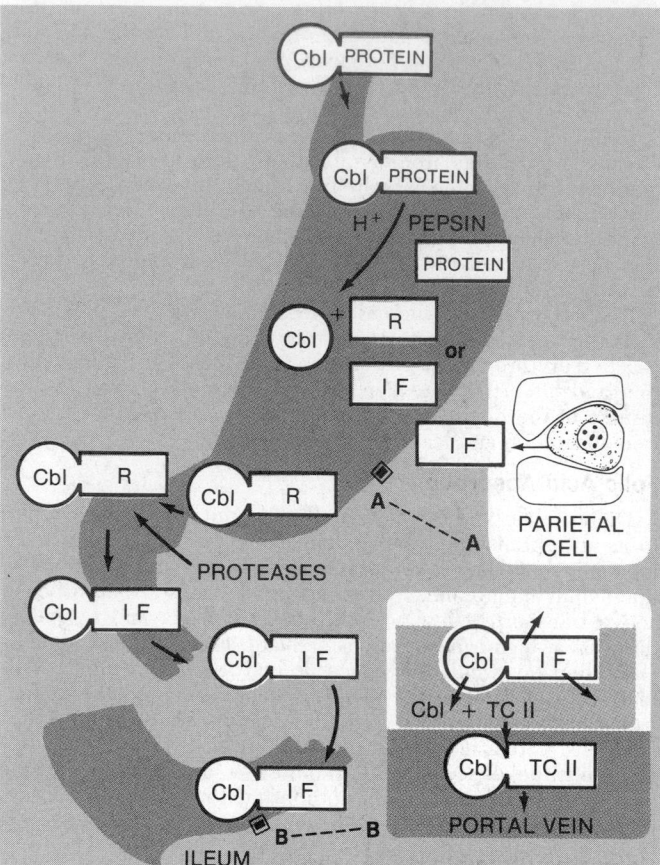

FIGURE 102–2. Cobalamin absorption and transport. Cbl = Cobalamin, R = R-protein or cobalophilin, IF = intrinsic factor, TC II = transcobalamin II. (From Toskes PP: J Clin Gastroenterol 2:287, 1980.)

but are arbitrarily classified under one major category. The differential features and management of important types of this syndrome are detailed later in the chapter.

Clinical Manifestations

Patients with the malabsorption syndrome usually present with diarrhea, weight loss, and malnutrition. These patients often complain that their stools are bulky, greasy, and excessively malodorous and that they float and are difficult to flush down the toilet. Steatorrheal stools float not because of their fat content but because of their high gas content. Patients with severe malabsorption, as exemplified by that secondary to pancreatic insufficiency, may complain of oil seeping out of the rectum. The symptoms and signs of malabsorption are varied and involve a number of organ systems. Patients may demonstrate one or more of these manifestations depending on the severity of their malabsorption. The different symptoms and signs that such patients may show and the causes of these symptoms and signs are detailed in Table 102–3. These aspects of the history and physical examination are crucial in evaluating a patient with malabsorption.

DIAGNOSIS OF MALABSORPTION

Although there may be selective malabsorption of nutrients, most patients with clinically relevant malabsorption have steatorrhea. Consequently, documentation of steatorrhea is important and is the cornerstone of the diagnostic evaluation of patients with malabsorption. The only truly reliable means to document the presence of steatorrhea is the quantitative chemical analysis of fat in a 72-hour stool collection while the patient is ingesting a high-fat diet (at least 100 grams per day). On such a diet normal subjects excrete less than 7 grams of fat per day (coefficient of absorption of >93 per cent). Unfortunately, the quantitative fecal fat determination is cumbersome to perform and difficult to

obtain in most hospitals. Furthermore, the documentation of steatorrhea only indicates that the patient has the malabsorption syndrome—it does not indicate the pathophysiology or confer a specific diagnosis.

Table 102–4 details some alternative tests (other than the quantitative fecal fat determination) that can be employed to detect the presence and the cause of malabsorption in a given patient. The tests are categorized into screening tests and those that are more specific in localizing the site of the malabsorption. It is usually necessary to utilize a number of malabsorptive tests to establish the cause of the malabsorption.

Qualitative Stool Fat

The microscopic examination of stool for the presence of fat is a helpful test if performed properly and if the patient is ingesting a high-fat diet. Two specimens of stool are placed on two slides. To the first slide, two drops of water and two drops of 95 per cent ethyl alcohol are added, followed by two drops of a fat stain (e.g., Sudan III). The specimen is microscopically examined for orange neutral fat (triglyceride) globules. The globules should be larger than a red cell and should be numerous per high-power field. To the second slide, several drops of 36 per cent acetic

TABLE 102–2. CLASSIFICATION OF THE MALABSORPTION SYNDROME

1. Impaired digestion
   a. Primary pancreatic exocrine insufficiency
   b. Gastric surgery (Billroth I and II, vagotomy, and pyloroplasty)*
   c. Gastrinoma*
2. Reduced bile salt concentration
   a. Liver disease
   b. Small intestine bacterial overgrowth (scleroderma, diabetes mellitus, primary motility disturbances, postgastrectomy, achlorhydria)*
   c. Ileal disease or resection*
3. Abnormalities of intestinal mucosa
   a. Disaccharidase deficiency
   b. Impaired monosaccharide transport
   c. Folate or cobalamin deficiency
   d. Nontropical sprue
   e. Nongranulomatous ileojejunitis
   f. Amyloidosis
   g. Crohn's disease*
   h. Eosinophilic enteritis
   i. Radiation enteritis*
   j. Abetalipoproteinemia
   k. Cystinuria
   l. Hartnup disease
4. Inadequate absorptive surface
   a. Short bowel syndrome
   b. Jejunoileal bypass*
5. Infection
   a. Tropical sprue
   b. Whipple's disease*
   c. Acute infectious enteritis
   d. Parasitic infections
6. Lymphatic obstruction
   a. Lymphoma*
   b. Tuberculosis
   c. Lymphangiectasia
7. Cardiovascular disorders
   a. Congestive heart failure
   b. Constrictive pericarditis
   c. Mesenteric vascular insufficiency
8. Drug-induced
   a. Cholestyramine
   b. Neomycin
   c. Colchicine
   d. Phenindione
   e. Irritant laxatives
9. Unexplained
   a. Carcinoid syndrome
   b. Diabetes mellitus*
   c. Adrenal insufficiency
   d. Hyper- and hypothyroidism
   e. Mastocytosis
   f. Hypogammaglobulinemia

* Multiple reasons for malabsorption.

TABLE 102–3. SYMPTOMS AND SIGNS OF MALABSORPTION

History	Pathophysiology	Physical Examination	Pathophysiology
Diarrhea	Increased secretion and impaired absorption of water and electrolytes, unabsorbed dihydroxy bile acids, unabsorbed fatty acids	Pallor	Anemia secondary to iron, folate, or cobalamin deficiency
		Glossitis, stomatitis, cheilosis	Iron, folate, cobalamin, and other vitamin deficiencies
Greasy, bulky, malodorous stools that are difficult to flush	Increased fat in stool		
Oil seeping from rectum	Unabsorbed triglyceride (pancreatic insufficiency)	Ecchymosis, purpura	Vitamin K malabsorption
		Acrodermatitis	Zinc and fatty acid deficiency
Weight loss despite good appetite	Loss of calories from malabsorption	Dehydration, hypotension	Water and electrolyte malabsorption
Excessive flatus	Fermentation of unabsorbed carbohydrates by colonic bacteria	Edema	Protein malabsorption (decreased serum albumin)
Diffuse abdominal pain	Inflammation or infiltration of tissue (pancreatic insufficiency, Crohn's disease, lymphoma)	Peripheral neuropathy	Cobalamin deficiency
Postprandial (30 minutes after eating) midabdominal pain	Intestinal ischemia		
Abnormal bruisability	Vitamin K malabsorption		
Weakness and fatigue	Protein, electrolyte, fat, iron, folate, cobalamin malabsorption		
Milk intolerance	Lactase deficiency		
Bone pain	Calcium and protein malabsorption		
Tetany, paresthesias	Calcium and magnesium malabsorption, cobalamin deficiency (paresthesias only)		
Night blindness	Vitamin A malabsorption		
Nocturia	Delayed absorption of water, hypokalemia		
Amenorrhea	Protein malabsorption		

TABLE 102–4. TESTS FOR MALABSORPTION

Test	Normal Values	Comments Relevant to Patients with Malabsorption
Screening Tests		
1. Serum carotene	>0.06 mg/dl	Decreased; very good test if poor oral intake has been excluded
2. Serum calcium	9.0 to 10.5 mg/dl	Decreased, not very sensitive
3. Serum cholesterol	150 to 250 mg/dl	Decreased, not very sensitive
4. Serum albumin	4.0 to 5.2 mg/dl	Decreased, not very sensitive
5. Serum magnesium	1.7 to 2.0 mEq/L	Decreased, not very sensitive
6. Prothrombin time	Control value	Increased, not very sensitive
7. Qualitative stool fat	No fat globules per hpf*	Numerous fat globules per hpf; part 1 for neutral fats, part 2 for split fats (see text)
Specific Tests		
1. Serum iron	80–150 μg/dl	Malabsorbed in proximal small bowel disease
2. Serum folate	5–21 ng/ml	Decreased in proximal small bowel disease, may be increased in bacterial overgrowth
3. Serum cobalamin (vitamin B_{12})	200–900 pg/ml	Malabsorbed in distal small bowel disease, pernicious anemia, bacterial overgrowth, chronic pancreatitis
4. Urinary D-xylose	>5 grams/5 hr	Decreased in small bowel disease and bacterial overgrowth, normal in pancreatic disease
5. Bentiromide test	Arylamine excretion >57% in 6 hr	A value of <50 per cent is diagnostic of pancreatic insufficiency
6. Serum trypsin–like immunoreactivity (TLI)	29–80 ng/ml	A value of <20 ng/ml is specific for pancreatic insufficiency
7. Secretin test	HCO_3^- conc >80 mEq/L Vol >1.8 ml/kg/hr	Most sensitive test of pancreatic function
8. ^{57}Cyanocobalamin urinary excretion test	>8%/24 hr	Decreased in pernicious anemia, chronic pancreatitis, bacterial overgrowth, ileal disease
9. Urine 5-HIAA*	1.7–8.0 mg/24 hr	Markedly elevated in carcinoid syndrome, minimally elevated in any kind of malabsorption
10. Breath tests		
a. ^{14}C-xylose	<0.0013% of administered dose as breath $^{14}CO_2$ at 30 min	Elevated in bacterial overgrowth
b. cholyl-1-^{14}C-glycine	<1% of administered dose as breath $^{14}CO_2$ at any interval over 4 hr	Elevated in bacterial overgrowth or bile acid malabsorption
c. Lactulose H_2	<10 ppm rise in breath H_2 over baseline at any interval for 120 min	Elevated in bacterial overgrowth; increase in fasting breath H_2 suggests bacterial overgrowth; up to 27% of subjects may not have flora that produces H_2
d. Lactose-H_2	<20 ppm rise in breath H_2 over baseline at any interval for 180 min	Elevated in lactase deficiency
11. Small intestinal culture	≤10^5 organisms per ml jejunal secretions	>10^5 organisms per ml jejunal secretions indicates bacterial overgrowth
12. Small intestinal biopsy	See Figure 102–4	See Table 102–7

*hpf = High-power field; 5-HIAA = 5-hydroxyindoleacetic acid.

acid are added, then several drops of Sudan III. The slide is heated until it begins to boil. Microscopically, the presence of large orange globules or spicules represents free fatty acids. Part 1 is positive in patients with pancreatic insufficiency, detecting undigested triglyceride; part 2, in patients with small bowel disease, detecting free fatty acids. Figure 102–3 demonstrates a positive part 1 test in a patient with pancreatic insufficiency. There is a 25 per cent false-negative rate when steatorrhea is mild, i.e., <10 grams per 24 hours. The false-positive rate is about 15 per cent. This test is simple to perform and inexpensive.

Urinary D-Xylose Test

The urinary xylose excretion test distinguishes between malabsorption due to small intestinal disease and that due to pancreatic exocrine insufficiency. A 5-hour urinary excretion of 5 grams or greater is normal following the oral administration of 25 grams of D-xylose to a well-hydrated subject. Decreased xylose absorption and excretion are found in patients with damage to the proximal small intestine and in bacterial overgrowth in the small intestine (the bacteria catabolize the xylose). Patients with pancreatic steatorrhea usually have normal xylose absorption. As with any urinary excretion test, decreased renal function or incomplete collection of the urine may invalidate the test. Impaired renal function is most important when evaluating an elderly patient who may not have obvious renal disease, but whose creatinine clearance may be low. Decreased urinary xylose values may also be seen in patients with ascites. Although a blood level of 30 mg per deciliter or greater 1 hour after ingestion of xylose may indicate normal absorption, there appears to be a great deal of overlap between control subjects and those with malabsorption.

Bentiromide Urinary Excretion Test

Bentiromide is a synthetic peptide attached to para-aminobenzoic acid (PABA). The bond between the peptide and PABA is easily split by chymotrypsin. Following the oral administration of 500 mg of bentiromide, PABA is absorbed in the proximal small intestine, partially conjugated in the liver, and excreted in the urine as arylamines. A cumulative 6-hour arylamine excretion of less than 50 per cent of that ingested as bentiromide is virtually diagnostic of pancreatic insufficiency. In a patient with symptomatic diarrhea or steatorrhea or both, a normal bentiromide test result virtually excludes pancreatic disease as the cause of the symptoms. The use of bentiromide offers a simple, reliable confirmatory test (high specificity, few false-positive results) for the diagnosis of pancreatic insufficiency. The test is not accurate when the serum creatinine level exceeds 2.0 mg per deciliter.

Serum Trypsin-like Immunoreactivity (TLI)

TLI, a radioimmunoassay, measures serum levels of this pancreas-derived protein. Although not as sensitive as the bentiro-

mide or secretin test, a decreased value appears to be completely specific for pancreatic insufficiency.

Secretin Test

The most sensitive tests of impaired pancreatic function are direct measurements of its exocrine function; unfortunately, these are the most complex to perform. The patient swallows a tube that is fluoroscopically placed, with the aspiration site within the second part of the duodenum near where the pancreatic duct enters the duodenum. A hormone is given intravenously, and a component of pancreatic secretion (bicarbonate after secretin; trypsin, amylase, or lipase after cholecystokinin) is measured. False-positive tests are virtually nonexistent if the tube has been properly positioned, and false-negative tests are not relevant because the secretin test will invariably be abnormal if the steatorrhea is secondary to pancreatic insufficiency.

Tests for Cobalamin (Vitamin B$_{12}$) Absorption (Ch. 132)

In the Schilling test, 1.0 μg of ^{57}Co-cyanocobalamin is administered orally, followed by 1000 μg of nonlabeled cobalamin given intramuscularly to help "wash out" that fraction of the isotope that has been absorbed. If the subsequent 24-hour urinary excretion of the radioactivity is less than 8 per cent of that administered, cobalamin malabsorption is present. There are four common clinical causes of cobalamin malabsorption, which can be sorted out by a differential Schilling test (Table 102–5). If an abnormal test result improves with the concomitant administration of hog intrinsic factor or pancreatic extract (six to eight conventional tablets or three enteric-coated microsphere capsules), the cobalamin malabsorption is secondary to pernicious anemia or exocrine pancreatic insufficiency, respectively. If cobalamin malabsorption still persists, the tests should be repeated after 4 days of antimicrobial therapy (metronidazole, 250 mg three times daily). If the malabsorption of labeled cobalamin is corrected by this therapy, bacterial overgrowth was the etiology. Metronidazole is the antimicrobial agent of choice because anaerobes such as *Bacteroides* are usually responsible for the cobalamin malabsorption. If the malabsorption still persists, damage to the ileal receptor (Crohn's disease, ileal resection, lymphoma, Imerslund's syndrome) is probably present and the patient must always receive a monthly injection of cobalamin (100 μg). In the face of renal impairment, 4 ml of plasma may be obtained 8 hours after the administration of labeled cobalamin. A value greater than 0.6 per cent of the orally administered dose is considered normal.

There are two caveats concerning the Schilling test: (1) Severe cobalamin deficiency itself may damage the ileum such that the ileal receptors may not bind the intrinsic factor–cobalamin complex. This may confuse interpretation of the Schilling test. Thus, it is advisable to wait until 1 week of cobalamin therapy (100 μg per day intramuscularly) has been completed before performing the differential Schilling test. (2) Two other clinical conditions

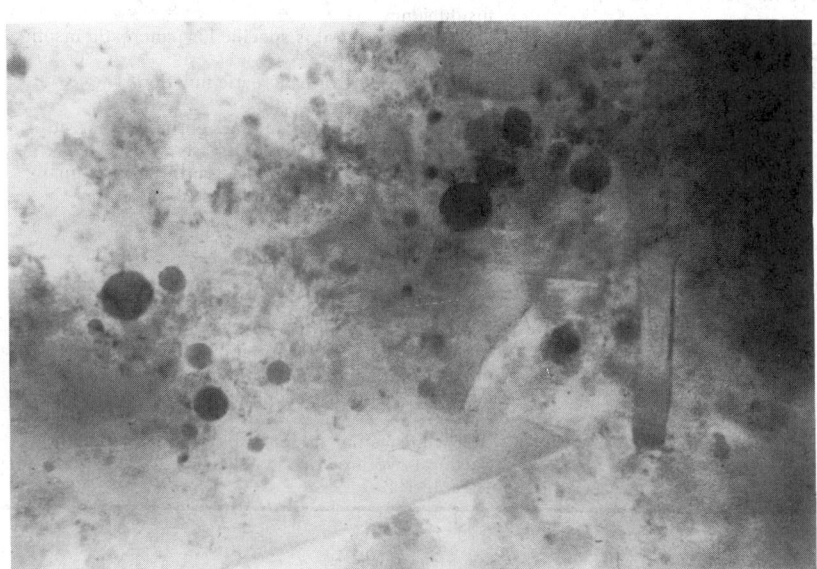

FIGURE 102–3. Positive fecal fat stain. Note the many globules of undigested triglycerides.

TABLE 102–5. THE DIFFERENTIAL SCHILLING (^{57}CO-CYANOCOBALAMIN) TEST

	Stage 1: Free Cobalamin	Stage 2: Free Cobalamin and Intrinsic Factor	Stage 3: Free Cobalamin and Pancreatic Extract	Stage 4: Free Cobalamin and Antibiotics	Comment
Pernicious anemia	Abnormal	Normal	Abnormal	Abnormal	In face of severe cobalamin deficiency, test should be performed only after a week of cobalamin therapy
Chronic pancreatitis	Abnormal	Abnormal	Normal	Abnormal	Although cobalamin malabsorption is common, cobalamin deficiency is rare
Bacterial overgrowth	Abnormal	Abnormal	Abnormal	Normal	Anaerobicidal antibiotic is needed
Ileal disease	Abnormal	Abnormal	Abnormal	Abnormal	Once receptor is permanently damaged, cobalamin malabsorption is permanent
Complete vegetarian* (vegan)	Normal	Normal	Normal	Normal	Cobalamin deficiency secondary to poor intake, absorption normal
Hypo- or achlorhydria*	Normal	Normal	Normal	Normal	Absorption of cyanocobalamin (free B_{12}) does not depend on acid; food B_{12} (protein-bound) does; must employ protein-bound cobalamin absorption test

*Cobalamin deficiency with normal Schilling test.

are associated with cobalamin deficiency—cobalamin deficiency secondary to lack of intake (as in complete vegetarians) and the failure to absorb food-bound cobalamin because of decreased acid secretion—that are not associated with an abnormal Schilling test (Table 102–5). The patient's history is the key to the former, and a test of protein-bound cobalamin absorption detects the latter.

Breath Tests

Two breath tests are reliable enough to receive routine clinical use—the lactose-H_2 breath test for detecting lactase deficiency and the ^{14}C-xylose breath test for the diagnosis of small intestine bacterial overgrowth.

The *lactose-H_2 breath test* has replaced the lactose intolerance test because of superior sensitivity and specificity. Lactose (1 gram per kilogram) is administered orally, and an increase in breath H_2 of more than 20 ppm over basal breath H_2 indicates lactose malabsorption. This test depends upon the release of H_2 from unabsorbed lactose by bacterial metabolism.

The *^{14}C-xylose breath test* is a sensitive and specific test for bacterial overgrowth. Following the oral administration of xylose (1 gram, 5 to 10 μCi), breath $^{14}CO_2$ concentration is monitored at 30 and 60 minutes, with an increase of $^{14}CO_2$ at 30 minutes being the most reliable assessment. Neither false-negative nor false-positive results appear to be a clinically significant problem. Xylose is catabolized by gram-negative aerobes, which are always part of the overgrowth flora, whereas other breath tests often utilize substrates that are catabolized by gram-negative anaerobes, which may or may not be present in the overgrowth of bacteria. The small dose of xylose (1 gram) is either catabolized by the overgrowth flora or absorbed in the proximal bowel, leaving very little xylose to "dump" into the colon, causing a possible false-positive result. An abnormal xylose breath test indicates, similar to a culture, the presence of increased numbers of bacteria within the lumen of the proximal small intestine. Whether or not the abnormal test indicates that therapy is necessary is a decision the clinician must make. Table 102–6 lists two other breath tests used to diagnose bacterial overgrowth, both of which suffer from inadequate sensitivity and specificity.

A ^{14}C-triolein breath test has received some use as a test of fat absorption, but it does not appear to separate control subjects from those with malabsorption very reliably, especially if the steatorrhea is not severe.

Culture of the Small Intestine

The proximal small intestine of normal subjects has fewer than 10^5 organisms per milliliter of jejunal fluid—usually fewer than 10^3, largely streptococci and staphylococci, and only an occasional coliform or *Bacteroides*. The ileocecal area is a transition zone with both a qualitative and a quantitative change toward the pattern that is found in the colon. In the colon, there is a marked increase in both aerobes (>10^7 organisms per milligram of stool) and anaerobes (>10^{10} organisms per milligram of stool). The qualitative change is also remarkable, with a preponderance of anaerobes (*Bacteroides, Clostridium,* enterococci) and coliforms (*Escherichia coli, Klebsiella*). In small intestine bacterial overgrowth, the small intestine becomes populated with a colon-like flora. Cultures should be considered suspicious if more than 10^3 organisms per milliliter are present (especially when anaerobes are identified) and clearly abnormal when more than 10^5 organisms per milliliter are present.

Biopsy of the Small Intestine

Biopsy of the small intestine is an important test in the evaluation of malabsorption presumed to be secondary to disease of the small intestine itself. Most instruments (Rubin's tube, Crosby's capsule, Carey's capsule) utilize a blind suction biopsy technique, but biopsies can be obtained endoscopically as well. Figure 102–4 illustrates the findings of a normal biopsy. Note the long, frondlike villi. The lining columnar epithelium is regular with basal orientation of the nuclei. There is not much cellular infiltration of lamina propria. The villus/crypt ratio favors the villus, with villus height normally being three to four times the height of the crypts.

For contrast, note Figure 102–5, which represents a biopsy from a patient with nontropical sprue (adult celiac disease). There is total villus atrophy, elongated crypts, and a dense infiltration

TABLE 102–6. BREATH TESTS FOR BACTERIAL OVERGROWTH

Procedure	Simplicity	Sensitivity	Specificity	Safety
^{14}C-xylose	Excellent	Excellent	Excellent	Good
Cholyl-1-^{14}C-glycine	Excellent	Fair	Poor	Good
Lactulose-H_2	Excellent	Fair–good	Fair	Excellent

Modified from King CE, Toskes PP: The use of breath tests in the study of malabsorption. Clin Gastroenterol 12:591, 1983.

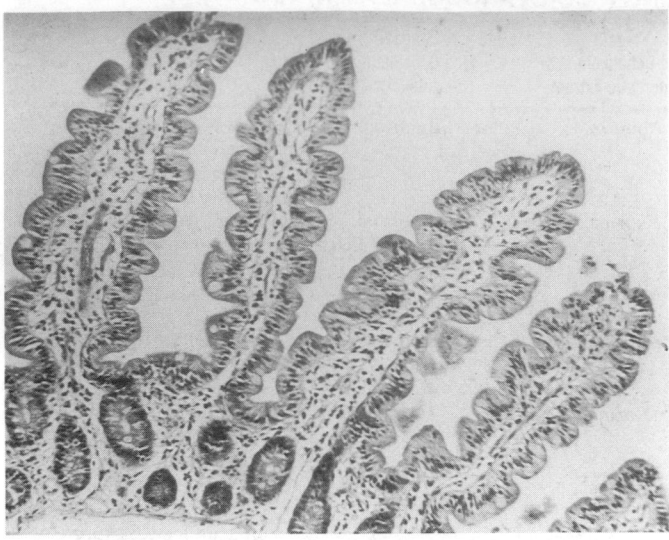

FIGURE 102–4. Appearance of normal small intestine on biopsy.

of chronic inflammatory cells in the lamina propria, and at higher magnification the surface epithelial cells are cuboidal, not columnar. Total villus atrophy, as shown in Figure 102–5, is almost always nontropical sprue (adult celiac disease), but it is not a specific lesion, since it may occasionally be observed in other diseases such as lymphoma, Whipple's disease, tropical sprue, ileojejunitis, or bacterial overgrowth. Table 102–7 lists disorders associated with abnormalities in the biopsy of the small intestine and points out that there are very few disorders in which multiple biopsies are consistently abnormal and diagnostic, i.e., a diagnostic diffuse lesion.

Gastrointestinal Radiology

With the possible exception of pancreatic calcification on plain film of the abdomen, radiographs of the intestinal tract do not play a primary role in the diagnostic evaluation of malabsorption. Function tests as described previously are more sensitive and more specific and afford the patient little, if any, radiation exposure. The radiation exposure received from a small bowel series may be considerable. The traditional signs of malabsorption on small bowel radiographs—segmentation or clumping of the barium (moulage sign)—were noted when thick barium was used in contrast to the thin barium commonly employed now. Small bowel radiographs are most frequently used now to determine why bacterial overgrowth has occurred (e.g., the presence of

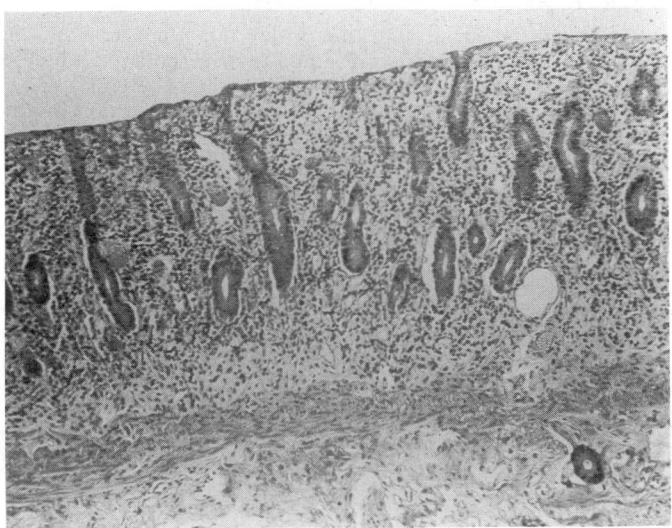

FIGURE 102–5. Small intestinal biopsy from a patient with nontropical sprue showing total villus atrophy.

TABLE 102–7. VALUE OF SMALL INTESTINAL BIOPSY

I. **Conditions in which the biopsy is consistently abnormal and diagnostic:**
 Abetalipoproteinemia
 Immunodeficiency syndrome
 Whipple's disease
II. **Conditions in which the biopsy is diagnostic but the lesion is often patchy:**
 Amyloidosis
 Capillariasis
 Coccidiosis
 Crohn's disease
 Cryptosporidiosis
 Eosinophilic enteritis
 Giardiasis
 Lymphangiectasia
 Lymphoma
 Mastocytosis
 Strongyloidiasis
III. **Conditions in which the biopsy is often abnormal but not diagnostic:**
 Bacterial overgrowth
 Cobalamin (vitamin B_{12}) deficiency
 Celiac sprue (nontropical)
 Drug enteritis
 Folate deficiency
 Infectious gastroenteritis
 Protein-calorie malnutrition
 Radiation enteritis
 Tropical sprue
 Unclassified sprue
 Zollinger-Ellison syndrome
IV. **Conditions in which the biopsy is invariably normal:**
 Functional bowel disease
 Liver disease
 Pancreatic disease
 Primary disaccharidase deficiency
 Ulcerative colitis

diverticula or dilation of the small intestine in scleroderma) or to confirm a clinical diagnosis of Crohn's disease.

Algorithm for Evaluation of Malabsorption

An algorithm for evaluating patients with malabsorption is presented in Table 102–8. The algorithm complements a thorough history and physical examination. A serum carotene determination and a microscopic fat stain of the stool are the best screening tests and together detect the presence of steatorrhea about 85 per cent of the time, especially if the patient is excreting more than 15 grams of fat per day. Once steatorrhea has been confirmed, the clinician should ask whether the steatorrhea is secondary to pancreatic disease or to small bowel disease. The urinary xylose test helps differentiate between these two categories. If xylose absorption is normal, tests of pancreatic function should be pursued. If diffuse calcification of the pancreas is present on a plain film of the abdomen, there is likely to be approximately 80 per cent damage to the exocrine pancreas. The bentiromide test has about the same sensitivity as plain film calcification and is abnormal 80 to 90 per cent of the time if the steatorrhea has a pancreatic cause. A serum trypsin level complements the bentiromide test, adding specificity to the evaluation. If these simple tubeless tests of pancreatic function are not diagnostic, a direct tube test like the secretin test should be performed.

If the xylose test is abnormal, small bowel tests should be performed. A breath test (^{14}C-xylose, lactulose H_2) detects bacterial overgrowth. If normal, a small bowel radiograph, culture, and biopsy should be done, with the radiograph suggesting the site to be biopsied. If steatorrhea is not present, tests designed to detect selective malabsorption of single nutrients can be pursued (lactose H_2 breath test, the Schilling test, and so on).

The algorithm is logical and cost effective, emphasizing inexpensive, noninvasive, outpatient evaluation. A specific diagnosis can often be made for less than $300 with minimal or no discomfort to the patient. If more complicated tests are needed, such as the secretin test or small bowel biopsy, the expense and discomfort to the patient increase. The algorithm also emphasizes initial testing for the more common causes of malabsorption (pancreatic insufficiency, bacterial overgrowth) and delayed testing for less common disorders (nontropical sprue, Whipple's disease, and so on).

DIFFERENTIAL FEATURES AND TREATMENT OF INDIVIDUAL FORMS OF THE MALABSORPTION SYNDROME

Numerous disorders can be associated with malabsorption (see Table 102–2). Although there may be specific therapy for individual disorders (gluten-free diet for nontropical sprue, pancreatic enzymes for pancreatic insufficiency), there are many nonspecific therapies for malabsorption (Table 102–9).

Impaired Digestion

PANCREATIC EXOCRINE INSUFFICIENCY (Ch. 106). Pancreatic exocrine insufficiency is a relatively common cause of severe malabsorption. It is not rare to note steatorrhea in excess of 50 grams of fat per day.

Steatorrhea in pancreatic disease is relatively well treated with administration of pancreatic extract. Large doses of pancreatic extract are required: six to eight conventional tablets (Viokase, Cotazym) or three enteric-coated, microsphere preparations (Creon, Pancrease MT, Entolase, Zymase) with each meal. Adjuvant therapy (sodium bicarbonate, H_2-receptor antagonists) along with conventional tablet therapy may lead to the best results by raising duodenal pH. The adjuvant of choice is sodium bicarbonate (650-mg tablet before and after each meal) because of its effectiveness, low cost, and lack of side effects at this dose. Antacids containing calcium or magnesium are not to be used as adjuvant therapy because they may increase steatorrhea. Adjuvant therapy is not recommended with enteric-coated preparations, for it may cause the enteric coat to open up within the stomach and the released enzymes may then be destroyed by gastric acid before they can enter the duodenum.

POSTGASTRECTOMY STATES (Ch. 98.4). The pathogenesis of the malabsorption noted in patients with gastric surgery (Billroth I, Billroth II, vagotomy and antrectomy, vagotomy and pyloroplasty) is multifactorial: (1) loss of reservoir function with rapid emptying and dispersion of food through the small intestine, thereby diluting the normal output of pancreatic enzymes; (2) postcibal asynchrony, i.e., in a patient who has undergone a Billroth II procedure, food may get to the jejunum before bile salts and pancreatic enzymes do; and (3) occurrence of stasis, leading to bacterial overgrowth of the small intestine. Postgastrectomy steatorrhea is usually mild (<10 grams of fat per day) but occasionally may be marked. Severe steatorrhea in this setting is usually the result of bacterial overgrowth or rarely is secondary to pancreatic insufficiency. Because the duodenum (the major site for calcium and iron absorption) is bypassed when a Billroth II procedure is performed, clinically significant problems related to calcium and iron malabsorption may result.

GASTRINOMA (Ch. 98.6). Multiple mechanisms contribute to the malabsorption observed in patients with a gastrinoma (Zollinger-Ellison syndrome). The extreme hypersecretion of acid irreversibly inactivates lipase, causing a secondary pancreatic insufficiency. In addition, this acid environment precipitates bile salts and may cause abnormal small bowel histologic findings. All of these abnormalities have been shown to revert to normal after effective therapy with large doses of H_2-receptor antagonists (cimetidine or ranitidine).

Reduced Concentration of Bile Salts

LIVER DISEASE. Steatorrhea (usually mild) may occur in acute or chronic liver disease, presumably owing to impaired synthesis and excretion of conjugated bile salts. Patients with liver disease who manifest clinically significant steatorrhea should have their pancreatic function evaluated, since these patients often have pancreatic exocrine insufficiency responsive to pancreatic extract therapy. Metabolic bone disease (bone pain, spontaneous pathologic fractures) resulting from malabsorption of calcium and vitamin D may occur, particularly in those with biliary cirrhosis (Ch. 234).

BACTERIAL OVERGROWTH. Overgrowth of bacteria within the small intestine accompanied by nutrient malabsorption is called the stasis, stagnant loop, or blind loop syndrome. The normal subject usually has sparse bacterial growth in the proximal small intestine (see section on Diagnosis—Culture of the Small Intestine). In the stasis syndrome, the proximal small intestinal flora resembles that of the colon and the overgrowth flora competes with the human host for ingested nutrients. The resultant malabsorption is due to a disturbed intraluminal environment (catabolism of carbohydrate by gram-negative aerobes, deconjugation of bile salts by anaerobes, binding of cobalamin by anaerobes) and patchy damage to the small intestinal enterocyte, perhaps secondary to toxins secreted by the overgrowth flora.

In healthy persons, bacteria within the small intestine are controlled by the cleansing motion of the small intestine, gastric acid secretion, and luminal immunoglobulins. Any alteration of these protective factors may lead to bacterial overgrowth (Table 102–10). In the past, bacterial overgrowth was thought to be related largely to blind loops and other structural abnormalities. Now the emphasis is on motor disturbances, often with no structural abnormality, and on states of decreased acid secretion. Indeed, bacterial overgrowth is one of the major, if not the major, cause of clinically significant malabsorption in the elderly, who often have both decreased acid secretion and a motility disturbance of the small intestine.

The diagnosis has become much more practical with the development of noninvasive breath tests (see section on Diagnosis—Breath Tests, Tables 102–4 and 102–6). This has greatly increased the awareness of this syndrome. Intestinal cultures have been expensive, awkward to perform, and usually not utilized extensively in clinical practice.

In the past, treatment was often empiric, not based on a firm diagnosis but dictated by a clinical impression. Broad-spectrum antibiotics (tetracycline) were prescribed for 7 to 10 days and the clinical response monitored. Up to 60 per cent of the anaerobes (*Bacteroides*) now may be resistant to tetracycline. It behooves the physician to establish the diagnosis firmly, for the antibiotics needed may have serious side effects.

The mainstays of therapy are antimicrobial therapy and nutritional support. If there is a surgically correctable cause of the overgrowth, surgery should be performed if possible. Most patients with overgrowth do not have a surgically correctable

TABLE 102–8. ALGORITHM FOR EVALUATION OF MALABSORPTION

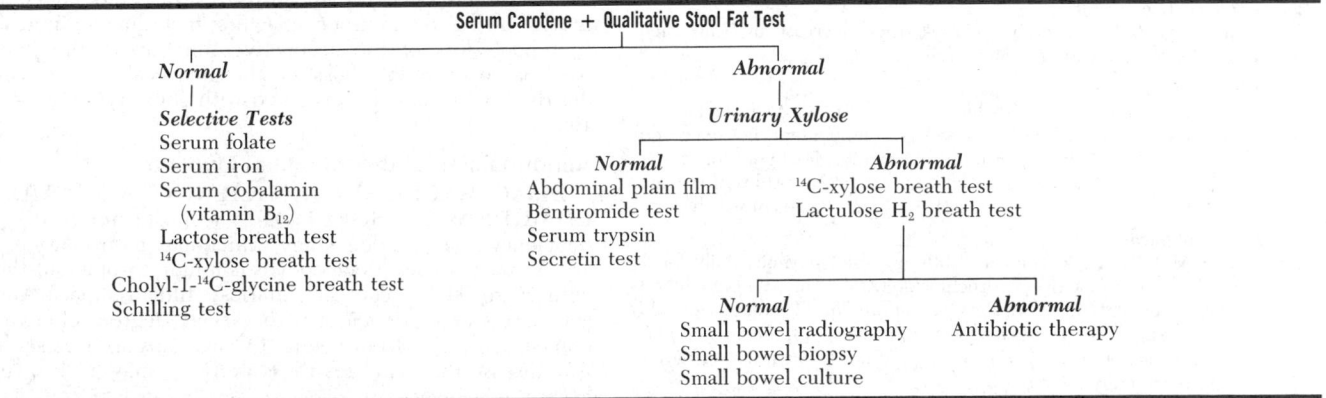

Serum Carotene + Qualitative Stool Fat Test

Normal → Selective Tests: Serum folate, Serum iron, Serum cobalamin (vitamin B_{12}), Lactose breath test, ^{14}C-xylose breath test, Cholyl-1-^{14}C-glycine breath test, Schilling test

Abnormal → Urinary Xylose

Normal: Abdominal plain film, Bentiromide test, Serum trypsin, Secretin test

Abnormal: ^{14}C-xylose breath test, Lactulose H_2 breath test

Normal: Small bowel radiography, Small bowel biopsy, Small bowel culture

Abnormal: Antibiotic therapy

TABLE 102–9. AGENTS USED IN THE TREATMENT OF MALABSORPTION

1. **Calcium**
   Oral: Requires 1200 mg elemental calcium daily. Preparations:
   a. Calcium gluconate (91 mg Ca^{2+}/gm), 5–10 gm 3 times per day
   b. Calcium carbonate (500 mg Ca^{2+}/tablet),1–2 gm per day in divided doses
   c. Calcium carbonate, 2 tablets supplied as Caltrate or 2½ tablets as Os-Cal 500
   Intravenous: Calcium gluconate injection (10% solution, 9.1 mg Ca^{2+}/ml), 10–30 ml administered slowly

2. **Magnesium**
   Oral: Magnesium gluconate, 500-mg tablets (20 mg Mg^{2+}/tablet), 1–4 gm daily in divided doses
   Intramuscular: (20% sol.) 10 ml 2–3 times daily
   Intravenous: Magnesium sulfate, 0.5 per cent sol., up to 1000 ml at a rate not faster than 1.0 mEq/min

3. **Iron**
   Oral: Ferrous sulfate, 325 mg (65 mg elemental iron) 3 times daily
   Intramuscular: Imferon must be calculated according to severity of anemia

4. **Cyanocobalamin** (vitamin B_{12})
   Intramuscular: 100 μg daily for 2 weeks, then 100 μg monthly

5. **Folic acid**
   Oral: 5 mg daily for 1 month; maintenance 1 mg daily

6. **Vitamin B complex**
   Any multivitamin preparation that contains US RDA amounts; use 2 tablets daily; intramuscular preparations are available

7. **Fat-soluble vitamins**
   a. Vitamin A
      Capsules (25,000 units of Vitamin A per capsule), 100,000–200,000 units daily in severe deficiencies; maintenance, 25,000–50,000 units daily. *Caution:* Vitamin A toxicity can occur with recommended doses if hypertriglyceridemia is present
   b. Vitamin D
      Vitamin D_2 or D_3, 30,000 units daily; dosage varies considerably depending on response as determined by level of serum calcium and urinary calcium
   c. Vitamin K
      Oral: Menadione, 4–12 mg daily; vitamin K tablets (Mephyton), 5–10 mg daily
      Intravenous: Acute bleeding episodes: vitamin K (Mephyton), 50-mg ampule administered slowly over 10-min period; repeat in 8–12 hr if prothrombin time has not returned to normal

8. **Cholestyramine**
   4-gm pk, 1–2 pk before breakfast and lunch

9. **Medium-chain triglyceride** (MCT oil)
   Administer 60% of fat intake as MCT oil

10. **Human albumin, salt poor** (0.25 gm/ml)
    Intravenous administration of 50–100 gm daily for 3–7 days to elevate a severely depressed serum albumin level

11. **Immune serum globulin** (0.165 gm/ml)
    Intramuscular injection of 0.05 ml/kg each 3–4 wk in patients with hypogammaglobulinemia and recurrent infection

12. **Adrenocorticosteroids**
    Prednisone, 40–60 mg daily for 2 wk, then decrease by 5 mg each week to maintenance of 5–15 mg daily

13. **Antidiarrheal agents**
    Oral: Diphenoxylate hydrochloride (Lomotil), 5.0 mg (2 tablets) initially and after each loose bowel movement, not to exceed 8 tablets daily; loperamide hydrochloride (Imodium), 2-mg capsules, 2 capsules initially and then 2 capsules after each loose bowel movement, not to exceed 8 capsules daily

14. **Drugs for parasites**
    Oral: Metronidazole (Flagyl), 250-mg tablet 3 times daily for 1 wk, or quinacrine hydrochloride (Atabrine), 100-mg tablet 3 times daily for 1 wk for *Giardia lamblia.* Thiabendazole (25 mg/kg/day): strongyloidiasis, 2–3 days; *Capillaria philippinensis,* 30 days; *A. duodenale, N. americanus,* 25 mg/kg/day twice daily for 2 days

TABLE 102–10. CLINICAL CONDITIONS ASSOCIATED WITH BACTERIAL OVERGROWTH

I. **Gastric proliferation of bacteria**
   Hypo- or achlorhydria, especially when combined with motor or anatomic disturbances

II. **Small intestinal stagnation**
   Anatomic
      Afferent loop of Billroth II partial gastrectomy
      Duodenal or jejunal diverticulosis
      Surgical blind loop (end-to-side anastomosis)
      Surgical recirculating loop (side-to-side anastomosis)
      Obstruction (stricture, adhesion, inflammation, cancer)
   Motor
      Scleroderma
      Idiopathic intestinal pseudo-obstruction
      Derangements of interdigestive motor complex
      Diabetic autonomic neuropathy

III. **Abnormal communication between proximal and distal gastrointestinal tract**
   Gastrocolic or jejunocolic fistula
   Resection of ileocecal valve

IV. **Miscellaneous**
   Hypogammaglobulinemia
   Chronic pancreatitis

Modified from King CE, Toskes PP: Small intestine bacterial overgrowth. Gastroenterology 76:1035, 1979.

cause (e.g., they have scleroderma, diverticulosis, or diabetes) and must receive lifelong antimicrobial and nutritional therapy.

A 10-day course of a cephalosporin (Keflex), 250 mg four times a day, and metronidazole (Flagyl), 250 mg three times a day, is very effective in suppressing the flora and correcting malabsorption, as is the clavulonic acid derivative Augmentin, 250 mg three times a day. Tetracycline is an alternative, but the resistance problem must be appreciated. If these fail, chloramphenicol (50 mg per kilogram per day in four divided doses) is also very effective. Anaerobicidal agents by themselves (metronidazole, clindamycin) do not seem to be as effective as the combination of an aerobicidal and an anaerobicidal agent.

Three therapeutic patterns occur. Usually a 10-day course of an effective antimicrobial program corrects the malabsorption for months; some patients may need cyclic therapy (1 week out of every 6); rarely a patient may need continuous therapy for several months. Antibiotic sensitivity assays of the overgrowth flora are not recommended because of the multitude of organisms present.

Nutritional therapy (especially with medium-chain triglyceride oil) is very important but often ignored. Medium-chain triglyceride administration is ideal therapy for this condition, since this form of fat does not need bile salts for absorption. Other agents such as cobalamin, vitamin D, and calcium are given in doses detailed in Table 102–9.

ILEAL DISEASE OR RESECTION. Disease of the distal ileum leads to an interruption of the enterohepatic circulation of conjugated bile acids, resulting in a diminished bile acid pool and steatorrhea. The degree of steatorrhea is proportional to the amount of diseased or resected intestine. When less than 100 cm of intestine is damaged or resected, proximal to the ileocecal valve, the steatorrhea is mild and choleretic diarrhea tends to be the most frequent problem. The malabsorbed bile acids dump into the colon and impair water and electrolyte absorption. When more than 100 cm of small intestine is resected, the steatorrhea is large owing to a number of factors, including a diminished bile acid pool, loss of the absorptive function of the ileum, and bacterial overgrowth (loss of the ileocecal valve). Choleretic diarrhea can usually be managed with cholestyramine (see Table 102–9).

Abnormalities of the Intestinal Mucosa

DISACCHARIDASE DEFICIENCY AND MONOSACCHARIDE MALABSORPTION. The most common disaccharide deficiency is lactase deficiency, which may be primary or secondary. Primary lactase deficiency is common throughout the world, with 60 to 90 per cent of American Indians, black Americans, and Asians being deficient with varying degrees of lactose intolerance. Only 5 to 15 per cent of Caucasians are lactase deficient. Any disease that damages the enterocyte may lead to secondary lactase deficiency.

Lactase-deficient subjects are intolerant to milk, experiencing bloating, abdominal cramps, and diarrhea. The lactose within milk cannot be hydrolyzed to glucose and galactose. It remains in the intestinal lumen, where it is fermented by bacteria, producing organic acids, which increase the osmotic load, inducing shifts of water into the intestinal tract. The end result is distention of the intestine and diarrhea.

Primary lactase deficiency may not manifest itself until adulthood, yet the reason for this delayed appearance is not clear. Subtotal gastrectomy or pyloroplasty and vagotomy may unmask the condition by increasing the load of ingested lactose on the jejunal mucosa. Although the diagnosis is often made by taking a history, the lactose-H_2 breath test is the best way to document lactose intolerance (see Diagnosis section and Table 102–4). Treatment of primary lactase deficiency is avoidance of milk products or the ingestion of one to two capsules of Lactrase when dairy products are ingested. Lactrase, derived from *Aspergillus oryzae*, is commercially available.

Sucrase deficiency is quite rare. In afflicted patients, diarrhea occurs after ingesting sucrose. Elimination of sucrose, dextrins, and starches from the diet is effective.

Monosaccharide (glucose-galactose) malabsorption is a rare disorder present from birth. All sugars metabolized to glucose or galactose cannot be tolerated. Therapy consists of utilizing fructose as a source of sugar.

NONTROPICAL SPRUE (ADULT CELIAC DISEASE, CELIAC SPRUE, GLUTEN-SENSITIVE ENTEROPATHY). Nontropical sprue is a disease of unknown etiology characterized by malabsorption resulting from gluten-induced damage to the differentiated villus epithelial cells of the small intestine. Gluten is a high molecular weight protein found in wheat, rye, oats, and barley. The mechanism for this toxic effect is not known, but the most accepted theory at present is that metabolites of gluten initiate an immunologic reaction in the enterocyte. The enterocyte is often strikingly damaged, and biopsy of the small intestine demonstrates characteristic changes (see Fig. 102–5 and discussion of small bowel biopsy in Diagnosis section). Malabsorption is secondary to the impaired transport of nutrients through the damaged enterocyte. In addition, a net secretory state for water and electrolytes has been noted in the jejunum, and pancreatic exocrine function may be secondarily diminished owing to a decreased release of secretin and cholecystokinin from the damaged small bowel mucosa.

Genetic factors appear important in this disease. Nontropical sprue is closely linked to two histocompatibility antigens, HLA-B8 and HLA-DRw3. These antigens are present in 60 to 90 per cent of patients with this disease and in only 20 to 30 per cent of the general population. An additional antigen has been found on the surface of B lymphocytes in 70 to 80 per cent of patients with nontropical sprue and in 15 per cent of normal controls. The same antigen is present in 100 per cent of the patients' parents. Perhaps these antigens evoke antibodies to gluten, which result in the binding of gluten to the enterocyte with subsequent mucosal damage.

Patients with nontropical sprue usually have severe malabsorption—steatorrhea, diarrhea, weight loss, and many of the other symptoms and signs detailed in Table 102–3. Symptoms typically begin in infancy, disappear in late childhood, and reappear in the third to sixth decade of life. The proximal small intestine is usually the most severely damaged organ, and the symptoms, signs, and laboratory evaluation reflect this (Tables 102–3 and 102–4). At times, the clinical presentation may be quite subtle, e.g., anemia secondary to iron deficiency or bone pain from osteomalacia without obvious diarrhea or steatorrhea. Small bowel biopsy is essential in this disease, for a diagnosis of nontropical sprue commits the patient to a very restricted diet indefinitely. Evidence is accumulating that increased levels of serum antibodies to gliadin may be of considerable diagnostic benefit. Elevated serum IgA antigliadin may spare patients unnecessary small bowel biopsies.

The cornerstone of therapy is the withdrawal of all gluten from the diet, i.e., all grains must be eliminated except rice and corn. Most patients respond to dietary restriction with a remarkable decrease in symptoms and signs within a few days to a week. In some patients, however, it may take months before a significant improvement is noted. Function tests such as urinary xylose excretion return to normal within a few weeks of gluten with-

drawal. Post-treatment biopsies demonstrate marked improvement in most patients and completely normal histologic findings in many. The patient with the characteristic syndrome and biopsy findings who does not respond to gluten withdrawal is usually not adhering to the diet. Some patients may have the characteristic clinical picture and flat biopsy and in reality are not responding because they have another disease such as Whipple's disease, nongranulomatous ileojejunitis, giardiasis, lymphoma, or collagenous sprue. Collagenous sprue, a variant of nontropical sprue, demonstrates not only the characteristic changes in the small intestinal biopsy but also masses of eosinophilic hyaline material in the lamina propria. Such patients have a poor prognosis. Corticosteroid therapy (see Table 102–9) or parenteral hyperalimentation may be needed in some patients.

Small bowel lymphoma and carcinoma in general seem to be increased in patients with nontropical sprue. The appearance of abdominal pain in a patient with sprue should suggest lymphoma. Whether or not these complications are fewer in those who adhere strictly to a gluten-free diet is controversial.

Two other associated abnormalities in patients with sprue are (1) ulcers of the jejunum and ileum with abdominal pain, bleeding, and perforation, which are unresponsive to therapy, and (2) dermatitis herpetiformis. Some patients with this skin lesion may have latent sprue. The dermatitis is pruritic, vesicular, and papular and responds to sulfone treatment. Sulfone does not improve the intestinal lesion, but some of these lesions may respond to gluten withdrawal.

NONGRANULOMATOUS ILEOJEJUNITIS. This disease has features of both Crohn's disease and nontropical sprue, even a flat small intestinal biopsy. There is an abrupt onset with fever, abdominal pain, at times splenomegaly, and elevated white count—all suggesting lymphoma. Malabsorption may be profound, resulting in a therapeutic trial of steroids and a gluten-free diet—often to no avail.

CROHN'S DISEASE (Ch. 103). Malabsorption in Crohn's disease results from several problems: (1) decreased absorptive surface from active disease or surgical resection, (2) bile salt depletion from ileal disease, and (3) bacterial overgrowth secondary to dilatation of the bowel and resection of the ileocecal valve.

EOSINOPHILIC ENTERITIS. Peripheral blood eosinophilia and infiltration of the gastrointestinal tract by eosinophils characterize this disease. Three patterns of involvement are seen: (1) involvement of the muscle layers of the stomach and small intestine causing obstruction, (2) involvement of the mucosa of the small intestine causing malabsorption, and (3) involvement of the subserosa causing ascites. Most patients have no evidence of allergy or food sensitivity. Corticosteroids and occasionally surgery are employed successfully.

RADIATION ENTERITIS (Ch. 112 and 530). Radiation injury to the intestine may lead to malabsorption from (1) extensive mucosal damage, (2) lymphangiectasia from lymphatic obstruction, and (3) bacterial overgrowth. Malabsorption may occur shortly after exposure to radiation or years later. Most patients with clinically significant malabsorption appear to respond to therapy for bacterial overgrowth.

ABETALIPOPROTEINEMIA (Ch. 172). This rare disease represents a defect in chylomicron formation. The intestinal cells are lacking apoprotein B, and therefore fat absorption cannot occur normally. Biopsy of the small intestine shows the epithelial cells to be engorged with fat even after an overnight fast. The clinical manifestations are steatorrhea, neurologic disease (ataxia, retinitis pigmentosa), very low serum cholesterol and triglyceride levels, and "spiny red cells" (acanthocytes). Therapy consists of substitution of dietary fat with medium-chain triglyceride and administration of fat-soluble vitamins, especially vitamin E.

Inadequate Absorptive Surface

SHORT BOWEL SYNDROME. Extensive resection of the small intestine is usually performed for Crohn's disease, intestinal infarction, or trauma. Acute hyperalimentation in these patients has been life-saving, and the ability of the remaining gut to adapt for increased nutrient absorption by hypertrophy of residual small intestinal villi is remarkable. Patients do rather well despite extensive resection if approximately 90 to 100 cm of duodenum and jejunum and the terminal ileum (intact ileocecal valve) remain.

Treatment consists of parenteral hyperalimentation for weeks to months until evidence exists that the remaining gut is functional. Gradual introduction of oral feedings, high in protein content, vitamins, and minerals, as well as medium-chain triglyceride (MCT), forms the basis for maintenance therapy. Antidiarrheal agents and cholestyramine may help (see Table 102–9). Occasionally, pancreatic extract therapy and H_2-receptor antagonists are necessary to treat the transient acid hypersecretion and secondary pancreatic insufficiency that may occur. Steroids may increase water absorption. Some patients must receive hyperalimentation at home indefinitely. Diarrhea resistant to all other therapy may respond to somatostatin analogues (Sandostatin).

JEJUNOILEAL BYPASS. Some patients with morbid obesity have had a surgical procedure performed (14 inches of proximal jejunum is anastomosed to 4 inches of terminal ileum) that induces malabsorption. In addition to many of the problems detailed above in the short bowel syndrome, other serious complications occur, such as oxalate kidney stones, intestinal pseudo-obstruction, cirrhosis, and arthritis. Because of these complications, the operation has been abandoned.

Infection

TROPICAL SPRUE. The pathogenesis of this malabsorptive disorder occurring in tropical regions (Far East, India, Caribbean) is poorly understood. An overgrowth of coliforms within the jejunum has been demonstrated in these patients. Such organisms have been shown to elaborate an enterotoxin that induces fluid secretion. Tropical sprue is not a true bacterial overgrowth, since anaerobes (particularly *Bacteroides*) are conspicuously absent. Malabsorption of many nutrients occurs, especially folic acid, cobalamin, and fat. The intestinal biopsy does not demonstrate total villus atrophy, but rather nonspecific changes in the villi (shortening, thickening) and cellular infiltration of the lamina propria. Successful therapy has been achieved with cobalamin, folic acid, or antibiotics. A two-month course of a broad-spectrum antibiotic (e.g., tetracycline, 250 mg orally four times daily) and folic acid, 5.0 mg daily, is most effective. In those patients with cobalamin deficiency, 1000 μg of cobalamin should be given intramuscularly for 2 consecutive days. Improvement of malabsorption following therapy with folic acid or cobalamin alone casts doubt upon infection as the sole etiology.

WHIPPLE'S DISEASE. Patients (usually male) who present with Whipple's disease manifest steatorrhea, weight loss, abdominal pain, nondeforming arthritis, fever, peripheral lymphadenopathy, and neurologic abnormalities (nystagmus, ophthalmoplegia, cranial nerve defects). Protein-losing enteropathy may be present because of lymphatic obstruction.

Small bowel biopsy is diagnostic, demonstrating heavy infiltration of the mucosa and lymph nodes by macrophages that stain positive with periodic acid–Schiff reagent (PAS). Biopsy of the small intestine also shows blunting of villi and dilated lymphatics. The macrophages are filled with rod-shaped bacilli, which disappear after antibiotic therapy and reappear prior to an exacerbation of the disease. Although these rodlike structures resemble bacilli, no bacteria have been consistently cultured from patients with this disease—hence the bacterial etiology of Whipple's disease has not been proved.

Untreated, this is a fatal disease. These patients should be treated for at least a year and probably indefinitely. The antibiotic of choice appears to be trimethoprim-sulfamethoxazole, 500 mg given orally four times daily.

Lymphatic Obstruction

LYMPHOMA (INTESTINAL). Malabsorption occurs in patients with intestinal lymphoma from (1) mucosal invasion, (2) lymphatic obstruction, and (3) bacterial overgrowth secondary to dilatation of the bowel with stasis. Antibiotic therapy often completely corrects the clinical manifestations of malabsorption (diarrhea, steatorrhea), suggesting that bacterial overgrowth is an important cause of malabsorption in these patients. Abdominal pain, fever, and steatorrhea are principal complaints; lymphadenopathy and hepatosplenomegaly are uncommon. The small

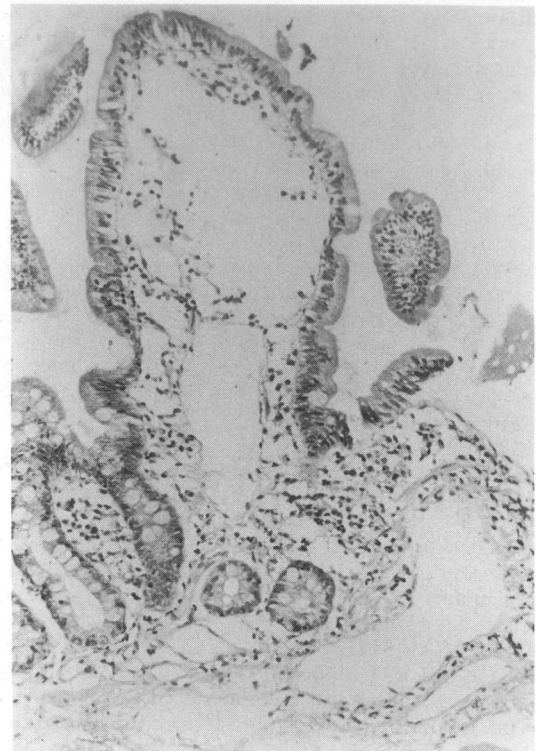

FIGURE 102–6. Small intestinal biopsy from a patient with intestinal lymphangiectasia. Note the dilated lymph channels (clear spaces).

bowel biopsy may mimic nontropical sprue but not respond to a gluten-free diet. The diagnosis is usually made by the finding of malignant lymphoid cells in the mucosa or submucosa via small bowel biopsy or by full-thickness biopsy at surgery. As many as 10 per cent of patients with nontropical sprue may develop lymphoma.

LYMPHANGIECTASIA. Primary or congenital lymphangiectasia is characterized by diarrhea, mild steatorrhea, edema, enteric loss of protein (protein-losing enteropathy), and abnormal dilated lymphatic channels on small intestinal biopsy (Fig. 102–6). The main clinical feature of this disorder, which affects primarily children and young adults, is asymmetric edema secondary to the hypoplastic peripheral lymphatics and chylous effusions. Lymphocytopenia and depressed serum protein levels are a result of the protein-losing enteropathy. The hypoplastic lymphatics lead to an obstruction in lymph flow, increased pressure within lymphatics, dilated lymphatic channels in the intestine, and finally rupture of the lymphatic channels, discharging lymph into the bowel lumen. Therapy is directed to decreasing lymph flow via a low-fat diet and substitution of dietary fat with medium-chain triglycerides (MCT), which are transported by the portal venous system rather than the lymphatic system.

Although protein-losing enteropathy is a hallmark of intestinal lymphangiectasia, many other disorders can also cause enteric protein loss. The mechanisms are multifactorial: (1) exudation of protein through inflamed or engorged mucosa (gastric cancer, hypertrophy of gastric mucosa, ulcerative colitis), (2) loss of protein because of abnormal enterocytes (nontropical sprue, scleroderma), and (3) passage of proteins into the intestine secondary to increased pressure within lymphatics (lymphangiectasia, constrictive pericarditis, lymphoma).

Enteric protein loss can be detected by intravenously administering various labeled macromolecules and measuring the radioactivity in the feces. These tests are cumbersome to perform and not readily available. Recently, α_1-antitrypsin has been used as a marker for this disorder. Alpha$_1$-antitrypsin (similar size as albumin) can be measured in the feces by immunodiffusion.

Cardiovascular Disorders

Any disorder causing poor perfusion of the intestine may lead to steatorrhea. Atherosclerosis and vasculitis may both affect the mesenteric blood supply.

Drug-Induced Malabsorption

This entity is not very common and usually produces clinically insignificant malabsorption. Steatorrhea secondary to therapy with cholestyramine and neomycin is thought to be a result of precipitation of bile salts. The mechanism or mechanisms of most drug-induced malabsorption are not well understood.

Unexplained Malabsorption

Other than that in diabetes and perhaps in the carcinoid syndrome, the malabsorption occasionally observed in endocrine disorders (adrenal insufficiency, thyroid disease) is not at all understood. In diabetes, malabsorption may result from neuropathic changes (diarrhea) or bacterial overgrowth (steatorrhea). In systemic mast cell disease, there may be massive infiltration of the small intestine with mast cells, blunting of intestinal villi, and marked acid hypersecretion (Ch. 252). Malabsorption, however, does not appear to correlate well with any of these abnormalities. Hypogammaglobulinemia is at times associated with severe malabsorption. Although the pathogenesis is not well defined, such patients may have giardiasis, bacterial overgrowth, and histologic abnormalities of the small intestine (patchy villus atrophy, nodular lymphoid hyperplasia). Plasma cells are absent within the intestine.

Malabsorption in the Elderly

Elderly patients may develop malabsorption from any of the disorders listed in Table 102–2, but bacterial overgrowth appears to be the most common cause of clinically significant steatorrhea in this population. The elderly often have decreased gastric acid secretion and abnormalities in intestinal motility that predispose them to malabsorption from bacterial overgrowth. The hypo- or achlorhydria may lead to cobalamin (vitamin B_{12}) deficiency from malabsorption of food-bound cobalamin (see Table 102–5). Such patients may be treated effectively just with tablets of cyanocobalamin (unbound B_{12}), since they have intrinsic factor in adequate amounts. Recognition of this problem may avoid parenteral administration of cobalamin.

Malabsorption in the Acquired Immunodeficiency Syndrome (AIDS) (Ch. 416)

Patients with AIDS often have diarrhea, malabsorption, and weight loss. A number of infectious agents, including *Giardia lamblia, Mycobacterium avium-intracellulare, Cryptosporidium, Microsporidium, Strongyloides stercoralis,* and *Isospora belli,* may cause malabsorption in patients with AIDS. Although these patients often have enteric infections and intestinal involvement with Kaposi's sarcoma, there are significant numbers of patients with AIDS who have malabsorption without these two abnormalities. In some patients with AIDS, biopsy of the small intestine demonstrates large numbers of histiocytes within the lamina propria. Although such findings on biopsy may be confused with Whipple's disease, in patients with AIDS these histiocytes contain acid-fast bacilli, representing *Mycobacterium avium-intracellulare.* Still other patients with AIDS have malabsorption with the only abnormality found being that of a nonspecific mild to moderate chronic inflammatory response in the small bowel biopsy. The malabsorption in this last group of patients may be due to bacterial overgrowth or other unidentified enteric infections.

Brasitus TA, Sitrin MD: Intestinal malabsorption syndromes. Ann Rev Med 41:339, 1990. *New developments in malabsorption associated with AIDS, celiac sprue, bacterial overgrowth, and old age.*

Donaldson RM, Toskes PP: The relation of enteric bacterial populations to gastrointestinal function and disease. *In* Sleisenger MH, Fordtran JS (eds.): Gastrointestinal Disease. 4th ed. Philadelphia, W. B. Saunders Company, 1989, p 107. *Thorough review of human intestinal flora.*

Keinath RD, Merrell DE, Vlitstra R, et al.: Antibiotic treatment and relapse in Whipple's disease. Long-term follow-up of 88 patients. Gastroenterology 88:1867, 1985. *Current discussion of therapy in this disease.*

Kelly CP, Feighery CF, Gallagher RB, et al.: Diagnosis and treatment of gluten-sensitive enteropathy. Adv Intern Med 35:341, 1990. *Current thorough review of clinical features of celiac disease.*

King CE, Toskes PP: Comparison of the 1-gram ^{14}C-xylose, 10-gram lactulose-H_2, and the 80-gram glucose-H_2 breath tests in patients with small intestine bacterial overgrowth. Gastroenterology 91:1447, 1986. *Direct comparison of ^{14}C breath tests and H_2 breath tests for diagnosing bacterial overgrowth.*

King CE, Toskes PP: The use of breath tests in the study of malabsorption. Clin Gastroenterol 12:591, 1983. *Thorough overall review of clinical usefulness of these tests.*

Ladefoged K, Christensen KC, Hegnhoj J, et al.: Effect of a long-acting somatostatin analogue SMS 201-995 on jejunostomy effluents in patients with severe short bowel syndrome. Gut 30:943, 1989. *Somatostatin analogues offer new therapy for intractable diarrhea of short bowel syndrome.*

Montgomery RD, Haboubi NY, Mike NH, et al.: Cause of malabsorption in the elderly. Age Ageing 15:235, 1986. *Points out importance of bacterial overgrowth in the elderly.*

Rich EJ, Christie DL: Anti-gliadin antibody panel and xylose absorption test in screening celiac disease. J Pediatr Gastroenterol Nutr 10:174, 1990. *Role of serum antibodies to gliadin in the diagnosis of celiac disease.*

Sleisenger MH, Fordtran JS (eds.): Gastrointestinal Disease. 4th ed. Philadelphia, W. B. Saunders Company, 1989, Ch. 18, 19, 57, 61, 66–68. *Normal absorption and malabsorption in well-referenced text of gastroenterology.*

Toskes PP: The bentiromide test for pancreatic endocrine insufficiency. Pharmacotherapy 4:74, 1984. *Review of worldwide experience with this noninvasive test of pancreatic function.*

Toskes PP, Donaldson RM: The blind loop syndrome. *In* Sleisenger MH, Fordtran JS (eds.): Gastrointestinal Disease. 4th ed. Philadelphia, W. B. Saunders Company, 1989, p 1289. *Complete review of pathophysiology, diagnosis, and treatment of small intestine bacterial overgrowth.*

103 Inflammatory Bowel Disease

Stephen B. Hanauer

DEFINITION

The term "inflammatory bowel disease" applies to the idiopathic, chronic inflammatory bowel diseases (IBD): Crohn's disease (CD) and ulcerative colitis (UC). These are distinguished from IBD of established origin such as viral, bacterial, and parasitic infections; diverticulitis; radiation enteritis or colitis; drug or toxin-induced enterocolitis; or vasculitis of the intestinal tract. CD and UC are disorders of unknown etiology involving genetic and immunologic influences on the gastrointestinal tract's ability to distinguish foreign from self-antigens and/or to down-regulate the mucosal immune response. They share many overlapping epidemiologic, clinical, and therapeutic features. Both are chronic, medically incurable conditions. Whereas a proctocolectomy cures UC, surgery for CD is limited to treatment of complications.

Ulcerative colitis encompasses a spectrum of diffuse, continuous, superficial inflammation of the colon, which begins within the rectum and extends to a variable proximal level. The inflammatory features are constant within the involved segment of the colon and, once established, the upward margin of inflammation usually remains constant in the same individual. Occasionally, the disease progresses to more proximal areas, usually within the first several years after diagnosis. The condition never involves the small intestine except when the distal terminal ileum is inflamed in a similar, superficial fashion (backwash ileitis) in patients with inflammation throughout the colon (pancolitis). The inflammation extends beneath the lamina propria only in severe cases, when submucosal involvement produces a thinning of the circular and longitudinal muscles leading to colonic distention (toxic megacolon). UC is primarily a mucosal process, and removal of the entire mucosa is curative.

Crohn's disease is characterized by focal, asymmetric, transmural inflammation affecting any portion of the gastrointestinal tract from the mouth to the anus. The ileum and right colon are most often involved, but any segment of the gastrointestinal tract can be inflamed. The focal, transmural inflammation and the potential for proximal gastrointestinal tract involvement distinguish CD from UC. The presence of noncaseating granuloma also distinguishes CD from UC but is not necessary for the diagnosis. Microscopic changes are present throughout the gastrointestinal tract, distant from grossly involved segments of intestine.

ETIOLOGY

The cause(s) of UC and CD is not known. Although genetic, biochemical, and immunologic patterns are recognized in patients, a definitive etiopathogenesis remains elusive. The absence of an appropriate animal model for chronic IBD has hampered progress in determining pathogenesis. Spontaneously occurring chronic colitis in the cotton-top tamarin, *Sanguinus oedipus*, shares many biochemical, pathologic, and chronic features with UC, including the increased frequency of colonic adenocarcinoma. Unfortunately, these animals are an endangered species, and their rarity and the difficulty of breeding them in captivity complicate investigations. An alternative animal model is needed.

No infectious agent has been linked to UC or to CD, although it is speculated that exposure to a common bacterial antigen stimulates an autoimmune reaction against a shared host antigen via molecular mimicry.

EPIDEMIOLOGY (Table 103–1)

UC and CD occur among all age groups but have a peak incidence in the second and third decades. The incidence of CD has risen over the past 20 years and now shares incidence and prevalence rates with UC of 5 per 100,000 and 50 per 100,000, respectively. The combined prevalence of the two diseases is approximately 100 per 100,000 population. These disorders are seen most commonly in Northern Europe and North America and in relatives of European immigrants in the cities of South Africa, Australia, and New Zealand. IBD is rare in Central America, South America, Africa, the Middle East, and Asia. Although IBD can be seen in all ethnic groups, there is an increased prevalence in Jews who have emigrated from Northern Europe. This Jewish predisposition is not seen in Sephardic (Mediterranean or Middle-Eastern) Jews. Although less common in the nonwhite population, more cases are being recognized in the black population in American cities and in Asian immigrants to Great Britain.

A presumed genetic influence is derived from family studies, in which approximately 20 per cent of individuals with IBD have a relative with UC or CD. The pattern of inheritance is more complicated than that of a simple mendelian trait, and the risk is spread across families. In children with IBD the likelihood of another family member having the diagnosis is greater than 40 per cent. Although the risk to a child of a parent with IBD is less than 5 per cent, when both parents have IBD the risk to offspring is greater than 50 per cent. There is a stronger concordance within families and in twin studies for CD than for UC. The only epidemiologic difference between UC and CD pertains to cigarette smoking. Cigarette smoking appears to protect against the development of UC and is associated with CD. More than 80 per cent of patients with UC are nonsmokers, whereas 80 per cent of patients with CD smoke cigarettes. Often, UC begins after a "predisposed" individual stops smoking.

Attempts have been made to implicate a number of environmental factors in the development of IBD, including atypical mycobacterium, diets high in refined sugar (including corn flakes), increased consumption of polysaturated fats (margarine), and oral contraceptive pills, but none has been proven.

PATHOGENESIS

The absence of an etiologic factor leaves a gap in our understanding of the pathogenesis of IBD. Although a number of potential factors may influence the *initiation* of the inflammatory response, a popular view is that there is a defect in the "downregulation" of immune events, allowing persistent *amplification* of the tissue-damaging process. The inflammatory reaction in IBD closely mimics infectious enterocolitis with the exception of the failure to halt progressive tissue destruction. Subtle differences exist between the immunologic findings of UC and CD,

TABLE 103–1. EPIDEMIOLOGY OF INFLAMMATORY BOWEL DISEASE

More common in whites than nonwhites
Increased frequency among European stock
More common among Jews (especially Ashkenazic)
    than non-Jews (three to six times)
Most frequent age of onset: 15 to 30 years
Aggregation in families (25–40%)
Concordance for Crohn's disease in twins
Cigarette smokers—Crohn's disease
Nonsmokers—ulcerative colitis

such as the production of immunoglobulin heavy-chain allotypes or neutrophil-cytoplasmic antibodies; however, pathognomonic findings to classify these disorders remain elusive. Nosology is currently based on descriptive clinical, endoscopic, and histologic criteria, and misclassification often is recognized as the clinicopathologic process evolves over time. When the diagnosis changes, it is almost always from UC to CD and virtually never the converse.

Potential initiating events in IBD include increased intestinal permeability, aberrant epithelial processing of antigen, improper epithelial utilization of short-chain fatty acids, and molecular mimicry between a luminal antigen and components of intestinal mucosa. There is evidence of increased intestinal permeability to small or medium-sized molecular particles in patients and relatives of patients with IBD, which may be affected by qualitative differences in intestinal mucus glycoprotein. Similar alterations in colonic mucin fraction IV from patients with UC are present in cotton-top tamarins with spontaneous colitis. Cigarette smoking can also influence mucin production and intestinal permeability, and nonsteroidal anti-inflammatory drugs damage proximal and distal intestinal epithelium, increase intestinal permeability, and tend to exacerbate IBD.

Intestinal epithelial cells stimulated by interferon express class II major histocompatibility complexes and become antigen-presenting cells. The processing and presentation of antigens to T8 (suppressor T cells) are altered in patients with IBD such that the presentation of antigen is preferentially directed toward the T4 (helper T cell) system. This could be a primary, genetically mediated event that stimulates the gut immune system rather than induces tolerance.

A defect in the ability of the gut epithelium to metabolize short-chain fatty acids derived from the intestinal lumen or injury to the epithelium by an infectious or toxic injury may alter or expose cell proteins that are perceived as foreign by the mucosal immune system. A conclusive target antigen has not been identified for either UC or CD. A variety of antibodies to epithelial cell components, some of which cross-react with enterobacterial antigens, are present but are not specific for IBD. In addition, serum antibodies against enteric bacteria or food-related antigens (e.g., milk protein) are increased in a nonspecific manner. There is also evidence of autoimmune lymphocyte-mediated cytotoxicity against epithelial cells, but a consistent abnormality in mucosal or systemic immune regulation has not been identified. Most of the local (mucosal) or systemic immunologic parameters represent secondary rather than primary changes.

Once initiated, many of the pathophysiologic events in IBD are related to amplification of the inflammatory process. When antigens are presented to mucosal macrophages, cytokines and other inflammatory mediators are activated and released. IL1 is released and induces T-cell activation and proliferation. Activated T cells become cytotoxic and/or release IL2, which induces clonal expansion of helper T cells, B-cell proliferation, and antibody synthesis. IgG production by B cells invokes complement activation and subsequent activation of the kinin system. The arachidonic acid cascade of inflammatory mediators is shifted toward the proinflammatory, lipoxygenase pathway with enhanced production of leukotriene B_4, a potent chemotactic agent for neutrophils, and platelet-activating factor (PAF) is produced. When neutrophils accumulate and are stimulated, they further damage tissue by releasing reactive oxygen species, amplifying the inflammatory process via recruitment of additional acute inflammatory cells, whether or not the primary initiating sequences have been halted.

The release of inflammatory mediators, including prostaglandins and leukotrienes, histamine from mast cells, and neuropeptides such as substance P or vasoactive intestinal peptide, alters epithelial function and contributes to the intestinal secretory process inducing diarrhea. The enteric nervous system participates in the regulation of the local and systemic immune system, linking the association of "stress" and psychological factors with flare-ups of disease activity.

PATHOLOGY

UC and CD encompass a spectrum of clinicopathologic findings. Many of the macroscopic and microscopic changes are not specific and overlap with those of acute and chronic infectious enteritides, toxin- or radiation-induced damage to the intestine, ischemic changes, and, on rare occasion, malignancy.

ULCERATIVE COLITIS. Ulcerative colitis, primarily a mucosal disease, begins in the anorectum and involves a variable contiguous proximal segment of colonic mucosa. In approximately one quarter of patients the disease is limited to the rectum (proctitis); in another 25 to 50 per cent the rectum and sigmoid (proctosigmoiditis) or the descending colon (left-sided colitis) is involved. In approximately one third of patients the inflammation extends proximal to the splenic flexure (extensive colitis) or involves the entire colon (pancolitis). The small intestine occasionally is involved by superficial inflammation (backwash ileitis) in a small group of patients with pancolitis. Once the upper demarcation of disease has been identified, it usually remains constant. Approximately 10 to 15 per cent of patients develop proximal extension of colonic involvement, usually within the first few years after diagnosis. With treatment, healing typically begins proximally, with the rectum being the last segment to improve. Occasionally, UC may heal in a patchy distribution, although interval segments demonstrate chronic histologic changes. Some patients with proctitis have patches of endoscopic or histologic changes in the cecum or right colon. The prognostic implications of these findings are uncertain.

The gross or endoscopic appearance of the colonic mucosa in UC ranges from normal-appearing mucosa to complete denudation. Mild inflammatory changes include absence of the mucosal vascular pattern, fine granularity of the mucosa, pinpoint hemorrhage to mucosal swabbing, and exudation of mucopus (see Color Plate 2A). Moderate changes include coarse granularity and pinpoint ulceration, confluent hemorrhage, confluent mucopus that progresses to gross ulcerations, spontaneous hemorrhage, and exudation of pus (see Color Plate 2A). With healing the mucosal vascular pattern remains distorted. Islands of postinflammatory "pseudopolyps" may appear as filamentous projections or mucosal bridges that may be quite friable or indistinguishable from adenomatous polyps (see Color Plate 2B).

Early histologic changes include vascular congestion, increased inflammatory cells in the lamina propria, and distortion of the crypts of Lieberkühn. The degree of the inflammatory reaction determines the "activity" of disease. In inactive colitis the mucosal architecture is distorted with branching or regenerating crypts, and epithelial cells are depleted of goblet cell mucus (see Color Plate 2C). In the active phase of inflammation, acute inflammatory cells, primarily polymorphonuclear leukocytes, accumulate near the epithelium, invade the crypts, and are concentrated within the crypt lumen (crypt abscess) (see Color Plate 2D). Progressive changes include degeneration or necrosis of the crypt epithelium with coalescence of crypt abscesses to produce shallow ulcerations extending to the lamina propria. Only rarely, in severe UC or toxic megacolon, do inflammation and necrosis extend below the lamina propria to involve the submucosa and circular or longitudinal muscles. Then the bowel wall may become "tissue paper" thin with a significant risk of spontaneous perforation.

Typically with acute disease, reversible changes in the colonic musculature lead to loss of haustrations, thickening of the smooth muscle of the colon, and the "lead pipe" appearance of the colon or, occasionally, the appearance of a stricture on radiographic examination.

Epithelial dysplasia may occur in longstanding UC and is highly associated with the presence of colonic malignancy as a long-term complication (see below).

CROHN'S DISEASE. CD involves any segment or combination of segments of the alimentary tract from the mouth to the anus. Unlike UC, microscopic changes often are identified distant from sites of macroscopic disease. These focal changes and the tendency of CD to recur after segmental resection suggest that subtle changes of CD exist throughout the alimentary tract. Most commonly the distal ileum and right colon are macroscopically inflamed (ileocolitis). The colon is involved, exclusively, in about 20 per cent of patients (Crohn's colitis or granulomatous colitis); approximately 15 to 20 per cent of individuals have gross disease limited to the small bowel (ileitis or regional enteritis). The stomach or duodenum is involved in fewer than 10 per cent of patients and usually in association with more distal disease. Diseases of the anal canal, including deep fissures, fistulas, and prominent "hemorrhoidal" skin tags, are common and distinguish CD confined to the colon from UC. Unlike UC, the mucosa in

CD is involved in a focal, discontinuous fashion, both microscopically and macroscopically. Rarely, lesions indistinguishable from those of CD occur in the skin or urogenital mucosal surfaces (miliary CD).

The earliest lesion of CD is the aphthoid ulcer (see Color Plate 2E), a minute ulceration that invariably occurs over a lymphoid aggregate. These ulcerations extend in a linear fashion (see Color Plate 2F), often isolating normal islands of mucosa to produce a "cobblestone appearance," or extend deep throughout the layers of the bowel wall, producing a fissure that can become a fistula into the mesentery or a contiguous organ. Inflammatory changes in CD are typically transmural, accounting for the thickening of the bowel wall and narrowing of the lumen. As CD heals, fibrotic changes replace acute inflammation, creating permanent, focal strictures. In gross specimens, changes include the thickened, "sausage-shaped" appearance of the bowel with serosal hyperemia, "creeping fat" along the antimesenteric border, and thickening and lymphoid hyperplasia of the adjacent mesentery. The inflammatory process is focal in all layers of the bowel (see Color Plate 2G). Acute and chronic inflammatory cells invade isolated or contiguous single crypts (including the production of crypt abscesses) with normal adjacent glands. Lymphoid aggregates are common throughout all layers of the mucosa, submucosa, and serosa, with characteristic aggregations of histiocytes forming noncaseating granulomas in up to 50 per cent of resected specimens. Mucosal biopsies, however, reveal granuloma formation in fewer than 20 per cent of patients. The presence of granulomas differentiates CD from UC, but they are not necessary to distinguish the two diseases. Rather, the focal, transmural involvement of CD associated with aphthoid or linear ulcers, fissures, fistulas, perianal disease, or small intestinal involvement morphologically distinguishes CD from UC. In approximately 20 per cent of patients with colitis, "indeterminant" features do not allow classification between UC and CD. In this setting, the response to therapy and repeated observations over the course usually allow eventual classification.

CLINICAL MANIFESTATIONS

ULCERATIVE COLITIS. The symptoms of UC depend upon the extent and severity of inflammation within the colon. UC always involves the rectum; patients with proctitis present with rectal bleeding, tenesmus, and the passage of mucopus. The consistency of stools is variable, and many patients with ulcerative proctitis are constipated. Abdominal cramping is common, but abdominal pain or tenderness is not a typical finding of UC. The inflammatory process is limited to the mucosa, while pain receptors are located on the serosa or peritoneum. The greater the extent of colon involved, the more likely the patient is to suffer from diarrhea. Rectal urgency reflects reduced compliance of the inflamed rectum.

As the severity of inflammation increases, the patient is more likely to suffer from systemic symptoms. Low-grade fever, malaise, occasional nausea and vomiting associated with defecation, night sweats, and arthralgias are frequent complaints. With severe UC, patients present with fever, dehydration, tachycardia, and symptoms of abdominal tenderness, reflecting progressive inflammation into deeper layers of the colon. A distended abdomen and tympanic bowel sounds accompanied by fever, tachycardia, and vomiting are ominous signs of fulminant colitis or toxic megacolon.

Patients with UC in remission have normal bowel habits, although many patients suffer from an accompanying irritable bowel syndrome with occasional cramping, irregular bowel habits, and the passage of mucus without blood or pus.

Laboratory studies reflect the severity of colitis. Iron deficiency anemia secondary to chronic blood loss is the most common abnormality. A low serum ferritin confirms the presence of iron deficiency anemia and better documents iron stores than do serum iron and iron-binding capacity, which are reduced by chronic disease. Elevation of the erythrocyte sedimentation rate and other acute phase reactants are inconstant features in UC and are of no value in the evaluation of individual patients. A low serum albumin occurs with extensive colitis as a manifestation of protein exudation from the inflamed colon. Serum alkaline phosphatase and GGTP may be modestly elevated (less than twice normal) in patients with pericholangitis; greater changes in bilirubin or hepatocellular enzymes suggest sclerosing cholangitis or chronic hepatitis.

CROHN'S DISEASE. The symptoms and signs of CD also are determined by the site and extent of inflammation. Gastroduodenal CD mimics peptic ulcer disease, with nausea, vomiting, and epigastric pain. Patients with small intestinal involvement present with abdominal cramping, diarrhea, and abdominal tenderness. The pain and tenderness of CD are due to transmural inflammation. Transmural inflammation leads to fibrosis and narrowing of the intestinal lumen, which produce symptoms of obstruction: nausea, vomiting, waves of abdominal pain, and a reduced output of stool. This is appreciated as a thickened, tender loop of bowel or an abdominal mass, if the mesentery is involved. Patients with colonic CD present with abdominal pain, cramping or localized pain, rectal bleeding, and diarrhea.

Weight loss is more common in CD than in ulcerative colitis due to small bowel–related malabsorption or a reduced intake of food to minimize postprandial symptoms. Systemic symptoms, including fever, night sweats, malaise, and arthralgias, are common.

Laboratory features in CD reflect blood loss, malabsorption, protein-losing enteropathy, and elevation of acute phase reactants. Anemia may be due to iron deficiency (blood loss or malabsorption), folic acid deficiency, or vitamin B_{12} deficiency. Serum albumin and total protein are reduced with either malnutrition or protein-losing enteropathy. Electrolyte abnormalities reflect the severity of diarrhea, and lowered serum calcium may reflect reduced serum albumin, calcium malabsorption, or vitamin D deficiency. Patients with ileal disease often malabsorb fat-soluble vitamins (A, D, E, and K), deficiency of which can produce clinically significant symptoms or signs.

COMPLICATIONS

INTESTINAL COMPLICATIONS. *Rectal bleeding* is a common manifestation of both UC and CD. In UC the superficial inflammation induces capillary hemorrhage, manifested as bright red coating of stool or blood-tinged mucopus. In severe UC the bleeding can be more prominent and on rare occasions is profuse. Iron deficiency anemia is a common secondary association due to the chronic blood loss. In CD, hemorrhage may be profuse as a result of deeper inflammation and ulceration into larger vessels. Recurrent bleeding occurs in a small subset of patients with CD and is sometimes the single indication for surgery.

Toxic megacolon, once thought only to occur with UC, also occurs in CD and infectious colitis. Toxic megacolon develops in seriously ill individuals when transmural inflammation extends into the muscular layer, thinning the intestinal wall. The entire colon, or segments of the colon, can dilate as a result of disruption of the neural and muscular elements that maintain normal tone. Dilatation of the diameter of the colon on a plain abdominal radiograph to greater than 6 cm (see Color Plate 2*H*), associated with clinical symptoms of increasing abdominal pain, distention, rebound tenderness, and signs of fever, tachycardia, dehydration, and a reduction in bowel sounds, is diagnostic of toxic megacolon. Even in the absence of prominent dilatation, similar symptoms and signs are sufficient to diagnose severe colitis with an identical risk of perforation and the hazard of peritonitis. Precipitating circumstances include severe colitis, instrumentation with barium studies or endoscopic procedures in severe inflammation, potassium depletion, anticholinergic medications, or narcotics, which are thought to reduce neuromuscular activity of the gut. Associated laboratory findings include leukocytosis, hypokalemia, anemia, and hypoalbuminemia.

Toxic megacolon should be anticipated in any patient with severe colitis, including segmental colitis, and these individuals require careful monitoring of vital signs, abdominal examinations for rebound tenderness, flat-plate abdominal radiographs for dilatation or free air, and laboratory studies to maintain an adequate hematocrit and electrolyte status. Toxic megacolon should be treated with intensive medical therapy, and failure to improve within 12 to 24 hours is an indication for colectomy.

Early colectomy can prevent the morbidity and mortality of a perforation, which may exceed 20 per cent.

Crohn's disease, being transmural, is associated with additional intestinal complications. Thickened segments of inflamed bowel become fibrotic, and stricturing is common. Whereas bowel narrowing in UC is due to reversible muscular hypertrophy, the scarring in CD is largely irreversible. Transmural fissures extend into adjacent structures, producing an inflammatory mass, abscess, or fistula. Entero-enteric, -vesicular, -mesenteric, or -cutaneous fistulas are common, as are rectovaginal fistulas, perianal fistulas, and abscesses.

CANCER (Table 103–2, also Ch. 105). Cancer of the colon not infrequently complicates longstanding UC, depending upon two factors: the extent of mucosal involvement (pancolitis greater than left-sided colitis) and the duration of disease. Severity of the initial attack, subsequent course, and specific medical therapies are not related to the cancer risk. Colonic adenocarcinomas may occur in patients who have had quiescent UC for decades. Indeed, these may be the patients at highest risk. In European countries where colectomy is performed earlier, the risk of cancer is reduced.

Mucosal dysplasia is a precursor of cancer. Dysplasia can be identified with colonoscopic biopsies by experienced pathologists (see Color Plate 2*I*) and must be distinguished from inflammatory or regenerative epithelial changes. Repeat biopsies and aggressive medical therapy should be considered when there is doubt about pathologic interpretation. Confirmed epithelial dysplasia is an indication for colectomy, as malignancies are often identified separate from the dysplastic foci. Routine screening for dysplasia and neoplasia is now recommended in longstanding UC. Surveillance colonoscopies and biopsies throughout the length of the colon should be initiated after 8 to 10 years of extensive colitis and repeated at 1- to 2-year intervals. The finding of dysplasia warrants confirmation by an experienced pathologist or repeat examination. Dysplasia in a nodular or polypoid lesion has an extremely high (greater than 50 per cent) association with concurrent malignancy. Dysplasia and cancers in UC can occur in normal flat mucosa, with ulceration or stricture formation, or within a polyp or mass.

CD also increases the incidence of adenocarcinomas of the intestine. The same risk factors (extent and duration) probably apply but have not been as clearly established for CD. Patients with inactive CD should be monitored for a change in symptoms, bleeding, or obstruction; endoscopic or radiographic evaluation should be pursued for a change in an otherwise inactive phase. There is also a small increased risk of leukemia, lymphoma, and bile duct carcinomas in patients with IBD.

EXTRAINTESTINAL COMPLICATIONS (Table 103–3). The extraintestinal manifestations of IBD can be divided into complications of gastrointestinal inflammation or diseases associated with IBD. The latter occur most often with "colitis" but can occur in either UC or CD when the colon is inflamed.

Nutritional and metabolic abnormalities occur with chronic disease, inadequate intake of calories, maldigestion, and malabsorption. Blood and protein loss contribute to iron deficiency anemia and hypoalbuminemia. Deficiencies of calcium, magnesium, or zinc are most often noted with small intestinal CD in the presence of active inflammation or extensive surgical resections. Calcium deficiency may be aggravated by milk-free diets or vitamin D deficiency. Deficiency of folic acid can be secondary to inadequate intake, proximal small bowel disease, or competitive inhibition of folate absorption by sulfasalazine. Treatments for these nutritional deficiencies require appropriate diagnosis,

TABLE 103–2. CANCER IN ULCERATIVE COLITIS

Risk factors
Extent of colon involved
Duration of disease after 10 years

Surveillance
Begin after 10 days
Increase frequency of surveillance with increased duration of disease

Warning
Dysplasia; low grade, low grade with mass, high grade; requires confirmation and follow-up in 3 to 6 months

Surgical indication
Confirmed high-grade dysplasia, or dysplasia-associated lesion or mass (DALM)

TABLE 103–3. EXTRAINTESTINAL MANIFESTATIONS OF THE INFLAMMATORY BOWEL DISEASES

Nutritional and metabolic abnormalities
Weight loss, growth retardation in children
Hypoalbuminemia—nutritional, protein-losing enteropathy
Vitamin deficiencies*
Deficiencies of calcium, magnesium, or zinc*

Hematologic abnormalities
Anemia—Fe, folate, B$_{12}$* deficiency
Leukocytosis, thrombocytosis

Skin and mucous membranes
Pyoderma gangrenosum
Erythema nodosum
Stomatitis with multiple aphthous ulcers

Musculoskeletal
Ankylosing spondylitis, sacroiliitis (HLA-B27 associated)
Peripheral arthritis of large joints
Osteoporosis
Osteomalacia*

Hepatic and biliary manifestations
Fatty liver
Pericholangitis
Sclerosing cholangitis
Gallstones*
Carcinoma of the bile ducts

Renal complications
Kidney stones
Uric acid
Calcium oxalate*
Obstructive uropathy*
Fistulas to urinary tract*
Amyloidosis (rare)

Eye complications
Conjunctivitis, episcleritis, iritis
Uveitis (HLA-B27)

*Crohn's disease.

treatment of the underlying inflammation, and enteral or parenteral repletion. Deficiencies in fat-soluble vitamins (vitamins A, D, E, and K) are most often produced by ileal disease or resection. Low vitamin D levels can aggravate metabolic bone disease and calcium malabsorption. Vitamin B$_{12}$ deficiency can be avoided by regular injections of intramuscular vitamin B$_{12}$ (Ch. 132).

Diarrhea is aggravated by malabsorption of fat or bile salts due to ileal disease or resection. Diarrhea with fat malabsorption is diagnosed by increased fecal fat (greater than 5 grams per day) and treated with a low-fat diet (Ch. 101). Additional calories can be supplied by medium-chain triglycerides, which are absorbed more proximally and do not require bile salts. Ileal resection also can deplete the bile salt pool owing to inadequate reabsorption and recirculation. Bile salt malabsorption induces diarrhea after bile salts are converted into bile acids in the colon, which stimulate secretion. Bile acid–induced diarrhea can be treated with small amounts of cholestyramine, which binds to bile salts and prevents its conversion to bile acids. Malabsorption of fat and bile salts in Crohn's disease increases the incidence of gallstones and kidney stones. Gallstones form because cholesterol levels are more saturated in the gallbladder secondary to a reduced bile salt pool. Calcium oxalate kidney stones are increased by fat malabsorption (Ch. 102). Normally dietary oxalate binds to calcium within the lumen of the small intestine and is excreted as insoluble calcium oxalate in the feces. With fat malabsorption, calcium alternatively binds to long-chain fatty acids rather than to oxalate. Free oxalate is then abnormally absorbed from the colon and excreted in the urine as "enteric hyperoxaluria." In CD kidney stones are due more often to hyperabsorption of oxalate than to increased urinary excretion of calcium. In addition, patients with IBD have low levels of urinary citrate, a nonspecific solubilizer that reduces mineral saturation in the urine. The treatment of calcium oxalate kidney stones includes reduction of fat intake to reduce fat malabsorption; maintenance of fluid intake and hydration; a low-oxalate diet; supplementation of citrate; supplementation with oral calcium as

an intestinal oxalate binder; and the addition of cholestyramine as an alternative binder for intestinal oxalate. Enteric hyperoxaluria is discussed further in Ch. 88.

Skin and mucous membrane changes are common in IBD. Oral aphthae occur in CD, and fissuring of the lips or mouth may be due to zinc deficiency or *Candida* infection. Inflammatory skin disorders associated with IBD, pyoderma gangrenosum and erythema nodosum, tend to correlate with the disease activity in the colon, although, on occasion, skin changes may precede symptomatic colitis. Erythema nodosum presents usually as a painful, tender, erythematous, or violaceous nodule, most commonly on the leg. The lesions may be multiple, may develop on any extremity, and may be induced by minor trauma. Erythema nodosum usually responds to treatment of the underlying inflammation in the bowel but may respond more rapidly to topical or systemic steroids. Pyoderma gangrenosum, a more serious, necrotizing ulceration, occasionally runs an independent course from the intestinal inflammation. It also typically occurs on the lower extremities but can be noted anywhere on the skin and occasionally on surgical incisions or adjacent to a stoma. These lesions should not be biopsied, since this may lead to cutaneous breakdown and ulceration. Effective treatment of the underlying IBD, as well as topical antibiotics and potent topical steroids, should be implemented immediately. Systemic steroids may be necessary; pyoderma gangrenosum also responds to oral sulfone therapy. On rare occasions resection of the active IBD is necessary to prevent progressive skin breakdown from extending into muscle or, rarely, into bone.

Ocular complications of IBD share many inflammatory components with the intestinal inflammation. Conjunctivitis, episcleritis, and iritis often occur in conjunction with active intestinal inflammation and respond to topical steroids. Uveitis, an HLA-B27–associated complication, may run an independent course from the IBD.

Hepatic and biliary complications of IBD are frequent. Gallstones are related to bile salt malabsorption in Crohn's disease, and steatosis may be secondary to malnutrition, corticosteroid therapy, or excessive parenteral carbohydrates from total parenteral nutrition solution. There is a spectrum of bile duct inflammation ranging from pericholangitis to sclerosing cholangitis and associated biliary cirrhosis. Pericholangitis (portal triaditis) is a nonprogressive inflammation of intrahepatic bile ductules manifested as a minor elevation of the alkaline phosphatase and GGTP with minimal elevation of the serum transaminases. Bilirubin remains normal, and inflammation is confined to the portal triads. Sclerosing cholangitis is a progressive form of bile duct inflammation involving the intrahepatic and/or extrahepatic biliary tree. Elevations of serum alkaline phosphatase and GGTP are greater than two times normal, and transaminase elevation can occur. Intermittent cholangitic episodes or asymptomatic jaundice may be the first manifestation. Visualization of the biliary tree via ERCP or transhepatic cholangiography confirms the extent of bile duct abnormalities. There are no proven therapies to limit the biliary inflammation, although preliminary studies using ursodeoxycholic acid or methotrexate are encouraging. Occasionally, endoscopic dilatation of a prominent stricture can relieve obstruction, although the disease is typically multifocal. Rarely, carcinoma of the bile duct mimics sclerosing cholangitis limited to the extrahepatic biliary system.

Kidney stones are a common complication of IBD. Hyperoxaluria and calcium oxalate stones are related to steatorrhea, whereas uric acid stones are more commonly associated with dehydration in patients with diarrhea or ileostomies. Obstructive uropathies can occur as a complication of an inflammatory mass. Fistula to the bladder occurs frequently with ileal CD in association with ileo-sigmoid-bladder communication, manifested as urinary frequency, dysuria, sterile pyuria, or recurrent cystitis. Amyloidosis is a rare, occasionally reversible complication of longstanding intestinal inflammation.

The metabolic bone diseases, osteoporosis and osteomalacia, occur commonly in chronic IBD. Osteoporosis is a frequent complication of long-term steroid therapy. Reduced bone mineralization also is a complication of malabsorption of vitamin D and calcium. Clubbing of the fingers and two distinct syndromes of enteric arthropathy may occur: (1) Peripheral arthritis frequently involves larger joints (knees, elbows, ankles) in an asymmetric fashion with swelling, erythema, and an inflammatory synovial analysis. It precedes or coincides with bowel symptoms and usually responds to treatment of the intestinal inflammation. Joint destruction does not occur, and serologic studies for rheumatoid factors are negative. (2) Central arthritis of the spine, ankylosing spondylitis, and sacroiliitis are HLA-B27–associated arthropathies that run an independent course from the bowel disorders. Progressive calcification and joint fusion proceed despite treatment of the IBD and require independent therapy (physical therapy and anti-inflammatory drugs). Nonsteroidal anti-inflammatory drugs must be used with caution in patients with IBD because of the potential for aggravating intestinal inflammation while attempting to treat arthritic symptoms.

Children are susceptible to several unique complications of IBD. Often the initial manifestations of IBD in children occur without intestinal symptoms. Growth retardation, delayed sexual maturation, peripheral arthritis, fevers of undetermined origin, or anemia can precede abdominal symptoms. Impairments of growth and development usually are associated with inadequate nutritional status. Improved caloric intake can reverse growth failure in conjunction with treatment of intestinal inflammation. Surgical resection is sometimes necessary to reverse growth failure. Children also are susceptible to delayed psychological development because of chronic illness and may require additional supportive therapy from the physician and other health care providers. Family counseling can also provide an important service for the patient and family.

Fertility, pregnancy, and lactation are important aspects for young adults with IBD. In general, IBD does not reduce fertility. Women with active IBD or high-dose steroid therapy, however, often have anovulatory menstrual cycles or secondary amenorrhea, which temporarily impairs fertility. Women with active IBD are more likely to miscarry, but usually fetal development is normal in those carried to term. Medicinal and nutritional support for the pregnant woman should be continued throughout pregnancy. Corticosteroids and sulfasalazine should not be discontinued if they are successful in managing the mother's intestinal symptoms. Occasionally, total parenteral nutrition may be necessary to supply adequate calories. Metronidazole and immunosuppressive agents are not recommended during pregnancy. Immunosuppressive therapies have been used with success in patients following transplantation and in several patients with IBD. Approximately one third of women with quiescent IBD experience flare-ups during the postpartum period. Corticosteroids and sulfasalazine are secreted in small quantities in breast milk, but nursing is generally safe during their use.

DIAGNOSIS

There are no pathognomonic clinical, endoscopic, or histologic features of the idiopathic IBD's. The physician must therefore consider the entire clinical picture and the evolution of the illness. It is particularly important to exclude other disorders that may mimic the broad range of symptoms and findings that may be present in IBD. It is important first of all to establish the presence of intestinal inflammation. A cardinal feature is the exudation of inflammatory cells into the lumen, reflected in the presence of fecal leukocytes or red blood cells on examination of the stool. Symptoms of rectal bleeding, tenesmus associated with the passage of pus, nocturnal pain and diarrhea, fever, night sweats, weight loss, or extraintestinal symptoms or signs generally exclude an uncomplicated "irritable bowel syndrome." The presence of anemia, electrolyte disorders, hypoalbuminemia, or an elevated erythrocyte sedimentation rate or C-reactive protein is sufficient, but not necessary, to suggest IBD. On physical examination, evidence of significant weight loss or extraintestinal signs, a palpable abdominal mass or tenderness, or significant perianal disease suggests IBD. When suspicion of the diagnosis warrants, endoscopic and radiographic studies, in conjunction with histologic interpretation of biopsy specimens, confirm the diagnosis. The degree of illness at the time of presentation should determine the aggressiveness of the diagnostic workup. Acutely ill patients should be stabilized before invasive studies are pursued.

ENDOSCOPY. Patients presenting with colitic symptoms of rectal bleeding, cramping, tenesmus, mucopus, or watery diarrhea in conjunction with fecal leukocytes warrant a colonic examination. A proctoscopic examination or flexible sigmoidoscopy reveals the presence and pattern of distal colonic inflammation. In the absence of perianal disease, diffuse, continuous mucosal changes with a distinct upper boundary to adjacent normal-appearing mucosa are typical of ulcerative proctitis or proctosigmoiditis. Focal inflammation with aphthoid ulcers, linear or stellate ulcers with normal intervening mucosa, or inflammatory changes beginning above the rectum (rectal sparing) in previously untreated patients suggest Crohn's disease. If the patient is not acutely ill, colonoscopy demonstrates more proximal colonic changes and allows examination and intubation of the ileocecal valve to evaluate terminal ileal findings. Patients with upper abdominal symptoms can be diagnosed with upper gastrointestinal endoscopy when typical mucosal changes of Crohn's disease involve this area. Findings can be correlated with mucosal biopsy studies and radiographic evaluation of the small and large intestine.

RADIOGRAPHY. Radiographic examination should begin with a supine and upright view of the abdomen. Associated findings of nephrolithiasis, cholelithiasis, or arthritis of the spine or sacroiliac joints may be identified. Intestinal dilatation or air-fluid levels suggesting obstruction preclude aggressive barium studies until the patient's clinical condition is stabilized. In colitis, a plain view of the abdomen often demonstrates a tubular, ahaustral segment of colon in the presence of distal UC with fecal matter proximal to diseased mucosa. Intestinal edema, ulceration, or thumb-printing may give a gross estimate of disease activity. Air-contrast barium studies of the colon reveal diffuse, contiguous granularity, superficial ulceration, and absent haustration in active UC (see Color Plate 2J). Pseudopolyps or a tubular-appearing "lead pipe" colon may be found in chronic UC. Focal, asymmetric ulceration with linear or fissuring ulcers, the presence of fistulas, rectal sparing, or a diseased terminal ileum with reflux of the barium defines the radiographic extent and severity of colonic CD (see Color Plate 3A). A small bowel follow-through or enteroclysis (small bowel enema) demonstrates the extent of small intestinal involvement in CD (see Color Plate 3B) and is normal in the absence of backwash ileitis in UC.

Specialized diagnostic imaging studies are occasionally useful to diagnosis the extent or complications of IBD. Ultrasonography or a computed tomography (CT) examination can clarify the presence of thickened bowel wall and mesentery versus an abscess cavity in an abdominal mass. Perineal CT scan or rectal ultrasonography demonstrates the degree of perianal involvement and the complexity of anorectal fistulas. Occasionally, ultrasound- or CT-guided aspiration of a cavity can reduce the morbidity of abdominal or retroperitoneal suppuration. Injected indium- or technetium-labeled leukocytes localize in sites of intestinal inflammation, and fecal excretion of radiolabeled leukocytes can be a measure of inflammatory activity.

DIFFERENTIAL DIAGNOSIS. Patients with irritable bowel syndrome rarely present with "inflammatory" features. Persistent symptoms despite therapy for presumed irritable bowel syndrome, especially in the presence of weight loss, bleeding attributed to "hemorrhoids," or a family history of IBD, deserve a more comprehensive evaluation to exclude IBD. Most enteric infections are self-limited. Viral gastroenteritis typically lasts 1 to 4 days without the presence of rectal bleeding or fecal leukocytes. Most bacterial pathogens produce self-limited disease lasting less than 7 to 14 days, despite the presence of intermittent rectal bleeding, fevers, fecal leukocytes, and a mucosal appearance that may be indistinguishable from that of UC or CD. Occasionally, Campylobacter jejuni produces protracted symptoms (Ch. 316), and Clostridium difficile toxin–induced colitis can mimic the symptoms, signs, and endoscopic appearance of UC or CD (Ch. 308). When a patient with IBD presents with new or exacerbated symptoms, stool cultures for enteric pathogens and studies for Clostridium difficile toxin should be obtained, especially if the patient has been recently treated with antibiotics. In Northern Europe and Canada, Yersinia enterocolitica infection can mimic terminal ileitis (Ch. 321). If the clinical suspicion warrants, cultures and serologic studies for Yersinia should be obtained. Similarly, tuberculosis of the gastrointestinal tract may mimic CD in areas where intestinal tuberculosis is endemic, and, rarely, actinomycosis simulates fistulizing CD.

TABLE 103–4. COMPARISON OF CLINICAL AND PATHOLOGIC FEATURES OF CROHN'S COLITIS AND ULCERATIVE COLITIS

Feature	Crohn's Colitis	Ulcerative Colitis
Clinical		
Smoker	+ +	+ / –
Malaise, fever	+ +	+
Rectal bleeding	+ +	+ + +
Abdominal tenderness	+ + +	+
Abdominal mass	+ +	–
Abdominal pain	+ + +	+
Perianal disease	+ + +	–
Endoscopic		
Rectal disease	+	+ + +
Diffuse, continuous, symmetric involvement	+	+ + +
Aphthous or linear ulcers	+ + +	–
Cobblestoning	+ +	–
Friability	+ +	+ + +
Radiologic		
Continuous disease	+	+ + +
Ileal involvement	+ +	–
Asymmetry	+ + +	–
Strictures	+ +	+
Fistulas	+ +	–
Pathologic		
Discontinuity	+ +	–
Transmural involvement	+ + +	+ / –
Lymphoid aggregates	+ + +	–
Crypt abscesses	+ + +	+ + +
Granulomas	+ +	–
Sinus tract/fistula	+ + +	–

+ + + = Always
+ + = Common
+ = Occasional
– = Never

Chronic intestinal infections usually are parasitic. Amebiasis may present with diarrhea, rectal bleeding, and a sigmoidoscopic appearance similar to that of idiopathic IBD (Ch. 431). Deep "collar button" ulcerations are similar to focal ulcerations of CD. Fresh stool specimens should be examined repeatedly for amebic cysts or trophozoites; and biopsies may be indicated in patients who have been exposed to endemic environments (including nursing homes and the homosexual population). Syphilis, gonorrhea, and lymphogranuloma venereum also induce proctitis in the gay population. HIV diarrhea should be excluded by serologic studies in patients with suspected exposure.

Occasionally, with an acute onset, Crohn's ileitis is diagnosed at laparotomy performed for presumed appendicitis. Likewise, in young individuals with acute right lower quadrant pain, mesenteric adenitis may mimic the symptoms of CD. In the older population, ischemic bowel disease, especially chronic mesenteric ischemia, or recurrent diverticulitis can mimic Crohn's colitis.

Persistent rectal bleeding should not be attributed to hemorrhoids unless a flexible sigmoidoscopy has excluded IBD (Ch. 94). In the older population, colonic carcinomas also can present with chronic symptoms and intermittent rectal bleeding (Ch. 111). Intestinal lymphoma may be very difficult to distinguish from CD and often requires a surgical diagnosis when suspected. Radiation enteritis is limited to patients with a history of that

therapy. Some patients receiving chemotherapy or gold develop diarrhea and mucosal ulceration. Nonsteroidal anti-inflammatory drug–induced ulceration of the ileum and colon mimics the aphthous ulcers of CD. Eosinophilic gastroenteritis presents with diarrhea, malabsorption, and protein-losing enteropathy, but the associated peripheral blood eosinophilia and biopsies are distinguishing. The diffuse, proximal malabsorptive pattern of celiac sprue, associated with diffuse villous atrophy, is distinct from the focal, distal small bowel changes of CD. Table 103–4 outlines the distinguishing features between UC and CD confined to the colon.

TREATMENT

The therapy of either UC or CD depends upon the extent and severity of intestinal involvement (Table 103–5). The patient/physician team must embark upon treatment with due consideration of the entire clinical picture and the chronic nature of the illness. Both the patient and the family should participate in the decision making, and this requires education and support. Although the therapies for UC and CD overlap in many ways, they are considered separately to clarify the differences. A primary difference is that UC can be cured by removing the colon and all colonic mucosa. CD is not cured by surgery and has a predictable tendency to recur after removal of an involved segment of intestine. Medical alternatives are discussed first, followed by specific IBD syndromes.

Medical Alternatives

SULFASALAZINE AND MESALAMINE. Sulfasalazine was developed 50 years ago to combine a known antibiotic (sulfapyridine) with a salicylate (5-aminosalicylic acid, mesalamine) for delivery into the connective tissue of the colon. It is now recognized that the azo bond between sulfapyridine and 5-aminosalicylic acid is split by colonic bacteria, releasing both separate components in the colon. The majority of the sulfapyridine is absorbed from the colon, acetylated by the liver in a genetically determined fashion, and excreted in the urine. The majority of the mesalamine remains within the colon and is excreted within the feces. Mesalamine delivered into the colon has therapeutic efficacy similar to that of sulfasalazine, but without the potential adverse consequences of the sulfa moiety.

Sulfasalazine is effective in a dose-dependent manner for the treatment of acute UC and for maintaining remission of quiescent UC. Sulfasalazine also has been effective for mild to moderate CD when the colon is involved. It has not been clearly shown that sulfasalazine maintains a remission in CD, although patients with CD who respond symptomatically to sulfasalazine may have flare-ups when the drug is discontinued.

Many patients develop side effects from sulfasalazine before achieving therapeutic doses. Nausea, malaise, headache, and myalgias are common side effects that reduce patient compliance. Sulfa-induced hemolysis, allergic reactions, and toxic pancreatitis, pneumonitis, hepatitis, or colitis are rare, but reversible abnormalities of sperm motility and morphology are seen in up to 80 per cent of males taking sulfasalazine. Sulfasalazine also competitively inhibits intestinal absorption of folate, occasionally producing folate deficiency (Ch. 132). Folic acid supplementation (1 mg daily) is therefore recommended for patients on long-term therapy. Sulfasalazine seems to be safe for both the mother and the infant during pregnancy and with breast feeding.

Because 5-ASA (mesalamine) is an active moiety of sulfasala-

TABLE 103–5. INFLAMMATORY BOWEL DISEASE: SEVERITY CRITERIA

	Mild	Severe	Fulminant / Toxic
Bowel frequency	<4/day	>6/day	>10/day
Blood in stool	+ / –	+ +	Continuous
Fever	Normal	>37.5° C	>37.5° C
Pulse	Normal	>90/min	>90/min
Hemoglobin	Normal	<75%	Transfusion required
Erythrocyte sedimentation rate	<30 mm/hr	>30 mm/hr	>30 mm/hr
Abdominal radiograph	Normal	Colonic edema, thumb-printing, air-fluid levels	Dilated colon or small bowel
Clinical sign		Abdominal tenderness	Rebound tenderness, distention, diminished bowel sounds

TABLE 103–6. ULCERATIVE COLITIS: MEDICAL THERAPY

Therapy	Mild/Moderate	Severe*	Fulminant*	Maintenance
Diet	Symptomatic	PO + PN	NPO/TPN	Symptomatic
Oral anti-inflammatory				
Sulfasalazine	2–6 g/day	2–6 g/day	—	2–4 g/day
Olsalazine	1.5–3.0 g/day	1.5–3.0 g/day	—	0.75–1.5 g/day
Mesalamine	1.5–4.8 g/day	1.5–4.8 g/day	—	1.5–3.0 g/day
Topical anti-inflammatory				
Mesalamine enema or suppository	1–4 g/day	—	—	—
Corticosteroid enema or foam	80–200 mg/day	100–200 mg/day	—	—
Systemic anti-inflammatory†				
Prednisone	20–60 mg/day	40–60 mg/day IV	40–60 mg/day	—
ACTH	—	80–120 U/day IV	80–120 U/day	—
Antibiotics	—	—	+	—
Surgical consultation	—	+	+ +	

*Avoid anticholinergics, antidiarrheals, narcotics, and invasive procedures.
†Not warranted for proctitis.

zine, topical mesalamine has been used as a substitute for sulfasalazine in the treatment of distal colitis. Mesalamine enemas are effective for active UC confined to the left colon when administered nightly, and they prolong remissions of left-sided UC if therapy is maintained. Mesalamine suppositories (500 mg administered two to three times daily) are also effective for ulcerative proctitis, and nightly therapy with 500-mg suppositories maintains remissions.

Free mesalamine is rapidly absorbed from the proximal gastrointestinal tract. Several delayed or sustained-release preparations are currently under development in the United States. Asacol, which contains 400 mg of mesalamine coated with a resin that breaks down at pH 7, supplies the same amount of mesalamine present in 1 gram of sulfasalazine. Pentasa, which contains mesalamine encapsulated into microgranules of ethylcellulose, releases mesalamine throughout the small and large intestine. Dipentum (olsalazine), an azo-bonded dimer of two 5-ASA molecules, releases two molecules of mesalamine in the colon in a manner similar to that of sulfasalazine.

Mesalamine has fewer side effects than sulfasalazine. Except for topical therapy with mesalamine enemas in distal UC, mesalamine has no therapeutic advantage over sulfasalazine. Mesalamine preparations are tolerated in 80 per cent of patients who cannot tolerate sulfasalazine. The sperm abnormalities associated with sulfasalazine are reversed when the patient is transferred to mesalamine treatment. Olsalazine may increase intestinal secretion to produce diarrhea that is sufficiently severe to stop therapy in approximately 6 per cent of patients. Diarrhea can be minimized or avoided by gradual titration of the therapeutic doses.

CORTICOSTEROIDS. Corticosteroids are indicated for the induction of remission in either UC or CD, but they should not be used for maintenance therapy because of their inability to prevent relapse and their associated side effects (Ch. 27). In UC, hydrocortisone enemas are useful for the treatment of distal colonic symptoms, and cortisone acetate foam can be applied for the relief of rectal inflammation. Oral prednisone is indicated for moderate to severe UC at doses of 40 mg daily initially, followed by gradual tapering according to the clinical course. Severe UC should be treated with parenteral corticosteroids in intravenous daily doses comparable to 40 mg of prednisone. Alternatively, intravenous ACTH may be administered for patients who have not previously received steroid therapy. In CD, corticosteroids are useful in similar doses for acute disease and, again, are not recommended for maintenance therapy.

Corticosteroid therapy is also limited by its well-recognized adverse effects. Cushingoid features, acne, facial hair, and elevations of blood pressure are common early side effects. Cataract formation, osteoporosis (aggravated by vitamin D deficiency and calcium malabsorption in CD), and aseptic necrosis limit high-dose or long-term therapy. In children, corticosteroid therapy may further aggravate growth retardation.

ANTIBIOTICS. Antibiotic therapy for UC is limited to the presurgical treatment of severe or toxic colitis. Antibiotics have not been useful for less severe UC or to prevent relapse. In CD, metronidazole is as effective as sulfasalazine for colonic CD and

may be more beneficial for small intestinal disease and perianal complications of CD. Metronidazole (10 to 20 mg per kilogram administered orally in divided doses) can relieve symptoms of CD, reduce acute phase reactants, and heal perianal disease. Metronidazole therapy is limited by coating of the tongue, nausea, alcohol intolerance, and peripheral neuropathy. The latter may be most troublesome, with documented abnormalities on neurologic examination and nerve conduction studies before clinical symptoms arise. Alternative antibiotics have not been adequately studied in CD, although many clinicians continue to use broad-spectrum antibiotics, such as tetracycline, sulfa-trimethoprim, or cephalexin, for symptomatic therapy of mild to moderate CD.

IMMUNOSUPPRESSIVES. 6-Mercaptopurine and azathioprine are effective in the long-term therapy of UC and CD. In both settings, these agents are useful in doses (50 to 150 mg per day) that are not immunosuppressive but probably have anti-inflammatory activity. There has been a reluctance to use these agents in UC because immunosuppressives have been found to be carcinogenic in patients who have received organ transplants. These medications, which require 3 to 6 months to have a maximal therapeutic effect, are largely useful for patients who are steroid-dependent, for disease refractory to standard medical therapies, for the healing of some intestinal and perianal fistulas, and possibly for maintenance therapy for patients who fail treatment or who cannot tolerate mesalamine. Allergic pancreatitis occurs in up to 15 per cent of patients receiving these drugs (Ch. 106). Blood counts should be monitored for the risk of neutropenia, although this is rarely found in patients receiving low-dose therapy for IBD. Immunosuppressives are not recommended during pregnancy, and the long-term potential carcinogenic effects should limit therapy to the above-stated indications.

Specific Syndromes

ULCERATIVE COLITIS

The medical therapy of UC depends upon the extent and severity of mucosal ulceration. It is advisable early in the course to define the colonic extent of disease with either colonoscopy or a combination of proctosigmoidoscopy and air-contrast barium enema. The treatment of UC can be divided into that for acute disease and that for maintaining remission (Table 103–6). Maintenance therapy is indicated because 80 per cent of patients who are seen to improve by endoscopic or histologic examination experience an exacerbation of their disease within a year after cessation of active therapy.

ULCERATIVE PROCTITIS. Mild ulcerative proctitis can be treated with topical corticosteroids or topical mesalamine. Hydrocortisone enemas (Cortenema) or cortisone acetate foam (Cortifoam), administered intrarectally at night, generally provides prompt relief. Patients should be treated until the symptoms resolve and the mucosa has healed (absence of granularity, friability, and mucopus at proctoscopy). After healing, the topical corticosteroids should be discontinued and used intermittently for mild relapses, or oral mesalamine* should be substituted for

---

*For purposes of discussion, sulfasalazine, olsalazine, and mesalamine preparations are all included as "mesalamine."

maintenance therapy. Some patients prefer oral mesalamine therapy as initial treatment for mild disease. Patients with more severe symptoms of proctitis with profound urgency, tenesmus, and frequent stooling may require a combination of topical corticosteroids and oral mesalamine or a combination of oral and topical mesalamine. Rarely, systemically active steroids are required for distal proctitis.

PROCTOSIGMOIDITIS. Proctosigmoiditis also responds to hydrocortisone or mesalamine enemas but more often requires combination therapy with oral mesalamine. Patients with severe symptoms require oral corticosteroids at a dose equivalent to 40 mg of prednisone daily. As the inflammation resolves and the mucosa heals, the steroids should be tapered with maintenance by either oral or topical mesalamine. Steroids generally can be withdrawn according to the acuteness of symptoms. A reduction by 5 to 10 mg per week from 40 down to 20 mg, followed by a reduction of 2.5 mg per week, is a reasonable approach that should be modified according to the individual's response. Again, mesalamine maintenance therapy is beneficial.

EXTENSIVE COLITIS. Patients with extensive colitis but mild symptoms should be treated with oral mesalamine. More severe symptoms (e.g., greater than 5 to 10 bowel movements per day, weight loss, abdominal tenderness, night sweats) require the addition of corticosteroids, with mesalamine as a maintenance therapy.

SEVERE COLITIS OR TOXIC MEGACOLON. Either of these conditions is a medical emergency. Patients presenting with more than 10 bowel movements per day accompanied by fever, leukocytosis, anemia, and tachycardia should be hospitalized. Appropriate fluid and electrolyte resuscitation should be instituted, and patients with significant anemia should receive transfusions to keep up with continued blood loss until the inflammation is stabilized. Patients who have not received prior corticosteroid therapy may be treated with parenteral ACTH or corticosteroids. Rectal application of steroid enemas or foam provides relief from severe tenesmus in conjunction with systemic steroids. Patients with a dilated colon should not be fed until their condition improves. Less severely ill patients may continue an oral intake of elemental feedings or a light diet, as tolerated, if there is no nausea or vomiting. Parenteral nutrition should be added for malnourished patients. Severely ill patients require constant monitoring because of the potential of toxic megacolon. Abdominal flat-plate examination should be performed at 12- to 24-hour intervals if there is evidence of colonic dilatation or any worsening. Patients with evidence of transmural disease, such as abdominal tenderness, fever, or leukocytosis, should receive broad-spectrum antibiotic treatment (e.g., metronidazole and an aminoglycoside) as if they had a bowel perforation. Failure to improve, evidence of rebound tenderness, or free air under the diaphragm requires surgical intervention.

MAINTENANCE THERAPY. Corticosteroids are not useful for the maintenance therapy of UC because they do not prevent relapse and they have many undesirable, long-term side effects. Sulfasalazine, olsalazine, and mesalamine are effective as maintenance therapies and should be continued "indefinitely" at the lowest dose that prevents relapse, with any withdrawal being carried out at a very gradual pace. Any recurrent symptoms require resumption of therapeutic doses.

SUPPORTIVE THERAPY. Dietary therapy has a limited role in the treatment of inflammation in UC, but diet should not be ignored as a symptomatic therapy. Patients who present with constipation improve with an increase in the fiber content of their diet. Patients with abdominal cramping or diarrhea have symptomatic improvement with a low-fiber diet with the exclusion of nonabsorbed carbohydrates (sorbitol, fructose, and lactose in lactose-intolerant patients). Iron replacement is necessary for patients with continued blood loss, and folic acid should be supplemented in patients taking sulfasalazine. In patients with mild disease, antispasmodics or antidiarrheal agents improve associated symptoms of bowel "irritability," but these should be used cautiously in severe disease because of the potential of inducing toxic megacolon.

SURGERY. UC can be cured by colectomy, which alleviates the symptoms, medication requirements, and potential long-term complications of colitis (cancer). Indications for surgery include toxic megacolon, perforation, intractable hemorrhage, complications of medical therapy, failure to improve with medical therapy, or evidence of confirmed dysplasia or cancer.

Surgical alternatives include proctocolectomy and ileostomy, which is the standard operation, or sphincter-saving operations, which remove the abdominal colon and rectal mucosa (saving the distal rectal musculature) and which create an ileal pouch and ileoanal anastomosis. This novel surgical approach is performed satisfactorily in two or three stages with an expected outcome of four to eight liquid bowel movements per day and full continence in 80 per cent of patients. The operation is limited to patients with confirmed UC and may be complicated by inflammation of the ileal pouch ("pouchitis"), which often requires therapy with metronidazole, sulfasalazine, or corticosteroids. The cause of pouchitis is not yet known, although it occurs only in patients with ileoanal anastomoses performed for IBD.

CROHN'S DISEASE

Medical therapy for CD must be individualized according to the disease location, severity, and complications. Unlike UC, nutritional therapies have a more prominent role in the treatment of CD and the prevention of complications. Furthermore, it has been difficult to prove any maintenance therapy effective in CD clinical trials. Corticosteroids should not be continued once clinical benefit has been obtained, because of their severe long-term sequelae and their lack of benefit in preventing relapse. Many patients who respond to sulfasalazine or mesalamine worsen upon withdrawal, and chronic therapy has a much larger benefit/risk ratio. Metronidazole has unique long-term toxicity (neuropathy), and other antibiotics can induce vitamin K deficiency or growth of *C. difficile*. Immunosuppressives have the best record in maintaining remission, but their long-term risks have not been established.

Symptomatic *gastroduodenal* CD is uncommon and usually responds to short-term corticosteroid therapy in conjunction with acid reduction with an H_2-receptor antagonist or omeprazole (Ch. 98.3). Gastric outlet obstruction unresponsive to corticosteroids requires surgical diversion with a gastrojejunostomy. *Jejunoileitis* often presents with diarrhea and protein-losing enteropathy. Mild symptoms respond to oral mesalamine or alternating antibiotics, which control associated small bowel bacterial overgrowth. Corticosteroids and an elemental diet have equal beneficial effects on persistent symptoms and laboratory studies, including albumin and acute phase reactants. Immunosuppressives are sometimes necessary for control of this diffuse form of small intestinal CD when steroids cannot be withdrawn. *Ileitis* and *ileocolitis* are more common variants of CD. Mild symptoms respond to adjustments in the diet to control diarrhea and abdominal cramping. If a low-residue diet is not sufficient, elemental feedings can be useful to reduce symptoms. Sulfasalazine, mesalamine, or antibiotics control mild symptoms, but patients presenting with fever, abdominal tenderness, or the presence of an inflammatory mass usually require short-term corticosteroids. Immunosuppressives or total parenteral nutrition can be useful for patients who cannot be tapered off steroids or who remain refractory with active disease. *Colonic* CD also responds to sulfasalazine, mesalamine, antibiotics, or, if necessary, corticosteroids. Immunosuppressives should be reserved for steroid-dependent or refractory patients.

NUTRITION IN CROHN'S DISEASE. The panenteric nature of CD can lead to a variety of nutritional deficiencies. Besides the enhanced requirements for iron due to blood loss and protein due to inflammatory exudation from the digestive tract, patients with small bowel CD who malabsorb calcium and magnesium, folic acid, and water-soluble vitamins require supplementation. Ileal CD requires monitoring and therapy for malabsorption of fat-soluble vitamins and vitamin B_{12}.

Some symptoms can be treated with dietary alterations, e.g., avoidance of fiber in patients with intestinal narrowing or diarrhea, the addition of fiber to patients who are constipated, avoidance of fat in patients with fat malabsorption, and avoidance of lactose for lactose-intolerance. Dietary modifications can also sometimes reduce the inflammatory features of CD. Elemental diets and corticosteroid therapy have equal therapeutic benefit. Elemental feedings can be administered by nasoenteric tube at night and are most beneficial for children with impaired growth. Total parenteral nutrition also benefits patients who cannot tolerate elemental feedings, who have a short bowel syndrome, or who have refractory symptoms despite medical therapy. Bowel rest does not affect the natural history of CD after therapy is discontinued.

SURGERY IN CROHN'S DISEASE. Active CD recurs at a predictable rate at the margins of a surgical resection. Virtually all patients develop some endoscopic and microscopic inflammation at an anastomotic site by 1 year after an operation. Usually, the course of a recurrence is similar to the initial manifestations; e.g., inflammatory or suppurative CD tends to recur as an inflammatory mass or fistula, whereas chronic, fibrosing CD recurs at a slower rate, evolving to intestinal obstruction. The recurrence rate is lower after exteriorization of the bowel with an ileostomy or colostomy than after reanastomosis.

Since surgery does not cure CD, the indications for surgery are for treatment of complications rather than as a "cure." Surgery is indicated for recurrent intestinal obstruction, complicated fistulas, intractable hemorrhage, disease refractory to medical therapy or complicated by inability to withdraw corticosteroids, growth retardation that does not respond to medical or nutritional intervention in children, or cancer. Unfortunately, the recurrence of CD cannot be prevented after resection, although mesalamine or immunosuppressives may possibly delay the time to recurrence.

PROGNOSIS

ULCERATIVE COLITIS. The course of UC depends upon the severity of the initial attack and the response to medical treatment. Fewer than 5 per cent of patients succumb to fulminant UC or require immediate colectomy, and a small percentage of patients have a single attack without recurrence. The majority of patients have periods of remission maintained by medical therapy interrupted by spontaneous, acute exacerbations induced by stress, intercurrent illness, pregnancy, infectious diarrhea, or the injudicious use of nonsteroidal anti-inflammatory drugs. Noncompliance or cessation of maintenance therapy may lead to recurrence. Approximately 15 per cent of patients have refractory UC with continuous symptoms, despite all attempts at medical therapy, and 20 per cent of patients in the United States require a colectomy at some time in their course.

Advances in medical and surgical therapies have greatly improved the prognosis for patients with UC. Patients who are properly managed rarely succumb to acute disease, and supportive long-term treatment can reduce chronic morbidity and mortality. Death, when it occurs, is usually due to complications of colonic perforation when surgery is deferred, to postoperative complications after colectomy, or to colonic carcinoma. The life expectancy after recovery from an initial attack of UC is no different from that of the general population. Long-term morbidity from UC is usually due to complications of medical therapy, especially when chronic corticosteroid therapy is required or abused. Changes in lifestyle may be required after colectomy and ileostomy, although, in general, there is an improvement in well-being after surgery undertaken for protracted or complicated illness. The long-term outcome of ileoanal anastomoses needs to be evaluated. By and large, patients who have undergone the sphincter-saving operations prefer to accommodate to frequent stooling and the occasional need for medical treatment of pouchitis rather than to life with a stoma.

CROHN'S DISEASE. The prognosis for CD depends upon the site and extent of intestinal involvement, as well as upon complications of the disease. Approximately 50 per cent of patients require surgical intervention, the risk being higher for patients with small intestinal disease than large bowel CD. Fifty per cent of patients undergoing an operation require a second operation, and 50 per cent of these, a third procedure. Periodic remissions and exacerbations are common, although disease-free intervals may extend for years or decades after surgery for chronic, fibrotic strictures. Relapses after acute inflammatory CD are more common and occur earlier. The tendency for recurrence is a frustrating psychosocial feature. Additionally, physical changes associated with surgical or medical therapy can greatly affect self-image, especially in adolescents or socially active patients. Perianal disease can be an especially troublesome feature.

Fortunately, recent advances in medical and supportive therapy have limited mortality in CD to that of the general population. Death usually occurs as a complication of surgical therapy, related to pulmonary emboli or sepsis. Morbidity, however, may be significant in patients requiring dietary modifications, frequent medical therapy, or recurrent surgeries or in individuals troubled by refractory diarrhea or perianal disease. The quality of life with CD is lower than with UC, often because of uncertainties related to recurrence after operations. Corticosteroid therapy adds significant morbidity to the long-term treatment of CD, and the increasing recognition of intestinal cancer as a long-term complication may have increasing significance as patients survive over longer intervals.

SUMMARY

Inflammatory bowel disease extracts a substantial cost in altered patient lifestyle and in regular, often intensive medical and surgical care. The outlook for patients with ulcerative colitis and Crohn's disease has improved steadily with advances in medical and surgical treatment, and further progress is anticipated as scientific advances in the understanding of the genetic influence on the gut immune response evolve. In the meantime, the treatment of patients with inflammatory bowel disease requires an optimistic physician working in conjunction with the patient and the family and with nursing, dietary, and psychosocial ancillary staff. Patient support groups and educational material from the Crohn's Disease and Colitis Foundation of America have offered substantial benefit to patients and their families.

Bayless TM: Current Therapy in Gastroenterology and Liver Disease. Philadelphia, B. C. Decker, Inc., Publishers, 1990. *Individual aspects of medical and surgical management are discussed by experts.*

Camilleri M, Proano M: Advances in the assessment of disease activity in inflammatory bowel disease. Mayo Clin Proc 64:800, 1989. *A review of methods of disease assessment.*

Ginsberg AL: Management of Inflammatory Bowel Disease. Gastroenterol Clin North Am 18(1):March, 1989. *Recent reference on inflammatory bowel disease.*

Hanauer SB, Kirsner JB: Inflammatory Bowel Disease: A Guide for Patients and Their Families. New York, Raven Press Publishers, 1985. *A helpful text for patient and family information.*

Hawthorne AB, Hawkey CJ: Immunosuppressive drugs in inflammatory bowel disease: A review of their mechanisms of efficacy and place in therapy. Drugs 38:267–288, 1989. *Discussion of immunosuppressives, possible mechanisms of action and efficacy.*

Peppercorn M: Therapy of Inflammatory Bowel Disease: New Medical and Surgical Approaches. New York, Marcel Dekker Publishers, 1990. *A thorough review of medical therapies for IBD.*

Riddell RH, Goldman H, Ransahoff DF, et al.: Dysplasia in inflammatory bowel disease: Standardized classification with provisional clinical implications. Human Pathol 14:931, 1983. *The outcome of a multispecialty work-group on classification and management of dysplasia and cancer in IBD.*

Shorter RG, Kirsner JB: Inflammatory Bowel Disease. 3rd ed. Philadelphia, Lea & Febiger, 1988. *A comprehensive, inclusive text covering all aspects of IBD.*

104 Vascular Diseases of the Intestine

James H. Grendell

ANATOMY, PHYSIOLOGY, AND PATHOPHYSIOLOGY OF THE MESENTERIC CIRCULATION

The intra-abdominal portions of the digestive tract receive their blood supply almost entirely from three relatively large arteries arising from the aorta. The anatomy of these vessels, including their anastomotic interrelationships and potential for collateral formation, determines the consequences of acute or chronic vascular occlusion.

The *celiac axis*, the most cephalad of the three major arteries, usually originates at a level between the twelfth thoracic and the first lumbar vertebrae, passing next to the median arcuate ligament of the diaphragm (Fig. 104–1). Its branches supply the liver and biliary structures (hepatic artery), the spleen (splenic artery), and the stomach (left gastric and gastroepiploic, short gastrics, and branches of the gastroduodenal, including the right gastroepiploic). The gastroduodenal artery gives rise to the superior

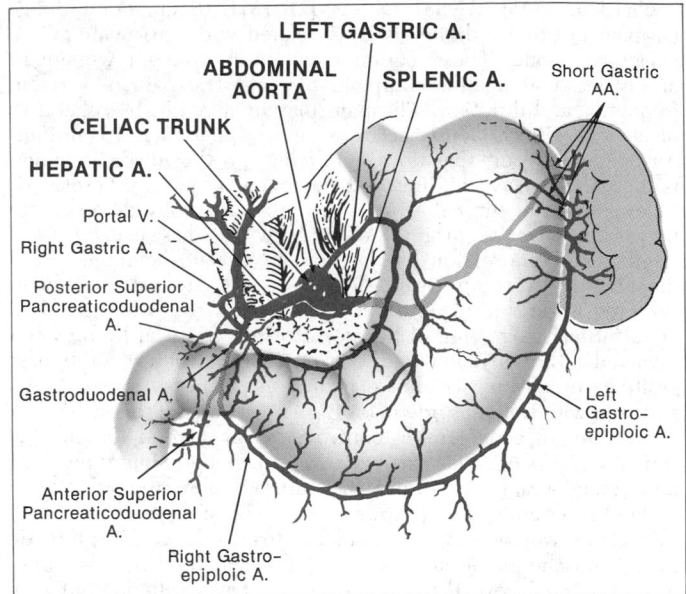

FIGURE 104–1. Arterial supply to the stomach and duodenum, showing major branches of the celiac axis and the superior portion of the pancreaticoduodenal arcades. (From Grendell JH, Ockner RK: *In* Sleisenger MH, Fordtran JS [eds.]: Gastrointestinal Disease. 3rd ed. Philadelphia, W. B. Saunders Company, 1983.)

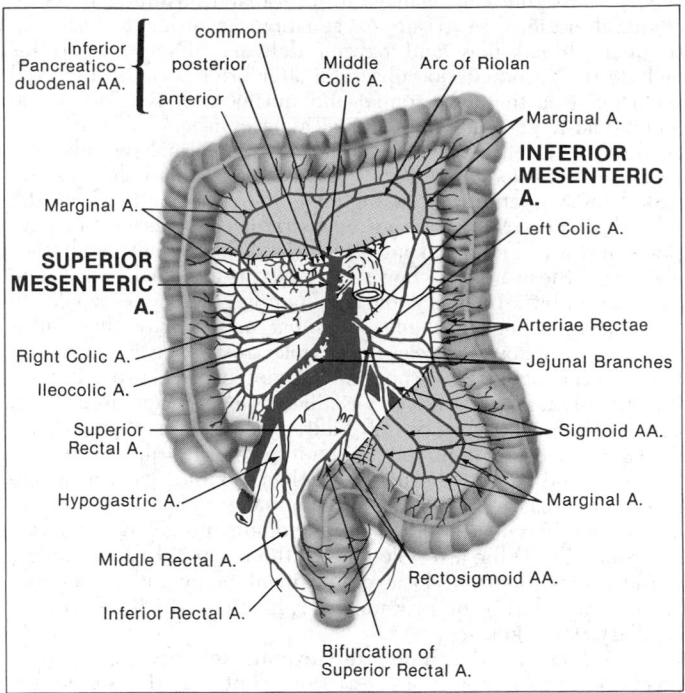

FIGURE 104–2. Arterial supply to the small and large intestines, showing the inferior portion of the pancreaticoduodenal arcades and the anastomoses between superior and inferior mesenteric arteries (arc of Riolan or "meandering mesenteric," and the marginal artery). (From Grendell JH, Ockner RK. *In* Sleisenger MH, Fordtran JS [eds.]: Gastrointestinal Disease. 3rd ed. Philadelphia, W. B. Saunders Company, 1983.)

pancreaticoduodenal arteries, which not only provide part of the blood supply to the pancreas and duodenum but also form anastomoses with the inferior pancreaticoduodenal arteries, which are derived from the superior mesenteric artery. These interconnections, the pancreaticoduodenal arcades, are an important potential route for collateral blood flow between the celiac and the superior mesenteric arteries.

The *superior mesenteric artery* originates behind the pancreas at the level of the first lumbar vertebra, just caudal to the celiac axis (Fig. 104–2). In addition to the inferior pancreaticoduodenal arteries, the superior mesenteric artery gives rise to branches supplying the small and large intestines from the distal duodenum to the distal transverse colon. These intestinal branches form a series of three or four arcades before entering the wall of the intestine as arteriae rectae. Although there is considerable potential for collateral flow within the primary and secondary arcades, the arteriae rectae appear to represent end-arteries, and few, if any, important anastomotic connections are present within the bowel wall itself. Accordingly, selective occlusion of these more distal vessels, as may occur in vasculitis, may lead to segmental infarction.

The *inferior mesenteric artery*, the smallest of the three major arteries, supplies the distal transverse colon, the descending and sigmoid colon, and the proximal portions of the rectum. Its branches form a series of arcades ending in arteriae rectae similar to what is found in the superior mesenteric artery's distribution. Branches of the inferior mesenteric artery connect with those of the superior mesenteric artery via the arc of Riolan ("meandering mesenteric artery") and the marginal artery (Fig. 104–2), and with the inferior and middle rectal branches of the hypogastric (internal iliac) arteries.

In general, veins parallel arteries in the smaller branches and for portions of the main mesenteric trunks (Fig. 104–3). However, rather than entering the vena cava directly, the superior mesenteric and splenic veins join to form the portal vein, which enters the liver after receiving additional blood from the gastric circulation via the coronary vein. The inferior mesenteric vein usually drains into the splenic vein.

The blood supply to the intra-abdominal portion of the gastrointestinal tract is richly endowed with anastomotic interconnections that help protect against the consequences of occlusive vascular disease. If the occlusive process is chronically progressive, these interconnections usually permit sufficient collateral flow to maintain intestinal viability. In fact, it is possible for *all* of the intra-abdominal digestive tract to be adequately supplied by only one of its three primary arterial sources. Conversely, the

collateral supply may be only marginally adequate or nonexistent in certain areas, such as the arteriae rectae and intramural arteries. Also potentially vulnerable are the "watershed" areas in the distal transverse colon and splenic flexure and at the junction of the superior and middle portions of the rectum, where branches of the inferior mesenteric artery anastomose with branches of the superior mesenteric and hypogastric arteries, respectively. This may, in part, explain why segmental infarction of the colon occurs most commonly in the region of the splenic flexure and rectosigmoid.

The *mesenteric circulation* is regulated by three different means: (1) *Intrinsic regulation* or local modulation of blood flow

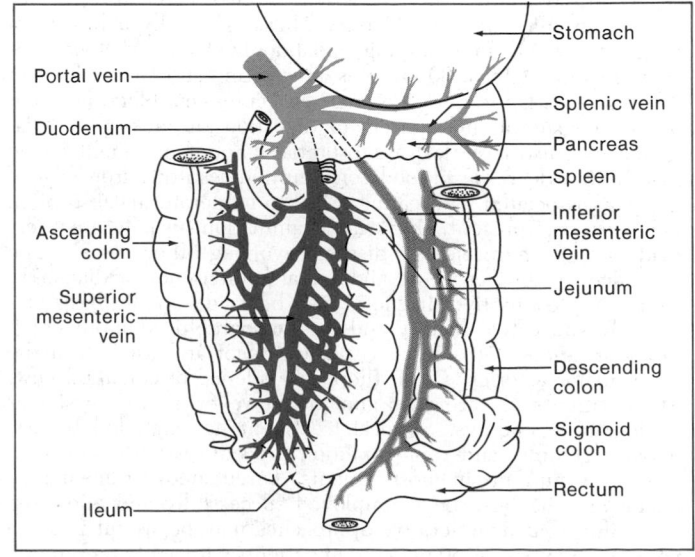

FIGURE 104–3. Venous drainage of the small intestine and colon showing the superior and inferior mesenteric veins, which, along with the splenic vein, constitute the major tributaries of the portal vein.

occurs in response to changes in arteriolar transmural pressure or to alterations in tissue oxygenation in order to maintain adequate blood flow and oxygen delivery. Examples of this include the vasodilatation observed after brief periods of arterial occlusion (reactive hyperemia) and during digestion of a meal (functional hyperemia). Functional hyperemia may also, in part, be due to the effects of regulatory gastrointestinal peptides. (2) *Extrinsic neurologic regulation* of intestinal blood flow is mediated by sympathetic postganglionic fibers originating from the splanchnic nerves, which cause constriction of arteries and arterioles and a reduction in intestinal blood flow. Continued stimulation of these nerves, however, leads to a partial or in some cases complete recovery of flow (autoregulatory escape). (3) *Circulating endogenous and exogenous agents* may affect mesenteric blood flow. Increased arteriolar resistance is caused by α-adrenergic agonists, vasopressin, angiotensin II, prostaglandin F_2, and digitalis glycosides. Vasodilatation and increased blood flow result from the actions of β-adrenergic agonists, prostaglandin E_2, papaverine, aminophylline, nitroglycerin, calcium channel blockers, and the gut hormones cholecystokinin, gastrin, glucagon, and vasoactive intestinal polypeptide.

The microcirculation of the intra-abdominal digestive organs is controlled by (1) the arteriole that, as the major site of resistance, is the most important local determinant of overall mesenteric blood flow, and (2) the precapillary sphincter, which determines capillary perfusion.

Several factors determine the extent, severity, or possible reversibility of ischemic processes or events: (1) the abruptness of a vascular occlusion; more gradually occlusive processes may permit development of collaterals; (2) size and configuration of a vessel; emboli most commonly enter the large, obliquely situated superior mesenteric artery; (3) the level of involvement of a localized occlusive process; vasculitis involving arteriae rectae or intramural arteries does not allow for development of collateral blood flow and may result in ischemia of a limited segment of intestine.

Intestinal ischemia may occur in hypoxic or low cardiac output states in the absence of an anatomic obstruction to blood flow (nonocclusive intestinal infarction). It is postulated that this may result from (1) the formation of toxic superoxide anions, (2) loss of the protective function of small intestinal brush border glycoproteins against the deleterious effects of luminal pancreatic proteases and bacterial toxins, or (3) shunting of oxygen from the villus tip caused by a countercurrent exhange resulting from the arrangement of blood vessels in the villus.

CHRONIC INTESTINAL ISCHEMIC SYNDROMES

ABDOMINAL ANGINA. This uncommon syndrome is due to severe atherosclerosis involving at least two of the three major arterial supplies to the intestine. There is usually a history of intermittent dull or cramping midabdominal pain characteristically beginning 15 to 30 minutes after eating and lasting for 1 to 2 hours. This is the period of increased intestinal blood flow and oxygen consumption required for digestion and absorption. Patients may also have lost a substantial amount of weight owing mainly to a decrease in food consumption resulting from fear of the pain associated with eating. Mild to moderate malabsorption may also be present. Physical examination usually uncovers evidence of atherosclerotic disease involving other vessels. The presence or absence of an abdominal bruit is not of diagnostic value. A presumptive diagnosis may be made on the basis of a strongly suggestive history and the angiographic demonstration of significant (> 50 per cent) narrowing of at least two of the three major arteries. Often there is evidence of collateral flow. Many patients who are asymptomatic, however, may show similar angiographic findings. Surgical treatment has included bypass, endarterectomy, and reimplantation procedures with significant relief of symptoms in most patients. Percutaneous transluminal angioplasty has also been employed successfully and offers the possibility that nonoperative approaches may be useful in some patients. As many as 50 per cent of patients with acute mesenteric arterial occlusion (see below) give a history suggestive of previous abdominal angina. Successful treatment of chronic intestinal ischemia may prevent such a catastrophic outcome.

CELIAC COMPRESSION SYNDROME. Recurrent abdominal pain in some individuals is associated with narrowing of the celiac axis alone. These patients, generally younger women in otherwise good health, complain of epigastric pain of variable frequency and duration. The pain may or may not be related to meals and is infrequently accompanied by nausea and vomiting. An epigastric bruit that does not radiate to the lower abdomen is the only physical finding that has been frequently described. Lateral views of the celiac axis during angiography demonstrate narrowing near its origin. At surgery this has usually been ascribed to compression by the median arcuate ligament of the diaphragm. In some cases, however, the stenosis has been reported to be due to neurofibrous tissue of the celiac ganglion or to intimal narrowing of the vessel itself. Surgical therapy has involved either division of the obstructing structure or bypass grafting, usually with relief of symptoms. The symptoms have recurred with time in some patients. The validity of this syndrome is a matter of considerable controversy for several reasons: (1) similar degrees of celiac axis narrowing have been found incidentally at angiography or autopsy in a substantial number of patients without symptoms of this syndrome, and (2) stenosis of the celiac axis alone would not be expected to result in symptomatic intestinal ischemia because of mesenteric collateral vessels. Some investigators believe that the pain is not truly ischemic but may arise in the celiac ganglion, which is removed or disrupted by most surgical treatments for this syndrome. In view of this controversy, surgery should be reserved for those patients with preoperative angiographic evidence of celiac stenosis who would otherwise undergo exploratory laparotomy for disabling and unexplained abdominal pain. At operation a thorough search for other disorders should precede treatment for presumed celiac compression syndrome.

CHRONIC RECTAL ISCHEMIA. A syndrome of rectal or sacral pain, at times associated with fecal incontinence, has been reported in some patients with occlusive disease involving both the inferior mesenteric artery *and* the internal iliac arteries.

ACUTE INTESTINAL ISCHEMIC SYNDROMES

ACUTE BOWEL INFARCTION: MESENTERIC ARTERIAL OCCLUSION. Gradual occlusion of one or sometimes even two of the three major mesenteric arteries may be asymptomatic because of the development of adequate collateral circulation. However, when intestinal blood flow falls below a critical level, ischemic necrosis of the supplied areas results. Most commonly this is due to advanced *atherosclerotic disease* affecting at least two of the major visceral branches of the aorta. Generally the most proximal segments of these arteries are most severely involved. In addition to *embolism*, which is discussed below, other causes of mesenteric arterial occlusion include dissecting *aortic aneurysm, fibromuscular hyperplasia,* and *systemic vasculitides,* which may involve the mesenteric arteries at any level from the major arterial trunks to the intramural arteries. An association has also been reported with the use of *oral contraceptives.*

Diagnosis. The early diagnosis of acute intestinal infarction is often difficult. The history usually is not very helpful, but evidence of "abdominal angina" (see above) or other conditions predisposing to thrombosis may aid in the evaluation. Patients frequently have *severe abdominal pain* that initially may be colicky in nature and periumbilical in location. Bowel sounds not only may be present but may even be hyperactive. At this stage the patient's complaint of pain often appears out of proportion to physical findings or laboratory studies. As ischemia progresses, pain becomes constant and poorly localized. Systemic manifestations become prominent and severe, including *tachycardia, hypotension, fever, leukocytosis, acidosis,* and the presence of *blood* in nasogastric aspirate, vomitus, or stool. It has been suggested that an elevation in serum and peritoneal fluid phosphate concentration may be a sensitive indicator of intestinal infarction. Because an elevation in serum phosphate concentration in this setting is often associated with extensive bowel injury, acute renal insufficiency, and acidosis, it implies a poor prognosis. Abdominal radiographs usually show evidence of an *ileus* with distended, thick-walled loops of bowel and air-fluid levels (Fig. 104-4). Gas in the intestinal wall or portal vein is a late finding. Ultimately, when ischemic necrosis becomes transmural, signs of

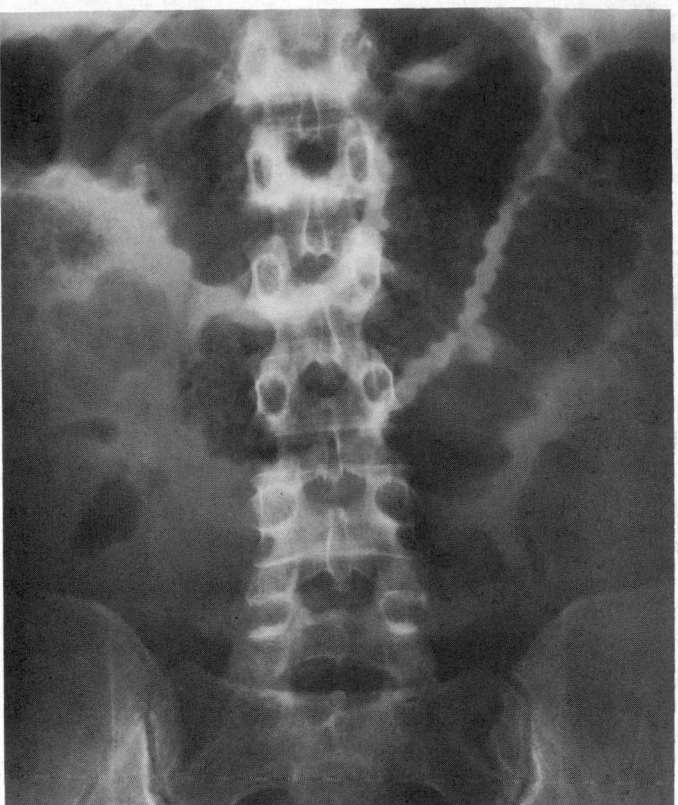

FIGURE 104–4. A supine abdominal radiograph in a patient with acute infarction of the small intestine showing dilated loops of small bowel with irregular thickening of the bowel wall.

peritonitis, including bloody peritoneal fluid, appear. At this point, the prognosis (with or without surgery) is extremely poor.

The early diagnosis of bowel infarction depends upon a high index of suspicion and exclusion of other intra-abdominal conditions that can manifest virtually identically (e.g., acute pancreatitis, perforated viscus, bowel obstruction). A decision regarding extensive radiographic studies, especially angiography, in patients with suspected bowel infarction must be individualized. For the patient in whom hypotension, acidosis, or signs of peritonitis are present, suggesting that perforation may have already occurred, the information to be obtained from further studies may not justify the necessary delay in surgical management. However, earlier in the course, angiography may help define the nature and extent of the occlusive process or, in the absence of major vessel occlusion, suggest the diagnosis of nonocclusive infarction. Interpretation, however, is often difficult, and clinical judgment is based only in part on angiographic findings. Abdominal sonography and, in particular, computed tomography show promise as rapid, noninvasive means of confirming the diagnosis of acute bowel infarction by identifying characteristic changes in the appearance of the bowel wall and mesentery. The sensitivity and specificity of these imaging techniques remain to be defined, however.

Treatment. Initial supportive therapy, aimed at stabilization of the patient's condition prior to surgery, includes nasogastric suction, replacement of fluid and electrolyte deficits, administration of broad-spectrum antibiotics after blood cultures have been obtained, and cardiopulmonary support, if needed. In the treatment of patients judged to be sufficiently stable to tolerate angiography, the use of vasodilators infused through a catheter placed at angiography has been advocated to treat the severe vasospasm frequently observed in the setting of intestinal ischemia. Papaverine is most commonly employed, although tolazoline has also been used in this setting. Although appealing on a theoretical basis, the efficacy of this use of vasodilators has not been conclusively established. As soon as the patient's condition is adequately stabilized and the diagnosis strongly suspected, prompt surgical exploration should be performed. At surgery, resection of necrotic bowel is the primary objective. An attempt

may be made to revascularize the remaining viable intestine by bypass graft or endarterectomy if the patient's condition is sufficiently stable to permit the additional surgery.

At the time of operation the limits of viable bowel must be defined in order to resect completely irreversibly diseased intestine while at the same time avoiding unnecessary development of the short bowel syndrome. It is often necessary to perform a "second-look" operation 12 to 36 hours after the initial exploration to identify and resect any additional bowel that in the interim proves to be nonviable. Infarction of large segments of intestine carries essentially a 100 per cent mortality rate without surgery. Even with surgery the mortality rate is greater than 50 per cent in most series because of delay in diagnosis or because of other complicating factors such as advanced age or atherosclerotic disease involving other vital organs.

Mesenteric vasculitis (e.g., as may occur in lupus erythematosus, polyarteritis nodosa, dermatomyositis, rheumatoid vasculitis, and Henoch-Schönlein purpura) may cause segmental intestinal infarction not conforming to the distribution of the major arteries. Vascular occlusion may not be demonstrable angiographically if only intramural arteries and arterioles are involved. Although some patients may require emergency surgery for intestinal necrosis and perforation, these complications are less common than with occlusions of the major arteries or their principal branches. In some cases the acute episode may resolve spontaneously, which may leave the patient with a segmental stricture demonstrable by barium contrast studies.

MESENTERIC ARTERY EMBOLISM. Emboli to the mesenteric circulation most commonly involve the superior mesenteric artery because of its size and the oblique angle of its origin from the aorta. These emboli usually arise from mural thrombi in the heart in patients with atherosclerotic or valvular heart disease but may also arise from vegetations of bacterial endocarditis, atrial myxomas, valvular prostheses, or atherosclerotic plaques in the thoracic or upper abdominal aorta, either spontaneously or during angiography. Patients may have a history of previous embolic episodes or exhibit evidence of simultaneous peripheral embolization (e.g., to the brain or extremities). Typically patients describe the *abrupt onset of severe midabdominal cramping pain*, accompanied by vomiting or diarrhea. Although patients may feel and appear severely ill, early in the course objective physical findings are sparse. If the diagnosis is not made promptly and appropriate treatment undertaken, a mesenteric embolus leads to bowel infarction. Angiography may demonstrate mesenteric artery occlusion in the absence of collateral circulation, indicating the acute nature of the process. The use of intraarterial infusion of vasodilators has been advocated, although its value has not been clearly proven. Computed tomography may also strongly suggest the diagnosis early in the course of the disease in a patient with acute onset of abdominal pain of unknown source. Following supportive measures as needed to stabilize the patient's condition, immediate exploration with embolectomy and resection of any infarcted bowel is indicated. A "second-look" procedure is sometimes necessary. The characteristic setting in which mesenteric embolism occurs, as well as its abrupt onset, offers a greater opportunity for early diagnosis and treatment. For this reason, and because the patients generally are younger, the prognosis is more favorable than for most nonembolic causes of bowel infarction. Some patients who are successfully treated by embolectomy without need for bowel resection may develop a transient malabsorption syndrome persisting for several months.

NONOCCLUSIVE INTESTINAL INFARCTION. In some patients clinical findings suggestive of mesenteric arterial occlusive disease or embolism occur without a demonstrable obstruction to arterial flow. This syndrome, now recognized with increasing frequency, usually occurs in the setting of severe congestive heart failure, shock, hypoxia, or a recent myocardial infarction. In addition, it has been reported following cocaine use, possibly related to α-adrenergic stimulation due to the drug. The clinical course often evolves more slowly than is seen with occlusive processes. Occasionally a precipitating event is not identifiable. The use of α-adrenergic vasoconstrictors (and possibly digitalis glycosides) may also contribute to the development of this process. Because of its high degree of metabolic activity, the mucosa has the greatest requirement for intestinal blood flow of the various layers of the bowel wall. Thus it shows the earliest evidence of ischemic injury. At times, it may be the only portion to undergo hemorrhagic infarction. However, infarction may ultimately become transmural and occur in a patchy and irregular distribution, not conforming to the area supplied by a major vessel. Early angiography is useful to exclude a major vessel occlusion, which would usually require vascular surgery. In at least 50 per cent of such patients angiography reveals irregular narrowing of the major arterial branches and arcades (due to spasm) and impaired filling of the intramural vessels. Therapy consists of supportive measures and surgical exploration to resect infarcted bowel if the patient's situation suggests the need for this. Selective infusion of vasodilators into the mesenteric circulation has been suggested, but its therapeutic efficacy remains to be established. This syndrome generally carries a very poor prognosis, primarily because it is usually associated with shock or severe cardiopulmonary disease.

ISCHEMIC COLITIS. Ischemic injury to the colon may be caused by advanced atherosclerosis or interruption of the colonic blood supply during surgery (e.g., abdominal aortic aneurysmectomy, aortoiliac reconstruction, abdominoperineal resection) or may occur in association with "hypercoagulable" states, amyloidosis, vasculitis, ruptured aortic aneurysm, colorectal cancer, or the use of oral contraceptive agents. In addition, nonocclusive colonic ischemia may occur in states of low cardiac output or hypoxia. Nonocclusive colonic ischemia may be mediated primarily by the renin-angiotensin system, to which the colonic vasculature appears to be remarkably sensitive. The syndrome of ischemic colitis may be quite variable in its extent, severity, and prognosis. However, extensive infarction and perforation appear to be infrequent. Localized or segmental ischemia is more common, particularly affecting those areas of the colon that lie on the "watershed" between two adjacent arterial supplies, i.e., the splenic flexure (superior and inferior mesenteric arteries) and the rectosigmoid (inferior mesenteric and internal iliac arteries). Characteristically, patients over the age of 50 are most often affected with *abrupt onset of lower abdominal cramping pain, rectal bleeding*, and, to variable degrees, *vomiting* and *fever*. Some patients give a history of similar symptoms occurring intermittently for weeks to months before presentation. Left-sided abdominal tenderness and peritoneal signs may be present, as well as evidence of generalized atherosclerotic disease. Sigmoidoscopy may be normal; may show evidence of mild, nonspecific proctitis; or may reveal a spectrum of findings, including multiple discrete ulcers, blue-black hemorrhagic submucosal blebs, or an adherent pseudomembrane. Angiography generally has not proved useful in the diagnosis of patients in this setting. The differentiation of ischemic colitis from infections of the colon,

diverticulitis, and idiopathic inflammatory bowel disease (ulcerative colitis, Crohn's disease of the colon) may be very difficult. Initial management consists of general supportive measures, including antibiotics. In those patients in whom perforation or infarction of the colon appears likely, early surgical exploration is indicated; however, many patients improve without surgery. Subsequent barium enema often shows a characteristic picture of intramural hemorrhage and edema, including "thumb-printing," tubular narrowing, and "sawtooth" irregularity (Fig. 104–5). Some patients proceed to complete resolution of the clinical process and radiographic abnormalities. Others develop a residual stricture that eventually may require surgical resection.

MESENTERIC VENOUS THROMBOSIS. This condition, which accounts for about 5 to 15 per cent of patients with intestinal ischemia, almost always involves the superior mesenteric vein. It is associated with a variety of conditions: stasis in the mesenteric venous bed (portal hypertension, congestive heart failure), abdominal neoplasms, intra-abdominal inflammation (peritonitis, abscess, inflammatory bowel disease), abdominal surgery and trauma, a variety of presumed hypercoagulable states (antithrombin III deficiency, polycythemia vera), and use of oral contraceptives. Occasionally a predisposing condition is absent. Patients may have abrupt onset of a clinical picture indicative of acute bowel infarction; however, many others have a more gradual course with development of progressive abdominal discomfort over a period of weeks. Physical findings are nonspecific. The presence of a small amount of bloody peritoneal fluid is typical and may be an important clue to the diagnosis in patients with a subacute clinical course. Selective superior mesenteric angiography shows intense spasm of the arteries to the involved segment of bowel and absence of venous drainage.

Following initial supportive care to stabilize the patient's condition, an operation should be performed to resect infarcted or severely ischemic bowel. Reconstructive venous surgery is not generally possible. Because there is about a 25 per cent rate of recurrent thrombosis within the first several weeks postoperatively, anticoagulation is recommended except in patients who have underlying disease processes that would make this too hazardous. A "second-look" operation to search for recurrent thrombosis may also be required if there is unexplained clinical deterioration following initial surgery. In general, the prognosis is more favorable than for patients with mesenteric arterial disease, with reported mortality as low as 20 per cent.

MISCELLANEOUS DISORDERS

INTRAMURAL INTESTINAL HEMORRHAGE. This may follow abdominal trauma or may occur in the setting of ischemic bowel injury, vasculitis, or bleeding diatheses. Some patients have a picture suggesting a perforated viscus (severe abdominal pain, tenderness, leukocytosis), but most have cramping abdom-

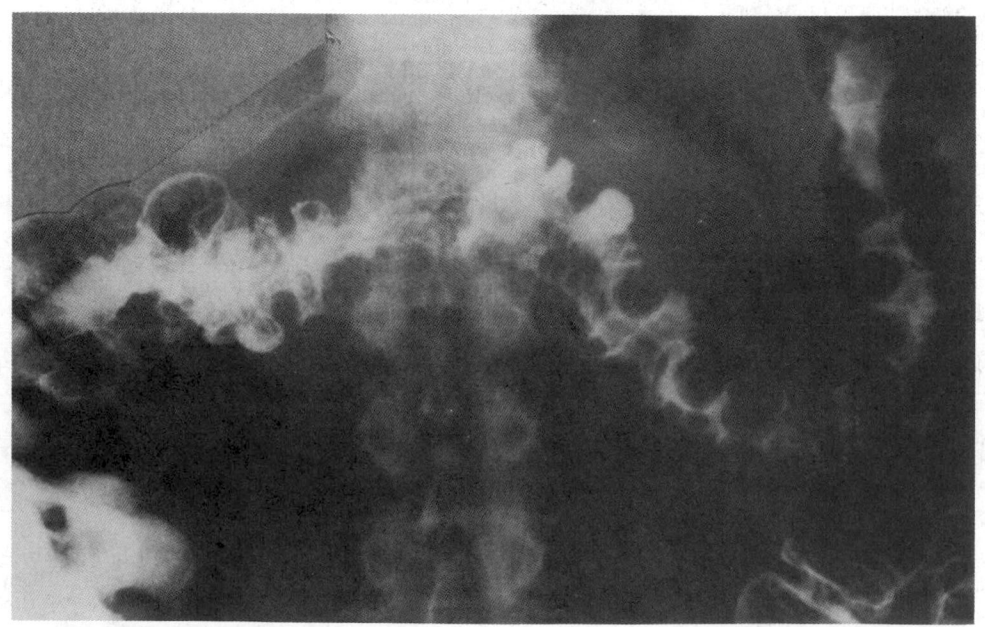

FIGURE 104–5. A barium enema in a patient with ischemic colitis showing narrowing and "thumb-printing" (nodular indentations of the bowel wall) in the distal transverse colon. This is one of the "watershed" areas of the colon between two adjacent arterial supplies (superior and inferior mesenteric arteries) where ischemia is more likely to develop.

inal pain and vomiting suggestive of partial or complete bowel obstruction. Hematemesis or melena and fever may be present. Occasionally a palpable abdominal mass caused by the presence of a hematoma may be noted. Barium studies of the small intestine typically show a "stacked coins" or "thumb-print" appearance. Usually intramural intestinal hemorrhage can be managed conservatively with nasogastric suction, intravenous hydration and electrolytes, and correction of any underlying coagulopathy, when possible. In those patients with high-grade or unremitting intestinal obstruction, or in whom signs of peritonitis develop (suggesting perforation), surgery is necessary.

PARAPROSTHETIC-ENTERIC AND AORTOENTERIC FISTULAS. Following aortic aneurysmectomy and other procedures in which vascular prostheses are placed in the abdomen or retroperitoneum, fistulas may form between the graft and adjacent bowel. This may occur as early as several weeks postoperatively but in most cases is delayed by at least 2 years. This complication usually results from local infection or damage to the intestine or its blood supply at surgery, with subsequent erosion of the bowel wall by the graft. Patients may present with massive upper or lower gastrointestinal bleeding or both that may be rapidly fatal without emergency surgery. In a number of patients, however, bleeding may be initially intermittent, resembling that from a number of more common lesions. In these patients, early consideration of this diagnosis with urgent evaluation by upper endoscopy to exclude other lesions and computed tomography, if the patient's condition permits, may be required to establish the diagnosis and need for surgical intervention.

Unoperated abdominal aortic aneurysms and aneurysmal dilatations of other major abdominal arteries may erode into the gastrointestinal tract, causing upper or lower gastrointestinal bleeding or both of various degrees of severity.

SUPERIOR MESENTERIC ARTERY SYNDROME. This uncommon syndrome of postprandial epigastric pain, distention, and vomiting has been attributed to compression of the third portion of the duodenum between the superior mesenteric artery anteriorly and the fixed retroperitoneal structures posteriorly. This has been described as occurring most commonly in individuals who have lost a substantial amount of weight or are of "asthenic habitus," and in children with rapid growth in the absence of corresponding weight gain or who have been fixed in a position of hyperextension by a cast following spinal injury or surgery. Barium contrast studies show distention of the proximal duodenum, and lateral aortograms or abdominal sonograms have shown a narrowing of the angle between the aorta and the superior mesenteric artery. The differential diagnosis includes generalized disorders of gastrointestinal motility, such as scleroderma, and anorexia nervosa. Recommended treatment has included the use of small feedings and elemental diets with the patient lying prone or on the left side in the knee-chest position after eating. In refractory cases duodenal mobilization or duodenal-jejunal bypass has reportedly been effective in relieving symptoms. Since apparent compression of the duodenum by the superior mesenteric artery does not prove to be a clinically significant obstruction, the diagnosis of this syndrome must be made only after other possible causes of duodenal stasis have been excluded. This entity is frequently overdiagnosed unless strict diagnostic criteria are employed.

VASCULAR MALFORMATIONS INCLUDING VASCULAR ECTASIA. Hemangiomas of the small intestine are very uncommon vascular tumors found throughout the bowel, particularly the jejunum. They represent one of the causes of gastrointestinal bleeding that may be very difficult to locate. These lesions are most reliably diagnosed by abdominal angiography. Surgical removal of the involved segment of bowel is the usual treatment.

Vascular malformations can occur in the gastrointestinal tract in association with diseases involving the skin, such as the *hereditary hemorrhagic telangiectasia (Osler-Weber-Rendu) syndrome, blue rubber bleb nevus syndrome,* and the *CREST syndrome* (calcinosis, Raynaud's phenomenon, esophageal hypomotility, sclerodactyly, and telangiectasia). In addition, vascular malformations may occur as a primary process (*vascular ectasia, angiodysplasia*) chiefly involving the colon but also occurring in the stomach or small intestine. This is a frequent cause of lower intestinal bleeding, especially in patients over the age of 60. An association of angiodysplasia with aortic stenosis has also been reported but not fully established. Vascular ectasias of the stom-

ach and small intestine may be the most common source of upper gastrointestinal bleeding in patients with chronic renal failure.

Vascular ectasias consist of ectatic, tortuous submucosal veins and groups of ectatic mucosal vessels lying just under the gastric, intestinal, or colonic epithelium or at times on the luminal surface unprotected by any intestinal epithelium. The etiology of these lesions remains uncertain. One theory suggests that they develop as a result of chronic low-grade obstruction of the submucosal veins as they penetrate the muscularis propria; another theory proposes that these lesions develop because of chronic mucosal ischemia.

Larger vascular malformations, including some vascular ectasias, may be visualized by selective mesenteric arteriography. However, most of these lesions are small and are best demonstrated by endoscopy. Such lesions are present in a large number of older individuals without apparent gastrointestinal blood loss. For those patients who have severe anemia due to chronic or recurrent gastrointestinal blood loss without other apparent cause, surgery has been recommended if vascular malformations could be identified and localized (e.g., right colectomy for lesions in the cecum). This approach is often unsatisfactory, and bleeding may recur either because some lesions in other parts of the gastrointestinal tract may not have been appreciated at the initial evaluation or because new lesions may subsequently develop. For these reasons, nonoperative endoscopic approaches have been developed to obliterate vascular malformations by such techniques as laser photocoagulation, electrocoagulation, or thermal coagulation (heater probe).

Baur CM, Millay DJ, Taylor CM, et al.: Treatment of chronic visceral ischemia. Am J Surg 148:138, 1984. *Illustrates the efficacy of surgical treatment for abdominal angina in properly selected patients.*

Cello JP, Grendell JH: Endoscopic laser treatment for gastrointestinal vascular ectasias. Ann Intern Med 104:352, 1986. *Demonstrates the effective use of nonoperative therapy for this disorder.*

Croft RJ, Menon GP, Marston A: Does "intestinal angina" exist? A critical study of obstructed visceral arteries. Br J Surg 68:316, 1981. *A provocative report demonstrating the difficulty in relating gastrointestinal symptoms to angiographic findings.*

Federle MP, Chun G, Jeffrey RB, et al.: Computed tomographic findings in bowel infarction. AJR 142:91, 1984. *This report demonstrates the potential value of computed tomography in the diagnosis of vascular diseases of the intestine.*

Fiddian-Green RG: Splanchnic ischaemia and multiple organ failure in the critically ill. Ann R Coll Surg Engl 70:128, 1988. *Interesting discussion of the pathophysiology, diagnosis, and treatment of nonocclusive intestinal ischemia.*

Grendell JH, Ockner RK: Vascular diseases of the bowel. *In* Sleisenger MH, Fordtran JS (eds.): Gastrointestinal Disease. 4th ed. Philadelphia, W.B. Saunders Company, 1989, p 1903. *A comprehensive survey including pathophysiology, diagnosis, and management.*

Hines JR, Gore RM, Ballantyne GH: Superior mesenteric artery syndrome: Diagnostic criteria and therapeutic approaches. Am J Surg 148:630, 1984. *Emphasizes the importance of strict diagnostic criteria to avoid overdiagnosis of this entity.*

Hunter GC, Guernsey JM: Mesenteric ischemia. Med Clin North Am 72:1091, 1988. *This review emphasizes diagnostic and therapeutic considerations in managing the different types of mesenteric ischemic processes.*

Kiernan PD, Pairolero PC, Hubert JP Jr, et al.: Aortic graft–enteric fistula. Mayo Clin Proc 55:731, 1980. *A detailed review of clinical features, management, and prognosis.*

Reinus JF, Brandt LJ, Boley SJ: Ischemic diseases of the bowel. Gastroenterol Clin North Am 19:319, 1990. *A thorough and up-to-date review emphasizing the approach to diagnosis and management.*

Zuckerman GR, Cornette GL, Clouse RE, et al.: Upper gastrointestinal bleeding in patients with chronic renal failure. Ann Intern Med 102:588, 1985. *Demonstrates the importance of angiodysplastic lesions as a source of upper gastrointestinal bleeding in patients with chronic renal failure.*

105 Neoplasms of the Large and Small Intestine

Bernard Levin

NEOPLASMS OF THE LARGE INTESTINE

Cancer of the large bowel (colon and rectum) is the most common malignancy of the gastrointestinal tract and together with breast and lung cancer is one of the three most frequent malignancies in the United States. It is also a worldwide health problem of great importance, particularly in other Western countries. Approximately 155,000 cases of cancer of the colon and rectum were diagnosed in the United States in 1990, only one half of whom will survive 5 years or longer. The mortality from colorectal cancer has slowly declined over the past 10 years while the incidence has been stable. New understanding about the genetics and molecular biology of this neoplasm has been recently gained, and advances have also been made in methods of prevention, diagnosis, and treatment.

The large bowel also may be involved by other malignant tumors. These include anal carcinoma (squamous or transitional types), lymphoma, leiomyosarcoma, malignant carcinoid tumor, and Kaposi's sarcoma. The large bowel may also be involved through direct invasion by malignancies from adjacent sites such as prostate, ovary, uterus, and stomach. The most frequent tumors that occur in the large intestine are benign adenomas (adenomatous polyps). Except for lipomas of the ileocecal valve, other benign tumors are very unusual.

POLYPS OF THE COLON

A polyp is any lesion that arises from the surface of the gastrointestinal tract and protrudes into the lumen. In the large intestine, polyps noted at sigmoidoscopy or colonoscopy or during barium enema may be single or multiple, pedunculated or sessile, and sporadic or part of an inherited syndrome. They become significant because of bleeding or because of their potential for malignant transformation.

PATHOLOGY. In addition to adenocarcinoma, which may present as a polypoid mass, three distinct types of benign polyps arise from colonic epithelium: hyperplastic (metaplastic), inflammatory, and neoplastic (adenomatous). Hyperplastic polyps, which tend to be small and asymptomatic, account for about one fifth of all polyps in the colon and for most of the polyps in the rectum and distal sigmoid. They are not considered neoplastic. Inflammatory polyps occur in chronic ulcerative colitis and also are not neoplastic (Ch. 103). Juvenile polyps are hamartomas of the lamina propria and may be single or multiple and occur most commonly in the rectum. They are susceptible to hemorrhage and autoamputation.

Adenomatous Polyps

PREVALENCE AND DISTRIBUTION. The incidence of colonic adenomas increases with age in countries with a high or intermediate risk for colorectal cancer, occurring in 40 to 50 per cent of individuals over the age of 60 in the United States. Adenomas are uncommon in areas where the incidence of cancer is low; for example, the prevalence of adenomas varies from almost zero among black South Africans to 10 per cent in Japan and in Cali, Colombia. The presence of adenomas does not necessarily convey a high risk because the propensity for neoplastic transformation is related to size. The low incidence of cancer in some countries, such as Japan, is probably related to the small number of large adenomas as well as to the total number of adenomas.

MACROSCOPIC AND MICROSCOPIC APPEARANCES. Adenomas may be separated into tubular, villous, and intermediate tubulovillous types. The typical tubular adenoma is small and spherical and has a stalk. Its surface is roughly separated into lobules by intercommunicating clefts. In contrast, the villous adenoma may be large and sessile with a velvety surface. Histologically the tubular adenoma consists of closely packed tubular glands that divide and branch. In the villous adenoma, finger-like projections of neoplastic epithelium project toward the bowel lumen. The tubulovillous lesions consist of a mixture of tubular and villous patterns. About 60 per cent of adenomas are tubular, 20 to 30 per cent are tubulovillous, and about 10 per cent are villous. All adenomas are dysplastic, and dysplasia in adenomas may be graded into mild, moderate, and severe. This classification is based on the presence of cytologic (mainly nuclear) abnormalities and glandular architectural changes.

DEVELOPMENT OF ADENOMAS. In the normal adult, the epithelial tissue of the colon actively renews itself with a turnover of about 3 to 8 days. DNA synthesis occurs primarily in cells in the lower one third of crypts. Normally cells replicate and migrate up the crypt to be subsequently exfoliated from the mucosal surface. In adenomas immature cells are found higher up the colonic crypt than normal, associated with unrepressed DNA synthesis, representing abnormal cell renewal along the surface of the crypt and the entire length of the crypt. DNA-synthesizing cells can accumulate on the luminal surface, thus forming new adenomatous tissue.

RELATIONSHIP OF COLONIC ADENOMAS TO CANCER. Colonic adenomas appear to have malignant potential: (1) The epidemiology of adenomas and carcinoma is similar; (2) adenocarcinomas and adenomas occur in the same anatomic distribution in the colon; (3) residual adenomatous tissue is observed quite commonly in small cancers; (4) the incidence of cancer increases as the size of the adenoma increases; (5) the adenoma-to-cancer transition has been observed in familial polyposis and in experimental animals treated with a carcinogen; (6) the risk for colorectal cancer is higher in patients with a history of adenomas and may be lessened if the adenoma is removed; (7) a period of approximately 5 years elapses between the diagnosis of adenoma and the development of carcinoma.

Less than 5 per cent of adenomas develop into carcinomas. Several important factors in this transformation can be identified, especially size, histologic type, and epithelial dysplasia. The frequency of cancer in adenomas under 1 cm is 1 to 3 per cent, those between 1 to 2 cm have a rate of 10 per cent, whereas those over 2 cm have a rate of malignancy over 40 per cent. The highest malignancy rate is associated with a villous growth pattern. Invasive neoplasm has been found in 40 per cent of the villous tumors, in less than 5 per cent of the tubular ones, and in 23 per cent of the tubulovillous variety. The malignant potential of adenomas increases with increasing degrees of dysplasia. Most adenomas smaller than 1 cm show only mild dysplasia and have a low malignant potential. With severe dysplasia, the rate of malignant transformation rises to 27 per cent.

Cancer in adenomas is usually well differentiated and occurs most commonly in the tip of a pedunculated adenoma without invasion of the muscularis mucosae. These lesions are usually satisfactorily treated by polypectomy. Occasionally cancers in adenomas invade the muscularis mucosae, grow down the stalk, invade lymphatics and adjacent lymph nodes, and metastasize. The roles of autocrine factors, tumor suppressor genes, and oncogenes in the development of adenomas and their malignant transformation are currently under study.

CLINICAL MANIFESTATIONS. Most adenomatous polyps are asymptomatic. Some adenomatous polyps are diagnosed by detection of occult blood loss in asymptomatic individuals being screened for colon cancer. Adenomas may also be detected by double contrast barium enema examination or by fiberoptic sigmoidoscopy or colonoscopy. Adenomas may also cause hematochezia and rarely iron deficiency anemia (Ch. 131). Large villous adenomas may very rarely cause watery diarrhea (with severe potassium depletion).

MANAGEMENT AND FOLLOW-UP. Because of the association of adenomas with the development of adenocarcinomas, colonic polyps should usually be removed or destroyed. In individual clinical circumstances (e.g., age of patient, location of lesion) this rule may rarely have to be modified. Pedunculated polyps, even if large, can be removed by electrocautery snare while small sessile polyps (1 to 8 mm in size) should be biopsied and destroyed with the "hot biopsy" forceps. For sessile polyps with a wide-based attachment to the colonic wall, several electrocautery sessions may be required for complete excision. Endoscopic removal may not be safe or possible if a sessile lesion is larger than 3 cm or if it is in a relatively inaccessible location. In general, benign-appearing polyps are removed by electrosurgery and not biopsied and the entire lesion is submitted for histopathologic examination.

The endoscopic appearance of a polyp that suggests carcinomatous invasion includes ulceration, an irregular surface contour, firm consistency, and friability. If a diagnosis of malignancy is made after polypectomy, a decision has to be made about the adequacy of the polypectomy. In the presence of a poorly differentiated histology, penetration of the muscularis mucosa, vascular or lymphatic invasion, and a resection margin containing cancer, the risk of regional lymph node involvement is approximately 5 per cent. The mortality from surgical resection is less than 2 per cent in patients aged 50 to 69 years and 4.4 per cent for those over 70 years, so any decision to recommend surgical resection must take into account individual operative risk.

FOLLOW-UP AFTER COLONOSCOPIC POLYPECTOMY. Ideally, the colon should be cleared of all synchronous adenomas at the time of the initial examination. A follow-up colonoscopy is appropriate at 1 year to evaluate for the presence of any lesions missed at the time of the previous procedure as well as new lesions that may have arisen. If this examination is normal, an interval of 2 to 3 years is appropriate for the next colonoscopy. Nutritional and chemotherapeutic strategies aimed at prevention of adenoma recurrence are being studied.

Inherited Polyposis Syndromes

Recent advances in genetics and molecular biology have accentuated our interest in the inherited risk of colorectal cancer. The polyposis syndromes account for approximately 1 per cent of colorectal cancer, whereas the nonpolyposis inherited conditions may be responsible for up to 6 per cent.

ADENOMATOUS POLYPOSIS SYNDROMES. The adenomatous polyposis syndromes include familial adenomatous polyposis and Gardner syndrome, in both of which hereditary disorders hundreds to thousands of colonic adenomas are present (Fig. 105–1). The adenomas begin to appear early in the second decade of life. Gastrointestinal symptoms occur in the third or fourth decade. Almost all patients with familial polyposis develop carcinoma of the colon by age 40 if the colon has not been removed.

Some cases occur without a family history and may represent spontaneous mutations.

Gardner syndrome differs from familial adenomatous polyposis in that affected individuals exhibit benign extraintestinal growths, including osteomas (especially mandibular) and soft tissue tumors (lipomas, sebaceous cysts, fibrosarcomas). Other associated features include supernumerary teeth, desmoid tumors, and mesenteric fibromatosis (Fig. 105–2). The colonic adenomas are similar to those of familial adenomatous polyposis and have the same potential for malignancy.

In both familial adenomatous polyposis and Gardner syndrome, upper gastrointestinal polyps are commonly found. Gastric polyps are hyperplastic and rarely cause symptoms. Adenomatous duodenal polyps are present in up to 80 per cent of individuals with familial adenomatous polyposis or Gardner syndrome, and approximately 10 per cent develop periampullary cancer. Adenomas occur in the small bowel distal to the duodenum but rarely undergo malignant transformation.

Familial adenomatous polyposis and Gardner syndrome are inherited as autosomal dominant disorders with incomplete penetrance. The mutant adenomatous polyposis coli (APC) gene on the long arm of chromosome 5 has recently been identified in both conditions. DNA markers can be used to ascertain whether a specific individual in a polyposis family is likely to express the phenotype.

For screening purposes, flexible proctosigmoidoscopy should

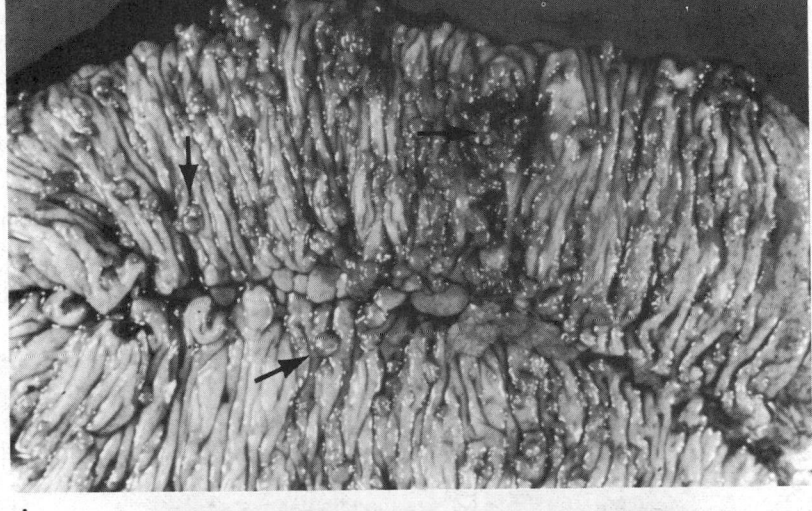

A

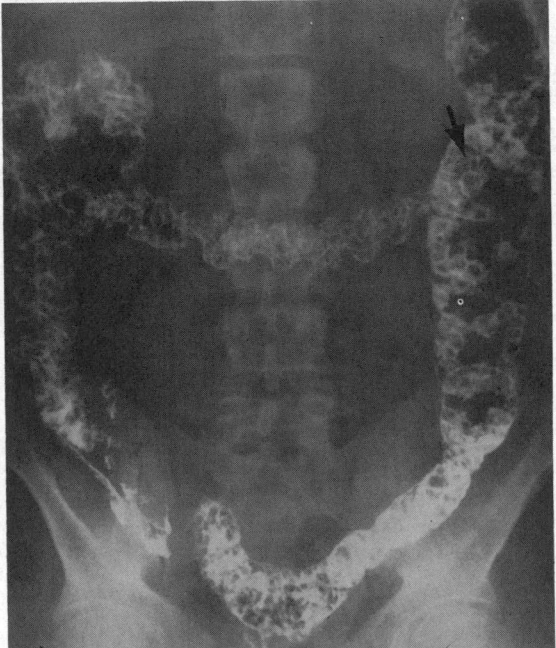

B

FIGURE 105–1. *A,* Patients with familial polyposis have multiple adenomatous polyps carpeting the colon, as demonstrated in this gross specimen. Note that the colon is diffusely studded with sessile and occasional pedunculated adenomatous polyps (*arrows*). Many of the larger polyps contain villous elements, and occasionally villous adenomas are found. Although no carcinoma was seen in this patient, nearly all patients eventually develop colorectal carcinoma if surgery is not performed. *B,* This barium enema examination of a patient with familial polyposis represents diffuse studding of the large bowel with adenomatous polyps. Note the marked variation in size of these polyps. Although this patient did not have osteomas or soft tissue tumors, the barium enema is similar to that seen in Gardner syndrome. (From Boland CR, Kim YS: *In* Sleisenger MH, Fordtran JS [eds.]: Gastrointestinal Disease. 3rd ed. Philadelphia, W. B. Saunders Company, 1983.)

be performed annually in all first-degree relatives, beginning at 12 years of age until age 40, and every 3 years thereafter. This screening is appropriate for those with the mutant gene. Until gene markers are 100 per cent specific and sensitive, screening is also indicated for those without the mutant gene, although less often. Surveillance with a side-viewing endoscope for gastric and duodenal polyps should begin when the diagnosis of colonic polyposis is made and should continue every 2 to 3 years thereafter.

HEREDITARY NONPOLYPOSIS COLORECTAL CANCER (LYNCH SYNDROMES I AND II). In both of the Lynch syndromes, colon cancer is inherited in a highly penetrant, autosomal dominant manner. Several adenomas, which are occasionally flat, may be present (in spite of the name), but myriads of adenomas are not found. The average age of diagnosis of cancer is in the mid 40's, and it is characteristic to find a majority of lesions proximal to the splenic flexure as well as multiple synchronous cancers. In Lynch syndrome I (site-specific colon cancer) only inherited colonic neoplasms occur, whereas Lynch syndrome II (cancer family syndrome) includes female genital (uterine, ovarian) and breast cancer. Individuals in families with hereditary nonpolyposis colorectal cancer should have colonoscopy every 2 years beginning at an age 5 years younger than the age of the earliest colon cancer diagnosed in the family. Mammography (at an earlier age than the general population) and ovarian ultrasonography are also appropriate in Lynch syndrome II families in whom there is a preponderance of breast or ovarian malignancies.

PEUTZ-JEGHERS SYNDROME. This syndrome is characterized by melanotic spots on the lips, buccal mucosa, and skin and by multiple hamartomatous polyps throughout the gastrointestinal tract from the stomach to the rectum (Fig. 105–3). It is generally believed to be inherited in an autosomal dominant fashion but with variable expressivity. Usually polyps are fewer in number than in familial adenomatous polyposis. Microscopically, these polyps consist of elongated branching glands lined by benign epithelium native to the location of the polyps. The most distinctive feature is the presence of an arborizing proliferation of smooth muscle in the lamina propria. Rarely, malignancies have been described in the intestine with a preponderance in the small intestine. Other manifestations include ovarian sex cord stromal tumors and polyps of the gallbladder, ureter, and nose. Intestinal symptoms of recurrent, colicky abdominal pain may appear in adolescence, and intussusception may require surgical removal of a polyp. Gastrointestinal bleeding may occur, causing iron deficiency anemia.

OTHER POLYPOSIS SYNDROMES. *Turcot's syndrome,* inherited as an autosomal recessive condition, is rare and is characterized by hereditary adenomatous polyposis with a low number of polyps (20 to 300) and tumors of the central nervous system. These neoplasms include medulloblastoma, glioblastoma, and ependymoma.

Juvenile polyposis is inherited as an autosomal dominant trait, with an occasional case occurring spontaneously. The number of polyps is less than in familial adenomatous polyposis, averaging 25 to 40. Polyps may be found throughout the gastrointestinal tract or may be restricted to the colon. Symptoms may begin in childhood or adolescence with rectal bleeding, anemia, abdominal pain, or intussusception. A variety of extraintestinal symptoms including congenital abnormalities and pulmonary arteriovenous malformations have been described in association with juvenile polyposis. Foci of adenomatous epithelium may be present in these polyps, or adenomas may coexist. The true risk of malignancy in these patients is unknown, but 10 per cent of the reported patients with juvenile polyposis have developed carcinoma of the gastrointestinal tract. Subtotal colectomy may occasionally be warranted in those with severely dysplastic adenomas.

Cronkite-Canada syndrome is a nonfamilial disorder of adults characterized by diffuse gastrointestinal polyposis, alopecia, dystrophy of the fingernails, and cutaneous hyperpigmentation. The polyps resemble juvenile polyps and are in greatest density in the stomach and colon. Watery diarrhea, anorexia, abdominal pain, cachexia, protein-losing enteropathy, and carcinoma of the gastrointestinal tract (in up to 14 per cent of cases) have been reported.

Cowden's syndrome (multiple hamartoma syndrome) is transmitted in an autosomal dominant manner and is characterized by multiple facial tricholemmomas, oral papillomas, keratoses of the hands and feet, and a high rate of associated systemic malignancies, particularly of thyroid and breast. The polyps are not dysplastic, and the risk of gastrointestinal malignancy is not increased.

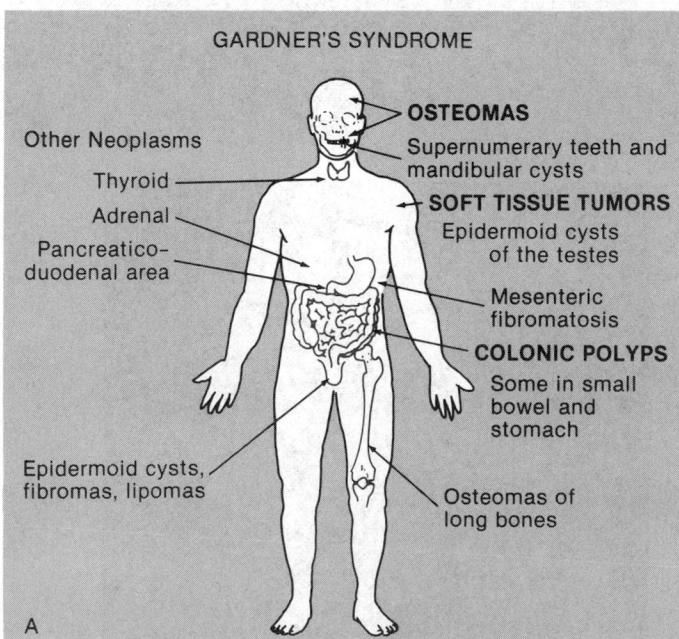

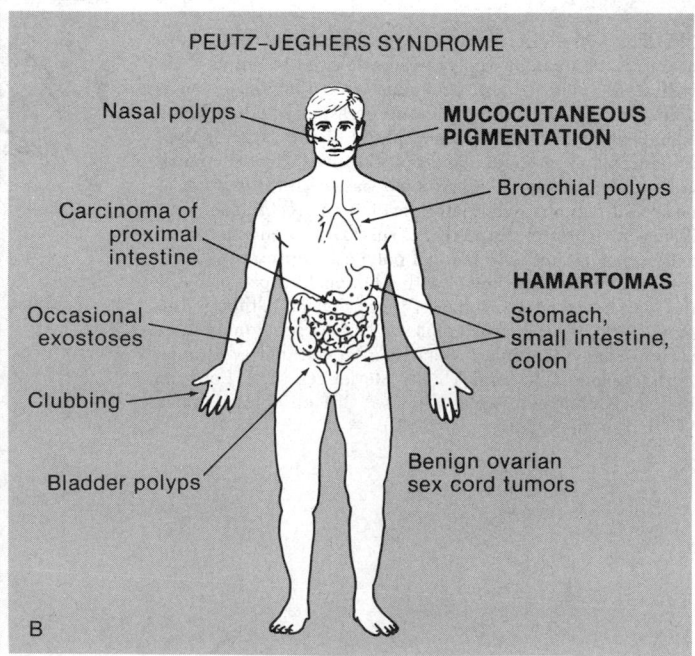

FIGURE 105–2. *A,* Schematic representation of Gardner syndrome. The triad of colonic polyposis, bone tumors, and soft tissue tumors (heavy print) constitutes the primary features; other features are indicated in lighter print. *B,* Schematic presentation of the Peutz-Jeghers syndrome. Mucocutaneous pigmentation and benign gastrointestinal polyposis (heavy print) are the primary features of this syndrome. Lighter print shows the secondary features. (From Boland CR, Kim YS: *In* Sleisenger MH, Fordtran JS [eds.]: Gastrointestinal Disease. 3rd ed. Philadelphia, W. B. Saunders Company, 1983.)

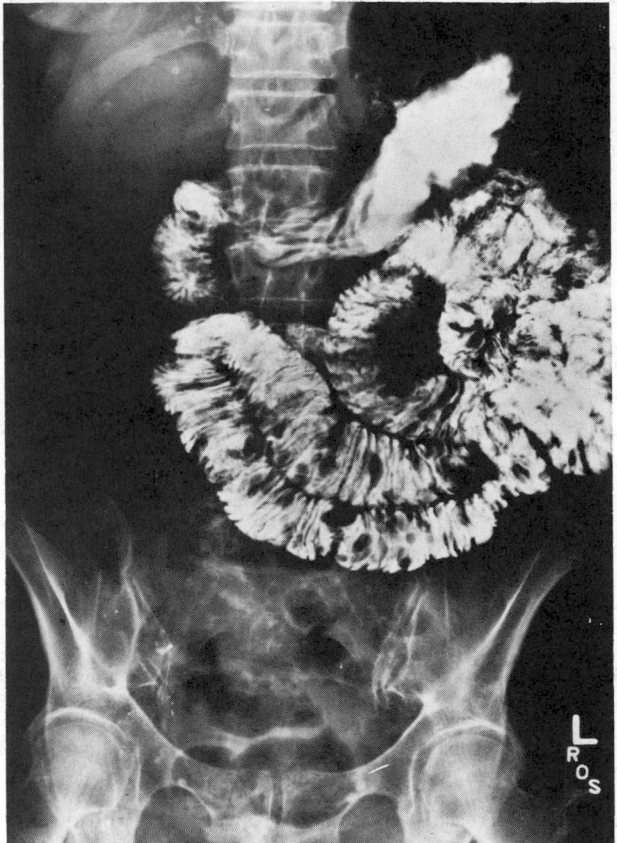

FIGURE 105–3. Barium study of the upper gastrointestinal tract showing multiple polyps of the small bowel in a patient with Peutz-Jeghers syndrome.

ADENOCARCINOMA OF THE LARGE BOWEL

Carcinoma of the colon and rectum varies widely in frequency in different parts of the world. Large bowel cancers occur commonly in North America, northwestern Europe, and New Zealand, whereas in South America, southwest Asia, equatorial Africa, and India the risk is much less. The incidence varies from 3.5 per 100,000 in India to 32.3 per 100,000 in Connecticut. Colorectal cancers display regional differences within the United States, with the highest incidence in the Northeast. Rectal cancer is more common in men in most, but not all, areas of the world. In the United States rectal cancer incidence has declined over the past 50 years.

Migrants from parts of the world with a low incidence to regions with a higher risk, such as the United States or Canada, show a rapid increase in incidence. This is exemplified by the higher incidence in Puerto Ricans who have migrated to the mainland compared with those in Puerto Rico and in first- and second-generation Chinese and Japanese immigrants to Hawaii and the mainland United States compared with Japanese in Japan and Chinese in the Peoples' Republic of China.

ETIOLOGY. Both inherited predisposition and environmental factors seem to be implicated in carcinogenesis in the colon and rectum, but in ways yet to be clearly delineated. Of the environmental factors, diet has been the most extensively studied. Fat intake, not only the amount, but also the type of fat, has been correlated with the risk for colorectal cancer in many but not all studies. Consumption of saturated fat (with a high content of animal fat) has been reported to be positively correlated with colon cancer incidence. Other studies suggest that monounsaturated fatty acids may exert a protective effect against the development of colon cancer. In countries with a high incidence of colon cancer, the average fat content in the diet is about 40 per cent of total calories, in contrast to the dietary fat content of 15 to 20 per cent or less of total calories in countries with a low cancer incidence. If fat in the colon does in fact promote cancer, the effect might be related to increased biliary sterol excretion,

leading to increased colonic epithelial proliferation, to modification of cell membranes, or to stimulation of the synthesis of prostaglandins that induce cellular proliferation. The possible role of *dietary fiber* in reducing colonic carcinogenesis has been suggested but not firmly established. Fiber is not a single chemical substance. Certain components of fiber found in cereals, fruits, and vegetables may be helpful in reducing the risk of cancer by diluting and binding carcinogens in the lumen, by modifying colonic bacterial flora, and by acidifying the colonic lumen by short-chain fatty acids. Naturally occurring anticarcinogens found in fruits and vegetables (indoles, thioethers, dithiothiones, retinoids) are being investigated. Other factors that have been postulated to play a role in colonic carcinogenesis are excess caloric intake and obesity and inadequate intake of calcium and vitamin D.

AGE. Risk factors for colorectal cancer are listed in Table 105–1. The relationship of age to adenomas has been previously discussed. The risk of colorectal cancer begins to increase from the age of 40 and rises sharply at age 50 to 55; with each succeeding decade the risk doubles, reaching a peak by age 75.

INFLAMMATORY BOWEL DISEASE (Ulcerative Colitis and Crohn's disease—Ch. 103). Among all patients diagnosed as having a large bowel adenocarcinoma, only about 1 per cent give an antecedent history of inflammatory bowel disease. In chronic ulcerative colitis, carcinoma of the colon occurs more commonly (approximately 10 to 20 times) than in the general population. The duration of disease and the extent of colonic involvement correlate with the subsequent development of colon cancer. Approximately 2 to 4 per cent of all patients with chronic ulcerative colitis develop colorectal carcinoma, with a cumulative incidence of about 12 per cent after 25 years. Patients with ulcerative proctitis have no increase in risk, and the risk for patients with left-sided colitis may be delayed until approximately 10 years later. In ulcerative colitis, mucosal dysplasia, defined as an unequivocal neoplastic alteration of the colonic epithelium, is the recognized precursor for the development of carcinoma. Dysplastic epithelium may itself overlie an area of malignancy associated with direct invasion into the submucosa. The dysplastic area may be flat or proliferative, and the likelihood of carcinoma increases significantly in the presence of a dysplasia-associated lesion or mass. Whether routine colonoscopic surveillance is useful in patients with inflammatory bowel disease is not settled. Nevertheless, many authorities favor periodic colonoscopy with multiple biopsies for dysplasia in individuals with over 8 years of symptoms and extensive colonic involvement. The availability of newer surgical procedures, such as ileoanal pouches, favors a trend toward earlier colectomy in high-risk individuals. The demonstration of high-grade dysplasia or a dysplasia-associated lesion or mass, even in the presence of low-grade dysplasia, warrants prophylactic colectomy because the risk of an associated carcinoma may be as high as 50 or 60 per cent. Newer epithelial markers, such as flow cytometry, lectins, oncogene mutations, and mucins, are being studied in an attempt to define the biology of neoplastic transformation and to identify individuals at high risk before cancer develops.

Patients with Crohn's colitis are also at higher risk (approximately 4 to 7 times that of the general population) for the development of colorectal cancer, but this is probably lower than

TABLE 105–1. RISK FACTORS FOR COLORECTAL CANCER

Standard Risk: Age over 40 years in men and women
Higher Risk
  Associated disease
    Ulcerative colitis
    Crohn's colitis
  Personal history
    Colorectal cancer
    Colorectal adenomas
    Female genital or breast cancer
  Family history
    Familial polyposis syndromes
    Hereditary nonpolyposis colorectal cancer
      (Lynch syndromes I and II)

in ulcerative colitis. Colonic surveillance has not been widely used.

HEREDITY AND COLONIC CANCER. Inherited risk has become very important in colonic cancer screening. The adenomatous polyposis syndromes and hereditary nonpolyposis colorectal cancer, previously discussed, together account for approximately 7 per cent of colon cancers. The remainder of colon cancers are referred to as "sporadic," but this term may be a misnomer. Population studies have demonstrated a two- or threefold increased risk for colon cancer in first-degree relatives of individuals with colon cancer. A similar risk is present in first-degree relatives of individuals with adenomatous polyps. In fact, as many as 50 per cent or more of "sporadic" adenomas and cancers may exhibit a partially penetrant autosomal dominant inheritance.

MOLECULAR GENETICS OF COLORECTAL CANCER. The genetic events surrounding the development of colorectal cancer are now being studied with increasing sophistication. The gene for familial adenomatous polyposis has been identified on chromosome 5. Deletions of DNA sequences at the same locus are also frequently observed in adenocarcinomas from "sporadic" cases. This may be the earliest change in the neoplastic process. K-*ras* mutations follow the chromosome 5 changes and are observed more commonly on larger adenomas and cancers (Ch. 157). Chromosome 17 (p53 gene) and chromosome 18 (DCC gene) deletions are often present and may be important in malignant transformation. Overexpression of the c-*myc* gene has also been reported in colonic cancers. The total accumulation of genetic changes (allelic deletions, oncogene mutations) may be more important than a particular sequence of events in the development of invasive cancer.

PATHOLOGY. The vast majority of colorectal cancers are adenocarcinomas. The tumors exhibit varying degrees of glandular differentiation and produce variable amounts of mucin. Cross morphologic features may be divided into two major groups, polypoid and annular constricting lesions. The polypoid lesion is most commonly found on the right side, and the annular constricting lesion is more common on the left side of the colon. Adenocarcinomas of the rectum may be sessile or polypoid. Approximately 75 per cent of colorectal cancers occur in the descending colon, rectosigmoid, and rectum. Approximately 50 per cent are within the reach of the 60-cm fiberoptic sigmoidoscope. The cecum and ascending colon are involved in 15 per cent and the transverse colon in 10 per cent (Fig. 105–4). Carcinoma of the colon spreads by direct extension through the wall of the bowel into the pericolonic fat and mesentery, by invasion of surrounding organs, by way of the lymphatics to the regional lymph nodes, and via the portal vein to the liver. Additionally, the tumor may spread throughout the peritoneal cavity and to the lungs and bones. Rectal cancers may directly invade the perirectal fat, vagina, prostate, bladder, ureters, and bony pelvis and may metastasize to the lungs and liver.

CLINICAL MANIFESTATIONS. The major symptoms of colorectal cancer are *rectal bleeding, pain,* and *change in bowel habit.* The clinical presentation in an individual patient is related to the size and location of the tumor. Those on the right side are often asymptomatic, and bleeding may be occult. Tumors of the cecum and ascending colon rarely obstruct early. Changes in bowel habit, with reduction in stool caliber or progressive constipation, and hematochezia are more common with left-sided lesions. Adenocarcinomas of the colon may present with a localized perforation and with signs of peritonitis. An abdominal mass or symptoms and signs of liver metastasis may be the earliest clinical manifestations of an underlying colorectal cancer.

Rectal or anal cancers may present with rectal bleeding, perineal pain, or change in bowel habit. Presenting symptoms may also include those referable to invasion of adjacent organs, including hematuria, renal insufficiency (obstructive uropathy), and vaginal fistulas.

Colorectal cancer must be suspected when patients present with rectal bleeding, a change in bowel habit, decrease in stool caliber, iron deficiency anemia, or unexplained abdominal pain. Rectal bleeding may be caused by other conditions, including hemorrhoids, angiodysplasia, diverticulosis, and other benign and malignant tumors (Ch. 111). Over the age of 40, the frequency

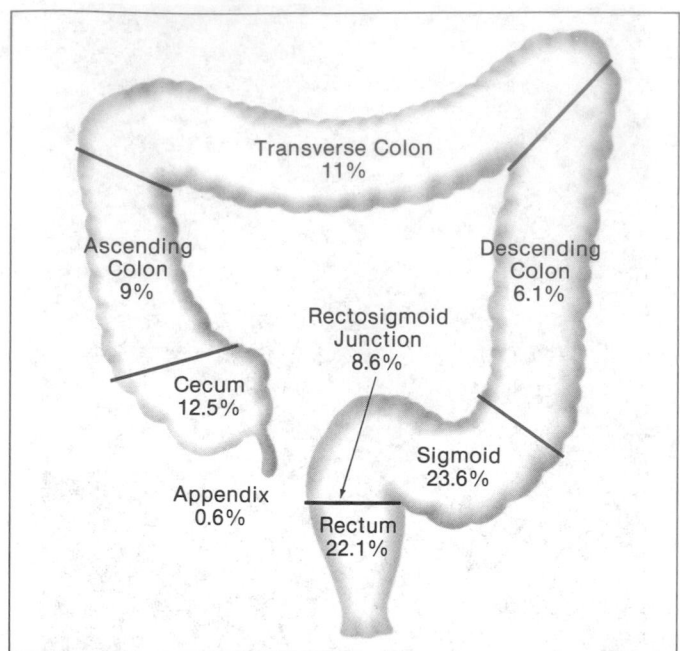

FIGURE 105–4. Distribution of large bowel cancer by anatomic segment according to the third national cancer survery (segment unspecified). (From Shottenfeld D, Fraumeni J Jr [eds.]: Cancer Epidemiology and Prevention. Philadelphia, W. B. Saunders Company, 1982, pp 703–727.)

of neoplasia increases significantly. Unexplained iron deficiency in both older men and women always requires a thorough evaluation to exclude gastrointestinal cancer (Ch. 131).

METASTATIC COLON CANCER. Metastases may be clinically apparent before or after resection of the primary colorectal cancer. Massive hepatomegaly may occur with pain due to distention of the liver capsule. Spread within the abdomen may cause small and large bowel obstruction and ascites. Pelvic spread may cause bladder dysfunction, sacral or sciatic nerve pain, and vaginal discharge or bleeding. Distant spread to lungs and bone may be silent until very advanced. Intestinal recurrences are uncommon and usually result from tumor implants related to the original resection growing from the serosa into the lumen.

DIAGNOSIS. A careful history, physical examination, and selected use of laboratory and radiologic tests facilitate the diagnosis of colorectal cancer. The history includes the patient's symptoms, prior removal of an adenoma or cancer, previous or present inflammatory bowel disease, or a family history of one of the inherited colorectal cancer syndromes. Special emphasis should be paid to first-degree relatives with a history of colorectal neoplasia. Physical examination may reveal evidence for Peutz-Jeghers or Gardner syndrome and may provide substantiation of spread to lymph nodes, liver, or peritoneal cavity. A digital rectal examination is essential in determining the presence of a distal rectal cancer or of perineal or pelvic spread. A complete pelvic examination should not be omitted. Laboratory tests may reveal iron deficiency anemia or an abnormality of liver enzymes. Radiologic studies may include a chest roentgenogram or computed tomographic scan of the abdomen and pelvis.

In the evaluation of patients with symptoms or signs of colorectal cancer, the digital rectal examination is followed by colonoscopy or double-contrast barium enema following sigmoidoscopy. Endoscopic ultrasonography is being used with increasing frequency to help in the staging of rectal cancers. Depth of invasion can often be accurately determined. Flexible sigmoidoscopy has replaced rigid proctoscopy and is particularly useful in evaluating a patient with a rectosigmoid neoplasm or an individual who presents with rectal bleeding and in whom active inflammatory bowel disease is suspected. In the latter case a barium enema or even colonoscopy may be undesirable.

Colonoscopy is more sensitive than double-contrast barium enema in detecting small adenomas and cancers and is also of value in evaluating patients who have had an abnormality detected by barium enema. In addition, the presence or absence of synchronous cancers and adenomas can be determined. Colonoscopy can be used to remove adenomas, to biopsy suspected cancers, and to obtain brush biopsy for cytology of suspected malignancies and colonic strictures.

MANAGEMENT. The modern approach to management is a multidisciplinary one and includes consideration not only of the immediate clinical problem but also a long-term approach to the patient. This may include postoperative adjuvant treatment, future plans for assessment of local recurrence or distant metastasis, and attention to family members at increased risk.

Surgery. The most important goal of treatment for primary malignancies of the colon and rectum is complete removal. Surgical resection of the affected segment, including omentum and lymph nodes, is performed. Cancers of the right and left colon are treated by hemicolectomies; cancer of the sigmoid and upper rectum above 6 cm from the anal verge are resected anteriorly with removal of a margin of normal colon above and below the tumor. Stapling techniques have facilitated anastomoses within the pelvis. While 3-cm proximal and distal margins have been previously emphasized, an adequate radial margin is equally important.

Lesions within 5 cm of the anal verge are usually treated by a combined abdominoperineal resection and permanent colostomy. Newer approaches for small, early rectal cancers include sphincter-saving procedures utilizing local excision followed in some instances by radiation therapy to the pelvis.

For anal cancers the standard approach is to utilize a combination of radiation and chemotherapy, which will usually shrink or obliterate the cancer. Surgical resection is now usually reserved for lesions that do not respond to chemoradiation or that recur.

Surgery may be required for palliation as well as for cure. Colonic obstruction may necessitate a palliative colostomy, although a primary resection and colostomy can often be accomplished at the same operation. A perforated carcinoma is usually managed by primary resection and colostomy with later closure of the colostomy. For selected medically fit patients with one to three hepatic metastases, surgical resection of part of the tumor-bearing liver is often possible. Careful preoperative radiologic staging as well as intraoperative ultrasonography facilitates these technically demanding procedures. Laser photoablation is being increasingly used to relieve colonic or rectal obstruction or bleeding in patients with unresectable tumors or those with extensive metastatic disease.

Radiation Therapy. Radiation therapy plays an important role in the postoperative management of rectal cancer. The combination of radiation (50 Gy) and chemotherapy, 5-fluorouracil (5-FU), is now standard therapy and has been shown to decrease local recurrence and distant metastasis. Preoperative radiation therapy decreases postoperative local recurrence but does not prolong overall survival. It may also be used to reduce tumor size and enable otherwise unresectable lesions to be resected. Radiation therapy is useful in palliating recurrent rectal cancer (pain or bleeding) or bone or brain metastases. Intraoperative radiation therapy is being evaluated in several centers.

Chemotherapy. Patients with resected colonic cancer with lymph node spread may have improved survival if treated with the combination of 5-FU and levamisole for a period of 1 year. For patients with metastatic spread, the combination of 5-FU and leucovorin increases tumor shrinkage compared to 5-FU alone. Combinations of chemotherapeutic agents and cytokines are under study.

In patients with liver metastases, hepatic arterial therapy with implantable pumps or via injection ports using floxuridine (FUDR) alone or in combination with other drugs such as leucovorin produces an enhanced tumor shrinkage in the liver, but increased survival has not been demonstrated.

PROGNOSIS AND FOLLOW-UP. The 10-year survival for patients with colorectal cancer after surgical resection is approximately 50 per cent. The survival correlates well with the stage of the disease: cancer confined to the mucosa, 80 to 90 per cent 10-year survival; cancer extending through all areas of the bowel wall, 70 to 80 per cent; and cancer involving the regional lymph nodes, 30 to 55 per cent. Cancers of the distal rectum with lymph node involvement have a poorer prognosis. Several histopathologic staging systems (e.g., Dukes' or TNM) are in use to describe the extent of the malignancy (Table 105–2).

Prior to surgical resection, the entire colon should be examined, preferably by colonoscopy, for the presence of synchronous

TABLE 105–2. AMERICAN JOINT COMMITTEE ON CANCER: CLASSIFICATION OF COLON/RECTAL CANCER

Stage 0	Carcinoma in situ; the cancer does not extend beyond the smooth muscle that separates the mucosa from the submucosa. (T_{is}, N_0, M_0)
Stage I	Cancer confined to the mucosa, submucosa, or external muscle; the cancer does not extend through the bowel wall. (T_1 or T_2, N_0, M_0)
Stage II	Cancer that penetrates all layers of the bowel wall, with or without invasion of adjacent tissues. (T_3, N_0, M_0)
Stage III	Cancer involving regional lymph nodes or extending into nearby tissues or organs without spread to lymph nodes. (Any T, N_1–N_3, M_0; or T_4, N_0, M_0)
Stage IV	Cancer that has spread to distant sites, usually the liver or lungs. (Any T, any N, M_1)

T = Tumor size; N = lymph node involvement; M = degree of metastasis.

adenomas. If not possible preoperatively, colonoscopy should be performed postoperatively, usually within 2 to 3 months of the surgical procedure. Colonoscopy should be repeated a year later and every 2 to 3 years thereafter because new adenomas require 3 years or more to develop into large adenomas with malignant potential.

After surgical resection, patients without known systemic metastases are evaluated for adjuvant therapy. Patients with colonic cancer and lymph node involvement should receive 5-FU and levamisole, and those with rectal cancer and spread through the wall or with lymph node involvement should receive radiation plus chemotherapy. While receiving chemotherapy or radiation therapy, patients are followed very carefully according to protocol guidelines. For those not receiving any specific therapy, periodic follow-up including interim history, physical examination, and laboratory tests (liver enzymes, hematocrit) are performed every 3 to 6 months for the first 3 years, then every 6 months until the fifth year. Controversy exists concerning the cost-effectiveness of obtaining periodic chest radiographs or computed tomography (CT) scans of the abdomen and pelvis as part of routine follow-up care in the absence of symptoms or laboratory test abnormalities.

Carcinoembryonic Antigen (CEA). CEA levels in the blood may rise before symptoms or other laboratory test abnormalities are evident in patients with recurrent or metastatic colonic cancer. Some authorities favor periodic CEA determinations (e.g., every 3 months) after colorectal cancer resection, but this is very expensive and helpful only in a minority of patients. Occasionally, a rising CEA may detect a localized, surgically resectable metastasis. In conjunction with conventional radiologic techniques (CT scan or MRI), radiolabeled monoclonal antibodies to CEA may be helpful in localizing such metastases. In the absence of defined lesions, a "second look" laparotomy based on a rising CEA has not been shown to prolong survival.

In screening large patient groups for colon cancer, CEA elevation was found to have a false-positive rate of 15 per cent and a false-negative rate of about 50 per cent in nonmetastatic disease. The test is thus unsuitable for screening, lacking both appropriate specificity and sensitivity.

PREVENTION OF COLORECTAL CANCER

Many colorectal cancers are first brought to medical attention by the patient's recognition of symptoms. For improved survival, the diagnosis should ideally be made earlier, in an asymptomatic phase. A greater emphasis is now being placed on preventive measures. Primary prevention is the identification of factors, either genetic or environmental, responsible for colorectal cancers. Secondary prevention refers to the identification and eradication of premalignant lesions and the detection and resection of cancer while still curable.

Although definitive evidence of effectiveness is still lacking, the National Cancer Institute has issued certain dietary guidelines to try to reduce the risk of colorectal cancer: (1) a reduction of fat intake to less than 30 per cent of calories; (2) an increase of dietary fiber to 20 to 30 grams per day; (3) inclusion in the diet of a variety of vegetables and fruits; (4) avoidance of obesity; and

(5) moderate consumption of alcohol, if at all. In addition, regular exercise may also reduce risk.

Implicit in the concept of secondary prevention is the need for improved techniques for screening for early cancer or premalignant adenomas. Effective screening requires the availability and application of simple and economic measures to a large number of asymptomatic individuals to identify those with these lesions. Screening for colorectal cancer can be classified as follows: general screening of patients at average risk and screening of patients in high-risk groups. (For discussion of high-risk groups see *Polyposis Syndromes* and *Ulcerative Colitis*.)

AVERAGE-RISK PATIENTS. Currently, testing for fecal occult blood and flexible sigmoidoscopy in asymptomatic individuals are used for detecting early colorectal cancer. Testing for occult blood using guaiac-based methods seems to detect earlier lesions in those screened compared to controls, but whether cancer mortality is reduced has not yet been demonstrated. Newer immunochemical tests for human hemoglobin in the stool, currently under clinical trial, are likely to be more specific. Randomized controlled trials of flexible sigmoidoscopy have not been performed on a large scale. Flexible sigmoidoscopy can not only identify and eradicate premalignant and malignant lesions in the area examined but also can identify individuals who may have more proximal synchronous adenomas and carcinomas.

In the absence of definitive data concerning the value of mass screening, many physicians have accepted interim guidelines for their own patients: (1) annual digital rectal examination after age 40; (2) testing for fecal occult blood annually after age 50; and (3) flexible sigmoidoscopy every 3 to 5 years after age 50. Patients with abnormal findings require careful diagnostic evaluation, including colonoscopy. A critical evaluation of a screening program for colorectal cancer requires that important issues be addressed: (1) What are the expected benefits in terms of survival of patients whose disease is discovered by screening tests and treated? (2) Is there a mortality reduction from colorectal cancer in the entire screened population? (3) What are the psychological, economic, and other factors influencing patient compliance? (4) Are there adequate health resources available for the diagnostic workup and treatment of patients with a positive screening test? (5) What are the costs and risks of such screening?

Adenomas

Haggitt RC, et al.: Prognostic factors in colorectal carcinomas arising in adenomas: Implications for lesions removed by endoscopic polypectomy. Gastroenterology 89:328, 1985. *A practical discussion of cancers arising in adenomas.*

Risk

Burt RW, et al.: Dominant inheritance of adenomatous colonic polyps and colorectal cancer. N Engl J Med 312:1540, 1985. Cannon-Albright LA, et al.: Common inheritance of susceptibility to colonic adenomatous polyps and associated colorectal cancers. N Engl J Med 319:533, 1988. *These two papers present data concerning the inheritance of sporadic adenomas and cancer.*

Levin B, et al.: Surveillance of patients with chronic ulcerative colitis. WHO Bulletin (in press). *A review of the current approach to surveillance for dysplasia in high-risk individuals and an evaluation of the relationship between inflammatory bowel disease and cancer.*

Lynch HT, et al.: Differential diagnosis of hereditary nonpolyposis colorectal cancer (Lynch syndrome I and Lynch syndrome II). Dis Colon Rectum 31:372, 1988. *A review of hereditary nonpolyposis colorectal cancer.*

Molecular Biology

Nishisha I, Nakamura Y, Miyoshi Y, et al.: Mutations of chromosome 5 q 21 genes in FAP and colorectal cancer patients. Science 253:665, 1991. *One of several exciting recent papers on the molecular biology of polyps and colon cancer.*

Therapy

Moertel CG, et al.: Levamisole and fluorouracil for adjuvant therapy of resected colon carcinoma. N Engl J Med 322:352, 1990. *An encouraging report of a trial of adjuvant therapy in 1300 patients, demonstrating a benefit for adjuvant therapy.*

Poon MA, et al.: Biochemical modulation of fluorouracil: Evidence of significant improvement of survival and quality of life in patients with advanced colorectal carcinoma. J Clin Oncol 7:1407, 1989. *A description of biochemical modulation with apparent clinical benefit.*

Rosenberg SA, et al.: Principles and applications of biologic therapy in cancer. *In* DeVita VT, Hellman S, Rosenberg SA (eds.): Principles and Practice of Oncology. Philadelphia, J. B. Lippincott Company, 1989, pp 301–347.

Dietary Factors

Garland C, Shekelle RB, Barrett-Connor E, et al.: Dietary vitamin D and calcium and risk of colorectal cancer: A 19 year prospective study in men. Lancet 1:307, 1985. *An intriguing epidemiologic study suggestive of an important role for calcium in the prevention of colorectal cancer.*

Physiological Effect and Health Consequences of Dietary Fiber. Federation of American Societies for Experimental Biology, Life Science Research Office, 1987. *A critical evaluation of the interactions of fiber and intestinal physiology.*

Wargovich MJ, et al.: Dietary factors and colorectal cancer. Gastroenterol Clin 17:727, 1988. *A review of naturally occurring anticarcinogens and other factors that may influence the development of colorectal cancer.*

Screening

Hardcastle JD, Pye G: Screening for colorectal cancer: A critical review. World J Surg 13:38, 1989.

Winawer SJ, St. John J, Bond J, et al.: Risks and screening of average risk individuals for colorectal cancer. WHO Bull 68:505, 1990. *These two papers evaluate current approaches to screening for large bowel cancers.*

NEOPLASMS OF THE SMALL BOWEL

Benign and malignant tumors of the lining epithelium and mesenchymal tissues may arise in the small intestine, or these areas may be secondarily involved by direct invasion from surrounding structures or by metastases. The small bowel represents almost 90 per cent of the mucosal surface of the gut, but small intestinal cancers account for only 1 to 2 per cent of all gastrointestinal neoplasms. Only about 2000 cases occur in the United States each year.

RISK FACTORS. Patients with regional enteritis, especially those who have had segments of intestine surgically bypassed, have an increased incidence of small bowel carcinoma. Individuals with Gardner syndrome have an increased risk of periampullary adenocarcinoma. In patients with Peutz-Jeghers syndrome, the relative risk of small intestinal adenocarcinoma is 16 times that expected, with a lifetime incidence of 2 per cent. Patients with celiac disease of long duration have an increased incidence of intestinal lymphoma, as do patients with the acquired immunodeficiency syndrome and other immunodeficiency states. Mediterranean abdominal lymphoma (immunoproliferative small intestinal disease) has been widely reported among Arabs and Jews of Middle Eastern origin and also occurs sporadically throughout the world, including blacks in southern Africa.

Why small bowel neoplasms, especially adenocarcinomas, are so uncommon compared with large bowel cancers is uncertain. It is possible that the rapid transit time with a resultant decreased exposure time to carcinogens, lower numbers of bacteria, and dilution of potential carcinogens by the large volume of enteric liquids may contribute.

PATHOLOGY. *Benign.* These lesions include adenomas, leiomyomas, lipomas, and angiomas. Brunner's gland adenomas are not neoplastic but represent a hyperplasia or hypertrophy of submucosal duodenal glands. These appear as small nodules in the duodenal mucosa detected at endoscopy or on barium radiographs.

Malignant. Adenocarcinomas, carcinoids, lymphomas, and leiomyosarcomas account for over 90 per cent of malignant small bowel tumors. Adenocarcinomas are most common in the proximal small intestine, whereas lymphomas and carcinoids are most common in the distal small intestine.

CLINICAL MANIFESTATIONS. Over one half of all benign bowel tumors remain asymptomatic and may only be discovered incidentally at laparotomy or autopsy. Lack of symptoms is attributable to the liquid contents of the small intestine and distensibility of the small intestine. Large tumors may lead to partial or complete mechanical obstruction from intussusception or volvulus. Adenocarcinomas account for about half of the malignant tumors of the small intestine, with a peak incidence in the sixth and seventh decades. The duodenum is the most frequently affected site. When postbulbar in location, adenocarcinoma may simulate peptic ulcer disease; when in the periampullary region, it may cause obstructive jaundice. More distally, adenocarcinomas may remain silent until symptoms of intestinal obstruction or gastrointestinal hemorrhage occur.

Carcinoids are the most frequent small intestinal neoplasm, with over half found incidentally either at autopsy or at operation for other diseases. Small carcinoid tumors may be asymptomatic, but larger carcinoid tumors can obstruct the lumen or bleed. Once metastasis occurs to the liver, features of the carcinoid syndrome become apparent (Ch. 230). Weight loss, intestinal obstruction, fever, bleeding, and evidence of malabsorption syndrome are features of lymphoma. Massive hemorrhage and intestinal perforation may be the presenting symptoms of large sarcomas.

SIGNS. Physical examination may be unremarkable in patients with benign tumors, unless the neoplasms are large enough to present with a mass. Loud borborygmi, visible peristalsis, and abdominal distention may be present in intestinal obstruction. In patients with malignant small bowel neoplasms, more obvious physical findings may be evident. Cachexia, hepatomegaly, ascites, and jaundice may be found. Peripheral lymphadenopathy or splenomegaly may be found in those with extensive lymphoma.

DIFFERENTIAL DIAGNOSIS. The initial symptoms may be vague and poorly defined. Once bleeding occurs, causes such as peptic ulceration, Meckel's diverticulum, and vascular anomalies need to be considered (Ch. 111). Obstructive jaundice may occur with periampullary neoplasms, bile duct cancer, impacted common duct stones, pancreatitis, and pancreatic cancer (Ch. 107). Intestinal obstruction may be due to adhesions, particularly in patients who have had prior abdominal operations, internal hernias, volvulus, or intussusception.

LABORATORY AND RADIOLOGIC STUDIES. A hypochromic, microcytic anemia is quite common. Elevation of alkaline phosphatase and bilirubin may recur if the ampulla of Vater is obstructed or if liver metastases are present. Elevated levels of plasma serotonin or urinary 5-hydroxyindoleacetic acid occur in the carcinoid syndrome (Ch. 230). Dysproteinemia is a typical feature of Mediterranean lymphoma and is characterized by the presence of abnormal fragments of IgA in the serum and urine that is devoid of light chains (Ch. 151).

Upper gastrointestinal barium radiographs and selective nasoenteric intubation (enteroclysis), which permits the introduction of barium and air into a relatively localized segment, may be useful in localizing tumors. Abdominal ultrasonography and computed tomography may determine the extent of hepatic involvement, aid in the workup of jaundice, and assess intraabdominal and retroperitoneal spread. Intestinal lymphoma may occasionally be diagnosed by peroral intestinal biopsy, but the disease mainly involves the lamina propria and usually requires a full-thickness surgical biopsy. A thorough staging of lymphoma involves bone marrow biopsy, laparotomy with splenectomy, and biopsies of regional lymph nodes and liver.

ENDOSCOPIC EVALUATION. Front-viewing and side-viewing fiberoptic endoscopes are used to examine the duodenum; suspicious lesions can be biopsied and brushed. Periampullary lesions can be well visualized; the pancreatic and biliary trees can be studied by contrast radiography after endoscopic cannulation. The terminal ileum can also be viewed at colonoscopy. Small bowel enteroscopy, a relatively new technique, is sometimes helpful in localizing a small bleeding lesion.

THERAPY. Treatment is primarily surgical for symptomatic benign tumors, adenocarcinomas, leiomyosarcomas, malignant carcinoids, and those with secondary involvement of the small intestine. Duodenal carcinomas or large villous adenomas are treated by pancreaticoduodenal resection (Whipple procedure). In patients with localized lymphoma (stage I) surgical excision is recommended. Combination chemotherapy is used for more extensive lymphoma (Ch. 147). Radiation therapy may be helpful for bulky tumors or localized recurrences.

PROGNOSIS AND PREVENTION. The prognosis for benign tumors of the intestine is good if surgical resection can alleviate bleeding and obstruction. The prognosis of small intestinal adenocarcinomas is generally poor. The prognosis for leiomyosarcoma and primary lymphomas is good if surgical resection is complete, but this is rarely possible. Patients with malignant carcinoid tumors may survive for long periods even in the presence of extensive hepatic involvement (Ch. 230).

Primary small intestinal lymphomas occurring in the Middle East could possibly be decreased by public health measures that decrease parasitic infestation. Earlier diagnosis and adequate treatment of celiac disease (gluten free diet) may reduce the frequency of malignancy. Surgical bypass should not be performed in patients with Crohn's disease. In patients with familial polyposis syndromes, duodenal and periampullary adenomas should be monitored periodically. Prophylactic endoscopic or surgical removal may be appropriate.

Ashley SW, Wells SA: Tumors of the small intestine. Semin Oncol 15:116, 1988. *An updated review of pathology, natural history, and epidemiology.*

Lightdale CJ, Koepsell TC, Sherlock P: Small intestinal cancer. In Schottenfeld D, Fraumeni J (eds.): Cancer Epidemiology and Prevention. Philadelphia, W. B. Saunders Company, 1982. *A comprehensive discussion of the topic, including epidemiologic and etiologic aspects.*

Moertel CG: An odyssey in the land of small tumors. J Clin Oncol 5:1503, 1987. *New insights into the biology, natural history, and management of carcinoid tumors.*

106 Pancreatitis
William M. Steinberg

Normal Anatomy and Physiology of the Pancreas

The dorsal pancreas forms in the fetus as an outpouching from the duodenum at approximately 4 weeks of gestation. Several days later, the ventral pancreas forms from the hepatic diverticulum. At 7 to 8 weeks of gestation, the rotation of the duodenum leads the two pancreatic buds and their main ducts to fuse. If the two buds fuse incompletely, the duct of Wirsung drains only the ventral pancreas and the duct of Santorini the dorsal pancreas. This common anomaly, termed pancreas divisum, is present in 5 to 10 per cent of the general population.

The exocrine pancreas consists of acinar, centroacinar, and ductular cells. The acinar cells, the majority of cells, synthesize approximately 20 digestive enzymes, which are secreted from zymogen granules in the apical portions of the cell into the central ductule of the acinus by exocytosis. The ductules coalesce to form larger ducts, which empty into the duodenum at the ampulla of Vater. The ductular cells exchange bicarbonate for chloride, especially at increased rates of secretion. This ensures an alkaline milieu in the duodenum, which is necessary for optimal activity of pancreatic enzymes. Pancreatic secretion is stimulated by the vagus nerve (cerebral, gastric, and intestinal phases) and by the action of two hormones secreted by the duodenum: (1) secretin, which is released in response to acid in the duodenum and stimulates a pancreatic juice high in bicarbonate concentration, and (2) cholecystokinin (CCK), which is released in response to fatty acids and amino acids in the duodenum and results in a secretion rich in enzymes.

The enzymes from the pancreas digest starch (amylase), fats (lipase), and protein (trypsin and many other proteolytic enzymes). Although amylase and lipase are secreted in active forms, the proteolytic enzymes are secreted as inactive zymogens that must be activated in the duodenum. Trypsinogen is activated by the small bowel mucosal enzyme enterokinase to form trypsin. Trypsin then activates the other proteolytic enzymes. The pancreas is protected from autodigestion by three mechanisms: (1) secretion of proteolytic enzymes in an inactive form; (2) packaging of pancreatic proenzymes and lysozomes in separate compartments, preventing premature activation, and (3) concomitant secretion of protease inhibitors to neutralize any prematurely activated enzyme.

ACUTE PANCREATITIS
Pathogenesis

The precise mechanisms that trigger the autodigestive processes causing acute pancreatitis are not known. Some of the factors that may play a role include transient obstruction of the pancreatic duct, reflux of duodenal contents into the pancreatic duct, ischemia, altered pancreatic duct permeability, and intracellular coalescence of zymogen granules with lysozomal enzymes, such as cathepsin B, causing premature acinar cell activation of trypsin. The autodigestive process starts with the intraacinar activation of trypsin, which in turn activates other enzymes, such as phospholipase A_2 and elastase. These active enzymes disrupt cellular membranes and cause intrapancreatic edema, peripancreatic fat necrosis, parenchymal hemorrhage, and necrosis of acinar cells. Furthermore, activated enzymes, liberated into the peritoneal space and systemic circulation, may overwhelm host defenses (α_1-antitrypsin and α_2-macroglobulin) and cause distant end-organ dysfunction by as yet unknown mechanisms.

Etiologic Associations (Table 106–1)

In the United States, acute pancreatitis is most commonly associated with *alcoholism* and *gallstones;* a large number of cases are also *idiopathic*. The pathogenesis of alcoholic pancreatitis is discussed in the section on chronic pancreatitis. Most alcoholics who present with a first attack of alcoholic pancreatitis probably already have superimposed chronic pancreatitis, as evidenced by reduced bicarbonate or enzyme secretion when tested with sensitive methods. In these patients the trigger for the acute attacks of pain is unknown.

Gallstone-associated pancreatitis, especially common in elderly women, is thought to occur when gallstones transiently obstruct the common bile duct in or near the orifice of the pancreatic duct. In fact, a gallstone can usually be found if stools are carefully collected and examined immediately after attacks of gallstone pancreatitis. The mechanism by which choledocholithiasis causes pancreatitis is unclear. Theories include (1) obstruction of the ampulla of Vater by a stone, allowing bile to reflux into the pancreatic duct, injuring the parenchyma, and (2) transient obstruction of the pancreatic duct without bile reflux.

TABLE 106–1. ETIOLOGIC ASSOCIATIONS WITH ACUTE PANCREATITIS

I. Obstructive causes
  A. Choledocholithiasis
  B. Ampullary or pancreatic tumors
  C. Worms or foreign bodies obstructing the papilla
  D. Pancreas divisum with accessory duct obstruction
  E. Choledochocele
  F. Periampullary duodenal diverticula
  G. Hypertensive sphincter of Oddi
  H. Duodenal loop obstruction
II. Toxin/drug causes
  A. Toxins
    1. Ethyl alcohol
    2. Methyl alcohol
    3. Scorpion venom
    4. Organophosphorus insecticides
  B. Drugs
    1. Definite association (documented with rechallenges): azathioprine/6-mercaptourine, valproic acid, estrogens, tetracycline, metronidazole, nitrofurantoin, pentamidine, furosemide, sulfonamides, methyldopa, cytarabine, cimetidine, sulindac
    2. Not definite (no rechallenges reported): thiazide diuretics, ethacrynic acid, phenformin, procainamide, chlorthalidone, L-asparaginase, acetaminophen
III. Metabolic causes
  A. Hypertriglyceridemia
  B. Hypercalcemia
IV. Trauma
  A. Accidental—blunt trauma to the abdomen
  B. Iatrogenic—postoperative, ERCP, endoscopic sphincterotomy, sphincter of Oddi manometry
V. Inherited
VI. Infection
  A. Parasitic—ascariasis, clonorchis
  B. Viral—mumps, hepatitis A, hepatitis B, coxsackie B, Epstein-Barr
  C. Bacterial—*Mycoplasma, Campylobacter jejuni*
VII. Vascular
  A. Ischemia—hypoperfusion (e.g., post–cardiac surgery).
  B. Atherosclerotic emboli
  C. Vasculitis—systemic lupus erythematosus, polyarteritis nodosa, malignant hypertension
VIII. Miscellaneous
  A. Penetrating peptic ulcer
  B. Crohn's disease of the duodenum
  C. Pregnancy associated
  D. Pediatric association—Reye's syndrome, cystic fibrosis
IX. Idiopathic

Whether pancreas divisum predisposes to acute pancreatitis is controversial. Some believe that both the congenital abnormality and stenosis of the accessory papilla (which obstructs the flow of juices draining the duct of Santorini) must be present to cause pancreatitis. Other conditions that obstruct the pancreatic duct (either Wirsung or Santorini) have been reported to cause acute pancreatitis (e.g., foreign bodies, parasites, tumors) (Table 106–1). Hypertensive sphincter of Oddi as determined by pressure measurements has been reported to be a cause of recurrent acute pancreatitis and based on this presumption has been treated by endoscopic sphincterotomy. In elderly patients, gallstones are usually the cause of a first attack of acute pancreatitis, but a small tumor of the ductular or periampullary region must also be considered.

Toxins other than ethanol that may cause acute pancreatitis include methyl alcohol (Ch. 28), scorpion stings, and organophosphorus insecticides.

Drug-induced pancreatitis usually reflects hypersensitivity rather than excessive dosage. Characteristically, it occurs within the first month of exposure and is usually mild and self-limited. The most commonly implicated drugs in adults are azathioprine and its congener 6-mercaptopurine. Three to 5 per cent of individuals taking these drugs develop pancreatitis. In children, valproic acid is most commonly implicated.

Hypertriglyceridemia with levels exceeding 1000 mg per deciliter may be associated with moderate to severe acute pancreatitis (Ch. 172). If triglyceride levels are reduced to below 500 mg per deciliter, recurrent attacks are greatly reduced in frequency. *Hypercalcemia* from any cause is another rare metabolic cause of acute pancreatitis (Ch. 235).

Trauma to the pancreas, either accidental (e.g., blunt abdominal trauma in an automobile accident) or iatrogenic (surgical abdominal trauma), can lead to pancreatitis. Postoperative acute pancreatitis can also follow extra-abdominal surgery and may occasionally be severe. The trauma of endoscopic retrograde cholangiopancreatography (ERCP) produces acute pancreatitis in about 1 to 5 per cent of patients.

A propensity for pancreatitis may be inherited as a rare autosomal dominant trait. Characteristically, attacks of acute pancreatitis begin in childhood or young adulthood and progress to chronic pancreatitis and pancreatic insufficiency. Pancreatolithiasis may be prominent, and an associated aminoaciduria has been described in some families.

Infections as precipitating events in initiating acute pancreatitis have been reported secondary to mumps, hepatitis A and B, and Epstein-Barr and coxsackie B viruses, as well as from *Mycoplasma* and *Campylobacter jejuni*. Further documentation to confirm many of these associations is needed.

Vascular insufficiency (hypoperfusion, atherosclerotic plaques) and vasculitis have also been implicated as causes of acute pancreatitis, consistent with experimental evidence that reducing blood flow to the pancreas can cause or exacerbate pancreatitis.

Clinical Presentation

Severe knifelike epigastric *pain* with radiation to the back associated with nausea and vomiting is the classic presentation of acute pancreatitis. The pain tends to come on rapidly over seconds to minutes, is constant, and can last from days to more than a week. The latter distinguishes acute pancreatitis from peptic ulcer and biliary colic, in which painful episodes are shorter. The pain of pancreatitis can sometimes be partially relieved by flexing the trunk. Rarely, acute pancreatitis may be painless.

Physical findings include mild fever, tachypnea, tachycardia, and hypo- or hypertension. The abdomen may be distended because of the presence of ileus or a pseudocyst or phlegmon (an inflammatory mass), which may be palpable. If ileus is present, the bowel sounds are hypoactive or absent. Epigastric tenderness is usually marked and occasionally is associated with rigidity and guarding suggestive of an acute surgical abdomen. Rarely, with hemorrhagic pancreatitis, blood dissects from the retroperitoneal location of the pancreas around fascial planes and appears as a large ecchymosis in the flanks (Grey Turner sign) or umbilical area (Cullen sign). With hemorrhagic or other forms of severe pancreatitis, patients may present in shock with marked hypotension due to loss of blood into the pancreas, or exudation of large amounts of plasma into the retroperitoneal space, or changes in vascular tone mediated in part by vasoactive peptides.

The differential diagnosis is that of the acute abdomen and includes peptic ulcer with or without perforation, biliary colic, renal colic, small bowel obstruction and infarction, and suppurative cholangitis.

Diagnosis

LABORATORY TESTS

AMYLASE. The diagnosis of acute pancreatitis relies heavily on the demonstration of an increased serum amylase activity. Serum amylase, however, can be mildly elevated in many diseases not affecting the pancreas (e.g., those involving the salivary glands, small intestine, biliary tract, and Fallopian tubes), as well as in macroamylasemia (aggregated circulating amylase with or without immunoglobulin A). Amylase elevations of more than two- or threefold above the upper limit of normal in the setting of acute abdominal pain most often indicate acute pancreatitis. The amylase returns to normal more rapidly than do other pancreatic enzymes (e.g., lipase) so that a normal amylase by no means excludes the diagnosis of pancreatitis. This is especially true in a patient with acute pancreatitis superimposed on chronic pancreatitis (e.g., a chronic alcoholic) in whom a normal amylase level presumably reflects a "burnt out" pancreas with extensive destruction of acinar cells. The height of the rise of the serum amylase does not correlate with the severity of the pancreatitis. Patients with alcoholic pancreatitis tend to have lower serum levels of amylase (usually < 1000 IU per liter) than patients with other forms of pancreatitis. Amylase can be fractionated into pancreatic and salivary isoamylase components by different techniques. Several simple-to-use chemical kits have been developed to semiquantitatively measure pancreatic isoamylase, but technical difficulties with these kits have limited their usefulness. In general, amylase fractionation gives no more useful clinical information than that which can be obtained from other enzyme markers such as the serum lipase.

In the typical attack of pancreatitis, the serum amylase tends to normalize 4 to 7 days after the onset of pain. If the amylase is elevated beyond 7 days, complications such as a pseudocyst may be present. Renal failure, in the absence of pancreatitis, may raise the serum amylase (as well as lipase and other enzyme markers) to as high as four to six times the upper limit of normal. Elevations above this level in a patient with renal failure suggest concurrent pancreatic inflammation. Hypertriglyceridemia associated with turbid serum can mask an elevated serum amylase, thus obscuring the diagnosis of acute pancreatitis. In these circumstances, diluting the serum leads to a paradoxical rise in the measured serum amylase value.

LIPASE. Serum lipase tests, especially those that employ colipase as a cofactor, have the advantage of greater sensitivity and specificity than the amylase levels. Lipase is elevated as early as amylase but stays elevated for much longer periods of time. This allows a diagnosis to be made after the amylase level may have returned to normal. An initial lipase determination is often helpful in confirming pancreatitis in patients who are hyperamylasemic or who have symptoms of pancreatitis but a normal serum amylase level.

OTHER BLOOD TESTS. Immunologic blood tests (radioimmunoassays and ELISA assays) of other enzymes or proenzymes such as trypsinogen or elastase are more sensitive and specific than amylase in detecting pancreatic injury. They offer few, if any, advantages over the lipase assay, however. Immunoassays are more helpful in detecting pancreatic exocrine insufficiency (see below) than are the enzymatic lipase or amylase assays.

The white blood cell count is frequently elevated moderately (< 20,000 per microliter). Acute pancreatitis characteristically lowers the serum calcium concentration (see below under complications). A patient presenting with a high normal level of serum calcium during acute pancreatitis may actually have an underlying hypercalcemia. Serum triglyceride levels should be obtained in all patients with acute pancreatitis because of potential etiologic importance and also to aid in interpreting amylase levels. Gallstone pancreatitis is suspected if patients with acute pancreatitis present with bilirubin levels greater than 2.5 mg per deciliter and alkaline phosphatase and aminotransferase levels greater than three times normal. Other blood tests are discussed under risk factors.

URINARY TESTS. Plasma amylase is filtered by the renal glomerulus; normally most is resorbed or metabolized by the renal tubules, and the remainder is excreted in the urine. During acute pancreatitis, increased amounts of amylase are excreted into the urine owing to inhibition of renal tubular resorption. Timed 2-hour or 24-hour measurements of urinary amylase content or of the amylase-to-creatinine clearance ratio have been used as diagnostic markers of acute pancreatitis. These urinary measurements, however, are not as sensitive or specific as the easier-to-obtain serum lipase or immunologic blood tests and add little clinical information.

OTHER DIAGNOSTIC TESTS. A diagnostic peritoneal tap with lavage can occasionally be helpful in diagnosing acute pancreatitis and in differentiating this condition from other intra-abdominal processes. Acute pancreatitis frequently is accompanied by sterile, straw- to prunish-colored peritoneal fluid with a high amylase content. Dark prune-colored fluid suggests severe necrotizing or hemorrhagic pancreatitis. Fluid that is foul smelling and has bacteria or vegetable matter on Gram's stain suggests a perforated viscus.

IMAGING TESTS

Plain and upright films of the abdomen are important in ruling out a perforated viscus, e.g., as suggested by the finding of free air under the diaphragm. Pancreatitis may sometimes be difficult to differentiate from small bowel obstruction because it may lead to diffuse or localized ileus (sentinel loop). In rare circumstances, an acutely inflamed pancreas may cause localized obstruction of the transverse or descending colon (colon "cutoff" sign). Calcification of the pancreas suggests that the bout of acute disease is superimposed on chronic pancreatitis. Later in the course of severe pancreatitis, a plain film may rarely detect air bubbles ("soap bubble sign") in the retroperitoneum, suggestive of a pancreatic abscess with gas-producing organisms.

Chest roentgenograms may show some of the pulmonary findings seen in association with pancreatitis, including pleural effusions (left side more often than right), atelectasis, and acute pulmonary edema patterns. Barium contrast studies of the upper gastrointestinal tract may show anterior displacement of the stomach due to a pancreatic phlegmon or edema and spiculation of the duodenal C loop due to the adjacent pancreatic inflammatory process.

The two most important imaging modalities in the field of pancreatitis are *ultrasonography* and *computed tomography* (CT scan) of the abdomen. These two techniques have important complementary roles in the diagnosis and management of acute pancreatitis (Figs. 106–1, 106–2, and 93–2). Ultrasonography is especially helpful in detecting the presence of cholelithiasis and in determining if there is dilatation of the biliary tree to suggest choledocholithiasis and gallstone pancreatitis (see Figs. 93–5 amd 93–6). Ultrasonography is less sensitive in detecting stones in the common bile duct and tends not to visualize the pancreas well because of overlying bowel gas. The CT scan does not visualize the gallbladder as completely as does ultrasonography, but it visualizes the pancreas and peripancreatic spaces with greater accuracy. A CT scan of the pancreas is frequently normal in mild cases of acute pancreatitis but is especially helpful in determining if phlegmonous pancreatitis is present or if extra- or intrapancreatic fluid collections are forming. Serial scans may delineate the formation of abscesses, which may require drainage. CT scanning with high-bolus intravenous contrast (dynamic CT scanning) may demonstrate areas of low or no perfusion, suggestive of necrosis. This may be helpful in prognosis, as greater than 50 per cent necrosis of the pancreas is associated with high mortality.

ASSESSMENT OF RISK FACTORS IN PROGNOSIS. Several blood tests alone or in combination (multiple criteria tests) are used to delineate severe forms of acute pancreatitis (Table 106–2). Ranson's criteria have been modified over time to separate those patients with gallstone from nongallstone pancreatitis. If three or more risk factors are present from the Ranson or Glasgow list (Table 106–2), the patient's course tends to have much greater morbidity and mortality. For instance, patients who have up to two Ranson risk factors have a mortality of less than 5 per cent; those with three to four risk factors, a mortality of 15 to 20 per cent; five to six risk factors, a mortality of 40 per

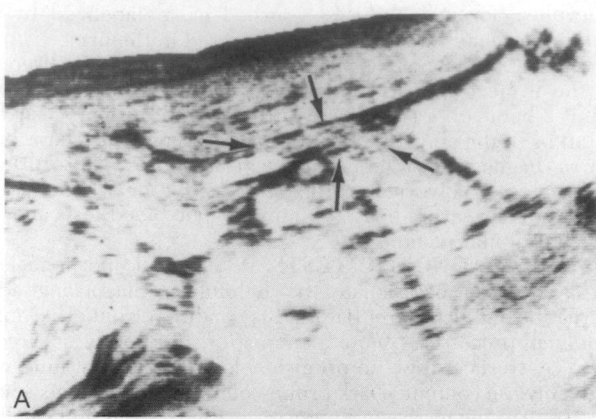

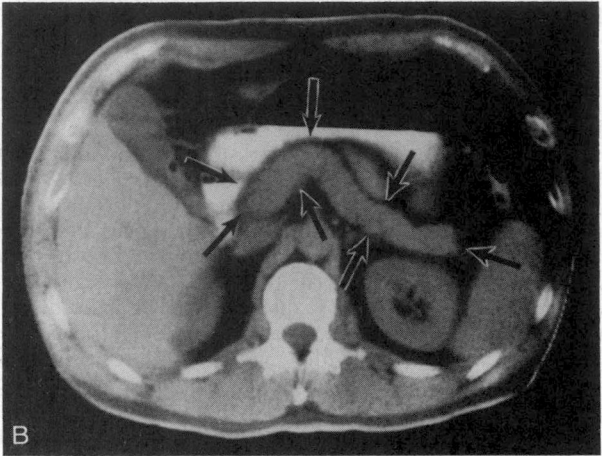

FIGURE 106–1. Normal pancreas demonstrated by ultrasound (A) and computed tomography (B). (Courtesy of Dr. Eugene P. DiMagno, Mayo Medical School, Rochester, Minnesota.)

cent; seven to eight risk factors, a mortality approaching 100 per cent.

Other blood tests, such as phospholipase A₂, methemalbumin, α₁-antitrypsin, α₂-macroglobulin, and, most recently, the C-reactive protein and trypsinogen-activated peptide, have been reported to be helpful in predicting severity of disease.

Course and Complications

In most patients acute pancreatitis is mild, requiring less than 1 week of hospitalization, but 5 to 25 per cent of patients have a more complicated course. The complications of pancreatitis (Table 106–3) can be divided into those that occur early (within the first week or two after admission) and those that occur late (more than 2 weeks after admission). The most serious of the early complications, usually found with necrotizing pancreatitis, are shock and pulmonary failure.

The pathogenesis of shock in acute pancreatitis can be hemorrhage into the substance of the pancreas or extravasation of massive amounts of plasma into the retroperitoneum. Release of vasoactive substances that cause vasodilation or myocardial depression may play an ancillary role. *The adult respiratory distress syndrome* (Ch. 70), the most serious of the pulmonary complications, is thought to be caused by injury of pulmonary capillaries and surfactant by circulating pancreatic enzymes, such as phospholipase A₂. The autodigested, necrotic pancreas may be sterile or secondarily infected with enteric organisms (infected necrosis). Severe hypocalcemia (serum calcium < 7 mg per deciliter) is associated with a more serious prognosis. The etiology of hypocalcemia is thought to be multifactorial, including concomitant hypoalbuminemia (the most prevalent cause), complexing of calcium to fatty acids released in the vicinity of the pancreas, and inadequate secretion or increased inactivation of parathyroid hormone or refractoriness to its action. Fluid collections and inflammatory debris may form between the pancreas and adjacent organs (Fig. 106–3). Most of these pseudocysts resolve sponta-

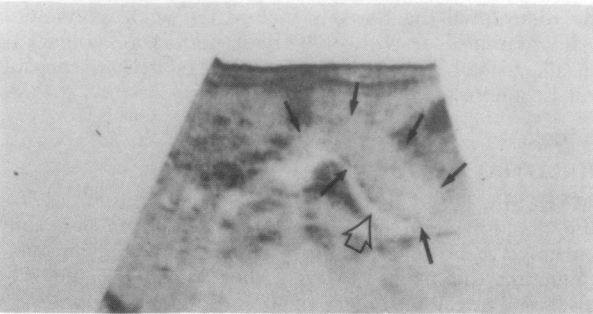

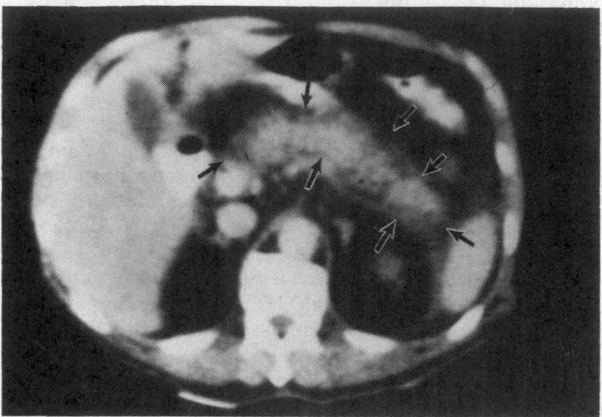

FIGURE 106–2. Diffusely enlarged pancreas of acute pancreatitis demonstrated by ultrasonography (*above*) and computed tomography (*below*). The large arrow on the sonogram points to the splenic vein. (Courtesy of Dr. Henry I. Goldberg, Department of Radiology, University of California at San Francisco.)

neously, but some may persist and become infected. Infected pseudocysts or abscesses, the most common causes of late morbidity and mortality in acute pancreatitis, should be suspected in patients who have recurrent or persistent fever into the second or third week of illness. Serial CT scans can detect most, but not all, fluid collections but cannot conclusively confirm or exclude infection. Fever spikes within the first week are common in severe pancreatitis and may be seen with either sterile or infected necrosis.

TABLE 106–2. ADVERSE PROGNOSTIC FACTORS IN SEVERE ACUTE PANCREATITIS

| Ranson's Criteria[1, 2] | | Modified Glasgow Criteria[3] |
Nongallstone	Gallstone	
On admission	**On admission**	**Within 48 hours**
Age >55	Age >70	Age >55
WBC >16,000/μl	WBC >18,000/μl	WBC >15,000/μl
Glu >200 mg/dl	Glu >220 mg/dl	Glu >180 mg/dl
LDH >350 IU/L	LDH >400 IU/L	BUN >96 mg/dl
AST >250 IU/L	AST >250 IU/L	LDH >600 IU/L
		Albumin <3.3 gm/dl
Within 48 hours	**Within 48 hours**	Calcium <8 mg/dl
HCT decrease >10 pts	HCT decrease >10 pts	Po₂ <60 mm Hg
BUN increase >5 mg/dl	BUN increase >2 mg/dl	
Calcium <8 mg/dl	Calcium <8 mg/dl	
Po₂ <60 mm Hg		
Base deficit >4 mEq/L	Base deficit >5 mEq/L	
Fluid deficit >6 L	Fluid deficit >4 L	

¹Ranson JH, Rifkind KM, Roses DF, et al.: Prognostic signs and the role of operative management in acute pancreatitis. Surg Gynecol Obstet 139:69, 1974.
²Ranson JHC: Etiological and prognostic factors in human acute pancreatitis: A review. Am J Gastroenterol 77:633, 1982.
³Blamey SL, Imrie CW, O'Neill J, et al.: Prognostic factors in acute pancreatitis. Gut 25:1340, 1984.
Glu = Glucose; LDH = lactic dehydrogenase; AST = aspartate aminotransferase; HCT = hematocrit; BUN = blood urea nitrogen.

TABLE 106–3. COMPLICATIONS OF ACUTE PANCREATITIS

Early
Vascular instability, shock
Pulmonary insufficiency—atelectasis, effusions, adult respiratory distress syndrome
Renal insufficiency—acute tubular necrosis
Metabolic disturbances—hypergylcemia, acidosis, hypocalcemia, hypomagnesemia
Acute fluid collections—pseudocysts
Infected necrosis
Colonic obstruction and necrosis
Pancreatic hemorrhage
Disseminated intravascular coagulation
Miscellaneous—metastatic fat necrosis (skin, bone, brain), psychosis, sudden blindness due to retinal artery occlusion

Late
Fluid collections—pseudocysts, abscess

Management

Patients with mild pancreatitis, who have few poor prognostic factors (see Table 106–2), are easily managed by avoidance of oral intake, intravenous hydration, and analgesia with meperidine. Pain usually subsides in 2 to 4 days and oral feedings can be resumed.

Patients with severe pancreatitis and more than three risk factors (see Table 106–2) frequently require close monitoring in an intensive care unit with specific attention to the complications that develop. Hypotension and vascular instability require intensive and frequently massive fluid resuscitation monitored by a central venous line. Metabolic complications such as hyperglycemia, hypocalcemia, and hypomagnesemia may require insulin and appropriate calcium or magnesium supplementation. Pulmonary failure may require mechanical ventilation with positive end-expiratory pressure therapy. When performed within the first few days of hospitalization, peritoneal dialysis has been reported to ameliorate and stabilize the severe vascular and pulmonary complications of early acute pancreatitis. Unfortunately, overall survival is not improved, as patients succumb from pancreatic abscess later in the course of their disease. The use of agents known to suppress pancreatic secretion, either directly or indirectly (e.g., glucagon, somatostatin, cimetidine, or nasogastric suction), or of enzyme inhibitors (e.g., aprotinin or gabexate mesilate) has also failed to improve the morbidity or mortality of acute pancreatitis in controlled studies. Whether antibiotics are useful in the treatment of acute pancreatitis has not been well defined. Many authorities use broad-spectrum antibiotics in patients having a complicated course, but without documentation of their effectiveness.

If gallstone pancreatitis is suspected (gallstones on sonogram, dilated common bile duct, elevated serum bilirubin and alkaline phosphatase), and the patient has severe disease (three or more Ranson criteria) without improvement within 48 hours, emergency endoscopic retrograde pancreatography should be considered. Emergent sphincterotomy with extraction of the common duct stone can improve the prognosis in this setting.

Patients with acute pancreatic fluid collections should be followed with serial CT scans. Most cysts subside spontaneously. Cysts that are greater than 5 to 6 cm in diameter after 6 weeks of observation usually do not resolve spontaneously. They should be drained percutaneously, endoscopically, or surgically to prevent complications such as perforation, infection, or hemorrhage. Early fluid collections accompanied by signs of sepsis in a toxic-appearing patient should be aspirated percutaneously under CT scan guidance. If bacteria are found on Gram's stain, prompt percutaneous or surgical drainage is indicated.

Surgery in acute pancreatitis is usually reserved for the following indications: (1) patients with an acute abdomen in whom a surgical emergency, such as a perforated viscus, cannot be excluded; (2) patients who require elective biliary surgery after gallstone pancreatitis has resolved (usually within 7 to 10 days after presentation); and (3) patients who require drainage of an infected fluid collection. In the absence of these indications, the role of surgery is more controversial. Patients with early pulmonary or vascular complications, who do not respond to intensive medical management, are sometimes operated upon with necrosectomy, total or partial pancreatectomy, wide debridement with sump drainage, multiple decompressions of adjacent organs, or a feeding jejunostomy. Dynamic CT scanning for evidence of extensive necrosis and percutaneous needle aspiration of pancreatic phlegmons for evidence of bacterial invasion may indicate which patients might benefit most from surgery.

CHRONIC PANCREATITIS

Pathogenesis

The pathogenesis of chronic pancreatitis is usually obscure, except for that of alcohol-induced disease. In an animal chronically fed large amounts of ethanol, the pancreas hypersecretes protein, which may precipitate as proteinaceous plugs in the small ductules. These plugs combine with the supersaturated solutions of calcium carbonate in pancreatic fluid to form small calcium carbonate stones, further obstructing the small ductules. There is some debate as to whether the pancreas normally secretes a

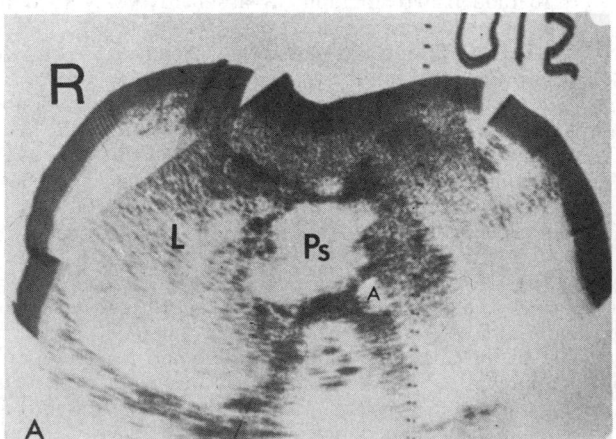
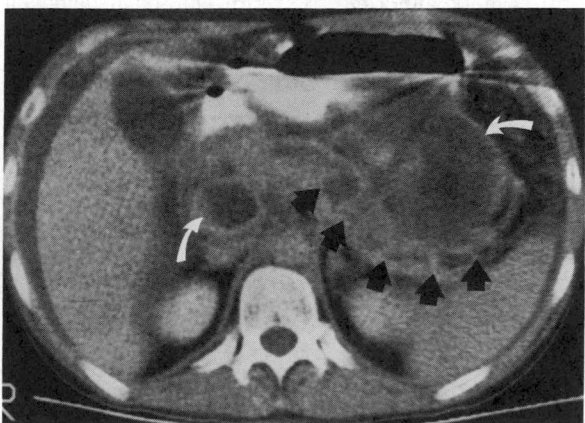

FIGURE 106–3. *A*, A pseudocyst demonstrated by ultrasonography. Ps = pseudocyst; A = aorta; L = liver; R = right of patient. (Courtesy of Dr. Dennis A. Sarti, Dept. of Radiological Sciences, University of California at Los Angeles, and Radiology 125:789, 1977.) *B*, A CT scan through the region of the tail, body, and head of the pancreas demonstrates the presence of two pancreatic pseudocysts (*curved white arrows*). The larger of the two extends from the tail of the pancreas anteriorly to compress a portion of the greater curvature of the stomach, here denoted by contrast material in the dependent portion and an air-fluid level. The smaller of the two is well circumscribed and located in the head of the pancreas. Both pseudocysts are of low CT density and well-described margins. In addition, the pancreatic duct (*black arrows*) is dilated and irregular in contour, a finding typical of a chronic pancreatitis. (Courtesy of Dr. Henry Goldberg, University of California at San Francisco.)

TABLE 106–4. ETIOLOGIC ASSOCIATIONS WITH CHRONIC PANCREATITIS

Nonobstructive
  Chronic alcoholism
  Tropical/nutritional
  Inherited
  Traumatic
  Metabolic—hypertriglyceridemia, hypercalcemia
  Idiopathic
Obstructive
  A. Benign obstruction—localized fibrosis of the duct, pancreas divisum with obstruction of accessory ampulla
  B. Neoplastic obstruction—tumors of the ampulla or ductal system

specific protein inhibitor of stone formation, insufficient secretion of which leads to a stone-forming diathesis. Blockage of the ductules, and later of the large ducts including the main pancreatic duct, leads to periductular and intralobular fibrosis, to loss of acinar parenchyma, and eventually to destruction of the islets of Langerhans. Chronic pancreatitis secondary to alcohol sometimes progresses even if alcohol ingestion is discontinued.

When the pancreatic ductal system is obstructed by other processes, such as by benign or malignant tumors, the duct distal to the obstruction becomes dilated and the acinar parenchyma becomes atrophic and fibrotic. This form of pancreatitis, termed obstructive pancreatitis, can be partially reversed if the obstruction is relieved.

Etiologic Associations (Table 106–4)

The most common cause of chronic pancreatitis is chronic alcoholism, usually present for more than 10 years by the time of presentation. Most alcoholics do not develop pancreatitis, so that unknown genetic, dietary, or environmental factors may play protective roles. Diets either high or low in fat content are thought by some to be additional risk factors in the development of alcoholic pancreatitis. Some alcoholics with pancreatitis develop hypertriglyceridemia after ingesting alcohol; possibly this metabolic aberration initiates pancreatitis in this subset of patients.

If alcoholism is excluded, most patients with chronic pancreatitis in the United States have no demonstrable cause, and therefore the disorder is classified as idiopathic. Idiopathic pancreatitis can present at any age and be associated with a spectrum of findings from mild functional disturbances of the pancreas with a normal ductal system to advanced calcific disease with markedly abnormal ducts. Notably, acute pancreatitis associated with gallstones rarely if ever leads to chronic pancreatitis.

Pancreatitis can be inherited as a rare autosomal dominant trait, presenting as acute or chronic pancreatitis with prominent pancreatolithiasis. Rarely, chronic pancreatitis may result from trauma or from metabolic disturbances, such as hypertriglyceridemia and hyperparathyroidism.

A form of calcific chronic pancreatitis, termed nutritional or tropical pancreatitis, occurs in children and young adults in southern India and some other parts of the developing world. It is speculated that this puzzling form of pancreatitis may be caused by a combination of factors, including genetic factors, protein and calorie deficiency, and/or ingestion of potentially injurious dietary factors, such as cassava. Affected individuals present most frequently with signs and symptoms of diabetes mellitus.

Clinical Presentation

Chronic pancreatitis presents most often with *abdominal pain*. Pain can occur either in discrete episodes lasting hours to days or can persist for months or even years at a time. On occasion, chronic pancreatitis is painless and patients present with the sequela of exocrine or endocrine insufficiency: steatorrhea, weight loss, or diabetes mellitus. Weight loss may also be due to avoidance of food, as pain is frequently exacerbated after eating. Pain may be due to (1) perineural irritation of the nerves supplying the pancreas, (2) dilatation of the pancreatic duct, (3) the presence of a pancreatic pseudocyst, or (4) a combination of these factors. Chronic pancreatitis and cancer of the pancreas

may present in a similar manner, making it difficult to differentiate between them.

Diagnosis

BLOOD TESTS. Serum amylase and lipase are often mildly elevated during acute exacerbations of abdominal pain in chronic pancreatitis, but not to the degree seen in acute pancreatitis. These enzyme markers are frequently normal, however, as a result of loss of pancreatic parenchyma. The immunoassays, such as the radioimmunoassay for trypsinogen, are better markers of pancreatic insufficiency. With severe pancreatic insufficiency leading to steatorrhea, the serum trypsinogen level falls below normal in 80 to 85 per cent of patients. With milder forms of the illness, trypsinogen levels are low in only 15 to 20 per cent of patients. A low trypsinogen level is highly specific for chronic pancreatic exocrine deficiency.

URINE TESTS. The bentiromide (Chymex) absorption test measures the chymotrypsin component of pancreatic exocrine function. This test, described in Ch. 102, can detect about 90 per cent of patients with steatorrhea, but its specificity is only about 80 per cent. The pancreo-lauryl test, similar in principle to the bentiromide test, is commonly employed in Europe, but not in the United States.

TUBED PANCREATIC FUNCTION TESTS. In the most sensitive test to detect chronic pancreatitis, a double-lumen tube is placed fluoroscopically into the C loop of the duodenum. Careful collection of pancreatic and intestinal juices is made after a stimulus (secretin or cholecystokinin) is given. Analysis of duodenal contents for bicarbonate or enzyme concentrations can determine mild, moderate, or severe exocrine insufficiency of the pancreas. In the simpler Lundh test, a defined liquid meal with various nutrients is used to stimulate pancreatic secretion, and trypsin concentrations are measured in duodenal secretions.

STOOL TESTS. The qualitative and quantitative tests for stool fat and the use of these and other tests for detecting pancreatic exocrine deficiency are described in Ch. 102.

IMAGING TESTS. The plain film of the abdomen can visualize calcifications within the pancreas. Calcifications, which may be localized or diffuse, represent calcium carbonate stones in the small or large ducts, not calcium in the parenchyma of the pancreas. Oblique views, as well as anteroposterior views, allow the calcifications to be seen best. Pancreatic calcification is usually diagnostic of chronic pancreatitis. Small amounts of calcium may be missed on plain films of the abdomen but detected on the more sensitive CT scans of the pancreas. Other findings on CT scan include masses within the organ and dilatations of the main pancreatic duct (see Fig. 94–3). The latter two findings can occur also with cancer of the pancreas (Ch. 107). Early in chronic pancreatitis the small secondary ductules become blunted and dilated, changes that later extend to the major ducts. Endoscopic retrograde pancreatography is a sensitive way to detect these diagnostic changes.

OTHER TESTS. An abnormal Schilling test (vitamin B_{12} absorption), corrected by pancreatic enzyme preparations, is a highly specific but not a sensitive test (sensitivity of about 30 to 40 per cent) for diagnosing chronic pancreatitis (Ch. 132). Clinical vitamin B_{12} deficiency in chronic pancreatitis is rare. The CA 19-9 radioimmunoassay blood test, a tumor-associated marker, may be helpful in differentiating chronic pancreatitis from cancer of the pancreas. Very high blood levels of this antigen suggest cancer of the pancreas.

SEQUENCE OF TESTS. A logical sequence in ordering these tests is to advance from the simple and less invasive ones to the more difficult and expensive tests, as deemed necessary. A plain film of the abdomen should be obtained from the patient presenting with chronic abdominal pain in order to detect calcification. A serum trypsinogen level and a urinary bentiromide test might also be considered simple, inexpensive, and noninvasive tests. Symptoms of steatorrhea suggest pancreatic exocrine insufficiency and may be evaluated as described in Ch. 102. If the simple tests are not diagnostic, CT scanning, endoscopic pancreatography, and/or tubed function tests may be employed as indicated.

Course and Complications

Usually in chronic pancreatitis, attacks of abdominal pain precede calcification of the gland. With time, calcification may become evident and with further progression, steatorrhea and/or diabetes may develop. Secretion of pancreatic lipase must be diminished by more than 90 per cent before steatorrhea develops. Despite fat malabsorption, deficiency of fat-soluble vitamins is uncommon. The painful attacks tend to diminish over time (5 to 10 years), as endocrine and exocrine insufficiencies worsen. Abstinence from alcohol also lessens the frequency of painful attacks, but exocrine and endocrine insufficiencies may progress notwithstanding. Diabetes secondary to pancreatitis may exhibit with time some of the microvascular complications seen with other causes of diabetes (Ch. 218).

Chronic pancreatitis may be complicated by pseudocysts, pancreatic ascites, or biliary obstruction. Pseudocysts usually occur anterior to the pancreas. If a pseudocyst develops posteriorly, however, it may dissect down or up fascial planes and appear in atypical locations, such as the mediastinum, neck, or pelvis. Moderate to large pseudocysts (>5 to 6 cm in diameter) that do not resolve by 6 weeks will probably not resolve spontaneously and drainage procedures are advised (Fig. 106–3). In practice, if a CT scan obtained within several days of a painful attack of pancreatitis demonstrates a large pseudocyst with a thick wall, it probably is chronic rather than acute. Percutaneous drainage usually results in recurrence unless drainage catheters are left in place for some time. Endoscopic techniques using electrocautery or laser can create drainage fistulas between the cyst and adjacent stomach or duodenum, but surgical drainage with anastomosis to an adjacent organ is usually the procedure of choice. If large pseudocysts are not drained, they may become infected or perforated or bleed internally or into adjacent structures, such as the stomach, intestine, or retroperitoneum.

Pancreatic ascites occurs when a tear in the pancreatic duct or pseudocyst communicates with the peritoneal cavity. This most frequently occurs gradually in the absence of significant abdominal pain. Analysis of peritoneal fluid shows an elevation in protein content and in amylase concentration (higher than its serum concentration).

Biliary obstruction, an insidious complication of chronic pancreatitis, is caused by compression of the distal common bile duct as it passes through the fibrotic head of the pancreas. It is suspected in patients with chronic pancreatitis who have persistent elevations of serum alkaline phosphatase activity. Some of these patients develop dilatation of the common bile duct, jaundice, pruritus, biliary sepsis, and, rarely, secondary biliary cirrhosis.

Management

The most difficult task in the treatment of chronic pancreatitis is the control of abdominal pain. Exacerbations of pain frequently require hospitalization. The acute attacks usually respond to abstinence from oral intake and the use of intravenous fluids and parenteral analgesics. Oral narcotic analgesics are usually required for chronic unremitting pain, and addiction is common. Abstinence from alcohol may lessen the frequency and severity of pain. In a few patients with mild forms of chronic pancreatitis, pain may be improved by the oral administration of large doses of oral pancreatic proteolytic enzyme preparations, which tend to reduce endogenous pancreatic secretion by a negative feedback mechanism, thus "putting the pancreas at rest." Non–enteric-coated pancreatic enzyme preparations, such as Viokase, Cotazyme, or Ilozyme, five to eight pills with meals, may be helpful. Failure of response may be due to destruction of the enzymes by gastric acid. Concomitant use of preparations to neutralize acid, such as sodium bicarbonate or aluminum antacids, or of histamine receptor blockers (e.g., cimetidine or ranitidine) to inhibit acid secretion, may improve results. Magnesium- and calcium-containing antacids should not be used, as these complex with fatty acids and interfere with their absorption. Alternatively, enteric-coated enzyme preparations, such as Pancrease, Entolase, or Creon, two to three pills with meals, may be tried. Unfortunately, pancreatic enzyme therapy is usually unsuccessful in managing the painful attacks of chronic pancreatitis. Percutaneous CT-guided celiac nerve blocks with phenol or alcohol have been tried to control pain with some degree of success, as have biofeedback and endoscopically placed pancreatic stents. Improvement of pain has been reported to result from endoscopic sphincterotomy followed by basket removal of pancreatic stones,

and from extracorporeal shock wave lithotripsy of large stones with subsequent endoscopic removal. For intractable pain, different surgical approaches are sometimes attempted after endoscopic retrograde pancreatography delineates the pancreatic ductal anatomy: celiac ganglionectomies, splanchnicectomies, various resections of the pancreas (distal pancreatectomy to 95 per cent or total pancreatectomy), drainage of pseudocysts, and lateral pancreaticojejunostomy (Puestow procedure). Surgical series report a 70 to 90 per cent success rate in alleviating abdominal pain.

Pancreatic steatorrhea is treated with adequate doses of oral pancreatic enzyme therapy as described above. If symptomatic steatorrhea persists, a low-fat diet (<40 grams per day) can improve symptoms. Supplementation of the diet with medium-chain triglycerides can improve caloric intake. The diabetes mellitus that accompanies chronic pancreatitis usually requires treatment with insulin.

Medical management of pancreatic ascites consists of large-volume paracentesis and total parenteral nutrition. If medical management is unsuccessful, an endoscopic retrograde pancreatogram should be performed to define the site of leakage for surgical repair. Internal drainage of pseudocysts, anastomosis between bowel and pancreas, or pancreatic resection is performed in this setting.

The need and timing of any intervention with regard to biliary obstruction depend on the level of symptoms (jaundice, pruritus, fever) and the fear of the possible development of the complications (sepsis, biliary cirrhosis). Endoscopic placement of biliary stents or surgical bypass of the obstructed ducts (e.g., choledochoduodenostomy, choledochojejunostomy) can successfully decompress the duct.

Bradley EL, Clements JL, Gonzalez AC: The natural history of pancreatic pseudocysts: A unified concept of management. Am J Surg 137:135, 1979. *The classic paper on the natural history of pseudocysts.*

DiMagno EP, Go VLW, Summerskill WHJ: Relations between pancreatic enzyme outputs and malabsorption in severe pancreatic insufficiency. N Engl J Med 288:813, 1973. *The classic paper on the pathophysiology of fat malabsorption in chronic pancreatitis.*

Neoptolemos JP, Carr-Locke DL, London NJ, et al.: Controlled trial of urgent endoscopic retrograde cholangiopancreatography and endoscopic sphincterotomy versus conservative treatment for acute pancreatitis due to gallstones. Lancet 2:979, 1988. *An important study delineating the usefulness of urgent endoscopic sphincterotomy in gallstone pancreatitis.*

Ranson JHC: Etiological and prognostic factors in human acute pancreatitis: A review. Am J Gastroenterol 77:633, 1982. *Ranson describes his classification of risk factors that guide the early prognosis of acute pancreatitis in a given patient.*

Rattner DW, Warshaw AL: Surgical intervention in acute pancreatitis. Crit Care Rev 16:89, 1988. *A good review of the surgical management of acute pancreatitis, its indications and limitations.*

Sarner M, Cotton PB: Classification of pancreatitis. Gut 25:756, 1984.

Singer MV, Gyr K: Revised classification of pancreatitis; report of the second international symposium on the classification of pancreatitis in Marseille, France, March 28–30, 1984. Gastroenterology 89:683, 1985. *Two important international meetings defined and classified the different forms of pancreatitis.*

Slaff J, Jacoson D, Tillman CR, et al.: Protease specific suppression of pancreatic exocrine secretion. Gastroenterology 87:44, 1984. *This paper explains the rationale for the use of oral enzymes to relieve the pain of chronic pancreatitis.*

Steer ML: Classification and pathogenesis of pancreatitis. Surg Clin North Am 69:467, 1989. *A good review of the different theories of the pathogenesis of acute pancreatitis.*

Steinberg WM, Schlesselman S: Treatment of acute pancreatitis: Comparison of animal vs. human studies. Gastroenterology 93:1420, 1987. *An analysis of the controlled medical trials in acute pancreatitis, giving the reasons for the negative results.*

107 Carcinoma of the Pancreas

Eugene P. DiMagno

DEFINITION

Ductal adenocarcinoma, comprising 90 per cent of pancreatic cancers, is a relentlessly progressive and fatal disease. Most tumors are moderately well differentiated mucinous carcinomas arising from the cuboid epithelium of pancreatic ducts. The remaining 10 per cent of pancreatic cancers are endocrine tumors (Ch. 220); acinar cell, giant cell, and epidermoid cancers; adenocanthomas; sarcomas; or cystadenocarcinomas.

INCIDENCE AND EPIDEMIOLOGY

Pancreatic cancer kills more Americans than any other neoplasm except breast, colorectal, lung, and prostate cancers. Each year approximately 27,000 Americans develop pancreatic cancer and 25,000 die. Median survival after diagnosis is only 4 to 8 months. Overall 5-year survival remains less than 1 per cent. Resection of the tumor improves median survival to 17 to 20 months, but 5-year survival remains less than 10 per cent. For reasons that are unclear, the incidence of pancreatic cancer has more than doubled during the past generation (from less than 5 to between 11 and 12 per 100,000 population).

Pancreatic cancer is associated with certain demographic characteristics and risk factors (Table 107–1). Pancreatic cancer occurs more frequently in men (1.5:1). Eighty per cent occur between ages 60 and 80; the disease is unusual under age 40. Patients with hereditary pancreatitis, members of families with the nonpolyposis colon cancer syndrome, and patients with diabetes mellitus of greater than 2 to 3 years' duration are at increased risk. The major environmental factors associated with an increased risk of pancreatic cancer are ingestion of a high-fat and cholesterol diet rich in linoleic acid and exposure to coal tar derivatives, coke, benzidine, and β-naphthylamine. It is unlikely that consumption of coffee, alcohol abuse, or a previous cholecystectomy or gastrectomy increases the risk of pancreatic cancer. The risk for pancreatic cancer may be reduced by eliminating cigarette smoking and eating a diet low in cholesterol and containing olive oil and fish as the main sources of fat.

PATHOPHYSIOLOGY AND CLINICAL MANIFESTATIONS (Table 107–2)

In pancreatic ductal adenocarcinoma, well-differentiated to poorly differentiated duct glands are embedded in a dense network of fibrous tissue. As it extends in the pancreas and surrounding tissue, the tumor envelops and fixes vessels and invades fat, lymph channels, and perineural areas. Symptoms and signs of pancreatic cancer are related to the location of the tumor within the gland and to the extension of the tumor to stomach, duodenum, bile duct, retroperitoneum, and porta hepatis. The presenting symptoms are nonspecific and most commonly consist of pain, jaundice, weight loss, and, rarely, diabetes mellitus.

Pain occurs in 90 per cent of patients. It may be vague and rather nonspecific and may occur up to 3 months before the onset of jaundice. Early in the course the pain may be ignored both by the patient and by the physician to whose attention it is brought. The tumor most commonly extends to the retroperitoneal space, producing visceral pain variously described as persistent, disagreeable, aching, increased by lying supine or by eating, and causing the patient to awaken at night. Relief is sometimes obtained by bending forward, lying on the side, and

TABLE 107–1. RISK FACTORS FOR PANCREATIC CANCER

Definite
Age >60
Male sex
Cigarette smoking
Hereditary pancreatitis
Nonpolyposis colon cancer syndrome
Diabetes mellitus

Probable
High-fat diet
Chemical exposure

Unlikely
Coffee
Alcohol
Prior cholecystectomy or gastrectomy

TABLE 107–2. CLINICAL MANIFESTATIONS OF PANCREATIC CANCER

Clinical Manifestations	Pancreatic Cancer of	
	Head (%)	Body and Tail (%)
Symptoms		
Weight loss	92	100
Jaundice	82	7
Pain	72	87
Anorexia	64	33
Dark urine	63	—
Light stools	62	—
Nausea	45	37
Vomiting	37	37
Weakness	35	43
Pruritus	24	—
Signs		
Jaundice	87	13
Palpable liver	83	33
Palpable gallbladder	29	—
Ascites	14	20
Abdominal mass	13	23

Data from Howard JM, Jordan GL: Cancer of the pancreas. Curr Probl Cancer 2(3):1, 1977; and DaVita VT Jr., Hellman S, Rosenberg SA (eds.): Cancer: Principles and Practice of Oncology. Philadelphia, J. B. Lippincott Company, 1985, p 100.

drawing the knees to the chest or chin and sometimes by crouching forward on four extremities.

Jaundice secondary to obstruction of the bile duct occurs early in the course of the disease in the 60 to 70 per cent of patients with carcinoma of the head of the pancreas. When carcinomas of the head of the pancreas arise in its central part or in the uncinate process, jaundice is usually not an early presentation. In cancer of the body and tail of the pancreas jaundice occurs late and is secondary to hepatic metastases or obstruction of the bile duct at the porta hepatis by lymphadenopathy. Painless jaundice is not a manifestation of pancreatic cancer.

Weight loss of more than 10 per cent of ideal body weight, almost universal, is usually due to both malabsorption and decreased food intake. Seventy-five per cent of patients malabsorb fat and 50 per cent malabsorb protein. Malabsorption occurs in patients who have a carcinoma of the head of the pancreas that obstructs the pancreatic duct and thereby produces pancreatic exocrine insufficiency. The particular features of pancreatic malabsorption are described in Ch. 102.

Glucose intolerance may be present in up to 80 per cent of patients with pancreatic cancer, but in most such patients diabetes is mild. Less than 5 per cent of patients have hyperphagia, polydipsia, and polyuria.

Other symptoms and signs include *depression, light-colored stools* (60 per cent of patients with carcinoma of the pancreatic head), *constipation,* and *emotional lability* (27 per cent of patient with carcinoma of the tail). *Vomiting* and *weakness* occur in one third of patients. More rarely patients exhibit superficial thrombophlebitis (Trousseau's syndrome) or gastrointestinal bleeding due either to direct extension of the tumor into the stomach or duodenum or to varices secondary to splenic vein obstruction. Metastases from pancreatic cancer of the body and tail may cause testicular enlargement and pain, whereas metastases to the temporal bone may produce sudden profound hearing loss, and metastases to the esophagus may lead to dysphagia.

Hepatomegaly and *jaundice* are present in 80 and 30 per cent of patients with pancreatic carcinoma of the head and body and tail, respectively. A palpable gallbladder (Courvoisier's sign) is present in 30 per cent of patients with carcinoma of the head of the pancreas. An abdominal mass or ascites is present in less than 20 per cent of patients. Ascites, splenomegaly, and peripheral edema may occur secondary to occlusion of the portal vein by tumors, whereas compression of the aorta or splenic artery may produce an abdominal bruit.

DIAGNOSIS

In patients suspected of having pancreatic cancer, an initial screening series of blood tests should be obtained, as well as a chest radiograph and an abdominal film to look for calcification

TABLE 107-3. DIAGNOSTIC ACCURACY OF IMAGING TESTS IN THE DIAGNOSIS OF PANCREATIC CANCER

	Sensitivity (%)	Specificity (%)	Predictive Value	
			Positive (%)	Negative (%)
Ultrasonography	74	84	78	79
Computed tomography	79	64	76	78
Endoscopic retrograde cholangiopancreatography	95	90	87	97

of the pancreas. As a group, patients with pancreatic cancer have higher values for serum lipase, amylase, and glucose than do other patients, but these tests do not distinguish between pancreatic cancer and pancreatitis. Similarly, serum alkaline phosphatase, aspartate aminotransferase, and bilirubin are commonly elevated, but these tests lack specificity in excluding hepatic disorders. Nonspecific findings on the chest radiograph and abdominal films may be present in patients with pancreatitis or pancreatic cancer. Pancreatic calcifications have a sensitivity of 95 per cent for the diagnosis of chronic pancreatitis, but primary ductal carcinomas, mucosal pancreatic cancers such as a mucinous cystadenocarcinoma (curvilinear calcification), and solid and papillary epithelial neoplasms can calcify. If obvious pulmonary or bony metastases are found, one may opt to perform no further diagnostic tests.

No sensitive serologic marker with tumor and organ specificity has been established as a routine diagnostic or screening test for pancreatic cancer. Currently available serologic tests include carcinoembryonic antigen (CEA), galactosyltransferase, monoclonal antibodies CA 19-9, CA-50, and DU-PAN-2, pancreatic oncofetal antigen, and pancreatic cancer–associated antigen. These tests have ranged in sensitivity from 50 to 85 per cent, but positive tests occur in up to 46 per cent of patients with benign diseases and in up to 65 per cent of those with other malignancies.

Pancreatic cancer is most readily diagnosed by imaging the pancreas with ultrasonography, computed tomography (CT), or endoscopic pancreatography. The diagnosis is usually confirmed by ultrasonographic or CT-guided percutaneous aspiration cytology of the pancreatic mass or biopsy of liver metastases. This technique is 90 per cent sensitive for the diagnosis of pancreatic cancer.

The sensitivity and specificity of ultrasonography and CT are approximately 80 per cent for the detection of a pancreatic mass or cancer (Table 107–3). Endoscopic retrograde cholangiopancreatography is 90 to 95 per cent sensitive and specific (Table 107–3). In practice, ultrasonography is commonly the first test used to diagnose pancreatic cancer (Fig. 107–1) because it is least expensive. When ultrasonography fails for technical reasons (10 per cent), or if the diagnosis is uncertain (20 per cent), CT is then performed. If doubt still exists, endoscopic retrograde pancreatography should be performed (see Fig. 94–2). Rarely is it necessary to perform an invasive pancreatic function test, in which either secretin or cholecystokinin is administered intravenously and pancreatic secretion is obtained through a tube placed into the duodenum. Patients with pancreatic cancer have a low volume of pancreatic secretion, but a normal bicarbonate concentration after secretin stimulation or reduced enzyme outputs after cholecystokinin stimulation. The algorithm in Figure 107–1 has a sensitivity and specificity of greater than 90 per cent.

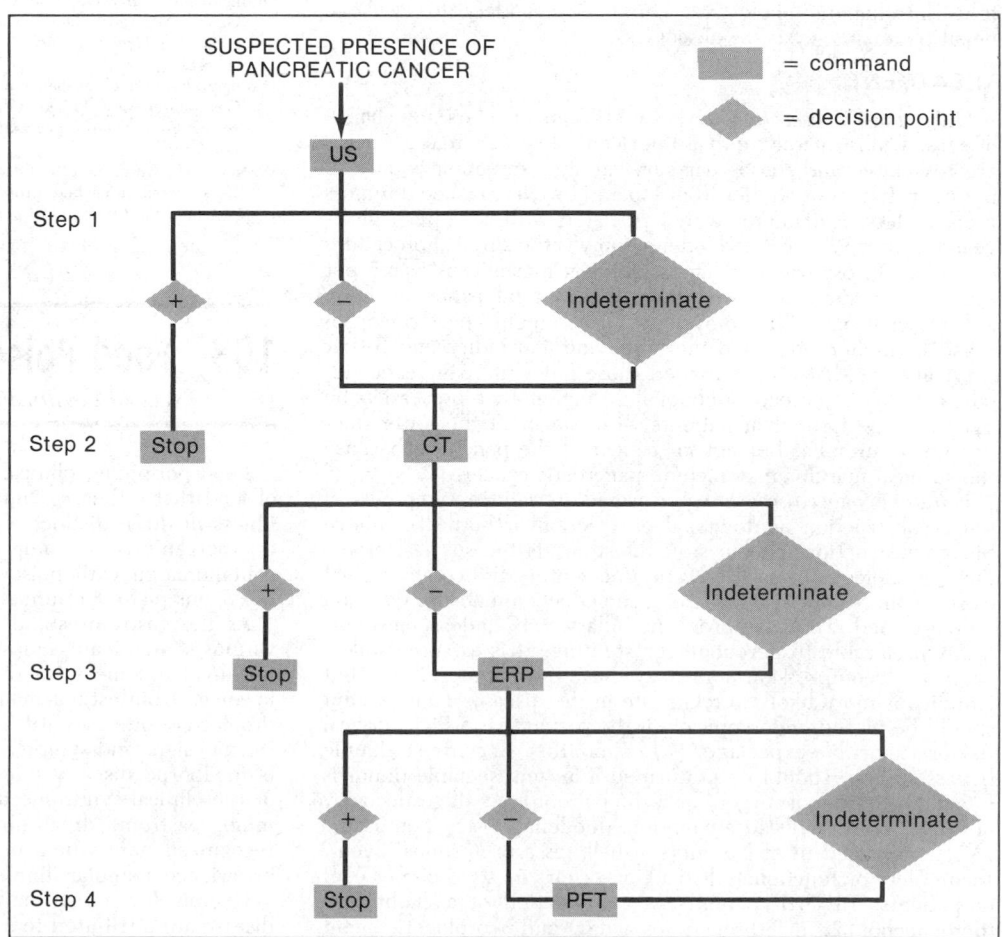

FIGURE 107–1. Algorithm for the diagnosis of pancreatic cancer. US = Ultrasonography; CT = computed tomography; ERP = endoscopic retrograde pancreatography; PFT = pancreatic function tests. (From DiMagno EP: Overview: Biology and diagnosis of pancreatic cancer. *In* Levin B [ed.]: Annual Clinical Conference on Cancer, Vol. 30, Gastrointestinal Cancer: Current Approaches to Diagnosis and Treatment. Houston, University of Texas Press, 1988, pp 299–308.)

TABLE 107–4. DIFFERENTIAL DIAGNOSIS OF PANCREATIC CANCER

Nonmalignant conditions
Chronic pancreatitis
Extrahepatic jaundice
    Common bile duct stones
    Bile duct stricture (secondary to previous biliary tract surgery or
        sclerosing cholangitis)
    Cholecystitis
Intrahepatic cholestatic jaundice
    Alcoholic hepatitis
    Toxins
    Cysts
    Abscess
Posterior penetrating duodenal or gastric ulcers
Depression
Functional bowel disorders

Malignant conditions
Retroperitoneal lymphomas
Bile duct cancer
Ampullary cancer
Gynecologic malignancies
Carcinoma of the duodenum or small intestine

DIFFERENTIAL DIAGNOSIS (Table 107–4)

The presenting symptoms and signs of pancreatic cancer are nonspecific. Indeed, most patients presenting with weight loss and abdominal pain, with or without jaundice, do not have pancreatic cancer. In patients without jaundice, the abdominal pain and weight loss of pancreatic cancer may be difficult to distinguish from an extensive list of disorders (Table 107–4). In jaundiced patients, it is extremely important to differentiate pancreatic cancer from potentially treatable conditions, such as common bile duct stones, chronic pancreatitis obstructing the common bile duct, bile duct stricture secondary to previous biliary tract surgery or sclerosing cholangitis, cholecystitis, and from intrahepatic cholestatic jaundice secondary to alcoholic hepatitis, toxins, cysts, or abscesses.

TREATMENT

Only *surgical resection* of pancreatic cancer offers any chance of cure. Unfortunately, only 10 per cent of all pancreatic cancers are resectable and the 5-year survival after resection is only 10 per cent. In recent studies from Japan, however, resected tumors 2 cm or less in diameter were associated with a 37 per cent 5-year survival. Pancreaticoduodenectomy is the surgical procedure of choice. In experienced hands, surgical mortality is 2 to 5 per cent. Other surgical procedures, such as total pancreatectomy and regional pancreatectomy, are not commonly performed because of higher operative mortality and morbidity and 5-year survival rates that do not exceed those following pancreaticoduodenectomy. Pancreaticoduodenal resection that preserves the pylorus is performed in patients with cancer of the lower duodenum or ampulla, but not for cancer of the pancreas, because the surgical margins may include pancreatic cancer.

Palliative procedures are performed to relieve symptoms of biliary obstruction or duodenal obstruction or both. To relieve biliary obstruction, cholecystojejunostomy is the surgical procedure of choice, unless the cystic duct enters the common duct close to the tumor. In this case, choledochojejunostomy should be performed. To decompress the biliary tree, endoscopic stenting is preferable to percutaneous stenting. It is as successful as surgical decompression and may have lower morbidity, but jaundice is more likely to recur late in the disease. Thus, a stent should be placed endoscopically if the patient has a high surgical risk or a short life expectancy (1 to 3 months). In contrast, double bypass surgery should be performed if an unresectable tumor is found at the time of surgery or if the patient has a life expectancy of 6 to 7 months, because complete duodenal obstruction occurs in 5 to 15 per cent of patients—usually as a preterminal event. Incomplete or functional obstruction occurs in 40 to 60 per cent of patients. In such patients, a combination of a cholinergic (bethanechol, 25 mg three times a day) and a prokinetic agent (metoclopramide, 10 mg four times a day) may alleviate symptoms of gastric stasis by enhancing gastric emptying.

No single agent or combination of *chemotherapeutic drugs* significantly prolongs or enhances the quality of life of patients with pancreatic cancer. 5-Fluorouracil (5-FU) produces a partial response rate in 10 to 15 per cent of patients, but its use is associated with a median survival of less than 20 weeks. Other agents have a similar limited effect (mitomycin C), even less effect (streptozotocin, doxorubicin, Epirubicin, ifosfamide, methyl-CCNU and high-dose methotrexate), or no effect (actinomycin D, carmustine, standard-dose methotrexate, cisplatin, melphalan, and L-asparaginase).

The combination of 5-FU or SMF (streptozotocin, mitomycin C, and 5-FU) and external beam radiation improves survival compared to radiation or chemotherapy alone. Intraoperative electron-beam radiation and ^{125}I implants do not improve survival in comparison to external-beam radiation. Even though these modalities may limit local tumor extension, they do not control liver and peritoneal metastases.

Pain can usually be successfully managed if analgesics are prescribed on a regular basis, adequate doses are used, and adjuvant drugs are used when necessary. Mild to moderate pain can be controlled with aspirin, acetaminophen, and nonsteroidal anti-inflammatory agents. If these drugs fail to relieve pain, opioid analgesics should be used (codeine or morphine). Addition of an antihistamine or an amphetamine to an opiate increases analgesia. Intraoperative or percutaneous neurolytic celiac plexus block is remarkably effective in controlling pain. If patients have intolerable pain, subcutaneous patient-controlled analgesia or epidural administration of narcotics affords pain relief.

Malabsorption can be reasonably well controlled by the ingestion of eight tablets of pancreatin with meals (total dose of lipase should be 30,000 IU). Two tablets should be taken immediately after eating a few bites, two tablets at the end of the meal, and four tablets interspersed during the meal (Ch. 102).

Cello JP: Carcinoma of the pancreas. *In* Sleisenger MH, Fordtran JS (eds.): Gastrointestinal Disease. Pathophysiology, Diagnosis, and Management. Philadelphia, W. B. Saunders Company, 1989, pp. 1872–1884. *A complete review of pancreatic cancer, with 67 references.*
DiMagno EP: Early diagnosis of chronic pancreatitis and pancreatic cancer. *In* Geokas MC (ed.): Difficult Diagnoses. Med. Clin. North Am. 72:979–992, 1988. *A review that includes the epidemiology and diagnosis of pancreatic cancer.*
DiMagno EP: Exocrine pancreatic neoplasia. *In* Yamada T (ed.): Textbook of Gastroenterology. Philadelphia, J. B. Lippincott Company, 1990. *This recent review is a general overview of pancreatic cancer and includes over 170 references.*
Warshaw AL, Swanson PS: What's new in general surgery. Pancreatic cancer in 1988. Possibilities and probabilities. Ann Surg 208:541, 1988. *A thorough review of the treatment of pancreatic cancer, with 164 references.*

108 Food Poisoning

David F. Altman

Food poisoning, clinical syndromes arising from the ingestion of food that either is contaminated or is itself toxic, may cause illness in three distinct ways: (1) by contamination of food with microorganisms or their products (most common); (2) by its contamination with poisonous chemicals; or (3) by ingestion of poisonous plants or animals.

As the gastrointestinal tract is the mode of entry for these various contaminants, most illnesses associated with food poisoning involve some form of gastroenteritis, with either upper or lower gastrointestinal manifestations predominating. Other syndromes are often identifiable by extraintestinal (particularly neurologic) signs and symptoms. It is difficult to identify single cases of foodborne disease unless the incubation period is very short or the clinical syndrome distinctive because of the frequency of minor gastrointestinal illnesses. Foodborne disease is usually recognized only when an outbreak occurs and several persons experience a similar illness after ingesting a common food.

Overall, fewer than half of the known outbreaks of foodborne disease are attributed to a specific etiologic agent. Nevertheless, it is important to attempt to define the etiology of such an outbreak. Prophylaxis against secondary spread of an infection may be important (e.g., in shigellosis). A more accurate prognosis for the victim may become available, as some illnesses are self-limited and short-lived, whereas others may have a chronic residual effect. Perhaps most important, faulty food handling or storage techniques may be identified and further outbreaks prevented.

To facilitate identification of possible agents in foodborne illness, such syndromes can be classified by their incubation period and the type of clinical symptoms (see Table 108–1). With the possibilities thus limited, specific sampling of food or bacteriologic cultures of blood or stool may quickly lead to the correct diagnosis.

BACTERIAL FOOD POISONING

As an aid to diagnosis and therapy, bacterial food poisoning can be conveniently classified as (1) that due to the ingestion of living microorganisms, (2) that due to the ingestion of a toxin produced by microorganisms in food prior to its ingestion, or (3) that due to enterotoxins produced in the gut by pathogens only after their ingestion.

The most important "infectious" types of food poisoning, requiring ingestion of living organisms, are *Salmonella* gastroenteritis and *Shigella* dysentery, which are dealt with in Ch. 314 and 315, respectively. Other organisms responsible in this way include *Campylobacter jejuni, Escherichia coli, Vibrio cholerae, Vibrio parahaemolyticus, Bacillus cereus,* and *Clostridium perfringens.* In addition, epidemics of listeriosis transmitted by food and a foodborne outbreak of streptococcal pharyngitis have both been reported.

The "toxin" type of food poisoning most often identified is due to *Staphylococcus aureus.* The syndrome of botulism caused by ingestion of the toxin produced by *Clostridium botulinum* is discussed in Ch. 309.

Staphylococcal Food Poisoning

ETIOLOGY. This form of food poisoning is caused by an enterotoxin produced by multiplying staphylococci before the contaminated food is ingested. Most but not all strains known to elaborate enterotoxins are coagulase-positive *Staphylococcus aureus.* The two major sources of contamination are human carriers (90 per cent, usually nasal or skin) and cows with mastitis. Staphylococcal food poisoning requires not only contamination of food with the microorganisms but also a period of some hours during which they may multiply, as may occur during slow cooling after cooking or if food is held at ambient temperature. Subsequent reheating may destroy the organism but not the remarkably heat-resistant toxin, the proximate cause of the clinical illness.

PATHOGENESIS, CLINICAL MANIFESTATIONS, AND TREATMENT. In experimental animals enterotoxins destroy gastrointestinal mucosal cells, evoke an inflammatory response, and may affect other organ systems, including the emetic centers in the brain. Symptoms usually begin 2 to 4 hours after ingestion of the toxin, heralded by salivation and followed rapidly by nausea, vomiting, abdominal cramping, and diarrhea. The illness usually is short, rarely lasting 24 hours, and often is subsiding by

the time medical attention is sought. It may occasionally be life-threatening, especially in the elderly or in persons with other serious illness. Therapy is supportive and symptomatic, the primary goal being to restore extracellular fluid volume with parenteral fluids as necessary. Antibiotic therapy may worsen the course of the illness.

PREVENTION. Proper food handling prevents staphylococcal food poisoning. Sanitary measures and personal hygiene can prevent contamination of the food to some degree. More importantly, enterotoxin is not produced at ordinary domestic refrigerator temperatures. Foods should not be left to cool slowly, especially in large containers, and should be taken from the refrigerator (and reheated, if required) immediately before serving.

Clostridial Food Poisoning

ETIOLOGY. *Clostridium perfringens* type A is the third most common bacterial cause of food poisoning in the United States. Clostridial poisoning typically occurs in fairly large outbreaks. The organism is ubiquitous, being found in most samples of raw meat, human and animal feces, flies, soil, and dirt from kitchens. Both heat-sensitive and heat-resistant strains can cause outbreaks. Usually outbreaks follow the cooking of meat, poultry, or beans at a temperature (usually less than 100°C) high enough to kill vegetative forms but insufficient to destroy heat-resistant spores. Oxygen is driven out of the food, thereby lowering the oxidation-reduction potential of the medium. During slow cooling the spores germinate, encouraged by the relatively anaerobic environment and the rich supply of amino acids and other growth factors. If the food is not reheated to a temperature high enough to inactivate the recently multiplied organism, ingestion may result in illness.

PATHOGENESIS AND CLINICAL MANIFESTATIONS. Clostridial food poisoning follows ingestion of living organisms, as the production of the enterotoxin responsible for the clinical manifestations occurs with sporulation in the alkaline environment of the small intestine. The incubation period is usually 7 to 15 hours after ingestion but may be as long as 24 hours. The usual symptoms are abdominal cramps and diarrhea; nausea, vomiting, and fever are much less common. The illness is self-limited, rarely lasting more than 24 hours. Treatment rarely is necessary and should always be confined to efforts at symptomatic relief. The few deaths recorded have been in elderly or debilitated patients.

PREVENTION. Food is best served immediately after cooking. If it is to be kept, it should be cooled rapidly. Cooked meat should always be kept either cold, below 5°C, or hot, over 60°C. This is especially true of food prepared in large batches.

Vibrio parahaemolyticus Food Poisoning

V. parahaemolyticus, a gram-negative facultative anaerobe found in marine water and fauna throughout the world, lives in sediment of coastal and estuarian waters during cold winter months. As the temperature rises in spring and summer, the organism leaves the sediment and colonizes animal life, especially shellfish and crustaceans. Not all strains are pathogenic.

TABLE 108–1. CLINICAL INDICATORS OF THE ETIOLOGY OF FOODBORNE ILLNESS

Predominant Symptomatology	Mean Incubation Period			
	< 2 Hours	2–7 Hours	8–14 Hours	> 14 hours
Upper intestinal	Heavy metals	S. aureus B. cereus		
Lower intestinal			C. perfringens B. cereus	V. cholerae Enterotoxic or invasive E. coli Shigella spp. V. parahaemolyticus Salmonella
Both upper and lower gastrointestinal				V. parahaemolyticus
Extragastrointestinal, i.e., some gastrointestinal plus others, usually paresthesias or other abnormal sensory complaint	Scombrotoxin Shellfish toxin Mushroom toxin (early)	Ciguatoxin	Mushroom toxin (delayed)	C. botulinum

The pathogenesis of the illness is not clearly defined, and different serotypes may produce disease by different mechanisms. The presence of fecal leukocytes and occasionally bloody diarrhea implies bacterial invasion and damage of the gut mucosa.

Virtually all outbreaks of *V. parahaemolyticus* food poisoning occur during warm months of the year and are associated with the ingestion of raw or improperly refrigerated seafood. Although originally described in Japan, cases have occurred in other parts of Asia and on the Atlantic, Gulf, and Pacific coasts of the United States. The incubation period is usually between 12 and 24 hours but has been as long as 96 hours. Explosive watery diarrhea is present in more than 90 per cent of cases, with nausea, vomiting, and abdominal cramps as common accompaniments. Fever, headache, and chills occur less often. The diagnosis is suspected when a typical illness occurs after eating seafood and is confirmed by recovery of the organism from stool. Treatment is rarely necessary, as the illness infrequently lasts more than 3 days. However, in protracted cases, antibiotic treatment with tetracycline or ampicillin may shorten the illness.

Prevention depends on the recognition both of the potential for contamination of seafood with *V. parahaemolyticus* during warm months and of the predisposition of organisms to multiply under conditions of inadequate refrigeration. Cooked seafood may also become cross-contaminated when stored under proper conditions with a raw source.

Bacillus cereus Food Poisoning

Bacillus cereus, an anaerobic, motile, spore-forming, gram-positive rod, causes two separate clinical forms of the foodborne disease. An emetic form, clinically identical to staphylococcal food poisoning, is associated with contaminated fried rice. A diarrheal form has a longer incubation period and predominantly lower gastrointestinal symptoms, reminiscent of *Clostridium perfringens* food poisoning. Cell-free filtrates derived from *B. cereus* strains responsible for this latter form of illness stimulate the adenylate cyclase–cyclic adenosine monophosphate (cAMP) system in intestinal epithelial cells. This activity is destroyed by heat, thus resembling cholera enterotoxin. The illnesses are usually mild and self-limited, and antibiotics are not indicated. No fatalities have been reported. As the organism commonly occurs in soil and in many dried or processed foods, careful food handling is most important in prevention of the disease. *B. cereus* may be found in uncooked rice, for example, and heat-resistant spores may survive boiling. If the rice is left unrefrigerated, the spores may then germinate and produce toxin. Flash frying or rewarming before serving is often not sufficient to destroy the preformed, heat-stable toxin. The disease thus can be prevented by prompt refrigeration of boiled rice.

Benenson AS (ed.): Foodborne intoxication. *In* Control of Communicable Diseases in Man. 14th ed. Washington, D.C., American Public Health Association, 1985, pp 142–152. *A brief compendium of information on foodborne illness, with emphasis on identification and prevention.*

Centers for Disease Control: Foodborne disease outbreaks, annual summary, 1982. *In* CDC Surveillance Summaries, 35:7ss, 1986. *An annual compendium of reports of foodborne diseases in the United States, with analysis of vehicles of transmission and contributing factors to contamination for each type of infection identified.*

Linnan MJ, Mascola L, Lou XD, et al.: Epidemic listeriosis associated with Mexican-style cheese. N Engl J Med 319:823, 1988. *A classic description of an epidemiologic investigation of a recently recognized cause of foodborne illness.*

Morris JG Jr., Black RE: Cholera and other vibrioses in the United States. N Engl J Med 312:343, 1985. *This article reviews both common and more obscure illnesses caused by these organisms.*

Shandera WX, Tacket CO, Blake PA: Food poisoning due to *Clostridium perfringens* in the United States. J Infect Dis 147:167, 1983. *This article provides a thorough review of the pathogenesis of this cause of food poisoning, as well as information on epidemiology and diagnosis.*

Terranova W, Blake PA: *Bacillus cereus* food poisoning. N Engl J Med 298:143, 1978. *A brief but comprehensive review of the various forms of this illness.*

CHEMICAL FOOD POISONING

Chemicals may cause food poisoning following accidental contamination of food prior to its preparation or during storage or as food additives or preservatives. Thus various forms of metallic poisoning, discussed in Ch. 533, can occur when food, particularly acid liquids, comes in contact with certain metals, especially cadmium, copper, tin, or zinc.

The so-called Chinese restaurant syndrome, in which individuals develop sensations of burning skin, facial pressure, chest pressure, and headaches 10 to 20 minutes after eating certain Chinese foods (especially won ton soup), has been attributed to the use of monosodium L-glutamate (MSG). The symptoms appear to be a pharmacologic effect of MSG, obeying a dose-effect relationship, but with a widely variable threshold for an oral dose.

Sodium nitrite, widely used as a preservative in smoked meats, has been blamed for the "hot dog headache" seen in some persons. In addition, because of its metabolism to nitrosamines it is suspected to be a potential carcinogen, although evidence for this is inconclusive.

L-Tryptophan, an essential amino acid, is available as an over-the-counter nutritional supplement and has been recommended for the treatment of depression, insomnia, and the premenstrual syndrome. It has now been associated with a potentially fatal disorder called the eosinophilia-myalgia syndrome. This illness is characterized by diffuse, severe myalgias and skin changes ranging from a morbilliform rash to scleroderma-like changes, all associated with peripheral blood eosinophilia. Some patients also develop a hypersensitivity pneumonitis, myocarditis, cerebral vasculitis, and a progressive polyneuropathy. Onset may be months to years after beginning use of L-tryptophan–containing products, and at least in some patients discontinuation leads to resolution of the symptoms. Some deaths have been reported, however. The syndrome is now believed to have been caused by the ingestion of a chemical constituent that arose from the manufacturing conditions of L-tryptophan at one company. This compound apparently decomposes to a carboxylic acid derivative in the presence of gastric acid. The syndrome is strikingly similar to the toxic oil syndrome that was epidemic in Spain in 1981 and that was linked to the consumption of denatured rapeseed oil sold as cooking oil.

Food additives such as aspartame and pesticides have been incriminated as a cause of foodborne disease. Although the former have not been conclusively identified as the source of illness, outbreaks of the latter have been documented. Contamination of watermelons by aldicarb caused gastrointestinal and neurologic symptoms in over 1000 individuals.

Martin RW, Duffy J, Engel AG, et al.: The clinical spectrum of the eosinophilia-myalgia syndrome associated with L-tryptophan ingestion. Ann Intern Med 113:124, 1990. *A description of a new syndrome, including clinical features and speculation on pathogenesis.*

Schaumburg HH, Byck R, Gerstil R, et al.: Monosodium L-glutamate: Its pharmacology and role in the Chinese restaurant syndrome. Science 163:826, 1969. *A careful analysis of MSG pharmacology and its dose-effect relationships.*

POISONOUS ANIMALS AND PLANTS

Fish and Shellfish Poisoning

Various toxins from vertebrate fish are capable of causing human illness. Most commonly this is due to toxin contained in musculature (ichthyosarcotoxins), of which nine types have been described. The most common fish poisonings worldwide—ciguatera, scombroid, and puffer fish poisoning—are attributable to ichthyosarcotoxins.

Two forms of shellfish poisoning, paralytic and neurotoxic, have been described. These are caused by toxins derived from dinoflagellates contaminating the shellfish.

CIGUATERA FISH POISONING. Ciguatera poisoning, the most common illness brought on by the ingestion of fish and seafood, follows the ingestion of ciguatoxin produced by the dinoflagellate *Gambierdiscus toxicus*. This marine organism is passed up the food chain, and more than 400 fish species, generally bottom-dwelling shore fish in temperate and tropical zones, have been implicated.

Ciguatoxin is a lipid-soluble, heat-stable substance that is resistant to gastric acid. It is believed to inhibit the calcium regulation of passive cell membrane sodium channels.

The onset of the illness usually occurs 1 to 6 hours after ingestion of toxic fish, but this time interval may vary from as soon as a few minutes to as long as 30 hours. Gastrointestinal symptoms, including abdominal cramps, nausea, vomiting, and diarrhea, predominate at the outset, along with numbness, pruritus, and paresthesias of the lips, tongue, and throat. Paresthesias may later involve the extremities, and in severe cases there may be abnormal temperature sensations, cranial nerve palsies, hypotension, bradycardia, and even respiratory paralysis. Acute symptoms usually subside within a few days and require only symptomatic, supportive therapy. Intravenous mannitol has been reported to provide rapid symptomatic relief, as has oral tocainide. Neither therapy has been subjected to careful clinical trials. The return of pruritus with alcohol ingestion is thought to be almost pathognomonic of this syndrome. Weakness and sensory disturbances may persist for months or years.

SCOMBROID FISH POISONING. Scombroid fish poisoning is the only form of ichthyosarcotoxism in which toxins are formed by the action of bacteria, in this case particularly *Proteus morgani*, on fish flesh. Scombrotoxin is thought to consist of histamine and related substances. Most fish that have caused outbreaks are members of the suborder Scombroidae, most commonly mahimahi, tuna, mackerel, and bonito. Symptoms begin within a few minutes of ingestion and resemble those of a histamine reaction: flushing, headache, dizziness, abdominal cramps, nausea, vomiting and diarrhea, and occasionally urticaria and generalized pruritus. The illness has a median duration of 4 hours in the reported outbreaks. Both intravenous cimetidine and antihistamines have provided symptomatic relief. Production of the toxin is inhibited by proper refrigeration, perhaps reflecting the temperature optimum of 20 to 30°C for the enzymatic conversion of histidine to histamine. Improper refrigeration of fresh-caught fish has been observed in most outbreaks of this illness.

PUFFER FISH POISONING (TETRODOTOXIN POISONING). Many puffer fish found in the Pacific, Atlantic, and Indian Oceans are inherently toxic. The tetrodotoxin found in their viscera is a neurotoxin, and its effects are nearly identical to the saxitoxin that produces paralytic shellfish poisoning (see below).

PARALYTIC SHELLFISH POISONING. Paralytic shellfish poisoning is caused by the ingestion of bivalve mollusks contaminated with the neurotoxin of the dinoflagellates *Gonyaulax catanella* or *Go. tamarensis*. Although a "red tide," related to "blooming" of the dinoflagellates, has been associated with paralytic shellfish poisoning, not all red tides are toxic, and some outbreaks have occurred in the absence of a red tide. The toxin of *Go. catanella*, saxitoxin, appears to act by inhibiting sodium channels on excitable membranes, thus blocking the propagation of nerve and muscle action potentials.

The illness begins within 30 minutes of ingestion of a toxic mollusk and is characterized by paresthesias of the mouth, lips, face, and extremities and by nausea, vomiting, and diarrhea. In more severe cases, muscle weakness or paralysis and respiratory embarrassment may occur. The fatality rate is 8 to 9 per cent, with deaths occurring within the first 12 hours. Treatment consists of a cathartic or enema in severe cases to remove unabsorbed toxin. Gastric lavage may be used if vomiting has not occurred. Mechanical ventilatory assistance may be required.

NEUROTOXIC SHELLFISH POISONING. *Ptychodiseus breve*, a toxic dinoflagellate, causes a red tide off both the Gulf and Atlantic coasts of Florida. Within 3 hours of the consumption of shellfish contaminated with this toxin, patients experience paresthesias, abnormal temperature sensations, ataxia, nausea, vomiting, and diarrhea. The disease is self-limited and milder than paralytic shellfish poisoning. No deaths have been reported.

MUSHROOM POISONING

Of the more than 2000 identified species of mushrooms, fewer than 50 are poisonous. However, even expert mycologists may have difficulty identifying poisonous species. Moreover, with the increased interest in "organic" foods and in the hallucinogenic substances found in certain species, poisoning from the ingestion of wild mushrooms has been increasing in frequency.

The principal toxin is α-amanitin, which contains cyclic octapeptides. It selectively inhibits nuclear ribonucleic acid (RNA) polymerase II. Phalloidin, another putative toxin, appears to have some hepatocellular toxicity, but probably is primarily responsible for the gastroenteritis seen early in the course. Mushrooms containing these toxins belong to the genera *Amanita* and *Galerina*. *Amanita verna* (the "destroying angel"), *A. virosa*, and *A. phalloides* (the "death cap") are the species most often associated with mushroom poisoning in the United States, and *A. phalloides* accounts for more than 90 per cent of such deaths in Europe.

Symptoms of *A. phalloides*–type mushroom poisoning characteristically occur in three stages. The first is characterized by the abrupt onset of abdominal pain, nausea, vomiting, and diarrhea 6 to 24 hours after ingestion. This may be accompanied by severe fluid and electrolyte disturbances and fever. The second stage, occurring during the next 24 to 48 hours, involves worsening of hepatic and renal function despite resolution of the initial symptoms. Finally, during the third and fourth days after ingestion, hepatic and renal functions rapidly deteriorate, accompanied occasionally by cardiomyopathy and coagulopathy, convulsions, coma, and death. The mortality rate is between 40 and 90 per cent.

The diagnosis of mushroom poisoning may be difficult. The delayed onset of symptoms may cause patients not to associate the illness with the ingestion of wild mushrooms. The mushroom toxins can be detected in blood, gastric aspirate, vomitus, or stool by thin-layer chromatography or by radioimmunoassay in some laboratories. Treatment remains supportive, including dialysis for the renal insufficiency. A number of medical therapies, including cytochrome C, sulfamethoxazole, penicillin G, thioctic acid, and silibinin, have been recommended, but none has been subjected to controlled trials. Careful attention to the complications of hepatic failure and consideration of orthotopic liver transplantation are particularly critical. Early identification of those patients at highest risk of fulminant hepatic failure—a rapidly rising prothrombin time or the development of stage II encephalopathy, for example—is critical, since early hepatic transplantation can be life-saving.

Plant Alkaloids, Mycotoxins, and Other Poisonings

These various forms of food poisoning remind us of historic knowledge of the pharmacologic effect of plant alkaloids and other toxicants found naturally in foods. Although formerly used with therapeutic intent, plant alkaloids are now more often ingested accidentally and often in large doses: e.g., digitalis intoxication from home-brewed teas made with foxglove or oleander; diarrhea from senna tea, which contains the stimulant cathartic anthraquinone; and liver failure from *Senecio longilobus*, which contains highly hepatotoxic pyrrolizidine alkaloids. Other highly toxic plants include *Atropa belladonna* (deadly nightshade) and *Datura stramonium* (thorn apple, jimson weed), whose berries and seeds can cause an atropine effect; *Conium maculatum* (hemlock), which contains several alkaloids with severe central nervous system depressant effects; and *Phytolacca americana* (pokeweed), whose leaves and berries have strong emetic properties. Finally, the ingestion of fava beans can trigger hemolysis in those with G6PD deficiency (Ch. 134).

Lathyrism, a slowly progressive spastic paraplegia, is associated with the ingestion of sweet peas of the species *Lathyrus sativus*. Large amounts of this may be ingested during famines in Africa and Asia. The toxic principle appears to be β-aminoproprionitrile. Interestingly, this substance, when given to poultry and other experimental animals, causes degeneration of the aortic media, with resulting dissecting aortic aneurysms or aortic rupture. This effect is not seen in humans.

Mycotoxins may contaminate some moldy foods. Ergotism, characterized by intense vasospasm, is the most familiar syndrome caused by this ingestion. Aflatoxin, a product of *Aspergillus flavus*, contaminates grains stored in warm, damp areas and has been associated with the development of hepatocellular carcinoma. Small amounts of aflatoxin have been found in commercial peanut butter in the United States.

Eastaugh J, Shepherd S: Infectious and toxic syndromes from fish and shellfish consumption. Arch Intern Med 149:1735, 1989. *An up-to-date review with thorough discussion of pathogenesis and treatment of these diseases.*

Klein A, Hart J, Brems JJ, et al.: *Amanita* poisoning: Treatment and the role of liver transplantation. Am J Med 86:187, 1989. *Case presentations and analysis of therapeutic options. Recommended treatment protocol explained in detail.*

Poisoning associated with herbal teas. MMWR 26:257, 1977. *Case reports and discussions of several types of herbal poisonings.*

Wogan GN: Mycotoxins. Ann Rev Pharmacol 15:437, 1975. *A review of the current understanding of the pharmacology and health impact of mycotoxins.*

109 Diseases of the Rectum and Anus

Theodore R. Schrock

ANATOMY

The rectum and anus fuse over a zone several centimeters long, and together these structures are termed the "anorectum" (Fig. 109–1). The distal anal canal is lined by modified skin (anoderm), the epithelium of the upper anal canal is columnar, and the transitional zone (cuboidal epithelium) lies between the two. The anoderm is exquisitely sensitive, but the upper anal canal is relatively insensitive.

At the dentate line, an important site of pathologic problems, anal papillae project into the lumen. Flaps of skin connecting anal papillae are termed anal valves; behind these valves lie anal crypts, each containing in its depths an anal gland.

The internal anal sphincter is the thickened lower portion of the circular smooth muscle layer of the gut. This involuntary muscle is encircled by skeletal muscle bundles comprising the external sphincters. The levators ani form the muscular floor of the pelvis. One of the levators, the puborectalis, passes around the rectum as a sling and is easily palpable posteriorly on digital rectal examination.

EXAMINATION OF THE ANORECTUM

The anorectum is examined with the patient in the left lateral decubitus position or in the prone jackknife position, if a special table is available for that purpose. Good lighting is essential. The buttocks are retracted to expose the anal orifice. Digital rectal examination is performed. Anoscopy is required for thorough evaluation of the anal canal. Rigid or flexible sigmoidoscopy completes the examination in some patients, but others (e.g., those with bleeding) need colonoscopy or a barium enema.

HEMORRHOIDS

Hemorrhoids are masses of areolar tissue containing numerous small arteries and veins. These congenital vascular cushions are located above the dentate line and are termed "internal hemorrhoids." External hemorrhoids are dilated vessels below the dentate line; they rarely cause symptoms by themselves, but they are enlarged in association with prolapsing internal hemorrhoids. Intrarectal pressure pushes hemorrhoids downward, the anchoring fibromuscular structures attenuate, and the tissues congest, bleed, and eventually prolapse. Small hemorrhoids that protrude a short distance into the anal canal are first-degree hemorrhoids. Second-degree hemorrhoids prolapse but reduce spontaneously. Third-degree hemorrhoids must be manually reduced, and fourth-degree hemorrhoids are irreducible. Internal hemorrhoids occur in three primary locations: right posterior, right anterior, and left lateral.

Bleeding and *prolapse* are the most common symptoms of internal hemorrhoids. Blood is typically bright red, and it may spurt or drip from the anus. Nonspecific discomfort is noted, but pain is usually caused by some other associated condition such as fissure or abscess.

Anoscopy reveals a mass of tissue above the dentate line; large hemorrhoids prolapse to the outside as the anoscope is withdrawn. Differential diagnosis includes skin tags, hypertrophied anal papillae, and rectal prolapse.

Acute prolapse and thrombosis of internal hemorrhoids are severely painful. The entire circumference of the anus appears to protrude, and there is extreme pain from the edema and inflammation.

Initial treatment of internal hemorrhoids involves a high-bulk diet and avoidance of prolonged sitting at stool. Proprietary remedies have little benefit. Small bleeding hemorrhoids can be treated by a "fixation procedure" that promotes adherence of the vascular cushions to the underlying sphincter. These outpatient procedures require no anesthetic. One popular method is the injection of a sclerosing agent (e.g., 5 per cent phenol in oil) into the submucosa of the hemorrhoid above the dentate line. This painless injection evokes fibrosis and eventual adherence of the sliding mucosa. Another method is rubber band ligation, in which tiny bands are slipped over each internal hemorrhoid using a special instrument. The banded tissue sloughs and fixation results. Photocoagulation using an infrared device is also effective. Lasers can be used for the same purpose, but they are more expensive and more hazardous. Electrocoagulation with a bipolar electrode or a direct current device and thermocoagulation with a "heater probe" are new alternatives. All of these procedures have the same objective, and they are similarly effective.

Fourth-degree hemorrhoids with large external components are not responsive to fixation procedures, and if the symptoms warrant, hemorrhoidectomy is advised. Surgical excision can be performed in an outpatient setting. Results are good, although the operation is painful, and there is loss of time from work. Complications are uncommon and recurrences are unusual.

Thrombosed external hemorrhoid is a blood clot within a complex of subcutaneous external veins. This problem develops in young adults, often related to heavy exercise. A painful bluish mass is present at the anal verge. If pain does not subside after 48 hours, the thrombosed hemorrhoid can be excised under local anesthesia.

ANAL FISSURE

Anal fissure (fissure in ano, anal ulcer) is a tear in the anoderm just inside the anal verge. Acute fissures are common, but in some patients the tiny laceration does not heal and it becomes chronic. Severe pain with defecation and spots of blood on the toilet tissue are the symptoms.

The diagnosis is made by inspection. Pain is so severe that the patient may not tolerate digital rectal examination. Lateral trac-

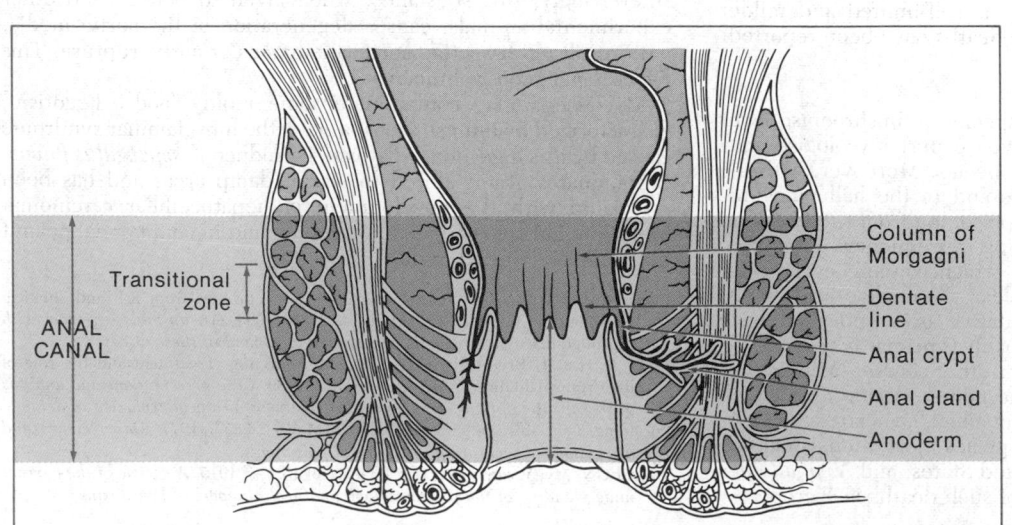

FIGURE 109–1. The lining of the anal canal. (Redrawn from Goldberg SM, Gordon PH, Nivatvongs S: Essentials of Anorectal Surgery. Philadelphia, J. B. Lippincott Company, 1980. Used by permission.)

Column of Morgagni

Dentate line

Anal crypt

Anal gland

Anoderm

ANAL CANAL

Transitional zone

tion on the buttocks exposes the fissure in nearly every instance. Acute fissures are red, but chronic fissures may have eroded completely through the anoderm to expose the white fibers of the internal sphincter in the base. The fissure triad seen in chronic lesions includes the fissure, an edematous sentinel tag at the anal verge, and a hypertrophied anal papilla at the dentate line.

Fissures are located in the posterior midline in 98 per cent of men and 90 per cent of women. The remaining fissures are in the anterior midline. A fissure off the midline should raise a suspicion of cancer, Crohn's disease, or a sexually transmitted infection.

Measures to improve bulk and softness of stools are important, and sitz baths are soothing. Acute fissures usually heal. Chronic fissures may require lateral subcutaneous internal anal sphincterotomy. This simple procedure reduces pressure in the anal canal and allows the fissure to heal. The long-term cure rate exceeds 95 per cent.

ANORECTAL ABSCESS

Infections arising in anal glands at the dentate line may develop into abscesses in the adjacent tissue spaces (Fig. 109–2). Abscesses near the skin surface cause throbbing pain that is worse with walking. Deeper abscesses may produce insidious symptoms including abdominal pain. Patients with large abscesses are febrile. An indurated tender mass is apparent on examination in a patient with a perianal or ischiorectal abscess, and the anus is pushed to one side. Intersphincteric abscesses are invisible on the outside, but they are palpable as a firm, tender area on digital rectal examination. Supralevator abscesses are also palpable.

Prompt surgical incision and drainage are required. A neglected abscess may extend, and necrotizing infections can be lethal. Abscesses in immunocompromised patients pose special problems, and standard treatment may not be appropriate.

ANORECTAL FISTULAS

A hollow fibrous tract lined by granulation tissue develops after spontaneous or surgical drainage of an anorectal abscess. The primary orifice is usually at the dentate line where the infection originated. The secondary orifice is most often external at the site of drainage. The patient has pus, blood, mucus, and discomfort. One or more reddish papules on the perianal skin mark the sites of secondary openings. Gentle pressure may produce a drop of pus from the orifice. A firm tract may be palpated with a well-lubricated finger as it travels from the secondary orifice toward the anal verge.

Anoscopy reveals the primary opening; a hooked probe confirms its patency. At times it is difficult to identify the primary orifice. Goodsall's rule describes the usual relationship of primary

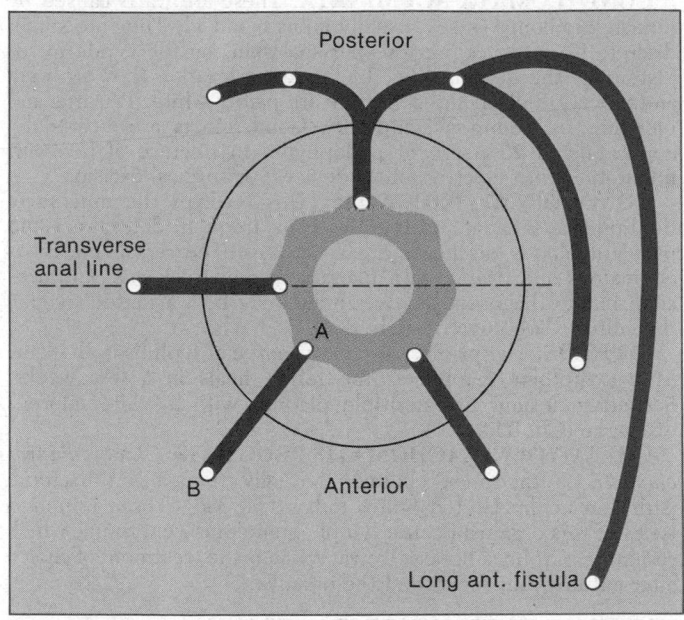

FIGURE 109–3. Goodsall's rule indicates the usual relationship of primary (A) and secondary (B) fistula orifices. The long anterior fistula is an exception to the rule. (Redrawn from Schrock TR: *In* Fromm D [ed.]: Gastrointestinal Surgery. New York, Churchill Livingstone, 1985. Used by permission.)

and secondary fistula orifices (Fig. 109–3). Crohn's disease, carcinoma, tuberculosis, and chlamydial infections should be considered in the differential diagnosis. Proctosigmoidoscopy is done routinely, and barium studies or even colonoscopy may be indicated in some cases.

Fistulas do not heal spontaneously, and operation is required (fistulotomy). The tissue overlying the tract is incised and the base is curetted. The defect heals secondarily. High fistulas encompass important sphincters and require special techniques.

Rectovaginal fistulas most commonly result from childbirth injuries. Fecal incontinence may be associated. The patient complains of passage of flatus and occasionally feces through the vagina. Surgical repair is usually successful.

PRURITUS ANI

Pruritus ani is perianal itching. It is a symptom, not a diagnosis, and the causes are many and varied. Responsible conditions include anorectal diseases, dermatologic diseases, contact dermatitis, infections by bacteria or fungi, parasites, oral antibiotics, systemic diseases (e.g., diabetes), poor or excessively zealous hygiene, warmth and moisture, dietary intolerance (coffee, cola, tomatoes, chocolate), and psychological problems. Leakage of mucus or tiny amounts of stool onto the perianal skin is perhaps the most frequent cause of pruritus, and usually there is no significant sphincter defect.

A thorough history should be obtained. Examination may disclose no abnormality, or at the other extreme there may be moist, macerated, excoriated perianal skin. Dermatologic diseases should be looked for elsewhere on the trunk and extremities. Parasites are rare.

If a specific cause of pruritus is identified, appropriate therapy is given. Antibiotics should be stopped, topical agents discontinued, and diet modified. Cleansing after defecation should be accomplished with moist cotton followed by gentle drying. Nonmedicated talcum powder is applied to combat moisture. A small bit of cotton applied to the anal verge may absorb excess moisture. More severe cases may require application of corticosteroid creams.

SEXUALLY TRANSMITTED DISEASES

Homosexually active men have a high incidence of anorectal infections, and women who practice anal intercourse also are at risk for development of these conditions.

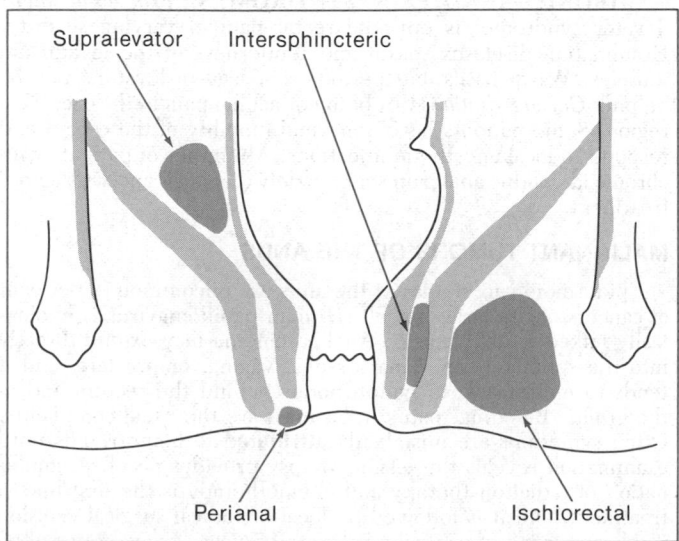

FIGURE 109–2. Classification of anorectal abscesses. (Redrawn from Gordon PH: Management of anorectal abscesses and fistulous disease. *In* Kodner IJ, Fry RD, Roe JP [eds.]: Colon, Rectal and Anal Surgery. St. Louis, The C. V. Mosby Company, 1986.)

CONDYLOMATA ACUMINATA. These are warts caused by human papillomaviruses, usually types 6 and 11. They are small, discrete excrescences on the perianal skin, on the anoderm, or just above the dentate line. In the latter location they are pink and velvety, but on the skin they are pearly white. Pruritus and bleeding are common symptoms. Condylomata are treated by application of 25 per cent podophyllin in tincture of benzoin, fulguration with electrocautery devices, or surgical excision.

GONOCOCCAL PROCTITIS. This involves the mucosa of the upper anal canal and rectum. Pain, frequent defecation, and purulent bloody discharge are symptoms. The rectal mucosa is edematous and friable with ulcerations and thick pus. Cultures confirm the diagnosis but treatment may be warranted even if the cultures are negative (Ch. 336).

SYPHILIS. The primary lesion of anorectal syphilis is an ulcer. Mild symptoms resolve as the lesion heals in a few weeks. Secondary lesions are multiple plaques with a white odorous discharge (Ch. 340).

CHLAMYDIA TRACHOMATIS PROCTITIS. *Chlamydia trachomatis* is the most common sexually transmitted bacterial pathogen in the United States today (Ch. 345). Three immunotypes of this organism cause lymphogranuloma venereum, which resembles Crohn's disease. Tetracycline is the treatment of choice after culture confirmation of the organism.

FOREIGN BODIES AND RECTAL TRAUMA

Foreign bodies are introduced into the anus for erotic purposes, for concealment, for self-treatment, accidentally, or by assault. Complications include perforation of the rectum or colon and injuries of the sphincters. Removal of a rectal foreign body can be difficult because the sphincters tighten and trap the slippery object in the rectal ampulla. Most objects can be removed through the rectum with the aid of local or occasionally general anesthesia.

DISORDERS OF THE PELVIC FLOOR

Disorders of the pelvic floor are a group of conditions arising from abnormal structure or function of the levators ani and anal sphincters.

ANAL INCONTINENCE. Anal incontinence has many causes (Table 109–1). Partial incontinence is occasional loss of flatus or loose stool, and major incontinence is abnormal control of stool of normal consistency. Thorough history should be obtained. The anus may be deformed and gaping, and an obvious anatomic defect may be visible and palpable. In other instances the

TABLE 109–1. CAUSES OF ANAL INCONTINENCE

Normal sphincters and pelvic floor
  Diarrhea
  Fistula
Abnormal function of sphincters and/or pelvic floor
  Partial incontinence
    Deficient internal sphincter
      Trauma
      Rectal prolapse
      Third-degree hemorrhoids
    Fecal impaction
      Elderly
      Neurologic disorders
    Minor external sphincter and pelvic floor denervation
  Major incontinence
    Congenital anomalies
    Trauma
    Complete rectal prolapse
    Rectal carcinoma
    Anorectal infection
    Idiopathic
    Drug intoxication
    Neurologic
    Upper motor neuron
      Cerebral
      Spinal
    Lower motor neuron

Modified from Henry MM, Swash M (eds.): Coloproctology and the Pelvic Floor. Pathophysiology and Management. Boston, Butterworths, 1985.

structures seem intact but function is inadequate. Special investigations include anorectal manometry and electromyography.

The underlying systemic intestinal disorder, if any, should be treated. Loose stools are managed with bulk agents and constipating drugs. Elderly patients who soil because of fecal impaction may need regular laxatives and/or enemas. Biofeedback may improve patients with organic neuromuscular impairment. Surgical repair is successful for traumatically disrupted sphincters.

SOLITARY RECTAL ULCER SYNDROME. Solitary rectal ulcer syndrome is a chronic, benign condition characterized by anal pain, bleeding, mucous discharge, and obsessive straining to defecate. It affects mainly young women. Excessive straining forces the anterior rectal mucosa downward where it becomes traumatized.

On examination the anterior rectal mucosa 6 to 10 cm above the anal verge is indurated and may be grossly ulcerated. Biopsies confirm the diagnosis. Treatment should be directed toward avoidance of straining by education of the patient and the use of bulk agents. Unfortunately, current methods of therapy are often disappointing, and patients must live with the chronic condition. Surgical repairs are unsatisfactory unless the patient has a true rectal prolapse.

DESCENDING PERINEUM SYNDROME. Some patients, mostly parous women, complain of a sense of incomplete evacuation and a constant desire to defecate. They are, in effect, attempting to evacuate their own rectal mucosa. The diagnosis is made if the patient strains and the plane of the perineum balloons downward below a line connecting the ischial tuberosities. Education, bulk agents, and occasionally local surgical procedures are helpful.

RECTAL PROLAPSE. Partial prolapse is protrusion of the mucosa alone, and complete rectal prolapse (procidentia) is protrusion of the entire thickness of the rectum. Prolapse is much more common in women than in men, and it appears with increasing frequency after age 40. Surgical or other traumatic injuries are causative in a few patients, but laxity of the pelvic musculature as a result of aging or neurologic disease is more commonly responsible.

With the patient sitting on the edge of the examining table or, even better, on a toilet seat, straining produces the prolapse. Mucosal prolapse is a small symmetric projection 2 to 4 cm long with radial folds. True procidentia may protrude as much as 12 cm from the anus, and the mucosal folds are concentric. Palpation reveals a large mass of tissue anteriorly. Proctosigmoidoscopy and barium enema are required.

Procidentia must be repaired surgically to avoid further weakening of the anal sphincters. Repairs can be accomplished abdominally or through the perineum, depending on the circumstances. Mucosal prolapse is managed by fixation procedures or excision, as described for hemorrhoids.

CHRONIC ANAL PAIN SYNDROMES. *Proctalgia fugax* (levator syndrome) is episodic rectal pain of varying severity. Examination discloses spasm and tenderness of the levator ani muscles. Warm baths and periodic massage of levators may be helpful. *Coccygodynia* is throbbing or aching pain in the coccygeal region. Some patients have abnormal mobility of the coccyx and respond to local anesthetic injections. A number of patients with chronic idiopathic anal pain seem to defy diagnosis and satisfactory treatment.

MALIGNANT TUMORS OF THE ANUS

Epidermoid carcinomas of the anus are uncommon (2 per cent of cancers of the large bowel). Human papillomavirus is etiologically linked to anal cancer. Anal carcinoma may extend directly into the sphincters, perianal tissues, vagina, or prostate, and it tends to metastasize to lymph nodes behind the rectum and in the groins. Bleeding, pain, and a mass are the usual complaints. Often symptoms are mistakenly attributed to hemorrhoids until examination reveals the lesion. Biopsy provides proof. A combination of radiation therapy and chemotherapy is the first line of treatment, and it is followed by local or radical surgical excision if the tumor is not controlled. Overall 5-year survival rates of 60 per cent are expected.

Malignant melanoma in the anorectum is rare but highly lethal. *Mucinous adenocarcinoma* in the glands is also rare. *Bowen's disease* is chronic squamous cell carcinoma in situ. Local excision is required to prevent progression to invasive cancer. Extramammary *Paget's disease* is an intraepithelial mucinous adenocarcinoma. It is treated by wide local excision. It tends to recur locally and can metastasize.

Adams YG, Efron G: Current concepts and controversies concerning the etiology, pathogenesis, diagnosis, and treatment of malignant tumors of the anus. Surgery 101:253, 1987. *A review of most of the current issues regarding anal malignancies.*

Gordon PH: Management of anorectal abscesses and fistulous disease. *In* Kodner IJ, Fry RD, Roe JP (eds.): Colon, Rectal and Anal Surgery. Current Techniques and Controversies. St. Louis, The C. V. Mosby Company, 1985, pp 91–107. *An authoritative discussion of a complex topic.*

Henry MM, Swash M (eds.): Coloproctology and the Pelvic Floor. Pathophysiology and Management. Boston, Butterworths, 1985, pp 193–392. *This monograph helped establish the importance of the pelvic floor in pathogenesis of anorectal diseases.*

Motson RW, Clifton MA: Pathogenesis and treatment of anal fissure. *In* Henry MM, Swash M (eds.): Coloproctology and the Pelvic Floor. Pathophysiology and Management. Boston, Butterworths, 1985, pp 340–349. *An excellent review of the pathophysiology and treatment of anal fissure.*

Rompao AM, Stamm WE: Anorectal and enteric infections in homosexual men. West J Med 142:647, 1985. *An excellent review of the myriad of sexually transmitted anorectal and enteric infections.*

Schrock TR: Hemorrhoids: Nonoperative and interventional management. *In* Barkin JS, O'Phelan CA (eds.): Advanced Therapeutic Endoscopy. New York, Raven Press, 1990. *A thorough review of the subject with details of therapeutic procedures.*

Smith LE, Henrichs D, McCullah RD: Prospective studies on the etiology and treatment of pruritus ani. Dis Colon Rectum 25:358, 1982. *Analysis of the causes and management of this symptom.*

110 Diseases of the Peritoneum, Mesentery, and Omentum

Michael D. Bender

ANATOMY AND PHYSIOLOGY. The peritoneum, a continuous mesothelial membrane, lines the abdominal cavity and its contained viscera. The peritoneal cavity is subdivided by peritoneal reflections and mesenteric attachments into several compartments or recesses, which are clinically important because they determine the location and spread of pathologic processes such as abscesses and metastases. The omentum, a double layer of fused peritoneum, plays an important role in peritoneal defense mechanisms by closing perforations, containing infection, and providing blood supply. The microvascular anatomy of the peritoneum consists of long, straight vessels arranged in two layers at right angles to each other, which helps account for the efficiency of the peritoneal membrane as an exchange interface.

The visceral peritoneum does not contain pain receptors; afferent stimuli are transmitted via the visceral autonomics. In contrast, the parietal peritoneum is supplied by spinal nerves that also innervate the abdominal wall. As a result, irritation of the parietal peritoneum produces well-localized somatic pain, whereas irritation of the visceral peritoneum produces a less well-defined discomfort that is poorly localized. The diaphragmatic portion of the peritoneum is supplied by the phrenic nerve centrally and by intercostal nerves peripherally. As a result, pain caused by diaphragmatic irritation may be referred either to the shoulder or to the thoracic and abdominal wall.

The peritoneal surface, a semipermeable membrane, allows for the passive diffusion of water and solutes between the abdominal cavity and the subperitoneal vascular (blood and lymphatic) channels. In general, water and solutes of molecular weight less than 2000 are absorbed from the peritoneal cavity via the blood vascular system; larger molecules and particulate substances enter the lymphatics. Movement of particles from the peritoneal cavity into the subdiaphragmatic lymphatics is facilitated by discontinuities that exist between the peritoneal mesothelial cells and the lymphatic endothelial cells. Basement membranes are scanty or absent so that particles of substantial size may move freely from the abdominal cavity into the subdiaphragmatic lymphatics, a process that may be facilitated by respiratory motion of the diaphragm itself. Water and electrolytes equilibrate rapidly (within 2 hours) between the blood vascular compartment and the free peritoneal cavity. Net fluid movement from the abdominal cavity into the plasma occurs at a maximal rate of approximately 30 to 35 ml per hour both in normal persons and in patients with portal hypertension and ascites. This rate cannot be exceeded despite vigorous diuresis; rather, such diuresis serves only to remove fluid from other body compartments and may cause hypovolemia. The importance of transperitoneal fluid exchange is also illustrated in peritonitis, in which fluid movement into the peritoneal cavity caused by increased vascular permeability can be rapid and massive and may lead to hypotension and shock.

The peritoneum heals readily after damage. Peritoneal injuries normally heal without the formation of adhesions, but in the presence of infection, ischemia, or foreign bodies, adhesions may result. In these situations, fibrinogen released into the peritoneal cavity is converted to fibrin, and then to fibrous adhesions.

DIAGNOSIS. The cardinal symptoms of peritoneal disease are *abdominal pain* and *ascites*. More variable in their occurrence are fever, distention, nausea and vomiting, and altered bowel habits. Direct tenderness, rebound tenderness, and involuntary spasm of the abdominal musculature are the major signs of peritoneal irritation. These signs and symptoms may be minimal or absent in the elderly or debilitated patient and vary, with the location, cause, and acuteness of the underlying process. Because of this, peritoneal disease should be considered in any patient whose abdominal pain is difficult to diagnose.

Radiographically, ascites may be manifested by abdominal haziness, separation of bowel loops, or widening of the flank stripe on plain abdominal films. Otherwise, peritoneal disease reflects itself indirectly on barium contrast studies. Angulation, separation, or rigidity of bowel loops may indicate visceral peritoneal involvement. *Ultrasonography* and *computed tomography* demonstrate inflammatory or neoplastic masses more directly, and may be useful in demonstrating relatively small amounts of peritoneal fluid, and especially in distinguishing free fluid from cystic masses. Computed tomography also has occasionally been successful in the demonstration of peritoneal implants and in the examination of the retroperitoneum. At present, magnetic resonance imaging is rarely indicated in evaluating ascites or peritoneal disease.

If ascites is present, *abdominal paracentesis* is essential to establish its cause (see below). *Peritoneal biopsy*, particularly with the Cope needle, is a relatively simple and safe bedside technique that may yield a positive diagnosis of neoplastic or infectious causes in 50 to 60 per cent of cases. *Peritoneoscopy*, performed under the proper circumstances by a physician experienced in this technique, can be accomplished with little morbidity or mortality. A successful examination may obviate the need for exploratory surgery and may permit biopsy under direct vision of involved portions of the peritoneum or liver. If a diagnosis cannot be made in a patient with obvious peritoneal disease by means of the aforementioned procedures, *exploratory laparotomy* may be necessary.

Patients with mesenteric disease usually have nonspecific symptoms such as abdominal pain, distention, or intestinal obstruction. The most frequent physical finding is a mass, which may be mobile. There are no specific laboratory findings, but mesenteric disease may be suspected if calcifications, displacement of bowel loops, or pressure deformities are observed radiographically. Ultrasonography and computed tomography are useful in identifying mesenteric and omental masses. However, definitive diagnosis usually depends on direct inspection and biopsy, either surgically or by peritoneoscopy.

ASCITES

CLINICAL FEATURES. The accumulation of fluid within the peritoneal cavity is a common clinical finding with a wide range of causes. Its pathophysiology varies with the cause; possible factors are outlined in Table 110–1. The pathophysiology of ascites associated with portal hypertension is considered in Ch. 122.

Small amounts of ascites may be asymptomatic, but as it increases the patient becomes aware of abdominal distention and a sense of fullness and discomfort. Larger amounts of ascites,

TABLE 110–1. FACTORS IN ASCITES FORMATION

Cirrhotic Ascites
Increased portal venous hydrostatic pressure
Decreased portal venous colloid osmotic pressure
Increased hepatic lymph formation
Decreased renal sodium excretion
Decreased renal free water excretion
Noncirrhotic Ascites
Increased subperitoneal capillary permeability
Decreased peritoneal lymphatic drainage
Leakage from disrupted abdominal viscera

especially if the abdomen is tensely distended, may cause respiratory distress, anorexia, nausea, early satiety, pyrosis, or frank pain. Body weight may vary, depending on the state of nutrition and the underlying disease process. On physical examination the flanks bulge, and a fluid wave may be demonstrable. Shifting dullness is somewhat more sensitive but may be nonspecific. Although it is difficult to detect less than 1.5 to 2 liters of fluid, placing the patient on his or her hands and knees and percussing flatness over the dependent abdomen (puddle sign) may demonstrate smaller amounts. Indirect evidence such as penile or scrotal edema, umbilical herniation, or pleural effusion may suggest the presence of ascites.

The diagnosis of ascites may be facilitated by plain abdominal films, ultrasonography, or computed tomography.

EVALUATION OF ASCITIC FLUID. Once the diagnosis of ascites is made by examination, imaging techniques, or paracentesis, laboratory analysis of the fluid removed is essential to determine its cause. Evaluation of ascitic fluid consists of routine studies to characterize the fluid and other studies that may be chosen depending on the clinical situation, as noted in Table 110–2.

Fluids with protein concentrations *exceeding 3 grams per 100 ml* are designated exudates, and below these values, transudates. Other characteristics that may help separate transudates from exudates include ascites–lactate dehydrogenase (LDH), and ascites–serum protein and LDH ratios. The *serum–ascites albumin gradient* (serum albumin – ascites albumin), which reflects the oncotic pressure gradient between the vascular bed and the ascitic fluid, is elevated in association with increased portal pressure, whereas a low gradient occurs in conditions in which portal hypertension is not a factor in the genesis of ascites. Conditions associated with a wide gradient usually are transudative, and conditions with a low gradient usually are exudative. Tests that help distinguish transudates from exudates, and their common causes, are listed in Table 110–3. Although this classification is useful, exceptions in both directions occur not infrequently. For this reason, ascitic fluid chemistries must be interpreted only in the context of all other clinical and laboratory findings.

A large number of red cells suggests the diagnosis of neoplasm, especially hepatocellular or ovarian carcinoma. Other causes of bloody ascites include tuberculosis, trauma, perforated viscus, and spontaneous bleeding associated with cirrhosis. An ascitic fluid leukocyte count of more than 500 per cubic millimeter is strongly suggestive of a peritoneal inflammatory process, such as infection or tumor infiltration. A predominance of polymorphonuclear leukocytes suggests acute bacterial infection, whereas lymphocytes and monocytes characterize chronic inflammatory disease, especially tuberculosis, but there are exceptions. Cytologic examination is essential if malignancy is suspected and may be expected to yield accurate results in more than half of cases. Samples of fluid should be cultured for bacteria, acid-fast bacilli, or fungi in the appropriate clinical setting, such as fever, undiagnosed pain, or deterioration in a patient with cirrhosis. Other chemical determinations that may be helpful in diagnosis are listed in Table 110–2.

TREATMENT: GENERAL CONSIDERATIONS. Although small or moderate amounts of ascites are often only esthetically displeasing, ascites frequently has a detrimental effect on the overall sense of well-being of the patient. Massive ascites may require urgent removal for severe abdominal discomfort, respiratory distress, cardiac dysfunction, or ulceration or impending

TABLE 110–2. LABORATORY ANALYSIS OF ASCITIC FLUID

Test	Abnormal Values	Clinical Situations
Red cell count	> 10,000/mm³	Routine
White cell count and differential	> 500/mm³	Routine
Total protein*	> 3 gm/dl	Routine
LDH*	> 200 IU/liter	Routine
Albumin†	< 1.1 gm/dl	Routine
Bacterial culture	+	Routine
Acid-fast, fungal culture	+	History or findings of Tbc; cirrhosis; immunosuppressed patient
Cytology	+	Neoplasm
Amylase‡	Ascites > serum	Pancreatitis, alcoholism, cirrhosis
Glucose‡	Ascites < serum	Tuberculosis, neoplasm, secondary bacterial peritonitis
Triglycerides‡	Ascites > serum	Chylous (milky) ascites
Starch granules (polarizing microscopy)	+	Postoperative abdominal pain
pH§	< 7.35	Spontaneous bacterial peritonitis
Lactate§	> 25 mg/dl	Spontaneous bacterial peritonitis
CEA	> 10 ng/ml	Adenocarcinoma
Hyaluronic acid¶	> 0.25 mg/ml	Mesothelioma

*Simultaneous blood value for ratio.
†Serum albumin – ascites albumin = gradient. See text.
‡Simultaneous blood value for comparison.
§Also abnormal in neoplastic, tuberculous, and pancreatic ascites.
¶Liquid chromatographic method.
LDH = lactate dehydrogenase; CEA = carcinoembryonic antigen; Tbc = tuberculosis.

rupture of an umbilical hernia. Paracentesis is the method of choice for rapid removal of fluid, as it rapidly reduces intraabdominal pressure and improves cardiac performance. The risk to the patient of a single, large paracentesis of 2 to 5 liters is minimal and is not associated with a change in plasma volume in cirrhotic patients with edema. One should not hesitate to remove ascites in sufficient volume to treat the complications of tense ascites noted above, but repeated paracentesis to control ascites is rarely warranted.

In patients with intractable, disabling, massive ascites that does not respond to repeated paracentesis or diuretic therapy, peritoneovenous shunting has been successful. Because of numerous complications, careful consideration must be given before recommending peritoneovenous shunting (see Ch. 122). Details of nutritional and diuretic management of ascites are discussed in Ch. 122.

DIFFERENTIAL DIAGNOSIS OF ASCITES. More than 90 per cent of patients with ascites have *cirrhosis, neoplasm, congestive heart failure,* or *tuberculosis.* Causes of ascites may be

TABLE 110–3. DIAGNOSIS OF TRANSUDATIVE VERSUS EXUDATIVE ASCITES

	Transudate	Exudate
Protein	< 3 gm/dl	> 3 gm/dl
LDH	< 200 IU/liter	> 200 IU/liter
Protein ascites/serum ratio	< 0.5	> 0.5
LDH ascites/serum ratio	< 0.6	> 0.6
Albumin gradient*	> 1.1	< 1.1
Common causes	Congestive heart failure	Neoplasm
	Constrictive pericarditis	Tuberculosis
	Inferior vena cava obstruction	Pancreatitis
	Budd-Chiari syndrome	Myxedema
	Cirrhosis	Vasculitis
	Nephrotic syndrome	
	Hypoalbuminemia	

*Serum albumin – ascites albumin.
LDH = lactate dehydrogenase.

TABLE 110–4. CAUSES OF ASCITES NOT ASSOCIATED WITH PERITONEAL DISEASE*

I. **Portal hypertension**
   A. Cirrhosis
   B. Hepatic congestion
      1. Congestive heart failure
      2. Constrictive pericarditis
      3. Inferior vena cava obstruction
      4. Hepatic vein obstruction (Budd-Chiari syndrome)
   C. Portal vein occlusion
II. **Hypoalbuminemia**
   A. Nephrotic syndrome
   B. Protein-losing enteropathy
   C. Malnutrition
III. **Endocrine**
   A. Myxedema
   B. Ovarian disease
      1. Meigs' syndrome
      2. Struma ovarii
      3. Ovarian overstimulation syndrome
IV. **Visceral leakage**
   A. Pancreatic ascites
   B. Bile ascites
   C. Chylous ascites
   D. Urine ascites and nephrogenic ascites

*Modified from Bender MD, Ockner RK: *In* Sleisenger MH, Fordtran JS (eds.): Gastrointestinal Disease. 4th ed. Philadelphia, W. B. Saunders Company, 1988.

divided into diseases not involving the peritoneum (Table 110–4) and diseases of the peritoneum (Table 110–5). Of those cases not associated with peritoneal disease, cirrhosis is by far the most common (Ch. 122). Portal hypertension caused by diseases of the heart and great veins accounts for a substantial number of patients with ascites of obscure origin. Included in this group are patients with congestive heart failure, constrictive pericarditis, and inferior vena cava and hepatic vein obstruction (Budd-Chiari syndrome). Clinically, patients with these conditions may not be readily distinguishable from those with hepatic cirrhosis; a high index of suspicion is necessary, and special procedures may be required in order to establish or exclude the diagnosis.

Hypoalbuminemia of any cause, including nephrotic syndrome and protein-losing enteropathy, may be associated with a classically transudative ascites. Ascites occurs only when the serum albumin is very low, usually less than 2 mg per deciliter.

Various endocrine conditions may be associated with ascites. These include *myxedema*, in which the fluid is typically protein rich, and diseases of the ovary, among them *Meigs' syndrome*, in which transudative ascites is associated with ovarian fibroma or cystadenoma, struma ovarii, ovarian edema, and "ovarian overstimulation syndrome."

Pancreatic ascites usually occurs in the presence of chronic pancreatitis or pseudocyst. The most common etiologic factors are alcohol and trauma. The ascitic fluid amylase concentration is elevated, often to extremely high levels. Diagnosis of ductal disruption and pseudocyst leakage is usually possible with endoscopic retrograde pancreatography. Drainage of the pseudocyst and repair of duct injury often have been effective in managing this complication, particularly in traumatic cases. In the chronic alcoholic with pancreatic ascites, a trial of conservative management is indicated before surgery is undertaken. Leakage of bile may be associated with the development of *bile ascites*, a condition for which surgical repair of the biliary tract is usually necessary. This situation is not necessarily associated with the fulminant clinical picture of fever, leukocytosis, and peritonitis, i.e., *bile peritonitis*, which appears to result from superimposed infection.

Chylous ascites is due to the presence of lipoproteins and chylomicrons in the peritoneal cavity and is the result of lymphatic obstruction or leakage. These lipid-rich particles impart a turbidity to the fluid that facilitates its diagnosis. However, not all turbid abdominal fluids are "chylous." Establishment of the diagnosis requires direct evidence that the turbidity is indeed the result of neutral lipid, a determination best made by analysis of the fluid for triglyceride concentration. Other turbid abdominal fluids may be due to cellular debris and are designated *pseudochylous ascites*, a condition occasionally associated with abdominal neoplasm or infection. The differential diagnosis of true chylous

ascites depends upon its chronicity and the age of the patient. *Chronic chylous ascites* in adults is caused in over 80 per cent of cases by abdominal neoplasm, usually lymphoma, with associated obstruction and disruption of the abdominal lymphatics resulting from extensive lymph node involvement. Inflammatory causes include tuberculosis, pancreatitis, cirrhosis, and adhesions. *Acute chylous ascites* ("chylous peritonitis") is associated with abrupt onset of abdominal pain. In some cases, this syndrome is due to trauma, intestinal obstruction, or rupture of a chylous cyst, but identifying a specific cause may not be possible even at laparotomy. In children, congenital malformations of the lymphatics, including intestinal lymphangiectasia, account for a higher proportion of the cases of chylous ascites. Treatment of chylous ascites depends on the underlying cause. General measures include (1) the use of low-fat diets with medium-chain triglyceride supplementation (these are transported by the portal vein rather than the lymphatics); (2) total parenteral nutrition, to achieve bowel rest and allow healing of damaged lymphatics; and occasionally (3) peritoneovenous shunting, if other measures are unsuccessful.

Urine ascites may result from trauma to the urinary tract, high-grade obstruction caused by posterior urethral valves in the neonate, or renal transplantation. Ascites also may occur in a few patients maintained on chronic hemodialysis. The cause appears to reflect a number of factors including prior peritoneal dialysis or infection, fluid overload, hypertension, poor nutrition, or hypoalbuminemia. Management may be difficult, but if aggressive dialysis does not help, renal transplantation seems to offer the best chance of relieving this form of chronic ascites.

TABLE 110–5. DISEASES OF THE PERITONEUM

I. **Infections**
   A. Bacterial peritonitis
   B. Tuberculous peritonitis
   C. Fungal diseases
      1. Candidiasis
      2. Histoplasmosis
      3. Coccidioidomycosis
      4. Cryptococcosis
   D. Parasitic diseases
      1. Schistosomiasis
      2. Enterobiasis
      3. Ascariasis
      4. Strongyloidiasis
      5. Amebiasis
II. **Neoplasms**
   A. Secondary malignancy
   B. Mesothelial hyperplasia and benign mesothelioma
   C. Primary malignant mesothelioma
   D. Pseudomyxoma peritonei
III. **Granulomatous peritonitis**
   A. Exogenous
   B. Endogenous
   C. Iatrogenic
IV. **Sclerosing peritonitis**
   A. Toxic
   B. Indwelling foreign bodies
   C. Idiopathic
V. **Miscellaneous**
   A. Vasculitis
   B. Familial paroxysmal peritonitis (familial Mediterranean fever)
   C. Eosinophilic gastroenteritis
   D. Whipple's disease
   E. Gynecologic disease
      1. Endometriosis
      2. Deciduosis
      3. Gliomatosis
      4. Leiomyomatosis
      5. Dermoid cyst
      6. Melanosis
   F. Splenosis
   G. Peritoneal lymphangiectasia
   H. Peritoneal cysts
   I. Peritoneal encapsulation

*Modified from Bender MD, Ockner RK: *In* Sleisenger MH, Fordtran JS (eds.): Gastrointestinal Disease. 4th ed. Philadelphia, W. B. Saunders Company, 1988.

INFECTIONS OF THE PERITONEUM

ACUTE BACTERIAL PERITONITIS. Bacterial peritonitis most commonly results from perforation of an abdominal viscus caused by trauma, obstruction, infarction, neoplasm, foreign bodies, or primary inflammatory disease (Ch. 51). Peritonitis may also be associated with chronic indwelling catheters used for chronic ambulatory peritoneal dialysis, peritoneovenous shunting, and intraperitoneal chemotherapy. The peritoneum has several defense mechanisms in response to bacterial contamination: (1) Bacteria may be cleared from the peritoneum via the diaphragmatic lymphatics. (2) Opsonins, polymorphonuclear leukocytes, and macrophages enter the peritoneal cavity, where phagocytosis of bacteria can occur. (3) The peritoneum and omentum can contain localized infections and enclose small visceral perforations, in part by exudation of fibrin-containing fluid.

Regardless of etiology, abdominal pain, nausea, vomiting, tachycardia, and fever are usually present. The severity of these symptoms is related to the extent of contamination; in generalized peritonitis, shock is often present and may be profound, whereas signs and symptoms may be minimal if infection is localized. In severe cases, there may be exquisite, diffuse, direct, and rebound tenderness and rigidity of the abdomen; bowel sounds are usually diminished or absent, and distention may be present. Despite its dramatic presentation, recognition of acute peritonitis may be difficult in those patients in whom the clinical manifestations are masked or suppressed, such as the elderly patient or those receiving corticosteroids. In these patients, a high index of suspicion is necessary, since minor or isolated signs such as tachycardia or unexplained hypotension may herald peritonitis.

Laboratory findings are nonspecific and may include leukocytosis, hemoconcentration (from fluid loss into the peritoneum), and subdiaphragmatic air or distended intestinal loops on plain abdominal films. In debilitated or obtunded elderly patients, *peritoneal lavage* may help establish or rule out the presence of peritonitis. One liter of fluid is instilled through a peritoneal dialysis catheter; a positive lavage fluid contains more than 500 white blood cells per cubic milliliter of fluid or more than 50,000 red blood cells per milliliter or, on Gram's stain, reveals bacteria.

The principal systemic complications of peritonitis are septicemia, shock, ileus, and widespread organ failure, including respiratory, renal, hepatic, and cardiac failure. Local complications include wound infection, abscess, anastomotic breakdown, and fistula formation.

The initial management of peritonitis includes restoration of fluid and electrolyte balance, institution of nasogastric suction to reduce distention and improve pulmonary function, oxygen, analgesics to control pain, and early antibiotic therapy. In advanced peritonitis, polymicrobial aerobic and anaerobic organisms are usually found, requiring broad-spectrum coverage. A frequently used regimen combines an aminoglycoside for aerobes with clindamycin or metronidazole for anaerobes. Cephalosporins are popular for their low toxicity and broad-spectrum coverage, especially the third-generation compounds such as cefoxitin and ceftazidime, which provide broad aerobic and anaerobic coverage. Total parenteral nutrition may be necessary in severe peritonitis with major catabolic losses.

In patients who are seen early after a recognized perforation of a viscus and who are good operative candidates, early surgery is usually indicated. In a few patients who are very poor operative risks, it may be desirable to attempt to control the process nonoperatively and to encourage its localization by antibiotic drugs and other conservative measures. Localized abscesses so formed may be drained later when circumstances are more favorable.

Despite the use of antibiotics, modern anesthesia, and intensive support systems, the mortality of generalized peritonitis remains at 50 per cent. Factors adversely affecting prognosis include older age, malnutrition, shock, and organ failure.

ABDOMINAL ABSCESSES. Intra-abdominal abscesses form from a collection of necrotic tissue, bacteria, and white blood cells contained in one of the spaces of the peritoneal cavity and walled off from the rest of the peritoneal cavity by inflammatory adhesions. The contamination is almost invariably derived from endogenous gut flora that escapes as a result of inflammatory perforation, ischemia, traumatic injury, or a surgical procedure. Abscesses within the abdomen localize in three distinct areas: the subphrenic spaces, the intermesenteric area (including the paracolic gutters and interloop areas), and the pelvis. The subphrenic and pelvic localizations reflect the dependent position of these spaces in the recumbent patient and the effect of diaphragmatic movement in drawing fluid up into the subphrenic spaces.

The diagnosis of intra-abdominal abscesses is often a difficult challenge, particularly in immunologically depressed patients with malignancy or malnutrition or patients receiving perioperative antibiotics; all of these may mask clinical signs of sepsis. Fever is the most reliable finding. Other signs and symptoms include malaise, pain, nausea, vomiting, anorexia, tachycardia, abdominal tenderness, and abdominal distention. A subphrenic localization is suggested by thoracic symptoms and signs, including dyspnea, chest pain, decreased breath sounds, dullness, and radiologic evidence of impaired diaphragmatic motion, pleural effusion, or atelectasis. Pelvic localization is suggested by urinary or rectal symptoms and careful vaginal or rectal examination. Leukocytosis with a left shift in the differential count, the usual finding, may be absent. Elevated bilirubin or hepatic enzymes may be a clue to the presence of intra-abdominal sepsis. In summary, a high degree of suspicion is important, and the possibility of an abdominal abscess should be suggested by otherwise unexplained fever, sepsis, leukocytosis, ileus, poor postoperative recovery, or organ dysfunction.

Diagnosis is facilitated by imaging procedures. Plain films may reveal nonmovable gas bubbles, often with air-fluid levels, and barium contrast studies may suggest a mass by displacement of normal structures. Ultrasonography, computed tomography, and gallium citrate-76 or indium-111 leukocyte labeling are newer modalities to diagnose and visualize abscesses. Of these, computed tomography is the most sensitive and specific. Occasionally the diagnosis is made only at the time of abdominal exploration.

Antimicrobial therapy usually suppresses the process and helps to contain it but may also obscure its recognition. Prior computed tomography–guided percutaneous aspiration, with Gram's stain and culture of the obtained fluid, may quickly confirm the presence or absence of an abscess and expedite selection of the proper antibiotic.

Appropriate drainage is indispensable for treatment of an intra-abdominal abscess. Computed tomography–guided percutaneous drainage has increasingly been utilized but may be less successful in complex abscesses associated with multiple cavities, viscous debris, or a source of continued contamination, such as a perforated viscus or fistula. If percutaneous drainage is inappropriate, surgical drainage should be undertaken.

PRIMARY (SPONTANEOUS) BACTERIAL PERITONITIS. Bacterial peritonitis may occur in the absence of an acute intra-abdominal precipitating factor. In this circumstance, the offending organism may not be enteric, and the syndrome is more likely to occur in patients who have pre-existing ascites, impaired immunologic defenses, or a cause for bacteremia such as localized infection elsewhere in the body or indwelling catheters. A widely recognized example of this circumstance is the child with nephrotic syndrome and ascites who develops primary peritonitis. The pathogenesis is probably hematogenous seeding of the peritoneum, particularly suggested by the frequent identification of extra-abdominal pathogens such as *Streptococcus pneumoniae*. The mortality rate associated with this entity has diminished considerably during recent decades because of the availability of antimicrobial drugs.

More common is spontaneous bacterial peritonitis in patients with advanced, decompensated cirrhosis and ascites. This syndrome is discussed in Ch. 122.

OTHER INFECTIONS. *Tuberculous peritonitis* is discussed in detail in Ch. 332. This disorder may present in a variety of ways, ranging from an acute abdomen to an insidiously developing, otherwise unexplained ascites resembling cirrhosis. Accordingly, its presence should be suspected in all patients with ascites, particularly in patients from endemic areas, in cirrhotic patients, and in immunosuppressed patients. Fewer than half of the patients have active disease elsewhere in the body, and tuberculosis skin testing and appropriate cultures of ascitic fluid for tubercle bacilli should be regarded as routine in the evaluation of ascites. The diagnosis is strongly suggested by a high percentage of lymphocytes in the abdominal fluid and may be confirmed by means of a positive culture, peritoneal biopsy, laparoscopy, or, if necessary, exploratory laparotomy. The very satisfactory response of this condition to appropriate chemotherapy adds to the importance of early diagnosis.

N. gonorrhoeae and *C. trachomatis* may enter the peritoneal cavity through the female genital tract and cause peritonitis, or rarely, ascites. This usually presents with right upper quadrant pain, tenderness, and fever (perihepatitis, Fitz-Hugh-Curtis syndrome) (see Ch. 336). *Fungal and parasitic diseases* may be associated with peritoneal involvement and occasionally with ascites. The most common fungal peritonitis is due to *candidiasis*, which may occur after contamination of the peritoneal cavity caused by perforated ulcer, trauma, surgery, or peritoneal dialysis. Other disorders, including histoplasmosis, coccidioidomycosis, cryptococcosis, ascariasis, amebiasis, and schistosomiasis, are quite uncommon, but deserve consideration in otherwise unexplained cases of peritoneal disease with or without ascites.

TUMORS OF THE PERITONEUM

SECONDARY CARCINOMATOSIS. Secondary malignancy is the most common form of neoplastic involvement of the peritoneum. More than 75 per cent of such tumors are classified as adenocarcinoma, mainly from ovary, pancreas, and colon, but peritoneal involvement by sarcoma, lymphoma, leukemia, carcinoid, and multiple myeloma has been described. Ascites formation in these patients appears to result from the combination of increased capillary permeability and obstruction of channels that drain the peritoneal cavity by way of the subdiaphragmatic lymphatics. The clinical picture is usually that associated with advancing malignancy, including weakness and weight loss, and variable complaints referable to the abdomen such as pain, distention, nausea, or vomiting. Radiographic findings may include angulation, fixation, or displacement of intestinal loops, or submucosal edema reflecting lymphatic obstruction. Ultrasonography or computed tomography may help confirm the presence of ascites and associated mass lesions. On abdominal paracentesis, the fluid obtained usually has a high LDH and protein content (more than 3.0 grams per deciliter) and low albumin gradient; cellular composition is variable, and occasionally the fluid is grossly bloody (see Tables 110–2 and 110–3). The diagnosis is made by cytology in approximately 50 per cent of patients, and, if that is negative, by computed tomography–guided percutaneous biopsy or peritoneoscopy. The diagnostic yield of fluid and tissue studies may be increased by new techniques such as flow cytometry and immunologic determination of a variety of tumor or tissue markers. Occasionally surgical exploration may be necessary.

Malignant ascites formation is a grave prognostic sign, with few patients surviving beyond 6 months after onset. Treatment of this condition involves the intraperitoneal administration of antitumor agents, including alkylators, antimetabolites, or radioactive isotopes. The standard intracavitary treatments use a small drug volume, but recent trials have used a large volume (2 liters) administered through a semipermanent indwelling catheter to allow for uniform drug distribution, high local drug levels, and repetitive treatments. Intra-abdominal quinicrine or other sclerosing agents have occasionally been successful in producing a fibrous serositis, thereby obliterating the free peritoneal space and reducing further fluid exudation, but the usefulness of this approach is limited by the frequent occurrence of fever, nausea, vomiting, and abdominal pain.

Salt restriction and diuretics may be tried but are often unsuccessful. Paracentesis is useful, and removal of large volumes may be well tolerated; although it may reduce body protein stores, it is often indispensable for patient comfort. In selected patients, peritoneovenous shunting affords palliation in 75 per cent of cases.

PRIMARY MESOTHELIOMA. The mesothelium may undergo hyperplasia or metaplasia, and rare benign cystic and papillary mesotheliomas have been described, but most mesothelial neoplasms are malignant. Primary mesotheliomas are tumors arising from the epithelial and mesenchymal elements of the mesothelium. Approximately 25 per cent involve the peritoneum, often in association with the more frequent pleural localization. Exposure to asbestos is the most established etiologic factor (see Ch. 527), although it is unclear if asbestos fibers produce peritoneal disease by passage from the intestinal lumen, penetration of the diaphragm, or via retrograde lymphatic transport.

Mesothelioma is most common in males over the age of 50 and is associated with the gradual onset of abdominal pain and distention, anorexia, nausea, vomiting, weight loss, and ascites. Blood counts and chemistries are rarely helpful, and barium contrast films reveal nonspecific findings. Ultrasonography and computed tomography demonstrate ascites and sheetlike masses that may suggest the diagnosis. Paracentesis yields an exudate that may be hemorrhagic, and high fluid hyaluronic acid concentrations suggest the diagnosis. Peritoneoscopy reveals extensive studding of peritoneal surfaces with nodules and plaques. However, laparotomy is often necessary to provide adequate biopsies and rule out a primary neoplasm. Even with biopsy or cytologic specimens, the variable histologic characteristics of epithelial and mesenchymal elements may make it difficult to differentiate from other malignancies.

The prognosis of peritoneal mesothelioma is exceedingly poor, with a median survival of about 1 year after diagnosis. Death usually results from cachexia or obstruction rather than metastatic disease. Tumor response and increased survival have been reported after chemotherapy (especially doxorubicin) and/or radiotherapy. Intensive combination therapy with surgical debulking, whole abdominal radiotherapy, and intraperitoneal doxorubicin and cisplatin may provide substantial palliation in selected, early cases.

PSEUDOMYXOMA PERITONEI. Pseudomyxoma peritonei is a rare condition in which the peritoneal cavity becomes distended with a mucinous, semisolid, translucent material. The two major causes of this "mucinous ascites" are mucinous cystadenomas and cystadenocarcinomas of the ovary and appendix, although other tumors of the genitourinary and gastrointestinal tract have been associated with the process. Extensive pseudomyxoma is invariably associated with cystadenocarcinomas, although they may be low grade.

The condition usually presents as an increase in abdominal girth with little in the way of other clinical signs of disease. At surgery, the abdominal cavity is found to contain gelatinous material existing in a variety of states, including cystic masses, lying freely without apparent attachment or anchored to the peritoneal surface. If the tumor is indeed malignant, it appears to be low grade and rarely metastasizes. As a result, the course of the disease is prolonged and is characterized by recurrent episodes of intestinal obstruction and fistula formation. Surgical removal of the ovary, appendix, and as much mucin as possible and intraperitoneal instillation of an alkylating agent are usually indicated. More aggressive combination therapy with surgical debulking and intra-peritoneal chemotherapy is also being investigated.

GRANULOMATOUS PERITONITIS. The peritoneum responds to a wide variety of stimuli with a granulomatous inflammatory reaction. *Exogenous* causes include mycobacteria, parasites, fungi, or organic material; *endogenous* causes are rare and include keratin in squamous tumors, meconium, sarcoidosis, and Crohn's disease. The most common etiology is *iatrogenic*, due to contamination at the time of surgery from starch, talc, cotton, or wood fibers used in surgical gloves, gowns, or drapes. *Starch granulomatous peritonitis* presents 2 to 9 weeks postoperatively with pain, tenderness, fever, distention, nausea, and vomiting and may suggest adhesions or abscesses. If it is considered, the diagnosis can be made by demonstrating starch granules in peritoneal fluid. Short-term indomethacin or corticosteroids often speed recovery.

SCLEROSING PERITONITIS. This unusual form of peritonitis manifests with symptoms of intestinal obstruction caused by the encasement of the entire small bowel in a fibrotic membrane or "cocoon." Several causes have been reported: (1) *Toxins*, such as practolol, a β-blocker; (2) *foreign bodies*, such as indwelling peritoneal catheters for shunts, chemotherapy, or dialysis, and (3) *idiopathic*, occurring in young females. The etiology is unclear but may involve toxins or subacute infections that stimulate fibroblast proliferation.

MISCELLANEOUS DISEASES OF THE PERITONEUM. The peritoneal membrane may be affected by a wide variety of systemic diseases, including systemic lupus erythematosus (see Ch. 261) and other collagen vascular diseases, Whipple's disease (see Ch. 102), familial Mediterranean fever (see Ch. 196), and eosinophilic gastroenteritis. Rarely, unusual tissues deposit on the peritoneum, which may cause low-grade peritoneal symptoms or be mistaken for metastatic carcinoma. Examples include endometrial, decidual, glial, and splenic tissue. Several other unusual conditions affecting the peritoneum have been described (Table 110–5).

MESENTERIC INFLAMMATORY DISEASE. This syndrome includes a spectrum of conditions ranging from acute inflammation to a chronic fibrosing process associated with intestinal obstruction, ascites, and steatorrhea. Included are such conditions as "mesenteric panniculitis" and "retractile mesenteritis." The cause of this syndrome is not known, but it is believed to represent the sequel to some inciting event such as trauma, infection, or ischemia in the mesentery. Fat necrosis occurs, evoking an inflammatory reaction with subsequent scarring and granuloma formation.

The condition is most commonly seen in males and in late adulthood. The acute syndrome ("mesenteric panniculitis"), which constitutes the presentation of 60 per cent of cases, is characterized by recurring abdominal pain, weight loss, nausea, vomiting, and fever. In most patients, a tender abdominal mass is palpable; leukocytosis may or may not be present. The remaining 40 per cent of cases are identified by the discovery of a mass on examination or at surgery. Radiographic examination is nonspecific, showing the effects of an abdominal mass and variable scarring that includes displacement and separation of intestinal loops with angulation, stenosis, and extrinsic compression. In some patients the condition evolves into a more chronic process ("retractile mesenteritis"), characterized by continuing pain, fever, weight loss, and various signs of intestinal obstruction, ascites, and steatorrhea. At surgery, the small bowel mesentery is found to be the principal site of involvement; it is thickened and fibrotic, particularly at the root. Resection of the mass is often not possible and generally should not be attempted. Microscopically in mesenteric panniculitis there is infiltration of adipose tissue by foamy macrophages and lymphocytes, with fat necrosis, fibrosis, and calcification. In retractile mesenteritis, the thickening and fibrosis are more pronounced, and there is less evidence of acute necrosis and inflammation. Infrequently, the mesocolon or parietal peritoneum may be involved, or the process may occur in association with retroperitoneal fibrosis.

Most patients seem to have prolonged survival and become asymptomatic after a period of months to years. A minority exhibits the more chronic symptoms noted earlier. The role of corticosteroids is uncertain; although they may be effective in the management of those patients in whom acute symptoms predominate, there is no evidence that they affect the long-term prognosis or progression of the disease. In 15 per cent of patients, malignant lymphomas develop; the basis for this apparent association is not known.

MESENTERIC AND OMENTAL CYSTS AND TUMORS. Mesenteric cysts usually develop as the result of anomalies in the mesenteric lymphatic system but may also be of mesothelial origin. They may spontaneously wax and wane in size; usually they do not cause symptoms in patients less than 10 years of age. Symptoms are related to the size and position of the cyst, which on physical examination is nontender, round, and mobile. Spontaneous rupture, hemorrhage, or infection may occur, but these complications are unusual. Treatment consists of surgical enucleation or excision.

Mesenteric tumors are rare and usually arise from the cellular elements normally present in the mesentery. They include fibromas, myxomas, lipomas, and other less common neoplasms of mesenchymal or neural origin. Most are well differentiated, low-grade fibrosarcomas that produce symptoms such as pain, weight loss, abdominal mass, and compression of adjacent organs. They may be treated successfully by surgical excision. Others are more highly malignant and may metastasize distantly. *Mesenteric lymphoid tumors* also occur, and certain of these have been associated with unexplained abnormalities in iron metabolism with hypochromic microcytic anemia. *Metastatic tumors* of the mesentery are more common than primary tumors and are usually due to enlarged lymphomatous or carcinomatous lymph nodes.

Tumors of the omentum, unlike those of the mesentery, are chiefly muscular in origin (leiomyomas, leiomyosarcomas). About 40 per cent of these are malignant and cause symptoms by virtue of local invasion and development of an abdominal mass; distant metastasis is unusual.

MISCELLANEOUS DISEASES OF OMENTUM AND MESENTERY. *Torsion of the omentum* is an acute surgical condition that mimics acute appendicitis or cholecystitis. It usually occurs in patients over age 30 and causes right-sided abdominal pain with nausea, vomiting, fever, leukocytosis, and occasionally a mass. Omentectomy is indicated. *Idiopathic primary omental infarction* presents a similar clinical picture and is invariably diagnosed only at laparotomy. *Mesenteric fibromatosis* (desmoid tumor) is a benign, noninflammatory fibrous proliferation of the mesentery, which occurs mainly in patients with familial polyposis of the colon or Gardner's syndrome.

Bender MD, Ockner RK: Ascites. *In* Sleisenger MH, Fordtran JS (eds.): Gastrointestinal Disease. 4th ed. Philadelphia, W. B. Saunders Company, 1989.
Bender MD, Ockner RK: Diseases of the peritoneum, mesentery and diaphragm. *In* Sleisenger MH, Fordtran JS (eds.): Gastrointestinal Disease. 4th ed. Philadelphia, W. B. Saunders Company, 1989. *A broad review, extensively referenced.*
Hoefs JC: Diagnostic paracentesis: A potent clinical tool. Gastroenterology 98:230, 1990. *A complete review of the role of paracentesis in the diagnosis of peritonitis and the differential diagnosis of ascites. The utility of the albumin gradient is thoroughly explained and stressed.*
Malangoni MA, Shumate CR, Thomas MA, et al.: Factors influencing the treatment of intra-abdominal abscesses. Am J Surg 159:167, 1990. *A comparison of radiologic and surgical drainage, and the best time to use each.*
Piceigallo E, Jeffer LJ, Reddy KJ, et al.: Malignant peritoneal mesothelioma. Dig Dis Sci 33:633, 1988. *An analysis of 10 cases collected over 20 years from two institutions. Laparoscopic findings are well described.*
Press OW, Press NO, Kaufman SD: Evaluation and management of chylous ascites. Ann Intern Med 96:358, 1982. *An analysis of 28 cases from one institution, seen over 20 years.*
Reddy KJ, DiPrima RE, Raskin JB, et al.: Tuberculous peritonitis: Laparoscopic diagnosis of an uncommon disease in the United States. Gastrointest Endosc 34:422, 1988. *Review of 15 cases found over 15 years from one institution.*
Rodgers PN, Wright IH, Ledingham IM: Critical abdominal sepsis. J R Coll Surg Edinb 34:1, 1989. *A thorough review of the pathophysiology and treatment of severe peritonitis.*
Vanek VW, Phillips AK: Retroperitoneal, mesenteric and omental cysts. Arch Surg 119:838, 1984. *Surveys the literature and gives a complete overview of cystic lesions.*
Weaver DW, Walt AJ, Sugawa C, et al.: A continuing appraisal of pancreatic ascites. Surg Gynecol Obstet 154:845, 1982. *Reviews a series of 42 alcoholic patients with chronic pancreatitis. Preoperative endoscopic retrograde cholangiopancreatography (ERCP) is emphasized to plan the surgical approach.*

111 Gastrointestinal Hemorrhage

John P. Cello

Bleeding from the gastrointestinal tract is one of the most common causes of admission to urban medical centers in the Western world. While in some countries the number of patients admitted for peptic ulcer disease has gradually decreased, the overall mortality for gastrointestinal tract hemorrhage has remained largely unchanged over the past several decades. A multiplicity of lesions can cause bleeding from the gastrointestinal tract (Tables 111–1 and 111–2). Although the specific bleeding lesion and pathophysiology of hemorrhage may vary considerably, the initial therapeutic and diagnostic approach to the bleeding patient remains largely the same (Fig. 111–1).

SIGNS AND SYMPTOMS

Gastrointestinal tract hemorrhage usually produces dramatic clinical signs and symptoms that bring patients to the attention of physicians. *Hematemesis* is the term applied to vomiting of gross blood. Usually, vomiting of bloody material is indicative of bleeding from the upper gastrointestinal tract, but blood passing into the gastrointestinal tract from anywhere proximal to the ligament of Treitz (duodenojejunal junction) can be vomited by the patient (Table 111–1). Hematemesis most frequently follows bleeding *from* the esophagus, stomach, or duodenum, but occasionally nasopharyngeal, pulmonary, and even pancreaticobiliary

TABLE 111–1. ETIOLOGY AND SEVERITY OF UPPER GASTROINTESTINAL TRACT HEMORRHAGE*

Source of Hemorrhage	Severity of Hemorrhage	
	Mild-Moderate (246 cases)	Severe (140 cases)
Esophagus		
Esophagitis	12%	7%
Ulcer	2%	2%
Mallory-Weiss tear	5%	19%
Esophageal varices	5%	31%
Total Esophagus	24%	59%
Stomach		
Gastric ulcer	15%	14%
Prepyloric ulcer	2%	4%
Pyloric channel ulcer	4%	2%
Gastric erosions	2%	0
Gastritis	7%	0
Varices	1%	2%
Portal-hypertensive gastropathy	2%	
Gastric cancer	2%	2%
Polyp	0	
Dieulafoy lesion	0	
Total Stomach	35%	24%
Duodenum		
Ulcer	31%	15%
Duodenitis	8%	
Diverticulum		
Aortoenteric fistula	2%	2%
Pancreatic pseudocyst		
Post-sphincterotomy		
Total Duodenum	41%	17%
	100%	100%

*All patients underwent diagnostic endoscopy at the San Francisco General Hospital over 3 years.

tract bleeding can be manifested initially by hematemesis. *Melenemesis,* or "coffee grounds" vomiting, occurs when blood has had an appreciable period of time in contact with gastric acid. Patients vomiting "coffee grounds" material are usually bleeding at a slower rate than those who have bloody emesis. As with hematemesis, "coffee grounds" emesis follows bleeding into the gastrointestinal tract from a site proximal to the duodenojejunal junction. As with hematemesis, however, it too can follow bleeding from the nasopharynx, tracheobronchial tree, liver, or pancreas. *Melena,* usually noted by patients with bleeding from the proximal gastrointestinal tract, is characterized by dark black, liquid, tarry, metallic-smelling stools. Melenic stools usually indicate upper gastrointestinal tract bleeding, but not infrequently mid- to distal small bowel and even proximal colonic bleeding can be manifested by dark, black, liquid stools. *Hematochezia,* bright red stools, is usually a sign of distal small bowel or colonic hemorrhage (Table 111–2). Brisk hemorrhage from the proximal gastrointestinal tract with accelerated transit may, however, present with dark red blood in the stools. Up to 10 per cent of patients with hemodynamically significant hematochezia are actually bleeding from an upper, not lower, gastrointestinal tract lesion. The remaining 90 per cent of patients with hemato-

TABLE 111–2. ETIOLOGY OF HEMATOCHEZIA IN 72 HOSPITALIZED PATIENTS*

Source of Hemorrhage	Per Cent
Colonic cancer	7
Colonic polyps	11
Diverticula	23
Colitis	11
Vascular ectasia	1
Large hemorrhoids only	12
Ulcer/tear (rectum)	10
Upper gastrointestinal or small bowel source	10
No site identified	15
	100

*Patients underwent colonoscopy (and endoscopy if colonoscopy was negative) at the San Francisco General Hospital

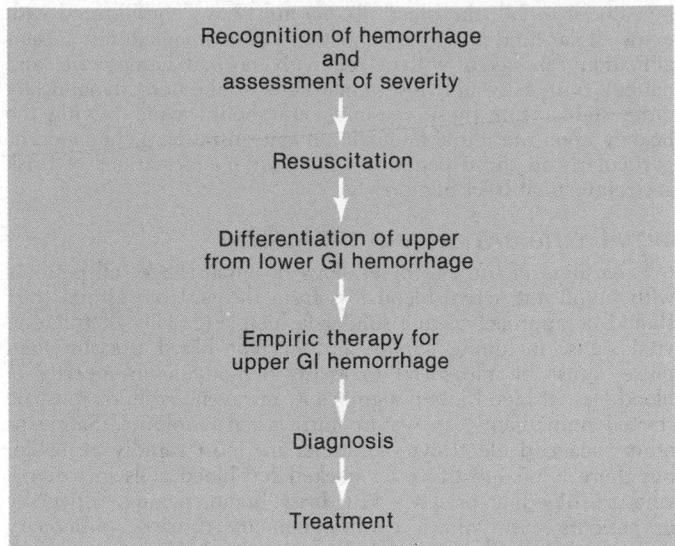

FIGURE 111–1. Approach to the patient with gastrointestinal hemorrhage.

chezia are bleeding from some site distal to the ileocecal valve, with the majority, particularly in those without orthostatic signs or symptoms, bleeding from superficial mucosal lesions in the sigmoid, rectum, or anorectal junction. In addition to signs of gross blood loss, patients with hemodynamically significant gastrointestinal tract bleeding often present with lightheadedness, dizziness, diaphoresis, or frank syncope if hypovolemia has occurred. Patients with slow but persistent gastrointestinal tract bleeding may present with signs and symptoms of profound iron deficiency anemia, including pallor, dyspnea, angina, and exertional weakness (Ch. 131).

DETERMINATION OF THE SEVERITY OF THE HEMORRHAGE

Patients with gastrointestinal tract bleeding often present very dramatically with the above-indicated signs and symptoms. First, the severity of bleeding must be rapidly assessed and resuscitation instituted. In all patients with brisk gastrointestinal tract hemorrhage, these measures take priority over any diagnostic or specific therapeutic approaches. The most accurate noninvasive indicator of the severity of blood loss is the presence of *shock* or changes in *postural vital signs.* Shock is indicative of an acute blood volume loss of at least 15 to 20 per cent. Postural vital sign changes, i.e., upright tachycardia, widening of the pulse pressure, and/or upright systolic hypotension, are indicative of acute intravascular volume loss of at least 10 to 15 per cent. It is therefore essential to determine the blood pressure and pulse in the sitting and standing positions in patients who report signs and symptoms of gastrointestinal tract blood loss but who have normal *supine* vital signs.

Other bedside diagnostic findings may indicate the severity of hemorrhage in patients with upper gastrointestinal tract bleeding. Brisk hemorrhage with hematemesis and/or "coffee grounds" emesis is usually associated with *increasing stool frequency, hyperactive bowel sounds,* and a *change in the color of the stools* from dark black to dark red color. With bleeding from a postpyloric duodenal ulcer, relatively small amounts of blood may be vomited or lavaged by nasogastric tube, most passing distally into the gastrointestinal tract. *Nasogastric lavage* is helpful but highly inaccurate in estimating the severity of upper gastrointestinal tract bleeding. Young patients with duodenal ulcers in particular may exhibit a small amount of bloody emesis and/or "coffee grounds" on nasogastric tube lavage. However, the absence of significant blood by nasogastric lavage (particularly when the lavage does not contain bile) does not rule out upper gastrointestinal tract bleeding. With profuse hematemesis, the return of large amounts of clots or bright red blood is obviously indicative of vigorous active upper gastrointestinal tract hemorrhage. In the face of fresh bleeding, the *hematocrit and hemoglobin levels* are not reliable indicators of the severity of bleeding. For the hematocrit to fall, the blood plasma must have equilibrated with extracellular fluid or with administered intravenous fluids. Exsanguination can occur with a relatively normal hematocrit, and patients with extremely low hematocrits can be hemodynamically quite stable. For these reasons, one should avoid relying too heavily upon the initial hemoglobin concentration or hematocrit, particularly in those patients with other manifestations of brisk gastrointestinal tract hemorrhage.

INITIAL EVALUATION AND TREATMENT

Regardless of the site or etiology of hemorrhage, all patients with significant active blood loss from the gastrointestinal tract should be approached in a similar fashion (Fig. 111–1). Initially, vital signs, including supine and upright blood pressure and pulse, must be measured to assess hemodynamic severity of blood loss. If blood loss is significant, intravenous fluids must be started immediately to restore intravascular volume. Saline or other balanced electrolyte solutions are most rapidly available, but there is no substitute for packed red blood cells in patients who are bleeding briskly. With brisk hemorrhaging, especially in patients with known cardiopulmonary disease, pulmonary artery and peripheral arterial catheters may be helpful in monitoring the severity of bleeding and the adequacy of resuscitation. Nasal oxygen should be administered to these patients to improve blood oxygen transport.

The history of the bleeding episode and of any previous gastrointestinal tract hemorrhage should be rapidly obtained after the initial evaluative and resuscitative measures noted above. A personal or family history of gastrointestinal tract illness, particularly from peptic ulcers, cancer, or vascular ectasias (e.g., Osler-Weber-Rendu syndrome) is helpful, as is a history of previously documented gastrointestinal tract disease as determined by radiography, endoscopy, or surgical procedures. Patients with a longstanding history of alcohol abuse or known or suspected chronic active liver disease may present with painless hematemesis from esophageal varices. Substernal burning pain, regurgitation, or reflux symptoms may indicate longstanding reflux esophagitis. Patients with forceful, dry retching or multiple episodes of vomiting of food prior to the onset of hematemesis may be bleeding from Mallory-Weiss tears of the gastroesophageal junction. A history of epigastric burning pain promptly relieved by food or antacids or nocturnal pain suggests peptic ulcer disease, particularly duodenal ulcer (Ch. 98). Dyspepsia may not always occur in patients with bleeding from peptic ulcer disease, however.

A history of known diverticular disease supports the possibility of colonic diverticular hemorrhage in patients with brisk hematochezia (Ch. 112). Colorectal malignancy is often suggested by a history of gradual weight loss, intermittent blood in the stools, or altered bowel habits (Ch. 105). Patients with idiopathic inflammatory bowel disease often have longstanding mucous and bloody diarrhea (Ch. 103). Hemorrhoidal bleeding is often suggested by the presence of bright red blood surrounding well-formed normal-appearing stools.

The physical examination is sometimes helpful in suggesting the etiology of hemorrhage. Patients with stigmata of chronic liver disease (e.g., spider angiomata, ascites, gynecomastia) and upper gastrointestinal tract bleeding often bleed from esophageal varices, but almost half are found to be bleeding from lesions other than varices. Localized epigastric tenderness to palpation may indicate peptic ulcer disease or gastritis. Occasionally patients with lower gastrointestinal tract bleeding from a malignancy have a palpable lower abdominal mass, signs of obvious weight loss, or adenopathy. A rectal examination is essential to document stool color as well as to palpate for gross anorectal mass lesions such as polyps, cancers, or large hemorrhoids.

Following rapid resuscitation and an expedited history and physical examination, nasogastric tube lavage should be carried out, not only for obvious signs and symptoms of upper gastrointestinal tract hemorrhage but also for hemodynamically significant hematochezia. Blood or "coffee grounds" material in a nasogastric lavage may indicate that bright red blood per rectum is coming from an upper gastrointestinal tract site. Nasogastric tube lavage using room temperature water may also decrease the bleeding rate by vasoconstricting smaller gastric vessels.

Following the initial evaluation, the hematocrit or hemoglobin, the prothrombin time, and the partial thromboplastin time should be measured and a specimen of blood obtained for typing and cross-matching for transfusions. For patients with shock or postural vital sign changes, four to six units of packed red cells should be cross-matched urgently. A serum electrolyte and chemistry panel should likewise be requested. A disproportionate elevation of the BUN:creatinine ratio may indicate bleeding from a proximal gastrointestinal site. In addition, gross abnormalities of liver function tests may suggest the presence of varices as the cause of hemorrhage.

UPPER GASTROINTESTINAL TRACT

Peptic ulcer disease, including both duodenal and gastric ulcers, is the most common cause of upper gastrointestinal tract bleeding (see Color Plate 1C). It is responsible for 50 per cent of moderately severe and 35 per cent of severe bleeding episodes (Table 111–1). Bleeding from peptic ulcers may not always be associated with heartburn or epigastric burning pain, especially in older patients. *Hemorrhage from esophageal or gastric varices* (responsible for nearly one third of the episodes of massive upper gastrointestinal hemorrhage) is usually, but not always, associated with known or suspected chronic liver disease (see Color Plate 1A and B). Most patients with variceal hemorrhage due to alcohol abuse have physical stigmata of liver disease such as a large, firm liver, gross ascites, scleral icterus, palmar erythema, and evidence of peripheral muscle wasting. However, patients with postnecrotic cirrhosis due to viral hepatitis often lack overt peripheral stigmata of chronic liver disease. Variceal hemorrhage usually presents with brisk bleeding, occasionally with regurgitation of large amounts of dark, clotted blood without emesis. However, variceal hemorrhage may present occasionally with only "coffee grounds" emesis and melena. *Mallory-Weiss tears* of the gastroesophageal junction (causing 5 per cent of minor and 20 per cent of severe upper gastrointestinal hemorrhage) are usually associated with antecedent, forceful retching. Nearly half of patients with Mallory-Weiss tears abuse alcohol and report "dry heaves" followed by small and then progressively larger amounts of bloody emesis. *Gastritis* due to alcohol or nonsteroidal anti-inflammatory agents is usually manifested by epigastric discomfort not relieved by food or antacids (Ch. 97). The signs and symptoms of gastritis-associated bleeding may be identical to those of gastric ulcer disease. *Esophagitis* (see Color Plate 1D), particularly in the patient with longstanding reflux or regurgitation, is suggested by substernal burning pain occasionally relieved by the ingestion of food or antacids (Ch. 96). Alcohol abusers or patients with prolonged recumbency may sometimes have brisk bleeding from esophagitis without any antecedent substernal burning. *Gastrointestinal tract malignancies*, such as esophageal, gastric, or duodenal cancer or carcinoma of the ampulla of Vater, rarely cause hemodynamically significant upper gastrointestinal tract bleeding (Table 111–1). Rare causes of upper gastrointestinal tract bleeding include (1) *aortoduodenal fistulae* in patients with atherosclerotic aneurysms of the abdominal aorta, usually following prosthetic grafting; (2) chronic renal disease and *acquired vascular ectasias*, or (3) ectasias associated with other systemic conditions, such as hereditary hemorrhagic telangiectasias (Osler-Weber-Rendu syndrome). Patients with trauma to the liver or with pancreatic pseudocysts may present with signs and symptoms suggestive of upper gastrointestinal tract bleeding but are actually bleeding from adjacent organs. Even rare causes include ectatic superficial arteries (Dieulafoy lesions), duodenal diverticula, and endoscopic sphincterotomy.

Diagnostic and Therapeutic Approach
ENDOSCOPY

Multiple diagnostic procedures are available to localize the site of hemorrhage in patients with upper gastrointestinal bleeding. For patients with hemodynamically significant upper gastrointestinal tract bleeding (bleeding associated with shock, postural vital sign changes, multiple units of transfusion), endoscopy is the diagnostic procedure of choice because of its high accuracy and immediate therapeutic potential. Endoscopy, however, must be performed only following adequate resuscitation and clinical assessment of the patient (Fig. 111–1). If bleeding is severe, the patient should be transferred to an intensive care unit or an operating room where adequate monitoring and resuscitation can be maintained. Endoscopy can document the site of brisk hemorrhage in at least 95 per cent of patients. In patients with significant cardiopulmonary disease, however, endoscopy is not without risk, since it does require sedation and analgesia. Furthermore, endoscopy is considerably more expensive than other means of evaluation, such as an upper gastrointestinal barium series. An endoscopic evaluation of a vigorously bleeding, unstable patient should be performed by an expert because it requires careful sedation, lavage, selection of instruments, and the use of accessory therapeutic endoscopic procedures. Although endoscopy is used in virtually all patients with manifestations of acute gastrointestinal tract hemorrhage, its urgent use is indicated primarily for patients with any of the following: postural vital sign changes or shock, multiple transfusions, hematocrits diluting below 30 per cent, a high index of suspicion of variceal hemorrhage, recurrent hemorrhage from unknown sources, and high risk for surgery (prior to undertaking a surgical procedure). Contraindications to endoscopy include acute myocardial infarction, severe chronic lung disease, hemodynamic instability, and patient agitation. Furthermore, endoscopy is strongly contraindicated in any patient whose underlying disease is so severe as to preclude effective treatment. This latter contraindication to endoscopy is the only absolute one, since patients with other contraindications can often undergo endoscopy safely with expert attention.

In addition to documenting the site and probable cause of hemorrhage, endoscopy may provide definitive short-term or long-term therapy. Acute variceal bleeding, for example, can be controlled with endoscopic sclerotherapy in nearly 90 per cent of patients and the likelihood of recurrent bleeding diminished. The long-term effect of this treatment on survival is less well established. Endoscopic multipolar (or bipolar or "bicap") electrocoagulation and heater probe coagulation are inexpensive, widely available, and highly reliable techniques for controlling upper gastrointestinal tract hemorrhage, particularly for patients with actively bleeding ulcers. These techniques, essentially comparable to one another in effectiveness, not only control acute hemorrhage but also decrease transfusion requirements, the necessity for surgery, and the duration and cost of hospitalization. Endoscopic injections of sclerosants or dilute solutions of epinephrine directly into the bleeding site of an ulcer also show early promise. Endoscopic laser photocoagulation has been advocated, but its expense, logistic constraints, lack of general availability, and absence of advantages over the use of contact coagulation probes have greatly reduced its employment. Endoscopic sclerotherapy for varices and coagulation and injection hemostasis for peptic ulcers are now widely accepted therapies, particularly for patients with hemodynamically significant bleeding.

BARIUM RADIOGRAPHY

An "upper G.I. series," when performed with a double-contrast technique, identifies at least 70 to 80 per cent of lesions confirmed to be associated with upper gastrointestinal tract bleeding. Barium radiography is noninvasive, lower in cost than endoscopy, and readily available but has significant disadvantages, particularly in patients who are bleeding briskly. Large amounts of retained blood in the upper gastrointestinal tract impede the mucosal coating by barium and therefore the localization of superficial mucosal lesions. In patients who are briskly bleeding and hemodynamically unstable, contrast radiography is also impractical. Moreover, on occasion, multiple lesions may be detected by barium radiography and the actual site of bleeding may be difficult to assess. Barium contrast radiography is an acceptable means of diagnosing upper gastrointestinal lesions, however, in patients who have not bled excessively, who have no stigmata of chronic liver disease, and who are not in need of endoscopic hemostasis.

ANGIOGRAPHY

The site of upper gastrointestinal tract bleeding may occasionally be missed on endoscopy. In these patients, angiography may localize the site of bleeding. In addition, selective infusion with vasopressin or coil embolization of actively bleeding arteries may control bleeding. In most instances, angiography localizes the bleeding site but does not establish its etiology. Bleeding must also be active because angiography detects only extravasation of contrast into the gastrointestinal tract. Angiography is expensive, time consuming, and invasive and requires transportation of the patient to a specialized unit, but it is particularly helpful if bleeding is brisk in the face of a negative evaluation of the upper or lower gastrointestinal tract.

NUCLEAR SCINTIGRAPHY

For patients with less active blood loss, technetium red cell nuclear scintigraphy ("red cell scan") can be helpful in localizing the site of bleeding, with a reported sensitivity of as little as 3 ml of blood loss per hour. Scintigraphy is noninvasive and can be performed with portable gamma cameras. As with angiography, the sensitivity of technetium scintigraphy is limited, since active hemorrhage is needed; therefore, frequent repeat scanning is necessary. Technetium red cell scanning is often performed prior to any angiographic evaluation to assist in the localization of the bleeding focus.

LOWER GASTROINTESTINAL TRACT (Table 111–2)

Colonic diverticula (see Color Plate 1*G*) are responsible for nearly one quarter of all episodes of hemodynamically significant bleeding from the lower gastrointestinal tract (Table 111–2). Diverticular hemorrhage is characteristically painless and associated with large-volume hematochezia. Patients with clinical diverticulitis rarely bleed significantly (Ch. 112). *Colonic cancers and polyps* (see Color Plate 1*E* and *H*) often present with gross blood loss, particularly with lesions in the distal sigmoid colon and rectum. Colonic neoplasms cause nearly 20 per cent of lower gastrointestinal bleeding episodes. Proximal colonic polyps and cancers, however, often present with iron deficiency anemia and less frequently with dark black or bloody stools. *Idiopathic ulcerative colitis and Crohn's colitis* commonly present with bloody diarrhea and tenesmus, and usually with a longstanding history of inflammatory bowel disease (Ch. 103). Significant lower gastrointestinal tract bleeding also occurs from abnormal, superficial vessels called *vascular ectasias*, previously called angiodysplasia (see Color Plate 1*F*). As noted above, up to 10 per cent of hemodynamically significant hematochezia is secondary to bleeding from upper gastrointestinal sites, particularly from duodenal bulbar ulcers (Table 111–2). Other uncommon causes of "lower" gastrointestinal blood loss include aortoenteric fistulae, Meckel's diverticula of the ileum, and mesenteric varices.

Diagnostic and Therapeutic Approach

Proctoscopy (whether by rigid or flexible instruments) with a careful evaluation of the anorectal junction is the initial diagnostic step for all patients with hematochezia. The anus and anorectal junction must be carefully examined for hemorrhoids or lacerations, since documented brisk bleeding from one of these sources can obviate the need for further invasive or noninvasive imaging. Blood from a very distal site in the rectum may retrogress into the colon and appear as blood coming from above the maximal depth of insertion of the proctoscope or sigmoidoscope. In addition to hemorrhoids, diverticula, and rectal lacerations, colitis and many polyps and cancers are found within reach of a sigmoidoscope.

Following anorectal and sigmoidoscopic examination, the evaluation of patients with lower gastrointestinal tract hemorrhage depends upon the clinical presentation. If blood loss is modest (as evidenced by a normal hematocrit and vital signs), sigmoidoscopy may be followed by *double-contrast barium radiography*, which is highly accurate for detecting even smaller polyps and superficial mucosal abnormalities such as colitis. Single-contrast barium enemas have a high false-negative rate, particularly for modest-sized polyps. If signs and symptoms indicate lower gastrointestinal tract hemorrhage together with anemia, *colonoscopy* should be performed as the next step in evaluation. The colon can be rapidly cleaned within a few hours, using oral, nonabsorbable electrolyte solutions, in order to make colonoscopy technically feasible. Colonoscopic evaluation not only allows the site of hemorrhage to be accurately determined but also allows for biopsy of suspicious mass lesions, polypectomy for modest-sized polyps, and the use of coagulation techniques for the control of bleeding from vascular ectasias. If brisk bleeding continues, as evidenced by profuse hematochezia, rapid *upper endoscopic evaluation* should be considered. Certainly this should be performed in all patients with "coffee grounds" nasogastric lavage and in patients with known or suspected peptic ulcer disease.

If bleeding is brisk, colonoscopy is usually not possible and other means of determining the site of hemorrhage are required. *Technetium red blood cell scintigraphy* can be employed in patients in whom there is substantial active bleeding (at least 3 to 10 ml per hour for a positive scan). Frequent repeat scanning may be needed over the first several hours. Technetium red cell scintigraphy usually localizes the site but not the etiology of active hemorrhage. If bleeding continues at a rate exceeding 30 to 50 ml per hour, *angiography* can be extremely helpful in localizing the site of hemorrhage. In addition, angiographic therapy is possible with vasopressin or embolization techniques. An obvious advantage for technetium scintigraphy or angiographic localization is that surgical resection of the site of hemorrhage, regardless of etiology, is usually very effective.

UNKNOWN ORIGIN

Rarely patients continue to bleed from the gastrointestinal tract without any lesion being detected by upper gastrointestinal endoscopy or pancolonoscopy. In these cases bleeding is usually from a lesion distal to the inferior duodenal angle and proximal to the ileocecal valve. In such patients, technetium scintigraphy, often repeated frequently, can be extremely helpful in localizing the site of hemorrhage. In addition, angiography may determine the site of active blood loss. Other techniques that are sometimes useful in patients with persistent gastrointestinal tract blood loss are *small bowel enteroclysis* and operative *panenteroscopy*. Small bowel enteroclysis, or small bowel enema, is performed by passing a nasoduodenal tube to facilitate the direct instillation of barium and methylcellulose. Radiographic evaluation of the entire small bowel can be completed by enteroclysis in less than 1 hour. Mass lesions such as polyps or cancers and diverticula such as Meckel's diverticula can thus be detected with a high degree of reliability. In patients who have bled repeatedly and profusely from the gastrointestinal tract and have negative evaluations by upper and lower endoscopy, operative panenteroscopy should be considered. At laparotomy, a sterilized endoscope is passed, usually through an enterotomy, and the entire small bowel is passed over the endoscope while the operator and assistant visualize the entire luminal surface. This is most commonly employed in detecting and treating patients with multiple vascular ectasias of the small bowel.

Cello JP, Grendell JH: Endoscopic laser treatment of gastrointestinal vascular ectasias. Ann Intern Med 104:352, 1986. *Review of clinical presentation, therapy, and outcome of patients with bleeding vascular ectasias.*

Cello JP, Grendell JH, Crass RA, et al.: Endoscopic sclerotherapy versus portacaval shunt in patients with severe cirrhosis and acute variceal hemorrhage. Long-term follow-up. N Engl J Med 316:11, 1987. *Randomized trial of endoscopic therapy and surgical shunting in cirrhotic patients with acute hemorrhage from esophageal varices.*

Cello JP, Thoeni RF: Gastrointestinal hemorrhage—comparative values of double-contrast upper gastrointestinal radiology and endoscopy. JAMA 243:685, 1980. *Study of endoscopy and radiography in diagnosing sites of acute upper gastrointestinal hemorrhage.*

Jensen DM, Machicado GA: Diagnosis and treatment of severe hematochezia. The role of urgent colonoscopy after purge. Gastroenterology 95:1569, 1988. *Prospective study of 80 patients admitted with severe rectal bleeding.*

Laine L: Multipolar electrocoagulation in the treatment of active upper gastrointestinal tract hemorrhage. A prospective controlled trial. N Engl J Med 316:1613, 1987. *Endoscopic coagulation reduces rebleeding, transfusions, duration of hospitalization, and hospital costs.*

Laine L: Multipolar electrocoagulation in the treatment of peptic ulcers with nonbleeding visible vessels. A prospective controlled trial. Ann Intern Med 110:510, 1989. *Endoscopic treatment of nonbleeding vessels in ulcer bases decreases morbidity, hospital stay, and hospital costs.*

Lewis BS, Waye JD: Chronic gastrointestinal bleeding of obscure origin: Role of small bowel enteroscopy. Gastroenterology 94:1117, 1988. *Endoscopic examination of the small bowel discloses additional lesions missed by standard endoscopy and colonoscopy.*

Rex DK, Lappas JC, Maglinte DD, et al.: Enteroclysis in the evaluation of suspected small intestinal bleeding. Gastroenterology 97:58, 1989. *Small bowel enemas may diagnose specific lesions in up to 20 per cent of patients with occult hemorrhage.*

112 Miscellaneous Inflammatory Diseases of the Intestine

Marvin H. Sleisenger

ACUTE APPENDICITIS (INCLUDING THE ACUTE ABDOMEN)

DEFINITION. Appendicitis is acute inflammation of the vermiform appendix. It is rare before the age of 2 and reaches a peak incidence in the second and third decades. The vast majority of patients are between the ages of 5 and 30. Although incidence of the disease declines after the age of 40, the annual incidence is about 1.5 per thousand for males and 1.9 per thousand for females between the ages of 17 and 64. The disease is important because it is common and curable; it therefore constitutes the most important entity in the differential diagnosis of the acute abdomen.

PATHOLOGY. Usually, the appendix is swollen, hyperemic, warm, and covered with exudate. However, in the early stages it may appear only slightly discolored and, in the late stages, gangrenous with perforation. Microscopically, the picture ranges from some acute inflammatory cells in the lumen and mucosa to acute inflammatory changes transmurally with superficial mucosal ulcerations; in advanced stages, one or more perforations may be noted, particularly in patients over the age of 60.

ETIOLOGY AND PATHOGENESIS. Although the vast majority of cases have no obvious cause for obstruction, identifiable etiologies include *calculi, Enterobius vermicularis, Kaposi's sarcoma, Burkitt's lymphoma, adenocarcinoma, schistosomiasis,* and *carcinoid tumors.* The initiating event in acute appendicitis appears to be obstruction, followed by increased intraluminal pressure, reduced venous drainage, thrombosis, hemorrhage, edema, and bacterial invasion of the wall. The appendiceal artery (an end-artery) becomes occluded and perforation results.

Calculi are thought to be the most common cause of the initial obstruction. A small percentage of inflamed appendices contain a radiologically demonstrable calculus, compared with 2.7 per cent of normal ones. Gangrene and perforation are more common in appendices with calculi. The calculi are composed of inspissated fecal material, calcium phosphate–rich mucus, and inorganic salts. Although fecaliths are more common in populations eating a low-fiber diet, the incidence of appendicitis is decreasing in the West, and 70 per cent of patients with acute appendicitis do not have calculi. Etiology when the lumen is not obstructed is unclear. Whether the increasing use of high-fiber diets underlies this reduction of incidence is not yet proved.

CLINICAL PICTURE AND DIAGNOSIS. The duration of appendicitis is usually 12 to 48 hours from onset to hospitalization. Over 95 per cent of patients complain of *pain* at onset, classically referred to the epigastric or periumbilical areas and later localizing in the right lower quadrant. This sequence, however, is not found in all patients and is notably absent in *retrocecal appendicitis.* Further, in a significant number of patients, particularly women in the late second or third trimester of pregnancy, the pain does not localize clearly to the right lower quadrant, being either diffuse or in the lower abdomen. In *pelvic appendicitis* the pain may be in the left lower quadrant. When retrocecal, the pain may be referred to the thigh or right testicle. Dysuria is present frequently in both types of appendicitis.

Pain referred to the mid-epigastrium is due to stretching of the organ during early inflammation. Initially it is vague and mild, but it gradually increases over about 4 hours and may be colicky. It tends to subside, and when the process has reached the serosa and the peritoneum, it localizes over the site of disease. In some patients distress appears to be alleviated at the time of perforation; after perforation, localization of pain depends on whether or not the process is quickly walled off locally. Thus if the spreading infection is not contained, generalized abdominal discomfort of variable severity results. *Anorexia* and *nausea* (with or without vomiting) are the second and third most frequent symptoms. In almost all instances, pain precedes the appearance of these other complaints, and its principal feature is *persistence*. About 10 per cent of patients have constipation; diarrhea is uncommon. Temperature usually ranges between 38 and 38.6°C; higher levels usually indicate perforation.

PHYSICAL EXAMINATION. The findings on physical examination depend not only upon the stage of the inflammation but also upon the age of the patient. Tenderness to palpation is the most common (99 per cent), important, and reliable sign; indeed, without it, diagnosis is unlikely. It is usually confined to McBurney's point (one finger) in the right lower quadrant, corresponding to the usual location of the organ. However, although rectal tenderness is present in about one third of patients, it may be so severe as to indicate pelvic peritonitis and thus probable *pelvic appendicitis*. On initial examination in a minority of patients, a mass may be felt in the right lower quadrant or in the pelvis or transrectally. Localized rebound pain is found in 75 per cent. Generalized rebound tenderness indicates diffuse peritonitis. Bowel sounds may be present or absent; absence associated with distention and generalized rebound tenderness is consistent with perforation and diffuse peritonitis. The patient with acute appendicitis often does not seem ill. The physician must not be deceived; the diagnosis rests upon persisting pain and localized tenderness.

On occasion, tenderness may be elicited in the case of retrocecal appendicitis by stretching the psoas by hip extension. Very rarely, because of the odd location of the appendix, tenderness may be in the right upper quadrant or even the left lower quadrant.

LABORATORY FINDINGS. Laboratory studies consistently show a leukocytosis with an increase in polymorphonuclear cells—over 10,000 per cubic millimeter and greater than 75 per cent, respectively. Urinalysis is usually normal; however, about 15 per cent of patients have either a slight amount of protein or mild pyuria or hematuria. Presence of a calcified fecalith in the right lower quadrant on flat film of the abdomen is helpful, but it is present in only a small percentage of patients. Other findings on flat film include possible obliteration of the right psoas shadow, right lower quadrant sentinel loop ileus, and a right lower quadrant soft tissue mass with or without gas bubbles. With perforation and generalized peritonitis, fluid in the peritoneal cavity and obliteration of the peritoneal lines may be noted.

DIFFERENTIAL DIAGNOSIS OF APPENDICITIS AND OF THE ACUTE ABDOMEN. Appendicitis is first on the list of conditions causing acute abdominal pain that require surgery or immediate consultation with a surgeon. Computed tomography (CT) is now increasingly used in diagnosis, demonstrating swelling, perforation, and fecaliths in a high proportion of cases, and appears to be more helpful than a plain film early in the disease. About 15 per cent of patients operated upon for acute appendicitis have a normal appendix; in view of the gravity of unoperated upon disease, this figure is entirely acceptable. Here a few principles regarding the acute surgical abdomen in the setting of the differential diagnosis of acute appendicitis are reviewed.

Pain Characteristics. Conditions associated with pain of sudden onset include *perforated viscus*, more commonly a *peptic ulcer* or a *colonic diverticulum*, or, rarely, a *carcinoma of the colon* or *acute ischemia* (although acute ischemia does not always cause acute or severe pain in the elderly). The onset of pain in *acute small bowel obstruction, choledocholithiasis, ureteral obstruction, rupture of an abdominal aortic aneurysm,* and *dissection of the abdominal aorta* may also be abrupt. The more gradual onset of pain usually indicates an inflammatory lesion—*cholecystitis, acute pancreatitis, diverticulitis,* and *appendicitis*. However, the pain of diffuse *inflammatory bowel disease* is not localized as it is in appendicitis, except as a consequence of perforation or fistulization in Crohn's disease. The pain of pelvic inflammatory disease is usually associated with menstruation and has been present for 24 or more hours, whereas appendicitis pain is more often intermenstrual and rarely persists so long except with perforation.

The type and radiation of the pain also help in differential diagnosis. For example, evidence of irritation of the diaphragm may be found on the right in *acute cholecystitis* and on the left in *acute pancreatitis*. Sudden, severe pain referred to the tips of the shoulders, associated with diffuse intra-abdominal pain and, later, distention, is more typical of perforated viscus, particularly *peptic ulcer*. *Ureteral obstruction* causes pain that is frequently

referred to the genitalia or groin. Steady, continuous pain is more characteristic of inflammation, as in appendicitis; on the other hand, intermittent or crampy pain is more characteristic of *obstruction of a hollow viscus* such as the gallbladder or small bowel.

Pain precedes nausea and vomiting in *appendicitis*; on the other hand, vomiting may be an early symptom of *acute cholecystitis* or *acute pancreatitis*. Bile-stained vomitus associated with acute cramping upper abdominal pain suggests *small bowel obstruction*; blood in the vomitus points toward a mucosal lesion proximal to the third portion of the duodenum. Relief of pain by vomiting suggests *gastric outlet obstruction*. Vomiting, of course, may accompany any intra-abdominal conditions, particularly if the patient is in great pain and has ileus or generalized peritonitis.

Physical Findings. Physical examination of the patient with an acute abdomen is of great importance, and the range of findings expected in acute appendicitis has been discussed. Unlike many causes of acute and severe abdominal pain, *mesenteric ischemia* is not associated with notable abdominal tenderness for 6 or more hours after onset. Localized tenderness and temperature elevation associated with continuing pain over a period of hours reflect either *localized peritonitis*, with or without perforation, or *vascular necrosis* of an ischemic organ. In such instances, the temperature is approximately 38.5 to 39.5°C. Higher temperatures are more often associated with urinary tract infections or bacterial pneumonias. Marked epigastric tenderness in a patient with a steadily increasing boring type of epigastric pain for several hours, particularly if accompanied by falling blood pressure, suggests *acute pancreatitis*. A rapidly rising pulse rate strengthens this possibility but is present with *perforation of a viscus*, a *gangrenous bowel*, or *rupture of an aneurysm*, as well.

Diffuse peritonitis is reflected by resistance of movement and change in position because of accentuation of pain; on the other hand, colic caused by *obstruction* of bile ducts, ureter, or small bowel early in its course is associated with restless movement. Later, in biliary tract and small bowel obstruction, infection and compromise of the blood supply may ensue and cause the appearance of signs of localized tissue necrosis and peritonitis. The abdomen should be carefully examined for scars of previous surgery that may now underlie an *intestinal obstruction* caused by adhesions; hernias must be sought. A succussion splash indicates marked *gastric outlet obstruction*. A large, pulsatile mid-abdominal mass points to *dissection of the abdominal aorta*. *Rupture of an aortic aneurysm* is usually very sudden; pain is brief, since shock quickly supervenes. Abdominal examination reveals distention.

In examining the patient with an acute abdomen, the physician should palpate in the quadrant farthest removed from the site of distress. The important findings that indicate a surgical condition include persistent, localized tenderness with unequivocal rebound, indicating localized peritonitis, and guarding. Guarding must be interpreted circumspectly, because it may be voluntary or involuntary. If it is the latter, underlying peritoneal irritation is likely. Generalized involuntary guarding is a classic finding for a perforated intra-abdominal viscus. The presence of an abdominal mass not previously noted, particularly when associated with other findings of inflammation, gangrene, or perforation, is very strong evidence for a surgical condition. Likewise, free air in the abdominal cavity, as evidenced by distention, absence of bowel sounds, and absence of liver dullness in the setting of acute abdominal pain, reflects a perforated viscus. Bowel sounds may be more active and high pitched in early obstruction or continuously active in diffuse acute inflammation (nonsurgical) of the small bowel. With increasing distention of small bowel loops, the sounds become less frequent and more high pitched. Bruits are an important finding, because they may reflect the presence of *arterial aneurysms*, the dissections of which may be the cause for the abdominal pain.

Rectal examination is crucial in differential diagnosis. Unequivocal tenderness indicates pelvic inflammation, and a mass usually reflects the presence of an abscess. As noted above, this examination often reveals positive findings in *acute appendicitis*. A glove specimen of stool must always be examined for occult blood. In females with acute abdominal pain, pelvic examination is essential to complement a careful gynecologic history.

Laboratory Aids in Diagnosis. The laboratory examination, consisting of urinalysis, complete blood count, serum electrolytes, blood urea nitrogen (BUN) and creatinine, serum amylase, radiographic examination of the abdomen and chest, and sonography of the abdomen, is essential in the differential diagnosis of the acute abdomen.

A *polymorphonuclear leukocytosis* strongly substantiates an acute intra-abdominal process with inflammation or necrosis; a low hematocrit reflects a disorder that is also capable of producing bleeding—*mucosal ulcerations, intestinal carcinoma, ischemia, dissecting aneurysms,* or, uncommonly, *acute hemolysis* associated with acute abdominal pain. An elevated hematocrit and BUN suggest dehydration, usually caused by vomiting and deficient fluid intake.

Urinalysis is vital in differential diagnosis, because the presence of pyuria, particularly white cell casts and bacteria on the smear of urinary sediment, is strong evidence for urinary tract infection and interdicts surgical exploration. Microscopic hematuria (numerous red cells) suggests stone or tumor of the genitourinary tract; red cell casts, on the other hand, suggest glomerulitis. A few scattered white and red cells may be seen in the sediment of about 20 per cent of patients with acute appendicitis. Examination of a *stool specimen* for blood and white blood cells is indicated in patients with right lower quadrant pain, fever, and *diarrhea*. *Salmonella* enterocolitis (and other bacterial infections) may be confused with acute appendicitis.

Important blood chemistries are *serum amylase*, elevation of which usually reflects acute pancreatitis; however, it may not be elevated in chronic relapsing pancreatitis, and it is elevated in other conditions such as *perforated peptic ulcer, strangulated obstruction* of the small bowel with perforation, *acute cholecystitis, cholangitis, acute renal failure,* and *ruptured tubal pregnancy*.

Visual Aids in Diagnosis. Roentgenologic examinations of importance include chest and flat films of the abdomen and CT scans, including contrast films with water-soluble, iodine (1 to 2 per cent)-containing substances. Radionuclide studies and ultrasonography are often useful as well. The flat and upright films of the abdomen may show free air in the peritoneal cavity, reflecting a perforation of a hollow viscus (80 per cent of cases are due to perforated ulcer, followed by perforated diverticulum and appendicitis). They also support the diagnosis of acute small bowel obstruction, indicate the likelihood of calculus disease of either gallbladder or urogenital tract, outline a large obstructed stomach, and reveal a variety of soft tissue masses that may reflect cysts or abscesses. Collections of extraintestinal gas often point to abscesses; occasionally, the biliary tree may be outlined by air, thus revealing a fistula to bowel. Diffuse calcification of the region of the pancreas indicates chronic pancreatitis. As noted, calculi in the right lower quadrant may rarely help in the diagnosis of acute appendicitis. Flat film of the abdomen also may yield findings characteristic of acute pancreatitis, including "sentinel" loops and a "cut-off" of the colon. A cross-table lateral view will outline an abdominal aortic aneurysm. A routine chest radiograph is essential in order to reveal free intraperitoneal air under the diaphragm, to demonstrate pneumonia, or to show an elevated diaphragm on the left with or without pleural effusion and partial atelectasis, as noted in acute pancreatitis, or on the right, reflecting subphrenic abscess.

Sonography is particularly helpful in demonstrating gallstones, obstruction of the extrahepatic biliary tract (dilated intrahepatic ducts), collections of fluid including abscesses, defects in the liver, and obstruction of the urinary tract. Compression sonography demonstrating a noncompressible appendix larger than 6 mm in diameter is very sensitive in the diagnosis of *acute appendicitis*. A diameter less than 6 mm accurately rules out *acute appendicitis*. Overall accuracy is about 90 per cent, limited, of course, by inability to visualize retrocecal appendices that are inflamed. Ultrasonography may also indicate *colonic diverticulitis, Crohn's disease, intramural hemorrhage,* or *intussusception* by revealing a thickened bowel wall. It may also help in diagnosing "*closed loop*" *obstruction*.

CT scans are increasingly used in difficult cases, especially when flat films and sonograms are not helpful. CT may detect choledocholithiasis, the swollen pancreas of acute pancreatitis; inflammatory pseudocyst of the pancreas; intra-abdominal and pancreatic abscess; enlarged lymph nodes; subcapsular hematomas of liver, spleen, or kidney; dissection of the aorta; colonic diverticulitis; and with contrast, perforated or thickened bowel of Crohn's disease or cancer.

Radionuclides given intravenously may help by visualizing the gallbladder (technetium-99m–labeled iminodiacetic acid or derivative compounds) or by localizing an intra-abdominal abscess (gallium citrate-67). Visualization of the gallbladder by technetium-99m scan renders the diagnosis of acute cholecystitis highly unlikely. Radiolabeled agents may also detect localized inflammation and abscess. Gallium-67 collects in granulocytes and mononuclear cells; indium-111-labeled white cells of the patient are given intravenously. These agents are most useful when CT scanning and ultrasonography yield negative findings in the search for an inflamed organ or mass.

Nonsurgical conditions that cause acute abdominal pain are important in the differential diagnosis of acute appendicitis. Chief among these are *pyelonephritis, pneumonia, pulmonary infarction, acute myocardial infarction,* and *pericarditis,* all of which may cause acute upper abdominal pain. Acute distention of the liver and its capsule resulting from *acute right heart failure* may stimulate *acute cholecystitis*. *Acute hepatitis,* viral or toxic (including alcohol), may closely stimulate acute biliary tract disease. In these instances, however, an enlarged, tender liver will be felt. Further, serum glutamic-oxaloacetic transaminase (SGOT) determinations will be markedly elevated when the liver has been acutely damaged by virus, carbon tetrachloride, or acetaminophen. Alcoholic hepatitis usually demonstrates only modest elevations of SGOT. (However, acute obstruction of the common duct with cholangitis may transiently raise SGOT to levels of 1000 units or more for 24 to 48 hours.)

Systemic diseases, such as *sickle cell disease, acute intermittent porphyria, tabes dorsalis, heavy metal poisoning,* and *diabetic neuropathy,* all may present pictures simulating an acute surgical abdomen.

Acute pancreatitis usually is characterized by pain of many hours' to days' duration, associated with a history suggestive of biliary tract disease or indicative of acute and chronic alcoholism, and in its early stages abdominal tenderness is usually localized to the epigastrium. Markedly elevated plasma amylase (within 48 hours of onset) will help establish the diagnosis. Elevation of serum bilirubin above 3.0 mg per deciliter and of alkaline phosphatase indicates obstruction of the common bile duct, and occasionally ultrasonography or CT scan, in addition to indicating obstruction, may help in establishing choledocholithiasis as the cause of the pancreatitis.

SPECIAL CONSIDERATIONS IN DIFFERENTIAL DIAGNOSIS OF ACUTE APPENDICITIS. Great care must be extended to establish the diagnosis of this condition in the very young and very old. Children with diffuse abdominal pain that is preceded by anorexia, nausea, and vomiting and is often associated with diarrhea are more likely to have *acute infectious gastroenteritis,* in some cases due to *Yersinia enterocolitica, Campylobacter,* or *Salmonella*. Acute enteric infection with *Salmonella* must always be suspected, particularly in young adults with right lower quadrant pain, fever, and diarrhea. *Acute mesenteric adenitis,* presumably caused by viral illnesses and often associated with diffuse abdominal pain, is frequently confused with acute appendicitis in children. The difficulty is in those patients in whom there is some right lower quadrant tenderness and slight elevation of the white count. In such instances a diagnosis must be established at operation, because it is far safer to undertake a negative exploration than to neglect removal of an acutely inflamed appendix. Clinical differentiation of acute appendicitis from *Meckel's diverticulitis* is impossible. The acute onset of *Crohn's disease* involving terminal ileum may be very difficult to distinguish from acute appendicitis, although such patients usually have cramping abdominal pain and diarrhea.

In young women diagnosis is confused by problems in the reproductive system, such as *ruptured graafian follicles, twisted ovarian cysts, ectopic pregnancy, dysmenorrhea, ruptured endometrioma,* and *acute pelvic inflammatory disease*. *Ruptured ectopic pregnancy* is usually of dramatic suddenness and is often associated with shock and massive blood loss; these findings in a pregnant woman make the diagnosis virtually certain. The *ruptured graafian follicle* is noted in mid-cycle; fever and leukocytosis are uncommon. Tenderness on moving of the cervix on vaginal examination points toward a *twisted ovarian cyst*, the pain of which is out of proportion to the general well-being of the patient. The pain of *gonococcal salpingitis* is more diffuse, and tenderness is not so well localized as in appendicitis. Localized pain and tenderness in a pregnant woman whose pregnancy remains normal and who is not bleeding indicate probable appendicitis.

The differential diagnosis of appendicitis in the elderly may also be difficult. The classic picture is seldom noted, the history may be inadequate or misleading because of infirmity or the effects of medication, and the appendix perforates early. Findings on physical examination are usually not as dramatic, and, despite complications, fever may be only slightly elevated. Accuracy in diagnosis of patients over 60 years of age is below 70 per cent, and the incidence of perforation without a localized or generalized peritonitis at surgery is nearly 70 per cent—more than twice as high as all other age groups combined.

In elderly patients the principal problems in differential diagnosis are *cholecystitis, diverticulitis, mesenteric thrombosis, intestinal obstruction, incarcerated hernia,* and *perforated ulcer.*

Right-sided acute diverticulitis, particularly *cecal diverticulitis*, may simulate acute appendicitis in every respect. In a few instances, *left-sided diverticulitis* may localize tenderness to the right lower quadrant, because the sigmoid is often more redundant in the elderly. Rarely perforation of a *cecal carcinoma* presents a picture indistinguishable from that of acute appendicitis. The patient also may have an episode of diarrhea associated with cramping or steady lower abdominal pain, slight temperature elevation, and, later, evidence of moderate-to-complete large bowel obstruction. When differential diagnosis is difficult, a cautiously administered barium enema or a CT scan with contrast may help greatly in excluding acute diverticulitis as the cause of the problem.

In all instances, elderly patients must not be subjected to the risk of exploration falsely. Accordingly, all efforts should be extended to make certain that *acute myocardial* or *pulmonary infarction, pneumonia,* or other systemic disease or toxin, in addition to intra-abdominal conditions that do not require immediate surgery, are not responsible for acute abdominal pain simulating appendicitis.

TREATMENT. Unless strongly contraindicated, the principal therapy for acute appendicitis is surgical removal of the appendix. Recently appendectomies via laparoscopy have been successfully performed. Since mortality correlates with perforation and, except in elderly patients, perforation correlates with duration of symptoms, early diagnosis and appendectomy are essential for the lowest acceptable morbidity and mortality for the disease. To avoid the catastrophe of unoperated-upon acute appendicitis, normal appendices may have to be removed in 10 to 15 per cent of patients.

In patients in whom complications (*perforation, peritonitis,* and *abscess*) have already occurred or are suspected, dehydration must be corrected; continuous nasogastric suction should be started; and gentamicin, 1.0 to 1.5 mg per kilogram, clindamycin, 1.6 to 2.5 grams, and metronidazole, 2.0 grams, given parenterally per day in divided doses, should be administered prior to surgery.

Patients with obvious acute appendicitis for whom no surgeon is available may be treated with head-up position of the bed; intravenous fluids; gentamicin, 1.0 to 1.5 mg per kilogram, clindamycin, 1.6 to 2.4 grams, and ampicillin, 2.0 grams, intravenously in divided doses daily; and nasogastric suction. The chance for recovery in otherwise healthy individuals with this program is surprisingly good. However, these patients must be scheduled for appendectomy 6 weeks later, or appendicitis is likely to recur.

MORBIDITY AND MORTALITY OF SURGERY. Overall, about 15 per cent of patients with acute appendicitis develop complications postoperatively; this figure is about 35 per cent in those with perforation and localized peritonitis at the time of surgery and is 70 per cent in those with perforation and generalized peritonitis. The complications include *wound infection, intra-abdominal abscess,* mechanical *small bowel obstruction, fecal fistula,* and, much more rarely, *intraperitoneal hemorrhage. Pylephlebitis* is extremely rare (1 in 1000).

The overall mortality of acute appendicitis ranges from 0.18 to 1.6 per cent and is due principally to the interrelated factors of age and perforation. Indeed, mortality over the age of 60 ranges from 6.4 to 14 per cent. The cause of death in this group may be attributed equally to septic and nonseptic complications.

Alvarado A: A practical score for the early diagnosis of acute appendicitis. Ann Emerg Med 15:557, 1986. *Predictive factors for diagnosis in order of importance are localized tenderness in the right lower quadrant, leukocytosis, migration of pain, shift to the left in the neutrophils, temperature elevation, nausea, vomiting, anorexia, and direct rebound pain.*

Jeffrey RB Jr., Laing FC, Townsend RR: Acute appendicitis; sonographic criteria based on 250 cases. Radiology 167:327, 1988. *A new compression technique shows an accuracy of about 90 per cent in ruling the diagnosis in or out.*

Lau WY, Fan ST, Yiu TF, et al.: Acute appendicitis in the elderly. Surg Gynecol Obstet 161:157, 1985. *A prospective study of 104 patients more than 60 years old with appendicitis showed clinical features similar to those of the younger patient; however, the elderly patient may have little or no pain, and the incidence of appendiceal perforation is increased.*

Schrock TR: Acute appendicitis. In Sleisenger MH, Fordtran JS (eds.): Gastrointestinal Disease. 4th ed. Philadelphia, W. B. Saunders Company, 1989. *A concise yet comprehensive article on every aspect of the subject. A handy reference.*

Way LW: Abdominal pain and the acute abdomen. In Sleisenger MH, Fordtran JS (eds.): Gastrointestinal Disease. 4th ed. Philadelphia, W. B. Saunders Company, 1989. *An excellent chapter containing all important information on diagnosis of the acute abdomen, identifying the cause and the accepted approaches to management.*

DIVERTICULITIS OF THE COLON

DEFINITION. *Diverticulitis* of the colon is a focal inflammation in the wall of the apex of a diverticulum, most commonly of the sigmoid, caused by inspissated feces. It is more common in those with multiple diverticula that have appeared at an early age. Peridiverticulitis results from necrosis with micro- or macroperforation. An abscess then forms, its size depending on the size of the rupture; small ones may subside with scarring, whereas larger abscesses involve pericolonic tissue and may even dissect along, or within, the bowel wall. Occasionally they rupture into contiguous organs (bladder, ureter, vagina, and small bowel).

CLINICAL PICTURE. The predominant clinical symptoms of diverticulitis are *pain* and *fever.* The pain is usually prominent and is frequently constant. Most commonly, it is localized in the left lower quadrant, because the sigmoid and descending colon are the sites of the largest number of diverticula; however, it may be suprapubic or in the right lower quadrant if the sigmoid is redundant or a right-sided diverticulum is involved. The patient may have a few loose stools or become constipated, and only rarely is rectal bleeding noted. Bleeding from diverticula is not associated with inflammation and perforation. It is usually bright red and may be copious. Bleeding colonic diverticula must be differentiated from ischemic colitis, acute amebic and *Shigella* dysenteries, *ulcerative colitis,* and *tumors of the colon* (see Ch. 111). When the perforation and sepsis are of sufficient magnitude, the patient may also have chills with fever as high as 39 to 39.5°C. Usually, however, the fever is low grade, between 38 and 39°C.

Although the pain may be somewhat intermittent and even colicky at onset, it usually becomes steady and is of the same quality as noted in acute appendicitis. Indeed, acute diverticulitis has often been referred to as "left-sided appendicitis." The patient may seek medical help after only a few hours or, when the situation is not so severe, after a few days of lingering but nagging lower quadrant pain and low-grade fever. Rarely, a *diverticulum of the right colon* perforates, causing right lower quadrant pain with fever, closely simulating appendicitis. Diagnosis is usually made at laparotomy.

Physical examination is extremely important in establishing the diagnosis. Since the process usually quickly involves the serosal surface and peritoneal cover, marked, localized tenderness is found, both direct and rebound. Frequently, a tender mass may be discerned. When present for more than a few days, this mass may be astonishingly firm, even hard, and the distinction grossly from carcinoma is almost impossible. The abdomen is often slightly distended. Rectal examination is also painful, because inflamed bowel is often within reach of the finger; also, a mass may be palpable if a sizable abscess has formed.

In some instances the patient presents with complications of diverticulitis; *dysuria, pyuria, pneumaturia,* or *passing gas or feces through the vagina.* These symptoms are due to perforation of bladder or vagina by the diverticulitis (colovesical and colovaginal fistulas). The vast majority of these patients, usually elderly, do not relate these symptoms to a prior attack of severe pain. The presenting symptom may be septic fever, caused by pericolic, pelvic, or subdiaphragmatic abscess. The inflammatory process may penetrate other pelvic organs, but such fistulization is often clinically undramatic. Rarely, the diverticulum perforates freely. In this instance the signs of free perforation are evident—that is, distention of the abdomen, generalized rebound tenderness, and absent bowel sounds. It is unusual also for diverticulitis to cause persistent colonic obstruction (see below). Very rarely arthritis and pyoderma gangrenosum accompany acute diverticulitis—symptoms more commonly associated with Crohn's disease (see below). The disease may also underlie *polymicrobial septicemia.*

DIAGNOSIS. Diverticulitis should be suspected particularly in patients with known diverticula who develop fever, leukocytosis, and signs of pericolic and peritoneal inflammation in the left lower quadrant. The diagnosis is even more likely if a mass is palpable. Fever between 38.5 and 39°C is also compatible with the diagnosis. When the process is more extensive and with formation of a *pericolic abscess* and its complications, the temperature is usually over 39°C, and the white count is proportionately higher. Urinalysis reflects varying degrees of involvement of the urinary tract by this septic process; that is, with mild ureteral irritation a few red and white cells may be seen in the urinary sediment, but with direct involvement of the ureter or invasion of the ureter or the bladder, the urine may be frankly septic and contain large numbers of red cells.

Some patients suffer much left flank pain owing to *hydronephrosis* resulting from obstruction of the ureter by a *pericolic abscess.* An intravenous pyelogram shows no function or an obstructed kidney on the left, and a sonogram or CT scan demonstrates unilateral hydronephrosis.

The use of radiographs is of crucial importance in the diagnosis, especially a flat film of the abdomen. Pericolic perforation and abscess formation may be suspected from collections of air and fluid in the left lower quadrant. Free air may be seen under the diaphragm in instances of free perforation. Sonography may reveal a localized thickening of the wall or pericolic abscess, particularly in the sigmoid abutting the wing of the ilium. CT scans are particularly helpful by showing inflamed pericolic fat, fistulas, and pericolic abscess in nearly all cases, the involved diverticula in 85 per cent, and thickening of the bowel wall in 75 per cent. A small volume of Hypaque (200 ml) may be instilled to enhance tomographic definition. A fistula to the bladder or ureteral obstruction may be seen with ultrasonography or by CT scan.

Flexible sigmoidoscopy, carefully performed without preparation and air insufflation, helps to exclude other conditions (see below). Usually with diverticulitis the instrument cannot be passed beyond the rectosigmoid junction, which is occluded by fixation, angulation, and spasm.

Clinicians debate the advisability of using a barium or Hypaque enema in the diagnosis of diverticulitis. The concern is that the increased intraluminal pressure may cause perforation. The history, physical examination, laboratory information, cautious Hypaque enema, and, in appropriate instances, ultrasonography or CT scan are sufficient to make the clinical diagnosis. Hypaque enema is safer than barium enema (in the event of extravasation) and, if cautiously performed, is a sensitive method for diagnosis of uncomplicated diverticulitis. It also helps to rule out *acute ischemic colitis* of the left colon and perforation of a left colonic carcinoma.

The roentgenographic features characteristic of diverticulitis are the presence of contrast agent outside a diverticulum, the delineation of a pericolic mass, or the demonstration of a fistula originating in the colon. In some instances the distinction between diverticulitis and carcinoma or Crohn's disease may be difficult (see below). The presence of irregularity, thickening, or even a sawtooth appearance of the bowel is not sufficient to make the diagnosis of diverticulitis, because these are typical for diverticula without perforation.

CT scan with contrast is a sensitive method for diagnosis of complications of diverticulitis, particularly *fistulas* and *pericolic abscess* (Fig. 112–1). It and sonography are also important in ascertaining *ureteral obstruction* or contiguous inflammation, particularly left sided.

DIFFERENTIAL DIAGNOSIS. For many years symptoms of *diverticulosis* have been attributed incorrectly to *diverticulitis.* *Diverticulosis* may periodically be associated with marked local tenderness, a palpable sigmoid loop, and some degree of large bowel obstruction, and thus the picture suggests diverticulitis. However, such patients do not have fever, the localized tenderness gradually recedes, the white count is not elevated, and there is no evidence of involvement of contiguous organs. Barium enema reveals an irregular luminal contour with a narrowed sigmoid, possibly even a so-called sawtooth appearance of the mucosa. Barium or Hypaque must be noted outside the diverticulum, a fistula seen, or evidences of a pericolic or intramural mass detected before the diagnosis of *diverticulitis* is definitely made.

Carcinoma of the colon must be distinguished from diverticulitis because of similarity of age during which both diverticulitis and cancer of the colon appear. The differential diagnosis is especially difficult, because in about 25 per cent of patients with diverticulitis the lumen is narrowed, suggesting carcinoma. Differentiation from cancer is more difficult if diverticulitis has appeared insidiously. Chronic obstruction, more persistent rectal bleeding, and weight loss are more characteristic of *cancer.* However, the tumor may be obscured on barium enema in 50 per cent of patients with diverticula. Localized tenderness with rebound, leukocytosis, and fever support the diagnosis of diverticulitis. In some cases, however, it may be impossible to

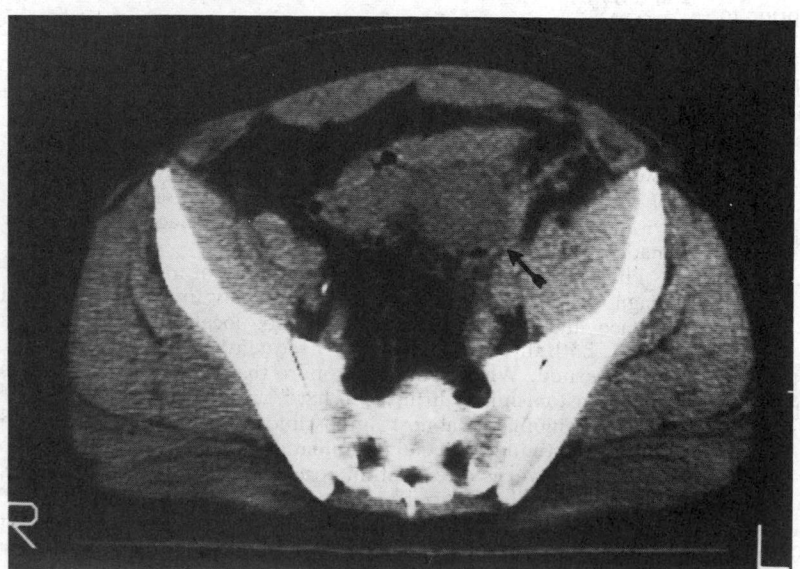

FIGURE 112–1. CT scan showing air-filled diverticula in a contracted segment of sigmoid colon lying just anterior to a paracolic abscess, indicated by a circumscribed area of uniform low density *(arrow).* (From Sleisenger MH, Fordtran JS (eds.): Gastrointestinal Disease. 4th ed. Philadelphia, W. B. Saunders Company, 1989.)

distinguish the two conditions, especially when the contrast enema has features common to both—i.e., a mass, luminal irregularities, and partial obstruction. In such patients CT scan with contrast and colonoscopy may be very helpful in excluding cancer. Rapid disappearance of the obstruction strongly suggests diverticulitis. In some patients correct diagnosis can be made only at surgery, and, in a few, only from surgical biopsy or by the disappearance of the occlusion following colostomy.

Crohn's disease of the colon may be difficult to exclude in the face of marked luminal narrowing or multiloculated channels parallel to the bowel wall on radiograph. Clinically, although both may produce pain, partial obstruction and lower abdominal mass, some rectal bleeding, fever, and leukocytosis, the past history differs. The patient with Crohn's colitis usually has had previous episodes of lower abdominal pain, fever, and diarrhea. Sigmoidoscopy may reveal the rectum to be involved with granulomatous disease. Also, evidence elsewhere in the bowel of granulomatous disease, such as cobblestoning, long intramucosal sinus tracts, and skip areas, help in the differential diagnosis (see Ch. 103).

Ischemic colitis of the left colon in elderly patients may produce signs and symptoms of bowel necrosis and localized peritonitis that are difficult to distinguish from diverticulitis. In these instances, gross rectal bleeding is prominent, and a barium enema is of crucial importance, because so-called thumb-printing is found in ischemic colitis, especially in the area of the splenic flexure and descending colon (see Ch. 104).

TREATMENT OF DIVERTICULITIS. Patients with low-grade fever and no evidence of mass, fistula, or obstruction may be treated with clear liquids by mouth and ampicillin (2.0 grams) or a cephalosporin (4.0 to 6.0 grams) per day in divided dosage intravenously. If the patient has fever of 39°C or more or has a tender mass or other evidence of greater extent of infection, gentamicin, 1.0 to 1.5 mg per kilogram, clindamycin, 1.6 to 2.4 grams, and metronidazole, 2.0 grams, are given parenterally in divided doses daily. In such patients nasogastric suction and intravenous fluids are given to maintain intravascular volume, urinary output, and electrolyte balance. About 50 per cent of complicated cases require surgery. Surgical consultation must be obtained early in all cases in which a mass is palpable or when there is suspicion of peritonitis or involvement of a contiguous organ.

Most patients respond well to this type of therapy with abatement of the fever, tenderness, and evidence of partial obstruction. Long-term therapy becomes identical with that for diverticulosis (see Ch. 100).

COMPLICATIONS AND INDICATIONS FOR SURGERY. Intervention is necessary for the complications of diverticulitis, such as an *enlarging mass* despite therapy, *generalized peritonitis*, *persisting intestinal obstruction*, or the development of a *fistula*. Fistulas extend most commonly to the urinary bladder, occasionally to the vagina, and rarely to other contiguous structures, such as the left hip, infecting joint or bone. Unresolving pericolic abscesses are best drained transabdominally by an interventional radiologist under sonographic or CT guidance. For more complicated or multiple abscesses, fistulas, or obstruction, surgery is recommended. If possible, a one-stage procedure is carried out; if not, a temporary colostomy is established after resection of a fistula or drainage of a septic area. More definitive resection and reanastomoses are carried out later. Elective surgery is indicated for recurrent attacks of diverticulitis and for the inability to exclude a carcinoma as the cause for persisting deformity after recovery from the acute phase.

Almy TP, Naitove A: Diverticula of the colon. *In* Sleisenger MH, Fordtran JS (eds.): Gastrointestinal Disease. 4th ed. Philadelphia, W. B. Saunders Company, 1989. *A complete description of etiology, pathogenesis, and clinical pictures and complications of colonic diverticula, including diverticulitis.*

Chappins CW, Cohn I Jr.: Acute colonic diverticulitis. Surg Clin North Am 68:301, 1988. *A comprehensive review of the disease with a good summary of the modern tools for diagnosis and of the evolving relationship of CT scanning, percutaneous drainage, and surgical management of complications.*

Johnson CD, Baker ME, Rice RP, et al.: Diagnosis of acute colonic diverticulitis: Comparison of barium enema and CT. AJR 148:541, 1987. *A careful analysis of the sensitivities of barium enema and CT in diagnosis of this disease and its complications.*

RADIATION ENTEROCOLITIS

Damage to the small intestine and colon may result from radiation therapy for abdominal and pelvic malignancy.

INCIDENCE. Incidence of severe radiation injury varies between 2.5 and 25 per cent of patients treated with radiotherapy for pelvic and intra-abdominal malignancy. Minor degrees of damage are common, as evidenced by impaired ileal absorption of conjugated bile acids in many women who are irradiated for pelvic cancer. It is noted most commonly after the total dosage exceeds 5000 rads. Transient histologic inflammatory change may, however, be found in the rectal mucosa of nearly 75 per cent of individuals receiving such therapeutic irradiation. The small intestine is more frequently affected than the rectum.

PATHOGENESIS AND PATHOLOGY. Damage results from interference with replication of radiosensitive epithelial cells, particularly of the crypt, leading to varying degrees of damage to the mucosal surface. Often it is reversible if dosage is not too great or treatment is not prolonged. Such damage may follow dosage of less than 5000 rads. Damage to the mesothelial cells of the small submucosal arterioles results in varying degrees of occlusion and mucosal transmural necrosis. Accordingly, hyperemia and ulceration of the mucosa are frequent. With extreme damage, diffuse edema is followed by extensive fibrosis with multiple strictures and irreversible damage. Such serious damage is more common in diabetics, in those with previous abdominal surgery, previous fixation of intestines, and serious vascular disease.

The pathologic changes range from diminution of crypt cell mitosis and shortening of villi of the small intestine to varying degrees of hyperemia, edema, and inflammatory cell infiltration of the mucosa. Mucosal thickness decreases. Progress of damage is marked by crypt abscesses, sloughing of epithelial cells, and, later, mucosal ulcerations, diffuse or localized, are found. Two to 12 months after radiotherapy, the damage to the blood vessels becomes prominent. In these instances, repair of acute damage does not ensue. The mucosa and submucosa become progressively ischemic and fibrotic. *Abscesses* and *fistulas* may form with sinus tracts between loops of intestine and between intestine and neighboring organs. A more general discussion of radiation injury is found in Ch. 530.

CLINICAL PICTURE. Symptoms may appear early, that is, during the first or second week of therapy, or late, that is, 6 months or more after completion of therapy. Early, diarrhea and mild rectal bleeding may appear, resembling ulcerative colitis. Sigmoidoscopy reveals acute proctitis with an edematous mucosa that may be friable; in more extreme instances, the acute changes also reveal a patchy or diffusely necrotic mucosa.

Later, symptoms of radiation include gross rectal bleeding, decrease in stool caliber, and progressive difficulty in defecation with marked constipation, all indicating severe rectal involvement. Small intestinal symptoms result from either fibrosis and obstruction or fistulization and abscess formation. These serious complications are clinically apparent, on the average, 20 to 24 months after the insult; however, serious symptoms due to obstruction, fistula, or abscess may appear 10 to 15 years after therapy. Those with fistulas are more likely to have synchronous lesions; areas most severely affected are the mid and distal small intestine and the rectosigmoid. If the damage is especially diffuse, malabsorption may be noted. Malabsorption also follows resections of small intestine, as described in Ch. 102. Impaired motility, in addition to mucosal damage, contributes to impaired absorption.

DIAGNOSIS. Diagnosis of *radiation enteritis* is suspected with any of the aforementioned symptoms in patients who have received significant radiation. Sigmoidoscopy shows a picture that ranges from variable degrees of edema to a markedly inflamed and necrotic mucosa. Multiple telangiectases are common, as is rectal stricture. Since most cases are fairly clear cut, biopsy is usually not indicated.

Barium studies of the intestine are not specific and range from changes of diffuse edema and spasm to diffuse fibrosis with strictures, fistulas, and ulceration in more severe cases. Thus the picture may resemble localized malignancy in the colon or diffuse granulomatous disease in the small intestine. Long strictured areas may also be noted, however, in the colon. CT scans are useful if complications such as fistulas or abscesses are suspected.

Differential diagnostic usefulness of small vessel angiography of the intestine in radiation enteritis remains to be confirmed.

TREATMENT. Improving methods for monitoring radiotherapy and delivering rads in small increments will probably reduce the incidence of this complication; however, the increasing incidence of malignancy and of the efficacy of radiotherapy will probably increase the total number of such patients.

Symptoms caused by early reaction consist of mild diarrhea and perhaps some minimal bleeding that can be managed by reduction of dose by 10 per cent, with the judicious use of tranquilizers, anticholinergic drugs, local analgesics, agents that increase stool bulk, and warm sitz baths for those with rectal involvement. An elemental diet free of gluten, milk protein, and lactose may benefit patients with early radiation reaction. If watery diarrhea is a problem, treatment with cholestyramine (4 to 6 grams per day) to bind bile salts may help greatly. If rectal bleeding is prominent, treatment with steroid retention enemas should be initiated as in ulcerative colitis (see Ch. 103). If the bleeding is more significant, transfusions may be required and even, possibly, surgery. Rectal strictures may be dilated, provided that it is early in their course and they are not extensive. Lubricants and stool softeners are often helpful; however, the progress to symptomatic occlusion of the lumen may necessitate proximal colostomy. Fistulas should be resected and abscesses drained. Resection of bowel and anastomoses are hazardous in view of the impaired blood supply, and anastomoses should always be made to uninvolved intestine.

In patients with malabsorption, treatment is as outlined in Ch. 102.

PROGNOSIS. Prognosis depends on the extent and degree of damage, the age of the patient, the course of the underlying malignancy, and whether or not the patient has systemic vascular disease. Unfortunately extensive disease of the colon usually means significant disease in the small intestine. The prognosis is guarded in those with ulceration, fibrosis, or fistulas in whom repeated resections or other major surgical procedures must be carried out. In such cases, age and cardiovascular status are also crucial determining factors. Life expectancy is shorter in those with perforation or fistulas than in those with stricture or bleeding.

Earnest DH, Trier JS: Radiation enterocolitis. In Sleisenger MH, Fordtran JS (eds.): Gastrointestinal Disease. 4th ed. Philadelphia, W. B. Saunders Company, 1989. A comprehensive discussion of the radiation damage to small and large gut.

Galland RB, Spencer J: Radiation-induced gastrointestinal fistulae. Ann R Coll Surg Engl 68:5, 1986. Of 70 patients with radiation enteritis, 10 (14 per cent) had 14 radiation-induced fistulas. The median latent period between radiotherapy and presentation of the fistula was 20 months. The fistulas were often multiple and/or associated with other radiation-induced lesions, patients presenting with fistulas being significantly more likely to have synchronous lesions compared with those who presented with strictures.

Harling H, Balslev I: Long-term prognosis of patients with severe radiation enteritis. Am J Surg 155:517, 1988. An important follow-up of 136 patients with radiation enteritis over nearly 5 years. Twelve died within 3 months of operation; 68 became asymptomatic. The remaining 56 continued to have problems.

Miholic J, Vogelsang H, Schlappack D: Small bowel function after surgery for chronic radiation enteritis. Digestion 42:30, 1989. A study of 22 patients with diarrhea, 16 of whom had resection of small intestine or terminal ileum for complications of radiation injury. Studies of absorption and motility indicate that impaired motility of intestine due to radiation injury contributes to malabsorption caused by resection.

SMALL INTESTINAL ULCERATION: ISOLATED AND DIFFUSE

ISOLATED NONSPECIFIC ULCERS

In most patients with this rare inflammatory disease, the etiology is unknown. About 75 per cent are ileal and 25 per cent jejunal. Often they are multiple. These ulcers may be caused by ingestion of enteric-coated potassium chloride. Such ulceration may also be associated with *vascular disease* (systemic lupus erythematosus, polyarteritis nodosa, rheumatoid arthritis), *hematologic disorders, granulomatous diseases, trauma, infections, Behçet's syndrome, neoplasia* (including acute leukemia), and *tuberculosis.* Rarely, they result from blunt abdominal trauma and are associated with strictures.

The clinical picture consists of periumbilical colicky pain and perhaps nausea and vomiting. Frequently, however, the patient presents with small bowel obstruction, bleeding, or perforation. Duration of illness is usually weeks to months but may be years. Accordingly, examination may show signs of obstruction, or peritonitis may be present.

Laboratory investigation is normal unless the patient has been bleeding or has had protracted vomiting; plain films of the abdomen are of great value if small bowel is obstructed or has perforated. Barium contrast studies in the uncomplicated cases are most often unrevealing, although in rare instances ulceration and narrowing may be noted. Upper endoscopy may reveal the ulcer or ulcers if located in the high jejunum.

Treatment for the disease is conservative if no complications have occurred. If the involved segment is bleeding, perforated, or stenotic, it should be resected.

Bayless T: Small intestinal ulcers and strictures. In Sleisenger MH, Fordtran JS (eds.): Gastrointestinal Disease. 4th ed. Philadelphia, W. B. Saunders Company, 1989. An up-to-date summary of all the types of cases.

Thomas WE, Williamson RC: Nonspecific small bowel ulceration. Postgrad Med J 61:587, 1985. Good report of clinical and radiologic features of this entity.

DIFFUSE ULCERATION OF JEJUNUM AND ILEUM

Diffuse ulceration of the small bowel may be found in *gluten-sensitive enteropathy (celiac sprue), lymphoma,* and *idiopathic chronic ulcerative enteritis* (also known as *chronic ulcerative nongranulomatous jejunoileitis*). It may also be found after oral administration of flucytosine. Patients with *gluten-sensitive enteropathy* may develop diffuse ulceration of jejunum and ileum, usually signaling a rapid decline in their clinical course despite elimination of gluten from the diet, with increased diarrhea, malabsorption, and, in some patients, perforation or hemorrhage. In instances of mild degrees of ulceration, steroids may induce remission; however, the majority are refractory to medical therapy. Mortality in this group is high. The condition in patients with *lymphoma* and diffuse ulceration also is often refractory to localized resection and radiotherapy.

Chronic ulcerative enteritis and *eosinophilic gastroenteritis* affect the small intestine, usually in patients under 50. They are characterized by diarrhea, weight loss, variable degrees of malabsorption, and protein-losing enteropathy. *Chronic ulcerative enteritis* is a much graver illness, often with fever, ascites and edema, a rapidly progressive course unresponsive to steroids, and a high mortality. It has been reported in association with skin rash, pancytopenia, and hepatitis. The etiology is unknown. Biopsy, peroral or at laparotomy, reveals nonspecific diffuse inflammation and mucosal ulcers. Prednisolone, 60 to 100 mg intravenously daily over 2 to 3 weeks, may be associated with remission in about one half of these patients. Infection, intraperitoneal or systemic, is the common cause of death.

Eosinophilic gastroenteritis may be localized to stomach, small intestine, or colon—so-called *eosinophilic granuloma*. It appears in the fourth to sixth decades and consists of infiltration by sheets of eosinophils into the submucosal and muscle layers. Epigastric pain, anorexia, and nausea are common complaints; it may obstruct the gastric outlet or even the duodenum and terminus of the common bile duct. It may be associated with other diseases, including malignancy. Steroids are often effective, but surgery may be indicated. *Universal eosinophilic gastroenteritis,* on the other hand, is a disease of younger persons, is often associated with allergies, always has a peripheral eosinophilia (greater than 20 per cent), affects stomach and small intestine diffusely, and is associated with diarrhea, crampy pain, weight loss, hypoalbuminemia, and often occult bleeding. Rarely, it responds to elimination of certain foods, particularly fish or meat. Most patients, however, require treatment with steroids, usually short-term (10 days to 2 weeks), but some may require long-term administration of 10 mg of prednisolone daily.

Bayless TR: Small intestinal ulceration: Isolated and diffuse. In Sleisenger MH, Fordtran JS (eds.): Gastrointestinal Disease. 4th ed. Philadelphia, W. B. Saunders Company, 1989. Excellent clarification and description of isolated and diffuse ulceration of the small gut.

Heyman IN: Allergic disorders of the intestine and eosinophilic gastroenteritis. In Sleisenger MH, Fordtran JS (eds.): Gastrointestinal Disease. 4th ed. Philadelphia, W. B. Saunders Company, 1989. A concise review of eosinophilic disease of the gut.

PART XI

DISEASES OF THE LIVER, GALLBLADDER, AND BILE DUCTS

113 Clinical Approach to Liver Disease

Robert K. Ockner

The liver plays a central and varied role in many essential physiologic processes. It is the sole source of albumin and many other plasma proteins, and of blood glucose in the postabsorptive state; it is the major site of lipid synthesis and source of plasma lipoproteins; and it is the principal organ in which a wide variety of endogenous and exogenous substances such as ammonia, steroid hormones, drugs, and toxins undergo biotransformation. To the extent that biotransformation "detoxifies" or inactivates a substance, the liver may be viewed as serving a regulatory or protective function for the whole organism. To the extent that such biotransformation results in the formation of toxic products, as in the case of certain drugs, the liver may bear the brunt of their adverse effects.

The clinical manifestations of liver diseases are also varied. Moreover, the clues by which the clinician may be first alerted to the existence of liver disease, even when advanced, may be subtle, consisting of seemingly trivial information gleaned during a careful history (e.g., increased fatigue, or the reversal of sleep pattern or personality change of early hepatic encephalopathy), physical examination (e.g., prominence of breast tissue and small testes in a man with cirrhosis, or excoriation reflecting pruritus), or routine laboratory screening tests (e.g., mild decreases in one or more of the formed elements of the blood because of portal hypertension-associated hypersplenism). Careful assessment is equally important in the patient with obvious liver disease, to address more complex questions. For example, does what seems to be acute hepatitis in fact represent relapse of previously subclinical chronic hepatitis, or delta-agent (hepatitis D) infection in a hepatitis B carrier? (See Ch. 117.) Or does the deteriorating course of a patient with known cirrhosis represent the natural progression of the disease, or a superimposed common bile duct stone, adverse drug reaction, or hepatocellular carcinoma?

HISTORY. Some very *nonspecific symptoms* may be important evidence of liver disease, including fatigue, malaise, fever, change in sleep pattern or behavior, diminished libido, anorexia, weight loss, nausea, and vomiting. *Pruritus* is an important symptom of *cholestasis* (impaired bile secretion), and may be present in the absence of jaundice. *Jaundice* is often first noted by family members or friends, and, especially in dark-skinned individuals, may appear first as a yellow discoloration of the conjunctivae, ("*scleral icterus*"). Since jaundice in most forms of liver and biliary disease reflects cholestasis (see below), such patients will often observe that stool color lightens; while urine gets darker as the excretion of "bile pigments" is diverted from bile to urine. Right upper quadrant *abdominal discomfort* or *pain* may reflect a rapidly enlarging liver with distention of Glisson's capsule because of acute hepatic inflammation or congestion, an acutely inflamed gallbladder, common bile duct obstruction by an im-pacted gallstone, or abscess or tumor in the liver or adjacent areas.

The history may provide important clues to the presence of *complications of liver disease*, especially those reflecting *portal hypertension* and *portal-systemic shunting*. Early hepatic *encephalopathy* may cause subtle changes in affect or sleep pattern. More overt symptoms include episodic somnolence, confusion, combativeness, ataxia, incoordination, or obtundation. A history of *abdominal swelling* suggests ascites and may be most easily recalled by the patient as a change in the fit of clothing, possibly associated with *edema*. Ascites may also occur in many other conditions, including hepatic vein or inferior vena cava occlusion, congestive cardiac failure, and constrictive pericarditis, and a wide variety of neoplastic and inflammatory processes (see Ch. 110). A history of *gastrointestinal bleeding* in a patient with liver disease may suggest esophageal varices but can also reflect other lesions such as *gastritis, Mallory-Weiss syndrome,* and *peptic ulcer.*

The history is of major importance in the identification of potentially significant *etiologic* or *predisposing factors*. Viral hepatitis is suggested by a history of contact with jaundiced persons, exposure to persons known to have hepatitis or to a common source of hepatitis, ingestion of uncooked or partially cooked shellfish, prior blood transfusion, work with subhuman primates, employment in certain health professions (especially in dialysis or transplantation units), accidental inoculation, sexual promiscuity (especially in the homosexual community), sharing of needles, travel to geographic areas with inadequate public health programs, and consumption of water or uncooked vegetables in such areas. Foreign travel may also suggest parasitic disease such as amebic liver abscess. Q fever hepatitis may occur in individuals in proximity to livestock. Exposure to drugs, ethanol, and other potential dietary, occupational, or environmental toxins must be reviewed in detail. The information obtained may require supplementation or corroboration by family members or other close associates, especially in regard to ethanol consumption. It is often possible to document previous liver function through recourse to *medical records*, and this is particularly useful in evaluating the chronicity of liver disease. A *family history* of jaundice, liver disease, or neonatal jaundice may suggest an inherited disorder such as Wilson's disease, α_1-antitrypsin deficiency, or hemochromatosis.

PHYSICAL EXAMINATION. Scleral *icterus* may be detected at a serum bilirubin concentration as low as 2.0 to 2.5 mg per deciliter. Although *spider telangiectasias*, most prominent around the shoulders and upper trunk, and *palmar erythema* are nonspecific and may be present to a limited extent in normal subjects (especially women in pregnancy), they are potentially important signs of liver disease and usually imply chronicity. Excoriations reflect pruritus and suggest significant cholestasis, not necessarily accompanied by jaundice. *Xanthomas* and *xanthelasmas* are not specific for hepatobiliary disease, but may be a sign of prolonged cholestatic hypercholesterolemia. Changes in hair pattern, gynecomastia, and small or soft testes may reflect the *hormonal changes* that accompany cirrhosis in men. Prominence of cutaneous veins in the epigastrium or around the umbilicus may indicate a *portal-systemic collateral circulation* and, therefore, portal hypertension.

Examination of the heart and lungs may provide evidence of congestive cardiac failure, constrictive pericarditis, or diseases of the lungs or pleura that may be associated with liver dysfunction, cause pain referred to the abdomen, or reflect processes involving the subdiaphragmatic regions such as tumor or abscess.

Examination of the *liver* should include documentation of its *size* and is best recorded both as the distance to which the lower edge extends below the costal margin and its overall vertical span as determined by percussion. These dimensions should be related to a reproducible landmark such as the mid-clavicular line. The *form* and *consistency* of the liver should be noted: e.g., smooth, with a sharp edge; nodular and rock-hard; firm with a rounded and irregular edge. A rapidly decreasing liver size during the course of severe acute hepatitis may be a sign of massive hepatic necrosis. An abdominal mass, tenderness, or muscular spasm may suggest secondary involvement of the liver or biliary passages by a neoplastic or inflammatory process. *Ascites*, most readily detected as dullness or bulging in the flanks, fluid wave, or shifting dullness, may be caused by advanced liver disease, or superimposed infectious or neoplastic processes. Unfortunately, physical findings of ascites may be unreliable, and in equivocal cases abdominal ultrasound may be helpful.

A diffusely tender and enlarged liver suggests hepatitis or congestion, whereas tenderness in a relatively limited area at or below the lower margin in the region of the interlobar fissure may reflect acute cholecystitis. A visible or palpable gallbladder is abnormal and may be an important sign of primary gallbladder pathology or of cystic or common bile duct obstruction, the latter usually neoplastic in jaundiced patients (Courvoisier's sign). Splenomegaly may be the first evidence of portal hypertension of any cause, or may reflect primary splenic pathology such as neoplasm or infection.

Neurologic evaluation is of particular importance with respect to signs of hepatic encephalopathy. These are discussed in detail in Ch. 123, but, as noted, these may be very subtle, consisting initially of a personality change, a mild confusional state, or lethargy. A *flapping tremor* (asterixis), characteristic of metabolic encephalopathy of any cause, is usually present in more obvious cases. In advanced hepatic encephalopathy almost any form of neurologic abnormality may be present, including seizures, lateralizing signs, and abnormal posturing. Despite this, it is essential in patients with liver disease to consider other causes of central nervous system pathology such as the effects of ethanol, sedatives or other toxins, hypoglycemia, trauma, hemorrhage, infection, and primary or secondary neoplasms.

LABORATORY AND IMAGING STUDIES. These special studies, which may play an essential role in the evaluation and management of diseases of the liver and biliary tract, are discussed in Ch. 116 and 126.

Schiff L, Schiff E (eds.): Diseases of the Liver. 6th ed. Philadelphia, J. B. Lippincott Company, 1987.
Sherlock S: Diseases of the Liver and Biliary System. 7th ed. Oxford, Blackwell Scientific Publications, Ltd., 1985.
Wright R, Millward Sadler GH, Alberti KGMM, et al. (eds.): Liver and Biliary Disease. 2nd ed. London, W. B. Saunders Company, 1985.
Zakim D, Boyer T (eds.): Hepatology: A Textbook of Liver Disease. 2nd ed. Philadelphia, W. B. Saunders Company, 1990. *Four current and comprehensive textbooks that serve to introduce the topic and provide literature references dealing with the broad field of hepatobiliary structure, function, and disease.*

114 Hepatic Metabolism in Liver Disease

Richard A. Weisiger

Intermediary metabolism may be profoundly disturbed in liver disease. In some instances, the resulting changes may overshadow the underlying disease process.

CARBOHYDRATE METABOLISM. Except during the absorption of dietary carbohydrate, maintenance of normal blood glucose levels depends entirely on the liver. Two distinct mechanisms are involved: *glycogenolysis* and *gluconeogenesis*. In glycogenolysis, glucose is released from hepatic glycogen by activated glycogen phosphorylase. The process is triggered by the action of glucagon or epinephrine on specific liver cell surface receptors, which activate glycogen phosphorylase kinase via the calcium messenger system. Conversely, insulin stimulates the incorporation of glucose into hepatic glycogen. Normal hepatic glycogen stores are sufficient to sustain blood glucose levels for only about 24 hours. Beyond that, maintenance of blood glucose in the fasting state depends entirely on hepatic gluconeogenesis: the de novo synthesis of glucose from precursors including lactate, pyruvate, and amino acids. This process is stimulated by glucagon and epinephrine and inhibited by insulin.

The normally functioning liver continually responds to changes in its nutritional and hormonal milieu. In the fed state (relative excess of insulin and glucose), glucose production by gluconeogenesis and glycogenolysis is minimal. Instead, dietary glucose is either stored as glycogen or converted to fatty acids (*lipogenesis*), largely to be secreted from the liver in the form of triglyceride-rich lipoproteins and destined for storage in adipose tissue. In the fasting state the process is reversed, resulting in mobilization rather than storage of energy substrates. High glucagon levels relative to insulin trigger glycogenolysis and gluconeogenesis. The resulting glucose is no longer diverted to lipogenesis but is released into the plasma. The decrease in fatty acid synthesis is associated with increased fatty acid oxidation, which becomes the principal energy source for the liver.

Failure of these homeostatic mechanisms in liver disease may produce *hypoglycemia* or *glucose intolerance*. Mild hypoglycemia (blood glucose concentrations between 45 and 60 mg per deciliter) occurs in about 50 per cent of patients with uncomplicated acute viral hepatitis. As a rule, these patients are not hyperinsulinemic. Instead, hypoglycemia may reflect several metabolic abnormalities, including diminished glycogen stores, diminished glycogenolytic response to glucagon, diminished gluconeogenesis, and impaired repletion of hepatic glycogen during the fed state. In most cases, the hypoglycemia is not clinically significant, but in severe acute liver injury of any cause, such as virus- or toxin-induced necrosis and Reye's syndrome, hypoglycemia may be profound and life threatening. Hepatic hypoglycemia may also occur in the absence of overt liver damage. For example, *alcoholic hypoglycemia* classically occurs in persons whose only important source of calories over a period of days is ethanol, which cannot be metabolically converted to glucose and may inhibit gluconeogenesis. Hypoglycemia should be considered in the differential diagnosis of altered mental status in any patient with significant acute liver disease or exposure to ethanol or other toxins.

Glucose intolerance, on the other hand, is more typically associated with chronic liver disease and cirrhosis. Plasma insulin concentrations tend to be high, suggesting a state of *insulin resistance*. Both the number of insulin receptors and their binding affinity may be diminished in peripheral blood monocytes in liver disease, suggesting a more generalized receptor defect. In addition, insulin resistance may in part reflect increased plasma glucagon concentrations and in part a diminished insulin effect on the liver owing to diversion of insulin from the liver by portal-systemic shunts. Regardless of the mechanism, the glucose intolerance associated with chronic liver disease is rarely of clinical significance. Occasionally, patients with chronic liver disease may also have other disorders such as *hemochromatosis* (Ch. 193) and *chronic pancreatitis* (Ch. 106), in which *diabetes mellitus* may contribute to glucose intolerance.

LIPID METABOLISM. The liver plays a central role in the metabolism of fatty acids and other lipids and lipoproteins. Of the total daily turnover of plasma nonesterified (free) fatty acids derived from adipose tissue, about one third enter the liver, where they are esterified to triglycerides or other esters or undergo oxidation. The balance between esterification and oxidation is closely regulated, as is the rate of de novo fatty acid synthesis. In the fasting state, fatty acid synthesis is inhibited, whereas fatty acid oxidation is increased at the expense of the esterification pathways. In the fed state, de novo fatty acid synthesis and esterification are favored, whereas oxidation is diminished. Exclusive of dietary sources and de novo synthesis, a total of approximately 60 to 70 grams of plasma nonesterified fatty acid (>200 mmol) is taken up by the liver each day in the average adult. This provides the major energy source for the liver in the fasting state. Interference with hepatic fatty acid metabolism may either cause or be caused by clinically significant abnormalities of hepatic structure and function.

Fatty liver usually reflects excess accumulation of triglyceride, which may be deposited as large vacuoles displacing the nucleus, or as small droplets surrounding a central nucleus. It usually reflects an imbalance between the rate of triglyceride biosynthesis and secretion into the plasma, primarily as very low density lipoproteins. This imbalance may result from many factors that can affect synthesis, secretion, or both. Conditions associated with large fat droplets in liver cells include obesity, protein-calorie malnutrition (e.g., kwashiorkor, jejunoileal bypass), diabetes mellitus, corticosteroid therapy, and ethanol ingestion (Ch. 118). Small-droplet fat accumulation (see below) is characteristic of acute fatty liver of pregnancy, Reye's syndrome, Jamaican vomiting sickness, and tetracycline and valproic acid hepatotoxicity but is occasionally ethanol related. Accumulation of triglyceride in the liver cell is usually associated with hepatomegaly and reflects abnormal liver function but does not *by itself* appear to cause severe, progressive, or lasting liver damage.

Conversely, interference with fatty acid oxidation at any of several stages may have profound consequences. For example, *alcoholic ketosis* is attributed to an ethanol- or acetaldehyde-mediated impairment of the tricarboxylic acid cycle, resulting in incomplete oxidation of the products derived from β-oxidation of fatty acids. Metabolites of hypoglycin, a low molecular weight compound present in the unripened fruit of the ackee tree and the cause of *Jamaican vomiting sickness,* are converted to coenzyme A thioesters and to carnitine derivatives. Since these cannot be metabolized further, they effectively sequester the cellular carnitine pool. Fatty acid oxidation is inhibited, and there is a corresponding decrease in ATP production and gluconeogenesis. Continuing fatty acid esterification under these conditions leads to a form of fatty liver characterized by *small-droplet fat* deposition, associated in severe cases with liver failure and hypoglycemia. This entity is clinically similar to *Reye's syndrome, obstetric fatty liver,* and *tetracycline* and *valproic acid hepatotoxicity,* but in none of these latter conditions has the pathogenesis been fully elucidated.

The liver is the major source of endogenously synthesized cholesterol (approximately 0.5 gram per day). Together with cholesterol of dietary origin, this newly synthesized cholesterol enters a "metabolically active" hepatic cholesterol pool, from which is derived the cholesterol destined for secretion into bile or into plasma (in lipoproteins), for synthesis of liver cell membranes, and for conversion to bile acids. Bile acid synthesis accounts for the disposition of approximately half of the total daily turnover of cholesterol and, as such, is an important determinant of body cholesterol stores. Relative rates of secretion of bile acids, cholesterol, and phosphatidyl choline (lecithin) into bile are important factors in the pathogenesis of cholesterol gallstones (Ch. 126), but the mechanism(s) by which the secretion of these substances is effected and controlled is incompletely understood.

AMINO ACID AND PROTEIN METABOLISM. Except for the immunoglobulins, most plasma proteins, including albumin, clotting factors, transferrin, α_1-antitrypsin, and the nonalimentary lipoproteins, are synthesized in the liver. The synthesis of each is controlled by specific regulatory mechanisms. In all cases, however, synthesis and secretion are dependent on the integrity of many aspects of cell function, including the transcriptional mechanisms in the nucleus, the translational mechanisms in the rough endoplasmic reticulum, and the secretory mechanisms in the Golgi apparatus. Despite these common features, individual proteins are affected differently in liver disease. This nonuniformity may result from several factors such as the availability of an essential *nutritional* component (e.g., the vitamin K–dependent clotting factors), *hormonal* influences (e.g., very low density lipoproteins), *genetic* determinants (e.g., ceruloplasmin or α_1-antitrypsin), the effects of drugs or toxins (e.g., the warfarin-like anticoagulants or ethanol), or the response of selected proteins such as fibrinogen (and other "acute phase reactants," including C-reactive proteins, ceruloplasmin, haptoglobin, and transferrin) to inflammatory processes. In addition, the *kinetics* of synthesis and turnover of a particular protein are major determinants of

response of its plasma concentration to acute liver injury. In general, plasma concentrations of proteins of which the turnover is rapid (e.g., clotting factors, plasma half-time of hours to days) are more likely to be depressed by severe acute liver injury than are those proteins that turn over more slowly (e.g., albumin, plasma half-time about 3 weeks). Finally, *catabolism* of certain plasma proteins may be accelerated (e.g., clotting factors in *disseminated intravascular coagulation,* or albumin in *protein-losing enteropathy*). For these reasons, although liver disease generally tends to depress the plasma concentration of proteins of hepatic origin, plasma concentrations of such proteins may not accurately reflect the severity of the liver disease in a given patient. Interpretation of the prothrombin time, partial thromboplastin time, and serum albumin concentrations in the evaluation of liver disease is discussed in Ch. 116.

Amino acids, in addition to their obvious importance in protein synthesis, also participate in other reactions in the liver. Of special significance is the role of certain amino acids as precursors for gluconeogenesis, as discussed above. Amino acids may undergo *transamination,* in which the α-amino group is transferred to an α-keto group, as in the alanine transaminase (ALT)–mediated deamination of alanine to pyruvate; the resulting transfer of the amino group to α-ketoglutarate converts this acceptor to glutamate. Alternatively, amino acids may undergo *oxidative deamination.* In this case, an α-keto acid is formed as the amino group is converted to ammonium ion and, ultimately, to urea (see below).

BIOTRANSFORMATION AND DETOXIFICATION. The liver is the major site of chemical modification of a wide variety of exogenous drugs and toxins, as well as endogenous substances such as hormones. The reactions potentially involved are numerous and, in many instances, involve the cytochrome P-450–dependent microsomal mixed function oxidase system. The basic principles of drug disposition are discussed in Ch. 118, but several aspects warrant special emphasis in the context of liver function disease. First, while biotransformation of an endogenous or exogenous substance may *inactivate* it or render it more suitable for urinary or biliary excretion, there are many examples of compounds that are rendered toxic by this process. A number of clinically significant hepatotoxins are *activated* in this way, and some "idiosyncratic" drug reactions may reflect individual differences in drug metabolism rather than an immunologic response (see Ch. 118). Second, diseases of the liver may seriously impair the biotransformation of exogenous substances, thereby resulting in an *increased sensitivity* to certain drugs (e.g., sedatives and opiates) or may enhance the biologic effect of endogenous hormones (e.g., contributing to the feminizing effects of chronic liver disease) or toxins (e.g., diminished hepatic conversion of ammonia to urea in hepatic encephalopathy). Finally, one substance may significantly influence the hepatic biotransformation of another. Examples of this particular form of *drug-drug interaction* include the well-recognized induction of the microsomal drug-metabolizing system by prior administration of phenobarbital and its inhibition by various toxins.

A particularly important hepatic detoxification pathway converts *ammonium ion* to urea via the Krebs-Henseleit *urea cycle,* in which ornithine, citrulline, argininosuccinate, and arginine are intermediates and which involves both mitochondrial and cytosolic components (see Fig. 180–1). Glutamate, formed from NH_4^+ and α-ketoglutarate, is the principal NH_2 donor. Ammonium ion is produced in abundance in the intestinal tract, especially the colon, by the bacterial degradation of luminal proteins and amino acids and of endogenous urea, 25 per cent of the daily production of which diffuses into the intestinal lumen. The NH_4^+ diffuses into the portal circulation and is transported to the liver, where it is converted to urea by the mechanism described above. *Hepatic encephalopathy* in part reflects the failure of this important detoxification process (or of analogous pathways for other *enterogenous toxins*) because of extensive acute liver cell necrosis or direct entry of portal blood into the peripheral circulation via spontaneous or surgically created portal-systemic shunts (Ch. 123).

Arias IM, Jakoby WB, Popper H, et al. (eds.): The Liver: Biology and Pathobiology. New York, Raven Press, 1988. *An in-depth and well-referenced presentation of many basic aspects of normal and abnormal hepatic structure and function.*

Arky RA: Hypoglycemia associated with liver disease and ethanol. Endocrinol Metab Clin North Am 18:75, 1989. *Comprehensive review of this important clinical complication.*

Howden CW, Birnie GG, Brodie MJ: Drug metabolism in liver disease. Pharmacol Ther 40:439, 1989. *Includes practical information on adjusting drug dosages in liver disease.*

Zakim D, Boyer T (eds.): Hepatology: A Textbook of Liver Disease. 2nd ed. Philadelphia, W. B. Saunders Company, 1990. *A comprehensive and well-written clinical text with a good foundation in basic metabolism.*

115 Bilirubin Metabolism and Hyperbilirubinemia

Bruce F. Scharschmidt

BILIRUBIN METABOLISM (See Fig. 115–1)

BILIRUBIN CHEMISTRY. Bilirubin consists of four pyrrole rings linked by three carbon bridges. Unconjugated bilirubin is virtually water-insoluble at physiologic pH because its —COOH and —NH groups are involved in strong intramolecular hydrogen bonds and are therefore unable to interact with water. These intramolecular hydrogen bonds are disrupted by conjugation of the —COOH groups with glucuronic acid as occurs in the liver cell, thus greatly enhancing the aqueous solubility of the molecule and altering its biologic properties. In contrast to the more polar water-soluble conjugates, relatively nonpolar unconjugated bilirubin diffuses across most biologic membranes such as the blood-brain barrier, placenta, and intestinal and gallbladder epithelium. It is excreted in bile in only trace amounts. Thus, hepatic conjugation confers upon bilirubin the properties that permit its elimination from the body and thereby prevents damage to the central nervous system. Exposure of unconjugated bilirubin to light causes the formation of polar photoisomers and "lumirubin," which results from intramolecular cyclization. These compounds are excreted by the liver without conjugation; their formation is the mechanism by which phototherapy lowers serum bilirubin concentration in neonatal hyperbilirubinemia.

BILIRUBIN FORMATION. Bilirubin is formed from the breakdown of heme. Daily bilirubin production in adults averages about 4 mg per kilogram. About 70 per cent is derived from the heme moiety of hemoglobin in senescent erythrocytes, which are sequestered and degraded in the mononuclear phagocytic cells of the spleen, liver, or bone marrow. Most of the remainder results from the breakdown of nonhemoglobin hemoproteins in the liver, principally the cytochromes P-450. A minor fraction of bilirubin production results from ineffective erythropoiesis; i.e., premature destruction of newly formed erythrocytes in the bone marrow or circulation.

Microsomal heme oxygenase, the heme-cleaving enzyme, is most abundant in the liver, spleen, and bone marrow and exhibits substrate-mediated induction by heme or hemoglobin. The conversion of heme to biliverdin, which is rate limiting for bilirubin formation, is followed by reduction of biliverdin to bilirubin by cytosolic biliverdin reductase. Tin-protoporphyrin, a synthetic metalloporphyrin, is a potent competitive inhibitor of heme oxygenase. This compound may prove useful in reducing bilirubin production and preventing kernicterus in selected infants with hyperbilirubinemia. Mammals, unlike birds, reptiles, and amphibia, convert nontoxic, water-soluble biliverdin to water-insoluble bilirubin. This may reflect the fact that bilirubin, unlike biliverdin, is able to cross the placenta. Moreover, bilirubin may be more than a waste product and serve as a potent physiologic antioxidant.

BILIRUBIN BINDING TO PLASMA PROTEINS. Unconjugated bilirubin is bound reversibly to albumin at a primary high-affinity site (10^8 M^{-1}). At plasma concentrations exceeding its molar equivalence with albumin (about 35 mg per deciliter), bilirubin also binds to at least two low-affinity sites. A variety of compounds, including certain sulfonamides, penicillin derivatives, furosemide, and radiographic contrast media, may displace bilirubin from its albumin-binding sites and increase the risk of kernicterus in neonates. Presumably because of its tight albumin binding and low water solubility, unconjugated bilirubin is not excreted in urine. Conjugated bilirubin is somewhat less tightly bound to albumin than is bilirubin. It is filtered to a greater extent at the glomerulus, is incompletely reabsorbed by the renal tubules, and therefore does appear in the urine in small amounts in patients with conjugated hyperbilirubinemia.

In addition to the reversible binding to albumin just described, another bilirubin fraction binds very tightly, perhaps covalently, to albumin. This pigment fraction has a serum half-life of about 17 days, similar to that of albumin. It has been detected only in patients with conjugated hyperbilirubinemia, in whom it accounts for a varying (8 to 90 per cent) fraction of total bilirubin (see below). The identification of this protein-bound fraction helps explain the occasionally slow resolution of hyperbilirubinemia in patients convalescing from hepatitis or in whom biliary obstruction has been relieved, as well as the disappearance of bilirubinuria in these patients prior to the resolution of jaundice.

HEPATIC BILIRUBIN TRANSPORT. Uptake of bilirubin and other substances tightly bound to protein is facilitated by large fenestrations in the cells of the sinusoidal lining that permit plasma proteins to enter the space of Disse and directly contact the hepatocyte plasma membrane. Uptake of bilirubin and other organic anions such as sulfobromophthalein across the sinusoidal membrane of the hepatocyte displays several features characteristic of carrier-mediated transport, including saturability and competition. Once inside the liver cell, bilirubin and other organic anions appear to bind to cytoplasmic proteins such as ligandin. Ligandin, which constitutes 2 per cent of cytoplasmic protein in human liver, may alter net uptake by reducing bilirubin efflux back into plasma. In addition to transport through the

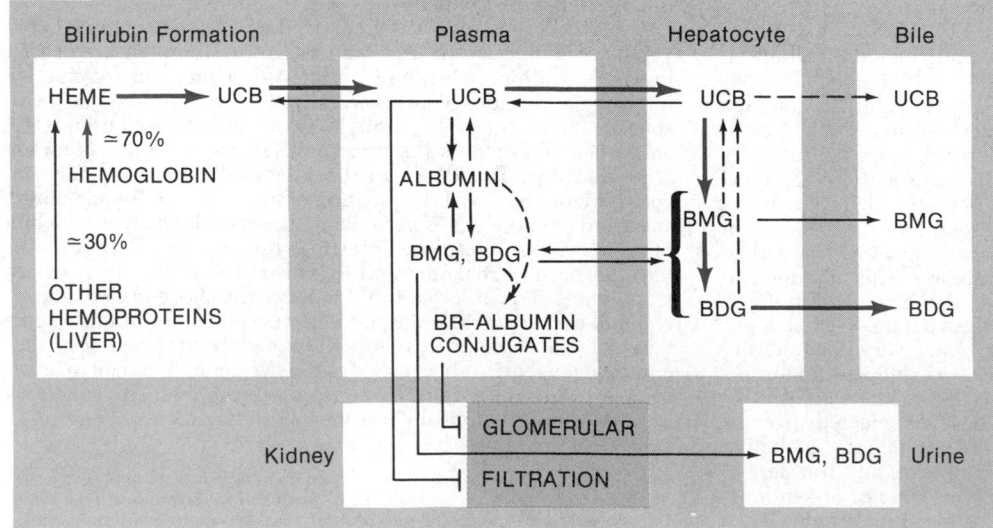

FIGURE 115–1. Overview of bilirubin metabolism. Unconjugated bilirubin (UCB) formed from the breakdown of hemoglobin heme and other hemoproteins is transported in plasma reversibly bound to albumin and is converted in the liver to bilirubin monoglucuronide (BMG) and diglucuronide (BDG), the latter being the predominant form secreted in bile. BMG and BDG together normally account for less than 5 per cent of serum bilirubin. In the presence of hepatobiliary disease, BMG and BDG accumulate in plasma and appear in urine. Bilirubin glucuronides in plasma also react nonenzymatically with albumin and possibly other serum proteins to form protein conjugates, which do not appear in urine and have a plasma half-life similar to that of albumin.

cytoplasm, bilirubin may be directly transferred from the plasma membrane to the membranes of the endoplasmic reticulum, where conjugation occurs.

In the process of conjugation, the carboxyl groups of one or both propionic acid side chains of bilirubin are esterified, usually with glucuronic acid. Glucose and xylose conjugates are formed in trace amounts only. Formation of bilirubin monoglucuronide and diglucuronide is catalyzed by microsomal UDP-glucuronyltransferase. Transport of conjugated bilirubin from the hepatocyte into bile, like the uptake step, exhibits saturability and competition and is presumably carrier mediated. The carrier responsible for excretion of conjugated bilirubin may also transport conjugated sulfobromophthalein as well as certain sulfate and glucuronide bile acid conjugates. Excretion and/or conjugation, but not uptake, appears to be rate limiting for overall bilirubin transport from blood to bile. Bilirubin diglucuronide predominates in human bile (70 to 80 per cent), with the isomeric monoglucuronides present in small amounts.

ENTEROHEPATIC CIRCULATION. Absorption of conjugated bilirubin from the gallbladder and small intestine is negligible. In the terminal ileum and colon, conjugated bilirubin is hydrolyzed by bacterial enzymes to form unconjugated bilirubin, which is converted into colorless urobilinogens and related products, including urobilins. Most urobilinogen that is absorbed from the intestine is re-excreted in bile and ultimately in feces; a small fraction appears in urine. Urobilinogen is absent from the bile and urine of patients with complete biliary obstruction; however, fecal and urinary urobilinogen levels correlate poorly with bilirubin production rate and are of little clinical utility. In addition to urobilins, the normal brown color of stool may reflect the presence of nonbilirubin pigments, perhaps of plant origin, which are also excreted in bile and undergo enterohepatic circulation.

CONCENTRATION IN PLASMA. Plasma bilirubin concentration, which ranges normally between 0.3 and 1.0 mg per deciliter, varies directly with bilirubin production and inversely with hepatic bilirubin clearance. About 95 per cent of circulating bilirubin in healthy adults is unconjugated. In contrast, circulating bilirubin in patients with hepatocellular or biliary tract disease consists predominantly of monoconjugates and diconjugates. The conventional diazoassay, which is employed in most clinical laboratories, tends to overestimate the conjugated fraction, particularly at low concentrations of total bilirubin. The tightly, perhaps covalently bound conjugated bilirubin fraction reacts directly with the diazoreagent but is often removed by the deproteinizing step used in many laboratories. Nonetheless, for practical clinical application, conventional laboratory techniques are generally adequate. While more accurate methods for measurement of conjugated and unconjugated serum bilirubin have been developed, they are not readily automated and therefore not widely available.

APPROACH TO THE PATIENT WITH HYPERBILIRUBINEMIA

Differential Diagnosis (Table 115–1)

The differential diagnosis of hyperbilirubinemia can be divided into two major pathophysiologic categories: bilirubin overproduction and decreased bilirubin clearance.

BILIRUBIN OVERPRODUCTION. Bilirubin overproduction

TABLE 115–1. DIFFERENTIAL DIAGNOSIS OF HYPERBILIRUBINEMIA

I. **Increased bilirubin production**
   Examples: hemolysis, ineffective erythropoiesis, resorption of hematomas
II. **Decreased bilirubin clearance**
   A. Inherited disorders of bilirubin metabolism
      Examples: Gilbert's syndrome, Crigler-Najjar syndrome, Dubin-Johnson syndrome, Rotor's syndrome
   B. Fasting hyperbilirubinemia
   C. Cholestasis
      1. Hepatocellular disease
         Examples: viral, drug-induced, or alcoholic hepatitis
      2. Biliary tract obstruction
         Examples: choledocholithiasis, tumor, sclerosing cholangitis, chronic pancreatitis

is most commonly caused by hemolysis (see also Ch. 133). Chronic steady-state hemolysis does not, by itself, usually account for a sustained bilirubin concentration greater than 4 to 5 mg per deciliter. Concentrations consistently above this level typically indicate the additional presence of hepatic dysfunction. In contrast to chronic hemolysis, acute hemolysis can result in a rate of bilirubin production that transiently exceeds the excretory capacity of even a normal liver and may cause striking bilirubin elevation and occasionally conjugated hyperbilirubinemia. Ineffective erythropoiesis may also be increased in certain disease states and can cause hyperbilirubinemia. Examples include megaloblastic anemia from either vitamin B_{12} or folic acid deficiency, iron deficiency anemia, sideroblastic anemia, thalassemia minor, polycythemia vera, aplasia, and lead poisoning. Markedly increased ineffective erythropoiesis is the basis of the rare disorder known as *shunt hyperbilirubinemia* or *idiopathic dyserythropoietic jaundice*. Bilirubin overproduction may also result from the resorption of large hematomas.

INHERITED DISORDERS OF BILIRUBIN METABOLISM. The hereditary disorders of hepatic bilirubin metabolism are characterized by impaired ability of the liver to transport or conjugate bilirubin (Table 115–2). The common, benign entity of *Gilbert's syndrome* and the rare, almost uniformly lethal type I *Crigler-Najjar syndrome* represent opposite ends of this spectrum. Routine tests of liver function are generally normal in all these disorders, but a variety of abnormalities in the hepatic handling of bilirubin and other compounds such as sulfobromophthalein have been described. Many of these disorders, including Gilbert's syndrome, the *Dubin-Johnson syndrome,* and *Rotor's syndrome,* may be mistaken for acquired hepatobiliary disease.

Gilbert's Syndrome. Because of its frequency (up to 7 per cent of the population), Gilbert's syndrome is the disorder most likely to be encountered by the clinician. Mild unconjugated hyperbilirubinemia is recognized most commonly during the second and third decades of life because of the presence of scleral icterus, often first noted with fasting or as an incidental laboratory finding. Although a variety of nonspecific symptoms have been described, it is unlikely that any significant symptoms are attributable to Gilbert's syndrome itself. Gilbert's syndrome results from a decrease in the hepatic clearance of unconjugated bilirubin, probably due to impaired conjugation. Up to one half of patients with Gilbert's syndrome have a very slight decrease in red cell survival detectable by ^{51}Cr labeling. The principal clinical importance of this disorder is that it may be confused with more serious acquired hepatobiliary disease. From a practical standpoint, the diagnosis of Gilbert's syndrome is made by demonstrating low-grade unconjugated hyperbilirubinemia in a patient with a normal physical examination and otherwise repeatedly normal laboratory tests of liver function. Liver biopsy to demonstrate normal histology is usually not necessary. An exaggerated hyperbilirubinemic response to fasting, lipid withdrawal, or nicotinic acid administration has been found to be helpful by some investigators, but these tests are neither sensitive nor specific enough to warrant routine use. In patients with overt hemolysis, direct measurement of hepatic bilirubin clearance may be necessary to establish the diagnosis. Gilbert's syndrome and the other inherited disorders of hepatic bilirubin metabolism are outlined in Table 115–2.

FASTING HYPERBILIRUBINEMIA. Fasting causes an increase in the plasma concentration of unconjugated, indirect-reacting bilirubin owing primarily to a decrease in hepatic bilirubin clearance. This effect may be particularly marked in patients with Gilbert's syndrome and the type II Crigler-Najjar syndrome. Both dietary composition and total caloric intake are important, since a normocaloric but lipid-free diet produces a response similar to that observed with complete fasting, and the effect of complete fasting is reversed by feeding small amounts of lipid. The mechanism of the decrease in hepatic bilirubin clearance with fasting is unclear. A slight increase in bilirubin production contributes to fasting hyperbilirubinemia.

CHOLESTASIS. In most patients, hyperbilirubinemia and jaundice reflect the presence of cholestasis, that is, impaired bile formation and/or bile flow resulting from extrahepatic biliary tract obstruction or hepatic parenchymal disease. Even in cholestasis, however, increased bilirubin production may be an important

TABLE 115–2. THE HEREDITARY DISORDERS OF HEPATIC BILIRUBIN METABOLISM

	Gilbert's Syndrome	Type I Crigler-Najjar Syndrome	Type II Crigler-Najjar Syndrome	Dubin-Johnson Syndrome	Rotor's Syndrome
Incidence	Up to 7% of population	Very rare	Uncommon	Uncommon	Rare
Inheritance	? Autosomal dominant	Autosomal recessive	? Autosomal dominant	Autosomal recessive	Autosomal recessive
Defect(s) in bilirubin metabolism	Decreased hepatic UDP-glucuronyltransferase activity, (?) slow hepatic bilirubin uptake, associated mild hemolysis in up to 50% of patients	Absence of hepatic UDP-glucuronyltransferase activity	Markedly decreased or undetectable UDP-glucuronyltransferase activity	Impaired biliary excretion of conjugated bilirubin	Impaired biliary excretion of conjugated bilirubin
Plasma bilirubin concentration (mg/dl)	≤3 in absence of fasting or hemolysis, predominantly unconjugated	17–50, usually >20, all unconjugated	6–45, usually <20, all unconjugated	1–25, usually <7, about 60% conjugated	1–20, usually <7, about 60% conjugated
Clinical sequelae	None	Death in infancy from kernicterus in almost all cases	Usually none, rarely kernicterus	Probably none	Probably none
Plasma sulfobromophthalein disappearance rate	Mildly abnormal in some patients (45-min retention <15%)	Usually normal	Usually normal	Slow initial disappearance with frequent secondary rise (45-min retention <20%)	Markedly slowed, no secondary rise (45-min retention 30–50%)
Oral cholecystography	Normal	Normal	Normal	Faint or nonvisualization	Usually normal
Hepatic histology (light microscopy)	Normal, occasionally increased lipofuscin	Normal	Normal	Coarse pigment in centrolobular cells	Normal
Reduction of plasma bilirubin concentration by phenobarbital	Yes	No	Yes	Minimal	Unknown
Diagnosis	Clinical and laboratory findings, response to fasting occasionally helpful, liver biopsy not usually necessary	Clinical and laboratory findings, lack of response to phenobarbital	Clinical and laboratory findings, response to phenobarbital	Clinical and laboratory findings, sulfobromophthalein disappearance, urinary coproporphyrin excretion	Clinical and laboratory findings, sulfobromophthalein disappearance, urinary coproporphyrin excretion
Treatment	None necessary	Liver transplantation; other measures not uniformly effective	Phenobarbital if bilirubin concentration markedly elevated	None available, avoid estrogens (may worsen jaundice)	None available

contributing factor (e.g., hemolysis complicating viral hepatitis or ineffective erythropoiesis caused by folate deficiency complicating alcoholic hepatitis).

Cholestasis can be subdivided into intrahepatic and extrahepatic causes. Intrahepatic causes include conditions in which the hepatocyte is unable to excrete bile even though the major ducts are patent. Included are acute and chronic viral hepatitis, drugs or toxins (in particular, alcohol, phenothiazines, and estrogens), primary biliary cirrhosis, congestive heart failure, sepsis, pregnancy, infiltrative diseases of the liver, and liver disease in infancy. The other major cause of cholestasis is extrahepatic biliary obstruction, most commonly due to gallstones or a neoplasm.

Evaluation of the Patient

CLINICAL EVALUATION. Most conditions causing hyperbilirubinemia can be diagnosed by means of the clinical history, physical examination, and routine laboratory tests. Certain aspects of the *patient history* may be particularly helpful in the differential diagnosis. Itching should alert one to the presence of cholestasis. Although the identity of the "pruritogen(s)" is controversial, bile salts in the skin are the most likely candidates. A history of dark urine implies an increased level of bilirubin conjugates in the serum and represents a clue to the presence of cholestasis, Rotor's syndrome, or Dubin-Johnson syndrome. The presence of clay-colored (acholic) stool implies severe cholestasis. Abdominal pain suggestive of biliary or pancreatic disease, previous biliary surgery, intermittent cholestasis, and abdominal pain all represent clues to the presence of biliary disease.

Physical examination is also important. A serum bilirubin concentration of 3 mg per deciliter or greater is usually required for the detection of scleral icterus; mucous membrane or cutaneous icterus generally requires higher concentrations. Chronic cholestasis also may produce markedly elevated cholesterol levels, which may result in cutaneous xanthomas. The presence of occult blood in the stool may represent a clue to a periampullary neoplasm or hemobilia. Additional clues to biliary obstruction include a palpable gallbladder or abdominal mass, fever suggestive of cholangitis, or abdominal tenderness.

Biochemical tests are of particular value and should include a complete blood count, reticulocyte count in selected cases, and hepatic function tests. If hepatic function tests apart from bilirubin

are normal, one should think of either hemolysis, ineffective erythropoiesis, or a selective defect in hepatic bilirubin transport, such as Gilbert's syndrome. If hepatic function tests are abnormal, the jaundice is very likely a manifestation of cholestasis. Cholestasis is characteristically accompanied by increased serum activities of γ-glutamyl transpeptidase, 5'-nucleotidase, leucine aminopeptidase, and alkaline phosphatase, and variable increases in alanine and aspartate aminotransferase. Unlike bilirubin or bile acids, an elevated alkaline phosphatase activity in serum does not reflect diminished biliary excretion, but rather increased synthesis and possibly increased release of this enzyme into the circulation. Alkaline phosphatase activity may also be increased in certain bone disorders and in pregnancy. γ-Glutamyl transpeptidase activity may be increased by certain enzyme-inducing drugs or alcohol, even in the absence of a hepatic disorder. It is not found in bone, and a normal value therefore suggests that an elevated alkaline phosphatase activity is of bony origin. Leucine aminopeptidase is also present in virtually all tissues, but elevated serum levels are seen only in hepatobiliary disease, particularly biliary obstruction, and pregnancy. Again, the primary use of this enzyme is in evaluating the significance of an elevated alkaline phosphatase activity. Elevated serum bile acids are a sensitive indicator of cholestasis, but this test is not widely available. Biochemical *clues to the presence of biliary obstruction* include a disproportionate elevation of bilirubin concentration and alkaline phosphatase activity with mildly abnormal transaminase activities, an elevated amylase suggestive of pancreatic disease, and normalization of a prolonged prothrombin time following vitamin K administration. The latter is indicative of vitamin K malabsorption due to intestinal bile acid deficiency, with normal hepatic synthetic function.

IMAGING STUDIES. If extrahepatic obstruction is suspected, further evaluation to determine the site and nature of the obstruction is warranted (Fig. 115–2). A reasonable next step is the use of a noninvasive study such as *ultrasonography* or *computed tomography* (CT) to determine whether the intra-and/or extrahepatic biliary system is dilated, implying mechanical obstruction. Because of its lesser expense and the lack of radiation exposure, ultrasonography is often preferred to CT as a first procedure. Ultrasonography and CT both demonstrate ductal dilatation in 85 per cent or more of patients with jaundice due to biliary obstruction. Both techniques may also yield additional

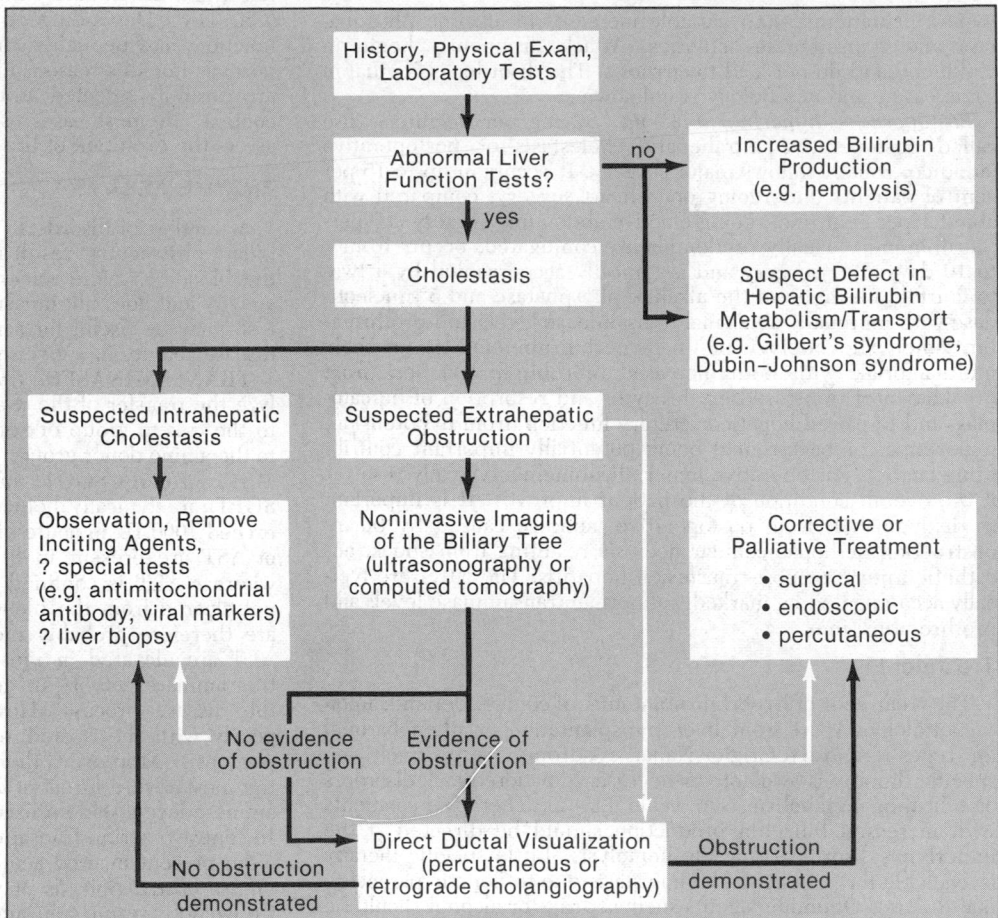

FIGURE 115–2. Approach to the patient with cholestasis. (From Scharschmidt BF, Way LW: The jaundiced patient: Differential diagnosis and clinical approach. *In* Way LW, Pellegrini CA (eds.): Surgery of the Gallbladder and Bile Ducts. Philadelphia, W.B. Saunders Company, 1987.)

information such as the presence of stones in the gallbladder or the presence of a pancreatic mass. CT may be preferable in instances in which precise definition of anatomic structures and level of obstruction is desired. False-negative examinations may occur in patients with sclerosing cholangitis or cirrhosis, presumably because of poor distensibility of the biliary tree, and in patients with gallstones, which commonly produce only partial or intermittent biliary obstruction.

If dilated bile ducts are detected, it is generally appropriate to further define the location and nature of the obstruction with direct cholangiography. Direct cholangiography is also appropriate even when noninvasive imaging studies are negative, if the clinical suspicion of biliary obstruction is high. Indeed, in selected situations such as the evaluation of a patient who has previously undergone biliary surgery, direct ductal visualization may be appropriate as a first procedure. Because of its lower morbidity, *endoscopic retrograde cholangiography* is often preferred to *percutaneous transhepatic cholangiography* as the initial procedure for direct visualization. In an individual patient, the choice between these procedures reflects a variety of factors, including the suspected location of the lesion (proximal versus distal); the presence of a coagulation disorder or prior gastroduodenal surgery which might, respectively, preclude a percutaneous or retrograde approach; anticipation of a therapeutic maneuver such as stent placement or sphincterotomy; and the availability of skilled personnel.

Other tests are occasionally employed in the evaluation of suspected biliary obstruction but are of lesser value. *Hepatobiliary scintigraphy* using derivatives of iminodiacetic acid, which are taken up by hepatocytes and excreted into bile, are of value primarily in the evaluation of cystic duct obstruction and acute cholecystitis (Ch. 126). However, radionuclide scans are unable to provide the resolution available with direct cholangiography and are of limited value in the evaluation of cholestasis. *Intravenous cholangiography* is also unreliable and usually fails to produce ductal visualization if the bilirubin concentration exceeds

3 mg per deciliter. *Oral cholecystography*, while useful in identifying gallbladder stones, is of little value in the evaluation of cholestasis. *Liver biopsy* is not indicated in the routine workup of suspected obstruction, because diagnostic histologic findings are often absent even in the presence of proven obstruction, and the biopsy generally provides no information regarding the location or nature of the obstruction. The principal role of a liver biopsy is in the differential diagnosis of difficult or confusing cases of intrahepatic cholestasis (Fig. 115–2).

HEPATIC DISORDERS THAT MAY MIMIC OBSTRUCTION. It is important for the clinician to be aware of certain hepatic disorders that may present with severe cholestasis suggestive of extrahepatic obstruction (Table 115–3). In some instances (e.g., alcoholic hepatitis, amyloidosis), liver biopsy usually permits a specific diagnosis. In other instances (e.g., cholestatic hepatitis, drug- or estrogen-induced cholestasis, benign recurrent cholestasis, cholestasis related to sepsis), liver biopsy typically demonstrates only cholestasis with variable hepatocellular necrosis, findings that by themselves do not permit a specific diagnosis.

Benign recurrent cholestasis is a particularly confusing disorder. Patients with this rare entity have recurrent episodes of cholestasis which last from weeks to months and recur at highly irregular intervals. These are manifested by pruritus, conjugated

TABLE 115–3. CHOLESTATIC DISORDERS THAT CAN MIMIC EXTRAHEPATIC OBSTRUCTION

Viral hepatitis	Primary biliary cirrhosis
Alcoholic hepatitis	Postoperative cholestasis
Benign recurrent cholestasis	Parenteral nutrition
Pregnancy	Hodgkin's disease
Sepsis	Drugs (e.g., estrogens,
Infiltrative liver disease (e.g.,	phenothiazines, rifampin)
amyloidosis, sarcoidosis)	Inherited disorders (e.g., arterio-
Hepatic neoplasia	hepatic dysplasia)
Hepatic abscess	Sickle cell disease

hyperbilirubinemia, and variable increases in alkaline phosphatase and transaminase activities. Attacks frequently begin in childhood and do not lead to cirrhosis. The disorder is familial in some cases, and its etiology is unknown.

Postoperative hyperbilirubinemia (>2 mg per deciliter), also called postoperative intrahepatic cholestasis or postoperative jaundice, usually follows major surgery. It occurs in up to 15 per cent of patients undergoing open heart surgery, compared with about 1 per cent undergoing elective abdominal surgery. Hyperbilirubinemia, usually predominantly conjugated, occurs from 1 to 10 days after surgery and is typically accompanied by a two- to fourfold elevation of the alkaline phosphatase and 5'-nucleotidase with minimally abnormal transaminase levels and prothrombin time. The etiology of the hyperbilirubinemia is probably multifactorial, with both increased bilirubin production (from breakdown of transfused erythrocytes and resorption of hematomas) and impaired hepatic excretory function (from hypotension, hypoxemia, or bacteremia) being potentially important contributing factors. Postoperative hyperbilirubinemia typically resolves if the overall condition of the patient improves. It is important to distinguish it from postoperative jaundice caused by biliary obstruction or hepatocellular necrosis resulting from shock, anesthetic injury, or post-transfusion hepatitis. The latter are typically accompanied by markedly abnormal transaminase levels and prothrombin time.

Treatment

The treatment of hyperbilirubinemia, of course, depends upon the etiology. Apart from liver transplantation or phenobarbital for types I and II Crigler-Najjar syndrome, respectively, no specific therapy is available or necessary for hereditary disorders of bilirubin metabolism (see Table 115–2). Therapy in patients with increased bilirubin production should be directed at the underlying disorder, typically hemolysis. Little specific therapy is available for patients with cholestasis due to hepatic parenchymal disease. Offending agents such as drugs or alcohol should be withdrawn when possible, and transplantation is appropriate for patients with progressive cholestasis and hepatic dysfunction due to primary biliary cirrhosis or other disorders. Biliary tract disease typically requires direct intervention via surgery or a percutaneous or endoscopic approach.

In patients with prolonged cholestasis and fat malabsorption, oral or parenteral administration of fat-soluble vitamins may be necessary, as well as alteration in the type or amount of dietary fat (Ch. 102). Mild pruritus may be relieved by less frequent bathing and the use of skin softeners. Cholestyramine should be tried in patients with more severe pruritus. Other agents (oral charcoal administration, rifampin, plasma exchange) have also been advocated for refractory pruritus but are not proven modalities.

Gollan JL (ed.): Pathobiology of bilirubin and jaundice. Semin Liver Dis 8:105, 1988. *An entire volume containing nine thoroughly referenced articles focusing on all aspects of bilirubin metabolism.*

La Russo NF (ed.): Medical and surgical aspects of biliary tract disease. Semin Liver Dis 7:311, 1987. *Six review articles outlining the evaluation and treatment of the patient with suspected biliary disease.*

Scharschmidt BF, Way LW: The jaundiced patient: Differential diagnosis and clinical approach. *In* Way LW, Pellegrini CA (eds.): Surgery of the Gallbladder and Bile Ducts. Philadelphia, W. B. Saunders Company, 1987. *A thoroughly referenced review of the diagnosis and treatment of the jaundiced patient.*

116 Laboratory Tests in Liver Disease

Richard A. Weisiger

Many "liver function" tests provide only indirect evidence of hepatic integrity, unlike most tests used for evaluating other organ systems. Specific functions of the liver include clearance of toxic substances from the blood (including drugs, metabolites,

and bacterial toxins), synthesis of plasma proteins and lipoproteins, and intermediary metabolism (e.g., glucose and ammonia) (Ch. 114). Depending on the disease process, some of these functions may be highly compromised while others remain nearly normal. For this reason, liver tests are most valuable when they are carefully selected and interpreted within the total clinical context. In most cases, serial determinations are required to assess the evolution of the disease.

ENZYME ASSAYS

A number of disorders, including inflammation, necrosis, and biliary obstruction, result in the release of hepatic enzymes into the blood. Enzyme release is an indirect indication of disease activity and does not measure liver function. Nevertheless, these tests may be useful for screening and for following the level of disease activity in a given patient.

TRANSAMINASES. *Transaminases (aminotransferases)* catalyze the transfer of the α-amino group from aspartate or alanine to the α-keto group of ketoglutarate; they are named according to the amino donor group. Serum levels of aspartate transaminase (AST, formerly SGOT) and alanine transferase (ALT, formerly SGPT) are typically below 40 IU per liter in normals but may exceed 1000 IU in acute viral or toxic injury. Different isozymes of AST are present in liver cell mitochondria and cytoplasm, whereas ALT is confined to the cytoplasm. Transaminases are not cleared from the blood by excretion into urine or bile and are therefore probably metabolized. Serum levels of AST and ALT are elevated in most hepatic diseases; the height of the transaminase activity in general reflects the current activity of the disease process. However, transaminase levels correlate poorly with the overall severity of the liver disease and with prognosis. Moreover, there are important exceptions. Even in the most severe forms of *alcoholic hepatitis*, for example, transaminase levels seldom exceed 200 to 300 IU per liter (Ch. 118). In contrast, serum transaminase activities of 1000 IU or more are often present in mild acute *viral hepatitis* or shortly after acute *biliary obstruction*, as may occur during passage of a gallstone. Conversely, serum transaminase levels may fall during the clinical course of massive hepatic necrosis, suggesting that the liver is so severely damaged that little enzyme activity remains (Ch. 123). Spuriously low transaminase levels may also occur in renal failure due to chemical interference with the assay.

Despite these caveats, serum transaminase activities may be helpful in certain circumstances. First, they are useful as *screening tests* for liver disease. Elevation of the ALT is relatively specific for hepatobiliary disease. Although AST levels may be increased in diseases of other organs (e.g., myocardium and skeletal muscle), values more than 10 times the upper limit of the normal range usually reflect hepatic or biliary pathology. In the context of other clinical and laboratory findings, identification of the source of increased serum transaminase activity is not usually difficult. Second, transaminase values are useful in monitoring the course of acute or chronic parenchymal liver disease, although they may be misleading in certain cases, as noted earlier. Finally, they may be useful diagnostically: It is distinctly uncommon for the AST to exceed 15 times the upper limit of normal in bile duct obstruction, except when it occurs suddenly or is associated with cholangitis. Because hepatic ALT is a cytoplasmic enzyme while most AST is sequestered in mitochondria, a high ratio of AST to ALT usually indicates severe hepatocellular necrosis (such as *alcoholic hepatitis*). Milder insults that cause leakage of cytoplasmic enzymes commonly produce a ratio of 1 or less.

ALKALINE PHOSPHATASE. *Alkaline phosphatases*, present in many tissues (e.g., liver, bile ducts, intestine, bone, kidney, placenta, and leukocytes), catalyze the release of orthophosphate from ester substrates at alkaline pH. The normal serum level of activity in adults is 25 to 85 IU per liter, although higher levels are normal in children and in pregnancy. The biologic function of alkaline phosphatase is unknown, except for an apparent role in the deposition of hydroxyapatite in osteoid to form bone. Normally, serum alkaline phosphatase activity reflects mainly the hepatic and bone isozymes, although occasionally the intestinal form may account for 20 to 60 per cent of the total. In the later stages of pregnancy, the placental contribution may be substantial. A less common variant, called the *Regan isozyme*, is associated with tumors (especially hepatoma and lung cancer) and appears identical to the placental form (Ch. 125).

Serum alkaline phosphatase activity may be increased in many conditions not associated with hepatobiliary disease, including bone disorders (e.g., Paget's disease, osteomalacia, metastases to bone), pregnancy, normal growth, and occasionally the presence of malignancy not involving bones or liver. In some cases, the source is obvious because of other clinical and laboratory findings. When the source is less apparent, several methods, such as heat stability and electrophoretic separation, are available to differentiate hepatobiliary from other isozymes. However, it is usually more practical to measure serum levels of 5'-nucleotidase, *leucine aminopeptidase*, or *γ-glutamyl transpeptidase*, which tend to parallel alkaline phosphatase in hepatobiliary disease but do not usually increase in bone disease (see below). The increased serum activity in liver disease reflects increased enzyme synthesis rather than decreased biliary excretion or leakage from damaged cells and may be triggered by high tissue bile salt concentrations.

Slight to moderate increases in serum alkaline phosphatase activity (one to two times normal) occur in many parenchymal disorders of the liver such as *hepatitis* and *cirrhosis*. In the absence of bone disease, larger increases (3 to 10 times normal) usually indicate obstruction of bile flow. Although the highest levels usually occur with extrahepatic bile duct obstruction, very high values may also be seen with *intrahepatic cholestasis* and with infiltrative or mass lesions (primary or metastatic *cancer*, *lymphoma*, *leukemia*, or *sarcoidosis*). The serum alkaline phosphatase level rarely remains normal in the presence of significant bile duct obstruction. Increased alkaline phosphatase may be the only clinically apparent abnormality in bile duct stricture or in lesions that produce obstruction of a single hepatic lobe or segment. Its measurement, therefore, offers a relatively sensitive screening test for tumors involving the liver. As many as one third of patients with isolated elevations of serum hepatobiliary alkaline phosphatase activity may have no demonstrable underlying liver or biliary disease.

OTHER HEPATIC ENZYMES. *Leucine aminopeptidase* (LAP) is an ubiquitous cellular peptidase, while 5'-nucleotidase (5'-NT) is a plasma membrane enzyme that cleaves orthophosphate from the 5' position on the pentose sugar of adenosine or inosine phosphate. The serum activity of both enzymes usually increases in cholestasis, and their major clinical value is to help determine if an elevated serum alkaline phosphatase activity originates from the liver. A parallel elevation of the serum activity of either of these enzymes suggests an hepatobiliary origin of the alkaline phosphatase, but the converse is not true. Serum levels of liver alkaline phosphatase may occasionally be increased while LAP and 5'-NT levels remain normal. Because both of these enzymes may be increased in late pregnancy, they are most useful in the nonpregnant patient.

γ-Glutamyl transpeptidase (GGTP), present in many tissues, increases in serum not only in hepatobiliary disease, but also after myocardial infarction, in neuromuscular diseases, in pancreatic disease (even in the absence of biliary obstruction), in pulmonary disease, in diabetes, and during the ingestion of ethanol and other inducers of microsomal enzymes. Measurement of GGTP has been proposed as a sensitive screening test for hepatobiliary disease and for the monitoring of abstinence from ethanol, but its high sensitivity ensures that many who test positive have no identifiable liver disease on further study. It offers no clear advantage over LAP or 5'-NT for identifying the source of increased serum alkaline phosphatase activity except in pregnancy.

Lactate dehydrogenase (LDH) is often elevated in liver disease but is usually not helpful in diagnosis because it is also found in most other body tissues.

CLEARANCE OF METABOLITES AND DRUGS

As a major function, the liver removes various metabolites and absorbed toxins from the blood (Ch. 118). In liver disease, clearance of these compounds may be impaired as a result of loss of parenchymal cells, obstruction of bile flow, reduced cellular transport, or reduced hepatic blood flow. When a metabolite is produced at a relatively constant rate (as is usually true for bilirubin), its serum level can be a sensitive indicator of liver function. The rate of clearance of certain drugs and dye com-

pounds from the plasma following a single dose can be used similarly.

BILIRUBIN. The metabolism of bilirubin and its measurement are discussed in detail in Ch. 115.

BILE ACIDS. Bile acids, absorbed from the ileum in an active recycling process, are nearly completely removed by the liver before they reach the systemic circulation. Impaired hepatic uptake or reflux from blocked bile ducts can lead to high plasma levels of bile acids and result in severe pruritus. Quantitation of serum bile acids has little proven clinical utility at present, however.

AMMONIA. The liver clears ammonia from blood by converting it to urea via the Krebs-Henseleit cycle for excretion by the kidney (Fig. 180–1). In the setting of severe hepatic dysfunction (e.g., fulminant hepatic failure) or portosystemic shunting, serum ammonia levels rise. The level of serum ammonia is widely used to confirm the diagnosis of hepatic encephalopathy and to monitor the success of therapy, but the correlation of the ammonia level with the degree of encephalopathy is only approximate (Ch. 123). Elevated ammonia levels may also be seen when ammonia production is increased by intestinal flora (e.g., following a high-protein meal or gastrointestinal bleeding), by the kidney (in response to metabolic alkalosis or hypokalemia), or in certain rare genetic diseases affecting the pathway of urea synthesis (Ch. 180). Arterial or cerebrospinal fluid levels of ammonia are not more useful than venous levels for clinical purposes.

DRUG CLEARANCE. The liver is primarily responsible for clearing many drugs from blood, particularly those that are poorly filtered by the kidney because of binding to albumin or to other blood components. Clearance of certain drugs has therefore been used to quantitate this function. Indocyanine green clearance provides a useful estimate of hepatic blood flow. The retention of sulfobromophthalein in blood 45 minutes following bolus injection is normally 5 per cent or less but is increased by even mild hepatic dysfunction. Unfortunately, this drug has produced occasional anaphylactic reactions and is no longer routinely available in the United States. Other drugs that have been used to quantitate hepatic function include antipyrene, caffeine, and rose bengal.

SYNTHETIC FUNCTIONS

PROTHROMBIN TIME. The prothrombin time, usually performed by the one-stage (Quick) method, measures the rate at which prothrombin in citrated plasma is converted to thrombin in the presence of added calcium, tissue thromboplastin, and activated clotting factors (Ch. 155). This test depends on the plasma concentration not only of prothrombin, but also of other clotting factors synthesized in the liver, including Factors V, VII, and IX, and fibrinogen. Results may be expressed in seconds, percentage of a standardized control sample, or prothrombin content. The test is abnormal in the setting of reduced synthesis (e.g., liver failure, vitamin K deficiency), increased consumption (e.g., disseminated intravascular coagulation), or both.

Synthesis of fibrinogen, prothrombin, and Factors II, V, IX, X, XI, XII, and XIII occurs in the liver. Synthesis of prothrombin and Factors VII, IX, and X depends on an adequate supply of *vitamin K*, which activates certain hepatic polypeptides by stimulating the synthesis of the calcium-binding residue, γ-carboxyglutamic acid. An abnormal prothrombin time is commonly caused by *vitamin K deficiency, liver disease*, or both and may rarely be seen with *inherited abnormalities*. Vitamin K, a fat-soluble vitamin that is found in many foods, is also produced by intestinal bacteria (Ch. 204). Deficiency is most commonly seen in *malabsorption syndromes*, including failure to absorb dietary fat due to biliary obstruction or other causes of cholestasis (Ch. 102). It may also be seen with antimicrobial suppression of intestinal bacteria, especially when the patient is receiving inadequate oral or parenteral vitamin K replacement.

Any acute or chronic liver disease may cause an abnormal prothrombin time if the synthesis of essential clotting factors is impaired. The plasma half-life of these factors is typically less than 1 day; the prothrombin time therefore responds rapidly to changes in hepatic synthetic function. This property makes the prothrombin time particularly useful for following the course of acute liver diseases; significant elevation often indicates an unfavorable prognosis.

An abnormal prothrombin time may be of diagnostic value in the evaluation of the jaundiced patient. In general, when it is prolonged on the basis of vitamin K deficiency alone (as in fat malabsorption due to cholestasis), it returns to normal within hours of parenteral administration of vitamin K. In contrast, when the synthesis of clotting factors is diminished because of parenchymal liver disease, response to vitamin K may be slight or absent. Both factors may coexist, however. In severe liver failure, elevation of the prothrombin time may also reflect disseminated intravascular coagulation (Ch. 155). Because of these shortcomings, the prothrombin time must be interpreted in the context of all available information.

The *partial thromboplastin time* is used to assess the "intrinsic" clotting mechanism and reflects the activity of all clotting factors except for platelet factor 3, Factor VII, and Factor XII. For this reason, the test is complementary to the prothrombin time and may indicate deficiencies of other clotting factors or the presence of a circulating anticoagulant (Ch. 155).

ALBUMIN. *Albumin*, synthesized exclusively in the liver at a rate of 100 to 200 mg per kilogram of body weight per day, has a long half-life in plasma (about 3 weeks in healthy adults). The synthesis rate is influenced by many factors, including nutritional state, the presence of systemic and/or liver disease, thyroid and glucocorticoid hormones, plasma colloid osmotic pressure, and toxins such as alcohol and carbon tetrachloride. The normal mechanism of albumin turnover is not well understood, although losses are increased in nephrotic syndrome, protein-losing enteropathy, severe burns, exfoliative dermatitis, and gastrointestinal bleeding.

The serum albumin concentration reflects a balance between synthesis and loss and is therefore not specific for the functional state of the liver. Because the serum half-life is long, abnormalities are slow to develop and may persist for weeks after correction of the underlying problem. On the other hand, when other factors can be excluded, hypoalbuminemia may be an important indicator of chronic liver disease. In patients with cirrhosis and ascites, hypoalbuminemia commonly reflects diminished synthesis, but in some cases synthesis is normal and hypoalbuminemia is caused by a redistribution among the extracellular fluid compartments, including the peritoneal cavity.

SERUM LIPIDS AND LIPOPROTEINS. Parenchymal liver disease and bile duct obstruction may produce significant abnormalities in serum lipids and lipoproteins. In acute parenchymal liver disease, the serum electrophoretic band of α_1-lipoprotein may be lost, reflecting an abnormal composition and altered physical properties of the high density lipoproteins. A transient hypertriglyceridemia may also occur because of the presence in serum of abnormal low density lipoproteins rich in triglycerides. These changes appear attributable in part to deficient activity of plasma lecithin–cholesterol acyltransferase (LCAT), an enzyme of hepatic origin that esterifies plasma cholesterol. The changes are transient, and with resolution of the acute liver injury plasma lipids and lipoproteins return to their previous state.

The liver is primarily responsible for removing cholesterol from the body by its direct secretion into bile or its conversion to bile acids. In cholestasis, the serum concentrations of unesterified cholesterol and phospholipids increase, and *xanthomas* and *xanthelasma* may develop if these abnormalities are severe and sustained. A major fraction of the increased plasma unesterified cholesterol is accounted for by an abnormal low density lipoprotein, designated LPX. LPX consists mainly of unesterified cholesterol and phosphatidyl choline (lecithin) with a small amount of protein, largely albumin and C apolipoproteins. LPX is not of value in the differential diagnosis of jaundice, but it may contribute to an elevated plasma cholesterol concentration in patients with liver disease.

IMMUNOLOGIC TESTS

GLOBULINS. *Serum globulins* are of limited diagnostic utility in hepatobiliary diseases. As a group, they are heterogeneous with respect to site and regulation of production, physical properties, and physiologic function. Their concentration, as measured by serum protein electrophoresis or salt fractionation, may be influenced by a wide variety of hepatic and extrahepatic factors and disease states. The mechanism of their increased serum concentration in liver disease is not fully understood but may include stimuli to increased antibody production resulting from decreased removal of bacterial antigens from the portal blood or release of antigenic material from damaged liver cells. An important exception is the finding of a diminished concentration of the α_1-globulin fraction as demonstrated by serum protein electrophoresis. Since approximately 85 per cent of this fraction is accounted for by α_1-antitrypsin, a decrease in its concentration may be an important sign of α_1-antitrypsin deficiency, an inherited disorder associated with neonatal hepatitis, cirrhosis, and pulmonary emphysema (Ch. 121). Elevated IgM concentrations are common in primary biliary cirrhosis, but other clinical, laboratory, and imaging procedures are of greater diagnostic value. Diffuse increases in globulin concentrations are commonly seen in cirrhosis and may be especially pronounced in chronic active hepatitis in the absence of serum markers for active infection by hepatitis B or C viruses.

MITOCHONDRIAL ANTIBODY. In approximately 90 per cent of patients with primary biliary cirrhosis, the serum contains antibodies directed against a lipoprotein component of the inner mitochondrial membrane (Ch. 122). The antibodies are neither organ nor species specific and are demonstrated by immunofluorescent techniques employing rat kidney, liver, and stomach and human thyroid, stomach, and kidney. These antibodies include the three main immunoglobulin classes, are complement fixing, and bind to at least seven different components of the inner and outer mitochondrial membranes. In patients with primary biliary cirrhosis, the titer is not related to the increased level of serum IgM or to the stage or severity of the disease.

Mitochondrial antibodies are also present in up to 25 per cent of patients with chronic active hepatitis and postnecrotic cirrhosis and in 7 to 8 per cent of asymptomatic relatives of patients with primary biliary cirrhosis. They are rarely present in extrahepatic biliary obstruction. A small percentage of patients with nonhepatic diseases may also exhibit positive tests; these include the collagen-vascular disorders, thyroiditis, myasthenia gravis, Addison's disease, autoimmune hemolytic anemia, and chronic biologic false-positive reactions for syphilis. Of the several types of mitochondrial antibodies thus far identified, M_2 is the type usually found in primary biliary cirrhosis. Mitochondrial antibodies are demonstrable in only 0.4 to 0.7 per cent of the general population.

The mitochondrial antibody is useful in the differential diagnosis of jaundice for two reasons. First, a negative result renders the diagnosis of primary biliary cirrhosis unlikely, although it does not exclude it. Second, because of its rarity in extrahepatic biliary obstruction, a positive result helps confirm parenchymal disease. Since the incidence of gallstones in patients with primary biliary cirrhosis is approximately 40 per cent and is also increased in other forms of cirrhosis, the mitochondrial antibody test does not reliably exclude extrahepatic obstruction.

ANTINUCLEAR AND SMOOTH MUSCLE ANTIBODIES. Either or both of these tests are positive in a variable percentage of patients with chronic active hepatitis, usually in cases not associated with hepatitis B or C infection. These antibodies also occur in a minority of patients with primary biliary cirrhosis. As is true of the mitochondrial antibody, these factors are neither organ nor species specific. They probably do not play a role in pathogenesis. The presence of these antibodies in serum does not exclude bile duct obstruction.

TESTS FOR HEPATITIS VIRUS INFECTION. These tests and their clinical significance are discussed in Ch. 117.

EXAMINATIONS OF URINE AND STOOL

The presence of bilirubin in urine indicates that a significant fraction of plasma bilirubin is conjugated and is strong evidence of hepatobiliary disease. Jaundice in the absence of bilirubinuria indicates an exclusively unconjugated hyperbilirubinemia, i.e., reflecting hemolysis, ineffective erythropoiesis, or an inherited disorder of bilirubin conjugation. For several reasons, urine and fecal urobilinogen determinations usually do not provide useful information in the evaluation of hepatobiliary disease (Ch. 115). Testing of stool for occult blood is essential and may provide the first evidence of an alimentary tract lesion related or unrelated to hepatobiliary disease, a bleeding diathesis, or an explanation for the appearance of hepatic encephalopathy. In selected cases, depending on the clinical circumstances, stool culture or examination for ova and parasites may provide information of importance in the diagnosis of liver disease.

HEMATOLOGIC TESTS IN LIVER DISEASE

Diseases of the liver may be associated with a wide variety of hematologic abnormalities, including qualitative and quantitative changes in the formed elements and in clotting function. The abnormalities depend not only on the etiology of the liver disorder but also on whether it is acute or chronic or associated with complications such as liver failure or portal hypertension.

In acute liver disease not associated with liver failure, major changes in the formed elements are uncommon and consist primarily of mild anemia, reflecting either low-grade hemolysis or marrow depression. Slight leukopenia is not uncommon and is often associated with atypical lymphocytes.

Severe aplastic anemia may sometimes complicate acute viral hepatitis, especially following liver transplantation for fulminant hepatitis C infection. In other forms of acute liver disease, hematologic abnormalities such as marrow suppression may be caused by toxins such as ethanol or drugs. In the alcoholic, Zieve's syndrome, consisting of hemolytic anemia and hypertriglyceridemia, may rarely be found. Coagulopathy may complicate massive hepatic necrosis, reflecting depressed hepatic synthesis of clotting factors and, frequently, disseminated intravascular coagulation.

In chronic liver disease, erythrocytic target cells, often associated with cholestasis, result from an expansion of the cell membrane, with relative preservation of the cholesterol-phospholipid ratio. Spur cells (acanthocytes), most often found in advanced alcoholic cirrhosis, reflect a more profound relative and absolute increase in membrane cholesterol.

Red cells, white cells, and platelets may be decreased in patients with portal hypertension, primarily because of hypersplenism (Ch. 152). A number of other abnormalities may be present, but to a large extent these are caused by associated nutritional, pathologic, or pharmacologic influences. Examples include iron deficiency, megaloblastic, and sideroblastic anemias.

LIVER BIOPSY

Liver biopsy is of value in the diagnosis of diffuse or localized parenchymal diseases, including cirrhosis, chronic hepatitis, and mass lesions. It is commonly performed by the blind percutaneous technique but may be done under direct visualization during laparoscopy or with sonographic or radiologic guidance when specific areas must be sampled. Because the histologic changes are usually nonspecific in acute hepatitis or acute cholestatic jaundice, the value of liver biopsy in this setting is primarily prognostic. Liver biopsy requires the cooperation of the patient, except in infants, and normal clotting function. Relative or absolute contraindications include the presence of biliary sepsis or high-grade biliary obstruction, ascites, severe coagulopathy, and right pleural disease.

IMAGING TECHNIQUES AND CHOLANGIOGRAPHY

These techniques are discussed in detail in Ch. 126.

McKenna JP, Moskovitz M, Cox JL: Abnormal liver function tests in asymptomatic patients. Am Fam Physician 39:117, 1989. *Many enzyme abnormalities are detected during routine screening, such as for blood donation. Here is a cost-effective method for evaluating these patients.*

Reichling JJ, Kaplan MM: Clinical use of serum enzymes in liver disease. Dig Dis Sci 33:1601, 1988. *Comprehensive review of the use of serum enzymes for diagnosis and monitoring liver disease. Over 150 references.*

Zakim D, T Boyer (eds.): Hepatology: A Textbook of Liver Disease. 2nd ed. Philadelphia, W. B. Saunders Company, 1990. *A comprehensive and well-written text covering all aspects of liver function and dysfunction.*

Zaloga GP, Prough DS: Monitoring hepatic function. Crit Care Clin 4:591–603, 1988. *Well-written review with an emphasis on clearance tests.*

117 Acute Viral Hepatitis

Robert K. Ockner

DEFINITION. Acute viral hepatitis is caused by any of several agents and presents as a spectrum of syndromes ranging from entirely subclinical and inapparent to rapidly progressive and fatal. In most cases, it is self-limited and uncomplicated, but, depending on the viral agent involved, there is a variable incidence of clinically significant extrahepatic manifestations or of progression to chronic liver disease. These diseases represent infections by viral agents with relative or absolute predilection for the hepatocyte. After a variable incubation period, viral replication in the liver cell approaches a maximum, leading to the appearance of viral components in body fluids and/or excreta, liver cell necrosis with an associated inflammatory response, changes in laboratory tests of liver function, and symptoms and signs of liver damage. The immunologic response of the host appears to play an important but not fully defined role in pathogenesis.

ETIOLOGY. Viral hepatitis is caused by five major agents which differ in structure and in the epidemiology and natural history of the diseases they cause, and several minor agents. The vast majority of cases in the United States are accounted for by hepatitis viruses A, B, C, and D. In addition hepatitis E has been identified as a cause of severe disease in Asia, Africa, and Mexico. Selected characteristics are summarized in Table 117–1, and each is considered in greater detail below. Other viral agents that cause an acute hepatitis syndrome include the Epstein-Barr virus (infectious mononucleosis), cytomegalovirus, herpes simplex, yellow fever, and rubella; the clinical disorders caused by these agents are considered in greater detail elsewhere in the text.

PATHOLOGY. The lesion of acute hepatitis consists of focal necrosis of individual hepatocytes associated with a mononuclear inflammatory response and expanded portal areas that are infiltrated predominantly by lymphocytes and in which bile ducts may be especially prominent (bile duct "proliferation"). There is often a variable, but usually minor, degree of necrosis of hepatocytes bordering the portal areas (so-called periportal hepatitis or piecemeal necrosis). Necrosis of an individual liver cell, whether periportal or within the lobule, is usually reflected in its replacement by a cluster of mononuclear cells, or it may be represented by balloon degeneration or by a shrunken cell with homogeneously eosinophilic cytoplasm and a condensed pyknotic nucleus ("acidophil body"). The regular pattern of the cords of hepatocytes is disrupted, mitotic figures and cholestasis are common, and Kupffer cells are prominent. Although these features are characteristic of typical acute viral hepatitis, they are not specific, individually or collectively. Thus, the same overall pattern of injury is seen in certain forms of drug-induced liver disease, and its individual components are seen in many processes of diverse etiology and duration. Mononuclear cell portal infiltrates, periportal hepatitis, and bridging or confluent necrosis may be especially prominent in chronic forms of hepatitis.

More severe variants of the acute necrotic process include "bridging" necrosis, "confluent" or "submassive" necrosis, and massive necrosis. In these, the necrotic process simultaneously involves contiguous groups of cells rather than single cells in isolation. As a result, there may be variable collapse or condensation of stroma. Bridging necrosis, so named because the continuous zones of necrosis may extend between (i.e., "bridge") adjacent portal and/or central areas, may be a necessary, if not sufficient, antecedent to evolution to a subacute form of hepatitis with progressive deterioration of liver function leading over several months to death in liver failure or to chronic hepatitis or to cirrhosis. Such a predisposition is not conclusively established, however. Thus, bridging necrosis is compatible with complete clinical and histologic recovery and therefore does not per se constitute evidence of chronic or progressive liver disease.

Submassive and massive forms of hepatic necrosis are reflected in a more severe clinical course and a less favorable prognosis. Massive necrosis, in which broad areas of hepatocytes are destroyed, with condensation of stromal elements and portal structures (bile ducts and vessels), is usually manifested clinically as fulminant hepatic failure (see Ch. 123). This syndrome is characterized by severely deranged liver function, hepatic encephalopathy, and a high case fatality rate. In survivors, however, despite the severity of the acute process, a chronic course is unusual, and liver histology typically returns nearly to normal.

In the recovery phase there is regeneration of hepatocytes and a largely complete restoration of normal lobular architecture. It

TABLE 117–1. CHARACTERISTICS OF COMMON CAUSATIVE AGENTS OF ACUTE VIRAL HEPATITIS

	Hepatitis A	Hepatitis B	Hepatitis D	Hepatitis C	Hepatitis E
Causative agent	27 nm RNA virus	42 nm DNA virus; core and surface components	36 nm hybrid particle with HBsAg coat	Flavivirus-like RNA agent	27–34 nm non-enveloped RNA virus
Transmission	Fecal-oral; H₂O-, foodborne	Parenteral inoculation, or equivalent; direct contact	Similar to HBV	Similar to HBV	Similar to HAV
Incubation period	2–6 weeks	4 weeks–6 months	Similar to HBV	5–10 weeks	2–9 weeks
Period of infectivity	2–3 weeks in late incubation and early clinical phases	During HBsAg positivity (occasionally only with anti-HBc positivity)	During HDV RNA or anti-HDV positivity	During anti-HCV positivity	Similar to HAV
Massive hepatic necrosis	Rare	Uncommon	Yes	Uncommon	Yes
Carrier state	No	Yes	Yes	Yes	No
Chronic hepatitis	No	Yes	Yes	Yes	No
Prophylaxis (see text)	Hygiene; immune serum globulin	Hygiene; hepatitis B immune globulin; vaccine	Hygiene; HBV vaccine	Hygiene; ? immune serum globulin	Hygiene, sanitation

is distinctly uncommon for the healing that follows a circumscribed acute hepatitis to be accompanied by fibrous scar formation or by nodular regeneration. In the latter, hepatocytes cluster in an abnormal configuration lacking a central vein and other components of the normal lobular architecture. These two manifestations of an *abnormal* healing process (fibrosis and nodular regeneration) are the essential components of cirrhosis, a form of chronic liver disease that almost always reflects ongoing injury and repair rather than a single acute event.

CLINICAL AND LABORATORY MANIFESTATIONS. The earliest symptoms of acute viral hepatitis typically are nonspecific, predominantly constitutional and gastrointestinal. They may include malaise, fatigue, anorexia, nausea, vomiting, and arthralgias and may suggest a "flu" or upper respiratory syndrome to both patient and physician. Classically, the patient may describe a loss of taste for coffee or cigarettes. Fever, if present, is usually mild. Abdominal discomfort may reflect an enlarged tender liver. Arthritis occurs in 10 to 15 per cent of cases; in hepatitis B it appears to represent immune complex deposition. Skin rash and arthritis occur with similar frequency in hepatitis A, in which circulatory immune complexes also have been demonstrated. Urticaria may occur occasionally.

After a period of several days to a week or more, the prodromal phase may lead to an icteric phase. The earliest clinical manifestation of a rising serum concentration of direct-reacting bilirubin is bilirubinuria, followed by a lightening of stool color, scleral icterus, and, in light-skinned individuals, frank jaundice. Constitutional symptoms often abate during the icteric phase, especially in children, in whom the disease is characteristically less severe. In adults, the gastrointestinal components of the prodrome may persist or even increase for a time. If cholestasis worsens, pruritus may cause increasing discomfort.

Physical findings are variable and depend on the stage of the illness. The only objective finding during the prodrome, apart from mild fever, may be an enlarged and tender liver, associated in perhaps 20 per cent with splenomegaly. Jaundice may or may not appear; indeed, it is likely that the majority of cases remain anicteric, especially among children with hepatitis A. Excoriations reflect the intensity of pruritus. Spider nevi occasionally develop during an acute hepatitis, but since this is unusual, it should suggest the possibility of a more chronic process.

Laboratory studies are highly variable, but almost by definition the clinical onset is accompanied by rising activities of serum aminotransferases; usually the ALT (SGPT) exceeds the AST (SGOT). An elevated serum bilirubin is predominantly direct reacting; very high concentrations, e.g., greater than 15 to 20 mg per deciliter, indicate a severe lesion or may reflect associated hemolysis. The alkaline phosphatase is usually moderately increased, whereas serum albumin concentration may decrease slightly. A diffuse hyperglobulinemia is common. Prothrombin time is prolonged in more severe cases, and a persisting or increasing prolongation is an unfavorable prognostic sign. Mild

and clinically insignificant hypoglycemia occurs in perhaps 50 per cent of cases; more profound hypoglycemia may complicate fulminant hepatic failure. Hematologic tests are also quite variable. Usually the total leukocyte count is normal or slightly decreased and atypical lymphocytes may be present. In more severe cases, total leukocytes may be increased, with relative or absolute neutrophilia. Hemoglobin and hematocrit are usually relatively normal, but occasionally there may be a coincidental hemolytic process, and rarely the course is complicated by aplastic anemia, especially following hepatitis C (non-A, non-B). Urinalysis is usually nonspecific except for the presence of bilirubin.

An important aspect of the laboratory approach to acute viral hepatitis is the etiologic serodiagnosis. Although establishing a specific etiologic diagnosis does not usually influence management, it may have a bearing on prognosis and is particularly useful epidemiologically and for preventing transmission. These tests are considered below, in the discussions of hepatitis A, B, C, and D, and of prevention.

After an icteric phase lasting usually from several days to several weeks, the patient enters a convalescent phase in which there is gradual improvement in symptoms and laboratory tests. The healing process may require several weeks, during which time residual weakness and malaise are common. Normalization of laboratory tests is usually complete within 4 months. Persistence of abnormalities beyond 6 to 12 months suggests that for hepatitis B, C, or D, the process may have become chronic; in this circumstance, liver biopsy may be indicated if there is no evidence of continuing improvement.

COMPLICATIONS AND EXTRAHEPATIC MANIFESTATIONS. The two most important complications of acute viral hepatitis are massive hepatic necrosis (fulminant hepatitis) and progression to chronic hepatitis. Fortunately, these are uncommon, especially in hepatitis A, in which chronicity does not occur and massive necrosis is less common and has a somewhat more favorable prognosis than in hepatitis B, C, and D.

Massive hepatic necrosis with fulminant hepatic failure occurs in fewer than 1 per cent of cases of acute viral hepatitis and is usually signaled by deepening jaundice, increasing prothrombin time, and hepatic encephalopathy, which, in its earliest stages, may appear only as a subtle personality change. Serum transaminase levels may remain high, but in many cases will fall, often in association with a decrease in liver size. These changes are assumed to reflect extensive loss of parenchymal mass and, in the presence of other evidence of a deteriorating course, are unfavorable prognostic signs suggesting fulminant hepatic failure, and the possible need to consider urgent orthotopic liver transplantation. The diagnosis and management of acute hepatic failure and encephalopathy are considered in greater detail in Ch. 123.

Evolution to chronic hepatitis is a more common complication of acute hepatitis B, C, and D. It is suggested by persistence of abnormal serum transaminases, with or without other laboratory abnormalities and clinical symptoms, beyond an arbitrarily selected endpoint. Authorities differ as to where that endpoint belongs; guidelines range from 4 to 12 months, but most would accept 6 months as reasonable. Clearly, however, judgments must be individualized as to when an acute process becomes chronic (or, more pragmatically, when investigations such as liver biopsy should be performed). For example, as long as the patient continues to show evidence of clinical and laboratory improvement, there is little to be gained from a more vigorous diagnostic or therapeutic approach. Conversely, evidence suggestive of chronic liver disease (e.g., signs of portal hypertension or progressive deterioration of laboratory tests) appearing before 6 months may justify earlier diagnostic intervention. Since many of the histopathologic features associated with chronic hepatitis also may be components of an acute process, however, liver biopsies obtained too early in the course may be difficult to interpret and potentially misleading. Chronic hepatitis is also considered in the discussions of hepatitis B, C, and D below, and in greater detail in Ch. 119.

The *cholestatic hepatitis syndrome* occurs occasionally as a complication of acute viral hepatitis, especially hepatitis A. Patients may exhibit a relatively prolonged course of several months dominated by cholestatic features, including pruritus, dark urine, light stools, direct-reacting hyperbilirubinemia, and elevation of alkaline phosphatase. Almost without exception, the prognosis is favorable. The major problem in management posed by this variant is the occasional need to exclude disorders such as biliary stones, stricture, and tumors by means of appropriate imaging and cholangiographic techniques. Brief corticosteroid therapy may be useful symptomatically.

Aplastic anemia may very rarely complicate the icteric or convalescent phase of acute viral hepatitis, especially non-A, non-B (presumably some of which are C). Its pathogenesis is unknown, and its prognosis is poor. Among the relatively few survivors, there is no clear evidence of a beneficial effect of glucocorticoids or anabolic steroid treatment. Other formed elements may also be depressed, and pancytopenia, agranulocytosis, and thrombocytopenia have been reported.

Extrahepatic manifestations of acute viral hepatitis also include *arthralgias* and *arthritis*, and *urticaria*. These are usually most prominent during the prodromal phase and, in hepatitis A and B, appear to reflect deposition of immune complexes. They also may occur in hepatitis C. Other manifestations of hepatitis B infection, such as *glomerulonephritis* and *vasculitis*, are also associated with immune complex deposition and are discussed in Ch. 79 and 60, respectively. A tentative association of *essential mixed cryoglobulinemia* with hepatitis B infection also has been reported. *Pancreatitis* is found in 12 to 40 per cent of cases of fatal acute viral hepatitis, and serum amylase activity may be elevated in up to 30 per cent of nonfatal cases; the true overall incidence and mechanism of pancreatitis in viral hepatitis are not known. Myocarditis, pneumonitis, and other extrahepatic manifestations are rare, and in their presence other systemic disorders should be considered.

SPECIFIC ETIOLOGIC CATEGORIES OF VIRAL HEPATITIS

HEPATITIS A. This form of hepatitis also has been referred to as infectious hepatitis, short-incubation hepatitis, or MS-I hepatitis. The causative agent (hepatitis A virus) is a 27-nm diameter RNA virus that is readily and almost exclusively transmitted via the fecal-oral route. In this important respect it differs significantly from other forms of hepatitis except E (see below). Accordingly, when the etiology of water-borne, point-source, food-handler-related, and institutional hepatitis outbreaks in North America and Europe has been defined, hepatitis A almost invariably has been implicated. In addition, hepatitis A occurs sporadically and is spread by direct person-to-person contact; there appears to be an increased incidence among promiscuous homosexuals. Spread of hepatitis A in day care centers may involve not only children but also the staff and the families of affected children. Although parenteral transmission is theoretically possible, it is rare. The incidence of the disease appears to correlate in a general way with personal hygiene and the efficacy of public health measures, as suggested by the apparent influence of socioeconomic status on the prevalence of hepatitis A antibodies (anti-HAV), which averaged 45 per cent in one study of an urban population in the United States and approximated 90 per cent in residents of Costa Rica. There is no evidence for the existence of a chronic form of hepatitis A or a carrier state. The "reservoir" for the virus appears to consist of clinically inapparent acute cases, in which the disease is not recognized at the time of viral shedding.

Hepatitis A infection typically has an incubation period of 2 to 6 weeks. Fecal shedding of virus occurs over a 2- to 3-week period beginning during the final week of the incubation period and the prodromal phase, and declines as serum transaminases reach maximal levels (Fig. 117–1 and Table 117–1). Although there is a transient viremia during this interval, parenteral transmission of the disease is very rare. Viral shedding in stool declines as antibody (anti-HAV) appears in serum. Initially, antibody is predominantly of the IgM class, but an IgG antibody soon appears. The IgG antibody persists in serum for many years; its exclusive presence indicates prior experience with, and immunity to, the hepatitis A virus. The presence of the IgM antibody, on the other hand, almost always indicates recent infection (within a few months) (Table 117–2), although occasionally this antibody may persist for up to 1 year or more. An IgA antibody to HAV appears in the feces of patients at about the time fecal shedding of virus ceases and persists for several weeks.

The acute illness itself is quite diverse in its clinical manifestations and course. The majority of cases probably are clinically inapparent, especially in children, or are perceived as a nonspecific "flu" syndrome. Jaundice, when it occurs, is usually mild. Symptoms usually subside, and serum transaminases return to normal within 3 to 4 months. Hepatitis A virus infection has been

FIGURE 117–1. Sequence of clinical and laboratory findings in a patient with hepatitis A. Fecal shedding of virus is brief in duration and ends with the appearance of anti-HAV in serum. IgM anti-HAV, usually present for a few months, may persist in serum for a year or more after the acute illness. (From Krugman S, Gocke DJ: Viral Hepatitis. Philadelphia, W. B. Saunders Company, 1978.)

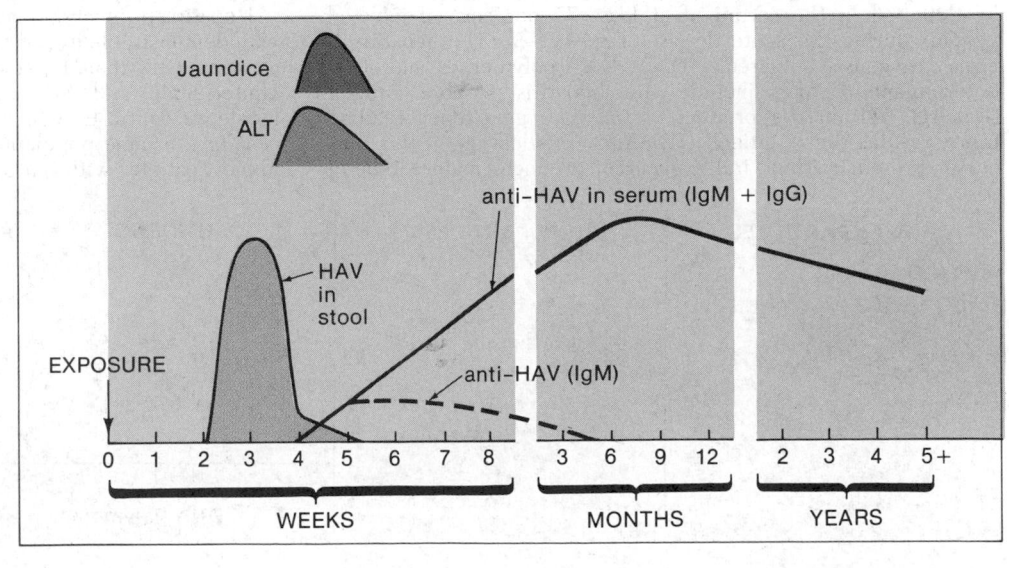

TABLE 117–2. SEROLOGIC TESTS IN VIRAL HEPATITIS

Agent	Terminology	Definition	Significance
Hepatitis A (HAV)	Anti-HAV IgM type	Antibody to HAV	Current or recent infection or convalescence
	IgG type		Current or previous infection; indicates immunity
Hepatitis B (HBV)	HBsAg	HBV surface antigen	Positive in most cases of acute or chronic infection
	HBeAg	e antigen; HBV core component	Transiently positive during active virus replication, acute hepatitis, and in some chronic cases; reflects Dane particle concentration and infectivity
	Anti-Hbc (IgM or IgG)	Antibody to HBV core antigen	Positive in all acute and chronic cases and in carriers; thus, marker of HBV infection; not protective; IgM anti-HBc may reflect active virus replication
	Anti-HBe	Antibody to e antigen	Transiently positive during convalescence and in some chronic cases and carriers; not protective; reflects low infectivity
	Anti-HBs	Antibody to surface antigen	Becomes positive late in convalescence in most acute cases; protective
Hepatitis C (HCV)	Anti-HCV	Antibody to cloned C100-3 polypeptide	Becomes positive on average 15 weeks after clinical onset; not protective; may be infectious
Hepatitis D (HDV)	Anti-HDV (IgM or IgG)	Antibody to HDV antigen	Similar to anti-HBc in indicating infection; not protective

implicated in some cases of acute cholestatic hepatitis and may exhibit a relapsing or protracted course. Rarely, hepatitis A causes massive hepatic necrosis and fulminant hepatic failure, but this complication is less common and more favorable in prognosis than that in hepatitis B and C.

The ease with which hepatitis A is transmitted among contacts and via water and food, as well as the demonstrated efficacy of immune serum globulin in prevention or amelioration of the disease, underscores the value of individual and public health measures to control the spread of infection. The application of these to the management of the individual patient and his or her contacts is discussed below.

HEPATITIS B. In contrast to hepatitis A, hepatitis B virus infection may cause a wide variety of acute or chronic hepatic and extrahepatic diseases, as well as a chronic carrier state. Its presentation as an acute hepatitis is typical of those cases that previously were designated serum hepatitis, homologous serum jaundice, long-incubation hepatitis, or MS-II hepatitis, although it is now apparent that some of these cases represented hepatitis C (see below). The hepatitis B virus (HBV) differs in almost every respect from hepatitis A (Tables 117–1 and 117–2; Fig. 117–2). The complete infective virion, or *Dane (HBV) particle*, is a DNA virus of 42 nm diameter, consisting of antigenically distinct surface and core components. The *surface coat* is largely lipid and protein and may exist in serum or other body fluids either as a component of the Dane particle or as separate 20-nm diameter spheres or cylinders. Its major antigenic determinant (hepatitis B surface antigen, HBsAg) includes several subtypes (d, y; w, r), and it can be detected in the serum of at least 75 per cent of infected persons during the acute disease (Fig. 117–2). The hepatitis B virus *core* consists of circular DNA, DNA polymerase, and other determinants, which include the hepatitis B core antigen (HBcAg). Within the product of the core gene open reading frame resides the e antigen (HBeAg). Self-cleavage of this precursor protein during viral replication produces mature HBcAg

and HBeAg. HBcAg remains an intrinsic part of the complete virion, while HBeAg is secreted from the hepatocyte and exists separately in plasma. Each elicits a humoral antibody response (anti-HBc and anti-HBe, respectively) during the course of the hepatitis B infection. HBV-DNA can be detected in serum by molecular hybridization techniques, including polymerase chain reaction, and is the most sensitive indicator of the presence of infective virus.

Also unlike hepatitis A, *transmission* of hepatitis B by the fecal-oral route is relatively unimportant; infection may follow oral ingestion, but large doses appear necessary. Instead, the virus is present in virtually all body fluids and excreta, and transmission of this disease occurs primarily via parenteral routes. Therefore, it usually requires either overt inoculation (e.g., transfusion, or injection via a contaminated needle) or intimate personal contact (e.g., between sexual partners, patients and health professionals, and mother and newborn infant). The disease occurs with an increased frequency among sexual partners of acutely infected individuals, as well as among chronically exposed persons, including health professionals and patients exposed to blood and blood products (e.g., workers and patients in clinical laboratories, dialysis and oncology units), the sexually promiscuous (especially male homosexuals), drug users who share needles, and handlers of primates (which are susceptible to infection). In urban centers, hepatitis B may account for up to 50 per cent of sporadic cases of acute hepatitis, even in the absence of documented parenteral inoculation. This attests to the importance of person-to-person contact in the spread of this disease.

Hepatitis B infection may become chronic, either in association with demonstrable liver disease or in otherwise seemingly healthy carriers. Less than 1 per cent of the general population of the United States and Western Europe is HBsAg-positive. This low incidence contrasts with incidence of anti-HBs of about 10 per cent in the same population, providing additional evidence that in most patients with acute hepatitis B the infection is self-limited

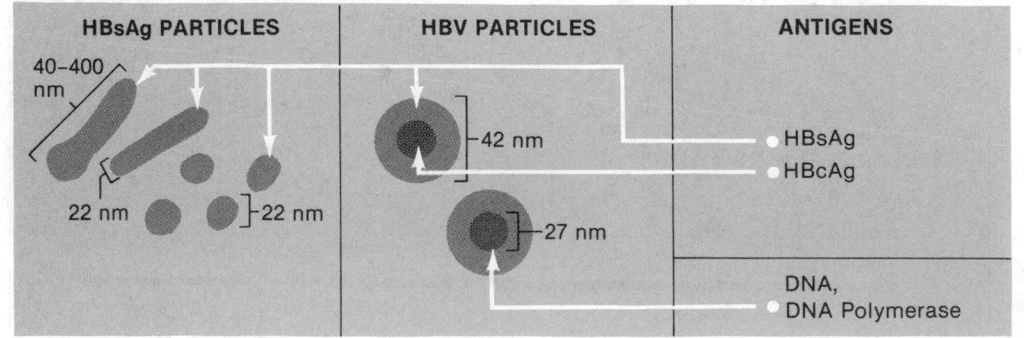

FIGURE 117–2. Forms of HBV in plasma, showing location of the various components and antigenic determinants. HBeAg, probably not a component of the complete virus particle, is not shown. (Adapted from Koff RS: *In* Sanford JP, Luby JP [eds.]: The Science and Clinical Practice of Medicine. Infectious Diseases. Vol. 8. New York, Grune & Stratton, 1981; by permission.)

and followed by immunity and only infrequently leads to chronic liver disease or a carrier state. The incidence of HBsAg positivity is much higher in less-developed areas (up to 15 per cent) and among certain subpopulations with increased exposure and/or impaired immunity, such as patients with Down's syndrome, leprosy, or lymphoproliferative disorders; addicts; and patients undergoing dialysis. In addition to acute cases, therefore, these chronically infected individuals constitute the "reservoir" that serves to perpetuate the virus. Historically, it is likely that transmission of the disease has occurred not so often via overt parenteral inoculation but rather via close personal and sexual contact or from mother to newborn. In the latter instance (*vertical transmission*), i.e., in infants born to mothers with acute or chronic infection, there is a high probability that the neonate will acquire the disease. This is especially likely when the mother develops acute hepatitis B in late pregnancy or in the early postpartum period or has chronic hepatitis. Transmission appears to correlate with the presence of HBeAg in maternal serum, reflecting the concentration of infective virions. Characteristically, these infants remain chronically infected for many years, either as "carriers" or with a persisting low-grade and chronic hepatitis. They are at increased risk of developing hepatocellular carcinoma (see Ch. 125). Vertical transmission may be an important mechanism by which the reservoir of the virus is sustained from generation to generation.

The *incubation period* of acute hepatitis B, as defined by the appearance of clinical symptoms, varies between 4 weeks and 6 months, with an average of about 50 days. If the incubation period is defined instead in terms of the interval between exposure and the first *serologic* evidence of viremia, it may be as brief as 2 weeks, especially after exposure to large parenteral doses. Two weeks to 2 months prior to the clinical onset, HBsAg becomes detectable in serum (see Fig. 117–3 and Table 117–2). At about the time of the clinical onset and the rise in serum transaminase activities, anti-HBc becomes detectable. Initially, an IgM anti-HBc is present in high titer and persists for several months to 1 year; thereafter IgG anti-HBc predominates. In chronic HBV infections, IgM anti-HBc may be detectable during periods in which the virus is actively replicating. IgG anti-HBc persists for up to several years after acute hepatitis and is present in all chronic carriers. It appears to play no role in host defenses; rather, it serves as a reliable marker of hepatitis B infection currently or within the preceding few years. The Dane particle markers (HBeAg and DNA polymerase) usually become detectable in serum prior to the increase in transaminase. The duration of HBsAg positivity is highly variable. It may persist for a few days to 2 to 3 months; persistence beyond this time may indicate a chronic course. Characteristically, HBsAg becomes undetectable prior to the appearance of anti-HBs. This antibody can be demonstrated in 80 to 90 per cent of patients, usually late in convalescence, and indicates relative or absolute immunity. Its appearance suggests a successful response to the infection, but there are exceptions to this in certain patients with chronic hepatitis (see Ch. 119).

Several important qualifications should be noted in interpreting the results of hepatitis B serologic tests. First, in a significant number of patients with acute hepatitis B the serum is negative for HBsAg, presumably because the antigen is very low in titer or evanescent. For this reason, a single negative HBsAg test does not exclude the diagnosis. Anti-HBc is more sensitive in this regard and may be the only serologic indication of hepatitis B infection. A negative test for anti-HBc effectively excludes the diagnosis. On the other hand, a positive test for anti-HBc in an HBsAg-negative serum could merely reflect a prior episode of hepatitis B. These HBsAg-negative, anti-HBc–positive patients may be classifiable on the basis of the anti-HBs: a positive test early in the course of an acute hepatitis is evidence against the diagnosis of acute hepatitis B. Detection of IgM anti-HBc suggests recent acute or chronic HBV infection during a phase of active virus replication, as noted above. In those IgM-anti-HBc–negative subjects in whom HBV infection appears to have antedated the acute illness, the possibility of superimposed infection by hepatitis D (delta-agent), a non-A, non-B virus, or other causes of an acute hepatitis syndrome must be considered. With the advent of more sensitive methods for detecting HBV-DNA, perceptions of the relationship of serology to host-virus interactions are evolving.

The *clinical course* of acute hepatitis B is more variable and usually more prolonged than that of hepatitis A. It is also associated with extrahepatic manifestations, including urticaria and other rashes, arthritis, and, much less commonly, glomerulonephritis and vasculitis. The immune complexes that appear to cause these extrahepatic manifestations consist of HBsAg, anti-HBs, and complement components. Glomerulonephritis and vasculitis are also associated with chronic hepatitis B infection and are not necessarily accompanied by apparent liver disease. Indeed, up to one third of all cases of polyarteritis nodosa may be associated with hepatitis B virus infection.

Approximately 90 per cent or more of otherwise healthy adult patients with acute hepatitis B recover completely and become HBsAg negative. Fewer than 1 per cent develop massive hepatic necrosis, but this complication is more common than in hepatitis A. The 5 to 10 per cent of patients who remain HBsAg positive beyond 4 to 6 months are at risk of developing chronic hepatitis (see Ch. 119).

HEPATITIS C ("NON-A, NON-B"). The ability to document hepatitis A and B virus infection made it clear that many cases of acute hepatitis were caused by one or more other agents,

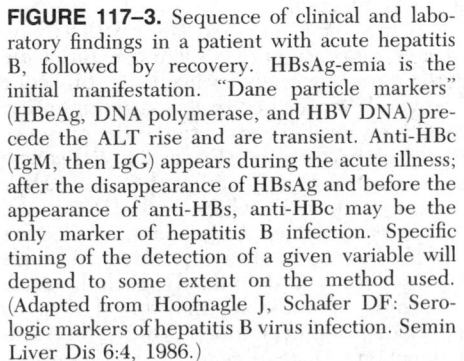

FIGURE 117–3. Sequence of clinical and laboratory findings in a patient with acute hepatitis B, followed by recovery. HBsAg-emia is the initial manifestation. "Dane particle markers" (HBeAg, DNA polymerase, and HBV DNA) precede the ALT rise and are transient. Anti-HBc (IgM, then IgG) appears during the acute illness; after the disappearance of HBsAg and before the appearance of anti-HBs, anti-HBc may be the only marker of hepatitis B infection. Specific timing of the detection of a given variable will depend to some extent on the method used. (Adapted from Hoofnagle J, Schafer DF: Serologic markers of hepatitis B virus infection. Semin Liver Dis 6:4, 1986.)

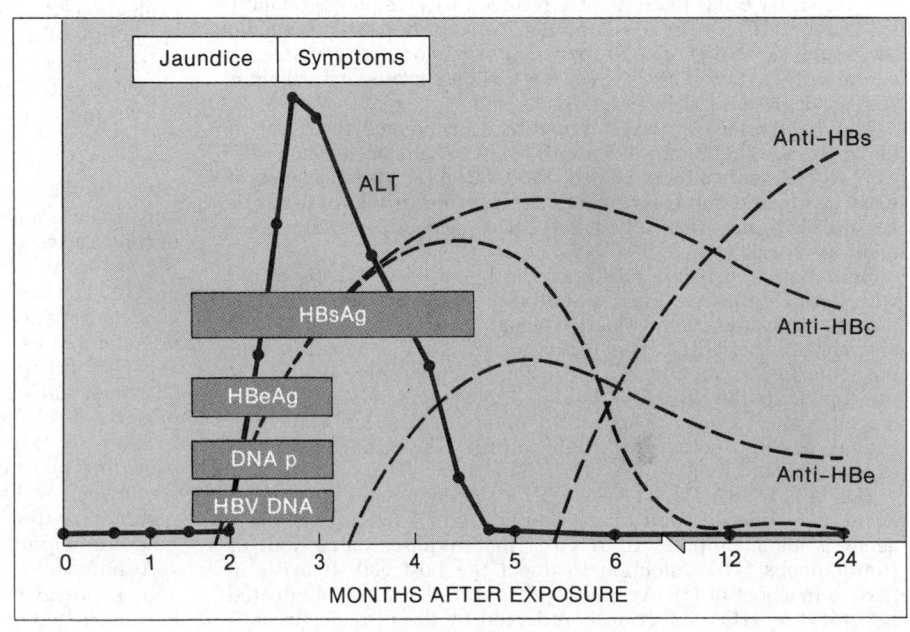

designated "non-A, non-B." One of these, hepatitis C virus, has been characterized and appears to account for the great majority of such cases. Accordingly, the designation hepatitis C, as used here, includes cases previously referred to as non-A, non-B (except for the water-borne epidemic disease now referred to as hepatitis E, noted below). It remains likely that a few cases of non-A, non-B hepatitis may ultimately be attributed to one or more as yet unidentified agents.

Hepatitis C virus (HCV) was identified by a novel and painstaking application of the techniques and concepts of molecular biology, initially utilizing the sera of chimpanzees known to carry post-transfusion non-A, non-B hepatitis infection in high titer. Nucleic acid sequences from chimpanzees' sera were cloned and screened for in vitro expression of a polypeptide antigen recognized by antibodies present in the sera of patients with well-characterized post-transfusion non-A, non-B hepatitis. These efforts led to the development of an assay for an antibody to one viral epitope (C100-3) and to the characterization of the virus itself. HCV is an RNA agent related to the flaviviruses, a family that includes dengue fever and yellow fever. The agent appears to be readily transmitted parenterally; vertical transmission probably occurs, and transmission to sexual and household contacts appears to occur less frequently than in hepatitis B. In adults, it causes an illness with an average incubation period of 7 weeks (range 5 to 10). The antibody test does not become positive until 15 weeks after the clinical onset; among acute resolving cases only 15 per cent were positive. Thus, the antibody test is not useful in the early diagnosis of acute resolving hepatitis, and additional assays are under development. These confirmatory tests are important for identifying false-positive standard tests for the anti–C100-3 antibody, which is commonly found during screening of normal populations, e.g., in blood donors, and in patients with hyperglobulinemia. They include a recombinant immunoblot assay (RIBA) for the C100-3 epitope and polymerase chain reaction assays for HCV-RNA. The latter may detect viral sequences in acute hepatitis and in many cases that are positive for anti–C100-3, indicating that this antibody may be present in the infectious serum of patients with ongoing disease. In chronic cases worldwide, the antibody test is positive in 70 to 100 per cent of post-transfusion and in 22 to 90 per cent of community-acquired non-A, non-B hepatitis. It is positive in 65 per cent or more of patients with hepatocellular carcinoma.

Hepatitis C is the major cause of *post-transfusion hepatitis*. It occurs in approximately five to ten cases per 1000 transfusions and can be transmitted in whole blood, packed cells, platelets, plasma, and especially clotting factor concentrates. The recent availability of tests to screen donor units for HCV antibodies, and eventually components of the virus itself, should decrease the incidence substantially, just as the incidence of post-transfusion hepatitis B has been greatly reduced by screening of donors for HBsAg. HCV also is a common cause of hepatitis in needle users and accounts for 50 per cent or more of sporadic or community-acquired cases, i.e., those not associated with obvious contact or parenteral inoculation.

The incubation period of hepatitis C is longer than that of hepatitis A, ranging from 5 to 10 weeks, with an average of 7 weeks. The acute illness is also quite variable. The incidence of massive hepatic necrosis appears comparable to that of hepatitis B, and together these two categories account for the great majority of cases.

Both post-transfusion and sporadic hepatitis C are associated with both an apparent carrier state (inferred from the fact that it may be transmitted by blood from apparently healthy donors) and chronic hepatitis. The incidence of chronic hepatitis after post-transfusion hepatitis C approaches 50 per cent. In some of these patients the disease is mild and may spontaneously subside or remit after a year or more. In others, a "carrier" state may evolve, or the process may exhibit a progressive course and lead to cirrhosis and liver failure (see Ch. 119).

HEPATITIS D (DELTA-AGENT). Infection with this unusual agent may be regarded as a complication of hepatitis B. The agent is an incomplete RNA virus that requires antecedent or simultaneous HBV infection to infect the host cell. It exists in plasma in a coat of HBsAg and is present in the nuclei of infected hepatocytes. HDV infection is reflected by the presence of anti-HDV antibody (IgM acutely; IgG chronically) or HDV-RNA in serum. Almost invariably the serum is positive for HBsAg and anti-HBc and, in most, anti-HBe. It is most commonly found among intravenous drug addicts and recipients of multiple transfusions. In subjects who are acutely and simultaneously infected with HBV and HDV there is no apparent increase in the probability that chronic hepatitis will ensue, but the likelihood of fulminant hepatic failure is greater than for acute hepatitis B alone. In individuals chronically infected with HBV, however, superimposed acute HDV infection usually also becomes chronic and is associated with the histopathologic findings of chronic active hepatitis.

HEPATITIS E. In recent years, an *epidemic form of non-A, non-B hepatitis* has been described, associated with outbreaks in India, Southeast Asia, Burma, North Africa, and the Soviet Union. The responsible agent is an RNA virus distinct from HAV and the enteroviruses. Serologic tests for it are not yet generally available. The illness affects young adults primarily and is associated with a mortality approaching 20 per cent in pregnant women. There is no evidence that this illness becomes chronic.

GENERAL APPROACHES TO DIAGNOSIS AND MANAGEMENT

DIAGNOSIS. In its classic presentation, the presumptive diagnosis of acute viral hepatitis is readily suggested by a compatible history and physical examination, in association with laboratory evidence of hepatocellular injury, i.e., significantly increased serum aminotransferase activities. Because all of these features are nonspecific, however, it is essential that other possible etiologic factors be considered, such as use of medications or illicit drugs, alcohol, exposure to environmental or industrial toxins, and the possible acquisition of unusual infections as suggested by travel or residence in rural or less well-developed areas. Exposure to viral hepatitis itself is suggested by contact with jaundiced persons or persons known to have developed hepatitis, sexual promiscuity (especially among male homosexuals), transfusion of blood or blood products, or the sharing of needles by drug users. Among health professionals, workers in dialysis and oncology units, surgeons, dentists, and clinical laboratory technicians are at increased risk, as is anyone in direct contact with blood, blood products, or other body fluids. Despite the importance of a careful inquiry into these possible risk factors, many patients with acute viral hepatitis report no significant exposures.

A careful and complete physical examination helps establish the diagnosis (tender hepatomegaly is the most common finding) and helps exclude other processes that occasionally mimic acute viral hepatitis, such as acute hepatic congestion, disseminated sepsis or liver abscess, or biliary tract disease with or without cholangitis.

Serodiagnosis of viral hepatitis is an important part of the initial evaluation. A positive test for the IgM class of anti-HAV or a rising titer of total anti-HAV is strong evidence for acute hepatitis A. Conversely, if the test for anti-HAV is negative well into the convalescent phase, the diagnosis is excluded. A single positive test for unfractionated anti-HAV is of little diagnostic value, since this could reflect a previous infection.

Although an acute hepatitis syndrome associated with HBsAg positivity has been taken as presumptive evidence for acute hepatitis B, none of the tests generally available at this time permits early and unequivocal diagnosis or exclusion of this entity. An important but not routinely available exception is the presence of HBV-DNA. Also, the presence of anti-HBs early in the course of acute hepatitis tends to suggest chronic rather than acute HBV infection. Since the classic pattern in which both HBsAg and anti-HBc are positive acutely may not be present in all cases (although anti-HBc itself is virtually always positive), a single negative test for HBsAg does not definitively exclude acute hepatitis B. Medical records, if available, may be of help by providing information about prior liver function tests, hepatitis serologies, or blood donation. Since donated blood has been screened routinely for HBsAg since 1972, such information may be quite helpful in the evaluation of hepatitis B serologies.

As noted above, early acute hepatitis C is not usually associated with a positive test for the C100-3 antibody, which does not become reactive until an average of 15 weeks after the clinical onset. Moreover, a positive result indicates only that the patient has been or is infected with HCV, possibly chronically, and does not necessarily reflect the etiology of an acute hepatitis syndrome. Serologic characterization of hepatitis C infection will be facilitated by the development of direct assays for viral components. Hepatitis D may be documented by a positive test for serum IgM anti-HDV or for HDV-RNA.

If a *liver biopsy* is performed, it may demonstrate the pathologic features of acute viral hepatitis. However, these are nonspecific, and in the vast majority of cases biopsy is not indicated. Its use should be reserved for patients in whom the diagnosis is uncertain or in whom there is concern regarding chronicity or a deteriorating course, or any circumstance in which documentation of the histopathology may influence management. In the most severely ill patients biopsy may not be possible because of abnormalities of clotting function.

DIFFERENTIAL DIAGNOSIS. Acute viral hepatitis may be mimicked by a large number of other acute infections and noninfectious processes. Infections include other viruses such as cytomegalovirus, Epstein-Barr virus (infectious mononucleosis), and yellow fever virus; and nonviral processes such as Q fever, secondary syphilis, leptospirosis, salmonellosis, pyogenic and amebic liver abscess, malaria, and toxoplasmosis. A wide variety of drugs and toxins may injure the liver and cause a clinical syndrome that can resemble viral hepatitis (see Ch. 118). Inborn errors of metabolism such as Wilson's disease may also lead to acute hepatic necrosis. Acute hepatic congestion secondary to cardiac failure or venous occlusion, cholecystitis, and acute biliary obstruction should also be excluded. Finally, the possibility that what appears to be acute hepatitis may in fact represent the exacerbation of chronic hepatitis should be considered.

MANAGEMENT. There is no specific treatment for acute viral hepatitis. Major emphasis is placed on symptomatic and supportive care and on the prevention of transmission. Prevention is considered in detail below.

Most patients with acute viral hepatitis do not require hospitalization and are appropriately managed at home. Rest is advisable, but strict confinement to bed is not necessary beyond what is dictated by the patient's own sense of fatigue and malaise. No specific dietary measures are indicated, but most patients find a low-fat, high-carbohydrate diet more palatable. During the most severe phases of the illness, anorexia and nausea may be so extreme that oral intake of any kind is minimal. In such instances, attention to fluid balance is important, and it may be necessary to advise the intake of small amounts of clear fluids at frequent intervals. Although there is an appropriate reluctance to administer medication to the patient with liver disease, judicious use of small doses of antinausea agents such as hydroxyzine, trimethobenzamide, and even prochlorperazine is occasionally necessary and usually well tolerated. As the patient's symptoms decrease and appetite improves, intake can be liberalized, usually according to taste. Alcoholic beverages should be avoided throughout the course of the acute illness. Ambulation and activity may be increased as symptoms and laboratory tests improve; the most useful advice is that such activity should be limited so as to avoid causing fatigue. The decision to return to employment or school must take into consideration the patient's symptoms, the strenuousness of the work, and the potential for transmission of the disease; this, in turn, is a function of the viral etiology and the closeness of contact with others. In general, transmission is quite unlikely after 2 to 3 weeks in hepatitis A, whereas spread of hepatitis B or C ordinarily requires direct person-to-person contact.

Hospitalization is indicated for those patients in whom severe nausea and vomiting prevent maintenance of adequate fluid balance, in whom there is evidence of progressive deterioration, especially with encephalopathy or prolongation of prothrombin time, or in whom invasive diagnostic studies are indicated.

There is no convincing evidence to justify the use of corticosteroids in acute hepatitis, regardless of its severity. The management of fulminant hepatitis poses special problems in patient monitoring and support and should take place in a center with liver transplantation capability. It is discussed in detail in Ch. 124.

PREVENTION. The entire area of hepatitis prophylaxis has been dramatically changed by the availability of an effective vaccine for hepatitis B. In this vaccine, the immunizing antigen is HBsAg, prepared from donor sera or, more recently, by recombinant DNA technology employing yeast. An appropriate immune response is reflected by the appearance of anti-HBs. Immunization for hepatitis B also prevents hepatitis C. Hepatitis A virus has been propagated in tissue culture, and a vaccine is undergoing clinical trials. Finally, continuing progress in the identification, isolation, and characterization of hepatitis C, D, and other non-A, non-B agents suggests the possibility of active immunization, although not for some time. Pending the advent of generally available and effective vaccines for all of the viral causes of acute hepatitis, prevention must depend mainly on personal hygiene and public health measures directed at minimizing the exposure of potentially susceptible individuals, and on the appropriate use of passive immunization.

The use of public health and hygienic measures rests on the premise that body fluids and excreta of infected individuals are potentially infective. Clearly there are certain exceptions, depending on the specific virus involved, the clinical stage of the infection, the amount of potentially infective material involved, and the nature of the exposure. For example, because of the ease with which hepatitis A and E are spread via the fecal-oral route, contact of such patients with others should be minimized, and their excreta and essentially all materials handled by them during their brief period of infectivity should be carefully disposed of. In contrast, hepatitis B, C, and D are not commonly spread via the fecal-oral route. Although excreta are to be regarded as infective in these patients, the more important concern is transmission via puncture by contaminated needles (or equivalent exposure to infective material) or intimate personal (sexual) contact, especially during the period of HBsAg positivity. Because of these differences among the agents and differences in the approach to passive immunization, serologic diagnosis of the acute viral hepatitis case is useful, even though most patients with these disorders may be expected to do well regardless of etiology. In practice, rapid serodiagnosis is not always possible, and for this reason certain generalizations regarding the early management of the patient and his or her contacts are appropriate and are discussed below, along with measures for specific agents.

Hepatitis A. Since the infection is spread primarily via the fecal-oral route, including transmission by handling food, in drinking water, and potentially by fomites, strict attention to hygiene on the part of the patient and his or her attendants, whether in home or hospital, is of utmost importance during the period of viral shedding (Fig. 117–1). Direct body contact should be limited to that necessary for care; attendants should wear gloves, and careful handwashing is appropriate. Food, utensils, clothing, linen, needles, and excreta should be handled separately and carefully, also by gloved attendants. The virus is readily inactivated by boiling or by exposure to formalin, chlorine, or ultraviolet irradiation. In the hospital setting, strict isolation is not usually required for cooperative and informed patients with hepatitis A. In the home, similar measures should be implemented to the extent possible.

Close contacts of patients with hepatitis A should receive passive immunization with immune serum globulin as soon as possible, preferably within the first few days. The official recommended dose is 0.02 ml per kilogram up to a maximum of 2 ml, although up to 5 ml has been advocated. This would apply to immediate family members, sexual contacts, or others with whom the patient has been in close contact during the presumed period of infectivity. Casual contacts in the workplace or school probably do not require passive immunization unless there is reason to suspect mutual handling of food, beverages, or contaminated items. On the other hand, it is important to inquire about other possible cases among work or classroom associates. If there is reason to suspect a possible point-source outbreak, then all similarly exposed persons should receive immune serum globulin and appropriate epidemiologic information should be obtained.

The mode of transmission of hepatitis A also renders its prevention a matter of concern for those who intend to travel in areas where public health and sanitation measures may be suboptimal. In such circumstances, drinking water, fresh fruits and vegetables, and shellfish may be contaminated and should be avoided if possible. For these persons, administration of a standard dose (0.02 ml per kilogram) of immune serum globulin may be expected to afford protection for up to 3 months; for longer periods, a dose of 0.06 ml per kilogram is recommended and should be repeated at 4 to 6 month intervals.

Hepatitis B. Although this agent is less readily transmitted via the fecal-oral route, due consideration should be given to the general hygienic measures outlined for hepatitis A, in both home and hospital. Transmission ordinarily requires direct contact with the patient or the equivalent of a parenteral inoculation of infective material. Thus, in the home, children are far less likely than the spouse to acquire hepatitis B from an acutely infected adult. In the hospital, strict isolation may not be necessary if excreta, needles and other medical supplies, and personal utensils are identified, carefully handled, and discarded.

Passive immunization with immune serum globulin enriched in anti-HBs (hepatitis B immune globulin, or HBIG) is protective against hepatitis B infection in certain circumstances and when used in accordance with established guidelines. Because this material is expensive, it should not be used indiscriminately. At present, its use is officially recommended in the following specific situations:

1. Inoculation of material known to be contaminated with the hepatitis B virus, e.g., inadvertent puncture of a health professional by a needle from an HBsAg-positive patient, or accidental transfusion of HBsAg-positive blood or blood products.

2. Splash of HBsAg-positive material into the eye or on an open skin wound or eruption, as may occur in a laboratory accident or during a surgical or diagnostic procedure.

3. Ingestion of HBsAg-positive material, as may occur during a laboratory pipetting accident.

4. Sexual partners of patients with *acute* hepatitis B (partners of patients with chronic hepatitis B presumably have been previously exposed) within 14 days of contact.

5. Infants born to HBsAg-positive mothers, especially those who have had acute hepatitis B during the final trimester of pregnancy or first 2 months post partum or who are positive for both HbsAg and HBeAg at the time of delivery.

The rational use of HBIG depends on two essential components. First, it must be documented that the material to which the person has been exposed contains HBsAg, and this requires identification of the source and appropriate serologic confirmation. For example, accidental puncture of the skin by one of several used needles in a disposal container effectively precludes meeting this requirement and, therefore, the use of HBIG. Second, the exposed person must actually be at risk. If, at the time of exposure, he or she is already positive for HBsAg (i.e., infected) or anti-HBs (i.e., immune if the s/n value by radioimmunoassay exceeds 10), nothing will be gained from the administration of anti-HBs (HBIG). Ideally, therefore, the serologic status of both "donor" and "recipient" should be documented before the decision to administer HBIG is made. In practice, however, this is not usually possible within the few days' interval after exposure in which HBIG appears to be most effective. As a practical alternative to this dilemma, one possible approach is to immediately obtain serum from both the "donor" and the person at risk. Pending results of the HBsAg assays, the latter may be given 5 ml of ordinary immune serum globulin. HBIG may be administered later, if indicated by the test results. This approach represents a compromise between the need to institute early passive immunization on the one hand and to avoid indiscriminate use of HBIG on the other, and at a cost that is small relative to that of the HBIG itself. Other approaches are possible. In the family situation, the value of administering HBIG to the spouse remains controversial, but it is generally accepted that its use is not required for children, since they are at low risk.

Hepatitis B Vaccine. Safe and effective vaccines have been developed for the prevention of hepatitis B, consisting either of highly purified and triple-inactivated HbsAg obtained from the serum of chronic carriers or a recombinant preparation utilizing HBsAg synthesized in yeast. The vaccine is administered in three doses: initially and 1 month and 6 months later, and usually elicits production of anti-HBs in the recipient. Intramuscular injection is important and is more likely effective with deltoid than with gluteal administration. (Smaller doses are used for children, and larger doses for dialysis and immunocompromised patients.) The recombinant vaccine is safe for use in pregnant

women. Although most subjects who have completed the three-dose immunization are protected against hepatitis B infection, there are important exceptions, especially among immunosuppressed subjects. The duration of this protection varies, but probably is of the order of 5 years. No firm recommendations exist regarding booster doses.

The vaccine is recommended for use in high-risk groups and individuals. These include, but are not limited to, health professionals (especially those with high exposure risk such as surgeons, dentists, and dialysis workers), susceptible dialysis patients, and those subject to multiple transfusions (e.g., hemophiliacs), certain residents and staff of custodial care institutions, parenteral illicit drug users, heterosexual and household contacts of HBsAg carriers, Alaskan Eskimos, and sexually active and promiscuous male homosexuals. Available evidence suggests that it is also effective, when the first vaccine dose is combined with HBIG, in the passive-active immunization of health professionals after accidental needle stick and of infants born to HBsAg-positive mothers. The cost-effectiveness of screening of potential vaccine recipients (e.g., anti-HBs determination) varies with the circumstance. In general, in those groups in which prevalence of hepatitis B is relatively low, screening is not cost effective, whereas it is useful in groups with a high prevalence (e.g., the homosexual community). For most health professionals, screening is marginally cost effective and depends on the prevalence of hepatitis B infection in the particular subgroup. In any case, it is established that administration of the vaccine to individuals already infected or immune is not harmful.

Hepatitis D. There is no established method for active or passive immunization. Since HDV infection requires simultaneous or antecedent HBV infection, prevention of HBV, e.g., by the vaccine, protects against HDV. Since previously infected HBV subjects are at risk for HDV infection, care should be taken to minimize exposure to HDV-containing materials, e.g., HBV-positive serum or secretions.

Hepatitis C. It appears to be transmitted in a manner that more closely resembles that of hepatitis B than hepatitis A. Thus close personal contact and parenteral inoculation appear necessary, suggesting that prophylactic measures suitable for hepatitis B are appropriate, although available evidence suggests that it is not as readily transmitted to sexual and household contacts.

A problem largely confined to hepatitis C at present is that of post-transfusion hepatitis. The single most effective means of reducing the incidence of this disorder has been the exclusion of blood obtained from commercial (paid donor) sources. There is a correlation between both elevated aminotransferase activity and anti-HBc positivity in donor unit plasma and the probability of post-transfusion hepatitis in a recipient, and exclusion of such units is desirable. The advent of wide-scale screening of donor units for anti-HCV is expected to diminish the incidence of post-transfusion hepatitis further. The possible role of pre-exposure (i.e., pretransfusion) immune serum globulin in the prevention of the disorder remains unclear, and at present immune serum globulin is not officially recommended for its prevention.

Advisory Committee on Immunization Practices: Recommendations for protection against viral hepatitis. MMWR 34:313, 1985. Ibid: Update on hepatitis B prevention. Ann Intern Med 107:353, 1987. Ibid: Prevention of perinatal transmission of hepatitis B virus: Prenatal screening of all pregnant women for hepatitis B surface antigen. MMWR 37:341, 1988. *Three papers that summarize current policy regarding hepatitis immunization, including the most recent revisions concerning vertical transmission.*

Alter MJ, Hadler SC, Judson FN, et al.: Risk factors for acute non-A, non-B hepatitis in the United States and association with hepatitis C virus infection. JAMA 264:2231, 1990. *Useful trends derived from sentinel counties survey.*

Alter HJ, Purcell RH, Shih JW: Detection of antibody to hepatitis C virus in prospectively followed transfusion recipients with acute and chronic non-A, non-B hepatitis. N Engl J Med 321:1494, 1989. *Important information regarding the natural history of hepatitis C infection and the utility of screening blood for hepatitis C antibody.*

Dienstag JL (ed.): Viral hepatitis. Semin Liver Dis, Vol. 11, May 1991. *A minisymposium in which clinically relevant aspects of acute and chronic hepatitis are critically reviewed by recognized experts.*

Everhart JE, DiBisceglie MD, Murray LM, et al.: Risk for non-A, non-B (type C) hepatitis through sexual or household contact with chronic carriers. Ann Intern Med 112:544, 1990. *Evidence suggesting that hepatitis C is less readily transmitted via these kinds of personal contact than is hepatitis B.*

Favero MS, Maynard JE, Leger RT, et al.: Guidelines for the care of patients hospitalized with viral hepatitis. Ann Intern Med 91:872, 1979. *Specific recommendations that provide a useful guide.*

Gocke D: Hepatitis A revisited. Ann Intern Med 105:960, 1986; Lemon SM: Type

A viral hepatitis. New developments in an old disease. N Engl J Med 313:1059, 1985. *Two useful reviews and summaries of some more recently recognized clinical features of the disease.*

Miller RH, Kaneko S, Chung CT, et al.: Compact organization of the hepatitis B virus genome. Hepatology 9:322, 1989. *Authoritative and comprehensive summary.*

Ramalingaswami V, Purcell RH: Waterborne non-A, non-B hepatitis. Lancet 1:571, 1988. *An authoritative review of epidemiologic and clinical aspects of hepatitis E.*

Reyes GR, Purdy MA, Kim JP, et al.: Isolation of a cDNA from the virus responsible for enterically transmitted non-A, non-B hepatitis. Science 247:1335, 1990. *Further progress in the characterization of hepatitis E and a useful summary of the status of the field.*

Zuckerman A (ed.): Viral Hepatitis and Liver Disease. New York, Alan R. Liss, 1988. *Proceedings of a recent symposium in which clinical and basic aspects of all forms of viral hepatitis are addressed.*

118 Toxic and Drug-Induced Liver Disease

Nathan M. Bass

In clearing and biotransforming xenobiotics, the liver is exposed to a large variety of potentially toxic chemical agents and metabolites: naturally occurring plant alkaloids and mycotoxins, industrial chemicals, and, most commonly, pharmacologic agents used in the treatment of disease. The manifestations of toxic and drug-induced liver disease also constitute a spectrum of clinical, laboratory, and histopathologic changes and prognoses virtually as broad as the entire range of acute and chronic hepatobiliary disorders. The severity may range, at one extreme, from asymptomatic abnormalities in liver function tests to fatal massive liver necrosis at the other. Viral hepatitis and biliary obstruction may be closely mimicked by several types of hepatotoxic drug reactions, and exposure to certain agents may also lead to chronic hepatitis, cirrhosis, and liver tumors.

PATHOGENESIS

It is rare for a parent chemical to be directly responsible for drug- and toxin-induced liver disease; more commonly a toxic metabolite(s) formed by the drug-metabolizing enzymes within the liver is the immediate causative agent. Drug biotransformation appears to be a common requirement in the pathogenesis of many different types of drug-induced liver injury. Individual susceptibility to the injury produced by some drugs varies considerably. Potentially hepatotoxic agents are therefore conventionally divided into two categories based on the predictability with which they produce liver disease: *intrinsic hepatotoxins* and *idiosyncratic hepatotoxins.*

Intrinsic hepatotoxins typically produce acute liver damage after a relatively brief latent period (usually a few days) in a predictable, dose-dependent fashion that is largely independent of host susceptibility factors and that is readily reproducible in experimental animals. Examples of this group include the industrial solvents *carbon tetrachloride, 2-nitropropane, trichloroethane,* the octapeptide toxins of the *Amanita* mushroom species, and the antipyretic *acetaminophen.* In most instances, toxic metabolites formed from the parent compound by the cytochrome P-450 drug-metabolizing enzymes produce liver damage by covalent modification of liver macromolecules, or through the generation of reactive oxygen species and subsequent peroxidation of cell membrane lipids.

Idiosyncratic hepatotoxins, in contrast, produce liver disease in an infrequent, unpredictable fashion after a variable latent period, often only after several months of administration of the drug. A large number of therapeutic agents are capable of producing idiosyncratic hepatotoxic reactions in a small proportion of patients who receive them (e.g., halothane, isoniazid, phenytoin, and chlorpromazine). Although severe liver disease occurs infrequently with these drugs, milder hepatic dysfunction may occur frequently (e.g., with isoniazid and chlorpromazine), or toxic liver disease may be reproduced in animal models (e.g., halothane) Many of these agents may therefore be "intrinsic hepatotoxins" which lead to severe "idiosyncratic" liver disease in a few susceptible individuals, possibly because of variations in the pathways of drug biotransformation, immune-mediated hypersensitivity ("drug allergy"), or both. In a given individual, genetic polymorphism in drug-metabolizing enzymes may increase activity of subsidiary pathways that form toxic metabolites and thereby increase the risk of severe toxicity from drugs that are processed in part via these pathways. In idiosyncratic drug-induced liver disease, fever, arthralgias, rash, and eosinophilia are often prominent, indicative of a hypersensitivity-based mechanism. Furthermore, in some cases of drug-induced hepatitis (e.g., halothane), antibodies that recognize liver cell macromolecules covalently modified by metabolites of the implicated drug antibodies have been detected. Adducts formed on the liver cell surface between drug metabolites and liver cell membrane proteins may therefore constitute neoantigens that are capable of provoking immune-mediated liver damage.

MORPHOLOGIC PATTERNS OF DRUG-INDUCED LIVER DISEASE

Drugs and toxins produce a wide variety of pathologic lesions in the liver (Table 118–1). Some agents may injure the liver in more than one way. For example, isoniazid may produce a nonspecific focal hepatitis, an acute viral hepatitis–like lesion, or chronic active hepatitis, whereas oral contraceptives may cause cholestasis or liver cell adenoma and have been implicated in hepatic vein thrombosis.

ZONAL NECROSIS. Intrinsic hepatotoxins typically cause liver cell necrosis, largely confined within a particular zone of the liver lobule. Centrilobular necrosis, the most common pattern of zonal injury, is produced by *carbon tetrachloride, acetaminophen,* and *Amanita* toxins (see Ch. 108). This pattern of injury is explained in part by the greater abundance of cytochrome P-450 drug-metabolizing enzymes in the central region of the liver lobule and possibly also by the relative hypoxemia of the centrilobular region. *Halothane,* despite its classification as an idiosyncratic hepatotoxic agent, also frequently produces centrilobular necrosis. Periportal zonal necrosis, a much rarer lesion, is produced by *allyl alcohol* and *yellow phosphorus.* Extremely high elevations of serum transaminases usually accompany this type of liver injury, and in severe cases, acute liver failure may result. Acute zonal necrosis is either fatal or is followed by complete recovery. Chronic exposure to some toxins may produce a similar lesion, but it is not certain that this ultimately progresses to cirrhosis.

NONSPECIFIC FOCAL HEPATITIS. Nonspecific focal hepatitis consists of scattered foci of liver cell necrosis with mononuclear cell infiltrates, without the characteristic features of viral hepatitis. Nonspecific hepatitis may result from many forms of drug injury including the dose-dependent, intrinsic hepatotoxicity of *aspirin* and *oxacillin.* This lesion has an excellent prognosis and resolves completely upon discontinuation of the responsible drug.

VIRAL HEPATITIS–LIKE REACTIONS. Diffuse hepatocellular degeneration and necrosis with variable inflammatory infiltration and acidophil bodies, resembling the acute pathologic lesion of viral hepatitis and producing similar clinical manifestations, is another common pattern of idiosyncratic injury. In severe

TABLE 118–1. CLASSIFICATION OF DRUG-INDUCED LIVER DISEASE

Category	Examples
Zonal necrosis	Acetaminophen, carbon tetrachloride
Nonspecific hepatitis	Aspirin, oxacillin
Viral hepatitis-like reactions	Halothane, isoniazid, phenytoin
Cholestasis	
Noninflammatory	Estrogens, 17α-substituted steroids
Inflammatory	Chlorpromazine, antithyroid agents
Fatty liver	
Large droplet	Ethanol, corticosteroids
Small droplet	Tetracycline, valproic acid
Granulomas	Phenylbutazone, allopurinol
Chronic hepatitis	Methyldopa, nitrofurantoin
Fibrosis	Methotrexate, hypervitaminosis A
Tumors	Estrogens, vinyl chloride
Vascular lesions	6-Thioguanine, anabolic steroids

cases this lesion may progress to bridging, submassive or massive liver necrosis, and fulminant liver failure. Drugs producing viral hepatitis–like reactions include *halothane, isoniazid, ketoconazole, methyldopa, sulfonamides,* and *phenytoin.* In some instances, the presence of fever, rash, and serum and tissue eosinophilia, as well as other evidence of immunologic dysfunction, are important clues to the drug etiology of the disease and also implicate a hypersensitivity-based mechanism. In other examples, such as halothane and isoniazid, features of hypersensitivity are highly variable or distinctly rare.

CHOLESTASIS. Cholestasis is characterized by clinical symptoms of pruritus and jaundice and biochemically by elevated serum alkaline phosphatase and minimal or modest increases in serum transaminases. Two distinct forms of this very common manifestation of drug-induced liver injury are recognized. In the first, caused principally by *natural and synthetic estrogens* and by *17α-substituted androgenic and anabolic steroids,* there is usually little or no evidence of hepatocellular necrosis or inflammation. The injury is most simply viewed as the impaired secretion of bile by the liver cell, probably reflecting a direct steroid effect on the physical properties of cellular membranes or the activities of enzymes involved in this process. The lesion is completely and rapidly reversible.

In the second form of cholestatic injury, there is significant hepatocellular necrosis and portal and lobular inflammation; acidophil bodies and eosinophils are variably present. Systemic features, including fever, rash, and arthralgias, are not uncommon. This form of injury is produced by a broad group of agents, including the *phenothiazines, oral hypoglycemic* and *antithyroid* agents, and the *macrolide antibiotics* (e.g., erythromycin estolate). Its prognosis is generally favorable and complete recovery may be expected, except in very few individuals in whom chlorpromazine leads to a prolonged but ultimately resolving cholestatic course; rarely, the reaction may prove fatal. Marked differences in individual susceptibility associated with systemic features have suggested drug allergy as the basis for this form of injury. Chlorpromazine, however, is converted to a number of variably toxic metabolic products; this may account not only for the frequently abnormal liver function observed in patients receiving large doses for prolonged periods but also for the smaller number who develop the overt inflammatory and necrosing cholestatic lesion.

FATTY LIVER. Triglycerides may accumulate within hepatocytes in two forms. Most commonly, fat accumulates as large droplets that displace the liver cell nucleus and confer an adipocyte-like appearance. Hepatomegaly and mildly elevated transaminases are typically found, but liver function is usually well preserved. This form of fatty liver typically occurs with direct hepatotoxins including *ethanol, halogenated hydrocarbons, acetaminophen,* and also with *corticosteroids* and is similar in appearance to the fatty liver seen in other systemic conditions such as *protein-calorie malnutrition, obesity,* and uncontrolled *diabetes mellitus.*

A much less common pattern is seen in association with *tetracycline* or *valproic acid* hepatotoxicity, and occasionally with *alcoholic liver disease,* and superficially resembles that seen in *Reye's syndrome, obstetric fatty liver,* and *Jamaican vomiting sickness.* It consists of fat deposited in smaller droplets throughout the liver cell, the nucleus remaining central. This pattern is usually associated with significant, occasionally fatal, disturbances in liver function. A distinctive type of hepatic lipid accumulation in the form of lysosomal phospholipid storage occurs as a direct effect of the drugs *amiodarone* and *perhexilene maleate.*

GRANULOMAS. Therapeutic agents are probably responsible for up to one third of cases of granulomatous hepatitis. Drug-induced granulomas are typically noncaseating and are often associated with extrahepatic granulomas and prominent systemic features of hypersensitivity. Responsible agents include *phenylbutazone, quinidine, allopurinol, phenytoin, hydralazine, sulfonamides,* and *sulfonylurea derivatives.*

CHRONIC HEPATITIS. Chronic hepatitis has been associated with an increasing number of drugs, including *amiodarone, dantrolene, isoniazid, methyldopa, nitrofurantoin, oxyphenisatin, perhexilene maleate, phenytoin, propylthiouracil, sulfonamides, acetaminophen,* and *aspirin.* Although these agents more often

cause acute liver injury, prolonged use may occasionally result in a chronic progressive process leading in some instances to cirrhosis. The histologic abnormalities usually resemble those seen in idiopathic autoimmune or viral chronic active hepatitis. In the case of amiodarone, a lesion strikingly similar to that of alcoholic hepatitis with prominent Mallory bodies may be produced. In many cases, the lesion is largely or completely reversible, but in severe cases this may require many months after the drug is discontinued. Rarely, progressive liver failure and death may ensue despite cessation of the drug.

FIBROSIS. Chronic liver injury from some agents increases collagen deposition, often with minimal or absent evidence of hepatocellular necrosis or inflammatory response. Fibrosis may progress to cirrhosis and portal hypertension, although the latter may occur as a result of hepatic portal fibrosis even in the absence of cirrhosis. This type of injury may occur following the chronic administration of *methotrexate* in the treatment of psoriasis or exposure to *inorganic arsenicals* and in *hypervitaminosis A.*

TUMORS. Tumors caused by drugs and other chemical agents may be of several types, including *hepatic adenoma (and possibly hepatocellular carcinoma)* associated with *oral contraceptive* use, and *angiosarcoma* caused by prolonged exposure to *vinyl chloride* monomer or Thorotrast. The mechanisms by which these tumors are produced are not known, but their clinical and laboratory features generally resemble those of similar tumors occurring "spontaneously." A possible exception is the apparently greater size, vascularity, and tendency to sudden hemorrhage of hepatic adenomas associated with oral contraceptive use (see Ch. 125).

VASCULAR LESIONS. Vascular lesions of several kinds occasionally are caused by drugs. Oral contraceptives have been implicated as a cause of hepatic vein thrombosis. Hepatic *veno-occlusive disease,* a process that affects the smaller tributaries of the hepatic veins, has been associated with the use of *antitumor agents,* including *6-thioguanine, cytarabine,* and *azathioprine,* as well as with ingestion of *pyrrolidizine alkaloids,* e.g., from plants of *Senecio* and *Crotalaria* species ("bush tea poisoning"). *Oral contraceptives* and *anabolic steroids* have been identified as causes of *peliosis hepatis,* a condition in which the liver lobule contains extrasinusoidal blood-filled spaces; this lesion is also seen in certain chronic wasting neoplastic and inflammatory diseases.

PRINCIPLES OF DIAGNOSIS AND MANAGEMENT

A causal relationship between the use of a drug and liver injury may be difficult to establish. Drugs may produce abnormalities very similar to those of other common disorders such as viral hepatitis or biliary disease, and some drugs may produce more than one kind of lesion. A detailed drug history is essential, and information about past exposure and the response to a suspect agent may be of considerable value in diagnosis. Because a number of industrial chemicals are potential hepatotoxins, details of the patient's occupation and work environment should be routinely obtained. The diagnosis of drug-induced liver disease ultimately depends on (1) a history of exposure, (2) consistent clinical, laboratory, and occasionally liver biopsy findings, and (3) resolution of the problem after the presumed toxin is discontinued. In some instances, when only a single agent is involved and a characteristic histologic type of injury is found, the diagnosis based on laboratory and biopsy findings is relatively straightforward. Examples include the small-droplet fatty liver caused by *tetracycline* or the centrilobular necrosis produced by *acetaminophen* (usually associated with significant blood levels of the drug). Conditions are more complex when several drugs are being used, any one of which or even the underlying disorder for which the drugs were prescribed may be responsible for a nonspecific or viral hepatitis–like type of liver injury. The causal role of a particular drug in idiosyncratic liver disease can usually be established through rechallenge with the drug. Rechallenge is rarely justified, however, because of the risk of a severe or even fatal outcome. Furthermore, it is not necessary to incriminate the drug unambiguously if alternative drugs are available.

Drug-induced liver disease is managed by discontinuing the implicated drug(s) and giving supportive care for acute hepatitis and hepatic failure as needed. In the case of severe, acute drug- or toxin-induced liver failure, urgent liver transplantation may be life-saving (Ch. 124). Specific pharmacologic intervention is generally limited to the administration of *N*-acetylcysteine in acetaminophen overdosage (see below). Corticosteroids have no established value in the treatment of drug-induced liver disease, although they may suppress the serum sickness–like syndrome associated with certain idiosyncratic reactions.

SELECTED EXAMPLES OF DRUG-INDUCED LIVER DISEASE

ACETAMINOPHEN. This readily available analgesic and antipyretic is a classic example of an intrinsic, dose-dependent hepatotoxin causing zonal necrosis and acute liver failure, often associated with renal failure. Significant liver injury usually occurs with doses in excess of 10 to 15 grams, most frequently taken in a suicide attempt. Within a few hours, patients develop nausea, vomiting, and diarrhea. These initial symptoms soon subside and are followed by a relatively asymptomatic phase. Clinical and laboratory signs of liver damage become evident 24 to 48 hours following ingestion. Serum transaminase levels in excess of 5000 U per liter are common, whereas severe liver injury may lead to progressive liver failure with encephalopathy, prolongation of the prothrombin time, hypoglycemia, and lactic acidosis.

The liver injury is caused by a toxic metabolite of acetaminophen formed by the cytochrome P-450–dependent drug-metabolizing system. Below threshold doses, this metabolite is efficiently detoxified by conjugation with glutathione. In the toxic dose range, glutathione stores are rapidly exhausted and the metabolite reacts with essential cellular constituents, leading to cell dysfunction and death. The rate at which reactive acetaminophen metabolites are formed is influenced not only by the dose ingested but also by the activity of the cytochrome P-450 enzymes (which may be stimulated by inducers such as phenobarbital and ethanol) and by the availability of glutathione, which may be reduced by fasting and ethanol. A combination of both enzyme induction and glutathione depletion may underlie the particular susceptibility of patients with chronic alcoholism to acetaminophen hepatotoxicity. In such individuals, doses of acetaminophen within the therapeutic range occasionally produce significant liver damage.

The initial treatment of acetaminophen overdose consists of supportive measures and gastric lavage. N-Acetylcysteine should be administered to high-risk patients, in whom it may significantly reduce the severity of liver necrosis and its attendant mortality. The plasma level of acetaminophen is the most reliable means for assessing prognosis. Levels in excess of 200 mg per liter at 4 hours, 100 mg per liter at 8 hours, or 50 mg per liter at 12 hours after ingestion are predictive of severe liver damage and are indications for treatment with N-acetylcysteine. This agent appears to act mainly by providing cysteine for glutathione synthesis and is most effective when given within 10 hours of acetaminophen ingestion. N-Acetylcysteine may afford some benefit after 10 hours, but not after 24 hours have elapsed. Intravenous preparations have been used in Britain, but only the oral form of N-acetylcysteine is currently available in the United States. The recommended oral dose is 140 mg per kilogram initially, followed by maintenance doses of 70 mg per kilogram every 4 hours for 72 hours.

Survivors of acute acetaminophen toxicity usually recover completely without progressive or residual liver damage. Chronic ingestion of acetaminophen at doses in the range of 3 to 8 grams per day may produce a largely subclinical liver injury with centrilobular necrosis or chronic hepatitis found on liver biopsy. This injury reverses fully after the drug is discontinued.

AMIODARONE. This iodinated benzofuran, used in the treatment of refractory arrythmias, is capable of producing an unusual form of liver injury, in addition to its recognized pulmonary, thyroid, ocular, and cutaneous toxicity. A number of patients who receive amiodarone develop mild increases in serum transaminases levels, which may normalize despite continuation of therapy, accompanied by engorgement of lysosomes with phospholipid. Between 1 and 3 per cent of patients receiving amiodarone develop a more severe liver injury that histologically resembles acute alcoholic hepatitis, with fat infiltration of hepatocytes, focal necrosis, fibrosis, polymorphonuclear leukocyte infiltrates, and Mallory bodies. This lesion may progress to micronodular cirrhosis, with portal hypertension and liver failure. The pseudoalcoholic lesion and its progression to cirrhosis often occur in a clinically insidious manner, with minimal elevation of serum transaminases. Hepatomegaly may be found, but jaundice is rare. Evidence of hepatotoxicity may persist for several months after the drug is discontinued.

Amiodarone concentrates in lysosomes and inhibits lysosomal phospholipases, causing the characteristic phospholipidosis. How amiodarone causes pseudoalcoholic hepatitis and how this relates to phospholipid accumulation are unknown; the processes appear to be independent. Liver biopsy is helpful in diagnosis and should be considered in patients receiving amiodarone who develop persistent or significant (greater than twofold) elevation of serum transaminases or hepatomegaly. The decision to discontinue amiodarone in the presence of histologic evidence of hepatotoxicity is often difficult in view of the more ominous risk of sudden death from cardiac arrhythmias which may be increased by abrupt withdrawal of the drug.

CHLORPROMAZINE. This agent, and less frequently other phenothiazines, produces a cholestatic reaction in approximately 1 per cent of patients after 3 to 5 weeks of treatment. Symptoms of fever, anorexia, nausea, upper abdominal pain, rash, and arthralgias may occur at the onset, preceding the development of pruritus and jaundice. Eosinophilia is commonly present. Liver biopsy reveals cholestasis with canalicular bile plugs, a prominent portal inflammatory cell infiltrate of mononuclear, polymorphonuclear, and eosinophilic leukocytes with variable focal liver cell necrosis. The systemic accompaniments of this idiosyncratic type of hepatotoxicity suggest a drug hypersensitivity mechanism, but chlorpromazine is also an intrinsic hepatotoxin. Thus, subclinical abnormalities of liver function tests occur frequently among patients treated with high doses or for prolonged periods with this drug. In addition, chlorpromazine impairs bile secretion in experimental animals at doses approximating those used clinically, and certain metabolites of this drug adversely affect several factors necessary for bile formation.

The symptoms of chlorpromazine cholestasis usually subside over a period of weeks following discontinuation of the drug. Rarely, a syndrome of prolonged cholestasis resembling primary biliary cirrhosis may occur, but eventual recovery, even after a period of years, is also the rule. Fatalities are rare. Apart from discontinuing the drug, treatment is supportive, with cholestyramine for severe pruritus and fat-soluble vitamin supplementation in cases of prolonged cholestasis.

ERYTHROMYCIN. A cholestatic reaction with components of inflammatory cell infiltration and liver cell necrosis may complicate the use of erythromycin. In most instances, this has occurred with erythromycin estolate; other erythromycins including the ethylsuccinate and lactobionate have been less frequently implicated. Hepatotoxicity typically presents as an acute syndrome of right upper quadrant pain, fever, and variable cholestatic symptoms. The clinical picture may closely mimic acute cholecystitis or cholangitis and has prompted surgical exploration in some instances. The prognosis is uniformly excellent, but the reaction may recur within days of readministration of the drug. The mechanism of the injury is unknown.

HALOTHANE. This halogenated alkane anesthetic rarely causes a viral hepatitis–like reaction which, in severe cases, may progress to fatal massive hepatic necrosis. Susceptibility to halothane hepatitis appears to be increased in older persons, women, and obese individuals, and severe reactions usually occur after previous or multiple exposures to this anesthetic. Symptoms usually indistinguishable from viral hepatitis occur between 7 and 10 days after anesthesia, but this interval may shorten considerably after repeated exposure. Fever, which may be hectic, with chills and sweats, commonly precedes the onset of jaundice; rash and eosinophilia are less consistent features. The course may terminate fatally within days, or recovery occurs, which is usually rapid and complete. Some patients run a more protracted course before either recovery or the development of liver failure. Metabolites of halothane formed by the cytochrome P-450 system are clearly important in the mechanism of the hepatic injury. Some of these metabolites may be directly toxic; others may form haptens with cell membrane proteins, provoking an immune-mediated attack on the liver. Cross-sensitization may occur between halothane, methoxyflurane, and enflurane, although hepatic injury appears to be less common with the latter two anesthetic agents.

ISONIAZID (INH). Among persons taking isoniazid (INH) for single-drug chemoprophylaxis against tuberculosis, there is approximately a 10 to 20 per cent incidence of subclinical liver injury. This manifests during the first few weeks of therapy as a mild to moderate increase in serum transaminase levels. These laboratory abnormalities, which reflect a focal nonspecific hepatitis, subside in the majority of patients despite continued administration of the drug. About 1 per cent of patients receiving isoniazid develop significant liver injury, which clinically and histologically resembles the wide spectrum of viral hepatitis. The liver disease may present as a relatively mild, acute process, a subacute or chronic hepatitis, or fatal massive liver necrosis. The onset usually occurs within 2 to 3 months after commencing the drug, and initial symptoms are often nonspecific, with malaise and anorexia preceding signs of liver disease. Clinical features of "drug allergy" are distinctly unusual. Age influences the incidence of severe isoniazid liver injury, which increases significantly after the age of 35, and probably exceeds 2 per cent among persons over the age of 50.

Isoniazid appears to injure the liver through the formation of a toxic metabolite. Liver injury is more frequent in persons who are slow acetylators (as opposed to rapid acetylators) of the drug. The conversion of the isoniazid metabolite acetylhydrazine to the nontoxic diacetylhydrazine may be impaired in slow acetylators, thus favoring the formation of a toxic derivative of acetylhydrazine via the cytochrome P-450–dependent drug-metabolizing system. Induction of P-450 enzymes by rifampin may account for occurrences of a precipitous and severe form of isoniazid hepatitis when the two drugs have been administered together.

Patients receiving isoniazid should be followed at regular intervals and advised to report intercurrent symptoms. If these are associated with evidence of disturbed liver function, the drug should be discontinued, pending further evaluation. Since liver enzyme abnormalities are common early in the course of isoniazid treatment and reflect, in the vast majority (especially in younger patients), a transient and self-limiting event, routine monitoring of liver function tests in patients taking isoniazid is not generally recommended. The risk:benefit ratio of isoniazid chemoprophylaxis rises rapidly after the age of 35, however, warranting a conservative approach to the institution of chemoprophylaxis in this group. A several-fold elevation in transaminases in a patient over 35 years of age, even in the absence of symptoms, should be regarded as potentially serious and may justify discontinuation of the drug.

METHYLDOPA. This antihypertensive drug is similar to isoniazid in that minor and apparently inconsequential abnormalities in liver function occur in up to 6 per cent of treated patients. Clinically overt hepatotoxicity is much less common and usually resembles acute viral hepatitis or chronic active hepatitis, as a rule developing within 20 weeks after methyldopa is started. The Coombs' test is not infrequently positive in users of this drug but does not correlate with the occurrence of hepatic injury. Furthermore, clinical manifestations of drug hypersensitivity are unusual in methyldopa-induced liver disease, which may be mediated by a toxic drug metabolite. Hepatitis usually abates when the drug is discontinued, but full recovery may be delayed by months while progression to a fatal outcome has occurred in some cases despite stopping the drug.

PHENYTOIN. This anticonvulsant has been rarely associated with a severe, viral hepatitis–like liver injury with pronounced accompanying hypersensitivity features. The onset, usually within 6 weeks of starting the drug, is characterized by malaise, marked fever, lymphadenopathy, and a striking rash. Leukocytosis may be marked, with atypical lymphocytosis and eosinophilia. Liver histology resembles that of acute viral hepatitis except with a greater abundance of eosinophils. In the most severe cases, progressive liver failure and death may ensue. In spite of the marked serum sickness–like syndrome that characterizes phenytoin hepatotoxicity, a toxic metabolite may participate in its pathogenesis. Phenytoin is partly converted in the liver to highly reactive arene oxides. A genetically determined impairment in the ability to detoxify arene oxides may underlie individual susceptibility to toxicity from these metabolites via their covalent and hence immunologic modification of hepatic macromolecules.

SODIUM VALPROATE. This branched, medium-chain fatty acid used principally in the treatment of petit mal epilepsy may produce severe hepatotoxicity, most commonly in children under the age of 10 years. Similar to isoniazid, sodium valproate treatment is accompanied by a high incidence of transient, slight, and asymptomatic increases in serum transaminase activity, usually after several weeks of therapy. In rarer cases of severe liver injury, nonspecific systemic and digestive symptoms are followed by jaundice and evidence of liver failure, including encephalopathy and coagulopathy. Rash and eosinophilia are absent. The liver injury is characterized histologically by centrilobular necrosis and small-droplet fat infiltration, and bile duct injury may also be evident. The clinical and histologic features of sodium valproate hepatotoxicity are, to a degree, reminiscent of Reye's syndrome, although the former is distinguished by a greater frequency of jaundice, bile duct injury, and liver necrosis. The mechanism of sodium valproate–induced liver disease is uncertain, but available evidence has implicated the impairment of mitochondrial oxidation of long-chain fatty acids by a metabolite of the drug. Spontaneous recovery after stopping sodium valproate is the rule; fatalities are rare.

ORAL CONTRACEPTIVES. These hormonal agents produce several adverse effects on the hepatobiliary system: (1) hepatocellular cholestasis, (2) liver cell neoplasms, (3) increased predisposition to cholesterol gallstone formation, and (4) hepatic vein thrombosis (Budd-Chiari syndrome). In many cases of hepatic vein thrombosis associated with oral contraceptives, a latent myeloproliferative disorder appears to be present and undoubtedly predisposes to the thrombogenic disorder.

The cholestatic effects of oral contraceptives are largely attributable to the estrogenic component. Estrogens appear to affect directly several aspects of the formation of bile. Indeed, most users of oral contraceptives exhibit subtle disturbances in hepatic excretory function as evidenced, for example, by impaired plasma clearance of sulfobromophthalein. A small number of patients develop clinical cholestasis with pruritus and jaundice in a matter of weeks to months after commencing the pill. Manifestations of drug hypersensitivity are absent, and histologically, cholestasis without inflammation or liver cell necrosis is found. This condition is highly analogous to the clinical syndrome of *intrahepatic cholestasis of pregnancy*, which manifests as subclinical to overt cholestasis in the later stages of gestation, resolving rapidly in the postpartum period. Women with either a personal or family history of cholestasis occurring during pregnancy are particularly susceptible to cholestasis induced by estrogenic preparations. A genetic predisposition to estrogen-induced cholestasis is also suggested by the high incidence of this disorder in certain populations (e.g., Scandinavian and Chilean women).

Treatment of oral contraceptive–induced cholestasis consists of discontinuation of the drug and symptomatic support (e.g., cholestyramine for pruritus) as needed. Complete resolution within 2 to 3 months is the rule. Abnormalities persisting or worsening beyond this period suggest the unmasking of a pre-existing subclinical condition such as primary biliary cirrhosis and indicate the need for additional diagnostic evaluation.

Bass NM, Ockner RK: Drug-induced liver disease. *In* Zakim D, Boyer TD (eds.): Hepatology: A Textbook of Liver Disease. 2nd ed. Philadelphia, W. B. Saunders Company, 1990, pp 754–791. *A detailed current classification and summary of pharmacologic agents that may cause liver injury, including consideration of mechanisms and clinical aspects.*

Gitlin N: Clinical aspects of liver diseases caused by industrial and environmental toxins. *In* Zakim D, Boyer TD (eds.): Hepatology. 2nd ed. Philadelphia, W. B. Saunders Company, 1990, pp 791–821. *A well-referenced summary of industrial and environmental agents that may cause liver disease, including clinical and pathophysiologic aspects.*

Kaplowitz N, Aw TY, Simon FR, et al.: Drug-induced hepatotoxicity. Ann Intern Med 104:826, 1986. *A useful review of mechanisms and clinical aspects of drug hepatotoxicity.*

Lewis JH, Ranard RC, Caruso A, et al.: Amiodarone hepatotoxicity: Prevalence and clinicopathologic correlations among 104 patients. Hepatology 9:679, 1989. *A careful prospective study of the prevalence, as well as clinical and histopathologic aspects, of amiodarone hepatotoxicity, with a detailed, well-referenced discussion.*

Lewis JH, Zimmerman HJ: Drug-induced liver disease. Med Clin North Am 73:775, 1989. *A concise summary of current perspectives on prevalence, mechanisms, and clinical aspects of drug hepatotoxicity.*

McMaster KR, Hennigas GR: Drug-induced granulomatous hepatitis. Lab Invest 44:61, 1981. *A summary of implicated agents, with histopathologic documentation.*

Seeff LB, Cuccherini BA, Zimmerman HJ, et al.: Acetaminophen hepatotoxicity in alcoholics. A therapeutic misadventure. Ann Intern Med 104:399, 1986. *This* paper and an accompanying editorial by M. Black and J. Raucy provide and review evidence regarding the mechanism by which alcohol use increases susceptibility to acetaminophen hepatotoxicity.

Zimmerman HJ: Hepatotoxicity. The Adverse Effects of Drugs and Other Chemicals on the Liver. New York, Appleton-Century-Crofts, 1978. Although this classic monograph is now outdated, it remains a comprehensive and authoritative source. Well organized, readable, and thoroughly referenced.

119 Chronic Hepatitis

Robert K. Ockner

GENERAL CONSIDERATIONS

DEFINITION. Chronic hepatitis, a syndrome characterized by liver cell necrosis and inflammation lasting more than 6 months to 1 year, encompasses a spectrum of disorders differing in etiology, pathogenesis, histopathology, and clinical manifestations. Patients with chronic hepatitis may be entirely asymptomatic and exhibit only minimal abnormalities on routine laboratory tests or may be incapacitated by progressive liver failure and the complications of portal hypertension. At any given time, the clinical and laboratory features may not correlate well with histopathology or long-term prognosis. On biopsy, there is variable hepatocellular necrosis and an inflammatory response that may be predominantly portal, periportal, or lobular in its distribution. When severe, this lesion may include collapse of stromal elements, distortion of the lobular architecture, and a reparative process consisting of fibrosis and nodular regeneration (i.e., cirrhosis). These disorders may be classified on the basis of either etiology or histopathology.

ETIOLOGIC CLASSIFICATION (Table 119–1). Chronic hepatitis can be caused by hepatitis B (with or without superimposed hepatitis D) and hepatitis C virus infection, drugs and toxins (see below and Ch. 118), and inborn errors of metabolism, such as Wilson's disease and α_1-antitrypsin deficiency. In addition, some types are of unknown etiology (idiopathic) in which clinical and laboratory features may suggest but do not prove an immunologically mediated process ("autoimmune"). The prevalence of these categories of chronic hepatitis varies and depends in part on the prevalence of hepatitis virus infection in the general population. Genetic hemochromatosis, while not typically associated with biopsy findings of chronic hepatitis, is a more common cause of chronic liver disease than had been appreciated and deserves consideration in the differential diagnosis.

HISTOPATHOLOGY AND HISTOPATHOLOGIC CLASSIFICATION. Because the clinical and laboratory features are nonspecific, the diagnosis of chronic hepatitis cannot be established without liver biopsy. In most forms of chronic hepatitis, hepatic portal areas are prominently inflamed and are infiltrated

TABLE 119–1. CAUSES OF CHRONIC HEPATITIS

Chronic viral infections
Hepatitis B
Hepatitis B with superimposed hepatitis D
Hepatitis C (non-A, non-B)
Drugs and toxins, including
Acetaminophen
Amiodarone
Aspirin
Dantrolene
Ethanol
Isoniazid
Methyldopa
Nitrofurantoin
Oxyphenisatin
Perhexilene maleate
Phenytoin
Propylthiouracil
Sulfonamides
Wilson's disease
α_1-**Antitrypsin deficiency**
Idiopathic ("autoimmune")

mainly by mononuclear cells, especially small lymphocytes and plasma cells. Necrosis and inflammation may also involve hepatocytes immediately adjacent to the portal area. In this *periportal hepatitis* (or *"piecemeal necrosis"*), the inflammatory process involves the peripheral portions of the hepatic lobule, so that individual liver cells or nests of cells become isolated. Periportal hepatitis is not specific for chronic hepatitis and often is present in uncomplicated acute hepatitis and several other processes. For this reason it does not necessarily reflect a chronic or progressive process, and its significance can be judged only in the context of associated histopathologic, laboratory, and clinical findings.

The lobular architecture may be substantially disrupted. The portal inflammatory and necrotic process may extend into the lobule to a depth sufficient to span adjacent portal and/or central areas, i.e., *"bridging necrosis."* Although bridging necrosis can occur as part of an otherwise uncomplicated and self-limited acute hepatitis, it reflects a more severe injury that may have a greater propensity to lead to progressive deterioration over a period of weeks to months (*"subacute hepatic necrosis"*) or to chronic active hepatitis and cirrhosis. Thus, its presence, or the presence of submassive necrosis or significant fibrosis, in a patient with liver disease lasting more than 6 to 12 months, suggests a chronic and progressive process. Paradoxically, among survivors of the most severe form of acute liver injury (i.e., massive hepatic necrosis) chronic progressive liver disease is uncommon. The histopathologic classification of chronic hepatitis that follows is useful for descriptive purposes, but overlap is common, and differentiation of one from the other may be difficult. Most importantly, any of the histopathologic types may be associated with any of the causes of chronic hepatitis, and its significance may vary among them.

Chronic Persistent Hepatitis. Chronic persistent hepatitis, the most common form of chronic hepatitis, is an inflammatory process largely confined to the portal areas. There is little or no periportal or lobular hepatitis; significant fibrosis and cirrhosis are absent. Of the small number of patients with acute hepatitis B whose illness becomes chronic, most are found to have this lesion. By definition, the diagnosis of persistent hepatitis is not appropriate if there is significant stromal collapse, fibrosis, or nodular regeneration.

Chronic persistent hepatitis of most etiologies is usually associated with mild clinical manifestations. Patients have nonspecific symptoms, including fatigue, anorexia, abdominal discomfort, or right upper quadrant pain. Extrahepatic manifestations such as arthritis, glomerulonephritis, and vasculitis are unusual. Jaundice, if present, is usually mild. Physical findings are usually limited to palmar erythema, a few spider telangiectasias, and mildly tender hepatomegaly; the spleen occasionally is slightly enlarged. By definition, complications of advanced liver disease and portal hypertension, such as evidence of a collateral circulation, ascites, and encephalopathy, are absent.

Laboratory abnormalities are also mild and include moderate increases in serum aminotransferase activities, bilirubin, and globulins. Albumin concentration and prothrombin time are usually normal.

The outlook for persistent hepatitis usually is favorable, in that progression to chronic active hepatitis, cirrhosis, or liver failure is uncommon. However, the syndrome may last for 10 years or more and may cause continuing or intermittent discomfort or disability. Because of the difficulties inherent in the biopsy diagnosis of this group of disorders, continuing observation is important. Evidence of significant clinical deterioration may indicate the presence of a more serious process such as chronic active hepatitis, cirrhosis, or hepatocellular carcinoma and would be reason to consider repeat liver biopsy. In chronic hepatitis B infection, for example, increased activity of virus replication may be associated with clinical and histopathologic deterioration (see below).

The possible role of antiviral therapy in chronic hepatitis B, C, and D has been examined in recent clinical trials (see below). Symptomatic and nutritional support is appropriate, and exposure to potential hepatotoxins should be avoided. For patients in whom alcohol has been excluded etiologically, small amounts of alcoholic beverages are permissible if these do not cause worsening of symptoms or laboratory tests. A form of chronic persistent hepatitis may be found in those patients in whom corticosteroid treatment of idiopathic or "autoimmune" chronic active hepatitis has induced a remission (see below).

Chronic Lobular Hepatitis. This is a less well-defined category of chronic hepatitis in which the predominant lesion is a scattered single-cell necrosis in the lobule, with a relatively minor portal inflammatory component. It is, in effect, a variant of chronic persistent hepatitis, appearing not to progress to cirrhosis or liver failure except in those subjects in whom the underlying disease becomes more active.

Chronic Active Hepatitis. This most serious form of chronic hepatitis has the potential for progression to cirrhosis and liver failure. Approximately 20 per cent of cases are associated with, and presumably caused by, *chronic hepatitis B infection,* with or without superimposed *hepatitis D* infection (see Ch. 117). Chronic active hepatitis may also follow post-transfusion or community-acquired *hepatitis C* or *non-A, non-B.* Drugs that can cause the syndrome include *amiodarone, dantrolene, isoniazid, methyldopa, nitrofurantoin, oxyphenisatin, perhexilene maleate, phenytoin, propylthiouracil,* and *sulfonamides* (Table 119–1). Long-term use of acetaminophen, aspirin, and ethanol occasionally may cause similar changes, as may *Wilson's disease* and α_1-*antitrypsin deficiency.* In a large number of cases, the etiology is unknown, although many patients in this group exhibit clinical features and serologic abnormalities suggestive of autoimmunity. Despite such suggestive evidence, however, a truly "autoimmune" basis for chronic hepatitis has not been established conclusively, and in many instances phenomena that might be considered to reflect such a mechanism are also found in those forms of the disease associated with chronic hepatitis virus infections. The syndrome is characterized by expansion of portal areas, which are infiltrated by lymphocytes and plasma cells, by periportal hepatitis, and by a variable degree of bridging necrosis, collapse, and fibrosis. In one third or more of patients, macronodular cirrhosis is present at the time of diagnosis. Except for the characteristic features of α_1-antitrypsin deficiency, which can be demonstrated histochemically, the various causes of chronic active hepatitis cannot be differentiated on the basis of histopathology.

The course of chronic active hepatitis may be highly variable. The onset is usually insidious but in perhaps one third of cases may resemble an acute hepatitis. It may affect all age groups and both sexes. However, HBsAg-negative cases, sometimes associated with a more severe course and "autoimmune" features, occur mainly in young adult females, whereas HBsAg-positive cases are more common in males and are often minimally symptomatic.

Patients with chronic active hepatitis may be asymptomatic or may exhibit a wide range of local or constitutional symptoms typical of liver disease, such as fatigue, malaise, fever, anorexia, jaundice, or ascites. *Extrahepatic manifestations* are often quite prominent, especially in young females with the idiopathic ("autoimmune") type. These include amenorrhea, various skin rashes, glomerulonephritis, polyserositis, thyroiditis, vasculitis, Sjögren's syndrome, pneumonitis, depression of the formed elements of the blood, and an apparently increased incidence of ulcerative colitis.

Physical findings may also be quite variable. Patients may exhibit only a few spider telangietasias, possibly with mild enlargement of liver and/or spleen, and may or may not be jaundiced. In advanced cases with cirrhosis, patients may have ascites, evidence of collateral circulation, or encephalopathy. In young women, acne and hirsutism may reflect the hormonal effects of chronic liver disease. Evidence of other extrahepatic manifestations may also be prominent, as noted above.

Serum aminotransferase activities are usually increased over a range from minimally abnormal to over 1000 IU per liter. Globulins usually are diffusely increased, and the albumin value often is low. The alkaline phosphatase is usually only slightly to moderately increased; major increases should suggest the possibility of biliary tract disease or infiltrative or mass lesions. Prothrombin time generally reflects the severity of the disease but may also be influenced by vitamin K deficiency. Because of their variability, the laboratory tests often poorly reflect the pathologic process; for this reason they do not always provide a reliable basis for the assessment of natural history or response to treatment. Serologic tests, including autoantibodies and viral antigen/antibody markers, are discussed below.

The diagnosis of chronic active hepatitis requires liver biopsy. In addition to the histopathology, it is essential to establish a specific etiology, if possible (e.g., chronic hepatitis B/D or C infection, drugs, ethanol, Wilson's disease, or α_1-antitrypsin deficiency). Exposure to drugs and toxins usually can be identified by means of a careful history, including, when appropriate, questioning of family members or friends. Tests for chronic viral hepatitis are discussed below. Wilson's disease should be excluded in any patient with chronic hepatitis who is under the age of 40. Appropriate tests for this purpose include slit-lamp examination for Kayser-Fleischer rings and measurement of serum ceruloplasmin and urinary copper excretion. If all tests are negative, additional studies are not necessary; when the suspicion persists, measurement of liver copper concentration or incorporation of radioactive copper into serum ceruloplasmin may be necessary (see Ch. 192). α_1-Antitrypsin deficiency can be demonstrated by protease-inhibitor phenotyping of serum and, in liver biopsy specimens, by the presence of PAS-positive material in hepatocytes after diastase treatment of the tissue section.

The differential diagnosis includes chronic persistent hepatitis, postnecrotic cirrhosis, and some cases of primary biliary cirrhosis in which clinical and pathologic features may resemble those of chronic active hepatitis. Treatment options for the various forms of chronic active hepatitis, which now include orthotopic liver transplantation, are discussed below.

IDIOPATHIC ("AUTOIMMUNE") CHRONIC ACTIVE HEPATITIS. The general characteristics of this syndrome, including its propensity to affect young women and to be associated with extrahepatic manifestations, have been noted above. The syndrome has been characterized in addition by the presence in serum of several autoantibodies, of uncertain role in etiology and pathogenesis. These include smooth-muscle antibodies (antiactin), positive in approximately two thirds of patients; antinuclear antibodies (SMA; anti–DNA–histone complex) in about one half; anti–double-stranded DNA; and anti–mitochondrial (AMA) antibodies in about one third each. These autoantibodies also occur with increased frequency in family members, although there is no evidence of a simple genetic basis for this observation. A high incidence of HLA-B8 and -DR3 has also been noted. Additional variants of the syndrome have been described, based on recognition of novel autoantibodies and, to a variable extent, distinctive clinical features. These autoantibodies include an anti–nuclear lamin antibody and an anti–liver/kidney microsomal (anti-LKM1) antibody in idiopathic chronic hepatitis, an anti-LKM2 associated with tricrynafen hepatitis, and an anti-LKM3 associated with chronic hepatitis D. Anti-LKM1 and anti-LKM2 are directed against the hepatic microsomal drug-metabolizing enzymes cytochrome P-450IID6 and P-450IIC, respectively; the significance of this is unknown. Also identified in autoimmune chronic hepatitis have been antibodies to liver-specific proteins (LSP), liver membrane antigen (LMAg), and soluble liver antigen (anti-SLA) or liver cytosol antigen (anti-LC1). Although there are some clinical differences among the syndromes associated with these autoantibodies, there is no clear evidence that they either reflect the etiology of the disease or are involved in its pathogenesis.

In fact, the syndrome of chronic hepatitis with autoimmune features can be caused by chemical agents such as nitrofurantoin. Moreover, an unexpectedly high incidence of antimeasles antibodies and of persistent measles virus genome in peripheral blood mononuclear cells has been reported in patients with autoimmune chronic active hepatitis, raising the possibility that some of these cases represent a persistent viral infection. Finally, chronic hepatitis C infection is present in some patients with autoimmune chronic active hepatitis, although the C100-3 antibody test may be falsely positive when serum globulins are highest, and a confirmatory test, such as the recombinant immunoblot assay (RIBA), may be required. Whether any cases of this syndrome are truly the result of a primary immune attack on a previously normal liver has not been established.

In the treatment of idiopathic chronic active hepatitis, *corticosteroids,* with or without low-dose azathioprine, usually reduce symptoms, improve laboratory test results, suppress the inflammatory process seen on biopsy, and decrease short-term and long-term morbidity and mortality. For example, in a Mayo Clinic study, a favorable clinical, biochemical, and histologic response was seen initially in 56 per cent of patients, whereas spontaneous improvement occurred in only 20 per cent of placebo controls; early mortality and progression to cirrhosis were also decreased.

Despite this seemingly beneficial overall response, several factors that importantly influence the natural history and response to treatment must be considered in making the decision to institute a chronic treatment plan with potentially significant adverse effects. First, chronic hepatitis does not usually progress to cirrhosis or liver failure in the absence of bridging necrosis on liver biopsy; the absence of such changes would weigh significantly against the use of corticosteroids. Second, there is no evidence that corticosteroids are of benefit in asymptomatic chronic active hepatitis. Third, since the reported series include an unknown number of patients with chronic hepatitis C, and since the natural history of this disorder is variable, it is difficult to assess the impact of corticosteroids in this subset. Fourth, the presence or absence of autoimmune features seemed to be of little consequence in the Mayo Clinic series, in regard to prognosis or response to treatment. Finally, since many patients with chronic active hepatitis would fail to meet the criteria for inclusion in some of the published series, any decision regarding their treatment is necessarily an extrapolation from a selected study population.

In view of this substantial uncertainty concerning the value of corticosteroids in certain subsets of chronic active hepatitis, it is very difficult to make broadly applicable recommendations concerning their use. In general, however, an initially favorable response would most likely be expected in a young symptomatic female with progressive disease and no recent transfusion or other exposure to or evidence for hepatitis B or C.

In the Mayo Clinic study, the following regimen was found to be most effective: an initial daily dose of 60 mg of prednisone or of 30 mg of prednisone combined with 50 mg of azathioprine, tapered gradually over several weeks to months to a daily maintenance dose of 20 mg of prednisone or 10 mg of prednisone plus 50 mg of azathioprine. Azathioprine was of no value when given alone but permitted use of the lower prednisone dose, thereby reducing the incidence of significant steroid-related complications, which otherwise approximated 60 per cent. Alternate-day treatment was less effective. If a favorable response is not observed within 2 to 3 months, treatment should be discontinued.

Patients being treated for chronic active hepatitis should be examined and have liver tests periodically. The possible side effects of drug treatment should be monitored, and liver biopsies may need to be repeated at intervals of 6 months to 1 year, depending on the circumstances. Repeated biopsies serve little purpose in a stable patient. Return of liver enzymes to a level less than twice the upper limit of normal, together with a liver biopsy showing subsidence of the inflammatory and necrotic process to a picture similar to that of persistent hepatitis, is considered a successful response and warrants an attempt gradually to discontinue treatment. In about 50 per cent of patients, this attempt succeeds and additional corticosteroid treatment is not needed. In the remainder, evidence of relapse may suggest the need for reinstitution of therapy.

Unfortunately, the disease may eventually progress to cirrhosis or liver failure despite an apparently favorable initial clinical response, especially in those patients in whom repeated recurrences of activity require treatment over a period of 3 years or longer. Over these longer intervals the advisability of continued corticosteroid therapy must be judged not only on the basis of symptoms and laboratory and biopsy findings but also in recognition of the successful treatment of many of these patients with orthotopic liver transplantation (Ch. 124).

CHRONIC HEPATITIS B. Up to 10 per cent of otherwise healthy individuals remain chronically infected with hepatitis B virus after acute hepatitis caused by this agent (Ch. 117). Approximately two thirds develop the lesion of chronic persistent hepatitis and the remainder chronic active hepatitis. Chronicity is more common in men than women, is predisposed to by immune suppression, and is, in general, a clinically more subdued disease process than its autoimmune counterpart. Nevertheless, chronic hepatitis B clearly may evolve to cirrhosis, liver failure, and hepatocellular carcinoma. The severity of the course is largely dependent on the activity of virus replication in the hepatocyte

and the response of the host immune system. In somewhat simplified terms, the process can be described as follows: Active replication of episomal (i.e., nonintegrated viral DNA) results in the presence in serum of markers of the complete virion, or Dane particle (i.e., HBeAg, DNA polymerase, and HBV DNA). Viral antigens are also expressed on the surface of the hepatocyte in association with Class I HLA determinants, thereby eliciting lymphocyte cytotoxicity and a resulting hepatitis. When replication subsides, fewer complete virions are produced; HBeAg gives way to anti-HBe (seroconversion); and a brief flare in the hepatitis ushers in a period of relative clinical and histopathologic quiescence. This may occur in 10 to 30 per cent of patients each year. The reverse may also occur, if an increase in viral replication leads to increases in the production of virions and markers and in the severity of the hepatitis (reactivation).

This dynamic host-virus interaction has important diagnostic implications. Thus, an HBsAg-positive patient with a syndrome of apparent acute hepatitis may in fact have chronic hepatitis B undergoing either seroconversion or reactivation. Other factors, such as superimposed viral or drug-induced hepatitis, may lead to similar confusion. Active HBV replication and chronic hepatitis B are suggested by HBsAg, HBeAg, and anti-HBc positivity and anti-HBs negativity. (In a small number of patients, usually with active disease, an heterotypic anti-HBs may be present simultaneously with HBsAg.) Definitive evidence of active replication would be provided by demonstration of DNA polymerase in serum or HBV DNA in serum, but these tests are not available routinely.

The treatment of chronic hepatitis B remains frustrating. Corticosteroids are not beneficial and may be harmful, possibly in part reflecting their demonstrated enhancement of HBV replication. In trials of antiviral therapy, patients selected have usually exhibited active viral replication (i.e., HBeAg, DNA polymerase, and HBV DNA positivity). In these trials adenine arabinoside (ara-A) and ara-AMP have proven to be unacceptably toxic. α-Interferon, however, has proven more promising in that about one third of patients respond to a variable extent by decreasing replicative activity (e.g., loss of HBeAg), although only approximately 10 per cent seem to eradicate the virus. Factors predisposing to a favorable response included female sex, a clinically mild course, relatively brief duration, high serum aminotransferase and HBV DNA levels, and immune competence (e.g., HIV negativity), whereas less favorable results have been obtained in male homosexuals, HIV-positive and Asian subjects, and individuals with neonatally acquired infections. Unfortunately, it is unclear in those patients in whom treatment appears successful whether the longer-term course of the disease is substantially altered; thus, α-interferon use at present should remain limited to controlled trials. Other antiviral and immunomodulatory agents are also undergoing clinical trials. Orthotopic liver transplantation has been successfully employed in the management of liver failure secondary to chronic hepatitis B (Ch. 123). Results thus far suggest that there is a somewhat increased early postoperative mortality, possibly related to sepsis, and virtually universal reinfection of the transplanted liver. In most centers, liver failure in chronic hepatitis B is considered an appropriate indication for liver transplantation despite the fact that the overall outlook for this group is less favorable.

CHRONIC HEPATITIS C. Acute post-transfusion or community-acquired hepatitis C becomes chronic in about 50 per cent of cases (Ch. 117). Typically, chronic hepatitis C exhibits an intermittent course, in which episodes of increased symptoms and laboratory abnormalities are separated by periods of relative quiescence, but 10 to 20 per cent of patients evolve to cirrhosis or progressive liver failure. Furthermore, 65 per cent or more of patients with primary hepatocellular carcinoma test positive for the antibody to HCV.

Treatment of chronic hepatitis C remains undefined. It seems likely but undocumented that a significant number of these patients were included in the various treatment trials of autoimmune hepatitis and responded to corticosteroids; α-interferon has been used with limited success and with an unknown overall effect on the natural history of the disease. Thus, normalization or near normalization of the serum aminotransferase activity was achieved in 46 per cent of patients with chronic post-transfusion hepatitis C treated with 3 million units three times weekly for 24 weeks, as compared with untreated controls, and was associated with histologic improvement. Unfortunately, 51 per cent of the responders relapsed within 6 months after the end of the treatment.

Patients with liver failure resulting from HCV-induced chronic active hepatitis or cirrhosis have successfully undergone orthotopic liver transplantation and are regarded as appropriate candidates for the procedure in virtually all centers. Unlike chronic hepatitis B, disease recurrence in the transplanted organ appears to be mild and evidently of limited clinical impact. The actual recurrence rate is not yet known and will require more sensitive assays such as polymerase chain reaction or immunologic tests for viral antigens.

CHRONIC HEPATITIS D. Hepatitis D infection depends on antecedent or simultaneous infection with the hepatitis B virus. When HDV infection is superimposed on pre-existing chronic hepatitis B, it also becomes chronic in most cases. Simultaneous infection with both HBV and HDV does not increase the probability of chronic disease but is associated with an increased incidence of fulminant hepatic failure. Trials involving α-interferon treatment of chronic HBV with HDV have met with limited temporary success and a high probability of relapse after cessation of treatment. There is also a high probability of recurrent disease after orthotopic liver transplantation.

SPECIAL CLINICAL PROBLEMS

Two circumstances are encountered in clinical practice with sufficient frequency that they deserve particular comment with reference to diagnostic approach and management.

UNEXPECTED INCREASE OF SERUM AMINOTRANSFERASE. The advent and common use of multiphasic laboratory screening techniques have led to the identification of individuals in whom aminotransferase activities are abnormal but who lack clinical evidence of liver disease. If the abnormal finding is confirmed, and if it does not reflect muscle or other extrahepatic disease, it may have either of two possible implications: (1) It may reflect a subclinical acute process (e.g., acute viral hepatitis) or (2) it may reflect a chronic process (e.g., chronic toxic or viral hepatitis or nonalcoholic steatohepatitis). If the patient is asymptomatic or nearly so, a period of observation is appropriate, and follow-up studies and hepatitis serologies should be obtained. Alcohol and potentially hepatotoxic drugs and toxins should be avoided. Improvement would presumably reflect resolution of a self-limited process or the response to removal of a toxin (e.g., ethanol). Worsening of the test results during observation may herald the onset of overt disease, the proper evaluation of which would depend on the circumstances. Persistence of the abnormality beyond 6 to 12 months may reflect a chronic hepatitis and may justify liver biopsy.

HEPATITIS B SURFACE ANTIGEN POSITIVITY. Approximately 0.1 to 0.2 per cent of the population of the United States is positive for HBsAg. At any given time, most of these persons exhibit no overt evidence of liver disease and are designated carriers. The meaning of the term *carrier* varies, however, and has been used to include all chronically positive individuals, or only those who have no apparent liver disease.

The practical question of significance concerns the management of the otherwise apparently healthy patient with a positive test. If the result is confirmed, it could indicate (1) a subclinical acute hepatitis B, (2) chronic hepatitis (persistent or active) or cirrhosis, or (3) a "healthy" carrier state. Although differentiation of these conditions may require liver biopsy, HBsAg-positive persons who have no other clinical or laboratory evidence of liver disease usually have normal or nonspecific biopsy findings. There is no conclusive evidence that treatment is indicated for the few among this group of asymptomatic persons with normal liver function tests who may have chronic active hepatitis on biopsy. Therefore, these individuals can be followed at intervals without first obtaining a liver biopsy. Those HBsAg-positive persons who do have clinical and/or laboratory signs of liver disease should be managed in accordance with the severity and duration of the process; persistence of the abnormalities beyond 6 months may suggest a chronic hepatitis and the need to consider liver biopsy.

Carman WF, Jacyma MR, Hadziyannis S, et al.: Mutation preventing formation of hepatitis B e antigen in patients with chronic hepatitis B infection. Lancet 2:588, 1989. *An important description of the molecular basis for a clinically severe variant of chronic hepatitis B.*

Czaja AJ, Hay, JE, Rakela J: Clinical features and prognostic implications of severe corticosteroid-treated cryptogenic chronic active hepatitis. Mayo Clin 65:23, 1990. *Recent demonstration, in a large series of cases, of the apparent lack of effect of autoimmune features on disease severity, histopathology, response to treatment, and survival.*

Czaja AJ, Taswell HF, Rakela J, et al.: Frequency and significance of antibody to hepatitis C virus in severe corticosteroid-treated cryptogenic chronic active hepatitis. Mayo Clin Proc 65:1303, 1990. *Evidence that hepatitis C virus infection is uncommon in this population.*

Davis GL, Balart LA, Schiff ER, et al.: Treatment of chronic hepatitis C with recombinant interferon alpha. N Engl J Med 321:1501, 1989; DiBisceglie AM, Martin P, Kassianides C, et al.: Recombinant interferon alpha therapy for chronic hepatitis C. N Engl J Med 321:1506, 1989. *Two controlled trials demonstrating a potential role for antiviral therapy.*

Dienstag JL (ed.): Viral hepatitis. Semin Liver Dis, Vol. 11, May 1991. *A minisymposium in which clinically relevant aspects of acute and chronic hepatitis are critically reviewed by recognized experts.*

Hoofnagle JH: Type D (delta) hepatitis. JAMA 261:1321, 1989. *A brief but well-referenced and informative review.*

Liaw Y-F, Chu C-M, Chen T-J, et al.: Chronic lobular hepatitis: A clinicopathological and prognostic study. Hepatology 2:258, 1982. *A histopathologic category with generally benign prognostic implications, but for which continuing observation is indicated.*

Maddrey WC: Chronic hepatitis. *In* Zakim D, Boyer T (eds.): Hepatology: A Textbook of Liver Disease. Philadelphia, W. B. Saunders Company, 1989, pp 1025–1061. *A comprehensive and well-referenced review, emphasizing clinical aspects.*

Meyer zum Buschenfelde K-H (ed.): Autoimmune hepatitis. Semin Liver Dis, Vol. 11, August 1991. *A collection of authoritative, critical reviews of autoimmunity and liver disease.*

Perillo RP, Schiff, Davis GL, et al.: A randomized, controlled trial of interferon alpha-2b alone and after prednisone withdrawal for the treatment of chronic hepatitis B. N Engl J Med 323:295, 1990. *Results of a multicenter trial demonstrating the efficacy of interferon in certain patients.*

Scott J, Gollan JL, Samourian S, et al.: Wilson's disease presenting as chronic active hepatitis. Gastroenterology 74:645, 1978. *A thorough clinical and pathologic description of 17 patients presenting with features of chronic active hepatitis. Emphasis is placed on the often difficult problem of differential diagnosis.*

Vitirski-Trepo L, Kay A, Pichoud C, et al.: Early and frequent detection of HBxAg and/or anti-HBx in hepatitis B infection. Hepatology 12:1278, 1990. *Useful information concerning detection of hepatitis B x-gene markers.*

Zuckerman A (ed.): Viral Hepatitis and Liver Disease. New York, Alan R. Liss, 1988. *Proceedings of a recent symposium in which clinical and basic aspects of all forms of viral hepatitis are addressed.*

120 Parasitic, Bacterial, Fungal, and Granulomatous Liver Disease

Teresa L. Wright

Fungal and parasitic diseases of the hepatobiliary system are more commonly associated with underdeveloped countries, but their frequency is increasing in the United States. Contributing factors include the growing number of patients with AIDS, as well as patients receiving cancer chemotherapy or immunosuppressive therapy following organ transplantation.

PARASITIC DISEASES OF THE LIVER AND BILIARY TRACT

Clinical features of parasitic infections that involve the liver and biliary tract are summarized in Table 120–1. A history of travel to areas where these infections are endemic should be obtained and the appropriate diagnostic tests ordered. Geographic distributions of these diseases, as well as specific therapies, are discussed elsewhere in this book.

Helminthic Infections

PATHOGENESIS. Humans are important intermediate hosts in the life cycles of many helminths, and the liver and biliary tract are commonly involved in both the larval stage (toxocariasis, ascariasis, strongyloidiasis, schistosomiasis, echinococcosis, and fascioliasis) and the adult stage (ascariasis, clonorchiasis, fascioliasis). In addition, adult worms residing in mesenteric vessels or the biliary tract lay eggs, which form a nidus for granuloma formation (schistosomiasis, ascariasis, clonorchiasis). The liver responds to the larvae in a variable manner. Ascariasis usually causes little tissue injury, whereas larval migration in toxocariasis results in a marked inflammatory response with tissue eosinophilia (visceral larva migrans). Damage from the adult worms is also variable. In ascariasis, migration of adult worms into the bile ducts may be accompanied by acute pain. Biliary tract obstruction, cholangitis, and biliary calculi may occur; treatment involves surgical or endoscopic removal of worms. In clonorchiasis, the adult worm migrates up the bile duct from the duodenum and lays its eggs in the intrahepatic ducts. Little inflammation occurs within the liver itself, and eosinophilia is rare. Infection may remain silent for years until patients present with cholangitis (recurrent Oriental cholangiohepatitis) or cholangiocarcinoma. Despite surgical drainage of the bile ducts, recurrent stone

formation is common. In schistosomiasis, adult worms migrate from the portal vein into the mesenteric vessels where they lay eggs (Ch. 434). Subsequently blood carries the eggs into portal venules, where they lodge and elicit an immune response from the host. Granuloma formation, fibrosis, and portal hypertension result. Treatment of chronic infection may include sclerosis of bleeding esophageal varices or portacaval shunt.

CLINICAL MANIFESTATIONS. The clinical features of helminthic infections are variable. Tender hepatomegaly and eosinophilia are common findings during larval migration. Fever, jaundice, and abdominal pain accompany the biliary tract obstruction caused by adult worms of ascariasis and clonorchiasis. Bleeding from esophageal varices is a common manifestation of the portal hypertension that results from infection with schistosomiasis.

DIAGNOSIS. Diagnosis of helminthic disorders relies on iden-

TABLE 120–1. COMMON PARASITIC DISEASES OF THE LIVER AND BILIARY TRACT

Disorder (Organism)	Predisposition to Infection*	Nature of Hepatic Involvement		
		Pathophysiology	*Manifestations*	*Diagnosis*
Helminthic disorders				
Ascariasis (*Ascaris lumbricoides*) (roundworm)	Ingestion of raw vegetables	Larval migration through portal vein to liver; later adult invasion of biliary tract with egg production	Abdominal pain, fever, jaundice during larval migration; bile duct obstruction, cholangitis, perforation later; granuloma formation around eggs	Ova or adult worm in stool; worms in duodenum on contrast studies or endoscopic examination
Toxocariasis (*Toxocara carris, cati*) (roundworm)	Contact with dogs and cats	Larval migration in hepatic parenchyma (visceral larva migrans)	Granuloma formation with eosinophilia	Demonstration of larvae in tissue; serology: ELISA
Strongyloidiasis (*Strongyloides stercoralis*)	Immunodeficiency (AIDS, organ transplant, cancer chemotherapy)	Larval penetration through intestine into liver	Occasional jaundice, hepatomegaly, larvae in portal tract and liver lobule	Larvae in stool or duodenal aspirate; serology not useful
Echinococcosis (*Echinococcus granulosa, multilocularis*) (tapeworm)	Sheep and cattle raising	Larval migration to liver where encystment occurs (hydatid cyst)	Asymptomatic; symptoms of hepatic mass lesions, biliary tract obstruction, cyst rupture	Serologic tests (indirect hemagglutination, ELISA); CT scans: hepatic cysts
Schistosomiasis (*Schistosoma mansoni, Japonicum*) (flatworm)		Host immune response to ova in portal vein, resulting in fibrosis	*Acute:* eosinophilic infiltrate *Chronic:* hepatosplenomegaly, complications of portal hypertension, granuloma formation	Identification of ova in stool or on liver biopsy
Clonorchiasis (*Clonorchis sinensis*) (flatworm)	Ingestion of raw fish	Migration of worms through ampulla of Vater; eggs produced in bile ducts	Bile duct obstruction, cholangitis, choledocholithiasis, cholangiocarcinoma	Ova in stool; multiple bile duct stones at ERCP
Fascioliasis (*Fasciola hepatica*) (flatworm)	Ingestion of fresh-water plants	Larval migration through liver, penetration of bile ducts	*Acute:* fever, abdominal pain, jaundice, hemobilia *Chronic:* asymptomatic hepatomegaly, choledocholithiasis	Eosinophilia, elevated liver tests; ova in stool; adult flukes in bile ducts at ERCP
Protozoan disorders				
Amebiasis (*Entamoeba histolytica*)	Poor sanitation, sexual contact	Hematogenous spread with tissue invasion; abscess formation	Fever, RUQ pain, peritonitis, elevated right hemidiaphragm	Cysts in stool; serologic tests (counterimmunoelectrophoresis, indirect hemagglutination); technetium-99 liver scan
Malaria (*Plasmodium vivax, falciparum, ovale, malariae*)	Blood transfusion, parenteral drug use	Sporozoites cleared from circulation by hepatocytes; exoerythrocytic replication in liver	Tender hepatomegaly; rarely hepatic failure (*P. falciparum*)	Identification of organism on blood smear
Cryptosporidiosis (*Cryptosporidium*)	Immunodeficiency (AIDS)	Unknown; biliary tract involvement only in immunodeficient patients	Fever, RUQ pain, cholecystitis	Elevated alkaline phosphatase; bile duct dilatation at ERCP
Toxoplasmosis (*Toxoplasma gondii*)	Intrauterine infection; immunodeficiency (AIDS, organ transplant)	Multiplication in liver causing necrosis and inflammation	Fever, hepatosplenomegaly	Transaminase elevation; isolation of organism from tissue; Sabin-Feldman dye test
Visceral leishmaniasis (*Leishmania donovani*)	Immunodeficiency (AIDS, organ transplant)	Infection of reticuloendothelial cells of liver	Fever, leukopenia, hepatosplenomegaly	Organism in bone marrow; immunoserologic tests
Trypanosomiasis (*Trypanosoma cruzi, rhodesiense, gambiense*)		*Acute:* parasites in reticuloendothelial cells of liver *Chronic:* passive congestion secondary to heart failure	*Acute:* fever, hepatosplenomegaly *Chronic:* hepatomegaly	Organisms in blood, tissue; immunofluorescent tests

*Travel in endemic areas predisposes to infection with all protozoa and helminths. Additional predisposing factors are listed.

tification of ova in stool. Serologic tests are usually unhelpful (except in the diagnosis of echinococcosis or toxocariasis). Occasionally liver biopsy demonstrates organisms. Adult worms may be found at laparotomy, performed for biliary tract obstruction (e.g., for clonorchiasis or ascariasis).

Protozoan Infections

Protozoa commonly infect the liver, with organisms in both reticuloendothelial cells (leishmaniasis and trypanosomiasis) and hepatocytes (toxoplasmosis and malaria).

CLINICAL MANIFESTATIONS. These are usually nonspecific and may resemble viral hepatitis (toxoplasmosis and malaria). In certain infections, extrahepatic manifestations predominate (e.g., cardiomyopathy with chronic trypanosomiasis, diarrhea with cryptosporidiosis). Extrahepatic features may be prominent early in the course (e.g., amebic colitis), and hepatic symptoms predominate later (e.g., with hepatic abscess formation).

DIAGNOSIS. In contrast to helminthic infections, serologic tests are useful in making a specific diagnosis (Table 120–1). Amebic liver abscess is discussed below.

FUNGAL INFECTIONS OF THE LIVER

The liver is frequently involved in disseminated fungal infection. Prevalence of these infections varies geographically. *Coccidioides immitis* is endemic in the southwest region of the United States, whereas *Histoplasma capsulatum* is endemic in the eastern and central regions.

CLINICAL MANIFESTATIONS. Patients present with fever, hepatomegaly, and an elevated serum level of alkaline phosphatase. Hepatic involvement in histoplasmosis, coccidioidomycosis, North American blastomycosis, and cryptococcosis occurs in immunocompetent patients, most commonly with granuloma formation (Table 120–2). In contrast, hepatic involvement in candidiasis, aspergillosis, and mucormycosis occurs in immunocompromised patients, often with abscess and granuloma formation.

DIAGNOSIS. The diagnosis of all fungal infections relies on identification of the organism on liver biopsy. Serologic tests are not helpful. Because of diagnostic difficulty with systemic fungal infections, antifungal therapy is frequently started empirically in an immunocompromised patient with persistent fever. The diagnosis may only be made at postmortem examination.

THERAPY. Despite therapy, mortality in disseminated fungal infection remains high (25 to 100 per cent). Amphotericin B (0.6 mg per kilogram per day intravenously for at least 42 days) may be effective in the treatment of candidiasis, histoplasmosis, coccidioidomycosis, and cryptococcosis. Newer antifungal agents (e.g., ketoconazole or fluconazole, 200 mg per day) may be as effective as amphotericin, with fewer side effects (Ch. 398). *Aspergillus* is poorly responsive to amphotericin and should be treated with miconazole or fluconazole.

HEPATIC MANIFESTATIONS OF SYSTEMIC BACTERIAL INFECTION

Liver abnormalities are associated with a wide variety of bacterial infections (Table 120–2). The mechanism by which jaundice occurs is unclear but has been postulated to be due to effects of bacterial endotoxin on hepatocyte function (e.g., *Escherichia coli*), direct mechanical effects (e.g., right lower lobe pneumonia), nonspecific inflammation and necrosis (e.g., typhoid fever), or associated hemolysis (e.g., pneumococcal pneumonia). Organisms may directly infect the liver (e.g., actinomycosis, tuberculosis, and syphilis) with granulomas or abscess formation. With successful antibiotic therapy, liver function abnormalities usually resolve.

LIVER ABSCESS

DEFINITION. Liver abscesses are focal collections of organisms and pus within the hepatic parenchyma. Although frequently multiple, abscesses may coalesce to form a single abscess. There is geographic variation in causative organisms, with amebae more prevalent in developing countries and pyogenic organisms more common in developed nations, including the United States.

Pyogenic Liver Abscess

ETIOLOGY. Multiple hepatic abscesses are most frequently due to underlying biliary tract infection (cholecystitis, cholangitis). Infection in organs drained by the portal vein (e.g., appendicitis, diverticulitis) may cause pylephlebitis and secondary abscess formation. Abscesses also result from seeding of the liver with bacteremia from a nonabdominal source as well as from abdominal trauma with hematoma formation. Causative organisms include enteric bacteria (*Escherichia coli, Klebsiella pneumoniae, Streptococcus faecalis*) and pyogenic gram-positive cocci (*Staphylococcus aureus*). Careful culture techniques have demonstrated anaerobic bacteria (*Bacteroides, Clostridium*) in approximately 50 per cent of abscesses.

CLINICAL MANIFESTATIONS. Hepatic abscesses present with fever, anorexia, and abdominal pain. No feature of the fever pattern distinguishes hepatic abscesses from any other intra-

TABLE 120–2. HEPATOBILIARY MANIFESTATIONS OF BACTERIAL INFECTIONS

Disease	Organism	Clinical Features	Liver Histology
Lobar pneumonia	*Pneumococcus*	Jaundice, hepatomegaly	Focal necrosis, inflammation
Toxic shock syndrome; osteomyelitis	*Staphylococcus*	Jaundice	Abscess formation; granulomas
Fitz-Hugh-Curtis syndrome	*Gonococcus*	RUQ pain, tender hepatomegaly, peritoneal adhesions	Perihepatitis; organism seen on liver biopsy
Neonatal infection	*Esherichia coli*	Jaundice	Focal necrosis, inflammation
Typhoid fever	*Salmonella typhi*	Hepatomegaly, jaundice; asymptomatic (carrier state)	Focal necrosis; chronic cholecystitis
Brucellosis	*Brucella abortis, melitensis, suls*	Tender hepatomegaly, splenomegaly	Granulomas
Gas gangrene; pylephlebitis	*Clostridium welchii*	Jaundice, high mortality	Abscess formation; portal vein gas
Melloidosis	*Pseudomonas pseudomallei*	Hepatomegaly only with septicemia	Focal necrosis, abscess formation
Legionnaire's disease	*Legionella pneumophilia*	Hepatosplenomegaly	Focal necrosis
Actinomycosis	*Actinomyces israelii, bovis*	Fever, abdominal pain	Multiloculated abscess with pus, organisms
Mycobacteria			
Miliary tuberculosis	*Mycobacterium tuberculosis*	Fever, weight loss, hepatomegaly	Caseating granulomas, tuberculomas, tuberculous cholangitis
Atypical mycobacterial infection	*Mycobacterium avium-intracellulare*	Fever, hepatomegaly, alkaline phosphatase elevation	Caseating granulomas, frequent organisms
Leprosy	*Mycobacterium leprae*	Asymptomatic	Granulomas, "foamy histiocytes," frequent organisms
Spirochetes			
Syphilis (congenital, secondary, tertiary)	*Treponema pallidum*	Hepatomegaly	Organisms, granulomas; gummatous necrosis
Leptospirosis (Weil's disease)	*Leptospira icterohaemorrhagiae*	Fever, jaundice, renal failure, hemolysis	Hemorrhagic necrosis, cholestasis

abdominal infection. Presentation may be insidious, with fever for weeks, or more acute. Jaundice occurs in 20 per cent of cases and is often associated with underlying biliary tract disease. Patients typically have hepatomegaly with point tenderness on palpation of the liver. Rales and percussion dullness may be found at the base of the right lung.

DIAGNOSIS. Leukocytosis, anemia, hypoalbuminemia, and elevation of serum alkaline phosphatase are invariably present. Other liver tests are usually only mildly abnormal. Blood cultures are positive in 60 per cent of patients with hepatic abscesses. Liver ultrasonography is highly sensitive in detecting hypoechoic mass lesions. Abcesses can usually be distinguished from cysts by their irregular borders and increased echogenicity within the lesion. Computed tomography (CT) scan with intravenous contrast can detect lesions of 1 cm or greater, which typically appear as low-density lesions with a surrounding "rim" of tissue. CT scan is also useful in identifying other intra-abdominal processes (e.g., diverticular abscess). However, neither ultrasonography nor CT scan can reliably distinguish abscesses from necrotic tumors in the liver. Diagnosis should be confirmed by ultrasound-guided fine-needle aspiration with Gram's stain, culture, and histology (Fig. 120–1).

TREATMENT. When the diagnosis of hepatic abscess is suspected, blood cultures should be drawn and ultrasound-guided fine-needle aspiration performed prior to institution of antibiotics. Aspiration should be both diagnostic and therapeutic. Initial therapy should include anaerobic coverage (e.g., with ampicillin, an aminoglycoside, and metronidazole). Treatment can be modified when results of cultures are obtained and should be continued for 10 to 14 days. Percutaneous catheter drainage of large abscesses plays an adjunctive role to antibiotics and may obviate surgical intervention. Although surgical drainage has been advocated in the past, this is necessary only if there is an associated intra-abdominal process (e.g., diverticular abscess, appendiceal abscess, or biliary tract disease). Patients with multiple small abscesses who fail to respond to an initial course of antibiotics may require treatment for months. With early diagnosis and aggressive treatment, mortality has improved from 80 per cent to less than 10 per cent.

Amebic Liver Abscess

ETIOLOGY. Although several types of amebae are found in the colon in man, only *Entamoeba histolytica* is known to be pathogenic (Ch. 431). Amebae may remain dormant in the colon for years before tissue invasion with hematogenous spread that results in hepatic abscess formation. The reason for the male predominance of this disease is unknown.

CLINICAL MANIFESTATIONS. Amebic liver abscess should be suspected in a patient with fever, malaise, right upper quadrant pain, and a history of travel to an endemic area. Signs of infection include tender hepatomegaly and percussion dullness at the base of the right lung. Jaundice is rare. A minority of patients have symptoms of amebic colitis (bloody diarrhea). Complications of amebic abscess include rupture into the chest (empyema), peritoneum, or pericardium and obstruction of the common bile duct or inferior vena cava. The development of complications carries a poor prognosis and may require surgical intervention.

DIAGNOSIS. Serologic tests are positive in the majority of patients with amebic liver abscess (Table 120–1). Because titers may remain elevated for years, they provide supportive rather than definitive evidence of acute infection. Liver function abnormalities are nonspecific. Imaging studies (ultrasonography, CT scan, and technetium-99 liver scan) demonstrate the abscess. In contrast to pyogenic abscesses, amebic abscesses are usually single. An elevated right hemidiaphragm and a pleural effusion are often present on chest radiography. Aspiration of the abscess is usually not required for diagnosis and carries the risk of causing bacterial superinfection.

TREATMENT AND PROGNOSIS (also see Ch. 431). Medical therapy with metronidazole (750 mg three times per day for 10 days) is usually adequate both for treatment of the abscess and for eradication of amebae from the colon. Concomitant treatment with the intestinal amebicide diiodoquine (650 mg three times daily for 20 days) has also been advocated. In the past, surgical drainage of amebic abscesses was routine but is now rarely required. Aspiration may be necessary for abscesses extending into the pleura, peritoneum, or pericardium but is not required routinely. Aspiration, if performed, reveals straw-colored fluid (described as "anchovy paste") and amebae on microscopic examination.

GRANULOMATOUS LIVER DISEASE

ETIOLOGY. Reticuloendothelial cells in the liver remove circulating antigens, microorganisms, and immune complexes from the systemic circulation. These in turn form the nidus of the inflammatory reaction that results in granulomas. The large number of Kupffer cells (tissue macrophages), as well as the strategic location of the liver, probably account for the frequent finding of granulomas in liver biopsy specimens (2 to 10 per cent). Some of the numerous causes of hepatic granulomas are listed in Table 120–3. The relative frequency of causes varies geographically. Sarcoidosis and tuberculosis account for approximately two thirds of all causes of hepatic granulomas in the United States. In endemic areas, the predominant granulomas are those surrounding the eggs of *Schistosoma mansoni* in portal vein tributaries (Ch. 434). Hepatic granulomas associated with lepromatous leprosy are also frequent in underdeveloped countries. Commonly, no specific cause of the granuloma can be identified.

PATHOLOGY AND PATHOGENESIS. As in other organs, granulomas in the liver are focal collections of inflammatory cells that are distinct from the adjacent tissue. As granulomas develop, macrophages, the predominant cell type in the granuloma, fuse to form multinucleate giant cells. Histologic features of the granuloma may point toward a specific etiology. For example, a fibrinoid ring in a fat granuloma is highly suggestive of *Coxiella burnetii* infection, Q fever; acid-fast organisms may be found in tuberculosis or *Mycobacterium avium-intracellulare* infection; ova may be present in schistosomiasis; and birefringent granules indicate starch granulomas associated with intravenous drug use. The presence of central necrosis or "caseation" within the granuloma, although suggestive of tuberculosis, is not pathognomonic. The location within the hepatic lobule may be suggestive of certain etiologies. For example, granulomas associated with primary biliary cirrhosis or sarcoidosis tend to be well circumscribed and are found in the periportal region, whereas those associated with lymphomas tend to be poorly formed and are scattered throughout the lobule.

CLINICAL MANIFESTATIONS. Most frequently hepatic granulomas are found in a patient with fever of unknown etiology and an elevated serum alkaline phosphatase. Patients have hepatomegaly but rarely have evidence of portal hypertension (splenomegaly, ascites, or esophageal varices).

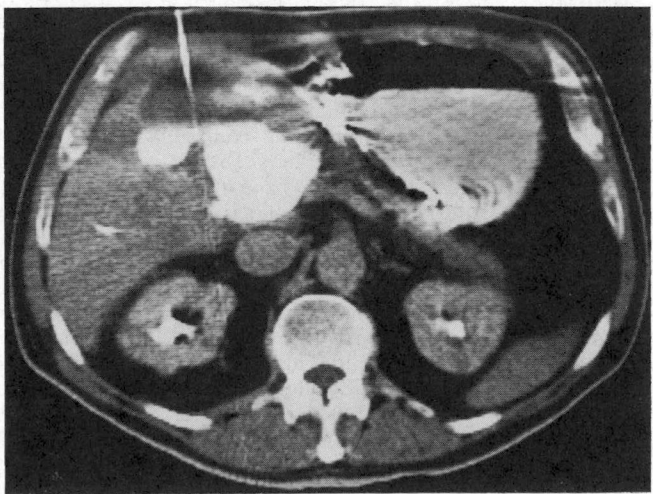

FIGURE 120–1. Computed tomogram showing CT-directed needle aspiration of a liver abscess. The needle is seen as the thin dense linear object entering the liver from the anterior abdominal wall. Contrast material has been introduced into the abscess cavity through the needle in order to outline the extent of the abscess.

TABLE 120–3. CAUSES OF HEPATIC GRANULOMAS

I. Infection
  A. Bacterial
    *Tuberculosis   Salmonellosis
    *Brucellosis   Listeriosis
    *Leprosy   Nocardiosis
    *Mycobacterium avium-   Melioidosis
      intracellulare
  B. Fungal
    *Histoplasmosis   Candidiasis
    *Coccidioidomycosis Blastomycosis
    Aspergillosis   Cryptococcosis
  C. Viral
    Mononucleosis   Lymphogranuloma venereum
    Cytomegalovirus   Influenza B
    Chickenpox   Psittacosis
  D. Parasitic
    *Schistosomiasis   Visceral larval migrans
    Ascariasis   Toxoplasmosis
    Stronglyloides   Giardiasis
    Clonorchiasis   Cryptosporidiosis
  E. Rickettsial
    *Q fever
  F. Spirochetal
    Secondary syphilis
II. Systemic diseases
    *Sarcoidosis   Lymphoma
    *Hodgkin's disease Polymyalgia rheumatica
    Crohn's disease   Systemic lupus erythematosus
    Wegener's granulomatosis
III. Drugs
    Sulfonamides   Halothane
    Penicillin   Allopurinol
    Cephalosporines   Carbamazepine
    Methyldopa   Phenytoin
    Hydralazine   Chlorpropamide
    Procainamide   Phenylbutazone
    Quinidine   Contraceptive pill
    Tocainide
IV. Miscellaneous conditions
    Berylliosis   Parenteral drug abuse
    Jejunoileal bypass Primary biliary cirrhosis

*Denotes more common causes.

DIAGNOSIS. Diagnosis ultimately depends on pathologic or culture confirmation. Serial sections of the biopsy should be examined and tissue cultured for mycobacteria and fungi. Determining a specific cause of hepatic granulomas often relies on demonstration of extrahepatic disease (e.g., granulomas of the uvea in sarcoidosis or acid-fast bacilli in sputum with tuberculosis). Thus, liver biopsy plays an adjunctive rather than a primary role in identifying a specific etiology in patients with fever of unknown origin. Serum angiotensin-converting enzyme is elevated in granulomatous liver disease of any etiology and is not specific for sarcoidosis.

TREATMENT. This is dependent on the etiology of the granulomas. Histologic or culture evidence of infection with a specific infectious agent (e.g., schistosomiasis, Q fever) should prompt specific therapy with praziquantel and tetracycline, respectively. The presence of hepatic granulomas in patients with tuberculosis is evidence of miliary disease, and if the suspicion of tuberculosis is high, therapy should be initiated prior to culture confirmation. Response to treatment of *Mycobacterium avium-intracellulare* in patients with AIDS has been disappointing. Demonstration of hepatic involvement in sarcoidosis, particularly in association with systemic symptoms, should prompt treatment with corticosteroids (Ch. 67). Although patients with hepatic sarcoidosis may develop symptoms of portal hypertension (e.g., bleeding esophageal varices), hepatic failure is rare. Treatment of systemic mycoses is discussed above.

PROGNOSIS. Prognosis is dependent on the underlying condition. With treatment and resolution of associated bacterial, viral, and rickettsial infections, prognosis is excellent. Disseminated fungal infections carry a poor prognosis despite therapy. Patients with hepatic sarcoidosis usually respond symptomatically

to steroid therapy, although progressive fibrosis and cirrhosis may occur. In patients with primary biliary cirrhosis, the presence of granulomas is indicative of improved prognosis.

Barnes PF, De Cock KM, Reynolds TN, et al.: A comparison of amebic and pyogenic abscess of the liver. Medicine 66:472, 1987. *Clinical and radiologic features, diagnosis, and outcome of 146 patients with hepatic abscesses admitted to a county hospital.*

Elliot DL, Tolle SW, Goldberg L, et al.: Pet-associated illness. N Engl J Med 313:985, 1985. *Review of parasitic, bacterial, and rickettsial illnesses acquired from cats and dogs.*

El-Rooby A: Management of hepatic schistosomiasis. Semin Liver Dis 5:263, 1985. *Summary of pathology, clinical manifestations, diagnosis, and treatment of acute and chronic schistosomiasis.*

Greenstein AJ, Sachar DB: Pyogenic and amebic abscesses of the liver. Semin Liver Dis 8:210, 1988. *Concise summary of clinical features, diagnosis, and current recommendations for treatment of pyogenic and amebic liver abscesses.*

Harrington PL, Gutierrez JJ, Ramirez-Rhondra CH, et al.: Granulomatous hepatitis. Rev Infect Dis 4:638, 1982. *Complete review of disorders associated with hepatic granulomas.*

Schneiderman DJ: Hepatobiliary abnormalities of AIDS. Gastroenterol Clin North Am 17:615, 1988. *Complete review of infectious agents causing liver and biliary tract disease in patients with AIDS, with a summary of the recent literature.*

Thaler M, Pastakia B, Shawker TH, et al.: Hepatic candidiasis in cancer patients: The evolving picture of the syndrome. Ann Intern Med 108:88, 1988. *Presentation, diagnosis, and treatment of eight patients with hepatic candidiasis, and review of 60 patients in the literature.*

---

121 Inherited, Infiltrative, and Metabolic Disorders Involving the Liver

Bruce F. Scharschmidt

The liver is involved in a variety of inherited, infiltrative, and metabolic disorders. Most of the disorders included in this chapter, e.g., Wilson's disease, hemochromatosis, the glycogen and lipid storage diseases, and amyloidosis, are discussed here only with respect to their hepatic involvement. A more comprehensive treatment of these entities can be found elsewhere in this textbook.

ALPHA₁-ANTITRYPSIN DEFICIENCY

Alpha₁-antitrypsin (A₁AT) deficiency is an inherited disorder associated with a decreased concentration of A₁AT in serum (see Ch. 58). This glycoprotein, which is found in other body fluids as well as in serum, inhibits a variety of proteolytic enzymes, including pancreatic trypsin, chymotrypsin, and elastase, as well as certain proteases produced by macrophages and leukocytes, in particular neutrophil elastase. It is produced primarily by the liver and released into the bloodstream, where it is normally present in a concentration of about 200 mg per deciliter and accounts for 90 per cent of total antitrypsin activity and a major portion of the α_1-globulin fraction.

A₁AT production is controlled by codominant alleles, with about 75 different alleles identified. There are four common (normal) "M" alleles. They differ from each other by a single amino acid substitution, have a collective allele frequency of about 0.95 in the United States, and are associated with normal plasma A₁AT levels. The deficiency state results from mutations that cause the A₁AT gene to encode for defective proteins. Homozygous and heterozygous combinations of at least 17 different mutations are associated with abnormally low serum levels and an increased risk of emphysema (Ch. 58), but only a subset of these mutant alleles (the "Z" allele, in particular) is associated with liver disease.

The pathogeneses of lung and liver disease in patients with A₁AT deficiency appear to differ from each other. Lung disease likely results from the deficiency state per se, possibly due to the lack of inhibition of neutrophil elastase. Liver disease, associated only with alleles encoding for proteins that cannot be effectively secreted, likely results from accumulation of defective α_1-antitrypsin within the endoplasmic reticulum of hepatocytes. This is supported by the observations that transgenic mice that express the abnormal human Z gene develop liver disease despite the presence of normal endogenous A_1AT levels and that patients with the "null" phenotype who have no α_1-antitrypsin in serum or in hepatocytes do not develop liver disease.

The presence of the mutant genes is not, by itself, sufficient to produce disease. Only up to 10 per cent of individuals with P_iZZ phenotype develop overt liver disease in childhood and have signs and symptoms of cholestasis in the first few days to weeks of life. In a minority of infants, cholestasis persists or worsens and is associated with liver failure and death in a few years. Cholestasis typically remits by 6 months in the remaining patients, about half of whom nevertheless develop cirrhosis. The long-term prognosis for these children is uncertain. An as yet undefined proportion of infants with P_iZZ phenotype who do not develop neonatal cholestasis have also been shown to have elevated transaminase levels in serum and fibrosis or cirrhosis on liver biopsy. Severe deficiency, P_iZZ phenotype, is associated with a several-fold increase in the risk of developing both cirrhosis and hepatocellular carcinoma, particularly in males. Heterozygous A_1AT deficiency (phenotypes MZ and SZ) may also be associated with an increased incidence of liver disease and cancer, although the link is less clear than for severe deficiency.

The diagnosis of A_1AT deficiency is made by measurement of A_1AT in serum either as trypsin inhibitory activity or by immunoassay. Individuals with heterozygous A_1AT deficiency may have serum levels of A_1AT in the low normal range. More definitive diagnosis requires determination of protease inhibitor phenotype by isoelectric focusing, and genotype can be determined using molecular biologic techniques including polymerase chain reaction to identify specific alleles. On liver biopsy, patients with the Z allele, with or without liver disease, also exhibit characteristic rounded eosinophilic cytoplasmic inclusions in periportal hepatocytes. These inclusion bodies are immunologically related to A_1AT but differ in certain amino acids as well as in their content of sialic acid and other sugars. Importantly, such eosinophilic inclusions occur as an apparently acquired defect in patients with alcoholic liver disease and are thus not diagnostic of inherited A_1AT deficiency.

There is currently no specific therapy for patients with A_1AT deficiency and liver disease. While direct administration of A_1AT or gene therapy to increase serum levels may help prevent or retard lung disease, it is unlikely to prevent liver disease. Liver transplantation (Ch. 124) should be considered in patients with progressive deterioration in hepatic function. Following transplantation, serum A_1AT levels increase and assume the genotype of the donor.

WILSON'S DISEASE

Wilson's disease is an autosomal recessive disorder with a prevalence worldwide of about 1 in 30,000 (Ch. 192). Its clinical and pathologic manifestations result from excessive accumulation of copper in many tissues, including the brain, liver, cornea, and kidneys. The abnormal gene responsible for Wilson's disease is on chromosome 13 and is manifested as impaired hepatic excretion of copper into bile, which is the cause of the copper accumulation. Unfortunately the diagnosis of this treatable disorder is often missed or delayed because of its rarity and diverse presentations. Hepatic disease is a common initial clinical manifestation in childhood and adolescence and may take the form of a self-limited illness resembling viral hepatitis, fulminant hepatic failure, or chronic active hepatitis; thus, biochemical screening for Wilson's disease is imperative in all patients under the age of 35 years who have liver disease of uncertain etiology. Biochemical clues to the presence of Wilson's disease include an alkaline phosphatase to bilirubin ratio of <2 and AST to ALT ratio of >4. Hemolysis represents an important clinical clue to the presence of Wilson's disease and predisposes to the development of cholelithiasis. Neurologic manifestations typically appear between the ages of 12 and 30 years and are almost invariably accompanied by the presence of Kayser-Fleischer rings.

The diagnosis and treatment of Wilson's disease are discussed in detail in Ch. 192; however, certain points merit special emphasis here. First, while the combination of an abnormally low ceruloplasmin level in serum and Kayser-Fleischer rings establishes the diagnosis, about 15 per cent of patients having Wilson's disease presenting with hepatic manifestations have serum ceruloplasmin concentrations in the low normal range, and low concentrations are seen in some heterozygotes as well as in occasional patients with severe hepatic dysfunction but without Wilson's disease. Moreover, about one half of patients who seek medical help with chronic active hepatitis or fulminant hepatic failure have not yet developed Kayser-Fleischer rings. If the diagnosis of Wilson's disease is uncertain, a liver biopsy should be performed for quantitative copper determination. If coagulation abnormalities preclude a biopsy, measurement of incorporation of orally administered radiolabeled copper into ceruloplasmin or measurement of serum copper or urinary copper excretion may be useful. Finally, patients with hepatic failure due to Wilson's disease frequently do not respond to chelation therapy, and liver transplantation should be considered. Because the genetic defect is expressed in the liver, successfully transplanted patients are effectively "cured" of their disease.

HEMOCHROMATOSIS

Hemochromatosis is among the more common genetic disorders, with a calculated homozygous frequency of about 1 in 300 to 1 in 400 in certain high-prevalence areas. The molecular basis of the underlying defect responsible for enhanced intestinal iron absorption remains undetermined. Males homozygous for the hemochromatosis allele, which is in close linkage with HLA-A3 on chromosome 6, show progressive accumulation of hepatic iron, and clinical evidence of disease usually develops in the fourth, fifth, or sixth decades of life. Most homozygous females do not develop clinical evidence of disease, presumably because of iron loss through menses and pregnancy. Heterozygotes may also show abnormal accumulation of hepatic iron, but the absolute amounts present are much less than in homozygotes, and clinical evidence of iron overload rarely develops.

Hepatic iron overload is most commonly manifested as moderate to marked hepatomegaly with initially well-preserved liver function. Esophageal varices, ascites, and impaired hepatic synthetic function are present in more advanced cases. Other important clinical features include abnormal skin pigmentation, glucose intolerance, cardiac involvement, hypogonadism, and arthropathy. Hepatocellular carcinoma develops in up to one third of patients. These classic manifestations are present in only a minority of homozygotes. Indeed, there is considerable variability in the expression of the disorder, and some homozygotes never develop overt disease. With appropriate phlebotomy therapy hepatic function frequently improves, and there are case reports that suggest regression of apparent cirrhosis.

Screening for hemochromatosis is probably best accomplished by measurement of transferrin saturation and serum ferritin. A saturation exceeding 50 per cent is present in nearly all homozygotes over 20 years of age, and a value less than 50 per cent largely precludes the diagnosis. However, the positive predictive value of a transferrin saturation exceeding 50 per cent is relatively low. In contrast, a transferrin saturation exceeding 80 per cent is a more reliable indicator of hemochromatosis, and a large study in Utah suggests that a transferrin saturation greater than 62 per cent most reliably separates homozygotes from heterozygotes and normal persons. Serum levels of ferritin are a generally accurate reflection of tissue iron stores and exceed 1000 ng per ml in most patients. However, occasional families with hemochromatosis and normal serum ferritin levels have been described and, conversely, serum ferritin is typically increased out of proportion to tissue iron stores in patients with hepatocellular necrosis. If either of these tests suggests iron overload, liver biopsy with quantitative iron determination and histochemical stains for iron should be performed.

Patients with alcohol-induced liver injury frequently have an abnormally elevated transferrin saturation and serum ferritin level and therefore represent a problem in differential diagnosis. Liver biopsies in such patients typically demonstrate hepatic iron levels well below those seen in patients with genetic hemochromatosis, and these patients are not benefited by phlebotomy. Conversely, an abnormally elevated hepatic iron level is indicative of genetic hemochromatosis, irrespective of a history of alcohol abuse.

A variety of noninvasive methods for measurement of hepatic iron have been proposed for use in patients who cannot undergo a liver biopsy. Dual-energy computed tomography appears particularly promising, and nuclear magnetic resonance and magnetic susceptibility measurement are also undergoing evaluation. Hemochromatosis is discussed in detail in Ch. 193.

STORAGE DISEASES

The *glycogen storage diseases* may present as disorders of the liver as well as of the heart and musculoskeletal system. Hepatomegaly is a prominent feature of most of these disorders, whereas splenomegaly is found primarily in type IV and less commonly in type III. Most of these disorders are not distinguishable on clinical grounds, and tissue analysis for glycogen content and enzyme activity are required for definitive diagnosis. Patients with type I or III glycogen storage disease frequently survive childhood and may be encountered by the physician treating adults. Patients with type I glycogen storage disease have an increased incidence of hepatic adenoma as well as hepatocellular carcinoma. Portacaval anastomosis may improve growth and reverse certain metabolic abnormalities in selected type I patients, although the mechanism for these beneficial effects is uncertain. Cirrhosis invariably develops in patients with type IV disease, as well as some patients with type III. The glycogen storage diseases are discussed in detail in Ch. 169. In addition to glycogen, the liver abnormally stores fatty acids, cholesterol, or complex lipids in the lipid storage disorders as well as various mucopolysaccharides and mucolipids. Although hepatomegaly is common to most of these disorders, the clinical consequences are attributable to involvement of the nervous and musculoskeletal systems.

PROTOPORPHYRIA

Protoporphyria is a disorder characterized by increased protoporphyrin content in erythrocytes, plasma, feces, and liver. It is usually classified as an autosomal dominant trait and results from a deficiency of heme synthase (ferrochelatase), the enzyme that catalyzes the formation of heme from protoporphyrin and iron. It is most conveniently diagnosed by demonstrating an elevated level of erythrocyte protoporphyrin. Protoporphyria is usually manifested by mild photosensitivity and, rarely, hemolysis. Hepatobiliary complications include pigment gallstones and, in less than 30 reported cases, hepatic failure. The hepatic failure, typically heralded by cholestasis, is associated with and presumably results from massive hepatic accumulation of birefringent crystals of protoporphyrin. Interruption of the enterohepatic circulation of protoporphyrin with cholestyramine or activated charcoal has been reported to deplete hepatic protoporphyrin deposits and restore liver function to normal in some patients with mild disease. Oral iron therapy has also been reported to decrease protoporphyrin production. The value of such treatments in patients with severe cholestasis and established hepatic failure is unknown, however, and hepatic transplantation should be considered in such instances. At present there is no way of identifying the small proportion of patients with protoporphyria who will develop significant hepatic disease.

CYSTIC FIBROSIS

In infants with cystic fibrosis, amorphous eosinophilic material in bile ducts and ductules, presumably representing inspissated secretions, may produce cholestasis (Ch. 64). Later manifestations include cholangitis, fibrosis, and obstructive biliary cirrhosis. Up to 20 per cent of patients who survive to adolescence have cirrhosis with portal hypertension, and bleeding from esophageal varices represents a significant cause of morbidity in this older age group. Patients who have bled from varices and have good pulmonary function are candidates for shunt surgery. Since liver disease with portal hypertension has even been reported as a first manifestation of cystic fibrosis, the diagnosis should be considered in a young patient with otherwise unexplained liver disease.

AMYLOIDOSIS

Amyloid deposition in the liver is common in amyloidosis of all types (Ch. 156). Hepatomegaly is present in approximately one half of patients with systemic amyloidosis; splenomegaly is present in about 10 per cent of patients; and mild elevation of the serum alkaline phosphatase is the most common biochemical abnormality. Cutaneous stigmata of chronic liver disease (e.g., spider angiomas, palmar erythema) and portal hypertension are unusual. Intrahepatic cholestasis with marked elevation of the serum bilirubin and alkaline phosphatase concentrations occurs in about 5 per cent of patients. The diagnosis of amyloidosis can usually be established without resorting to liver biopsy.

SARCOIDOSIS

Hepatic involvement in sarcoidosis represents a continuum from the presence of asymptomatic granulomas to cases in which hepatic involvement represents a prominent part of the overall clinical picture (Ch. 67). Approximately two thirds to three quarters of patients with sarcoidosis have hepatic granulomas, making the liver one of the most commonly involved organs in this disease, and liver biopsy is often of value in establishing the diagnosis of sarcoidosis.

About 20 per cent of patients with sarcoidosis have hepatomegaly. A higher proportion have abnormal liver function tests, most commonly elevation of alkaline phosphatase. Overt hepatic involvement is present in fewer than 20 per cent of patients. This may take several forms, including (1) hepatomegaly, generally with splenomegaly, and multiple abnormal liver function tests; (2) portal hypertension and its manifestations; and (3) chronic cholestasis, which may closely mimic primary biliary cirrhosis. Primary biliary cirrhosis can usually be distinguished from sarcoidosis based on the absence of systemic disease and presence of antimitochondrial antibody. The characteristic histologic feature of hepatic sarcoidosis is the presence of granulomas, frequently located in portal tracts. Chronic portal tract inflammation, hepatocyte poikilocytosis and anisocytosis, fibrosis, and even cirrhosis may be accompanying findings. Fever and systemic symptoms typically respond to corticosteroid treatment. It is less certain whether corticosteroids retard hepatic fibrosis and progression to portal hypertension, but a therapeutic trial is justified if significant symptoms are present and tuberculosis and other disorders producing hepatic granuloma have been excluded.

ENTERIC BYPASS

Hepatic disease related to enteric bypass surgery has typically been reported in patients who have had extensive bypass procedures for treatment of marked obesity. Jejunocolic bypass, an early operation, has now largely been abandoned because of a high incidence of complications, including cirrhosis and hepatic failure. Hepatic abnormalities are also common following jejunoileal bypass and may take several forms. Fatty change is present in up to two thirds of markedly obese patients prior to bypass surgery, and hepatic lipid content increases during the period of weight loss. Cirrhosis ensues in up to 5 per cent of patients, and death from liver failure accounts for a substantial proportion of the early postoperative mortality of 2 to 4 per cent. Histologic features may mimic those of alcoholic liver disease, including the presence of alcoholic hyalin. Longer-term follow-up studies suggest that hepatic abnormalities may not appear until several years after surgery in some patients.

The pathogenesis of these hepatic changes is unclear. Weight loss itself does not account for the progressive postoperative fat accumulation, since this does not occur in nonoperated obese patients who lose weight through dietary measures. However, hepatic disease resembling alcoholic hepatitis and even cirrhosis have been described in abstinent patients with obesity who have not undergone bypass surgery. Protein depletion, leading to a kwashiorkor-like state, may contribute to the fatty change. Increased production in the gut of potentially toxic substances may also play a role. For example, increased delivery of chenodeoxycholate to the colon results in increased production of the potentially hepatotoxic bile salt, lithocholate. The bypassed segment may also serve as a site for bacterial overgrowth and production of potentially toxic bacterial products.

Laboratory studies of hepatic function are frequently abnormal in the first few postoperative months following bypass surgery even in the absence of serious liver disease. Conversely, the absence of abnormal hepatic function tests or clinical evidence of liver disease during the first postoperative year does not preclude the possible later development of significant liver disease. Deterioration of synthetic or excretory function as evidenced by an abnormal prothrombin time that does not respond to vitamin K administration, hypoalbuminemia, or hyperbilirubinemia is an ominous sign. Biopsy is the only reliable way of assessing the severity of hepatic disease, and some advocate follow-up biopsies in all patients. Serious and persistent hepatic disease is an indication for re-establishing normal bowel continuity, which may be required in up to 25 per cent of patients. Currently, alternative procedures such as gastroplasty, which are associated with fewer hepatic and metabolic complications, are preferred in the morbidly obese patients.

INFLAMMATORY BOWEL DISEASE

Liver function tests may be transiently abnormal in up to one half of patients with chronic ulcerative colitis and less commonly in Crohn's disease, but significant and persistent biochemical abnormalities are present in fewer than 10 per cent of patients (Ch. 103).

A variety of hepatic abnormalities occur in patients with inflammatory bowel disease, the most important of which is *primary sclerosing cholangitis* (PSC). With increasing use of direct cholangiography, bile duct abnormalities characteristic of PSC have been identified in up to 5 per cent of patients with ulcerative colitis (much less commonly in Crohn's disease), and many hepatic histopathologic abnormalities in these patients appear to be manifestations of PSC. *Pericholangitis*, a histologic diagnosis, denotes a spectrum of acute and chronic portal tract changes including edema, inflammatory infiltration, bile duct damage, periductal and periportal fibrosis, and cirrhosis. Most patients with these findings have radiologic evidence of PSC. In those patients without abnormalities in radiologically demonstrable ducts, pericholangitis may represent *small duct sclerosing cholangitis*. Although PSC has been postulated to be secondary to inflammatory bowel disease or to the accompanying presence of bacteria or other toxins in portal blood, the high frequency of HLA-B8 and -DR3 in PSC and occasional association with thyroiditis implicate an immune pathogenesis in genetically predisposed individuals. There is evidence that more than 90 per cent of patients with PSC have, or will develop, ulcerative colitis. Apart from the tendency of PSC to accompany inflammatory bowel disease with extensive colonic involvement, there is no clear relationship between the severity of PSC and the accompanying inflammatory bowel disease. Similarly, treatment of the inflammatory bowel or colectomy does not predictably alter the course of PSC.

Patients with radiologically documented PSC have highly variable biochemical and clinical manifestations ranging from asymptomatic, in which case the disorder may be accompanied only by elevation of alkaline phosphatase activity, to deeply jaundiced with clinical and biochemical features of cirrhosis and hepatic decompensation. Although a variety of medical and surgical treatments have been tried, none has been proven to be effective for this disorder, and liver transplantation should be considered for patients with advanced disease.

Chronic active hepatitis also occurs in patients with inflammatory bowel disease, but the histologic changes of PSC can mimic those of chronic active hepatitis, and the latter diagnosis should not be made unless a cholangiogram is normal. Even then, the distinction between small duct PSC and chronic active hepatitis is difficult. Other hepatic abnormalities in patients with inflammatory bowel disease include fatty liver (which often parallels disease severity), amyloidosis (present in a small percentage of patients with Crohn's disease), and cholangiocarcinoma (closely linked to PSC).

TOTAL PARENTERAL NUTRITION

Total parenteral nutrition has been associated with a spectrum of hepatic abnormalities, including mild elevations in alkaline phosphatase and transaminase levels, cholestasis with jaundice, and, rarely, progressive hepatic disease resulting in death. Liver biopsy in these patients has frequently revealed fatty change, cholestasis, and mild periportal inflammation, with fibrosis or cirrhosis found in a minority. Some of these abnormalities have been due to the underlying disease or complicating infection, but total parenteral nutrition, by itself, can produce elevated serum bile salt levels and occasionally hyperbilirubinemia in both infants

and adults. The degree of abnormality appears related to the duration, type, and amount of parenteral alimentation. In infants, cholestasis associated with parenteral nutrition also increases in frequency with decreasing gestational age and birth weight, and adults with the short-bowel syndrome appear particularly at risk for severe liver disease. Hepatic function generally returns gradually to normal after total parenteral nutrition is discontinued. Modifying the infusate by lowering the calorie:nitrogen ratio or decreasing the total caloric intake has reportedly produced improvement in some patients, but this has not been systematically studied, and no one component of the parenteral formula has been clearly implicated as causative. Total parenteral nutrition also appears to predispose patients to the development of gallstones and both calculous and acalculous cholecystitis, and these possibilities should be kept in mind when one is evaluating a patient receiving parenteral nutrition for hepatobiliary disease.

In patients with mild biochemical abnormalities, adjustments in the infusion regimen may be helpful, including increasing the proportion of nonprotein calories supplied as lipid (versus glucose) or cyclic parenteral nutrition, in which the infusion is stopped for 8 to 12 hours per day. Copper and manganese, which are secreted in bile, should be decreased or eliminated in patients with cholestasis. Progressive liver disease in patients requiring chronic parenteral nutrition is a serious problem. While alteration of the infusion regimen or antibiotics such as metronidazole to alter gut flora may be tried, their usefulness is unproven. Finally, daily stimulation of gallbladder contraction by infusion of cholecystokinin or (if possible) oral administration of lipid and protein meals may be useful in preventing complications with biliary stasis.

PREGNANCY

Liver size and liver histology remain normal during uncomplicated pregnancy. Serum levels of alkaline phosphatase and leucine aminopeptidase typically rise in the second and third trimesters and are of placental origin; aminotransferase and bilirubin levels are normal.

EFFECT OF PREGNANCY ON COEXISTING LIVER DISEASE. In the United States and Western Europe, pregnancy does not appear to alter the course of acute viral hepatitis. In underdeveloped countries, however, an epidemic form of non-A, non-B viral hepatitis appears to run a more severe course in pregnancy, particularly during the third trimester, and is associated with an unusually high incidence of fulminant hepatic failure with high fetal and maternal mortality. Pregnancy has not been shown to alter the course of chronic persistent or chronic active hepatitis, although maternal and fetal morbidity and mortality may be increased because of variceal bleeding and postpartum hemorrhage. Vertical transmission of hepatitis B virus infection occurs commonly when the mother contracts acute hepatitis B during the third trimester or is a chronic carrier (particularly if she also is HBeAg positive), and it is important that the infant receive appropriate passive and active prophylaxis at delivery (Ch. 117).

LIVER DISEASES ASSOCIATED WITH PREGNANCY. *Hyperemesis gravidarum* of sufficient severity to require hospitalization may be accompanied by minor abnormalities in standard liver function tests. *Acute fatty liver of pregnancy* can be defined as a syndrome of acute hepatic dysfunction that develops in late pregnancy, is associated with microvesicular fat accumulation in hepatocytes, and resolves with delivery. It is more common in twin gestations and is associated with pre-eclampsia in up to one half of cases. It typically becomes apparent after the 30th week of gestation and is manifested initially by constitutional symptoms, often with abdominal pain, followed in many instances by overt evidence of hepatic failure, including encephalopathy and jaundice. In the past, intravenous tetracycline therapy was incriminated in some cases, but this is rarely true at present. The only known treatment is termination of the pregnancy. Early reports suggested that the disorder was associated with a very high mortality rate, but more recent reports suggest that there is a spectrum of disease severity and that milder cases without frank hepatic failure occur and have a favorable prognosis. At least 15 women who survived this disorder have had normal subsequent pregnancies. It also appears that acute fatty liver may, at least in some instances, fall within the spectrum of hepatic dysfunction associated with *pre-eclampsia* or *eclampsia*, as these two disorders occasionally share certain features, including onset in late pregnancy, increased incidence in young primiparas, the presence of coagulopathy, hypertension, and proteinuria, and resolution upon delivery. Focal necrosis and, rarely, hepatic rupture may occur in women with *eclampsia*. *Cholestasis of pregnancy* generally occurs in the last 4 months of gestation (range 27 to 39 weeks). It is characterized by pruritus, sometimes followed by jaundice. It typically resolves within 2 weeks of delivery and frequently recurs in subsequent pregnancies or with administration of oral contraceptives. Serum alkaline phosphatase and bile salts are increased, and hyperbilirubinemia may be present. Serum transaminase is also frequently mildly increased. Although generally considered a benign condition, cholestasis of pregnancy has been associated with an increased incidence of premature labor and postpartum hemorrhage.

CIRCULATORY DISTURBANCE

Hepatic function and histology are commonly altered in patients with cardiovascular disease. Disorders associated with an elevation of systemic venous pressure typically produce hepatic venous congestion manifested by hepatomegaly, minor abnormalities of liver function tests, and centrolobular congestion without necrosis. Longstanding hepatic congestion may lead to cardiac cirrhosis with fibrous bands joining centrilobular areas (Ch. 122). When hypotension is superimposed, even transiently, on hepatic congestion, severe centrilobular to midzonal necrosis, transaminase levels exceeding 1000 units, marked hyperbilirubinemia, and hypoprothrombinemia may result. Differentiating this disorder from viral hepatitis may be difficult, since the clinical features are similar and hepatic dysfunction often is not recognized until several days after the resolution of the circulatory failure. Unlike viral hepatitis, however, serum transaminase levels frequently fall very rapidly and may approach normal within days. If the circulatory insult is brief, patients usually recover from their hepatic injury uneventfully. Fatal fulminant hepatic failure has been reported, however. A similar form of acute hepatic injury is occasionally seen in persons without preexisting cardiovascular disease who suffer severe or prolonged hypotension or in patients with severe isolated left-sided heart failure.

Adams PC, Halliday JW, Powell LW: Early diagnosis and treatment of hemochromatosis. Adv Intern Med 34:111, 1989. *A comprehensive review with a practical orientation.*

Crystal RG: Alpha-1-antitrypsin deficiency, emphysema and liver disease: Genetic basis and strategies for therapy. J Clin Invest (In press, 1990). *A thoroughly referenced and current review which focuses on the pathogenesis and prospects for treatment.*

Faloon WW: Hepatobiliary effects of obesity and weight-reducing surgery. Semin Liver Dis 8:229, 1988. *A concise review with 77 references.*

Klein S, Nealon WH: Hepatobiliary abnormalities associated with total parenteral nutrition. Semin Liver Dis 8:237, 1986. *A well-written review dealing with practical aspects of diagnosis and management.*

Shrumpf E, Fausa O, Elgjo K, et al.: Hepatobiliary complications of inflammatory bowel disease. Semin Liver Dis 8:201, 1988. *A well-referenced review focusing in particular on primary sclerosing cholangitis and its pathologic and clinical manifestations.*

Smith LH Jr: Overview of hemochromatosis. West J Med 153:296, 1990.

van Theil DH: Effects of pregnancy and sex hormones on the liver. Semin Liver Dis 7:1, 1987. *An entire volume with eight chapters covering various liver problems associated with pregnancy and steroid hormones.*

122 Cirrhosis of the Liver and Its Major Sequelae

Thomas D. Boyer

GENERAL CONSIDERATIONS. Cirrhosis is an irreversible alteration of the liver architecture, consisting of hepatic fibrosis and areas of nodular regeneration. When the nodules are small

(less than 3 mm), uniform, and encompass one lobule, the term micronodular or unilobular cirrhosis is applied. In macronodular or multilobular cirrhosis the nodules exceed 3 mm, vary in size, and encompass more than one lobule. Frequently, features of both micronodular and macronodular cirrhosis are present in the same liver. Etiologic diagnosis may be impossible from the gross and microscopic appearance of the cirrhotic liver and must therefore be based on history, physical examination, biochemical and serologic tests, and histochemical stains. The causes of cirrhosis are listed in Table 122–1.

Patients with cirrhosis may have one of two general types of manifestations: (1) signs or symptoms related to hepatocellular necrosis, which are similar to those of acute hepatitis and include jaundice, nausea and vomiting, and tender hepatomegaly; or (2) signs or symptoms of the complications of cirrhosis, which are largely due to the rise in intrahepatic vascular resistance that leads to portal hypertension and its complications (ascites, formation of portal-systemic collaterals, encephalopathy, splenomegaly, and bleeding esophageal and gastric varices). Other, less specific manifestations of cirrhosis include gynecomastia, spider angiomas, parotid hypertrophy, and testicular atrophy. Patients frequently present a mixed picture with features of both hepatocellular necrosis and portal hypertension.

Agents that cause cirrhosis may have systemic effects as well. Extrahepatic features may dominate the clinical picture with little or no evidence of liver disease. For example, patients with alcoholic liver disease frequently have complaints referable to the central nervous system, peripheral nerves, heart, muscles, and gastrointestinal tract. Patients with disease such as primary biliary cirrhosis may have prominent eye and skin disorders. Patients with hemochromatosis may present with diabetes mellitus or arthritis, and patients with Wilson's disease, with central nervous system dysfunction, before liver disease becomes apparent. Thus, cirrhosis is frequently a subclinical illness, and a high index of suspicion may be necessary to establish a correct diagnosis.

ALCOHOLIC LIVER DISEASE

DEFINITION AND INCIDENCE. Alcoholic liver disease, a frequent and serious sequela of the chronic abuse of ethanol, occurs singly or intermingled in three forms: *fatty liver, alcoholic hepatitis*, and *cirrhosis*. Alcohol is the most common cause of liver disease in the Western world. Alcoholic cirrhosis is discovered in 1.6 to 9.9 per cent of all necropsies in the United States. The peak incidence is in patients 40 to 55 years of age; however, patients in their 20's may be seen with advanced alcoholic liver disease. The male to female ratio is 2:1.

ETIOLOGY AND PATHOGENESIS. *The relationship between alcohol abuse and cirrhosis* is well established. The incidence of cirrhosis and the per capita consumption of alcohol are directly related; countries with the greatest alcohol consumption also have the highest incidence of cirrhosis. Neither the pattern

TABLE 122–1. CAUSES OF CIRRHOSIS

Drugs and Toxins	Metabolic
Alcohol	Wilson's disease
Methyldopa	Hemochromatosis
Methotrexate	Erythropoietic protoporphyria
Isoniazid	Pediatric—α_1-antitrypsin
Perhexiline maleate	deficiency, galactosemia,
Amiodarone	hereditary fructose
Oxyphenisatin	intolerance, glycogen storage
Vitamin A	disease type IV, tyrosinosis
Carbon tetrachloride	**Cardiovascular**
Infections	Chronic right heart failure
Hepatitis B and C	Budd-Chiari syndrome
Syphilis (tertiary)	Veno-occlusive disease
Schistosoma japonicum	**Miscellaneous**
Biliary Obstruction	Chronic active hepatitis
Carcinoma (pancreatic or bile duct)	Primary biliary cirrhosis
	Sarcoidosis
Chronic pancreatitis	Jejunoileal bypass
Common duct stones	Neonatal hepatitis
Strictures	Indian childhood cirrhosis
Cystic fibrosis	Hereditary hemorrhagic
Biliary atresia	telangiectasia
Sclerosing cholangitis	**Cryptogenic**

of drinking (spree versus daily) nor the type of alcoholic beverage consumed appears to be important in the genesis of liver disease. The single most important factor is the average daily consumption of ethanol. Levels of daily ethanol consumption exceeding 40 to 80 grams (36 to 72 oz of beer, 4.5 to 9 oz liquor, 15 to 30 oz of wine) for 10 to 15 years are associated with an increase in the incidence of cirrhosis. Women may be more susceptible to the toxic effects of ethanol than men, and a lower (20 grams) daily consumption of ethanol by women may lead to cirrhosis. As the daily level of alcohol consumed rises, the time required for the development of cirrhosis is reduced.

Ethanol is a hepatotoxin. Administration of alcohol to humans or animals leads to the development of fatty liver (hepatic steatosis). The mitochondria and endoplasmic reticulum of hepatocytes are altered morphologically and functionally. Many of the effects of ethanol reflect its metabolism, which is catalyzed primarily by the cytosolic enzyme alcohol dehydrogenase as shown:

$$CH_3CH_2OH \xrightarrow[]{\text{Alcohol dehydrogenase}} CH_3CHO$$
$$\text{Ethanol} \quad NAD \longrightarrow NADH + H^+ \quad \text{Acetaldehyde}$$

(Other metabolic pathways via a microsomal ethanol oxidizing system or a catalase system appear to be of minor importance, except perhaps at high ethanol concentrations.) The acetaldehyde formed from ethanol is then oxidized to acetate by acetaldehyde dehydrogenase with NAD^+ as a cofactor. The lack of the active high-affinity form of acetaldehyde dehydrogenase (50 per cent of Japanese) leads to high blood levels of acetaldehyde following ethanol ingestion. The high levels of acetaldehyde in these individuals are associated with flushing, vasodilatation, tachycardia, and aversion to ethanol. A similar but more severe reaction is seen in patients who ingest ethanol while taking the acetaldehyde dehydrogenase inhibitor disulfiram. The limiting step in the rate of metabolism of ethanol is the availability of the cofactor NAD^+, which is converted to NADH during the aforementioned two reactions. This increased reducing potential in the cell favors the conversion of pyruvate to lactate. When blood levels of ethanol are high (more than 200 mg per deciliter), the resulting lactic acidemia decreases the clearance of urate by the kidneys and hyperuricemia develops. Inhibition of gluconeogenesis and fasting hypoglycemia may also follow ethanol abuse (Ch. 114). Fatty acid oxidation is impaired, and the esterification of fatty acids to triglycerides is increased. The latter effects, acting in concert with less well defined events, lead to the development of a fatty liver. Chronic use of ethanol also leads to an increase in the activity of some P-450 isozymes, and alcoholics may manifest altered metabolism of drugs that are normally degraded by these P-450 isozymes (Ch. 24).

The metabolic effects of ethanol are relatively well understood, but the mechanism by which it causes chronic liver disease is not. There is evidence for impaired protein synthesis and secretion, mitochondrial injury, lipid peroxidation, interaction of acetaldehyde with cellular proteins and membrane lipids, cellular hypoxia, and cell-mediated and antibody-mediated cytotoxicity, but the relative importance of each of these in producing sustained cell injury is unknown.

Ethanol fed to animals receiving an otherwise balanced diet has not been shown to cause alcoholic hepatitis. In addition, only 10 to 20 per cent of alcoholics and about 30 per cent of ethanol-fed baboons develop cirrhosis despite similar levels of ethanol ingestion. Thus, *genetic, nutritional,* or *environmental* factors may act in concert with ethanol to cause liver disease.

Malnutrition is a common finding in alcoholics who have both poor diet and reduced intestinal absorption of dietary nutrients. Lesions identical to those of alcoholic hepatitis may develop following jejunoileal bypass for obesity, a condition in which protein malnutrition is common. Thus, malnutrition appears to potentiate the adverse effects of alcohol. Other factors, such as simultaneous exposure to other hepatotoxins, may also be important in the genesis of liver injury. For example, because of the effects of alcohol on drug metabolism, alcoholics are more susceptible to injury by direct hepatotoxins such as acetaminophen. Alcoholism and alcoholic liver disease are more common in certain populations, in twins, and within families, but there is no

evidence of a genetically determined abnormality in the metabolism of ethanol that renders them more susceptible to liver injury.

DIAGNOSIS. The diagnosis of alcoholic liver disease should be considered in any patient who consumes more than 40 grams of ethanol daily. Tender hepatomegaly, fever, and jaundice are suggestive of alcoholic hepatitis, whereas ascites and venous collaterals suggest cirrhosis. Many patients, however, lack any distinctive clinical features such that a firm diagnosis cannot be established without liver biopsy. In addition, up to 20 per cent of patients with clinical features of alcoholic liver disease are found on liver biopsy to have another type of hepatic disorder.

PATHOLOGY, CLINICAL PRESENTATION, AND THERAPY. Alcohol causes three major pathologic lesions and clinical illnesses: *fatty liver, alcoholic hepatitis, and cirrhosis.* Each of these may occur as an isolated event, or they may be present in any combination in a single patient. Therefore, although the three lesions are described as single entities, many patients have all three and have a mixed clinical picture. The histologic pattern is not specific for alcohol alone but may also be found in the livers of patients who have undergone jejunoileal bypass for obesity or as an unusual accompaniment of obesity or diabetes mellitus. Patients treated with the vasodilator perhexiline maleate or the antiarrhythmic drug amiodarone also may develop a lesion identical to alcoholic liver disease (Ch. 118).

Fatty Liver. Fatty liver is the most common biopsy finding in alcoholics. The fat, either centrilobular or diffuse in location, is present in large droplets, which occupy most of the volume of the hepatocyte. Occasionally the fat is present in small droplets, resembling the lesion of Reye's syndrome or fatty liver of pregnancy. Patients with fatty liver are usually asymptomatic, but on occasion they may have abdominal pain, icterus, or vague gastrointestinal complaints. The liver is enlarged and may be tender but is of normal consistency. Ascites, venous collaterals, and the stigmata of chronic liver disease, if present, are not attributable to the fatty liver per se but reflect more serious lesions. The laboratory tests are only mildly abnormal in fatty liver. Jaundice, when present, is usually mild (bilirubin below 5 mg per deciliter), although intense cholestasis occasionally develops in patients with fatty liver. The AST, if elevated, is only modestly so (less than five times normal). The serum albumin and globulin levels are abnormal in about 25 per cent of patients. Patients with alcoholic fatty liver alone have an excellent prognosis unless there is fibrosis around the central veins. Withdrawal of the alcohol leads to a rapid resolution of the clinical illness and histologic lesion (fat disappears within 3 to 6 weeks). On rare occasions, these patients die suddenly from multiple fat emboli to the lungs (Ch. 66).

Alcoholic Hepatitis. Alcoholic hepatitis (acute sclerosing hyaline necrosis) is a serious sequela of alcoholism because it may lead to hepatic failure or to cirrhosis. The pathologic lesion is most severe in central areas and consists of hepatocellular necrosis and the triad of (1) *alcoholic hyalin,* (2) *infiltration by polymorphonuclear leukocytes,* and (3) *increased intralobular connective tissue* in the space of Disse and sclerosis of terminal hepatic (central) veins. Alcoholic hyalin (Mallory body), an eosinophilic intracellular aggregate of proteinaceous material characteristically perinuclear in location, is present in only 30 per cent of liver biopsies in which the diagnosis of alcoholic hepatitis can be made on clinical and other histologic criteria. Alcoholic hyalin is not specific for alcoholic liver disease, since it has also been found in the livers of patients with Wilson's disease, primary biliary cirrhosis, hepatocellular carcinoma, and diabetes mellitus, as well as following jejunoileal bypass. Central vein sclerosis may be severe enough to cause a severe outflow block and portal hypertension in the absence of cirrhosis.

The clinical features of alcoholic hepatitis range from absence of symptoms to hepatic failure. Patients commonly complain of anorexia, nausea, vomiting, abdominal pain, and weight loss. Tender hepatomegaly is present in at least 80 per cent of hospitalized patients. Ascites, jaundice, fever (temperature 37.2 to 39.4°C), splenomegaly, and encephalopathy are common but not invariable. Although fever is common, bacterial infection should be excluded, since such patients are at an increased risk for developing pneumonia, urinary tract infections, sepsis, and bacterial peritonitis. The AST is elevated frequently; however, the degree of elevation is modest (less than 10 times normal) although on occasion it can exceed 15 times normal. The ALT may be normal and is almost always less than the AST. The AST/ALT ratio frequently exceeds two. This is in contrast to viral hepatitis, in which the AST frequently exceeds 15 to 25 times normal and the ALT is equal to or greater than the AST. Hyperbilirubinemia is common (60 to 90 per cent) in alcoholic hepatitis, and it may be marked (20 to 30 mg per deciliter). The alkaline phosphatase is usually elevated to less than three times normal, but an occasional patient has a cholestatic picture in which the alkaline phosphatase is unusually high. Prolongation of the prothrombin time, hypoalbuminemia, and hyperglobulinemia may be present. The white blood cell count frequently is elevated (>10,000) and may exceed 30,000 to 40,000 per cubic millimeter. Patients with alcoholic hepatitis may develop the hepatorenal syndrome, and a rising BUN and creatinine are poor prognostic signs.

Treatment for alcoholic hepatitis is nonspecific. Patients should receive a well-balanced diet, high in calories (2500 to 3000 kcal). Protein should be included in the diets unless encephalopathy is present. Anorexia is frequent, and tube or intravenous alimentation may be necessary. Improvement in the patient's nutritional state may be associated with more rapid resolution of the liver test abnormalities; however, the effect of nutritional support on survival is unclear. Prednisone has not been shown to decrease the morbidity or mortality in patients with mild to moderate disease. Use of steroids to treat patients with severe alcoholic hepatitis is controversial and cannot be recommended on the basis of available evidence. Propylthiouracil, penicillamine, anabolic steroids, and colchicine also have been used in the treatment of alcoholic hepatitis, but without clear success.

The *prognosis* for patients with alcoholic hepatitis is much worse than for those with fatty liver. Some patients who stop drinking may have complete resolution of the lesion. In most patients, however, alcoholic hepatitis persists (with clinical improvement), progresses to diffuse fibrosis or cirrhosis, or leads to hepatic failure and death. The hospital mortality for patients with severe disease (who cannot have a biopsy or who have encephalopathy) exceeds 40 per cent, whereas for those with milder disease the expected death rate is 10 per cent or less.

Alcoholic Cirrhosis. *Alcoholic cirrhosis* usually consists of micronodules of regular size, but it can be macronodular or of a mixed type. Micronodular cirrhosis is not specific for alcoholic liver disease. Histologically, dense bands of connective tissue join portal and central areas. Scarring is most severe in the central regions, and collagen may deposit in the space of Disse. In addition, alcoholic hepatitis frequently coexists, as well as varying amounts of cholestasis, iron, and fat.

Clinically, cirrhosis is an asymptomatic disease in 10 to 20 per cent of patients. It is also commonly present in association with alcoholic hepatitis, and signs of acute liver injury may dominate the clinical picture. Patients may also have ascites, gastrointestinal bleeding, or encephalopathy, to be discussed later. The liver may be large or small and usually has a firm consistency. Spider angiomas, palmar erythema, parotid enlargement, testicular atrophy and gynnecomastia (men), menstrual irregularities (women), and muscle wasting are found frequently; however, these findings are not specific for alcoholic cirrhosis. Upper abdominal pain associated with bloody ascitic fluid, right upper quadrant bruit, or a friction rub over the liver suggests hepatocellular carcinoma.

The *laboratory abnormalities* present in patients with cirrhosis may be similar to those of alcoholic hepatitis. The AST is normal to mildly elevated, and bilirubin is only slightly increased unless the picture is complicated by alcoholic hepatitis, hemolysis, sepsis, hepatic failure, or carcinoma. Anemia is a common finding. The cause of the anemia is multifactorial, including blood loss, folate and pyridoxine deficiency, hemolysis, and the toxic effect of ethanol on the bone marrow. Hypersplenism or bone marrow suppression by ethanol may lead to thrombocytopenia or leukopenia. The serum sodium and potassium may be low in patients with ascites. Hypomagnesemia and hypophosphatemia are common, as is a mild respiratory alkalosis. The BUN and creatinine are increased in patients who have been treated with excessive diuretics or who are developing hepatorenal failure.

The *treatment* of alcoholic cirrhosis is also nonspecific. Colchicine, when used for several years, may improve survival, but further study is warranted before its use can be recommended. Deficiencies of vitamins (folate, thiamine, pyridoxine, vitamin K) and minerals (magnesium, phosphate) should be corrected. The sodium content of the diet need not be reduced unless there is sodium retention by the kidneys. Protein restriction is necessary only when there is clinical evidence of hepatic encephalopathy.

The *prognosis* for patients with alcoholic cirrhosis depends upon two features: presence of complications and continued abuse of alcohol. Patients without ascites, jaundice, or gastrointestinal bleeding have a better prognosis than those with these complications. Continued alcohol abuse reduces the expected 5-year survival to only 40 per cent, whereas it is 60 per cent or greater in those who abstain.

D'Amico G, Morabito A, Pagliaro L, et al.: Survival and prognostic indicators in compensated and decompensated cirrhosis. Dig Dis Sci 31:468, 1986. *Analysis of variables associated with a poor prognosis in alcoholic and nonalcoholic cirrhosis.*

Kershenobich D, Vargas F, Garcia-Tsao G, et al.: Colchicine in the treatment of cirrhosis of the liver. N Engl J Med 318:1709, 1988. *This paper describes the treatment of alcoholic liver disease with colchicine. The results of this study were encouraging, but the accompanying editorial should be read, as it discusses some of the difficulties with the study.*

Rothschild MA, Oratz M (eds.): Alcohol, alcoholism and alcoholic liver disease. Semin Liver Dis 8:1, 1988. *Contains a series of articles that discuss the metabolism of ethanol, the genetics of alcoholism, and the diagnosis and management of alcoholic liver disease.*

Zakim D, Boyer TD, Montgomery C: Alcoholic liver disease. *In* Zakim D, Boyer TD (eds.): Hepatology: A Textbook of Liver Disease. 2nd ed. Philadelphia, W. B. Saunders Company, 1990, pp 821–869. *A complete review of the pathogenesis, diagnosis, and treatment of alcoholic liver disease.*

PRIMARY BILIARY CIRRHOSIS

DEFINITION AND ETIOLOGY. Primary biliary cirrhosis, a cholestatic disorder, develops because of progressive destruction of small and intermediate-sized intrahepatic bile ducts. The extrahepatic biliary tree and larger intrahepatic bile ducts are patent. The cause of primary biliary cirrhosis is unknown. The injury to the bile ducts is thought to be on an immunologic basis, as there is a high frequency of serum autoantibodies, elevated levels of immunoglobulins (especially IgM), circulating immune complexes, and a reduced cell-mediated immune response in patients with this disease. In addition, the injured bile ducts are surrounded by lymphocytes and, on occasion, by granulomas. These findings, however, are nonspecific and do not establish the etiologic agent or agents responsible for the disease. Genetic factors may also be important, as the disease has been described in a mother and daughter, in siblings, and in twins. In addition, the incidence of positive tests for antimitochondrial antibodies in relatives of patients with primary biliary cirrhosis is increased. The high female preponderance suggests that estrogens or progesterone may be important in the pathogenesis of this disease.

PATHOLOGY. Primary biliary cirrhosis is characterized by progressive, nonsuppurative, destructive cholangitis, which occurs in four histopathologic stages: *ductal, ductular, scarring,* and *cirrhotic.* The lesions in the first two stages are distributed unevenly and may therefore be absent in needle biopsies of the liver. The characteristic lesion (ductal or Stage 1) consists of damaged interlobular and septal bile ducts surrounded by a dense infiltrate of lymphocytes and plasma cells. Well-formed granulomas are seen frequently near the injured bile ducts. In Stage 2 (ductular) of the disease, bile ductules proliferate and bile ducts are reduced in number. Portal fibrosis may be present or absent, and granulomata are found less often than in Stage 1. Later, as the inflammation subsides, scarring increases, most marked in portal areas with fibrous septa extending into the lobule (Stage 3). When cirrhotic (Stage 4), the liver may lose all of the characteristic lesions. Bile ducts are few in both Stages 3 and 4, and this paucity of bile ducts may be the only clue to the diagnosis of primary biliary cirrhosis. In one quarter of the cases, alcoholic hyalin is identifiable in the biopsy. Histologic features of chronic active hepatitis may also be present, leading to difficulties in diagnosis.

CLINICAL MANIFESTATIONS (Table 122–2). Ninety per cent of patients with primary biliary cirrhosis are female. The disease has been found in patients as young as 23 and as old as 72; however, the majority of patients are of ages 40 to 60. The

TABLE 122–2. CLINICAL FEATURES OF PRIMARY BILIARY CIRRHOSIS

Signs and Symptoms	Laboratory
Female preponderance (> 90%)	Antimitochondrial antibodies (> 90%)
Pruritus	
Jaundice (late)	Elevated alkaline phosphatase, cholesterol, IgM, serum bile acids, and bilirubin
Skin hyperpigmentation	
Hepatosplenomegaly	
Xanthelasma/xanthoma	**Associated Diseases**
Bleeding diathesis (vitamin K deficiency)	Sjögren's syndrome
	Scleroderma/CREST syndrome
Bone pain (osteoporosis/ osteomalacia)	Arthritis
	Autoimmune thyroiditis
Ascites/variceal hemorrhage (late)	Renal tubular acidosis

onset is usually marked by *pruritus* or by discovery of asymptomatic hepatomegaly. Sometimes the first abnormality is an elevated alkaline phosphatase noted on an automated screening panel. The itching may start during pregnancy or with the use of birth control pills. Following delivery or withdrawal of the medication, the itching usually continues; this is in contrast to *cholestasis of pregnancy,* in which pruritus resolves following parturition. Itching leads to excoriative dermatitis and thickening and darkening of the skin. Hepatomegaly and less frequently splenomegaly may be found at the time of diagnosis. *Jaundice* rarely precedes the onset of pruritus and may follow it by several years. *Portal hypertension* and *hepatic failure* are usually late events, and ascites or bleeding esophageal varices are uncommon presenting features. *Hypercholesterolemia,* secondary to the decreased biliary excretion of cholesterol, may be severe enough to produce xanthomas. *Osteomalacia* or more commonly *osteoporosis* may develop in these patients. The cause of the bone disease is incompletely understood; however, malabsorption of vitamin D and calcium are important pathogenic factors. Copper accumulates in the livers of patients with primary biliary cirrhosis because it cannot be efficiently secreted into the bile. The levels of hepatic copper may reach levels equal to those found in Wilson's disease, and rarely *Kayser-Fleischer rings* have been described.

ASSOCIATED DISEASES. Primarily biliary cirrhosis is associated with a variety of disorders. *Sjögren's syndrome* with dryness of the eyes and mouth is present in at least 70 per cent of patients when specific tests (Schirmer test, buccal biopsy, and others) are used (Ch. 263). These same patients may have hyposecretion by the pancreas. *Scleroderma* and the *CREST syndrome* (calcinosis, Reynaud's phenomenon, esophageal hypomotility, sclerodactyly, telangiectasia) are both increased in frequency in patients with primary biliary cirrhosis. The prevalence of *arthritis,* both seropositive and seronegative, is increased in these patients. *Thyroid autoantibodies* are found in about 25 per cent of patients, and in the antibody-positive patients thyroid dysfunction (primarily hypothyroidism) is common. *Renal tubular acidosis* also is present in patients with primary biliary cirrhosis. The pathogenesis of the renal tubular acidosis is unknown, but it may be secondary to deposition of copper in renal tubules. There also appears to be an increase in the frequency of breast cancer and celiac disease in these patients.

LABORATORY FINDINGS. The *alkaline phosphatase* is elevated in almost all patients with primary biliary cirrhosis, although it may be normal in asymptomatic patients. The elevation is usually two to six times normal, but can be more than 10 times normal. The serum bilirubin is usually normal or mildly elevated until the later stages of the disease are reached. Serum bile acids and cholesterol are increased frequently. Serum *immunoglobulin M* levels are increased in 75 per cent of patients with primary biliary cirrhosis. The finding, however, is not specific. Hypoprothrombinemia and hypocalcemia may be present and reflect deficiencies of vitamins K and D. The serum transaminases are normal to mildly elevated. Eighty-four to 98 per cent of patients with primary biliary cirrhosis have *circulating antimitochondrial antibodies.* There are a number of different antimitochondrial antibodies, but the one most specific for primary biliary cirrhosis is termed M2 and is directed toward an antigen in the inner mitochondrial membrane. The antibody is neither species nor organ specific. Antimitochondrial antibodies

may be present in patients with HBsAg-negative chronic active hepatitis, cryptogenic cirrhosis, and collagen vascular diseases; however, test results are normal in patients with extrahepatic obstruction unless they also have primary biliary cirrhosis or chronic active hepatitis. A small percentage of patients (5 to 30 per cent) with primary biliary cirrhosis have antinuclear antibodies in their serum.

DIAGNOSIS. The diagnosis of primary biliary cirrhosis is established by finding a positive antimitochondrial antibody test and the characteristic pathology (Stage 1 or 2) on liver biopsy. It may be necessary to exclude extrahepatic obstruction in some patients in whom the diagnosis of primary biliary cirrhosis cannot be made with certainty, as *extrahepatic biliary obstruction* can clinically mimic primary biliary cirrhosis. Also, patients with primary biliary cirrhosis have an increased incidence of gallstones, which may cause biliary obstruction. Biliary tract disease may be excluded by either transhepatic or endoscopic retrograde cholangiography.

THERAPY AND PROGNOSIS. No specific therapy for primary biliary cirrhosis is available. Corticosteroids are not known to be effective in this disease and will aggravate the bone disease. D-Penicillamine, azathioprine, ursodeoxycholic acid and colchicine have been used in the treatment of primary biliary cirrhosis. D-Penicillamine cannot be recommended because its use is associated with numerous complications without improvement in survival. Treatment with colchicine has been shown to improve liver tests but not hepatic histology as compared to placebo-treated controls. Similarly, treatment with ursodeoxycholic acid improves liver tests but not symptoms, and its effects on survival are unclear. Further experience is required in the use of colchicine and ursodeoxycholic acid before they can be recommended. Patients with advanced clinical disease (e.g., jaundice, ascites) are excellent candidates for liver transplantation (Ch. 124). Successful transplantation is associated with resolution of all hepatic symptoms.

The treatment of primary biliary cirrhosis is directed toward its complications and includes correction of specific deficiency states and reduction in the pruritus. Dietary fat may be reduced to 40 grams daily to decrease steatorrhea and improve calcium absorption. Medium-chain triglycerides, which are absorbed directly into the portal vein without the requirement for intraluminal bile salts, may be given as a dietary supplement. If the prothrombin time is prolonged, vitamin K (10 mg) is given intramuscularly every 4 weeks. Osteomalacia can be prevented by exposure to sunlight (10 to 20 minutes daily) and dietary supplementation with vitamin D and calcium. The serum 25(OH)D level should be measured, and, if low, it should be increased to the normal range with oral vitamin D (Ch. 233). Hepatic osteomalacia, but not the more common osteoporosis, responds to treatment with metabolites of vitamin D. Patients with thyroid antibodies should be tested for hypothyroidism.

The cause of the pruritus is unknown, but it may be secondary to increased tissue levels of bile salts. Cholestyramine and colestipol are anion exchange resins that bind bile salts in the intestines, preventing their reabsorption in the terminal ileum. Eight to 12 grams of cholestyramine is given daily in divided doses with breakfast and dinner. Fat-soluble vitamins should not be given at the same time as the resin. The hypercholesterolemia may also respond to cholestyramine therapy. Clofibrate should not be used in these patients, as there may be a paradoxical increase in the serum cholesterol.

Asymptomatic patients with primary biliary cirrhosis have a good prognosis, with a 10-year survival similar to age-matched controls. Patients who present with symptoms have, in contrast, an average life expectancy of 5.5 to 11 years. The development of jaundice, ascites, or cirrhosis is associated with a poor prognosis.

Dickson ER, Grambsch PM, Fleming TR, et al.: Prognosis in primary biliary cirrhosis: Model for decision making. Hepatology 9:1, 1989. *The prognosis of individual patients with primary biliary cirrhosis can be determined with reasonable accuracy by using symptoms and laboratory test results. This study has developed a model for this type of analysis.*

Gershwin ME, Mackay IR (eds.): Primary biliary cirrhosis. Semin Liver Dis 9:1, 1989. *A series of articles about primary biliary cirrhosis including discussions of antimitochondrial antibody tests, medical therapy, and liver transplantation.*

Kaplan M: Primary biliary cirrhosis. N Engl J Med 316:521, 1987. *A succinct Medical Progress article with an excellent bibliography of 124 references. A good place to start.*

Leuschner U, Fischer H, Kurtz W, et al.: Ursodeoxycholic acid in primary biliary cirrhosis: Results of a controlled double-blind trial. Gastroenterology 97:1268, 1989. *One of the first controlled trials on the use of ursodeoxycholic acid in the treatment of primary biliary cirrhosis. There was a significant improvement in some liver tests during treatment with ursodeoxycholic acid, and following withdrawal of therapy liver tests worsened.*

Vierling J: Primary biliary cirrhosis. In Zakim D, Boyer TD (eds.): Hepatology: A Textbook of Liver Disease. 2nd ed. Philadelphia, W. B. Saunders Company, 1990, pp 1158–1205. *An up-to-date review of the pathogenesis, diagnosis, and treatment of primary biliary cirrhosis.*

SECONDARY BILIARY CIRRHOSIS

DEFINITION, ETIOLOGY, AND PATHOLOGY. Secondary biliary cirrhosis is an uncommon sequela of longstanding obstruction of the biliary tree. Obstruction is usually present for more than 1 year (mean of about 6 years) before cirrhosis develops; however, intervals as short as 4 months from the onset of obstruction (jaundice) to the diagnosis of cirrhosis have been reported. Cirrhosis or fibrosis may also develop in the absence of jaundice in patients with prolonged partial biliary tract obstruction, as may be seen in chronic pancreatitis. In adults, obstruction is due most commonly to gallstones, strictures, carcinoma, chronic pancreatitis, or sclerosing cholangitis. In children, biliary atresia and cystic fibrosis are common causes of secondary biliary cirrhosis.

The liver is usually enlarged and dark green. The surface is granular or occasionally nodular. The lobular pattern is usually preserved until the cirrhosis is advanced. The portal tracts are widened owing to fibrosis and proliferation of bile ducts. The hepatic parenchyma may contain bile plugs, infarcts, or lakes. There is focal hepatocellular necrosis. As the cirrhosis progresses, the fibrous septa extend into the hepatic parenchyma, forming pseudolobules. In advanced cirrhosis, there is nodular regeneration.

CLINICAL MANIFESTATIONS. *Jaundice* is common but not invariable, and the level of jaundice may fluctuate. Patients with strictures or stones may have suffered recurrent bouts of cholangitis or biliary colic. *Pruritus* is also a common complaint and may precede the onset of icterus. If the pruritus is severe, itching may lead to thickening and darkening of the skin. Xanthelasma and xanthomas may appear. *Steatorrhea* with diarrhea may be a major complaint, and *bone disease* may develop owing to malabsorption of vitamin D and calcium. Splenomegaly is common. Ascites and gastrointestinal bleeding develop later in the course of the disease and are uncommon presenting complaints.

LABORATORY TESTS. The serum bilirubin is usually moderately increased (3 to 15 mg per deciliter). The alkaline phosphatase is also almost always increased; however, in 25 to 30 per cent, the elevation is less than twice normal. The AST is usually elevated, but the elevations are moderate. The prothrombin time may be prolonged and may improve with vitamin K administration. Hypoalbuminemia and hyperglobulinemia may also be present. Serum cholesterol and bile acids are frequently increased. *Lipoprotein X*, an abnormal lipoprotein, is found commonly in patients with extrahepatic obstruction (see Ch. 116). Lipoprotein X is also present in other forms of liver disease, and its absence does not exclude extrahepatic obstruction. Elevations of the white blood cell count in patients with extrahepatic obstruction suggest the presence of cholangitis or a hepatic abscess.

THERAPY AND PROGNOSIS. Relief of the biliary obstruction is the only specific form of treatment. In patients in whom the obstruction cannot be relieved, the correction of vitamin deficiencies and the use of cholestyramine to relieve itching, as outlined for the treatment of primary biliary cirrhosis, is warranted. In addition, there may be recurrent episodes of cholangitis requiring antibiotic treatment. Liver transplantation is an excellent option for patients with benign diseases such as sclerosing cholangitis and biliary atresia.

The prognosis for patients with carcinoma is poor, with most dying because of the malignancy and not because of the liver disease. The mortality for patients with benign obstructions (stone or stricture) depends on whether or not the obstruction can be relieved. When the obstruction cannot be relieved, mortality is high; however, survival may be prolonged (years) before the patient dies from hepatic failure or bleeding esophageal varices. Surgical relief of the biliary obstruction improves survival, although ascites and esophageal varices may develop later. The development of these complications, usually many years after apparently successful surgery, may be due to subclinical recurrence of partial biliary obstruction.

Littenberg G, Afroudakis A, Kaplowitz N: Common bile duct stenosis from chronic pancreatitis: Clinical and pathologic spectrum. Medicine 58:385, 1979. *Reviews the effects on the liver of biliary obstruction secondary to chronic pancreatitis.*

CRYPTOGENIC CIRRHOSIS

DEFINITION AND ETIOLOGY. Cryptogenic (macronodular or postnecrotic) cirrhosis is any cirrhosis for which the etiology is unknown. The liver contains little or no necrosis or inflammation and has no diagnostic pathologic lesions (for example, alcoholic hepatitis). It lacks any specific lesions demonstrable by histochemical stains, e.g., α_1-antitrypsin or iron; and specific serologic tests, e.g., HBsAg, anti-HBc, AMA, and ceruloplasmin, are normal. It is assumed that most cases represent the end stage of a previously active, chronic, or recurrent hepatitis, but alcoholic and other chronic liver diseases give rise to a very similar form of coarsely nodular cirrhosis. At least half of patients with cryptogenic cirrhosis have antibodies against the recently identified hepatitis C virus, and it may be that the development of cirrhosis in these patients is due to chronic infection with this virus. Cryptogenic cirrhosis should become a less frequent diagnosis as our understanding of the causes of liver disease increases and we develop tests for agents such as the hepatitis C virus.

PATHOLOGY. The size of the liver is variable and its surface distorted by large regenerative nodules (macronodular), which may be several centimeters in diameter. The liver between the nodules appears to be collapsed and fibrotic. The microscopic appearance of the liver is one of regenerative nodules separated by connective tissue. The portal areas may be infiltrated by mononuclear cells, but the liver cells are well preserved, and active hepatocellular necrosis or hepatic steatosis is minimal or absent.

CLINICAL MANIFESTATIONS. Cryptogenic cirrhosis may remain clinically silent for many years and frequently is discovered unexpectedly, often during the evaluation of an unrelated condition. When the disease becomes "clinically manifest," its signs and symptoms are usually nonspecific (malaise, lethargy) or related to portal hypertension and include ascites, splenomegaly, hypersplenism, or bleeding esophageal varices. The liver frequently is of normal size or small. Splenomegaly is common; spider angiomas, ascites, and abdominal wall venous collaterals may also be present. Serum transaminases and bilirubin are usually normal to slightly increased. Hyperglobulinemia is common and may be the only laboratory abnormality.

DIAGNOSIS. Cryptogenic cirrhosis is a diagnosis of exclusion and is based on histologic and clinical evidence of cirrhosis in the absence of a definable etiology (see Table 122–1). Wilson's disease and hemochromatosis are specifically treatable and should therefore be carefully excluded (see Ch. 192 and 193). Hepatitis B and C should be excluded by appropriate serologic tests. A small number of patients with cryptogenic cirrhosis may have chronic hepatitis B infection despite the absence in the serum of detectable levels of HB$_s$Ag. Measurement of anti-HB$_c$ may be helpful in identifying these patients. Testing for antimitochondrial antibodies, ANA, and an LE preparation helps exclude primary biliary cirrhosis and chronic active hepatitis. Alpha$_1$-antitrypsin deficiency may be excluded by appropriate histochemical stains and serologic tests (see Ch. 121). Findings of hepatic congestion on biopsy may be indicative of occult cardiac disease or hepatic vein occlusion. A previous history of alcoholism may be the only evidence for alcohol as the cause of the cirrhosis.

TREATMENT AND PROGNOSIS. Specific therapy for this type of cirrhosis is lacking. Complications such as ascites, encephalopathy, and gastrointestinal bleeding should be managed as discussed in Ch. 110, 111, and 123. Patients who have asymptomatic cirrhosis may do quite well with a good 5-year prognosis; however, the onset of ascites or bleeding esophageal varices is a poor prognostic sign.

Bruix J, Barrera J, Calvet X, et al.: Prevalence of antibodies to hepatitis C virus in Spanish patients with hepatocellular carcinoma and hepatic cirrhosis. Lancet

CARDIAC CIRRHOSIS

ETIOLOGY. Cardiac cirrhosis is an uncommon complication of severe, prolonged, recurrent right heart failure of any cause, although it is usually due to rheumatic heart disease (mitral or aortic stenosis with tricuspid regurgitation), cardiomyopathy, or constrictive pericarditis.

PATHOLOGY. The gross appearance of the liver in acute hepatic failure is one of alternating red and pale areas (nutmeg liver). The red areas are congested central areas of the hepatic lobule, whereas the pale areas are the preserved hepatocytes. With recurrent bouts of heart failure, the centrilobular hepatocytes atrophy and fibrosis develops. The fibrosis is most marked in the central areas, and with time fibrous septa extend out into the rest of the lobule. Regenerative nodules develop later, and they arise from the periphery of the hepatic lobule.

CLINICAL MANIFESTATIONS, DIAGNOSIS, AND THERAPY. The clinical picture is usually dominated by the cardiac disease. Differentiation of patients with acute hepatic congestion from those with cardiac cirrhosis is difficult, as the clinical features are similar (see Ch. 121). The liver may be small or enlarged and firm. When tricuspid regurgitation is present, the absence of hepatic pulsation suggests cirrhosis. Ascites and splenomegaly are common. The bilirubin is usually only mildly increased, and either the unconjugated or conjugated pigment may predominate. The AST is often moderately elevated but may be normal if the heart failure is controlled. The prothrombin time may be prolonged, and in the presence of significant liver disease coumarin anticoagulants should be used with caution. The diagnosis of cardiac cirrhosis is established by performing a liver biopsy. However, in most situations, this is not warranted.

Reduction in the incidence of rheumatic fever and tuberculosis as well as advances in cardiovascular surgery in the Western world have made cardiac cirrhosis an uncommon disease. Its prognosis depends largely upon the course of the cardiac disease. If the latter can be successfully treated, hepatic function improves and liver disease stabilizes.

Cello JP, Grendell J: The liver in systemic conditions. *In* Zakim D, Boyer TD (eds.): Hepatology: A Textbook of Liver Disease. 2nd ed. Philadelphia, W. B. Saunders Company, 1990, pp 1415–1422. *A portion of this chapter reviews the effects of acute and chronic heart failure on the liver.*

MAJOR SEQUELAE OF CIRRHOSIS

The major sequelae of cirrhosis are summarized in Table 122–3. Portal hypertension, bleeding esophageal and gastric varices, ascites, and the hepatorenal syndrome are discussed here. Liver failure, portosystemic encephalopathy, hepatocellular carcinoma, and hypersplenism are discussed elsewhere (Ch. 123 and 125).

Portal Hypertension

ANATOMY AND PHYSIOLOGY OF PORTAL VENOUS SYSTEM. The portal venous system begins in the capillaries of the intestines and terminates in the hepatic sinusoids. The portal vein is formed by the confluence of the superior and inferior mesenteric veins and splenic vein.

The liver receives about 1500 ml of blood each minute, two thirds of which is provided by the portal vein. The hepatic artery provides 40 to 60 per cent of the oxygen supply to the liver. The liver offers little resistance to the flow of blood, and the pressure within the sinusoids is low (less than 5 mm Hg above the pressure in the inferior vena cava). Since the veins in the portal system lack valves, increased resistance to flow at any point between the splanchnic venules and the heart increases pressure in all vessels on the intestinal side of the obstruction.

DEFINITION AND PATHOGENESIS. Portal hypertension represents an increase in the hydrostatic pressure within the portal vein or its tributaries. This is manifested clinically by the development of *portal-systemic collaterals, splenomegaly,* and/or *ascites.* Since portal hypertension may be present in the absence of clinical findings, it may be detectable only by measurement of pressures in the portal system. Pressures within the hepatic sinusoids may be measured by catheterizing the hepatic veins (wedged hepatic vein pressure), or the portal vein pressure may be measured directly by transhepatic or umbilical vein catheterization or at surgery. Portal hypertension is present when the wedged hepatic vein pressure is more than 5 mm Hg higher than the inferior vena cava pressure. Although generally considered to be a progressive disorder, portal hypertension may in fact decrease as the liver disease improves, i.e., alcoholic hepatitis. Portal hypertension also can be an acute and transient phenomenon, as may occur with acute right heart failure. Since the pressure in any vascular system is directly proportional not only to resistance but also to flow, portal hypertension may result from either increased blood flow in the portal vein or increased resistance to flow within the portal venous system.

Increased portal venous blood flow is an unusual cause of portal hypertension for two reasons: (1) Increases in portal vein flow cause a reflex decrease in hepatic artery blood flow, thereby tending to maintain relatively normal sinusoidal pressure. (2) The outflow resistance from the liver is so low that increases in portal vein flow must be very large to cause a significant increase in portal venous pressure.

Increased resistance to venous flow is the most common mechanism for the development of portal hypertension. Liver disease accounts for the majority of cases; however, occlusion of the portal or hepatic veins and cardiac disease also cause increased resistance to flow and increases in portal pressure. The diseases causing portal hypertension are listed in Table 122–4 and are discussed below.

CLINICAL MANIFESTATIONS. The clinical presentation of portal hypertension depends to a certain extent upon its cause. Essentially all forms may present with either *bleeding esophageal varices* or *splenomegaly* with or without *hypersplenism*. In portal vein thrombosis, as the liver is normal, ascites and jaundice are unusual. *Ascites* and other signs of hepatic disease (jaundice, spiders, encephalopathy) are common clinical features of cirrhosis. Occlusion of the hepatic veins almost always leads to development of ascites and varying degrees of hepatic dysfunction. Thus, the clinical findings may be important clues to the cause of the portal hypertension.

The development of portal-systemic collaterals is the major complication of portal hypertension. Several vessels may form collaterals. The veins that lie in the mucosa of the gastric fundus and esophagus are of greatest clinical interest because, when

TABLE 122–3. MAJOR SEQUELAE OF CIRRHOSIS

1. Portal hypertension
   a. Bleeding esophageal and gastric varices
   b. Splenomegaly and hypersplenism (Ch. 152)
   c. Ascites
   d. Spontaneous bacterial peritonitis
2. Hepatorenal syndrome
3. Liver failure (Ch. 123)
4. Portosystemic (hepatic) encephalopathy (Ch. 123)
5. Hepatocellular carcinoma (Ch. 125)

TABLE 122–4. CAUSES OF PORTAL HYPERTENSION

I. Increased resistance to flow
    Liver diseases
        Cirrhosis—all causes
        Congenital hepatic fibrosis
        Schistosomiasis
        Idiopathic portal hypertension
        Sarcoidosis
        Alcoholic hepatitis
        Partial nodular transformation
    Diseases of cardiovascular system
        Portal vein occlusion
        Splenic vein occlusion
        Hepatic vein occlusion
        Veno-occlusive disease
        Web lesion or thrombosis of inferior vena cava
        Congestive heart failure—constrictive pericarditis
II. Increased portal blood flow
    Splenomegaly not due to liver disease
    Arteriovenous fistula

dilated, they form gastric and esophageal varices (Fig. 122–1 and Color Plate 1A and B). The remnant of the umbilical vein may also dilate. If flow through this vessel becomes great enough, a loud venous hum may be audible over the path of the umbilical vein (Cruveilhier-Baumgarten syndrome). The umbilical vein enters the left portal vein, and therefore, if a venous hum is present, the cause of the portal hypertension must be intrahepatic or in the hepatic veins or inferior vena cava. Large collaterals also may form between the splenic and renal (chiefly left) veins. Dilated abdominal wall veins are common in patients with portal hypertension and are especially prominent when the patient stands. The hemorrhoidal veins may also act as collaterals. Varices may also form in unusual locations within the intestines (e.g., ileostomies, upper small bowel, and ascending, descending, and sigmoid colons), and these may bleed.

DISEASES CAUSING PORTAL HYPERTENSION (see Table 122–4). *Arteriovenous fistulas* may form between an artery and the portal vein or one of its tributaries as a consequence of abdominal trauma, liver biopsy, carcinoma (either intrahepatic or extrahepatic), or rupture of an arterial aneurysm (e.g., splenic). An upper abdominal bruit or a palpable thrill at surgery suggests this diagnosis in any patient with portal hypertension. The fistula can be localized by celiac angiography and is usually surgically correctable.

Splenomegaly resulting from hematologic diseases such as polycythemia rubra vera and myelofibrosis or an infiltrative process such as Gaucher's disease may, in rare instances, lead to portal hypertension. The enlarged spleen receives high blood flow from the splenic artery, leading to high flow within the splenic vein which is thought to cause the rise in portal pressure. These diseases also frequently involve the liver, and the infiltrative process may increase intrahepatic resistance. However, the principal event in the genesis of the portal hypertension appears to be the high portal vein blood flow, since splenectomy usually cures the portal hypertension.

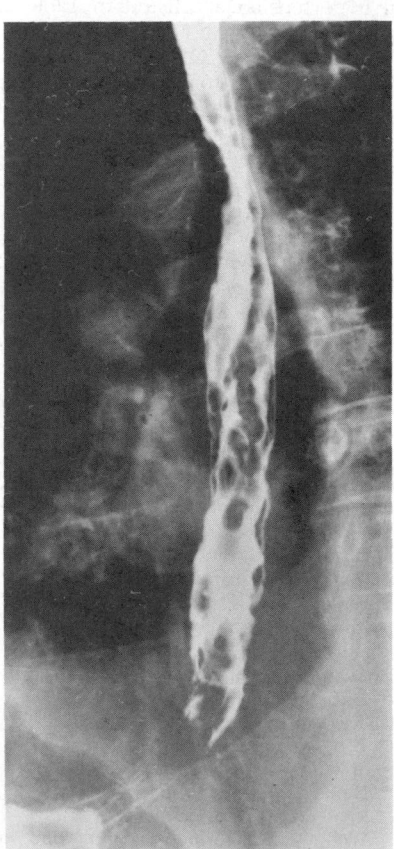

FIGURE 122–1. Barium esophagogram, demonstrating large varices involving the lower two thirds of the esophagus. (Courtesy of T. Munyer. *From* Zakim D, Boyer TD [eds.]: Hepatology: A Textbook of Liver Diseases, 2nd ed. Philadelphia, W. B. Saunders Company, 1990.)

Splenic vein thrombosis may be caused by pancreatitis, abdominal trauma, or a locally invasive tumor. Pressure is increased only in areas drained by the splenic vein, whereas pressure in the portal vein is normal. The diagnosis should be suspected in a patient with gastric or esophageal varices but a normal liver biopsy and is established by celiac angiography. Splenectomy is curative.

Portal vein thrombosis may develop following abdominal trauma or intra-abdominal sepsis, or in association with cirrhosis or hepatocellular carcinoma. In the majority of cases, however, the cause is unknown. This is primarily a disease of children, although adults may also develop portal vein thrombosis. The diagnosis again is suggested by the presence of portal hypertension in a patient with a normal liver biopsy. The diagnosis is established by angiography. Thrombi also may be identified by ultrasonography or CT scan. The surgical management of these patients may be difficult because of the absence of a patent vein to use for making a portal-systemic shunt.

Thrombosis of the hepatic veins (Budd-Chiari syndrome) may follow abdominal trauma or the use of birth control pills or may occur in patients with diseases such as polycythemia rubra vera, myeloproliferative disorders, and paroxysmal nocturnal hemoglobinuria, which have an associated hypercoagulable state. Patients with hepatic vein thrombosis may develop an acute, subacute, or chronic illness in which abdominal pain and ascites are the major features. The liver is usually enlarged and tender. Elevations of the serum transaminases and bilirubin are usually mild, although they can be increased significantly in patients who have an acute illness. The initial clinical diagnosis is usually cirrhosis, and the correct diagnosis is not suspected until centrilobular congestion is seen on liver biopsy. Catheterization of the inferior vena cava and hepatic veins is a useful test in the evaluation of this condition. The presence of thrombi in the inferior vena cava can be established. The diagnosis of hepatic vein thrombosis is made by finding the characteristic pathology on liver biopsy, excluding cardiac disease that causes a similar histologic lesion, and inability to catheterize the hepatic veins. The outlook for patients with hepatic vein thrombosis is poor, with mortality of 50 to 90 per cent. The use of side-to-side portacaval shunts in these patients has been thought to prolong survival. Further experience is required before the proper role of this procedure can be evaluated. The use of anticoagulants has not been shown to affect survival. Liver transplantation is an effective therapy, but anticoagulation is required to prevent recurrent hepatic vein thrombosis.

Veno-occlusive disease (nonthrombotic occlusion of hepatic venules) also causes a Budd-Chiari–like syndrome. Veno-occlusive disease develops in patients who have ingested plants containing pyrrolidizine alkaloids, who have been treated for malignant disease with certain chemotherapeutic agents, or following bone marrow transplantation. It also is a common pathologic finding in patients with alcoholic hepatitis and cirrhosis. The disease is thought to be due to a toxic injury to the endothelium of the affected vessels. The occluded venules may be present in a liver biopsy, and an abnormal vascular pattern is found when contrast material is injected into the hepatic veins.

Thrombi, tumor, or a membrane in the inferior vena cava may obstruct the hepatic veins and give a clinical picture similar to that of hepatic vein thrombosis, with the additional features of peripheral edema and stasis dermatitis. Membranous obstruction near the terminus of the inferior vena cava has been described in all areas of the world but is most frequently observed in South Africa and Asia. These patients also have a high incidence of hepatocellular carcinoma. The reasons for this latter association are unclear. Catheterization of the inferior vena cava identifies the obstructing lesion. Removal of the membrane surgically is sometimes possible and leads to resolution of the portal hypertension. Thrombectomy is usually not helpful.

Cirrhosis causes portal hypertension by increasing the intrahepatic vascular resistance. The increased resistance is thought to occur because of compression of vessels by regenerative nodules, distortion and reduction of the sinusoidal bed, and narrowing of portal vessels by the fibrous tissue. In alcoholic liver disease, serious portal hypertension may develop without cirrhosis. In some patients with acute alcoholic hepatitis, there is progressive obliteration of the central veins with resultant centrilobular fibrosis. These patients develop a severe outflow block, which leads to the formation of ascites or esophageal varices.

Portal hypertension due to noncirrhotic portal fibrosis may occur in four conditions. In *schistosomiasis*, the adult worm resides in the intestinal venules. The eggs are shed into these vessels and are swept into the portal vein and into the liver, where they lodge in and obstruct the portal venules. The host's immune response to the eggs leads to periportal fibrosis and the development of portal hypertension. (Schistosomiasis is discussed more fully in Ch. 434). *Idiopathic portal hypertension* (Banti's syndrome) is a disease in which there is portal hypertension, no cirrhosis, and a patent portal vein. The liver biopsy may be normal, or there may be fibrosis in the periportal areas and in the space of Disse. The disease process is progressive, with the liver eventually becoming small and fibrotic. A similar clinical picture may be seen in patients exposed to arsenic, vinyl chloride, and copper salts. *Congenital hepatic fibrosis* also causes portal hypertension without cirrhosis. In the portal areas, there is marked hyperplasia of the bile ducts and stellate fibrosis. This condition may be present in association with cystic liver disease and Caroli's disease (intrahepatic ductal ectasia), with an associated polycystic renal lesion in many patients. The development of portal hypertension is the major consequence of this form of liver disease, as hepatic function is well maintained. Hepatic *sarcoidosis* may rarely lead to hepatic fibrosis and portal hypertension.

DIAGNOSTIC APPROACH TO PORTAL HYPERTENSION. Portal hypertension should be suspected in any patient with ascites or splenomegaly, and its presence is established when portal-systemic collaterals are found. One may find collaterals on physical examination (dilated abdominal wall or umbilical veins), or they may be identified in the esophagus or stomach by a gastrointestinal series or by endoscopy. It is important that the etiology of portal hypertension be identified, since some causes (splenic vein thrombosis) may be curable. A liver biopsy will provide useful information as to the presence of liver disease; central venous congestion suggests hepatic vein thrombosis or cardiac disease. If the biopsy is not diagnostic, then catheterization of the hepatic veins may be performed. Elevated pressure establishes the presence of liver disease. Also, inferior vena cava or hepatic vein thrombosis may be found during catheterization of the hepatic veins. If the wedge pressure and right atrial pressure are normal, then the cause of the portal hypertension is (1) occlusion of the portal vein or its tributaries, (2) liver disease that involves the periportal areas and portal venules (schistosomiasis or idiopathic portal hypertension) and therefore does not increase the wedge pressure, or (3) increased flow in the portal vein. Celiac angiography usually differentiates among this group of patients. Ultrasonography or CT also may be used to identify thrombi in the portal vein.

Bleeding Esophageal and Gastric Varices

PATHOGENESIS. Hemorrhage from esophageal varices is a major complication of portal hypertension. The mortality in adult patients with cirrhosis varies from 30 to 60 per cent for each bleeding episode. The varices form because of increased pressure in the portal vein. Bleeding from varices may occur when the portal pressure exceeds 11 to 12 mm Hg above inferior vena cava pressure. However, not all patients with pressures above these levels have bleeding varices. The tension on the vessel wall is greater in large than in small varices for a given level of pressure. Therefore, large varices are more likely to rupture and bleed than are smaller ones; reflux esophagitis and ascites do not appear to be important in the genesis of bleeding.

CLINICAL MANIFESTATIONS. The most common presentation is hematemesis. The bleeding may be massive with the rapid development of shock, or the bleeding may stop spontaneously only to recur later. On occasion, the patient may only complain of hematochezia or melena without an antecedent history of hematemesis. Features suggesting underlying liver disease such as hepatomegaly, ascites, or jaundice may be present or absent, depending on the etiology of the portal hypertension and the activity of the underlying hepatic disease.

DIAGNOSIS AND TREATMENT. The care of the patient with gastrointestinal bleeding is discussed in detail in Ch. 111. The restoration of the patient's blood volume takes precedence

over all other therapy and diagnostic tests. The blood volume should be corrected rapidly but not excessively, since overexpansion may lead to the development of ascites or renewed bleeding. Proof that esophageal or gastric varices are the source of hemorrhage depends on endoscopy, since, even in those with known varices, 30 to 50 per cent are bleeding from other lesions (especially gastritis).

The bleeding from varices in many patients stops without any specific therapy. The *medical management* of patients who continue to bleed includes *vasopressin, endoscopic sclerosis of varices,* and *balloon tamponade.* Long-term therapy with *propranolol* for the prevention of variceal hemorrhage is controversial and cannot be recommended.

Vasopressin, a potent vasoconstrictor, is believed to act by constricting the splanchnic arterioles, which results in a fall in portal flow and thus a drop in portal pressure. This drug should be given only to patients who can be carefully monitored, preferably in an intensive care unit. Vasopressin is infused into a peripheral vein at a rate of 0.2 to 0.4 unit per minute. This therapy provides temporary control in about 60 per cent of patients. Unfortunately, about half of those initially controlled have rebleeding, and the use of vasopressin has little effect on morbidity or mortality. The intravenous use of somatostatin or combined use of vasopressin and nitroglycerin may be as effective as vasopressin alone in controlling variceal hemorrhage, with fewer side effects. The gastric and esophageal varices lie in the mucosa of the gastric fundus and esophagus and are therefore susceptible to *balloon tamponade.* Tamponade is best accomplished by inserting a tube that has a gastric balloon with or without an esophageal balloon (Sengstaken-Blakemore tube). Once placed in the stomach, the gastric balloon is inflated and pulled into the cardia of the stomach, tamponading the varices. If bleeding does not stop, then the esophageal balloon is inflated. This therapy is effective in controlling hemorrhage in 70 to 90 per cent of patients. There is a significant risk of aspiration during balloon tamponade, and 50 to 60 per cent of the patients hemorrhage again. During endoscopy, the *direct injection of esophageal varices* with sclerosing agents has been described as a method for the control of acute bleeding and for the long-term management of these patients. Repeated injections over several weeks are required to obliterate the varices, and rebleeding during this period is common. Once they are obliterated the rate of rebleeding from the varices is reduced, and survival may be improved. Endoscopic sclerotherapy is associated with serious side effects (esophageal ulcers and strictures, pleural effusions), but it is an important form of therapy for the management of recurrent bleeding esophageal varices.

In *surgical therapy* for portal hypertension the high-pressure portal system is anastomosed to the low-pressure systemic venous system to create a *portal-systemic shunt.* There are two basic types of shunts. One is *nonselective,* in that the entire portal-venous system is decompressed. The end-to-side and side-to-side portacaval and mesocaval shunts are nonselective. *Selective* shunts decompress only the varices. The pressure remains high in the portal vein, and portal flow into the liver is preserved. Thus the varices are decompressed with minimal disruption of the normal hepatic circulation. The distal splenorenal shunt is of this type. The selective shunt may cause less encephalopathy than the nonselective types of shunts without improving survival.

Portal-systemic shunts have been used in four clinical situations: (1) *Hypersplenism* is not an indication for a portal-systemic shunt, because the reduction in formed elements in the blood is usually not of clinical significance. (2) The *prophylactic shunt* is made in patients with cirrhosis and varices who have never bled. Prophylactic shunts shorten survival compared to unoperated controls, with death from hepatic encephalopathy and liver failure. Thus prophylactic shunts should not be performed. (3) *Emergency shunts* may be used to control hemorrhage in actively bleeding patients. However, the operative mortality may exceed 50 per cent, so that emergency shunts should be used rarely and in a select group of patients. The indications for this operation are still controversial. (4) *Therapeutic portal-systemic shunts* are used in patients who have bled at least once from varices. Operations in these patients have been shown to effectively stop further bleeding from varices. Unfortunately, the patient's survival is not improved significantly because of an increased incidence of hepatic encephalopathy and liver failure when compared to unoperated controls. Possibly these results could be improved by better selection of patients for the operations. As might be expected, the majority of patients with poor hepatocellular function, i.e., those who are jaundiced with hypoalbuminemia, ascites, encephalopathy, and poor nutrition, tolerate a portal-systemic shunt less well than do patients without these complications of liver disease. Patients with more severe liver disease may well be better managed by sclerosis of their varices or liver transplantation than by shunt operations. The choice of therapy (sclerosis or shunt) for bleeding varices in patients with well-compensated cirrhosis is controversial. The morbidity and mortality from bleeding esophageal varices will remain high until current therapies are refined and new ones developed.

Bass NM: Preventing variceal hemorrhage. N Engl J Med 317:893, 1987. *An editorial that reviews the controversy of the effectiveness of β-blockers in preventing variceal hemorrhage.*

Boyer TD: Portal hypertension and bleeding esophageal varices. *In* Zakim D, Boyer TD (eds.): Hepatology: A Textbook of Liver Disease. 2nd ed. Philadelphia, W. B. Saunders Company, 1990, pp 572–615. *A current review of portal hypertension and treatment of bleeding varices.*

de Franchis R, et al.: Prediction of the first variceal hemorrhage in patients with cirrhosis of liver and esophageal varices. N Engl J Med 319:983, 1988. *Patients at greatest risk of hemorrhage had poor hepatic function and large varices.*

Groszman RJ (ed): Portal hypertension: Circulatory and renal abnormalities. Semin Liver Dis 6:277, 1986. *Contains a number of excellent articles on the portal circulation and the changes in portal hemodynamics that occur with liver disease.*

Smith JL, Graham D: Variceal hemorrhage: A critical evaluation of survival analysis. Gastroenterology 82:968, 1983. *A careful evaluation of survival following an episode of hemorrhage from varices.*

Ascites

DEFINITION. Ascites is the presence of excess fluid in the peritoneal cavity. It is most frequently due to cirrhosis, but there are numerous other causes (see Ch. 110), and it cannot be assumed that the appearance of ascites is indicative of cirrhosis. For this reason, patients with a recent onset of ascites must be thoroughly evaluated to establish its cause.

PATHOGENESIS (Table 122–5). Ascites forms in patients with portal hypertension because of changes in the formation and reabsorption of hepatic and splanchnic lymph and because of alterations in the metabolism of salt and water by the kidneys.

Splanchnic Lymph Formation. Increases in portal venous pressure cause a rise in the pressure within the splanchnic capillaries, resulting in loss of fluid into the interstitial space. The capillaries of the intestine restrict the loss of protein to the interstitial space, and an oncotic gradient develops between the capillary and the extravascular space. This oncotic gradient returns the majority of the fluid to capillary, and any fluid loss is usually removed by the intestinal lymphatics. For this reason, diseases that elevate the pressure only in the splanchnic bed, e.g., portal vein thrombosis, cause ascites uncommonly.

Hepatic Lymph Formation. In the noncirrhotic liver the endothelial lining of the hepatic sinusoids is discontinuous and does not effectively restrict plasma protein loss with even slight increases in sinusoidal pressure. Thus, in contrast to the intestines, the oncotic gradient between the sinusoids and extravascular space is small, and much of the fluid entering the interstitial space is not returned to the vascular space. These large amounts of fluid lost into the interstitial space must be returned to the

TABLE 122–5. FACTORS IN THE PATHOGENESIS OF CIRRHOTIC ASCITES

1. Increased hydrostatic pressure in hepatic sinusoids and splanchnic capillaries.
2. Overproduction of hepatic and splanchnic lymph secondary to (1), leading to a transudation of lymph into peritoneal space.
3. Limited or reduced reabsorption of water and protein by peritoneal lymphatics.
4. Sodium retention by the kidney secondary to hyperaldosteronism, increased sympathetic activity, alterations in metabolism of prostaglandins and kinins, and altered renal hemodynamics.
5. Impaired renal water excretion, in part caused by increased levels of ADH.

vascular space via hepatic lymphatics. When the rate of formation of lymph exceeds the rate of removal, then fluid "weeps" out of the lymphatics and into the peritoneal cavity. Diseases that cause marked elevations of the sinusoidal pressure in an otherwise normal liver, e.g., congestive heart failure and hepatic vein thrombosis, therefore commonly cause ascites. With cirrhosis the situation is more complex in that there is "capillarization" of the sinusoids such that an oncotic gradient forms between plasma and lymph. Large amounts of lymph are formed by the cirrhotic liver with overflow into the peritoneal space; however, the protein content of this fluid is low.

Peritoneal Reabsorption. The peritoneum plays an active role in the reabsorption of the ascitic fluid. Water and protein are reabsorbed by the lymphatics in the peritoneal membrane. The intra-abdominal pressure and character of the peritoneum are important factors in determining the rate of ascitic fluid removal. The amount of fluid removed by the peritoneal lymphatics is variable but usually does not exceed 800 to 1000 ml every 24 hours.

Renal Function. An important factor in the genesis of ascites is the *retention of sodium* by the kidney. During the formation of ascites there is a positive sodium balance despite a total body sodium that is greater than normal. The pathogenesis of the sodium retention by the kidney is understood poorly; however, there is increased reabsorption of sodium by both proximal and distal tubules. The increased reabsorption of sodium may be mediated, in part, by increased plasma levels of aldosterone, increased sympathetic activity, and alterations in the renal production of prostaglandins and kinins. Reduced renal blood flow resulting from vasoconstriction also leads to enhanced sodium reabsorption.

CLINICAL MANIFESTATIONS AND DIAGNOSIS. Patients with ascites complain of increasing abdominal girth. The presence of ascites on physical examination is suggested by the findings of shifting dullness, a ballotable liver, or a fluid wave. Small amounts of ascites may be identified by abdominal ultrasonography. Once the presence of ascites is suspected, diagnostic paracentesis should be performed. The character of the ascitic fluid in cirrhosis is variable; however, 80 to 90 per cent of patients have an ascitic fluid protein concentration of less than 2.5 grams per deciliter. The ascitic fluid lactic dehydrogenase is low, and the difference between the serum and ascitic albumin exceeds 1.1 grams per deciliter. The ascitic fluid white blood cell count is less than 500 per cubic millimeter in 90 per cent of patients with cirrhosis, and mononuclear cells predominate (>75 per cent). Patients with cirrhosis who have high protein ascites and a low serum/ascites albumin difference or a high ascitic fluid white blood cell count require further evaluation.

MANAGEMENT. Resolution of the acute hepatic injury, following withdrawal of ethanol or a specific course of therapy, may reduce portal pressure, and ascites may resolve spontaneously. In many patients, however, ascites is chronic and specific therapy is warranted. Accumulation of ascitic fluid occurs only in patients who are in positive sodium balance; therefore, *restricting sodium intake* diminishes or stops the accumulation of ascitic fluid. Diets containing 250 to 500 mg of sodium (10 to 20 mEq) are adequate to achieve sodium balance in most patients. The kidney is also unable to excrete a water load normally in some patients with ascites, in part because of high blood levels of antidiuretic hormone. *Fluid restriction* (1000 to 1500 ml daily) is sometimes necessary, therefore, to prevent hyponatremia. Many patients do not lose their ascites or edema with sodium restriction, and the use of *diuretics* becomes necessary. Spironolactone, amiloride, and triamterene act on the distal tubule and cause natriuresis with sparing of potassium. Spironolactone, 150 to 400 mg daily, causes diuresis in patients with mild to moderate sodium retention and is used as initial therapy. Furosemide, thiazides, and ethacrynic acid are more potent diuretics and cause both natriuresis and potassium wasting. If the patient fails to respond to treatment with spironolactone, furosemide, 40 to 80 mg daily, is added to the diuretic regimen. All diuretics cause a loss of fluid from the plasma. This fluid is then replaced by the reabsorption of ascitic or edema fluid. The rate of fluid lost should therefore not exceed the rate at which the ascites and edema fluids may be reabsorbed. The maximal rate of reabsorption of ascitic fluid varies widely; however, fluid losses of 1 kg daily in patients with edema and ascites and 0.3 to 0.5 kg daily in those with only ascites are well tolerated. The BUN and electrolytes must be monitored for the development of azotemia and hypokalemia. The use of diets very low in sodium (250 to 500 mg) is possible in the hospital; however, this is rarely possible in an outpatient setting. Therefore, preceding discharge from the hospital, the patient's sodium intake should be increased (1 to 2 grams daily) and diuretics adjusted so that he or she is still in negative sodium balance.

A few patients with cirrhosis do not respond to diuretic therapy. It is important to establish that failure is not due to an inappropriately high sodium intake. This can be determined by measuring the urine sodium. If this value is high (greater than prescribed sodium intake), the patient's diet requires adjustment. Alternately, if the urine sodium is low and treatment in the hospital with increasing doses of diuretics leads to azotemia or hepatic encephalopathy, the patient is resistant to diuretic therapy. Repeated large-volume (4 to 5 liters) paracentesis in combination with an infusion of albumin (40 grams) to maintain plasma volume has been used to manage patients with cirrhotic ascites. Although relief of ascites is more rapid and complications fewer than are observed with diuretic therapy, survival and frequency of readmission to the hospital for recurrent ascites are unaffected. The use of repeated large-volume abdominal paracentesis should be limited to patients who are refractory to diuretic therapy or who require relief of tense ascites because of difficulty in breathing. If these refractory patients are incapacitated by the ascites, they may be candidates for other therapies. The *peritoneovenous (LeVeen) shunt* consists of a tube placed subcutaneously between the peritoneal cavity and the superior vena cava. There is a pressure-activated one-way valve that allows peritoneal fluid to enter the vascular space but prevents the backflow of blood into the tube. This shunt may be effective in controlling ascites; however, its use is associated with episodes of disseminated intravascular coagulation, sepsis, and frequent shunt thrombosis, thus limiting its application only to patients who have severe and incapacitating ascites. The shunt should not be used in patients whose condition can be managed by other therapies including repeated paracentesis. Attempts to increase the venous oncotic pressure by infusions of albumin or plasma are not likely to cause sustained diuresis and are an expensive form of therapy.

SPONTANEOUS BACTERIAL PERITONITIS. Patients with cirrhosis and ascites may develop spontaneous bacterial peritonitis without obvious cause, i.e., perforation of the bowel. Possibly peritonitis occurs because of bacterial seeding of the ascitic fluid via the lymph or blood or by bacteria traversing the bowel wall. The frequency of this complication in patients with ascites may be increasing, and its early recognition is essential (mortality exceeds 60 to 90 per cent even if treated). Patients with very low ascitic fluid protein levels (less than 1 gram per deciliter) appear to be at greater risk for developing peritonitis because of a low level of opsonic activity in the fluid. The clues to the diagnosis are the presence of fever, abdominal pain or tenderness, or decreased bowel sounds in a patient with ascites. The diagnosis should also be suspected in patients with the sudden onset of hepatic encephalopathy or hypotension. Patients may be asymptomatic and the diagnosis suggested only by finding an elevated ascitic fluid white blood cell count, or by a positive ascitic fluid culture. The diagnosis is established by abdominal paracentesis, which should be performed in patients with onset of new ascites or in those with a change in their clinical course. The ascitic fluid white blood cell count in peritonitis is usually above 500 per cubic millimeter (93 per cent of cases), and more than 50 per cent of the cells are polymorphonuclear leukocytes. The ascitic fluid pH also is lower than the blood pH. Bacteria may be identified on Gram's stain. The ascitic fluid and blood should be cultured and treatment instituted before the results of culture are known, as delays in therapy may increase mortality. The organisms most frequently cultured are Enterobacteriaceae (mainly *E. coli*) and Group D streptococci, *Streptococcus pneumoniae*, and *Streptococcus viridans*. Other bacteria are cultured less frequently, and anaerobic bacteria are uncommon isolates. Initial antibiotic therapy should therefore include both an aminoglycoside and ampicillin or a newer cephalosporin antibiotic such as cefotaxime. When using an aminoglycoside, blood levels of the drug must be obtained to minimize the risk of renal injury. The response to therapy is monitored by the fever pattern and by changes in the ascitic fluid leukocyte count. If therapy is effective, the ascitic fluid leukocyte count falls and the predominant cell again becomes mononuclear. Antibiotic therapy is continued for 7 to 10 days.

Hepatorenal Syndrome

DEFINITION AND PATHOGENESIS. The hepatorenal syndrome (functional renal failure) is a decrease in renal function that develops in a patient with serious liver disease in whom all other causes of renal dysfunction are excluded. The kidneys lack serious pathologic lesions. If the liver disease improves, normal renal function returns. The pathogenesis of the hepatorenal syndrome is unknown. There is intense intrarenal vasoconstriction and redistribution of blood flow. In addition, the plasma levels of renin, aldosterone, and prostaglandins are increased, and there is increased sympathetic activity. These changes may be due to reduced "effective" plasma volume in some patients.

CLINICAL MANIFESTATIONS. Patients developing the hepatorenal syndrome frequently have severe hepatic disease and therefore are jaundiced and have other signs and symptoms of liver disease. Almost all of the patients with this syndrome have ascites. The illness is marked by oliguria. The urine is usually free of protein, and the urine sediment is normal. The urine sodium level is low (<10 mEq per liter), the urine:plasma creatinine ratio is high (>30:1), and the urine:plasma osmolality ratio is greater than 1.0. These urine findings are different from those of acute tubular necrosis, in which the urine sodium content is high (>30 mEq per liter), the urine:plasma creatinine ratio is low (<20:1), and the urine is isosmotic to plasma. The progression of the renal failure is variable, with some patients having a complete loss of renal function over several days, whereas in others the serum creatinine slowly increases over several weeks as the liver function gradually worsens.

DIFFERENTIAL DIAGNOSIS (Ch. 76). Patients with liver disease may develop renal failure for a variety of reasons. These patients commonly receive diuretics and may develop prerenal azotemia. Renal function will improve with withdrawal of the medication. Acute tubular necrosis may occur following an episode of hypotension (bleeding or sepsis) or during fulminant hepatitis and can be distinguished from hepatorenal failure by the urine findings. Drugs (antibiotics, especially aminoglycosides, and nonsteroidal anti-inflammatory medications) may cause worsening of renal function in patients with cirrhosis. Acute pyelonephritis, with or without papillary necrosis, may also cause renal failure in patients with liver disease.

THERAPY AND PROGNOSIS. Specific causes of renal failure should be looked for and excluded. Any medications that are potential nephrotoxins should be withdrawn. A brief trial of plasma expansion with monitoring of urine output and serum creatinine may be attempted, to exclude hypovolemia as a cause of the renal failure. The volume of fluid infused should be limited (1000 ml), as overexpansion of the plasma volume may precipitate variceal hemorrhage. Infusions of vasodilators may transiently improve renal function; however, this does not improve survival. Uremia may be treated by dialysis; again, overall survival is not improved. The use of peritoneovenous shunts in these patients is being investigated, but their efficacy is as yet unproven. The prognosis for patients with the hepatorenal syndrome is poor, with over 90 per cent dying during hospitalization, usually from liver failure or complications of portal hypertension. Definitive therapies must await a better understanding of the pathogenesis of this syndrome.

Akriviadis EA, Runyon BA: Utility of an algorithm in differentiating spontaneous from secondary bacterial peritonitis. Gastroenterology 98:127, 1990. *Reviews the criteria used to diagnose spontaneous bacterial peritonitis and how to tell it from secondary bacterial peritonitis.*

Epstein M: Functional renal abnormalities in cirrhosis: Pathophysiology and management. *In* Zakim D, Boyer TD (eds.): Hepatology: A Textbook of Liver Disease. 2nd ed. Philadelphia, W. B. Saunders Company, 1990, pp 493–513. *A review of the renal abnormalities present in patients with cirrhotic ascites.*

Schrier RW: Pathogenesis of sodium and water retention in high-output and low-output cardiac failure, nephrotic syndrome, cirrhosis, and pregnancy. N Engl J Med 319:1127, 1988. *A brief discussion of some of the factors thought to be important in the formation of cirrhotic ascites.*

Tito L, Gines P, Arroyo V, et al.: Total paracentesis associated with intravenous albumin in management of patients with cirrhosis and ascites. Gastroenterology 98:146, 1990. *Describes the use of a single large-volume paracentesis to remove all of a patient's ascitic fluid. This therapy was associated with few side-effects and rapid relief of the ascites.*

Wright TL, Boyer TD: Diagnosis and management of cirrhotic ascites. *In* Zakim D, Boyer TD (eds.): Hepatology: A Textbook of Liver Disease. 2nd ed. Philadelphia, W. B. Saunders Company, 1990, pp 616–636. *Discusses the pathogenesis and treatment of cirrhotic ascites and spontaneous bacterial peritonitis.*

123 Acute and Chronic Hepatic Failure

Bruce F. Scharschmidt

This chapter begins with a discussion of hepatic encephalopathy, one of the most characteristic features of liver failure. This is followed by discussions of the approach to the patient with acute or chronic hepatic failure.

THE SYNDROME OF HEPATIC ENCEPHALOPATHY

DEFINITION AND SIGNIFICANCE. Hepatic encephalopathy (also called hepatic coma or portal-systemic encephalopathy) is a reversible neuropsychiatric syndrome which can accompany advanced, decompensated liver disease of all types and/or extensive portal-systemic shunting. Recognition of the signs and symptoms of encephalopathy represents an important clue to the presence of deteriorating liver function or superimposed complications. In addition, repeated neurologic evaluation of the encephalopathic patient provides valuable information regarding the patient's course and prognosis.

PATHOGENESIS. The pathogenesis of hepatic encephalopathy remains unclear, and possible mechanisms are outlined in Table 123–1. The encephalopathy is at least partially attributable to toxic materials that are derived from the metabolism of nitrogenous substrate in the gut and that bypass the liver through anatomic or functional shunts. This is the origin of the term *portal-systemic encephalopathy*, often used interchangeably with hepatic encephalopathy. *Ammonia* and *mercaptans* result from the degradation of urea or protein and sulfur-containing compounds, respectively, and both can produce coma when administered in large doses to animals. The presence of mercaptans in the breath of some encephalopathic patients probably accounts for the characteristic sweetish musty odor termed *fetor hepaticus*. While often present in increased amounts in the blood or cerebrospinal fluid or both, the absolute concentration of ammonia, ammonia metabolites including glutamine, and mercaptans correlates only roughly with the presence or severity of encephalopathy. *Gamma-aminobutyric acid* (GABA), the principal inhibitory neurotransmitter in the mammalian brain, is also produced in the gut and is present in increased amounts in the blood of patients and animals with hepatic failure. A role for GABA in hepatic encephalopathy is supported by the observation that visual evoked potentials in animals with hepatic failure mimic those produced by benzodiazepines or barbiturates, both of which act on the GABA receptor, but differ from those of comatose states caused by administration of ether, ammonia, or mercaptans. Moreover, recent studies suggest a beneficial effect of GABA receptor antagonists. Their use should still be regarded as experimental, however. A separate hypothesis holds that accelerated entry of *aromatic amino acids* into the central nervous system results in decreased synthesis of normal neurotransmitters such as norepinephrine and enhanced synthesis of *false neurotransmitters* such as octopamine. Other compounds such as short-chain *fatty acids* are also present in blood in increased amounts and have been proposed as potentially toxic. Finally, there is impaired integrity of the *blood-brain barrier* in animals with acute hepatic failure. It is possible that hepatic encephalopathy may represent the synergistic effects of a number of toxins acting on an unusually susceptible nervous system.

NEUROLOGIC MANIFESTATIONS. Patients with hepatic encephalopathy display a characteristic spectrum of mental and motor changes which are frequently divided into stages (Table 123–2). Although useful, individual variations occur, and many patients do not show an orderly progression of symptoms. Moreover, the clinical grading scale is relatively insensitive. Standardized testing has revealed psychomotor abnormalities in a high proportion of patients with cirrhosis in whom conventional neurologic examination is normal. Such *subclinical encephalopathy* is potentially important inasmuch as it may be associated with impaired functional capacity, including job performance and ability to drive an automobile.

In addition to the acute, reversible signs and symptoms already mentioned, rare patients with longstanding liver disease and portal-systemic shunting develop *irreversible neurologic dysfunction*. Acquired *hepatocerebral degeneration* is characterized by tremor, rigidity, dysarthria, oral-facial dyskinesia, choreoathetosis, and ataxic gait. *Myelopathy* is another rare manifestation of advanced chronic liver disease and portal-systemic shunting and may be manifested by spastic paraparesis, hyperreflexia, and incontinence.

As with other types of metabolic encephalopathy, asymmetric neurologic findings are unusual, and brain stem reflexes such as the pupillary light response, oculovestibular response, and oculocephalic response are typically preserved. Thus, asymmetric

TABLE 123–1. HEPATIC ENCEPHALOPATHY: PROPOSED PATHOGENIC MECHANISMS

Mechanism	Hypothesis	Evidence For	Evidence Against	Therapeutic Implications
Toxins (ammonia and mercaptans)	Produced by action of intestinal bacteria on urea, protein; decreased clearance from portal blood by diseased liver	Increased levels of these substances or their metabolites in blood, CSF; administration can produce coma	Poor correlation of plasma levels with encephalopathy; EEG changes produced by administration of these agents differ from those in hepatic encephalopathy	Oral administration of poorly absorbable antibiotics, lactulose
False neurotransmitters (increased brain octopamine and phenylephrine; decreased dopamine and norepinephrine)	Increased brain influx of aromatic amino acid precursors for false neurotransmitters	Increased ratio of plasma aromatic amino acids to branched-chain amino acids	Inconsistent findings regarding brain levels of neurotransmitters; lack of effect of false neurotransmitter administration on neurologic function	Administration of branched-chain amino acids (no consistent benefit in clinical trials)
Enhanced GABA (-ergic) neurotransmission	Decreased hepatic clearance of gut bacteria-derived GABA, which enters brain and inhibits neurotransmission	Increased plasma levels of GABA; increased brain entry of GABA-like substances; visual evoked responses in encephalopathy mimic those produced by GABA; increased brain GABA receptors	Inconsistent evidence regarding serum GABA levels and GABA receptor density in brain	Administration of poorly absorbable antibiotics; improved mental status with experimental use of GABA receptor antagonists

neurologic signs or abnormal brain stem reflexes may suggest a structural lesion of the central nervous system such as a subdural hematoma. Seizures are also uncommon in the absence of alcohol withdrawal and should alert the clinician to the possibility of a structural lesion or hypoglycemia. The disappearance of pupillary reactivity, of the oculocephalic or oculovestibular response, or of deep tendon reflexes is associated with a very poor prognosis in all types of metabolic encephalopathy, including hepatic encephalopathy (but excluding drug overdose). Electroencephalographic changes are sensitive indicators of hepatic encephalopathy, being present in most patients with subclinical disease (Table 123–2), but are not specific for this disorder. They include symmetric slowing observed initially over the frontal areas with later spreading laterally and posteriorly.

DIAGNOSIS. The diagnosis of hepatic encephalopathy is based upon the presence of compatible neurologic signs and symptoms in a patient with advanced liver disease and exclusion of other possible causes of the neurologic abnormalities. The diagnosis is most difficult when liver disease is not obvious. Routine laboratory studies, including electrolytes, calcium, blood urea nitrogen, creatinine, glucose, and standard liver function tests, are of help primarily in excluding other causes of metabolic encephalopathy and evaluating the presence and severity of hepatic disease. Toxicologic screening is also appropriate when ingestion of sedatives or toxins capable of altering neurologic function is suspected. Blood ammonia and cerebrospinal fluid levels of glutamine correlate only roughly with mental status and are therefore of limited value in most circumstances. Structural lesions such as a subdural hematoma are often a consideration and may require special radiologic studies. Other causes of encephalopathy such as the Wernicke-Korsakoff syndrome, sepsis, or meningitis must also be excluded, depending on the clinical circumstances.

TREATMENT. The management of patients with hepatic encephalopathy is largely supportive and has as its goals (1) improvement, when possible, of hepatic function, (2) prevention or correction of factors that may precipitate or aggravate encephalopathy (Table 123–3), and (3) decreasing the production of putative toxins that result from enteric bacterial metabolism of nitrogenous substrates. All nonessential drugs should be stopped—particularly sedatives and potentially hepatotoxic agents. For the occasional patient who demonstrates manic disorientation as an early manifestation of encephalopathy, soft restraints are preferable to sedative hypnotic agents.

Decreasing Production and Absorption of Enteric Toxins. Gut cleansing should be accomplished by enema, and oral administration of cathartics such as magnesium citrate is appropriate unless lactulose (see below) is administered. It is also generally appropriate to restrict dietary protein to about 40 grams per day in mildly encephalopathic patients and eliminate it in patients

TABLE 123–2. STAGES OF HEPATIC ENCEPHALOPATHY

Stage	Mental Status	Motor Changes
Subclinical	No changes on routine examination; may be associated with impaired work performance or driving ability	Impaired performance on standardized psychomotor tests or bedside tests such as figure drawing or number connection
I	Mild confusion, apathy, agitation, anxiety, euphoria, restlessness, sleep disorder	Fine tremor, slowed coordination, asterixis
II	Drowsiness, lethargy, disorientation, inappropriate behavior	Asterixis, dysarthria, primitive reflexes (suck and snout), ataxic paratonia
III	Somnolent but rousable, marked confusion, incomprehensible speech	Hyperreflexia, Babinski's sign, incontinence, myoclonus, hyperventilation
IV	Coma	Decerebrate posturing; brisk oculocephalic reflexes; response to painful stimuli present early; may progress to flaccidity and absence of response to stimuli

TABLE 123–3. HEPATIC ENCEPHALOPATHY—COMMON PRECIPITATING FACTORS

Deterioration in hepatic function
Drugs (sedative or potentially hepatotoxic agents)
Gastrointestinal hemorrhage
Increased dietary protein
Azotemia
Hypokalemia
Infection
Constipation
Anesthesia and surgery
Hypoxia
Diuretics (hypokalemia, alkalosis, and hypovolemia)

with more advanced or progressive encephalopathy. *Vegetable protein* appears somewhat less likely to induce encephalopathy than animal protein and may be useful in the long-term management of patients with chronic or recurrent encephalopathy. While oral or parenteral administration of *branched-chain amino acids* has been reported to be beneficial in the treatment of hepatic encephalopathy, controlled trials have not provided clear evidence of efficacy, and their use is not generally recommended (see Table 123–1).

In addition to these measures aimed at decreasing nitrogenous substrate, production of enteric toxins should be further inhibited by oral administration of a poorly absorbable antibiotic, such as neomycin in a dose of 1 to 2 grams every 6 hours, or by administration of lactulose. Lactulose is neither metabolized nor absorbed in the upper small bowel and is metabolized by ileal and colonic bacteria to organic acids. It is as effective as neomycin in lowering blood ammonia and reversing encephalopathy in patients with chronic liver disease. Because prolonged neomycin administration may produce ototoxicity or malabsorption, lactulose is preferable as chronic therapy. The mechanisms of action of lactulose may include increased bacterial assimilation of ammonia, decreased ammonia production, and possibly trapping of ammonia as NH_4^+ in the bowel lumen. Therapy is commonly initiated by administering 30 to 45 ml of the syrup orally every 2 hours until diarrhea ensues. Thereafter, the dose is decreased to that amount necessary to produce two to four soft stools per day. Lactulose can also be given by retention enema. Concomitant administration of neomycin and lactulose may be useful in selected patients.

FULMINANT HEPATIC FAILURE

DEFINITION. *Fulminant hepatic failure* is defined as hepatic failure with encephalopathy developing in less than 8 weeks in a patient without pre-existing liver disease. *Subacute* or *late-onset hepatic failure* refers to a slightly slower-paced illness, also occurring in patients without pre-existing disease, in whom the time from jaundice to onset of encephalopathy ranges from 8 weeks to 6 months.

ETIOLOGY. Among the various causes of hepatic failure (Table 123–4), acute viral hepatitis, particularly hepatitis B with or

TABLE 123–4. CAUSES OF FULMINANT HEPATIC FAILURE

Common	Uncommon
Viral hepatitis	Ischemia
A	Hepatic vein obstruction
B	Veno-occlusive disease
D (coinfection with B or superinfection)	Malignant infiltration
Non-A, non-B (presumed)	Wilson's disease
Drugs	Fatty liver of pregnancy
Necrosis: acetaminophen, halothane, isoniazid, methyldopa;	Reye's syndrome
Steatosis: tetracycline, valproate	Hyperthermia
Toxins	
Amanita phalloides, chlorinated hydrocarbons, phosphorus, aflatoxins	

without coexistent D hepatitis, is the most common both in the United States and elsewhere. Many cases are attributed to non-A, non-B hepatitis based on an absence of known causes and negative serologic tests for hepatitis A and B. Recently developed serologic tests for hepatitis C are just beginning to be used in these patients. The course of the illness differs depending on the cause. Acetaminophen overdose, exposure to toxins, *Amanita phalloides* ingestion, and ischemia typically produce a fulminant illness with encephalopathy in less than a week. Most patients with late-onset hepatic failure, by contrast, have presumed non-A, non-B hepatitis. Finally, combined hepatic and renal failure should alert one to the possibility of toxic exposure.

DIAGNOSIS. The diagnosis of fulminant hepatic failure requires the presence of encephalopathy in a patient with severe, acute liver disease. Synthetic function of the liver as reflected by the prothrombin time is nearly always markedly abnormal. Serum bilirubin concentration is less helpful, since some patients may become very ill rapidly and progress to coma before the serum bilirubin is markedly elevated. Serum transaminase levels are usually elevated early in the illness but do not reliably distinguish between fulminant hepatic failure and acute hepatitis without encephalopathy.

TREATMENT. *Supportive Measures.* A thorough search should be made to detect and correct factors that may precipitate (Table 123–3) or complicate hepatic failure (Table 123–5); several points merit emphasis. Encephalopathy in fulminant hepatic failure primarily reflects the severe nature of the underlying liver injury, and correcting potential precipitating factors is less likely to produce objective benefit than it is in patients with encephalopathy complicating chronic liver disease. *Cerebral edema* is present in over half of patients dying of fulminant hepatic failure. It is often detectable on CT scan and may result in intracranial herniation. Moreover, in conjunction with systemic hypotension, it reduces cerebral perfusion and may cause brain death. Treatment of clinically evident intracranial hypertension, manifested by unequal or abnormally reactive pupils, myoclonus, and/or decerebrate posturing, is certainly appropriate. Unfortunately, clinical signs may be an insensitive way of detecting intracranial hypertension, and invasive monitoring of intracranial pressure is advocated by some. The decision regarding invasive intracranial pressure monitoring must thus be carefully individualized. Coagulation abnormalities should be corrected before monitor insertion.

Experimental Measures. Because the mortality of fulminant hepatic failure is high even with optimal supportive care, a variety of other forms of therapy have been tried. These include *corticosteroid administration, exchange transfusion,* administra-tion of L-*dopa* or *hepatitis B hyperimmune globulin* (for hepatitis B), *charcoal hemoperfusion, amino acid infusion, plasmapheresis, hemodialysis, total body washout, cross circulation* with a human volunteer or baboon, or *extracorporeal perfusion* through a human cadaver liver, pig liver, or baboon liver. However, these experimental forms of therapy offer *no advantage* over conventional supportive care. Thiopental, as well as osmotic agents such as mannitol, are effective at least temporarily in reducing intracranial pressure. The utility of these agents and intracranial pressure monitoring are still under evaluation.

Liver Transplantation. Liver transplantation may yield favorable results (60 to 70 per cent survival) in patients with fulminant hepatic failure. While the follow-up in such patients is limited, most deaths following liver transplantation occur in the first 3 postoperative months. Physicians caring for patients with fulminant and late-onset hepatic failure who are likely to have a poor prognosis with supportive care alone should therefore contact a liver transplant center as soon as possible for consideration of transfer (Ch. 124).

PROGNOSIS. The short-term prognosis for patients with fulminant hepatic failure that progresses to coma is poor, the average reported survival being 10 to 40 per cent. Factors associated with an especially poor prognosis include age of less than 10 or greater than 40 years, illness due to presumed non-A, non-B hepatitis or idiosyncratic drug reaction, a slow course with encephalopathy following jaundice by more than 7 days, Stage IV encephalopathy, marked biochemical abnormalities (bilirubin exceeding 20 mg per deciliter, prothrombin time exceeding 30 seconds), or the presence of complications (Table 123–5). In contrast, the outlook for those patients who do survive an episode of fulminant hepatic failure with coma is quite good. Virtually all patients have returned to their previous state of health within 2 to 3 months, and follow-up liver biopsies have usually demonstrated no or minimal abnormalities. Patients with persistent biochemical or histologic abnormalities have frequently been found to have had pre-existing liver disease or to have continuing exposure to toxic or infectious agents.

CHRONIC LIVER DISEASE WITH ENCEPHALOPATHY

ETIOLOGY. Hepatic encephalopathy may also occur in patients with chronic liver disease, usually cirrhosis with portal-systemic shunting. Some patients with cirrhosis may be chronically encephalopathic. In most, however, encephalopathy tends to occur acutely and intermittently. In this latter group, the occurrence of encephalopathy reflects a worsening of hepatic function and/or the presence of one or more precipitating factors (Table 123–3).

DIAGNOSIS. As with fulminant hepatic failure, diagnosis requires the presence of signs and symptoms compatible with

TABLE 123–5. HEPATIC FAILURE: COMPLICATIONS AND MANAGEMENT

Complications	Pathophysiology	Management
Aspiration	Decreased mental status, emesis	Endotracheal intubation with onset of coma
Azotemia	Volume depletion, acute tubular necrosis, hepatorenal syndrome	Assess volume (may require invasive monitoring or fluid challenge), fluid administration if appropriate
Cerebral edema	?Altered vascular permeability, circulating toxins	Clinical assessment insensitive; intracranial pressure monitoring advocated by some, but entails risk and not of proven value; elevation of head of bed; hyperventilation; mannitol; barbiturates
Encephalopathy	See Table 123–1	See Table 123–1
Gastrointestinal bleeding	Stress gastritis aggravated by coagulopathy and portal hypertension	Prophylaxis (e.g., with H_2-receptor antagonists, antacids or sucralfate); fresh frozen plasma if overt bleeding occurs
Hypoxemia	Right to left shunting, noncardiogenic pulmonary edema	Increased inspired O_2; intubation with positive end-expiratory pressure
Hypotension	Decreased vascular resistance, sepsis, gastrointestinal bleeding	Identify and treat underlying cause, pressors if necessary
Infection	Via intravenous lines, enteric origin	Blood cultures, empiric treatment if infection suspected
Metabolic		
Acidosis	Decreased perfusion, decreased hepatic clearance of organic acids	Identify and treat underlying cause; administration of HCO_3^-
Alkalosis	Hyperventilation, presumably central	No treatment necessary
Hypoglycemia	Decreased glycogenolysis and gluconeogenesis	Frequent glucose monitoring, 1–2 liters of 5% or 10% glucose daily
Hypokalemia	Renal or gastrointestinal K^+ loss	KCl administration
Hyponatremia	Decreased renal free water clearance, fluid administration	Minimize administration of free water

hepatic encephalopathy in a patient with underlying chronic liver disease. Routine tests of liver function are typically abnormal but are of little value in differential diagnosis. Unlike fulminant hepatic failure, encephalopathy in patients with chronic liver disease may be accompanied by only minimally abnormal liver function tests. A markedly elevated or rising prothrombin time in an encephalopathic patient with known chronic liver disease suggests superimposed acute hepatocellular necrosis. It is extremely important in patients with chronic alcoholic liver disease to exclude other causes of metabolic encephalopathy (e.g., hypoglycemia, alcohol intoxication, Wernicke-Korsakoff syndrome), meningitis, or structural lesions such as subdural hematoma.

TREATMENT. *Supportive Measures.* Unlike fulminant hepatic failure, encephalopathy in the patient with chronic liver disease frequently results from one or more potentially reversible precipitating factors. These should be sought and, when possible, corrected (Table 123–3). Additional general measures as outlined earlier for the treatment of hepatic encephalopathy should be undertaken.

The complications and additional supportive care required for these patients are similar to those described for fulminant hepatic failure. Overall, however, the severity and frequency of complications (e.g., hypoglycemia) are less than with fulminant hepatic failure. The various forms of experimental therapy that have been tried in fulminant hepatic failure also have no established role in the management of patients with chronic liver disease with encephalopathy.

Liver Transplantation. Patients with chronic, progressive liver disease of all types may be candidates for transplantation. The presence of encephalopathy or other complications should prompt the physician to consider this option and contact a transplant center (Ch. 124).

PROGNOSIS. Because encephalopathy in patients with chronic liver disease is frequently precipitated by potentially reversible factors, the short-term prognosis is better than in fulminant hepatic failure, particularly if the encephalopathy is not attributable to a sudden deterioration of hepatic function. However, because the underlying chronic liver disease is commonly irreversible and slowly progressive, the long-term prognosis is guarded.

Gammal SH, Jones EA: Hepatic encephalopathy. Med Clin North Am 73:793, 1989. *A comprehensive review with a particular focus on manifestations and pathogenesis.*

Katelaris PH, Jones DB: Fulminant hepatic failure. Med Clin North Am 73:955, 1989. *A complete treatment of this topic, including the role of transplantation.*

Munoz SJ, Maddrey WC: Major complications of acute and chronic liver disease. Gastroenterol Clin North Am 17:265, 1989. *An exhaustive review with over 150 references focusing on prevention, diagnosis, and management of complications.*

O'Grady J, Alexander GJM, Hayllar KM, et al.: Early indicators of prognosis in fulminant hepatic failure. Gastroenterology 97:439, 1989. *A very important article summarizing information on nearly 600 patients, the largest series reported.*

Rothstein JD, Herlong HF: Neurologic manifestations of hepatic disease. Neurol Clin 7:563, 1989. *A thoroughly referenced review that deals with neurologic manifestations of specific hepatic disorders as well as hepatic encephalopathy.*

124 Liver Transplantation

John Paul Roberts

In the last 25 years liver transplantation has moved from an experimental procedure to an accepted medical therapy for patients with both acute and chronic liver failure. Survival following liver transplantation has improved from approximately 30 per cent in the 1970's to 80 per cent or better in the closing years of the 1980's. The procedure is currently underwritten by many states and most private insurance companies, and recently Medicare has decided to pay for liver transplantation for specific indications. Although liver transplantation is still an expensive procedure, the cost has decreased such that it now offers a better outcome and lower cost than many therapies for acute and chronic liver failure.

More than 1800 liver transplantations were carried out in the United States during 1989. The improvement in patient and graft survival following liver transplantation has resulted from changes in (1) patient selection, (2) operative techniques, and (3) immunosuppressive drugs and their use. As newer immunosuppressive medications become available, it appears likely that the morbidity, mortality, and costs of liver transplantation will continue to decrease. With improvement in survival and with more patients undergoing liver transplantation, availability of donor organs has become rate-limiting in its use.

PATIENT SELECTION

The indications for liver transplantation have broadened with improved postoperative survival. When 1-year survival was 50 per cent, liver transplantation was indicated only in those patients who were expected to have less than a 50 per cent 1-year survival from their primary disease. Predictability for survival based on natural history data has been reasonably well established for primary biliary cirrhosis and for fulminant liver failure, but the natural histories of other liver diseases (e.g., chronic active hepatitis with cirrhosis or sclerosing cholangitis) vary widely, making it difficult to select patients with a less than 50 per cent 1-year survival. Fortunately, the current marked improvement in survival after liver transplantation has made it possible to broaden the criteria and to include quality-of-life issues in making the decision for liver transplantation. These issues include extreme fatigue or pruritus in patients with chronic liver disease, recurrent cholangitis in patients with sclerosing cholangitis, portal-systemic encephalopathy, ascites refractory to medical management, and correction of certain metabolic diseases.

Liver transplantation has also changed the indications for or replaced many of the operations previously done for complications of chronic liver disease, such as portal-systemic shunting for recurrent variceal hemorrhage, LeVeen shunting for intractable ascites, and radical biliary tract surgery for patients with sclerosing cholangitis. These operations, which were once the only option for the patient with liver disease, are now assuming a secondary role. As an example, portacaval shunting has a poor outcome in patients with severe liver dysfunction, whereas these patients can do very well following liver transplantation. It is therefore important that patients who would otherwise be suitable candidates for transplantation and in whom another surgical procedure is contemplated be discussed with a liver transplantation center regarding the appropriateness of the planned procedure.

Early referral is extremely important in patients with *fulminant liver failure* (Ch. 123). This diagnosis can only be made in patients with evidence of hepatic failure, including Stage III or IV encephalopathy developing less than 8 weeks after onset in the absence of pre-existing liver disease (Table 124–1). Viral hepatitis is the most common cause of fulminant liver failure, but other etiologies include toxins (e.g., *Amanita phalloides*), medications (e.g., acetaminophen), or metabolic disorders (e.g., fulminant Wilson's disease). If a patient has reached Stage IV coma or has a prothrombin time greater than 20 seconds, limited survival without hepatic replacement can be expected. These patients are at high risk for developing cerebral edema followed by brain herniation if not properly managed. Pretransplantation management includes elevation of the head, monitoring intracranial pressure, and aggressive therapy using mannitol, hyperventilation, and barbiturate coma for increased intracranial pressure.

The most common indication for liver transplantation is chronic active hepatitis (Table 124–1). The role of the hepatitis C virus in this group of disorders is becoming increasingly clear as the ability to identify this infection has improved. Other common diseases for which transplantation is performed include primary biliary cirrhosis, autoimmune hepatitis, sclerosing cholangitis, Wilson's disease, extrahepatic biliary atresia, α_1-antitrypsin deficiency, alcoholic liver disease, cholangiocarcinoma, and primary hepatic malignancy. Contraindications to liver transplantation include systemic sepsis, active substance abuse, extrahepatic malignancy, and advanced cardiopulmonary disease. Transplantation for cholangiocarcinoma is controversial because survival of these patients following transplantation is poor, although disease limited to the extrahepatic ducts without lymph node involvement

TABLE 124-1. INDICATIONS FOR LIVER TRANSPLANTATION AND POSTOPERATIVE SURVIVAL*

Disease	Per Cent of Patients	(n)	6-month Actuarial Survival	12-month Actuarial Survival
Chronic active hepatitis/cryptogenic cirrhosis	22	(37)	97%	88%
Alcoholic liver disease	16	(26)	100%	100%
Fulminant liver failure	13	(21)	95%	95%
Subacute fulminant liver failure	2	(3)	100%	100%
Primary biliary cirrhosis	10	(17)	94%	85%
Sclerosing cholangitis	8.5	(14)	100%	92%
Chronic active hepatitis B	9	(15)	80%	69%
α_1-Antitrypsin disease	3	(5)	100%	100%
Extrahepatic biliary atresia	3	(5)	60%	60%
Cancer	3	(5)	80%	60%
Hemochromatosis	2	(4)	100%	100%
Autoimmune hepatitis	2	(4)	100%	100%
Miscellaneous†	5	(8)	50%	50%

*Based on 164 patients who underwent liver transplantation at the University of California, San Francisco.
†Includes Budd-Chiari, Crigler-Najjar, fatty liver, Wilson's disease, unknown etiology.

has a more favorable prognosis. Although theoretically liver transplantation is a logical therapy for hepatocellular carcinoma, (Ch. 125), an effective adjuvant chemotherapy is lacking, and hepatic and systemic relapse of the disease is common. Thus, only 20 per cent of patients with hepatocellular carcinoma survive 3 years following liver transplantation. As an exception, the fibrolamellar variant of hepatocellular carcinoma carries a much better prognosis. End-stage liver disease caused by chronic ethanol abuse has been increasingly recognized as an appropriate indication for transplantation; results in these patients are the same as those for patients with chronic liver failure of other causes. The 6- and 12-month actuarial survival is given for different disease entities in Table 124-1. The overall patient survival is given in Figure 124-1.

Liver transplantation has also been performed for a variety of metabolic conditions, including those that directly lead to chronic liver disease (e.g., Wilson's disease) and those that do not produce liver disease but for which transplantation removes all or much of the metabolic defect leading to disease expression systemically (e.g., primary hyperoxaluria). At this time liver transplantation has been carried out for the following genetic diseases: α_1-antitrypsin deficiency, Wilson's disease, hemochromatosis, homozygous familial hypercholesterolemia, Crigler-Najjar syndrome, erythropoietic protoporphyria, glycogen storage disease types I and IV, tyrosinemia, primary hyperoxaluria, and genetic diseases of the urea cycle.

DONOR SELECTION

Selection of the appropriate organ donor for liver transplantation is primarily based on ABO blood type and body size compatibility between donor and recipient. In general, donors for large non-O recipients tend to be more available than for small O recipients. This discrepancy reflects a higher accident rate for young adult males, and the ability to utilize type O livers in recipients of other blood types. In October, 1987, a nationwide organ-sharing system was instituted in the United States. In this system potential organs are first offered to local transplantation programs; if no local recipient is available, the organ is offered to centers within a defined geographic region. If no regional recipient is available, the organs are then offered nationally. Selection of a recipient is based upon criteria that include the level of care that potential recipients currently require. Those in intensive care or with fulminant hepatic failure are assigned the highest priority; those still able to work, the lowest.

IMPROVEMENTS IN OPERATIVE TECHNIQUE

A number of operative advances have contributed to the improved results seen with liver transplantation. The use of choledochocholedochostomy or choledochojejunostomy has decreased the incidence of biliary leak and sepsis. The liver from a large donor can be pared down to fit a smaller recipient; this procedure has increased the donor pool for small recipients. Further, this technique has led to the recent use of liver segments from living related donors. Finally, the use of multiple organ transplants in patients with multiorgan disease involvement has increased the access of patients who otherwise would not be candidates for transplantation.

POST-TRANSPLANTATION COMPLICATIONS

Complications of liver transplantation are primarily vascular (e.g., thrombosis of the anastomosed hepatic artery or portal vein), biliary (relating to reconstruction of the biliary tract), infectious, or those relating to organ rejection. Early postoperative hepatic artery thrombosis requires retransplantation, since it usually results in necrosis of the liver and/or biliary tree. Portal vein thrombosis can be asymptomatic or present with complications of portal hypertension. Biliary tract complications usually appear as strictures within the biliary tree or as leakage of bile from the biliary reconstruction. Renal failure may complicate the post-transplantation period, resulting from pre-existing renal dysfunction, intraoperative renal ischemia, postoperative cyclosporine toxicity, or a combination of these factors.

Postoperative infections commonly occur. The average patient develops at least one episode of bacterial infection and has a 40 to 50 per cent chance of developing a fungal or viral infection following liver transplantation. Bacterial infections may involve the biliary tree, intra-abdominal abscesses, pneumonia, or may be related to central venous catheters. Fungal infections include systemic candidiasis, usually occurring during the early transplant period and related to intravascular catheters or intra-abdominal candidal abscesses. Other opportunistic fungal infections, such as aspergillosis, predominate later, and all can represent a serious threat to the patient's life. Viral infections following liver transplantation are most often caused by members of the Herpesvirus family. Mucocutaneous herpes simplex and varicella zoster can

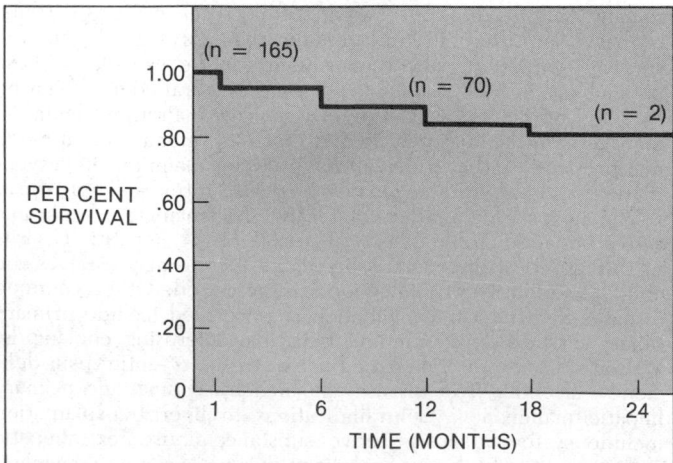

FIGURE 124-1. Survival following hepatic transplantation (adult and pediatric) at the University of California, San Francisco, from January 31, 1988 to June 27, 1990.

occur following transplantation, and either prophylactic or therapeutic acyclovir is effective in preventing and treating these infections. Post-transplantation cytomegalovirus (CMV) infections represent either a reactivation of disease in a previously infected, immunosuppressed recipient or a primary infection arising from transmission of the agent via the donor liver or a blood transfusion. In general, primary disease appears to be more serious than reactivation. In renal transplantation recipients, high doses (3200 mg per day) of acyclovir are effective prophylaxis for CMV infections, and it is hoped that this approach will also prove effective in liver transplantation recipients. Gancyclovir, a congener of acyclovir, appears to be effective in treatment of systemic CMV disease in liver recipients. As one of the major complications of immunosuppression is infection, the use of prophylactic anti-infectives is a method of improving the therapeutic index of the immunosuppressive agents. *Pneumocystis carinii* infection was previously a problem in all forms of solid organ transplantation, but with the use of prophylactic trimethoprim-sulfamethoxazole, it is expected that morbidity and mortality related to this protozoal agent will be eliminated in transplantation recipients.

IMMUNOSUPPRESSION

Immunosuppression in the liver transplantation recipient is largely based on the use of cyclosporine, a cyclic polypeptide that binds to and inhibits the action of an intracellular prolyl peptidyl isomerase. As a result the production of interleukin-2 (IL-2) by T helper cells is sharply diminished; this in turn prevents cell proliferation and the generation of cytotoxic T cells. Cyclosporine is usually started in the early post-transplantation period and is continued indefinitely. Because the intestinal absorption of oral cyclosporine depends on the presence of bile, external biliary diversion or postoperative liver dysfunction can interfere with this process. Cyclosporine is metabolized by the cytochrome P-450–dependent mono-oxygenases and, therefore, systemic levels can be decreased by drugs that induce this pathway, such as rifampin, barbiturates, or phenytoin. Major side effects of cyclosporine include neurotoxicity, manifested by headache and tremor; nephrotoxicity, manifested by increase in BUN and creatinine; sensitivity to volume depletion; hypertension; and hyperkalemia. Chronic cyclosporine administration can result in renal interstitial fibrosis and an increased risk of post-transplantation lymphoproliferative disorders.

Prednisone is generally used in combination with cyclosporine to prevent rejection. Prednisone reduces the release of interleukin-1 (IL-1) by macrophages and in this fashion inhibits IL-1's amplification of IL-2 production. The complications of the use of glucocorticoids are described elsewhere (Ch. 27).

Azathioprine, a third agent used for post-transplantation immunosuppression, blocks proliferation of white blood cells and thereby decreases the proliferative or amplification response of the rejection process. The major adverse effect of azathioprine is marrow depression.

Several new drugs are being evaluated for use in liver transplantation. The most promising of these, FK-506, appears to act similarly to cyclosporine, but through binding to a different intracellular peptidyl prolyl isomerase in the cell. This results in a marked increase in potency. Its primary benefits appear to be less nephrotoxicity and its ability to achieve adequate immunosuppression without concomitant azathioprine and with relatively small doses of prednisone.

Rejection occurs commonly after liver transplantation, but with prompt diagnosis and therapy it is rarely a cause of graft loss. Its histologic features include periportal infiltrate, bile duct epithelial damage, and endothelialitis. Treatment for rejection includes additional steroids or the use of antilymphocyte preparations.

Kusne S, Dummer JS, Singh N, et al.: Infections after liver transplantation. An analysis of 101 consecutive cases. Medicine 67:132, 1988. *Compilation of infectious complications at the University of Pittsburgh.*

Roberts JP, Forsmark C, Lake JR, et al.: Liver transplantation today. Ann Rev Med 40:287, 1989. *Report from a single institution performing liver transplantation.*

Starzl TE, Demetris AJ, Van Thiel DH: Liver transplantation. N Engl J Med 321:1014, 1092, 1989. *A comprehensive review of the history of clinical liver transplantation and a summary of advances in the field.*

125 Hepatic Tumors

Bruce F. Scharschmidt

Characteristic aspects of hepatic neoplasms encountered commonly in adults are summarized in Table 125–1 and selectively described in more detail below. The approach to the patient with a neoplasm and the role of imaging studies are outlined at the end of this section.

BENIGN HEPATIC TUMORS

Hepatocellular Adenoma

Hepatocellular adenomas occur almost exclusively in women. These tumors are most frequently detected during the third and fourth decades of life but are occasionally found in postmenopausal women as well. Adenomas most commonly occur in the right lobe of the liver, are frequently solitary, and are often quite large, with up to one half being 10 cm or more in diameter. Hepatocellular adenomas are usually well circumscribed, may be surrounded by a pseudocapsule, and often show areas of bile stasis, hemorrhage, and necrosis. Microscopically, these tumors consist of a monotonous sheet of normal to slightly atypical hepatocytes without portal tracts or bile ducts. Kupffer cells are markedly reduced in number or absent, and a few arteries and thin-walled veins are present.

The preponderance of this tumor in women suggests a hormonal role in its pathogenesis, and there is strong evidence implicating oral contraceptives. Nearly 90 per cent of cases are associated with oral contraceptive use, and some adenomas have regressed in a period of months to years after use of oral contraceptives was discontinued. The annual incidence is estimated to be 3 to 4 per 100,000 in women who have taken oral contraceptives continuously for several years. Although not generally regarded as a premalignant lesion, there are instances in which hepatocellular carcinoma appears to have arisen in an hepatocellular adenoma.

Symptomatic patients with hepatocellular adenomas present with signs and symptoms of an abdominal mass, tumor infarction, intratumor hemorrhage (pain, fever, leukocytosis), or, in about one third of cases, tumor rupture (pain, hemoperitoneum, circulatory collapse). The mortality in this last group is approximately 20 per cent. Because the true incidence of these tumors is unknown, the actual proportion that ruptures cannot be determined.

The management of hepatocellular adenomas is a matter of some debate. In patients taking oral contraceptives that can be discontinued, a several-month period of observation with repeated imaging studies is justifiable, particularly if the location, size, or number of tumors would make resection hazardous. Surgery is appropriate for most persistent resectable lesions.

Focal Nodular Hyperplasia

Focal nodular hyperplasia, which shows a female to male predominance of 2:1 to 7:1, has also been referred to as pseudotumor, focal cirrhosis, and hepatic hamartoma. Unlike hepatocellular adenoma, a firm link between focal nodular hyperplasia and oral contraceptives has not been established. Focal nodular hyperplasia generally is a solitary tumor in the right lobe measuring 5 cm or less in diameter. On cut section it has a characteristic grossly lobulated appearance, which is produced by a central fibrous core with septa radiating in a stellate pattern. Hemorrhage and necrosis are rare. Microscopically, these fibrous septa contain bile ductules and inflammatory cells and are surrounded by normal or slightly atypical hepatocytes as well as Kupffer cells.

Unlike hepatocellular adenomas, focal nodular hyperplasia does not usually produce symptoms and is generally found incidentally at surgery or necropsy. In up to 20 per cent of the cases, it presents as an upper abdominal mass. Portal hypertension has been reported in association with multiple lesions, and rupture is rare. Since focal nodular hyperplasia has no known malignant potential, asymptomatic lesions can be followed nonoperatively. If the lesion is encountered unexpectedly at surgery, simple wedge biopsy is appropriate if complete excision would be difficult.

Hemangioma

Cavernous hemangioma is probably the most common benign hepatic tumor, occurring in up to 7.3 per cent of necropsies with a predominance in females. The great majority are asymptomatic and are found incidentally at surgery or necroscopy. These lesions can, however, present with signs and symptoms of an abdominal mass, infarction, rupture, or thrombocytopenia and hypofibrinogenemia. Because of the accuracy of current imaging techniques in distinguishing hemangioma from other tumors (Table 125–1),

resection is not usually necessary to establish a diagnosis and is appropriate only for large symptomatic lesions. There are also case reports of regression following radiotherapy or hepatic artery ligation.

Other Benign Tumors

A variety of less common benign liver tumors may also occur in adults. They usually produce no symptoms unless very large. Included in this group are *bile duct adenomas, bile duct cystadenomas, fibromas, lipomas, leiomyomas, mesotheliomas, teratomas,* and *myxomas. Nodular regenerative hyperplasia* (also called *nodular transformation* or *multiple adenomatosis*) is a condition characterized by multiple nodules of varying size typically occurring throughout a noncirrhotic liver. The nodules are composed

TABLE 125–1. CHARACTERISTICS OF HEPATIC NEOPLASMS

	Predisposing Factors	M/F Ratio	Manifestations and Complications	Imaging/Diagnostic Studies	Treatment
Benign tumors					
Hepatocellular adenoma	Oral contraceptives; glycogen storage disease type I	<1:10	Abdominal mass; intratumor or intraperitoneal hemorrhage; rare transition to malignancy	Detectable by US, CT, or MRI and may show areas of hemorrhage or necrosis; cold spot on colloid scan; typically hypervascular on AG; may be difficult to diagnose on biopsy	Must be individualized: discontinue oral contraceptives and observe if no symptoms; resection if symptomatic or diagnosis uncertain
Focal nodular hyperplasia	None established	1:2–7	Typically none; occasionally mass effect and rarely portal hypertension	Detectable by US, CT, or MRI and may show central scar; has Kupffer cells and may not be visible on colloid scan; typically hypervascular on AG; may be difficult to diagnose on biopsy	Usually none; resection if symptomatic
Hemangioma	None established	<1:1	Typically none; occasionally mass effect, rarely infarction, rupture, or thrombocytopenia	Characteristic appearance on MRI, CT with bolus contrast, or radionuclide blood pool scan; typically hyperechoic on US; biopsy not necessary if imaging studies show typical findings and probably associated with increased risk of hemorrhage	None if asymptomatic; resection if symptomatic; radiotherapy or hepatic artery ligation in unusual circumstances
Malignant tumors					
Hepatocellular carcinoma	Cirrhosis; hepatitis B or C virus infection; hemochromatosis; mycotoxin exposure; α_1-antitrypsin deficiency; androgenic steroids; Thorotrast; possibly oral contraceptives; tyrosinemia; glycogen storage disease type II	3:1	Abdominal mass; tumor infarction, intratumor or intraperitoneal hemorrhage; portal or hepatic vein occlusion; rarely hypercalcemia, hypercholesterolemia, carcinoid syndrome, hypoglycemia, acquired porphyria	Detectable by US, CT, MRI, or colloid scan (cold spot); often multicentric with vascular invasion; takes up gallium; biopsy or aspiration cytology often diagnostic; elevated or rising α-fetoprotein suggestive	Resection if technically feasible and permitted by hepatic function; transplantation curative in less than one third of even selected cases; palliative chemotherapy
Fibrolamellar carcinoma (variant of hepatocellular carcinoma)	None established	About equal	Mass effect	Detectable by US, CT, MRI (may show calcifications on CT and central scar); cold spot on colloid scan; α-fetoprotein typically not elevated	As for hepatocellular carcinoma; resection or transplantation more likely to result in cure
Cholangiocarcinoma	Primary sclerosing cholangitis; clonorchiasis or opisthorciasis	—	Mass effect; obstructive jaundice	Direct cholangiography often helpful in jaundiced patients; also detectable by US or CT, which may show dilated biliary radicles; aspiration cytology may be diagnostic	As for hepatocellular carcinoma; resection or transplantation rarely curative
Angiosarcoma	Exposure to vinyl chloride, arsenic, or Thorotrast	>1:1	Mass effect; intraperitoneal hemorrhage; thrombocytopenia	Detectable by US, CT; MRI or AG particularly helpful; biopsy	As for heptocellular carcinoma; resection or transplantation rarely curative

Abbreviations: US = ultrasonography; CT = computed tomography; MRI = magnetic resonance imaging; AG = angiography.

of liver plates that are two cells thick. An association with rheumatoid arthritis, Felty's syndrome, CREST syndrome, oral contraceptives, and a variety of drugs is reported. The most common manifestation of nodular regenerative hyperplasia is portal hypertension.

MALIGNANT HEPATIC TUMORS

Hepatocellular Carcinoma

EPIDEMIOLOGY. Hepatocellular carcinoma (hepatoma) is relatively uncommon (less than 2.5 per cent of all malignancies) in the United States and Western Europe. In certain other areas of the world, including parts of sub-Saharan Africa, Southeast Asia, Japan, Oceania, and Greece, hepatocellular carcinoma is among the most frequent malignancies. Hepatocellular carcinoma is predominantly a disease of males and usually arises in a cirrhotic liver. The risk appears to be greatest in cirrhosis associated with hemochromatosis and hepatitis B and C virus infection, low in primary biliary cirrhosis and Wilson's disease, and intermediate in alcoholic and cryptogenic cirrhosis. There is a particularly strong association between chronic hepatitis B virus infection and hepatocellular carcinoma, and prospective epidemiologic studies suggest that the incidence of hepatocellular carcinoma is about 100-fold higher in individuals with hepatitis B virus infection than in noninfected controls. Moreover, tumor tissue in patients with serologic evidence of hepatitis B virus infection frequently has hepatitis B virus integrated into the genome, and woodchucks and ducks infected with viruses that are related to the human hepatitis B virus also develop hepatocellular carcinoma. Infection with the recently identified hepatitis C virus is also associated with an increased prevalence of hepatocellular carcinoma.

Epidemiologic evidence has also suggested a link between hepatocellular carcinoma and ingestion of aflatoxins, mycotoxins produced by *Aspergillus flavus*, a mold that can grow in warm moist areas and contaminate peanuts and stored grains. Case reports also suggest a link between hepatocellular carcinoma and α_1-antitrypsin deficiency and administration of androgenic steroids, Thorotrast, and possibly estrogenic steroids in the form of oral contraceptives (Table 125–1).

CLINICAL FEATURES. The most common presenting features of hepatocellular carcinoma are *abdominal pain,* the presence of an *abdominal mass,* and *weight loss.* Hepatocellular carcinoma may also present with rupture and hemoperitoneum, obstructive jaundice, unexplained deterioration in a patient with cirrhosis, or a variety of paraneoplastic syndromes, including erythrocytosis, persistent fever, hypercalcemia, and hypoglycemia. Hepatomegaly is present in about two thirds of patients. Other suggestive physical findings include the presence of a bruit, hepatic friction rub, or bloody ascites. Hepatocellular carcinoma may invade and obstruct the portal and hepatic veins and metastasizes most often to regional lymph nodes and the lungs. Alpha-fetoprotein levels in serum greater than 1000 ng per milliliter or progressively rising levels are highly suggestive of hepatocellular carcinoma. Unfortunately, only a minority of patients with asymptomatic hepatocellular carcinoma in most parts of the world, including the United States, have elevations of this magnitude. Elevations up to about 200 ng per milliliter are a more sensitive indicator of early tumors but are also less specific. For this reason, α-fetoprotein has proved disappointing in the screening of high-risk populations. Ultrasonography is also used for screening in certain centers throughout the world. While these screening modalities do identify some tumors at an early stage, they have not yet been proven to improve survival in high-risk populations.

TREATMENT AND PROGNOSIS. The results of current treatment for hepatocellular carcinoma are discouraging. In the United States, median survival from the time of diagnosis is about 6 months. Because of the advanced stage of the disease at the time of diagnosis and the frequent coexistence of severe liver disease, less than 20 per cent of patients are candidates for hepatic resection. The presence of coexisting cirrhosis in a patient with well-preserved hepatic function does not altogether preclude surgery; however, such patients may not tolerate more than limited resection of a localized tumor. Adriamycin alone or in combination with other agents has produced objective tumor response in up to 50 per cent of patients but has minimally affected survival. Radiation therapy has also yielded disappointing results. Other approaches (e.g., hormonal therapy, hepatic artery ligation or embolization, radiolabeled antibodies to tumor-specific antigens) have been tried but have not yet been shown to improve survival. As discussed in Ch. 123, liver transplantation for unresectable hepatocellular carcinoma is curative in only a minority of patients.

A variant of typical hepatocellular carcinoma termed *fibrolamellar carcinoma* differs from the typical form of the disease in that it usually occurs in young adults without underlying cirrhosis, lacks the usual male predominance, is associated with a longer survival (32 to 68 months) when untreated, and has been cured surgically in between 10 and 30 per cent of cases.

Other Primary Hepatic Malignancies

Cholangiocarcinoma occurs much less frequently than hepatocellular carcinoma and shows an association with sclerosing cholangitis and with clonorchiasis and opisthorchiasis in the Far East. It may present with obstructive jaundice when it involves major ducts in the area of the hepatic hilum. Truly mixed hepatocellular cholangiocarcinomas are rare. Angiosarcoma, an unusual tumor associated with vinyl chloride exposure as well as arsenic and Thorotrast administration, frequently causes thrombocytopenia and has a propensity to rupture, causing hemoperitoneum and circulatory collapse. Other unusual primary hepatic malignant tumors of adults include cystadenocarcinoma, squamous carcinoma, and hepatoblastoma.

As with hepatocellular carcinoma, treatment of these malignant hepatic tumors has been unsatisfactory. Resection is seldom possible. Of patients with cholangiocarcinoma who have undergone liver transplantation, the 3-year survival is less than among patients with hepatocellular carcinoma.

Tumors Metastatic to Liver

The liver and lung are the most frequent sites of metastatic cancer, and metastases constitute the largest group of hepatic tumors in adults. Necropsy studies have demonstrated hepatic metastases in more than half of patients with primary malignant tumors having portal venous drainage (e.g., stomach, colon, and pancreas). Other solid tumors that frequently metastasize to the liver include melanoma and tumors of the lung, oropharynx, and bladder. Next to the spleen, the liver is also the most common extranodal site of involvement by Hodgkin's disease, the non-Hodgkin's lymphomas, and malignant histiocytosis (histiocytic medullary reticulosis).

Pseudotumors

A variety of nonneoplastic lesions may mimic hepatic tumors. These include regenerative nodules, anomalous hepatic lobulation, cysts, and focal fatty deposits. In many cases, imaging studies can distinguish these from true neoplasms.

DIAGNOSTIC APPROACH TO THE PATIENT WITH A SUSPECTED HEPATIC NEOPLASM

CLINICAL EVALUATION. Most hepatic neoplasms present as a right upper quadrant or epigastric mass. Additional clinical features that may provide clues regarding the specific type of tumor are summarized above and in Table 125–1. Cholangiocarcinoma and hepatocellular carcinoma can cause biliary obstruction, but this may potentially result from strategically located tumors of all types. Physical examination most commonly reveals hepatomegaly or a discrete mass. The presence of a bruit or friction rub may suggest hepatocellular carcinoma but is not specific. Elevations of alkaline phosphatase and transaminase levels are the most common biochemical abnormalities; however, liver function tests are not particularly helpful in diagnosis and may be entirely normal in some patients. A markedly elevated and/or rising α-fetoprotein level is strongly suggestive of hepatocellular carcinoma.

IMAGING TECHNIQUES. The detection of hepatic neoplasms has been improved by modern imaging modalities. Ultrasonography (US), computed tomography (CT), and magnetic resonance imaging (MRI) have gradually replaced hepatic scintigraphy. Unlike scintigraphy, these other modalities visualize structures outside the liver, and US and CT can be used for directed biopsy. Because of its lesser expense and lack of radiation exposure, US is often a useful initial study. As compared with US, CT provides sharper definition of other abdominal structures, is not hindered by bowel gas, and probably detects smaller hepatic lesions. MRI appears comparable to CT, but its role in hepatic imaging is still being defined. Angiography, which entails more risk and discomfort for the patient, may be particularly helpful in planning surgical resection. Because of the rapidly evolving capabilities of current imaging modalities, radiologic consultation is often appropriate.

METASTATIC TUMORS. In a patient with a known extrahepatic malignant tumor and clinical or biochemical evidence of hepatic metastases, US is a reasonable screening study. The finding of single or multiple defects is consistent with metastatic disease, and a percutaneous biopsy can be expected to recover tumor in 50 to 75 per cent of such cases. Two biopsies performed through the same skin site and cytologic examination of the tissue core and aspirated fluid appear to enhance the yield without increasing the risk of bleeding. In patients with lymphoreticular malignant disease, percutaneous biopsy is less sensitive in demonstrating hepatic involvement than wedge biopsy obtained at laparotomy, and histologic evidence of hepatic involvement may be found even in the absence of clinical, biochemical, or radionuclide scan abnormalities.

PRIMARY TUMORS. The workup in suspected primary hepatic tumor must be individualized on the basis of the relative risks and benefits of establishing a diagnosis. Asymptomatic patients in whom imaging studies yield findings characteristic of hemangioma (Table 125–1) may not require additional evaluation. In most other instances, however, examination of tissue is appropriate. In a patient who is a candidate for operation and who has an apparently resectable lesion of uncertain or suspicious nature based on imaging studies, preoperative biopsy may not be necessary. In the patient who is not a candidate for surgery or in whom information regarding tumor type will importantly influence decisions regarding further evaluation and therapy, biopsy is usually appropriate. Several factors should be considered in this regard. First, needle biopsy of lesions such as hemangioma, angiosarcoma, and possibly hepatocellular adenoma is probably associated with increased risk of hemorrhage, and biopsy of a possible echinococcal cyst is contraindicated. Second, definitive diagnosis of hepatocellular adenoma and focal nodular hyperplasia, which consist predominantly of normal or minimally abnormal hepatocytes, may be difficult from examination of a needle biopsy alone. Third, compared with percutaneous biopsy, laparoscopic approach permits directed biopsy of visible tumor deposits and may facilitate control of bleeding. Finally, a CT- or US-directed fine needle percutaneous aspiration biopsy has yielded excellent results in many centers and appears to be associated with a lower risk of hemorrhage than standard biopsy. It is particularly helpful for lesions not accessible to blind percutaneous biopsy.

Colombo M, Choo QL, Del Ninno E, et al.: Prevalence of antibodies to hepatitis C virus in Italian patients with hepatocellular carcinoma. Lancet 2:1006, 1989. *This is one of two companion articles in the same issue that implicates hepatitis C in the pathogenesis of hepatocellular carcinoma.*

DiBiscegli AM, Rustgi VK, Hoofnagle JH, et al.: Hepatocellular carcinoma. Ann Intern Med 108:390, 1988. *Proceedings of a National Institutes of Health Conference dealing with all aspects of this topic.*

Ishak KG: Benign tumors and pseudotumors of the liver. J Appl Pathol 6:82, 1988. *A review oriented toward histopathology drawn from the uniquely rich experience of the Armed Forces Institute of Pathology.*

Reading NG, Forbes A, Nunnerly HB, et al.: Hepatic hemangioma: A critical review of diagnosis and management. Q J Med 67:431, 1988. *An excellent recent review of this most common hepatic neoplasm.*

Regan LS: Screening for hepatocellular carcinoma in high-risk individuals: A clinical review. Arch Intern Med 149:1741, 1989. *A brief review of an important topic.*

Rothschild MA, Oratz M: Hepatic imaging. Semin Liver Dis 9:1, 1989. *An entire issue with nine thoroughly referenced chapters dealing with all aspects of hepatic imaging.*

126 Diseases of the Gallbladder and Bile Ducts

Peter F. Malet and Roger D. Soloway

Biliary tract disorders result from a variety of congenital, inflammatory, metabolic, infectious, and neoplastic conditions. These conditions often present in subtle ways and can pose challenging diagnostic problems. Ongoing improvements in diagnostic and therapeutic techniques have allowed the clinician to diagnose biliary tract disease more quickly and to treat patients more effectively.

NORMAL PHYSIOLOGY OF BILE FORMATION

Bile is an isotonic aqueous mixture consisting primarily of electrolytes, proteins, bile salts, cholesterol, phospholipids, and bilirubin. Secretion across the canalicular membrane of the hepatocyte accounts for about two thirds of total bile flow. Bile salt-dependent secretion comprises about one half of canalicular bile formation, while the other half is termed bile salt independent and consists mainly of electrolytes. The remaining one third of bile flow is an alkaline fraction generated by the epithelial cells lining the bile ducts; ductular secretion is stimulated by secretin, cholecystokinin, and gastrin. An as yet unquantitated contribution to canalicular bile flow consisting mainly of water and electrolytes occurs by way of the interhepatocytic space (paracellular pathway). The total volume of bile produced ranges from 500 to 800 ml per day.

Under basal (fasting) conditions, tonic contraction of the sphincter of Oddi diverts about half of the flow of hepatic bile into the gallbladder; the other half flows into the duodenum assisted by phasic peristaltic action of the sphincter. The gallbladder actively reabsorbs Na^+, Cl^-, and HCO_3^+ and passively resorbs H_2O. It is capable of concentrating bile 10-fold within about 4 hours. The gallbladder mucosa secretes H^+ and mucin.

Cholecystokinin, released from the intestinal mucosa after meals by fat, amino acids, and H^+, simultaneously stimulates the gallbladder to contract and the sphincter of Oddi to relax, emptying bile into the duodenum.

Bile salts are synthesized by hepatocytes (Fig. 126–1) from cholesterol by a multistep process, the rate-limiting step of which is catalyzed by 7α-hydroxylase, which is under inhibitory feedback control. Cholate and chenodeoxycholate, the two *primary* bile salts (that is, they are synthesized in the liver), are conjugated with either glycine or taurine before secretion to improve solubility. Bile salts are secreted by active transport across the biliary canalicular membrane. After entering the proximal small intestine, bile salts aid in fat absorption by forming *micelles* (Ch. 102) and then are largely reabsorbed in the mid and distal small intestine. Bile salts that reach the colon are partially deconjugated, which makes them more lipid soluble and facilitates their reabsorption. Cholate and chenodeoxycholate are also partially converted by bacterial 7α-dehydroxylation to the *secondary* bile salts, deoxycholate and lithocholate, respectively. Deoxycholate is absorbed from the colon, reconjugated in the liver, and excreted in bile. Lithocholate is poorly reabsorbed; it is sulfated as well as reconjugated during hepatic transfer. Sulfation increases aqueous solubility and further reduces intestinal reabsorption. The average bile salt composition of bile is 35 per cent chenodeoxycholate, 35 per cent cholate, 25 per cent deoxycholate, 2 per cent ursodeoxycholate, and 2 per cent lithocholate. Each is conjugated with either glycine or taurine in a ratio of 2 to 3:1. Bile salts are secreted in the form of micelles containing phospholipids (mainly lecithin), and cholesterol. These lipids account for 90 per cent of biliary solids.

Intestinal reabsorption of bile salts, which is about 95 per cent for a single passage, occurs by passive diffusion throughout the intestine and by active transport within the terminal ileum. The reabsorbed bile salts are largely bound to albumin in portal blood and are then almost completely removed by the hepatocytes in a single passage through the liver sinusoids. The bile salt pool, normally 1.8 to 3.0 grams, passes through the liver and intestine two or three times during each meal, producing six to nine cycles

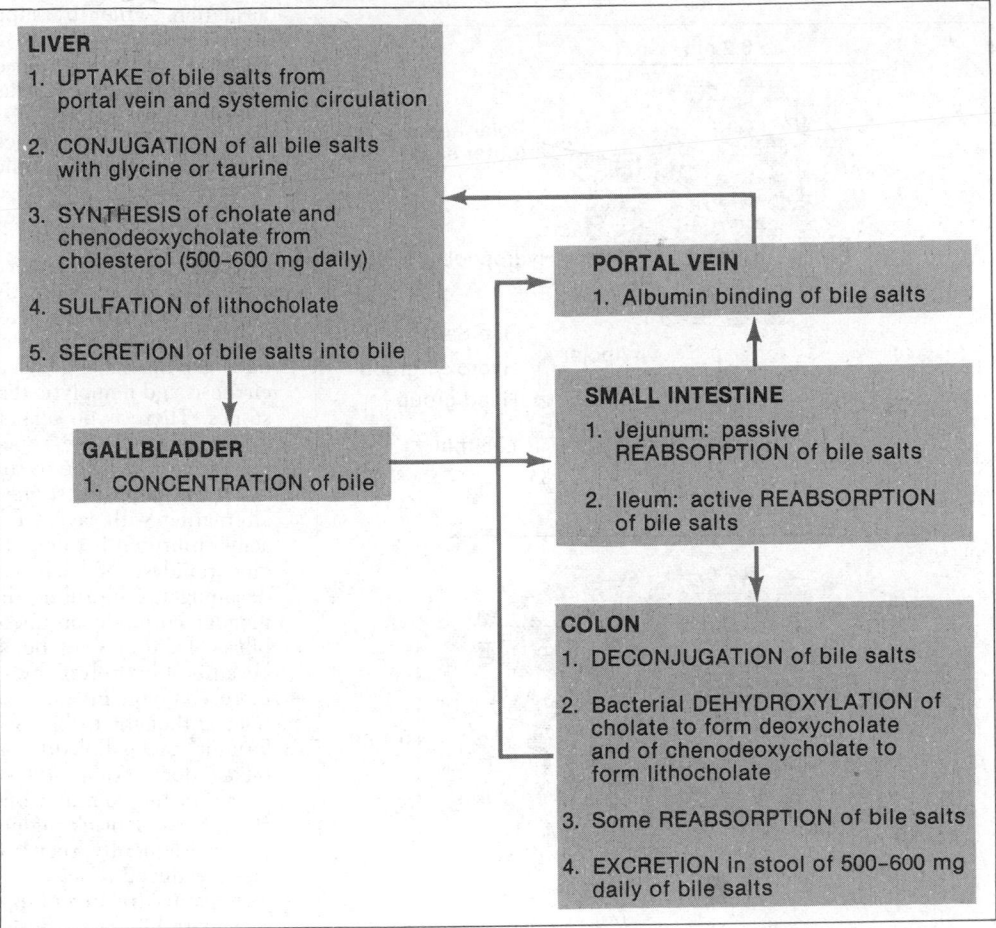

LIVER

1. UPTAKE of bile salts from portal vein and systemic circulation

2. CONJUGATION of all bile salts with glycine or taurine

3. SYNTHESIS of cholate and chenodeoxycholate from cholesterol (500–600 mg daily)

4. SULFATION of lithocholate

5. SECRETION of bile salts into bile

GALLBLADDER

1. CONCENTRATION of bile

PORTAL VEIN

1. Albumin binding of bile salts

SMALL INTESTINE

1. Jejunum: passive REABSORPTION of bile salts

2. Ileum: active REABSORPTION of bile salts

COLON

1. DECONJUGATION of bile salts

2. Bacterial DEHYDROXYLATION of cholate to form deoxycholate and of chenodeoxycholate to form lithocholate

3. Some REABSORPTION of bile salts

4. EXCRETION in stool of 500–600 mg daily of bile salts

FIGURE 126–1. The major steps in the enterohepatic circulation of bile salts. This cycle provides for conservation of bile salts by an effective reabsorption mechanism in the intestine.

daily (i.e., each day about 20 to 25 grams of bile salts enter the duodenum); this cycling is termed the *enterohepatic circulation*. During an average day involving three meals, bile salts are in continuous motion with peaks of secretion during and following meals. At night, when the majority of the secreted hepatic bile eventually enters the gallbladder, and there is no stimulus for gallbladder contraction, the intestinal concentration of bile salts is much lower. Conservation of bile salts in this enterohepatic circulation is so efficient that only 15 to 25 per cent (500 to 600 mg) of the bile salt pool must be replaced by hepatic synthesis of new bile salts daily. If the efficiency of enterohepatic conservation is impaired by conditions such as biliary fistula, ileal Crohn's disease, or ileal resection, hepatic synthesis of bile salts increases. The maximal synthetic rate (5 grams per day) is insufficient to restore intraluminal concentrations to normal if external losses exceed this amount.

Bile salts are *amphophiles*, possessing water-soluble and fat-soluble sides. In an aqueous medium they are distributed randomly until a critical concentration (about 2 mM) is reached, at which point spontaneous aggregation forms multimolecular structures called micelles. In micelles the bile salt molecules line up with their hydrophilic portions facing the solvent (water) and their hydrophobic portions facing each other (Fig. 126–2). The hydrocarbon center of the micelle can incorporate biliary lecithin and cholesterol, and the entire aggregate remains water soluble. The addition of lecithin expands micellar size and enhances the ability of bile salt micelles to incorporate other lipids. In addition, a variable amount of cholesterol is carried in lecithin-cholesterol vesicles. The ultimate cholesterol-carrying capacity of bile depends on the relative amounts of bile salts and lecithin as well as the total lipid concentration.

Besides electrolytes, other solutes in bile are bilirubin that has been conjugated in the liver with glucuronic acid (Ch. 115), proteins, and cations such as calcium, iron, copper, and zinc, and low concentrations of the end-products of drug and hormone metabolism.

PATHOPHYSIOLOGY OF GALLSTONE DISEASE

In Western nations about 75 per cent of gallstones are composed principally of cholesterol (*cholesterol gallstones*) and 25 per cent of calcium bilirubinate and other calcium salts (*pigment gallstones*). Overall, about 15 per cent of gallstones are radiopaque, about two thirds of which are pigment and one third are cholesterol stones. The symptoms caused by gallstones are the same regardless of the chemical composition and to a large extent are independent of size. Stones can cause pain and jaundice by passage into the common bile duct or can cause pain by intermittently becoming impacted in the neck of the gallbladder.

CHOLESTEROL GALLSTONES. Cholesterol stones are usually yellow-green to tan or brown and are round or faceted. They may be single or multiple; most range in size from 1 mm to 3 to 4 cm. Cholesterol accounts for 50 to 100 per cent of stone weight, the remainder consisting of mucin glycoproteins and less than 10 per cent calcium bilirubinate and/or other calcium salts. These stones occur two to three times as frequently in women as men, the difference beginning at puberty and declining after menopause. In the United States, 20 per cent of 75-year-old men and 35 per cent of 75-year-old women have stones at autopsy. The incidence is higher with multiparity and with the use of birth control pills. About 75 per cent of American Indian women over the age of 25 years and 90 per cent of those over age 60 are affected. Obesity and hereditary influences are also important in stone formation.

Cholesterol, which is insoluble in water, is normally carried in bile within bile salt–lecithin micelles and lecithin-cholesterol vesicles. A completely clear micellar solution of bile is one in which cholesterol is completely solubilized. A prerequisite for cholesterol gallstone formation is an excess of cholesterol in relation to carrying capacity, a condition that may result from decreased bile salt or increased cholesterol concentration in bile. When the cholesterol-solubilization capacity of bile is exceeded, bile is termed *supersaturated* or *lithogenic*.

Bile of patients with gallstones has relatively more cholesterol

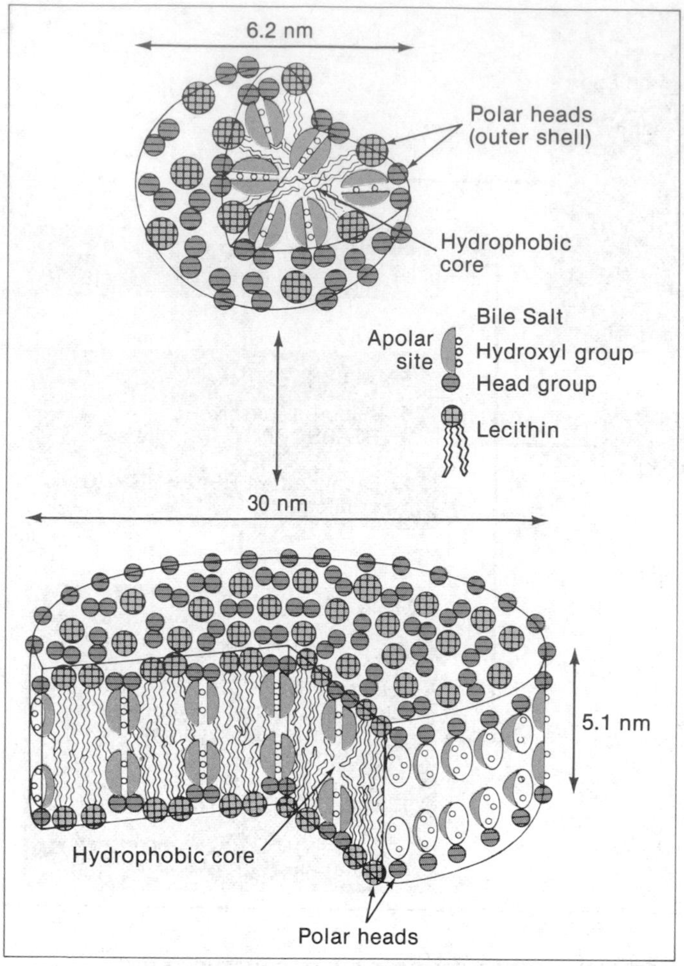

FIGURE 126–2. Dimorphic structure of a biliary mixed lipid micelle, which has been shown to exhibit a sphere → disc transition, depending upon whether the solution is bile salt-rich (*sphere*) or lecithin-rich (*disc*). The lecithin-rich micelle is larger and capable of dissolving and transporting a much larger amount of cholesterol. The transition depends upon the bile salt–lecithin molar ratio present in the micelle but may also be influenced by other constituents present in native bile. Bile salt molecules in both micellar forms are thought to form pairs (dimers) to avoid contact of the hydroxyl groups (*small clear circles*) with the nonpolar environment of the micellar core. (Adapted with permission from Muller K: Biochemistry 20:404, 1981. Copyright 1981 American Chemical Society.)

than that of normal persons, although the overlap is great. In patients with gallstones, bile is supersaturated with cholesterol as it emerges from the liver, implicating the hepatocytes as the cause of the abnormality. In some patients with gallstones the total bile salt pool is decreased in size, and the hepatocytes have decreased amounts of the enzyme 7α-hydroxylase. Another factor, particularly associated with obesity, is increased cholesterol secretion into hepatic bile.

The relationship between cholesterol and bile salt output is hyperbolic, so that when bile salt secretion declines, the cholesterol–bile salt ratio climbs and the bile becomes more supersaturated. During fasting, bile salts are sequestered in the gallbladder, hepatic secretion of bile salts declines, the rate of cholesterol secretion persists, and the bile becomes more lithogenic. Supersaturation of bile with cholesterol is therefore common even in normal persons after overnight or prolonged fasting.

Cholesterol saturation of bile appears to be a necessary but not a sufficient condition for cholesterol gallstone formation. Supersaturated bile from patients without gallstones forms cholesterol crystals slowly on prolonged incubation (long nucleation time), while bile of identical lipid composition from patients with stones usually forms such crystals quickly (short nucleation time). Normal human bile contains *solubilizing* or *antinucleating factors*,

for example, apolipoprotein A-1, that inhibit cholesterol crystallization. The gallbladder is considered to be important in gallstone formation, either by supplying a nidus (*nucleating factor*) for crystallization, such as mucin glycoproteins or other smaller proteins secreted by the epithelium, or by providing an area of stasis to facilitate precipitation.

PIGMENT GALLSTONES. Pigment stones are subdivided into two categories, black and brown stones, on the basis of differing compositional and microstructural characteristics.

Black pigment stones, much more common in the West, are usually under 1 cm, irregular in shape, and homogeneous on cross-section. They form in the gallbladder and are composed of calcium bilirubinate, bilirubin polymers, calcium phosphate and carbonate, and mucin glycoproteins. There is no relationship between black stones and obesity, parity, or saturation of bile with cholesterol. The great majority of patients with black stones have no underlying disease, but the elderly or patients with cirrhosis and hemolytic diseases are predisposed to develop these stones. There is no sexual predisposition. American Indians are rarely affected. The concentration of unconjugated bilirubin is increased in the bile of some patients with these stones.

Brown pigment stones have layers of calcium bilirubinate alternating with layers of cholesterol and calcium salts of fatty acids. Bilirubin is thought to precipitate with calcium because β-glucuronidase of bacterial, biliary epithelial, or hepatic origin deconjugates bilirubin diglucuronide to less soluble bilirubin monoglucuronide or unconjugated bilirubin. The fatty acids of biliary lecithin may be similarly precipitated as calcium salts because of hydrolysis by phospholipases. These stones are much more common in Asia, where bacterial infection of the biliary tract is thought to be involved in their pathogenesis. They can form in the gallbladder and/or in intrahepatic or extrahepatic biliary ducts (Table 126–1). In Western nations they form primarily in the common bile duct years after cholecystectomy for cholesterol or black pigment stones. Unlike in the West, in Asia stones frequently recur after removal and are associated with massive dilatation of the biliary tract and accompanying cholangiohepatitis (recurrent pyogenic cholangitis), often resulting in secondary biliary cirrhosis and hepatic failure.

DISSOLUTION OF GALLSTONES. Cholesterol gallstones can be dissolved by reversing some of the above pathogenetic mechanisms. Ursodeoxycholate (urso), 10 to 12 mg per kilogram per day orally, dissolves a proportion of radiolucent cholesterol gallbladder stones within 2 years. Urso causes the bile to become unsaturated, thereby allowing absorption of cholesterol from the surface of the stone. Minor problems with urso therapy include diarrhea and elevation of serum ALT in about 1 per cent of patients. Urso is ineffective for dissolution of stones greater than 20 mm diameter, of pigment stones, radiopaque stones, and stones in gallbladders nonopacified by oral cholecystography. Candidates for dissolution treatment are mildly to moderately symptomatic patients who wish to avoid surgery or are bad risks for surgery because of other illnesses. Stones usually dissolve in 1 or 2 years in 30 to 40 per cent of patients. Higher success rates

TABLE 126–1. CONDITIONS ASSOCIATED WITH A PROPENSITY FOR GALLSTONE FORMATION

1. **Cholesterol**
   Obesity
   Ileal disease or resection
   Multiparity
   Drugs: clofibrate, estrogens
   Race: American Indian
   Cystic fibrosis
   Rapid weight loss
2. **Black pigment**
   Old age
   Cirrhosis
   Hemolysis
   Intravenous hyperalimentation
3. **Brown pigment**
   Oriental cholangiohepatitis
   Sclerosing cholangitis
   Caroli's disease
   Choledochal cysts
   Duodenal diverticula (perivaterian)

are seen in patients with small (less than 5 mm diameter) floating gallstones. Women who may become pregnant should not be treated because of the potential (though not proven) for harmful effects of urso on the fetus. When treatment is discontinued after initial dissolution, gallstones re-form in about two thirds of patients within 12 years. Prophylactic therapy with urso (300 mg per day orally) can halve this recurrence rate.

Current research into new methods of gallstone dissolution includes direct instillation of methyl-tert-butyl ether into the gallbladder lumen by percutaneous transhepatic catheter placement. This technique usually dissolves cholesterol gallstones within 1 to 2 days. Another technique undergoing study is extracorporeal shock-wave lithotripsy in which gallstones are fragmented into fine particles. These particles are easier to dissolve with urso than are the intact stones.

PATHOPHYSIOLOGY OF BILIARY OBSTRUCTION

Obstruction caused by a stone is the primary cause of all manifestations of gallstone disease. Obstruction of the cystic duct by gallbladder stones distends the gallbladder, producing biliary pain. If the obstruction persists, acute cholecystitis or hydrops may ensue. Whether complications such as empyema or perforation develop depends on whether secondary infection occurs. Cholecystectomy cures cholecystitis, but cholecystostomy, which only relieves the obstruction, eliminates all the clinical manifestations of the disease.

Obstruction of the common duct may produce pain, jaundice, pruritus, infection, and biliary cirrhosis. Surgical procedures that decompress the duct upstream from the stone eliminate these manifestations. The situation in the ductal system differs from that in the gallbladder, however, because when ductal pressure exceeds about 25 cm/H_2O, bile is refluxed into blood. Pressures in this range and even higher commonly accompany mechanical obstruction. Regurgitation of ductal bacteria into the systemic circulation may explain why cholangitis is often accompanied by systemic bacteremia, chills, and high fever. Fortunately obstruction of the common duct by stones is rarely complete. With unrelieved ductal obstruction, biliary cirrhosis gradually develops. Three months is the shortest time in which cirrhosis occurs, and the earliest cases follow neoplastic (high-grade) obstruction.

OBSTRUCTIVE JAUNDICE. Patients with biliary obstruction often present with jaundice. The approach to the clinical evaluation of jaundice is described in detail in Ch. 115.

ROENTGENOLOGIC AND OTHER IMAGING TESTS

Since biliary disease usually results from obstructive lesions, radiologic techniques, if successful in outlining the system, are often diagnostic. The choice and timing of these direct and indirect procedures depend upon the diagnostic strategy of the clinician. They are discussed in greater detail in Ch. 93 and 113.

Plain roentgenograms can demonstrate the 10 to 15 per cent of gallstones that contain enough calcium to be radiopaque, but the relationship of the stones to the gallbladder or bile ducts is not always obvious. Emphysematous cholecystitis, air in the bile ducts, and calcium in the wall of the gallbladder also have diagnostic appearances on plain films.

Oral cholecystography requires that the night prior to the examination the patient swallow tablets of iopanoic or tyropanoic acid, which are then absorbed from the gut, excreted in bile, and concentrated in the gallbladder. If the gallbladder is opacified, stones in the lumen are shown as radiolucent defects (Fig. 126–3). Oral cholecystography is 90 to 95 per cent accurate in detecting gallstones. Nonopacification of the gallbladder occurs if the cystic duct is blocked or if the diseased gallbladder mucosa cannot concentrate the contrast material. The gallbladder may not be opacified for several reasons not related to gallbladder disease: if the patient has been vomiting, if the patient has been fasting for several days immediately before taking the tablets, or if absorption by the gut or excretion by the liver is faulty. If extrabiliary causes of a nonopacified gallbladder are excluded, nonopacification is 95 per cent reliable in indicating gallbladder disease.

Ultrasonography of the biliary tree may demonstrate gallstones or dilatation of the intrahepatic or extrahepatic ductal system (Fig. 126–4). It also has the advantage of being able to examine the liver and pancreas at the same time. Real-time ultrasonog-

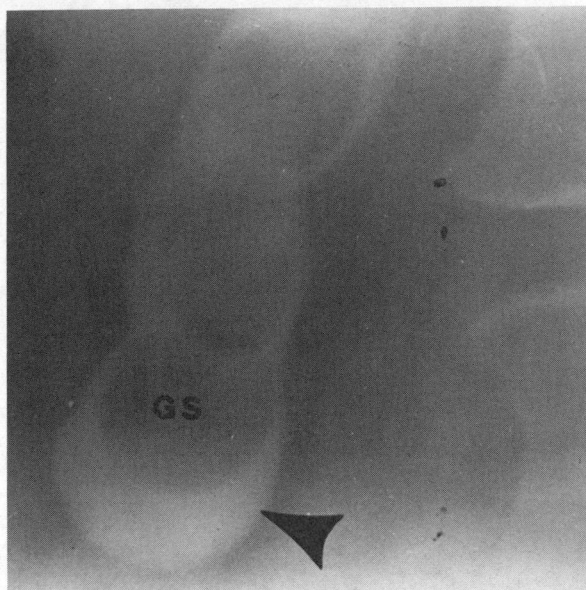

FIGURE 126–3. Oral cholecytogram showing a gallbladder (*arrowhead*) opacified by an orally administered contrast agent. The gallbladder is filled with four large round gallstones (GS).

raphy is very reliable in detecting gallbladder stones (false positives are uncommon); it should be used as the first test for screening for gallstones. Ductal dilatation is detected in about 90 per cent of cases of proven obstruction. Unfortunately, less than one third of common duct stones are actually identified. Ductal dilatation usually indicates distal obstruction by neoplasm, stricture, or stone. The correlation between dilatation and obstruction is inexact because (1) the ducts may be dilated from previous disease or surgery although currently unobstructed, (2) cirrhosis or scarring from previous cholangitis may stiffen the ducts enough to prevent dilatation, and (3) lesions characterized by intermittent obstruction (e.g., common duct stones, stricture) may result in dilatation followed by spontaneous decompression; ducts may appear undilated if the patient is examined after such decompression.

Percutaneous transhepatic cholangiography (PTC) involves direct percutaneous puncture of an intrahepatic duct by a needle inserted through the eighth or ninth right intercostal space into the center of the liver. An abnormal clotting mechanism, significant ascites, and severe cholangitis are contraindications. PTC has proved particularly valuable in diagnosing gallstones within the intrahepatic biliary tract, biliary strictures, and neoplastic obstruction of the bile ducts (Fig. 126–5). A technically successful study can be obtained in nearly all patients with dilated ducts and in 70 per cent of patients with normal-sized ducts.

Endoscopic retrograde cholangiopancreatography (ERCP) involves cannulation of the common bile duct and pancreatic duct through the ampulla of Vater via the endoscope (see Fig. 93–7). With experience, a successful study of one or both ducts is possible in 90 per cent of attempts. ERCP is particularly useful in patients with normal-sized bile ducts or in whom pancreatic disease as a cause of bile duct obstruction is strongly suspected.

Both PTC and ERCP are usually contraindicated in active cholangitis unless a therapeutic maneuver is planned because as ductal pressure increases during injection of the contrast material, severe uncontrollable sepsis may be produced. Patients undergoing either of these procedures should usually receive premedication with antimicrobial agents if biliary obstruction is known or suspected.

Radionuclide imaging of the biliary tree may be accomplished by intravenous injection of a ^{99m}Tc-labeled derivative of iminodiacetic acid (e.g., HIDA or DISIDA). Normally, a high-quality image of the biliary tree appears within 30 minutes after administration of the radionuclide agent (see Fig. 93–9). This test is the procedure of choice in verifying the diagnosis of acute cholecystitis. Filling of the ducts but not of the gallbladder

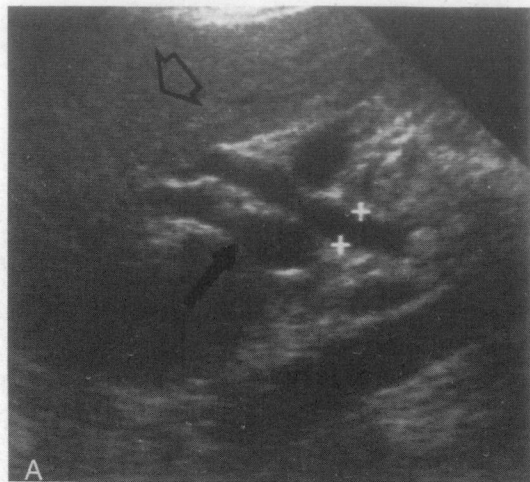

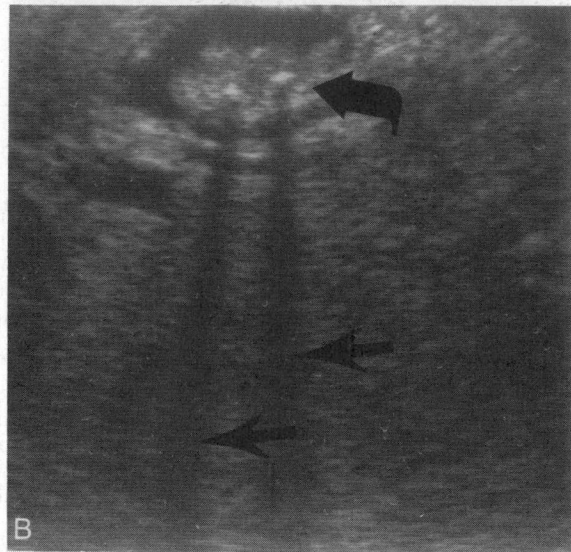

FIGURE 126–4. *A,* Real-time ultrasonography of the extrahepatic biliary tract showing a dilated common bile duct (the width of the duct measured between the two white crosses is 9 mm); the portal vein is seen as the anechoic area *(solid arrow)* directly beneath the common bile duct. The liver parenchyma is indicated by the arrowhead. *B,* Ultrasonography of a gallbladder containing gallstones and sludge *(curved arrow)* that appear as echogenic foci within the gallbladder lumen. The gallstones exhibit acoustic shadowing *(lower two arrows),* that is, paucity of echoes distal to the stones due to blockage of the echo waves by the solid stones. (Courtesy of Dr. Peter Arger.)

supports the diagnosis of cholecystitis due to obstruction of the cystic duct by a stone or edema. A false-negative study is rare; however, false-positive (nonfilling) studies are seen in patients with severe illnesses such as pancreatitis and in those receiving intravenous hyperalimentation. Ultrasonography is more useful in detecting common bile duct obstruction than is radionuclide imaging.

Computed tomography is usually performed after evidence of biliary ductal disease has been ascertained by ultrasonography or cholangiography. It is useful in defining pancreatic causes of biliary tract obstruction, in detecting paraductal lymph node enlargement, and in examining the liver for abscesses, intrahepatic ductal dilatation, and neoplasms.

CLINICAL CATEGORIES OF GALLBLADDER AND BILIARY TRACT DISEASES

Asymptomatic Gallstones

Approximately 60 to 80 per cent of patients with gallstones are asymptomatic, based on surveys using ultrasonography. In the past, patients with asymptomatic gallstones were advised to have a cholecystectomy. The trend now is to observe such patients

and not to recommend surgery unless they develop biliary pain. Prophylactic cholecystectomy is reserved for patients with *calcified gallbladders,* often associated with carcinoma of the gallbladder. Asymptomatic patients with gallstones have approximately a 20 per cent chance of developing biliary pain in 20 years. Even with symptomatic patients, the decision to perform surgery is not always clear-cut. Patients with infrequent mild pain may prefer not to undergo cholecystectomy, or the physician may be hesitant to recommend surgery because of serious coexisting illnesses. Such patients are suitable candidates to consider for medical dissolution with ursodeoxycholate.

Symptomatic Gallstones

PATHOLOGY. The pathologic findings in the gallbladder wall and the clinical manifestations of gallstone disease often correlate poorly. In some patients the gallbladder is severely affected as the result of previous attacks of acute cholecystitis, with shrinking, scarring, and thickening of the wall, adhesions to adjacent viscera, and patchy replacement of the mucosa by granulation tissue or collagen. Nonopacification following oral cholecystography is frequent in such patients. At the other extreme the gallbladder may be grossly normal with only slight thinning of the mucosa, mild patchy scarring and inflammation, and a normally visualized oral cholecystogram. The term *chronic cholecystitis* is a descriptive pathologic term for such changes, although it has been used to describe the clinical manifestations of chronically symptomatic gallstones.

CLINICAL MANIFESTATIONS. Symptomatic gallstones commonly produce a steady pain most often located in the epigastrium or right upper quadrant, thought to be caused by gallbladder distention arising from transient obstruction of the cystic duct by a stone. The onset of pain takes only a few minutes; it quickly reaches a plateau in intensity that may range from mild to moderate to excruciating. After 30 minutes to several hours the pain subsides gradually. The pain does not wax and wane like intestinal colic; hence the preferred term is *biliary pain,* not biliary colic. Nausea and vomiting may accompany the attack, and a vague residual ache or soreness may remain after the acute pain has dissipated. Tenderness, muscular guarding, a palpable mass, fever, and leukocytosis are absent, distinguishing this condition from acute cholecystitis. Many patients have simultaneous pain referred to the back near the scapula or to the right shoulder area. Attacks may occur daily or as seldom as once every few years. Not uncommonly, patients with symptomatic gallstones have pain that does not exactly fit this "textbook description." Dyspepsia, intolerance to fatty food, flatulence, heartburn, and belching may occur but are not helpful diagnostically because they often occur in persons with normal gallbladders.

Hydrops (mucocele) of the gallbladder refers to its distention with mucus (white bile) and gallstones; it may develop from cystic duct obstruction. Hydrops produces constant discomfort in the right upper quadrant and a palpable mass without the clinical findings of acute cholecystitis.

DIAGNOSIS. Real-time *ultrasonography* is the preferred test because it is 95 to 99 per cent sensitive in detecting gallbladder stones. It also has the advantage of allowing examination of the common bile duct, pancreas, and liver at the same time without radiation exposure. An oral cholecystogram after a double dose of contrast material (that is, taken on the two nights prior to the examination) identifies 90 to 95 per cent of gallstones. In about 5 to 10 per cent of patients with gallstones, opacification of the gallbladder is adequate during oral cholecystography, but calculi are not demonstrated, usually because the stones are too small to be seen.

In patients with typical biliary pain in the absence of demonstrable gallstones by cholecystography or ultrasonography, examination of bile for crystals may prove helpful. A sample of bile is obtained from an orally placed duodenal tube or via endoscopy and is examined microscopically for the presence of cholesterol crystals. The significance of calcium bilirubinate crystals is uncertain. In the presence of what seems to be biliary pain, a positive duodenal drainage test is highly suggestive that tiny stones are present or, in rare cases, that cholesterolosis is present.

The *differential diagnosis* includes other common causes of chronic abdominal symptoms such as peptic ulcer, gastroesophageal reflux, esophageal spasm, and pancreatitis, which may have manifestations similar to those of gallstones. Radicular pain from spinal lesions or rib pain from bone lesions may mimic biliary pain. Angina pectoris may cause pain thought to be abdominal, just as biliary pain may be felt in the precordial region. Postprandial pain or discomfort may result from the irritable bowel syndrome or intestinal infection.

COMPLICATIONS. *Choledocholithiasis* is the most common complication, affecting about 15 per cent of patients with cholecystolithiasis. The incidence of common duct stones increases with advancing age. Patients with symptomatic gallstones may eventually develop an attack of *acute cholecystitis.* About two thirds of patients with acute cholecystitis have previously had symptomatic gallstones. *Acute pancreatitis* may develop when stones migrate through the distal common bile duct. *Mirizzi's syndrome* results from extrinsic compression of the common hepatic or common bile duct by a large stone in the cystic duct. Obstructive jaundice may develop. Calcification of the gallbladder *(porcelain gallbladder)* is an uncommon condition, but of special significance because of its frequent association with carcinoma of the gallbladder. The diagnosis is made from the radiographic demonstration of an eggshell-like rim of calcium in the gallbladder wall. *Adenocarcinoma* of the gallbladder is found mainly in elderly patients with cholelithiasis, most of whom have had biliary symptoms for many years.

TREATMENT. Dietary changes, anticholinergics, and antispasmodics have no effect on the course of the disease, but they sometimes provide temporary symptomatic relief. Analgesics should be used for relief of pain. *Cholecystectomy* is the treatment of choice. An attempt to dissolve the stones with urso is an appropriate alternative in selected cases. At operation the common bile duct is inspected, a cholangiogram is obtained, and the duct is explored if there is evidence of choledocholithiasis.

Cholecystectomy relieves symptoms from gallstones; the postcholecystectomy syndrome is discussed later in this chapter. Removal of the gallbladder does not impair gastrointestinal function. The mortality in elective cholecystectomy is less than 0.5 per cent. In patients over 70 years of age, however, mortality rises to 2 to 3 per cent; most of the postoperative deaths are a result of pre-existing cardiopulmonary diseases.

Acute Cholecystitis

PATHOGENESIS. Acute cholecystitis is the result of cystic duct obstruction and chemical inflammation rather than of bacterial infection. Filling the gallbladder of a dog with concentrated bile and obstructing the cystic duct produce acute inflammation. If the gallbladder is empty or distended with physiologic saline solution instead of bile, cystic duct obstruction is tolerated without inflammation. Obstruction is associated with the release of phospholipase from the gallbladder epithelium that can hydrolyze lecithin, resulting in lysolecithin, an epithelial toxin. Simultaneously the epithelial barrier coating of mucin glycoproteins may be acutely disrupted, making the epithelium susceptible to injury by the detergent action of the concentrated bile salts.

Bacterial infection is secondary to biliary obstruction rather than being primary. Bacteria are not present in the gallbladders of asymptomatic or chronically symptomatic patients with cholesterol or black pigment gallstones. Early in acute cholecystitis, the gallbladder bile is sterile, but within a week after onset, bacteria may be present in bile in over 50 per cent of cases. Although infection is secondary, it may be ultimately responsible for the most serious sequelae of acute cholecystitis—empyema, gangrene, and perforation.

Acalculous cholecystitis accounts for less than 5 per cent of cases. Most cases have been associated with prolonged fasting after major trauma, e.g., war or automobile accident injuries, surgical operations, multisystem organ failure, sepsis, or severe burns. Rare cases are caused by *Salmonella typhosa,* polyarteritis nodosa, or ischemia of other causes. At operation the bile is viscous and full of sludge. Gangrene and perforation are more frequent, and the outcome is worse than in acute calculous cholecystitis.

PATHOLOGY. Early inflammation with subserosal edema, mucosal ulcerations, and submucosal hemorrhages progresses slowly to cellular infiltration of the wall after 3 to 4 days, which reaches its greatest intensity at the end of the first week. During the second week, patchy mural gangrene, small intramural ab-

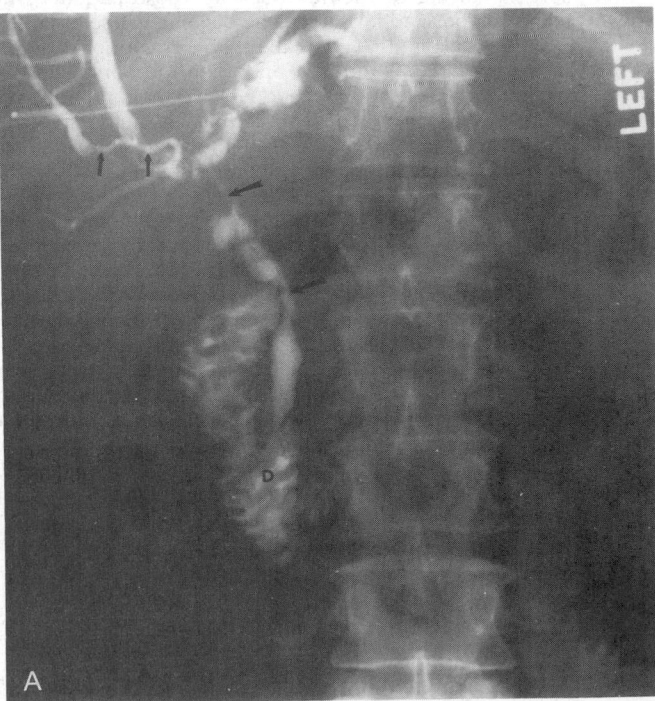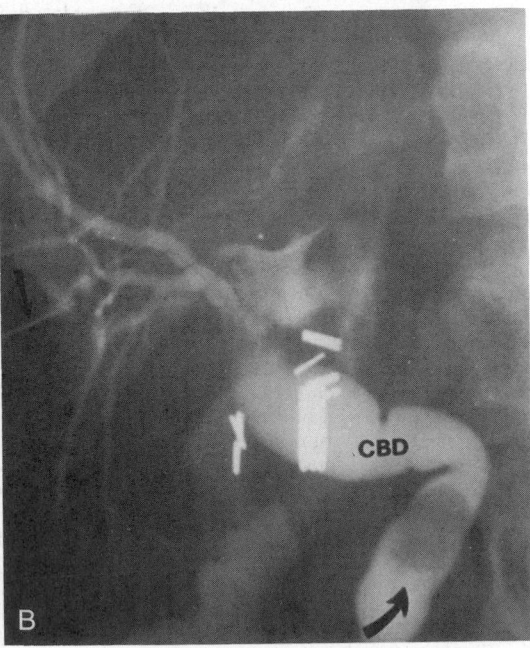

FIGURE 126–5. *A,* Percutaneous transhepatic cholangiogram demonstrating primary sclerosing cholangitis in a 54-year-old woman with a long history of Crohn's disease and biochemical evidence of cholestasis. There are strictures *(arrows)* scattered throughout her intra- and extrahepatic biliary tract; dye is seen to flow into the duodenum (D). *B,* Percutaneous transhepatic cholangiogram (skinny needle used for dye injection is indicated by arrow on left) showing a 1.5 × 2.0 cm gallstone *(curved arrow)* in the distal common bile duct (CBD) causing dilatation of the extrahepatic biliary tract. The metallic clips are from a prior cholecystectomy. The patient presented with a 3-day history of RUQ pain and jaundice with a total bilirubin of 5.6 mg per deciliter. (Courtesy of Dr. Gordon McLean.)

scesses, and collagen deposition appear. Resolution of the acute changes takes another week or more.

The term *empyema* describes the rare entity of a pus-filled gallbladder characterized clinically by a septic form of acute cholecystitis. Gangrene and perforation are most common in the fundus where the blood supply is meager or in the neck where stones become impacted. With perforation, gallbladder contents may spill into the free abdominal cavity (bile peritonitis) or, more often, are confined by adhesions (pericholecystic abscess). Sometimes an adherent viscus is penetrated, forming a cholecystenteric fistula through which the gallstones and pus may be discharged. Fistulization is most frequent with the duodenum, but jejunal and colonic fistulas have been described.

CLINICAL MANIFESTATIONS. An attack of acute cholecystitis begins with *abdominal pain* that increases gradually in severity. The pain is usually located in the right subcostal region from the start, but it sometimes begins in the epigastrium or left upper quadrant and then shifts to the region of the gallbladder as inflammation progresses. Two thirds or more of patients have had previous episodes of typical biliary pain. Early in the attack the patient may expect the symptoms to subside spontaneously as had happened before with similar pain, and medical aid is often not sought until 24 to 48 hours or more. Referred pain may be experienced in the back at the scapular level. Patients in their 70's and 80's may have few or no localizing symptoms.

Anorexia, nausea, and vomiting are often present, but vomiting is rarely severe enough to be confused with bowel obstruction and is generally less than in acute pancreatitis. In the absence of complications, chills are rare, and the temperature is about 38°C. Chills and high temperature suggest suppurative cholecystitis or associated cholangitis.

The right subcostal region is tender to palpation, and involuntary muscle spasm generally limits the examination. If the patient takes a deep breath while the subhepatic area is being palpated, heightened tenderness arrests inspiration *(Murphy's sign)*.

In somewhat less than a quarter of the patients, a distended, tender gallbladder can be distinctly felt, an important finding that confirms the suspected diagnosis. The gallbladder cannot be felt in the rest of the patients because of obesity, rigidity of the abdominal wall, or deep subhepatic location or because it is small and shrunken from previous inflammation. Other related conditions characterized by a tender mass in the same area are pericholecystic abscess, acute cholecystitis complicating carcinoma of the gallbladder, or gallbladder distention in obstructive cholangitis.

About 10 per cent of patients with acute cholecystitis have *mild jaundice* caused by edema of the nearby common duct or by common duct stones.

With treatment, improvement is usually noticeable within the first 12 to 24 hours, and the signs and symptoms gradually subside over 3 to 7 days. Persistent severe pain, a rise in temperature or leukocyte count (>10,000 per cubic millimeter), and appearance of shaking chills or of more severe local or generalized abdominal tenderness all indicate progression of the disease and the need for immediate surgery.

Empyema (suppurative cholecystitis) can produce systemic toxicity and mild increases in bilirubin, alkaline phosphatase, and the transaminases and may herald perforation.

DIAGNOSIS. The diagnosis is strongly suggested by the clinical manifestations just described. Roentgenograms of the abdomen may show calcified gallstones. Ultrasonography is the simplest and most reliable method of detecting gallbladder stones in these patients.

Radionuclide scanning following intravenous administration of ^{99m}Tc DISIDA or related compounds is the procedure of choice to verify a clinical impression of acute cholecystitis. If the gallbladder fills, the diagnosis of acute cholecystitis is quite unlikely. If the bile duct fills but the gallbladder does not, the diagnosis is strongly supported.

In the differential diagnosis, acute pancreatitis, acute appendicitis, and penetrated or perforated peptic ulcer are the conditions that most often cause major problems. Furthermore, acute cholecystitis and acute pancreatitis may coexist.

In women, *gonococcal perihepatitis* (Fitz-Hugh-Curtis syndrome), caused by intra-abdominal spread of the infection from the reproductive tract to the right upper quadrant, may be mistaken for acute cholecystitis, but adnexal tenderness is usually present on pelvic examination. A cervical smear usually reveals gonococci, and the patients are younger, often have higher temperature, and are in less distress than would be expected with cholecystitis.

Acute hepatitis, either viral or alcoholic, sometimes produces marked right upper quadrant pain and tenderness. A history of recent binge drinking, high transaminase levels, and liver biopsy aid differentiation. Pneumonitis, pyelonephritis, and acute cardiac disease (particularly right-sided failure) all on occasion may cause acute pain suggestive of cholecystitis. The use of ^{99m}Tc DISIDA distinguishes between the unusual location of pain in these disorders and acute cholecystitis.

TREATMENT. Most patients with acute cholecystitis improve with either expectant treatment or cholecystectomy performed during the acute attack. In general, the decision regarding the kind of treatment should include the following considerations (Fig. 126–6): (1) whether the diagnosis is secure, (2) whether biliary complications have occurred or appear imminent, and (3) the overall condition of the patient (operative risk).

Upon the patient's admission to the hospital, nasogastric suction should be started if the patient has significant vomiting, and fluids should be given intravenously to correct dehydration. In many elderly patients the acute biliary condition may aggravate pre-existing cardiac, pulmonary, or renal disease and produce a more ominous prognosis if surgery is delayed or if adequate treatment is not given.

Antimicrobials are of principal value to prevent bacteremia and to treat suppurative complications. If the patient is seen shortly after symptoms begin, and if local signs and symptoms are mild, antimicrobial therapy need not be given. Otherwise, an antimicrobial regimen with coverage for gram-negative aerobes as well as enterococci is preferred. One that is often used is ampicillin plus gentamicin given parenterally. In seriously ill patients, such as those with empyema or perforation, it is wise to also add an antimicrobial with anaerobic coverage, such as clindamycin.

Cholecystectomy is the optimal therapy for acute cholecystitis, but only after the diagnosis is secure and the patient adequately prepared for operation. Some physicians still prefer to reserve surgery during the acute attack for those patients who develop complications and for those who become worse or fail to improve. Although this is still done, about 25 per cent of patients managed in this way require urgent operation for worsening disease. For patients who respond to nonoperative management, cholecystectomy is recommended. The timing of cholecystectomy in such patients has been debated, but the trend is to perform surgery early on during the same hospitalization.

In about 30 per cent of patients, the diagnosis is obvious within 12 to 24 hours, they are good operative risks, and cholecystectomy can be scheduled promptly. Another 30 per cent are good surgical candidates, but the diagnosis is not quite firm. In this situation, a ^{99m}Tc DISIDA scan should be obtained to verify the clinical impression. Another 30 per cent of patients have serious coexistent cardiac, respiratory, or other disease for which treatment takes precedence. The cholecystitis should be treated expectantly while the other problems are being corrected. Progression of local abdominal findings requires continued re-evaluation, balancing the risks of operation with the risks of continued delay.

About 10 per cent of patients require emergency intervention for complications present on admission or that appear later during observation and medical management. When emergency operation becomes necessary, cholecystostomy may sometimes be preferable to cholecystectomy in the seriously ill patient. In this procedure the fundus is incised, stones and pus are removed from the lumen, and the organ is decompressed by catheter drainage, allowing the acute infection to resolve. Cholecystostomy can also be performed using radiologic techniques. Patients who recover should undergo cholecystectomy 6 to 8 weeks later. Those who continue to be poor surgical risks may be followed expectantly if postoperative cholecystography shows that the gallbladder and common duct contain no residual stones. If stones are present, interventional radiologic techniques can be used to remove gallbladder stones through the cholecystostomy tract after 4 to 6 weeks of tract maturation, and endoscopic sphincterotomy can be utilized to remove ductal stones. In seriously debilitated patients the cholecystostomy tube can be left in place indefinitely.

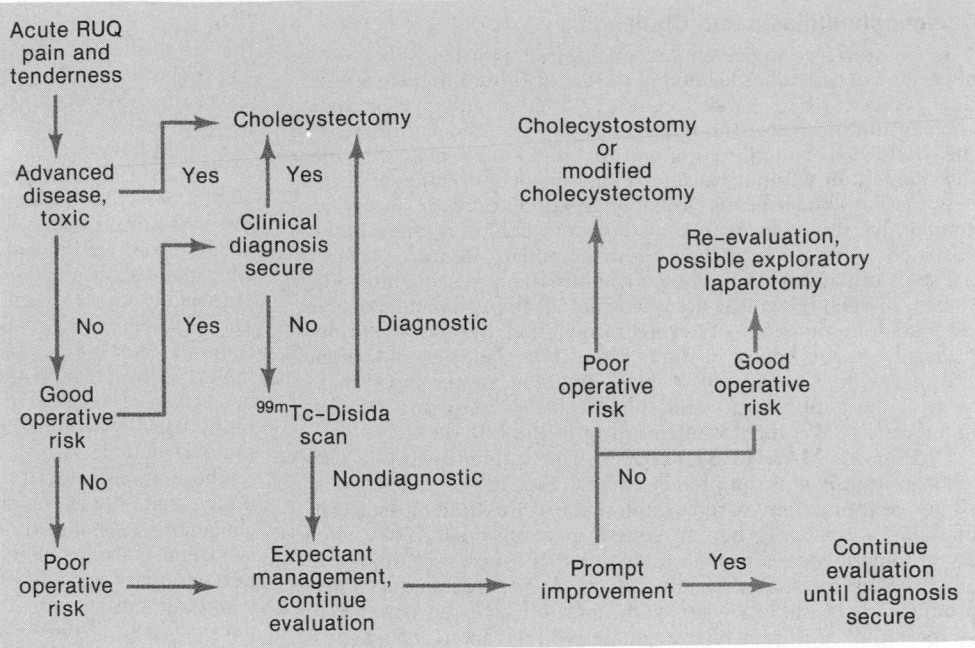

FIGURE 126–6. Schema for managing patients with right upper quadrant pain and tenderness who are thought possibly to have acute cholecystitis. This approach is based on a policy of early operation for appropriate patients and distinguishes between patients who are good versus poor operative risks.

After the cholecystostomy tube is removed from a patient whose biliary system contains no calculi, within several years about 50 per cent of patients develop new stones.

COMPLICATIONS. *Emphysematous Cholecystitis.* In emphysematous cholecystitis, a rare variant of acute cholecystitis, gas of bacterial origin can be seen in the gallbladder lumen and adjacent tissues. Clinically, emphysematous cholecystitis causes the same signs and symptoms as acute cholecystitis. About 30 per cent of patients have diabetes mellitus, and the gallbladder is acalculous in about half the cases. Gas does not develop until 24 to 48 hours after the attack begins, at which time a radiolucent halo outlines the lumen, and an air-fluid level may be seen on upright films. Subserosal and then pericholecystic emphysema appear with time. Differential diagnosis of the radiographic findings includes cholecystenteric fistula and appendiceal, perinephric, or subhepatic abscess. In about half the cases the gas-forming organisms are clostridia, and the rest are *Escherichia coli*, streptococci, and other bacteria of intestinal origin. Treatment is the same as for acute cholecystitis, but the more aggressive nature of emphysematous cholecystitis mandates prompt surgery.

Perforation. Perforation is usually manifested by greater sepsis and more marked abdominal signs. Perforation may take any of three forms: (1) free perforation into the abdominal cavity, (2) localized (contained) perforation with pericholecystic abscess, and (3) perforation into another viscus with fistula formation.

Free perforation, which has a 25 per cent mortality, is the least common type. It usually occurs early in the attack, often within the first 3 days, suggesting that when gangrene develops this quickly it cannot be walled off by adjacent viscera or the omentum. Clinically, free perforation classically causes toxicity with high temperatures (greater than 39°C), leukocytosis (over 15,000 per cubic millimeter), and diffuse abdominal tenderness and rigidity. In more than half the cases the correct diagnosis is unsuspected until laparotomy or autopsy, because a clear-cut history of preliminary right upper quadrant pain is often lacking. Treatment consists of intravenous antimicrobial therapy and emergency cholecystectomy.

Localized perforation most often appears in the second week of the attack at the peak of the inflammatory reaction. The diagnosis should be suspected with increasing local signs, especially when a mass suddenly appears. In most cases cholecystectomy can be performed, but in a severely ill patient cholecystostomy and drainage of the abscess may be wiser.

Fistula formation usually involves the nearby second portion of the duodenum or, less commonly, the colon, jejunum, stomach, or common bile duct. Rare fistulas have entered the renal pelvis or bronchus or extended through the abdominal wall (empyema necessitatis). After intestinal fistulization the contents of the gallbladder are discharged into the gut, often aborting the acute attack. Clinically, the fistula itself may not be suspected because it produces no unique findings; many are discovered incidentally later. In the absence of biliary obstruction a cholecystenteric fistula is not necessarily of pathophysiologic significance. Cholecystocolonic fistulas may cause malabsorption from diversion of bile or from bacterial overgrowth in the upper gut.

Gallstone Ileus. If a particularly large gallstone enters through the fistula, it may obstruct the intestine, a condition called gallstone ileus. The stone, passing through a cholecystenteric fistula, most often enters the gut in the duodenum, less commonly in the jejunum, ileum, colon, or stomach. It is often assumed that the initial event responsible for fistula formation is an attack of acute cholecystitis, but only 30 per cent of patients with gallstone ileus give a history of recent right upper quadrant pain. After entering the gut, the gallstone moves downstream until it encounters an area of intestinal lumen too narrow to accommodate it. Gallstones, usually more than 2.5 cm in diameter, most frequently obstruct the terminal ileum; they block the colon only if its lumen has been narrowed by intrinsic disease.

On physical examination the findings are those of small-bowel obstruction. Rarely can the stone be felt as a mass on abdominal, vaginal, or rectal examination. Roentgenograms usually show air in the biliary tree if the films are carefully examined, and in some cases a radiopaque gallstone can be identified at the leading edge of the obstruction. Treatment consists of removing the obstructing gallstone through a small enterotomy. It is generally wise to leave the biliary disease undisturbed initially, because these often elderly patients tolerate long procedures poorly, and nothing much is gained by repairing the fistula primarily. Postoperatively, many patients remain asymptomatic, and the fistula may even close spontaneously; for them, expectant management is best. Some patients may require cholecystectomy later because of symptoms related to gallstones.

The mortality is 15 to 20 per cent because of delay in diagnosis and because of cardiopulmonary complications.

PROGNOSIS. The mortality in acute cholecystitis of 5 to 10 per cent is almost totally confined to patients over 60 years of age with serious associated disease. Suppurative complications are more common in the elderly, who can tolerate them least. In most instances, localized perforation can be managed satisfactorily at operation. Free perforation is considerably more ominous (25 per cent mortality) but is rare.

Choledocholithiasis and Cholangitis

In Western countries choledocholithiasis is usually the result of passage of gallstones formed in the gallbladder into the common duct. About 10 to 15 per cent of patients with symptomatic cholecystolithiasis are thought to develop choledocholithiasis on this basis. Once in the common duct the stones may pass into the duodenum without causing symptoms. The frequency of this event is not known but is probably greatly underestimated. Less commonly, stones form in a dilated duct behind a longstanding obstruction caused by a stricture or ampullary stenosis. About 5 per cent of patients with choledocholithiasis have no gallbladder stones; in such cases it is assumed that all the gallbladder stones escaped into the duct or, more rarely, that the stones formed primarily in the common duct. Stone type helps to determine site of origin: Cholesterol or black pigment stones more likely form in the gallbladder, while almost all brown pigment stones in patients in Western countries form in the bile ducts.

CLINICAL MANIFESTATIONS. The natural history of choledocholithiasis is incompletely known (Fig. 126–7). About 30 to 40 per cent of patients are asymptomatic at the time of diagnosis, implying a relatively benign course in many cases. How often asymptomatic stones remain undetected is, of course, unknown. Obstruction by stones of the biliary or pancreatic ducts may produce any of the following syndromes: biliary pain, jaundice or increased alkaline phosphatase alone (without pain), cholangitis, pancreatitis, or a combination of these. Secondary hepatic effects of persistent obstruction include biliary cirrhosis or hepatic abscesses.

Intermittent *cholangitis*, consisting of biliary pain, jaundice, and fever and chills (*Charcot's triad*), is a common presenting symptom complex. In the absence of previous biliary surgery it is almost diagnostic of choledocholithiasis. Intermittency of symptoms is quite characteristic, a manifestation of intermittent partial obstruction. Whenever pain, chills with fever, and jaundice fluctuate together over a span of a few days or a week, cholangitis from biliary obstruction is almost certainly the cause. In a typical attack, chills may precede the other symptoms, and bilirubinuria may follow. Epigastric or right upper quadrant pain, indistinguishable from biliary pain caused by gallbladder stones, is steady and severe. Pain may be referred to the right infrascapular area, the upper back, the right shoulder, or even the precordium, suggesting coronary artery or esophageal disease.

The severity of cholangitis varies widely from the usual mild transient illness to overwhelming sepsis with shock (see Suppurative Cholangitis, below). In the average case, the temperature rises to 38.5 to 40°C, preceded by chills and positive blood cultures. Localized tenderness in the subcostal region may be associated with extreme guarding and rigidity, but more often

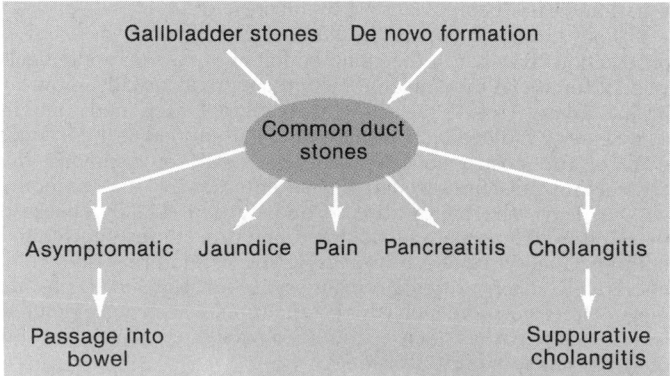

FIGURE 126–7. Natural history of choledocholithiasis. In most cases, common duct gallstones originate in the gallbladder. In some cases, particularly after the gallbladder has been surgically removed, stones may form in the common duct. The majority of stones in the common duct remain asymptomatic and may either remain in the duct without causing symptoms, pass into the bowel through the ampulla of Vater and be excreted in stool, or eventually result in symptoms, the most common of which are indicated. The exact frequency of each of these occurrences is not known.

the local findings are minimal or intermittent and are usually less severe than in acute cholecystitis.

In most cases of common duct obstruction caused by stones the gallbladder does not become distended, because it is scarred and inelastic, and the obstruction is recent, partial, or transient. This is the obverse of Courvoisier's law; i.e., a distended nontender gallbladder in a jaundiced patient signifies neoplastic obstruction of the bile duct.

DIAGNOSIS. In cholangitis the leukocyte count averages 15,000 per cubic millimeter but may go much higher in severe cases. Bilirubin values are usually in the range of 2 to 4 mg per deciliter and are uncommonly higher than 10 mg per deciliter. Elevated serum alkaline phosphatase and 5'-nucleotidase levels are usually greater than three times the upper limit of normal. The ALT generally remains below 200 units; however, transiently it may exceed 1000 units. In these instances the prompt drop of the ALT level within 48 hours allows differentiation from viral hepatitis and suggests the diagnosis of obstruction. Ultrasonography usually demonstrates a dilated ductal system proximal to the obstruction.

The demonstration of gallbladder stones does not necessarily imply that stones in the bile ducts are responsible for the cholangitis, although this is usually true. When the presenting syndrome is painless cholestatic jaundice, other causes, especially periampullary and biliary neoplasms, must be considered. With neoplastic obstruction, the bilirubin averages about 15 to 20 mg per deciliter and rarely fluctuates. Although jaundice from stones may be as intense, the level of bilirubin is characteristically less than 10 mg per deciliter, and it may rise and fall episodically. The diagnosis of intrahepatic cholestasis from causes such as drugs, viral hepatitis, or pregnancy should follow the schema outlined in Ch. 115. In such cases, opacification of normal bile ducts by PTC or ERCP may ultimately be required. Gallstone disease is common in cirrhosis, so choledocholithiasis and liver disease may coexist. In patients who have had cholecystectomy, differentiation between choledocholithiasis and biliary stricture as the cause of cholangitis depends on direct radiologic demonstration of the ducts.

Common duct stones may cause acute pancreatitis indistinguishable clinically from that resulting from alcohol or other causes and unaccompanied by specific signs of biliary disease (Ch. 106). Pancreatitis caused by biliary calculi, despite numerous attacks, rarely progresses to pancreatic calcification, chronic pain, and pancreatic insufficiency, as often occurs in the alcoholic variety. Gallstone disease should be ruled out in every patient with acute pancreatitis, because further damage during such an episode and future attacks can be avoided if the gallstones are removed.

TREATMENT. The potential seriousness of cholangitis necessitates hospitalization for diagnosis and treatment. After blood cultures are obtained, antimicrobial drugs effective against enteric organisms are given by the parenteral route. A regimen consisting of an aminoglycoside plus ampicillin for mild attacks with the addition of clindamycin in severe infection is usually successful. A shift from the initial regimen on the basis of the result of cultures and drug susceptibility tests may be necessary. The margin between mild and severe illness is small; antimicrobial therapy should be expected to control the acute attack within 24 to 48 hours, and if there is no improvement or worsening after this period, emergency surgery or endoscopic sphincterotomy must be considered seriously.

More than 90 per cent of patients respond satisfactorily to treatment, allowing an orderly attempt at diagnosis. Ultrasonography should be performed first to detect ductal dilatation. Direct opacification of the ducts can be attempted by PTC or ERCP. Both kinds of direct cholangiography are potentially hazardous in active cholangitis and should be postponed if possible until infection is well controlled; then one proceeds only under the protection of antimicrobial therapy. However, rapid decompression of the bile duct using a percutaneous transhepatic catheter or by endoscopic sphincterotomy may provide the control needed in advanced cases.

Deciding between endoscopic and surgical approaches to the management of choledocholithiasis should be on a case-by-case basis. If the gallbladder is present, cholecystectomy is performed and the common duct is opened and emptied of stones. A T tube is left in the duct to decompress biliary pressure in the postop-

Selected patients with choledocholithiasis such as the elderly, poor operative risks, or those who have already had a cholecystectomy may be satisfactorily treated by endoscopic sphincterotomy. By means of the side-viewing duodenoscope, a wire (papillotome) is passed into the bile duct and the sphincter divided by electrocautery. Common duct stones 1.5 cm or smaller usually pass into the duodenum. This technique may be unsuccessful with very large stones. Bleeding and pancreatitis are the principal complications but are infrequent. Mortality in the procedure is less than 1 per cent in experienced hands. When endoscopic sphincterotomy is successfully used for cholangitis in patients with gallbladder stones, there is debate about whether to perform cholecystectomy at a later date. In our opinion this decision should be based on whether the patient subsequently develops symptoms referable to the gallbladder stones.

RETAINED COMMON DUCT STONES. The methods for detecting duct stones at operation are about 95 per cent reliable, which means, unfortunately, that a few are overlooked only to be discovered on postoperative T-tube cholangiograms. There are several approaches to remove residual stones without another laparotomy. Instrumental extraction is the treatment of choice. Under image-intensification fluoroscopy the T tube is pulled out, a basket is passed into the duct, and the stone is grasped and withdrawn. This method should not be tried until 4 to 6 weeks postoperatively to allow for maturation of the T-tube tract. If mechanical extraction is not successful, endoscopic sphincterotomy may allow the stone to pass into the duodenum. Another uncommonly used technique depends on the ability of mono-octanoin (glyceryl-1-mono-octanoate) to dissolve cholesterol gallstones. Mono-octanoin is infused into the duct at 2 to 5 ml per hour. The retained stones disappear in about one half of patients within a 4- to 8-day treatment period. If all these are unsuccessful, reoperation is necessary.

SUPPURATIVE CHOLANGITIS. The most severe form of cholangitis, suppurative cholangitis, involves the same causative factors as the "nonsuppurative" form but differs in that obstruction is complete, ductal contents become purulent, and clinically the manifestations of sepsis overshadow those of cholestasis. Hypotension and mental changes such as lethargy or confusion appear in addition to right upper quadrant pain, chills, fever, and jaundice. Some elderly patients may be hypothermic and have minimal clinical signs. Because infection in the face of the high-grade obstruction progresses so rapidly, the serum bilirubin does not reach very high levels before the patient becomes moribund from sepsis. Costly delays in diagnosis are frequent, a consequence of failure to recognize the significance of mild icterus and abdominal pain in a patient with sepsis. All but a few cases involve complications of choledocholithiasis, the others occurring with biliary stricture or neoplastic obstruction, usually from bile duct carcinoma.

Laboratory tests reveal evidence of cholestasis with bilirubin values between 2 and 5 mg per deciliter and elevated serum levels of alkaline phosphatase, 5'-nucleotidase, and transaminases. The leukocyte count varies from subnormal to 40,000 per cubic millimeter. Hypoglycemia may sometimes be present.

Tenderness to palpation is present in the right upper quadrant, but rigidity is uncommon. In some cases secondary cholecystitis develops, and an enlarged tender gallbladder may be found on abdominal examination. Ultrasonography shows dilated bile ducts. Diagnosis rests on recognizing the evidence of biliary obstruction and its relationship to the sepsis and on verifying the initial impression by ultrasonography. After initial resuscitation—consisting of intravenous infusions, antimicrobial drugs (gentamicin plus ampicillin and clindamycin parenterally), and measures to restore cardiac, pulmonary, or renal function—decompression of the duct by emergency laparotomy, percutaneous transhepatic catheter placement, or endoscopic sphincterotomy offers the only hope of saving the patient. Biliary stents have also been placed endoscopically to reduce obstruction and systemic sepsis.

At surgery when choledochotomy is performed, pus often squirts from the duct as a result of the high pressure. If the patient's condition permits, thorough exploration can be carried out to correct the obstruction by removing stones, repairing a stricture, or bypassing a tumor. Insertion of a T tube proximal to the obstruction is sufficient in patients who are unable to tolerate

a longer operation, but sometime later it will be necessary to perform a second, more definitive procedure before the T tube can be removed. The mortality is about 50 per cent, resulting from septic shock, renal or respiratory failure, acute hepatic insufficiency, or a combination of these complications.

Other Causes of Bile Duct Obstruction

Duodenal and pancreatic tumors are common causes of obstruction in the middle-aged or elderly (Ch. 105 and 107). Common bile duct obstruction may also be caused by a variety of uncommon disorders such as sclerosing cholangitis or by Oriental cholangiohepatitis. Rare causes are compression by neoplastic paraductal lymph nodes or by duodenal Crohn's disease.

SCLEROSING CHOLANGITIS. Sclerosing cholangitis, a condition of unknown cause, consists of benign nonbacterial chronic inflammatory narrowing of the bile ducts. The entire ductal system is involved in most cases; less commonly the process may be confined to the extrahepatic or intrahepatic portion. The ratio of males to females is 3:2, and the peak incidence occurs in the third and fourth decades. More than half of the cases are associated with *ulcerative colitis* (Ch. 103) or *regional enteritis*. The severity of sclerosing cholangitis does not parallel the activity of the colitis, and colectomy does not improve the cholangitis. Other rarely associated diseases are retroperitoneal fibrosis and Riedel's thyroiditis.

The initial complaint may be jaundice or pruritus, although more cases are being discovered at an asymptomatic stage. There may be mild upper abdominal pain and sometimes fever, but a clinical picture resembling bacterial cholangitis is uncommon in the absence of previous surgical exploration or instrumentation of the ducts. Hepatomegaly may be present in some cases; when secondary cirrhosis develops, ascites or splenomegaly may be found.

Jaundice may be constant or fluctuating, and bilirubin values are usually in the range of 2 to 10 mg per deciliter. The alkaline phosphatase is always increased, usually greater than three times the upper limit of normal, and remains increased despite variations in clinical manifestations. Transaminases are usually mildly increased. Antimitochondrial antibodies are normal.

Percutaneous transhepatic cholangiography or preferably endoscopic retrograde cholangiopancreatography is required to establish the diagnosis. The radiographs show diffuse or focal irregular ductal narrowing with intervening areas of normal caliber or dilatation; this "beaded" appearance is characteristic. Some patients develop gallstones behind the strictured areas as a result of stasis; these are usually brown pigment gallstones. Localized strictures may be difficult to distinguish from ductal carcinoma. A radiographic appearance similar to that of sclerosing cholangitis may be seen in some patients with AIDS and CMV infection of the biliary tract and in some patients after intra-arterial infusion of FUDR for liver metastases.

In asymptomatic patients, no therapy is warranted. Treatment with corticosteroids or immunosuppressants has not been proved to be generally effective. Cholestyramine is useful for pruritus. Antimicrobials are necessary if bacterial cholangitis develops.

In symptomatic patients the aim of therapy is to relieve biliary obstruction if technically possible and if the benefit is thought to outweigh the risk. If a segmental stricture is present, balloon dilatation can be attempted either percutaneously or, if the lesion is in the common bile duct, endoscopically. This involves the insertion into the bile duct of a balloon-tipped catheter; inflation of the balloon stretches the narrowed area and allows greater bile flow. Balloon dilatation may have to be repeated intermittently to provide sustained relief of obstruction; there is the risk of inducing bacterial cholangitis, particularly with the endoscopic approach. Percutaneous catheter drainage is another option but often does not provide adequate drainage of all obstructed areas in diffuse disease. Surgical therapy is warranted in some cases to provide stenting in diffuse disease or to bypass severe distal common bile duct disease. Significant palliation follows surgery in most cases, but is not usually permanent. Most patients have episodic remissions and exacerbations, during which secondary biliary cirrhosis develops. Death may follow uncontrollable biliary sepsis with hepatic abscesses, liver failure, or bleeding from esophageal varices. Liver transplantation is now an option for those with advanced disease.

STRUCTURAL ABNORMALITIES. *Choledochal cysts* occasionally produce their initial clinical manifestations in young adults, presenting with jaundice, pain, or cholangitis. Diagnosis requires direct ductal visualization with PTC or ERCP; computed tomography or ultrasonography can provide information about surrounding structures. The most definitive surgical procedure is excision of the cyst, followed by Roux-en-Y choledochojejunostomy.

Caroli's disease, consisting of saccular intrahepatic bile duct dilations, most often becomes symptomatic in patients between the ages of 20 and 50 years, because of intrahepatic stone formation and cholangitis. Two forms are recognized: (1) disease of the ducts only and (2) ductal disease associated with hepatic fibrosis and medullary sponge kidney (more common). The latter patients often have complications of portal hypertension before cholangitis or obstructive jaundice appears. Antimicrobial therapy may control attacks of cholangitis, and surgical procedures to facilitate ductal emptying or to extract stones may help in some cases, but the intrahepatic anomaly cannot be definitively corrected unless lobectomy is possible for single lobe involvement.

PANCREATITIS. Acute pancreatitis can produce transient jaundice by obstruction of the distal common duct where it is surrounded by pancreatic tissue. Prolonged obstruction can result from pressure by an adjacent *pseudocyst* or entrapment of the distal common bile duct in severe pancreatic scarring from *chronic pancreatitis.* Diagnosis may be delayed in alcoholic patients in whom elevated alkaline phosphatase or bilirubin values are usually attributed to hepatocellular disease. Persistent elevation of the alkaline phosphatase value in an alcoholic should raise suspicion of the possibility of biliary obstruction, particularly if pancreatic calcification is present on plain abdominal radiographs. Jaundice resulting from chronic pancreatitis requires choledochoduodenostomy or Roux-en-Y anastomosis of the jejunum to the common bile duct.

HEMOBILIA. Hemobilia classically presents with biliary pain, obstructive jaundice, and occult or gross intestinal bleeding. Most cases are caused by hepatic injury from external or operative trauma, with secondary bleeding into the ductal system. Other causes include biliary or hepatic neoplasms, ductal rupture of a hepatic artery aneurysm, hepatic abscess, and gallstones, or it may follow percutaneous needle biopsy of the liver or cholangiography. Hemobilia following trauma is best treated by hepatic artery ligation, which is well tolerated except when there is advanced parenchymal disease; otherwise, direct management of the causative lesion is necessary.

PARASITIC DISEASE. An *echinococcal hepatic cyst* can rupture into the ducts and can give rise to biliary colic, jaundice, and cholangitis (Ch. 433). *Ascariasis* may produce biliary colic, jaundice, and cholangitis by worm invasion into the bile ducts from the duodenum (Ch. 433).

ORIENTAL CHOLANGIOHEPATITIS. Oriental cholangiohepatitis or *recurrent pyogenic cholangitis* is a common form of recurrent cholangitis in Asia associated with brown pigment gallstone formation throughout the biliary tract. The cause is unclear, but the parasite *Clonorchis sinensis* is found in very few cases so does not seem to be a major causative factor. Most patients present with acute cholangitis; those with recurrent cholangitis may develop liver abscesses, biliary-enteric fistulas, or sepsis. In advanced cases, one (usually the left) or both lobar ducts may become honeycombed with scars or abscesses, producing atrophy of the hepatic parenchyma.

Direct cholangiography is necessary for a definitive diagnosis. Sphincteroplasty or choledochojejunostomy is usually performed to remove stones and sludge and provide adequate biliary drainage. Cholecystectomy or partial hepatic resection is required when the gallbladder or localized hepatic segments are involved.

BILIARY STRICTURE. Biliary stricture almost always results from *surgical injury* to the duct and usually follows cholecystectomy rather than procedures on the duct itself such as common duct exploration. Biliary stricture may also result from external trauma or scarring produced by choledocholithiasis.

The symptoms resemble those of cholangitis with choledocholithiasis. Differential diagnosis includes all the various causes of obstructive jaundice and cholangitis. Laboratory evidence consists of leukocytosis and elevated serum levels of bilirubin, alkaline phosphatase, and transaminases. The jaundice and cholangitis are generally mild and transient, and infection generally responds promptly to antimicrobial therapy. Diagnosis can be made with visualization of the biliary tract by either PTC or ERCP. With persistent obstruction over several years, secondary biliary cirrhosis or multiple intrahepatic abscesses may develop.

In almost all cases an attempt should be made to repair the stricture surgically by creating a new unobstructed conduit between normal duct on the hepatic side of the lesion and the proximal intestine rather than attempting direct end-to-end anastomosis of the duct after excision of the lesion. The overall success rate of these operations is about 75 per cent with an operative mortality of 10 per cent.

Balloon catheter dilatation of a short stricture at the time of either PTC or ERCP may be useful in some patients, particularly those who are poor operative risks.

Carcinoma of the Gallbladder

In the United States there are approximately 2500 deaths annually from carcinoma of the gallbladder, a number equal to the mortality from benign disease of the biliary tract. Women are affected more frequently than men by a ratio of 3:1, and the average age is 70 years. Because 70 to 80 per cent of cases occur in patients with gallstones, cholelithiasis or lithogenic bile is thought to be etiologically important, but the mechanism involved is unclear. Gallbladder cancer develops in fewer than 1 per cent of patients with cholelithiasis. The disease is 5 to 10 times more frequent in American Indian populations.

Almost all gallbladder carcinomas are *adenocarcinomas;* the earliest spread is usually by metastasis to the hilar lymph nodes and adjacent hepatic parenchyma followed by direct extension to the liver and hilar structures. Distant metastases appear relatively late.

Patients have one of the following clinical pictures: (1) unremitting deep jaundice from common duct and hepatic involvement; (2) acute cholecystitis, often with a palpable mass; (3) chronic intermittent right upper quadrant pain; and (4) advanced disseminated carcinoma. The diagnosis is not often considered preoperatively, but in some instances clinical clues are present. In about two thirds of patients a mass can be felt, and in one third there is local tenderness. In all but a few cases the gallbladder is not opacified during oral cholecystography, and even when it is, the tumor can rarely be demonstrated. The diagnosis can be suspected on ultrasound study if an intraluminal gallbladder mass is identified that does not change with position. The differential diagnosis is that of a cholesterol polyp or of a stone adherent to the gallbladder wall. Pathologic studies indicate that all apparent tumor would be removed in 25 per cent of cases by cholecystectomy, resection of a rim of adjacent liver, and dissection of the common duct lymph node chain. Even in this favorable group the 5-year survival rate is 5 per cent. Most patients live for only a few months after the diagnosis.

Benign Tumors and Pseudotumors of the Gallbladder

Adenomyomatous hyperplasia, also called *adenomyomatosis,* is the most common of the benign conditions of the gallbladder; there is hyperplasia of the mucosa with formation of intramural diverticula. The cause is unknown. Typically, neoplastic or inflammatory changes are absent. Adenomyomatosis is usually diagnosed by oral cholecystography as a diffuse, segmental, or focal sessile filling defect with a central umbilication and small peripheral opaque areas representing diverticula. Most often adenomyomatosis is asymptomatic. Rare cases are associated with biliary pain that can be cured by cholecystectomy.

Cholesterolosis (strawberry gallbladder) is a condition of unknown cause characterized by an accumulation of cholesterol and other lipids in macrophages in the gallbladder mucosa. Unlike cholesterol gallstones, it does not appear to be necessarily related to biliary supersaturation with cholesterol. *Cholesterol polyps* are a focal form of cholesterolosis consisting of a core of macrophages filled with cholesterol covered with epithelium located at a villous tip. Generally, multiple polyps are present. The polyp is attached to the mucosa by a fragile stalk that can easily be broken. Cholesterol polyps appear on oral cholecystography or ultrasonography as a fixed filling defect on the gallbladder wall that does not change with position; in contrast to gallstones, no acoustic shadowing is seen on ultrasonography. Unless cholesterol polyps are present, cholesterolosis is difficult to detect by oral cholecystography. Most patients with cholesterolosis are asymptomatic. Some patients have concomitant gallstones and, if symptoms are present, they are attributed to the stones. Those few patients with cholesterolosis without gallstones who have typical biliary pain are often relieved by cholecystectomy.

Papillary and nonpapillary adenomas are benign neoplasms of the gallbladder. They are much less common than cholesterol polyps. Most adenomas are pedunculated; about two thirds are multiple. They appear as filling defects on oral cholecystography. Carcinoma in situ is found in about 5 per cent of adenomas, but the relationship between gallbladder adenomas and carcinoma is not clear.

Tumors of the Bile Duct

The main cause of early morbidity from tumors of the bile duct is biliary obstruction with gradual hepatocellular damage or secondary hepatobiliary infection. Tumors of the bile ducts are rarely benign. Papilloma, the most frequent benign tumor, is often multifocal and therefore difficult to cure. Adenomas and granular cell tumors are localized, but are often difficult to treat surgically without radical excision. This section is directed primarily to discussion of malignant tumors, but many of the same principles of pathophysiology and diagnosis apply to the rare benign tumors.

Except for a rare squamous cell tumor, malignant bile duct tumors are adenocarcinomas with either a scirrhous or a papillary pattern. Grossly, three types of pathologic presentations occur: *focal stricture, diffuse thickening,* and *nodular mass.* The first two varieties can easily be mistaken for a benign process such as post-traumatic stricture or sclerosing cholangitis. In many cases, spread is confined to local lymph node metastases or hepatic invasion for months or years before there is more widespread abdominal or systemic involvement. The common hepatic duct or common bile duct is the site of origin in about two thirds of the cases. The eponym *Klatskin tumor* is often used to refer to adenocarcinoma at the bifurcation of the common hepatic duct. In contrast with carcinoma of the gallbladder, cholelithiasis is found in only one third of patients, and men slightly outnumber women. The average age at diagnosis is 70 years. A number of cases have been reported in younger patients with ulcerative colitis. Since some of these patients have previously undergone colectomy, it is thought that elimination of the diseased colon is not protective. Sclerosing cholangitis is a complication in these same patients and may have identical clinical features, especially when it primarily affects the extrahepatic bile ducts. Caroli's disease and choledochal cysts are also associated with the development of carcinoma in a small percentage of cases. In Asia, infestation with *Clonorchis sinensis* probably contributes to the higher incidence of bile duct carcinoma.

CLINICAL MANIFESTATIONS. The typical patient presents with unremitting severe jaundice, mild deep-seated upper abdominal pain, and weight loss. Pruritus is reported by many, usually but not always after the onset of jaundice. Pain, present in more than half the patients, is not colicky and tends to be steady; fever and chills are absent. Hepatomegaly without splenomegaly is found on abdominal examination. Tumors of the common duct sparing the cystic duct often produce in addition to jaundice a distended nontender palpable gallbladder (*Courvoisier's law*).

The serum bilirubin value exceeds 10 mg per deciliter in most cases, with a mean between 15 and 20 mg per deciliter. Complete obstruction of the ductal system results in a bilirubin value of 30 mg per deciliter or higher. The alkaline phosphatase is almost always increased, often more than 10-fold, and ALT may be slightly elevated, although rarely higher than 200 units per liter. Obstruction of the right or left hepatic system alone causes a 10- to 30-fold increase in alkaline phosphatase with normal levels of bilirubin. The prothrombin time may be prolonged, but responds to parenteral vitamin K.

DIAGNOSIS. Ultrasonography or computed tomography shows dilatation of the bile ducts. Transhepatic or retrograde cholangiography can demonstrate the site of the block.

The differential diagnosis includes primary biliary cirrhosis and drug-induced cholestatic jaundice. Antimitochondrial antibodies can be demonstrated in the serum of 95 per cent of patients with primary biliary cirrhosis. Sclerosing cholangitis shows a characteristic pattern on cholangiography, although it may be difficult to distinguish focal disease from carcinoma. Choledocholithiasis and postoperative biliary stricture are less likely to present with deepening jaundice and weight loss. The jaundice fluctuates, is milder, and is usually associated with fever. PTC or ERCP helps to differentiate these diseases from carcinoma.

Cytologic examination of tissue obtained by brushing the suspected tumor at the time of PTC or ERCP or by radiologically guided skinny needle aspiration may reveal malignant cells. Not uncommonly, however, a preoperative tissue diagnosis may not be made because of the scirrhous nature of many of these carcinomas.

TREATMENT. Unfortunately, complete excision of the tumor is often impossible, because nonexpendable anatomic structures are involved early. Nevertheless, a few cures can be expected when radical surgery is judiciously employed, and palliation is often lengthy and of excellent quality.

Distal lesions require pancreaticoduodenectomy (Whipple's procedure) for complete removal. Because this operation has a 10 to 15 per cent mortality, it should be performed only if no gross tumor would be left behind. Tumors of the midportion of the common bile duct are sometimes amenable to complete resection. Localized tumors of the bifurcation of the hepatic duct can sometimes be treated by excision, even though microscopic deposits of tumor usually remain in the bed of the dissection. Reconstruction involves use of a Roux-en-Y hepaticojejunostomy. Radiotherapy with either external beam or intraluminal rods may provide some benefit.

For tumors with local or distant spread the goal is palliation. The treatment of choice is percutaneous or endoscopic stenting of the biliary tract with catheters having multiple portholes above and below the point of bile duct obstruction. Either type of tube can be changed periodically to prevent clogging. Distal tumors can be bypassed by cholecystojejunostomy or other types of biliary-enteric anastomoses.

PROGNOSIS. Cure is achieved in 5 to 10 per cent, and many patients survive in good condition for several years or more following palliative surgery. If biliary drainage can be maintained with a catheter, patients with unresectable lesions occasionally do well for a year or two. Death eventually results from hepatic replacement with tumor or intrahepatic sepsis from ductal obstruction.

Postcholecystectomy Syndrome

After cholecystectomy, 10 per cent of patients continue to have significant abdominal symptoms. In most patients the explanation for continued postoperative symptoms is that the gallstone disease was not the cause of their preoperative complaints. Patients with typical biliary pain are more often relieved by cholecystectomy than are those with atypical pain or vague symptoms such as fatty food intolerance, dyspepsia, or flatulence. Postcholecystectomy complaints can often be attributed to overlooked disease such as choledocholithiasis, pancreatitis, peptic ulcer, esophageal or small-bowel disease, or irritable bowel syndrome. These possibilities must be investigated by appropriate studies.

Neuroma of the cystic duct stump and other cystic duct remnant lesions are uncommon conditions that may be responsible for postcholecystectomy symptoms. A few patients with episodic typical biliary pain in the absence of stones or other bile duct abnormalities have hypertension, dysmotility, and/or stenosis of the sphincter of Oddi. The appearance of a narrowed sphincter alone is insufficient to document either stenosis or dyskinesia. Dyskinesia of the sphincter without stenosis is very difficult to establish as a cause of the syndrome. Clinicians should remain skeptical about a diagnosis of ampullary stenosis or dyskinesia when the principal finding is abdominal pain. The diagnosis is more secure in patients with recurrent pancreatitis, increase of transaminases, cholangitis, and/or a dilated bile duct whose sphincter appears tight radiographically and will accept only a small probe.

The usual evaluation of such patients, after other more common conditions have been ruled out, starts with ultrasonography of the right upper quadrant. Typically, ERCP is performed next. Manometric recordings of sphincter of Oddi pressures obtained transendoscopically show hypertension or dysmotility in some but not all cases.

In the management of such patients with chronic abdominal pain thought to be due to dyskinesia, treatment can be tried with nitrates, antispasmodics, anticholinergics, or calcium channel blockers. If this is unsuccessful, consideration can be given to endoscopic sphincterotomy, although its efficacy remains uncertain. Exploratory laparotomy has a very low rate of success for diagnosis, and surgical correction of minor variations in the gut anatomy usually fails to cure.

Barkun ANG, Ponchon T: Extracorporeal biliary lithotripsy. Review of experimental studies and a clinical update. Ann Intern Med 112:126, 1990. *Excellent review of this topic, with 72 references.*

Carey MC, Cahalane MJ: Whither biliary sludge? Gastroenterology 95:508, 1988. *An in-depth treatise on the biochemical and physicochemical events leading to cholesterol stone formation.*

Duane WC: Pathogenesis of gallstones: Implications for management. Hosp Pract 25:65, 1990. *Succinct review of cholesterol and pigment gallstone formation.*

Neoptolemos JP, Carr-Locke DL, Fossard DP: Prospective randomised study of preoperative endoscopic sphincterotomy versus surgery alone for common bile duct stones. Br Med J 294:470, 1987. *Routine precholecystectomy endoscopic sphincterotomy for removal of concomitant common bile duct stones was not shown to be better (or worse) than conventional surgery.*

Neoptolemos JP, Carr-Locke DL, London NJ, et al.: Controlled trial of urgent endoscopic retrograde cholangiopancreatography and endoscopic sphincterotomy versus conservative treatment for acute pancreatitis due to gallstones. Lancet 2:979, 1988. *This prospective study of 121 patients demonstrated that urgent ERCP with endoscopic sphincterotomy was safe and effective for acute gallstone pancreatitis; the decision to perform ERCP in this setting remains an individualized one, however.*

Pessa ME, Hawkins IF, Vogel SB: The treatment of acute cholangitis. Percutaneous transhepatic biliary drainage before definitive therapy. Ann Surg 205:389, 1987. *Percutaneous cholangiography performed early can provide an accurate diagnosis and allow stabilization of the patient before definitive therapy.*

Podda M, Battezzati PM, Ghezzi C, et al.: Efficacy and safety of a combination of chenodeoxycholic acid and ursodeoxycholic acid for gallstone dissolution: A comparison with ursodeoxycholic acid alone. Gastroenterology 96:222, 1989. *Comprehensive study of bile salt dissolution of gallstones in 120 patients; 53 references.*

Ransohoff DF, Gracie WA: Management of patients with symptomatic gallstones: A quantitative analysis. Am J Med 88:154, 1990. *An erudite analysis of strategies for treating symptomatic patients.*

Savoca PE, Longo WE, Zucker KA, et al.: The increasing prevalence of acalculous cholecystitis in outpatients. Results of a 7-year study. Ann Surg 211:433, 1990. *Although most often thought of as a problem associated with sepsis, burns, severe trauma, and the postoperative period, acalculous cholecystitis can also be seen in outpatients. Thirty-six of 47 patients seen over a 7-year period developed it at home without evidence of these predisposing conditions; most were elderly with vascular disease.*

Sievert W, Vakil NB: Emergencies of the biliary tract. Gastroenterol Clin North Am 17:245, 1988. *Good review of acute cholecystitis, cholangitis, and gallstone pancreatitis, with 83 references.*

Sivak MV: Endoscopic management of bile duct stones. Am J Surg 158:228, 1989. *An extensive, authoritative review of the use of endoscopic sphincterotomy, with 105 references.*

van Erpecum KJ, van Gerge Henegouwen GP, Stoelwinder B, et al.: Bile concentration is a key factor for nucleation of cholesterol crystals and cholesterol saturation index in gallbladder bile of gallstone patients. Hepatology 11:1, 1990. *An important contribution to our understanding of cholesterol crystal nucleation from supersaturated bile.*

PART XII

HEMATOLOGIC DISEASES

127 Introduction to Hematologic Diseases

David G. Nathan

This introduction is primarily intended to provide a general background to diagnostic hematology and marrow function. The remaining chapters in Part XII emphasize fundamental physiologic principles and provide descriptions of relatively common hematologic disorders. It is hoped that the entire part will influence the reader to consider such diseases broadly and systematically.

The nonmalignant disorders of erythrocytes, phagocytes, and platelets, including their precursors and progenitors, are initially discussed. Then follows a description of the acute and chronic proliferative disorders that involve the cells of the marrow and lymphoid systems, a series of chapters that ends with a discussion of bone marrow transplantation. The final chapters of Part XII are devoted to a review of the disorders of the fluid phase of blood coagulation and the vascular purpuras.

DIAGNOSTIC HEMATOLOGY. The circulating blood cells are the products of the terminal differentiation of recognizable precursors. In fetal life, hematopoiesis occurs throughout the reticuloendothelial system. In the normal adult, terminal differentiation of the recognizable precursors of erythrocytes, granulocytes, and platelets occurs exclusively in the marrow cavities of the axial skeleton, with some extension into the proximal femora and humeri. The space is highly expandable, however, when the demand for blood cell production is accelerated (Fig. 127–1).

Observations of differentiated blood cells by enumeration and relatively simple morphologic studies of properly prepared blood films provide the essential cornerstone of diagnostic hematology.

Automated blood counts and cell sizing now provide both reproducibility and enhanced diagnostic capacity. For example, early failure of red cell production may be heralded by unexpected macrocytosis. Peripheral blood cell counts and morphology offer insight into the rate of effective hematopoiesis; the state of marrow nutrition with respect to vitamin B_{12}, folic acid, and iron; the presence of acquired and congenital disorders of the erythrocyte membrane; the energy metabolism or the hemoglobin of erythrocytes, which influences the rate of their destruction; the differential diagnosis of infections; the presence of allergic reactions; the acquired or congenital abnormalities of intracellular organelles; and the invasion of the marrow by malignant cells or infectious agents. The contributions of morphologic techniques to hematologic diagnosis depend entirely upon the adequacy of specimen preparation and the skill of the observer. Egregious errors are made when diagnostic pronouncements are based on inadequate material. The slavish enumeration of individual cells is rarely of aid without careful overall inspection and positive searches for diagnostic clues that are relevant to the case at hand. Morphology can be particularly misleading if the observer does not understand that many kinds of disorders induce similar changes in shape, particularly in the red cells.

Although circulating lymphocytes appear to be terminally differentiated cells, they are instead capable of rapid proliferative responses to appropriate stimuli, during which they resume the appearance of relatively undifferentiated precursors. At this stage, they are often called atypical. The functional subsets of lymphoid cells are not readily demonstrable by inspection, although "killer" lymphocyte function may be associated with larger cells that contain granules. Obtaining useful information about lymphocyte subsets requires studies of lymphocyte function and measurements with specially prepared antibodies reactive with lymphocytes.

Well-prepared marrow films and biopsy specimens also contribute important information, such as total marrow cellularity, the presence of invading malignant cells or infectious granulomas,

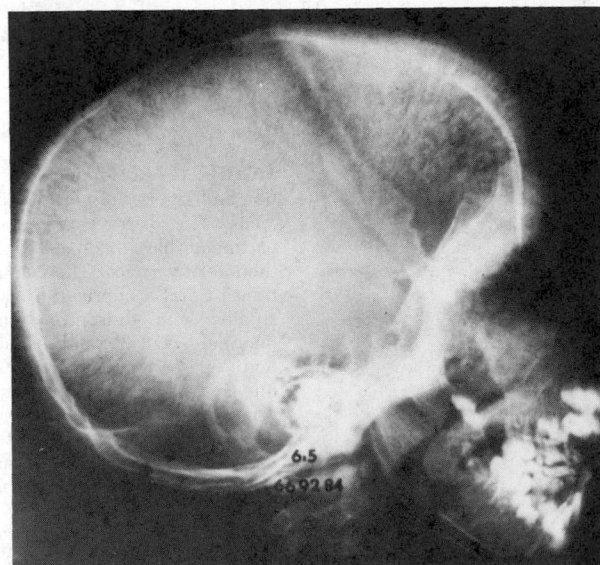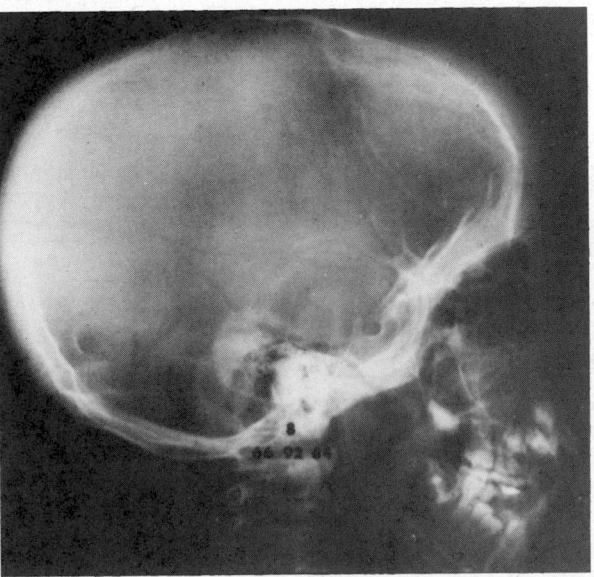

FIGURE 127–1. Roentgenograms of the skull of a patient with homozygous beta-thalassemia at the age of 6½ years *(left)*, before splenectomy and transfusion therapy, and at the age of 8 years *(right)*, after splenectomy and transfusion therapy to control anemia. Note the marked "hair-on-end" appearance in the left-hand radiograph, signifying expansion of the marrow space. (From Nathan DG: N Engl J Med 286:586, 1972. Reprinted by permission of the New England Journal of Medicine.)

the adequacy of the numbers of megakaryocytes, the ratio of myeloid to erythroid precursors, the state of marrow cell nutrition, the presence of abnormal storage cells, and even the deposition of abnormal crystals in metabolic diseases. In brief, the blood and marrow lend themselves to biopsy and to structural, chemical, and functional studies far more readily than do any other human organs. Their mature cellular elements are diverse, bearing in common only a joint ancestral cell, origin in the marrow, and the property of being transported through vessels suspended in plasma.

PRECURSORS OF CIRCULATING BLOOD CELLS. *Erythrocytes.*

Much of the progress of differentiation of erythroid precursors can be appreciated morphologically, particularly the onset of hemoglobin synthesis and the maturation and extrusion of the nucleus. During this process, each proerythroblast may give rise to approximately eight erythrocytes. The transit time from proerythroblast to emergence of reticulocytes is approximately 5 days. The transit time may decrease during anemic stress to as few as 2 days by means of skipped divisions. The red cells that emerge under conditions of stress are macrocytic and may contain as much as 25 per cent fetal hemoglobin (F cells). They may also bear additional fetal characteristics, particularly the presence of i antigen on their surfaces. More quantitative analyses of the transit of erythroid precursors during the process of maturation may be appreciated from the use of radioactive iron that, when injected intravenously, accumulates preferentially in the newly synthesized ferritin of proerythroblasts and ultimately emerges in peripheral blood incorporated into reticulocyte hemoglobin. The use of surface scanning following infusion of ^{59}Fe-labeled transferrin reveals the site as well as the rate of intramedullary erythropoiesis, and the rate of erythropoiesis may be estimated from the level of transferrin receptors in plasma. The use of ^{59}Fe transferrin is largely an investigative and not a clinical tool, except for cases in which the anatomic site of erythropoiesis needs to be determined, such as in myeloid metaplasia. A qualitative clinical assessment of erythroid precursor activity throughout the body may be gained from injection of indium chloride and marrow scintigraphy. Indium–111 binds to transferrin and is incorporated into immature marrow erythroid precursors. Body scanning then reveals the distribution of marrow.

Granulocytes. The process of intramedullary granulocyte maturation involves changes in nuclear configuration and the accumulation of specific intracytoplasmic granules. A model that describes the production and kinetics of neutrophils is shown in Figure 127–2 (see also Ch. 138). It is highly compartmentalized. The relatively small peripheral blood pool is divided into two compartments in equilibrium, the circulating and the marginated pools. These pools provide entrance into the tissues. The level

of peripheral cells is buffered by an immense marrow reserve of identifiable precursors, some of which are in the mitotic compartment and some in the maturing and storage compartment. The kinetics of proliferation of these recognizable precursors have been studied using labeled precursors of DNA. These so-called labeling indices, from which estimates of cell cycle times can be derived, have served as important approaches to the study of pharmacology and toxicity of chemotherapeutic agents.

Platelets. The differentiation of committed megakaryocytes, the precursors of platelets, involves a nuclear endoreduplication phenomenon that produces 16N and 32N megakaryoblasts. The endoreduplication ceases at the stage of the mature megakaryocyte. Platelet shedding from megakaryocytes is accomplished by the formation of multiple demarcation membranes within the cytoplasm of the cell, usually visible only by electron microscopy. Although the platelet appears to be a simple tissue fragment, its functions are diverse and hemostatically versatile. It must selectively adhere to abnormal surfaces and then sequentially secrete, aggregate, fuse, and retract to ensure a firm platelet-fibrin plug. In the process, it assists in the coagulation cascade, synthesizes prostaglandins, and releases adenosine diphosphate (ADP) and a variety of other substances of known and unknown function (Ch. 154).

Lymphocytes. The geography of lymphocyte precursor maturation and differentiation is considerably more complex than that of the other hematopoietic cells. Primitive lymphoid precursors of B cell origin arise in the marrow, spleen, and lymph nodes, where they continue their maturation and differentiation. Primitive T cell precursors arise in the marrow; travel to the thymus, where they undergo further differentiation; and are finally exported to the spleen, lymph nodes, and marrow, where they establish their final residence and perform many of their functions. Both T and B cells enter the peripheral blood circulation, which delivers them to tissue sites at which their functions may be required or their unbridled activity may cause disease. T cells previously "educated" in the thymus give rise to progeny that may survive for the life of the individual. Circulating lymphocytes represent only a tiny fraction of the total lymphocyte pool. Therefore, analysis of these circulating cells may not reflect the nature of the total pool.

THE HEMATOPOIETIC MICROENVIRONMENT.

For clarity, we have separately described each class of blood precursor cells, but in reality they are closely packed together. The bone marrow is a vast mesh that is best described as millions of fronds of fibroblasts and endothelial cells (to be described below), which provide a lacy framework in which are embedded differentiating progenitor cells, developing precursors bound by fibronectin to the mesh, tissue macrophages, and T cells.

The fronds of developing marrow cells float in a bog of sluggishly moving venous blood, the so-called sinusoids. Figure 127–3 demonstrates one of the least understood, but most dra-

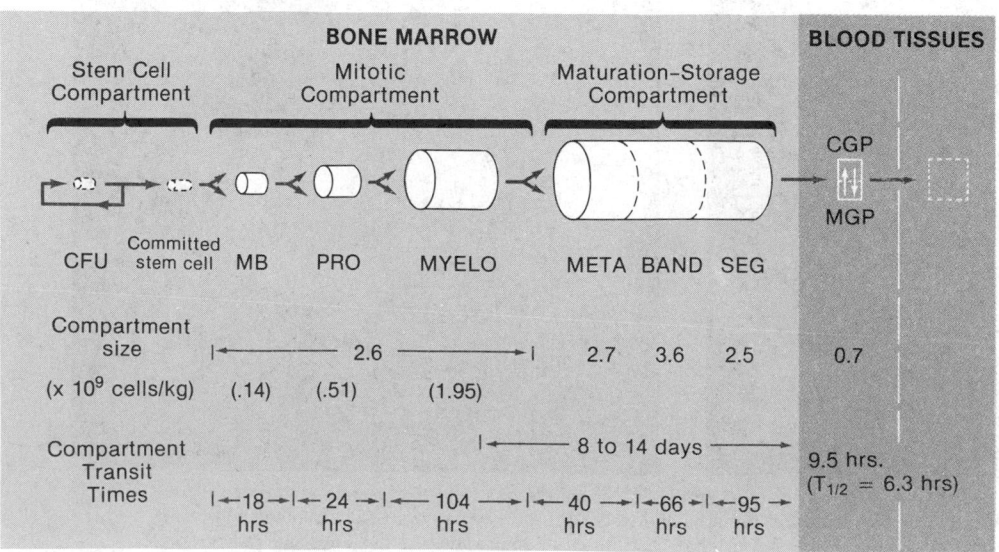

FIGURE 127–2. Model of the production and kinetics of neutrophils in humans. The marrow and blood compartments have been drawn to show their relative sizes. The compartment transit times, as derived from labeling studies with di-isopropyl phosphofluoridate (DF^{32}P) and tritiated thymidine, are shown on the next to last line and the last line. The less obvious symbols in the figure include CGP, the circulating granulocyte pool; MGP, the marginating granulocyte pool; CFU (colony-forming unit), the tripotential stem cell; MB, myeloblast; and PRO, promyelocyte. (From Wintrobe MM, Lee RG, et al.: Clinical Hematology. 7th ed. Philadelphia, Lea & Febiger, 1974, p 244.)

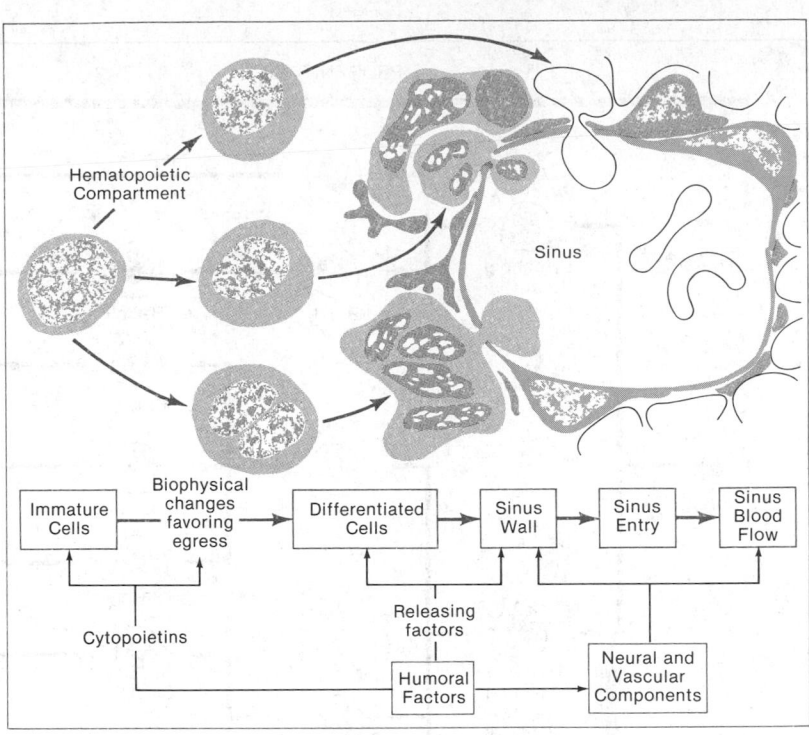

FIGURE 127–3. A schematic diagram of the factors that may be involved in controlling the release of marrow cells. The central relationship between the hematopoietic compartment and the marrow sinus is depicted. The drawing highlights the similarity of the egress process for the three major hematopoietic cells: reticulocytes in the top pathway, granulocytes and monocytes in the center pathway, and platelets in the lower pathway. Immature cells undergo biophysical changes under the influence of cytopoietins that favor egress. In the case of reticulocytes, enucleation precedes egress. This is shown by the solid black inclusion in the perisinal macrophage, representing nucleophagocytosis antecedent to digestion of the erythroblast nucleus. The cytoplasmic protrusion of the megakaryocyte presumably detaches itself from the cell and will further fragment into platelets in the circulation. (From Lichtman MA, Chamberlain JK, Santillo PA: *In* Silber R, LoBue J, Gordon AS [eds.]: The Year in Hematology, 1978. New York, Plenum Medical Book Company, 1978, p 274.)

matic, aspects of hematopoiesis, the migration of completed blood cells in the fronds through gaps that exist between endothelial cells and fibroblasts to gain access to the sinusoids and on to the general circulation. Bone marrow aspiration disrupts the fronds and eliminates a view of this microanatomy, while marrow biopsy provides only a two-dimensional aspect that sacrifices cytology for a better, albeit imperfect, representation of architecture. The fronds of hematopoietic tissue are lined by reticular cells that form the adventitial surfaces of the vascular sinuses and extend cytoplasmic processes to create a lattice for the mesh of endothelial cells and fibroblasts on which blood cells reside. The lattice is revealed by reticulin stains of marrow sections and scanning electron photomicrographs. To escape the fronds, the developing blood cells must lose their adhesiveness and do so, at least with respect to the erythroid system, by shedding fibronectin receptors to escape the sticky embrace of the microenvironment and pass into the circulation. Clumps of megakaryocytes are found adjacent to marrow sinuses. They shed platelets, the products of their cytoplasm, directly into the lumen. This situation avoids the requirement for movement of bulky megakaryocytes, a mobility characteristic of the granuloid and erythroid differentiated precursors as they approach the point at which they egress from the marrow.

KINETICS OF HEMATOPOIESIS. The marrow microenvironment supporting the progenitors and precursors must provide for the normal steady-state rates of renewal of the cellular elements of blood. Under homeostatic conditions, the production rates precisely equal destruction rates. The average lifespan of a human red cell is approximately 120 days. This means that approximately 5×10^4 red cells must be produced per day per microliter of blood in an adult. The average lifespan of platelets is 7 to 10 days, for a daily production rate of 2×10^4 platelets per microliter of blood. The white blood cell compartment exhibits more complex kinetics. Granulocytes are rapidly turned over, with an approximate intravascular lifespan of 6 to 12 hours in humans. To maintain a level of circulating granulocytes of 5×10^3 per microliter requires a daily production that is roughly comparable to that of red cells and platelets, approximately 2×10^4 cells per microliter of blood. At the opposite extreme in terms of lifespan are lymphocytes, some of which can exhibit lifetimes measured in months, or even years. This long lifespan of lymphocytes suggests that the daily renewal of certain lymphocyte progenitors occurs at a rate substantially lower than that of the

progenitors of the other formed elements of blood. The various symptoms of complete marrow failure are closely related to the lifespan and the turnover of the peripheral cells of the blood. Thus, patients with complete marrow failure initially lose granulocytes and therefore usually present with enhanced susceptibility to infection. Bleeding caused by platelet deficiency rapidly follows, and finally pallor and symptoms of anemia occur. Loss of circulating lymphocytes and cellular immune function is an unusual event in such circumstances and represents severe and longstanding marrow failure.

The turnover of red cells and platelets can be measured for diagnostic purposes, using $Na_2{}^{51}CrO_4$ as a labeling agent. Both the red cell and the platelet lifespans can be estimated and the site of the red cell destruction determined. This can be a useful maneuver in decisions regarding splenectomy.

HEMATOPOIETIC PROGENITORS. The recognizable marrow precursors of the differentiated peripheral blood cells tend to occupy the attention of hematologists, but they are rarely primary causes of the hematopoietic cytopenias. It is true that various toxins, cytotoxic antibodies, or nutritional deficiencies can so seriously damage the orderly progression of precursor differentiation that effective production of fully differentiated cells is embarrassed. In general, however, deficient or excessive production of blood cells is due to abnormalities of *undifferentiated progenitor cells.* They must themselves undergo vital processes of maturation and amplification to give rise to the recognizable precursors of circulating differentiated blood cells.

Progenitor Maturation. The hematopoietic progenitor system can be envisaged as a continuum of functional compartments (Fig. 127–4). The most primitive compartment is made up of very rare cells with high self-renewal capacity. These are so-called pluripotent stem cells (PSC's). These PSC's randomly (or stochastically) give rise to more mature stem cells that are committed to either lymphoid or myeloid development. But the fidelity of these commitments is not absolute. Hence, lymphoid surface markers may be expressed on myeloid leukemic cells. Lymphoid stem cells give rise to T and B cell precursors and their mature progeny (see Ch. 242). Trilineage myeloid stem cells are called CFU-S, for the spleen colony-forming unit first described in mice. Hematopoietic colonies were observed in the spleens of lethally irradiated mice rescued with bone marrow cells of histoidentical donors. The spleen colonies contained megakaryocyte, granulocyte, and erythroid precursors. Following

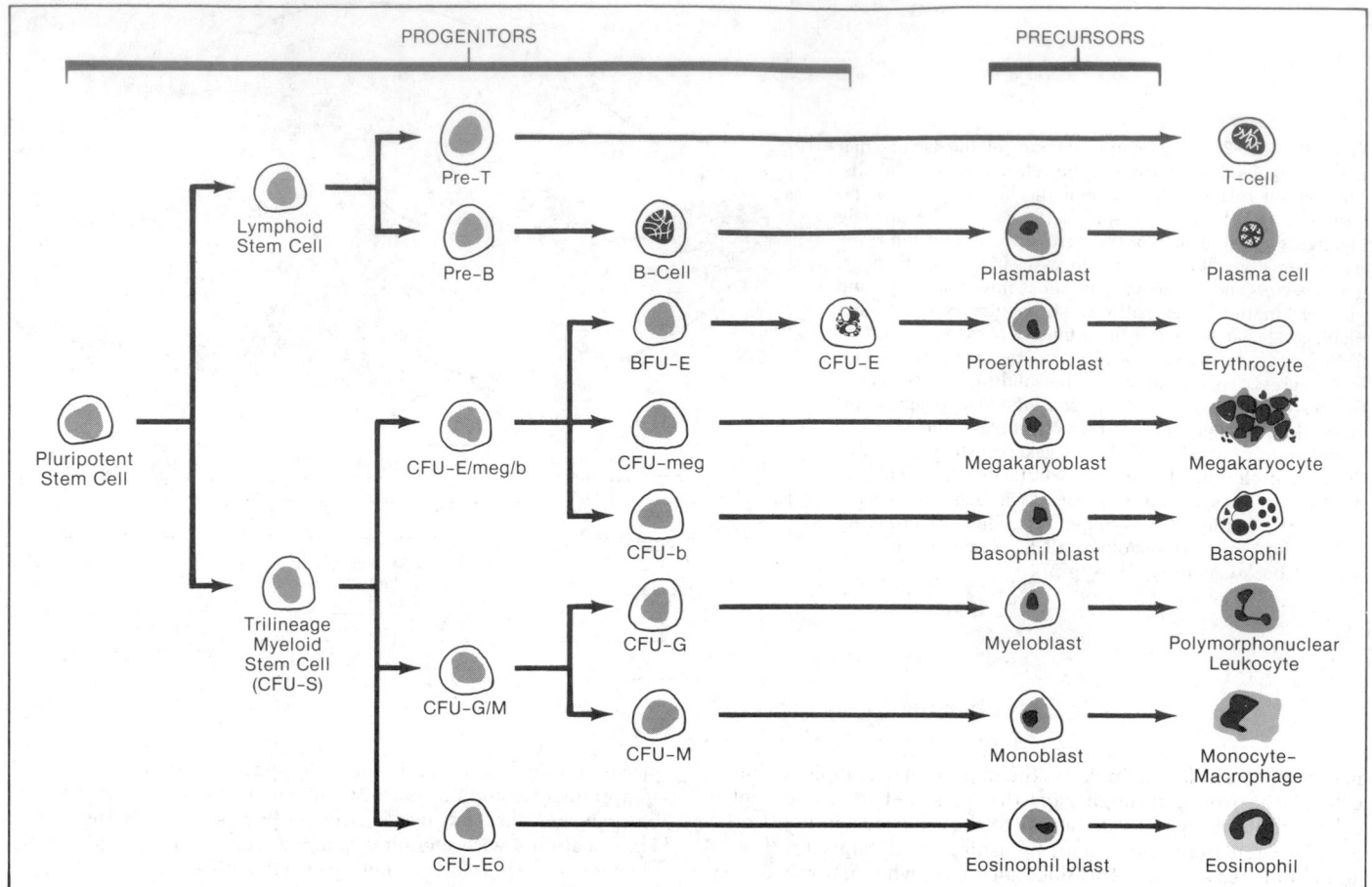

FIGURE 127-4. A schematic outline of the progenitor basis of hematopoiesis. Note the progressive restriction in the potential for terminal differentiation of the progenitors as they mature from left to right in the drawing. They finally form the recognizable marrow precursors from which the circulating blood cells, shown on the far right, are derived. Not shown in this outline is the process of self-renewal of fractions of the progenitor cell populations, particularly the immature progenitors. Also not shown is the progressive amplification of progenitors and precursors as they mature and differentiate. The bipotential erythroid-megakaryocyte progenitor shown in this drawing and referred to in the text has been demonstrated in the mouse, but not definitely in humans.

bone marrow transplantation in mice with a limited number of PSC's, a process of so-called clonal equilibration takes place, in which the progeny of some PSC's are extinguished while other PSC's begin to populate the marrow. A subset of the grafted pluripotent stem cells then dominates hematopoiesis.

Trilineage myeloid stem cells (CFU-S) eventually give rise to the committed single-lineage progenitors of the recognizable precursors through a random process of lineage restriction, shown in Figure 127–4 as a stepwise process. Actually, this represents a random set of choices that eventuate in progenitors that are restricted to single-lineage development. The restriction is probably due to the cell-surface expression of lineage-specific growth factor receptors. These single-lineage progenitors, including erythroid burst-forming units (BFU-E), erythroid colony-forming units (CFU-E), megakaryocyte colony-forming units (CFU-Meg), and basophil, granulocyte, monocyte, and eosinophil colony-forming units (CFU-Baso, CFU-G, CFU-M, and CFU-Eo, respectively), proliferate and differentiate to their respective precursors in response to the growth factors that bind to their unique receptors. The capacity of lineage-specific committed progenitors

TABLE 127-1. CHARACTERISTICS OF HUMAN HEMATOPOIETIC GROWTH FACTORS

Growth Factor	Cellular Source	Progenitor Cell Target*	Mature Cell Target
Interleukin 3 (IL3)	T lymphocytes	CFU-Blast, CFR-GEMM, CFU-GM, CFU-G, CFU-M, CFU-Eo, CFU-Meg, CFU-Baso, BFU-E	Eosinophils, monocytes
GM-CSF	T lymphocytes, monocytes, fibroblasts, endothelial cells	CFU-Blast, CFU-GEMM, CFU-GM, CFU-G, CFU-M, CFU-Eo, CFU-Meg, BFU-E	Granulocytes, eosinophils, monocytes
G-CSF	Monocytes, fibroblasts, endothelial cells	CFU-G	Granulocytes
M-CSF	Monocytes, fibroblasts, endothelial cells, uterus	CFU-M	Monocytes
Erythropoietin	Peritubular cells of the kidney, Kupffer cells	CFU-E, late BFU-E?, CFU-Meg	None
IL5	T lymphocytes	CFU-Eo	Eosinophils

*CFU-Blast = colony-forming unit—blast; CFU-GEMM = colony-forming unit—granulocyte, erythrocyte, monocyte, and megakaryocyte; CFU-GM = colony-forming unit—granulocyte and macrophage; CFU-Eo = colony-forming unit—eosinophil; CFU-Meg = colony-forming unit—megakaryocyte; BFU-E = burst-forming unit—erythroid; CFU-G = colony-forming unit—granulocyte; CFU-M = colony-forming unit—macrophage; CFU-E = colony-forming unit—erythroid; and CFU-Baso = colony-forming unit —basophil.

to proliferate and differentiate in response to demand constitutes the most important buffer of the hematopoietic system against increased requirement for mature blood cell production. Little is known about the cell biology of progenitors because their rarity makes their purification extremely difficult. Such purification has been recently accomplished to a considerable extent in mice, and the antibody to the cell-surface antigen CD–34 has been useful in achieving partial purification of progenitors in humans.

Hematopoietic Growth Factors. The proliferation, differentiation, and survival of immature hematopoietic progenitor cells are sustained by a family of glycoproteins, the hematopoietic growth factors (HGF's) (see Table 127–1). In addition to their effect on the proliferation and differentiation of progenitors, these factors also influence the survival and function of mature blood cells. The HGF's are also known collectively as the colony-stimulating factors (CSF's), a term derived from the in vitro observation that they stimulate progenitor cells to form colonies of recognizable maturing cells. It is important to recognize that the lineage-specific HGF's, erythropoietin, G-CSF, M-CSF, and interleukin 5 (IL5), are not active alone except in their interactions with the most mature committed progenitor cells. The majority of lineage-specific progenitors demand the presence of either IL3 or GM-CSF in addition to a lineage-specific HGF to produce the colonies for which they are programmed. Hence, immature committed

progenitors bear receptors for both IL3 and GM-CSF. They differ from one another with respect to their lineage-specific receptors.

The genes for several human HGF's have been cloned, and this, in turn, has led to the production and purification of the respective recombinant proteins. This advance in molecular biology has allowed intensive investigations of the actions of purified HGF's, their cellular origins, and their regulatory mechanisms (Fig. 127–5), while the availability of large quantities of highly purified HGF's has led to preclinical and clinical evaluation of their effectiveness in vivo. In general, IL3 and GM-CSF stimulate the survival, proliferation, and differentiation of a broad range of progenitors, if lineage-specific HGF's are also present. Stem cells may also be stimulated by three other interleukins, IL1, IL4, and IL6, but the actions of these factors may be indirect or may require the presence of other cytokines. Interleukin 6 is particularly interesting because in combination with IL3 it reduces the time during which blast cells in culture begin to divide to form colonies, suggesting that the combination influences stem cell cycling. It may also synergize with IL3 or GM-CSF to induce megakaryocyte differentiation. Figure 127–5 emphasizes the interaction of the most important HGF's with progenitor cells. Note the requirement for combinations of IL3 and/or GM-CSF

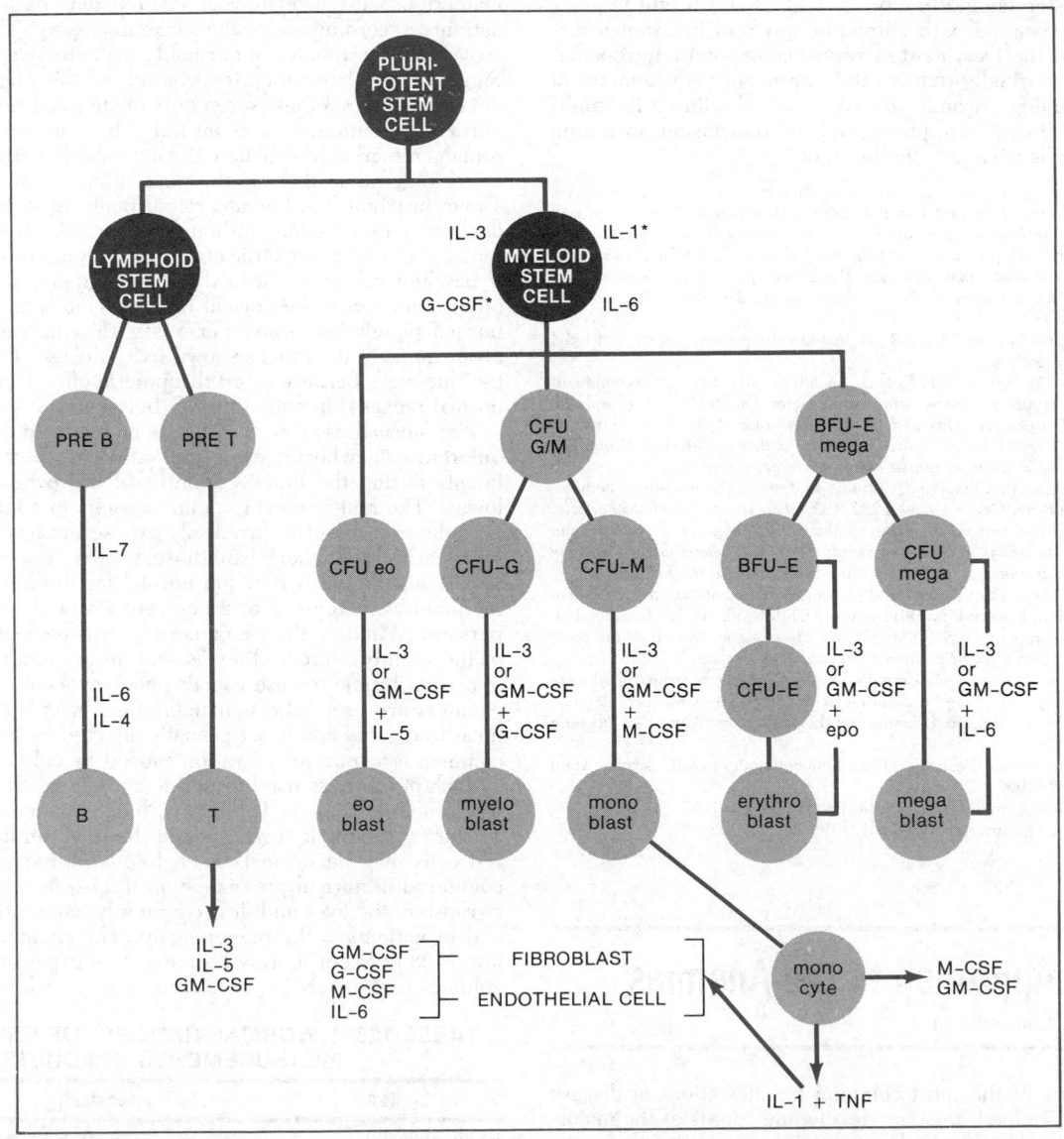

FIGURE 127–5. The hematopoietic progenitors and growth factors. The differentiation of hematopoietic progenitors is shown, beginning with the pluripotent stem cell. The myeloid stem cell differentiates randomly into the CFU-G/M, BFU-E/mega, and CFU-Eo lineages. The rate of differentiation is influenced by IL3 (interleukin 3) and IL6 and perhaps by G-CSF (colony-stimulating factor) and IL1. The synergistic effects of IL5, G-CSF, M-CSF, and IL6 with either IL3 or GM-CSF are shown. The production of growth factors is demonstrated at the bottom of the figure. See footnote to Table 127–1 for definition of the growth factors.

with lineage-specific growth factors for the induction of specific precursors.

The bottom of Figure 127–5 summarizes the cells of origin of the HGF's and demonstrates that the monocyte and T cell play an important role in progenitor differentiation. Monocytes produce IL1 and tumor necrosis factor (TNF) in response to bacterial products. These in turn stimulate fibroblasts and endothelial cells to produce all of the HGF's except IL3 and IL5. Antigens of various kinds stimulate T cells to produce IL3 and IL5, as well as GM-CSF. All of these growth factors in turn interact with their specific progenitors to produce the developing blood cells. As mentioned above, fibroblasts and endothelial cells are not merely factories of growth factors. They also provide a critically important adherent layer on which progenitor differentiation must take place. Fibronectin is a key component of the microenvironment because it binds progenitors to fibroblasts and endothelial cells through fibronectin receptors.

THERAPEUTIC APPLICATIONS. Thus far, three HGF's have shown promise in clinical trials. GM-CSF regularly elevates the granulocyte count in a dose-dependent fashion in patients with acquired immunodeficiency syndrome (AIDS) and shows promise as well in the management of aplastic anemia in children. It may also be useful in protocols involving autotransplantation following intensive chemotherapy. G-CSF is also useful in granulocytopenia associated with chemotherapy and has shown distinct promise in the treatment of severe congenital neutropenia. Erythropoietin markedly reduces the transfusion requirements of patients undergoing chronic dialysis for renal failure. Its application in other disorders requiring red cell transfusion, including autotransfusion, is currently under study.

Cannistra SA, Griffin JD: Regulation of the production and function of granulocytes and monocytes. Semin Hematol 25:173, 1988. *This article and the second and sixth through tenth references offer excellent reviews of the status of the hematopoietic growth factors as the field evolved between 1987 and 1990. The article by Strober and James discusses the growth factors that interact with progenitors and precursors of the lymphoid system. The others focus on the myeloid system.*

Groopman JE, Molina JM, Scadden DT: Hematopoietic growth factors. N Engl J Med 321:1449, 1989.

Guinan EC, Sieff CA, Oette DH, et al.: A Phase I/II trial of recombinant granulocyte-macrophage colony stimulating factor for children with aplastic anemia. Blood, in press. *This article represents one of the more optimistic results of the treatment of aplastic anemia patients with GM-CSF. The bibliography is also useful in that it describes other clinical trials.*

Jordan CT, Lemischka IR: Clonal and systemic analysis of the long-term hematopoiesis in the mouse. Genes Devel 4:220, 1990. *This is a very technical article, but it explores the various theories of the contribution of stem cells and progenitors to hematopoiesis in the steady state and immediately following bone marrow transplantation. It is an important article in the field.*

Lipton JM, Nathan, DG: The anatomy and physiology of hematopoiesis. In Nathan DG, Oski F (eds.): Hematology of Infancy and Childhood. 3rd ed. Philadelphia, WB Saunders Company, 1987. *This chapter offers a good review of the basic anatomy and physiology of the human hematopoietic system.*

Nathan DG, Sieff CA: The biological activities and uses of recombinant granulocyte macrophage and multi-colony stimulating factors. Prog Hematol 15:1, 1987.

Nicola NA: Hemopoietic cell growth factors and their receptors. Annu Rev Biochem 58:45, 1989.

Sieff CA: Biology and clinical aspects of the hematopoietic growth factors. Annu Rev Med 41:483, 1990.

Sieff C: Hematopoietic growth factors. J Clin Invest 79:1549, 1987.

Strober W, James S: The interleukins. Pediatr Res 24:549, 1988.

128 An Approach to the Anemias

John Lindenbaum

Anemia is one of the most common manifestations of disease the world over. Indeed, in some developing countries the majority of apparently normal people in certain population groups are anemic. Even in technologically advanced nations, a third or more of patients admitted to the medical service of a hospital are anemic. Yet a low hematocrit is often ignored or is put aside to be dealt with at a later time while other, more pressing medical problems are managed on an urgent basis. This practice is frequently a mistake, since anemia is usually a clue that should not be ignored. In fact, the clinician should almost always think of anemia in a manner similar to the way in which he or she regards symptoms like chest pain or diarrhea—as an indicator or a manifestation of an underlying disease, rather than an entity in itself.

Physicians often use laboratory tests inappropriately in the evaluation of anemic patients. In some instances, the small number of crucial tests needed to diagnose the cause of any anemia is not obtained. In others, blood is withdrawn for a long list of unnecessary tests, often worsening the anemia without elucidating it. In this chapter a logical and orderly approach to anemia is advocated. Commonly encountered diagnostic challenges receive greater emphasis than the rarer entities. The strategy outlined allows the clinician to diagnose the cause of anemia in the great majority of patients, using a small number of laboratory tests (since most anemias are caused by only a handful of conditions). The strategy also furnishes clues to the less common or more esoteric causes of anemia.

DEFINITION OF ANEMIA

In Table 128–1, normal ranges are listed for the hematocrit, hemoglobin concentration, and red blood cell count in adults. Any of these three tests can be used as an estimate of the presence or absence of anemia. Since the hemoglobin and hematocrit usually correlate very strongly with each other in anemic patients, recording both values is unnecessary. The ranges shown are arbitrary estimates of normality (as is the case for the normal range for any laboratory test) based on the mean ±2 standard deviations (SD's) of measurements made in a presumably healthy normal population. In a given individual, however, these values remain remarkably constant during health within a much narrower range than that for the population. Thus, for example, in a man in whom the hematocrit normally is 48 to 50 per cent, a decline to 40 per cent—although still within the normal range—may be an important indicator of underlying disease. Therefore, if baseline values are available, they are often useful. On the other hand, since the normal range excludes 2.5 per cent of the normal population, some persons with a hematocrit below the lower limits of the ranges shown in Table 128–1 may not actually be "anemic." Because of erythropoietic effects of androgens, the normal ranges differ significantly between the sexes.

The normal ranges for the hematocrit and the MCV are different in newborns (when the values are higher) as well as in infants during the first 24 months of life (when the values are lower). The ranges used to define anemia in adults living at high altitudes and thereby chronically exposed to low ambient oxygen levels are also higher than those shown. For reasons that are uncertain, the lower limits of normal for the hematocrit in black men and women are 1 to 2 per cent lower than those for white persons. Whether the hematocrit normally declines with aging or the slightly decreased levels seen in the elderly are indicators of occult chronic disease remains controversial. When electronic counters are used, the hematocrit is a calculated rather than a measured value and is occasionally affected by artifacts; the most common is a spurious elevation caused by cold agglutinins.

Each of the tests used to define anemia is affected by changes in the *plasma volume*. Patients with an expanded plasma volume appear to be anemic, even though the total number of circulating red cells may be normal. Such hemodilution is frequently encountered in normal pregnancy; in fluid-retaining states, such as cirrhosis of the liver and, less commonly, congestive heart failure; and in patients with splenomegaly. The hematocrit may fall as low as 28 per cent merely because of an expansion of the plasma volume. Conversely, in an anemic patient who has a decreased

TABLE 128–1. NORMAL RANGES* OF ERYTHROCYTE MEASUREMENTS IN ADULTS

Test	Females	Males
Hematocrit (%)	36–48	40–52
Hemoglobin (grams/dl)	12.0–16.0	13.5–17.7
Red blood cells (× 10⁶/μl)	4.0–5.4	4.5–6.0
Mean cell volume (fl)	80–100	80–100

*Ranges of values measured by Coulter electronic counting, representing 2 SD's above and below the mean for healthy white adults living at sea level.

plasma volume (e.g., due to dehydration), the hematocrit may lie within the normal range. If necessary, the total number of circulating red cells can be measured by a radioisotope dilution method, yielding a value known as the "red cell mass." This test is usually not necessary clinically and is more often employed in the evaluation of polycythemia.

CARDIOVASCULAR ADJUSTMENTS TO ANEMIA

The circulating erythrocyte is a nonreplicating, differentiated cell with a normal average lifespan of 120 days. Its function is to deliver oxygen to the tissues. Therefore, the main consequence of anemia is tissue hypoxia. When anemia develops slowly, several adjustments tend to maintain tissue oxygenation. The plasma volume increases, tending to maintain the total blood volume at a normal or only slightly reduced level. Early in the development of anemia, there is increased generation of the glycolytic intermediate, 2,3-diphosphoglycerate (2,3-DPG), in erythrocytes. The 2,3-DPG binds to hemoglobin, causing a rightward shift in the oxyhemoglobin dissociation curve, which allows more oxygen to be unloaded from the erythrocyte at any given blood oxygen tension.

As anemia becomes more severe, compensatory peripheral vascular dilatation increases blood flow to the tissues, through a fall in the systemic vascular resistance and an increase in the cardiac output. The latter mainly results from an increased cardiac stroke volume, since the heart rate increases only slightly, if at all, in most anemic patients. An increase in cardiac output is usually seen only in severe anemia, when the hematocrit falls to levels of about 20 per cent or less. As a result of the decrease in peripheral resistance, the blood pressure falls modestly, especially the diastolic component, leading to an increased pulse pressure. The systolic pressure, although often reduced from the normal baseline of the patient, typically remains normal. Not infrequently, a patient with previous hypertension who develops severe anemia (due, for example, to deficiency of iron or vitamin B_{12}) becomes unexpectedly normotensive; hypertension then recurs after the anemia is corrected. Similarly, correction of anemia due to renal failure by treatment with erythropoietin may cause or exacerbate hypertension. In a minority of anemic patients (usually but not invariably those with underlying cardiovascular disease), the demands of the high output state coupled with impaired coronary oxygenation lead to circulatory congestion, in some cases without an associated fall in output ("high output failure").

The cardiovascular adjustments described above are those seen when anemia develops slowly. In patients with acute blood loss, however (e.g., massive gastrointestinal bleeding), there is no time for them to occur. Instead, there is a sudden marked contraction of the intravascular volume, which may result in severe postural hypotension, a fall in cardiac output, the shunting of blood from the skin to central organs, sweating, restlessness, thirst, and air hunger (Ch. 111). This life-threatening emergency must be managed by immediate restoration of the intravascular volume, usually by transfusion of red cells. In contrast, in the chronically anemic patient, who often has a relatively well maintained central intravascular volume, blood transfusions (particularly if given rapidly to an elderly patient with underlying heart disease) may expand the central blood volume and precipitate or worsen congestive heart failure.

SYMPTOMS AND SIGNS OF ANEMIA

The complaints caused by anemia are related to tissue hypoxia. In patients with chronically developing anemia, the hematocrit level at which symptoms appear varies widely, influenced by the rate of development of anemia, the age of the patient, and the presence of underlying vascular disease. Frequent symptoms include dyspnea with exertion, dizziness, light-headedness, throbbing headaches, tinnitus, palpitations, syncope, easy fatigability, disruption of sleep patterns, decrease in libido, disturbances of mood, and impaired ability to concentrate. In elderly patients with vascular disease, angina pectoris may be a prominent complaint, even with only modest reductions in hematocrit. Anemia also frequently worsens or precipitates dementia or intermittent claudication. Anorexia is common and may be accompanied by significant weight loss. *Common physical findings in severely anemic patients include pallor of the skin and mucous membranes* (a sign of limited sensitivity and specificity), modest tachycardia and increased pulse pressure, systolic ejection murmurs, venous hums, and mild peripheral edema. Retinal hemorrhages, often flamelike, may occur in severe anemia, most commonly in association with thrombocytopenia.

THE HISTORY

As in almost all other clinical disorders, *a careful history usually provides information crucial to diagnosing the underlying cause of anemia.* The duration and time of onset of anemia or its symptoms should be determined. Onset during childhood is seen with congenital hemolytic disorders, although when anemia is not severe, these conditions may first manifest in adult life. A history of scleral icterus or gallstones, or the presence of jaundice, gallstones, or anemia in a sibling or a parent, suggests hemolysis. A history of blood loss or blood donation should be sought. Onset of the anemia during or soon after pregnancy is consistent with iron or folate deficiency. Recurrences and remissions of anemia are frequent in iron, cobalamin (vitamin B_{12}), and folate deficiencies. Pica, or excessive craving for certain (sometimes bizarre) food items, occurs with lack of iron. A history of alcohol intoxication raises a number of diagnostic considerations (see below). Paresthesia or ataxia suggests cobalamin deficiency; a sore tongue may indicate lack of cobalamin, folate, or iron. If these deficiencies are caused by celiac or tropical sprue, diarrhea or other gastrointestinal symptoms are commonly present. The patient

TABLE 128–2. DRUGS AND OTHER AGENTS THAT MAY CAUSE ANEMIA

Anemia	Type of Agent	Example
Marrow aplasias	Anticancer	Antimetabolites, alkylating agents
	Anti-inflammatory	Phenylbutazone, gold
	Antibiotic	Chloramphenicol
	Anticonvulsant	Phenytoin
	Other	Benzene, insecticides
Macrocytic or megaloblastic states	Dihydrofolate reductase inhibitors	Methotrexate, pyrimethamine, trimethoprim, triamterene, pentamidine
	Antiviral	Zidovudine
	Anticancer	Hydroxyurea, cytosine arabinoside, alkylating agents
	Immunosuppressive	Azathioprine
	Other	Alcohol, sulfasalazine
Hemolytic	Antibiotic	Penicillin,* cephalosporins,* sulfonamides*†
	Antiarrhythmic	Procainamide,* quinidine*
	Antihypertensive	Alpha-methyldopa*
	Antimalarials	Primaquine*
	Other	Fava beans,† naphthalene,† dapsone†
Blood loss	Anti-inflammatory	Aspirin, nonsteroidal drugs
	Anticoagulants	Warfarin, heparin

*Causes antibody-induced hemolysis.

†Causes hemolysis in glucose-6-phosphate dehydrogenase (G6PD)–deficient persons. Sulfonamides also cause hemolysis in patients with unstable hemoglobins.

TABLE 128–3. THE INITIAL LABORATORY DATA BASE IN THE EVALUATION OF ANEMIA

Hematocrit
Reticulocyte count (absolute)
MCV
Blood smear
Serum ferritin level
White blood cell count and differential
Platelet count (or estimate)

MCV = mean cell volume.

must be questioned, sometimes repeatedly, about the possible intake of various medications (Table 128–2). The most important aspect of the history in an anemic patient, however, is often the search for underlying disease: for evidence of renal, liver, or endocrine disturbances; the acquired immunodeficiency syndrome (AIDS), tuberculosis, or other infections; chronic inflammatory disorders, such as rheumatoid arthritis or lupus erythematosus; or malignancies.

THE PHYSICAL EXAMINATION

Findings on physical examination that point to specific underlying etiologic mechanisms include atrophy of the tongue (in cobalamin, folate, or iron deficiencies); abnormal gait or impaired vibration sense or other sensory modalities (in cobalamin lack); scleral icterus, splenomegaly, or leg ulcers (in certain hemolytic anemias); petechiae (with thrombocytopenia of any cause, e.g., acute leukemia); and the myriad signs of primary diseases (e.g., infections, malignancies, liver disorders, hypothyroidism) that may cause a secondary anemia.

THE INITIAL LABORATORY DATA BASE

A small number of tests should be obtained on every anemic patient: the complete blood count (CBC), including the white blood cell count and differential, a platelet count, or an estimate on the smear of the numbers of platelets; a careful evaluation of red blood cell morphology on the Wright-stained blood smear; the reticulocyte count; the mean cell volume (MCV); and some measure of iron stores—the serum ferritin (preferably) or the combined determination of the serum iron and total iron-binding capacity (Table 128–3). In at least three quarters of patients, the cause of the anemia will be apparent when the results of these tests are combined with the history, physical examination, and other diagnostic studies that are guided by complaints not caused by the anemia.

THE BLOOD SMEAR. In the current era of automation and high technology, the value of careful, expert assessment of the red cell morphology on the peripheral blood smear tends to be forgotten. The blood smear, however, is essential to the diagnosis of many anemias and virtually always provides useful information, even when unremarkable or normal. Proper identification of the full range of clinically useful abnormalities requires a certain expertise. Blood smears are subject to both *overinterpretation* (usually because of frequent artifacts in poorly prepared smears

or in inappropriate areas of well-prepared ones) and *underinterpretation* (most frequently the result of hurried interpretation by an overwhelmed routine laboratory). Therefore, the clinician must take the time to develop expertise in this area or, in most instances, demand that the hospital laboratory provide an expert assessment of the blood smear.

Some characteristic red cell abnormalities useful in the diagnosis of various anemias are listed in Table 128–4. The *context* in which a particular morphologic finding is noted must be emphasized. If red cell fragmentation is the most striking abnormality on the blood smear of a patient with a high reticulocyte count, hemoglobinuria, and a poorly functioning aortic valve prosthesis, the morphologic changes strongly support the diagnosis of a traumatic hemolytic anemia. In contrast, an occasional fragmented cell in the blood smear of a patient with marked hypochromia, microcytosis, a low reticulocyte count, and a history of recent blood loss is much more likely to be caused by iron deficiency. The widely used term *poikilocytosis*, to indicate variation in cell shape, is of limited usefulness. The clinician really desires to know precisely which abnormalities in shape have been noted, e.g., sickle cells, oval macrocytes, elliptocytes, or fragments. Although *polychromasia* (see Color Plate 5F, left) is indicative of the presence of young reticulocytes (see below), the abundance of polychromatic cells is important. An occasional polychromatic cell is often seen in severe anemias due to bone marrow failure (e.g., megaloblastic anemia, marrow infiltration by tumor). The presence of blasts in the differential white count suggests acute leukemia as the cause of a patient's anemia; decreased numbers of platelets or white cells point toward conditions in which anemia is associated with other cytopenias (e.g., megaloblastic anemia, hypersplenism, acute leukemia, aplastic anemia).

ERYTHROPOIETIC RESPONSE TO ANEMIA. As tissue hypoxia develops with increasing anemia, a major homeostatic system attempts to return the number of circulating red cells to normal. Although a number of other hormones and growth factors may influence erythrocyte production, erythropoietin, a glycoprotein, is probably the most important. Erythropoietin appears to be predominantly produced by peritubular cells of the kidney (most likely capillary endothelial cells). Other cells, possibly including hepatocytes and macrophages, may be less important sources of the hormone. A heme protein present in cells sensitive to hypoxia may undergo a conformational change that in some way activates the gene for erythropoietin production. Erythropoietin released into the circulation acts mainly to stimulate the differentiation of erythroid stem cells in the bone marrow, cells that are already committed to form red cells (so-called CFU-E, or colony-forming units–erythroid). The hormone also acts on later erythroid precursors. The result is the enhanced production and release of young red cells, or *reticulocytes* (see Color Plate 5F, right).

THE RETICULOCYTE COUNT. A key test that should be included as part of the initial workup of every anemic patient is the reticulocyte count. The reticulocyte, a 1- to 2-day-old cell that is continuing to synthesize protein (unlike more elderly erythrocytes), contains aggregates of ribosomes, demonstrated by a supravital stain (new methylene blue). The reticulocyte count is the percentage of such cells per 500 or 1000 cells counted,

TABLE 128–4. ABNORMALITIES ON BLOOD SMEARS IN ANEMIC PATIENTS

Abnormality	Characteristic Disorder	Found Also in Other Conditions
Hypochromia, microcytosis	Iron deficiency, thalassemias	Anemia of chronic disease, sideroblastic anemias
Macro-ovalocytes	Cobalamin and folate deficiencies	Myelodysplasias, myelofibrosis, autoimmune hemolysis
Hypersegmented neutrophils	Cobalamin and folate deficiencies	Renal failure, iron deficiency, chronic myelocytic leukemia, congenital hypersegmentation
Teardrop cells, nucleated red blood cells	Myelofibrosis	Marrow replacement by tumor, autoimmune hemolysis, megaloblastic anemias, thalassemia major
Microspherocytes	Autoimmune hemolysis, hereditary spherocytosis	Microangiopathic hemolysis, hypophosphatemia
Sickle cells	Hemoglobin SS, SC, S-thalassemia	Hemoglobin C$_{Harlem}$
Red cell fragments (schistocytes)	Microangiopathic or traumatic hemolysis	Iron deficiency, megaloblastic anemias, cancer chemotherapy
Target cells	Hemoglobin C, SC, thalassemias, liver disease	Artifact, SS disease, iron deficiency, splenectomy
Elliptocytes	Hereditary elliptocytosis	Iron deficiency, myelofibrosis, megaloblastic anemias
Burr cells (echinocytes)	Renal failure	Artifact, pyruvate kinase deficiency
Spur cells (acanthocytes)	Liver disease, abetalipoproteinemia	

TABLE 128–5. CAUSES OF ANEMIA

Cause	Absolute Reticulocyte Count
Bone marrow failure	Low or normal
Acute blood loss	High
Hemolysis	High

TABLE 128–6. CLASSIFICATION OF ANEMIAS DUE TO MARROW FAILURE

Type	MCV (fl)
Normocytic	80–100
Microcytic	<80
Macrocytic	>100

rather than an absolute number. It therefore needs to be "corrected" to make it a better index of total production of young cells. This can be done by multiplying the reticulocyte percentage times the red blood cell count. Thus, for example, in a normal person with a reticulocyte count of 1 per cent and a red cell count of 5 million per microliter, the absolute numbers of circulating reticulocytes would be $0.01 \times 5,000,000 = 50,000$ reticulocytes per microliter. The upper limit of normal is approximately 100,000 per microliter. In contrast, in an anemic patient with a red cell count of 2 million per microliter and a reticulocyte count of 1 per cent, the number of circulating reticulocytes would be $0.01 \times 2,000,000$, or 20,000 per microliter. Although the reticulocyte percentage is the same (1 per cent) in this instance, the absolute number is markedly below normal, indicating that the bone marrow has failed to respond to the severe anemia by increasing its production of young cells.

INITIAL EVALUATION OF ANEMIA

Calculation of the absolute numbers of reticulocytes allows the clinician to make an important early decision that will shape further diagnostic thinking (Table 128–5). Anemias can be divided into those in which the marrow response to the anemia is appropriate, that is, red cell production is increased, and those in which there is an inappropriate failure of the marrow to augment cell output. An anemia in which the absolute number of reticulocytes is not increased is defined as one in which *bone marrow failure* is present (Table 128–5). *In most anemic patients encountered in clinical medicine, the underlying cause of the anemia is marrow failure.* The subsequent diagnostic workup of the patient with marrow failure differs markedly from that of one in whom the reticulocyte count is elevated.

The classification shown in Table 128–5, although extremely useful clinically, is an oversimplification. It emphasizes the *predominant* cause of the anemia. In many anemias, more than one mechanism is operative. Thus, for example, in the anemia of chronic disease, the red cell lifespan is modestly shortened, although the primary cause of the anemia is the failure of the bone marrow to increase the number of circulating reticulocytes. Similarly, in severe anemias due to deficiencies of iron, vitamin B_{12}, or folate, or in beta-thalassemia major, the red cell lifespan may be shortened, although the primary problem is one of cell production. In addition, in many chronic hemolytic anemias, even though the bone marrow has increased its output of new cells, the marrow response is less than maximal and an element of inadequate marrow compensation may contribute to the anemia. Furthermore, when acute hemolysis or blood loss develops, the maximal reticulocyte response may be delayed for several days or as long as a week. Thus, approximately 20 per cent of patients with an acute episode of autoimmune hemolytic anemia do not have an elevated absolute reticulocyte count at the time of admission to the hospital, although reticulocytosis develops subsequently. In patients hospitalized for several weeks, the equivalent of a unit of whole blood is often obtained as part of an intensive diagnostic workup for various disorders. In this situation, acute blood loss caused by multiple venesections may be superimposed upon a marrow failure anemia, frequently without an adequate reticulocyte response.

ANEMIA DUE TO BONE MARROW FAILURE

RED CELL SIZE IN PATIENTS WITH MARROW FAILURE. The first question that should be asked about a patient with a marrow failure anemia is, *what is the average size of the red cells?* The MCV is measured directly by electronic counters and is usually available as part of the initial hemogram. Although the mean cell hemoglobin (MCH) and mean cell hemoglobin concentration (MCHC) are also routinely provided, they add little information of diagnostic value. The MCH varies in the same direction as the MCV in microcytic or macrocytic anemias. The MCHC is of very limited value and is often normal in

patients with frank microcytic anemias. The normal range for the MCV in adults is 80 to 100 fl (femtoliters), a better working range in the classification of anemias than the more narrow ones often reported by hospital laboratories. The MCV determination may be falsely elevated by laboratory artifacts, which may be caused by cold agglutinins, marked hyperglycemia, and extreme leukocytosis.

On the basis of the MCV, anemias due to marrow failure should be classified as normocytic, microcytic, or macrocytic (Table 128–6). In normocytic or microcytic anemias, the subsequent diagnostic evaluation differs markedly from that in macrocytic anemias.

Normocytic Anemias Due to Marrow Failure

Normocytic anemias due to marrow failure account for the largest group of patients with anemia seen in clinical practice. The most common causes of normocytic anemia due to decreased cell production (Table 128–7) are iron deficiency, the anemia of chronic disease, and anemias secondary to renal, hepatic, and endocrine disorders. Less frequently, a normocytic marrow failure anemia may result from one of a variety of "primary" marrow disturbances.

IRON DEFICIENCY ANEMIA (Ch. 131). Iron deficiency anemia is usually considered microcytic and hypochromic. As iron deficiency develops, however, the hematocrit often falls before the MCV becomes subnormal. Therefore, iron lack (especially when the hematocrit is above 30 per cent) must always be considered in patients with normocytic marrow failure anemia. In outpatient practice, iron deficiency is a frequent cause of such an anemia. Blood smears may be entirely normal except for mild anisocytosis; or there may be a minority population of microcytic cells, even though the MCV is still normal. Since most of the iron in the body is found in red cells, loss of blood (commonly from gastrointestinal or uterine sources) is usually the underlying cause of iron deficiency. Imbalances between demand and dietary supply frequently cause iron deficiency anemia in normal pregnancy, infancy, and adolescence. Rare causes include loss of hemoglobin and hemosiderin in the urine in certain hemolytic anemias (e.g., with malfunctioning valve prostheses or in paroxysmal nocturnal hemoglobinuria), intrapulmonary hemorrhage (in idiopathic pulmonary hemosiderosis), and malabsorption of iron (usually secondary to gastrectomy or to celiac or tropical sprue). Iron deficiency anemia due to primary inadequacy of iron intake in the diet is an unusual cause of anemia in adults in industrialized countries. In many developing nations, however, in addition to blood loss, anemia may be caused by a diet that is adequate in total iron content but that contains iron in poorly bioavailable form.

ANEMIA OF CHRONIC DISEASE (Ch. 131). In patients who have chronic infections (e.g., tuberculosis, lung abscess), chronic inflammation (e.g., rheumatoid arthritis, systemic lupus

TABLE 128–7. CAUSES OF NORMOCYTIC MARROW FAILURE ANEMIAS

Iron deficiency
Anemia of chronic disease
Renal failure
Liver disease
Endocrine disorders
"Primary" marrow disorders*
   Aplasias
   Myelodysplasias
   Myelofibrosis
   Hematologic or solid tumors
   Granulomas
   HIV infection

*Marrow aspiration and biopsy are useful.

erythematosus, inflammatory bowel disease), or underlying malignancies that are not necessarily metastatic to the bone marrow, or who have recently had major trauma or surgery, a characteristic anemia that is gradual in onset and is usually normocytic often develops. Typically, the anemia is mild, although in 10 per cent of patients (usually with very severe chronic illnesses) the hematocrit may be below 20 per cent. Red cell morphology is little changed from normal, although there may be modest anisocytosis with a few microcytes. Marked anisocytosis, poikilocytosis, or nucleated red blood cells are not seen. The primary problem is failure of cell production. Relative lack of erythropoietin, sequestration of iron in macrophages, and inhibitory effects of cytokines are among the postulated causes of the marrow failure. The anemia remits when the underlying disorder clears. The presence of one of the associated chronic disorders is usually obvious. Occasionally, however, the anemia of chronic disease is the only apparent illness, and a careful search for an occult disorder, such as a malignancy or polymyalgia rheumatica, is indicated. The anemia of chronic disease does not occur in all chronic conditions, however. Uncomplicated diabetes mellitus, hypertension, asthma, ischemic heart disease, or congestive heart failure should not be considered a satisfactory explanation for an anemia of this type.

DIFFERENTIATION OF IRON DEFICIENCY ANEMIA FROM THE ANEMIA OF CHRONIC DISEASE. Since iron deficiency is usually accompanied by greater variation in red cell size than is seen in the anemia of chronic disease, it has been proposed that a quantitative assessment of the degree of anisocytosis, as measured by electronic cell sizing (the "red cell distribution width," or RDW), can be helpful in distinguishing these two common causes of marrow failure anemia. This assessment has not proved to be reliable. The differentiation is often aided, however, by serum tests that are influenced by the amount of iron in body stores. The most useful screening measure for this purpose is the *serum ferritin* level (Ch. 131), which is low in the majority of patients with iron deficiency and normal or elevated in the anemia of chronic disease. A low serum ferritin value virtually always indicates iron deficiency. Unfortunately, there is an overlap zone (approximately 20 to 150 ng per milliliter) in the lower end of the normal range that is compatible with *either* condition. Other tests frequently used for estimating iron stores are the *serum iron* and the *serum total iron-binding capacity* (TIBC). The serum iron level is typically low in both disorders, however. In chronic disease, the TIBC (an indicator of circulating levels of the iron-binding protein transferrin) is usually depressed, and in iron deficiency it is often elevated. Unfortunately, many patients with iron deficiency anemia, especially if complicated by a chronic disease, may have normal or even low levels of the TIBC. In both conditions, *the per cent saturation of serum transferrin* (i.e., the serum iron divided by the TIBC × 100) is low. The test is not helpful unless the value is higher than 25 per cent, which argues against iron deficiency. The interpretation of these laboratory measures is summarized in Table 128–8. If these tests are equivocal, direct examination of the bone marrow with histochemical staining of iron stores in macrophages is needed to exclude iron deficiency definitely. Alternatively, a therapeutic trial of iron can be given, repeating the hematocrit after 3 to 4 weeks. This practice may be reasonable

TABLE 128–8. RELIABILITY OF SERUM TESTS IN PREDICTING IRON STORES

Test	Interpretation
Definitive	
Low ferritin	Deficient
High TIBC	Deficient
High normal or high ferritin	Not deficient*
Equivocal	
Low normal ferritin	Uncertain
Low serum iron	Uncertain
Low or normal TIBC	Uncertain
Low per cent of transferrin saturation	Uncertain

*Even if inflammation, malignancy, liver disease, or renal failure is present.
TIBC = total iron-binding capacity.

in a patient with uncomplicated iron deficiency anemia (for example, a menstruating woman who is otherwise well but with a serum ferritin level of 35 ng per milliliter). In a patient with an underlying chronic disorder, however, if iron is given at the same time as the chronic disease is treated or spontaneously improves, the "response" of the hematocrit to iron will be difficult to interpret. It is preferable to assess marrow iron stores directly before treatment, since once lack of iron is proved, a search for an underlying cause of blood loss is mandated.

The serum ferritin is an acute phase reactant; it is elevated out of proportion to the amount of iron in stores in acute and chronic inflammatory disorders or malignancies (as well as liver and kidney disease). Nonetheless, the presence of some iron in stores appears to be necessary for a marked increase in the serum ferritin level to occur in association with these conditions. Therefore, *an elevated or high normal serum ferritin is not seen in patients who are iron deficient*, even though they have associated inflammation, malignancy, liver disease, or renal failure. Such a value rules out the presence of coexistent iron deficiency.

ANEMIAS SECONDARY TO OTHER SYSTEMIC CONDITIONS. In addition to iron deficiency and the anemia of chronic disease, normocytic marrow failure anemias are frequently encountered in association with renal failure, hepatic disease, and a variety of endocrine disturbances. The anemia in such patients often resembles the anemia of chronic disease but is commonly of multifactorial etiology.

Renal Failure. A normocytic marrow failure anemia occurs in chronic renal insufficiency. Its severity is roughly (but not invariably) proportional to the degree of the renal failure. Erythrocyte survival is modestly decreased, although the absolute reticulocyte count is not elevated. Serum iron levels and TIBC are either low or normal, and the serum ferritin level is typically increased. Red cells with scalloped outlines ("burr" cells) (see Color Plate 6F, right) may be seen on blood smears. Failure of the kidney to elaborate erythropoietin in amounts appropriate to the degree of anemia appears to be a major (if not the principal) cause of the anemia. In most cases, the anemia responds completely to the regular parenteral administration of recombinant human erythropoietin, thereby obviating blood transfusions. Resistance to erythropoietin is also likely to contribute to the marrow failure state, although circulating inhibitors of erythropoiesis have not been clearly identified. In individual patients with renal failure, however, other mechanisms may contribute to anemia, such as iron deficiency. A serum ferritin level below 60 ng per milliliter in the presence of renal insufficiency strongly suggests lack of iron. Anemia in renal disease may also be caused by folate deficiency (much less frequently); aluminum toxicity, in which case the anemia is typically *microcytic;* partial fibrous replacement of the bone marrow in patients with severe hyperparathyroidism and osteitis fibrosa, which may be associated with leukopenia and thrombocytopenia; hypersplenism, which occasionally develops with chronic hemodialysis; and "microangiopathic hemolytic anemia" accompanied by fragmentation on blood smears and an elevated absolute reticulocyte count (with malignant hypertension, vasomotor nephropathy, acute glomerulonephritis, thrombotic thrombocytopenic purpura, and the hemolytic-uremic syndrome).

Liver Disease. Any chronic liver disease may cause an associated anemia of the type seen in other chronic diseases, but additional mechanisms are also often important. For example, anemia caused by acute blood loss may occur, and iron deficiency may eventually supervene owing to continuing hemorrhage. A variety of hemolytic states are also seen, including "spur cell" anemia, in which irregularly contracted red cells, or *acanthocytes*, are seen on blood smears in tandem with brisk hemolysis in advanced liver disease; autoimmune hemolytic anemia accompanying acute viral or chronic active hepatitis; acute hemolysis caused by profound hypophosphatemia in alcoholics; and, rarely, acute hemolytic states associated with alcoholic hepatitis. Chronic alcoholics (independent of the presence of liver disease) are highly prone to develop megaloblastic anemia due to folate deficiency, as well as sideroblastic anemia. Chronic infections, such as tuberculosis and lung abscesses, may cause an anemia of chronic disease. Therefore, in anemic patients with liver disease, careful evaluation of the patient, with particular attention to the MCV, reticulocyte count, and blood smear, is essential to determine the likely contributory factors. In alcoholics the anemia is *usually* multifactorial. The clinician should avoid the casual attribution of

PLATE 5   HEMATOLOGY

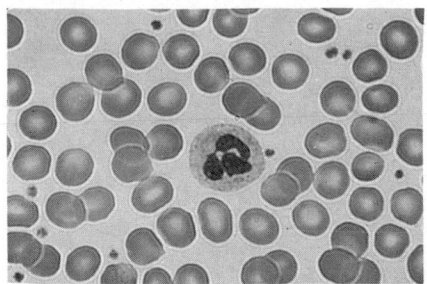

A, A normal peripheral blood smear. The red cells are normocytic with a good hemoglobin content. A normal segmented neutrophil is in the center of the field. A normal platelet is immediately adjacent. (L.O.)

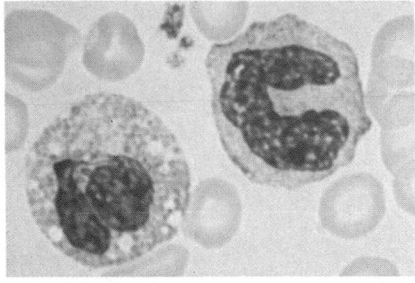

B, A normal eosinophil *(left)* and band *(right)*. The eosinophil shows orange granules, vacuoles, and a segmented nucleus. The band has gray-pink cytoplasm and a reticular, horseshoe-shaped nucleus. (V.H.O.)

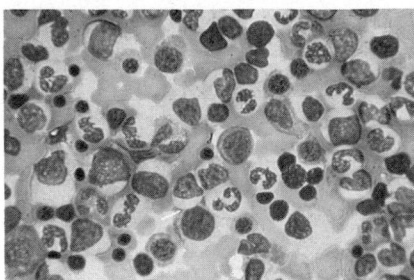

C, Normal bone marrow aspirate seen at low power. There is a 2:1 ratio between myeloid and erythroid precursors. The latter are identified by their shrunken, pyknotic ("coal black") nuclei. (L.P.)

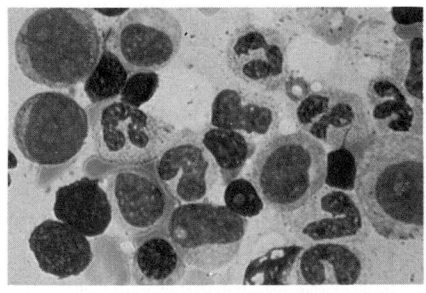

D, A bone marrow aspirate. Five erythroid precursors (with pyknotic nuclei) are present. The remaining cells are myeloid precursors in various stages of maturation, ranging from myeloblast to segmented neutrophil. (L.O.)

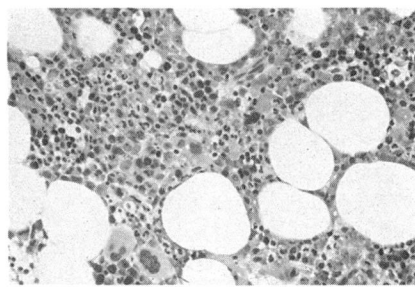

E, A hematoxylin and eosin (H & E)-stained normal bone marrow biopsy. Normal distribution and cellularity are seen. Several distinct megakaryocytes can be recognized because of their large size and multiple nuclear lobes. (L.P.)

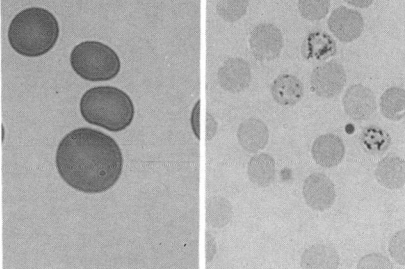

F, Left, The larger, gray-pink erythrocyte in the center of this field is called a polychromatophilic or "shift" cell. (H.O.) Right, Reticulocytes. The dark purple reticulin in red cells newly entering the blood is demonstrated by this new methylene blue stain. (L.O.)

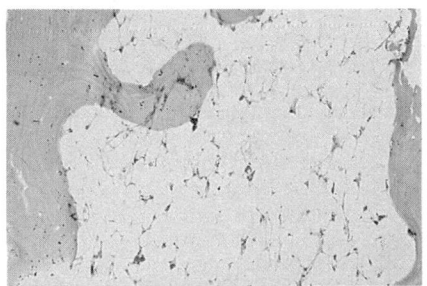

G, This low-power view of an H & E-stained bone marrow biopsy is from a patient with severe aplastic anemia. The virtually empty marrow can be appreciated by comparing with frame E. Even the marrow stroma is scanty. (L.P.)

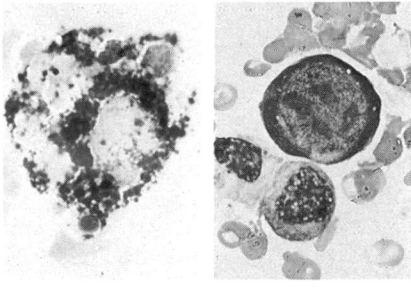

H, Left, Anemia of chronic disease; iron-stained bone marrow aspirate. Heavy dark blue globules of iron are seen in the storage cells. Right, Giant pronormoblast is from the bone marrow aspirate of a patient with red cell aplasia due to parvovirus infection. (H.O.)

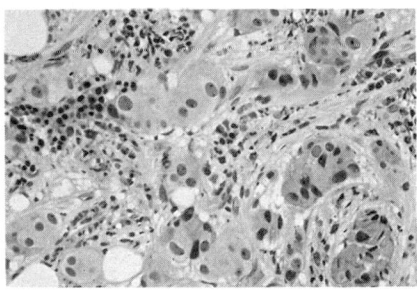

I, Metastatic breast carcinoma is seen in this view of an H & E-stained bone marrow biopsy. The malignancy has virtually replaced normal marrow elements. (L.P.)

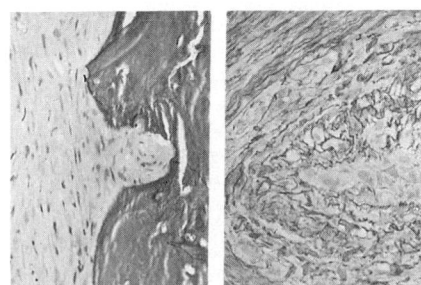

J, Agnogenic myeloid metaplasia with myelofibrosis. *Left,* This H & E-stained preparation shows virtual replacement of the marrow cavity with light pink-staining fibrous tissue. *Right,* A reticulin stain demonstrates the fibrosis as well. (L.P.)

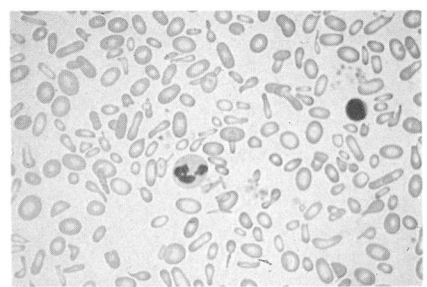

K, The peripheral blood in a patient with severe iron deficiency anemia. A normal lymphocyte is present (for comparison purposes) to the right of center. Marked anisocytosis and poikilocytosis can be appreciated, as can microcytosis and hypochromia. (L.P.)

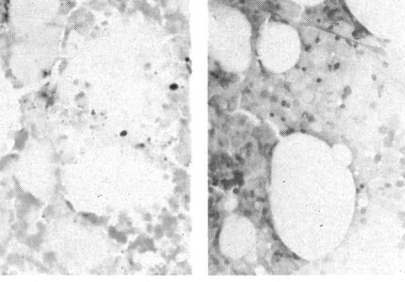

L, These are views of iron-stained bone marrow. *Left,* Normal iron stores are seen as dark blue-staining material. *Right,* The absence of iron is a characteristic finding in iron deficiency anemia. (L.P.)

PLATE 6   HEMATOLOGY

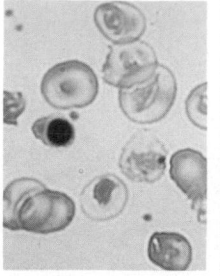 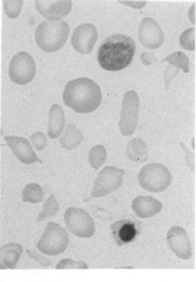

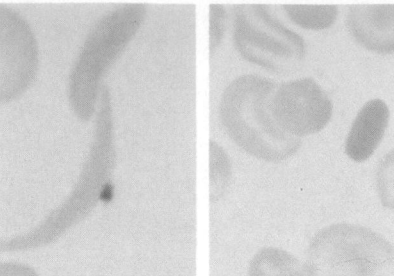

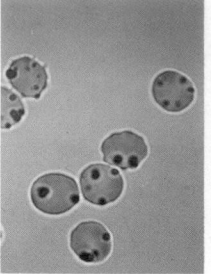 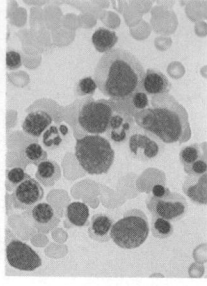

A, Left, Beta-thalassemia. Smear shows an orthochromic normoblast to the left. Also seen are targeting, hypochromia, and a Howell-Jolly body. (H.O.) *Right,* Alpha-thalassemia, E hemoglobinopathy. A normoblast and lymphocyte and anisocytosis are present. (L.O.)

B, Left, Sickle cell disease. A classic sickle cell is seen in this field. *Right,* The cell to the right of center is a classic finding in hemoglobin C disease. It represents crystallized hemoglobin C. Also present are targeting and anisocytosis. (V.H.O.)

C, Hemolytic anemia. *Left,* Heinz body preparation showing dark-staining denatured globin intraerythrocytic particles. (H.O.) *Right,* The ratio of erythroid to myeloid cells in the bone marrow aspirate is less than 1, indicating increased erythroid activity. (L.O.)

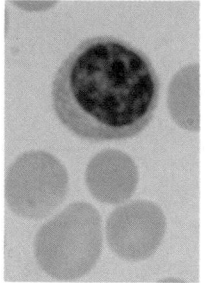 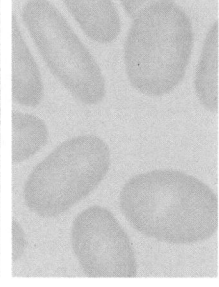

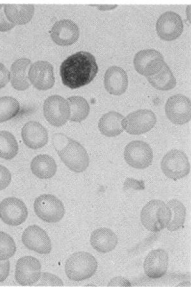

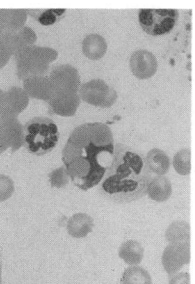 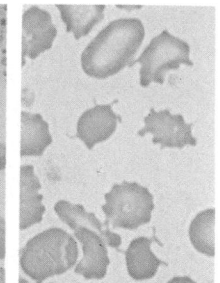

D, Left, This view of the peripheral blood in a patient with hereditary spherocytosis (HS) shows microspherocytes and a normal lymphocyte. *Right,* Hereditary elliptocytosis. Significant numbers of elliptocytes (oval erythrocytes) are seen in this field. (V.H.O.)

E, Left, G6PD deficiency. Central to the normal lymphocyte is a red cell with a blistered appearance secondary to portions of denatured hemoglobin being "bitten" off. *Right,* Microangiopathy. A shift cell and fragments are seen centrally. (L.O.)

F, Hemolytic anemia. *Left,* Erythrophagocytosis. Four red blood cells (center) have been engulfed by a cell of the monocyte-macrophage line. *Right,* Marked red cell membrane abnormalities in severe hepatorenal failure, with burr cells and spur cells. (L.O., H.O.)

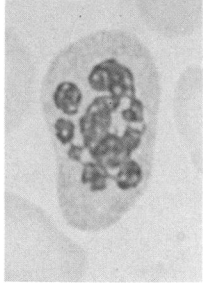 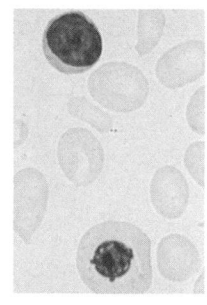

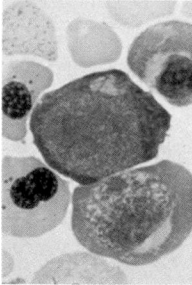

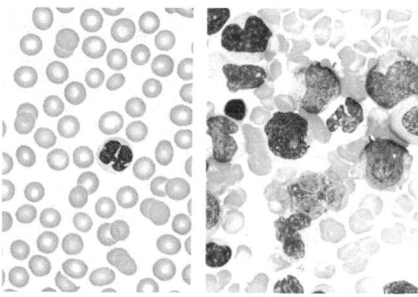

G, Pernicious anemia. *Left,* Marked neutrophil hypersegmentation. *Right,* Peripheral blood with large lymphocyte (top), macrocytosis, and orthochromic megaloblast (bottom). The latter has nuclear-cytoplasmic disproportion and beaded nuclear chromatin. (V.H.O.)

H, Pernicious anemia megaloblasts. Typical nuclear chromatin changes are seen in both frames. *Left,* Large central cell is a promegaloblast. *Right,* Large cell below is a basophilic megaloblast. Two cells above are polychromatophilic megaloblasts. (V.H.O.)

I, Myelodysplasia. *Left,* Therapy-related myelodysplasia. Dysmorphic red cells and a markedly abnormal granulocyte are seen. *Right,* Refractory anemia with excess blasts in transition (RAEBT). Several blasts and other dyspoietic changes are seen. (H.P.)

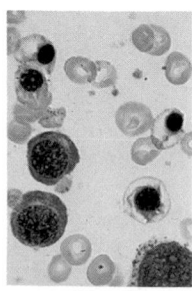 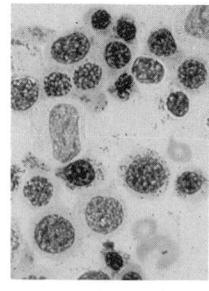

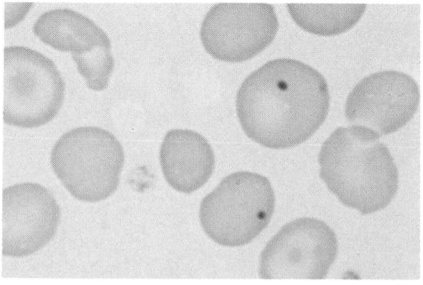

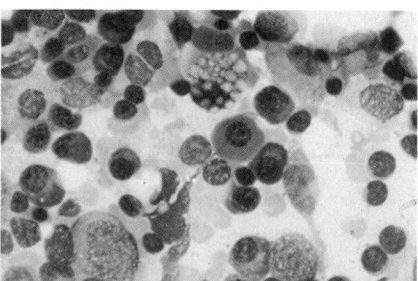

J, Myelodysplasia. *Left,* Marked erythroid dyspoiesis. Diagnosis was refractory anemia with ring sideroblasts (RARB). *Right,* An iron stain in the same patient showing perinuclear rings of iron-laden mitochondria. (L.O.)

K, Postsplenectomy changes. This view of the peripheral blood shows three deeply basophilic granules peripherally in three different red cells—Howell-Jolly bodies. Targeting is also seen. (V.H.O.)

L, A bone marrow aspirate in a patient with Felty's syndrome. Maturation arrest is at the metamyelocyte stage. There is significant reactive plasmacytosis (30 per cent). A "Mott cell" with grapelike inclusions is seen top center. (L.O.)

PLATE 7   HEMATOLOGY

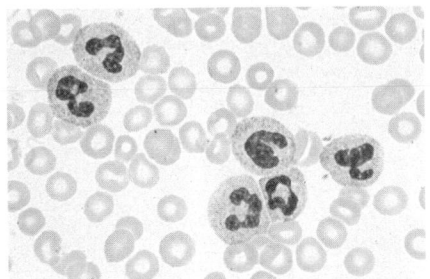

A, Neutrophilia. Four segmented and two band neutrophils are seen in this view of the peripheral blood. Some red blood cells are slightly hypochromic. (L.O.)

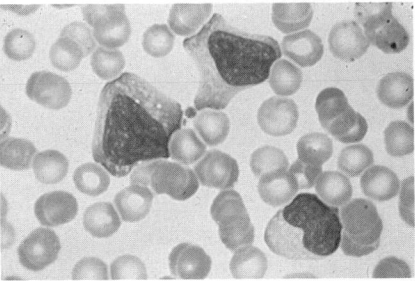

B, Infectious mononucleosis. Reactive (or atypical) lymphocytosis is seen in this peripheral blood smear. Pleomorphic reticular nuclei, peripheral basophilia of cytoplasm, and scalloped cell borders are characteristic. Slight rouleaux are also present. (H.O.)

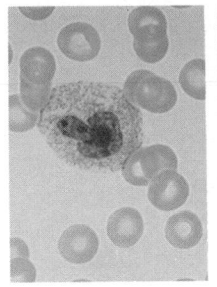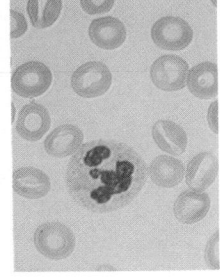

C, Left, This band neutrophil shows basophilic or toxic granulation. Right, This segmented neutrophil shows some toxic granulation and a grayish Döhle body at 7 o'clock. Both are blood changes seen in bacterial infection. (H.O.)

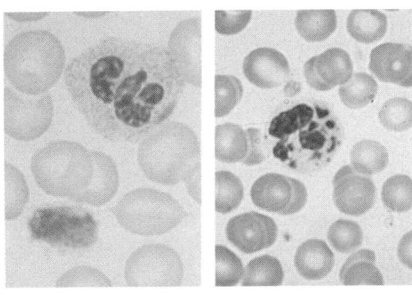

D, Left, May-Hegglin anomaly. The segmented neutrophil at the top of this field has a gray, spindle-shaped Döhle body at 4 o'clock. A giant platelet is seen at the bottom. (V.H.O.) Right, Chédiak-Higashi syndrome. Characteristic giant neutrophilic lysozymes are seen. (H.O.)

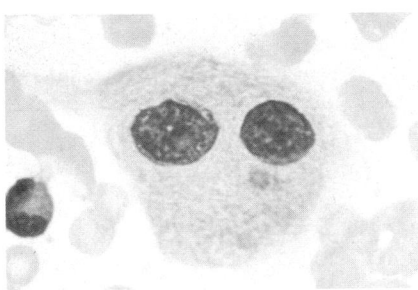

E, Gaucher's disease. This bone marrow aspirate shows a giant binucleate storage cell filled with glucocerebrosides. The fibrillar pattern is characteristic. (H.O.)

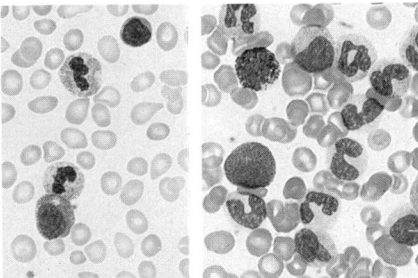

F, Left, Agnogenic myeloid metaplasia. This blood smear shows some teardrop-shaped red cells and a characteristic leukoerythroblastic reaction. Right, Chronic myelogenous leukemia (CML). Marked neutrophilia with left shift and two abnormal eosinophils are seen. (H.P.)

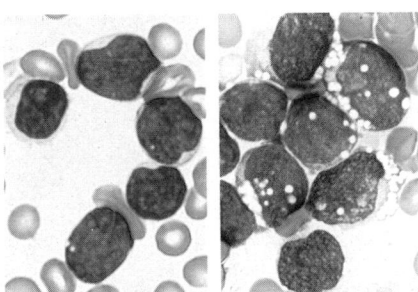

G, Left, Chronic myelogenous leukemia, blast crisis. The blasts have very immature nuclear chromatin. The patient was Ph-1 chromosome positive. Right, Ph-1 chromosome–positive acute lymphoblastic leukemia. These blasts are shown for comparison. (H.O.)

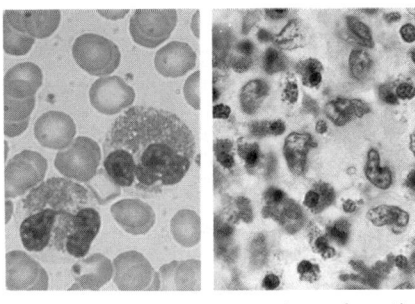

H, Left, Two eosinophils are shown from the peripheral blood of a patient with the hypereosinophilic syndrome. (H.O.) Right, Eosinophilic granuloma. In this lymph node, eosinophils and histiocytes are seen. (H.P.)

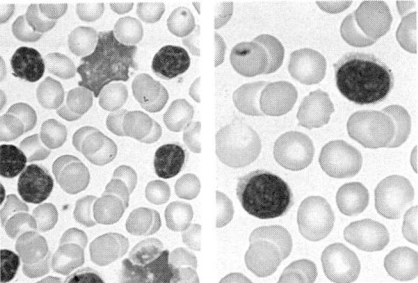

I, Left, Chronic B cell lymphocytic leukemia. The neoplastic lymphocytes are B cells. Two destroyed lymphocytes are in the center. (L.O.) Right, Chronic T cell lymphocytic leukemia. The neoplastic lymphocytes have been identified as T cells. (H.O.)

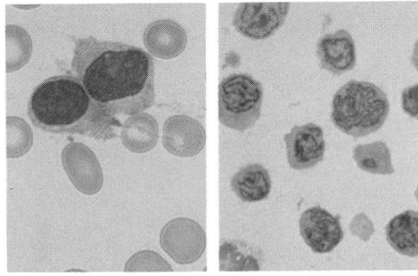

J, Left, Hairy cell leukemia (HCL). This frame shows two "hairy cells" with thin cytoplasmic projections and reticular nuclear chromatin. (H.O.) Right, Sézary's syndrome. This buffy coat preparation shows nuclear pleomorphism and convolutions.

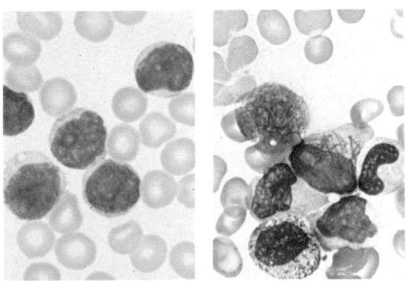

K, Acute nonlymphoblastic leukemia (ANLL). Left, M-1 type. The blasts have round or slightly indented nuclei, fine nuclear chromatin, and very little cytoplasmic granulation. Right, M-3 type. Three leukemic promyelocytes with multiple Auer rods and cytoplasmic inclusions are seen. (H.O.)

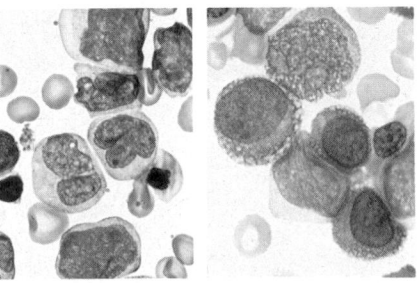

L, ANLL (continued). Left, M-4 type. Blasts in the center of this field have both monocytic and myeloid features. Right, M-6 type. This field shows abnormalities seen in erythroleukemia. Most blasts have marked nuclear dyspoiesis. The central blast could be myeloid. (H.O.)

PLATE 8 HEMATOLOGY

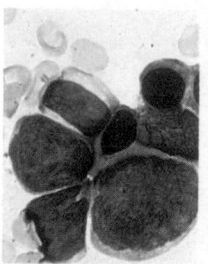 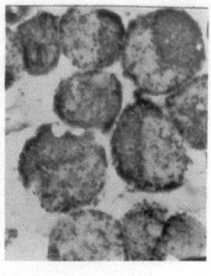

A, ANLL (continued). *Left,* M-7 type. This bone marrow aspirate shows characteristic large blasts. *Right,* The myeloperoxidase stain is often useful in identifying myeloid blasts. Dark granules are characteristic of a positive reaction. (H.O.)

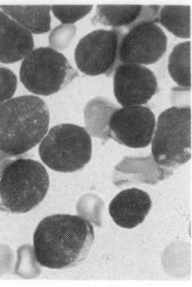 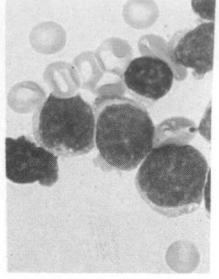

B, Acute lymphoblastic leukemia (ALL). *Left,* L-1 type. This bone marrow aspirate shows L-1 lymphoblasts that are moderately uniform in size. *Right,* L-2 type. In this bone marrow aspirate, the pleomorphism of the blasts is apparent. (H.O.)

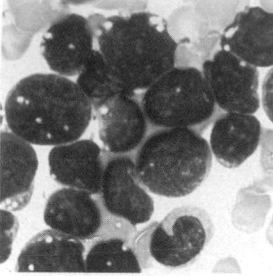

C, ALL (continued). *Left,* L-3 type. This bone marrow aspirate shows characteristic blasts. Cytoplasmic and nuclear vacuoles are seen. *Right,* Coarse, red-pink cytoplasmic granules characterize periodic acid–Schiff (PAS)–positive lymphoblasts.

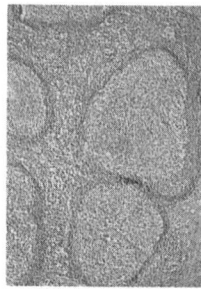 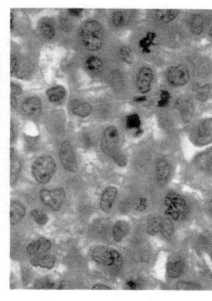

D, *Left,* Non-Hodgkin's lymphoma (follicular, small cleaved cell type). Lymph node. The follicular pattern is seen. (L.P.) *Right,* Non-Hodgkin's lymphoma (diffuse, T immunoblastic type). Lymph node, H & E stain. A diffuse pattern of large neoplastic cells is seen. (H.P.)

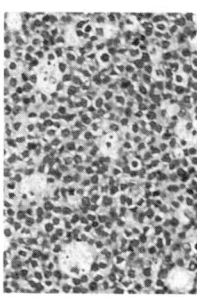

E, *Left,* Non-Hodgkin's lymphoma (B cell type) in a patient with AIDS. Lymph node biopsy, H & E stain. *Right,* Non-Hodgkin's lymphoma in a patient with AIDS. Brain involvement is present. (L.P.)

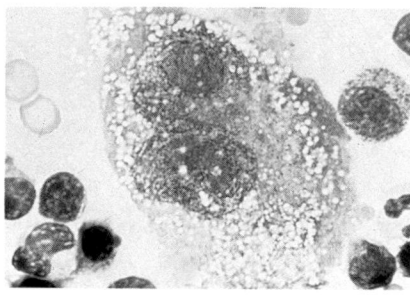

F, Hodgkin's disease. This bone marrow aspirate shows a classic Reed-Sternberg cell. The "mirror-image" nuclei are characteristic, as are the large nucleoli. It is unusual to find these cells in the bone marrow aspirate. (H.O.)

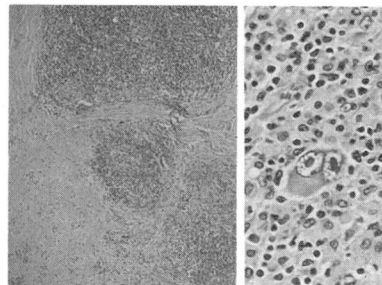

G, *Left,* Hodgkin's disease (nodular sclerosis type). Large fibrotic nodules enclose the cellular areas of Hodgkin's disease. (L.P.) *Right,* Hodgkin's disease (lymphocyte-depleted type). Lymph node biopsy. A Reed-Sternberg cell is near the center of the field. (H.P.)

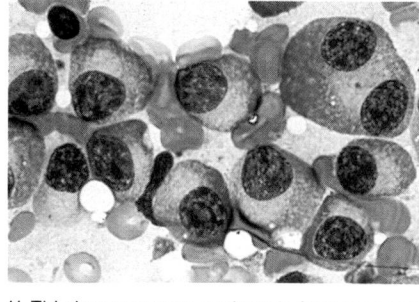

H, This bone marrow aspirate is from a patient with multiple myeloma. All plasma cells in this field are neoplastic myeloma cells. The nuclei are pleomorphic and eccentric, and the cytoplasm is gray-blue. One cell is binucleate. (H.O.)

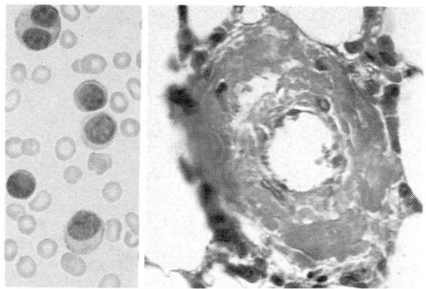

I, *Left,* Plasma cell leukemia. Five neoplastic plasma cells (one of which is binucleate) are seen in this field. (L.O.) *Right,* Amyloid. Bone marrow biopsy. A small blood vessel is heavily infiltrated with the pink-staining, waxy amyloid material. (H.P.)

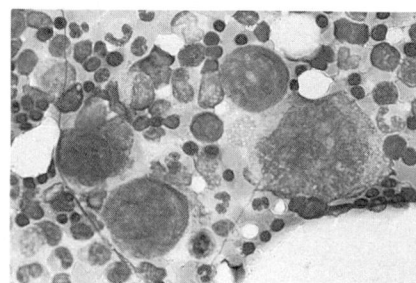

J, Immune thrombocytopenic purpura (ITP). Bone marrow aspirate. Megakaryocytosis is reflected in this field, where four are seen. These range from a megakaryoblast (top) to a mature megakaryocyte (middle right).

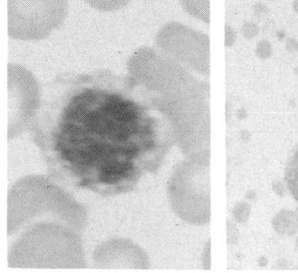

K, *Left,* Bernard-Soulier syndrome. A typical giant platelet is seen in the center of the field. *Right,* Essential thrombocythemia. Massive thrombocytosis is noted, as is variation in platelet size and a giant platelet. (H.O.)

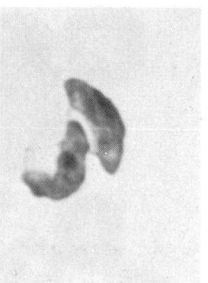 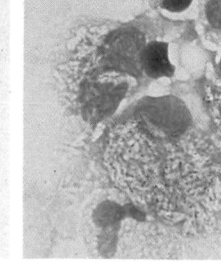

L, *Left,* Falciparum malaria. Peripheral blood showing two crescent-shaped gametocytes. *Right,* AIDS, *Mycobacterium avium-intracellulare* infection. Massive numbers of red, acid-fast organisms are seen in the macrophages of this marrow aspirate. (H.O.)

anemia in a patient with hepatic dysfunction to "the anemia of liver disease." The term should be abandoned in favor of more precise diagnostic thinking. In addition, in many patients with portal hypertension and an expanded plasma volume, the hematocrit may be moderately decreased, even though the number of circulating red cells is normal ("hemodilution").

Endocrine Disorders. A mild normocytic anemia occurs in some patients with endocrine disturbances. One quarter of patients with *hypothyroidism* are anemic. The red cell lifespan is normal, and there is no reticulocytosis. In many patients the anemia responds to hormone replacement therapy. Such anemias are usually normocytic, although in a minority the MCV may be mildly elevated and may return to normal after treatment with thyroid preparations. Another cause of macrocytic marrow failure anemia in hypothyroidism is pernicious anemia due to associated autoimmune gastritis. When microcytic anemia is seen, iron deficiency is the rule. Ferritin synthesis may be depressed as a result of insufficient thyroid hormone action, and the serum ferritin level may not be a reliable indicator of iron stores in hypothyroid patients.

A mild normocytic marrow failure anemia is a characteristic feature of *hypopituitarism* and may also occur in *primary adrenal insufficiency*, although it is often masked by a contracted plasma volume due to dehydration. A normocytic marrow failure anemia is also encountered in a few patients with *thyrotoxicosis*, although in some the MCV may be low. In either event, the anemia remits after suppression of thyroid hyperactivity. An occasional patient with *hyperparathyroidism* has a mild normocytic anemia due to marrow failure.

"PRIMARY MARROW DISORDERS." When iron deficiency and anemia related to systemic diseases have been excluded, there remains a minority of normocytic marrow failure anemias that are caused by primary disturbances of the bone marrow (see Table 128–7). These include rare disorders in which developing red cells are absent or markedly diminished in the bone marrow (aplastic anemia, pure red cell aplasia) or in which there are increased marrow erythroid precursors that fail to mature normally, so-called "ineffective erythropoiesis" (sideroblastic anemias, other myelodysplasias); replacement of the bone marrow by fibrosis or a variety of hematologic and solid tumors or granulomas; and a poorly understood marrow failure state that may be associated with AIDS. In many patients with AIDS, the anemia is typical of that seen with other chronic infections; in others, ineffective erythropoiesis (often associated with neutropenia) is present, possibly related to human immunodeficiency virus (HIV) infection of marrow stem cells. In most patients with these marrow disturbances, certain features of the initial laboratory data base strongly suggest that the patient has something other than iron deficiency, the anemia of chronic disease, or anemia secondary to renal, hepatic, or endocrine dysfunction. These clues include depression of the platelet count, white blood cell count, or both; abnormalities in the white cell differential; significant numbers of nucleated erythrocytes on the blood smear; marked abnormalities in red cell morphology, especially significant poikilocytosis; and a normal or increased serum iron level with a per cent saturation of transferrin that is above normal. In the normocytic anemias due to primary disturbances of marrow function, *bone marrow aspiration* and *biopsy* (see Color Plates 5 to 8) often provide highly useful diagnostic information, whereas in the previously discussed causes of normocytic anemia, marrow examination is rarely useful (except for the estimation of iron stores when the serum indicators of iron status give equivocal results). These primary marrow disorders may, on occasion, also present as a *macrocytic* marrow failure anemia.

Microcytic Anemias Due to Marrow Failure

In contrast to the potentially complex considerations in normocytic anemias, the differential diagnosis of marrow failure associated with a low MCV is relatively straightforward (Table 128–9). Two major conditions commonly cause marrow failure with microcytic anemia—iron deficiency and the anemia of chronic disease. Although most patients with the anemia of chronic disease have a normal MCV, in approximately 30 per cent, mean red cell size is slightly decreased, with the MCV in the range of 70 to 80 fl. An MCV lower than 70 fl is almost always due to iron deficiency or thalassemia. With severe iron

TABLE 128–9. CAUSES OF MICROCYTIC MARROW FAILURE ANEMIAS

Common	Rare
Iron deficiency	Aluminum toxicity
Anemia of chronic disease	Thyrotoxicosis
Thalassemias	Hereditary sideroblastic anemias

deficiency, the MCV may fall as low as 50 fl, and marked anisocytosis and poikilocytosis may be seen. The results of the serum tests of iron status are similar to those seen when iron deficiency and the anemia of chronic disease manifest with a normal MCV (Table 128–8).

THALASSEMIAS (Ch. 136). In these disorders, decreased synthesis of either the alpha or the beta chain of hemoglobin occurs, with the resultant imbalance in globin chain formation leading to a decreased rate of hemoglobin production as well as microcytosis. In *homozygous beta-thalassemia*, which manifests in childhood, a severe microcytic anemia results owing to a combination of ineffective erythropoiesis and a shortened red cell lifespan. Reticulocytosis is modest, although grossly inadequate. In *heterozygous beta-thalassemia*, anemia is frequently absent, or only mild in degree, although the MCV is low. In some patients the blood smear may show target cells, basophilic stippling, anisocytosis, and poikilocytosis; in others the smear is unremarkable because there is a uniform population of small red cells with little anisocytosis. The reticulocyte count is normal or minimally elevated, and the serum ferritin, iron, and TIBC values are normal. The disorder is usually detected when a CBC, including an MCV, is obtained during the evaluation of some other medical problem. *Alpha-thalassemia* is more varied because there are four genes for alpha globin chain synthesis. When three alpha chain genes are deleted or abnormal, a moderate hemolytic anemia develops, with microcytosis and the formation of "β_4" tetramers (hemoglobin H disease). This anemia sometimes occurs as an acquired disorder in association with acute leukemia or myelodysplastic states. Much more commonly, *heterozygous alpha-thalassemia* with two-chain deletion is encountered, particularly in American blacks, 3 per cent of whom are affected. Typically, these patients have a low MCV, have a normal blood smear and iron studies, and are not anemic, although in some the hematocrit may be slightly decreased. A common error in attempting to diagnose heterozygous thalassemic states is to obtain a routine hemoglobin electrophoresis, which is normal. Instead, the conditions can be differentiated by specific measurement of the hemoglobin A_2 concentration, which is usually elevated in patients with beta-thalassemia but is normal or reduced in those with alpha-thalassemia. There is no readily available test for alpha-thalassemia. It should be suspected in blacks and patients from Southeast Asia with microcytosis. Family members also often have microcytosis without anemia. Even though, as a rule, anisocytosis is more striking in iron deficiency than in the heterozygous thalassemias, there are so many exceptions that measurement of the RDW is not a useful screening test.

RARE CAUSES OF MARROW FAILURE WITH MICROCYTIC ANEMIAS. *Aluminum toxicity* in patients with renal failure who receive aluminum-containing phosphate binders can result in a microcytic marrow failure anemia by an unknown mechanism. Aluminum overload may cause resistance to erythropoietin therapy in chronically hemodialyzed patients (even those with a normal MCV). *Thyrotoxicosis* may occasionally result in a mild microcytic anemia. Although in most sideroblastic anemias (which are almost always acquired in nature) the MCV is normal or elevated, mean red cell size is decreased in the much rarer *hereditary sideroblastic anemias*, which may present in childhood or adult life.

Macrocytic Anemias Due to Marrow Failure

Macrocytic anemias due to bone marrow failure (Table 128–10) are common. The history, physical examination, and blood smear are the cornerstones of the initial approach to a patient with an elevated MCV and in most cases indicate its cause. Major clues include the recent use of alcohol, exposure to chemother-

TABLE 128–10. CAUSES OF MACROCYTIC MARROW FAILURE ANEMIAS

Megaloblastic anemias
    Cobalamin and folate deficiencies
    Congenital disorders
Alcoholism
Drugs (see Table 128–2)
Liver disease
"Primary" marrow disorders (see Table 128–7)
Hypothyroidism
Splenectomy
Artifactual MCV elevations

apeutic or immunosuppressive drugs, and evidence of liver disease, glossitis, or neurologic signs and symptoms. In most macrocytic anemias, the blood smear contains round macrocytes without multilobed granulocytes. On the other hand, *the combination of macro-ovalocytes and hypersegmented neutrophils strongly suggests the presence of cobalamin or folate deficiency* (although rarely this dual abnormality may be seen after chemotherapy with methotrexate or cytosine arabinoside, in myelodysplasias, or in acute myelocytic leukemia) (see Color Plate 6G and H). The reticulocyte count is also a useful early test in patients with macrocytosis. Because of the slightly increased size of young erythrocytes, brisk *reticulocytosis* (an uncorrected count of ≥10 per cent) caused by hemolysis or blood loss often causes a modest elevation of the MCV.

MEGALOBLASTIC ANEMIAS (Ch. 132). Megaloblastic anemias due to a disturbance in DNA synthesis caused by cobalamin or folate deficiency account for only 5 to 10 per cent of macrocytic anemias with marrow failure. Early recognition is extremely important, however, because of their responsiveness to therapy and the need to prevent irreversible neurologic damage caused by lack of cobalamin. As with most other causes of macrocytic anemia, the MCV becomes elevated early in the development of cobalamin or folate deficiency, before a lowered hematocrit is evident. A distinction should be made between the hematologic and biochemical profiles of patients with *early* cobalamin or folate deficiency (with little or no anemia) and the classic textbook manifestations of severe megaloblastic anemia. With severe anemia, marked anisocytosis and poikilocytosis (often including teardrop erythrocytes, microcytes, and red cell fragments) are found on blood smears. The consequences of ineffective erythropoiesis (destruction of red cell precursors in the bone marrow) may simulate a hemolytic anemia, with decreased or absent plasma haptoglobin values, elevated serum unconjugated bilirubin levels, sometimes exceptionally high serum lactate dehydrogenase (LDH) levels, and an elevated serum iron level with an increased transferrin saturation. In such severely deficient patients, marrow failure often causes thrombocytopenia and (sometimes) neutropenia. In any moderately or severely anemic patient with pancytopenia, cobalamin and folate deficiency should always be considered. In contrast, patients with deficiency of cobalamin or folate who have little or no anemia often have minimal changes on the blood smear, with few macro-ovalocytes and only rare hypersegmented neutrophils that may not be identified by routine hospital laboratories. In addition, there may be normal values for serum LDH, bilirubin, haptoglobin, white cell count, and platelet count. In cobalamin deficiency, severe involvement of the tongue or nervous system may occur early or late relative to the hematologic manifestations, so that a patient with advanced neurologic impairment may not have developed anemia or even a clear-cut elevation of the MCV.

Radioisotopic assays of serum cobalamin and folate levels are valuable in the diagnosis (Ch. 132). A serum cobalamin level should be measured in any patient with neutrophil hypersegmentation, macro-ovalocytes, atrophic glossitis, or a neurologic disorder compatible with cobalamin deficiency, as well as in virtually all patients with an elevated MCV in the absence of reticulocytosis. Possible exceptions to this rule are those treated with drugs that interfere with DNA synthesis (e.g., zidovudine, azathioprine, methotrexate) in whom the MCV has been clearly documented to be normal immediately prior to beginning drug therapy. There are problems with both the specificity and the sensitivity of the vitamin assays. The serum cobalamin level is often low in patients who are not deficient in the vitamin, and it may also be depressed as a result of folate deficiency. At least 5 per cent of patients with unequivocal clinical evidence of cobalamin deficiency have normal serum cobalamin concentrations (usually in the range of 200 to 350 pg per milliliter). The measurement of *methylmalonic acid* and *total homocysteine* in serum is very useful in the interpretation of low or low-normal serum cobalamin values when the presence of deficiency of the vitamin is not clinically obvious (Ch. 132). There are similar problems with the *serum folate* level. The *red cell folate* concentration is a better indicator of tissue folate stores; however, it is diminished in 50 per cent of patients with primary cobalamin deficiency and may be normal in some patients deficient in folate. Serum total homocysteine levels are almost always elevated in clinically significant folate depletion (as well as in cobalamin deficiency); however, the serum methylmalonic acid value remains normal in deficiency of folate. With the combined use of a careful history and physical examination, as well as examination of the blood smear, serum vitamin levels, and (if needed) serum metabolites, it is rarely necessary to perform a bone marrow examination to show the presence of a megaloblastic anemia. The determination of *antibodies to intrinsic factor* in serum is a useful early test in patients with cobalamin deficiency, since it is positive in approximately half of those with pernicious anemia (the most common cause of lack of cobalamin) and is specific for that diagnosis, eliminating the need for a Schilling test when such antibodies are present.

Iron deficiency frequently coexists with lack of cobalamin (e.g., in patients with pernicious anemia) or folate (e.g., in pregnant patients or alcoholics). In such combined deficiency states, the MCV may be low, normal, or high, and macro-ovalocytes and hypersegmented neutrophils on blood smear may be the most important clues to the presence of a "masked" megaloblastic anemia when the MCV is low or normal.

MACROCYTOSIS OF ALCOHOLISM. The most common cause of an elevated MCV in chronic alcoholic patients is not folate deficiency, but the *macrocytosis of alcoholism*. This condition appears to be an effect of chronic alcohol intoxication that is not related to the presence of liver disease, reticulocytosis, or vitamin deficiency (which are all part of the differential diagnosis of an elevated MCV in an alcoholic). The macrocytosis of alcoholism does not respond to vitamin B_{12} or folic acid and will disappear only after months of abstinence. The degree of MCV elevation is modest (usually ≤110 fl), and anemia is often absent. Round macrocytes are seen on blood smears. In many anemic patients with the macrocytosis of alcoholism, the anemia is due to some other cause (e.g., lung abscess, hepatic inflammation, or even iron deficiency), and the patient only apparently has a macrocytic anemia.

DRUG-INDUCED MACROCYTOSIS. In current clinical practice, this is the most common cause of an elevated MCV in nonalcoholic patients. Frequent offending agents are listed in Table 128–2. Most of the drugs that cause macrocytosis interfere with DNA synthesis by erythroid precursors. These agents most commonly cause macrocytosis without anemia; a low hematocrit is typically seen only after prolonged high dosage. The reticulocyte count is characteristically not increased, although slight elevations are not uncommon with sulfasalazine and azathioprine.

LIVER DISEASE. In patients with hepatic dysfunction, because of a poorly understood abnormality in serum lipoproteins, increased amounts of cholesterol and phospholipids are deposited on the membranes of circulating erythrocytes, causing an increase in surface area, which results in macrocytosis. Blood smears typically show round macrocytes and target cells. This is a benign abnormality that does not affect the red cell lifespan and is unrelated to any of the causes of anemia seen in liver disease.

PRIMARY MARROW DISTURBANCES. All of the derangements involving the bone marrow that are occasional causes of normocytic anemias resulting from decreased cell production (see Table 128–7) may also cause a macrocytic marrow failure anemia. The mechanisms underlying the macrocytosis in such diverse disorders as marrow aplasia, sideroblastic anemia, myelodysplasias, acute myeloblastic leukemia, and infiltration of the marrow by myeloma, lymphoma, or solid tumors have not been established. Macro-ovalocytes may be present in these conditions, but neutrophil hypersegmentation is extremely unusual. Aspiration and biopsy of the marrow are often crucial to establishing the cause of macrocytosis in this group of patients. Cytogenetic studies on material obtained by marrow aspiration may also be useful.

ANEMIAS ASSOCIATED WITH INCREASED RED CELL PRODUCTION

Assuming that recovery from marrow failure (e.g., pernicious anemia recently treated with an injection of vitamin B$_{12}$) has been excluded, the patient with an absolute reticulocytosis usually has underlying blood loss or hemolysis. In these conditions, the MCV is normal or increased, although very rarely in hemolytic anemias it may be low. Owing to the presence of reticulocytes, modest increments in red cell volume (usually MCV's in the range of 100 to 110 fl) are common in patients with increased cell production. Rarely, an even higher MCV is caused by artifactual clumping of red cells by a cold agglutinin. Elevations in the MCV are more common in hemolytic anemias than in acute blood loss. The diagnostic approach to the patient with an elevated reticulocyte count differs from that in patients with marrow failure. The very first consideration is to rule out obvious or occult blood loss. In the absence of bleeding, evidence of an underlying hemolytic disorder must be sought utilizing a different set of diagnostic tests than are used in the patient with marrow failure. Even in the absence of reticulocytosis, a rapidly developing anemia cannot be due primarily to marrow failure, because of the long lifespan of the red cell. When the marrow fails, anemia develops gradually over many weeks. Thus, if a marked fall in hematocrit (e.g., 10 per cent over a period of a few days) is noted, a search for blood loss or hemolysis should be initiated, regardless of the reticulocyte count.

HEMOLYTIC ANEMIAS (Ch. 133)

Anemias primarily due to red cell destruction are much less common than those caused by marrow failure or blood loss. Nonetheless, after blood loss has been excluded, the possibility of a hemolytic anemia takes center stage in the patient with an absolute reticulocytosis. At this point, a very long list of laboratory tests might be ordered. Therefore, the clinician needs to make a fundamental distinction. One group of tests (Table 128–11) attempts to answer the question, *is hemolysis present?* An entirely separate set of laboratory determinations, to be obtained only subsequently, addresses the question, *what is the cause of hemolysis?* Examples of the latter type would include the Coombs test or a hemoglobin electrophoresis. Such studies are often inappropriately ordered in the assessment of marrow failure or blood loss anemias. It is much more rational to obtain evidence first that the patient is actually hemolyzing before undertaking a search for various disorders that are known to cause hemolysis.

IS HEMOLYSIS PRESENT? Unfortunately, no one measure has been shown to be 100 per cent sensitive in detecting clinically significant hemolysis. Therefore, to answer the first question, a number of tests should be obtained (Table 128–11). Hemoglobin liberated into the circulation after red cells are damaged forms a complex with circulating haptoglobin, which is rapidly removed by hepatocytes. If the capacity of the liver to compensate by synthesizing new haptoglobin is exceeded, the plasma concentration will fall. Once the plasma haptoglobin reaches zero, free hemoglobin circulates and is filtered by the kidney. Modest amounts of filtered hemoglobin are taken up by renal tubular cells, which convert the iron in hemoglobin to a storage form, hemosiderin. This can be detected days later by histochemical staining of renal tubular cells that have been shed in the urine. If the amount of hemoglobin filtered exceeds the renal tubular uptake capacity, hemoglobin itself will appear in the urine. This hemoglobin may be detected by specific laboratory assays or may

be suspected when a routine urinalysis is positive for occult blood in the absence of hematuria. If the amount of hemoglobin excreted is great, the patient will pass urine that is red, reddish-purple, or even black. In contrast, when red cells are engulfed by macrophages and digested intracellularly, the heme moiety of hemoglobin is processed to unconjugated bilirubin, which is transferred to the circulation (Ch. 115). Lactate dehydrogenase is also released from hemolyzed cells. A distinction is sometimes made between *intravascular* and *extravascular* hemolytic states, but this is only occasionally useful. Acute intravascular hemolysis certainly occurs with a severe hemolytic transfusion reaction after ABO-incompatible blood is given. The plasma haptoglobin, however, is often decreased in states such as hereditary spherocytosis, in which red cell destruction is believed to occur primarily in splenic macrophages. Probably most hemolytic anemias reflect a combination of intravascular and extravascular events. The presence of hemoglobin or hemosiderin in the urine may reflect the *rate* of hemolysis as much as its location.

Any of the tests listed in Table 128–11 may be normal in patients with a clear-cut hemolytic anemia. The ability of the liver to clear a load of unconjugated bilirubin is greater in some individuals than in others. The plasma haptoglobin level is often normal in acutely hemolyzing patients who have an associated illness, since it is an acute phase reactant and hepatic synthesis may be markedly stimulated. Many of the tests are also not specific for hemolysis. The LDH may be released from many different injured organs; unconjugated bilirubin elevations are commonly due to Gilbert's disease; the plasma haptoglobin may be reduced on a genetic basis or due to liver dysfunction; myoglobin may cause a positive urine test for occult blood. It is possible to demonstrate that the red cell lifespan is shortened by performing a cumbersome and time-consuming study with radioisotopically labeled erythrocytes, but this is rarely necessary. In almost all patients with a hemolytic anemia, one or more of the tests listed in Table 128–11 are positive.

WHAT IS THE CAUSE OF HEMOLYSIS? Once there is a positive answer to one or more of the tests that determine whether hemolysis is present, the clinician must then ask, what is the cause of hemolysis? The list of possible causes of hemolytic states is formidably long. Many of these disorders are discussed in Ch. 134 to 136. For example, deficiencies of 14 different red cell enzymes may lead to a congenital hemolytic anemia. Table 128–12 lists some hemolytic conditions that are likely to be encountered over the course of a year in an adult medical service. It is representative but not necessarily exhaustive. With so many possible causes of hemolytic anemia, the clinician must be judicious in the choice of laboratory tests to answer this second question. Diagnostic strategy must be based on clues provided by the history, physical examination, and blood smear. For example, a young black man with a history of episodes of bone

TABLE 128–11. COMMONLY USED TESTS INDICATING THE PRESENCE OF HEMOLYSIS

Test	Result
Plasma haptoglobin	Decreased
Urine hemosiderin	Present
Urine hemoglobin	Present
Serum unconjugated bilirubin	Increased
Serum lactate dehydrogenase	Increased

TABLE 128–12. SOME RELATIVELY COMMON CAUSES OF HEMOLYTIC ANEMIA

Mechanism	Examples
Congenital	
Enzyme deficiency	Glucose-6-phosphate dehydrogenase, pyruvate kinase
Membrane skeletal protein abnormalities (e.g., spectrin)	Hereditary spherocytosis, hereditary elliptocytosis
Hemoglobinopathies	Hemoglobin SS, SC, CC, S-thalassemia
Acquired	
Antibody-induced	Autoimmune hemolysis (warm antibodies), cold agglutinin disease, hemolytic transfusion reaction
Mechanical fragmentation	Intravascular coagulation, malignant hypertension, cancer chemotherapy, malfunctioning valve prosthesis, thrombotic thrombocytopenic purpura
Membrane protein anchoring abnormality	Paroxysmal nocturnal hemoglobinuria

pain and sickle cells on the smear needs a hemoglobin electrophoresis, not a Coombs test or sucrose hemolysis determination. A previously healthy middle-aged woman who suddenly develops a severe anemia with many microspherocytes on the smear should have a Coombs test, not a hemoglobin electrophoresis, as part of the initial evaluation. In a man with malignant hypertension, evidence of hemolysis, and many red cell fragments on the blood smear, no further diagnostic studies may be required to conclude that a microangiopathic hemolytic anemia has developed secondary to damage to small blood vessels. Therefore, rather than following a rigid algorithm, the physician is guided by the clinical context and the blood smear in ordering laboratory tests for the individual patient. Morphologic abnormalities (see Table 128–4) often provide highly useful clues, although in some hemolytic anemias (e.g., glucose-6-phosphate dehydrogenase [G6PD] deficiency, paroxysmal nocturnal hemoglobinuria), the blood smear may be unremarkable or nondiagnostic. In some cases, clinical judgment may supersede the laboratory results. About 10 per cent of patients with autoimmune hemolytic anemias have a negative Coombs test but this diagnosis may still be considered on the basis of clinical and morphologic findings.

Hemolytic anemias may appear in deceptive disguises. Hereditary spherocytosis, a common congenital disorder that can be caused by a variety of abnormalities of the major red cell skeletal protein, spectrin, is frequently so mild that there is little or no anemia (Ch. 134). Only an elevated reticulocyte count, microspherocytes on smear, and minimal splenomegaly may bear witness to a state of *compensated hemolysis*. Such a patient may present as an adult with bilirubin gallstones or may develop anemia for the first time when a parvovirus B19 infection of committed red cell marrow precursors (CFU-E) causes an *aplastic crisis* with a sudden loss of the compensatory reticulocytosis. This virus is the most common cause of aplastic crisis, which may occur in a number of hemolytic anemias, including sickle cell disease. Continuing hemolysis that is no longer accompanied by reticulocytosis may rapidly lead to a life-threatening worsening of the anemia and require immediate transfusion. In the most common type of G6PD deficiency, the A-variant seen in 11 per cent of American blacks, there is no chronic hemolytic state. Anemia and hemolysis occur only acutely, after exposure to an oxidant stress, such as infection, acidosis, or certain drugs, e.g., antimalarials or sulfonamides.

ANEMIA DUE TO ACUTE BLOOD LOSS

The causes and management of blood loss are discussed in other chapters. A few points are worth noting here. In the bleeding patient, a reticulocytosis will be sustained until iron stores are depleted by continued chronic blood loss. In acute blood loss, however, a high reticulocyte count may not occur until a few days after the onset of bleeding. In most patients, the source of hemorrhage is clinically obvious, e.g., the gastrointestinal or genitourinary tract. The clinician must be alert to more occult sites of potentially massive blood loss, e.g., into a fractured hip or the retroperitoneal area, especially in patients with coagulation disorders or those receiving anticoagulants. Even though hemorrhage may be documented, it is worthwhile to obtain the entire initial laboratory base. The blood smear may reveal unexpected findings. It is not unusual in a bleeding alcoholic to find evidence of other coexistent causes of anemia (e.g., macroovalocytes and hypersegmented neutrophils). In the hemorrhaging patient with AIDS, absence of reticulocytosis may point to a coexistent marrow failure anemia.

Since red cells are lost from the body in most bleeding patients, the tests used to determine whether hemolysis is present are usually negative. With hemorrhage into an internal space, however, (as with a hemothorax, hemoperitoneum, or hip fracture), the decomposed blood in the body cavity is handled in similar ways to red cells that are hemolyzed. The plasma haptoglobin may be absent and the LDH and unconjugated bilirubin elevated in patients bleeding internally. Combined with the increased reticulocyte count, these findings may lead the unwary clinician to misdiagnose a hemolytic anemia.

EXAMINATION OF THE BONE MARROW IN ANEMIC PATIENTS

In more than 90 per cent of patients with anemia, it is unnecessary to obtain a bone marrow aspiration or biopsy if the approach advocated here is followed. In certain situations, however, the test is quite useful, such as in marrow failure anemias for definitive estimation of marrow iron stores when serum tests of iron status are equivocal. In all of the primary marrow disorders that cause normocytic and macrocytic marrow failure states (see Table 128–7), marrow aspiration and biopsy are often diagnostic. In a pancytopenia of unknown cause, it is wise to obtain an early marrow examination. If aplasia, marrow infiltration by tumor, myelofibrosis, or granulomatous infection is suspected, a greater diagnostic yield is obtained by biopsy than by aspiration (see Color Plate 5). A marrow aspirate may resolve diagnostic conundrums in patients suspected of having combined or dimorphic anemias (e.g., simultaneous iron and cobalamin deficiency, megaloblastic anemia accompanying the anemia of chronic disease). Marrow aspiration and biopsy are also indicated in monoclonal gammopathies and in any patient with a severe or unexplained anemia.

BLOOD TRANSFUSION

In contrast to patients with acute hemorrhage, those with chronic anemia often have few symptoms, particularly while at rest in the hospital, and the physician should always think twice before exposing them to the many risks of blood transfusion, some of them potentially fatal, which are discussed in Ch. 137. There is no threshold level of hematocrit that mandates transfusion, and the decision to administer red blood cells must be based on the functional status and symptomatology of the patient. Transfusion should never be used as a substitute for careful diagnostic evaluation that may lead to more definitive and less dangerous therapy. However, it may be necessary to transfuse elderly anemic patients before they undergo rigorous procedures, such as colonoscopy or barium enema.

ABNORMAL MEAN CELL VOLUMES IN THE ABSENCE OF ANEMIA

With the widespread availability of electronic cell counting, patients are frequently seen with increased or decreased MCV's in the absence of anemia. Not uncommonly, the MCV elevation is ignored because the hematocrit is normal—a potentially dangerous practice, especially in patients with macrocytosis. In some instances, a minimal increase or decrease in the MCV may be compatible with no underlying disorder, since the normal range excludes 2.5 per cent of healthy individuals at either extreme. However, an *elevated MCV* in the absence of anemia is most commonly a sign of chronic alcoholism (often in patients who deny it). Cobalamin or folate deficiency is another frequent cause of such an MCV increment; correct diagnosis may prevent subsequent hospitalization for anemia, or may avert serious nervous system damage (in the case of lack of cobalamin). Therefore, it is worth obtaining a serum cobalamin level in any patient with an unexplained increase in the MCV. Another common cause of nonanemic macrocytosis is the administration of drugs (Table 128–2). An MCV elevation may precede the development of anemia in a patient with a myelodysplasia (e.g., a sideroblastic anemia or refractory anemia following antimetabolite therapy) or marrow aplasia (e.g., a congenital Fanconi anemia manifesting in a young adult) (see Color Plate 6*I* and *J*). Occasionally, a modest rise in the MCV without anemia is caused by reticulocytosis in a compensated hemolytic state.

A *decreased MCV* associated with a normal hematocrit is almost always caused by heterozygous alpha- or beta-thalassemia. In some patients with polycythemia vera or polycythemia secondary to chronic hypoxia, iron stores may be outstripped by the expanding erythroid marrow. The previously elevated hematocrit then falls to the normal range as the MCV decreases. Studies of iron status are typically diagnostic of iron deficiency in these patients, and iron administration causes a return of the hematocrit to polycythemic levels. Blood loss should be ruled out, however, before the iron depletion is merely attributed to increased internal demands. Occasionally, a patient with microcytosis and a normal hematocrit is recovering from a self-limited or treated episode of iron deficiency anemia.

Cook JK: Clinical evaluation of iron deficiency. Semin Hematol 19:6, 1982. *A clinically sophisticated review of the use of laboratory tests in the diagnosis of iron deficiency and related conditions.*

Erslev AJ, Schuster SJ, Caro J: Erythropoietin and its clinical promise. Eur J Hematol 43:367, 1989. *An excellent review of the physiology of erythropoietin and the therapeutic use of the recombinant hormone.*

Liesveld JL, Rowe JM, Lichtman MA: Variability of the erythropoietic response in autoimmune hemolytic anemia: Analysis of 109 cases. Blood 3:820, 1987. *An interesting series of antibody-induced anemias with a focus on the lag in the response of the erythroid marrow to hemolytic stress.*

Lindenbaum J: Hematologic complications of alcohol abuse. Semin Liver Dis 7:169, 1987. *A comprehensive review of the pathophysiology and clinical features of the effects of ethanol on blood cells and the hematologic syndromes seen in liver disease.*

Petz LD, Swisher SW (eds.): Clinical Practice of Transfusion Medicine. 2nd ed. New York, Churchill Livingstone, 1989. *An up-to-date and well-written text centered on the transfusion of blood components. Contains many nuggets of clinical wisdom and a number of interesting chapters on the pathophysiology and immunologic aspects of various anemias.*

Stabler SP, Allen RH, Savage DG, et al.: Clinical spectrum and diagnosis of cobalamin deficiency. Blood 76:871, 1990. *A large series of patients with clinically significant cobalamin deficiency as seen in current practice, including many with "atypical" presentations. Data are presented that support the use of serum metabolite values as ancillary tests in the diagnosis of deficiency of this vitamin.*

129 Aplastic Anemia and Related Bone Marrow Failure Syndromes

Neal S. Young

Blood counts may be low because cells are prematurely removed from the peripheral circulation or are inadequately produced in the bone marrow. Bone marrow failure occurs commonly but is often classified by other dominant clinical or morphologic features (like the leukemias) or by specific etiology (like pernicious anemia). The term "bone marrow failure" is vague and inclusive, and it awaits redefinition with more precise understanding of pathophysiologic processes. By default, therefore, the disorders discussed in this chapter are currently defined by their marrow pathology: the fatty bone marrow of aplastic anemia, the disordered hematopoiesis of the myelodysplasias, and the fibrosis of myelofibrosis. Making inferences about disease processes from the appearance of the bone marrow is as misleading as it is inevitable, and an effort is made here to distinguish what is understood from what is conjecture.

APLASTIC ANEMIA

Definition (Table 129–1)

APLASTIC ANEMIA. Aplastic anemia is a disease of the young, with a median incidence at about 25 years of age (excluding aplasia secondary to cancer chemotherapy). It must be a leading diagnosis in the pancytopenic adolescent or young adult. The bone marrow is usually readily aspirated but appears dilute on smear. The biopsy specimen (see Color Plate 5G), often grossly pale, shows mainly fat under the microscope, with hematopoietic cells occupying by definition less than 25 per cent of the marrow space and, in the most serious cases, 0 to 5 per cent (Fig. 129–1). Prognosis is determined by the degree of blood count depression. The commonly accepted standard for severe disease requires two of the following three values: (1) absolute neutrophil count (percentage of polymorphonuclear and band forms multiplied by the total white blood cell count) of less than 500 per cubic millimeter; (2) platelets less than 20,000 per cubic millimeter; and (3) reticulocyte count (corrected for hematocrit) in the presence of anemia of less than 1 per cent (or an absolute reticulocyte count less than 40,000 per cubic millimeter).

BICYTOPENIA AND SINGLE-LINEAGE FAILURE STATES. Some patients present with bone marrow hypocellularity and depression of only two of the three major blood lines; many progress to typical aplastic anemia. Failure of a single lineage also occurs, as in pure red blood cell aplasia (rare), amegakaryocytic thrombocytopenia (extremely rare), and agranulocytosis (not rare but usually an idiosyncratic drug reaction). Single-lineage failures show a characteristic absence of a single set of recognizable precursor cells in an otherwise cellular bone marrow, and in this way they are differentiated from the much more common causes of anemia (such as vitamin or iron deficiency

TABLE 129–1. CLASSIFICATION OF APLASTIC ANEMIA AND SINGLE CYTOPENIAS

I. Acquired aplastic anemia
- Radiation
- Drugs and chemicals
  - Regular effects
  - Idiosyncratic reactions
- Viruses
  - Epstein-Barr virus (infectious mononucleosis)
  - Hepatitis C virus (non-A non-B hepatitis)
  - Parvovirus (transient aplastic crisis, pure red cell aplasia [PRCA])
  - Human immunodeficiency virus (AIDS)
- Immune diseases
  - Eosinophilic fasciitis
  - Hypoimmunoglobulinemia
  - Thymoma and thymic carcinoma
  - Graft-versus-host disease in immunodeficiency
- Paroxysmal nocturnal hemoglobinuria
- Pregnancy
- Idiopathic—the most frequent diagnosis

II. Inherited aplastic anemia
- Fanconi's anemia
- Dyskeratosis congenita
- Schwachman-Diamond syndrome
- Reticular dysgenesis
- Amegakaryocytic thrombocytopenia
- Familial aplastic anemias
  - Preleukemia (e.g., monosomy 7)
- Nonhematologic syndromes (Down's, Dubovitz's, Seckel's)

I. Acquired cytopenias
- *Anemias*
  - Pure red cell aplasia (see Table 129–3)
  - Transient erythroblastopenia of childhood
- *Neutropenias*
  - Idiopathic
  - Drugs, toxins
- *Thrombocytopenias*
  - Drugs, toxins

II. Inherited cytopenias
- *Anemias*
  - Congenital pure red cell aplasia
- *Neutropenias*
  - Kostmann's syndrome
  - Schwachman-Diamond syndrome
  - Reticular dysgenesis
- *Thrombocytopenias*
  - Thrombocytopenia with absent radii
  - Idiopathic amegakaryocytic

and hemolysis) or thrombocytopenia (from peripheral destruction of platelets). The pathophysiology of the more restricted marrow failure states is probably similar to that of general bone marrow failure, but with a more mature target cell.

CONSTITUTIONAL (FANCONI'S) ANEMIA. Fanconi described children with inherited pancytopenia and marrow hypocellularity with associated anomalies of the skeletal and urogenital systems. Fanconi's anemia now is defined by specific chromosomal aberrations in cultured cells after clastogenic stress. Indeed, cytogenetic analysis of families of children with Fanconi's anemia has shown that the majority of patients lack associated anomalies and that the disease can manifest in adults, in the third and fourth decades or even later. Congenital pure red cell aplasia (Diamond-Blackfan syndrome) lacks a cytogenetic marker or associated physical abnormalities, and distinction from acquired aplastic anemia after infancy is possible only by family history. Isolated neutropenia or thrombocytopenia occurs in a number of pediatric syndromes.

Etiology

In the majority of patients, aplastic anemia is diagnosed as "idiopathic." There is little to distinguish these cases clinically from those with a presumed etiology, like exposure to a drug or chemical. Even when clinical associations are established, they should not automatically be equated with etiology and pathophysiology: Association is not equivalent to cause, nor does it define a mechanism.

RADIATION. Marrow aplasia is a major acute sequela of radiation exposure. Radiant energy damages DNA. The bone marrow, as a tissue dependent on active mitosis, is particularly susceptible to its effects. Nuclear accidents and radiation injury

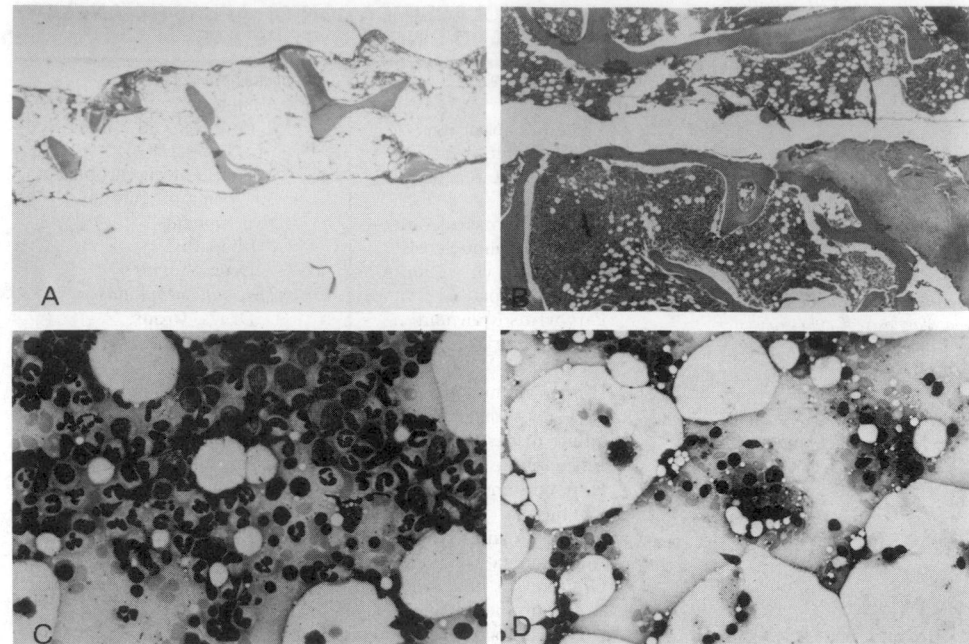

FIGURE 129–1. The bone marrow is normally 30 to 70 per cent cellular, and there is a heterogeneous mix of myeloid, erythroid, and lymphoid cells. Marrow biopsies show (A) severe hypocellularity of aplastic anemia and (B) hypercellularity of myelodysplasia. Normal aspirate smear (C) shows variety of hematopoietic precursor cell types, replaced in aplastic anemia (D) by fat and only residual stromal and lymphoid cells.

can involve not only power plant workers but also employees of hospitals, laboratories, and industry (e.g., food sterilization, metal radiography, and so forth), as well as those innocent persons exposed to stolen, misplaced, or misused radiation sources. The radiation dose can be approximated from the rate and degree of decline in blood counts; dosimetry by reconstruction of the exposure can help to estimate the patient's prognosis and also to protect medical personnel from contact with radioactive tissue and excreta. Myelodysplasia and leukemia, but not aplastic anemia, are late effects of irradiation.

CHEMICALS (Table 129–2). Benzene has been clearly linked to bone marrow failure, including aplastic anemia, acute leukemias, and probably multiple myeloma. The occurrence of hematologic abnormalities is roughly correlated with cumulative exposure, but there must also be an important element of susceptibility, as only a minority of even heavily exposed workers develop evidence of benzene myelotoxicity. A history of past employment is important, especially in "open" industries in which benzene is used for a secondary purpose (usually as a solvent) rather than in "closed" industries for chemical production. Benzene-related blood diseases have declined with regulation of industrial exposure, and benzene is not generally available as a household solvent. However, the benzene content of gasoline has been increased with its unleading. The association of marrow failure with other chemicals that contain a benzene ring is much less well substantiated; some, like the insecticide lindane, were probably contaminated with benzene during manufacture.

DRUGS (Table 129–2). Many of the common cancer chemotherapeutic drugs suppress the bone marrow. The mechanisms by which these drugs act offer useful clues to the pathophysiology of "idiopathic" aplastic anemia (see below). A very large and diverse group of drugs is related to aplastic anemia by rare but serious idiosyncratic reactions. These associations, which rest mainly on case reports, are tenuous at best. For example, some incriminated drugs may have been used to treat the first symptoms of bone marrow failure (antibiotics for fever or the preceding viral illness) or may have provoked the first symptom of a pre-existing disease (petechiae produced by nonsteroidal anti-inflammatory agents administered to a thrombocytopenic individual). In the context of total drug employment, idiosyncratic reactions, while individually devastating, are very rare events.

Chloramphenicol, the most infamous culprit, reportedly produced aplasia in only about 1 of 60,000 therapeutic courses, and even this number is almost certainly an overestimate. Chloramphenicol also consistently causes a dose-related, rather modest marrow depression, mainly reticulocytopenia and altered marrow morphology and iron kinetics. This effect of chloramphenicol use is mechanistically unrelated to and clinically not predictive of the rare, severe reaction, which occurs 1 to 2 months or longer after its routine use. The introduction of chloramphenicol was thought to have produced a notable increase in the number of cases of aplastic anemia, but its diminished use has not been followed by a reduced frequency of aplastic anemia. Chloramphenicol remains a popular antibiotic in less developed countries.

Suspected drug reactions account for only about 20 per cent of cases of aplastic anemia, while virtually all instances of agranulocytosis in the adult are drug related. The drugs associated with agranulocytosis are similar but not identical to those related to generalized bone marrow failure. Myeloid cells may be uniquely susceptible because of their ability to metabolize drugs, often to toxic intermediate compounds. In contrast to drug-associated aplastic anemia, agranulocytosis should spontaneously resolve with removal of the drug, and the severely neutropenic patient should survive if infection is adequately treated.

INFECTIONS. Hepatitis is the most common infection preceding aplastic anemia, accounting for about 5 per cent of Western cases and perhaps twice that proportion in Asian series. Typically,

TABLE 129–2. SOME DRUGS AND CHEMICALS ASSOCIATED WITH APLASTIC ANEMIA

I. Agents that regularly produce marrow depression as the major toxicity in commonly employed dose or normal exposures:
  Cytotoxic drugs used in cancer chemotherapy: alkylating agents, antimetabolites, antimitotics
  Some antibiotics

II. Agents that frequently but not inevitably produce marrow aplasia:
  Benzene (and benzene-containing chemicals like kerosene, carbon tetrachloride, Stoddard's solvent, chlorophenols)

III. Agents probably associated with aplastic anemia but with a relatively low probability:
  Chloramphenicol
  Insecticides
  Antiprotozoals: quinacrine and chloroquine, mepacrine
  Nonsteroidal anti-inflammatory drugs (including phenylbutazone, indomethacin, ibuprofen, sulindac, aspirin)
  Anticonvulsants (hydantoins, carbamazepine, phenacemide)
  Heavy metals (gold, arsenic, bismuth, mercury)
  Sulfonamides: some antibiotics, antithyroid drugs (methimazole, methylthiouracil, propylthiouracil), antidiabetes drugs (tolbutamide, chlorpropamide), carbonic anhydrase inhibitors (acetazolamide and methazolamide)
  Antihistamines (cimetidine, chlorpheniramine)
  D-Penicillamine
  Estrogens (in pregnancy and in high doses in animals)

severe aplasia occurs in a young man who has recovered from a mild bout of hepatitis 1 to 2 months earlier. The hepatitis is most often the non-A, non-B type, and some cases may represent aberrant responses to hepatitis C virus infection. Aplastic anemia can rarely follow infectious mononucleosis, and Epstein-Barr virus has been found in the marrow of some patients with aplastic anemia, with or without a suggestive preceding history. Parvovirus B19 has not been associated with generalized bone marrow failure. Moderate marrow depression occurs commonly in the course of many viral and bacterial infections, but the primary disease is usually overt.

IMMUNOLOGIC DISEASE. Aplasia occurs in immunodeficient children who develop graft-versus-host disease after infusion of unirradiated blood products. Pure red blood cell aplasia is associated with thymoma, and patients with red cell aplasia or pancytopenia may be hypoimmunoglobulinemic. Immunologic aspects of aplastic anemia are discussed in greater detail below.

OTHER ASSOCIATIONS. Aplastic anemia may occur during pregnancy and has sometimes resolved with delivery or with spontaneous or induced abortion. Pancytopenia occurs in about one third of patients with paroxysmal nocturnal hemoglobinuria (Ch. 135), and perhaps 5 per cent of patients with aplastic anemia have a positive Ham's test, often with hematopoietic recovery.

Pathophysiology

TYPES OF INJURY. Most bone marrow failure almost certainly results from damage to the hematopoietic stem cell compartment; little evidence exists that aplastic anemia results from defective stroma or from inadequate production of growth factors. Two different routes to stem cell damage are derived from animal experiments and models of the stem cell compartment. The paradigm for type I damage is the effect of drugs that directly damage DNA. The administration of busulfan in the mouse is followed by a long latent period and then severe aplasia. DNA damage is random and will affect late precursor cells and primitive stem cells alike; the consequences for the earlier cell may be graver, owing to its necessity to transit more mitotic cycles to mature. In humans, examples of type I aplasia are Fanconi's anemia, the result of defective DNA repair (the same chromosomal phenotype and recessive inheritance might result from genetic defects in different DNA repair enzymes), and aplasia caused by irradiation, benzene, and perhaps also chloramphenicol. Type I aplasia is associated with both early aplasia (immediate, direct cytotoxicity) and later myelodysplasia and leukemia (the sequelae of mutational events).

Type II aplasia is illustrated by the effect of a cycle-active agent like 5-fluorouracil, which mainly depletes later progenitor cells and leaves relatively intact the most quiescent and also most proliferatively capable stem cells. Most environmental damage would be expected to affect preferentially the mitotically and metabolically active cells, although massive disruption of hematopoiesis may severely dysregulate the spared stem cells. The drug- and virus-associated marrow failure syndromes are probably type II, mediated either by chemical injury to the hematopoietic cell's metabolic machinery or by immunologic injury to the cell membrane.

Cases of aplastic anemia can be apportioned roughly equally between types I and II, based on indirect evidence (the failure to cure about half of identical twins with simple bone marrow infusion, the 50 per cent response rate to nonreplacement therapies like antithymocyte globulin [ATG]). The severity of injury in both types is probably related to the duration, repetition, or specific type of the damaging agent.

METABOLIC DRUG INJURY. Many drugs and chemicals, especially if they are polar and have limited water solubility, are metabolized to highly reactive electrophilic intermediates that bind to cellular macromolecules. Excessive generation of such toxic intermediates or failure to detoxify them may be genetically determined and apparent only on drug challenge. The complexity and specificity of the pathways imply multiple susceptible loci. In one case of phenytoin-associated aplastic anemia, a defect in detoxification of that drug's metabolites was detected in the patient after recovery, and cells from the patient's mother were intermediately susceptible; cells from both normally detoxified metabolites generated from closely related drugs.

IMMUNE-MEDIATED INJURY. The recovery of their own marrow function by some patients being prepared for bone marrow transplantation with immunosuppressive horse antilymphocyte globulin first suggested that aplastic anemia might be immune mediated. Blood and bone marrow of patients often suppress normal bone marrow growth in progenitor assays, and removal of T cells from the bone marrow of those with aplastic anemia can improve colony formation in vitro. Patients with aplastic anemia may have increased numbers of activated cytotoxic lymphocytes (CD8+ cells bearing HLA-DR and interleukin 2 [IL2] receptors) that overproduce lymphokines (particularly gamma-interferon), and these abnormalities usually improve with successful immunosuppressive therapy. The clinical effectiveness of cyclosporine is further evidence that T cells play a pathogenic role in many cases of bone marrow failure.

In some cases, the inciting cause of the immune response may be an antecedent viral infection. Hepatitis C is a member of the flavivirus family, and other similar viruses, like that causing dengue, can both infect hematopoietic cells and stimulate a lymphocyte-lymphokine reaction similar to that observed in aplastic anemia. A similar final immune pathway may occur following infections with herpesviruses and retroviruses. Presumably, disease is the result of genetically determined features of the immune response that convert a normal physiologic response to a sustained and abnormal pathologic process.

PURE RED BLOOD CELL APLASIA (Table 129–3). Like aplastic anemia, pure red blood cell aplasia results from diverse mechanisms. Immune mechanisms have been implicated when pure red cell aplasia is associated with thymoma, systemic lupus erythematosus, and chronic lymphocytic leukemia, but not in failed erythropoiesis secondary to myelodysplasia, myeloproliferative diseases, and distinct cytogenetic abnormalities. Antibodies to red blood cell precursors can be detected in the blood of some patients, but T cell inhibition is probably the more common mechanism. Cytotoxic lymphocyte activity restricted by histocompatibility locus or specific for cells infected by human T cell lymphotropic virus (HTLV1) has been demonstrated in particularly well studied individual cases.

Parvovirus B19 (see Color Plate 5H, right) represents the best example of the interaction of virus, host hematologic target cell, and immune response. This common virus causes "fifth disease," a benign exanthema of childhood and a polyarthralgia syndrome in adults. In persons with underlying hemolysis, parvovirus infection causes abrupt but temporary worsening of anemia resulting from failed erythropoiesis, a syndrome called transient aplastic crisis. Parvovirus B19 has extraordinary tropism for human erythroid progenitor cells. Direct cytotoxicity of the virus causes anemia if demands on erythrocyte production are high. In normal individuals, the temporary cessation of red cell production is not clinically apparent, and disease is mediated entirely by immune complex deposition. In persons unable to mount an

TABLE 129–3. CLASSIFICATION OF PURE RED BLOOD CELL APLASIA

Self-limited
Transient erythroblastopenia of childhood
Transient aplastic crisis of hemolysis (B19 parvovirus infection)

Fetal red blood cell aplasia
Nonimmune hydrops fetalis (in utero parvovirus infection)

Hereditary pure red cell aplasia
Congenital pure red cell aplasia (Diamond-Blackfan syndrome)

Acquired pure red cell aplasia
   I. Thymoma and malignancy: thymoma, lymphoid malignancies (and more rarely other hematologic diseases), paraneoplastic to solid tumors
  II. Connective tissue disorders with immunologic abnormalities: systemic lupus erythematosus, juvenile rheumatoid arthritis, rheumatoid arthritis, multiple endocrine gland insufficiency
 III. Virus: B19 parvovirus, hepatitis, adult T cell leukemia virus, Epstein-Barr virus
  IV. Pregnancy
   V. Drugs: especially phenytoin, azathioprine, chloramphenicol, procainamide, isoniazid
  VI. Idiopathic

adequate antibody response, parvovirus B19 persists in the bone marrow and causes a chronic anemia that resembles pure red blood cell aplasia. The presence of giant pronormoblasts (Fig. 129–2), the cytopathic sign of the virus, should suggest the diagnosis. Persistent parvovirus infection should be sought in anemic patients with congenital and acquired immunodeficiency syndromes and in patients iatrogenically immunosuppressed because it can be effectively treated with immunoglobulin infusions.

Incidence and Epidemiology

The incidence of aplastic anemia is approximately 1.5 to 2 per million, but the disease may be more frequent in Asia. Mortality statistics indicate an equal sex ratio and a preponderance of older persons, but at referral centers the median age is about 24 years.

Agranulocytosis has an incidence of 3.4 per million. Pure red blood cell aplasia is a very rare disease, with only a few hundred reported cases, and amegakaryocytic thrombocytopenia is rarer still, with fewer than 20 cases in the literature.

Clinical Description

HISTORY. Bleeding is the most common early symptom of aplastic anemia: A complaint of days to weeks of easy bruising, including oozing from the gums, nose bleeds, or heavy menstrual flow is made, and sometimes petechiae will have been noticed. With thrombocytopenia, massive hemorrhage is unusual, but small amounts of bleeding in the central nervous system can result in serious intracranial or retinal hemorrhage. In cases of more gradual onset, symptoms of anemia are also described, usually lassitude, weakness, shortness of breath, and a pounding sensation in the ears. Infection is unusual as a first symptom in aplastic anemia, in contrast to agranulocytosis, in which pharyngitis, anorectal infection, or frank sepsis may be presenting syndromes. A striking feature of aplastic anemia is the restriction of symptoms to the hematologic system. Patients often feel and look remarkably well despite drastically reduced blood counts; systemic complaints and weight loss should point to other etiologies of pancytopenia. Drug use, chemical exposure, and preceding viral illnesses must often be elicited with repeated questioning; prompt cessation of drug or chemical exposure is especially important in agranulocytosis, which is usually self-limited.

PHYSICAL EXAMINATION. Petechiae and ecchymoses are frequently present, and there may be retinal hemorrhages. Pelvic and rectal examinations should be performed infrequently and gently to avoid trauma; these examinations often show bleeding from the cervical os and blood in the stool. Pallor of the skin and mucous membranes is also common except in the most acute cases or in those patients already transfused. Although infection on presentation is uncommon, by the time the patient reaches a referral center, fever and signs of systemic or local infection may well be present. Lymphadenopathy and splenomegaly are very unusual in aplastic anemia. Café au lait spots and short stature point to Fanconi's anemia; peculiar nails suggest dyskeratosis congenita.

Diagnosis and Differential Diagnosis (Table 129–4)

The diagnosis of aplastic anemia is usually straightforward, based on the combination of pancytopenia with a fatty, empty bone marrow. Prompt arrival at the appropriate diagnosis is part of the effective management of the patient with aplastic anemia.

BLOOD. The smear typically shows large erythrocytes and a paucity of platelets and granulocytes. Macrocytosis determined by automated cell counting is very common. Lymphocyte numbers may be normal or also reduced. The presence of immature myeloid forms should suggest leukemia or myelodysplasia; nucleated red blood cells suggest marrow fibrosis or invasion; and abnormal platelets suggest either peripheral destruction or dysplasia.

BONE MARROW (Fig. 129–2). "Watery" marrow can almost always be obtained, and a "dry tap" occurs in fibrotic or myelophthisic disease. In severe aplasia, the smear of the aspirated specimen shows only residual lymphocytes and stromal cells; in milder cases, the remaining hematopoietic cells can show "megaloblastoid" erythropoiesis. Megakaryocytes are invariably greatly reduced, usually absent. The areas adjacent to the spicule should be searched for myeloblasts. Total cellularity is assessed by biopsy (see Color Plate 5G) of a core more than 1 cm in length, which in the most severe cases is virtually 100 per cent fat and in more moderate disease less than 20 per cent cellular. Nonetheless, the correlation between marrow cellularity and severity is imperfect: Some patients with moderate disease according to blood counts have empty iliac crest biopsies, and there may be "hot spots" of hematopoiesis in severe cases. In unilineage failure states, the bone marrow reflects the absence of a specific morphologic subtype, but in both pure red blood cell aplasia and agranulocytosis, early and midmature precursor cells may be present. Granulomas (in cellular specimens) may indicate an infectious cause of the marrow failure.

ANCILLARY STUDIES. Cytogenetic studies of peripheral blood should be performed on patients younger than 35 years (at least) to exclude Fanconi's anemia. Testing for abnormal sensitivity of erythrocytes to complement (Ham's test) establishes paroxysmal nocturnal hemoglobinuria (Ch. 135). Serologic studies may show evidence of viral infection, especially antibodies to human immunodeficiency virus, Epstein-Barr virus, and hepatitis viruses. Parvovirus should be sought by DNA hybridization in chronic pure red cell aplasia. Hypoimmunoglobulinemia and thymoma are also associated with pure red blood cell aplasia; a thymoma should be sought by computed tomography, less because the hematologic disease remits with thymectomy (it often does not) than because a potentially malignant tumor should be removed. The size of the spleen should be determined by scanning if the physical examination of the abdomen is unsatisfactory.

DIFFERENTIAL DIAGNOSIS. Pancytopenia occurs in many

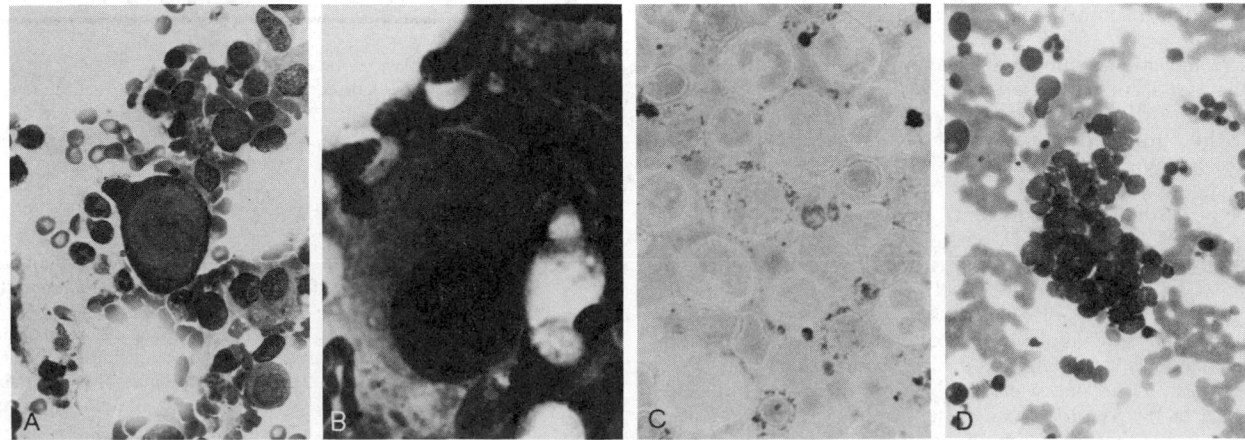

FIGURE 129–2. Four pathognomonic cells in the bone marrow. *A*, Giant pronormoblast, the cytopathic effect of B19 parvovirus infection of the erythroid progenitor cell. *B*, Uninuclear megakaryocyte and microblastic erythroid precursors typical of the 5q-myelodysplasia syndrome. *C*, Ringed sideroblast showing perinuclear iron granules. *D*, Clump of nonhematopoietic cells forming syncytium of metastatic tumor cells.

TABLE 129–4. DIFFERENTIAL DIAGNOSIS OF PANCYTOPENIA

Pancytopenia with hypocellular bone marrow
  Acquired aplastic anemia
  Inherited aplastic anemia (Fanconi's anemia)
  Some myelodysplasia syndromes
  Rare aleukemic leukemia (acute myelogenous leukemia [AML])
  Some acute lymphoblastic leukemias
  Some lymphomas of bone marrow

Pancytopenia with cellular bone marrow
  Myelodysplasia syndromes
  Paroxysmal nocturnal
    hemoglobinuria
  Myelofibrosis   } Primary bone marrow diseases
  Some aleukemic leukemias
  Myelophthisis
  Bone marrow lymphoma
  Hairy cell leukemia

  Systemic lupus erythematosus
  Hypersplenism
  Vitamin B₁₂, folate deficiency
  Overwhelming infection   } Secondary to systemic diseases
  Alcohol
  Brucellosis
  Sarcoidosis
  Tuberculosis

Hypocellular bone marrow ± cytopenia
  Q fever
  Legionnaires' disease
  Anorexia nervosa, starvation
  Mycobacterial infection

---

diseases, but when secondary blood count depression rivals that of severe aplastic anemia, the primary diagnosis is usually obvious from either the history or the physical examination (e.g., the massive spleen of alcoholic cirrhosis, the history of metastatic cancer or systemic lupus erythematosus, or obvious miliary tuberculosis on the chest radiograph).

Treatment

BONE MARROW TRANSPLANTATION (Ch. 153). This offers the best therapy for a young patient with a fully histocompatible sibling donor. Survival of patients younger than 20 years old following bone marrow transplantation is about 80 per cent. Early consideration of the transplantation option in a child or adolescent can avoid unnecessary transfusions. Transfusions increase the risk of graft rejection, already peculiarly high in patients with aplastic anemia, and graft rejection is the major determinant of a successful clinical outcome. Survival of minimally transfused patients approximates that of patients who have had an identical twin as donor. Graft-versus-host disease increases progressively with age and occurs in about 90 per cent of adults over 30 years old. In older persons, marrow transplantation also carries significant risks from interstitial pneumonitis and opportunistic infections secondary to the conditioning regimen. As a result, it is usually not recommended for patients with aplastic anemia who are more than 40 years old. Management of patients in the intermediate range, 20 to 40 years old, depends on their transfusion history, on their general clinical condition, and, unfortunately, often on their medical insurance. Use of alternative donors, unrelated histocompatible volunteers or closely but not perfectly matched family members, remains experimental but has been occasionally successful.

IMMUNOSUPPRESSION. Most patients with aplastic anemia lack a suitable marrow donor. Antithymocyte globulin therapy leads to recovery of autologous bone marrow function in about 50 per cent of patients, usually with independence from transfusion and a leukocyte count adequate to prevent infection. Improvement in granulocyte number is generally apparent within 2 months of treatment. In most patients who recover with this treatment, the blood counts remain somewhat depressed, the mean corpuscular volume continues to be high, and the bone marrow cellularity returns only very slowly toward normal, if at all. Relapse is infrequent, although 5 to 10 per cent of patients may suffer recurrent severe pancytopenia or myelodysplasia, paroxysmal nocturnal hemoglobinuria, or acute leukemia. Bone

marrow examinations should therefore be performed annually or when there is an unfavorable change in blood counts, and a Ham test should be obtained periodically. About 50 per cent of patients in whom therapy with ATG fails will respond to a 3- to 6-month course of cyclosporine. The combination of ATG and cyclosporine may be superior to ATG alone as initial therapy for severe aplastic anemia.

Antithymocyte globulin can be given intravenously in a regimen of 40 mg per kilogram per day for 4 days. Anaphylaxis is a rare but occasionally fatal complication of ATG treatment; allergy should be tested for by a prick test with an undiluted solution and immediate observation. Antithymocyte globulin binds to peripheral blood cells, and therefore platelet and granulocyte numbers may fall further during active treatment. Serum sickness often develops about 10 days after initiating treatment (Ch. 249). Most patients receive methylprednisolone (1 mg per kilogram per day for 2 weeks) to ameliorate the immune consequences of heterologous protein infusion. Cyclosporine is administered orally at an initial dose of 12 mg per kilogram per day in adults and 15 mg per kilogram per day in children, with subsequent adjustment according to blood levels obtained every 2 weeks. Nephrotoxicity, hypertension, seizures, and opportunistic infections, especially *Pneumocystis carinii* pneumonia, are the most serious complications of cyclosporine treatment.

Immunosuppression is also effective in pure red blood cell aplasia and probably in amegakaryocytic thrombocytopenia as well. Treatments include corticosteroids, azathioprine, or cyclophosphamide, followed by ATG or cyclosporine.

OTHER THERAPIES. Androgen therapy has not been verified as effective in controlled trials, but occasional patients respond or even demonstrate blood count dependence on continued therapy. For patients with moderate disease or for those with severe pancytopenia in whom immunosupression has failed, a 3- to 4-month trial of an androgen is appropriate: nandrolone decanoate at 5 mg per kilogram per week given intramuscularly (with firm pressure at the injection site to prevent hemorrhage) or oxymetholone at 150 mg per day by mouth.

Hematopoietic growth factors, GM-CSF and G-CSF, have not been shown to induce remissions in aplastic anemia, although they may increase the white blood cell count during the period of administration in some patients.

PRINCIPLES OF SUPPORT. Meticulous medical care is required so that the patient can survive to benefit from definitive therapy or, having experienced a treatment failure, can maintain a reasonable existence in the face of pancytopenia. First and most important, infection in the patient with severe neutropenia must be aggressively treated (see also Ch. 140). Parenteral, broad-spectrum antibiotics should be started promptly, usually a combination of an aminoglycoside, cephalosporin, and semisynthetic penicillin (monotherapy with ceftazidime is a reasonable alternative). Therapy is empiric and must not await results of culture, although specific foci of infection, like oropharyngeal or anorectal abscesses, pneumonia, sinusitis, and typhlitis, should be sought on physical examination and with suitable radiographic studies. When indwelling plastic catheters become contaminated, vancomycin should be added. Persistent or recrudescent fever implies fungal disease; candidiasis and aspergillosis are common, especially after several courses of antibacterial antibiotics, and a progressive course may be averted by the timely initiation of amphotericin. Granulocyte transfusions are seldom indicated (Ch. 140). Handwashing, the single most effective method of preventing the spread of infection in the hospital, remains a neglected practice. Nonabsorbed antibiotics for gut decontamination may be effective but are rarely tolerated because of their gastrointestinal side effects. Total reverse isolation is difficult, expensive, psychologically debilitating, inhibitory of nursing and medical attention, and not clearly beneficial in reducing mortality from infections.

Platelets and erythrocytes can be maintained by transfusion. Candidates for bone marrow transplantation should be transfused sparingly and, of course, never with blood products from a family member. Alloimmunization limits the usefulness of prophylactic platelet transfusions, and single-donor platelets from which leukocytes have been removed by filtration are the best product (Ch. 140). There are no direct studies of the value of prophylaxis versus demand platelet transfusions in chronic bone marrow failure. Any rational regimen of prophylaxis requires transfusions once or twice weekly to maintain the platelet count above 10,000 per microliter (oozing from the gut, and presumably also from other vascular beds, increases precipitously at values lower than 5000 per microliter). About one third of patients become refractory to platelet transfusions, sometimes to HLA-matched as well as to random-donor platelets. Inhibitors of fibrinolysis, like aminocaproic acid, may help reduce mucosal oozing. Menstruation should be suppressed by either oral estrogens or nasal follicle-stimulating hormone (FSH)/luteinizing hormone (LH) antagonists. Aspirin and other nonsteroidal anti-inflammatory agents that inhibit platelet function must be avoided.

Red blood cells should be transfused to allow a normal level of activity, usually to a hemoglobin value of 70 grams per liter (90 grams per liter if there is underlying cardiac disease). A regimen of 2 units every 2 weeks replaces the normal loss of erythrocytes in a patient without a functioning bone marrow. In chronic anemia, the iron chelator deferoxamine should be added at about the time the patient receives the fiftieth transfusion to avoid secondary hemochromatosis.

Prognosis

The natural course of untreated severe aplastic anemia is rapid deterioration and death resulting from infection or hemorrhage. Survival in patients with severe disease treated with transfusions only is poor, probably about 20 per cent at 1 year. In most large unselected series, bone marrow transplantation leads to a 60 to 80 per cent survival rate at 1 year. In Europe, immunosuppression has given overall results equivalent to marrow transplantation in adults, although survival was better with transplantation if severe neutropenia (<200 per microliter) was present. The physician has the responsibility of informing the patient of the relative values of bone marrow transplantation, which cures the hematologic disease but at great cost and often with significant morbidity, and immunosuppressive therapy, which is easier but often not completely effective.

Red cell aplasia is compatible with long life. Patients with congenital anemias have survived for decades with a combination of transfusions and iron chelation. Probably more than half of patients with acquired red cell aplasia can be cured by immunosuppression.

MYELODYSPLASIA

Definition

Myelodysplasia describes a heterogeneous group of hematologic disorders that are defined only broadly by cytopenias associated with a dysmorphic or abnormal-appearing bone marrow (Table 129–5) (see Color Plate 6I and J). The classification scheme marks the convergence of two areas of investigation: preleukemia, the cytopenic phase sometimes observed to precede frank malignancy, and refractory anemia, states that resemble megaloblastic anemia but without evidence of vitamin deficiency. The French-American-British nomenclature, while based on morphologic features, has real predictive value. (Sideroblastic anemia is also discussed in Ch. 131 as an example of hypochromic anemias.)

Etiology and Pathophysiology

The myelodysplastic syndromes are clonal disorders and have been convincingly linked to exposure to radiation, benzene, and many drugs employed in the treatment of cancer, particularly the radiomimetic alkylating agents. Cytogenetic abnormalities are common in patients with myelodysplasia. Some of the same specific chromosomal lesions also occur in frank leukemia and can be a transient stage in the development of a fully malignant phenotype. The presence and number of gross cytogenetic abnormalities in myelodysplasia are strongly correlated with the probability of leukemic transformation and therefore inversely with survival. One stereotypical karyotypic finding is deletion of a portion of the short arm of the fifth chromosome, or 5q-syndrome (Fig. 129–2), particularly provocative because the genes for multiple hematopoietic growth factors and their receptors are found in the affected region (including granulocyte-macrophage and macrophage colony-stimulating factors; interleukins 3, 4, 5, and 9; and the cell-surface receptors for macrophage colony-stimulating factor [the c-fms gene] and platelet-derived growth factor). Mutations that activate the ras oncogene and the c-fms gene have also been implicated in other cases of myelodysplasia. A mutation in a cell-surface receptor might result in a continuous proliferative stimulus and the uncoupling of signal transduction required for normal differentiation. The dysfunction measured in erythrocyte enzyme pathways for heme synthesis or in platelet aggregation in myelodysplasia is likely a secondary effect of mutations that dysregulate progenitor cell growth.

Incidence and Epidemiology

Idiopathic myelodysplasia is a disease of the elderly; the average mean age at onset is approximately 68 years, with a slight male preponderance. The exact incidence of myelodysplasia is unknown, but this is not a rare syndrome in our aging population. Therapy-related myelodysplasia, which is not age-related, may occur in 10 to 15 per cent of patients within a decade following intensive treatment, especially following a combination of irradiation and drugs like busulfan, nitrosourea, or procarbazine.

Clinical Description

Anemia dominates the early course. Most symptomatic patients complain of the gradual onset of fatigue and weakness, dyspnea, and pallor, but half are asymptomatic, with the myelodysplasia being discovered only incidentally. Previous chemotherapy or radiation exposure is an important historical fact. Fever and weight loss are more indicative of a myeloproliferative than of a myelodysplastic process. A family history may indicate a hereditary form of sideroblastic anemia. The physical examination is remarkable for signs of anemia and, in about 20 per cent of cases, splenomegaly. In addition, some unusual skin lesions, like those of Sweet's syndrome (febrile neutrophilic dermatosis), have been associated with myelodysplasia.

Diagnosis and Differential Diagnosis

BLOOD. Anemia is present in the majority of cases, either alone or as part of bicytopenia or pancytopenia, but isolated neutropenia or thrombocytopenia is unusual. Macrocytosis is common, and the smear may be dimorphic with a distinctive population of large cells. Platelets are large and lack granules. Neutrophils may be hypogranulated, show Pelger-Huët, ringed, or abnormally segmented nuclei, and contain Döhle's bodies. Circulating myeloblasts usually correlate with the number of marrow blasts, and their quantitation is important for classification and prognosis. The total white blood cell count is usually normal or low, with the exception of the monocytosis observed in chronic myelomonocytic leukemia.

TABLE 129–5. CLASSIFICATION OF MYELODYSPLASIA

Subtype	Blood	Marrow	Per Cent of Cases	Median Survival (mo)	Leukemic Evolution (%)
Refractory anemia	Blasts <1%	Blasts <5%	27	50	16
Refractory anemia with ringed sideroblasts	Blasts <1%	Blasts <5%	20	65	15
Refractory anemia with excess blasts	Blasts ≤5%	Blasts 5–20%	26	15	48
Refractory anemia with excess blasts in transformation	Blasts >5%	Blasts 20–30% or Auer rods	13	9	62
Chronic myelomonocytic leukemia	≥1 × 10⁹/L monocytes	Any number	14	23	29

By definition, the bone marrow of acute myelogenous leukemia contains more than 30 per cent blasts. Leukemic evolution refers to the percentage of cases that transform into acute myelogenous leukemia. Data derived from published series after Dunbar and Nienhuis.

A. **Neoplastic infiltration of the marrow**
   1. Hematologic malignancies
      Leukemias—acute and chronic
      Lymphomas—Hodgkin's and non-Hodgkin's
      Plasma cell myeloma
      Hairy cell leukemia
   2. Nonhematologic malignancies
      Carcinomas—especially breast, prostate, lung, stomach
      Neuroblastoma
B. **Myelofibrosis**
   1. Primary (idiopathic)
   2. Secondary—chronic myeloid leukemia, cancers, vasculitis (lupus, rheumatoid arthritis)
C. **Granulomatous infections**
   1. Tuberculosis
   2. Fungi
D. **Metabolic abnormalities**
   1. Lipid storage diseases, e.g., Gaucher's disease
   2. Osteopetrosis

BONE MARROW. The bone marrow is usually normocellular or hypercellular, but in 20 per cent of patients with myelodysplasia, it is sufficiently hypocellular to be confused with aplasia. No single characteristic feature of marrow morphology distinguishes myelodysplasia. Megaloblastoid and dyserythropoietic changes in the red blood cell precursors, a left shift with an increase in myeloblasts, and abnormal megakaryocytes with reduced numbers of disorganized nuclei are common features. The specific diagnosis is based on the presence of ringed sideroblasts (Fig. 129–2), the percentage of blasts, and increased immature myelomonocytic forms. A hematologist helps delineate myelodysplasia from acute myelogenous leukemia on the one hand and aplastic anemia on the other. Analysis of chromosomes from cultured bone marrow cells should always be performed, as cytogenetic abnormalities are unusual in aplasia and common in myelodysplasia. Complex chromosomal abnormalities imply poor survival.

Treatment

Therapy for myelodysplasia has generally been unsatisfactory. Occasional patients with sideroblastic anemia, usually hereditary, respond to pyridoxine. Androgens and corticosteroids may improve blood counts but have not been shown to influence survival. Older patients suffer a high mortality during induction with high-dose chemotherapy for leukemia and have a lower remission rate than do patients with acute myelogenous leukemia. Reported good responses using low-dose chemotherapy (in particular, cytosine arabinoside) or retinoids to induce marrow differentiation have not been widely confirmed.

A substantial proportion of patients with myelodysplasia have been found to respond with significant blood count improvement to granulocyte or granulocyte-macrophage colony-stimulating growth factors. Leukocytes almost always increase during factor therapy, and in some cases blast numbers have been significantly reduced and cytogenetic abnormalities have resolved. Unfortunately, sometimes progression to acute leukemia has also occurred. Platelet and reticulocyte numbers respond less consistently. Current long-term trials of these factors, as well as interleukin 3 and factors in combination, should provide an indication of optimal regimens and long-term benefits.

The same principles of supportive care described for aplastic anemia apply to myelodysplasia. Because many patients will be anemic for years, erythrocyte transfusion support should be accompanied by iron chelation to prevent hemochromatotic damage to the heart, liver, and pancreas.

Prognosis

The median survival for a patient with myelodysplasia is about 2 years, but survival varies greatly with the specific subtype. Most patients die as a result of complications of pancytopenia and not because of leukemic transformation. Approximately one third succumb to other diseases unrelated to myelodysplasia. Precipitous worsening of pancytopenia, acquisition of new chromosomal abnormalities detected on serial cytogenetic determination, and increase in the number of blasts are all obviously poor prognostic indicators. The outlook in therapy-related myelodysplasia is particularly poor, with many patients rapidly progressing to refractory acute myelogenous leukemia.

MYELOPHTHISIC ANEMIAS AND MYELOFIBROSIS

Marrow fibrosis, usually accompanied by a characteristic blood smear presentation called leukoerythroblastosis (see Color Plate 7F, left), can occur as a primary hematologic disease, called myelofibrosis or myeloid metaplasia (see Color Plate 5J), and as a secondary process, called myelophthisis, which represents reaction to invading tumor cells (see Color Plate 5I), infectious agents like mycobacteria or fungi, intracellular lipid deposition in Gaucher's disease (see Color Plate 7E), and the granulomas of sarcoidosis (Table 129–6). In secondary fibrosis, the infectious or malignant underlying processes are usually obvious. The pancytopenia of human immunodeficiency virus may be associated with moderate marrow fibrosis. Modest degrees of fibrosis can also be a feature of a variety of other hematologic syndromes, especially chronic myelogenous leukemia, poorly differentiated lymphomas, myeloma, and hairy cell leukemia. Marrow fibrosis also occurs in the bony proliferative disease of childhood called osteopetrosis.

The pathophysiology of myelofibrosis has three distinct features: proliferation of fibroblasts in the marrow space; extension of hematopoiesis into the long bones and most peculiarly into extramedullary sites, usually the spleen, liver, and lymph nodes (myeloid metaplasia); and ineffective erythropoiesis. The etiology of fibrosis is unknown but most likely involves dysregulated production of growth factors. Many cell types in the marrow produce growth factors for fibroblasts: Platelet-derived growth factor is one example, and profuse megakaryocytopoiesis and thrombocytosis are often seen early in the course of idiopathic myelofibrosis. Abnormal regulation of other hematopoietins would lead to the localization of blood-producing cells in nonhematopoietic tissues and uncoupling of the usually balanced processes of stem cell proliferation and differentiation. Myelofibrosis is remarkable for pancytopenia despite extraordinarily large numbers of circulating hematopoietic progenitor cells.

Idiopathic (or agnogenic) myelofibrosis is one of the myeloproliferative syndromes, a category that also includes polycythemia vera, essential thrombocythemia, and chronic myelogenous leukemia. It is discussed in Ch. 143 in the context of the myeloproliferative disorders.

Deeg HJ, Klingemann H-G, Phillips GL: A Guide to Bone Marrow Transplantation. Berlin, Springer-Verlag, 1988. *Multifaceted and balanced approach.*

Dunbar C, Nienhuis A: The myelodysplastic syndromes. *In* Handin R, Lux S, Stossel T (eds.): Blood, Principles and Practice of Hematology. Philadelphia, J.B. Lippincott, in press. *Good clinical descriptions and in-depth considerations of mechanisms.*

Young NS: Drugs and chemicals as agents of bone marrow failure. *In* Testa NG, Gale RP (eds.): Hematopoiesis: Long-term Effects of Chemotherapy and Radiation. New York, Marcel Dekker, 1988, 131 pp. *Detailed review of epidemiologic and mechanistic aspects.*

Young NS: Hematologic and hematopoietic consequences of B19 parvovirus infection. Semin Hematol 25:159, 1988. *The story of this virus, from its discovery to the genetic engineering of a vaccine, should make good reading.*

Young NS, Alter BA: Bone marrow failure. *In* Handin R, Lux S, Stossel T (eds.): Blood, Principles and Practice of Hematology. Philadelphia, J.B. Lippincott, in press. *Exhaustive review of aplastic anemia, both acquired and constitutional, and single-lineage failures.*

130 Normochromic, Normocytic Anemias

James P. Kushner

The normocytic, normochromic anemias are those in which the average cell size (mean corpuscular volume [MCV]) and the average cell hemoglobin concentration (mean corpuscular hemoglobin concentration [MCHC]) are normal. These anemias occur in association with a large number of diseases, and the mechanisms responsible for the anemia are quite diverse. Frequently, the anemia is only a minor manifestation of a systemic disease.

The anemia, however, may be the first detected evidence of disease, and the finding of anemia may lead to studies resulting in correct diagnosis of an underlying disorder.

In spite of their highly variable causes, it is possible to approach normocytic, normochromic anemias with a classification scheme that can direct the diagnostic investigation (Table 130–1). Central to this classification is the determination of whether the bone marrow is responding appropriately to a given degree of anemia. Normally functioning bone marrow can accelerate the rate of erythropoiesis up to eightfold. Accelerated erythropoiesis is reflected by an increase in the reticulocyte count. Reticulocytosis can be detected on routinely stained smears by the finding of a population of large polychromatophilic red cells. When reticulocytosis is pronounced, the MCV may be moderately elevated because of the contribution of the large young erythrocytes to the measurement of the average cell size. Reticulocytosis (see Color Plate 5F, right) is a manifestation of an appropriate marrow response to hemolytic anemia (see Ch. 133) and to acute posthemorrhagic anemia. These two conditions can generally be differentiated on clinical grounds.

When evidence of accelerated erythropoiesis in response to anemia is *not* found, it is likely that the underlying disorder is directly or indirectly affecting the bone marrow. Intrinsic marrow disease should be strongly suspected when leukopenia and thrombocytopenia are also found, or when morphologic abnormalities are found on the blood smear. These morphologic abnormalities include nucleated red cells, teardrop-shaped poikilocytes, immature granulocytes, and large platelets or megakaryocyte fragments (dwarf megakaryocytes). Marrow aspiration and biopsy are nearly always indicated when these findings are present.

When anemia is found in association with an impaired marrow response and no signs of intrinsic marrow disease are detected, it is likely that an underlying disease is producing an indirect effect on red cell production. Renal disease, liver disease, and a variety of endocrine disorders indirectly affect erythropoiesis in association with a reduction of erythropoietin production. The pathogenesis of the anemia of chronic disease may also involve this mechanism, in addition to the defect in the mobilization of reticuloendothelial iron stores (Ch. 131).

ACUTE POSTHEMORRHAGIC ANEMIA

DEFINITION. The anemia caused by loss of a large volume of blood may occur as a result of trauma or because of an underlying disease that affects blood vessels or the coagulation mechanism. Bleeding may be obvious when profuse hemorrhage occurs from a body orifice or from an external wound. If bleeding occurs within a body cavity, tissue space, or the gastrointestinal tract, the nature of the problem may not be immediately appreciated (Ch. 111). The manifestation of hemorrhage depends on the rate and magnitude of the bleeding and the time elapsed between the acute hemorrhage and the first clinical observations.

CLINICAL MANIFESTATIONS AND DIAGNOSIS. The events following a single acute hemorrhage can be divided into two phases. The first, lasting up to 3 days, reflects the volume of blood loss and is dominated by the manifestations of hypovolemia. Anemia may not be detected by measurement of the hematocrit or hemoglobin. The second phase occurs after the body has restored the blood volume to normal or nearly normal and is characterized by the findings of anemia and reticulocytosis.

As outlined in Table 130–2, a normal individual can rapidly lose up to 20 per cent of the blood volume without any signs or symptoms. Limited signs of cardiovascular distress appear with losses up to 30 per cent of the blood volume, but shock gradually appears only when the blood loss exceeds 30 to 40 per cent of the blood volume. As the plasma volume and red cell mass are reduced in proportional amounts, the hematocrit and hemoglobin fail to reflect the magnitude of blood lost. Clinical signs and symptoms must be used initially to estimate the degree of blood volume depletion and to plan emergency treatment. When blood loss is more gradual, the plasma volume may be restored by endogenous mechanisms, and very large volumes of blood can be lost without clinical manifestations of shock.

Anemia is first detected following expansion of the plasma volume. In recumbent patients most of the plasma volume expansion has occurred by 24 hours; this expansion mainly is caused by movement of water and electrolytes into the intravascular space. In ambulatory patients plasma volume expansion occurs more slowly, mainly through the mobilization of albumin from extravascular sites. The hematocrit may not reach the minimum value until 3 or 4 days after the hemorrhagic episode. Erythropoietin secretion is stimulated shortly after the appearance of the anemia, and hyperplasia of marrow erythroid elements then begins.

Reticulocytosis is usually detected 3 to 5 days after the hemorrhagic episode, and maximal reticulocyte counts are reached at 6 to 11 days. The degree of reticulocytosis is related to the magnitude of hemorrhage but rarely exceeds 14 per cent. During the period of maximal reticulocytosis, polychromatophilia and macrocytosis can be detected on the peripheral blood smear, and the MCV may become transiently increased. If the initial evaluation is done during this state, the findings may be mistaken for those of hemolytic anemia. Differentiation from hemolytic anemia may be difficult if bleeding has occurred into a body cavity or tissue space, because resorption of blood from these areas often results in an increased production of unconjugated bilirubin and even mild jaundice. In contrast to the reticulocyte response, both the platelet count and the leukocyte count may rise dramatically within hours of hemorrhage. Platelet counts as great as 1000×10^9 per liter may be detected within 1 to 2 hours, and leukocyte counts of 20 to 35×10^9 per liter may be reached by 2 to 5 hours. Elevated platelet and leukocyte counts generally return to normal within 3 to 5 days.

TREATMENT. During the hypovolemic phase, therapy should be directed at stopping the hemorrhage, combating shock,

TABLE 130–1. CLASSIFICATION OF THE NORMOCYTIC, NORMOCHROMIC ANEMIAS

I. **Anemia with appropriate marrow response**
  A. Acute posthemorrhagic anemia
  B. Hemolytic anemia (may be macrocytic when there is pronounced reticulocytosis) (Ch. 133–135)
II. **Anemia with impaired marrow response**
  A. Marrow hypoplasia
    1. Aplastic anemia (Ch. 129)
    2. Pure red cell aplasia (Ch. 129)
  B. Marrow infiltration
    1. Infiltration by malignant cells
    2. Myelofibrosis (Ch. 143)
    3. Inherited storage diseases
  C. Decreased erythropoietin production
    1. Kidney disease
    2. Liver disease
    3. Endocrine deficiencies
    4. Malnutrition
    5. Anemia of chronic disease (Ch. 131)

TABLE 130–2. CLINICAL MANIFESTATIONS OF ACUTE BLOOD LOSS IN OTHERWISE HEALTHY INDIVIDUALS

Percentage of Blood Volume Lost	Amount Lost (ml)	Clinical Manifestations
10–20	500–1000	Usually none; vasovagal syncope may occur in 5%; tachycardia in response to exercise; mild postural hypotension may be noted
20–30	1000–1500	Few changes in the supine position; light-headedness and hypotension commonly occur when the patient is upright; marked tachycardia in response to exertion
30–40	1500–2000	Blood pressure, cardiac output, central venous pressure, urine volume reduced even when supine; thirst, shortness of breath, clammy skin, sweating, clouding of consciousness and rapid, thready pulse may be noted
40–50	2000–2500	Severe shock, often resulting in death

and restoring the blood volume. Restoration of the blood volume may be achieved by intravenous infusion of crystalloid (electrolyte) solutions; colloid solutions of plasma protein, albumin, or dextran; or fresh whole blood. Complete reliance on fresh whole blood in the emergency situation is unwise for several reasons. First, large amounts of type O Rh-negative whole blood are required. If typing and crossmatching are done prior to transfusion, there may be a dangerous delay in therapy. Second, allergic transfusion reactions may restrict volume expansion or even produce plasma volume contraction. For the emergency situation, crystalloid solutions are preferred.

A nonprotein crystalloid solution with a sodium concentration approximating that of plasma is the most widely used fluid therapy for hemorrhagic shock. Ringer's lactate, Ringer's acetate, or normal saline supplemented with 90 mmol of sodium bicarbonate (2 ampules) per liter may be used. Crystalloid solutions containing large amounts of glucose should be avoided, as they may induce osmotic diuresis, further depleting the vascular volume. An initial infusion of two to three times the volume of the estimated blood loss is administered. When larger volumes of crystalloid solutions are administered, peripheral edema often develops, as these solutions are rapidly distributed throughout the intravascular and extravascular compartments.

The use of protein-containing solutions (albumin or fresh frozen plasma) has been supported by some who claim that increasing the oncotic pressure within the vascular space is beneficial. There is little evidence to support this contention, as protein is extravasated into interstitial spaces throughout the body in patients in shock. Dextran solutions have been widely used in the treatment of hemorrhagic shock, but there is no convincing evidence to suggest they are superior to crystalloid solutions in acute emergencies. Acute renal failure has occurred in a few patients receiving dextran solutions. Dextran may cause difficulty in crossmatching and may interfere with platelet adhesiveness and the normal coagulation cascade.

The administration of 3 liters of a crystalloid solution over 15 to 20 minutes generally resuscitates any patient in hemorrhagic shock if the hemorrhage has been arrested. Continued signs and symptoms of hypovolemia indicate continued bleeding and usually indicate the need for surgical intervention to control the hemorrhage.

Once the emergency has been dealt with, the bleeding lesion identified, and the bleeding stopped, attention can be directed to the anemia. The anemia itself rarely requires specific therapy, and provision of a high-protein diet and oral iron supplementation suffices in most cases. Blood transfusions may be reserved for those situations in which rapid correction of the anemia is required, as in preparation of the patient for surgery.

Billhardt RA, Rosenbush SW: Cardiogenic and hypovolemic shock. Med Clin North Am 70:853, 1986. *A useful review of the crystalloid versus colloid controversy in the acute management of hypovolemic shock.*

Mollison PL: Blood Transfusion in Clinical Medicine. 8th ed. St. Louis, C.V. Mosby, 1988. *The "bible" for detailed analysis of the measurement of blood volume and its restoration by transfusions.*

OTHER NORMOCYTIC, NORMOCHROMIC ANEMIAS

ANEMIA OF CHRONIC RENAL INSUFFICIENCY. In contrast to the anemia found in association with most chronic diseases, the anemia associated with renal failure may be quite severe. Many factors may contribute to the anemia. Folate may be lost into the dialysate in patients receiving long-term dialysis therapy. Iron deficiency may develop because of blood loss from the genitourinary or gastrointestinal tracts or into the hemodialysis coil. Microangiopathic hemolytic anemia (see Color Plate 6E, right) may occur in patients with renal failure because of malignant hypertension, or in the hemolytic-uremic syndrome. In the absence of any of these mechanisms, the degree of anemia correlates roughly with the increase in the blood urea nitrogen and creatinine levels. Although red cell survival may be moderately shortened, the mechanism underlying the anemia is mainly reduced red cell production. Failure of the erythropoietin-secreting function of the kidney appears to be responsible for the impaired marrow response to the anemia.

Blood transfusions are infrequently required. The hematocrit rarely drops below 15 per cent, and most patients tolerate this degree of anemia remarkably well. Long-term dialysis therapy may result in a modest reduction in the degree of anemia,

provided that folate or iron deficiency does not develop as a complicating factor. Human erythropoietin derived from recombinant DNA is extremely effective in treating the anemia of chronic renal disease in patients maintained by hemodialysis. An initial intravenous dose of 150 units per kilogram of body weight three times per week usually raises the hematocrit to 35 per cent or greater in 6 to 8 weeks. Most patients require a maintenance dose between 50 and 125 units per kilogram of body weight three times per week. Intravenous injections of erythropoietin are generally administered after each dialysis treatment. Following a successful renal homograft, normal and even supranormal hematocrit values may be achieved.

ANEMIA IN CIRRHOSIS AND OTHER LIVER DISEASE. Anemia is a frequent manifestation of liver disease; the pathogenetic mechanisms responsible may be more varied than those underlying the anemia of chronic disease. The anemia is generally normocytic and normochromic, but occasionally it may be mildly macrocytic. It is unusual for the MCV to exceed 115 fl in the absence of advanced folate deficiency with frank megaloblastic changes in the marrow. Etiologic factors implicated in the pathogenesis of the anemia associated with liver disease include chronic alcoholism and its effect on erythropoiesis; iron deficiency due to blood loss from gastritis, peptic ulcer, varices, and deficient coagulation factors; sequestration of erythrocytes and other formed elements of the blood by the enlarged spleen resulting from portal hypertension; exaggeration of the degree of anemia because of the increased plasma volume associated with cirrhosis; and alterations in the lipid composition of erythrocyte membranes.

ANEMIAS ASSOCIATED WITH ENDOCRINE DISORDERS. Anemia frequently accompanies disorders of the pituitary gland, the thyroid gland, the adrenal glands, and the gonads. In general, the anemia is mild and by itself produces few symptoms. Reduced tissue oxygen requirements as a result of the endocrine disturbance may result in diminished renal production of erythropoietin. Loss of the stimulating effect of androgens on erythrocyte production may be a factor in some cases. Endocrine disorders tend to begin insidiously; the early symptoms are generally no more specific than fatigue and lassitude. When initial laboratory testing reveals anemia, the diagnostic studies may be directed to the hematopoietic system. Unless endocrine disease is included in the differential diagnosis of a normocytic, normochromic anemia, the primary diagnosis may be overlooked.

Anagnostou A, Kurtzman NA: Hematological consequences of renal failure. *In* Brenner BM, Rector FC (eds.): The Kidney. 3rd ed. Philadelphia, W. B. Saunders Company, 1986. *A comprehensive treatise on the subject, with over 500 references.*

Eschbach JW: The anemia of chronic renal failure: Pathophysiology and the effects of recombinant erythropoietin. Kidney Int 35:134, 1989. *Clinical features and the application of erythropoietin in the treatment of the anemia of chronic renal failure presented in the format of a clinical conference.*

Savage D, Lindenbaum J: Anemia in alcoholics. Medicine 65:322, 1986. *A review of factors causing anemia in alcoholics, the group of patients most likely to manifest advanced liver disease.*

Williams WJ, Beutler E, Erslev AJ, et al. (eds.): Hematology. 4th ed. New York, McGraw-Hill Book Company, 1990. *Extensive references to the anemias associated with renal and endocrine disorders.*

131 Hypochromic Anemias

James P. Kushner

Anemias associated with a subnormal average cell hemoglobin concentration (mean corpuscular hemoglobin concentration [MCHC]) are classified as hypochromic. When the average cell size (mean corpuscular volume [MCV]) is also reduced, the anemia is classified as hypochromic, microcytic. Hypochromia and microcytosis can be detected either by examination of the stained blood smear (see Color Plate 5K) or by calculation of the erythrocyte indices (Table 131–1). The widespread use of electronic cell counting equipment makes available the erythrocyte

TABLE 131-1. RED CELL INDICES*
IN HYPOCHROMIC AND MICROCYTIC ANEMIAS

	MCV (fl)	MCHC (gm/dl)	MCH (pg)
Normal	83–96	32–36	28–34
Hypochromic	83–100	28–31	23–31
Microcytic	70–82	32–36	22–27
Hypochromic-microcytic	50–79	24–31	11–29

*Variations in the methods for measuring the red blood cell count, the volume of packed red cells, and the hemoglobin concentration could change the values slightly.

indices at the same time that anemia is usually detected by the finding of subnormal values for the hemoglobin concentration and the hematocrit.

The developing erythrocyte requires iron, protoporphyrin, and globin for the biosynthesis of hemoglobin. Hypochromic anemias, characterized by deficient hemoglobin synthesis, can be divided into three groups, depending on which of the three components required for hemoglobin biosynthesis is deficient (Table 131-2).

IRON DEFICIENCY ANEMIA

DEFINITIONS. Iron deficiency anemia occurs when body iron stores become inadequate for the needs of normal erythropoiesis. Body iron stores must be exhausted before red cell production is restricted; therefore, anemia occurs at a late stage of iron deficiency. In its fully developed form, iron-deficient erythropoiesis is characterized by hypochromia and microcytosis of the circulating erythrocytes, low plasma iron and ferritin concentrations, and a transferrin saturation of about 15 per cent or less. Iron deficiency anemia is a sign of disease and is not in itself a complete diagnosis.

PREVALENCE. Iron deficiency is the most common cause of anemia throughout the world, although it is difficult to define its prevalence precisely. In parts of Africa and India, where marginal dietary intake and excessive iron loss due to intestinal parasites are present together, over half the population may suffer from iron deficiency anemia.

In most developed countries, about 3 per cent of men, 20 per cent of women, and over 50 per cent of pregnant women are deficient in iron, as judged by plasma iron levels. As judged by serum ferritin levels, iron stores are greatly reduced in about 25 per cent of children, 30 per cent of adolescents, 30 per cent of menstruating women, 60 per cent of pregnant women, and 3 per cent of men.

IRON METABOLISM. The total iron content of a healthy human subject remains within relatively narrow limits. Loss of iron from the body is precisely matched by absorption of iron from food. Iron loss is not due to "excretion" in the usual sense but rather to loss of intact cells containing iron. Epithelial cells

TABLE 131-2. CLASSIFICATION OF ANEMIAS CHARACTERIZED BY DEFICIENT HEMOGLOBIN SYNTHESIS AND THE PRESENCE OF HYPOCHROMIC ERYTHROCYTES

I. Disorders of iron metabolism
  A. Iron deficiency anemia
  B. Anemia of chronic disease
  C. Hereditary atransferrinemia
  D. Congenital hypochromic-microcytic anemia with iron overload (Shahidi-Nathan-Diamond syndrome)
II. Disorders of porphyrin and heme synthesis: sideroblastic anemias
  A. Acquired sideroblastic anemias
    1. Idiopathic refractory sideroblastic anemia
    2. Complicating other diseases
    3. Associated with drugs or toxins—ethanol, INH, lead
  B. Hereditary sideroblastic anemias
    1. X chromosome–linked
    2. Autosomal recessive
III. Disorders of globin synthesis
  A. The thalassemias (Ch. 136)
  B. Hemoglobinopathies characterized by unstable hemoglobins (Ch. 136)

from the gastrointestinal and urinary tracts, and from the skin, account for the normal daily iron loss in men of about 1 mg. In women, menstrual flow, childbearing, and lactation are additional routes of iron loss.

The body iron content in normal adult men is about 50 to 55 mg per kilogram of body weight and in women is about 35 to 40 mg per kilogram. This difference reflects the high incidence of iron deficiency in women and does not indicate any fundamental differences in iron metabolism between the sexes. Most of the body iron is found in hemoglobin, with smaller amounts in myoglobin and iron storage compounds (Table 131-3). Only a minute portion is found in plasma, where it is bound to transferrin.

The metabolism of iron is dominated by its role in hemoglobin synthesis. Iron incorporated into hemoglobin is utilized over and over again through an internal cycle, the *iron cycle* (Fig. 131-1). The plasma iron compartment, in which iron is bound to the transport protein transferrin, is central to this cycle. Iron moves from the plasma to erythroid precursor cells in the marrow. These cells synthesize hemoglobin and, with maturation, are released into the circulation. At the end of their 120-day lifespan, the red cells are ingested by macrophages, principally in the splenic sinusoids, and the iron is extracted from hemoglobin by the enzyme heme oxygenase. A small portion of this iron is stored in macrophages as ferritin, but most is returned to the plasma, where it becomes bound to transferrin, completing the cycle. In the normal adult male about 30 mg of iron completes the iron cycle daily. One to 2 mg of iron leaves the plasma daily and enters the liver and other tissues, where it is utilized for the synthesis of other hemoproteins such as cytochromes and myoglobin.

ABSORPTION. The average intake of iron in the meat-containing diet in the United States is about 10 to 30 mg per day, but much greater variations occur in different parts of the world. Only 5 to 10 per cent of dietary iron (about 1 mg) is absorbed daily to balance precisely the amount lost. The amount of iron absorbed can increase up to fivefold if body iron stores are depleted or if erythropoiesis is accelerated. The amount absorbed decreases in states of iron overload or if there is erythroid hypoplasia. Total body iron balance is thus regulated at the absorptive step; the precise mechanism by which this control is accomplished has not been defined. Iron is absorbed chiefly in portions of the intestine proximal to the mid-jejunum, and very little is absorbed in more caudal intestinal segments.

Iron is absorbed by two distinct pathways in humans, one for iron in heme and the other for iron in ferrous and ferric iron salts. Heme iron is derived from the hemoglobin, myoglobin, and other heme proteins in foods of animal origin. Exposure to the acid and proteases of gastric juice liberates the heme from its apoprotein. Heme is rapidly taken up by gastrointestinal epithelial cells, and the iron is made available by enzymatic degradation of the porphyrin macrocycle. The absorption of heme iron is influenced very little by other dietary components.

The "bioavailability" of nonheme dietary iron, however, varies greatly. Availability is dependent on the oxidation state and solubility of the iron and the presence of chelating substances in the diet. Factors modifying the form in which iron is presented to the intestinal mucosal cell play an important role in the amount of iron that can be absorbed. At the acidic pH normally found in the stomach, both ferrous and ferric iron are soluble. Patients who have undergone gastrectomy, or who are achlorhydric for other reasons, demonstrate impaired absorption of iron. In the duodenum, as the pH rises, ferric iron is readily converted to

TABLE 131-3. DISTRIBUTION OF IRON IN THE BODY

Compound	Iron Content (mg) Men (70 kg)	Iron Content (mg) Women (50 kg)	Per Cent of Total Body Iron Men	Per Cent of Total Body Iron Women
Hemoglobin	2670	1500	69.6	73.1
Myoglobin	350	220	9.1	10.7
Heme enzymes	8	7	0.2	0.3
Transferrin	6	5	0.2	0.2
Ferritin-hemosiderin	800	320	20.9	15.7
Total	3834	2052	100.0	100.0

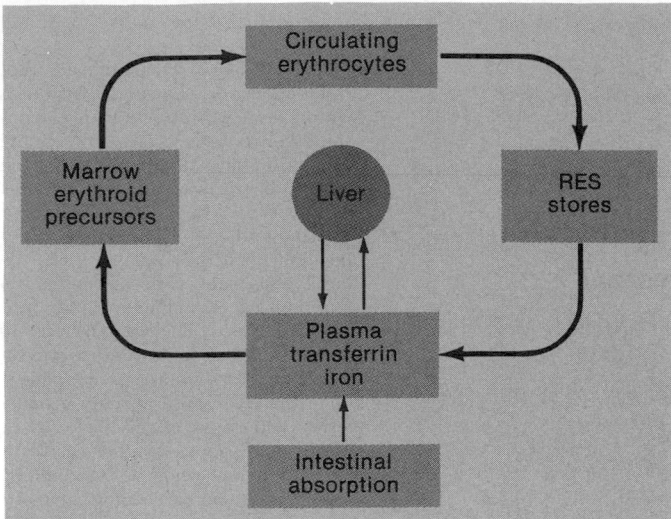

FIGURE 131–1. The internal iron cycle. In the plasma, iron bound to transferrin is transported to the marrow where it is transferred to developing red blood cells and incorporated into hemoglobin. The mature red blood cells are released into the circulation and after 120 days are ingested by macrophages in the reticuloendothelial system (RES). Here the iron is extracted from hemoglobin and returned to plasma, completing the cycle.

insoluble ferric hydroxides. Agents such as ascorbic acid may promote iron absorption by reducing some ferric iron to ferrous iron, which remains soluble at neutral pH. Dietary constituents such as citrate may enhance the solubility of inorganic iron and hence enhance absorption. Phytates, neutral detergent fibers, and other substances present in cereals, grain, and corn impair iron absorption by binding iron as relatively insoluble complexes.

The clinical significance of the various luminal factors that influence iron absorption may be minimal in U.S. society, where the diet provides relatively large amounts of heme iron. In developing countries, however, diets are generally characterized by low meat content and high content of grains and vegetables. Such diets, with low heme iron content and high content of substances that impair nonheme iron absorption, may not meet the iron demands of many individuals. The manipulation of dietary iron content by large-scale iron supplementation programs has been instituted in both developed and underdeveloped countries. The incidence of iron deficiency in the population is decreased by such programs, but the risks to individuals predisposed to iron loading remain to be determined (Ch. 193).

The uptake of iron from the intestinal lumen is both energy dependent and regulated. The uptake of ^{59}Fe by duodenal mucosal cells in iron-deficient individuals exceeds that in normal subjects by twofold or threefold. Although correction of the anemia in iron-deficient subjects by red cell transfusion does not decrease iron uptake, repletion of body iron stores restores the kinetics of iron uptake to normal. Once iron enters the mucosal cell, it must be transported to the serosal surface of the intestine, where iron enters the plasma. Iron within the mucosal cell can have two fates. One is to be incorporated into ferritin within the cytosol of the mucosal cell. Most ferritin iron does not ultimately reach the plasma but is lost from the body when the intestinal mucosal cell is sloughed after its 3- to 4-day lifespan. Iron not incorporated into mucosal cell ferritin is transported across the cell and ultimately appears in plasma as ferric iron bound to transferrin. The process of intracellular transport is unclear. Although transferrin plays a central role in transporting iron from sites of entry into plasma to tissue sites of utilization, it may not play an important role in iron absorption. Rare patients with congenital atransferrinemia show no evidence of deficient iron absorption.

TRANSPORT. Transferrin, the iron transport protein in plasma, is a glycoprotein with an approximate molecular weight of 80,000. The liver is the major source of transferrin synthesis, and the protein is equally distributed in the intravascular and extravascular spaces. Transferrin is capable of binding two iron atoms in the ferric state. In normal subjects the plasma

concentration of transferrin is about 2.5 to 3.0 grams per liter. Plasma transferrin is usually quantified in terms of the amount of iron it will bind, a measure called the *total iron-binding capacity* (TIBC). In normal subjects only about one third of the available transferrin binding sites are occupied (transferrin saturation = 33 per cent). Plasma iron concentration varies diurnally, with the highest values in the morning and the lowest in the evening, but no diurnal variation occurs in the TIBC. Transferrin has no known function other than as a transport protein and is reused for many cycles of iron transport. With the exception of very small amounts of iron in ferritin, all the iron in plasma is carried by transferrin. The affinity of transferrin for iron is sufficiently high that, theoretically, less than one free iron atom might be present in a liter of blood.

CELLULAR UPTAKE. The initial event in the transfer of iron to cells is binding of diferric transferrin to specific, high-affinity receptors on the cell surface. When receptors are lost because of cell maturation (as occurs in developing erythrocytes in vivo) or artificial manipulations in vitro, the ability of the cell to take up iron from transferrin is lost. Cellular iron uptake is directly proportional to the number of transferrin cell-surface receptors. The biosynthesis of hemoglobin by erythroid cells has a high iron requirement, and the human reticulocyte may have as many as 300,000 receptors per cell. Developing erythroid cells in the bone marrow may have even more.

In the process of iron uptake by cells, the transferrin receptor–diferric transferrin complex is internalized into an acidic, nonlysosomal vesicle (Fig. 131–2). At the acidic pH of the vesicle, iron is readily dissociated from diferric transferrin, but the resulting apotransferrin remains bound to the receptor. The transferrin receptor–apotransferrin complex is transported back to the cell surface, where, at neutral pH, the apotransferrin is liberated and becomes available for another cycle of iron binding and release.

Once iron enters the cell, two events occur. One is the delivery of iron to the mitochondria, where it is enzymatically incorporated into protoporphyrin to form heme. The other is the incorporation of iron into ferritin. Ferritin iron is a storage form of iron and is probably not utilized by the cell for heme synthesis. Ferritin iron may, however, be recycled for use by other cells.

STORAGE. Iron-free apoferritin is a spherical protein made up of 24 subunits that surround a central cavity. The central cavity of each apoferritin molecule can potentially store more than 4000 molecules of iron. When iron is present in the central cavity, the protein is termed ferritin. The importance of ferritin as an iron storage compound is emphasized by the wide distribution of structurally similar ferritins in both plant and animal tissues. Two different ferritin subunits exist, termed H (the major subunit of heart ferritin) and L (the major subunit of liver ferritin). These may be present in differing quantities within a given ferritin molecule, leading to heterogeneity. The H and L subunits are derived from different genetic loci.

Ferritin meets the requirement of cells for an efficient form of iron storage. It has a large capacity to store iron, maintains a reserve storage capacity (few ferritin molecules are iron replete), and can quickly both take up and release iron. Ferritin aggregates are visible by light microscopy in developing erythroid cells when bone marrow smears are stained with Prussian blue. These "siderotic granules" are found in the cytosol of normal developing erythroblasts and are absent in erythroblasts obtained from subjects with iron deficiency anemia (see Color Plate 5L).

Small amounts of iron-poor ferritin (mostly apoferritin) circulate in plasma and can be accurately measured by a widely available radioimmunoassay. Under most conditions, the concentration of ferritin in the plasma correlates directly with body iron stores. Normal values range from 12 to 325 ng per milliliter, with a mean of about 125 ng for men and 55 ng for women. The concentration of ferritin in iron-deficient individuals is less than 10 ng per milliliter, whereas in individuals with iron overload, the concentration is proportional to the increase in tissue storage iron.

Hemosiderin is an insoluble iron aggregate with a ratio of iron to protein that is high. It is derived from ferritin; however, the reactions leading from ferritin to hemosiderin have not been resolved. Iron in hemosiderin disappears from tissues after repeated venesections, but the mechanism by which iron is mobilized is unknown.

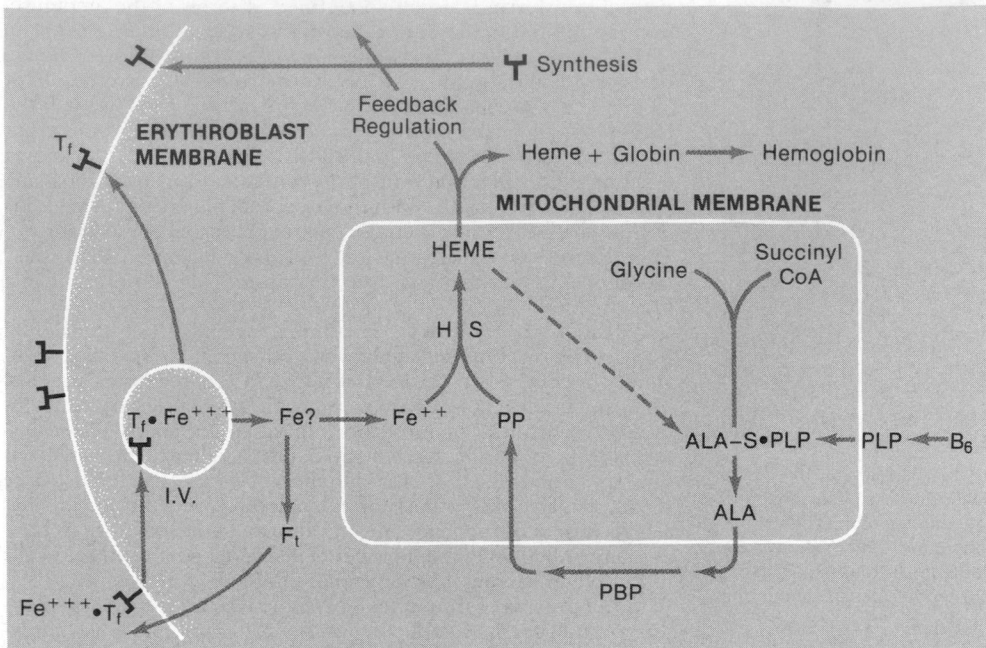

FIGURE 131–2. Diagrammatic representation of heme biosynthesis within the erythroblast. The relationships between the iron pathway, the porphyrin biosynthetic pathway, the vitamin B_6 pathway, and the synthesis of transferrin receptors are illustrated. The biosynthesis of porphyrins is dependent upon the availability of pyridoxal phosphate as a cofactor at the rate-limiting Δ-aminolevulinic acid synthase step. The biosynthesis of heme requires both protoporphyrin and iron. Iron uptake is dependent upon the interaction of diferric transferrin with high affinity cell-surface receptors. Receptor synthesis is regulated by heme; when heme synthesis is impaired, more receptors are synthesized and the cell takes up more iron. T_f = transferrin ⊤ receptors for diferric T_f; I.V. = the acidic, non-lysosomal intermediate vesicle; Fe^{+++} = ferric iron; PP = protoporphyrin; PBP = porphyrin biosynthetic pathway; ALA = Δ-aminolevulinic acid; ALA-s = Δ-aminolevulinic acid synthase; PLP = pyridoxal-5'-phosphate; and B_6 = vitamin B_6.

THE MACROPHAGE. While net iron uptake occurs through the intestinal mucosa, most transferrin-bound iron (over 95 per cent) reflects iron recycled from damaged or aged red blood cells by macrophages in the spleen and other organs. Within the macrophage, the membrane of ingested erythrocytes is disrupted and the iron in hemoglobin is oxidized to the trivalent state, forming methemoglobin. The heme and globin are dissociated, and the iron is liberated from hemin (ferric-protoporphyrin) by the microsomal enzyme heme oxygenase, yielding iron and biliverdin. To meet a variable demand for iron, macrophages maintain a storage pool in ferritin and hemosiderin. Under normal conditions, the amount of iron entering the macrophage approximates that leaving, and there is little interchange between iron newly liberated from hemin and iron in the storage pool. Iron from recently destroyed erythrocytes passes quickly through the macrophage and appears in the plasma bound to transferrin.

When the red cell mass is expanding and erythrocytes are being produced more rapidly than they are being destroyed (e.g., following an acute hemorrhage), iron is mobilized from macrophages. The amount of iron leaving the macrophage under these conditions exceeds that entering. When red cell destruction exceeds production (e.g., in aplastic anemia), the amount of iron entering the macrophage exceeds that leaving and iron is deposited in stores. The control mechanism coupling the rate at which iron leaves the macrophage to the rate of erythrocyte production is unknown. Mobilization of iron from the storage pool is interfered with by infection, inflammation, and malignancy; such interference may be responsible for the anemia associated with chronic disease (see Color Plate 5H, left).

FERROKINETICS. Ferrokinetic studies, based on tracking ^{59}Fe as it moves from the plasma transferrin to the bone marrow and into circulating erythrocytes, make it possible to assess rates of both effective erythropoiesis and ineffective erythropoiesis. The term *ineffective erythropoiesis* refers to the production of defective erythrocytes that are destroyed before they leave the marrow (or very shortly thereafter). A small proportion of erythropoiesis is ineffective even in normal subjects, but in conditions such as megaloblastic anemia, thalassemia, and sideroblastic anemias, ineffective erythropoiesis becomes greatly exaggerated. The plasma ^{59}Fe disappearance, expressed as the half-life ($t\frac{1}{2}$), is normally between 60 and 120 minutes. More rapid disappearance (a shorter $t\frac{1}{2}$) is found in iron deficiency and conditions with accelerated erythropoiesis (such as polycythemia and hemolytic anemias). A long $t\frac{1}{2}$ indicates erythroid hypoplasia. The *plasma iron transport* (PIT) rate is a measure of the rate at which iron

leaves the plasma. The PIT is a good index of total erythropoiesis, whether effective or ineffective. The PIT correlates well with the total nucleated red cell mass and the rate of red cell production. However, when erythropoiesis is reduced, or when the degree of transferrin saturation is high, the interpretation of the PIT is complicated by transfer of iron to tissues other than marrow.

The *erythrocyte iron turnover* (EIT) rate measures the rate at which iron moves from marrow to circulating red cells and correlates well with the reticulocyte index.

The *marrow transit time* (MTT) evaluates the responsiveness of the marrow to erythropoietin. In general, there is an inverse correlation between the MTT and the degree of erythropoietic stimulation. In situations characterized by an appropriate marrow response to anemia, the MTT may be less than 24 hours.

Ferrokinetic measurements are useful for clinical and investigational purposes but are only approximations. Sophisticated computer analysis of plasma iron disappearance curves, coupled with body surface counting over the liver, spleen, and sacrum, may yield a more accurate assessment of the rates at which iron moves through the iron cycle, but such analyses are not routinely employed for clinical purposes.

PATHOGENESIS. Iron deficiency comes about as a late manifestation of prolonged negative iron balance caused by one or a combination of the following factors: inadequate dietary intake, malabsorption, blood loss, repeated pregnancies, and rapid growth during childhood. As daily iron loss under normal conditions is very small (about 1 mg), assigning the cause of iron deficiency in adults to inadequate intake or malabsorption implies chronicity measured in years. Iron losses that occur from the gastrointestinal tract or through excessive menstrual bleeding are far more important factors. Factors leading to negative iron balance can be divided into two broad categories: decreased iron uptake and increased iron loss (Table 131–4).

Decreased Iron Uptake. The daily dietary iron requirement for healthy adult men is about 5 to 10 mg. For premenopausal women the daily dietary requirement is higher, roughly 7 to 20 mg per day. In the United States the average diet contains about 6 mg per 1000 calories. The average man therefore consumes more iron than needed, but many women subsist on a marginal iron uptake. Because of the adequacy of their diets and their larger iron stores, men in the United States rarely develop iron deficiency solely on the basis of an inadequate dietary intake of iron. Even in women, some factor in addition to poor diet is usually necessary before overt anemia develops.

Gastric acid facilitates the absorption of ferric iron in the diet

TABLE 131–4. FACTORS PRODUCING NEGATIVE IRON BALANCE AND IRON DEFICIENCY

I. **Decreased iron uptake**
  A. Inadequate diet
  B. Impaired absorption
    1. Achlorhydria
    2. Gastric surgery
    3. Celiac disease
    4. Pica

II. **Increased iron loss**
  A. Gastrointestinal bleeding (Ch. 111)
    1. Neoplasm
    2. Duodenal and gastric ulcers
    3. Hiatal hernia
    4. Gastritis from salicylates, other drugs, or toxins
    5. Diverticulosis
    6. Ulcerative colitis and regional enteritis
    7. Hookworm
    8. Meckel's diverticulum
    9. Hemorrhoids
    10. Arteriovenous malformations
  B. Menometrorrhagia
  C. Repeated blood donations
  D. Repeated pregnancies
  E. Hemoglobinuria due to chronic intravascular hemolysis
  F. Hereditary hemorrhagic telangiectasia
  G. Idiopathic pulmonary hemosiderosis
  H. Disorders of hemostasis

(although it has little effect on heme iron or ferrous iron), and iron deficiency is a frequent complication following gastric operations. Additional factors that impair iron absorption after gastrectomy include rapid intestinal transit and bypass of the most active sites of iron absorption in the duodenum (as occurs in the Billroth II or Polya procedures). Malabsorption of iron may also occur in patients with adult celiac disease, and rarely iron deficiency anemia may be the dominant manifestation of celiac disease.

Impaired absorption of iron because of interactions with food substances such as phytates and vegetable fibers has been discussed. The ingestion of unusual substances, a practice known as *pica*, may also impair iron absorption. Although pica may be a manifestation of iron deficiency, in certain cultural groups the compulsive ingestion of substances such as clay (geophagia) or starch (amylophagia) may lead to iron deficiency. Clay interferes with iron absorption by acting in the gut as an ion exchange resin. Laundry starch is a carbohydrate with a very low iron content. When it is consumed in large quantities to the exclusion of other foods, a dietary deficiency of iron results.

Increased Iron Loss. Gastrointestinal bleeding is by far the most common cause of iron deficiency in men and is second only to menstrual loss as a cause in women. Repeated pregnancies without iron supplementation are a less common cause of iron deficiency in women.

Although any hemorrhagic lesion of the gastrointestinal tract may cause iron deficiency (Table 131–4), those most likely to do so are associated with chronic occult bleeding and the steady loss of small amounts of blood. To estimate the effect of blood loss on iron balance, it is convenient to consider that 1.0 ml of blood contains about 0.4 mg of iron. A steady blood loss of as little as 4 to 5 ml per day (1.6 to 2.0 mg of iron) can result in negative iron balance and depletion of iron stores over several years. Failure to detect occult blood in the stool, even after repetitive testing, does not exclude gastrointestinal blood loss as the cause of iron deficiency. *Iron deficiency in men and in postmenopausal women must be considered to result from blood loss unless some other cause can be proved.* This is a critical dictum because iron deficiency anemia may be the first sign of a cancer of the gastrointestinal tract, and the anemia may lead to the diagnosis when the tumor is in an operable stage. Carcinoma of the cecum, for example, is often clinically silent until the symptoms of anemia appear.

Blood loss from erosive gastritis due to aspirin ingestion is a frequent cause of iron deficiency. Chronic ingestion of as few as two aspirin tablets daily may lead to blood loss of up to 4.5 ml per day.

CLINICAL MANIFESTATIONS. Iron deficiency anemia is not a disease; it is a sign of disease. In some patients, iron deficiency anemia is discovered incidentally when the presenting signs and symptoms are those of the disease that led to the deficiency. In some patients, signs and symptoms of both the underlying disease and the iron deficiency are found together. In others, only the symptoms of iron deficiency are present, and the disease leading to the deficiency is occult.

The onset of iron deficiency anemia is insidious, and the progression of symptoms is gradual. Patients are often able to accommodate quite well to the anemia and may continue to perform strenuous work with few symptoms. Fatigue, irritability, palpitations, dizziness, breathlessness, and headache are all common complaints of symptomatic individuals with anemia of any type and do not in themselves suggest iron deficiency as the cause of the anemia. However, some clinical findings do specifically suggest the presence of iron deficiency.

Chlorosis, a peculiar greenish pallor of iron-deficient adolescent girls, was frequently described in the decades between 1890 and 1910, although now is rarely noted. Oral lesions associated with iron deficiency include angular stomatitis (ulcerations or fissures at the corners of the mouth), atrophy of the lingual papillae, and varying degrees of glossitis. *Ozena* (chronic atrophy of the nasal mucosa associated with a foul-smelling discharge) occurs in some patients with iron deficiency anemia, particularly in southeastern Europe. Thinning and flattening of nails and finally the development of spoon-shaped nails (koilonychia) have been described in patients with advanced iron deficiency.

The association of dysphagia, angular stomatitis, and lingual abnormalities with iron deficiency anemia (Plummer-Vinson or Paterson-Kelly syndrome) is rarely noted in the United States but is quite common in Great Britain and Scandinavia. The dysphagia is due to the development of a mucosal web at the juncture of the hypopharynx and esophagus. Multiple webs may develop, usually extending from the anterior wall of the esophagus into the lumen. Occasionally, they may encircle the lumen, forming a cufflike structure. In other patients a stricture with or without a web may be found, drastically constricting the opening into the esophagus at the level of the cricoid cartilage. Relief of the dysphagia requires rupturing of the webs or dilatation of the stenosis, because repletion of the iron stores alone is not effective. Other gastrointestinal complaints, such as anorexia, pyrosis, flatulence, nausea, belching, and constipation, are common in association with advanced iron deficiency anemia.

Pica, as already mentioned, can be a cause of iron deficiency but it also may be a striking manifestation of iron deficiency. The ingestion of ice (pagophagia) is particularly common. Many patients compulsively eat one or other food items; oddly, the object of the unnatural dietary craving usually contains very little iron.

The spleen is slightly enlarged in about 10 per cent of patients with iron deficiency anemia. There are no specific pathologic changes in the organ, and the splenomegaly recedes with correction of the iron deficiency. Neuralgic pains, numbness, and tingling without objective neurologic abnormalities are reported by 15 to 30 per cent of patients, and rarely iron deficiency anemia may lead to increased intracranial pressure, papilledema, and the clinical picture of pseudotumor cerebri.

LABORATORY FINDINGS. The degree of anemia is variable and depends upon the duration of iron-limited erythropoiesis. Because of the hypochromia, the hemoglobin concentration is usually reduced to a greater degree than the hematocrit. The mean corpuscular volume (MCV), mean corpuscular hemoglobin (MCH), and mean corpuscular hemoglobin concentration (MCHC) are all usually reduced. The degree of change in the red cell indices is related to both the duration and the severity of the anemia. Average values for patients with hemoglobin concentrations of 8 to 9 grams per deciliter are MCV of 74 fl, MCHC of 28 grams per deciliter, and MCH of 20 pg.

A well-stained blood smear reveals an increase in the area of central pallor in the individual red corpuscles (hypochromia), microcytes, and marked variations in cell size (anisocytosis) and shape (poikilocytosis) (Fig. 131–3 and Color Plate 5K). The plasma iron concentration is generally less than 50 μg per deciliter, and the plasma TIBC (the transferrin concentration) is greater than 350 μg per deciliter. As a result, the transferrin saturation is less

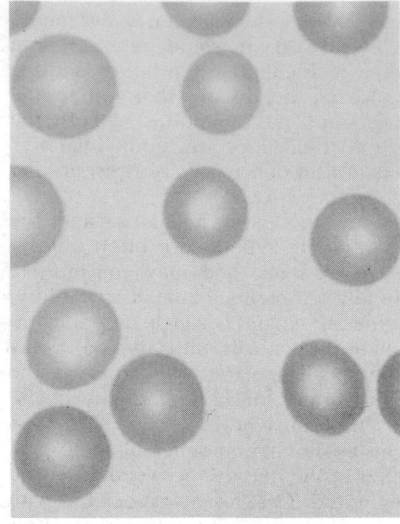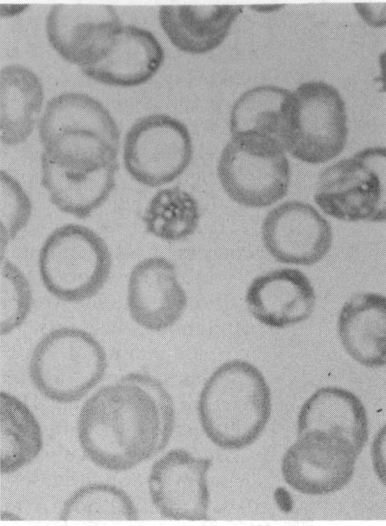

FIGURE 131–3. Blood smear from a patient with advanced iron deficiency anemia (*right*) and from a normal subject (*left*). The red cells from the iron-deficient subject are poorly hemoglobinized (hypochromic), are smaller than normal (microcytic), and vary in size and shape (anisocytosis and poikilocytosis). (Wright's stain, ×1000.)

than 15 per cent. The plasma ferritin concentration is generally less than 10 ng per milliliter. The last enzymatic reaction leading to the biosynthesis of heme (the ferrochelatase or heme synthase reaction) requires both iron and protoporphyrin as substrates. In iron deficiency excess protoporphyrin accumulates in the developing erythrocyte and is retained by the circulating erythrocytes. As a result, the free erythrocyte protoporphyrin (FEP) is increased, generally about five times normal (normal range, 30 to 80 μg per deciliter of red cells).

Both the percentage and the absolute number of reticulocytes are usually normal. The osmotic fragility of the erythrocytes may be normal, but more often there is increased resistance to hemolysis in hypotonic salt solutions. Although the leukocyte count is usually normal, in very chronic iron deficiency a slight decrease in the absolute number of granulocytes may be seen. The platelet count is usually elevated to levels of about two to three times normal and returns to normal after therapy. Rarely, in severe, longstanding iron deficiency anemia, mild thrombocytopenia may be noted.

Examination of the bone marrow is generally not required to establish a diagnosis of iron deficiency anemia. An exception is the clinical situation when suspected iron deficiency coexists with a chronic disease. Although anemias associated with chronic disease may mimic iron deficiency (see below), they can be distinguished by examination of the marrow. In iron deficiency the marrow is usually normocellular and there is mild erythroid hyperplasia. Macrophage iron is absent or severely reduced. Fewer than 10 per cent of the marrow normoblasts contain siderotic granules visible with Prussian blue staining. In the anemia of chronic disease, macrophage iron stores are normal or increased; however, as in iron deficiency, very few normoblasts contain siderotic granules.

The sequence of laboratory changes in slowly developing iron deficiency is fairly predictable. Initially, as iron stores are depleted, the serum ferritin concentration falls. At the earliest stage of iron deficiency, the transferrin concentration rises, the plasma iron concentration falls, and the FEP increases. When anemia first appears, the morphology of the circulating erythrocytes and the erythrocyte indices are generally normal. As the anemia progresses, the morphology becomes clearly hypochromic and microcytic, and the indices reflect this.

TREATMENT. *Every effort must be made to recognize and, if possible, correct the underlying cause.* This should be possible in most patients. A simpler goal is correcting the anemia and replenishing body iron stores.

Iron is highly effective in treating iron deficiency but has no other legitimate therapeutic use. Iron exerts no beneficial effect on any of the anemias not caused by iron deficiency. A large number of preparations containing iron have been promoted for the oral treatment of iron deficiency, but none has any advantage over simple ferrous salts (ferrous sulfate, ferrous gluconate, and ferrous fumarate). Ferrous sulfate is the standard preparation for oral use. A daily dose of about 200 mg of elemental iron produces an optimal response. This dose is achieved with three ferrous sulfate tablets (each tablet contains 60 mg of elemental iron) given in divided doses with or just after a meal. Iron is best absorbed when the stomach is empty, but gastric irritation is extremely common when iron is taken this way. In spite of some reduction in absorption when iron is taken with meals, the gain in patient compliance is worth this slight disadvantage. Enteric-coated preparations, designed to reduce gastric irritation by retarding dissolution of the iron, cannot be recommended because with them the most actively absorbing regions of the intestine are bypassed and absorption is markedly reduced. Although large doses of ascorbic or succinic acid increase iron absorption as much as 20 to 30 per cent, they add greatly to the expense of therapy.

Some patients given oral iron therapy complain of gastrointestinal symptoms (nausea, epigastric pain, cramps, diarrhea); however, it is rare that these symptoms are severe enough to require discontinuation of therapy. Gastric symptoms appear to be dose related, and patients intolerant of full therapeutic doses may be able to take a dose of 120 mg per day. Gastric symptoms may be minimized by gradually increasing the dose during the first week of therapy. Regardless of the form of oral therapy used, it is important to continue treatment for 6 to 12 months after the anemia has been corrected. The prolonged therapy allows for repletion of iron stores.

When adequate doses of iron are given, there is often a rapid subjective improvement with a reduction of fatigue, lassitude, and other nonspecific symptoms. This response may occur within 2 or 3 days, before any evidence of a hematologic response can be detected. An increase in the number of reticulocytes is the first sign of hematologic response, and a maximal value of 5 to 10 per cent is usually achieved after about 10 days of therapy. The height of the reticulocyte peak and the rate of hemoglobin regeneration are proportional to the severity of the anemia. With only slight to moderate degrees of anemia, a pronounced reticulocyte response cannot be expected. Although the hemoglobin concentration increases more rapidly at low levels than at high, it takes about 2 months to reach normal values regardless of the starting level.

It is not rare to encounter patients said to have iron deficiency anemia unresponsive to oral iron therapy. The following possible explanations for failure to respond to iron should be considered: (1) The diagnosis is incorrect and the anemia is not due to iron deficiency; (2) a complicating illness is present that dampens the expected response to iron therapy; (3) the patient failed to take the iron preparation as prescribed; (4) an ineffective iron preparation was prescribed; (5) the patient is continuing to lose iron in excess of intake; and rarely (6) there is malabsorption of iron.

Parenteral iron therapy should be reserved for patients who

(1) are unable to tolerate iron compounds given orally, (2) repeatedly fail to heed instructions or are incapable of following them, (3) are losing blood at a rate too rapid to be compensated for by oral iron intake, (4) have a disorder such as ulcerative colitis or regional enteritis in which symptoms may be aggravated by oral iron therapy, or (5) are unable to absorb iron from the gastrointestinal tract.

Iron-dextran complex (Imferon) containing 50 mg of iron per milliliter is the preparation of choice for parenteral administration. The total dose required to correct the anemia and to replenish stores can be calculated by the following formula:

$$\text{Iron to be injected (mg)} = [15 - \text{patient's Hb (gm/dl)}] \times \text{body weight (kg)} \times 3$$

Iron-dextran can be given intramuscularly or intravenously. Intravenous administration does not appear to have a higher incidence of adverse effects than the intramuscular route. Anaphylactic reactions are rare (0.1 to 0.6 per cent), but fever, arthralgia, myalgia, and regional adenopathy occur in about 5 per cent of patients. Intramuscular injections should be made into the upper outer quadrant of the buttock, and the skin displaced laterally prior to injection to prevent staining of the skin by reflux of the dark-brown iron solution along the injection path. A test dose of 0.5 ml should be given initially to test for hypersensitivity. Generally, 2.5 ml is injected into each buttock (total of 5 ml or 250 mg of iron) daily. Intravenous administration permits larger doses to be given in a single injection; thus, the discomfort and inconvenience of repeated intramuscular injections can be avoided. After testing for hypersensitivity, 10 ml (500 mg of iron) of undiluted iron-dextran may be administered over about a 5-minute period. In Great Britain and Europe, it is usual to administer the entire dose calculated by the formula in a single intravenous infusion. A 1:20 dilution of iron-dextran in saline is prepared and administered at an initial flow rate of 20 drops per minute. After 5 minutes, if no side effects are observed, the rate is increased to 40 to 60 drops per minute. Dextrose solutions should not be used as a diluent because the incidence of superficial phlebitis may be as high as 25 per cent with this vehicle.

PROGNOSIS. The prognosis in iron deficiency relates only to the underlying disorder causing the anemia. Patients rarely, if ever, die of iron deficiency anemia itself, but they may die of the underlying cause. Recurrence of iron deficiency anemia after treatment is common, emphasizing the importance of identifying and effectively treating the cause of the iron deficiency.

HYPOCHROMIC ANEMIAS NOT CAUSED BY IRON DEFICIENCY

Once iron deficiency has been excluded as the cause of a hypochromic anemia, a limited number of diagnostic possibilities remain. A presumptive diagnosis is generally possible after analysis of the history and physical examination and the basic hematologic parameters. If the diagnosis remains obscure, a useful approach is to segregate the diagnostic possibilities on the basis of an accurate determination of the serum iron level. When the serum iron is reduced to levels at which the transferrin saturation is less than about 15 per cent, only iron deficiency and the anemia of chronic disease need be considered.

Hypochromic anemias due to defects in globin biosynthesis (the thalassemias and hemoglobinopathies characterized by unstable hemoglobins) are discussed in Ch. 136.

THE ANEMIA OF CHRONIC DISEASE

The anemia of chronic disease is not always hypochromic; however, because of its association with hypoferremia, it is best discussed under the heading of hypochromic anemias. Although the anemia of chronic disease is usually normocytic and normochromic, hypochromia and even microcytosis may be the dominant morphologic abnormalities. When microcytosis is present, it is usually not as marked as in iron deficiency. The MCV rarely falls below 72 fl.

DEFINITION. A mild to moderate anemia frequently accompanies chronic infections, inflammatory diseases such as rheumatoid arthritis, and cancers. Since these are so common, the anemia of chronic disease is frequently encountered and may be second only to iron deficiency anemia in overall incidence. The anemia of chronic disease is defined by the presence of a chronic disease, anemia, and hypoferremia despite abundant quantities of iron in macrophage stores.

ETIOLOGY AND PATHOGENESIS. Three factors seem to interact in the pathogenesis of the anemia: (1) impaired flow of iron from macrophages to plasma, (2) decreased erythrocyte lifespan, and (3) inadequate marrow response to the mild hemolysis.

Characteristically, the serum iron level is decreased, TIBC is reduced (a point often useful in differentiating the anemia from iron deficiency anemia), and transferrin saturation is subnormal. Injection of ^{59}Fe-labeled red cells (or labeled hemoglobin) reveals rapid clearance by reticuloendothelial cells but defective reutilization of the iron for new hemoglobin synthesis. In bone marrow aspirates stained for iron, there is an increase in hemosiderin and ferritin in the macrophages; however, the number of red cell precursors containing siderotic granules is reduced. A decrease in the amount of iron available for heme biosynthesis results in the production of hypochromic erythrocytes and, as in iron deficiency, an increase in FEP to levels of three to five times normal. In contrast to iron deficiency anemia, in the anemia of chronic disease, the FEP increases slowly and does not become clearly abnormal until significant anemia has developed. Humoral factors are probably involved in the pathogenesis of the abnormal iron metabolism. These factors include the cytokines interleukin 1, interleukin 6, and tumor necrosis factor–alpha (TNF-α). TNF-α, when injected into humans, produces the abnormalities of iron metabolism that characterize the anemia of chronic disease. It is not known if this is a direct effect or an indirect effect mediated through other factors produced in response to TNF-α.

The erythrocyte lifespan is about 80 days rather than the normal 120 days. When red cells from a patient with the anemia of chronic disease are transfused into normal subjects, they survive normally. Conversely, normal red cells have a shortened survival when transfused into patients with anemia. This finding suggests that an extracorpuscular factor is involved in the pathogenesis of the hemolysis. However, no such factor has yet been identified. Normally, the bone marrow should be able to compensate for such a modest reduction in erythrocyte survival. Failure of the marrow to do so implies that impaired production capacity is important in the pathogenesis of the anemia. The marrow response to anemia is under the control of erythropoietin. In patients with the anemia of chronic disorders, erythropoietin levels are usually lower than expected for the degree of anemia. The marrow, however, is capable of responding appropriately to erythropoietin when the hormone is injected or when erythropoietin production is stimulated by hypoxia or cobalt administration. The precise mechanism causing failure of erythropoietin release in response to the slowly developing anemia is unknown.

The three basic abnormalities are interrelated in the pathogenesis of the anemia. For example, the response to erythropoietin suggests that the hormone directly or indirectly affects the block in iron metabolism. It appears that balance is eventually reached among the three factors, and thus the anemia is only mild to moderate and does not generally progress to the point at which transfusion therapy is required.

CLINICAL MANIFESTATIONS. Because this type of anemia occurs in association with so many diseases, the clinical manifestations vary widely. Although the signs and symptoms of the underlying disorder usually overshadow those of the anemia, in occasional patients the anemia is the first sign of the underlying disease.

DIAGNOSIS. The anemia develops during the first few months of the underlying illness and rarely progresses thereafter. The hematocrit generally remains constant in a range between 25 and 40 per cent. The red cell morphology is usually normal, as is the reticulocyte count. The characteristic iron determinations are a transferrin saturation less than 15 per cent and a normal serum ferritin level. In the marrow the number of erythroid precursors containing cytoplasmic iron granules (sideroblasts) is decreased, but reticuloendothelial cells contain normal or increased iron stores (see Color Plate 5H, left). Despite the hemolysis, the usual manifestations of increased blood destruction are absent. The serum bilirubin and the excretion of urobilinogen are generally normal.

TREATMENT. Correction of the anemia depends upon successful treatment of the underlying disease. Blood transfusions are not usually necessary because the anemia is generally mild to moderate and is not progressive. Therapy with cobalt, androgenic steroids, and corticosteroids offers more potential for harm than good. The block to iron flow cannot be bypassed, and the administration of oral or parenteral iron is of no benefit. When bleeding causes superimposed iron deficiency, the administration of iron will restore hemoglobin levels to those of the underlying chronic disorder but not back to normal.

SIDEROBLASTIC ANEMIA

DEFINITION. When hypochromic anemia is associated with hyperferremia and increased transferrin saturation, a diagnosis of sideroblastic anemia is suggested. The sideroblastic anemias are a heterogeneous group of disorders associated with various defects in the porphyrin biosynthetic pathway. Porphyrin biosynthetic defects lead to diminished synthesis of heme, which in turn may be associated with an increase in cellular iron uptake (Fig. 131–2). The sideroblastic anemias are characterized by the association of anemia with the presence of an abnormal erythroid precursor in the marrow. The abnormal precursor, the ringed sideroblast, is a normoblast containing excessive deposits of iron within mitochondria. These iron-laden mitochondria, because of their perinuclear distribution, account for the Prussian blue–positive granules forming a full or partial ring around the nucleus of the ringed sideroblast (see Color Plate 6J, right). Normal sideroblasts contain one to four Prussian blue–positive ferritin aggregates in the cytoplasm and no visible iron in mitochondria.

PATHOGENESIS AND CLASSIFICATION. Mitochondrial iron excess appears to be a consequence of defective heme synthesis. A population of hypochromic erythrocytes, common to all the sideroblastic anemias, is morphologic evidence of the synthetic defect. Other common characteristics include abnormalities in porphyrin biosynthesis; an increase in total body iron stores; an increase in the serum iron concentration, often to the point of complete saturation of transferrin; and kinetic evidence of ineffective erythropoiesis. It is customary to divide the sideroblastic anemias into two groups, depending on whether the disorder appears to be acquired or inherited (see Table 131–2).

Acquired Sideroblastic Anemias

IDIOPATHIC REFRACTORY SIDEROBLASTIC ANEMIA. This acquired disease of older adults has an unknown pathogenesis. The anemia develops insidiously and is often discovered during a routine examination. The anemia is usually slightly macrocytic. Examination of the peripheral blood smear reveals two populations of erythrocytes. One is entirely normal, and the other is macrocytic and quite hypochromic with prominent basophilic stippling. Leukocyte and platelet counts are usually normal, but leukopenia is occasionally noted, and either moderate thrombocytopenia or thrombocytosis has been reported. The FEP is increased, but the precise enzymatic defect (or defects) in porphyrin biosynthesis has (or have) not been defined. About 30 to 40 per cent of patients have a palpable spleen. Therapy with pyridoxine or folic acid is not successful, and only rare patients respond to androgens. The median survival for patients with idiopathic refractory sideroblastic anemia is about 10 years; most patients require no therapy. Transfusion therapy should be kept to a minimum because the chronic administration of erythrocytes has led to transfusional hemochromatosis. Therapy with daily subcutaneous infusions of deferoxamine may be of value to selected patients who require repeated transfusion. The condition in about 10 per cent of patients eventually shows evidence of transformation to acute leukemia. No reliable indicators predict the likelihood of leukemic transformation. The closest association between the development of leukemia and the presence of ringed sideroblasts is noted when sideroblastic anemia occurs following chemotherapy for a variety of malignant disorders. Alkylating drugs such as cyclophosphamide, nitrogen mustard, and melphalan are the most common offenders.

SIDEROBLASTIC ANEMIA COMPLICATING OTHER DISEASES. Acquired sideroblastic anemia associated with other diseases and with drugs or toxins is quite common; however, the anemia is usually only mild. Inflammatory diseases such as rheumatoid arthritis, neoplasms, and a variety of primary hematologic disorders have all been associated with a secondary sideroblastic anemia. The treatment, course, and prognosis are all related to the nature of the associated disease.

SIDEROBLASTIC ANEMIA ASSOCIATED WITH DRUGS OR TOXINS. Sideroblastic anemia is a common complication in hospitalized alcoholics. Withdrawal of alcohol results in a reticulocytosis and disappearance of the ringed sideroblasts within 5 to 10 days. *Alcohol* may cause sideroblastic anemia by interfering with pyridoxine metabolism and thus indirectly affecting the activity of Δ-aminolevulinic acid synthetase, the rate-limiting enzyme in the porphyrin biosynthetic pathway. This mechanism likely also underlies the sideroblastic anemia occasionally seen in association with the administration of the antituberculous agent *isonicotinic acid hydrazide* (INH). The sideroblastic anemia that occurs in *lead poisoning* is caused by the inhibition by lead of the enzyme that converts Δ-aminolevulinic acid to porphobilinogen (Δ-aminolevulinic dehydratase) and the enzyme heme synthetase (ferrochelatase). As a result of these two enzymatic defects, it is possible to screen for lead poisoning by detecting either increased urinary excretion of Δ-aminolevulinic acid or a markedly increased FEP.

Hereditary Sideroblastic Anemias

Hereditary sideroblastic anemia is almost always a disease of males and is most likely inherited as an X-linked recessive trait. Although the anemia is usually detected in the late teenage years, in rare cases the anemia is found first in either infancy or adult life. The anemia is severe (average blood hemoglobin, 6.5 grams per deciliter), and the red cell indices indicate marked microcytosis and hypochromia. The inherited defect in some way involves the interaction between Δ-aminolevulinic acid synthetase and its cofactor pyridoxal phosphate. Individuals with hereditary sideroblastic anemia are not pyridoxine deficient; however, large amounts of vitamin B_6 produce partial correction of the anemia. There is an erythroid-specific form of Δ-aminolevulinic acid synthetase that is coded for by a gene on the X chromosome. It seems likely that mutations at this locus will prove to be the cause of many cases of hereditary sideroblastic anemia.

Beutler E, Fairbanks VF: The effects of iron deficiency. *In* Jacobs A, Worwood M (eds.): Iron in Biochemistry and Medicine II. New York, Academic Press, 1980, pp 394–428. *An extensive review of both the hematologic and the nonhematologic manifestations of iron deficiency.*

Miescher PA, Jaffe ER, Finch CA (eds.): Semin Hematol, vol. 19, no. 1, 1984. *An issue of a respected review journal devoted to the clinical aspects of iron deficiency and excess.*

Ward JH, Kushner JP, Kaplan J: Iron: Metabolism and clinical disorders. *In* Fairbanks VF (ed.): Current Hematology and Oncology. Vol. 3. New York, John Wiley & Sons, 1984, pp 1–50. *A review of basic iron metabolism with an extensive list of references.*

Williams WJ, Beutler E, Erslev AJ, et al. (eds.): Hematology. 4th ed. New York, McGraw-Hill Book Company, 1990. *A comprehensive textbook of hematology with an excellent presentation of basic iron metabolism and its application to clinical medicine.*

Wintrobe MM, Lee GR, Boggs DR, et al. (eds.): Clinical Hematology. 8th ed. Philadelphia, Lea & Febiger, 1981. *The oldest standard textbook of hematology with an exhaustive description of the clinical manifestations of iron deficiency anemia.*

132 Megaloblastic Anemias

Robert H. Allen

DEFINITION

The megaloblastic anemias are caused by various defects in DNA synthesis that lead to a common set of hematologic abnormalities of the bone marrow and peripheral blood. The term "megaloblastic" refers to a morphologic abnormality of cell nuclei that is readily recognizable but difficult to describe (see Color Plate 6G and H). The erythrocytic, granulocytic, and megakaryocytic cell lines are all involved, and a pancytopenia may develop. Recognition of megaloblastic anemia is important because two of its most common causes, cobalamin (vitamin B_{12}) deficiency and folate deficiency, are completely corrected with appropriate therapy. The recognition of cobalamin deficiency is of particular importance because it also causes a wide variety of neurologic and psychiatric abnormalities that are preventable or reversible if the diagnosis is made at an early stage.

ETIOLOGY

The four major etiologic categories of megaloblastic anemia are (1) cobalamin deficiency, (2) folate deficiency, (3) drugs, and (4) miscellaneous, which includes rare enzyme deficiencies and unexplained disorders (Table 132–1). The etiology of cobalamin deficiency can be subdivided into causes of decreased ingestion, impaired absorption, or impaired utilization of the vitamin. Folate deficiency can also be caused by decreased intake, by impaired absorption, by impaired utilization, and, in addition, by a number of conditions in which there is an increased requirement for folic acid or an increased loss of folic acid. Drugs that cause megaloblastosis can be categorized as those that are purine or pyrimidine antagonists and those that inhibit some other aspect of DNA synthesis. The miscellaneous category includes enzyme defects and some cases of myelodysplastic syndrome and acute leukemia.

It is important to determine the correct etiology of megalo-

blastic anemia. For example, if a cobalamin-deficient patient is misdiagnosed as having a myelodysplastic syndrome, the use of chemotherapy for the latter condition might result in the early death of a patient who could have been completely cured with cobalamin therapy. Similarly, some causes of cobalamin and folate deficiency require therapy for the underlying disease in addition to replacement therapy with the appropriate vitamin.

INCIDENCE AND PREVALENCE
Cobalamin Deficiency

The term "pernicious anemia," often used as a synonym for cobalamin deficiency, should be reserved for conditions in which a gastric mucosal defect results in insufficient intrinsic factor to facilitate the absorption of physiologic amounts of cobalamin. It is by far the most common cause of cobalamin deficiency in the Western Hemisphere. Pernicious anemia was originally believed to be primarily a disease of elderly individuals of northern European ancestry. It is now clear that it also occurs in individuals in their 20's and in all ethnic groups, including blacks and Hispanics. Before the discovery of liver therapy in 1926, perni-

TABLE 132–1. ETIOLOGIC CLASSIFICATION OF THE MEGALOBLASTIC ANEMIAS

Category	Etiologic Mechanisms
I. Cobalamin deficiency	
A. Decreased ingestion	Poor diet, lack of animal products, strict vegetarianism
B. Impaired absorption	1. Failure to release cobalamin from food protein
	Old age
	Gastrectomy (partial)
	2. Intrinsic factor (IF) deficiency
	Pernicious anemia
	Gastrectomy (total)
	Destruction of gastric mucosa by caustics
	Congenital abnormal or absent IF molecule
	3. Chronic pancreatic disease
	4. Competitive parasites
	Bacteria in diverticula of bowel, blind loops
	Fish tapeworm infestations (*Diphyllobothrium latum*)
	5. Intrinsic intestinal disease
	Ileal resection, Crohn's disease, radiation ileitis
	Tropical sprue, celiac disease
	Infiltrative intestinal disease (e.g., lymphoma, scleroderma)
	Drug-induced malabsorption
	Congenital selective malabsorption (Imerslund-Gräsbeck syndrome)
C. Impaired utilization	Congenital enzyme deficiencies
	Lack of transcobalamin II
	Nitrous oxide administration
II. Folate deficiency	
A. Decreased ingestion	Poor diet, lack of vegetables
	Alcoholism
	Infancy
B. Impaired absorption	Intestinal short circuits
	Tropical sprue, celiac disease
	Anticonvulsants, sulfasalazine, other drugs
	Congenital malabsorption
C. Impaired utilization	Folic acid antagonists: methotrexate, triamterene, trimethoprim, pyrimethamine, ethanol
	Congenital enzyme deficiencies
D. Increased requirement	Pregnancy, infancy
	Hyperthyroidism
	Chronic hemolytic disease
	Neoplastic disease, exfoliative skin disease
E. Increased loss	Hemodialysis
III. Drugs—metabolic inhibitors	Purine synthesis: methotrexate, 6-mercaptopurine, 6-thioguanine, azathioprine
	Pyrimidine synthesis: methotrexate, 6-azauridine
	Thymidylate synthesis: methotrexate, 5-fluorouracil
	Deoxyribonucleotide synthesis: hydroxyurea, cytosine arabinoside
IV. Miscellaneous	
A. Inborn errors	Lesch-Nyhan syndrome
	Hereditary orotic aciduria
	Others
B. Unexplained disorders	Pyridoxine-responsive megaloblastic anemia
	Thiamine-responsive megaloblastic anemia
	Some cases of myelodysplastic syndrome
	Some cases of acute myelogenous leukemia

cious anemia was invariably fatal. About 1.0 per cent of individuals in the United States will develop pernicious anemia at some time during their life. With a population of 250 million, an average lifetime of 75 years, and the assumption that cobalamin deficiency exists for an average of 5 years before it is treated or the patient dies, there should be about 150,000 patients at various stages of cobalamin deficiency in the United States at any point in time. Approximately 10 per cent of the U.S. population over age 70 have low or low-normal serum cobalamin levels *and* metabolic evidence of cobalamin deficiency (elevated levels of serum methylmalonic acid and homocysteine that fall to normal with cobalamin therapy). The etiology and the hematologic and neuropsychiatric significance of these findings are unknown at the present time. These estimates of the actual and potential incidence of cobalamin deficiency further emphasize the importance of recognizing this eminently treatable disease.

Folate Deficiency, Drugs, and Other Causes

The incidence of folate deficiency and of drug-related megaloblastic anemia is less well established. Through its association with alcoholism, folate deficiency is far from a rare condition. The marked increase in the use of chemotherapeutic agents to treat malignancies and immune disorders suggests that these drugs may now be the most common cause of megaloblastic anemia in the Western Hemisphere.

PATHOGENESIS AND PATHOLOGY

Mechanism of Megaloblastosis

FOLATE DEFICIENCY. Folate functions to transfer one-carbon units, such as methyl, methylene, and formyl groups, to various substrates in a variety of enzymatic reactions that are intimately related to the synthesis of DNA, RNA, and proteins. In folate deficiency, all forms of folate are reduced within cells, which impairs the growth and maturation of rapidly growing cells, such as those in the bone marrow. For example, thymidylate synthase catalyzes the synthesis of thymidine (dTMP) from deoxyuridine (dUMP) and 5,10-methylenetetrahydrofolate. Inhibition of thymidylate synthase leads to increased intracellular concentrations of deoxyuridine triphosphate (dUTP), which is incorporated into DNA in positions that normally arise from deoxythymidine triphosphate (dTTP). Attempts to repair this abnormal DNA increase DNA fragmentation, which may play a major role in causing the abnormalities of cell growth and maturation that are present in folate deficiency.

COBALAMIN DEFICIENCY. Cobalamin functions as an essential cofactor for only two enzymes in human cells, methionine synthase and L-methylmalonyl-CoA (coenzyme A) mutase (Figs. 132–1 and 132–2). Methionine synthase catalyzes the recycling of homocysteine to methionine, using 5-methyltetrahydrofolate as a required coenzyme (Fig. 132–1). Methionine, an essential amino acid for protein synthesis, also serves in the form of S-adenosylmethionine as the major methyl donor in numerous important enzymatic reactions. In cobalamin deficiency, increasing amounts of intracellular folate are converted to 5-methyltetrahydrofolate in an attempt to prevent intracellular methionine deficiency. The "trapping" of intracellular folate as 5-methyltetrahydrofolate is augmented by the fact that this is the major component of plasma folate and is the form that enters cells and must be converted to tetrahydrofolate by methionine synthase before it can enter the folate pool. Thus, cobalamin deficiency results in a secondary intracellular deficiency of all forms of folate except for 5-methyltetrahydrofolate. As a result, the activities of all of the enzymes that utilize folate to transfer one-carbon moieties, including thymidylate synthase, are impaired. This concept of "methylfolate trapping" explains why cobalamin deficiency and folate deficiency produce indistinguishable hematologic abnormalities and why the hematologic abnormalities seen in cobalamin deficiency can be completely reversed by pharmacologic amounts of folic acid. The latter oxidized, nonphysiologic form of folate can be reduced directly to tetrahydrofolate without first being converted to 5-methyltetrahydrofolate. This concept also explains why the hematologic abnormalities caused by folate deficiency respond only slightly, if at all, to large amounts of cobalamin.

DRUGS AND OTHER CAUSES. Drugs that cause megaloblastic anemia inhibit a variety of enzymes involved in DNA synthesis. 5-Fluorouracil (5-FU) inhibits thymidylate synthase directly. The addition of 5-formyltetrahydrofolate (Leucovorin) to 5-FU regimens actually increases the inhibition of thymidylate synthase, since 5-formyltetrahydrofolate is readily converted to 5,10-methylenetetrahydrofolate, which is involved in the formation of inhibitory ternary complexes between 5,10-methylenetetrahydrofolate, 5-FU, and thymidylate synthase. Why megaloblastic changes occur in some cases of the myelodysplastic syndrome and acute leukemias is unknown, but this is probably due to a variety of mutations that alter DNA synthesis.

Mechanism of Neuropsychiatric Abnormalities in Cobalamin Deficiency

A wide variety of neuropsychiatric abnormalities are seen in cobalamin deficiency and appear to be due to an undefined defect involving myelin synthesis. These abnormalities are not seen in folate deficiency. It has therefore been tempting to ascribe them to deficient activity of the second cobalamin-dependent enzyme, L-methylmalonyl-CoA mutase, which is unrelated to any folate-dependent enzyme or pathway. This enzyme catalyzes the conversion of L-methylmalonyl-CoA to succinyl-CoA, utilizing adenosylcobalamin as a required coenzyme (Fig. 132–2). Abnormal odd-carbon and branched-chain fatty acids are formed when the mutase is impaired. The neuropsychiatric abnormalities of cobalamin deficiency are not seen, however, in individuals with genetic defects of the mutase reaction, caused either by primary defects in the enzyme itself or by defects in the formation of adenosylcobalamin. Impairment of methionine synthase has also been postulated as the cause of the neuropsychiatric abnormalities because of the importance of methionine and s-adenosylmethionine for the many methylation reactions that take place in the nervous system. As noted, however, the neuropsychiatric abnormalities caused by cobalamin deficiency are not seen in folate deficiency, even though methionine synthase appears to be equally impaired in both vitamin deficiencies (based on similar marked elevations in serum homocysteine concentrations). Genetic defects in which the synthesis of adenosylcobalamin and methylcobalamin are both impaired do lead to neuropsychiatric abnormalities of the kind seen in cobalamin deficiency. These observations suggest that both cobalamin-dependent enzymes must be impaired for the neuropsychiatric abnormalities to develop and that the two cobalamin-dependent enzymes or pathways are connected or interrelated in some way that has not yet been discovered.

Mechanisms of Cobalamin Deficiency

Cobalamin is not present in plants; until recently, humans obtained their cobalamin exclusively from animal products. Cobalamin is synthesized only by certain microorganisms. During the past 40 years, humans have received increasing amounts of their dietary cobalamin from multivitamin supplements taken in the form of pills and as additives to many food preparations. Most

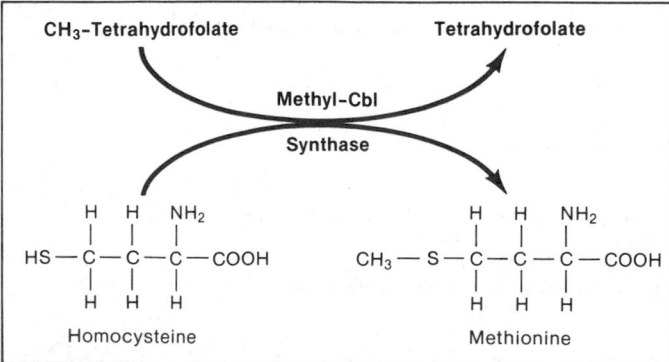

FIGURE 132–1. Reaction catalyzed by methionine synthase that requires methylcobalamin (methyl-Cbl) and transfers the methyl group of 5-methyltetrahydrofolate (CH$_3$-tetrahydrofolate) to homocysteine to form methionine and tetrahydrofolate. Homocysteine accumulates in cobalamin deficiency owing to a lack of methylcobalamin and in folate deficiency owing to a lack of 5-methyltetrahydrofolate.

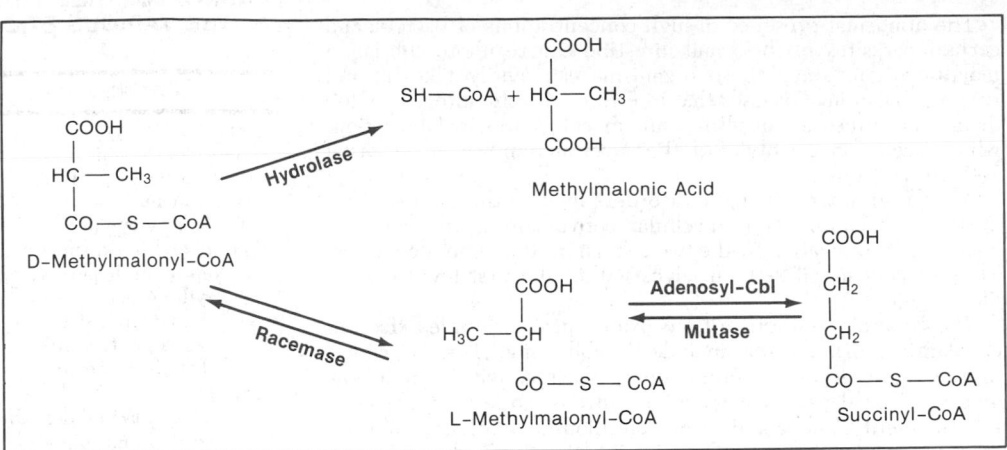

FIGURE 132–2. Reactions involved in the metabolism of D- and L-methyl-malonyl-CoA (CoA = coenzyme A). Methylmalonic acid accumulates in cobalamin deficiency owing to a lack of adenosylcobalamin (adenosyl-Cbl), which leads to an increase of L-methylmalonyl-CoA, which is converted to D-methylmalonyl-CoA and hydrolyzed to methylmalonic acid.

cobalamin in animal products is tightly bound to proteins, i.e., the two cobalamin-dependent enzymes, and is released from them in the stomach by the concerted action of HCl and pepsin. The stomach is also the site of synthesis of intrinsic factor (IF), which binds free cobalamin with high affinity and plays an essential role in cobalamin absorption (Fig. 102–2). Gastric juice contains another cobalamin-binding protein that originates in saliva and has a more rapid or "R"-type electrophoretic mobility than does IF. R protein binds cobalamin with a higher affinity than does IF, particularly at an acid pH. Thus, under normal conditions of gastric acidity, dietary cobalamin enters the duodenum bound to R protein. Additional cobalamin bound to R protein enters the duodenum after it is secreted into bile by the liver (this is the only significant route by which cobalamin is lost from the body). Pancreatic proteases partially degrade salivary and biliary R protein–cobalamin complexes in the jejunum, and only after this occurs is cobalamin bound to IF. The IF-cobalamin complex remains intact until it reaches the distal ileum, where it binds with high affinity to specific receptors located on ileal mucosal cells. Cobalamin then enters these cells and reaches the portal plasma, which contains three cobalamin-binding proteins known as transcobalamin I (TC I), transcobalamin II (TC II), and transcobalamin III (TC III). Their roles are summarized in Table 132–2. Although it contains only about 10 per cent of the plasma cobalamin, TC II is the important transport protein because of its rapid clearance and its ability to deliver cobalamin to all cells within the body. TC II–cobalamin is taken up by cells by endocytosis during a process in which the TC II moiety is degraded and the cobalamin is reduced and eventually converted to its two coenzyme forms, i.e., methylcobalamin and adenosylcobalamin. Cobalamin is not stored intracellularly; all of the intracellular vitamin is bound to the two enzymes, which are present in greater amounts than is cobalamin. Additional information concerning the gastrointestinal phase of cobalamin absorption is found in Ch. 102.

A large number of acquired and genetic diseases affect the pathway of cobalamin absorption and transport and result in cobalamin deficiency (see Table 132–1). Strict vegans, i.e., those who ingest neither meat nor other animal products, such as milk, cheese, and eggs, and who do not ingest multivitamin supplements, become cobalamin deficient on a dietary basis. Approximately 10 to 15 years are required for clinical signs to develop, since the absorption of biliary cobalamin remains intact. The secretion of biliary cobalamin ranges from 5 to 10 µg per day, and approximately 90 per cent is reabsorbed by strict vegans and other normal individuals. Thus, only 0.5 to 1.0 µg of the 5 to 10 µg of cobalamin present in a normal diet must be absorbed each day to maintain the total body content of cobalamin in the normal range of 2000 to 5000 µg.

Achlorhydria and the loss of pepsin secretion are very common in elderly subjects (>50 per cent of individuals > age 70) and in those with partial gastrectomies. These individuals develop cobalamin deficiency because of an inability to liberate cobalamin from its protein-bound form in foods of animal origin. Secretion of IF is reduced, but because it is normally formed in vast excess, sufficient IF usually remains for the reabsorption of biliary R protein–cobalamin, which is not dependent upon HCl and pepsin. The same time span of 10 to 15 years is required for these subjects to develop clinical signs of cobalamin deficiency as for those with dietary lack. Many of them never develop cobalamin deficiency, apparently because of the availability of free, non–protein-bound cobalamin in multivitamin pills and supplements and because some natural animal products contain small amounts of free cobalamin.

A complete lack of IF occurs in individuals who have undergone total gastrectomy or who have pernicious anemia, in which there is an idiopathic and essentially complete atrophy of the gastric mucosa in association with autoantibodies to parietal cells and IF. Only about 3 to 5 years are required for clinical signs of cobalamin deficiency to develop because these individuals malabsorb biliary as well as all forms of dietary cobalamin.

Cobalamin malabsorption occurs commonly in severe pancreatic exocrine insufficiency because of an inability to degrade R protein–cobalamin complexes in the jejunum. Clinically evident cobalamin deficiency rarely occurs, however, probably because oral therapy with pancreatic extract is usually instituted in these patients during the 3 to 5 years that are necessary for the signs of cobalamin deficiency to develop.

TABLE 132–2. DISTRIBUTION OF ENDOGENOUS COBALAMIN AMONG THE VARIOUS TRANSCOBALAMINS AND THEIR RELATIVE IMPORTANCE TO COBALAMIN TRANSPORT*

Cobalamin Transport Protein	Endogenous Cobalamin (pg/ml)	T½ for Cobalamin Clearance (hr)	Cobalamin Clearance (pg/ml/24 hr)	Site of Specific Uptake
R proteins†:				
Transcobalamin I	425–450	240.0	30	None
Transcobalamin III	0–25	0.1	0–4000	Hepatocytes
Transcobalamin II‡	50	0.1	8000	All cells

*In a typical normal subject with a serum cobalamin level of 500 pg per milliliter.

†In congenital R protein deficiency, the total serum cobalamin level is very low, but no hematologic abnormalities are present because R proteins do not transport cobalamin to rapidly dividing cells, such as those in the bone marrow.

‡In congenital transcobalamin II deficiency, the total serum cobalamin level is well within the normal range, but severe megaloblastic anemia develops because only transcobalamin II transports cobalamin to rapidly dividing cells, such as those in the bone marrow.

The abnormal presence of high concentrations of bacteria and certain parasites in the small intestine can result in cobalamin malabsorption, since these organisms can avidly take up and retain cobalamin. Diseases that interfere with the integrity of the distal ileal mucosa can also result in cobalamin malabsorption, which occurs invariably after the surgical removal of the distal 100 cm of ileum.

A large number of genetic disorders involve the plasma transport of cobalamin, its intracellular conversion to its coenzyme forms, or its utilization by the two cobalamin-dependent enzymes. They usually manifest themselves within the first few weeks of life.

The general anesthetic nitrous oxide causes multiple defects in cobalamin utilization that include the following: (1) rapid (within minutes) inhibition of methionine synthase activity, with a slow (over several days) recovery when nitrous oxide is stopped; (2) displacement of cobalamin from methionine synthase; (3) a decrease in the level of methylcobalamin; (4) irreversible conversion of cobalamin to inactive and inhibitory cobalamin analogues; (5) the gradual (over many weeks) development of cobalamin deficiency; (6) an eventual decrease in L-methylmalonyl-CoA mutase activity; and (7) a further decrease in methionine synthase activity.

Mechanisms of Folate Deficiency

Folate is widely distributed in plants and products of animal origin. Green vegetables are particularly rich sources of folate. Excessive cooking can destroy or remove a high percentage of folate in foods. Folate either is missing or is present in relatively small amounts (≤ 400 μg) in nonprescription multivitamin pills and supplements because of the justified concern that its presence in larger amounts could mask the diagnosis of cobalamin deficiency by correcting its hematologic abnormalities without having any beneficial effect on the neuropsychiatric abnormalities. Folates in natural foods are conjugated to chains of polyglutamic acid. Enzymes in the lumen of the small intestine convert the polyglutamate forms of folate to the monoglutamate and diglutamate forms, which are much more readily absorbed in the proximal jejunum. Absorption involves active and passive transport. Most of the folate in plasma is present as 5-methyltetrahydrofolate in the monoglutamate form. The majority is loosely bound to albumin, from which it is readily taken up by high-affinity folate receptors that are present on cells throughout the body. Once it enters the cell, the 5-methyltetrahydrofolate must be converted to tetrahydrofolate by the cobalamin-dependent enzyme methionine synthase before it can be converted to the polyglutamate form and take part in the other folate-dependent enzymatic reactions (Fig. 132–1). In addition to being secreted in the bile and reabsorbed in the small intestine, folates are also degraded and excreted in the urine.

Decreased intake is by far the most common cause of folate deficiency. Normal individuals have about 5000 to 20,000 μg of folate in body stores. Because folate is degraded within the body and is excreted in both the bile and the urine, approximately 50 to 100 μg must be absorbed each day from the average Western diet, which contains about 200 to 500 μg of folate. Clinical signs of folate deficiency develop in about 4 months of decreased intake, as can occur readily in chronic alcoholics.

Absorption of folate is impaired in a variety of diseases that affect the mucosa of the jejunum, including tropical sprue and celiac disease. Certain drugs, such as anticonvulsants and sulfasalazine, may impair folate absorption in some individuals. Ethanol and drugs such as triamterene impair the utilization of folate. Certain conditions associated with hypermetabolism or rapid cell growth lead to an increased requirement for folate that often cannot be met by a normal diet. These conditions include hyperthyroidism, pregnancy, chronic hemolytic disease, and various exfoliative skin diseases. An increased loss of folate from the body is caused by hemodialysis.

CLINICAL MANIFESTATIONS OF MEGALOBLASTIC ANEMIA

Hematologic Manifestations

All of the causes of megaloblastic anemia produce a common set of hematologic, laboratory, and other abnormalities that are

TABLE 132–3. HEMATOLOGIC AND OTHER ABNORMALITIES THAT MAY BE CAUSED BY ANY OF THE VARIOUS ETIOLOGIES OF MEGALOBLASTIC ANEMIA*

Hematologic	Other
Anemia	Glossitis
Reticulocytopenia	Stomatitis
Macrocytosis ($\uparrow$ MCV)	Gastrointestinal symptoms
Neutropenia	Hyperpigmentation
Thrombocytopenia	Infertility
Peripheral blood smear:	Orthostatic hypotension
Neutrophil hypersegmentation	Weight loss
Erythrocytes:	
Variation in size	
Variation in shape	
Macro-ovalocytes	
Serum:	
Elevated lactate dehydrogenase	
Elevated bilirubin	
Elevated iron	
Decreased haptoglobin	
Bone marrow:	
Hypercellular	
Megaloblastic morphology	
Giant bands and metamyelocytes	

*These abnormalities may be present in any number or combination in a given patient. The absence of any one or more of them occurs commonly in individual patients with all causes of megaloblastic anemia, including cobalamin deficiency and folate deficiency.

summarized in Table 132–3. None of the abnormalities are specific for the various diseases that cause megaloblastic anemia. The abnormalities may also be present in any combination, which can vary greatly from patient to patient. In addition, none of the abnormalities are always seen in conditions that cause megaloblastic anemia, and the absence of any one or more of them cannot be used to exclude any of the diseases that cause megaloblastic anemia, including cobalamin or folate deficiency, in a given patient.

The anemia typically develops slowly over many months and may not cause symptoms until the hematocrit is less than 20 per cent. The reticulocyte count is not elevated, in either absolute or relative (percentage) terms, even when the anemia is severe. The mean cell volume (MCV) is often increased (normal, 80 to 100 fl), and values as high as 140 fl may be seen. A review of previous blood counts often reveals a steady increase in the MCV over several months or years, often within the normal range. Neutropenia and thrombocytopenia occur less commonly than anemia and are usually not severe. On occasion, however, neutrophil counts less than 1000 per microliter and platelet counts less than 50,000 per microliter are seen. The peripheral blood smear frequently shows neutrophil hypersegmentation (Fig. 132–3 and Color Plate 6G, left), which can be documented by

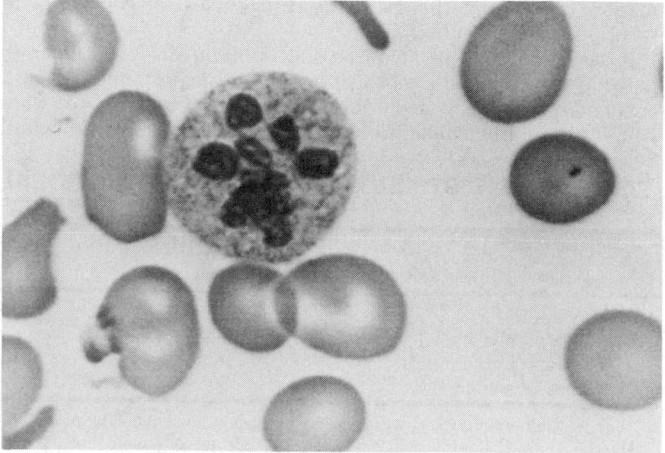

FIGURE 132–3. A hypersegmented neutrophil on a peripheral blood smear from a patient with megaloblastic anemia.

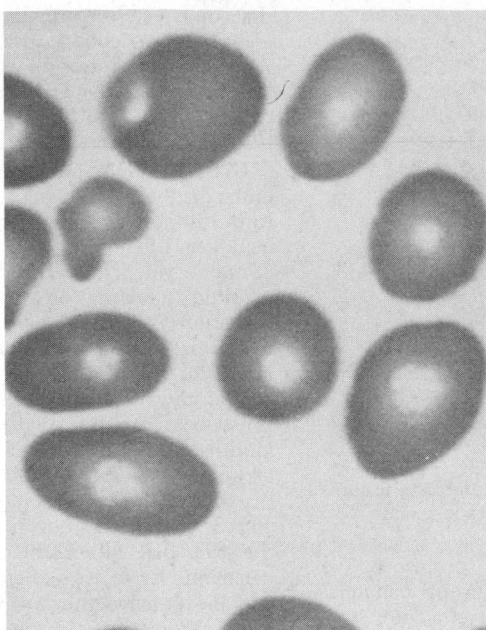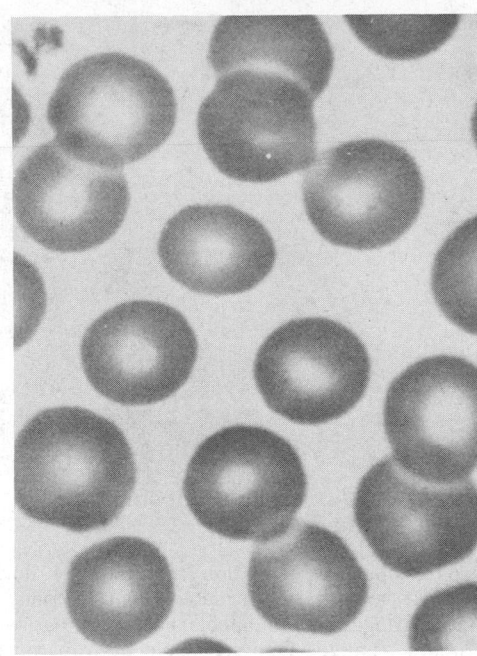

FIGURE 132-4. Peripheral blood smears from a patient with megaloblastic anemia *(left)* and from a normal subject *(right)*, both at the same magnification. The smear from the patient shows variation in the size and shape of erythrocytes and the presence of macro-ovalocytes.

observing one or more of the following: (1) the presence of at least one neutrophil containing 6 or more lobes; (2) the presence of 5 per cent or more of 5-lobe neutrophils; or (3) an increased neutrophil lobe average, which is normally fewer than 3.4 lobes per neutrophil. Erythrocytes often vary markedly in size and shape, and macroovalocytes, large, oval erythrocytes, are frequently present (Fig. 132–4 and Color Plate 6G, right). When the hematocrit is low, nucleated red cells may be seen on the peripheral smear, and then the megaloblastic morphology of the nuclei can be observed without performing a bone marrow aspiration or biopsy.

Although the reticulocyte count is normal or low, a number of serum abnormalities are often present that are usually seen and associated with hemolytic anemia. These include elevated serum levels of lactate dehydrogenase, indirect bilirubin, and iron and decreased levels of haptoglobin. Red cell production and destruction can be markedly increased in megaloblastic anemia, but both are confined to the bone marrow, described as "intramedullary hemolysis" or "ineffective erythropoiesis."

The bone marrow is usually hypercellular with an increase in all cellular elements. Megaloblastic morphologic changes are often seen in all cells within the bone marrow but are usually more prominent in the erythroid series. All cells in the erythroid series are larger than their normal counterparts, their cytoplasm appears more mature than their nuclei (nuclear-cytoplasmic asynchrony), and the nuclear chromatin has a distinctive open and fine-grained texture (Fig. 132–5 and Color Plate 6H). Similar abnormalities are seen in neutrophil precursors and are usually most striking at the metamyelocyte and band stage, in which "giant metamyelocytes" and "giant bands" are seen. All of these features are much more prominent in the Wright stain smear of bone marrow aspirates than in fixed sections of the bone marrow biopsy. The use of the latter alone can lead to disastrous clinical consequences because even the most experienced hematopathologist can, on the basis of fixed bone marrow sections only, have difficulty in distinguishing the hypercellularity and abnormal morphology of megaloblastosis from the changes seen in the myelodysplastic syndromes and some cases of acute leukemia. Coexisting iron deficiency may also cause diagnostic problems, since all of the erythroid megaloblastic changes may be absent even in the Wright stain smears of aspirated bone marrow. Thus, the diagnosis of megaloblastic anemia should never be excluded after a bone marrow examination has been performed unless bone marrow aspirates have been examined and the presence of bone marrow iron has been established.

Megaloblastic abnormalities may occur in other proliferating body cells, all of which share the underlying defect in DNA synthesis. These changes have been documented in the epithelial cells of the buccal mucosa, stomach, intestine, and vagina and account for such phenomena as glossitis, stomatitis, and secondary malabsorption. Similar changes may account for the infertility that is sometimes seen.

Few, if any, patients with cobalamin or folate deficiency or other causes of megaloblastic anemia have all or even most of the hematologic and other abnormalities listed in Table 132–3. Even the classic abnormalities, such as anemia and an elevated MCV, are frequently absent, even in patients with otherwise severe deficiencies of cobalamin or folate. This point is often overlooked despite being well documented by several studies, including a recent prospective study of 86 consecutive patients with low serum cobalamin levels (<200 pg per milliliter) *and* one or more objective hematologic and/or neuropsychiatric responses to cobalamin therapy. These patients failed to display the abnormalities listed in Table 132–3 with the following frequencies: (1) lack of anemia (44 per cent); (2) MCV of 100 fl or less (36 per cent); (3) normal white blood cell count (86 per cent); (4) normal platelet count (79 per cent); (5) normal peripheral smear on routine laboratory study (33 per cent); (6) normal serum lactate dehydrogenase (43 per cent); and (7) normal serum bilirubin level (83 per cent).

Neuropsychiatric Abnormalities Caused by Cobalamin Deficiency

Cobalamin deficiency, unlike folate deficiency and other causes of megaloblastic anemia, produces a wide variety of neuropsychiatric abnormalities (Table 132–4). None of these abnormalities are specific for cobalamin deficiency, and they may be present alone or in any combination, which can vary greatly from patient to patient. In addition, none of the abnormalities are always seen in cobalamin deficiency, and the absence of any one or combination of them does not rule out cobalamin deficiency. The neuropsychiatric abnormalities may occur early or late in the course of cobalamin deficiency and with or without any of the hematologic or other abnormalities listed in Table 132–3. How the deficiency of a single substance, such as cobalamin, can produce a clinical picture with such wide differences in the severity and dissociation of various hematologic and neuropsychiatric abnormalities is unknown.

Pathologic studies show loss of myelin with axonal degeneration, most frequently in the dorsal and lateral columns of the spinal cord but also in peripheral and cranial nerves and the cerebral cortex. *Combined systems disease* designates a spinal cord disorder marked by an insidiously beginning and a gradually

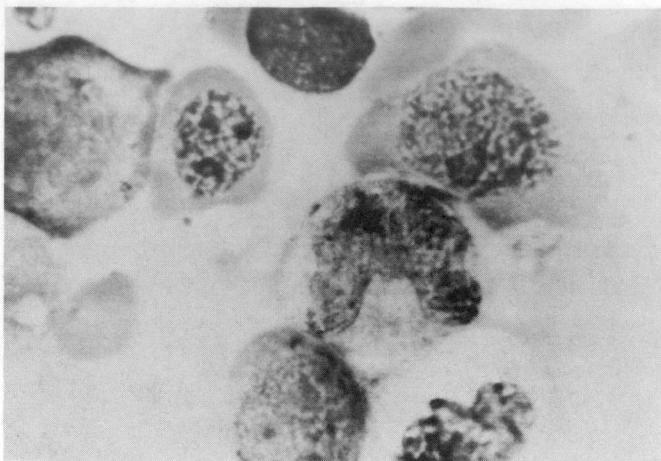

FIGURE 132–5. Erythroid precursors with marked megaloblastic features on a bone marrow smear from a patient with megaloblastic anemia.

progressing demyelination of, first, the dorsal (proprioceptive afferent) and, later, the lateral (corticospinal efferent) columns. Axonal degeneration affects the same pathways as a late, irreversible change. Demyelinative neuropathy of large peripheral fibers may precede or develop concurrently with the cord changes. Signs and symptoms are usually symmetric and often include paresthesias in the extremities, together with impaired vibration and position sense, which may progress to an abnormal gait, spastic ataxia, and quadriparesis. Urinary and fecal incontinence may be seen, as well as impotence. Cerebral and cranial nerve abnormalities include irritability, memory loss, disorientation, obtundation, and changes of taste, smell, and vision, with the last-named sometimes progressing to severe optic atrophy and near-blindness. Psychiatric abnormalities may be prominent and isolated. They include depression, hallucinations, agitation, marked personality change, abnormal behavior, and suicide.

The neuropsychiatric abnormalities caused by cobalamin deficiency frequently bear no relationship to the presence or degree of hematologic abnormalities. The severity of neuropsychiatric abnormalities actually bears a striking *inverse correlation* to the degree of anemia. The frequency with which hematologic and neuropsychiatric abnormalities are dissociated is often unappreciated. For example, several clinical studies document that a

TABLE 132–4. NEUROPSYCHIATRIC ABNORMALITIES* THAT MAY BE CAUSED BY COBALAMIN DEFICIENCY

Neurologic Abnormalities:	Psychiatric Abnormalities:
Paresthesia	Depression
Impaired vibration sense	Paranoia
Impaired position sense	Listlessness
Impaired touch or pain perception	Acute confusional state
Ataxia	Hallucinations
Abnormal gait	Delusions
Fatigue	Insomnia
Memory loss	Apprehensiveness
Disorientation	Psychosis
Obtundation	Slow mentation
Decreased reflexes	Paraphrenia
Weakness	Mania
Decreased muscle strength	Panic attacks
Romberg's sign	Suicide
Increased reflexes	
Spasticity	
Babinski's sign	
Lhermitte's phenomenon	
Urinary or fecal incontinence	
Urinary urgency or nocturia	
Impotence	
Abnormal smell or taste	
Decreased vision or optic atrophy	

*These abnormalities may be present in any number or combination in a given patient. They are seen frequently with *or without* any of the hematologic or other abnormalities listed in Table 132–3.

normal hematocrit, MCV, or both occur in at least 25 per cent to 50 per cent of patients with neuropsychiatric abnormalities that are caused by cobalamin deficiency *and* respond partially or completely to cobalamin therapy. Other hematologic and laboratory abnormalities of the kind outlined in Table 132–3 are lacking in a similar or even higher percentage of these patients.

DIAGNOSIS

INDICATIONS. If drugs are excluded as a cause, the differential diagnosis of megaloblastic anemia in adults is usually limited to the important task of distinguishing between cobalamin deficiency and folate deficiency and firmly establishing the presence of one or the other. The diagnostic approach to the patient with possible cobalamin or folate deficiency is outlined in Table 132–5. Patients should always be evaluated for these two conditions in the presence of any unexplained hematologic or other abnormality of the kind listed in Table 132–3. In addition, patients should always be evaluated for cobalamin deficiency in the presence of any unexplained neuropsychiatric abnormality of the kind listed in Table 132–4, regardless of the presence or absence of hematologic abnormalities. The yield may be relatively low because of the nonspecific nature of the abnormalities in Tables 132–3 and 132–4, but such evaluations are clearly justified by the fact that all of the hematologic abnormalities caused by cobalamin or folate deficiency are completely corrected by safe and inexpensive therapy with the proper vitamin. In addition, the neuropsychiatric abnormalities caused by cobalamin deficiency are usually partially or completely corrected by cobalamin therapy, and in the small minority of patients who do not improve, cobalamin therapy always prevents them from getting worse. It is particularly important that the diagnosis of cobalamin deficiency be established with a high degree of certainty because parenteral cobalamin therapy must almost always be given for the lifetime of the patient. The distinction between cobalamin deficiency and folate deficiency is also very important because the treatment of cobalamin deficiency with folate does not improve the neuropsychiatric abnormalities, even though hematologic responses often occur.

SERUM COBALAMIN AND FOLATE. Radiodilution assays for serum cobalamin and serum folate are used as the initial screening tests because they are widely available and relatively inexpensive. Essentially all serum cobalamin assays today utilize cobalt-57–cobalamin and purified IF, which does not bind and measure the serum cobalamin analogues that caused problems with earlier assays. Radiodilution assays for serum folate utilize iodine-125–folate and a milk folate-binding protein. Because of the composition of commercial assay kits, and because cobalt-57 and iodine-125 are readily distinguished from each other, assays for serum cobalamin and serum folate are almost always performed in the same test tube. Values for serum levels of both vitamins are thereby recorded by laboratories, even though they

TABLE 132–5. DIAGNOSTIC APPROACH TO THE PATIENT WITH COBALAMIN OR FOLATE DEFICIENCY

I. **Initial approach**
   A. Indications
      1. Any unexplained hematologic or other abnormality of the kind listed in Table 132–3 (cobalamin and folate deficiency)
      2. Any unexplained neuropsychiatric abnormality of the kind listed in Table 132–4 (cobalamin deficiency)
   B. Initial tests
      1. Serum cobalamin (normal, 200–900 pg/ml)
      2. Serum folate (normal, 2.5–20 ng/ml)
II. **Follow-up**
   A. Indications
      1. Serum cobalamin <300 pg/ml, *or*
      2. Serum folate <5 ng/ml, *or*
      3. Clinical condition:
         a. Serious unexplained hematologic or neuropsychiatric abnormalities, *or*
         b. Very suggestive of cobalamin or folate deficiency
   B. Follow-up tests
      1. Serum methylmalonic acid (normal, 70–270 nM)—elevated in cobalamin deficiency
      2. Serum homocysteine (normal, 5–16 μM)—elevated in cobalamin and folate deficiency

will report only the cobalamin or the folate level if only one was ordered by the physician. This point can be of practical importance because the physician can usually obtain the value for the other vitamin many weeks or months later if questions arise about the possible deficiency of the other vitamin and the original serum is no longer available.

Normal ranges are defined as the mean ±2 standard deviations for normal subjects and thus include only 95 per cent of normal individuals. Such normal ranges for serum cobalamin are approximately 200 to 900 pg per milliliter and for serum folate, approximately 2.5 to 20 ng per milliliter. By definition, 2.5 per cent of normal subjects who have no evidence of cobalamin deficiency and who will not benefit in any way from cobalamin therapy have low values for serum cobalamin of less than 200 pg per milliter (false-positive readings). One can calculate that approximately 6,250,000 normal subjects in the United States have serum cobalamin levels lower than 200 pg per milliliter (2.5 per cent × 250,000,000 = 6,250,000). This number is much greater than the estimate of approximately 150,000 cobalamin-deficient patients who are present in the United States at any point in time (see above). The number of false-positive readings will remain large even if cobalamin testing is restricted, as it should be, to individuals with one or more unexplained abnormalities of the kind contained in Tables 132–3 and 132–4. Similar calculations can be made with respect to serum folate values. Serum cobalamin and folate levels cannot, therefore, be used alone to establish unequivocally the diagnosis of cobalamin or folate deficiency. The problem is compounded by the fact that not all patients with clinically confirmed cobalamin or folate deficiency (defined as those who have objective clinical responses to appropriate therapy) have low values for serum cobalamin or folate (false-negative readings). The following distribution of serum cobalamin levels has been noted in clinically confirmed cobalamin-deficient patients: less than 100 pg per milliliter, approximately 50 per cent; 100 to 200 pg per milliliter, approximately 40 per cent; 200 to 300 pg per milliliter, approximately 10 per cent; and higher than 300 pg per milliliter, approximately 0.1 to 1 per cent. The distribution of serum folate levels in patients with clinically confirmed folate deficiency has been less well studied, but currently available data indicate that only about 75 per cent of such patients have serum folate levels lower than 2.5 ng per milliliter, with almost all of the remaining 25 per cent being in the 2.5 to 5.0 ng per milliliter range.

Perhaps it is not surprising that many patients with clinically confirmed cobalamin or folate deficiency have serum vitamin levels within the normal range. Both vitamins, after all, function within cells and not in plasma. In the case of cobalamin, furthermore, serum levels of the vitamin are greatly influenced by levels of plasma binding proteins, which bear no relationship to cellular cobalamin levels. In fact, TC I has no apparent function (Table 132–2). Thus, the assays for serum cobalamin and serum folate are useful as initial screening tests that allow the physician to exclude from consideration almost all patients with serum cobalamin levels of 300 pg per milliter or higher and serum folate levels of 5.0 ng per milliliter or higher. Additional follow-up tests are required for serum cobalamin levels lower than 300 pg per milliliter, serum folate levels less than 5.0 ng per milliliter, or clinical conditions that are serious or very suggestive of cobalamin or folate deficiency. Examples of such conditions include (1) a patient with marked myelodysplasia who is about to be started on chemotherapy; (2) a young patient with incapacitating urinary and fecal incontinence of unknown cause; (3) a patient with pancytopenia and an elevated MCV and serum lactate dehydrogenase level; and (4) a patient with symmetric paresthesias in the hands and feet who also has spastic ataxia and a recent change in personality.

SERUM METHYLMALONIC ACID AND HOMOCYSTEINE. The most useful follow-up tests for diagnosing and distinguishing between cobalamin and folate deficiency are serum levels of methylmalonic acid (normal, 70 to 270 nM) and homocysteine* (normal, 5 to 16 μM). These tests, which can be performed on serum that remains after cobalamin and folate levels have been determined, are now widely available in the United States through a number of laboratories, including all of the large national reference laboratories. The combined cost of the two tests, which are usually performed together, is similar to the cost of a Schilling test or a bone marrow examination. The serum methylmalonic acid level is elevated in more than 95 per cent of patients with clinically confirmed cobalamin deficiency (Fig. 132–2). Values as high as 2,000,000 nM have been observed, with a median value in the range of 3500 nM. Serum methylmalonic acid levels are not elevated in folate deficiency. In contrast, serum homocysteine concentrations are elevated in both cobalamin and folate deficiency (Fig. 132–1). Values as high as 500 μM have been observed in cobalamin deficiency, with a median value of 70 μM. Values as high as 250 μM have been observed in folate deficiency, with a median value of 50 μM. Except for rare inborn errors of metabolism involving cobalamin- and folate-dependent enzymes or pathways, the only other conditions that also give rise to elevations of serum methylmalonic acid or serum homocysteine are renal failure and intravascular volume depletion. Broad-spectrum antibiotics can lower an elevated serum methylmalonic acid level to normal in patients with cobalamin deficiency by inhibiting the gut microflora, an important source of precursors of methylmalonic acid. Antibiotics do not affect elevated homocysteine levels in these patients, nor do they change any clinical parameters.

Elevated levels of methylmalonic acid and homocysteine due to cobalamin deficiency return to normal within 5 to 10 days of starting cobalamin therapy. Elevated levels of homocysteine due to folate deficiency fall to normal during the same period following folate therapy. Elevations of serum methylmalonic acid and homocysteine due to cobalamin deficiency do not respond to pharmacologic doses of folate therapy even in cobalamin-deficient patients in whom folate causes a marked hematologic improvement (together with no response or a worsening of neuropsychiatric abnormalities). Elevations of homocysteine due to folate deficiency do not respond to pharmacologic doses of cobalamin therapy. Elevations of methylmalonic acid and homocysteine due to renal insufficiency or intravascular volume depletion are not corrected with therapy with either vitamin unless vitamin deficiency coexists. Thus, repeat determinations of serum methylmalonic acid and homocysteine levels after a short course of therapy with a single vitamin may provide additional information of diagnostic usefulness.

With few exceptions, patients with serum cobalamin levels lower than 300 pg per milliliter or serum folate levels less than 5.0 ng per milliliter do not show objective hematologic or neuropsychiatric responses to cobalamin or folate therapy if their serum levels of methylmalonic acid and homocysteine are normal. Thus, the use of serum levels of cobalamin and folate as initial screening tests, together with the use of serum methylmalonic acid and homocysteine determinations as follow-up tests, makes it possible to diagnose cobalamin or folate deficiency and to distinguish between them in the vast majority of patients (Table 132–5). If in doubt, one can always start empiric therapy, but such therapeutic trials can be difficult to perform (see below) and should be monitored carefully in an attempt to establish a definitive diagnosis. As an alternative, patients can be followed carefully with repeat determinations of methylmalonic acid and homocysteine after 6 months or a year. The usual patterns of serum cobalamin, folate, methylmalonic acid, and homocysteine concentrations in cobalamin and folate deficiency are summarized in Table 132–6.

OTHER TESTS. A number of other tests have been used as diagnostic or follow-up tests in cobalamin deficiency. Serum antibodies to IF are present in about 50 per cent of patients with pernicious anemia and are highly specific for that condition. They fail to diagnose about 50 per cent of such patients, however, as well as all patients with other causes of cobalamin deficiency. The standard Schilling test (see Ch. 102) for a complete description of this test) requires a reliable 24-hour urine collection, and since it uses free, i.e., non–protein-bound, cobalamin, it fails to diagnose cobalamin deficiency not only in patients who are strict vegans but also the much more common patients who malabsorb cobalamin from food sources. Both the IF antibody test and the

---

* What is actually measured is "total homocysteine," which consists of the sum of homocysteine and the homocysteine that is linked via disulfide bond formation in a variety of compounds that include homocystine (homocysteine–homocysteine disulfide), homocysteine-cysteine mixed disulfide, proteins via their cysteine moieties, and peptides such as glutathione via their cysteine moieties.

TABLE 132–6. TYPICAL SERUM FINDINGS IN MEGALOBLASTIC ANEMIA

	Normal Levels	Deficiency of Cobalamin	Folate
Cobalamin	200–900 pg/ml	↓ *	N
Folate	2.5–20 ng/ml	N	↓ *
Methylmalonic acid	70–270 nM	↑ ↑	N
Homocysteine	5–16 μM	↑ ↑	↑ ↑

*A significant number of patients with cobalamin deficiency will have serum cobalamin levels in the lower portion of the normal range (see text). The same is true with respect to folate deficiency and serum folate levels.

Schilling test actually provide information about the etiology of cobalamin deficiency rather than information about the presence or absence of cobalamin deficiency per se. The etiology of cobalamin deficiency (and of folate deficiency) should be pursued in unusual patients and those with gastrointestinal symptoms that do not respond to cobalamin therapy because such studies may disclose the presence of a disease that requires additional therapy. It is acceptable practice to institute lifetime cobalamin therapy in individuals with anti-IF antibodies or abnormal Schilling tests who lack evidence of current cobalamin deficiency, since they will likely become deficient in the future. A normal result with either test should never be used, however, to exclude the diagnosis of cobalamin deficiency or to withhold lifetime therapy.

RESPONSE TO THERAPY. Therapeutic trials with cobalamin or folate must be performed with physiologic levels of either vitamin (1 μg per day for cobalamin and 100 μg per day for folate), since larger amounts can give hematologic responses even if the incorrect vitamin is employed. Such trials may require months before responses can be completely evaluated. They can be particularly difficult to interpret in patients with neuropsychiatric abnormalities, since these do not always respond to even large doses of cobalamin, even if cobalamin deficiency is the cause of the abnormalities. Therapeutic trials with pharmacologic doses of folate are potentially dangerous, since partial or even complete hematologic responses may be seen in cobalamin-deficient patients. The continuation of folate therapy in such patients is extremely dangerous, since folate does nothing for the neuropsychiatric abnormalities, which may progress or develop during folate therapy.

THERAPY

COBALAMIN DEFICIENCY. Therapy consists of the intramuscular or subcutaneous administration of either cyanocobalamin or hydroxocobalamin. Because cobalamin is inexpensive and free of any side effects, it is better to give too much than too little. The regimen used in our clinic consists of injections of 1000 μg of cyanocobalamin given once a week for 8 weeks and then once a month for life. More frequent injections are often used in hospitalized patients or those with marked neuropsychiatric abnormalities, but there is no evidence that this is beneficial. Once the weekly injections are completed, one can often teach the patient or a family member or friend to give the injections. The absolute requirement of lifetime therapy must be well understood by the patient. Oral therapy with cobalamin in a dose of 10 μg per day can be used with strict vegans. In theory, such therapy could also be used in individuals who malabsorb food cobalamin, but this is not recommended, since their IF production is often precarious and may decrease further over the years. Oral therapy with cobalamin in doses of 500 to 1000 μg per day should be reserved for the occasional patient who, for some reason, cannot receive cobalamin injections. Future measurements of serum levels of methylmalonic acid and homocysteine under various treatment and maintenance regimens may lead to changes in these recommendations.

FOLATE DEFICIENCY. Therapy is usually administered orally in the form of 1-mg tablets of folic acid. Oral therapy is almost always satisfactory, even in the presence of intestinal malabsorption. The usual dose is 1 to 2 mg daily. Therapy limited to several weeks is usually adequate in an alcoholic who begins to eat a normal diet. In patients with chronic conditions, such as malabsorption, hemolysis, exfoliative skin diseases, or renal fail-

ure requiring hemodialysis, oral folate is continued indefinitely and usually given prophylactically.

COBALAMIN OR FOLATE DEFICIENCY. Red cell transfusions are rarely required because of the well-compensated state of moderately, and even severely, anemic patients. Such transfusions should be avoided if at all possible because of the cost and risk associated with them. If transfusions are required, they should be given very slowly, since fluid overload occurs commonly and can precipitate lethal congestive heart failure. The only additional therapy is that required for certain underlying causes of cobalamin or folate deficiency, such as antibiotics in bacterial overgrowth or dietary changes in celiac disease.

DRUGS OR OTHER CAUSES. When drugs are responsible, either they can be stopped or the dosages can be reduced if necessary. In other cases, pyridoxine or thiamine can be tried in pharmacologic doses, since an occasional patient will respond.

PROGNOSIS

The hematologic abnormalities due to cobalamin or folate deficiency respond rapidly to therapy with the appropriate vitamin. Reticulocytosis begins by day 5, followed shortly by an increase in the hematocrit, which returns to normal within several months. Neutrophil and platelet counts and other laboratory abnormalities usually return to normal within a week to 10 days. If a complete correction of all hematologic abnormalities does not occur, a search should be made for other conditions, such as iron deficiency or hypothyroidism.

The response of the neuropsychiatric abnormalities caused by cobalamin deficiency is less predictable. Cobalamin therapy always prevents such patients from getting worse and most often results in a partial or complete correction. Responses may be seen within several days but may take as long as 12 or 18 months before improvement can be ruled out or is maximal. Patients with pernicious anemia have an approximately twofold elevated risk of developing gastric carcinoma, an increased association with hyperthyroidism and hypothyroidism, and other manifestations of the polyglandular failure syndrome (Ch. 228).

Allen RH, Stabler SP, Savage DG, et al.: Diagnosis of cobalamin deficiency I: Usefulness of serum methylmalonic acid and total homocysteine concentrations; II: Sensitivity of serum cobalamin, methylmalonic acid and total homocysteine concentrations. Am J Hematol 34:90, 1990. *A review of the development of serum cobalamin, methylmalonic acid, and homocysteine assays and their use in diagnosing cobalamin deficiency and distinguishing it from folate deficiency.*

Babior BM: Metabolic aspects of folic acid and cobalamin. Erythrocyte disorders—anemias related to disturbance of DNA synthesis (megaloblastic anemias). *In* Williams WJ, Beutler E, Erslev AJ, et al. (eds.): Hematology. 4th ed. New York, McGraw-Hill Book Company, 1990, pp 339–355, 453–481. *Sections of a leading hematology text that cover the megaloblastic anemias in detail. Extensive bibliographies through part of 1988.*

Carmel R: Pernicious anemia—the expected findings of very low serum cobalamin levels, anemia, and macrocytosis are often lacking. Arch Intern Med 148:1712, 1988. *The important message of this article is stated in its title.*

Carmel R, Sinow RM, Siegel ME, et al.: Food cobalamin malabsorption occurs frequently in patients with unexplained low serum cobalamin levels. Arch Intern Med 148:1715, 1988. *This article provides a convincing explanation for the normal results that are frequently obtained with standard Schilling tests in patients with proven cobalamin deficiency and underscores the important point that a normal Schilling test should never be used to exclude the diagnosis of cobalamin deficiency.*

Castle WB: The conquest of pernicious anemia. *In* Wintrobe MM (ed.): Blood, Pure and Eloquent: A Story of Discovery, of People, and of Ideas. New York, McGraw-Hill Book Company, 1980, pp 283–318. *An engrossing historical essay by the one who, in 1929, discovered intrinsic factor.*

Healton EB, Savage DG, Brust JCM, et al.: Neurologic aspects of cobalamin deficiency. Medicine 70:229, 1991. *Detailed description of 143 patients seen from 1968 to 1985, together with an excellent review of the literature; 57 references.*

Hector M, Burton J: What are the psychiatric manifestations of vitamin B_{12} deficiency? J Am Geriatr Soc 36:1105, 1988. *An excellent review of the psychiatric abnormalities that are caused by cobalamin deficiency and respond to cobalamin therapy, although I disagree with the definition of and conclusions about dementia; 85 references.*

Lindenbaum J, Healton EB, Savage DG, et al.: Neuropsychiatric disorders caused by cobalamin deficiency in the absence of anemia or macrocytosis. N Engl J Med 318:1720, 1988. *Detailed description of 42 patients with serious neuropsychiatric abnormalities that responded to cobalamin therapy despite the lack of one or more of the classic hematologic abnormalities that are also caused by cobalamin deficiency.*

Stabler SP, Allen RH, Savage DG, et al.: Clinical spectrum and diagnosis of cobalamin deficiency. Blood 76:871, 1990. *A total of 145 patients with serum cobalamin levels lower than 200 pg per milliliter were studied before and after cobalamin therapy; 86 had objective clinical responses and 59 did not. The two groups are compared in detail.*

133 Hemolytic Disorders: Introduction

Manuel E. Kaplan

PATHOPHYSIOLOGY OF HEMOLYSIS. Human red blood cells normally survive for approximately 120 days after they are released from the bone marrow as reticulocytes, being destroyed only after they have become senescent. With advancing cell age the activities of various red cell enzymes decline, and the cells become denser and less deformable. Phagocytic cells of the spleen and liver are believed to recognize and destroy effete red cells, although splenectomy does not extend the red cell lifespan beyond 120 days.

A hemolytic disorder is defined by premature destruction of red cells, which may occur either because inherently defective red cells are produced or because noxious factors are present in the intravascular environment. Intrinsic abnormalities that predispose to hemolysis may occur in the red cell membrane or in its contained hemoglobin or enzymes. These are, for the most part, genetically determined. In contrast, the environmental abnormalities that curtail red cell survival are almost all acquired. A classification of the causes of hemolytic anemia is given in Table 133–1.

To measure red cell survival, anticoagulated venous blood is incubated with radioactive chromium (^{51}Cr), which combines primarily with intracellular hemoglobin, and is then reinfused. Normally, 50 per cent of the injected ^{51}Cr activity disappears from the blood ($t\frac{1}{2}$) in 29 ± 3 days rather than at 60 days, because ^{51}Cr is an imperfect label and slowly elutes from the red cells. Nevertheless, the results of such studies are clinically informative because rates of hemolysis are reliably quantified and the sites of red cell destruction can be identified by external scanning utilizing a collimated gamma scintillation counter.

CONSEQUENCES OF HEMOLYSIS. Accelerated destruction of red cells may occur intravascularly or, much more commonly, after the cells have been culled from the circulation (sequestered).

Intravascular Hemolysis. Following intravascular hemolysis, hemoglobin is released into the plasma and is bound by haptoglobin, an alpha globulin synthesized by the liver. The haptoglobin concentration of blood, normally about 100 mg per 100 ml, reflects the rate of haptoglobin synthesis and catabolism. Haptoglobin synthesis is usually diminished in patients with parenchymal liver disease and may be increased in various inflammatory disorders, since it acts as an acute-phase protein. Free (uncomplexed) haptoglobin has a half-life of approximately 4 days. In contrast, hemoglobin-haptoglobin complexes are removed from the plasma within minutes, primarily by hepatic reticuloendothelial cells that catabolize both components of the complex. Haptoglobin catabolism usually exceeds haptoglobin synthesis in patients with intravascular hemolysis, and plasma haptoglobin levels fall, frequently to undetectable levels. If the quantity of hemoglobin entering the plasma exceeds the binding capacity of haptoglobin, hemoglobin appears in the glomerular filtrate, primarily as a 32,000-dalton alpha-beta dimer. The dimers are readily absorbed by cells of the proximal tubules, which convert heme iron into ferritin and hemosiderin. After the tubular cells are sloughed, hemosiderin can be detected in the urinary sediment with a Prussian blue stain. Hemoglobinuria, which occurs only when the filtered load of alpha-beta dimer exceeds the absorptive capacity of the tubular cells, connotes very rapid intravascular hemolysis. Persistent urinary loss of hemosiderin or hemoglobin may result in iron deficiency.

Hemoglobin in the plasma is unstable. Its ferrous (Fe^{2+}) heme prosthetic groups tend to dissociate, oxidize to metheme (Fe^{3+}), and bind either to hemopexin, a beta globulin, or to albumin, forming methemalbumin. Neither of these heme-protein complexes appears in the urine unless significant proteinuria is present. Because heme-hemopexin complexes are cleared rapidly from the blood, serum levels of hemopexin, like haptoglobin, are typically reduced or absent in the presence of significant intravascular hemolysis.

Since erythrocytes are rich in the enzyme lactate dehydrogenase (LDH), very high serum LDH levels are found in patients with intravascular hemolysis.

Extravascular Destruction. In most hemolytic disorders red cell destruction occurs extravascularly rather than intravascularly. Red cells are sequestered primarily within the spleen and/or liver and are phagocytized in situ. Although only a small fraction of the hemoglobin they contain escapes into the plasma, plasma haptoglobin levels characteristically fall, particularly when hemolysis is longstanding. Because plasma hemoglobin levels do not rise significantly, no hemoglobinuria or hemosiderinuria occurs. Serum LDH levels may be elevated, but not to the degree seen in intravascular hemolysis.

Hemoglobin derived from destroyed red cells is normally catabolized by reticuloendothelial cells to unconjugated, indirect-reacting bilirubin. As each heme tetrapyrrole ring is opened, one molecule of carbon monoxide is elaborated. Thus, the rate of formation of endogenously produced carbon monoxide can be used to quantify red cell destruction in vivo. However, this may not accurately reflect the rapidity of hemolysis, since ineffective erythropoiesis (destruction of immature red cells in the bone marrow) also contributes to carbon monoxide formation. The unconjugated bilirubin produced by phagocytic cells is bound by albumin, and its concentration in the patient's serum reflects the quantity of heme catabolized and the rate at which the liver is able to convert it into the direct-reacting, water-soluble product (Ch. 115). Serum levels of conjugated bilirubin are typically normal in patients with uncomplicated hemolysis, and bilirubinuria does not occur unless there is concomitant hepatocellular or biliary disease.

Bone Marrow Response. The loss of circulating red cells results in an erythropoietic stimulus to the bone marrow proportional to the decline in the oxygen-carrying capacity of the blood. The normal bone marrow responds by increasing commensurately its erythropoietic activity. When examined morphologically, the bone marrow of patients with hemolysis characteristically exhibits erythroid hyperplasia (see Color Plate 6C, right). Consequently, unless an underlying neoplastic disorder such as leukemia or lymphoma is suspected, bone marrow studies are usually not informative. The marrow's effective erythropoietic response to hemolysis, which may reach a maximum of approximately eight times normal, is reflected by the number of reticulocytes in the peripheral blood. The reticulocyte percentage alone does not adequately mirror the degree of marrow compensation (see Color Plate 5F, right). This may be more reliably gauged by calculating the reticulocyte index (patient's hematocrit times the percentage of reticulocytes/normal hematocrit). In some patients, a sustained reticulocytosis may compensate fully for the increased red cell destruction, and there is no anemia. More commonly, bone marrow compensation is incomplete, so that anemia, of greater or lesser severity, supervenes. If, in the presence of hemolysis, bone marrow function is compromised by such factors as infection or folate deficiency, the resultant reticulocytopenia will herald a rapidly worsening anemia.

TABLE 133–1. CLASSIFICATION OF THE CAUSES OF HEMOLYTIC ANEMIA

I. **Congenital hemolytic disorders** (see Ch. 134)
  A. Membrane defects
  B. Enzyme defects
    1. Embden-Meyerhof pathway defects
    2. Hexose monophosphate shunt defects
  C. Hemoglobin defects
    1. Structural (hemoglobinopathies) (see Ch. 136)
    2. Synthetic (thalassemias) (see Ch. 136)
  D. Other
II. **Acquired hemolytic disorders** (see Ch. 135)
  A. Sequestrational hemolysis (hypersplenism)
  B. Immune hemolytic disorders
    1. Alloimmune
    2. Autoimmune
    3. Drug-induced
  C. Paroxysmal nocturnal hemoglobinuria
  D. Due to toxins and metabolic abnormalities
  E. Due to red cell parasites
  F. Due to red cell trauma

DIFFERENTIAL DIAGNOSIS OF HEMOLYTIC DISORDERS. *Recognition and Diagnosis of Hemolysis.* The recognition of clinically significant hemolysis is generally not difficult. Commonly, a nonbleeding patient presents with a sustained reticulocytosis but exhibits no evidence of a rising hemoglobin or hematocrit. Some or all of the following findings may be seen:

1. *Evidence of enhanced marrow response:* reticulocytosis, polychromasia, erythroid hyperplasia of the bone marrow
2. *Evidence for excessive release and catabolism of red cell constituents:*
   a. in plasma—unconjugated bilirubin ↑, LDH ↑, haptoglobin ↓, hemopexin ↓, methemalbumin +, free hemoglobin ↑;
   b. in urine—hemosiderin +, methemalbumin +, hemoglobin +
3. *Decreased ^{51}Cr red cell survival*

The problem remains to determine the etiology of the hemolytic process (see Table 133–1). Hemolysis is caused either by an intrinsic abnormality of the red cell or an abnormality in its environment, the circulatory system in which the red cell resides. Red cell abnormalities that predispose to hemolysis may be congenital (genetically determined) or acquired. The congenital red cell defects may involve the membrane, the cellular enzymes, or the contained hemoglobin. Acquired red cell defects that predispose to hemolysis occur less commonly (1) under conditions of grossly abnormal (dysplastic) red cell maturation within the marrow (such as occurs in marked deficiencies of iron, vitamin B$_{12}$, or folate) with resultant release into the circulation of severely misshapen erythrocytes and (2) in paroxysmal nocturnal hemoglobinuria (Ch. 135). More commonly, acquired hemolytic disorders are due to the presence in the circulation of such noxious factors as red cell antibodies, immune complexes that provoke complement activation, microthrombi, chemical or metabolic "toxins," or parasites.

Clinical Findings. A patient with hemolysis may present with diverse complaints and physical findings that reflect the rapidity, underlying etiology, and pathophysiologic mechanism of red cell destruction. Patients with congenital hemolytic disorders are commonly anemic and intermittently jaundiced early in life. A suggestive family history of anemia, jaundice, cholelithiasis, splenomegaly, and/or therapeutic splenectomy can usually be elicited. A significant proportion of patients with acquired hemolysis have an identifiable underlying disease such as systemic lupus erythematosus (SLE) or chronic lymphocytic leukemia (CLL). A patient with rapidly falling hemoglobin due to hemolysis, whatever its cause, frequently presents with fatigue, palpitations, breathlessness, postural dizziness, and worsening of pre-existing angina. Physical examination commonly discloses pallor, mild jaundice, and splenomegaly. When hemolysis occurs secondary to an underlying disease, signs and symptoms of the latter may also be present: joint discomfort, rash, and pleuritis in SLE and lymphadenopathy in CLL.

Laboratory Findings. As previously noted, patients with significant hemolysis typically exhibit reticulocytosis with polychromasia on peripheral smear, unconjugated hyperbilirubinemia, serum haptoglobin levels ranging from decreased to absent, erythroid hyperplasia of the bone marrow, and elevated serum LDH levels. Indeed, these findings form the basis of recognizing a hemolytic anemia. Hemoglobinemia, hemoglobinuria, and hemosiderinuria occur only as a result of rapid intravascular hemolysis, which occurs in relatively rare situations, e.g., glucose-6-phosphate dehydrogenase (G6PD) deficiency exacerbated by oxidant drugs, certain infections (*Clostridium welchii*, falciparum malaria), paroxysmal nocturnal hemoglobinuria, paroxysmal cold hemoglobinuria, incompatible transfusions, and as a result of

TABLE 133–2. MORPHOLOGIC ABNORMALITIES OF RED CELLS IN VARIOUS HEMOLYTIC DISORDERS

Abnormality	Hemolytic Disorder	
	Congenital	Acquired
Permanently sickled cells	Sickle cell anemia	—
Fragmented cells (schistocytes)	Unstable hemoglobins (Heinz body anemias)	Microangiopathic processes Prosthetic heart valves
Spur cells (acanthocytes)	Abetalipoproteinemia	Severe liver disease
Spherocytes	Hereditary spherocytosis	Immune, warm antibody (immunoglobulin G, IgG) type
Target cells	Thalassemia Hemoglobinopathies (Hb C)	Liver disease
Agglutinated cells	—	Immune (immunoglobulin M, IgM), cold agglutinin disease

traumatic disruption of red cell membranes by excessive heat or mechanical stress.

Frequently, the morphologic appearance of red cells is abnormal in patients with hemolysis. Occasionally, the abnormalities are so typical that they indicate the correct diagnosis (Table 133–2).

Further Studies. The overall clinical picture in an individual hemolyzing patient is usually sufficiently informative to suggest a rational diagnostic approach. Laboratory studies that are frequently useful in elucidating the cause of a putative congenital hemolytic process include measurement of osmotic fragility, G6PD and pyruvate kinase screening, and hemoglobin electrophoresis. Where the hemolytic disorder is presumably acquired, a direct antiglobulin (Coombs') test should always be performed.

TREATMENT OF HEMOLYTIC ANEMIA. Only general supportive measures are discussed here, since optimal therapy requires precise definition of the etiology and pathophysiologic mechanism underlying the hemolytic process in the individual patient, as described in the subsequent two chapters.

Poorly compensated anemic patients should limit their activities to reduce cardiac output. Bed rest and nasal oxygen may afford symptomatic relief. Transfusions with packed red cells should be utilized to correct hemodynamic abnormalities rather than to treat low hemoglobin or hematocrit values. Transfusions, when necessary, should be administered slowly to avoid iatrogenically induced hypervolemia. The physician must consider the potential dangers of transfusion, particularly in patients with autoimmune hemolytic disorders (see Ch. 135).

To maintain maximal erythropoietic activity in patients with chronic hemolysis, supranormal quantities of folic acid are required. Therefore, daily oral supplementation with folic acid, 1 to 2 mg per day, is recommended. Serum cobalamin concentrations should also be measured if concomitant vitamin B$_{12}$ deficiency is suspected; when low, parenteral vitamin B$_{12}$ should also be administered.

SPECIFIC HEMOLYTIC DISORDERS. The purpose of this brief introduction is only to provide a pathophysiologic background to the hemolytic anemias and their general classification (Table 133–1). The anemias are discussed more extensively in Ch. 131 and 132. Specific hemolytic diseases resulting from intracorpuscular abnormalities caused by genetic abnormalities of the red cell membrane, of red cell enzymes, or of hemoglobin are presented in the following chapter. Ch. 135 summarizes the acquired hemolytic disorders.

134 Hereditary Defects in the Membrane or Metabolism of the Red Cell

Samuel E. Lux

MEMBRANE DISORDERS

Normal Red Cell Membrane

STRUCTURE

Membrane Lipids. The red cell membrane, or *ghost*, is a mixture of phospholipids, unesterified cholesterol, and glycolipids, arranged in a bilayer, and traversed randomly by transmembrane protein channels and receptors. The phospholipids are asymmetrically arranged. Choline phospholipids (phosphatidyl choline and sphingomyelin) are found primarily in the outer half of the bilayer; amino phospholipids (phosphatidyl serine and phosphatidyl ethanolamine) and phosphatidyl inositols are confined to the inner half. The mechanism that maintains this arrangement is poorly understood, but there is evidence that an adenosine triphosphate (ATP)–dependent aminophospholipid translocase ("flippase") is involved. It is probably important to sequester amino phospholipids, since their exposure triggers coagulation and causes red cells to adhere to phagocytes. The lipids are mobile in the plane of the membrane. This gives the membrane properties of a viscous two-dimensional fluid.

Membrane Proteins. The red cell membrane contains 10 to 15 major proteins and innumerable minor ones (Fig. 134–1). The proteins fall into two classes. (1) *Integral membrane proteins* traverse the bilayer, interact with the hydrophobic lipid core, and are tightly bound. They include functionally important transport proteins (e.g., the anion exchange protein) and glycoprotein surface antigens (e.g., glycophorin). (2) *Peripheral membrane proteins* are confined to the cytoplasmic membrane surface and include structural proteins, such as spectrin and actin, and some red cell enzymes (e.g., glyceraldehyde-3-phosphate dehydrogenase). These proteins bind to each other and to anchoring sites on integral proteins.

The major peripheral membrane proteins form a two-dimensional protein network that laminates the cytoplasmic membrane surface (Fig. 134–1). The principal components of this *membrane skeleton* are spectrin, actin, protein 4.1, and ankyrin. *Spectrin*, the major skeletal protein, is composed of two long, flexible chains, the alpha and beta subunits. The chains are mostly a series of successive 106 amino acid repeats, the result of ancient gene duplications. The two subunits are aligned antiparallel and are twisted about each other. These heterodimers interact at their "head" end to form heterotetramers or higher order oligo-

mers (spectrin self-association) (Fig. 134–1). At the opposite ("tail") end, spectrin binds to *short filaments of actin*. This interaction is greatly strengthened by *protein 4.1*, which attaches to beta spectrin near the actin-binding site. Because multiple spectrins can bind to each actin filament, the spectrin-actin-4.1 complex is a molecular junction that allows spectrin filaments to branch and form a two-dimensional membrane skeleton.

The skeleton is anchored to the overlying lipid bilayer by *ankyrin*, which binds to spectrin near the self-association site and links it to the cytoplasmic portion of protein 3, the anion exchange protein. Protein 4.2, which binds to both ankyrin and protein 3, may strengthen this interaction (Fig. 134–1). Interactions between protein 4.1 and some of the glycophorins and between various skeletal proteins and membrane lipids also occur but are less well characterized.

MAJOR FUNCTIONS

Membrane Strength and Durability. In humans the red cell must be flexible enough to negotiate splenic and capillary channels less than half its diameter and still be strong and durable enough to survive the turbulent journey through the heart approximately 500,000 times during its 120-day lifespan. These properties are *determined by the membrane skeleton*. The membrane spontaneously vesiculates when spectrin and actin are selectively extracted or when spectrin is denatured (at 49°C). Mice with hereditary deficiencies of alpha or beta spectrin or ankyrin have extremely fragile red cells that rapidly fragment in the circulation, leading to marked spherocytosis and severe hemolysis.

Maintenance of Cell Volume. The red cell controls its volume and water content by regulating its intracellular concentration of Na^+ and K^+. This is possible because the membrane is relatively impermeable to cations. Normally, small passive cation leaks are balanced by the active transport of Na^+ outward and K^+ inward. These ion movements are powered by a pump that is fueled by the membrane enzyme Na^+-K^+-ATPase. Normally, this system maintains intracellular Na^+ and K^+ at about 10 mEq per liter and 100 mEq per liter, respectively. The pump is regulated by the intracellular Na^+ concentration and has considerable ability to compensate for an increased leak of Na^+ into the cell. If this capacity is surpassed and the inward leak of Na^+ exceeds the K^+ leak out, red cells gain cations and water and swell. Unfortunately, the pump does not compensate nearly as well to a decrease in intracellular K^+. Any increase in the outward leak of K^+ relative to Na^+ leads to loss of total monovalent cations and water and results in cellular dehydration.

Calcium Homeostasis. Excessive intracellular Ca^{2+} is very deleterious, and the red cell actively extrudes it with an efficient, calmodulin-regulated calcium pump that is driven by a Ca^{2+}-ATPase. Intracellular Ca^{2+} is normally almost undetectable (about 0.1 μM). If ATP levels fall below about 20 per cent of normal or if Ca^{2+} leakage exceeds the capacity of the pump, Ca^{2+} accumulates and changes the red cell from a biconcave disc to an echinocyte—a spiculated sphere with numerous short, regular projections. Elevated intracellular Ca^{2+} also causes a selective loss of K^+ and water. The result is a crenated, dehydrated, almost indeformable cell that is highly susceptible to splenic sequestration and destruction.

Anion Exchange. Physiologically, the red cell is a critical component of CO_2 transport. Red cells normally convert tissue CO_2 to HCO_3^- and carry the HCO_3^- to the lungs, where they exchange it for Cl^-. The process is massive and requires a large number of transport channels (~1 million per red cell). These are formed by *protein 3* (Fig. 134–1).

Interactions Between Red Cells and the Spleen

Red cells that enter the spleen must squeeze their 7-μ wide bodies through narrow elliptical fenestrations that separate the splenic cords and sinuses to return to the circulation (Ch. 152). Normal red cells make this journey about 120 times per day and complete it in about 30 seconds, but abnormal cells may be detained for minutes to hours in the hypoxic, acidic, hypoglycemic environment of the splenic cords. This taxing metabolic stress is often fatal for old or defective erythrocytes.

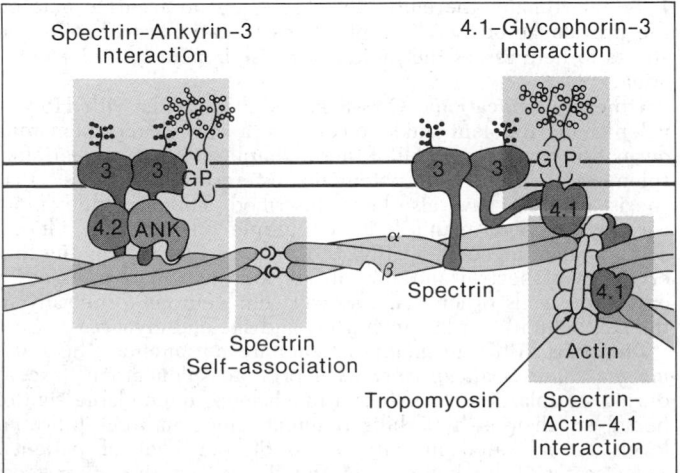

FIGURE 134–1. Schematic illustration of the organization of the major proteins of the red cell membrane and membrane skeleton. ANK = ankyrin; GP = glycophorin.

Red cells are detained in the spleen if they are rigid or if they are coated with proteins such as immunoglobulin G1 (IgG1), immunoglobulin G3 (IgG3), or C3b that bind to receptors on splenic macrophages. Probably other, less well defined, changes in the red cell surface also attract phagocytes and lead to red cell death. Increased rigidity may result from (1) increased cytoplasmic viscosity (e.g., sickled cells and other dehydrated red cells); (2) intracellular rubbish (e.g., Heinz bodies); (3) membrane rigidity (e.g., secondary to oxidative crosslinking of the membrane skeleton); or (4) a decrease in the red cell surface-volume ratio.

SURFACE-VOLUME RATIO: OSMOTIC FRAGILITY TEST

Spherocytes are caused by a decrease in the surface-volume ratio of the red cell. Target cells form when this ratio is increased. Because the area of the red cell membrane is fixed (i.e., the membrane is not stretchable), the cell becomes progressively more rigid as its spheroidicity increases. Surface-volume ratio is assessed clinically by the *unincubated osmotic fragility test*. This test measures the ability of red cells to swell in a graded series of hypotonic solutions. Spherocytes are osmotically fragile; that is, they can tolerate less osmotic swelling than normal cells before they hemolyze. Target cells are osmotically resistant.

Hereditary Spherocytosis (HS)

Hereditary spherocytosis is an inherited hemolytic anemia characterized by osmotically fragile, partially spherical, spectrin-deficient red cells that are selectively trapped by the spleen (see Color Plate 6D, left). The disease occurs in all races but is particularly common in northern Europeans, in whom the prevalence is about 1 in 5000. There are at least two patterns of inheritance: 75 per cent of the families show a classic autosomal dominant pattern. Most of the remainder have a nondominant (probably autosomal recessive) form.

Pathogenesis. Hereditary spherocytes transfused into normal subjects show impairment of survival, demonstrating clearly that they are intrinsically defective. The primary physiologic defect appears to be membrane instability. Red cell membranes from most HS patients fragment more easily than normal when stressed. This weakness suggests defects of the membrane skeleton.

Most HS red cells are spectrin deficient, and many are also ankyrin deficient. The degree of spectrin deficiency correlates closely with the degree of spherocytosis, as measured by osmotic fragility, and with the severity of hemolysis and response to splenectomy. In general, patients with dominant HS have only mild deficiency (spectrin content is 75 to 90 per cent of normal) and mild to moderate hemolysis. Patients with recessive HS often have a more severe deficit—rarely so severe (30 to 50 per cent of normal) that it produces life-threatening, transfusion-dependent hemolysis.

The causes of spectrin and ankyrin deficiency are an active topic of investigation. Preliminary evidence suggests that alpha spectrin defects are common in recessive HS, while ankyrin and beta spectrin defects predominate in the dominant form of the disease. Recessive HS associated with *absence of protein 4.2* and dominant HS with partial *deficiency of protein 3* also occur. However, in these variants, red cell spectrin content is normal.

It is speculated that HS red cells gradually lose portions of the lipid bilayer and become progressively more spherocytic as they age in the circulation (Fig. 134–2). Eventually, they are detained in the splenic cords, where, for unknown reasons, their membrane loss is accentuated by the toxic cordal environment. This *"splenic conditioning"* can be mimicked in vitro by incubating red cells in the absence of glucose for 24 hours. Under these conditions, hereditary spherocytes lose membrane fragments more rapidly than do normal red cells. This is the basis of the *incubated osmotic fragility test*. In vivo, conditioned spherocytes are prevalent in the splenic pulp, and some escape into the peripheral circulation as the characteristic HS hyperchromic microspherocytes. These impaired cells form the hyperspherical tail on osmotic fragility curves. Undoubtedly, many HS red cells never escape the conditioning process. Those that do are especially susceptible to recapture and destruction by the spleen.

Clinical Features (Table 134–1). The hallmarks of HS are *anemia, jaundice,* and *splenomegaly.* The disease may present at any age. In neonates, excessive jaundice is frequent (~50 per cent) and sometimes requires an exchange transfusion. In addition, some HS infants respond sluggishly to their anemia during the first few months of life and require intermittent booster transfusions. After the neonatal period most patients develop partially compensated hemolysis with only mild to moderate anemia (hemoglobin [Hb] = 9 to 11.5 grams per deciliter), intermittent mild jaundice (especially during viral infections), and splenomegaly. *Clinical severity can vary widely,* sometimes even within the same family. A small proportion of patients have life-threatening hemolysis and are transfusion dependent. A much larger proportion, roughly 25 per cent, have unusually mild disease. In these patients marrow erythropoiesis is sufficient to balance the modest rate of spherocyte destruction, and there is no anemia, little or no jaundice, and minimal splenomegaly. However, severe hemolysis and anemia may develop with illnesses that cause the spleen to hypertrophy, such as infectious mononucleosis. Hemolysis may also be exacerbated by long-term intensive physical activity, possibly because of increased splenic blood flow. Finally, in old age, when bone marrow function becomes sluggish, previously well compensated nonsplenectomized patients may become dangerously anemic.

Complications. Crises. The clinical course is interrupted in most patients by occasional crises, characterized by worsening anemia. *Hemolytic crises* are the most frequent but usually are mild and clinically insignificant. They are presumably secondary to the reticuloendothelial hyperplasia that accompanies many infections. *Aplastic crises* are less prevalent but are often severe enough to threaten heart failure and require transfusion. They are frequently caused by a human parvovirus (see Color Plate 5H, right) (Ch. 129) that invades erythropoietic stem cells and inhibits their growth. The infection typically presents in young children as a febrile illness or as fifth disease, a viral exantham; however, some older children and adults are also susceptible to the virus and aplastic crises. Parvovirus is contagious and is especially dangerous to the fetus. All patients with aplastic crises should be isolated from contact with women who are or might be pregnant. *Megaloblastic crises* (see Color Plate 6H) occur when dietary intake of folic acid is inadequate for the increased needs of the erythroid HS bone marrow. This need is particularly acute during pregnancy. To prevent megaloblastic crises, all HS patients should receive daily supplements of folic acid (1 mg per day).

Gallstones. Untreated older children and adults with HS often develop bilirubinate gallstones secondary to increased bilirubin production. Only 5 per cent of children less than 10 years old are affected, but the prevalence rises to 40 to 50 per cent in the second to fifth decades and 55 to 75 per cent thereafter. The frequency after age 30 parallels the frequency in the general population, which suggests that gallstones in HS patients form primarily in the second and third decades. Ultrasonography is the most reliable method for detecting bilirubin stones. Only 50 per cent are radiopaque. Concern about cholecystitis and biliary obstruction is the major impetus for splenectomy in most patients. It is unfortunate, therefore, that there are no accurate data on the prevalence of these complications in patients with bilirubin stones to help assess the indications (risk-benefit ratio) for operation.

Other Complications. Occasional adult patients with HS develop gout, indolent ankle ulcers, or a chronic erythematous dermatitis on the legs. All of these complications disappear after splenectomy. Rarer but potentially interesting syndromes that coexist with HS have also been described. These include spinal cord dysfunction, manifest as a multiple sclerosis–like illness, and a familial myocardiopathy. In this regard it is intriguing that erythrocyte spectrin and ankyrin are known to be expressed in only three cells other than the red cell: neurons (especially in the cerebellum), cardiac myocytes, and skeletal myocytes.

Diagnosis. Although many patients are not anemic, the *reticulocyte count is always increased* prior to splenectomy (except during an aplastic crisis). It is a much more dependable sign of hemolysis than is hyperbilirubinemia, since indirect bilirubin levels are elevated in only 50 to 60 per cent of patients. *Spherocytosis,* the hallmark of the disease, is the other most reliable finding (see Color Plate 6D, left). However, spherocytes are a frequent artifact in normal blood smears, so the physician must take care to examine only areas of the smear in which the

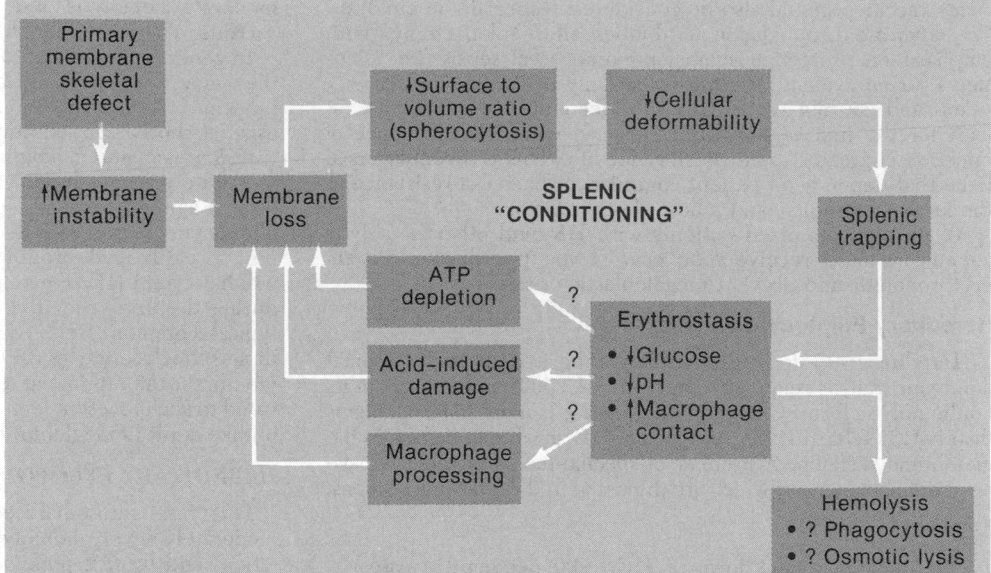

FIGURE 134–2. Currently favored model of the pathophysiology of hereditary spherocytosis. ATP = adenosine triphosphate.

red cells are well separated and some cells with central pallor are evident. Spherocytosis is also observed in a variety of other conditions (Table 134–2); however, with the exception of certain *immunohemolytic anemias* (which can be excluded with a Coombs test), most of these do not present any diagnostic difficulty.

In 20 to 25 per cent of patients, classic microspherocytes are sparse, and it may be difficult to recognize spherocytosis from the blood smear alone. In these patients, the *unincubated* osmotic fragility (OF) test is sometimes normal or only slightly increased, since it simply quantifies what is visible on the smear. The *incubated* OF, however, is almost always abnormal and is the most reliable available diagnostic test. HS red cells are quite dehydrated and therefore have an *increased mean corpuscular hemoglobin concentration (MCHC)*. An MCHC level of 36 or greater is present in 50 per cent of HS patients and is useful confirmatory evidence of the disease. Since deficiencies of spectrin, ankyrin, protein 3, or protein 4.2 appear to be the primary defects in HS, quantitation of these proteins should provide the most accurate diagnostic test; however, at present these measurements are available in only a few research laboratories.

Once HS is diagnosed, *a careful search for the disease should always be made in all close relatives.* It is tragic to see HS become symptomatic in elderly patients with a poor operative risk, in whom this condition could have been discovered earlier.

Treatment. *Splenectomy* dependably blunts both red cell conditioning and hemolysis in HS and is the recommended therapy. Following surgery, spherocytosis persists because the basic red cell defect is unchanged, but conditioned microspherocytes disappear and changes typical of the postsplenectomy state (Howell-Jolly bodies, target cells, siderocytes, and acanthocytes) become evident on the blood smear (see Color Plate 6K). During the

operation the surgeon must be careful to search for accessory spleens, which occur in 20 to 30 per cent of patients. Recurrence of hemolysis due to regrowth of an accessory spleen is occasionally observed after years or even decades and should be suspected if reticulocytosis recurs or Howell-Jolly bodies disappear from the blood smear.

Splenectomy increases susceptibility to sepsis from pneumococci and certain other encapsulated bacteria. The major issues today are who should undergo splenectomy and how should they be treated postoperatively. It is impossible to answer either question absolutely. In general, *we recommend splenectomy for all HS patients with either anemia or significant hemolysis* (reticulocyte counts repeatedly greater than 5 per cent). We defer splenectomy in patients with mild compensated hemolysis, but if these patients subsequently develop bilirubin gallstones and require cholecystectomy, we advocate splenectomy to prevent the recurrence of common duct stones. The risk of sepsis after splenectomy is very high in infancy and early childhood; splenectomy should therefore be delayed until the age of 6 or 7 years if possible and to at least 2 to 3 years in all cases, even if chronic transfusion is required in the interim. There is no evidence that delay beyond 7 years is useful, and it may be harmful, since the risk of gallstones increases dramatically after the age of 10 years.

It is difficult to estimate accurately the risk of postsplenectomy sepsis in older children and adults. The incidence of fulminant infection in splenectomized adults appears to be about 0.2 cases per 100 person-years, and the incidence of all serious infections is about 7 cases per 100 person-years.

All splenectomized patients should receive *polyvalent pneumococcal vaccine* (Pnu-Immune 23 or equivalent, 0.5 ml given subcutaneously or intramuscularly), preferably given preoperatively. Immunization with meningococcal and *Haemophilus influ-*

TABLE 134–1. HEREDITARY SPHEROCYTOSIS

Clinical Manifestations	Laboratory Features
Anemia	Reticulocytosis
Splenomegaly	Spherocytosis
Intermittent jaundice	Elevated MCHC
From hemolysis	Increased osmotic fragility
From biliary obstruction	(especially incubated osmotic
	fragility test)
Aplastic crises	Normal Coombs' test
Often dominant inheritance	Decreased red cell spectrin or
	spectrin and ankyrin or protein
	3 or protein 4.2
Rare manifestations	
Leg ulcers	
Spinal cord dysfunction	
Myocardiopathy	
Good response to splenectomy	

TABLE 134–2. DISEASES WITH SPHEROCYTOSIS AS THE PREDOMINANT MORPHOLOGIC ABNORMALITY ON THE BLOOD SMEAR

Common
  Hereditary spherocytosis
  Immunohemolytic anemias (warm antibody type)
  ABO incompatibility in neonates
Uncommon to rare
  Hemolytic transfusion reactions
  Clostridial sepsis
  Severe burns and other red cell thermal injuries
  Spider, bee, and snake venoms
  Acute red cell oxidant injury*
  Severe hypophosphatemia
  Hawkinsinuria

*Acute red cell oxidant injury is common, but spherocytosis is rarely the predominant morphology.

enzae vaccines should also be considered, especially in children. We advocate prophylactic antibiotics after splenectomy, with emphasis on protection against pneumococcal sepsis (i.e., Pen-Vee K or equivalent, 125 mg twice daily in young children [<7 years] and 250 mg twice daily in older children and adults), at least for the first 2 years after surgery, when the incidence of infection is greatest, and possibly for life. This is a controversial issue that depends on patient compliance, bacterial resistance in the local community, and a host of other factors.

All unsplenectomized patients with HS (and other hemolytic anemias) should receive *folic acid* (1 mg per day) to sustain erythropoiesis and prevent megaloblastic crises.

Hereditary Elliptocytosis (HE)

Hereditary elliptocytosis, usually inherited as an autosomal dominant trait, is relatively common (~1:2500), particularly in its nonhemolytic form. Clinically, the disease is more heterogeneous than is HS (Table 134–3). All types of HE are due to defects in the membrane skeleton. A number of specific molecular defects have been defined, some of which are discussed in the following sections.

MILD HE

This most prevalent form of HE (~90 per cent of cases) is usually caused either by defects in the head end of spectrin that interfere with spectrin self-association or by the partial absence or dysfunction of protein 4.1. Practically, it is little more than a morphologic curiosity. Most patients have no anemia or splenomegaly and only mild hemolysis (reticulocyte counts of 1 to 3 per cent). The blood smear shows prominent elliptocytosis (usually

TABLE 134–3. HEREDITARY ELLIPTOCYTOSIS

Clinical Manifestations	Laboratory Features
Mild HE	
Asymptomatic	Blood smear: elliptocytes, few or no poikilocytes
Dominant inheritance: one parent with HE	No anemia, little or no hemolysis (reticulocytes = 1 to 3%)
Variants:	Normal osmotic fragility
Some neonates with moderately severe hemolytic anemia and HPP-like smear. Converts to typical common HE by 1 to 2 years	Often defect in spectrin self-association or partial deficiency or dysfunction of protein 4.1
Some patients with mild chronic hemolysis	
Hereditary Pyropoikilocytosis (HPP)	
Anemia	Blood smear: bizarre poikilocytes, fragments, spherocytes, ± elliptocytes
Splenomegaly	
Intermittent jaundice	Reticulocytosis
Aplastic crises	Decreased MCV due to red cell fragmentation
Recessive inheritance: both parents normal or one or both parents with HE	Increased osmotic fragility
Good response to splenectomy	Decreased red cell heat stability
	Marked defect in spectrin self-association
Spherocytic HE	
Anemia	Blood smear: rounded elliptocytes, ± spherocytes
Splenomegaly	
Intermittent jaundice	Reticulocytosis
Dominant inheritance pattern	Increased osmotic fragility
Good response to splenectomy	Primary defect unknown
Southeast Asian Ovalocytosis	
Asymptomatic	Blood smear: rounded elliptocytes, some with a transverse bar that divides the central clear space
Dominant inheritance	
Lowland aboriginal tribes in Melanesia and Malaysia	No anemia or hemolysis
	Very rigid red cells that resist invasion by malarial parasites
	Increased ankyrin binding to a mutant protein 3 molecule

>40 per cent; normal <15 per cent) (see Color Plate 6D, right). Osmotic fragility is normal. A few cases (10 to 20 per cent) have moderate hemolysis and are classified as sporadic hemolytic variants. The reason for this variation is unknown.

In general, patients with common HE require no therapy; but they may develop significant hemolysis if the spleen hypertrophies in response to various stimuli (e.g., infectious mononucleosis, cirrhosis). In addition, the physician must be alert for *transient neonatal hemolysis.* Neonates in some HE families have moderately severe hemolytic anemia with marked red cell budding, fragmentation, and poikilocytosis. The relative paucity of elliptocytes may create diagnostic confusion; however, the diagnosis is easily made from family studies, since one of the parents will have mild HE. Hemolysis gradually declines in these infants during the first year or so of life, and the disorder evolves into typical common HE. This susceptibility may be due to 2,3-diphosphoglycerate (2,3-DPG), which destabilizes the red cell membrane at millimolar concentrations. Free 2,3-DPG is elevated to such levels in fetal erythrocytes because fetal hemoglobin (unlike adult hemoglobin) does not bind 2,3-DPG.

HEREDITARY PYROPOIKILOCYTOSIS (HPP)

This rare autosomal recessive disorder is characterized by moderately severe hemolytic anemia, marked red cell fragmentation, and *bizarre poikilocytosis.* It is most common in blacks. When heated for short periods, HPP red cells fragment (and their isolated spectrin denatures) at 45 to 46°C instead of the normal 49°C. This *exceptional heat sensitivity* is one of the primary tests for the disease. Hemolysis decreases after splenectomy, the treatment of choice, but the bizarre red cell morphology and heat sensitivity are unchanged. HPP is related to common HE in that all HPP patients have a *defect in spectrin self-association* that is qualitatively identical to the defect in common HE, but more severe. In addition, patients with HPP often have first-degree relatives with HE. A current hypothesis is that HPP patients are homozygous or compound heterozygous for mild HE, homozygous for a related "silent" mutation, or doubly heterozygous for mild HE and the putative silent gene defect.

SPHEROCYTIC HE

This variant (~10 per cent of cases) is clinically and pathophysiologically similar to hereditary spherocytosis. It is inherited in an autosomal dominant pattern. The primary molecular defect is unknown. Patients typically have moderate hemolysis, mild anemia, and splenomegaly. Elliptocytes are less prominent and are more rounded than in typical common HE. Spherocytes are often evident and occasionally may predominate; however, at least one family member will usually have clear-cut elliptocytosis. Patients with this form of HE, like those with HS, have osmotically fragile red cells and respond dramatically to splenectomy. The indications for splenectomy are the same as for HS.

SOUTHEAST ASIAN OVALOCYTOSIS

This curious autosomal dominant disorder is very prevalent in Melanesian and Malaysian aborigines but is rarely seen in other populations. It is characterized by *extraordinarily rigid* red cells that resist invasion by a variety of malarial parasites. The rigidity appears to be caused by increased binding of ankyrin to a mutant protein 3. Surprisingly, the red cells circulate freely, despite their rheology, and there is no associated hemolysis or anemia. Blood smears show rounded elliptocytes, some of which have a characteristic transverse bar that crosses the long axis of the cells and divides the area of central pallor.

Hereditary Defects in Membrane Permeability

HEREDITARY XEROCYTOSIS

In this rare autosomal dominant disorder of red cell membrane permeability, the ratio of K^+ loss to Na^+ gain exceeds the normal ratio of 2:3; as a result, total cation content and cell water decrease. This occurs as a secondary event in a variety of conditions (e.g., sickle cell disease, hereditary spherocytosis, hemoglobin C disease, and glycolytic enzyme deficiencies). Morphologically, dehydrated red cells are typically either targeted or contracted and spiculated. Because dehydration increases intracellular viscosity, these cells are relatively rigid and risk splenic sequestration and hemolysis.

HEREDITARY HYDROCYTOSIS (HEREDITARY STOMATOCYTOSIS)

In this rare autosomal dominant disease, an inherited defect in Na^+ permeability causes massive Na^+ influx, which overwhelms the Na-K pump and leads to an increase in intracellular cations and water. In some families this results in severe hemolysis. In others, for unknown reasons, hemolysis is much milder. Patients with the severe variant respond well to splenectomy. The partially swollen red cells appear on blood smears as stomatocytes (i.e., red cells with a mouthlike band of pallor across the center of the stained cell). Stomatocytes are much more frequently seen as an acquired defect, without hydrocytosis, cation changes, or hemolysis, in patients with acute alcoholism or with various types of liver disease.

ENZYME DEFICIENCIES
Normal Red Cell Metabolism

Reticulocytes have no nuclei and lose their mitochondria and microsomes as they mature; consequently, mature red cells consume little oxygen and do not synthesize protein. Glucose, the main metabolic substrate of the cells, is metabolized via two major pathways: the *Embden-Meyerhof pathway* and the *hexose monophosphate shunt* (Fig. 134–3).

THE EMBDEN-MEYERHOF (EM) PATHWAY

Approximately 90 to 95 per cent of metabolized glucose is converted to lactate via the EM pathway. This is the *major pathway of ATP synthesis in mature red cells.* Only two moles of ATP are generated from glycolysis per mole of glucose consumed, very inefficient compared with cells that possess mitochondria and an active Krebs cycle (that generates 38 moles of ATP per mole of glucose). Nevertheless, the meager amount of ATP produced permits renewal of 150 to 200 per cent of the total red cell ATP every hour. Red cell ATP is used to transport monovalent cations and calcium, to phosphorylate various proteins, to synthesize glutathione, to salvage nucleotides, and to produce the hexose phosphates needed to fuel glycolysis.

The EM pathway is also the major source of red cell nicotinamide-adenine dinucleotide, reduced form (NADH). This cofactor is essential for the maintenance of heme iron in the reduced state, an enzymatic process that is mediated by *NADH methemoglobin reductase.* Oxidation of heme iron to Fe^{3+} produces methemoglobin, which does not transport oxygen (Ch. 136).

Red cells have a uniquely high concentration of *2,3-DPG;* only traces of this metabolic intermediate are present in other cells. This intermediate, formed by the Rapaport-Luebering shunt (Fig. 134–3), decreases the oxygen affinity of hemoglobin and increases oxygen delivery to peripheral tissues (Ch. 136).

HEXOSE MONOPHOSPHATE (HMP) SHUNT

Approximately 5 to 10 per cent of utilized glucose is normally directed through the HMP shunt. This pathway is the *major source of nicotinamide-adenine dinucleotide phosphate, reduced form (NADPH)* in human red cells: Two moles of NADPH are produced for each mole of glucose metabolized. Under conditions in which the oxidation of NADPH is accelerated, diversion of glucose through the shunt can increase up to 10- or 20-fold.

The most important reactions associated with NADPH oxidation are those related to glutathione. Red cells contain relatively high concentrations (2 mM) of *reduced glutathione (GSH)*, a tripeptide (gamma-glutamylcysteinylglycine) that is synthesized by mature red cells (Fig. 134–3). GSH protects red cells from injury by oxidants such as superoxide anion (O_2^-), hydrogen peroxide (H_2O_2), and hydroxyl radical (OH•), which are produced continuously in normal red cells as by-products of the oxidation of heme by its dangerous oxygen cargo. Large amounts of oxidants are generated by activated phagocytes (e.g., during infections) and by red cells in the presence of certain drugs. Injury to cell lipids and proteins occurs if these agents accumulate. Normally, this is prevented by GSH. Detoxification of H_2O_2 can occur spontaneously, but it is enhanced by *glutathione peroxidase.* Catalase also degrades H_2O_2, but under physiologic conditions it is less important. In these reactions GSH is converted to *oxidized glutathione (GSSG)* and to mixed disulfides with protein thiols (Fig. 134–3). GSH levels are restored by *glutathione reductase.* In the process, NADPH is oxidized to NADP, which stimulates the HMP shunt, regenerating NADPH. This tight coupling of

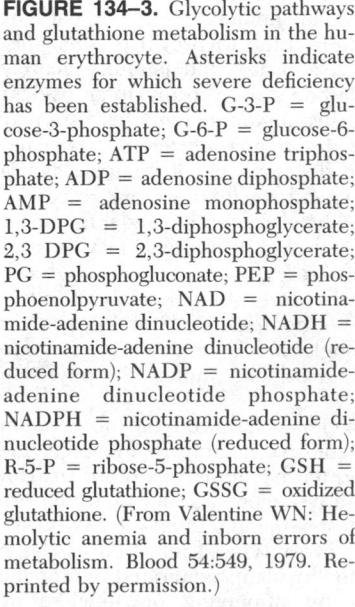

FIGURE 134–3. Glycolytic pathways and glutathione metabolism in the human erythrocyte. Asterisks indicate enzymes for which severe deficiency has been established. G-3-P = glucose-3-phosphate; G-6-P = glucose-6-phosphate; ATP = adenosine triphosphate; ADP = adenosine diphosphate; AMP = adenosine monophosphate; 1,3-DPG = 1,3-diphosphoglycerate; 2,3 DPG = 2,3-diphosphoglycerate; PG = phosphogluconate; PEP = phosphoenolpyruvate; NAD = nicotinamide-adenine dinucleotide; NADH = nicotinamide-adenine dinucleotide (reduced form); NADP = nicotinamide-adenine dinucleotide phosphate; NADPH = nicotinamide-adenine dinucleotide phosphate (reduced form); R-5-P = ribose-5-phosphate; GSH = reduced glutathione; GSSG = oxidized glutathione. (From Valentine WN: Hemolytic anemia and inborn errors of metabolism. Blood 54:549, 1979. Reprinted by permission.)

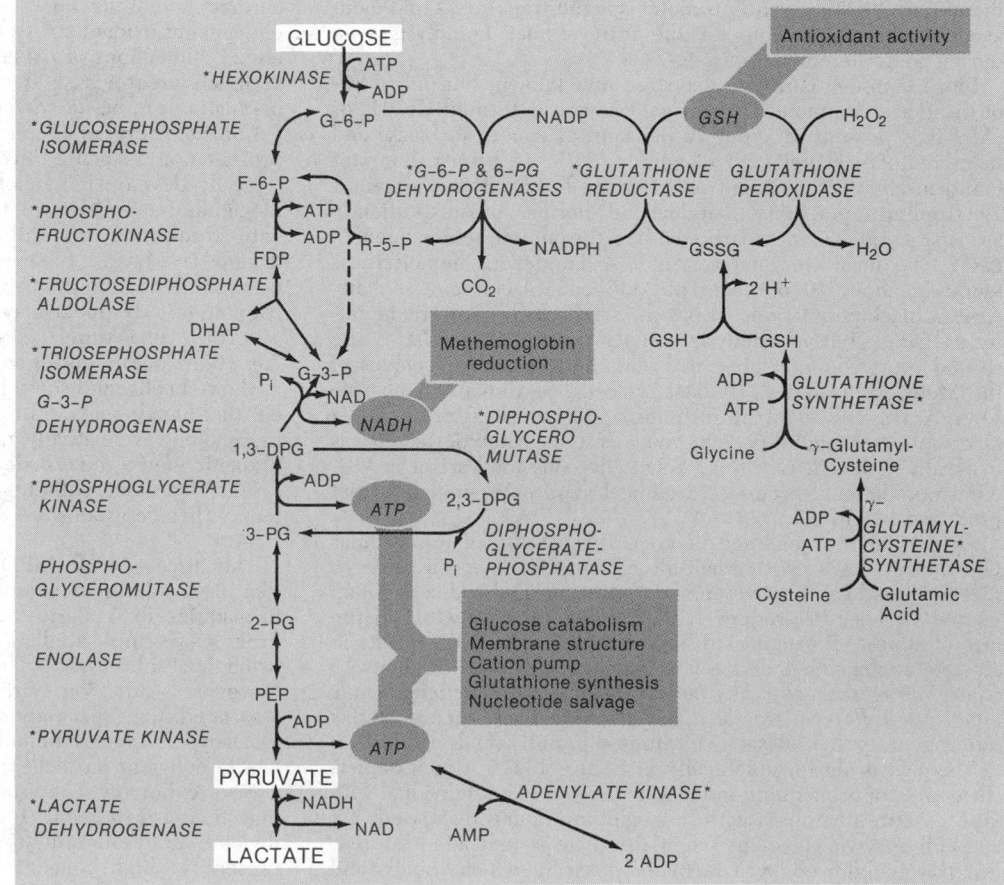

the HMP shunt with glutathione metabolism normally protects red cells from oxidant injury.

Defects in the HMP Shunt or Glutathione Metabolism

Almost all HMP shunt defects are due to *glucose-6-phosphate dehydrogenase (G6PD)* deficiency, the most common enzyme abnormality associated with hemolytic anemia. It affects millions of people throughout the world. In contrast, pyruvate kinase deficiency, the most common glycolytic defect, affects only hundreds to thousands of patients.

GLUCOSE-6-PHOSPHATE DEHYDROGENASE (G6PD) DEFICIENCY

Pathophysiology. Defects in the HMP shunt or glutathione metabolic pathways impair the ability of red cells to defend themselves against oxidative assault. Oxidants produced by infections or oxidant drugs are normally detoxified by GSH, but GSH levels are not maintained in G6PD deficiency because of the diminished ability to generate NADPH. As a consequence, the oxidants are free to damage vital cell constituents. Oxidation of hemoglobin produces the functionless *methemoglobin* and intracellular precipitates of denatured hemoglobin that are known as *Heinz bodies* (see Color Plate 6C, left). Heinz bodies are not visible in ordinary Wright's-stained blood smears but are revealed with supravital stains such as *methyl violet*. They attach to the membrane and damage it in various ways. Among other things, they cause protein 3 molecules and immunoglobulin to cluster on the cell surface, opsonizing the cells for phagocytes. In vitro, they also increase membrane leakiness to cations and decrease osmotic fragility and cellular deformability. In vivo, Heinz bodies are "pitted" from circulating red cells by the spleen and thus are more plentiful in splenectomized patients. *"Bite cells"*—that is, red cells with a localized invagination, possibly at the site of Heinz body damage or removal—appear in the circulation during acute hemolytic episodes. Red cells with a submembranous hemoglobin-free area, *"blister cells,"* may also be seen (see Color Plate 6E, left). In addition to damage from Heinz bodies, G6PD-deficient red cells suffer oxidative crosslinking of spectrin and peroxidation of membrane lipids. Spectrin crosslinking decreases membrane flexibility and promotes splenic trapping. Lipid damage may be responsible for the intravascular hemolysis seen during acute hemolytic episodes.

More than 300 G6PD variants are now known, but only a few of these are common. The normal enzyme is termed G6PD^B or *Gd^B*. It is present in about 70 per cent of American blacks and in more than 99 per cent of whites. *Gd^{A+}* is a normal variant found in about 20 per cent of American blacks. It has a greater electrophoretic mobility than does Gd^B because of substitution of an asparagine for an aspartic acid in the amino acid sequence. *Gd^{A-}*, the most common variant associated with hemolysis, is found in about 10 per cent of American blacks and in many African black populations. It has the same electrophoretic mobility as Gd^{A+}, but its catalytic activity is decreased. *Gd^{Med}*, the second most common abnormal variant, is found in peoples of the Mediterranean area (Italians, Greeks, Sardinians, Sephardic Jews, Arabs, and so forth), in India, and in southeastern Asia. Its electrophoretic mobility is normal, but its catalytic activity is markedly reduced. *Gd^{Canton}*, a relatively common variant in Oriental populations, produces a clinical syndrome similar to that produced by Gd^{A-}.

As normal red cells age in vivo, the activity of intracellular Gd^B decays slowly, with a half-life of about 60 days (Fig. 134–4). Despite this loss of active enzyme, older normal red cells retain enough activity to produce NADPH and maintain GSH in the face of almost all oxidant stresses. The defect in Gd^{A-} results in a *labile enzyme* that disappears and has a half-life of about 13 days. *Young red cells thus have normal enzyme activity, while older red cells are grossly deficient.* As a consequence of this heterogeneity, hemolysis is self-limited in individuals with Gd^{A-}.

This fact is shown graphically in Figure 134–5, which depicts the course of primaquine-induced hemolysis in an individual with Gd^{A-}. Acute hemolysis with hemoglobinuria and decreased ^{51}Cr red cell survival develops when the drug is first administered, but this is followed by a recovery phase in which anemia and

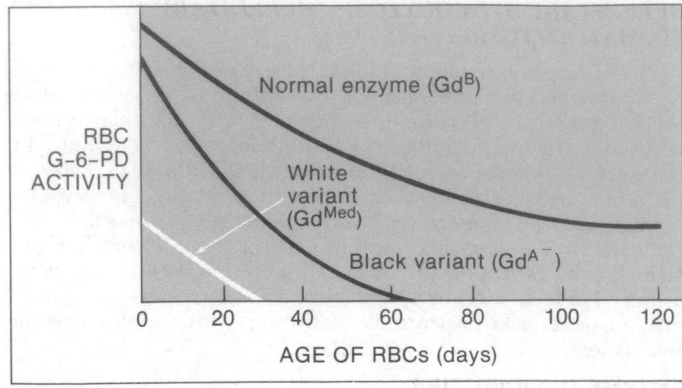

FIGURE 134–4. Intracellular decay of red cell G6PD as a function of cell age. The top curve shows the decay rate for Gd^B, the normal enzyme. The middle and lower curves show the greater than normal decay rates for the unstable Gd^{A-} and Gd^{Med} variants. Note that only the oldest Gd^{A-} red cells are markedly G6PD deficient and susceptible to hemolysis, whereas nearly all Gd^{Med} erythrocytes are vulnerable. Note also that after the most deficient Gd^{A-} red cells have been destroyed, the average G6PD level in the remaining cells will be near normal. This explains why G6PD assays after a hemolytic episode often fail to disclose the defect in Gd^{A-} males. (Modified from Lux SE: Hemolytic anemias. Metabolic disorders. In Beck WS [ed.]: Hematology. 4th ed. Cambridge, MA, The MIT Press, 1985, p 223. Reprinted with permission.)

reticulocytosis abate and red cell survival improves despite continued administration of the drug. The reason is that once the oxidant-sensitive older red cells are destroyed, the remaining young cells are oxidant resistant. Since only about 50 per cent of the cells are oxidant sensitive to begin with in Gd^{A-}, the bone marrow can compensate by simply doubling its output. This apparent drug resistance persists as long as the offending drug is continuously administered. Note, however, that if the drug is stopped for 2 to 3 months, older red cells will survive and accumulate, and the patient will again become drug sensitive.

Gd^{Med} is considerably more unstable than Gd^{A-} (Fig. 134–4). Very little activity is present in mature red cells. Despite this, chronic hemolysis does not occur, which must indicate that endogenous oxidant stresses are normally very low. When threatened by infections or oxidant drugs, however, these patients are at much greater risk because virtually their entire red cell population can be destroyed.

Clinical Features (Table 134–4). The most dramatic clinical presentation is acute intravascular hemolysis. These patients typically develop hemoglobinemia (pink to brown plasma), hemoglobinuria (red-brown to black urine), and jaundice acutely with an infection or within 1 to 3 days of exposure to an oxidant drug or fava beans. In severe cases, abdominal or back pain may be prominent. Symptoms of acute anemia (dizziness, headache, palpitations, dyspnea) may also develop, and if hemoglobinuria is severe, renal tubular necrosis and renal failure are risks (Ch. 76). Heinz bodies and increased levels of methemoglobin appear in the red cells, and some bite cells and blister cells may be seen on the blood smear. In many cases, however, the red cell morphology is relatively normal. More often, hemolysis is less dramatic, and a modest decline of hemoglobin (3 to 4 grams per deciliter) occurs, without hemoglobinuria or prominent symptoms. These episodes are easily overlooked unless the physician is alert.

The discovery of G6PD deficiency followed the observation that black soldiers developed explosive hemolysis after receiving primaquine for malaria. Subsequently, numerous other oxidant drugs were implicated as causative agents, some of which are listed in Table 134–5. The most common cause of hemolysis, however, is *infection*. Virtually every type of infection has been associated. One speculation is that oxidants generated by warring phagocytes trigger hemolysis by impinging on neighboring G6PD-deficient red cells.

Severe hemolytic episodes occur in some patients following ingestion of *fava beans* (Italian broad beans), probably caused by divicine and isouramil, oxidant pyrimidine derivatives that are present in high concentrations in the beans. This dangerous

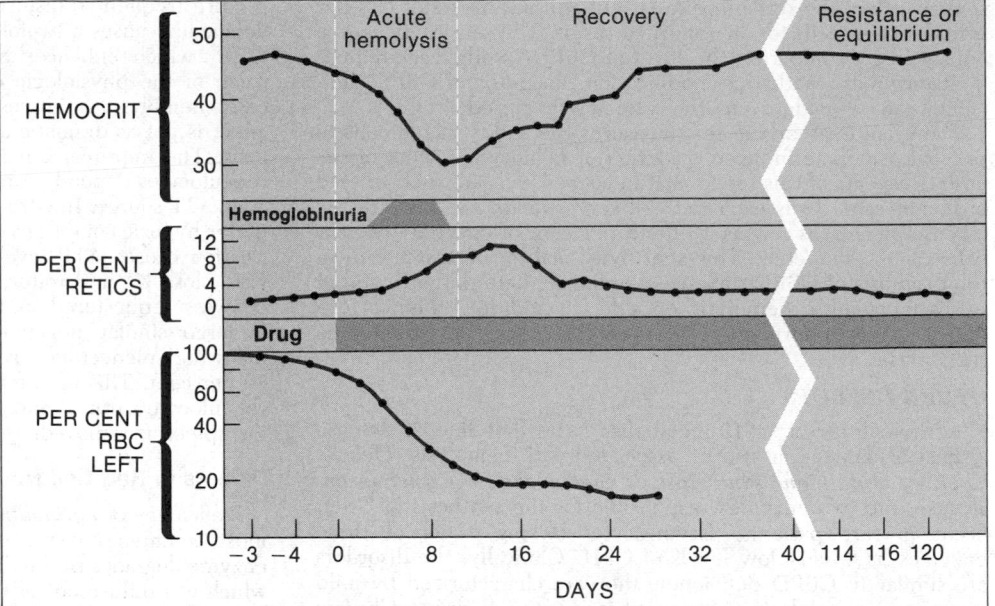

FIGURE 134–5. Course of drug-induced hemolysis in an individual with Gd^{A-}. Note that hemolysis abates and apparent resistance to the drug develops after the initial hemolytic episode owing to repopulation with young red cells. (Adapted from Alving AS: Bull World Health Organ 22:621, 1960. Reprinted with permission.)

phenomenon occurs mainly in individuals with Gd^{Med}; it is not seen in Gd^{A-}. This, and the fact that not all patients with Gd^{Med} are susceptible, indicates that other unknown factors must be involved.

Neonatal jaundice is a common complication of G6PD deficiency. It typically develops at 1 to 4 days of age and may require an exchange transfusion. In most cases, however, the jaundice is adequately controlled with phototherapy.

In some patients with rare variants of G6PD, *chronic hemolysis* occurs in the absence of obvious oxidants. These cases are characterized by enzymes that are unable to maintain basal NADPH production. Variants generally have a low substrate affinity for G6P or nicotinamide-adenine dinucleotide phosphate (NADP) and decreased affinity for the inhibitor, NADPH.

Genetics. The gene for G6PD is located on the X chromosome, so its inheritance is sex linked. Males have one type of G6PD; females can have two types. For example, 70 per cent of black males have Gd^B, 20 per cent have Gd^{A+}, and 10 per cent have Gd^{A-}. Black females, however, can be heterozygous for any two of these enzymes. According to the *Lyon hypothesis*, only one X chromosome is active in any somatic cell; thus any given red cell in heterozygous females is either normal or deficient. Mean enzyme activity in females who are heterozygous for G6PD deficiency may be normal, moderately reduced (usual), or grossly deficient, depending on the degree of lyonization. Deficient cells in heterozygous females are just as susceptible to oxidant injury as enzyme-deficient cells in males; however, the overall magnitude of hemolysis is less because of the smaller population of vulnerable cells.

Despite the disadvantages of a gene for G6PD deficiency, it remains common in many geographic areas. Its prevalence has been attributed to a selective advantage heterozygotes are believed to enjoy against malaria caused by *Plasmodium falciparum.* This proposal is supported by a large body of data, including epidemiologic studies, observations in heterozygous females demonstrating the resistance of cells containing the abnormal enzyme to malarial infection, and poor growth of *P. falciparum* parasites in G6PD-deficient red cells in vitro.

Diagnosis. Several tests for the diagnosis of G6PD deficiency are currently available. Their sensitivity varies, and their usefulness is determined by the clinical situation (sex of patient, type of G6PD deficiency, and proximity to the hemolytic episode).

Commonly used screening tests are based on NADPH-mediated dye decolorization or on the reduction of methemoglobin in the presence of methylene blue. These tests are of limited sensitivity, since 30 to 40 per cent of the cells must be abnormal for the deficient state to be detected. This criterion may not be met in patients with Gd^{A-} or Gd^{Canton} after a severe hemolytic episode, since most of their enzyme-deficient, older red cells will have been destroyed.

Definitive assay of the enzyme depends on direct spectrophotometric measurement of NADPH production. This test is more

TABLE 134–4. CLINICAL COMPARISON OF THE TWO COMMON FORMS OF G6PD DEFICIENCY

	Gd^{A-}	Gd^{Med}
Frequency	Common in black populations	Common in Mediterranean populations
Chronic hemolysis	None	None
Degree of acute hemolysis	Moderate	Severe
G6PD defect	Old red cells	All red cells
Hemolysis with:		
Drugs	Unusual	Common
Infection	Common	Common
Need for transfusions	Rare	Sometimes

TABLE 134–5. DRUGS COMMONLY LEADING TO HEMOLYSIS IN G6PD DEFICIENCY*

Antimalarials
  Primaquine
  Quinacrine (Atabrine)

Sulfonamides
  Sulfanilamide
  Salicylazosulfapyridine
    (Azulfidine)
  Sulfisoxazole (Gantrisin)†

Other Antibacterials
  Nitrofurantoin (Furadantin)
  Nitrofurazone (Furacin)
  Chloramphenicol†
  Para-aminosalicylic acid
  Nalidixic acid

Analgesics
  Acetanilid
  Acetylsalicylic acid†
  Acetophenetidin (Phenacetin)†

Sulfones
  Diaminodiphenylsulfone
    (Dapsone)

Miscellaneous
  Dimercaprol (BAL)
  Naphthalene (moth balls)
  Methylene blue†
  Vitamin K (water-soluble
    analogues)†
  Ascorbic acid†

*A more comprehensive list of drugs implicated in oxidant hemolysis appears in Beutler E: Pharmacol Rev 21:73, 1969.

†Hemolysis is infrequent and generally requires a high concentration of the drug. Probably a risk in Gd^{Med} but not in Gd^{A-} or Gd^{Canton}.

sensitive than the screening tests, but still requires 20 to 30 per cent deficient cells for an abnormal result. The sensitivity can be enhanced by comparing the level of G6PD to other age-dependent enzymes. With this modification, diagnosis of G6PD deficiency can be made even after a hemolytic episode.

The cyanide-ascorbate test measures the ability of red cells to prevent ascorbate-induced oxidation of hemoglobin. One of the unique aspects of this test is that intact red cells are used instead of hemolysate. Thus each red cell serves as its own cuvette. As a consequence, as few as 10 to 15 per cent of enzyme-deficient cells can be detected. This sensitivity makes the test useful in the diagnosis of G6PD deficiency in female heterozygotes and in males following a hemolytic episode. In addition, this test can detect other abnormalities of the HMP shunt or glutathione metabolism.

OTHER DEFECTS

Abnormalities of GSH metabolism, the first line of defense against oxidants, can also be associated with hemolysis. Defects in either *glutathione synthetase* or *gamma-glutamylcysteine synthetase,* the two enzymes responsible for the synthesis of GSH, occur in rare patients. Erythrocytes lacking either of these enzymes have very low levels of GSH. Clinically, the disorders are similar to G6PD deficiency; they are characterized by mild to moderate hemolytic anemia that is sensitive to drugs. Chronic neurologic disease also occurs in some patients with glutathione synthetase deficiency, but it is not certain that the enzyme disorder and neurologic defect are causally related.

Inherited deficiencies of *GSSG reductase* are thought to exist, but they are rare, and no case of hemolysis due to this disorder has been proved. Many individuals (including all newborn infants) are relatively deficient in *GSH peroxidase,* but they do not have excessive hemolysis. This probably reflects the fact that nonenzymatic reduction of peroxide by GSH occurs at a significant rate.

Defects in Glycolysis

General Features. Abnormalities in most glycolytic enzymes have been described, but pyruvate kinase (PK) deficiency accounts for about 90 per cent of the cases associated with hemolysis.

Almost all of the glycolytic defects are inherited in an autosomal recessive pattern. Hemolysis is observed in homozygotes. Heterozygotes are normal, although their red cells contain less than normal amounts of enzyme. Phosphoglycerate kinase (PGK) deficiency is an exception, since this enzyme is located on the X chromosome.

Hemolysis caused by glycolytic defects is thought to be due to lack of ATP. However, red cell ATP concentrations are often not decreased because (1) the mean cell age is very young and reticulocytes have high ATP levels; (2) defective cells with low ATP content are probably removed promptly from the circulation; and (3) ATP may be compartmentalized within reticulocytes, in which case a decline in ATP at one critical locus may be sufficient to cause cell injury.

Clinical Features. Hemolysis is chronic and is not affected by drugs. *Splenomegaly* is usually present because of stagnation of red cells in this organ. The acidic, hypoxic, and nutrient-poor environment of the spleen is an added insult to the metabolically abnormal cells. Thus the hemolytic rate often decreases after splenectomy. In most cases red cell morphology is relatively unremarkable prior to splenectomy. After splenectomy the blood smear typically contains a small number of *dense, spiculated red cells,* but this is not invariable or unique to these disorders.

Diagnosis. Definitive diagnosis requires spectrophotometric enzyme assays performed under a variety of conditions (i.e., with varying substrate and cofactor concentrations) to detect enzymes with abnormal kinetics. Measurements of glycolytic intermediates may reveal subtle enzyme abnormalities, since the concentration of an intermediate usually increases proximal to a defect and decreases distal to it.

PYRUVATE KINASE (PK) DEFICIENCY

PK catalyzes one of the major reactions responsible for ATP production in glycolysis; it is not surprising, therefore, that deficiency of this enzyme causes hemolytic anemia. Hemolysis can be mild and completely compensated or severe enough to require frequent transfusions. The distal glycolytic block in PK deficiency causes a twofold to threefold increase in red cell 2,3-DPG, which enhances tissue oxygenation and may minimize some of the physiologic consequences of the anemia. In most cases hemolysis improves following splenectomy, although the effect is not as dramatic as in diseases like hereditary spherocytosis. The improvement is related to the fact that PK-deficient reticulocytes depend on mitochondrial oxidative phosphorylation as an ATP source. In vitro incubation of PK-deficient reticulocytes under hypoxic conditions or with inhibitors of oxidative phosphorylation causes ATP levels to fall. The cells subsequently gain Ca^{2+}, lose K^+ and water, and become rigid. PK-deficient reticulocytes sequestered in the hypoxic splenic cords presumably undergo similar degeneration. Even when anemia improves following splenectomy, reticulocytes may rise to levels of 50 to 70 per cent. This *paradoxical reticulocytosis* is due to increased reticulocyte survival once the adverse metabolic environment of the spleen is removed.

Defects in Red Cell Nucleotide Metabolism

Deficiency of *pyrimidine-5'-nucleotidase* is the third or fourth most common enzyme deficiency leading to hemolysis. This enzyme degrades pyrimidine nucleotides to cytidine and uridine, which can diffuse out of the cell. Lacking this activity, red cells accumulate partially degraded messenger and ribosomal RNA, and up to 5 per cent of the cells develop *prominent basophilic stippling.* Apparently, the basophilic stippling in lead poisoning is produced by a similar mechanism, since pyrimidine-5'-nucleotidase is markedly inhibited by lead. Patients with an inherited (autosomal recessive) deficiency of this enzyme have chronic, moderately severe hemolytic anemia. The mechanism of hemolysis is unknown. Splenomegaly is common, but splenectomy produces little discernible benefit.

Finally, a rare disorder characterized by *overproduction of adenosine deaminase* illustrates the importance of ATP in red cell integrity. In affected patients, excessive deamination of adenosine apparently reduces the amount of this purine sufficiently to impair ATP synthesis. A chronic hemolytic anemia results. The disorder seems to be caused by hyperefficient translation of an adenosine deaminase mRNA that is present in normal amounts and produces a qualitatively normal enzyme. This extraordinary result suggests that a defect will be found in the 5' untranslated region of the mRNA that enhances binding of the message to ribosomes or initiation factors.

Agre P, Asimos A, Casella JF, et al.: Inheritance pattern and clinical response to splenectomy as a reflection of erythrocyte spectrin deficiency in hereditary spherocytosis. N Engl J Med 315:1579, 1986. *By comparing red cell spectrin content with clinical manifestations in 33 HS patients, the authors find that the dominant form of the disease is milder than the nondominant form and that spectrin content correlates closely with spheroidicity, hemolytic rate, and response to splenectomy.*

Arese P, DeFlora A: Pathophysiology of hemolysis in glucose-6-phosphate dehydrogenase deficiency. Semin Hematol 27:1, 1990. *Review of the mechanisms of red cell damage in G6PD deficiency, with an emphasis on favism.*

Bennett V: The spectrin-actin junction of erythrocyte membrane skeletons. Biochim Biophys Acta 988:107, 1989. *Recent review of the structure of the normal red cell membrane skeleton by one of the most accomplished investigators in the field.*

Beutler E: Current concepts: Glucose-6-phosphate dehydrogenase deficiency. N Engl J Med 324:169, 1991. *Review of the molecular defects responsible for G6PD deficiency and the insight they provide about the structure and function of the normal enzyme.*

Delaunay J, Alloisio N, Morle L, et al.: The red cell skeleton and its genetic disorders. Mol Aspects Med 11:161, 1990. *Comprehensive review of the structure of the normal red cell membrane skeleton and its derangement in HS and HE.*

Lux SE, Becker PS: Disorders of the red cell membrane skeleton: Hereditary spherocytosis and hereditary elliptocytosis. *In* Scriver CR, Beaudet AI, Sly WS, et al. (eds.): The Metabolic Basis of Inherited Disease. 6th ed. New York, McGraw-Hill, 1989, pp 2367–2408. *Comprehensive review of the etiology and clinical features of HS and HE.*

Lux SE, Tse WT, Menninger JC, et al.: Hereditary spherocytosis associated with deletion of human erythrocyte ankyrin gene on chromosome 8. Nature 345:736, 1990. *First direct evidence that ankyrin deficiency causes HS.*

Palek J: Hereditary elliptocytosis, spherocytosis and related disorders: Consequences of a deficiency or a mutation of membrane skeleton proteins. Blood Rev 1:147, 1987. *Review of membrane skeleton disorders with an emphasis on molecular defects responsible for HE.*

Schwartz PE, Sterioff S, Mucha P, et al.: Postsplenectomy sepsis and mortality in adults. JAMA 248:2279, 1982. *The only good epidemiologic study of postsplenectomy sepsis. Indicates that the risk of serious infection is much lower than previously thought.*

Valentine WN, Tanaka KR, Paglia DE: Hemolytic anemias and erythrocyte enzymopathies. Ann Intern Med 103:245, 1985. *One of the best recent reviews of the biochemical and clinical abnormalities in glycolytic enzyme deficiency.*

135 Acquired Hemolytic Disorders

Manuel E. Kaplan

Hemolysis resulting from congenital, intrinsic defects of the red cell has been discussed in Ch. 134. Hemolysis can also result from a variety of acquired abnormalities of the erythrocyte or of its extracellular environment (see Table 133–1). In these disorders, red cells are destroyed prematurely as a result of immunologic, physical, or chemical injury. The general manifestations of the acquired hemolytic anemias do not differ from those resulting from inherited intracorpuscular defects.

SEQUESTRATIONAL HEMOLYSIS (HYPERSPLENISM)

By virtue of its unique vascular architecture, the normal spleen carefully sieves circulating red cells (Ch. 152). Arterial blood enters the spleen via arterioles in the white pulp. In the red pulp these arterioles communicate with either endothelium-lined sinuses which communicate directly with the splenic venous system or with closed, nonendothelialized cords that end blindly and contain numerous fixed macrophages. To enter the splenic venous circulation, red cells in the cords must squeeze through narrow (3 μ) fenestrations between the endothelial cells that line the splenic sinuses. Poorly deformable red cells are unable to meet this challenge and are destroyed by splenic cord macrophages. The splenic filtration barrier does not significantly jeopardize the survival of normal nonsenescent red cells. However, when the spleen becomes enlarged, it may randomly entrap and destroy normal red cells. This pathologic process is called *hypersplenism*. The differential diagnosis of splenomegaly is discussed in Ch. 152. In patients with hypersplenism the rapidity of hemolysis is poorly correlated with overall spleen size. Indeed, patients with marked splenomegaly may exhibit little evidence of hemolysis.

Hypersplenism is best treated by effectively managing the underlying disease process. Splenectomy is rarely indicated; the procedure should be limited to transfusion-dependent patients who are reasonable operative risks and whose condition is refractory to medical therapy. Splenectomized individuals, particularly the young (under age 10), are statistically more likely to develop fulminant bacterial or protozoal infections and are less able to mount an effective primary IgM immune response to certain antigens. Consequently, the indications for splenectomy and its inherent risks should be carefully weighed before it is recommended.

IMMUNOHEMOLYTIC DISORDERS: PATHOPHYSIOLOGY

In patients with immune hemolysis, red cell destruction results from the binding of antibodies and/or complement components to the erythrocyte membrane. This may occur as a result of autoimmunization, alloimmunization, or exposure to certain drugs.

TYPES OF ANTIBODIES. Antibodies induce red cell destruction in vivo by mechanisms that are largely determined by their structure, concentration, and immunologic properties (complement-fixing activity, the optimal temperature at which they are active) as well as by the density and topographic distribution of the membrane antigens with which they combine. IgM red cell antibodies are generally agglutinating ("complete"), complement fixing, and active at colder temperatures. In contrast, most IgG red cell antibodies are fully active at 37°C ("warm"), have little or no agglutinating activity ("incomplete"), and vary in their ability to fix complement. IgA red cell antibodies usually occur in conjunction with IgG and/or IgM, have little complement-fixing activity, and rarely cause red cell destruction.

ROLE OF COMPLEMENT. Most IgM and some IgG red cell antibodies, after combining with membrane antigens, activate the classic complement pathway. After C1 binds to the Fc region of immunoglobulin heavy chains, it develops proteolytic C1 esterase (1S) activity, splits C4 into two fragments, C4a and C4b (Ch. 243). Nascent C4b may covalently attach to the red cell membrane and bind C2, which is then cleaved by C1s into C2a and C2b. The C4b, 2a membrane complex acts as the classic pathway C3 convertase, binding and cleaving C3 into C3a and C3b. Nascent C3b may also be covalently bound to the red cell membrane, where it completes assembly of the classic pathway C5 convertase (C4b,2a,3b). C5, after binding to C3b, is cleaved by C2a, thereby activating the terminal "membrane attack complex" (C5–9) of the complement cascade. Insertion of activated C9 into the red cell membrane produces its osmotic destabilization, resulting in egress of hemoglobin. If unopposed complement activation were to occur, life-threatening intravascular hemolysis could ensue. However, the process is restrained by inhibitors and inactivators of complement normally present in the plasma (Factor I, Factor H, C4-binding protein) and within the red cell membrane itself, i.e., CR1 (the receptor for C3b), DAF (decay-accelerating factor), HFR (homologous restriction factor or C8-binding protein), and MIRL (membrane inhibitor of reactive lysis). Red cells bearing covalently bound fragments of activated complement, i.e., C4b, C3b, and C3bi (C3b cleaved by Factor I), are prematurely removed from the circulation and destroyed, primarily by hepatic macrophages bearing complement receptors (CR1 and CR3). A more detailed description of complement is given in Ch. 243.

HEMOLYSIS WITHOUT COMPLEMENT ACTIVATION. Red cells sensitized with IgG antibodies without complement are sequestered and destroyed primarily within the splenic cords. Here they come into prolonged and intimate contact with macrophages bearing membrane receptors (FcγR) for the Fc portion of the IgG molecule. The sensitized cells may be damaged by a cytotoxic process (antibody-dependent cell-mediated cytotoxicity, or ADCC), be totally engulfed, or undergo partial phagocytosis. Incompletely phagocytized red cells may reseal their membranes and, having lost proportionately more membrane than cytoplasm, become microspherocytic. If these cells re-enter the systemic circulation, their spherocytic shape testifies to their previous encounter with splenic macrophages. They are particularly vulnerable to resequestration, since their deformability has been impaired and they retain significant membrane antibody.

DETECTION OF ANTIBODIES. The presence of red cell antibodies may be suspected from the appearance of the patient's anticoagulated venous blood and perusal of the peripheral blood film. IgM antibodies may induce such marked red cell agglutination at room temperature that anticoagulated blood samples may appear "clotted." Red cell clumping is readily apparent in the blood smear. Although IgG antibodies are usually nonagglutinating, they may so markedly reduce the negative charge (zeta potential) of the red cell that the cells are aggregated by fibrinogen and other plasma macromolecules. This condition appears as rouleaux in the blood film.

The *direct antiglobulin (Coombs') test* is most frequently used to detect immunoproteins present on the red cell membrane. A polyspecific antiserum containing antibodies against human immunoglobulins and complement components is added to a washed, dilute suspension of the patient's red cells. If agglutination is observed, the test is positive. More precise identification of the membrane-bound immunoprotein may help to delineate the etiology and pathophysiologic mechanisms underlying the hemolytic disorder. This is accomplished by exposing the patient's red cells to monospecific antisera reactive with individual immunoglobulin classes or complement components. Almost all patients with immunohemolytic disorders exhibit positive direct antiglobulin tests. In the small number of patients (< 5 per cent) in whom this test is negative, more sensitive immunologic techniques may disclose increased concentrations of red cell–associated immunoproteins.

The *indirect antiglobulin test,* important when considering red cell transfusions, detects serum antibodies capable of attaching to normal red cells. The patient's serum is incubated with a panel of serologically defined normal red cells; the cells are then washed, and membrane-associated immunoprotein is sought by the antiglobulin reaction. Although in clinical situations, both direct and indirect Coombs' tests are frequently ordered simultaneously, only the former provides unequivocal evidence of an immune hemolytic process.

HEMOLYSIS DUE TO ALLOANTIBODIES. Alloantibodies capable of destroying transfused, but not autologous, red cells are products of immunologic responses to (1) bacteria that normally colonize the large intestine (giving rise to so-called natural antibodies that cross-react with allogeneic erythrocyte antigens), (2) transfused, imperfectly matched red cells, or (3) antigens of fetal red cells that entered the maternal circulation during pregnancy or at delivery.

Alloimmune red cell antibodies present in a patient's serum may be detected by agglutination of normal cells or by the indirect antiglobulin reaction. Since these antibodies have specificity for nonself antigens, they are harmless unless the patient receives red cells that contain the immunizing antigen, or is pregnant. In the latter situation, the IgG red cell alloantibodies that gain access to the fetal circulation may induce erythroblastosis fetalis.

AUTOIMMUNE HEMOLYTIC ANEMIAS. Autoimmune hemolytic disorders are characterized by antibodies directed against autologous red cell antigens. The pathophysiologic mechanisms that result in autoantibody production are not fully understood. B lymphocyte clones capable of producing red cell autoantibodies probably are present normally. However, in health, they fail to synthesize detectable quantities of autoantibody because their activities are suppressed by immunoregulatory T lymphocytes. If this mechanism is deranged, such autoantibodies may be produced in quantities sufficient to trigger red cell destruction. Certain diseases—infections, neoplasms, or collagen vascular disorders—appear to predispose to increased synthesis of red cell autoantibodies. The hemolytic disorders that result are therefore categorized as secondary. In primary or idiopathic autoimmune hemolytic anemia, no underlying disease can be detected.

AUTOIMMUNE HEMOLYTIC DISEASE DUE TO IgG WARM-REACTING ANTIBODIES

CLINICAL MANIFESTATIONS. *Disease Associations.* In approximately 40 per cent of patients with IgG-mediated autoimmune hemolytic anemia, the process is secondary to an underlying disease, usually neoplastic or collagen vascular in origin. Chronic lymphocytic leukemia (see Color Plate 7*I*, left) and, less frequently, other lymphoproliferative disorders are the most commonly associated malignancies. There is a well-documented relationship between warm autoimmune hemolytic anemia and ovarian teratoma as well as adenocarcinoma of the stomach. Systemic lupus erythematosus is the most frequently associated collagen vascular disorder; less common are systemic sclerosis and rheumatoid arthritis. Occasional patients with ulcerative colitis present with warm autoimmune hemolysis. Certain drugs, the most commonly used being methyldopa, may give rise to this problem as well.

Symptoms and Signs. Since the rate of red cell destruction, degree of anemia, and presence of underlying disease differ from patient to patient, a highly variable clinical picture can result. If hemolysis is sudden in onset and rapid, the patient usually presents with symptoms and signs related to severe anemia, i.e., pallor, fatigue, exertional dyspnea, dizziness, and palpitations. When hemolysis starts more gradually, the anemia is usually less severe, and the patient may be relatively asymptomatic. On physical examination mild jaundice and splenomegaly are commonly present.

Laboratory Findings. The degree of anemia is variable, and there are usually normal numbers of white cells and platelets. In occasional patients significant thrombocytopenia or neutropenia, or both, occurs in conjunction with immune hemolysis (*Evans' syndrome*). The mean corpuscular volume (MCV) may be increased, sometimes strikingly so (> 115 fl). When spherocytosis is prominent, the mean corpuscular hemoglobin concentration (MCHC) is usually elevated. In addition to rouleaux formation, the peripheral blood film typically discloses significant anisocy-

tosis with numerous microspherocytes and increased numbers of large polychromatophilic reticulocytes. Normoblasts may be present, particularly when hemolysis is rapid. The reticulocyte count is almost always elevated. Reticulocytopenia may be encountered in occasional patients and requires additional diagnostic evaluation, including bone marrow aspiration and biopsy as well as search for an infectious etiology, including parvovirus (B19) (see Color Plate 5*H*, right). Other typical laboratory findings include hyperbilirubinemia of the unconjugated type, diminished to absent serum haptoglobin, normal or slightly elevated plasma hemoglobin levels, and no urine hemosiderin. The direct antiglobulin test discloses only IgG or IgG and complement (C3dg). The indirect antiglobulin test may be positive or negative, a positive result generally indicating that excess red cell autoantibody has been produced. Antibody eluted from the patient's red cells may occasionally exhibit specificity for a well-defined antigen, particularly Rh. More commonly, the eluted antibody is found to be a "panagglutinin," reacting with all normal red cells tested.

DIFFERENTIAL DIAGNOSIS. Since identifiable underlying disorders are present in about half the patients with warm autoimmune hemolytic anemia, appropriate diagnostic studies should be undertaken. If hemolysis appears to be acquired but the direct antiglobulin test is negative, a previously undiagnosed congenital hemolytic process, paroxysmal nocturnal hemoglobinuria, and various nonimmunologic causes (hypersplenism, microangiopathy, and so on) must be considered (Table 135–1). If there is no evidence for these, the patient may have an immunohemolytic process that can be demonstrated only by immunologic studies more sensitive than the antiglobulin test. Alternatively, this process may be inferred from a patient's objective clinical response to an empiric therapeutic trial of steroids.

TREATMENT. If an underlying disease process is identified and treated, marked improvement of the accompanying hemolysis frequently results. Slow, well-compensated hemolysis may require no therapy.

Glucocorticoids. Patients with more rapid hemolysis should be treated with oral steroids equivalent to 1 to 1.5 mg prednisone per kilogram per day, in daily single or divided doses. If the patient is very symptomatic because of severe anemia, initial treatment with intravenous hydrocortisone, 400 to 800 mg per day, may be preferred, followed by daily oral prednisone in divided doses. Improvement usually occurs within 5 to 10 days, evidenced by increasing hemoglobin and hematocrit levels and decreasing reticulocytosis. At this time steroid therapy can be consolidated into a single daily dose. Over the succeeding 3 to 4 weeks, as hemoglobin levels approach normal, the daily steroid dosage can usually be tapered, at 5- to 7-day intervals, to a daily prednisone dose of approximately 20 mg. Blood counts and reticulocyte counts should be checked periodically. Thereafter, the dose of steroids should be decreased more slowly, every 2 to 3 weeks, by 5 mg per day as long as the reticulocyte count does not rise significantly and the hemoglobin level remains stable. In occasional patients it may be possible to discontinue steroids

TABLE 135–1. DIAGNOSTIC APPROACH TO ACQUIRED COOMBS-NEGATIVE HEMOLYTIC ANEMIA

Reassess patient's history
Re-evaluate red cell morphology
Deduce most likely site(s) of hemolysis,
    i.e., extravascular (E), intravascular (I)

Morphology	*Site(s)*	*Possible diagnosis*
Fragments	I	Microangiopathy (TTP/HUS)
		Cardiac/valvular abnormality
		DIC
Spherocytes*	E	Hypersplenism
		Immunohemolytic anemia†
	I(E)	Paroxysmal cold hemoglobinuria†
		Toxins (clostridial, drugs, etc.)
Inclusions		
Parasites	E(I)	Malaria, etc.
Heinz bodies‡	I(E)	Oxidant drugs/toxins (consider G6PD deficiency)
Normal	I	Paroxysmal nocturnal hemoglobinuria

*Hereditary spherocytosis must always be considered.
†Characteristically Coombs-positive.
‡Requires special stain.

entirely without exacerbating the hemolysis. More commonly, significant hemolysis persists and patients require daily mainte- nance steroid therapy, 5 to 15 mg of prednisone, or 10 to 30 mg on alternate days, which results in fewer undesirable side effects.

The mechanism of the corticosteroid effect in warm autoim- mune hemolytic disorders is not fully understood. Steroids appear to diminish the number, and possibly the binding strength, of monocyte and macrophage Fcγ receptors, thereby decreasing the ability of these cells to bind and destroy IgG-sensitized red cells. Prolonged therapy with steroids suppresses antibody synthesis; however, this effect certainly does not explain the prompt, frequently dramatic clinical improvement seen in most patients.

If the response to corticosteroid therapy is unsatisfactory, i.e., if (1) hemolysis and anemia are not significantly improved within 2 weeks after initiating high-dose steroid therapy or (2) unac- ceptably large daily doses of steroids (> 15 to 20 mg of predni- sone) are required to maintain hematologic improvement, other therapeutic approaches must be considered.

Splenectomy. ^{51}Cr red cell survival and sequestration studies should be performed, if possible, before splenectomy is under- taken. Typically, they disclose significantly reduced red blood cell survival (t ½ = 5 to 15 days), and the spleen will be the major, if not exclusive, site of red cell destruction. In such a patient splenectomy is advisable and should result in marked hematologic improvement. Occasionally, significant hemolysis persists after splenectomy. This results from intense red cell sensitization with IgG autoantibody and usually responds to small maintenance doses of steroids. If ^{51}Cr sequestration studies reveal the liver to be a major site of red cell destruction, the direct antiglobulin test usually discloses complement (C3dg) as well as IgG. Splenectomy results in less effective control of hemolysis in such patients, favorable responses being achieved in only 30 per cent. Consequently, a trial of an immunosuppressive drug and/ or high-dose intravenous gamma globulin may be preferred prior to splenectomy.

Immunosuppressive Drugs. Oral azathioprine* (Imuran), 50 to 200 mg per day, and cyclophosphamide* (Cytoxan), 50 to 150 mg per day, are frequently employed in patients with refractory, warm immunohemolytic anemia. Responses are variable and usually not very dramatic. However, their use in patients whose hemolysis is resistant to steroids may permit reduction in the excessive steroid dosages required for maintenance. Significant toxicities include marrow suppression evidenced by leukopenia, thrombocytopenia, or reticulocytopenia with worsening anemia. Chronic treatment with immunosuppressive agents predisposes to development of malignancies.

Large amounts of intravenously administered gamma globulin (0.5 to 1.0 gram per kilogram), when infused daily for 5 consec- utive days, has been shown to mitigate hemolysis in a small number of well-studied patients with IgG-mediated immunohe- molytic anemia. The observed therapeutic responses have not been striking, appear slowly (7 to 10 days), and have been transient. Indeed, the majority of patients so treated have failed to respond. High-dose gamma globulin therapy induces hemolysis in some patients with immune thrombocytopenia or immunode- ficiency disorders, probably because of its anti-Rh antibody content.

Transfusion. Before hemolysis is adequately controlled by steroid therapy, severely anemic patients may require red cell transfusions. Transfusion carries an increased risk when the patient has a positive indirect antiglobulin test because donor- patient compatibility cannot be ensured by crossmatching tech- niques. The serum of such a patient frequently contains a panagglutinating autoantibody reactive with red cells from all prospective donors. More important, the serum autoantibody may mask the presence of a red cell alloantibody that may be capable of provoking intravascular hemolysis of transfused red cells. To distinguish these possibilities, the patient's red cells from which autoantibody has been eluted are used to absorb all autoantibody from the patient's serum. The absorbed serum is then tested for alloantibody activity with potential donor cells. In addition, blood banks usually attempt to identify possible blood group specificity of antibody eluted from a patient's red cells and of the serum antibody. Following these studies, donor

---

*This use is not listed in the manufacturer's directive.

red cells "most compatible" with the patient are selected for transfusion. Usually, patients with warm autoimmune hemolysis can be safely transfused when these precautions are taken. Donor cells should be administered slowly, with the patient being closely observed for symptoms and signs suggestive of a possible hemo- lytic transfusion reaction, the diagnosis and treatment of which are described in Ch. 137.

COURSE AND PROGNOSIS. In patients with secondary IgG- mediated autoimmune hemolytic disorders, the clinical course and ultimate prognosis are generally determined by how effec- tively the underlying disease process can be controlled. In 75 per cent of patients with primary (idiopathic) immune hemolysis due to IgG autoantibodies, anemia can be abrogated with corti- costeroid therapy or splenectomy or both. Uncontrollable he- molysis resulting in death rarely occurs. All evidence of hemolysis may disappear in rare patients. More commonly, a positive direct antiglobulin test persists, and the patient may experience recur- rent episodes of mild hemolysis requiring intermittent steroid therapy. Splenectomized patients are generally more stable he- matologically than are patients managed by medical therapy alone. Major causes of death include thromboembolic complica- tions and sequelae of chronically impaired host defense mecha- nisms caused by corticosteroids, splenectomy, or immunosup- pressive drugs.

AUTOIMMUNE HEMOLYTIC DISEASE DUE TO COLD-REACTING ANTIBODIES

Cold-reacting red cell antibodies combine most avidly with erythrocyte membrane antigens at grossly subphysiologic tem- peratures (0 to 4°C). They exhibit characteristic "thermal ampli- tudes," i.e., maximum temperatures beyond which they are unable to combine effectively with their antigens. Pathologically significant cold antibodies produce clinical hemolysis because they retain significant immunologic reactivity at temperatures that are achievable in vivo (30 to 32°C). Thus, if the thermal amplitude of a red cell antibody does not extend to 30°C, the antibody will have no pathophysiologic relevance. IgM cold- reacting antibodies occur most commonly. Because they strongly agglutinate red cells in the cold, they are designated *cold agglutinins*. Rare IgA cold agglutinins have been described; however, these antibodies do not produce hemolysis in vivo because they lack complement-fixing activity. Cold-reacting IgG red cell autoantibodies are occasionally encountered. They are intensely complement fixing and produce the disease picture of paroxysmal cold hemoglobinuria.

COLD AGGLUTININ DISEASE. Pathophysiology. IgM cold agglutinins are normally present in low concentrations in human serum. They have no known function and may represent by- products of polyclonal immunologic responses to viruses and other microorganisms. They are quantified by the cold agglutinin titer, i.e., the maximal serum dilution, at 4°C, that induces red cell agglutination. Normal cold agglutinins are harmless because they are present in low titer (≤ 1:32) and exhibit low thermal amplitude. Usually, but not always, the higher the patient's titer, the higher the thermal amplitude of the cold agglutinin, and the greater the probability that the patient will experience hemolysis.

The synthesis of polyclonal cold agglutinins may increase in response to certain infections, especially with mycoplasma, var- ious viruses (Epstein-Barr [EB] cytomegalovirus), and protozoans (trypanosomiasis, malaria). Cold agglutinin titers usually peak within 2 to 3 weeks of onset, but rarely do they rise sufficiently to provoke clinically apparent hemolysis.

Secondary cold agglutinin disease occasionally appears in pa- tients with lymphoproliferative disorders (see Color Plates 6 to 8), particularly large cell lymphomas. Indeed, hemolytic anemia may be the initial manifestation of the lymphoma. In these patients the cold agglutinins are predictably monoclonal, contain- ing either kappa or lambda light chains. Occasionally, the anti- body may be present in such high concentrations that it is detectable as a monoclonal spike on serum protein electropho- resis.

Idiopathic cold agglutinin disease occurs most frequently in elderly patients in whom, by definition, no underlying infectious or neoplastic process can be identified. The cold agglutinin is almost always monoclonal kappa IgM.

Cold agglutinins react with polysaccharide constituents of red cell membranes, glycolipids and glycoproteins immunochemically related to human ABO blood group antigens. One of these polysaccharide antigens (I) is better expressed on adult erythrocytes and another (i) on fetal red cells. Cold agglutinins that react more strongly with adult red cells are said to exhibit anti-I specificity, whereas those that preferentially combine with fetal (cord) erythrocytes are designated anti-i. I and i are not alleles, and both antigens are usually expressed on adult, as well as on fetal, red cells. However, infrequently, the red cells of otherwise normal individuals express only I or i. Rare patients with cold agglutinin disease have antibodies that exhibit exclusive anti-I or anti-i reactivity. Some cold antibodies that react equally well with adult and cord cells fail to agglutinate red cells pretreated with proteolytic enzymes; they are said to show anti-PR specificity. Identification of the major reactivity of a cold agglutinin (anti-I, -i, or -PR) and its clonal diversity may be clinically informative, since cold agglutinins produced in various diseases show different characteristic patterns of reactivity (Table 135–2).

Mechanisms of Hemolysis. When high thermal amplitude cold agglutinins bind to red cells in the cooler portions of the circulation, they initiate agglutination and complement activation via the classic pathway so that intra-vascular hemolysis may ensue. However, in most patients, this occurs minimally, or not at all, because propagation of the complement cascade is effectively aborted before membrane damage occurs. Activation of the earlier components of the classic pathway (C1, 4, 2, and 3), as previously described, results in the binding of nascent C3b to the red cell membrane (EC3b). EC3b is usually so rapidly cleaved by the plasma C3 inactivator (Factor I) that it is unable to support effective activation of the membrane attack components of complement (C5–9). Factor I activity is greatly enhanced by cofactors in the plasma (Factor H) and in the red cell membrane itself (CR1). EC3b is sequentially cleaved into EC3bi and ECdg, which are incapable of supporting further complement activation. Indeed, EC3dg appears to inhibit binding of additional cold agglutinin to the red cell membrane. Although significant intravascular hemolysis is prevented, red cells bearing C3b or C3bi are sequestered primarily within the liver and destroyed by hepatic macrophages.

Clinical Manifestations. In patients with cold agglutinin disease secondary to infections, hemolysis is usually self-limited and mild. In contrast, idiopathic and lymphoma-associated cold agglutinin syndromes are characterized by persistent hemolysis that is usually worse in winter. After exposure to cold, the patient may experience painful acrocyanosis, resembling Raynaud's phenomenon, induced by intense red cell agglutination. Unlike Raynaud's, there is usually no antecedent blanching or reactive hyperemia, and local gangrene does not occur. Severe chilling may accelerate hemolysis to such a degree that hemoglobinuria results.

Diagnosis. On physical examination the patient may be mildly jaundiced. When the patient's blood is drawn, the red cells may clump so rapidly that it appears to clot despite the presence of an anticoagulant. Warming the anticoagulated blood to 37°C rapidly restores its normal appearance. Electronically measured

TABLE 135–2. RELATIONSHIP BETWEEN COLD AGGLUTININ STRUCTURE AND SPECIFICITY IN VARIOUS DISEASES

Structure	Specificity		
	Anti-I	Anti-i	Anti-PR
Polyclonal/ oligoclonal ($\alpha + \lambda$)	Mycoplasma pneumoniae	Infectious mononucleosis	—
Monoclonal κ	Idiopathic cold agglutinin disease	Lymphoma	Idiopathic cold agglutinin disease
λ	—	Lymphoma	—

blood counts are frequently inaccurate because of the intense autoagglutination at room temperature. The red count and MCV are particularly affected, leading to distortion of the calculated hematocrit. This situation should be recognized by alert laboratory personnel. Not uncommonly, the reticulocyte count is only mildly increased, indicating suboptimal bone marrow compensation. The cold agglutinin titer is invariably elevated, and the direct antiglobulin test discloses only EC3dg. Typically, serum haptoglobin levels are decreased, and lactate dehydrogenase (LDH) concentrations are increased.

Treatment. An underlying disease process should be sought and, when identified, should be treated appropriately. Patients must avoid exposure to the cold and dress warmly. Treatment with daily chlorambucil,* 2 to 4 mg orally, decreases the rate of hemolysis in some patients, probably by reducing the synthesis of cold agglutinin. Glucocorticoids and splenectomy are generally of no benefit. If rapid hemolysis persists, the daily chlorambucil dosage may be increased to as much as 10 mg, with careful monitoring for toxicity. It may be advisable for the patient to move to a warmer climate. Although transfusions are not absolutely contraindicated, they should be avoided unless the patient is critically ill, i.e., exhibiting evidence of cardiovascular decompensation (tachyarrhythmias, angina, congestive failure) or cerebral hypoxia (e.g., confusion and visual disturbances) that responds poorly to bed rest and oxygen therapy. In addition to the transfusion-associated risks previously described in patients with warm autoimmune hemolysis, the following must be considered: (1) Transfused compatible red cells will be hemolyzed as rapidly, or even more rapidly, than the patient's own cells; the latter, having membrane-associated C3dg, appear to be more resistant to additional IgM cold agglutinin binding. By increasing the circulating red cells at risk of complement-mediated destruction, transfusion may exacerbate intravascular hemolysis, resulting in hemoglobinemia and hemoglobinuria. This situation may further jeopardize the patient's renal function and predispose to thromboembolic complications, red cell stroma being thrombogenic. (2) Although theoretically hazardous, the actual danger of administering refrigerated donor blood to a patient with cold agglutinin disease has been debated. Some experts strongly advise that a properly functioning, in-line blood warmer be utilized. Uncontrolled warming of donor erythrocytes must be avoided, since this is more hazardous than the slow administration of refrigerated blood. (3) The usual risks of transfusion therapy (Ch. 137) must be considered. By expanding the patient's blood volume, transfusion may exacerbate congestive heart failure. Transmission of hepatitis, cytomegalovirus, or human immunodeficiency virus (HIV) infections may occur. When transfusions are administered, the patient must be kept warm, a limited volume of red cells (designed to alleviate life-threatening symptoms, not simply to improve the hemoglobin concentration) should be infused slowly, and the patient's response monitored carefully. In life-threatening situations, plasmapheresis with plasma exchange should be considered. When this procedure is performed, the blood tubing and centrifugation apparatus should be maintained at 37°C.

PAROXYSMAL COLD HEMOGLOBINURIA (DONATH-LANDSTEINER HEMOLYTIC ANEMIA). Paroxysmal cold hemoglobinuria (PCH) is an exceedingly rare autoimmune hemolytic disorder caused by IgG cold-reacting antibodies directed against the ubiquitous P blood group antigen. It was first described in patients with tertiary syphilis who, following exposure to cold, developed paroxysms of chills, fever, headache, and diffuse pain in the abdomen, back, and legs accompanied by hemoglobinuria. PCH now more commonly occurs as a complication of certain viral infections, particularly infectious mononucleosis, measles, or mumps. In this context, hemolysis is rarely paroxysmal, and a history of cold exposure is seldom obtained. Consequently, it has been proposed that the syndrome be renamed Donath-Landsteiner (DL) hemolytic anemia to honor the investigators who first described the offending antibody. The diagnosis of PCH is made by demonstrating in the patient's serum the biphasic DL cold hemolysin. This IgG, nonagglutinating autoantibody activates complement so efficiently that intravascular hemolysis results. Normal red cells are mixed with the patient's serum and a source of complement, briefly chilled (0 to 4°C) and then warmed to

---

*This use is not listed in the manufacturer's directive.

37°C. If hemolysis is observed, this is presumptive evidence of the DL antibody. The patient's direct Coombs' test may be negative or may disclose only small amounts of complement, with or without traces of IgG. When PCH occurs secondary to a viral infection, hemolysis is usually transient, requiring only supportive therapy. If hemolysis recurs or becomes chronic, it may respond to treatment with glucocorticoids or to immunosuppressive drugs, such as cyclophosphamide.*

IMMUNOHEMOLYTIC ANEMIA DUE TO DRUGS. A number of drugs, or their in vivo metabolic derivatives, may induce immune hemolysis. Three distinct mechanisms have been described (Fig. 135–1):

1. *Drug binding to red cells.* When administered intravenously, certain immunogenic drugs, exemplified by penicillin, bind tightly to erythrocyte membranes. If drug-specific antibodies are produced, they attach to the cells at membrane sites containing the drug, triggering red cell destruction. In the case of penicillin-induced immune hemolysis, a non–complement-fixing, IgG antipenicillin antibody is characteristically involved. In vivo, it binds to penicillin-modified red cells and causes their destruction by a mechanism essentially identical to that seen in warm autoimmune hemolytic anemia, i.e., IgG-sensitized red cells are sequestered primarily within the spleen and destroyed by Fcγ receptor–bearing macrophages. The direct antiglobulin test discloses only IgG, whereas the indirect Coombs test is characteristically negative. The antipenicillin specificity of the red cell antibody can be demonstrated by eluting it and showing that it fails to combine with normal erythrocytes unless they have been pretreated with penicillin. Since hemolysis promptly ceases soon after penicillin is discontinued, corticosteroid therapy is usually unnecessary.

2. *Innocent bystander hemolysis.* Other drugs that induce immune hemolytic anemia in humans (e.g., sulfonamides, phenothiazines, quinine and quinidine) are bound primarily by plasma proteins rather than red cells. Although they are weakly immunogenic, they stimulate the synthesis of drug-specific, complement-fixing antibodies in some patients. As a result, the patient's erythrocytes are bathed in plasma containing drug-antibody immune complexes that may bind to the cells and activate complement. Nascent C3b may covalently bind to the red cell membrane and facilitate activation of the alternative complement pathway by binding factor B, which is then cleaved into Bb by factor D, a proteolytic enzyme normally present in plasma. C3b,Bb, the alternative pathway C3 convertase, cleaves additional C3, generating more nascent C3b that is available to bind to the red cell membrane. C3b,Bb,C3b complexes, acting as the alternative pathway C5 convertase, cleave C5, thereby triggering activation of the terminal (C5–9) membrane attack complex of complement. If inadequately restrained by the complement inactivators and inhibitors previously described, this process will result in life-threatening intravascular hemolysis. Even if activation of the membrane attack complex is effectively prevented, red cells bearing C4b, C3b, and C3bi are at risk of sequestration and destruction by hepatic macrophages. The direct antiglobulin test reveals only membrane-associated complement cleavage products, primarily C3dg. Efforts to elute immunoprotein from the patient's red cells are usually unsuccessful. The indirect antiglobulin test is characteristically negative. However, when the offending drug, or an appropriate metabolic derivative thereof, is added to normal erythrocytes that have been suspended in the patient's serum with a source of complement, hemolysis may be provoked. Coombs' testing of the nonhemolyzed cells may disclose membrane-associated complement fragments. After the patient discontinues the drug, hemolysis usually subsides promptly, and no additional therapy is required.

3. *Drug-induced autoimmune hemolytic anemia.* A pure IgG direct antiglobulin test appears in approximately 15 per cent of patients undergoing long-term treatment with methyldopa (Aldomet). However, only 10 per cent of these Coombs-positive patients develop clinically apparent hemolysis. The IgG eluted from patient's red cells combines readily with normal erythrocytes in the absence of methyldopa, thereby displaying true autoimmune reactivity. Patients treated with levodopa or mefenamic

---

*This use is not listed in the manufacturer's directive.

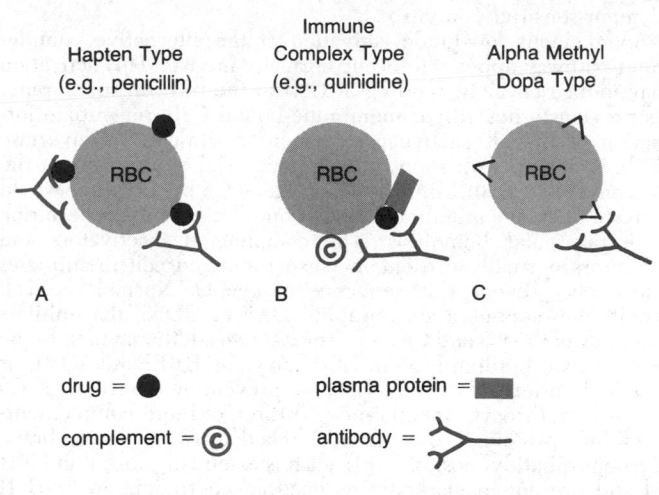

FIGURE 135–1. Mechanisms of drug-induced, immune hemolysis. *A,* The drug, or its metabolite, binds to the red cell membrane and acts as a hapten. Antibodies to the drug-membrane complex can induce red cell destruction either via FcγR-mediated sequestration by macrophages or by activating complement. *B,* A drug capable of acting as a hapten binds to plasma protein(s). After antibodies are formed, the Ab-drug-protein complex binds to the red cell membrane and activates complement, resulting in lysis. *C,* Long-term treatment with drug appears to induce a change in the red cell membrane, often altering its Rh specificity. Antibodies that develop bind to the altered membrane, producing a positive direct Coombs test and, rarely, hemolysis. (Adapted from Andreoli TE, Carpenter CCJ, Plum F, et al. [eds.]: Cecil Essentials of Medicine. 2nd ed. Philadelphia, W. B. Saunders Company, 1990, p 357.)

acid (Ponstel), a nonsteroidal anti-inflammatory drug, may develop similar erythrocyte autoantibodies. By unknown mechanisms these agents may interfere with immunoregulatory processes that suppress synthesis of red cell autoantibodies. Moreover, it is not clear why hemolysis occurs in only a small percentage of Coombs-positive, methyldopa-treated patients. The mechanism of cell destruction appears identical to that seen in warm autoimmune hemolytic anemia, i.e., splenic sequestration and red cell destruction by Fcγ receptor–positive macrophages. Hemolysis usually subsides within 1 to 3 weeks after methyldopa is discontinued, but a positive direct antiglobulin test may persist for many months. Although the hemolysis responds to steroid therapy, it is rarely required. If methyldopa is readministered to a patient who has fully recovered from methyldopa-induced hemolysis, no anamnestic autoimmune response usually occurs. Hemolysis may recur, but only after a prolonged treatment period.

PAROXYSMAL NOCTURNAL HEMOGLOBINURIA

Paroxysmal nocturnal hemoglobinuria (PNH) is an acquired hemolytic disorder resulting from the proliferation of an abnormal clone of stem cells whose progeny are uniquely susceptible to complement-mediated membrane damage. Its etiology is not known. Since patients with PNH are unusually prone to develop aplastic anemia or acute leukemia, the disease may represent a "preneoplastic" transformation of hematopoietic stem cells. PNH is quite rare; however, it is probably underdiagnosed because of its frequently protean manifestations. It occurs with greatest frequency in early adulthood but has been described in young children and in the very elderly.

PATHOPHYSIOLOGY. PNH red cells are inordinately sensitive to the lytic effects of complement. A patient's peripheral blood usually contains two or three subpopulations of red cells differing in their complement sensitivity (I = normally sensitive cells, II = cells of intermediate sensitivity, and III = very sensitive cells). In vitro, when PNH red cells are exposed to complement activated by either the classic or the alternative pathway, PNH II and III cells bind more C3b than do normal red cells. The in vivo rate of red cell destruction correlates well with the percentages of erythrocytes that exhibit extreme complement-sensitivity in vitro.

Spontaneous low-grade activation of the alternative complement pathway appears to occur normally in vivo. This activation may induce covalent binding of C3b to the red cell membrane. As previously described, membrane-bound C3b can initiate formation of the alternative complement pathway C3 convertase (C3b, Bb). This formation, in turn, may lead to assembly of the C5 convertase (C3b,Bb,C3b). Cleavage of C5 by the latter would activate the C5–9 membrane attack complex, potentially resulting in intravascular hemolysis. The complement inactivators and inhibitors normally present in plasma and red cell membranes effectively prevent this sequence of events. Normal red cell membranes contain a glycoprotein, DAF or CD55, that inhibits assembly of the C3 and C5 convertases. Two additional membrane proteins, C8 binding protein (also known as HRF) and MIRL or CD59, interfere with hemolysis by preventing insertion of C9 into the erythrocyte membrane. All three of these complement-inhibitory proteins are covalently linked to red cell membrane glycophosphatidylinositol (GPI): each is essentially absent in PNH III and present in markedly reduced concentrations in PNH II red cells. This situation accounts for the marked susceptibility of these cells to complement-mediated hemolysis.

Platelets and granulocytes in paroxysmal nocturnal hemoglobinuria are also deficient in these GPI-anchored, complement-regulatory proteins. These cells also exhibit increased vulnerability to complement activation in vitro. Although the in vivo survival of PNH platelets has been reported to be normal, their enhanced susceptibility to complement activation may underlie the thrombotic diathesis commonly seen in these patients. Functional abnormalities of the PNH granulocyte, which has been found to be deficient in the GPI-linked Fcγ receptor (type III), have also been described.

CLINICAL MANIFESTATIONS. The diagnosis of PNH must be considered in all patients with chronic hemolysis, particularly when associated with hemoglobinuria, pancytopenia, or unusual veno-occlusive events. During episodes of rapid hemolysis, patients commonly experience diffuse abdominal and back pain that has been attributed to ischemia resulting from microcirculatory thrombi. Not infrequently, major thromboses occur, involving the hepatic, splenic, portal, or cerebral veins. On physical examination, pallor and scleral icterus are common. The degree of anemia is highly variable, ranging from mild to severe. The reticulocyte count may be inappropriately low, given the severity of the anemia. The MCV may be normal, slightly increased, or diminished, depending upon the degree of reticulocytosis and the presence of accompanying iron deficiency due to prolonged urinary loss. Mild thrombocytopenia and granulocytopenia occur commonly. The peripheral blood smear reveals no autoagglutination, spherocytosis, or red cell fragmentation. The direct antiglobulin test is usually negative. Bone marrow cellularity varies from markedly hypoplastic to profoundly hyperplastic, and iron stores are usually reduced or absent. Erythroid elements predominate, and cell maturation is typically normoblastic.

Because red cell destruction occurs intravascularly, the serum LDH is elevated, serum haptoglobin levels are reduced or absent, and hemosiderinuria is present. Frank hemoglobinuria usually occurs only intermittently and is most apparent after periods of sleep.

DIAGNOSIS. The diagnosis of PNH requires that the patient's red cells show excessive susceptibility to complement-mediated hemolysis in vitro, usually demonstrated by mixing the patient's red cells with freshly collected normal human serum that has been mildly acidified (Ham's test). The hemolysis observed results from activation of the alternative pathway. The Ham test is highly specific but is too insensitive to detect all patients with PNH. The simpler sucrose hemolysis test, which induces complement activation via the classic pathway, is much more sensitive than Ham's test. However, it is less specific, false-positive results occurring in some patients with myeloproliferative disorders. Neutrophil alkaline phosphatase and erythrocyte acetylcholinesterase are characteristically reduced in PNH. Although these findings are not specific for PNH, both enzymes are GPI linked, strengthening the concept that PNH results from defective anchoring of various membrane constituents to GPI.

Other causes of intravascular hemolysis and hemoglobinuria that should be considered in the differential diagnosis include (1) drug-induced immunohemolytic anemia; (2) paroxysmal cold hemoglobinuria; (3) red cell hemolysins such as those present in snake venoms and *Clostridium welchii* exotoxin; (4) traumatic intravascular hemolysis as occurs in thrombotic thrombocytopenic purpura, hemolytic-uremic syndrome, and march hemoglobinuria; and (5) glucose-6-phosphate dehydrogenase (G6PD) deficiency exacerbated by oxidant drugs (Ch. 134).

TREATMENT. Erythropoiesis may be enhanced with folic acid, iron, and androgen therapy. In some patients iron administration may provoke increased hemolysis and hemoglobinuria. This situation may be prevented by prior transfusion and probably results from the destruction of increased numbers of newly produced, complement-sensitive reticulocytes. Androgen administration may significantly improve the anemia. A 6- to 8-week trial of oral fluoxymesterone or oxymesterone (5 to 50 mg per day), or of intramuscular nandrolone decanoate (25 to 200 mg once weekly), is usually sufficient to identify androgen-responsive patients.

Glucocorticoids (equivalent to 0.25 to 1 mg of prednisone per kilogram per day) slow the acute hemolytic episodes in some patients. Continuous treatment with low-dose steroids may reduce chronic hemolysis. However, daily steroids should not be administered except in life-threatening situations because of their unacceptable side effects and the increased danger of overwhelming bacterial or fungal sepsis. Alternate-day prednisone, in doses ranging from 15 to 40 mg, has been reported to improve the majority of patients so treated.

Most patients with PNH eventually require blood transfusions. Initially, donor red cells survive normally and suppress the production of the patient's abnormal red cells, resulting in marked clinical improvement. Following repetitive transfusions, however, patients are prone to develop hemosiderosis and to produce alloantibodies to red cell, neutrophil, platelet, and even plasma protein antigens. Once alloimmunization has occurred, further transfusion therapy is difficult, since in vivo complement activation triggered by alloantigen administration may result in rapid destruction of the patient's red cells. Even compatible transfusions may accelerate hemolysis of the patient's red cells and induce hemoglobinuria, probably because the donor material contains small quantities of activated complement. If evidence of increased hemolysis follows transfusion of packed donor red cells, administration of washed or frozen and reconstituted red cells may circumvent this problem.

Patients with PNH are predisposed to major venous thromboses and therefore require anticoagulation not infrequently. Since heparin therapy has been reported to exacerbate hemolysis in some patients, it must be used with caution. Vitamin K antagonists can usually be employed without difficulty, but it is not clear whether continuous prophylactic anticoagulation with warfarin (Coumadin) derivatives is clinically beneficial.

Bone marrow transplantation has successfully eradicated the PNH clone in a small number of patients.

PROGNOSIS. The course of PNH is exceedingly variable. Most patients die within 10 years of diagnosis. In a small percentage of patients, all disease manifestations spontaneously subside, possibly reflecting disappearance of the aberrant clone. More commonly, patients experience waxing and waning hemolysis, which may be exacerbated by immunologic stress, such as infection, transfusion, and immunization. Thrombotic events, primarily venous, account for much of the morbidity and mortality. With time, marrow function progressively deteriorates, not infrequently evolving into a clinical picture of aplastic anemia. In approximately 5 per cent of patients, acute myeloblastic leukemia develops.

HEMOLYSIS CAUSED BY CHEMICALS

A number of chemical toxins may directly injure and destroy red cells. These range in complexity from inorganic cations (arsenic and copper) and simple organic compounds such as chloramine to complex biologic substances produced by microorganisms, plants, and lower animals. Arsenic and copper damage red cells probably by binding to membrane sulfhydryl groups. Copper-induced hemolysis has been observed in hemodialyzed patients and may be responsible for the transient hemolytic episodes observed in patients with Wilson's disease.

Purification of urban water supplies with alum and chlorine results in the generation of chloramine, a potent oxidant. If chloramine is not effectively removed from tap water used for hemodialysis, it may swiftly oxidize hemoglobin to methemoglobin, resulting in Heinz body formation and rapid hemolysis.

Amphotericin B is a lipophilic fungal product that binds avidly to red cell membrane lipids rendering them more permeable to sodium. In occasional patients it may provoke hemolysis.

Clostridium welchii, spiders, and snakes produce potent lipolytic toxins capable of damaging red cell membrane integrity. They provoke rapid intravascular hemolysis characterized by marked spherocytosis. Hemolysis of uncertain etiology may accompany severe infections with other bacteria (*Streptococcus pneumoniae, Escherichia coli, Staphylococcus aureus*). Castor beans and certain species of mushrooms contain hemolysis-inducing toxins.

HEMOLYSIS CAUSED BY METABOLIC ABNORMALITIES

SPUR CELL HEMOLYTIC ANEMIA. Patients with a significant hepatocellular disease are frequently anemic. Blood loss, folate deficiency, alcohol-induced marrow dysfunction, and hypersplenism may contribute to the etiology of the anemia. However, in a small percentage of patients with end-stage cirrhosis, a clinical picture of rapid hemolysis develops with the appearance of numerous acanthocytes (spiculated, spur-shaped red cells).

Pathophysiology. Red cell membrane cholesterol and phospholipids exist in dynamic equilibrium with plasma lipids. In many patients with severe parenchymal liver disease, plasma lipoproteins appear to unload excessive cholesterol and phospholipid onto the erythrocyte membrane. As a result, the membranes spread and the cells thin, becoming target cells. However, the molar ratio of cholesterol to phospholipids in target cells remains normal, and the cells usually survive normally in vivo. In patients with spur cell hemolytic anemia, excess cholesterol relative to phospholipid accumulates in the red cell membrane. This condition may be caused by an abnormal high-density plasma lipoprotein. Red cell deformability becomes markedly reduced and hemolysis results.

Clinical Manifestations. Patients with spur-cell hemolytic anemia characteristically exhibit marked splenomegaly and signs of advanced cirrhosis, including jaundice, ascites, varices, and neurologic manifestations of hepatic encephalopathy. The anemia is usually severe, and the peripheral smear contains numerous acanthocytes and polychromatophilic reticulocytes. The direct antiglobulin test is negative. Red cell survival is short, the cells being sequestered by the spleen.

Diagnosis. The presence of a significantly elevated reticulocyte count and numerous spur cells on peripheral smear in a patient with end-stage cirrhosis is diagnostic of this syndrome. When normal compatible red cells are incubated with the patient's plasma in vitro, they become echinocytic in shape.

Prognosis and Treatment. Spur cell hemolytic anemia carries an exceedingly poor prognosis, almost all patients dying within months as a result of underlying liver disease. The benefits of transfusion are limited, since normal erythrocytes survive no better than patient's cells. Splenectomy may slow the rate of hemolysis but is exceedingly hazardous because of the severe liver disease.

HYPOPHOSPHATEMIA. Hemolysis may occur in patients with profoundly depressed serum phosphorus levels (< 1 mg per 100 ml) (Ch. 194). Hypophosphatemia of this degree occurs primarily in severely malnourished patients, particularly when they ingest excessive quantities of phosphate-binding antacids. Erythrocyte adenosine triphosphate (ATP) levels fall, the cells become poorly deformable, and hemolysis occurs primarily within the spleen.

HEMOLYSIS CAUSED BY RED CELL PARASITES

MALARIA. *Malarial infections*, particularly with *Plasmodium falciparum*, are probably the most common cause of hemolytic anemia worldwide (see Color Plate 8L, left) (Ch. 424). Merozoites invade red cells and utilize for their own purposes the contained hemoglobin, enzymes, and substrates. The metabolically deprived erythrocytes are unable to maintain normal cation fluxes and become osmotically fragile. Moreover, infected red cells may display new membrane antigens that incite host immune responses, resulting in positive direct antiglobulin tests. IgG antibodies eluted from the Coombs-positive red cells exhibit specificity for malarial antigens. Red cell destruction appears to occur primarily in the spleen, and splenomegaly is almost universally present in patients with chronic malarial infection. Rarely, rapid intravascular hemolysis with hemoglobinuria (blackwater fever) occurs soon after antimalarial therapy is initiated. It is not clear whether the infection or the drug plays the more important role in this phenomenon.

BABESIOSIS. *Babesia* are protozoans that parasitize red cells of many animal species (Ch. 432). Several cases of babesia-induced hemolytic anemia have been reported in humans, the disease being particularly fulminant in previously splenectomized individuals. Such patients may present with thrombocytopenia, disseminated intravascular coagulation, and renal insufficiency. Although deer ticks are the usual vector, the disease may be transmitted by transfusion of infected red cells. The disease has been reported most frequently in the northeastern United States (Martha's Vineyard and Nantucket). Intraerythrocytic parasites can usually be seen in Giemsa-stained peripheral blood films.

BARTONELLOSIS. *Bartonella bacilliformis*, a gram-negative pleomorphic bacterium, is endemic to Peru, Ecuador, and Columbia. It grows on the surface of red cells rather than within them (Ch. 331). The disease is transmitted by the bite of the sand fly and usually appears 3 weeks thereafter. The patient develops hectic fever and chills, headache, and musculoskeletal pain before hemolysis begins. The hemolytic episode is acute in onset and rapid. The red cells are Coombs-negative and are sequestered by both liver and spleen. The peripheral blood smear typically discloses rod-shaped organisms on the erythrocyte surface and large numbers of spherocytes, normoblasts, and reticulocytes. The infection responds well to various antibiotics.

HEMOLYSIS RESULTING FROM TRAUMA TO RED CELLS

When subjected to excessive mechanical stress, circulating red cells may undergo fragmentation and hemolyze. The forces responsible may be generated extracorporeally or intravascularly. For example, fragmentational hemolysis may result from excessive intravascular shear stress originating around critically narrowed heart valves, pathologic shunts (arterial or arteriovenous), cardiac valve prostheses, poorly endothelialized vascular surfaces, or microvascular thrombi. In these situations hemolysis is accompanied by characteristic morphologic evidence of red cell fragmentation. Similarly, red cells may be injured by excessive heat, resulting in hemolysis. Temperatures exceeding 49°C destabilize the human red cell membrane. In vitro, they are observed to undergo budding and fragmentation. Patients who have suffered extensive third-degree burns may show prominent spherocytosis on the peripheral smear, and in some cases hemoglobinemia and hemoglobinuria may occur acutely. The major syndromes associated with traumatic hemolysis are summarized briefly.

MARCH HEMOGLOBINURIA. As red cells circulate through narrow vessels overlying the bones of the hands and feet, they may be traumatized by repetitive, relatively uncushioned forces generated, for example, by prolonged marching, running, and karate blows. Intravascular hemolysis accompanied by hemoglobinemia and hemoglobinuria may result. Interestingly, no red cell morphologic abnormalities are apparent in the peripheral blood film during, or immediately following, the physical activity that precipitated the hemolytic episode.

FRAGMENTATIONAL HEMOLYSIS DUE TO CARDIAC PATHOLOGY OR ABNORMALITIES OF LARGE VESSELS. Cardiac abnormalities primarily involving the left side of the heart, where pressures are high, may predispose to hemolysis. These include severe aortic stenosis or regurgitation and ruptured sinus of Valsalva. Significant red cell fragmentation may also result from traumatic arteriovenous fistulas or therapeutic aorto-femoral bypass procedures. In such patients the hemolysis is usually low grade.

More rapid hemolysis may occur in patients with prosthetic heart valves. It occurs more frequently with aortic than mitral prostheses, with artificial valves rather than those of biologic (porcine) origin, with metallic rather than Silastic valves, and with defective or poorly functioning valves that exhibit ball variance or paravalvular leaks.

Clinical Manifestations. Patients rarely present with rapid intravascular hemolysis. A common clinical picture is one of increasing anemia, low-grade reticulocytosis, and numerous fragmented red cells (schistocytes) on peripheral blood film (see Color Plate 6E, right). Some findings typical of significant intravascular hemolysis are usually present, i.e., low to absent haptoglobin levels, increased serum LDH concentrations, and hemosiderinuria. Chronic urinary iron loss may result in iron deficiency. Although the direct Coombs test is usually negative, a poorly understood positive result has been observed in a few patients.

Treatment. Patients should be advised to limit their physical activity in an effort to reduce cardiac output and, thereby, to slow the rate of hemolysis. Oral iron, 300 mg of ferrous sulfate three times a day, should be given to correct iron deficiency. Rarely, parenteral iron (iron-dextran) or transfusions may be required. If the rate of hemolysis necessitates repeated transfusion, replacement of the prosthesis should be considered.

FRAGMENTATIONAL HEMOLYSIS DUE TO ABNORMALITIES WITHIN THE MICROCIRCULATION (MICROANGIOPATHIC HEMOLYTIC DISORDERS). Pathophysiology. Red cells may be fragmented by being forced to flow through small vessels partially occluded by microthrombi. Excessive shear forces are generated as the cells encounter and become tethered to fibrin strands that bisect and fragment the erythrocytes. The microthrombi may result from (1) an underlying coagulopathy, i.e., disseminated intravascular coagulation (DIC), (2) injury to the vascular endothelium, or (3) unknown mechanisms. Pathophysiologic processes that trigger DIC commonly induce endothelial injury as well; however, the reverse is frequently not true. Diseases accompanied by diffuse microvascular pathology may present with none of the laboratory findings characteristic of DIC. Consequently, in many patients with microangiopathic hemolytic anemia, the predominant etiologic factor (i.e., coagulation or vascular injury) can be discerned.

Disseminated intravascular coagulation results when procoagulant is introduced into the systemic circulation (Ch. 155). Coagulation factors are consumed, thrombus formation occurs, and fibrinolytic mechanisms are secondarily activated. Patients with significant DIC typically present with thrombocytopenia and abnormal plasma coagulation studies, i.e., prolonged prothrombin, activated partial thromboplastin, and thrombin times, reflecting decreased concentrations of certain clotting factors (particularly V, VIII, and fibrinogen) and increased plasma concentrations of fibrin degradation products. These abnormalities are generally poorly corrected by addition of normal plasma to that of the patient. DIC may be triggered by infections, particularly with gram-negative endotoxin-containing bacteria, amniotic fluid embolism, and disseminated neoplasms (Trousseau's syndrome) that elaborate potent procoagulants such as mucin, tissue factor, or cysteine proteases that activate clotting Factors VII or X. Although patients with severe DIC may be critically ill, rapid hemolysis is unusual.

Diffuse or localized vascular lesions associated with a variety of diseases may induce red cell fragmentation, e.g., cavernous hemangiomas (Kasabach-Merritt syndrome), renal allografts undergoing rejection, malignant hypertension, eclampsia, diseases associated with vasculitis (rickettsial infections, periarteritis nodosa, Wegener's granulomatosis), and certain disseminated neoplasms. The severity of hemolysis ranges from mild to severe. Coagulation abnormalities mimicking those of DIC are frequently absent.

Thrombotic thrombocytopenic purpura (TTP) (Ch 154), the hemolytic uremic syndrome (HUS) (Ch. 79), and mitomycin C–induced HUS of cancer patients are life-threatening disorders of unknown etiology. They closely resemble one another clinically, and are characterized by fragmentational hemolysis, thrombocytopenia, and renal failure. The patients are frequently febrile, manifest mild to moderate jaundice reflecting unconjugated hyperbilirubinemia, have petechiae and ecchymoses, and exhibit a variety of CNS abnormalities, including seizures. Gastrointestinal bleeding is commonly present. In patients presenting with bloody diarrhea, infections with verotoxin-producing *Escherichia coli* may be responsible for the clinical picture of HUS/TTP. Biopsies disclose characteristic microscopic findings of hyaline thrombi within small arterioles and capillaries.

Diagnosis. The diagnosis of a microangiopathic hemolytic disorder is based on the demonstration of schistocytes, grossly misshapen, sharply angulated erythrocytes that occasionally appear helmet shaped (see Color Plate 6E, right), usually in association with reticulocytosis, unconjugated hyperbilirubinemia, serum haptoglobin levels that are diminished to absent, increased serum LDH concentrations, and hemosiderinuria. Hemoglobinemia and hemoglobinuria occur much less frequently. The direct Coombs test is characteristically negative. If significant thrombocytopenia is present, laboratory evidence of DIC should be sought but is frequently absent.

Treatment. Treatment of the patient with microangiopathic hemolysis must be highly individualized. Efforts should be made to reverse the underlying triggering mechanism (i.e., withdrawal of potentially offending drugs or treatment with antibiotics or chemotherapeutic agents) and the patient supported with red cell transfusions, platelet packs, and cryoprecipitate as required. Occasional patients may benefit from anticoagulation with heparin. Although antiplatelet drugs and high-dose adrenocorticoid therapy are frequently employed, their efficacy is less certain. Vigorous plasma exchange (plasmapheresis combined with infusion of normal plasma) may induce dramatic remissions in TTP. TTP, HUS, and mitomycin-associated microangiopathy have also been reported to respond to intravenous administration of high-dose gamma globulin.

Jandl JH: Blood: Textbook of Hematology. Boston, Little Brown and Company, 1987. *Contains crystal clear, succinct expositions of the various topics covered in this chapter—especially recommended for its discussions of the hemolytic anemias associated with red cell trauma, liver disease (spur cell hemolysis), and infections (malaria, Babesia, Bartonella).*

Moake JL: Hypercoagulable states. Adv Intern Med 35:235, 1990. *A brief, incisive review of the pathophysiology of this complex and confusing topic—includes discussion of DIC.*

Rosse WF: Clinical Immunohematology: Basic Concepts and Clinical Applications. Boston, Blackwell Scientific Publications, 1990. *This authoritative treatise, encyclopedic in scope and lucidly written, includes masterful discussions of all the immunohemolytic anemias as well as paroxysmal nocturnal hemoglobinuria. Enthusiastically recommended as a primary reference.*

Ruggenenti P, Remuzzi G: Thrombotic thrombocytopenic purpura and related disorders. Hematol/Oncol Clin North Am 4:219, 1990. *A thorough, beautifully organized discourse on the pathophysiology, diagnosis, and treatment of these disorders.*

136 Hemoglobin and Hemoglobinopathies

136.1 STRUCTURE, FUNCTION, AND SYNTHESIS OF THE HUMAN HEMOGLOBINS

Edward J. Benz, Jr.

The structure, genetics, physiology, and pathology of human hemoglobins are topics important to the internist for several reasons. First, hemoglobins and the erythrocytes in which they circulate are well characterized at the cellular, biochemical, and genetic levels. Second, hemoglobinopathies are extremely common disorders in many areas of the world. Third, elucidation of the molecular basis of hemoglobinopathies has been the result of the most thorough and successful application to date of recombinant DNA technology to the understanding of human disease. The derived principles have enhanced the understanding of many other clinical conditions. Finally, the mechanisms by which abnormal amounts or functions of hemoglobin derange other organ systems demonstrate uniquely well the pathophysiologic principles by which disordered function of a single gene can lead to multisystem disease.

THE STRUCTURE OF HEMOGLOBIN

Each human hemoglobin consists of a tetramer of globin polypeptide chains: a pair of "α-like" and a pair of "non-α" chains (Table 136–1). The major adult hemoglobin (Hb), Hb A, for example, has the following structure: $\alpha_2\beta_2$. Each chain enfolds a single heme moiety, consisting of a protoporphyrin IX ring complexed with a single ferrous ion atom (Fe^{2+}). The heme moiety resides within each polypeptide chain in a configuration optimal for reversible binding of oxygen. One heme moiety can bind a single oxygen molecule, so that every molecule of hemoglobin can transport up to four oxygen molecules. The α-like globin chains (α and ζ) are 141 amino acids long, whereas the non-α chains (ε, γ, δ, β) are 146 amino acids long.

The *primary structures* (amino acid sequences) of globins are highly homologous to one another, suggesting that all of the proteins arose from a common ancestral gene.

Each globin has a largely helical *secondary structure*. About 80 per cent of each polypeptide exists in the form of α helix. The non-α chains contain eight helical segments, designated A to H, separated from one another by short nonhelical stretches. The α-like chains contain seven helices; D helix is absent. The helices fold into three-dimensional globular *tertiary structures* (Fig. 136–1).

Each globin chain folds in a manner that causes the exterior surface to be rich in polar (hydrophilic) amino acids that enhance solubility; the hydrophobic interior forms a cleft between the E and F helices into which the heme ring is deeply buried. This "heme pocket" excludes water from the vicinity of the heme, allowing numerous noncovalent hydrophobic "weak" bonds to form. These in turn stabilize the interaction between heme and globin chains. In particular, a histidine in the F helix forms a strong covalent bond with the iron atom; in the presence of oxygen, the iron also bonds with a histidine in the E helix. These histidine iron-oxygen bonds are critical for reversible oxygenation.

The *quaternary structure* of normal adult Hb A is also complex and clinically important. The tetramer consists of two αβ dimers. The two α chains in the complete tetramer interact indirectly by means of numerous tight interactions ($\alpha_1\beta_1$ contacts) between the α and β chain within each dimer. The tetramer is held together by noncovalent bonds ($\alpha_1\beta_2$ contacts) between the α-like chain of one dimer and the non-α chain of the other dimer. These contact points undergo major conformational shifts during binding and release of oxygen.

In its oxygen transport function, hemoglobin undergoes complex conformational and solubility changes secondary to the changes that occur within the heme groups, the globin chains, and the contact points between dimers during binding and release of oxygen. The hydrophilic surface amino acids, the hydrophobic amino acids lining the heme pocket, the F8 and E7 histidines, the $\alpha_1\beta_1$ and $\alpha_1\beta_2$ contact points, and the contacts between αβ dimers represent particularly critical regions within the globin polypeptide chains. Mutations in residues that influence these strategic sites tend to be the ones associated with significant changes in clinical phenotype.

OXYGEN-CARRYING FUNCTION OF HEMOGLOBIN

Hemoglobins are physiologically useful oxygen transport proteins because of their reversible interaction with oxygen. They bind avidly to oxygen at the Po_2 of the alveolar capillary bed, retain the bound oxygen as the red cells traverse the circulation, and unload the ligand to the tissues at the lower oxygen tensions of tissue capillary beds. Hemoglobins provide for the necessary

TABLE 136–1. COMPOSITION OF NORMAL HUMAN HEMOGLOBINS

Name of Hemoglobin	Subunit Structure	Time of Expression
Hemoglobin Portland	$\zeta_2\gamma_2$	Embryonic life
Hemoglobin Gower I	$\zeta_2\epsilon_2$	Embryonic life
Hemoglobin Gower II	$\alpha_2\epsilon_2$	Embryonic life
Hemoglobin F	$\alpha_2G\gamma_2$	Fetal life*
	$\alpha_2A\gamma_2$	
Hemoglobin A$_2$	$\alpha_2\delta_2$	Minor adult hemoglobin
Hemoglobin A	$\alpha_2\beta_2$	Major adult hemoglobin

*Produced in small amounts in a limited subpopulation of cells (F cells) in adults.

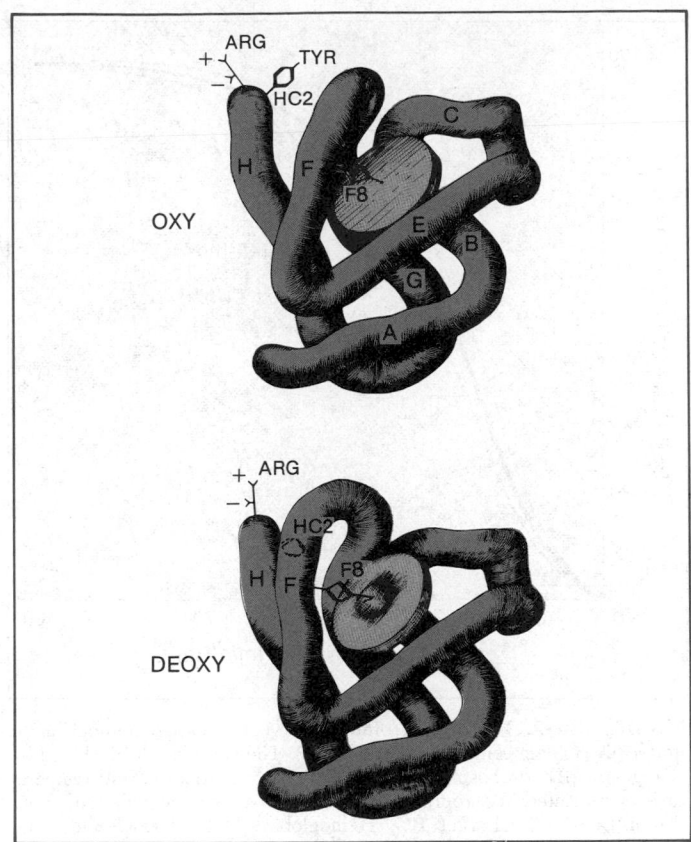

FIGURE 136–1. Structure of the oxy and deoxy states of a globin chain. Note that the amino acid sequence of globin dictates folding of eight helical segments (A–H) around the "heme" pocket in which the heme residue resides. In the deoxy state, the "F8" histidine is bound to the heme group, but this bond is broken in the oxy state. Also shown is an allosteric effect of this change on the topology of the arginine and tyrosine residues in the H helix (not discussed in the text).

amounts of oxygen acquisition and delivery over a relatively narrow range of oxygen tensions because of a property called "cooperativity" or "heme-heme interaction." This property is inherent in the tetrameric arrangement of the heme and globin subunits.

Monomeric globin-like peptides, e.g., individual globin subunits or myoglobin, acquire oxygen readily but cannot release it except at very low oxygen pressures incompatible with life. In contrast, complete hemoglobin tetramers exhibit an **S**-shaped oxygen dissociation curve (Fig. 136–2). At low oxygen tensions, the hemoglobin is deoxygenated. As the oxygen tension rises, oxygen binds to the tetramer; each heme group in the tetramer can bind one oxygen moiety. The binding of the first oxygen to deoxyhemoglobin requires a considerable amount of free energy (see below). Fully deoxygenated hemoglobin is thus said to be in the T (tense) state. As soon as one oxygen has been bound by the hemoglobin molecule, however, affinity for the binding of the remaining oxygen moieties increases, causing an increased slope in the binding curve. In other words, oxygen binding begets more oxygen binding. Oxyhemoglobin is said to be in the "R," or relaxed, state.

The cooperative mechanism of oxygen binding has been clarified by x-ray crystallography. The completely deoxy form is stabilized in its T state by the formation of several strong salt bonds (electrostatic bonds), especially within each α chain. To bind the first oxygen, these bonds must be broken. The first oxygen to bind must overcome significant resistance. As the bonds are broken, the oxygen affinity approaches that of the individual subunits, resulting in a marked increase in the affinity for the remaining oxygen molecules. This situation results in the physiologically more useful **S**-shaped oxygen equilibrium curve. Substantial amounts of oxygen are thus loaded and unloaded over a narrow range of oxygen tensions.

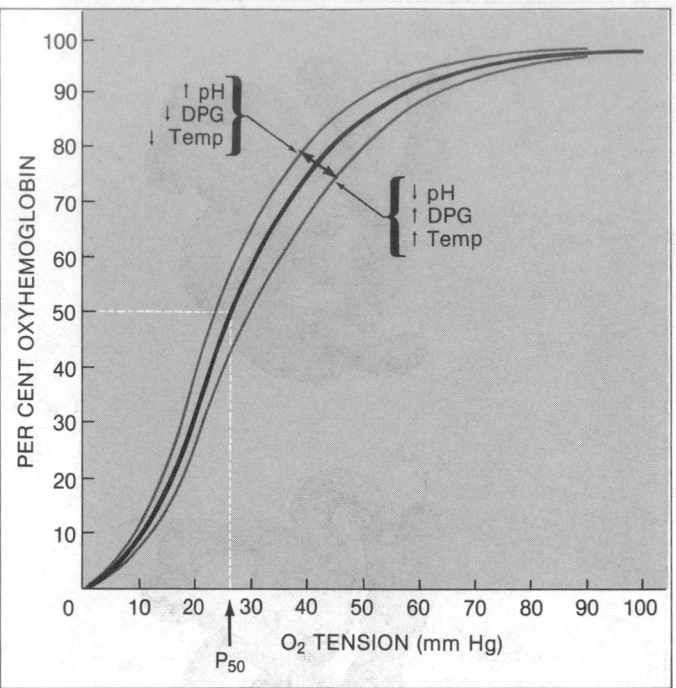

FIGURE 136–2. The oxygen binding curve for human hemoglobin A under physiologic conditions (*dark curve*). The affinity will be shifted by changes in pH, diphosphoglycerate (DPG) concentration, and temperature as indicated. P_{50} represents the oxygen tension at half saturation. (From Bunn HF, Forget BG: Hemoglobin: Molecular, Genetic, and Clinical Aspects. Philadelphia, W. B. Saunders Company, 1986.)

The oxygen affinity of normal hemoglobin is affected by many factors. Maintenance of the iron in the ferrous (Fe^{2+}) rather than the ferric (Fe^{3+}) form is critical. Hemoglobin carrying ferric iron is called methemoglobin. The classic effect of pH on oxygen affinity, known as the Bohr effect, arises from the stabilizing action of protons on the deoxy confirmation. Deoxyhemoglobin binds protons more readily than oxyhemoglobin because it is a weaker acid. Protons tend to stabilize the salt bonds that make deoxyhemoglobin more resistant to oxygen binding. Hemoglobin thus has a lower oxygen affinity at lower pH.

Allosteric effectors are small molecules that bind hemoglobin and alter oxygen affinity. The best characterized of these is 2,3-diphosphoglycerate (2,3-DPG), generated and destroyed enzymatically as an intermediate of glycolysis in red cells. In its interaction with deoxyhemoglobin, 2,3-DPG stabilizes the deoxy state. High levels of 2,3-DPG or other conditions that increase the affinity of hemoglobin for 2,3-DPG tend to result in *lower* oxygen affinity.

The major adult hemoglobin, Hb A, has a reasonably high affinity for 2,3-DPG. The oxygen affinity of Hb A is thus sensitive to the presence of 2,3-DPG. In contrast, Hb F, the major fetal hemoglobin, has very little ability to bind 2,3-DPG. Thus, Hb F and Hb A exhibit identical oxygen binding curves when analyzed as "stripped" hemoglobins in solution, but Hb F tends to have a higher oxygen affinity than does Hb A in vivo because Hb F does not interact with 2,3-DPG very well.

In brief, the structure-function features just outlined provide an exquisitely adaptive form of oxygen binding. Proper oxygen transport depends on the tetrameric structure of the proteins, the proper arrangement of charged and hydrophobic amino acids, and interaction with low molecular weight substances, such as protons or 2,3-DPG.

ONTOGENY OF HUMAN HEMOGLOBINS

Hemoglobin synthesis begins during the second month of gestation. Red cells first appear in yolk sac erythroblastic islands; these erythrocytes, called the primitive cell line, are large and nucleated. The predominant hemoglobins produced are Hb Portland ($\zeta_2\gamma_2$), Hb Gower I ($\zeta_2\epsilon_2$), and Hb Gower II ($\alpha_2\epsilon_2$), but small amounts of Hb F and Hb A can be detected even at these early stages. At about 10 to 11 weeks of gestation, erythropoiesis moves to the liver and spleen. Coincidentally, the embryonic hemoglobins decline (Fig. 136–3), to be replaced by fetal hemoglobin (Hb F: $\alpha_2\gamma_2$), a mixture of two hemoglobins differing in the composition of the γ chain component. $^A\gamma$ chains have alanine and $^G\gamma$ chains have glycine at position 136. Red cell production shifts to bone marrow during the sixth to seventh month of gestation, but Hb F continues to predominate until late in the third trimester (about 38 weeks of gestation). At that time, a switch (Hb F $\rightarrow$ Hb A switch) to the predominant synthesis of Hb A (Hb A: $\alpha_2\beta_2$) occurs. The switch causes an abrupt increase in Hb A production accompanied by a reciprocal rapid decline in Hb F production (Fig. 136–3). Synthesis of a minor Hb (Hb A_2: $\alpha_2\delta_2$) also commences at this time. Hb A (95 to 98 per cent) predominates throughout the rest of life under normal conditions. Hb F is usually present in minute amounts of 0.5 to 1.5 per cent, while Hb A_2 comprises 1.5 to 3.5 per cent of total hemoglobin in normal subjects.

Fetal and adult erythrocytes differ from each other in several ways, in addition to hemoglobin content. Fetal red cells tend to be larger (macrocytes) and have shorter circulating lifespans. Fetal red cells express the i, rather than the I (adult), surface antigen; lack the β isozyme of carbonic anhydrase present in adult cells; and produce the $^G\gamma$ and $^A\gamma$ forms of Hb F at a $^G\gamma$:$^A\gamma$ ratio of 7:3, whereas the adult $^G\gamma$:$^A\gamma$ ratio is 2:3.

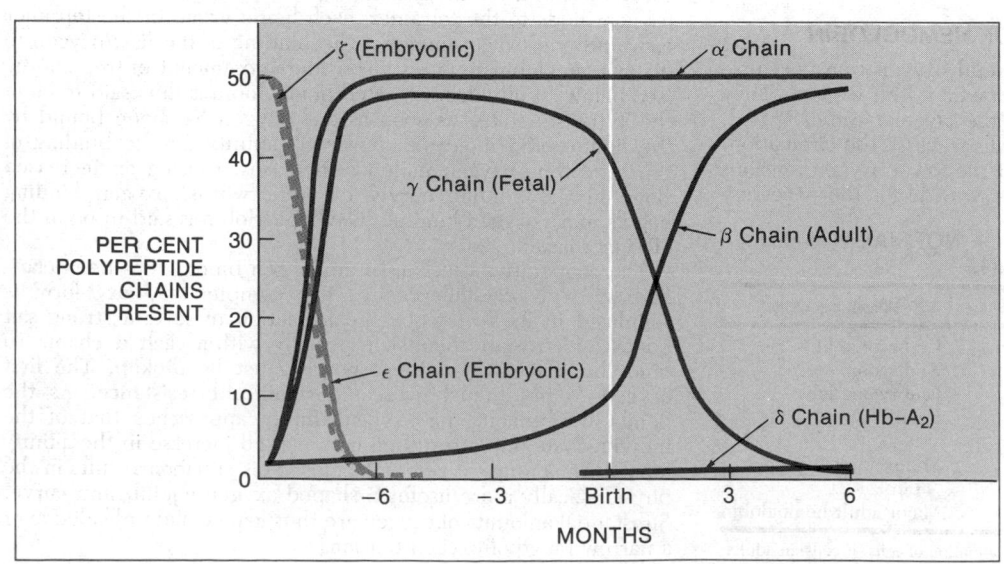

FIGURE 136–3. A diagram of the relative abundance of various human globin chains during development. (From Bunn HF, Forget BG: Hemoglobin: Molecular, Genetic, and Clinical Aspects. Philadelphia, W. B. Saunders Company, 1986.)

How hemoglobin switching is regulated is unclear. The potential of a given primitive erythroid stem cell (burst-forming unit–erythrocyte, or BFU-E) to express a particular globin gene is determined early in differentiation. By the time the stem cell has differentiated to the proerythroblast stage, when globin gene expression begins, the genetic program has been fixed and is not particularly susceptible to further modulation. The regulation of hemoglobin switching appears to result from a complex series of events. Changes in stem cell pools with varying potential for Hb F expression have profound effects, as does the chromatin configuration of the γ and β genes. The latter genes modulate transcriptional potential during the erythroblast phase of erythropoiesis. Gene expression of Hb F and Hb A is regulated largely at the stage of the primitive stem cell rather than the maturing erythroblast. Elevated Hb F levels in adults are thus often encountered in states of disordered erythropoiesis.

Small amounts of Hb F are produced during postnatal life but are confined to a small subpopulation of red cells called "F" cells. Both the numbers of F cells produced and the Hb F content of each F cell appear to be genetic polymorphisms. F cells are not truly fetal cells; they express other features of fetal cells incompletely. Changes in Hb F after birth result from altered stem cell dynamics. The most immature committed erythroid stem cell precursors (BFU-E) proceed through a series of proliferative and differentiating cell divisions before they actually form a pool of more fully differentiated progenitors (colony-forming units–erythrocyte, or CFU-E) ready to become proerythroblasts (Fig. 136–4). To a first approximation, the most immature or undifferentiated BFU-E's retain the highest potential to express Hb F in adult subjects. Under normal conditions of erythropoiesis, these cells continue to proliferate slowly and to differentiate into more mature BFU-E's before being "recruited" into the pool of maturing progenitors (CFU-E's and proerythroblasts). By this time, they have largely lost their ability to produce Hb F. Only a small number of "early" BFU-E's are actually recruited into the maturing pool, thus accounting for the small number of F cells produced under normal conditions.

Under conditions of marked erythroid stress or deranged erythropoiesis (e.g., as in chronic congenital hemolytic anemias, recovery from bone marrow transplantation or chemotherapy, or certain myelodysplastic syndromes), many BFU-E's are recruited into the pool of maturing progenitors before they have undergone their normal series of differentiating cell divisions. These cells still retain considerable potential to produce Hb F, resulting in higher than normal levels of F cells and Hb F. The molecular mechanisms mediating these complex events remain poorly understood.

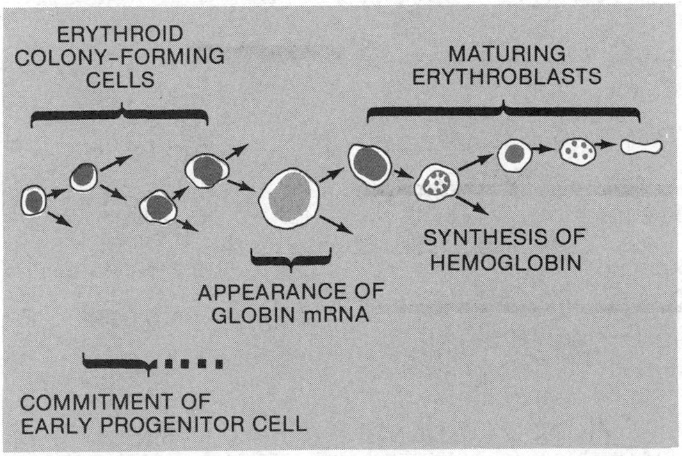

GENETICS AND BIOSYNTHESIS OF HUMAN HEMOGLOBIN

The production of the various human hemoglobins is controlled by two tightly linked gene clusters (Fig. 136–5). The α-like globin genes are clustered on the short arm of chromosome 16, between band 13.2 and the telomere, and the non-α genes are found on chromosome 11 at band P15, near the terminus of the short arm. The α-like cluster consists of two α globin genes and a single copy of the ζ gene. The non-α gene cluster consists of a single ε gene, the $^G\gamma$ and $^A\gamma$ fetal globin genes, and the adult δ and β genes. The functional anatomy of globin genes is typical of most eukaryotic genes. Each globin gene contains three blocks of nucleotide sequences (exons) that ultimately code for mature messenger RNA (mRNA); these are arrayed in tandem with two intervening sequences (introns). The non-α globin genes contain a small (130 bases) and large (900 to 1100 bases) intervening sequence, whereas both of the intervening sequences in the α and ζ globin genes are small (100 to 200 bases).

Flanking sequences at each end of the globin genes are important for regulating their activity. Immediately upstream (30 to 70 base pairs [bp]) are typical eukaryotic promoter elements facilitating entry of mRNA polymerase (Fig. 136–6). Regions 100 to 500 bases upstream are important for proper developmental expression. Sequences in the 5′ flanking region of the γ genes and the β genes influence, but do not exclusively control, the developmental regulation of these genes.

Important regulatory elements are also found in the 3′ flanking regions. The regions in which these regulatory sequences exist exhibit the structural features of highly active genes in bulk chromatin, such as DNase hypersensitivity. The methylation state of the γ globin genes also changes during development. In fetal erythroblasts, the promoter regions are relatively devoid of methyl group modification of cytosines (hypomethylation). In general, this characteristic correlates with higher levels of gene activity. In adult erythroblasts, the genes are heavily methylated, a feature associated with inactivity. Whether this correlation is causally related to the level of γ gene expression in fetuses and adults is unclear.

In proerythroblasts, globin synthesis comprises at most 0.5 to 1 per cent of total protein synthesis. During the subsequent maturation steps, globin gene expression increases enormously. For example, in reticulocytes generated during this 3- to 5-day period, globin mRNA and globin synthesis comprise 90 to 95 per cent of total mRNA content and protein synthesis, respectively. To achieve this remarkable degree of activation, globin genes are highly adapted for expression in erythroid cells.

Tissue and developmental activation of individual globin genes depends in part upon short DNA sequences called enhancers. These are located in the 5′ and 3′ flanking sequences and possibly in the introns of the genes. An important enhancer activating the entire non-α gene complex (called the "locus activating region" [LAR] or "dominant control region" [DCR]) has been tentatively identified several thousand bases upstream of the ε gene. These regulatory DNA sequences are called "cis" acting elements. They achieve their biologic effects via their interaction with "trans" acting factors, i.e., nuclear DNA binding proteins that specifically bind to these sequences, thereby promoting or inhibiting transcription.

Several "transcription factors" have been found to bind the globin gene promoters and enhancers. Many of these protein factors appear to be nonspecific in that they can activate a number of genes in many tissues if they gain access to their binding sites. At least one factor, however, called NFe-1 or GF-1, is largely erythroid specific (it is also found in megakaryocytes). It recognizes a consensus DNA sequence called "AGATAAG" found near many genes that are expressed specifically in erythroid cells, including the globin genes and the erythropoietin receptor gene. Although *important* for activation of the erythroid program of gene expression, GF-1 alone is probably not sufficient to trigger the process. The activity of GF-1 may depend on interaction with other transcription factors.

Each globin gene possesses structural features that are essential for the normal function of most genes (Fig. 136–6). These include the presence of a "CAP" site necessary to mark the beginning of

FIGURE 136–4. Regulation of hemoglobin synthesis during erythropoiesis. Two general classes of cells are the precursors of circulating red cells. Erythroblasts at various stages of maturation may be recognized within the bone marrow; these cells and circulating reticulocytes are engaged in hemoglobin synthesis. Erythroid stem cells, the progenitors of erythroblasts, are present within the bone marrow in very small numbers but may be detected by virtue of their ability to form colonies of erythroblasts in semisolid media in vitro. Current evidence suggests that commitment to expression of either the γ or the β globin genes occurs in erythroid stem cells prior to the initial appearance of globin messenger RNA (mRNA).

Within the figure:

ERYTHROID COLONY-FORMING CELLS

MATURING ERYTHROBLASTS

SYNTHESIS OF HEMOGLOBIN

APPEARANCE OF GLOBIN mRNA

COMMITMENT OF EARLY PROGENITOR CELL

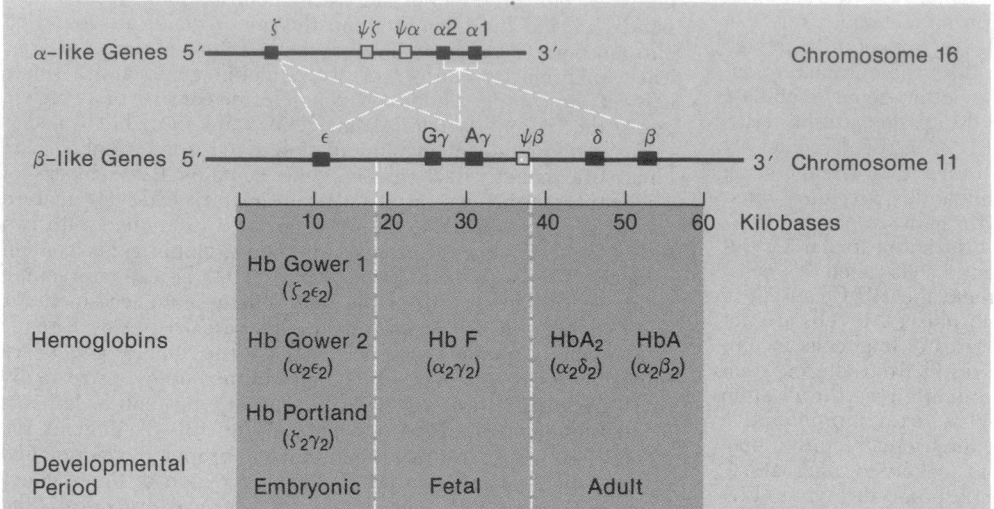

FIGURE 136–5. A diagram of the arrangement of the clusters of human α-like and β-like globin genes on chromosomes 16 and 11 and the embryonic, fetal, and adult hemoglobins that result from the combinations of the various globin chains encoded by these genes. The ψ genes are similar to globin genes but do not code for protein. Distances along the chromosome are expressed in terms of 1000 nucleotide pairs (a kilobase).

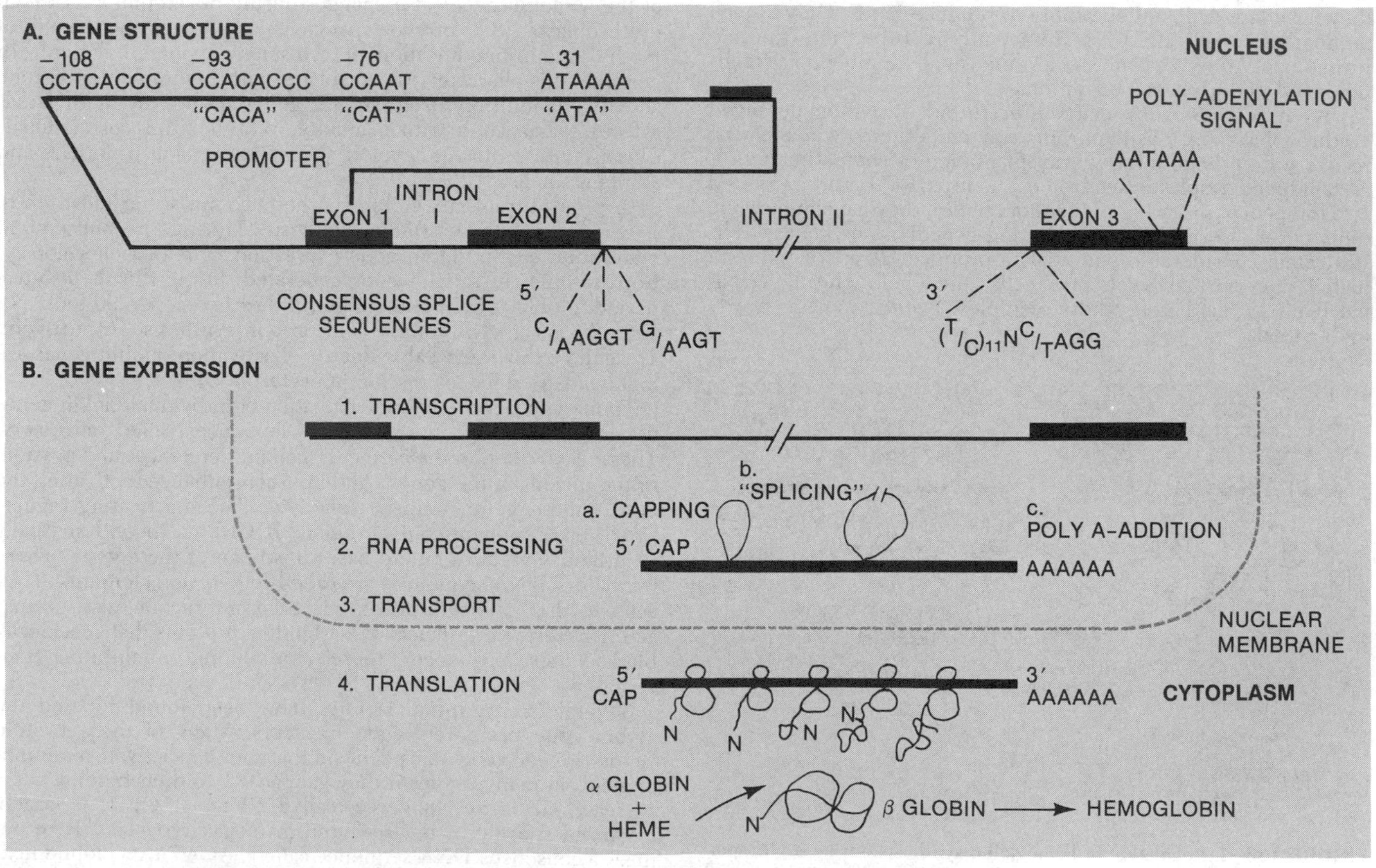

A. GENE STRUCTURE

NUCLEUS

POLY-ADENYLATION SIGNAL

−108 CCTCACCC   −93 CCACACCC   −76 CCAAT   −31 ATAAAA

"CACA"   "CAT"   "ATA"

PROMOTER

AATAAA

EXON 1   INTRON I   EXON 2   INTRON II   EXON 3

CONSENSUS SPLICE SEQUENCES $5'$ $^C/_A AGGT$ $^G/_A AGT$ $3'$ $(^T/_C)_{11} N ^C/_T AGG$

B. GENE EXPRESSION

1. TRANSCRIPTION

2. RNA PROCESSING

   a. CAPPING   5′ CAP

   b. "SPLICING"

   c. POLY A-ADDITION   AAAAAA

3. TRANSPORT

NUCLEAR MEMBRANE

4. TRANSLATION   5′ CAP   3′ AAAAAA   **CYTOPLASM**

N   N   N   N

α GLOBIN + HEME   N   β GLOBIN ⟶ HEMOGLOBIN

FIGURE 136–6. Structure and expression of the normal human β globin gene. The three exons encode for β globin; these coding sequences are interrupted by two introns or intervening sequences. Certain segments of the promoter region ("boxes") are conserved in many globin genes. The actual sequence of these "boxes" in the β globin gene promoter is shown. The splice sequences shown represent the consensus of those found at many exon-intron boundaries. Those actually found in the β globin gene resemble the consensus sequence but are not identical. The processes involved in gene expression include transcription of the gene, processing of the primary RNA transcript, transport of the mRNA from nucleus to cytoplasm, and translation of the mRNA into β globin. C = cytosine; T = thymine; A = adenine; G = guanine.

transcription of the mRNA precursor; properly located initiation and termination codons to signal the beginning and end of translation of the mature mRNA; the presence in the appropriate locations, but nowhere else, of the donor (GT) and acceptor (AG) splicing sites that mark the points in the mRNA precursor at which the introns should be removed while the exons are ligated together; "consensus" sequences surrounding the donor and acceptor dinucleotides that form the functional splicing signal; and the presence of 5' and 3' untranslated sequences whose significance remains unclear. Like many other eukaryotic mRNA's, globin RNA's are polyadenylated. Their 3' untranslated sequences contain appropriate polyadenylation signals. As discussed in Ch. 136.4, these regions are mutated in various forms of thalassemia.

The pathway of globin gene expression is typical of most eukaryotic genes (Fig. 136–6). Each gene is initially transcribed into an mRNA precursor. Through a series of splicing reactions, the introns are removed and the exons are spliced together. At an early step in this process, the mRNA is modified at the 5' end by the "5' CAP" structure and the addition of a poly A tail. Mature mRNA is then transported from nucleus to cytoplasm. It associates with ribosomes, transfer RNA's (tRNA's), and proteinaceous initiation and elongation factors needed for translation on polyribosomes. The newly synthesized globin polypeptide chains combine rapidly with heme and then with one another to form hemoglobin tetramers. These posttranslational steps proceed rapidly and spontaneously (i.e., nonenzymatically). As hemoglobin "ages" in circulating erythrocytes, it is susceptible to further modification, such as acetylation (especially Hb F) and nonenzymatic glycosylation (Hb A_{1-C}). The latter has been used to follow control of diabetes mellitus, since A_{1-C} levels increase when the blood glucose level is high.

The hemoglobin tetramer, the final product of this complex process, is a highly soluble molecule. In contrast, the individual globin chains are rather insoluble. To prevent the globin chains from precipitating, it is essential that α and non-α globins be synthesized in approximately equal, or balanced, amounts. Each newly synthesized α or non-α globin chain will then have a "mate" with which to pair. The pathophysiology of severe thalassemia syndromes involves imbalance of globin chain synthesis and precipitation of the unpaired chains.

RELATIONSHIP OF IRON ACCUMULATION AND HEME SYNTHESIS TO HEMOGLOBIN PRODUCTION

The successful synthesis of hemoglobin requires coordination and regulation of the expression not only of the globin genes but also of the many genes responsible for heme and iron metabolism. The considerable amount of iron required for hemoglobin synthesis is provided to the erythroblast via membrane receptors specific for the iron transport protein transferrin. Iron is ultimately inserted into protoporphyrin to form heme. Synthesis of protoporphyrin IX occurs by a series of reactions catalyzed by enzymes found in relatively high concentrations in erythroblasts (Ch. 191). Excess iron is stored as ferritin and may later become available for heme synthesis or may be transferred from erythroid to phagocytic cells in bone marrow.

Heme has important roles in the process of hemoglobin synthesis in addition to being an essential component of the hemoglobin molecule. Heme deficiency leads to inactivation of a critically required initiation factor, thereby markedly reducing the rate of protein synthesis. Furthermore, heme may stimulate the synthesis and accumulation of globin mRNA directly and thus may have a regulatory role in modulating globin gene expression.

Globin biosynthesis and heme biosynthesis are coupled and cross-regulated in a poorly understood fashion. Disorders in which either iron or the protoporphyrin component of heme accumulates in inadequate amounts generally result in a secondary reduction in the amount of hemoglobin being synthesized. For complex reasons, a mild imbalance in globin chain synthesis also occurs: α Chain synthesis is more impaired by heme or iron deficiency than is β chain synthesis. Anemias characterized by inadequate iron or heme accumulation thus tend to be *mildly* α-thalassemic. With the exception of this phenomenon, interactions among heme and globin biosynthetic pathways remain poorly understood. The mechanisms whereby heme, α, and non-α globin are constrained to be expressed in equal amounts remain totally obscure. Since imbalances in this regulatory scheme occur reg-

ularly in the thalassemic syndromes, iron deficiency anemia, and disorders of heme biosynthesis, it can be inferred that the normal regulatory mechanisms are rather easily overcome.

Rodgers GP, Schechter AN: Molecular pathology of the hemoglobin molecule. *In* Hoffman R, Benz EJ Jr, Cohen H (eds.): Hematology: Basic Principles and Practice. New York, Churchill Livingstone, 1991, pp 441–449.

Steinberg MH, Benz EJ Jr: Hemoglobin synthesis, structure, and function. *In* Hoffman R, Benz EJ Jr, Cohen H (eds.): Hematology: Basic Principles and Practice. New York, Churchill Livingstone, 1991, pp 291–302.

136.2 CLASSIFICATION AND BASIC PATHOPHYSIOLOGY OF THE HEMOGLOBINOPATHIES

Edward J. Benz, Jr.

In patients with hemoglobinopathies, clinical abnormalities are attributable to altered structure, function, or production of hemoglobin. These disorders are usually inherited disorders that arise from mutations within the globin gene clusters described above (Ch. 136.1), but "acquired hemoglobinopathies" can occur as the result of toxic exposures (e.g., methemoglobinemia) or hematologic neoplasms. Hemoglobinopathies range in clinical severity from asymptomatic laboratory abnormalities to profound multisystem syndromes that result in death in utero or in early childhood. Hemoglobinopathies are the most common inherited disorders in humans. In many geographic areas, they constitute significant public health problems because of their prevalence and chronicity. The hemoglobinopathies demonstrate extremely well the complex pathophysiologic consequences that can arise from deranged function of single genes. Hemoglobinopathies frequently manifest as clinical syndromes in childhood, but with improved supportive care, many of these patients now survive well into adult life. The molecular basis, pathophysiology, epidemiology, and clinical features of the major hemoglobin disorders are therefore issues of increasing importance to internists.

CLASSIFICATION OF HEMOGLOBINOPATHIES

Hemoglobinopathies can be classified into five major groups:

1. *Structural hemoglobinopathies* (Table 136–2) are due to mutations altering the amino acid sequence and, thereby, the physiochemical properties of a particular globin polypeptide chain. The altered properties of the resulting abnormal hemoglobin produce the characteristic clinical syndrome. Some hemoglobins polymerize abnormally, e.g., those in sickle cell anemia (see Color Plate 6B, left); others exhibit abnormal solubility, while others have altered oxygen affinity.

2. The *thalassemia syndromes* are characterized by defective *biosynthesis* of globin chains, caused by mutations that impair production and/or translation of globin messenger RNA (mRNA). Symptoms result from the inadequate supply of hemoglobin and from imbalances in the production of individual globin chains.

3. *Thalassemic hemoglobin variants* exhibit features of both thalassemia, i.e., defective globin biosynthesis, and structural hemoglobinopathies, i.e., an abnormal amino acid sequence (see Color Plate 6A, left).

4. *Hereditary persistence of fetal hemoglobin*, as the name implies, represents continued synthesis of Hb F at high rates after the perinatal period.

5. *Acquired hemoglobinopathies* are secondary to other disease processes, rather than resulting from genetic derangements of hemoglobin structure or synthesis. Common examples include modifications of the hemoglobin molecule by toxins (acquired methemoglobinemia). Abnormal hemoglobin synthesis, e.g., high levels of Hb F production in preleukemia, also occurs sporadically in blood cell dyscrasias.

More than 400 structural variants and 100 thalassemia mutations have been identified. Only a few cause significant morbidity. Most of these involve the α and β globin chains that constitute the major adult hemoglobin, Hb A ($\alpha_2\beta_2$). Disorders of fetal and embryonic hemoglobins that are not lethal in utero are asymp-

TABLE 136–2. CLASSIFICATION OF HEMOGLOBINOPATHIES

I. Structural hemoglobinopathies—hemoglobins with altered amino acid sequences that result in deranged function or altered physical or chemical properties
  Abnormal hemoglobin polymerization—Hb S
  Altered O$_2$ affinity
    High affinity—polycythemia
    Low affinity—cyanosis, pseudoanemia
  Hemoglobins that oxidize readily
  Unstable hemoglobins, hemolytic anemia, jaundice
  M hemoglobins—methemoglobinemia, cyanosis

II. Thalassemias—defective production of globin chains
  α-Thalassemias
  β-Thalassemias
  δβ-, γδβ-, αβ-Thalassemias

III. Structural hemoglobinopathies—structurally abnormal Hb associated with co-inherited thalassemia phenotype
  Hb E
  Hb Constant Spring
  Hb Lepore

IV. Hereditary persistence of fetal hemoglobin—persistence of high levels of Hb F into adult life
  Pancellular—all red cells contain elevated Hb F levels
    Nondeletion forms
    Deletion forms
    Hb Kenya
  Heterocellular—only specific subpopulations of red cells contain elevated levels of Hb F
  Acquired—see below

V. Acquired hemoglobinopathies
  Methemoglobin due to toxic exposures
  Sulfhemoglobin due to toxic exposures
  Carbonoxyhemoglobin
  Hb H in erythroleukemia
  Elevated Hb F in states of erythroid stress and bone marrow dysplasia, usually heterocellular

tomatic after birth because these hemoglobins are not normally expressed then.

DISTRIBUTION AND EPIDEMIOLOGY OF HEMOGLOBINOPATHIES

Hemoglobinopathies are especially common in areas where malaria is endemic. The clustering of hemoglobinopathies in the "malaria belt" suggests that heterozygotes enjoy a selective advantage if infected with the malaria parasite. Presumably, their erythrocytes provide a less hospitable environment during the obligate intraerythrocytic stages of the parasitic life cycle (Ch. 424). For example, malarial parasites grow poorly in sickle cell trait erythrocytes. This selective advantage fixes the mutant genes in the population. One should thus be especially alert to the presence of hemoglobinopathies in Asians, blacks, and ethnic groups derived from the Mediterranean basin. Hemoglobinopathies do occur in every ethnic group, however.

INHERITANCE OF HEMOGLOBINOPATHIES

Hemoglobinopathies are "autosomal co-dominant" traits; thus, compound heterozygotes, who inherit a different abnormal globin allele from each parent, exhibit composite features of each abnormal allele. For example, patients inheriting a β-thalassemia gene from one parent and a β^s (sickle cell) allele from the other have sickle cell/β-thalassemia, which exhibits features of both β-thalassemia and sickle cell anemia. Each hemoglobinopathy is transmitted in families as a tightly linked allele of a globin gene. A thorough family history is thus an important part of the general approach to hemoglobinopathies, regardless of type.

Globin gene mutations behave like "co-dominant" traits in that some evidence of the abnormality, even if it be only laboratory evidence, can be detected in the heterozygote. The dominance of individual mutations with respect to clinical symptoms varies in different types of hemoglobinopathies. For example, patients with thalassemia trait and sickle cell anemia are, for the most part, asymptomatic. In each case, the amount of normal Hb A generated by the normal β globin allele, coupled with the lessened impact of abnormal globin production from the affected allele, protects patients from the complications of these diseases under normal conditions. Certain provocative stresses, such as very high altitude (low partial pressure of oxygen) for the patient with sickle cell trait, or pregnancy (for the patient with thalassemia trait), can occasionally produce symptoms characteristic of these disorders, i.e., sickling or anemia.

Some hemoglobinopathies behave like dominant traits, especially the structural mutations causing reduced solubility or profoundly altered oxygen affinity of the hemoglobin. In these cases, the absolute amount of the abnormal hemoglobin arising from the single affected allele is often sufficient to alter the behavior of the red cell.

In some hemoglobinopathies, the homozygous state is clinically benign, but compound heterozygous states are associated with severe disease. For example, homozygous hemoglobin C disease is only minimally symptomatic, but inheritance of β^s on one chromosome and β^c on the other (hemoglobin sickle cell [SC] disease) behaves like a moderately severe form of sickle cell anemia, exhibiting certain unique and distinctive features, to be described subsequently. Similarly, homozygous Hb E disease is very mild, but co-inheritance of Hb E and β-thalassemia produces a moderately severe β-thalassemia–like syndrome. These considerations illustrate the complexity of hemoglobin genetics. The ultimate clinical phenotype is determined not only by the type of change resulting from the globin gene mutation but also by a composite effect of the altered properties of the abnormal chain, the amount produced (or the severity of the production deficit), and the interaction between the product of one abnormal allele and that of the normal allele or of a different type of abnormal allele present on the complementary chromosome. These principles, important for understanding individual syndromes, also offer the best existing examples of gene interactions in determining the ultimate clinical phenotype.

Spontaneous mutations occur at a measurable frequency within the globin gene cluster, producing symptomatic or asymptomatic hemoglobinopathies in patients with negative family histories. The unstable (insoluble) hemoglobin disorders seem especially prone to arise by de novo spontaneous mutation. Thus, while family history is an extremely important part of the evaluation of patients with potential hemoglobinopathies, a negative family history does not necessarily rule out the diagnosis.

BASIC PRINCIPLES OF PATHOPHYSIOLOGY

The α globin genes are duplicated; the β gene is a single-copy locus. In the diploid erythroblast, there are thus four copies of the α and only two copies of the β gene. Mutation of a single α globin gene thus affects only about 25 per cent of the hemoglobin produced, while β mutations affect about 50 per cent. Consequently, β chain mutations tend to be encountered more frequently than α variants as causes of symptomatic hemoglobinopathies.

Globin genes are expressed exclusively in developing erythroid cells. During the terminal stages of erythroid maturation, one might expect symptoms to be confined to the red cell compartment, e.g., anemia. The clinical manifestations of hemoglobinopathies are protean, however. In most cases, it has been possible to trace these changes to the impact of specific mutations on particular properties of the hemoglobin molecule. Homeostasis of hemoglobin and the homeostasis of the red cells in which it circulates are closely linked. Deranged production or function of globin frequently deranges erythropoiesis, and the converse is also often true. Hemoglobin accumulates to extremely high concentrations within red cells, where it must remain soluble and chemically reduced. Individual globin chains are insoluble and have extraordinarily high oxygen affinities. If globin or hemoglobin molecules precipitate within red cells, the resulting inclusions cause premature destruction of the red cells (hemolytic anemia) with all of its attendant stigmata. Lesions affecting oxygen affinity perturb the erythropoietin circuit by which red cell production is regulated. The signal for release of erythropoietin is based upon *oxygen delivery* to cells within the kidney rather than to the *red cell mass*. Inappropriate secretion of erythropoietin as well as premature destruction of red cells can thus be caused by hemoglobinopathies. These consequences of deranged hemoglobin structures, amount, or structure-function relationships, rather than mere reduction in the amount or normal function of hemoglobin, tend to dominate the pathophysiology of the disorders.

The behavior of particular hemoglobinopathies is also influenced by the ontogeny of hemoglobin synthesis. α Chain hemoglobinopathies cause abnormalities of Hb A, Hb A$_2$, and Hb F, because the α chain is present in all of these hemoglobins. The α globin hemoglobinopathies are symptomatic both in utero and after birth because normal function of the α globin gene is required throughout gestation as well as adult life. In contrast, β globin gene expression is not abundant until after birth. Infants with β globin hemoglobinopathies thus tend to be asymptomatic until 3 to 9 months of age, the time at which Hb F is largely replaced by Hb A.

Schecter AN: Molecular pathology of the hemoglobin molecule. *In* Hoffman R, Benz EJ Jr, Cohen H (eds.): Hematology: Basic Principles and Practice. New York, Churchill Livingstone, 1990, in press.
Steinberg MH, Benz EJ Jr: Hemoglobin: Structure and synthesis. *In* Hoffman R, Benz EJ Jr, Cohen H (eds.): Hematology: Basic Principles and Practice. New York, Churchill Livingstone, 1990, in press.

136.3 HEMOGLOBINOPATHIES WITH ALTERED SOLUBILITY OR OXYGEN AFFINITY

Edward J. Benz, Jr.

Structural hemoglobinopathies are due to mutations that alter the amino acid sequence and, thereby, the functional properties of the hemoglobin molecule: (1) mutations causing abnormal polymerization, of which hemoglobin (Hb) S (sickle cell hemoglobin) is the most important example; (2) mutations causing altered solubility of hemoglobin within circulating erythrocytes; (3) mutations causing altered affinity of the hemoglobin molecule for oxygen; and (4) methemoglobinemia, which represents a subclass of hemoglobins with altered oxygen affinity. Sickle cell syndromes are so common, serious, and protean in their manifestations that they merit extended separate coverage (Ch. 136.5). In this chapter, we shall consider hemoglobins exhibiting abnormal solubility and altered oxygen affinity. Methemoglobins are considered a separate category within this chapter, even though they could be considered a subclass of hemoglobins with altered oxygen affinity. The altered interaction with oxygen is far more severe in methemoglobin than in most other types of oxygen affinity mutations; moreover, methemoglobin is important as one of the few acquired hemoglobinopathies (carbon monoxyhemoglobin being another) that can develop by exposure to selected toxins. Finally, methemoglobins can arise by inherited mechanisms in other genes as well as globin genes. Therefore, these syndromes receive special consideration.

HEMOGLOBINS EXHIBITING REDUCED SOLUBILITY— UNSTABLE HEMOGLOBINS

Pathogenesis and Clinical Manifestations

"Unstable" hemoglobins arise from amino acid substitutions that render the hemoglobin less soluble or more susceptible to oxidation of its amino acid residues (Fig. 136–7). Both α and β globin variants can cause this condition; about 100 such variants have been described. The mutations that produce insoluble hemoglobins tend to disrupt hydrogen bonding and hydrophobic interactions holding the tetramer together. Some alter the helical segments [Hb Geneva, ($\beta^{28leu \rightarrow pro}$)]; others disrupt contact points between the α- and β-subunits [Hb Philadelphia, ($\beta^{35Tyr \rightarrow Phe}$)], while others disrupt interactions of the hydrophobic pockets of the globin subunits for heme [e.g., Hb Köln, ($\beta^{98Val \rightarrow Met}$)]. The most common biochemical basis for reduced solubility is reduced strength of the binding of heme to globin. An actual loss of heme groups can occur, e.g., in Hb Gun Hill, in which five amino acids, including the F8 histidine, are deleted.

Precipitation of hemoglobin in circulating red cells produces intracellular inclusions called "Heinz bodies" (see Color Plate 6C, left). The spleen attempts to remove these inclusions, leading to formation of pitted, rigid cells that eventually become seques-

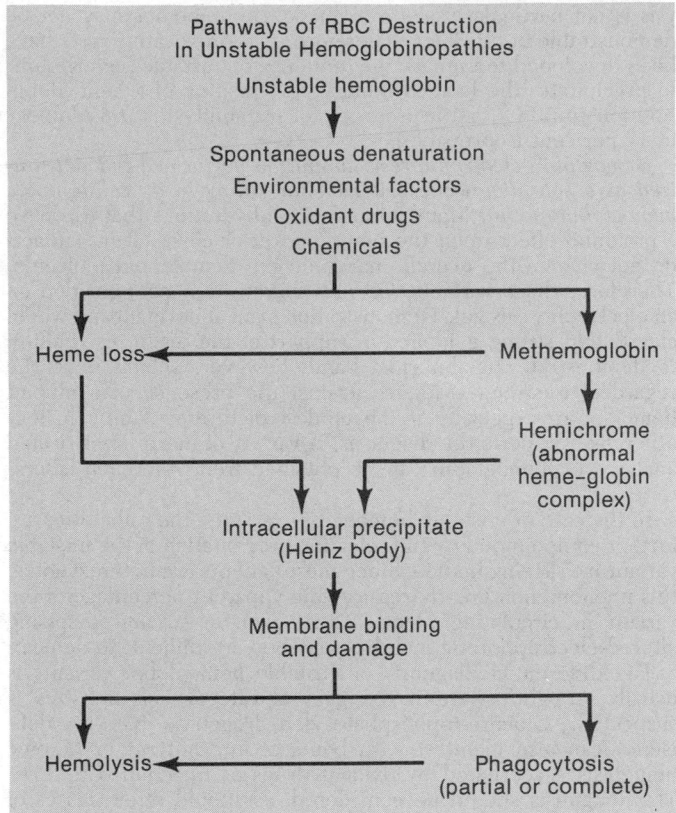

FIGURE 136–7. The presumed mechanisms by which denaturation of hemoglobin leads to erythrocyte destruction are outlined. The rate of travel through the various pathways probably differs for different hemoglobin variants and for a variety of stresses to which the protein is subjected.

tered, thus producing a hemolytic anemia. In severely affected patients, the anemia may require chronic transfusion therapy. Splenectomy is often effective for relief of anemia. Leg ulcers and premature gallbladder disease occur with high frequency.

Unstable hemoglobins are quite rare in comparison to sickle cell anemia and the thalassemias. They occur sporadically in many ethnic groups, often by spontaneous mutation. The heterozygous state is usually symptomatic ("dominant") because significant numbers of Heinz bodies form even when the unstable variant accounts for only half of the total hemoglobin. Most of the symptomatic unstable hemoglobins are β globin variants, since sporadic mutations affecting the α globin loci would usually involve only one of the four alleles, thus generating only 20 to 30 per cent abnormal hemoglobin. The propensity of unstable hemoglobins to precipitate is exaggerated by "oxidative" stress, such as infection or exposure to oxidizing drugs (e.g., quinine). Indeed, some of these variants are symptomatic only when oxidant stress occurs.

Diagnosis

The presence of an unstable hemoglobin should be suspected in individuals with chronic hemolytic anemia, unexplained jaundice, premature biliary tract disease (caused by bilirubin gallstones generated by excess red cell turnover), unexplained reticulocytosis, or bouts of intermittent hemolysis that can be related to exposure to oxidant drugs or infections. Other suggestive symptoms include dark urine, transient jaundice, or leg ulcers. These findings are stigmata of chronic or intermittent hemolysis.

Laboratory diagnosis is based upon identification of a mutant hemoglobin that precipitates more easily than normal hemoglobin. The in vivo evidence for precipitated hemoglobin is the Heinz body, which is an intraerythrocytic inclusion body detectable by staining of a peripheral blood film with a supravital dye, usually brilliant cresyl blue or new methylene blue. Since the spleen can remove Heinz bodies efficiently, especially if hemolysis is not particularly acute or brisk, Heinz bodies may not be demonstrable at all times. Therefore, two provocative tests have been developed to unmask the tendency of unstable hemoglobins to precipitate: the heat instability test (heating of a hemoglobin solution to 50°C) or the isopropanol instability test (insolubility in 17 per cent isopropanol).

Hemoglobin electrophoresis should be performed but not utilized as a sole diagnostic criterion for ruling in or ruling out a hemoglobinopathy. Many amino acid substitutions that can have a profound effect upon the heme pocket or chain-chain contacts do not change the overall charge on the hemoglobin molecule. Therefore, these variants will not migrate to a new position on an electrophoresis gel. Demonstration of an abnormal band would clearly add strong evidence in support of the diagnosis. Failure to demonstrate an abnormal band, however, should never be regarded as strong evidence against the presence of a mutant hemoglobin, especially if the clinical picture or family history otherwise supports the diagnosis. A variety of more sophisticated analyses of hemoglobin can be obtained from reference laboratories.

In the case of unstable hemoglobin variants, the difficulties are further compounded by the selective precipitation of the unstable variant into Heinz bodies. Since most patients are heterozygotes, this phenomenon greatly reduces the apparent percentage of the variant in circulating blood. Thus, even a variant possessing altered electrophoretic mobility may be very difficult to detect.

The differential diagnosis of unstable hemoglobin variants is usually straightforward if the general category of diagnosis is suspected. Glucose-6-phosphate dehydrogenase (G6PD) deficiency can also manifest with bouts of intermittent or chronic hemolysis exacerbated by oxidant drugs or infection (Ch. 134). This diagnosis should be considered, as should other causes of chronic or intermittent hemolytic anemia, such as red cell membrane disorders (e.g., hereditary spherocytosis) or immune hemolytic anemias. Spherocytes are relatively rare in unstable hemoglobin disorders; this is sometimes a useful discriminant.

Management

The severity of the clinical complications of unstable hemoglobins varies enormously. Many patients can be managed adequately by expectant monitoring and avoidance of drugs provoking hemolysis. Occasional patients may require transfusions during bouts of severe acute hemolytic anemia. Individuals who suffer significant morbidity because of chronic anemia or repeated episodes of severe hemolysis should be considered candidates for splenectomy, especially if hypersplenism has developed. Finally, the tendency of infection to exacerbate hemolysis should prompt one to monitor these patients closely during those episodes.

HEMOGLOBINS WITH INCREASED OXYGEN AFFINITY

Hemoglobin functions as a biologically useful oxygen transport pigment because of the sigmoidal shape of its oxygen affinity curve. In the transition from the fully deoxygenated (tense, or T) to the fully oxygenated (relaxed, or R) state, the initial oxygenation steps occur with difficulty. In fact, the act of binding the first oxygen molecule increases the affinity of the molecule for subsequent oxygen binding events, thus creating the sigmoidal shape of the curve. The necessary intramolecular reorganization occurs only when the proper arrangement of hydrogen bonds, hydrophobic interactions, and salt bridges is broken and formed in the proper sequence during R-T transitions.

Mutant hemoglobins exhibiting altered oxygen affinity usually arise when amino acid substitutions occur at the interface between α and β chains or in regions affecting the hydrogen bonds, hydrophobic interactions, or salt bridges. A second major class of mutations comprises those affecting interaction with 2,3-diphosphoglycerate (2,3-DPG) (Ch. 136.1), which alters oxygen affinity when bound to hemoglobin.

Pathogenesis and Clinical Manifestations

"High-affinity" hemoglobins exhibit higher avidity for oxygen, causing the oxygen dissociation curve to "shift to the left"; an example is Hb Zurich ($\beta^{63\text{his}\rightarrow\text{arg}}$) (Fig. 136–8). These hemoglobins bind oxygen more readily but are less able to deliver the oxygen

to tissues at normal capillary oxygen pressures. Since the Po_2 in the lung ($Po_2 = 90$ to 100 mm Hg) is normally well above that needed to saturate hemoglobin fully with oxygen (60 mm Hg), these variant hemoglobins cannot acquire any additional oxygen in the lung despite their higher affinity. At capillary Po_2 (35 to 45 mm Hg), however, high-affinity hemoglobins deliver less oxygen. The resultant mild tissue hypoxia stimulates erythropoietin release and leads to inappropriately high red cell production and polycythemia (Ch. 142). In extreme cases, hematocrits of 60 to 65 per cent can be encountered.

High-affinity variants arise from several forms of mutations. Some alter interactions within the heme pocket, others disrupt the Bohr effect or the salt-bond site, and others impair the interaction of Hb A with 2,3-DPG. The 2,3-DPG binding lowers the oxygen affinity of Hb A. Reduced 2,3-DPG binding results in an effective increase in oxygen affinity. As a good example of a high-affinity hemoglobin, a single amino acid substitution in Hb Kempsey blocks the hydrogen bond formation with the tyrosine at α^{42} needed to stabilize the T (deoxy) state. This and numerous other examples that have been analyzed at the molecular level have greatly aided our understanding of the molecular basis for reversible oxygen binding.

Diagnosis

"High-affinity" hemoglobins should be considered in patients with unexplained erythrocytosis, especially if there is a positive family history (Ch. 142). Oxygen affinity is usually measured as the P-50, the partial pressure of oxygen at which a hemoglobin preparation (either in the form of a red cell suspension or in the form of a hemoglobin solution) is 50 per cent saturated with oxygen (Fig. 136–2). The hemoglobin preparation is exposed to increasing oxygen pressures in the laboratory, and the relative percentages of oxyhemoglobin and deoxyhemoglobin are determined optically, forming a curve from which the 50 per cent saturation point is determined. A "shift to the left" means that the hemoglobin reaches 50 per cent saturation at a *lower* partial pressure of oxygen. *High-affinity variants are thus associated with a lower than normal P-50 value.* Hemoglobin electrophoresis should be performed but may not be revealing.

The most common cause of a low P-50 value is carbon monoxide poisoning. Hemoglobin–carbon monoxide has an extremely "left-shifted" oxygen affinity curve, which reflects stabilization of hemoglobin in the R state without benefit of oxygen binding. The clinical impact is the same as that of a very high oxygen affinity hemoglobin. The most common cause of hemoglobin–carbon monoxide is cigarette smoking, although chronic carbon monoxide exposure in individuals such as caisson workers or tunnel toll booth collectors is encountered sporadically.

P-50 curves should be performed with both whole-blood suspensions and isolated hemoglobin solutions. In the latter circumstance, the contribution of 2,3-DPG is eliminated. This can eliminate the potential confounding artifact and reveal those variants arising from abnormal interaction with this ligand.

Management

Most patients with high-affinity hemoglobins have mild erythrocytosis not requiring treatment. Very rarely, the hematocrit and, therefore, the blood viscosity are sufficiently elevated to warrant treatment by phlebotomy.

HEMOGLOBINS WITH DECREASED OXYGEN AFFINITY

Pathogenesis and Clinical Manifestations

Low-affinity hemoglobin variants, such as Hb Kansas ($\beta^{102\text{Asn}\rightarrow\text{Thr}}$), represent the pathophysiologic "mirror image" of the high-affinity hemoglobins (Fig. 136–8). In Hb Kansas, the threonine position β^{102} cannot form a hydrogen bond with aspartic acid at position α^{94}, which normally stabilizes the R (oxy) state. Thus, Hb Kansas has less tendency to bind oxygen and exhibits a "right-shifted" P-50 value.

In all but the most severe examples of low-affinity variants, oxygen affinity remains high enough that the hemoglobin becomes fully saturated in the highly oxygen-abundant environment of the pulmonary capillary. At the Po_2 of the capillary bed in most tissues, however, these hemoglobins "dump" excessive amounts of oxygen and become more desaturated than normal hemoglobin. There are two pathophysiologic consequences of this higher than normal level of oxygen delivery. First, since tissue oxygen delivery is so efficient, the erythropoietin "thermostat" can be set lower, resulting in normal oxygen transport at lower than normal hematocrits. This situation produces a state of "pseudo-anemia." In other words, the hematocrit appears to be abnormally low, even though homeostasis of oxygen transport and the patient are completely normal. Second, the amount of desaturated hemoglobin circulating in capillaries can be greater than 5 grams per deciliter, producing clinically apparent cyanosis. In contrast to most other causes of cyanosis, this usually ominous finding is entirely benign in these individuals.

Diagnosis

A low-affinity variant should be suspected in patients with unexplained anemia or cyanosis who, by all other criteria, appear to be entirely well, especially if there is a positive family history. Testing for the abnormal variant follows the same reasoning as that just described for high-affinity variants, except that the P-50 value will be shifted to the right.

Management

Patients with low-affinity hemoglobins are usually asymptomatic. No treatment is required. It is important to document that a low-affinity hemoglobin is the cause of an apparent anemia and that this finding is only a physiologic response to the altered oxygen affinity. Cyanosis in some individuals can pose a cosmetic problem, but correction with transfusions is rarely, if ever, justified.

METHEMOGLOBINEMIAS

Methemoglobin is generated by oxidation of the iron moieties in hemoglobin from the ferrous (Fe^{2+}) to the ferric (Fe^{3+}) state. Oxygen transport by hemoglobin requires that iron be present in the ferrous state in deoxyhemoglobin. Yet oxygenation of hemoglobin causes a partial transfer of an electron from the iron to the bound oxygen; iron in this state thus resembles ferric iron. The oxygen resembles superoxide (O_2^-). Deoxygenation returns the

electron to the iron, with release of oxygen. When this electron return fails to occur, methemoglobin forms. Normally methemoglobin constitutes 3 per cent or less of the total hemoglobin content. Indeed, reduction of methemoglobin levels to less than 1 per cent is routinely accomplished in vivo by the activity of an enzyme called methemoglobin reductase (nicotinamide-adenine dinucleotide [NADH]–dehydratase, NADH-diaphorase, erythrocyte cytochrome b_3). This enzyme reduces hemoglobin iron by transfer of an electron from NADH to oxidize cytochrome b_3; cytochrome b_3 then converts ferric to ferrous iron by direct interaction with hemoglobin. The generation of NADH depends on the glycolytic pathway.

A second reducing enzyme, nicotinamide-adenine dinucleotide phosphate (NADPH)–dependent methemoglobin reductase, does not normally function in erythrocytes because there is no electron carrier available to interact with NADPH as the "go-between" with hemoglobin iron. Artificial electron carriers, such as methylene blue, can provide this missing link. As discussed later, methylene blue is therefore an important agent for the treatment of methemoglobinemia. Reduced glutathione and ascorbic acid can also reduce methemoglobin directly; however, these nonenzymatic reactions are considerably slower than the reductase pathways.

Pathogenesis and Clinical Manifestations

Methemoglobinemias of clinical import arise by one of three distinct mechanisms: (1) globin chain mutations that result in increased formation of methemoglobin; (2) deficiencies in the reductase pathways described above; and (3) "toxic" methemoglobinemia in which even normal red cells endowed with normal hemoglobin and normal methemoglobin reductase can be "overwhelmed" by exposure to substances that oxidize hemoglobin iron (Table 136–3).

Abnormal hemoglobins causing methemoglobinemia ("M hemoglobins") tend to arise from mutations that alter the heme

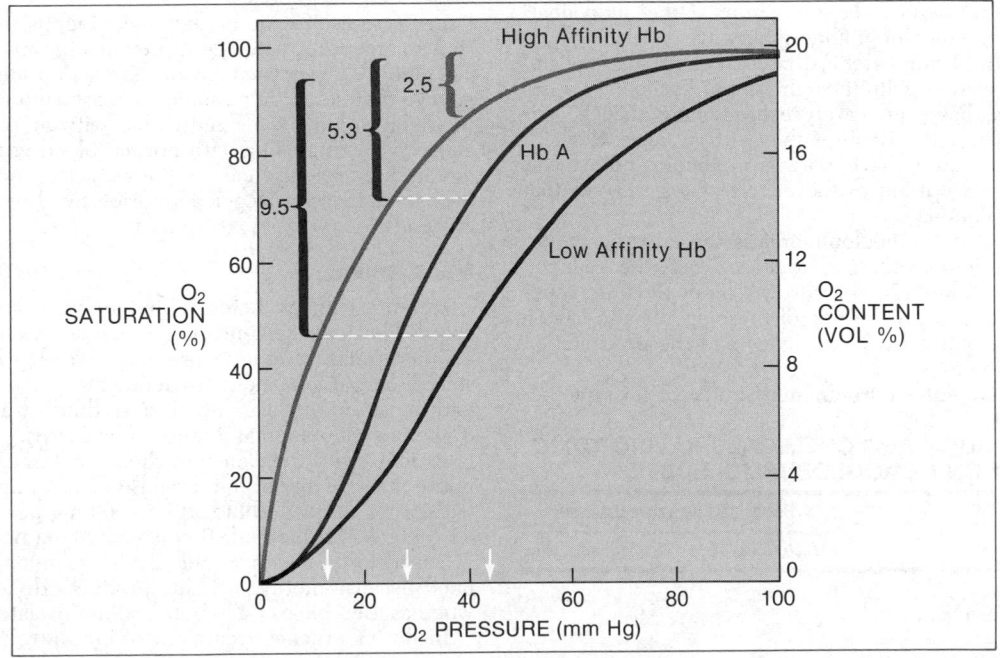

FIGURE 136–8. Hemoglobin-oxygen dissociation curves are illustrated for normal hemoglobin (Hb A) and for model abnormal hemoglobins with high and low oxygen affinities. On the abscissa the partial pressure of oxygen is indicated in millimeters of mercury. On the left ordinate the saturation of hemoglobin with oxygen is indicated as a percentage; on the right ordinate the oxygen content of the hemoglobin is expressed as volumes per cent. The three inverted arrows show the P_{50} for the three hemoglobins (the partial pressure of oxygen at which the hemoglobin is 50 per cent saturated). This value is lowest for the high-affinity hemoglobin. As the partial pressure of oxygen drops from 100 (arterial) to 40 (tissues), hemoglobin desaturates, giving up a portion of its bound oxygen; the numbers on the brackets indicate the amount of oxygen unloaded by the three hemoglobin types expressed in volumes per cent. Note that the high-affinity hemoglobin delivers less than half the oxygen that Hb A gives to the tissues, resulting in tissue anoxia, increased erythropoietin secretion, and erythrocytosis. Conversely, the low-affinity hemoglobin is even more efficient than Hb A in supplying the tissues with oxygen, resulting in diminished erythropoietin production and anemia.

TABLE 136–3. TYPES OF METHEMOGLOBINEMIA

A. Congenital
1. Defective enzymatic reduction of Fe^{+3}-hemoglobin to Fe^{+2}-hemoglobin
   a. NADH–methemoglobin reductase (cytochrome b_5 reductase) deficiency
   b. Cytochrome b_5 deficiency
2. Abnormal hemoglobins resistant to enzymatic reduction (M hemoglobins)
B. Acquired
1. Excessive (toxic) oxidation of Fe^{+2}-hemoglobin
   a. Environmental chemicals
   b. Drugs

pocket in a fashion that favors stabilization of the iron in the ferric state. In the majority of these, a histidine is replaced by a tyrosine; the hydroxyl group of the tyrosine forms a complex that stabilizes the iron in the ferric state in a fashion resistant to reduction by the methemoglobin reductase system. A few of the variants tend to lose heme and thus also exhibit features of a mildly unstable hemoglobin disorder.

Methemoglobin has a brownish to blue color, which does not become red upon exposure to oxygen. These individuals thus appear to be cyanotic. In contrast to truly cyanotic individuals, however, arterial Po_2 values are normal. These individuals are otherwise asymptomatic, because methemoglobin is rarely above 30 to 50 per cent, the levels at which symptomatology becomes apparent, as described below.

Hereditary methemoglobinemia resulting from methemoglobin reductase deficiency is rare; 100 to 200 cases have been described. Numerous recessive mutations cause a variety of defects in the resulting variant enzymes, including catalytic activity, electrophoretic mobility, and structural stability. Hispanics, Eskimos, and Native Americans in particular are frequently affected. In some individuals, neurologic defects are also present, suggesting that the mutation affects isoforms of the enzyme common to both erythrocytes and other tissues, including brain. Other individuals exhibit only the methemoglobin abnormality.

Like patients with M hemoglobins, patients with methemoglobin reductase deficiency exhibit slight gray "pseudocyanosis." Even homozygotes, however, rarely exhibit more than 25 per cent methemoglobin, a level compatible with absence of symptoms. Heterozygotes often have normal methemoglobin levels but are especially susceptible to the effects of toxic agents that cause methemoglobinemia.

The third form of methemoglobinemia is caused by exposure to certain chemical agents and drugs that accelerate the oxidation of methemoglobin (Table 136–4). Nitrite compounds are especially notorious in this regard. Some of these agents also have a propensity to exacerbate G6PD deficiency and the precipitation of unstable hemoglobins.

Nitrates are a frequent environmental source of toxic methe-

TABLE 136–4. DRUGS AND CHEMICALS HAVING TOXIC EFFECT ON HEMOGLOBIN MOLECULE

Agent	Hemoglobin Derivative Observed	
	Methemoglobin	Sulfhemoglobin
Acetanilid, phenacetin	+	+
Nitrites (amyl, sodium, potassium, nitroglycerin)	+	+
Trinitrotoluene, nitrobenzene	+	+
Aniline, hydroxylamine, dimethylamine	+	+
Sulfanilamide	+	+
Para-aminosalicylic acid	+	
Dapsone	+	
Primaquine, chloroquine	+	
Prilocaine, benzocaine, lidocaine	+	
Menadione, naphthoquinone	+	
Naphthalene	+	
Resorcinol	+	
Phenylhydrazine	+	+

moglobinemia, even though nitrates do not directly interact with either hemoglobin or the reductase system. Rather, nitrates are converted to nitrites in the gut. Well water is the most frequently encountered source of excessive nitrates. In general, substantial intake of these agents is required before significant amounts of methemoglobin are generated. Very young infants are more susceptible to these agents than are adults, but all age groups are at risk if exposure is sufficient.

Toxic or acquired methemoglobinemia is virtually the only situation in which life-threatening amounts of methemoglobin accumulate. In general, the only symptom produced when methemoglobin comprises less than 30 per cent of total hemoglobin is the cosmetic effect of cyanosis. As levels of methemoglobin rise above 30 per cent, however, patients begin to exhibit symptoms of oxygen deprivation, such as malaise, giddiness, and other alterations of mental status. The symptoms reflect a true lack of oxygen availability at the tissue level, since a substantial number of hemoglobin molecules are no longer delivering oxygen to the tissues. At levels of methemoglobin greater than 50 per cent, loss of consciousness, coma, and death can ensue rapidly. At this level of methemoglobin, "cyanosis" is severe, and the blood is chocolate brown.

Diagnosis

Methemoglobinemia should be suspected in patients with unexplained cyanosis. One should be especially alert to the potential medical emergency inherent in a patient with cyanosis and altered mental status, despite a normal arterial Po_2. The ingestion of nitrites as a suicide gesture, especially in individuals knowledgeable with respect to chemistry, medicine, or pharmacology, is not uncommon. The diagnosis of methemoglobinemia can be suspected from the brownish color of blood when it is drawn. In the laboratory, methemoglobin exhibits characteristic peaks of absorption at 630 and 502 nm, rendering it easily distinguishable from normal hemoglobin. In addition, the inherited M hemoglobins are frequently detectable by altered electrophoretic mobility, especially if ferricyanide treatment in vitro is used to convert all of the hemoglobin solution to methemoglobin prior to electrophoresis.

In the case of toxic methemoglobinemia, recognition of exposure to an appropriate agent provides the most important historical clue. Acute poisoning can represent a life-threatening emergency; therefore, one should request laboratory evaluation for methemoglobin in any individual with atypical cyanosis or cyanosis occurring along with normal blood gas values. Methemoglobin due to deficiencies of the reductase system can be further evaluated in reference laboratories by direct analysis of these enzymes.

Management

Patients with M hemoglobins are usually asymptomatic and require no management. The secondary cyanosis can represent an unfortunate cosmetic problem, which cannot be reversed, since ascorbic acid and methylene blue (see below) are ineffective with most of these variants despite their utility in the treatment of methemoglobinemia due to other causes.

Patients with deficiency of the reductase system generally do not require treatment, but cyanosis can be improved by treatment with oral methylene blue, 100 to 300 mg per day, or 500 mg per day of oral ascorbic acid. Riboflavin (20 mg per day) has also been reported to be effective. Riboflavin treatment has been championed because methylene blue produces discolored (blue) urine, whereas ascorbic can generate sodium oxalate stones.

In the emergency treatment of high levels of toxic methemoglobinemia, 1 to 2 mg per kilogram of methylene blue is given as a 1 per cent solution in saline, usually administered rapidly (10 to 15 minutes) intravenously. The dose may be repeated if necessary. This treatment is usually effective. As noted above, methylene blue acts via the NADPH reductase system, which in turn requires G6PD activity. The method is thus not effective in patients who also have G6PD deficiency. These patients, or patients who are severely affected, may require exchange transfusion. Oral ascorbic acid, at doses noted earlier, is not useful in emergency situations because it acts too slowly. Follow-up maintenance management, however, can be accomplished with either ascorbic acid or oral methylene blue.

Mild cases of methemoglobin intoxication do not require treatment. The patient can be monitored for 1 to 3 days, during which time methemoglobin levels will gradually return to normal if the offending agent is eliminated. The most important follow-up therapy of patients with toxic methemoglobinemia involves a thorough search for the offending agent and its removal from the environment.

Bunn HF, Forget BG: Hemoglobin: Molecular, Genetic and Clinical Aspects. Philadelphia, W.B. Saunders Company, 1986. *Chapter 13 discusses unstable hemoglobins; Chapter 14, hemoglobins with altered oxygen affinity; and Chapters 15 and 16, various forms of methemoglobinemia.*

Mansouri A: Methemoglobinemia. Am J Med Sci 289:200, 1985.

Weatherall DJ, Clegg JB, Higgs DR, et al.: The hemoglobinopathies. *In* Scriver CR, Beaudet AL, Sly WS, et al. (eds.): The Metabolic Basis of Inherited Disease. 6th ed. New York, McGraw-Hill Book Company, 1989, pp 2281–2339.

136.4 THE THALASSEMIAS

Arthur W. Nienhuis

The thalassemias are hereditary anemias that occur because of mutations that affect the synthesis of hemoglobin. In β-thalassemia there is deficient synthesis of β globin, whereas in α-thalassemia there is deficient synthesis of α globin (see Color Plate 6A). Reduced synthesis of one of the two globin polypeptides leads to deficient hemoglobin accumulation, resulting in hypochromic and microcytic red cells. These red cell abnormalities are the most constant and characteristic features of this group of disorders. Table 136–5 contains a clinical classification of the thalassemias presented in the order in which they are discussed in this chapter.

The incidence and prevalence of these conditions are highly variable. Most common is thalassemia trait, a mild, clinically insignificant anemia that apparently protects individuals from malaria (see below), and therefore through natural selection it has become extremely common in certain parts of the world. Thalassemia trait generally represents the heterozygous form of either α- or β-thalassemia. Hence where thalassemia trait is common, homozygous, more severely affected patients will be found frequently. In the United States, the incidence of β-thalassemia is highest among ethnic groups originating from the Mediterranean area, parts of Africa, and Asia, whereas the incidence of α-thalassemia is highest among those from Asia. Generally, the incidence of thalassemia trait in these ethnic groups is 3 to 5 per cent. Approximately 1000 patients with more severe forms of thalassemia are known in the United States.

SEVERE β-THALASSEMIA (Cooley's Anemia)

Severe β-thalassemia occurs in patients who are homozygous for mutations that lead to a decrease in β globin synthesis. Because both β globin genes are affected, there is marked deficiency in β globin synthesis, but α globin synthesis continues at an approximately normal rate. Accumulation of a large excess of α chains for which there are no β chains with which to combine has several serious deleterious effects. α Globin is highly insoluble and forms large intracellular inclusions. These interfere with the cell cycle in the bone marrow, retard the passage of red cells

TABLE 136–5. CLINICAL CLASSIFICATION OF THE THALASSEMIAS

I. Severe β-thalassemia (Cooley's anemia)	Severe anemia, growth retardation, hepatosplenomegaly, bone marrow expansion, and bone deformities
A. Thalassemia major	Transfusion dependent
B. Thalassemia intermedia	No regular transfusion requirement
II. Thalassemia trait (α or β)	Mild anemia with microcytosis and hypochromia
III. Hb H disease (α-thal)	Moderately severe hemolytic anemia, icterus, and splenomegaly
IV. Hydrops fetalis (α-thal)	Death in utero caused by severe anemia
V. Silent carrier (α or β)	Hematologically normal

from the bone marrow, and reduce the survival of red cells in the circulation by virtue of membrane damage and splenic trapping. Marked ineffective erythropoiesis is the hallmark of this disorder because α inclusions interfere with erythroblast maturation, leading to intramedullary death of many red cell precursors. Severe anemia stimulates erythropoietin production, leading to erythroid stem cell and erythroblast proliferation. The vastly expanded erythroid cell mass results in osteoporosis with a potential for pathologic fractures. Extramedullary hematopoiesis is also often seen, and compression of vital structures, particularly the spinal cord, may occur as a consequence. Because of marrow expansion and deformities of the skull and facial bones, patients with severe β-thalassemia often have an abnormal appearance with prominent epicanthal folds, referred to as a chipmunk facies.

Patients with severe β-thalassemia may be divided into two groups on the basis of their requirement for blood transfusion. Those with thalassemia major have an absolute requirement for blood without which severe anemia leads to death in infancy or early childhood. In contrast, patients with thalassemia intermedia are able to maintain their hemoglobin at 6 to 7 grams per deciliter without transfusion. This level is compatible with fairly normal growth and development, and many of these patients survive into adulthood.

Thalassemia Major

CLINICAL FEATURES. At birth patients with thalassemia major are nearly normal hematologically, since γ globin synthesis is normal and hemoglobin (Hb) F production is therefore adequate. However, as the switch from Hb F to Hb A is completed during the first year of life, the deficiency in β globin production becomes evident. By 6 to 9 months of age, severe anemia reflected by pallor, poor growth, or inadequate food intake leads the anxious parents to bring the infant to the physician, at which time examination reveals the presence of marked hepatosplenomegaly. The hemoglobin may be 3 to 6 grams per deciliter, and the red cells exhibit the characteristic severe microcytosis, hypochromia, and fragmentation (see Color Plate 6A, left). Demonstration of thalassemia trait (see below) in both parents is usually sufficient to establish the diagnosis. Study of the infant's blood shows absence of or low Hb A, a large amount of Hb F, and an increase in the amount of Hb A_2 to 4 to 10 per cent of the total (normal <2.5 per cent). Biosynthetic studies, a tool of the research laboratory, may be employed to show the deficiency of β globin production.

CLINICAL COURSE. Prior to the use of regular blood transfusions, these children were grossly deformed because of expansion of the marrow spaces of the skull (see Fig. 127–1). Severe osteoporosis led to pathologic fractures, and anemia caused weakness and inanition. Death by 2 to 3 years of age was common. Blood transfusions were initially given infrequently for palliation, but gradually physicians interested in this condition came to recognize that regular transfusion to nearly normal hemoglobin levels could be used to suppress all disease manifestations. Growth and bone development are normal in children who have undergone hypertransfusion, and in fact they are virtually indistinguishable from other children if the hypertransfusion regimen is started at a very early age. If transfusions are given less frequently, the patient may exhibit some stigmata of the untreated disorder—bone deformities, growth retardation, and hepatosplenomegaly.

THE PROBLEM OF IRON OVERLOAD. Because humans have a very limited ability to excrete iron, regular blood transfusions inevitably lead to a vast accumulation. Each unit of packed red cells contains approximately 200 mg of iron, so that by the age of 12 the average thalassemic, having received 125 to 150 units of packed cells, will have accumulated 25 to 30 grams of excess iron. This amount compares with the normal 3 to 4 grams found in adults, 75 per cent of which is present in red cells as hemoglobin. Even in the patient with thalassemia intermedia who has not had transfusions, excess iron absorption leads inevitably to the manifestations of hemochromatosis, although at a later age than in the patient with transfusion-dependent thalassemia. Excess iron deposition occurs in virtually all organs. Most cells have a considerable ability to cope with this extra iron by making ferritin and its partial degradation product hemosiderin. Nonetheless, cell damage occurs by virtue of iron-catalyzed peroxidation of membrane lipids and release of the enzymes from lysosomes rendered labile by their content of hemosiderin granules. Thus tissue hemosiderosis (excess iron) leads ultimately to the clinical condition of secondary hemochromatosis. The liver, endocrine glands, and particularly the heart are the primary target organs (see Ch. 193).

Liver dysfunction is mild in the thalassemic patient with secondary hemochromatosis. Typically the liver is enlarged several centimeters below the right costal margin, and the transaminases are two to four times above the normal limits. Despite a 20- to 30-fold increase in iron concentration over normal, liver biosynthetic function as reflected by the concentration of serum albumin and various clotting factors is preserved. Fibrosis, invariably present on liver biopsy, may progress to frank cirrhosis anatomically, but clinical evidence of cirrhosis is rare.

As noted above, the course of adequately tranfused thalassemic patients is essentially normal until the age of 10 to 12. Then growth failure is a frequent and distressing complication for both the child and parents. The mechanism for this growth failure is not known; growth hormone levels are generally normal, but the serum somatomedin concentration may be low. Failure of growth is accompanied by lack of pubescence. Primary hypogonadism is exceedingly common. The mechanism is usually a failure of the pituitary to produce adequate amounts of follicle-stimulating hormone (FSH) and luteinizing hormone (LH). Diabetes mellitus, hypothyroidism, and, rarely, hypoparathyroidism with tetany are additional complications that may occur, particularly in patients who are in their late teenage years or early 20's.

Cardiac disease in the patients with severe β-thalassemia may take three forms: pericarditis, congestive heart failure, and cardiac arrhythmias. Recurrent attacks of acute pericarditis are manifested by chest pain, often pleuritic and affected by a change of position, accompanied by fever and occasionally a pericardial friction rub. These attacks are usually self-limited, lasting 4 to 7 days. Treatment consists of bed rest, aspirin, and other anti-inflammatory agents, such as indomethacin in appropriate doses. Rarely, constrictive pericarditis may require a pericardiectomy.

Congestive heart failure is to be expected ultimately in patients with secondary hemochromatosis unless death occurs early by virtue of cardiac arrhythmias. Careful echocardiographic studies have suggested that iron deposition begins by the age of 5 to 6 years. By 10 or 12 years, when the patient has received more than 100 units of blood, left ventricular dysfunction may be demonstrated by radionuclide cineangiography during the physiologic stress of exercise. Clinical congestive heart failure is usually a late complication; most patients die within 12 months of the onset of definite evidence of heart failure. Treatment with digoxin in doses adequate to achieve therapeutic blood levels may be quite helpful. Appropriate use of diuretics and vasodilator therapy may be extremely useful in providing palliation and extending the lifespan of these patients.

Atrial and ventricular ectopy is present in 24-hour electrocardiographic recordings in virtually all patients who have received more than 150 units of packed red cells. High-grade ventricular ectopy with couplets, short runs of ventricular tachycardia, and multiple ventricular foci are of ominous prognostic significance. Ectopy may be extremely distressful to the patient, particularly at night, when it is often most severe. Tachyrhythmias such as ventricular tachycardia and/or ventricular fibrillation occur despite therapy and are frequent causes of death in patients with severe thalassemia who are undergoing regular transfusions. The pharmacologic treatment of cardiac arrhythmias is described in Ch. 42.

The prognosis of patients with thalassemia major is determined by the cardiac disease. The average age of death is 17 years, although a few patients may survive to their mid-20's. Because of this grim prognosis, a considerable effort has been focused on attempts to reduce the iron burden in these patients.

THE ROLE OF SPLENECTOMY. Splenic enlargement is frequent and often causes functional hypersplenism as manifested by an increasing transfusion requirement. Careful documentation of the patient's needs often alerts the physician to the development of hypersplenism as the need for blood rises. An average patient on a hypertransfusion regimen designed to maintain the hemoglobin at a level greater than 10 grams per deciliter requires 250 ml of packed cells per kilogram per year. If substantially more blood is required, the spleen should be removed. Leukopenia and thrombocytopenia, if present, are indicators of the presence of hypersplenism and should lead to prompt splenectomy.

The complication of splenectomy in this patient population is a risk of sudden overwhelming sepsis by encapsulated organisms. For this reason, delay of splenectomy until after the age of 4 is highly desirable. Splenectomized patients should receive Pneumovax and may be placed on a regimen of daily penicillin prophylaxis. More important, each patient should be given a small supply of a broad-spectrum antibiotic, such as ampicillin, to be taken orally in appropriate doses if a high temperature develops and immediate medical attention cannot be obtained.

CHELATION THERAPY. The only drug available for use in removal of iron is deferoxamine (Desferal). This drug has an extremely high affinity for trivalent iron, and despite extensive clinical use it appears to be relatively free of serious toxicity when given subcutaneously. It must be given parenterally and it has a very short serum half-life. Thus, most of the drug, given as a single intramuscular injection, is rapidly excreted without binding any iron. To maximize the efficacy of the drug, a technique has been devised to administer it subcutaneously by using a small mechanical infusion pump. A needle is inserted into the subcutaneous tissue of the abdomen, and the drug is infused very slowly over a period of 8 to 12 hours. With 1.5 to 2.0 grams of Desferal, two to three times more iron may be removed than by a single daily intramuscular injection. Often daily excretion of 30 to 40 mg of iron may be achieved in older patients and may lead to overall negative iron balance despite continued transfusion therapy, provided that the drug is used at least five times per week. This regimen retards the rate of iron accumulation in the liver and reduces liver fibrosis.

Clinical evidence indicates that cardiac disease may be delayed. Indeed, reversal of established congestive heart failure with documented left ventricular dysfunction has been observed in patients treated intensively with intravenous deferoxamine. This may be accomplished by placement of a Hickman catheter. Well-motivated patients may be taught to administer the drug daily by the intravenous route in doses of 3 to 4 grams per day given over 18 to 20 hours. Gastrointestinal disturbances and reversible renal dysfunction have been observed. Reduction of dose eliminates these complications. Significant neurosensory toxicity affecting sight and auditory function has been observed at high intravenous doses. The greatest probability of successfully preventing iron damage is in patients in whom treatment is begun early, preferably by the age of 5 years. Vitamin C in small doses (150 to 250 mg per day) given orally may increase the amount of iron excretion in response to deferoxamine infusions, although some evidence suggests that this agent may enhance tissue iron toxicity, particularly to the heart, and therefore it should be used with caution in older patients.

Various oral chelations have been developed, and two have reached the stage of clinical trials in limited numbers of patients. The efficacy of Desferal is well established, however, and therefore substitution of untested therapy is problematic, since the outcome cannot be known for several years.

Thalassemia Intermedia

Those patients with severe β-thalassemia who maintain their hemoglobin levels above 6.0 to 7.0 grams per deciliter have a generally better prognosis. Individual patients with thalassemia intermedia generally have large amounts of Hb F, significant amounts of Hb A₂, and variable amounts of Hb A in their red cells. Iron accumulation may occur because of increased gastrointestinal absorption and ultimately may lead to secondary hemochromatosis with endocrine and cardiac dysfunction, but most patients with thalassemia intermedia survive into adulthood and many have children. Splenectomy may become necessary if evidence of hypersplenism is present. Osteoporosis may be severe, as these patients' erythroid mass is not suppressed. A disabling form of arthritis has been described. Large masses of erythroid tissue in extramedullary sites may cause organ dysfunction. Particularly distressing is spinal cord compression with paraplegia, although usually local radiation reverses this condition. Any or all of these complications may ultimately lead to the use of a regular transfusion regimen in patients with thalassemia intermedia despite their marginally adequate hemoglobin levels. Such treatment has the added benefit of preventing the disfiguring facial abnormalities.

Genetically this condition is heterogeneous. Often the red cells of both parents exhibit stigmata of thalassemia trait, although frequently one parent may be a silent carrier of the thalassemia gene (see below). In such persons the impairment of β globin synthesis is so mild that the red cells are normal, but when the abnormal β gene is paired with another affected by a more severe β-thalassemia mutation, thalassemia intermedia results. Elucidation of any thalassemia mutations at the molecular level has revealed marked quantitative variability ranging from 50 to 100 per cent reduction of β globin messenger RNA (mRNA) production (see below). Many patients are doubly heterozygous for two different mutations. The clinical heterogeneity of the β-thalassemias reflects the many combinations of mutations that may be present in individual patients. Other genetic modifiers of the β-thalassemia phenotype include α-thalassemia mutations and genetic variants characterized by increased Hb F production. Co-inheritance of an α-thalassemia gene decreases α globin production, leading to partial correction of the highly deleterious imbalance in α and β biosynthesis. Increased γ globin synthesis, resulting in increased Hb F production, compensates directly for deficient β globin production.

THALASSEMIA TRAIT

CLINICAL CHARACTERISTICS. Common to both α- and β-thalassemia is a condition referred to as thalassemia minor or trait. This condition generally occurs in individuals who are heterozygous for a mutation affecting α or β globin synthesis (see below). Characteristically the red blood cells are small and contain less hemoglobin than normal; the mean corpuscular volume averages 65 μm^3 (range, 56 to 74), whereas the mean corpuscular hemoglobin averages 21 pg (range, 20 to 23). Normal values for these parameters are 88 ± 5 and 30 ± 2, respectively. The total red cell count is often increased to 10 to 20 per cent above the normal range, so that anemia, if present, is mild. Rarely the packed cell volume may be as low as 30 per cent; values of 32 to 38 per cent are more typical. Splenomegaly is said to occur but is distinctly unusual, and other causes should be sought if this physical finding is present. No clinical symptoms may be attributed to the presence of thalassemia trait.

DIFFERENTIAL DIAGNOSIS. A characteristic feature of β-thalassemia trait is an elevation of the level of Hb A_2. This minor hemoglobin accounts for only 2 or 3 per cent of the total in normal red cells, but in thalassemia trait it may be elevated in the range of 4 to 8 per cent in more than 90 per cent of persons with this condition. Similarly, the level of Hb F is often elevated to 1.5 to 2.5 per cent, although in rare types of thalassemia trait it may be as high as 10 to 15 per cent. In normal red cells, Hb F accounts for less than 1 per cent of the total. The minor hemoglobins, Hb A_2 and Hb F, are either normal or slightly decreased in patients with α-thalassemia.

The differential diagnosis of thalassemia trait includes a consideration of iron deficiency. This diagnosis can be excluded only by measurement of the serum iron, total iron-binding capacity, and serum ferritin. If these values are normal in patients whose red cells are severely microcytic, but in whom anemia, if present, is mild, the diagnosis of thalassemia trait can be considered established. The distinction between α- and β-thalassemia depends on the measurement of the minor hemoglobins. If these are normal, the diagnosis of α-thalassemia is most likely, although rare subjects with β-thalassemia also have normal levels of Hb A_2 and Hb F.

GENE FREQUENCY. Thalassemia trait is thought to protect persons from malaria, particularly during the early years of life when immunity is not yet established and fatal cerebral malaria caused by *Plasmodium falciparum* may occur. This selective advantage accounts for the high frequency of thalassemia genes in regions where malaria has been endemic for the past two millennia. These include the Mediterranean basin particularly, but also large parts of Asia and Africa. The gene frequency may be as high as 20 per cent in certain populations.

HEMOGLOBIN H DISEASE

PATHOPHYSIOLOGY. An anemia of moderate severity characterized by hypochromia, microcytosis, striking red cell frag-

mentation, and the presence of a fast migrating hemoglobin on electrophoresis occurs in patients who have a moderately severe deficiency in α globin production. The genetics of this condition are considered later in this chapter. The fast migrating "hemoglobin" has the globin subunit composition $β_4$. It may account for up to 30 per cent of the total hemoglobin in these patients. Because the $β_4$ tetramer exhibits no cooperativeness and has an extremely high oxygen affinity, it is functionally useless in oxygen transport. Thus patients with a significant amount of Hb H functionally have a more severe anemia than measurement of the hemoglobin concentration might suggest.

Hb H is an unstable tetramer. Thus as the red cell ages and loses its ability to withstand oxidative stress, Hb H may precipitate, forming inclusions that cause hemolysis (see Color Plate 6C, left). Oxidant drugs such as the sulfonamides may exacerbate hemolysis. Because the $β_4$ tetramer is soluble during the early phases of the red cell's lifespan, erythropoiesis in the bone marrow is effective and the anemia is generally not as severe as that seen in patients with β-thalassemia who have an equivalent impairment in β globin production.

CLINICAL FEATURES. The average patient with Hb H disease maintains gainful employment, marries, and reproduces. Usually the anemia is moderate, with a hemoglobin concentration of 7 to 10 grams per deciliter, although occasional patients may have more severe anemia. Moderate splenomegaly is often present. Splenectomy may be considered, but the occurrence of severe postoperative thrombocytosis with a propensity for recurrent pulmonary emboli makes this procedure inadvisable except in patients with unequivocal clinical evidence of hypersplenism, as manifested by leukopenia, thrombocytopenia, and a worsening anemia or a transfusion requirement in a previously stable patient. Other therapeutic measures include prescription of folic acid, avoidance of oxidant drugs and iron salts, prompt treatment of infection, and judicious use of transfusions. Acquired Hb H disease has been described as a complication in patients with various forms of myeloproliferative and myelodysplastic disorders. In such patients, treatment and prognosis are related to the primary disorder.

HYDROPS FETALIS

The birth of stillborn infants from parents who both have α-thalassemia trait reflects the severest form of α-thalassemia. These infants are grossly edematous or hydropic because of the congestive heart failure that occurs as a result of severe anemia. Their failure to produce any α globin results in the production of only Hb Barts ($γ_4$) and Hb H ($β_4$) during the later parts of gestation. Both these hemoglobins are nonfunctional in oxygen transport, so that once the embryonic hemoglobins disappear from the circulation early in fetal development, life is no longer possible. A high incidence of toxemia of pregnancy has been noted in mothers of hydropic infants. Prenatal diagnosis of this condition is possible (see below) and should be followed by prompt termination of the pregnancy.

SILENT CARRIER

The silent carrier state was first recognized among the α-thalassemia syndromes. One parent of a patient with Hb H disease usually has all the features of α-thalassemia trait, whereas the other has normal-appearing red cells with no anemia. Similarly, progeny of persons with Hb H disease fall into two groups: those having α-thalassemia trait and those with apparently normal hemoglobin production. In the silent carrier, the defect in α globin synthesis is so mild that no impairment in hemoglobin synthesis is evident, although when the mutation is paired genetically with a more severe impairment of globin synthesis, e.g., α-thalassemia trait, Hb H disease occurs. A similar silent carrier state has also been described among the β-thalassemia syndromes. Thalassemia intermedia occurs in those who inherit one thalassemia gene from a silent carrier and a second from a person with thalassemia trait.

THE GENETICS OF THE α THALASSEMIA SYNDROMES

As described in Ch. 136.1, the α globin genes in humans are duplicated. Thus two genes are found on each chromosome 16, making a total of four in each diploid cell. Four clinical states are seen in α-thalassemia: silent carrier, thalassemia trait, Hb H disease, and hydrops fetalis. These conditions occur in persons who have, respectively, one, two, three, or four α globin genes affected by mutations that reduce α globin synthesis.

The most frequent mutation that leads to α-thalassemia is gene deletion. In the silent carrier one of the two genes on one chromosome 16 is missing, whereas the other two genes on the other chromosome 16 are normal. α-Thalassemia trait can occur by two mechanisms. Persons who have two chromosomes with only one α gene exhibit α-thalassemia trait. This form is most common in the black population. Hb H disease is distinctly uncommon in this population, since offspring of two persons each of whom is homozygous for the one α gene chromosome can have only α-thalassemia trait and not Hb H disease. In the Asian population, α-thalassemia trait occurs most commonly in those who lack both α genes on one chromosome and have the normal two on the other. Mating of such a person with a silent carrier who has one chromosome having only one α gene can lead to children with Hb H disease. Hydrops fetalis occurs among offspring of parents both of whom are heterozygous for chromosomes lacking both normal α globin genes.

In addition to the deletion mutations, many nondeletional types of α-thalassemia have been described. Molecular characterization of several has revealed a diversity of defects involving RNA splicing, polyadenylation, mRNA translation, or α globin stability. These mutations are similar to those in β-thalassemia globin genes; their effects on RNA metabolism are discussed in more detail in the next section.

THE MOLECULAR GENETICS OF THALASSEMIA

The β-thalassemia mutations may be separated into two classes: β^+-thalassemia, in which there is synthesis of a small amount of normal β globin, and β^0-thalassemia, which in the homozygote is manifested by no β globin production at all. Similarly, nondeletional types of α-thalassemia may abolish (α^0) or decrease (α^+) α globin production. Many mutations having specific effects on gene expression have been characterized by molecular cloning, DNA sequencing, and functional characterization. Each of the several steps in RNA metabolism—transcription, processing, transport, and mRNA translation—has been found to be affected by one or more individual mutations. The variable quantitative effect of the individual mutations on globin production has been clarified by these molecular studies.

PROMOTER MUTATIONS. Five globin genes, each of which has a single nucleotide substitution in the promoter region, have been isolated from different individuals with β-thalassemia. Three of the mutant genes have substitutions in the "ATA" box (see Fig. 136–6). These mutations reduce promoter function to 20 to 25 per cent of normal, but some β mRNA is produced from these genes; hence they cause β^+-thalassemia. The other two promoter mutants characterized to date have substitutions at 86 or 87 nucleotides from the start site for transcription in the first of the conserved "CACA" boxes.

SPLICING MUTATIONS. These are among the most common of mutations that cause thalassemia. Figure 136–9 contains a few illustrative examples classified by the manner in which they affect splicing of the globin mRNA precursor. Mutations that occur within the splice junction sequence decrease or abolish normal splicing at that site and often are accompanied by splicing at other sites that are not normally used. A substitution in the invariant GT, as shown in the example (Fig. 136–9A), abolishes splicing, making this a β^0 gene, whereas substitutions in consensus nucleotides at the splice junction have a quantitative effect on splicing and hence are β^+ mutations.

An interesting class of mutations consists of those that create an alternate site for splicing. These may occur within introns or, as shown in the examples in Figure 136–9B, within coding sequence (exons). These substitutions occur within regions of the precursor RNA molecule that resemble the consensus splice junction sequence (see Fig. 136–6) but lack some critical element necessary for splicing. Nucleotide substitutions that add that element to the potential splice junction sequence lead to its activation, causing abnormal splicing and hence a thalassemic

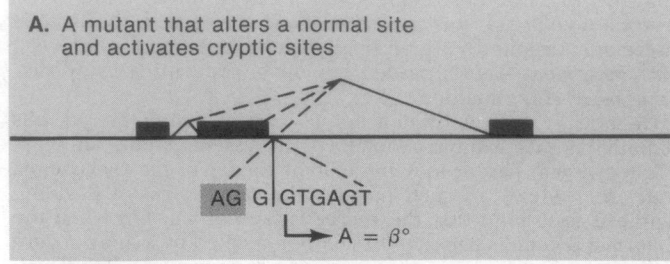

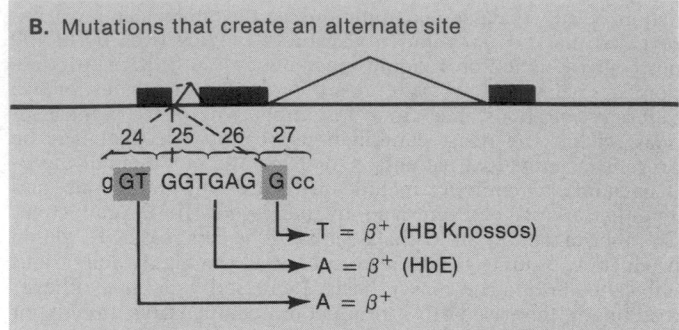

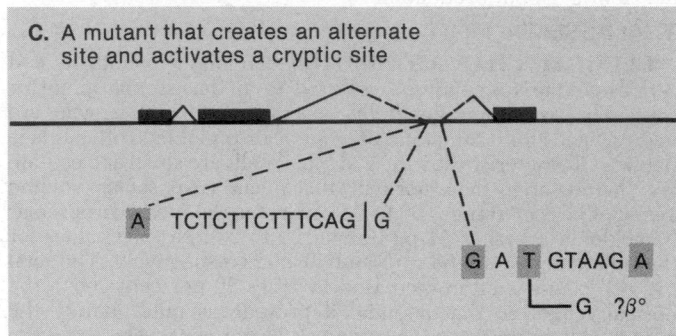

FIGURE 136–9. Thalassemia mutations that alter the splicing of the β globin gene transcript. *A*, The nucleotides guanine (G) and thymine (T) are obligatory for normal splicing. Replacement of the G with adenine (A) abolishes normal splicing and leads to abnormal splicing at otherwise cryptic sites. *B*, Several different mutations at this position in the transcript create an alternate site that leads to abnormal splicing. This segment of the normal transcript includes the obligatory dinucleotide, GT, and matches the consensus sequence in all but the nucleotides in the boxes. Single nucleotide substitutions activate this otherwise inactive site. *C*, A substitution toward the end of intron II creates an alternate splice site. A normally cryptic site farther upstream in the intron is also involved in a splicing reaction with exon 2–intron II splice junction, resulting in formation of a processed globin RNA that retains a portion of the sequence transcribed from intron II. Therefore, it cannot be translated into β globin.

effect. Substitution of A for T in codon 24 of the β globin gene does not alter the amino acid sequence (GGT and GGA both encode for glycine) but creates an alternative splicing site. The other two mutations illustrated in Figure 136–9B (Hb E and Hb Knossos) alter both protein structure and the splicing pattern. Such structural mutants that are also characterized by decreased synthesis are referred to as *thalassemic hemoglobinopathies*.

A class of mutations that has interesting implications for control of splicing is made up of those that create an alternate site and also activate cryptic splice sites remote from the mutation. There is a potential for a cryptic splice site in the β globin gene transcript that matches the consensus splice junction sequence nearly perfectly, and yet this site is used rarely, if ever, during normal splicing. Use of an alternative site, created by a thalassemia mutation, apparently alters the secondary structure of the precursor RNA molecule, leading to splicing at the otherwise cryptic site (Fig. 136–9C).

A POLYADENYLATION MUTATION. The sequence "AA-TAAA" is one of the signals that leads to cleavage of the globin gene transcript and addition of the poly-A tail (see Fig. 136–9). An α-thalassemia gene isolated from an individual with Hb H disease has G substituted for A, altering the polyadenylation signal to "AATAGA." Most of the RNA transcript is not processed correctly and is prematurely degraded, although a small amount of normal α globin mRNA is produced by this mutant gene. Thus it is an α⁺ thalassemia gene.

MUTATIONS THAT AFFECT mRNA TRANSLATION. Among the more common mutations in thalassemia genes are those that lead to premature termination of mRNA translation. Single nucleotide substitutions or small deletions that alter the mRNA reading frame introduce codons that signal the termination of protein synthesis on the abnormal mRNA. For example, substitution of thymine for cytosine in codon 39 introduces the stop codon UAG at that position. This abnormal β globin mRNA can be read only through codon 38, yielding a small, nonfunctional remnant of β globin. Premature termination mutations cause β⁰- (or α⁰-) thalassemia.

Common mutations that cause α-thalassemia are chain termination mutations. As described in Ch. 136.2, the completed globin molecule is released from the polyribosome when the protein synthetic apparatus encounters the normal terminator codon UAA. A single nucleotide change in this terminator codon converts it to a codon that is functional for the insertion of any one of several amino acids, depending on the exact nucleotide that is substituted. In this case protein synthesis continues into the part of the mRNA that is usually untranslated, leading to the synthesis of a protein that may be as many as 30 amino acids longer than normal. Such an elongated α globin is found in Hb Constant Spring. This protein accounts for only 1 to 2 per cent of the total α globin in the cells of patients with Hb Constant Spring, and their red cells exhibit the stigmata of thalassemia trait.

MUTATIONS THAT AFFECT GLOBIN STABILITY. Certain mutations may alter globin sequence and lead to instability and thus have a thalassemic effect despite a normal rate of synthesis of the mutant globin. Among the more dramatic of this class of mutations is one that leads to substitution of leucine for proline at position 125 of the α globin found in Hb Quong Sze. This mutation was discovered upon sequencing of the abnormal α gene and evidence of α^Quong Sze instability was subsequently obtained in vitro. Because of its marked instability, α^Quong Sze could not be detected in the red cells of the affected individual. Hb Quong Sze, like Hb E, is another of the thalassemic hemoglobinopathies characterized by both deficient net globin production and a structural abnormality.

DELETION MUTATIONS. Deletions causing α-thalassemia have been described earlier. Small deletions that leave one of the two α-globin genes intact on a chromosome are classified as α⁺ mutations, while large deletions that remove both α genes are considered α⁰ mutations. In contrast to α-thalassemia, in which gene deletion is the most common mutation, gene deletion is rarely the mechanism for β-thalassemia. A few patients of Indian ancestry have been found to have a deletion that has removed the 3′ half of the β globin gene and a small amount of flanking DNA. A special kind of deletion has resulted in the δβ fusion gene present in a few Italian patients who produce Hb Lepore. An unequal crossover during meiosis has led to the fusion gene that encodes for a globin that has the N-terminal sequence of δ globin and the C-terminal sequence of β globin. This globin is produced in very small amounts; hence this gene leads to thalassemia trait or thalassemia major in heterozygotes or homozygotes, respectively.

Several large deletions that have removed two or more genes from the β cluster have been characterized. The β-thalassemia mutations have resulted in loss of the δ and β genes; the ^Aγδβ-thalassemia deletions include the ^Aγ gene in addition. Two interesting forms of γδβ-thalassemia have resulted in loss of all but the β gene, and yet this β gene does not function. These observations suggest that the DNA sequences remote from a gene can nonetheless influence its expression. Two deletions have resulted in loss of the entire β-like gene cluster.

MUTATIONS THAT INCREASE Hb F PRODUCTION

About 1 per cent of the hemoglobin in adult blood is Hb F. This fetal hemoglobin is found in 2 to 10 per cent of red cells; these cells—called F cells—contain roughly 4 to 8 pg of Hb F and 24 to 28 pg of adult hemoglobin. As discussed in Ch. 136.2, these F cells originate during the differentiation of erythroid progenitor cells. F cell number and therefore Hb F levels are genetically determined in humans.

Increased Hb F in individuals who are homozygous for β-thalassemia mainly reflects amplification of the F cell population. In the bone marrow, those erythroblasts producing small amounts of γ globin have less of an excess in α globin synthesis and therefore are more likely to survive and leave the bone marrow. By this mechanism, the 1 per cent of γ synthesis in the bone marrow cell population may be amplified 10- to 40-fold in the peripheral blood. Of more interest from the aspect of gene control are those mutations that alter Hb F production by genetic mechanisms.

There are two general classes of deletion mutations that increase Hb F production in adults. The δβ-thalassemia mutations are characterized by production of 5 to 12 per cent of Hb F in heterozygotes, while *hereditary persistence of fetal hemoglobin* (HPFH) deletion mutations are characterized by production of 25 to 30 per cent. Most of the red cells in heterozygous individuals with HPFH contain Hb F, whereas heterozygotes with δβ-thalassemia mutations have Hb F in only 30 to 70 per cent of their red cells. These mutations have been carefully characterized structurally in an attempt to define the basis at the DNA level for these differing phenotypes. Twenty-eight mutations have been studied, but no common patterns have emerged, with one exception. Deletions that remove the left side of the cluster (ε and γ genes) also inactivate the remaining intact β gene, whereas deletions that remove the right-hand portion of the cluster (δ and β genes) increase expression of the remaining γ globin genes. The removal of sequences within the cluster that normally modulate gene expression and the movement of "activating" sequences into the cluster by virtue of deletion are other possible mechanisms that may lead to increased Hb F production as a consequence of these deletions.

Another category of mutations that cause HPFH leave the β-like gene cluster intact and therefore are referred to as *nondeletion mutations*. Nondeletion HPFH mutations are often characterized by a heterogeneous distribution of Hb F in red cells (heterocellular) in contrast to the pancellular distribution of Hb F in heterozygotes with the deletion types of HPFH. There may be many different heterocellular HPFH mutations; genetic studies indicate that at least some are not linked to the β-like gene cluster. Ten different point mutations within the γ globin gene promoter region have been discovered in individuals with nondeletion HPFH.

PRENATAL DIAGNOSIS

Because of the serious consequences of severe β-thalassemia (Cooley's anemia), prenatal diagnosis of this condition with subsequent therapeutic abortion is thought by many to be highly desirable. Two general strategies have made this a feasible undertaking. The first approach is based on the fact that small amounts of β globin synthesis may be detected in the early midtrimester fetus. In fetuses who have inherited two genes for β-thalassemia, no β globin or very small amounts are produced at a time when normal fetuses are producing approximately 10 per cent β globin. By using sophisticated obstetric techniques, blood may be obtained from the umbilical vein and used for biosynthetic measurements of the globin synthetic pattern. Absence of or low β globin synthesis occurs in homozygous fetuses, whereas intermediate levels are found in heterozygotes. This strategy has been widely applied in parts of Greece and Italy and has led to a significant reduction in the incidence of the severe form of β-thalassemia in certain populations.

A second and now more widely applied strategy relies on the use of fetal DNA for analysis. A chorionic villus biopsy late in the first trimester of pregnancy provides a simple noninvasive method to obtain DNA. Alternatively, amniotic fluid obtained at mid-pregnancy provides sufficient cells for extraction of fetal DNA. Major advances in our knowledge of mutations that cause thalassemia and in methods of detection of such mutations make DNA analysis the most useful approach for prenatal diagnosis.

More than 60 point mutations that cause β-thalassemia have been described. However, each ethnic group has two or three common mutations and three or four mutations that occur with lower frequency and that together account for the majority of disease in that ethnic group. Since the spectrum of mutations has been defined for each of the ethnic groups in which thalassemia is common, prenatal diagnosis can be directed to detection of a specific subset of known mutations.

The polymerase chain reaction has revolutionized DNA diagnosis. With the use of sequence-specific primers, a small segment of the entire genome can be amplified more than a million-fold within a few hours. Nanogram quantities of the amplified DNA are obtained. Usually the entire β globin gene is amplified in two segments. Detection of specific mutations is accomplished by annealing aliquots of the amplified DNA, immobilized on filter paper, to a series of mutation-specific oligonucleotides and the corresponding oligonucleotides having the normal sequence. Occasionally, it is necessary to sequence the amplified DNA if the patient carries a rare or new mutation. The parents can be prescreened with this methodology so that prenatal diagnosis can focus on the mutation or mutations for which the fetus is at risk.

Prenatal diagnosis of α-thalassemia often requires Southern blot analysis to detect deletion mutations. Again, the spectrum of mutations in individual ethnic groups has been defined so that probes and enzymes can be chosen that readily define the deletion breakpoint. Southern blot analysis is occasionally also required for β-thalassemia if the phenotype in the parents suggests the presence of a δβ-thalassemia mutation. Red cell microcytosis combined with Hb F of 5 per cent or greater is suggestive of this diagnosis.

The application of prenatal diagnosis requires appropriate screening and identification of persons at risk. Thalassemia trait can usually readily be identified by virtue of the morphologic changes in the red cells. Confirmation of the diagnosis depends on measurement of hemoglobin A_2 and Hb F.

EXPERIMENTAL THERAPY

Knowledge of globin gene structure and regulation has suggested a means to activate the structurally normal but inactive γ globin genes in individuals with severe β-thalassemia. Increased γ globin synthesis is desirable because it partially compensates for the deficiency of β globin production and decreases the relative excess of α globin. DNA is modified after synthesis by methylation of cytosine residues. Expressed genes are relatively undermethylated compared with unexpressed DNA sequences. For example, the γ globin genes are undermethylated in fetal erythroid cells, but after the switch to adult hemoglobin synthesis the γ globin genes are fully methylated in adult erythroid cells. 5-Azacytidine* inhibits DNA methylation and has been shown to activate genes in tissue culture cells and in experimental animals. Administration of 5-azacytidine to patients with severe β-thalassemia under defined experimental protocols has resulted in increased γ globin synthesis and improvement in red cell production and survival. The effect is transient, lasting only 2 to 3 weeks. Reluctance to administer a potentially carcinogenic and toxic drug for longer periods has limited the use of 5-azacytidine to experimental studies of a few severely affected patients. Nonetheless these encouraging results have prompted a search for other effective and less toxic drugs that may make pharmacologic stimulation of the γ globin genes a useful approach for treatment of severe β-thalassemia.

Cure of severe β-thalassemia can be achieved by bone marrow transplantation from an HLA-identical, unaffected sibling. Several patients have already been cured by this method. This procedure carries a 5 to 20 per cent risk of death or significant graft-versus-host disease (GVHD). Transplantation in infancy, preferably before transfusions are given, increases the probability of successful engraftment, although a high cure rate has also been achieved in older patients. However, adequate transfusion therapy and effective chelation may provide 20 or more years of good-quality life for newborns. Thus, the availability of bone marrow transplantation raises a significant ethical dilemma for parents and physicians. In the future, refinements in the treatment of GVHD and transplantation techniques may permit wider appli-

---

*Available from the National Cancer Institute.

cation of bone marrow transplantation as treatment for patients with severe β-thalassemia.

Insertion of intact globin genes into the bone marrow cells of patients with severe forms of thalassemia has become a feasible research objective. Gene transfer mediated by retroviral vectors is highly efficient and has resulted in the insertion and expression of genes in experimental animals. Many problems remain to be overcome before this strategy becomes clinically feasible, however.

Hershko C, Weatherall DJ: Iron-chelating therapy. Crit Rev Clin Lab Sci 26:303, 1988; Fosburg MT, Nathan DG: Treatment of Cooley's anemia. Blood 76:435, 1990; Nathan DG, Piomelli S: Oral iron chelators. Semin Hematol 27:83, 1990. *This series of articles provides a detailed account of current therapeutic recommendations for severe β-thalassemia, including the status of iron chelation therapy and new oral iron chelators.*

Kazazian HH Jr, Boehm CD: Molecular basis and prenatal diagnosis of beta-thalassemia. Blood 72:1107, 1988. *This is a definitive account of the mutations that could cause β-thalassemia and the modern strategies used for prenatal diagnosis.*

Lucarelli G, Galimberti M, Polchi P, et al.: Bone marrow transplantation in patients with thalassemia. N Engl J Med 322:417, 1990. *This article summarizes the most extensive experience with transplantation for severe β-thalassemia and provides a guide to patient selection and predicted outcomes.*

McDonagh KT, Nienhuis AW: The thalassemias: Disorders of hemoglobin synthesis. In Nathan DG, Oski F (eds.): Hematology of Infancy and Childhood. Philadelphia, W. B. Saunders Company, 1991. *This chapter contains a more detailed exposition of the thalassemia syndromes with a comprehensive account of the molecular basis of these disorders and the current status of prenatal diagnosis.*

Nienhuis AW, Ley TJ, Humphries RK, et al.: Pharmacological manipulation of fetal hemoglobin synthesis in patients with severe beta-thalassemia. Ann NY Acad Sci 445:198, 1985. Ley TJ, Nienhuis AW: Induction of hemoglobin F synthesis in patients with beta thalassemia. Ann Rev Med 36:485, 1985. *Reviews of the results achieved by using drugs in an effort to stimulate fetal hemoglobin synthesis for therapeutic benefit in patients with thalassemia.*

136.5 SICKLE CELL ANEMIA AND ASSOCIATED HEMOGLOBINOPATHIES

Bernard G. Forget

DEFINITION. The sickle cell syndromes are due to the inheritance of a gene for a structurally abnormal β globin chain subunit of adult hemoglobin (Hb), the $β^s$ chain of Hb S ($α_2β_2^s$). The structural abnormality of the $β^s$ globin chain consists of a single amino acid substitution or replacement: valine instead of the normal glutamic acid at position number 6 of the β polypeptide chain. Hb S can be found in the heterozygous state (Hb AS or sickle cell trait), in the homozygous state (Hb SS, sickle cell anemia, or sickle cell disease) (see Color Plate 6B, left), in association with other structural hemoglobin variants (i.e., Hb SC and SD disease), in association with β-thalassemia (Hb S/β-thalassemia or sickle/β-thalassemia syndromes), or in association with the thalassemia-like disorder termed hereditary persistence of fetal hemoglobin (Hb SF or Hb S/HPFH). The structural abnormality of Hb C, a nonsickling hemoglobin, also consists of a single amino acid substitution at residue number 6 of the β globin chain: in the $β^c$ chain lysine replaces glutamic acid. Clinical syndromes associated with the inheritance of Hb C include Hb SC disease and homozygous Hb C disease (see Color Plate 6B, right).

PREVALENCE AND GENETICS. The sickle cell syndromes are particularly prevalent in black persons of African or Afro-American ancestry. However, the gene is also found at a lower frequency in persons of Mediterranean ancestry (southern Italians, Sicilians, and Greeks), in Saudi Arabia, and in India. The highest gene frequencies occur in equatorial Africa, in the so-called malaria belt. The heterozygous state for Hb S (sickle cell trait) probably confers a biologic advantage against infection with *Plasmodium falciparum* malaria, and for this reason the gene frequency for Hb S has achieved high levels through natural selection in geographic areas of endemic malaria. In the United States the prevalence of the sickle cell trait in blacks is 8 to 10 per cent and the number of homozygous persons approaches 50,000, or 1 in 400 births. In certain areas of western Africa (Ghana and Nigeria), the prevalence of Hb AS can reach 25 to 30 per cent. The prevalence of Hb AC in black Americans is approximately 3 per cent. Gene mapping studies, using restriction endonuclease analysis of cellular DNA to identify polymorphisms of nucleotide sequence in the DNA around the β^s globin gene, have disclosed an unexpected heterogeneity of polymorphisms linked to the sickle β globin genes in different individuals, suggesting multiple independent origins of the sickle gene.

PATHOPHYSIOLOGY. Disease in the sickle syndromes results from aggregation or polymerization of Hb S molecules inside erythrocytes, which causes (1) chronic compensated hemolytic anemia, (2) chronic and progressive tissue and organ damage, and (3) acute painful vaso-occlusive crises. These clinical phenomena are directly related to the physicochemical behavior of the intracellular Hb S molecules and result from alterations of red cell rheology and, possibly, changes in the red cell membrane.

The polymerization process occurs only when the Hb S molecule is in the deoxy conformation (see Ch. 136.1). When Hb S is in the oxy conformation it has essentially normal physicochemical properties. In the deoxy conformation, Hb S molecules can aggregate with one another into long polymers and are aligned to form a gel of liquid crystals that are also called tactoids. The polymerization process goes through a number of stages, as illustrated diagrammatically in Figure 136–10. In the process of nucleation, Hb S molecules form small aggregates, which then grow by addition of successive Hb S molecules. The larger aggregates then align themselves to form linearly arranged fibers that constitute a paracrystalline gel. These fibers can be detected as helical electron-dense tube-like structures by electron microscopy (Fig. 136–10). The end result of the polymerization process is the transformation of the intracellular contents of the red cell from a fluid liquid to a viscous gel. The amount of Hb S polymer within red cells increases progressively as the percentage of oxygen saturation of the hemoglobin decreases. The viscous polymer decreases the flexibility of the erythrocyte and thus impairs its transit through the microcirculation. When the amount of polymer is sufficiently high, the red cells may assume the typical sickle or holly leaf shape associated with sickled erythro-

cytes (Fig. 136–11). The shape change of the erythrocyte is a passive phenomenon in which the red cell membrane conforms to the shape that is assumed by the intracellular gel of polymerized hemoglobin. The polymerization phenomenon is reversible: With reoxygenation of the Hb S molecules the aggregated molecules disassociate, the gel becomes liquid, and the erythrocyte, if it has sickled, can return to its normal shape, as long as the red cell membrane has not become altered to form an irreversibly sickled cell (see below).

A number of factors can influence the rate and degree of Hb S aggregation in red cells. One of the most important determinants is the concentration of Hb S and of total hemoglobin within the red cell. In general, the higher the percentage of Hb S, the more severe the sickle syndrome. Factors such as cellular dehydration that increase the mean corpuscular hemoglobin concentration (MCHC) greatly facilitate polymerization by increasing the opportunity and frequency of contact between Hb S molecules. The importance of hemoglobin concentration on polymerization is underscored by the clinical observation that the co-inheritance of α-thalassemia together with sickle cell anemia is generally (but not universally) associated with less severe hemolysis. The milder clinical course of Hb S/β-thalassemia is also thought to be due in part to the associated hypochromia. The length of time during which Hb S remains deoxygenated is also very important; Hb S polymerization is enhanced with any increase in the transit time of the red cell through the microcirculation. The presence of other hemoglobins within the red cell can also influence sickling. In general, at a constant MCHC, any other non-S hemoglobin molecules in the red cell, by a simple dilution effect, decrease the opportunity of contact between Hb S molecules. In addition, the type of non-S hemoglobin present can differentially affect polymerization: Fetal hemoglobin (Hb F)

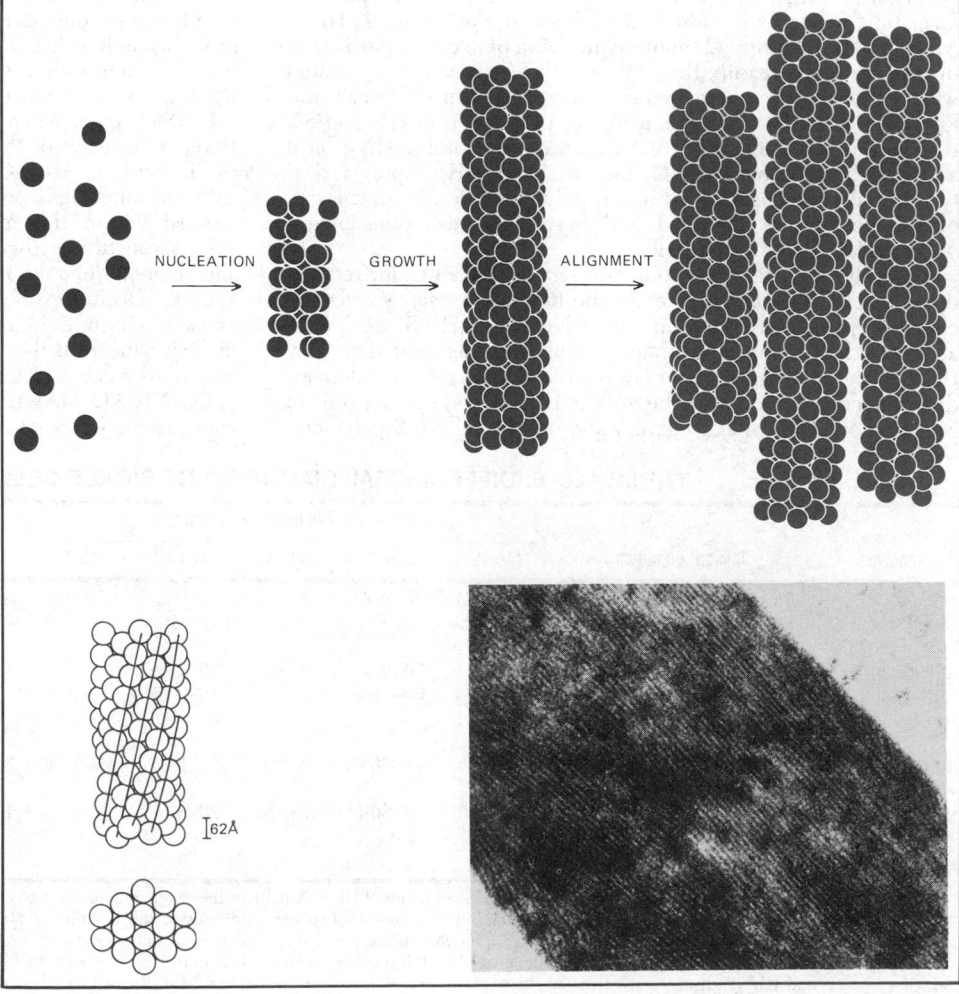

FIGURE 136–10. *Top,* Schematic representation of mechanism of deoxyhemoglobin S polymerization. Each circle represents a deoxyhemoglobin S tetramer: α_2β_2^s. *Lower left,* Molecular model, based on electron microscopy, of the helical arrangement of deoxyhemoglobin S tetramers in a fiber of polymerized Hb S molecules; side view *(above)* and cross-section or end-on view *(below)*. *Lower right,* Electron micrograph (longitudinal section) of deoxyhemoglobin S gel in a sickled erythrocyte.

NUCLEATION → GROWTH → ALIGNMENT

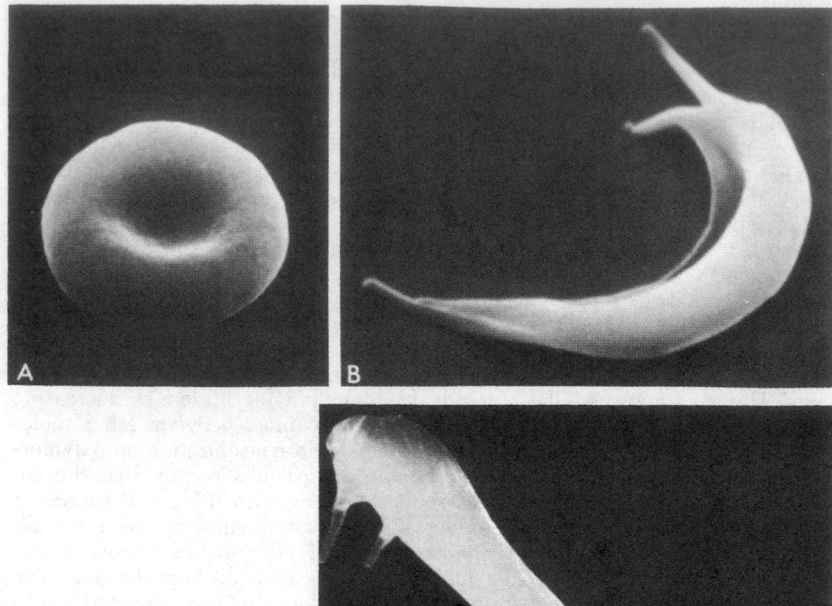

FIGURE 136–11. Scanning electron micrographs of oxygenated (*A*) and deoxygenated (*B* and *C*) SS erythrocytes. (Courtesy of Dr. James White. *In* Bunn HF, Forget BG: Hemoglobin: Molecular, Genetic, and Clinical Aspects. Philadelphia, W. B. Saunders Company, 1986.)

participates much less readily than normal Hb A in polymer formation, whereas certain mutant hemoglobins, such as Hb O Arab and Hb D, although nonpolymerizing per se, will participate in gelation more readily than Hb A. Hb SC disease is associated with a more severe clinical course than is seen in sickle cell trait for two reasons: (1) There is a higher proportion of Hb S in SC than in AS cells (Table 136–6); and (2) cells containing Hb C have a higher than normal MCHC, thus facilitating Hb S polymerization. Finally, acidosis can enhance polymerization by decreasing oxygen affinity (see Ch. 136.1) and thereby increasing the amount of deoxy Hb S in the red cell.

The polymerization phenomenon results in two major red cell disturbances. The first relates to the flow properties of red cells containing substantial amounts of polymerized Hb S. Such cells are much less deformable than normal red cells, and their flow through the microcirculation is greatly retarded. A second major disturbance is damage to the red cell membrane as a result of repeated episodes of aggregation and melting of Hb S polymers.

Sickle red cells are "leaky." They tend to lose K^+ and water and eventually become dehydrated, the resulting increase in MCHC probably enhancing further polymerization. The red cell membrane becomes altered in other ways, so that it may assume a rigid, abnormal conformation, thus forming an irreversibly sickled cell (ISC), even when the hemoglobin is not in the aggregated state. As a result of the intracellular polymerization of Hb S, of the increase in MCHC, and of the membrane changes, the red cells become rigid and are sequestered and prematurely destroyed within the reticuloendothelial system. This series of events constitutes the basis for the shortened red cell survival and hemolytic anemia that invariably accompany sickle cell anemia. Occlusion of the microvasculature by viscous erythrocytes leads to ischemia and eventual infarction of the tissue downstream from the obstruction, results in organ damage, and may be the cause of the characteristic painful "crises."

CLINICAL MANIFESTATIONS. *Sickle Cell Trait.* Persons who are heterozygous for Hb S are essentially asymptomatic.

TABLE 136–6. DIFFERENTIAL DIAGNOSIS OF SICKLE CELL SYNDROMES

Genotype	Clinical Condition	Hemoglobin Electrophoresis Findings					Other Associated Findings
		Hb A	*Hb S*	*Hb A$_2$*	*Hb F*	*Hb C*	
AS	Sickle cell trait	55–60%	40–45%*	2–3%	~1%	—	Asymptomatic; no anemia
SS†	Sickle cell anemia	0	85–95%	2–3%	5–15%	—	Usually clinically severe; Hb F distributed heterogeneously among red blood cells
S/β⁰-thal	Sickle cell/β-thalassemia	0	70–80%	3–5%	10–20%	—	Moderate severity; splenomegaly in over half of
S/β⁺-thal	Sickle cell/β-thalassemia	10–20%	60–75%	3–5%	10–20%	—	the cases; Hb F distributed heterogeneously among red blood cells; hypochromia and microcytosis
SC‡	Hb SC disease	0	45–50%	2–3%	~1%	45–50%	Moderate severity; splenomegaly; many target cells on blood smear
SF (S/HPFH)	Sickle/hereditary persistence of fetal hemoglobin	0	70–80%	1.5–2%	20–30%	—	Uniform distribution of Hb F among all red cells; asymptomatic; no anemia

*Persons with associated α-thalassemia trait (-α/-α) have lower levels of Hb S, usually in the range of 25 to 30 per cent; those with concomitant heterozygous α-thalassemia 2(-α/αα) have Hb S levels of 30 to 36 per cent. The finding of a (nonsickling) hemoglobin with the mobility of Hb S but in much lower amounts (5 to 15 per cent) is suggestive of the Hb Lepore trait (see Ch. 136.4). Except for the (-α/αα) genotype, hypochromia and microcytosis are usually associated with these conditions.

†Hb SD disease gives similar electrophoretic findings at pH 8.6 but can be distinguished from Hb SS disease by hemoglobin electrophoresis in citrate agar at pH 6.1.

‡Hb S/O-Arab and Hb SE diseases give similar electrophoretic findings at pH 8.6 but can be distinguished from Hb SC disease by hemoglobin electrophoresis in citrate agar at pH 6.1. Hb A$_2$ co-migrates with Hb C at pH 8.6 and can be quantitated only by column chromatography.

They should not have any anemia attributable to the hemoglobinopathy. Any anemia in such persons should be investigated for other secondary causes. Symptoms resulting from vaso-occlusion occur only in extreme circumstances of severe hypoxia such as flying in unpressurized aircraft. However, a universal finding in sickle cell trait is microinfarction of the renal medulla presumably owing to the ambient hyperosmolarity that is thought to lead to dehydration of the red cells, an increased MCHC, and sickling; as a result, in affected persons the urine is unconcentrated and isosthenuria is manifested. Painless hematuria can also occasionally be attributed to microinfarction of the renal medulla, although the other usual causes should be ruled out before painless hematuria in persons with sickle cell trait is attributed to the sickling phenomenon.

Sickle Cell Disease. The Anemia. Patients homozygous for Hb S invariably have a chronic compensated hemolytic anemia of variable severity. In general, the hematocrit ranges between 20 and 30 per cent and the hemoglobin between 6.5 and 10 grams per deciliter. The hemolysis is compensated for by increased erythropoiesis, manifested as an elevated reticulocyte count in the range of 10 to 25 per cent. Mild jaundice and indirect hyperbilirubinemia are also present as a reflection of the hemolysis. The degree of the anemia is usually stable in a given patient, although occasional hypoplastic or aplastic crises can occur owing to suppression of erythropoiesis at the time of infectious episodes and can result in a rapid decrease in the reticulocyte count and a precipitous drop in the hemoglobin and hematocrit levels. Infection with parvovirus B19 has been implicated in the pathogenesis of aplastic crises. Another cause of rapid worsening of the anemia is the acute splenic sequestration crisis (a sudden pooling of large volumes of blood in the spleen) that can occur in younger patients with sickle cell anemia before autoinfarction of the spleen or in older patients with Hb SC disease and Hb S/β-thalassemia in whom the spleen is not infarcted and may in fact be enlarged. There is some controversy whether or not a hyperhemolytic state can be associated with sickle cell anemia. From what is known of the basis for the hemolysis in this condition, there is no pathophysiologic mechanism for variable or accelerated hemolysis resulting from sickling alone. In general, the anemia and hemolysis in sickle cell disease do not increase or worsen during vaso-occlusive painful crises. If hemolysis suddenly worsens, one should look to other secondary causes that may be responsible, such as an associated glucose-6-phosphate dehydrogenase deficiency and exposure to an oxidant stress from drugs or an acute infection. Finally, in patients with marginal nutritional status and increased requirements, such as during pregnancy, folic acid deficiency can develop and aggravate the anemia—the so-called megaloblastic crisis of sickle cell disease.

Vaso-occlusive Crises. The major disabilities suffered by patients with sickle cell anemia are related to painful vaso-occlusive crises and to secondary end-organ damage as a direct consequence of the sickling phenomenon and occlusion of the microvasculature of one or another organ, most commonly the bones of the trunk and extremities. The episodes are characterized by sudden onset of excruciating pain in the back, chest, or extremities. There is frequently no identifiable precipitating event, although infections may be associated with the onset of the episode. Other predisposing factors include dehydration, acidosis, or increased hypoxia, as during a pulmonary infection. A low-grade fever may be associated with the painful attacks, although not necessarily. In general, the onset of fever occurs 1 or 2 days after the onset of pain and parallels the degree of tissue necrosis resulting from the ischemic infarction. The painful attacks last for variable periods, ranging from a few hours to a few days, depending on the extent of the vaso-occlusive phenomenon and the rapidity with which treatment is initiated and is successful in reversing the occlusive episode. In general there are no external signs, such as heat, swelling, or tenderness of the soft tissues over the affected bones. However, if the bone infarction occurs in proximity to a joint, an effusion can develop. Bone infarction may be difficult to differentiate from osteomyelitis, and definitive diagnosis of the latter must ultimately rely on positive bacterial cultures from aspirated material.

When the vaso-occlusive process occurs in the vasculature (including large vessels) of organs other than bones, the clinical manifestations are primarily related to damage of the affected organ. Common acute vaso-occlusive clinical syndromes include cerebrovascular accidents (i.e., hemiplegia and seizures) caused by involvement of the cerebral vasculature; the acute chest syndrome associated with occlusion of the pulmonary vessels, which can be difficult to differentiate from acute pulmonary infarction caused by emboli or from acute pulmonary infections; hepatic crisis, with marked hyperbilirubinemia and other abnormal liver function tests, which can be difficult to differentiate from acute hepatitis or choledocholithiasis; priapism resulting from vaso-occlusion within the corpus cavernosum; and acute renal papillary infarction with hematuria and/or obstruction of the urinary collecting system.

More chronic complications include refractory skin ulcers of the leg, usually in the vicinity of the medial malleolus, an area that has poor collateral circulation, and variable degrees of renal insufficiency resulting from the combination of repeated infarctions and infectious episodes. All patients manifest the inability to concentrate the urine and have isosthenuria. Microinfarction in the peripheral retina is initially asymptomatic but may lead to the formation of new blood vessels that are fragile and can hemorrhage, causing retinal detachment and blindness. For this reason periodic eye examinations are important so that the early asymptomatic lesion may be recognized and treated before it progresses to the point of causing visual disturbances. Finally, repeated bone infarcts in the vicinity of joints can lead to secondary degenerative arthritis, and gradual infarction of the head of the femur results in aseptic necrosis of the hip.

Other Clinical Manifestations. Clinical manifestations of sickle cell anemia not directly related to the sickling phenomenon include increased susceptibility to infections, cholelithiasis, and abnormal growth and development. The increased susceptibility to infections is probably related at least in part to absence of splenic function and in some cases to an abnormality of the properdin opsonization pathway. In early childhood, septicemia and meningitis caused by encapsulated organisms such as *Streptococcus pneumoniae* and *Haemophilus influenzae* are common. In later life common infectious episodes include recurrent pneumonias, urinary tract infections, and osteomyelitis. The predisposition to osteomyelitis is probably related to the repeated bone infarcts that can form a nidus for infection. Although osteomyelitis caused by *Salmonella* occurs almost exclusively in patients with sickle cell anemia or one of the other sickle cell syndromes, *Staphylococcus aureus* is still the most common causative organism of osteomyelitis in these syndromes.

Cholelithiasis is very common and can be manifested at a young age; it is caused by the chronic hemolysis that results in increased bilirubin production. Episodes of cholecystitis and choledocholithiasis can easily be confused with abdominal and hepatic sickle cell crises. The causes of delayed growth and development are poorly understood. Delayed puberty can result in late closure of the epiphyses and an asthenic habitus.

Sickle/β-Thalassemia and Hb SC Disease. The anemia and the hemolysis are less severe in the other sickle syndromes, such as Hb SC disease and sickle/β-thalassemia, in which there is somewhat less propensity for sickling than in homozygous Hb SS disease. The degree of anemia is strongly related to the extent of intracellular Hb S polymerization. In these conditions the anemia frequently ranges between hemoglobin levels of 10 and 12 grams per deciliter, and the reticulocyte counts are usually less than 10 per cent, frequently in the range of 5 per cent.

In general the vaso-occlusive manifestations resulting from sickling are also less frequent and less severe in Hb SC disease and in sickle/β-thalassemia than in sickle cell anemia, although all of the complications previously described for sickle cell anemia can also occur in these conditions. However, in contrast to sickle cell anemia, splenomegaly in adults is usually present in these syndromes, and splenic infarcts and acute splenic sequestration crises can occur. The ocular complications of sickling also tend to occur more frequently in Hb SC disease than in sickle cell anemia and can in fact be the presenting symptoms. There is also increased frequency of aseptic necrosis of the femoral head in Hb SC disease. Sickle/β0-thalassemia, in which Hb A is totally absent, is generally more severe than sickle/β+-thalassemia and can be as clinically severe as sickle cell anemia.

DIAGNOSIS. The diagnosis of the various sickle syndromes relies on two types of tests: (1) screening tests to detect the presence of Hb S on the basis of its physicochemical properties, and (2) more definitive tests for the precise diagnosis of the particular genetic syndrome involved.

Two types of screening tests for the detection of Hb S are in current use. Both tests simply detect the presence of some Hb S in erythroid cells but do not differentiate sickle cell trait from the other sickle syndromes. The standard "sickle cell preparation" consists of mixing blood with a solution of sodium metabisulfate, which totally deoxygenates the blood and thus induces sickling that can be observed under the microscope. A second screening test is a solubility test that consists of mixing blood with a solution of high ionic strength and observing the mixtures for turbidity; normal hemoglobin gives a clear solution, whereas any Hb S in the solution precipitates to give a turbid solution through which one cannot see the lines of an indicator card. Both tests, if properly done, are highly specific and accurate. The solubility test has the advantages that a microscope is not needed and that the test solution is relatively stable.

Once Hb S is detected by screening tests, hemoglobin electrophoresis should be carried out for precise diagnosis of the sickle syndrome. Table 136–6 summarizes the results obtained by hemoglobin electrophoresis in the various sickle cell syndromes as well as other associated clinical and laboratory findings that are useful in the differential diagnosis. In general, routine hemoglobin electrophoresis at pH 8.6 will suffice to establish the diagnosis. However, a few exceptions to this rule require additional tests to confirm or establish the suspected diagnosis. Because other hemoglobin variants can have the same electrophoretic mobility as Hb S at pH 8.6, electrophoresis in citrate agar at pH 6.1 should be performed to confirm the diagnosis (see Table 136–6). The distinction between Hb SS disease and Hb S/β^0-thalassemia can be very difficult to establish, since electrophoretic findings are similar in both cases. The Hb A_2 level should be elevated in Hb S/β-thalassemia, but precise quantitation of Hb A_2 in the presence of Hb S is sometimes unreliable. Findings that should establish the diagnosis of Hb S/β^0-thalassemia rather than Hb SS disease include (1) the presence of hypochromia and microcytosis indicated by low mean corpuscular volume (MCV) and MCH; (2) family study showing that one parent or an offspring has β-thalassemia trait rather than sickle cell trait; (3) experimental studies of globin chain synthesis using labeled amino acid precursors (see Ch. 136.4), demonstrating decreased synthesis of β^s chains relative to α chains ($\beta^s/\alpha = 0.5$ to 0.6); and (4) gene mapping studies to distinguish between β^A and β^s globin genes in the patient's DNA (Fig. 136–12). The rare but interesting syndrome of Hb S/HPFH also gives hemoglobin electrophoretic findings similar to those of Hb SS disease, but with an unusually high level of Hb F in the range of 30 per cent. Such patients, however, are not anemic and should be asymptomatic. The diagnosis can be confirmed by family study showing the absence

of sickle cell trait and the presence of heterozygosity for HPFH in a parent or offspring. Study of the distribution of Hb F in individual red cells, using the acid elution test of Betke and Kleihauer, shows uniform distribution of Hb F in Hb S/HPFH but heterogeneous distribution of Hb F in Hb SS disease. Inheritance of Hb D (another relatively common β chain hemoglobinopathy in blacks) along with Hb S can also mimic homozygosity for Hb S, since Hb D co-migrates with Hb S on electrophoresis at pH 8.6. Hb SD disease is not as clinically severe as sickle cell disease, and the diagnosis can be established by performing hemoglobin electrophoresis at neutral or acid pH, which separates the two hemoglobins. Similarly, Hb SC disease can be confused with the inheritance of Hb S along with a second hemoglobin variant that has an electrophoretic mobility similar to that of Hb C at pH 8.6, such as Hb O Arab or Hb E. These syndromes can be distinguished from Hb SC disease by electrophoresis in citrate agar at pH 6 to 7.

The peripheral blood smear in individuals with Hb SS disease shows variable numbers of ISC's, usually ranging between 5 and 10 per cent. In general, the number of ISC's is relatively stable for a given patient, and there is a rough correlation between the numbers of ISC's and the severity of the hemolytic anemia. There is no correlation between the number of ISC's and the frequency or presence of vaso-occlusive crises. The peripheral blood smear, in addition to ISC's, usually shows variable numbers of target cells and occasional Howell-Jolly bodies owing to absence of spleen function. Other hematologic findings related to functional asplenia include the presence of somewhat elevated leukocyte counts and platelet counts. Examination of the peripheral blood smear can also be helpful in the differential diagnosis of the sickle syndromes. In general, significant numbers of ISC's are found essentially only in homozygous SS disease and not in the other sickle syndromes. Large numbers of target cells are characteristic of the inheritance of Hb C in either the heterozygous or the homozygous state (see Color Plate 6B, right).

TREATMENT. Despite extensive knowledge of the molecular basis and physical chemistry of the polymerization and sickling phenomena, there is still no specific molecular therapy available for the treatment or prevention of sickling. A number of compounds have been tested, and new compounds continue to be sought, that might interfere with sickling in vivo and be useful clinically. Unfortunately no such compound is currently available. Another potential molecular approach to the prevention of sickling would be to reactivate or increase fetal hemoglobin synthesis in the majority of the erythroid cells of affected patients to render them similar to the red cells of patients with Hb S/HPFH, a clinically mild syndrome. Successful enhancement of Hb F levels in patients with sickle cell anemia and homozygous β-thalassemia (see Ch. 136.4) has been accomplished by the administration of the chemotherapeutic agents 5-azacytidine* and hydroxyurea to a number of patients. The rationale for 5-azacytidine therapy resided in the findings that the drug causes demethylation of DNA and that active genes are usually hypomethylated, whereas the inactive fetal γ globin genes of adults are hypermethylated. However, other mechanisms related to cell toxicity and depletion followed by regeneration, cell selection, and changes in gene expression resulting from disruption of the cell cycle probably also contribute to the increased levels of Hb F following administration of chemotherapeutic agents. These therapies should be considered investigational at this time and restricted in their general applicability until the long-term efficacy and toxicity of these drugs, including carcinogenicity, is established. Hydroxyurea is likely to be a less toxic agent for chronic administration. Clinical trials of the drug have revealed that it is effective in raising the Hb F levels of many, though not all, patients with sickle cell anemia. However, controlled clinical trials have not yet been carried out to determine the efficacy of the drug in decreasing the frequency of painful vaso-occlusive crises.

The cornerstones of therapy in sickle cell anemia have therefore not changed in recent years and continue to consist of the administration of the following supportive measures: large volumes of intravenous fluids (preferably hypotonic and alkaline); analgesics to control the pain; when indicated, antibiotics to treat any associated bacterial infection; and oxygen to treat hypoxemia.

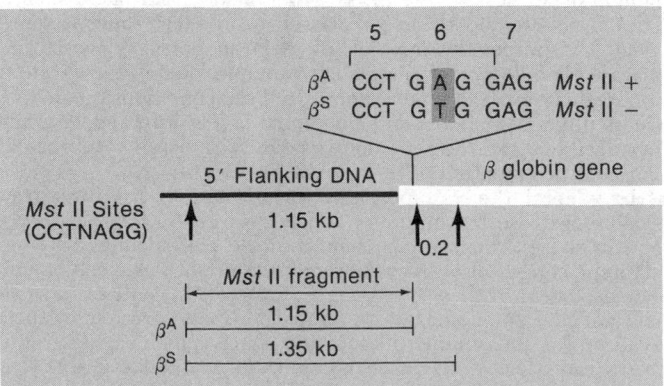

FIGURE 136–12. Direct identification of the sickle cell mutation in cellular DNA by restriction endonuclease digestion using the enzyme *Mst* II. The diagram shows the flanking region and 5' portion of the β globin structural gene. Arrows indicate the *Mst* II sites, including the one corresponding to amino acid portions 5, 6, and 7. The 1.15-kilobase (kb) fragment is seen in normal DNA, and the 1.35-kb fragment is seen in sickle DNA.

---

*Investigational agent available from the National Cancer Institute.

When administering fluids to patients with sickle cell anemia, one should remember that these patients have a fixed renal water loss owing to inability to concentrate urine and that they are frequently dehydrated on presentation because of associated infection and fever. The amounts of intravenous fluids administered should therefore be increased to two to three times what would be considered a normal maintenance volume. Patients with sickle cell disease are frequently hypoxic because of chronic pulmonary disease. Even though they do not appear to be cyanotic, monitoring of arterial Po_2 is important, especially if there is an associated chest syndrome, and oxygen should be administered if there is significant hypoxemia. In the absence of arterial hypoxemia, oxygen therapy is probably not beneficial in the treatment of vaso-occlusive crises and may result in suppression of erythropoiesis. The role of alkali is controversial, and certainly if the patient is mildly acidotic, this acidosis should be corrected, since it can potentiate the propensity of deoxy Hb S molecules to aggregate.

The role of blood transfusions and partial exchange transfusions is controversial in the treatment of acute vaso-occlusive crises of sickle cell disease. In general there is very little rationale for performing partial exchange transfusions simply for a painful vaso-occlusive crisis in a nonvital organ. Nevertheless such treatment may be occasionally indicated to interrupt an unusually prolonged painful crisis or when a patient is virtually continually disabled by frequent recurrent crises. In cases of life-threatening vaso-occlusive episodes or when there is a threat of severe organ damage, as in acute cerebrovascular accidents and priapism, partial exchange transfusions should be promptly carried out because no other effective form of therapy is available. It is also generally agreed that patients who have suffered one cerebrovascular accident are likely to have recurrent life-threatening or debilitating episodes, and a course of long-term maintenance blood transfusions to prevent recurrent sickling is indicated in such cases. Such a program should probably be associated with phlebotomies prior to transfusion and/or the institution of an iron chelation program to prevent or delay the complications of iron overload (see Ch. 136.4). Use of transfusions during pregnancy is controversial. It is common practice in many centers to give transfusions to pregnant women with sickle cell syndromes during the latter half of pregnancy to prevent fetal loss and postpartum complications. However, a controlled study has not documented that this practice is clearly beneficial. Finally, it is also general practice for patients with clinically significant sickle cell syndromes to receive a partial exchange transfusion to lower the Hb S value to less than 50 per cent prior to general anesthesia for surgical procedures because of the risk of a fatal or incapacitating sickling episode in the event of an anesthetic accident or transient hypoxia. With the exception of the hypoplastic crises and acute sequestration crises, blood transfusions are not usually required to maintain hemoglobin levels above 6.5 to 7 grams per deciliter, and transfusions are not required on a long-term basis simply to treat the anemia.

Because of the high risk of septicemia and other serious infections caused by *Streptococcus pneumoniae*, young children with sickle cell anemia should receive prophylactic oral penicillin. This approach has been shown to be highly effective in reducing morbidity and mortality in pediatric populations. Pneumococcal and *Haemophilus influenzae* vaccines may provide additional protection against such infections.

PROGNOSIS. The prognosis of patients with sickle cell syndromes is variable. A significant number of infants with sickle cell anemia and Hb SC disease may die in the first 2 to 3 years because of overwhelming sepsis and/or acute splenic sequestration crises. Cord blood screening programs and identification of affected individuals with subsequent close medical follow-up, including prophylactic penicillin and vaccinations, should prevent or decrease the incidence of these early fatalities. For the group of patients who survive the early years, improved general medical care has substantially prolonged survival in the past two decades. There are reports of patients surviving to the fifth and sixth decades, although the mean survival is probably to the fourth decade, with death resulting from cardiopulmonary complications and/or renal insufficiency. Other causes of death include sepsis and cerebrovascular accidents. In general, patients with Hb S/β-thalassemia and Hb SC disease have longer survival than do patients with sickle cell disease, although there are unexplained cases of relatively mild disease with homozygous inheritance of Hb S.

PREVENTION. Sickle cell disease and other clinically significant sickle syndromes can be prevented in two general ways. First, genetic counseling of identified heterozygotes can alert couples at risk about the possibility of having affected offspring. However, no matter how good the program of genetic counseling and education, it rarely significantly affects the reproductive behavior of identified carriers and generally has little impact on the overall incidence of the disease.

An alternative approach is the availability of prenatal diagnostic services for pregnancies at risk for sickle cell anemia and other sickle hemoglobinopathies. Prenatal diagnosis for sickle cell anemia has gone through many stages in recent years, including fetal blood sampling by fetoscopy for assays of hemoglobin synthesis and analysis by gene mapping techniques of DNA from amniotic fluid cells, obtained after amniocentesis, for restriction fragment length polymorphisms shown to be linked to the sickle gene by prior study of DNA from family members. A restriction endonuclease enzyme (*Mst* II) can distinguish between a sickle and a nonsickle β globin gene because the recognition site for this enzyme is specifically abolished by the nucleotide base substitution that is associated with the sickle mutation (Fig. 136–10). Thus the most reliable and acceptable method for prenatal diagnosis of sickle cell anemia is analysis of fetal DNA by the enzyme *Mst* II. The source of DNA may be amniotic fluid cells obtained by amniocentesis between 14 and 20 weeks of gestation, or chorionic villi obtained by transcervical biopsy between 8 and 10 weeks of gestation. The latter has the advantage of allowing diagnosis, counseling, and decision making to occur much earlier in the pregnancy. Although DNA analysis may be accomplished by standard gene mapping techniques (Southern gel blotting), it is much more quickly and efficiently achieved by use of the polymerase chain reaction procedure, as in the case of prenatal diagnosis of β-thalassemia (see Ch. 136.4).

HOMOZYGOUS Hb C DISEASE. Individuals homozygous for Hb C usually have a mild to moderate hemolytic anemia characterized by splenomegaly and large numbers of target cells on peripheral blood smear. Occasionally, intraerythrocytic crystals of Hb C can be visualized in fixed blood smears. The clinical manifestations and general laboratory findings are those of any mild chronic hemolytic anemia. Diagnosis is established by hemoglobin electrophoresis (see Color Plate 6B, right).

Bunn HF, Forget BG: Sickle cell disease—clinical and epidemiological aspects; and molecular basis of sickle cell disease. *In* Hemoglobin: Molecular, Genetic and Clinical Aspects. Philadelphia, W. B. Saunders Company, 1986, pp 502–554. Platt OS, Nathan DG: Sickle cell disease. *In* Nathan DG, Oski FA (eds.): Hematology of Infancy and Childhood. 3rd ed. Philadelphia, W. B. Saunders Company, 1987, pp 655–698. *Comprehensive chapters in hematology textbooks covering the pathophysiology as well as the clinical manifestations and therapy of sickle cell disease.*

Fleming AF (ed.): Sickle Cell Disease: A Handbook for the General Clinician. New York, Churchill Livingstone, 1982. Serjeant GR: Sickle Cell Disease. New York, Oxford University Press, 1985. *Comprehensive and detailed clinical descriptions of the manifestations of sickle cell anemia.*

Francis RB Jr, Johnson CS: Vascular occlusion in sickle cell disease: Current concepts and unanswered questions. Blood 77:1405, 1991. *An up-to-date review of this major and serious complication of sickle cell disease.*

137 Blood Transfusion

Jay E. Menitove

Whole blood collected for transfusion contains approximately 450 ml of anticoagulated blood. From this, red blood cells (or packed cells) are separated from plasma to achieve a hematocrit of 65 to 80 per cent in 250 to 300 ml. Solutions containing adenine and saline, added to blood shortly after collection, extend the permissible storage time from 21 or 35 days to 42 days. Red blood cells, adenine-saline added, have a hematocrit of 55 to 65 per cent and a volume of approximately 325 ml.

TABLE 137–1. INDICATIONS FOR RED BLOOD CELL COMPONENTS

Whole blood
  Symptomatic deficit in oxygen-carrying capacity and significant
    hypovolemia
Red blood cells (packed cells)
  Symptomatic deficit of oxygen-carrying capacity in anemic patients
Leukocyte-depleted red blood cells
  Symptomatic anemia, prevention of recurrent febrile, nonhemolytic
    transfusion reactions
Washed red blood cells
  Symptomatic anemia, prevention of severe urticarial reactions and
    anaphylaxis in IgA-deficient patients
Frozen/thawed red blood cells
  Symptomatic anemia, inventory maintenance for rare blood types

Blood donors are questioned extensively, and their blood is tested to decrease the risk of transmitting retroviruses, hepatitis, syphilis, and, in some instances, cytomegalovirus. All hazards cannot be eliminated, however. Transfusion therapy must therefore be used appropriately to ensure that the benefit outweighs potential risk (Table 137–1).

INDICATIONS FOR WHOLE-BLOOD TRANSFUSION

Whole blood is indicated for patients with a symptomatic deficit in oxygen-carrying capacity and hypotension as a result of hypovolemia. Crystalloid or colloid solutions are used to restore intravascular volume in patients with moderate hemorrhage. It is appropriate to use whole blood when blood loss exceeds 25 to 30 per cent of blood volume.

Factors V and VIII are labile, but the activity of other coagulation factors is stable during the shelf-life of whole blood (Ch. 155). Since Factor V or VIII deficiency is unusual in patients resuscitated after massive blood loss, whole blood is appropriate replacement therapy for patients with coagulation factor deficiency who also require red cell augmentation. Currently, whole blood accounts for approximately 5 per cent of red cell component transfusions in the United States.

INDICATIONS FOR RED BLOOD CELLS

Red blood cells are indicated for anemic patients who require an increase in oxygen-carrying capacity. The hemoglobin/hematocrit level at which tissue oxygenation is compromised is the subject of debate. In the perioperative period, a hemoglobin concentration of 7 grams per deciliter (hematocrit of approximately 21 per cent) is usually tolerated in the absence of depleted intravascular volume. In patients with chronic anemia, decreased oxygen delivery is compensated for by an increase in cardiac output, redistribution of blood away from renal and splanchnic beds to muscle tissue, and enhanced oxygen extraction by tissues (Ch. 111). In addition, coronary artery blood flow increases, ventilatory volume and respiratory rates rise, and oxygen unloading is more rapid, since erythrocyte levels of 2,3-diphosphoglycerate (2,3-DPG) are elevated. Anemic patients are susceptible to fatigue, dyspnea on exertion, decreased exercise capacity, decreased mental acuity, and breathlessness. These symptoms usually become significant when the hemoglobin concentration is between 7 and 10 grams per deciliter but vary according to the patient's cardiac, respiratory, and cerebrovascular status. Increasing cardiac and respiratory rate, congestive heart failure, angina, or confusion may indicate that compensatory mechanisms are not able to meet tissue oxygen demands.

Symptomatic patients with chronic anemia should receive two to three units of red blood cells at 2- to 3-week intervals. One unit of red cells raises the hemoglobin by approximately 1 gram per deciliter (or a hematocrit increase of 3 per cent) in the average-size adult. In general, the "transfusion trigger" is a hemoglobin concentration of 8 or 9 grams per deciliter (hematocrit of 24 or 27 per cent). The efficacy of compensatory mechanisms is uncertain when the hemoglobin is lower than 7 grams per deciliter.

LEUKOCYTE-DEPLETED RED BLOOD CELLS. Leukocyte-depleted red blood cells are used to prevent the recurrence of nonhemolytic febrile transfusion reactions in patients who have a history of two or more such reactions.

Leukocytes are removed from red blood cells by filtration or centrifugation. Certain filters withhold more than 95 per cent of white cells while allowing 90 per cent of red cells to pass. In contrast, there is a 70 to 80 per cent decrease in leukocyte content and a 20 to 30 per cent red cell loss when leukocyte depletion is accomplished by centrifugation.

WASHED RED BLOOD CELLS. Washed red blood cells are indicated for patients with a history of severe allergic or anaphylactic reactions. Plasma is effectively removed from red cells by adding saline to blood, sedimenting the red cells by centrifugation, and decanting the supernatant. Washed blood cells are not currently recommended for patients with paroxysmal nocturnal hemoglobinuria.

RED BLOOD CELLS STORED IN THE FROZEN STATE. Frozen red blood cells are used to create repositories of "rare" red blood cell units for patients with alloantibodies directed against red cell antigens that occur at high frequency in the population. They may be used for patients who have febrile nonhemolytic transfusion reactions but leukocyte-depleted red blood cells by filtration are preferred.

Red blood cells are prepared for frozen storage for up to 10 years by adding glycerol as a cryoprotective agent. Prior to transfusion, red cells are thawed and washed to remove glycerol. Only minimal amounts of leukocytes and plasma remain.

AUTOLOGOUS TRANSFUSION

The procedure of collecting and reinfusing a patient's own blood is a recommended alternative to homologous transfusion for patients who have at least 2 weeks' notice prior to scheduled surgery, who are likely to need a transfusion during or after surgery, and who have a hemoglobin higher than 11 grams per deciliter. Patients providing autologous blood should receive oral iron supplementation. They may donate as frequently as every 3 days but no later than 72 hours before surgery.

Perioperative blood salvage is another approach for reducing homologous transfusion. Blood lost during and immediately after surgery is collected and reinfused. Intraoperative blood salvage is contraindicated if the operative field is contaminated with bacteria or tumor.

Acute normovolemic hemodilution is also an alternative to homologous transfusion. Blood is removed prior to anesthesia induction, concomitant with crystalloid/colloid infusion. Hence, patients must be able to tolerate rapid blood withdrawal. The removed blood is reinfused at the completion of surgery, or sooner if needed.

Used alone or in combination, these methods are effective in decreasing homologous blood use and should be considered for appropriate patients. Recombinant erythropoietin has been used to augment hemoglobin concentration in patients initiating autologous blood collections 3 weeks before surgery. It is effective in ameliorating transfusion requirements in patients with renal insufficiency and may increase erythropoiesis in the perioperative setting.

DIRECTED DONATIONS

A directed donation refers to blood provided by a donor (usually a family member or friend) selected by the patient. There is an impression that these donors are "safer" than those donating to the general blood supply. This hypothesis is not supported by data.

MINIMAL EXPOSURE TRANSFUSION CONCEPT

Reducing the number of donors to whom a patient is exposed has a theoretical advantage of decreasing transfusion-associated risk. For example, donor exposures are reduced by use of whole blood in lieu of red blood cells from one donor and fresh frozen plasma from another or by providing apheresis platelet transfusions collected from one donor instead of an equivalent dose of pooled platelet concentrates from six to eight donors. Minimal exposure transfusion is potentially more adaptable for pediatric patients, who use less blood than adults, or for supplying platelets to those with a self-limited condition (such as extensive coronary artery bypass surgery).

BLOOD GROUPS. Red blood cell antigenic determinants are under genetic control. Allelic relationships are assigned on the basis of family studies and population statistics that demonstrate different antigens or through gene mapping and biochemical analysis. The clinical importance of a particular blood group depends on its frequency in the population, the immunogenicity of the antigen, and whether alloantibodies directed against it are immunoglobulin G (IgG) or immunoglobulin M (IgM) or whether they activate complement.

Blood group nomenclature has been revised into systems, collections, and series. Each of the 19 distinct systems refers to red cell antigens controlled by a single gene or continuous homologous genes and include ABO, MNS, P, Rh, Lutheran (Lu), Kell (Kk), Lewis (Le), Duffy (Fy), Kidd (Jk), and so on. The nine collections comprise specificities that have serologic, biochemical, or genetic connections, e.g., Gerbich (Ge), Cromer (Cr), Auberger (Au), and Ii. Two series have determinants that cannot be assigned to systems or collections: One consists of 38 specificities of low incidence (<1 per cent in a random Caucasian population), and the other contains 13 specificities of high incidence (>90 per cent in a random Caucasian population). Examples of such low-incidence antigens are Wright (Wr ^{a}), Batty (By ^{a}), and Christiansen (Chr ^{a}), and high-incidence markers include Vel, Langreis (Lan), JMH, Fritz (Wr ^{b}), and Sid (Sd ^{a}).

ABO is the most important blood group system, because anti-A and anti-B are found in all persons lacking the corresponding antigen (Table 137–2). Intravascular hemolysis is a significant hazard if these antibodies are present at high titer and incompatible blood is infused. Anti-A and anti-B are "naturally occurring" antibodies, i.e., are present in the absence of previous transfusion or pregnancy. They are probably formed in response to bacterial antigens.

The Rh system is next in importance. Approximately 70 per cent of Rh-negative persons exposed to Rh-positive blood form anti-Rh antibodies. Anti-Rh antibodies are implicated in hemolytic reactions and cross the placenta to cause hemolytic disease of the newborn. For practical purposes, the Rh system is divided into Rh-positive and Rh-negative types by testing red cells with the most frequent Rh antibody, anti-D. A commonly used classification further subdivides the Rh system into three pairs of closely linked allelic genes: Cc, Dd, Ee. For example, a person may inherit C, D, e from one parent and c, d, e from another. Although the symbol "d" is used, it is an amorph; i.e., there is no allele for D.

A, B, and D are the most immunogenic red cell antigens. Kell (K), c, and E are less potent immunogens, and Fy ^{a} and Jk ^{a} are even less immunogenic. As a result of differences in antigenic strength and the frequency that patients are exposed to non-self antigens, Rh antibodies other than anti-D account for approximately 50 per cent and anti-K, anti-Fy ^{a}, and anti-Jk ^{a} for approximately 45 per cent of alloantibodies detected by hospital transfusion services.

COMPATIBILITY TESTING. Compatibility testing involves confirming the donor's blood group, determining the recipient's ABO and Rh types, screening the patient's serum for unexpected antibodies (i.e., antibodies other than anti-A and anti-B), and performing a major crossmatch.

Recipients of whole blood must receive blood from a donor with the same ABO group, since anti-A and/or anti-B present in the plasma may cause destruction of recipient red cells. For example, group O whole blood must be given only to group O patients, and group AB patients must receive only group AB whole blood. Since the amount of plasma is reduced in red blood cells, the blood type of donor and recipient of packed cell transfusions may be compatible rather than identical; i.e., group O (universal donor) red cells may be given to group A, B, or AB patients, and group AB patients (universal recipients) may receive group O, A, or B red blood cells. Rh-negative patients should receive Rh-negative whole blood or red blood cells. Rh-positive recipients may receive either Rh-positive or Rh-negative blood.

The test for unexpected antibodies must include antiglobulin reagents to detect agglutinating and nonagglutinating antibodies.

The crossmatch detects incompatibility between donor red cells and antibodies in the recipient's serum or plasma. Donor cells and the patient's serum are incubated; subsequently, antiglobulin reagents are added. Incompatibility is recognized by red cell agglutination or hemolysis. An abbreviated or "type and screen" procedure is used in some laboratories to determine incompatibility. The patient's blood is typed for ABO and Rh, and the serum or plasma is screened for unexpected antibodies. In the absence of unexpected antibodies or a record of such antibodies, the patient's serum is made to react with donor red cells and centrifuged briefly. If agglutination or hemolysis does not occur, the blood is released for transfusion. The centrifugation step, or "immediate spin," is used to detect ABO incompatibility. If unexpected antibodies are present, blood that does not contain the corresponding antigen should be selected, and a crossmatch should be performed.

When there is an urgent requirement for blood, such as when a delay in transfusion may jeopardize the patient unduly, blood may be issued without performing compatibility testing. If the ABO type of the recipient is not known, group O red cells should be provided. If the ABO group was determined by the hospital transfusion service, ABO group–compatible red cells may be given. Whole blood must be ABO group identical. In these circumstances, the patient's record should contain a statement from the attending physician explaining the urgent nature of the clinical situation and the requirement to transfuse blood before completion of the compatibility testing.

ADVERSE EVENTS ASSOCIATED WITH BLOOD TRANSFUSION

Complications of blood transfusion are categorized into acute, delayed, or transfusion-transmitted disease-related events (Table 137–3).

ACUTE REACTIONS. Acute adverse events caused by transfusion occur within minutes or hours after infusing red blood cells or other components. The presenting signs and symptoms are not always sufficiently specific to indicate a definite diagnosis. Correlation of clinical findings and laboratory test results is needed to establish the pathogenic mechanisms and treatment plan.

Acute Hemolytic Transfusion Reactions. These serious complications of blood transfusion occur infrequently—1 per 6000 to 25,000 component infusions. Intravascular destruction of red cells is the result of complete complement activation. Osmotic red cell lysis occurs, and free hemoglobin and antibody-coated red cell stroma are released into the plasma. If this situation is caused by anti-A or anti-B, the associated mortality approaches 10 per cent.

TABLE 137–2. FREQUENCY (%) OF BLOOD GROUPS IN SELECTED POPULATIONS

	Whites‡	Blacks‡	Hispanics§	Asians§	Native Americans§	Antibody in Plasma
O*	40	51	57	34	60	Anti-A, anti-B
A	44	25	32	35	35	Anti-B
B	12	20	9	23	4	Anti-A
AB†	5	4	2	8	1	None
Rh-positive	84	95	97	99+	97	—
Rh-negative	16	5	3	<1	3	—

*Universal donor of red blood cells.
†Universal recipient of red blood cells.
‡Derived from unpublished observations, Blood Center of Southeastern Wisconsin, Milwaukee.
§Estimates based on selected populations.

Extravascular hemolysis is associated with antibodies that coat red cells without complement activation beyond C3b. Opsonized red cells are removed by tissue macrophages. Most antibodies directed against Rh, Kell, Kidd, and Duffy antigens behave in this manner.

Fever is observed in almost all patients suffering a hemolytic reaction. Nausea, vomiting, and chest pain occur less often. Also reported are wheezing and dyspnea, back pain, restlessness, and discomfort at the infusion site. Hypotension may be a prelude to disseminated intravascular coagulation (DIC).

Major adverse sequelae are a consequence of vasomotor instability, hypotension, bleeding diatheses, and renal impairment. Hypotension is caused by release of C3a, C4a, and C5a into plasma as a result of antibody-antigen interaction. The thromboplastic activity of red cell stroma activates the intrinsic clotting cascade and gives rise, in some patients, to DIC. Renal insufficiency and oliguria are caused by changes in renal blood flow brought about by hypotension and vasoconstriction.

Most hemolytic reactions are a consequence of clerical error or failure to observe proper procedures, such as misidentification of blood samples, donor units, or patients. The blood infusion must be stopped as soon as a hemolytic transfusion reaction is suspected. Therapy is directed at correction of hypotension, control of bleeding, and prevention of acute renal failure. Blood pressure maintenance is important, since hypotension is a prelude to DIC and acute renal failure. Intravenous fluids, mannitol, or other diuretics such as furosemide or ethacrynic acid are used to increase renal blood flow and maintain urine output at 100 ml per hour. If oliguria or anuria ensues, standard measures for renal failure management must be instituted (Ch. 76).

Febrile Nonhemolytic Transfusion Reactions. These chill-fever reactions occur at a frequency of approximately 1 per 200 component infusions. They are characterized by a posttransfusion temperature rise of 1°C or more in the absence of hemolysis. They are caused by cytotoxic or agglutinating antibodies stimulated by previous transfusions or pregnancies against antigens on donor lymphocytes, granulocytes, or platelets.

These reactions occur in three phases. Initially, there is a transient episode of flushing, palpitation, tachycardia, cough, chest discomfort, or neutropenia that often is unnoticed. A 15- to 60-minute latent period intervenes. The third part consists of a rise in diastolic blood pressure, headache, chilliness, or a frank rigor. The reactions cannot be distinguished from hemolytic reactions on the basis of clinical presentation. Hence, the infusion should be stopped immediately. Most febrile nonhemolytic reactions are self-limited, however, and subside with supportive measures and orally administered antipyretics. Fewer than 15

per cent of patients suffer a recurrence when transfused subsequently. After a second reaction, it is advisable to provide further transfusions with red blood cells that have been leukocyte depleted by filtration.

Transfusion-Related Acute Lung Injury. This occurs infrequently but has significant clinical consequences. It is probably caused by passive infusion of donor antibody directed against recipient leukocytes (anti–human leukocyte antigen [HLA] antibody). The symptom complex is marked by fever, substernal chest pain, severe dyspnea, cyanosis, cough, blood-tinged sputum, and hypoxemia that occur within 4 hours (usually 1 to 2 hours) after plasma-containing components are given. The presentation resembles pulmonary edema, but hemodynamic measurements indicate a noncardiogenic etiology. Rapid intervention with respiratory support and mechanical ventilation is required. If the pulmonary capillary wedge pressure is low and hypotension is present, fluid replacement may be indicated. Recovery usually ensues within 48 hours.

Allergic Reactions. Urticarial eruptions and pruritus occur in 1 to 3 per cent of transfused patients. They are caused by an interaction between donor plasma proteins and recipient immunoglobulin E (IgE) antibody. The reactions are usually mild and respond to antihistamines. The transfusion may be continued after hives subside.

Anaphylactic reactions occur with a frequency of 1 per 150,000 component transfusions, usually in immunoglobulin A (IgA)–deficient patients (approximately 1 per 1000 of the population) who have anti-IgA that is reacting against IgA in donor plasma. The dramatic clinical presentation includes apprehension, a feeling of doom, chest or lumbar pain, facial flushing, generalized urticaria, laryngeal or facial edema with bronchospasm, wheezing, dyspnea, hypotension, loss of consciousness, vomiting, or diarrhea. These reactions require urgent treatment with intravenous epinephrine. If subsequent transfusions are required, cellular components should be washed to remove plasma.

Hypervolemia. Patients with impaired myocardial reserve are at risk of congestive heart failure caused by overexpansion of intravascular volume. An average unit of whole blood contains 56 mEq of sodium; a unit of red cells, 8 to 20 mEq of sodium; and a unit of red cells with additive solutions, 24 to 30 mEq of sodium.

Bacterial Sepsis. Septicemia is a rare complication of blood transfusion. In these cases blood has been contaminated at the time of phlebotomy, and bacteria have proliferated during storage. Following infusion of as little as 50 to 70 ml of blood, patients develop chills or frank rigors, which may be associated with nausea, vomiting, and lethargy. Subsequently, fever, hypotension, shock, and DIC may occur. Profound symptoms are compatible with endotoxin produced by gram-negative organisms.

TABLE 137–3. SIGNS AND SYMPTOMS OF ACUTE AND DELAYED ADVERSE CONSEQUENCES OF TRANSFUSION

Fever
  Acute and delayed hemolytic transfusion reactions
  Febrile, nonhemolytic reactions
  Acute lung injury
  Anaphylaxis
  Septic transfusions
Chills/rigors
  Acute hemolysis
  Febrile, nonhemolytic reactions
  Anaphylaxis
  Septic transfusions
Nausea/vomiting
  Acute hemolysis
  Anaphylaxis
  Septic transfusions
Chest discomfort/pain
  Acute hemolysis
  Febrile, nonhemolytic reactions
  Acute lung injury
  Anaphylaxis
  Air embolus
Facial flushing
  Brisk, acute hemolysis
  Febrile, nonhemolytic reactions
  Anaphylaxis

Wheezing/dyspnea
  Acute hemolysis
  Acute lung injury
  Anaphylaxis
  Hypervolemia
  Air embolus
Back/lumbar pain
  Acute hemolysis
  Anaphylaxis
  Septic transfusions
Discomfort at infusion site
  Acute hemolysis
  Septic transfusions
Hypotension
  Acute hemolysis
  Anaphylaxis
  Septic tranfusions
Bleeding/DIC
  Acute hemolysis
  Complication of massive transfusion
Hemoglobinuria
  Acute hemolysis
  Nonimmune hemolysis
Hives/pruritus
  Allergic reactions

Less dramatic clinical presentations occur when gram-positive organisms are involved. The infusion must be stopped. Samples for microbacteriologic examination and a Gram stain of an aliquot of noninfused blood should be obtained, and broad-spectrum antibiotics must be started immediately.

DELAYED REACTIONS. Delayed or nonimmediate adverse consequences of blood transfusion occur days to years after the transfusion is given.

Delayed Hemolytic Transfusion Reactions. Destruction of red cells by an antibody not detected by compatibility testing occurs at a frequency between 1 in 300 and 1 in 1600 transfusions. Only 20 per cent of these patients experience clinical symptoms, however. The antibodies are a result of a secondary or amnestic response. Clinical symptoms appear 6 to 8 days (range, 3 to 21 days) after transfusion. The triad of anemia, fever, and a history of recent transfusion in a patient previously immunized by transfusion or pregnancy should alert the clinician to suspect a delayed hemolytic transfusion reaction. Jaundice is present in approximately two thirds of those who are symptomatic. The direct antiglobulin test is usually positive. Anti-E, anti-Jk^a, anti-K, anti-D, anti-C, anti-c, and anti-Fy^a are commonly associated with these reactions. Severe sequelae are uncommon, and specific therapy is rarely needed.

Graft-Versus-Host Disease. This reaction occurs when transfused lymphocytes recognize and react against the "host" (recipient). Graft-versus-host disease requires the transfer of viable immunocompetent T lymphocytes that are disparate in HLA type from those of the patient but are sufficiently similar to permit initial engraftment. Most patients developing graft-versus-host disease have severely impaired cellular immune function; however, this syndrome has occurred in patients undergoing therapy for Hodgkin's disease, non-Hodgkin's lymphoma, acute leukemia, and neuroblastoma. Immunocompetent patients recovering from cardiac surgery have also been affected. Transfusion-associated graft-versus-host disease occurs 4 to 30 days after transfusion. Patients develop fever that may be accompanied by erythema, diarrhea, liver function abnormalities, and bone marrow suppression marked by pancytopenia. Treatment is usually unsuccessful; the mortality rate is approximately 90 per cent. Hence, prevention, accomplished by gamma irradiation (1500 to 3000 cGy, 15 to 30 Gy) of blood and components, is the primary strategy.

Iron Overload. Endocrine, cardiac, and liver dysfunction occurs in adults who receive 60 to 210 (mean, 120) units of blood. Iron chelation therapy has been used successfully to reduce iron stores.

Posttransfusion Purpura. This syndrome is manifested by profound thrombocytopenia 5 to 9 days after transfusion. Most cases occur in multiparous women receiving their first blood transfusion, but nulliparous women as well as previously transfused women and men have had this complication. The etiology is not known precisely, but more than 90 per cent of patients are Pl^{Al} negative and make an anti-Pl^{Al} alloantibody. Pl^{Al} is a platelet-specific antigen present on the platelets of 98 per cent of the population. It is unclear why a Pl^{Al}-negative patient with Pl^{Al} alloantibody becomes thrombocytopenic. Potential mechanisms relate to production of autoantibodies in addition to alloantibodies, formation of immune complexes that bind to autologous platelets, or binding of soluble alloantigen to autologous platelets, which are destroyed subsequently by alloantibody. The syndrome also occurs in association with alloantibodies directed against Pl^{A2}, Bak^a, Bak^b, and other platelet-specific antigens. Posttransfusion purpura is a self-limited condition but may be fatal. Therapy involves corticosteroids, plasma exchange, whole blood exchange transfusions, or intravenous gamma globulin infusion.

TRANSFUSION-TRANSMITTED DISEASES. These complications are among the most feared consequences of transfusion. The recent introduction of screening tests for retroviruses and hepatitis has decreased the incidence of these infections.

Hepatitis (Ch. 117). Posttransfusion hepatitis A and hepatitis B are reported occasionally, and posttransfusion hepatitis C (previously non-A, non-B hepatitis) occurs most frequently. Recently introduced screening tests to detect potentially infectious donors should reduce the frequency of posttransfusion hepatitis C to 1 per 1000 to 1500 components transfused. Clinical illness, described in Ch. 117, occurs an average of 7 to 8 weeks after transfusion. Approximately 50 per cent of patients with hepatitis C develop chronic hepatitis and, of these, 10 to 20 per cent are

at risk for cirrhosis or hepatocellular carcinoma, which may occur several decades after transfusion.

Retroviral Infections. Approximately 3 per cent of acquired immunodeficiency syndrome (AIDS) cases are transfusion related, and 1 per cent have appeared in patients treated with coagulation factor concentrates. The median latent period between transfusion with an infected unit and clinical evidence of AIDS is at least 7 years. Screening tests to detect human immunodeficiency virus–1 (HIV-1) carriers, combined with donor screening measures, have reduced the risk of HIV infection to less than 1 per 150,000 components transfused.

HIV-2 is closely related to HIV-1 and causes a similar illness. The infection is endemic in West Africa; very few cases have been reported in the United States. Concern that transfusion could be a vector for further spread throughout the population led to development of screening tests combining anti–HIV-1 and anti–HIV-2 reagents.

The human T lymphotropic virus I (HTLV-I) is a transforming retrovirus associated with adult T cell leukemia/lymphoma and tropical spastic paraparesis. This cell-associated virus is transmitted to 60 to 70 per cent of recipients of infected units of whole blood, red cells, or platelet concentrates. Serologic tests for anti–HTLV-I are used routinely to identify donors at risk of transmitting the virus through transfusion. The HTLV-I screening test also detects donors infected with HTLV-II, an agent not currently linked to a specific disease entity. Confirmatory testing indicates the majority of volunteer blood donors found reactive by the screening test are infected with HTLV-II rather than HTLV-I.

Cytomegalovirus (CMV) (Ch. 372). This latent virus is found predominantly in polymorphonuclear (PMN) leukocytes and lymphocytes. Most immunocompetent patients exposed to CMV become infected but are rarely symptomatic. In contrast, bone marrow transplant recipients and low birth weight neonates are at risk for fever, arthralgias, enteritis, hepatitis, thrombocytopenia, leukopenia, encephalitis, and interstitial pneumonitis that may be fatal. Blood components from donors who are anti–CMV antibody negative do not transmit the virus and are indicated for seronegative bone marrow transplant patients who receive bone marrow from seronegative donors and neonates who weigh less than 1200 grams and who are born to seronegative women. Preliminary results indicate that CMV is not transmitted by blood passed through newly developed, highly effective blood filters.

Malaria (Ch. 424). This is an uncommon complication of transfusion. It occurs approximately 3 weeks (range, 7 to 50 days) following transfusion from an asymptomatic infected donor. Deferral of donors who are residents of geographic regions where malaria is endemic is an appropriate method for reducing the risk of this complication.

Chagas' Disease (Ch. 426). This infection, caused by *Trypanosoma cruzi*, may cause transfusion-associated illness in immunocompromised patients. The incubation period between transfusion and onset of symptoms is approximately 2 months. Epidemiologic studies to determine the prevalence of infection in U.S. blood donors are in progress.

Syphilis (Ch. 340). Syphilis is an extremely uncommon complication of blood transfusion because donors are screened by serologic tests for syphilis and spirochetes remain viable in blood stored at 4°C for only a few days. The period between infusion of spirochete-infected blood and symptoms is 1 to 4½ months.

Other Infectious Agents. Other infectious agents that are transmitted infrequently by blood transfusion include *Babesia*, *Bartonella*, Epstein-Barr virus, parvovirus, and *Toxoplasma*. It is possible, but unlikely, that *Borrelia* is transmitted by transfusion.

SUMMARY

Red blood cell transfusions are indicated when there is a clinical need to increase oxygen-carrying capacity in anemic patients. Transfusion of one unit of red cells increases the hemoglobin concentration by 1 gram per deciliter in the average adult patient. The "transfusion trigger" in the perioperative period may be as low as 7 grams per deciliter if physiologic compensatory mechanisms are adequate. In chronically anemic patients, transfusions should be given only if clinical symptoms are present or eminent. Since transfusion is associated with risks that are unavoidable, it must be used appropriately. Alternatives to homologous transfusion, such as autologous transfusion, should be considered and used whenever possible.

Huestis DW, Bove JR, Case S: Practical Blood Transfusion. 4th ed. Boston, MA, Little, Brown and Company, 1988. *Answers to day-to-day questions arising in hospital-based transfusion services are provided in this quick-reading text.*

Mollison PL, Engelfriet CP, Contreras M.: Blood Transfusion in Clinical Medicine. 8th ed. Oxford, Great Britain, Blackwell Scientific Publications, 1987. *This is an encyclopedic compendium about transfusion medicine and is considered the primary reference on this subject.*

Petz LD, Swisher SN: Clinical Practice of Blood Transfusion. 2nd ed. New York, Churchill Livingstone, 1988. *This text provides excellent in-depth discussions of clinical aspects of transfusion medicine.*

138 Function of Neutrophils and Mononuclear Phagocytes

Bernard M. Babior

Neutrophils and mononuclear phagocytes (see Color Plate 5*A* and *B*) are essential components of the host defense system. Both are made in the bone marrow, and both accomplish most of their purposes through the act of eating (Greek *phagein*, to eat). Mononuclear phagocytes are versatile cells whose functions include the destruction of invading pathogens, the elimination of debris from the bloodstream and from sites of tissue damage, the remodeling of normal tissues, and the assignment of targets to lymphocytes. Neutrophils, on the other hand, are singlemindedly dedicated to the destruction of invading pathogens.

THE NEUTROPHIL

ORIGIN. Like other cells in the circulation, neutrophils originate from pluripotential stem cells that reside in the bone marrow. Depending on environmental influences, a pluripotential stem cell may give rise to the committed progenitors of any of the blood cells. Under the influence of certain *colony-stimulating factors* (CSF's), this stem cell will give rise to a population of neutrophils.

Colony-stimulating factors are proteins that control the proliferation and differentiation of particular types of cells. Table 138–1 lists the four CSF's that promote the formation of neutrophils and monocytes. Multi-CSF (interleukin 3) and GM-CSF act on early as well as late progenitors and show broad specificity, stimulating the production of phagocytes, red cells, platelets, and eosinophils. The other two act only on late progenitors, M-CSF stimulating the production of monocytes and G-CSF of neutrophils. The four CSF's also function as partial activators of the mature cells.

The route from a committed progenitor to a neutrophil involves a series of precursors, some of which can be recognized under the microscope. The earliest identifiable neutrophil precursor is a myeloblast, a relatively large cell with a rim of pale blue cytoplasm surrounding a large nucleus containing dispersed chromatin and multiple nucleoli. As the cell progresses through later stages of differentiation, the chromatin condenses and the nucleoli are lost, while at the same time the cytoplasm acquires its characteristic granules. The various neutrophil precursors are listed in Figure 138–1 (see Color Plate 5*D*).

Through the myelocyte stage, neutrophil precursors divide as well as differentiate (Fig. 138–1). These proliferative forms constitute the *mitotic compartment* of the neutrophil precursor pool. Later precursors, which do not divide, constitute the *nonmitotic* or *storage compartment*. Cells in this compartment can be released into the bloodstream in response to infections or other stresses. As a rule, the only cells released from the storage compartment are neutrophils and bands, but if the stress is sufficiently severe, a few metamyelocytes may be liberated as well.

A newly committed stem cell requires 8 to 10 days to become a mature neutrophil. In the bloodstream, neutrophils are distributed evenly between two rapidly exchanging pools: the *circulating pool*, composed of neutrophils suspended in the circulation, and the *marginated pool*, consisting of cells that have settled onto the endothelium of the capillaries and postcapillary venules. Neutrophils in the circulation leave for the tissues randomly and rapidly; their half-time in the bloodstream is only 6 hours. In the tissues, however, the cells may sojourn for days.

STRUCTURE. The neutrophil is a terminally differentiated, nondividing cell that is well equipped for killing microorganisms. The cell is packed with granules whose contents are used to kill and degrade target microorganisms. The granules are of two types: *azurophil*, which contain proteases and other hydrolytic enzymes, defensins and other microbicidal peptides, and myeloperoxidase, a Cl^--oxidizing enzyme; and *specific*, which contain, among other things, a collagenase and an enzyme that releases C5a from the complement component C5. The nucleus is a vestigial structure that can no longer replicate its DNA. The plasma membrane contains some of the neutrophil's killing equipment as well as sensors that locate the microorganisms against which the neutrophil acts. The cytoskeleton of the neutrophil is a complex system of tubes and fibers that is responsible for the orderly movement of this highly motile cell.

FUNCTION. Neutrophils undergo radical changes in behavior in response to external stimuli. These changes include aggregation, degranulation (i.e., the discharge of granule contents through the plasma membrane), and the initiation of oxidant production. They are provoked by many stimuli, the most important of which are target microorganisms and chemotactic factors at high concentration (see below). These behavioral changes convert the neutrophil from a placid resident of the bloodstream to a powerful weapon. A cell that has undergone these changes is known as an *activated neutrophil*. The destruction of a microorganism by a neutrophil can be divided into three stages: finding the microorganism, ingesting it, and finally killing it and disposing of its remains.

Adhesion. Because neutrophils move by crawling, they must adhere to surfaces to migrate through the tissues to an inflammatory site. Adhesion is accomplished through a group of neutrophil surface glycoproteins known as the *CD11/CD18* family. Neutrophils bind to other cells through an interaction between CD11/CD18 and *ICAM-1* (intercellular adhesion molecule), a protein expressed on the surfaces of a variety of cells, including fibroblasts, epithelia, and vascular endothelium. Endothelium also expresses *ELAM-1* (endothelial leukocyte adhesion molecule), which binds neutrophils through an unknown mechanism not involving CD11/CD18. The activities of these adhesion molecules increase when cells bearing them are activated by inflammatory mediators, explaining the increase in neutrophil adhesiveness at sites of inflammation.

Chemotaxis. The neutrophil finds its target through a chemical sense that enables the cell to detect certain substances known as

TABLE 138–1. COLONY-STIMULATING FACTORS

CSF	Sources	Targets
Multi-CSF	T lymphocytes	Early and late progenitors (broad specificity)
GM-CSF	T lymphocytes	Early and late progenitors (broad specificity)
	Fibroblasts, monocytes, endothelium	
M-CSF	Fibroblasts, monocytes, endothelium	Late monocyte progenitors
G-CSF	Fibroblasts, monocytes, endothelium	Late neutrophil progenitors

Data from Groopman JE, Molina J-M, Scadden DT: Hematopoietic growth factors. N Engl J Med 321:1449, 1989. By permission of the New England Journal of Medicine.

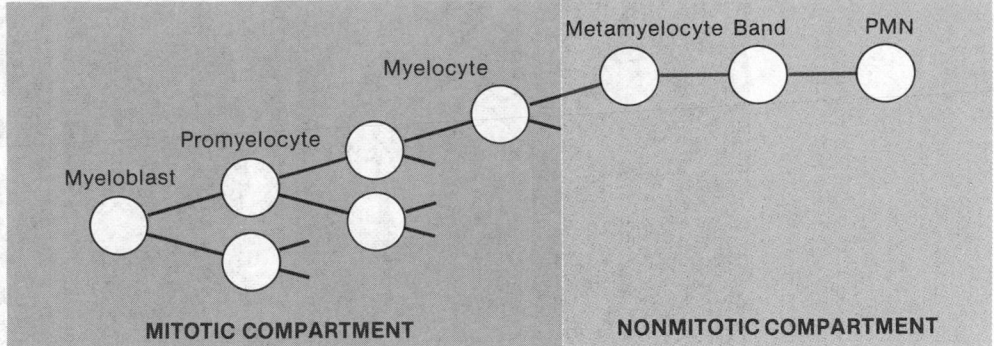

FIGURE 138–1. Neutrophil precursor pool.

chemotactic factors. These chemotactic factors are continuously released at sites where microorganisms have invaded tissues, diffusing away to set up a concentration gradient. Neutrophils in the circulation sense this gradient and travel toward its source. They begin their journey by marginating on the capillary and postcapillary endothelium. They then migrate outward through the vessel walls, penetrating the subendothelial basement membrane by local digestion, presumably with collagenase. Once outside the capillaries, they continue their directed migration, eventually reaching the site of origin of chemotactic factors—that is, the region of tissue that has been invaded by microorganisms. This process of migrating toward the source of a chemical attractant is known as *chemotaxis* (Fig. 138–2).

Neutrophils respond to a large number of chemotactic factors, but three are of primary importance: (1) *N-formylated oligopeptides,* (2) the complement fragment *C5a,* and (3), *leukotriene B₄* (LTB₄), a product of arachidonate oxidation. These chemotactic factors are produced both by the invading microorganisms (N-formylated oligopeptides and C5a) and by the neutrophils themselves (C5a and LTB₄). N-formylated oligopeptides are intermediates in bacterial protein synthesis and are released from damaged bacteria. C5a is produced by the complement system when it interacts with microorganisms and also by activated neutrophils through the release of the C5-splitting enzyme of the specific granules. LTB₄ is also produced by activated neutrophils, which manufacture it from arachidonic acid released from endogenous phospholipids. The production of C5a and LTB₄ by activated neutrophils lends a self-reinforcing character to the process of chemotaxis, since neutrophils at a site of inflammation generate chemotactic factors that attract more neutrophils to the inflamed region.

Bacteria in the circulation are thought to be handled primarily by the mononuclear phagocytes (see below). Neutrophils, however, may play a role in clearing the circulation of microorganisms that enter the bloodstream suddenly and in large numbers. During such episodes of bacteremia, the complement system is

activated, releasing C5a into the circulation. Neutrophils react to this surge of C5a by marginating in the pulmonary capillaries, where they may act temporarily (15 to 30 minutes) as a filtration system, removing microorganisms from the blood as they pass through the pulmonary circulation. In this special situation, chemotaxis is not needed to help the neutrophils find their targets, because the targets are brought directly to the phagocytes by the flow of blood.

Ingestion. Once the neutrophil has come into contact with the microorganism, the stage is set for ingestion. For this to occur, the cell has to recognize the microorganisms as an edible target, not just a piece of random debris. Often it is not the microorganism itself that the cell recognizes, but certain plasma proteins that coat the microorganism once it has entered the bloodstream or tissue. These proteins are called *opsonins* (Greek, *opson,* seasoning), and their attachment to the surface of the microorganism is called *opsonization* (Fig. 138–3).

The proteins that are able to opsonize targets for ingestion by neutrophils include antibodies belonging to certain of the immunoglobulin G (IgG) subclasses (opsonizing antibodies) and the complement component C3b. These bind to the surface of the microorganism by mechanisms discussed elsewhere (see Ch. 243). The opsonized target then attaches to the neutrophil surface by means of these opsonins, which are recognized and bound by receptors in the neutrophil membrane: the Fc receptors, which recognize complexes between antigen and opsonizing antibody, and the C3 receptors, which recognize particle-associated C3b.

The attachment of the target to the neutrophil surface is the signal for ingestion (Fig. 138–4). The membrane in the region of the attached particle invaginates into the cell, carrying the particle in with it. When the particle is fully internalized, the invagination closes at its neck to form a vesicle that breaks away from the cell membrane. The end result is that a particle initially attached to the surface of the neutrophil is transferred to the cell's interior in a vesicle lined with what was originally neutrophil plasma membrane. This vesicle, known as the *phagocytic vesicle,* is the site of killing of the ingested organism.

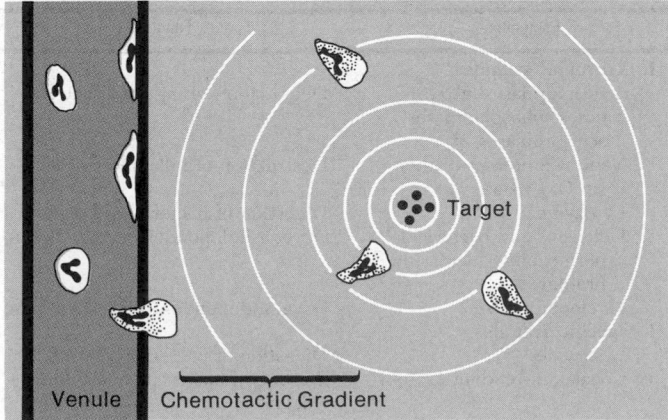

FIGURE 138–2. Chemotaxis. Neutrophils in the venule undergo margination in response to chemotactic factor, then leave the vessel by migrating between the endothelial cells (diapedesis) and travel up the chemotactic gradient toward the target.

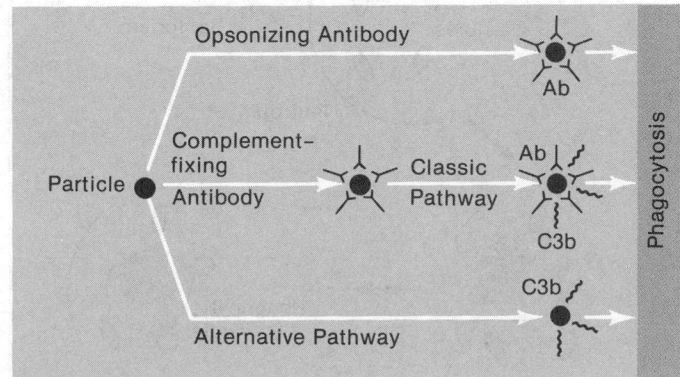

FIGURE 138–3. Opsonization. The coating of a particle by a plasma protein that is recognized by neutrophil receptors as a signal for ingestion is termed *opsonization.* Two classes of proteins are capable of opsonizing particles for ingestion by neutrophils: opsonizing antibodies and complement component C3b.

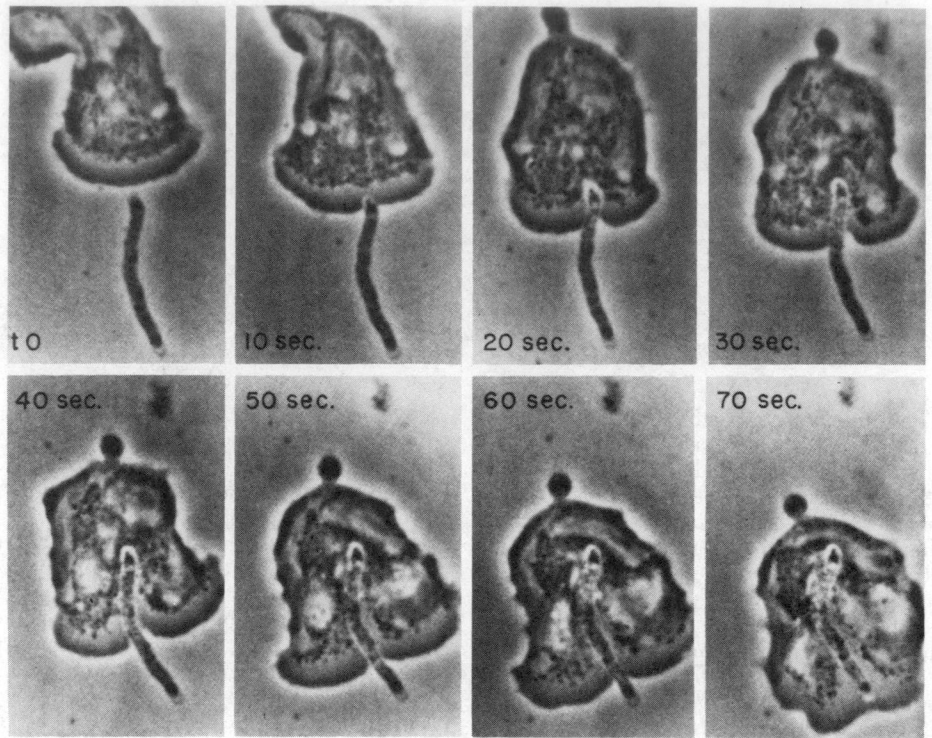

FIGURE 138–4. Ingestion of a target microorganism by a neutrophil. (Reproduced from Hirsch JG: Cinemicrophotographic observations of granule lysis in polymorphonuclear leucocytes during phagocytosis. J Exp Med 116:827, 1962, by copyright permission of the Rockefeller University Press.)

Killing. Killing involves two separate actions on the part of the neutrophils: *degranulation* and the *activation of the respiratory burst*. Degranulation refers to a process whereby the granule membrane fuses with the plasma membrane, releasing the granule contents into a transmembrane compartment—either a phagocytic vesicle (Fig. 138–5) or the external environment. Azurophil granules degranulate almost exclusively into the phagocytic vesicles, so their contents act principally against the ingested microorganism. Specific granules degranulate into both the phagocytic vesicles and the external environment, so their contents act exterior to the neutrophils as well as on the ingested microorganisms. Some of the constitutents of each of these granules are listed in Table 138–2, together with their actions.

The respiratory burst refers to a metabolic event whose purpose is the production of potent microbicidal oxidants through the partial reduction of oxygen. The burst is activated by the same stimuli that provoke degranulation of the specific granules—primarily contact with ingestible particles and exposure to chemotactic factors at high concentrations. These stimuli activate a plasma membrane–bound oxidase that catalyzes the reduction of oxygen to superoxide (O_2^-) at the expense of nicotinamide-adenine dinucleotide phosphate (NADPH) (Fig. 138–6). Most of the O_2^- reacts with itself to yield H_2O_2 while at the same time NADPH is regenerated by way of the hexosemonophosphate shunt.

The microbicidal oxidants are derived from the H_2O_2: (1) A portion of the H_2O_2 is used to oxidize Cl^- to the highly microbicidal hypochlorite ion (OCl^-), a reaction catalyzed by myeloperoxidase, an enzyme delivered into the phagocytic vesicle from the azurophil granules. (2) Another portion of the H_2O_2 is converted to the exceedingly reactive hydroxyl radical ($OH\cdot$) in a metal-catalyzed reaction with O_2^-. These and related oxidants

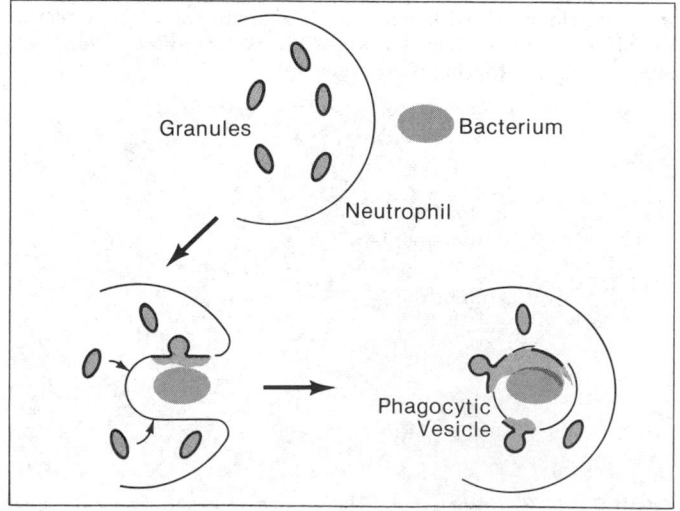

FIGURE 138–5. Degranulation into a phagocytic vesicle. Granules migrate toward a phagocytic vesicle, eventually fusing with it. Upon fusion, the contents of the granule are released into the vesicle, while the granule membrane becomes incorporated into the vesicle wall.

Table 138–2. CONTENTS OF NEUTROPHIL GRANULES

Compound	Function
I. Azurophil granules	
Acid hydrolases (glycosidases, phospholipases, acid proteases)	Degradation of ingested material
Neutral proteases (cathepsin G, elastase)	Destruction of inflamed tissue?
Lysozyme	Digestion of bacterial cell wall
Defensins and bactericidal/permeability-increasing protein	Oxygen-independent bacterial killing
Myeloperoxidase	Oxygen-dependent bacterial killing
II. Specific granules	
Lysozyme	Digestion of bacterial cell wall
Cobalamin-binding protein	Binding of bacterial cobalamin analogues
Apolactoferrin	Binding of free iron, control of granulopoiesis
Collagenase	Digestion of connective tissue
C5-splitting enzyme	Release of C5a

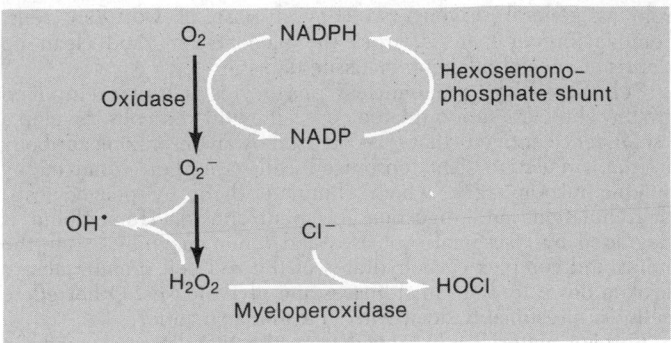

FIGURE 138–6. The respiratory burst.

TABLE 138–3. TISSUE MACROPHAGES

Fixed
  Kupffer cells
  Microglial cells (central nervous system)
  Macrophages of spleen, lymph nodes, and bone marrow sinusoids
  Mesangial cells (kidney)
  Osteoclasts
Wandering
  Macrophages of serosal cavities (pleural, peritoneal, pericardial)
  Alveolar macrophages

attack and kill ingested microorganisms by oxidizing their cellular constituents.

MONONUCLEAR PHAGOCYTES

Mononuclear phagocytes and neutrophils (see Color Plate 5A and B) are closely related. Both are descended from the same progenitor, and both share many functions, including the unusual ability to ingest particles as large as half or more their own diameter. There is, however, only one type of neutrophil, whereas there are many varieties of mononuclear phagocytes.

ORIGIN AND STRUCTURE. All mononuclear phagocytes are derived from a single circulating precursor: the monocyte. This cell and the neutrophil both arise from a single pluripotential stem cell. During differentiation, this stem cell first makes a general commitment to the phagocyte lineage. Later its descendants commit themselves further, some to the neutrophil and others to the monocyte line.

The first recognizable monocyte precursor is the *monoblast*. In normal marrow, this cell is indistinguishable from a myeloblast; it can be identified, however, in marrow from patients with monocytic leukemia. The next stage is the *promonocyte*, a somewhat larger cell with cytoplasmic granules and an indented nucleus containing finely divided chromatin. Finally, the fully developed *monocyte* appears. Larger than the neutrophil, and with a large horseshoe-shaped nucleus containing dispersed chromatin, the mature monocyte has cytoplasm that is filled with granules whose contents include hydrolytic enzymes and other proteins necessary for the cell's activities. It requires about 5 days to go from a monoblast to a mature circulating monocyte.

FURTHER DIFFERENTIATION. Unlike neutrophils, monocytes retain a limited capacity to divide and, in addition, undergo considerable further differentiation. After circulating briefly in the bloodstream ($t_{1/2} \sim 12$ hours), they enter the tissues, where they differentiate into mature macrophages that live for weeks to months. The properties of these macrophages depend on the tissues in which they reside. Those in the liver, for example, are the Kupffer cells, spidery phagocytes that bridge the sinusoids separating adjacent plates of hepatocytes (Fig. 138–7A). Those in the lungs are the large ellipsoidal alveolar macrophages (Fig. 138–7B). These and other tissue macrophages are listed in Table 138–3.

Macrophages are important components of the inflammatory reactions elicited by noxious agents (e.g., microorganisms or foreign bodies). Some of the macrophages that appear at a site of inflammation are recruited from surrounding tissues, while others are derived from monocytes that have migrated there from the bloodstream. Once at the inflamed site, macrophages are exposed to certain stimuli (e.g., *gamma-interferon*, a T lymphocyte product, and *lipopolysaccharide* from the bacterial cell walls) that induce them to undergo functional and morphologic changes that enable them to deal more effectively with the inciting agent. Initially, the cells enlarge, accumulate many new granules, and begin to secrete large quantities of certain specific proteases, including collagenase, elastase, and plasminogen activator, a component of the fibrinolytic system (see Ch. 146). CD11/CD18 increases on their surfaces. Their capacity for phagocytosis is increased, as is their ability to degrade ingested material. The cells become stickier and more motile and develop the ability to manufacture lethal oxidizing agents. Most important, their microbicidal power is greatly increased, so they can kill pathogens that they were unable to deal with in their former state. Cells that have attained this heightened degree of microbicidal potency are known as *activated macrophages*.

If the inciting agent has not been eliminated within the first few days, the activated macrophages begin to aggregate into a

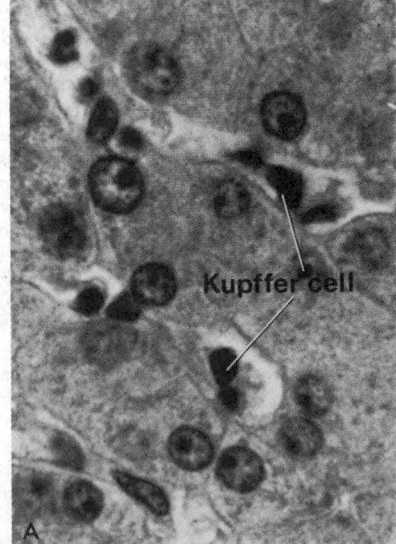

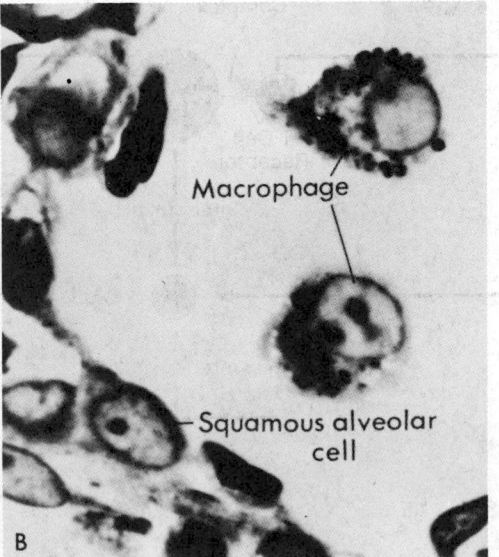

FIGURE 138–7. Some tissue macrophages. *A*, Kupffer cell. (Reprinted with permission from Popper H: Liver Structure and Function. New York, McGraw-Hill Book Company, 1957, p 97.) *B*, Alveolar macrophage. (From Sorokin SP: The respiratory system. *In* Weiss L, Greep RO: Histology. 4th ed., p 765. Copyright © 1977 by McGraw-Hill Inc. Used by permission of McGraw-Hill Book Company.)

TABLE 138–4. SUBSTANCES SECRETED BY MACROPHAGES

Substance	State of Macrophage	Additional Stimulus Needed
Lysozyme	Resident, activated	None
Neutral proteases	Activated	None
Collagenase		
Elastase		
Plasminogen activator		
Interleukin 1	Resident, activated	Lymphokine, endotoxin, others
Superoxide	Activated	Contact with particles or
Leukotrienes	Resident, activated	appropriate soluble stimulus
Complement components		

granuloma. Continued stimulation leads to additional growth of the aggregated cells and further augmentation in secretory capacity; the phagocytes have now turned into epithelioid cells, the characteristic constituents of mature granulomas. Eventually, giant cells appear, arising through the fusion of epithelioid cells with each other and with newly arrived macrophages. With the elimination of the inciting agent, the inflammatory process resolves and the macrophages disappear.

FUNCTIONS. Mononuclear phagocytes carry out three basic functions: secretion, ingestion, and interaction with lymphocytes.

Secretion. Mononuclear phagocytes secrete a large number of substances, some protein and others nonprotein in nature (Table 138–4). Lysozyme is secreted by mononuclear phagocytes regardless of their state of activation, but proteases active at neutral pH ("neutral proteases") are secreted only by activated cells. Activated cells also produce interleukin 8, a neutrophil chemotaxin. Other substances such as O_2^- and leukotrienes are secreted under even more specialized circumstances.

Ingestion. Mononuclear phagocytes (see Color Plate *6F*, left) eat for two purposes: to eliminate waste and debris (scavenging) and to kill invading pathogens.

Scavenging. Mononuclear phagocytes play a highly important role as general scavengers. They dispose of worn-out cells, remove foreign material from the bloodstream, and clean up debris at sites of infection or tissue damage.

Cell disposal by mononuclear phagocytes is best exemplified by the elimination of outdated red cells. Old red cells develop a "senescence antigen" that is recognized by an opsonizing antibody in the circulation. The opsonized cells are then removed by splenic macrophages, which eliminate them by phagocytosis, degranulation, and digestion (cf. neutrophils). Hemoglobin is degraded by lysosomal proteases and other enzymes, while the lipids and complex carbohydrates of the red cell membrane are broken down by lysosomal lipases and glycosidases. Other effete cells are presumably dealt with in a similar manner.

Foreign material is removed from the bloodstream chiefly in the liver and spleen. In these two organs, the blood is forced to pass through a dense network of mononuclear phagocytes, which ingest foreign matter encountered in the flow. Bacteria and bacterial breakdown products (e.g., lipopolysaccharide) that enter the bloodstream from the large intestine are removed principally by the Kupffer cells of the liver, because these are the first mononuclear phagocytes encountered by the gastrointestinal venous drainage.

Dead cells and tissue fragments at sites of infection or injury are disposed of by macrophages recruited to the damaged area. Ingestion may be aided by circulating fibronectin, which opsonizes denatured collagen for phagocytosis by macrophages. The activated macrophages also secrete neutral proteases that break down damaged connective tissue (collagenase, elastase) and fibrin mesh (plasminogen activator), clearing the way for the reconstruction of injured tissues.

Mononuclear phagocytes also eliminate from the circulation denatured proteins, protein fragments, and certain native proteins (e.g., activated clotting factors). Some proteins are eliminated through *pinocytosis*, a process in which the material to be eliminated is taken into the cell along with a minuscule quantity of plasma via a tiny invagination of the cell membrane that buds off and enters the cytoplasm as a pinocytotic vesicle. (Mononuclear phagocytes are constantly engaged in pinocytosis; they take in and process several times their own volume of plasma every day.) Other proteins are eliminated by *receptor-mediated endocytosis*, a process similar to pinocytosis except that the ingested protein is bound to a surface receptor before internalization. The lipids of atherosclerotic lesions are derived in part from lipopro-

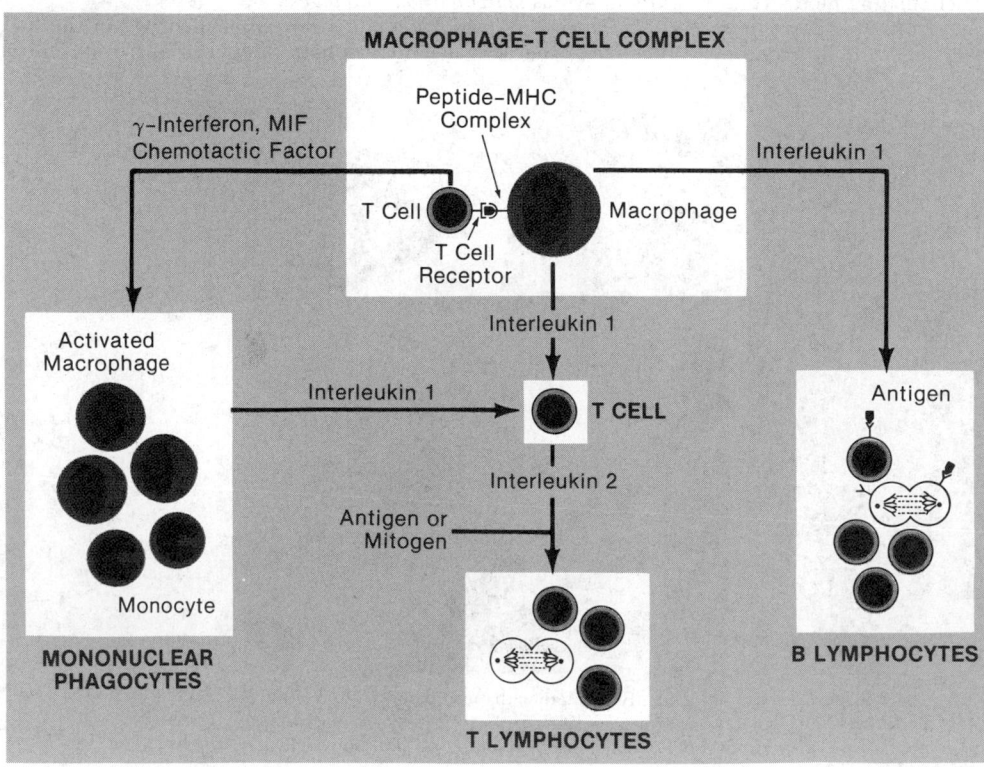

FIGURE 138–8. Macrophage-lymphocyte interactions. The macrophage, acting in its capacity as an "accessory cell," presents a peptide to a T cell equipped with specific receptors that recognize the complex between the peptide and a class II MHC molecule on the macrophage surface. The T cell to which the antigen has been presented undergoes activation and begins to secrete lymphokines. These lymphokines include γ-interferon, macrophage-immobilizing factor (MIF), and monocyte chemotactic factor; they cause macrophages to accumulate and undergo activation at the site of the initial macrophage–T cell interaction. Macrophages so activated secrete interleukin 1, a potent mediator capable, among other things, of inducing the proliferation of both B and T cells. B cells are directly stimulated by interleukin 1 to proliferate and to differentiate into antibody-secreting plasma cells. T cells, however, proliferate under the influence of a mediator known as interleukin 2 (T cell growth factor), itself a T cell product; interleukin 1 promotes the proliferation of T cells indirectly by inducing them to secrete interleukin 2.

TABLE 138–5. INTRACELLULAR PATHOGENS AGAINST WHICH MACROPHAGES PLAY A SPECIAL ROLE

Bacteria	*Chlamydia*
Brucella	*Rickettsia*
Listeria	Protozoan parasites
Legionella	*Leishmania*
Salmonella	*Trypanosoma*
Mycobacteria and systemic fungi	*Toxoplasma*
Coccidioides immitis	
Histoplasma capsulatum	
Mycobacterium tuberculosis	
Others	

teins that had been taken into macrophages by receptor-mediated endocytosis.

Killing. Like neutrophils, mononuclear phagocytes can kill invading microorganisms. Killing by both types of phagocytes involves the same general sequence of events—an initial encounter between the phagocyte and the target microorganism, ingestion, and finally the destruction of the target—but the events differ in detail between the two cell types. Monocytes, for example, attach to three endothelial adhesion molecules. *ICAM-1, ELAM-1,* and *VCAM-1* (vascular cell adhesion molecule, which binds to *VLA-4,* a molecule found on monocytes but not neutrophils); neutrophils attach only to the first two. Neutrophils generally find their targets by migrating up a chemotactic gradient, while many mononuclear phagocytes (the fixed-tissue varieties, such as Kupffer cells and splenic macrophages) have their targets brought to them by the bloodstream. Those mononuclear phagocytes that find their targets by chemotaxis (e.g., monocytes) respond to a wider variety of attractants than neutrophils do. Monocytes, for instance, are attracted by lymphocyte-generated chemotactic factors that have no effect on neutrophils. With respect to ingestion, mononuclear phagocytes can take up particles opsonized by immunoglobulin E (IgE) as well as IgG; neutrophils will take up only the latter. Mononuclear phagocytes are also equipped with a mannose receptor that enables them to take up certain bacteria and other particles without the need for opsonization. With regard to microbial killing, mononuclear phagocytes lose their myeloperoxidase as they develop from monocytes into macrophages, so that oxygen-dependent killing by mature macrophages is accomplished by oxidants that can be generated in the absence of myeloperoxidase (e.g., hydroxyl radical).

Mononuclear phagocytes play a particularly important role in defending against nonviral pathogens that live and grow intracellularly (Table 138–5). For the destruction of these pathogens, macrophage activation is critical. The pathogens are readily killed by activated macrophages, but they are able to infect and multiply within unactivated macrophages, eventually killing them and spreading to infect fresh macrophages. Little is known about how the pathogens evade the microbicidal system of the unactivated macrophages.

Mononuclear phagocytes, particularly activated macrophages, are also able to kill malignant cells in vitro. The extent to which they perform this antitumor function in vivo is unknown.

Interactions Between Mononuclear Phagocytes and Lymphocytes. The activation of mononuclear phagocytes by gamma-interferon is one of a series of mutually potentiating interactions between mononuclear phagocytes and lymphocytes that take place at sites of inflammation (Fig. 138–8). Both T lymphocytes and B lymphocytes participate in these interactions.

The interaction with T lymphocytes begins with a special physical encounter between a T lymphocyte and a mononuclear phagocyte. When an antigen-bearing particle is ingested by a mononuclear phagocyte, the antigen is degraded to small peptides, some of which are transferred to the phagocyte surface bound to class II proteins of the major histocompatibility complex (MHC; the MHC controls immune responses to such challenges as foreign proteins, virally infected cells, and tissue allografts [see Ch. 250]). If a T lymphocyte bearing a suitable receptor should encounter this peptide-bearing mononuclear phagocyte, it will recognize the peptide-MHC complex and bind to the phagocyte, and both cells will begin to secrete immunologic mediators. In this interaction, the mononuclear phagocyte is referred to as an *accessory cell* and is said to have "presented" the antigen to the lymphocyte.

Immunologic mediators secreted by T lymphocytes (*lymphokines*) include gamma-interferon, macrophage inhibitory factor, and monocyte chemotactic factor. Their net effect is to cause the accumulation and activation of mononuclear phagocytes in the vicinity of the initial interaction between the peptide-bearing phagocyte and its complementary T lymphocyte. Mediators secreted by mononuclear phagocytes are known as *monokines.* One of these is *interleukin 1;* among its other effects (for a list, see Table 138–6), it stimulates the proliferation of T lymphocytes indirectly by causing them to secrete *interleukin 2,* a substance that promotes their own growth. Another monokine, *tumor necrosis factor,* causes many of the manifestations of endotoxin shock, and may be responsible for the weight loss seen in patients with chronic wasting illnesses, such as tuberculosis and certain forms of cancer.

Macrophages also act upon B lymphocytes. They are not needed for the presentation of antigen to B lymphocytes, because B lymphocytes carry surface immunoglobulins that directly recognize the antigens against which the cells are programmed. Rather, the macrophages exert their effects after the antigen-recognition step. They operate through interleukin 1, which helps the antigen-primed B lymphocytes proliferate and differentiate into antibody-secreting plasma cells.

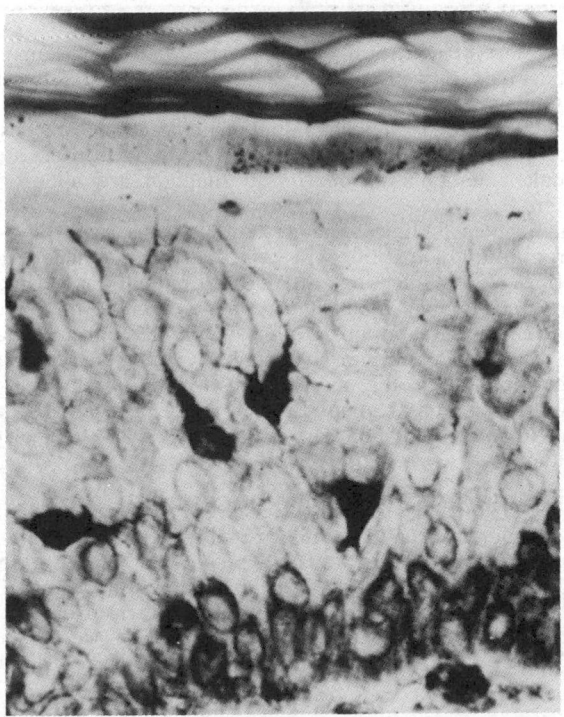

FIGURE 138–9. Langerhans cells in the skin. The darkly stained cells in the acanthocyte layer are the Langerhans cells. Their characteristic branching dendrites are easily seen. (Reproduced with permission from Breathnach AS, Wolff K: Structure and development of the skin. *In* Fitzpatrick TB, Eisen AZ, Wolff K, et al.: Dermatology in General Medicine. 2nd ed., p 56. Copyright © 1979 by McGraw-Hill, Inc. Used by permission of McGraw-Hill Book Company.)

TABLE 138–6. SOME ACTIONS OF INTERLEUKIN 1

Site of Action	Effect
T lymphocytes	Secretion of interleukin 2 (T cell growth factor)
B lymphocytes	Proliferation, secretion of immunoglobulins
Hepatocytes	Production of acute phase reactants
Hypothalamus	Fever
Muscle	Catabolism of protein

Dendritic Cells. Antigens are also presented by *dendritic cells.* These cells are found in the follicles of the lymph nodes and spleen, in the thymus, and in the skin, where they are known as *Langerhans' cells* (Fig. 138–9). Like mononuclear phagocytes, they carry class II MHC molecules on their surfaces but are thought to be incapable of phagocytosis. Their major role seems to be to present new antigens to the T lymphocytes.

Adams DO, Hamilton TA: The cell biology of macrophage activation. Annu Rev Immunol 2:283, 1984. *A complete and clearly written review of this sometimes confusing topic.*

Gallin JI, Goldstein IM, Synderman R (eds.): Inflammation: Basic Principles and Clinical Correlates. New York, Raven Press, 1988. *A multiauthor text providing comprehensive coverage of all aspects of inflammation.*

Ganz T, Selsted ME, Szklarnek D, et al.: Defensins. Natural peptide antibiotics of human neutrophils. J Clin Invest 76:1427, 1985. *The structure and properties of these recently discovered antimicrobial agents.*

Groopman JE, Molina J-M, Scadden DT: Hematopoietic growth factors. Biology and clinical applications. N Engl J Med 321:1449, 1989. *An up-to-date survey of this rapidly moving field.*

Murray HW: Interferon-gamma, the activated macrophage, and host defense against microbial challenge. Ann Intern Med 108:595, 1988. *A recent review of macrophage activation, emphasizing the role of gamma-interferon.*

Patarroyo M, Makgoba MW: Leucocyte adhesion to cells in immune and inflammatory responses. Lancet: 2:1139, 1989. *A succinct discussion of the leukocyte adhesion molecules.*

Steinman RM: Dendritic cells. Transplantation 31:151, 1981. *A short review of dendritic cell structure and function.*

Unanue ER, Cerottini J-C: Antigen presentation. FASEB J 3:2496, 1989. *Recent developments in this area, including current views of antigen processing.*

Williams GT, Williams WJ: Granulomatous inflammation: A review. J Clin Pathol 36:723, 1983. *An excellent review of the development and function of granuloma.*

139 Disorders of Neutrophil Function

Bernard M. Babior

Disorders of neutrophil function are relatively common. For the most part, they are minor manifestations of systemic diseases, rarely diagnosed and of little clinical significance. In a few disorders, however, defective neutrophil function leads to serious clinical problems. Most of these are inherited disorders in which particular elements of neutrophil function are almost totally deficient.

The principal clinical manifestation of a serious disorder of neutrophil function is the repeated occurrence of major bacterial infections. Such infections are most commonly associated with severe neutropenia (<500 neutrophils per cubic millimeter) or an abnormality of immunoglobulins or complement. Occasionally, however, repeated bacterial infections cannot be accounted for by abnormalities in the neutrophil count, the immunoglobulins, or the complement system. In such a case, a qualitative abnormality in neutrophil function is likely to be at the root of the problem.

EVALUATING NEUTROPHIL FUNCTION

A complete evaluation of neutrophil function, including motility, granule content and function, respiratory burst activity, and bacterial killing, requires a specialized laboratory. Screening for functional abnormalities, however, can be carried out relatively simply (Table 139–1). Morphologic abnormalities (see Color Plate 7D), such as the large malformed granules of Chédiak-Higashi

TABLE 139–1. SCREENING FOR ABNORMALITIES OF NEUTROPHIL FUNCTION

Examination of blood film
Rebuck skin window test
NBT test
Special stains: myeloperoxidase, alkaline phosphatase

TABLE 139–2. ACQUIRED ALTERATIONS OF NEUTROPHIL ADHESIVENESS

1. Decreased ashesiveness
   A. With demargination
      Corticosteroids
      Epinephrine
   B. Without demargination
      Aspirin
      Alcohol
2. Increased adhesiveness
   A. Bacteremia
   B. Hemodialysis

disease, can be detected by *examination of a blood film* under the microscope. Chemotaxis and locomotion can be estimated by a *Rebuck skin window,* a test that measures the migration of phagocytes onto a glass coverslip applied to a superficial abrasion. The respiratory burst is evaluated by the *NBT test,* in which cells are activated in the presence of nitroblue tetrazolium (NBT), a dye that forms a dark precipitate on any cell engaged in the production of O_2^- (superoxide). Neutrophil enzymes can be detected by *special stains for myeloperoxidase and alkaline phosphatase.* One or more of these tests are abnormal in most symptomatic disorders of neutrophil function.

ACQUIRED DISORDERS

In acquired disorders of neutrophils, functional abnormalities are generally incomplete. Accordingly, signs and symptoms caused by neutrophil dysfunction are uncommon in these conditions.

ADHESION (Table 139–2). Neutrophils undergo frequent alterations in adhesiveness, with resulting changes in the size of the marginated pool (see Ch. 138). *Corticosteroids* and *epinephrine* reduce neutrophil adhesiveness, releasing the cells from the marginated pool into the circulation. Conversely, C5a and agents that release C5a (e.g., gram-negative bacteremia) increase neutrophil adhesiveness, causing cells to aggregate into clumps. These tend to be trapped in small vessels, particularly in the lungs.

Besides corticosteroids and epinephrine, *aspirin* and *alcohol* cause decreased adhesiveness of neutrophils. With these agents the decrease in adhesiveness occurs in vitro but is not associated with demargination. Evidently, neutrophil adhesiveness covers a broader range of functions than merely the ability to attach to an endothelial cell.

In patients undergoing *hemodialysis,* neutrophil counts fall sharply, rising a few minutes later to values that exceed the predialysis counts. Pulmonary symptoms may accompany these changes in neutrophil counts. The fall in the neutrophil count and the accompanying pulmonary symptoms occur because C5a is released when the complement system is activated by the passage of blood over the dialysis membrane, causing neutrophils to marginate and be trapped in the lungs. The subsequent neutrophilia reflects the release of cells from the marrow storage pool.

CHEMOTAXIS. Depressed neutrophil chemotaxis is seen in a large number of conditions (Table 139–3). In some of these conditions, chemotactic depression is caused by a circulating inhibitor, while in others the neutrophils themselves are defective. These chemotactic abnormalities contribute in only a minor way to the decreased resistance to bacterial infections characteristic of many of these disorders.

TABLE 139–3. CONDITIONS ASSOCIATED WITH DEPRESSED NEUTROPHIL CHEMOTAXIS

Diabetes mellitus	Anergy
Uremia	Hodgkin's disease
Cirrhosis of liver	Leprosy
Severe burns	Sarcoidosis
Bacterial infections	Hypophosphatemia
	Neonates

Various functional abnormalities are seen in neutrophils from patients with these conditions. Cells in *chronic myelogenous leukemia* are very sluggish, showing markedly reduced motility and chemotaxis. Granules are often abnormal in number and type (specific granules, for example, may be absent), the respiratory burst is frequently attenuated, and bacterial killing may be depressed. These cells, however, make up in numbers what they lack in function, so infections are unusual in patients with chronic myelogenous leukemia.

In patients with *acute myelogenous leukemia*, neutrophils may arise from residual normal stem cells or by differentiation of the leukemic clone; in the latter case, the neutrophils may show abnormalities similar to those seen in chronic myelogenous leukemia. *Myelodysplasia* (see Color Plate 6*I* and *J*) is a disease in which hematopoiesis is taken over by a nonmalignant but defective stem cell that gives rise to inadequate numbers of functionally abnormal blood cells. Bilobed nuclei (pseudo Pelger-Huët anomaly) and abnormal granulation are typical of myelodysplastic neutrophils. In both acute myelogenous leukemia and myelodysplasia, bacterial infections are frequent, but their frequency is due more to neutropenia than to functional abnormalities of the phagocytes.

CONGENITAL DISORDERS

CHRONIC GRANULOMATOUS DISEASE. Chronic granulomatous disease (CGD) refers to a group of inherited disorders in which phagocytes cannot express a respiratory burst (Ch. 138). The disease is caused by a major defect in the O_2^--forming nicotinamide-adenine dinucleotide phosphate (NADPH) oxidase of phagocytes. The oxidase consists of several components, and different types of CGD occur when different components are defective. The most common type of CGD, affecting two thirds of patients, is due to a mutation in an X chromosomal gene encoding a protein that forms part of a membrane-associated cytochrome found only in leukocytes. Patients with this type of CGD lack the leukocyte cytochrome, and transmission of the disease is X linked. Most of the remaining patients lack a cytosolic oxidase-activating protein; in these patients, the leukocyte cytochrome is present, and CGD is transmitted as an autosomal recessive trait.

Clinical Picture. The clinical picture of CGD is one of recurrent, severe bacterial infections that are slow to heal and difficult to treat. The infections include sinusitis, pneumonia, and abscesses that usually involve the deep subcutaneous tissues, lymph nodes, or liver. Infections generally begin in infancy or early childhood, although the disease occasionally presents in adolescence or later. In its unmodified form, the course of CGD is characterized by frequent hospitalizations for repeated infections caused by bacteria that the defective phagocytes are unable to kill (mostly *Staphylococcus aureus* and enterobacteria), with death from infection in the first or second decade. With chronic antibiotic prophylaxis, however, the course of the disease has changed. Hospitalization is much less frequent, and survival seems to be prolonged, but patients develop serious complications owing to imperfectly suppressed infections—e.g., strictures of the bladder and gastrointestinal tract and chronic lung disease with fibrosis and bronchiectasis. Death often results from infections by fungi, particularly *Aspergillus*.

Diagnosis. The diagnosis is made by neutrophil function studies. Most of these are normal, but those that measure the respiratory burst are severely deranged: the NBT test is negative (Fig. 139–1), and O_2^- production and other manifestations of the respiratory burst are greatly reduced or absent. Many microorganisms are handled in a normal fashion by CGD neutrophils (including pneumococci and streptococci, accounting for the rarity of pneumococcal and streptococcal infections in patients with CGD), but those such as *S. aureus* or *Pseudomonas cepacia*, whose destruction is particularly dependent on oxidant production by phagocytes, are poorly killed by the defective cells. In CGD carriers the size of the respiratory burst is decreased by about half, so suspected carriers can often be identified by quantitation of the burst. Because carriers of X-linked CGD are mosaics, only a fraction of their neutrophils are able to make O_2^-; the NBT test stains only that fraction, leaving the rest of the cells unstained (Fig. 139–1).

A condition similar to CGD has been seen in a few patients with exceptionally severe *glucose-6-phosphate dehydrogenase (G6PD) deficiency*. G6PD is essential for the production of NADPH, the reducing agent used by the O_2^--forming oxidase. In neutrophils that are severely deficient in G6PD, the levels of NADPH may be so low that the O_2^--forming oxidase is starved for substrate, so the cells cannot express an adequate respiratory burst.

Treatment. Management of CGD consists of long-term antibiotic prophylaxis (trimethoprim-sulfamethoxazole at 5 to 10 mg

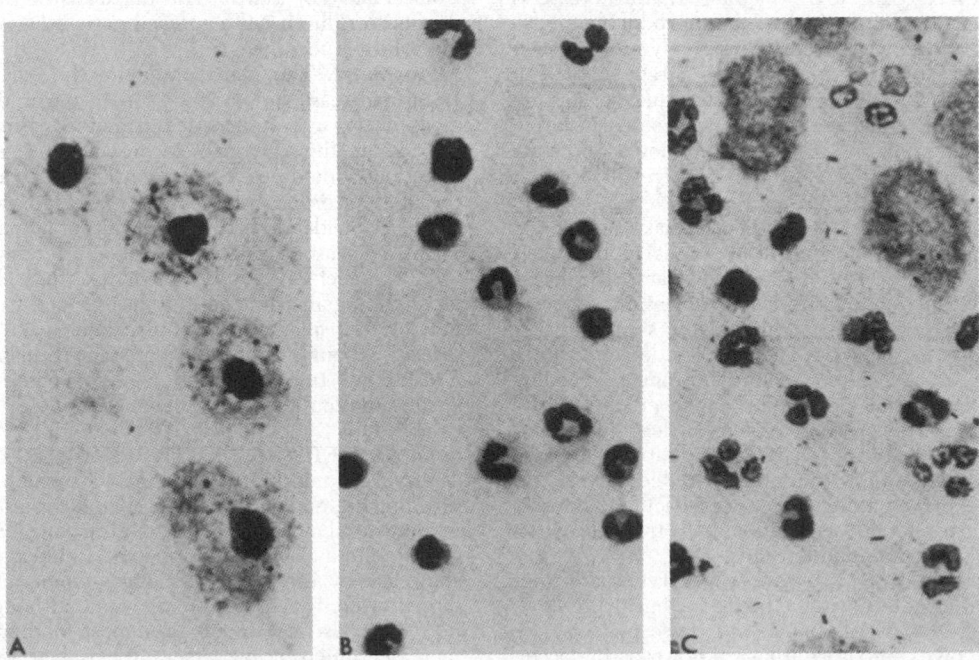

FIGURE 139–1. The NBT test in CGD. *A*, Normal. *B*, CGD. *C*, Carrier of X-linked CGD, showing an NBT-positive and an NBT-negative population of neutrophils. (From Babior BM, Crawley CA: Chronic granulomatous disease and other disorders of oxidative killing by phagocytes. *In* Stanbury JB, Wyngaarden JB, Fredrickson DS, et al. [eds.]: The Metabolic Basis of Inherited Disease. 5th ed., p 1972. Copyright © 1983 by McGraw-Hill Inc. Used by permission of McGraw-Hill Book Company.)

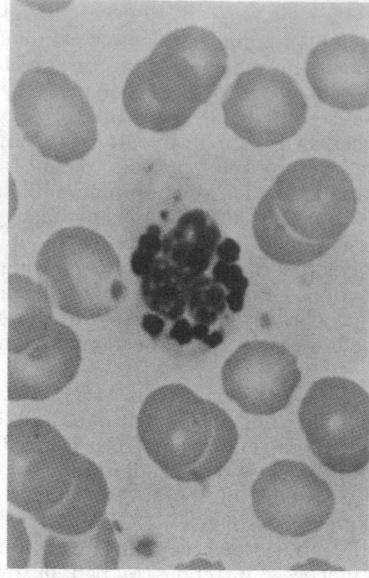 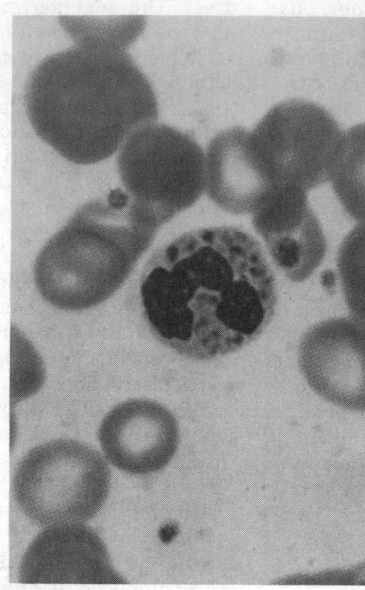

FIGURE 139–2. Neutrophils in Chédiak-Higashi disease, showing the giant granules that are the hallmark of the disease. *A*, A cell with unusually large and prominent granules. *B*, A more typical Chédiak-Higashi neutrophil. (Reprinted with permission from Miwa S, Watanabe Y [eds.]: Atlas of Blood Cells. 4th ed. Tokyo, Bunkodo Press, 1990.)

of trimethoprim per kilogram per day), long-term gamma-interferon (50 µg per square meter in adults or 1.5 µg per kilogram in children, given three times a week), and vigorous treatment of acute infections with antibiotics in adequate doses, plus surgery if indicated. Leukocyte transfusions may be helpful. Complications should be treated as conservatively as possible, although surgery may be required. Bone marrow transplantation has been performed in a few instances, but with its widely known hazards and the improvement in the outlook of CGD resulting from the use of long-term prophylaxis, marrow transplantation must be regarded as a last resort. Families of patients with CGD should be investigated to ascertain the mode of transmission of the disease, and genetic counseling should be offered to them. In pregnant carriers, CGD may be diagnosed prenatally through NBT tests of fetal blood or, in X-linked disease, through a restriction fragment length polymorphism in DNA obtained by amniocentesis or chorionic villus biopsy.

CHÉDIAK-HIGASHI DISEASE. Chédiak-Higashi disease is an autosomally inherited defect in lysosome production. Normally, these organelles are oval bodies of relatively uniform size, but in Chédiak-Higashi disease they are very irregular both in size and in shape, ranging from tiny spheres to huge, malformed bodies many times larger than normal. The molecular lesion responsible for Chédiak-Higashi disease is unknown, although there is some evidence that the condition may result from an abnormality in microtubule function.

Clinical Picture. The clinical features of Chédiak-Higashi disease result from the malfunction of three types of lysosome-containing cells: the melanocytes, the platelets, and the phagocytes. Melanocyte dysfunction leads to *partial albinism,* a uniform but incomplete loss of pigment from the irises, skin, and hair that can be detected even at birth. The platelet defect causes a mild *bleeding disorder* associated with a prolonged bleeding time. The most serious clinical problems, however, are caused by the abnormalities in the phagocytes. These lead to *marked lowering of resistance to bacterial infections,* so that patients with Chédiak-Higashi disease suffer from frequent deep tissue abscesses as well as recurrent attacks of severe bacterial sinusitis and pneumonia. These infections are difficult to treat and often lead to death in the first or second decade.

Patients with Chédiak-Higashi disease who survive into their teens or later are confronted with a further clinical problem, probably the most serious of all. In most of these patients, the disease ultimately evolves into a fatal form known as the accelerated phase. This is a peculiar lymphoma-like illness possibly caused by an out-of-control Epstein-Barr virus infection (see Ch. 373). The lymph nodes, liver, spleen, and bone marrow become infiltrated with small lymphocytes and histiocytes that look perfectly benign but behave in a malignant fashion, causing the infiltrated organs to enlarge and producing through marrow infiltration and splenomegaly a rapid, relentless, and ultimately fatal progression of the mild granulocytopenia seen in the stable phase of the disease. Death from pancytopenia generally occurs within a few months after the onset of the accelerated phase.

In Chédiak-Higashi disease, the white blood cell count is typically low (2000 to 3000 per cubic millimeter), a result of ineffective granulopoiesis. The low white cell count is an important factor in the low resistance to infection that characterizes this condition. Neutrophil chemotaxis and degranulation are depressed, but phagocytosis and the respiratory burst are normal. Bacterial killing is defective, probably because the abnormality in degranulation hinders the delivery of microbicidal substances into the phagocytic vesicles.

Diagnosis. The diagnosis is made by demonstrating giant granules in neutrophils and eosinophils, a feature that is virtually pathognomonic of Chédiak-Higashi disease (Fig. 139–2) (see Color Plate 7D, right). The diagnosis of the accelerated phase depends on finding the characteristic infiltrate in a biopsy of the involved tissue.

Treatment. The management of the early stage of Chédiak-Higashi disease amounts to the management of the infectious complications. Prophylactic antibiotics (trimethoprim-sulfamethoxazole at the dose given previously) should be used, and infections should be treated vigorously with appropriate antibiotic therapy. Ascorbic acid (20 mg per kilogram per day) has corrected the microbicidal defect in some but not all patients with Chédiak-Higashi disease. Treatment of the accelerated phase is unsatisfactory; splenectomy has been tried, as has chemotherapy with a variety of agents, but nothing has proved to be of much benefit. Marrow transplantation has also been used in Chédiak-Higashi disease, though the indications for transplantation (e.g., the question of transplantation in early childhood as opposed to transplantation for the accelerated phase) are not yet clearly established.

DISORDERS OF NEUTROPHIL MOTILITY (Table 139–4). There are a number of conditions in which recurrent abscesses or other bacterial infections occur because of severe impairment in neutrophil mobility. Neutrophils from affected patients migrate poorly onto a glass coverslip in the Rebuck skin window test and show grossly impaired chemotaxis when tested in vitro. These disorders are thought to be inherited, although evidence for their heritability is often weak. For most of them (e.g., congenitally increased microtubule assembly), only one or two cases have been reported. A few, however, have been seen in several patients. These are discussed here.

Hyper-IgE Syndrome. In this condition, reduced neutrophil motility is associated with bacterial respiratory tract infections and cold staphylococcal abscesses (i.e., abscesses lacking much

TABLE 139–4. DISORDERS OF NEUTROPHIL MOTILITY

Disorder	Distinguishing Features
Job's syndrome	Cold abscesses, eosinophilia, greatly increased IgE
Juvenile periodontitis	Early severe gingival inflammation, systemic infections only in occasional patients
Leukocyte glycoprotein deficiency	Omphalitis or other infections in newborn, delayed separation of umbilical stump, leukemoid reactions
Congenital absence of specific granules	Abnormal segmentation of nucleus, alkaline phosphatase decreased or absent

of the swelling and redness associated with inflammation), eosinophilia, and greatly increased levels of IgE. Patients characteristically have very high blood levels of an antistaphylococcal IgE antibody. Neutrophils from these patients show greatly reduced chemotaxis if assayed immediately after isolation, but chemotaxis returns to normal if the cells are stored for a few hours in the absence of serum prior to assay. The abnormalities in leukocyte function and IgE production may be related to a defect in gamma-interferon production by T cells from affected patients.

Juvenile Periodontitis. In this familial disease, neutrophils show a chemotactic defect that is thought to be caused by a serum abnormality. Serious gingival inflammation develops in late childhood or adolescence, similar to but more severe than that seen in normal middle-aged adults with poor dental hygiene. Affected individuals will often have lost many of their teeth by the time they are 30 years old. Among the organisms infecting the gums of such patients is *Capnocytophaga*, an anaerobic bacillus that secretes a potent inhibitor of neutrophil chemotaxis. The antichemotactic agent enters the bloodstream, where, in a few patients with juvenile peridontitis, it reaches concentrations that impair systemic host defenses and result in repeated bacterial infections. Elimination of the *Capnocytophaga* organisms by long-term administration of antibiotics and vigorous local therapy corrects the impairment in host defenses and normalizes the patient's resistance to bacterial infections.

Leukocyte Adhesion Deficiency. In this inherited disease, a chemotactic defect is caused by a defect involving the CD11/CD18 adhesion glycoproteins. The first indication of this condition may be delayed separation of the umbilical stump. Patients are subject to recurrent infections, particularly with *Pseudomonas*. The first infection may occur in the newborn as an omphalitis. Infections are generally accompanied by a neutrophilic leukemoid reaction in which the white count may exceed 100,000. The diagnosis can be made with commercially available anti-CD11/CD18 antibodies, which bind to normal but not glycoprotein-deficient white cells. Vigorous and prolonged therapy is necessary for successful treatment of infections in leukocyte adhesion deficiency. Prophylactic antibodies are indicated in this condition; they maintain the patient's health and keep the white cell count at normal or near-normal levels.

Congenital Absence of Specific Granules. In this disorder a chemotactic defect results in recurrent, severe bacterial infections. The neutrophils show abnormalities in nuclear segmentation, most frequently a grotesque bilobed nucleus, and stain poorly for alkaline phosphatase. Certain granule-associated proteins (e.g., defensins, cobalamin-binding protein) are absent, and bacterial killing is impaired. Under the electron microscope, the neutrophils show normal azurophil granules, but specific granules are rare or absent.

MYELOPEROXIDASE DEFICIENCY. Deficiency of myeloperoxidase (MPO) is the most common inherited disorder of neutrophil function. Transmitted as an autosomal recessive trait, it affects 1 person in ~2000. Once thought rare, its true incidence was revealed through automated white cell differential counters that rely on the peroxidase stain to identify neutrophils.

Clinically, MPO deficiency is almost completely silent. The most frequent problem is an increase in *Candida* infections in occasional MPO-deficient patients with coincident diabetes mellitus. The original misconception about the incidence of MPO deficiency can probably be explained by the low incidence of clinical disease in patients with this condition.

MPO-deficient neutrophils show characteristic functional abnormalities. Chemotaxis, phagocytosis, and degranulation are normal, but the respiratory burst is prolonged because of an increase in the lifespan of the O_2^--forming oxidase, which is normally destroyed by myeloperoxidase during the course of the respiratory burst. Bacterial killing by MPO-deficient cells is delayed but eventually reaches completion, indicating that the myeloperoxidase-independent oxidants generated by the deficient cells kill more slowly but just as effectively as the myeloperoxidase-dependent oxidants of normal cells. The completeness of bacterial killing by MPO-deficient cells contrasts with the extensive failure of bacterial killing in CGD, and it explains why bacterial infections are such a serious problem in the latter but not the former condition.

The diagnosis is made from a peroxidase stain of the blood film. The stain normally shows activity in neutrophils, monocytes, and eosinophils. In MPO deficiency the activity is missing from neutrophils and monocytes. Eosinophils, however, stain normally, since their peroxidase, which is different from myeloperoxidase, is not affected in myeloperoxidase deficiency. Peroxidase levels can be quantitated spectrophotometrically if desired, but this is usually unnecessary. Treatment is generally not required for MPO deficiency.

Babior BM, Woodman RC: Chronic granulomatous disease. Semin Hematol 27:247, 1990. *The latest on CGD and the respiratory burst oxidase.*

Boogaerts MA, Nelissen V, Roelant C, et al.: Blood neutrophil function in primary myelodysplastic syndromes. Br J Haematol 55:217, 1983. *A thorough study of neutrophil dysfunction in myelodysplasia.*

Curnutte JT (ed.): Phagocytic defects. Hematol/Oncol Clin North Am, 1988, Vols. 1 and 2. *A series of reviews on the inherited disorders of phagocytes.*

Donabedian H, Gallin JI: The hyperimmunoglobulin E recurrent infection (Job's) syndrome. A review of the NIH experience and the literature. Medicine 62:195, 1983. *A detailed clinical study of Job's syndrome.*

Lehrer RI, Ganz T: Antimicrobial polypeptides of human neutrophils. Blood 76:2169, 1990. *A recent and excellent review of this important but rarely discussed topic.*

Lomax KJ, Malech HL, Gallin JI: The molecular biology of selected phagocyte defects. Blood Rev 3:94, 1989. *A clearly written and up-to-date review of the molecular defects in several inherited disorders of phagocytes.*

140 Leukopenia

Grover C. Bagby, Jr.

The peripheral blood white cell count ranges from 5.0 to 10.0 $\times 10^9$ per liter in normal individuals. Circulating leukocytes consist of heterogeneous cell types (neutrophils, monocytes, basophils, eosinophils, and lymphocytes), each of which serves a unique purpose and each of which represents a different fractional component of the total peripheral leukocyte population. A rational discussion of leukopenia must therefore focus on specific leukocyte types. Nor can a normal white blood cell count ensure that substantial and serious deficiencies of leukocyte components do not exist. Patients may be severely neutropenic or lymphocytopenic despite total white blood counts that fall within the normal range. If there is a reason to order a white blood count, that reason is generally sufficient to justify performance of a differential count as well.

NEUTROPENIA

DEFINITION. Neutropenia exists when the peripheral neutrophil count is less than 2.0×10^9 per liter. Because the normal range in blacks and Yemenite Jews is somewhat lower, neutropenia in these populations is defined as counts less than 1.5×10^9 per liter. The role of the neutrophil in phagocytic defense of the host is generally met if the neutrophil count is above 1.0×10^9 per liter. If the neutrophil count drops below this number, particularly when the count falls below 0.5×10^9 per liter, the incidence of serious, recurrent, and difficult-to-treat infections rises markedly.

ETIOLOGY AND PATHOGENESIS. The multiple causes of neutropenia in pathophysiologic terms are best described in the context of the normal processes of neutrophil production and traffic. Such a description also simplifies the diagnostic and therapeutic approaches to patients with neutropenia. Neutrophils arise from a pool of marrow precursor cells through serial divisions and synchronous maturation steps (Fig. 140–1). The rate of neutrophil production is astonishingly high: more than 10^{11} cells per day. The bone marrow component of the neutrophil's life consists of a mitotic pool and a storage pool, the latter containing cells that no longer divide. Released after a few days in the bone marrow, neutrophils circulate freely for only a matter of hours before crawling into the extravascular space. For unknown reasons, half of the neutrophils in the peripheral blood are "marginated" along the endothelium and therefore are not measured in the white blood cell count. Accordingly, the true peripheral blood content of neutrophils, consisting of the circulating and the marginated pools, is ordinarily twice that measured by the neutrophil count (Fig. 140–1).

A simple etiologic classification of neutropenia can be derived from the three-compartment model, representing abnormalities in (1) the marrow compartment, (2) the peripheral blood compartment, (3) the extravascular compartment, or (4) combinations of the above (Fig. 140–2).

Abnormalities in the Marrow Compartment. Abnormalities in the marrow account for the majority of neutropenias in clinical practice. Failure of the marrow compartment can occur as a result of direct injury, in which case the marrow usually contains fewer than normal hematopoietic cells, or from maturation defects of hematopoietic cells, principally characterized by normal or increased numbers of morphologically abnormal hematopoietic cells. In either case, neutropenia most frequently occurs along with abnormalities in the number of platelets and red cells. Marrow injury can occur as a consequence of a variety of diseases (Fig. 140–2).

Drug-induced injury is most common (Table 140–1). Antineoplastic and immunosuppressive agents are generally *designed* to inflict injury on a proliferative population of cells; myelosuppressive toxicity is the rule but is generally predictable and dose related. Drugs that are well tolerated in the majority of patients, however, can induce either marrow injury or peripheral neutrophil destruction in certain patients. These drug-induced reactions can result from direct drug-mediated cytotoxicity or from an immune mechanism in which (1) neutrophils are destroyed in extramedullary sites (e.g., the penicillins) or (2) the marrow compartment is injured (e.g., procainamide, chloramphenicol, dapsone).

Radiation may result in acute self-limited and chronic marrow injury. Chronic radiation-induced injury can also result in the later development of myelodysplasia and nonlymphocytic leukemia, both of which often present with neutropenia. *Benzene* toxicity can also result in acute or chronic neutropenia and, like radiation-induced marrow failure, is associated with a high risk of acute nonlymphocytic leukemia.

Immune-mediated abnormalities may injure the marrow, either by autoantibody-mediated or by T lymphocyte–mediated mechanisms. Most patients with immune-mediated leukopenia have concurrent rheumatic or autoimmune diseases (see Color Plate 6L). *Infection* of the marrow per se is unusual and most often does not result in neutropenia; some exceptions include mycobacterial infection (especially those caused by *Mycobacterium tuberculosis* and *M. kansasii*) and certain viral infections.

Marrow invasion by abnormal cells can result in neutropenia. Carcinoma of the prostate, breast, stomach, and lung, as well as malignant hematopoietic disorders, can occupy enough of the medullary space to cause global marrow failure. Similarly, fibroblasts can proliferate in certain disease states to the extent that they dominate the marrow (Fig. 140–2).

Maturation arrest can result in bone marrow failure in the absence of granulopoietic hypocellularity. In *folate* and *vitamin* B_{12} *deficiency*, for example, the marrow is loaded with granulocyte precursors that, because of the effects of the deficiency states on nuclear replication, fail to mature normally and therefore suffer a high rate of intramedullary death (Ch. 132). The marrow is hypercellular, and hematopoiesis goes on actively, but this activity belies the inability of the marrow to deliver mature cells effectively—hence the term *ineffective hematopoiesis*. Certain congenital neutropenias also represent maturation abnormalities, as do the acute nonlymphocytic leukemias, myelodysplastic syndromes, and paroxysmal nocturnal hemoglobinuria.

Abnormalities in the Peripheral Blood Compartment. Perturbations of the peripheral blood compartment result from shifts in the circulating pool (Figs. 140–1 and 140–2). In *pseudoneutropenia*, neutrophil production and utilization are normal, but the size of the marginated pool is unusually large and substantially greater in size than the circulating pool. Patients with stable hereditary or constitutional pseudoneutropenia are not at increased risk of infection unless a neutrophil function abnormality coexists. Acquired pseudoneutropenia often occurs as an acute or subacute response to systemic infections. It is generally associated with acute changes in other compartments (Fig. 140–3) and

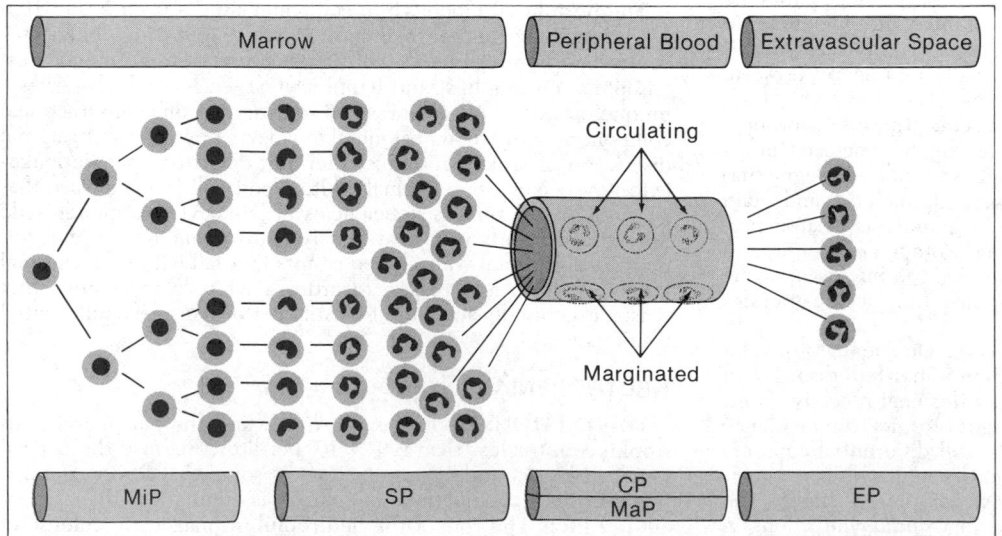

FIGURE 140–1. Production and distribution of neutrophils involve three compartments. Stem cells, committed progenitor cells, and morphologically recognizable precursor cells proliferate and mature (differentiate) under the influence of a variety of humoral regulatory factors, including GM-CSF (colony-stimulating factor) and G-CSF. These phenomena occur in the "mitotic pool" (MiP). Once the cells reach the intermediate maturation stage known as the metamyelocyte, they stop proliferating but continue differentiating to bands and segmented neutrophils. These cells, although capable of leaving the marrow if needed, generally spend about 5 days in the marrow, in the "storage pool" (SP). The neutrophils then enter the blood. Half of those cells in the blood circulate and can be measured in a blood sample by counting—the "circulating pool" (CP)—but the other half move about out of the main column of flowing blood, probably in close association with vascular endothelial cells. These latter cells are components of the "marginated pool" (MaP). After their brief sojourn in the peripheral blood, the neutrophils invade the extravascular compartments of most organs, where they either are utilized as defenders or garbage disposal systems or die within 1 or 2 days.

Marrow | Peripheral Blood | Extravascular Space

Circulating

Marginated

MiP | SP | CP / MaP | EP

THE CAUSES OF NEUTROPENIA

Marrow

ABNORMALITIES IN THE BONE MARROW COMPARTMENT

1. Bone Marrow Injury
   A. Drugs
      Cytotoxic and noncytotoxic agents
   B. Radiation
   C. Chemicals
      Benzene, DDT, dinitrophenol, arsenic, bismuth, nitrous oxide
   D. Certain congenital and hereditary neutropenias
   E. Immunologically mediated (largely seen in patients with rheumatic disorders)
      Cytotoxic T cell-mediated (T)
      Antibody-mediated (Ab)
      Mechanisms that require both T and Ab
   F. Infection
      Viral (hepatitis, parvovirus, AIDS)
      Bacterial (*M. tuberculosis, M. kansasii*)
   G. Bone marrow replacement (infiltrative diseases)
      Malignancies (lung, breast, prostate, stomach, lymphomas, and lymphoid leukemias)
      Fibrosis
      Agnogenic myeloid metaplasia
      Long-standing polycythemia vera
      Chronic myelogenous leukemia
      Radiation injury
      Injury from chronic cytotoxic drug therapy
      Acute megakaryocytic leukemia

2. Maturation Defects
   A. Acquired
      Folic acid deficiency
      Vitamin B_{12} deficiency
   B. Neoplastic and other clonal disorders
      Congenital neutropenias
      Acute nonlymphocytic leukemia
      Myelodysplastic syndromes
      Paroxysmal nocturnal hemoglobinuria

Peripheral Blood

ABNORMALITIES IN THE PERIPHERAL BLOOD COMPARTMENT

1. Shift of neutrophils from the circulating to the marginated pool (known as pseudoneutropenia)
   A. Hereditary or constitutional benign pseudoneutropenia
   B. Acquired
      Acute: Severe bacterial infection, frequently associated with endotoxemia
      Chronic: Protein-calorie malnutrition, malaria
2. Intravascular sequestration
   A. In lung (complement-mediated leukoagglutination)
   B. In spleen (hypersplenism)

Extravascular

ABNORMALITIES IN THE EXTRAVASCULAR COMPARTMENT

1. Increased utilization
   A. Severe bacterial, fungal, viral, or rickettsial infection
   B. Anaphylaxis

FIGURE 140–2. The causes of neutropenia have been arranged according to the compartment in which the abnormality usually resides. The approach to the neutropenic patient should begin by determining which of the three major compartments is likely at fault.

resolves when the infection is appropriately treated or spontaneously abates.

Demands of the Extravascular Compartment. Neutrophils and their precursors respond to infections in a highly coordinated and regulated fashion. The cellular responses are largely controlled by two granulopoietic factors, GM-CSF and G-CSF, and include (1) a rather prompt increase in the rate of production of neutrophils in the mitotic compartment, a response mediated by a complex network of cellular and humoral regulatory interactions, (2) the early release of neutrophils from the marrow storage pool to the peripheral blood pool, (3) an increase in the rate of neutrophil egress from the peripheral blood pool to the invaded tissue or tissues, and (4) increased phagocytic and bactericidal activity of the neutrophils. Rarely, increased demand for neutrophils in the extravascular compartment can lead to transient neutropenia, especially in patients with severe acute infections (Fig. 140–3). In such cases, the immediate demand for neutrophils completely utilizes the marrow storage pool before it can be restored by increased proliferative activity. The neutrophil count generally rises within a few days. The bone marrow is highly effective in responding to infectious events, so that the demand for neutrophils almost never exceeds the capacity of the mitotic pool to supply them. In contrast, neutrophil consumption in patients with autoimmune neutropenia and hypersplenism can

outstrip marrow production. Whether this reflects absence in such patients of the complete humoral stimulatory mechanisms that evolve in the infected host, or whether the rate of destruction in these patients actually exceeds the rate of utilization in patients with infections, is not known.

In summary, the causes of neutropenia are heterogeneous and best categorized in pathophysiologic terms (Fig. 140–3).

CLINICAL MANIFESTATIONS. Neutropenia can occur in a wide variety of systemic diseases (Fig. 140–2), the manifestations of which may dominate the clinical picture. Many neutropenic patients remain asymptomatic, most often those whose neutrophil count exceeds 1.0×10^9 per liter or those whose neutropenia is acute and self-limited in duration. When symptoms do occur, they generally result from recurrent, often severe, bacterial infections. This is not surprising in view of the pivotal importance of the neutrophil in the defense of the host against microorganisms (Ch. 138).

This risk of bacterial infection increases significantly as the peripheral neutrophil count falls below 1.0×10^9 per liter but is greatly increased at levels below 0.5×10^9 per liter. The degree to which monocytosis compensates for neutropenia may modify the risk. I have observed a patient with such severe congenital neutropenia that no neutrophil has ever been seen in her blood smears over an 18-year period. Her leukocyte count is, however,

TABLE 140–1. DRUGS THAT CAUSE NEUTROPENIA

Antiarrhythmics
  Procainamide, propranolol, quinidine
Antibiotics
  Chloramphenicol, penicillins, sulfonamides, trimethoprim-methoxa-
    zole, para-aminosalicylic acid (PAS), rifampin, vancomycin, isonia-
    zid, nitrofurantoin
Antimalarials
  Dapsone, quinine, pyrimethamine
Anticonvulsants
  Phenytoin, mephenytoin, trimethadione, ethosuximide, carbamaze-
    pine
Hypoglycemic agents
  Tolbutamide, chlorpropamide
Antihistamines
  Cimetidine, brompheniramine, tripelennamine
Antihypertensives
  Methyldopa, captopril
Anti-inflammatory agents
  Aminopyrine, phenylbutazone, gold salts, ibuprofen, indomethacin
Antithyroid agents
  Propylthiouracil, methimazole, thiouracil
Diuretics
  Acetazolamide, hydrochlorothiazide, chlorthalidone
Phenothiazines
  Chlorpromazine, promazine, prochlorperazine
Immunosuppressive agents
  Antimetabolites
Cytotoxic agents
  Alkylating agents, antimetabolites, anthracyclines, vinca alkaloids,
    cis-platinum, hydroxyurea, actinomycin D
Other agents
  Recombinant alpha- and gamma-interferon, allopurinol, ethanol, lev-
    amisole, penicillamine

normal because of marked monocytosis; the frequency of infections in this patient has been low.

Lungs, genitourinary system, oropharynx, and skin are the most frequent sites of infection in neutropenic patients. The infecting organisms are the expected pathogens for the given anatomic site. In patients who have recurrent infections and require prolonged and recurrent antibacterial therapy, unusual

organisms can colonize and subsequently cause infection. The antibiotic history of infected neutropenic patients is important to obtain. *The usual signs and symptoms of infection are often diminished or absent in patients with neutropenia because the cell that mediates much of the inflammatory response to infection is absent.* Thus, neutropenic patients with severe bilateral bacterial pneumonia can present with minimal infiltrates demonstrable by the chest radiograph and nonpurulent sputum; patients with pyelonephritis may not exhibit pyuria; patients with bacterial pharyngitis may not have purulence in the oropharynx; and patients with severe bacterial infection of the skin may present only with erythroderma rather than furunculosis. In the neutropenic patient, infections that in an otherwise normal individual might have been well localized become quickly disseminated. Therefore, not only is the infected neutropenic patient a diagnostic problem but, in addition, because any given infection is more apt to be widespread at the time of diagnosis, these patients are often dangerously ill.

DIAGNOSIS. The diagnostic evaluation of neutropenia is influenced by its severity and the clinical setting in which it occurs. The assessment of patients with neutrophil counts of less than 0.5 to 1.0 $\times 10^9$ per liter should obviously proceed briskly. The patient with fever, sepsis, or both, in whom neutropenia is discovered for the first time, presents a particularly difficult problem. In such patients it is impossible to determine immediately whether the neutropenia antedated sepsis, a situation with both prognostic and therapeutic implications, or whether the neutropenia is merely a short-lived response to the infection itself (Fig. 140–3). Examination of the peripheral blood smear and differential white blood count can be helpful in such cases. If the blood film has been prepared promptly after obtaining the sample, vacuolization of neutrophil cytoplasm suggests the presence of bacterial infection. An increase in the fraction of circulating band forms to levels above 20 per cent suggests that marrow granulopoietic activity is responding appropriately (Fig. 140–4). It is then presumed either that the marrow is recovering from injury or that the neutropenia is derived from a transient shift to the marginated pool or to the extravascular compartment.

The diagnostic evaluation of neutropenia must first address the question of the severity of the disorder and then whether the patient has fever, sepsis, or both. The patient with sepsis and severe neutropenia should be treated promptly with intravenous antibiotics following appropriate cultures, but *without waiting* for the results of those cultures. Once these important initial questions are answered, the remainder of the diagnostic evaluation

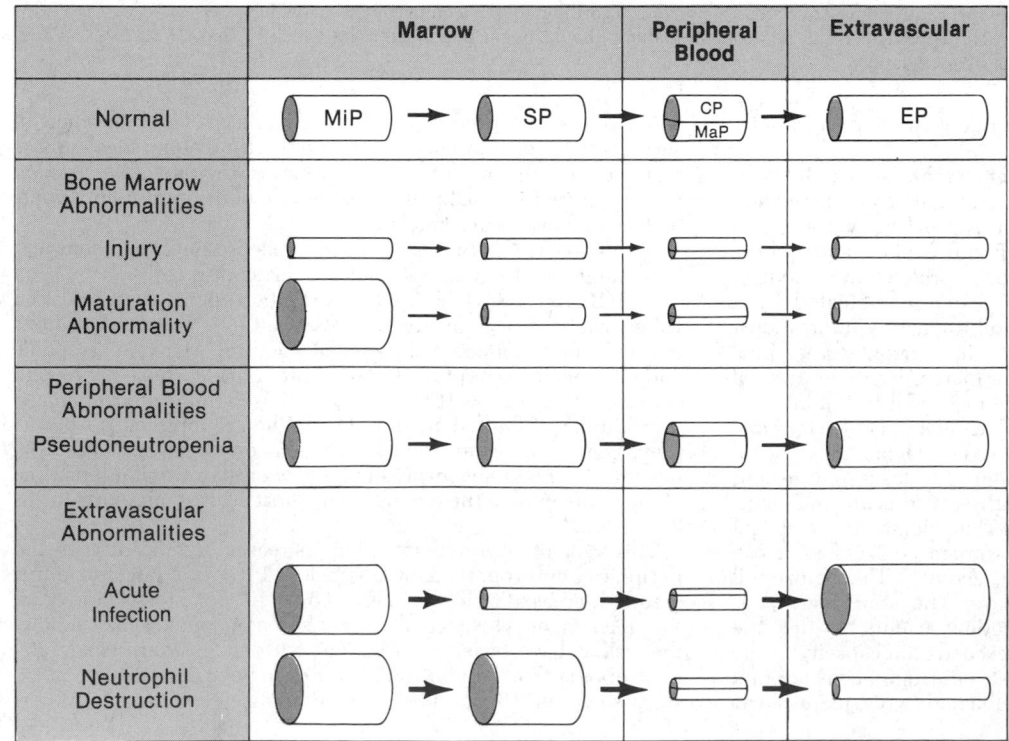

	Marrow		Peripheral Blood		Extravascular
Normal	MiP →	SP →	CP / MaP →		EP
Bone Marrow Abnormalities					
Injury					
Maturation Abnormality					
Peripheral Blood Abnormalities					
Pseudoneutropenia					
Extravascular Abnormalities					
Acute Infection					
Neutrophil Destruction					

FIGURE 140–3. Pathophysiologic mechanisms of neutropenia. The size of a given compartment is represented by the size of the corresponding cylinder. The number of cells leaving a compartment for the next compartment can vary substantially, but flow between compartments is unidirectional. Notice that in every case the circulating neutrophil pool is small, but the size of the other pools is variable. In marrow injury there is a global decline in the size of all pools. A maturation abnormality, however, is characterized by an increase in the number of precursor cells that do not mature. Pseudoneutropenia is characterized by a movement of circulating neutrophils to the marginated pool. In severe infections the acute demand for neutrophils in the infected extravascular site results in a transient loss of storage pool neutrophils before the hypercellular (but as yet immature) mitotic compartments can renew the storage pool. Finally, excessive destruction of neutrophils can result in neutropenia. MiP = mitotic pool; SP = storage pool; CP = circulating pool; MaP = marginated pool; EP = extravascular pool.

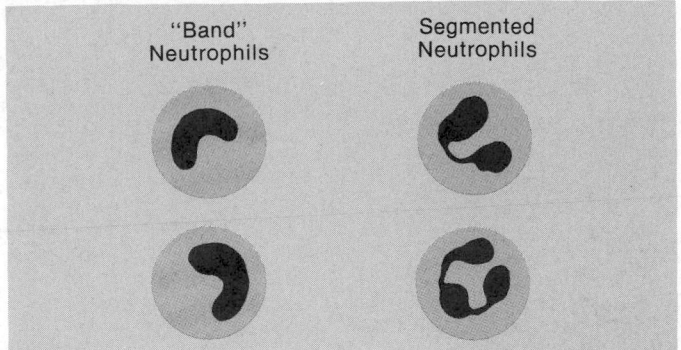

FIGURE 140–4. Band neutrophils are somewhat "younger" forms than segmented neutrophils. The nuclear lobes in a segmented form are separated by fine filaments absent in the band.

can proceed (Fig. 140–5): (1) identifying any potential drugs and toxins to which the patient might have been exposed; (2) determining, if possible, the chronicity of the neutropenia; (3) ascertaining whether there have been recurrent infections; (4) identifying any underlying systemic disease that might be causative; and (5) examining the blood counts and blood morphology and bone marrow (the latter is usually indicated) to determine the most likely pathophysiologic explanation. The latter is important even if a specific, likely causative, underlying disease is promptly identified. Felty's syndrome, for example, is a well-recognized cause of neutropenia, but there are at least two separate pathophysiologic mechanisms in groups of these patients, one mediated by antineutrophil antibodies, the other by T lymphocyte–mediated bone marrow failure. Each mechanism has different therapeutic implications.

One approach to the neutropenic patient is shown in algorithmic form in Figure 140–5. Once the severity of the neutropenia is determined, careful examination of the peripheral blood counts and blood smear is in order. Patients with selective neutropenia are approached differently from those with additional deficiencies of platelets and red cells, although drugs or toxins may be involved in either category. Patients with selective neutropenia but with no drug or toxin exposure, no history of recurrent sepsis, and no underlying chronic inflammatory or autoimmune disease may have stable and benign neutropenia. This category includes some cases of familial and congenital neutropenia and pseudoneutropenia. Any patient with selective neutropenia with a history of sepsis or toxin exposure should have a bone marrow examination to assess (1) the degree of cellularity of each compartment (storage and mitotic pools), (2) the distribution of differentiation stages found in each pool, and (3) whether any morphologic abnormality exists in the hematopoietic cells.

In patients with pancytopenia or bicytopenia, bone marrow examination, which must include not only aspiration but biopsy as well, is almost always indicated. The only regular exception to this rule would include patients with unambiguous evidence of vitamin B_{12} or folate deficiency (Ch. 132).

TREATMENT. Rational treatment of the neutropenic patient follows diagnosis and generally involves treatment of the underlying disease or discontinuation of suspected toxins or drugs. The nature of the specific therapy naturally depends on the pathophysiology of the neutropenia in a given patient.

Treatments Specifically Designed to Increase the Neutrophil Count. Trials of the few agents available for the purpose of increasing the neutrophil count must be considered only in patients with severe neutropenia and a history of infections and should be attempted only after the potential risks involved are explained to the patient.

Lithium carbonate, an agent that increases the neutrophil production rate in normal individuals, rarely has been effective in the management of chronic bone marrow failure. The dose used in adults is 300 mg by mouth three times daily. In view of the frequency of toxicity, trials of therapy should be considered only as a last resort. No test to predict individual responsiveness has yet been developed.

Immunosuppressive therapy, including glucocorticoids or azathioprine, almost always elicits a favorable response in patients with marrow failure mediated by cytotoxic T lymphocytes. In vitro clonogenic cultures of bone marrow cells in severely neutropenic patients can aid in the identification of patients apt to respond to such therapy. Some responses to immunosuppressive therapy have also occurred in patients whose neutropenia resulted from antineutrophil antibodies. Splenectomy is rarely helpful in the management of neutropenic patients, even those with Felty's syndrome. It is now reserved for patients with unambiguous hypersplenism in whom bone marrow function is normal.

Recombinant Human Granulopoietic Factors. The genes of many hematopoietic growth factors have been cloned, their sequences reported, and the biologic activities of the proteins encoded by them characterized in humans. Some of these recombinant proteins, including GM-CSF (colony-stimulating factor, granulocyte and macrophage) and G-CSF (colony-stimulating factor, granulocyte), are now in clinical trials for management of bone marrow failure. Both GM-CSF and G-CSF induce neutrophilic leukocytosis; GM-CSF also induces the appearance of eosinophils. GM-CSF and G-CSF have many similar therapeutic effects, but there are some differences. (1) Used in high doses, some GM-CSF preparations may induce fever and local thrombophlebitis (in the vein of administration) more frequently than does G-CSF. (2) G-CSF is effective in the treatment of children and adults with cyclic neutropenia and of children with severe congenital agranulocytosis. These growth factors have recently been approved by the Food and Drug Administration for use in selected clinical settings. However, they will probably be beneficial in the management of patients with neutropenia in specific clinical settings such as bone marrow transplantation. These clinical settings have yet to be defined completely. An important unresolved issue is the theoretical potential of these factors to worsen the underlying disease. Some in vitro models, for example, predict that therapy with certain recombinant granulopoietic factors might hasten the development of leukemia in selected types of myelodysplasia and may stimulate the growth of certain cancer cells. GM-CSF by itself might possibly induce the release of HIV-1 from latently infected cells, but in combination therapy GM-CSF enhances the net anti-HIV effect of azidothymidine. Recombinant granulopoietic factors can undoubtedly play an important therapeutic role in the near future, but the underlying cause of the neutropenia must be taken into account to ensure that short-term benefits are not ultimately complicated by acceleration of the primary disease process.

Bone Marrow Transplantation. In severe aplastic anemia the role of bone marrow transplantation is well established (Ch. 153). Other marrow failure states (e.g., myelodysplastic syndromes and congenital neutropenias) may also prove to respond to transplantation. Allogeneic transplantation is associated with high mortality; its use in patients with selective neutropenia is therefore uncertain. Before transplantation is seriously considered, the duration and severity of the neutropenia must be assessed; marrow failure must be established as the primary cause; and immunologically mediated marrow failure should be ruled out. If the patient has an identical twin, transplantation might be attempted with fewer constraints, but allogeneic transplantation should always be reserved for individuals with severe and symptomatic neutropenia caused by marrow failure.

Treatment of the Infected Neutropenic Patient. Each patient with neutropenia should understand the function of neutrophils, the consequences of neutrophil deficiency, and the importance of communicating with his or her physician the moment signs and symptoms of infection occur. If a neutropenic patient is afebrile and there is no sepsis, the diagnostic workup should generally take place in the outpatient clinic to avoid unnecessary exposure to nosocomial infections. Patients with severe neutropenia and fever, however, should be hospitalized. Cultures of urine, blood, and other relevant sites should be obtained, but broad-spectrum antibiotics should be given without waiting for the results of these cultures. One of three responses will be seen. (1) A causative organism will be identified, in which case the spectrum of antimicrobial agents can be appropriately narrowed.

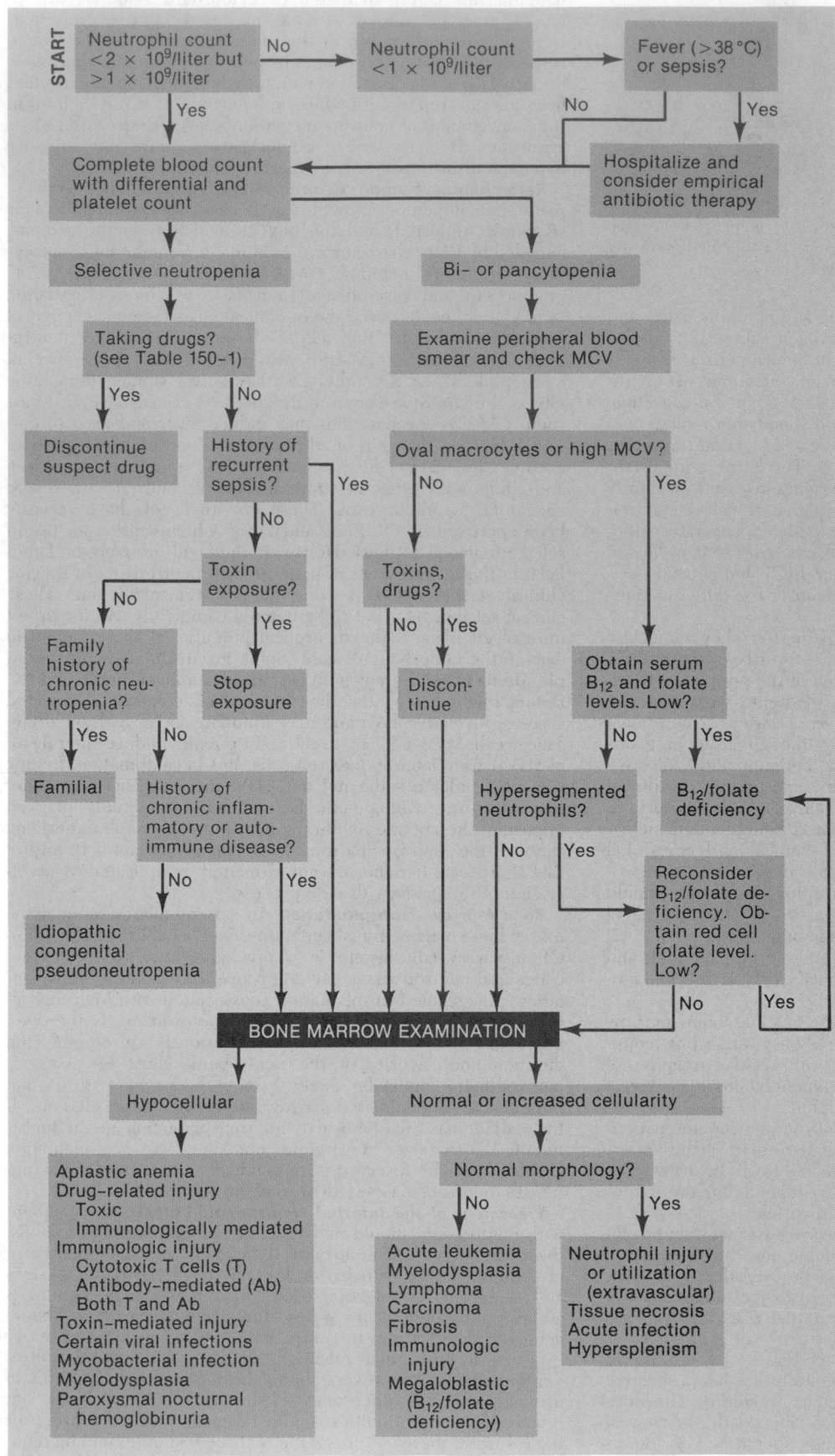

FIGURE 140–5. An algorithm for the evaluation of patients with neutropenia.

(2) A candidate organism will not be found, but the patient still improves with empiric therapy. In this type of setting a full course of broad-spectrum antibiotics should be given. Moreover, after a full course of parenteral antibiotics has been given, another 7 to 14 days of oral antibiotics should be considered, especially in patients with invasive infections associated with necrosis, in those whose initial response was slow, or in those with infections that have recurred in the same anatomic site. (3) No organism is found, and the clinical picture is not altered after 3 days of empiric treatment. This unsettling situation occurs with some regularity in practice. The approach to a patient at this point depends on the seriousness of the infection. For a patient with localized disease who is not critically ill, it is sometimes helpful for empiric therapy to be discontinued and for repeat cultures to be obtained. If the patient is critically ill, however, antibiotics should be discontinued *only* if other antibiotics are substituted. Among those antibiotics to consider in this situation is amphotericin B. Amphotericin B should be strongly considered for the therapeutic regimen in certain clinical settings, i.e., for patients with acute leukemia, diabetes, dysphagia and/or esophagitis, endophthalmitis, or defective cell-mediated immunity (including those receiving immunosuppressive therapy) and for those who have received prolonged treatment with broad-spectrum antibacterial agents in the recent past.

Neutrophil transfusions, when used specifically for the treatment of seriously infected neutropenic patients, are capable of providing enough phagocytes to make a difference in the course of some infections. They should not, however, be used prophylactically in uninfected neutropenic patients. Neutrophils survive briefly in the peripheral circulation and tissues, so that they must be given at least daily, probably for at least 3 days. The decision to use neutrophil transfusions is not a trivial one. White cells for transfusion are expensive, and if preformed antibodies exist in the recipient, a number of transfusion reactions can occur, including fever, chills, myalgia, and acute dyspnea with or without transient bilateral pulmonary infiltration. These same clinical manifestations can also result from invasion of the sites of infection by the transfused neutrophils and their subsequent release of mediators of inflammation that have hitherto been absent in the infected patient. In the absence of clear-cut signs of hypersensitivity (e.g., urticaria), therefore, one cannot be sure whether the infection is being better controlled or whether the transfused cells are being destroyed. For this reason, a decision to discontinue neutrophil transfusions cannot be made on the grounds that such reactions have occurred. Each patient's adverse response must be approached individually.

DEFICIENCIES OF OTHER CIRCULATING PHAGOCYTES

Monocytopenia, eosinopenia, and basophilopenia are seen in most of the bone marrow failure states associated with neutropenia. Selective *monocytopenia*, however, is very unusual. In view of the heterogeneous and critical roles played by the monocyte-macrophage in normal physiology (Ch. 138), complete failure of monocyte production for a period of more than 9 to 10 months (the estimated lifespan of tissue macrophages) may be incompatible with life.

Eosinopenia and *basophilopenia* are more common than monocytopenia in clinical practice and most often represent redistributional mechanisms resulting from stress, including acute infections, widespread neoplasms, and severe injury (e.g., burns). A variety of humoral factors, including glucocorticoids, prostaglandins, and epinephrine, are released in such settings and are known to induce eosinopenia. In view of the consistency of this stress response, if a patient with sepsis does not have eosinopenia, one should consider that adrenocortical insufficiency or a primary myeloproliferative syndrome may coexist.

LYMPHOCYTOPENIA. The life cycle of the neutrophil involves a well-defined and limited set of compartments and a unidirectional flow of cells from the marrow to the blood and from the blood to the tissues. Lymphocyte production and traffic are difficult to assess: (1) Both T and B lymphocytes replicate in heterogeneous anatomic sites, including the lymph nodes, spleen, tonsils, and bone marrow; (2) lymphocytes are capable of leaving and then later re-entering a given compartment. Given these variables, it is surprising that the lymphocyte counts in the

peripheral blood are so tightly regulated; normal counts range from 2 to 4 × 10^9 per liter. Approximately 20 per cent of these are B lymphocytes, and 70 per cent are T lymphocytes. Lymphocytopenia is defined as a peripheral blood lymphocyte count below 1.5 × 10^9 per liter.

ETIOLOGY AND PATHOGENESIS. Lymphocytopenia can result from three types of abnormalities: (1) those of lymphocyte production, (2) those of lymphocyte traffic, and (3) those of lymphocyte loss and destruction (Table 140–2).

Reduced Production of Lymphocytes. The most common cause of reduced lymphocyte production in the world is *protein-calorie malnutrition* (Ch. 201). The immunologic paresis resulting from malnutrition contributes substantially to the high incidence of infection in malnourished populations. *Radiation* and *immunosuppressive agents*, including alkylating agents and antithymocyte globulin, can induce lymphocytopenia by injuring the progenitor pool and inhibiting replication of more well differentiated cells. A variety of *congenital lymphocytopenic immunodeficiency states* exist, some of which result in selective deficiencies of B lymphocytes, some of T cells, and, in other cases, combined deficiencies of both T cells and B cells (Ch. 244). The mechanisms by which production and maturation of B and T lymphocytes are impaired in these patients are heterogeneous; many are ill defined. Immunodeficiency states can clearly exist even in the absence of lymphocytopenia, because of abnormal lymphocyte function or selective deficiency of one component of the circulating lymphocyte population. Certain *viruses* are capable of inducing lymphocytopenia; some of these agents infect lymphoid cells and cause their destruction. Such viruses include measles, polio, varicella zoster, and HIV (human immunodeficiency virus, the acquired immunodeficiency syndrome [AIDS] virus) (Part XXI). HIV does not frequently cause lymphocytopenia but does infect the helper (T4$^+$) subset of T lymphocytes and destroys them, a process that results in a marked decline in the absolute numbers of helper (T4$^+$) T cells in the peripheral circulation. Patients with untreated Hodgkin's disease occasionally have lymphocytopenia, especially during the late stages of the disease and with the least favorable histologic subtypes (Ch. 148).

Alterations in Lymphocyte Traffic. Alterations are common and most frequently represent transient responses to a variety of stressful events, including bacterial infections and trauma. These responses are likely mediated by high levels of endogenous glucocorticoids that induce rapid declines in circulating levels of B and T lymphocytes. The lymphocytopenic response to this type of steroid results from a self-limited shift of lymphocytes away from the peripheral blood compartment. Lymphocyte values generally return to normal within 24 to 48 hours. For this reason, the transient declines induced by endogenous steroid production

TABLE 140–2. CAUSES OF LYMPHOCYTOPENIA

Abnormalities of lymphocyte production
  Protein-calorie malnutrition
  Radiation
  Immunosuppressive therapeutic agents
  Congenital immunodeficiency states
    Wiskott-Aldrich syndrome
    Nezelof's syndrome
    Adenosine deaminase deficiency
  Viral infections
  Hodgkin's lymphoma (?)
  Widespread granulomatous infection (mycobacterial, fungal)
Alterations in lymphocyte traffic
  Acute bacterial infection, trauma, stress, glucocorticoids
  Viral infection
  Widespread granulomatous infection
  Hodgkin's lymphoma (?)
Lymphocyte destruction or loss
  Viral infection
  Antibody-mediated lymphocyte destruction
  Protein-losing enteropathy
  Chronic right ventricular failure
  Thoracic duct drainage or rupture

are not associated with functional immunologic deficiency. Certain viruses can also bind to lymphocyte populations and cause their departure from the blood compartment into other sites.

More persistent lymphocytopenia has been described in patients with widespread granulomatous disease, a phenomenon that is likely multifactorial, deriving from both inhibition of production and alterations of traffic. Patients with these disorders are often difficult to treat. Establishing a cause-and-effect relationship between the infection and lymphocytopenia is difficult when one considers that the reverse might just as easily be true; consider, for example, the frequency of mycobacterial infection in patients with AIDS.

Increased Destruction of Lymphocytes. Lymphocytopenia can occur as a result of *viral infection*, as outlined above. In some patients lymphocytopenia results from *antilymphocyte antibodies*. As was the case in patients with immunologically mediated neutropenia, the majority of such individuals have underlying autoimmune or rheumatic diseases. Losses of viable lymphocytes can also occur because of *structural defects* in sites of high-density lymphocyte traffic, e.g., via thoracic duct fistulas. In such patients, both T cells and B cells decline in the peripheral blood. Loss of lymphocytes from intestinal lymphatics can occur in protein-losing enteropathies, severe congestive heart failure, or primary diseases of the gut or intestinal lymphatics (Table 140–2).

CLINICAL MANIFESTATIONS AND DIAGNOSIS. There are no specific clinical manifestations of lymphocytopenia per se. The signs and symptoms present in patients with lymphocytopenia are those characteristic of the disease with which the cytopenia is associated. Whether the patient exhibits signs of immunologic deficiency depends on the pathophysiology of the disorder, the duration of the disease, which subsets of lymphocytes are affected most significantly, and the degree to which cellular or humoral immunity is functionally perturbed. Accordingly, unless the clinical setting is clearly one in which transient lymphocytopenia is likely, the approach to diagnosis should involve comprehensive assessment of the integrity of the immune apparatus. Specifically, the subsets of lymphocytes remaining in the circulating blood should be identified and should at least include B cells, helper-inducer T cells, and cytotoxic-suppressor T cells. In addition, quantitative immunoglobulin levels should be measured in the serum, and a series of skin tests performed to detect deficiencies of cell-mediated immunity.

TREATMENT. Because lymphocytopenia ordinarily represents a response to an underlying disease, primary attention must be paid to establishing the nature of that disease and instituting therapy for it. Patients whose lymphocytopenia is accompanied by hypogammaglobulinemia may require immune globulin replacement therapy (Ch. 244). The treatment of severe deficiencies of cell-mediated immunity remains experimental. Responses have been described with transplantation of allogeneic marrow, fetal liver, or thymic epithelial cells.

Brandt SJ, Peters WP, Atwater SK, et al.: Effect of recombinant human granulocyte-macrophage colony-stimulating factor on hematopoietic reconstitution after high-dose chemotherapy and autologous bone marrow transplantation. N Engl J Med 318:869, 1988. Neta R, Oppenheim JJ: Cytokines in therapy of radiation injury. Blood 72:1093, 1988. Pluda JM, Yarchoan R, Smith PD, et al.: Subcutaneous recombinant granulocyte-macrophage colony-stimulating factor used as a single agent and in an alternating regimen with azidothymidine in leukopenic patients with severe human immunodeficiency virus infection. Blood 76:463, 1990. *The first paper provides good evidence that GM-CSF therapy can reduce the period of marrow failure in patients who have received high-dose chemotherapy followed by autologous bone marrow reinfusion. The second paper, one of many by this group, indicates that interleukin 1 (IL1) is radioprotective in mice and is capable of protecting mice from life-threatening marrow failure even when administered after radiation exposure. It is likely that clinical trials in humans will begin soon. The third paper supports, in a clinical study, the legitimacy of the concern that GM-CSF, used as a single agent, may activate proviral expression in latently infected cells and also demonstrates that GM-CSF enhances the antiviral activity of azidothymidine.*

Gabrilove JL, Jakubowski A, Scher H, et al.: Effect of granulocyte colony-stimulating factor on neutropenia and associated morbidity due to chemotherapy for transitional-cell carcinoma of the urothelium. N Engl J Med 318:1414, 1988. Bonilla MA, Gillio AP, Ruggeiro M, et al.: Effects of recombinant human granulocyte colony-stimulating factor on neutropenia in patients with congenital agranulocytosis. N Engl J Med 320:1574, 1989. Negrin RS, Haeuber DH, Nagler A, et al.: Maintenance treatment of patients with myelodysplastic

syndromes using recombinant human granulocyte colony-stimulating factor. Blood 76:36, 1990. *These three papers provide convincing evidence that G-CSF therapy will likely be part of future standard therapy for selected patients with the disorders discussed by the respective authors. GM-CSF and G-CSF not only stimulate granulocyte production but also activate neutrophils to become more potently phagocytic, another advantage for the neutropenic patient.*

Hoffman R, Benz EJ, Shattil FJ, et al.: Hematology: Basic Principles and Practice. New York, Churchill Livingstone, 1991. *This new textbook of hematology includes a number of informative and well-referenced chapters on phagocyte and lymphocyte production, granulopoietic factors, and phagocyte traffic and function.*

Jacob HS, Craddock PR, Hammerschmidt D, et al.: Complement-induced granulocyte aggregation. An unsuspected mechanism of disease. N Engl J Med 302:789, 1980. *This work documents very well the rapidity with which complement-induced aggregation can account not only for neutropenia but for significant respiratory dysfunction as well.*

Lelezari P, Jiang A-F, Yegen L, et al.: Chronic autoimmune neutropenia due to anti-NA2 antibody. N Engl J Med 293:744, 1975. *Despite the difficulties in documenting shortened survival of a cell whose survival is intrinsically short, this paper presents good evidence that chronic neutropenia can be mediated by antibodies directed at antigens expressed by neutrophils.*

Metcalf D: The molecular control of cell division, differentiation, commitment and maturation in haemopoietic cells. Nature 339:27, 1989. Clark SC, Kamen R: The human hematopoietic colony-stimulating factors. Science 236:1229, 1987. *These are two comprehensive reviews by investigators who have themselves contributed mightily to the development of new knowledge on the structure, function, and biologic activity of heterogeneous hematopoietic growth factors. Potential readers should not be daunted by the breadth of Metcalf's title; the article is short and focuses almost exclusively on humoral control.*

Vincent PC: Drug induced aplastic anaemia and agranulocytosis. Incidence and mechanisms. Drugs 31:52, 1986. *This comprehensive review is informative and is easy to read.*

141 Leukocytosis and Leukemoid Reactions

Grover C. Bagby, Jr.

Circulating leukocytes consist of neutrophils, monocytes, eosinophils, basophils, and lymphocytes. Any one or all of these cell types can rise to abnormal levels in peripheral blood in response to various stimuli. Each type of leukocyte is produced by the bone marrow in response to specific growth factors. The term *leukocytosis*, an increase in the total leukocyte count to a level above 11.0×10^9 per liter, is less meaningful clinically than are terms that identify the type of leukocyte that is predominantly increased. The terms *neutrophilia* (neutrophilic leukocytosis), *monocytosis, lymphocytosis, eosinophilia,* and *basophilia* suggest specific diagnostic considerations.

Leukocytosis is a common finding in acutely ill patients. When the leukocyte count exceeds 25 to 30×10^9 per liter, it is termed a *leukemoid reaction*. Leukemoid reactions generally reflect the response of healthy bone marrow to signals that evolve in the patient under the influence of trauma, inflammation, and similar stresses. Leukemoid reactions are *not* synonymous with *leukoerythroblastosis*, which indicates the presence of immature white cells and nucleated red cells in the peripheral blood irrespective of the total leukocyte count. Leukoerythroblastosis is less common than leukemoid reactions but often, especially in the adult patient, reflects serious marrow dysfunction (Table 141–1). Consequently, the finding of leukoerythroblastosis (see Color Plate 7F, left) represents a clear indication to perform bone marrow aspiration and biopsy, unless the clinical setting is acute severe hemolytic anemia, sepsis in a patient with hyposplenism, or massive trauma (with multiple fractures).

NEUTROPHILIA

PATHOPHYSIOLOGY. There are three major anatomic sites of neutrophil traffic: the bone marrow, the peripheral blood, and the extravascular space (Fig. 141–1). Traffic moves unidirectionally from marrow to blood to extravascular space. The number of neutrophils within each site can be independently regulated. The number of neutrophil precursors in the marrow mitotic pool (MiP) is largely influenced by the granulopoietic growth factors:

TABLE 141–1. CAUSES OF LEUKOERYTHROBLASTOSIS

Normal marrow
  Severe acute hemolytic anemia
  Acute infection in hyposplenic patients
Abnormal marrow
  Multiple fractures
  Marrow infiltration
    Tuberculosis
    Fungal disease
    Fibrosis
    Malignant cells (carcinoma, sarcoma, lymphoma,
      myeloma, acute leukemia)
  Chronic myeloproliferative disorders
    Agnogenic myeloid metaplasia
    Chronic myelogenous leukemia
  Other disorders
    Osteopetrosis
    Gaucher's disease
    Amyloidosis
    Paget's disease of bone
    Severe tissue hypoxia

granulocyte-macrophage colony-stimulating factor (GM-CSF) and granulocyte colony-stimulating factor (G-CSF). These factors, the products of separate genes, not only function to stimulate the growth and differentiation of granulocyte and/or macrophage progenitor cells but also functionally activate neutrophils. The marrow storage pool is sufficient to provide the periphery with neutrophils for about 5 days in the steady state, even if it were unsupported by the MiP. Neutrophils are released from the storage pool into the circulating pool in response to a variety of physiologic stresses, including endogenous glucocorticoids (Fig. 141–1B). Peripheral neutrophils are normally equally divided between the circulating pool and the marginated pool. Neutrophilia can therefore result from a shift of neutrophils from the marginated to the circulating pool—"demargination" (Fig. 141–1C). This response is rapid and can be induced by injections of epinephrine. In patients with acute inflammatory illnesses, storage pool release and demargination usually occur together (Fig. 141–1D).

A complex regulatory network of mononuclear phagocytes, stromal cells, lymphocytes, and granulocyte progenitors and their progeny responds to acute inflammatory events by augmenting production of the critically important CSF's (Fig. 141–2). The CSF's act on the granulopoietic progenitors to increase mitosis, which expands the storage pool and consequently increases the size of the blood and extravascular pools (Fig. 141–1E). This new state persists until the inflammatory process is resolved.

CAUSES. Neutrophilia (neutrophil counts greater than 7.5×10^9 per liter), a common finding in clinical practice, usually reflects the inflammatory response to acute or subacute infection (Fig. 141–2, Table 141–2) (see Color Plate 7A). Indeed, while the presence of neutrophilia should initiate a search for the cause of this response, it should also be viewed as a sign that the patient is likely responding appropriately to the stimulus.

When neutrophilia occurs in the absence of evidence of acute inflammation or illness, three conditions should be considered: (1) Certain agents such as glucocorticoids, lithium chloride, or epinephrine commonly produce neutrophilia. (2) Malignant tumors may express certain of the CSF genes inappropriately and thereby increase CSF blood levels. When such cancers are effectively treated, the neutrophilia resolves. (3) The chronic myeloproliferative disorders—chronic myelogenous leukemia, agnogenic myeloid metaplasia, essential thrombocytosis, and polycythemia rubra vera—may result in substantial neutrophilia. Patients with these diseases can present with few symptoms. When there is an acute inflammatory illness, it is most prudent to await its resolution before seeking to rule out one of the myeloproliferative disorders.

DIAGNOSIS. The diagnostic approach to patients with neutrophilia is presented as an algorithm in Figure 141–3. Notice that the diagnostic path leads quickly to the performance of bone marrow aspiration and biopsy for patients with leukoerythroblastosis. In patients without leukoerythroblastosis, neutrophilic leu-

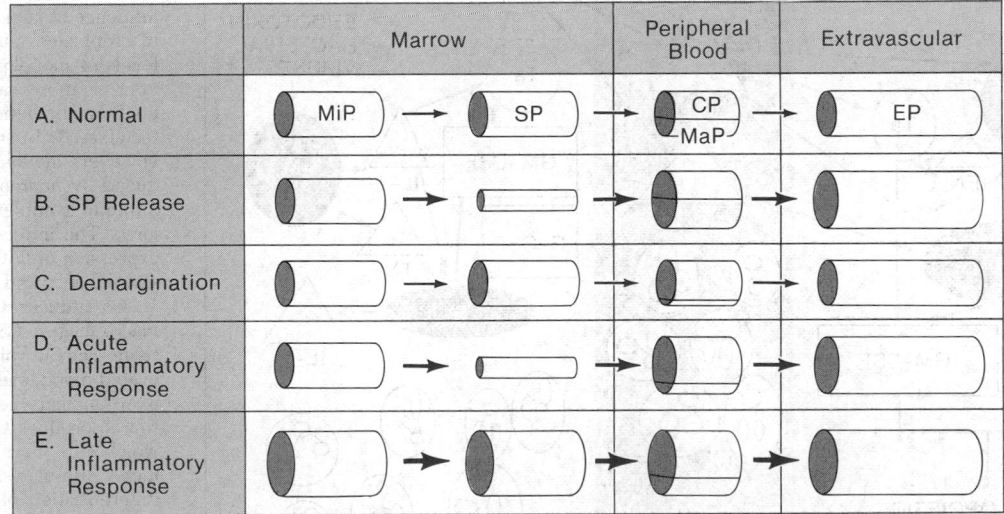

	Marrow	Peripheral Blood	Extravascular
A. Normal	MiP → SP	CP / MaP	EP
B. SP Release			
C. Demargination			
D. Acute Inflammatory Response			
E. Late Inflammatory Response			

FIGURE 141–1. Pathophysiologic mechanisms of neutrophilia. In this figure the size of a given compartment is represented by the size of a given cylinder. The number of cells leaving a compartment for the next compartment is reflected by the size of the arrows between compartments. A, MiP = the mitotic pool of granulocyte precursor cells; SP = the granulocyte storage pool; CP = the circulating granulocyte pool; MaP = the marginated pool; EP = the extravascular pool. Notice that in every case the circulating neutrophil pool is large, but the size of the other pools is variable. B, A variety of stresses on the organism can result, perhaps through the action of glucocorticoid hormones, in the release of storage pool granulocytes. This occurs commonly as an acute response to acute infections. C, The circulating granulocyte pool can also increase in size by virtue of a shift of neutrophils from the marginated to the circulating pool. The demargination response can be regularly elicited by the administration of epinephrine and can also result from a variety of stresses, including acute infection. D, With most bacterial infections and other inflammatory processes, the acute demand for neutrophils in the infected extravascular sites results in the simultaneous release of storage pool neutrophils and demargination. E, Once the hematopoietic growth factor released in response to the inflammatory stimulus (see Fig. 141–2) has induced a few days of proliferation in the mitotic pool, the content of granulocytes in all pools increases, and delivery to the tissues becomes maximal.

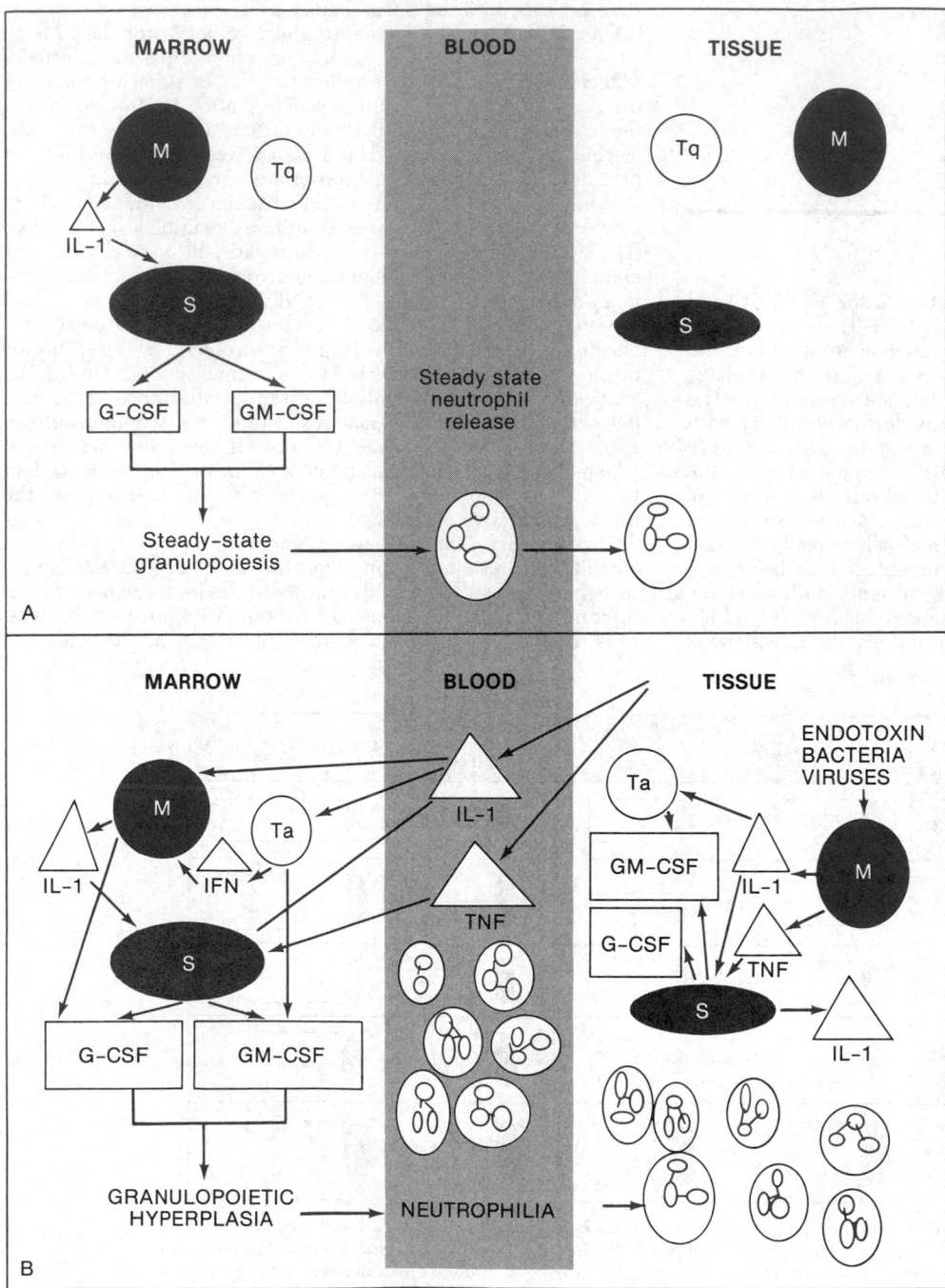

FIGURE 141–2. An intercellular regulatory network controls the production and function of phagocytes in inflammation. The figure represents the likely mechanisms by which neutrophil production and function are enhanced during the inflammatory response. The cells (*circles*) labeled M, S, and T represent monocytes/macrophages, stromal cells (e.g., fibroblasts and endothelial cells), and T lymphocytes, respectively. Tq are quiescent T cells (not activated), and Ta are activated T cells. Neutrophils have segmented trilobed nuclei. Two monokines, interleukin 1 (IL-1) and tumor necrosis factor–alpha (TNF), are depicted by triangles labeled IL-1 or TNF. The two granulopoietic factors—granulocyte colony-stimulating factor (G-CSF) and granulocyte-macrophage CSF (GM-CSF)—are symbolized by rectangles. Relative concentrations of monokines and CSF's are reflected by the size of the triangles or rectangles, respectively. *A*, In the steady state, stromal cells of the marrow produce both CSF's. The production of G-CSF and GM-CSF by stromal cells even in the steady state may be under the influence of IL-1 produced by marrow macrophages and monocytes. Blood levels of monokines are low. Production of these factors in uninflamed nonhematopoietic tissues is barely detectable. *B*, In states of inflammation, however, monokine production is induced by microorganisms, endotoxin, immune complexes, crystals, and so forth. The induced monokines induce expression of G-CSF and GM-CSF by stromal cells and activated T cells. IL-1 also induces G-CSF expression in macrophages. CSF's produced in the tissue activate phagocytes locally. Elevated blood levels of monokines stimulate auxiliary cells in the bone marrow to produce G-CSF and GM-CSF, which, in that microenvironmental niche, stimulate increased growth and differentiation of granulocyte precursors, with consequent granulocytic hyperplasia and neutrophilic leukocytosis.

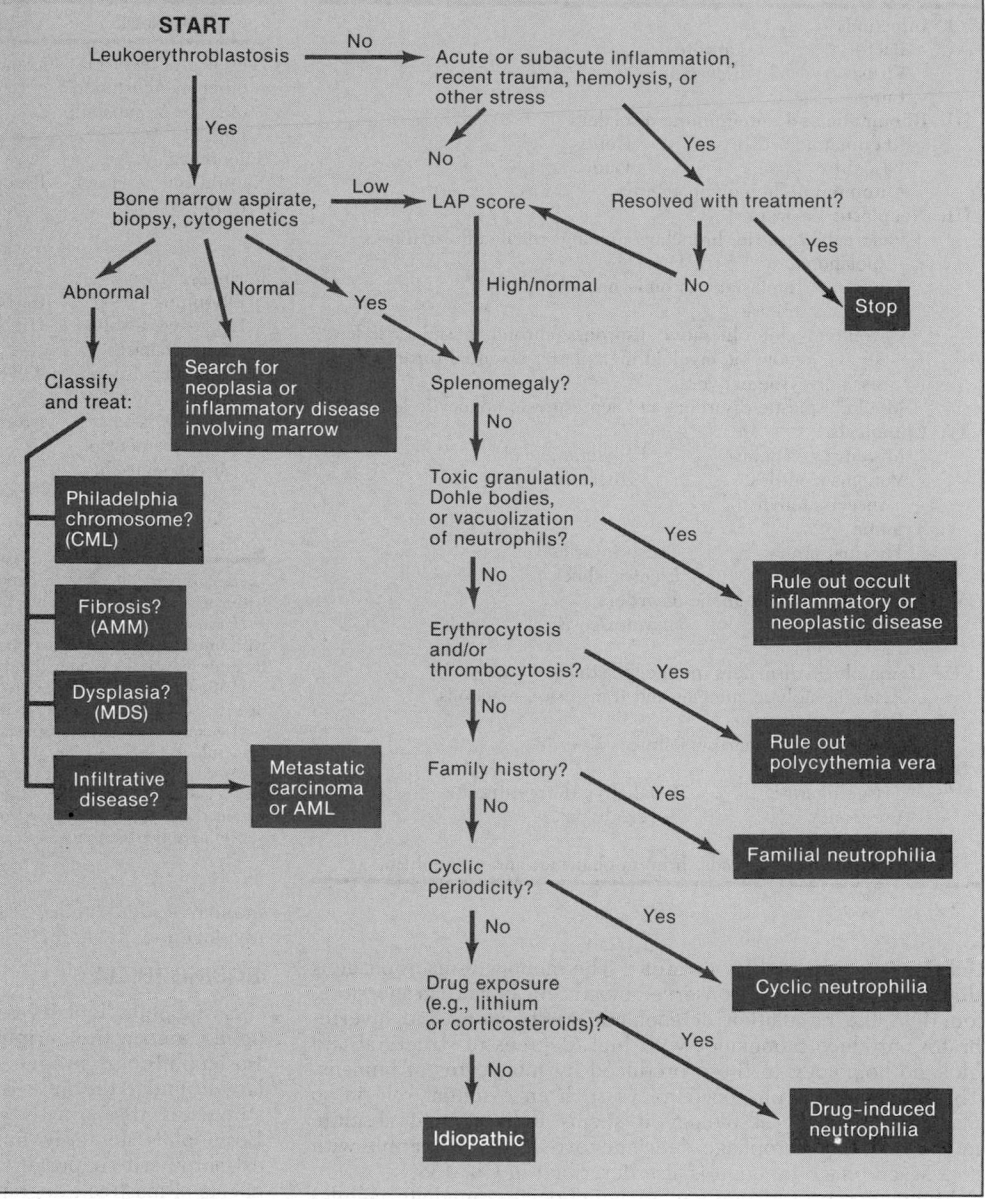

FIGURE 141–3. An algorithm for the evaluation of patients with neutrophilic leukocytosis (NL). LAP = leukocyte alkaline phosphatase; CML = chronic myelogenous leukemia; AMM = agnogenic myeloid metaplasia; MDS = myelodysplastic syndromes; AML = acute myelogenous leukemia. Branch termini are enclosed in boxes.

kocytosis generally results from acute toxic, inflammatory, or traumatic stresses, and it is usually best simply to observe the course of neutrophilia to determine its degree of linkage with the underlying disease. If the underlying disease resolves and the neutrophilia does not, other, less common, explanations must be pursued.

Neutrophil Morphology. Neutrophil morphology can lead to early diagnosis (Fig. 141–3). Toxic granulation of neutrophils, the presence of Döhle bodies (see Color Plate 7C), and the presence of vacuoles in the neutrophil cytoplasm suggest that overt or subclinical inflammation, exposure to a toxin, trauma, or neoplasia exists. Because glucocorticoids induce prompt eosinopenia and basophilopenia, these cells are almost universally absent in the blood of the acutely injured or infected patient. Thus their presence should indicate that (1) the acutely ill patient may have concomitant adrenocortical insufficiency, (2) the neutrophilia derives from the inappropriate production of GM-CSF (generally by malignant cells), or (3) the neutrophilia is one manifestation of a hematopoietic neoplasm (a chronic myeloproliferative disorder, myelodysplastic syndrome, or certain of the acute nonlymphocytic leukemias).

Leukocyte Alkaline Phosphatase. Leukocyte alkaline phosphatase (LAP) activity is restricted to the neutrophil. Simple histochemical techniques are used to measure LAP levels in neutrophils of the peripheral blood. When neutrophilia represents a reaction to an acute illness, the LAP levels usually increase substantially. In chronic myelogenous leukemia (CML), however, the LAP score is markedly decreased. A low LAP level in a patient with neutrophilia should therefore lead to a diagnostic evaluation designed to rule out CML (Table 141–3 and Fig. 141–3).

Differential Diagnosis of Neutrophilic Leukemoid Reactions. Neutrophilic leukemoid reactions generally occur in patients who are obviously systemically ill. When the neutrophil count exceeds 80×10^9 per liter, or when the mildness of the systemic illness seems discordant with the extremely high level of neutrophils in the peripheral blood, the diagnosis most often considered is CML. A number of additional features distinguish leukemoid reactions from CML (Table 141–3). In the past, the most definitive test for CML has been a marrow chromosome analysis for the Philadelphia chromosome (see Ch. 144). In the near future, even more sensitive tests may be direct DNA analyses to detect structural changes in the bcr (breakpoint cluster region) locus on chromosome 22 or immunoassay for the abnormal c-abl gene product p210 (Table 141–3).

MONOCYTOSIS

Monocytosis is defined as absolute peripheral blood monocyte counts greater than 0.80×10^9 per liter in children and greater

TABLE 141–2. COMMON CAUSES OF NEUTROPHILIA

I. **Infections**
   Bacteria   Parasites
   Viruses   *Rickettsiae*
   Fungi
II. **Rheumatic and autoimmune disorders**
   Rheumatoid arthritis   Colitis
   Vasculitis   Gout
   Autoimmune hemolytic anemia
III. **Neoplastic disorders**
   Pancreatic, gastric, bronchogenic, and renal cell carcinoma;
      melanoma
   Any cancer metastatic to bone marrow
   Hodgkin's disease
   Chronic myeloproliferative disorders (chronic granulocytic leu-
      kemia, agnogenic myeloid metaplasia, essential thrombocyto-
      sis, polycythemia vera)
   Myelodysplastic disorders and acute myelomonocytic leukemia
IV. **Chemicals**
   Mercury poisoning   Ethylene glycol
   Venoms (reptiles,   Histamine
      insects, jellyfish)
V. **Trauma**
   Thermal injury   Crush injuries
   Hypothermia   Electric shock
VI. **Endocrine and metabolic disorders**
   Ketoacidosis   Thyrotoxicosis
   Lactic acidosis
VII. **Hematologic disorders (nonneoplastic)**
   Acute hemolytic anemias and transfusion reactions
   Postsplenectomy
   Recovery from marrow failure
VIII. **Other disorders**
   Tissue necrosis   Exfoliative dermatitis
   Pregnancy   Severe hypoxia
   Eclampsia
   Drugs: corticosteroids, lithium chloride, and epinephrine

TABLE 141–3. DISTINCTIONS BETWEEN NEUTROPHILIC LEUKEMOID REACTIONS AND CHRONIC MYELOGENOUS LEUKEMIA (CML)

Finding/Result	Leukemoid Reaction	CML
Presence of fever or other manifestations of acute or subacute illness	Usual*	Infrequent†
Splenomegaly	Rare	Frequent
Natural course of neutrophilia	Resolution linked temporally with abatement of underlying disease	Progressive slow increase over time
Peripheral blood:		
Basophilia	Rare‡	Common
Leukocyte alkaline phosphatase	High	Low§
Philadelphia chromosome	Never	Frequent (85%)
Abnormal DNA: Rearrangement of breakpoint cluster region in DNA (chromosome 22)	Absent‖	Frequent (>85%)

*Regular exceptions to this rule are patients with leukemoid reactions associated with certain carcinomas (Table 141–1).
†Patients with CML are not exempt from developing infections. Some patients with infectious processes may be found to have CML. The ideal time to evaluate them diagnostically is after the inflammatory process resolves.
‡Patients with acute allergic reactions and patients with widespread parasitic diseases are frequently exceptions to this rule.
§Leukocyte alkaline phosphatase scores are sometimes normal in CML patients after splenectomy.
‖As described in Ch. 144, the Philadelphia chromosome forms when chromosome 22 breaks in a region called the breakpoint cluster region (bcr). There are some patients with CML who have no Philadelphia chromosome on karyotypic analysis, yet do have bcr rearrangement on DNA analysis.

than 0.50×10^9 per liter in adults. The monocyte-macrophage is the most evolutionarily conserved blood cell. In fact, its ancestors, found in the circulation or coelomic cavity of marine invertebrates, produce monokines with high degrees of structural and biologic homology to those produced by monocytes of humans. The mononuclear phagocyte plays such an essential role in so many components of biology it seems unlikely that absolute monocyte and macrophage deficiency would be compatible with life. Macrophage function is also described in Ch. 138.

Monocytes present antigen to lymphocytes, mediate cellular cytotoxicity, release procoagulants, participate in bone remodeling and wound repair, dispose of damaged cells, and regulate immune and hematopoietic responses by producing interleukin 1 (IL1), tumor necrosis factor (TNF)–alpha, G-CSF, and certain alpha-interferons. Two factors stimulate the growth and differentiation of mononuclear phagocytes: M-CSF and GM-CSF (Fig. 141–3). Stromal cells, including endothelial cells and fibroblasts, constitutively produce M-CSF, a protein that acts only on cells of the monocyte lineage to stimulate their differentiation and survival. Steady-state monocyte production probably depends upon GM-CSF production. M-CSF production is not clearly inducible by factors released during the inflammatory response, but GM-CSF production is induced during inflammation (Fig. 141–2).

The mononuclear phagocyte is more sluggish than the neutrophil in moving toward and killing bacteria but is as effective, if not more so, in killing obligate intracellular parasites such as fungi, yeast, and viruses. In addition, it participates substantially in all types of granulomatous inflammation. Accordingly, monocytosis is often seen in patients with tuberculosis, syphilis, fungal infections, ulcerative and granulomatous colitis, and sarcoidosis (Table 141–4). Mild monocytosis is common in patients with Hodgkin's disease and a variety of cancers. High levels of monocytes in the blood are most often seen in patients with myeloid malignant diseases, including acute and chronic myelo-

monocytic leukemia, acute monocytic leukemia, and chronic myelogenous leukemia of the juvenile type.

EOSINOPHILIA

Eosinophilic leukocytosis (eosinophilia) exists when the eosinophil count in the peripheral blood exceeds 0.4×10^9 per liter. Eosinophils are produced by progenitor cells in the marrow largely under the influence of interleukin 5, a protein that also stimulates the growth and differentiation of B lymphocytes. Eosinophils not only function as phagocytes but also play an extraordinarily important role in modulating the potentially toxic effects of mast cell degranulation in hypersensitivity reactions.

The eosinophilic syndromes and the causes of eosinophilia are described in Ch. 150.

TABLE 141–4. CAUSES OF MONOCYTOSIS

I. **Infections**
   Tuberculosis   Syphilis
   Brucellosis   Fungal infections
   Bacterial endocarditis   Recovery from acute infections
   Typhoid and paratyphoid   Protozoal infections
      fevers
   Listeriosis
II. **Neoplastic disorders**
   Hodgkin's disease
   Carcinoma (many)
   Acute and chronic myelomonocytic leukemia, myelodysplastic
      syndromes, and chronic myelogenous leukemia of the juvenile
      type
III. **Gastrointestinal disorders**
   Ulcerative colitis   Cirrhosis
   Granulomatous colitis
IV. **Sarcoidosis**
V. **Drug reactions**
VI. **Recovery from marrow suppression**
VII. **Congenital neutropenia**

LYMPHOCYTOSIS

Lymphocytosis is defined as any lymphocyte count in excess of 5.0×10^9 per liter. Atypical lymphocytosis is present when atypical lymphocytes account for more than 20 per cent of the total peripheral blood lymphocyte population (see Color Plate 7B). The production and traffic of lymphocytes are clearly under tight control. A number of factors induce growth of T lymphocytes (IL2 and IL3), natural killer cells (IL2), and B lymphocytes (IL2, B cell stimulatory factor [BSF]-1, BSF-2, and B cell growth factor II).

DIAGNOSIS. Mild to moderate lymphocytosis (lymphocyte counts $< 12 \times 10^9$ per liter) is most commonly caused by viral infections, notably infectious mononucleosis and infectious hepatitis. Careful examination of the peripheral blood lymphocyte morphology can help distinguish between these two disorders. In infectious mononucleosis (see Ch. 373), many of the lymphocytes are large, with abundant cytoplasm and a ballerina skirt–like cytoplasmic border. These are the characteristic "atypical" lymphocytes that exceed 20 per cent of the total lymphocyte population during the course of this disease. Interestingly, while the B lymphocyte is the target of the causative Epstein-Barr (EB) virus, the majority of the cells in the peripheral blood of patients with this disease are T lymphocytes. This proliferative response of T cells probably plays a major role in coordinating the process of recovery from the viral infection.

Acute bacterial infections rarely cause lymphocytosis. One exception is pertussis (in children), in which profound lymphocytosis (up to 60×10^9 per liter) is sometimes seen. Interestingly, specific soluble factors derived from the causative organism, *Bordetella pertussis*, induce lymphocytosis in experimental ani-

mals. In Table 141–5 are listed a variety of additional disorders associated with mild to moderate lymphocytosis. Perhaps with the exception of those with early chronic lymphocytic leukemia, most patients have overt signs of an underlying illness involving anatomic sites other than the lymphohematopoietic system. This

TABLE 141–5. CAUSES OF LYMPHOCYTOSIS

I. High (>15 × 10⁹ per liter)

Infectious mononucleosis	Chronic lymphocytic leukemia
Pertussis	Acute lymphocytic leukemia
Acute infectious lymphocytosis	

II. Moderate (<15 × 10⁹ per liter)

Many viral infections

Infectious mononucleosis	Coxsackie
Measles	Adenovirus
Varicella	Mumps
Hepatitis	Cytomegalovirus

Other infectious diseases

Toxoplasmosis	Typhoid fever
Brucellosis	Syphilis (secondary)
Tuberculosis	

Neoplastic disorders
   Carcinoma
   Hodgkin's disease
   Acute lymphocytic leukemia (early)
   Chronic lymphocytic leukemia (early)
Other disorders
   Graves' disease

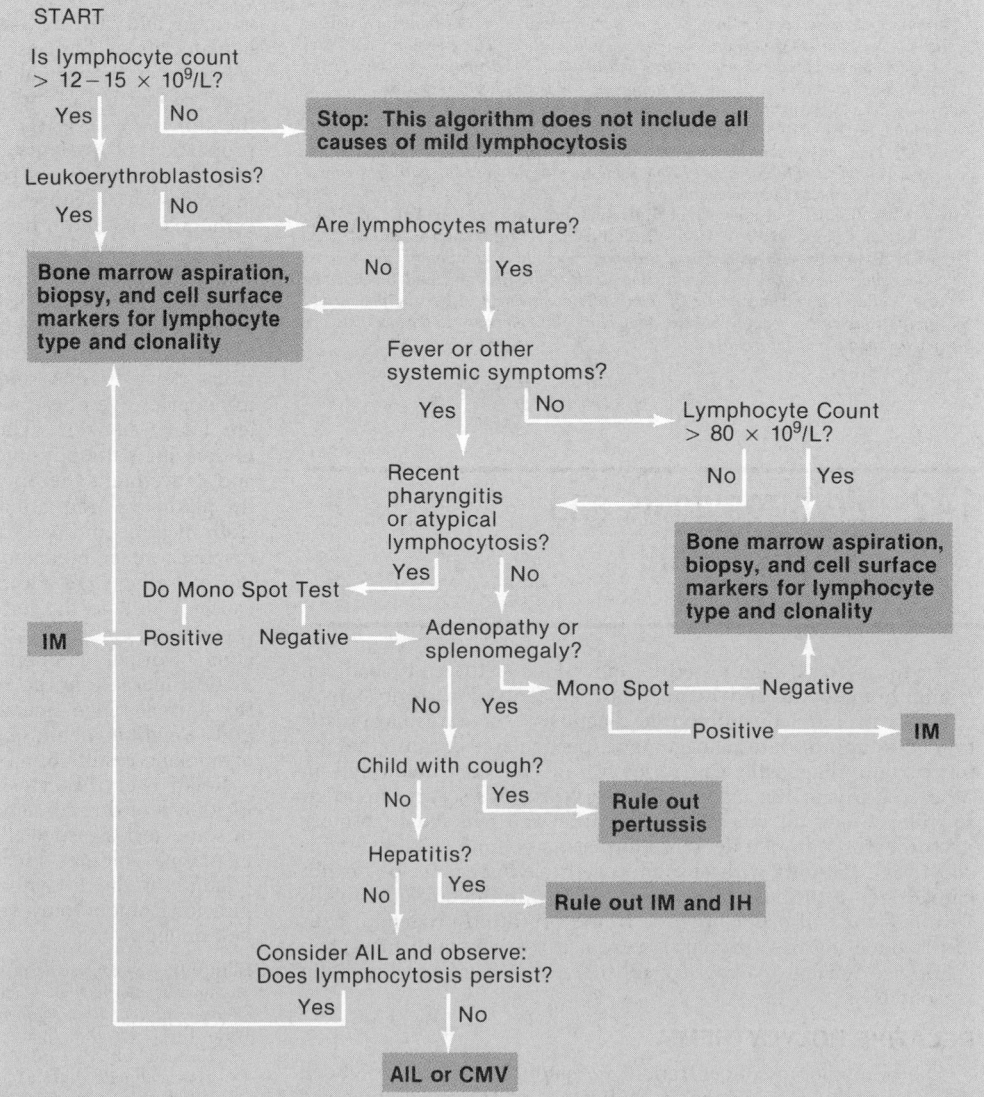

FIGURE 141–4. An algorithm for the evaluation of patients with lymphocytosis in excess of 12×10^9 per liter. IM = infectious mononucleosis; CMV = cytomegalovirus infection; AIL = acute infectious lymphocytosis; IH = infectious hepatitis. Branch termini are enclosed in boxes.

rule also holds true for patients with substantial lymphocytosis (>12 to 15 × 10⁹ per liter), the differential diagnosis of which is limited (Table 141–5). The diagnostic approach presented as an algorithm in Figure 141–4 depends simply upon establishing a tissue diagnosis to rule out malignant disease in patients who do not have clear-cut evidence of one of the benign disorders.

An important adjunct to histologic diagnosis is immunophenotypic analysis of the lymphocyte surface. Not only will such studies provide evidence for or against dominance of one lymphocyte type, but they are also capable of determining whether B lymphocytes in the circulation are all members of a single (therefore, likely neoplastic) clone.

Bagby GC, Dinarello CA, Wallace P, et al.: Interleukin 1 stimulates granulocyte macrophage colony-stimulating activity release by vascular endothelial cells. J Clin Invest 78:1316, 1986. Broudy VC, Kaushansky K, Segal G, et al.: Tumor necrosis factor type alpha stimulates human endothelial cells to produce granulocyte/macrophage colony-stimulating factor. Proc Natl Acad Sci USA 83:7467, 1986. Zucali J, Dinarello C, Oblon D, et al.: Interleukin 1 stimulates fibroblasts to produce granulocyte-macrophage colony-stimulating activity and prostaglandin E₂. J Clin Invest 77:1857, 1986. *These three papers provide important evidence that the production of granulopoietic factors by stromal cells can be stimulated by the monokines IL1 and TNF-alpha. These in vitro observations provide insight into the importance of mononuclear phagocytes, the producers of monokines, as regulators of phagocyte production and function in inflammatory states. The reader is also referred to Figure 141–2.*

Clark SC: Biological activities of human granulocyte-macrophage colony-stimulating factor. Int J Cell Cloning 6:365, 1988. Metcalf D: The molecular control of cell division, differentiation, commitment and maturation in haemopoietic cells. Nature 339:27, 1989. Herrmann F, Schulz G, Lindemann A, et al.: Hematopoietic responses in patients with advanced malignancy treated with recombinant human granulocyte-macrophage colony-stimulating factor. J Clin Oncol 7:159, 1989. Sullivan R, Fredette JP, Socinski M, et al.: Enhancement of superoxide anion release by granulocytes harvested from patients receiving granulocyte-macrophage colony-stimulating factor. Br J Haematol 71:475, 1989. *For those readers interested in a short course on the biologic activities of G-CSF and GM-CSF, these papers will suffice. The first two are good reviews by two leaders in the field. The third and fourth papers provide direct experimental evidence of the two major in vivo activities of GM-CSF.*

Daley GQ, Van Etten RA, Baltimore D: Induction of chronic myelogenous leukemia in mice by the p210bcr/abl gene of the Philadelphia chromosome. Science 247:824, 1990. *This outstanding work provides the most up-to-date clarification of the exact role of the Philadelphia chromosome translocation in the pathophysiology of chronic myelogenous leukemia.*

Williams WJ, Beutler E, Erslev AJ, et al.: Hematology. 4th ed. New York, McGraw-Hill Book Company, 1990. Paul WE: Fundamental Immunology. 2nd ed. New York, Raven Press, 1989. *These textbooks include a number of chapters on phagocyte and lymphocyte production, traffic, distribution, and function. In the Williams text, the reviews of neutrophilia, monocytosis, eosinophilia, and lymphocytosis are comprehensive and clinically relevant. Reference lists are encyclopedic and informative.*

142 Erythrocytosis and Polycythemia

Paul D. Berk

Erythrocytosis, manifested by elevations of the red blood cell count, hematocrit, and hemoglobin concentration, represents a complex problem in differential diagnosis. Accurate diagnosis is crucial to appropriate management, particularly because therapy for certain diagnostic categories would be contraindicated in others. Early in the evaluation of erythrocytosis it is important to differentiate an increase in the total red cell mass (absolute erythrocytosis) from a decrease in plasma volume (relative erythrocytosis). Patients with absolute erythrocytosis must be further categorized into those in whom excessive production of red cells results from a disorder intrinsic to the erythroid progenitor cells of the bone marrow (primary) or from excessive stimulation of an otherwise normal marrow by substances such as erythropoietin (secondary).

RELATIVE POLYCYTHEMIA

The hemoglobin concentration, hematocrit, and red blood cell count, usually interpreted as indicators of the circulating red blood cell or hemoglobin masses, are in fact, merely measures of the extent to which the red cell mass is diluted in the plasma volume. The red cell mass and the plasma volume are regulated independently. Hence, a patient with an elevated hemoglobin concentration, hematocrit, or red cell count may have (1) an increase in the red cell mass, i.e., an absolute erythrocytosis; (2) a reduction in the plasma volume; or (3) a combination of a red cell mass at the upper end of the normal range and plasma volume at the lower end of the normal range. These last two situations have been termed relative or spurious polycythemia, since the elevated hemoglobin concentration, hematocrit, and red cell count do not reflect an absolute increase in the mass of circulating erythrocytes. Strictly speaking, the designation polycythemia should be reserved for conditions involving increased levels of other formed elements (granulocytes, platelets) in addition to erythrocytes; in fact, the term *polycythemia* is also widely applied to disorders characterized solely by abnormalities in erythroid parameters and is therefore employed in this chapter.

The most frequent cause of relative polycythemia is dehydration. Accordingly, fluid balance should be corrected before a hematologic evaluation of an elevated hematocrit is done. As an important first step, after dehydration is ruled out, patients with absolute polycythemia can be accurately distinguished from those with relative polycythemia by measurement of both the red cell mass and the plasma volume, using ⁵¹Cr-labeled erythrocytes and ¹²⁵I-albumin, respectively. This is especially important because, in the absence of arterial hypoxemia (e.g., cyanotic congenital heart disease, chronic pulmonary disease), cases of relative polycythemia are at least as common as cases of absolute polycythemia but need not be subjected to the extensive and expensive investigations required to determine the cause of an absolute increase in the circulating red cell mass.

The normal red cell mass averages 30 ± 3 (SD) ml per kilogram in men and 27 ± 2 ml per kilogram in women. Although hematocrits as high as 54 per cent in men or 48 per cent in women may be normal, increased red cell masses are found in a small proportion of individuals of either sex with hematocrits in the upper 40's. As the hematocrit increases into the 50's, the proportion of patients with an increased red cell mass also increases but does not reach 100 per cent until the hematocrit is in excess of 60. Since approximately half of patients with polycythemia vera and other forms of true erythrocytosis and a large majority of those with spurious erythrocytosis present with hematocrits between 50 and 60, the need for direct measurement of the red cell mass to distinguish true polycythemia from spurious erythrocytosis is apparent.

Relative erythrocytosis, also called spurious polycythemia, stress polycythemia, and Gaisböck's syndrome, typically occurs in hypertensive obese middle-aged men, especially in those who are heavy smokers. The male-female ratio is at least 5:1. Its underlying pathophysiology remains obscure. Both hypertension and its frequent therapy with diuretics may lead to reduction in the plasma volume. Smoking may contribute by two mechanisms. Both nicotine and carboxyhemoglobin, which circulates in smokers because of inhalation of carbon monoxide, may have mild diuretic effects. In addition, the presence of carboxyhemoglobin causes a shift to the left in the oxygen dissociation curve of the remaining hemoglobin, leading to mildly impaired tissue oxygenation. Normal compensatory mechanisms, in turn, lead to a modest increase in the red cell mass that may not always exceed the normal range, particularly when expressed per kilogram of body weight in an obese patient. In some smokers discontinuation of smoking results in cure of the erythrocytosis.

Relative erythrocytosis is not always a benign condition, the incidence of thromboembolic events reaching almost 30 per cent in some series, especially in patients with an absolute reduction in plasma volume. Treatment remains controversial, but maintenance of the hematocrit at no more than 50 per cent by a judicious phlebotomy regimen is often recommended and may be beneficial.

Isbister JP: The contracted plasma volume syndromes (relative polycythemias) and their haemorheological significance. Clin Haematol 1:665, 1987. *A lucid review of a subject with a confusing and often contradictory literature.*

Watts EJ, Lewis SM: Spurious polycythemia—a study of 35 patients. Scand J Haematol 31:241, 1983. *An evaluation of factors, such as smoking and obesity, associated with spurious polycythemia. The authors argue in favor of treating the underlying condition rather than the hematocrit.*

ABSOLUTE POLYCYTHEMIA: PATHOPHYSIOLOGY AND CLINICAL EVALUATION

Regulation of the Red Cell Mass

The circulating red cell mass is determined by a balance between the rate at which new erythrocytes are produced and released from the bone marrow and the rate of peripheral red cell destruction. The latter, as measured by studies of the red cell lifespan, is ordinarily fixed, with a normal mean value of about 100 days. While red cell lifespan may be reduced in pathologic states, there are no mechanisms by which it may be increased. Hence, physiologic regulation of the red cell mass occurs entirely by changes in the rate of red cell production.

Alterations in the red cell mass are effected to provide for a critical level of tissue oxygenation (Fig. 142–1). The principal sensors of the state of tissue oxygenation in adults are probably located in the kidney, although the existence of extrarenal oxygen sensors has also been proposed. The kidney responds to the perceived adequacy of oxygen delivery by modulating the output of the hormone erythropoietin. The gene for this carbohydrate-rich glycoprotein has been successfully cloned, and its biologic activity has been found to reside in a polypeptide chain of 166 amino acids.

Normal hematopoiesis is regulated by a complex network of interactions between a hierarchy of bone marrow stem cells of differing proliferative capacity and potential to differentiate (see Ch. 127 and 143). The network includes a variety of soluble mediators (erythropoietin; granulocyte-macrophage colony-stimulating factor, granulocyte colony-stimulating factor, and macrophage colony-stimulating factor [GM-CSF, G-CSF, and M-CSF, respectively]; interleukins 1, 3, 5, and 6 [IL1,3,5, and 6]; insulin-like growth factor I; γ-interferon; and tumor necrosis factor [TNF]) as well as nonhematopoietic regulatory cells with both stimulatory and suppressor functions. The functions of each of these mediators in regulating hematopoiesis are still being elucidated.

Pluripotent bone marrow stem cells differentiate to the earliest erythroid-committed progenitors, the *erythroid burst-forming units* (BFU$_E$), under the influence of a T cell–derived growth regulator called *burst-promoting activity*. In vitro, such burst-promoting activity can be provided by IL3 and GM-CSF. By contrast, erythropoietin, the principal regulator of the subsequent stages of erythropoiesis, stimulates proliferation of the *erythroid colony-forming units* (CFU$_E$), the more differentiated but still morphologically unrecognizable progeny of the BFU$_E$. CFU$_E$ are primitive blastlike cells with large nuclei, a prominent nucleolus, a perinuclear clear zone, and an absence of granules. Since further differentiation of the CFU$_E$ to early, recognizable proerythroblasts is a stochastic process, expansion of the pool of CFU$_E$ results in an increase in the production of recognizable erythroid precursors in the marrow. Erythropoietin also shortens the overall maturation time of developing erythroid precursors and accelerates the release of reticulocytes into the circulation. Hence its net effect is to increase the output of red cells from the marrow and ultimately to expand the circulating red cell mass.

Mechanisms Producing Erythrocytosis

Erythrocytosis, or "polycythemia" reflects an increase in marrow red cell production caused by increased proliferation of erythroid progenitors. This proliferation could be either "autonomous," as a result of an intrinsic cellular defect permitting escape from normal regulatory mechanisms, or secondary to an external stimulus.

AUTONOMOUS PROLIFERATION. The increased erythroid activity in the primary polycythemias, including polycythemia rubra vera and the more recently described entity of primary erythrocytosis, is seemingly autonomous in that increased red cell production occurs despite low or undetectable levels of erythropoietin as measured by in vivo bioassay techniques. Moreover, "endogenous colonies" of erythroid progenitors from such patients may be successfully grown in various in vitro tissue culture systems without added erythropoietin, which is otherwise essential for erythroid progenitor growth in vitro. Finally, phlebotomy to low normal or anemic levels produces an increase in erythropoietin production, indicating that the "servomechanism" relating erythropoietin output to tissue oxygen delivery is intact. The apparent independence of erythropoiesis from erythropoietin in the primary polycythemias has been postulated to reflect a markedly increased sensitivity of erythroid progenitors to minute amounts of the hormone, rather than total independence from erythropoietin.

SECONDARY PROLIFERATION. Alternatively, the proliferation could result from abnormalities in the erythropoietic regulatory mechanism extrinsic to the erythroid progenitors themselves. The increased red cell production in these circumstances is driven by increased levels of erythropoietin or other erythroid stimulatory substances, and erythroid progenitors require exogenous erythropoietin to grow successfully in vitro. These features characterize the various secondary polycythemias.

The secondary polycythemias can be further subdivided into three categories. The *first* is disorders in which the signal resulting in erythrocytosis, most often an increase in erythropoietin production, represents a physiologically appropriate response to poor tissue oxygenation caused by arterial hypoxemia, genetically determined or "acquired" high-affinity hemoglobins that release oxygen to tissue inadequately, or reduced tissue perfusion. For these conditions, reduction of the red cell mass by phlebotomy, even to values still substantially greater than normal, may reduce tissue oxygen delivery and result in a further increase in erythropoietin output. The *second* category comprises disorders characterized by excessive autonomous production of erythropoietic stimulatory substances (erythropoietin, androgens, adrenal corticosteroids). Increased, autonomous erythropoietin production may occur in certain neoplasms, as a result of nonneoplastic lesions in the kidney (hydronephrosis, cysts, tumors, vascular lesions) that produce local ischemia involving the renal oxygen-sensing mechanism, or in certain rare familial syndromes, without a demonstrable anatomic lesion. For the disorders in this category, erythropoietin production is not influenced by phlebot-

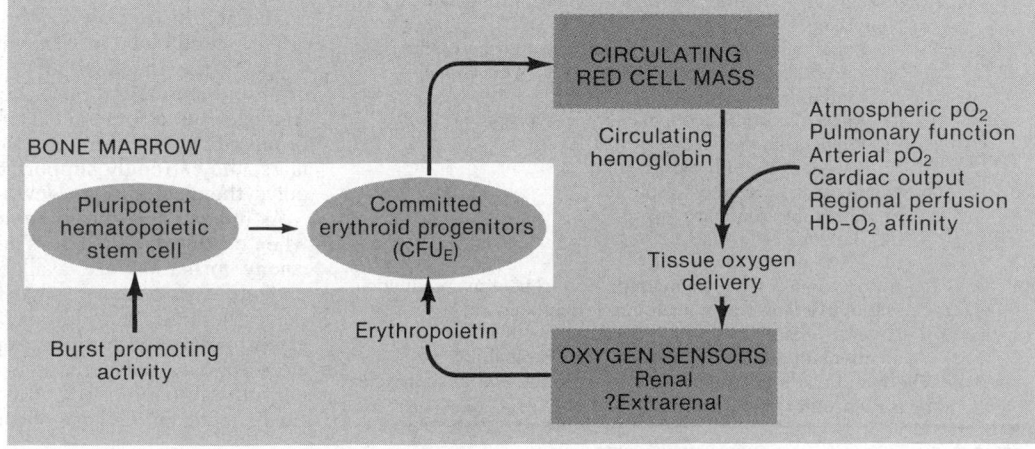

FIGURE 142–1. Relationship between tissue oxygen delivery, erythropoietin output, and the circulating red cell mass.

omy-induced changes in the red cell mass. The *third* category is the entity in which erythropoietin secretion remains under physiologic control in that it responds to phlebotomy, but at a level of production inappropriately high for the level of tissue oxygenation. A classification of the various absolute erythrocytoses, based on underlying mechanisms, is presented in Table 142–1.

Pathophysiology of Absolute Erythrocytosis

Irrespective of underlying etiology, all disorders characterized by an absolute erythrocytosis share certain common clinical manifestations resulting from the expanded blood volume and increased blood viscosity. The increased blood volume leads to generalized vascular expansion and venous engorgement, which are reflected by the characteristic ruddy cyanosis of the skin and mucous membranes. These factors are magnified by the marked decrease in cerebral blood flow that accompanies elevation of the hematocrit and in turn contributes to headaches, tinnitus, a frequently described feeling of fullness in the head and neck, and light-headedness. There appears to be an increase in thrombotic complications, particularly involving the cerebrovascular circulation, in patients with markedly elevated hematocrit and expanded blood volume. Epistaxis and upper gastrointestinal hemorrhage are also more frequent in the hypervolemic patient. The increase in viscosity accompanying hypervolemia and erythrocytosis may result in a decrease in cardiac output, in a reduction in regional blood flow, and ultimately in an impairment of tissue oxygenation, even in cases in which the underlying initial stimulus was poor oxygen delivery.

In contrast to the consequences of expanded blood volume and blood viscosity, the consequences of bone marrow hyperactivity and of increased red cell destruction are minimal. Because expansion of the red cell mass often occurs very slowly, increases in bone marrow volume, alterations in the myeloid-erythroid ratio, and changes in reticulocyte count or plasma iron turnover

TABLE 142–1. CAUSES OF ERYTHROCYTOSIS

I. Relative erythrocytosis (stress, spurious, or pseudopolycythemia; Gaisböck's syndrome)
II. Absolute erythrocytosis
  A. Primary (proliferative bone marrow disorder)
    1. Polycythemia vera
    2. Primary erythrocytosis
  B. Secondary (e.g., increased marrow stimulation by erythropoietin)
    1. Physiologically appropriate increased erythropoietin production
      a. Arterial hypoxemia
        i. High altitude
        ii. Chronic pulmonary disease
        iii. Cardiovascular shunt (right-to-left)
        iv. Massive obesity (pickwickian syndrome)
        v. Postural hypoxemia
      b. Abnormal release of oxygen from hemoglobin
        i. Hereditary hemoglobin with high oxygen affinity
        ii. Congenitally decreased red cell 2,3-DPG
        iii. Smoker's polycythemia (carboxyhemoglobinemia)
      c. Interference with tissue oxygen metabolism
        i. Cobalt
    2. Physiologically inappropriate erythropoietin production
      a. Neoplasms
        i. Renal, adrenal, hepatocellular, and ovarian carcinomas
        ii. Cerebellar hemangioblastomas (e.g., von Hippel–Lindau syndrome)
        iii. Adrenal cortical adenoma and/or hyperplasia
        iv. Pheochromocytoma
        v. Large uterine fibroids (rare)
      b. Nonneoplastic renal diseases
        i. Cysts, hydronephrosis
        ii. Bartter's syndrome
        iii. Posttransplantation
      c. Autonomous, fixed increased erythropoietin production without demonstrable anatomic lesion (familial)
      d. Excessive basal erythropoietin output with further augmentation following phlebotomy (familial)
    3. Therapeutic administration or excess production of androgens or certain other corticosteroids

may be difficult to appreciate. Similarly, although a doubling of the red cell mass results in a doubling of bilirubin production, this may be insufficient to drive the plasma unconjugated bilirubin concentration outside its relatively wide normal range.

Clinical Evaluation of the Patient with Erythrocytosis

ROLE OF CONVENTIONAL DIAGNOSTIC METHODS. A systematic approach to the evaluation of the patient with erythrocytosis is illustrated in Figure 142–2. This algorithm ensures the correct classification of patients with relative as opposed to absolute erythrocytosis. In the majority of instances, patients with absolute erythrocytosis can also be appropriately classified as having primary or secondary erythrocytosis, and in the latter case, the specific underlying cause can be identified on the basis of conventional, widely available diagnostic studies. The diagnosis of polycythemia vera is discussed later in this chapter.

SPECIAL STUDIES: ASSAY OF ERYTHROPOIETIN AND ENDOGENOUS COLONY FORMATION. Erythropoietin may be estimated by an in vivo bioassay in polycythemic mice. Injection of plasma or urine preparations from the patient into such animals stimulates the incorporation of ^{59}Fe into newly produced erythrocytes, to a degree proportional to the erythropoietin content of the injected material. When this assay is applied to urine samples, normal individuals have basal levels of erythropoietin excretion within a well-defined normal range. After phlebotomy, urinary erythropoietin excretion increases, and an inverse logarithmic relationship is observed between the hematocrit and the erythropoietin excretion rate. Patients with hypoxic secondary erythrocytosis have variable basal values ranging from normal to increased, but all have increased values following reduction of the hematocrit to normal by means of phlebotomy. In contrast, basal urinary erythropoietin excretion is very low in patients with polycythemia vera. Normal human plasma contains a mean of 25 mIU of erythropoietin per milliliter, as determined by current radioimmunoassay procedures. The lower limit of sensitivity of the polycythemic mouse assay is approximately 50 mIU per milliliter. Hence, when applied to plasma, this bioassay cannot distinguish normal subjects from those with polycythemia vera, since both groups fall below this sensitivity limit. The assay can detect the elevated levels seen in some cases of secondary polycythemia. After concentrating the plasma to increase the sensitivity of this technique, patients with polycythemia vera still had undetectable plasma levels of erythropoietin by bioassay, whereas most (but not all) normal subjects had detectable values, and the majority of patients with a clinical diagnosis of secondary polycythemia had elevated levels. Unfortunately, the concentration procedure is cumbersome and may introduce artifacts into the in vivo bioassay.

Several alternative procedures for measuring erythropoietin are now available. Radioimmunoassays (RIA's) give a well-defined normal range (typically, approximately 17 to 38 mIU per milliliter of plasma). Patients with polycythemia vera usually have significantly reduced values, and some patients with secondary erythrocytosis have appreciably elevated values, although there is overlap with the normal range in both groups. The problem of immunoreactive but biologically inert erythropoietin fractions or of other cross-reacting materials remains of concern with available RIA procedures. A hemagglutination inhibition assay is also commercially available, but its specificity has been questioned.

The ability to grow erythroid progenitors from bone marrow or peripheral blood in vitro without added erythropoietin strongly supports the diagnosis of a primary bone marrow disorder of erythroid regulation. Such seemingly erythropoietin-independent "endogenous colonies" have been reported in all of the myeloproliferative disorders. In the setting of an expanded red cell mass, they strongly support the diagnosis of one of the primary polycythemias, e.g., polycythemia vera.

As indicated in the foregoing discussion and in Figure 142–2, when erythropoietin assays and/or studies of in vitro endogenous colony formation are available, they may help to distinguish patients with primary polycythemias from those with secondary polycythemias. In addition, the influence of phlebotomy on erythropoietin output may separate the physiologically appropriate secondary polycythemias from those in which erythropoietin output is autonomous. In the majority of cases, these distinctions can be made on the basis of conventional diagnostic investigations.

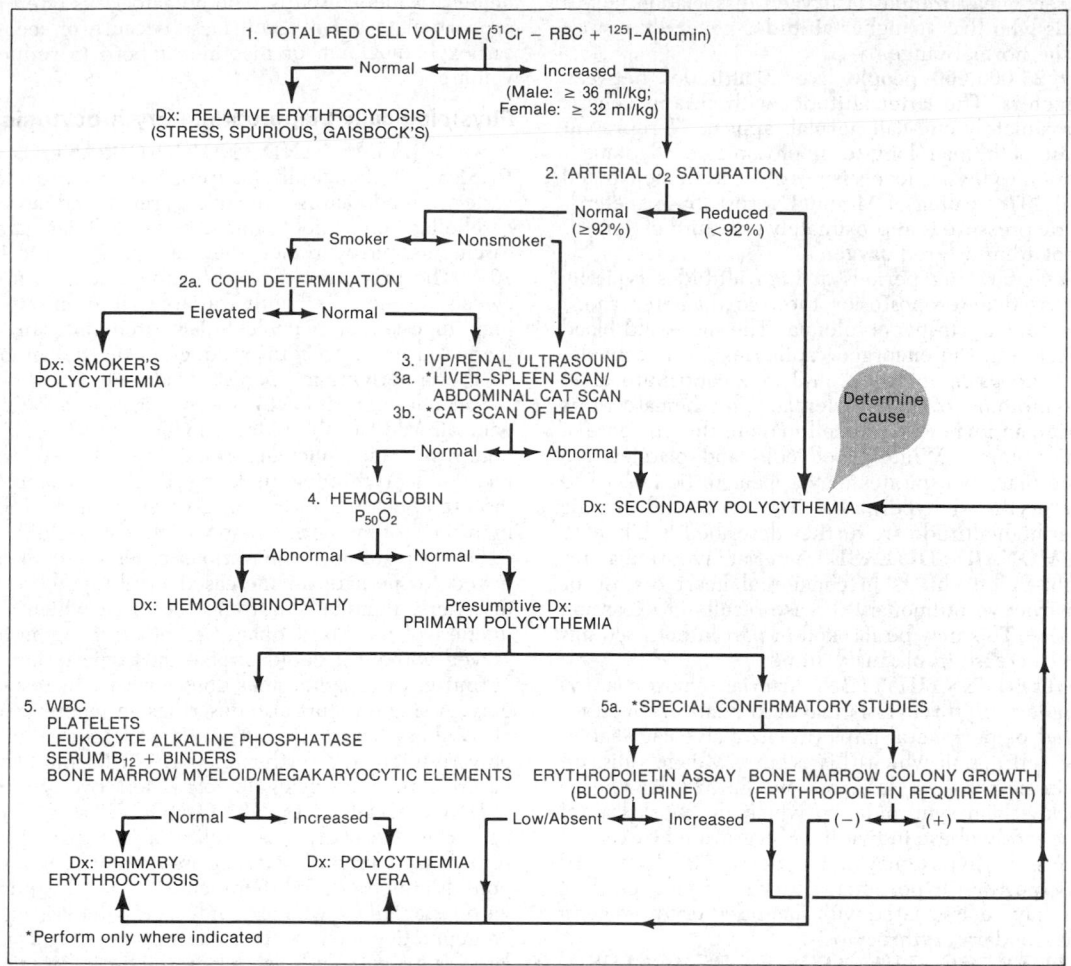

FIGURE 142–2. Algorithm for evaluation of an elevated hematocrit. Laboratory features suggestive of a myeloproliferative disease include elevated platelet and white blood cell counts and increased reticulin and clustered atypical megakaryocytes in a bone marrow biopsy. A careful history (e.g., ? family history of elevated hematocrit, ? heavy smoking) and physical examination (? splenomegaly, evidence of cardiac or pulmonary disease) provide indispensable information.

Cotes PM, Doré CJ, Liu Yin JA, et al.: Determination of serum immunoreactive erythropoietin in the investigation of erythrocytosis. N Engl J Med 315:283, 1986. *A careful examination of the value of measuring serum immunoreactive erythropoietin levels in patients with elevated hematocrits, with a useful bibliography.*

Erslev AJ, Caro J: Pure erythrocytosis classified according to erythropoietin titers. Am J Med 76:57, 1984. *Clear demonstration of both the uses and limitations of erythropoietin bioassays in diagnosis of polycythemic states.*

Groopman JE, Molina J-M, Scadden DT: Hematopoietic growth factors: Biology and clinical applications. N Engl J Med 321:1449, 1989. *An excellent review of the complex biology of hematopoietic regulation, indicating clinical applications of the five hematopoietic growth factors that have already been cloned and produced on a large scale through recombinant DNA technology: erythropoietin, GM-, G-, and M-CSF and IL3.*

Quesenberry PJ: Hemopoietic stem cells, progenitor cells and growth factors. *In* Williams WJ, Beutler E, Erslev AJ, et al. (eds.): Hematology. 4th ed. New York, McGraw-Hill, 1990, pp 129–147. *Another excellent review with the focus more on cell biology than clinical application. Outstanding bibliography.*

SECONDARY POLYCYTHEMIAS

In the secondary polycythemias, a normal bone marrow is stimulated to produce increased numbers of red blood cells, leading to an increase in the circulating red cell mass, as a result of increased production of erythropoietin or of other erythrostimulatory substances. These disorders all have in common the diverse symptomatic consequences of hypervolemia and increased blood viscosity described earlier. The secondary polycythemias may be classified into those in which the polycythemia is an appropriate physiologic response to inadequate tissue oxygenation and those in which the development of erythrocytosis is inappropriate to the oxygen balance of the patient (Table 142–1).

Physiologically Appropriate Polycythemias

HIGH ALTITUDE. In the presence of normal hemoglobin A and appropriate intraerythrocytic levels of 2,3-diphosphoglyceric acid (2,3-DPG), the partial pressure of oxygen in capillaries must be maintained close to 40 mm Hg to ensure adequate off-loading of oxygen to tissues. At sea level, where the atmospheric partial pressure of oxygen is approximately 160 mm Hg, oxygen is readily loaded onto the hemoglobin molecule, and the steep oxygen pressure gradient from the alveoli to the tissue capillaries ensures an adequate driving force for tissue oxygenation. In contrast, at elevated altitudes the atmospheric oxygen tension diminishes, and at approximately 5400 meters, the altitude of the highest permanent human settlement, atmospheric oxygen pressure is only 80 mm Hg, providing a much smaller alveolar-capillary oxygen pressure gradient. To provide adequate tissue oxygenation in the face of this reduced driving force, individuals constantly exposed to high altitude are acclimatized by two principal mechanisms, hyperventilation and the development of erythrocytosis. Hyperventilation causes a reduction in the pulmonary dead space and an increase in the surface area of adequately perfused alveoli. Erythrocytosis increases the oxygen-carrying capacity of circulating blood. Together, these two alterations permit acclimatization to occur without the need for a significant increase in cardiac output. In general, although a shift in the oxygen-hemoglobin dissociation curve to the right would also increase tissue oxygenation at a given capillary oxygen tension, such a change would also impair the on-loading of oxygen in the lungs at high altitudes. The latter appears to take precedence in that direct measurement of oxygen dissociation curves among individuals who live at higher altitudes generally reveals patterns within the normal range.

Approximately 25,000,000 people live at altitudes between 3000 and 5400 meters. The latter altitude, with an atmospheric pressure of approximately one-half normal, appears to represent the extreme limit of human long-term physiologic adaptation. Transient adaptation to higher levels is possible, as demonstrated by the successful 1978 scaling of Mount Everest (8848 meters), where atmospheric pressure is approximately one third of normal, without the use of administered oxygen.

Those who dwell for long periods at high altitudes typically develop an increased anteroposterior thoracic diameter and a ruddy cyanosis secondary to hypervolemia. The increased blood volume is manifested in the engorged capillaries of the conjunctivae, skin, and mucous membranes, and may contribute to all of the classic symptoms of hypervolemia. The hematocrit is elevated, reflecting an increased red cell mass in the presence of a normal plasma volume. White blood cells and platelets are normal, and bone marrow aspirates may appear to be normal or to show modest erythroid hyperplasia. The acute and chronic effects of living at high altitude are further described in Ch. 528.

CARDIOPULMONARY DISEASE. Arterial hypoxemia, resulting from right-to-left shunts in congenital heart disease or from chronic obstructive pulmonary disease results in expansion of the red cell mass. This may be masked in part in both settings by a concomitant increase in plasma volume.

ALVEOLAR HYPOVENTILATION. Arterial hypoxemia, cyanosis, and secondary erythrocytosis may also result from either centrally mediated or peripheral impairment of alveolar ventilation. One of the settings in which this occurs, Monge's disease (chronic mountain sickness), is described in Ch. 528. Another is the so-called pickwickian syndrome, in which the work load of ventilation in a severely obese individual is aggravated by central hyporesponsiveness to hypoxemia and hypercapnia. In a third group of patients, postural hypoxemia occurs during sleep. All of these conditions may be associated with increased erythropoietin production and secondary erythrocytosis.

ABNORMALITIES OF THE OXYGEN-HEMOGLOBIN DISSOCIATION CURVE. Abnormalities in the ability of hemoglobin to release oxygen to tissues, manifested by a shift in the oxyhemoglobin dissociation curve to the left, may occur on either a congenital or an acquired basis. At least 42 such hemoglobins have been described in association with erythrocytosis (Ch. 136.3). In most an amino acid substitution occurring in the contact area between the α and β chains interferes with the normal conformational changes that facilitate oxygen release from the molecule. The resulting hemoglobin with high oxygen affinity results in noncyanotic tissue hypo-oxygenation and ultimately in secondary erythrocytosis. High-affinity variants involving both α chain substitutions (hemoglobin Capetown, hemoglobin Chesapeake) and β chain substitutions (hemoglobin Ranier, hemoglobin Yakima) have been described. Most of these high-affinity mutations are electrophoretically silent because there is no charge difference between the normal and variant hemoglobin. Hence, determination of an oxygen-hemoglobin dissociation curve or determination of the P_{50} is essential in the evaluation of patients suspected of having a hemoglobin with high oxygen affinity. This suspicion particularly should be directed toward individuals in whom familial erythrocytosis is observed.

Secondary erythrocytosis may also occur in the presence of certain hereditary methemoglobinemias, disorders in which amino acid substitutions occur in the regions of the heme pockets. Most of these conditions are associated with hemolysis, but in the few in which the rate of red cell destruction is nearly normal, compensatory mechanisms may result in a secondary erythrocytosis. Several different congenital disorders involving a decreased ability to synthesize 2,3-DPG have been described. Since reductions in red cell 2,3-DPG content are associated with an increased oxygen affinity for hemoglobin, such patients may behave clinically as if they had a high-affinity hemoglobin disorder with resulting secondary erythrocytosis, even though they in fact have hemoglobin A. Finally, prolonged exposure to carbon monoxide, occasionally on an industrial basis but more frequently in chain

smokers, results in erythrocytosis because carboxyhemoglobin has the effect of increasing the oxygen affinity of the remaining heme prosthetic groups. The hematocrit is often increased out of proportion to the red cell mass because of secondary effects of carboxyhemoglobin or nicotine or both in reducing the plasma volume.

Physiologically Inappropriate Erythrocytosis

NEOPLASMS AND NONNEOPLASTIC RENAL DISEASES. Physiologically inappropriate erythrocytosis is seen in a variety of neoplasms, including renal and adrenal carcinoma, cerebellar hemangioblastoma, hepatocellular carcinoma, ovarian carcinoma, pheochromocytoma, and massive uterine fibroids (Ch. 161). The proportion of each of these tumors in which erythrocytosis develops is highly variable. It seems to be particularly high in cases of hepatocellular carcinoma. In most instances, increased erythropoietin production by the tumor is believed to be the underlying mechanism leading to erythrocytosis.

Secondary erythrocytosis also occurs in a variety of nonmalignant disorders of the kidney, including cystic disease and hydronephrosis, and following renal transplantation. Production of increased erythropoietin levels in the presence of renal cystic disease appears likely in view of the frequent documentation of high titers of the hormone in aspirated cyst fluid. Local intrarenal ischemia resulting from various types of renal pathology is believed to mediate an increased erythropoietin output in these disorders. Familial syndromes occur in which autonomous production of increased quantities of erythropoietin has been observed without a demonstrable anatomic lesion. Erythropoietin output in these syndromes does not vary in response to phlebotomy. A single report also describes an inappropriately high level of basal erythropoietin output in an individual in whom phlebotomy resulted in a further increase in hormone production. The nature of the underlying defect in these two syndromes is unclear.

DRUG-INDUCED ERYTHROCYTOSIS. Testosterone and its various derivatives, as well as a variety of adrenal corticosteroids, may stimulate red cell production. Testosterone-like compounds are often used therapeutically for this purpose in patients with renal failure who are undergoing dialysis or in patients with aregenerative anemia. In some instances, androgens also stimulate granulocyte and platelet production. Occasionally, increased levels of steroid hormones, whether administered therapeutically or produced in the course of adrenal disorders, may result in secondary erythrocytosis.

Treatment of the Secondary Polycythemias

Hypervolemia and increased blood viscosity accompany the development of erythrocytosis. Accordingly, when a secondary erythrocytosis is not in response to an appropriate physiologic stimulus, reduction of hematocrit to less than 50 per cent by means of phlebotomy is an appropriate part of the treatment regimen, which should also address itself to the underlying disorder.

The issue is more complex in those secondary erythrocytoses that represent a physiologic response to poor tissue oxygenation. The beneficial effect of expansion of the red cell mass may ultimately be offset by the detrimental effect of increasing blood viscosity on cardiac output, systemic oxygen transport, and local tissue oxygen delivery. In a normovolemic state, oxygen transport is optimal at a hematocrit of 40 to 45 per cent. In the presence of hypervolemia, optimal oxygen delivery may occur at hematocrits close to 60 per cent. However, hematocrits higher than this inevitably impair oxygen delivery. Nevertheless, in a given patient, if an increase in the hematocrit to the region of 60 per cent does not achieve normal tissue oxygenation, a continued increase in erythropoietin output may result in overcompensation. This overcompensation may not only decrease net tissue oxygen delivery but may also impair regional blood flow in a number of organs, particularly within the cerebral circulation. In summary, in the physiologic secondary polycythemias, there is a balance between the beneficial effects of an increasing hematocrit and the negative consequences of an excessive increase in blood viscosity. In general, hematocrits in excess of 60 per cent are detrimental and should be reduced by phlebotomy. In patients with arterial hypoxemia resulting from pulmonary disease or right-to-left cardiac shunts, the optimal level of hemoglobin and hematocrit may be difficult to determine except by trial and error. In some cases, improvement in cerebral function and decrease in congestive heart failure may follow a reduction in blood volume to hematocrits in the mid 50's or even lower.

Bunn HF, Forget B: Hemoglobin: Molecular, Genetic and Clinical Aspects. Philadelphia, W. B. Saunders Company, 1986, pp 595–622. *This chapter presents an outstanding review of hemoglobin variants with abnormal oxygen binding and their clinical consequences, as well as a comprehensive bibliography.*

Chetty KG, Brown SE, Light RW: Improved exercise tolerance of the polycythemic lung patient following phlebotomy. Am J Med 74:415, 1983. *A detailed clinicophysiologic study documenting that patients with polycythemia due to chronic obstructive pulmonary disease benefit from reduction of hematocrit to the mid 50's by phlebotomy.*

Erslev AJ: Blood and mountains. *In* Wintrobe MM (ed.): Blood, Pure and Eloquent. New York, McGraw-Hill, 1980, pp 257–280. *A lucid and fascinating review of the evolution of current concepts of human adaptation to the hypoxemia of high altitudes. Excellent bibliography.*

Erslev AJ: Secondary polycythemia (erythrocytosis). *In* Williams WJ, Beutler E, Erslev AJ, et al. (eds.): Hematology. 4th ed. New York, McGraw-Hill, 1990, pp 705–715. *A detailed review of the causes, pathophysiology, and treatment of the different forms of secondary polycythemia. Good discussion of the rare familial syndromes associated with hypererythropoietinemia. Comprehensive bibliography.*

Wallis PJW: Effects of erythropheresis on pulmonary haemodynamics and oxygen transport in patients with secondary polycythemia and cor pulmonale. Clin Sci 70:91, 1986. *Outstanding clinical physiologic study of the benefits of phlebotomy in this setting.*

POLYCYTHEMIA VERA: A CLONAL STEM CELL DISORDER

Nature of the Defect in Polycythemia Vera

Polycythemia vera is a hematologic malignant disorder characterized by excessive proliferation of erythroid, myeloid, and megakaryocytic elements within the bone marrow, resulting in an increased red blood cell mass and, frequently, elevated peripheral granulocyte and platelet counts. Several lines of evidence, including cytogenetic observations and isoenzyme marker studies in glucose-6-phosphate dehydrogenase (G6PD) heterozygotes, indicate that the increased proliferation of all three hematopoietic cell lines can trace its origin to a single abnormal clone, which has presumably developed at the level of the pluripotent stem cell. B lymphocytes are also derived from the abnormal stem cell clone. Studies of the growth of both erythroid progenitors and granulocyte-macrophage progenitors (CFU-GM) in vitro have demonstrated the presence of residual normal stem cells in the marrow early in the disease, but a steady decline in the proportion of the normal elements as the duration of the illness lengthens.

Thrombotic episodes that are usually attributed to increased blood viscosity and/or thrombocytosis; hemorrhagic episodes associated with thrombopathy and/or the elevated platelet and erythrocyte counts; the development of a "spent" phase characterized by cytopenias, myelofibrosis, and myeloid metaplasia; and the transformation to acute leukemia are among the principal complications of this disorder. Polycythemia vera shares several clinical, pathophysiologic, and histologic features with agnogenic myeloid metaplasia, chronic myelogenous leukemia, and primary (essential) thrombocythemia, which are collectively classified as the myeloproliferative disorders (Ch. 143).

The excessive rate of erythropoiesis in polycythemia vera occurs despite bioassayable erythropoietin levels that are low or absent; endogenous erythroid colonies in this disorder can grow in vitro without added erythropoietin. These observations led to the concept that erythropoiesis in polycythemia vera was "autonomous." The growth of endogenous colonies from patients with polycythemia vera can be markedly reduced or eliminated by adding antierythropoietin antibody to the culture, however, and can be restored by the re-addition of minute quantities of the hormone. This suggests that erythroid progenitors in polycythemia vera, rather than being independent of the hormone, may be uniquely sensitive to trace levels of erythropoietin. However, studies of erythropoietin receptors on erythroid progenitors in polycythemia vera have not demonstrated an increase in either receptor number or hormone affinity, which could account for this observation. In blood and bone marrow of patients with polycythemia vera, increased numbers of pluripotent colony-forming stem cells give rise to mixed colonies of granulocytic, erythroid, macrophage, and megakaryocytic elements (CFU-

GEMM). These CFU-GEMM undergo erythroid differentiation without added erythropoietin and, compared with normal CFU-GEMM, exhibit increased megakaryocyte formation. The "endogenous" erythroid differentiation is abolished with antibodies to erythropoietin. Hence, both the increased "erythropoietin-independent" erythropoiesis and the increased megakaryopoiesis characteristic of polycythemia vera reflect functional features of an identifiable abnormal pluripotent stem cell population. Long-term tissue cultures of bone marrow from patients with polycythemia vera demonstrate a population of abnormally replicating erythroid progenitors. These cells fail to respond to the normal inhibitory signals derived from nonhematopoietic elements within the marrow.

The mechanism of malignant transformation in polycythemia vera is unknown. The rare occurrence of documented polycythemia vera in monozygotic twins and the only marginally increased incidence in first-degree relatives of affected patients suggest a minimal genetic role in most cases, and neither toxic chemicals nor exposure to radiation is established as an etiologic factor. Although two documented cases occurred among exposed observers of a 1957 nuclear test explosion, the incidence of polycythemia vera has not been appreciably increased in survivors of the Hiroshima and Nagasaki atomic bomb explosions. Preliminary reports of reverse transcriptase activity and of retrovirus-like particles in platelets of patients with myeloproliferative disorders are intriguing, particularly in view of the murine polycythemia produced by one strain of Friend mouse erythroleukemia virus. These studies require extensive confirmation.

Clinical Manifestations

Polycythemia vera is typically a disease of later life, with the median age at presentation being close to 60 years. Nevertheless, patients in their second through fourth decades are not rare. The disorder is characterized by a slight preponderance in males and a propensity to occur with somewhat increased frequency in patients of Jewish ancestry.

Multiphasic screening is currently resulting in an increasing percentage of cases being detected prior to the development of symptoms. Alternatively, a routine blood count may demonstrate increased hematocrit and other abnormalities in patients who present with only mild headaches and plethoric facies. Further symptoms as they develop usually are referable to the combination of hypervolemia and hyperviscosity resulting from the increased red cell mass and blood volume, frequently aggravated by thrombocytosis and platelet dysfunction; to the local consequences of panhyperplasia of the bone marrow; or to the metabolic consequences of increased cell turnover.

SYMPTOMS. Headaches, tinnitus, light-headedness and vertigo, and blurred vision appear to result principally from increased blood viscosity and hypervolemia. Thrombotic complications, which may involve both arterial and venous occlusive events, are usually attributed to a combination of hyperviscosity, thrombocytosis, and platelet dysfunction. An increased incidence of epistaxis, spontaneous bruising, and upper gastrointestinal hemorrhage is also ascribed to the effects of hypervolemia and platelet dysfunction. Peptic ulcer disease seems to occur with increased frequency in patients with polycythemia vera, as does pruritus, sometimes aggravated after a hot bath or shower, and occasionally so severe as to be disabling. The increased frequency of both peptic ulcer and pruritus may be related to the increased histamine release caused by excessive turnover of granulocytes and, more specifically, basophils. Approximately one third of patients complain of sweating and weight loss, presumed to be on the basis of a hypermetabolic state. Patients with polycythemia vera often complain of severe pain in their feet, which is characteristically relieved by very low doses of aspirin or nonsteroidal anti-inflammatory agents.

PHYSICAL FINDINGS. In established cases, physical examination typically reveals plethora or dusky cyanosis of the face, hands, feet, and mucous membranes. Engorgement of the conjunctivae and retinal veins is frequently present, and in patients with markedly increased hematocrit, retinal hemorrhages are occasionally seen. Mild hypertension is noted in approximately one third of patients. Ecchymoses are not infrequently observed.

The most useful physical finding in terms of differential diagnosis is splenomegaly, which is present in approximately 75 per cent of patients with polycythemia vera and tends to exclude the diagnosis of most of the secondary polycythemias. Procedures such as abdominal computed tomography demonstrate splenomegaly in a percentage of those patients in whom the spleen is not palpably enlarged. Splenic enlargement appears to reflect principally the development of extramedullary hematopoiesis. Hepatomegaly is present in approximately 40 per cent of patients.

Symptomatic bone pain and tenderness on physical examination, particularly in the ribs and sternum, are occasionally severe and reflect intense panhyperplasia of the bone marrow. In addition to hyperhistaminemia, the cellular proliferation of polycythemia vera results in overproduction of uric acid, leading, not infrequently, to either uric acid stone diathesis or overt secondary gout.

Laboratory Data

The characteristic laboratory findings in polycythemia vera reflect the various consequences of increased bone marrow activity.

ERYTHROCYTES. Patients with this disorder typically present with an elevation of the hemoglobin concentration, hematocrit, and red blood cell count. Red blood cell morphology usually reveals hypochromic microcytic cells with a reduced mean corpuscular volume, suggestive of iron-deficient erythropoiesis (see Color Plate 5K). This suggestion is frequently confirmed by a low serum iron level and absence of bone marrow iron stores. These features may occur prior to the onset of therapeutic phlebotomy and without any history of gastrointestinal blood loss and result from the shift of iron from various body storage pools into the circulating erythron as the red cell mass is expanded. This phenomenon may of course be exaggerated in patients who have gastrointestinal bleeding or in whom therapeutic phlebotomies have been initiated. Of the three conventional parameters reflecting the red cell mass, the red blood cell count is often most strikingly elevated, and red cell counts of 10×10^6 per microliter may be seen in the newly diagnosed case. In contrast, the hematocrit probably provides the best, although imperfect, simple guide to the size of the circulating red cell mass and to blood viscosity. It is difficult to define the precise upper limit for the normal hematocrit. As noted earlier, increased red cell masses may be found in a small percentage of patients with hematocrits of 48 per cent or above, and an increase in the hematocrit to greater than 60 per cent is required before the hematocrit alone can be taken positively as evidence for an absolute erythrocytosis. The plasma volume in polycythemia vera has variously been reported to be normal, reduced, or increased and thus has no direct correlation with the red cell mass. The red cell lifespan is normal in the early phases of polycythemia vera, even in the presence of moderate splenomegaly. As the disease evolves, the development of increasingly ineffective erythropoiesis, as well as a larger element of extramedullary hematopoiesis with hepatomegaly and splenomegaly, results in progressive shortening of the red cell lifespan in some patients. This development is usually associated with the appearance of anisocytosis and poikilocytosis, nucleated red blood cells, and teardrop cells in the peripheral blood. When such studies are available, patients with untreated polycythemia vera will invariably demonstrate very low levels of plasma and urine erythropoietin and the ability to grow endogenous, erythropoietin-independent colonies of erythroid progenitors in vitro from either peripheral blood or bone marrow samples.

LEUKOCYTES. Sixty per cent of patients with polycythemia vera have an increased granulocyte count in the peripheral blood at the time of diagnosis. Early in the disease, elevations are usually modest and involve the presence of only normal granulocytes and bands. Subsequently, striking elevations in total white cell count may achieve leukemoid proportions, associated with the appearance of early myeloid forms, particularly myelocytes and metamyelocytes. When the appearance of these cells is accompanied by increasing splenomegaly and the appearance of abnormal erythroid elements in the periphery, a significant element of myeloid metaplasia is likely. The alkaline phosphatase

activity of circulating granulocytes is increased in polycythemia vera, in contrast to the reduction observed in chronic granulocytic leukemia. Increased granulocyte turnover is reflected by high serum and urine muramidase (lysozyme) levels and by an increase in serum B_{12} and unbound B_{12} binding capacity that results from high levels of transcobalamins 1 and 3. The basophil count and, to a lesser extent, the eosinophil count may also be increased in polycythemia vera. Increased excretion of histamine metabolites reflects increased turnover of the former cell line. Total lymphocyte counts in polycythemia vera are normal. However, a decreased number of suppressor T lymphocytes and an increase in the helper/suppressor T lymphocyte ratio have been reported.

PLATELETS. At diagnosis, the platelet count exceeds 500,000 per microliter in approximately half of patients with polycythemia vera, and striking elevations into the millions have been recorded. There is a tendency for the platelet count to increase with time, particularly in patients who are treated principally with phlebotomy. The platelets in polycythemia vera frequently appear morphologically abnormal, with megathrombocytes and megakaryocytic fragments being observed in the peripheral blood smear. As determined by electronic particle sizing, both the mean platelet volume and the platelet distribution width are increased in patients with polycythemia vera and other myeloproliferative disorders who have thrombocytosis. By contrast, the platelet distribution width is generally normal in reactive thrombocytosis. An appreciable fraction of patients with polycythemia vera also have abnormalities of conventional studies of platelet function, including aggregation; a prolonged bleeding time may be present. Studies of prostaglandin metabolism also demonstrate decreased lipoxygenase activity and increased thromboxane A_2 production by the platelets of patients with polycythemia vera and other myeloproliferative diseases. However, it has not been possible to correlate either the height of the platelet count or the presence of platelet functional abnormalities with the propensity to thrombosis in these patients. In contrast, there seems to be a crude association between the extent of the elevation of the platelet count and the propensity to hemorrhagic complications.

BONE MARROW. The bone marrow in polycythemia vera is typically hyperplastic and reveals a panmyelosis. Because of the parallel increase in all three cell lines, the myeloid/erythroid ratio may be normal. Megakaryocytes are not merely increased but typically are seen in sheets or clumps (Fig. 142–3), either in biopsy sections or in the spicules of bone marrow aspirates; this finding is strongly supportive of the diagnosis of a myeloproliferative disease. Bone marrow biopsy as well as aspirate is useful in the assessment of polycythemia vera, both because it gives a better indication of the extent of hypercellularity and because connective tissue staining illustrates the extent of myelofibrosis. Serum levels of the procollagen III amino terminal peptide, now

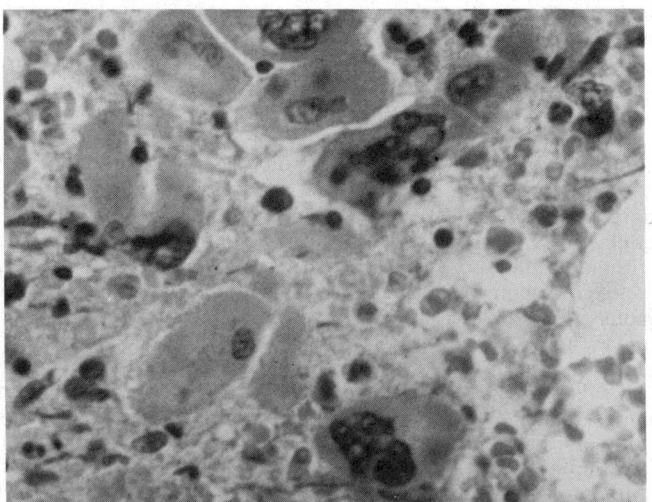

FIGURE 142–3. Bone marrow biopsy specimen from a patient with polycythemia vera. Increased numbers of atypical megakaryocytes present in clusters, as shown here, are indicative of a myeloproliferative disorder and, in the presence of an increased red cell mass, strongly support a diagnosis of polycythemia vera. Such megakaryocytic clusters may also be observed within the spicules obtained from a bone marrow aspirate.

measurable by commercially available RIA, also reflect the extent of myelofibrosis. Cytogenetic studies reveal various abnormalities in as many as 50 per cent of patients with polycythemia vera. Trisomy of chromosomes 8 and 9 and loss of chromosome 7 or its long arm (7q−) are the abnormalities most frequently observed in untreated patients; loss of chromosome 5 or of the long arms of chromosome 5 (5q−) or 20 (20q−) has been observed in some patients, especially those treated with myelosuppressives. However, no abnormality is either specific for or diagnostic of polycythemia vera. Interestingly, the presence of cytogenetic abnormalities at the time of diagnosis appears to be of no prognostic significance.

MISCELLANEOUS. Low serum cholesterol concentrations are frequently observed in patients with polycythemia vera; these reflect accelerated catabolism of low density lipoproteins, presumably by the spleen. Hyperuricemia, reflecting a general increase in cell turnover, and an increase in lactate dehydrogenase and the indirect serum bilirubin concentration, reflecting accelerated erythroid turnover, are other commonly found abnormalities.

Diagnosis and Differential Diagnosis

The diagnosis of polycythemia vera is based on the demonstration of an increased red cell mass that is not associated with excessive erythropoietin production, as well as evidence of a concomitant increase in bone marrow production of granulocytes and thrombocytes. Polycythemia is one of two disorders characterized by "autonomous" erythropoiesis. It differs from the entity designated *primary erythrocytosis* in its associated increase in granulocyte and megakaryocytic proliferation and the presence of related abnormalities such as elevated levels of leukocyte alkaline phosphatase and serum B_{12}–binding proteins. The abnormalities in primary erythrocytosis are limited to the erythroid series, but within this sphere the low bioassayable erythropoietin levels and the presence of endogenous colonies are similar to those seen in polycythemia vera. Some argue that primary erythrocytosis represents a disorder arising in the committed erythroid stem cell compartment, i.e., at a later stage than the pluripotent stem cell affected in polycythemia vera, but primary erythrocytosis has not yet been demonstrated to be a clonal disorder. Others believe that these patients represent a forme fruste of typical polycythemia vera and that granulocytic or thrombocytic abnormalities will be revealed if patients are observed for sufficient periods.

The diagnosis of a primary bone marrow disorder with autonomous erythropoiesis may be made in accordance with the algorithm illustrated in Figure 142–2 by systematically excluding the various secondary causes of an absolute erythrocytosis. Patients appearing to have increased erythroid proliferation due to a primary bone marrow defect would be classified as having polycythemia vera if they have concomitant granulocytic or platelet abnormalities in the peripheral blood, evidence of a panmyelosis in the bone marrow, or splenomegaly. In the absence of these features, when abnormalities are restricted solely to the erythroid series, the diagnosis of primary erythrocytosis would be made.

The Polycythemia Vera Study Group has developed a set of empiric criteria that permit the diagnosis of polycythemia vera to be established in many patients within one to two office visits (Table 142–2). In patients who meet these criteria, the diagnosis of polycythemia vera is highly likely, the false-positive rate having been found to be less than 0.5 per cent. False-positive results are most likely in patients who are excessive users of both alcohol and tobacco. In this setting, excessive erythroid proliferation associated with carboxyhemoglobinemia and splenomegaly, leukocytosis, and increased leukocyte alkaline phosphatase activity and serum B_{12} associated with alcoholic liver disease may confound the diagnosis. The false-negative rate for the Polycythemia Vera Study Group criteria is unknown. Patients with early disease who do not yet meet these criteria may ultimately prove to have polycythemia vera, or at least a form of primary erythrocytosis, when more extensive evaluation is carried out in accordance with the criteria of Figure 142–2.

Course

In the absence of treatment, polycythemia vera is a serious disease in which a high incidence of fatal thrombotic or hemor-

rhagic complications historically has led to a median survival of 6 to 18 months from diagnosis. Current treatment programs designed to maintain peripheral blood counts and the red cell mass at close to normal levels have achieved median survivals approximating 10 years, during the course of which aspects of the natural history of the disease have become more evident. In many patients, polycythemia vera is a readily managed disorder that remains asymptomatic for long periods. However, inadequate control of the red cell mass predisposes to both thrombotic and hemorrhagic complications, of which cerebrovascular, coronary, and abdominal vascular occlusions involving both arterial (e.g., mesenteric artery) and venous (Budd-Chiari syndrome) thromboses are most frequent. Expansion of the red cell mass is clearly not the only factor predisposing to thrombosis in polycythemia vera. The presence of endogenous erythroid progenitor colonies may be the only laboratory indicator of incipient myeloproliferative disease in young patients presenting initially with the Budd-Chiari syndrome. Thrombosis is the major cause of death overall in polycythemia vera, accounting for approximately one third of all fatalities. Some patients are particularly prone to thrombosis, suffering repeated events, one of which may ultimately prove fatal; others are spared. Unfortunately, there is no way at present to identify this thrombosis-prone subset prior to a thrombotic event. Transformation to acute leukemia, the development of other neoplasms, hemorrhage, and myelofibrosis are other major causes of fatality and collectively, along with thrombosis, account for 75 per cent of all deaths. Acute leukemia is clearly a part of the natural history of polycythemia vera, occurring with an incidence of up to 2 to 4 per cent even in patients who have not been exposed either to radiotherapy or to radiomimetic drugs.

Upper gastrointestinal hemorrhage, particularly from bleeding peptic ulcers, occurs with an increased incidence in patients with polycythemia vera. Underlying etiologic factors are believed to be increased acid secretion stimulated by hyperhistaminemia and vascular mucosal ischemia caused by increased blood viscosity and poor regional perfusion.

The complete natural history of polycythemia vera involves the ultimate transition from the proliferative phase, during which therapy is aimed at reducing peripheral blood counts, to a stable phase in which relatively normal blood counts may be maintained without therapy, to the so-called *burned out* or *spent phase*. Transition results predominantly from the gradual development of progressive myelofibrosis and, possibly, from a gradual reduction in the proliferative capacity of the abnormal hematopoietic clone. That myelofibrosis is a complication of polycythemia vera has long been recognized, but the nature of the association has been uncertain. The bulk of current evidence suggests that bone marrow fibroblasts in this setting are not part of the hematopoietic malignant clone. Similar conclusions have been reached in studies of the bone marrow fibroblast following transplantation. Hence, the increasing proliferation of fibroblasts and increased collagen deposition leading to myelofibrosis appear to be reactive phenomena rather than an intrinsic component of the neoplastic process. The clinical features and the management of postpolycythemic myelofibrosis do not differ appreciably from those of idiopathic myelofibrosis with myeloid metaplasia except that the incidence of acute leukemic transformation is markedly increased in the postpolycythemic setting, especially if the myelofibrosis follows

TABLE 142–2. PARAMETERS FOR THE DIAGNOSIS OF POLYCYTHEMIA VERA

A1 ↑ Red cell mass Male: ≥36 ml/kg Female: ≥32 ml/kg	B1 Thrombocytosis Platelet count >400,000/μl
A2 Normal arterial O_2 saturation (≥92%)	B2 Leukocytosis: >12,000/μl (no fever or infection)
A3 Splenomegaly	B3 ↑ Leukocyte alkaline phosphatase (LAP) (>100)
	B4 ↑ Serum B_{12} (>900 pg/ml) or ↑ $UB_{12}BC$ (>2200 pg/ml)*

Dx acceptable if following combinations are present:
  A1 + A2 + A3
  A1 + A2 + any two from category B
*$UB_{12}BC$ = unbound serum B_{12} binding capacity

treatment with radioactive phosphorus or chlorambucil (see Ch. 143).

Treatment

The initial treatment in any newly diagnosed case of polycythemia vera is phlebotomy. Efforts should be made to reduce the hematocrit to approximately 45 per cent, a level at which the complications of hypervolemia and hyperviscosity are minimized. In patients with appreciable splenomegaly, the hematocrit no longer reliably reflects the red cell mass, which may continue to be significantly increased despite hematocrits in the upper 40's. The initial phlebotomy regimen may involve removal of 500-ml aliquots of whole blood as often as every 2 to 3 days until a normal hematocrit is achieved. Subsequent phlebotomies should be carried out as frequently as necessary to maintain the hematocrit at or below 45 per cent. As iron deficiency supervenes, red cell production will be retarded, so that patients managed by phlebotomy alone may require as few as two or three phlebotomies per year.

Some investigators believe that phlebotomy alone, at rates sufficient to maintain a normal hematocrit and blood viscosity, is adequate to prevent the thrombotic complications of the disease and provides a minimal incidence of leukemic transformation. Others argue that some form of myelosuppression is preferable, in part because this offers an approach to the control of the thrombocytosis that is often a major clinical feature of the illness. Myelosuppression in this disorder has most often been carried out with radioactive phosphorus (^{32}P), with alkylating agents such as chlorambucil or busulfan and, more recently, with the nonalkylating myelosuppressive agent hydroxyurea.

In an ongoing randomized, controlled study in 431 patients, median survivals of 13.9 years with phlebotomy or 11.8 years with radioactive phosphorus therapy were significantly better than those achieved with chlorambucil (8.9 years), although the difference achieved statistical significance only after more than 10 years of treatment. Causes of death varied appreciably as a function of the treatment administered. Patients managed with phlebotomy alone had a significant excess incidence of severe and often fatal thrombotic complications, particularly in the first 2 to 4 years of treatment. Thrombotic complications were particularly frequent in more elderly patients (e.g., older than 70 years), in those with a high phlebotomy requirement (more than four to six per year), and in those who had had a prior history of a thrombotic event. Beyond 3 years, the incidence of thrombotic complications became the same in patients treated with phlebotomy alone as in those treated with myelosuppression, suggesting that a subset of patients particularly susceptible to thrombosis had been selected out by this time. By contrast, myelosuppression with either ^{32}P or alkylating agents effectively decreased the risk of thrombotic complications in thrombosis-prone patients early in the disease. However, both chlorambucil and ^{32}P were associated with a statistically significant increased risk of acute leukemia, which became particularly prominent after 5 to 7 years of treatment, and a somewhat later increased incidence of carcinomas of the skin and gastrointestinal tract. Thus, long-term myelosuppression with either of these agents is associated with an increased propensity for malignant transformation of the three rapidly proliferating tissues of the body: bone marrow, skin, and gastrointestinal mucosa. In addition, an increased incidence of intra-abdominal lymphocytic lymphoma has followed long-term treatment of polycythemia vera with chlorambucil.

Radioactive phosphorus, preferably given as an intravenous dose of 3 to 5 mCi, reliably produces a reduction in bone marrow proliferation with few immediate side effects. Chlorambucil or busulfan, administered either continuously or intermittently, also successfully controls peripheral counts in a high proportion of patients. In contrast to ^{32}P, myelosuppression with alkylating agents results in an appreciable incidence of cytopenias, which in the case of busulfan may be prolonged and troublesome. Because of these drug-related cytopenias and the fact that malignant complications occur both earlier and more frequently with chlorambucil than with ^{32}P, long-term treatment of polycythemia vera with alkylating agents can no longer be recommended. Although some argue that complications observed with chlorambucil should not preclude use of other alkylating agents, especially busulfan, there are sufficient anecdotal cases of leukemic transformation with all of the alkylating drugs that the burden of proof must be on those who argue for the safety of any such agent.

Hydroxyurea,* administered at a dose of 0.5 to 1.5 grams per day, has recently been shown to be an effective nonalkylating chemotherapeutic agent in the management of polycythemia vera. To date, this regimen has not been associated with an increased incidence of malignant transformation. However, the maximal follow-up with this agent, now approximately 10 years, is still too short for its full mutagenic potential to have been realized.

In patients with marked thrombocytosis refractory to conventional management, successful control of the platelet count has been achieved with experimental protocols employing either anagrelide or interferon.

Since no form of treatment for polycythemia vera is without some risks, the following recommendations would appear to provide the best control of the disease with the fewest treatment-related complications. Because of the increased risk of thrombosis associated with age, patients over 70 are most effectively treated with a combination of ^{32}P and supplemental phlebotomy. Patients below the age of 50, particularly those in the childbearing years, should be treated with phlebotomy alone whenever possible. Myelosuppression with hydroxyurea would seem advisable in such younger patients if they are particularly at risk for thrombotic complications because of a high phlebotomy requirement or a history of prior thrombotic events. The role of myelosuppression is most uncertain in the age group between 50 and 70. In the absence of thrombosis-associated risk factors, it is probably preferable to attempt to manage such patients by phlebotomy alone. If chemotherapy is deemed advisable, hydroxyurea would appear to be the agent of choice. Chlorambucil would now seem to be contraindicated for long-term therapy of polycythemia vera in view of its unacceptably high risk of leukemic and carcinogenic transformation, which may apply as well to other alkylating agents.

Although conclusive data are lacking, many physicians believe that a substantial increase in platelet count (i.e., in excess of 10^6 per microliter) is an indication for myelosuppressive therapy. Excessive splenic enlargement with local symptoms, bone tenderness, intractable pruritus, and poor veins may be other indications for the addition of myelosuppression to the treatment regimen. H_1 (cyproheptadine, 4 mg by mouth three times daily) and H_2 blockers (cimetidine, 300 mg by mouth three times daily), alone or in combination, provide relief from pruritus in some patients.

The results of attempts to reduce the incidence of thrombotic complications with the prophylactic use of platelet-antiaggregating agents have been controversial. Some investigators have reported a reduced incidence of such complications with the use of low-dose aspirin. A randomized, controlled trial of aspirin and dipyridamole, however, found not only no significant benefit from these agents in terms of thrombosis but also a statistically significant increase in the incidence of gastrointestinal hemorrhage, particularly with prolonged administration to patients with platelet counts greater than 1 million. Hence, long-term prophylactic use of this group of agents cannot be recommended at this time. Short-term use of platelet-antiaggregating agents may be helpful during transient attacks of digital or cerebral ischemia, but such episodes are an indication for, and often respond to, myelosuppression.

Patients with polycythemia vera are at increased risk for complications associated with surgery, including an appreciably increased surgical mortality rate. The incidence of complications appears to decrease with good control of the underlying disorder. Therefore, elective surgery in such patients should be undertaken only after careful consideration of the risk-benefit ratio and should always be delayed until optimal control of the peripheral blood counts has been achieved.

Treatment of the burned-out myelofibrotic stage of polycythemia vera can be extremely difficult but does not differ from that described for idiopathic myelofibrosis. The acute leukemias that develop in polycythemia vera, either spontaneously or following

---

*This use is not listed in the manufacturer's directive.

myelosuppressive therapy, may be myeloid, myelomonocytic, lymphoid, or biphenotypic in morphology. In those patients with lymphoid morphology and/or increased levels of terminal deoxyribonucleotidyl transferase (TdT), a trial of vincristine and prednisone is indicated. Nevertheless, response to any form of treatment in these patients is infrequent, and median survival in a relatively recent series of postpolycythemic acute leukemias was approximately 30 days.

Meticulous control of blood volume and viscosity with the use of phlebotomy, supplemented when specifically indicated by judicious use of myelosuppression, can ensure most patients with polycythemia vera a prolonged period of relatively symptom-free survival. Median survival in recent series has exceeded 10 years, and symptom-free survival of 15 to 20 years is no longer uncommon. The longest documented survival following a well-founded diagnosis is 34 years.

Berk PD, Goldberg JD, Donovan PB, et al.: Therapeutic recommendations in polycythemia vera based on Polycythemia Vera Study Group protocols. Semin Hematol 23:132, 1986. *A detailed report on a continuous 19-year randomized control study of a large cohort of patients with polycythemia vera and the therapeutic recommendations derived from it. Part of a useful eight-article symposium on polycythemia vera.*

Caldwell GG, Kelley DB, Heath CW Jr, et al.: Polycythemia vera among participants of a nuclear weapons test. JAMA 252:662, 1984. *A provocative report that illustrates some of the difficulties in conclusively linking relatively uncommon disorders to radiation exposure.*

Cashman JD, Eaves CJ, Eaves AC: Unregulated proliferation of primitive neoplastic progenitor cells in long-term polycythemia vera marrow cultures. J Clin Invest 81:87, 1988. *An interesting and important study emphasizing both the abnormal replicative potential of the primitive stem cells in polycythemia and the existence of inhibitory signals derived from nonhematopoietic marrow elements to which these stem cells fail to respond.*

Conley CL: Polycythemia vera, diagnosis and treatment. Hosp Practice 22:107, 1987. *An excellent overview by a senior hematologist with great experience.*

Ellis JT, Peterson P, Geller SA, et al.: Studies of the bone marrow in polycythemia vera and the evolution of myelofibrosis and second hematologic malignancies. Semin Hematol 23:144, 1986. *An important review of bone marrow findings in polycythemia vera, exploring such issues as the evolution of fibrosis and second malignant disorders.*

Malmaeus J, Akre T, Adami HO, et al.: Early postoperative course following elective splenectomy in haematological diseases: A high complication rate in patients with myeloproliferative disorders. Br J Surg 73:720, 1986. *A recent review that underscores the increased risks of surgery in patients with myeloproliferative disorders.*

Means RT Jr, Krantz SB, Sawyer ST, et al.: Erythropoietin receptors in polycythemia vera. J Clin Invest 84:1340, 1989. *One of the first studies employing purified erythropoietin to examine the state of receptors on erythroid progenitors in polycythemia vera. It provides no support for the hypothesis that abnormalities in receptor number or affinity explain the apparent increased sensitivity to erythropoietin observed in polycythemia vera.*

Murphy S: Polycythemia vera. In Williams WJ, Beutler E, Erslev AJ, et al. (eds.): Hematology. 4th ed. New York, McGraw-Hill, 1990, pp 193–202. *An excellent and comprehensive review of the pathophysiology, clinical features, and treatment, with an especially complete bibliography.*

Najean Y, Mugnier P, Dresch C, et al.: Polycythemia vera in young people: An analysis of 58 cases diagnosed before 40 years. Br J Haematol 67:285, 1987. *An important review that emphasizes the somewhat different biologic behavior of polycythemia in younger patients.*

Silverstein MM, Petitt RM, Solberg LA Jr, et al.: Anagrelide: A new drug for treating thrombocytosis. N Engl J Med 318:1292, 1988. *Preliminary report on a promising new agent with highly selective effects in controlling thrombocytosis in myeloproliferative disorders.*

143 Myeloproliferative Disorders

Paul D. Berk

The normal bone marrow contains self-replicating pools of morphologically undifferentiated stem cells, recognizable hematopoietic cells undergoing differentiation and maturation, as well as vascular and connective tissue stromal elements. There is a hierarchy of hematopoietic stem cell populations: (1) a pluripotent stem cell capable, under appropriate conditions, of producing erythroid, myeloid, megakaryocytic, macrophage, and B lymphocyte progeny; (2) intermediate stem cells capable of producing several but not all of these lineages; and (3) committed, unipotent stem cells giving rise exclusively to erythroid, myeloid, or megakaryocytic offspring. The rate of proliferation, pool size, and rate of transition from less restricted to more restricted potential are carefully regulated so that the bone marrow can respond to the body's need for blood elements in a manner that is both selective in terms of the cell types produced and restricted or self-limited in duration (see Fig. 127–2). These selective responses are mediated by a complex and incompletely understood network of endocrine, paracrine, and possibly autocrine factors, including erythropoietin, various interleukins, interferons, and growth factors (Ch. 127 and 142), of which macrophages, as well as the endothelial cells lining the marrow vascular channels, may be the major sources. As a result, in hemolysis, pyogenic infection, and immune platelet destruction, specific needs for increased production of erythrocytes, granulocytes, and platelets, respectively, are met ordinarily by selective erythroid, myeloid, or megakaryocytic hyperplasia of the marrow. Stromal cells such as fibroblasts do not appear to play a significant role in these physiologic responses.

In the myeloproliferative disorders, in contrast, each of the three major marrow cell lines proliferates in an unregulated, essentially autonomous and self-perpetuating manner. Four disorders—polycythemia vera, agnogenic myeloid metaplasia, chronic myelogenous leukemia, and essential thrombocythemia—can usefully be classified under this heading. Although the proliferation of one particular cell line may dominate the clinical picture, each of these is a clonal hematopoietic malignant disorder arising at the level of the pluripotent stem cell. In each disorder, erythroid, myeloid, and megakaryocytic elements proliferate excessively, but to varying degrees, in the bone marrow and in sites of extramedullary hematopoiesis (often resulting in splenomegaly). In each disorder there is a variable tendency for reactive proliferation of the otherwise normal bone marrow fibroblast—which both cytogenetic and glucose-6-phosphate dehydrogenase (G6PD) isoenzyme studies confirm is not a part of the malignant clone—with the development of myelofibrosis, and for termination in an acute blastic leukemia. Despite differences in the predominant cell line released into the periphery, bone marrows at the time of presentation show many similarities and may be indistinguishable, with clumps or sheets of abnormal megakaryocytes being common to all. Hyperuricemia secondary to increased cell turnover and abnormal levels of serum B_{12} and its binding proteins and of leukocyte alkaline phosphatase activity are also common to this group. Some investigators include acute leukemias of various types (notably erythroleukemia) and paroxysmal nocturnal hemoglobinuria within the myeloproliferative syndromes; others consider these disorders sufficiently different from the basic four to warrant their exclusion.

The myeloproliferative syndromes have long been considered to exhibit transitions between the various entities. The evolution of polycythemia vera into a disorder characterized by myelofibrosis with myeloid metaplasia is well documented, as is the transition of all entities—albeit with varying frequency—to acute leukemia. Other transitions have been harder to document. Thus, Philadelphia chromosome (Ph[1])–positive chronic myelogenous leukemia may present transiently with elevated red cell and platelet counts but does not at this stage represent polycythemia vera. Similarly, a patient with polycythemia vera who has suffered a gastrointestinal hemorrhage may at initial examination have only an elevated platelet count, resembling essential thrombocythemia. Repletion of iron stores with resulting erythrocytosis does not represent a true transition from essential thrombocythemia to polycythemia vera.

Despite the failure to confirm true transitions among several of these disorders, the concept of a myeloproliferative syndrome involving the four basic entities just listed is now firmly supported by their clonal, morphologic, pathophysiologic, and clinical similarities. Various nonspecific cytogenetic abnormalities are also observed in each of these entities. The appearance of the Ph[1] chromosome, characteristic of chronic myelogenous leukemia, is a late event in the pathogenetic evolution of the disorder and follows the initial development of the malignant clone of pluripotent stem cells.

Gilbert HS: Myeloproliferative disorders. Clin Geriatr Med 1:773, 1985. *A reassessment of the myeloproliferative disease concept on its fortieth anniversary by an astute clinical observer.*

Lichtman MA: Classification and clinical manifestations of the hematopoietic stem cell disorders. *In* Williams WJ, Beutler E, Erslev AJ, et al. (eds.): Hematology. 4th ed. New York, McGraw-Hill, 1990, pp 148–157. *A useful classification of various types of hematopoietic stem cell disorders that places the chronic myeloproliferative disorders in proper perspective.*

Nathan CF: Secretory products of macrophages. J Clin Invest 79:319, 1987. *A concise yet lucid review of the diverse biologic properties of the numerous regulatory molecules now known to derive, at least in part, from macrophages, including modulation of cellular replication and differentiation.*

MYELOFIBROSIS WITH MYELOID METAPLASIA

Definition and Pathogenesis

Myelofibrosis with myeloid metaplasia is a syndrome in which morphologic evidence of excessive fibroblast proliferation and collagen deposition in the bone marrow is accompanied by myeloid metaplasia of organs such as the liver, spleen, and lymph nodes. These organs, involved normally in fetal but not adult erythropoiesis, become active sites of extramedullary hematopoiesis. Similar clinical syndromes may be seen in three distinct settings. The first of these is progressive hepatosplenomegaly and the evolution of a leukoerythroblastic peripheral blood picture indicative of myeloid metaplasia occurring in the absence of an apparent inciting cause. This disorder, termed *agnogenic myeloid metaplasia* (see Color Plates 5J and 7F, left), is a clonal stem cell hemopathy constituting one of the primary myeloproliferative syndromes. Second, a similar picture of myelofibrosis with myeloid metaplasia may evolve in the course of polycythemia vera or chronic granulocytic leukemia, either as a part of the natural history of the illness or as a consequence of the myelosuppressive therapies administered. The third setting is myeloid metaplasia with varying degrees of reactive myelofibrosis that may occur secondary to a wide spectrum of clinical disorders, including, among others, severe hemolytic anemia, Hodgkin's disease, various nonhematopoietic neoplasms metastatic to the bone marrow, infections such as tuberculosis, or following bone marrow injury caused by radiation, benzol, fluorine, phosphorus, or strontium.

In myelofibrosis with myeloid metaplasia, the extent of extramedullary hematopoiesis tends to parallel the extent of bone marrow fibrosis. Indeed, it was previously believed that the mesenchymal cells in the liver, spleen, and lymph nodes resumed their embryonic potential for hematopoiesis in an attempt to compensate for myelophthisis. However, in some cases there is a dissociation between the degree of marrow fibrosis and extramedullary hematopoiesis, resulting in (1) marrow fibrosis without evidence of significant myeloid metaplasia or (2) progressive hepatosplenomegaly with a leukoerythroblastic peripheral blood picture in the absence of significant fibrosis. Pluripotent hematopoietic stem cells, presumably of bone marrow origin, are constantly present in the circulation of normal individuals and appear in increased numbers in the peripheral blood of patients with myelofibrosis. It is more likely that these circulating stem cells take up residence in organs such as the liver and spleen to produce extramedullary hematopoiesis than that this represents the reactivation of hematopoietic capabilities in local mesenchymal cells.

Except in the secondary setting noted above, the primary pathogenetic event is believed to be a mutation leading to a malignant pluripotent hematopoietic stem cell clone. In black women with agnogenic myeloid metaplasia who are also heterozygous for two different G6PD isoenzymes, the presence of only one G6PD isoenzyme in all of their erythroid, myeloid megakaryocytic, macrophage, and B lymphoid cells and/or progenitor colonies confirms that all of these cells are derived from a single, mutated pluripotent stem cell. A similar cellular distribution of acquired cytogenetic abnormalities in the significant proportion of patients with abnormal karyotypes suggests the same conclusion. Endogenous colonies of erythroid progenitor cells can be grown from peripheral blood or bone marrow.

The development of myelofibrosis appears to be a reaction to the presence of this abnormal, proliferating hematopoietic clone. Marrow fibrosis in agnogenic myeloid metaplasia, as in the other myeloproliferative disorders, correlates with the presence in the marrow of increased numbers of often dysplastic megakaryocytes (Fig. 142–3). The release of increased quantities of megakaryocyte- and platelet-derived growth factor, and of transforming growth factor–β (TGF-β), from the markedly expanded bone marrow megakaryocyte pool appears to be primarily responsible for the increased fibroblast proliferation and collagen deposition that characterize these disorders. Possible roles for tumor necrosis factor–α and interleukin 1 (IL1), also potent stimulators of fibroplasia, remain to be established. Colonization of the liver, spleen, and lymph nodes may, in this setting, represent a form of metastasis of abnormal stem cells to organs that retain an intrinsic potential to support hematopoiesis.

Clinical Features

Myelofibrosis with myeloid metaplasia, whether agnogenic or secondary to another myeloproliferative syndrome, is primarily a disorder of the middle-aged or older adult. Although reported to occur as early as infancy, at least 60 per cent of cases occur in those between the ages of 50 and 70, with no predilection for either sex. The onset of symptoms is usually insidious over several years, and in most cases disease progression is slow. One quarter of cases are asymptomatic at diagnosis. Most commonly presenting symptoms are referable to anemia with its cardiovascular consequences or to increased abdominal girth or discomfort resulting from splenic and hepatic enlargement. Bone pain, often migratory, and gouty arthritis occasionally bring the patient to medical attention. Osteosclerosis is common; deafness resulting from otosclerosis occurs in a small minority of cases. Increasing numbers of asymptomatic patients are being detected today in the course of routine screening laboratory or physical examinations.

On physical examination, splenomegaly is an almost universal finding. In approximately 85 per cent of cases, the spleen extends 8 cm or more below the left costal margin and in one third of cases is enlarged more than 16 cm. Occasional patients without palpable splenomegaly are demonstrated to have splenic enlargement by means of an isotopic or computed tomographic (CT) imaging study. Rarely, significant myelofibrosis with cytopenia occurs, at least initially, without myeloid metaplasia and with no evidence of splenic enlargement. Hepatomegaly occurs in approximately 50 per cent of cases, frequently with mild abnormalities of liver function tests—especially elevation of alkaline phosphatase levels. Hepatomegaly in the absence of splenomegaly is extremely rare in agnogenic myeloid metaplasia or when the syndrome occurs secondary to another myeloproliferative disease and points to a diagnosis of secondary myeloid metaplasia. Extramedullary hematopoiesis is frequently demonstrable histologically in lymph nodes, but clinically significant lymph node enlargement occurs in only 10 per cent of cases. Extramedullary tumors of hematopoietic tissue, often with intense fibrosis, may occur virtually anywhere but are most commonly reported in the adrenal glands, kidneys, intestinal tract, lungs, mediastinum, breast, and skin. When they occur in the intracranial or intraspinal epidural spaces, they may lead to serious neurologic consequences. Ascites and pleural or pericardial effusions, often containing immature hematopoietic cells, may result from the implantation of hematopoietic foci on various serosal surfaces. A combination of increased splenic and portal blood flow, due to proliferation of extramedullary hematopoietic tissue within the spleen, and decreased intrahepatic vascular compliance, caused by both intrasinusoidal extramedullary hematopoiesis and perisinusoidal fibrosis, may lead to clinically significant portal hypertension, with consequent ascites, esophageal varices, and gastrointestinal hemorrhage. Jaundice, edema, and ascites occur in 10 to 20 per cent of cases. Petechiae, caused by both thrombocytopenia and platelet dysfunction, have been reported in up to 25 per cent of patients.

Laboratory Data

At diagnosis, a mild to moderate degree of anemia is typical, with the hemoglobin ranging between 9 and 13 grams per deciliter. Red cells are initially normocytic and normochromic with mild poikilocytosis. Polychromatophilia, a modest reticulocytosis of 2 to 5 per cent, and occasional teardrop erythrocytes are seen (see Color Plate 7F, left). The presence of at least a few normoblasts and occasionally even earlier erythroid precursors is extremely common. As the disease progresses and the spleen enlarges, more severe anisocytosis, poikilocytosis, polychromasia, basophilic stippling, and normoblastosis may be sufficiently characteristic to indicate the diagnosis. Red cell autoantibodies, with autoimmune hemolysis, may contribute to the anemia in some cases. The white blood cell count is initially normal in about one third of patients, elevated in approximately one half, and low in the remaining 15 per cent. Most typically, the count is in the range of 15,000 to 30,000 per cubic millimeter, but counts as high as 70,000 per cubic millimeter are observed. The white count tends to fluctuate with time and often does not show the downward trend observed for the hemoglobin concentration and platelet count. A degree of granulocyte immaturity in the peripheral blood is typical, including the presence of as many as 10 per cent blasts. This condition does not necessarily suggest the evolution of acute leukemia, particularly when there are proportionate numbers of promyelocytes, myelocytes, and metamyelocytes as well. Basophilia and an acquired Pelger-Huët anomaly are other typical features of the peripheral blood smear. The leukocyte alkaline phosphatase score is variable but is most often normal or increased. The platelet count initially is most often normal, although reduced or elevated counts are not uncommon. Exceedingly high counts in excess of 10^6 per microliter may cause this condition to be confused with the entity of primary thrombocytosis. Morphologically, megathrombocytes and megakaryocytic fragments are extremely common. Over time, the platelet count gradually tends to decrease, and thrombocytopenia is common late in the disorder. Overall, a peripheral blood smear demonstrating striking teardrop poikilocytosis, leukoerythroblastic nucleated cells, and megathrombocytes and megakaryocytic fragments is highly suggestive of the syndrome of myelofibrosis with myeloid metaplasia. Erythrocyte survival is almost invariably reduced, and splenic sequestration often is present. Erythrokinetic studies demonstrate markedly ineffective erythropoiesis. Platelet production is usually increased even in patients with thrombocytopenia, associated with a marked increase in splenic pooling.

Normal or slightly elevated serum levels of vitamin B_{12} and B_{12}-binding proteins occur both in agnogenic myeloid metaplasia and postpolycythemia myelofibrosis, but the values are not as striking in those seen in chronic granulocytic leukemia. Hyperuricemia, caused by increased uric acid production, is common. Miscellaneous laboratory abnormalities include high levels of lactate dehydrogenase (LDH), modest elevations of serum transaminase and bilirubin levels, increased serum alkaline phosphatase activity caused by both hepatic and bone isoenzyme fractions, and modest increases in muramidase (lysozyme). A variety of autoantibodies, circulating immune complexes, and complement activation have been reported, as have associations with systemic lupus erythematosus, periarteritis nodosa, scleroderma, and nonspecific vasculitis. These reports have suggested a possible autoimmune pathogenesis in some cases.

Cytogenetic abnormalities occur in up to 50 per cent of patients with agnogenic myeloid metaplasia, with trisomy of chromosomes 7, 8, and 9 being most commonly found. Abnormalities of chromosomes 1, 5, and 20 also occur with increased frequency. The Ph¹ chromosome is not present; cases in which this abnormality was reported most likely represent atypical examples of chronic myelogenous leukemia.

Osteosclerosis distributed primarily in the flat bones of the axial skeleton and in the metaphyseal ends of the femur and humerus may be recognized radiographically in up to 70 per cent of patients. The typical radiographic finding is the loss of definition of individual bony trabeculae, leading to a ground glass appearance.

Attempts to aspirate bone marrow almost invariably lead to a dry tap, even when the marrow is very cellular. Accordingly, bone marrow biopsy, either percutaneous or surgical, is usually required for diagnosis. Demonstration of bone marrow fibrosis (see Color Plate 5J), often with accompanying osteosclerosis, is the sine qua non, and the marrow content of types I, III, and IV collagen is increased. The bone marrow may sometimes be hypercellular, frequently demonstrating a panhyperplasia, in residual focal areas. Even in these areas, in which mature collagen may not be evident, an increase in reticulin fibers can usually be demonstrated by silver impregnation. Extramedullary hematopoiesis is demonstrable in both liver and spleen, but because of the risks involved in percutaneous biopsy of these organs, its diagnosis usually is based on the typical leukoerythroblastic blood picture and occasionally on isotopic erythrokinetic studies. The

increase of bone marrow collagen content in myelofibrosis is principally the result of excessive collagen deposition and is reflected in an increase in the serum level of procollagen III amino-terminal peptide. Serum prolyl hydroxylase and plasma fibronectin are also increased.

Course of the Disease

The course of both agnogenic and postpolycythemic myelofibrosis is characterized by progressive splenic enlargement and, typically, by slightly less striking enlargement of the liver. The spleen often fills the entire left side of the abdomen, extending beyond the midline to the right and down into the pelvis. The resulting early satiety, associated with a hypermetabolic state from increased cell turnover, may result in appreciable weight loss. Painful splenic infarcts may also complicate the disease. The marked splenic enlargement and consequent increase in splenic blood flow, coupled with increased resistance to flow within the liver caused by extramedullary hematopoiesis, lead to portal hypertension and its various complications, including ascites, edema, and variceal hemorrhage in a small proportion of patients. Hepatic vein thrombosis with the Budd-Chiari syndrome is another recognized complication. The progressive splenomegaly is accompanied almost inevitably by progressive anemia and thrombocytopenia, the former occasionally complicated by iron deficiency of blood loss or, less frequently, by folic acid deficiency. Although granulocyte counts are usually better maintained than those of other blood cellular elements, eventually granulocytopenia may develop. In this setting, bacterial infections occur with increased frequency and may be a major factor leading to death. The association of myelofibrosis with tuberculosis is well documented, and this infection should be excluded by histologic and bacteriologic examination. Because of the almost inevitable hyperuricemia, attacks of gouty arthritis may develop in untreated patients.

Acute leukemic transformation is an occasional terminal event in agnogenic myeloid metaplasia. About 10 per cent of patients with polycythemia vera will develop a spent phase with advanced myelofibrosis. The likelihood of developing postpolycythemic myelofibrosis does not seem to be influenced by the type of therapy given for the underlying polycythemia, but evolution to the spent phase is a risk factor for subsequent development of acute leukemia. Once myelofibrosis has developed in this setting, the incidence of subsequent leukemic transformation (6 per cent in phlebotomy-treated patients, 45 per cent in those taking chlorambucil, and 25 per cent in those treated with ³²P) is 2½ to 4 times greater than in similarly treated polycythemic patients who have not developed myelofibrosis.

Treatment and Prognosis

No agreement has been reached concerning the optimal treatment of agnogenic myeloid metaplasia or of postpolycythemic myelofibrosis. There is thus far no effective treatment that inhibits the fibrotic process. Moreover, none of the conventional forms of treatment, including androgen therapy to stimulate erythropoiesis, chemotherapy, or splenectomy, has been shown to prolong life. Because of the relatively indolent progression of the disorder in most patients, a majority of hematologists undertake no specific treatment in the asymptomatic patient except for the administration of allopurinol at doses of 200 to 400 mg per day to avoid the complications of hyperuricemia.

In the presence of symptomatic anemia, androgens may be employed: testosterone enanthate, 200 to 600 mg weekly given intramuscularly, or oxymetholone, 50 to 150 mg daily by mouth. Treatment must be continued for at least 3 months to establish whether a particular preparation is effective, and some hematologists argue that patients who fail to respond to one androgen preparation may ultimately respond to another. Androgens seem most effective in women who have been splenectomized previously or who have never had massive splenomegaly. The doses employed inevitably lead to excessive fluid accumulation and, in female patients, to significant masculinization. Except in patients with a documented autoimmune component, the hemolytic anemia almost never responds to corticosteroids; these drugs may, however, increase the risk of infection in granulocytopenic patients. In patients with marked thrombocytosis, busulfan, in an initial dosage of 4 mg per day, followed by lower doses as the platelet count normalizes, or hydroxyurea, at a dosage of 500 to 1500 mg per day, is often effective in gaining control of the platelet count. Although busulfan is widely used in this setting, its potential mutagenic risks are a cause for concern. These agents may occasionally produce a beneficial reduction in spleen size and/or increase the hemoglobin concentration but equally frequently result in suppression of erythropoiesis and thrombopoiesis. Anagrelide and alpha- and gamma-interferons have also been used experimentally to reduce thrombocytosis (Ch. 142). Radiation therapy to the spleen has largely been abandoned because the doses required to produce a meaningful reduction in spleen size often cause severe leukopenia and thrombocytopenia. Radiotherapy remains useful for the treatment of areas of localized bone pain, serosal hematopoietic implants leading to serous effusions, or symptomatic extramedullary hematopoietic tumors, especially those compressing the brain or spinal cord.

The role of splenectomy in patients with agnogenic myeloid metaplasia or postpolycythemic myelofibrosis is highly controversial. As a high-risk procedure, it should probably be reserved for patients with severe hemolytic anemia, thrombocytopenia sufficient to produce bleeding, portal hypertension, or severe discomfort secondary to pressure symptoms or infarction. Striking thrombocytosis with thrombosis or hemorrhage or both may develop postoperatively and may require aggressive myelosuppression. In some patients splenectomy is followed by progressive and massive enlargement of the liver, with recurrent hemolysis and thrombocytopenia. The diagnosis of acute leukemia is often difficult to make in these patients, in whom the percentage of blasts in the peripheral blood may increase slowly and progressively for years.

Survival in agnogenic myeloid metaplasia and in postpolycythemic myelofibrosis is difficult to define with certainty. Several authors suggest that median survival in agnogenic myeloid metaplasia is approximately 10 years from the onset of the disease and 5 years from the time of diagnosis. However, there is considerable heterogeneity, with both shorter and longer survival frequently observed.

Bone marrow transplantation has been attempted both by conventional techniques and after surgical manipulation of bone marrow cavity spaces in attempts to provide an improved microenvironment for the transplanted marrow. Only occasional successes have been reported, and this procedure must be considered highly experimental.

Several additional suggested approaches to the treatment of myelofibrosis include the use of inhibitors of collagen synthesis (such as monoamine oxidase inhibitors and colchicine) and the vitamin D analogues 1,25-dihydroxyvitamin D and 1,25-dihydroxycholecalciferol. The latter are reported to decrease proliferation of megakaryocytes and, presumably, the consequent release of platelet- and megakaryocyte-derived fibroproliferative factors. The clinical value of these experimental approaches has not been established.

The syndrome of acute myelofibrosis, which is a rapidly progressive and fatal variant, has been shown by various cytologic marker studies to represent a form of acute megakaryocytic leukemia. It is believed that the release of platelet-megakaryocyte–derived growth factor from the malignant megakaryoblasts is responsible for the rapidly progressive marrow fibrosis. Induction chemotherapy may produce temporary hematologic remission, but only partial reversal of marrrow fibrosis. This is the one setting with myelofibrosis in which bone marrow transplantation deserves early consideration, particularly in patients under 40 years of age who have a suitable bone marrow donor.

Berk PD, Castro-Malaspina H, Wasserman LR (eds.): Myelofibrosis and the Biology of Connective Tissue. New York, Alan R. Liss, 1984. *This book contains 29 concise chapters by multiple authors who review the available information about the regulation of fibroblast proliferation, collagen biosynthesis, cell biology of marrow stromal cells, and other aspects of basic biologic science believed to be relevant to the pathogenesis of myelofibrosis.*

Carlo-Stella C, Cazzola M, Gasner A, et al.: Effects of recombinant α and γ interferons on the in vitro growth of circulating hematopoietic progenitor cells (CFU-GEMM, CFU-Mk, BFU-E and CFU-GM) from patients with myelofibrosis with myeloid metaplasia. Blood 70:1014, 1987. *An interesting study demonstrating an inhibitory effect of recombinant interferons on proliferation of abnormal hematopoietic progenitors in myelofibrosis with myeloid metaplasia. In concert with other studies showing that interferons decrease collagen synthesis, this study sets the stage for clinical trials of interferon therapy.*

Lichtman MA: Agnogenic myeloid metaplasia. *In* Williams WJ, Beutler E, Erslev AJ, et al. (eds.): Hematology. 4th ed. New York, McGraw-Hill, 1990, pp 223–232. *A comprehensive review of the pathogenesis, clinical features, and management of the myelofibrosis syndromes, with a thorough and up-to-date bibliography.*

McCarthy DM: Fibrosis of the bone marrow: Content and causes. Br J Haematol 59:1, 1985. *An examination of the pathobiology of marrow fibrosis and of experimental approaches to its prevention and treatment.*

ESSENTIAL THROMBOCYTHEMIA

Essential (primary) thrombocythemia, also known as a hemorrhagic thrombocythemia or essential thrombocytosis, is a primary myeloproliferative disorder of the pluripotent hematopoietic stem cell in which the predominant laboratory feature is a persistent, striking elevation of the platelet count to values in excess of 1×10^6 per microliter (see Color Plate 8K, right). Megakaryocytic colony-forming units (CFU-M) in peripheral blood and bone marrow are both quantitatively increased and qualitatively altered, in that they can be grown in vitro in the absence of various normally required growth factors. The disorder shows many features of polycythemia vera, including an almost identical distribution of patient ages at the time of diagnosis, similar degrees of leukocytosis, morphologically similar bone marrow abnormalities, and the presence of endogenous erythroid progenitors in peripheral blood and bone marrow. Splenomegaly has been reported to occur in 30 to 75 per cent of cases. The criteria outlined in the following paragraph would restrict the diagnosis to patients who have either normal or reduced hemoglobin concentrations, those with concomitant erythrocytosis being classified as having polycythemia vera.

The Polycythemia Vera Study Group has proposed the following diagnostic criteria for essential thrombocythemia: (1) platelet count persistently greater than 1×10^6 per microliter in the absence of an identifiable cause, such as malignant disease, infection, chronic inflammatory disease, or previous splenectomy; (2) normal total red cell volume, the measurement of which may be omitted if the hemoglobin concentration is less than 13 grams per 100 ml; (3) presence of iron in the bone marrow; if iron is absent, failure of the hemoglobin concentration to increase by more than 1 gram per deciliter after a 1-month trial of oral iron therapy; (4) absence of collagen fibrosis in bone marrow biopsy; and (5) absence of the Ph[1] from unstimulated metaphases obtained from a bone marrow aspirate. Because of both morphologic and clinical similarities, criteria 2 and 3 are necessary to exclude a diagnosis of polycythemia vera, whereas criteria 4 and 5 distinguish the disorder from agnogenic myeloid metaplasia and chronic myelogenous leukemia, respectively.

Clinical Features

Essential thrombocythemia is generally a disease of later life, diagnosed most often in those between the ages of 50 and 70, and affecting both sexes equally, but a distinct second peak of incidence occurs in younger patients, particularly females, and childhood cases have been reported.

The predominant clinical manifestations of essential thrombocythemia result from hemorrhagic and/or thrombotic events. Some patients have easy bruising, epistaxis, unexplained gastrointestinal bleeding, and an excessive tendency to postoperative hemorrhage. Conversely, other patients present evidence for microvascular occlusion in sites such as the extremities, the central nervous system, and the coronary circulation. The most common manifestation of microvascular occlusion is burning pain in the feet, hands, and digits, which may progress to frank gangrene. Although these symptoms are striking when they occur, approximately two thirds of patients are asymptomatic at diagnosis, and large numbers of patients, particularly younger patients, may remain asymptomatic for long periods. Hence, the precise incidence of these complications is unknown. Similarly, transition to acute leukemia has been clearly documented, but there is no accurate estimate of its frequency, particularly in patients not previously exposed to mutagenic agents.

Course and Prognosis

The natural history of this disease is poorly appreciated, and most reports in the literature describe very small series of patients with a focus on a particular complication. Neurologic manifestations, ranging from headaches and paresthesias to visual disturbances, transient ischemic attacks, and strokes, are especially worrisome, but their overall frequency remains unclear. The most typical manifestation is erythromelalgia, a vaso-occlusive syndrome characterized by localized pain, burning, redness, and warmth of one or more distal extremities. It may progress to frank necrosis of a digit. When present, erythromelalgia typically responds dramatically to rapid reduction of the platelet count or to administration of nonsteroidal anti-inflammatory agents. These responses are consistent with a proposed pathogenesis involving the arteriolar vasospastic effects of metabolites of platelet arachidonic acid. Descriptions emphasizing hemorrhagic, thrombotic, and embolic episodes and a high fatality rate are directly contradicted by others emphasizing prolonged periods without complications. The largest series suggest a life expectancy perhaps analogous to that of polycythemia vera.

Therapy

Because of uncertainties about its natural history, there is a substantial lack of agreement about appropriate therapy for essential thrombocythemia. Despite strikingly high platelet counts, many hematologists recommend expectant management in asymptomatic patients under the age of 60, while others recommend the use of only platelet-antiaggregating agents (e.g., aspirin, 300 mg per day, with or without dipyridamole, 50 mg three times per day). However, the experience in polycythemia vera suggests that prolonged administration of platelet-antiaggregating agents may increase the risk of gastrointestinal hemorrhage. Chronic myelosuppression should be attempted in older patients and those who have a history of significant thrombotic episodes. In these cases, prevention of neurologic damage takes precedence over concern about long-term mutagenic effects of myelosuppression. Control of the thrombocytosis can usually be achieved with hydroxyurea* at an initial dose of 500 to 1500 mg per day, tapered to an individualized maintenance dose as the platelet count falls. Concerns about the long-term mutagenic effects of alkylating agents and of radioactive phosphorus have made hydroxyurea the initial drug of choice in this setting. Its short duration of action, however, requires strict adherence to the prescribed regimen to maintain control of the platelet count. In less compliant patients, adequate control can be obtained with a longer acting agent, such as melphalan,* 6 to 10 mg per day by mouth for 1 week, followed by 4 to 6 mg per day until the platelet count is in the normal range. Subsequent maintenance with 2 to 6 mg per week is continued indefinitely, the dose being adjusted according to the platelet count. Alternatively, particularly in the elderly patient, radioactive phosphorus, 2.9 mCi per square meter of body surface area given intravenously, repeated as necessary at intervals of not less than 3 months, is highly effective. Both anagrelide and interferons have been used experimentally to control the platelet count is essential thrombocythemia, as they have in polycythemia vera (Ch. 142), but their precise roles remain to be established. Patients presenting with serious thrombotic or hemorrhagic manifestations and uncontrolled thrombocytosis should be treated with platelet-antiaggregating agents, urgent plateletpheresis, and the initiation of a myelosuppressive regimen. Every effort should be made to avoid splenectomy in patients with essential thrombocythemia because of the extreme thrombocytosis and serious complications that often follow this procedure.

Barbui T, Buelli M, Cortelazzo S, et al.: Aspirin and risk of bleeding in patients with thrombocythemia. Am J Med 83:265, 1987. *A clinical study demonstrating that aspirin may excessively prolong the bleeding time in some patients with thrombocythemia associated with myeloproliferative disorders. The message is that chronic administration of aspirin as a platelet antiaggregating agent in this setting may be hazardous.*
Jabaily J, Iland HJ, Laszlo J, et al.: Neurologic manifestations of essential thrombocythemia. Ann Intern Med 99:513, 1983. *A contrary report suggesting that approximately two thirds have evidence of at least transient neurologic dysfunction.*
Kessler CM, Klein HG, Havlik RJ: Uncontrolled thrombocytosis in chronic myeloproliferative disorders. Br J Haematol 50:157, 1982. *A retrospective study suggesting that, at least in the younger patient, severe thrombocytosis in myeloproliferative disease may have fewer complications than previously believed.*

*This use is not listed in the manufacturer's directive.

Mazur EM, Cohen JL, Bogart L: Growth characteristics of circulating hematopoietic progenitor cells from patients with essential thrombocythemia. Blood 71:1554, 1988. *One of several recent studies demonstrating quantitative and qualitative abnormalities in both megakaryocytic and erythroid progenitor cells in essential thrombocythemia.*
Murphy S: Primary thrombocythemia. *In* Williams WJ, Beutler E, Erslev AJ, et al. (eds.): Hematology. 4th ed. New York, McGraw-Hill, 1990, pp 231–236. *A balanced critique of the often contradictory literature about this uncommon yet fascinating disease.*

144 The Chronic Leukemias
Michael J. Keating

CHRONIC MYELOGENOUS LEUKEMIA (Chronic Myeloid Leukemia, Chronic Myelocytic Leukemia, Chronic Granulocytic Leukemia)

Definition

Chronic myelogenous leukemia (CML) is a disease characterized by an overproduction of cells of the granulocytic, especially the neutrophilic, series and occasionally the monocytic series (see Color Plate 7F, right), leading to marked splenomegaly and very high white blood cell counts. Basophilia and thrombocytosis are common. A characteristic cytogenetic abnormality, the Philadelphia (Ph¹) chromosome, is present in the bone marrow cells in more than 95 per cent of cases. The granulocytes usually appear relatively normal, although many patients exhibit dysplastic changes, including Pelger-Huët anomalies. Neutrophil functions, such as phagocytosis and bactericidal activity, are largely preserved. Before effective treatment was available, patients survived, on the average, approximately 2 years after diagnosis.

Etiology

Usually, no etiologic agent can be incriminated in CML. Exposure to ionizing radiation increases the risk of subsequent CML. Survivors of the atomic bomb explosions in Japan in 1945 have had an increased incidence of CML, with a peak occurring 5 to 12 years after exposure and seemingly dose related. The relative risk has been falling since that time but is still above the expected rate for Japan. Radiation treatment of ankylosing spondylitis and cervical cancer has increased the incidence of CML. No increase in the risk of CML has been demonstrated in individuals working in the nuclear industry. Radiologists working without adequate protection prior to 1940 were more likely to develop myeloid leukemia, but no such association has been found in recent studies. Benzene exposure increases the risk of acute myelogenous leukemia (AML) but not of CML. Patients with CML have an increased frequency of the Cw3 and Cw4 human leukocyte antigens (HLA's). Chronic myelogenous leukemia is not a frequent secondary leukemia following the treatment of other cancers with radiation and/or alkylating agents.

Incidence

Chronic myelogenous leukemia constitutes one fifth of all cases of leukemia in the United States. One or 2 persons per 100,000 are diagnosed as having CML per year, with a slight male preponderance. This incidence has not changed significantly in the past few decades. The incidence of CML increases with age; the median age at diagnosis is approximately 45 to 50 years. Ph¹-positive CML is uncommon in children and adolescents. Patients who are older than 60 years have a poorer prognosis. No familial association of CML has been noted.

Molecular Pathogenesis

The striking feature in CML is the presence of Ph¹ chromosome in the bone marrow cells of more than 90 per cent of patients with typical CML. The Ph¹ chromosome results from a balanced translocation of material between the long arms of chromosomes 9 and 22. As more chromosomal material is lost from chromosome 22 than is gained from chromosome 9, the Ph¹ chromosome is a shortened chromosome 22 containing approximately 60 per cent of its normal complement of DNA. The break, which occurs at band q34 of the long arm of chromosome 9, allows translocation of the cellular oncogene *C-ABL* to a position on chromosome 22 called the breakage cluster region (bcr). The breakpoint in the bcr varies from patient to patient but is identical in all cells of any one patient. *C-ABL* is a homologue of *V-ABL*, the Abelson virus that causes leukemia in mice (Ch. 157). The apposition of these two genetic sequences produces a new hybrid gene (*abl/bcr*), which codes for a novel protein of molecular weight 210,000 kD (P210). The P210 protein, a tyrosine kinase, may play a role in triggering the uncontrolled proliferation of CML cells. The Ph¹ chromosome occurs in erythroid, myeloid, monocytic, and megakaryocytic cells, less commonly in B lymphocytes, rarely in T lymphocytes, but not in marrow fibroblasts. This extensive cellular distribution places the abnormality in CML close to the pluripotent stem cell. Studies of glucose-6-phosphate dehydrogenase (G6PD) isoenzymes support the finding of multilineage monoclonal proliferation, since a single isoenzyme is present in the above-mentioned cells in informative patients with CML. *C-sis*, the homologue of the simian sarcoma virus, is also translocated from chromosome 22 to chromosome 9 in CML but is distant from the breakpoint and not expressed in benign-phase CML. *C-sis* encodes for a protein identical to platelet-derived growth factor (PDGF). Insertion of a retrovirus encoding P210 (*abl/bcr*) into cells of mice has led to the development of a disease closely resembling CML in some of these animals, giving credence to the hypothesis that the (*abl/bcr*) hybrid gene is sufficient to cause CML.

The fusion *abl/bcr* gene and the P210 protein can be found in many cases of typical CML in which no cytogenetic abnormality occurs or in which changes other than typical t(9;22)(q34;q11) are identified. These patients have a survival rate and a response to therapy that are similar to those in Ph¹-positive patients. Patients with atypical CML who are Ph¹ and *abl/bcr* negative have a different natural history than do patients who are either Ph¹ positive or Ph¹ negative with *abl/bcr* positivity. They resemble more closely patients with myelodysplastic syndrome (MDS) (Ch. 129). Thus, three groups of patients with CML can be identified: (a) positive for Ph¹ and *abl/bcr*, (b) Ph¹ negative and *abl/bcr* positive, and (c) negative for Ph¹ and *abl/bcr* (Table 144–1).

Although 100 per cent of the metaphases on cytogenetic analysis usually show the presence of the Ph¹ chromosome, some normal stem cells must remain. Normal diploid cells appear on long-term bone marrow culture and following treatment with interferon, high-dose chemotherapy, and autologous bone marrow transplantation.

Symptoms and Signs

Many asymptomatic patients are diagnosed as having CML because of the use of hematologic studies in routine annual physical examinations or in evaluations for other illnesses. In these patients, the white blood cell (WBC) count may be relatively low at the time of diagnosis. The WBC count correlates well with tumor mass as defined by spleen size. Patients with higher WBC counts and larger spleens have more symptoms. The symptomatology of CML, usually nonspecific, is secondary to anemia, spleen size, or an increased basal metabolic rate, but most patients are asymptomatic or only mildly symptomatic. Fatigue, weight loss, malaise, easy satiety, and a sense of left upper quadrant fullness are the major symptoms of CML. Rarely, bleeding (associated with a low platelet count and/or platelet dysfunction) or thrombosis (associated with thrombocytosis and/ or marked leukocytosis) occurs. The serum uric acid level is commonly elevated at diagnosis, and acute gouty arthritis may follow treatment. An elevated blood histamine level (related to the basophil cell mass) can cause upper gastrointestinal ulceration and bleeding. Neutrophil function is usually normal or only modestly impaired, and neutrophil numbers are markedly increased; infections are therefore uncommon at the time of diagnosis. Headaches, bone pain, arthralgias, pain from splenic infarction, and fever are uncommon in the early stages of CML but become more common as the disease progresses. Priapism is occasionally noted, usually in patients with marked leukocytosis or thrombocytosis. Leukostatic symptoms, such as dyspnea, drowsiness, loss of coordination, or confusion, which are due to sludging in the pulmonary or cerebral vessels, are uncommon in the benign phase of CML despite WBC counts that may exceed 400,000 per microliter. These symptoms appear more frequently in later stages of the disease (i.e., in the accelerated or blast crisis phases, in which more premature cells predominate). All symptoms subside as the WBC count falls and the splenomegaly decreases as a result of effective treatment.

Splenomegaly, by far the most consistent physical sign in CML, occurs in more than 90 per cent of cases. The spleen may extend to the pelvic brim and across the midline of the abdomen in some cases. Hepatomegaly is less common and is usually minor (1 to 3 cm below the right costal margin). Lymphadenopathy is very uncommon, as is infiltration of skin and other tissues. If present, these findings suggest a Ph¹-negative CML or an accelerated or blastic transformation of CML. Rarely, patients present initially with a blast crisis; these patients can have any of the clinical manifestations of acute leukemia.

Natural History

More than 90 per cent of patients present with CML in the benign phase, in which the disease behaves in a predictable fashion, with the symptoms, abnormal physical signs, and abnormal blood findings returning to normal following treatment. This satisfactory response is transient; all patients eventually develop a variety of changes in the behavior of the disease. Most frequently, there is a "blast crisis," a clinical picture resembling that of acute leukemia. This change can be abrupt, but more frequently it is preceded by a period of progressively greater difficulty in maintaining the WBC count at a level of less than 20,000 per microliter and of other manifestations, such as increasing splenomegaly, hepatomegaly, and infiltration of nodes, skin, bones, or other tissues; the appearance of blast cells or basophils in the peripheral blood; development of anemia and/or thrombocytopenia; or fever, malaise, and weight loss. This last group of features, termed the accelerated phase of CML, demands reevaluation of the bone marrow, which, in the accelerated phase, shows dysplastic changes in the myeloid and other cell lineages and may show an increase in the percentage of blast cells (5 to 29 per cent) and an increase in basophils. Aspiration of bone marrow may be difficult, especially in patients who have developed myelofibrosis subsequent to the CML. Chromosomal abnormalities, in addition to the Ph¹ chromosome, occur in both the accelerated and the blastic phases of CML. Blast crisis is diagnosed when 30 per cent or more blast cells are present in the bone marrow and/or peripheral blood.

When the accelerated phase or blast crisis is suspected (i.e., 10 to 40 per cent blasts in bone marrow), the patient should be further evaluated in 2 to 4 weeks, since the percentage of blasts in the blood and bone marrow can increase transiently after the treatment of CML is discontinued, especially with hydroxyurea or interferon. It is important to be cautious in classifying patients as having blast crisis or accelerated phase because of the adverse prognostic implications (Fig. 144–1). Criteria for the accelerated phase are the following: an increase in blast cells (>15 per cent or basophils (>20 per cent) in the blood or bone marrow, thrombocytopenia (<100,000 per microliter), serious anemia (hemoglobin [Hb] < 7 grams per deciliter); documented extramedullary leukemia, or development of clonal evolution (new chromosomal changes in addition to the Ph¹ chromosome).

The risk of developing accelerated phase or blast crisis in CML is relatively low in the first 2 years after diagnosis (~10 per cent per year) but then increases and remains constant (15 to 20 per cent per year) after that unless therapy such as bone marrow transplantation is used.

TABLE 144–1. CLASSIFICATION OF CHRONIC MYELOGENOUS LEUKEMIA (CML)

Disease	Ph¹ Present	abl/bcr Rearrangement	Prognosis
Classic CML	Yes	Yes	Median, 4 yr
bcr⁺, Ph¹⁻	No	Most	Median, 4 yr
CMML/CMoL/bcr-CML	No	No	18–24 mo

bcr = Break cluster region; *abl/bcr* = a hybrid gene (see text); CMML = chronic myelomonocytic leukemia; CMoL = chronic monocytic leukemia.

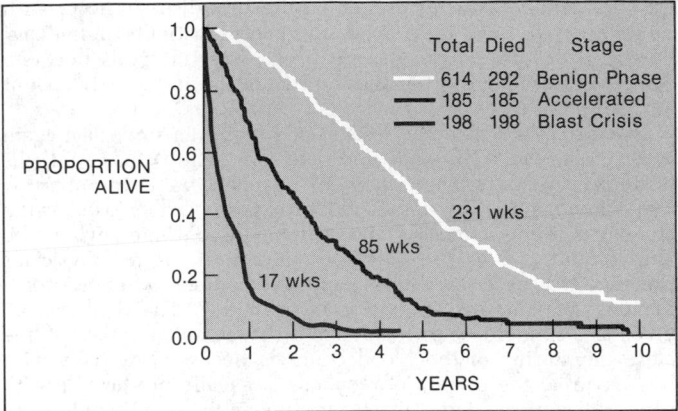

FIGURE 144–1. Survival of M. D. Anderson Cancer Center patients with chronic myelogenous leukemia (CML) by phase of disease.

Laboratory Findings

All patients with untreated CML have an elevated WBC count ranging from 10,000 per microliter to more than 1,000,000 per microliter. The predominant cells are of the neutrophil series, with a left shift extending to blast cells (see Color Plate 7F, right). In addition, eosinophils and basophils are commonly increased in number. Monocytes may be slightly increased in some cases that overlap with chronic myelomocytic leukemia (CMML). The bone marrow is hypercellular with marked myeloid hyperplasia and sometimes shows evidence of increased reticulin or collagen fibrosis. The myeloid-erythroid ratio is 15:1 to 20:1. About 15 per cent of patients have 5 per cent or more blast cells in the peripheral blood or bone marrow at diagnosis. T cells (both T-helper and T-suppressor), but not B cells, are increased in number in CML. A hemoglobin of less than 11 grams per deciliter is present in one third of patients. The red cells are usually normochromic and normocytic, but nucleated red cells are present in the blood of one quarter of the patients at diagnosis. Autoimmune hemolytic anemia and thrombocytopenia (<100,000 per microliter) are rare in CML, but thrombocytosis (>450,000 per microliter) occurs in almost half of the patients.

Biochemical abnormalities in CML include a markedly decreased leukocyte alkaline phosphatase (LAP) score in the neutrophils of 90 per cent or more of patients, being completely absent in 5 to 10 per cent of cases. A low LAP score also occurs in some patients with agnogenic myeloid metaplasia, which is sometimes difficult to differentiate from CML (Ch. 143). The serum levels of transcobalamins I and III, cobalamin-binding glycoproteins produced by neutrophils, are elevated in accord with the increased neutrophils (Ch. 132). This elevation leads to extremely high serum cobalamin values (e.g., vitamin B_{12} levels >10 times normal). Serum levels of lactate dehydrogenase, uric acid, and lysozyme are often increased. The lysozyme levels are modestly increased in CML compared with CMML, in which the levels in blood and urine are often markedly increased. Kinetic studies show an increased neutrophil production rate related to a markedly expanded myeloid mass. The number of colony-forming cells in the blood in CML is increased, but the number in the bone marrow is in the normal range. Defective feedback control of WBC production is common in CML; some patients demonstrate a cyclic oscillation of the WBC count. The labeling index of myeloblasts in CML is lower than in normal bone marrow, and the generation time is prolonged, confirming the concept that CML is an accumulative rather than a proliferative disease. Neutrophils in CML survive intravascularly slightly longer than do normal granulocytes.

Diagnosis

The diagnosis of typical CML is not difficult. The presence of unexplained myeloid leukocytosis with splenomegaly should lead to a LAP test on the peripheral blood neutrophils and a bone marrow examination with a cytogenetic analysis. Marrow myeloid hyperplasia and hypercellularity further suggest the diagnosis. The ultimate test, however, remains the cytogenetic analysis; the

presence of the Ph^1 chromosome in this clinical setting establishes the diagnosis. When the Ph^1 chromosome is not found in a patient with suspected CML, molecular evidence for the presence of the hybrid *abl/bcr* gene should be sought, as 40 to 50 per cent of Ph^1-negative patients with CML have *abl/bcr* rearrangement. The Ph^1 chromosome is usually present in 100 per cent of metaphases, ordinarily as the sole abnormality. Ten to 15 per cent of patients at initial presentation have an additional chromosomal change, such as loss of the Y chromosome, trisomy 8, an additional 22q−, or an atypical translocation. The patients who have atypical complex chromosomal changes, which may or may not involve chromosome 9 or 22 morphologically, demonstrate evidence of the hybrid *abl/bcr* gene when techniques of molecular biology are used.

Chronic myelogenous leukemia must be differentiated from leukemoid reactions, which usually produce WBC counts lower than 50,000 per microliter, toxic granulation vacuolation, Döhle bodies in the granulocytes, absent basophilia, a normal or increased LAP level, and a clinical history and physical examination suggesting the origin of the leukemoid reaction (Ch. 141). Corticosteroids can rarely cause extreme neutrophilia together with the left shift, but this response is self-limited and short in duration and thus seldom a cause of diagnostic difficulty.

Chronic myelogenous leukemia may be more difficult to differentiate from other myelodysplastic or myeloproliferative syndromes. Patients having agnogenic myeloid metaplasia with or without myelofibrosis present with splenomegaly and often with neutrophilia and thrombocytosis (Ch. 143). Polycythemia rubra vera with associated iron deficiency, which allows a normal hemoglobin level and hematocrit value, can manifest with an elevated neutrophil and platelet count (Ch. 142). Such patients usually have a normal or increased LAP score and a WBC count less than 25,000 per microliter, and the Ph^1 chromosome is not present.

The greatest diagnostic difficulty lies with patients who have splenomegaly and leukocytosis but who do not have the Ph^1 chromosome. Many of these patients have the usual blood and marrow findings of Ph^1-positive CML, and the *abl/bcr* hybrid gene can be demonstrated despite a normal or atypical cytogenetic pattern. Patients who are Ph^1 negative and *abl/bcr* negative are considered to have Ph^1-negative CML or CMML (Table 144–1). The cytogenetic findings in patients with CMML are normal or involve an additional chromosome 8 or findings other than the Ph^1 chromosome. Patients with CMML have *ras* mutations in 50 to 60 per cent of cases. Rarely, patients present with myeloid hyperplasia, which involves almost exclusively the neutrophil, eosinophil, or basophilic cell lineage. These patients are described as having chronic neutrophilic, eosinophilic, or basophilic leukemia and do not have evidence of the Ph^1 chromosome or *abl/bcr* gene. Isolated megakaryocytic hyperplasia can give rise to a syndrome called idiopathic thrombocythemia with marked thrombocytosis and splenomegaly (Ch. 143, 154). These conditions are considered to fall under the general category of myeloproliferative disorders and have a better prognosis than does CML.

Evolution of CML

Death occurs rarely during the chronic phase of CML, but over time the clinical behavior of the disease changes. One third of patients abruptly develop an acute transformation (blast crisis of CML); the other two thirds respond progressively less well in the control of the WBC count and spleen size with conventional agents such as busulfan and hydroxyurea. This loss of control (accelerated phase) is often associated with an increased proportion of blasts, promyelocytes, and basophils in the peripheral blood and bone marrow and is often accompanied by anemia and thrombocytopenia. Some patients develop bone marrow failure in which anemia and thrombocytopenia are accompanied by increasing evidence of dysplastic changes in the marrow and myelofibrosis. The median survival after developing a blast crisis of CML is only 3 months (Fig. 144–1). The survival after development of the accelerated phase of CML is 12 to 18 months if the blood and bone marrow contain more than 30 per cent blasts plus promyelocytes or more than 20 per cent basophils or if the platelet count falls to less than 100,000 per microliter. Most patients with blast crisis or accelerated phase have additional chromosomal abnormalities (clonal evolution), such as duplication of the Ph[1] chromosome, trisomy of chromosome number 8, or development of an isochromosome number 17. Clonal evolution usually presages the accelerated phase or blast crisis of CML. The blast cells in blast crisis are usually myeloblasts, but less commonly erythroid, monocytoid, or megakaryoblastic transformations occur. In one-quarter of cases, the blast cells are lymphoid in origin, as demonstrated by cytochemical stains (terminal deoxynucleotidyl transferase), immunophenotyping, and immunoglobulin heavy-chain rearrangement studies. In 10 per cent of cases, the blast cells are completely undifferentiated. Some patients who present with acute leukemia and the Ph[1] chromosome abnormality presumably have blast crisis that occurred before the diagnosis of CML was made. These cases have the P210 protein and 8.5-kb fusion messenger RNA. Patients with acute lymphoblastic leukemia (ALL) with a Ph[1] usually have a P190 protein or a 7.1-k fusion messenger RNA probably restricted to the lymphoid cells. Extramedullary blast crisis of CML can occur in the spleen, lymph nodes, skin, meninges, bone, and other sites. This initial extramedullary transformation is usually shortly followed by evidence of marrow involvement.

Chronic myelomonocytic leukemia and Ph[1]- and *abl/bcr*-negative CML appear to overlap clinically in some instances, and their clinical behavior, progress, and response to therapy resemble those of the MDS more than Ph[1]-positive CML. A male preponderance is noted, splenomegaly is common (60 to 70 per cent), and the WBC count, while elevated, is usually in the 25,000 to 100,000 per microliter range. Anemia and thrombocytopenia are more common than in Ph[1]-positive CML, and eosinophilia and basophilia are less common. The median survival is 18 to 24 months, with patients dying of infection, bleeding, or transformation to acute leukemia.

Treatment

Immediate treatment of CML is not necessary unless the WBC count exceeds 200,000 per microliter or there is evidence of leukostasis (priapism, venous thrombosis, confusion, or dyspnea) or unless painful splenomegaly suggests splenic infarction. Hyperuricemia is common at the diagnosis of CML and should be treated with allopurinol, 100 mg three times a day, and adequate hydration while the WBC count is higher than 25,000 per microliter to prevent renal dysfunction. Acute gouty arthritis is rare.

Palliative Treatment

Chronic myelogenous leukemia has been treated traditionally with oral busulfan, which, if used prudently, gives smooth, sustained control of the WBC count, platelet count, and spleen size. Since overdosage with busulfan can cause prolonged myelosuppression, another active oral agent, hydroxyurea, has been increasingly used. Both agents have a high level of acceptance by the patient, and both control the manifestations of the disease in 90 per cent of cases when first used, but over time they produce progressively shorter and less complete reductions in the WBC count and spleen size.

Busulfan is usually started at a dosage of 4 to 8 mg per day, depending on the WBC count and the patient's body size. Use of higher dosages of 12 to 16 mg per day should be restricted to patients with WBC counts greater than 200,000 per microliter. Leukapheresis can also be used on a short-term basis to decrease the leukocyte or platelet counts rapidly. When the initial WBC count halves, the starting dose should be decreased by 50 per cent. The leukocyte count decreases exponentially and is closely correlated with a reduction in spleen size. Since the WBC count continues to fall for 2 to 4 weeks after cessation of busulfan, the drug should be discontinued when the WBC count reaches 20,000 to 25,000 per microliter to prevent severe pancytopenia from marrow hypoplasia. The WBC count may not begin to rise again for several months or for more than a year, at which time a lower dose (2 to 4 mg per day) should be reinstituted. Few acute side effects are noted with busulfan, although premature menopause does occur in 20 to 40 per cent of young women and sterility is frequent in both men and women. Hyperpigmentation, weight loss, and fatigue, which can mimic Addison's disease, occur with prolonged use, and in a small number of patients pulmonary fibrosis develops. As the disease progresses, intervals between courses of busulfan shorten and the rate of rise in the WBC count at relapse increases.

Hydroxyurea is given at dosages of 1 to 4 grams per day, again according to the WBC count and body size. The WBC count falls in similar fashion to that induced by busulfan, but severe marrow hypoplasia is rare. The dosage of hydroxyurea is decreased as the leukocyte count decreases and can be discontinued when the WBC count is 5 to 10 × 10³ per microliter. Some physicians prefer to treat patients with intermittent courses, whereas others maintain patients on 0.5 to 2 grams per day. The drug can be given as a single dose or fractionated throughout the day. While close monitoring of the blood count is necessary initially with hydroxyurea, the pattern of response is usually predictable with repeated courses. Side effects are uncommon, although rash, mucositis, and diarrhea can occur. The survival of patients treated with busulfan or hydroxyurea is similar. Splenic irradiation is not recommended for the treatment of CML.

Cytogenetically Directed Therapy

Busulfan and conventional-dose hydroxyurea rarely eliminates the Ph[1] chromosome from marrow cells. With high-dose hydroxyurea, however, diploid metaphases have been observed in several patients. A return to a normal chromosomal pattern would seem to be a reasonable therapeutic goal, and it might be anticipated that patients who achieve a normal karyotype may survive better than those who do not. Three therapeutic initiatives have been developed based on this concept: the use of interferons, intensive chemotherapy, and bone marrow transplantation.

INTERFERON THERAPY. Both human leukocyte interferon and recombinant alpha-interferon (r-IFnα) have been demonstrated to produce hematologic and cytogenetic remissions in CML. Complete hematologic remissions are obtained in 75 to 80 per cent of patients treated with r-IFnα, and 30 to 40 per cent of the patients have a complete or partial suppression in the Ph[1] chromosome. Gamma-interferon alone or combined with alpha-interferon does not have a significant therapeutic effect. Return of normal metaphases following the use of r-IFnα is associated with a longer survival than is seen in patients without a cytogenetic response. The dosage of r-IFnα is 2 to 5 million units per square meter per day, administered subcutaneously or intramuscularly. The response rate is higher with the higher dose. The most common acute side effects—musculoskeletal discomfort, fever, and chills—subside in most patients but are often replaced by symptoms of fatigue, depression, lethargy, inattention, loss of weight, lack of libido, and mild alopecia. These toxicities are more common in patients over 60 years of age. Reactions at the injection site occur in approximately 5 per cent of patients. Thrombocytopenia, anemia, arthritis, nephrotic syndrome, and seizures occur rarely. Loss of disease control, together with lack of side effects, may signal the development of neutralizing antibodies to interferon.

AGGRESSIVE CHEMOTHERAPY. Regimens commonly employed for the treatment of acute myelogenous leukemia (AML) have been used in an attempt to suppress the Ph[1] chromosome. In more than 50 per cent of the treated patients, the percentage of Ph[1]-positive metaphases is greatly reduced, and about one third become transiently diploid for 2 to 12 months. Research protocols using chemotherapy induction therapy followed by r-IFnα maintenance are now under way.

ALLOGENEIC BONE MARROW TRANSPLANTATION. Marrow transplantation has been performed in patients with benign-phase CML (Ch. 153). The risk of early death due to complications of transplantation (20 to 30 per cent) is balanced against the observation that 50 to 60 per cent of patients will be in hematologic or cytogenetic remission 3 to 5 years after transplantation. Favorable factors for survival are age lower than 30 years, transplantation within 1 year of diagnosis, and absence of severe graft-versus-host disease (GVHD). Long-term survival rates after transplantation in accelerated and blast phases of CML are only approximately 10 to 15 per cent. After syngeneic (identical twin) bone marrow transplantations, 84 per cent of patients treated at the Fred Hutchinson Cancer Center (Seattle, Washington) are alive and 75 per cent continue in complete hematologic and cytogenetic remission. The possibility exists that many of these patients will be cured. Autologous marrow and peripheral blood stem cell support following ablative chemotherapy and radiation therapy is currently being evaluated.

Treatment of Accelerated and Blast Crisis of CML

Loss of control of CML with agents such as busulfan, hydroxyurea, or interferon is marked by development of increasing splenomegaly, leukocytosis, and thrombocytosis. Many of these patients developed additional cytogenetic abnormalities (clonal evolution). Some patients develop severe anemia and thrombocytopenia. Splenectomy occasionally corrects the thrombocytopenia. The bone marrow often develops increasing dysplasia of one or multiple cell lines, together with an increasing left shift (5 to 29 per cent blast cells), eosinophilia, and basophilia. Change of therapy from busulfan to hydroxyurea or vice versa is successful for a short time (3 to 6 months) in 10 to 25 per cent of patients. These patients are considered to have an accelerated phase of the disease. If the proportion of blast cells in bone marrow exceeds 30 per cent, the patient is considered to be in blast crisis (acute transformation of CML) (see Color Plate 7G). The blast crisis or refractory accelerated phase of CML is usually treated with regimens designed for the treatment of acute leukemia (Ch. 145). Treatment of myeloid, undifferentiated, or mixed-lineage blast crisis is usually unsatisfactory, with only 25 to 30 per cent of patients achieving a complete remission. Patients with a lymphoid blast crisis phenotype have a better chance (50 to 65 per cent) of achieving a complete remission on regimens utilizing vincristine, corticosteroids, asparaginase, and/or anthracyclines. The Ph[1] chromosome persists, and the duration of response is usually short (2 to 6 months), with no prospect of cure. Only 10 to 15 per cent of patients with blast crisis survive for more than 1 year (Fig. 144–1). Allogeneic marrow transplantation should be offered to patients with blast crisis (with active disease or after remission is obtained) if a suitable donor is available, since few of these patients have survived more than 5 years. The mortality rate and relapse rate after allogenic transplantation for CML blast crisis are much higher than for CML in the benign phase. Patients who have an HLA-compatible sibling should have an allogeneic transplantation performed before the accelerated or blast phases of CML develop.

Prognosis

The median survival of Ph[1]-positive CML was 3 to 4 years for patients treated in the 1970's, with a range of 1 to 20 years (Fig. 144–2). The median survival at the M. D. Anderson Cancer Center in Houston, Texas, for patients diagnosed after 1980 is greater than 5 years. The risk of death is 5 to 8 per cent per year for the first 24 months and increases to 15 to 20 per cent per year for the next 2 years and 25 per cent per year thereafter. No

TABLE 144–2. ADVERSE PROGNOSTIC FACTORS IN CHRONIC MYELOGENOUS LEUKEMIA

Older age
Large spleen size
Large liver size
Increase or decrease in platelets
High white count
Basophilia
Clonal evolution

From Kantarjian HM, Keating MJ, Smith TL, et al.: Proposal for a simple synthesis prognostic staging system in chronic myelogenous leukemia. Am J Med 88:1, 1990; with permission.

patients are projected to be cured with a palliative use of busulfan and/or hydroxyurea. The influence of treatment with interferon, aggressive chemotherapy, and allogeneic transplantation on the improved survival of patients diagnosed after 1980 is not certain at this time. Large spleen, increased liver size, elevated platelet counts, high marrow and blood blast and basophil percentages, advanced age, and clonal evolution are consistent adverse prognostic factors (Table 144–2) and have been combined into a simple staging system. This system identifies a high-risk group (30 to 40 per cent) of patients with a median survival of only 2 years. The quality of life of patients in the benign phase is usually excellent.

Bos JL: *Ras* oncogenes in hematopoietic malignancies. Hematol Pathol 2:55, 1988. *A review illustrating the frequency and pattern of mutations in the* ras *oncogene family in acute and chronic leukemias.*

Butturini A, Keating A, Goldman J, et al.: Autotransplants in chronic myelogenous leukemia: Strategies and results. Lancet 335:1255, 1990. *A recent review of the results and problems of autologous transplantation in CML.*

Daley GQ, Van Etten RA, Baltimore D: Induction of chronic myelogenous leukemia in mice by the P210abl/bcr gene of the Philadelphia chromosome. Science 247:824, 1990. *A seminal report of the role of the abl/bcr gene as a causative factor in CML.*

Fefer A, Thomas ED: Bone marrow transplantation for the treatment of chronic myelogenous leukemia. *In* DeVita VT, Hellman S (eds.): Important Advances in Oncology. Philadelphia, J.B. Lippincott, 1990, p 143. *A comprehensive overview of the results of allogeneic transplantation in CML.*

Kantarjian HM, Dixon D, Keating MJ, et al.: Characteristics of accelerated disease in chronic myelogenous leukemia. Cancer 61:1441, 1988. *A quantitative analysis of the impact on survival of various features of accelerated-phase CML.*

Kantarjian HM, Keating MJ, Walters RS, et al.: Clinical and prognostic features of Philadelphia chromosome–negative chronic myelogenous leukemia. Cancer 58:2023, 1986. *An analysis of the prognostic factors and clinical features of Ph[1] chromosome–negative CML, illustrating differences from Ph[1]-positive CML and similarities to the MDS.*

Kurzrock R, Gutterman JU, Talpaz M: The molecular genetics of Philadelphia chromosome–positive leukemias. N Engl J Med 319:990, 1988. *A detailed analysis of the current relevance of molecular genetic data in Ph[1] chromosome-positive acute and chronic leukemias.*

Strife A, Lambek C, Wisniewski D, et al.: Discordant maturation as the primary biological defect in chronic myelogenous leukemia. Cancer Res 48:1035, 1988. *An analysis of the morphologic changes associated with the various clinical stages of CML.*

Talpaz M, Kantarjian HM, McCredie K, et al.: Hematologic remission and cytogenetic improvement induced by recombinant human interferon alpha A in chronic myelogenous leukemia. N Engl J Med 314:1065, 1986. *Initial demonstration of the ability of interferon to induce cytogenetic remissions in CML.*

HAIRY CELL LEUKEMIA

Clinical Features

Hairy cell leukemia (HCL) is uncommon (1 to 2 per cent of all leukemias). The median age at diagnosis is 50 years, with a 4:1 male preponderance. Patients present with symptoms of fatigue due to anemia, fever, weight loss, and/or abdominal discomfort produced by splenomegaly. Sometimes the disease is diagnosed when patients present with infection secondary to granulocytopenia or monocytopenia. The only consistent physical findings are slight to marked splenomegaly (75 to 80 per cent of cases) caused by massive infiltration by hairy cells and slight to moderate hepatomegaly (33 per cent of cases). Clinical lymphadenopathy is very uncommon, although retroperitoneal lymphadenopathy is noted on computed tomography (CT) scans in 20 to 25 per cent of cases. More than two thirds of patients present with anemia (<10 grams per deciliter), neutropenia (<1500 per microliter),

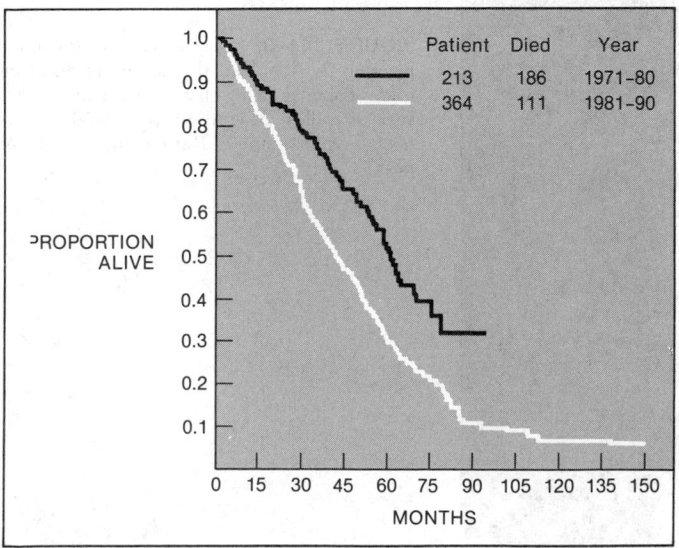

FIGURE 144–2. Survival of M. D. Anderson Cancer Center patients with benign-phase CML by year of diagnosis.

thrombocytopenia (<100,000 per microliter), and monocytopenia (<100 per microliter). The WBC count is usually lower than 4000 per microliter at diagnosis, but marked thrombocytopenia is rare. The cytopenias are due to a combination of bone marrow production failure caused by leukemic infiltration and of hypersplenism. Marrow failure may be due in part to inhibitory factors (e.g., tumor necrosis factor) produced by the leukemic infiltrate, since the pancytopenia is often much more marked than would be anticipated from the degree of leukemic infiltration. During the course of the illness, patients often experience repeated infections and more rarely a systemic vasculitis resembling polyarteritis nodosa or osteolytic bone lesions, usually affecting the upper femora. Although gram-positive or gram-negative infections occur as expected with neutropenia, patients with HCL have a predilection to develop tuberculosis, atypical mycobacterial infections, or fungal infections, perhaps related to the severe monocytopenia that is characteristic of this disorder. Pneumonia and septicemia are common causes of death in HCL.

Diagnosis

In conjunction with the described clinical features, examination of the blood often suggests the diagnosis of HCL. In addition to the cytopenias described above, the peripheral blood film usually demonstrates a relative or absolute lymphocytosis, composed of cells with cytoplasmic projections, giving rise to the name "hairy cell" leukemia (Fig. 144–3) (see Color Plate 7J, left). The cytoplasmic projections are best seen using phase contrast or electron microscopy. The hairy cells are 10 to 15 μm in diameter with pale blue cytoplasm and a nucleus with a loose chromatin structure and one or two indistinct nucleoli. Bone marrow aspiration is usually inadequate owing to increased reticulin, collagen, and fibrin deposition, and a bone marrow biopsy is necessary. The biopsy demonstrates an increased cellularity with a diffuse or occasionally patchy infiltrate with hairy cells. The infiltrate is loose and spongy, with pale-staining cytoplasm surrounding bland, monotonous round or ovoid nuclei.

Hairy cells exhibit a strong acid phosphatase (isoenzyme 5) cytochemical reaction in 95 per cent of cases, a reaction that is resistant to the inhibitory effect of tartaric acid (TRAP). Other lymphoproliferative diseases are rarely TRAP positive. Electron microscopy exquisitely demonstrates the microvillar projections. Often, ribosomal-lamellar complexes can be identified; these are characteristic, but not diagnostic, of HCL. The peroxidase stain is negative, and lysozyme activity is absent in hairy cells, differentiating the cells from monocytes.

The cell of origin of HCL is the B lymphocyte, as documented by the demonstration of heavy- and light-chain immunoglobulin gene rearrangements. Hairy cells express CD19 and CD20, FMC7, and CD22, but not CD21 or CD5. Cell-surface immunoglobulins can be immunoglobulin G (IgG) or immunoglobulin A (IgA), which are rare in chronic lymphocytic leukemia (CLL). The cells demonstrate a kappa or lambda light-chain phenotype excess. The cells are CD25 (TAC or low-affinity interleukin 2 [IL + 2] receptor) positive and anti-HC2 positive, and they are positive for an early plasma cell antigen PCA-1, but not a late plasma cell antigen PCl. These findings suggest that hairy cells are late B lymphocytes or early plasma cells. High levels of soluble IL-2 receptors (>5 times normal) are present in the sera of almost all patients with HCL, with extremely high levels being noted in many cases. Some cases of HCL have a 14q + cytogenetic abnormality with a breakpoint at 14q32 (the locus of the Ig heavy-chain gene). Hairy cells have a low proliferative index, with fewer than 1 per cent being in the S phase of the cell cycle. Immune dysfunction is wide ranging in HCL. Monocytopenia is universal, B and T lymphocytes are decreased in number; the CD4/CD8 ratio is often inverted; and skin test reactivity to recall antigens is impaired, as is antibody-dependent cellular cytotoxicity. Humoral immunity is relatively preserved with normal immunoglobulin levels. A markedly impaired ability of patients with HCL to produce alpha-interferon has been reported.

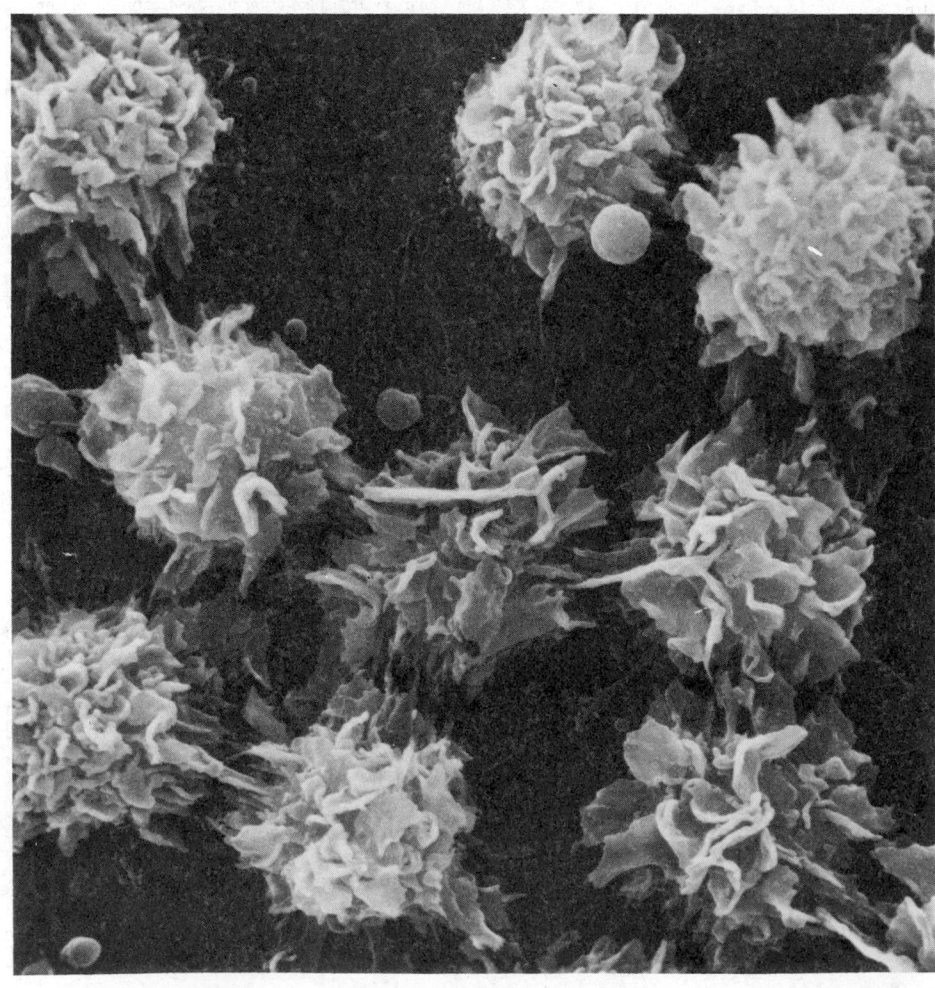

FIGURE 144–3. Hairy cells from the bone marrow as seen in the scanning electron microscope, showing characteristic prominent surface ruffles. Magnification ×8750. (Courtesy of Dr. Etienne deHarven and Nina Lampen.)

The differential diagnosis is most difficult between HCL and patients with lymphoma or CLL who have predominant splenomegaly and minimal lymphadenopathy. Some patients with a myelodysplastic or myeloproliferative syndrome have marked splenomegaly and pancytopenia with only a few atypical cells. Patients with other diseases, such as systemic lupus erythematosus and other autoimmune diseases, infiltrative splenomegaly, or tuberculosis, may present with splenomegaly and cytopenia, but these diagnoses can usually be made by history, physical examination, and appropriate blood and bone marrow tests. Splenomegaly, cytopenia, and an inaspirable marrow in a male should create a very high index of suspicion for HCL.

Other pathologic conditions to be differentiated from HCL requiring special tests are HCL variant, splenic lymphoma with villous lymphocytes, B cell and T cell prolymphocytic leukemia, and CLL with splenomegaly and no lymphadenopathy. Splenectomy and lymph node biopsy are sometimes necessary to establish the diagnosis in difficult cases. Cases of HCL variant manifest with higher WBC counts, are TRAP negative, have prominent nucleoli, and are only occasionally positive for antibodies against CD25. HCL variant responds poorly to interferon or deoxycoformycin, which are very effective agents in the management of typical HCL.

Prognosis and Treatment

A small proportion (<5 per cent) of patients with HCL do not require therapy. These patients have mild cytopenias, are not transfusion dependent, have no history of infections, and have a low level of marrow infiltration by hairy cells.

SPLENECTOMY. Because splenomegaly can itself cause pancytopenia, splenectomy was used in the past as the first treatment of most patients with HCL when complications such as splenic infarction or abdominal discomfort occurred, when infections became frequent, or when anemia, neutropenia, or thrombocytopenia worsened. Splenectomy was temporarily effective in improving blood counts in two thirds of patients, with improvement usually noted within 1 to 4 weeks. Splenectomy was usually ineffective if the spleen was not palpable. Removal of the spleen does not decrease the infiltration of hairy cells in the marrow or reduce the incidence of infections. Usually within 2 years, pancytopenia recurs owing to progressive marrow infiltration. The median survival of most patients in whom splenectomy alone was utilized was 4 to 5 years. Splenectomy is now recommended mainly for patients with splenic infarcts or massive splenomegaly.

INTERFERON. Chemotherapy for HCL with alkylating agents, corticosteroids, androgens, and anthracyclines is not effective and, when used in the past, was associated not infrequently with prolonged myelosuppression and severe infections. Low-dose chlorambucil was better tolerated but seldom resulted in significant clinical improvement. The use of human leukocyte interferon (HuIFn), however, has revolutionized the present approach to therapy. The use of HuIFn or r-IFnα rapidly improves (1 to 3 months) granulocyte, platelet, and hemoglobin levels; reduces spleen size; and consistently decreases marrow infiltration. Peripheral blood counts return to normal in 80 per cent of cases, and these patients achieve a complete remission (no hairy cells in the marrow) or a partial remission (>50 per cent reduction in marrow HCL infiltration). The most commonly used dosage of IFn is 3×10^6 units given subcutaneously three times a week, although daily schedules for 6 months reduce the marrow HCL infiltration more effectively. Higher doses (3 to 5 $\times 10^6$ units daily) increase the complete remission rate from 5 to 10 per cent to 25 per cent, with a partial remission rate of 55 to 65 per cent and a total failure rate of less than 5 per cent. Most patients achieve a partial remission by 6 months and a complete remission by 12 to 18 months. Response to therapy is most satisfactory in patients who are less anemic and monocytopenic and who have lower marrow cellularity. Lack of response or loss of an initial response may result from the development of neutralizing antibodies to r-IFnα, especially if the antibody titer is high. When treatment is discontinued, most patients relapse within 1 to 2 years, but most will again respond to treatment. Relapse occurs more quickly in patients who achieve only a partial remission than in those who respond completely. Treatment is usually reintroduced when patients become granulocytopenic. The presence of active, severe infection is not a contraindication to treatment with interferon. Indeed, the response to therapy provides patients with the best chance to recover from the infection.

INVESTIGATIONAL AGENTS. *Pentostatin* (2-deoxycoformycin), an adenosine deaminase inhibitor, has marked activity in HCL. At the low dosages used to treat HCL (4 mg per square meter every 2 weeks), pentostatin produces complete remissions in 50 to 60 per cent of patients and partial remissions in 40 per cent. Higher dosages of pentostatin are associated with a high rate of infections, usually with opportunistic infections, since the agent is very immunosuppressive, decreasing both T cell number and function. The response rate of the higher dose regimen is 80 to 90 per cent, with more than 60 per cent of patients achieving a complete response. The response to treatment is more rapid than for interferon, occurring within 2 to 4 months following the initiation of therapy. Pentostatin is active in patients previously treated with interferon. Responses appear to be more durable than those seen in interferon-treated patients. Toxicity includes nausea and vomiting, infection, renal and hepatic dysfunction, conjunctivitis, and photosensitivity.

2-Chlorodeoxyadenosine (2-CDA), an adenosine analogue, has been reported to produce complete remissions in more than 90 per cent of HCL patients with a single course of 0.1 mg per kilogram per day for 7 days by continuous intravenous infusion. Since the remissions appear to be very durable, 2-CDA promises to be the most effective agent developed to treat HCL. The drug is very well tolerated, with a low infection rate. *Granulocyte colony-stimulating factor (G-CSF)* has been reported to correct the granulocytopenia in HCL.

PROGNOSIS. The median survival of patients with HCL prior to interferon was 2 to 3 years. A return to normal leukocyte counts in HCL diminishes the risk of infection and is certain to improve the survival of patients with HCL. More than 90 per cent of interferon-treated patients are projected to be alive at 5 years.

Chilosi M, Semanzato G, Cetto G, et al.: Soluble interleukin-2 receptors in the sera of patients with hairy cell leukemia: Relationship with the effect of recombinant alpha-interferon therapy on clinical parameters and natural killer in vitro activity. Blood 70:1530, 1987. *Description of a clinically useful serum marker in the diagnosis and management of HCL.*

Piro LD, Carrera CJ, Carson DA, et al.: Lasting remissions in hairy-cell leukemia induced by a single infusion of 2-chlorodeoxyadenosine. N Engl J Med 322:1117, 1990. *Report of dramatic clinical activity of a purine analogue, 2-chlorodeoxyadenosine, in HCL, resulting in a high frequency of complete remissions.*

Quesada J: Hairy cell leukemia. In Freireich EJ, Kantarjian HM (eds.): Therapy of Hematopoietic Neoplasia. New York, Marcel Dekker, in press. *A balanced analysis of the biology, clinical features, treatment, and prognosis of HCL.*

Van Norman AS, Nagorney DM, Martin JK, et al.: Splenectomy for hairy cell leukemia. A clinical review of 63 patients. Cancer 57:644, 1986. *Describes the features associated with response to splenectomy in HCL.*

CHRONIC LYMPHOCYTIC LEUKEMIA

Chronic lymphocytic leukemia (CLL) is a neoplasm characterized by accumulation of monoclonal lymphocytes, usually of B cell immunophenotype (>95 per cent of cases), more rarely of T cell immunophenotype (see Color Plate 7I). The cells accumulate in the bone marrow, lymph nodes, liver, spleen, and occasionally other organs. Chronic lymphocyte leukemia is the most common leukemia (one third of all cases) in the Western world and is twice as common as CML. The disease occurs rarely in those below the age of 30; most patients with CLL are over 60 years of age. Chronic lymphocytic leukemia increases in incidence exponentially with age; by age 80 the incidence rate is 20 cases per 100,000 persons per year. The male-female ratio is approximately 2:1. Asian countries such as Japan and China have an incidence of CLL only 10 per cent of that in the United States and other Western countries. Intermediate incidence rates exist for persons of Hispanic origin.

Etiology

The cause of CLL is unknown. Ionizing radiation and viruses have not been associated with CLL. Familial clustering in CLL is more common than in other leukemias; first-degree relatives of patients have a twofold to fourfold higher risk than does the general population. Farmers have a higher incidence of CLL than do those in other occupations, raising the question of the possible etiologic role of herbicidal or pesticidal chemicals. No specific leukemogenic role of chemicals, including benzene, has been established for CLL.

Pathogenesis

Leukemia cells in CLL are usually remarkably homogeneous. The cells express monoclonal surface immunoglobulin (SmIg, usually immunoglobulin M [IgM] ± immunoglobulin D [IgD]) of a single kappa or lambda light-chain phenotype. A number of patients with CLL have SmIg molecules that cross-react with IgM rheumatoid factor paraprotein. CLL cells are early B cells and have lost terminal deoxynucleotidyl transferase activity. The CLL cells express the pan B antigens CD19, CD20, and CD24 in almost all cases and CD21 (which includes the receptor for the Epstein-Barr virus and the C3D component of complement) in more than 75 per cent of cases. In fewer than 20 per cent of cases is the C3B complement component receptor expressed. The vast majority of cells exhibit Ia antigen, have receptors for the Fc fragment of IgG, and spontaneously form rosettes with mouse erythrocytes. In 95 per cent of cases, the CLL cells coexpress pan B cell antigens and CD5 (Leu 1, T1, and T101), a pan T cell antigen. Other T cell antigens and common acute lymphocytic leukemia antigen (CALLA) (CD10) are absent. CD25 (TAC, IL2 receptor) antigen is positive in more than 20 per cent of cells in 20 per cent of cases.

Monoclonality of the B cells is demonstrated by a marked preponderance of kappa or lambda light chains, by evidence of immunoglobulin gene rearrangement, by the presence of monoclonal serum Ig peaks in some cases, and by glucose-6-phosphate dehydrogenase isoenzyme studies.

Chronic lymphocytic leukemia is an accumulative rather than a proliferative disease, since the CLL cells have a low proliferative index. Patients with higher WBC counts and more advanced stages have higher proliferative indices and shorter survivals. Most of the CLL cells in the blood and bone marrow are in the Go phase of the cell cycle, with only a small proportion of larger cells in the marrow and lymph nodes being in the other phases. The CLL cells have a longer lifespan in the blood than do normal B cells and have impaired egress from the blood. The CLL B cells have impaired responses to B cell mitogens and to B cell growth factors. The cells appear to be blocked in differentiation, with a high content of cytoplasmic IgM but a low surface IgM. Although most of the cells do not secrete immunoglobulins, in about 5 per cent of cases, a paraprotein of the same type as that on the surface of the CLL cells is present in the plasma or urine. The CLL cells have a low or absent stimulatory effect in allogeneic or autologous mixed lymphocyte cultures. The CLL cells can be stimulated to differentiate into cells resembling hairy cells or plasma cells under the influence of phorbol esters, B cell mitogens, or growth factors.

T cell function is invariably abnormal in CLL. T cells are increased in number in the blood, bone marrow, and lymph nodes of patients with CLL, but they are polyclonal, and T cell receptor gene rearrangement is rare. The CD4/CD8 (T-helper/T-suppressor) ratio is often close to unity or is inverted owing to a relatively greater increase in the CD8-positive cells. The T cells have a blunted response to T cell mitogens in unseparated blood and decreased delayed hypersensitivity reactions to recall antigens. The T cell defects worsen as the disease progresses to a more advanced stage. Purified T cells have a normal response to T cell mitogens.

Clinical Features

Many patients with CLL are asymptomatic, and the disease is diagnosed when an absolute lymphocytosis is noted in the peripheral blood during evaluation for other illnesses or when the patient undergoes a routine physical examination. Symptoms such as fatigue, lethargy, loss of appetite, weight loss, or reduced exercise tolerance are nonspecific. These features are occasionally greater than can be explained by the degree of anemia or extent of tumor burden. Many patients present with enlarged lymph nodes, usually cervical, noted by themselves or others. Fever and night sweats, or documented infections, are uncommon initial symptoms (<5 per cent) but become more prominent as the disease progresses. Sinopulmonary infections are most common during the early phase of the disease, but as the disease progresses, the frequency of neutropenia, T cell deficiency, and hypogammaglobulinemia increases, resulting in gram-negative bacterial, fungal, and viral infections. Herpes zoster, herpes simplex, and cytomegalovirus infections usually occur later in the disease. An intriguing but unexplained common feature of CLL is an exuberant reaction to insect bites.

The major physical findings relate to infiltration of the reticuloendothelial system. Lymphadenopathy with discrete, rubbery, mobile lymph nodes is present in two thirds of patients at diagnosis. Later, as the lymph nodes enlarge, they become matted. Enlargement of the liver or spleen is less common at diagnosis (approximately 10 per cent and 40 per cent of cases, respectively). Less commonly, and usually late in the disease, clinically significant infiltration of skin, eyelids, heart, lungs, pleura, or gastrointestinal tract may occur. Organ failure due to infiltration with CLL is uncommon, with pulmonary symptoms being most likely to cause clinical problems. Infiltration of the central nervous system in CLL is rare, and central nervous system symptomatology is more likely to be due to opportunistic infections, such as cryptococcosis or listeriosis. The extent of involvement varies from only a single node or node group to enlargement of virtually all nodes. Later in the disease, massive adenopathy may develop and cause luminal obstruction, such as obstructive jaundice, obstructive uropathy, dysphagia, or partial bowel obstruction. Unilateral or bilateral leg edema can occur owing to obstruction of the lymphatic and/or venous systems. Pleural effusions and ascites can also develop and are associated with a poor prognosis.

Diagnostic Features

Chronic lymphocytic leukemia is characterized by an absolute lymphocytosis in the peripheral blood, a minimal level of more than 5000 per microliter, but more usually in the range of 40,000 to 150,000 per microliter. Extreme leukocytosis approaching 1 × 10⁶ per microliter occurs only late in the disease, and hyperviscosity symptoms can occur if the WBC count is higher than 500,000 per microliter. If the lymphocyte count is 5000 to 15,000 per microliter, supportive evidence for clonality (kappa or lambda light chain excess or immunoglobulin gene rearrangement) should be present before the diagnosis is made. Most physicians also document a lymphocytosis in the bone marrow (>30 per cent lymphocytes) and perform a bone marrow biopsy. Anemia (<11 grams per deciliter) is present in 15 to 20 per cent of patients at diagnosis and thrombocytopenia (<100,000 per microliter) in 10 per cent. Bone marrow replacement and hypersplenism contribute to the anemia and thrombocytopenia in most cases. The anemia is usually normochromic and normocytic, and the reticulocyte count is normal unless the patient has autoimmune hemolytic anemia, which usually results from the development of a warm-reacting IGg antibody (Ch. 135). The diagnosis of autoimmune hemolytic anemia, which occurs in the course of 8 to 10 per cent of cases, is confirmed by a positive direct Coombs test, reticulocytosis, a low serum haptoglobulin value, and an elevated unconjugated serum bilirubin level. In such patients, reactive erythroid hyperplasia as a response to the hemolysis may be masked in the bone marrow by the marked lymphocytic infiltration. Autoimmune thrombocytopenia can be diagnosed in some cases with a positive test for platelet antibodies. Cold agglutinin hemolysis occurs rarely in CLL. The antibodies causing the red cell and platelet destruction are not produced by the CLL cells, and the mechanism for the autoimmune diseases is not known. Pure red cell aplasia associated with T-suppressor cell activity is an additional reported cause of anemia in CLL.

The lymphocytes in CLL are indistinguishable on light or electron microscopy from normal small B lymphocytes. On bone marrow aspiration, the proportion of lymphocytes is greater than 30 per cent and may extend up to 100 per cent in newly diagnosed patients with CLL. The rest of the cells are normal myeloid and erythroid cells. Four patterns of lymphocyte infiltration on bone marrow biopsy occur and have prognostic value in CLL: (a) nodular (15 per cent), (b) infiltrative (30 per cent), (c) mixed nodular and infiltrative (30 per cent), and (d) diffuse (35 per cent).

Most early-stage patients have patterns a, b, or c; a diffuse histology is most common in advanced-stage disease and becomes more prominent as the disease evolves. A diffuse histologic pattern confers a poor prognosis regardless of the stage of disease. Hypogammaglobulinemia is common in CLL and predisposes to infections, especially with encapsulated microorganisms. Low levels of IgG, IgA, or IgM occur in 25 per cent of newly diagnosed patients, are more common in advanced stages, and increase in frequency to 50 to 70 per cent as the disease progresses.

Nonrandom cytogenetic abnormalities in CLL include trisomy 12 (40 per cent), 14q+ abnormalities (25 per cent), and abnormalities in the long arm of chromosomes 6 and 11. Single abnormalities are more common in early and recently diagnosed diseases, and additional changes develop with time (clonal evolution). The site of the breakpoint on chromosome 14 (q32) is close to the site of the Ig heavy-chain gene.

Staging Systems

Two major staging systems are used. The Rai staging system (1975) defines five stages and is most frequently used in the United States, whereas the Binet system (1981) defines three stages and is most frequently used in Europe (Table 144–3). Both systems have the advantage of simplicity, low cost, and reproducibility and have been prospectively validated (Figs. 144–4 and 144–5). Within the stages, outcome is variable and other prognostic factors, such as the bone marrow histologic pattern, provide additional prognostic information. Patients with anemia and thrombocytopenia (Rai stages III and IV, Binet C) have, on the average, a poor prognosis; patients with lymphocytosis alone (Rai 0, some Binet A patients) have an excellent prognosis. The prognosis of the other patients is heterogeneous and, as might be expected, is worse in patients with a greater tumor burden. Rai stage II patients who have splenomegaly without lymphadenopathy (pure splenic form) have a better prognosis than do other stage II patients. While useful in the design and analysis of clinical trials, the staging systems are not particularly useful for individual patients because of the heterogeneity of outcome. A group of patients with a lymphocyte count of less than 30,000 per microliter, a hemoglobin higher than 11 grams per deciliter, a platelet count lower than 100,000 per microliter, with fewer than three involved node areas, and a lymphocyte doubling time of greater than 12 months has been described as having "smoldering" CLL, with a survival equal to that of an age- and sex-matched population.

Patients tend to progress through stages, with many patients developing more sites of involvement with time and eventually experiencing marrow failure, but anemia and thrombocytopenia can develop abruptly even without antibody-mediated destruction or increasing tumor burden.

Differential Diagnosis

Many diseases can cause a lymphocytosis: pertussis, infectious lymphocytosis, cytomegalovirus and Epstein-Barr virus mononucleosis, tuberculosis, toxoplasmosis, chronic inflammatory disorders, and autoimmune syndromes. Although they may superficially resemble CLL, their clinical pictures seldom are confused with that of B cell CLL. Many of these patients are younger and

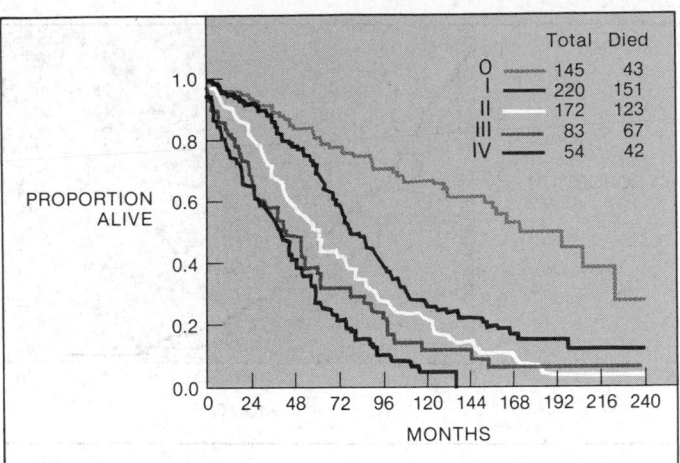

FIGURE 144–4. Survival of untreated patients with chronic lymphocytic leukemia (CLL) by Rai stage.

have fever or other acute symptoms, or exhibit other clinical features, such as rash and joint symptoms, that are uncommon in CLL. The lymphocytosis is usually less than 15,000 per microliter and not sustained. If doubt persists, monoclonal antibodies will distinguish the monoclonal lymphocytosis in CLL from the polyclonal B cell proliferation in the other disorders. The more difficult differential diagnosis is from other lymphoproliferative disorders, such as prolymphocytic leukemia, HCL, the leukemic phase of lymphoma, Waldenström's macroglobulinemia, and T cell CLL. While certain clinical features are more common in some of these disorders—for example, marked splenomegaly with minimal or no lymphadenopathy in prolymphocytic leukemia and HCL versus extensive lymphadenopathy with or without splenomegaly in CLL—none of these differential features is specific. The differential diagnosis therefore depends largely on histopathologic and more specifically immunophenotypic features (Table 144–4).

Small lymphocytic lymphoma (SLL) shares histopathologic and immunophenotypic features with CLL, differing only in lacking an absolute monoclonal lymphocytosis in the peripheral blood. The bone marrow in SLL may or may not have more than 30 per cent lymphocytes. LFA-1 adhesion protein is much more commonly expressed on SLL cells than CLL cells. Occasionally, other lymphomas, such as follicular small cleaved cell lymphoma (FSCCL), manifest in a leukemic phase. These cells are often cleaved on light microscopy, have bright staining for SmIg, and are commonly FMC7 and CD10 positive. Lymph node biopsy should be performed to identify these cases with greater precision. The presence of lymphoma cells in the blood in SLL and FSCCL is more common later in the disease. The WBC count in Waldenström's macroglobulinemia at diagnosis is usually much lower than in CLL (<10,000 per microliter), and many patients

TABLE 144–3. RAI AND BINET STAGING SYSTEMS IN CHRONIC LYMPHOCYTIC LEUKEMIA (CLL)

	Lymphocytosis	Lymphadenopathy	Hepatomegaly or Splenomegaly	Hemoglobin (grams/dl)	Platelets × 10³/μl
Rai stage					
0	+	—	—	≥11	≥100
I	+	+	—	≥11	≥100
II	+	±	+	≥11	≥100
III	+	±	±	<11	≥100
IV	+	±	±	Any	<100
Binet stage					
A	+	±	±	≥10	≥100
		(<3 Lymphatic groups* positive)			
B	+	±	±	≥10	≥100
		(≥3 Lymphatic groups* positive)			
C	+	±	±	<10 or	<100

*(1) Cervical, axillary, and inguinal nodes; (2) liver; and (3) spleen; each group is considered one group whether unilateral or bilateral.

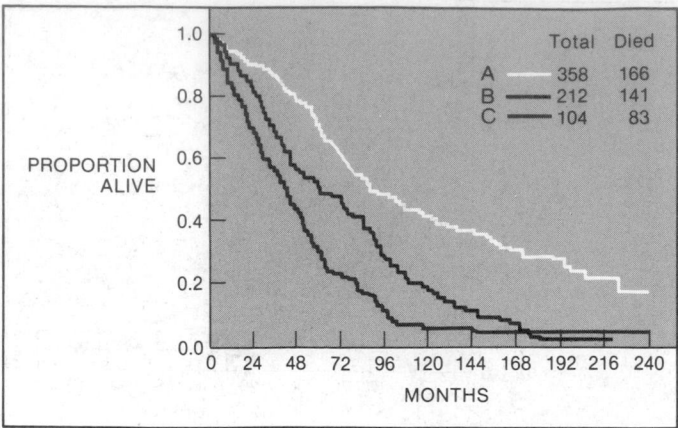

FIGURE 144–5. Survival of untreated patients with CLL by Binet stage.

are leukopenic (Ch. 151). The cells have a plasmacytoid appearance, CD38 and PCA-1 positivity, and more SmIg and cytoplasmic Ig. A monoclonal IgM plasma peak is present in almost all cases of Waldenström's macroglobulinemia but is rare in CLL. Prolymphocytic leukemia (PLL) is an uncommon disease (10 per cent of the incidence of CLL), and its characteristics of massive splenomegaly, minimal lymphadenopathy, WBC count commonly greater than 100,000 per microliter, with 10 to 90 per cent of the cells being prolymphocytes, distinguish this disease from typical B cell CLL. Prolymphocytes are larger cells than typical CLL lymphocytes; they have a distinct nucleolus and are often FMC7 positive. The male-female ratio is 4:1, and the median age at diagnosis is 70 years. Survival is shorter than in CLL (median, 3 years), and response is poor to therapies usually applied in CLL. A monoclonal spike, usually IgG or IgA, is present in one third of cases. The immunoglobulin on the surface of the cells is usually IgG or IgA, not IgM ± IgD, as in CLL. A specific karyotypic abnormality, t(6;12) (q15;q13), has been reported in PLL. One fifth of the cases are of T cell phenotype. The predominant clinical manifestation in Sézary's syndrome (a CD4+ T cell malignancy related to mycosis fungoides) is chronic exfoliative erythroderma with a low number of circulating monoclonal T cells. The clinical and laboratory differential diagnosis from CLL is not difficult. Other T cell malignancies with peripheral blood involvement are adult T cell leukemia-lymphoma and large granular lymphocytosis (LGL). Adult T cell leukemia-lymphoma is associated with a retrovirus (human T cell leukemia/lymphoma virus [HTLV-1]) and is common in Japan and the Caribbean. It is frequently manifested by lytic bone lesions and hypercalcemia. In LGL the absolute lymphocyte count is usually low (<5000 per microliter), with a CD2+, CD3+, and CD8+ (T-suppressor) phenotype (T-gamma cells). These patients often have spleno-

megaly, neutropenia, and rheumatoid arthritis–like symptomatology and serology. The lymphocytes have abundant cytoplasm with azurophilic granules. In most patients a benign course is noted, although repeated infections can occur.

Prognostic Factors

In addition to the impact of tumor burden and marrow function on prognosis, as reflected in the Rai and Binet staging systems, other adverse factors are as follows: (a) a diffuse pattern of lymphocytic infiltration observed on bone marrow biopsy; (b) an abnormal karyotype (e.g., trisomy 12 or multiple chromosomal abnormalities); (c) advanced age; (d) male sex; (e) elevated serum levels of thymidine kinase, uric acid, alkaline phosphatase, or lactate dehydrogenase; (f) rapid lymphocyte doubling time; and (g) an increased proportion of large or atypical lymphocytes in the peripheral blood. A poor response to therapy is an adverse factor in all phases of the disease. As the disease progresses, a worsening of stage and the development of a prolymphocytic leukemia (10 per cent of cases), large cell lymphoma, or myelomatous or acute lymphocytic leukemia (rare) are grave prognostic features. Multiple chromosomal abnormalities identify patients at risk of developing a large cell lymphomatous transformation (Richter's syndrome), which occurs in 5 to 10 per cent of CLL patients as a terminal event. Richter's syndrome should be suspected whenever a single lymph node area or the spleen begins to enlarge in CLL or when unexplained clinical deterioration occurs. The transformation does not always share immunophenotypic or cytogenetic features with the original CLL clone and may be a coincidental second tumor. Response to therapy in Richter's transformation is not usually as satisfactory as for de novo large cell lymphoma. A high incidence of second malignancies (10 to 20 per cent of patients) either precedes or follows the diagnosis of CLL, with the roles of therapy versus impaired immune surveillance as causative factors being unclear. Skin cancer, including melanoma, colorectal and lung cancers, and sarcomas are common in patients with CLL. Hypogammaglobulinemia may have an adverse impact on survival. Patients who develop repeated infections fare less well than other patients.

Treatment

The major therapeutic questions for CLL are when to treat and which therapeutic agent or agents to use.

WHEN TO TREAT. Patients with CLL are usually in later life, and the prognosis of the disease is variable (with some early-stage patients being stable for 5 to 20 years). It is traditional, therefore, to delay treatment of early-stage CLL (Rai 0, Binet A) until the disease progresses. Early treatment with alkylating agents does not prolong survival and may be associated with a heightened risk of developing second malignancies. Treatment of Rai stages III and IV (Binet stage C) patients is recommended at the time of diagnosis because of the poor survival of these patients (median, 2 years). Treatment of intermediate-stage disease (Rai stages I and II, Binet stage B) is recommended if symptomatic disease (fever, sweats, weight loss, severe fatigue), massive lymphadenopathy, or hepatosplenomegaly is present. Progressive

TABLE 144–4. DIFFERENTIAL DIAGNOSIS OF INDOLENT LYMPHOPROLIFERATIVE DISORDERS

Disease	Lymphadenopathy (%)	Splenomegaly (%)	Cell of Origin (B/T)	SmIg	CD5	CD19, 20 (%)	Other Positive
CLL	75	50	B(20:1)	Weak	>90%	≥90	Mouse red blood cell (RBC) receptors
Prolymphocytic leukemia	33	95	B(4:1)	Bright	T cell PLL	75	FMC-7
Hairy cell leukemia	<10	80	B(T rare)	Bright	—	>90	CD25, CD11C
Lymphoma (leukemic phase)	90	80	B(T rare)	Bright	Some	>90	CD10
Waldenström's macroglobulinemia	33	33	All B	Weak	Some	Many	CD38, PCA-1
Large granular lymphocytosis	10	10	All T	Absent	—	—	CD2, CD3, CD8

*CD5 —pan T cell, B CLL   CD8 —T cell (suppressor-cytotoxic)
  CD19 —early pan B cell   CD10 —early B cell
  CD20 —pan B cell   CD11C—hairy cells, activated T cell, NK cell
  FMC7—PLL and hairy cells   CD38 —activated B cell, thymocytes, plasma cells
  CD2 —pan T cell   PCA1 —plasma cell
  CD3 —pan mature T cell   CD25 —low-affinity interleukin 2 (IL2) receptor

organ and/or node enlargement and lymphocytosis (>100,000 per microliter) are other common indications for treatment. Development of anemia, thrombocytopenia, or neutropenia associated with infections is usually an indication for systemic antileukemic therapy unless an autoimmune cause of the cytopenia (positive direct Coombs' test, antiplatelet or antineutrophil antibodies) is found. In the latter group of cases, the use of corticosteroids, such as prednisone, should be tried prior to the initiation of cytotoxic therapy. A doubling of blood lymphocytes in less than 12 months is an adverse prognostic factor and suggests that treatment is indicated.

CHEMOTHERAPY. *Chlorambucil* (less commonly, cyclophosphamide) is usually the first chemotherapeutic agent used. Corticosteroids are often used concurrently, but with no clearly demonstrated advantage in therapeutic response or survival. Chlorambucil regimens vary widely. In the chronic low-dosage daily regimen, 0.1 to 0.2 mg per kilogram per day of chlorambucil is continued for 3 to 6 weeks until the desired effect is obtained or until thrombocytopenia or neutropenia develops. The dosage is then adjusted for maintenance and is continued for 6 to 12 months. For intermittent high-dosage (pulse) schedules, chlorambucil (0.5 to 2 mg per kilogram) is given over 1 to 4 days every 4 weeks or given at half dosage every 2 weeks. Neither dosage schedule for chlorambucil has been established as definitely superior. If prednisone is given concurrently with chlorambucil, the dosage is 60 to 100 mg per day in the pulse schedule. Continuous prednisone is not recommended in this elderly population but can be given at a dosage of 40 to 60 mg per day for 4 weeks initially, tapering to 10 to 20 mg per day when combined with chlorambucil in the continuous-therapy schedule. Following therapy, many patients remain stable for months to years before disease progression indicates the need for further treatment. The endpoints for response to therapy have not been well defined, since treatment is usually strictly palliative. Most physicians try to achieve the disappearance of lymphadenopathy and splenomegaly and the return to a normal WBC count, but rarely a normal bone marrow. Myelosuppression is the most common toxicity with chlorambucil, although occasionally rash, nausea, or pulmonary toxicity occurs.

The COP regimen (cyclophosphamide, 100 to 300 mg per square meter per day given orally on days 1 through 5; vincristine [Oncovin], 2 mg given intravenously on day 1; and prednisone, 100 mg administered orally on days 1 through 5) does not appear to have any advantage over chlorambucil. Indeed, vincristine has never been demonstrated to have activity in CLL. Sixty to 75 per cent of patients obtain at least a partial clinical response with these alkylating agents, but a complete remission, including fewer than 30 per cent lymphocytes in the bone marrow aspirate, is achieved in only 10 to 15 per cent of the cases. Repeated rechallenge with the same drug combinations is usually associated with less satisfactory and shorter responses. Damage to DNA gives rise to concern regarding the role of alkylating agents as contributory factors to the high incidence of second malignancies in CLL. Two recent sets of recommendations address response and eligibility criteria in CLL studies (Table 144–5).

Regimens utilizing cyclophosphamide, doxorubicin (Adriamycin), and prednisone with vincristine (CHOP) or without vincristine (CAP) have produced response rates of 50 to 70 per cent in previously untreated Binet stage C patients and are well tolerated in CLL despite the advanced age of most patients. The CAP regimen resulted in a complete remission rate of 45 per cent in CLL, with a median survival of 7 years in the Binet C patients.

CORTICOSTEROID THERAPY. Corticosteroids, usually prednisone (60 to 100 mg per day), are indicated as treatment for Coombs-positive autoimmune hemolytic anemia and for some cases of immune-mediated thrombocytopenia in CLL. If there is no response in 3 to 4 weeks, the treatment has failed and the dose should then be tapered over 1 to 2 weeks. If a response is obtained, the dose is usually reduced by 25 per cent each week over 4 weeks. Autoimmune hemolytic anemia and immune-mediated thrombocytopenia do not correlate closely with the activity of CLL.

RADIATION THERAPY. In CLL, radiation therapy is usually restricted to external irradiation of localized nodal masses or an enlarged spleen that has been refractory to chemotherapy. Repeated leukapheresis and extracorporeal irradiation of blood can decrease the tumor burden in CLL and occasionally increase hemoglobin and platelet levels but are not practical for long periods.

EXPERIMENTAL THERAPIES. Two adenosine analogues, fludarabine monophosphate and 2-CDA, and pentostatin (deoxycoformycin), an adenosine deaminase inhibitor, have exhibited therapeutic potential in CLL. Fludarabine monophosphate (25 to 30 mg per square meter per day for 5 days every 4 weeks) leads to complete remission in 70 per cent of untreated patients and 35 per cent of those previously treated with alkylating agents. The dose-limiting toxicity is myelosuppression. The course of therapy may be complicated by infections with organisms usually associated with immunodeficiency syndromes involving T lymphocytes (e.g., those caused by *Pneumocystis carinii*, herpesviruses). 2-CDA and deoxycoformycin have not been as widely studied in CLL.

Intravenous immunoglobulin (400 mg per kilogram every 3 to 4 weeks) significantly decreases the incidence of infections of minor to moderate severity in CLL patients with hypogammaglobulinemia, but the cost of this therapy is substantial. Although ineffective in patients with advanced-stage CLL, alpha-interferon may significantly decrease the lymphocyte count in 50 to 70 per

TABLE 144–5. DEFINITION OF REMISSION IN CLL: COMPARISON OF THE INTERNATIONAL WORKSHOP IN CLL (IWCLL) AND THE NATIONAL CANCER INSTITUTE WORKING GROUP (NCI-WG) CRITERIA

Criteria	Complete Remission (CR)		Partial Remission (PR)	
	IWCLL	*NCI-WG*	*IWCLL*	*NCI-WG*
Physical examination				
Nodes	None	None	Shift to a lower Binet stage, e.g., C → A or B, B → A	≥50% decrease
Liver/spleen	Not palpable	Not palpable		≥50% decrease
Symptoms	None	None		N/A
Peripheral blood				
Neutrophils	≥1500/μl	≥1500/μl		>1500/μl or ≥50% ↑ from baseline
Platelets	>100,000/μl	>100,000/μl		100,000/μl or >50% ↑ from baseline
Hemoglobin	Not specified	>11 grams/dl		>11 grams/dl or >50% ↑ from baseline
Lymphocytes	<4000/μl	<4000/μl		>50% decrease
Bone marrow				
Lymphocytes	Normal aspirate and biopsy*	<30%		N/A
		Normal*		N/A

*Nodules or focal aggregates of lymphocytes are comparable to CR.

cent of early-stage patients as well as increase the absolute granulocyte count, improve the serum immunoglobulin level, and improve T-helper/T-suppressor ratios. Interleukin 2 has been administered sparingly to patients with refractory CLL, with no consistent improvement in disease parameters. Similarly, monoclonal antibodies directed against CLL cells have not as yet resulted in consistent benefit to patients.

Prognosis in CLL (Figs. 144–4 and 144–5)

The median survival of patients with CLL is 4 to 5 years following the initiation of treatment. As expected, early-stage patients (Rai 0 to II) survive significantly longer, a median of 7 to 8 years. No current treatment strategy has demonstrated a survival advantage over conventional therapy with chlorambucil.

Chronic lymphocytic leukemia tends to develop in elderly patients; death often occurs, therefore, from other intercurrent illnesses of this age group. Younger patients (<60 years of age) almost all die as a result of CLL or one of its complications, especially infections. Gram-positive organisms usually cause nonfatal infections early in CLL, but most deaths due to infection are associated with gram-negative bacterial or fungal infections. Other opportunistic organisms such as *Mycobacterium tuberculosis*, herpesvirus, and *Pneumocystis carinii* may also contribute to death.

Bennett JM, Catovsky D, Daniel M-T, et al.: Proposals for the classification of chronic (mature) B and T lymphoid leukaemias. J Clin Pathol 42:567, 1989. *Classification of common and less common chronic leukemias using an integrated clinical, morphologic and immunophenotypic approach.*

Cheson BD, Bennett JM, Rai KR, et al.: Guidelines for clinical protocols for chronic lymphocytic leukemia: Recommendations of the National Cancer Institute–sponsored Working Group. Am J Hematol 29:152, 1988. *Standard guidelines for eligibility criteria, indications for treatment, and response criteria in B cell CLL.*

Foon KA, Rai KR, Gale RP: Chronic lymphocytic leukemia: New insights into biology and therapy. Ann Intern Med 113:525, 1990. *This is a useful general review of recent advances in our understanding of the pathogenesis of CLL and of new approaches to therapy; 227 references.*

Freedman AS, Boyd AW, Bieber FR, et al.: Normal cellular counterparts of B cell chronic lymphocytic leukemia. Blood 70:418, 1987. *Surface markers are used to indicate the differentiation arrest in CLL and to address the question of the cell of origin of the disease.*

French Cooperative Group on Chronic Lymphocytic Leukemia: Effects of chlorambucil and therapeutic decision in initial forms of chronic lymphocytic leukemia (Stage A): Results of a randomized clinical trial on 612 patients. Blood 75:1414, 1990. *Randomized trial comparing the outcome of early versus late treatment with chlorambucil in CLL. Disturbing data on second malignancies in the early treatment group.*

Juliusson G, Oscier DG, Fitchett M, et al.: Prognostic subgroups in B-cell chronic lymphocytic leukemia defined by specific chromosomal abnormalities. N Engl J Med 323(11):720, 1990. *A major report on the prognostic and biologic importance of cytogenetic abnormalities in CLL.*

Keating MJ, Kantarjian H, Talpaz M, et al.: Fludarabine: A new agent with major activity against chronic lymphocytic leukemia. Blood 74:19, 1989. *Report of the marked clinical activity of fludarabine, a new purine analogue, in refractory CLL.*

Montserrat E, Vinolas N, Reverte JC, et al.: Natural history of chronic lymphocytic leukemia: On the progression and prognosis of early clinical stages. Nouv Rev Fr Hematol 30:359, 1988. *Illustrates the features associated with risk of progression in early-stage CLL.*

Rozman C, Montserrat E, Rodriguez-Fernandez JM, et al.: Bone marrow histologic pattern—the best single prognostic parameter in chronic lymphocytic leukemia: A multivariate analysis of 329 cases. Blood 64: 642, 1984. *The bone marrow histologic pattern in CLL is shown to be a major prognostic factor for survival in all stages of disease.*

Ziegler-Heitbrock HWL, Schlag R, Flieger D, et al.: Favorable response of early stage B CLL patients to treatment with IFN-α₂. Blood 73:1426, 1989. *Despite modest antitumor activity in CLL, interferon enhances a variety of immune functions, including gamma globulin levels.*

145 The Acute Leukemias

Frederick R. Appelbaum

DEFINITION

Normal hematopoiesis requires the tightly regulated proliferation and differentiation of pluripotent hematopoietic stem cells to become mature peripheral blood cells. Acute leukemia is the result of a malignant event, or events, occurring in an early hematopoietic precursor. Instead of proliferating and differentiating normally, the affected cell gives rise to progeny that fail to differentiate and instead continue to proliferate in an uncontrolled fashion. As a result, immature myeloid cells (in acute myelogenous leukemia) or lymphoid cells (in acute lymphocytic leukemia), often called "blasts," rapidly accumulate and progressively replace the bone marrow, leading to diminished production of normal red cells, white cells, and platelets. This loss of normal marrow function in turn gives rise to the common clinical complications of leukemia: anemia, infection, and bleeding. With time the leukemic blasts pour out into the bloodstream and eventually occupy the lymph nodes, spleen, and other vital organs. If untreated, acute leukemia is rapidly fatal; most patients die within several months of diagnosis. With appropriate therapy, the natural history of acute leukemia can be markedly altered and many patients can be cured.

ETIOLOGY

In most cases acute leukemia develops for no known reason, but sometimes a possible cause can be identified.

Radiation

Ionizing radiation is leukemogenic. Acute lymphocytic leukemia (ALL), acute myelogenous leukemia (AML), and chronic myelogenous leukemia (CML) are all increased in incidence in patients given radiation therapy for ankylosing spondylitis and in survivors of the atomic bomb blasts of Hiroshima and Nagasaki. The magnitude of the risk depends on the dose of radiation, its distribution in time, and the age of the individual. Greater risk results from higher dose radiation delivered over shorter periods to younger patients. An increased incidence of leukemia is seen within several years of exposure and appears to peak between five and ten years after exposure. In areas of high natural background radiation (often due to radon), chromosomal aberrations have been reported to be more frequent, but an increase in acute leukemia has not been consistently found. Recently, concern has been raised about possible leukemogenic effects of extremely low-frequency nonionizing electromagnetic fields emitted by electrical installations. If such an effect exists at all, the magnitude of the effect is small.

Oncogenic Viruses

The search for a viral cause of leukemia has been intensely pursued, but not found, except for two rare leukemias associated with retroviruses. Human T cell lymphotropic virus type I (HTLV-I), an enveloped, single-stranded RNA virus, is considered the causative agent of adult T cell leukemia (ATL). This distinct form of leukemia is found within geographic clusters in southwestern Japan, the Caribbean basin, and Africa. The virus can be spread vertically from mother to fetus or horizontally by sexual contact or through blood products. In areas where ATL is found, infection with the virus is endemic, but only 1 to 2 per cent of those infected with HTLV-I develop ATL, and the latency period seems to be quite long (perhaps 10 to 30 years). Although previously rare in the United States, HTLV-I seropositivity has been found with increasing frequency among chronically transfused patients and intravenous drug users. Screening of blood products for antibodies to HTLV-I is now a routine practice in blood banks in the United States. A second human retrovirus, genetically distinct from HTLV-I, termed HTLV-II, has been isolated from several patients with a syndrome resembling hairy cell leukemia. The etiologic link between HTLV-II and malignancy is uncertain.

Genetics and Congenital Factors

A genetic predisposition to leukemia exists in some individuals. If leukemia develops before age 10 in a patient with an identical twin, the unaffected twin has a one in five chance of subsequently developing leukemia. In occasional families, multiple members have developed an identical form of leukemia. Several autosomal recessive disorders associated with chromosomal instability are prone to terminate in acute leukemia, including Bloom syndrome, Fanconi anemia, and ataxic telangiectasia. Other congenital disorders associated with an increased incidence of leukemia are Down syndrome and infantile X-linked agammaglobulinemia.

Chemicals

Heavy occupational exposure to benzene frequently results in marrow hypoplasia, which sometimes evolves into acute leukemia. Other associations between occupational exposure to chemicals and subsequent leukemia are not persuasive.

Prior exposure to alkylating agents, such as chlorambucil, melphalan, and nitrogen mustard, is associated with an increased risk of AML. The risk of secondary AML is greater with increasing exposure to the agent and with increased patient age. Patients often present with a myelodysplastic syndrome before developing secondary AML. Cytogenetic studies of secondary leukemias frequently reveal abnormalities of chromosomes 5, 7, and 8.

INCIDENCE

The annual new case incidence of all leukemias is 8 to 10 per 100,000. This rate has remained static over the past three decades. The relative incidences for the four categories of leukemia are as follows: ALL, 11 per cent; CLL, 29 per cent; AML, 46 per cent; and CML, 14 per cent. The leukemias account for about 3 per cent of all cancers in the United States. The impact of leukemia is heightened because of the young age of some patients. For example, ALL is the most common cancer and the second leading cause of death in children under 15 years of age. Acute lymphocytic leukemia has a maximal incidence between 2 and 10 years of age, with a second, more gradual rise in frequency in later life. The incidence of AML gradually increases with age, without an early peak. Approximately half of AML cases occur in patients under age 50.

PATHOPHYSIOLOGY

The precise molecular event or events that cause leukemic transformation are unknown; the end result, however, is the relentless proliferation of immature hematopoietic cells that have lost their capacity to differentiate normally. The development of leukemia may be a multistep process, as demonstrated by the fact that in many cases acute leukemia develops in patients with a pre-existing myelodysplastic disorder. The disease is monoclonal, i.e., the final leukemic event occurs in a single cell. The level of differentiation at which the malignancy becomes evident is variable. In some cases of AML, it appears that the malignancy occurs in a very undifferentiated cell similar to the normal hematopoietic stem cell, in that red cell, platelet, and myeloid precursors are all products of the malignant clone. In other cases of AML, the malignant event may occur in a more differentiated cell, and only granulocyte and monocyte precursors develop from the malignant cell, while red cell and platelet precursors do not. In almost all cases of ALL, the myeloid lineage is not malignant, suggesting that in ALL, the malignant event occurs in a cell that is at least partially differentiated. Although the majority of leukemic cells are relatively undifferentiated, some mature circulating cells may be products of the malignant clone.

As the malignant clone expands, it does so at the expense of normal hematopoiesis. The mechanism of normal marrow suppression in leukemia is complex; in many patients with hypercellular marrows, pancytopenia is probably the result, at least in part, of physical replacement of normal marrow precursors by leukemic cells. Some patients with acute leukemia develop pancytopenia with a hypocellular marrow, however, suggesting that marrow failure is not simply due to physical replacement of the marrow space but also may be due to substances released by the malignant cells.

CLASSIFICATION

The acute leukemias can be classified in a variety of ways, including morphology, cytochemistry, cell-surface markers, cytoplasmic markers, cytogenetics, and oncogene expression. The most important distinction is between AML and ALL, since these two diseases differ considerably in their clinical behavior, prognosis, and response to therapy. Within the various subgroups of AML or ALL, there are also some important differences. A summary of the major subtypes of acute leukemia is provided in Table 145–1.

Morphology

Leukemic cells in AML typically are 12 to 20 μm in diameter, with discrete nuclear chromatin, multiple nucleoli, and cytoplasm that usually contains azurophilic granules. Auer rods, which are slender, fusiform cytoplasmic inclusions that stain red with Wright-Giemsa Stain, are virtually pathognomonic of AML. The French-American-British (FAB) collaborative group has subdivided AML into eight subtypes based on morphology and histochemistry (Table 145–1). M0, M1, M2, and M3 reflect increasing degrees of differentiation of myeloid leukemic cells. M4 and M5 leukemias have features of the monocytic lineage, M6 has features of the erythroid cell lineage, and M7 is acute megakaryocytic leukemia (see Color Plates 7K and L and 8A).

The leukemic cells in ALL tend to be smaller than AML blasts and relatively devoid of granules. Acute lymphocytic leukemia can be divided, using FAB criteria, into L1, L2, and L3 subgroups. L1 blasts are uniform in size, with homogeneous nuclear chromatin, indistinct nucleoli, and scanty cytoplasm with few, if any, granules. L2 blasts are larger and more variable in size and may have nucleoli. L3 blasts are quite distinct, with prominent nucleoli and deeply basophilic cytoplasm with vacuoles (see Color Plate 8B and C).

Cell-Surface Markers

Monoclonal antibodies reactive with cell-surface antigens have been used to classify acute leukemias. Antibodies that react with antigens found on normal immature myeloid cells, including CD13, CD14, CD33, and CD34, also react with blast cells from most patients with AML. Exceptions are the M6 and M7 variants, which have antigens restricted to the red cell and platelet lineages, respectively. Myeloid leukemia blasts also express Ia antigens but usually lack T cell, B cell, and other lymphoid antigens. In 10 to 20 per cent of patients, however, the leukemic cells have characteristics of both myeloid and lymphoid cells. Such cases are termed "hybrid" leukemias. Although sometimes useful in discriminating myeloid from lymphoid leukemias and in defining M6 and M7 variants, cell-surface markers do not have other clearly defined, important clinical correlations in AML.

Acute lymphocytic leukemia can be divided into several forms based on cell-surface antigen expression. Approximately 60 per cent of cases of ALL express the common ALL antigen, or CALLA, on the cell surface. CALLA (CD10) is a glycoprotein also found on occasional normal early lymphocytes and other nonhematopoietic tissues. CALLA-positive ALL's are felt to represent a very early B cell differentiative state. About 20 per cent of CALLA-positive ALL's have intracytoplasmic immunoglobulin and are termed pre–B cell ALL. B cell ALL is signified by the presence of immunoglobulin on the cell surface and accounts for fewer than 5 per cent of cases of ALL. About 20 per cent of cases of ALL are of the T cell phenotype, expressing antigens found on normal early T cells, such as CD5, CD3, or CD2. Approximately 15 per cent of cases of ALL fail to express CALLA, B, or T cell markers and are termed null cell ALL. Leukemic cells in about 25 per cent of patients with ALL also express myeloid antigens.

Cytoplasmic Markers

Of the cytoplasmic markers identified, only one is commonly used clinically, deoxynucleotidyl transferase (TdT), a nuclear enzyme that is not found on normal mature myeloid or lymphoid cells. In more than 90 per cent of cases of ALL, however, the lymphoblasts contain large amounts of the enzyme. Only 4 per cent of cases of AML stain positively for TdT. Other cytoplasmic enzymes of occasional relevance include adenosine deaminase, which is elevated in T cell ALL; 5-nucleosidase, which is low in T cell ALL; and lysozyme, which is produced by monocytic leukemia cells.

Cytogenetics

In most cases of acute leukemia, there is a numerical or structural chromosomal abnormality within the leukemic cell population. The simplest chromosomal change is a gain or loss of a whole chromosome. Other common structural changes include translocations, which involve the exchange of material between two chromosomes; deletions, in which part of a chromosome is lost; or inversions, in which a single chromosome is broken in two places and the middle piece is inverted and rejoined. When

TABLE 145–1. CLASSIFICATION OF ACUTE LEUKEMIAS

| Subtype | Morphology | Histochemistry | | | Monoclonal Reactivity | Cytogenetic Abnormalities |
		Myeloperoxidase	Nonspecific Esterase	PAS		
M0, Acute undifferentiated leukemia	Uniform, very undifferentiated	−	−	−	For subtypes M0–M5b, approximately 90% of cases will react with at least one of the following antimyeloid antibodies: Anti-CD13 Anti-CD14 Anti-CD33 Anti-CD34	Various
M1, Acute myeloid leukemia with minimal differentiation	Very undifferentiated, few azurophilic granules	+/−	+/−	−		Various
M2, Acute myeloid leukemia with differentiation	Granulated blasts predominate; Auer rods may be seen	+++	+/−	+		Various
M3, Acute promyelocytic leukemia	Hypergranular promyelocytes predominate	+++	+	+		t(15;17)
M4, Acute myelomonocytic leukemia M4E	Both monoblasts and myeloblasts present; like M4 but with eosinophils	++	+++	++		Various inv/del(16)
M5, Acute monocytic leukemia M5a M5b	Monoblasts predominate type a >80% monoblasts type b >20% promonocytes	+/−	+++	++		t(9;11)
M6, Acute erythroleukemia	Erythroblasts and megaloblastic red cell precursors seen	−	−	++	Antiglycophorin, antispectrin	Various
M7, Acute megakaryocytic leukemia	Undifferentiated blasts	−	+/−	+	Antiplatelet GpIIb/IIIa	Various
L1, Acute lymphoid leukemia Childhood variant	Small, uniform blasts, nucleoli indistinct	−	−	+++	65% react with anti-CD10 (anti-CALLA)	Various
L2, Acute lymphoid leukemia Adult variant	Larger, more irregular nucleoli present	−	−	++	20% react with anti-CD5, 3, or 2 (anti–T cell)	Various
L3, Burkitt-like acute lymphoid leukemia	Large with strongly basophilic cytoplasm and vacuoles	−	−	−	Antisurface immunoglobulin, anti-CD19, anti-CD20	t(8;14)

PAS = periodic acid–Schiff.

patients with acute leukemia and a chromosomal abnormality are treated and enter a complete remission, the chromosomal abnormality disappears, but it reappears when patients relapse.

In more than 80 per cent of cases of AML, a clonal chromosomal abnormality is found. The most frequent changes are a gain of chromosome 8 or loss of part or all of chromosome 7 or 5. These abnormalities are each seen in approximately 7 to 12 per cent of cases of AML and are not associated either with a particular subtype of AML or with a particularly good or bad prognosis. Other chromosomal abnormalities are associated with specific syndromes of AML. Acute promyelocytic leukemia virtually always has a translocation involving chromosomes 15 and 17 [(t(15;17)]. Acute myelomonocytic (M4) leukemia with abnormal eosinophilia is associated with an inversion in chromosome 16. Patients with M2 AML who have t(8;21) have a particularly good outcome with chemotherapy.

Between 15 and 20 per cent of adults with ALL have a Philadelphia (Ph) chromosome [t(9;22)]; the precise breakpoint of the translocation in ALL differs from that in CML. The other two most common changes in ALL are t(4;11), an abnormality seen mostly in neonatal ALL, and t(8;14), an abnormality associated with the L3 variant of ALL. The leukemic cells in about 20 per cent of patients with ALL have a propensity to gain many chromosomes, often reaching an average of 50 to 60 chromosomes per cell. Patients with such hyperdiploid leukemias tend to respond well to chemotherapy.

Oncogenes (Ch. 157)

It is generally believed that the above-mentioned abnormalities in chromosomal structure are important in the development of leukemia, either by altering the expression of a normal gene (a proto-oncogene) necessary for cell growth and development or by causing the loss or inactivation of certain "tumor suppressor genes" (anti-oncogenes). To date, the specific changes caused by these chromosomal abnormalities have not been identified, but it is known that the abl proto-oncogene is affected in the t(9;22) translocation, while the myc proto-oncogene is altered with t(8;14). Approximately 25 per cent of AML samples and 10 per cent of ALL cases exhibit point mutations in the N-ras oncogene.

CLINICAL MANIFESTATIONS

The signs and symptoms of acute leukemia result from decreased normal marrow function and invasion of normal organs by leukemic blasts. Anemia is present at diagnosis in most patients, causing fatigue, pallor, and headache and, in predisposed patients, angina or heart failure. Thrombocytopenia is usually present, and approximately one third of patients have clinically evident bleeding at diagnosis, usually in the form of petechiae, ecchymoses, bleeding gums, epistaxis, or hemorrhage. Most patients with acute leukemia are significantly granulocytopenic at diagnosis. As a result, approximately one third of patients with AML, and slightly fewer patients with ALL, have significant or life-threatening infections at presentation, most of which are bacterial in origin.

In addition to suppressing normal marrow function, leukemic cells can infiltrate normal organs. The prevalence and degree of organ infiltration differ between ALL and AML. In general, ALL tends to infiltrate normal organs more often than AML. Enlargement of lymph nodes, liver, and spleen is common at diagnosis. Bone pain, thought to result from leukemic infiltration of the periosteum or expansion of the medullary cavity, is a common complaint, particularly in children with ALL, many of whom are originally diagnosed as having juvenile rheumatoid arthritis. Leukemic cells may infiltrate the leptomeninges, causing leukemic meningitis. Signs of leukemic meningitis are headache and nausea. As the disease progresses, central nervous system palsies and seizures may develop. Although fewer than 5 per cent of patients have central nervous system involvement at diagnosis, the central nervous system is a frequent site of relapse, particularly with ALL, and because of the so-called blood-brain barrier, the central nervous system requires special therapy, as will be discussed. Testicular involvement is also seen in ALL and is a frequent site of relapse. In AML, collections of leukemic blast cells, often referred to as chloromas or myeloblastomas, can occur in virtually any soft tissue, presenting as rubbery, fast-growing masses.

Certain clinical manifestations are unique to specific subtypes of leukemia. Patients with acute promyelocytic leukemia (M3) commonly present with subclinical or clinically evident disseminated intravascular coagulation, caused by tissue thromboplastins present in the leukemic cells, which are released as the leukemic cells die. Acute monocytic or myelomonocytic leukemias are the forms of AML most likely to have extramedullary involvement. M6 leukemia often has a long prodromal phase. Patients with T cell ALL often have mediastinal masses.

LABORATORY MANIFESTATIONS

Abnormalities of peripheral blood counts are usually the initial laboratory evidence of acute leukemia. Anemia is present in most patients. Most are also at least mildly thrombocytopenic, and up to one quarter have severe thrombocytopenia (<20,000 per microliter). Although most patients are granulocytopenic at diagnosis, the total peripheral white cell count is more variable, with approximately 25 per cent of patients presenting with very high white cell counts (>50,000 per microliter), approximately 50 per cent presenting with white cell counts between 5000 and 50,000, and 25 per cent presenting with a low white cell count (<5000 per microliter). In most cases, blasts are present in the peripheral blood, although in some patients the percentage of blasts may be quite low, or blasts may be absent.

The diagnosis of acute leukemia is generally established by marrow aspiration and biopsy, usually from the posterior iliac crest. Marrow aspirates and biopsy specimens are usually hypercellular and contain 30 to 100 per cent blast cells, which largely replace the normal marrow. Occasionally, in addition to the blast cell infiltrate, other findings are present, including marrow fibrosis (especially with M7 AML) or bone marrow necrosis.

Other laboratory abnormalities often seen are hyperuricemia, especially in ALL, and increased serum lactate dehydrogenase (LDH). Increased serum or urinary levels of muramidase, a hydrolytic enzyme present in the primary granules of primitive granulocytes and especially monocytes, are sometimes seen with M4 and M5 AML. Rarely, lactic acidosis may complicate acute leukemia, especially in patients with extreme hyperleukocytosis and L3 ALL.

DIFFERENTIAL DIAGNOSIS

The diagnosis of acute leukemia is usually straightforward but occasionally can be more difficult. Leukemia and aplastic anemia can both manifest with peripheral pancytopenia, but the finding of a hypoplastic marrow without blasts usually distinguishes aplastic anemia. Occasionally, a patient may present with a hypocellular marrow and a clonal cytogenetic abnormality, which establishes the diagnosis of myelodysplasia or hypocellular leukemia. A number of processes other than leukemia can lead to the appearance of immature cells in the peripheral blood. Although other small round cell neoplasms can infiltrate the marrow and sometimes mimic leukemia, immunologic markers are effective in differentiating between the two. Leukemoid reactions to infections such as tuberculosis can result in the outpouring of large numbers of young myeloid cells, but virtually never does the percentage of blasts in marrow or peripheral blood reach 30 per cent in a leukemoid reaction (Ch. 141). Infectious mononucleosis and other viral illnesses can sometimes resemble ALL, particularly when large numbers of atypical lymphocytes are present in the peripheral blood and when the disease is accompanied by immune thrombocytopenia or hemolytic anemia.

TREATMENT

With the development of effective programs of combination chemotherapy and advances in marrow transplantation, many

patients with acute leukemia can be cured. These therapies are complex and therefore are best carried out at centers with appropriate support services and experience in treating leukemia. Because leukemia is a rapidly progressive disease, specific antileukemic therapy should be started as soon after diagnosis as possible, usually within 48 hours. Before starting therapy, hemorrhage and infection should be brought under control, if possible. To prevent uric acid nephropathy, patients should be hydrated and placed on allopurinol, 100 to 200 mg given orally, three times per day. The diagnosis of leukemia usually comes as a profound psychological shock to the patient and family. In addition to stabilizing the patient hematologically and metabolically, therefore, it is worthwhile having at least one formalized conference before treatment is initiated in which the patient and the family are advised about the meaning of the diagnosis of leukemia and the consequences of therapy.

Management of Emergencies

Patients sometimes present with treatable emergencies that require immediate attention before specific antileukemic therapy is begun. Severe bleeding usually results from thrombocytopenia, which can be reversed with platelet transfusions. Once thrombocytopenic bleeding is stopped, continued prophylactic transfusions of platelets to maintain the platelet count above 20,000 per microliter are warranted. Occasionally, patients also have evidence of disseminated intravascular coagulation (DIC), usually associated with the diagnosis of M3 AML. If active bleeding is due to DIC, the use of low doses of heparin (50 units per kilogram) given intravenously every 6 hours can often be of benefit. Whether heparin should be given prophylactically to patients with laboratory evidence of DIC but no active bleeding is an often debated, but unsettled, question. Patients who present with fever and granulocytopenia should have cultures, but infection should be assumed, and broad-spectrum antibiotics should be begun empirically. It is preferable to bring an infection under control before starting initial chemotherapy if the patient has an adequate granulocyte count. Patients often present with infection and essentially no granulocytes, and delaying chemotherapy in such patients is unlikely to be of benefit. Patients with very high blast counts (>150,000 per microliter) may develop symptoms attributable to the effect of masses of these immature cells on blood flow. The leukostasis may evolve into vascular injury and local hemorrhage. If this situation occurs in the central nervous system, the outcome may be fatal. Leukapheresis, immediate whole-brain irradiation (600 cGy in one dose), and administration of hydroxyurea, 3 grams per square meter given orally for 2 or 3 days, can usually prevent this complication. Patients with very high white cell counts may also present with uremia and anuria secondary to greatly increased serum uric acid levels, with subsequent intratubular crystallization. Rehydration, urine alkalinization with acetazolamide (500 mg per day), and prevention of uric acid production with allopurinol may lead to improved renal function. If patients do not respond and remain uremic, dialysis should be begun before instituting chemotherapy.

Treatment of ALL

After patients have been stabilized, antileukemic therapy should be started as soon as possible. Initial therapy for ALL can be divided into three phases: remission induction, postremission therapy, and central nervous system prophylaxis.

REMISSION INDUCTION. The initial goal of treatment is to induce a complete remission, which is usually defined as the reduction of leukemic blasts to undetectable levels and restoration of normal marrow function. A number of different chemotherapeutic combinations can be used to induce remission; all include vincristine and prednisone, and most add L-asparaginase and/or daunorubicin, administered over 3 to 4 weeks. With such regimens, 90 per cent of children and 75 per cent of adults achieve complete remission. Since vincristine, prednisone, and L-asparaginase are relatively nontoxic to normal marrow precursors, patients often enter complete remission after a relatively brief period of myelosuppression. Failure to achieve complete remission is usually due either to resistance of the leukemic cells to the drugs used or to progressive infection. These two complications occur with approximately equal frequency.

POSTREMISSION CHEMOTHERAPY. If no further therapy is given after induction of complete remission, virtually all patients relapse, most within several months. This fact demonstrates the need for further postremission therapy. Chemotherapy after complete remission can be given in a variety of combinations, dosages, and schedules. The term "consolidation chemotherapy" generally refers to short courses of further chemotherapy given at doses similar to those used for initial induction and thus requiring rehospitalization. Attempts are usually made to select drugs for consolidation that were not used in inducing the initial remission. In the case of ALL, such drugs include high-dose methotrexate, cyclophosphamide, and cytarabine, among others. "Maintenance" involves the administration of low-dose chemotherapy on a daily or weekly outpatient basis for long periods. The most commonly used maintenance regimens in ALL are daily 6-mercaptopurine and weekly or biweekly methotrexate. The optimal duration of maintenance chemotherapy is unknown, but maintenance is usually given for 2 to 3 years. Optimal chemotherapy for ALL requires both consolidation and maintenance chemotherapy.

CENTRAL NERVOUS SYSTEM PROPHYLAXIS. Most chemotherapeutic agents, when given intravenously or orally, do not penetrate the central nervous system well, making the central nervous system a common site of relapse unless specific measures are taken. Effective regimens for central nervous system prophylaxis include the use of intrathecal methotrexate alone, intrathecal methotrexate combined with 2400 cGy to the cranium, or 2400 cGy to the craniospinal axis.

PROGNOSIS AFTER INITIAL CHEMOTHERAPY. A number of factors are predictive of outcome in ALL, the two most consistent of which are age and white cell count at diagnosis. With currently available treatment regimens, 50 to 70 per cent of children and 25 to 45 per cent of adults who achieve a complete remission remain in complete remission for longer than 5 years and thus are probably cured of their disease. In both children and adults, a low white cell count at diagnosis predicts a favorable outcome, while a high white cell count at diagnosis does the reverse. Specific syndromes of ALL with a poor prognosis include the L3 variant of ALL or the presence of the Philadelphia chromosome or the t(4;11) chromosomal abnormality.

TREATMENT OF RELAPSED ALL. Most relapses occur within 2 years of diagnosis, and most occur in the marrow. Occasionally, a relapse may first be found in an extramedullary site, such as the central nervous system or testes. Extramedullary relapse is usually followed shortly by systemic (marrow) relapse and so should be considered part of a systemic recurrence. With the use of chemotherapeutic regimens similar to those used for initial induction, 50 to 70 per cent of patients achieve at least short-lived second remissions. A small percentage of patients whose first remission was longer than 2 years may be cured with salvage chemotherapy. If the central nervous system or testes were the initial site of the relapse, specific therapy to that site is also required along with systemic retreatment. Since the prognosis of relapsed leukemia treated with chemotherapy is so poor, marrow transplantation is now generally recommended in this setting.

MARROW TRANSPLANTATION (Ch. 153). The use of high-dose chemoradiotherapy followed by marrow transplantation from a human leukocyte antigen (HLA)–identical sibling can cure 20 to 40 per cent of patients with ALL who fail to achieve an initial remission or who relapse after an initial complete remission. The major limitations of transplantation are graft-versus-host disease, interstitial pneumonia, and disease recurrence. If an HLA-identical sibling is not available, alternative sources of marrow are from a partially matched family member; from an HLA-matched unrelated donor; or autologous marrow that has been removed during remission, treated in vitro to remove contaminating tumor cells, and then subsequently stored. The outcome of transplantation using either autologous marrow or alternative sources of marrow has not been as favorable as that using matched allogeneic family member donors.

Treatment of AML

REMISSION INDUCTION. Treatment with a combination of daunomycin and cytarabine leads to complete remission in 60 to 80 per cent of patients with AML. Profound myelosuppression always follows when these agents are used at doses capable of achieving complete remission. Failure to achieve complete remission is usually due either to drug resistance or to fatal complications of myelosuppression.

POSTREMISSION THERAPY. Intensive consolidation chemotherapy using repeated courses of daunomycin and cytarabine at conventional doses, high-dose cytarabine, or other agents prolongs the average remission duration and improves the chances for long-term disease-free survival. Unlike the situation in ALL, low-dose maintenance therapy is of no benefit after intensive consolidation treatment. In AML, leukemic recurrence occurs less often in the central nervous system, being seen in only approximately 10 per cent of cases, most commonly in patients with M4 or M5 variants. There is no evidence that central nervous system prophylaxis improves overall disease-free survival in AML.

PROGNOSIS AFTER INITIAL CHEMOTHERAPY. Among those patients who achieve complete remission, 15 to 30 per cent remain alive in continuous complete remission for more than 5 years, suggesting probable cure. As with ALL, younger patients and those with a low white cell count at diagnosis have a more favorable outcome. Patients whose disease is characterized by certain chromosomal abnormalities, particularly t(8;21), t(15;17), and inv 16, do somewhat better, whereas those with t(4;11) and t(9;22) do worse. Patients who have a long preleukemic phase before their condition evolves into acute leukemia and those whose leukemia is secondary to prior exposure to alkylating agents or radiation respond poorly to chemotherapy.

TREATMENT OF RECURRENT AML. Patients whose AML recurs after initial chemotherapy can achieve second remission in about 50 per cent of cases following retreatment with daunomycin-cytarabine or high-dose cytarabine. Unfortunately, these remissions tend to be short lived, and few patients who relapse after first-line chemotherapy are cured by salvage chemotherapy.

BONE MARROW TRANSPLANTATION (Ch. 153). For patients with AML who fail to achieve an initial remission or who relapse after chemotherapy, marrow transplantation from an HLA-identical sibling offers the best chance for cure. If carried out when patients have end-stage disease, approximately 15 per cent of patients can be saved. If the procedure is applied earlier, the outcome with marrow transplantation improves, with approximately 30 per cent of patients transplanted at first relapse or second remission being cured, and with cure rates of 50 to 60 per cent if transplantation is carried out in the first remission. Several studies have prospectively compared the outcome of marrow transplantation with that of chemotherapy in patients with AML in first remission. The trend in all of these studies has been in favor of transplantation, although in not all the studies was there a statistically significant difference. Currently, transplantation is the treatment of choice for patients with AML who have suffered an initial relapse, and it should be strongly considered for most patients while in first remission. The major limitations to transplantation are graft-versus-host disease, interstitial pneumonia, and disease recurrence. Since the incidence of graft-versus-host disease increases with age, most centers limit transplantation to patients age 50 or less. Alternative sources of marrow include the use of partially matched family members, matched unrelated donors, and autologous transplantation. As with ALL, these alternative sources of marrow, while sometimes successful, do not yield results as good as those obtained using a matched family member.

Supportive Care

Treatment of acute leukemia, especially AML, is accompanied by a number of complications, the two most serious and frequent being infection and bleeding. During the granulocytopenic period following induction and consolidation chemotherapy, most patients become febrile, and in approximately 50 per cent of cases, a bacterial infection can be documented. The most commonly isolated organisms vary somewhat from medical center to medical center, but usually gram-positive organisms, such as *Staphylococcus epidermidis,* and gram-negative enteric organisms, such as *Pseudomonas aeruginosa, Escherichia coli,* and *Klebsiella aerobacter,* are the most commonly isolated bacteria. Even if no cause for fever is found, bacterial infection should be assumed, and in general, all patients with fever and neutropenia should begin receiving broad-spectrum antibiotics. Commonly used antibiotic combinations include a cephalosporin and a semisynthetic penicillin or a semisynthetic penicillin and an aminoglycoside. Once begun, antibiotics should be continued until patients recover their granulocyte count, even if the patients become afebrile first. If documented bacterial infections persist despite appropriate antibiotics, removal of indwelling catheters and granulocyte transfusions should be considered. It may be possible to reduce the incidence of bacterial infection through the use of selective gastrointestinal decontamination, using, for example, ciprofloxacin or a combination of trimethoprim-sulfamethoxazole plus colistin. The use of protective environments can also reduce the incidence of infection, but it is costly and has not been shown to influence overall survival.

Frequently, patients on broad-spectrum antibiotics become afebrile for a time, only to develop a second fever. Such patients should be carefully reassessed with a high index of suspicion for fungal infection. Granulocytopenic patients who remain febrile for more than a week on broad-spectrum antibiotics should be treated empirically with amphotericin for presumed fungal infection.

In addition to being granulocytopenic, patients undergoing induction chemotherapy for leukemia have deficient cellular and humoral immunity, at least temporarily, and so are subject to those infections common in other immunodeficiency states, including *Pneumocystis carinii* infection and a variety of viral infections. *Pneumocystis carinii* infection can be prevented by prophylactic use of trimethoprim-sulfamethoxazole. Cytomegalovirus (CMV) infection can be prevented in the CMV-seronegative patient by the sole use of CMV-seronegative blood products. Herpes simplex can often complicate existing mucositis and can be treated successfully with acyclovir. Acyclovir is also useful for the treatment of disseminated varicella zoster.

Platelet transfusions from random donors often suffice to maintain platelet counts above 20,000 per microliter. In 30 to 50 per cent of cases, however, patients eventually become alloimmunized and require the use of HLA-matched platelets. Occasionally, cells (presumably T cells) within the blood product can engraft in the immunosuppressed leukemic patient and cause a graft-versus-host reaction. Transfusion-induced graft-versus-host disease manifests with a rash, low-grade fever, elevated values in liver function tests, and falling blood counts. This syndrome can be prevented by irradiating all blood products with at least 1500 cGy before transfusion.

Appelbaum FR, Fisher LD, Thomas ED, et al.: Chemotherapy and marrow transplantation for adults with acute nonlymphocytic leukemia: A five-year follow-up. Blood 72:179, 1988. *A comparison of the outcome of marrow transplantation with that of continued chemotherapy for adults with AML.*

Bennett JM, Catovsky D, Daniel MT, et al.: Proposed revised criteria for the classification of acute myeloid leukemia. Ann Intern Med 103:626, 1985. *An update of the French-American-British (FAB) classification of acute leukemia.*

Champlin R, Gale RP: Acute myelogenous leukemia: Recent advances in therapy. Blood 69:1551, 1987. *Very good review of therapy for AML with an excellent bibliography.*

Champlin R, Gale RP: Acute lymphoblastic leukemia: Recent advances in biology and therapy. Blood 73:2051, 1989. *Like above reference, but this time directed at ALL.*

Cheson BD, Cassileth PA, Head DR, et al.: Report of the National Cancer Institute–sponsored workshop on definitions of diagnosis and response in acute myeloid leukemia. J Clin Oncol 8:813, 1990. *A report of the recently adopted NCI definitions of diagnostic and response criteria for AML.*

Clarkson B, Ellis S, Little C, et al.: Acute lymphoblastic leukemia in adults. Semin Oncol 12:160, 1985. *A review of chemotherapy for adult ALL centering on the Sloan-Kettering experience.*

Mayer RJ: Current chemotherapeutic treatment approaches to the management of previously untreated adults with de novo acute myelogenous leukemia. Semin Oncol 14:384, 1987. *A comprehensive, balanced review of chemotherapy for adult AML.*

Rowley JD: Recurring chromosome abnormalities in leukemia and lymphoma. Semin Hematol 27:122, 1990. *Updated review of the chromosomal abnormalities seen in the hematologic malignancies.*

146 Introduction to Neoplasms of the Immune System

Carol S. Portlock

Neoplasms of the immune system are a heterogeneous group of tumors whose cells of origin may be the lymphocyte, the histiocyte, or other cell components of the immune system. Each neoplasm is thought to be a monoclonal expansion of malignant cells, although this has only been conclusively demonstrated for lymphocytic tumors. It is interesting that these neoplasms often retain many morphologic, functional, and migratory characteristics common to their normal cell counterparts.

With increasing understanding of the normal immune system, it has become possible to classify many malignant immune disorders according to their cell of origin. Monoclonal antibodies to cell-surface antigens permit the identification of B or T lymphocyte proliferations. By such immunophenotyping, malignant lymphocytic neoplasms can be related to stages of normal B or T lymphocyte development and maturation. Table 146–1 lists these diseases according to their normal cell lineage counterpart.

Establishing clonality of a B lymphocyte proliferation is usually accomplished by the demonstration of a single class of heavy-and/or light-chain cell-surface immunoglobulin. At the DNA level, clonality can be confirmed by the presence of a single immunoglobulin gene rearrangement. In precursor B lymphocyte neoplasms where surface immunoglobulin is not present, gene rearrangement studies are necessary to demonstrate clonality.

For T lymphocyte proliferations, clonality can be conclusively shown only by T lymphocyte receptor gene rearrangement studies. Studies of cell-surface antigens alone are not sufficient. Clonal lymphocyte proliferations are not always malignant, as exemplified by the chronic monoclonal T lymphocyte disorder of lymphomatoid papulosis.

Tumors of histiocytic lineage have not yet been shown to be monoclonal. These cells lack endogenous immunoglobulin but may acquire exogenous immunoglobulin on their cell surface. They may be rich in lysozyme or muramidase, and as phagocytic cells, they can be shown to ingest latex particles or sensitized erythrocytes. The cell lineage of the Reed-Sternberg cell in Hodgkin's disease is not known with certainty. It has in vitro characteristics in common with both histiocytes and lymphocytes. Recent molecular studies demonstrating immunoglobulin gene rearrangement and the presence of *bcl-2* oncogene suggest a B lymphocyte origin.

TABLE 146–1. LYMPHOMAS AS NEOPLASMS OF THE IMMUNE SYSTEM

Cell of Origin	Neoplasm
I. B cell	
Medullary B cell	Chronic lymphocytic leukemia, diffuse small lymphocytic lymphoma
Follicular B cell	Follicular lymphomas, diffuse mixed lymphoma, diffuse large cell lymphoma, Burkitt's lymphoma
Immunoblastic B cell	Diffuse immunoblastic lymphoma
II. T cell	
Thymic T cell	Lymphoblastic lymphoma
Mature T cell	Peripheral T cell lymphomas, chronic lymphocytic leukemia (rare), HTLV-I–associated lymphoma, mycosis fungoides, Sézary's syndrome
Immunoblastic T cell	Diffuse immunoblastic lymphoma
III. Histiocytic	
Histiocyte	Malignant histiocytosis, true histiocytic lymphoma (rare)
IV. Unknown	Hodgkin's disease

In addition to a specific immunotype and genotype, chromosomal abnormalities can be detected in the majority of immune system neoplasms. In many, the recurring karyotypic abnormality appears to be specific. Among B lymphocyte lymphomas, these abnormalities most often include translocations involving chromosome 14 q 32 (the heavy-chain immunoglobulin gene locus) and the cellular oncogenes c-myc (chromosome 8), bcl-1 (chromosome 11), or bcl-2 (chromosome 18). The 14;18 and 11;14 translocations are primarily associated with follicular lymphomas and t8;14 with Burkitt's lymphoma. Similarly, specific translocations of the T lymphocyte receptor gene loci appear to be involved in the recurring karyotypic changes identified among T-cell lymphocyte lymphomas. These include chromosome 14 q 11 (lymphocyte receptor alpha- and delta-chain genes) or chromosome 7 q 34–36 or chromosome 7 p 15 (T lymphocyte receptor beta- and gamma-chain genes). The presumed oncogene translocation partner is yet to be identified for the majority of T lymphocyte neoplasms. No specific chromosomal changes have been identified thus far in Hodgkin's disease. Reed-Sternberg cells are difficult to isolate, are few in number, and have complex hyperdiploid karyotypes. Another marker that appears to be specific is the presence of antibodies to the human retrovirus HTLV-1 (human T cell leukemia/lymphoma virus) found in patients with adult T cell leukemia/lymphoma. These and other in vitro methods may provide additional information for defining prognostically important patient subsets.

Each neoplasm of the immune system is a distinct clinicopathologic entity. However, these disorders tend to share some common clinical features. For example, systemic symptoms of fever, night sweats, and weight loss may be present and tend to correlate with advanced stage of disease. The neoplasm usually arises in one or more organs of the hematopoietic system (lymph nodes, spleen, liver, bone marrow), and if untreated or ineffectively treated, it tends to disseminate to all those organs, as well as to other sites. Bone marrow involvement with or without peripheral blood manifestation is common in certain disorders and may be the predominant feature. Meningeal infiltration is often present when aggressive neoplasms involve the bone marrow.

PATHOLOGY AND CLASSIFICATION

Neoplasms of B or T lymphocytic lineage are termed non-Hodgkin's lymphomas. They are a diverse group of diseases with varying clinical presentations, responses to therapy, and prognoses. The Rappaport histopathologic classification of non-Hodgkin's lymphomas (Table 146–2) has been used successfully in clinical trials and practice. It has permitted the identification of specific clinicopathologic entities and of favorable and unfavorable

TABLE 146–2. CLASSIFICATION OF NON-HODGKIN'S LYMPHOMAS

NCI Working Formulation (1982)	Rappaport Classification (1966)
Low-grade	
Small lymphocytic (SLL)	Diffuse lymphocytic, well differentiated (DLWD)
Follicular, small cleaved cell (FSCL)	Nodular lymphocytic, poorly differentiated (NLPD)
Follicular, mixed small cleaved and large cell (FML)	Nodular mixed lymphocytic-histiocytic (NML)
Intermediate-grade	
Follicular, large cell (FLCL)	Nodular histiocytic (NHL)
Diffuse, small cleaved cell (DSCL)	Diffuse lymphocytic, poorly differentiated (DLPD)
Diffuse, mixed small cleaved and large cell (DML)	Diffuse, mixed lymphocytic-histiocytic (DML)
Diffuse, large cell (cleaved and noncleaved) (DLCL)	Diffuse histiocytic (DHL)
High-grade	
Large cell immunoblastic (IBL)	Diffuse histiocytic (DHL)
Lymphoblastic (convoluted and nonconvoluted) (LL)	
Small noncleaved cell (Burkitt and non-Burkitt) (SNCL)	Diffuse undifferentiated (DUL)

prognostic groups since 1956. Nevertheless, the Rappaport classification, based exclusively upon morphologic concepts, does not take into account recent information regarding the immune system. For example, the term "histiocytic" lymphoma is generally incorrect because virtually all non-Hodgkin's lymphomas are of lymphocytic origin.

Table 146–2 juxtaposes a more recent National Cancer Institute Working Formulation with the Rappaport classification. Tumor architecture is an important feature in both: Rappaport's "nodular" is replaced by the more immunologically accurate term "follicular." Cell morphology is more descriptive in the Working Formulation, and "histiocytic" is replaced by "large cell." Prognostically favorable and unfavorable groups are termed low, intermediate, and high grade. The low-grade category includes small lymphocytic consistent with chronic lymphocytic leukemia; a miscellaneous category includes mycosis fungoides and true histiocytic lymphoma.

Many non-Hodgkin's lymphomas may exhibit two distinct histologic subtypes. Both the architecture and the cell type may change, usually evolving from a low-grade lymphoma to an intermediate- or high-grade lymphoma. Rarely, two histologic subtypes may be present at diagnosis in the same lymph node (composite lymphoma). More often, two histologic subtypes may be seen at diagnosis in two separate biopsy specimens; most frequently, one is seen at diagnosis and a second at relapse or autopsy. It is thought that such "transformation" represents clonal expansion of a more aggressive cell line. Its clinical importance is that both therapy and prognosis may be dramatically altered by its emergence.

In contrast to non-Hodgkin's lymphomas, the diagnostic malignant cells (Reed-Sternberg cells) of Hodgkin's disease appear similar in all four histologic subtypes of the neoplasm. Instead, distinguishing pathologic features include the number of Reed-Sternberg cells and the composition of normal background cells and stroma. The pathologic classification of Hodgkin's disease is fully discussed in Ch. 148.

DIAGNOSIS AND STAGING

The diagnosis of a neoplasm of the immune system is based upon pathologic classification of biopsy material. This classification requires adequate tissue (preferably lymph node, so that both architecture and cell type may be assessed), proper handling, and excellent hematopathologic interpretation. Special studies, such as imprints, immunotyping, gene rearrangement, karyotyping, deoxynucleotidyl transferase (TdT) determination, and electron microscopy, may provide additional information for classification. Since these latter studies require fresh tissue and special handling, it is important that the pathologist be involved *before* biopsy. Similarly, it is important that each case be evaluated jointly by a medical oncologist, radiation therapist, surgeon, and radiologist from the outset.

With the diagnosis established, the extent of disease should be completely defined. Since each neoplasm has distinct clinicopathologic features, the choice of staging studies will be based on that information. All patients should have a complete history, particularly assessing the presence or absence of systemic symptoms, and physical examination. All nodal areas should be examined, including Waldeyer's ring and preauricular, epitrochlear, and popliteal lymph nodes. In addition to liver and spleen, epigastric or other abdominal masses may be found. The lungs, skin, breasts, testicles, and central nervous system should be carefully examined for extranodal involvement. Blood counts and liver and renal function tests are necessary in all patients. In addition to chest radiography, computed tomography (CT) may be indicated in an abnormal chest. Abdominal CT and lymphography are often complementary and not mutually exclusive. Gallium-67 scanning may be useful but is not a diagnostic method. Liver and spleen scans are of minimal value. Studies of bone or gastrointestinal tract should be performed when symptoms are present. However, with Waldeyer's ring involvement, associated upper gastrointestinal disease may be asymptomatic, and therefore it should be screened for routinely. Bone marrow biopsy is often indicated, particularly if advanced clinical disease is present or the patient has a low-grade lymphoma. Cerebrospinal fluid cytology should be determined in all patients with intermediate- and high-grade lymphomas who have bone marrow involvement and in all patients with Burkitt's lymphoma, lymphoblastic lymphoma, or malignant histiocytosis.

Several different staging systems are applied to neoplasms of the immune system. Their purpose is to define disease extent, to assist in treatment strategies, to evaluate therapeutic results, and to determine prognosis. In Hodgkin's disease the utility of staging has been elegantly demonstrated, and excellent clinical care demands careful clinical and often pathologic staging. Staging laparotomy with splenectomy and biopsy of liver, lymph nodes, and bone marrow was developed for adequate intra-abdominal assessment of Hodgkin's disease. It accurately identifies pathologic stage, and its results often dictate treatment strategy. The Ann Arbor staging system for Hodgkin's disease has also been applied to non-Hodgkin's lymphomas. In this setting it has less value in determining therapy but remains an important prognostic variable. Modified staging systems are used in pediatric lymphomas, chronic lymphocytic leukemia, Burkitt's and lymphoblastic lymphomas, and mycosis fungoides. Since pathologic intra-abdominal assessment is rarely needed to determine treatment in non-Hodgkin's lymphomas, staging laparotomy is usually unnecessary. Nonetheless, careful clinical staging is imperative in all cases.

DIFFERENTIAL DIAGNOSIS

The differential diagnosis of neoplasms of the immune system is usually that of lymphadenopathy. Reactive processes, infections, other malignant tumors, and collagen vascular disorders may all cause enlarged lymph nodes or hepatosplenomegaly or both. The location or locations of the lymph nodes, their size, shape, consistency, rapidity of onset, and other characteristics may aid in determining etiology.

Regional lymph node hyperplasia may be seen with acute or chronic infections of the extremities and with vaccinations or insect bites. Diffuse lymphadenopathy may occur following ingestion of phenytoin. Other diffuse reactive processes, such as acquired immunodeficiency syndrome (AIDS) angioimmunoblastic lymphadenopathy, and collagen vascular disorders, may be associated with an increased likelihood of developing lymphoma. Consequently, a single lymph node biopsy may not solve the diagnostic dilemma. That is why pathologic consultation before biopsy is recommended.

Among infectious etiologic factors, viral illnesses predominate and often produce bizarre pathologic material. Infectious mononucleosis may present with features common to Hodgkin's disease. Cytomegalovirus, cat-scratch disease, toxoplasmosis, tuberculosis, syphilis, and sarcoidosis are other considerations. Other malignant neoplasms usually involve lymph nodes by regional spread. For example, cervical lymphadenopathy may be the first symptom of a malignant tumor involving the oropharynx or nasopharynx. Similarly, breast cancer may manifest with axillary adenopathy and a microscopic primary tumor.

In virtually all instances, the only way to determine conclusively the cause of lymphadenopathy is by pathologic tissue examination. Low cervical and supraclavicular lymph nodes are more likely to yield diagnostic material than are axillary and inguinal nodes. When only intrathoracic or abdominal disease is present, bone marrow biopsy may provide diagnostic information and obviate surgery. Fine-needle aspiration is of lesser value in neoplasms of the immune system than in solid tumors, because cell morphology and architecture are both important diagnostic parameters.

Lippman ME, Yee D (eds.): The lymphomas: Current concepts in pathogenesis and management. J Natl Cancer Inst Monogr 10:1–82, 1990. *This monograph reviews basic science and clinical aspects of non-Hodgkin's lymphomas and Hodgkin's disease.*

Non-Hodgkin's lymphoma pathologic classification project. National Cancer Institute sponsored study of classifications of non-Hodgkin's lymphomas: Summary and description of a working formulation for clinical usage. Cancer 49:2112, 1982. *The Working Formulation is presented, and six pathologic classifications are compared.*

Simon R, Durrleman S, Hoppe RT, et al.: The non-Hodgkin's lymphoma pathologic classification project: Long-term follow up of 1153 patients with non-Hodgkin's lymphomas. Ann Intern Med 109:939, 1988. *A median follow-up of 11 years, again demonstrating the clinical relevance of the Working Formulation.*

147 Non-Hodgkin's Lymphomas
Carol S. Portlock

Non-Hodgkin's lymphomas are the single largest group of neoplasms of the immune system. Composed of more than 10 distinct disease entities, non-Hodgkin's lymphomas are best understood as a heterogeneous group of malignant diseases whose common link is a characteristic monoclonal expansion of malignant B or T cells.

EPIDEMIOLOGY

Non-Hodgkin's lymphomas may occur at any age, although they are rarely diagnosed during the first year of life. They occur with increasing frequency throughout adulthood. The incidence is estimated to be approximately 33,000 cases per year in the United States (1989), with males affected more often than females. Moreover, male predominance is most evident among young patients in association with the aggressive histologic subtypes of lymphoblastic and Burkitt's lymphomas.

Geographic clustering is characteristic of some non-Hodgkin's lymphomas: Burkitt's lymphoma in central Africa; adult T cell leukemia/lymphoma in southwestern Japan and the Caribbean; and small intestinal lymphoma with associated immunoglobulin disorders in the Middle East.

Preceding immune dysfunction has been associated with the development of aggressive non-Hodgkin's lymphomas. Congenital immunodeficiency states associated with lymphoma include severe combined immunodeficiency, ataxia-telangiectasia, Wiskott-Aldrich syndrome, X-linked lymphoproliferative syndrome, and common variable immunodeficiency (Ch. 244). Transplant recipients, patients with autoimmune states, and patients with AIDS (acquired immunodeficiency syndrome) also have increased risk of developing lymphoma.

ETIOLOGY AND PATHOGENESIS

The etiology of non-Hodgkin's lymphomas is unclear. Perhaps the best studied lymphoma is Burkitt's with which the Epstein-Barr virus (EBV) has been associated and for which specific chromosomal and oncogene translocations have been implicated in its pathogenesis.

Burkitt's lymphoma is the most common childhood malignant disorder in Uganda. The disease is found along a "lymphoma belt" lying approximately 10 degrees north and 10 degrees south of the African equator. Within the belt there are altitude, temperature, and rainfall restrictions; these climatic conditions are similar to those of Papua, New Guinea, where Burkitt's lymphoma is also commonly identified. Holoendemic or hyperendemic malaria follows the geographic distribution of the lymphoma belt and originally suggested to Burkitt a mosquito-borne vector and/or associated host immune dysfunction.

In addition to its geographic restrictions, endemic Burkitt's lymphoma is associated with time-space clustering. Nonendemic Burkitt's lymphoma, a similar disease occurring rarely and sporadically in other areas of the world (less than one case per million annually in the United States), has also been reported to occur in time-space clusters. Moreover, nonendemic Burkitt's lymphomas may be associated with preceding immune dysfunction (e.g., organ transplantation and AIDS).

The EBV is present in almost 90 per cent of African Burkitt's lymphoma but fewer than half of nonendemic cases. Whether the virus plays an etiologic role or is merely a passenger in Burkitt's lymphoma remains controversial. Typically, primary EBV infection precedes the development of Burkitt's lymphoma by at least 7 or more months. Ugandan children with high EBV capsid antigen titers have a 30-fold greater risk of developing Burkitt's lymphoma than do control subjects. Elevated EBV/VCA (viral capsid antigen) titers are also associated with a favorable prognosis in both African and nonendemic tumors.

Adult T cell leukemia/lymphoma (ATL), a rare and recently discovered disorder, is associated with a unique human retrovirus, HTLV-I (human T cell leukemia/lymphoma virus). This disease is endemic to southwestern Japan, where 12 to 15 per cent of normal persons have HTLV-I antibodies; it is also found in the Caribbean basin.

The specific chromosomal translocations seen in Burkitt's lymphoma have uniformly involved the *c-myc* oncogene on chromosome 8 and the immunoglobulin heavy- or light-chain genes on chromosomes 14, 2, or 22. These chromosomal translocations— t(8;14), t(8;2), and t(8;22)—deregulate the *myc* gene and result in the constitutive production of a DNA binding protein that appears to control aspects of gene expression or DNA replication. The biologic correlate of this molecular event is the finding of spontaneous B cell lymphomas in transgenic mice carrying DNA sequences from the 8;14 translocation breakpoint. Specific chromosomal translocations have also been reported in follicular lymphomas, involving chromosomes 11 and 14 or 18 and 14. The translocation site on chromosome 14 also involves the immunoglobulin heavy-chain locus and, by analogy, suggests that a transforming gene on chromosome 11 or 18 is activated when brought into proximity with this locus. These oncogenes, *bcl-1* (on chromosome 11) and *bcl-2* (on chromosome 18), have been identified and cloned.

In addition to the etiologic considerations of oncogenic viruses and oncogene transformation, other factors that have been associated with an increased incidence of lymphoma include ionizing radiation (whole-body dose greater than 100 cGy), hereditary predisposition, congenital or acquired immunodeficiency, and exposure to pesticides.

PATHOLOGY AND CLINICAL FEATURES

Many different pathologic classifications have been proposed for non-Hodgkin's lymphomas (Ch. 146). Rappaport's classification (see Table 147–2) has been the most successfully utilized and applied in clinical trials, while that of Lukes and Collins is more immunologically correct, classifying diseases based on their cell of origin. The National Cancer Institute Working Formulation (1982) is being increasingly accepted, since it is proving both clinically useful and immunologically correct.

Pathologic interpretation of non-Hodgkin's lymphomas can be supplemented with a variety of complementary studies. Immunophenotyping may identify the cell of origin by demonstrating B cell monoclonal surface immunoglobulin, T cell sheep erythrocyte rosettes (E rosettes), and B or T cell differentiation antigens. Clonality may also be ascertained by detection of the rearrangement of the B cell immunoglobulin genes or of the T cell receptor gene loci. Moreover, the karyotype may reveal a specific chromosomal translocation. The presence of antibody against HTLV-I suggests a T cell lymphoma, whereas human immunodeficiency virus (HIV) antibody suggests an aggressive B cell neoplasm (see Color Plate 8E).

Each disease entity of the Working Formulation has a distinct clinical presentation and prognosis, as noted below. The pathologic appearance and some of the clinical characteristics of each category, as outlined in the Working Formulation, are listed in Tables 147–1 and 147–2.

LOW GRADE (see Color Plate 8D, left). The low-grade lymphomas (small lymphocytic [SLL]; follicular, predominantly small cleaved cell [FSCL]; and follicular, mixed, small cleaved and large cell [FML]) have several clinical characteristics in common: (1) Each has a history of waxing and waning or of slowly progressive adenopathy. (2) These are rubbery, mobile lymph nodes that are rarely fixed and have no overlying skin infiltration; lymph nodes may be very bulky but are rarely painful. (3) Liver and spleen are frequently involved pathologically and may be enlarged; liver function tests are usually normal, although the alkaline phosphatase level may be mildly increased. (4) Bone marrow involvement is common; circulating lymphoma cells may be identified on smear or by cell-sorting techniques. (5) Blood counts are usually normal at diagnosis. Elevation of the white blood cell count with circulating cells, anemia with autoimmune hemolytic anemia, and cytopenias secondary to hypersplenism or bone marrow replacement are uncommon complications. (6) Other extranodal disease sites may include pleura, lung, skin, breast, and gastrointestinal tract. (7) Enlarged lymph nodes may cause lymphedema, ureteral obstruction, or epidural cord com-

pression. (8) Central nervous system (meningeal or parenchymal), renal, or testicular infiltration rarely occurs.

INTERMEDIATE GRADE AND HIGH GRADE (see Color Plate 8D, right). As a group, the intermediate (follicular, predominantly large cell [FLCL]; diffuse, small cleaved cell [DSCL]; diffuse, mixed small and large cell [DML]; and diffuse, large cell [DLCL]) and high-grade lymphomas (large cell immunoblastic [IBL]; lymphoblastic [LBL]; and small noncleaved cell, including Burkitt's lymphoma and diffuse and undifferentiated lymphoma, non-Burkitt's type [SNCL]) have several general clinical features in common: (1) There is a history of abrupt onset with rapidly enlarging lymph node masses. (2) Lymph nodes may be rubbery and mobile but may also be hard, fixed, and with overlying skin infiltration. Masses may be warm, erythematous, and painful. (3) Bulky lymph node masses (>10 cm) may be present in the mediastinum, retroperitoneum, and/or mesentery. (4) Waldeyer's ring may be involved and is often associated with extranodal disease of the stomach or small bowel or both. (5) Hepatosplenomegaly may be present, and liver function tests may be abnormal. Porta hepatis or even intrahepatic obstructive patterns may be seen. (6) Extranodal involvement is common: stomach, small bowel, lung, skin, bone, and central nervous system (particularly meningeal disease in association with bone marrow involvement). Rarely ovarian, testicular, or renal disease may be present. (7) Bone marrow involvement and circulating cells are less commonly seen at diagnosis than in low-grade lymphomas. A leukemic picture may emerge, however, when progressive disease develops. (8) Lymph node masses may cause lymphedema, ureteral obstruction, vascular obstruction (superior vena cava syndrome, thrombophlebitis), and epidural cord compression.

MISCELLANEOUS. A miscellaneous category of the Working Formulation includes mycosis fungoides (see Color Plate 7J, right)—a rare helper T cell lymphoma of the skin; composite lymphoma—multiple histologic subtypes (e.g., FSCL and IBL) occurring simultaneously; and true histiocytic lymphoma.

Since the Formulation's publication in 1982, additional mature T cell lymphomas have been recognized. The peripheral T cell lymphomas are a diverse group of "postthymic" neoplasms, whose cell of origin is the differentiated T cell. Their morphology includes diffuse small cell, mixed cell, large cell, or immunoblastic lymphoma, as well as subgroups with histologic features of angioimmunoblastic lymphadenopathy, lymphomatoid granulomatosis, Hodgkin's-like disease, or Lennert's lymphoma. Clinical features include a 2:1 male predominance, prominent extranodal disease (particularly lung involvement) in the majority, systemic symptoms, and skin rash. In general, response to treatment and

TABLE 147–1. PATHOLOGIC CHARACTERISTICS OF NON-HODGKIN'S LYMPHOMAS

Subtype	Architectural Pattern	Malignant Lymphocyte Cytology	Immunophenotype/ Immunogenotype
SLL	Diffuse	Small round cells	B cell; rarely T cell
FSCL	Follicular	Small cleaved cells	B cell
FML	Follicular	Small cleaved cells admixed with large cells, cleaved or noncleaved	B cell
FLCL	Follicular	Large cells cleaved or noncleaved	B cell
DSCL	Diffuse	Small cleaved cells	B cell; occasionally T cell
DML	Diffuse	Admixture of small and large cells cleaved or noncleaved	B cell; T cell
DLCL	Diffuse	Large cells cleaved or noncleaved	B cell; T cell
IBL	Diffuse	Large cells; plasmacytoid, clear, or polymorphic cell variants	B cell; T cell
LBL	Diffuse "starry sky"	Lymphoblasts, convoluted or nonconvoluted nuclei	Thymic T cell
SNCL	Diffuse "starry sky"	Noncleaved cells, round nuclei with prominent nucleoli	B cell

TABLE 147-2. CLINICAL CHARACTERISTICS OF NON-HODGKIN'S LYMPHOMAS*

Subtype	% All Lymphomas	Median Age (yr)	Sex Ratio M:F	% PS I, II	% PS III, IV	% Bone Marrow Involvement
SLL	3.6	61	1.2:1	11	89	71
FSCL	22.5	54	1.3:1	18	82	51
FML	7.7	56	0.8:1	27	73	30
FLCL	3.8	55	1.8:1	27	73	34
DSCL	6.9	58	2:1	28	72	32
DML	6.7	58	1.1:1	45	55	14
DLCL	19.7	57	1:1	46	54	10
IBL	7.9	51	1.5:1	52	49	12
LBL	4.2	17	1.9:1	27	74	50
SNCL	0.5	30	2.6:1	34	66	14

*PS = pathologic stage (according to the Working Formulation, 1982).

survival appear to parallel their counterparts in the Working Formulation.

HTLV-I–associated adult T cell leukemia/lymphoma is characterized by geographic clustering, the presence of antibody to HTLV-I, and a rapidly fatal clinical course. Clinical features include abrupt onset of generalized lymphadenopathy, hepatosplenomegaly, skin infiltration, lytic bone disease, bone marrow involvement with circulating cells, and hypercalcemia. In spite of intensive chemotherapy, median survival is less than 1 year. Although clinically distinct, this rare T cell lymphoma is not easily distinguishable pathologically from other T cell lymphomas. Diffuse small cell, mixed cell, large cell, and undifferentiated cell types have all been described. Therefore, clinical suspicion and the presence of HTLV-I antibody are necessary to confirm the diagnosis.

DIAGNOSIS AND STAGING

As discussed in Ch. 146, the diagnosis of non-Hodgkin's lymphoma requires skilled interpretation of adequate tumor tissue, preferably from an involved lymph node, so that tumor architecture as well as cell type may be assessed. B cell and T cell typing studies may complement the pathologic interpretation but do not supplant it. The clinical history and ancillary studies, e.g., HTLV-I or HIV antibody, may also contribute. Once a diagnosis has been established, then it is useful to determine the extent of disease through staging.

The Ann Arbor staging system utilized for Hodgkin's disease (see Ch. 148) is also used in the management of non-Hodgkin's lymphomas. Although of clinical value, this staging system has several shortcomings when applied to non-Hodgkin's lymphomas: Factors such as disease site, disease bulk, and extent of extranodal involvement are not considered. In addition, the presence of systemic symptoms plays a lesser role in influencing treatment planning and prognosis in non-Hodgkin's lymphoma. Nevertheless, thorough pretreatment staging is necessary in all patients.

Noninvasive studies, which should be obtained in all patients, are listed in Table 147-3.

On the basis of this information, the clinical stage of the lymphoma can be determined. Since bone marrow involvement is so common, particularly in low-grade lymphoma, bilateral percutaneous bone marrow biopsies are often the simplest way to establish pathologic stage IV disease.

Pathologic confirmation of other extranodal sites may be appropriate, as when gastroscopic biopsy, pleural cytology, or skin biopsy is obtained. Laparotomy or thoracotomy is indicated only in those patients with no other evident disease or when a gastrointestinal tumor is removed prior to treatment. Staging laparotomy as performed for Hodgkin's disease is rarely, if ever, indicated.

TREATMENT

In defining a treatment approach for the patient with non-Hodgkin's lymphoma, it is necessary to consider such factors as histologic subtype, stage, sites of disease, tumor bulk, thoroughness of initial staging, general medical condition, and age, as well as the goals and effectiveness of therapy. In practical terms, non-Hodgkin's lymphomas can be considered in two broad categories: those diseases that progress slowly and have an indolent natural history (the low-grade lymphomas) and those diseases that present aggressively, progress rapidly, and, if unsuccessfully treated, are soon fatal (the intermediate- and high-grade lymphomas).

LOW-GRADE LYMPHOMAS. As outlined above, low-grade lymphomas infrequently present with truly localized disease (pathologic stage I or II). Only 11 to 27 per cent, depending upon histologic subtype, are therefore eligible for regional treatment with radiation therapy. Although uncommon, this disease presentation appears to be highly favorable, with more than 75 per cent of patients remaining free of disease for 10 years or longer after irradiation alone (3500 to 4400 cGy to the region).

Many more patients appear to have clinically localized disease after noninvasive staging and bone marrow biopsy but have not undergone complete laparotomy staging. Under these circumstances, radiation therapy may still accomplish good local control. Many patients, however, have undetected microscopic disease outside the treatment portal that will slowly progress and lead to disease recurrence several years after initial therapy. Nevertheless, irradiation may still be a reasonable choice, since relapse may occur years later, and salvage treatment at relapse may be effective. Patients eligible for this approach are those with peripheral lymph node presentations (stages I and II) involving cervical, supraclavicular, axillary, or inguinal regions. Abdominal masses usually require whole-abdominal irradiation in which this approach may not be justified. Thoracic presentations are rare.

The majority (74 to 89 per cent) of patients with low-grade lymphomas have advanced stage (III or IV) disease and are therefore ineligible for localized treatment approaches. Optimal management of such patients remains controversial. Complete disappearance of all known tumor (including bone marrow biopsy) may be induced in more than 80 per cent of patients with single-

TABLE 147-3. NONINVASIVE STUDIES IN NON-HODGKIN'S LYMPHOMA

History with assessment of systemic symptoms, predisposing epidemiologic factors
Physical examination
Complete blood count and platelet count; Coombs' test if anemic
Liver and renal function tests
Serum immunoglobulins in low-grade lymphomas
Antibody for HTLV-I or HIV, if indicated
Chest radiograph, posteroanterior and lateral
Chest computed tomography, if indicated
Abdominal and pelvic computed tomography
  If unavailable, abdominal ultrasound study
  If normal, lymphography possibly indicated
Bone scan and bone radiographs if clinical involvement suspected
Upper gastrointestinal series, if clinical involvement suspected or if Waldeyer's ring involved
Gallium scan, optional in aggressive histologies
Cerebrospinal fluid cytology (in all patients with intermediate- or high-grade lymphomas and known bone marrow disease)

agent or multiagent chemotherapy, with whole-body irradiation, or with combined chemotherapy-irradiation. Unfortunately, median remission durations are usually limited to 2½ to 5 years. Complete responders actually have persistent lymphoma cells in their peripheral blood and bone marrow that may be detected by sensitive methods. The presence of such cells correlates with subsequent relapse.

The most promising combination chemotherapy program is ProMACE-MOPP* followed by a total lymphoid irradiation of 2400 cGy in complete responders. Preliminary results reveal a high complete response rate, with more than 70 per cent remaining in remission at 4 years. It is premature to speculate on the ultimate remission durability of such combined-modality regimens. Sensitive molecular methods (utilizing the polymerase chain reaction) to detect residual cells may be helpful in assessing whether such programs can eliminate the malignant clone.

In summary, a standard treatment regimen in advanced low-grade lymphoma has not been established. Daily single-agent cyclophosphamide; daily or pulse chlorambucil; or combinations of cyclophosphamide, vincristine, prednisone with or without procarbazine or doxorubicin (Adriamycin) are reasonable choices, depending upon the clinical circumstances. Enrollment in a protocol regimen is encouraged whenever possible, since an optimal treatment regimen has not been identified.

Another management approach in patients with advanced low-grade non-Hodgkin's lymphomas is initial treatment deferral, with institution of therapy when there is disease progression. This approach is based on the premise that treatment at diagnosis does not appear curative. Many patients have indolent, slowly progressive disease, and treatment deferral does not appear to compromise therapeutic outcome. Approximately one half of all patients may be eligible for observation at diagnosis; the median treatment-free period correlates with histology: more than 8 years for SLL, 5 years for FSCL, and 10 months for FML.

Biologic therapies have also been investigated in low-grade lymphomas and appear to have transient efficacy. These include monoclonal antibody therapy directed specifically against the malignant B cell immunoglobulin idiotype, antibody against B cell differentiation antigens, and alpha-interferon.

In up to 50 per cent of patients, low-grade lymphomas may change with or without treatment from an indolent to an aggressive form by the eighth year following diagnosis. Most often the transformation manifests as rapidly growing disease in one or more sites, while the low-grade component remains stable or progresses slowly. Pathologic study reveals DLCL, IBL, or other aggressive subtypes, and studies of clonality are consistent with the low-grade histology (B cell primarily). Most transformations represent the emergence of an aggressive subclone from the original indolent disease, but some cases appear to represent the emergence of a completely new second neoplasm that is a clonally distinct, aggressive lymphoma in the setting of indolent lymphoma.

Histologic transformation is important to recognize, since it has prognostic and therapeutic implications. Median survival is less than 1 year following its emergence, and intensive treatment programs are necessary to gain disease control. Some patients appear to have the aggressive component eradicated by such measures, often with persistence or later relapse of the indolent histology.

INTERMEDIATE- AND HIGH-GRADE LYMPHOMAS. Intensive combination chemotherapy is the mainstay of curative treatment in aggressive non-Hodgkin's lymphomas. Of the half of all patients who may present with regional disease alone, only that small subset with pathologic stage I presentation may be eligible for radiation therapy alone. This is because the intent and realistic goal of treatment in the aggressive lymphomas is always cure, and relapse must be avoided whenever possible.

The expectation of cure in the majority of patients with aggressive lymphomas, regardless of stage, is based upon the

following observations in advanced disease: (1) Tumors are rapidly proliferating and initially very sensitive to combination chemotherapy. (2) Survival curves in advanced disease are biphasic, revealing a rapid death rate during the 2 first years (composed of partially responding and nonresponding patients) and then a plateau of cured cases (composed of complete responders). (3) With intensifying drug regimens, the proportion of complete responders may be increased and, similarly, the proportion cured. (4) Increasing tumor bulk correlates with decreased complete response, the emergence of drug resistance, and poor survival. (5) The highest complete response rates to combination chemotherapy are achieved in patients with regional or disseminated nonbulky disease.

Commonly used agents in combination regimens include cyclophosphamide, doxorubicin (Adriamycin), vincristine, prednisone, methotrexate, bleomycin, etoposide, and cytosine arabinoside. Representative regimens are listed in Table 147–4. Treatment should be initiated promptly after diagnosis and appropriate noninvasive staging; the regimen must be intensive (leading to at least moderate toxicity), administered in high and often escalating doses, on a rigorous schedule; attention must be paid to rapidity of response and any evidence of early drug resistance; and after a defined treatment course, complete restaging is undertaken. With these guidelines, at least 60 per cent of patients with advanced disease and more than 80 per cent with localized disease achieve complete response. The majority of complete responses (>70 per cent) are durable, and maintenance chemotherapy is unnecessary.

By increasing the relative dose intensity of combination chemotherapy regimens utilized in the treatment of aggressive lymphomas, the number of complete responders appears to have increased. To establish the validity of this concept, a national intergroup study is currently testing the relative efficacy of the four most commonly utilized regimens (each with a different dose intensity).

Another investigative approach has been the use of potentially lethal doses of chemotherapeutic agents with autologous bone marrow rescue in high-risk patients. Preliminary reports suggest that this approach is superior to standard combination chemotherapy.

SPECIAL CONSIDERATIONS. *Histopathologic Subtype.* Lymphoblastic lymphoma and SNCL are often treated with modified intensive drug programs, and all patients require central nervous system prophylaxis.

Mediastinal Disease. Superior vena cava syndrome may be present and is effectively managed with chemotherapy and/or irradiation. Biopsy of undetermined mediastinal masses must be accomplished with less than 750 to 1000 cGy (200 to 250 cGy fractions) of irradiation before biopsy.

Gastrointestinal Disease. Perforation and/or bleeding may be complications prior to or following treatment. To avoid this, surgical resection of the involved region is often recommended, prior to therapy.

Central Nervous System. All patients with lymphoblastic lymphoma and SNCL, as well as those with other aggressive histologic types and bone marrow involvement, are at risk for meningeal disease. Cerebrospinal fluid cytology is determined before therapy, and meningeal prophylaxis is given.

Primary brain lymphoma, as often identified in immunodeficient patients, requires high-dose whole-brain irradiation with or without chemotherapy.

Tumor Masses Larger than 10 cm. Supplementary irradiation is sometimes administered concurrently with or following chemotherapy. Residual fibrosis may occasionally persist after therapy. Surgical resection of tumor masses has been shown to be of value only with intra-abdominal Burkitt's lymphoma.

Tumor Lysis Syndrome. Rapid tumor shrinkage with excess urate production should be anticipated in all patients and allopurinol administered. With bulky or disseminated tumor or both, rapid cell lysis may lead to hyperkalemia, hypocalcemia, hyperphosphatemia, hyperuricemia, and acute renal failure. Patients with SNCL and lymphoblastic lymphoma are most often affected.

AIDS-Associated Lymphomas. The presence of significant immunodeficiency, multiple infections, and extranodal disease may make standard chemotherapy regimens excessively toxic and unsuccessful in this group of patients (see Color Plate 8E).

---

*ProMACE = prednisone, methotrexate, doxorubicin (Adriamycin), cyclophosphamide, etoposide; MOPP = Mechlorethamine (Mustargen), vincristine (Oncovin), procarbazine, prednisone.

TABLE 147–4. REPRESENTATIVE DRUG COMBINATIONS FOR INTERMEDIATE AND HIGH-GRADE NON-HODGKIN'S LYMPHOMAS

MACOP-B

Methotrexate	400 mg/m² IV	Weeks 2, 6, 10 with leucovorin
Adriamycin (doxorubicin)	50 mg/m² IV	Weeks 1, 3, 5, 7, 9, 11
Cyclophosphamide	350 mg/m² IV	Weeks 1, 3, 5, 7, 9, 11
Oncovin (vincristine)	1.4 mg/m² IV	Weeks 2, 4, 6, 8, 10, 12
Prednisone	75 mg PO	Daily, dose tapered over the last 15 days
Bleomycin	10 U/m² IV	Weeks 4, 8, 12
Co-trimoxazole	2 tab PO	Twice daily throughout

ProMACE-CytaBOM (21-day cycles)

Prednisone	60 mg/m² PO	Days 1–14
Adriamycin (doxorubicin)	25 mg/m² IV	Days 1 and 8
Cyclophosphamide	650 mg/m² IV	Day 1
Etoposide (VP-16)	120 mg/m² IV	Day 1
Cytarabine	300 mg/m² IV	Day 8
Bleomycin	5 mg/m² IV	Day 8
Oncovin (vincristine)	1.4 mg/m² IV	Day 8
Methotrexate	120 mg/m² IV	Day 8 with leucovorin
Co-trimoxazole	2 tab PO	Twice daily throughout

m-BACOD (28-day cycles)

Methotrexate	200 mg/m² IV	Days 8 and 15 with leucovorin
Bleomycin	4 mg/m² IV	Day 1
Adriamycin (doxorubicin)	45 mg/m² IV	Day 1
Cyclophosphamide	600 mg/m² IV	Day 1
Oncovin (vincristine)	1 mg/m² IV	Day 1
Dexamethasone	6 mg/m² PO	Days 1–5

CHOP (21- to 28-day cycles)

Cyclophosphamide	750 mg/m² IV	Day 1
Hydroxydaunomycin/ Adriamycin (doxorubicin)	50 mg/m² IV	Day 1
Oncovin	1.4 mg/m² IV	Day 1
Prednisone	100 mg PO	Days 1–5

IV = intravenous; PO = by mouth.

PROGNOSIS

The Working Formulation identifies more than 10 distinct disease entities and groups them according to prognosis. The survival curves upon which these prognostic groups were initially based are no longer entirely valid because of improved treatment methods. Nevertheless, it is still important to recognize a low-grade category in which the lymphoma progresses slowly and has an indolent natural history, as well as intermediate- and high-grade categories in which the disease presents aggressively, progresses rapidly, and, if unsuccessfully treated, is soon fatal.

In Figure 147–1A are the overall survival curves of the original Working Formulation (based on 1975 data) according to prognostic category. The median survivals are approximately 6½ years for the low-grade, 2½ years for the intermediate-grade, and 1½ years for the high-grade categories. Figure 147–1B illustrates representative overall survival curves based on 1985 data, according to prognostic category. The median survival in the low-grade category is 6½ years, unchanged from the original Working Formulation, whereas the median survival for the intermediate- and high-grade categories has not yet been reached, and at least 60 per cent of all patients remain alive and disease free at 5 years. Followed to 8 years, the curves overlap as patients in the low-grade category succumb to progressive lymphoma, while patients in the intermediate- and high-grade categories continue to be disease free.

This, then, is the prognostic paradox of non-Hodgkin's lymphomas: Initially favorable and indolent, the low-grade histologic types are, in fact, the unfavorable category with longer observation; and initially unfavorable and aggressive intermediate- and high-grade histologic types are, in fact, the favorable categories, since cure may be regularly achieved.

Armitage JO: Bone marrow transplantation in the treatment of patients with lymphoma. Blood 73:1749, 1989. *An excellent review of the topic of transplantation in lymphomas.*

DeVita VT Jr, Hubbard SM, Young RC, et al.: The role of chemotherapy in diffuse aggressive lymphomas. Semin Hematol 25 (Suppl 2):2, 1988. *A review of combination chemotherapy regimens, emphasizing the importance of prognostic factors and relative dose intensity in analyzing results.*

Haber DA, Mayer RJ: Primary gastrointestinal lymphoma. Semin Oncol 15:154, 1988. *A comprehensive review of pathology, clinical aspects, and therapeutic strategies.*

Knowles DM, Chamulak GA, Subar M, et al.: Lymphoid neoplasia associated with the acquired immunodeficiency syndrome (AIDS): The New York University

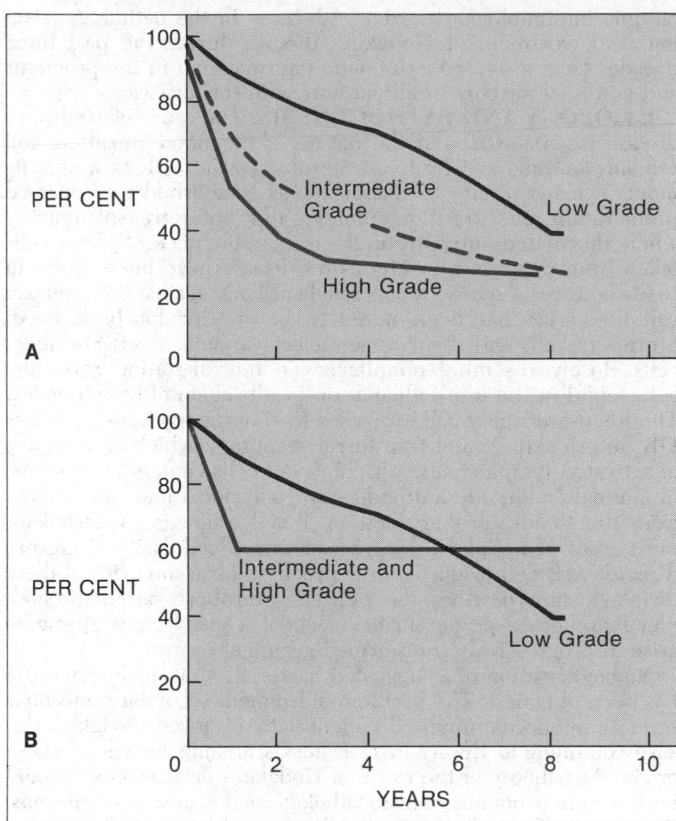

FIGURE 147–1. *A,* Actuarial survival according to histologic grade, based on 1975 data, as reported in the Working Formulation (1982). *B,* Hypothetical actuarial survival according to histologic grade, based on 1985 data (see text).

Medical Center experience with 105 patients (1981–1986). Ann Intern Med 108:744, 1988. *A comprehensive study of the epidemiology, clinical features, and treatment outcome of 105 patients with AIDS-associated lymphomas.*

The Non-Hodgkin's Lymphoma Pathologic Classification Project: National Cancer Institute sponsored study of classifications of non-Hodgkin's lymphomas: Summary and description of a working formulation for clinical usage. Cancer 49:2112, 1982. *The Working Formulation is presented in detail with pathologic and clinical analyses.*

Williams SF, Golomb HM (eds.): Non-Hodgkin's lymphoma. Semin Oncol 17:1–132, 1990. *A complete journal issue devoted to all aspects of non-Hodgkin's lymphomas: Pathology, basic science, clinical management, and complications of disease and therapy.*

Young RC, Longo DC, Glatstein E, et al.: The treatment of indolent lymphomas: Watchful waiting versus aggressive combined modality treatment. Semin Hematol 25 (Suppl 2):11, 1988. *The results of ProMACE-MOPP plus irradiation are presented in this preliminary report of a randomized trial.*

148 Hodgkin's Disease

John H. Glick

DEFINITION. Hodgkin's disease is a unique malignant disorder, usually arising in lymph nodes, with a characteristic histopathologic appearance. It is defined by the presence of the virtually pathognomonic Reed-Sternberg giant cell in an appropriate cellular background. The disease was first recognized as a distinct clinicopathologic entity in 1832 by Thomas Hodgkin, who described seven patients with a fatal illness involving "hypertrophy of the lymphatic system." Although the etiology is unknown, definitive evidence has emerged that Hodgkin's disease is indeed a malignant neoplasm and not a granulomatous infection or a chronic immunologic disorder. Advances in the pathology, staging, and treatment of Hodgkin's disease during the past three decades have provided a dramatic improvement in the prognosis and potential for cure of all patients with this disease.

ETIOLOGY AND PATHOGENESIS. The cause of Hodgkin's disease is unknown, and the nature of the Reed-Sternberg cell remains an enigma. The Reed-Sternberg giant cell, as well as its mononuclear variants, is malignant, as established by sustained proliferation in vitro, aneuploidy, and heterotransplantability when inoculated intracerebrally into nude mice. Spleen cells taken from patients with Hodgkin's disease have been grown in tissue culture. A mouse monoclonal antibody against the Hodgkin cell line L428 has been noted to be specific for both Reed-Sternberg cells and their mononuclear variants. Reed-Sternberg cells closely resemble nonphagocytic interdigitating reticulum cells found in the interfollicular or T cell region of lymph nodes. The Reed-Sternberg cell expresses Ki–1 antigens, Leu-Ml, HLA-DR, interleukin 2, and transferrin receptors, which are features of activated lymphocytes. Although the cells contain cytoplasmic immunoglobulin, the antibodies are polyclonal and not derived from the Reed-Sternberg cell. A T cell origin is suggested for most cases of nodular sclerosis and mixed cellularity Hodgkin's disease. A B cell origin is most probable for a minority of these histologic subtypes, and for the Reed-Sternberg variants in nodular lymphocyte predominance, which in many cases appear to arise in progressively transformed germinal centers.

No confirmation of a suggested bacterial, viral, or fungal cause has been obtained. The problem of frequent secondary infections in the immunocompromised patient with advanced Hodgkin's disease continues to thwart investigators searching for an infectious origin. Any theory of the cause of Hodgkin's disease must account for the wide panorama of histopathologic and clinical presentations, the variety of neoplastic giant cells, the signs of an inflammatory reaction and infection-like symptoms, the characteristic immunologic defects, and the specific epidemiologic patterns.

EPIDEMIOLOGY. Approximately 8000 new cases of Hodgkin's disease are diagnosed each year in the United States, with only 1600 deaths. These patients average 32 years of age and are more commonly male than female. The age-specific distribution curve is an unusual bimodal pattern for both sexes, with the first peak at ages 15 to 35 and the second after age 50. Hodgkin's disease is distributed throughout the world, but the age-specific rates differ markedly in different countries. The developed areas of the United States and Northern Europe have a prominent young adult peak, which is lower in less developed countries and absent in Japan.

There is an inverse risk with family size, with a rate 2.5 times greater among persons without siblings than those with four or more siblings. There is up to a sevenfold increased risk among siblings of young adults with Hodgkin's disease. Increased risk also occurs with early birth order position and improved living conditions. All these factors tend to decrease and delay exposure to infectious agents. It has been suggested that Hodgkin's disease may be an age-dependent host response to a common infection. Population-based studies have failed to document significant "clustering" of cases. No increased risk in medical personnel exposed to large numbers of patients with Hodgkin's disease has been observed. Thus, at the present time, there is no firm evidence for a contagious etiology.

PATHOLOGY. Histologic diagnosis of Hodgkin's disease requires the presence of characteristic Reed-Sternberg giant cells in association with an appropriate stromal background or cellular milieu. The classic Reed-Sternberg cell (Fig. 148–1A) is a large, bilobed cell with prominent eosinophilic nucleoli, perinucleolar clearing, thick nuclear membrane, and relatively abundant cytoplasm (see Color Plate 8F). Distinctive multinuclear giant cells in lacunar-like spaces (Fig. 148–1B) are associated with the nodular sclerosis subtype and are considered Reed-Sternberg variants. Mononuclear variants are also found on biopsy but cannot be considered as reliably diagnostic. Although the diagnosis of Hodgkin's disease is rarely made in the absence of Reed-Sternberg cells, the presence of such a cell is not pathognomonic of the disease. Cells indistinguishable from or closely resembling Reed-Sternberg cells may be found in reactive conditions such as infectious mononucleosis, in which immunoblasts, or trans-

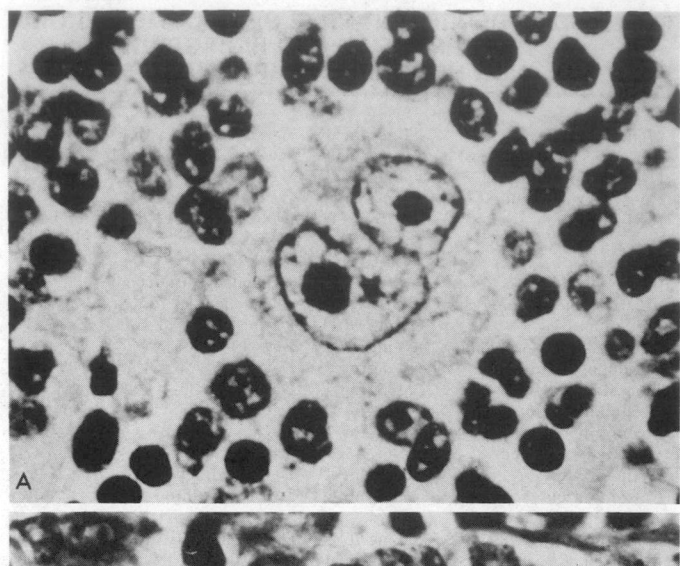

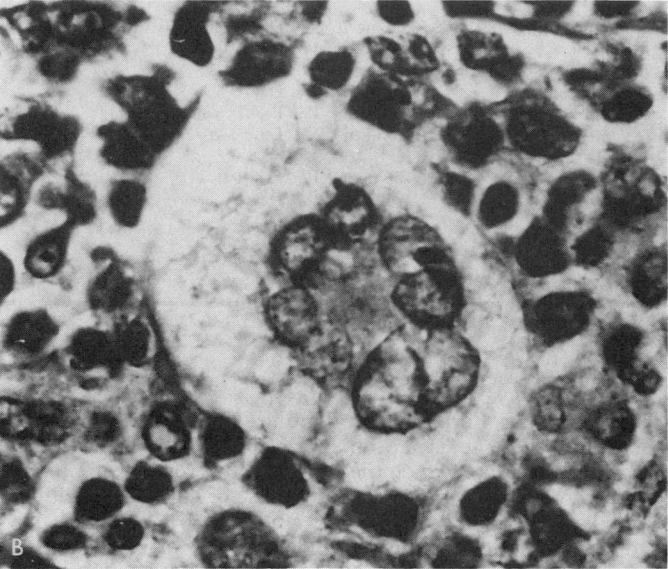

FIGURE 148–1. Pathologic diagnosis. A, Diagnostic Reed-Sternberg cell with large inclusion-like nucleoli, high power. B, Reed-Sternberg cell variant, lacunar cell type, high power. (Reprinted by permission from Tindle BH: Pathology of Lymphomas. In Bennett JM [ed.]: Lymphomas I. The Hague, Martinus Nijhoff, 1981, p. 70.)

formed lymphocytes, may mimic Reed-Sternberg cells. The character of the stromal background is as important for the diagnosis of Hodgkin's disease as is the Reed-Sternberg cell. This background consists of a mixed population of cytologically benign cells, including reactive lymphocytes, benign histiocytes, plasma cells, and eosinophils.

Frozen section material should not be used to make a definitive diagnosis when Hodgkin's disease is suspected because of the presence of artifacts. Formalin-fixed tissue is required for careful histologic review. If any uncertainty of diagnosis exists, consultation with an experienced hematopathologist is required. The monoclonal antibody Leu-M1, which reacts with granulocytes, stains Reed-Sternberg cells and their mononuclear variants. This immunodiagnostic marker may be particularly useful in distinguishing Hodgkin's disease from other lymphoproliferative disorders, such as peripheral T cell lymphomas. Needle aspiration of lymph nodes for diagnostic purposes is generally not reliable because insufficient tissue is obtained for accurate evaluation.

Hodgkin's disease is subclassified histopathologically into four subtypes according to the Rye classification (Table 148–1) (see Color Plate 8G). The relative frequency of the four groups is variable in different series, depending on epidemiologic and patient referral factors. The natural history of Hodgkin's disease correlates well with the histopathologic groups. The *lymphocyte predominance type* is the most favorable and is associated with early-stage disease in asymptomatic patients with nodal presentations. The *nodular sclerosis variety* has a relatively

TABLE 148–1. RYE HISTOPATHOLOGIC CLASSIFICATION OF HODGKIN'S DISEASE

Subgroup	Major Histologic Features	Relative Frequency
Lymphocyte predominance	Abundant normal-appearing lymphocyte infiltrate with or without benign histiocytes; occasionally nodular; rare Reed-Sternberg (R-S) cells	5–15%
Nodular sclerosis	Nodules of lymphoid infiltrate of varying size, separated by bands of collagen and containing numerous "lacunar" cell variants of R-S cells	40–75%
Mixed cellularity	Pleomorphic infiltrate of eosinophils, plasma cells, histiocytes, and lymphocytes with numerous R-S cells	20–40%
Lymphocyte depletion	Paucity of lymphocytes with numerous R-S cells, often bizarre in appearance; may have diffuse fiberosis or reticulum fibers	5%

favorable prognosis, usually occurs in young women with supradiaphragmatic nodes, and frequently involves the mediastinum. The *mixed cellularity pattern* tends to occur in middle-aged patients with systemic symptoms and more extensive disease than is first evident on initial presentation. The *lymphocyte depletion subtype* has the least favorable prognosis, as it generally occurs in patients with advanced-stage disease and systemic symptoms and frequently involves the bone marrow. Recent studies have indicated a lower incidence of lymphocyte depletion Hodgkin's disease than previously reported and have suggested that some cases formerly diagnosed as this histologic subtype may have represented large cell immunoblastic lymphomas. Advances in aggressive therapy, after precise staging, have obscured the prognostic value of histopathologic classification.

CLINICAL MANIFESTATIONS. The initial presentation and subsequent clinical course of patients with Hodgkin's disease can be extremely variable, depending on when in the natural history the patient first seeks medical attention.

Adenopathy. The majority of patients present with a painless and enlarging mass, most commonly in the neck, but occasionally in the axilla or inguinal-femoral region. This lymphadenopathy is usually discovered accidentally by the patient and is often the only manifestation of the disease at the time of diagnosis. Upon examination, this mass is found to be a discrete, rubbery, usually nontender lymph node or group of surrounding enlarged and matted lymph nodes. Asymptomatic lymphadenopathy may also be noted by the physician on a routine physical examination. In other instances, a chest roentgenogram, obtained either for a routine purpose or because of a persistent, dry, nonproductive cough, may demonstrate a mediastinal mass. Physical examination may then disclose lymphadenopathy of which the patient had been unaware. Although these typical presentations may occur at any age with any histopathologic type, they are more common in young patients, usually between 15 and 35 years of age with the nodular sclerosis histologic pattern.

The duration of lymphadenopathy prior to diagnosis is extremely variable. Typically, several weeks to several months elapse between the time of the patient's first observation of an asymptomatic mass and the diagnostic biopsy. However, some patients report that a particular mass has been present for many months to several years, with intermittent waxing and waning in size.

Fever and Systemic Symptoms. Although the asymptomatic presentation is most common, one quarter to one third of patients present with unexplained and persistent fever and/or night sweats as initial symptoms. Fatigue and weight loss may be associated complaints. Patients with these symptoms tend to be in the older age group, are more often men than women, and are generally discovered to have more widespread disease than the usual patient presenting without symptoms. Although superficial lymphadenopathy is present in most such patients, occasionally palpable lymphadenopathy is absent in the patient past the age

of 40 with severe systemic symptoms. These patients present with fever of undetermined origin. Extensive diagnostic efforts may be required to discover the presence of Hodgkin's disease, including lymphangiography, abdominal computed tomographic (CT) scanning, bone marrow biopsies, or even exploratory laparotomy.

The presence of fever, drenching night sweats requiring the changing of bed clothing, and weight loss exceeding 10 per cent of baseline body weight during the 6 months preceding diagnosis constitute systemic or B symptoms for staging purposes and confer an adverse prognosis.

Although fever secondary to Hodgkin's disease is usually low grade, occasional patients have intermittent evening fever lasting several days, alternating with afebrile periods lasting days or weeks. This cyclic fever has been labeled the *Pel-Ebstein type* but is rarely the presenting manifestation of the disease.

Pruritus. Pruritus is another characteristic systemic symptom of Hodgkin's disease. It may be mild and localized, but usually progresses and becomes generalized. Severe pruritus may result in extensive excoriations and inability to sleep. It is rarely relieved by topical medications or antihistamines. The prognostic significance of pruritus itself is unclear. It rarely occurs in the absence of fever and/or night sweats but is no longer considered a B symptom because its presence does not correlate with an adverse prognosis. Generalized, severe pruritus may occur in patients with non-Hodgkin's lymphomas and in other medical and dermatologic conditions, but its presence should always suggest Hodgkin's disease. Its cause is unknown.

SELECTED CLINICAL PROBLEMS. A wide variety of other symptoms may initially call the attention of patients and their physicians to the disease. These same problems occur more commonly as the course of Hodgkin's disease progresses. In addition, almost all patients receive treatment that profoundly affects the natural history of their illness, resulting in either apparent cure or persistent, relapsing Hodgkin's disease, or frequently in complications that become difficult to separate from the manifestations of the disease itself.

Pulmonary involvement occurs in only 10 to 20 per cent of patients at presentation. It appears to arise by spread along lymphatics from ipsilateral hilar lymph nodes. Hodgkin's disease frequently involves the lungs with a patchy pulmonary infiltrate without circumscribed borders. Its appearance is variable, and it must be distinguished from radiation effects, drug reactions, and the wide variety of pulmonary infections that occur in these immunocompromised patients. In a severely ill patient in whom the diagnosis is uncertain, the therapeutic significance of these lesions is so great that bronchoscopy with transbronchial biopsy or diagnostic thoracotomy may be justified. Pleural effusions—transudates, exudates, or chylous—are most frequently caused by central lymphatic and venous obstruction resulting from Hodgkin's disease in the mediastinum or obstruction of the thoracic duct. These effusions are rarely caused by direct pleural involvement, and cytologic examination of the fluid or pleural biopsy infrequently reveals diagnostic Reed-Sternberg cells.

Superior vena caval obstruction, upper airway compression, and recurrent laryngeal nerve involvement are rare despite bulky intrathoracic disease presentations. Myocardial involvement is extremely unusual, but pericardial effusions may occur from direct invasion by adjacent mediastinal Hodgkin's disease. Effusions rarely produce cardiac tamponade, and this complication is more often a consequence of radiation-induced pericarditis.

Spinal cord compression, usually caused by epidural spread of tumor from paravertebral lymph nodes through intervertebral foramina in the thoracic or lumbar regions, may be a devastating acute complication. This syndrome may be seen in patients with an otherwise favorable prognosis, although it usually occurs in patients with progressive tumor in whom primary treatment has failed. Back or neck pain, either directly over the vertebral body or occurring in a radicular pattern, should promptly raise the suspicion of cord compression. Symptoms suggestive of more advanced cord compression include numbness, tingling or weakness of an extremity, motor weakness, and bladder or bowel dysfunction. Prompt diagnostic evaluation, including magnetic resonance imaging (MRI) and/or CT scanning is mandatory, as is prompt therapeutic intervention with immediate radiotherapy to prevent permanent neurologic damage. Surgical decompression is rarely indicated.

Bone involvement may occur from hematogenous spread in advanced disease or by local nodal spread to adjacent bone. Bone involvement often produces pain but rarely fracture, since the bone lesion is generally osteoblastic or mixed osteoblastic and osteolytic.

Hepatic involvement is present in fewer than 5 per cent of patients at the time of diagnosis and is generally focal in nature. Liver involvement in Hodgkin's disease is almost always associated with splenic involvement. Massive hepatomegaly or jaundice is rarely seen at the time of initial presentation. However, as the liver becomes progressively involved, diffuse infiltration of the portal spaces may be associated with serious hepatic dysfunction and laboratory features of intrahepatic biliary obstruction. Rarely, enlarged lymph nodes in the porta hepatis may produce extrahepatic biliary obstruction. Direct *renal involvement* is rarely a clinically significant problem, and ureteral obstruction and hydronephrosis, secondary to massive retroperitoneal lymphadenopathy, suggest a non-Hodgkin's lymphoma. The nephrotic syndrome, presenting as lipoid nephrosis, is a rare manifestation of Hodgkin's disease and is occasionally accompanied by evidence of glomerular immune complex deposition.

Infectious complications are common in patients with Hodgkin's disease and may or may not be temporarily related to concurrent treatment. Virtually all patients with uncontrolled Hodgkin's disease who succumb to this disorder have episodes of serious infections at some point in the course of their disease. Localized or disseminated herpes zoster is the most frequently diagnosed serious viral infection, while cryptococcosis, especially of the lungs and meninges, is the most virulent of the fungal complications. *Pneumocystis carinii* pneumonia causes diffuse pulmonary infiltrates and may appear in patients whose disease is in remission between cycles of chemotherapy, as well as in patients in whom relapse occurs. Toxoplasmosis is being recognized with increasing frequency, while tuberculosis has become distinctly uncommon in this population. Children who have undergone splenectomy are particularly predisposed to overwhelming pneumococcal infections unless prophylactic antibiotics or pneumococcal vaccine is administered.

Immunologic abnormalities are common in patients with Hodgkin's disease even at the time of initial diagnosis and prior to initiation of any treatment. A significantly higher frequency of cutaneous anergy is observed than in a control population. The presence or absence of anergy, however, has been shown to have no influence on the prognosis within a specific stage, given the effectiveness of modern therapy. Thus, there is no role for the routine anergy panel. With refined immunologic techniques, a defect in delayed hypersensitivity and T cell transformation can be detected even in early stage I disease. These deficits are aggravated by therapy and persist for many years even after successful curative treatment. In addition, T cell number, T cell helper (CD4)/suppressor (CD8) ratio, and T cell in vitro response to antigen may also be reduced. Decreased production of interleukin 2 (IL2) by peripheral blood mononuclear cells and decreased natural killer cell activity have been reported. Although cell-mediated immunity may be abnormal, patients with Hodgkin's disease rarely develop opportunistic infections prior to treatment. Therapy for Hodgkin's disease undoubtedly accentuates the T cell abnormality. However, it is still unknown whether the observed immunologic abnormalities contribute to the pathogenesis of the disease or are merely secondary phenomena. B cell function and B cell numbers appear to be normal in Hodgkin's disease at the time of diagnosis. Pneumococcal vaccine, for example, results in normal antibody response as long as subsequent treatment is delayed 10 to 14 days. However, overwhelming bacterial sepsis with encapsulated organisms is still a potential risk following splenectomy, especially in children.

STAGING. The progress achieved in the treatment of Hodgkin's disease has paralleled the improvement in techniques for identifying the extent or stage of disease in the untreated patient. In view of the current choices of therapy, it is essential that all cases of Hodgkin's disease be completely evaluated before therapeutic decisions are made. The primary goals of staging are to assess the extent of disease, facilitate the selection of an appropriate treatment program, provide an accurate determination of prognosis, and establish a baseline for re-evaluation following completion of therapy.

The staging classification in current use is outlined in Table 148–2. Patients are assigned a *clinical stage* (CS) on the basis of their initial biopsy, systemic symptoms, physical examination, laboratory results, and radiologic procedures. However, treatment decisions are generally based on a *pathologic stage* (PS), after the extent of involvement has been documented with appropriate biopsies. The basic staging classification is modified by the adverse prognostic significance of systemic symptoms (B disease) and by the realization that localized contiguous extranodal extension (E disease) generally does not carry the same poor prognosis as hematogenous extranodal involvement (stage IV disease).

Within each stage of Hodgkin's disease there is a spectrum of patients who have a more or less favorable prognosis, depending on the site or sites of disease, size of the tumor masses, and degree of symptoms. The importance of these prognostic factors and substages within the Ann Arbor classification has become increasingly recognized, because treatment methods are now tailored to individual clinical situations. Controversy exists over the prognostic and therapeutic significance of the E lesion and the substaging of IIIA patients. Pathologic stage IIIA disease, for example, may be subdivided into a prognostically favorable III$_1$ group, in which abdominal disease is confined to the upper abdominal nodes and/or the spleen, and a less favorable III$_2$ group, with disease extending to the lower abdomen, including the para-aortic, iliac, or inguinal lymph nodes.

Further modifications in the Ann Arbor staging system have been recommended to reflect changes in clinical staging criteria, newly recognized prognostic factors, and their impact on therapeutic decisions. The value of CT scanning and other imaging modalities in defining the extent of lymph node, liver, and splenic involvement is now recognized. In regional disease, the number of involved sites is denoted by a subscript (e.g., II$_3$). Bulky disease is defined by maximal dimension (> 10 cm) or by mass to thorax ratio ($\geq$ one third at T5–T6). In the setting of bulky intrathoracic disease, contiguous spread to adjacent extranodal tissues is clearly distinguished from disseminated extranodal involvement (such as multiple lung nodules). A complete knowledge of staging is vital to guide an efficient but thorough diagnostic evaluation. The tests performed as part of a staging evaluation must be individualized rather than obtained automatically.

DIAGNOSTIC EVALUATION. Recommended staging procedures are outlined in Table 148–3. This evaluation should

TABLE 148–2. MODIFIED ANN ARBOR STAGING CLASSIFICATION

Stage	
I	Involvement of a single lymph node region (I) or of a single extralymphatic organ or site (I$_E$)
II	Involvement of two or more lymph node regions on the same side of the diaphragm (II) or localized involvement of an extralymphatic organ or site and of one or more lymph node regions on the same side of the diaphragm (II$_E$)
III	Involvement of lymph node regions on both sides of the diaphragm (III), which may also be accompanied by involvement of the spleen (III$_S$) or by localized involvement of an extralymphatic organ or site (III$_E$) or both (III$_{SE}$)
III$_1$	Involvement limited to the lymphatic structures in the upper abdomen, that is, spleen, or splenic, celiac, or hepatic portal nodes, or any combination of these
III$_2$	Involvement of lower abdominal nodes, that is, para-aortic, iliac, inguinal, or mesenteric nodes, with or without involvement of the splenic, celiac, or hepatic portal nodes
IV	Diffuse or disseminated involvement of one or more extralymphatic organs or tissues, with or without associated lymph node involvement

E = extralymphatic site; S = splenic involvement

Note: The presence of fever, night sweats, and/or unexplained loss of 10 per cent or more of body weight in the 6 months preceding diagnosis is denoted by the suffix letter B. The letter A indicates the absence of these symptoms. Each patient is assigned a clinical stage (CS) on the basis of the initial biopsy, physical examination, and laboratory and radiologic results and a pathologic stage (PS) on the basis of subsequent biopsy results, whether normal or abnormal.

TABLE 148–3. DIAGNOSTIC EVALUATION

A. Required procedures
  1. Histologic confirmation by biopsy
  2. Detailed history for unexplained fever, weight loss, night sweats, and pruritus
  3. Physical examination to document all areas of lymphadenopathy, including Waldeyer's ring, size of liver and spleen, bone tenderness; neurologic evaluation
  4. Laboratory studies
    a. CBC and platelet count, ESR
    b. Serum alkaline phosphatase, LDH
    c. Renal function, including uric acid
    d. Liver function
  5. Radiologic studies
    a. Chest roentgenogram
    b. Bipedal lymphangiogram
    c. CT of the chest and whole abdomen, including the pelvis
B. Frequently performed procedures under specific clinical conditions
  1. Bone marrow biopsy (needle or open surgical technique)
  2. Bone roentgenography and scanning for areas of bone pain or tenderness
  3. Gallium whole-body scanning
  4. Staging laparotomy and splenectomy, if therapeutic decisions will depend on the identification of subdiaphragmatic disease

CBC = complete blood count; ESR = erythrocyte sedimentation rate; LDH = lactate dehydrogenase.

commence promptly after the initial biopsy establishes the diagnosis.

History and Physical Examination. A careful history and physical examination are essential to discover characteristic systemic symptoms and to describe all the lymph node areas of the body. Enlarged lymph nodes are not necessarily involved by disease; reactive lymphoid hyperplasia occasionally occurs in some patients with Hodgkin's disease. If confirmation of Hodgkin's disease in suspicious lymph nodes will change the therapeutic approach, then additional biopsies should be obtained. Although Waldeyer's ring involvement is uncommon in Hodgkin's disease, the lymphoid tissues in this region should be evaluated by physical examination. The size of the liver and spleen should be carefully determined, although mild enlargement of either organ may merely be a sign of nonspecific hypertrophy rather than involvement by Hodgkin's disease. A palpable abdominal mass caused by enlarged mesenteric or para-aortic lymph nodes is a rare initial finding. The bones should be examined for areas of tenderness, and a careful baseline neurologic examination performed.

Laboratory Studies. Routine laboratory tests include a complete blood count, erythrocyte sedimentation rate (ESR), urine analysis, renal and liver function tests, and serum alkaline phosphatase. Mild to moderate anemia may be found in patients with widespread disease and is often associated with normal indices, normal or low reticulocyte count, and a negative Coombs test. Anemia in a patient with Hodgkin's disease is usually caused by the typical chronic anemia of malignancy and rarely is secondary to hypersplenism, marrow involvement, or a Coombs-positive hemolytic anemia. A moderate to marked neutrophilic leukocytosis and thrombocytosis are characteristic of active, symptomatic Hodgkin's disease. Eosinophilia of a mild degree is common. In patients with severe and longstanding pruritus, moderate or marked eosinophilia frequently occurs. Absolute lymphopenia (<1000 per cubic millimeter) may be seen in a small percentage of patients with more advanced disease and is usually a poor prognostic sign.

The ESR is commonly elevated in patients with active disease but has limited sensitivity. An elevated serum alkaline phosphatase level may be a nonspecific finding or secondary to involvement of bone, bone marrow, or liver with Hodgkin's disease. Elevation of the serum uric acid level is rare at the time of initial presentation, except in advanced stages of disease with massive nodal or bone marrow involvement.

Radiologic Studies. Radiologic examinations should include routine chest roentgenograms, which demonstrate mediastinal involvement in 50 to 60 per cent of patients. In contrast, hilar disease is seen at presentation in fewer than 20 per cent of cases. In the absence of mediastinal involvement, hilar disease is unusual. Computed tomography of the chest provides better definition of mediastinal, hilar, and paravertebral adenopathy, and pulmonary involvement, and is indicated for all patients. Its role is to define more precisely the extent of disease, including possible localized extension into the pulmonary parenchyma, as well as to assist in radiation treatment planning. The presence of a small pleural effusion in the patient with a mediastinal mass does not necessarily indicate malignant involvement of the pleura. Thoracentesis or pleural biopsy is rarely diagnostic of Hodgkin's disease in these situations.

Subdiaphragmatic sites are best evaluated by performing both bipedal lymphangiography and abdominal-pelvic CT. These examinations are complementary, and neither procedure should replace the other. Recently, with the advent of CT, the routine use of the lymphangiogram has been questioned. However, the specificity appears better for lymphangiography, in that abnormalities of intranodal architecture can be demonstrated in up to 25 per cent of cases at presentation (Fig. 148–2). The overall accuracy of this procedure is 80 to 90 per cent. Lymphangiography is also valuable in preparation for exploratory laparotomy, in that it directs the surgeon to potentially abnormal areas for lymph node biopsy.

Abdominal CT complements lymphangiography by demonstrating lymphadenopathy in the mesentery, porta hepatis, celiac nodes, and para-aortic nodes above the level of those opacified by the lymphangiogram. Computed tomography can assess nodal involvement only when there is an increase in lymph node size (Fig. 148–3). In contrast, lymphangiography provides information

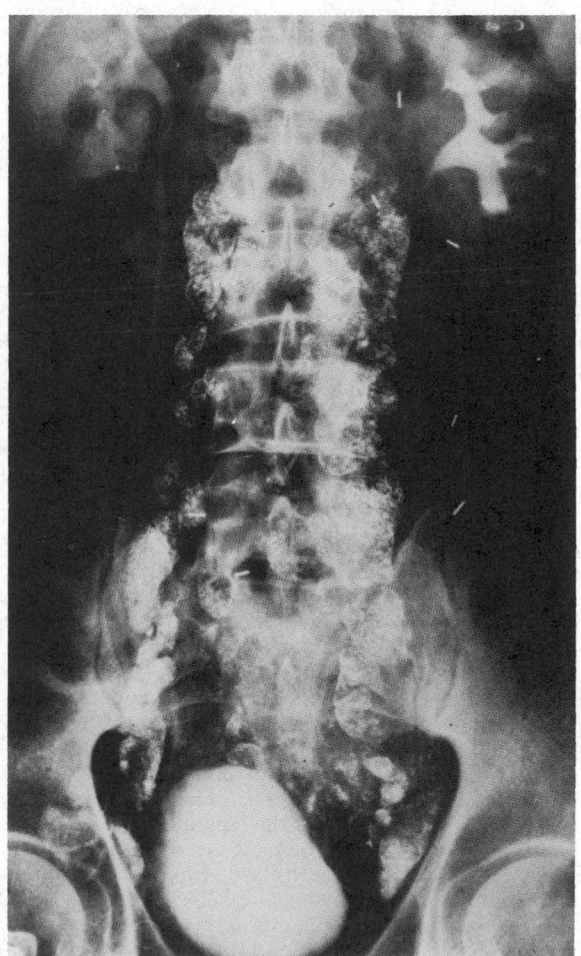

FIGURE 148–2. Abnormal lymphangiogram with enlargement and distortion of the internal architecture in the pelvic, iliac, and para-aortic lymph nodes. Despite the extensive lymphadenopathy, little displacement of the ureters and no obstruction of the upper urinary tracts were seen. (Reprinted, by permission of the publishers, from Hodgkin's Disease by Henry S. Kaplan, Cambridge, MA, Harvard University Press. Copyright © 1972, 1980, by the President and Fellows of Harvard College.)

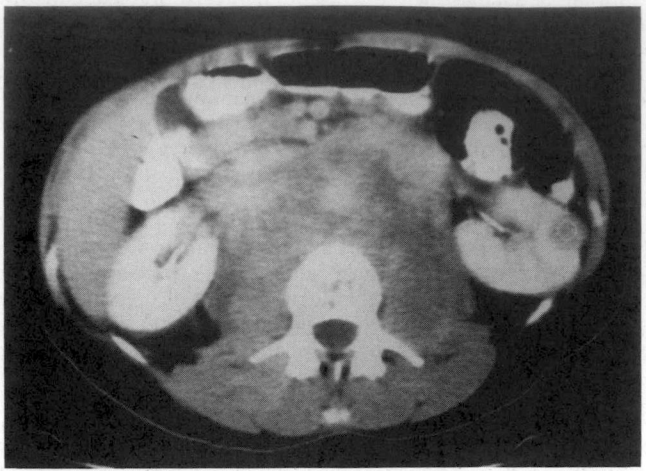

FIGURE 148–3. Abnormal abdominal CT scan with massive enlargement of retroperitoneal nodes.

on abnormal architecture even in unenlarged nodes. Thus, reliance on CT alone may lead to understaging.

Routine bone scans or skeletal radiographic examinations are not indicated in the asymptomatic patient with a normal alkaline phosphatase level. However, in those patients with areas of bone pain or tenderness, bone scans complemented by selective radiographic examinations are indicated to detect osseous lesions.

The liver is considered involved if multiple focal defects are detected by CT scan. A single percutaneous needle biopsy of the liver is rarely diagnostic, because of the focal nature of hepatic involvement. Gallium whole-body scans, particularly with higher dose (7 to 10 mCi) imaging on a triple-peak camera, may be occasionally helpful in determining sites of initial disease but is more useful in evaluating response to therapy (e.g., in the mediastinum) and in detecting areas of recurrence after therapy. Magnetic resonance imaging has not proved more useful than CT in determining sites of initial involvement, but MRI may be able to distinguish lymphomatous involvement from residual fibrosis of lymph nodes after treatment.

Bone Marrow Biopsy. This procedure should be performed in all patients with systemic symptoms or CS III disease or both. It is also useful in patients with significant peripheral blood count abnormalities, increased serum alkaline phosphatase level of bone origin, and abnormal bone roentgenograms or scans. Hodgkin's disease in the bone marrow is rarely demonstrable by simple marrow aspiration. Involvement is usually focal, is often associated with fibrosis, and is diagnosed more readily by either a unilateral or a bilateral bone marrow biopsy.

Staging Laparotomy. In the absence of medical contraindications, an exploratory laparotomy with splenectomy is frequently employed as part of the staging evaluation to identify and confirm the presence of Hodgkin's disease below the diaphragm. The purpose of the laparotomy is diagnostic, the results of which may alter treatment selection significantly. Laparotomy findings that frequently influence both the staging and the subsequent treatment include detection of Hodgkin's disease in the spleen, detection of the extent of splenic involvement, and detection of the presence of disease in the celiac or retroperitoneal lymph nodes. Secondary benefits from the laparotomy include attempting to preserve ovarian function by means of an oophoropexy when pelvic irradiation is to be utilized in young women, reducing required irradiation fields when the spleen is treated, and improving the peripheral blood counts in the occasional patient with hypersplenism. In one quarter of patients with normal-sized spleens on physical examination, Hodgkin's disease is found in the spleen removed at surgery. Conversely, approximately 50 per cent of patients with clinical or radiologic enlargement of the spleen do not have histologic involvement. The identification of Hodgkin's disease in the liver is especially difficult. Physical examination, routine liver function tests, and liver scans correlate poorly, if at all, with histologic verification. Liver involvement can be demonstrated at laparotomy on wedge or needle biopsy

and is more often found in patients with significant splenomegaly and/or abnormal lymphangiograms.

Staging laparotomy is not a routine diagnostic procedure and should be performed only in those patients in whom the results will potentially modify treatment selection. Discussion of potential treatment options with the radiotherapist or medical oncologist for each stage of Hodgkin's disease should be held prior to the decision to perform a laparotomy. Thus, staging laparotomy with splenectomy is generally recommended for patients with CS I to IIA/B or IIIA disease. Patients with stage IIIB or IV disease are not candidates for laparotomy because combination chemotherapy is used as their primary method of treatment.

Certain subgroups have a very low likelihood of change in stage with laparotomy. Female patients with CS IA at a single supradiaphragmatic site and patients with CS IA limited to a small mediastinal mass have less than a 10 per cent risk of intra-abdominal involvement. In other cases, such as patients with massive mediastinal disease, laporotomy is omitted because chemotherapy is employed as the primary treatment, eliminating the need for precise staging below the diaphragm.

As a result of staging laparotomy and splenectomy, approximately one third of patients with CS I and II are found to have either subdiaphragmatic lymph node disease or splenic involvement. The factors most likely to be associated with upstaging include male gender, B symptoms, and two or more sites of disease above the diaphragm. If extensive splenic involvement (> four nodules) is documented, either combination chemotherapy alone or a combined-modality program is required. Approximately one third of CS IIIA patients (i.e., those with suspicious lymphangiograms or abdominal CT scans) have a negative staging laparotomy that allows their pathologic stage to be downgraded to I or II. Although the results of the laparotomy allow change in the stage in as many as 35 per cent of patients, this change modifies the treatment plan in approximately 25 per cent, depending on the extent of disease found below the diaphragm. Even in the hands of experienced surgeons, staging laparotomy is associated with a small risk of perioperative morbidity, including infection, fever, and phlebitis. Rare fatalities have been reported. Because of occasional severe bacterial infections occurring after splenectomy, pneumococcal vaccine should be administered preoperatively.

MODE OF SPREAD. Careful mapping of initial sites of involvement of Hodgkin's disease and the use of lymphangiography, staging laparotomy, and splenectomy provide evidence that involvement of various lymph node groups is distinctly nonrandom. Two different theories have been proposed to account for the nonrandom patterns of spread: (1) The *contiguity theory* (Rosenberg and Kaplan) postulates that the disease is unifocal in origin, beginning in an initial focus within the lymphatic system and spreading via lymphatic channels to contiguous lymphatic structures. The contiguity theory has been challenged because of the frequency of cervical, supraclavicular, and retroperitoneal lymph node involvement without intervening mediastinal disease, as well as the common involvement of the spleen, which has no afferent lymphatics. (2) The *susceptibility theory* (Smithers) postulates that the disease is multifocal in origin. The giant cells of Hodgkin's disease are thought to migrate in and out of lymph nodes from the bloodstream but are thought to grow only in preferential sites, presenting an appearance of contiguous spread. Noncontiguous spread is more common in the mixed cellularity and lymphocyte depletion subtypes, when multiple sites are present and when vascular invasion is present. However, the role of vascular invasion in the spread of Hodgkin's disease is not fully understood. Vascular invasion in the spleen may lead to hematogenous dissemination, since the spleen is almost invariably involved when Hodgkin's disease is present in the liver or bone marrow.

TREATMENT. The prognosis for patients with Hodgkin's disease has improved dramatically during the past three decades because of (1) the advances in precise staging and an awareness of the important prognostic factors previously described, (2) the development of supervoltage radiotherapeutic techniques, and (3) the use of effective combination chemotherapy programs.

Radiotherapy. Important factors in determining the success of radiation therapy include the radiation dose per field, the extent of the fields employed, the beam energy, and precision of treatment planning. A tumoricidal dose of 3600 to 4400 cGy is required to eradicate the lesions of Hodgkin's disease. Lymphoid regions adjacent to areas of known disease or those that are contiguous via lymphatic channels are usually treated to full dose. Apparently uninvolved areas are treated prophylactically for subclinical disease with doses of 3600 cGy. Large fields, shaped to conform to the patient's anatomy, are designed to treat multiple contiguous lymph node regions. A *mantle* port covers the cervical, supraclavicular, infraclavicular, axillary, mediastinal, and hilar lymph nodes. The *para-aortic* field includes the para-aortic lymph nodes from the level of the diaphragm down to the aortic bifurcation but omits the pelvis and treats the splenic hilar lymph nodes in a patient with a prior splenectomy. An inverted-**Y** port in one field not only includes the para-aortic and splenic hilar lymph nodes but also extends into the pelvis to encompass the iliac and inguinal-femoral lymph nodes. The combination of a mantle and para-aortic field is also referred to as subtotal nodal or extended-field irradiation. *Total lymphoid irradiation* implies sequential treatment to both a mantle and an inverted-**Y** field.

The use of sequential large-field irradiation minimizes the risk of either overlap or underdosage, which could result in either undue normal tissue toxicity or inadequate therapy, respectively. Treatment of these large fields requires supervoltage radiation. This capability is available primarily with contemporary linear accelerators, which have the advantages over cobalt of skin sparing, increased depth dose, and sharp beam edges with reduced lateral scatter. The use of a treatment simulator to plan the radiotherapy fields and proper field verification (portal films) during the treatment process is essential.

Definitive radiation therapy alone is appropriate initial management for the majority of patients with PS I and II Hodgkin's disease. Mantle and para-aortic irradiation is the treatment of choice for most patients with PS IA and IIA disease, providing an 80 to 85 per cent chance of cure with irradiation alone. Selected patients with PS IA and IIA supradiaphragmatic disease of the nodular sclerosis or lymphocyte predominance histology who do not have mediastinal involvement can be treated with mantle radiotherapy alone. Many patients with stage IB and IIB disease can be treated effectively with mantle and para-aortic radiotherapy alone, with a 70 to 75 per cent chance of cure, provided they do not have both fever and weight loss and/or a large mediastinal mass. Controversy exists over the indications for using both radiotherapy and chemotherapy in stage I or II patients who present with large mediastinal masses, limited contiguous extranodal disease (the E lesion of the Ann Arbor system), or systemic symptoms. In each of these disease settings, the use of radiation alone results in a lower disease-free survival rate than when a combined-modality program is employed as the initial treatment, although the use of chemotherapy at relapse may provide an equivalent chance of cure. Patients with III$_S$A or III$_1$A Hodgkin's disease and minimal splenic involvement are usually treated with either mantle and para-aortic radiotherapy or total lymphoid irradiation alone. Controversy exists over whether prophylactic hepatic irradiation should be delivered to those patients with splenic involvement.

Subdiaphragmatic early-stage Hodgkin's disease is a relatively rare clinical presentation. These patients tend to be older and male and to have mixed cellularity pathology. Staging laparotomy is generally indicated with treatment based on pathologic findings. Patients with subdiaphragmatic stage IA are generally treated with inverted-**Y** radiotherapy. In patients with PS IIA, with or without limited splenic involvement, total lymphoid irradiation and combined-modality therapy appear to be of comparable efficacy, based on limited data.

Complications of radiation treatment are related to the technique employed, dosage administered, and irradiated volume. Acute side effects of radiotherapy include transient nausea and vomiting, dysphagia, and marrow suppression. These effects subside shortly after radiation therapy is completed. Late potential side effects of radiation include hypothyroidism, pneumonitis, transient myelitis (generally manifested as electric-like shocks in limbs on neck flexion known as *Lhermitte's sign*), and rarely pericarditis. Persistent myelosuppression is a rare late complication. Radiation-induced decreased bone growth has been noted in children.

Chemotherapy. The major advance in the treatment of stage IIIB and IV Hodgkin's disease was the development of curative combination chemotherapy. The initial studies from the National Cancer Institute demonstrated that a four-drug combination known as MOPP (nitrogen mustard [Mustargen], vincristine [Oncovin], procarbazine, and prednisone) was capable of producing documented complete remissions in 70 to 80 per cent of patients with advanced Hodgkin's disease. At least one half to two thirds of the patients who achieved complete remission with MOPP have not had recurrence after more than 10 to 20 years of observation. Thus, 50 per cent of all patients with stage IIIB and IV who underwent treatment were cured with MOPP chemotherapy alone.

The potential for clinical cure of Hodgkin's disease with chemotherapy exists for all histologic subtypes, stages, and extranodal sites of disease. Patients who have received prior radiotherapy and in whom relapse subsequently occurs have an equivalent chance of being cured with "salvage" chemotherapy. Older patients and those with bone marrow involvement, systemic symptoms, bulky disease, and poor performance status have a less favorable long-term response with chemotherapy. The best results have been reported for asymptomatic patients with disease limited to the lymph nodes and/or lung.

It is essential to administer the drugs in the MOPP regimen at full doses and in a timely fashion. Therapy is repeated every 4 weeks, for a minimum of six cycles. An additional two cycles are administered after a complete clinical remission is obtained. At that time, chemotherapy is discontinued only when repeat restaging studies document that a true complete remission has been obtained. The restaging diagnostic evaluation includes repeat radiologic procedures and biopsies as indicated to verify the complete response status. Maintenance chemotherapy beyond the documentation of a restaged complete remission is of no advantage in improving either disease-free or overall survival. Patients who have relapsed after definitive radiation treatment for early-stage disease are often salvaged and cured with the same chemotherapy regimens used for patients with previously untreated advanced disease.

No alternative four- or five-drug combinations have been demonstrated conclusively to be superior to MOPP, considering differences in patient selection, prognostic factors, restaging evaluation, and adequate follow-up. However, results comparable to those with MOPP have been achieved with a variety of alternative chemotherapy programs that offer significantly less toxicity than MOPP. Combinations that contain cyclophosphamide or chlorambucil instead of nitrogen mustard, vinblastine in place of vincristine, and/or the addition of a nitrosourea appear to be as efficacious as MOPP in producing durable complete responses but have substantially fewer side effects.

The identification of the active non–cross-resistant combination ABVD (doxorubicin [Adriamycin], bleomycin, vinblastine, and dacarbazine [DTIC]) in the patient who has had a relapse led to the investigation of sequential alternating chemotherapy regimens (i.e., MOPP alternating monthly with ABVD or a hybrid of seven drugs, MOPP/ABV, in one monthly cycle) as primary induction therapy. By exposing tumor cells to more drugs early in the course of disease, drug-resistant clones might be eradicated before growing too large to be cured. Recent randomized trials have demonstrated significantly improved relapse-free and overall survival with either alternating monthly MOPP/ABVD or the MOPP/ABV hybrid regimens compared with MOPP alone as first-line therapy. Thus, at the present time it now appears that MOPP can no longer be considered standard initial therapy for advanced-stage Hodgkin's disease. The use of ABVD alone is intriguing because of its apparently reduced long-term toxicity, but this regimen cannot be routinely recommended, as it is still being evaluated in controlled clinical trials.

The major complication of chemotherapy is bone marrow suppression with increased risk of infection and, rarely, hemorrhage. The peripheral blood counts are monitored carefully during chemotherapy, and drug doses are adjusted depending on the degree of myelosuppression. However, drug dose reductions made simply for the purpose of decreasing subjective toxicity are inappropriate because the opportunity for cure is also reduced. Sterility, more commonly seen in male patients, is a permanent side effect of chemotherapy. Significant nausea and vomiting are seen with the MOPP and ABVD regimens, requiring the use of antiemetic agents. These drug programs also often produce serious psychological problems that require effective counseling. Mild peripheral neuropathy is commonly seen with vincristine, but paresthesias are not an indication to reduce drug dosage. Acute leukemia as a late effect of chemotherapy alone is a recognized complication.

Combined-Modality Therapy. Combinations of irradiation and chemotherapy in the treatment of Hodgkin's disease have been utilized during the past 20 years with the goal of increasing the cure rate. It is logical to assume that combination chemotherapy, effective in curing a significant percentage of patients with advanced disease, should be even more effective for occult disease that might be present after radiation therapy. Patients who have recurrence after receiving MOPP chemotherapy frequently have relapse in sites of major pretreatment involvement, including bulky lymph node areas. An additional rationale for combined-modality therapy includes improved management of childhood Hodgkin's disease by reduction of radiation fields that may cause bone growth retardation, decreased requirement for staging laparotomy, and reduced complications from newer radiotherapy techniques involving larger treatment fields.

Adjuvant chemotherapy can substitute effectively for prophylactic irradiation of apparently uninvolved sites, but to date there is no clear justification for the routine use of a combined-modality approach for the overwhelming majority of patients with PS I or II disease. However, there are certain subsets of patients with early-stage Hodgkin's disease for whom combined-modality treatment is indicated because of an unacceptably high relapse rate, that is, patients with large mediastinal masses or contiguous extranodal involvement. In this subgroup of patients with early-stage disease who receive initial combined-modality therapy, staging laparotomy is not indicated, and treatment is initiated with one of the currently accepted regimens for advanced disease (e.g., MOPP/ABVD or the MOPP/ABV hybrid). Once maximal benefit from chemotherapy has been obtained, limited radiation therapy (generally to the mediastinum alone or a mantle field) is utilized. With this approach, approximately 80 to 85 per cent of patients remain relapse free beyond 5 years.

The treatment of PS IIIA Hodgkin's disease remains controversial. Retrospective studies have concentrated on identifying prognostic subgroups in which there is an unacceptably low disease-free survival with radiotherapy alone. At the present time, it would be premature for radiation therapists to abandon definitive irradiation in III₁A patients in whom the prognosis is favorable and who at laparotomy are found to have minimal involvement of the spleen or upper abdominal nodes. In this subgroup, mantle and para-aortic irradiation and total nodal irradiation appear equally effective as initial treatment, with chemotherapy reserved for those who relapse. However, for the majority of stage IIIA patients, chemotherapy alone or combined-modality therapy should be utilized. Patients to be treated in this manner should meet one or more of the following criteria: extensive splenic involvement (i.e., more than four splenic nodules), PS III₂A disease, unequivocal CS III₂A (grossly positive lymphangiogram and/or CT scan), and CS IIIA patients with large mediastinal masses. Although combination chemotherapy remains the mainstay for stage IIIB disease, both improved disease-free and overall survival may be obtained for those patients in whom initial chemotherapy followed by or sequenced with total nodal irradiation is utilized.

Significant improvement in survival rates as a result of combined-modality programs has not been clearly demonstrated for certain subsets of patients. In part, this is because of the long time (10 or more years) required to establish an overall survival benefit. Combined-modality programs generally demonstrate improved disease-free survival, but interpretation of current clinical trials must be tempered by the observation that patients who relapse after radiation alone are frequently salvaged or cured with chemotherapy administered only at the time of relapse. It may be more acceptable to treat patients conservatively at the onset of their disease with one method, reserving the more complicated combined-modality programs for those patients with poor prognostic factors and an unacceptably high relapse rate after primary irradiation alone.

The complications and morbidity of combined-modality programs are significant. The potential risk of acute complications, including profound and prolonged myelosuppression, sterility of both men and women, and demonstrated risk of second malignant tumors, has modified the enthusiasm for a combined-modality approach.

Second Neoplasms. Patients cured of their Hodgkin's disease are at an increased risk of developing second primary cancers. The most widely reported neoplasm is acute nonlymphocytic leukemia. The risk of leukemia is lowest in patients treated with radiotherapy alone, while the development of nonhematologic second neoplasms (e.g., lung cancer) increases significantly over time with this modality. The incidence of leukemia is approximately 3 to 9 per cent at 10 years in patients treated with chemotherapy alone using a MOPP-like regimen, with initial combined-modality therapy using adjuvant MOPP, and with salvage chemotherapy following relapse after radiotherapy. It is interesting that there does not appear to be an increased risk of leukemia after ABVD chemotherapy with or without radiotherapy.

Salvage Therapy for Advanced Disease. The choice of salvage therapy for patients relapsing after initial treatment must be individualized to the specific clinical circumstances of the relapse. Patients with early-stage disease relapsing after primary radiotherapy have a greater than 50 per cent chance of being cured with one of the accepted chemotherapy regimens used as initial treatment for stage III and IV disease (e.g., MOPP/ABVD or MOPP/ABV hybrid). For patients whose initial complete remission on chemotherapy lasted more than 1 year, retreatment with the same regimen results in a high rate of second complete response. Patients whose initial response to chemotherapy lasted less than 1 year and those who failed to achieve a complete response with initial chemotherapy represent a poor prognostic group. Recent experience with high-dose chemotherapy followed by autologous bone marrow transplantation now offers these patients a significant survival advantage and the possibility of cure.

Hodgkin's Disease in Acquired Immunodeficiency Syndrome (AIDS) Patients. There are increasing reports of Hodgkin's disease in AIDS patients. In these cases, Hodgkin's disease usually presents as stage IV, frequently with B symptoms and extranodal sites of involvement. Absence of mediastinal adenopathy is common, and marrow involvement in the absence of splenic disease has been reported. The presence of extranodal Hodgkin's disease alone should raise the suspicion of human immunodeficiency virus (HIV) infection. Although Hodgkin's disease in the AIDS patients responds to chemotherapy, these remissions are usually brief, and patients die of opportunistic infections or progressive Hodgkin's disease.

Recommended Therapy. The recommended therapy for a patient with Hodgkin's disease must be individualized. Important management considerations include stage and bulk of disease, age, prior therapy, medical complications, and availability of modern skills in radiotherapy and chemotherapy. The improved results of aggressive therapy after accurate clinical evaluation and pathologic staging are achievable only by experienced teams of physicians working closely together to achieve the excellent cure rates now possible while avoiding the risks of excesses in treatment. The recommended therapeutic approaches for the previously untreated adult patient with various stages of Hodgkin's disease are listed in Table 148–4. Estimated results are expressed as the percentage of patients likely to achieve a disease-free interval of 5 years. Careful evaluation of their condition and observation of a high proportion of patients, perhaps 90 or 95 per cent, who have survived free from relapse for 5 years demonstrate that they are cured of their disease.

A patient with early-stage disease who has relapsed after radiation therapy alone may be cured with salvage chemotherapy. Thus, freedom from a first or even second relapse must be considered in the evaluation of both disease-free and overall survival when the results of current clinical trials are analyzed. With dramatically improved treatment results, the challenge facing physicians and investigators caring for patients with all stages of Hodgkin's disease is to weigh carefully the toxicity-benefit ratio for each new recommended regimen.

PROGNOSIS. Hodgkin's disease is a curable malignant condition. Advances in histopathologic classification, precise diagnostic evaluation, and selection of appropriate aggressive therapy have led to continuous improvement in both disease-free and

TABLE 148-4. THE TREATMENT OF HODGKIN'S DISEASE IN ADULTS

Ann Arbor Pathologic Stage	Recommended Therapy	Estimated 5-Year Disease-Free Survival (%)
IA, I$_E$A, IIA, II$_E$A*†	Mantle and para-aortic radiotherapy	80–90
IB, I$_E$B, IIB, II$_E$B*	Mantle and para-aortic or total lymphoid radiotherapy	70–75
III$_1$A, III$_S$A*‡	Mantle and para-aortic radiotherapy ± chemotherapy or chemotherapy alone	60–85
III$_2$A	Combination chemotherapy (i.e., MOPP/ABVD or MOPP/ABV hybrid) ± total lymphoid radiotherapy	70–85
IIIB, III$_S$B, III$_E$B	Combination chemotherapy (i.e., MOPP/ABVD or MOPP/ABV hybrid) ± total lymphoid radiotherapy	60–80
IVA, IVB	Combination chemotherapy (i.e., MOPP/ABVD or MOPP/ABV hybrid)	55–70

*Patients with large mediastinal masses (>0.33 of the transverse diameter of the chest) are controlled by irradiation alone in approximately 40 to 50 per cent of cases and should receive combined-modality therapy (chemotherapy followed by irradiation) as primary management, with 5-year disease-free survival of 80 to 85 per cent.

†Patients with subdiaphragmatic state IA should receive inverted-Y radiotherapy, while patients with subdiaphragmatic stage IIA or II$_S$A with minimal splenic involvement are treated with either total lymphoid radiotherapy or chemotherapy plus inverted-Y radiotherapy.

‡Patients with extensive involvement of the spleen (> four nodules) are controlled by irradiation alone in approximately 40 per cent of cases and should receive combined-modality therapy (chemotherapy and irradiation) or chemotherapy alone as primary management.

overall survival. Survival figures and prognostic factors that were acceptable 10 or even 20 years ago are not acceptable today. The 5-year survival rate has increased from approximately 25 to 50 per cent 20 years ago to at least 75 per cent today.

The success of modern radiotherapy, chemotherapy, or combined-modality programs has obscured the significance of such important prognostic factors as histologic subtype, stage of disease, and the presence of systemic symptoms. In recent years, newer prognostic factors have been identified, including anatomic substage III$_2$A, extensive splenic disease, bulky mediastinal lymphadenopathy, and contiguous extranodal extension. Combined-modality treatment programs or chemotherapy alone is recommended for patients with these unfavorable prognostic factors. However, any potential disease-free survival advantage seen after combined-modality therapy must be balanced by the potential risk of late complications, particularly second malignant conditions, and must be translated into an overall survival benefit before general acceptance.

Table 148–4 presents a reasonable estimate of prognosis, recommended therapy, and current appropriate investigative approaches for the various stages of Hodgkin's disease. These treatment recommendations provide only the broadest of guidelines. Therapy must be individualized, depending on the specific clinical situation and the skill and experience of physicians treating the patient. Any treatment recommendations and estimates of cure must be viewed with the understanding that the management of Hodgkin's disease is dynamic, constantly undergoing change and refinement, and is designed to provide each patient with the best probability of cure and the least possibility of long-term toxicity.

Bonadonna G, Valagussa P, Santoro A: Alternating non–cross-resistant chemotherapy or MOPP in stage IV Hodgkin's disease: A report of 8-year results. Ann Intern Med 104:739, 1986. *The first report of the superiority of the MOPP/ABVD regimen over conventional chemotherapy. These results have now been confirmed.*

Crnkovich MJ, Leopold K, Hoppe RT, et al.: Stage I and IIB Hodgkin's disease: The combined experience at Stanford University and the Joint Center for Radiation Therapy. J Clin Oncol 5:1041, 1987. *The combined experience from two major institutions in the treatment of stage IB and IIB is reported, indicating that definitive radiotherapy is the preferred treatment for these patients.*

Glick JH, Portlock C: Hodgkin's disease: Clincial manifestations, staging, and treatment. *In* Benz EJ, Cohen HJ, Furie B, et al. (eds.): Hematology: Basic Principles and Practice. New York, Churchill Livingstone, 1991. *A thorough*

analysis and current review of staging and treatment for all stages of Hodgkin's disease are presented.

Jagannath S, Armitage JO, Dicke KA, et al.: Prognostic factors for response and survival after high-dose cyclophosphamide, carmustine, and etoposide with autologous bone marrow transplantation for relapsed Hodgkin's disease. J Clin Oncol 7:179, 1989. *An important summary of the benefits of high-dose chemotherapy and autologous bone marrow transplantation for relapsed Hodgkin's disease, indicating that prolonged disease-free survival can be obtained in this subset of patients.*

Kadin ME: Pathology and origin of Hodgkin's disease. *In* Benz EJ, Cohen HJ, Furie B, et al. (eds.): Hematology: Basic Principles and Practice. New York, Churchill Livingstone, 1991. *A complete review of current concepts in the histopathology of Hodgkin's disease, as well as a thoughtful discussion of the controversies surrounding the origin of the Reed-Sternberg cell.*

Kaplan H: Hodgkin's Disease. 2nd ed. Cambridge, MA, Harvard University Press, 1980. *A detailed, extensively illustrated and referenced volume covering every aspect of the disease as seen by one of the acknowledged experts and pioneers in the field.*

Klimo P, Connors JM: An update on the Vancouver experience in the management of advanced Hodgkin's disease treated with the MOPP/ABV hybrid program. Semin Hematol 25:34, 1988. *A report on an important new chemotherapy regimen, MOPP/ABV hybrid, for advanced disease. The results from this single institution trial await long-term follow-up but are being confirmed in large multi-institutional trials.*

Lister TA, Crowther D, Sutcliffe SB, et al.: Report of a committee convened to discuss the evaluation and staging of patients with Hodgkin's disease: Cotswolds meeting. J Clin Oncol 7:1630, 1989. *Report of an international multidisciplinary committee recommending modifications in the Ann Arbor staging classification to reflect changes in clinical staging criteria, newly recognized prognostic factors, and their impact on therapeutic decisions.*

Longo D, Young R, Wesley M, et al.: Twenty years of MOPP therapy for Hodgkin's disease. J Clin Oncol 4:1295, 1986. *A classic and important long-term follow-up report of MOPP-treated patients by the National Cancer Institute group.*

Mauch P, Larson D, Osteen R, et al.: Prognostic factors for positive surgical staging in patients with Hodgkin's disease. J Clin Oncol 8:257, 1990. *An important retrospective analysis correlating clinical stage and histopathology with pathologic stage as documented by staging laparotomy. This analysis suggests that certain subgroups of patients can be treated with limited-field radiotherapy without staging laparotomy.*

Mauch P, Tarbell N, Weinstein H, et al.: Stage IA and IIA supradiaphragmatic Hodgkin's disease: Prognostic factors in surgically staged patients treated with mantle and para-aortic irradiation. J Clin Oncol 6:1576, 1988. *A retrospective analysis of a large series of PS IA and IIA patients treated with mantle and para-aortic irradiation. Correlation with prognostic factors, including large mediastinal masses, is reported with long follow-up.*

Rosenberg S, Kaplan H: The evolution and summary results of the Stanford randomized clinical trials of the management of Hodgkin's disease. Int J Radiat Oncol Biol Phys 11:5, 1985. *The long-term follow-up on the important Stanford controlled trials of the use of radiotherapy with or without adjuvant chemotherapy.*

Young RC, Bookman MA, Longo DL: Late complications of Hodgkin's disease management. Monogr J Natl Cancer Inst 10:55, 1990. *A concise but detailed review of the late complications of radiotherapy, chemotherapy, and combined-modality treatment for Hodgkin's disease.*

149 Langerhans Cell (Eosinophilic) Granulomatosis

Jerome E. Groopman

The numerous and sometimes confusing classifications of clinical disorders associated with Langerhans cell proliferation reflect our ignorance of both the cause and the pathophysiology of many of these diseases. The Langerhans cell belongs to the larger family of cells termed *histiocytes*. Histiocytes are tissue macrophages and include the hepatic Kupffer cell, the alveolar macrophage of the lung, the giant cell of granulomas, and the osteoclast, in addition to the dermal Langerhans cell. The microglial cell of the brain is probably of macrophage origin as well. All of these tissue macrophages derive from precursor cells that normally reside in bone marrow, mature into circulating blood monocytes, and then egress into tissues and differentiate into a particular type of histiocyte.

A number of benign disorders are associated with proliferation of histiocytes and their fusion into multinucleated giant cells that form granulomas. Langerhans cell (eosinophilic) granulomatosis is an idiopathic benign disease characterized by proliferation and infiltration of tissue by histiocytes and eosinophils. Although this disorder was previously termed eosinophilic granuloma, the proliferating cell that appears primarily responsible for the clinical manifestations of the disorder is the Langerhans cell. The eosinophils may take residence in the lesion because of potent eosinophilic chemotactic factors released secondarily by the histiocytes. Langerhans cell granulomatosis is a distinct disorder unrelated to the eosinophilic syndromes (Ch. 150).

The interaction of "activated macrophages" with surrounding normal tissues may form the pathophysiologic substructure of many of the clinical features of Langerhans cell granulomatosis.

Clinical conditions of unknown cause characterized pathologically by proliferation of tissue macrophages in sheetlike masses with interspersed eosinophils have been difficult to define as specific disease entities. There is great histologic variability within these disorders, and lesions taken from different sites in the same patient may differ pathologically. The clinical course and prognosis do not correlate with histopathologic findings. The concept of Langerhans cell granulomatosis, Hand-Schüller-Christian disease (the classic triad of exophthalmos, diabetes insipidus, and bone destruction) and Letterer-Siwe disease as elements of a continuum termed histiocytosis X fails to recognize important differences in clinical course, organ involvement, and therapeutic response. This chapter discusses unifocal Langerhans cell granulomatosis, multifocal Langerhans cell granulomatosis, and Letterer-Siwe disease. These are the best characterized idiopathic histiocytoses, yet in clinical practice many cases do not readily fit into these categories.

UNIFOCAL LANGERHANS CELL (EOSINOPHILIC) GRANULOMATOSIS

Unifocal Langerhans cell granulomatosis is a benign disorder generally occurring in males during childhood or early adult life. It may occur as late as the sixth or seventh decade of life.

CLINICAL MANIFESTATIONS. The most common presentation of the disorder is a single osteolytic lesion in a long or flat bone, most frequently in the calvarium or femur in children and in a rib in adults. The predilection for skull, femur, rib, pelvis, vertebra, and mandible is not understood. The small bones of the distal extremities are not generally involved. Although the lesions are usually purely lytic, mixed blastic and lytic lesions occur. Pain and swelling over the affected area are common presenting symptoms, although disruption of teeth with mandibular disease, fracture, and otitis media due to mastoid involvement are not infrequent. Many lesions are asymptomatic and diagnosed serendipitously during radiologic evaluation for unrelated problems. Unifocal Langerhans cell granulomatosis of lymph nodes, thymus, or salivary glands is very rare and has the same benign course as that of the more frequent bone lesions. Unifocal Langerhans cell granulomatosis is rarely associated with systemic symptoms, and there are no characteristic laboratory findings. Diagnosis is established by biopsy.

DIAGNOSIS. The bone scan is very useful in determining that the lesion is indeed unifocal and in following patients over time for development of new osteolytic lesions. An open biopsy should be performed for diagnosis. Pathologically, an infiltrate with foamy macrophage and admixed eosinophils favors the diagnosis of Langerhans cell granulomatosis. Langerhans histiocytes contain a cytoplasmic inclusion of unknown composition but with constant thickness and striation termed an X body. They also stain by immunoperoxidase for a cytoplasmic protein termed S–100; detection of S–100 assists the histopathologic diagnosis of Langerhans cell granulomatosis.

TREATMENT. At the time of biopsy, curettage, with or without bone chip packing, should be carried out. This simple surgical approach is almost uniformly successful as definitive therapy for an individual lesion. Lesions in anatomic sites that are difficult to approach surgically, such as weight-bearing bones or cervical vertebrae, are best treated by low-dose (300 to 600 cGy fractioned total dose) local supervoltage irradiation. This low-dose radiotherapy generally eradicates the proliferating histiocytes and allows for normal bone repair, while high-dose radiotherapy leads to tissue damage and resultant poor healing. Surgical decompression followed by low-dose irradiation is some-

times indicated for lesions requiring emergency intervention, such as those compressing the spinal cord. Patients should be carefully followed after therapy for the development of new lesions, which generally arise within the first year after diagnosis. Individuals with a lesion in the bones of the head, neck, or pelvis are more likely to have subsequent disease. Bone scans to detect new lesions and plain films to follow the known site of involvement should be obtained every 6 months for 1 to 2 years after therapy. Extraosseous Langerhans cell granulomatosis involving soft tissue is generally successfully managed by complete surgical excision, if possible, or by low-dose irradiation.

MULTIFOCAL LANGERHANS CELL (EOSINOPHILIC) GRANULOMATOSIS

CLINICAL MANIFESTATIONS. Similar to the unifocal form, multifocal Langerhans cell granulomatosis generally presents in children, predominantly in males, and often with bone lesions. In addition to the calvarium, the sphenoid bone, sella turcica, mandible, and long bones of the upper extremities may be involved. This tropism for the head is unexplained but may indicate local reaction to an inciting agent that enters via the nasopharynx or oropharynx. Complications of this disorder include chronic otitis media caused by destruction of temporal and mastoid bones, proptosis with orbital masses, loose teeth with infiltration of maxilla or mandible, and both anterior and posterior pituitary dysfunction with involvement of the sella turcica. This last complication may occur with focal disease of the hypothalamus or pituitary without bone involvement, and growth retardation of the patient may occur. Diabetes insipidus is caused by granulomatous involvement of the hypothalamus or pituitary and may be either transient or permanent. The classic triad of lytic skull lesions, exophthalmos, and diabetes insipidus, called Hand-Schüller-Christian disease, is best viewed as a subset of multifocal Langerhans cell (eosinophilic) granulomatosis. Dermal lesions may appear papulosquamous, seborrheic, eczematous, and rarely xanthomatous. Vulvar lesions with ulceration are not uncommon. Hepatosplenomegaly and lymphadenopathy are unusual in multifocal Langerhans cell granulomatosis.

In Langerhans cell granulomatosis the lung is an important extraosseous site of involvement. The disorder mainly affects young adult men and often manifests with a chronic cough, pneumothorax, and constitutional symptoms. The chest radiograph usually shows a diffuse micronodular and interstitial infiltrate involving the mid-zones and bases of the lungs with relative sparing of the costophrenic angles. Ultimately, a honeycomb appearance may occur; it is caused by coalescence of small parenchymal pulmonary cysts. Fibrosis is a late finding that may lead to chronic cor pulmonale. Pulmonary function tests may show restrictive impairment. Diagnosis is best made by biopsy that shows the mixed histiocytic-eosinophilic infiltrate with a variable degree of fibrosis. Pulmonary Langerhans cell granulomatosis has a highly variable natural history. Spontaneous remissions are not infrequent, but prognosis is poorer at the extremes of age and with involvement of extrapulmonary organs.

DIAGNOSIS. There are no distinctive laboratory abnormalities in multifocal Langerhans cell granulomatosis. The leukocyte count is generally normal, and eosinophilia is not present unless it is from another cause. Hypercalcemia generally does not result from bone lesions.

The diagnosis of multifocal Langerhans cell granulomatosis is definitively made by biopsy (see Color Plate 7H, right), usually of a bone lesion. Again, S–100 detected by the immunoperoxidase method may be useful in confirming the diagnosis. The extent of multifocal involvement is established by physical examination, chest radiography, bone scanning, and, if indicated, computed tomography of the brain. This last test is useful for hypothalamic or pituitary lesions associated with diabetes insipidus.

TREATMENT. The natural history of multifocal Langerhans cell granulomatosis is relatively favorable when cases best diagnosed as Letterer-Siwe disease (see below) are excluded. Destructive lesions of bone, when present early in the clinical course, may predict a better outcome. The therapy is guided by the particular organs involved. Diabetes insipidus and growth retardation should be treated by hormonal replacement with vasopressin (Ch. 213) and human growth hormone, respectively. Low-dose irradiation to the suprasellar area may restore endocrine function in certain individuals. The seborrheic dermal eruption is responsive to tar treatments. X-irradiation using doses generally below 600 cGy to symptomatic bone lesions is nearly always effective. Surgery may be necessary to relieve spinal cord compression and mastoid problems and to excise skull lesions eroding through skin. Oral granulomatosis can be treated with dexamethasone elixir used as a mouth rinse three times a day. Similarly, topical steroid creams may accelerate the healing of vulvar lesions.

Systemic therapy is indicated when either radiation fails or multiple sites demand treatment. Corticosteroids alone may achieve dramatic results. Prednisone at a single dose of 0.5 to 1.0 mg per kilogram can be used in the acute phase. Alternate-day corticosteroid therapy can be initiated after remission is achieved. Use of cytotoxic agents, such as vinblastine or methotrexate, is generally reserved for aggressive and refractory disease.

There is insufficient experience to recommend a single first-line chemotherapeutic regimen. Addition of vinblastine at a dose of 0.1 mg per kilogram intravenously every week for 4 to 8 weeks is generally successful in achieving remission. It is unclear whether maintenance chemotherapy with weekly vinblastine or prednisone is required to sustain remission. Should disease recur within several months after discontinuation of therapy for the acute phase, the patient should be re-treated with the initially successful regimen and receive maintenance therapy. The striking variability in clinical course makes it difficult to generalize with regard to therapeutic guidelines.

LETTERER-SIWE SYNDROME

In 1924 Letterer described a 6-month-old child with diffuse purpura, fever, otitis media, lymphadenopathy, and hepatosplenomegaly. Nine years later, Siwe included this case in a series of six similar cases. In all instances, there was diffuse tissue infiltration by histiocytes. The histiocytes of Letterer-Siwe disease have abundant acidophilic cytoplasm and are often vacuolated. There may be prominent hemophagocytosis. Generally, there is a relative paucity of eosinophils in the histiocytic infiltrates.

CLINICAL MANIFESTATIONS. Children are usually affected in the first years of life, although an adult form of the syndrome may exist. Liver, spleen, lymph nodes, lung, and bone are the most commonly affected areas. Laboratory evaluation often demonstrates leukocytosis, although pancytopenia caused by hypersplenism or bone marrow infiltration may be seen. The dermal lesion of Letterer-Siwe disease is generally a brown-red, scaly eczematoid or seborrheic eruption, and purpura secondary to thrombocytopenia may be present. Hepatosplenomegaly may occur with or without jaundice or elevated levels of hepatic parenchymal enzymes. There is no familial or hereditary predisposition, and that distinguishes Letterer-Siwe disease from another histiocytic disorder of infants, familial erythrophagocytic lymphohistiocytosis. A clinical pathologic syndrome nearly identical to Letterer-Siwe disease has been described in immunologically compromised children infected with a variety of viruses. In addition, certain cases termed Letterer-Siwe disease may actually be unusual forms of malignant lymphoma.

TREATMENT. The course of Letterer-Siwe disease is commonly fulminant and fatal. Spontaneous remissions are rare. It is important to distinguish Letterer-Siwe disease from disorders of infectious or clearly neoplastic origin before initiating therapy. Systemic symptoms of Letterer-Siwe disease often improve with corticosteroids, and focal lesions may be palliated with radiotherapy. Occasionally, clinical remission has been achieved with chemotherapy, particularly vinblastine and prednisone. If this regimen fails, methotrexate and 6-mercaptopurine may be used. Successful allogeneic bone marrow transplantation has been reported in a single case.

Chu T, D'Angio GJ, Favara, B, et al.: Histiocytosis syndromes in children. Lancet 1:208, 1987. *This brief article offers an up-to-date classification of this group of disorders "not only as a standard for diagnosis and patient management but also for research and for use in publications on the subject."*

Greenberger JS, Crocker AC, Vawter G, et al.: Results of treatment of 27 patients with systemic histiocytosis (Letterer-Siwe syndrome, Schuller-Christian syndrome and multifocal eosinophilic granuloma). Medicine 60:311, 1981. *A detailed analysis of therapy of histiocytic disorders at a single academic medical center.*

Groopman JE, Golde DW: The histiocytic disorder: A pathophysiologic analysis.

Ann Intern Med 94:95, 1981. *Comprehensive review of the histiocytic disorders, with emphasis on pathophysiologic mechanisms; extensive bibliography.*

Komp DM: Langerhans cell histiocytosis. N Engl J Med 316:747, 1987. *An informative editorial with an excellent bibliography.*

Novice FM, Collison DW, Kleinsmith DM, et al.: Letterer-Siwe disease in adults. Cancer 63:166, 1989. *An illustrative case report and comprehensive review of adult cases, with emphasis on treatment options; extensive bibliography.*

Sims DG: Histiocytosis X: Follow-up of 43 cases. Arch Dis Child 52:433, 1977. *A large series followed over a long period; illustrates the striking variability in clinical course.*

Zinkham WH: Multifocal eosinophilic granuloma: Natural history, etiology and management. Am J Med 60:457, 1976. *A comprehensive and well-written clinical paper; of great assistance in clinical management.*

---

150 Eosinophilic Syndromes

Peter F. Weller

Eosinophilia, often with heightened production of eosinophils as well as increased blood and tissue eosinophil accumulations, is associated with distinctive disease processes that include helminthic parasitic infections, allergic diseases, and a diversity of diseases of often ill-defined etiologies. Several eosinophil-related diseases are discussed in other chapters. This chapter provides an overview on eosinophils as a distinct class of leukocytes and considers the variety of diseases associated with eosinophilia.

STRUCTURE OF EOSINOPHILS. Eosinophils are distinguished from other leukocytes by their morphologies, constituents, products, and associations with specific diseases. Eosinophils are produced in the bone marrow. The cytokine interleukin 5, which specifically promotes the development and terminal differentiation of eosinophils, is principally responsible for increases in eosinophilopoiesis. Eosinophils normally dwell primarily in tissues, especially in tissues with an epithelial interface with the environment, including the respiratory, gastrointestinal, and lower genitourinary tracts. The lifespan of eosinophils, longer than that of neutrophils, may extend for weeks within tissues. Eosinophils, of a size similar to neutrophils but with usually bilobed nuclei, are morphologically characterized by their cytoplasmic granules. Specific granules, the most numerous of several types of cytoplasmic granules, have unique crystalloid cores and contain eosinophil-specific cationic proteins. These cationic granule proteins, which bind acidic dyes like eosin, are responsible both for the tinctorial properties and for many of the functional properties of eosinophils. The four eosinophil cationic proteins are major basic protein, eosinophil peroxidase, eosinophil cationic protein, and eosinophil-derived neurotoxin. Lysophospholipase, another predominant eosinophil protein, forms bipyramidal Charcot-Leyden crystals, often found in sputum, feces, and tissues as a hallmark of eosinophil-related diseases. In addition to their content of preformed granule proteins, eosinophils also elaborate newly synthesized lipid mediators, including the 5-lipoxygenase pathway–derived eicosanoid, leukotriene C_4, and platelet activating factor.

FUNCTION OF EOSINOPHILS. Eosinophils serve several immunologic functions. Eosinophils are capable of phagocytosing and killing bacteria and other small microbes. In vivo however, eosinophils do not have a major role in host defense against such microbial pathogens and cannot constitute an effective defense against bacterial infections when neutrophil function is deficient. Rather, eosinophils primarily defend against large, nonphagocytosable organisms, most notably the multicellular, helminthic parasites, utilizing several mechanisms, including their cytotoxic cationic granule proteins. In allergic diseases, including asthma, eosinophils elaborate specific lipid mediators, leukotriene C_4 and platelet activating factor, which can contract airway smooth muscle, promote mucus secretion, alter vascular permeability, and elicit eosinophil and neutrophil infiltration. Eosinophils can also elicit the release of allergic mediators from mast cells and from basophils. Some of the mechanisms beneficial in the eosinophil's role in host defense can prove detrimental to the host. Released eosinophil cationic proteins are toxic to host cells and may contribute to the pathogenesis of diseases in which heightened numbers of eosinophils are found within involved tissues. The effector functions of mature eosinophils, whether they be mediated by release of preformed granule proteins or by the synthesis of new lipid mediators, can be stimulated by cytokines, including interleukin 5 and granulocyte macrophage colony-stimulating factor. Additional immunologic functions, based on the eosinophil's capabilities to interact collaboratively with lymphocytes and other cells, are beginning to be defined, which may further contribute to our understanding of how eosinophils participate in normal mucosal immune responses and in eosinophil-related diseases.

Blood eosinophil numbers do not always reflect the extent of eosinophil involvement in affected tissues in various diseases. Eosinophils usually number less than 450 per microliter in the blood, with a mild diurnal variation, being higher in the early morning and falling as endogenous glucocorticosteroid levels rise. Eosinopenia occurs with corticosteroid administration and also is frequent with active bacterial and viral infections. Some patients with sustained blood eosinophilia develop organ damage, especially cardiac damage, as found in the idiopathic hypereosinophilic syndrome. Why this complication of sustained eosinophilia occurs in some patients but not others is unclear. It suggests that some other activating events, as yet ill-defined, promote eosinophil-mediated tissue damage in the face of eosinophilia. Patients with sustained eosinophilia should be monitored for evidence of cardiac disease (see below).

DISEASES ASSOCIATED WITH EOSINOPHILIA
(Table 150–1)

PARASITIC DISEASES. Eosinophilia is not elicited by infections with single-celled protozoan parasites (with the exception of the intestinal coccidian parasite *Isospora belli*), but rather by the multicellular helminthic parasites. The level of eosinophilia tends to parallel the magnitude and extent of tissue invasion, especially by larvae. Eosinophilia may be absent in established infections that are well contained within tissues or are solely intraluminal in the gastrointestinal tract (e.g., *Ascaris*, tapeworms). Even with helminthic diseases, superimposed bacterial infections (e.g., in disseminated strongyloidiasis) can suppress eosinophilia. In evaluating a patient with unexplained eosinophilia, geographic and dietary histories are germane in indicating potential exposures to helminthic parasites. The stool should be examined for diagnostic ova and larvae, although with some infections more than the usual three examinations may be needed. In addition, for a number of the helminthic parasites that cause eosinophilia, diagnostic parasite stages are never present in feces. Hence, normal stool examinations do not necessarily exclude a helminthic etiology for eosinophilia, and examination of appropriate blood or tissue biopsy specimens, as guided by the clinical findings and exposure histories, may be needed. Specific tissue or blood-dwelling infections capable of causing eosinophilia include trichinosis, filarial infections, and, in children, visceral larva migrans.

OTHER INFECTIOUS DISEASES. Acute bacterial and viral infections usually cause eosinopenia, although in the convalescent phase of these diseases eosinophil numbers return to normal and at times to above normal, as seen with scarlet fever. Two fungal

TABLE 150–1. DISEASES ASSOCIATED WITH EOSINOPHILIA

I. Infectious diseases
   A. Tissue-invasive helminths
      1. Principally outside North America
         a. Filariasis (especially in those from nonendemic regions)
         b. Schistosomiasis, acute and chronic
         c. Fascioliasis, acute
         d. Paragonimiasis
         e. Clonorchiasis
         f. Echinococcosis (often absent unless cyst fluid leakage)
      2. Indigenous to North America and other regions
         a. Trichinosis
         b. Toxocariasis (visceral larva migrans)
         c. Strongyloidiasis (may be suppressed with sepsis in hyperinfection syndrome)
         d. Ascariasis and hookworm disease (especially with early lung and tissue invasive stages)
   B. Other infections
      1. Coccidioidomycosis (acute and less commonly chronic)
      2. Bronchopulmonary aspergillosis
      3. Afebrile tuberculosis
      4. Convalescent phase of some infections, especially scarlet fever
      5. Chlamydial pneumonia of infancy
II. Allergic diseases
   A. Allergic rhinitis
   B. Asthma
   C. Atopic dermatitis
   D. Acute urticaria
   E. Hypersensitivity drug reactions
III. Myeloproliferative and neoplastic diseases
   A. Idiopathic hypereosinophilic syndrome
   B. Solid tumors, principally of mucin-secreting, epithelial cell origin, when metastatic to serosa or bone
   C. Lymphoid
      1. Lymphomas, especially T cell type and Hodgkin's disease
      2. Acute lymphoblastic leukemia, only uncommonly
      3. Occasionally with myeloma (heavy-chain disease)
   D. Myelogenous
      1. Eosinophilic leukemia—rare
      2. Chronic myelogenous leukemia
      3. Acute myelogenous leukemia, with some subtypes
   E. Other
      1. Angioimmunoblastic lymphadenopathy
      2. Histiocytosis with cutaneous involvement
      3. Angiolymphoid hyperplasia (Kimura's disease)

IV. Other cutaneous disease
   A. Bullous pemphigoid
   B. Herpes gestationis
   C. Scabies
   D. Eosinophilic cellulitis (Well's disease)
   E. Episodic angioedema with eosinophilia
   F. Pruritic urticarial papules and plaques of pregnancy
V. Other pulmonary diseases
   A. Transient pulmonary eosinophilic infiltrates (Löffler's syndrome)
   B. Hypersensitivity pneumonitis
   C. Allergic bronchopulmonary aspergillosis
   D. Tropical pulmonary eosinophilia
   E. Eosinophilic pneumonia—acute and chronic
VI. Connective tissue diseases
   A. Vasculitis
      1. Allergic granulomatosis with angiitis (Churg-Strauss syndrome)
      2. Hypersensitivity vasculitis
   B. Rheumatoid arthritis (severe)
   C. Eosinophilic fasciitis
VII. Immunodeficiency diseases
   A. Hyper-IgE syndrome
   B. Wiskott-Aldrich syndrome
   C. Nezelof's syndrome with thymic dysplasia and increased IgE
   D. Selective IgA deficiency, when associated with increased IgE
   E. Graft-versus-host reactions
VIII. Gastrointestinal diseases
   A. Eosinophilic gastroenteritis
   B. Inflammatory bowel disease
IX. Occasional causes of eosinophilia
   A. Cholesterol embolization
   B. Long-term peritoneal dialysis
   C. Postirradiation
   D. Hypoadrenocorticosteroidism: Addison's disease, hypopituitarism
   E. Other localized disorders with occasional blood eosinophilia
      1. Eosinophilic lymphadenitis
      2. Eosinophilic cystitis
      3. Eosinophilic cholecystitis
      4. Eosinophilic meningitis
   F. Toxic: L-tryptophan, toxic oil syndrome (Spain)

diseases may be associated with eosinophilia: aspergillosis, but only in the form of allergic bronchopulmonary aspergillosis and not as invasive disease (Ch. 406), and coccidioidomycosis, following primary infection, especially in conjunction with erythema nodosum and at times with progressive disseminated disease (Ch. 400). On occasion, eosinophilia may be present in chronic tuberculosis.

ALLERGIC DISEASES. These diseases, including allergic rhinitis and asthma, are discussed elsewhere (Ch. 246 and 57). Hypersensitivity drug reactions can elicit eosinophilia, not necessarily accompanied by other manifestations, such as drug fever or organ dysfunction. When organ dysfunction develops, the drug must be stopped. Drug-induced interstitial nephritis (Ch. 80) may be accompanied by blood eosinophilia, and eosinophils may be found in the urine.

MYELOPROLIFERATIVE DISEASES. The idiopathic hypereosinophilic syndrome (see Color Plate 7H, left) is a myeloproliferative disease characterized by sustained overproduction of eosinophils. The three diagnostic criteria for this disorder are (1) eosinophilia in excess of 1500 per microliter of blood persisting for longer than 6 months, (2) lack of an identifiable parasitic, allergic, or other etiologic cause for eosinophilia; and (3) signs and symptoms of organ involvement. Not all patients with prolonged eosinophilia develop organ involvement, and many have benign courses. Moreover, the above diagnostic criteria are sufficiently broad to include, potentially, eosinophilic disorders of other etiologies, currently unrecognized, that may have more favorable courses. The presence of angioedema was recognized as a good prognostic sign in hypereosinophilic patients, and this finding may be related to the more recent identification of a distinct clinical syndrome of recurrent episodic angioedema with eosinophilia, not complicated by the development of hypereosinophilic cardiac disease. The clinical signs and symptoms of the hypereosinophilic syndrome can be heterogeneous, since patients reflect the diversity of potential organ involvement. One of the most serious and more frequent complications in this disorder is cardiac disease due to endomyocardial thrombosis and fibrosis. Chordae tendineae may sustain progressive fibrotic damage, leading to mitral and tricuspid regurgitation and congestive heart failure from valvular incompetence and endomyocardial fibrosis. Echocardiography can facilitate detection and monitoring of these changes. Neurologic involvement can take three forms: embolic disease originating from the heart, diffuse encephalopathy, and peripheral neuropathy, especially mononeuritis multiplex. Other organ systems that can be involved include the skin, liver, spleen, gastrointestinal tract, and lungs. For patients with prominent organ involvement and no therapy, mortality is about 75 per cent after 3 years. Therapy is aimed at suppressing eosinophilia and is initiated with corticosteroids, to which about one third of patients respond. In those unresponsive to corticosteroids, hydroxyurea may be beneficial. For those unresponsive to or intolerant of hydroxyurea, vincristine or chlorambucil, alone or with lower doses of hydroxyurea, can control the disease. Similar cardiac involvement to that seen in the hypereosinophilic syndrome, which may require surgical valve replacement, may occur rarely with eosinophilias of other etiologies, including parasitic infections. A pathologically similar disease, Löffler's endocarditis and endomyocardial fibrosis, occurs in tropical regions, where it is possible that antecedent parasite-elicited eosinophilias are responsible for the development of this cardiac disease.

NEOPLASTIC DISEASES. Eosinophilic leukemia is distinctly uncommon. Eosinophilia may accompany chronic myelogenous leukemia (often with basophilia) and some subtypes of acute myelogenous leukemia but is uncommon with acute lymphoblastic leukemia. In a minority of patients with Hodgkin's disease, blood eosinophil levels are elevated, occasionally to high values. Increases in marrow and lymph node eosinophilia are more common. A small proportion of patients with carcinomas, especially those of mucin-producing epithelial cell origins, have associated blood eosinophilia. About a third of patients with angioimmunoblastic lymphadenopathy have eosinophilia. Eosinophilia may accompany mycosis fungoides, Sézary's syndrome, and lymphomatoid papulosis.

CUTANEOUS DISEASES. In addition to the neoplastic involvement of skin noted above, a number of cutaneous diseases can be associated with eosinophilia, including scabies, bullous pemphigoid, and two diseases associated with pregnancy, herpes gestationis and the syndrome of pruritic urticarial papules and plaques of pregnancy. In episodic angioedema with eosinophilia, recurrences are marked by blood eosinophilia; by prominent angioedema, at times with significant weight gain from fluid retention; and less frequently by fever. This entity is responsive to corticosteroids.

PULMONARY EOSINOPHILIAS (see Ch. 60). Blood eosinophilia can infrequently accompany pleural fluid eosinophilia, which is a nonspecific response seen with various disorders, including trauma and even repeated thoracenteses.

GASTROINTESTINAL DISEASES. Eosinophilic gastroenteritis (Ch. 112) and inflammatory bowel diseases (Ch. 103) are considered elsewhere. Although eosinophils are present in the lesions of ulcerative colitis, on occasion increased blood eosinophilia can accompany both ulcerative colitis and Crohn's disease.

IMMUNE DISEASES. Of the various forms of vasculitis (Ch. 264), only two are commonly associated with eosinophilia: hypersensitivity vasculitis and allergic granulomatous angiitis, the Churg-Strauss syndrome, in which asthma, eosinophilia, and pulmonary and neurologic involvement are frequent. Cholesterol embolization is at times associated with eosinophilia and hypocomplementemia, suggesting a secondarily elicited immunologic component. Some primary immunodeficiency syndromes are associated with eosinophilia, either commonly with the hyper–immunoglobulin E (IgE) syndrome, the Wiskott-Aldrich syndrome, and graft-versus-host disease or more selectively with Nezelof's syndrome and selective immunoglobulin A (IgA) deficiency when these are accompanied by increased levels of IgE. Eosinophilic fasciitis (Ch. 262) and rheumatoid arthritis (Ch. 258) are considered elsewhere. Eosinophilia may uncommonly accompany rheumatoid arthritis itself but is more commonly due to treatment medications.

OTHER DISEASES. Irritation of serosal surfaces can be associated with eosinophilia, e.g., Dressler's syndrome, eosinophilic pleural effusions, peritoneal and, at times, blood eosinophilia that develops during chronic peritoneal dialysis, and perhaps the eosinophilia that follows abdominal irradiation. Two notable apparently toxic diseases, the eosinophilia-myalgia syndrome due to contaminated L-tryptophan and the earlier toxic oil syndrome in Spain, were prominently associated with eosinophilia. Loss of normal adrenoglucocorticosteroid production in Addison's disease, adrenal hemorrhage, or hypopituitarism can cause modest eosinophilia (Ch. 217.6).

Fauci AS, Harley JB, Roberts WC, et al.: NIH Conference. The idiopathic hypereosinophilic syndrome. Clinical, pathophysiologic, and therapeutic considerations. Ann Intern Med 97:78, 1982. *Provides a review of the idiopathic hypereosinophilic syndrome with considerations of the prognosis and therapy for this disorder, based on experience at a referral center that has had the opportunity to evaluate many eosinophilic patients.*

Nutman TB, Ottesen EA, Cohen SG: The eosinophil, eosinophilia, and eosinophil-related disorders. III. Clinical assessments and eosinophil-related disorders. Allergy Proc 10:33, 1989.

Nutman TB, Ottesen EA, Cohen SG: The eosinophil, eosinophilia, and eosinophil-related disorders. IV. Eosinophil-related disorders (continued). Allergy Proc 10:47, 1989. *These articles discuss the approach to the patient with eosinophilia and provide a thorough consideration of the various diseases associated with eosinophilia.*

Weller PF: The immunobiology of eosinophils. N Engl J Med 324:1110, 1991. *A brief review of the structure and immunologic functions of eosinophilic leukocytes.*

151 Plasma Cell Disorders*

Robert A. Kyle

The plasma cell disorders are a group of neoplastic or potentially neoplastic diseases associated with proliferation of a single clone of immunoglobulin-secreting plasma cells derived from the B cell series of immunocytes. This group of disorders has been

*Copyright 1990, The Mayo Foundation, Rochester, MN.

referred to as monoclonal gammopathies, immunoglobulinopathies, paraproteinemias, and dysproteinemias.

The plasma cell disorders are characterized by the secretion of electrophoretically and immunologically homogeneous (monoclonal) proteins. Each monoclonal protein (M-protein, myeloma protein, or paraprotein) consists of two heavy (H) polypeptide chains of the same class and subclass and two light (L) polypeptide chains of the same type (Fig. 242–1). The heavy polypeptide chains are designated by Greek letters: γ in immunoglobulin G (IgG), α in immunoglobulin A (IgA), μ in immunoglobulin M (IgM), δ in immunoglobulin D (IgD), and ε in immunoglobulin E (IgE). The subclasses of IgG are IgG1, IgG2, IgG3, and IgG4. There are two subclasses of IgA—IgA1 and IgA2. No subclasses of IgM, IgD, or IgE have been recognized. The light-chain types are kappa (κ) and lambda (λ). Both heavy chains and light chains have "constant" and "variable" regions with respect to amino acid sequence. Class specificity of each immunoglobulin is defined by a series of antigenic determinants on the constant regions of the heavy chains (γ, α, μ, δ, and ε) and the two major classes of light chains (κ and λ). The amino acid sequence in the variable regions of the immunoglobulin molecule corresponds to the active antigen-combining site of the antibody, whereas the constant regions convey other biologic properties (see Ch. 242).

RECOGNITION OF MONOCLONAL PROTEINS

Electrophoresis with cellulose acetate membrane is satisfactory for screening. High-resolution agarose gel electrophoresis is more sensitive for the detection of small monoclonal proteins. Immunoelectrophoresis or immunofixation with agarose gel or both should be used to confirm the presence of a monoclonal protein and to distinguish the immunoglobulin class and its light-chain type.

Analysis of Serum for Protein

Serum protein electrophoresis should be done when multiple myeloma, macroglobulinemia, or amyloidosis is suspected. Electrophoresis is also indicated in any patient with unexplained weakness or fatigue, anemia, back pain, osteoporosis, osteolytic lesions or spontaneous fracture, elevation of the erythrocyte sedimentation rate, hypercalcemia, Bence Jones proteinuria, renal insufficiency, immunoglobulin deficiency, or recurrent infections. It should also be performed in adults with sensorimotor peripheral neuropathy, carpal tunnel syndrome, refractory congestive heart failure, nephrotic syndrome, orthostatic hypotension, or malabsorption, because a spike or localized band is strongly suggestive of primary systemic amyloidosis (AL).

A monoclonal protein (M-protein) is usually seen as a narrow peak (like a church spire) in the densitometer tracing or as a dense, discrete band on the cellulose acetate membrane (Fig. 151–1A). Although the immunoglobulins (IgG, IgA, IgM, IgD, and IgE) compose the gamma component, they are also found in the β-γ or β region, and IgG may actually extend to the α_2-globulin area. Consequently, an IgG monoclonal protein may range from the slow gamma (cathode) to the α_2-globulin region. In contrast, an excess of polyclonal immunoglobulins (having one or more heavy-chain types and both κ and λ light chains) produces a broad-based peak or broad band. It is usually limited to the γ region (Fig. 151–1B). It is important to differentiate between a monoclonal protein and a polyclonal increase because the former is associated with a malignant process or a potentially neoplastic condition, whereas a polyclonal increase in immunoglobulins is associated with a reactive or inflammatory process. In 2 to 3 per cent of sera with a monoclonal peak, there is an additional monoclonal protein of a different immunoglobulin class. This condition is designated as a biclonal (double) gammopathy.

The presence of an M-protein is most suggestive of monoclonal gammopathy of undetermined significance (MGUS), multiple myeloma, primary amyloidosis, Waldenström's macroglobulinemia, or other lymphoproliferative disease. Rarely, other conditions may also simulate the presence of an M-protein in the serum, e.g., free hemoglobin-haptoglobin complexes resulting from hemolysis, large amounts of transferrin in patients with iron deficiency anemia, or the presence of fibrinogen. On the other hand, a monoclonal protein may appear as a rather broad band

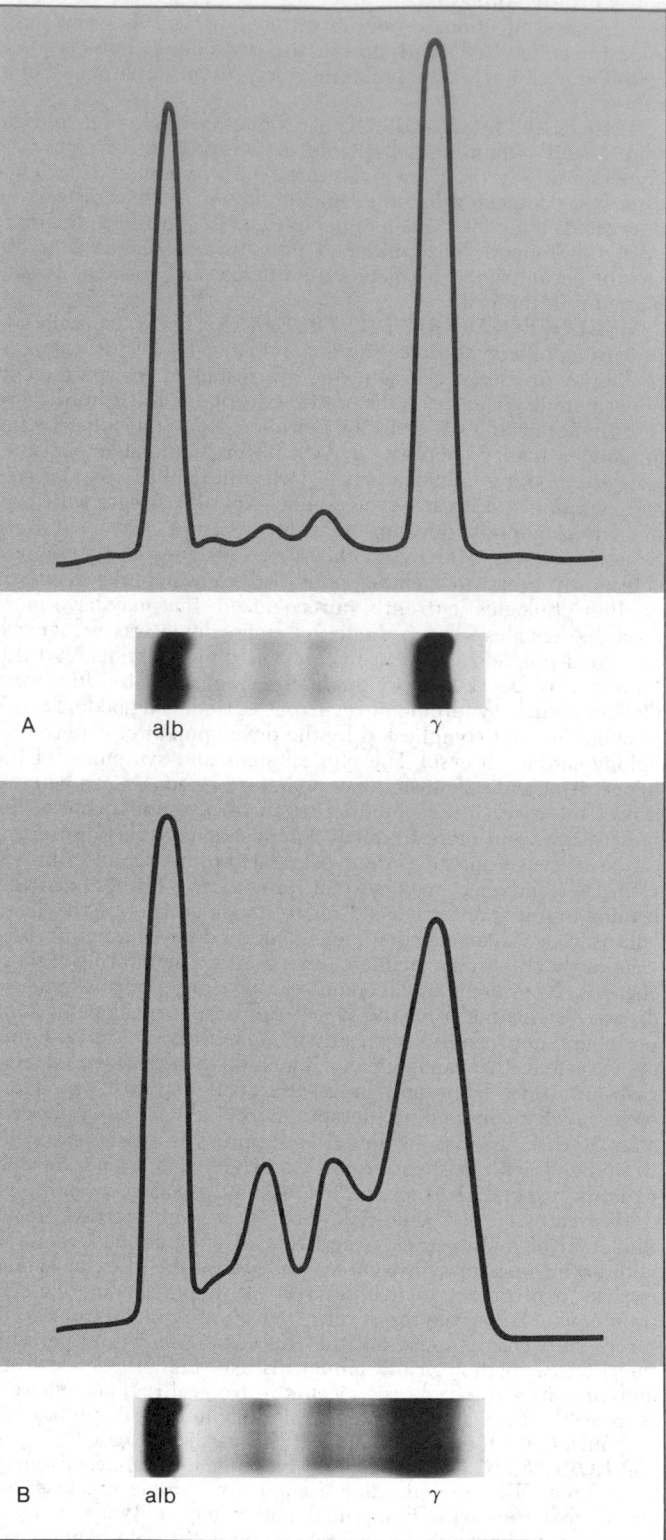

FIGURE 151–1. *A, top,* Monoclonal pattern of serum protein from densitometer tracing after electrophoresis on cellulose acetate (anode on left): tall, narrow-based peak of γ mobility. *Bottom,* Monoclonal pattern from electrophoresis of serum on cellulose acetate (anode on left): dense, localized band representing monoclonal protein in γ area. *B, top,* Polyclonal pattern of serum protein from densitometer tracing after electrophoresis on cellulose acetate (anode on left): broad-based peak of γ mobility. *Bottom,* Polyclonal pattern from electrophoresis of serum on cellulose acetate (anode on left): γ band is broad. (*A* and *B* from Kyle RA, Garton JP: Laboratory monitoring of myeloma proteins. Semin Oncol 13:310, 1986; with permission of W. B. Saunders Company.)

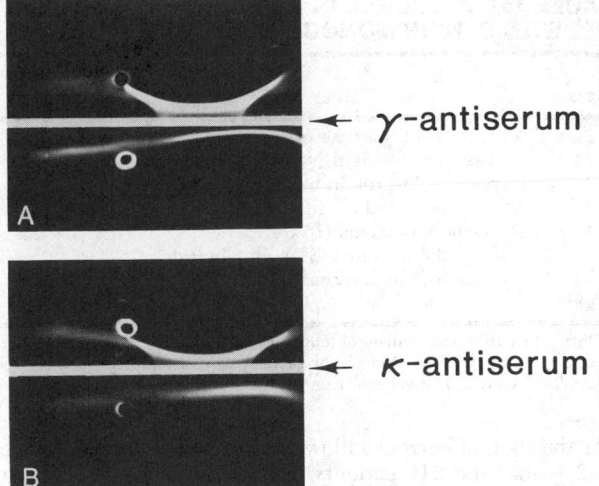

← γ-antiserum

← κ-antiserum

FIGURE 151–2. Immunoelectrophoretic pattern of serum. *A, top,* Antiserum to IgG (γ) shows a thickened arc. *B, top,* Antiserum to κ chains shows a thickened arc similar to the IgG arc. *A* and *B, bottom,* Antiserum to γ and to κ chains shows a faint normal arc. Patient's serum contains a monoclonal IgG κ protein. (From Kyle RA, Greipp PR: 3. The laboratory investigation of monoclonal gammopathies. Mayo Clin Proc 53:719, 1978; with permission of the Mayo Foundation, Rochester, MN.)

on the cellulose acetate membrane or as a broad peak in the densitometer tracing, owing to the complexing of a monoclonal protein with other plasma components or aggregates of IgG, polymers of IgA, or dimers of IgM.

An M-protein can be present when the total protein concentration, β and γ globulin levels, and quantitative immunoglobulin values are all within normal limits. A small M-protein may be concealed in the normal β or γ areas and may be overlooked. In addition, the presence of a monoclonal light chain (Bence Jones proteinemia) is rarely seen in the cellulose acetate tracing. In the heavy-chain diseases, the M-component is usually not apparent. Immunoelectrophoresis, a useful technique for identifying an M-protein, should be performed when a peak or band is seen in the cellulose acetate tracing or when multiple myeloma or related disorders are suspected (Fig. 151–2). Immunofixation, which is more sensitive, is useful when results of immunoelectrophoresis are equivocal or when one is searching for a small M-protein in primary amyloidosis, solitary plasmacytoma, or extramedullary plasmacytoma, or after successful treatment of multiple myeloma or macroglobulinemia.

Quantitation of Immunoglobulins

This procedure is more useful than immunoelectrophoresis or immunofixation for the detection of hypogammaglobulinemia. Quantitation can be performed by radial immunodiffusion, but this is tedious and subject to spurious abnormalities. Rate nephelometry is the preferred method for quantitation of immunoglobulins. The degree of turbidity produced by antigen-antibody interaction is measured by nephelometry in the near-ultraviolet region.

Serum Viscometry

Serum viscometry should be measured when the IgM monoclonal level is more than 3 grams per deciliter, when the IgA or IgG value is more than 4 grams per deciliter, or when the patient has oronasal bleeding, blurred vision, or other symptoms suggestive of a hyperviscosity syndrome.

Analysis of Urine

Dipstick tests are used in many laboratories to screen for protein, but unfortunately they are often insensitive to Bence Jones protein. Consequently, sulfosalicylic acid or Exton's reagent is best for the detection of protein.

Screening tests for Bence Jones proteins (monoclonal light chain in the urine) that utilize their unique thermal properties are not recommended because of their serious shortcomings. Characteristically, Bence Jones protein precipitates at 40°C to

60°C, dissolves at 100°C, and reprecipitates with cooling. Both false-positive and false-negative results occur. Immunoelectrophoresis or immunofixation of an adequately concentrated 24-hour urine specimen reliably detects Bence Jones protein, however. An M-protein appears as a dense, localized band on the cellulose acetate strip or a tall, narrow, homogeneous peak in the densitometer tracing, and its amount can be calculated on the basis of the size of the spike and the amount of total protein in the 24-hour specimen. It is not uncommon to have a negative reaction for protein and no obvious spike on electrophoresis and yet for immunoelectrophoresis or immunofixation of a concentrated urine specimen to show a monoclonal light chain. Immunoelectrophoresis or immunofixation should also be done on the urine of every adult older than 40 years who develops a nephrotic syndrome of unknown cause. The presence of a monoclonal light chain in a nephrotic urine is strongly suggestive of primary amyloidosis.

The differential diagnosis of a monoclonal protein in the serum or urine is given in Table 151–1.

Kyle RA, Garton JP: Laboratory monitoring of myeloma proteins. Semin Oncol 13:310, 1986. *This is a guide for the analysis of serum and urine for monoclonal proteins. Multiple illustrations of immunoelectrophoresis and immunofixation are provided.*

MONOCLONAL GAMMOPATHY OF UNDETERMINED SIGNIFICANCE (MGUS)

The term "monoclonal gammopathy of undetermined significance" (MGUS) (benign monoclonal gammopathy) denotes the presence of a monoclonal protein (M-protein) in persons without evidence of multiple myeloma, macroglobulinemia, amyloidosis, or other related diseases. The term "benign monoclonal gammopathy" is misleading because one does not know at the time of diagnosis whether a process producing a monoclonal protein will remain stable and benign or will develop into symptomatic multiple myeloma, macroglobulinemia, amyloidosis, or a related disorder. MGUS is characterized by a serum M-protein concentration less than 3 grams per deciliter; fewer than 5 per cent plasma cells in the bone marrow; no or only small amounts of M-protein in the urine; absence of lytic bone lesions, anemia, hypercalcemia, and renal insufficiency; and, most important, the stability of the presence of the M-protein and the failure of other abnormalities to develop.

Incidence

During 1989, 764 patients with a serum M-protein were found at the Mayo Clinic. The most frequent clinical diagnosis was MGUS (benign monoclonal gammopathy), occurring in two thirds of patients (Fig. 151–3).

TABLE 151–1. CLASSIFICATION OF PLASMA CELL PROLIFERATIVE DISORDERS

  I. Monoclonal gammopathies of undetermined significance (MGUS)
   A. Benign (IgG, IgA, IgD, IgM, and, rarely, free light chains)
   B. Associated neoplasms or other diseases not known to produce monoclonal proteins
   C. Biclonal gammopathies
   D. Idiopathic Bence Jones proteinuria
 II. Malignant monoclonal gammopathies
   A. Multiple myeloma (IgG, IgA, IgD, IgE, and free light chains)
     1. Overt multiple myeloma
     2. Smoldering multiple myeloma
     3. Plasma cell leukemia
     4. Nonsecretory myeloma
     5. IgD myeloma
     6. Osteosclerotic myeloma
     7. Solitary plasmacytoma of bone
     8. Extramedullary plasmacytoma
   B. Waldenström's macroglobulinemia
     1. Other lymphoproliferative diseases
III. Heavy-chain diseases (HCD's)
   A. γ HCD
   B. α HCD
   C. μ HCD
IV. Cryoglobulinemia
 V. Primary amyloidosis (AL)

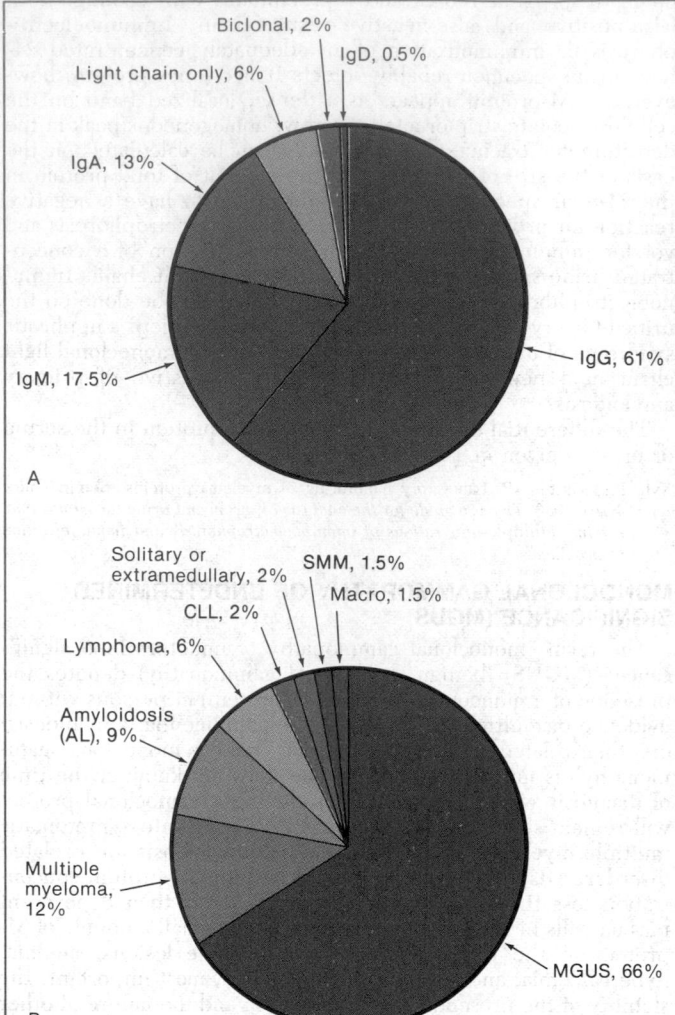

FIGURE 151–3. *A,* Distribution of monoclonal serum proteins in 764 patients seen at the Mayo Clinic during 1989. *B,* Diagnoses in 838 cases of monoclonal gammopathy seen at the Mayo Clinic during 1989.

The prevalence of MGUS is 1 per cent of patients older than 50 years and 3 per cent of those older than 70 years. Because of this high prevalence, it is of great importance for both the patient and the physician that it be determined whether the M-protein will remain benign or will evolve to multiple myeloma, amyloidosis, macroglobulinemia, or other lymphoproliferative disease.

Prognosis

At the Mayo Clinic, a long-term study of 241 patients with benign monoclonal gammopathy (i.e., patients in whom multiple myeloma, macroglobulinemia, amyloidosis, lymphoma, or related diseases were excluded) has been carried out. At the time when the M-protein was recognized, some of the characteristics of the patient group were as follows:

1. The median age was 64 years.
2. Approximately three fourths of the patients had other conditions seemingly unrelated to the monoclonal gammopathy that brought them to medical attention.
3. Anemia, leukopenia, leukocytosis, thrombocytopenia, renal insufficiency, and hypercalcemia, when present, were unrelated to the monoclonal protein.
4. Laboratory findings were as follows: The M-protein level ranged from 0.3 to 3.2 grams per deciliter (median, 1.7 grams per deciliter) and consisted of IgG (74 per cent), IgA (10 per cent), and IgM (16 per cent); an M-protein was found in the urine in only 15 patients; bone marrow plasma cells ranged from 1 to 10 per cent (median, 3.0 per cent).

TABLE 151–2. COURSE IN A SERIES OF 241 PATIENTS WITH BENIGN MONOCLONAL GAMMOPATHY*

Group	Status	Percentage of Patients
1	No significant increase of serum or urine M-protein (benign)	24
2	Increase of M-protein to >3 grams/dl	3
3	Died of unrelated cause	51
4	Developed myeloma (15%), macroglobulinemia (3%), amyloidosis (3%), or related diseases (1%)	22
Total		100

*During first 19 years (median) of follow-up.

Modified from Kyle RA: Monoclonal gammopathy of undetermined significance and smoldering multiple myeloma. Eur J Haematol 43(Suppl 51):70, 1989.

At the time of current follow-up (median, 19 years; range, 11 to 32 years), the 241 patients can be divided into four groups (Table 151–2). Approximately one fourth of the patients have remained stable and can be classified as having benign monoclonal gammopathy, although they must continue to be observed because serious disease may still develop. No initial laboratory measurements or clinical factors were predictive of which patients would remain in this stable or benign group. In 3 per cent of the patients, the M-protein level increased to more than 3 grams per deciliter, but they did not develop symptomatic multiple myeloma, macroglobulinemia, or related disorders. Their condition remains clinically "benign," although with an M-protein that occasions concern. Approximately half of the patients died of seemingly unrelated causes without developing multiple myeloma, macroglobulinemia, or related disorders. Approximately one fourth of the patients (22 per cent) developed multiple myeloma (15 per cent), macroglobulinemia (3 per cent), amyloidosis (3 per cent), or related disorders (1 per cent) (Table 151–2), with an actuarial rate of 17 per cent at 10 years and 33 per cent at 20 years (Fig. 151–4). The interval from the time of recognition of the M-protein to the diagnosis of serious disease ranged from 2 to 22 years (median, 8 years).

Differentiation of MGUS from Multiple Myeloma and Macroglobulinemia

Differentiation of the patient with benign monoclonal gammopathy from one in whom multiple myeloma, macroglobulinemia, or a related disorder eventually develops is very difficult when the M-protein is first recognized. The size of the monoclonal protein is of some help—levels greater than 3 grams per deciliter usually indicate overt multiple myeloma or macroglobulinemia, but some exceptions, such as smoldering multiple myeloma (SMM), exist. Levels of immunoglobulin classes not associated with the M-protein (normal polyclonal or background immunoglobulins) are almost always reduced in multiple myeloma or

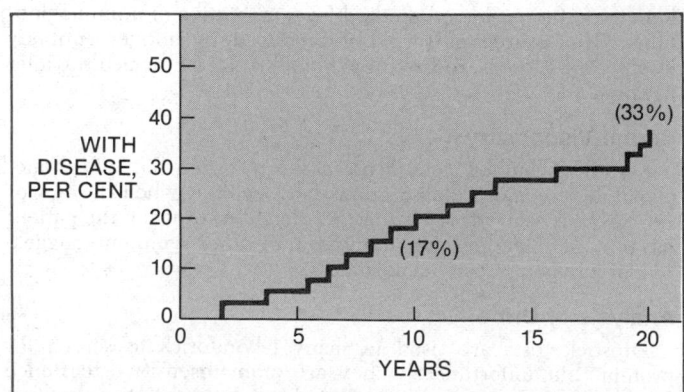

FIGURE 151–4. Incidence of multiple myeloma, macroglobulinemia, amyloidosis, or lymphoproliferative disease after recognition of monoclonal proteins. (From Kyle RA, Lust JA: The monoclonal gammopathies [paraproteins]. Adv Clin Chem, 28:145, 1990, with permission of Academic Press.)

Waldenström's macroglobulinemia, but a reduction may also occur in benign monoclonal gammopathy. The association of a monoclonal light chain (Bence Jones proteinuria) with a serum monoclonal gammopathy is suggestive of multiple myeloma or macroglobulinemia, but in many patients with small amounts of monoclonal light chain in the urine, the M-protein in the serum remains stable for many years. The presence of more than 10 per cent plasma cells in the bone marrow suggests multiple myeloma, but some patients with more plasma cells have remained stable for long periods. The presence of osteolytic lesions strongly suggests multiple myeloma, but metastatic carcinoma may produce lytic lesions as well as plasmacytosis and may be associated with an unrelated monoclonal gammopathy.

Certain research procedures show promise in differentiating the patient with MGUS or SMM from the patient with multiple myeloma. The plasma cell labeling index measures the synthesis of DNA, and when elevated it is good evidence that the patient has multiple myeloma or will soon have symptomatic disease. The use of a monoclonal antibody (BU-1) reactive with 5-bromo-2-deoxyuridine (BrdUrd) detects those cells synthesizing DNA, and the test can be performed in 4 to 5 hours.

In summary, no single technique reliably differentiates a patient with a benign monoclonal gammopathy from one who will subsequently have symptomatic multiple myeloma or other malignant disease. The M-protein level in the serum and urine should be serially measured, together with periodic re-evaluation of clinical and other laboratory features, to determine whether multiple myeloma or another related disorder is present.

If the serum M-protein is less than 2.0 grams per deciliter, electrophoresis should be repeated 6 months later, and if it is stable, it should be checked annually. If the serum M-protein is 2.0 grams per deciliter or more without evidence of myeloma or related disorders, electrophoresis should be repeated in 3 months, and if it is stable, the test should be repeated at 6 months. If there is no progression, electrophoresis should be performed annually thereafter. If an M-protein is present in the urine, the patient should be followed more closely.

Association of Monoclonal Gammopathies with Other Diseases

Monoclonal gammopathy frequently exists without other abnormalities, but certain diseases are associated with it, as would be expected in an older population. The association of two diseases depends on the frequency with which each occurs independently. Furthermore, an association may be biased because of differences in a referral pattern or in other selected patient groups. Of the myriads of associations that have been described, those listed below are the best established.

LYMPHOPROLIFERATIVE DISORDERS. An M-protein is found in 3 to 4 per cent of patients with a diffuse lymphoproliferative process but in fewer than 1 per cent of those with a nodular lymphoma. IgM monoclonal gammopathies are more common than IgG or IgA in lymphoproliferative diseases.

In a large series of patients in whom a serum IgM monoclonal gammopathy had been identified at the Mayo Clinic, more than half were originally considered to have MGUS (Table 151–3). During follow-up, 17 per cent of patients with MGUS of the IgM class developed a malignant lymphoid disease, most frequently Waldenström's macroglobulinemia.

An M-protein may be seen in angioimmunoblastic lymphade-

TABLE 151–3. CLASSIFICATION OF IgM MONOCLONAL GAMMOPATHIES AMONG 430 PATIENTS

Classification	Percentage of Patients
Monoclonal gammopathy of undetermined significance	56
Waldenström's macroglobulinemia	17
Lymphoma	7
Chronic lymphocytic leukemia	5
Primary amyloidosis (AL)	1
Lymphoproliferative disease	14
Total	100

From Kyle RA, Garton JP: The spectrum of IgM monoclonal gammopathy in 430 cases. Mayo Clin Proc 62:719, 1987; with permission of the Mayo Foundation, Rochester, MN.

nopathy, angiofollicular lymph node hyperplasia (Castleman's disease), Sjögren's syndrome, and Kaposi's sarcoma.

LEUKEMIA. M-proteins occur in the sera of some patients with chronic lymphocytic leukemia (Table 151–3), but with no recognizable effect on the clinical course. M-proteins have also been recognized in hairy cell, adult T cell, chronic myelogenous, acute promyelocytic, and acute myelomonocytic leukemias, but without a documented increased incidence over that in the normal population.

NEUROLOGIC DISORDERS. Approximately 5 per cent of patients with sensorimotor peripheral neuropathy of unknown cause have an associated monoclonal gammopathy. In half of those with an IgM monoclonal gammopathy and peripheral neuropathy, the M-protein binds to myelin-associated glycoprotein (MAG). These patients have a slowly progressive sensorimotor neuropathy beginning in the distal extremities and extending proximally. Sensory involvement is more prominent than motor involvement. Cranial nerves and autonomic function are intact. The clinical and electrodiagnostic manifestations resemble those of chronic inflammatory demyelinating polyneuropathy. The relationship of the M-protein to the peripheral neuropathy is not clear.

DERMATOLOGIC DISEASES. Lichen myxedematosus (papular mucinosis, scleromyxedema) is characterized by papules, macules, and plaques infiltrating the skin and is associated with a cathodal IgG λ protein. Scleredema (Buschke's disease), pyoderma gangrenosum, and necrobiotic xanthogranuloma have also been associated with a monoclonal protein.

Monoclonal Gammopathies with Antibody Activity

In miscellaneous patients with MGUS, myeloma, or macroglobulinemia, the monoclonal protein has exhibited unusual specificity to one of various antigens. Examples include actin, dextran, antistreptolysin O, antinuclear activity, riboflavin, von Willebrand factor, thyroglobulin, insulin, double-stranded DNA, and apolipoprotein.

The binding of calcium by an M-protein may produce hypercalcemia without symptomatic or pathologic consequences. Affected patients should not be treated for hypercalcemia. Monoclonal proteins have also been found to bind to copper and to phosphate.

BICLONAL GAMMOPATHIES

Biclonal gammopathies occur in 2 to 3 per cent of patients with monoclonal gammopathies. Biclonal gammopathy of undetermined significance accounts for about two thirds of patients. The remainder have multiple myeloma, macroglobulinemia, or other lymphoproliferative diseases. Triclonal gammopathies may also occur.

IDIOPATHIC BENCE JONES PROTEINURIA

Bence Jones proteinuria is a recognized feature of multiple myeloma, primary amyloidosis, Waldenström's macroglobulinemia, and other malignant lymphoproliferative disorders. A benign Bence Jones proteinuria may also occur. Patients have been documented to have a stable serum level of M-protein and Bence Jones proteinuria for more than 15 years without developing multiple myeloma or related disorders.

Kyle RA, Lust JA: Monoclonal gammopathies of undetermined significance. Semin Hematol 26:176, 1989. *This is a comprehensive review of the pathogenesis of monoclonal gammopathies as well as the results of a long-term follow-up of benign monoclonal gammopathy. The association of monoclonal gammopathies with various diseases is emphasized.*

Merlini G, Farhangi M, Osserman EF: Monoclonal immunoglobulins with antibody activity in myeloma, macroglobulinemia and related plasma cell dyscrasias. Semin Oncol 13:350, 1986. *Monoclonal gammopathies with antibody activity are reviewed in detail. Many useful references are included.*

MULTIPLE MYELOMA

Multiple myeloma (myelomatosis, plasma cell myeloma, or Kahler's disease) is characterized by the neoplastic proliferation of a single clone of plasma cells engaged in the production of a monoclonal immunoglobulin. This clone of plasma cells proliferates in the bone marrow and frequently invades the adjacent bone, producing extensive skeletal destruction that results in bone pain and fractures. Anemia, hypercalcemia, and renal insufficiency are other important features.

Etiology

The cause of multiple myeloma is unknown. Radiation may play a role in some cases. The incidence of multiple myeloma increased modestly in atomic bomb survivors 20 years after exposure to more than 50 rads. Patients with ankylosing spondylitis who were given radiation therapy and workers exposed to radiation in nuclear plants have also exhibited modest increases in the incidence of this disease.

There is little evidence that chemicals cause myeloma. Increased risk of multiple myeloma has been reported in farmers, grain workers, furniture workers, and those exposed to pesticides, benzene, or asbestos. The number of cases is small, however, and more data are necessary. There is little evidence that repeated antigenic stimulation plays a role.

Multiple myeloma has occurred in familial clusters of two or more first-degree relatives as well as in monozygotic twins. Epstein-Barr virus (EBV) may be an etiologic agent in some cases. Myeloma has also been seen in patients with acquired immunodeficiency syndrome (AIDS).

Incidence and Epidemiology

Multiple myeloma accounts for 1 per cent of all malignant disease and slightly more than 10 per cent of hematologic malignancies in the United States. The annual incidence of multiple myeloma is 3 per 100,000. An apparent increase of incidence in recent years is probably related to increased availability and use of medical facilities. Multiple myeloma occurs in all races and all geographic locations. Its incidence in blacks is almost twice that in whites. Multiple myeloma is slightly more common in men than in women. The median age of patients at the time of diagnosis is 61 years; only 2 per cent of patients are younger than 40 years.

Biologic Aspects

T cells play an important role in normal B cell differentiation. When compared with normal controls, patients with multiple myeloma have a reduced percentage of CD4 cells and an increased percentage of CD8 cells.

An aneuploid myeloma cell population is found in approximately 80 per cent of cases. The pre-B common acute lymphoblastic leukemia antigen (CALLA) is expressed on some aneuploid myeloma cells. A myeloma pre-B–like malignant hybrid with coexpression of cytoplasmic μ, CALLA, terminal deoxynucleotidyl transferase (TDT), and plasma cell antigens (PCA-1 and PC-1) has been found in direct and cultured bone marrow specimens. Heavy- and light-chain immunoglobulin gene rearrangements demonstrated monoclonality of these cells, and double-labeling experiments (immunophenotype and labeling index) showed that the cells had a proliferative component exceeding that of myeloma, suggesting that they may represent the stem cell population of myeloma.

There is good evidence that plasma cell precursors of myeloma circulate in the peripheral blood. Several lymphoid growth factors are involved in the differentiation of normal B cells. Resting B cells enter into DNA synthesis stimulated by interleukin 4 (IL4), proliferate with IL5, and differentiate into plasma cells with IL6. Interleukin 6 appears to be an important growth factor for myeloma cells. Elevated levels of IL6 have been found in patients with progressive multiple myeloma, in contrast to those with MGUS. It has been postulated that expression of IL6 induces a polyclonal proliferation of plasma cells and that a second event, such as an altered oncogene expression, may transform the cells into a monoclonal process.

Cytogenetic Abnormalities

Chromosome abnormalities have been detected in about half of patients with multiple myeloma, but no specific abnormality has been demonstrated. Structural changes of chromosomes 1, 11, and 14, monosomies and trisomies, and translocations have been observed. Alterations in the expression of c-myc and H-ras have also been reported in myeloma.

TABLE 151–4. CLINICAL MANIFESTATIONS OF MULTIPLE MYELOMA

Skeletal involvement: pain, reduced height, pathologic fractures, hypercalcemia
Anemia: due mainly to decreased erythropoiesis; produces weakness and fatigue
Renal insufficiency: mainly due to "myeloma kidney" from light chains or hypercalcemia; rarely from amyloidosis
Recurrent infections: respiratory and urinary tract infections or septicemia due to gram-positive or gram-negative organisms
Bleeding diathesis: from thrombocytopenia or coating of platelets with M-protein
Amyloidosis: develops in 10% to 15%
Extramedullary plasmacytomas: occurs late in the disease
Cryoglobulinemia type I: rarely symptomatic

Clinical Manifestations (Table 151–4)

SYMPTOMS. Bone pain, particularly in the back or chest and less often in the extremities, is present at the time of diagnosis in more than two thirds of patients. The pain is usually induced by movement and does not occur at night except with change of position. The patient's height may be reduced by several inches because of vertebral collapse. Weakness and fatigue are common and often are associated with anemia. Fever is rare and, when present, is most often caused by an infection. The major symptoms may result from an acute infection, renal insufficiency, hypercalcemia, or amyloidosis.

PHYSICAL FINDINGS. Pallor is the most frequent physical finding. The liver is palpable in about 20 per cent of patients and the spleen in 5 per cent. Occasionally, extramedullary plasmacytomas may appear.

Laboratory Findings

A normocytic, normochromic anemia is present initially in two thirds of patients but eventually occurs in nearly every patient with multiple myeloma. The erythrocyte sedimentation rate is typically increased but is normal in 10 per cent of cases.

The serum protein electrophoretic pattern (cellulose acetate) shows a peak or localized band in 80 per cent of patients (see Fig. 151–1), hypogammaglobulinemia in almost 10 per cent, and no apparent abnormality in the remainder. IgG monoclonal protein is found in 50 per cent, IgA in 20 per cent, light chain only (Bence Jones proteinemia) in 17 per cent, IgD in 2 per cent, and biclonal gammopathy in 1 per cent, and 10 per cent have no serum M-protein at the time of diagnosis.

Immunoelectrophoresis or immunofixation of the urine reveals a monoclonal protein in approximately 80 per cent of patients. The κ/λ ratio is 2:1. Ninety-nine per cent of patients with multiple myeloma have an M-protein in the serum or urine at the time of diagnosis.

In the bone marrow of patients with multiple myeloma, plasma cells usually account for 10 per cent or more of all nucleated

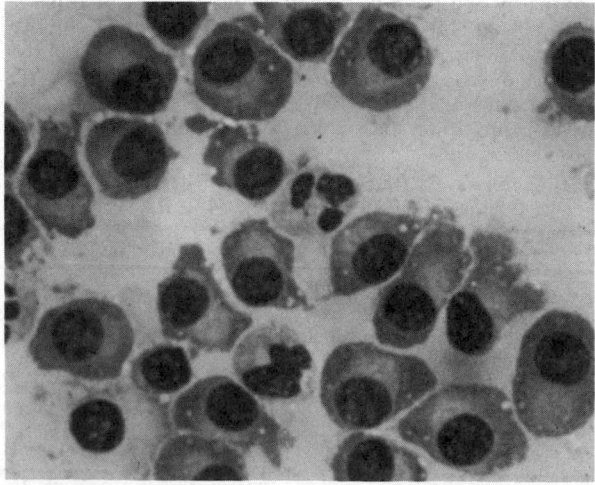

FIGURE 151–5. Bone marrow aspirate containing increased numbers of abnormal plasma cells.

cells, but they may range from less than 5 per cent to almost 100 per cent (Fig. 151–5) (see Color Plate 8H). Bone marrow involvement may be focal rather than diffuse, requiring repeated bone marrow examinations for diagnosis. Identification of a monoclonal immunoglobulin in the cytoplasm of plasma cells by immunoperoxidase staining is helpful for differentiating monoclonal plasma cell proliferation in multiple myeloma from reactive plasmacytosis (see Color Plate 6L) due to connective tissue disease, metastatic carcinoma, liver disease, and infections. The immunoperoxidase technique is also useful in recognizing neoplastic plasma cells that have atypical features.

Radiologic Findings

Conventional roentgenograms reveal abnormalities consisting of punched-out lytic lesions (Fig. 151–6), osteoporosis, or fractures in 80 per cent of patients at diagnosis. The vertebrae, skull, thoracic cage, pelvis, and proximal humeri and femora are the most frequent sites of involvement. Technetium-99m bone scanning is inferior to conventional roentgenography and should not be used. Computed tomography (CT) or magnetic resonance imaging (MRI) is helpful in patients who have skeletal pain but no abnormality on roentgenograms.

Diagnostic Criteria

Minimal criteria for the diagnosis of multiple myeloma are a bone marrow containing more than 10 per cent plasma cells or a plasmacytoma plus at least one of the following: (1) M-protein in the serum (usually greater than 3 grams per deciliter, (2) M-protein in the urine, and (3) lytic bone lesions. These findings must not be from metastatic carcinoma, connective tissue diseases, chronic infection, or lymphoma. Patients with multiple myeloma must be differentiated from those with MGUS and smoldering multiple myeloma.

Organ Involvement

RENAL. Proteinuria is present in almost 90 per cent of patients with multiple myeloma. Bence Jones proteinuria detected by immunoelectrophoresis or immunofixation is present in 80 per cent. The serum creatinine value is increased initially in almost half of patients.

The two major causes of renal insufficiency are "myeloma kidney" and hypercalcemia. Myeloma kidney is characterized by the presence of large, waxy, laminated casts in the distal and collecting tubules. The casts are composed mainly of precipitated monoclonal light chain. The extent of cast formation correlates directly with the amount of free urinary light chain and with the severity of renal insufficiency. With dehydration, acute renal failure may occur.

Hypercalcemia, which is present in 30 per cent of patients initially, is a major and treatable cause of renal insufficiency. Hyperuricemia may contribute to renal failure. Amyloidosis occurs in 10 to 15 per cent of patients and may produce a nephrotic syndrome or renal insufficiency or both. Acquired Fanconi's

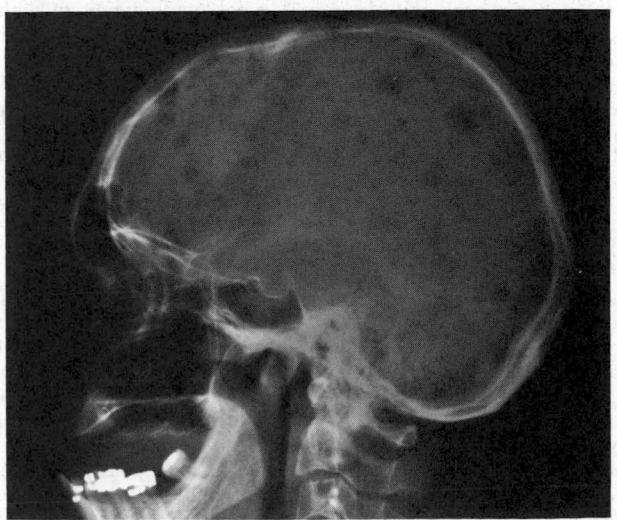

FIGURE 151–6. Skull roentgenogram showing multiple lytic lesions.

syndrome, characterized by proximal tubular dysfunction, results in glycosuria, phosphaturia, and aminoaciduria (see Ch. 82). Deposition of monoclonal light chains in the renal glomerulus (light-chain deposition disease) may produce renal insufficiency and the nephrotic syndrome.

NEUROLOGIC. Radiculopathy, the single most frequent neurologic complication, is usually in the thoracic or lumbosacral area and results from compression of the nerve by the vertebral lesion or by the collapsed bone itself. Compression of the spinal cord occurs in approximately 10 per cent of patients. Peripheral neuropathy is uncommon in multiple myeloma and, when present, is usually caused by amyloidosis. Rarely, myeloma cells diffusely infiltrate the meninges. Intracranial plasmacytomas almost always represent extensions of myelomatous lesions of the skull.

Other Systemic Involvement

Hepatomegaly from plasma cell infiltration is uncommon. Ascites is rare. Plasmacytomas of the ribs are common and present either as expanding bone lesions or as soft tissue masses. The incidence of infections is increased in multiple myeloma. *Diplococcus pneumoniae* and *Staphylococcus aureus* organisms have been the most frequent pathogens, but gram-negative organisms now account for more than half of all infections. Propensity to infection results from impairment of antibody response, deficiency of normal immunoglobulins, and neutropenia. Bleeding from coating of the platelets by the M-protein may occur. Occasionally, a tendency to thrombosis is present.

Treatment

Not all patients who fulfill the minimal criteria for the diagnosis of multiple myeloma should be treated. The patient's symptoms, physical findings, and all laboratory data must be considered. If there are doubts about whether to begin chemotherapy, treatment should be withheld and the patient re-evaluated in 2 or 3 months.

Chemotherapy is the preferred initial therapy for overt symptomatic multiple myeloma. Palliative irradiation should be limited to patients with disabling pain from a well-defined focal process that has not responded to chemotherapy. In most cases, analgesics together with chemotherapy control the pain.

The major controversy in chemotherapy is whether melphalan and prednisone or a combination of alkylating agents should be used. The oral administration of melphalan (L-phenylalanine mustard, Alkeran) and prednisone, a standard form of therapy, produces objective response in 50 to 60 per cent of patients. Melphalan may be given orally in a daily dose of 0.15 mg per kilogram for 7 days (8 to 10 mg per day), with 20 mg of prednisone given three times daily for the same period. Leukocyte and platelet levels should be determined at 3-week intervals, and the melphalan and prednisone therapy repeated in cycles every 6 weeks. The dose of melphalan should be adjusted until modest midcycle cytopenia occurs.

Many combinations of chemotherapeutic agents have been used. The best-known combination, the M2 protocol, includes melphalan, cyclophosphamide, carmustine (bischloroethylnitrosourea, or BCNU), vincristine, and prednisone. This regimen produces an objective response in 70 to 75 per cent of patients, but the median survival is approximately 2.5 years, which is not significantly different from that produced by melphalan and prednisone. The M2 and various other drug combinations have not clearly been shown to produce longer survival than does melphalan-prednisone.

The ideal duration of chemotherapy is unknown. Cessation of chemotherapy usually results in relapse, but continued chemotherapy may lead to the development of a myelodysplastic syndrome or acute leukemia. The peak incidence of acute leukemia occurs 3 to 5 years after initiation of therapy; the 5-year incidence is approximately 5 per cent, and the 10-year incidence is about 10 per cent in those who survive. Chemotherapy should be continued for 1 to 2 years and then discontinued if the M-protein levels in the serum and urine have been stable for at least 6 months and the patient has no other evidence of active disease. Patients should be followed closely, and the same chemotherapy should be reinstituted when relapse occurs.

α_2-Interferon appears to be beneficial in prolonging the duration of remission in patients with multiple myeloma.

Treatment of Refractory Multiple Myeloma

Almost all patients with multiple myeloma who respond to chemotherapy eventually relapse. The highest response rates for patients with multiple myeloma resistant to alkylating agents have been with VAD (vincristine, Adriamycin [doxorubicin], and dexamethasone). VAD has induced remission in two thirds of patients who had relapse from a chemotherapeutic response. VBAP—vincristine, carmustine (BCNU), and doxorubicin (Adriamycin) on day 1 and prednisone daily for 5 days every 3 to 4 weeks—benefits approximately 40 per cent of patients. α_2-Interferon has been disappointing in the treatment of patients with multiple myeloma refractory to alkylating agents.

Management of Complications

HYPERCALCEMIA. Hypercalcemia, present in almost one third of patients at the time of diagnosis, should be suspected in the presence of anorexia, nausea, vomiting, polyuria, polydipsia, increased constipation, weakness, confusion, or stupor. If it is untreated, renal insufficiency usually develops. Hydration, preferably with isotonic saline plus prednisone (25 mg four times per day), relieves the hypercalcemia in most cases. The dosage of prednisone must be reduced and its use discontinued as soon as possible. If these measures fail, mithramycin, diphosphonates, calcitonin, or gallium nitrate may be beneficial. Patients with myeloma should be encouraged to be as active as possible because prolonged bed rest contributes to hypercalcemia. The manifestations and treatment of hypercalcemia are also discussed in Ch. 235.

RENAL INSUFFICIENCY. This occurs in half of patients with multiple myeloma and may develop insidiously or rapidly (acute renal failure). Hydration and prednisone are necessary if there is an accompanying hypercalcemia. Furosemide is helpful for maintaining a high urine flow rate (100 ml per hour). Hemodialysis is necessary in the event of symptomatic azotemia. Plasmapheresis may be helpful for regaining renal function, but patients with severe myeloma cast formation or other irreversible changes are unlikely to benefit from plasmapheresis. Allopurinol is necessary if hyperuricemia is present. For a more general discussion of renal insufficiency, see Ch. 76 and 77.

INFECTION. Prompt, appropriate therapy for bacterial infections is necessary. Prophylactic penicillin often benefits patients with recurrent gram-positive infections. Intravenously administered gamma globulin is helpful but expensive. Pneumococcal and influenza immunizations should be given to all patients (see Ch. 16).

SKELETAL LESIONS. Patients should be encouraged to be as active as possible but to avoid trauma. Fixation of fractures or impending fractures of long bones with an intramedullary rod and methyl methacrylate has produced good results.

MISCELLANEOUS COMPLICATIONS. Symptomatic hyperviscosity should be treated with plasmapheresis. The presence of an extradural plasmacytoma must be recognized and treated with radiation therapy and dexamethasone. If the neurologic deficit increases, surgical decompression is necessary.

Prognosis

Multiple myeloma has a progressive course, with a median survival of 6 months when no treatment is given. The serum β_2-microglobulin (β_2-M) level is the single most reliable prognostic factor in previously untreated multiple myeloma. The bone marrow plasma cell labeling index and age of the patient are also additional prognostic factors. Plasmablastic morphology, circulating myeloma cells in the peripheral blood, increased myeloma colony growth, and increased levels of IL6 are all associated with more aggressive disease. Patients who respond rapidly to chemotherapy and who have an elevated plasma cell labeling index have a shorter remission and survival.

Future Directions

A combination of alternating cycles of α_2-interferon with VBMCP (vincristine, BCNU, melphalan, cyclophosphamide, and prednisone) has produced an objective response in 80 per cent of previously untreated patients with myeloma. Forty per cent had a complete or nearly complete response. High-dose melphalan produced a complete response in 27 per cent of previously untreated patients, but most have relapsed.

Bone marrow transplantation from an identical twin (syngeneic) or a human leukocyte antigen (HLA)–compatible donor (allogeneic) has been performed (see Ch. 153). Utilization of high-dose cyclophosphamide or melphalan plus total-body irradiation followed by autologous or allogeneic bone marrow transplantation for multiple myeloma refractory to chemotherapy has been described. Unfortunately, the relapse rate is high, and graft-versus-host reaction can be a serious problem in allogeneic transplantation.

Autologous bone marrow transplantation is potentially applicable to more patients. The two major problems are (1) eradication of multiple myeloma from the patient and (2) the removal of myeloma cells and their precursors from the autologous marrow. Purging of the marrow with monoclonal antibodies or chemotherapy is being investigated. The use of stem cells from autologous peripheral blood has successfully reconstituted the marrow of multiple myeloma patients treated with high-dose chemotherapy and total-body irradiation. The use of agents such as verapamil or quinine to reverse the resistance to doxorubicin is another interesting approach.

Anderson KC, Barut BA, Ritz J, et al.: Monoclonal antibody–purged autologous bone marrow transplantation therapy for multiple myeloma. Blood 77:712, 1991.
Barlogie B, Epstein J, Selvanayagam P, et al.: Plasma cell myeloma—new biological insights and advances in therapy. Blood 73:865, 1989. *This excellent review includes advances in the molecular biology and immunologic aspects of multiple myeloma.*
Bergsagel DE: Is aggressive chemotherapy more effective in the treatment of plasma cell myeloma? Eur J Cancer Clin Oncol 25:159, 1989. *This is a summary of prospective studies comparing single and multiple alkylating agents for the treatment of myeloma. The author concludes that aggressive chemotherapy does not significantly prolong survival when compared with single-agent therapy.*
Buzaid AC, Durie BGM: Management of refractory myeloma: A review. J Clin Oncol 6:889, 1988. *This is a comprehensive review of the therapy of refractory myeloma. The authors provide information on a wide variety of chemotherapeutic approaches to the refractory patient.*
Jagannath S, Barlogie B, Dicke K, et al.: Autologous bone marrow transplantation in multiple myeloma: Identification of prognostic factors. Blood 76:1860, 1990.
Kyle RA: Multiple myeloma: Review of 869 cases. Mayo Clin Proc 50:29, 1975. *The clinical and laboratory findings in a large series of multiple myeloma cases are presented. Results of long-term follow-up are emphasized.*
Kyle RA: Monoclonal gammopathies and the kidney. Ann Rev Med 40:53, 1989. *A review of the renal aspects of multiple myeloma, Waldenström's macroglobulinemia, acquired Fanconi's syndrome, light-chain deposition disease, and primary systemic amyloidosis is presented.*
Kyle RA, Greipp PR: Plasma cell dyscrasias: Current status. CRC Crit Rev Oncol Hematol 8:93, 1988. *This is a comprehensive review of monoclonal gammopathies with more than 450 references.*
Mandelli F, Avvisati G, Amadori S, et al.: Maintenance treatment with recombinant interferon alpha-2b in patients with multiple myeloma responding to conventional induction chemotherapy. N Eng J Med 322:1430, 1990.

VARIANT FORMS OF MULTIPLE MYELOMA
(Table 151–1)

Smoldering Myeloma

The diagnosis of smoldering multiple myeloma (SMM) depends on the presence of an M-protein level greater than 3 grams per deciliter in the serum and greater than 10 per cent plasma cells in the bone marrow, but no anemia, renal insufficiency, or skeletal lesions. Often, a small amount of M-protein is found in the urine, and the concentration of normal immunoglobulins in the serum is decreased. The plasma cell labeling index is low. Patients with SMM should be recognized because they must not be treated unless progression occurs. Biologically, patients with SMM have a benign monoclonal gammopathy (MGUS), but it is difficult to accept that diagnosis initially when the M-protein level is greater than 3 grams per deciliter and the bone marrow contains more than 10 per cent plasma cells.

Plasma Cell Leukemia

Patients with plasma cell leukemia (see Color Plate 8I, left) have greater than 20 per cent plasma cells in the peripheral blood and an absolute plasma cell count of at least 2000 per microliter. Plasma cell leukemia is classified as primary when it is diagnosed in the leukemic phase (60 per cent) or as secondary when there is leukemic transformation of a previously recognized multiple myeloma (40 per cent). Patients with primary plasma cell leukemia are younger and have a greater incidence of hepatosplenomegaly and lymphadenopathy, a higher platelet count, fewer bone lesions, a smaller serum M-protein component, and a longer survival (median, 6.8 versus 1.3 months) than patients with secondary plasma cell leukemia. Treatment of plasma cell leukemia is unsatisfactory, but partial responses do occur with melphalan and prednisone or with a combination of alkylating agents. Secondary plasma cell leukemia rarely responds to chemotherapy because the patients have already received chemotherapy and are resistant.

Nonsecretory Myeloma

Patients with nonsecretory myeloma have no M-protein in either the serum or the urine and account for only 1 per cent of patients with myeloma. For certainty of diagnosis, a monoclonal protein should be identified in the plasma cells by immunoperoxidase or immunofluorescence methods. More than a dozen patients in whom no monoclonal protein could be found within the myeloma cell have been described.

IgD Myeloma

The M-protein is smaller than in IgG and IgA myelomas, and Bence Jones proteinuria of the λ type is more common. Plasma cell leukemia, amyloidosis, and extramedullary plasmacytomas are more frequent with IgD myeloma. Survival is generally believed to be shorter than with other myeloma types, but IgD myeloma is often not diagnosed until later in its course.

Osteosclerotic Myeloma (POEMS Syndrome)

This syndrome is characterized by polyneuropathy, organomegaly, endocrinopathy, M-protein, and skin changes (POEMS). The major clinical features are a chronic inflammatory-demyelinating polyneuropathy with predominantly motor disability and sclerotic skeletal lesions. Except for the presence of papilledema, the cranial nerves are not involved. The autonomic nervous system is intact. Hepatomegaly occurs in almost one half of patients, but splenomegaly and lymphadenopathy occur in a minority. Hyperpigmentation and hypertrichosis are usually evident. Gynecomastia and atrophic testes as well as clubbing of the fingers and toes may be seen. In contrast to multiple myeloma, the hemoglobin level is usually normal or elevated, and thrombocytosis is common. The bone marrow usually contains fewer than 5 per cent plasma cells, and hypercalcemia and renal insufficiency rarely occur. Most patients have a λ M-protein. Evidence of Castleman's disease may be found. Diagnosis is confirmed by the identification of monoclonal plasma cells obtained at biopsy of an osteosclerotic lesion.

If the lesions are in a limited area, radiation therapy will produce substantial improvement of the neuropathy in more than half of the patients. If the patient has widespread osteosclerotic lesions, chemotherapy with melphalan and prednisone may be helpful.

Solitary Plasmacytoma (Solitary Myeloma) of Bone

The diagnosis of this disease is based on histologic evidence of a tumor consisting of monoclonal plasma cells identical to those seen in multiple myeloma. In addition, complete skeletal roentgenograms must show no other lesions of myeloma, the bone marrow aspirate must contain no evidence of multiple myeloma, and immunoelectrophoresis or immunofixation of the serum and concentrated urine should show no M-protein. Exceptions to the last-mentioned criterion occur, but therapy for the solitary lesion usually results in disappearance of the M-protein. Disease-free survival at 10 years ranges from 15 to 25 per cent. Almost 50 per cent of patients with solitary plasmacytoma are alive at 10 years. Treatment consists of radiation in the range of 4000 to 5000 rads (40 to 50 Gy). The most uncertain criterion for diagnosis is the length of observation necessary before it can be assured that the disease will not become generalized.

Extramedullary Plasmacytoma

Extramedullary plasmacytoma is a plasma cell tumor that arises outside the bone marrow. The tumor is found in the upper respiratory tract in approximately 85 per cent of cases, especially in the nasal cavity and sinuses, nasopharynx, and larynx. Extramedullary plasmacytomas may also occur in the gastrointestinal tract, central nervous system, urinary bladder, thyroid, breast, testes, parotid gland, and lymph nodes. The diagnosis is based on the finding of a plasma cell tumor in an extramedullary site and the absence of multiple myeloma on bone marrow examination, roentgenography, and appropriate studies of blood and urine. Treatment consists of tumoricidal irradiation. The plasmacytoma may occur locally, metastasize to regional nodes, or develop into multiple myeloma.

WALDENSTRÖM'S MACROGLOBULINEMIA (PRIMARY MACROGLOBULINEMIA)

Macroglobulinemia is the result of an uncontrolled proliferation of lymphocytes and plasma cells in which a large monoclonal IgM protein is produced. The cause is unknown, but it does occur more frequently in certain families. The median age of patients at the time of diagnosis is 60 years, and about 60 per cent are male.

Clinical Presentations

Weakness, fatigue, and bleeding (especially oozing from the oronasal area) are common presenting symptoms. Blurred or impaired vision, dyspnea, loss of weight, neurologic symptoms, recurrent infections, and congestive heart failure may occur. In contrast to multiple myeloma, lytic bone lesions, renal insufficiency, and amyloidosis are rare. Physical findings include pallor, hepatosplenomegaly, and lymphadenopathy. Retinal hemorrhages, exudates, and venous congestion with vascular segmentation ("sausage" formation) may occur. Sensorimotor peripheral neuropathy is common. Pulmonary involvement is manifested by diffuse pulmonary infiltrates and isolated masses. Pleural effusion may occur. Diarrhea and steatorrhea are uncommon.

Laboratory Evaluation

Almost all patients have moderate to severe normocytic, normochromic anemia. Coombs-positive hemolytic anemia is uncommon. The serum cholesterol value is often low. The serum electrophoretic pattern is characterized by a tall, narrow peak or dense band and is almost always of γ mobility. Seventy-five per cent of the IgM proteins have a κ light chain. Low molecular weight IgM (7S) is present and may account for a significant part of the elevated IgM level. A monoclonal light chain is present in the urine of 80 per cent of patients. The amount of urinary protein is usually modest.

The bone marrow aspirate is often hypocellular, but the biopsy is hypercellular and extensively infiltrated with lymphoid cells and plasma cells. The number of mast cells is frequently increased. Rouleaux formation is prominent, and the sedimentation rate is markedly increased unless gelation of the plasma occurs. About 10 per cent of macroglobulins have cryoproperties.

Diagnosis

The combination of typical symptoms and physical findings, the presence of a large monoclonal IgM protein (usually greater than 3 grams per deciliter), and lymphoid–plasma cell infiltration of the bone marrow provides the diagnosis. Multiple myeloma, chronic lymphocytic leukemia, and MGUS of the IgM type must be differentiated.

Treatment

Patients should not be treated unless they have anemia; constitutional symptoms such as weakness, fatigue, night sweats, or weight loss; hyperviscosity; or significant hepatosplenomegaly or lymphadenopathy. Chlorambucil (Leukeran) is usually given orally in a dosage of 6 to 8 mg per day and is reduced when the leukocyte or platelet value decreases. Patients should be treated for 2 years, and if the disease has reached a plateau state, the treatment can be discontinued and the patients followed closely. Chemotherapy should be reinstituted when the disease relapses. Combinations of alkylating agents, such as the M2 protocol (vincristine, BCNU, melphalan, cyclophosphamide, and prednisone), may be beneficial. α_2-Interferon may be of some use.

Transfusions of packed red blood cells should be given for symptomatic anemia. Spuriously low hemoglobin and hematocrit levels may occur because of the increased plasma volume from the large amount of M-protein. Consequently, transfusions should not be given solely on the basis of the hemoglobin or hematocrit value. Symptomatic hyperviscosity should be treated with plasmapheresis. The median survival in macroglobulinemia is 5 years.

HYPERVISCOSITY SYNDROME

Chronic nasal bleeding and oozing from the gums are frequent, but postsurgical or gastrointestinal bleeding may occur. Retinal hemorrhages are common, and papilledema may be seen. The patient occasionally complains of blurring or a loss of vision. Dizziness, headache, vertigo, nystagmus, decreased hearing, ataxia, paresthesias, diplopia, somnolence, and coma may occur. Hyperviscosity can precipitate or aggravate congestive heart failure. Most patients have symptoms when the relative viscosity is greater than 4 centipoises (cp), but the relationship between serum viscosity and clinical manifestations is not precise. Patients with symptomatic hyperviscosity should be treated with plasmapheresis. Plasma exchange of 3 to 4 liters should be performed daily until the patient is asymptomatic. The plasma should be replaced with albumin rather than plasma.

Fibbe WE, Jansen J: Prognostic factors in IgD myeloma: A study of 21 cases. Scand J Haematol 33:471, 1984. *Twenty-one patients with IgD myeloma from the Netherlands are described.*

Franchi F, Seminara P, Teodori L, et al.: The non-producer plasma cell myeloma: Report of a case and review of the literature. Blut 52:281, 1986. *The authors describe a case of nonsecretory (nonproducer) multiple myeloma and present an excellent review of the literature.*

Frassica DA, Frassica FJ, Schray MF, et al.: Solitary plasmacytoma of bone: Mayo Clinic experience. Int J Radiat Oncol Biol Phys 16:43, 1989. *This is a review of 46 cases of solitary plasmacytoma of bone. The presence of an M-protein did not significantly alter the survival or duration of disease-free survival.*

Jackson A, Scarffe JH: Prognostic significance of osteopenia and immunoparesis at presentation in patients with solitary myeloma of bone. Eur J Cancer 26:363, 1990.

Knowling MA, Harwood AR, Bergsagel DE: Comparison of extramedullary plasmacytomas with solitary and multiple plasma cell tumors of bone. J Clin Oncol 1:255, 1983. *This is a helpful review of extramedullary plasmacytomas and gives the reader a well-balanced report.*

Kyle RA, Garton JP: The spectrum of IgM monoclonal gammopathy in 430 cases. Mayo Clin Proc 62:719, 1987. *This study of 430 patients with an IgM monoclonal protein emphasizes the variable clinical patterns of disease. Sixty-three patients with Waldenström's macroglobulinemia are reviewed, and the clinical and laboratory features are provided.*

Kyle RA, Greipp PR: Smoldering multiple myeloma. N Engl J Med 302:1347, 1980. *This is a report of six patients who fulfilled the criteria for the diagnosis of multiple myeloma but whose conditions behaved like a benign monoclonal gammopathy. The authors emphasize that such patients must be recognized and not treated.*

Noel P, Kyle RA: Plasma cell leukemia: An evaluation of response to therapy. Am J Med 83:1062, 1987. *This review of 43 patients with plasma cell leukemia differentiates primary and secondary plasma cell leukemia. The short survival is emphasized.*

Takatsuki K, Sanada I: Plasma cell dyscrasia with polyneuropathy and endocrine disorder: Clinical and laboratory features of 109 reported cases. Jpn J Clin Oncol 13:543, 1983. *This provides an excellent picture of the clinical and laboratory features of a large number of patients with osteosclerotic myeloma (POEMS syndrome) from Japan.*

HEAVY-CHAIN DISEASES

The heavy-chain diseases (HCD's) are characterized by the presence of a monoclonal protein consisting of a portion of the immunoglobulin heavy chain in the serum or urine or both. These heavy chains are devoid of light chains and represent a lymphoplasma cell proliferative process. There are three major types: γ HCD, α HCD, and μ HCD.

Gamma Heavy-Chain Disease (γ HCD)

The abnormal protein consists of a γ chain with significant deletions of amino acids, including the C_{H1} domain of the constant region.

The median age of patients is approximately 60 years, although the condition has been noted in persons younger than 20 years. Patients with γ HCD often present with a lymphoma-like illness, but the clinical findings are diverse and range from an aggressive lymphoproliferative process to an asymptomatic state. Hepatosplenomegaly and lymphadenopathy occur in about 60 per cent of patients. Anemia is found in about 80 per cent of patients initially and in nearly all eventually. A few patients have had a Coombs-positive hemolytic anemia. The electrophoretic pattern often shows a broad-based band more suggestive of a polyclonal than a monoclonal protein. The urinary heavy-chain protein value ranges from a trace to 20 grams daily, but it is usually less than 1 gram per 24 hours.

Increased numbers of lymphocytes, plasma cells, or plasma-

cytoid lymphocytes are seen in the bone marrow and lymph nodes. The histologic pattern is variable and usually includes generalized or localized lymphoma or myeloma, but in some cases there is no evidence of a lymphoplasmacytic proliferative process.

Treatment is indicated only for symptomatic patients. Many different drugs have been used, but the results have been inconsistent and generally disappointing. Therapy with cyclophosphamide, vincristine, and prednisone is a reasonable choice. If there is no response to this regimen, doxorubicin should be added.

The prognosis of γ HCD is variable and ranges from a rapidly progressive downhill course of a few weeks' duration to the asymptomatic presence of a stable monoclonal heavy chain in the serum or urine.

Alpha Heavy-Chain Disease (α HCD)

This most common HCD occurs in patients from the Mediterranean region or Middle East, usually in the second or third decade of life. About 60 per cent are men. Most commonly, the gastrointestinal tract is involved, resulting in severe malabsorption with diarrhea, steatorrhea, and loss of weight. Plasma cell infiltration of the jejunal mucosa is the most frequent pathologic feature.

The serum protein electrophoretic pattern is normal in half the cases, and in the remainder an unimpressive broad band may appear in the α_2 or β regions. The diagnosis depends on the recognition of a monoclonal α heavy chain. The amount of α heavy chain in the urine is small, and Bence Jones proteinuria has never been reported.

Most often, α HCD is progressive and fatal, but response to melphalan or cyclophosphamide and prednisone may occur. Unexpectedly, antibiotics may also produce a remission.

Mu Heavy-Chain Disease (μ HCD)

This disease is characterized by the demonstration of a monoclonal μ chain fragment in the serum. The patient may present with chronic lymphocytic leukemia or lymphoma, but it is likely that the clinical spectrum will broaden when more cases are recognized.

The serum protein electrophoretic pattern is usually normal except for hypogammaglobulinemia. Bence Jones proteinuria has been found in two thirds of cases. The course of μ HCD is variable, and survival ranges from a few months to many years. Treatment with corticosteroids and alkylating agents has produced some benefit.

Brouet J-C, Seligmann M, Danon F, et al.: μ-Chain disease: Report of two new cases. Arch Intern Med 139:672, 1979. *This is a report of two cases of μ HCD and an excellent review of the literature.*

Haghighi P, Wolf PL: Alpha–heavy chain disease. Clin Lab Med 6:477, 1986. *This is a review of α HCD that emphasizes the histologic features.*

Kyle RA, Greipp PR, Banks PM: The diverse picture of gamma heavy-chain disease: Report of seven cases and review of literature. Mayo Clin Proc 56:439, 1981. *This report of seven cases of γ HCD from a single institution includes a detailed review of 49 cases from the literature. The clinical picture is emphasized.*

CRYOGLOBULINEMIA

Cryoglobulins are proteins that precipitate when cooled and dissolve when heated. They are designated as idiopathic or essential when they are not associated with any recognizable disease. Cryoglobulins are classified into three types: type I (monoclonal), type II (mixed), and type III (polyclonal).

Type I (monoclonal) cryoglobulinemia is most commonly of the IgM or IgG class, but IgA and Bence Jones cryoglobulins have been reported. Most patients, even with large amounts of type I cryoglobulin, are completely asymptomatic from this source. Others with monoclonal cryoglobulins in the range of 1 to 2 grams per deciliter may have pain, purpura, Raynaud's phenomenon, cyanosis, and even ulceration and sloughing of skin and subcutaneous tissue on exposure to the cold because their cryoglobulins precipitate at relatively high temperatures. Type I cryoglobulins are associated with macroglobulinemia, multiple myeloma, or MGUS.

Type II (mixed) cryoglobulinemia typically consists of a monoclonal IgM protein and polyclonal IgG, although monoclonal IgG or monoclonal IgA may also be seen with polyclonal IgM. Serum protein electrophoresis usually shows a normal pattern or a diffuse, polyclonal hypergammaglobulinemia pattern. The quantity of mixed cryoglobulin is usually less than 0.2 gram per deciliter. Vasculitis, glomerulonephritis, lymphoproliferative dis-

TABLE 151–5. CLINICAL CLASSIFICATION OF AMYLOIDOSIS

Amyloid Type	Classification	Major Protein Component
AL	Primary	κ or λ light chain
AA	Secondary	Protein A
AL	Localized	κ or λ light chain
AF	Familial	
	Neurologic	Transthyretin (prealbumin)
	Cardiopathic	Transthyretin (prealbumin)
	Nephropathic	
	Familial Mediterranean fever	Protein A
ASC_1	Senile cardiac amyloid	Transthyretin (prealbumin)
AB	Dialysis arthropathy	β_2-Microglobulin

ease, and chronic infectious processes are common. Purpura and polyarthralgias are frequently seen. Involvement of the joints is symmetric, but joint deformities rarely develop. Raynaud's phenomenon, necrosis of the skin, and neurologic involvement may be present. In almost 80 per cent of renal biopsy specimens, glomerular damage can be identified. Nephrotic syndrome may result, but severe renal insufficiency is uncommon. Hepatic dysfunction and serologic evidence of infection with hepatitis B virus are common.

Early administration of corticosteroids is the most frequent therapy. Cyclophosphamide, chlorambucil, or azathioprine should be used if there is no response. Plasmapheresis has been effective in some instances. α_2-Interferon has been of benefit.

Type III (polyclonal) cryoglobulinemia is not associated with a monoclonal component. Type III cryoglobulins are found in many patients with infections or inflammatory diseases and are of no clinical significance.

Montagnino G: Reappraisal of the clinical expression of mixed cryoglobulinemia. Springer Semin Immunopathol 10:1, 1988. *This is an important review summarizing the findings of four previous series of patients with type II cryoglobulinemia. Clinical features are emphasized, and therapy is described.*

PRIMARY AMYLOIDOSIS (AL) (see Ch. 197)

Amyloid (see Color Plate 8*I*, right), stained with Congo red, produces an apple-green birefringence under polarized light. It is a fibrous protein that consists of rigid, linear, nonbranching, aggregated fibrils of 7.5 to 10 nm width and of indefinite length. The type of amyloid cannot be differentiated by organ distribution or by electron microscopy. The amyloid fibrils in AL consist of the variable portion of a monoclonal light chain or, in some instances, the intact light chain (Table 151–5). The light-chain class is more frequently λ than κ (2:1), with a predominance of the λ_{VI} subclass. Patients with AL may have aberrant de novo synthesis or abnormal proteolytic processing of light chains. Amyloid P-component (AP) is a glycoprotein found in all types of amyloid, but its function is

unknown. The catabolism, or breakdown, of amyloid fibrils is an important factor in pathogenesis.

Clinical Features

The median age at diagnosis is 61 years, and only 3 per cent of patients are younger than 40 years. Two thirds are male. Weakness or fatigue and loss of weight are the most frequent symptoms. Dyspnea, pedal edema, paresthesias, light-headedness, and syncope are frequently seen in patients with congestive heart failure or peripheral neuropathy. Hoarseness or change of voice as well as jaw claudication may occur.

The liver is palpable in 20 per cent of patients, but splenomegaly occurs in only 5 per cent. Macroglossia is present in 10 per cent of patients. Purpura often involves the neck, face, and eyes. Ankle edema is common.

Almost one third of patients have a nephrotic syndrome. Carpal tunnel syndrome, congestive heart failure, peripheral neuropathy, and orthostatic hypotension are other major presenting syndromes (Fig. 151–7). The presence of one of these syndromes and an M-protein in the serum or urine is a strong indication of AL, for which appropriate biopsy specimens must be taken for diagnosis.

Laboratory Findings

Anemia is not a prominent feature, but, when present, it is usually due to renal insufficiency, multiple myeloma, or gastrointestinal bleeding. Thrombocytosis occurs in 5 to 10 per cent of patients. Proteinuria is present initially in 80 per cent and renal insufficiency in almost 50 per cent of patients. Elevation of the serum alkaline phosphatase value is not uncommon. Hyperbilirubinemia is infrequent, but, when present, it is an ominous sign. Hypoalbuminemia and elevation of the cholesterol and triglyceride values are common with the nephrotic syndrome. The Factor X level is decreased in fewer than 5 per cent of patients and is rarely the cause of bleeding. The prothrombin time is increased in about 15 per cent of patients, and the thrombin time is prolonged in 60 per cent.

Immunoelectrophoresis or immunofixation reveals a monoclonal protein in the serum and in the urine of two thirds of patients. A monoclonal protein is found in the serum or urine in 85 per cent of patients.

Bone marrow plasma cells are usually only modestly increased. Only 15 per cent of patients have more than 20 per cent plasma cells in the marrow. Roentgenograms of the bones are normal unless the patient has multiple myeloma.

Organ System Involvement

CARDIAC AND CIRCULATORY. Congestive heart failure is present in approximately 25 per cent of patients at the time of diagnosis and develops during the course of the disease in an additional 10 per cent. The electrocardiogram frequently shows either low voltage in the limb leads or features consistent with

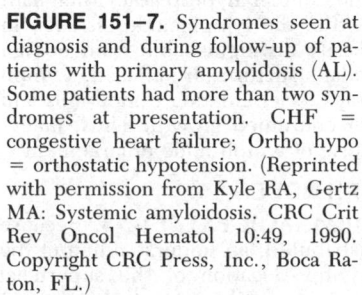

FIGURE 151–7. Syndromes seen at diagnosis and during follow-up of patients with primary amyloidosis (AL). Some patients had more than two syndromes at presentation. CHF = congestive heart failure; Ortho hypo = orthostatic hypotension. (Reprinted with permission from Kyle RA, Gertz MA: Systemic amyloidosis. CRC Crit Rev Oncol Hematol 10:49, 1990. Copyright CRC Press, Inc., Boca Raton, FL.)

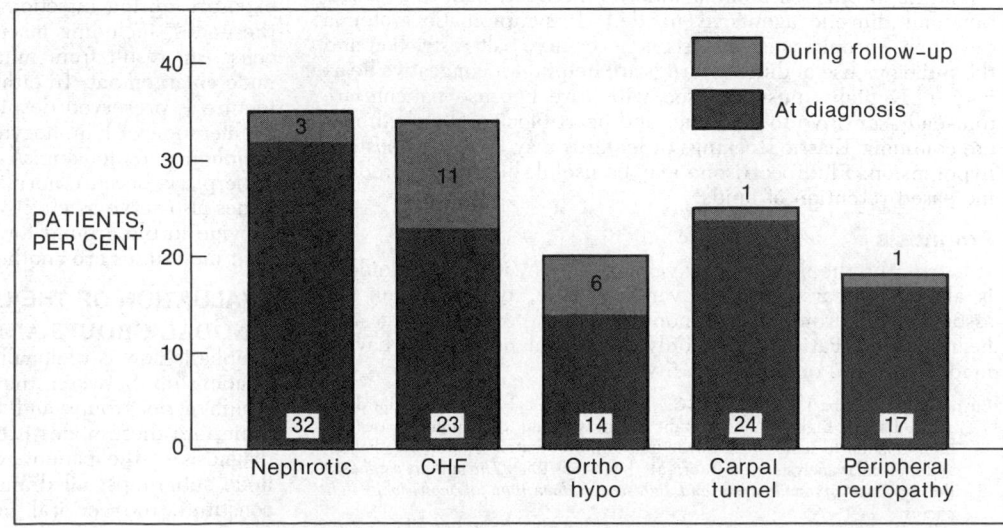

an anteroseptal infarction (loss of anterior forces). Atrial fibrillation, atrial or junctional tachycardia, ventricular premature complexes, and heart block are common electrocardiographic features.

Echocardiography is a valuable technique for the evaluation of amyloid heart disease. Increased thickness of the ventricular wall and septum correlates with an increased incidence of congestive heart failure. Early cardiac amyloidosis is characterized by abnormal relaxation, whereas advanced involvement is characterized by restrictive hemodynamics. Intermittent claudication of the lower extremities, the upper extremities, or the jaw may be a prominent feature.

OTHER ORGANS. Nephrotic syndrome is present in one third of patients at the time of diagnosis. The degree of proteinuria does not correlate well with the extent of amyloid deposition in the kidney. Gross hematuria is rare. Other organ involvement includes the lungs and gastrointestinal tract, but it is asymptomatic in most instances. Sensorimotor peripheral neuropathy characterized by dysesthetic numbness involving the lower extremities occurs in one sixth of patients. Autonomic dysfunction may be a prominent feature and is usually manifested by orthostatic hypotension, diarrhea, or impotence. Amyloidosis can involve the periarticular structures and produce the shoulder pad syndrome. Rarely, osteolytic lesions from amyloid may occur. Pseudohypertrophy of skeletal muscles from amyloid deposition may be impressive. Petechiae, ecchymoses, papules, plaques, nodules, tumors, bullous lesions, thickening of the skin, and dystrophy of the nails may occur.

The diagnosis of amyloidosis depends on histologic proof. The initial diagnostic procedure should be abdominal fat aspiration, which is positive in more than 70 per cent of patients. A bone marrow aspiration and biopsy should be done to determine the degree of plasmacytosis, and results are positive for amyloid in about one half of patients. If the abdominal fat and bone marrow biopsy results are negative, a rectal biopsy specimen, including the submucosa, should be taken. If these sites yield negative findings, biopsy of the kidney, liver, carpal tunnel tissue, sural nerve, or endomyocardium should be performed.

Specific antisera are helpful for identifying the type of systemic amyloidosis. Antiserum to AP reacts with all amyloid types and is useful in demonstrating the presence of amyloid.

Treatment

Therapy of AL amyloidosis is not satisfactory. In a prospective study of treatment with melphalan and prednisone compared with colchicine, no significant difference in survival was noted (25 and 18 months, respectively). When the survival of patients who received only one regimen was analyzed, or when survival was determined from the time of entry into the study to the time of death or progression of disease, significant differences favoring melphalan and prednisone therapy were evident.

Supportive Measures

The nephrotic syndrome should be managed with salt restriction and diuretic agents as needed. If symptomatic azotemia develops, chronic renal dialysis is necessary. Salt restriction and the judicious use of diuretic drugs are helpful for congestive heart failure. Digitalis must be used with care because patients are unusually sensitive to the drug, and heart block and arrhythmias are common. Elastic stockings or leotards may benefit orthostatic hypotension. Fludrocortisone may be useful, but it does produce increased retention of fluids.

Prognosis

Currently, the median survival of patients with AL amyloidosis is almost 2 years. Survival varies greatly, depending on the associated syndrome; it is 6 months from the onset of congestive heart failure. Patients with only peripheral neuropathy have a median survival of more than 5 years.

Buxbaum JN, Chuba JV, Hellman GC, et al.: Monoclonal immunoglobulin deposition disease: Light chain and light and heavy chain deposition diseases and their relation to light chain amyloidosis: Clinical features, immunopathology, and molecular analysis. Ann Intern Med 112:455, 1990. *The authors emphasize the presence of amyloidosis and light-chain deposition of monoclonal light chains.*

Kyle RA, Gertz MA: Systemic amyloidosis. CRC Crit Rev Oncol Hematol 10:49, 1990. *This is a comprehensive review of primary, secondary, localized, hereditary, senile, and endocrine amyloidoses. More than 550 references are given.*

Kyle RA, Greipp PR: Amyloidosis (AL). Clinical and laboratory features in 229 cases. Mayo Clin Proc 58:665, 1983. *This is a review of the clinical and laboratory aspects of 229 patients with primary amyloidosis. Survival of the various syndromes is emphasized.*

Stone MJ: Amyloidosis: A final common pathway for protein deposition in tissues. Blood 75:531, 1990. *This is an excellent overview of systemic amyloidosis.*

152 Diseases of the Lymph Nodes and Spleen

Douglas V. Faller

PHYSIOLOGY AND FUNCTIONS OF THE LYMPH NODES

The lymph node is divided structurally into three primary areas: the cortex, paracortex, and medulla (Fig. 152–1). These areas are physically and functionally interlaced and surrounded by a series of sinuses. The *cortex* is the outermost portion of the lymph node, located immediately beneath the subcapsular sinus, and is the major site of B cell (antibody-producing lymphocyte) localization in the node. *Afferent lymphatic* drainage, carrying antigens and microorganisms, flows into this space and into immediate contact with lymphocytes, antigen-presenting nonphagocytic cells (histiocytes), and phagocytic cells (macrophages) of the cortex. Such immune stimulation results in enlargement of *lymphoid follicles* in the cortex, producing *germinal centers*, sites of intense B cell proliferation and antibody production. The *paracortex* lies between the cortex and medulla and is the primary site of localization of T cells. It additionally contains macrophages and histiocytes. The paracortex is also the site of lymphocyte trafficking, where recirculating T and B cells enter the lymphatics from the venous system. The *medulla* of the lymph node is made up of a tortuous network of endothelial cell–lined sinuses that coalesce at the hilus to form the *efferent lymphatic*. Antigens are effectively trapped during the slow percolation of lymphatic fluid through the node. In addition, the sinuses are decked with macrophages, which actively scavenge particulate matter and microorganisms.

The lymph node functions as the major site of interaction of antigen with cells of the immune system. Macrophages and histiocytes, which are capable of taking up and presenting antigen, are placed in intimate contact with helper T cells and B cells to facilitate lymphocyte stimulation and production of antibody. Antigen can reach the node in two ways. Antigen can flow in passively via the afferent lymphatics or be actively carried into the node by recirculating lymphocytes and macrophages.

Enlargement of lymph nodes (*lymphadenopathy*) can thus result from proliferation of resident lymphocytes following antigen exposure during infection. Hyperplasia of nonlymphoid cells in the nodes, including macrophages and circulating inflammatory cells, can result from inflammation or infection and also cause node enlargement. In either of these situations, the nodal architecture is preserved despite the cellular hyperplasia. Malignant proliferation of lymphocytes within the lymph node, as seen in lymphomas or leukemias, is easily distinguishable from benign hyperplasia because normal nodal structures are effaced. Lymph nodes also serve as effective traps for circulating tumor cells and provide fertile ground for their continued growth. Thus, malignant metastases are another cause of lymph node enlargement.

EVALUATION OF THE LYMPH NODES

NODAL GROUPS AND DRAINAGE PATTERNS. Because lymphatic flow is regionally distributed, an understanding of the relationship between the anatomic location of the superficial lymph node groups and the origin of afferent lymphatics that drain into these nodes is critical for examination and differential diagnosis of the patient with lymphadenopathy. Several lymph node subgroups, all draining structures in the head and neck, constitute the cervical nodes. The submental nodes, located

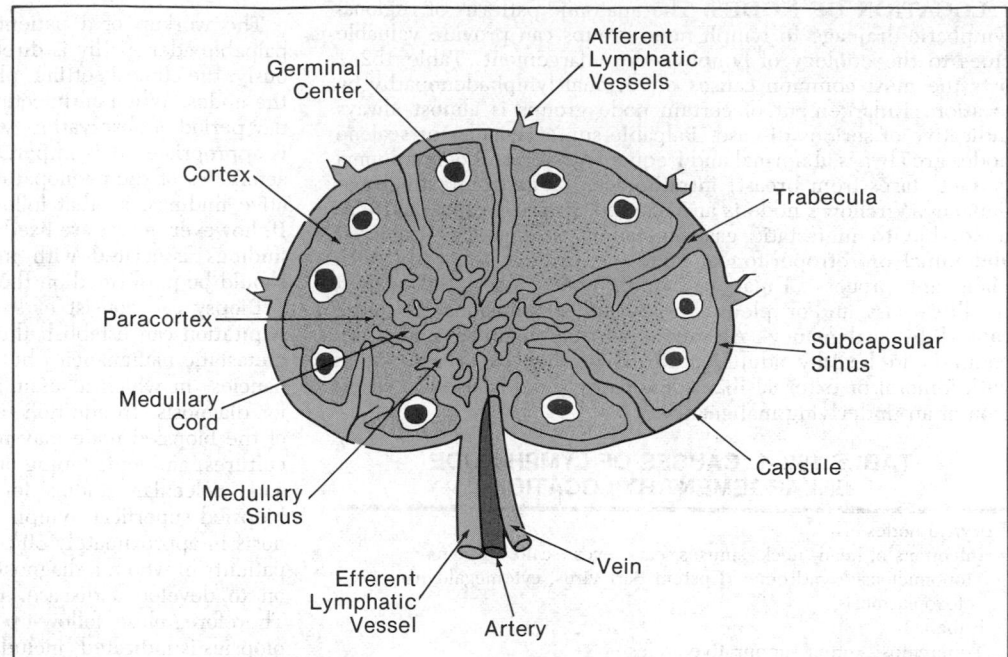

FIGURE 152–1. Diagrammatic representation of the structure of a lymph node.

under the chin, and the submandibular nodes, near the angles of the jaw, receive drainage from structures in the mouth and salivary glands. The jugular nodes, which lie along the anterior border of the sternocleidomastoid muscle, the supraclavicular nodes, found behind the midportion of the clavicle, and the suboccipital nodes, which lie in the posterior cervical triangle, receive lymphatics from many head and neck structures. In addition, the supraclavicular nodes also drain intrathoracic and intra-abdominal organ systems. Lymphatic flow from the eyes, the ears, and the scalp is directed toward the preauricular and postauricular node groups, which lie in front of and behind the ear, respectively. The central and lateral axillary node groups, which are located in the chest wall and along the upper humerus, respectively, receive drainage from the upper extremity, chest wall, breast, and intrathoracic structures. Other node groups with similar drainage patterns include the subscapular nodes, lying anterior to the latissimus dorsi muscle, the pectoral nodes, lying under the edge of the pectoralis major muscle, and the infraclavicular nodes, lying under the distal clavicle. The epitrochlear nodes, located just above the medial humeral epicondyle, receive lymphatic flow from the forearm and hand. The inguinal nodes lie along the inguinal ligament and drain the lower extremity and genitalia. The external iliac and femoral nodes, found in the femoral triangle, have a similar drainage pattern but also receive afferents from pelvic structures.

The deep node systems of the thorax and abdomen, including the hilar, mediastinal, abdominal, retroperitoneal, and pelvic nodes, receive afferent lymphatic flow directly from organs of the thorax, abdomen, and pelvis. In addition, they receive secondary drainage from the superficial node groups. Discovery of enlargement of these deep node groups is usually the result of a directed diagnostic workup or is occasionally made from surveillance roentgenography. However, the mass effect resulting from enlargement of deep node groups can result in distinctive symptoms that should suggest to the clinician a disease process producing internal adenopathy. Enlargement of thoracic nodes (hilar or mediastinal) can compress the trachea or mainstem bronchi (producing cough, dyspnea, or wheezing), the esophagus (resulting in dysphagia), the superior vena cava or subclavian vein (causing venous congestion in the face, neck, and arm), the phrenic nerve (causing paralysis of the diaphragm), or the recurrent laryngeal nerve (producing hoarseness). Because the abdomen and pelvis are less rigidly enclosed than the thorax, compression syndromes resulting from enlargement of deep node groups here are less common, but internal iliac or pelvic node enlargement can lead to venous or lymphatic congestion in the leg or external genitalia. Extremely large abdominal and pelvic nodes are occasionally detectable by deep palpation.

SIGNIFICANCE OF LYMPH NODE ENLARGEMENT

Lymph node enlargement is a common finding on physical examination. Certain lymph nodes are palpable under normal circumstances. Submandibular nodes less than 1 cm in diameter are common in children and young adults, and inguinal nodes 0.5 to 2 cm in diameter are frequently found in healthy adults. The first component of an efficient approach to lymphadenopathy is evaluation of its significance. Assessment of three factors permits interpretation of the importance of the finding of lymphadenopathy and, in addition, begins to establish a differential diagnosis.

CLINICAL SETTING. The age of the patient is of major importance in evaluating lymphadenopathy, with lymph node enlargement more often reflecting serious disease in adults. Lymphadenopathy in patients less than 30 years of age is due to benign (and usually infectious) causes in at least 80 per cent of cases. In those more than 30 years of age, however, lymphadenopathy is due to a benign process only 40 per cent of the time. Clinical features and the setting frequently guide and direct the workup. For example, coexistence of fever and signs of localized or systemic infection, especially in a younger patient, usually suggests an infectious etiology. Alternatively, the presence of constitutional symptoms, such as weight loss, night sweats, or low-grade fevers, points to a malignant cause of localized adenopathy. The differential diagnosis of mediastinal adenopathy in a young patient from an endemic area must include histoplasmosis as well as lymphoma. Generalized lymphadenopathy in a homosexual, hemophiliac, or intravenous drug abuser suggests a human immunodeficiency virus (HIV)–related syndrome.

PHYSICAL CHARACTERISTICS. Palpation of lymph nodes is best performed with the fingertips, using a circular motion and gradually increasing pressure. Examination of enlarged lymph nodes reveals physical characteristics, such as firmness, mobility, and tenderness, that are helpful in narrowing the diagnostic choices. Because of rapid enlargement and stretching of the joint capsule, lymphadenopathy due to infectious processes is often tender. Nodes enlarged by infection can be matted or asymmetric, and the overlying skin may be inflamed and tender. The nodes may be suppurative, especially when the infectious agent is a mycobacterium or a pyogenic bacterium like staphylococcus. Metastatic tumor produces enlarged nodes that are firm, nontender, and frequently fixed to underlying tissue. Lymphomatous processes result in large, often symmetric lymph nodes that are firm, mobile, nontender, and rubbery.

LOCATION OF NODES. The anatomic patterns of regional lymphatic drainage to lymph node groups can provide valuable clues to the etiology of lymph node enlargement. Table 152–1 lists the most common causes of regional lymphadenopathy by location. Enlargement of certain node groups is almost always indicative of serious disease. Palpable supraclavicular or scalene nodes are always abnormal and frequently the result of lymphoma or metastases from breast, intrathoracic, or gastrointestinal malignancy. Virchow's node is an enlarged, firm left supraclavicular node due to metastatic gastrointestinal malignancy. Enlarged abdominal or retroperitoneal nodes are usually the result of a malignant process. Enlarged lymph nodes associated with a satellite mass and/or pleural or peritoneal effusions are often caused by malignancy. Although palpable inguinal nodes are common in healthy adults, progressive changes or association with femoral or external iliac adenopathy should raise the suspicion of an underlying malignancy.

TABLE 152–1. CAUSES OF LYMPH NODE ENLARGEMENT BY LOCATION

Cervical nodes
　Infections of head, neck, sinuses, ears, eyes, scalp, pharynx
　Mononucleosis syndromes (Epstein-Barr virus, cytomegalovirus, toxoplasmosis)
　Rubella
　Tuberculosis (often suppurative nodes)
　Lymphoma (often unilateral)
　Head and neck malignancy (often unilateral)
Scalene/supraclavicular nodes
　Lung, retroperitoneal, or gastrointestinal malignancy (e.g., Virchow's node)
　Lymphoma
　Thoracic or retroperitoneal bacterial or fungal infections
Axillary nodes
　Infections, bites, trauma to hands or arms
　Cat-scratch disease
　Lymphoma
　Breast carcinoma
　Brucellosis
　Melanoma
Epitrochlear nodes
　Infections of hand (unilateral)
　Lymphoma (unilateral)
　Sarcoidosis (bilateral)
　Tularemia (often unilateral)
　Secondary syphilis (bilateral)
Inguinal nodes
　Infections of leg or foot
　Lymphoma
　Pelvic malignancy
　Venereal diseases (lymphogranuloma venereum, syphilis)
　Pasteurella pestis
Hilar nodes
　Sarcoidosis
　Tuberculosis
　Systemic fungal infections
　Lung carcinoma (unilateral)
Mediastinal nodes
　Mononucleosis syndromes
　Sarcoidosis
　Tuberculosis
　Histoplasmosis
　Lung carcinoma
　Lymphoma
Abdominal/retroperitoneal nodes
　Mesenteric lymphadenitis (tuberculosis)
　Lymphoma
　Germ cell tumors/seminoma
　Prostatic carcinoma and other malignancies
Generalized lymphadenopathy (more than two separate sites)
　Infections (EBV, CMV, toxoplasmosis, tuberculosis, hepatitis, syphilis, HIV/AIDS, histoplasmosis)
　Malignancy (lymphoma, chronic myelogenous leukemia, chronic lymphocytic leukemia, acute leukemia)
　Drug reactions
　Systemic lymphadenopathy syndromes

DIAGNOSTIC APPROACH TO LYMPH NODE ENLARGEMENT

The workup of a patient presenting with newly discovered palpable adenopathy is directed by the factors mentioned previously: the clinical setting, physical characteristics, and location of the nodes. When an infectious cause is strongly suspected, a 14-day period of observation, with or without antimicrobial therapy, is appropriate. It is imperative to record the location and characteristics of the adenopathy carefully, including pertinent negative findings, so that follow-up observations can be validated. If, however, nodes are fixed or firm, or any of the aforementioned findings associated with malignancy are discovered, a biopsy should be performed on the node immediately.

Biopsy can consist of surgical excision or needle aspiration. Aspiration can establish the diagnosis in infectious processes or metastatic malignancies but is rarely helpful in lymphoid malignancies, in which assessment of nodal architecture is required for diagnosis. In addition to routine pathologic studies, analysis of the biopsied node may include (where appropriate) microbial cultures, antigenic typing of lymphocytes, chromosomal analysis, and molecular studies for gene rearrangements. Analysis of biopsied superficial lymph nodes in adults establishes the diagnosis in approximately 50 per cent of cases. One fourth of those patients in whom a diagnosis cannot be established by biopsy go on to develop a disease, usually a lymphoma, within a year. Therefore, close follow-up of patients with nondiagnostic first biopsies is indicated, including repeat biopsies if adenopathy and symptoms persist, as well as consultation with experienced hematopathologists.

Evaluation of deep lymph node groups for enlargement usually requires roentgenography or ultrasonography. Enlarged nodes deep in the axilla may be visualized by mammographic or xerographic techniques. Hilar and mediastinal nodes can be evaluated by standard chest radiographs or computed tomography (CT). Lymphangiography was formerly the standard for evaluation of pelvic, retroperitoneal and abdominal nodes but is being rapidly supplanted by CT.

DISEASE PROCESSES RESULTING IN LYMPHADENOPATHY

A number of mechanisms can produce enlargement of the lymph nodes: (1) hyperplasia of benign lymphocytes in response to infection and/or antigenic stimulation; (2) proliferation of circulating inflammatory and phagocytic cells in response to infection; (3) proliferation and infiltration of phagocytic cells in the lipid storage disorders; (4) neoplastic proliferation of malignant lymphocytes or phagocytes; and (5) infiltration by metastatic malignant cells.

Table 152–2 lists the most common diseases associated with lymphadenopathy and the pathophysiologic mechanism responsible for nodal enlargement. Infectious, inflammatory, and neoplastic disorders account for the vast majority of lymphadenopathy encountered in practice. In addition, there are a number of other uncommon diseases of unknown etiology that primarily involve the lymph nodes, or in which lymphadenopathy is prominent or even the cardinal manifestation of the disease.

Amyloidosis is a condition manifested by deposition of fibrillar material in various organs, including the lymph nodes (Ch. 197). The disease states associated with this deposition may be inflammatory, neoplastic, or hereditary. If the function of internal organs is not compromised by the deposited amyloid, lymphadenopathy, which is characteristically firm, nontender, and diffuse or localized may be the first manifestation of the condition. Analysis of sections from a biopsied node reveals the characteristic staining and ultrastructural properties of the amyloid material.

Sarcoidosis (Ch. 67) is a granulomatous disease of young adults involving multiple organ systems, most commonly the lungs, skin, eyes, and nervous system. Bilateral symmetric hilar adenopathy, often associated with paratracheal adenopathy in an asymptomatic patient, is characteristic of the disease. Peripheral lymphadenopathy is modest or absent. The differential diagnosis of hilar adenopathy must include lymphoma, lung carcinoma, histoplasmosis, and tuberculosis, although the symmetry of the

Infection (lymphoid and/or phagocytic hyperplasia)
   Viral (herpesviruses [CMV, EBV, varicella zoster (V-Z)], rubella, HIV, hepatitis A, vaccinia)
   Bacterial (streptococcal, staphylococcal, *Brucella*, tularemia, *Listeria*, cat-scratch disease, *Pasteurella pestis, Haemophilus ducreyi*, syphilis, leptospirosis)
   Fungal (histoplasmosis, coccidioidomycosis)
   Mycobacterial (tuberculosis, leprosy)
   Chlamydial (trachoma, lymphogranuloma venereum)
   Parasitic (toxoplasmosis, trypanosomiasis, filariasis)

Inflammation (lymphoid hyperplasia)
   Rheumatoid arthritis, sarcoidosis, systemic lupus erythematosus, dermatomyositis, immune complex disease/serum sickness, angioimmunoblastic lymphadenopathy, drug reactions

Neoplasms
   Hematologic (myeloproliferative or lymphoproliferative): lymphomas, Hodgkin's disease, acute or chronic myeloid and lymphoid leukemias, malignant histiocytosis
   Metastatic (infiltrative): tumors of breast, lung, kidney, prostate, head and neck, and gastrointestinal tract; melanoma; germ cell tumors; seminoma; neuroblastoma; sarcoma

Infiltration
   Gaucher's disease, Niemann-Pick disease, amyloidosis

Endocrine (lymphoid hyperplasia)
   Hyperthyroidism

Disease of unknown cause with prominent lymphadenopathy
   Mucocutaneous lymph node syndrome
   Lymphomatoid granulomatosis
   Dermatopathic lymphadenitis
   Histiocytic disorder (Letterer-Siwe disease, erythrophagocytic lymphohistiocytosis, sinus histiocytosis, histiocytic medullary reticulosis, malignant histiocytosis)
   Giant follicular lymph node hyperplasia

adenopathy and frequent lack of associated symptoms in sarcoidosis are distinctive.

Mucocutaneous lymph node syndrome (Kawasaki's syndrome) is a disease of children and occasionally young adults, manifested by a distinctive erythematous and desquamative exanthem, conjunctivitis, and fever, with asymmetric cervical adenopathy found in 75 per cent of patients.

Lymphomatoid granulomatosis (Ch. 264) is an infiltration of blood vessel walls with atypical lymphoid and plasmacytoid cells that form granulomas. The vessels of the lung, skin, kidneys, and central nervous system are most often involved, and the intrathoracic lymph nodes are enlarged in 40 per cent of cases. The invading lymphocytes are most likely premalignant T cells, as up to half of patients will go on to develop a T cell lymphoma.

Angioimmunoblastic lymphadenopathy is characterized by a distinctive proliferation of immature and mature plasma cells in a setting of neovasculature. Hepatosplenomegaly and generalized lymphadenopathy are accompanied by a polyclonal hyperglobulinemia, hemolytic anemia, and systemic symptoms. Diagnosis can usually be established by lymph node biopsy, although the disease can be confused with the immunoblastic lymphadenopathy associated with drug reactions, especially phenytoin and allopurinol. One quarter to one half of patients with angioimmunoblastic lymphadenopathy go on to develop a B cell lymphoma (immunoblastic sarcoma).

HISTIOCYTIC DISORDERS

An array of diseases characterized by proliferation of normal or malignant histiocytes (antigen-presenting and antigen-processing mononuclear phagocytes) can manifest with lymphadenopathy as a prominent finding. The benign proliferative disorders can be subdivided according to whether or not the proliferating cell is a Langerhans (or Langerhans-like) histiocyte. The *Langerhans cell histiocytoses* (Ch. 149) occur most often in children with three overlapping presentations. In the past, they were collectively designated *histiocytosis X* (X for unknown etiology). The presentations include the following: (1) *eosinophilic granuloma* occurs in older children and adults and presents as solitary or multiple bone lesions; (2) *Hand-Schüller-Christian syndrome*, defined as the triad of lytic skull lesions, exophthalmos, and diabetes insipidus, usually affects young children; (3) *Letterer-Siwe disease*, a systemic histiocytosis disorder, occurs in infants and is manifested

by fever, eczematoid rash, otitis, lymphadenopathy, hepatosplenomegaly, and other visceral involvement.

The non–Langerhans cell histiocytoses are also nonmalignant proliferative disorders and can all result in regional or generalized lymphadenopathy. *Familial erythrophagocytic lymphohistiocytosis* and *infection-associated hemophagocytic syndrome* are both characterized by constitutional symptoms, pancytopenia, hepatosplenomegaly, lymphadenopathy, and the distinctive pathologic finding of phagocytosed erythrocytes in bone marrow or lymph node specimens. *Sinus histiocytosis* frequently manifests with massive cervical lymphadenopathy, fever, leukocytosis, and, less often, generalized lymphadenopathy. *Malignant histiocytosis (histiocytic medullary reticulosis)* is a progressive proliferation of atypical (but not clearly malignant) histiocytes and immature monocytoid cells, producing severe constitutional symptoms, generalized lymphadenopathy in 50 per cent of cases, hepatosplenomegaly, pancytopenia, and papulonodular skin lesions. True malignancies of histiocytes are rare. They include histiocytic sarcoma, true malignant histiocytosis, and monocytic leukemia, all of which produce prominent lymphadenopathy.

PHYSIOLOGY AND FUNCTIONS OF THE SPLEEN

The spleen, the largest lymphoid organ in the body, plays a major role in the cellular and humoral immune response to infection and inflammation. In addition, with its unique architecture and network of fixed phagocytic cells, the spleen is the primary filter for circulating senescent cells, antigens, and microorganisms in the blood. Unlike the lymph nodes, the spleen receives no direct lymphatic drainage. A spleen of average size (135 grams) receives a blood flow of 300 ml per minute. Splenic vessels from the hilus penetrate trabeculations formed by invaginations of the splenic capsule (Fig. 152–2). The central arterioles, surrounded by sheaths of lymphoid tissue, have branches (follicular arterioles) that take off at right angles, effectively skimming plasma and circulating antigens from the blood and delivering them directly to the splenic immune system. The terminal arterioles are open ended and dump the remaining concentrated blood cells into the splenic cords. Some cells are shunted rapidly into the venous collection system, but many percolate slowly through the open splenic cords for several minutes before squeezing through 0.5- to 2.5-μm slits between the endothelial cells and the discontinuous basement membrane of the venous sinusoids and re-entering the splenic venous system. The cut surface

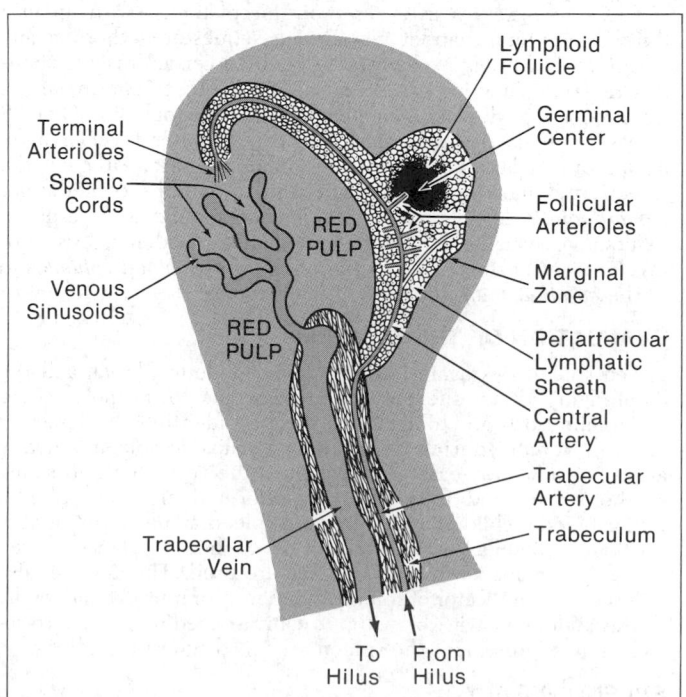

FIGURE 152–2. Diagrammatic representation of the structure of the spleen.

of the spleen displays a prominent red pulp, dotted with islands of white pulp, which serve to compartmentalize the filtrative and immunologic functions of the spleen, respectively.

THE WHITE PULP. The white pulp consists of periarteriolar lymphatic sheaths, with a mantle layer of small lymphocytes (predominantly T lymphocytes) surrounding lymphoid germinal centers, which contain B cells and plasmablasts. Blood-borne antigens and pathogens are concentrated and contact immune responder cells in the white pulp. Circulating particulate antigens and opsonized microorganisms are rapidly phagocytized by macrophages in both the white and the red pulp and are presented to the lymphocytes surrounding the germinal centers in the white pulp. Reactive plasmablasts secreting immunoglobulin M (IgM) appear, and the germinal centers enlarge within 24 hours. Consequently, the white pulp component of the spleen hypertrophies in response to infection and antigenic stimulation. The spleen is therefore important in mounting a response to new immune challenges and serves as the major source of IgM production in the body. The marginal zone of the spleen surrounds these periarteriolar lymphatic sheaths of the white pulp with a dense reticulum in which the terminal arterioles end. This marginal zone blends into the red pulp.

THE RED PULP. The splenic cords (of Billroth) make up the red pulp. Erythrocytes slowly traverse these nonendothelialized cords and are subjected to metabolic conditions (including hypoxia, glucose deprivation, and low pH) that stress senescent or even mildly damaged cells. Defective erythrocytes with abnormally stiff cytoplasm (as in the sickle cell hemoglobinopathies), deficient cellular membrane (as in the spherocytic hemolytic diseases), or excessive rigidity of membrane and cytoskeleton (as in the thalassemia syndromes) are then *culled* from this retarded microcirculation by the avidly phagocytic macrophages, reticular cells, and littoral cells that line the cords. *Pitting* of inclusions from erythrocytes is also performed by these phagocytes as the red cells are squeezed through narrow fenestrations into the venous sinuses. This pitting function removes Howell-Jolly bodies (nuclear remnants), Heinz bodies (denatured hemoglobin), and intraerythrocytic parasites, such as *Plasmodium* and *Bartonella*. New reticulocytes are *conditioned* in this environment, losing up to 30 per cent of their cell membrane and any remaining mitochondria. Iron from ingested red blood cells is stored by the splenic phagocytes and released to the plasma for *reutilization of iron*. In states of abnormal hemolysis, a buildup of hemosiderin occurs in these cells.

The spleen serves as a *reservoir* for platelets, with up to a third of the total platelet mass being sequestered there at any one time in a freely exchangeable pool. In certain disease states this reservoir function can be exaggerated. Acute entrapment of erythrocytes in the splenomegalic crisis of hemoglobin SC or SS disease (*splenic sequestration*) or the blackwater fever crisis of falciparum malaria can result in profound shock. Although the spleen is a blood-forming organ until 5 months of gestation, *hematopoiesis* in the adult spleen occurs only as a result of pathologic, usually neoplastic, conditions. Evidence exists for involvement of the spleen in the *regulation of blood volume* and in the *catabolism of low density lipoproteins*.

EVALUATION OF THE SPLEEN

The spleen lies against the posterior abdominal wall and the diaphragm. When the spleen enlarges, its lower pole moves down, anteriorly and to the right. It is best identified by detection of its movement during respiration. A palpable spleen is nearly always significantly enlarged, except in the very young. Imaging of the spleen and liver can be performed after injection of radiolabeled colloid. To visualize the spleen alone, or to identify accessory spleens, heat-damaged or chemically damaged red blood cells tagged with ^{51}Cr or ^{99m}Tc are used. This test can also be used as an indicator of splenic function. Computed tomography of the abdomen (with or without contrast medium) and ultrasonography complement the spleen scan as diagnostic studies.

SPLENOMEGALY

Five general mechanisms may enlarge the spleen: (1) reactive proliferation of lymphoid cells, (2) infiltration by neoplastic cells

TABLE 152–3. CAUSES OF SPLENOMEGALY

Infection (lymphoid hyperplasia)
  Viral, parasitic, bacterial, fungal
Inflammation (lymphoid hyperplasia)
  Rheumatoid arthritis, sarcoidosis, systemic lupus erythematosus, renal dialysis, beryllium, serum sickness
Neoplasms (infiltrative or myeloproliferative)
  Leukemia, lymphoma, polycythemia vera, myeloid metaplasia, Hodgkin's disease, metastatic tumors, primary tumors
Hemolytic diseases (phagocytic hyperplasia)
  Spherocytosis, thalassemia major, pyruvate kinase deficiency, paroxysmal nocturnal hemoglobinuria, hemoglobinopathies, immune cytopenias
Deficiency diseases
  Iron deficiency, pernicious anemia
Infiltration
  Gaucher's disease, Neimann-Pick disease, amyloidosis, extramedullary hematopoiesis
Splenic vein hypertension (vascular congestion)
  Cirrhosis, splenic or portal vein thrombosis, hepatic schistosomiasis, congestive heart failure
Endocrine
  Graves' disease, Hashimoto's thyroiditis
Hemophilia (subsequent to intensive therapy with clotting factor concentrate)
Other
  Cysts, angioimmunoblastic lymphadenopathy, histiocytoses, hyperlipidemias

or lipid-laden macrophages, (3) extramedullary hematopoiesis, (4) proliferation of phagocytic cells, and (5) vascular congestion. Diseases may cause splenomegaly by one or by a combination of these mechanisms (Table 152–3). The causes of massive splenomegaly (greater than 3000 grams) are somewhat more limited (Table 152–4). The myelodysplastic disorders and malignant lymphoid disorders are the most common causes of chronic massive splenomegaly in nontropical countries. Splenomegaly can be present as an isolated finding on physical examination, can exist in association with a systemic disorder, or can be discovered as a consequence of the secondary hematologic effects of splenic enlargement—the hypersplenism syndrome. Symptoms arising from splenomegaly may include pain from the stretched capsule of an acutely enlarged spleen or shock from atraumatic rupture of a tense capsule.

Evaluation of splenomegaly should include examination of the peripheral blood and frequently the bone marrow. A spleen scan is recommended to determine the size and shape of the spleen and to look for defects suggestive of tumors, cysts, or extrasplenic masses displacing the spleen. In general, diagnostic tests are not

TABLE 152–4. CAUSES OF MASSIVE SPLENOMEGALY

Acute
  Malaria (falciparum) with splenic sequestration crisis
  Sickle cell anemia with splenic sequestration crisis
Chronic
  Myelodysplastic
    Chronic myelogenous leukemia
    Myeloid metaplasia/myelofibrosis
    Polycythemia vera (end-stage)
    Primary thrombocythemia
  Neoplastic
    Lymphoma
    Malignant reticuloendotheliosis
    Hodgkin's disease
    Hairy cell leukemia
    Chronic lymphocytic leukemia
  Hematologic
    Thalassemia major
    Sickle cell anemia (rarely)
  Inflammatory-infiltrative
    Gaucher's disease
    Sarcoidosis
    Felty's syndrome
  Infectious
    Malaria
    Kala-azar

performed on the spleen itself; they are oriented toward the diagnosis of disease states producing splenomegaly. Chest radiography or liver function tests may reveal the etiology of the splenic enlargement. If lymphadenopathy is present, lymph node biopsy may yield a diagnosis. When systemic symptoms accompany splenomegaly but no lymphadenopathy is appreciated, a laparotomy with biopsies of liver, spleen, and lymph nodes is sometimes indicated. Such a study will produce a diagnosis of lymphoma in one third of cases, congestive splenomegaly in one quarter, and an inflammatory state in one fifth.

INFECTION. Systemic infections are the most common causes of moderate and transient splenomegaly. Splenic enlargement is the rule in mononucleosis due to Epstein-Barr virus infection but is less frequent in the heterophil-negative mononucleosis syndromes associated with cytomegalovirus, adenovirus, or acquired toxoplasmosis. Splenomegaly can be massive, however, in congenital toxoplasmosis or other infectious causes of the TORCH (toxoplasmosis, rubella, cytomegalovirus, and herpes simplex) syndrome. A palpable spleen is often detected in the course of viral hepatitis and influenza and less often in association with infectious lymphocytosis, pertussis, and roseola infantum. Bacterial infections causing splenomegaly include secondary syphilis, subacute bacterial endocarditis, and acute brucellosis. Hematogenous spread of tuberculosis or histoplasmosis can involve the spleen. Splenomegaly is common in tropical populations and is due to malaria, schistosomiasis, leishmaniasis (kala-azar), chronic worm infestation, and other disorders. Rickettsial infection can produce splenic enlargement, with a palpable spleen being noted in up to 40 per cent of patients with Rocky Mountain spotted fever. Modest splenomegaly is appreciated in 30 to 80 per cent of patients with the lymphadenopathy accompanying the HIV disease–related complex (ARC).

INFLAMMATION. Splenomegaly is found in systemic lupus erythematosus (20 per cent), rheumatoid arthritis (5 to 10 per cent), and Behçet's disease and frequently results in production of cytopenias by hypersplenism. Angioimmunoblastic lymphadenopathy, sometimes associated with anticonvulsant administration, is characterized by splenomegaly, autoimmune hemolytic anemia, and dysproteinemia. Regional ileitis is occasionally accompanied by a histiocytic infiltration of the spleen.

NEOPLASMS. The myelodysplastic disorders and leukemias (acute and chronic) commonly infiltrate the spleen, causing modest to massive enlargement. Splenic involvement is noted in 30 to 40 per cent of adult non-Hodgkin's lymphoma at presentation. Primary malignant tumors of the spleen are rare and include lymphangiosarcomas, hemangiosarcomas, fibrosarcomas, and leiomyosarcomas. They may present with local or systemic problems and are diagnosed by CT, spleen scan, and angiography. Metastatic tumor is a rare cause of splenomegaly.

STORAGE DISEASES. Previously undiagnosed Gaucher's disease is a cause of asymptomatic splenomegaly. Niemann-Pick disease and the sea-blue histiocyte syndrome can also present in this way. Diagnosis can often be made by bone marrow biopsy.

CHRONIC CONGESTIVE SPLENOMEGALY (BANTI'S SYNDROME). This complex is characterized by splenomegaly, pancytopenia as a consequence of hypersplenism, and gastrointestinal bleeding secondary to portal hypertension. The splenic vein hypertension is due to either intrahepatic disease (e.g., cirrhosis or schistosomiasis) or extrahepatic disease (such as portal or splenic vein thrombosis). Splenic vein thrombosis is most commonly caused by compression of the splenic vein by tumor or fibrosis. Pregnancy, trauma, or intravascular coagulation can predispose to portal vein thrombosis. The spleen is markedly enlarged and congested, with distended veins and venous sinuses. Periarteriolar hemorrhage, siderotic nodules, hyperplasia of the red pulp, and progressive fibrosis occur. Symptoms can range from vague gastrointestinal complaints to catastrophic bleeding from esophageal or gastric varices. Hematologic cytopenias may be severe but are rarely the major medical concern. Etiologic studies of congestive splenomegaly should include evaluation for alcoholism, liver function tests, liver-spleen scan, liver biopsy, and a search for varices. If no liver disease is found, venous obstruction should be considered and splenoportal venography performed. Splenic or hepatic vein thrombosis may be the initial presentation in an occult myeloproliferative disease, particularly polycythemia vera.

HYPERSPLENISM

Hypersplenism is an exaggeration of normal splenic function, with enhanced filtration and phagocytosis of the cellular elements of the blood. The hyperplastic spleen can sequester as much as 90 per cent of the total platelet pool or 45 per cent of the red cell mass. Four criteria support the diagnosis of hypersplenism: (1) cytopenia of one or more hematologic cell lines, (2) compensatory reactive marrow hyperplasia, (3) splenomegaly, and (4) correction of abnormalities by splenectomy.

Hypersplenism is frequently secondary to splenic enlargement. Splenomegaly due to infiltrative diseases (lymphoma, chronic leukemia, Gaucher's disease, amyloidosis) is not usually associated with the severe cytopenias of hypersplenism. Enlargement of the spleen due to hypertrophy of the phagocytic elements (inflammatory diseases) or secondary to congestive splenomegaly with slowing of the cellular transit time through the spleen, however, is frequently accompanied by anemia, thrombocytopenia, or granulocytopenia of varying degrees. The erythrostatic environment of hypersplenism is especially threatening to red blood cells with mild intrinsic abnormalities. The patient with well-compensated hereditary spherocytosis or elliptocytosis may experience acute, severe hemolysis from the transient splenic enlargement accompanying mononucleosis. Similarly, the anemia of chronic liver disease may worsen as the increasing pressure in the portal system causes stasis and destruction of acanthocytes in the spleen. The harsh metabolic environment of the splenic cords (hypoxia, low glucose levels, and low pH) is exaggerated in the enlarged and congested spleen. In addition, phagocytosis of red cells or platelets stimulates more reactive hyperplasia of splenic histiocytes, begetting more hypersplenism. This is the mechanism underlying *primary hypersplenism*, in which the spleen hypertrophies because of phagocytosis of defective red cells (hereditary spherocytosis), antibody-coated red cells (autoimmune hemolytic anemia), or antibody-coated platelets (autoimmune thrombocytopenia). Hypersplenism can be documented and quantified by demonstrating a decrease in the circulating half-life of labeled erythrocytes along with an increase in the spleen-liver uptake ratio.

INDICATIONS FOR SPLENECTOMY

Splenectomy may be indicated for either of two medical conditions: (1) to stage or control a basic disease process (Hodgkin's disease, hereditary spherocytosis, autoimmune cytopenias) or (2) to alleviate the consequences of hypersplenism secondary to other disease processes. In addition, the spleen may have to be removed because of traumatic or, rarely, spontaneous rupture causing intra-abdominal hemorrhage.

THROMBOCYTOPENIA. *Chronic autoimmune thrombocytopenia* (ITP) refractory to corticosteroid therapy usually improves (in 70 to 90 per cent of patients) after splenectomy, with the platelet count becoming normal in 60 per cent of patients. Those who do not respond completely can often be maintained on a lower corticosteroid dose. The thrombocytopenia accompanying *systemic* or *discoid lupus* responds poorly to splenectomy. *Thrombotic thrombocytopenic purpura* has been treated in the past with splenectomy and steroid therapy, but newer modalities, including plasmapheresis or plasma exchange, appear more promising (Ch. 154).

HEMOLYTIC ANEMIAS. *Autoimmune hemolytic anemia* caused by warm-reacting antibodies that does not resolve after 2 months of corticosteroid therapy may be treated by splenectomy. Two thirds of such patients have complete or partial remission, but the relapse rate is high. Splenectomy is a uniformly effective treatment for the anemia of *hereditary spherocytosis* (Ch. 134). Surgery should be delayed until the age of 5 years, if possible, to decrease the risk of overwhelming sepsis. Other congenital hemolytic anemias do not respond as consistently to splenectomy, and the decision to remove the spleen should be based on the severity of the anemia and lack of response to alternative treatments.

LEUKEMIAS. Splenectomy is routinely performed for symptomatic cytopenias or splenomegaly in *hairy cell leukemia* (leukemic reticuloendotheliosis). Improvement occurs in up to 85 per cent of patients, but recurrence of cytopenias is common.

Early splenectomy is no longer recommended, and the advent of alpha-interferon therapy for this disease may relegate splenectomy to a secondary role (Ch. 144). In the past, splenectomy was commonly carried out in patients with *chronic myelogenous leukemia* for relief of symptoms or prior to bone marrow transplantation. Any benefit is transient, however; survival is not affected, and the operation in this setting is associated with a high mortality. Splenectomy can provide useful palliation in patients with *prolymphocytic leukemia* and *chronic lymphocytic leukemia* who have symptomatic splenomegaly or autoimmune hemolytic anemia. Splenectomy improves the hematologic status and the quality of life in cases of severe *agnogenic myeloid metaplasia* (Ch. 143).

STORAGE DISEASES. Splenectomy can be performed in *Gaucher's disease* when splenomegaly produces mechanical or cytopenic problems. The spleen serves as a storage area for undigested cerebroside, so it is possible that splenectomy might accelerate the disease (Ch. 174).

FELTY'S SYNDROME. Neutropenia of variable degrees and splenomegaly, occasionally accompanied by thrombocytopenia or anemia, occur in about 1 per cent of patients with rheumatoid arthritis. The spleen appears to be both the source of the antibody coating the neutrophils and the means of their destruction. If the neutropenia is severe enough to cause frequent infections or skin ulcerations, splenectomy is beneficial in 60 to 80 per cent of patients.

THALASSEMIA MAJOR. In the setting of longstanding thalassemia, therapeutic splenectomy is often required. It appears, however, that aggressive transfusion regimens combined with iron chelation therapy may reduce the incidence of severe hypersplenism.

RENAL DIALYSIS HYPERSPLENISM. Up to 10 per cent of uremic patients undergoing long-term dialysis develop signs of hypersplenism. Splenectomy may decrease bleeding tendencies and transfusion requirements in this setting.

ALTERNATIVES TO SPLENECTOMY. Therapy with glucocorticoids inhibits phagocytosis and can provide a useful "chemical splenectomy" in short-term situations. Partial splenectomy is sometimes advocated in children to reduce the risk of postsplenectomy complications. Partial or complete embolization of the spleen using percutaneous catheterization is a relatively safe, effective, and noninvasive approach when surgery is contraindicated. Splenic irradiation (100 to 500 cGy) can provide transient therapy for hypersplenism or splenomegaly due to infiltrative diseases.

POSTSPLENECTOMY SYNDROMES AND HYPOSPLENISM

HEMATOLOGIC SEQUELAE. The hyposplenic or postsplenectomy state can often be diagnosed by examination of the peripheral blood smear (see Color Plate 6K). In the absence of splenic culling and pitting functions, nucleated red blood cells, Howell-Jolly and Heinz body inclusions, siderocytes, and acanthocytes are found in the circulation. Reticulocytes are no longer conditioned, and their redundant cell membrane produces target cells upon drying and staining.

A transient and modest increase in the leukocyte count occurs after splenectomy and lasts 1 to 2 weeks. The bulk of this *leukocytosis* is accounted for by early *neutrophilia*. Later, *lymphocytosis* and *monocytosis* become more prominent.

Splenectomy routinely results in prominent postoperative *thrombocytosis*, often producing platelet counts of 1 million or more per cubic millimeter for weeks to months following surgery. This elevation may persist in 40 per cent of patients. The risk of consequent thromboembolic phenomena after splenectomy is high only in the setting of myeloproliferative disease or paroxysmal nocturnal hemoglobinuria. Attempts should be made to decrease the platelet count with chemotherapy before surgery in such cases. Following surgery, therapy with anticoagulants and antiplatelet agents should be considered, especially if the patient is bedridden.

INFECTION. In the absence of the spleen, or in the setting of functional hyposplenism, certain inadequacies of immune function can be demonstrated. IgM levels fall, and complement-mediated opsonization is decreased. This is in part due to a fall in the levels of tuftsin and properdin, two opsonic proteins produced by the spleen. The ability to phagocytose circulating antigens is compromised, as is cell-mediated immunity.

The risk of *overwhelming sepsis* following splenectomy or in functional hyposplenism is especially high in children, up to 10 per cent per year in debilitated infants. The incidence falls to 1 per cent per year in older children and is rare, but reported, in adults. The etiologic organisms are encapsulated bacteria, predominantly pneumococcus and less commonly meningococcus or *Haemophilus influenzae*. These are poorly opsonized in the body, and the intact spleen, with its slow, tortuous blood flow past avid phagocytes, appears to be the primary site for clearance of these pathogens. All patients with decreased splenic function, whether due to functional hyposplenism or to splenectomy (traumatic or therapeutic), must be warned to take any febrile illness seriously. Prophylaxis with penicillin is recommended for all children with asplenia or splenic hypofunction (e.g., sickle cell anemia). Immunization with polyvalent vaccines to pneumococci, meningococci, and *H. influenzae* is advised for patients over the age of 3 years. Serologic response to these vaccines may not be normal in hyposplenia or asplenia. The optimal timing of vaccine administration (with respect to splenectomy) is not established, but vaccination should precede splenectomy and any chemotherapy, if possible. Serious infections with unusual organisms like *Babesia* or *Bartonella* also occur in hyposplenic individuals. A concurrent viral infection may predispose hyposplenic patients to fulminant bacteremias.

FUNCTIONAL HYPOSPLENISM. Repeated symptomatic or silent infarction of the spleen in the course of veno-occlusive diseases, like the sickle cell syndromes, results in substantial or total loss of splenic tissue (*autosplenectomy*). The spleen is shrunken and fibrosed. Circulating erythrocytes reflect the loss of the splenic filtration function and are found to contain mitochondrial remnants and inclusions of nuclear fragments (Howell-Jolly bodies) and denatured hemoglobin (Heinz bodies). Bizarrely shaped red cells, target cells, and large platelets are observed. Hyposplenism can occur even with a large or normal-sized spleen if splenic tissue has been replaced by sarcoid granulomas, amyloid, or multiple myeloma or if splenic phagocytes have been paralyzed by high-dose corticosteroid therapy. Other diseases linked with hyposplenism include ulcerative colitis, celiac disease, dermatitis herpetiformis, systemic lupus erythematosus, primary thrombocythemia, and Graves' disease. Such patients run the same risk of fulminant bacteremia as do those who have had their spleen surgically removed.

CONGENITAL ASPLENIA. This uncommon condition is associated with symmetric development of normally asymmetric organs or pairs of organs. Complex and multiple cardiovascular anomalies are the rule.

OTHER DISEASES OF THE SPLEEN

SPLENIC RUPTURE. Rupture of the capsule may be precipitated by trauma, by overly zealous palpation of an enlarged spleen (secondary to mononucleosis, sepsis, or leukemia), or rarely by dissection of a pancreatic pseudocyst into the spleen. The patient presents with left upper quadrant pain, sometimes radiating to the left scapular region, and abdominal guarding and rigidity, quickly progressing to hypovolemic shock. Usually, emergency splenectomy is indicated. In selected cases, nonoperative management or splenorrhaphy, including gluing or wrapping of the ruptured capsule ("hair netting"), is a treatment alternative to splenectomy.

SPLENIC INFARCTION. Infarction usually occurs in the setting of splenic enlargement secondary to myeloproliferative disease or vascular occlusive phenomena (sickle hemoglobinopathies, including SS, Sβ thalassemia, and SC diseases). These may be silent infarctions or present with severe left upper quadrant pain.

ARTERIAL ANEURYSMS. These lesions are most common in women beyond middle age. They may be asymptomatic or cause left upper quadrant pain or vague gastrointestinal complaints. The aneurysm of the spleen is sometimes palpable, and a bruit may be appreciated. Radiologic studies can reveal a calcified aneurysmal wall, and the diagnosis is made by sonography or angiography. Embolization of such aneurysms has been successful in situations in which surgery is contraindicated.

SPLENIC HEMANGIOMATOSIS. Diffuse cavernous hemangiomatosis of the spleen is rare, but the cavernous hemangioma is the most common benign tumor involving the spleen. The patient can present with splenic infarctions, splenomegaly, or thrombocytopenia secondary to platelet destruction within the hemangiomas, or the finding of hemangiomatosis may be incidental. The diagnosis can usually be made by CT or sonography.

SPLENIC CYSTS. Echinococcal infection should be suspected in a patient with an appropriate travel history, single or multiple splenic cysts with calcified walls, and eosinophilia. Serologic studies may be helpful in establishing the diagnosis. True splenic cysts (dermoids and mesenchymal inclusion cysts) are embryonic rests and may be diagnosed by CT, sonography, and angiography.

SPLENIC ABSCESS. An occult, deep-seated infection, splenic abscess usually follows a bacteremic episode. The source of the septicemia can be infected endocardium, lung (pneumonia, lung abscess, empyema), skin or soft tissue, pelvis (pelvic inflammatory disease or septic abortion), nasopharynx, or ear. Predisposing factors include previous splenic damage by infarction (secondary to sickle cell disease or leukemia), trauma, and infection (malaria, typhoid, ameba, cysts). Extension of an abscess into the spleen from adjacent perforated abdominal organs (stomach, transverse colon, tail of pancreas) can occur. In most series, streptococci are the most common etiologic agents, followed by staphylococci and, with increasing frequency, by gram-negative organisms (*Salmonella*, Enterobacteriaceae, *Pseudomonas*, *Serratia*, *Bacteroides*) and anaerobes. Presenting symptoms include fever, chills, and left upper quadrant pain, often accompanied by tenderness, muscle spasm, and subcutaneous edema over the spleen. Infection localized to the upper pole of the spleen can produce pleuritic pain and even left pleural effusion. An abscess in the lower pole may result in signs of peritoneal inflammation. A splenic friction rub may be appreciated. Splenic scan, sonography, and CT aid in the diagnosis. The differential diagnosis must include subphrenic abscess, pulmonary empyema, splenic infarction, perinephric abscess, neoplasms, and pancreatic pseudocyst. A combination of antibiotics and surgical intervention, usually splenectomy, is indicated. Single abscesses respond well, but multiple abscesses, often the result of generalized sepsis in a debilitated or immunocompromised patient, are associated with a high mortality.

Cahill CG, Wastell C: Splenic conservation. Surg Annu 22:379, 1990. *A comprehensive review of current surgical techniques aimed at preserving splenic function.*

Chaikof EL, McCabe CT: Fatal overwhelming postsplenectomy infection. Am J Surg 149:534, 1985. *A review of infection patterns in 776 splenectomized adults and children.*

Chun CH, Raff MJ, Contreras L, et al.: Splenic abscess. Medicine, 59:50, 1980. *Comprehensive review of this often fatal disease, discussing etiology, predisposing factors, diagnosis, and treatment.*

Hibberd PL, Rubin RH: Approach to immunization in the immunosuppressed host. Infect Dis Clin North Am 4:124, 1989. *A discussion of the roles of vaccines and adjunctive measures, such as antimicrobials and immunoglobulin, in the asplenic patient.*

Knecht H: Angioimmunoblastic lymphadenopathy: Ten years' experience and state of current knowledge. Semin Hematol 26:208, 1989. *A review of the idiopathic and drug-related forms of this disease and their natural history.*

Pochedly C, Sills RH, Schwartz AD (eds.): Disorders of the Spleen: Pathophysiology and Management. New York, Marcel Dekker, 1989. *Detailed description of splenic anatomy, physiology, and pathophysiology, with extensive discussion of the causes and sequelae of splenic hypofunction and hyperfunction.*

Shaw JH, Print CG: Postsplenectomy sepsis. Br J Surg 76:1074, 1989. *A review of the infectious consequences of elective and emergency splenectomy, with discussion of the role of immunization and prophylaxis.*

153 Bone Marrow Transplantation

Rainer Storb

PRINCIPLES OF MARROW TRANSPLANTATION

Transplantation of marrow from a donor identical with the recipient at the major histocompatibility complex reduces graft-versus-host disease (GVHD) and improves survival of the recipient. Successful human transplantation using allogeneic, human leukocyte antigen (HLA)–identical sibling donors was carried out first in children with immunodeficiency diseases and subsequently in patients with severe aplastic anemia and leukemia.

Marrow transplantation differs in several respects from transplantation of solid organs, in particular the kidney: (1) The host-versus-graft reaction can generally be abrogated by a single short course of high-dose immunosuppressive therapy given immediately before transplantation; (2) preceding blood transfusions are not beneficial but rather can interfere with subsequent marrow engraftment, particularly in patients with aplastic anemia; (3) until recently, donors have mostly been HLA-identical family members; (4) donors do not suffer a permanent organ loss, since the removed marrow is replaced within weeks; and (5) postgrafting immunosuppression of recipients can generally be terminated after 3 to 12 months.

To prepare for marrow transplantation, the recipient's immune system must first be destroyed. This is effectively accomplished by use of cyclophosphamide (CY), at 50 mg per kilogram per day for 4 days, or total body irradiation (TBI), at 800 to 1500 rads in midline tissue doses (4 to 25 rads per minute), either alone or combined with CY or other chemotherapeutic agents. An alternative has been to combine CY with busulfan. These programs not only set the stage for establishment of the allogeneic graft but also serve to kill leukemic cells, if that is the patient's basic disease.

After the conditioning regimen, 2 to 6 $\times$ 10^8 donor marrow cells per kilogram are infused intravenously. Most grafts are initially successful, so that within 2 to 4 weeks marrow cellularity increases and peripheral blood counts of donor origin rise. Over time, all hematopoietic and immune cells of the recipient are replaced by those from the marrow donor, including plasma cells and tissue macrophages.

COMPLICATIONS

Graft-versus-host disease may occur when genetically foreign, immunologically active lymphocytes are transferred into an immunosuppressed recipient incapable of rejecting the lymphocytes. This condition is found in all allogeneic marrow transplant recipients (donors are other than monozygous twins). Donor T lymphocytes present in the marrow inoculum recognize histocompatibility antigens of the host as foreign, become sensitized, proliferate, and attack recipient tissue, thereby producing the clinical syndrome of GVHD. The main targets of GVHD are skin, gastrointestinal tract, and liver. As perhaps the most effective immunosuppressive agent to prevent GVHD, methotrexate or cyclosporine is given within the first 3 to 12 months after grafting. The best results seem to be achieved when the drugs are combined. Once the drugs are discontinued, many patients do well with persisting graft-host tolerance. However, acute GVHD occurs in approximately 35 to 60 per cent of the patients, and as many as 40 per cent of afflicted patients die of associated infections. Xenogeneic antihuman thymocyte globulin (ATG), prednisone, or cyclosporine has been used to treat acute GVHD with some success. Better approaches to prevent or treat acute GVHD are necessary, such as the more imaginative use of known immunosuppressive agents, the use of "germ-free" isolation, or the removal of T lymphocytes from the marrow inoculum by antibodies to human T lymphocytes.

Chronic GVHD affects approximately 25 to 45 per cent of patients surviving more than 180 days. Most frequent in older patients and those who had acute GVHD, it may affect the same organs that are involved in acute GVHD and, additionally, mucous membranes. It resembles collagen vascular diseases and is characterized by severe immunodeficiency, impaired granulocyte chemotaxis, and recurrent, sometimes life-threatening bacterial infections. Combination therapy with prednisone and cyclosporine, azathioprine, CY, or procarbazine is effective in most patients with chronic GVHD.

Interstitial pneumonias, either of unknown etiology or associated with infectious agents such as cytomegalovirus, cause morbidity and fatality during the first 4 months after grafting. They are a major problem in patients who are treated with TBI and then receive transplants for leukemia, but a minor problem in

CY-treated patients receiving transplants for aplastic anemia. Probably these infections are the result of deficient immune reactivity of the compromised host, although radiation effects may also play a role. Effective methods of accelerating the immune reconstitution and/or the use of antiviral agents or hyperimmune globulin might be of value in eliminating the problem of interstitial pneumonia. Patients with cultures negative for cytomegalovirus should receive blood products from cytomegalovirus-negative donors.

CLINICAL RESULTS

SEVERE APLASTIC ANEMIA (Ch. 129). Aplastic anemia is most frequently attributable to a stem cell defect. In many cases, infusion of marrow from a monozygotic twin (syngeneic transplant) has been successful in reconstituting the marrow without immunosuppression of the recipient. Some syngeneic grafts have been successful only after preparation with CY and a second transplant, suggesting that these cases may involve other mechanisms, perhaps of autoimmune etiology, which can be overcome by CY. Allogeneic marrow transplantation (donors are HLA-identical family members) is often effective therapy for severe aplastic anemia, with significantly better survival.

Marrow graft rejection has been a major problem in aplastic anemia, most frequently caused by transfusion-induced sensitization. When transplantation is carried out in patients who have not received transfusions before transplantation, graft failure is the exception. Eighty-three per cent of our first 43 patients are alive between 6 and 16½ (median, 9) years after grafting (Fig. 153–1). We believe that the immunologic mechanisms involved in graft failure are, for the most part, iatrogenic (i.e., induced by previous blood transfusion).

Many programs are being carried out to avoid rejection in multiply transfused patients by using more intensive immunosuppressive conditioning regimens. In all programs, CY is used, but other features of the conditioning regimens vary. In Seattle, methotrexate and cyclosporine are used after grafting, and viable donor buffy coat cells have been infused together with the marrow inoculum. The donor's peripheral blood is a potential source of additional pluripotent hematopoietic stem cells and/or lymphoid cells capable of overcoming rejection. As a rule, the rejection rates have decreased and survival has increased. Of 65 Seattle patients with aplastic anemia who received marrow grafts from HLA-identical siblings following multiple transfusions, 70 per cent are alive after follow-up periods of 6 to 12½ years.

Most of the regimens have associated risks. The addition of buffy coat cells has led to an increased risk of chronic GVHD. Radiation regimens carry the potential risk for late malignant

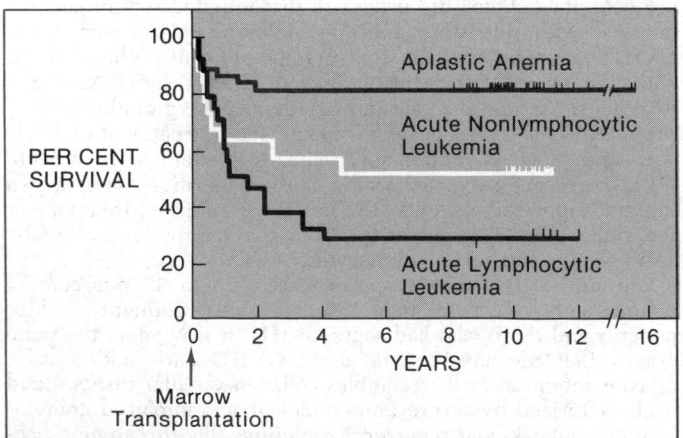

FIGURE 153–1. The survival of 43 untransfused patients with aplastic anemia, 22 patients with acute nonlymphoblastic leukemia having transplants in first remission, and 22 patients with acute lymphoblastic leukemia having transplants in second or subsequent remission after marrow grafts from HLA-identical family members. The surviving patients with leukemia remain in unmaintained remission. Day "0" is the day of marrow transplantation. The tick marks indicate living patients. Survival is as of May 1988.

disease. A recent Seattle regimen combining CY and ATG appears effective in reducing the risk of graft rejection without the use of buffy coat cells. Nevertheless, emphasis should be placed on measures to prevent rather than to overcome the sensitization caused by blood transfusions. For this the physician should be aware of the possibility of marrow transplantation when aplastic anemia is first diagnosed. If an HLA-identical family member is available, early transplantation before transfusions is the therapy of choice. If transfusions are necessary, white blood cells should be removed as much as possible to reduce the chance of sensitization. Treatment of blood products with gamma radiation may prove effective in preventing sensitization.

LEUKEMIA (Ch. 144 and 145). Marrow grafting for leukemia presents the same general transplantation problems encountered with aplastic anemia. Graft rejection is rare, however. The unique problem is recurrence of leukemia. Formerly, marrow transplantation was carried out only after failure of all other therapies, when patients were undergoing advanced relapse. Of the first 100 patients with acute leukemia receiving grafts in Seattle after CY and TBI, 12 per cent are alive with the disease in remission between 12 and 18 years without any maintenance therapy. Approximately 75 per cent of all patients could be expected to have recurrent leukemia unless they died of other causes. Leukemic recurrence usually originated from host-type cells, indicating that it is difficult to kill every leukemic cell once the patient has reached the end stage of the disease. Currently, attempts are being made to reduce the rate of leukemic relapse and increase long-term survival in patients with leukemia receiving transplants in the end stage of their disease. Higher doses of TBI, by means of fractionating the radiation, and additional chemotherapeutic agents are being used. Most recently, monoclonal antibodies, to which short-lived high-energy beta-emitting radioactive isotopes have been coupled, have been used to increase the effect of the conditioning programs. These attempts may be doomed to failure, since, in an exponential cell kill process, it is difficult to kill the last leukemic cell. Some of the apparent cures may have occurred because of leukemic cell kill by immune mechanisms directed at non-HLA antigens expressed on leukemic cells. This theory is suggested by the observation of a graft-versus-leukemia effect in humans.

It is advisable to carry out marrow transplantation earlier in the course of leukemia while the disease is in remission. At this time, the number of leukemic cells in the body is small and the cells are not yet resistant to therapy. In addition, the patient is in a better clinical condition and therefore better able to tolerate the therapy. Accordingly, we began in 1976 to treat patients with acute nonlymphoblastic leukemia by marrow grafting when the disease was in first or subsequent remission and those with acute lymphoblastic leukemia when it was in second or subsequent remission after conditioning with CY and TBI.

Patients with acute nonlymphoblastic leukemia who receive chemotherapy have an approximate median duration of survival of 2 years. Only 15 to 20 per cent of patients who receive chemotherapy are alive at 5 years. Of the first 22 patients with acute nonlymphoblastic leukemia treated by marrow transplantation during first remission, 12 are alive with the disease in unmaintained remission between 10 and 12 years after transplantation. The survival curve shows a plateau at 55 per cent (Fig. 153–1).

Approximately 50 per cent of patients with acute lymphoblastic leukemia, especially children, can be cured by chemotherapy. Once relapse has occurred, another remission can often be induced with chemotherapy, but long-term survival of patients who have relapsed is poor, with very few alive at 2 years. Treatment of patients with acute lymphoblastic leukemia during second or subsequent remission by marrow transplantation seems justified in an attempt to change the otherwise grim outlook and perhaps "cure" some of these patients.

The survival curve of the first 22 patients with acute lymphoblastic leukemia in second or subsequent remission receiving marrow grafts in Seattle shows a plateau at 27 per cent, 11 to 12 years after transplantation (Fig. 153–1).

The results of marrow transplantation for the treatment of patients with chronic granulocytic leukemia in blast crisis have been similar to those in patients with leukemia in relapse. The projected survival is approximately 15 per cent (Fig. 153–2). The patients' marrows show absence of the Philadelphia chromosome, a unique result.

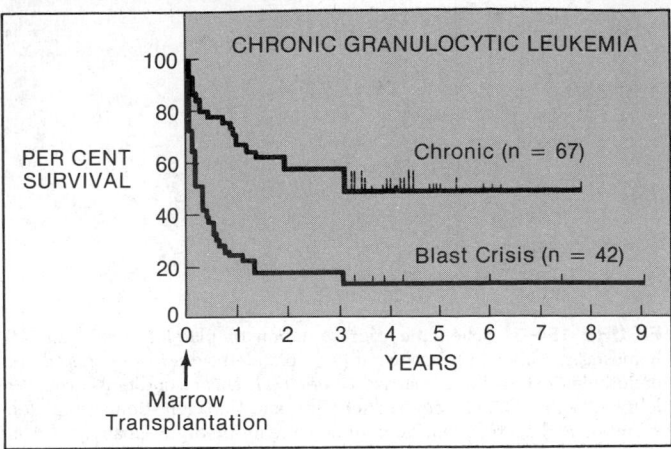

FIGURE 153–2. Survival after marrow grafting in patients with chronic granulocytic leukemia having transplants either in blast crisis or in chronic phase. The tick marks indicate living patients. Survival is as of March 1987.

Transplantation during the chronic phase of chronic granulocytic leukemia promises to improve these results. Although follow-up is still short, it appears that long-term disease-free survival will be on the order of 50 per cent (Fig. 153–2). Over the past 7 years, with the introduction of methotrexate and cyclosporine for GVHD prophylaxis, disease-free survival has increased to more than 70 per cent.

Marrow transplantation has now also been successfully applied to the treatment of patients with non-Hodgkin's lymphoma, myelofibrosis, multiple myeloma, preleukemia, and hairy cell leukemia.

Common to all results of marrow grafting for leukemia and lymphoma is the problem of recurrence of disease due to host cells that have survived the high-dose chemoradiation therapy. New treatment programs being explored in a number of centers are aimed at more effectively destroying the malignant cells, thereby increasing the success of marrow transplantation.

CONCLUSION

Marrow transplantation, once considered a desperate form of therapy in patients with end-stage disease, has now become increasingly successful when used early in the course of aplastic anemia or leukemia. The current success now obliges the physician to identify, soon after diagnosis, those patients who have suitable donors and who may be candidates for transplantation. Marrow grafting has now been extended to the therapy of patients with other hematologic malignant diseases and genetic disorders of hematopoiesis. In the longest survivor with malignant non-Hodgkin's lymphoma, the disease is now in unmaintained remission 16 years after marrow grafting. Cures of congenital Fanconi's anemia, paroxysmal nocturnal hemoglobinuria, thalassemia major, osteopetrosis, and certain genetic storage diseases have been achieved by marrow transplantation.

Many patients do not have HLA-identical siblings, and very few have monozygotic twins. To extend marrow transplantation to a larger number of patients, the use of less well matched family members has been explored, with remarkable success. Successful human transplants from unrelated donors for the treatment of patients with acute and chronic leukemias and aplastic anemia have been carried out. This work has been facilitated by the establishment of national bone marrow donor registries.

With the development of techniques to "purge" marrow from unwanted malignant cells and to cryopreserve marrow for indefinite periods, a renaissance of autologous marrow transplantation for the treatment of malignant diseases has occurred. Autologous marrow is an attractive option, since it avoids the problem of GVHD.

Ferrara JLM, Deeg HJ: Mechanisms of disease: Graft-versus-host disease. N Engl J Med 324:667, 1991. *This is a valuable, up-to-date, brief review of GVHD; with 55 references.*

Moller G (ed.): Graft-versus-host reaction. Immunol Rev 88:1, 1985. *Reviews by multiple authors of the pathophysiology, immunology, treatment, and prevention of acute and chronic GVHD in experimental animals and in humans.*

Storb R: Bone marrow transplantation. In DeVita VT Jr, Hellman S, Rosenberg SA (eds.): *Cancer: Principles and Practice of Oncology.* Vol. 2. 3rd ed. Philadelphia, JB Lippincott, 1989, pp 2474–2489. *Review of marrow transplantation as treatment for hematologic malignancies.*

Van Rood J, Zwaan F (eds.): Bone marrow transplantation. Semin Hematol 21:1, 1984. *Multiple-author reviews of marrow transplantation for malignant and nonmalignant hematologic diseases, including late complications and immune reconstitution.*

154 Hemorrhagic Disorders: Abnormalities of Platelet and Vascular Function

Marc Shuman

MECHANISMS OF HEMOSTASIS

Normal Hemostasis

Normally, blood clots in response to vascular damage to form a local seal. The mechanisms involved can be divided into three categories:

1. Vasoconstriction
2. Platelet adhesion and aggregation
3. Fibrin formation and stabilization

All three processes are intimately related and are initiated simultaneously. Once the clot is formed and tissue repair has started, digestion of the clot (fibrinolysis) begins, eventually leading to vascular patency. Blood coagulation and fibrinolysis are largely described in Ch. 155.

The normal sequence of events leading to clotting is initiated by trauma to the vessel, which constricts reflexly to reduce blood flow (Fig. 154–1). With damage to the vascular endothelium, platelets adhere to the subendothclial matrix (Fig. 154–2). Tissue factor, a protein-phospholipid complex, is exposed in the vessel wall and activates clotting by binding Factor VII.

The tissue factor–Factor VIIa complex activates coagulation Factor X ("extrinsic pathway") and Factor IX ("intrinsic pathway"). The intrinsic pathway can also be entrained by activation of coagulation Factor XII; however, it is unclear whether or how this is initiated in vivo, under physiologic conditions (Ch. 155).

After the first platelets adhere to the injured vessel, platelet aggregation begins, initiated probably through multifactorial mechanisms (Fig. 154–2). Collagen fibers bind to platelet surface receptors, which activate aggregation and stimulate secretion of intracellular granular contents, including adenosine diphosphate (ADP), prostaglandin G_2 (PGG_2), and thromboxane A_2. These secreted substances mediate and further amplify aggregation. Besides collagen, thrombin in minute concentrations ($\cong$ 1nM) aggregates platelets. Presumably, this is an additional stimulus to aggregation once the soluble clotting factors have been activated.

Platelets secrete serotonin and thromboxane A_2, which enhance vasoconstriction and expose surface sites that bind and accelerate the activation of Factors X and II (prothrombin) (Fig. 154–2). In addition to aggregating platelets, thrombin converts fibrinogen to fibrin, which becomes incorporated into the platelet plug. With crosslinking of fibrin strands by Factor XIIIa, a stable clot is formed.

Normally, activation of clotting and platelets is inhibited by an intact vascular endothelium and continuous blood flow (Fig. 154–3A). Endothelium makes PGI_2, which inhibits platelet activation and is vasodilatory. Thrombomodulin, an integral membrane endothelial protein, serves as a receptor for thrombin, which in this way activates protein C, a potent inhibitor of coagulation (Ch. 155). Activated protein C inactivates coagulation Factors Va and VIIIa. Endothelial cells also make tissue plasminogen activator, the primary activator of intravascular fibrinolysis. Platelets

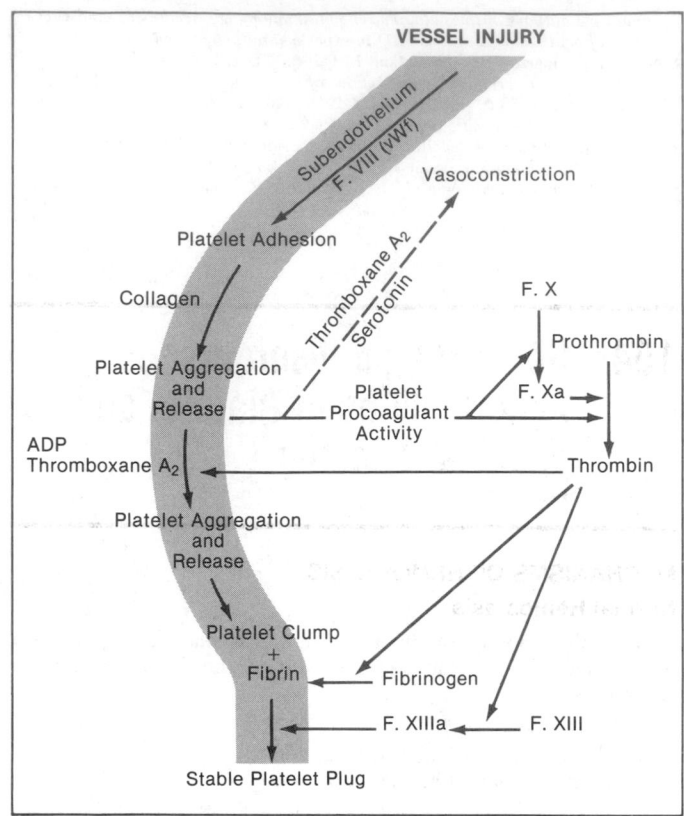

FIGURE 154–1. Schematic representation of platelet participation in hemostasis. Following vascular injury, platelets adhere to exposed subendothelial extracellular matrix. Under high shear conditions, von Willebrand factor (vWf) is required for adhesion. Collagen stimulates platelet secretion and aggregation. Secretion of adenosine diphosphate (ADP) and thromboxane A_2 further amplifies aggregation. Secretion of serotonin and thromboxane A_2 stimulates vasoconstriction. Factors IXa and VIIIa bind to specific platelet receptors, amplifying activation of Factor X. Factors Xa and Va bind to platelet receptors, amplifying thrombin formation. Thrombin aggregates platelets and converts Factor XIIIa and fibrinogen to fibrin. The end-product of these reactions is a crosslinked platelet-fibrin thrombus.

do not bind to the surface of normal endothelial cells. Vascular endothelium contains large amounts of heparan sulfate, a glycosaminoglycan, on its luminal surface. Antithrombin III binds with high affinity to heparan, thus providing a rapid and potent mechanism for inhibiting activated clotting factors. Clearly, the inner lining of blood vessels has a critical function in maintaining vascular patency by inhibiting activation of hemostasis.

Pathologic Hemostasis

Thrombi formed by platelets in the arterial system, called white thrombi, are composed primarily of fibrin and platelets. Red thrombi, found in the venous circulation, are composed of red blood cells trapped in the fibrin meshwork and usually contain few platelets. Clotting is activated pathologically in response to abnormalities in (1) the vessel wall, e.g., atherosclerosis; (2)

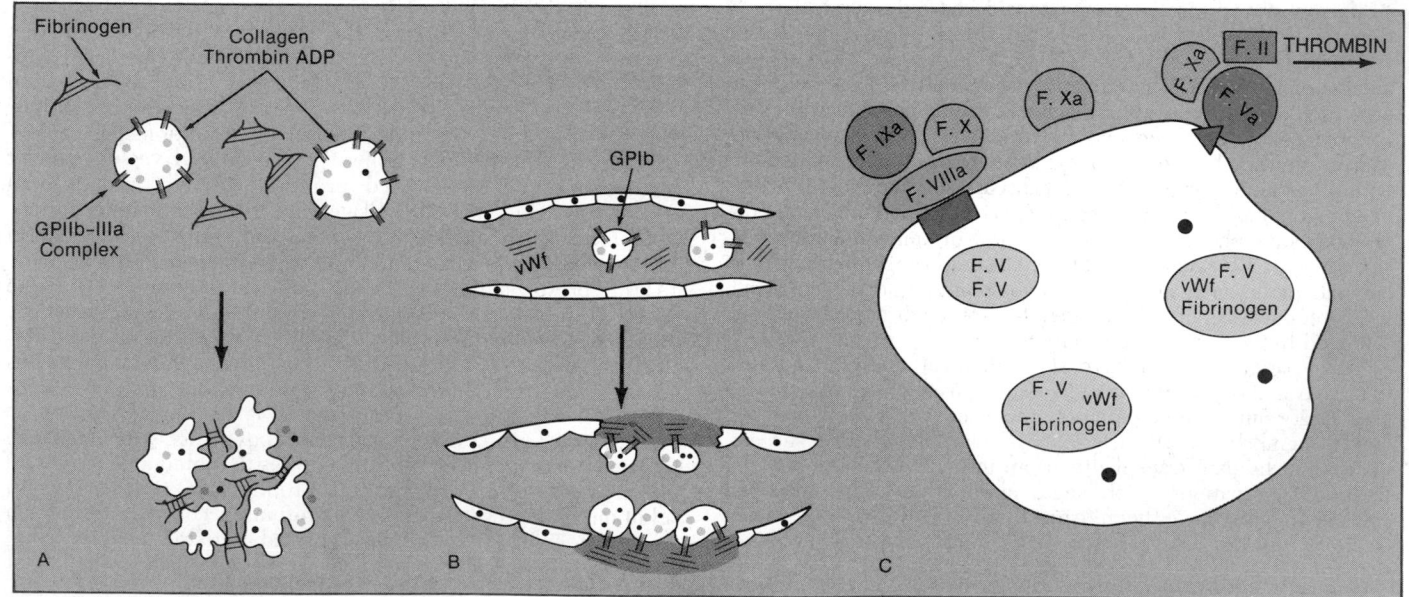

FIGURE 154–2. Platelet aggregation, adhesion, and enhancement of coagulation. *A*, Platelet aggregation. Several physiologic stimuli activate platelets, resulting in fibrinogen binding to specific receptors, GPIIb–IIIa. Binding of fibrinogen is followed by platelet aggregation. *B*, Platelet adhesion. Injury to the vascular endothelium results in exposure of extracellular matrix. Under high shear, von Willebrand factor binds to the platelet receptor GPIb. The platelet-vWf complex then binds to the subendothelium. *C*, Amplification of thrombin formation by platelets. Coagulation Factors IXa, VIIIa, and X form a Ca^{2+}-dependent trimolecular complex on the platelet surface. Activation of Factor X is amplified several hundred thousand-fold. Coagulation Factors Xa, Va, and prothrombin form a Ca^{2+}-dependent trimolecular complex on platelets. Thrombin formation is amplified several hundred thousand–fold.

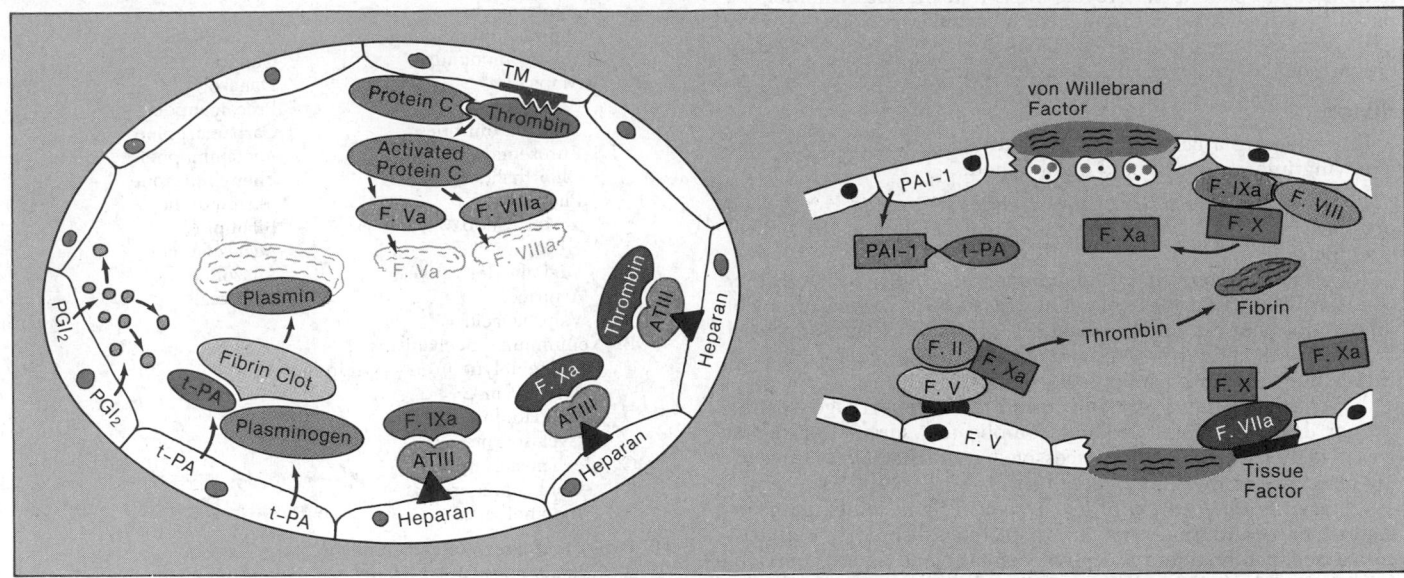

FIGURE 154–3. Regulation of coagulation by vascular endothelium. *Left,* Inhibition of activation of clotting by endothelium. Endothelial cells make substances that inhibit platelet secretion and aggregation and activate clotting factors. In addition, endothelium initiates degradation of the fibrin clot. *Right,* Activation of clotting by vascular endothelium. Injury to endothelium exposes tissue factor, which initiates the extrinsic pathway of clotting. Receptors for activation of Factor X and prothrombin amplify coagulation on the endothelial surface. Endothelium also secretes an inhibitor of clot lysis. PGI_2 = prostaglandin I_2; t-PA = tissue-plasminogen activator; PAI–1 = plasminogen activator inhibitor–1; TM = thrombomodulin; AT III = antithrombin III.

platelets, e.g., myeloproliferative disorders; and (3) the coagulation system, e.g., antithrombin III deficiency. Anatomic and/or biochemical alterations of the vascular intima are by far the most frequent causes of pathologic thrombosis. A variety of pathologic alterations of the vessel wall modify endothelial function in a prothrombotic fashion (Fig. 154–3B). At one extreme, the endothelial lining may be physically disrupted, with exposure of circulating blood to extracellular matrix and tissue factor. On the other hand, several substances may induce intact endothelium to promote thrombosis. Thus, interleukin 1, tumor necrosis factor, and endotoxin increase both endothelial plasminogen activator inhibitor–1, an inhibitor of fibrinolysis, and endothelial tissue factor. Moreover, endothelial cells express receptors for several of the coagulation factors, including Factors Va, IXa, Xa, so that once coagulation is initiated, it can be amplified on the endothelial cell surface. It is not difficult to imagine how rupture of an atherosclerotic plaque results in pathologic initiation of clotting, terminating in vascular occlusion. Thrombosis is clearly an important event in atherosclerotic vascular disease: (1) Platelet thrombi are found in the coronary circulation in fatal myocardial infarction; (2) fibrinolytic therapy can restore blood flow early in coronary occlusion; and (3) thrombin inhibitors prevent reocclusion of vessels after lysis of intracoronary thrombi (experimental studies in animals).

APPROACH TO THE PATIENT WITH A POSSIBLE BLEEDING DISORDER

When evaluating whether a bleeding disorder is present and, if so, its likely cause, very useful information may be obtained from the patient. The history may strongly suggest whether a bleeding diathesis is congenital or acquired and, if the latter, the most likely category into which it falls. Moreover, careful exam-

TABLE 154–1. DIFFERENTIAL DIAGNOSIS OF BLEEDING DISORDERS

	Hemophilia	Von Willebrand's Disease	Qualitative Platelet Abnormalities	Blood Vessel Disorders
Hereditary				
Genetics	X-Linked recessive	Autosomal dominant	Autosomal dominant Autosomal recessive	Autosomal dominant
Type of Bleeding	Hemarthrosis Visceral CNS Soft tissues	Mucocutaneous	Mucocutaneous	Mucocutaneous Arterial rupture (Connective tissue disorders)
Onset of Bleeding	Delayed	Immediate	Immediate	Immediate
Physical Examination	Joint deformities Hematomas Ecchymoses	Ecchymoses	Petechiae Ecchymoses	Ecchymoses Telangiectasia (HHT) Skin, joint, and eye abnormalities (Connective tissue disorders)
Coagulation Tests	aPTT: Abn	aPTT: Abn/N	N	N
Bleeding Time	N	Abn	Abn	N/Abn

	Coagulation	Platelet	Blood Vessel Disorders	
Acquired				
Type of Bleeding	Visceral Soft tissues	Mucocutaneous	Mucocutaneous	
Onset of Bleeding	Delayed	Immediate	Immediate	
Physical Examination	Hematomas Ecchymoses	Petechiae Ecchymoses	Ecchymoses Perifollicular hemorrhage (scurvy)	
Coagulation Tests	PT: Abn/N aPTT: Abn/N	N	N	
Bleeding Time	N	Abn	N/Abn	

CNS = central nervous system; HHT = hereditary hemorrhagic telangiectasia; N = normal; Abn = abnormal; aPTT = activated partial thromboplastin time; PT = prothrombin time.

ination of the patient may reveal signs that indicate whether the patient has a platelet, a vascular, or a coagulation defect. On the basis of this information, one can focus the laboratory investigation on particular types of disorders of hemostasis (Table 154–1).

History

In evaluating a patient with a putative bleeding disorder, the following information should be obtained:

1. *What is the duration of the bleeding tendency?* Has it been present since birth? Was there excessive bleeding at the time of circumcision?

2. *What are the frequency and duration of episodes?* A history of intermittent episodes (bleeding on some occasions, but not others) does not exclude the diagnosis of a hemorrhagic diathesis. Patients with mild von Willebrand's disease or Factor XI deficiency may give this type of history.

3. *What are the triggering events?* Is hemorrhage spontaneous? Has excessive bleeding complicated surgery or dental work? Is menstrual bleeding excessive (menorrhagia)? Was bleeding abnormal at the time of childbirth?

4. *What is the location of hemorrhage?* Skin, joints, gastrointestinal or genitourinary tracts? In platelet disorders, epistaxis, cutaneous bleeding, and excessive vaginal bleeding are common. Joint hemorrhage is common in hemophilia but rare in platelet disorders.

5. *What medication or medications is the patient taking?* (See Table 154–2.)

6. *What is the family history?* Are only males affected? Is there an X-linked recessive maternal pattern of transmission (hemophilia)?

Physical Examination

In platelet abnormalities or vascular defects, hemorrhage is usually mucosal and/or cutaneous. Bleeding from a clotting factor deficiency is often intramuscular or intra-articular. The presence of *petechiae*, small (<3 mm) hemorrhages in the skin or mucous membranes, indicates a platelet or vascular defect. Petechiae are not present in deficiencies of clotting factors. *Purpura*, larger cutaneous hemorrhages, are found more commonly in platelet than in blood clotting disorders. *Hematoma* refers to bleeding into tissues and occurs more commonly in coagulation disorders. Punctate *telangiectasia* on the tongue, nasal mucosa, lips, or fingertips is found in hereditary hemorrhagic telangiectasia.

The history and physical examination alone may strongly indicate into which category a bleeding diathesis falls (Table 154–1).

Laboratory Evaluation

Laboratory evaluation should be directed toward disorders suggested by the patient's history and physical examination. For example, a strong family history of a mild bleeding disorder affecting both sexes raises the possibility of von Willebrand's disease. The finding of petechiae suggests a platelet or blood vessel disorder. When the patient's history and physical examination are not helpful in focusing the investigation, the prothrombin time (PT), activated partial thromboplastin time (aPTT), and platelet count are helpful initial screening tests. An algorithm for proceeding with further evaluation, depending on some common patterns in the initial results, is shown in Figure 154–4.

BLOOD PLATELETS
Formation and Kinetics

Platelets are disc-shaped cells, 2 to 4 μm in diameter, normally found in the peripheral blood (150,000 to 300,000 per microliter). In Wright's-stained blood smears, they are identified by their blue-gray cytoplasm and red (lysosomal) granules and by lack of a nucleus (see Color Plate 5A). Their physiologic role in hemostasis has been described above (Fig. 154–2).

Platelets are formed in the bone marrow from giant polyploid cells called megakaryocytes. Megakaryocytes mature by a series of nuclear replications within a common cytoplasm (endomitosis), leading to four to six lobed nuclei, and by elaboration of specific granules in the cytoplasm. Following maturation, the megakaryocyte cytoplasm becomes demarcated into platelet subunits, and the platelets are released into the circulation through the marrow

TABLE 154–2. DRUGS THAT MAY ALTER HEMOSTASIS

I. **Drugs reported to cause thrombocytopenia**
   A. Immune mechanism proposed[*]

Quinine/quinidine	Ranitidine
Sulfa compounds	Cimetidine
Ampicillin	Danazol
Penicillin	Procainamide
Thiazide diuretics	Carbamazepine
Furosemide	Acetaminophen
Chlorthalidone	Phenylbutazone
Phenytoin	p-Aminosalicylate
α-Methyldopa	Rifampin
Heparin	Acetazolamide
Digitalis derivatives	Anazoline
Aspirin	Arsenicals
Valproic acid	

   B. Nonimmune mechanisms
      (Hemolytic-uremic syndrome)
      Mitomycin C
      cis-Platinum
      Cyclosporine
   C. Mechanism undefined
      Gold compounds
      Indomethacin

II. **Drugs that alter platelet function**
   A. Primary antiplatelet agents

Aspirin	Sulfinpyrazone
Dextran	Ticlopidine
Dipyridamole	

   B. Drugs in which inhibition of platelet function is associated with prolongation of the bleeding time
      Nonsteroidal anti-inflammatory agents
      β-Lactam antibiotics
      ε-Aminocaproic acid (>24 grams/day)
      Heparin
      Plasminogen activators (streptokinase, urokinase, tissue plasminogen activator)

III. **Drugs that affect coagulation factors**
   A. Induction of antibodies inhibiting function
      Lupus anticoagulant[†][‡]
         Phenothiazines
         Procainamide
      Factor VIII antibodies
         Penicillin
      Factor V antibodies
         Aminoglycosides
      Factor XIII antibodies
         Isoniazid
   B. Inhibitors of synthesis of vitamin K–dependent clotting factors
      (Factors II, VII, IX, X, proteins C and S)
      Coumarin compounds
      Moxalactam
   C. Inhibitor of fibrinogen synthesis
      L-Asparaginase[‡]

[*]List is limited to drugs for which there are multiple reports and there is in vitro or in vivo evidence for antiplatelet antibodies.
[†]Does not cause bleeding.
[‡]May cause thrombosis.

sinusoids. Two hematopoietic growth factors—interleukin 6 (IL6) and granulocyte/macrophage colony-stimulating factor—stimulate megakaryocyte maturation. Interleukin 6 also stimulates platelet production. Both growth factors also stimulate growth of other hematopoietic cells, however, and therefore are not specific.

Ordinarily, 1000 to 3000 platelets are produced from each megakaryocyte. Normally, 3 to 10 megakaryocytes are seen in bone marrow smears under low-power magnification, but none are seen in the peripheral blood smear. Platelets circulate for 9 to 10 days. Approximately one third reside in a splenic pool, which exchanges freely with the circulating pool. In diseases associated with platelet antibodies, the spleen is frequently the site of destruction. In addition, in disorders in which there is secondary splenic enlargement, thrombocytopenia may result from splenic sequestration (Ch. 152). Similarly, following splenectomy, the platelet count may increase to 1×10^6 per microliter.

An estimate of platelet number in the peripheral blood film (normal, increased, decreased) is quite useful in detecting patients with significantly low platelet counts. Normally, there are 3 to 10 platelets per high-power (oil immersion) field on the peripheral smear. Platelets are counted directly by phase microscopy using a counting chamber and a standard dilution of blood or by using an automated particle counter.

Platelet Function

Platelets contain three types of secretory granules: *lysosomes, α-granules,* and *dense bodies* (electron-dense organelles) (Fig. 154–5). Lysosomes in platelets, as in all other cells, contain acid hydrolases. α-Granules contain platelet-specific proteins: platelet Factor 4, which neutralizes heparin; β-thromboglobulin; and several growth factors, including platelet-derived growth factor (PDGF), endothelial cell growth factor (PD-ECGF), and transforming growth factor-β (TGF-β). (PDGF and PD-ECGF have also been identified in other tissues since their discovery in platelets.) α-Granules also contain several hemostatic proteins (fibrinogen, Factor V, and Factor VIII:vWf), but why these clotting factors are present in platelets in addition to plasma is unclear. Some of these proteins, such as fibrinogen, are endocytosed by megakaryocytes. Others (von Willebrand factor) are synthesized by megakaryocytes. Dense bodies (δ-granules) contain adenosine triphosphate (ATP), ADP, Ca^{2+}, and serotonin.

In hemostasis, platelets (1) release potent vasoconstrictors—thromboxane A_2 and serotonin—from their intracellular granules, (2) aggregate and form a plug at the site of vessel injury, and (3) provide a surface for the activation of soluble coagulation factors (Fig. 154–2C).

At high shear rates, platelets require a plasma protein, von Willebrand factor, to adhere to subendothelial extracellular matrix (Fig. 154–2). Platelets aggregate and secrete their granular contents in response to a variety of substances. With striking morphologic changes, platelets discharge the contents of their secretory granules into the canalicular system and then extracellularly. At the same time, the platelet becomes irregularly spherical and develops multiple finger-like projections.

Platelets contain a membrane phospholipase C, which, upon stimulation by activating agents, hydrolyzes endogenous phosphatidylinositol to form a diglyceride. The diglyceride, in turn, is converted to arachidonic acid by a diglyceride lipase. Arachi-

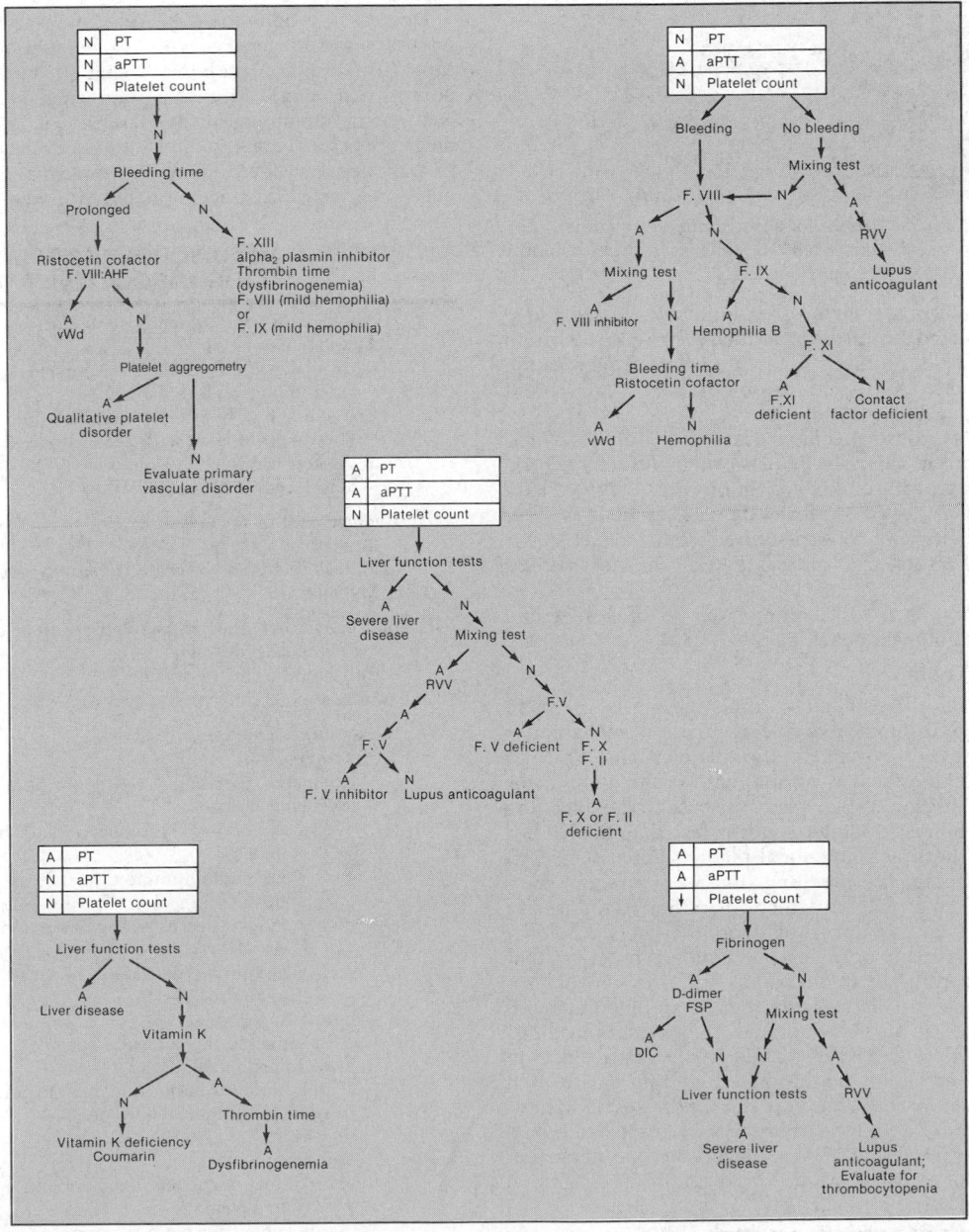

FIGURE 154–4. Algorithm for laboratory evaluation of bleeding disorders. vWd = von Willebrand's disease; A = abnormal; N = normal; RVV = Russell viper venom test; FSP = fibrin split products; PT = prothrombin time; aPTT = activated partial thromboplastin time; AHF = antihemophilic factor; DIC = disseminated intravascular coagulation.

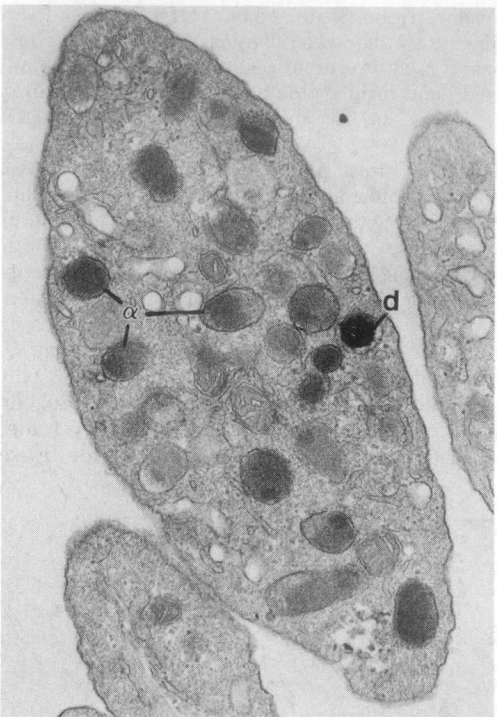

FIGURE 154–5. Electron micrograph of an unstimulated platelet. α = alpha granule; d = dense body (×24000). (Courtesy of Dr. Dorothy Bainton, University of California, San Francisco.)

donic acid acts as a substrate for prostaglandin synthetase and is subsequently converted to prostaglandins. The prostaglandin endoperoxide, PGG_2, is required for ADP-induced aggregation and release, and both PGG_2 and thromboxane A_2 are potent platelet aggregating agents.

Activated platelets expose specific surface receptors that bind Factor Xa and Va and in this way increase their local concentration, thus accelerating prothrombin activation (Fig. 154–2). Platelet procoagulant activity has been termed "platelet factor 3," but this refers to an activity, not to a specific substance. Factor X is also activated by Factors IXa and VIII:AHF on the platelet surface.

Platelet dysfunction is a less common cause of a bleeding diathesis than is thrombocytopenia.

Platelet Function Tests

BLEEDING TIME. The bleeding time measures the time required for bleeding to stop from a shallow incision, made under standardized conditions. It reflects the platelet and vascular components of coagulation and is normal with coagulation factor deficiencies (except in von Willebrand's disease). The bleeding time is prolonged when the platelet count is less than 90,000 per microliter or when there is a functional platelet abnormality. In von Willebrand's disease, the bleeding time is prolonged; however, this is not due to a platelet defect but rather to the lack of a plasma factor important for normal platelet function (see below). The bleeding time is the only test of platelet function that correlates with susceptibility to bleeding. Patients with a prolonged bleeding time are at risk for increased bleeding with surgery; however, not all such patients have abnormal bleeding.

PLATELET AGGREGOMETRY. The response of platelets to a variety of aggregating agents can be quantitated in platelet-rich plasma or whole blood. The aggregometer measures temporal, semiquantitative, and qualitative parameters of in vitro aggregation. Agents typically used are ADP, collagen, and epinephrine. This technique is of greatest value in diagnosing congenital qualitative platelet disorders.

ABNORMALITIES IN PLATELET COUNT

Thrombocytopenia

Low platelet counts (thrombocytopenia) can be caused by disturbances in production, in distribution, or in destruction.

The consequences of thrombocytopenia are entirely hemostatic. With normally functioning platelets, the following is expected:

1. Platelet count ≥ 100,000 per microliter—patients have no abnormal bleeding even with major surgery.
2. Platelet count, 50,000 to 100,000 per microliter—patients may bleed longer than normal with severe trauma.
3. Platelet count 20,000 to 50,000 per microliter—bleeding occurs with minor trauma, but spontaneous bleeding is unusual.
4. Platelet count < 20,000 per microliter—patients may have spontaneous bleeding.
5. Platelet count < 10,000 per microliter—patients are at high risk for severe bleeding.

DECREASED PRODUCTION OF PLATELETS

Hypoplasia of hematopoietic stem cells due to a variety of disorders may cause thrombocytopenia (Table 154–3); most of these disorders are discussed in other chapters. These include decreased numbers of megakaryoblasts and replacement of the bone marrow by abnormal tissue. Examination of the bone marrow reveals decreased numbers of megakaryocytes and either an overall decrease in cellularity or an infiltration by abnormal cells.

Decreased production of platelets may also be due to abnormal maturation of megakaryocytes. Deficiency of either B_{12} or folate can cause thrombocytopenia owing to ineffective thrombocytopoiesis (Ch. 132). Similarly, abnormal platelet production is common in hematopoietic dysplasias (Ch. 129). In both disorders, megakaryocytes are usually increased. In hematopoietic dysplasia, megakaryocytes may be abnormal in appearance, e.g., micromegakaryocytes occasionally with a single-lobed nucleus.

TABLE 154–3. DISORDERS ASSOCIATED WITH THROMBOCYTOPENIA

I. **Hypoplasia of hematopoietic stem cells**
Aplastic anemia
Marrow damage from drugs, chemicals, ionizing radiation, alcohol, infection
Congenital and hereditary thrombocytopenias
Thrombocytopenia with absent radii syndrome
Wiskott-Aldrich syndrome
May-Hegglin anomaly

II. **Replacement of normal marrow**
Leukemias
Metastatic tumor (prostate, breast, lymphoma)
Myelofibrosis

III. **Ineffective thrombocytopoiesis (normal or increased numbers of megakaryocytes)**
Cobalamin or folate deficiency
Hematopoietic dysplastic syndromes

IV. **Increased destruction of platelets**
A. Immune disorders
Idiopathic thrombocytopenic purpura (ITP)
Secondary causes:
Cancer: chronic lymphocytic leukemia, lymphoma, and so on
Systemic autoimmune disorders: SLE, polyarteritis nodosa
Infectious diseases: infectious mononucleosis, CMV, HIV
Drugs: quinine/quinidine, heparin, sulfa compounds (see Table 154–1)
B. Nonimmune disorders
Disseminated intravascular coagulation
Cavernous hemangioma
Thrombotic thrombocytopenic purpura
Hemolytic-uremic syndrome
Sepsis
Malaria
Paroxysmal nocturnal hemoglobinuria
Congenital cyanotic heart disease
Acute renal transplant rejection

V. **Disorders of distribution**
Hypersplenism

VI. **Dilutional: secondary to transfusion**

IMMUNE DISORDERS. Three types of immunologic reactions result in the premature destruction of platelets: (1) the development of autoantibodies against platelet membrane antigens, (2) the binding of immune complexes to platelet Fc receptors, and (3) the lysis of platelets due to fixation of complement on their surface.

Idiopathic Thrombocytopenic Purpura (ITP). Idiopathic thrombocytopenic purpura is an autoimmune bleeding disorder characterized by the development of antibodies to one's own platelets, which are then destroyed by phagocytosis in the spleen and, to a lesser extent, the liver. Childhood ITP is usually acute and follows recovery from a viral infection. The incidence is equal in boys and girls. In adults, the onset is usually more gradual, without a preceding illness and with a chronic course. In a small percentage of adult cases, the disease has an acute onset. Ninety per cent of adults with ITP are under the age of 40, and the ratio of women to men is 3–4:1. In some patients' sera, antibodies against platelet glycoproteins IIb and IIIa have been observed. Patients develop petechiae, ecchymoses, and epistaxis. Women may develop menorrhagia. Death due to hemorrhage is unusual in chronic ITP, approximately 5 per cent of cases. Cerebral bleeding occurs in ~1 per cent of cases.

The diagnosis of ITP is usually one of exclusion of underlying systemic disorders that result in increased peripheral destruction or decreased production of platelets. On physical examination, the spleen is not enlarged, although it may be in childhood ITP as a consequence of viral infection. In ITP, the hemoglobin is normal unless the patient has significant bleeding. The peripheral blood smear reveals normochromic, normocytic red blood cells. Similarly, the leukocyte count and differential are normal, although these values may continue to reflect a preceding viral illness in children. Several assays for detecting antiplatelet antibodies on the platelet surface have been proposed. The value of these assays in diagnosing ITP, analogous to the direct Coombs test used to detect antibodies against red blood cells, is unclear. Most of these tests do not distinguish between autoantibodies and immune complexes that bind to the platelet Fc receptor. Furthermore, these assays do not differentiate between specific antiplatelet antibodies, and nonspecifically absorbed immunoglobulin G (IgG). In most cases of ITP, the diagnosis is clear-cut, and confirming the presence of antiplatelet antibodies is unnecessary. In complex cases, the antibody test may be helpful. The level of platelet-associated IgG does not correlate with the severity of thrombocytopenia. In more than 90 per cent of cases of chronic ITP, the antibody is IgG; most are IgG1.

If the general clinical evaluation and blood tests do not confirm the diagnosis of systemic disorders causing thrombocytopenia, the bone marrow should be examined. In ITP, the marrow is normal, although megakaryocytes may be increased in number (see Color Plate 8*J*).

In children, the disease is self-limited. Approximately 70 per cent recover within 4 to 6 weeks. In adults, indications for treatment depend on the severity of bleeding and the degree of thrombocytopenia. Asymptomatic patients with platelet counts above 40,000 per microliter can be observed with periodic evaluation to determine the natural fluctuations of their disease. On the other hand, patients with platelet counts below 20,000 per microliter are usually symptomatic and require treatment. Patients with platelet counts above 30,000 per microliter who have bleeding may have an acquired platelet function abnormality due to the antibody. Initially, bleeding associated with ITP is treated with prednisone or a similar corticosteroid at a dose of 1 to 2 mg per kilogram per day. Prednisone inhibits macrophage ingestion of antibody-coated platelets, in addition to suppressing antibody synthesis. Prednisone has also been shown to have a stabilizing effect on small blood vessels in thrombocytopenic animals. In 80 to 90 per cent of patients, the platelet count rises to hemostatic levels within 2 to 3 weeks. Failure to respond to steroids is indicated by a platelet count below 50,000 per microliter after 4 weeks of treatment. A subnormal platelet count after 6 weeks of treatment indicates steroid failure also. Once the platelet count has reached its apex and is stable, steroids should be tapered slowly. When the dose of prednisone is tapered, however, most patients (~90 per cent) exhibit a relapse of thrombocytopenia. Thus, the primary benefit of prednisone is in the acute management of bleeding.

Another effective approach to managing patients who are actively bleeding or for whom major surgery is necessary is the use of intravenous γ globulin. Immunoglobulin G concentrates raise the platelet count within 3 to 5 days in most patients and thus is the most rapidly active agent. Unfortunately, the therapeutic effect is usually transient, since the platelet count falls to baseline levels over the next month. In a few instances, repeated infusions of γ globulin lead to sustained remissions after discontinuation of therapy. It is proposed that IgG works by blocking Fc receptors on macrophages, thereby inhibiting phagocytosis. The dosage is 1 gram per kilogram per day on 2 successive days. In 80 per cent of patients, the platelet count rises above 50,000 per microliter with this therapy. Owing to the lack of a sustained remission in most patients with severe thrombocytopenia treated with steroids or IgG, a more definitive approach is necessary. Splenectomy results in improvement of the platelet count in ~70 per cent of patients and in sustained remission in approximately 60 per cent of patients with ITP, but there are no reliable tests to predict which patients will respond. The platelet count rises within a few days after splenectomy, or at most in 1 to 2 weeks. Benefit from splenectomy appears to be due to at least two mechanisms. As indicated, the spleen is the principal reticuloendothelial site of platelet destruction in ITP. In addition, the spleen appears to be the major site of synthesis of antibody production in ITP, with sufficient amounts made to account for the degree of thrombocytopenia seen.

A variety of other therapies have been shown to be efficacious in inducing partial or complete remissions in patients with chronic ITP in whom splenectomy has failed. Danazol, 200 mg three times per day, induces a remission in approximately 40 per cent of patients with chronic ITP. Response is delayed and takes anywhere from 4 to 6 weeks. The mechanism by which danazol induces a remission is unknown. Intravenous vincristine and vinblastine also raise the platelet count in ITP, usually within 1 to 2 weeks. Responses are transient, and remissions are not sustained.

Immunosuppressive agents—cyclophosphamide and azathioprine—have also been used to induce remissions in chronic ITP. Because of the small numbers of patients reported, the relative efficacy of these two drugs is unclear. Success in improving the platelet count has been reported in 20 to 30 per cent of cases. The potential benefit of these drugs must be weighed against the risks of toxicity, immunosuppression, suppression of hematopoiesis, and, in the case of cyclophosphamide, acute leukemia.

Management of ITP in pregnancy is complicated by the additional risk to the fetus of developing thrombocytopenia secondary to maternal antibodies. Intraventricular hemorrhage, gastrointestinal bleeding, and death have been reported in these newborns. Whether the mother had ITP prior to pregnancy is critical. When women first develop ITP during pregnancy, the risk of serious bleeding in the newborn is negligible. However, neonates born to women with a history of ITP preceding pregnancy have a 20 per cent risk of severe thrombocytopenia. Therefore, in addition to treating the underlying ITP, cesarean delivery is recommended to decrease the risk of intracranial bleeding in these newborns.

Berchtold P, McMillan R: Therapy of chronic idiopathic thrombocytopenic purpura in adults. Blood 74: 2309, 1989. *Reviews current experience with therapeutic options in ITP as well as experimental approaches.*

Platelet Antibodies Associated with Systemic Disorders. Antibodies directed against platelets and causing thrombocytopenia occur in several types of disorders, in all of which bone marrow megakaryocytes are normal or increased in number.

Immune Thrombocytopenia Due to Cancer. Antibody-mediated destruction of platelets occurs in lymphoproliferative disorders, such as chronic lymphocytic leukemia and lymphoma. Generally, thrombocytopenia improves with treatment of the underlying malignancy. Immune thrombocytopenia has also been associated with nonhematologic tumors, but it is unclear whether or not these have been chance associations. The platelet count improves with immunosuppressive therapy such as prednisone.

Thrombocytopenia Associated with Systemic Autoimmune Disorders. Immune thrombocytopenia is common in systemic lupus erythematosus (SLE) (Ch. 261). Whether this is due to specific antiplatelet antibodies, to antibodies against common antigens also found on platelets, or to immune complexes is unclear. The platelet count is usually mildly to moderately decreased. Treatment is usually directed at SLE, as other manifestations of the disease are present in most cases.

Occasionally, immune thrombocytopenia occurs in patients who have serologic evidence of lupus but who do not meet all of the criteria for the diagnosis of SLE. The decision to treat such patients with splenectomy is a difficult one, since other manifestations of SLE may appear subsequently. If the platelet count is severely decreased (less than 30,000 per microliter) and the patient has no other complications of SLE, splenectomy is a reasonable course of action. However, if the platelet count is moderately decreased ($\geq$30,000 to 40,000 per microliter) and the patient does not have major bleeding problems, careful observation may be the best course.

Monthly intravenous cyclophosphamide, 0.75 to 1.0 gram per square meter of body surface area, has recently been shown to normalize platelet counts within 2 to 18 weeks in patients with SLE who were also taking prednisone. This therapy also allowed significant reduction in steroid dosage in these patients.

Immune thrombocytopenia occurs less commonly in other systemic autoimmune disorders.

Immune Thrombocytopenia with Viral Illnesses. Thrombocytopenia associated with antiplatelet antibodies has been reported in patients with infectious mononucleosis, with human immunodeficiency virus (HIV) infection, and with cytomegalovirus (CMV) infection. In the case of infectious mononucleosis and CMV infection, thrombocytopenia is usually self-limiting, with recovery in 3 to 4 weeks. In patients with severe thrombocytopenia, a short course of glucocorticoids may be indicated. The nature of the immune reaction has not been characterized.

HIV Thrombocytopenia (Ch. 419). Thrombocytopenia occurs frequently in patients infected with HIV, whether or not the illness has progressed to acquired immunodeficiency syndrome (AIDS). Patients are usually asymptomatic. Frequently, the causes are multifactorial: (1) infection causing increased platelet destruction and/or inhibition of platelet production due to granulomatous replacement of the bone marrow, (2) suppression of hematopoiesis by drugs used to treat AIDS or associated infections, and (3) immune destruction of the patient's own platelets. Antibodies associated with platelets have been demonstrated in these patients, although it is unclear whether thrombocytopenia is due to immune complexes bound to platelets or to specific antiplatelet antibodies. Treatment with prednisone is hazardous owing to the immunocompromised status of these patients. Similarly, splenectomy has the disadvantage of further compromising the immune system. Azidothymidine (AZT) treatment may raise the platelet count in some patients with mild to moderate thrombocytopenia. For acute bleeding, intravenous γ globulin raises the platelet count within a few days.

Immune Thrombocytopenia Due to Drug-Induced Antibodies (Table 154–2). More than 50 drugs have been reported to cause immune thrombocytopenia, but infrequently with conclusive in vitro confirmation. Quinine and quinidine often cause immune thrombocytopenia, and drug-dependent antibodies have been demonstrated conclusively. Sulfa compounds, including sulfisoxazole, sulfonamide, sulfamethoxypyridazine, and sulfamethazene, have also been demonstrated to cause immune thrombocytopenia. There are also multiple reports of immune thrombocytopenia caused by hydrochlorothiazide, phenytoin, methyldopa, heparin, and digitalis derivatives. In most instances, the drug must be present for antibody binding and thrombocytopenia to occur. Therefore, the platelet count returns to normal within a few days after discontinuation of the drug. Glucocorticoids do not accelerate recovery in drug-induced thrombocytopenia. Platelet antibody tests with and without the putative offending agent are useful in determining the cause of thrombocytopenia. Unfortunately, the test cannot be performed until the drug has been cleared from the plasma. In addition, a drug metabolite may be responsible for antibody formation and binding to platelets rather than the parent compound. Unless the metabolite is specifically tested, a negative result will be obtained.

Heparin-Induced Thrombocytopenia. The incidence of thrombocytopenia associated with heparin therapy appears to be 3 to 5 per cent, with a higher percentage of cases associated with bovine

TABLE 154–4. DIFFERENTIAL DIAGNOSIS OF ANEMIA AND THROMBOCYTOPENIA

Diagnostic Study	Autoimmune Disorders (Evans' Syndrome, Collagen-Vascular Disease)	Disseminated Intravascular Coagulation	Thrombotic Thrombocytopenic Purpura/Hemolytic-Uremic Syndrome
Peripheral blood smear	Microspherocytes	Schistocytes (+)	Schistocytes (+ + +)
Reticulocyte count	Increased (+ + +)	N/Increased (+)	Increased (+ + +)
Coombs' test	Positive	Negative	Negative
Coagulation tests	N	Abn (+ + +)	N/Abn (+)

N = normal; Abn = abnormal.

than with porcine preparations. The platelet count usually decreases after the first few days of treatment; the decline is gradual and is not usually associated with bleeding. The platelet count is rapidly corrected after heparin is discontinued. If the platelet count falls below 50,000 per microliter, heparin should be discontinued. Thrombocytopenia has been reported with the usual therapeutic doses as well as with the very low doses used for procedures such as hemodialysis.

NONIMMUNE DISORDERS ASSOCIATED WITH INCREASED CONSUMPTION OF PLATELETS. Disseminated Intravascular Coagulation (DIC) (Ch. 155). In this syndrome, discussed elsewhere, coagulation is pathologically activated, resulting in thrombin formation and the subsequent removal of platelets from the circulation.

Thrombotic Thrombocytopenic Purpura (TTP). This is a rare disease of unknown etiology, characterized by severe thrombocytopenia, microangiopathic hemolytic anemia (>96 per cent of patients), and neurologic abnormalities (>92 per cent of patients). Fever and renal involvement—proteinuria, hematuria, azotemia, and casts—are present in 98 per cent and 88 per cent of patients, respectively. Renal abnormalities are usually mild; the creatinine rarely exceeds 3.0 mg per deciliter. Azotemia is usually reversible, concomitant with remission, in contrast to the hemolytic-uremic syndrome (see below), in which renal failure is common and patients frequently have chronic renal insufficiency. In the involved organs, small vessels—i.e., arterioles and capillaries—are occluded by a hyaline material consisting principally of platelet thrombi. In addition, fibrin is detected in the vessel wall. Virtually any organ may be involved. Symptoms frequently wax and wane, presumably owing to aggregation and disaggregation of platelets. Thus, patients may have evanescent headache or aphasia or may be stuporous one moment and alert the next.

Thrombotic thrombocytopenic purpura must be considered when there is the acute onset of thrombocytopenia and anemia with microangiopathic changes of red blood cells on the peripheral blood smear in the absence of evidence of other disorders (Tables 154–4 and 154–5) (see Color Plate 6E, right). Although similar findings are present in DIC, patients with TTP have minimal changes in coagulation tests. Evans' syndrome, autoimmune hemolytic anemia and thrombocytopenia, is characterized by microspherocytes on peripheral smear, rather than by schistocytes, and by a positive Coombs test. Rarely, TTP has been reported to complicate SLE. More

TABLE 154–5. DISORDERS ASSOCIATED WITH THROMBOCYTOPENIA AND MICROANGIOPATHIC ANEMIA

Thrombotic thrombocytopenic purpura
Hemolytic-uremic syndrome
Disseminated intravascular coagulation
Malignant hypertension
Eclampsia
Vasculitis
  SLE
  Polyarteritis nodosa
Cavernous hemangioma
  (Kasabach-Merritt syndrome)
Disseminated carcinoma
Renal allograft rejection
Prosthetic heart valves
Malignant angioendotheliomatosis

commonly, patients with SLE have immune thrombocytopenia and anemia of chronic disease or immune hemolytic anemia (Ch. 261). Some patients with SLE, however, have microangiopathic hemolysis due to vasculitis. Thrombotic thrombocytopenic purpura has also been reported in association with oral contraceptives and pregnancy. In most cases, the diagnosis of TTP is straightforward. When the diagnosis is uncertain, gum, skin, or bone marrow biopsy may be helpful, with positive results reported in 40 to 60 per cent of cases. It is extremely important to establish the diagnosis and begin treatment rapidly, as delay in treatment can result in severe morbidity or in mortality. If untreated, most patients die within 3 months. Large-volume plasmapheresis, approximately two plasma volumes, with replacement infusion of normal plasma, is the treatment of choice for TTP, with a cure of approximately 70 per cent of patients. Infusion of large volumes of plasma without pheresis has induced remission in some patients also. However, not all patients respond to plasma infusion alone, and concomitant plasmapheresis becomes necessary. Since repeated courses of plasma infusion are usually necessary, the practical management of TTP is facilitated by plasmapheresis, which prevents excessive expansion of the blood volume and the subsequent risk of cardiovascular compromise. The best indication of the response to treatment is the platelet count, as a rise in platelets is the first sign of improvement. Plasmapheresis/plasma infusion should be continued until the platelet count is normal and stable. Complete correction of anemia and of neurologic signs and symptoms usually follows normalization of the platelet count. Why these treatments work is unknown. Approximately 10 per cent of patients have a chronic, relapsing form of TTP. In chronic TTP, abnormally large multimers of von Willebrand factor are present in the plasma of patients in remission.

Eisenstaedt RS, Colman RW, Marder VJ: Thrombotic thrombocytopenic purpura. In Colman RW, Hirsh J, Marder VJ, et al. (eds.): Hemostasis and Thrombosis: Basic Principles and Clinical Practice. 2nd ed. Philadelphia, JB Lippincott, 1987, pp 1016–1025. *A comprehensive review of the clinical manifestations; also includes current theories of pathogenesis and a review of therapeutic options.*

Hemolytic-Uremic Syndrome (HUS). Primarily a disorder of infants and young children, HUS rarely occurs in adults. Like those with TTP, patients with HUS have microangiopathic hemolytic anemia, but thrombocytopenia is mild to moderate and neurologic symptoms and signs are not present. In HUS, acute renal failure is a prominent feature, frequently requiring hemodialysis, while in TTP, the serum creatinine level is rarely higher than 2.5 mg per deciliter at presentation. Severe hypertension is a prominent feature also. Children typically present with gastrointestinal signs and symptoms, abdominal pain, and diarrhea. Hemolytic-uremic syndrome may occur in women who are in the postpartum period or who are taking oral contraceptives. In addition, HUS has been reported in patients with cancer who are receiving mitomycin C or cis-platinum chemotherapy.

Sepsis. In gram-negative (more commonly than gram-positive) sepsis, there is increased destruction of platelets apart from possible DIC. Binding of immune complexes of bacteria to the platelet may account for their accelerated destruction. Severe thrombocytopenia may occur.

DISORDERS OF DISTRIBUTION OF PLATELETS

With splenic enlargement, platelet pooling increases (e.g., Gaucher's disease, congestive splenomegaly, lymphoma) and may cause thrombocytopenia (Ch. 152). Platelet counts below 30,000 to 50,000 per microliter are unusual, however.

DILUTIONAL THROMBOCYTOPENIA

When packed erythrocytes or whole blood that is not fresh is transfused to replace blood loss, thrombocytopenia may occur. Approximately 35 to 40 per cent of platelets remain after replacement of one blood volume; microvascular bleeding due to thrombocytopenia occurs rarely after replacement of one to two blood volumes. Platelets should not be transfused unless thrombocytopenia and bleeding are documented. An algorithm for evaluating thrombocytopenia is shown in Figure 154–6.

Thrombocytosis

Elevation of the platelet count above the normal range is due to increased production and either is reactive or results from a myeloproliferative disorder. Most frequently, thrombocytosis is a secondary effect of an underlying disorder and not associated with complications. However, when it is due to a primary disorder of hematopoiesis, serious bleeding and/or thrombotic complications may result. Therefore, it is important to determine the cause of thrombocytosis.

ESSENTIAL THROMBOCYTHEMIA. Essential thrombocythemia is a myeloproliferative disorder in which the platelet count is elevated, frequently over 1×10^6 per microliter, and may be greater than 2×10^6 per microliter (see Color Plate 8K, right). In this disorder, platelet production is increased owing to a primary abnormality in megakaryocytopoiesis, with increased production of megakaryocytes and, consequently, of platelets. Complications may include thrombosis and/or bleeding. The former is the most common cause of death. In addition to increased numbers of platelets, abnormalities in platelet function have been demonstrated. Other myeloproliferative diseases, such as *agnogenic myeloid metaphasia* and *polycythemia vera*, are also associated with an elevated platelet count. The platelet count may be elevated in chronic myelogenous leukemia but rarely results in complications. Essential thrombocytopenia is discussed in detail in Ch. 143, which covers the myeloproliferative disorders.

REACTIVE THROMBOCYTOSIS. Elevated platelet counts occur secondarily in a number of unrelated disorders, but counts higher than 1×10^6 per microliter are unusual: *iron deficiency anemia; hemorrhage; post splenectomy* (Ch. 152); *inflammatory disorders, particularly inflammatory bowel disease; neoplasms (e.g., lung, gastrointestinal); leukemoid reaction* (Ch. 141).

No convincing evidence exists that reactive thrombocytosis increases the risk of thrombosis. Therefore, it should not be treated. With successful treatment of the primary disease, the count returns to normal.

Mitus AJ, Schafer AI: Thrombocytosis and thrombocythemia. In Colman RW, Rao AK (eds.): Platelets in health and disease. Hematol Clin North Am 4:157, 1990. *Complete discussion of the pathophysiology of thrombocytosis and its complications in myeloproliferative disorders as well as its differentiation from secondary causes.*

ABNORMALITIES IN PLATELET FUNCTION

Acquired Disorders of Platelet Function

DRUGS THAT INHIBIT PLATELET FUNCTION (Table 154–2). *Nonsteroidal anti-inflammatory agents* inhibit platelet function by blocking platelet synthesis of prostaglandins. Aspirin (acetylsalicylic acid, or ASA) irreversibly acetylates prostaglandin synthetase and, as a result, platelet function is impaired for its lifespan. One ASA tablet (300 mg) is sufficient to cause this effect. Fortunately, in normal people, this does not result in excessive bleeding, but in patients with von Willebrand's disease or with severe coagulation factor deficiency (Factor VIII or IX), serious bleeding can result. For this reason, aspirin is contraindicated in these disorders.

High doses of the β-*lactam antibiotics*, i.e., penicillin and related compounds, induce a significant abnormality in platelet function that persists for 2 to 3 days after the drug is discontinued. The mechanism is unclear. The bleeding time is prolonged, and patients may have increased bleeding.

Renal Failure. Platelets function abnormally in patients with renal failure. The uremic metabolites responsible for this dysfunction are uncertain. Guanidinosuccinic acid and phenolic compounds that accumulate in uremia may inhibit platelet aggregation. Abnormal platelet adhesion and activation may occur in uremia as well as thrombocytopenia. The latter is usually mild and may be due to the underlying cause of renal disease.

Uremic bleeding is usually mucocutaneous and reflects abnormal platelet and/or vascular hemostatic functions. The bleeding time is commonly prolonged, but other causes of prolongation must be excluded (e.g., medication, congenital platelet disorders, and von Willebrand's disease). Moreover, a low hematocrit (<24 per cent) prolongs the bleeding time in uremia. Transfusion of packed red blood cells to a hematocrit above 26 per cent improves the bleeding time. Tests of coagulation are normal.

When a uremic patient is bleeding, the possibility of a structural lesion or other hemostatic abnormalities must be evaluated. When the hemostatic defect of renal failure is believed to be a significant contributing factor in bleeding, the patient should be dialyzed. Either peritoneal dialysis or hemodialysis is usually effective in reversing the hemostatic defect. If the bleeding time remains prolonged, and the patient is bleeding, other agents that have been reported to improve or correct the bleeding time can be tried: low-dose estrogens, 1-deamino-8-D-arginine vasopressin (DDAVP), or cryoprecipitate. The efficacy of these agents in managing uremic bleeding has not been firmly established. All three raise the plasma levels of Factor VIII:AHF/vWf, but uremic patients usually already have normal concentrations of these proteins. Because the abnormalities in renal disease are extracellular, i.e., in the plasma, platelet transfusion is not usually beneficial.

HEPATIC FAILURE (Ch. 123). Platelet function is sometimes abnormal in liver disease, but why this is so and the extent to which this dysfunction contributes to bleeding in these patients are unclear. The bleeding time may be prolonged in moderately severe liver disease when the platelet count is above 90,000 per microliter. DDAVP has been reported to improve the bleeding time in these circumstances. More commonly in hepatic failure, a bleeding diathesis is due to deficiencies of coagulation factors (Ch. 123).

PARAPROTEINEMIAS (Ch. 151). Abnormal platelet function occurs in a subset of patients with multiple myeloma, or Waldenström's macroglobulinemia. The bleeding time is usually prolonged in these patients, and bleeding can be moderately severe. If the level of the paraprotein is lowered by plasmapheresis and/or chemotherapy, the bleeding time and bleeding improve, suggesting a direct effect of the paraprotein on platelet function.

Paraproteins may impair platelet function by inhibiting platelet-fibrinogen interaction.

ACQUIRED STORAGE POOL DISEASE. Patients may develop mild platelet function abnormalities from loss of storage granules. Some of the situations or disorders in which this has been reported include cardiopulmonary bypass surgery, hairy cell leukemia, and disorders with antiplatelet autoantibodies. Platelet dysfunction following bypass surgery is transient and not of clinical importance once the first 24 hours after surgery have elapsed.

MYELOPROLIFERATIVE DISORDERS. Patients with essential thrombocythemia and, less commonly, agnogenic myeloid metaplasia, may have abnormalities of platelet function. In essential thrombocythemia, abnormalities usually occur at platelet counts greater than 1×10^6 per microliter and may lead to abnormal bleeding, thrombosis, or both. Although the functional abnormalities are not specific, a prolonged bleeding time indicates that the patient is at risk for bleeding. Treatment of bleeding patients with thrombocytosis should be directed at lowering the platelet count as rapidly as possible.

George JN, Shattil SJ: Medical progress: The clinical importance of acquired abnormalities of platelet function. N Engl J Med 324:27, 1991. *An excellent recent review of this important topic.*

Hereditary Disorders of Platelet Function

In general, the bleeding history is similar for these diseases: a lifelong history of easy bruising, epistaxis, and prolonged oozing after venipuncture, dental extractions, and other challenges to hemostasis. All hereditary platelet disorders are quite rare.

GLANZMANN'S THROMBASTHENIA. This autosomal re-

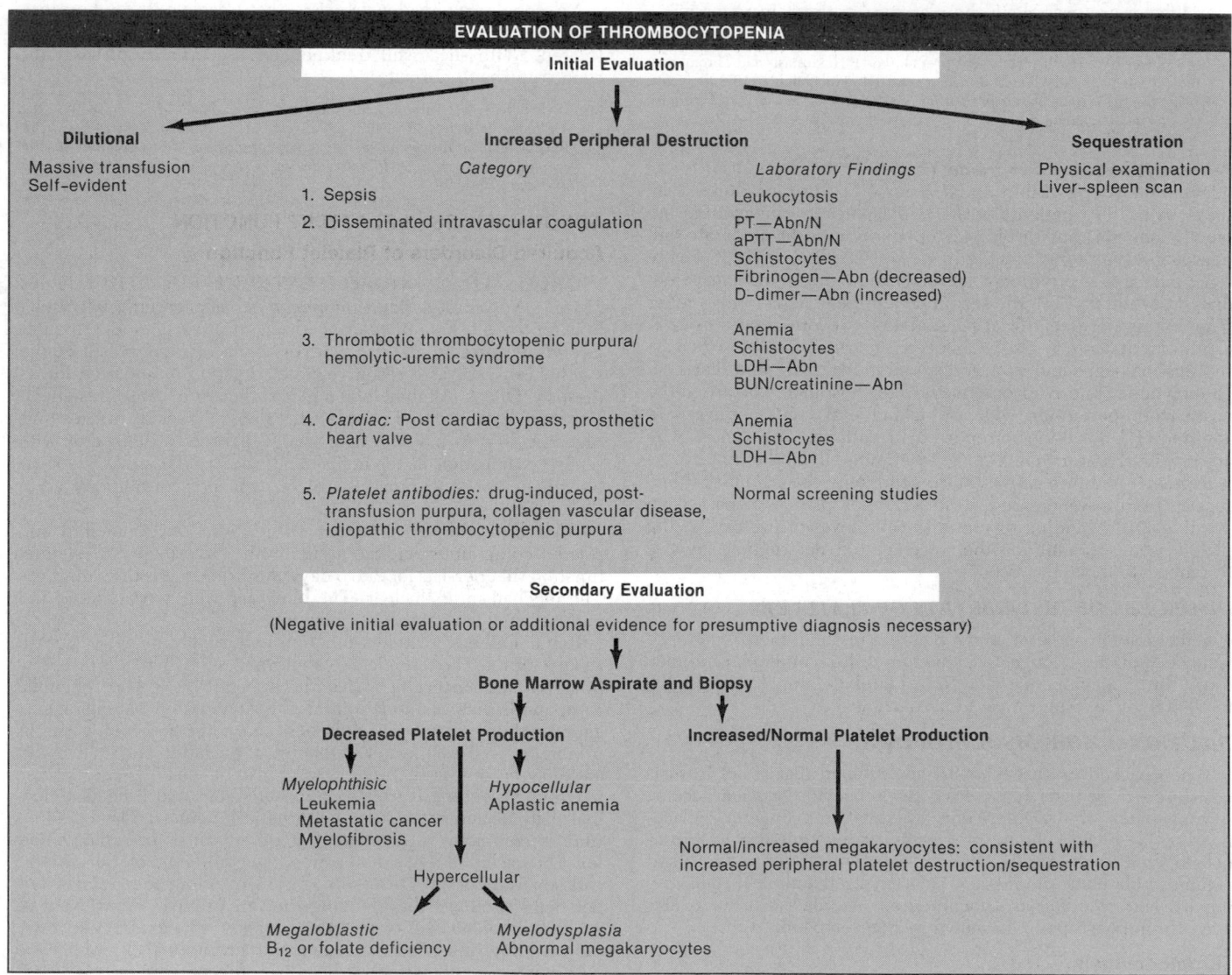

FIGURE 154–6. Evaluation of thrombocytopenia. Abn = abnormal; N = normal; PT = prothrombin time; aPTT = activated partial thromboplastin time; LDH = lactate dehydrogenase; BUN = blood urea nitrogen.

cessive bleeding disorder is characterized by a prolonged bleeding time and platelets that do not aggregate normally when stimulated with ADP, epinephrine, collagen, or thrombin. In Glanzmann's thrombocytopenia, two membrane glycoproteins (GPIIb-IIIa) that normally serve as the receptor for fibrinogen in activated platelets are markedly deficient (Fig. 154–2). Fibrinogen binding to platelets is required for normal platelet aggregation. The diagnosis is confirmed by demonstrating deficiency of platelet GPIIb-IIIa. The platelet count is always normal in this disease.

BERNARD-SOULIER SYNDROME. This autosomal recessive disorder is associated with "giant" platelets seen in the peripheral blood smear (see Color Plate 8K, left). Membrane protein abnormalities have also been demonstrated in this disease. Frequently, the platelet count is mildly decreased. In laboratory studies, platelets aggregate normally in response to ADP, collagen, or epinephrine but fail to aggregate in response to ristocetin. Physiologically, platelets fail to adhere normally to subendothelial connective tissue. This failure to adhere is due to defective binding of von Willebrand factor to a platelet membrane glycoprotein complex, GPIb-IX, which is deficient in this disease.

STORAGE POOL DISEASE (SPD). In this autosomal dominant disorder, platelet storage granules are decreased in number and/or content, presumably because of abnormal granule formation in megakaryocytes. The bleeding diathesis is mild and is found mostly in women. In SPD, with absent or decreased dense granules, platelets aggregate abnormally owing to inadequate secretion of ADP. Dense granule SPD is also associated with several other congenital disorders, including oculocutaneous albinism in both the Hermansky-Pudlak and Chédiak-Higashi syndromes, the Wiskott-Aldrich syndrome, and a syndrome in which there is thrombocytopenia and absent radii (TAR). Patients may also be deficient in α-granules, either in combination with dense granule deficiency or independently. The gray platelet syndrome refers to the latter situation, in which the absence of granule staining confers a gray color on the platelets. Mild thrombocytopenia may also be present in this disorder.

Bennett JS, Shattil SJ: Congenital qualitative platelet disorders. In Williams WJ, Beutler E, Erslev AJ, et al. (eds.): Hematology. 4th ed. New York, McGraw-Hill, 1990, pp 1407–1419.

VON WILLEBRAND'S DISEASE (see also Ch. 155). Von Willebrand's disease (vWd) is the most common congenital bleeding disorder, with an estimated incidence ranging from 0.1 to 2 per cent of the population in the United States. Several different types of vWd occur. Most commonly, vWd is an autosomal dominant disorder. Rarely, it is autosomal recessive, the most severe form. In the classic disorder, patients are deficient in both Factor VIII:AHF and vWf. The latter is a plasma glycoprotein necessary for adhesion of platelets to subendothelial connective tissue in blood flowing at high shear rates. Von Willebrand factor circulates in a noncovalent complex with Factor VIII:AHF. Unbound Factor VIII:AHF has a markedly shortened half-life; deficiency of vWf therefore results secondarily in Factor VIII:AHF deficiency. In vWd, Factor VIII:AHF levels are rarely below 5 per cent—hence the mild symptoms in this disorder, compared with hemophilia. The manifestations of this disease differ from hemophilia in that bleeding is predominantly in the skin and mucous membranes (epistaxis, bruising, and menorrhagia). The pattern of bleeding resembles that seen in platelet disorders rather than coagulation disorders. In contrast to hemophilia, hemarthrosis is rare. Von Willebrand's disease is discussed in detail in Ch. 155.

Acquired von Willebrand's Disease. Von Willebrand's disease secondary to SLE and lymphoproliferative disorders has been described. In some cases, deficiency of vWf is mediated by specific antibodies. Low levels of vWf have also been demonstrated in some patients with Wilms' tumor.

Pseudo von Willebrand's Disease. In this rare bleeding disorder, synthesis of plasma vWf is normal; however, because of a primary abnormality in the patients' platelets, high molecular weight vWf is bound spontaneously with high affinity. Consequently, plasma is depleted of high molecular weight multimers of vWf, resulting in an electrophoretic pattern similar to type II vWd. Addition of normal plasma to the patient's platelets results in spontaneous platelet aggregation in vitro. Moreover, patients are frequently thrombocytopenic owing to accelerated clearance of platelets bound with vWf. Transfusion of plasma or cryoprecipitate may result in worsening thrombocytopenia.

Ruggeri ZM, Zimmerman TS: Von Willebrand factor and von Willebrand disease. Blood 70:895, 1987. A review of the disease and its pathogenesis.

PLATELET TRANSFUSIONS

Indications

In general, when serious bleeding is a complication of thrombocytopenia, platelet transfusions are effective only when the cause is decreased production. When thrombocytopenia is due to increased peripheral destruction, or sequestration, the condition is usually refractory to platelet transfusion. Bleeding due to qualitative platelet disorders ordinarily responds to platelet transfusions except when it is secondary to uremia or hepatic failure or when an offending drug is still present in the circulation.

For patients with congenital platelet disorders, platelet transfusion must be given judiciously. With repeated transfusion, alloantibodies are formed. Eventually, it may become impossible to obtain a significant rise in the platelet count through transfusion. Therefore, platelet transfusions should be given only for serious bleeding or in preparation for surgery on patients with moderately severe platelet defects.

Platelet transfusions are indicated for patients who are bleeding actively and who have either a platelet count below ~50,000 per microliter or a qualitative platelet abnormality as manifested by a prolonged bleeding time. Platelet transfusions may also be indicated prophylactically before surgery or other invasive procedures. Prior to surgery, the platelet count should be above ~50,000 per microliter in most cases, and above 90,000 per microliter for surgery in which any abnormal bleeding will have unacceptable morbidity, as, for example, in surgery of the central nervous system or of the eye. For invasive procedures, such as kidney or liver biopsies, a platelet count above 50,000 per microliter is probably sufficient, but this recommendation assumes that platelet function is relatively normal.

Chronic Thrombocytopenia

For patients who are not bleeding, recommendations are based on the cause of thrombocytopenia. When thrombocytopenia is due to decreased production, the platelet count should be maintained above 10,000 to 20,000 per microliter. In patients with accelerated destruction of platelets, transfusion is generally not effective. In addition, in ITP, patients frequently tolerate low platelet counts with little bleeding.

Dosage

For patients who require platelet transfusions chronically, platelets should be obtained from a single donor for each transfusion (generally six to seven units) to reduce the risk of forming multiple alloantibodies (see below). In a 70-kg patient, one unit of platelets usually raises the platelet count by approximately 10,000 per microliter. The platelet count should be repeated 10 to 60 minutes after transfusion to assess the compatibility of the transfused platelets and to determine whether the desired platelet count has been achieved. In a patient who is actively bleeding, the platelet count should be maintained above ~50,000 per microliter.

Alloantibodies Against Platelets

In approximately 50 to 60 per cent of patients whose condition becomes refractory to random donor platelets, anti-HLA (human leukocyte antigen) antibodies appear to be responsible. The other presumed antigens have not yet been identified. In one rare form of alloimmunization, antibodies develop against the PL^A1 antigen, an epitope on platelet glycoprotein IIIa. The difference between PL^A1 positive and negative (PL^A2) is a single amino acid. Ninety-eight per cent of the normal population have PL^A1-positive platelets.

When PL^A1-negative patients are transfused with PL^A1-positive blood, they may develop anti-PL^A1 antibodies. This syndrome, posttransfusion purpura (PTP), occurs primarily in women. Previous immunization is necessary, either by transfusion or by pregnancy. Why this syndrome is rare in spite of the frequency of PL^A1-minus in the population is unknown. Moreover, these patients not only rapidly clear transfused platelets from their circulation but also destroy their own platelets, becoming thrombocytopenic usually 5 to 10 days after transfusion. If patients with antibodies against the PL^Al antigen become severely thrombocytopenic, treatment with plasmapheresis or exchange transfusion is necessary, as bleeding from thrombocytopenia can be life-threatening.

NEONATAL ALLOIMMUNE THROMBOCYTOPENIA. Thrombocytopenia due to maternal alloantibodies against fetal platelet antigens occurs in approximately 1 in 2000 to 1 in 4000 fetuses. Affected infants may have intracranial hemorrhages (estimated ranges between 10 and 30 per cent), and in families with an affected infant, the risk of recurrence is at least 75 per cent.

PL^Al antibodies have been identified in most cases as being responsible for thrombocytopenia. Affected infants are treated by transfusion with washed maternal platelets. Women with a prior history of an affected infant should be delivered by cesarean section. Recently, in pregnant mothers with a prior affected infant, intravenous γ globulin was shown to raise fetal platelet counts with a reduction in the rate of intracranial hemorrhage.

Tomasulo PA, Petz LD: Platelet transfusion. *In* Petz LD, Swisher SN (eds.): Clinical Practice of Transfusion Medicine. 2nd ed. New York, Churchill Livingston 1989, pp 427–467. *Excellent review of specific indications for platelet transfusion and of managing alloimmunized patients.*

VASCULAR DISORDERS (Table 154–6)

Normal vascular function is necessary for effective hemostasis (Fig. 154–1). Alteration in the integrity or structure of blood vessels can lead to a bleeding diathesis, the symptoms and signs of which are indistinguishable from those of a platelet disorder.

Congenital Vascular Disorders Associated with Bleeding

HEREDITARY HEMORRHAGIC TELANGIECTASIA (RENDU-OSLER-WEBER DISEASE). This disorder, the most common genetic cause of vascular bleeding, is inherited as an autosomal dominant trait. The most common problem is spontaneous epistaxis. More than half of the patients have epistaxis by age 20 and 90 per cent by age 45. Telangiectasia occurs most frequently on the face in two thirds of patients, on the mouth in one half of patients, and on the cheeks, tongue, nose, and lower lip in approximately one third of patients. In about 40 per cent of patients, the hands and wrists are also involved. Beyond this cutaneous or mucosal involvement, the organ system affected most often is the gastrointestinal tract (~12 per cent). Death from intestinal bleeding occurs in 12 to 15 per cent of symptomatic patients. The liver, lungs, central nervous system, and urinary tract are involved in decreasing order of frequency. Pulmonary arteriovenous fistulas, present in ~5 per cent of patients, are manifested by cyanoses, dyspnea, clubbing, and thoracic murmurs. Hemoptysis is unusual. Surgical resection is successful in managing this complication in most patients. Stroke may occur in patients with central nervous system involvement, a complication that tends to occur in younger patients (mean age, 33). Careful inspection of the nose and mouth usually reveals the

TABLE 154–6. VASCULAR DISORDERS ASSOCIATED WITH BLEEDING

Congenital
  Hereditary hemorrhagic telangiectasia
  Cavernous hemangioma
  Connective tissue disorders
    Ehlers-Danlos syndrome
    Osteogenesis imperfecta
    Pseudoxanthoma elasticum
Acquired disorders affecting vascular hemostatic function
  Scurvy
  Immunoglobulin disorders
    Cryoglobulinemia
    Benign hyperglobulinemia
    Waldenström's macroglobulinemia
    Multiple myeloma
    Henoch-Schönlein purpura
  Glucocorticoid excess
    Cushing's syndrome
    Glucocorticoid therapy

diagnosis. In other cases, endoscopy or angiography may be necessary. Pathologic examination of involved tissue demonstrates dilated capillaries with loss of subendothelial structures.

Tests of platelet function and the bleeding time are normal. There is no consistently effective therapy, but the prognosis is relatively good.

CAVERNOUS HEMANGIOMA (KASABACH-MERRITT SYNDROME). Congenital subcutaneous and visceral hemangiomas may be associated with thrombocytopenia and bleeding in infants and children with this syndrome. Bleeding occurs at the site of the lesions or systemically owing to thrombocytopenia. Platelets are activated within the hemangioma and subsequently removed from the circulation. In addition, mild DIC may occur with consumption of fibrinogen. Thrombocytopenia is severer than the coagulation abnormalities. Spontaneous regression of hemangiomas may occur over a period of years. In cases in which thrombocytopenia is severe and tumors are few in number, surgery and/or radiation therapy may be effective. Intentional thrombosis of hemangiomas by administration of inhibitors of fibrinolysis, with or without cryoprecipitate, has been successful in managing thrombocytopenia in a few cases.

DISORDERS OF CONNECTIVE TISSUE. Genetic abnormalities in structural glycoproteins such as collagen can result in vascular fragility caused by weakening of the vessel wall. Bleeding may be limited to increased bruising or may manifest as internal hemorrhaging. Ehlers-Danlos syndrome, osteogenesis imperfecta, and pseudoxanthoma elasticum, discussed elsewhere in this book, are examples of inherited disorders of connective tissue that may be associated with a bleeding diathesis on this basis.

Acquired Disorders of Blood Vessels Causing Bleeding

SCURVY (Ch. 204). Severe vitamin C deficiency results in defective collagen formation in small blood vessels. Bleeding may occur in any tissue but is prominent in the lower extremities and is perifollicular in distribution. Other sites where bleeding is common include the gums, the subperiosteum in children, and into the muscles.

PURPURA ASSOCIATED WITH IMMUNOGLOBULIN DISORDERS. *Cryoglobulinemia* (Ch. 151). Patients with all three types of cryoglobulinemia have purpura as a complication of their disease. In type I cryoglobulinemia, bleeding may be due to obstruction of blood flow in the microcirculation at cold temperatures by cryoprecipitates, resulting in increased vascular fragility. In type II and III cryoglobulinemia, bleeding may be due to leukocytoclastic vasculitis associated with the immune complexes. Purpura occurs most commonly in the distal extremities.

Benign Hyperglobulinemia (Waldenström's Purpura). In this syndrome, patients have polyclonal hyperglobulinemia associated with purpura of the lower extremities. Leukocytoclastic involvement of the vessel wall may account for increased vascular fragility and bleeding. Commonly, the onset of purpura is preceded by a stinging sensation in areas of involvement. While there is generally no evidence of systemic vasculitis, this disorder may evolve into Sjögren's syndrome or SLE.

Amyloidosis (Ch. 197). Amyloid deposition in the skin and subcutaneous tissues alters the normal structural support for small blood vessels, resulting in increased vascular fragility (see Color Plate 8*I*, right). Purpura can occur at any site; but for unclear reasons, periorbital hemorrhage is a characteristic finding in systemic amyloidosis.

Waldenström's Macroglobulinemia and Multiple Myeloma (Ch. 151). Abnormalities in platelet function may occur with M proteins, as noted above. An additional contributing factor is hyperviscosity when it complicates these diseases. Slowing of blood flow and increased hydrostatic pressure may increase vascular fragility, leading to purpura.

Henoch-Schönlein Purpura. This childhood disorder is characterized by symmetric purpura and arthralgias of the lower extremities, abdominal pain, and melena. Rarely, adults are affected. Patients may give a history of a recent infectious illness. The disease has an acute onset with a maculopapular rash evolving into palpable purpura. Other complications include glomerulonephritis and hypertension (both of which are self-limiting) and intussusception. Involved tissues, including the skin, demonstrate vasculitis with immunoglobulin A (IgA) and complement deposition.

Henoch-Schönlein purpura usually remits spontaneously over a period of 1 to 2 months, although the course is often punctuated by flaring of symptoms and signs. Symptomatic improvement is obtained with glucocorticoids.

Miscellaneous Disorders

CUSHING'S SYNDROME. Cushing's disease or chronic administration of glucocorticoids results in increased bruising, particularly in the extremities. Abnormal bleeding probably results from alterations in the structure of the perivascular matrix, with loss of normal elasticity.

AUTOERYTHROCYTE SENSITIZATION (GARDNER-DIAMOND SYNDROME). This bizarre syndrome is charaterized by the development of purpura at any site on the body, preceded by pain and burning. It occurs almost exclusively in women. Usually, affected women have a history of severe stress and emotional problems. Tests for abnormalities in hemostasis are all normal.

The diagnostic test is the development of large ecchymoses within 24 to 48 hours at the site of subcutaneous injection of a small amount (~0.1 ml) of the patient's own blood or erythrocytes. Injection should be at sites inaccessible to the patient, and a concurrent control injection should be administered. The primary differential diagnosis is factitious purpura.

PURPURA SIMPLEX. Purpura simplex is the term used to describe the phenomenon commonly observed in young children and middle-aged women of easy bruisability, primarily of the lower extremities. Laboratory evaluation, including the bleeding time, is normal, and there is no evidence of vascular abnormalities. Other than bruising, affected women do not experience excessive bleeding with surgery and do not have internal bleeding.

155 Disorders of Blood Coagulation

Deane F. Mosher

Normal hemostasis requires interactions among blood vessels, the formed elements of blood, especially platelets and monocytes, and blood coagulation proteins. The general biology of hemostasis and the approach to a patient suspected of having a hemorrhagic diathesis have been discussed in Ch. 154, Hemorrhagic Disorders: Abnormalities of Platelet and Vascular Function. In the present chapter, attention is focused on hemorrhagic and thrombotic disorders that occur as a consequence of abnormalities of blood coagulation proteins.

REVIEW OF BLOOD COAGULATION

Blood coagulation, initiated by substances in injured tissues, is propagated by an interlocking network of enzymic events, the so-called coagulation cascade. These controlled reactions ensure that blood coagulation happens quickly and yet remains localized. Blood coagulation results in the formation of a protein scaffolding, the fibrin clot, that controls bleeding and serves as a nidus for subsequent cellular ingrowth and tissue repair. After several days the fibrin clot is lysed and replaced by a more permanent scaffolding of connective tissue matrix molecules. Abnormalities that result in delay of clot formation or in premature lysis of clots are associated with a bleeding tendency. Abnormalities that result in inappropriate activation or localization of blood coagulation are associated with thrombosis.

COAGULATION MOLECULES. Coagulation and fibrinolysis involve many blood plasma proteins (Table 155–1). This list grows longer as blood coagulation mechanisms are studied in greater depth. Structural and functional similarities allow one to put the proteins into one of several groups. Some are zymogens of serine proteinases and hence members of the serine proteinase family of proteins. Among the serine proteinase family are five proteins (Factors II, VII, IX, and X and protein C) that are modified by vitamin K–dependent posttranslational carboxylation of glutamic acid residues. A sixth plasma protein, protein S, is also modified

by this reaction. The modification allows the six proteins to bind Ca^{2+} and phospholipids and thereby participate efficiently in blood coagulation. Factors V and VIII function as helper proteins during blood coagulation and are homologous to each other and to ceruloplasmin, a Cu^{2+}-binding plasma protein. Other proteins are *ser*ine *p*roteinase *in*hibitors and hence members of the "serpin" family of proteins. Most of the proteins listed in Table 155–1, including the vitamin K–dependent factors, are synthesized by hepatocytes. A number of the proteins, however, can also be synthesized by other cell types such as megakaryocytes, monocyte-macrophages, and endothelial cells.

There are also key molecules that are embedded in the external membrane of cells (tissue factor, thrombomodulin, urokinase receptor) or deposited in extracellular matrix (*e.g.*, heparan sulfate and dermatan sulfate). The molecules interact specifically with components of blood to initiate and modulate coagulation and fibrinolysis.

GENERAL MECHANISMS. Blood coagulation is activated, propagated, and controlled by mechanisms found in other proteolytic effector systems (*e.g.*, complement). These mechanisms include the following:

1. Sequential activation by limited proteolytic cleavage
2. Amplification of the response by feedback loops
3. Use of binding or helper proteins to bring reactants together
4. Destruction of activated proteins by further proteolytic cleavage
5. Inhibition of activated proteinases by stoichiometric complex formation with specific inhibitor proteins, *i.e.*, the serpins

In addition, there is a mechanism that is, so far, unique to blood coagulation:

6. Formation of a five-part complex of an activated vitamin K–dependent factor, to-be-activated vitamin K–dependent zymogen, helper protein, Ca^{2+}, and phospholipid surface.

EXTRINSIC AND INTRINSIC PATHWAYS. Blood coagulation can be initiated by exposure of blood to tissue factor (the "extrinsic system") or by activation of contact factors of plasma (the "intrinsic system"). Both of these initiation pathways lead to a common pathway, which results in the elaboration of thrombin, the master coagulation enzyme. As shown in Figure 155–1A, the concept of the two initiation pathways and the common pathway is useful in understanding two major coagulation tests, the activated partial thromboplastin time (APTT), in which blood plasma is activated by the intrinsic pathway, and the prothrombin time (PT), in which tissue factor is added to plasma so that activation proceeds by the extrinsic pathway. It is unlikely that the two initiation pathways are so clearly delineated in vivo. Activation of Factor IX, an intrinsic factor, by Factor VII, an extrinsic factor, must be of considerable importance because deficiencies of Factors VII and IX, as well as the factors that follow Factor IX in the intrinsic and common pathways, *i.e.*, Factors VIII, X, V, II, and I, all are associated with a bleeding tendency. In contrast, deficiency of Factor XII, prekallikrein, or high molecular weight kininogen (HMWK) does not cause a bleeding problem, and Factor XI deficiency is associated with a bleeding tendency in only a minority of cases.

Tissue Factor and the Extrinsic Pathway. Factor VII is unique among coagulation factors because it circulates in an active configuration. To initiate coagulation, however, Factor VII requires tissue factor. Sites rich in tissue factor include brain, adventitia of blood vessels, organ capsules, epidermis, and mucosal epithelium. Therefore, tissue factor is not exposed to blood unless there is an anatomic disruption that allows blood access to the hemostatic envelope around blood vessels, organs, or the body itself. Tissue factor is present in many types of cells, including endothelial cells and monocytes. In response to a variety of stimuli, such as exposure to lymphokines or monokines, tissue factor becomes expressed on cell surfaces.

In the presence of tissue factor, phospholipid, and Ca^{2+}, Factor VII can activate Factors IX and X (Fig. 155–1B). Activated Factor X (X_a) then activates Factor II, and Factor II$_a$ (thrombin) cleaves fibrinogen to fibrin. The time to clot formation after addition of tissue factor, phospholipid, and Ca^{2+} to citrated platelet-poor plasma is called the prothrombin time or PT, the single most important clotting test. When determined with an excess of tissue factor (as is generally done), the PT measures only factors of the extrinsic and common pathways and does not measure Factor IX.

Control of Factor VII/Tissue Factor by Extrinsic Pathway Inhibitor. Extrinsic pathway inhibitor (EPI) is a double-headed protease inhibitor of the pancreatic trypsin inhibitor class. One head of EPI binds to Factor X_a, and the second head inhibits Factor VII in association with tissue factor. Therefore, EPI extinguishes the Factor VII/tissue factor "match" that "ignites" blood coagulation (Fig. 155–1B). The "fuse" that propagates coagulation begins with Factor IX_a, not Factor X_a. This is why, when the concentration of tissue factor is low, most of Factor VII's clot-promoting activity is generated through Factor IX.

Contact Factors and the Intrinsic System. Activation of contact factors constitutes a second pathway for activating Factor X. Negatively charged surfaces, such as sulfatide micelles, glass, kaolin, and celite, bind Factor XII and HMWK. HMWK, in turn, binds prekallikrein and Factor XI. Binding to surfaces initiates a series of reciprocal cleavages of Factor XI and prekallikrein by activated Factor XII and of Factor XII by activated Factor XI and kallikrein (Fig. 155–1C). Activated Factor XI activates Factor IX in a reaction that requires Ca^{2+}. Kallikrein also releases bradykinin, a vasoactive and pain-causing octapeptide, from HMWK and low molecular weight kininogen. In the APTT, platelet-poor citrated plasma is allowed to incubate for 3 to 5 minutes with kaolin or ellagic acid to activate Factor XI optimally. Ca^{2+} and phospholipid are then added so that Factor XI_a can activate Factor IX, Factor IX_a can activate Factor X, and so on.

Amplification of Activation Pathways. Three analogous five-part propagating reactions take place (Fig. 155–1C): (1) Factor VII activates Factor X or IX in the presence of tissue factor, Ca^{2+}, and phospholipid; (2) Factor IX_a activates Factor X in the presence of Factor VIII, Ca^{2+}, and phospholipid; and (3) Factor X_a activates Factor II in the presence of Factor V, Ca^{2+}, and phospholipid. The phospholipid requirement for reaction 1 is

TABLE 155–1. PROTEINS INVOLVED IN BLOOD COAGULATION AND FIBRINOLYSIS

Protein	Synonym	Size in Kilodaltons*	Plasma Concentration in mg/dl (μM)*	Kind of Protein	Function†
Fibrinogen	Factor I	340	300(9)	Structural protein	Gels to form clot
Factor II	Prothrombin	72	15(2)	Vitamin K–dependent zymogen of serine proteinase	Activates I, V, VIII, XIII, protein C, and platelets
Factor V	Proaccelerin	350	2(0.05)	Ceruloplasmin-like binding protein	Supports X_a activation of II
Factor VII	Stable factor	50	0.01(0.002)	Vitamin K–dependent zymogen of serine proteinase	Activates IX and X
Factor VIII	Antihemophilic factor	350	0.01(0.0003)	Ceruloplasmin-like binding protein	Supports IX_a activation of X
Factor IX	Christmas factor	57	1(0.2)	Vitamin K–dependent zymogen of serine proteinase	Activates X
Factor X	Stuart-Prower factor	59	1(0.2)	Vitamin K–dependent zymogen of serine proteinase	Activates II
Factor XI	Plasma thromboplastin antecedent	160	0.5(0.03)	Zymogen of serine proteinase	Activates XII and prekallikrein
Factor XII	Hageman factor	75	2(0.2)	Zymogen of serine proteinase	Activates XI and prekallikrein
Factor XIII	Fibrin-stabilizing factor	320	3(0.08)	Zymogen of transglutaminase	Crosslinks fibrin and other proteins
von Willebrand factor	Factor VIII–related antigen	800–20,000	2(0.05)	Structural protein	Binds VIII, mediates platelet adhesion
Prekallikrein	—	88	2(0.3)	Zymogen of serine proteinase	Activates XII and prekallikrein, cleaves HMWK
High molecular weight kininogen (HMWK)	—	150	2(0.2)	Binding protein, unique	Supports reciprocal activation of XII, XI, and prekallikrein
Fibronectin	—	450	40(1)	Structural protein, unique	Mediates cell adhesion
Extrinsic pathway inhibitor	EPI, LACI	46	0.1(0.02)	Kunitz-type inhibitor	Inhibits VII/tissue factor in concert with X_a
Antithrombin III	Major antithrombin	60	20(2.5)	Serpin	Inhibits II_a, X_a, and other proteinases; cofactor for heparin
Heparin cofactor II	Minor antithrombin	55	5(0.6)	Serpin	Inhibits II_a, cofactor for heparin and dermatan sulfate
Protein C	—	62	0.4(0.06)	Vitamin K–dependent zymogen of serine proteinase	Inactivates V and VIII
Protein S	—	69	3(0.4)	Vitamin K–dependent binding protein	Cofactor for protein C_a, binds C4b-binding protein
Plasminogen	—	86	10(1.2)	Zymogen of serine proteinase	Lyses fibrin and other proteins
Alpha$_2$-antiplasmin	—	60	3(0.5)	Serpin	Inhibits plasmin
Prourokinase	—	50	tr	Zymogen of serine proteinase	Activates plasminogen
Tissue plasminogen activator	TPA	55	tr	Serine proteinase	Activates plasminogen
Plasminogen activator inhibitor 1	PAI1	52	tr	Serpin	Inactivates TPA and urokinase
Plasminogen activator inhibitor 2	PAI2	55	tr	Serpin	Inactivates TPA and urokinase

*For comparison, the size of albumin is 68 kilodaltons, and the plasma concentration of albumin is 3500 mg/dl (510 μM).
†For zymogens, the function after activation is given.
tr = trace.

satisfied by the surface of the tissue factor–containing cell. For the reactions involving Factor VIII or V, the phospholipid requirement is satisfied by platelet phospholipid.

The vitamin K–dependent factors (VII, IX, X, II) bind to the phospholipid surface in interactions that require gamma-carboxyl glutamic acid residues; the binding is Ca^{2+} dependent. Factors V and VIII contain domains for binding protease and zymogen, Ca^{2+}, and the phospholipid surface. Stimulated platelets contain discrete binding sites for Factor V. The accelerating role of platelets in the X_a-V-II reaction is called platelet factor 3 activity. Formation of the five-part complex dramatically increases the rate constant (K_{cat}) for activation of zymogen by protease. In the five-part complex, Factor V or VIII is most effective after it has been cleaved by Factor II_a (thrombin). Thus, thrombin is initially generated at a sluggish rate, but once a small amount of thrombin is generated so that it can cleave Factor V or VIII to a more active form, subsequent thrombin generation is "explosively" rapid and efficient, consuming almost all of the Factor II in plasma.

LOCALIZATION AND INHIBITION OF BLOOD COAGULATION. Blood coagulation is efficiently activated only on a phospholipid surface (Fig. 155–1C), and thus activation is localized to the area of injury. In addition to EPI described above, several mechanisms dampen activation by "snuffing out the fuse"

and thereby ensure that activated factors do not escape and cause thrombosis at a distant site (Fig. 155–1B).

Thrombin exhibits acquired altered specificity when complexed to thrombomodulin; rather than acting upon fibrinogen or Factors V and VIII, thrombin activates protein C (Fig. 155–1B). Activated protein C, in turn, inactivates thrombin-activated Factors V and VIII. In addition, activated protein C enhances fibrinolysis. Activation of protein C by thrombin-thrombomodulin complex, therefore, is a powerful anticoagulant event, just as the activation of Factors V and VIII by thrombin is a powerful procoagulant event. The cleavage of Factors V and VIII by activated protein C requires the sixth vitamin K–dependent protein of plasma, protein S. Protein S serves as a cofactor for activated protein C rather than acting as a proteinase. A portion of circulating protein S is complexed to C4 binding protein (C4bp).

Two antithrombins in plasma, called antithrombin III and heparin cofactor II, inhibit thrombin and other serine proteinases that are generated during blood coagulation. The antithrombins, members of the serpin family, are substrates for the proteinases. Upon cleavage the antithrombins undergo a structural rearrangement that allows them to form tight one-to-one complexes with the proteinases. As a result, the proteinases are irreversibly

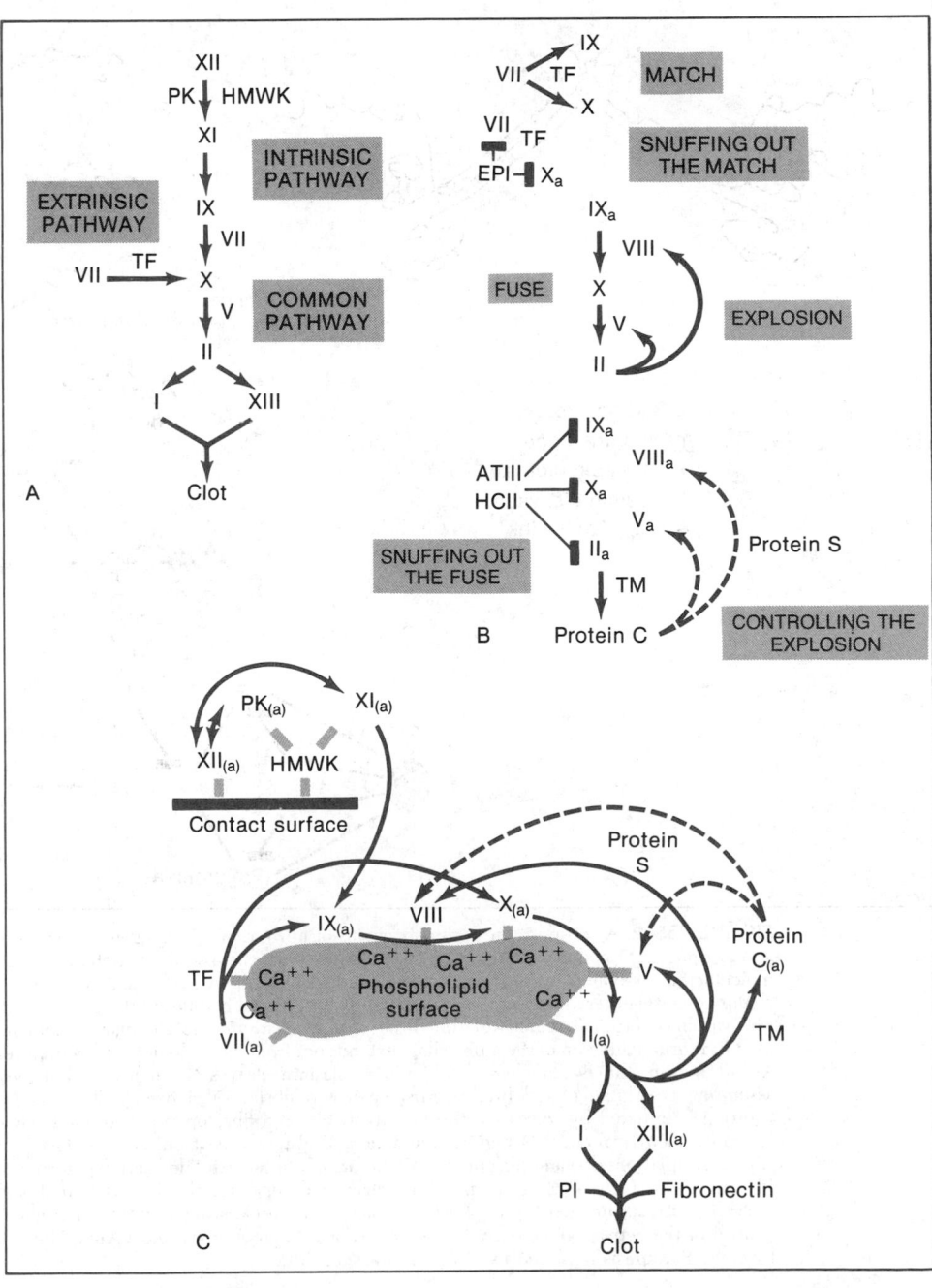

FIGURE 155–1. Diagrams of interactions among coagulation factors. *A* depicts the intrinsic, extrinsic, and common pathways in their simplest forms. *B* emphasizes critical stages in activation and control of blood coagulation. *C* is organized around the contact surface and the phospholipid surface. Solid lines with arrows indicate proteolytic activation. Broken lines with arrows indicate proteolytic inactivation. Solid lines with bars indicate complex formation and inactivation. The stippled patches indicate binding of proteins to surfaces or to one another. The subscript a indicates proteins that are zymogens and can be converted to active enzymes. PK = prekallikrein; HMWK = high molecular weight kininogen; TF = tissue factors; PI = alpha$_2$-antiplasmin; TM = thrombomodulin; EPI = extrinsic pathway inhibitor; ATIII = antithrombin III; HCII = heparin cofactor II.

inhibited. The rates at which both antithrombins combine with coagulation proteinases are accelerated many-fold by heparin and by heparan sulfate proteoglycan on the luminal surface of endothelial cells. The acceleration explains the anticoagulant action of heparin. The rate at which the heparin cofactor II combines with thrombin is accelerated by dermatan sulfate, a glycosaminoglycan found in the vessel wall.

As described in more detail below, inherited deficiency states of protein C, protein S, and antithrombin III have all been associated with thrombotic diatheses.

STRUCTURE OF FIBRINOGEN AND FIBRIN. Fibrinogen and fibrin monomer are extended trinodular molecules made up of pairs of three polypeptide chains (Fig. 155–2A). The three chains run through half of the molecule, that is, through half of the central E nodule and the whole of one of the two peripheral D nodules. The chains are thought to adopt a coiled-spring structure between the E and D nodules. This portion of the molecule is particularly susceptible to degradation by the principal fibrinolytic enzyme, plasmin. The nodules resist degradation

by plasmin. Thus the products of complete lysis of a clot by plasmin are one E nodule, two D nodules, and small fragments (Fig. 155–2B).

Thrombin cleaves negatively charged small peptides to convert fibrinogen to a clottable derivative called fibrin monomer. Fibrin monomer assembles to form an infinite branching network of fibrils (Fig. 155–2B). At physiologic fibrin concentrations, this network constitutes a strong gel and immobilizes blood. Fibrinogen is usually completely converted to fibrin during blood coagulation. Thus the concentration of fibrinogen antigen in serum is about 0.02 mg per deciliter, compared with 200 mg per deciliter in plasma. Fibrinogen, however, forms soluble complexes with fibrin monomer when the concentration of thrombin is low. The soluble complexes can escape from areas of active coagulation and be detected in the circulation.

The fibrin gel is modified by thrombin-activated Factor XIII. This enzyme, a transglutaminase, catalyzes covalent protein-protein crosslinking. Crosslinks are introduced between gamma chains of adjacent D domains, thus ligating the fibrin fibril end to end (Fig. 155–2B). Crosslinking of gamma chains renders the clot insoluble in protein denaturants such as 6M urea. The alpha

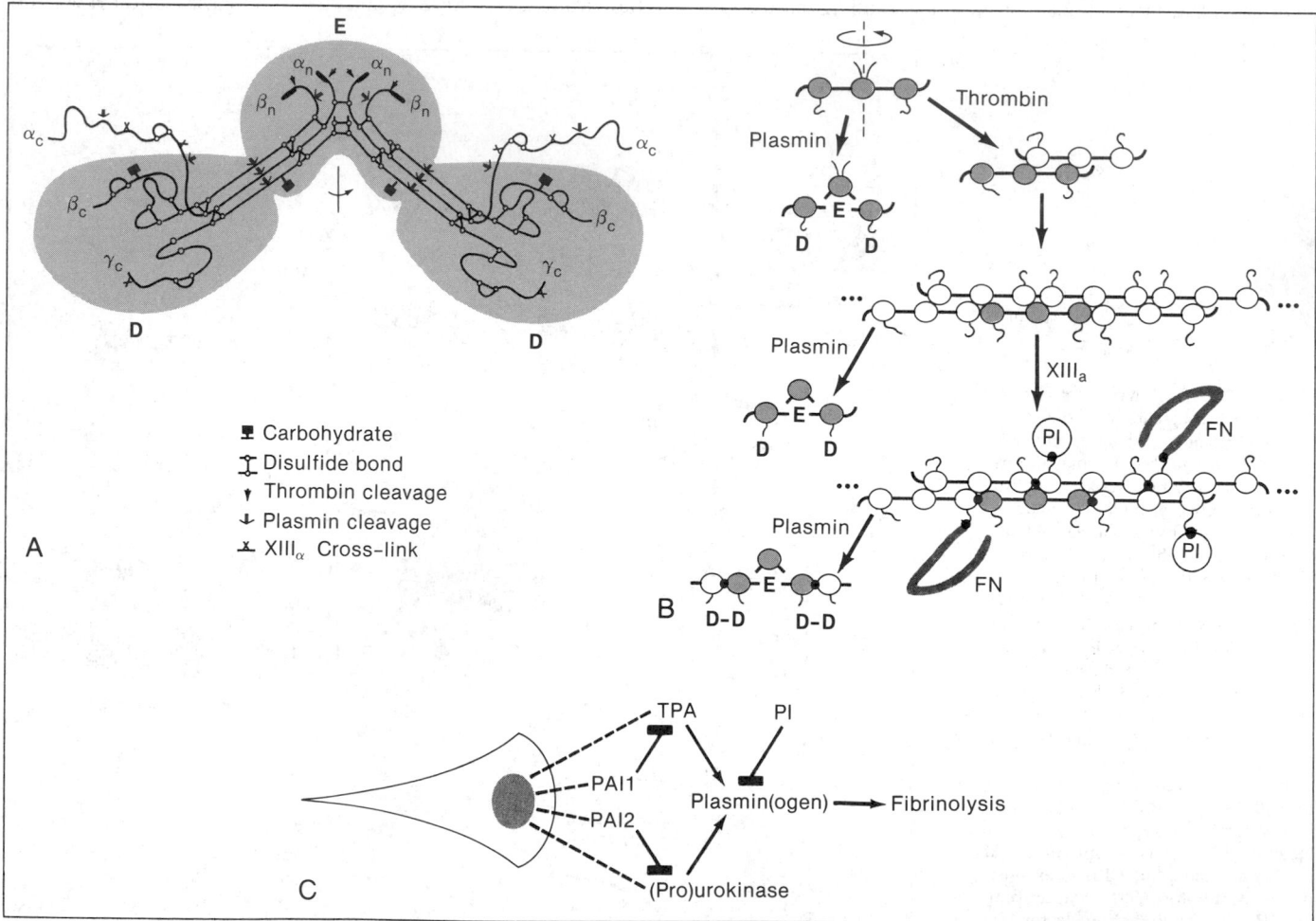

FIGURE 155–2. *A,* Disposition of the six chains of fibrinogen. Fibrinogen is composed of a central E nodule and two peripheral D nodules. One set of three nonidentical chains—alpha, beta, and gamma—runs through half the molecule and is bound to the other set by disulfide linkages in the E domain, where the amino termini of all six chains come together. The strands connecting the peripheral nodules to the central nodule contain all three chains. The carboxyl terminal regions of the three chains constitute the globular D domain. In addition, the extreme carboxyl terminal region of the alpha chain extends out from the D domain. Thrombin releases acidic fibrinopeptides A and B from the E domain to yield fibrin; plasmin cleaves the molecule between E and D. *B,* Activation, assembly, crosslinking, and lysis of fibrinogen and fibrin. Fibrinogen and fibrin are both trinodular proteins. Clotting is initiated by release of the negatively charged fibrinopeptides from the E nodule. Assembly is driven by noncovalent E nodule–D nodule interaction. End-to-end covalent crosslinking occurs between gamma chains. Alpha$_2$-antiplasmin (PI) and fibronectin (FN) crosslink to the extended carboxyl terminal portion of the alpha chain. Plasmin cleaves this portion of the alpha chain and separates the D and E nodules. *C* depicts the proteolytic activation of plasminogen by its physiologic activators, urokinase and tissue plasminogen activator (TPA), and the control of the activation by plasminogen activator inhibitors (PAI1 and PAI2). These four molecules are secreted by cells. Plasmin is inhibited by alpha$_2$-antiplasmin (PI).

chains can ligate side to side among themselves or be crosslinked to fibronectin or alpha$_2$-antiplasmin. Both the "hardening" of the fibrin clot by crosslinking and the incorporation of other proteins into the clot are probably important. Deficiency of Factor XIII or of alpha$_2$-antiplasmin is associated with a bleeding tendency, and some patients with Factor XIII deficiency suffer from poor wound healing.

FIBRINOLYSIS. Cleavage of plasminogen to the active proteinase plasmin is carried out by two plasminogen activators: tissue plasminogen activator (TPA) and urokinase (Fig. 155–2C). TPA is secreted as an active serine proteinase, whereas urokinase can be activated from a somewhat active precursor, prourokinase. Among the activators of prourokinase is plasmin. TPA, plasminogen, and plasmin all bind to fibrin, and it is in a fibrin clot that TPA can activate plasminogen to plasmin most efficiently. Prourokinase does not bind to fibrin. However, small amounts of plasmin already bound to fibrin can activate prourokinase to urokinase, which then can activate more plasminogen to plasmin.

Localization of fibrinolysis to the fibrin clot is further ensured by binding of the activators, especially urokinase, to cells and an efficient array of inhibitors. Cells secrete specific inhibitors of TPA and urokinase, called plasminogen activator inhibitors 1 and 2, to regulate fibrinolysis in their local environment. Indeed, tightly controlled secretion of activator and inhibitor may allow a cell to localize plasminogen activation to volumes that are only nanometers across. Anti-TPA is present in the circulation in low concentrations. Also in the circulation is alpha$_2$-antiplasmin, which inhibits plasmin extremely rapidly and efficiently.

Plasmin degrades a variety of proteins in addition to fibrin, especially connective tissue proteins and undoubtedly has other physiologic functions besides lysis of fibrin clots. For instance, ovarian follicular cells secrete plasminogen activator in response to hormonal stimulation just prior to ovulation and thereby initiate degradation of the follicular wall.

Epsilon-aminocaproic acid (EACA) and its cyclic analogue, tranexamic acid, bind to plasminogen and plasmin and inhibit binding of these molecules to fibrin. As a result, the molecules are good inhibitors of plasminogen activation.

Streptokinase, a bacterial protein, forms a complex with plasminogen and causes a conformational change that opens up the active site of plasminogen. The streptokinase-plasminogen complex can degrade fibrin and activate free plasminogen to plasmin. The complex is not inhibited by alpha$_2$-antiplasmin.

Colman RW, Hirsh J, Marder VJ, et al. (eds.): Hemostasis and Thrombosis: Basic Principles and Clinical Practice. 2nd ed. Philadelphia, J. B. Lippincott Company, 1987. *Extensive information about the structure and function of blood coagulation proteins with earnest attempts to relate biochemical facts to clinical problems.*

Drake TA, Morrissey JH, Edgington TS: Selective cellular expression of tissue factor in human tissues. Am J Pathol 134:1087, 1989. *Immunohistochemical localization of the hemostatic envelope.*

Furie B, Furie BC: The molecular basis of blood coagulation. Cell 53:505, 1988. *Short review of mechanisms.*

APPROACH TO PATIENTS WITH COAGULATION DISORDERS

HISTORY AND PHYSICAL EXAMINATION. There are three components to effective hemostasis: the blood vessel, the platelets, and the network of soluble factors. Abnormal bleeding occurs with much greater frequency when two of the three components are compromised as, for example, in a hemophilic patient who suffers trauma or takes aspirin or in a patient with peptic ulcer and thrombocytopenia. Disorders of platelets or blood vessels often cause mucosal or superficial bleeding; deficiency of a coagulation factor results in a tendency to form soft tissue hematomas or to suffer from repeated hemarthroses. Thrombosis tends to occur when there is inflammation, abnormalities of the luminal surface of a large blood vessel, or stasis.

A personal history, family history, and physical examination are important parts of the evaluation of a possible coagulation problem. In taking a history, it is not enough simply to ask, "Do you or your close relatives bleed or clot abnormally?" One must also determine how the hemostatic system has been stressed: "Have you had any operations or tooth extractions? If so, did you bleed abnormally or require blood transfusions afterward? Are your menstrual periods heavy? Do you bruise easily? Do you take iron tablets? Have you ever had a limb immobilized?" And

so on. A formal family tree indicating how many family members are at risk and which ones have symptoms or laboratory evidence of a coagulation disorder should be constructed.

LABORATORY SCREENING TESTS. When a bleeding disorder is suspected, a group of reproducible and fairly inexpensive laboratory tests should detect most clinically significant abnormalities of platelets, blood vessels, and the coagulation factor network:

1. A complete blood count and examination of the blood smear screen for abnormalities in bone marrow function or platelet number and morphologic changes in red cells caused by intravascular thrombosis or microangiopathy.

2. A quantitative platelet count provides more definitive information about platelet number.

3. A template bleeding time screens for abnormalities of blood vessels and platelets.

4. The PT and APTT screen for abnormalities of the extrinsic and intrinsic coagulation pathways, respectively. Both tests are sensitive to abnormalities of the common pathway. The PT or APTT should be abnormally long if a single factor is below 20 to 40 per cent of its normal plasma concentration.

5. The solubility of the fibrin clot in concentrated (6M) urea detects clinically significant deficiency of Factor XIII. In the absence of Factor XIII, the clot is not covalently crosslinked and therefore is soluble.

Evaluation of a Prolonged PT or APTT. The first step is to perform mixing experiments of normal plasma and the abnormal plasma to decide whether the abnormal plasma is deficient in a coagulation factor or contains an inhibitor of coagulation. If the screening test of the mixture is normal, it is likely that the abnormal plasma is deficient in one or more factors, and specific factor assays can be done to identify the deficiency. If the screening test of the mixture is abnormal, it is likely that the abnormal plasma contains an inhibitor. Inhibitors may be of the so-called lupus type and directed against the phospholipid used in the assays or more rarely may be directed against a single coagulation factor. Lupus-type inhibitors rarely cause clinical bleeding. Indeed, as described below, some patients with lupus-type inhibitors suffer from repeated episodes of venous and arterial thrombosis. Inhibitors directed against single factors, especially VIII and IX, may cause serious bleeding.

SPECIFIC TESTS OF INDIVIDUAL PROTEINS. A plasma protein can be measured as the protein per se, usually with an immunoassay, or for protein activity. Plasma contains many different proteins, some of which influence the activity of the coagulation factor of interest and others of which may influence the endpoint of the assay. Activity assays for coagulation proteins are therefore less straightforward than many laboratory measurements. In general, there are two approaches for such activity assays: use of factor-deficient plasmas and use of chromogenic substrates.

Use of Factor-Deficient Plasmas. Normal plasma and the patient's plasma are compared for their ability to correct the PT or APTT of plasma from an individual severely deficient in the factor of interest. Thus Factor VIII can be measured, using plasma from an individual with severe classic hemophilia. If the patient has a Factor VIII deficiency, the patient's plasma should correct the APTT of the hemophilic patient's plasma less well than does normal plasma. By convention, the normal plasma is said to have 100 per cent, or 1 unit per milliliter, of activity. If a 1/10 dilution of the patient's plasma has the correcting power of a 1/100 dilution of normal plasma, the patient is said to have a Factor VIII activity of 10 per cent, or 0.1 unit per milliliter. Such an assay should be accurate to within 10 to 20 per cent of the reported value.

Use of Chromogenic Substrates. A chromogenic substrate is a small peptide that is cleaved by an activated proteinase to yield a colored product. The rate of cleavage can be measured with high precision in a spectrophotometer, using dilute solutions of plasma. As an example, plasminogen can be assayed by the addition of streptokinase to diluted plasma and quantification of cleavage of a chromogenic substrate by streptokinase-plasminogen complexes. Alternatively, antiplasmin can be assayed by addition of plasmin to diluted plasma and quantification of the loss of the ability of plasmin to cleave the same substrate due to formation of plasmin-inhibitor complexes. Such assays should be accurate to within 3 to 5 per cent of the reported value but may be subject to artifact. For instance, a patient with a recent streptococcal infection could have artifactually low apparent plasminogen activity because of neutralizing antibodies to streptokinase.

Indications for Specific Tests. When there is a suspicious bleeding history but normal screening tests, several specific assays should be considered. Mild Factor VIII or IX deficiency (10 to 40 per cent of normal) is clinically significant but may result in a screening APTT that is at the upper limits of normal but still within the normal range. Deficiency of plasma alpha$_2$-antiplasmin can be diagnosed only with a specific assay.

Evaluation of a possible thrombotic diathesis, at present, can be done only with specific assays for proteins C and S, antithrombin III, plasminogen, and perhaps other components of the fibrinolytic system.

Diagnosis of a 50 Per Cent Deficiency State. Laboratory studies of family members are often crucial to the evaluation, especially when the diagnosis centers on a heterozygous (50 per cent of normal) deficiency. The normal level (i.e., the value in 99 per cent of normal individuals) of a coagulation factor is typically 70 to 140 per cent; the level of the factor in individuals with heterozygous deficiency is typically 35 to 70 per cent; and the assay for the factor is accurate to within only 5 to 10 per cent of the reported value. The problem of distinguishing the 50 per cent deficiency state from normal is therefore a formidable one. If the apparent deficiency is found in other family members at risk, one can be much more confident that a true deficiency state exists. For example, a random woman with a 50 per cent Factor VIII level is probably not a carrier of classic hemophilia. If the sister of a hemophilic patient has a 50 per cent Factor VIII level, however, the sister has a 95 per cent chance of being a carrier. Heterozygous deficiency states associated with thrombosis (i.e., deficiency of antithrombin III, protein C, or protein S) present a similar problem. The most important facet of the care of a patient with heterozygote deficiency is appropriate counseling. Therefore, a physician should not be reluctant to arrange extensive family studies. To give an example, it would be much more efficient (and cost effective) to identify a patient with antithrombin deficiency as part of a family study and counsel that patient that he or she is at risk for thrombosis after surgery than to screen all patients prior to surgery with a specific assay for antithrombin. In the future it is likely that informative protein or restriction fragment length polymorphisms will be identified that will allow most deficiency states to be traced in families with more than 99 per cent confidence.

Suchman AL, Griner PF: Diagnostic uses of the activated partial thromboplastin time and prothrombin time. Ann Intern Med 104:810, 1986. *Critical evaluation of when these tests should be ordered and how the tests should be interpreted.*

INHERITED DISORDERS OF BLOOD COAGULATION
General Comments

The plasma protein coagulation factors that are named with Roman numerals, with the exception of Factor XII, were identified as a consequence of patients presenting with bleeding disorders that were eventually recognized as unique and familial. Bleeding may be due to a structural defect in a coagulation factor or to a lack of its synthesis. In the former situation there is immunologically cross-reacting material (CRM) present in the patient's plasma, and the patient is said to be CRM+. In the latter situation the patient is said to be CRM−.

GENETICS. Genetic material for the coagulation factors has been cloned, and considerable information about the exact genetic defects that underlie inherited bleeding disorders has been generated. Deficiencies of Factors VIII and IX are inherited as X-linked traits, with bleeding occurring in the male hemizygotes. Von Willebrand disease is usually an autosomal dominant disorder, although rare patients have severe autosomal recessive disease. Deficiencies of all of the other coagulation factors are transmitted as autosomal recessive traits, with clinically significant bleeding usually manifested only in patients with homozygous or double heterozygous deficiency. Heterozygous carriers may have

reduced plasma levels of a coagulation factor activity, but the deficiency seldom affects hemostasis. In the case of protein deficiencies associated with familial tendency to thrombosis, however, heterozygotes with 50 per cent of the normal level of the protein are at risk.

McKusick VA: Mendelian Inheritance in Man. 9th ed. Baltimore, The Johns Hopkins University Press, 1990. *Catalogs genetic defects.*

TREATMENT STRATEGIES. The most obvious treatment is replacement of the missing factor. Concentrates of Factors VIII and IX are readily available at a cost of 50 to 70 cents per unit. Because of its large size, Factor VIII distributes mainly in the blood plasma. There is approximately 40 ml of plasma per kilogram of body weight. Thus it would take 1400 units of Factor VIII to raise the plasma Factor VIII level of a 70-kg patient with severe classic hemophilia from less than 1 per cent (<0.01 unit per milliliter) to 50 per cent (0.5 unit per milliliter) as calculated by the following formula:

$$0.5 \text{ unit/ml} \times 40 \text{ ml/kg} \times 70 \text{ kg} = 1400 \text{ units}$$

Because of its smaller size, Factor IX is distributed in a volume 1½-fold to 2-fold greater than the plasma volume. Thus, proportionately more Factor IX than Factor VIII must be infused to achieve a similar response in a patient with hemophilia B. Because of its longer half-life in the body, however, Factor IX needs to be given less often than Factor VIII to maintain a therapeutic level.

The most important, indeed overriding, problem with purified factor concentrates is with contaminating viruses. Each batch of concentrate is made from thousands of units of plasma, some of which come from commercial plasmapheresis centers. There is a high likelihood that recipients are infected with hepatitis B, non-A, non-B hepatitis, and/or human immunodeficiency virus (HIV). This likelihood can be minimized by use of source plasma that does not contain antibodies to the viruses and has a normal level of transaminase. The infectivity of concentrates can be further decreased or eliminated by subjecting the concentrates to treatment (e.g., heating or extraction with an organic solvent) that will inactivate the viruses but preserve the activity of the factor of interest or by use of pure factor. In addition, products made by recombinant DNA techniques are coming on the market. These products, however, are significantly more expensive than former concentrates. Several treatment strategies do not require exposure to blood products at all (e.g., use of desmopressin to raise transiently the level of factor VIII and EACA to minimize mucosal bleeding).

When elective procedures that require prophylactic therapy to raise factor levels are contemplated, it is wise to test the proposed therapy prior to the procedure to be sure that target levels can be achieved.

HEMOPHILIA A (Factor VIII Deficiency)

Hemophilia A, the most frequently encountered serious inherited disorder of blood coagulation, occurs in 1 of 10,000 males. The majority of hemophilic patients give a positive family history with an X-linked inheritance pattern. In the remainder the mutation of the Factor VIII gene may be new. A hemophilic patient's daughters will all be carriers, but all his sons will be normal. A carrier woman has a 50 per cent chance of producing a hemophilic male or a female carrier. Because of random inactivation (lyonization) of the X chromosome, the carrier is a genetic mosaic with two populations of cells containing either a normal X chromosome or an abnormal X chromosome (bearing the hemophilic gene). Therefore, a carrier should have about 50 per cent of the normal level of Factor VIII activity. The range of Factor VIII levels in carriers is broad, probably because inactivation of one of the X chromosomes is often disproportionate. If extreme lyonization occurs, so that the preponderance of cells in the carrier female contains the X chromosome with the hemophilic gene, and the Factor VIII level is less than 40 per cent of normal, the woman may have clinical features of mild hemophilia.

CLINICAL MANIFESTATIONS. In general, the degree of Factor VIII deficiency correlates with the frequency of clinically significant bleeding. Furthermore, the degree of deficiency and bleeding severity tends to be similar in affected members of a given family. Hemophilia, therefore, is often classified as severe

(<1 per cent of normal activity), moderate (1 to 5 per cent of normal activity), or mild (5 to 25 per cent of normal activity).

Hematomas and Internal Hemorrhage. Bleeding from the umbilical cord is rare at birth. Soft tissue hematomas may develop in early infancy. More difficulties begin when the child becomes physically active, and these continue throughout life. Hematomas often occur in muscles and soft tissues. Considerable blood loss can occur into thigh muscles or the retroperitoneum; the extent of blood loss in these areas may be difficult to discern clinically and is frequently underestimated. The bleeding of hemophilia can involve virtually any anatomic area and give rise to secondary symptoms and signs caused by compression. If bleeding occurs in the pharynx or neck, airway obstruction can result. Severe bleeding may occur from peptic ulcerations. Partial intestinal obstruction may result from hemorrhage into the bowel wall. Mesenteric bleeding can lead to the development of bowel ischemia and necrosis. Hematuria can be painless or may manifest as ureteral colic produced by the formation of clots that obstruct the ureter. Subdural hematomas and other central nervous system hemorrhages are uncommon but represent a major cause of death and disability. Many bleeding episodes appear to develop spontaneously without a history of trauma or other provoking causes. Such spontaneous bleeding may occur during periods of stress, as before school examinations or following family dissension. When bleeding follows trauma, it may be delayed, since the primary hemostasis furnished by vessels and platelets is intact (see Ch. 154).

Hemarthroses. Bleeding occurs in joints, usually in the elbows, knees, and ankles and less often in the wrist and hand. In about half of hemophilic patients, repeated hemarthroses result in eventual deformity and crippling. These patients have Factor VIII activity levels well below 5 per cent of normal and usually less than 1 per cent of normal. The patient experiences considerable pain with bleeding into joints because of distention of the joint capsule. Movement is severely limited, causing disuse atrophy of the muscles about the joint. Pressure erodes the ends of long bones, causing periosteal pain, eventual necrosis, and pseudocyst formation. Hemarthrosis causes proliferation of the synovium. Thus a vicious circle is set into play in which a joint, once weakened, may experience hemorrhage again and again in a seemingly spontaneous manner.

Bleeding After Surgery. Major or minor surgery, including dental extractions, can result in marked blood loss in a hemophilic patient and therefore must be carried out in conjunction with Factor VIII replacement therapy to assure adequate hemostasis. Even those patients with mild hemophilia, Factor VIII levels of 5 to 25 per cent of normal, may develop clinically significant bleeding with surgery or trauma and require replacement therapy.

DIAGNOSIS. A history of joint and soft tissue bleeding, a family history compatible with X-linked inheritance, and the presence of arthropathy on physical examination all point to the diagnosis of X-linked hemophilia. Factor VIII deficiency is most likely, although Factor IX deficiency (hemophilia B) must also be considered. Laboratory screening tests should show a normal PT and prolonged APTT. The abnormal APTT should be corrected by all deficient plasmas except those from individuals with known Factor VIII deficiency. In particular, the abnormal APTT should be corrected by plasma from a patient with factor IX deficiency. If plasmas from patients with known deficiencies are not available, correction can be attempted with normal plasma absorbed with barium salts (which removes Factor IX but not Factor VIII) and serum (which contains Factor IX but not active Factor VIII). Absorbed plasma, but not serum, corrects the abnormal APTT of a patient with Factor VIII deficiency. A quantitative assay for Factor VIII can be done by testing the ability of dilutions of the patient's plasma to correct the defect in Factor VIII–deficient plasma.

Von Willebrand factor (see below) stabilizes Factor VIII in the circulation; severe deficiency of von Willebrand factor is therefore accompanied by severe deficiency of Factor VIII, and hemophilia A can be confused with von Willebrand disease. Unlike hemophilia, however, von Willebrand disease is inherited as an autosomal dominant trait, and the patient may present with a history of vascular-type bleeding. Upon screening, the bleeding time should be grossly prolonged in von Willebrand disease, whereas the bleeding time is usually at the upper limit of normal or only slightly prolonged in hemophilia. Further investigation should demonstrate deficiency or abnormality of von Willebrand factor and defective platelet aggregation mediated by the antibiotic ristocetin in von Willebrand disease but not in hemophilia. If the diagnosis remains in doubt, it may be helpful to perform laboratory tests on family members to determine the inheritance pattern of the deficiency.

TREATMENT. The patient and family must learn about the nature of hemophilia, the anticipated severity of the patient's disease, the recognition and management of various types of bleeding episodes, the difference the disorder may make in the patient's future lifestyle, and the genetics of its transmission.

General Considerations. A major goal of patient, family, and physician is to have the patient lead as normal a life as possible. This will entail some restrictions of activities for the affected child and limitations on career choices. The physician, guided by the medical history, the degree of physical impairment, the severity of bleeding in affected family members, and the plasma level of Factor VIII, should advise the patient to participate in activities commensurate with the severity of his disease. A hemophilic child should be reared in a protective environment until he understands the consequences of hemophilia and can take responsibility for his actions. The physician should be alert for denial mechanisms sometimes constructed by patient and parents about the disease. For example, the patient may develop a willingness and receive unconscious encouragement from the parents to participate in dangerous activities or to forgo needed treatments. With maturity, the patient usually accepts the constraints imposed by his disease. He should be encouraged to develop his education and interests as fully as possible and counseled to adopt a career that does not expose him to undue hazards, is compatible with his physical capabilities, and allows him access to adequate health insurance coverage.

To be free to develop as normal a life as possible, the patient must participate in a major way in his medical care. This has led to the widespread adoption of home care programs in which the patient treats himself at home with the backup of a primary physician, a nurse coordinator, and a multidisciplinary team of a hematologist, orthopedic surgeon, dentist, social worker, financial counselor, and so on. It is reasonable to expect a responsible patient in a home care program to work or go to school full time, to require a minimum of emergency room visits, and to be hospitalized only for major trauma, medical illness, or elective surgery. The major cost of such a program is replacement therapy: A patient may consume many thousands of dollars in blood products each year. Home care programs, however, are cost effective because bleeding episodes are treated when first symptomatic and do not proceed to the point at which hospitalization is required for aggressive replacement therapy and pain management. About 50 per cent of patients with hemophilia A have enough problems to make home care worthwhile.

Patients receiving long-term replacement therapy need regular evaluation at 6- to 12-month intervals. The clinic visit should include a physical examination, with special attention paid to joints, an inhibitor screen, a chemistry panel including tests of liver function, and tests for antibodies to hepatitis viruses and HIV.

Factor VIII Preparations. Bleeding episodes are managed primarily by administration of Factor VIII, either in the form of cryoprecipitate or as a commercially prepared lyophilized concentrate. The use of cryoprecipitate or Factor VIII concentrate avoids the complication of volume overload that would occur with the large amount of plasma that would be necessary to attain acceptable levels of Factor VIII activity.

Blood banks prepare cryoprecipitate by freezing individual bags of fresh normal plasma, each containing approximately 200 units of Factor VIII activity in 200 ml of plasma, at $-20°C$ and then thawing at $4°C$. Approximately 50 per cent of the Factor VIII contained in the plasma remains as a precipitate, which is separated from the bulk of the plasma and stored frozen in individual bags containing approximately 100 units of Factor VIII activity in 20 to 40 ml of residual plasma. When needed, the appropriate number of bags is thawed at $37°C$, and the contents are pooled and administered intravenously to the patient.

Lyophilized Factor VIII concentrate is available in vials containing different amounts of Factor VIII activity (exact amounts stated on the labels). The concentrates are readily soluble upon addition of diluent and thus can be prepared and administered intravenously within 30 minutes.

The major advantage of cryoprecipitate in the past is that it exposed the recipient to fewer donors and thus minimized the chance of blood-transmitted viral infection. Indeed, individuals have been supported from infancy to young adulthood with cryoprecipitate prepared from plasma donated sequentially by the same donor. The major disadvantages of cryoprecipitate are the inconvenience of thawing and pooling bags prior to administration and the need for the bags to stay frozen at $-20°C$ until the time of administration.

The major advantages of lyophilized concentrates are stability on storage and convenience of administration. The current generation of concentrates have been processed to eliminate or inactivate HIV totally and possibly also hepatitis B and C.

Patients should be vaccinated against hepatitis B at the time of diagnosis and will be prime candidates for vaccines that may be developed in the future for non-A, non-B hepatitis viruses and HIV.

Replacement Therapy. Intensity of replacement therapy depends on the estimated plasma level of Factor VIII required to halt the bleeding and the disappearance rate of the infused Factor VIII. Very early hemarthrosis can be managed with a single infusion to attain a peak Factor VIII level of 25 to 50 per cent of normal. For more extensive hemorrhage or hematuria, Factor VIII infusions are usually continued for 2 days after cessation of symptoms or signs of bleeding. Muscle hematomas require a longer period of sustained Factor VIII levels, in the range of 40 to 60 per cent of normal for 4 to 6 days. Major trauma or surgery requires that the Factor VIII level be maintained at more than 70 per cent of normal until hemostasis is achieved and then in the range of 25 to 50 per cent of normal for 10 to 14 days. Plasma Factor VIII can be measured after administration of the calculated dose to document that the desired level has been achieved and prior to subsequent scheduled doses to determine whether desired levels have been sustained. If a low Factor VIII level persists despite replacement therapy, it may be that simply not enough Factor VIII is being given or that the patient has developed an inhibitor that neutralizes infused Factor VIII.

The amount of concentrate needed to achieve and maintain a desired level of Factor VIII activity can be estimated by knowing (1) that the patient's plasma volume is about 40 ml per kilogram of body weight, (2) the amount of Factor VIII activity in the average bag of cryoprecipitate (usually about 100 units) or in available vials of lyophilized concentrate Factor VIII activity, and (3) that Factor VIII has a half-life of about 10 to 12 hours in the circulation. Therefore, replacement therapy is ordinarily given three times a day when tight control of the level is needed and twice a day when deeper troughs in the level can be tolerated. Alternatively, a constant infusion of 1 to 2 units per kilogram per hour can be given after a loading dose.

Treatment of Hemarthroses. Joint bleeding is helped initially by immobilization of the affected limb and application of ice packs to diminish swelling and discomfort. Hemarthroses should not be aspirated unless such acute pain and tension are present that pressure necrosis is a major possibility. Aspiration should be performed only after administration of replacement Factor VIII. When pain and swelling have subsided, the patient should begin rehabilitation to regain motion and strength in conjunction with prophylactic replacement therapy. Patients with joint disease may benefit from periodic assessment by an orthopedic surgeon. In properly selected patients, synovectomy and artificial joint replacement have been very successful in improving the usefulness of severe chronic joint deformity.

Dental Care. The patient should be instructed about the importance of dental hygiene and should have frequent dental examinations. Bleeding in deep tissues of the oropharynx can be life threatening. Therefore, a local anesthetic should be administered by needle puncture only after prophylactic administration of Factor VIII concentrate. Extraction also requires prior administration of Factor VIII concentrate. For patients with mild or moderate hemophilia, it is likely that adequate levels of Factor VIII can be achieved with use of desmopressin, as described

below for patients with von Willebrand disease. Administration of EACA by mouth, also described below, is useful in prevention of rebleeding after tooth extraction.

Use of Analgesics. Bleeding can cause extraordinary pain. Injudicious use of narcotics can lead to addiction in hemophilic patients. Aspirin must be avoided by the hemophilic because it decreases platelet aggregation and accentuates bleeding. Acetaminophen and codeine are recommended as the first choices of analgesics. In selected cases, ibuprofen can be given for chronic joint pain. The likelihood that ibuprofen will cause increased bleeding can be assessed by a template bleeding time after the patient has received the drug for several days. If the bleeding time is prolonged compared with the bleeding time before therapy, the drug should be discontinued.

Factor VIII Inhibitors. The possibility that the patient has acquired neutralizing antibodies to Factor VIII (Factor VIII inhibitor) should be of constant concern. An inhibitor may initially appear at almost any time in the life of a hemophilic patient and need not be associated with any obvious change in the clinical severity of the disorder. Patients with inhibitors present special problems. Much depends on the titer of the inhibitor, which is commonly expressed in Bethesda units: 1 Bethesda unit, by definition, inhibits 1 unit of Factor VIII, i.e., the Factor VIII in 1 ml of normal plasma. If one calculates the amount of Factor VIII required to neutralize the inhibitor and achieve a 50 per cent normal level of circulating Factor VIII in a patient who weighs 70 kg and has a plasma volume of 2800 ml and an inhibitor titer of 10 Bethesda units per milliliter, the amount is immense:

$$2800 \text{ ml} \times 10.5 \text{ units/ml} = 29,400 \text{ units}$$

Several strategies are available, all expensive and none totally adequate. Because some inhibitors take up to several hours to complex with and inhibit Factor VIII, it may be possible to maintain Factor VIII levels at a therapeutic level by constant infusion. If the inhibitor is of modest titer (1 to 10 Bethesda units per milliliter), it may be possible to remove enough inhibitor by plasmapheresis to make therapy feasible with lower amounts of Factor VIII. A patient receiving Factor VIII concentrate may have an anamnestic immune response with an increase in the titer and avidity of his inhibitor. Therefore, everything possible should be done to achieve permanent hemostasis in the 4- to 6-day "golden period" during which replacement therapy is possible. Patients with high titers of rapidly acting inhibitor can be given porcine Factor VIII concentrate or activated Factor IX concentrate that also contains activated Factor X and therefore "bypasses" Factor VIII in the coagulation cascade. Both concentrates are expensive, and the activated Factor IX concentrate has considerable thrombogenic potential.

ACQUIRED IMMUNODEFICIENCY SYNDROME (AIDS). Regardless of whether they have antibodies to HIV, patients who have used significant quantities of blood products in the 1980's must take proper precautions to protect their close contacts and loved ones. They can be assured that the virus is not transmitted by casual household contact. They must be taught safe disposal procedures for needles and other injection paraphernalia. It should be strongly recommended that condoms be used during all sexual intercourse. This raises an irreconcilable conflict for couples considering pregnancy. There is a high likelihood of transmission of HIV to the newborn of a virus-positive mother. Thus, wives of men with hemophilia who are considering pregnancy should receive specific education and counseling and be tested for antibodies to HIV before pregnancy occurs.

PROGNOSIS. The major long-term complications of moderate and severe hemophilia are (1) progressive joint deformity and crippling, (2) development of inhibitors to Factor VIII activity, (3) hepatitis and cirrhosis, and (4) AIDS.

Despite the availability of replacement therapy, many hemophiliacs, for a variety of reasons, are treated inadequately or haphazardly and become severely crippled and, ultimately, chronic invalids. The last three of the four complications listed above are seen more often in patients who receive frequent replacement therapy. Up to 15 per cent of hemophilic patients develop inhibitory antibodies to Factor VIII activity, usually in childhood. Most patients who have received Factor VIII concentrate in the past have been exposed to hepatitis viruses and HIV. The risks of chronic hepatitis and AIDS in exposed individuals are both high. Newer concentrates are much safer. On the whole, the availability of concentrates has been beneficial and has improved the prognosis of all forms of hemophilia A—mild, moderate, and severe. It is reasonable to hope that future cohorts of hemophiliacs will enjoy the benefits of replacement therapy without the complications.

CARRIER DETECTION. Women who have relatives with hemophilia frequently seek help to determine whether they may pass the disorder to their children. Daughters of men with the disorder, mothers of more than one hemophilic son, and mothers who have a hemophilic son and another hemophilic male relative in their pedigree are obligate carriers of the hemophilic gene. Only about 15 per cent of the instances of hemophilia arise because of spontaneous mutation. Determination of Factor VIII procoagulant activity is of limited usefulness in the identification of carrier women, because low-normal levels overlap with Factor VIII levels found in obligate heterozygotes. A major reason for scatter in Factor VIII levels is scatter in the levels of von Willebrand factor, which functions as a carrier protein for Factor VIII. Therefore, the overlap between normal persons and obligate carriers is decreased considerably if the Factor VIII level is corrected for the level of immunoreactive von Willebrand factor (sometimes called Factor VIII–related antigen). When the ratios of these two proteins are analyzed by logarithmic discriminant analysis, greater than 95 per cent of carriers can be identified. Such an analysis is best done by a laboratory that is highly experienced with the assays and has proved the validity of the analysis in an adequate number of obligate carriers.

Several restriction fragment length polymorphisms close to the gene for Factor VIII have been shown to be useful in tracing hemophilia A in families. In families in which the polymorphisms segregate with hemophilia, the polymorphisms can identify carriers with greater than 99 per cent confidence. The polymorphisms can also be used to diagnose hemophilia in fetuses in the first trimester, whereas assays of Factor VIII per se can be done only in the second trimester when the fetal circulation is accessible for blood sampling by fetoscopy.

Brettler DB, Forsberg AD, Levine PH, et al.: The use of porcine factor VIII concentrate (Hyate:C) in the treatment of patients with inhibitor antibodies to factor VIII. Arch Intern Med 149:1381, 1989. *Describes a favorable response when compared with other modalities.*

Levine PH: The clinical manifestations and therapy of hemophilias A and B. In Colman RW, Hirsh J, Marder VJ, et al. (eds.): Hemostasis and Thrombosis: Basic Principles and Clinical Practice. 2nd ed. Philadelphia, J. B. Lippincott Company, 1987, pp 97–111.

White GC II, Shoemaker CB: Factor VIII gene and hemophilia A. Blood 73:1, 1989. *Update on genetic defects and potential applications of new knolwedge.*

VON WILLEBRAND DISEASE

This disorder is due to a deficiency or abnormality of a plasma protein, von Willebrand factor, that is required for the stabilization of Factor VIII in the circulation and for the normal adherence of platelets to sites of vascular injury. The gene for von Willebrand factor is on chromosome 12. The hallmarks of von Willebrand disease historically have been a low Factor VIII level, a long bleeding time, and autosomal inheritance. The last two characteristics distinguish von Willebrand disease from hemophilia A. With extensive characterization of von Willebrand factor over the past decade has come a broadening of the definition of von Willebrand disease, so that the name now encompasses a heterogeneous group of defects of von Willebrand factor.

FUNCTION OF VON WILLEBRAND FACTOR. Factor VIII and von Willebrand factor circulate in normal plasma as a complex. Endothelial cells and megakaryocytes-platelets synthesize, store, and secrete von Willebrand factor. Secretion increases when endothelial cells are stimulated or injured. Therefore the concentration of plasma von Willebrand factor is labile and can be increased by stimuli as innocuous as a vigorous Valsalva maneuver, and it is common to find levels of von Willebrand factor elevated 2-fold to 10-fold in ill patients. Von Willebrand factor exists as a series of multimers ranging in size from 850,000 to 12,000,000 daltons. The largest multimers, which have a half-life in the circulation of only several hours, are most active in mediation of platelet adhesion. Both large and small multimers complex with Factor VIII. Von Willebrand factor can interact with platelets in two different ways. It binds to platelet glycoprotein Ib in a reaction that is greatly enhanced by ristocetin (an

antibiotic that cannot be used because it causes thrombocytopenia). It also binds to platelet glycoprotein IIb-IIIa complex, but only when platelets are activated. Von Willebrand factor binds to collagen and other components of the vessel wall and thus mediates attachment and spreading of platelets to the subendothelium of damaged vessels. The role of von Willebrand factor in platelet adhesion is especially important when blood passes through the blood vessel at a high shear rate and the red blood cell count is normal or increased.

PATHOGENESIS OF VON WILLEBRAND DISEASE. In classic (type I) von Willebrand disease, patients have prolonged bleeding time, abnormal platelet aggregation in response to ristocetin, and parallel decreases in plasma Factor VIII activity, immunoreactive von Willebrand factor, and ristocetin cofactor activity. Patients with severe, usually homozygous, disease can have less than 1 per cent of normal von Willebrand factor in plasma and platelets and no detectable von Willebrand antigen in endothelial cells. Their Factor VIII levels may be less than 5 per cent of normal. Intravenous infusion of small amounts of normal plasma, hemophilic plasma, or normal serum into patients with severe von Willebrand disease results in a prolonged increase in Factor VIII that is out of proportion to the Factor VIII content of the transfused plasma or serum. This probably results from stabilization of the patients' endogenously produced factor VIII by infused von Willebrand factor.

A number of qualitative abnormalities of von Willebrand factor result in variant diseases called type IIA, type IIB, and so on. In type IIA disease the large and intermediate-sized multimers are not present in plasma or platelets. Von Willebrand factor function (e.g., ristocetin cofactor activity) is decreased more than von Willebrand factor antigen. These patients have abnormal platelet adhesion and long bleeding times, but normal Factor VIII activity. Abnormal multimer patterns can be ascertained by probing separated plasma proteins with antibodies to von Willebrand factors after agarose gel electrophoresis. Subtypes IIC, IID, etc., of von Willebrand disease have been identified, based on additional subtle abnormalities in the electrophoretic pattern of the multimers. In type IIB disease the largest multimers are missing from plasma but not from platelets, and the abnormal von Willebrand factor causes platelet aggregation at lower than usual ristocetin concentration. It is thought that the largest multimers are missing from plasma because the multimers bind spontaneously to platelets. In principle, such a spontaneous interaction could be due to defects in the patient's von Willebrand factor or in the patient's platelets ("pseudo von Willebrand disease"), and indeed patients have been identified in whom the defect is in the platelets (Ch. 154).

CLINICAL MANIFESTATIONS. Von Willebrand disease has a broad spectrum of clinical and laboratory features. It can range from a severe hemorrhagic disorder, in which the level of Factor VIII is low enough and the bleeding problems severe enough that the disease must be differentiated from classic hemophilia, to an asymptomatic condition that is a laboratory curiosity. The severity of symptoms due to von Willebrand disease can vary considerably even among afflicted family members, probably because there are a number of factors that control the synthesis and secretion of von Willebrand factor.

Patients with severe disease usually have inherited it from both parents, either as a true homozygous or as a double heterozygous disease. The principal bleeding problems are of the superficial type. Epistaxis is a frequent complaint, especially early in life, as is easy bruising. Hematuria and gastrointestinal bleeding occur less frequently, and hemarthroses are quite rare. Without adequate replacement therapy, postoperative bleeding is a major hazard. In patients with heterozygous type I or II disease, the hemorrhagic tendency usually becomes evident or troublesome only with trauma, surgery, or dental extractions. Women with the disorder commonly experience excessive menses and postpartum bleeding. In all forms of the disease, the frequency and severity of bleeding tend to lessen with age.

DIAGNOSIS. The classic findings in type I von Willebrand disease are prolonged bleeding time and a low level of Factor VIII. Confirmatory testing should reveal a low level of immunoreactive von Willebrand factor and absent or diminished platelet aggregation when ristocetin is added to the patient's platelet-rich plasma. The analysis using ristocetin can be made more sensitive and quantitative by testing the ability of dilutions of the patient's plasma to support agglutination of washed platelets; this is often called the ristocetin cofactor titer.

Electrophoretic analysis of the site distribution of von Willebrand factor multimers should be done in patients who are suspected of having type II von Willebrand disease on the basis of bleeding problems, prolonged bleeding time, and abnormal ristocetin-induced platelet aggregation but normal or only slightly decreased levels of von Willebrand factor and Factor VIII. In type IIA disease, the larger multimers are missing in both plasma and platelets. In type IIB disease (hypersensitivity to ristocetin), the larger multimers are missing in plasma but not in platelets.

It may be very difficult to know for sure whether someone with mild decreases in von Willebrand factor and Factor VIII, say, to 50 per cent of normal, has von Willebrand disease. A number of factors influence the plasma concentration of von Willebrand factor. People with type O blood have lower levels than do people with types A and B. Hypothyroidism causes the level of von Willebrand factor to fall. As mentioned above, endothelial cells can be stimulated to release von Willebrand factor. Thus, one must worry about both overdiagnosis and underdiagnosis. Serial studies of the same patient and studies of other family members can be helpful. Because symptoms in such patients are mild and tend to decrease with age, however, it may suffice to be honest with such patients about the ambiguities of the laboratory tests and counsel them to alert their physician about the possibility of von Willebrand disease in the event of trauma or major surgery.

TREATMENT. Indications for therapy in von Willebrand disease include surgery, severe epistaxis, severe menorrhagia, and recurrent gastrointestinal bleeding.

Replacement Therapy. Cryoprecipitate is equally rich in Factor VIII and von Willebrand factor and therefore corrects both the deficiency of Factor VIII and the long bleeding time of type I von Willebrand disease. Factor VIII concentrates are poor in von Willebrand factor and do not correct the bleeding time defect. Hence, replacement therapy in von Willebrand disease should be with cryoprecipitate rather than Factor VIII concentrate. Because the largest multimers of von Willebrand factor are cleared rapidly after infusion, the bleeding time is usually corrected only transiently. The smaller multimers allow the patient's own Factor VIII to circulate, and the Factor VIII level may remain elevated for considerably longer than would be predicted, based on the amount of infused Factor VIII. In the case of ongoing hemorrhage or major surgery, cryoprecipitate should be given, using the guidelines described above for Factor VIII replacement in hemophilia A. The infusion should be given immediately prior to maneuvers designed to achieve hemostasis. This practice will ensure that the bleeding time as well as the Factor VIII level is maximally corrected. It is not practical to give cryoprecipitate often enough to keep the bleeding time continuously corrected or to quantify the correction with serial bleeding times. Therefore, once hemostasis is achieved, therapy should be directed toward keeping the level of Factor VIII in the appropriate therapeutic ranges as described above for hemophilia A. This probably requires less cryoprecipitate than if one were treating a hemophiliac.

Desmopressin. Because there is not an effective virus-free purified concentrate of von Willebrand factor, considerable attention has been devoted to the therapeutic potential of desmopressin (1-deamino-8-D-arginine vasopressin, DDAVP), especially in patients with mild von Willebrand disease. Desmopressin causes release of von Willebrand factor and plasminogen activator from endothelial cells. EACA suppresses baseline and desmopressin-stimulated fibrinolysis and may be useful as an adjunctive therapy. Desmopressin, 0.3 μg per kilogram of body weight in 50 ml of saline, is given over 15 minutes. In type I disease, several-fold increases of both Factor VIII and von Willebrand protein occur 15 to 30 minutes after infusion, with a concomitant decrease in the bleeding time. The effect may last for several hours. The magnitude and duration of the response vary among individual patients, especially among those with type IIA disease. Desmopressin is contraindicated in type IIB disease because appearance of the large multimers in the circulation can cause thrombocytopenia.

To learn if the treatment is feasible in a given patient, one should quantify the response to a test dose of desmopressin at the time of diagnosis or 5 to 7 days prior to a planned procedure. For oral surgical procedures, EACA is given orally in a dosage of 75 mg per kilogram every 6 hours for 7 to 10 days beginning the evening before the procedure. It is controversial whether an antifibrinolytic agent should be given with major surgery.

Menstruation and Pregnancy. Excessive menstrual blood loss can be managed with hormonal suppression. Levels of Factor VIII, von Willebrand factor, and ristocetin cofactor activity may become normal during pregnancy. Therefore, these tests, along with determination of the bleeding time, should be repeated during the third trimester to plan for replacement therapy during delivery. Cryoprecipitate should be given if the Factor VIII level remains low. If the Factor VIII level is greater than 50 per cent, but the bleeding time remains long, cryoprecipitate should be on call, because postpartum blood loss is frequently severe enough to require replacement infusion.

Complications of Therapy. Chronic arthropathy is less common in von Willebrand disease than in hemophilia A. The complications of replacement therapy for severe von Willebrand disease are the same as those described above for hemophilia A. Rarely, antibodies that inhibit the activity of von Willebrand protein develop. Patients receiving blood products should be vaccinated against hepatitis B and monitored for the acquisition of hepatitis viruses and HIV.

Mannucci PM: Desmopressin. A nontransfusional form of treatment for congenital and acquired blood disorders. Blood 72:1449, 1988. *Review of therapeutic applications.*

Ruggeri ZM, Zimmerman TS: Von Willebrand factor and von Willebrand disease. Blood 70:895, 1987. *A review of the disease and its pathogenesis.*

HEMOPHILIA B (Factor IX Deficiency)

Factor IX deficiency is inherited as an X-linked disorder that presents with the historical and clinical features of classic hemophilia (hemophilia A). The severity of bleeding is usually similar in members of a single family. Factor IX–deficient patients have fewer symptoms than do patients with Factor VIII deficiency; patients with severe (<1 per cent of normal) Factor IX deficiency have the symptoms of patients with mild (1 to 5 per cent of normal) Factor VIII deficiency. Nevertheless, Factor IX deficiency causes serious bleeding problems. Patients with Factor IX deficiency can be more cavalier about their disease than can patients with Factor VIII deficiency, and therefore they are not as quick to seek medical attention when they need it—sometimes to their detriment.

CLINICAL MANIFESTATIONS. Many patients are asymptomatic until the hemostatic system is stressed by surgery or trauma. Patients with the most severe disease may develop muscle hematomas, gastrointestinal hemorrhage, and bleeding into large joints with progression to crippling joint deformities.

DIAGNOSIS. This disorder is suspected with the finding of a normal PT and prolonged APTT that can be corrected by normal serum but not by barium sulfate–adsorbed plasma. The inability of the patient's plasma to correct the prolonged APTT of plasma from a patient with known Factor IX deficiency establishes the diagnosis.

TREATMENT. The care and long-term goals of therapy for the patient with Factor IX deficiency are similar to those described above for the patient with hemophilia A. Most patients need less care than if they had hemophilia A, but they require the same intensity of education and counseling.

Replacement Therapy. Fresh frozen plasma is used to treat mild to moderate bleeding, especially in those patients who have hemorrhagic episodes infrequently. Ordinarily, transfusion of 500 ml of plasma twice daily is sufficient to maintain a level of Factor IX activity 10 to 12 per cent above baseline. EACA can be used as an adjunct to transfusions of plasma in patients with mucosal bleeding or dental work.

Patients with moderate to severe hemorrhage, such as large hemarthroses or muscle hematomas, and patients being prepared for surgery can be treated with commercially prepared Factor IX concentrate, aiming for levels that are approximately two thirds as high as those described above for Factor VIII replacement therapy. Because the volume of distribution and the half-life of Factor IX are both greater than for Factor VIII, a greater loading dose of Factor IX must be given than for Factor VIII, but subsequent doses can be given less frequently. The length of therapy is dependent on the severity of the hemorrhage and the patient's response. Therapy is generally continued for 2 days after bleeding and related symptoms have subsided.

Complications of Therapy. Currently available Factor IX concentrates are a mixture of all of the vitamin K–dependent factors—Factors II, VII, IX, and X and proteins C and S—and are heat treated. Factor IX stands up to heat treatment better than does Factor VIII, and therefore the concentrates are heated more vigorously and should be freer of infectious HIV than are Factor VIII concentrates. However, the concentrates are not free of infectious hepatitis viruses. Patients therefore should be immunized against hepatitis B.

Factor IX concentrates contain trace amounts of activated vitamin K–dependent factors and therefore are thrombogenic and carry a risk for thromboembolism, especially when used in high dosage in patients who have liver disease or are immobilized after surgery. EACA greatly enhances the risk of thromboembolism and should never be used as an adjunct to Factor IX concentrates. Indeed, some advocate that low-dosage heparin (5000 units every 12 hours) and plasma (as a source of antithrombins) be given to surgical patients receiving Factor IX concentrate. Because of these potential complications, it is advisable to reserve the use of Factor IX concentrates for patients who have acquired antibody to hepatitis B surface antigen as a result of prior exposure or immunization and for whom the benefits of treatment outweigh the risks of thromboembolism. In a situation in which levels greater than 10 to 15 per cent above baseline are desired but use of Factor IX concentrate is contraindicated, plasmapheresis can be used to prevent volume overload.

Antibody inhibitors to Factor IX occur in 5 to 10 per cent of treated patients.

CARRIER DETECTION. The normal range for Factor IX is narrower than the normal range for Factor VIII, and therefore carrier testing based on coagulation assays is better for hemophilia B than for hemophilia A. Nevertheless, laboratory definition of the carrier state is still an exercise in probabilities and is best done with genetic markers. The Factor IX gene exhibits considerable polymorphism, and informative genetic markers are found in most families. However, it is worthwhile doing Factor IX activity assays in known and potential carriers, because women who are carriers may have Factor IX levels that are sufficiently low to cause mild bleeding, especially after trauma or surgery.

Giannelli F, Green PM, High KA, et al.: Haemophilia B: Database of point mutations and short additions and deletions. Nucleic Acids Res 18:4053, 1990. *The only other specific group of inherited diseases with as many characterized mutations are the hemoglobinopathies.*

Thompson AR: Structure, function, and molecular defects of factor IX. Blood 67:565, 1986. *Comprehensive summary of information about Factor IX and hemophilia B.*

DEFICIENCIES OF CONTACT FACTORS

Deficiencies of Factor XII, prekallikrein, or HMWK are clinically benign, and deficiency of Factor XI may sometimes be benign. Patients with these abnormalities, however, have APTT's that are as prolonged as are those of patients with Factor VIII or IX deficiency. Therefore it is important to establish the correct diagnosis and to counsel the patient that he or she has a laboratory abnormality that carries little risk for bleeding.

Deficiency of Factor XII, Prekallikrein, or High Molecular Weight Kininogen

These autosomal recessive disorders are almost always asymptomatic and are usually identified as an abnormality in a routine APTT. The APTT of a mixture of patient's plasma and normal plasma should be normal, i.e., with no inhibitor demonstrable. The plasma concentrations of Factors VIII and IX should be normal. The coagulation defect can be identified by the inability of the patient's plasma to correct the APTT of the appropriately deficient plasma.

Deficiency of Factor XI

Factor XI deficiency is common among Ashkenazi Jews, and the prevalence of homozygous Factor XI deficiency in cities with a sizable Jewish population is comparable to the prevalence of hemophilia A. The defect is usually asymptomatic, but it is occasionally associated with bleeding. Major bleeding into mus-

cles or joints is rare. The inheritance pattern is autosomal recessive, so that the deficiency is found with equal frequency in men and women. The APTT is prolonged. The PT and bleeding time are normal. Normal serum or barium sulfate–adsorbed plasma both correct the APTT. Specific assays for Factors VIII and IX are normal. The diagnosis is established by demonstrating that the patient's plasma does not correct the APTT of Factor XI–deficient plasma.

Clinically significant bleeding usually occurs in association with trauma, surgery, or dental extractions. Fresh frozen plasma, 10 to 20 ml per kilogram, should be given as treatment of bleeding or as prophylaxis for surgery. One infusion should suffice, because Factor XI has a half-life of about 72 hours.

Silverberg M, Kaplan AP, Colman RW: Contact activation and its abnormalities. *In* Colman RW, Hirsh J, Marder VJ, et al. (eds.): Hemostasis and Thrombosis: Basic Principles and Clinical Practice. 2nd ed. Philadelphia, J. B. Lippincott Company, 1987, pp 18–38. *Well-referenced description of the biochemistry of Factor XI and the deficiency state.*

DEFICIENCIES OF THE EXTRINSIC AND COMMON PATHWAYS

Deficiencies of Factors VII, X, V, and II are all associated with clinically significant bleeding. The hemorrhagic diathesis is not as predictable or severe as in hemophilia A, but replacement therapy will probably be required at some point in a patient's lifetime, especially to control bleeding from mucous membranes, after dental extractions, or during menses.

Deficiency of Factor VII

CLINICAL MANIFESTATIONS. This is a rare autosomal recessive defect. Patients have a history of bleeding, usually beginning in infancy or early childhood. Bleeding, however, is frequently mild, even in patients with severe deficiency. Heterozygous relatives have no bleeding tendency. Mucous membrane bleeding, epistaxis, intramuscular hemorrhage, hemarthroses, and menorrhagia are the most common problems; gastrointestinal bleeding is less common, hematuria occurs only occasionally, and central nervous system bleeding is rare. Bleeding after dental extractions is predictable, and such extractions should be done with prophylactic replacement therapy. Clinical manifestations of bleeding can vary from mild to severe in the same patient. In fact, patients with impressive bleeding histories have undergone major surgery without accompanying hemorrhage. This phenomenon is unexplained and not consistent with the central role assigned to Factor VII in the physiologic initiation of blood coagulation. Also incongruent are observations of thromboembolism in Factor VII–deficient patients.

DIAGNOSIS. A diagnosis of Factor VII deficiency should be considered if the PT is prolonged whereas the APTT is normal. The coagulation time of the patient's plasma in response to Russell's viper venom, which directly activates Factor X, is normal. The diagnosis is established by the inability to correct the patient's PT with Factor VII–deficient plasma.

TREATMENT. Bleeding is treated with plasma, not necessarily fresh frozen, because Factor VII is very stable. The half-life of Factor VII is 2 to 6 hours, and therefore frequent treatment is needed during a bleeding episode. Levels of 15 to 20 per cent of normal can be obtained with a loading dose of plasma of 10 to 20 ml per kilogram followed by 3 to 6 ml per kilogram every 12 hours and should suffice to stop bleeding or as prophylaxis for surgery. Commercially available Factor IX concentrates, which contain Factors VII, IX, X, and II, can be used if it is essential to avoid any possibility of intravascular volume overload; such concentrates carry the risk of thromboembolism and hepatitis. Menorrhagia may require treatment with oral contraceptive agents.

Deficiency of Factor X

This deficiency is also a rare autosomal recessive disorder. Clinical symptoms include epistaxis; occasional mucous membrane, joint, and muscle hemorrhages; and gastrointestinal bleeding. Women may have severe, life-threatening menses and postpartum hemorrhage. The diagnosis is suspected when both the PT and APTT are prolonged. The abnormal tests are corrected with normal serum, but not with barium sulfate–adsorbed plasma. The clotting time of plasma in response to Russell's viper venom is usually prolonged, although an abnormal Factor X has been described that is activated normally by Russell's viper venom but not by the intrinsic or extrinsic systems of blood coagulation. The diagnosis is established by demonstration that the abnormal plasma does not correct Factor X–deficient plasma. Bleeding episodes are treated with plasma as described above for Factor VII deficiency; plasma needs to be given less often because the plasma half-life of Factor X is 24 to 48 hours.

Deficiency of Factor II (Prothrombin Deficiency)

Like deficiency of Factors VII and X, Factor II deficiency (hypoprothrombinemia) is a rare recessive disorder. Bleeding ranges from mild to severe and generally occurs only if the Factor II activity level is less than 20 per cent of normal. Symptoms include umbilical bleeding at birth, epistaxis, menorrhagia, postpartum hemorrhage, and bleeding after trauma or minor surgical procedures. The diagnosis is suspected if the PT and APTT are prolonged and the thrombin time is normal. Neither serum nor barium sulfate–adsorbed plasma corrects the abnormalities. A specific assay can be done based on the relative ability of the unknown to correct the PT of known factor II–deficient plasma. Alternatively, a test can be done in which clotting of plasma is initiated with Taipan viper venom, a specific activator of Factor II. Bleeding is treated with infusions of fresh frozen plasma, as described above for Factor VII deficiency. Infusions are necessary only every 2 days, since the half-life of Factor II is about 72 hours.

Global Deficiency of Vitamin K–Dependent Factors

These patients present as infants with bleeding, grossly prolonged PT and APTT, and low levels (<5 per cent of normal) of Factors II, VII, IX, and X, even though there is no evidence of liver disease, malabsorption, or ingestion of coumarin drugs. The levels of the vitamin K–dependent factors increase to 30 to 40 per cent of normal when the patients are given pharmacologic dosages (10 mg per day) of vitamin K, and the patients do well, with minimal symptoms. This syndrome is probably due to some abnormality of vitamin K metabolism, such as an abnormality of vitamin K epoxide reductase.

Deficiency of Factor V

CLINICAL MANIFESTATIONS. This disorder usually is inherited as an autosomal recessive trait. As with deficiencies of the other common pathway components, the severity of bleeding symptoms is variable, and hemorrhage most often involves the mucous membranes of the nose and oral cavity. Hemarthroses are unusual. Menorrhagia may be so severe as to be life threatening. Some women with Factor V deficiency, however, have normal menses or only mild menorrhagia. Obstetric deliveries may occur with little or no bleeding, but postpartum hemorrhage is frequent and requires replacement therapy.

DIAGNOSIS. Both the APTT and the PT are prolonged. The PT can be corrected by barium sulfate–adsorbed fresh plasma, but not by serum. Definitive diagnosis is established if the patient's plasma does not correct the deficiency of a patient known to lack Factor V activity. For unknown reasons, the bleeding time is prolonged in about one third of Factor V–deficient patients.

THERAPY. Factor V is an extremely labile protein. Treatment, therefore, should be with plasma that either is fresh or was frozen while fresh and has not been stored for more than several months. The therapeutic goal should be a Factor V activity level greater than 25 per cent of normal. Because Factor V is larger than the vitamin K–dependent factors, it should be possible to achieve such a level with the doses of plasma described above for Factor VII deficiency. The plasma half-life of Factor V activity is 12 to 36 hours. Cryoprecipitate and Factor VIII concentrate are not enriched in Factor V. Surgery should be done under the "cover" of prophylactic replacement therapy.

Platelets contain 10 to 20 per cent of the Factor V in blood, and therefore platelet concentrates are a good source of Factor

V. Several patients have responded well to platelet transfusion after developing neutralizing antibodies to Factor V.

Combined Deficiencies of Factors V and VIII

A number of patients have mild deficiencies of both Factors V and VIII inherited as an autosomal recessive trait. The basis of the syndrome is unknown, but it probably is related to some posttranslational modification of the two homologous proteins, which is necessary for their function. Therapy should be directed toward replacement of both proteins.

Roberts HR, Foster PA: Inherited disorders of prothrombin conversion. *In* Colman RW, Hirsh J, Marder VJ, et al. (eds.): Hemostasis and Thrombosis: Basic Principles and Clinical Practice. 2nd ed. Philadelphia, J. B. Lippincott Company, 1987, pp 162–181. *Thoroughly referenced, and an excellent source of more detailed information about the diagnosis and management of patients with rare but clinically important factor deficiencies.*

ABNORMALITIES IN CONVERSION OF FIBRINOGEN TO FIBRIN

Disorders of Fibrinogen

These disorders fall into two categories: absence (afibrinogenemia) or a low content (hypofibrinogenemia) of plasma fibrinogen and abnormally functioning plasma fibrinogen (dysfibrinogenemia). Afibrinogenemia and hypofibrinogenemia are autosomally recessive traits. Dysfibrinogenemia can be autosomally dominant or recessive.

AFIBRINOGENEMIA. In patients with absence of or low content of fibrinogen, the bleeding tendency may be noted at birth as continued oozing from the umbilical stump. The intensity and frequency of bleeding after trauma or surgery vary from mild to severe. Death from intracranial hemorrhage may occur in infancy or early childhood. It is not understood why some patients have a minimal bleeding tendency whereas others are very symptomatic. All assays that require formation of fibrin as an endpoint are abnormal. Plasma fibrinogen cannot be detected by immunologic or chemical (salting out) methods. The bleeding time may be markedly prolonged. Bleeding episodes should be treated with cryoprecipitate, which contains 8-fold to 10-fold more fibrinogen than does an equivalent amount of plasma. Plasma fibrinogen concentrations greater than 100 mg per deciliter are generally adequate and can be achieved by administration of one bag of cryoprecipitate for each 10 kg of body weight.

DYSFIBRINOGENEMIA. Dysfibrinogenemias are usually named after the cities in which they were discovered. The clinical features are very variable. Most individuals are asymptomatic. Some have mild to moderate bleeding tendencies, usually manifest only after surgery or trauma. Wound dehiscence is a problem in some. Some have a tendency for thrombosis. The abnormal proteins have a fascinating array of defects. For instance, several of the abnormal fibrinogens are poor substrates for thrombin, so that the fibrinopeptides are released slowly. Other abnormal fibrinogens, once converted to fibrin monomer by thrombin, display impaired aggregation into a fibrin gel. The diagnosis of these disorders should be suspected when delayed or poorly formed fibrin endpoints are observed in the PT, APTT, and thrombin time assays. The fibrinogen level, measured immunologically or chemically, is normal to low-normal. The majority of patients do not require treatment. In instances of bleeding or before surgical procedures on a patient known to have a propensity to bleed, replacement therapy in the form of cryoprecipitate should be given to attain a functioning plasma fibrinogen level of 100 to 150 mg per deciliter. Because the half-life of fibrinogen is 4 days, such infusions need to be given only once every several days. There are no absolute guidelines for how long therapy must be continued, but infusions of cryoprecipitate should be administered for 2 days after bleeding stops.

Deficiency of Factor XIII

Bleeding symptoms in Factor XIII deficiency occur in individuals with less than 1 to 2 per cent of normal plasma Factor XIII activity. The symptomatic deficiency state is an autosomal recessive trait. The bleeding diathesis is commonly apparent at birth as umbilical stump hemorrhage and continues throughout life. Wounds ooze slowly for days and heal poorly with scar formation. Intracranial hemorrhage after inapparent or only minor trauma is common. Males tend to be sterile, and women with the disorder have a high incidence of fetal loss unless they receive replacement therapy during pregnancy. Thrombin formation or conversion of fibrinogen to fibrin is not impaired. Consequently, the PT and APTT are normal. Platelet function tests are also normal. The laboratory diagnosis consists of demonstrating that a fibrin clot, made by recalcification of the patient's plasma, dissolves overnight at room temperature in 5M urea or 1 per cent monochloroacetic acid. Fibrin clots formed in the presence of greater than 1 to 2 per cent of the normal concentration of Factor XIII remain intact indefinitely in these solvents.

Treatment consists of giving fresh frozen plasma. Correction of the plasma concentration of Factor XIII to 5 to 10 per cent of normal provides normal hemostasis. The half-life of Factor XIII is approximately 12 days, and thus prophylactic replacement therapy is feasible. Because central nervous system hemorrhage is a major risk, Factor XIII–deficient patients are commonly given 5 to 10 ml per kilogram of fresh frozen plasma every 3 weeks. Extra plasma should be given in preparation for surgery or after head trauma. Development of inhibitory antibody to Factor XIII as a consequence of transfusion therapy is apparently rare.

Deficiency of Alpha₂-Antiplasmin

Congenital homozygous deficiency of alpha$_2$-antiplasmin is associated with a severe, hemophilia-like bleeding tendency. Heterozygous family members with plasma concentrations of the inhibitor 50 per cent of normal have a mild bleeding tendency characterized by postoperative bleeding, excessive bleeding after tooth extraction, and easy bruising after trauma. Levels of alpha$_2$-antiplasmin can be quantified with an activity assay. Patients with severe homozygous deficiency have fewer bleeding episodes when they receive long-term treatment with tranexamic acid. Heterozygotes would probably also benefit from treatment with tranexamic acid or EACA when symptomatic or when their antiplasmin level is depleted by stresses such as major surgery.

Leebeek FWG, Stibbe J, Knot EAR, et al.: Mild haemostatic problems associated with congenital heterozygous α$_2$-antiplasmin deficiency. Thromb Haemost 59:96, 1988. *Update on hemorrhagic diathesis associated with 50 per cent deficiency state.*
McDonagh J, Carrell N: Disorders of fibrinogen structure and function. *In* Colman RW, Hirsh J, Marder VJ, et al. (eds.): Hemostasis and Thrombosis: Basic Principles and Clinical Practice. 2nd ed. Philadelphia, J.B. Lippincott Company, 1987, pp 301–317. *Description of interesting and diverse set of disorders.*

INHERITED TENDENCIES TOWARD THROMBOSIS

There has been considerable progress in the biochemical definition of hypercoagulability. Quantitative or functional deficiencies of three plasma proteins—protein C, protein S, and antithrombin III—have been reported to be associated with a tendency toward thrombosis in affected families. Abnormalities of homocysteine metabolism have been shown to be associated with arterial thrombosis (Ch. 182). As more is learned about fibrinolysis, it is likely that genetic abnormalities of plasminogen, plasminogen activators, and plasminogen activator inhibitors that are associated with a thrombotic diathesis will be identified.

APPROACH TO THE PATIENT WITH A SUSPECTED THROMBOTIC TENDENCY. Patients with the recently described deficiency syndromes are fairly rare. It is therefore difficult to make firm guidelines about when or how to search for deficiency states and how to treat or counsel affected individuals. In general, it is worthwhile to evaluate the status of patients with family histories of thrombosis, young (<40 years old) patients, and patients with rare types of thrombosis (e.g., dural sinus or mesenteric vein thrombosis). Patients should be questioned and their status evaluated to ascertain whether they or family members have or have had conditions that would put them at risk for thrombosis (obesity, prolonged immobilization, injury to or abnormalities of vessels) or causes for secondary hypercoagulability (myeloproliferative syndrome, paroxysmal nocturnal hemoglobinuria, malignant disease, lupus anticoagulant). It has been estimated that of patients with "unexpected thrombosis," 1 to 2 per cent have deficiency of antithrombin III, 5 per cent have deficiency of protein C, and 5 per cent have deficiency of protein S. In my practice, the laboratory evaluation in individuals with a possible thrombotic diathesis includes activity assays of total antithrombin and plasminogen (readily available), activity and immunologic assays of protein C, and immunoassay of protein S

(available in coagulation reference laboratories). Plasma is also frozen at −70°C, with the anticipation that new tests may become available in the future. Patients with premature peripheral or cerebral occlusive arterial disease should be screened for excessive homocysteine accumulation after a standardized methionine-loading test.

Deficiency of Protein C

Two syndromes of hereditary protein C deficiency have been described: (1) heterozygous deficiency, in which half-normal concentrations of protein C are associated with an increased risk of venous thromboembolism, and (2) homozygous deficiency, in which total lack (<1 per cent of normal) of protein C is associated with neonatal purpura fulminans (ischemic necrosis of skin and digits) and massive venous thrombosis. Not all individuals with heterozygous deficiency have thrombosis. In families in which there is thrombosis, some family members with 50 per cent levels are asymptomatic, i.e., the phenotype displays autosomal dominance with incomplete penetrance. Heterozygous deficient individuals in other kindreds ascertained because of infants with homozygous deficiency do not seem at risk for thrombosis at all. It is likely, however, that homozygous deficiency is invariably associated with problems.

The diagnosis of protein C deficiency is based on decreased amounts of antigen or activity in plasma. For patients receiving long-term therapy with warfarin, other vitamin K–dependent proteins, e.g., Factors X and II, are also measured with an immunoassay to correct for the 35 to 50 per cent drop in the level of circulating vitamin K–dependent proteins caused by undercarboxylation. The antigenic measurements do not detect individuals with dysfunctional protein C.

Because not everyone with heterozygous protein C deficiency has thrombosis, long-term anticoagulation should be reserved for individuals who have had a thrombotic episode unless the family history is so striking that the physicians and affected members agree that prophylactic treatment is warranted. Asymptomatic family members should be counseled that they are at greater risk for thrombosis and advised about the dangers of prolonged immobilization of limbs, obesity, and smoking. When warfarin therapy is started in a patient with heterozygous deficiency, the anticoagulant effect should be achieved at a leisurely pace by daily administration of the predicted maintenance dose rather than by administration of a "loading dose" of drug. It is preferable to begin warfarin therapy while the patient is being treated with heparin. However, one should be aware that heparin induces thrombocytopenia and thrombosis in some patients, especially those who have received heparin for more than 10 days.

Infants with homozygous protein C deficiency respond acutely to administration of plasma or Factor IX concentrate, which is rich in protein C. Oral anticoagulants can be used to decrease the frequency of thrombotic events.

Deficiency of Protein S

Decreased levels of plasma protein S antigen or activity are associated with venous thrombosis. Correlation between antigen and activity is poor, because a fraction of protein S in plasma is complexed with C4b-binding protein, and only the fraction of protein S that is free has anticoagulant activity. The proportion of complexed and free protein S can be ascertained by crossed immunoelectrophoresis. The tendency toward thrombosis is inherited as an autosomal dominant trait with incomplete penetrance. Affected individuals tend to have levels of protein S that are 50 per cent of normal, i.e., they are heterozygous for the deficiency. The incidence of symptomatic heterozygous protein S deficiency is probably the same as the incidence of symptomatic protein C deficiency. Pending further information about this recently described syndrome, it seems reasonable to approach and treat heterozygous protein S deficiency using the guidelines described above for heterozygous protein C deficiency.

Deficiency of Antithrombin III

The average concentration of antithrombin III in deficient patients is approximately 50 per cent of normal. The most frequent manifestation of thromboembolism is lower extremity thrombophlebitis, often bilateral and recurrent and often with pulmonary embolism. Patients may develop venous insufficiency and chronic leg ulcers. Upper extremity thrombophlebitis and mesenteric vein thrombosis are less common. Rare patients may develop retinal or cerebral vein thrombosis, thrombosis of the renal vein or inferior vena cava, Budd-Chiari syndrome, priapism, or widespread clotting and defibrination syndrome. The cumulative incidences of thromboembolism are estimated to be 15 per cent by age 19, 50 per cent by age 29, and 85 per cent in individuals over 40 years. Complete, i.e., homozygous, lack of the major antithrombin has not been described. Patients homozygous for a dysfunctional antithrombin, however, have been reported.

Antithrombin deficiency can be ascertained by an activity assay in which diluted plasma and heparin are mixed with a known concentration of thrombin and the amount of uninhibited thrombin is quantified with a chromogenic substrate. Ongoing thrombosis and heparin therapy both lower the concentration of plasma antithrombin. Therefore, the diagnosis of antithrombin deficiency is best made after the patient has recovered from a thrombotic event.

A patient with acute thrombosis should be treated with heparin. Because of depletion of the major antithrombin, the level of antithrombin may become so low that the patient is resistant to heparin. In this case, a source of antithrombin should be infused, in the form of either fresh frozen plasma or, if available, antithrombin concentrate. The half-life of antithrombin is 16 to 24 hours. Administration of warfarin should be started promptly, and the patient probably should receive warfarin indefinitely.

Prophylactic use of anticoagulants should be considered in view of the spontaneous and unpredictable occurrence of thromboembolism with the potential for a fatal outcome. At the very least, affected individuals should be counseled about the risks of the disorder. Pregnancies should be managed in high-risk clinics prepared to cope with the difficult questions of how, when, or whether anticoagulants should be administered during the pregnancy.

Bovill EG, Bauer KA, Dickerman JD, et al.: The clinical spectrum of heterozygous protein C deficiency in a large New England kindred. Blood 73:712, 1989. Engesser L, Broekmans AW, Briët E, et al.: Hereditary protein S deficiency: Clinical manifestations. Ann Intern Med 106:677, 1987. *Good descriptions of the spectrum of clinical problems in these deficiency states.*

Menache D, O'Malley JP, Schorr JB, et al.: Evaluation of the safety, recovery, half-life, and clinical efficacy of antithrombin III (human) in patients with hereditary antithrombin III deficiency. Blood 75:33, 1990. *Phase I and II studies of a potentially valuable treatment modality.*

ACQUIRED ABNORMALITIES OF BLOOD COAGULATION

GENERAL COMMENTS. In a number of clinical situations, the APTT and/or PT become prolonged: use of heparin, use of fibrinolytic agents, vitamin K deficiency secondary to malabsorption or dietary deficiency, severe liver disease, use of coumarin anticoagulants to lower the activity of vitamin K–dependent factors, and consumption coagulopathy associated with severe illness. Rarer causes of acquired deficiencies include selective urinary loss of a coagulation factor in nephrotic syndrome, selective adsorption of a coagulation factor, especially Factor X, to amyloid, and selective neutralization or depletion of a clotting factor due to development of an antibody to the factor.

Heparin

Heparin is used commonly for its anticoagulant properties in the prevention of and therapy for thromboembolism and to keep blood fluid during extracorporeal circulation. By definition, 1 unit of heparin renders 1 ml of sheep blood incoagulable. The therapeutic concentration in a human (i.e., a patient with an APTT 1½ times longer than normal) is 0.1 to 0.3 units per milliliter.

Bleeding is the most common complication of heparin therapy. This can be minimized by (1) administration of the drug by continuous infusion rather than in boluses; (2) quantification of the anticoagulant effect at regular intervals by whole-blood clotting times or APTT; (3) selection of patients who do not have an occult bleeding site or underlying bleeding diathesis; and (4) prohibition of aspirin and intramuscular injections. Despite this, purpura, ecchymoses, hematomas, gastrointestinal hemorrhage, hematuria, retroperitoneal bleeding, or bleeding at sites of invasive procedures may occur. Heparin is cleared from the circulation within 2 to 4 hours. Therefore, if bleeding is minimal and can be controlled by local measures, discontinuation of heparin may be all that is necessary. If bleeding is severe, the effects of heparin can be counteracted by giving 1 mg of protamine sulfate for each 100 units of heparin estimated to be in the patient's circulation.

After 7 to 10 days of heparin therapy, thrombocytopenia sometimes occurs, subsiding when heparin is discontinued. Mild thrombocytopenia is likely due to a direct effect of heparin on platelets. In some patients, the thrombocytopenia can be severe and associated with venous and/or arterial thrombosis and disseminated intravascular coagulation (DIC). In these patients the thrombocytopenia is probably immunologically mediated. It is important to be alert for such a patient, because one's tendency is to treat the thrombosis by increasing the dose of heparin, only to make the situation worse. Heparin therefore should be discontinued if the platelet count drops precipitously. Low molecular weight heparin holds the promise of providing anticoagulant activity without undesirable reactions with platelets and may be a therapeutic option in the future for patients with heparin-induced thrombocytopenia. For the present, however, the best defense is prophylactic, i.e., to initiate warfarin therapy early so that a stable anticoagulant effect is achieved during the first week of heparin therapy.

Several patients with neoplastic plasma cell disorders have had clinical bleeding caused by a circulating heparin-like proteoglycan that required the major antithrombin for its function and could be neutralized by protamine sulfate.

Turpie AGG, Levine MN, Hirsh J, et al.: A randomized controlled trial of a low-molecular-weight heparin (enoxaparin) to prevent deep-vein thrombosis in patients undergoing elective hip surgery. N Engl J Med 315:925, 1986. Salzman EW: Low-molecular-weight heparin: Is small beautiful? N Engl J Med 315:957, 1986. *Good update and review of trends in heparin therapy.*

Therapeutic Fibrinolysis (Thrombolysis)

Intravenous administration of streptokinase, urokinase, or tissue plasminogen activator is accepted useful therapy for deep vein thrombosis, pulmonary embolism, acute myocardial infarction, and peripheral arterial thromboembolism. These agents reestablish patency of vessels more quickly than does heparin. The dosage and method of administration of the agents are specific for the different conditions, and in some instances the agent is administered by selective catheterization of the involved vessel.

In the case of streptokinase or urokinase administered systemically, therapeutic effectiveness requires that systemic fibrinolysis be achieved, i.e., that the patients develop iatrogenic primary fibrinolysis. Prolongation of the thrombin time to twice normal is often taken as evidence that the desired effect has been achieved. Such patients also have decreased plasma fibrinogen, plasminogen, and alpha$_2$-antiplasmin. In the case of streptokinase administered locally or TPA administered systemically or locally, thrombi can be lysed with variable and sometimes minimal evidence of systemic fibrinolysis.

If the level of plasminogen falls to zero, the patient will be relatively resistant to further infusion of fibrinolytic agents. At that point, or at the end of the planned infusion, there is hypercoagulability, and anticoagulation with heparin should be carried out.

The main complication of fibrinolytic therapy is hemorrhage, usually in the form of continuous, slow oozing at sites of invasive procedures. If a pressure dressing does not control this bleeding, administration of the agent can be discontinued with the anticipation that fibrinolytic activity will subside within a few hours. Fresh frozen plasma can be given if the bleeding is severe.

Marder VJ, Bell WR: Fibrinolytic therapy. *In* Colman RW, Hirsh J, Marder VJ, et al. (eds.): Hemostasis and Thrombosis: Basic Principles and Clinical Practice. 2nd ed. Philadelphia, J. B. Lippincott Company, 1987, pp 1393–1437. *Comprehensive review of indications and strategies.*

Vitamin K Deficiency and Coumarin Anticoagulants

Metabolism and Function of Vitamin K. Vitamin K is required for the posttranslational gamma-carboxylation of specific glutamyl residues in Factors VII, IX, X, and II and of proteins C and S and certain other proteins, e.g., osteocalcin, which constitutes 1 per cent of the protein in bone. In vitamin K–deficient states, levels of the vitamin K–dependent plasma proteins are near normal; however, the functions of these proteins in reactions and assays (e.g., the PT) that require a phospholipid surface are severely impaired. As vitamin K deficiency develops, the activities of Factor VII and protein C decrease rapidly, followed by diminished activities of Factors IX, X, and II.

There are limited body stores of vitamin K. A normal diet containing green, leafy vegetables provides 300 to 500 μg of vitamin K, more than enough to meet the adult daily requirement of 1 μg per kilogram of body weight. In addition, vitamin K synthesized by normal gastrointestinal bacterial flora contributes to the daily requirement. Vitamin K is a fat-soluble vitamin, and solubilization of fat must occur before vitamin K can be absorbed (Ch. 102). Hence, vitamin K deficiency may occur in bile salt–deficient states, in all malabsorptive disorders, or with an inadequate dietary intake combined with gastrointestinal sterilization by orally administered antibiotics. Vitamin K occurs naturally in two forms, vitamin K_1 (phylloquinone) and vitamin K_2 (menaquinone), both of which require lipid for absorption. A synthetic water-soluble form, vitamin K_3 (menadione), is commercially available. Despite its ready absorption from intestine, menadione must be converted to vitamin K_2 by the liver and therefore is not as rapidly effective as vitamin K_1 in promoting the gamma-carboxylation reaction.

VITAMIN K DEFICIENCY OF THE NEWBORN.
At birth, vitamin K levels are low, and production of vitamin K by intestinal bacteria is insufficient to meet an infant's requirements for production of normally functioning coagulation factors. The vitamin K–deficient state lasts for 3 to 5 days and may be the reason Israelites did not circumcise their babies until the eighth day (Leviticus 12:3). Cow's milk contains some vitamin K, but human milk contains essentially none (1 to 2 μg per liter). Unless vitamin K is given, the physiologic state of neonatal hypoprothrombinemia can lead to hemorrhagic disease of the newborn in the following high-risk groups: premature infants; breast-fed infants; infants of mothers who are receiving vitamin K antagonists, especially hydantoin anticonvulsants; and infants with malabsorption. If the PT is prolonged to greater than twice normal, it is common to encounter bleeding from the umbilicus, ecchymoses and hematomas, hematuria, and, most important, intracranial hemorrhage. Prophylactic intramuscular administration of a 1-mg dose of vitamin K_1 at delivery virtually eliminates the risk of subsequent hemorrhage. Excessive administration (5 mg or more) of vitamin K_3 may cause hemolytic anemia and kernicterus in the newborn and should be avoided.

MALABSORPTION SYNDROMES.
Malabsorptive states (Ch. 102) with impaired absorption of fat, such as adult celiac disease, regional enteritis, use of cholestyramine or neomycin, or deficient intraluminal bile salts (obstruction of biliary ducts, cholestatic liver disease), are often associated with vitamin K deficiency. Similarly, various chronic diarrheas can cause vitamin K deficiency, presumably because of decreased transit time and relative malabsorption of fats. The hallmark of vitamin K deficiency is prolonged PT. If the PT is longer than twice normal, the patient likely will have ecchymoses, gingival bleeding, hematomas, hematuria, and/or melena. Daily oral administration of vitamin K_1 in supraphysiologic doses (2 to 10 mg) prevents the deficiency and should be routine in patients with malabsorption of fat. The bleeding tendency, once developed, is easily corrected by giving 10 to 25 mg of vitamin K_1 intramuscularly. In cases in which the bleeding diathesis is so severe that intramuscular injections are contraindicated, 20 to 40 mg of vitamin K_1 may be infused intravenously. It should be infused slowly at a rate of 1 mg per minute because the vehicle in which the vitamin is dissolved can cause an adverse reaction. If this does not correct the PT, it is unlikely that additional vitamin K will have any effect.

DEBILITATED PATIENTS WHO MAY BE RECEIVING ANTIBIOTICS.
Patients who are without oral intake for more than several days and receiving antibiotics should be given parenteral vitamin K_1 at a dosage of 150 μg per day because they are likely to become vitamin K deficient. Patients with uremia or malignant disease are at special risk and may become vitamin K deficient on the basis of poor oral intake alone.

Some third-generation cephalosporins have a hypothrombi-

nemic effect that is greater than would be expected from elimination of bowel flora. It has been suggested that the N-methylthiotetrazole side chain shared by cefamandole, moxalactam, and cefoperazone is cleaved from the antibiotic and interferes with the action of vitamin K, especially in patients who are borderline deficient in vitamin K.

COUMARIN ANTICOAGULANTS.
Warfarin and other coumarin anticoagulants competitively inhibit the effects of vitamin K in the posttranslational gamma-carboxylation of vitamin K–dependent plasma proteins. Coumarin anticoagulants are administered for a long time for the prevention of recurrent thromboembolism in patients who have experienced deep vein thrombosis and pulmonary embolism or myocardial infarction. Patients should be reliable, able to be supervised, and without known potential sources of hemorrhage in the central nervous, gastrointestinal, or genitourinary systems.

Upon initiation of therapy, the activities of the proteins with the most rapid half-lives are lost first. Thus the activities of the vitamin K–dependent proteins become depressed in the following order: Factor VII and protein C, Factor IX, Factor X, and Factor II. The art of administration of warfarin involves balancing drug intake against vitamin K intake to prolong the PT about 1½ times as that of a normal control, e.g., 17 to 19 seconds compared with a control of 12 seconds. Ratios below this value are less effective in preventing thrombosis, whereas values twice normal or greater carry a high risk for hemorrhage. An adult receiving a normal diet usually needs 5 to 10 mg of warfarin per day to achieve the desired ratio. After initiation of therapy, it takes 3 to 4 days before the chosen dose of warfarin causes its maximal effect on the PT. The dose can then be altered to maintain the PT in the therapeutic range.

The syndrome of coumarin-induced skin necrosis recapitulates the syndrome of homozygous protein C deficiency. Upon initiation of warfarin therapy, the plasma concentration of protein C, which has a half-life of 6 hours, falls more quickly than the concentrations of Factors II, IX, and X, thus causing a hypercoagulable state. Therefore, therapy should be initiated with the predicted maintenance dose (rather than a "loading dose"), preferably while the patient is receiving heparin.

Once the PT is stabilized, it needs to be checked only every three to four weeks if the patient is on a stable diet and is in usual health. The therapeutic dose of warfarin may change dramatically if the diet is changed or if changes are made in the intake of one of the many drugs that enhance or depress the effect of warfarin (Table 155–2). Patients should wear a bracelet or neck tag stating that they are receiving an oral anticoagulant. They should not take aspirin in any of its forms.

It is not uncommon for patients to experience slight gingival bleeding, purpura with minimal trauma, or trace hematuria while receiving anticoagulants in the therapeutic range. These sympoms become more marked when there is overanticoagulation, and the patient is at risk for severe gastrointestinal or genitourinary hemorrhage, bleeding or hematoma formation after trauma, and intracranial bleeding. If the PT is prolonged and increased bleeding is not a clinical problem, warfarin, which has a half-life of 35 hours, can be omitted until the desired PT is obtained. When overanticoagulation results in clinically significant bleeding, the physician can give fresh frozen plasma, 10 to 20 ml per kilogram, as a source of normal vitamin K–dependent proteins, and/or give vitamin K, depending on the immediacy of the problem and whether continuation of warfarin is necessary. The effect of plasma on the PT is immediate but temporary. The use of Factor IX concentrates to treat warfarin overdose should be avoided because of occasional thrombotic complications and the risk of hepatitis. Oral or intramuscular vitamin K_1, 5 to 25 mg, should correct the PT within 8 to 24 hours. Slow intravenous infusion of vitamin K, 20 to 40 mg, should correct the PT in 4 to 6 hours. Administration of more than 5 mg of vitamin K makes the patient warfarin resistant and necessitates a round of re-anticoagulation. Therefore, the best strategy for the patient who needs continued anticoagulation is to give plasma and small doses (1 to 2 mg) of vitamin K while closely monitoring the PT and clinical state.

Patients occasionally present with bleeding complications after ingestion of a coumarin compound, either surreptitiously or as a

TABLE 155–2. DRUGS AND CONDITIONS THAT INFLUENCE RESPONSE TO WARFARIN

Increased Resistance to Warfarin

Hereditary warfarin resistance	Increased warfarin metabolism
Increase in dietary vitamin K	Barbiturates
Reduced drug absorption	Primidone
Malabsorption syndrome	Carbamazepine
Liquid paraffin laxatives	Ethchlorvynol
Cholestyramine resin	Glutethimide
Magnesium trisilicate	Meprobamate
	Griseofulvin
	Rifampin
	Nafcillin

Increased Sensitivity to Warfarin

Vitamin K deficiency	Synergism with warfarin
Malabsorption syndrome	Vitamin E
Wide-spectrum antibiotics	Anabolic steroids
Liquid paraffin	Danazol
Clofibrate	Blocking of warfarin metabolism
Displacement of albumin	Phenytoin sodium
binding	Chloramphenicol
Phenylbutazone	Clofibrate
Aspirin	Tricyclic antidepressants
Indomethacin	Erythromycin
Sulindac	Cimetidine
Mefenamic acid	Sulfamethoxazole-trimethoprim
Tolmetin	Sulfinpyrazone
Ibuprofen	Unknown mechanism
Naproxen	Quinine
Fenoprofen	Quinidine
Phenytoin sodium	Phenothiazine
Oral hypoglycemic agents	Disulfiram
Nalidixic acid	Sulfisoxazole
Estrogen	Amiodarone
Miconazole	

Adapted with permission from Peterson CE, Kwaan HC: Current concepts of warfarin therapy. Arch Intern Med 146:581, 1986. Copyright 1986, American Medical Association.

suicide attempt. Patients who take coumarins surreptitiously are usually depressed and receive gain from medical attention. They may belong to a health profession. The coumarin compounds in rat poisons are much more powerful than warfarin and can cause extreme resistance to vitamin K for weeks and even months.

Coumarin anticoagulants should not be given from the sixth to the twelfth week of gestation because of the high likelihood that characteristic facial and skeletal malformations, the so-called coumarin embryopathy, will be induced. Use of coumarin drugs in the second and third trimesters is associated with an increased incidence of central nervous system malformations presumed to be due to sporadic intracranial hemorrhages. If anticoagulation is needed during pregnancy, one approach is to switch to subcutaneous heparin between the sixth and twelfth week and after the thirty-eighth week.

Furie B, Furie BC: Molecular basis of vitamin K–dependent α-carboxylation. Blood 75:1753, 1990. *Update on the biochemistry of vitamin K action and the opposing effect of the coumarins.*

Hirsh J: Is the dose of warfarin prescribed by American physicians unnecessarily high? Arch Intern Med 147:769, 1987. *Recommendations on intensity of therapy in different situations. Good data in support of less intensive therapy.*

Iturbe-Alessio I, Fonseca MC, Mutchinik O, et al.: Risks of anticoagulant therapy in pregnant women with artificial heart valves. N Engl J Med 315:1390, 1986. *One group's approach to a difficult subject.*

Lipton RA, Klass EM: Human ingestion of a "superwarfarin" rodenticide resulting in a prolonged anticoagulant effect. JAMA 252:3004, 1984. Jones EC, Growe GH, Naiman SC: Prolonged anticoagulation in rat poisoning. JAMA 252:3005, 1984. *Illustrative case reports.*

O'Reilly RA: Vitamin K antagonists. *In* Colman RW, Hirsh J, Marder VJ, et al. (eds.): Hemostasis and Thrombosis: Basic Principles and Clinical Practice. 2nd ed. Philadelphia, J. B. Lippincott Company, 1987, pp 1367–1372.

Peterson CE, Kwaan HC: Current concepts of warfarin therapy. Arch Intern Med 146:581, 1986. *A concise review.*

Liver Disease

The liver is the major site of synthesis of fibrinogen, plasminogen, the vitamin K–dependent proteins, the antithrombins, and most other plasma proteins. The mechanisms by which steady-state concentrations of these proteins in plasma are regulated are obscure. As part of the "acute phase reaction" in response to interleukin 1, interleukin 6, and tumor necrosis factor, the synthesis of many plasma proteins, especially fibrinogen, increases at the expense of albumin synthesis. The normal liver seems to have a considerable reserve for production of fibrinogen but to be working at near-maximal capacity in the synthesis of vitamin K–dependent proteins.

Patients with liver disease occasionally develop petechiae, ecchymoses, prolonged bleeding after venipuncture, and/or gastrointestinal hemorrhage. Clinically significant bleeding may occur with biopsies and surgery. The causes of these problems are diverse.

In patients with alcoholic liver disease, bleeding can be secondary to dietary *vitamin K deficiency* and responds promptly to oral vitamin K. With more advanced disease, patients may become vitamin K deficient on the basis of fat malabsorption as well as poor nutrition, and parenteral vitamin K must be given. The synthesis of vitamin K–dependent factors becomes impaired as hepatocytes are lost, rendering the patient resistant to parenteral vitamin K. A poor prognosis is associated with a prolonged PT (greater than 1½ times normal) that does not become corrected after intravenous vitamin K. If the patient no longer responds to parenteral vitamin K, abnormal bleeding or correction of the PT prior to invasive procedures will require transfusions of fresh frozen plasma. In fulminant hepatocellular disease, *hypofibrinogenemia* can be profound enough to be considered the cause of bleeding; in such cases, both fresh frozen plasma and cryoprecipitate should be given.

Acquired dysfibrinogenemia, manifested by abnormal fibrin polymerization, has been observed in a number of patients having hepatic diseases such as alcoholic cirrhosis, postnecrotic cirrhosis of unknown cause, drug-induced hepatic failure, and hepatoma. The fibrinogen in these patients has an increased content of sialic acid. The clotting of these fibrinogens by thrombin is delayed in proportion to the increase of sialic acid. If the liver disease improves, the defect may disappear.

Patients with liver disease commonly have *increased fibrinolysis*, because of an inability to maintain normal levels of alpha₂-antiplasmin and/or decreased hepatic clearance of plasminogen activators. Enhanced fibrinolysis, however, is rarely the primary cause of bleeding. Occasionally, chronic, smoldering *disseminated intravascular coagulation* (DIC) may develop, in which case the platelet count is decreased and levels of several coagulation factors fall because of consumption. These patients do not require therapy unless they exhibit clinically significant bleeding, in which case the approach should be the same as for patients with other causes of diffuse intravascular coagulation (see below). Patients in whom LeVeen peritoneovenous shunts have been placed and women with acute fatty liver of pregnancy and marked deficiency of antithrombin III (<25 per cent of normal) are at particular risk of developing DIC.

Efforts should be made to normalize the PT, fibrinogen concentration, and platelet count in patients with liver disease prior to surgery, biopsy, or other invasive procedures. Factor IX concentrates are not recommended for prophylaxis in patients in whom the PT will not be corrected with parenteral vitamin K because such patients are likely to be deficient in plasma antithrombin, to have decreased hepatic clearance of activated clotting factors, and therefore to be at risk for thromboembolism. Platelet concentrates should be given if the platelet count is less than 75,000 per microliter. If hypersplenism is the cause of thrombocytopenia, however, it may be difficult to achieve a satisfactory platelet count.

Joist JH: Hemostatic abnormalities in liver disease. *In* Colman RW, Hirsh J, Marder VJ, et al. (eds.): Hemostasis and Thrombosis: Basic Principles and Clinical Practice. 2nd ed. Philadelphia, J. B. Lippincott Company, 1987, pp 861–872. *Review with good references.*

Renal Disease

Patients with uremia occasionally develop purpura, mucous membrane bleeding, gastrointestinal hemorrhage, and prolonged bleeding from venous and arterial needle puncture sites. Such patients usually have a prolonged bleeding time. The pathogenesis of the bleeding tendency is complex. The platelet count may be low. More important, platelet function is abnormal because of accumulation of a dialyzable substance in the circulation (Ch. 154). Anemia contributes to platelet dysfunction in vivo, because the stirring action of red cells causes a large increase in the diffusivity of platelets and allows platelets to be transported efficiently to areas where the vessel wall is injured. Erythropoietin therapy, therefore, normalizes the bleeding time. Daily infusion of cryoprecipitate has been useful in correcting the bleeding tendency in uremia. Although uncertain, the correction may be related to the high molecular weight von Willebrand factor multimers contained in cryoprecipitate. Desmopressin, which is effective in raising the plasma level of von Willebrand factor in patients with von Willebrand disease (see above), temporarily corrects the bleeding time in patients with uremia. Daily intravenous administration of conjugated estrogens may also correct the bleeding time over a period of days. Thus a number of therapeutic maneuvers can be tried in a symptomatic uremic patient: dialysis to restore platelet function; transfusion to normalize red cell and platelet number; and administration of cryoprecipitate, desmopressin, or conjugated estrogens.

Coagulation factors, especially vitamin K–dependent factors and Factor V, tend to be at low concentration in chronic renal disease, although not to levels that should cause bleeding. Some of these deficiencies probably result from hepatic insufficiency or from vitamin K deficiency secondary to oral antibiotic therapy, malabsorption caused by uremic enteritis, and diminished dietary intake. Very low plasma Factor IX levels (10 per cent of normal) have been observed in patients with severe nephrotic syndrome and preferential loss of Factor IX into the urine. Subclinical DIC occasionally occurs in patients with chronic renal disease, as evidenced by elevated amounts of fibrin degradation products in serum and urine. It has been suggested that loss of antithrombin III in nephrotic syndrome may cause renal vein thrombosis. There are no clear guidelines on when and how to treat such deficiencies. If the PT is long or the Factor IX level is low in a patient who is bleeding, fresh frozen plasma is the replacement product of choice, although it may be difficult to give enough to someone who cannot compensate for the large volume.

Di Minno G, Martinez J, McKean, M-L, et al.: Platelet dysfunction in uremia: Multifaceted defect partially corrected by dialysis. Am J Med 79:552, 1985. Castillo R, Lozano T, Escolar G, et al.: Defective platelet adhesion on vessel subendothelium in uremic patients. Blood 68:337, 1986. *Two studies of platelet function in uremic patients.*
Janson PA, Jubelirer SJ, Weinstein MJ, et al.: Treatment of the bleeding tendency in uremia with cryoprecipitate. N Engl J Med 303:1318, 1980. Mannucci PM, Remuzzi C, Pusineri F, et al.: Deamino-8-D-arginine vasopressin shortens the bleeding time in uremia. N Engl J Med 308:8, 1983. Livio M, Mannucci PM, Vigano G, et al.: Conjugated estrogens for the management of bleeding associated with renal failure. N Engl J Med 315:731, 1985. *Contain results of three different but possibly related approaches to improvement of the bleeding time in uremic patients. The mechanisms of the favorable clinical effects are enigmas.*
Van Geet C, Hauglustaine D, Verresen L, et al.: Haemostatic effects of recombinant human erythropoietin in chronic haemodialysis patients. Thromb Haemost 61:117, 1989. *Documents favorable effect of erythropoietin on the bleeding time.*

Factor VIII Inhibitors

An endogenously produced anticoagulant, usually referred to as a circulating anticoagulant or a circulating inhibitor, is an antibody that interacts with a clotting factor in a manner that neutralizes the functional activity of the factor. Production of such an antibody is pathologic and often results in hemorrhage. Factor VIII inhibitors are commonly observed in hemophilia A (Factor VIII deficiency) but are rare in nonhemophilic patients. Conditions in which sporadic Factor VIII inhibitors occur include the postpartum state, diseases of immunologic dysfunction, and old age. The sporadic inhibitors induce a hemophilia-like state, i.e., a significant bleeding diathesis, but are unlike the inhibitors of hemophilic patients in several ways. They tend to be of low titer (<1 to 20 Bethesda units) and to bind Factor VIII weakly. Titers often drop when patients are treated with cytoxan, 1 gram given intravenously, and prednisone, 80 mg per day, to be tapered once an effect is seen. Such a therapeutic response is rare in patients with hemophilia and an inhibitor. Acute bleeding episodes can be managed with variable success by continuous infusion of Factor VIII concentrate or cryoprecipitate.

When a Factor VIII inhibitor is present, the PT is normal but the APTT is prolonged. If the patient's plasma is incubated for

several hours with an equal quantity of normal plasma, the APTT of the mixture should be prolonged. The Factor VIII level in the patient's plasma and in the mixture of patient's plasma and normal plasma should be low no matter what dilutions are tested, whereas the Factor IX level should be normal. These characteristics distinguish Factor VIII inhibitors from the antiphospholipid inhibitors associated with lupus erythematosus (lupus-type inhibitors). A lupus-type inhibitor may cause prolongation of the PT, especially when the test is done with diluted thromboplastin; does not require an incubation period to express inhibitory activity in mixtures of patient's and normal plasma; and may interfere with the assays for both Factors VIII and IX when the patient's plasma is tested at a 1:10 dilution but not when the patient's plasma is tested at a 1:200 or 1:500 dilution. The implications of having a Factor VIII inhibitor versus a lupus-type inhibitor are very different, and the physician and laboratory must be sure that the correct diagnosis is made, even though there is no single test with which to make the distinction.

Lian ECY, Larcada AF, Chiu AYZ: Combination immunosuppressive therapy after Factor VIII infusion for acquired factor VIII inhibitor. Ann Intern Med 110:774, 1989. *Description of 12 nonhemophilic patients with inhibitors.*

Lupus-Type Inhibitors

Patients with systemic lupus erythematosus sometimes develop a circulating anticoagulant unrelated to the severity or duration of disease. A similar inhibitor sometimes occurs in patients who do not have lupus. Patients who have the lupus-type inhibitor may also have anticardiolipin antibodies and thrombocytopenia. Only rarely is the inhibitor associated with clinically significant bleeding. When patients with the inhibitor do bleed, it is due to thrombocytopenia, platelet dysfunction, and/or acquired Factor II deficiency. Instead, patients with the lupus-type inhibitor are at increased risk of having recurrent thromboembolic events. Thrombosis can involve both veins and arteries. There is probably accelerated atherosclerosis. Women with the inhibitor have a greatly increased incidence of spontaneous abortion. Some patients have neurologic abnormalities that may be due to cerebral thrombosis or myelitis or both. In short, the problems associated with a lupus-like inhibitor can be devastating.

Inhibition of clotting tests is thought to be a consequence of binding of the inhibitor to the acidic phospholipids used in the PT and APTT. The prolongations of both assays can be very impressive. Presumably, platelet membranes, rather than phospholipid micelles, provide the surface for activation of Factors X and II, thus accounting for the fact that clinically significant bleeding does not occur. The pathogenesis of the thrombotic diathesis associated with lupus-type inhibitors is unknown. A reasonable hypothesis is that the lupus-type inhibitor and the anticardiolipin are members of a cross-reacting family of antiphospholipid antibodies, and within the family are antibodies that react in a noxious fashion with endothelial cells, e.g., to block prostacyclin production or to inhibit the cofactor activity of thrombomodulin in the protein C–protein S pathway.

Without knowledge of the pathogenesis of the thromboembolism, there is no rational approach to treatment. Anticoagulants should be given but may not be effective. It also is reasonable to try immunosuppressive therapy or plasmapheresis. Administration of corticosteroids and low-dose aspirin during pregnancy had favorable laboratory and clinical effects in a group of women with the inhibitor and impressive histories of spontaneous abortion.

Love PE, Santoro SA: Antiphospholipid antibodies: Anticardiolipin and the lupus anticoagulant in systemic lupus erythematosus (SLE) and non-SLE disorders. Ann Intern Med 112:682, 1990. *Illustrates well the dilemmas of lupus-type inhibitors.*

Miscellaneous Inhibitors of Clotting Factors

Approximately 5 per cent of patients with Factor IX deficiency (hemophilia B) develop inhibitors to Factor IX after repeated transfusion. Inhibitors to Factor V have been reported in about eight patients, only one of these being a Factor V–deficient patient. Acquired inhibitors to von Willebrand factor activity have developed in very few patients. An IgG inhibitor was found in a Factor XIII–deficient patient following transfusion. A few patients receiving isoniazid have developed an inhibitor directed toward the fibrin crosslinking sites; this results in defective fibrin polymerization.

Myeloma or macroglobulinemia may give rise to defective fibrin polymerization as a result of interference by high concentrations of immunoglobulin. If overt bleeding occurs, plasmapheresis may restore adequate hemostasis by reducing plasma protein concentration.

A very interesting inborn error of alpha₁-antiproteinase (alpha₁-antitrypsin) has been reported in which the mutant serpin is a rapid, specific inhibitor of thrombin, thus causing a severe hemorrhagic diathesis.

Sporadic Acquired Factor Deficiency

A number of patients with amyloidosis have Factor X deficiency because of its removal from the circulation through binding of zymogen Factor X to the amyloid deposits. Patients present with mild to severe bleeding, just as do individuals with the inherited form of Factor X deficiency. Replacement therapy can be given with plasma or factor concentrates. However, the in vivo half-life of Factor X is shortened.

Occasionally, a patient is seen with isolated factor deficiency but no evidence of a neutralizing antibody, e.g., when the patient's plasma is mixed 1:1 with normal plasma, the factor level in the mixture is 50 per cent. Such a patient with Factor II deficiency was studied in depth and shown to have a nonneutralizing antibody to Factor II. Administration of corticosteroids was associated with a rise in Factor II activity and cessation of bleeding, but circulating Factor II was bound to antibody. These observations suggested that nonneutralizing antibodies to Factor II cause plasma Factor II deficiency because of rapid clearance of the antigen-antibody complexes, which is slowed by corticosteroids. Demonstration of nonneutralizing antibodies requires special techniques and takes some time. Therefore, in a patient who is bleeding seriously, one may need to begin administration of corticosteroids, possibly supplemented with fresh frozen plasma, before the diagnosis is established.

Bajaj SP, Rapaport SI, Barclay S, et al.: Acquired hypoprothrombinemia due to nonneutralizing antibodies to prothrombin: Mechanism and management. Blood 65:1538, 1985. *Although this paper describes only one patient, it illustrates what may be a fairly common happening.*

Greipp PR, Kyle RA, Bowie EJ: Factor X deficiency in amyloidosis: A critical review. Am J Hematol 11:443, 1981. *Well-documented description of the cause of this deficiency.*

Syndromes of Disseminated Intravascular Coagulation (DIC)

GENERAL COMMENTS. In the following discussion, DIC is divided into four clinical syndromes: (1) *compensated DIC*, which may be associated with thrombosis but does not result in bleeding; (2) *defibrination syndrome*, in which the mechanisms that localize blood coagulation are overwhelmed by release of tissue factor, leading to massive utilization and depletion of fibrinogen, other clotting factors, and platelets and resultant thrombosis and/or bleeding; (3) *primary fibrinolysis*, in which the mechanisms that localize fibrinolysis are overwhelmed by release of plasminogen activators, leading to bleeding; and (4) *microangiopathic thrombocytopenia*, in which platelet microthrombi are widespread, leading to depletion of platelets, ischemic necrosis of tissues, and microangiopathic changes in red cells. The causes of DIC syndromes are many, and there is considerable overlap among syndromes. Patients with DIC often have multiple medical problems, including bone marrow failure, liver failure, renal failure, vitamin K deficiency, and the like, which may complicate the clinical and laboratory analysis in a given patient. Much of the controversy that surrounds DIC undoubtedly stems from attempts to lump diverse conditions and patients together. Despite its oversimplicity, the following scheme is useful because the treatments of the four paradigm syndromes are quite different. For many of the diseases associated with DIC, specific descriptions of the DIC and recommendations for treatment can be found under individual diseases elsewhere in this textbook.

COMPENSATED DIC. Patients with serious underlying diseases (trauma, infection, malignant tumor, and so on) usually have increased production and consumption of platelets, fibrinogen, and other coagulation proteins. Patients with traumatized or inflamed tissues manifest the "acute phase reaction," and a number of plasma alpha₁, alpha₂, and beta globulins, including alpha₂-antiplasmin and fibrinogen, increase in concentration, whereas other plasma proteins, including transferrin and albumin, decrease in concentration. In areas of trauma or inflammation, there is ongoing coagulation and fibrinolysis. Under such conditions, unclottable fibrin degradation products can be detected by immunoassay in serum. However, the PT is normal, the platelet count is normal or only minimally decreased, and plasma fibrinogen concentration is elevated. There is speculation that low-grade DIC is associated with microemboli and microthrombi that contribute to the organ failure commonly found in patients with severe illnesses. At this point, however, the only indication to use heparin or other anticoagulants in such patients is as prophylaxis or treatment of thrombosis in large vessels. An outstanding example of the need for anticoagulation is in the Trousseau syndrome of "migratory" venous thrombosis in patients with malignant disease (Ch. 159). Warfarin therapy is often ineffective in such patients, and they must instead be started on a long-term regimen of heparin therapy.

DEFIBRINATION SYNDROME. The prototype of defibrination syndrome is the rapid onset of generalized bleeding that occurs when tissue factor is released into the circulation after massive brain trauma or during amniotic fluid embolization. Laboratory tests in such patients demonstrate gross depletion of platelets and fibrinogen, increase in fibrin degradation products, prolongation of PT, and variable decreases in Factors V and VIII, Factor II and the other vitamin K–dependent factors, the antithrombins, and plasminogen. Defibrination syndrome occurs most frequently with shock, sepsis, cancer, burns, and obstetric complications. Patients with sepsis, especially due to meningococcus, may develop purpura fulminans or the Waterhouse-Friderichsen syndrome (hemorrhagic necrosis of vital organs, including the adrenals). The patient's hemostatic system must be supported while the patient is resuscitated and the underlying cause is treated. Thus the patient should receive platelet concentrates, cryoprecipitate as a source of fibrinogen, and fresh frozen plasma as a source of other plasma proteins, especially the antithrombins. An appropriate mix is 10 bags of cryoprecipitate for every 2 to 3 units of plasma. One's goals should be a platelet count of more than 50,000 per microliter, a fibrinogen concentration greater than 100 mg per deciliter, a PT that is within 2 to 3 seconds of normal, and a concentration of antithrombins that is greater than 40 per cent of normal. The role of heparin is controversial. It is my view that unless the patient improves quickly or active bleeding cannot be controlled, heparin should be infused in low dosages (10 to 15 units per kilogram per hour after a loading dose of 30 to 40 units per kilogram) with the goal of dampening further defibrination as the patient's clotting components are replenished with cryoprecipitate and plasma. If the patient has overt thrombosis, the dose of heparin can be increased. The low dose of heparin should not cause lengthening of the PT or APTT or exacerbate the bleeding diathesis. Patients who are severely ill and have defibrination syndrome are at high risk of becoming vitamin K deficient and therefore should receive parenteral vitamin K.

PRIMARY FIBRINOLYSIS. Primary fibrinolysis, in its pure form, results from massive release of plasminogen activator. Conditions associated with DIC that cause "primarily" fibrinolysis, if not primary fibrinolysis, include carcinoma of the prostate, acute promyelocytic leukemia, hemangiomas, and sustained release of plasminogen activator by endothelial cells produced by injection of venoms. A critical point is reached when enough plasmin is activated to deplete the circulation of alpha₂-antiplasmin. This allows plasmin to work unopposed on a variety of substrates in blood. Fibrinogen is lysed to fibrinogen degradation products. Because of the lack of fibrinogen and the inhibitory effect of degradation products on fibrin polymerization, the PT is prolonged. The platelet count, however, is appropriate for the state of the bone marrow, and antithrombin levels are normal. Ecchymoses, mucosal bleeding, and bleeding from needle puncture sites can be extensive. It is usually possible to give enough cryoprecipitate to keep plasma fibrinogen at a concentration greater than 100 mg per deciliter. There is, however, no concentrated source of alpha₂-antiplasmin. EACA, 1 gram per hour in an adult, may be effective in minimization of bleeding and should be given a therapeutic trial in a symptomatic patient if the activity of alpha$_2$-antiplasmin in plasma is less than 35 to 40 per cent of normal. If there is a worry about induction of thrombosis with EACA, heparin in a low dose can be infused simultaneously as described above.

MICROANGIOPATHIC THROMBOCYTOPENIA. The hallmarks of microangiopathic thrombocytopenia are a low platelet count and fragmented red cells on blood smear. Although the serum may contain fibrin degradation products, the PT is generally not elevated, and the fibrinogen concentration is normal or increased. Microangiopathic thrombocytopenia can be seen in patients with sepsis, malignant disease, immune complex disease, vasculitis, malignant hypertension, eclampsia, vascular malformations, and intravascular aspergillosis. The prototype conditions, however, are hemolytic-uremic syndrome (HUS) and thrombotic thrombocytopenic purpura (TTP) (Ch. 154). HUS involves mainly the vessels of the kidney, usually occurs in children, and ordinarily is self-limited. TTP involves many organs, including the brain, ordinarily occurs in adults, and usually causes death unless aggressively treated. Acute neurologic symptoms are the most striking feature of full-blown TTP. The pathogenesis of HUS and TTP is obscure. It has been suggested that patients lack prostacyclin; have von Willebrand factor multimers that are extra large and cause spontaneous platelet aggregation; have autoantibodies that damage endothelial cells; or have a circulating substance, possibly of microbial origin, that causes spontaneous platelet aggregation and that is neutralized by immunoglobulin present in normal plasma. There are intriguing instances in which HUS or TTP occurs in small clusters, is recurrent, or is familial. Whatever the cause (or causes), both HUS and TTP respond in the majority of cases to infusion of fresh frozen plasma. In some cases the requirement for plasma is so great that plasma exchange is necessary. In other cases, occasional infusion of 1 to 2 units of plasma suffices. If extensive plasmapheresis fails, therapeutic options include use of drugs that inhibit platelet aggregation, splenectomy, and use of vincristine.

SNAKE BITES. Venoms from various snakes, especially the vipers and rattlesnakes, contain proteins that can, depending on the species, clot fibrinogen, activate Factor II, Factor X, protein C, or platelets; or cause release of plasminogen activator from endothelial cells. Fortunately, the clinical problems associated with DIC syndromes from venoms are not as striking as the laboratory abnormalities displayed by the victims. Treatment in most instances can be conservative: administration of antivenoms, transfusion of platelets and/or plasma, and general supportive therapy. In some instances, hypofibrinogenemia and thrombocytopenia persist for weeks.

Williams EC, Mosher DF: Disseminated intravascular coagulation. *In* Benz E, Cohen H, Furie B, et al. (eds.): Hematology: Basic Principles and Practice. New York, Churchill Livingstone, 1990, pp 1394–1405. *More detailed exposition.*

PART XIII
ONCOLOGY

156 Introduction
Bruce A. Chabner

HISTORICAL BACKGROUND AND DEFINITIONS

The term "cancer" is derived from *karkinos*, the Greek word for crab. Cancer as a clinical entity is described in the early writings of Greeks and Romans and has assumed a position of special significance as a much-feared disease and as an object of intensive biomedical investigation.

Peyton Rous, a Nobel laureate for his pioneering work on viral oncology, wrote, "Tumors destroy man in an unique and appalling way, as flesh of his own flesh, which had somehow been rendered proliferative, rampant, predatory and ungovernable."

About 1 million new cases of invasive cancer, excluding superficial skin cancers, are diagnosed each year, and half that number die each year of cancer. Cancer ranks second only to heart disease among the leading causes of death in the United States. Important trends have occurred in the incidence and mortality of cancer in the past two decades, with marked increases in deaths due to lung cancer in women and malignant melanoma, myeloma, brain tumors, and non-Hodgkin's lymphoma in men and women (Fig. 156–1). At the same time, mortality due to cancer has declined for the population less than 65 years of age, primarily as the result of improvements in treatment and early detection. There are also marked differences in the incidence rates of various cancers in different parts of the globe; esophageal, hepatocellular, and stomach cancer occur with much greater frequency in developing countries, undoubtedly as a function of exposure to hepatitis B and to carcinogens in the diet and the environment. Lung, breast, and colon cancer predominate in industrialized countries.

As a pathologic entity, cancer is defined by its properties of uncontrolled local proliferation of cells, with invasion of adjacent normal structure and by distant spread, or metastasis, via the bloodstream or lymphatics or within a body cavity. As a biologic entity, the malignant cell is defined by its ability to grow in tissue culture without the need for attachment to a firm surface and by its loss of responsiveness to growth regulatory signals that cause differentiation and suppress proliferation. Many malignant cells preserve the growth and antigenic properties characteristic of fetal cells, secrete proteins characteristic of fetal tissues (such as the α-fetoprotein of hepatocellular carcinomas and germ-cell tissues), and appear to be frozen in an early state of differentiation that recapitulates a specific stage in normal organ development.

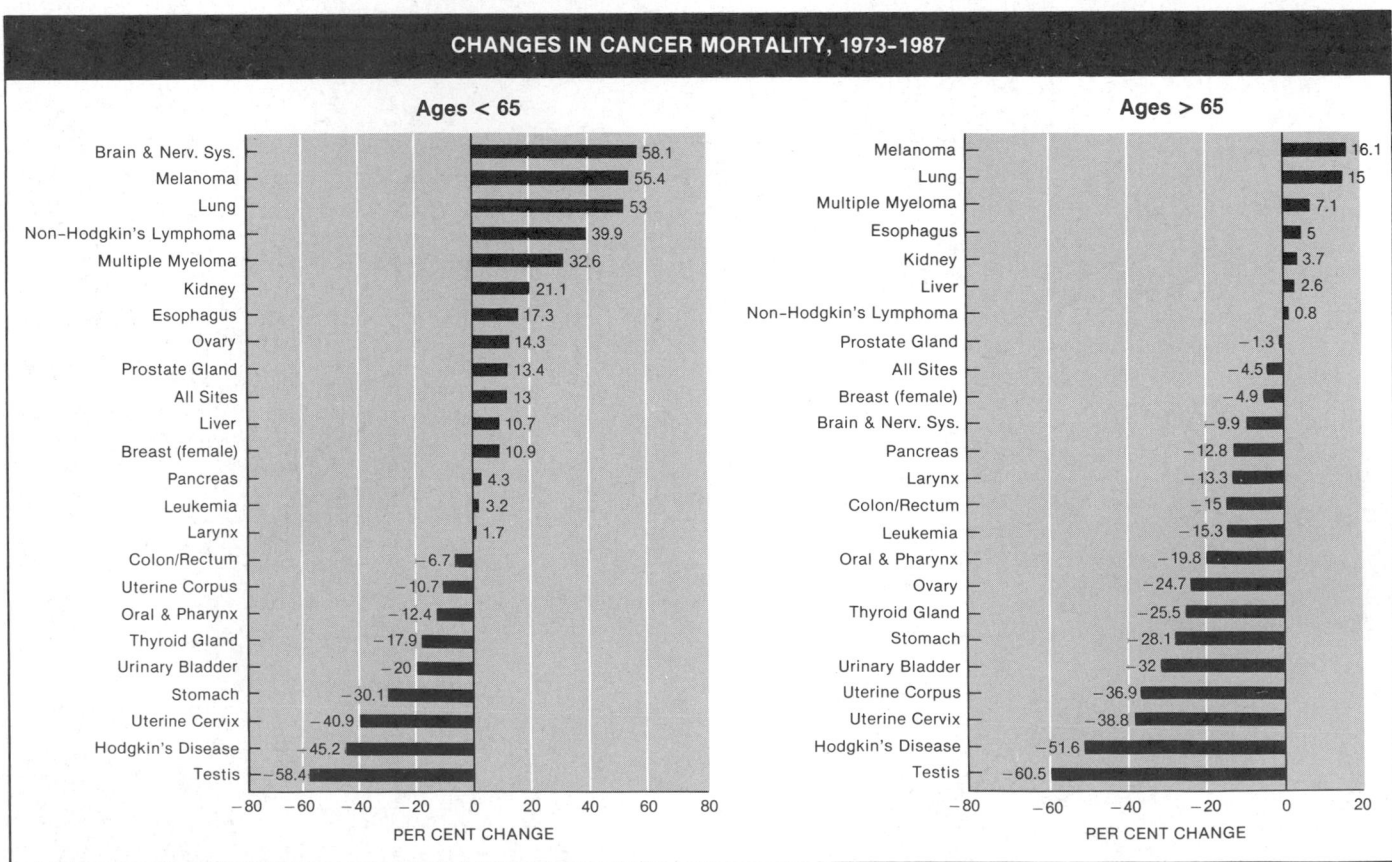

FIGURE 156–1. Changes in mortality rates for persons under and over 65 years of age. Note greater than 50 per cent increase in mortality due to cancers of the lung and bronchus and malignant melanoma in persons under 65. Also note the consistent decrease in mortality in most types of cancer affecting persons less than 65 years of age. (From Cancer Statistics Review: National Cancer Institute, Division of Cancer Prevention and Control, Surveillance Program. Bethesda, MD, National Institutes of Health, NIH Publ. No. 90-2789.)

TABLE 156–1. LYMPHOCYTIC LEUKEMIAS REFLECT PROGRESSIVE STAGES OF NORMAL LYMPHOID DIFFERENTIATION

Type of Leukemia	Phenotype and Molecular Features						
	Pan-B	Pan-T	TCR Re	CALLA	SIg	CIg	IgRe
Common type ALL:							
Early pre-B	+	–	–	+	–	–	H
Late pre-B	+	–	–	+	–	+	H
Mature B-cell ALL	+	–	–	+	+	+	H + L
B-cell CLL	+	–	–	+	+	+	H + L
Lymphoblastic ALL	–	+	β + γ	–	–	–	–
T-cell CLL	–	+	α, β, γ	–	–	–	–

ALL = acute lymphocytic leukemia; CLL = chronic lymphocytic leukemia; Pan-B = pan B-cell antigens; Pan-T = pan T-cell antigen; TCR Re = rearrangement of T-cell receptor genes (α, β, or γ chains) as indicated; CALLA = common ALL antigen (CD-10); SIg = surface immunoglobulin; CIg = cytoplasmic immunoglobulin; IgRe = immunoglobulin rearrangement, heavy (H) or light (L) chain. (From Greaves MF: Differentiation-linked leukemogenesis in lymphocytes. Science 234:697–704, 1986; with permission. Copyright 1987 by the American Association for the Advancement of Science.)

For example, malignancies arising from the lymphoid system reflect all stages and types of B- and T-lymphocyte development and preserve the same complex of immunoglobulin and T-cell receptor gene rearrangements and cell surface proteins (and in some cases potential for further differentiation) found in normal counterparts of the immune system (Table 156–1). These properties have become the basis for classification, diagnosis, and even treatment of tumors, as, for example, classification of lymphoid tumors based on reactivity with monoclonal antibodies. While the above characteristics are typical of most cancer cells, they are not universal. Some endocrine-related tumors, for example, not only maintain well-differentiated morphologic features of their tissue of origin but also retain endocrine function and produce bioactive hormonal substances typical of the mature tissue, as in pheochromocytomas.

Shimkin MB: Contrary to Nature. Washington, D.C., US Department of Health, Education and Welfare, 1977. *An outstanding and eminently readable work on the development of knowledge about cancer from earliest records to modern times. This well-illustrated book traces the impact of the scientists and institutions that have contributed to cancer research throughout the world.*

ETIOLOGY

A broad array of chemical, biologic, and physical agents can cause cancer either directly or indirectly. Most of the directly causative agents damage or alter DNA; these include chemicals—such as benzpyrene, benzene, aflatoxin, and nitrosamines—that form chemical adducts with DNA. Many such chemical carcinogens require activation by cytochrome P-450 enzymes found in liver and epithelial cells. DNA damage can also be caused by physical agents, such as ionizing radiation or ultraviolet light (see Ch. 158).

The precise manner in which these agents damage DNA and lead to cancer is under intensive investigation. One unifying hypothesis proposes that DNA damage results in breaks, translocations, or deletions that activate specific *oncogenes*, i.e., genes that have the potential to cause unrestrained growth if mutated in crucial ways. The biology underlying such mutation has been partially explained by studies of the transforming genes of certain animal RNA viruses (retroviruses) that produce tumors through activation of growth-factor receptors, G proteins, or other important regulatory steps. This topic is more fully discussed in Ch. 157. Analogous activation of oncogenes, such as of members of the *ras* and *myc* families, has been detected in human tumor cell lines and in tumors taken directly from patients with neuroblastoma, Burkitt's lymphoma, and colon cancer, but the precise cause of most human neoplasms remains uncertain at this time. Recently, certain viruses, such as the human T-cell leukemia virus, papilloma viruses, and the Epstein-Barr virus, have been implicated as the cause of human cancers, as have dietary factors such as saturated fats and the absence of fiber. The role of diet in cancer causation, although incompletely defined, is frequently the subject of patient inquiry and is discussed in further detail in Ch. 12.

Substances that are not themselves carcinogens may serve as tumor promoters when given in conjunction with or following exposure to specific carcinogens. These agents appear to work by promoting proliferation of cells already mutated by a primary carcinogen.

The major public health hazard relating to cancer in the United States is *tobacco. The incidence, time to occurrence, and site of cancer depend upon the frequency and mode of tobacco use (smoking, chewing), as well as on exposure to potentiating factors such as alcohol or asbestos.* About one third of cancers in the United States and Europe are related to the use of tobacco products, including those that occur in lung, esophagus, head and neck, and bladder. While specific dietary carcinogens have not been implicated as direct causes of common cancers in the United States, diets that contain high amounts of animal fat and are low in fiber and vegetables are associated with an increased risk of cancer of the colon and rectum. High alcohol intake increases esophageal and head and neck cancer. Sexual behavior patterns influence cancer risk, as reflected in the high incidence of cervical cancer (presumably due to papilloma virus) among women who have multiple sexual partners.

Some cancers are iatrogenic in origin, as in patients who develop acute leukemia or other cancers years after the use of cytotoxic chemotherapeutic drugs or radiotherapy, or in patients who receive immunosuppressive therapy following renal or cardiac transplantation. The most highly carcinogenic agents used in cancer chemotherapy are alkylating agents such as melphalan, cyclophosphamide, and chlorambucil, as well as certain drugs that form DNA adducts after metabolic activation, such as procarbazine.

In addition to environmental factors, *host susceptibility* is a critical determinant in the carcinogenic process. This is partly explained by genetic (or acquired) differences in the ability to metabolize a precursor to the proximate carcinogen, by differences in hormonal milieu and immunologic resistance, and by inherited or acquired mutation or deletion of specific genes, such as the retinoblastoma tumor suppressor gene, that protect against the development of cancer (so-called tumor suppressor genes). The high incidence of malignancy in certain kindreds, as observed in the inherited form of retinoblastoma, in familial polyposis, in the dysplastic nevus syndrome, and in kindreds with high incidence of various epithelial malignancies, is believed to result from inheritance of mutations in genes that protect normal cells against growth signals and proliferation (see Ch. 158). The alert clinician must always be attentive to clues of a predisposition to malignancy provided by a careful family and occupational history.

National Research Council: Diet and Health: Implications for reducing chronic disease risk. Washington, D.C., National Academy Press, 1989. *A definitive summary of the evidence for a relationship between diet and cancer.*

CANCER CELL GROWTH AND METASTASIS

A central concept in the understanding of cancer as a disease is its origin as a clonal proliferation of abnormal cells. Clonality of malignancies has been verified by chromosomal analysis and by molecular probes that identify unique DNA translocations or rearrangements in lymphomas, leukemias, and other tumors. Certain tumors, such as colon cancer, are believed to arise from pre-existing benign polyps, which are well-differentiated and noninvasive tumors confined to the mucosal surface; mutational events in these benign tumors lead to a site of malignant degeneration within the polyp and the emergence of a malignant, invasive tumor. These histologic events are paralleled by the acquisition of a sequence of specific genetic changes, such as loss of the p53 tumor suppressor gene on chromosome 17 and activation of the k-ras oncogene. Even after their establishment, malignant clones undergo further biologic evolution. Thus the clinically apparent tumors in man demonstrate multiple molecular and biochemical features, such as activation of oncogenes and deletion of suppressor genes, any one of which might be sufficient to cause malignant transformation. For example, small cell lung cancer in man is characterized by deletions of the 3p chromosome, activation of the l-myc oncogene, and deletion of the p53 and Rb tumor suppressor genes. Which of these events initiates the malignant transformation is uncertain, nor is the precise role of each abnormality in the final expression of the malignant phenotype understood.

Clonal evolution of malignancies is manifested in the natural history of many malignancies: (1) the transformation from the chronic to the acute phase (blastic crisis) of chronic granulocytic leukemia; (2) the transformation of nodular lymphomas to a diffuse histiocytic lymphoma; (3) the development of rapidly progressive metastases in a patient who had a slowly growing primary malignant melanoma; (4) the development of highly drug-resistant relapse in a patient with acute leukemia previously responsive to chemotherapy.

In general, clonal evolution proceeds along pathways that provide a growth advantage for the malignancy and allow for survival in a hostile environment. Thus, tumor cells elaborate autocrine (self-acting) growth factors and angiogenesis factors, secrete metalloproteinase and collagenases that digest basement membrane and allow invasion of adjacent structures, and express receptors that allow the attachment to laminin, a basement membrane protein. The digestion of collagen and basement membrane proteins allows tumor cells to invade through the walls of capillaries and lymphatics and thus to spread to distant sites. The ability to metastasize to distant sites is a consequence of these general properties, but in addition there is evidence that the ability to implant and survive in specific sites (such as lymph node, lung, or liver) results from the presence of additional biochemical factors elaborated by metastatic subclones. The pioneering work of Fidler and colleagues with the murine B-16 melanoma has demonstrated the existence of metastases that "home" and survive specifically in liver, lung, and other organs.

Although the survival and continuous proliferation of malignancy depend on the ability of a tumor cell to adapt to its milieu and to develop the specialized machinery for invasion and metastases, host factors play an important role in determining the fate of a malignant clone. Foremost among the host defenses is the immune system. Lymph nodes act as a barrier to metastases by filtering out tumor cells. For most malignancies, such as colon cancer and breast cancer, there is a finite, but small cure rate achieved by resection of a primary tumor and its draining lymph nodes when the nodes are involved with cancer, demonstrating that the lymph nodes represent a first line of defense. Several immune mechanisms are capable of killing tumor cells, including natural killer cells and the closely related lymphokine-activated killer cells (LAK cells) found in the mononuclear leukocyte fraction of the peripheral blood, T-lymphocyte–mediated cell killing as exemplified by tumor-infiltrating lymphocytes (TIL cells), and activated macrophages (see Ch. 159). The importance of an intact immune system in preventing cancer is graphically indicated by the high incidence of neoplasms in patients with primary immune deficiency states or in those receiving immunosuppressive therapy. These natural surveillance mechanisms are being exploited in new attempts to treat metastatic cancer.

Benign tumors may show a spectrum of variation from normal, and on occasion the distinction between a benign and a malignant lesion on the basis of histology alone may be subtle. A spectrum of morphologic findings may reflect progressive stages in neoplastic transformation. Dysplastic changes of bronchial epithelium or of the cervix are considered to be premalignant, although not necessarily destined to become cancerous, particularly if the inciting stimulus is removed. With the development of effective cancer-preventing agents, such as compounds of the retinoic acid class, the identification of dysplastic changes may allow early intervention to prevent progression to malignancy. As cells become more anaplastic in appearance, they may begin to show

microscopic invasion, progressing from carcinoma in situ to microscopic invasion and finally to overt invasive disease. *Dysplastic* changes in other organs also precede frank carcinomatous changes, but once malignant tumors are established they are programmed for continuing survival and growth except in rare cases of spontaneous regression.

CYTOGENETICS. Many types of cytogenetic abnormalities have been observed in leukemias and other cancers by study of metaphase preparations, by in situ hybridization with DNA probes, by high-resolution banding with the use of fluorescent acridine stains, and by other new techniques. The most common types of defects are inversions, deletions, and reciprocal translocations (exchanges of DNA between two chromosomes). Increasingly unique chromosomal abnormalities characteristic of particular tumors are being recognized, e.g., the Philadelphia chromosome (Ph[1]) in chronic myelogenous leukemia (CML), a translocation of a piece of chromosome 9, containing the c-abl oncogene, to the breakpoint cluster region (bcr) of chromosome 22. The Philadelphia chromosome is visibly detectable in karyotype preparations of 85 per cent of patients, and the translocation of the c-abl oncogene to the bcr of chromosome 22 is detectable by molecular techniques in most of the other 15 per cent of patients with clinical CML (see Ch. 144). The same clonal abnormalities also occur in myeloid, erythroid, and megakaryo-

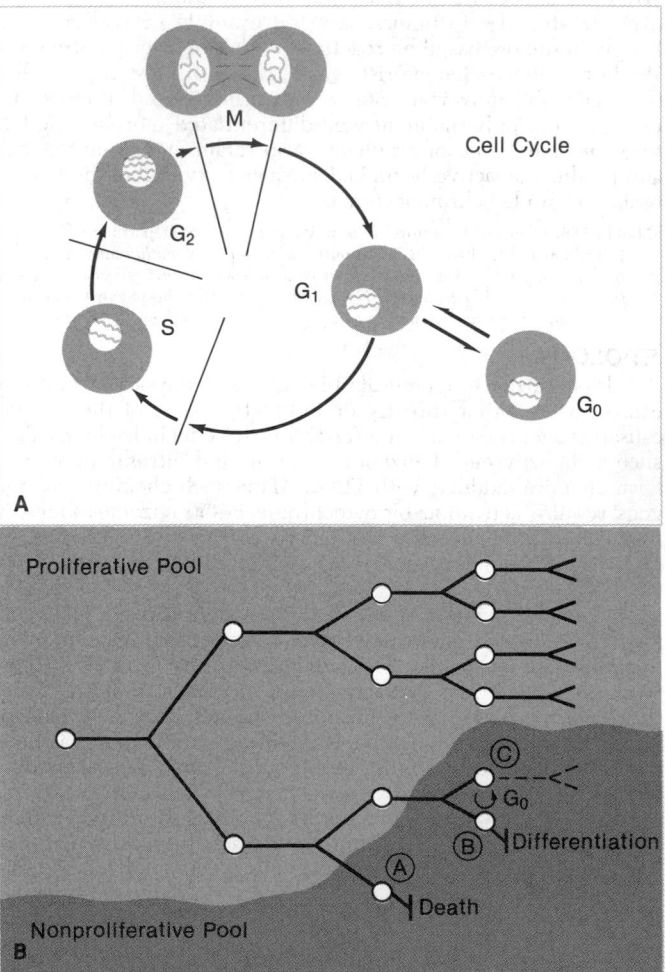

FIGURE 156–2. *A,* A diagrammatic representation of the events during the cell cycle. M is the period of mitosis—approximately 1 hour from prophase to cell division. G_1 reflects normal cell metabolism prior to DNA synthesis and usually constitutes more than half of the total cell generation time. Cells not actively undergoing replication are described as being G_0, where they may remain indefinitely or may be recruited back into the cycle. The DNA synthetic (S) phase is generally 6 to 12 hours. *B,* A schematic representation of tumor growth. As the cell population expands, a progressively higher percentage of cells leave the proliferative pool by death (A), by differentiation (B), or by entering resting phase G_0 (C), from which they may be recruited back into the proliferative pool if the population size is reduced.

cytic cells of CML patients, indicating an earlier common progenitor cell as the source of this clonal malignancy.

GROWTH KINETICS. Oncologists endeavor to quantify the growth rate of tumors as objectively as possible, using such parameters as the growth fraction of tumors, the duration of the cell cycle, the number of cells in the resting (G_O) phase, and the rate of cell death and removal (Fig. 156–2). The kinetics of tumor growth are crucial in determining prognosis and response to chemotherapy. "Doubling time" tends to be characteristic of particular tumors. *A tumor that has reached the size of clinical detectability (approximately 1 cm³) has already undergone approximately 30 doublings to reach 10^9 cells. Only 10 further doubling cycles are required to produce a tumor burden of approximately 1 kg, which is usually lethal.*

A simple exponential growth curve describes the early phase of growth of tumors (Fig. 156–3). As most tumors grow, the time required to complete a full cell cycle remains fairly constant, but an ever-increasing percentage of daughter cells enters a nonproliferating state, G_O, from which they may (potentially) be recruited back into cell cycle if the tumor cell population is reduced (see Fig. 156–2). The reasons for the progressive attenuation of proliferative rate are not completely understood but likely relate to progressive insufficiency of blood supply and hypoxia. For solid tumors, less than 30 per cent of the cells constituting the tumor mass are actively traversing the cell cycle by the time the tumor is detected; the remaining 70 per cent of cells are nonproliferating and are insensitive to most antimetabolites because they are not engaged in DNA synthesis. The progressive movement of cells into G_O and the increasing relative death rate of cells as the tumor grows larger combine to produce a slowing of the relative growth rate, reflected in a deviation of the growth curve away from a simple exponential function.

The later, clinical phases of tumor growth are best described by the Gompertz equation, which accommodates a continuous deceleration of the rate of increase in cell number with increase in tumor size. Tumors described by the Gompertz curve initially grow at a nearly exponential rate over a short span of observation, up to three or four doublings. Observation over a longer time span reveals the gradual slowing of relative growth rate (Fig. 156–3) to an eventual plateau level at which the rate of new cell production just equals the rate of cell loss. Such curves do not accommodate the heterogeneity of tumor cell population generated by mutations and the outgrowth of rapidly proliferating tumor subclones often observed in later stages of malignancy.

Strategies for cancer treatment are based on cell kinetic models (see Ch. 164). Both theoretical considerations and experimental evidence suggest that tumors are most susceptible to cytotoxic chemotherapy when their rate of proliferation is greatest, i.e., when the cell number is smallest (farthest to the left on the gompertzian curve in Fig. 156–3). Thus chemotherapy is most effective against rapidly proliferating tumors (lymphomas, leu-

kemias, testicular cancers) and when used after surgical removal of the primary tumor, as in adjuvant chemotherapy of breast cancer and colon cancer. Bulk reduction of tumor by surgery or radiation therapy is followed by a wave of increased proliferation of residual tumor cells, creating opportunities for effective introduction of chemotherapeutic modalities. The fraction of cells killed by a given exposure to chemotherapy or radiation therapy is greatest when treatment is introduced at the earliest stages in the natural history of a malignancy, thus accounting for the cure of tumors in the adjuvant setting by a therapy ineffective against metastatic disease. Even in patients with overt metastatic cancer, surgical debulking is associated with an improved response to chemotherapy in some settings, as in patients with ovarian cancer.

DeVita VT, Hellman S, Rosenberg SA (eds.): Cancer: Principles and Practice of Oncology. Philadelphia, J. B. Lippincott Company, 1989. *The introductory chapters to this standard text contain very complete background information for the clinician on the general subjects of cancer etiology, biology, and metastases.*

Fidler JJ: Origin and biology of cancer metastasis. Cytometry 10:673–680, 1990. *Presents basic concepts of the clonal origin and organ predilection of cancer metastases.*

Franks LM, Teich N (eds.): Introduction to the Cellular and Molecular Biology of Cancer. New York, Oxford University Press, 1986. *Contains excellent chapters on lineages of hematologic malignancies, phenotypic markers of differentiation, and growth regulation in normal and malignant cells.*

Ruddon RW: Cancer Biology, 2nd ed. New York, Oxford University Press, 1987. *A very readable review of all aspects of cancer biology, including epidemiology, causation, genetics, and metastases.*

STAGING, CLASSIFICATION, MARKERS, AND PROGNOSIS

Staging and biologic characterization of clinical neoplasms are essential for providing prognostic information, guiding therapy, designing and evaluating clinical trials, and communicating information among physicians. The TNM system (Table 156–2) stages tumors according to three elements: size of the primary *tumor*, involvement of regional *nodes*, and presence or absence of *metastasis*. TNM staging is particularly useful in epithelial cancers such as cancer of the head and neck, breast cancer, and most types of lung cancer. In these tumors, the orderly progression of malignancy to involve lymph nodes and later distant sites lends itself to the TNM system. Other, more simplified systems are used for hematologic malignancies, sarcomas, and pediatric tumors, which lack the same orderly progression. There is no doubt that the complex TNM system, although difficult to use and remember, provides more specific prognostic information than do the simple staging systems often used in breast cancer (Ch. 227), colon cancer (Ch. 105), and prostate cancer.

In addition to anatomic extent of disease, other determinants affect prognosis and response to treatment. Thus, immunologic and molecular probes and karyotyping have defined subsets of

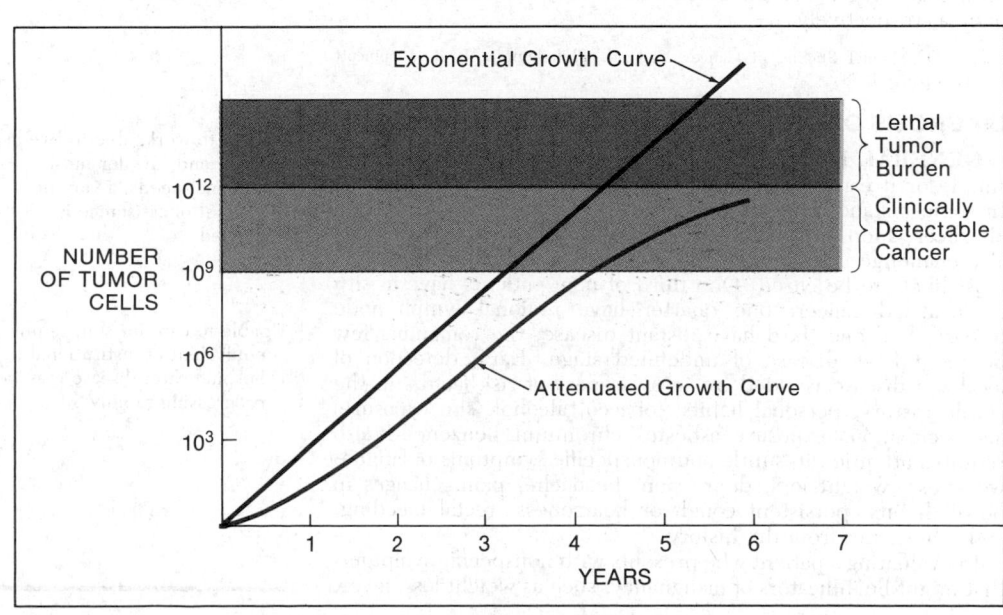

FIGURE 156–3. Schematic plot of exponential and attenuated (gompertzian) growth curves for hypothetical tumors. The clinical burden at the time of detection is probably 1 to 10 grams, depending on location and symptoms produced by the mass. The lethal body burden is also dependent on sites of involvement and impact on vital organ function. Note the slow period of tumor growth during the early preclinical phase, as the tumor establishes its blood supply and undergoes mutations that allow for unrestricted growth.

TABLE 156–2. THE TNM SYSTEM

Primary Tumor (T)

T_O	No evidence of primary tumor
T_{1b}	Carcinoma in situ
T_1, T_2, T_3, T_4	Progressive increase in tumor size and involvement, e.g., for breast cancer, 0–2 cm, 2–5, >5, any size plus skin or chest wall

Regional Lymph Nodes (N)

N_O	Regional nodes not demonstrable
N_{1a}, N_{1b}	Homolateral regional nodes (breast): metastases not suspected (a), suspected (b)
N_2, N_3	Homolateral regional nodes: fixed axillary (N_2), homolateral supraclavicular (N_3), or edema of arm; metastases suspected
N_x	Regional lymph nodes cannot be assessed clinically

Distant Metastasis (M)

M_O	No known distant metastasis
M_1	Distant metastasis present
Specific site_____	

The Manual for Staging of Cancer may be obtained free of charge from the American Joint Committee, 55 East Erie Street, Chicago, Ill. 60611.

patients with non-Hodgkin's lymphoma and with acute myelocytic leukemia who have unique clinical courses and responses to treatment. Immunophenotyping is now a standard step in defining prognosis and selecting therapy for childhood acute leukemia (Table 156–1). In breast cancer management, the clinician uses not only TNM information but also estrogen or progesterone receptor status and various measures of tumor proliferative capacity (Table 156–3) in defining prognosis and in selecting adjuvant therapy.

In addition to anatomic and biologic factors, the cancer patient's general condition influences prognosis and choice of therapy. The Karnofsky scale (Table 156–4) is the most widely used shorthand measure of a patient's performance status and, for many tumors, correlates closely with response to treatment and survival.

Other types of tumor markers may be useful in diagnosing or following the response to treatment of various cancers (see Ch. 160). Some of these are relatively specific markers such as the β-subunit of human chorionic gonadotropin and α-fetoprotein (germ-cell tumors of the testes and ovary), thyrocalcitonin (medullary carcinoma of the thyroid), serum acid phosphatase and prostate-specific antigen (prostate cancer), and monoclonal immunoglobulins (multiple myeloma). Others such as carcinoembryonic antigen (CEA) and serum lactate dehydrogenase (LDH) are less disease-specific but may nevertheless be useful indicators of disease progression for colon cancer and non-Hodgkin's lymphoma, respectively.

Beahrs O: Manual Staging of Cancer, 3rd ed. Philadelphia, J. B. Lippincott Company, 1988.

DIAGNOSIS OF CANCER AND ITS COMPLICATIONS

GENERAL EVALUATION. The diagnosis of cancer can be simple or it can challenge all the skills of clinical investigation. In some instances metastatic tumors may be the first indication of cancer, and the primary lesion may escape efforts at detection. The challenge is to detect cancer as early as possible, when it is most likely to be cured. One third of new patients have in situ or localized cancer, one quarter have regional lymph node disease, and one third have distant disease; the remaining few per cent have disease of undefined stage. Early detection of localized disease is aided by an awareness of risk factors in the family history, personal habits (tobacco, alcohol, sun exposure) and occupational exposure (asbestos, chromium, benzene). It also requires attention to subtle and nonspecific symptoms of fatigue, weakness, weight loss, depression, headache, pain, changes in bowel habits, persistent cough or hoarseness, rectal bleeding, and other clues from the history.

In evaluating a patient who presents with nonspecific symptoms that might be indicators of malignancy, such as weight loss, fever,

TABLE 156–3. TUMOR FEATURES PREDICTING HIGH RISK OF RELAPSE FOR PATIENTS WITH NODE-NEGATIVE BREAST CANCER*

Factor	High-Risk Values	5-Year Recurrence Rate	
		Low Risk	High Risk
Tumor size	> 2 cm	12%	20%
Hormonal status			
Estrogen receptor	< 10 fmol/mg protein	25%	34%
Nuclear grade	Qualitative	20%	36%
Proliferative rate			
S-phase fraction	> 7%	10%	29%
Protein expression			
Cathepsin D	Qualitative	29%	60%
Her-2/Neu	Qualitative	20%	60%

*Adapted from McGuire WL, Tandon AK, Allred DC, et al.: How to use prognostic factors in axillary node–negative breast cancer patients. J Natl Cancer Inst 82:1006, 1990.

or fatigue, the physician should carefully examine all mucosal surfaces, the sigmoid colon, and the rectum for masses or ulcerated lesions. In addition to elements of a routine examination, stool should be tested for occult blood. More subtle clues may be seen in the skin with findings such as petechiae, hyperpigmentation of skin folds (acanthosis nigricans), or atypical moles (dysplastic nevi). Attention should be paid to the presence of systemic cancer–associated effects, such as neuromyopathies (see Ch. 162 and 163). Leads from laboratory testing may be found in unexplained anemia, thrombocytopenia, hypercalcemia, or elevation of serum LDH and acid or alkaline phosphatase levels. Other frequent harbingers of cancer are pulmonary nodules or radiolucent bone lesions associated with new bone pain.

For the general internist, of equal importance is the strategy for early detection of occult malignancy in patients without complaints. Considerations of cost-effectiveness are still not resolved for many of the cancer screening tests, but their use undoubtedly saves lives. Those recommended for the average-risk individual are given in Table 156–5. For individuals from high-risk backgrounds, more frequent and earlier screening and additional tests may be indicated.

INITIAL DIAGNOSIS. Two major categories of diagnostic problems are associated with the management of cancer: obtaining the original diagnosis and correctly identifying the complications or intercurrent illnesses that may arise during the course of the

TABLE 156–4. "PERFORMANCE STATUS" (KARNOFSKY SCALE)

Criteria of Performance Status (PS)

Able to carry on normal activity; no special care is needed	100	Normal; no complaints; no evidence of disease
	90	Able to carry on normal activity; minor signs or symptoms of disease
	80	Normal activity with effort; some signs or symptoms of disease
Unable to work; able to live at home and care for most personal needs; a varying amount of assistance is needed	70	Cares for self; unable to carry on normal activity or to do active work
	60	Requires occasional assistance but is able to care for most needs
	50	Requires considerable assistance and frequent medical care
Unable to care for self; requires equivalent of institutional or hospital care; disease may be progressing rapidly	40	Disabled; requires special care and assistance
	30	Severely disabled; hospitalization is indicated although death not imminent
	20	Very sick; hospitalization necessary; active supportive treatment is necessary
	10	Moribund, fatal processes progressing rapidly
	0	Dead

TABLE 156–5. EARLY DETECTION OF OCCULT MALIGNANCY

Disease	Test Population	Screening Test	Frequency	Reduction in Cancer
Breast cancer	Women >50	Mammography	Yearly	20% reduction in deaths
Colon cancer	Men and women >50	Sigmoidoscopy	Every fifth year	Benefit unknown; 20% reduction
		Stool for occult blood	Yearly	in mortality is estimated*
Cervical cancer	Women >20	Pap smear	Yearly	>90% reduction in incidence

*See DeVita VT, Hellman S, Rosenberg SA (eds.): Cancer: Principles and Practice of Oncology. Philadelphia, J. B. Lippincott Company, 1989, pp 483–485; and Schottenfeld D, Fraumeni JF: Cancer Epidemiology and Prevention. Philadelphia, W. B. Saunders Company, 1982.

disease. A tissue diagnosis, usually from the primary site, is required in order to allow the patient and physician the certainty to embark on a plan of treatment. Although for most patients with lung, breast, or colon cancer the initial diagnosis is straightforward, some patients may present with metastatic disease but with no apparent primary lesion, or the primary mass may not be easily accessible to needle biopsy. In these patients, identification of the primary lesion and its biopsy are mandatory steps in patient management. *Indirect diagnostic techniques are not a substitute for a histologic or cytologic diagnosis of cancer.* Rarely it may not be possible to obtain tissue for histologic diagnosis, e.g., when there is a deep-seated brain tumor or when the patient's general condition is so poor that the malignancy has little bearing on prognosis.

Physicians often face the diagnostic dilemma posed by the discovery of a metastatic lesion of unknown primary site. In searching for the primary, two rules apply: *The clinician must consider the most common type of cancer in the given subject, taking into account age, sex, site of disease, and personal and family history, and must rule out the most treatable lesions, such as breast cancer in women and testicular cancer in young males.* Special immunohistologic or electron microscopic studies may be required to rule out malignant melanoma or lymphoma. The finding of mediastinal, retroperitoneal, or lymph node involvement and high human chorionic gonadotropin or α-fetoprotein levels are indicative of germ-cell tumors. Cisplatin-based chemotherapy programs may cure such patients.

DIAGNOSTIC PROBLEMS DURING CONTINUING CARE OF THE PATIENT WITH CANCER. The physician who undertakes the continuing care of a patient with cancer must be vigilant in promptly identifying complications arising from the progression of tumor and in detecting curable intercurrent illness that may be mistaken for manifestations of cancer itself. The patient with a known tumor who develops anorexia, weight loss, and jaundice may have cholecystitis and biliary obstruction rather than metastatic cancer and may die from that disorder unless the correct diagnosis is established. Furthermore, some potentially treatable conditions are actually caused by the cancer therapy—postoperative adhesions or radiation-induced strictures leading to bowel obstruction or chemotherapy-induced immunosuppression leading to an opportunistic fungal infection. Certain drugs may even produce complications that simulate paraneoplastic syndromes, such as inappropriate secretion of ADH, neuromyopathy, or cerebellar degeneration. Although errors in diagnosis of intercurrent medical and surgical illness sometimes seem almost inevitable, the best way to minimize these problems is to *assume that each new condition is due to a nonmalignant process, until it is proven otherwise. First recurrences of cancer must always be confirmed by biopsy because of their profound implications.*

PRINCIPLES OF MANAGEMENT OF THE PATIENT WITH CANCER

Subsequent chapters will outline strategies for the use of chemotherapy in patients with cancer, in addition to discussions of approaches to specific types of cancer. In this chapter, general principles of value in choosing therapies and in management of patients will be considered.

APPROACHES TO TREATMENT. A therapeutic strategy should be clearly defined for each patient with cancer, once the diagnosis has been firmly established, staging of the tumor has been carried out, and careful assessment has been made of the patient's overall physical, physiologic, and social situation. Such a strategy is often best devised by a multidisciplinary team,

including medical, surgical, and radiation oncologists who will weigh the possibilities of cure or significant palliation, consider the various treatment options and their expected untoward effects, and then define the best therapy for that patient. *Wherever possible, cancer treatment should be given according to standard protocols or as part of a peer-reviewed therapeutic trial, such as offered by the cooperative group program of the National Cancer Institute.* Detailed information about such trials and state-of-the-art therapies for specific types of cancer is available through the PDQ (Physicians Data Query) computer base, which is available at all medical school libraries and most tertiary-care hospitals in the United States. Trials information is also available through the National Cancer Institute's Cancer Information Service (1–800–4–CANCER). Improvisation, such as dosage attenuation, drug substitution, or changes in treatment schedule should not be undertaken unless there are compelling reasons for such changes.

Fortunately, the therapeutic horizons are constantly changing and improving. For example, patients with disseminated testicular cancer, acute lymphocytic leukemia, Ewing's sarcoma, Wilms' tumor, ovarian carcinoma, Hodgkin's disease, and histiocytic lymphoma now have an excellent chance for a cure. Cure is possible for a smaller fraction of patients with acute myelocytic leukemias, advanced ovarian cancer, and childhood sarcomas, and significantly palliative therapy is available for many additional patients with advanced cancer. Effective adjuvant therapies have been defined for early stages of breast cancer and colorectal cancer. Surgery or radiation therapy are the predominant forms of primary treatment. Although surgery is the sole initial treatment for over 50 per cent of patients with localized cancer, the use of adjuvant chemotherapy either before or after surgery is increasing. *Neoadjuvant chemotherapy*—defined as the use of drugs prior to surgery or radiotherapy to reduce the bulk of a primary tumor and thereby to render it more amenable to surgical removal or cure by radiotherapy—is being used with increasing frequency for head and neck, esophageal, and breast cancers. Combined-modality therapies reduce the extent of primary surgery required to cure limb sarcomas, bladder cancer, anal cancer, breast cancer, and head and neck cancer, thus preserving organ function and avoiding debilitation. The difficulty of attempting to predict tumor response to chemotherapy may one day be overcome through sensitivity tests in vitro, but for the present the selection process for drug regimens depends upon prior reports of clinical trials for particular types of cancer.

For patients with metastatic cancer, chemotherapy presents the only well-studied and well-understood alternative, although there is increasing experience with experimental biologic therapies. Chemotherapy should be administered only by physicians who have training and experience in its use and who are willing to use it with sufficient intensity to achieve optimal results. A thorough knowledge of the mechanisms of action, pharmacokinetics, routes of elimination, side effects, and interactions of the various chemotherapeutic drugs and irradiation is necessary to administer these agents with optimal safety and effectiveness. The risk of serious side effects may be much more acceptable to a patient who stands a good chance for a cure than to one who does not. After careful explanation by the physician of all options, the patient and his or her family must make the ultimate decisions about treatment. Therefore, good patient-doctor communication is essential for weighing treatment options.

One of the most difficult ethical dilemmas faced in cancer chemotherapy is the consideration of bone marrow transplantation, an expensive and dangerous procedure, in patients who have exhausted standard treatment alternatives. This decision requires a candid assessment of costs, likely therapeutic benefits, possible side effects, and the ability of the patient to withstand the emotional and physical stress of high-dose chemotherapy, the prolonged leukopenic interval, and in allogeneic transplants the immunosuppression required following transplant. No other setting in clinical practice more graphically poses the dilemma of a high-risk, potentially fatal, but possibly curative therapy as an alternative to a certain fatal outcome.

SUPPORTIVE CARE. In its broadest sense, "supportive care" refers to all types of medical care required to provide for the needs of the patient with cancer. Certain specific supportive-care programs for patients receiving aggressive chemotherapy for leukemia and other conditions have led to gratifying improvements in cure rates by anticipating and/or counteracting potentially fatal complications such as *infection* and *bleeding*. Early detection and vigorous antibacterial and antifungal treatment can be lifesaving for infected patients during periods of severe granulocytopenia. Similarly, platelet transfusions can minimize the risk of hemorrhage during periods of profound thrombocytopenia (platelet count less than 20,000 per cubic millimeter). These two advances, together with aggressive systemic and intrathecal chemotherapy, are responsible for the greater than 50 per cent cure rate that can now be achieved in childhood leukemia, for example. Most recently the availability of bone marrow colony-stimulating factors has allowed for abrogation of leukopenia and escalation of treatment dosage in conjunction with chemotherapy.

Severe *nausea* and *vomiting* induced by combination chemotherapy may be major, even limiting, factors in patient compliance because of the serious deterioration in the quality of life induced by these potent drugs. These side effects can largely be suppressed by newer antiemetics, such as the 5-hydroxytryptophan receptor antagonists. Anxiety, a very important part of the symptom complex, can be alleviated by benzodiazepines such as lorazepam.

General supportive care requires attention to nutritional, rehabilitative, psychosocial, and analgesic needs (see below). Anorexia and weight loss are almost invariably associated with advanced cancer; occasionally profound *cachexia* may occur in a patient with only a small and apparently localized lesion such as lung cancer. There are several potential explanations for nutritional problems—anatomic obstructions to chewing, swallowing, or digestion; liver disease; paraneoplastic syndromes; effects of chemotherapy; depression, or the release of peptides such as cachectin. In the individual patient it is often difficult to sort out the factors that contribute to anorexia and hypercatabolism. Regardless of etiology it is important to reverse this catabolic trend, since malnourished patients tolerate the usual courses of chemotherapy or radiation therapy very poorly and may die prematurely of complications related to treatment toxicity. Thus, in the case of a patient with recurrent cancer of the head and neck, improvement in nutrition is often a necessary prerequisite to the use of chemotherapeutic drugs. Increasingly, oncologists employ parenteral or tube feedings prior to major cancer surgery, radiation therapy, or chemotherapy. The dietitian familiar with the practical problems faced by these patients is an essential member of the team working with the patient and family.

The *psychosocial problems* that may be encountered by patients with cancer are profound and varied. Many of these are not unique to cancer and occur in age-matched patients with other types of chronic illness and shortened life expectancy. Shock, bereavement, anger, denial, withdrawal, and depression are common responses of people faced with such overwhelming problems. Disfigurement, feelings of shame and disgrace, loss of sexual activity, and job discrimination are problems that are more prevalent in patients with cancer than in those with many other illnesses. *The attitude of the physician and staff* is of key importance in helping the patient make the best possible adjustment, given all of the premorbid factors and limitations imposed by the illness. The physician who (verbally or nonverbally) conveys the impression that "There is nothing further that I can do" is sentencing his patient to untold misery or forcing him into the waiting arms of enthusiastic cancer quacks. All patients need help. Most patients respond positively to it, and they appreciate a gently supportive role that stresses honesty, trust, and a willingness simply to be available to help both patient and family with their fears and needs.

The *care of the patient who is dying of cancer* is the most sensitive issue for both patient and family. This is also commonly the period in which patients feel abandoned by physicians who themselves are frustrated by their inability to cure or cause remission of the illness and by the tragic human circumstances that often accompany such illnesses. Indeed, these take their toll on doctors and nurses as well as on relatives and friends, and busy cancer clinics recognize the need for support groups for their staff. (Indeed, unless there is an active self-renewing effort, oncology workers are subject to "burnout," an insidious syndrome difficult to recognize.) The physician must always prepare a reassuring setting so that when specific therapy is no longer warranted, patient comfort will be attended to in a considerate and thoughtful manner. In the final weeks of the illness, family members may require even more attention than the patient, and the team of doctor, nurse, social worker, and chaplain should provide the necessary support for all concerned, including staff.

Patients fear *pain* perhaps more than any other aspect of cancer, and there are many misconceptions about this subject by the public. Yet adequate techniques are available to control pain in most patients, if these are used in a timely and appropriate manner (see Ch. 8 and 26). Here, again, a careful history is an important initial step in diagnosis, for a patient with pain may have anything from cord compression to bone metastasis to a nonmalignant condition such as arthritis. Pain suppression is not a substitute for identification and treatment of a specific lesion. Relatively simple radiotherapy or neurosurgical procedures employed sufficiently early for localized pain and the *liberal use of narcotics for severe generalized pain* are usually successful in alleviating symptoms. One need not be concerned with potential narcotic addiction in dying patients. Patients themselves are often reluctant to take adequate doses of analgesics because of fears of addiction and should be encouraged to take them with sufficient frequency to alleviate pain *before* it becomes very severe.

Depending on the wishes of the family, it is often preferable to provide for the care of the dying patient in his or her own home. This can be done with a home care program supplemented by visiting nurses and volunteers. *Hospice programs* are rapidly developing in the United States, and these can provide the supportive ingredients for both the patient and family that others cannot supply. The patient is often much more comfortable in familiar surroundings near loved ones. Family and friends usually respond willingly to their duties when properly directed. Finally, the savings in costly hospitalizations can conserve already depleted financial resources. Indeed, careful curbing of unnecessary costly tests and interventions can make an enormous financial difference over the course of the illness.

Bonadonna G: Does chemotherapy fulfill its expectations in cancer treatment? Ann Oncol 1:11–21, 1990. *A thoughtful appraisal of the contributions of chemotherapy to cancer treatment by one of the pioneers of modern combination therapy regimens.*

Chabner BA, Collins JM (eds.): Cancer Chemotherapy, Principles and Practice. Philadelphia, J. B. Lippincott Company, 1990. *A detailed presentation of all pertinent aspects of anticancer drugs, including pharmacokinetics, dose adjustments for renal and hepatic dysfunction, drug interactions, and the rational design of protocols.*

McGuire WL, Tandon AK, Allred DC, et al.: How to use prognostic factors in axillary node–negative breast cancer patients. J Natl Cancer Inst 82:1006–1015, 1990. *A landmark paper summarizing the use of biochemical and molecular markers for prognosis in breast cancer.*

Physician Data Query (PDQ), National Cancer Institute: *PDQ is available to physicians at most medical libraries, at many hospitals, or through private computer software vendors* and contains information on state-of-the-art treatments for each pathologic type of cancer, as well as a listing of experimental protocols for each disease.*

---

*PDQ vendors for health professional inquiries as of November 1988: MEDLARS Management Section, National Library of Medicine, Bldg. 38, Rm 4N421, 8600 Rockville Pike, Bethesda, MD 20894, (301) 496–6193, (800) 638–8480; BRS/Saunders COLLEAGUE, 1350 Avenue of the Americas, Suite 1802, New York, NY 10019, 1–800–468–0908, in Pennsylvania or outside continental USA (215) 527–4155; Mead Data Central, MEDIS, 9333 Springboro Pike, Dayton, OH 45401, 1–800–277–4908; TELMED, Jakob Fugli Strasse 18, Postfach, CH-8048 Zurich, Switzerland; MEDIMATICA, Heemraadssingel, 3021 DM Rotterdam, The Netherlands.

157 Oncogenes

J. Michael Bishop

CANCER AS A GENETIC DISEASE

Astute observers have long nurtured the thought that cancer might be at its heart a genetic disease. The thought was at first vague and arose from seemingly disparate discoveries that included the existence of heritable diatheses to cancer, the presence of abnormal chromosomes in cancer cells, and the likelihood that many carcinogens act by inducing mutations in cellular DNA. Medical geneticists and epidemiologists first conceived the possibility of "cancer genes," prompted by occasional examples of human tumors whose occurrence seemed dictated by recessive or dominant inherited traits. Now the long-imagined cancer genes have been brought to view, first unearthed by two experimental strategies: the use of viruses that cause tumors in animals and the search for tumorigenic genes in the DNA of cancer cells. From these studies we have learned that the human genome contains a set of several dozen genes that may lie at the heart of every cancer. These genes take two forms. Some act in a dominant manner when mutated and are known as either proto-oncogenes or cellular oncogenes. Others are recessive when mutated and are known variously as tumor suppressor genes, recessive oncogenes, or (least desirably) anti-oncogenes. The discovery and isolation of these genes represent our present best hope of achieving an understanding of the molecular mechanisms by which cancer arises. We now have in view a keyboard on which many different carcinogens may play, the possible components of a final common pathway to neoplastic growth.

FIRST DESCRIPTIONS: VIRAL ONCOGENES

Documentation that specific genes can elicit cancerous growth emerged first from the study of viruses that cause tumors in animals. By the use of formal genetic analyses, and later of recombinant DNA, investigators were able to show that the tumorigenicity of many viruses can be attributed to viral germs now known as oncogenes.

The most decisive paradigm for the genetic origins of cancer came from the study of retroviruses, whose genes are carried in RNA but are copied into DNA by reverse transcriptase early in viral replication. The life cycle of retroviruses provides a microcosm of carcinogenesis (Fig. 157–1). The viral DNA produced by reverse transcriptase is inserted (or "integrated") into the chromosomal DNA of the host cell. Thereafter, the cell uses its own machinery to express the integrated viral genes. These events hold two possibilities for carcinogenesis.

First, the integration of viral DNA is potentially mutagenic: It can damage vital cellular genes, and it can influence their expression by bringing them under the sway of powerful viral signals. Virologists call this *insertional mutagenesis;* it may indeed be tumorigenic (see below), and the cellular genes perverted by viral DNA are candidate "proto-oncogenes."

Second, some (but not all) retroviruses carry oncogenes whose expression is sufficient to give rise to cancerous growth. The oncogenes of retroviruses make no apparent contribution to viral replication; therefore, their presence in viral genomes posed a puzzle. The puzzle was solved with the discovery that retroviral oncogenes are not viral genes at all, but wayward copies of cellular genes acquired during the course of viral replication by a process known formally as transduction, and carried as mere passengers in the viral genome. It is likely that transduction by retroviruses is a rare accident of nature, without design for the virus, and attributable to details of the curious means by which retroviruses replicate. There is no reason to believe that the transduction is limited to genes with tumorigenic potential. However, transduction of proto-oncogenes by retroviruses is of particular importance because it has brought to view cellular genes whose activities may be central to all forms of carcinogenesis.

THE PATHOGENIC MECHANISMS OF RETROVIRAL ONCOGENES

The study of viral oncogenes began with the hope that the mechanisms by which these genes act might help to reveal the

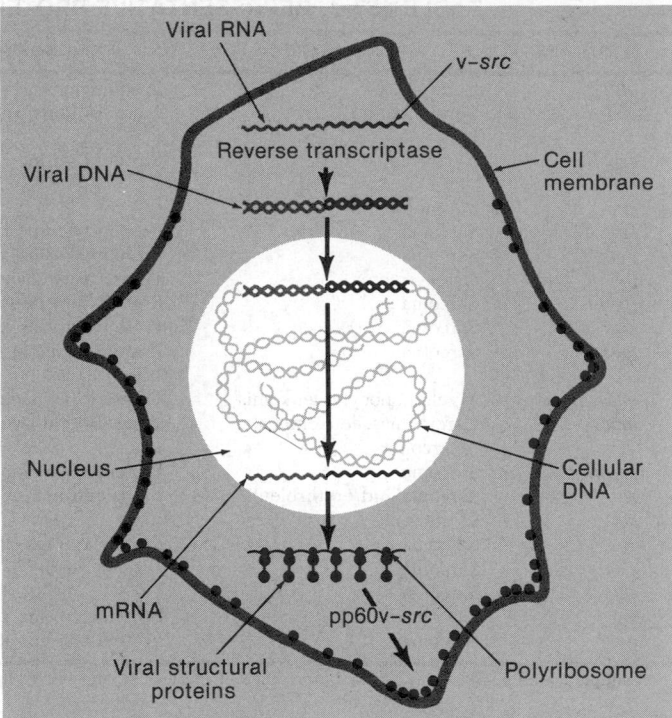

FIGURE 157–1. The molecular life cycle of retroviruses leads to insertion of viral genes into the chromosome of the host cell and the subsequent production of viral proteins that can transform the cell to neoplastic growth. In the example illustrated, the protein encoded by the *src* oncogene of the Rous sarcoma virus attaches to the inner surface of the plasma membrane and catalyzes phosphorylation of tyrosine residues in cellular proteins. (Modified from Bishop JM: Oncogenes and proto-oncogenes. Hosp Pract *18:*68, 1983, with permission from HP Publishing Co., Inc.)

inner workings of the cancer cell, to elucidate the biochemical abnormalities that prompt cancerous growth. This is now a burgeoning prospect because the number of retroviral oncogenes has grown to at least 20, each inducing specific forms of malignancy, each encoding a protein whose action apparently causes harm (Table 157–1). The first hint of how informative these genes might be came with the discovery that several retroviral oncogenes encode protein kinases, located on the plasma membrane of the cell and possessing a previously unencountered substrate specificity for tyrosine. Phosphorylation of tyrosine was discovered first through the study of retroviral oncogenes. But we now know that this same reaction is represented by hundreds, perhaps thousands, of enzymes within normal cells and that it plays a vital role in the governance of normal cellular phenotype. It would be difficult to envision a better explanation for neoplastic transformation: By phosphorylating numerous cellular proteins, a single enzyme could rapidly change myriad aspects of cellular structure and function. As the phosphorylated proteins are found (only a few have been, to date), doors are opened to the secrets of neoplastic growth.

Protein phosphorylation is not the only means by which retroviral oncogenes may act (Table 157–1). As more and more of the proteins encoded by oncogenes came into view, a provocative diversity emerged: Some of the proteins are protein kinases, others are GTP-binding proteins or transcription factors; some act in the nucleus of the cell, some in the cytoplasm, some at the plasma membrane (Fig. 157–2); and there is little correlation between what we now know of how oncogenes function and the character of their tumorigenicities. What does this diversity signify? The growth of cells is regulated by an interdigitating network that spans from the surface of the plasma membrane to the depths of the nucleus. If that network were to be touched at any point by an adverse influence and tilted out of balance, cancerous growth might ensue. It is now clear that the diverse means by which different oncogenes act mirror various components of the regulatory network, revealing how the network

TABLE 157–1. REPRESENTATIVE PROTEINS ENCODED BY RETROVIRAL ONCOGENES

Oncogenes	Tumorigenicity	Biochemical Properties	Subcellular Location	Cellular Homologue
abl	Lymphoma	Protein tyrosine kinase	Plasma membrane	
erb-A	Supplemental	Transcriptional repressor	Nucleus	Receptor for thyroid hormone
erb-B	Erythroleukemia	Protein tyrosine kinase	Intracellular and plasma membranes	Receptor for EGF
ets	Supplemental	?	Nucleus	
fgr	Sarcoma	Protein tyrosine kinase	Plasma membrane	
fims	Sarcoma	Protein tyrosine kinase	Plasma membrane	Receptor for CSF-1
fos	Osteosarcoma	Transcription factor	Nucleus	Transcription factor AP-1
fps/fes*	Sarcoma	Protein tyrosine kinase	Plasma membrane	
kit	Sarcoma	Protein tyrosine kinase	Plasma membrane	
mos	Sarcoma	Protein serine kinase	Cytoplasm	Embryonic cytostatic factor
myb	Myelomonocytic leukemia	Transcription factor	Nucleus	
myc	Carcinomas, leukemia and sarcoma	Transcription factor	Nucleus	
raf/mht/mil*	Sarcoma	Protein serine kinase	Membranes	
ras	Sarcoma and erythroleukemia	Binds and hydrolyzes GTP	Plasma membrane	GTPase regulatory proteins
rel	Lymphoma	?	?	
ros	Sarcoma	Protein tyrosine kinase	Plasma membrane	
sis	Sarcoma	Growth factor	Cytoplasm	Subunit β of PDGF
ski	Sarcoma	?	Nucleus	
src	Sarcoma	Protein tyrosine kinase	Plasma membrane	
yes	Sarcoma	Protein tyrosine kinase	Plasma membrane	

*Multiple names denote genes isolated from different species but later proved to be homologous.

performs its task. By studying oncogenes, we are learning of both cancerous and normal growth at one and the same time. It is an old adage of medical science that study of the abnormal can reveal the normal.

PROTO-ONCOGENES AND ONCOGENES

The cellular genes whose transduction engenders retroviral oncogenes provided the first glimpse and the first definition of proto-oncogenes. By all available criteria, these are cellular genes, not viral genes in disguise. They can be found in every member of every vertebrate species examined, probably in all metazoan organisms. Evolutionary conservation of this magnitude signifies that the proto-oncogenes serve essential functions for the species in which they are harbored. Proto-oncogenes are expressed in normal cells and tissues, and their expression can vary from one tissue to another, from one embryologic lineage to another, from one time in embryogenesis to another. It is widely assumed that, in their normal guise, proto-oncogenes help to control the growth and development of cells and organisms. This assumption has been strengthened by two discoveries. First, a number of proto-

oncogenes encode proteins known to participate in the regulation of cellular proliferation and differentiation, including platelet-derived growth factor (PDGF) and the receptors for epidermal growth factor (EGF) and colony-stimulating factor I (CSF-I) (Table 157–1). Second, mutations in the proto-oncogenes of fruit flies (*Drosophila melanogaster*) and laboratory mice cause profound disturbances of growth and development.

Why are the transduced forms of proto-oncogenes tumorigenic? What converts a proto-oncogene, a compliant member of the cellular citizenry, to an oncogene—an unruly and potentially lethal enemy? The possible answers to these questions have taken two general forms: Transduction may have unleashed the genes from their usual controls and inappropriate expression of otherwise normal genes might be the fatal flaw; alternatively, mutation during or after transduction could change the structure of the genes and the proteins they encode, giving rise to abnormal function. For the moment, it appears that either explanation may on occasion apply.

PROTO-ONCOGENES AS CANCER GENES

Do proto-oncogenes participate in many or all forms of tumorigenesis? Are they a common keyboard for all the players in carcinogenesis? Since these questions were first raised, the pertinent evidence has grown from a thin thread to a rich and provocative fabric of experimental observation.

1. Direct manipulation of proto-oncogenes isolated by molecular cloning has revealed that some (but not all) of these ostensibly normal genes can elicit neoplastic growth if they are first attached to viral signals that command vigorous gene expression and then inserted into cells in culture or used to create transgenic mice.

2. There is evidence that retroviruses without oncogenes of their own initiate tumorigenesis by the mutation of proto-oncogenes. The mutations may be of two sorts: those that enhance expression of a gene and those that change the structure of the protein(s) encoded by a gene.

3. Some human tumors (the exact number is not yet clear) display karyotypic evidence of gene amplification (double-minute chromosomes and homogeneously staining regions in marker chromosomes) and contain one or another proto-oncogene whose number has been multiplied as much as 200-fold over normal. As a consequence of amplification, the proto-oncogene is expressed in inordinately large amounts. Amplification of proto-oncogenes has been found in two patterns: as sporadic and occasional features of diverse tumors and as a common feature of particular tumors. The latter pattern gives promise of being

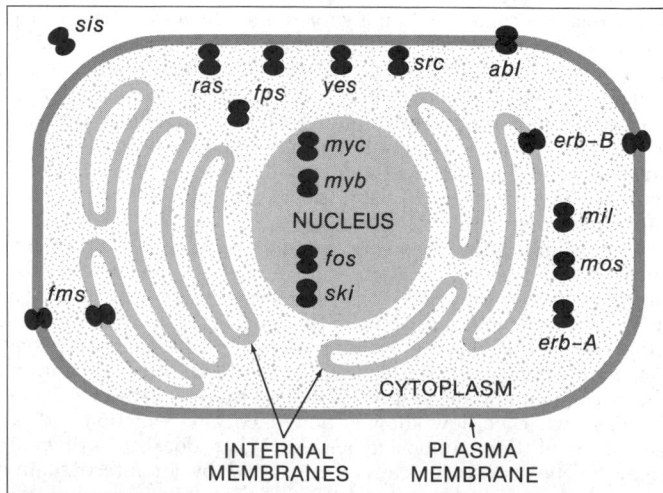

FIGURE 157–2. The products of oncogenes assume diverse locations within the cell, where they perform functions involved in the regulation of cellular growth and differentiation. (Modified from The Proteins of Oncogenes, by T. Hunter. Copyright © 1984 by Scientific American, Inc. All rights reserved.)

clinically useful. For example, amplification of the proto-oncogenes NMYC and NEU are common features of neuroblastoma and carcinoma of the breast, respectively, and apparently connote a poor prognosis.

4. At least several of the chromosomal translocations that typify a substantial variety of human tumors affect a proto-oncogene. As a consequence, expression of the proto-oncogene may be altered, or the gene may sustain mutations within the domain that encodes a protein. Representative examples include Burkitt's lymphoma (translocation of the proto-oncogene c-myc) and the Philadelphia chromosome (Ph¹) of chronic myelogenous leukemia (translocation of c-abl).

5. Application of DNA from a variety of human tumors to cells in culture can elicit neoplastic growth, as if the DNA contained oncogenes of the sort once found only in viruses. Approximately 20 per cent of all human tumors demonstrate activity of this type, no matter what their histopathology. The responsible genes have now been identified for a substantial variety of tumors. With remarkable frequency, they have proved to be one or another member of a family of proto-oncogenes known as *ras* genes and already familiar to us from the study of retroviruses. The *ras* genes have transforming activity because they have suffered mutations that change single amino acids in the protein products of the genes.

RECESSIVE GENETIC DAMAGE IN TUMORS

The oncogenes considered so far are thought to be genetically dominant: Their abnormalities have an impact even when a normal allele of the same gene is also present in the cell. But most if not all human tumors also bear lesions that are recessive, that make their presence known only when no normal counterpart is present. By inference from karyotypes and by the use of restriction endonucleases, substantial evidence has been obtained for the presence of recessive mutations in a variety of tumors. In each instance, the tumor is presumed to be entirely deficient in the function of at least one gene whose activity helps to regulate cellular proliferation. The examples of retinoblastoma and Wilms' tumor are the most celebrated, but other (and more common) examples are now also in view (Table 157–2). Four of the genes affected by recessive damage have been isolated to date: RB1, a gene first associated with the genesis and inheritance of retinoblastoma but now incriminated in a variety of other malignancies as well; a gene known as P53, named for the protein that it encodes and recessively damaged in a variety of human tumors; DCC, a gene deleted from a majority of adenocarcinomas of the colon; and WT1, a gene reputed to be involved in Wilms' tumor. Isolation of these "tumor suppressor genes" is a difficult endeavor and represents one form of medical research that would be greatly facilitated by having a complete physical map of the human genome—the first step in the controversial Human Genome Project.

Inheritance of recessive mutations can explain hereditary diatheses to several forms of neoplasm (again, retinoblastoma and Wilms' tumor are the seminal examples). By contrast, there is as yet no evidence to implicate any of the dominant oncogenes in the inheritance of cancer.

ONCOGENES AND THE MULTIPLE STEPS IN CARCINOGENESIS

The attribution of tumorigenesis to genetic damage seemed at first glance simplistic, since the genesis of tumors has long been described as a protracted and complex sequence of events. However, the identification of oncogenes and the proto-oncogenes from which they are derived has given us a tool with which to recognize several separate steps in tumorigenesis. Catalogues of genetic damage within individual tumors are taking shape, revealing how the malfunction of several different genes might combine to produce the malignant phenotype. For example, carcinomas of the colon contain no less than five different yet prevalent lesions—some genetically dominant, others recessive—and a similar plurality of lesions has emerged in carcinomas of the breast (five) and lung (four) and in neuroblastoma (three). It has even been possible to decipher the approximate order in which genetic lesions accumulate during the genesis of carcinoma of the colon. The phenomenon of tumor progression is moving rapidly from the realm of mystery to the realm of molecular

TABLE 157–2. REPRESENTATIVE RECESSIVE GENETIC LESIONS IN HUMAN CANCER

Tumor	Chromosomal Locus	Gene Incriminated
Retinoblastoma	13(q14)	RB1
Wilms' tumor	11(p13)	WT1
	11(p15)	?
Beckwith-Wiedemann syndrome (embryonal tumors)	11(p15)	?
Carcinoma of lung	3(p21)	?
	13(q14)	RB1
	17(p12–p13)	P53
Carcinoma of breast	3p	?
	11p	?
	13(q14)	RB1
Carcinoma of colon	5(q21–q22)	?
	17(p12–p13)	P53
	18(q21)	DCC
Neuroblastoma	1(p36.1)	?

reality. Moreover, detection of the lesions responsible for progression is likely to provide information useful for prognosis and therapeutic management.

THE FUTURE

By one means or another, more than a dozen genes have been implicated in the genesis of human tumors. In some instances, expression of the gene is enhanced or the structure of the gene product is changed, giving a dominant effect on function; in other instances, mutations eliminate the function of the gene in a recessive manner. Combinations of these events apparently lead to most if not all human tumors. These are remarkable conclusions, reached within a decade of the discovery of proto-oncogenes. However, the unknown still outweighs the known. How extensive is the role of proto-oncogenes in tumorigenesis? How are we to explain those human tumors that as yet offer no evidence of genetic lesions? How important are recessive genetic traits in tumorigenesis, how are they to be identified, and by what means do they act? What is the nature of heritable susceptibility to carcinogenesis and does this diathesis ever originate from proto-oncogenes? How do the proteins encoded by oncogenes conduct their nefarious business? Will we be able to parlay the growing information about oncogenes into devices for the prevention, diagnosis, and treatment of human cancer? It is too early to foretell how quickly the answers to these questions may come, but there now seems little reason to doubt that we have laid hold of cancer with a grip that should eventually extract the deadly secrets of the disease.

Bishop JM: The molecular biology of RNA tumor viruses: A physician's guide. N Engl J Med 303:675, 1980.

Bishop JM: Oncogenes. Sci Am 246(3):80, 1982.

Bishop JM: Trends in oncogenes. Trends Genet 1:245, 1985.

Bishop JM: The molecular genetics of cancer. Science 235:305, 1987.

Bishop JM: Oncogenes and clinical cancer. In Weinberg RA (ed.): Oncogenes and the Molecular Origins of Cancer. New York, Cold Spring Harbor Press, 1989, pp 327–358.

Hunter T: The proteins of oncogenes. Sci Am 251(2):70, 1984.

Sager R: Tumor suppressor genes: The puzzle and the promise. Science 246:1406, 1989.

Varmus HE: The molecular genetics of cellular oncogenes. Ann Rev Genet 18:553, 1984.

Weinberg RA: A molecular basis of cancer. Sci Am 249(5):126, 1983.

All of these references offer general reviews of this rapidly expanding area of medical research.

158 The Epidemiology of Cancer

William J. Blot

This chapter describes the distribution and causes of cancer in human populations. Through increased understanding of the patterns and determinants of the specific tumors, strategies can

TABLE 158–1. INTERNATIONAL VARIATION IN AGE-ADJUSTED INCIDENCE RATES FOR SELECTED CANCERS

Cancer Site	High-Rate Areas*	Rate†	Baseline Rate‡
Oral cavity	France, India	35–45	1–2
Nasopharynx	China, Hong Kong	30	<1
Esophagus	China, Iran	100+	1–2
Stomach	Japan	80	5
Colon/rectum	U.S., Australia	50–60	6
Liver	China	30	1
Pancreas	U.S. blacks	15	1
Larynx	Brazil	20	2
Lung	U.S. blacks	100	6
Skin melanoma	Australia	30	<1
Breast	U.S.	90	20
Uterine cervix	Brazil, Colombia, India	40–80	4
Ovary	Norway, Pacific Islands	15–25	4
Prostate	U.S. blacks	90	2
Bladder	U.S. whites, Spain	25–30	2
Non-Hodgkin's lymphoma	Switzerland	10	1
Hodgkin's disease	Canada	5	<1
Multiple myeloma	U.S. blacks	10	<1
Leukemia	Canada	12	2–3
Total	U.S. blacks	**400**	**100**

*Country in which high-rate areas occur is listed. The high rates do not necessarily persist throughout the country.

†Approximate age-adjusted (world standard) incidence rate per year per 100,000 population among males (except for breast, cervix, and ovarian cancers). Data collection periods vary by area but typically center on 1980.

‡Approximate age-adjusted incidence rate in typical low-rate area.

be developed to prevent cancer. Astute clinical observations can play a key role in this process, providing etiologic clues that can be evaluated by systematic epidemiologic investigations.

DESCRIPTIVE PATTERNS

THE GEOGRAPHY OF CANCER. Cancer affects all the world's populations, with about a threefold difference between areas with the highest and lowest age-adjusted rates. For certain cancers, the difference exceeds 100-fold (Table 158–1). Perhaps the most distinctive geographic patterns are seen for esophageal cancer. Pockets of exceptionally high mortality exist in areas of north central China, the Caspian littoral of Iran, and South Africa. In Linxian, China, for as yet unknown reasons, esophageal/gastric cardia cancer is the most common cause of death, causing over 30 per cent of all fatalities among adults. Clustering of elevated esophageal cancer rates has also been observed in parts of Europe and the United States. Heavy alcohol intake has been implicated in western populations, most recently in coastal South Carolina, where high rates of esophageal cancer among black men have been linked to consumption of moonshine whiskeys.

Geographic variation for other tumors is also noteworthy. Rates of oral cancer are highest in India and parts of south central Asia. Within the United States, elevated oral cancer mortality among females is found in the southern states, especially in rural areas. In both instances the cause is the same—high use of smokeless tobacco. Indeed, it was the observation of excess oral cancer mortality rates in several southern states, combined with clinical case descriptions, that led to epidemiologic investigations that in the early 1980's conclusively showed that snuff use can induce oral tumors. Among long-term users, risks of cancers of the gums and buccal mucosa, tissues in direct contact with the tobacco powder, were increased nearly 50-fold over those for tobacco abstainers.

In southeastern China, nasopharyngeal cancer is the most common malignancy. It is also a leading cancer among Alaskan Aleuts and Eskimos and occurs more frequently among Chinese than caucasian or black Americans. The primary cause of the cancer in southern China appears to be consumption of salted fish, especially during weaning and early childhood. The importance of early life events is also suggested by the up to threefold higher rates of nasopharyngeal cancer among Chinese-Americans

born and raised in China than among those born and raised in the United States. Similar migrant effects are seen for stomach cancer. Japanese-Americans born in Japan, where rates of stomach cancer are among the highest in the world, have a two- to threefold higher incidence of this cancer than Japanese-Americans born in the United States. American-born Japanese in turn experience more than twice the incidence of stomach cancer of white Americans. Such differences in rates suggest the strong influence of environmental factors.

The most common cancers in western countries, those of the lung, large bowel, and breast, also vary geographically. Within the United States, the highest rates of lung cancer are now found in the south. In the 1980's lung cancer mortality in southern rural counties surpassed that in northern cities, reversing a longstanding pattern. The shifts in lung cancer follow changes in cigarette smoking, now more prevalent in the south than elsewhere in the country. In addition, certain southern port and coastal areas still maintain excess lung cancer rates among males as a legacy of occupational exposures to asbestos in shipyards during World War II, when shipbuilding was the largest manufacturing industry in the United States. Colon and breast cancer show a contrasting pattern, with high rates in the northeast and low rates in the south, but the differentials are not large.

U.S. CANCER RATES AND TRENDS. It is estimated that in 1990 nearly 1,000,000 Americans developed and 500,000 died from cancer. Table 158–2 presents age-adjusted incidence rates during 1983 to 1987 (the most recent 5-year period for which complete data are available) for 28 cancers. The data derive from areas of the country participating in the SEER program of cancer registries (covering approximately 10 per cent of the U.S. population). Cancer, excluding basal and squamous cell skin cancers, was newly diagnosed in 429 of every 100,000 American males and 330 of every 100,000 American females each year during this period. The leading cancers among men are those of the prostate, lung, and colon/rectum, while among women the top three are breast, colon/rectum, and lung cancers. If mortality rather than incidence data are considered, the order shifts. Among males, lung cancer is by far the leading cause of cancer death (66.2 deaths per year per 100,000), followed by colon/rectum (24.1 per 100,000) and prostate (24.1 per 100,000) cancer. Among females, breast cancer death rates (27.4 per 100,000) were slightly higher than lung (26.0 per 100,000) and colon/rectum (17.0 per 100,000)

TABLE 158–2. AGE-ADJUSTED CANCER INCIDENCE RATES* IN THE UNITED STATES, 1983–1987, BY SEX

Cancer Site	Males	Females
Oral and pharynx	17.3	6.5
Esophagus	6.2	1.9
Stomach	12.1	5.4
Small intestine	1.3	0.8
Colon/rectum	61.2	43.4
Gallbladder and biliary	2.2	2.4
Pancreas	11.2	8.3
Larynx	8.4	1.6
Lung	84.2	35.6
Bone	1.0	0.7
Soft tissue	2.5	1.8
Skin melanoma	11.5	8.9
Breast	0.8	102.0
Uterine cervix	—	8.7
Uterus, corpus	—	21.9
Ovary	—	13.7
Prostate	89.3	—
Testis	4.1	—
Bladder	29.5	7.4
Kidney and renal pelvis	11.3	5.3
Eye	0.8	0.6
Brain and nervous system	7.1	5.0
Thyroid	2.5	6.0
Hodgkin's disease	3.3	2.3
Non-Hodgkin's lymphomas	15.3	10.4
Multiple myeloma	5.1	3.5
Leukemia	13.1	7.7
Total	**428.5**	**329.9**

*Age-adjusted (1970 U.S. population) incidence rates per year per 100,000 population.

cancer death rates during 1983 to 1987. However, by the late 1980's death rates from lung cancer had passed death rates from breast cancer among women in the United States.

For nearly all cancers, the incidence rates are higher among men than women, the exceptions being gallbladder and thyroid cancers. For some cancers, explanations for the male excess are evident (e.g., higher tobacco and alcohol intake account for most of the higher rates of oral, esophageal, laryngeal, and lung cancer among males), but for others (e.g., stomach cancer, leukemia) the reasons are enigmatic.

Rates of most cancers, particularly those deriving from epithelial tissue, rise steadily with advancing age, often exponentially. There are bimodal distributions for some cancers, however. Leukemia and nervous system tumors display an early childhood (age <5 years) peak, then rates decline before rising again in late middle age. Testis cancer occurs primarily between the ages of 20 and 40, while Hodgkin's disease incidence is highest at ages 20 to 30, declines somewhat, then rises again after age 50.

Racial differences in cancer occurrence are sometimes marked. Total cancer incidence during 1983 to 1987 was higher among black than white males by 22 per cent, while rates were higher among white than black females by 4 per cent. The black/white differences among males were particularly pronounced for esophageal, stomach, pancreas, lung, and prostate cancer and multiple myeloma, with age-adjusted incidence from 50 to 300 per cent higher among blacks than whites.

Rates of mortality of several cancers have been changing over the past decades (Fig. 158–1). Most notable has been the rise in lung cancer. Lung tumors were rarely diagnosed prior to the early 1900's, but incidence and mortality began a notable rise in the 1920's which has continued until today. The epidemic increase in lung cancer, almost entirely attributable to cigarette smoking, is beginning to end, however. Indeed, mortality from lung cancer between the mid 1970's and mid 1980's declined by nearly 30 per cent among white males below age 45, with smaller declines also noted for white females and nonwhites of both sexes. As younger Americans age and their more favorable lung cancer experience extends to older age groups, the overall rates of lung cancer should begin to decline. For white males the total age-adjusted rates have already plateaued, but the leveling off and subsequent decrease in lung cancer rates among females will not take place until after the year 2000. Rates of stomach and cervical cancers, the leading tumors early in this century, have declined in all groups, the former for reasons not yet fully understood, the latter at least in part due to cytologic screening for cervical pathology. The decreases in these tumors are beginning to end, however, and rates of gastric cardia cancer are now on the rise.

Although not shown in Figure 158–1, there has been nearly a doubling in incidence of melanoma and a 50 per cent rise in non-Hodgkin's lymphomas among whites since the early 1970's. In addition, the excess among blacks for certain cancers has been increasing over time. This is occurring for lung, oral, and laryngeal cancer but is particularly evident for esophageal cancer, rising rates of which have now made esophageal cancer the second leading cancer among black males below the age of 60. By contrast, rates of esophageal cancer have been stable or declining among whites. Reasons for the growing racial disparity are not entirely evident, although higher prevalences of cigarette smoking, heavy alcohol consumption, and nutritional disadvantages are suspect.

THE CAUSES OF CANCER

Cancer is believed to be a largely preventable disease. Clear knowledge now exists of the causes of most occurrences for several cancers, including those of the oral cavity and pharynx, esophagus, liver, larynx, lung, and uterine cervix. Agents influencing risk also have been identified for other cancers, but the search continues in order to clarify the etiologic factors that account for the bulk of malignancies in the United States and around the world. Most of the information currently available on risk factors for cancer has come from case-control studies assessing various characteristics and exposures of patients with individual cancers and from cohort studies determining rates of cancer among groups exposed to particular agents suspected of carcinogenic potential. Often the leads for these epidemiologic investigations were generated from descriptive studies of cancer rates and statistics and from alert clinical observations.

The striking variation in cancer rates within and between countries, the differing rates among migrants from one place to another, and the often marked trends over time suggest that most cancers are environmentally induced. Estimates of the per cent of cancer that is caused by environmental determinants are typically 75 per cent or higher, although it is likely that most tumors arise from the complex interplay of environmental and host, possibly genetic, factors. Those factors known to be related to the risk of cancer in humans are summarized below.

TOBACCO. Cigarette smoking is the dominant cause of the leading cancer (i.e., lung cancer) in the United States and many other western nations. The association was first suspected by clinical observation that new lung cancer patients were often smokers, then confirmed in the 1950's by case-control and cohort studies in the United States and Great Britain. In the years since the first U.S. Surgeon General's report on smoking in 1964, additional evidence has documented that risks of lung cancer rise in proportion to both duration of smoking and amount smoked per day, with risks of lung cancer more than 20 times greater among long-term heavy smokers than among nonsmokers. Life-long filter smokers have experienced a somewhat smaller increase in risk than life-long nonfilter smokers, but the greatest protection comes from smoking cessation. Risks 10 years after quitting are typically only one third or less those of continuing cigarette smokers. Smoking affects all the major types of lung cancers, although squamous and small cell carcinomas more than adenocarcinomas. Cigarette smoking also increases risk of other cancers. It is a principal cause of cancers of the oral cavity and pharynx, esophagus, larynx, and renal pelvis; a major contributor to cancers of the pancreas, bladder, and kidney; and implicated to a moderate degree in cancers of the stomach and uterine cervix. In addition, smokeless tobacco is the predominant cause of buccal mucosa cancers in some populations. In total, tobacco use is thought to account for nearly one third of all cancers in the United States and thus is the largest single preventable cause of cancer.

While the effects of smoking are far greater for smokers themselves, the consensus of evidence from nearly 20 epidemiologic studies conducted around the world in the past decade is that long-term exposure to environmental tobacco smoke can also increase risk of lung cancer among nonsmokers. The excess risk of lung cancer among nonsmoking women married to smokers has averaged 30 per cent. Because of tobacco's harmful effects, efforts to induce smokers to quit and to encourage nonsmokers, particularly adolescents, not to start smoking must be continued. Smoking prevalence among adult men in the United States has declined from a peak of nearly 60 per cent in the 1950's to about 30 per cent today, but further reductions are attainable and critical to the nation's public health.

ALCOHOL. Alcohol combines with tobacco to cause cancers of the oral cavity and pharynx, esophagus, and larynx. Alcoholic beverages have also been implicated in the etiology of liver, rectal, and breast cancers, although the associations with the latter remain to be verified. In a large recent case-control study involving over 1100 oral and pharyngeal cancer patients in the United States, cancer risk was shown to increase progressively with increasing intake of alcoholic beverages among nonsmokers as well as smokers. Smoking and drinking tended to multiply the effects of each other, so that risk of oral cancer was increased over 35-fold among two-pack-a-day smokers who consumed more than four alcoholic drinks per day, compared with abstainers of both products. Similar tobacco-alcohol interactions have been observed for esophageal and laryngeal cancer. Ethanol has generally not been shown to be carcinogenic in experimental studies using animal models but seems likely to be the etiologic agent in humans, since all types of alcoholic beverages—beer, wine, dark and light spirits—have been linked with increased risk in epidemiologic studies.

OCCUPATIONAL HAZARDS. Occupational exposures have long been recognized as causes of cancer, beginning with the observation in the 1700's of scrotal cancer among chimney sweeps in London. Today at least 20 substances in the workplace have been associated with increased cancer risk (Table 158–3). About one half have been implicated in lung cancer, occasionally in an interactive manner with cigarette smoking. The exposure accounting for the largest number of occupational cancers is asbestos. Increased rates of lung cancer and mesothelioma have been found among asbestos miners and millers; factory workers handling asbestos textile and other products; shipyard, railroad, and construction workers; and other employees working in industries where asbestos was manufactured or used. Although exposure to asbestos can induce lung cancer among nonsmokers, smoking and asbestos combine in a multiplicative fashion to enhance lung cancer risk, so that removing either agent significantly lowers the cancer burden. Asbestos also has been associated with gastrointestinal and urinary (kidney) tumors.

Another potent occupational lung carcinogen is radon and its daughter products, found in high levels in underground mines throughout much of the world. Over 20-fold increases of lung

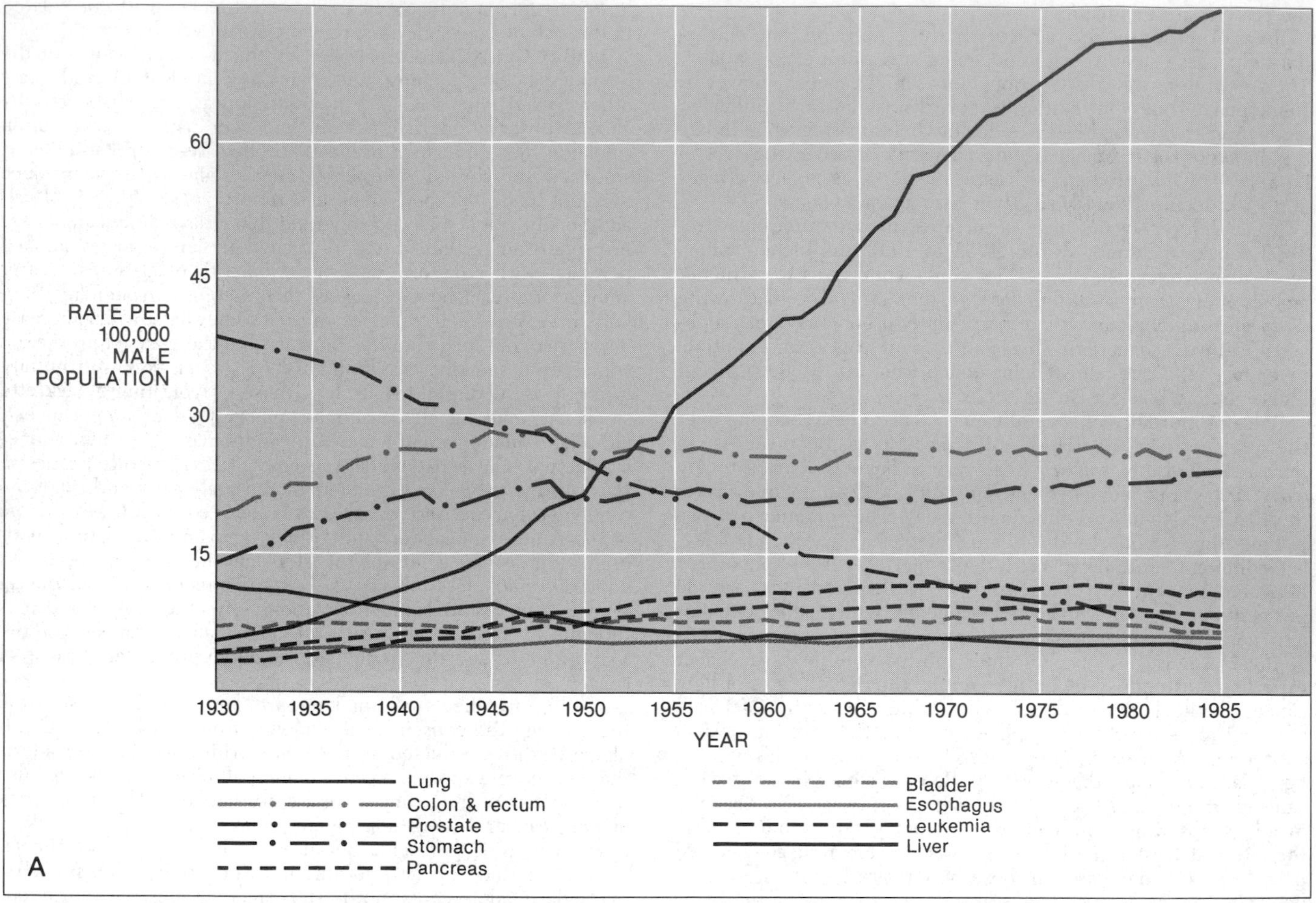

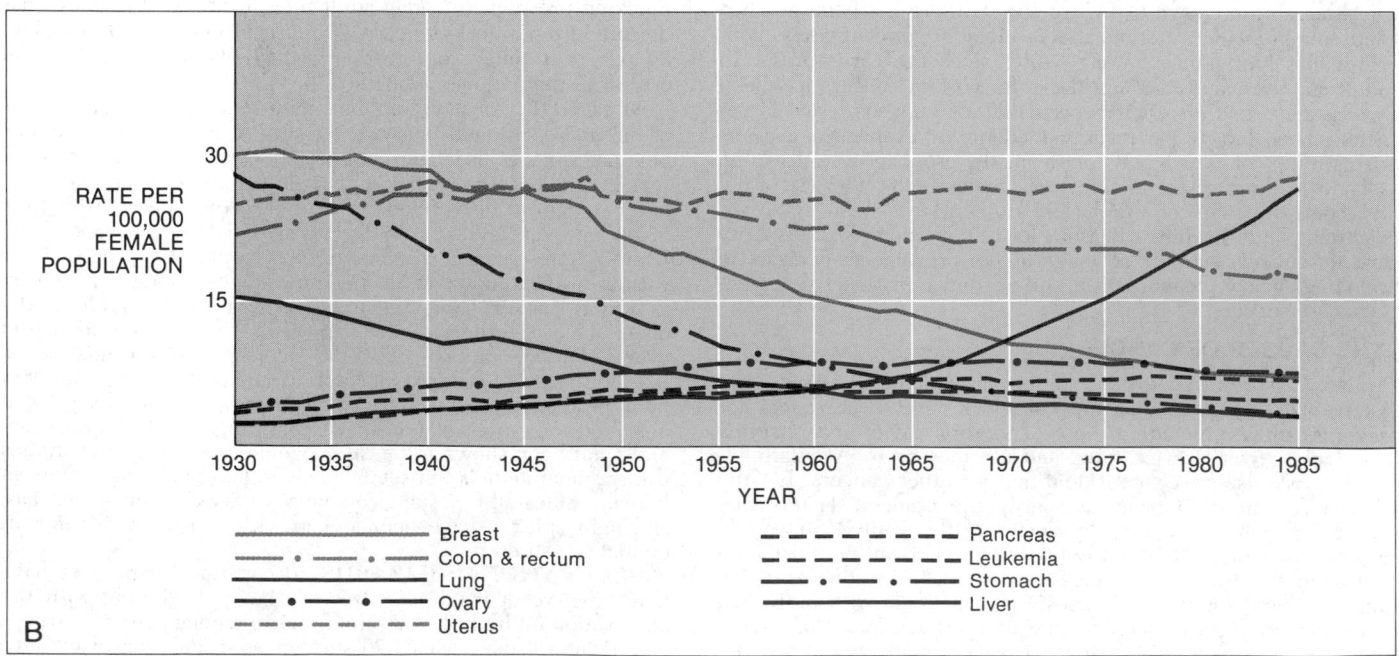

FIGURE 158–1. Trends during 1930–1985 in age-adjusted mortality rates for selected cancers in the United States. (Reproduced with permission from Silverberg E, Boring CC, Squires TS: Cancer statistics, 1990. Ca 40:9–26, 1990.)

TABLE 158–3. OCCUPATIONAL EXPOSURES RECOGNIZED AS HUMAN CARCINOGENS

Exposure	Site of Cancer
Aluminum production	Lung
4-Aminobiphenyl	Bladder
Arsenic	Lung, skin
Asbestos	Lung, pleura, peritoneum, GI tract, kidney
Auramine manufacture	Bladder
Benzene	Leukemia
Benzidine	Bladder
β-Naphthylamine	Bladder
Bischloromethylether	Lung
Boot and shoe manufacture	Bladder, nasal sinuses
Chromium (hexavalent) compounds	Lung
Coal gasification, coke production	Lung
Erionite	Mesothelioma
Isopropyl alcohol manufacture	Nasal sinuses
Magenta manufacture	Bladder
Mineral oils	Skin, other cancers
Mustard gas	Lung
Nickel compounds	Lung, nasal sinuses
Radon	Lung
Soots, tars, and oils (polycyclic hydrocarbons)	Lung, skin
Vinyl chloride	Liver
Wood dusts (furniture)	Nasal sinuses

cancer have been reported in some groups of radon-exposed miners, most of whom are also smokers, with the excesses most pronounced for small cell anaplastic carcinomas. Several chemicals, including inorganic arsenic, benzene, β-napthylamine and other aromatic amines, bischloromethyl ether, mustard gas, certain nickel compounds, and polycyclic hydrocarbons, have induced cancer in exposed workers (Table 158–3). Except for arsenic, there is confirmatory evidence of carcinogenicity from animal bioassays, often (but not always) with the carcinogen inducing similar tumors in the animals as in humans.

Among all cancers, those of the nasal cavity and sinuses and the urinary bladder have the highest proportion related to occupational exposures. In a nationwide survey of all nasal adenocarcinomas in Sweden over a recent 19-year period, nearly 25 per cent occurred among furniture makers as a result of wood dust exposures. It has been estimated that among American men up to 25 per cent of all bladder cancers are occupationally related. The percentages for other tumors are less, and for all cancers combined, it is generally thought that fewer than 5 per cent have been induced by workplace exposures.

ENVIRONMENTAL POLLUTION. Carcinogens have in some instances been identified in the air we breathe and water we drink. Quantifying the effects of air and water pollution has been extremely difficult, however, because of uncertainty over the amount and characteristics of exposures actually received by individuals. Air pollution, primarily from combustion products, earlier in this century was thought to be involved in the rise in lung cancer in Great Britain, the United States, and other countries, but now air pollution as found in most urban areas is considered to contribute to a small fraction (<10 per cent) of cases of this cancer. The percentage is higher in some areas of the world, including parts of China where excessive rates of lung cancer have been found among nonsmokers living in chimneyless houses and in homes heavily polluted by coal-burning heating systems. Increased risks of lung cancer have also been found among residents living near copper smelters, with industrial air emissions of inorganic arsenic suspected. Mesotheliomas have been diagnosed among women married to asbestos workers, presumably from handling clothing or otherwise being exposed to fibers brought home by their husbands. Since there are nearly linear dose-response relations between occupational asbestos exposure and mesothelioma and lung cancer, concern has arisen over possible health risks from lower levels of exposure that may occur in homes, schools, and other public places, although few such environmentally induced cancer cases have been documented. Pollutants in drinking water have also aroused concern.

Rates of bladder cancer have correlated with levels of halogenated compounds, some of which are carcinogenic in animal experiments, in some municipal water supplies. Recent laboratory tests also indicate an increased risk of osteogenic sarcomas following high levels of exposure to flouride in some subgroups of exposed animals, but epidemiologic investigations have found few or no unexpected changes in cancer rates following flouridation of water supplies.

MEDICINAL AGENTS. Among the chemicals considered to be causally associated with cancer in humans, nearly one half are medications (Table 158–4). These include drugs used in cancer treatment, especially alkylating agents, which have been found to induce acute nonlymphocytic leukemias and other cancers. The occurrence of second primary cancers in 5 to 10 per cent or more of those on therapy suggests that risks as well as benefits of chemotherapy with carcinogenic agents must be carefully assessed, particularly for patients whose long-term prognosis is otherwise highly favorable.

Exogenous estrogens have been implicated in cancer risk. Diethylstilbestrol (DES) taken during pregnancy has resulted in vaginal adenocarcinomas in offspring who were exposed in utero. The rising rates of endometrial cancer among American women in the 1970's were precipitated by use of conjugated estrogens for menopausal symptoms. Rates dropped abruptly following curtailment of use when the association with cancer became known. The link to breast cancer is less clear, although several investigations have found an increased risk among women receiving long-term estrogen replacement therapy for menopausal symptoms. Extended use of oral contraceptives prior to first pregnancy also has been reported to increase subsequent risk of breast cancer in some investigations, but as yet the widespread introduction of oral contraceptives in the 1960's has not been shown to have significantly influenced national rates of breast cancer in the United States. Combined (estrogen plus progestogen) oral contraceptives have been associated with a reduced risk of endometrial and ovarian cancer.

Certain immunosuppressive agents sharply increase risk of cancer. Indeed, among renal transplant recipients, the risk of subsequent lymphomas is increased over 30-fold, with the excesses occurring within months of immunosuppressive therapy—the fastest onset of any environmentally induced cancer.

RADIATION. Follow-up of survivors of the atomic bombs of Hiroshima and Nagasaki and of groups of patients receiving radiotherapy for ankylosing spondylitis, cancer, and certain other conditions provides conclusive evidence that ionizing radiation can induce cancer in humans as it does in lower animals. Leukemia is the initial carcinogenic consequence, occurring most frequently 5 to 10 years after exposure, with increased risks of a variety of solid tumors, particularly breast, thyroid, and lung cancers, following thereafter. Cancer risk tends to increase in proportion to radiation dose, in a linear fashion for some tumors

TABLE 158–4. MEDICINAL AGENTS RECOGNIZED AS HUMAN CARCINOGENS

Drug	Site of Cancer
Azathiopine	Lymphoma, skin, soft tissue sarcoma
Chlornaphazine	Bladder
1,4-Butanediol dimethanesulfonate (Myleran)	Leukemia
Combined chemotherapy for lymphoma, including MOPP*	Leukemia
Chlorambucil	Leukemia
Cyclophosphamide	Leukemia, bladder
Estrogens—conjugated	Endometrium
Estrogens—synthetic (DES)	Vagina, cervix
Estrogens—steroid contraceptives	Benign liver tumors
Melphalan	Leukemia
Methoxsalen with ultraviolet A therapy (PUVA)	Skin
Phenacetin-containing analgesics	Renal pelvis
Treosulphan	Leukemia

*MOPP: procarbazine, nitrogen mustard, vincristine, and prednisone

such as breast cancer, raising the possibility that some increase in risk may result from low-dose therapeutic or repeated diagnostic radiologic procedures. Significantly increased risks of breast cancer have been detected among atomic bomb survivors at doses somewhat below 50 rad, and head and neck tumors have followed less than 10 rad of scalp irradiation for tinea capitis in Israeli children. The findings suggest the need for prudence in the use of medical irradiation. Improvements in radiologic equipment, however, have resulted in lower radiation doses. Thus, for example, risks associated with mammography are now believed to be low enough to justify routine periodic screening for breast cancer among American women as young as age 40.

Ultraviolet radiation from sun exposure is the dominant cause of basal and squamous cell carcinoma and melanoma of the skin. The key to prevention is reduced solar exposure, even though there is uncertainty regarding variations in effect according to extent and timing of exposure. For melanoma, intermittent heavy sun exposures, particularly during childhood and adolescence, may carry the greatest risk.

DIET AND NUTRITION. Consistent evidence has arisen from around the world that diet and nutrition can influence cancer risk. Clearest are the inverse associations between risk of certain epithelial cancers, particularly oral, esophageal, stomach, and lung cancers, and intake of fresh fruits and vegetables. Risk of these cancers among persons in the highest quartile of consumption is lower, sometimes by more than one half, than among those in the lowest quartile of intake. Studies in experimental animals have shown that several compounds in these foods can inhibit carcinogenesis, but the ingredients responsible for the protective effects in people still remain to be clarified. Epidemiologic studies have shown that carotenoids, but not animal sources of vitamin A (retinols), are fairly consistently linked to reduced cancer risk, but vitamins C and E, which can inhibit the formation of carcinogenic N-nitroso compounds in vivo, and other possibly protective nutrients have also been identified. Recent studies in China and Italy suggest that garlic, onions, and other allium vegetables may significantly reduce the risk of stomach cancer, an intriguing finding because of the potent inhibitory properties of compounds in these vegetables documented in experimental animals. Some food contaminants, including aflatoxins sometimes found in moldy peanuts or grains, are also strong animal carcinogens. Rates of liver cancer tend to be high in parts of Asia and Africa where aflatoxin contamination is common.

Dietary fat, particularly saturated fat, and calories have been implicated in the risk of colon, breast, and other cancers, although the etiologic nature of the associations is still not well established. Dietary fiber has been reported to reduce the risk of colon cancer, but its role vis-à-vis that of other constituents in vegetables, grains, and other fiber-rich foods is not clear. Despite these uncertainties, it has been estimated that a high percentage of colorectal and breast cancers have a dietary etiology, in part because of the much higher rates of these cancers in western nations with high-fat, low-fiber diets. In total, some estimates suggest that one third or more of all cancers may be related to dietary and nutritional practices.

INFECTIOUS AGENTS. Several viral agents have been associated with human cancer, particularly cancers of the liver in endemic areas and of the uterine cervix worldwide. Hepatitis B virus (HBV) is the primary cause of hepatocellular carcinoma in China and other areas where infections are prevalent. Prospective follow-up studies show large increases in risk, with nearly all liver cancers arising among persons with prediagnosis HBV surface antigen positivity. The epidemiologic patterns of cervical cancer (with risks elevated among those with multiple sexual partners, early age at coitus) have long suggested a venereal component to etiology, but only recently have improvements in laboratory techniques enabled detection of human papillomavirus (HPV) as a likely etiologic agent in a high percentage of cases. Herpes simplex virus type 2 has also been associated with cervical cancer, but its independent or interactive role with HPV remains to be clarified. The Epstein-Barr virus has been implicated in both nasopharyngeal cancer and Burkitt's lymphoma, while certain human retroviruses have been associated with adult T-cell leukemias in Japan and the Caribbean. The human immunode-

ficiency virus, the cause of AIDS, is associated not only with Kaposi's sarcomas reported at the clinical diagnosis of nearly 5 per cent of AIDS patients, but also with increased risk of lymphoma among survivors of AIDS.

GENETIC SUSCEPTIBILITY. Risk of cancer is often increased when there is a history of cancer in the family. The increases for common cancers such as those of the lung, colon, and breast are typically on the order of two- to threefold. Shared environmental factors often may contribute to the familial clustering, but strong associations among subgroups with early age at onset of cancer or bilateral presentation of breast cancer indicate a genetic predisposition in some instances. The most marked genetic effects are seen for skin cancer, with tumors rarely appearing in persons inheriting darkly pigmented skin. A few cancers show mendelian inheritance patterns, including melanomas arising from familial dysplastic nevi and retinoblastomas. In addition, certain hereditary precancerous syndromes have been linked to increased cancer risk. Included are neurofibromatosis and other phacomatoses (associated with nervous system cancer), xeroderma pigmentosum and albinism (skin cancer), ataxia telangiectasia and certain other immunodeficiency syndromes (lymphoma, leukemia, and other cancers), Bloom's syndrome (lymphoma, leukemia, and other cancers), and Fanconi's anemia (leukemia). Investigations of families with unusually large numbers of members with the same or different cancers have provided insight into genetic patterns. In larger epidemiologic studies, increasing attention is being paid to systematic evaluations of genetic factors as reliable markers of host susceptibility become available. Lung cancer risk, for example, has recently been associated with the genetically controlled ability to metabolize the antihypertensive drug debrisoquine. Information on susceptibility factors will be crucial in understanding the mechanisms of carcinogenesis as well as delineating groups and individuals at high risk for targeted interventions.

International Agency for Research on Cancer: Overall Evaluations of Carcinogenicity: An updating of IARC Monographs Volumes 1 to 42. Monographs on the Evaluation of Carcinogenic Risks to Humans. Supplement 7. Lyon, World Health Organization, 1987. *A systematic review of epidemiologic and experimental evidence regarding carcinogenicity of over 150 substances.*

Ries LA, Hankey BF, Edwards BK (eds.): Cancer Statistics Review 1973–1987. Bethesda, MD, US Department of Health and Human Services, NIH Publication No. 90–2789, 1990. *Up-to-date listing of cancer incidence, mortality, and survival rates in the United States.*

Schottenfeld D, Fraumeni JF Jr (eds.): Cancer Epidemiology and Prevention. Philadelphia, W. B. Saunders Company, 1982. *A comprehensive review of cancer epidemiology, with individual chapters assessing 34 cancers and 16 causative agents, as well as basic concepts in cancer etiology and control.*

159 Paraneoplastic Syndromes

Paul A. Bunn, Jr.

The paraneoplastic syndromes are a heterogenous group of signs and symptoms indirectly caused by cancers at a distance from the primary tumor or its metastases. These "remote" or "biologic" effects of malignancy must be distinguished from direct effects of tumor or its metastases. The majority of paraneoplastic syndromes are caused by proteins secreted by these tumors. In some instances (e.g., endocrine paraneoplastic syndromes), the proteins (hormones) are well characterized, and the pathophysiology is well understood. These paraneoplastic syndromes invariably improve with effective antineoplastic therapy. In addition, drugs that interfere with the hormone action may be useful in severe cases or when the tumor fails to respond to therapy. An increasing number of paraneoplastic syndromes, especially those with neurologic manifestations, appear to be caused by immunologic reactions to tumor antigens that are shared with normal cells. These neurologic syndromes often do not improve even with effective antitumor therapy, perhaps because the nervous system cannot regenerate and damage is often permanent.

Recognizable paraneoplastic syndromes, other than wasting of the host or tumor cachexia, occur in a minority of cancer patients. They may be extremely important, however, in the early detection of the original cancer or may be the first sign of recurrence. They may also simulate metastatic disease and thus prevent patients from receiving curative therapy. Conversely, signs and symptoms of metastatic disease may be falsely ascribed to a paraneoplastic syndrome and thus lead to the withholding of systemic therapy. Paraneoplastic syndromes may be disabling but treatable with proper recognition. Thus, establishing a diagnosis is extremely important. True paraneoplastic syndromes must be distinguished from those caused by the primary tumor or its metastases, infections, toxicities of therapy, vascular abnormalities, obstruction caused by a tumor or its products, and fluid and electrolyte abnormalities. It is also important to understand which paraneoplastic syndromes respond to primary antitumor therapy. Alternative forms of therapy aimed at symptomatic control should be considered in those syndromes in which response to primary antitumor therapy is unlikely.

WASTING OF THE HOST. Wasting of the host, sometimes called tumor cachexia or the cachexia of malignant disease, is the most common of the paraneoplastic syndromes. The catabolic phase that usually accompanies malignant disease may be out of keeping with the size of the tumor and may be complex in its pathogenesis—decreased caloric intake (there is often a perverted sense of taste and smell with aversion to specific foods), malabsorption, loss of protein (e.g., hemorrhage or effusions), fever, and possibly a change in metabolic pathways. For example, increased anaerobic glycolysis with enhanced gluconeogenesis from amino acids and partial insulin resistance have been described. Possibly factors capable of distorting metabolism are secreted by the tumor, for example, tumor necrosis factor/cachectin, a macrophage-derived factor that is capable of inhibiting the activity of certain lipogenic enzymes. Certainly the caloric expenditure tends to remain high, and the basal metabolic rate is increased, despite the reduced intake of calories, suggesting a deranged metabolism.

Treatment of the underlying tumor is the major approach to therapy. Replacement alimentation is reserved for patients undergoing surgical treatment or for patients with severe nutritional deficiency but for whom there is hope for significant remission or cure. Progestational hormones (e.g., Megace) may stimulate appetite and increase weight in patients.

ENDOCRINE PARANEOPLASTIC SYNDROMES. The original description of a paraneoplastic syndrome was that of ectopic Cushing's syndrome, as reported by Brown in 1928. The endocrine neoplastic syndromes are listed in Table 161–1 and are described in detail in Ch. 161, to which the reader is referred.

NEUROLOGIC PARANEOPLASTIC SYNDROMES (Table 159–1). Neurologic signs and symptoms appear frequently in cancer patients and are most often directly related to metastases, fluid and electrolyte abnormalities, vascular abnormalities, infections, or toxicity of therapy. True paraneoplastic syndromes are generally diagnosed by exclusion of these other conditions (Ch. 162). Subacute cerebellar degeneration, subacute motor neuropathy, sensory neuropathy, Eaton-Lambert syndrome, and dermatomyositis in older males are so strongly associated with cancer that their presence should lead to a search for a primary tumor when none is evident. Many of these syndromes are caused by immunologic reactions to cross-reacting antibodies, as mentioned above.

HEMATOLOGIC PARANEOPLASTIC SYNDROMES. Cancers may indirectly affect any of the hematopoietic cell lines, producing increases or decreases in either individual cell lineages or multiple lineages. Increased cell numbers are generally produced when the tumor secretes a stimulatory hormone/growth factor.

Erythrocytosis most often results from erythropoietin production by renal or liver tumors. In a large review, paraneoplastic erythrocytosis when found was most often associated with hypernephromas (35 per cent), benign renal abnormalities (14 per cent), hepatomas (19 per cent), cerebellar hemangioblastomas (15 per cent), uterine tumors (7 per cent), adrenal tumors and pheochromocytomas (3 per cent), and miscellaneous tumors (3 per cent). In rare cases, induction of local kidney or systemic hypoxia by tumors may also result in erythrocytosis.

Leukemoid reactions, granulocytosis, eosinophilia, and/or basophilia are most often produced when the tumor secretes a colony-stimulating factor (CSF) and thus are corrected by effective treatment of the primary tumor. Granulocytosis is most often

TABLE 159–1. PARANEOPLASTIC SYNDROMES

1. Wasting of the host—"tumor cachexia"
2. Endocrine/hormone—see Table 161–1
3. Neuromyopathies—see Table 162–1
4. Hematologic
   - Erythrocytosis, granulocytosis, thrombocytosis
   - Anemia (chronic disease, pure red cell aplasia, hypersplenic, autoimmune hemolytic anemia, microangiopathic hemolytic anemia)
   - Granulocytopenia, thrombocytopenia
5. Thromboembolic
   - Venous thrombosis (Trousseau's syndrome)
   - Disseminated intravascular coagulation
   - Nonbacterial thrombotic endocarditis (marantic endocarditis)
6. Renal
   - Secondary to hormonal or metabolic effects
   - Glomerulopathies—including the nephrotic syndrome
   - Miscellaneous—myeloma kidney, amyloidosis, uric acid nephropathy, etc.
7. Dermatologic—see Table 163–4
8. Gastrointestinal
   - Anorexia, nausea, vomiting
   - Protein-losing enteropathy
   - Malignant hepatopathy
9. Miscellaneous
   - Lactic acidosis
   - Clubbing/hypertrophic pulmonary osteoarthropathy
   - Hyperlipidemia
   - Hypertension—hypotension
   - Hyperamylasemia
   - Amyloidosis
   - Arthritis

associated with lung, gastric, pancreatic, and brain cancers; melanomas; and Hodgkin's and non-Hodgkin's lymphomas. Eosinophilia is most often associated with lymphomas, especially Hodgkin's disease, and gastrointestinal carcinomas. These syndromes must be differentiated from chronic myelogenous leukemia and other causes of leukemoid reactions such as infection, inflammatory diseases, metabolic diseases, and certain drugs (Ch. 141).

Anemia is frequently associated with malignant disease, and granulocytopenia and thrombocytopenia may also be paraneoplastic in nature. *Autoimmune hemolytic anemia* is most often associated with B-cell lymphoproliferative neoplasms and less often with ovarian and lung cancers (Ch. 135). Successful treatment of the primary tumor often leads to improvement; corticosteroids are usually unsuccessful. *Pure red cell aplasia* is found in association with thymomas (50 per cent) and a variety of other cancers.

Microangiopathic hemolytic anemia, a rare cause of anemia in patients with cancer, is diagnosed by the presence of severe hemolytic anemia with fragmented erythrocytes seen in the blood smear and a negative Coombs test. Most often this syndrome is associated with mucin-producing adenocarcinomas, especially those from the stomach (55 per cent), breast (13 per cent), lung (7 per cent), and unknown primary site (10 per cent). It is often abrupt in onset and associated with thrombocytopenia and disseminated intravascular coagulation.

Granulocytopenia is usually the result of chemotherapy, radiation therapy, severe infection, or marrow involvement, but has been reported rarely in association with thymoma. A syndrome resembling *idiopathic thrombocytopenic purpura (ITP)* may occur in association with lymphomas (especially chronic lymphocytic leukemia, Hodgkin's disease, and immunoblastic lymphadenopathy) and less frequently with other malignant disorders.

THROMBOEMBOLIC PARANEOPLASTIC SYNDROMES. A *hypercoagulable* state is frequent in cancer patients and may manifest as (1) *migratory thrombophlebitis* (Trousseau's syndrome); (2) subacute or overt *disseminated intravascular coagulation* (DIC); and (3) *nonbacterial thrombotic endocarditis* (NBTE, marantic endocarditis); or (4) a combination of these three.

Thrombophlebitis occurs in as many as 1 to 11 per cent of cancer patients and is most often associated with mucin-producing adenocarcinomas of the gastrointestinal tract. It may also be seen with lung, breast, ovarian, and prostate cancers. The treatment of migratory thrombophlebitis is difficult; acute episodes require heparin. Long-term therapy with warfarin is generally unsuccessful, but long-term administration of subcutaneous heparin has had some limited success.

DIC may present as an acute hemorrhagic diathesis or be discovered incidentally as chronic laboratory abnormalities. Coagulation abnormalities by laboratory test may be seen in as many as 90 per cent of patients with cancer, but most of these never develop overt bleeding episodes. Acute episodes are most frequently associated with acute promyelocytic leukemia (APL) and adenocarcinomas (especially prostatic). Identification and treatment of all precipitating factors are the keystones to the management of DIC. This includes therapy for the primary tumor as well as for infection, acidosis, and other factors. Heparin is often used prophylactically in APL, although this is not mandatory if all coagulation parameters are normal and are monitored closely. For overt DIC, heparin appears to be superior to warfarin; spontaneous remission of DIC may occur in adenocarcinomas without any therapy.

NBTE is characterized by sterile verrucous lesions on the left-sided heart valves; these thrombi may embolize to the brain and other vital organs. These occur most often with mucin-producing adenocarcinomas. Therapy is directed to the primary tumor. The therapeutic role of heparin and warfarin is uncertain.

RENAL PARANEOPLASTIC SYNDROMES. Most renal abnormalities that occur in patients with cancer are due to metastases, obstruction, electrolyte and fluid imbalances, toxicity of therapy, or infection. The most common renal paraneoplastic syndrome, other than those linked to hormones (e.g., SIADH), is the nephrotic syndrome. In one report 10 per cent of patients with nephrotic syndrome had underlying malignant disease, with Hodgkin's disease being the most frequently associated disorder. Most of these patients have lipoid nephrosis (minimal change glomerulopathy). In contrast, patients with non-Hodgkin's lymphomas often have immunoglobulin deposits suggesting an immune complex etiology. In both instances the nephrotic syndrome resolves if there is a response to antitumor therapy. Patients with carcinomas most often have membranous glomerulonephritis with subepithelial electron-dense deposits. Other renal abnormalities associated with cancer include (1) the host of abnormalities associated with multiple myeloma and amyloidosis (Ch. 151); (2) the potassium wasting and hypokalemia syndrome caused by lysozyme secreted by patients with acute myelogenous leukemia (M4 or M5); (3) the syndrome of intrarenal obstruction preceded by mucoprotein secreted by patients with pancreatic carcinoma; and (4) the syndrome of nephrogenic diabetes insipidus found in some patients with leiomyosarcoma.

DERMATOLOGIC PARANEOPLASTIC SYNDROMES. This group of syndromes is summarized in Ch. 163. The strongest dermatologic associations with malignant disease are with acanthosis nigricans, erythema gyratum repens, tylosis, dermatomyositis in older males, flushing in the carcinoid syndrome and with the hereditary syndromes (Gardner's syndrome, Peutz-Jegher's syndrome, etc). Some of these syndromes may be caused by overexpression of epidermal growth factor.

GASTROINTESTINAL PARANEOPLASTIC SYNDROMES. *Protein-losing enteropathy* may be produced by inflammation and ulceration of the mucosa, obstruction of intestinal lymphatics (lymphomas), congestive heart failure (carcinoid, pericardial constriction), and undefined mechanisms. Although hypoalbuminemia is common in cancer patients, true protein-losing enteropathy is rare.

Malignant *hepatopathy* (Stauffer's syndrome) is characterized by biochemical abnormalities (increased alkaline phosphatase, hypercholesterolemia, prolonged prothrombin time) and hepatosplenomegaly in association with hypernephroma or malignant schwannoma without liver metastases. These abnormalities improve following resection of the primary tumor.

MISCELLANEOUS PARANEOPLASTIC SYNDROMES. *Fever* is a common finding in cancer patients and is often idiopathic. This is most common in lymphomas (where it is associated with a poor prognosis), hypernephromas, osteogenic sarcomas, and myxomas, although it may be found with other tumors. It almost always disappears with successful antitumor therapy. *Lactic acidosis* may be associated with acute leukemias and lymphomas and responds to successful antitumor therapy. *Hyperlipidemias* have been reported in association with multiple myeloma, hepatoma, and colon cancer.

Hypokalemia and hypertension with tumor production of renin have been reported with lung cancer, hypernephroma, and Wilms' tumor. *Hypotension* has been reported in association with a prostaglandin A-secreting hypernephroma and with intrathoracic tumors secondary to abnormal baroreceptor responses. *Hyperamylasemia* may be caused by lung cancers, especially adenocarcinomas, and is generally not associated with symptoms.

Hypertrophic pulmonary osteoarthropathy is characterized by clubbing, periostitis of the long bones, and occasionally polyarthritis. Involved bones include the distal ends of the tibia, fibula, humerus, radius, or ulna. It is associated most frequently with lung cancer (except small cell), mesothelioma (especially the benign form), and other cancers when they metastasize to the lungs or mediastinum. The abnormalities improve with successful treatment of the primary tumor. The etiology is unknown.

Amyloidosis occurs in association with multiple myeloma, lymphoma, or carcinomas (especially hypernephroma) in about 15 per cent of cases. The amyloidogenic protein is monoclonal light-chain (AL) in the case of B-cell tumors; other proteins (AA) are associated with other tumors (Ch. 197). Amyloidosis causes signs and symptoms by deposition in nerves, heart, kidney, and joints. Prognosis is poor, and there is no specific therapy. *Polyarthritis* has been reported in association with breast and other cancers. *Polymyalgia rheumatica* may precede development of several forms of cancer, and *systemic lupus erythematosus* (SLE) is associated with lymphomas, leukemias, thymomas, and testicular, lung, and ovarian cancers. Remission of SLE may occur with successful antitumor therapy.

Antman KH, Skarin AT, Mayer RJ, et al.: Microangiopathic hemolytic anemia and cancer: A review. Medicine 58:377, 1979. *Reviews the clinical manifestations and etiology of this syndrome.*

Barnes BE: Dermatomyositis and malignancy. A review of the literature. Ann Intern Med 84:68, 1976. *This review evaluates the association of dermatomyositis and malignant disease and shows the strong association in older males.*

Bunn PA Jr, Minna JD: Paraneoplastic syndromes. In DeVita VT, Hellman S, Rosenberg SA (eds.): The Principles and Practice of Oncology. Philadelphia, JB Lippincott Company, 1985, pp 1797–1842. *This chapter is an extensive review of all types of paraneoplastic syndromes with a complete bibliography.*

Crowthers D, Bateman CJT: Hematologic aspects of systemic disease—malignant disease. Clin Hematol 1:447, 1972. *This review discusses the various hematologic paraneoplastic syndromes in more detail.*

Furneaux HM, Rosenblum MK, Dalmau J, et al.: Selective expression of Purkinje-cell antigens in tumor tissue from patients with paraneoplastic cerebellar degeneration. N Engl J Med 322:1844, 1990. *Describes the mechanisms of neurologic paraneoplastic syndrome.*

Markham M: Response of paraneoplastic syndromes to antineoplastic therapy. West J Med 144:5, 1986. *A thorough review of the paraneoplastic syndromes that improve or disappear in response to effective antitumor therapy.*

McKinney TD (ed.): Renal Complications of Neoplasia. New York, Praeger, 1986. *A thorough review of all of the renal paraneoplastic syndromes.*

Rickles FR, Edwards RL: Activation of blood coagulation in cancer: Trousseau's syndrome revisited. Blood 63:14, 1983. *Reviews the possible causes of the hypercoagulable state in cancer.*

Sack GH, Levin J, Bell WR: Trousseau's syndrome and other manifestations of chronic disseminated coagulopathy in patients with neoplasms. Medicine 56:1, 1977. *A thorough review of the various manifestations of the hypercoagulable state associated with cancer.*

Torti FM, Dieckmann B, Beutler B, et al.: A macrophage factor inhibits adipocyte gene expression: An in vitro model of cachexia. Science 229:867, 1985.

Theologides A: Anorexins, asthenins, and cachectins in cancer. Am J Med 81:696, 1986. *These two articles suggest that "cachectin"—"tumor necrosis factor" and/or other monokines may play a role in the cachexia of malignant disease.*

Thirkill CE, Fitzgerald P, Sergott RC, et al.: Cancer associated retinopathy (CAR syndrome) with antibodies reacting with retinal, optic-nerve, and cancer cells. N Engl J Med 321:1589, 1989. *Describes the mechanisms of neurologic paraneoplastic syndrome.*

160 Tumor Markers

Paul A. Bunn, Jr.

In malignant disease there is aberrant expression of a number of genes. Many of the products of these genes, including hormones, enzymes, immunoglobulins, and a variety of other proteins, may be overexpressed on the cell surface of the cancer cell and are often secreted by the tumor cell. Cell surface antigens are usually assayed using monoclonal antibodies. Expression of specific antigens is useful for establishing a diagnosis and classification and providing prognostic information. Secreted proteins or biomarkers are potentially useful for (1) screening populations, (2) early detection of patients with suspected disease, (3) assessing tumor burden and prognosis, (4) assessing response to therapy, and (5) evaluating early recurrence. Currently available radioimmunoassays can often detect minute amounts (nanograms) of the marker substance. All of the marker proteins, however, are products of normal cells and may be present in small amounts in normal serum. Furthermore, the levels of some marker proteins may also increase with inflammation. Thus, to determine the clinical utility of each marker, the specificity, sensitivity, positive and negative predictive values, and accuracy must be considered. The sensitivity is defined as the number of positive tests divided by the number of true positives. The specificity is defined as the number of negative tests divided by the number of true negatives. The positive and negative predictive values are defined as the true positives divided by the true positives plus false positives and the true negatives divided by the true negatives plus false negatives, respectively. These reflect the confidence with which a positive test is correlated with malignancy or a negative test excludes malignancy. The accuracy (true positive plus true negative/number evaluated) gives an overall assessment of the marker's value. Very few tumor markers are sufficiently sensitive and specific to be useful for each of these purposes. The most established tumor markers include the β subunit of human chorionic gonadotropin (β-hCG), α fetoprotein (AFP), idiotypic immunoglobulins, and carcinoembryonic antigen (CEA).

CELL SURFACE ANTIGENS/TUMOR MARKERS

Evaluation of the expression of cell surface antigens is being used increasingly by pathologists to assist in securing a pathologic diagnosis and to provide prognostic information. Most often these tumor antigens are on the cell surface; however, cytoplasmic and nuclear antigens may also be assessed. Generally, monoclonal antibodies are used in immunohistochemical or immunocytochemical reactions to determine antigen expression. Flow cytometry and biologic assays may also be employed. Table 160–1 shows the most commonly employed antigens by tumor type. The panel of antigens screened for each tumor type is undergoing rapid evolution as new antigens are evaluated. The reader is referred to chapters on each specific malignancy for more information.

The non-Hodgkin's lymphomas always express panleukocyte antigens such as CD45 (T200, LCA). B-cell non-Hodgkin's lymphomas express cell surface immunoglobulin and B-cell antigens such as CD20, 21, and 22. Low-grade B-cell lymphomas usually express the CD5 antigen, which is generally present on mature T cells. Mycosis fungoides and the Sezary syndrome express mature helper T-cell antigens, including the T-cell receptor (CD3), sheep red blood cell receptor (CD2), and helper antigen (CD4), and lack CD8, IL-2 receptor (CD25), and CD7 antigens. Peripheral T-cell lymphomas usually express T-cell receptor antigens (e.g., CD3) and helper antigens (CD4) and have low expression of IL-2 receptors (CD25). By contrast, adult T-cell leukemia/lymphomas express IL-2 receptors (CD25) in addition to HTLV-1 viral antigens, T-cell receptors (CD3), and helper (CD4) antigens. Lymphoblastic lymphomas are of early T-cell lineage and therefore have rearranged T-cell receptor genes,

TABLE 160–1. CELL SURFACE TUMOR MARKERS

Tumor Type	Characteristic Cell Surface Antigens
Lymphomas	
B-cell	
Low grade	Idiotypic Ig, CD5, CD20-22, panleukocyte (CD45, T200, LCA)
Intermediate/high grade	Idiotypic Ig, CD20-22, panleukocyte (CD45, T200, LCA)
T-cell	
Mycosis fungoides/Sézary syndrome	TCR+, CD3+, CD4+, CD8−, CD25−, CD7−
Peripheral T-cell lymphoma	TCR+, CD4+, CD8−, CD3+, CD7−
Adult T-cell leukemia/lymphoma	TCR+, CD25+, CD4+, CD8−, HTLV-1+
Lymphoblastic lymphoma	TCR+, Tdt, CD2, CD7
Hodgkin's disease	Ki-1 (CD30), Leu M1 (CD15)
Leukemias	
Acute lymphoblastic leukemia (ALL)	
Common (80%)	Ig gene rearrangements, CALLA (CD10)
T-cell (15%)	CD7, CD2, TCR, Tdt
B-cell (5%)	Surface Ig, CD20-22
Acute nonlymphocytic leukemia (ANLL)	Myeloid (My) and monocyte (Mo) antigens
Chronic lymphocytic leukemia (CLL)	
B-cell (98%)	Surface Ig, CD20-22, CD5
T-cell (2%)	CD2, 3, 5 (CD4+8− or CD4−8+), TCR
Chronic myelogenous leukemia (CML)	LAP, B12, BCR/Abl
Myeloma	Cytoplasmic Ig, β₂ microglobulin, PCA-1
Carcinomas	
Lung cancers	
Non–small cell	CEA, Ca125, Ca19-9, blood group, HMFG
Small cell	NCAM, CKBB, NSE, GRP, chromogranin
Breast cancer	ER, PR, EGF receptors, cathepsin D, Her-2/neu oncogene
Gastrointestinal cancers	CEA, HMFG, other mucins, blood group antigens
Testicular cancer	β-hCG, AFP
Malignant melanoma	GD₂, GD₃, S100
Hepatoma	AFP
Sarcomas	Desmin, vimentin
Astrocytomas	Glial fibrillary proteins
Thyroid cancer	
Follicular/papillary	Thyroglobulin T₃, T₄
Medullary	Calcitonin, chromogranin, histaminase
Prostate cancer	PSA, PAP, NSE, HMFG's
Ovarian cancer	Ca125, Ca19-9
Pheochromocytoma	Calcitonin, chromogranin

Abbreviations: Ig = immunoglobulin; TcR = T-cell receptor gene rearrangements; LAP = leukocyte alkaline phosphatase; β-hCG = β subunit of human chorionic gonadotropin; AFP = α-fetoprotein; CEA = carcinoembryonic antigen; HMFG = human milk fat globulin; ER = estrogen receptor; PR = progesterone receptor; EGF = epidermal growth factor receptor; NCAM = neural cell adhesion molecule; CK-BB = creatine kinase BB isoenzyme; NSE = neuron-specific enolase; GRP = gastrin-releasing peptide (bombesin); PSA = prostate-specific antigen; PAP = prostatic acid phosphatase.

terminal deoxynucleotidyl transferase (Tdt), and CD2 and CD7 antigens. The cell of origin of Hodgkin's disease remains controversial, but these cells generally express LNFPIII (Leu-M1, CD15) and Ki-I (CD30).

The majority of patients with acute lymphoblastic leukemia have the "common" variety, which has characteristics of early B cells, including rearranged immunoglobulin genes and lack of surface Ig. These cells express the CALLA antigen (CD10). T-cell acute lymphoblastic leukemias, like the lymphoblastic lymphomas, are early T cells with rearranged T-cell receptor genes and the T-cell antigens (CD2 and CD7), and terminal deoxynucleotidyl transferase (Tdt). Myeloid markers are observed in about 25 per cent of ALL's. These biphenotypic cases may have a worse prognosis. ALL's with the Philadelphia chromosome and the BCR/Abl gene products also have a poor prognosis. B-cell ALL's express surface Ig and have a poor prognosis. Acute nonlymphocytic leukemias may express one or more myeloid (My) or monocyte (Mo) antigens depending on the FAB classification.

The vast majority of chronic lymphocytic leukemias (CLL) are of B-cell origin. These express surface immunoglobulin, CD20, 21, and 22 antigens, and the CD5 antigen (generally a T-cell marker). A few per cent of CLL's are of T-cell origin, expressing CD2 and CD3 antigens with rearranged T-cell receptor genes. These T-cell CLL's may have a helper (CD4+, CD8−) or a suppressor (CD4−, CD8+) phenotype. Chronic myelogenous leukemias have increased expression of leukocyte alkaline phosphatase and B12 and express the BCR/Abl oncogene product.

Multiple myeloma was initially thought to be a malignancy of mature plasma cells because of the large amount of cytoplasmic Ig. The finding of β_2 microglobulin and CALLA (CD10) in addition to Ig and TcR gene rearrangements in many cases suggests that the cell may be of primitive lymphoid origin.

Carcinomas nearly always express cytokeratins and lack pan–leukocyte and neural antigens. Non–small cell lung cancers often express CEA, human milk fat globule antigens, other glycolipid antigens, blood group antigens, the EGF receptor and abnormal ras protein. The latter may imply a poor prognosis in adenocarcinomas, although none of these is totally specific for lung cancer. Small cell lung cancers express a variety of neuroendocrine markers such as neural cell adhesion molecule (NCAM), neuron specific enolase (NSE), gastrin-releasing peptide (bombesin-like peptides), chromogranin, and the BB isoenzyme of creatine kinase.

Breast cancers may express estrogen (ER) or progesterone (PR) receptors, the Her2/neu oncogene product, epidermal growth factor receptors (EGF-R), and cathepsin D. Each of these has been reported to have prognostic implications.

Gastrointestinal adenocarcinomas (stomach, pancreas, colon, rectum) often express CEA, Ca125, Ca19-9, other HMFG, and mucin antigens. There are no site-specific antigens, and the clinical relevance of most antigens is undefined. Prostate cancers express prostate-specific antigen, which has a high sensitivity and specificity. NSE, CEA, and other mucin antigens may be expressed but are of less certain clinical relevance. Ovarian adenocarcinomas often express Ca125 and CA19-9, but these are not specific for ovarian cancer.

Testicular germ cell cancers express β-hCG and/or α-AFP in more than 90 per cent of cases. It is extremely important to look for these markers in cases of midline undifferentiated carcinomas, since these may be cured by chemotherapy.

Malignant melanomas nearly always express the S100 protein, although this may also be expressed in schwannomas, chordomas, and cartilaginous tumors. Melanomas usually express GD_2 and GD_3 antigens. Most primary hepatic carcinomas express AFP. Sarcomas express vimentin and dismin. Malignant astrocytomas express glial fibrillary proteins. Neuroblastomas express NCAM and other neural markers.

SERUM TUMOR MARKERS

A list of currently used markers is shown in Table 160–2.

HORMONES. Human chorionic gonadotropin (hCG) is a two-chain (α and β subunits) glycoprotein hormone secreted by the trophoblastic epithelium of the placenta. The β subunit is normally present in maternal serum during pregnancy, but its presence in males and nonpregnant females is indicative of cancer. Measurement of hCG has been used for the diagnosis and management of trophoblastic tumors (choriocarcinoma, hydatidiform mole) and certain germ cell tumors of the testes. Its level has prognostic importance. The rate of decline may be used to assess the effectiveness of therapy, and its reappearance is direct evidence of tumor recurrence. Extragonadal germ cell tumors often secrete β-hCG, and it can be used to help confirm the origin of undifferentiated mediastinal or retroperitoneal tumors. β-hCG may also be secreted by adenocarcinomas of the ovary, pancreas, stomach, and lung and by hepatomas.

A variety of other hormones may be useful tumor markers. Human placental lactogen is secreted by the majority of trophoblastic tumors and a minority of lung cancers, hepatomas, endocrine tumors, leukemias, and lymphomas.

Polypeptide hormones such as *adrenocorticotropic hormone (ACTH)* and *arginine vasopressin (AVP)* may be useful markers when produced by small cell lung cancer or other tumors with properties of amine precursor uptake and decarboxylation (APUD tumors). Similarly, *calcitonin* is used to predict medullary carcinoma of the thyroid in families or it can be used as a marker in APUD tumors that secrete it. *Gastrin-releasing peptide* (bombesin-like protein) is produced by the majority of small cell lung cancers. It is not an ideal tumor marker, however, because it is rapidly degraded in plasma. Elevated levels in the cerebrospinal fluid (CSF) may be useful for predicting leptomeningeal metastases.

TABLE 160–2. SERUM TUMOR CELL MARKERS

Marker	Tumor Types
Hormones	
β subunit of chorionic gonadotropin	Testicular cancers, choriocarcinoma, hydatidiform mole
AVP, ACTH	Small cell lung; APUD tumors
Calcitonin	Medullary thyroid carcinoma, small cell lung and APUD tumors
Gastrin-releasing peptide (bombesin)	Small cell lung cancer
Placental lactogen	Trophoblastic tumors, various carcinomas
Oncofetal Proteins	
α-Fetoprotein	Hepatoma, testicular cancers
Carcinoembryonic antigen (CEA)	Gastrointestinal tract, breast, lung, ovarian cancers
Enzymes	
L-dopa decarboxylase	Small cell lung cancer
Creatine phosphokinase (BB)	Prostate cancer, small cell lung cancer
Neuron-specific enolase	Prostate cancer, small cell lung cancer, others
Acid phosphatase (prostate specific)	Prostate cancer
Placental alkaline phosphatase	Uterus, ovary, breast, lung cancers
Lysozyme	Acute nonlymphatic leukemia (myelomonocytic and monocytic types)
Serum galactosyltransferase	Gastrointestinal carcinomas, breast and prostate cancers
Lactic dehydrogenase (LDH)	Lymphomas, Ewing's sarcoma, various carcinomas
Secreted Tumor Antigens	
CA 125	Ovarian cancer, other epithelial cancers
CA 19-9	Various carcinomas
Prostate-specific antigen	Prostate cancer
Other glycosphingolipids	Various carcinomas
β₂ microglobulin	Multiple myeloma
Miscellaneous	
Vitamin B₂–binding proteins	Acute or chronic myelogenous leukemia, myeloproliferative disease
Immunoglobulin	B-cell lymphoproliferative diseases
Polyamines	Various carcinomas
Chromogranin A	Small cell lung cancer; pheochromocytoma

ONCOFETAL PROTEINS. α-*Fetoprotein (AFP)* is normally secreted in large amounts during the twelfth through fifteenth weeks of gestation and then declines to low levels (<40 ng per milliliter) by the age of 1 year. Elevated levels occur in the majority (75 per cent) of patients with embryonal and teratocarcinomas of the testes and ovary, as well as in those with extragonadal germ cell tumors. Like β-hCG, the level has prognostic implications; the rate of decline predicts the effectiveness of therapy, and a rising titer is direct evidence of tumor progression. Elevated AFP levels are present in 70 to 95 per cent of hepatomas. The incidence is highest in areas where hepatoma is endemic. AFP is increased in a minority of patients with cancers of the pancreas, stomach, colon, and lung. Since AFP is produced by normal cells, there are instances of "false positives." AFP may be produced by benign liver tumors, by cirrhotic livers, or during hepatitis, although these entities usually produce levels less than 500 ng per milliliter. AFP may be increased in patients with ataxia-telangiectasia.

Carcinoembryonic antigen (CEA) is normally secreted during the second to sixth months of gestation. In nonsmoking adults, serum levels are less than 2.5 ng per milliliter, whereas smokers have normal levels up to 5 ng per milliliter. Serum levels of CEA may increase in a variety of inflammatory conditions (e.g., cirrhosis, pancreatitis, inflammatory bowel disease, and rectal polyps) as well as in a variety of human cancers.

Elevated levels of CEA are reported in patients with colon cancer (60 to 90 per cent), pancreatic cancer (80 per cent), gastric cancer (60 per cent), lung cancer (75 per cent), breast cancer (50 per cent), and many other malignant tumors in lower frequency. The frequency with which the level of CEA is elevated and the level attained are dependent on the extent of disease, the degree of differentiation (well-differentiated tumors produce more), and the presence of liver metastases. Because of the high false-positive rate in inflammatory diseases, the principal use of CEA is in monitoring response to therapy and disease progression, especially for carcinoma of the colon (Ch. 105). Elevated levels should return to normal following complete resection of the primary tumor. A persistent elevation or an increasing concentration is highly suggestive of residual or recurrent tumor. Surgical re-exploration in the face of increasing CEA without clinical evidence of disease may lead to discovery of surgically resectable recurrences. These resected patients may then have a long disease-free survival.

Radiolabeled antibodies to CEA and AFP are being evaluated for their ability to detect metastatic disease and for therapy. Preliminary studies show sensitivities in the range of 60 to 80 per cent.

ENZYMES. A variety of enzymes are also useful tumor markers in some settings. The key APUD enzyme, L-dopa decarboxylase, is often increased in patients with small cell lung cancer and other APUD tumors. The serum level of the BB isoenzyme of creatine phosphokinase is elevated in the majority of patients with small cell lung cancer or cancer of the prostate. Serum levels of neuron-specific enolase are often elevated in patients with these same tumors.

Prostatic epithelium also produces a specific *acid phosphatase (prostatic acid phosphatase)* whose serum level is elevated in about one third of patients with occult prostatic cancer and in 75 per cent of patients with more advanced prostatic cancers. *Placental alkaline phosphatase* is secreted by a minority of cancers of the female reproductive organs and breast and lung cancers. *Lysozyme,* a monocyte-derived enzyme, is frequently increased in patients with acute monocytic and myelomonocytic leukemia. An isoenzyme of *serum galactosyltransferase* is present in the serum of patients with gastrointestinal carcinomas (75 per cent) and breast cancer (78 per cent), as well as in a minority of patients with prostatic cancer and lymphoproliferative cancers. Serum lactic dehydrogenase (LDH) levels are elevated in a variety of malignant diseases, including lymphomas (especially Burkitt's), Ewing's sarcomas, and a variety of carcinomas. The extent of elevation may provide prognostic information as well as a useful measure of antitumor response.

SECRETED TUMOR ANTIGENS. The development of monoclonal antibody technology has led to recognition of many new glycoprotein and glycolipid antigens on tumor cells that may be secreted into the plasma. The antigen recognized by the monoclonal antibody *CA 125* is a useful marker for the majority of patients with ovarian cancer. *CA 19-9* recognizes an antigen secreted by many epithelial carcinomas, including colon cancer, but this marker is probably less useful than CEA. Many epithelial carcinomas, especially adenocarcinomas, secrete glycosphingolipids such as Lewis blood group antigens and human milk fat globule antigens. The value of these markers remains to be established. β₂ microglobulin, an HLA class I antigen, is present on the cell surface of most nucleated cells. It is secreted into the plasma in excess amounts in patients with multiple myeloma, where its level has prognostic value and may be useful in assessing response to therapy.

MISCELLANEOUS. *Vitamin B₁₂*-binding proteins are frequently increased in myeloproliferative disorders and occasionally in acute or chronic myelogenous leukemias. The idiotypic *immunoglobulins* produced by B-cell lymphoproliferative malignant disorders are excellent tumor markers and may be used to assess tumor burden as well as to follow response to therapy. More than 99 per cent of patients with multiple myelomas and Waldenström's macroglobulinemia secrete a heavy chain or a light chain (Ch. 151). Occasionally these tumors secrete globulins of more than one idiotype. Monoclonal antibodies to the idiotypic immunoglobulin are being evaluated as therapeutic agents. *Polyamines* are generally secreted in direct relation to the rate of proliferation. In many malignant diseases their quantitation has proven to be useful for prognosis and in assessing response. They are not sufficiently sensitive or specific for widespread use. *Chromogranin A* is a 68,000-dalton protein found in the neurosecretory granules of normal and malignant APUD cells. Serum measurement by radioimmunoassay may be a useful marker of small cell lung cancer disease activity and may be useful for the diagnosis of pheochromocytoma.

Aroney RS, Dermody WC, Alderndorfer P, et al.: Multiple sequential biomarkers in monitoring patients with carcinoma of the lung. Cancer Treat Rep 68:859, 1984. *Reviews the variety of proteins secreted by small cell lung cancers that can be used as tumor markers.*

Hakomori S: Glycosphingolipids. Sci Am 254(5):44, 1986. *This article reviews the various glycosphingolipid antigens present on cancer cells.*

Novis BH, Gluck E, Thomas P, et al.: Serial levels of CA 19-9 and CEA in colonic cancer. J Clin Oncol 4:987, 1986. *An article comparing the utility of these markers.*

Rosen SW, Weintraub BD, Vaitukaitus JL, et al.: Placental proteins and their subunits as tumor markers. Ann Intern Med 82:71, 1975. *A review of the value of placental proteins as tumor markers.*

Sobol RE, O'Connor DT, Addison J, et al.: Elevated serum chromogranin A concentrations in small cell lung cancer. Ann Intern Med 105:698, 1986. *This article is an example of one of several markers of neuroendocrine cells that are useful in following the course of small cell lung cancer patients.*

Wanebo HJ, Rao B, Pinsky CM, et al.: Preoperative carcinoembryonic antigen level as a prognostic indicator in colorectal cancer. N Engl J Med 299:448, 1978. *This article shows the value of oncofetal markers as prognostic indicators.*

161 Endocrine Manifestations of Tumors: "Ectopic" Hormone Production

Stephen B. Baylin

The clinical manifestations of cancer arise not only through the consequences of the invasive properties of primary and metastatic lesions, but also through the hormonal activity of proteins and small peptides secreted by tumor cells. Even though the tumor-associated production of these protein products is common, the incidence of paraneoplastic syndromes is less frequent. This is because these hormones are made, in tumors, either in amounts too small to result in a biologic response or in forms that are biologically inactive. For a given cancer, the spectrum of hormones produced often appears "foreign" with respect to the tissue of origin for the neoplasm. Hence, the term "ectopic" has been applied to this cancer-associated activity. In reality, studies over the past decade have increasingly demonstrated that such basic aspects of normal tissue development as cell lineage relationships and steps in embryogenesis and in cell differentiation during renewal of adult tissues often provide logical explanations for patterns of hormone production by specific cancer types. Also, the rapid elucidation of molecular events regulating gene expression is bringing further understanding of cellular relationships underlying hormonal production patterns in cancer.

Before considering individual endocrine syndromes associated with tumors, it is helpful to broadly classify cancer-associated hormone production patterns according to biologic concepts thought to underlie this phenomenon (Table 161–1). Much of this activity can be associated with the small polypeptide hormones normally secreted by cells that constitute classic endocrine tissues. Common neuroendocrine characteristics of these cells have been recognized and encompassed in the eponym *amine precursor uptake decarboxylase*, or "APUD" cells. Much of the "ectopic" hormone production by tumors involves the peptides from such cells, and the cancer most frequently represented— small cell lung carcinoma—has direct links to cells with APUD features. A common pattern of gene expression events in these cells during development may explain why APUD-associated tumors may often produce more than one small polypeptide hormone at a time.

A group of larger molecular weight glycoprotein hormones is more often produced by non–APUD-associated cancers (Table 161–1). Also, non-APUD tumors are more often associated with products of peptides which result in disorders of calcium homeostasis. The association of tumors and these gene expression events is much less well understood than that outlined above for APUD-cell tumors.

ECTOPIC ACTH PRODUCTION

Cushing's syndrome resulting from tumor cell production of ACTH is one of the first recognized and most common cancer-associated endocrine disorders. This disease is prototypical for the ectopic hormone syndromes associated with APUD cells and almost always occurs in tumors that arise from cells with endocrine features (Table 161–1). The cancer most commonly responsible for tumor-associated Cushing's syndrome is small cell lung carcinoma (SCLC), a common pulmonary neoplasm long recognized to have APUD features similar to those found in normal lung endocrine cells.

The expression of ACTH and related peptides by tumors, as was noted earlier for tumor-associated hormone production in general, is much more frequent than the actual occurrence of Cushing's syndrome. Thus, among all patients with SCLC, the incidence of clinical evidence of excess ACTH production is only 3 to 5 per cent. The biosynthetic events underlying production of biologically active ACTH are complex and involve a series of post-translational steps that cleave biologically active ACTH and other peptides from the precursor gene product, pro-opiomelanocortin (POMC). Normal pituitary cells contain all of the enzymes required for this processing. However, most cancer cells, even SCLC, cannot fully process the precursor POMC molecule even though they express, to variable levels, the POMC gene. In rare but well-documented situations, tumor-associated Cushing's syndrome can result from production of corticotropin-releasing factor (CRF) by cancer cells. The excess CRF then stimulates pituitary cells to release excess ACTH.

The symptoms of Cushing's syndrome in patients with cancer are much more varied and subtle than those in patients with pituitary-adrenal Cushing's disease (Ch. 217). The virulent behavior of the cancer most frequently involved, SCLC, means that the patients do not have time to develop the full spectrum of symptoms associated with Cushing's disease. The most prominent manifestations are therefore those associated with the early metabolic consequences of excessive glucocorticoid production, including generalized weakness, carbohydrate intolerance, and mental changes, and problems secondary to mineralocorticoid excess, including edema, hypertension, and hypokalemic alkalosis. Hypokalemia, especially, is more prominent in patients with tumor-associated ACTH excess than in patients with pituitary Cushing's disease. These symptoms and/or electrolyte changes in patients with cancer, and especially those with SCLC, should alert the physician to the possibility of ectopic Cushing's syndrome.

The diagnostic questions in ectopic Cushing's syndrome relate to documenting the source of excess ACTH secretion. A first clue for a nonpituitary tumor–related source is the finding of an extraordinarily high plasma ACTH value, much in excess of those found in pituitary Cushing's disease. Urinary free cortisol levels are always elevated and, unlike in Cushing's disease (Ch. 217), are usually *not* suppressible during a high-dose (8 mg per day) dexamethasone suppression test. Only in some patients with carcinoid tumors, and in the rare situation of tumors producing CRF, does this high-dose suppression test lower urinary cortisol in patients with "ectopic" Cushing's syndrome.

The treatment of tumor-associated Cushing's syndrome is often frustrating because of the aggressive nature of the cancers most frequently associated with this condition. An exception to this is

TABLE 161–1. HORMONE-SECRETING TUMORS

	Hormones Secreted
Tumors most frequently secreting APUD hormones	
Small cell lung carcinoma	ACTH,* CRF,* ADH,* calcitonin, GRP, GRF
Carcinoid tumors (lung, pancreas, GI tract, thymus, ovary)	ACTH,* GRF
Islet cell tumors of pancreas	ACTH,* GRF
Medullary thyroid carcinoma	ACTH,* GRF, GRP, somatostatin
Pheochromocytoma	ACTH,* GRF
Neural tumors (ganglioneuroma)	ACTH,* VIP,* GRF
Melanoma	ACTH*
Prostate	ACTH*
Tumors most frequently secreting large glycoprotein hormones	
Non–small cell lung carcinomas	hCG*
Testicular carcinomas (embryonal components)	hCG*
Sarcomas	hCG*
Tumors most frequently causing hormonally mediated hypercalcemia	
Squamous cell carcinoma (lung, head, and neck)	PTH RP*
Renal carcinomas	PTH RP*
Bladder carcinomas	PTH RP*
Adenocarcinomas	PTH RP*
Lymphomas	PTH RP*

*Responsible for producing a clinical syndrome.
  ACTH = adrenocorticopic hormone
  ADH = vasopressin
  CRF = corticotropin-releasing factor
  GRF = growth hormone–releasing factor
  GRP = gastrin-releasing peptide
  VIP = vasoactive intestinal polypeptide
  hCG = human chorionic gonadotropin
  PTH RP = parathyroid hormone–related peptide

carcinoid tumors, in which the clinical course is often protracted. The most efficacious therapy is primary eradication of the responsible neoplasm, either through chemotherapy or surgery. For SCLC, such complete tumor ablation is not usually possible. Alternatively, transient improvement may be obtained by using drugs, discussed in Ch. 217, which block steroid synthesis in the adrenal gland (such as metyrapone, aminoglutethimide, or ketoconazole).

CANCER-ASSOCIATED HYPERCALCEMIA

Hypercalcemia in patients with cancer is probably the most frequently seen paraneoplastic syndrome. In turn, cancer is the most commonly recognized cause of hypercalcemia in hospitalized patients. It is then imperative to rule out the presence of a tumor in any patient, especially one in the older age range, who has documented hypercalcemia.

The etiologies of tumor-associated hypercalcemia are varied. Direct effects of tumor metastases on bone resorption must always be considered, but it has become increasingly apparent that hormonal factors are more often involved. For many years, it was believed that parathyroid hormone (PTH), synthesized and secreted by tumor cells, was the etiologic agent. This hypothesis was based on detection of PTH immunoreactivity in sera of patients with tumors and hypercalcemia and presence of increased cyclic AMP levels in urine of such individuals.

However, during recent years, several groups have reported that a different small peptide, PTH-like peptide (PLP), which has partial homology to PTH only in the first 13 amino acids, is probably the humoral agent most frequently responsible for tumor-associated hypercalcemia. Interestingly, the gene for this hormone is normally ubiquitously expressed, and is not, as are other small polypeptide hormones, especially associated with normal cells having APUD endocrine features. Levels are especially high in normal keratinocytes, lactating mammary tissue, placenta, and other sites where the peptide appears to have a physiologic role. This distribution may explain why non-APUD tumors such as squamous cell, bladder, ovarian, and renal carcinomas have been most frequently associated to date with PLP secretion and hypercalcemia (Table 161–1).

Other humoral factors also play a variable role in producing hypercalcemia in patients with cancer. Growth factors, such as transforming growth factor (TGF-β), bone resorbing factors such as are found in hematologic malignancies, prostaglandins, and, occasionally, active vitamin D metabolites have all been documented as tumor products that can cause hypercalcemia. It is apparent, then, that multiple factors can be simultaneously active to cause the hypercalcemia associated with tumors.

The diagnosis of tumor-associated hypercalcemia should be suspected in any patient with hypercalcemia. The suspicion is obviously highest for a patient with known cancer who develops or presents with this metabolic abnormality. The most important alternative and treatable etiology for hypercalcemia is primary hyperparathyroidism (Ch. 235). Features favoring this latter condition include a longstanding history of hypercalcemia and presence of subperiosteal bone resorption and renal stones. High circulating PTH levels with high urinary cyclic AMP levels are characteristic of patients with primary hyperparathyroidism. In contrast, patients with cancer and hypercalcemia have relatively low PTH levels in conjunction with high urine cyclic AMP.

The treatment for tumor-associated hypercalcemia can be difficult because the cancers most frequently associated are often extensive and aggressive at the time of diagnosis. Direct ablation of, or reduction in, tumor mass is the optimal treatment when feasible. When this is not possible, treatment of the hypercalcemia depends upon its severity and consequences for the patient. The simplest therapeutic approaches employ combinations of hydration and diuretics. For more refractory and severe hypercalcemia, drugs such as mithramycin or diphosphonates may have to be added to this regimen. These treatments for hypercalcemia are discussed in more detail in Ch. 165.

TUMOR PRODUCTION OF HUMAN CHORIONIC GONADOTROPIN

The production by tumors of chorionic gonadotropin (hCG), a large molecular weight glycoprotein, is another example of hormonal activity most associated with the non-APUD group of

cancers (Table 161–1). As for other hormones, asymptomatic production of hCG is far more frequent than the situation in which enough biologically active hCG is produced to cause symptoms in the patient. hCG is composed of α and β subunits, which are often discordantly produced by neoplasms. Production of the α subunit is particularly common, and elevated circulating levels of this peptide are often found in patients with multiple types of cancer. Production of intact hCG is common in tumors of trophoblastic origin (i.e., choriocarcinomas, testicular embryonal carcinomas, and seminomas), the normal source for hCG, and less often seen in cancers of the lung, pancreas, and other types.

The infrequent symptoms associated with tumor-associated secretion of hCG include precocious puberty in children and gynecomastia in adult males, usually associated with advanced tumors such as lung carcinoma. The treatment for these syndromes, especially in adults, is usually ineffective given the advanced nature of the tumors.

HYPOGLYCEMIA AND TUMORS

A long-recognized syndrome, most often associated with mesenchymal tumors (retroperitoneal fibrosarcomas, hemangiopericytomas and leiomyosarcomas, adrenocortical carcinomas, and hepatomas), is hormonally induced hypoglycemia. This metabolic disorder, first thought to be secondary to excess insulin produced by tumor cells, has subsequently been linked to production of insulin-like factors or so-called nonsuppressible insulin-like activity. Recently, the association of one such factor, insulin-like growth factor II (IGF-II), with tumor-related hypoglycemia has been strengthened by the demonstration of IGF-II mRNA and peptide in mesenchymal tumors associated with hypoglycemia. However, the physiologic role of IGF-II remains uncertain, since serum IGF-II levels in patients with these tumors have not been found to be uniformly elevated. The interpretation of these studies is made difficult by the presence of serum-binding proteins, and further studies are needed to establish convincingly the role of IGF-II in tumor hypoglycemia.

HYPONATREMIA, INAPPROPRIATE ANTIDIURETIC HORMONE SYNDROME (SIADH), AND CANCER

An important metabolic abnormality occurring in patients with cancer is hyponatremia. The classic syndrome is associated with the presence of hyponatremia, increased urine osmolality, increased urine sodium (>20 mEq per liter), and decreased serum osmolality (<275 mOsm per liter). A series of investigators over the years, using first biologic assays and later immunoassays, has established that these electrolyte imbalances result from production and secretion by tumor cells of a polypeptide hormone, vasopressin or antidiuretic hormone (ADH). As for other "ectopic" hormone syndromes associated with small polypeptide hormones, inappropriate secretion of ADH is most often associated with, but not restricted to, the APUD tumor, SCLC (Table 161–1). Such tumors most frequently have the cellular features necessary to synthesize a 20,000-dalton glycosylated prohormone, provasopressin, and to process this peptide to the smaller biologically active ADH molecule.

Recognition of SIADH is important because the symptoms of hyponatremia, such as lethargy and mental changes, can present severe problems for patients with cancer. Also, the hyponatremia can be successfully managed by fluid restriction, careful administration of saline solutions, and/or treatment with drugs such as demeclocycline.

OTHER TUMOR-ASSOCIATED HORMONE SYNDROMES

While the syndromes discussed above constitute the majority of cancer-related endocrine diseases, there are other less frequent tumor-associated hormonal states that are important for the clinician to recognize.

ONCOGENIC OSTEOMALACIA

A syndrome associated with bone pain and muscle weakness, together with the radiologic features of osteomalacia, can occur in patients with mesenchymal tumors such as benign osteoblastomas, giant cell osteosarcomas, hemangiomas, and occasionally epithelial tumors such as prostate and SCLC. Biochemical studies show hypophosphatemia and subnormal 1,25-dihydroxyvitamin D levels. The pathophysiology of this disorder is unclear but appears to involve a hormonally mediated and severe renal phosphate loss as the primary event. The tumor origin of the inciting factor is inferred from the observations that the syndrome can remit dramatically with irradiation of the neoplasm. When primary treatment of the tumor is not feasible, treatment with phosphorus replacement and vitamin D can provide substantial improvement of symptoms and hypophosphatemia.

POLYCYTHEMIA

Tumors such as hepatomas, hemangiomas, and renal carcinomas can cause polycythemia. Recently, such tumors have been shown to produce erythropoietin mRNA, and patients with this syndrome have been found to have elevated erythropoietin levels in their serum by immunoassay. In general, no treatment is required. However, intermittent phlebotomy is occasionally required to alleviate symptoms.

TROPHOBLASTIC HYPERTHYROIDISM

The thyrotropic activity inherent to the choriogonadotropin (hCG) molecule can occasionally account for appearance of a small goiter and mild hyperthyroidism in patients with choriocarcinomas or hydatidiform moles. Occasionally, the hyperthyroidism can be severe enough to require treatment with antithyroid drugs.

HYPERTENSION

Renin-secreting tumors must be considered in the differential diagnosis of hypertension and hypokalemia. Most commonly, these tumors arise in the juxtaglomerular cells, the normal source of renin. Extrarenal renin-secreting tumors are rare and include pancreatic, ovarian, and pulmonary tumors. In general, hypertension subsides upon removal of the tumors. However, extrarenal renin-secreting tumors are usually aggressive and quite advanced at the time of presentation. In these situations, angiotensin-converting enzyme inhibitors such as captopril may be required for treatment of hypertension.

ACROMEGALY

The production of growth hormone or, more rarely, growth hormone–releasing factor (GRF), has been documented in nonpituitary tumors such as carcinoids, pancreatic islet cell neoplasms, pulmonary carcinomas, and gastric, ovarian, and breast carcinomas. Uncommonly, this can produce the full manifestations of acromegaly. For production of GRF (Table 161–1), the associated tumors generally arise from endocrine cells. The treatment of tumor-associated acromegaly is, when feasible, removal of the causative neoplasm.

OTHER HORMONES PRODUCED BY TUMORS

A number of other hormones, often in the small polypeptide hormone category (some are shown in Table 161–1), may be found in tumor tissue and/or secreted by the tumor. Examples include calcitonin, somatostatin, and GRP in endocrine tumors. These hormones have not been associated with clinical syndromes in patients with these diseases but in some instances may be useful tumor markers to follow in monitoring disease course.

Baylin SB, Mendelsohn G: Ectopic (inappropriate) hormone production by tumors: Mechanisms involved and the biological and clinical implications. Endocr Rev 1:45, 1980. *This review concentrates on the biology of tumor-associated hormone production.*

de Bustros A, Baylin SB: Ectopic hormone production by tumors. *In* Moore WT, Eastman R (eds.): Diagnostic Endocrinology. Ontario, B.C. Decker, Inc., 1990, p 283. *This more recent review both discusses current concepts of the biology of tumor-associated hormone production and outlines the clinical syndromes that result.*

Odell WD: Humoral manifestations of cancer. *In* Williams RH (ed.): Textbook of Endocrinology, 7th ed. Philadelphia, W.B. Saunders Company, 1984.

Ectopic ACTH Production

Carey RM, Varma SK, Drake CR Jr, et al.: Ectopic secretion of corticotropin-releasing factor as a cause of Cushing's syndrome: A clinical, morphological and biochemical study. N Engl J Med 311:13, 1984. *This study provides an example of a patient with Cushing's syndrome caused by tumor production of CRF.*

Gerwirtz G, Yallow RS: Ectopic ACTH production in carcinoma of the lung. J Clin Invest 53:1022, 1974. *This paper is the classic first description of the presence of ACTH immunoreactivity, most in a biologically inactive form, in all lung carcinomas.*

Hypercalcemia and Cancer

Broadus AE, Mangin M, Insogna KL, et al.: Humoral hypercalcemia of cancer. N Engl J Med 319:556, 1988. *This is a good overall review of the biology and clinical aspects of the humorally mediated hypercalcemia of cancer.*

Burtis WJ, Brady TG, Orloff JJ, et al.: Immunochemical characterization of circulating parathyroid hormone–related protein in patients with humoral hypercalcemia of cancer. N Engl J Med 322:1106–1112, 1990. *This paper defines the incidence of increased circulating parathyroid hormone–related protein levels in patients with neoplasms.*

Chorionic Gonadotropin and Cancer

Braunstein GD, Vaitukaitis JL, Carbone PP, et al.: Ectopic production of human chorionic gonadotropin by neoplasms. Ann Intern Med 78:39, 1973. *This is a classic paper for defining the incidence of ectopic production of hCG.*

Hypoglycemia and Cancer

Gorden P, Hendricks CM, Kahn CR, et al.: Hypoglycemia associated with non-islet-cell tumor and insulin-like growth factors: A study of the tumor types. N Engl J Med 305:1452, 1981. *This paper reviews the tumor types associated with hormonally mediated hypoglycemia.*

Widmer V, Zapf J, Froesch ER: Is extrapancreatic tumor hypoglycemia associated with elevated levels of insulin-like growth factor II? J Clin Endocrinol Metab 55:833, 1982. *Some of the questions about the role of IGF-II in tumor-associated hypoglycemia are addressed.*

Vasopressin and Cancer

Amatruda TT Jr, Mulrow PJ, Gallagher JC, et al.: Carcinoma of the lung with inappropriate antidiuresis. Demonstration of antidiuretic-hormone–like activity in tumor extracts. N Engl J Med 269:544, 1963. *This paper is the classic description of ADH production by a lung carcinoma.*

Yamaji T, Ishibashi M, Katayama S, et al.: Neurophysin biosynthesis in vitro in oat cell carcinoma of the lung with ectopic vasopressin production. J Clin Invest 68:1441, 1981.

Osteomalacia and Cancer

Nuovo MA, Dorfman HD, Sun C-C, Chalew SA: Tumor-induced osteomalacia and rickets. Am J Surg Pathol 13:588, 1989. *This is a good overall review.*

Ryan EA, Reiss E: Oncogenous osteomalacia: Review of the world literature of 42 cases and report of two new cases. Am J Med 77:501, 1984. *This is another extensive review of this syndrome.*

Polycythemia and Cancer

DaSilva J-L, Lacombe C, Bruneval P, et al.: Tumor cells are the site of erythropoietin synthesis in human renal cancers associated with polycythemia. Blood 75:577, 1990. *This paper documents erythropoietin production from tumor cells.*

Hammond D, Winnick S: Paraneoplastic erythrocytosis and ectopic erythropoietins. Ann NY Acad Sci 230:219, 1974. *This paper reviews this association.*

Trophoblastic Hyperthyroidism

Nisula BC, Ketelslegers J-M: Thyroid-stimulating activity and chorionic gonadotropin. J Clin Invest 54:494, 1974.

Wilber JF, Spinella P: Identification of immunoreactive thyrotropin-releasing hormone in human neoplasia. J Clin Endocrinol Metab 59:432, 1984. *These above two papers describe the syndrome and the role of hCG.*

Hypertension and Cancer

Atlas SA, Hesson TE, Sealey JE, et al.: Characterization of inactive renin ("prorenin") from renin-secreting tumors of non-renal origin. J Clin Invest 73:437, 1984.

Ruddy MC, Atlas SA, Salerno FG: Hypertension associated with a renin-secreting adenocarcinoma of the pancreas. N Engl J Med 307:993, 1982.

Acromegaly and Cancer

Asa SI, Kovacs K, Thorner MO, et al.: Immunohistological localization of growth hormone-releasing hormone in human tumors. J Clin Endocrinol Metab 60:423, 1985.

Gubler U, Monahan JJ, Lomedico PT, et al.: Cloning and sequence analysis of cDNA for the precursor of human growth hormone-releasing factor, somatocrinin. Proc Natl Acad Sci USA 80:4311, 1983.

Mayo KE, Vale W, Rivier J, et al.: Expression-cloning and sequencing of a cDNA encoding human growth hormone-releasing factor. Nature 306:86, 1983. *This paper documents growth hormone "production" by tumors.*

Rivier J, Spiess J, Thorner M, et al.: Characterization of a growth hormone releasing factor from a human pancreatic islet tumor. Nature 300:276, 1982. *This paper documents GRF from neoplasms.*

162 Nonmetastatic Effects of Cancer on the Nervous System

Jerome B. Posner

When patients with systemic cancer develop nervous system dysfunction, metastasis is usually the cause. However, cancer can exert deleterious effects on the nervous system by mechanisms other than metastasis. Recognition of these nonmetastatic neurologic complications can prevent inappropriate and perhaps harmful therapy directed at a nonexistent metastasis. Sometimes nervous system symptoms precede the discovery of the cancer and can, if correctly interpreted, lead the physician to the diagnosis of an otherwise occult neoplasm.

An almost bewildering variety of neurologic disorders have been ascribed to effects of systemic cancer (Table 162–1). Most patients with nervous system dysfunction not caused by metastases are eventually found to be suffering from infection, vascular or metabolic disorders, or neurotoxicity of chemotherapy. This chapter discusses two other types of nervous system damage related to cancer not described elsewhere in this book: "remote effects" or paraneoplastic syndromes (Table 162–2) and radiation injury.

REMOTE EFFECTS

Remote effects of cancer on the nervous system (paraneoplastic syndromes) refer to neurologic disorders of unknown cause that occur at higher frequency in patients with cancer than in the general population. These syndromes are not common. Excluding patients with mild peripheral neuropathy or myopathy possibly associated with cachexia, remote effects of cancer affect less than 1 per cent of unselected patients with cancer. Lung cancer accounts for more than 50 per cent of cases; the incidence is greatest among patients with ovarian and small cell lung cancer and Hodgkin's disease. Because of its rarity, the diagnosis of paraneoplastic syndrome should never be accepted until a thorough evaluation has excluded metastatic or other nonmetastatic causes of neurologic dysfunction. In particular, infiltration of nerve roots by tumor in the leptomeninges may mimic paraneoplastic peripheral neuropathy.

Increasing evidence suggests that the etiology of most or all remote effects is autoimmune. Patients with the Lambert-Eaton myasthenic syndrome (see below) harbor an IgG antibody that reacts with voltage-gated calcium channels on the presynaptic neuromuscular junction. Complexing of these channels by the antibody prevents normal release of acetylcholine, which, in turn, causes the clinical symptoms of the disorder. About two thirds of patients with the Lambert-Eaton myasthenic syndrome have, or will shortly develop, evidence of small cell lung cancer. The tumors possess a protein antigen homologous with or identical to the calcium channels in the neuromuscular junction against which the antibody response is presumed to be directed.

TABLE 162–1. NONMETASTATIC EFFECTS OF CANCER ON THE NERVOUS SYSTEM

Remote effects or paraneoplastic syndromes (see Table 162–2)
Side effects of therapy
  Chemotherapy
  Radiation therapy (see Table 162–3)
Metabolic and nutritional abnormalities
  Destruction of vital organs (e.g., liver)
  Elaboration of hormonal substances by tumor
  Competition between tumor and brain for essential substrates (e.g., glucose)
  Malnutrition
Infections (usually associated with lymphomas)
  Parasites (e.g., toxoplasmosis)
  Fungi (e.g., cryptococcosis, aspergillosis, mucormycosis)
  Bacteria (e.g., *Listeria monocytogenes*)
  Viruses (e.g., herpes zoster)
Vascular disease
  Intracranial hemorrhage
  Cerebral infarction

TABLE 162–2. REMOTE EFFECTS OF CANCER ON THE NERVOUS SYSTEM (PARANEOPLASTIC SYNDROMES)

Brain and cranial nerves
  Dementia—limbic encephalitis
  Retinal degeneration
  Optic neuritis
  Opsoclonus-myoclonus
  Subacute cerebellar degeneration
  Brain stem encephalitis
Spinal cord
  Subacute motor neuronopathy
  Necrotizing myelopathy
  Myelitis
  Motor neuron disease
Dorsal root ganglia
  Subacute sensory neuronopathy
Peripheral nerve
  Subacute or chronic sensorimotor peripheral neuropathy
  Acute polyradiculoneuropathy (Guillain-Barré syndrome)
  Remitting and relapsing peripheral neuropathy
  Mononeuropathies
  Mononeuritis multiplex
  Brachial neuritis
  Autonomic neuropathy
  Peripheral neuropathy associated with paraproteinemia
Neuromuscular junction and muscle
  Lambert-Eaton myasthenic syndrome
  Myasthenia gravis
  Dermatomyositis, polymyositis
  Acute necrotizing myopathy
  Carcinoid myopathies
  Myotonia
  Cachectic myopathy
  "Neuromyopathy"

Removal of IgG from the serum of a patient with Lambert-Eaton myasthenic syndrome ameliorates the neuromuscular symptoms, and injection of that IgG into experimental animals reproduces the neurologic disorder. High titers of antibodies against other onconeural antigens (antigens shared between tumor and nervous system) are found in several other paraneoplastic syndromes (see below), suggesting a mechanism similar to that in the Lambert-Eaton syndrome. However, paraneoplastic syndromes may be a heterogeneous group of disorders in which other etiologies, such as opportunistic viral infections, competition between tumor in the nervous system for essential metabolites, and secretion by tumor of neurotoxins, may also play a role.

Paraneoplastic syndromes are usually classified by the anatomic site of neurologic disability (Table 162–2). However, it is common for more than one anatomic site to be involved (e.g., Lambert-Eaton syndrome and cerebellar degeneration, dementia and myelopathy, limbic encephalitis and sensory neuronopathy). When more than one symptom is present, the disorder can be called paraneoplastic encephalomyelitis or paraneoplastic encephalomyeloneuritis. Some of the more characteristic paraneoplastic syndromes are described in the paragraphs below.

Brain and Cranial Nerves

CEREBRUM. Cerebral remote effects are usually characterized by dementia with or without other neurologic findings. Loss of recent memory and affective alterations, either anxiety or depression, are the usual findings. Seizures are prominent in some patients; others have a fluctuating confusional state. When other abnormal neurologic signs are present, they usually point to the brain stem, cerebellum, or peripheral nerves (encephalomyelitis). The cerebrospinal fluid usually contains 10 to 40 lymphocytes per cubic milliliter, with a slight elevation of the protein concentration. Computed tomography (CT) and magnetic resonance imaging (MRI) are usually normal, but in occasional patients abnormalities can be found in the medial temporal areas. Antibodies reacting with neuronal nuclei can be found in patients with limbic encephalitis associated with small cell lung cancer.

Pathologically, there are two main groups: In some patients, no significant pathologic changes are found in the cerebrum despite clinical dementia. Other patients demonstrate widespread cerebral neuronal loss, gliosis, and perivascular collections of lymphocytes, particularly in the medial temporal lobes (limbic encephalitis) or the thalamus. In those patients who have antineuronal antibodies in blood and spinal fluid, the same antibodies can also be identified in the brain. The differential diagnosis includes brain or leptomeningeal metastases; fungal, parasitic, or viral infections (including multifocal leukoencephalopathy); and metabolic encephalopathy. Appropriate imaging, cerebrospinal fluid (CSF) examination, and other laboratory tests usually identify these disorders. The rapid onset of dementia in middle age accompanied by cerebellar, brain stem, or peripheral nerve dysfunction, but no other focal cerebral signs, suggests paraneoplastic dementia as a remote effect of cancer. Degenerative dementias such as Alzheimer's disease usually are slower in onset and have a more protracted course. However, paraneoplastic dementia may be confused with Creutzfeldt-Jakob disease (see Ch. 478.6). There is no specific treatment for paraneoplastic dementias, but they occasionally improve with successful therapy of the cancer.

CEREBELLUM. Paraneoplastic cerebellar degeneration is clinically sufficiently characteristic to suggest cancer even when neurologic symptoms predate diagnosis of the tumor. Symptoms usually evolve over weeks, with bilateral and symmetric cerebellar dysfunction, the patient being equally ataxic in arms and legs. Severe dysarthria is usually present, vertigo and diplopia are common, but nystagmus may be absent. Some patients have neurologic signs pointing to disease outside the cerebellum (e.g., extensor plantar responses, diminished or exaggerated tendon reflexes, dementia). Early in the disorder there is a cerebrospinal fluid pleocytosis, and an elevated IgG content is common. The disease, which may be associated with any cancer, precedes the discovery of the neoplasm by a few weeks to 3 years in more than half the patients. Cerebellar atrophy may be seen on MR scan, particularly late in the course of the illness. In a subset of patients with gynecologic cancers (ovarian, uterine, fallopian tube, breast), an antibody reacting exclusively with cerebellar Purkinje cells and with the underlying tumor allows a definitive diagnosis to be made before the tumor is discovered. Other antibodies may be present in some other patients with nongynecologic tumors. The role of the antibody in the pathogenesis of the disease is not established.

Characteristic pathologic changes consist of diffuse or patchy loss of cerebellar Purkinje cells. There may be lymphocytic cuffs around blood vessels, particularly in the deep nuclei. The illness can be distinguished from cerebellar or leptomeningeal metastases by the symmetry of its signs and the absence of increased intracranial pressure as well as by MR and CSF examination. *Listeria* meningitis and progressive multifocal leukoencephalopathy may present with cerebellar signs also distinguishable by MR and CSF examination. In alcohol-nutritional cerebellar degeneration, truncal and lower extremity ataxia are prominent, but nystagmus, dysarthria, and upper extremity ataxia are mild or absent. Sporadic or familial cerebellar degenerative disorders are much slower in onset. Cerebellar dysfunction associated with viral infections (varicella, infectious mononucleosis) or with chemotherapy (5-fluorouracil, cytosine arabinoside) may mimic paraneoplastic cerebellar degeneration. Paraneoplastic cerebellar degeneration usually runs a subacute course and then stabilizes or, on rare occasions, improves with successful treatment of the tumor.

Cranial Nerves

Two rare but striking paraneoplastic syndromes affect the eyes. The first is characterized by rapid onset of blindness associated with retinal degeneration, usually of photoreceptors. In some such patients, antibodies that react with cells in the retina can be identified in the serum, suggesting that the disorder is an immune one. Optic neuritis, which does not differ clinically in any way from the idiopathic disorder, has also been described in some patients with underlying neoplasms. Opsoclonus (saccadic conjugate involuntary movement of the eyes), also called saccadomania, is often a paraneoplastic disorder. About 50 per cent of infants and children with opsoclonus have underlying neuroblastoma. In adults about 20 per cent of patients with opsoclonus probably have an underlying cancer, usually breast cancer. The disorder in adults may be associated with an antibody different from that found in encephalomyelitis associated with small cell lung cancer. Except when the autoantibody is present, there is no way of clinically distinguishing paraneoplastic opsoclonus from opsoclonus caused by metabolic or structural abnormalities of the brain stem or cerebellum.

Spinal Cord

Two rare but distinct myelopathies complicate cancer: The first, *subacute motor neuronopathy*, affects anterior horn cells, usually in patients with Hodgkin's disease or other lymphomas. The course is subacute, with progressive painless asymmetric lower motor neuron weakness of legs and arms. Some patients complain of sensory symptoms, but sensory loss is mild or absent despite profound weakness. The major pathologic finding is degeneration of anterior horn cells. Sometimes there is inflammation in the anterior horns and demyelination in the white matter of the spinal cord. The clinical course is different from most remote effects in that many patients improve spontaneously, independently of the course of the underlying lymphoma. The etiology is unknown, but a similar disorder in mice harboring lymphomas appears to be caused by a retrovirus. Rarely, gray matter myelopathies with clinical courses resembling syringomyelia or autonomic insufficiency complicate systemic cancer.

The second condition is *subacute necrotic destruction of the spinal cord*, a myelopathy in which both gray and white matter are affected equally. Clinically, there is rapidly ascending sensory and motor loss, usually to midthoracic levels, the patient becoming paraplegic and incontinent within hours or days. The neurologic symptoms often precede the discovery of the neoplasm, and the illness is clinically and pathologically indistinguishable from idiopathic subacute necrotic myelopathy. Since epidural spinal cord compression from metastatic tumor or arteriovenous spinal cord anomalies may present similar clinical signs, a myelogram or MR scan is essential. Amyotrophic lateral sclerosis has been reported as a remote effect of cancer, but it is doubtful that it occurs in patients with cancer more often than in the general population.

Peripheral Nerves and Dorsal Root Ganglia

Four clinical peripheral nerve disorders occur in association with cancer. Characteristic of carcinoma is *subacute sensory neuronopathy* marked by loss of sensation with relative preservation of motor power. The illness usually precedes the appearance of the carcinoma and progresses over a few months, leaving the patient with moderate or severe disability. Cerebrospinal fluid pleocytosis and increased IgG content are common. Pathologically, there is destruction of posterior root ganglia with perivascular lymphocytic cuffing and wallerian degeneration of sensory nerves. Many of the patients have inflammatory and degenerative changes in brain and spinal cord as well (encephalomyelitis). The disorder, when associated with small cell carcinoma, is characterized by serum antibodies reacting against neuronal nuclei and small cell lung cancer cells. There is no treatment.

More common than sensory neuronopathy is a *distal sensorimotor polyneuropathy* characterized by motor weakness, sensory loss, and absence of distal reflexes in the extremities. The illness is pathologically characterized by either segmental demyelination or wallerian degeneration (or both) of sensory and motor peripheral nerves. Pathologically and clinically, the sensorimotor neuropathy is indistinguishable from polyneuropathies not associated with cancer. Indeed, some have suggested that late or terminal polyneuropathy may be due to nutritional deprivation associated with cancer. Its etiology, however, is not clear, and it does not respond to treatment with vitamins or other nutritional supplements.

A *polyneuritis* clinically and pathologically indistinguishable from acute postinfectious polyneuropathy (Guillain-Barré syndrome) also complicates cancers, particularly Hodgkin's disease. A few patients with *neuropathy limited to the autonomic nervous system* have been reported.

Neuromuscular Junction and Muscles

NEUROMUSCULAR JUNCTION. *Myasthenia gravis* is associated with thymomas but usually not other systemic tumors.

The Lambert-Eaton myasthenic syndrome is characterized by weakness and fatigability of proximal muscles, particularly of the pelvic girdle and thighs. The cranial nerves and respiratory muscles are usually spared. Patients often complain of dryness of the mouth, impotence, pain in the thighs, and peripheral paresthesias. On examination there is weakness of the proximal muscles, but strength increases over several seconds of sustained contraction. The deep tendon reflexes are diminished or absent. The diagnosis is made by electromyographic studies in which repeated nerve stimulations at rates above 10 per second cause a progressive *increase* in the size of the muscle action potential (the opposite of myasthenia gravis). About two thirds of patients with this syndrome either have or will develop cancer, usually small cell carcinoma of the lung. The neuromuscular defect in this illness is believed to be deficient release of acetylcholine. Similar findings have been produced in experimental animals by injection of either serum IgG or extract of tumor in patients with the disorder. Plasmapheresis and immunosuppressant drugs may relieve symptoms, as may successful treatment of the neoplasm. The illness responds poorly to anticholinesterase drugs but does respond to 3,4-diaminopyridine in doses up to 100 mg per day.

MUSCLE. Typical *dermatomyositis* or *polymyositis* may occur as a remote effect of cancer (see Ch. 268). Fewer than 10 per cent of patients with this disorder have cancer, but the figure is higher in older patients. The clinical picture of polymyositis associated with cancer (i.e., subacute development of weakness, particularly involving proximal muscles and sometimes bulbar muscles) is indistinguishable from that of dermatomyositis or polymyositis not associated with cancer. Pathologically, there may be two groups: one with the typical inflammatory lesions of polymyositis and one with little inflammation but severe muscle necrosis. The latter group may suffer an explosive clinical course. The patients respond somewhat less well to corticosteroid therapy than do those with dermatomyositis unaccompanied by cancer, although substantial improvement with steroid treatment does occur in some.

Muscle Weakness. Some patients with cancer complain of *weakness* and *fatigability* that seem worse than can be accounted for by their cancer alone. Cachexia and weight loss alone do not usually cause measurable muscle weakness. The weakness is usually proximal and produces particular difficulty climbing stairs or getting out of low chairs. Ankle reflexes may be diminished or absent. Further neurologic evaluation does not yield findings diagnostic of one of the remote effects of cancer described above. Brain and his colleagues have labeled this entity neuromyopathy because its exact anatomic locus is unclear, but others have suggested that it is a nonspecific accompaniment of cachexia and systemic illness. Specific (type II) muscle fiber atrophy develops early in patients with systemic cancer. The cause and treatment of the weakness are unknown.

Henson RA, Urich H: Cancer and the Nervous System. Oxford, Blackwell Scientific Publications Ltd., 1982. *Comprehensive clinical and pathologic descriptions of all the paraneoplastic disorders.*
Posner JB, Furneaux HM: Paraneoplastic syndromes. *In* Waksman BH (ed.): Immunologic Mechanisms in Neurologic and Psychiatric Disease. New York, Raven Press, 1990, pp 187–219. *A review of paraneoplastic syndromes, with emphasis on the evidence for autoimmune pathogenesis.*

NERVOUS SYSTEM INJURY FROM THERAPEUTIC RADIATION

Adverse effects of ionizing radiation on the nervous system (Table 162–3) are related to the total dose of radiation, the size of each fraction, the total duration over which the dose is received, and the volume of nervous system tissue irradiated. Other factors, such as underlying nervous system disease (e.g., brain tumor, cerebral edema), previous surgery, concomitant use of chemotherapeutic agents, and individual susceptibility, make it impossible to define precisely a safe dose of radiation therapy for a given individual. However, guidelines allow the radiation therapist to calculate generally safe nervous system doses. Adverse effects may involve any portion of the central or peripheral nervous system and may occur acutely or be delayed weeks to years following irradiation.

CLINICAL MANIFESTATIONS. *Acute encephalopathy* may follow large radiation doses to the brains of patients with increased intracranial pressure, particularly in the absence of corticosteroid prophylaxis. Immediately following treatment, susceptible patients develop headache, nausea and vomiting, somnolence, fever, and occasionally worsening of neurologic signs, rarely culminating in cerebral herniation and death. Acute encephalopathy usually follows the first radiation fraction and becomes progressively less severe with each ensuing fraction. This disorder is believed to result from increased intracranial pressure or brain edema from radiation-induced alteration of the blood-brain barrier. It responds to corticosteroids. Acute worsening of neurologic symptoms does not occur after spinal cord irradiation.

Early delayed reactions appear 6 to 16 weeks after therapy and persist for days to months. A transient, diffuse encephalopathy commonly follows prophylactic irradiation of the brain for leukemia in children and for small cell lung cancer in adults. The disorder is characterized by somnolence, often associated with headache, nausea, vomiting, and sometimes fever. The electroencephalogram may be slow, but there are no focal signs. Whole-brain irradiation for brain tumor sometimes causes lethargy and worsening of focal neurologic signs, simulating progression of the brain tumor. CT and MR scans may also suggest worsening. Both disorders usually respond to steroids, but resolve spontaneously even if untreated. Rarely, a brain stem disorder characterized by diplopia, ataxia, dysarthria, and dysphagia, and associated with foci of demyelination resembling acute multiple sclerosis, follows irradiation to the brain stem. *Early delayed myelopathy* follows radiation therapy to the neck or upper thorax and is characterized by Lhermitte's sign (an electric shock–like sensation radiating into various parts of the body when the neck is flexed). The symptoms resolve spontaneously. Early delayed radiation syndromes are believed to result from demyelination, possibly due to radiation-induced damage to oligodendroglia.

Late delayed radiation injury appears after months to years and may affect any part of the nervous system. In the brain, there are two clinical syndromes. The first follows whole-brain irradiation that has been administered either prophylactically or in some patients with primary and metastatic brain tumors. The disorder is characterized by dementia without focal signs. There is cerebral atrophy on CT or MR scan; pathologic changes are nonspecific, and there is no treatment. The second disorder affects patients who receive either focal brain irradiation during therapy of extracranial neoplasms or whole-brain irradiation for intracranial neoplasms. Neurologic signs suggest a tumor and include headache, focal or generalized seizures, and hemiparesis. MR or CT scans reveal a hypodense mass, sometimes with contrast enhancement. Neuropathologic features include coagulative necrosis of white matter, telangiectasia, fibrinoid necrosis

TABLE 162–3. RADIATION INJURY TO THE NERVOUS SYSTEM

Time After RT	Organ Affected	Clinical Findings
Primary injury		
Immediate (minutes to hours)	Brain	Acute encephalopathy
Early delayed (6 to 16 weeks)	Brain	Somnolence, focal signs
	Spinal cord	Lhermitte's sign
Late delayed (months to years)	Brain	Dementia, focal signs
	Spinal cord	Transverse myelopathy
	Peripheral nerves	Paralysis, sensory loss
Secondary injury (years)	Several	Brain, cranial and/or peripheral nerve sheath tumors
	Arteries (atherosclerosis)	Cerebral infarction
	Endocrine organs	Metabolic encephalopathy

of blood vessels with thrombus formation, glial proliferation, and bizarre multinucleated astrocytes. The clinical and imaging findings cannot be distinguished from those of brain tumor, and the diagnosis can be made only by biopsy. Positron emission tomography, using radiolabeled glucose, generally shows decreased metabolism in areas of radiation damage, whereas most tumors show increased metabolism. Corticosteroids sometimes ameliorate symptoms. Improvement in symptoms may be sustained even after corticosteroid withdrawal, but if symptoms recur, the treatment of the disorder, if focal, is surgical removal.

Late delayed myelopathy is characterized by progressive paralysis, sensory changes, and sometimes pain. A Brown-Séquard syndrome (weakness and loss of proprioception in the extremities of one side with loss of pain and temperature sensation on the other) is often present at onset. Patients occasionally respond transiently to steroids, and the disorder may stop progressing, but generally patients become paraplegic or quadriplegic. Pathologic changes include necrosis of the spinal cord. *Late delayed neuropathy* may affect any cranial or peripheral nerve. Common disorders are blindness from optic neuropathy and paralysis of an upper extremity from brachial plexopathy after therapy for lung or breast cancer. The pathogenesis is probably fibrosis and ischemia of the plexus. There is no treatment.

Radiation-induced tumors, including meningiomas, sarcomas, or, less commonly, gliomas, may appear years to decades after cranial irradiation and may follow low-dose irradiation. Malignant or atypical nerve sheath tumors may follow irradiation of the brachial, cervical, and lumbar plexuses. The central nervous system may also be damaged when radiation alters extraneural structures. Radiation therapy accelerates *atherosclerosis,* and cerebral infarction associated with carotid artery occlusion in the neck may occur many years after neck irradiation. *Endocrine* (pituitary, thyroid, parathyroid) dysfunction from radiation may be associated with neurologic signs. Hypothyroidism often presents as a neurologic disorder, and hyperthyroidism or hyperparathyroidism from radiation may also cause an encephalopathy.

Delattre JY, Posner JB: Neurologic complications of chemotherapy and radiation therapy. *In* Aminoff MJ (ed.): Neurology and General Medicine. New York, Churchill Livingston, Inc., 1989, pp 365–387. *A general review of common complications of cancer therapy.*

Gutin P, Leibel S, Sheline G (eds.): Radiation Injury to the Nervous System. New York, Raven Press, in press. *A comprehensive description of all of the nervous system side effects of therapeutic irradiation.*

Hildebrand J (ed.): Neurological Adverse Reactions to Anticancer Drugs. Berlin, Springer-Verlag, 1990. *Detailed descriptions of clinical findings and mechanisms of neurotoxicity of anticancer drugs.*

163 Cutaneous Manifestations of Internal Malignancy

Frank Parker

Cutaneous changes associated with internal malignant disease are diverse. Some skin alterations are clear indicators of underlying malignant disease. Others, less specific, arise in either the presence or absence of malignancy, but occur with sufficient frequency to arouse suspicion and the need to search for underlying carcinoma or lymphoma. These various skin findings may precede any signs associated with the internal malignant disease; they are therefore of crucial importance in early identification and cure of internal neoplasms.

Skin manifestations of internal malignant disease can be classified into two major groups: (1) those in which malignant cells can be found in the skin on biopsy (specific skin lesions) and (2) those in which malignant cells cannot be identified on a skin biopsy (nonspecific skin lesions). The specific lesions are diagnostic of the internal malignant disease, while the nonspecific skin alterations may or may not be associated with an internal neoplasm. Some of the nonspecific skin changes are clear indicators of underlying tumor; others merely arouse concern.

SPECIFIC SKIN LESIONS ASSOCIATED WITH INTERNAL MALIGNANT DISEASE

Carcinomas, leukemia, lymphoma, plasma cell dyscrasias, and sarcomas can all affect the skin specifically in clinically identifiable patterns. A biopsy of a suspicious skin lesion is helpful because the tissue of origin (primary underlying neoplasm) can often be identified.

Skin Metastases (Table 163–1 and Color Plate 16A)

Metastases to the skin are comparatively rare (approximately 1 to 5 per cent of internal malignancies), but when present are readily diagnosed by biopsy. Cutaneous metastases usually appear as flesh-colored to red-purple or brownish solitary papules or nodules, stony-hard to the touch, and often innocent in appearance. There is no relationship between site of origin and size, color, and consistency of the metastatic deposit. Lung cancer in men and breast cancer in women most commonly involve the skin; other sources include malignant tumors of the gastrointestinal tract, kidney, ovary, uterus, and urinary bladder and oral cavity carcinomas.

Clinical patterns of metastatic spread to skin depend on several factors such as the organ of origin and whether tumor is disseminated by lymphatics or blood. In general, those neoplasms that spread via lymphatics, such as breast and oral cavity carcinoma, localize in the skin late in the clinical course. Tumors that often embolize through venous channels, such as those arising in the lung, kidney, and ovary, can appear early in the skin and thus may be the first indication of the internal malignant disease.

Certain areas of the skin are predisposed to metastases, localizing near the site of the primary cancer (Table 163–1). Thus, abdominal wall metastases, especially around the umbilicus (Sister Mary Joseph's nodules), arise from neoplasms of the stomach, kidney, and ovary. The lower abdominal wall and external genitalia metastases arise from cancers of the genitourinary systems; face and neck skin metastases, from carcinomas of the oropharynx; and the scalp is a favorite site for metastases from breast, lung, and the genitourinary system.

Some patterns of metastatic disease are characteristic. For example, metastases to the scalp simulate wens or turban (pilar) tumors that may ulcerate. More distinctive is "alopecia neoplastica"—that is, areas of scarring alopecia in the scalp with induration and atrophy that simulate alopecia areata. Metastases from the breast and, less commonly, from the stomach, prostate, lung,

TABLE 163–1. INTERNAL MALIGNANCIES METASTATIC TO SKIN: CLINICAL FEATURES AND AREAS OF DISTRIBUTION

Primary Internal Malignancy	Cutaneous Clinical Features	Areas of Distribution
Breast	Papules, nodules—rock hard En cuirasse—scirrhous form Erysipelatoides—cellulitis form Alopecia neoplastica	Chest wall Trunk Scalp
Lung	Papules, nodules Scirrhous—morpheic form Erysipeloides—cellulitis form Alopecia neoplastica	Chest wall Scalp Face
Kidney	Angiomatous, pulsatile nodules Scirrhous—en cuirasse form Alopecia neoplastica	Abdominal wall, trunk Scalp Face External genitalia
Stomach, bowel, pancreas	Nodules Scirrhous—en cuirasse form Cellulitis—erysipelatoides	Anterior abdomen Periumbilical
Ovary, uterus	Nodules Cellulitis form—erysipelatoides	Umbilicus, abdomen
Oral cavity	Nodules	Face and neck
Thyroid	Pulsatile angiomatous nodules	Anywhere

uterus, and pancreas can produce dramatic changes in the chest wall: carcinoma en cuirasse. This scirrhous form of cutaneous metastatic spread produces extensive fibrosis of the dermis as a result of lymphatic involvement and obstruction by the cancer cells so that large areas of the chest are girdled by a thick, rigid encasement on which pink to flesh-colored papules and nodules evolve to form morphea-like plaques. The distinctive skin lesion of inflammatory carcinoma, or "carcinoma erysipeloides," is usually caused by breast cancer (less frequently by malignant tumors of the uterus, lung, and gastrointestinal tract) and simulates cellulitis over the ipsilateral chest wall anteriorly. Renal cell carcinoma and medullary and anaplastic forms of thyroid cancer, which are highly vascularized tumors, may simulate hemangiomatous nodules that pulsate on palpation when deposited in the skin. *Inflammatory oncotaxis* is a term describing the attraction of cancer cells to an area of tissue trauma resulting presumably because trauma (surgery and radiation) causes inflammation and capillary disruption, thus predisposing cancer cells to settle in these areas. For example, cutaneous metastases from colon, kidney, and cervix have been known to localize in abdominal wall surgical incisions.

Prognosis among patients with cutaneous metastases is poor, as they imply metastases elsewhere internally. If a cutaneous metastatic lesion is discovered years after the primary cancer is diagnosed, a second internal cancer should be ruled out, since only 10 per cent of internal cancers (mostly breast carcinoma) spread to the skin after 5 years' time. Clearly any skin nodule or papule of obscure origin and uncertain diagnosis should undergo biopsy, especially if there are reasons to suspect malignancy.

Lymphomas

Specific cutaneous involvement (neoplastic cellular proliferation in the skin) is seen less frequently in the lymphoma-leukemia group of neoplasms when compared with carcinomas. Rather, cutaneous manifestations are more often nonspecific (i.e., pruritus, petechiae, purpura, infections) in patients with leukemias and lymphomas, occurring in 25 to 40 per cent of such patients (see below, Nonspecific Skin Lesions Associated with Internal Malignant Disease). The specific skin lesions that are seen are similar in patients with lymphoma and leukemia, regardless of the various types of these neoplasms. Thus, skin lesions in all forms of lymphomas and leukemias appear as red, blue, and violaceous asymptomatic macules, nodules, and plaques that may ulcerate. Particularly suggestive are thickened, beefy-red arcuate lesions as well as poikilodermatous plaques (hyperpigmentation and hypopigmentation with telangiectasis throughout the thickened patches).

CUTANEOUS T-CELL LYMPHOMAS (Table 163–2)

These lymphomas are lymphoproliferative disorders of helper T lymphocytes with an affinity for skin (epidermotropism) in which atypical lymphocytes accumulate in clusters in the epidermis to form so-called Pautrier's abscesses. They represent at least three types of lymphoma: mycosis fungoides, Sézary syndrome, and adult T-cell lymphoma, each of which presents with variable clinical characteristics and biologic behavior.

Mycosis fungoides (see Color Plate 16B) usually follows a prolonged course, beginning with nonspecific skin lesions (so-called premycotic stage) that, after a variable number of years, evolve into histologically specific skin lesions (cutaneous patches, plaques—the mycotic stage) and then into ulcerative nodules and tumors (tumor stage).

Extracutaneous disseminated disease involves first lymph nodes and then, in advanced stages, liver and spleen and other internal organs. Less commonly the disease may begin with cutaneous nodules and tumors without evolving from patches and plaques. Several types of clinical lesions (patches, plaques, and tumors) may coexist in any one patient. The premycotic stage (biopsy of lesions is nonspecific) can persist from a few months to more than 40 years, the morphology of the skin lesions resembling a number of banal dermatoses: psoriasis or eczema or poikilodermatous telangiectatic, stippled pigmented patches. In the plaque stage the premycotic lesions become infiltrated, although indurated, red-purple plaques also arise from previously uninvolved skin. The lesions usually are oval to round, but they may also be arciform or annular or assume a horseshoe shape, or the entire

TABLE 163–2. CUTANEOUS T-CELL LYMPHOMAS

Lymphoma	Skin Lesions	Other Features
Mycosis fungoides	Erythematous patches, plaques, tumors, erythroderma	Late involvement of lymph nodes, internal organs
Sézary syndrome	Erythroderma with ectropion and leonine facies; often spares body folds	Sézary cells in blood with high WBC, hepatosplenomegaly, lymphadenopathy
Adult T-cell lymphoma	Erythroderma, papules, nodules	HTLV 1 virus antibodies, hepatosplenomegaly, osteolytic bone lesions, hypercalcemia
T immunoblastic lymphoma	Plaques, tumors	Arise from pre-existing mycosis fungoides or Sézary syndrome
Chronic lymphoblastic leukemia, T-cell type	Erythroderma, plaques, nodules	Prolonged course
T lymphoblastic lymphoma	Tumors of skin	Rapidly fatal with bone marrow and mediastinal involvement

integument may be infiltrated, producing a thickened, red hide (erythroderma). In the final stage, tumors develop from pre-existing plaques, erythroderma, or previously uninvolved skin. Tumors may be a few centimeters to 10 cm in size and often ulcerate. It is difficult to diagnose mycosis fungoides in the premycotic stage; it requires multiple skin biopsies over extended periods. However, the detection of rearranged T-cell receptor genes can be readily demonstrated in skin lesions of mycosis fungoides, and this may prove to be a sensitive and practical method for the early diagnosis of T-cell neoplasms (including mycosis fungoides, human T-cell lymphomas, and chronic lymphocytic leukemia). Clonal rearrangements for the β T-cell receptor genes are also found in lymph nodes removed from patients with mycosis fungoides and considered histologically to contain only benign lymphadenopathy.

The *Sézary syndrome* (see Color Plate 16C), the leukemic variant of mycosis fungoides, consists of generalized exfoliative dermatitis with edema, redness, and thickening of the skin associated with ectropion, leonine facies, keratoderma of the palms and soles, hepatosplenomegaly, and lymphadenopathy associated with large numbers of atypical T lymphocytes in the circulation. The latter, so-called Sézary cells, represent T cells with highly convoluted nuclei identical to the cells infiltrating the skin in mycosis fungoides. The immediate source of the circulating Sézary cells appears to be the skin, as the bone marrow is rarely involved. In many patients mycosis fungoides pursues a chronic course, and the patients die of unrelated causes; some experience rapid progression to cutaneous tumors and ulcerative lesions and disseminated disease (visceral involvement is frequently diffuse and resembles leukemic infiltrates). Sézary syndrome has a particularly poor prognosis. Staphylococcal or *Pseudomonas* septicemia is the most common terminal event, accounting for half of the deaths.

Adult T-cell lymphoma, which is associated with a retrovirus, human T-cell lymphoma virus (HTLV), occurs mainly in blacks in the United States. Cutaneous findings are prominent in 70 per cent of patients and may be the presenting feature. Flesh-colored papules, nodules, and tumors as well as generalized erythroderma may be present. The papules are diffusely disseminated over the trunk and coalesce to form plaques. Patients also display peripheral and mediastinal lymphadenopathy, and hepatosplenomegaly is found in half of the patients. A unique feature of this lymphoma is trabecular and bone marrow involvement with multiple "punched-out" osteolytic lesions in the axial skeleton and long bones associated with extreme hypercalcemia.

Several other forms of T-cell lymphomas occur with skin involvement and are outlined in Table 163–2.

NON-HODGKIN'S LYMPHOMAS AND CUTANEOUS B-CELL LYMPHOMAS (see Ch. 147)

Red, blue, or violaceous skin lesions occur in all forms of non-Hodgkin's lymphoma. They appear as papules, nodules, and plaques with occasional large, ulcerated tumors that evolve in the skin after lymph node involvement. Skin involvement can be seen as the initial presentation, or it may occur late in the course of the disease. It appears to have no impact on prognosis.

HODGKIN'S DISEASE (see Ch. 148)

The skin is not commonly involved in a specific way, but when it is, the erythematous papules, nodules, and plaques that often ulcerate are indistinguishable from the skin lesions found in non-Hodgkin's lymphoma. The site of predilection is the thoracic wall, spread being via retrograde lymphatic drainage pathways from massively enlarged axillary and cervical lymph nodes. Specific cutaneous involvement is seen in those patients with extensive and highly aggressive Hodgkin's disease.

Leukemias

Leukemia cutis usually develops months after the diagnosis of leukemia (55 per cent of patients) or at the time of diagnosis (38 per cent), but it can occasionally precede systemic disease and be the first sign of the underlying condition. Red to violaceous papules, nodules, and thickened plaques are the usual forms that leukemic infiltrates take, but rarely erythroderma is found. When chronic myelogenous leukemia (CML) enters the blast phase, greenish tumors may develop in the skin, forming chloromas or granulocytic sarcomas (see Ch. 144). Skin lesions in acute leukemias and chronic lymphocytic leukemia (CLL) are found on the face and extremities, while those associated with CML are more commonly seen on the trunk. In monocytic leukemia, widespread leukemia skin infiltrates occur, and oral mucosal involvement (gingival hyperplasia) is commonplace. In general, the histology of leukemic cells in skin for various forms of leukemia mimics that seen in the blood and bone marrow, but it is difficult to diagnose the type of leukemia from skin biopsies.

Plasma Cell Dyscrasias

Specific skin manifestations of multiple myeloma, extramedullary plasmacytoma, and Waldenström's macroglobulinemia consist of lymphoplasmacytoid cell infiltrates or deposition of monoclonal paraprotein immunoglobulins (see Ch. 151). Bluish red and flesh-colored nonulcerated nodules and plaques on the trunk are observed in 4 per cent of patients with multiple myeloma, representing in most instances extensions from underlying medullary plasma cell proliferation.

Cutaneous Histiocytic Malignant Tumors

Malignant tumors of histiocytes may be solitary or present as disseminated disease. Malignant histiocytosis (histiocytic medullary reticulosis), a systemic, progressive proliferation of atypical histiocytes, produces wasting, fever, lymphadenopathy, hepatosplenomegaly, pancytopenia, and skin lesions. Children and adults are affected, and skin lesions are an integral part of the disease, especially in children (up to 90 per cent have cutaneous changes). The reddish purple papulonodular and ulcerative plaques occur over the trunk and face early in the clinical course. Malignant histiocytosis is fatal in adults but is somewhat less aggressive in children.

Angioblastic Lymphadenopathy

Immunologically mediated, this often fatal disorder is characterized by proliferation of plasmacytoid immunoblasts and plasma cells. Fever, malaise, weight loss, hepatosplenomegaly, and generalized lymphadenopathy are accompanied in 40 per cent of cases by generalized, maculopapular, purpuric, and, at times, exfoliative erythroderma. Biopsy findings of involved lymph nodes are diagnostic (proliferation of plasma cells, arborizing vessels, and deposition of amorphous material), while skin biopsy reveals a lymphohistiocytic vasculitis composed of plasma and immunoblast-like cells.

Neuroblastoma

Neuroblastoma, a poorly differentiated tumor derived from primordial neural crest cells, arises within the sympathetic ganglion (cervical, thoracic, and pelvic tumors) and adrenal glands of children. It frequently metastasizes to bone, lymph nodes, liver, and skin. Bluish nodules appear over a wide area (causing these children to be called blueberry-muffin children). A helpful clinical sign occurs after rubbing these lesions: They blanch with a halo of surrounding erythema, probably related to the release of catechols contained in the cells of the tumors. Even though patients with neuroblastoma are not hypertensive, 85 per cent have increased urinary catecholamine metabolites.

Kaposi's Sarcoma (see Color Plates 12D and 16D)

Kaposi's sarcoma, a multifocal, vascular malignant tumor, can occur in four major clinical settings: African Kaposi's, classic Kaposi's in elderly Jewish or Mediterranean males, Kaposi's secondary to immunodeficiency conditions, and Kaposi's sarcoma occurring as a complication of acquired immunodeficiency syndrome (AIDS). In each instance the skin lesions are identical histologically and clinically; they present as purplish brown macules, plaques, papules, or nodules. The distribution and course of these sarcomatous lesions, however, vary according to the clinical setting (Table 163-3). Thus, classic Kaposi's sarcoma occurs in elderly males of Mediterranean background as purplish

TABLE 163-3. KAPOSI'S SARCOMA: COMPARISON OF VARIOUS FORMS

	Classic Form	African Form	Immunologic Deficiency State	AIDS Associated
Age	40–70 years	Middle age	Any age	20–50 years
Sex	M:F, 10–15:1	—	M or F	Mostly males
Social characteristics	Mediterranean or Jewish ancestry	Blacks in equatorial Africa	Patients taking immuno-suppressive drugs—renal transplant, etc.	Homosexuals, drug addicts, hemophiliacs
Occurrence	0.2% cancers in USA	10% of all malignant tumors in Africa	400% greater incidence than population at large	Increasing; 35% of AIDS patients
Clinical appearance of skin lesion	Multiple purple-brown macules, papules, plaques, nodules	Nodules, exophytic lesions, infiltrative, burrowing plaques	Papules, nodules	Multiple purple-brown macules, papules, nodules; follow cleavage lines of skin
Cutaneous location	Lower legs most often, occasionally arms	Extremities	Trunk, neck—widespread lesions	Widespread—upper body, face, neck
Mucosal involvement	Rare	Rare	—	Common
Node and systemic involvement	Rare—occasionally nodes, GI tract, liver in 10% of patients	Uncommon	—	Frequent; 75% with visceral involvement; 5% visceral lesions only
Course and prognosis	Indolent course, 15% mortality within 10 years	Indolent course	Good; may regress if immunosuppressive drugs can be stopped	Fulminant condition, poor prognosis
Response to therapy	Excellent	—	Good	Poor

macules that may progress to infiltrative plaques and nodules on the distal extremities, following an indolent course. The Kaposi's sarcoma occurring in young homosexuals and others with AIDS is characterized by widely distributed, red-brown macules, papules, and nodules over the upper body and progresses in a fulminant course. The Kaposi's lesions in AIDS often follow skin cleavage lines and frequently involve the oropharyngeal mucosa, appearing as purple hemorrhagic plaques. The importance of the immune status in the evolution of Kaposi's sarcoma is dramatically illustrated in renal transplant patients who are immunosuppressed. Kaposi's sarcoma develops after 9 to 16 months following transplantation and initiation of immunosuppressive drugs. Rapidly progressive, widespread, red to purple papules ensue, but they may regress when immunosuppressive therapy is withdrawn.

NONSPECIFIC SKIN LESIONS ASSOCIATED WITH INTERNAL MALIGNANT DISEASE (Table 163–4)

Malignant cells cannot be identified in the skin in a wide variety of cutaneous manifestations of internal malignant disease. The pathogenesis of these disparate skin reactions is obscure. Often the only evidence that malignancy and cutaneous changes are related is the observation that following removal of the tumor or treatment of the neoplasm the skin change subsides or disappears and may subsequently exacerbate if the neoplasm recurs. Skin manifestations may coincide with, antedate, or follow the clinical diagnosis of internal malignant disease.

Although nonspecific manifestations are often highly suggestive of underlying malignant disease, they are more frequently seen with other nonmalignant conditions. When these skin changes are observed, therefore, an internal neoplasm is only one of several possibilities in the differential diagnosis.

Nonspecific skin manifestations can be considered under two major headings: (1) skin changes common to many skin diseases, including internal malignancy and (2) syndromes and entities commonly associated with internal neoplasia.

Skin Changes Common to Many Skin Conditions, Including Internal Malignancy

Pruritus, unassociated with detectable abnormalities of the skin except for secondary lesions such as excoriations or prurigo-like papules, may be an important manifestation of various internal malignant diseases, including Hodgkin's disease, lymphocytic

TABLE 163–4. NONSPECIFIC SKIN LESIONS ASSOCIATED WITH INTERNAL MALIGNANCIES

I. Skin lesions common to many skin conditions, including internal malignancy
II. Syndromes and entities commonly associated with internal malignancy
  A. Nongenetic syndromes
    1. High incidence of association with internal malignancy
      Paget's disease
      Stewart-Treves syndrome
      Acanthosis nigricans
      Dermatomyositis
      Leser-Trélat syndrome
      Glucagonoma syndrome
      Bazex syndrome
      Pulmonary osteoarthropathy
      Carcinoid syndrome
    2. Low incidence of association with malignancy
      Sweet's syndrome
      Amyloid
      Urticaria pigmentosa and mastocytosis syndrome
      Bowen's disease
  B. Genetic syndromes
    1. High incidence of association with malignancy
      Torre's syndrome
      Gardner's syndrome
      Cowden's syndrome
      Multiple endocrine neoplasia 2b
      Ataxia-telangiectasia
    2. Low incidence of association with malignancy
      Neurofibroma
      Peutz-Jeghers syndrome
      Basal cell carcinoma nevus syndrome
      Bloom's syndrome

leukemia, carcinoid, polycythemia vera (in which pruritus often occurs after exposure to heat), and, less commonly, carcinoma. The itching may be mild or severe, localized or generalized, intermittent or constant. In Hodgkin's disease, itching is usually continuous and may be localized to the feet and lower part of the body, only later to become generalized. Up to 30 per cent of patients with Hodgkin's disease may itch. Pruritus of leukemia has a greater tendency to be generalized and may evolve into generalized erythroderma. Carcinomas of the gastrointestinal tract, lung, ovary, and prostate may also be associated with itching, which may precede recognition of these cancers by a year. Although dry skin (xerosis) is the most common cause of pruritus, other systemic causes of this bothersome symptom should be sought in addition to malignant disease, including drug reactions, cholestatic liver disease, uremia, diabetes, and thyroid disease.

Erythroderma, or exfoliative dermatitis, is a cutaneous reaction pattern with various causes. In 10 per cent of patients, total-body cutaneous redness, edema, scaling, and lichenification are associated with malignancy. In clinical practice the usual cause of exfoliative dermatitis is either a drug reaction or a generalized exacerbation of a pre-existing dermatosis such as atopic dermatitis, psoriasis, or contact dermatitis. When it is due to malignant disease, erythroderma is most pathognomonic of Hodgkin's disease, less frequently seen in lymphocytic leukemia, or rarely associated with underlying carcinoma. Erythroderma may be the first sign of Hodgkin's disease or leukemia. Skin biopsies do not reveal lymphomatous or leukemic infiltrates, although the patients clinically look similar to those with Sézary's syndrome (in which skin biopsies display diagnostic Sézary cells).

Figurate erythemas are red, gyrate, serpiginous, and annular bands that take on a pattern reminiscent of a wood grain and have been given descriptive names such as erythema gyratum repens and erythema annular centrifugum. These lesions are occasionally associated with neoplasia, especially breast and lung cancer.

Urticaria-like lesions, flesh-colored to red pruritic papules, nodules, and plaques, at times accompany leukemia, so-called leukemids. They may precede the development of leukemia by many months, and biopsy of the lesions does not show malignant cells. Treatment and control of leukemia often result in clearing.

Acquired hypertrichosis lanuginosa (malignant down), the sudden onset of excessive growth of fine, long, unpigmented fetal hair (lanugo) over the face, trunk, and limbs, has been associated with breast, uterine, pancreatic, pulmonary, and gastrointestinal carcinomas as well as lymphomas.

Herpes zoster is increased in incidence in patients with Hodgkin's disease and chronic lymphocytic leukemia as well as with a variety of neoplasms that are being managed with chemotherapy. This is evidence of the important role that impaired cellular immunity plays in activating viral replication. The painful, unilateral, grouped, clear, and often hemorrhagic umbilicated vesicles in a dermatomal distribution are readily recognized (see Ch. 374).

A number of miscellaneous dermatoses have occasionally been associated with internal malignant disease, but it is not entirely clear whether these associations are real or fortuitous. Table 163–5 lists some of these.

TABLE 163–5. DERMATOSES ASSOCIATED WITH INTERNAL MALIGNANT DISEASE

Dermatosis	Associated Cancer
Bullous lesions: pemphigoid, pemphigus, dermatitis herpetiformis	Rectal, breast, larynx, lymphoma
Tylosis: palmar hyperkeratosis	Esophagus
Acquired ichthyosis	GI leiomyosarcoma, lymphoma, multiple myeloma, lung, breast
Palmar fasciitis and polyarthritis: palmar fascial thickening with erythema, swelling of palms and dorsum of hands	Ovary

Syndromes and Entities Associated with Internal Neoplasia

A number of unique cutaneous syndromes, both genetic and nongenetic, are associated with internal neoplasms with sufficient frequency to alert the clinician to look for these potentially curable neoplasms early in their evolution. In some instances there is a high incidence of associated neoplasms, while in others this association is less clear.

NONGENETIC SYNDROMES AND ENTITIES ASSOCIATED WITH INTERNAL MALIGNANT DISEASE

HIGH INCIDENCE OF CUTANEOUS LESIONS ASSOCIATED WITH MALIGNANCY. *Paget's disease* of the breast is invariably found with an underlying intraductal mammary carcinoma. Erythematous scaling or weeping, sharply marginated patches on the nipple and areola of one breast should alert the clinician to examine the breast carefully. A breast mass may not be palpable or may not be definitely found with mammography, but in virtually every case an underlying carcinoma is present. Paget's disease can also occur in the anogenital region (extramammary Paget's disease). In this disorder, eczematous, pruritic, crusted, lichenified, well-demarcated patches may involve the lower abdominal wall, inguinal regions, genitalia, or perianal area. In up to 50 per cent of such patients, an underlying carcinoma of the rectum, prostate, urethra, other parts of the genitourinary tract, or apocrine gland is found. Biopsies taken from mammary and extramammary Paget's disease show the same diagnostic features, namely, large, round cells with clear cytoplasm in the epidermis (Paget's cells).

Stewart-Treves syndrome is the occasional occurrence of lymphoangiosarcoma as a complication of chronic lymphedema of the arm after radical mastectomy for carcinoma of the breast. Angiomatous, livid, or dusky red blebs and nodules exuding fluid may evolve from 2 to 20 years following mastectomy and the onset of the lymphedema. Angiosarcoma has also developed in congenital lymphedema as well as in lymphedema of the legs following surgery for cervical cancer.

Acanthosis nigricans (see Color Plate 16G) presents as soft, velvety, verrucous, brown hyperpigmentation of the body folds, especially those of the neck, axillae, and groin. When it occurs in patients over the age of 40 years, it is often a sign of an underlying malignant tumor, usually adenocarcinoma (most often stomach, gastrointestinal tract, and uterus; less commonly, ovary, prostate, breast, and lung) and rarely lymphoma. Acanthosis nigricans involving the tongue and oral mucosa is highly suggestive of underlying malignancy. Acanthosis nigricans may appear before the malignant neoplasm 20 per cent of the time. Regression of the skin sign following therapy for the tumor and reappearance with reactivation of the tumor have been observed, suggesting that the underlying tumor secretes an as yet unidentified substance that is responsible for the verrucoid skin lesions. Acanthosis nigricans is more commonly found in individuals under 40 years of age, and then it is not usually associated with malignancy but rather with obesity or a variety of endocrinopathies (Cushing's disease, acromegaly, polycystic ovaries, hypothyroidism and hyperthyroidism, insulin-resistant diabetes). It also occurs on a familial basis. Special concern must be given to nonobese adults who have recently developed the verrucous areas in body folds. In 80 to 90 per cent of all instances the cancer arises in the stomach.

Dermatomyositis (see Color Plate 16H) developing in individuals over 40 years of age also calls for a careful search for underlying carcinoma (see Ch. 268). Although there is disagreement whether the incidence of internal malignant disease is increased in dermatomyositis, numerous cases have been reported with this association. Not uncommonly the dermatomyositis resolves upon removal of the carcinoma, but the syndrome recurs if the tumor reappears. In some instances the dermatomyositis precedes the cancer by several years. The search for neoplasm should be continued, therefore, even if the initial evaluation fails to find it, especially with (1) failure of the dermatomyositis to respond to conventional therapy (i.e., after systemic steroids), (2) a history of previous malignant disease, or (3) presence of atypical symptoms of the dermatomyositis. Malignant tumors of the breast and lung are those most commonly associated with dermatomyositis. Dermatomyositis is recognized by proximal muscle pain and weakness and a characteristic dermatitis that includes heliotrope rash (edematous, dusky, violaceous discoloration of the eyelids) along with a brilliant violaceous, erythematous telangiectatic scaling rash over the cheeks, forehead, V of the neck, elbows, and knees. Gottron's papules, slightly elevated red to violaceous papules or small plaques over the knuckles, are also an important finding in dermatomyositis.

The *Leser-Trélet sign*, the sudden appearance and growth of multiple seborrheic keratoses, occurs with underlying cancer in the elderly. This sign has been the subject of controversy, since seborrheic keratoses of the same histologic type are common in the elderly. Nevertheless, several case reports have described new and enlarging keratoses in association with cancer of the lung, adenocarcinoma of the bowel, mycosis fungoides, and Sézary's syndrome and, in some of these patients, the keratoses regressed when the malignant tumor was treated.

Necrolytic migratory erythema, associated with α-cell tumors of the pancreas and elevated glucagon levels, evolves as gradually enlarging erythematous patches with central, superficial blister formation progressing to central crusting and healing. Annular and figurate lesions result, with exudative, erosive, and crusting areas most pronounced in the perineum, groin, and perioral areas. Painful glossitis may be another prominent sign of the glucagonoma syndrome. The skin rash and stomatitis often resolve within a week after the tumor is removed. The pathogenesis of the skin and mucous membrane lesions is unclear. The glucagonoma syndrome is discussed more completely in Ch. 220. Similar skin lesions may be seen in association with severe zinc deficiency.

Bazex syndrome, or acrokeratosis paraneoplastica, is a unique cutaneous marker of carcinomas of the upper respiratory tract, especially seen with squamous cell carcinomas of the oral, pharyngeal, laryngeal, esophageal, and bronchial areas, primarily in males. When the tumor is asymptomatic, red to violaceous, scaling, psoriasis-like patches are found confined to the bridge of the nose, the fingers, toes, and margins of the ear helices. The nail folds are often red, scaling, and tender with grooving of the nails and onycholysis. Later the eruption on the acral areas becomes more extensive, spreading from the fingers to the palms and soles, which, in turn, become red and scaling and form a honeycomb-like thickening. The fingers and toes become violaceous and bulbous, and the rash evolves on the nose. In the last stage, if the tumor has not been treated and has progressed, new scaling lesions resembling psoriasis spread over the face, trunk, knees, arms, and scalp. Nail dystrophy (ridged, brittle, crumbling nails) is extensive.

Clubbing of the fingers is a well-known manifestation of bronchogenic carcinoma, mesothelioma, metastatic carcinoma to the thorax (from the colon, larynx, breast, or ovary) and occasionally Hodgkin's disease. *Hypertrophic pulmonary osteoarthropathy* is the term used when clubbing is accompanied by subperiosteal new bone formation along the shafts of the long bones of the extremities and digits. Joints of the ankle, knees, wrists, and hand may be painful and swollen. In some patients cutaneous thickening of the forearms and legs produces cylindric enlargement of the limbs, and the facial features become coarse with deep facial furrows simulating acromegaly. At times, deep confluent skin wrinkles evolve over the forehead and scalp, a condition termed *pachydermoperiostosis* when the skin changes accompany acromegaloid features.

Carcinoid, malignant tumor of the chromaffin cells of the gastrointestinal tract and, less frequently, the bronchus, may be associated with intermittent scarlet to violet red flushing of the head, neck, and upper part of the trunk. Eventually the erythema becomes permanent, and telangiectasis and tortuous veins evolve in the flushed areas. This syndrome and its cutaneous manifestations are described more fully in Ch. 230.

LOW INCIDENCE OF CUTANEOUS LESIONS ASSOCIATED WITH MALIGNANCY. *Amyloid deposits* in the skin may occur without obvious cause (cutaneous amyloidosis) as part of an inherited syndrome or secondary to plasma cell dyscrasias—either primary systemic amyloidosis or multiple myeloma. In the case of plasma cell dyscrasias, shiny, translucent, waxy, firm purpuric papules and plaques occur on the mucocutaneous junctions of the eyes, nose, and mouth along with macroglossia. Occasionally, infiltrated papules are not apparent, and only purpuric lesions evolve around the eyes ("raccoon eyes").

Urticaria pigmentosa consists of skin lesions that appear as numerous red-brown macules and papules on the trunk and extremities. Light stroking of the skin lesions causes urtication with edema and a red flare due to the release of histamine from the mast cells infiltrating the skin (Darier's sign). These skin lesions are sometimes associated with systemic mastocytosis (see Ch. 252) or, more rarely, with mast cell leukemia or myeloproliferative disorders (myelofibrosis, myeloid metaplasia, polycythemia, and granulocytic leukemia) with extensive infiltration of mature mast cells in the marrow and mast cells or basophils in the peripheral blood.

Bowen's disease of the skin consists of multiple superficial squamous cell cancers occurring in non–sun-exposed areas of the body, particularly in individuals with a history of long-term ingestion or exposure to arsenicals (drinking of well water, exposure to insecticides or industrial arsenicals). Bowen's skin lesions appear as discrete, red, scaling, flat to slightly raised patches that mimic eczematous or psoriatic patches. These skin lesions should be removed to prevent progression to invasive squamous cell carcinoma. The relationship of these lesions to internal malignancy is controversial, but a careful search for cancers of the larynx, lung, esophagus, liver, and bladder is warranted.

Sweet's syndrome (acute febrile neutrophilic dermatosis) is associated rarely with underlying chronic myelogenous leukemia. Red, tender, infiltrated plaques and annular lesions are distributed asymmetrically on the face, neck, and upper arms. The skin lesions consist of massive polymorphonuclear infiltration of the dermis, of unknown cause. Patients with Sweet's syndrome also suffer from fever, malaise, peripheral leukocytosis, arthralgias and arthritis, and conjunctivitis and episcleritis. Peripheral leukocyte counts generally range from 15,000 to 20,000 with 80 to 90 per cent mature polymorphonuclear leukocytes. Careful evaluation of the peripheral cells and occasionally of the bone marrow is indicated because of the possibility of coincident myelogenous leukemia.

GENETIC SYNDROMES ASSOCIATED WITH INTERNAL MALIGNANT DISEASE

HIGH INCIDENCE OF ASSOCIATION WITH INTERNAL MALIGNANCY. *Gardner's syndrome* consists of multiple epidermoid and sebaceous cysts of the face and scalp, fibrous tissue tumors of the skin (desmoid tumors, fibromas and fibrosarcomas), osteomas of the membranous bones of the face and head, and polyps of the colon and rectum (Ch. 105). No patients with this syndrome live beyond the seventh decade without developing adenocarcinoma of the bowel.

Cowden's disease, a condition in which there are numerous hamartomas of the skin, mucous membranes, and internal organs, is associated with malignant neoplasms of the breast and thyroid in a high percentage of patients. The hamartomas present on the skin as keratotic, warty papules and nodules on the central area of the face and on the hands and arms. Papular, cobblestone lesions may appear on the gingiva, palate, tongue, and larynx.

Torre's syndrome, another autosomal dominant condition, consists of multiple sebaceous gland tumors, sebaceous adenomas, sebaceous hyperplasia, and basal cell cancers with sebaceous differentiation. It is associated with cancers of the colon, duodenum, ampulla of Vater, uterus, and genitourinary tract. The skin tumors in this condition are yellowish or red papules and nodules.

Multiple Endocrine Neoplasia Type 2b (see Ch. 228). Medullary carcinoma of the thyroid and pheochromocytoma are found in association with a marfanoid habitus and multiple whitish to pink papular mucosal neuromas studding the lips, tip of the tongue, and, less often, the buccal mucosa, gingivae, palate, and pharynx. Neuromas also develop on the conjunctivae and corneas, and thickened corneal nerves may be found with slit-lamp examination.

Ataxia-telangiectasia, an autosomal recessive disorder associated with lymphomas, is recognized by telangiectasias over the ears, eyelids, nose, butterfly area of the face, and conjunctivae in association with progressive cerebellar ataxia, profound im-

munologic deficiency, and sinopulmonary infections (see Ch. 244). Hodgkin's disease, non-Hodgkin's lymphoma, or leukemia develops in 10 per cent of patients, with other malignant neoplasms such as ovarian dysgerminomas, gliomas, cerebellar medulloblastomas, and gastric adenocarcinomas occurring less frequently. Persons with *Wiskott-Aldrich syndrome* also display a propensity to malignant lymphomas (79 per cent) or leukemias (13 per cent) by the age of 10 years, probably related to widespread immunologic abnormalities of both the humoral and cell-mediated systems found in this condition. The skin changes are similar to atopic dermatitis (and are associated with petechiae due to thrombocytopenia).

LOW INCIDENCE OF ASSOCIATION WITH INTERNAL MALIGNANCY. Some dominant inherited conditions are associated with internal malignancy, but the relationship is not frequently found. Thus, patients with *neurofibromatosis* have café-au-lait spots, axillary freckles, and multiple neurofibromas. They are prone to develop pheochromocytomas (10 per cent of patients by the age of 60 years), acoustic neuromas, and neurofibrosarcomas.

Patients with the *Peutz-Jeghers syndrome* have numerous brown-black macules on the lips, perioral regions, hands, and feet in association with hamartomatous polyps of the small bowel, stomach, and, less commonly, colon (see Ch. 105). Malignancy occasionally develops in the polyps. *Nevoid basal cell carcinoma syndrome* is occasionally associated with the development of medulloblastoma or fibrosarcoma of the jaw.

Bloom's syndrome (telangiectatic redness of the skin in photoexposed areas and stunted growth) and the *Chédiak-Higashi syndrome* (light coloration of skin and hair) are autosomal recessive conditions associated with a propensity to develop leukemias and lymphomas.

Braverman IM: Skin Signs of Systemic Disease. Philadelphia, W. B. Saunders Company, 1981. *This classic book, on all skin signs associated with systemic disease, has many useful pictures of the cutaneous lesions related to internal malignant disease.*

Callen JP: Cutaneous Aspects of Internal Disease. Chicago, Year Book Medical Publishers, 1981. *This book, written by a number of authoritative authors, reviews in detail the varied manifestations of cutaneous signs of internal malignancy. Part 3 is especially useful in covering the hematologic and oncologic cutaneous signs of systemic lymphomas and carcinomas.*

Thiers BH, Maize C (eds.): Symposium on Cutaneous T Cell Lymphoma and Related Disorders. Dermatol Clin Vol. 3, No. 4, 1985. *A series of articles relating to the basic scientific and clinical features of cutaneous lymphomas by a number of authorities in the field.*

164 Principles of Cancer Therapy

Sydney E. Salmon

The treatment of hematologic malignancies and solid tumors is now an integral component of internal medicine. Over the past few decades the development of effective anticancer drugs has resulted in the progressive integration of medical management with surgery and radiotherapy into the initial multimodal treatment of cancer. The approaches to medical management have expanded with the development of new cytotoxic and endocrine agents and with the introduction of biologic therapy based on recombinant synthesis of interferons and cytokines. Medical management of complications of cancer represents an additional important aspect of the care of the cancer patient. It is therefore essential that the internist also be familiar with palliative aspects of cancer care, including management of pain syndromes (see Ch. 26) and treatment of life-threatening complications of cancer (see Ch. 165).

Although systemic therapy is currently curative in relatively few forms of metastatic cancer, it is now increasingly effective as a component of multimodal management of apparently localized cancers known to have a high frequency of occult micrometastatic spread. This approach has generally been predicted on the availability of specific systemic agents with antitumor activity in advanced cancers of the same histopathology. Not all patients are candidates for attempts at curative cancer therapy because of limitations in the available anticancer drugs and also because of comorbidity from other medical problems associated with increasing age. To a significant extent, cancer is a disease of the elderly, and treatment for many types of cancer in patients over the age of 65 remains quite difficult, perhaps owing to reduced host tolerance to the toxicities of many cancer chemotherapeutic agents. Thus it is important that the patient and his or her family be fully informed about the nature of the treatment planned, whether it is of curative or palliative intent. Inasmuch as prognosis for individual patients is currently based on statistical estimates, the physician must evaluate each patient individually in relation to relevant prognostic factors in attempting to establish prognosis and develop a treatment plan.

This chapter highlights the general principles, modalities, and therapeutic agents currently used in "comprehensive cancer management." At present, systemic therapy as the sole therapeutic approach is most effective against some of the hematologic malignancies and more rapidly proliferating solid tumors. For many types of cancer, current therapy other than surgery and/or radiotherapy is of only limited efficacy. However, identification and effective use of systemic agents accounts for most of the progress made in cancer treatment over the past two decades. The successes achieved provide impetus for additional basic and clinical cancer treatment research. At the basic science level there is increased understanding of the molecular abnormalities in cancer. As a result, a new era is beginning in which the

paradigms for cancer treatment are changing to more fully integrate fundamental understanding of cancer into approaches to both cancer treatment and cancer prevention.

DEVELOPMENT OF A TREATMENT PLAN

The major clinical features of cancer to be considered in developing a treatment plan include (1) specific histologic diagnosis of the neoplasm, (2) tumor burden (stage) and extent of specific organ involvement, and (3) biologic characteristics and other prognostic factors relevant to the specific type of cancer.

DIAGNOSIS. Accurate histologic diagnosis and staging critically influence treatment selection. Increasingly, immunohistochemical analysis is of help in subtyping lymphomas and in distinguishing among various morphologically "undifferentiated" neoplasms. In individual patients, undifferentiated or poorly differentiated tumors can be proven with immunohistochemistry to be lymphoma, melanoma, germ cell neoplasm, sarcoma, and so on (Fig. 164–1). Tumors of such diverse histogenesis can have markedly different prognosis and treatment. On occasion, electron microscopy is also helpful by identifying specific morphologic features such as melanosomes (in melanoma) or desmosomes (in carcinomas) that permit more specific classification. For some specific neoplasms, other distinctive biologic markers can be of value and identified with immunohistochemistry, hormone receptor expression, serum or urinary tumor markers (e.g., β-hCG, α-fetoprotein, carcinoembryonic antigen, CA-125, myeloma proteins, urinary 5-hydroxyindole acetic acid), karyotype, or molecular analysis. Increasingly, molecular biologic methods for DNA analysis are also playing a role in diagnosis by identifying characteristic gene rearrangements (e.g., Southern blots), gene dele-

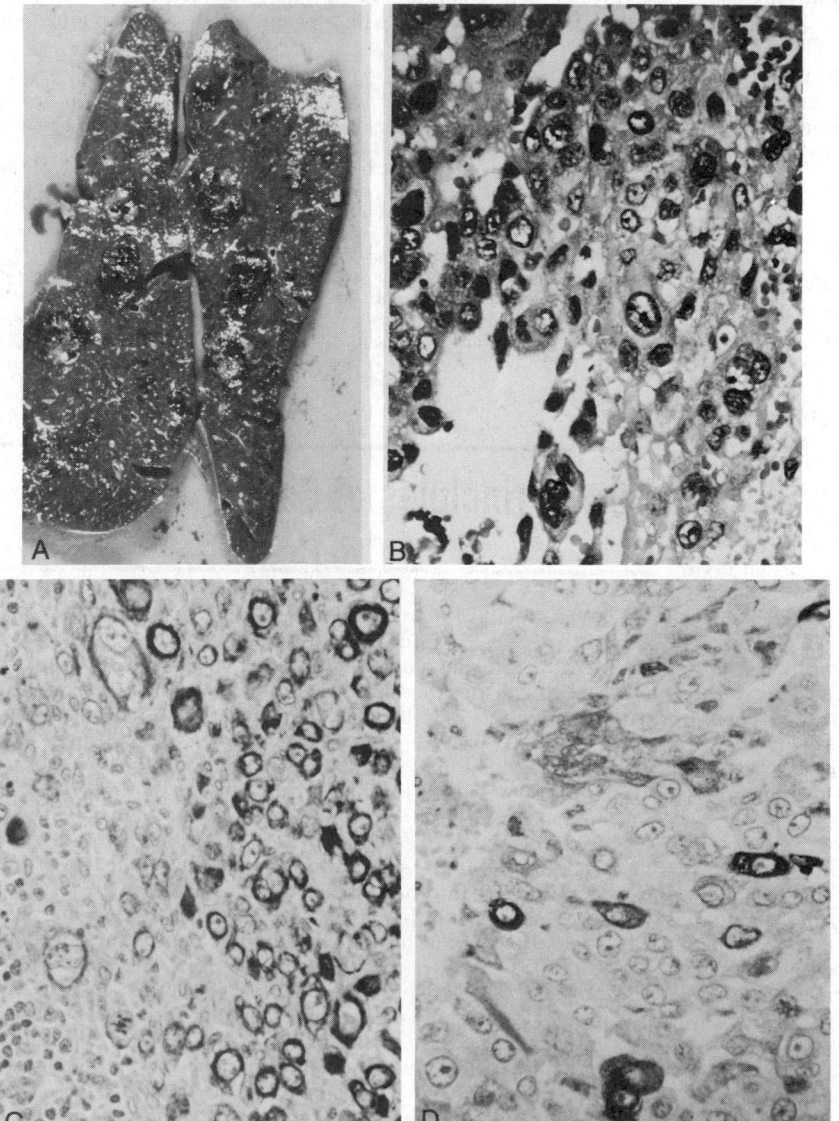

FIGURE 164–1. Example of the value of immunohistochemistry for cancer diagnosis. A 70-year-old man presented in shock with an acute abdomen. At emergency laparotomy he was found to have a ruptured spleen and hemoperitoneum as well as multiple metastatic lesions in the liver, spleen, and omentum. *A,* Gross appearance of spleen on cut section. *B,* By light microscopy the routine H & E–stained sections were interpreted as showing an undifferentiated large cell neoplasm. *C,* Positive immunoperoxidase stain for keratin established that the neoplasm was a carcinoma and excluded both large cell lymphoma and metastatic melanoma. Pertinent negative immunohistochemical findings (not shown) included stains for the S-100 antigen (melanoma) and leukocyte common antigen or anti-CD45 (lymphoma). *D,* Positive immunoperoxidase stain for β-hCG suggests the diagnosis of metastatic choriocarcinoma. The patient was then found to have a blood titer of 40,000 units per milliliter for β-hCG. Thus specialized testing changed the diagnosis from an undifferentiated cancer of unknown origin to a potentially treatable metastatic germ cell neoplasm. In this specific patient, clinical examination of the testes was negative for neoplasm. (Immunopathologic study by Dr. Raymond Nagle, University of Arizona College of Medicine, Tucson.)

TABLE 164–1. PROTO-ONCOGENE EXPRESSION OF IMPORTANCE IN PATHOGENESIS OF HUMAN NEOPLASMS

Neoplasm	Oncogene
Burkitt's lymphoma	c-myc
Follicular lymphoma	bcl-2
Chronic myelogenous leukemia	c-abl
Breast cancer	Her-2/neu
Ovarian cancer	Her-2/neu
Neuroblastoma	n-myc

tions, or oncogene expression. In recent years, cellular proto-oncogene amplification and expression have been linked to the pathogenesis of various neoplasms (Table 164–1).

In the leukemias and lymphomas, such information can prove important for selecting appropriate treatment approaches. For example, the approach to treatment of T-cell or B-cell lymphomas differs as a function of cell lineage, and this often cannot be identified with standard histologic approaches. Accordingly, it is important that the surgeon provide fresh tissue to the pathologist for cytogenetic or flow cytometric analysis; for touch preparations; or for cryopreservation for immunohistochemistry, receptor, or DNA analysis. Many of these specialized tests cannot be performed on tumor tissue that has been fixed. These specialized studies can in some instances provide evidence for a treatable or curable form of cancer that otherwise might go unrecognized. It is therefore very useful to obtain specialized pathologic studies prior to initiation of treatment.

STAGING. Assessment of the body burden of cancer by clinical means (staging) is important in developing the patient's treatment plan. Most staging systems assess the size of the primary tumor and define regional lymph node involvement, as well as the presence or absence of distant metastatic disease. It is important to distinguish between clinical and pathologic staging and to recognize that pathologic staging employing surgical biopsy is generally more accurate. Increasingly, staging can be accomplished by using noninvasive imaging procedures such as chest radiography and magnetic resonance imaging (MRI) or computerized tomography (CT) scanning. In the diagnostic workup of specific forms of cancer, such as breast or prostate cancer, a bone scan can be very useful when the tumor appears to be advanced but is of minimal use in early localized disease unless the patient has skeletal symptoms. For multiple myeloma, bone scans are of less use than skeletal radiographs. The temptation to use a variety of redundant and expensive tests such as CT, MRI, and ultrasonography for the same site in the same patient should be avoided. When invasive procedures such as staging laparotomy are considered, it is important to focus on the benefit-to-risk ratio of the procedure. In this appraisal the patient's age, performance status, concomitant medical problems, and histologic diagnosis all must be considered and the procedure carried out only if it appears likely to make a major and favorable improvement in the treatment plan. For patients who present with life-threatening local complications of cancer (e.g., spinal cord compression, upper airway obstruction, the superior vena cava syndrome, or obstructive jaundice), it is usually necessary first to treat the local complication on an urgent basis with irradiation, surgery, or chemotherapy before tumor staging can be completed.

OVERALL ASSESSMENT. Once diagnosis and staging have been performed, the information must be integrated to develop an optimal treatment plan for the individual patient. For patients with apparently localized cancers, multidisciplinary input is important, as a combined-modality approach to treatment may be indicated. The biologic characteristics of the specific cancer must also be considered. For many tumor types, histopathologic features such as grade of tumor cell differentiation are important, with a less differentiated or undifferentiated phenotype indicating a more aggressive neoplasm. For some sites, other biologic tests are of greater value than histologic grade. For example, in breast cancer, the presence or absence of estrogen or progesterone receptors and the DNA-index and ploidy status as determined by flow cytometry provide information that is useful in developing a treatment plan related to the aggressiveness of the neoplasm. Some patients with a minimal tumor burden (e.g., stage I) of currently incurable B-cell neoplasms (e.g., chronic lymphocytic

leukemia [CLL] and multiple myeloma) are best watched expectantly rather than treated. On the other hand, almost all patients with diffuse large cell (intermediate or high grade) lymphoma should be treated aggressively with curative intent irrespective of stage unless they are very elderly with other major medical problems. It is also important to recognize the severe limitations of current therapy for advanced or metastatic melanoma, pancreatic cancer, and non–small cell lung cancer.

Overall, the physician must synthesize a wide variety of pathologic, staging, and biologic information to reach a decision on therapy for the specific patient. In this context, it is important to decide whether curative therapy is available or not, and if so, whether the patient's age and overall medical condition permit a curative approach to be taken. If cure is not an option with available therapy, one must consider whether significant palliation with prolongation of survival (and relief of symptoms) can be achieved. For old and infirm patients a palliative approach may be preferable—particularly if there is significant morbidity associated with the treatment approach under consideration. On the other hand, some forms of cancer therapy are very effective and well tolerated even with advanced age (e.g., use of tamoxifen in adjuvant therapy of postmenopausal breast cancer or of chlorambucil for CLL). For many tumor types it is important to examine results of recent prospective clinical trials relevant to the patient's diagnosis and clinical setting.

THERAPEUTIC MODALITIES

There are currently three primary therapeutic approaches in the treatment of cancer: surgery, radiation therapy, and medical therapy.

Surgery

Cancer surgery is most useful to establish a tissue diagnosis, to excise the primary tumor with clear surgical margins free of tumor, and to determine the extent of cancer with surgical staging procedures. Surgery is a simple and safe means to remove solid tumors when the tumor is confined to a specific anatomic site of origin. However, in the case of some solid tumors, most patients already have metastatic disease at the time of presentation. In evaluating major surgery for an individual patient it is important to assess the operative risk-to-benefit ratio for the procedure in light of the patient's general health status, the extent of the tumor, and the likelihood that it can be completely removed. Additionally, the technical complexity of the surgical procedure, the type of anesthesia needed, and the experience of the personnel must also be considered. There are a number of specific roles that surgery can play in cancer treatment (Table 164–2).

With advances in both radiation and chemotherapy, the need for radical surgery has diminished. However, it remains a major primary approach to curative cancer therapy. For testicular cancer, even in the presence of limited metastatic disease, regional lymphadenectomy following radical orchiectomy can be curative and eliminate the need for chemotherapy in some patients who have metastases only to retroperitoneal lymph nodes. For many other sites, surgical resection of regional lymph nodes is carried out for diagnostic rather than therapeutic purposes, as involved regional nodes usually signify that the cancer has already disseminated. For example, in breast cancer, the presence or absence of axillary lymph node involvement is the

TABLE 164–2. APPLICATIONS OF SURGERY IN THE TREATMENT OF CANCER

1. Definitive treatment for primary cancer as a single modality
2. Use in combination with radiation and/or chemotherapy
3. Debulking residual disease (e.g., ovarian cancer) after resection of the primary
4. Resection of metastatic disease with curative intent (testicular cancer, pulmonary metastases in sarcoma)
5. Determining the extent of cancer, including regional node involvement (pathologic staging)
6. Treatment of emergency complications (e.g., obstructed viscus)
7. Palliation of symptoms and signs of locally invasive or metastatic cancer
8. Reconstruction and rehabilitation

single most important factor in evaluating the likelihood of distant recurrence, and this information is currently not obtainable by nonsurgical means. Similarly, surgical staging of nodal involvement in colorectal cancer plays an important role in deciding on whether adjuvant systemic chemotherapy is indicated.

Initial cancer therapy often requires a multimodal approach to maximize the chance of cure while simultaneously reducing the extent of surgery required and preventing the development of distant metastases. Multimodal approaches necessarily require close communication between the involved physicians prior to surgery. The opportunity for early communication is improved with histopathologic diagnosis by needle biopsy or local excision of the primary cancer before more extensive therapy. Two examples are of note in this regard: (1) the management of osteogenic sarcoma with limb salvage surgery, irradiation, and adjuvant chemotherapy and (2) the management of early breast cancer with lumpectomy, axillary staging followed by primary irradiation, and adjuvant systemic administration of cytotoxic or endocrine agents. In both instances, the combined approach yields a better cosmetic and functional outcome. With advances in breast conservation surgery, screening mammography is now more widely utilized, as a diagnosis of breast cancer is no longer tantamount to a subsequent mastectomy. The result is an increased ability to establish a diagnosis of breast cancer when the tumor is less extensive and when likelihood of cure is greater. Improved plastic surgical techniques have also made breast reconstruction possible for women who either require or prefer mastectomy.

In addition to its use in diagnosis, staging, and primary therapy, cancer surgery also plays an important role in the management of some patients with more extensive cancer. In ovarian cancer, when the gynecologic oncologist "debulks" peritoneal and omental spread to the status of minimal residual disease, patients become better candidates for systemic chemotherapy and have a better survival. Additionally, early resection of pulmonary metastases of soft tissue sarcomas, and of solitary brain metastases in melanoma, colon, or breast cancer, may provide marked palliation and improved survival of patients, albeit with only occasional cures.

Radiation Therapy

From the time of its initial development in the early 1900's, radiation therapy has made major strides in instrumentation, physics, radiobiology, treatment planning, and applications to curative and palliative cancer therapy. In general, the term "radiation" refers to ionizing radiation that is either electromagnetic or particulate (e.g., γ rays). Compared to surgery, there are distinct advantages in the use of radiotherapy in the locoregional treatment of cancer. Radiation causes less acute morbidity and can provide curative therapy for some specific sites while preserving organ or tissue structure and function. An excellent example is the use of radiation for the curative treatment of early-stage laryngeal cancer wherein vocal function can be preserved.

The basic unit of ionizing irradiation is the **gray** (Gy) which has superseded the rad (1 Gy = 100 rads). By interaction with molecular oxygen, radiation induces the formation of superoxide, hydrogen peroxide, or hydroxyl radicals that then damage or break cellular DNA, which is considered to be the critical target for radiation-induced cell death. Both single- and double-strand breaks of the DNA helix can be induced, with the latter constituting lethal damage. Single strand breaks, if not repaired by the cell, can also result in cell death. With high linear transfer (LET) radiation, direct damage to the molecular structure of DNA can be induced.

Radiation has limitations in treatment of bulky tumors. Large tumors frequently have poorly perfused and hypoxic zones in which radiation often fails to give rise to needed reactive intermediaries. Various forms of irradiation are used for differing therapeutic objectives. For example, electron beam irradiation deposits most of its energy in the skin and soft tissues and can be useful for superficial therapy in mycosis fungoides. Low energy (kilovoltage) x-rays expend most of their effects on the overlying tissues above a deep-seated tumor and therefore cause considerable normal tissue damage. By contrast, higher energy x-rays

(megavoltage) or γ-irradiation from a cobalt 60 source spare the skin and deposit their energy at greater depth and provide a better approach to treating deep-seated neoplasms. Use of radioactive implants can also be useful in some settings (e.g., cervical cancer). The use of multiple irradiation fields reduces the dose to normal tissue while increasing the dose to the tumor. The use of fractionated doses or radiation causes less cumulative damage to normal tissues than to the tumor, as the normal tissues are often able to repair sublethal damage more quickly. Additionally, as a tumor shrinks with therapy, its oxygenation can improve and thereby render it more radiosensitive. The selection of treatment is based on the relative radiosensitivity of the tumor and of the normal organs and tissues within the radiation field (Table 164–3).

The combined use of multiple fields, fractionated irradiation, and megavoltage radiation equipment is optimized by detailed treatment planning individualized to the patient's tumor. Although the major uses of radiotherapy involve local irradiation of sites of tumor involvement, total body irradiation is a valuable part of a preparative regimen together with high-dose chemotherapy for allogeneic or autologous bone marrow transplantation for leukemia or lymphoma. Total body irradiation in doses in the range of 10 Gy induces permanent aplasia of normal bone marrow and profound immunosuppression and is used only in conjunction with marrow transplantation.

Radiation therapy also has important palliative applications. One of these is for bone pain due to metastatic involvement of the skeleton. Irradiation can also cause sufficient cytoreduction of tumor in bone to permit healing of osteolytic lesions and thereby prevent pathologic fractures of weight-bearing bones. Other examples include tumor shrinkage to relieve postobstructive infection in lung cancer and to suppress bronchial or gastric bleeding secondary to cancer.

Although modern radiotherapy with megavoltage equipment has proven to be extremely useful, some even higher energy radiation approaches are currently in development. These include the use of higher LET sources of irradiation (e.g., neutrons, charged particles, heavy ions) which may also provide selective advantages for specific tumor sites and reduce the need for oxygenation of tumor tissue. Additionally, several classes of compounds are under study as **radiosensitizers** to enhance the cytotoxic effects of radiation on tumor cells. One class is the halopyrimidines, including bromodeoxyuridine, fluorouracil, and fluorodeoxyuridine, which sensitize DNA to strand breakage by radiation. A second class includes the nitroimidazoles (structural analogues of metronidazole [Flagyl]), which can enhance radiation damage to hypoxic cells by accepting free electrons and forming free radicals with oxygen. Several sulfhydryl compounds are also under investigation as potential radioprotective agents. Such compounds would need to exhibit selective uptake in normal cells in order to increase the therapeutic index of radiation for tumor cells, and this approach also remains experimental.

Although the term "radiation" normally refers to ionizing irradiation, there are also several other forms of radiation used in cancer treatment. These include hyperthermia and photodynamic therapy, both of which are still undergoing development. Some tumors show thermal sensitivity to temperatures in the range of 41 to 43°C and may be more sensitive than surrounding normal tissues. Hyperthermia appears to work best on bulky

TABLE 164–3. TOLERANCE OF NORMAL TISSUES TO IRRADIATION

Tissue	Toxic Effect	Limiting Dose (Gy)*
Bone marrow	Aplasia	2.5
Lung	Pneumonitis, fibrosis	15.0
Kidney	Nephrosclerosis	20.0
Liver	Hepatitis	25.0
Spinal cord	Infarction, necrosis	45.0
Intestine	Ulceration, fibrosis	45.0
Heart	Pericarditis, myocarditis	45.0
Brain	Infarction, necrosis	50.0
Skin	Dermatitis, sclerosis	55.0

*Radiation in 2.0-Gy fractions to the whole organ for 5 days weekly produces a 5 per cent incidence of the listed toxicities at the limiting doses listed.

TABLE 164–4. RESPONSIVENESS OF CANCER TO CHEMOTHERAPY*

Tumor Type	Useful Agents
A. Curable with chemotherapy in some patients and exhibiting improved survival in those not cured	
Choriocarcinoma (adjuvant, advanced)	MTX, VCR, Plat, Etop
Acute lymphocytic leukemia	VCR, Pred, Daun, MP, MTX
Acute nonlymphocytic leukemia	Ara-C, Daun, Mitox
Malignant lymphoma (Hodgkin's disease, diffuse high or intermediate grade non-Hodgkin's lymphoma)	Adr, Alk, VCR, Pred, Pro
Testicular carcinoma (advanced)	Plat, Etop, Bleo, VBL
Childhood sarcomas (adjuvant)	Adr, VCR, Alk, Act-D
Wilms' tumor (adjuvant)	VCR, Act-D
Osteosarcoma (adjuvant)	Adr, MTX, Alk, Plat
Rectal carcinoma (adjuvant)	FU, Mito, Nit
B. Improved survival after chemotherapy	
Breast carcinoma (adjuvant, advanced)	Alk, MTX, FU, Adr, Mito, VCR, Mitox, Tam
Ovarian carcinoma (adjuvant, advanced)	Plat, Alk
Multiple myeloma	Alk, Pred, VCR, Adr, IFN
Small cell lung carcinoma	Alk, Plat, Etop, Adr
Colon carcinoma (adjuvant)	FU, Lev
C. Useful palliation of symptoms of advanced cancer with chemotherapy but with limited or no improvement in survival	
Chronic myeloid leukemia	Alk, HU, IFN
Non-Hodgkin's lymphomas—low grade	Alk, Pred, IFN
Prostatic carcinoma	Endo, Sur
Thyroid carcinoma	Plat, FU, Adr
Soft tissue sarcomas	Adr, Dac
Head and neck carcinoma (combined modality)	Plat, FU
Bladder carcinoma	Plat, VBL, MTX, Adr
Esophageal (combined modality)	Plat, FU
D. Only occasionally responsive to current chemotherapy	
Primary brain tumors	Nit
Non–small cell lung carcinoma	Alk, Plat, Etop, MTX, FU, Adr
Melanoma	Dac, IFN
Gastric carcinoma	Plat, FU, Mito, Adr
Renal carcinoma	IFN, IL-2, VBL

*When indicated, favorable results obtained with adjuvant therapy are better than with surgery and/or radiation therapy. When annotated as "advanced," indicated results are obtained in the setting of overt metastatic cancer.

Act D = Actinomycin D; Adr = Adriamycin (doxorubicin); Alk = alkylating agent; Ara-C = cytarabine; Bleo = bleomycin; Dac = dacarbazine; Daun = daunorubicin; Endo = endocrine agent; Etop = Etoposide; FU = 5-fluorouracil; HU = hydroxyurea; IFN = interferon; IL-2 = interleukin-2; Lev = levamisole; Mito = mitomycin; Mitox = mitoxantrone; MP = 6-mercaptopurine; MTX = methotrexate; Nit = nitrogen mustard; Plat = platinum compound; Pred = prednisone; Pro = procarbazine; Sur = suramin; Tam = tamoxifen; VCR = vincristine; VBL = vinblastine.

tumors with poor blood supply in which the tumor cells are in an acidic environment. A variety of approaches is used to induce local or regional hyperthermia (e.g., ultrasonography, microwaves, regional perfusion) and may enhance the effects of ionizing irradiation or chemotherapy on local tumors.

Photodynamic therapy (PDT) is yet another form of nonionizing radiation therapy. PDT involves the preliminary systemic administration of a photosensitizing compound such as a hematoporphyrin derivative (e.g., dihematoporphyrin ether, Photofrin II). Such hematoporphyrins are concentrated in the vicinity of local tumors and can be activated with local exposure to visible red light (usually 630 nm), with a resulting preferential toxicity to cancer cells. The intense light used for PDT can be delivered via a fiberoptic probe, and therefore it can be used for various internal sites as well as on the skin. The mechanism of action of PDT is poorly understood but may involve vascular damage or a direct toxic effect on tumor cells. Side effects of photodynamic therapy include hypersensitivity to light (skin and eyes). Locally PDT induces transient sunburn and hyperpigmentation as well as local tumor necrosis. Tumor sites amenable to PDT include skin recurrences of breast cancer (e.g., chest wall) and malignant lesions in the endobronchus, peritoneal cavity, and bladder. Photodynamic therapy has not been approved by the Food and Drug Administration in the United States and therefore remains investigational.

Medical Therapy

As cancer may disseminate beyond its site of origin prior to diagnosis and because local treatment is frequently not curative, effective systemic drug therapy is needed. Limited clinical success with cytotoxic chemotherapy was first achieved about 40 years ago. Some of these early successes included findings that cytotoxic drugs could cure metastatic choriocarcinoma and induce complete remissions in children with acute leukemia. Subsequently, curative therapy was developed for a series of relatively uncommon neoplasms, and useful palliative therapy has been developed for some common forms of cancer (Table 164–4). With rare exceptions, effective therapy has utilized combinations of anticancer drugs. Increasingly, anticancer drugs are used in concert with surgery and/or irradiation.

Efforts to develop cytoxic and endocrine anticancer agents have been vigorous over the past two decades. Ideally, anticancer drugs should eradicate cancer without harming normal tissues; however, this goal has not been achieved, and most useful drugs have significant side effects. The introduction of anticancer drugs for clinical use has largely been predicted from animal tumor models. Perhaps because the initial murine models were for acute leukemia, many of the drugs that have been discovered are relatively general antiproliferative agents. Accordingly, they have greater efficacy in more rapidly proliferating tumors than in some of the more slowly growing solid tumors and are more toxic to rapidly growing tumors than to normal host tissues of the same histology. However, such generally antiproliferative agents can have significant toxic side effects on normal tissues that divide rapidly such as bone marrow, gastrointestinal mucosa, and skin.

CELL KINETICS AND RESPONSE TO CHEMOTHERAPY. A number of related factors, including total tumor burden, cell kinetics, and intrinsic sensitivity, influence the response to anticancer drugs. In both animal models and human tumors, growth occurs in accord with gompertzian kinetics. Initially growth occurs rapidly, and most tumor cells traverse the complete cell cycle. As the tumor burden grows larger, the rate of tumor cell doubling progressively slows (Fig. 164–2), and the fraction of cells traversing the cell cycle decreases as more and more cells remain "hung up" in a G_0 phase. Whereas the population doubling time may be in the range of 1 to 2 days at the subclinical phase (with less than 1 gram of tumor), by the time the tumor burden has reached 1 kg or more, the tumor cell population doubling time may be 3 to 6 months. A significant problem in the treatment of high tumor burden leukemias and metastatic solid tumors is that the tumor exhibits a significant degree of heterogeneity and subpopulations of cells exhibit differing biologic, kinetic, antigenic, and drug-sensitivity profiles.

Several important features related to cell kinetics and tumor burden are important with respect to drug dose, scheduling, and response to chemotherapy. Anticancer drugs can be classified as either cell cycle specific (CCS) or cell cycle nonspecific (CCNS) (Table 164–5). CCNS agents have greater effects on cycling than on noncycling cells but nonetheless can exert anticancer effects on noncycling cells, whereas CCS agents do not. Endocrine agents are also in a sense cycle-active, as they block the transition of tumor cells from G_1 to the S phase of the cell cycle. However, endocrine agents (e.g., prednisone, tamoxifen, progestins) are noncytotoxic and are considered to suppress growth rather than kill tumor cells. Endocrine agents are therefore often given for many years, whereas cytotoxic agents are usually given over a time course measured in months.

An important concept in cancer chemotherapy is that cellular killing with cytotoxic agents follows first-order kinetics, with a given dose of drug killing only a fraction of the tumor cells. This "fractional kill hypothesis" is particularly relevant to CCNS agents and predicts that the greater the dose of drug administered, the greater the "log kill" of tumor cells which will occur.

The concept of combination chemotherapy was developed to take advantage of the fact that many anticancer agents have

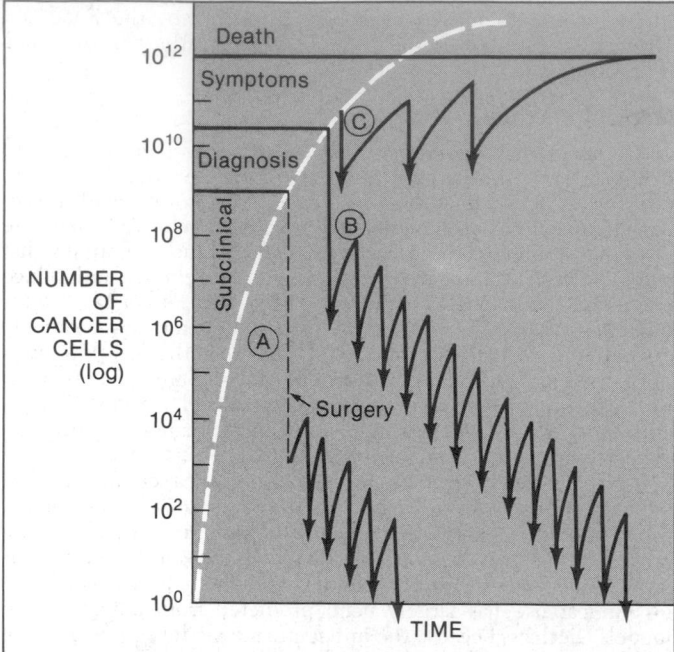

FIGURE 164–2. The relationship of tumor growth and tumor burden to treatment strategies and outcome with systemic chemotherapy. Human tumors grow in accord with the "Gompertz curve" *(dashed line)*, with a decreasing doubling time as tumor burden increases. Treatment interventions relate to tumor type and extent of disease. *A,* Surgery followed by pulse courses of adjuvant chemotherapy. *B,* Systemic chemotherapy for stage III Hodgkin's disease. *C,* Palliative chemotherapy for advanced non–small cell cancer. In *A,* combined modality has curative potential with the addition of chemotherapy after surgery. Cure is also possible in *B* with prolonged administration of combination chemotherapy. In *C,* the patient's tumor burden is too great and potency of the drugs for this specific form of cancer is inadequate. (Modified from Salmon SE, Sartorelli AC: Cancer chemotherapy. *In* Katzung BG (ed.): Basic and Clinical Pharmacology, 4th ed. Norwalk, CT, Appleton and Lange Co., 1989, p 685.)

differing mechanisms of action and side effects. This concept was based on the hypothesis that giving drugs with differing mechanisms of action may achieve synergistic antitumor effects while simultaneously retarding the rate of development of drug resistance. Additionally, by careful selection of drugs in a combination to include those with known single-agent activity against the tumor and different normal tissue toxicities, the side effects would be "spread" across different tissues and organs. The validity of this concept has been born out clinically, and optimal results for most tumor types sensitive to chemotherapy have been achieved with drug combinations, often employing CCNS and CCS agents with decidedly different mechanisms of action. For example, cisplatin has demonstrated clear-cut synergy with eto-

TABLE 164–5. RELATIONSHIP OF TUMOR CELL CYCLE TO ACTIVITY OF MAJOR CLASSES OF CYTOTOXIC ANTICANCER DRUGS

Cell Cycle–Specific (CCS) Agents	Cell Cycle–Nonspecific (CCNS) Agents
Antimetabolites (cytarabine, fluorouracil, methotrexate, mercaptopurine, hydroxyurea)	Alkylating agents (busulfan, cyclophosphamide, mechlorethamine, melphalan, thiotepa, chlorambucil)
Bleomycin	Antibiotics (dactinomycin, daunorubicin, doxorubicin, mitomycin)
Plant alkaloids (vincristine, vinblastine, etoposide, taxol)	Platinum compounds (cisplatin, carboplatin)
	Nitrosoureas (BCNU, CCNU)
	Dacarbazine
	Mitoxantrone
	L-Asparaginase

poside in testicular cancer and small cell lung cancer and with fluorouracil in both head and neck and esophageal cancer. The major potential toxicity for cisplatin is renal, whereas myelosuppression is the major side effect for both etoposide and fluorouracil.

New drugs entering clinical trials are normally first tested in patients with a large tumor burden of metastatic cancer who have relapsed from known effective chemotherapy regimens. Although this approach is ethically most acceptable, it nonetheless represents a significant obstacle to new drug development, as these patients have a lower probability of response to a new drug than those with a lower tumor burden or those who have not been previously treated. Additionally, some metastatic cells can gain access to pharmacologic sanctuaries (e.g., the central nervous system). The presence of the blood-brain barrier has been a major obstacle to the development of chemotherapy for primary or metastatic tumors in the brain. At present brain tumors are treated chiefly with surgery and radiation therapy.

DRUG RESISTANCE. For many of the drug-responsive tumor types listed in Table 164–3, major cytoreduction occurs with initial chemotherapy. However, some months to years thereafter, tumor regrowth occurs and continues even though therapy with the same drugs is reinstituted. This clinical observation usually reflects the acquisition of drug resistance by the tumor to the specific drugs used. In general, the development of drug resistance is considered to result from the high spontaneous mutation rate of cancer cells, which leads to the development of heterogeneous subpopulations, some of which exhibit resistance to various drugs. A variety of drug-resistance mechanisms has been identified in the laboratory, several of which have been documented to be clinically important. Perhaps the most important is a form of **multidrug resistance (MDR)**. MDR is mediated by a cell membrane glycoprotein (the **P-glycoprotein**), which functions as an energy-dependent efflux pump that actively extrudes a variety of cytotoxic agents from the cell (Fig. 164–3).

Drugs pumped out of the cancer cell by the P-glycoprotein include natural products such as plant alkaloids (vincas, podophyllotoxins), antibiotics (dactinomycin, doxorubicin, daunorubicin) and some synthetic agents (e.g., melphalan, mitoxantrone). The P-glycoprotein is normally expressed in tissues such as the gut and the kidney, perhaps to deal with toxic products in the environment. Cancer cells with mutations to "switch on" the expression of the gene responsible for encoding the P-glycoprotein show resistance to a wide variety of useful anticancer drugs. Techniques such as immunohistochemistry, Western blots, and

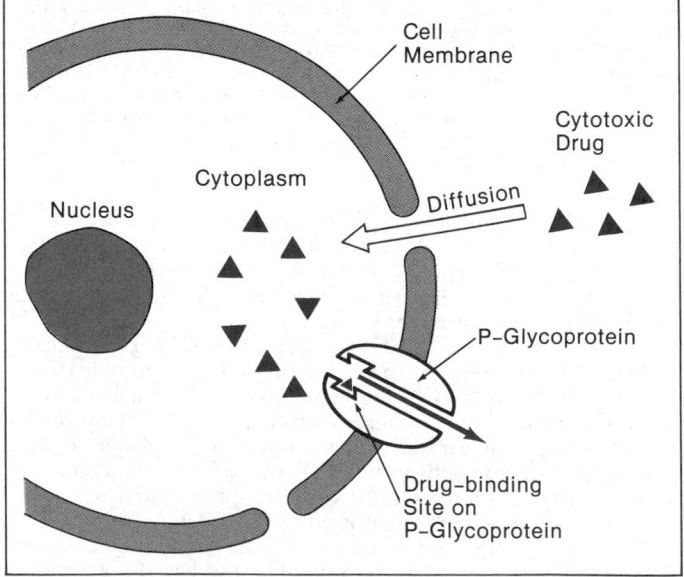

FIGURE 164–3. Model of cancer cell expressing P-glycoprotein. This transmembrane protein functions as an energy-dependent efflux pump or drug transporter. It has acceptor sites to which various natural product anticancer drugs bind, after which they are pumped out of the cell. Chemosensitizers such as verapamil also bind to the drug acceptor sites on P-glycoprotein and can competitively inhibit its function.

Northern blots can be used to detect the presence of P-glycoprotein in tumor tissues. Clinical studies suggest that patients whose tumors express P-glycoprotein have a poor prognosis. Culture studies performed on biopsy specimens in vitro have documented that P-glycoprotein–positive tumors usually exhibit resistance to doxorubicin. Tumor types such as sarcoma, neuroblastoma, malignant lymphoma, and myeloma are usually P-glycoprotein–negative at the time of diagnosis but are frequently positive for P-glycoprotein when the patient relapses from chemotherapy. A series of noncytotoxic drugs has been identified which are also subject to efflux by the P-glycoprotein (e.g., verapamil, cyclosporine, progestins). Such agents are now classified as **chemosensitizers** because they can competitively inhibit the function of P-glycoprotein in vitro by binding to the drug acceptor sites on the P-glycoprotein, inhibiting the efflux of the cytotoxic drug and thereby circumventing the drug resistance. In drug-resistant patients with malignant lymphoma and multiple myeloma, high doses of verapamil given simultaneously with vincristine and doxorubicin can reverse resistance to these agents, with some patients regaining remission. Although verapamil is not an ideal chemosensitizer (owing to its cardiovascular side effects), other potential chemosensitizers (quinidine, quinine, cyclosporine, nontoxic verapamil analogues) are now being tested in an effort to identify more effective and less toxic chemosensitizers. In the long run, such chemosensitizers may find their major use to prevent development of MDR expression.

An example of a more drug-specific mechanism of resistance has been identified for the antimetabolite methotrexate (MTX). MTX and its polyglutamated metabolites inhibit the function of the enzyme dihydrofolate reductase (DHFR). The normal function of DHRF in nucleic acid synthesis is to reduce inactive dihydrofolate to its active tetrahydrofolate form, which serves as a one-carbon donor for the synthesis of purine nucleotides and thymidylate. Some tumor cells that acquire MTX resistance have been found to have an increased number of DNA gene copies encoding for DHFR. This form of multiple gene reduplication is called **gene amplification.** The amplified DHFR genes in MTX-resistant cells produce a markedly increased number of copies of the DHFR enzyme, far exceeding the amount of MTX that can be delivered to the cell, and thereby allow tumor cell DNA synthesis and proliferation to continue. Gene amplification in mammalian cells has been observed only in tumor cells, but the phenomenon is not unique to MTX resistance.

PREDICTIVE TESTING IN VITRO. A variety of approaches has been developed to assess the probability of a patient's relapsing after primary therapy or responding to a given type or class of endocrine or cytotoxic agent. The goal of such efforts is to identify which patients might benefit from a planned treatment. The "S-phase" fraction of the tumor cell population undergoing DNA synthesis as well as DNA ploidy can be determined by flow cytometry. For several tumor types, patients with a high percentage of tumor cells in DNA synthesis and/or hyperdiploidy have a high likelihood of relapsing early after local primary cancer therapy. Taken with other prognostic characteristics, such flow cytometry assays may aid in identifying patients who should receive adjuvant chemotherapy. This approach is currently being applied in patients with stage I breast cancer in an effort to decide which patients are at higher risk for recurrence.

The results of S-phase and DNA ploidy analysis are often provided by diagnostic laboratories on breast cancer specimens along with the findings from estrogen and progesterone receptor testing. Estrogen and progesterone receptor assays in breast cancer have their primary use in identifying patients who are likely to respond to endocrine agents in either the adjuvant or recurrent cancer setting. These sex steroid hormone receptors are located in the cell nucleus and must bind the hormone and translocate it to cellular DNA to exert endocrine action via gene activation or suppression. Additionally, in the absence of adjuvant therapy, patients whose tumors are estrogen or progesterone receptor–positive have longer times to recurrence and a better overall prognosis than do patients whose tumors are receptor negative. Recent studies of another tumor cell constituent, the HER-2/neu oncogene, can be of prognostic value. Amplification of the number of copies of the HER-2/neu gene or increased expression of the gene product by RNA or protein analysis appears to predict a poor prognosis in both breast and ovarian cancer. The protein product of HER-2/neu is expressed on the surface of

tumor cells and structurally appears to be a hormone receptor analogous to the epidermal growth factor (EGF) receptor. However, the ligand for this presumed receptor has not yet been identified.

For specific anticancer drug testing, clonogenic and dye exclusion assays in vitro have been developed and applied with increasing success. Assays of this type are potentially of considerable value, because a critical factor regarding response to chemotherapy is the intrinsic sensitivity of the specific tumor to the agents being used for treatment. However, available techniques are labor intensive and must be applied to freshly biopsied and viable tumor specimens rapidly transferred to the testing laboratory. Chemosensitivity assays appear to be highly predictive of drug resistance but somewhat less accurate for predicting which drugs will be useful for an individual patient. Another type of testing for drug resistance that is now being applied to fresh frozen (and in some instances to fixed tissues) is immunohistochemical testing for P-glycoprotein expression.

PHARMACOKINETIC CONSIDERATIONS. Although intrinsic drug sensitivity appears to be the most critical determinant of response to chemotherapy, pharmacokinetic factors related to the route of administration, bioavailability, metabolism, and elimination are probably of greater importance in cancer therapy than in other areas of medicine. Many of the cytotoxic agents have a steep dose-response curve and a resulting narrow therapeutic index. Thus at too low an available dose level within the tumor, no response is seen. On the other hand, at higher doses, significant host toxicity supervenes and is usually dose-limiting. Because of the steep dose-response relationship, doses of most cytotoxic agents are calculated in relation to body surface area. This approach is more accurate than dose calculations based on body weight. The oral route of drug administration is often desired by patients but is not generally emphasized in cancer therapy, not only because of problems with compliance but also because of extremely marked variations in bioavailability in the blood after administration of oral formulations. For example, with the alkylating agent melphalan, more than a 10-fold variation in plasma levels has been documented after standard dosing. Unfortunately, plasma assays are not routinely available for most anticancer drugs, and the only semiquantitative indicator of bioavailability of cytotoxic agents is the occurrence of myelosuppression after drug administration. For patients presenting with hypercalcemia or other dire complications of myeloma, oral melphalan would therefore seem undesirable, as such patients need good drug bioavailability immediately. Similar difficulties are faced with oral administration of fluorouracil, methotrexate, and 6-mercaptopurine. On the other hand, for agents such as tamoxifen and cyclophosphamide, bioavailability is good after oral administration.

The intravenous route of drug administration is clearly preferable for most cytotoxic anticancer drugs, as it assures that adequate plasma levels can be achieved while minimizing problems with compliance. For some agents, continuous intravenous drug administration for 4 days or longer provides better results and less toxicity than do bolus or short-duration infusions. This is because tumor response for many agents can be related to the "area under the plasma disappearance curve (AUC)" for the drug, whereas toxicity generally relates more directly to peak plasma concentrations than to the AUC. With the advent of vascular access devices such as subcutaneous ports or external catheters and of sophisticated battery-powered infusion pumps, outpatient continuous infusion chemotherapy can now be used for stable drugs such as fluorinated pyrimidines, anthracyclines, and vinca alkaloids. Subcutaneous administration can be used effectively with drugs such as cytarabine, interferon-α, and erythropoietin. Subcutaneous dosing provides more sustained plasma levels than can be obtained with intravenous administration. Depot intramuscular formulations are available for a variety of endocrine agents used in treatment of breast or prostate cancer.

Regional administration of chemotherapy can also be used effectively for several tumor sites. One of these is metastatic colon cancer limited to the liver. Hepatic artery catheterization for arterial infusion of 5-fluorodeoxyuridine or 5-fluorouracil can be used effectively by connection of the catheter to an external pump or to an implantable perfusion pump. In either instance, arterial infusions are often administered for 14 days followed by a similar rest period. A relatively high objective response rate of metastatic colon cancer in the liver can be obtained by this means, but this route is ineffective for metastases outside the liver. Hepatic artery chemotherapy is expensive and associated with complications, including arterial thrombosis, biliary sclerosis, and chemical hepatitis. Nonetheless, it can induce sustained remissions for a year or more in selected patients with liver metastases. Regional infusion or isolated perfusion has been used with melanomas or sarcomas of the lower extremity. With intransit melanoma metastases of the lower extremity, melphalan or cisplatin has been administered in this fashion with or without regional hyperthermia.

Intracavitary drug administration has long been used in the bladder with instillation of a biologic agent such as BCG (bacille Calmette-Guérin) or interferon or a variety of cytotoxic agents (e.g., thiotepa, doxorubicin, mitomycin, cisplatin). Intraperitoneal drug administration has also gained increasing popularity and appears to show particular promise for patients with peritoneal carcinomatosis. It can induce remissions of established metastatic disease. In ovarian cancer intraperitoneal chemotherapy is being studied as a follow-up to cytoreductive surgery. Diffusion of intraperitoneally administered drugs is limited to a few millimeters of tumor tissue. Accordingly, intraperitoneal chemotherapy is seldom warranted in patients with bulky tumor masses. For optimal distribution, the drug is usually diluted in 2 liters of parenteral fluid for injection. Preferred drugs for intraperitoneal administration are those that tend to be largely limited to the peritoneal cavity and have good properties for tumor penetration. Mitoxantrone has these favorable characteristics, and cisplatin can also be quite useful. With both of these drugs, the intraperitoneal concentration of drug can be 1000-fold higher than measured in the systemic circulation. Other agents sometimes used in intraperitoneal administration include thiotepa, fluorouracil, and methotrexate. Intraperitoneal drug administration can be performed at repeated intervals with relative ease if a surgically implanted Tenkoff catheter is connected to a subcutaneous port. Mild to moderate chemical peritonitis and the development of peritoneal adhesions are common complications of intraperitoneal chemotherapy and limit repeated use.

The intrathecal route can be used to deliver therapy to the meninges. Both methotrexate and cytarabine can be given by this route for prevention of meningeal leukemia and for treatment of central nervous system leukemia or lymphoma. Intrathecal methotrexate has been used effectively for acute lymphoblastic leukemia as an adjuvant to initial systemic chemotherapy and has reduced the frequency of central nervous system relapse in patients in complete peripheral remission.

EVALUATION OF RESPONSE. Objective measurement of tumor shrinkage with medical or radiation therapy has prognostic importance. Subjective improvement alone is not evidence of response. Cure or significant prolongation of survival is seen in patients who achieve complete response (disappearance of all evidence of cancer). Whenever possible, confirmation of response should be obtained pathologically through the use of restaging procedures. Many patients achieve only a partial response, defined as a reduction of tumor burden by 50 per cent or more. Patients achieving partial responses generally have palliation of symptoms and usually have a prolonged period without tumor growth. Modest improvements in survival are seen in some patients with partial responses.

Tumor markers in the blood or urine can be useful in monitoring response to therapy (Table 164–6). Patients with testicular germ cell tumors and gestational choriocarcinoma cannot be considered potentially cured unless the titer of marker substance falls below the limit of detection. Tumor marker studies are also useful in judging responses in ovarian cancer, prostatic carcinoma, multiple myeloma, neuroblastoma, and the carcinoid syndrome. Markers of lesser predictive value are also available for colon and pancreatic cancer.

Response to adjuvant chemotherapy cannot be evaluated by these methods, as in this circumstance there is insufficient tumor present for assessment by physical or imaging studies or with tumor markers. However, in the neoadjuvant setting wherein chemotherapy is used prior to local surgery, the response to

TABLE 164–6. APPLICATIONS OF TUMOR MARKERS TO CANCER DIAGNOSIS AND THERAPY

Tumor Type	Marker*	Applications
Choriocarcinoma	hCG	Diagnosis, response
Testicular cancer	hCG, AFP	Diagnosis, response
Hepatoma	AFP	Diagnosis
Prostate cancer	PSA	Diagnosis, response
Multiple myeloma	M-proteins	Diagnosis, response
Carcinoid	5-HIAA	Diagnosis, response
Neuroblastoma	VMA	Diagnosis, response
Colon cancer	CEA	Response
Ovarian cancer	CA-125	Response
Pancreatic cancer	CA-19-9	Investigational

*hCG = human chorionic gonadotropin; AFP = α-fetoprotein; PSA = prostatic specific antigen; M-protein = monoclonal immunoglobulins; 5-HIAA = 5-hydroxyindoleacetic acid; VMA = vanillylmandelic acid; CEA = carcinoembryonic antigen.

chemotherapy provides an "in vivo sensitivity test" to determine whether the agents employed will be useful in adjuvant therapy after surgery. This approach has been used effectively in osteosarcoma even though calcified bone tumors do not shrink with therapy. This is because neovascularization, as detected by pre- and post-therapy angiography, regresses with effective chemotherapy. Furthermore, pathologic findings at the time of surgical resection after neoadjuvant chemotherapy can be important. In general, cure of osteosarcoma is achieved in patients whose tumors exhibit at least 90 per cent necrosis.

CYTOTOXIC ANTICANCER DRUGS. Safe and effective use of cytotoxic cancer chemotherapy requires considerable understanding of the pharmacology and toxicology of these drugs. This section provides a brief synopsis of some of the more important agents. The drug doses cited are for single-agent chemotherapy. When drugs are used in combinations, lower doses may be required for some agents. Therefore, it is generally wise to use effective and well-established combination protocols with known side-effect profiles rather than improvising combinations. The development of new combinations of standard drugs is best done in the research setting.

Alkylating Agents. The major clinically useful alkylating agents kill cells by binding to and crosslinking DNA via a bis(chloroethyl)amine, ethylenimine, or nitrosourea moiety. Although these agents likely kill cells by alkylating DNA (primarily at the N7 position of guanine), they also react chemically with sulfhydryl, amino, hydroxyl, and phosphate groups of all cellular nucleophilic (electron-rich) sites. The mechanism of action of alkylating agents involves intramolecular cyclization to form an ethylenimmonium ion that can transfer an alkyl group to a cellular target either directly or via formation of a carbonium ion. The interactions of alkylating agents with DNA can occur with one or both strands, as most alkylating agents contain two reactive groups. Alkylation of guanine can lead to abnormal base pairing with thymine or to depurination by excision of guanine residues. This effect results in DNA strand breakage. When crosslinking occurs between guanine residues on opposite strands, excision repair can disrupt the integrity of the DNA helix and result in a lethal mutation.

The initial alkylating agent introduced in clinical oncology was nitrogen mustard, an agent still used in treatment of Hodgkin's disease and mycosis fungoides. Nitrosoureas are a subset of alkylating agents that have an additional secondary mechanism of action involving carbamoylation of lysine residues of proteins by forming isocyanates. Alkylating agents are CCNS agents, but cells are most susceptible to alkylation in late G_1 and S phase, and the damage is manifest by a blockage in division after the G_2 phase. The mechanism of acquired resistance to alkylating agents may be a decreased retention of the alkylating agent, increased production of low molecular weight sulfhydryl compounds, and increased capacity to repair DNA damage. Although all alkylating agents have similar mechanisms of action, differences in their molecular structures reduce the degree of cross-resistance between various major subclasses. Alkylating agents also differ in the severity of early and late side effects. The major acute side effects are gastrointestinal (nausea and vomiting) and hematologic (myelosuppression). Most alkylating agents have strong vesicant action and can cause local tissue injury when infiltrated into the skin. All alkylating agents can potentially induce ovarian or testicular failure as well as acute leukemia. Agents such as melphalan and chlorambucil appear to be more leukemogenic than cyclophosphamide, whereas busulfan and the nitrosoureas cause more persistent damage to hemopoietic stem cells and more prolonged myelosuppression. The structures of some major alkylating agents are depicted in Figure 164–4.

Cyclophosphamide (Cytoxan) and Ifosfamide (Ifex). Cyclophosphamide is the most widely used alkylating agent and is effective in the treatment of both hematologic malignancies and solid tumors. It does not have significant vesicant effects, as it is a prodrug and must be biotransformed in the liver. Hepatic activation of cyclophosphamide via the microsomal P-450 mixed function oxidase system results in the generation of 4-hydroxycyclophosphamide and aldophosphamide. Thereafter, in both normal and tumor tissue, aldophosphamide breaks down nonenzymatically to the active metabolite phosphoramide mustard plus acrolein. Cyclophosphamide is available in both intravenous and oral formulations and is well absorbed by the oral route. A commonly used single-agent dosage schedule for intravenous cyclophosphamide is 1.0 gram per square meter every 3 weeks. By either route cyclophosphamide produces a somewhat different and less severe pattern of myelosuppressive toxicity than other alkylating agents, as it appears to spare noncycling hematopoietic stem cells. Cyclophosphamide can cause severe neutropenia, but it is usually of relatively short duration. Thrombocytopenia is significantly less severe than with other alkylators, and this platelet-sparing effect is a useful feature. Other toxicities of cyclophosphamide include alopecia and immunosuppression. When high doses are used (e.g., for bone marrow transplantation), cyclophosphamide can also cause myocardial necrosis or inappropriate renal water retention. Although cyclophosphamide can cause acute nonlymphocytic leukemia and pulmonary fibrosis, these toxicities are more common with other alkylating agents. Both cyclophosphamide and a related analogue ifosfamide (Ifex) can cause hemorrhagic cystitis. Bladder toxicity can be blocked by administration of the uroprotective agent mesna (Mesnex), which is concentrated in the urine and neutralizes active moieties causing bladder toxicity. Mesna is particularly valuable with ifosfamide, which otherwise routinely causes bladder toxicity. Mesna is given with ifosfamide at 20 per cent of the ifosfamide dosage. Ifosfamide causes somewhat less hematologic toxicity than other alkylating agents. At present ifosfamide is used mostly for second-line therapy (e.g., for second-line therapy of testicular cancer or metastatic sarcomas).

Chlorambucil (Leukeran). Chlorambucil has antitumor activity similar to that of cyclophosphamide and is also well absorbed after oral administration. It is used primarily in the treatment of chronic lymphocytic leukemia, low-grade lymphomas, macroglob-

ulinemia, and polycythemia vera. Chlorambucil does not cause hemorrhagic cystitis or alopecia, and gastrointestinal side effects are mild. However, it is myelosuppressive. Acute nonlymphocytic leukemia has been reported in patients treated with chlorambucil for polycythemia vera or other disorders.

Melphalan (Alkeran). Melphalan is L-phenylalanine mustard and gains access to cells through an amino acid transport system. Unlike cyclophosphamide and chlorambucil, oral melphalan absorption can be erratic and affected by food intake, gastric acidity, and other factors. Melphalan is commonly given orally in a dosage of 10 mg per square meter per day for 4 days every 3 to 4 weeks. It is essential to follow serial CBC's closely, as some patients do not absorb the drug and the only clue to this is the absence of myelosuppression. If myelosuppression does not occur, melphalan dosage should be increased in subsequent courses until moderate myelosuppression is induced. Melphalan is commonly used in the treatment of multiple myeloma and ovarian cancer and occasionally for other tumor types. Melphalan induces acute nonlymphocytic leukemia in some patients treated for myeloma or ovarian cancer.

Busulfan (Myleran). Busulfan is a methane-sulfonate–based alkylating agent that has specificity for myeloid neoplasms and appears to have lesser antitumor activity in other forms of cancer. It is available only for oral administration and is used primarily for treatment of chronic myeloid leukemia (CML). Busulfan can produce protracted myelosuppression, and hematologic recovery should be complete before the next course is administered, or cumulative myelosuppressive toxicity may develop with severe or permanent bone marrow aplasia as a consequence. In addition to its myelosuppressive toxicity, myleran can cause pulmonary fibrosis, hyperpigmentation, weakness, and wasting. Although these last three features suggest adrenal insufficiency, adrenal function is normal.

Nitrosoureas. Carmustine (BCNU) and **lomustine (CCNU)** are the two FDA-approved nitrosoureas available for clinical use. Nitrosoureas are rapidly biotransformed via nonenzymatic hydrolysis to release moieties with alkylating and carbamoylating activities. Carmustine is available for intravenous use and lomustine for oral administration. The major toxicity of nitrosoureas at standard dosage levels is on hematopoietic stem cells, and prolonged myelosuppression can result. At high dosage (e.g., in preparative regimens for bone marrow transplantation) nitrosoureas can induce a chemical hepatitis or pneumonitis. Prolonged use of nitrosoureas with total doses greater than 1500 mg per square meter can also result in pulmonary fibrosis or renal failure. Because of their high lipid solubility and ability to cross the blood-brain barrier, the nitrosoureas have some activity against primary brain tumors. The nitrosoureas also are useful in the management of Hodgkin's disease and multiple myeloma and as part of combined modality therapy for cancers of the anal canal.

Platinum Compounds. Cisplatin and **carboplatin** are platinum-coordination compounds with broad-spectrum antitumor activity and synergistic interactions with a variety of other cytotoxic agents, including alkylating agents, antimetabolites, and natural products. Although the mechanism of action of the platinum compounds is not completely understood, they act similarly to alkylating agents in terms of their ability to bind to the N7 position of guanine and crosslink DNA. However, crosslinking with adenine and cytosine also occurs, as does binding to RNA and protein.

Cisplatin and carboplatin differ significantly in their toxicity profiles. Both drugs are administered intravenously. Cisplatin is commonly given in a dose of 100 mg per square meter every 3 weeks, whereas the dose of carboplatin is in the range of 450 mg per square meter at similar intervals, although larger doses may be tolerated. After intravenous infusion, the major acute toxicity for both cisplatin and carboplatin is nausea and vomiting. Satisfactory suppression of the gastrointestinal side effects of platinum compounds requires use of extremely potent antiemetic agents, often in combination. Cisplatin has the additional potentials of renal toxicity and a progressive neuropathy with large cumulative doses of drug. The nephropathy can be largely prevented if the patient is well hydrated with simultaneous saline infusions and diuretics are given with cisplatin. Myelosuppression is minimal with cisplatin but is dose-limiting with carboplatin. Although

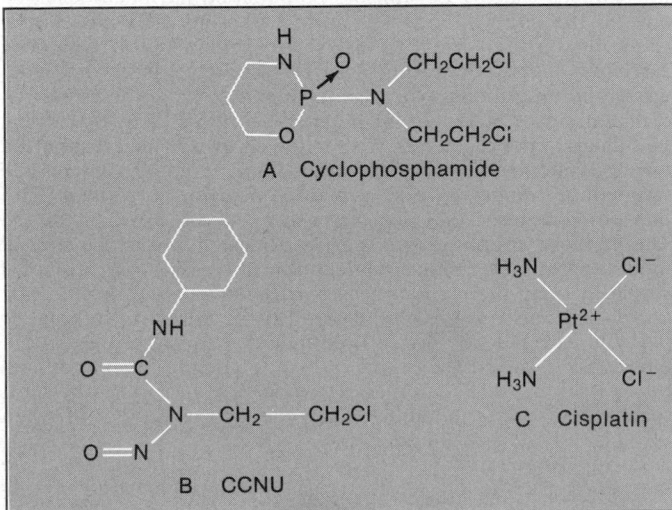

FIGURE 164–4. Alkylating agents. This figure depicts the structures of several prototypes representing subclasses within the general category of alkylating agents. A, Cyclophosphamide with bischlorethyl radical. B, CCNU, a nitrosourea. C, Cisplatin, one of the platinum-coordination complexes.

carboplatin is less toxic than cisplatin, its efficacy is equivalent. However, the lack of myelosuppression favors cisplatin for use in some drug combinations with myelosuppressive agents.

Antimetabolites. The antimetabolites are structural analogues of normal biochemical compounds, most of which are involved in DNA or RNA synthesis and generally function as CCS agents. Antimetabolites are classed in relation to their mechanisms of action. Structures of some major antimetabolites are shown in Figure 164–5.

Pyrimidine Antagonists. *Cytarabine (Cytosine Arabinoside, Cytosar-U, Ara-C).* Cytarabine is an S-phase–specific agent that is particularly useful in acute nonlymphocytic leukemia and to a lesser extent in other hematologic malignancies. Cytarabine is metabolized intracellularly to its active form, ara-CTP, which competitively inhibits DNA polymerase, blocking DNA synthesis. Ara-C is also incorporated into DNA, where it blocks chain elongation and ligation of fragments into newly synthesized DNA. Ara-C is given intravenously and has good CNS uptake into spinal fluid. It is administered either by continuous infusion in doses of at least 100 mg per square meter per day or in bolus doses of 50 to 100 mg every 8 to 12 hours by the intravenous or subcutaneous route for 5 to 7 days. In an alternative dosage schedule which exceeds the manufacturer's recommended maximum dose, high-dose ara-C is administered in doses of 1 to 3 grams every 12 hours for 5 to 6 days and causes higher response rates than do the standard dosage regimens. The duration of intracellular retention of ara-CTP appears to predict ara-C antileukemic effects, with best results in patients who have the longest ara-CTP retention times. The primary toxicity of both standard and high-dose ara-C is severe myelosuppression. With the high-dose regimen, chemical conjunctivitis is common and can be ameliorated with steroid ophthalmic drops. With rare exception, in order to achieve complete remissions in acute leukemia, ara-C must be administered with sufficient intensity to drive the bone marrow to severe hypocellularity and destroy the leukemic blast population. Thereafter the marrow is repopulated by residual normal progenitors that were suppressed by the leukemia. Ara-C is generally used in combination with daunorubicin in the

treatment of acute nonlymphocytic leukemia but also acts synergistically with other drugs including cisplatin. Cytarabine can also be given intrathecally in doses of 75 to 100 mg as treatment for leukemic or carcinomatous meningitis.

Another structural analogue related to cytidine is 5-azacytidine (5-azaC). 5-AzaC is a second-line antileukemic agent that has yet to be approved in the United States by the Food and Drug Administration. 5-AzaC is metabolized intracellularly to 5-azaCTP and is incorporated into DNA and RNA, impairing protein synthesis. As with cytarabine, the primary toxicity of 5-azaC is prolonged myelosuppression, but protracted nausea and vomiting also occur. 5-AzaC is unstable and sensitive to light and to alkaline or neutral pH, leading to ring opening and inactivation. Therefore solutions of 5-azaC must be freshly mixed, preferably in Ringer's lactate, prior to administration.

Fluorouracil (5-FU) and Fluorodeoxyurine (5-FUDR). 5-FU is an important anticancer agent in the treatment of a variety of solid tumors, including cancers of the head and neck, breast, and colon. It acts synergistically with a variety of agents, including platinum compounds and radiation therapy. 5-FU undergoes biotransformation to ribosyl and deoxyribosyl nucleotide metabolites. 5-Fluorouridine triphosphate is incorporated into RNA and interferes with RNA processing and function. An additional metabolite, 5-fluorodeoxyuridine phosphate, forms a ternary complex that binds covalently to thymidylate synthetase and its cofactor, N5,10-methylenetetrahydrofolate. This in turn inhibits DNA synthesis, resulting in "thymineless death." 5-FU is usually given intravenously by bolus or infusion schedules but can also be used in intra-arterial, intracavitary, and topical therapy. An optimal schedule for 5-FU administration is a 5-day continuous infusion at a dose rate of 1.0 gram per square meter per day. This schedule causes some gastrointestinal toxicity but only a mild degree of myelosuppression. With this dosage schedule, full doses of cisplatin can be administered additionally, and this treatment program is very active in the neoadjuvant chemotherapy of head and neck and esophageal cancer. When 5-FU is administered on a weekly intravenous bolus schedule there is greater hematologic toxicity and mucositis with lower total doses. Less common toxicities observed with 5-FU include a neurologic syndrome associated with ataxia, chemical conjunctivitis, and a syndrome including chest pain and cardiac enzyme elevation consistent with myocardial ischemia. The bioavailability of 5-FU after oral administration is erratic, and the drug is metabolized mostly during its first pass through the liver.

Both the gastrointestinal toxicity and the antitumor activity of 5-FU can be enhanced by administration of leucovorin, which increases the binding of fluorodeoxyuridine phosphate to thymidylate synthetase. This combination appears to increase the antitumor activity of 5-FU in breast and colon cancer. Both interferon-α and levamisole also appear to enhance 5-FU activity in colorectal cancer. Levamisole potentiation has been observed only in the adjuvant setting. Both 5-FU and 5-FUDR can be given by hepatic artery infusion for patients with colorectal carcinoma metastatic to the liver. This approach is generally not warranted for patients who also have extrahepatic metastases. A commonly used schedule for hepatic artery 5-FUDR is 0.15 mg per kilogram per day for 14 days followed by a 14-day rest period during which saline infusions are administered. This schedule can induce tumor regression in the majority of patients with hepatic metastases of colorectal cancer if the anatomy of the arterial blood supply provides good drug delivery to the sites of metastasis as determined angiographically. With the use of a surgically placed vascular access catheter, outpatient hepatic artery infusions can be administered using either an internal or portable external pump. One limitation of this approach is that either 5-FU or 5-FUDR can induce a chemical hepatitis and biliary sclerosis with jaundice. Hepatic dysfunction can be most readily detected by obtaining liver chemistries on day 14 when 5-FU is to be discontinued.

Purine Antagonists. *6-Mercaptopurine and 6-Thioguanine.* The first thiopurine found to be a useful anticancer drug was **6-mercaptopurine** (Purinethol, 6-MP). A related agent, **6-thioguanine** (6-TG) is also in use. Both 6-MP and 6-TG are converted to nucleotide form by hypoxanthine-guanine phosphoribosyl transferase (HGPRT), and their metabolites inhibit a number of enzymes in the purine pathway. In contrast to 6-MP, some 6-TG metabolites are incorporated into both DNA and RNA. 6-TG has

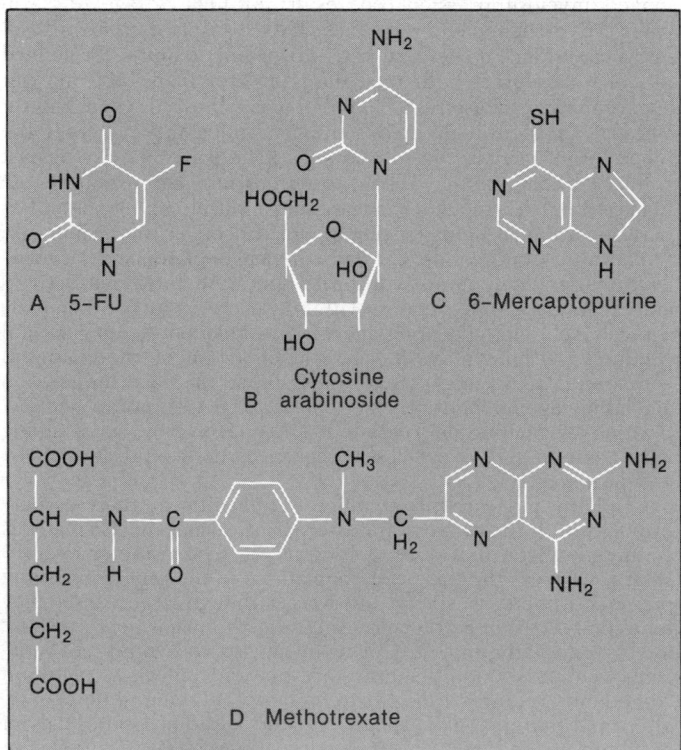

FIGURE / 164–5. Antimetabolites. Depicted here are several antimetabolites that are structural analogues of molecules relevant to nucleic acid metabolism. *A*, 5-Fluorouracil. *B*, Cytarabine. *C*, 6-Mercaptopurine. *D*, Methotrexate.

some uses in acute nonlymphocytic leukemia in combination with cytarabine, whereas 6-MP is used primarily in acute lymphoblastic leukemia, particularly in childhood. Absorption of 6-MP is variable, and recent studies indicate that plasma monitoring of 6-MP concentration can identify poor absorbers who have a high likelihood of developing recurrent leukemia, presumably because of inadequate bioavailability of 6-MP. The 6-MP analogue azathioprine is a useful immunosuppressive agent. Because both 6-MP and azathioprine are catabolized by xanthine oxidase, patients must have their thiopurine doses reduced to 25 per cent of their standard doses if they are also receiving the xanthine oxidase inhibitor allopurinol. 6-TG is not catabolized by xanthine oxidase, and dose correction is not required for allopurinol.

Fludarabine (Fludara, 5-Fluoroadenosine Monophosphate). Fludarabine is an analogue of adenine which appears to act through inhibition of DNA polymerase and ribonuceotide reductase by its phosphorylated product fludarabine triphosphate and by incorporation into DNA. Fludarabine is the single most active agent available in the treatment of chronic lymphocytic leukemia and also exhibits some antitumor activity in other indolent lymphomas and macroglobulinemia. Fludarabine is often given intravenously in a dose of 30 mg per square meter per day over 30 minutes for 5 days every 4 weeks. The major toxicity is myelosuppression. In higher doses in early trials in patients with acute nonlymphocytic leukemia, it produced cortical blindness in some patients. In the lower-dosage schedule used in chronic lymphocytic leukemia and other lymphoid neoplasms, the side effects are usually mild and reversible. Fludarabine has not yet been approved by the Food and Drug Administration.

Additional purine antagonists are deoxycoformycin (DCF) and 2-chloroadenosine (2-CA). Both DCF and 2-CA are extremely active agents in the treatment of hairy cell leukemia and can produce prolonged complete remissions after a single course of treatment. Both agents also exhibit some antitumor activity in other lymphoid neoplasms (e.g., CLL). 2-CA and DCF have not been approved by the Food and Drug Administration and remain investigational.

Folic Acid Antagonists. The first antifol to be used clinically about 40 years ago was aminopterine, which was superseded by **methotrexate** (MTX). Both agents are structural analogues of folic acid. Other antifols have been developed (e.g., trimetrexate), but none has proven superior to MTX. Methotrexate can be administered orally, intramuscularly, or intravenously and is a useful agent primarily as a component of chemotherapy combinations for various types of cancer, including acute lymphoblastic leukemia, small cell lung cancer, and breast cancer. When used in high dosage with leucovorin rescue, it has definite antitumor activity in osteogenic sarcoma. MTX binds tightly to the catalytic site on dihydrofolate reductase (DHFR) and inhibits the synthesis of thymidylate and purine nucleotides, as well as of serine and methionine, by interfering with the ability of DHFR to be reduced and accept one-carbon units. Intracellular formation of polyglutamated forms of MTX is important to the action of MTX, as the polyglutamated forms have equivalent ability to inhibit DHFR action but have a longer intracellular retention time than MTX. The polyglutamates also inhibit other folate-dependent enzymes, including thymidylate synthetase. MTX is excreted unchanged in the urine within 12 hours of administration as long as hydration status and renal function are satisfactory.

The major toxicities of MTX are manifest in rapidly dividing tissues, including the bone marrow and the gastrointestinal mucosa, and to a lesser extent in the skin. At high dosages or in patients with impaired renal function, MTX can also induce renal toxicity. The toxic effects of MTX on the rapidly dividing tissues can be circumvented by administration of the reduced folate leucovorin (folinic acid) within 36 hours after MTX administration. Leucovorin rescue can also be used when methotrexate is intentionally administered in higher than manufacturer's recommended maximum dose (e.g., 1500 mg per square meter or more). When high-dose MTX is administered, leucovorin must be administered in dosage of 15 to 50 mg per square meter every 6 hours for 48 hours, with the duration of leucovorin rescue contingent on the serum methotrexate level. Increased leucovorin dosage and longer periods of rescue are needed in patients with impaired renal function. The high-dose MTX/leucovorin rescue regimen therefore requires good renal function.

NATURAL PRODUCT ANTICANCER DRUGS. The two main classes of natural antitumor products are plant alkaloids and antibiotics. Resistance to the natural products discussed below (with the exception of bleomycin) can be mediated by the P-glycoprotein multidrug resistance mechanism. Structures of some of the major natural product anticancer drugs are depicted in Figure 164–6.

Plant Alkaloids. Vincristine and Vinblastine. The vinca alkaloids were isolated from the common periwinkle (*Vinca rosacea*). The major vincas in clinical use, vincristine (Oncovin) and vinblastine (Velban), result in precipitation of tubulin and disruption of cellular microtubules. Whereas the primary toxicity of vinblastine is hemopoietic, vincristine's major toxicity is to peripheral nerves, resulting in sensorimotor and autonomic neuropathies. Common symptoms of vincristine toxicity are paresthesias ("pins and needles sensation") in the digits and progressive muscular weakness, particularly in the lower extremities and associated with hyporeflexia. Foot drop can develop, as can occasional cranial, bladder, or bowel neuropathies. In general, individual bolus doses of greater than 2 mg are not recommended because of neurotoxicity. The neurotoxicity subsides slowly after the drug is discontinued, with improvement occurring over months. The lack of bone marrow toxicity of vincristine has made it useful for combination chemotherapy regimens. The vincas have vesicant effects and can be administered only intravenously. Both vincas have significant antitumor activity in leukemias and lymphomas as well as for selected solid tumors, including small cell lung cancer and breast cancer. Vincristine is used in various combinations, including "MOPP," "CHOP," "MACOP-B," and "M-BACOD" used in the treatment of lymphomas and "VMCP" and "VAD" used in the treatment of multiple myeloma. Vinblastine's most significant use has been in its incorporation into the "PVB" regimen for the treatment of nonseminomatous testicular cancers. Vinblastine is also used in combination with cisplatin in non–small cell lung cancer and with mitomycin in metastatic breast cancer.

Podophyllotoxins. Etoposide (VP-16, VePesid), a semisynthetic glucoside, is produced from extracts of the root of the mayapple or mandrake (*Podophyllum peltatum*). A closely related analogue, teniposide (VM-26) has not been approved in the United States by the Food and Drug Administration. The podophyllotoxins are CCS agents and block cells in the late S phase and early G_2 phase. Mechanistically, podophyllotoxins are thought to act as inhibitors of nuclear topoisomerase II, leading to DNA strand breaks. Additional effects include inhibition of nucleoside transport and mitochondrial electron transport. Etoposide is highly lipid soluble and water insoluble and requires a special formulation for intravenous administration. An oral formulation is also available. There is extensive protein binding of the drug, and good tissue distribution is achieved in all sites other than the brain. In one commonly used schedule, etoposide is administered intravenously for 3 days at a dose level of 150 to 200 mg per square meter per day. Etoposide is excreted primarily in the urine and to a lesser extent in the bile. Its dosage should be reduced by 50 per cent in patients with impaired renal function (serum creatinine greater than 2 mg per deciliter). The main side effect of etoposide is myelosuppression, although some gastrointestinal toxicity and alopecia are also associated with its use. Etoposide is used primarily in the treatment of metastatic testicular cancer in combination with cisplatin and bleomycin. In this combination etoposide is substituted for vinblastine, yielding a less toxic but equally effective regimen. Etoposide is also a potent agent in the treatment of small cell lung cancer, lymphomas, and monocytic leukemia.

Taxol. Taxol is a promising investigational anticancer agent derived from the bark of the western yew tree (*Taxus brevifolia*) but is not yet approved by the Food and Drug Administration and must be obtained through the National Cancer Institute. Taxol stabilizes cellular microtubules, thereby preventing cell division. It is water insoluble and is formulated for intravenous administration. The major toxicities are myelosuppressive and gastrointestinal. Taxol has confirmed activity in the treatment of refractory ovarian cancer and some activity against other tumor types as well. Because of the extremely low content of taxol in bark, efforts are now underway to develop a semisynthetic derivative.

ANTIBIOTICS. Doxorubicin and Daunorubicin. These two red anthracycline antibiotics were isolated from a variant of *Streptomyces peucetius* and are extremely useful in cancer chemotherapy. Daunorubicin (daunomycin) was the first agent in this class and is active in the treatment of acute leukemia. Its congener, doxorubicin (Adriamycin) has a broader spectrum of antitumor activity, including both hematologic malignancies and a variety of solid tumors such as carcinoma of the breast and thyroid, lymphoma, and myeloma, as well as osteogenic and soft tissue sarcomas. Daunorubicin is frequently used in combination with cytarabine in the treatment of acute leukemia, whereas doxorubicin is incorporated into regimens for solid tumors along with cyclophosphamide, fluorouracil, etoposide, vincristine, or cisplatin. Mechanistically, the anthracyclines intercalate with high affinity into DNA and inhibit the action of topoisomerase II, resulting in DNA strand breaks. Anthracycline cytotoxicity may also be related in part to the generation of free radicals. This appears to result from the chelation of divalent cations including Fe^{2+} and production of superoxide and other oxygen radicals. Both doxorubicin and daunorubicin must be administered intravenously by either bolus injection or prolonged infusion. Extravasation of anthracyclines can lead to severe tissue injury. Topical application of 1.5 ml of 99 per cent dimethylsulfoxide (DMSO)* has been reported to prevent the development of ulceration. For prolonged anthracycline infusions, use of a vascular access catheter is advisable to avoid drug extravasation. When ulceration and necrosis occur after an anthracycline extravasation, surgical debridement of the damaged tissues followed by skin grafting is usually required.

The most common acute toxicities of the anthracyclines include alopecia, nausea, vomiting, mucositis, and myelosuppression. A dose-dependent cardiomyopathy with reduced cardiac contractil-

---

* While commercially available, DMSO has not been approved for use by the United States Food and Drug Administration.

ity can develop as a delayed toxicity in patients who receive large cumulative doses of doxorubicin or daunorubicin. The cardiomyopathy can be serious and irreversible and is usually manifest as congestive heart failure. Acute cardiac arrhythmias are uncommon. The cardiac toxicity of anthracyclines is considered to result from the heart's lack of enzymes such as glutathione peroxidase which serve as free-radical scavengers. While various drugs have been tried in efforts to block free radical generation or to serve as free radical scavengers in the heart, there are currently no approved agents to block the development of anthracycline-induced cardiomyopathy. Several anthracycline analogues considered to have lesser cardiotoxicity have been evaluated clinically but have not yet shown sufficient advantage to be approved for licensure in the United States.

Monitoring for cardiac effects of anthracyclines is conducted serially by determining the left ventricular ejection fraction using radionuclide techniques. Endomyocardial biopsy can also be used. Periodic monitoring is normally initiated when a patient has received a total doxorubicin dose of 350 to 400 mg per square meter. Significant cardiac toxicity is uncommon with cumulative bolus doses of doxorubicin of less than 550 mg per square meter, above which the incidence rises progressively. Elderly patients and others with risk factors for cardiac disease (e.g., hypertension) are at somewhat higher risk for anthracycline cardiomyopathy. Use of anthracyclines is not recommended for patients who have major pre-existing heart disease. When doxorubicin is administered by continuous infusion (e.g., for 4 to 5 days), a significantly larger cumulative dose in the range of 1000 mg per square meter can usually be administered. However, regular monitoring of the ejection fraction is required, and doxorubicin should be discontinued if the left ventricular ejection fraction falls below 50 per cent.

Bleomycin. Bleomycin (Blenoxane) comprises 11 closely related glycopeptide moieties produced by *Streptomyces verticillus*. The major components are bleomycins A2 and B2. The mechanism of bleomycin action involves its binding to DNA and generation of superoxide and other reactive oxygen species, including hydroxyl radicals. These reactive species induce both single- and double-

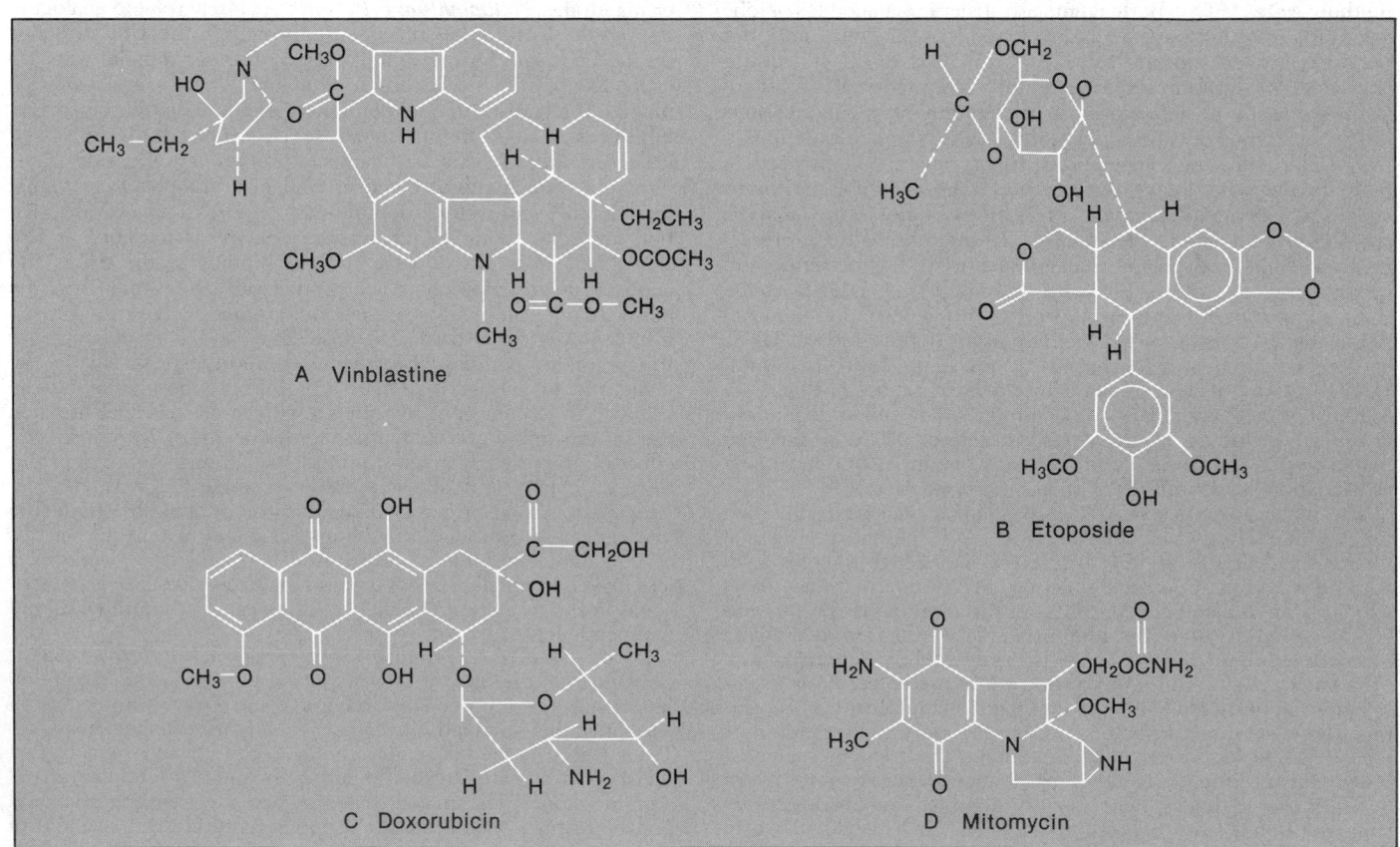

FIGURE 164–6. Natural product anticancer drugs. Commonly used plant alkaloids include (*A*) vinblastine (and its congener, vincristine) and (*B*) etoposide. Widely used antibiotics include (*C*) doxorubicin (and its congener, daunorubicin) and (*D*) mitomycin.

strand breaks. DNA fragmentation appears to result from the oxidation of a DNA-bleomycin-Fe^{2+} complex. Bleomycin's anti-tumor activity is schedule-dependent, and it is a CCS agent. It can be administered by subcutaneous, intramuscular, and intravenous routes. Bleomycin is synergistic with vinblastine or etoposide and with cisplatin, and its major uses are in carcinoma of the testis as well as squamous cell carcinomas of the head and neck, cervix, skin, penis, and rectum. It is also used in combination regimens for treatment of lymphomas.

One advantage of bleomycin is that it has minimal myelosuppressive effects and is useful in combination with drugs that cause leukopenia. Acute toxicities of bleomycin include anaphylactoid reactions and fever associated with hypotension and dehydration. Patients who have not previously been treated with bleomycin should receive a test dose (e.g., 1 to 2 mg) to see that they are not subject to this reaction. Individual therapeutic doses of bleomycin are usually in the range of 15 mg per square meter.

The most serious chronic reaction to bleomycin is pulmonary fibrosis related to the cumulative dose of drug and manifested by cough, dyspnea, and bilateral basilar infiltrates on chest radiography. It is possible to screen for earlier pulmonary abnormalities such as a decline in the diffusion capacity, which is usually detectable at total doses of bleomycin above 250 units. It is wise to discontinue use of bleomycin when the pulmonary diffusion capacity falls significantly. The incidence of pulmonary fibrosis rises at total doses above 450 units and is higher in patients with pre-existing pulmonary disease, after lung irradiation, and in the elderly. Unfortunately, there are no effective agents to reverse this toxicity and it is steroid insensitive. Other reactions to bleomycin include skin toxicity with blistering, desquamation, and hyperkeratosis of the palms and hyperpigmentation of skin creases.

Mitomycin. Mitomycin (Mutamycin, Mitocin-C, Mitomycin C) is isolated from *Streptomyces caespitosus*. The structure of this agent includes quinone, carbamate, and aziridine groups, which may play roles in its antitumor activity. Mitomycin functions as a CCNS alkylating agent after it has been activated in various tissues by the cytochrome P-450 system. Thereafter it can alkylate DNA to form intrastrand and interstrand crosslinks resulting in cell death. Mitomycin has "bioreductive" properties, with increased cytotoxic effects on poorly oxygenated tumor cells present in solid tumors. Mitomycin's clinical spectrum of antitumor activity includes breast, lung, gastrointestinal, genitourinary, and gynecologic cancers. Mitomycin has been incorporated into a variety of cytotoxic drug combinations for systemic administration, often in second-line therapy for patients who relapse from initial chemotherapy. It is usually administered intravenously, but it can be used for intravesical therapy of superficial bladder cancer. When used in combinations by the intravenous route, its normal dosage range is 10 to 15 mg per square meter.

The major toxicity of systemically administered mitomycin is myelosuppression, which is usually delayed until 4 to 6 weeks after injection. Mitomycin has a cumulative effect on bone marrow stem cells, which can lead to protracted marrow hypoplasia for 3 to 6 months after the drug has been discontinued. Nausea and vomiting and anorexia often occur at the time of drug administration but can usually be managed effectively with antiemetic agents. Occasionally, mitomycin can induce other serious reactions such as interstitial pneumonitis, nephrotoxicity, or hemolytic-uremic syndrome.

Actinomycin D. Actinomycin D (dactinomycin, Cosmegen) is the first effective antitumor antibiotic isolated from *Streptomyces*. It binds to the DNA helix by intercalation between adjacent guanine-cytosine base pairs and inhibits DNA-dependent RNA synthesis. It can also cause single-strand breaks. Actinomycin D has its greatest effect on ribosomal RNA synthesis, and this leads to cessation of most protein synthesis in sensitive cells. The drug is administered intravenously, and its major toxicity is myelosuppression, which is usually manifest in 7 to 10 days after injection. However, actinomycin D also causes significant gastrointestinal toxicity with abdominal cramps and diarrhea as well as mucositis. Actinomycin D commonly causes a radiation "recall" reaction wherein cutaneous erythema redevelops at a site of prior irradiation. The main clinical uses of actinomycin D are in pediatric oncology in combination chemotherapy for the treatment of Wilms' tumor, Ewing's sarcoma, and embryonal rhabdomyosarcoma. It also has some utility in adults in third-line therapy of germ cell tumors of the testis or ovary, gestational choriocarcinoma, and soft tissue sarcomas.

Miscellaneous Agents

PROCARBAZINE. Procarbazine (Matulane) is an orally administered methylhydrazine derivative that has antitumor activity in Hodgkin's disease (as part of "MOPP" combination chemotherapy) and some use also in non-Hodgkin's lymphomas, lung cancer, and brain tumors. Procarbazine is usually given in a dose of 100 mg per square meter per day for 10 to 14 days in each chemotherapy cycle. Procarbazine is activated metabolically to provide a methyldiazonium ion that binds to nucleic acids and proteins as well as phospholipids and inhibits macromolecular synthesis. Its mechanism of cytotoxicity is thought to involve DNA strand scission, possibly via generation of H_2O_2. Procarbazine's principal toxicities are nausea, vomiting, and myelosuppression. One of procarbazine's metabolites is a monoamine oxidase (MAO) inhibitor that can cause toxicity when the patient is taking other MAO inhibitors. Patients taking procarbazine are potentially subject to hypertension if they ingest tyramine-rich foods such as ripe cheese, wine, and bananas. Disulfiram-like reactions are also seen, with sweating and headache after alcohol ingestion. Other infrequent reactions include hemolytic anemia and pulmonary reactions. Procarbazine is also known to be leukemogenic, carcinogenic, and mutagenic and is considered to play a significant role in the late leukemias and other second malignancies in patients with Hodgkin's disease. Procarbazine also produces azospermia and anovulation. As alternative combinations lacking procarbazine can be used in the treatment of Hodgkin's disease, the benefits versus risks of using this agent must be carefully considered.

DACARBAZINE. Dacarbazine (DTIC, dimethylimidazole carboxamide) is activated by oxidative *N*-demethylation. A methyl carbonium ion metabolite is thought to be the cytotoxic intermediate with alkylating activity. Dacarbazine is administered intravenously either in a single-day infusion schedule of 750 mg per square meter or in fractionated bolus doses over 5 days or more. DTIC causes severe nausea and vomiting, and potent antiemetic agents are required. Myelosuppression is relatively mild. Dacarbazine is used in combination chemotherapy for Hodgkin's disease ("ABVD"), for soft tissue sarcomas in combination with doxorubicin and other agents, and in single-agent chemotherapy for metastatic melanoma.

HEXAMETHYLMELAMINE (HMM). This investigational agent is available only in an oral formulation because of its sparing solubility. However, oral bioavailability of HMM is quite variable, and it produces nausea and vomiting as its dose-limiting toxicity. The severity of gastrointestinal toxicity increases with daily use, limiting the length of treatment courses (at doses of up to 12 mg per kilogram per day) to 2 to 3 weeks. Myelosuppression occurs, but it is mild. Additionally, hexamethylmelamine can induce both central and peripheral neurotoxicities, including altered mood, hallucinations, and peripheral neuropathy. HMM is thought to act as an alkylating agent, possibly via the enzymatic hydroxylation of its demethyl metabolites to cytotoxic methylol compounds. HMM exhibits antitumor activity in alkylating agent–resistant ovarian cancer and to a lesser extent in several other neoplasms (lung, breast cancer, lymphomas) but has not yet been approved for use in the United States by the Food and Drug Administration.

HYDROXYUREA (HYDREA, HU). Hydroxyurea acts as an inhibitor of ribonucleotide reductase, resulting in intracellular depletion of deoxynucleoside triphosphates and inhibition of DNA synthesis. It is available for clinical use in oral formulation. HU's major toxicity is to the bone marrow, and it causes transient dose-related myelosuppression. At high dosage, a megaloblastic anemia can develop which is nonresponsive to vitamin B_{12} or folic acid. Gastrointestinal side effects of nausea and vomiting are also common with high-dose therapy. HU is used as a secondary agent for palliative treatment of chronic myeloid leukemia, but it also has some use in head and neck cancer and metastatic melanoma.

MITOXANTRONE (NOVANTRONE). Mitoxantrone is an anthracenedione with a structure that appears analogous to that of the anthracyclines. It has been approved by the Food and Drug Administration as a second-line agent for treatment of acute leukemia in relapse but is also useful in the treatment of breast cancer and lymphoma. Mitoxantrone binds to DNA and causes strand breaks as well as inhibits DNA and RNA synthesis. In terms of cellular response by tumor cells, there is not complete cross-reactivity between mitoxantrone and the anthracyclines. Mitoxantrone dosage for acute leukemia is significantly higher than for solid tumors. Comparative studies in patients with advanced breast cancer suggest that it is slightly less active and less toxic than doxorubicin. Its major acute toxicity is myelosuppression. Gastrointestinal side effects, including nausea, vomiting, and mucositis as well as alopecia, are less severe than with the anthracyclines. Mitoxantrone can cause some cardiac toxicities, usually manifest by development of arrhythmia at the time of injection, and can exacerbate pre-existing anthracycline-induced cardiomyopathy. It can be used intraperitoneally in patients with ovarian cancer, as most of the drug remains in the peritoneal cavity. This reduces systemic toxicity, although it can induce chemical peritonitis with subsequent adhesions.

ASPARAGINASE (CRASNITIN, ELSPAR). L-Asparaginase is a bacterial enzyme that is isolated from *Escherichia coli* or *Erwinia carotovora*. Its major use is in the treatment of lymphoblastic leukemias and some lymphomas with a deficiency in asparagine synthetase and cellular dependence on exogenous asparagine. L-Asparagine is a nonessential amino acid, and most normal cells can synthesize their required asparagine. Therapeutically, L-asparaginase acts by depleting the plasma of asparagine by catalyzing its degradation to aspartic acid and ammonia. Blood glutamine levels are also reduced. Most patients develop fever and chills as well as nausea and vomiting after asparaginase administration, but these symptoms can usually be reduced or prevented by premedication with antiemetics and anti-inflammatory agents. Toxicities of asparaginase occur in the liver and result in abnormal liver function test results (SGOT, alkaline phosphatase, and bilirubin) as well as in hypoalbuminemia, and reductions in plasma levels of clotting factors and insulin. Other occasional toxicities include pancreatitis and central nervous system abnormalities, which can include confusion or coma. Repeated use of asparaginase leads to the development of antibodies to the bacterial enzyme that can inhibit its activity and accelerate its clearance as well as induce hypersensitivity reactions. Patients developing hypersensitivity after asparaginase administration may exhibit hypotension, laryngeal edema, bronchospasm, and urticaria. Switching to an asparaginase derived from a different bacterial species can bypass neutralizing antibodies that have developed in hypersensitive patients. The lack of myelosuppressive or gastrointestinal toxicity has facilitated incorporation of L-asparaginase into drug combinations for the treatment of acute lymphocytic leukemia.

Management of Toxicity

Most cytotoxic drugs have significant toxicities on host cells. Nonetheless, there are methods to reduce the toxicity for a variety of antitumor agents. Because of the steep dose-response curve of cytotoxic agents, it is desirable to administer them at the maximally tolerated doses.

DOSE ADJUSTMENTS FOR BONE MARROW TOXICITY. It is often necessary to make downward adjustments of myelosuppressive agents in order to avoid serious or life-threatening side effects such as granulocytopenic fever and thrombocytopenic bleeding. For most drugs, empiric schedules have been developed for drug administration with single agents or combinations of myelosuppressive drugs normally given every 3 to 4 weeks. The interval between treatments provides time for hematopoietic recovery of normal myeloid progenitors in the bone marrow and avoids cumulative myelosuppression. It is essential to check the patient's CBC, differential, and platelet count immediately prior to each course of myelosuppressive chemotherapy. During the first few cycles of chemotherapy, and at intervals thereafter, it is useful to check counts between treatment courses, particularly in order to determine the nadir of absolute granulocyte count (AGC). Nadir AGC's are determined by multiplying the total WBC by the percentage of granulocytes plus band forms. If the

patient's AGC falls below 1000 per microliter, there is an increased risk of infection; AGC's below 500 are often associated with life-threatening infection. As hematopoietic recovery can occur rapidly after the nadir, the AGC immediately prior to the next course can be normal even though the nadir count may have been very low. For some drug combinations with low but brief AGC nadirs, prophylactic anti-infective agents (e.g., sulfamethoxazole-trimethoprim) are prescribed to bracket the AGC nadir to protect against infection secondary to neutropenia. In general, if the AGC immediately prior to the next course of chemotherapy is less than 2000 per microliter, the dose of myelosuppressive drugs should be reduced by 50 per cent. With an AGC of less than 1500 per microliter, the dosages should be reduced by 75 per cent. If the AGC is less than 1000, the dose of drug should be withheld until hematologic recovery has occurred. An additional approach to problems of myelosuppression involves the use of bone marrow growth factors as discussed below under "Biological Agents."

DOSE ADJUSTMENTS FOR IMPAIRED HEPATIC OR RENAL FUNCTION. The effects of altered hepatic or renal function on the clearance rates for anticancer drugs are not always predictable. Nonetheless, it is important to make downward dosage adjustments for specific drugs when altered hepatic or renal function plays a major role. The metabolism of doxorubicin depends upon good hepatobiliary function. Patients with a serum bilirubin of greater than 3.0 mg per deciliter should have their doxorubicin dose reduced by at least 50 per cent until drug tolerance is established.

Cisplatin, methotrexate, etoposide, hydroxyurea, and bleomycin are all cleared predominantly by renal excretion. In general, doses of these agents should be decreased in proportion to the decline in renal function as determined by creatinine clearance and reflected by the serum creatinine. These guidelines are at best approximate. It is very important to renormalize dosages if toxicity is not observed with myelosuppressive agents.

Endocrine Agents

Cancer cells often exhibit susceptibility to hormonal control mechanisms that regulate growth of the normal organ or tissue from which the neoplasm arose. Endocrine therapy appears generally to work through cytostatic rather than cytotoxic mechanisms and in most instances requires long-term suppression. Endocrine therapy includes the use of both hormones and "antihormones," which are either antagonists or partial agonists for a given endocrine mechanism. Inasmuch as the effects of hormones are receptor mediated, evaluation of receptors capable of binding hormones has played an important role in assessing both tumor types and individual patients for susceptibility to endocrine therapy. Dose schedules and applications of some major endocrine agents are summarized in Table 164–7.

STEROID HORMONES AND ANTIHORMONES. Cancers arising from endocrine organs and from the immune system show significant susceptibility to the effects of steroid hormones and steroid hormone antagonists and of hormone deprivation. The sex steroids and their antagonists represent major agents for the treatment of common cancers arising from the breast, prostate gland, and uterus. The role of endocrine ablation procedures (hypophysectomy, adrenalectomy, oophorectomy, orchiectomy) has diminished as systemic agents have been identified which can replace surgical procedures. Nonetheless, oophorectomy and orchiectomy are still useful in the treatment of endocrine-sensitive cancers of the breast and prostate, respectively.

Estrogens and Antiestrogens. Pharmacologic doses of estrogen have therapeutic effects in cancers of the prostate and the breast. Estrogen therapy remains a mainstay in the treatment of metastatic prostate cancer. Orchiectomy is an excellent alternative to estrogen therapy for prostate cancer, as it does not have feminizing side effects. Orchiectomy and estrogen therapy for prostate cancer are equally efficacious. There is no evidence to suggest an additive effect of the two.

For breast cancer, the use of the antiestrogen tamoxifen (Nolvadex) has largely replaced high-dose estrogen therapy because it is better tolerated. Tamoxifen improves survival of postmenopausal women with estrogen and/or progesterone receptor–positive breast cancer in both the adjuvant and metastatic settings. Some recent studies also suggest that tamoxifen may be a useful adjuvant drug for hormone receptor–negative cancers in postmenopausal women, but this finding is still controversial. In general, cytotoxic chemotherapy rather than endocrine therapy is recommended for women with hormone-receptor–negative breast cancer. Tamoxifen is available only in 10 mg tablets for oral administration, with a manufacturer's recommended dose of 10 mg twice daily. There is not a good scientific rationale for this schedule, because with chronic therapy, tamoxifen and its active metabolite dihydroxytamoxifen achieve a steady state with a large deep tissue reservoir. Accordingly, use of a single dose of 20 mg should be an acceptable alternative schedule with fewer problems with compliance. Serious or life-threatening toxicities of tamoxifen (thromboembolic disease, retinitis) are rare. Common side effects include hot flashes and weight gain, sometimes due to fluid retention. Mild nausea also occurs occasionally. In premenopausal women with hormone receptor–positive neoplasms and overt metastatic disease, both oophorectomy and antiestrogen therapy can be useful. However, in the adjuvant setting, the use of cytotoxic chemotherapy remains indicated irrespective of hormone receptor status, as it appears to have curative potential. The role of ovarian ablation or antiestrogen therapy added to chemotherapy in the adjuvant setting remains to be defined. Occasional palliative benefits have been reported for the use of tamoxifen in other neoplasms such as ovarian or endometrial cancer.

Androgens and Antiandrogens. Androgen therapy is contraindicated in prostate cancer because it is a growth stimulant. Virilizing androgens such as testosterone propionate, fluoxymesterone (Halotestin), and testosterone enanthate (Delatestryl) have all been used in the treatment of metastatic breast cancer with definite beneficial effects in hormone receptor–positive disease. However, androgen therapy has largely been replaced with antiestrogen therapy because the antiestrogen does not cause hirsutism, deepening of the voice, or changes in libido. Additionally, the oral halogenated androgens (e.g., fluoxymesterone) also can cause cholestatic jaundice. The antiandrogen flutamide (Eulexin) is a useful agent in the treatment of prostate cancer in combination with one of the gonadotropin-releasing hormone agonists (Lupron, Zoladex), and these combinations function as a "medical orchiectomy."

Progestins. Progestins are useful in palliative management of patients with metastatic breast or endometrial cancer and can cause tumor regression in patients with endocrine-sensitive disease. There is no evidence to suggest their utility in the adjuvant setting in either of these neoplasms. Occasional patients with prostate cancer also appear to benefit from progestational therapy. The most commonly used progestins include megestrol acetate (Megace), medroxyprogesterone (Provera), and hydroxyprogesterone caproate (Delalutin). Megestrol acetate is a useful oral progestin for second-line endocrine therapy for patients with metastatic breast cancer who show initial responsiveness to tamoxifen. In patients who experience disturbing side effects from tamoxifen (e.g., severe hot flashes), megestrol acetate may represent a reasonable alternative. In addition to its antitumor effects, megestrol acetate improves appetite in some patients with cancer-induced cachexia.

Glucocorticoids. Adrenal steroid hormones of the glucocorticoid class (e.g., prednisone, methylprednisolone, dexamethasone) are very useful anticancer agents in the treatment of lymphoid malignancies and may also potentiate the effects of cytotoxic agents in these tumor types as well as in breast cancer and perhaps other neoplasms. The glucocorticoids also play an important role in the treatment of complications of cancer (hypercalcemia, cerebral edema). Glucocorticoids are lympholytic and

TABLE 164–7. HORMONALLY ACTIVE AGENTS IN CANCER TREATMENT

Representative Agents	Dose (oral unless specified)	Toxicity A = Acute D = Delayed	Uses
Glucocorticoids			
Prednisone	20–100 mg/day or 50 mg qod (single dose)	A: Fluid retention, hyperglycemia, euphoria, depression, hypokalemia	Leukemia Lymphoma Myeloma Breast cancer Brain metastases
Dexamethasone	4–16 mg/day or 40 mg/day for 4-day pulses every 2–4 weeks	D: Osteoporosis, immunosuppression, gastrointestinal ulcers, cushingoid appearance, cataracts	
Estrogen			
Diethylstilbestrol	5 mg tid (breast) 1–3 mg qd (prostate)	A: Nausea, vomiting, fluid retention, hypercalcemia (flare reaction with bone metastases), uterine bleeding D: Feminization, accelerated coronary artery disease	Breast cancer Prostate cancer
Antiestrogen			
Tamoxifen	20 mg qd	A: Occasional nausea, fluid retention, hot flashes D: Retinal degeneration	Breast cancer
Aromatase Inhibitor			
Aminoglutethimide (plus hydrocortisone 20 mg bid)	250 mg bid (breast) 250 mg qid (prostate)	A: Dizziness D: Rash (transient)	Breast cancer Prostate cancer
Progestins			
Megestrol acetate Hydroxyprogesterone	40 mg qid 1 gm IM biw	A: Increased appetite (Megestrol), fluid retention D: Weight gain, thromboembolism	Breast cancer Endometrial cancer Renal cancer
Androgens			
Fluoxymesterone Testosterone	10–20 mg qd 600 mg IM q 4–6 wks	A: Cholestatic jaundice (with oral drug) D: Virilization	Breast cancer
Antiandrogen			
Flutamide	250 mg tid	D: Gynecomastia	Prostate cancer
Gonadotropin-releasing hormone agonists (depot formulations)			
Leuprolide acetate Goserelin acetate	7.5 mg SQ monthly 3.6 mg SQ monthly	A: Transient flare of symptoms	Prostate cancer Breast cancer (?)

nonmyelosuppressive and have therefore been incorporated into combination chemotherapy for acute and chronic lymphocytic leukemia, malignant lymphoma, and multiple myeloma.

AROMATASE INHIBITORS. Aminoglutethimide (Cytodren) inhibits the first step in adrenal steroid synthesis. Additionally, and probably more importantly, aminoglutethimide also inhibits the extra-adrenal conversion of the adrenal androgen androstenedione to estrone by the enzyme aromatase. Aromatase is found in body fat and some other tissues and provides an explanation for the presence of the weak estrogen estrone in the plasma of postmenopausal women. Aminoglutethimide is a useful agent in the palliative treatment of recurrent breast cancer in hormone receptor–positive patients. It is used in combination with hydrocortisone both to suppress endogenous steroid hormone synthesis (including androstenedione) as well as ACTH production and to slow the catabolism of aminoglutethimide. Aminoglutethimide is commonly administered in a dose of 250 mg twice daily along with 20 mg of hydrocortisone. Somewhat higher doses of aminoglutethimide have been employed for second-line endocrine therapy for metastatic prostate cancer. Patients receiving aminoglutethimide and hydrocortisone should be cautioned to avoid abrupt cessation of therapy to avoid symptoms of adrenal insufficiency.

GONADOTROPIN-RELEASING HORMONE (GnRH, LHRH) AGONISTS. Several synthetic analogues of natural GnRH (LHRH) are now clinically available. Both leuprolide acetate (Lupron) and goserelin acetate (Zoladex) are available in long-acting parenteral-depot formulations. These analogues are more potent than natural GnRH and function as GnRH agonists but also have an unusual effect on the pituitary, consisting of initial stimulation followed by long-term inhibition of the release of FSH and LH. This initial increase in gonadotropins can cause a transient increase in symptoms in patients with bone metastases. The inhibition of release of the gonadotropin reduces testicular androgen synthesis in males and ovarian estrogen production in women. The effects on testicular androgen production led to use of a GnRH agonist as an alternative to surgical orchiectomy in patients with prostate cancer. In comparative trials, GnRH agonists are as effective as estrogen therapy, and the two show comparable suppression of androgen synthesis and prostatic acid phosphatase. However, gynecomastia, nausea, vomiting, edema, and thromboembolic disease are not significant problems with the GnRH agonists. The effectiveness of GNRH agonists is enhanced by administration in combination with an antiandrogen (flutamide), and the combination has been reported to be more effective than a GnRH agonist alone in patients with Duke's D_2 metastatic prostate cancer. However, impotence results from this form of "medical orchiectomy," so it does not differ in that regard from surgical orchiectomy except that the effects of medical therapy are potentially reversible if treatment is discontinued. Medical orchiectomy is more expensive but acceptable to patients who decline surgical orchiectomy. GnRH agonists now show promise in combination with antiestrogens as endocrine therapy for premenopausal women with hormone receptor–positive breast cancer. The GnRH agonists are abortifacients in animals and should not be given to women who are or may become pregnant.

BIOLOGIC THERAPY

A major new form of cancer therapy, still early in its evolution, is the use of recombinant cytokines, growth factors, and monoclonal antibodies for the treatment of cancer. It is already clear that a number of biologic agents are directly useful as anticancer agents and that others play a supportive role. Thus, biologic therapy can now be considered the fourth major modality in cancer therapy. The term "biologic therapy" was developed to describe this heterogeneous group of agents that either are normal mammalian mediators or achieve antitumor effects through endogenous host defense mechanisms. Thus, the underlying concept is that the various biologic agents stimulate or participate in host immune defense mechanisms for the elimination of foreign molecules or cells, including transformed cells in neoplastic disease.

The biologic agents have also been termed "biologic response modifiers" (BRM's). Both the cellular and humoral limbs of

immunity can be exploited in cancer therapy. The cellular defenses include several classes of cytotoxic lymphocytes (natural killer [NK] cells), lymphokine-activated killer (LAK) cells, tumor infiltrating lymphoma (TIL), and cytotoxic T-lymphocytes (CTL), as well as antibody-dependent cytotoxic cells (ADCC). Additionally, the nonspecific cells of the reticuloendothelial system including activated macrophages may be important. Humoral agents with antitumor activities include cytokines such as interferons and interleukins as well as specific antibodies. Most of these humoral agents interact with specific immune effector cells in coordinated and synergistic fashion. The general availability of cytokines and growth factors has been facilitated by the development of recombinant DNA technology. Antibodies are highly specific and generally interact directly with their tumor targets when they are directed against cell surface constituents. Some humoral agents including the tumor necrosis factors α and β have potent local antitumor properties in preclinical models but have yet to be shown to be clinically useful.

Vaccines based on specific bacterial agents or extracts from bacteria can nonspecifically activate the host immune system. Using BCG, this approach has been applied successfully to intravesical therapy of in situ cancer of the urinary bladder. Specific cancer-associated antigen vaccines have been under active investigation for many years but have yet to be proven effective in cancer treatment. Approaches to biologic therapy of cancer are summarized in Table 164–8 and are discussed below.

INTERFERONS. The interferons (IFN's) are a family of antiviral proteins that differ in their cellular origin and polypeptide structure as well as in their clinical applications. The three major molecular species are IFN-α, -β, and -γ. IFN-α and -β mediate their action by binding to the same cell surface receptor, whereas a second cell surface receptor mediates the action of IFN-γ. IFN-α is the major IFN species for use in the treatment of hematologic malignancies and solid tumors. At present it is unclear whether IFN-β or -γ will have sufficient advantage over IFN-α in any specific cancer indication to gain regulatory approval. IFN-γ enhances granulocyte microbicidal function and macrophage activity and has definite value in the treatment of chronic granulomatous disease of children. IFN-γ may also prove useful in other infectious or inflammatory disorders as well.

Interferon-α. Recombinant IFN-α (IFN-α_2, Intron-A, Roferon) is a polypeptide cytokine with antiviral properties which is also useful for single-agent treatment of selected hematologic malignancies and solid tumors. The precise mechanism of antitumor action of IFN is still poorly understood, but it is known to activate the transcription of a number of cellular genes. IFN-inducible genes include those encoding for 2',5'-oligoadenylate synthetases, RNase, and RNA-activated initiation factor 2 kinase, as well as for cellular proteins such as class I and II MHC antigens, β_2-microglobulin, metallothionein IIA, and Fc receptors. Additionally, IFN action inhibits the synthesis of a number of proteins in

TABLE 164–8. BIOLOGIC THERAPY OF CANCER: APPROACHES AND AGENTS

Approach	Agents
Active immunotherapy	
Nonspecific	Adjuvants: BCG, levamisole
	Cytokines: Interferons
	Interleukin-2
	Interleukin-4
	Tumor necrosis factors
Specific	Tumor cell vaccines
Passive serotherapy	
Antibodies	Polyclonal or monoclonal antibodies (alone or conjugated with drugs, radionuclides, or toxins)
Adoptive cellular therapy	Lymphokine-activated killer cells
	Tumor-infiltrating lymphocytes
Immunomodulators	Levamisole, thymic hormones
Bone marrow growth factors (see Table 164–10)	GCSF, GMCSF, MCSF, IL-3, EPO
Growth factor antagonists	Suramin
	Antibodies to growth factor receptors (e.g., EGF, HER-2/neu, IL-2 receptors)

sensitive tumor target cells including ornithine decarboxylase, a rate-limiting enzyme in polyamine metabolism. Although IFN-α also has antiviral and immunoregulatory properties that alter the biologic function of many cell types involved in humoral and cellular immunity, it is unclear whether these additional functions have any bearing on its antitumor properties above and beyond its direct receptor-mediated effects on sensitive tumor cells. The antitumor properties of IFN-α also appear to be schedule-dependent with a cytostatic mode of action. Most remissions induced by IFN are only partial.

IFN-α can be administered parenterally by intravenous, intramuscular, subcutaneous, and intracavitary routes. Its preferred route of systemic use is by subcutaneous administration, which provides the longest duration of action. The dosage schedules of IFN-α are quite variable, and higher dosages may be required for some tumor types than for others. The tumor type most sensitive to IFN-α is hairy cell leukemia (HCL). Usual dosages are in the range of 3 million IU administered subcutaneously three times weekly. At these low dosage levels, IFN usually causes only mild side effects such as fever and chills with the first few doses. On the other hand, for Kaposi's sarcoma, far more aggressive and toxic IFN schedules are required and can cause significant anorexia, weight loss, failure in concentration, and profound weakness. High-dose IFN can also induce occasional cardiac arrhythmias, nausea, vomiting, leukopenia, myalgias, proteinuria, and hepatic dysfunction ("transaminitis"). Dosages thus have been derived in relation to their effects on specific forms of cancer and individualized to patient tolerance. Optimal biologic and antitumor effects appear to be more related to tumor type and perhaps biologic response modification than to dose alone. At all dosage schedules examined, elderly patients appear to develop more marked side effects. Some of the major current uses and dosage levels for IFN-α are summarized in Table 164–9.

IFN-α is also useful in the treatment of chronic myeloid leukemia, multiple myeloma, and some of the low-grade non-Hodgkin's lymphomas, and in some patients with metastatic melanoma or renal cell carcinoma. In myeloma, IFN-α appears to play a valuable role in maintaining remissions induced by chemotherapy. Patients receiving recombinant IFN-α for HCL, CML, or renal cancer have developed neutralizing antibodies to the recombinant product at the time of disease progression after an IFN-induced remission. A limited number of patients with neutralizing antibodies have been successfully retreated by switching to nonrecombinant IFN-α. IFN-α has recently been incorporated into combination therapy with various cytotoxic and endocrine agents. At present, use of IFN-α in combination with 5-FU is being explored in the treatment of metastatic colorectal cancer based on encouraging preliminary reports with an active but toxic regimen. Although the clinical indications for IFN therapy continue to grow gradually, it clearly does not have the type of broad-spectrum anticancer effects that were initially envisioned.

INTERLEUKIN-2 (IL-2, PROLEUKIN). IL-2 is an immunomodulatory cytokine that acts on T-cell progenitors to produce LAK cells that have cytotoxic effects in specific forms of cancer. Recombinant IL-2 has not yet been approved for therapeutic use by the United States Food and Drug Administration, although its use in renal cancer has been approved in some European countries. IL-2 has been used by direct intravenous infusion to induce LAK cells in the patient, or additionally after leukopheresis of the patient to obtain circulating lymphocytes that can then be exposed to IL-2 in vitro for activation of lymphoid progenitors in tissue culture to form LAK cells. During the several days of culture in vitro there is marked cellular proliferation of activated LAK cells. The LAK cells are then reinfused into the patient over several days along with additional dosages of IL-2 as a form of "adoptive immunotherapy." After the initial reports of very high response rates to IL-2/LAK by investigators at the National Cancer Institute, a number of other investigators have explored the use of IL-2 alone or of IL-2 plus LAK cells. There is general agreement that either IL-2 or IL-2/LAK can induce tumor regression in 10 to 20 per cent of patients with renal carcinoma, melanoma, lymphoma, or other neoplasms.

Whereas the infusion of LAK cells causes relatively few side effects, IL-2 induces considerable toxicity. Patients receiving high-dose IL-2 must be in an intensive care unit with very close management of blood pressure, fluids, and electrolytes. The high-dose regimens are suitable only for younger patients without other significant disease or impairment of cardiac, pulmonary, hepatic, or renal function. Common side effects of high-dose LAK/IL-2 are probably due to lymphoid infiltrates in major organs and a capillary leak syndrome induced by IL-2. Shortly after initiation of high-dose IL-2 therapy, tachycardia develops, and a significant drop in arterial blood pressure occurs. As IL-2 administration continues, compensatory fluid retention occurs, and the patient develops significant weight gain as well as oliguria and azotemia. Vasopressors are often needed. However, weight gain and hepatic and renal dysfunction remain quite common with the high-dose IL-2 regimens. Even at lower doses that can be used in a conventional hospital or outpatient setting (e.g., 3 million IU per square meter daily by intravenous infusion for 2 weeks), hypotension and fluid retention are not uncommon.

Pulmonary metastases appear to be somewhat more sensitive to IL-2 or IL-2/LAK therapy than are other tumors. With the adoptive immunotherapy approach using IL-2/LAK, a small percentage of patients treated at the National Cancer Institute who had undergone prior removal of the primary tumor achieved complete remission with all evidence of metastatic disease disappearing for prolonged periods of time. Some controversy nonetheless remains as to whether the use of high-dose IL-2/LAK has any advantage over administration of IL-2 alone at a lower and better-tolerated dosage level.

The National Cancer Institute group has moved on from IL-2/LAK to the collection of another subset of T-lymphoid cells called tumor-infiltrating lymphocytes (TIL). These are obtained by extracting lymphocytes from tumor biopsies from the patient and activating them in vitro with IL-2. Subsequently they are reinfused along with IL-2. In the initial clinical studies, activated TIL cells appear to have greater antitumor activity (e.g., in melanoma) than LAK cells, with 50 per cent of patients responding to TIL/IL2 therapy. The findings with IL-2, IL-2/LAK, and IL-2/TIL provide the first clear indication that endogenous cells in the immune system are capable of being activated to manifest anticancer properties. Thus, the findings to date are perhaps less important as a specific treatment than as an indication that this approach to biologic therapy with cytokines may serve as the basis for even more effective immunologic approaches to treatment of cancer.

LEVAMISOLE (ERGAMISOLE). Levamisole is an anthelmintic agent that was found to have immunopotentiating properties.

TABLE 164–9. SOME CURRENT USES OF INTERFERON-α IN CLINICAL ONCOLOGY

Tumor Type	Dose (mU)	Response Rate (%)
Hairy cell leukemia	3/day or 3 times weekly	75–90
Chronic myeloid leukemia	5/m²/day	50–80
Multiple myeloma	3/m²/day or 3 times weekly	20–30*
Cutaneous T-cell lymphoma	10/day or 3 times weekly	45
Follicular (B-cell) lymphoma	5/day or 3 times weekly	30–50*
Kaposi's sarcoma	10/m²/day or 3 times weekly	30
Metastatic melanoma	5–10/m² 3 times weekly	10–20
Renal cell carcinoma	5–10/m² 3 times weekly	10–30
Carcinoid syndrome	5/m² 3 times weekly	20–30†

*Also being used for remission maintenance therapy.
†Reduction in symptomatology and 5-HIAA excretion.

Administration of levamisole to patients with Hodgkin's disease has been reported to enhance various tests of cell-mediated immunity but has not been shown to have a beneficial therapeutic effect in those patients. However, when combined with 5-FU, levamisole has recently been reported to play a significant role in adjuvant chemotherapy of patients with Duke's C colon cancer. With use of the combination after surgery the recurrence rate is one third less than with surgery alone. The mechanism of potentiation of 5-FU effectiveness remains obscure. In patients with overt metastatic colon cancer, the combination of 5-FU and levamisole does not appear to be any more useful than 5-FU alone.

ANTITUMOR ANTIBODY THERAPY. The use of antibodies as therapeutic agents for cancer has been a longstanding dream, as antibodies have the ability to home to tumor-associated antigens and to bind to tumor cells and lyse them either directly via complement fixation or through cooperative mechanisms also involving cellular immunity (e.g., ADCC). The selective binding of antibodies to tumor cells has led to their use as carriers for highly potent therapeutic agents. In addition, diagnostic uses have included radionuclide conjugates for tumor imaging. Within the past decade, considerable effort has been expended to evaluate polyclonal and monoclonal antibodies from different mammalian species as potential therapeutic agents for patients with cancer. Antibody therapy has incorporated both unconjugated and radionuclide-, drug-, and toxin-conjugated antibodies. A number of problems have beset the development of antibody therapy, the first of which has been to identify antigens that are expressed uniquely on malignant cells and either not at all or to a far lesser extent on normal host cells. At the present time, antibody-based therapy for cancer remains investigational and has not been approved by the Food and Drug Administration.

Antibody therapy has shown some encouraging results in malignant B-cell lymphoma (both Hodgkin's disease and non-Hodgkin's lymphomas as well as chronic lymphocytic leukemia) and perhaps in hepatocellular carcinoma. Objective tumor regressions have been observed after administration of unconjugated, radionuclide-conjugated, and toxin-conjugated antibodies directed at lymphoma cells. One of the most impressive pilot observations used murine anti-idiotypic antibodies to the cell surface Ig on neoplastic B cells, and at least one prolonged complete remission was achieved using this technique. However, development of anti-idiotypic antibodies has required preparing a specific antibody for each individual patient. More recently, increasing efforts in lymphoma have been focused on employing antibodies that recognize "shared idiotypes" or other lymphoid-associated antigens as targets for antibodies that can be developed through more conventional methods. For other tumor types, results with antibody-based therapy have been disappointing.

The logistics of heterologous murine antibody therapy remain difficult. For most tumor types studied in patients there is a relatively "narrow window" of 1 to 2 weeks of therapy before the recipient develops a vigorous human antimurine antibody (HAMA) response that renders further antibody administration difficult owing to rapid inactivation and clearance of the administered antibody. Attempts to block this HAMA reaction with immunosuppressive agents have thus far been unsuccessful. Perhaps in part because of associated defects in immunologic responsiveness, patients with monoclonal B-lymphoid neoplasms can sometimes be treated for a longer time before the HAMA response becomes significant. In efforts to minimize the HAMA reaction, molecular biologic techniques are now being used to either "chimerize" or "humanize" the murine antibodies so that the constant regions of their murine structural components are replaced with human immunoglobulin sequences. Another specialized application of antitumor antibodies has been for the purging ex vivo of tumor cells from the bone marrow to be reinfused into patients who are to receive high-dose chemotherapy and autologous bone marrow rescue. This application has been used with success in lymphoma, neuroblastoma, and some other tumor types.

GROWTH FACTOR ANTAGONISTS. The use of antagonists to polypeptide growth factors is in a sense an extension of endocrine therapy but represents a form of biologic therapy as well. One growth factor antagonist that has recently been rec-

ognized to have anticancer properties is suramin, which has been used since the 1920's for the treatment of African sleeping sickness. Suramin is a polysulfonated naphthylurea that binds tightly to heparin-binding growth factors such as fibroblast growth factor (FGF), platelet-derived growth factor (PDGF), and insulin-like growth factor (IGF-1). Exclusion of growth factors from their receptors can result in "programmed cell death." Suramin is active in the treatment of prostate cancer, presumably by blocking the action of FGF and other growth factors. However, suramin also inhibits the function of a variety of enzymes and other proteins, so its precise mechanism of antitumor action remains to be defined. The multiple actions of suramin also account for a broad range of toxicities, which can be severe or irreversible. One of these is adrenal insufficiency, which requires long-term adrenal steroid replacement. Frequent plasma monitoring of suramin concentrations is essential, because there is the potential for serious neuropathy when suramin concentrations exceed 300 μg per milliliter. The use of suramin in cancer therapy is currently investigational. Suramin represents the first member of a new class of investigational agents that are active as BRM's for cancer therapy. Another approach to growth factor receptor blockade involves use of monoclonal antibodies to epidermal growth factor (EGF) receptor and to the IL-2 receptor.

BONE MARROW GROWTH FACTORS. A new approach to supportive care for bone marrow failure associated with cancer and for maintaining adequate hematopoietic function between courses of myelosuppressive chemotherapy is to administer bone marrow growth factors to stimulate an increased rate of production of myeloid progenitors. The bone marrow growth factors are glycoproteins that function in overlapping and hierarchical fashion on bone marrow progenitors and not only result in cell proliferation but also activate differentiation and cell trafficking. The factors currently in clinical trials in cancer patients are summarized in Table 164–10. The major factors also potently stimulate the proliferation of myeloid precursors. Several of these recombinant proteins, including granulocyte colony–stimulating factor (GCSF), granulocyte-macrophage colony–stimulating factor (GMCSF), and erythropoietin (Epogen, EPO) (see Table 164–6), are now entering general use for cancer treatment. Both IL-3 and macrophage colony–stimulating factor are at an earlier stage of development and their role in supportive care is currently uncertain. GCSF and GMCSF are approaching approval by the Food and Drug Administration. EPO was recently approved for the anemia associated with renal failure. Clinical trials using subcutaneously administered GCSF or GMCSF have shown that use of either can shorten the duration of granulocytopenia, the frequency of infectious complications, and the duration of hospitalization after chemotherapy combinations that are normally given on an inpatient setting. With bone marrow transplantation (wherein high-dose chemotherapy and/or total body radiation is employed) both myelosuppressive and nonmyelosuppressive side effects can be diminished with the use of GCSF or GMCSF. Although IL-3 (multi-CSF) is only in early clinical trial, preliminary evidence suggests that this bone marrow growth factor can stimulate platelet and red blood cell as well as granulocyte production.

In preclinical studies, IL-3 also appears to act synergistically with GMCSF to produce more complete and rapid recovery of circulating granulocytes and platelets than can be obtained with either factor alone. The major toxicities of the growth factors that

TABLE 164–10. RECOMBINANT BONE MARROW GROWTH FACTORS OF POTENTIAL IMPORTANCE IN SUPPORTIVE CARE OF CANCER PATIENTS

Growth Factor*	Effects
GCSF	Stimulates granulocyte production
GMCSF	Stimulates granulocyte, macrophage, and eosinophil production
MCSF	Stimulates macrophage production and activation
IL-3	Stimulates granulocyte, macrophage, and platelet production
EPO	Stimulates production of RBC's

*GCSF = granulocyte colony–stimulating factor; GMCSF = granulocyte-macrophage colony–stimulating factor; MCSF = macrophage colony–stimulating factor; IL-3 = interleukin-3; EPO = erythropoietin.

stimulate white cell production include fever, myalgias, and occasional skin rashes. Pericarditis has been reported with high-dose GMCSF or GCSF. Recombinant erythropoietin is already in general clinical use for the anemia of renal failure. Preliminary studies also suggest that when used in pharmacologic doses, EPO can restore normal red blood cell counts in some patients with multiple myeloma and perhaps in some other hematologic malignancies as well. EPO also has promise for reducing the degree of anemia induced by cytotoxic chemotherapy.

SUMMARY

Medical management of cancer is a complex task that requires extensive knowledge and clinical experience. The requisite knowledge includes not only the pharmacology and toxicology of and indications for cytotoxic, endocrine, and biologic agents but also an appreciation of the important roles of surgery and radiation therapy. Increasingly, the medical specialist plays a role in the patient's primary treatment, and the major modalities must be combined effectively for success. The steep dose-response curves for cytotoxic drugs leave little margin for error, and effective doses are very close to toxic levels. The practitioner who reduces drug doses a priori in an attempt to reduce toxicities that occur with standard protocols markedly reduces the likelihood that treatment will be successful. It is particularly important that standard protocol dosage regimens be used in initial therapy for patients with tumor types listed in sections A and B of Table 164–4, as they have the most to lose if they receive reduced and ineffective dosage regimens. Physicians are encouraged to have their patients participate in formal clinical trials of cancer therapy that are conducted at major cancer centers or through the clinical trials cooperative groups. Current therapy for many forms of cancer is in need of improvement, and this goal requires active participation by oncologic specialists and patients in large-scale clinical research.

Chabner BA, Collins JM: Cancer Chemotherapy: Principles and Practice. Philadelphia, J.P. Lippincott Company, 1990. *An excellent reference on cancer chemotherapy, including detailed discussion of the pharmacology of anticancer drugs.*

DeVita VT, Hellman S, Rosenberg SA: Cancer: Principles and Practice of Oncology, 3rd ed. Philadelphia, J.B. Lippincott Company, 1989. *A comprehensive textbook covering clinical, diagnostic, and therapeutic approaches for all major forms of cancer. Major modalities of treatment as well as drug combination schedules are delineated in detail in relation to relevant tumor types.*

Salmon SE (ed.): Adjuvant Therapy of Cancer 6. Philadelphia, W.B. Saunders Company, 1990. *An up-to-date summary of results of the most recent clinical trials of adjuvant and neoadjuvant chemotherapy for most forms of cancer.*

165 Oncologic Emergencies

Stephen M. Hahn and Angelo Russo

The care of patients with cancer is an exercise in the management of chronic disease. However, when acute oncologic emergencies occur, rapid evaluation and institution of therapy are required. Since several cancer types are now routinely cured and there is a general increase in the quality of life and survival time in patients with cancer, the early recognition and treatment of oncologic emergencies have a definite role in medical management.

FEVER AND NEUTROPENIA

The most common emergency encountered in clinical oncology is fever (temperature greater than 38°C or 100.5°F) and neutropenia (absolute neutrophil count less than 1000 per cubic millimeter). Neutropenic cancer patients have an increased risk of systemic infection and rapid development of the septic syndrome. Empiric emergency antibiotic therapy is crucial.

Infection risk increases once the neutrophil count drops below 1000 per cubic millimeter. Disruption of the patient's other host defenses also predisposes to infection. Paramount among these is disruption of the gastrointestinal barrier with mucositis. Additional factors include the presence of indwelling catheters, invasive procedures, and abnormal cellular and humoral immunity.

The patient usually presents with few signs or symptoms other than fever. Localized infection may be present but not clinically apparent. A careful history and physical examination must be performed focusing on common sites of infection. The oral cavity should be inspected for evidence of mucositis. Lesions suggestive of anaerobic, viral (especially herpes simplex), and fungal (especially *Candida* species) infection may be present. Odynophagia strongly suggests esophagitis. Examination of soft tissue and skin, especially at catheter sites, may show early cellulitis or septic phlebitis. A perirectal abscess should be sought by careful palpation of the anorectal area for induration, fluctuance, or tenderness.

Cultures should be performed on all patients prior to the initiation of antibiotic therapy and routinely sent for isolation of bacteria and fungi. Blood cultures should be obtained both from the port of an indwelling central catheter and from peripheral veins. If an indwelling catheter is suspected to be the source of infection, it should be removed and the tip sent for Gram's stain and culture. Sputum examination by Gram's stain and culture is usually not helpful but should be obtained if sputum is produced. Gram's stain and bacterial, fungal, and viral cultures should be performed on all oral, skin, and soft tissue lesions. Biopsies of cutaneous lesions may be especially helpful in the diagnosis of systemic viral and fungal infections and can be safely performed in the neutropenic patient. Chest radiography, urinalysis with microscopy, and evaluation of ascites and pleural fluid should be performed. Although meningitis is not typically encountered in febrile neutropenic cancer patients, a lumbar puncture is indicated in those patients with suggestive clinical signs or symptoms.

Indwelling urinary tract catheters and unnecessary intravenous catheters are to be avoided. Strict handwashing by all hospital personnel is required. Aggressive prophylactic or therapeutic mouth care (suggested regimen: Nystatin suspension, benadryl/antacid/lidocaine mixture, and 5 per cent sodium bicarbonate solution, alternating each every 2 hours, administered as swish and spit) provides relief of symptoms and may improve the patient's course.

Once evaluated and hospitalized, the patient should be started without delay on broad-spectrum antibiotics that include coverage for *Pseudomonas* species and other gram-negative organisms. Based upon the isolate patterns at an individual institution, coverage for gram-positive organisms may be necessary. Suggested regimens are (1) a third-generation cephalosporin (ceftazidime, 1 gram every 4 hours intravenously) or (2) a semisynthetic penicillin (piperacillin or mezlocillin, 3 to 4 grams every 4 hours intravenously) plus an aminoglycoside (gentamicin or tobramycin, 2 mg per kilogram loading dose followed by one to three divided doses daily depending upon renal function). If a specific organism is suspected, appropriate antibiotics should be added to the initial regimen. For example, if infection of an indwelling catheter is likely, additional gram-positive coverage with vancomycin (500 mg every 6 hours intravenously) should be added for *Staphylococcus aureus* and *Staphylococcus epidermidis*. Anaerobic coverage with clindamycin (250 to 750 mg intravenously every 6 hours) is strongly recommended for patients with mucositis or periodontal infections.

If fever persists after the initiation of antibiotics, cultures and diagnostic studies should again be performed daily and broader gram-positive coverage should be added to the patient's regimen. Patients with prolonged neutropenia on broad-spectrum antibiotics are at high risk for fungal infection. Early institution of antifungal therapy may be life saving. If the patient remains febrile after 5 to 7 days, empiric antifungal therapy with amphotericin B should be started (0.5 to 1.0 mg per kilogram per day intravenously). In general, if the neutropenic patient remains febrile despite broad-spectrum therapy, one should consider the following diagnostic possibilities: a second bacterial isolate, abscess, anaerobic infection, gram-positive bacteria, atypical organisms, fungi, and viruses.

Approximately 50 per cent of patients with fever and neutropenia have a documented infection. If a causative organism or a specific infection is discovered, specific therapy should be initiated; however, broad-spectrum antibiotics should not be discontinued, since there is a 40 per cent chance of developing infection with a second isolate when antibiotic therapy is narrowed.

Patients with documented infections should be treated until the infection resolves (usually a 2-week course of antibiotic therapy). Antibiotics may be discontinued when the absolute neutrophil count exceeds 1000 per cubic millimeter if the patient is afebrile and no specific infection has been documented. Antibiotics should be continued in the patient who remains neutropenic even if he or she becomes afebrile. Clinical deterioration or the return of fever occurs in a significant proportion of these patients.

At one time, white cell transfusions were thought to be indicated in the patient with gram-negative infection and prolonged neutropenia. However, it is unclear whether this benefits the patient, and the risk of morbidity or mortality (infectious diseases, alloimmunization, and pulmonary toxicity) is significant. Therefore, white cell transfusions are not recommended as routine care of the febrile neutropenic patient. Prophylaxis with absorbable or nonabsorbable antibiotics is controversial and not routinely recommended. Prophylactic antibiotic regimens may actually prolong cytopenias or lead to the development of infection with resistant organisms. *Clostridium difficile* infection and vitamin K deficiency may occur in the setting of broad-spectrum antibiotic use.

SPINAL CORD COMPRESSION

Back or neck pain is a frequent complaint in the general population; in a cancer patient it can be a harbinger of neurologic disaster and merits immediate, careful evaluation. The pain is worsened by straining, sneezing, coughing, movement, and recumbency. Complaints may precede diagnosis by days to months; however, once neurologic signs are present, progression is usually rapid. Typically, back pain progresses to radicular pain followed by weakness, sensory loss, paralysis, and/or loss of sphincter control (manifested as urinary or fecal retention or incontinence). Early recognition is important, as ambulatory ability and maintenance of sphincter control at initiation of therapy are highly correlated with successful outcome. Less than 15 per cent of patients with paraplegia or loss of sphincter tone regain function. The site frequency of spinal cord involvement corresponds to the volume and number of vertebral bodies (thoracic>lumbar>cervical>sacral). Although any malignancy can metastasize to and encroach upon the epidural space, tumors of lung or breast, lymphoma, carcinoma of unknown primary, myeloma, sarcoma, carcinoma of the prostate or kidney, melanoma, and gastrointestinal and thyroid carcinomas are commonly associated with spinal cord compression.

Evaluation and treatment tempo are determined by physical examination (Fig. 165–1). The patient with signs of spinal compression deserves immediate treatment with dexamethasone (10 mg intravenously followed by 4 mg every 6 hours) and emergency evaluation. Patients with no neurologic findings may be expeditiously evaluated as outpatients. In two thirds of patients with spinal cord compression, plain film radiographs of the spine show erosion or loss of pedicles, partial or complete collapse of vertebral bodies, or paraspinous mass. Metrizamide myelography is the diagnostic gold standard. The test is quickly performed and more easily tolerated than magnetic resonance imaging (MRI). If after a lumbar injection, a myelographic block is identified, a C1-C2 puncture should be performed to visualize fully the extent of the block, as well as to define other rostral lesions (15 per cent). A computed tomography (CT) scan focused on the spinal block is often useful to further delineate the lesion. MRI is particularly helpful in delineating intramedullary, extramedullary, intradural, and extradural lesions. Encroachment (myeloma, lymphoma) on the cord through spinal foramina is particularly well demonstrated by MRI. Likewise, MRI avoids the risk (14 per cent) of neurologic deterioration with myelography in a patient having complete obstruction.

Although treatment should be individualized, radiation therapy is the treatment of choice in patients having radioresponsive tumors who have slowly evolving neurologic symptoms, incomplete block, cauda equina involvement, or widely metastatic disease. For the most part, treatment is considered palliative. Treatment is initiated with high-dose fractions, followed by lower-dose fractions. Steroids can be reduced judiciously as radiation therapy proceeds. The role of surgery in spinal cord compression

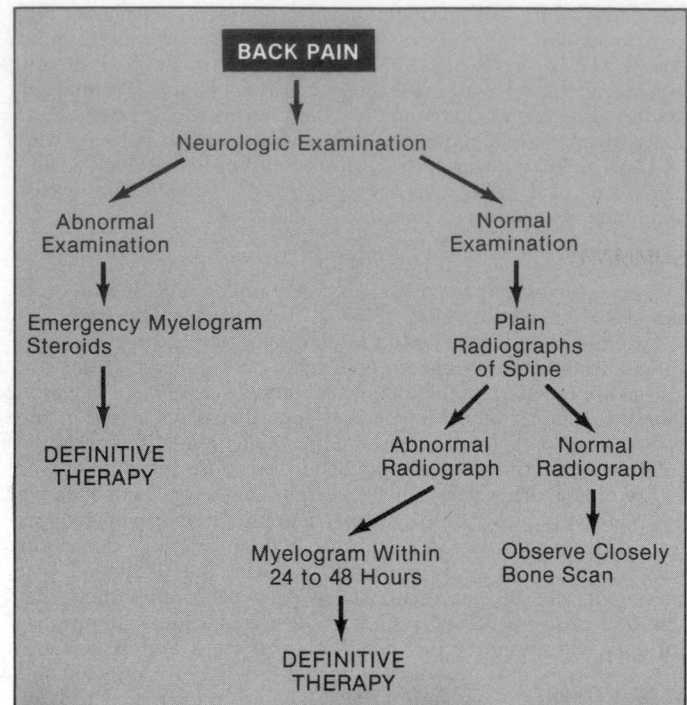

FIGURE 165–1. Flow diagram for evaluation of spinal cord compression in the cancer patient.

is evolving. Its use is recommended if a tissue diagnosis is needed, if neurologic dysfunction progresses during radiation treatment, if there is recurrent spinal cord compression in an area of previous radiation therapy, if there is spinal instability resulting from vertebral body collapse or bony protrusion into the spinal cord, or if the malignancy is considered radiation resistant (such as hypernephroma or melanoma). Simple laminectomy is not usually effective. The surgical procedure is dictated by tumor location and surgical experience and expertise. Radiation therapy should be used postoperatively. Chemotherapy for chemosensitive malignancies is used in addition to radiation or surgery.

INTRACRANIAL METASTASES

In the cancer patient, complaints of headache, altered mental status, and seizures may signal intracranial metastases. These processes are amenable to treatment and, if left untreated, could result in death. The differential diagnosis of altered mental status, seizures, and headache in a cancer patient includes iatrogenic causes (chemotherapy agents, narcotic analgesics, hypnotics, and antiemetics), metabolic disorders (hypercalcemia, hyponatremia, hypoglycemia, hypomagnesemia, hyperviscosity, hepatic encephalopathy), paraneoplastic syndromes (subacute cerebral degeneration, dementia, limbic encephalitis, optic neuritis, angioendotheliosis, progressive multifocal leukoencephalopathy), strokes (coagulation abnormalities, thrombocytopenia, Trousseau's syndrome), sepsis, and intracranial metastasis. Careful history and physical examination and laboratory evaluation are primary and should guide decision as to further workup. In the acutely ill cancer patient cranial CT should be done to define the presence and characteristics of the intracerebral lesion. MRI is more sensitive in defining metastatic lesions and differentiating between vascular and malignant lesions and should be considered if there is need to clarify CT scan findings. MRI requires more acquisition time, is highly sensitive to motion artifact, and is restricted to patients not requiring respiratory or cardiac monitoring and support. If no mass lesion is demonstrable, leptomeningeal carcinomatosis as the etiology of neurologic signs and symptoms is sought by examination of spinal fluid.

If there are signs of impending intracerebral herniation the patient should immediately have an endotracheal tube placed and be hyperventilated to maintain the P_{CO_2} between 25 and 30 mm Hg. Mannitol, up to 1.5 grams per kilogram, should be administered immediately and may be repeated every 6 hours. If there are signs of increased intracranial pressure without impending herniation, high-dose intravenous dexamethasone (10 mg every 6 hours) should be administered immediately to lessen cerebral edema. Status epilepticus requires immediate-acting drugs such as benzodiazepines and close attention to respiratory status. Seizures other than status epilepticus caused by intracranial metastasis are managed by phenytoin in an oral loading dose of 15 mg per kilogram followed by 300 mg per day. Drug levels should be monitored, since accompanying dexamethasone therapy can induce increased metabolism of phenytoin.

Radiation therapy for intracranial metastasis is usually palliative. A total dose of 30 Gy delivered over 10 to 15 fractions decreases motor deficits in approximately 33 per cent of patients and reduces or stops headaches in 50 per cent of patients. For patients with controlled or no evidence of systemic disease and a radioresponsive solitary intracranial metastasis in a site not amenable to surgery, radiation at higher doses (60 Gy) to the site of disease is justified to prolong survival. A surgically accessible solitary lesion in a patient with controlled systemic disease merits consideration of surgical removal of the tumor.

SUPERIOR VENA CAVA SYNDROME

Superior vena cava (SVC) syndrome is caused by either partial or complete obstruction of the superior vena cava. Obstruction results from extrinsic compression (90 per cent) or, less likely, fibrosis, thrombosis, or invasion. Both signs and symptoms can be subtle and evolve slowly (over 2 to 5 weeks). A spectrum of signs can be associated with the SVC syndrome, including cyanosis, edema, venous engorgement of the head, neck, arms, chest, and upper abdomen, varying degrees of airway obstruction, pleural and pericardial effusions, and tracheal edema. Nonpitting edema of the neck (Stokes' collar) can also be found. Symptoms, which frequently worsen when the patient lies down or leans forward, may include fullness or stuffiness in the ears or nose, eye disturbances, facial swelling, shortness of breath, cough, chest pain, voice changes (hoarseness), dysphagia, headache, stupor, seizures, and syncope. Back pain may herald simultaneous spinal cord compression by contiguously extending tumor. Upper extremity venography complements either CT scan or MRI with contrast in defining the obstruction.

In the past, malignancy-associated SVC syndrome was considered an oncologic emergency that merited immediate radiation treatment to avoid death from respiratory arrest or intracranial hemorrhage. Immediate therapy is indicated for impending airway obstruction (stridor) or increased intracranial pressure (stupor, seizure), particularly in a thrombocytopenic patient. Given the array of benign causes of SVC syndrome and the frequency of chemosensitive malignancies (small cell lung cancer and lymphomas), the etiology of SVC syndrome should be determined while judiciously managing the patient with diuretics and elevation of the head. Sputum cytology, bone marrow and lymph node biopsy, thoracentesis, bronchoscopy, and thoracotomy may confirm the etiology. The difference between a clotted and/or engorged vein with elevated pressures and a lymph node should be appreciated.

Once a neoplastic cause of SVC syndrome has been established, appropriate treatment should be initiated. In the majority of cases, radiation therapy remains the primary treatment with initial doses of 3 to 4 Gy per day followed by conventional doses of 1.5 to 2.0 Gy per day to a total dose of 30 to 50 Gy. The vast majority of patients (>85 per cent) experience relief within 3 weeks; however, symptoms usually recur. If small cell lung cancer, testicular cancer, or lymphoma is etiologic, appropriate chemotherapy should be administered through a lower extremity vein. Corticosteroids should be used for cerebral or laryngeal edema. The role of anticoagulants concurrent with radiation therapy remains undefined. As the use of indwelling, subclavian catheters for delivery of chemotherapy increases, the incidence of thrombosis as the etiology of SVC syndrome in cancer patients increases. Fibrinolytic therapy with urokinase (1000 U per square meter per hour during the first 24 hours; if no response, increase to 2000 U per square meter per hour for 48 hours) should be considered in those patients who have recently developed SVC syndrome and are not at high risk of dangerous bleeding. After successful fibrinolysis, heparin and subsequent coumadin therapy should be instituted to prevent recurrent SVC syndrome and to maintain the indwelling catheter.

CARDIAC TAMPONADE

Cardiac tamponade in a cancer patient may have a noncancerous etiology, may be the first manifestation of malignancy, or may signify disease progression. Diagnosis is necessary because tamponade is life threatening and successful treatment improves survival. Cardiac tamponade may result from primary tumors of the pericardium (mesothelioma, sarcoma, and teratoma) or more frequently from metastatic disease (carcinoma of the breast or lung, leukemia, lymphoma, melanoma, epidemic or nonepidemic Kaposi's sarcoma). When fluid pressure within the pericardial sac equals right atrial and ventricular diastolic pressure, cardiac tamponade occurs. As intrapericardial pressure increases, heart rate, myocardial contractility, and systemic resistance increase. If intrapericardial pressure increases rapidly, between 150 and 250 ml of fluid (normal volume <50 ml) may cause tamponade; however, if fluid accumulates slowly, more than 1 liter may be accommodated without decompensation. Symptoms are nonspecific and include shortness of breath, chest pain, cough, hoarseness, nausea, abdominal pain, hiccoughs, and distress. Signs associated with rapid effusion are a falling systolic pressure, elevated jugular venous pressure, a small, quiet heart (Beck's triad), and a narrowed arterial pulse pressure. If there has been chronic evolution of pericardial fluid, additional signs include percussion of an enlarged heart, most frequently on the left anteriorly but occasionally on the right in the fifth intercostal space (Rotch's sign), as well as a patch of dullness posteriorly below the angle of the left scapula (Ewart's sign) with bronchial breathing over this area. Pulsus paradoxicus is a classic but not constant sign of tamponade. The chest radiograph may show an enlarged globular (water bottle) heart and possibly pleural effusions. The pathognomonic finding on electrocardiogram of electrical alternans is rare; decreased voltage is frequently found. Two-dimensional echocardiography is the noninvasive, preferred diagnostic study and provides both anatomic and physiologic information. Right heart catheterization is the diagnostic gold standard and allows monitoring during therapeutic maneuvers (Fig. 165–2).

Pericardiocentesis provides immediate lifesaving treatment, allows fluid to be obtained for diagnosis, and, with insertion of a pigtail catheter, permits subsequent determination of the rate of fluid reaccumulation and instillation of drugs for treatment. Fluid can be serous, serosanguineous, or frankly hemorrhagic. In the case of hemorrhagic fluid, the absence of clot and a hematocrit lower than systemic levels weigh against the fluid resulting from

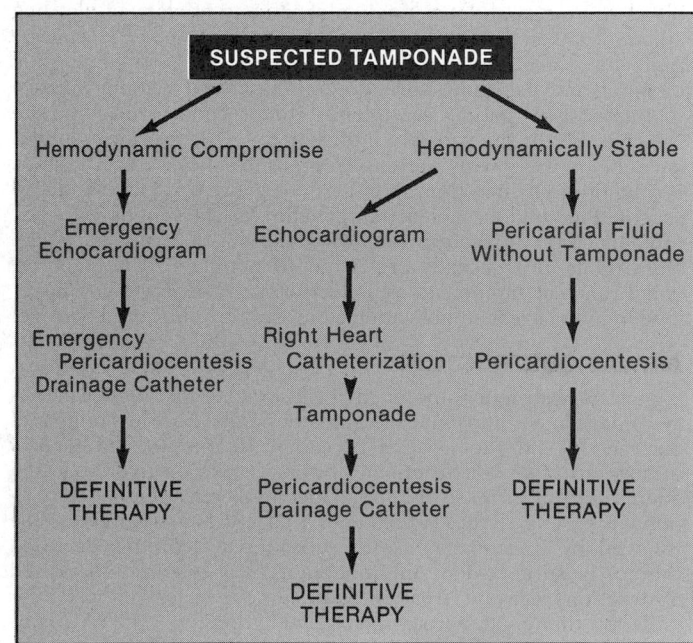

FIGURE 165–2. Flow diagram for evaluation of cardiac tamponade in the cancer patient.

puncture of the myocardium. Fluid should be sent for cultures and cytology. Once it has been established that the fluid is caused by a malignancy, there are three approaches to treatment: radiation, chemotherapy, and surgery. Radiation therapy up to 40 Gy is highly successful (approaching 100 per cent) in treating effusion caused by leukemias or lymphomas; however, unless all known disease can be encompassed within the radiation field, systemic chemotherapy is the treatment of choice for leukemic and lymphomatous pericardial effusions. Success rate for radiation control of melanoma, lung, and breast carcinoma is much lower. Surgical approaches to effusion include pericardiectomy, pleuro-pericardial window, and subxiphoid pericardiotomy. Pericardiectomy is the treatment of choice for radiation-induced constrictive pericarditis. Its use for malignant effusions is effective but carries more morbidity than either a window or subxiphoid pericardiotomy. A pleuropericardial window has a low complication rate (<5 per cent) and a relatively low recurrence rate. Subxiphoid pericardiotomy, unlike the window procedure, requires only local anesthesia and has virtually no complication or recurrence rate; however, there is an increased incidence of tumor cell dissemination. Drug instillation into the pericardial sac has been tried with various chemotherapeutic agents (thiotepa, methotrexate, nitrogen mustard), radioisotopes, and tetracycline. Tetracycline is highly effective in obliterating the pericardial space and eliminating fluid recurrence. However, there can be a period of transient fevers, arrhythmias, and chest pain. If tetracycline fails, surgical management is undertaken.

HEMOPTYSIS

The most common causes (tuberculosis, fungal infections, lung abscess, bronchiectasis, bronchial adenoma) of hemoptysis are not neoplastic; however, with increasing age, malignancies, especially of bronchogenic origin, are most common. Cancer patients who are immunocompromised and have underlying coagulation defects or thrombocytopenia and obstructing lung lesions are susceptible to infections that can cause hemoptysis. Greater than 600 ml of blood per 24 hours defines massive hemoptysis and is life threatening; however, because blood may be swallowed or aspirated, making volume determination difficult, hemoptysis associated with respiratory compromise should be considered an emergency.

Minor hemoptysis often presages massive hemoptysis; therefore, while the etiology of hemoptysis is pursued, observation, oxygen, and prevention of aspiration are prudent. The patient with massive hemoptysis is admitted to the intensive care unit. Correction of coagulopathy and thrombocytopenia, repletion of blood volume, and determination of site and etiology of bleeding are undertaken simultaneously. Bronchoscopy is the diagnostic procedure of choice for determination of site and etiology of bleeding and also allows direct therapeutic intervention. Surgical resection, if the patient can tolerate the procedure and if the site is localizable, is the procedure of choice. Other less ideal options have been used with varying degrees of success and include neodymium:yttrium-aluminum-garnet (Nd:YAG) laser-induced coagulation, endobronchial tamponade with a venous catheter, bronchial artery catheterization with embolization, and ice lavage. Nd:YAG laser is usually restricted to nonmassive hemoptysis; endobronchial tamponade should not be used for right upper lobe hemorrhages; embolization can result in spinal cord damage.

AIRWAY OBSTRUCTION

Airway obstruction by an intrinsic or extrinsic malignancy is an emergency, and management depends on the tempo of obstruction and the location, previous treatment, and type of tumor causing the obstruction. Steroids should be given to lessen edema and, in the case of lymphomas, begin treatment. Obstruction at or above the larynx and high tracheal region can be relieved by tracheostomy with subsequent definitive radiation therapy or surgery done in a nonemergency setting. More distal obstructions can be treated with surgery when indicated or radiation therapy (external and/or brachytherapy). Nd:YAG laser has found use in the care of high-grade, incomplete, centrally obstructing airway lesions. It is quick and safe and provides immediate relief. Restrictions to its use include lobar or segmental

level lesions, extraluminal compression, total obstruction, upper lobe lesions, and tracheoesophageal fistula. The Nd:YAG laser treatment results in incomplete removal of tumor, and therefore high dose-rate brachytherapy (interstitial endobronchial radiation therapy) combined with laser treatment may be most useful. The use of visible light lasers and fiberoptics with photosensitizers (photodynamic therapy [PDT]) has also been used extensively for relief of obstructed airway lesions. In this case, even a lesion totally obstructing the airway can be completely removed because cylindric light-emitting fibers are used. Furthermore, PDT can be repeated. Repeat bronchoscopy 2 to 3 days following endobronchial PDT should be performed to remove necrotic tissue and evaluate the status of treatment.

HYPERCALCEMIA

Other than hyperparathyroidism, cancer is the second most frequent cause of hypercalcemia. It occurs in approximately 10 per cent of all cancer patients. Lung, particularly squamous cell, and breast cancers account for 40 to 60 per cent of all cases. Other primary malignancies frequently associated with hypercalcemia include multiple myeloma (approximately 50 per cent develop hypercalcemia at some time during disease), carcinoma of unknown primary, lymphoma (adult T-cell lymphoma), and gastrointestinal (cholangiocarcinoma and hepatoma), renal, head and neck, and prostate carcinomas. The metabolic disorder frequently occurs with metastases to bone but may occur without bone metastases. Calcium homeostasis is usually regulated between 9 and 10.6 mg per deciliter, 45 per cent of which is ionized (nonprotein bound) (see Ch. 232). In multiple myeloma associated with high immunoglobulin levels, the total serum calcium level can be exceedingly high, yet the ionized fraction can be within the normal range.

Malignancy-associated hypercalcemia can be caused by tumor secretion of parathyroid-like hormone, which results in increased bone and renal tubular calcium reabsorption. Likewise, osteolytic metastases can act directly on bone to cause calcium resorption or can secrete factors that result in bone resorption (prostaglandins) or activation of osteoclasts (osteoclast-activating factor).

The clinical manifestations may be manifold and nonspecific and depend in part on the general metabolic condition and associated illness of the patient, as well as the degree and rapidity of calcium elevation. Symptoms include polyuria, nocturia, polydipsia, anorexia, nausea, vomiting, abdominal pain, fatigue, lethargy, confusion, psychosis, agitation, stupor, obtundation, and coma. Laboratory values usually show an elevated serum calcium, commonly above 12 mg per deciliter. Electrocardiography may show narrowed QT, widened T wave, and elongated PR interval.

For patients who are symptomatic or who have serum calcium levels above 13 mg per deciliter, treatment should be immediate and aggressive. Because of the reversible defects of renal tubular absorption and subsequent loss of fluid coupled with decreased fluid intake, the patient is invariably volume depleted. Volume repletion followed by normal saline at a rate of 200 to 300 ml per hour results in calciuresis. Once rehydration is accomplished, urinary output should be maintained at 200 to 300 ml per hour. Saline-induced calciuresis can be augmented by furosemide. Electrolytes, including magnesium and phosphate, should be checked frequently and, when necessary, repleted. Salmon calcitonin (4 IU per kilogram every 12 hours increased to 8 IU per kilogram every 8 hours) can lower the serum calcium by 2 to 3 mg per deciliter within a few hours. Unfortunately, natriuresis and calcitonin are only temporizing measures. Once the patient is initially stabilized, the optimal choice is treatment of the underlying malignancy. Steroids can be effective in reducing hypercalcemia in multiple myeloma, lymphoma, and breast cancer. For chronic management of hypercalcemia, intravenous mithramycin (10 to 25 μg per kilogram) may be given every 48 hours up to three doses. The response to mithramycin may last up to 3 weeks. After the initial course, mithramycin may be administered up to twice weekly to maintain normocalcemia. Mithramycin can cause hypotension, hepatic and renal dysfunction, and bone marrow suppression, especially thrombocytopenia. Etidronate disodium is a diphosphonate that blocks osteoclast bone resorption and is approved for use in the United States. Initial administration is intravenous, 7.5 mg per kilogram per day for 3 days, and then orally, 20 mg per kilogram per day. In the future severe hypercalcemia may be treated with diphosphonates like aminohydroxypropylidene diphosphonate (APD). A single infusion of APD (45 mg) for severe malignant hypercalcemia has resulted in a response rate of 96 per cent, with normocalcemia achieved in 75 per cent of cases.

TUMOR LYSIS SYNDROME

Tumor lysis syndrome is a metabolic emergency that can be anticipated and prevented. Rapid tumor lysis is usually encountered upon initiation of chemotherapy in the setting of rapidly proliferating malignancies such as high-grade lymphomas or acute leukemias. Rarely it has been reported to occur in solid tumors. The syndrome can occur within 48 hours after arterial embolization of large tumors within the liver. Tumor lysis syndrome causes rapid and severe metabolic changes, including hyperkalemia, hyperuricemia, hyperphosphatemia, and hypocalcemia. End-organ dysfunction may also ensue. Hyperuricemia or hyperphosphatemia can cause renal failure secondary to uric acid or calcium phosphate crystallization in the tubules. Hypocalcemia caused by precipitation of calcium phosphate and lowered calcitriol levels can result in neuromuscular irritability, tetany, and obtundation. Hyperkalemia can be profound and cause cardiac arrhythmias and sudden death.

Treatment begins with identification of the patient at risk and prevention of the metabolic and end-organ changes. If a patient is likely to develop rapid tumor lysis associated with chemotherapy, hospital admission and initiation of measures to circumvent the syndrome are necessary. Volume status, electrolytes, blood urea nitrogen, creatinine, uric acid, phosphorus, and calcium serum levels are obtained before beginning chemotherapy. If the patient presents with evidence of tumor lysis syndrome prior to chemotherapy, every effort should be made to correct the metabolic abnormalities before starting chemotherapy. However, it is not always possible to postpone chemotherapy, and in such a setting, hemodialysis may be necessary. Hyperkalemia must be treated aggressively with sodium polystyrene sulfonate (Kayexalate) or if electrocardiographic changes are noted, calcium chloride, insulin, dextrose, and sodium bicarbonate. The next treatment priority is to avoid uric acid precipitation in the renal tubules. This is done by alkalinizing the urine with 0.25N sodium chloride containing two ampules (100 mEq) of sodium bicarbonate and maintaining a urinary output between 100 and 200 ml per hour. Additional bicarbonate is titrated to maintain urine pH greater than 7.0. Acetazolamide (250 mg by mouth once or twice daily) may be administered in the first days to further hasten urine alkalinization. Allopurinol (500 mg per square meter on day one and 300 mg by mouth on subsequent days) decreases uric acid production by inhibiting xanthine oxidase. Loop diuretics (furosemide) may be necessary to maintain urine flow. It should be noted that calcium phosphate crystal formation theoretically can be increased by alkalinization of the urine. However, practical considerations dictate that excretion of uric acid is of primary importance, and high-volume urinary output, even when alkaline, dilutes calcium phosphate in the urine and lessens the danger of phosphate crystalluria. Hypocalcemia occasionally requires therapy with intravenous calcium. Rarely, calcitriol replacement is necessary to obviate persistent hypocalcemia caused by low calcitriol levels. Hemodialysis is initiated when volume status, urinary output, acid-base status, and electrolyte changes signal its necessity.

HEMORRHAGIC CYSTITIS

Patients who have or are receiving cyclophosphamide or ifosfamide may present with a life-threatening urologic emergency, hemorrhagic cystitis. The cystitis results from metabolites (chlorethylazeridine, chloroacetic acid, and acrolein) of either chemotherapy agent. Because the metabolites are excreted by the kidney, high concentrations can accumulate in the bladder. If there is bladder outlet obstruction, ureteral hemorrhage may occur. The bladder grossly appears hyperemic and edematous with areas of punctate hemorrhage; mucosal erosions and sloughing are common. The best management entails prevention by maintaining a high urinary output to decrease the concentration of metabolites in the bladder and by correcting any coagulation defect. Systemic use of sodium 2-mercaptoethanesulfonate (Mesna) prevents mucosal irritation by detoxifying the metabolites

within the bladder. Once hemorrhagic cystitis occurs, conservative management with care to ensure excellent urinary output is often adequate. Blood product replacement may be necessary. The use of urethral catheters to remove metabolites and rest the bladder is controversial because catheters can provoke spasm and may prevent passage of clots. If conservative management is not effective, the bladder may be irrigated by N-acetylcysteine. If that fails, irrigation with 0.37 to 0.74 per cent formalin solution for 10 minutes frequently (85 per cent) stops bleeding after one treatment. To avoid ureteral reflux of formalin, the formalin-containing irrigation bag should not be elevated more than 15 cm above the pubis. If formalin fails to control hemorrhage, diversion of hypogastric arteries with ureteral diversion and cystectomy may be necessary.

HEMATOLOGIC EMERGENCIES

Thrombocytopenia is a common finding in patients who are undergoing chemotherapy. When the platelet count is 20,000 per cubic millimeter or less, platelets should be administered prophylactically. If the platelet count is less than 50,000 per cubic millimeter, platelets should be transfused for active bleeding or before surgery or an invasive procedure. When the patient is symptomatic or has a hemoglobin of less than 8.0 grams per deciliter, red blood cells should also be administered, but platelet infusion should underpin treatment.

Disseminated intravascular coagulation (DIC) is a coagulopathic state in which there is prolongation of prothrombin, thrombin, and partial thromboplastin times, an increase in fibrinogen degradation products, and a decrease in platelets, fibrinogen, and clotting factors. DIC resulting in life-threatening hemorrhage should be anticipated in patients with acute promyelocytic leukemia, and anticoagulation with heparin should be started before antineoplastic treatment is begun. For DIC associated with other underlying malignancies (gastrointestinal, lung, breast, and prostate), the treatment of choice is cytoreduction of the underlying cancer by appropriate antineoplastic treatment. If treatment of DIC is necessary before the underlying malignancy responds, then heparin administration should be titrated to control DIC. Coagulation factors should be administered and fibrinogen levels should be maintained well above 100 mg per deciliter by infusion of cryoprecipitate (titrate cryoprecipitate to keep plasma fibrinogen above 100 mg per deciliter).

Leukostasis may result when the white blood cell count exceeds 100,000 per cubic millimeter. An oncologic emergency is not defined by the degree of leukocytosis but rather by the symptoms associated with elevated white blood count. The problem is most often seen in all phases of chronic myelogenous leukemia as well as acute myelogenous leukemia. The dysfunction results from the lack of deformability of white blood cell blasts, with subsequent plugging of small vessels. The leukostasis syndrome manifests primarily in the central nervous system (stupor, dizziness, visual problems, ataxia, coma, intracranial hemorrhage, and sudden death) and pulmonary circuit (pulmonary infiltrates, hypoxia progressing to pulmonary failure with a scenario similar to that of the adult respiratory distress syndrome). Because extreme leukocytosis results in hyperviscosity, diuresis with volume contraction should be avoided. The primary goal of treatment is reduction of white blood cell count by leukapheresis (decrease white blood count by 20 to 60 per cent over 3 to 4 hours), followed by immediate effective therapy of the underlying leukemia. Because of the potential of leukemic cell lysis, measures should be instituted to prevent tumor lysis syndrome.

Cohen LF, Balow JE, Magrath IT, et al.: Acute tumor lysis syndrome: A review of 37 patients with Burkitt's lymphoma. Am J Med 68:486, 1980. *Description of the metabolic sequelae and management of acute tumor lysis.*

Delaney TF, Oldfield EH: Spinal cord compression. *In* DeVita VT, Hellman JS, Rosenberg SA (eds.): Cancer: Principles and Practice of Oncology. Philadelphia, J. B. Lippincott, 1989, pp 1978–1986. *A broad review of diagnosis and radiotherapy, surgical, and chemotherapy management of spinal cord compression.*

Kaufman D, Rosen N, Young RC: Clinical consequences and management of antineoplastic agents (pp 265–304) and Medical emergencies in patients with solid tumors (pp 481–498). *In* Parrillo JE, Masur H (eds.): The Critically Ill Immunosuppressed Patient—Diagnosis and Management. Rockville, Maryland, Aspen Publishers, Inc., 1987. *Excellent and practical discussions regarding the general topic of oncologic emergencies.*

Nieto AF, Doty DB: Superior vena cava obstruction: Clinical syndrome, etiology, and treatment. Curr Probl Cancer 10:443–484, 1986. *Classic review of the topic of SVC syndrome.*

Pizzo PA, Robichaud KJ, Gill FA, et al.: Duration of empiric antibiotic therapy in granulocytopenic patients with cancer. Am J Med 67:194, 1979. *Prospective study with diagnostic and treatment algorithms.*

166 Approach to the Patient with Metastatic Cancer, Primary Site Unknown

Daniel C. Ihde

DEFINITION

For a malignant neoplastic disease first to manifest itself by the appearance of visceral or nodal metastases, without any clue to the location of the primary cancer on initial assessment, is not an uncommon occurrence. Patients presenting in this fashion are said to have metastatic cancer, primary site unknown (MCPSU). Other terms employed to denote this clinical entity include cancer (or carcinoma) of unknown primary site and metastases of unknown origin. This syndrome has been heterogeneously defined both clinically and, as discussed later, pathologically. There is no concensus regarding the extent of evaluation required before the conclusion is reached that the site of primary cancer cannot be readily ascertained, but most authorities agree that complete history and physical examination, blood count and chemistry screening panel, tests of urine and stool for occult blood, chest radiograph, and routine histologic evaluation of the diagnostic pathologic specimen should be performed.

ETIOLOGY

The syndrome of MCPSU by definition results from occult but metastatic primary cancer, the etiology of which varies markedly depending upon the organ of origin of the malignant process. Interestingly, in a minority of patients the underlying primary site is not apparent even at autopsy. In 302 patients with MCPSU who eventually had postmortem examination, the primary site of cancer was identified in 27 per cent during life and in an additional 57 per cent at autopsy, with a residual 16 per cent in whom even autopsy did not disclose the primary neoplasm. If autopsy is not performed, the fraction of patients in whom the origin of cancer is not discovered is as high as 70 to 80 per cent.

INCIDENCE

Since there is no standard definition of the MCPSU syndrome, its incidence can only be estimated. Various authorities suggest that 2 to 12 per cent of all cancer patients present in this fashion, with the higher estimates generally based on case series from tertiary care centers. Since the incidence of malignant neoplasms in the United States is approximately 1,000,000 persons per year, it is likely that the MCPSU syndrome is diagnosed in as many as 50,000 to 60,000 patients annually.

PATHOGENESIS AND PATHOLOGY

The primary pathogenesis of the MCPSU syndrome is the sequence of events which led to the formation and dissemination of the primary cancer. This of course differs greatly depending upon the causative primary neoplasm. Why the primary cancer is not discovered by routine diagnostic evaluation is a question of major interest. The most common explanation is that the tumor is simply too small to be detected by physical examination and imaging studies. Other possibilities include prior surgical excision of the primary, as can occasionally be established in malignant melanoma presenting as MCPSU; hemorrhagic infarction with resultant necrosis and scarring, as is thought to occur in some testicular choriocarcinomas; and spontaneous regression, perhaps mediated by immunologic mechanisms.

Since pathologic confirmation of malignant neoplasm must be obtained and a search for the primary cancer by routine evaluation must be unrewarding before a tentative diagnosis of MCPSU is made, further scrutiny of the pathologic specimen assumes critical importance in the subsequent approach to the patient. Discussion between clinician and pathologist should always occur and may reveal that available pathologic material is inadequate for a more specific diagnosis because of suboptimal amount or preparation. This is more often the case with pathologically undifferentiated neoplasms or when the diagnosis of malignancy rests solely on cytologic material obtained by fine-needle aspiration, which provides little information on tissue architecture and is often insufficient for the detailed immunohistochemical or electron microscopic studies that can help elucidate the primary site or type of malignancy. If the pathologist believes examination of more tissue could be beneficial, careful communication among pathologist, clinician, and surgeon is essential to ensure that repeat biopsy yields sufficient, properly processed material.

Once an adequate pathologic specimen is available, routine light microscopic examination reveals adenocarcinoma in approximately 40 per cent of MCPSU patients, undifferentiated carcinoma or malignant neoplasm in 40 per cent, squamous carcinoma in 10 to 15 per cent, and, in fewer than 5 per cent each, melanoma, neuroblastoma, or other types of cancer. The pathologist must determine that the presumed metastasis is not the primary site of cancer. Carcinoma occurring in a setting of adjacent epithelial dysplasia suggests a primary neoplasm, whereas types of cells not normally present in the biopsy site, such as epithelial acinar structures in lymph nodes, confirm that the tumor is metastatic. Light microscopic examination can sometimes reveal structural features that suggest the origin of the cancer. For example, papillary adenocarcinoma most often arises in the thyroid, ovary, or lung, and signet ring adenocarcinoma in the gastrointestinal tract. Rosetting malignant cells are characteristic of neuroblastoma and psammoma bodies of thyroid or ovarian carcinoma.

More specialized studies are especially helpful in evaluating undifferentiated carcinomas or malignant neoplasms, which can prove to be poorly differentiated squamous cell carcinoma or adenocarcinoma, lymphoma, amelanotic melanoma, germ cell carcinoma, or undifferentiated sarcoma, and can also identify the organ of origin of some carcinomas. Immunohistochemical techniques are now more widely utilized than electron microscopy. Analysis with panels of monoclonal or polyclonal antibodies can suggest specific diagnoses, such as lymphoma with leukocyte common antigen positivity, melanoma or sarcoma with neuroectodermal S-100 antigen positivity, carcinoma with cytokeratin or epithelial membrane antigen positivity, prostatic carcinoma with prostate-specific antigen (PSA) positivity, thyroid carcinoma with thyroglobulin positivity, and germ cell carcinoma with reactivity to antibodies against human chorionic gonadotropin (hCG) or α-fetoprotein (AFP). However, it is not firmly established that the clinical behavior and response to therapy of malignancies, particularly undifferentiated neoplasms, diagnosed solely by immunohistochemical means are identical to the behavior and response of corresponding neoplasms diagnosed by light microscopy.

Electron microscopic findings may likewise be of value, particularly in undifferentiated neoplasms. Ultrastructural demonstration of microvilli is characteristic of adenocarcinoma, desmosomes of squamous carcinoma, premelanosomes or melanosomes of malignant melanoma, and cytoplasmic dense-core granules of neuroendocrine carcinomas such as small cell lung cancer.

Differing degrees of certainty which individual pathologists require to make a more specific diagnosis and differing numbers and types of specialized pathologic studies employed before the diagnosis of MCPSU is made account for the second major source of heterogeneity in patients reported to have the MCPSU syndrome.

CLINICAL MANIFESTATIONS

The first clinical manifestation and site of initial pathologic diagnosis of cancer in patients with MCPSU most often occurs in the lung or pleural space, liver, bone, or lymph nodes. Other presentations include cancer in the peritoneal space and pelvis, brain, epidural space, and skin. The distribution of metastases is clearly different in patients with MCPSU and those with an obvious primary site. For example, bone metastases are not common in overt pancreatic cancer but are frequent in pancreatic cancer presenting as MCPSU. Liver and lung metastases are uncommon in overt prostatic cancer but occur much more frequently in prostatic cancer with a clinically undetected primary site.

The most common eventually detected primary sites of cancer in MCPSU patients are the pancreas, lung, colon, and hepatobiliary structures. In MCPSU cases presenting above the diaphragm, the lung is the most common primary cancer site which is later discovered, while for infradiaphragmatic presentations, the pancreas is the most frequently documented primary site.

The distribution of eventually proven sites of cancer origin in patients with MCPSU is somewhat different from that of various cancers in the general population. Germ cell, adrenal, hepatobiliary, pancreatic, and renal cancers are relatively overrepresented among patients with the MCPSU syndrome, whereas malignancies of breast, uterus and uterine cervix, lung, and prostate are relatively underrepresented. Cancers in the latter group are more readily diagnosed by simple means such as physical examination and chest radiograph than are malignancies in the former group.

STAGING EVALUATION

The oncologic staging evaluation, or determination of the extent of tumor dissemination, is somewhat atypical in patients with MCPSU. With the presence of metastatic cancer already proven, considerable effort is often expended in attempting to document the site of the primary malignancy. However, this is frequently inappropriate, since most MCPSU patients prove to have advanced carcinoma refractory to therapy, and performing extensive testing to locate the primary tumor site could occupy a considerable fraction of the patient's life expectancy with only minimal prospects of affecting the ultimate outcome.

Identifying the primary tumor site benefits the patient in only three circumstances. First, tumor confined to a single peripheral lymph node region may be potentially completely eradicated, making control of the primary cancer in the area drained by affected nodes the dominant determinant of survival. An example is occult primary squamous carcinoma of the head and neck region presenting in cervical lymph nodes. Second, documenting that the primary tumor arises in an organ for cancers of which effective systemic treatment is available, such as breast cancer, strongly supports the administration of such therapy. Finally, localizing a primary tumor producing or about to produce disabling symptoms may allow institution of palliative therapy.

Identification of additional asymptomatic visceral metastatic sites of tumor is of no value in a patient with known visceral metastases. However, in patients whose MCPSU arises in a single peripheral lymph node region, discovery of visceral or distant nodal metastases may prevent unnecessarily radical locoregional therapy.

There is universal agreement that radiographic barium studies of the upper gastrointestinal tract and colon and intravenous pyelography are of no value in the absence of symptoms or signs suggestive of an occult primary cancer in the region being imaged, since false-positive studies occur more frequently than the uncommon true-positive result. Computed tomographic (CT) scans of the abdomen and chest probably have a higher yield, but in most cases detect only an untreatable primary malignancy, especially pancreatic and non–small cell lung cancer. In all patients with MCPSU, any imaging studies suggested by the comprehensive evaluation of the pathologic specimen which might support the diagnosis of a treatable malignancy, such as prostatic ultrasonography in an adenocarcinoma reacting with antibodies to PSA or CT scan to detect retroperitoneal lymphadenopathy in an undifferentiated neoplasm reacting with antibodies to leukocyte common antigen, should be performed. Imaging studies for evaluation of symptoms are always appropriate, since detection of a primary or metastatic tumor that requires palliative treatment, such as intestinal bypass for impending obstruction, may result.

Serum biochemical studies that may help diagnose a treatable neoplasm, such as hCG and AFP (germ cell carcinoma) and PSA and prostatic acid phosphatase (prostatic cancer), should be obtained in the appropriate clinical and pathologic setting. However, only markedly elevated values of these biomarkers are specific for germ cell (or hepatocellular in the case of AFP) carcinoma and prostatic cancer, respectively, since other cancers and benign conditions, such as liver disease and prostatic hypertrophy, are associated with more modest elevations. Moderate elevations do, however, support further evaluation for the specific treatable neoplasm in question. Estrogen receptor determinations can be performed on an appropriately prepared tumor biopsy, but only markedly elevated values strongly support the diagnosis of hormonally responsive breast or endometrial cancer, as many types of carcinoma can exhibit modestly elevated receptor protein levels.

The remainder of the staging evaluation in patients with MCPSU should be closely tailored to the specific clinical presentation. It is most useful to segregate patients into two groups, those with known tumor confined to lymph nodes and those with tumor in visceral site(s) with or without node involvement.

MCPSU CONFINED TO LYMPH NODES. Malignant melanoma and lymphoma can present as isolated lymphadenopathy in any node-bearing region, and, if neither is excluded by pathologic evaluation, a primary cutaneous melanoma (along with pathologic review of previously excised skin lesions) or other sites of adenopathy (and possibly evidence of bone marrow involvement), respectively, should be sought. Likely sites of origin of other primary cancers vary markedly by nodal area.

In patients with middle and upper cervical adenopathy in whom biopsy reveals squamous or poorly differentiated carcinoma, complete endoscopic examination with blind biopsies and CT scan to identify areas of submucosal thickening may disclose a primary cancer of the upper aerodigestive tract. Patients with supraclavicular adenopathy more often prove to have adenocarcinoma, which is likely to originate in the lung, breast, or (only in the left fossa) the gastrointestinal tract.

Adenocarcinoma presenting as isolated axillary adenopathy most likely originates in the breast in the female, with lung cancer another possibility in both sexes. Careful breast examination and mammography are always performed in this setting. With other pathologic diagnoses, lung and skin of the upper extremity should be considered as possible primary sites. Isolated inguinal malignant adenopathy may be either squamous cell carcinoma or adenocarcinoma, and the primary cancer often originates in the genitalia, skin of the lower extremity, and anorectal structures, which should be carefully examined. A fraction of MCPSU patients with poorly differentiated tumor confined to the mediastinal or retroperitoneal nodes prove to have germ cell carcinoma, and testicular examination and ultrasonography are appropriate.

MCPSU IN VISCERAL SITES. Approximately 85 per cent of MCPSU patients present with visceral metastases, and no reproducibly effective systemic therapy is currently available for the great majority. The clinician should focus on identifying neoplasms for which effective systemic treatment exists, specifically chemotherapy-responsive breast and ovarian cancer, pulmonary and extrapulmonary small cell carcinoma, germ cell carcinoma, and lymphoma; hormone-responsive prostatic, breast, and endometrial carcinoma; and papillary carcinoma of the thyroid, which is responsive to radioactive iodine administration. Unfortunately, no more than 10 per cent of MCPSU patients with visceral metastases are found to have one of these neoplasms.

In women, pelvic examination should be performed and mammography obtained if pathologic evaluation does not exclude breast cancer. Any suspicion of gynecologic neoplasm should lead to abdominal and pelvic CT scan or pelvic ultrasonography. Some women who present with malignant ascites revealing adenocarcinoma on cytologic examination and no evidence of metastases outside the peritoneal cavity have tumors with clinical behavior similar to that of ovarian carcinoma and may be candidates for exploratory laparotomy. The thyroid gland should be carefully palpated in both sexes.

In men, prostatic examination and perhaps ultrasonography should be performed, and blind prostatic biopsy may be appropriate if suspicion of prostate cancer is high. The possibility of an overlooked subareolar mass due to male breast cancer should not be forgotten. In younger men with predominant midline nodal presentations and minimal visceral tumor, especially confined to the lung, historical evidence of rapid tumor growth or response to previous therapy suggestive of the recently described and incompletely characterized syndrome of "poorly differentiated carcinoma of unknown primary site" should be sought, and testicular examination and ultrasonography performed.

TREATMENT

MCPSU CONFINED TO LYMPH NODES. Patients who, after the staging evaluation outlined above, have all known tumor confined to a single lymph-node bearing region should be approached aggressively, as a fraction of them will attain 5-year survival and even cure. Those with melanoma should undergo radical lymphadenectomy, with the expectation of 5-year survival of 15 to 35 per cent, depending upon the number and volume of nodal metastases, an outcome similar to Stage III melanoma managed with excision of the primary skin lesion and radical lymphadenectomy. If malignant lymphoma is the suspected diagnosis, combination chemotherapy appropriate for lymphoma followed by local irradiation is a reasonable approach.

Squamous and undifferentiated carcinoma in middle to upper cervical nodes is most often managed with radical neck dissection and irradiation, although irradiation alone may be sufficient for low-volume disease. The radiation field often includes the nasopharynx, oropharynx, and laryngopharynx to treat possible primary tumor sites. Five-year survival of 25 to 50 per cent can be anticipated, depending upon tumor volume. The outlook for patients with adenocarcinoma and supraclavicular node metastases is much more grim, with only occasional patients living 5 years after irradiation.

Isolated axillary adenopathy in women with biopsy-proven adenocarcinoma is often treated as breast cancer. Axillary node dissection and modified radical mastectomy are usually advocated in this setting and yield 5-year survival rates of 30 to 70 per cent, results as least as good as in overt Stage II breast cancer. Only half of mastectomy specimens reveal a primary tumor. More recently, similar survival has been reported in patients treated only with axillary dissection or excision, often in conjunction with breast irradiation. Since a fraction of patients clearly have breast cancer, systemic adjuvant therapy appropriate for Stage II breast cancer, either chemotherapy or tamoxifen depending upon the individual patient, should be considered. Men and women with squamous or undifferentiated carcinoma confined to axillary nodes should be evaluated for node dissection, since approximately 20 per cent will live 5 years after surgery. Although physical examination usually reveals the primary cancer in patients with malignancy in inguinal nodes, surgical extirpation or irradiation alone yields 5-year survival of approximately 25 per cent in patients without a documented primary site.

If MCPSU of undifferentiated pathology is confined to mediastinal or retroperitoneal nodes, a trial of aggressive combination chemotherapy, especially in younger patients, may be appropriate, since these nodal regions are common areas in which extragonadal germ cell tumors and lymphomas arise.

MCPSU IN VISCERAL SITES. Palliative or supportive care is often the major focus of management in MCPSU patients with visceral metastases, since most have widely disseminated cancer for which no effective systemic treatment is available. Occasionally, surgical resection of metastases may be beneficial, as in the case of a solitary brain metastasis or an obstructing intestinal lesion. Palliative irradiation, to brain or bone metastases, for example, is often effective. Chemotherapy (or in some instances hormonal therapy or radioactive iodine), which are the only

maneuvers that address the problem of distant metastatic disease, can be administered with realistic expectation of success in only a few subgroups of patients.

If either detailed review of the pathologic material or the staging evaluation raises reasonable suspicion of one of the primary cancers discussed above which might be expected to respond to systemic treatment, a trial of appropriate therapy should be initiated, provided that a favorable risk-benefit ratio is thought to exist in the individual patient.

Two other clinical settings also merit strong consideration of chemotherapy. In women with isolated malignant ascites, laparotomy with maximum feasible resection of tumor masses, provided they are confined to the peritoneal cavity, may be appropriate. Whether or not a primary ovarian tumor is identified, a recent study reports a relatively indolent clinical course in these patients, with some complete responses to chemotherapy regimens utilized in ovarian cancer.

The syndrome of "poorly differentiated carcinoma of unknown primary site" is not well defined but is of importance because a fraction of patients with some or all of the characteristics enumerated above have complete remissions, some of which are durable, with cisplatin-containing chemotherapy regimens utilized for testicular cancer. Originally these cases were thought to represent germ cell carcinomas in which a definitive pathologic diagnosis could not be rendered, but in one series of patients in whom more than one fourth completely responded to chemotherapy, even detailed retrospective pathologic review suggested that no more than 5 per cent of patients had initially unrecognized germ cell tumors. Thus, the pathogenesis of this syndrome remains obscure, and until therapeutic results are obtained after the prospective application of strict diagnostic criteria, utilized to select a group of patients that is then uniformly treated, the proportion that derives substantial benefit from chemotherapy will remain uncertain.

For the remaining patients with visceral MCPSU, there is no evidence that any treatment improves survival. Close observation with palliation of symptoms as they arise is an appropriate management strategy. Chemotherapy regimens for which responses in the MCPSU syndrome have been reported or investigational treatments may be given to fully ambulatory patients who understand the limitations of therapy but still desire it.

PROGNOSIS

The prognosis of most patients with MCPSU is poor. Median and 5-year survival in several large series of consecutive patients accrued in single institutions is approximately 5 to 6 months and 3 to 7 per cent, respectively. The most important prognostic features, as in most other cancers, are sites and volume of tumor involvement, ambulatory status, and degree of weight loss. Five-year survival is reported to be 25 to 50 per cent for patients whose tumor is confined to peripheral lymph nodes and less than 3 per cent for all other patients.

Greco FA, Vaughn WK, Hainsworth JD: Advanced poorly differentiated carcinoma of unknown primary site: Recognition of a treatable syndrome. Ann Intern Med 104:547, 1986. *The initial detailed description of the clinical characteristics and prognostic features of a subgroup of MCPSU patients surprisingly responsive to combination chemotherapy.*

Haskell CM, Cochran AJ, Barsky SH, et al.: Metastasis of unknown origin. Curr Probl Cancer 12:1, 1988. *A comprehensive and critical review of the MCPSU syndrome.*

Kirsten F, Chi CH, Leary JA, et al.: Metastatic adeno or undifferentiated carcinoma from an unknown primary site: Natural history and guidelines for identification of treatable subsets. Q J Med 62:143, 1987. *Analysis of a large consecutive series of MCPSU patients, with emphasis on identification of the small number of patients for whom potentially effective therapy is available.*

PART XIV
METABOLIC DISEASES

167 Introduction

James B. Wyngaarden

The term *metabolism* encompasses the numerous chemical transformations that occur within living organisms. These are often divided into two large categories. Those reactions or processes that are synthetic, and in general result in a larger molecule than any of the reactants, are called *anabolic*. Such reactions are usually energy requiring. Those reactions that are degradative and involve the breakdown of large molecules into smaller products are termed *catabolic*. Such processes are essentially energy yielding. The term *intermediary metabolism* refers to all changes that take place between the moment of entry of a nutrient into the organism and the discharge of all of the chemical products into the environment. It is customary to consider separately the intermediary metabolism of carbohydrates, lipids, and proteins, although no sharp lines can be drawn between the metabolic reactions of these three classes of compounds. The term *basal metabolism* refers to energy requirements for maintenance and conduct of cellular and tissue processes under conditions in which the effects of muscular activity and the work of digestion and metabolism of foodstuffs are minimal.

Part XIV of this textbook is concerned with metabolic diseases. A disorder is classified as a metabolic disease when the fundamental pathogenetic mechanism involves a chemical transformation or process. Many diseases of metabolism involve specific enzyme or other protein abnormalities. When these can be attributed to an underlying genetic abnormality, they are termed *inborn errors of metabolism* (see Ch. 31). There are now over 350 human genetic diseases whose biochemical defects have been defined. Most of these are described somewhere in this textbook or listed in Tables 31–1 and 176–1, but only a fraction has been collected into Part XIV. For example, hemolytic anemias attributable to specific enzyme defects are included with the other hemolytic anemias in Part XII, Hematologic Diseases, and adrenal hyperplasia attributable to specific enzyme defects is discussed in Part XVI, Endocrine and Reproductive Diseases. The disorders included in Part XIV are chiefly those whose manifestations are multisystemic or those in which the biochemical and genetic factors dominate the description.

PATHOGENESIS OF HEREDITARY METABOLIC DISEASES. The etiology of an inborn error of metabolism is a mutant gene. The alteration in DNA structure produces a disturbance in protein structure and function, which in turn affects cell and organ function. Hereditary metabolic diseases can be considered in terms of these three sequential levels.

Altered DNA Structure. The nature of mutations can be deduced from changes in amino acid sequences in the mutant proteins and the genetic codes (see Ch. 30). This approach has been applied most extensively in studies of variant hemoglobins and glucose-6-phosphate dehydrogenases. DNA restriction enzyme analyses and DNA sequencing techniques permit direct analysis of alterations in DNA structure. By these methods, point mutations, deletions, and insertions are readily identified, and hybrid proteins or prematurely terminated or aberrantly extended proteins or totally deleted proteins explained in terms of genetic mechanisms. Restriction endonucleases identify many variations in gene structure as fragment-length polymorphisms. The latter approach provided the first clues to the genetic abnormality in cystic fibrosis and provided the starting point that eventually led to the identification of the abnormal gene and its product. With

the availability of DNA cloning techniques it is possible to study directly the altered DNA sequence in many human mutations, even those that involve genes that code for quantitatively minor proteins, such as enzymes. These techniques also disclose mutations in noncoding regions of DNA that affect rate of synthesis, processing, or stability of specific messenger RNA's.

Altered Protein Function. Abnormalities in the synthesis or structure of a specific enzyme protein result in absence of or reduced or (occasionally) enhanced rates of a specific enzyme-catalyzed reaction. In many genetic enzyme deficiency states, a reduced but detectable level of enzymatic activity can be measured by sensitive assays. The residual enzyme activity can frequently be attributed to a catalytically abnormal enzyme, which may exhibit decreased affinity for substrates, cofactors, or inhibitors. In the most extensively studied series of enzyme defects, those involving glucose-6-phosphate dehydrogenase, most of the enzyme deficiencies reflect unstable enzymes whose activities decay as the erythrocyte ages. This is a common mechanism of enzyme deficiency in the anucleated red blood cell but has not been demonstrated to be an important cause of enzyme deficiency in disorders that affect primarily nucleated cells. The most interesting example of mutations leading to increased enzyme activities involves phosphoribosylpyrophosphate synthetase. Different mutations in an X-linked structural gene lead to four discrete subtypes exhibiting (1) reduced sensitivity to nucleotide regulators, (2) increased affinity for substrate, (3) increased specific activity per enzyme molecule, or (4) a combination of (1) and (3). Relatively few lesions, other than hemoglobinopathies, have been attributed to mutations in genes coding for nonenzymatic proteins. One example is the ZZ variant of alpha$_1$-antitrypsin deficiency, in which an altered protein is not susceptible to normal posttranslational processing (glycosylation), with the result that the defective glycoprotein cannot be secreted by the liver. In some nonenzymatic proteins, a structural abnormality leads to aggregation (e.g., sickle cell hemoglobin). In others, the mutation affects the affinity of a receptor for a specific ligand (e.g., the low density lipoprotein [LDL] receptor in familial hypercholesterolemia and the cytoplasmic androgen receptor in complete testicular feminization).

Disrupted Cell and Organ Function. Most genetic diseases first come to clinical attention because of disturbances at the level of cell and organ function. Several types of derangements occur:

1. Altered flux through metabolic pathways. This is the most frequent basis of recognition of an inborn error of metabolism. The product may be missing (albinism), or a precursor may accumulate (mucopolysaccharidoses) or be shunted into a toxic metabolite (phenylketonuria).

2. Disordered feedback regulation of synthetic pathways. Decreased synthesis of a regulatory end-product may result in faulty control of an early step of the pathway leading to excessive production of intermediates. The classic example is acute intermittent porphyria, in which a deficiency of porphobilinogen deaminase leads to diminished production of heme, a normal feedback inhibitor of porphyrin synthesis. Decreased production of heme leads to overactivity of δ-aminolevulinic acid synthetase, overproduction of nonheme porphyrins, and acute intermittent porphyria.

3. Disordered membrane function. This is the basis for a large group of genetic diseases in which there is impairment of a specific function of a plasma membrane protein. In one type, transmembrane transport of specific small molecules is defective, apparently because a membrane carrier protein is nonfunctional. The affected substrates can be amino acids (cystinuria), carbohydrates (renal glycosuria), or ions (renal tubular acidosis). In

another type, receptor-mediated endocytosis of a macromolecule is defective. In familial hypercholesterolemia a mutation in the gene that codes for a receptor results in defective uptake and degradation of LDL by body cells, resulting in accumulation of LDL and its cholesterol in plasma and arterial walls. Still another type involves a defect in a plasma membrane protein whose action is required for hormone action. In pseudohypoparathyroidism, the guanosine triphosphate (GTP)–sensitive N-protein is defective, and parathyroid hormone cannot stimulate adenylate cyclase in the target cell. The latter two types of defects are inherited as dominant traits, in contrast to those that involve transmembrane transport of small molecules, which behave like recessive traits.

4. Disordered intracellular compartmentation. A few examples of primary genetic defects in cell compartmentation are known. The ZZ variant of alpha$_1$-antitrypsin deficiency, discussed above, is one. Another is I-cell disease, in which there is a deficiency of a processing enzyme that is normally responsible for the occurrence of mannose-6-phosphate residues in lysosomal enzymes. In the absence of mannose-6-phosphate residues, enzymes do not bind to a specific receptor that directs them to the lysosome, and these enzymes pass through the cell into the plasma like a secretory protein. An additional example is a rare form of familial hypercholesterolemia in which there is an abnormal cell-surface receptor that can bind LDL but cannot transport it into the cell.

5. Distorted cell or tissue architecture. The distorted shapes of erythrocytes in sickle cell diseases and in hereditary spherocytosis are examples of this type. Another example is illustrated by the immotile cilia syndrome (Kartagener's syndrome), in which a structural protein of cilia, dynein, is defective. In consequence, the "dynein arms" that crosslink microtubules are missing, they cannot slide properly, and cilia cannot undulate. Still another type is exemplified by type VI Ehlers-Danlos syndrome, in which collagen is deficient in hydroxylysine and does not crosslink normally.

ACQUIRED METABOLIC DISEASES. There are many examples of metabolic diseases that are acquired rather than hereditary. Gout exists in primary and secondary varieties. The secondary types occur because of excessive nucleic acid turnover in myeloproliferative diseases or chronic hemolytic anemias, or because of impaired renal excretion of uric acid resulting from drug effects upon the kidney or acquired renal disease. Certain varieties of porphyria can be attributed to acquired intoxications. Hyperlipoproteinurias are common accompaniments of other diseases: hypothyroidism, the nephrotic syndrome, acute and chronic alcoholism, biliary obstruction. In many conditions there is a prominent interaction between hereditary and environmental factors: obesity and diabetes mellitus, ingestion of phenylalanine-containing proteins in phenylketonuria, ingestion of milk in galactosemia. Without the environmental stress, these conditions would remain silent.

Some of the diseases of metabolism are very common, such as diabetes, with a prevalence in the United States of about 2.5 per cent, and the hyperlipidemias. Others are quite rare, and a few are perhaps more properly regarded as biochemical anomalies rather than diseases—pentosuria, for example. The study of rare metabolic disorders has provided a better understanding of normal metabolic processes and, in some instances, has allowed early recognition of a disorder whose manifestations are preventable simply by adjustment of diet (galactosemia, phenylketonuria). The identification of specific enzyme defects has led to attempts at replacement therapy with inklings of success following enzyme infusion (Gaucher's disease, Fabry's disease) or organ transplantation (bone marrow in immunologic deficiency states; kidney in cystinosis, Fabry's disease, Gaucher's disease).

Becker KL: Principles and Practices of Endocrinology and Metabolism. Philadelphia, J.B. Lippincott, 1990.

Scriver CR, Beaudet AL, Sly WS, et al. (eds.): The Metabolic Basis of Inherited Disease. 6th ed. New York, McGraw-Hill, Inc., 1989. *An authoritative text that presents detailed discussions of various hereditary diseases of metabolism by recognized experts on each topic.*

DISORDERS OF CARBOHYDRATE METABOLISM

168 Galactosemia

Stanton Segal

The galactosemias are toxicity syndromes exhibited by patients with an inherited inability to metabolize the sugar galactose, which is a constituent of the disaccharide lactose found in milk and milk products. There are three disorders, each of which results from a deficiency of one of the enzymes that catalyze the normal conversion of galactose to glucose: galactokinase, galactose-1-phosphate uridyltransferase, and uridine diphosphate-4-epimerase. A defect in galactokinase is manifested primarily by cataract formation early in life. Uridyltransferase deficiency, which is the most prevalent and is commonly referred to as classic galactosemia, results in a syndrome of nutritional failure, liver disease, abnormal renal tubule function, cataracts, mental retardation, and ovarian abnormalities in affected females. A deficiency of epimerase activity clinically resembles transferase deficiency but may exist in a more benign form when the enzyme defect is limited to red blood cells. For all three disorders, the elevations of the level of galactose and its metabolites in blood, urine, and tissues can be corrected and the clinical manifestations alleviated by omission of dietary galactose.

ETIOLOGY. Galactokinase, galactose-1-phosphate uridyl-transferase, and uridine diphosphate-4-epimerase deficiencies are all autosomal recessive genetic disorders. The individual human genes have been located on chromosomes 17, 9, and 1, respectively. The tissues of obligate heterozygotes contain about 50 per cent of the normal enzyme activity, while homozygotes exhibit absence of or very little activity. Immunoelectrophoretic analysis has shown that patients with transferase deficiency produce a protein similar to the normal, but with severely reduced enzyme activity or reduced stability, suggesting single amino acid substitution defects in the majority rather than deletion mutations.

PREVALENCE. Uridyltransferase deficiency has a prevalence of 1 per 40,000 births and a carrier rate of about 1 per cent in the U.S. population. A gene known as the Duarte variant is allelic to the normal transferase and codes for a protein that is electrophoretically different and enzymatically less active. The gene frequency of the Duarte variant is about 0.05 per cent, and homozygotes for the Duarte variant have about 50 per cent of normal transferase activity in their red blood cells. Widespread neonatal screening has detected a number of babies with low red cell transferase activity who are compound heterozygotes with one gene for defective transferase and another for the Duarte variant. Such infants have only 10 to 25 per cent of red cell enzyme activity but rarely have impaired galactose utilization that requires treatment.

Galactokinase deficiency is quite rare, having a prevalence of 1 in 500,000 to 1 in 1 million births. Epimerase deficiency is also rare. The benign type has mainly been described in Swiss and Japanese populations, while only a few cases of symptomatic epimerase deficiency have been detected.

PATHOGENESIS. Galactose is converted to glucose by a unique series of three enzyme reactions. The first enzyme in the pathway, galactokinase, causes galactose to react with adenosine triphosphate (ATP) to form galactose-1-phosphate:

$$\text{Galactose} + \text{ATP} \rightarrow \text{Galactose-1-P}$$

Next, galactose-1-phosphate reacts with uridine diphosphate (UDP)–glucose to form UDP-galactose in a reaction catalyzed by uridyltransferase:

$$\text{Galactose-1-P} + \text{UDP-glucose} \rightleftharpoons \text{Glucose-1-P} + \text{UDP-galactose}$$

The third enzyme, epimerase, performs the spatial change of the hydroxyl group about the fourth carbon to convert galactose to glucose:

$$\text{UDP-galactose} \rightleftharpoons \text{UDP-glucose}$$

In the presence of pyrophosphate, UDP-glucose pyrophosphorylase cleaves UDP-glucose to glucose-1-phosphate, which is converted to glucose-6-phosphate by phosphoglucomutase and then enters various other pathways of glucose metabolism. Normally, this pathway functions efficiently. Galactose rapidly disappears from blood after intravenous infusion, even faster than a comparable amount of glucose. In normal individuals, liver extraction of galactose results in a rise in the level of blood glucose.

In each of the three forms of galactosemia, diminished enzyme activity produces an accumulation of the substrates proximal to the metabolic block: galactose in galactokinase deficiency, galactose and galactose-1-phosphate in transferase deficiency, and galactose, galactose-1-phosphate plus UDP-galactose in epimerase deficiency. When galactose is increased, alternative pathways form large amounts of otherwise trace metabolites. In one reaction galactose is reduced to form the sugar alcohol, galactitol, while in another, galactose is oxidized to galactonic acid. These metabolites accumulate in tissues and are excreted in considerable amounts in the urine.

Identification of accumulated metabolites and the elucidation of alternative pathways have provided insights into the relationship of biochemical toxicity and clinical manifestations of the disorders. In galactokinase deficiency, in which galactose and metabolites of alternative pathways are increased, the principal clinical finding is cataracts, without multiple organ involvement. These findings implicate galactose-1-phosphate as causing the severe multisystem disease of transferase deficiency and systemic epimerase deficiency. Cataract formation appears to be due to the formation of galactitol by lens aldose reductase. Galactitol, which cannot be further metabolized, accumulates in the lens and produces osmotic changes with imbibition of fluid, lens swelling, and protein precipitation. The exact biochemical alterations in target organs affected by transferase deficiency have not been defined. There are no structural alterations of the brain associated with mental retardation in cases of transferase deficiency, but liver dysfunction is accompanied by altered architecture of the liver characterized by pseudoacinar formation of hepatic cells. The ovaries of females afflicted with hypogonadism may be small, fibrotic, or streaked.

The fact that galactose-1-phosphate can be increased in red cells of transferase-deficient patients and that mental retardation and ovarian abnormalities can occur in patients with no exposure to galactose has fostered the concept that there is continuous self-intoxication in this disorder. This self-intoxication could occur as a result of the formation of UDP-galactose from UDP-glucose via epimerase activity and subsequent pyrophosphorolysis of UDP-galactose to liberate galactose-1-phosphate. The pyrophosphorylase plays a dual role in the process, since it is also responsible for the formation of UDP-glucose from uridine triphosphate and glucose-1-phosphate.

CLINICAL MANIFESTATIONS. Cataracts are the principal finding in patients with galactokinase deficiency, who otherwise are healthy. The cataracts are usually discovered in infants and children examined for other medical reasons. Pseudotumor cerebri has been described in some galactokinase-deficient patients as well as those with transferase deficiency. Cataracts have been observed in some heterozygous carriers, and patients under 40

years with cataracts frequently have lower than normal red cell galactokinase levels.

Uridyltransferase deficiency usually manifests itself shortly after birth or within the first few weeks of life with growth failure, vomiting, diarrhea, hepatomegaly, ascites, jaundice, hemolytic anemia, hypoglycemia, proteinuria, and a renal Fanconi syndrome. Cataracts may not be easily observed with an ophthalmoscope in young infants but are found on slit-lamp examination. Infants with this disease may die in the first few days of life from overwhelming *Escherichia coli* sepsis before other manifestations are evident. Without elimination of galactose from the diet, severely affected infants will die of inanition and liver failure. Occasionally, because of vomiting, the infant's formula is changed to one that is galactose free, with subsequent cessation of the toxicity syndrome. Later in childhood these patients have severe mental retardation and cataracts after milk is reintroduced into the diet. Mental retardation is frequent if therapy is not initiated within the first 2 to 3 months of life. Postpubertal females have a high incidence of hypergonadotropic hypogonadism expressed as either primary or secondary amenorrhea, but the testes of male patients are normal. There is no correlation of the clinical course with ovarian function, but the frequency of hypogonadism appears to correlate with undetectable red cell transferase activity.

Black patients with transferase deficiency may have a milder toxicity syndrome and in some cases have no symptoms. This has been called the Negro variant. Such patients have been found to metabolize some galactose because of the presence of 10 per cent of normal transferase activity in liver and intestinal mucosa. A toxicity syndrome resembling transferase deficiency occurs in cases of systemic epimerase deficiency.

DIAGNOSIS. Galactokinase deficiency should be suspected in any infant or child with cataracts and the diagnosis confirmed by assay of red blood cell or cultured fibroblast galactokinase. A presumptive diagnosis is possible by detection of reducing sugar in urine that is glucose oxidase negative (galactose) or by chromatographic analysis for galactitol in the urine. These urinary findings also obtain in transferase deficiency, whose definitive diagnosis requires the assay of red cell transferase activity. Since severely affected babies may be given blood transfusions before a diagnosis of galactosemia is considered, red cell transferase assay should be delayed until transfused blood has been replaced by the infant's own cells. However, assay of transferase in parents' red cells and the findings of 50 per cent of normal activity in both may be helpful in making a presumptive diagnosis in such infants or in those who may have died before specimens for assay were obtained.

In the differential diagnosis, hereditary fructose intolerance with hepatomegaly, liver dysfunction, hypoglycemia, renal Fanconi syndrome, and nonglucose reducing substance in the urine should be considered. Lactosuria, a common finding in a variety of gastrointestinal disorders, also causes a positive test result for reducing substance. However, many laboratories use glucose oxidase–based tests for blood and urinary sugar determination, and in such instances, galactosemia and galactosuria would go undetected. The greatest confusion in differential diagnosis is the distinction between transferase deficiency and primary liver disease. Because the liver is the major organ metabolizing galactose, any disruption of hepatocellular function may result in galactosemia and galactosuria. Red cell transferase assay should be employed to make the distinction. Patients with clinical findings resembling classic transferase deficiency galactosemia who have normal red cell transferase activity should also be tested for red cell epimerase activity.

Besides the quantitative assay of red cell transferase, the performance of starch gel electrophoresis or isoelectric focusing to determine isoenzyme banding may be useful in distinguishing the carrier for classic galactosemia, the homozygous Duarte variant, whose red cell enzyme activity is comparable to that of carriers for the classic disease, and mixed Duarte variant–classic galactosemia carriers, who have 10 to 25 per cent of normal activity, as well as the Rennes and Chicago variants of transferase deficiency. In addition to these variants with diminished red cell activity and electrophoretic abnormalities, there are other variant forms. The Indiana variant has typical symptoms of transferase deficiency galactosemia and unstable red cell activity, while clinical disease in the Münster variant is caused by abnormal inhibition of transferase by glucose-1-phosphate, the product of the reaction.

Many cases are currently diagnosed as a result of neonatal screening. More than one half of the states in the United States and several foreign countries test all newborns by analysis of heel-stick-blood spots on filter paper. All of the procedures used detect transferase deficiency. Some also detect galactokinase or epimerase deficiency. All positive test results require confirmation by quantitative assay of the individual enzymes. Such screening has resulted in delineation of the benign form of epimerase deficiency, in which galactose-1-phosphate appears to accumulate only in red blood cells. Subsequent studies have indicated that the epimerase in such cases is unstable because of increased requirement for cofactor NAD, which can be supplied by other cells but not red blood cells.

TREATMENT. The institution of a galactose-free diet is the cornerstone of treatment. With galactose elimination, early cataracts may regress. Liver dysfunction and renal tubule abnormalities disappear, and growth and development may be normal. Besides the banning of milk and all milk products, care should be taken to eliminate foods in which milk is used in cooking and baking or lactose has been added. There is no indication that the ability to metabolize galactose increases with age, so that dietary restrictions should not be relaxed in older children.

PROGNOSIS. Dietary galactose restriction does not ensure a normal outcome. Despite excellent treatment from birth, many patients with transferase deficiency have below average mental development with learning deficits, diminished attention span, visual perceptual difficulties, and speech abnormalities. Eighty per cent of affected females have hypergonadotropic hypogonadism. The outcome in patients without symptoms who are treated at birth does not differ from that in patients who are recognized within the first several weeks of life on the basis of the acute galactose toxicity syndrome caused by ingestion of galactose-containing feeds. Untreated infants, however, may not survive. Older patients may develop an ataxic neurologic syndrome while on galactose-restricted diets.

PREVENTION. The insufficiency of the galactose-restricted diet may be due to continuous self-intoxication with endogenously produced galactose metabolites, which may start in utero. Galactose restriction during pregnancy in cases in which the fetus is at risk has not altered the prognosis. Prenatal diagnosis can be performed by assay of transferase of a chorionic villus biopsy specimen or cultured amniotic cells or by determination of galactitol in amniotic fluid.

Fishler K, Koch R, Donnell GN, et al.: Developmental aspects of galactosemia from infancy to childhood. Clin Pediatr 19:38, 1980. *Data describing outcome of dietary treatment of uridyltransferase-deficient patients in relation to age at diagnosis reveal normal IQ but abnormal visual-perceptual status and electroencephalogram (EEG) in patients well treated before 3 months of age.*

Kaufman FR, Kogut MD, Donnell GN, et al.: Hypergonadotropic hypogonadism in female patients with galactosemia. N Engl J Med 304:944, 1981. *Describes amenorrhea and ovarian abnormalities in patients with uridyltransferase deficiency.*

Segal S: Disorders of galactose metabolism. *In* Scriver CH, Beaudet AL, Sly WS, et al. (eds.): The Metabolic Basis of Inherited Disease. 6th ed. New York, McGraw-Hill, 1989, pp 453–480. *Survey of outcome of more than 300 classic uridyltransferase-deficient patients reveals frequency of developmental delay, speech abnormalities, and ovarian dysfunction.*

Waggoner D, Buist NRM, Donnell GN: Long term prognosis in galactosemia: Results of a survey of 350 cases. J Inherited Metab Dis 13:802, 1990. *Most informative data yet published on long-term outcome, which indicate that dietary therapy, even when started at birth, does not necessarily prevent mental retardation or ovarian failure.*

169 The Glycogen Storage Diseases

Harry L. Greene

Glycogen is the storage form of glucose and is present in varying amounts in virtually all cells, although the liver is the primary organ for storage and subsequent release of glucose into the circulation. Glycogen formation from glucose along with the release of glucose from glycogen is highly regulated, a process that aids in the maintenance of normal blood glucose concentrations during fasting. At least eight enzymes involved in glycogen synthesis and the hydrolysis to glucose are utilized in this control.

Glycogen storage diseases are characterized by an abnormal tissue concentration (>70 mg per gram of liver or >15 mg per gram of muscle) and/or an abnormal structure of the glycogen molecule. During the past 40 years, patients who have deficient activity in virtually every enzyme important in the normal synthesis or degradation of glycogen have been identified. With the exception of phosphorylase kinase deficiency, all are inherited in an autosomal recessive manner. Although the enzyme deficiency may vary among patients, the clinical expression of the disease can usually be traced to either the liver or the muscle.

HEPATIC FORMS OF GLYCOGENESIS

The various hepatic enzymatic deficiencies are expressed primarily as hypoglycemia and hepatomegaly, and three defects (branching enzyme, glycogen synthetase, and debranching enzyme) result in the accumulation of abnormally structured glycogen and may cause progressive hepatic cirrhosis and associated splenomegaly. Conversely, the accumulation of normally structured glycogen, as seen with deficiency of phosphorylase, phosphorylase b kinase, acid alpha-glucosidase, or glucose-6-phosphatase, is usually not associated with hepatic fibrosis and splenomegaly. Figure 169–1 summarizes the general location of enzymatic defects resulting in the hepatic forms of glycogenesis. With the exception of lysosomal acid glucosidase deficiency, hypoglycemia is a common presenting feature. Clinical and biochemical expressions of the various types of glycogen storage diseases are summarized in Table 169–1, and the more commonly diagnosed types are discussed below.

GLUCOSE-6-PHOSPHATASE DEFICIENCY (TYPE I GLYCOGEN STORAGE DISEASE). With the recent development of antibodies to several of the five components of glucose-6-phosphatase, this disorder has been subcategorized into types a, b, or c, with type a the most common; but all types have similar clinical features. As noted in Figure 169–1, all other enzymatic defects directly affect the formation or degradation of glycogen, with the exception of glucose-6-phosphatase. Similarly, the clinical expression of this defect is distinctly different from that of the other forms of glycogenosis. For example, fasting-induced

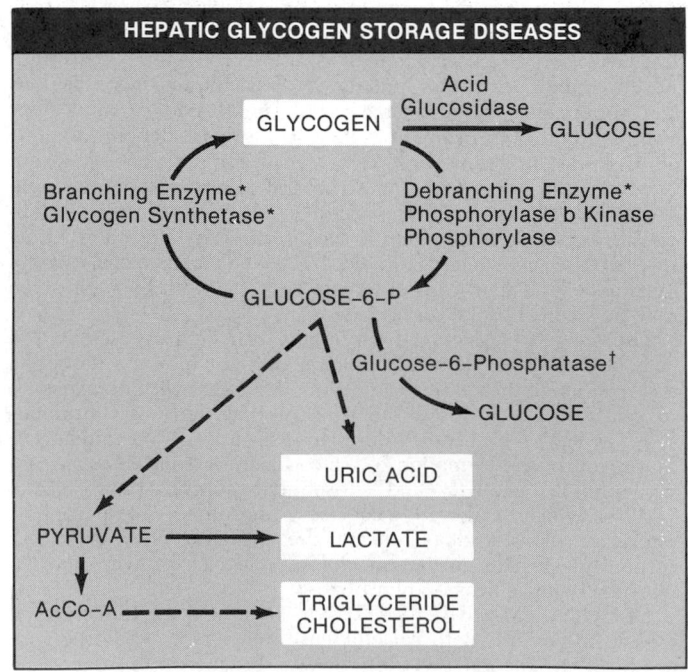

FIGURE 169–1. Mechanism for abnormalities in lipid, purine, and carbohydrate metabolism in the hepatic glycogen storage diseases. * = associated with hepatic cirrhosis. † = associated with elevated serum uric acid, lactate, and lipid levels and with hepatic adenoma.

hypoglycemia may be extreme, and, in combination with lactic acidosis, hyperlipidemia, and hyperuricemia, characterizes patients with type I. The mechanism for the striking abnormalities in lipid and purine metabolism as well as carbohydrate metabolism has been reviewed recently and results primarily from overproduction of substrate in response to a decline in blood glucose, as indicated in Figure 169–1. The documented reversal of these abnormalities by treatment that maintains the blood glucose level between 80 and 90 mg per deciliter supports the postulate that these changes are the result of hormonal responses to the hypoglycemia. Therapeutic intervention has been evaluated more extensively in patients with this defect than any other. As a result, it has been possible to devise reasonably effective dietary control for these patients that results in favorable development into adulthood.

Late Complications. As more patients have survived and developed into active, functioning adults, two subsequent, unexpected complications have become apparent: (1) single or multiple hepatic adenomas and (2) progressive glomerulosclerosis with renal failure. Adenomas usually develop in patients between 16 and 22 years of age, and it is unusual for a patient not to have adenomas by age 25 years. Since there is a tendency for subsequent malignant transformation of an adenoma, annual monitoring by ultrasound is recommended. Any rapidly expanding lesion should be considered potentially malignant and should undergo surgical biopsy, since serum alpha-fetoprotein measurements have been an unreliable marker for malignant transformation. There has been some indication that the adenomas could be prevented or reduced in younger children by more stringent dietary control; however, this hypothesis has not been substantiated in older individuals.

The development of progressive glomerulosclerosis, proteinuria, hypertension, and renal failure has been a recent observation and usually occurs in older patients (>18 years) who are less well managed and exhibit recurrent hypoglycemic episodes, chronic hypertriglyceridemia, and lactic acidosis. The mechanism causing the renal lesion is not defined, although some improvement in proteinuria has been seen following treatment with angiotensin-converting enzyme inhibitors.

DEBRANCHING ENZYME DEFICIENCY (TYPE III GLY- COGEN STORAGE DISEASE). This disease most often affects only the liver but may affect muscle as well. With muscle involvement, the serum creatine phosphokinase (CPK) level is elevated, and patients are usually classified as having type IIIb disease. Some patients may not show elevated CPK levels during early life, so evaluation during later childhood or adolescence should be performed. Hypoglycemia with fasting is less severe (usually 40 to 50 mg per deciliter) than in patients with type I, although hepatic enlargement may be substantially greater. Serum aspartate aminotransferase (AST) and alanine aminotransaminase (ALT) concentrations are commonly above 500 units per milliliter. Correspondingly, hepatic fibrosis of varying degrees is usually present during childhood and may be progressive. At least two adult patients (ages 43 and 55 years) presenting with "cryptogenic cirrhosis" and bleeding esophageal varices have been diagnosed as having debrancher enzyme deficiency.

Treatment of these patients has not been advocated, since the natural course of the disease has been thought to be benign. However, since growth retardation and cirrhosis may be serious complications, several patients have been treated with frequent feedings and raw cornstarch to maintain blood glucose levels between 75 and 100 mg per deciliter. Treated patients often show a significant reduction in serum transaminase levels and improvements in growth, and they may demonstrate improved muscle strength, although serum CPK activities remain elevated.

Clinical and laboratory features of the other, more unusual forms of hepatic glycogenoses are presented in Table 169–1.

MUSCULAR FORMS OF GLYCOGEN STORAGE

ACID ALPHA-GLUCOSIDASE DEFICIENCY (POMPE'S DISEASE, TYPE II GLYCOGEN STORAGE DISEASE). In this condition, virtually all tissues have an increased glycogen content. However, presenting clinical manifestations of the illness are cardiac enlargement, myocardial failure, and generalized muscle hypotonia without muscle wasting. The classic infantile form manifests during the first months of life, and few survive past the first year. The juvenile variant presents in later infancy or early childhood and progresses more slowly, with death in the

TABLE 169–1. CLASSIFICATION OF GLYCOGEN STORAGE DISEASES

Type	Enzyme Affected	Primary Organ Involved	Manifestations
O	Glycogen synthetase	Liver	Hypoglycemia, hyperketonia, FFT, early death
Ia	Glucose-6-phosphatase	Liver	Enlarged liver and kidney growth failure, fasting hypoglycemia, acidosis, thrombocyte dysfunction
Ib	Microsomal membrane G-6-P translocase	Liver	As in Ia; in addition, recurrent neutropenia, bacterial infections
Ic	Microsomal membrane P-transporter	Liver	As in Ia
II	Lysosomal acid glucosidase	Skeletal and cardiac muscle	*Infantile form:* early-onset, progressive muscle hypotonia, cardiac failure, death before 2 years *Juvenile form:* late-onset myopathy with variable cardiac involvement *Adult form:* limb-girdle muscular dystrophy–like feature
III	Amylo-1,6-glucosidase (debrancher enzyme)	Liver, skeletal muscle, heart	Fasting hypoglycemia, hepatomegaly in infancy; some have myopathic features, rarely clinical cardiac features
IV	Amylo-1,4-1,6-transglucosidase (brancher enzyme)	Liver, muscle	Hepatosplenomegaly, cirrhosis; may have late-onset myopathy
V	Muscle phosphorylase	Skeletal muscle	Exercise-induced muscular pain, cramps, and progressive weakness, sometimes with myoglobinuria; symptoms usually begin during adolescence or early adulthood
VI	Liver phosphorylase	Liver	Hepatomegaly, mild hypoglycemia, good prognosis
VII	Phosphofructokinase	Muscle, red blood cells	As in V; in addition, mild hemolytic anemia
Formerly VIb, VIII, or IX	Phosphorylase b kinase	Liver, leukocytes, (?) muscle	As in VI; X-linked inheritance
X	Cyclic AMP–dependent kinase	Liver, muscle	Hepatomegaly, mild hypoglycemia

second or third decade. The adult type manifests as a slowly developing adult-onset myopathy. In each case, the diagnosis is dependent on finding deficient activity of acid alpha-1, 4-glucosidase in muscle specimens or cultured fibroblasts. No treatment, including bone marrow transplantation and systemic enzyme infusion, has proved to be of long-term benefit to these patients.

MYOPHOSPHORYLASE DEFICIENCY (TYPE V GLYCOGEN STORAGE DISEASE, McARDLE'S DISEASE). Most of these patients are asymptomatic during early childhood and escape diagnosis until the second or third decade of life. Presentation with a history of muscle pain and cramps after exercise, signs of myoglobinuria, and painful cramping on an ischemic exercise test are characteristic. The diagnosis is suggested by an elevation in serum muscle CPK isoenzyme activity and by failure to elevate the serum lactate level with exercise. The diagnosis is established by documenting elevated muscle glycogen in the sarcolemmal regions and reduced muscle phosphorylase activity. Glucose or fructose ingestion prior to exercise is said to reduce the symptoms.

MUSCLE PHOSPHOFRUCTOKINASE DEFICIENCY (MUSCLE PHOSPHOGLYCERATE MUTASE DEFICIENCY, LACTATE DEHYDROGENASE [LDH-M] SUBUNIT DEFICIENCY, TYPE VII GLYCOGEN STORAGE DISEASE). These muscle glycogeneses are rare and clinically similar to myophosphorylase deficiency. Patients with phosphofructokinase deficiency may also show a mild hemolytic anemia. Diagnosis is dependent on muscle enzyme analysis. Treatment is aimed at avoiding strenuous exercise.

DIAGNOSIS AND PRENATAL DIAGNOSIS OF GLYCOGEN STORAGE DISEASE

Diagnostic enzyme analysis on hepatic or muscle tissue for all types of glycogen storage diseases is currently funded at Duke Medical Center, Division of Genetics. Prenatal diagnosis of three types of glycogen storage diseases (types II, III, and IV) is also possible and is performed on cultured amniotic cells in this laboratory.

Burchell A: Molecular pathology of glucose-6-phosphatase. FASEB J 4:2978, 1990. *This article provides the most up-to-date studies on the enzyme glucose-6-phosphatase and clears some of the confusion concerning the enzyme. It also describes a series of children with "partial" defects in the enzyme who experienced sudden infant death syndrome.*

Chen YT, Cornblath M, Sidbury JB: Cornstarch therapy in type I glycogen storage disease. N Engl J Med 310:171, 1984. *The usefulness of dietary raw cornstarch to maintain blood glucose concentrations is demonstrated.*

Ding JH, deBarsy T, Brown B, et al.: Immunoblot analyses of glycogen debranching enzyme in different subtypes of glycogen storage disease type III. J Pediatr 116:95, 1990. *This article provides newer insights into the molecular basis of type III glycogeneses.*

Folk CC, Greene HL: Dietary management of type I glycogen storage disease. J Am Diet Assoc 84:293, 1984. *This article provides a practical application of foods and food exchanges to management of glycogen storage diseases.*

Ghishan FK, Greene HL: Inborn errors of metabolism that lead to permanent liver injury. In Zakim D, Boyer TD (eds.): Hepatology: A Textbook of Liver Disease. 2nd ed. Philadelphia, W.B. Saunders Company, 1990. *An extensively referenced review that focuses on the altered metabolism treatment and outcome of the hepatic forms of glycogenesis.*

Hers HG, Van Hoof F, deBarsy T: The glycogen storage diseases. In Scriver CR, Beaudet AL, Sly WS, Valle D (eds.): The Metabolic Basis of Inherited Disease. 6th ed. New York, McGraw-Hill, 1989. *This is an extensively referenced article that provides information on the clinical and biochemical aspects of the glycogen storage diseases.*

170 Fructose Intolerance

Harry L. Greene

Fructose, a normal dietary constituent of fruits, vegetables, honey, and the disaccharide sucrose (table sugar), is present at a level of 50 to 100 grams in the average Western diet. It is rapidly absorbed in the proximal small intestine by a specific transport mechanism and extracted on first pass from the portal vein, with no appearance in the urine. Three defects in fructose metabolism have been identified: (1) essential fructosuria, (2) hereditary fructose intolerance, and (3) fructose-1, 6-diphosphatase deficiency. The major pathway for fructose metabolism and the three defects in fructose metabolism are illustrated in Figure 170–1.

ESSENTIAL FRUCTOSURIA. This is a rare (about 1 in 130,000 births), asymptomatic autosomal recessive condition caused by deficient activity of fructokinase, the first reaction in fructose utilization. Since no pathologic condition results from the defect, the primary concern relates to the fact that fructose is a reducing sugar. Thus, the finding of a positive reaction with urinary Clinitest tablets may result in the erroneous suggestion of diabetes unless the glucose oxidase is determined with a dipstick.

HEREDITARY FRUCTOSE INTOLERANCE (HFI). This is a potentially life-threatening autosomal recessive disorder that can be very effectively treated by elimination of dietary fructose. It has a prevalence of 1 in 20,000 and is due to deficiency of fructose-1-phosphate aldolase (aldolase B). The enzyme is normally present in large amounts in liver, intestine, and renal cortex, and the excessive intake of fructose by patients with HFI adversely affects each of these organs. Patients with the disorder exhibit profoundly deficient activity of fructose-1-phosphate aldolase and a modest reduction in the activity of fructose-1, 6-diphosphate aldolase.

Symptoms develop only after ingestion of fructose, and since lactose is the carbohydrate source in mammalian milk, infants do not develop symptoms until the introduction of dietary fruits or other fructose-containing foods or medication, i.e., fruits, fruit juices, medicinal syrups, sucrose-containing infant formulas, and so forth. The primary symptoms are vomiting and symptoms of hypoglycemia within 20 to 30 minutes after fructose ingestion. Concomitant laboratory findings include an acute decrease in serum glucose and phosphate levels and an elevation in the uric acid level. With continued exposure to fructose, hyperbilirubinemia, lactic acidosis, hepatosplenomegaly, and liver failure develop in conjunction with renal tubular dysfunction (bicarbonaturia, aminoaciduria, phosphaturia). At this stage, liver biopsy shows fatty infiltration of histiocytes with cellular necrosis and mild bile duct proliferation with fibrosis. If exposure to fructose continues, progressive fibrosis, cirrhosis, and death from liver failure follow. The brain may also show diminished neurons.

The diagnosis is suggested by the presence of urinary reducing sugar that is detected by Clinitest tablets and that is not detectable by urinary dipstick, since this test is specific for glucose. Since similar clinical features may be present with galactosemia or tyrosinemia, confirmation of the diagnosis can be made by measurement of fructose-1-phosphate aldolase activity in liver or intestinal biopsy specimens. An intravenous fructose tolerance test (0.2 to 0.3 gram per kilogram in adults or 3 grams per square meter in children) after restriction of dietary fructose for several weeks has been used for confirmatory evidence of the illness but may cause hypoglycemia.

In spite of recurrent bouts of hypoglycemia and substantial liver disease, restriction of dietary fructose usually results in almost complete recovery during a 3- to 5-week period, and affected adults have normal intelligence. Older children and adults are protected from large dietary intakes of fructose by an aversion to sweets, although small amounts taken chronically may result in isolated, reversible somatic growth retardation.

FRUCTOSE-1, 6-DIPHOSPHATASE DEFICIENCY. This rare disorder was first described in 1970. Patients usually present before the age of 6 months with fasting-induced lactic acidosis, hypoglycemia, and hepatomegaly. The reaction to glycerol is similar to that with fructose ingestion but is less severe than in patients with HFI. The condition is due to a defect of hepatic fructose-1, 6-diphosphatase, a gluconeogenic enzyme (see Fig. 170–1). Thus, when hepatic glycogen stores are depleted, fasting hypoglycemia develops.

The diagnosis is suspected when, after some 12 to 16 hours of fasting, the blood sugar concentration falls and is not restored by glucagon administration, and acidosis (lactate) is present. Loading tests with fructose or glycerol may be dangerous because they lead to hypoglycemia and lactic acidosis. The diagnosis is confirmed by measurement of the enzyme in hepatic biopsy material.

Baker L, Winegrad AI: Fasting hypoglycemia and metabolic acidosis associated with deficiency of hepatic fructose-1, 6-diphosphatase activity. Lancet 2:13, 1970. *The first description of a patient with deficient fructose-1, 6-diphosphatase activity.*

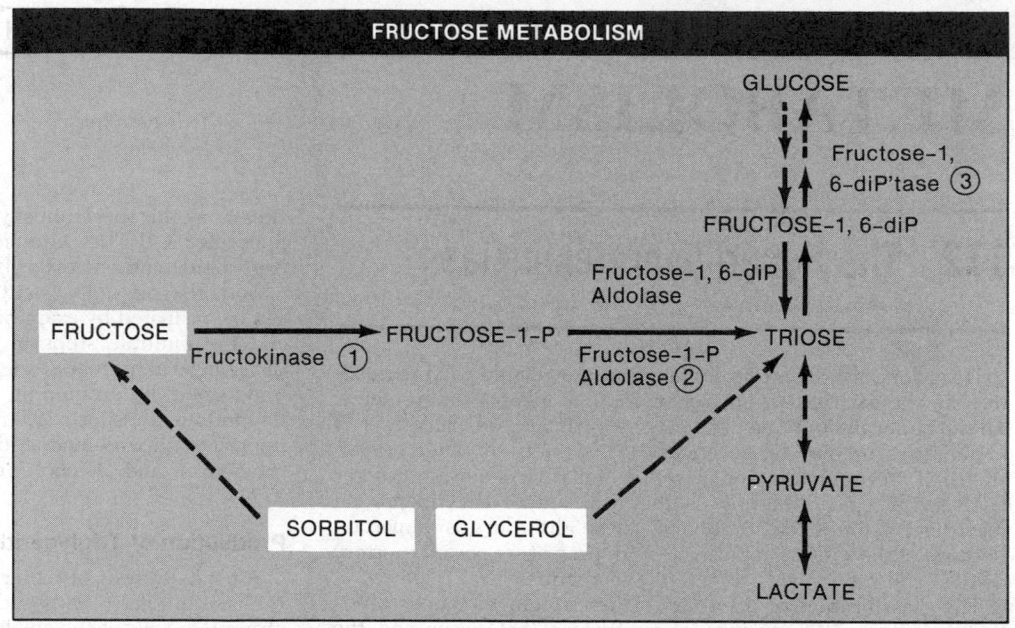

FIGURE 170–1. The major pathway for fructose metabolism and the three defects in fructose metabolism. 1 = Fructokinase deficiency results in asymptomatic fructosuria following ingestion of fructose or sorbitol. 2 = Fructose-1-phosphate aldolase deficiency results in hypoglycemia, lactic acidosis, and liver disease following ingestion of fructose or sorbitol. 3 = Fructose-1, 6-diphosphatase deficiency results in lactic acidosis and hypoglycemia with fasting, or hypoglycemia and acidosis following glycerol ingestion.

Ghishan FK, Greene HL: Inborn errors of metabolism that lead to permanent liver injury. *In* Zakim D, Boyer TD (eds): Hepatology: A Textbook of Liver Disease. 2nd ed. Philadelphia, W. B. Saunders Company, 1990. *An extensively referenced review that focuses on the altered metabolism, treatment, and outcome of patients with fructose intolerance.*

Odievre M, Gentil C, Gautier M, et al.: Hereditary fructose intolerance in childhood. Am J Dis Child 132:605, 1978. *This article is an excellent presentation of the clinical, hepatic, and biochemical changes that can be expected in children with HFI.*

Schulte MJ, Lenz W: Fatal sorbitol infusion in a patient with fructose-sorbitol intolerance. Lancet 2:188, 1977. *This paper illustrates the need to restrict sorbitol as well as fructose in patients with HFI.*

171 Primary Hyperoxaluria

Lloyd H. Smith, Jr.

Primary hyperoxaluria, a general term for two rare genetic disorders of glyoxylate metabolism, is characterized by excessive synthesis and urinary excretion of oxalic acid. Both disorders are transmitted as autosomal recessive traits. The diseases are usually clinically manifested in childhood by recurrent calcium oxalate nephrolithiasis or nephrocalcinosis, or both, leading to early renal failure. In addition to the usual clinical features of uremia, severe peripheral vascular insufficiency may complicate the course of the disease. At postmortem examination, calcium oxalate may be found widely deposited in extrarenal sites, a condition known as *oxalosis*. More rarely, milder forms of the disease may be found in adults. Although oxalate is an important constituent in approximately two thirds of all kidney stones, most adult patients with calcium oxalate nephrolithiasis excrete normal amounts of urinary oxalate (Ch. 88).

Primary hyperoxaluria type I (glycolic aciduria) represents a genetic defect in the activity of peroxisomal alanine: glyoxylate aminotransferase. As a result, glyoxylate accumulates and is excessively oxidized to oxalate and reduced to glycolate, both of which are excreted in increased amounts in the urine (more than 60 mg per 1.73 square meters per 24 hours each). In *primary hyperoxaluria type II* (L-glyceric aciduria), there is a defect in the enzyme D-glyceric dehydrogenase. Hydroxypyruvate accumulates and is reduced by lactate dehydrogenase (LDH) to L-glyceric acid, a compound that is undetectable in normal urine. The reduction of hydroxypyruvate to L-glycerate is probably coupled to the oxidation of glyoxylate to oxalate, both catalyzed by LDH. Each disease can be diagnosed by the characteristic pattern of metabolites in urine: type I, oxalate and glycolate; type

II, oxalate and L-glycerate. Pyridoxine deficiency in laboratory animals and humans also leads to hyperoxaluria and even oxalosis with a urinary pattern similar to that of the genetic disease type I. With the onset of renal failure, the clearance of oxalate is reduced (its clearance is normally about 1.2 times that of creatinine), so that its urinary excretion may return to normal. The diagnosis may then be difficult to establish because measurements of serum oxalate are not readily available and, furthermore, serum oxalate levels rise in all forms of uremia.

No specific methods of treatment are now available. Efforts are directed toward reducing the amount of oxalate excreted and increasing its solubility. Large amounts of pyridoxine (200 to 400 mg per 24 hours) may decrease oxalate excretion in type I disease. More physiologic doses of pyridoxine (2 to 10 mg) may be effective in some patients. Dilute urine should be maintained by forcing fluids, and a phosphate or magnesium oxide supplement may offer partial protection against stone formation (Ch. 88). Renal homotransplantation has been disappointing because of rapid deposition of calcium oxalate in the transplanted kidney, but there have been some reports of success. Long-term dialysis and pyridoxine are therefore indicated when renal failure is severe. Recently, several patients have been successfully treated by combined renal and liver transplantations, which effectively reverse the metabolic abnormalities. Nitroglycerin may improve the peripheral vascular insufficiency associated with oxalosis. A search for an inhibitor of oxalate synthesis is highly indicated.

Increased urinary excretion of oxalate and stone diathesis (in the absence of glycolic aciduria or L-glyceric aciduria) occur in many patients who have small bowel disease and malabsorption (Ch. 102). Normally, oxalate and fatty acids of the small intestine compete for available calcium ion, and calcium oxalate is poorly absorbed. This important form of acquired hyperoxaluria results from excessive colonic absorption of dietary oxalate in the presence of significant steatorrhea. It can be controlled by a low-oxalate diet.

Danpure CJ, Jennings PR, Watts RWE: Enzymological diagnosis of primary hyperoxaluria type I by measurement of hepatic alanine: glyoxylate aminotransferase activity. Lancet 1:289, 1987. *This study established primary hyperoxaluria type I as a specific transaminase defect, a finding consistent with the therapeutic response to pyridoxine exhibited by some patients.*

Hillman RE: Primary hyperoxalurias. *In* Scriver CR, Beaudet AL, Sly WS, et al. (eds.): The Metabolic Basis of Inherited Disease. 6th ed. New York, McGraw-Hill, 1989, pp 933–944. *An excellent summary of oxalate metabolism and of current knowledge about the primary hyperoxalurias; 197 references are supplied.*

Yendt ER, Cohanim M: Response to a physiological dose of pyridoxine in Type I primary hyperoxaluria. N Engl J Med 312:953, 1985. *This article describes varying degrees of sensitivity in the reduction in oxalate excretion during pyridoxine therapy and raises the intriguing possibility that in some patients the diagnosis may be obscured by small amounts of the vitamin.*

DISORDERS OF LIPOPROTEIN METABOLISM

172 The Hyperlipoproteinemias

John D. Brunzell

Disorders of lipoprotein metabolism are related to abnormalities in the synthesis and degradation of plasma lipoproteins. These abnormalities may result from primary inborn errors of metabolism or may be secondary to a variety of other disease states. Hyperlipidemia, the elevation of plasma cholesterol and/or triglyceride concentrations, is the hallmark of the lipoprotein disorders. Clinical delineation of these disorders is important because of the association of some with premature coronary artery disease and others with recurrent pancreatitis.

The classification of disorders of lipoprotein metabolism was first based on the varieties of xanthomas that occur and the appearance of plasma turbidity caused by the accumulation of large, light-scattering lipoprotein particles in plasma. With the discovery of relatively discrete lipoprotein species, classification of these disorders was based on separation of lipoproteins by ultracentrifugation or by electrophoresis. Understanding of lipoprotein physiology has allowed classification of lipoprotein disorders according to pathophysiologic defects, with specific discrete apoprotein, enzyme, or receptor abnormalities identified in some disorders.

PHYSIOLOGY OF LIPOPROTEIN TRANSPORT

Structure and Function of Lipoproteins

The structure of the lipoprotein macromolecule is well suited for the solubilization of lipids in plasma. The nonpolar lipids—cholesteryl ester and triglyceride—are present in the lipoprotein core surrounded by a monolayer composed of specific proteins and the polar lipids, unesterified cholesterol and phospholipid. This monolayer allows the lipoprotein to remain miscible in plasma.

The lipoproteins function as an efficient vehicle for site-to-site transport of triglyceride and cholesterol of both exogenous and endogenous origin. Although caloric need is fairly constant throughout the day, food is ingested only periodically. The excess calories that enter the circulation with each meal are transported mainly as triglyceride to be stored in adipose tissue for future utilization between meals as free fatty acids. Ingested and synthesized cholesterol also needs to be transported to extrahepatic tissues to serve as a source of membrane cholesterol and as substrate for steroid hormone synthesis. The transport of triglyceride and cholesterol is accomplished by a spectrum of lipoproteins that have been classified by arbitrary operational boundaries according to either their density by ultracentrifugation or mobility by electrophoresis (Fig. 172–1). Fortunately, the lipoproteins, as separated by ultracentrifugation or electrophoresis, are so similar that the synonyms based on each of these methods of separation are essentially interchangeable.

The triglyceride-rich lipoproteins can enter the plasma as chylomicrons derived from dietary fat adsorbed from the gut or endogenously as triglyceride-rich very low density lipoprotein (VLDL) synthesized in the liver from glucose or circulating free fatty acids. After removal of some of their triglycerides and surface components, the remaining lipoprotein remnant of the chylomicron is taken up by the liver and degraded. The remnant of endogenous triglyceride-rich lipoprotein probably also requires the liver for further processing. In contrast to the chylomicron, however, only some components of VLDL are removed, resulting in formation of the low density cholesterol-rich lipoprotein.

This is likely to be an oversimplification, as there is a continuous spectrum of particles, and lipoproteins enter and exit at many sites along this spectrum of varying lipoprotein sizes. High density lipoproteins (HDL) interact with this system for transport of triglyceride and cholesteryl ester, as is noted later.

Both the physiology and the pathophysiology of lipoproteins can be evaluated by examining the sites of lipoprotein production and the multiple steps in lipoprotein catabolism. Most pathophysiologic abnormalities leading to hyperlipidemic states can be understood by examining four sites of regulation of plasma lipoprotein transport: (1) triglyceride-rich lipoprotein input, (2) lipoprotein lipase–mediated triglyceride catabolism, (3) remnant catabolism, and (4) cholesterol-rich lipoprotein catabolism (Fig. 172–2).

Production of Triglyceride-Rich Lipoproteins

After hydrolysis of dietary triglycerides in the small intestine, the resulting fatty acids and monoglycerides are taken up by the absorptive cells of the small intestine and incorporated into large triglyceride-rich lipoproteins with a specific form of apoprotein B (apo B-48), phospholipid, and a small amount of cholesterol. These chylomicrons are secreted from the absorptive cells into the lymphatics and subsequently enter the plasma via the thoracic duct. Chylomicron secretion and transport represent a system of high-capacity energy transport, allowing calories ingested at one time, over and above immediate needs, to be transferred to sites of storage for use between meals. The chylomicron remnant taken up and degraded by the liver suppresses synthesis of components of endogenous triglyceride-rich lipoproteins.

Input into plasma of triglyceride-rich lipoproteins also occurs from endogenous sources. During meals, plasma free fatty acids enter the liver, where they may be esterified with glycerol to form triglyceride. Between meals, free fatty acids are mobilized from adipose tissue triglyceride stores. These serve as a potential source for hepatic triglyceride synthesis. Lipogenesis, synthesis of fatty acids de novo from carbohydrate, also occurs in the liver. Fatty acids in the cytosol of the hepatocyte either can enter mitochondria, when oxidation occurs, or can remain in the cytosol, where they are esterified to form triglyceride. These processes appear to be regulated by changes in insulin and glucagon levels that occur with feeding: Glucagon enhances and insulin prevents mitochondrial fatty acid uptake by regulating long-chain acyl carnitine transferase. Insulin also induces lipogenic enzymes in the hepatocytes that regulate the synthesis of fatty acids.

Triglyceride synthesized in the liver, together with cholesteryl ester, is combined with the lipoprotein monolayer composed of phospholipid, unesterified cholesterol, and apoprotein B and is secreted into the hepatic venous outflow as triglyceride-rich VLDL. Hepatic apoprotein B (apo B-100) in VLDL has a larger molecular weight than does intestinal apoprotein B (apo B-48) found in chylomicrons.

In normal individuals, the majority of triglyceride input into the plasma is of dietary origin. Whereas the average American diet contains about 100 grams of triglyceride per day, less than 30 grams of triglyceride is secreted endogenously.

Lipoprotein Lipase–Mediated Triglyceride Catabolism

The triglyceride that enters the plasma in chylomicrons and endogenously synthesized triglyceride-rich lipoproteins is transported to adipose tissue for storage or to muscle for utilization. The enzyme in adipose tissue and muscle that catalyzes this triglyceride uptake is lipoprotein lipase (LPL). In adipose tissue the enzyme is synthesized in the fat cell, and following secretion and transport to the capillary endothelial cell, it hydrolyzes the triglyceride in these lipoproteins at the endothelial surface. At least two of the three fatty acids potentially releasable from triglyceride hydrolysis are then transported to the fat cell, where

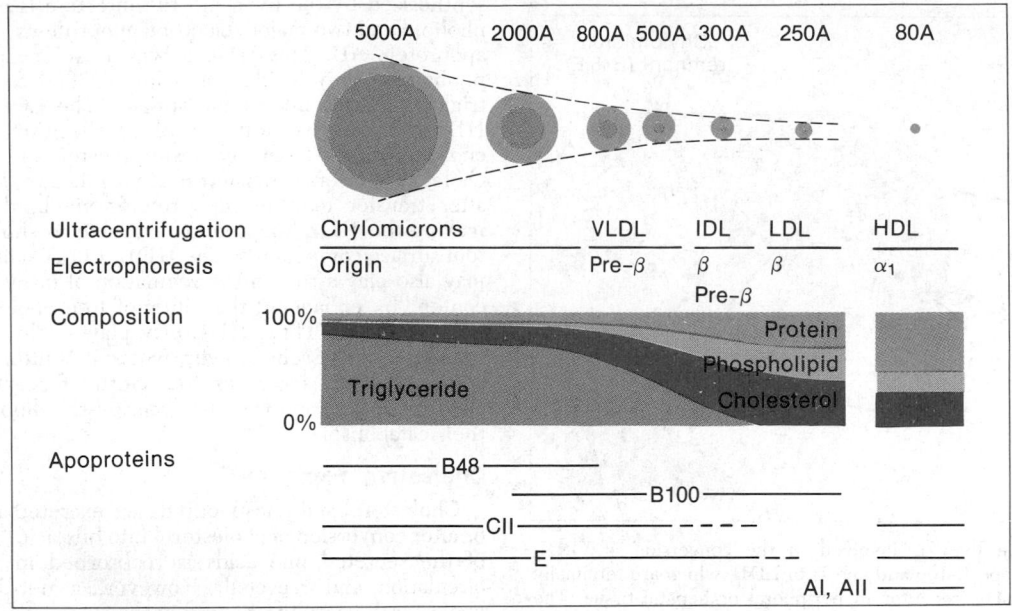

FIGURE 172–1. Classification of plasma lipoproteins by physical and chemical properties. (Modified from Bierman EL: Current Concepts: Hyperlipoproteinemia. The Upjohn Company, 1984.)

they are re-esterified with glycerol and stored as intracellular adipocyte triglyceride. The vast majority of the triglyceride in the adipocyte enters by this mechanism; little lipogenesis occurs de novo from glucose in adipose tissue in humans. The functional activity of LPL in adipose tissue is increased during and after meals. In humans, most of this increase in function is due to the increase in triglyceride-rich lipoproteins that serve as enzyme substrate. Although insulin is required to maintain LPL levels in adipose tissue, little change in enzyme levels occurs with normal meals. Between meals, calories stored as triglyceride are released from the adipocyte as free fatty acids. This hydrolysis of intracellular adipocyte triglyceride is mediated by "hormone-sensitive" lipase of the fat cells. Between meals, when insulin levels are low and glucagon is increasing, hormone-sensitive lipase activity increases, and free fatty acids are released to be used for energy utilization by most tissues of the body.

The interaction of LPL with triglyceride in triglyceride-rich lipoproteins requires a cofactor, apoprotein CII. When secreted from the absorptive cell of the gut and from the liver, chylomicrons and VLDL do not contain this activator. Shortly after entering plasma these lipoproteins pick up apoprotein CII from a reservoir in circulating HDL. Thus the triglyceride-rich lipoproteins contain both substrate and activator for their hydrolysis by LPL. Following hydrolysis of the triglyceride in these lipoproteins, the apoprotein CII is released and again picked up by HDL. Thus, HDL appears to serve as a shuttle for apoprotein CII (as well as other lipoprotein components) (see below). Other apoproteins (CI and CIII) are transferred bidirectionally between triglyceride-rich lipoproteins and HDL and may play a role in LPL triglyceride hydrolysis, as well as other lipoprotein interactions.

Remnant Lipoprotein Catabolism

Following hydrolysis of the triglyceride in triglyceride-rich lipoproteins and the simultaneous removal of surface components, "remnant" lipoproteins are formed from chylomicrons and endogenous triglyceride-rich lipoproteins. The intermediate density lipoprotein fraction isolated by ultracentrifugation consists largely of remnant particles of VLDL. Those remnants formed from chylomicrons and large endogenous VLDL are often distributed, however, in the density range of small VLDL. Thus, remnants and endogenously synthesized triglyceride-rich lipoproteins cannot be separated completely by ultracentrifugation. Once formed, the remnant has a short half-life in plasma and appears to be taken up by the liver (Fig. 172–3). The endogenous triglyceride-rich lipoprotein remnant is further processed into the cholesterol-rich low density lipoprotein (LDL). During this catabolic process, further triglyceride and cholesterol as well as some surface proteins are removed. The remnant lipoprotein contains apoprotein B and several forms of apoprotein C and apoprotein E. The apoprotein E that accumulates as the remnant lipoproteins are formed appears to be important for hepatic uptake of those remnants. There is a complex interaction of hepatic receptors specific for apoprotein E and other receptors that bind both apoprotein B and apoprotein E, with the apoproteins in the

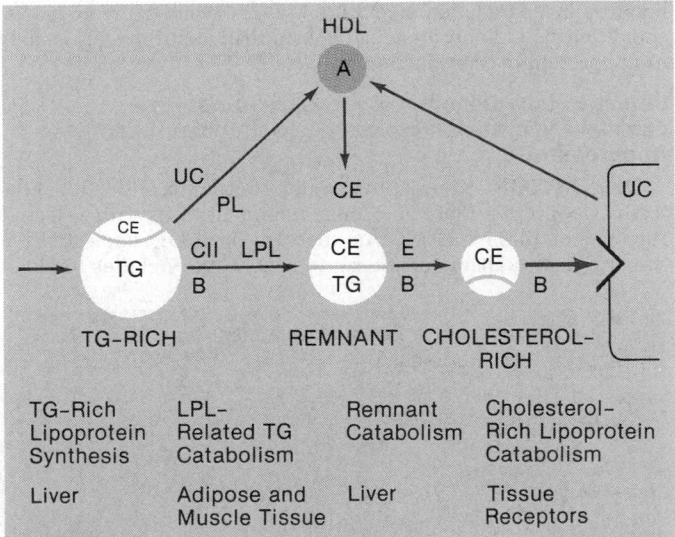

FIGURE 172–2. The triglyceride-rich very low density lipoprotein (VLDL) is synthesized in the liver and contains apo B, which remains with the particle through its subsequent catabolism. The triglyceride-rich lipoprotein core contains triglyceride (TG) and cholesteryl ester (CE) and surface unesterified cholesterol (UC) and phospholipid (PL). Upon entering plasma, acquired apo CII activates lipoprotein lipase (LPL) to catabolize TG core. The resulting remnant acquires apo E, which interacts with hepatic receptors to catabolize remnant to cholesterol-rich low density lipoprotein (LDL). The LDL binds to high-affinity receptor, with subsequent intracellular degradation of the lipoprotein. High density lipoproteins with apo AI and AII (A) acquire surface components of lipoproteins and plasma membranes of cells and form cholesteryl esters. These cholesteryl esters exchange with other lipoproteins or are delivered directly to the liver and may be the primary source of biliary cholesterol and bile acids.

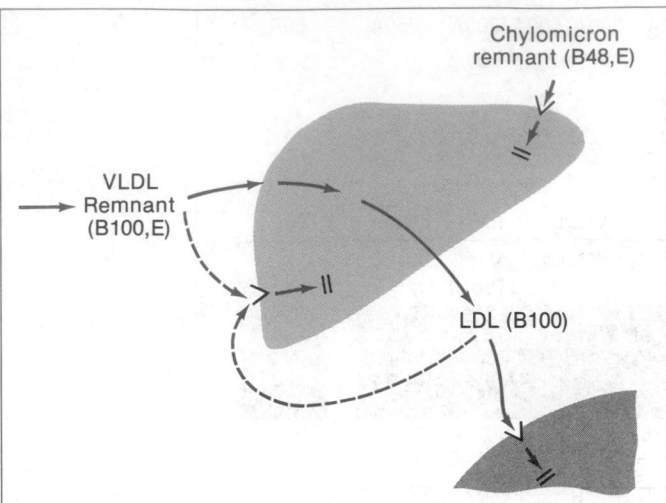

FIGURE 172–3. The liver is involved in the conversion of VLDL remnants containing apo B-100 and apo E to LDL, which are terminally catabolized via the LDL receptor in peripheral or hepatic tissue. The chylomicron remnant containing apo B-48 and apo E is processed completely in the liver via the apo E or chylomicron receptor.

remnant lipoproteins regulating their hepatic uptake. By the time the cholesterol-rich LDL has been formed, apoprotein B is the only apoprotein of the triglyceride-rich lipoproteins remaining.

Cholesterol-Rich Low Density Lipoprotein Catabolism

As the cholesterol-rich LDL normally arises from the remnant lipoprotein of VLDL, it contains the same amount of apoprotein B per lipoprotein particle as endogenous triglyceride-rich VLDL. Other apoproteins have been almost entirely removed, together with much of the phospholipid and some cholesterol. The cholesterol-rich lipoprotein can be removed from plasma by extrahepatic tissues, where it functions as the chief source of cholesterol for membrane synthesis or steroid hormone synthesis by these tissues. Alternatively, the lipoprotein may be taken up by the liver and degraded if not utilized peripherally. Apoprotein B in the cholesterol-rich lipoprotein appears to be recognized by a specific, high-affinity binding site in tissues (Fig. 172–4). Once bound, the lipoprotein is internalized by the cell in an endocytotic vesicle that fuses with a primary or pre-existing secondary lysosome. The protein moiety is degraded, and the cholesteryl ester is hydrolyzed to unesterified cholesterol by a lysosomal acid cholesteryl ester hydrolase. Hydrolysis of the triglyceride and phospholipid may also occur in the lysosome. The cell is able to regulate its own cholesterol content through a feedback control system in which intracellular free cholesterol suppresses endogenous cholesterol production by inhibiting the rate-limiting enzyme in cholesterol synthesis (HMG-CoA reductase). Furthermore, accumulation of intracellular free cholesterol limits the further uptake of cholesterol-rich lipoproteins by inhibiting synthesis of the lipoprotein receptor itself and stimulates its own re-esterification to cholesteryl ester by activating an acyl CoA:cholesterol transferase in the cytosol. Cholesterol content in the cell also is regulated by a receptor-mediated system involving HDL as a vehicle for cholesterol.

Apoprotein B containing lipoproteins may also be degraded by a scavenger system other than the high-affinity LDL receptor. This scavenger pathway involves the macrophage system and assumes greater importance in lipoprotein catabolism when defects in the LDL receptor or other abnormalities in lipoprotein catabolism exist.

Lipoprotein Surface Catabolism

Newly synthesized lipoproteins with their hydrophobic triglyceride and cholesteryl ester core are surrounded by a monolayer composed of protein, unesterified cholesterol, and phospholipid. As the core is removed and the lipoprotein decreases in size, several mechanisms process the resulting "excess" surface. The

catabolism of these surface components involves HDL and the enzyme lecithin-cholesterol acyl transferase (LCAT). The HDL synthesized by the liver and the intestine is composed of phospholipid and two major structural apoproteins, apoprotein AI and apoprotein AII. This HDL serves as an acceptor for the phospholipid (mainly lecithin) and unesterified cholesterol from the triglyceride-rich lipoprotein surface. The LCAT associated with HDL then removes a fatty acid from lecithin and transfers it to cholesterol, producing cholesteryl ester and lysolecithin. The cholesteryl ester is transferred from HDL to the liver directly or after transfer to other lipoproteins via lipid transfer protein, making the HDL apoproteins available to shuttle more lipoprotein surface components. The HDL, LCAT, and transfer proteins may also play a role in the regulation of intracellular cholesterol content by enhancing the efflux of free cholesterol from extrahepatic tissues. Thus, HDL may play a role in the transport of cholesterol from cells to liver, where it is ultimately excreted. In addition, HDL serves as the shuttle for apoprotein CII and apoprotein E to and from triglyceride-rich lipoproteins as part of their catabolism.

Cholesterol Excretion

Cholesterol and phospholipids are excreted as such in the bile, or after conversion of cholesterol into bile acid. A large proportion of the secreted bile acids is reabsorbed in the enterohepatic circulation and recycled. However, a net loss of bile acid, cholesterol, and phospholipid in the stool occurs by this pathway.

The definitive source of the cholesterol for output in the bile and for bile acid formation has not been determined. Cholesterol excreted into the bile may be synthesized directly in the liver. Alternatively, cholesterol may be secreted from the liver and gut in triglyceride-rich lipoproteins and may be esterified by the LCAT-HDL system, and it may re-enter the liver directly with HDL or via remnant lipoproteins.

INBORN ERRORS OF LIPOPROTEIN METABOLISM

The primary, or inborn, errors of lipoprotein metabolism leading to hyperlipidemia generally can be grouped into disorders associated with overproduction of triglyceride-rich lipoproteins or disorders due to defects in one of three catabolic steps in lipoprotein degradation (see Fig. 172–2). Much more is known about defects in lipoprotein catabolism than about defects leading to lipoprotein overproduction (Table 172–1).

Defective Low Density Lipoprotein Catabolism: Familial Hypercholesterolemia and Familial Defective Apoprotein B

DEFINITION. Familial hypercholesterolemia and familial defective apoprotein B are autosomal dominant traits with defective removal of plasma LDL. An increase in LDL cholesterol is associated with characteristic xanthomas in the Achilles tendons,

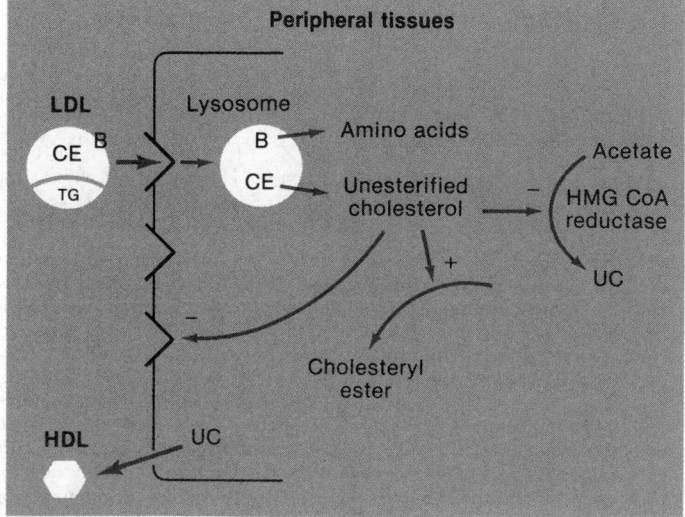

FIGURE 172–4. LDL containing apo B are removed from plasma by a high-affinity receptor and are processed in the lysosome. The resulting unesterified cholesterol regulates the cellular homeostatic mechanisms.

TABLE 172–1. INBORN ERRORS OF LIPOPROTEIN METABOLISM

Name	Prevalence	Physiologic Abnormality	Protein Abnormality	Lipoprotein Phenotype	Lipoproteins That Accumulate
Familial hypercholesterolemia	1/500	↓ LDL catabolism	Abnormal LDL receptor	IIA (IIB)	LDL ± VLDL
Familial dysbetalipoproteinemia	1/10,000	↓ Remnant catabolism	Abnormal apoprotein E	III	β VLDL
Lipoprotein lipase or apoprotein CII deficiency	Very rare	↓ TG catabolism	Absence of LPL or apo-protein CII	I (V)	Chylo ± VLDL
Familial hypertriglyceridemia	? 1/200	↑ VLDL-TG and bile acid synthesis	?	IV (V)	VLDL ± chylo
Familial combined hyperlipid-emia	? 1/100	↑ Apoprotein B synthesis	Probably heterogeneous	IIA, IIB, IV	LDL and/or VLDL

Phenotypes based on World Health Organization recommendations.
Chylo = chylomicron; TG = triglyceride.

the patellar tendons, and the extensor tendons of the hands and with early coronary artery disease.

ETIOLOGY AND PATHOGENESIS. This disorder in LDL catabolism is caused by one of several alleles producing an abnormal LDL receptor or the ligand for that receptor, apoprotein B-100. One receptor allele is associated with the absence of LDL receptor synthesis and the others with the production of receptors of abnormal composition. These nonfunctional receptors are associated with decreased LDL catabolism and, in the heterozygote, with an approximate twofold increase in LDL levels. In the very rare homozygote, no receptor degradation occurs, and LDL is removed by a lower affinity "scavenger" pathway with a sixfold or greater increase of cholesterol-rich lipoproteins in plasma. In familial defective apoprotein B, amino acid 3500 of apoprotein B is mutated, impairing binding to the LDL receptor.

CLINICAL MANIFESTATIONS. This disorder often manifests as coronary artery disease in a young man, who then is noted to have elevated cholesterol levels. The mean age of the first myocardial infarction in men with heterozygous familial hypercholesterolemia who develop atherosclerosis is about 41 years. Affected women without additional risk factors may go through life without clinical manifestations of atherosclerosis. Low HDL cholesterol levels and cigarette smoking have marked effects on accelerating coronary artery disease and may be the major determinants of clinical disease in women. Peripheral vascular disease and cerebrovascular disease do not seem to be increased as much as coronary artery disease in this disorder. Lipid deposits in tendons are pathognomonic for this disorder. These xanthomas, usually bilateral, may be nodular irregularities in the Achilles tendons or extensor tendons of the hands but can extend to diffuse, generalized thickening. Corneal arcus and xanthelasma may occur but are found with other lipoprotein abnormalities as well.

DIAGNOSIS. Plasma cholesterol levels in familial hypercholesterolemia are in the upper 1 per cent of levels seen in the general population (e.g., 300 to 500 mg per deciliter). Since this disease seems to be present in 1 in 500 individuals, at least 1 person in 5 with such plasma cholesterol levels (and normal triglyceride levels) would be expected to have this disease. Patients with defective remnant removal and those with chylomicronemia may also have markedly elevated cholesterol levels, but they can be distinguished by the degree of coincident hypertriglyceridemia. Hypothyroidism and the nephrotic syndrome are also associated with elevated cholesterol levels. The increase in LDL in familial hypercholesterolemia uniquely is persistent, is almost always present in a parent, and is detectable at birth. The coexistence of tendon xanthomas and hypercholesterolemia is diagnostic of this disorder. Unilateral Achilles tendon thickening may be the result of injury.

TREATMENT. Discontinuation of smoking should be the first consideration for those who smoke. A diet low in saturated fat and cholesterol should be initiated in all affected individuals with this disorder, even though only a 5 to 15 per cent reduction in LDL levels occurs. Normalization of LDL levels may occur with the combination of a bile acid–binding resin (15 to 30 grams per day in divided doses with meals) combined with high-dose nicotinic acid with meals and at bedtime (1.0 to 4.0 grams per day). Compliance with each drug regimen has been poor. Fat-soluble vitamins should be given at bedtime, since the resins (colestipol or cholestyramine) prevent their absorption. Some recommend therapy with nicotinic acid and resins for all affected individuals. More conservatively, treatment can be restricted to postadolescent males and women with additional risk factors for coronary artery disease. Lovastatin, a drug that suppresses hepatic HMG-CoA reductase and hepatic cholesterol synthesis (at 20 to 80 mg per day), may be combined with a bile acid–binding resin for effective lowering of LDL levels.

Remnant Removal Disease: Dysbetalipoproteinemia

DEFINITION. This disorder is due to the interaction between (1) an autosomal recessive defect in apoprotein E with abnormal remnant catabolism and (2) independent overproduction of triglyceride-rich lipoproteins. This situation results in the accumulation of post-LPL remnants from both chylomicrons and endogenously synthesized VLDL that lead to xanthomas and coronary artery and peripheral vascular disease.

ETIOLOGY AND PATHOGENESIS. About 1 per cent of individuals have two genes leading to an abnormal apoprotein E. Multiple alleles exist for apoprotein E; those producing amino acid substitutions in a critical region of the apoprotein have abnormal apoprotein E binding to hepatic membranes. Affected individuals either have two identical abnormal genes or are compound heterozygotes with two different abnormal genes. Most of these individuals do not have hyperlipidemia but rather have low plasma cholesterol and LDL levels, presumably because of defective conversion of VLDL remnants to LDL. VLDL remnants that are cholesteryl ester enriched are present, but plasma triglyceride levels are usually normal. About 1 in 100 individuals with this abnormal apoprotein E has hyperlipidemia with remnant removal disease. These individuals appear to have an independent abnormality leading to hypertriglyceridemia in addition to the defect in apoprotein E, and they accumulate significant levels of chylomicron and VLDL remnants. Much rarer forms of remnant removal disease are caused by total absence of apoprotein E.

CLINICAL MANIFESTATIONS. This disorder may present initially as premature clinical atherosclerosis or as planar or tuberous xanthomas, or it may be detected as hyperlipidemia on routine laboratory screen. This disorder is usually not manifested as an abnormality in triglyceride or cholesterol levels in men until the third or fourth decade or in women until after menopause. The coexistent apoprotein E abnormality can be detected at birth. The onset of the xanthomas also is late. Planar xanthomas of the palmar crease and tuberous or tuberoeruptive xanthomas are highly suggestive of this disorder, although both can occur in severe, chronic obstructive liver disease with residual hepatocellular function. Atherosclerosis often is first noted in men around age 50 years. Peripheral vascular disease often predominates, but coronary artery disease is increased as well. In women, development of peripheral vascular and coronary artery disease after menopause is rapid compared with that in nonaffected females. The presence of estrogen in the premenopausal state seems to minimize the defect in remnant catabolism.

DIAGNOSIS. The presence of palmar or tuberous xanthomas in the absence of liver disease is diagnostic. Plasma cholesterol and triglyceride are increased to similar levels. A method for separation of VLDL from the remainder of the more dense lipoproteins is necessary to demonstrate that these VLDL are cholesteryl ester enriched and have beta mobility on electrophoresis ("beta VLDL") rather than the typical pre-beta mobility of

VLDL. An abnormal apoprotein E can usually be demonstrated by isoelectric focusing. The concentration of LDL is typically low, and HDL is often normal or slightly depressed. Hypothyroidism can aggravate this disorder or rarely can lead to remnant accumulation by itself.

TREATMENT. In obese individuals with this disorder, weight loss should be considered in lowering triglyceride and cholesterol levels. In postmenopausal women, low-dose ethinyl estradiol seems to normalize the defect in remnant removal and to correct the hypercholesterolemia. Clofibrate (1 gram twice a day) or gemfibrozil (0.6 gram twice a day) also is effective in decreasing lipid levels. Alternatively, high-dose nicotinic acid is considered by some investigators to be the drug of choice for treatment of this disorder. There is evidence that the form of atherosclerosis occurring with this disorder is partially reversible with treatment.

Defective Lipoprotein Lipase–Related Triglyceride Catabolism

DEFINITION. Familial LPL deficiency is a rare autosomal recessive trait characterized by complete absence of active enzyme protein in all tissues, leading to massive hypertriglyceridemia from birth and recurrent episodes of pancreatitis. Similar syndromes also are caused by inborn defects in other aspects of the LPL system.

ETIOLOGY AND PATHOGENESIS. Hydrolysis of triglyceride from chylomicrons and endogenous VLDL in vivo requires both LPL and its activator apoprotein CII. A defect of either of these proteins is associated with severely decreased triglyceride removal and massive hypertriglyceridemia. In infants and young children, the triglyceride accumulates primarily as chylomicron triglyceride of dietary origin. As the patient gets older, a defect in VLDL triglyceride removal becomes more apparent as well. Both LPL and apoprotein CII deficiency are autosomal recessive disorders; often consanguinity can be documented. A number of defects in the genes for LPL and apoprotein CII have been described. Individuals also exist who have LPL activity missing from only selected tissues or who have a familial inhibitor of LPL activity. These latter groups usually have less severe hypertriglyceridemia and become symptomatic later in life than in the classic form of LPL deficiency.

CLINICAL MANIFESTATIONS. Infants with LPL deficiency rapidly manifest intolerance to fatty foods. As these children grow, they learn to avoid certain high-fat foods, such as whole milk. Abdominal pain, often with pancreatitis, occurs in association with the high levels of chylomicron triglyceride. Eruptive xanthomas occur on extensor surfaces, notably the elbows, knees, and the buttocks, and are pathognomonic for chronic chylomicronemia. Hepatomegaly and occasionally splenomegaly occur because of the accumulation of lipid-laden foam cells. The hepatosplenomegaly rapidly diminishes on a fat-free diet, which clears the chylomicronemia. Eruptive xanthomas also disappear with time after lowering of chylomicron levels. Other signs and symptoms seen with chronic chylomicronemia may also occur (see below).

DIAGNOSIS. A young child with abdominal pain and milky, lactescent plasma should be studied for a genetic abnormality in LPL. Other causes of chylomicronemia before adulthood relate to the occurrence of a common form of hypertriglyceridemia with diabetes or glucocorticoid therapy. Absent or diminished activity of LPL can be demonstrated in adipose tissue or muscle tissue, or in plasma after administration of intravenous heparin. Apoprotein CII deficiency can be detected by radioimmunoassay or by gel electrophoresis of the protein components of lipoproteins or by testing the ability of the patient's plasma to activate purified LPL.

TREATMENT. In all the inborn errors of the LPL-related triglyceride removal system associated with chylomicronemia, a decrease in total dietary fat is absolutely indicated. A total of polyunsaturated and saturated fat as low as 10 to 20 per cent of calories is often required. Medium-chain triglycerides can be used to prepare some foods, since their fatty acids leave the gut unesterified via the portal vein rather than via the thoracic duct, as does chylomicron triglyceride. The goal is to decrease the amount of dietary fat to a level low enough to eliminate the

occurrence of abdominal pain. These individuals can also be sensitive to agents that raise endogenous VLDL levels, such as alcohol or glucocorticoids, and to the effects of pregnancy.

Other Genetic Disorders with Mild to Moderate Hypertriglyceridemia

A number of less well characterized disorders associated with persistent or intermittent elevated VLDL levels exist. Some may be associated with increased hepatic secretion of VLDL, others with defective VLDL catabolism. It has been useful to classify those conditions into several relatively homogeneous groups on the basis of the existence of large, well-characterized families for each.

FAMILIAL HYPERTRIGLYCERIDEMIA. This apparently autosomal dominant trait may be quite common. Individuals with familial hypertriglyceridemia appear to have a defect leading to enhanced hepatic triglyceride synthesis with subsequent secretion of triglyceride-enriched, large VLDL. These individuals may also have increased cholesterol and cholic acid synthesis. LPL-related triglyceride removal and remnant lipoprotein catabolism appear to be normal. The LDL levels are normal, while HDL is triglyceride enriched with depletion of HDL cholesterol.

Most individuals with this disorder do not have an increased predisposition for coronary artery disease, remain asymptomatic, and are detected by routine lipid screen. Occasionally, with the onset of another disorder associated with elevated triglyceride levels, they develop the chylomicronemia syndrome (see below). These individuals develop no characteristic xanthomas. There is no increase in obesity in this disorder and no increase in the frequency of diabetes.

Persons with this disorder have persistent hypertriglyceridemia once they become adults. Below the age of 20, the abnormality usually is not manifested. Some of the increase in VLDL may persist after weight loss. Increased levels of LDL do not occur. One parent is characteristically affected, as are half of the siblings. These individuals appear to be quite sensitive to other factors that cause only mild hypertriglyceridemia in normal adults: obesity and alcohol, as well as estrogen, diuretic, beta-adrenergic blocker, and glucocorticoid therapy.

Treatment with clofibrate or gemfibrozil usually leads to significant decreases in VLDL levels. In families without evidence of increased atherosclerosis, no known benefit accrues from this therapy, and it should be discouraged. Drugs causing elevation of triglyceride levels should be avoided because they may precipitate massive chylomicronemia and pancreatitis.

FAMILIAL COMBINED HYPERLIPIDEMIA. It was first pointed out in 1973 that this disorder is very common in those with premature coronary artery disease, is inherited as an autosomal dominant trait, and is characterized by different "combinations" of hyperlipidemia: elevated cholesterol level alone, elevated triglyceride level alone, or elevations in levels of both lipids (familial multiple lipoprotein–type hyperlipidemia). It now appears that this disorder is better characterized as one with elevated plasma apoprotein B levels with variable lipid phenotype even in the same individual at different times, in contrast to familial hypercholesterolemia. The increase in apoprotein B, whether in VLDL or in LDL, appears to be caused by increased hepatic synthesis of the apoprotein. These individuals also have abnormalities in HDL, with a mild decrease in HDL cholesterol and apoprotein AI.

Men with this disorder have premature coronary artery disease with a mean age of infarct at about 40 years. Smoking has a marked effect on the prevalence of clinical heart disease. Individuals with this disorder are slightly more obese and may have more systemic hypertension. They have no characteristic xanthomas but occasionally have nonspecific xanthelasma.

OTHER FORMS OF HYPERTRIGLYCERIDEMIA. Individuals with chylomicronemia and triglyceride levels between 1000 and 2000 mg per deciliter are said to aggregate in families. In addition, there are individuals with primary hypertriglyceridemia who are noted to have a defect in VLDL removal not characterized by one of the above defects in the LPL system.

APPROACH TO THE PATIENT WITH MILD TO MODERATE HYPERTRIGLYCERIDEMIA. The major concern for the individual with hypertriglyceridemia relates to a possible increase in risk for atherosclerosis. When an individual is identified with elevated plasma triglyceride levels, acquired forms of hyperlipidemia should be identified and treated, and the primary forms of hypertriglyceridemia associated with defective remnant catabolism or LPL deficiency should be ruled out.

Elevations in plasma triglyceride levels often serve as a marker for associated abnormalities potentially related to atherosclerosis. A strong family history of early coronary artery disease in the father or mother's male relatives helps to identify such a hypertriglyceridemic individual at risk for early atherosclerosis.

The hypertriglyceridemic individuals who intermittently develop hypercholesterolemia caused by increased LDL levels as well as those who have elevated LDL apoprotein B levels with normal LDL cholesterol also seem to be ones at increased risk for atherosclerosis.

The level of HDL cholesterol is often low in the presence of hypertriglyceridemia. This situation can occur with familial LPL deficiency and with familial hypertriglyceridemia and does not seem to be associated with the increase in coronary risk seen with a low HDL cholesterol level in the absence of hypertriglyceridemia. However, a decrease in the level of the major apoprotein of HDL, apoprotein AI, seems to be a good predictor of risk, even in the presence of hypertriglyceridemia.

The aforementioned abnormalities characteristic of the hypertriglyceridemic subject at risk for atherosclerosis are similar to those in familial combined hyperlipidemia, which may account for a significant portion of this group.

While weight loss and clofibrate (or gemfibrozil) therapy lower VLDL levels, those at risk for early coronary artery disease may respond with an increase in LDL levels. Preferred therapy for the hypertriglyceridemic individual at risk, in particular the one with familial combined hyperlipidemia, may be like that used to treat elevated LDL levels in familial hypercholesterolemia: combined bile acid resin and high-dose nicotinic acid therapy, in addition to a diet low in saturated fat and cholesterol. Because of the uncertainty of the significance of elevated triglyceride levels and the unknown risks of lifelong drug therapy, many authorities have recommended diet therapy alone for hypertriglyceridemia.

ACQUIRED DISORDERS OF LIPOPROTEIN METABOLISM

Some disease states are associated with mild to moderate hyperlipidemia in the absence of primary forms of hyperlipidemia, while others seem to have a significant effect only in the presence of a familial form of hyperlipidemia. In general, these can be divided into conditions associated with increased levels of triglyceride-rich lipoproteins and those associated with multiple lipoprotein-type expression (acquired combined hyperlipidemia) (Table 172–2).

TABLE 172–2. ACQUIRED DISORDERS OF LIPOPROTEIN METABOLISM

A. Hypertriglyceridemia
  1. Mild to moderate hypertriglyceridemia
    a. Diabetes mellitus*
    b. Uremia and/or dialysis*
  2. Minimal hypertriglyceridemia alone
    a. Obesity
    b. Estrogen*
    c. Alcohol*
    d. Beta-adrenergic blocking agents*
  3. Rare forms of moderate to marked hypertriglyceridemia
    a. Systemic lupus erythematosus
    b. Dysgammaglobulinemias
    c. Glycogenosis type I
    d. Lipodystrophy
B. Combined hyperlipidemia
  1. Hypothyroidism*
  2. Nephrotic syndrome
  3. Glucocorticoid excess*
  4. Diuretics*
C. Hypercholesterolemia
  1. Acute intermittent porphyria
  2. Anorexia nervosa

*Can be associated with chylomicronemia syndrome when it occurs with the familial forms of hypertriglyceridemia.

Hypertriglyceridemia

DIABETES MELLITUS. Persons with untreated insulin-dependent diabetes and untreated symptomatic non–insulin-dependent diabetes have low adipose tissue or muscle LPL activity with a mild to moderate increase in triglyceride levels and decreased HDL cholesterol levels. With insulin resistance and milder degrees of insulin deficiency, hypertriglyceridemia is caused by excess free fatty acids mobilized from adipose tissue that are re-esterified in the liver and secreted as endogenous VLDL. Treatment with insulin or oral sulfonylurea agents will correct the abnormality in LPL over a period of weeks. In the treated diabetic, variability in free fatty acid mobilization and hepatic triglyceride synthesis, related to the degree of diabetic control, accounts for most of the variation in triglyceride levels.

CHRONIC UREMIA AND DIALYSIS. Many individuals with chronic uremia have elevated VLDL levels with hypertriglyceridemia and low HDL cholesterol levels. This condition persists after initiation of maintenance hemodialysis or peritoneal dialysis. These lipoprotein abnormalities appear to be related to defects in LPL-mediated triglyceride removal and, with smoking and hypertension, account for the marked atherosclerosis in the dialysis population.

OTHER. Obesity, estrogen use, and alcohol are associated with minimal to mild increases in triglyceride levels, usually not to levels considered abnormal, which appear to be caused by modest increases in hepatic VLDL secretion. Diuretic agents and beta-adrenergic blocking agents are also associated with small increases in triglyceride levels. The diuretics often raise LDL levels, while the beta-blocking agents decrease HDL.

Moderate to marked hypertriglyceridemia occurs extremely rarely in systemic lupus erythematosus or dysgammaglobulinemia caused by an immunoglobulin-lipoprotein interaction. Moderate hypertriglyceridemia can also occur in rare disorders such as glycogenosis (type I), lipodystrophy, and carnitine-palmitoyl transferase deficiency.

Combined Hyperlipidemia

HYPOTHYROIDISM. Thyroid hormone appears to be necessary for proper functioning of most steps in lipoprotein metabolism. Thyroxine is necessary for maintenance of the LDL receptor; in hypothyroidism LDL levels are elevated because of defective catabolism. Remnant removal is impaired, resulting in the accumulation of chylomicron with VLDL remnants, and finally the LPL level is low, resulting in hypertriglyceridemia. Thyroxine replacement corrects all of these defects.

NEPHROTIC SYNDROME. With urinary loss of albumin and the development of hypoalbuminemia, increases in the levels of VLDL or LDL or both occur. These lipoprotein abnormalities are associated with increased hepatic lipid synthesis and defective catabolism of triglyceride-rich lipoproteins. The latter defect may be related to the loss in the urine of cofactors required for LPL function.

GLUCOCORTICOID EXCESS. Excess glucocorticoid levels caused by Cushing's syndrome or exogenous steroid therapy are associated with elevated VLDL and/or LDL levels. The best studied situation is in the glucocorticoid-treated renal transplant subject, who in the absence of uremia or proteinuria has combined hyperlipidemia.

Hypercholesterolemia

Elevated LDL levels may occur in occasional individuals in response to high saturated fat and cholesterol feeding. Much of the hypercholesterolemia in the population has remained unexplained and has been termed multifactorial, suggesting that it is due to the interaction of multiple genes (polygenic) with the environment. Elevated LDL levels occur in acute intermittent porphyria and have been reported with hepatomas and in anorexia nervosa.

HYPERLIPIDEMIA AND ATHEROSCLEROTIC VASCULAR DISEASE

Although the etiology of atherosclerosis is multifactorial, the development of premature coronary artery disease and peripheral vascular disease is strongly dependent on abnormalities in plasma lipoprotein metabolism. Thus, coronary artery disease in men under the age of 60 years and in women of any age is more likely to occur in the presence of an inborn error or acquired form of hyperlipidemia. HDL may independently protect against atherosclerosis. Differences in HDL cholesterol levels between men and women may explain a large part of the sex difference in the risk for atherosclerosis.

Familial hypercholesterolemia is unequivocally associated with premature coronary artery disease, the expression of which is aggravated by cigarette smoking and low HDL cholesterol levels. Remnant removal disease is also associated with peripheral vascular and coronary artery disease. The increased atherosclerosis seen in patients with diabetes and in patients on long-term hemodialysis may also be related in part to abnormalities in lipoprotein metabolism. Nonetheless, all of these disorders still account for only a minor part of premature atherosclerosis. Mildly elevated levels of LDL, apoprotein B, or triglyceride, as well as low levels of HDL cholesterol and apoprotein AI, are likely to be present in the majority of patients with premature coronary artery disease. The frequency of familial combined hyperlipidemia or of other, as yet undefined, genetic forms of hyperlipidemia in this heterogeneous group of individuals has to be determined.

An increased risk for atherosclerosis that is independent of other lipoprotein abnormalties has been associated with elevated levels of lipoprotein (a) (Lp[a]). This lipoprotein consists of LDL with an additional large protein of varying molecular weight, apoprotein (a), attached to the apolipoprotein B. Lp(a) is higher than normal in familial hypercholesterolemia but is low or normal in homozygous LPL deficiency and remnant removal disease. This finding implies that the particle is not processed through the VLDL-LDL cascade and that it is removed via the LDL receptor. Increased lipoprotein (a) levels are associated with increased coronary artery disease, particularly in the presence of other risk factors for atherosclerosis. At present, no effective method lowers Lp(a) levels.

THE NATIONAL CHOLESTEROL EDUCATION PROGRAM

The National Cholesterol Education Program (NCEP) has devised a protocol based on total or LDL cholesterol levels for the detection, evaluation, and treatment of hyperlipidemia. Total cholesterol levels should be screened in young and middle-aged adults and in the children of high-risk families. This initial measurement may be made on a nonfasting plasma sample. The first decision is to determine which individuals are candidates for measurement of fasting plasma lipoproteins (Fig. 172–5). On the basis of data from the Multiple Risk Factor Intervention Trial (MRFIT) on one third of a million middle-aged men, a total cholesterol level above 240 mg per deciliter was arbitrarily called high and that below 200 per deciliter was regarded as desirable. The values between 200 and 240 mg per deciliter were termed borderline. By these criteria, about 15 per cent of the MRFIT men had high total cholesterol levels, 40 per cent had desirable levels, and the remaining 45 per cent had borderline levels. A major goal of the NCEP is to differentiate those borderline individuals who are at risk for premature atherosclerosis from those not at risk. Factors that were defined as indicating increased risk were male sex, a positive family history of premature atherosclerosis, cigarette smoking, hypertension, diabetes, truncal obesity, and an HDL cholesterol level below 35 mg per deciliter. Borderline individuals with two or more of these risk factors, individuals with pre-existing premature atherosclerosis, as well as those with high total cholesterol levels, are candidates for the measurement of fasting total cholesterol, HDL cholesterol, and triglyceride levels. To detect individuals with low HDL levels on a familial basis, individuals with desirable total cholesterol levels who have a strong family history of premature atherosclerosis should also be included.

The second NCEP decision, i.e., the identification of candidates for specific dietary therapy, is based on the LDL cholesterol level (Fig. 172–5). The LDL is calculated as follows:

$$\frac{\text{LDL}}{\text{cholesterol}} = \frac{\text{total}}{\text{cholesterol}} - \frac{\text{HDL}}{\text{cholesterol}} - \frac{\text{triglyceride}}{5}$$

Individuals with high LDL cholesterol levels (above 160 mg per deciliter) and those with borderline levels (130 to 160 mg per deciliter along with other atherosclerotic risk factors should be considered for the American Heart Association Step 1 or Step 2 diets, which restrict dietary saturated fat and cholesterol. While institution of the Step 1 diet can often be accomplished by the physician and staff through elimination of selected foods from the diet, the Step 2 diet usually needs the expertise of a nutrition specialist. The diet can be applied to a wide spectrum of age groups, from those as young as 2 years of age to the elderly, and often works best when based on the family unit. Individuals with desirable LDL levels or borderline levels without other risk factors for atherosclerosis require no specific dietary therapy. When a patient is considered for dietary therapy, the detection and subsequent treatment of causes of hyperlipidemia secondary to other diseases or drugs is essential, such as the replacement of diuretics and beta-adrenergic blocking agents with lipid-neutral medications, if possible.

The third NCEP decision, i.e., the initiation of drug therapy for elevated LDL cholesterol levels, can be considered after the patient has been on a diet low in saturated fat and cholesterol for 3 to 6 months (Fig. 172–5). The LDL level required before drug therapy should be considered is higher than that for dietary intervention. Because of biologic and laboratory variation in cholesterol levels, LDL cholesterol should be measured two or three times before drug therapy is initiated. Drug therapy should ideally be restricted to young and middle aged adults or to those who developed clinical atherosclerosis while middle aged. With rare exceptions, the use of drugs as a form of primary intervention in individuals over 65 years of age who do not have atherosclerosis is not recommended.

A young or middle-aged adult who has been on a diet low in saturated fat and cholesterol diet for 3 to 6 months and who continues to have an LDL cholesterol level higher than 190 mg per deciliter on several occasions is a candidate for drug therapy. Individuals with premature atherosclerosis or those who have high LDL cholesterol levels of 160 to 190 mg per deciliter with other risk factors as noted earlier are also candidates for drug therapy. If an individual has another disease that limits survival, drug therapy for hyperlipidemia should be questioned.

Once the decision has been made to initiate drug therapy, several protocols with single or combined drugs are possible. For milder increases in LDL cholesterol levels (perhaps in the range of 190 to 220 mg per deciliter), low-dose therapy with one to two scoops of bile acid–binding resin once or twice a day with major meals can be effective. Alternatively, 500 mg of crystalline nicotinic acid three times a day or 20 mg of lovastatin in the evening may be used. Higher doses of nicotinic acid (up to 1.0 gram four times a day) or lovastatin (up to 40 mg twice a day) can be used alone, or each can be combined with resin therapy in highly effective programs for lowering of LDL levels. Because of the high risk for muscle necrosis, lovastatin should not be combined with nicotinic acid, cyclosporine, erythromycin, or the fibric acids (clofibrate and gemfibrozil). When using nicotinic acid or lovastatin, it is recommended that liver function be monitored with serum glutamic-oxaloacetic transaminase (SGOT) levels every 6 to 12 weeks initially and then semiannually when treatment has been stabilized. Creatine kinase (CK) levels should be measured during lovastatin therapy. Contraindications to nicotinic acid therapy include liver disease, migraine headache, and insulin-resistant diabetes. The use of slow-release nicotinic acid should be discouraged because the incidence of hepatic dysfunction is high compared with that occurring when regular nicotinic acid is used. Another form of niacin, nicotinamide, does not affect lipid levels. The bile acid–binding resins also bind coumarin derivatives, digoxin, thyroxine, and possibly other drugs. In addition, the resins are contraindicated in patients in whom the increase in cholesterol is associated with triglyceride levels above 400 mg per deciliter, since resins markedly increase the plasma triglyceride toward levels that can cause pancreatitis.

The NCEP guidelines do not directly address the issue of hypertriglyceridemia. Most patients with mildly to moderately elevated triglyceride levels who are at risk for premature atherosclerosis can be treated under the NCEP guidelines by following estimated LDL cholesterol levels. This group of patients includes those with familial combined hyperlipidemia, those with remnant removal disease, and those at risk for atherosclerosis who have

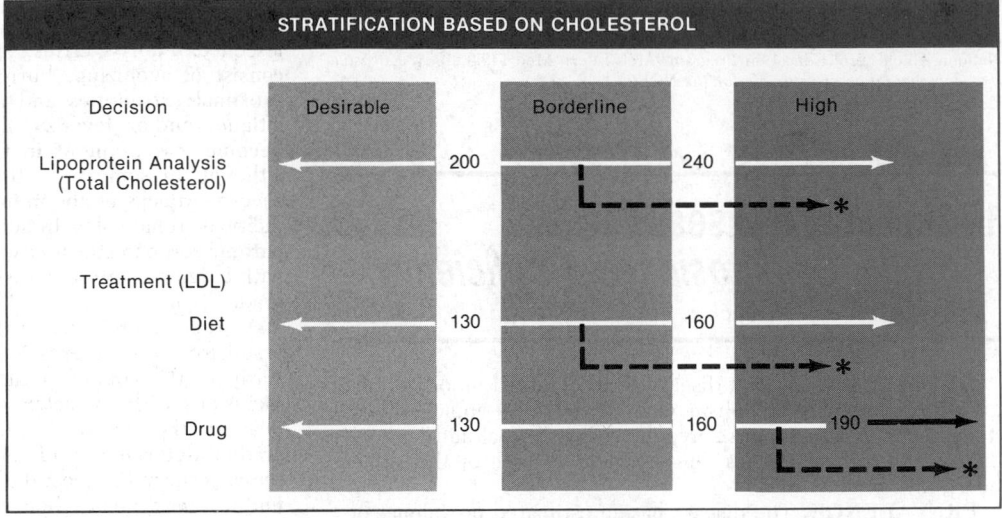

FIGURE 172–5. Stratification based on cholesterol for treatment of hyperlipidemia in patients at risk for premature atherosclerosis. The symbol * and dashed lines indicate high-risk patient; solid lines indicate cholesterol levels at which next step is considered.

other forms of hypertriglyceridemia. The fibric acid drugs (clofibrate and gemfibrozil) are drugs to be used for massive hypertriglyceridemia. They are also useful in remnant removal disease and in the treatment of selected individuals with milder hypertriglyceridemia, such as the patient who simultaneously has elevated triglyceride and LDL levels, as well as low HDL cholesterol levels (lipoprotein phenotype IIB with low HDL). The use of fibric acid drugs should be restricted to these three situations because of the limited benefit and the increased risk of gastrointestinal complications in other forms of hyperlipidemia.

This approach with drug therapy is conservative, focusing on those young to middle-aged men who are at very high risk for premature coronary artery disease due to hyperlipidemia. In North America, little evidence exists that total or LDL cholesterol levels are related to the development of new atherosclerosis in men after the age of 65 years, except at extreme levels, as seen in familial hypercholesterolemia. Therefore, we need to avoid aggressive use of either drug therapy or extremes of dietary modification because of the potential for harm. The majority of coronary artery disease becomes manifest after the age of 65, and we have yet to determine what role lipoproteins play in the risk of this disease in the elderly.

CHYLOMICRONEMIA SYNDROME

DEFINITION. Marked chylomicronemia with plasma triglyceride levels in excess of 2000 mg per deciliter is associated with a constellation of signs and symptoms called the chylomicronemia syndrome.

ETIOLOGY AND PATHOGENESIS. This syndrome can occur because of one of several inborn errors in the LPL system for plasma triglyceride removal as noted earlier. Much more commonly, the marked hypertriglyceridemia occurs as a result of the interaction of two common forms of hypertriglyceridemia, usually one genetic and one acquired. Untreated symptomatic diabetes mellitus in the presence of familial hypertriglyceridemia, familial combined hyperlipidemia, or, less commonly, remnant removal disease is a frequent cause of chylomicronemia. Commonly used drugs that interact with these inborn errors are the estrogens, diuretics, beta-adrenergic blocking agents, alcohol, and glucocorticoids. The effects of these drugs are often markedly exaggerated in patients with pre-existing hyperlipidemia. Hypothyroidism and uremia may also occasionally contribute.

CLINICAL MANIFESTATIONS. For unexplained reasons, some individuals are asymptomatic with plasma triglyceride levels as high as 29,000 mg per deciliter. More commonly, abdominal pain and/or pancreatitis or even chest pain is present. Impairment of recent memory can often be detected, and the patient may complain of paresthesias of the extremities, similar to the carpal tunnel syndrome. Lipemia retinalis can often be observed, hepatomegaly is common, splenomegaly can occur, and eruptive xanthomas are evidence of chronic chylomicronemia. All of these symptoms and signs clear when triglyceride levels are decreased

below 1000 or 2000 mg per deciliter. Marked hypertriglyceridemia may cause insulin resistance and impair control of diabetes. Also, many routine laboratory tests are invalid in the presence of milky plasma. Simple removal of chylomicrons from plasma by short-term ultracentrifugation helps to avoid this problem.

DIAGNOSIS. It is very simple to make a presumptive diagnosis of chylomicronemia syndrome by visual examination of the patient's plasma. Milky plasma always indicates the presence of chylomicrons, as does a plasma triglyceride level above 1000 mg per deciliter. In the presence of symptoms and signs of the chylomicronemia syndrome, a definitive diagnosis is made if these clear when the triglyceride level is lowered.

TREATMENT. With pancreatitis, the discontinuation of oral intake rapidly decreases triglyceride levels. With refeeding, fat must be avoided initially and replaced slowly. Often, mild to moderate abdominal pain can be treated by lowering dietary fat content and avoiding alcohol. The mainstay of treatment is to identify the causes of the elevation in triglyceride levels. A genetic form of hypertriglyceridemia is invariably present and may need to be treated with clofibrate, gemfibrozil, or nicotinic acid. The last drug is difficult to use in diabetic patients because it impairs insulin sensitivity. The acquired disease or agent contributing to the hypertriglyceridemia should be treated or removed, respectively. Slowly, the patient can be refed while the plasma is watched for turbidity and the patient's symptoms and signs are observed. With appropriate therapy, the chylomicronemia syndrome should rarely recur.

RARE DISORDERS OF LIPOPROTEIN METABOLISM

Several rare inherited disorders of lipoprotein metabolism are of considerable theoretical importance because they assist in the understanding of normal lipoprotein physiology. Each of these disorders is an autosomal recessive trait.

Abetalipoproteinemia presents in early childhood and is associated with the absence of apoprotein B–containing lipoproteins because of defective synthesis. Intestinal fat malabsorption, ataxia, neuropathy, retinitis pigmentosa, and acanthocytosis result. *Tangier disease* presents in childhood with absence of HDL and extremely low levels of apoproteins AI and AII. Cholesteryl esters are deposited in tonsils and other lymphoid tissues, and corneal opacities develop. *Lecithin-cholesterol acyl transferase deficiency* presents in the young adult as hemolytic anemia and renal failure. Although the free cholesterol level in plasma is variable, the cholesteryl ester level is very low. Other, even rarer disorders are described in recent reviews.

Diet and Health. Implications for Reducing Chronic Disease Risk. Committee on Diet and Health, Food and Nutrition Board, Commission on Life Sciences, National Research Council. Washington, D.C., National Academy Press, 1989. *Well-referenced reviews concerning dietary therapy and atherosclerosis.*

LaRosa JC: Lipid disorders. Endocrinol Metab Clin North Am 19:211, Philadelphia, W. B. Saunders Company, 1990. *Twelve short clinical articles about hyperlipidemia and its complications.*

Lipoprotein and lipid metabolism disorders. *In* Scriver CR, Beaudet AL, Sly WS, et al. (eds.): The Metabolic Basis of Inherited Disease. 6th ed. New York, McGraw-Hill, 1989, pp 1129–1302. *Nine detailed, extensive reviews about inborn errors of lipoprotein metabolism.*

National Cholesterol Education Program. Arch Intern Med 148:3, 1988. *Extensive documentation of rationale for the NCEP.*

173 Fabry's Disease (α-Galactosidase A Deficiency)

Robert J. Desnick

DEFINITION. Fabry's disease is an X-linked inborn error of glycosphingolipid metabolism characterized by angiokeratomas (telangiectatic skin lesions), hypohidrosis, corneal and lenticular opacities, acroparesthesias, and vascular disease of the kidney, heart, and brain.

PREVALENCE. The disease has an estimated prevalence of 1 in 40,000 males.

ETIOLOGY AND PATHOGENESIS. Fabry's disease is an X-linked recessive trait that is manifested in affected males. Heterozygous females are usually asymptomatic or exhibit mild disease manifestations.

The disease results from the deficient activity of α-galactosidase A, a lysosomal enzyme encoded by a gene located on the long arm of the X chromosome (Xq21.33–Xq22). The enzymatic defect leads to the systemic accumulation of the neutral glycosphingolipid globotriaosylceramide, particularly in the plasma and lysosomes of vascular endothelial and smooth muscle cells. The progressive vascular glycosphingolipid deposition in affected males results in ischemia and infarction, leading to the major disease manifestations. Affected males who are in blood group B or AB have a more severe disease course, as these blood group substances also accumulate because of the enzyme deficiency. The complementary DNA (cDNA) and genomic sequences encoding α-galactosidase A have been isolated and characterized. Molecular studies have identified a variety of different mutations in the α-galactosidase A gene that are responsible for this lysosomal storage disease; these mutations include amino acid substitutions, gene rearrangements, and messenger RNA (mRNA) splicing defects.

PATHOLOGY. Fabry's disease is characterized by the marked deposition of globotriaosylceramide and related glycosphingolipids with terminal α-galactosyl moieties in the lysosomes of endothelial, perithelial, and smooth muscle cells of blood vessels. These glycosphingolipid deposits are also prominent in epithelial cells of the cornea, in glomeruli and tubules of the kidney, in muscle fibers of the heart, and in ganglion cells of the dorsal roots and autonomic nervous system. The skin lesions are telangiectases. Capillaries, venules, and arterioles show pathologic lipid storage, and there is marked dilatation of the capillaries of the dermal papillae just below the epidermis. The larger lesions are usually located in the upper dermis, where they may produce elevation, flattening, or hypertrophy of the epithelium, with keratosis—hence the term *angiokeratoma*. Ultrastructurally, the glycosphingolipid inclusions in lysosomes have a concentrically arranged lamellar or myelin-like structure.

CLINICAL MANIFESTATIONS. The angiokeratomas usually occur in childhood and may lead to early diagnosis. They increase in size and number with age and range from barely visible to several millimeters in diameter. The lesions are punctate, dark red to blue-black, and flat or slightly raised. They do not blanch with pressure, and the larger ones may show slight hyperkeratosis. Characteristically, the lesions are most dense between the umbilicus and knees, in the "bathing trunk area," but may occur anywhere, including the oral mucosa. The hips, thighs, buttocks, umbilicus, lower abdomen, scrotum, and glans penis are common sites, and there is a tendency toward bilateral symmetry. Variants without skin lesions have been described. Sweating is usually decreased or absent. Corneal opacities and characteristic lenticular lesions, observed on slit-lamp examination, are present in affected males as well as in about 70 per cent of asymptomatic heterozygotes. Conjunctival and retinal vascular lesions are common and result from the systemic vascular involvement.

Pain is the most debilitating symptom in childhood and adolescence. Fabry's crises, lasting from minutes to several days, consist of agonizing, burning pain in the hands and feet and proximal extremities and are usually associated with exercise, fatigue, and/or fevers. These painful acroparesthesias usually become less frequent in the third and fourth decades of life, although in some men they may become more frequent and severe. Attacks of abdominal or flank pain may simulate appendicitis or renal colic. In addition, many affected men experience chronic acroparesthesias, which may occur daily, often associated with fatigue, exercise, stress, changes in the weather, and/or low-grade fevers.

As the patient's age increases, the major morbid symptoms result from the progressive involvement of the vascular system. Early in the course of the disease, casts, red cells, and lipid inclusions with characteristic birefringent "Maltese crosses" appear in the urinary sediment. Proteinuria, isothenuria, and gradual deterioration of renal function and development of azotemia occur in the second to fourth decades of life. Cardiovascular findings may include hypertension, left ventricular hypertrophy, anginal chest pain, myocardial ischemia or infarction, and congestive heart failure. Mitral insufficiency is the most common valvular lesion. Abnormal electrocardiographic and echocardiographic findings are common. Cerebrovascular manifestations result primarily from multifocal small vessel involvement. Other features may include chronic bronchitis and dyspnea, lymphedema of the legs without hypoproteinemia, episodic diarrhea, osteoporosis, retarded growth, and delayed puberty. Death most often results from uremia or vascular disease of the heart or brain. Prior to hemodialysis or renal transplantation, the mean age of death for affected men was 41 years. Atypical male variants with residual α-galactosidase A activity who are asymptomatic or mildly affected have been described.

DIAGNOSIS AND DIFFERENTIAL DIAGNOSIS. The diagnosis in affected males is most readily made from the history of painful acroparesthesias and hypohidrosis, the presence of characteristic skin lesions, and the observation of the corneal opacities and lenticular lesions. The disorder is often misdiagnosed as rheumatic fever, erythromelalgia, or neurosis. The skin lesions must be differentiated from the benign angiokeratomas of the scrotum in older men (Fordyce's disease) or from angiokeratoma circumscriptum. Angiokeratomas identical to those of Fabry's disease have been reported in fucosidosis, aspartylglycosaminuria, galactosialidosis, α-N-acetylgalactosaminidase deficiency, and sialidosis. The diagnosis is confirmed biochemically by the demonstration of markedly decreased α-galactosidase A activity in plasma, isolated leukocytes, or cultured fibroblasts or lymphoblasts.

Heterozygous females may have corneal opacities, isolated skin lesions, and intermediate activities of α-galactosidase A in plasma or cell sources. Rare female heterozygotes may have manifestations as severe as those in affected males. However, at-risk females in families affected by Fabry's disease who are asymptomatic should be studied by DNA diagnostic techniques, including the analysis of restriction fragment length polymorphisms (RFLP's) in and near the α-galactosidase A gene as well as the direct detection of the specific mutation in each family. Prenatal detection of affected males can be accomplished by the demonstration of deficient α-galactosidase A activity in chorionic villi obtained in the first trimester or in cultured amniocytes obtained by amniocentesis in the second trimester of pregnancy.

TREATMENT. Phenyltoin and carbamazepine have been shown to decrease the frequency and severity of the chronic acroparesthesias and the periodic crises of excruciating pain. Otherwise, treatment of the disease complications is supportive and nonspecific. Renal transplantation and chronic hemodialysis have become life-saving procedures. Replacement therapy using partially purified human enzyme has proved to be biochemically effective in pilot trials; however, sufficient enzyme has not been available to evaluate the clinical effectiveness of long-term replacement therapy. The recent availability of the cDNA encoding human α-galactosidase A should permit the future expression of sufficient quantities of recombinantly produced, active enzyme for further trials of enzyme replacement therapy.

Bernstein HS, Bishop DF, Astrin KH, et al.: Fabry disease: Six gene rearrangements and an exonic point mutation in the α-galactosidase A gene. J Clin Invest 83:1390, 1989. *Description of the first mutations in classic and variant cases.*

Desnick RJ, Bishop DF: Fabry disease: α-Galactosidase deficiency and Schindler disease: α-N-acetylgalactosaminidase deficiency. *In* Scriver CR, Beaudet AL, Sly WS, et al. (eds.): The Metabolic Basis of Inherited Disease. 6th ed. New York, McGraw-Hill, 1989. *A definitive chapter describing clinical, pathologic, biochemical, and molecular manifestations of Fabry's disease; more than 400 references.*

Desnick RJ, Dean KJ, Grabowski GA, et al.: Enzyme therapy XII: Enzyme therapy in Fabry disease: Differential *in vivo* plasma clearance and metabolic effectiveness of plasma and splenic α-galactosidase A isozymes. Proc Natl Acad Sci USA 76:5326, 1979. *Demonstration of the biochemical effectiveness and immunologic safety of enzyme replacement therapy.*

Sher NA, Letson RD, Desnick RJ: The ocular manifestations of Fabry's disease. Arch Ophthalmol 97:671, 1979. *A comprehensive and well-illustrated article on the ocular lesions in affected males and carrier females.*

Von Scheidt W, Eng CD, Fitzmaurice TF, et al.: An atypical variant of Fabry's disease confined to the heart. N Engl J Med 324:395, 1991. *A recently recognized mild variant of Fabry's disease with manifestations limited to the heart.*

174 Gaucher Disease

Edwin H. Kolodny

DEFINITION. This relatively common familial disorder results from progressive accumulation of glucocerebroside within phagocytic cells of the monocyte-macrophage system involving principally the liver, spleen, bone marrow, and lymph nodes. Three genetically distinct clinical types have been differentiated: type 1, a chronic nonneuronopathic or "adult" form that may appear at any age and is associated with hypersplenism and bone lesions; type 2, an acute neuronopathic or "infantile" form that presents in infancy with multiple brain stem signs; and type 3, a "juvenile" subacute neuronopathic form that presents in childhood and causes seizures, ataxia, and mental deterioration. The activity of glucocerebrosidase is deficient in all three types, but different mutations are responsible.

PATHOLOGIC PHYSIOLOGY AND PATHOGENESIS. Glucocerebroside contains equimolar amounts of sphingosine, fatty acid, and glucose. Considerable quantities of this compound are generated daily by the turnover of senescent red and white blood cells. In the central nervous system, glucocerebroside is produced in the course of ganglioside metabolism. A deacylated derivative, glucosylsphingosine, also accumulates in Gaucher disease. This highly cytotoxic compound is probably responsible for the nerve cell destruction that occurs in the neuropathic forms of the disease. Both of these glycolipids are degraded by the lysosomal enzyme glucosylceramide-β-D-glucosidase (glucocerebrosidase; E.C. 3.5.1.2.1). Its catalytic efficiency is increased by two low molecular weight, heat-stable proteins, SAP-2 and saposin A, that combine with the enzyme-lipid complex. Both the gene for active glucocerebrosidase and a pseudogene have been mapped to the q21→q31 region of chromosome 1.

Several mutations in the glucocerebrosidase gene have been characterized. The most common of these is a single base change in nucleotide 1226 of the complementary DNA (cDNA) causing an Asn[370] → Ser substitution. This mutation is present in about 70 per cent of Jewish patients and is associated with type 1 disease. Another mutation in nucleotide 1448 of the cDNA produces a Leu[444] → Pro change. This point mutation is found in all three forms of Gaucher disease and may be associated with other mutations in a complex allele resulting from recombination between the active gene and the pseudogene. Patients homoallelic for the nucleotide 1226 mutation have a milder phenotype than do those with a mixed 1226/1448 genotype. Homozygosity for the 1448 mutation results in neurologic forms of Gaucher disease.

A distinctive morphologic feature is the *Gaucher cell*, a large round or polyhedral phagocyte, 20 to 100 μm in diameter, containing one or more small eccentrically placed nuclei and a pale, striated cytoplasm resembling wrinkled tissue paper or crumpled silk (Fig. 174–1A). Under the electron microscope, this

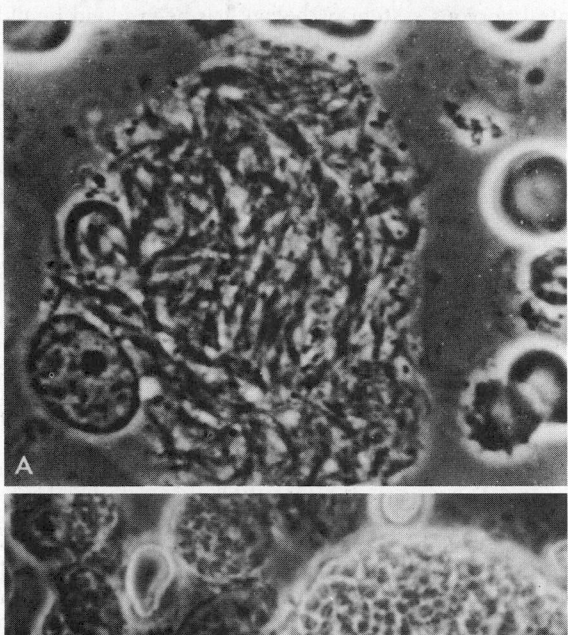
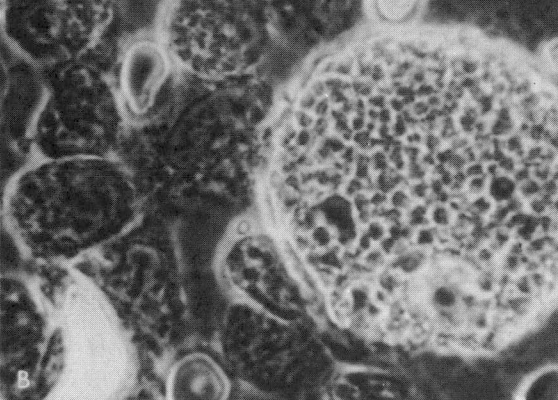

FIGURE 174–1. Appearance of the typical Gaucher cell (A) and a foam cell seen in Niemann-Pick disease (B). Both are viewed under phase microscopy in unstained smears of aspirated bone marrow. Magnification can be estimated from adjacent red cells.

fibrillary network consists of numerous dilated saclike structures resembling lysosomes containing tubules; these are similar to the twisted bilayers characteristic of glucocerebroside deposits. The reaction of the Gaucher cell cytoplasm with the periodic acid–Schiff stain is strongly positive. Stains for iron and acid phosphatase are also positive, but the reaction with lipid stains is weak. The bone marrow of patients with chronic myelogenous leukemia often contains cells with a similar appearance; the deposits in these "pseudo-Gaucher" cells are linear rather than twisted.

Glucosylceramide is increased 2- to 3-fold in plasma and more than 200-fold in the spleen and liver. Gaucher cells are present in virtually all organs surrounding small blood vessels and as sheets infiltrating their parenchyma. The spleen may become massively enlarged and develop multiple infarcts and fibrosis. The red pulp of the spleen appears white because of lipid infiltration by Gaucher cells; foci of extramedullary hematopoiesis can occur. In most patients the liver is also enlarged, the Kupffer cells of their sinusoids transformed into Gaucher cells. Fibrosis is present, but there is no proliferation of the bile ducts, and liver failure is rare. Excretion of glucosylceramide into the bile probably prevents more massive accumulation within the liver. In some cases, portal hypertension develops.

Gaucher cells may completely fill the medullary cavity of bone and may cause thinning of the cortex, loss of its normal trabeculation, patchy myelosclerosis, bone infarcts, and osteonecrosis. The metaphyseal plate in the long bones is especially prone to damage. An *Erlenmeyer flask deformity* of the distal femur is an early radiographic sign of bone involvement. With progression of the disease, spontaneous fractures and painful lytic lesions are found. Diffuse pulmonary infiltration can occur, with direct involvement of the alveoli, pleura, and interstitium, resulting in dyspnea and cor pulmonale. Renal involvement with severe proteinuric nephropathy and glomerulonephritis occurs in a few cases.

Central nervous system pathology has been found in all three types. Perivascular collections of Gaucher cells, nerve cell loss, neuronophagia, and infiltration of microglia are the principal changes observed. The most affected areas in type 2 are the deeper layers of the frontal cortex and the nuclei of the basal ganglia, mid-brain, and brain stem. The high concentrations of glucosylsphingosine, a cytotoxic compound, present in the brain, liver, and spleen of type 2 patients probably contribute to the necrosis that occurs in these tissues.

The activity of tartrate-resistant acid phosphatase and angiotensin-converting enzyme and concentrations of several serum proteins, including the immunoglobulins, are increased, especially in type 1 patients. The increased acid phosphatase is the type 5 isozyme and therefore is of osteoclastic origin and indicative of bone involvement. Some older patients develop a monoclonal gammopathy with multiple myeloma. Leukemias and other forms of malignant neoplasms are also more frequent in elderly patients with type 1 disease.

CLINICAL MANIFESTATIONS. Type 1: Chronic Nonneuronopathic Type. This disease is transmitted as an autosomal recessive trait and affects both sexes equally. It has been observed in whites, blacks, and Asians, but more than one half of cases are found in Ashkenazic Jews. As many as 1 in 13 of this population is probably a carrier, so that it is not unusual for the disease to appear in two successive generations of the same family. Clinical symptoms in this so-called adult form may appear at any age, from the first year of life to the ninth decade. One third of all cases are diagnosed in the first decade; the majority of these patients are not of Jewish ancestry. They develop massive enlargement of the spleen and evidence a delay in somatic growth that may severely hamper their intellectual and social development. The condition in another 25 per cent of patients is not diagnosed until after age 30. These patients have a much more benign course. Only rarely do these individuals have serious hematologic or osseous complications.

The most common presenting symptom is excessive fatigue associated with a hypochromic anemia and splenomegaly. Frequently there is a long history of bleeding tendency, such as repeated epistaxis and ecchymoses, but this rarely attracts medical attention unless it is associated with significant hemorrhage, such as splenic rupture, bleeding from esophageal varices, subdural hematoma, or hemopericardium. The first indication in some patients may be the appearance of bone or joint pain or a pathologic fracture. Lytic lesions develop in the shafts of the long bones, vertebrae, ribs, and pelvis. This condition produces osteosclerosis and, in the most virulent cases, osteonecrosis and eventually collapse of bone. In the acute crises affecting bone or joints, there is severe, incapacitating pain, erythema, swelling, tenderness, and occasionally joint effusion. While only 20 per cent of all type 1 patients have significant clinical involvement of bone, more than one half have radiologic evidence of the Erlenmeyer flask deformity, with tapering of the midshaft of the femur and failure of normal trabeculation causing a widening of the distal end.

The clinical course is variable. In response to an acute infection, the size of the spleen may increase dramatically and then regress, but slowly progressive splenomegaly is the usual pattern. Anemia, thrombocytopenia, and leukemia are frequent but rarely cause significant morbidity. Bleeding may occur if the platelet count falls below 50,000 to 70,000 per cubic millimeter; however, the count usually rises again spontaneously within a few weeks. Hepatomegaly with a firm liver edge is common, and in a few severe cases liver failure and portal hypertension occur.

Type 2: Acute Neuronopathic Type. This form of the disease is much rarer than the adult type 1 variety. It is observed in infants of different ethnic groups and does not show any predilection for Jews. The disease usually presents a few months after birth with retroflexion of the head, strabismus, increasing muscular hypertonicity, and marked increase in the size of the liver and spleen. In some cases, developmental milestones are normal until the second or third year. The major central nervous system signs reflect brain stem and cranial nerve involvement. Extreme arching of the neck, retraction of the lips, trismus, laryngeal spasm with a chronic cough and stridor, and spastic rigidity of the extremities are present. Seizures and psychomotor retardation

also occur. Death results from respiratory infection within a few months to 2 years after signs appear.

Type 3: Juvenile Type. This includes a heterogeneous group of patients with signs of the chronic adult type combined with progressive neurologic disease that begins in childhood or adolescence. A subtype of this disease occurs in youngsters from the northern Swedish provinces Norbotten and Vsterbotten. Their growth is retarded, and there are hypersplenism and skeletal changes of the type that occurs in the chronic nonneuropathic form. In addition, they develop oculomotor apraxia, convergent squint, spasticity, clumsiness, seizures, and a decline in mental abilities. In splenectomized patients, white retinal infiltrates may appear, the infiltration of glucosylceramide into the central nervous system is accelerated, and the pace of mental deterioration is faster than in nonsplenectomized patients.

DIAGNOSIS. Gaucher disease should be suspected in any patient with unexplained splenomegaly and a bleeding tendency, bone or joint pains, or pathologic fractures. A radioisotope scan of the liver and spleen reveals the extent of the hepatosplenomegaly and the presence of infarcts. Radionuclide scintigraphy or magnetic resonance imaging (MRI) is useful for locating lytic changes in bone. The bone marrow may demonstrate Gaucher cells. The diagnosis is established by assaying the activity of glucosylceramide-β-D-glucosidase in leukocytes or cultured fibroblasts. The artificial fluorogenic substrate, 4-methylumbelliferyl-β-glucoside, is commonly employed as a substitute for the natural lipid substrate. The degree of enzyme deficiency is similar in all three clinical subtypes of Gaucher disease. Within the same family, expression of the disease may vary considerably, so that enzyme assays should be done on all close relatives of the patient, whether or not they are symptomatic. Heterozygotes have approximately one-half the normal enzyme activity; however, with current methods the range of values overlaps the normal range. Therefore, carrier detection cannot be done with 100 per cent certainty. Prenatal diagnosis is possible using cultured amniotic cells. DNA diagnosis is useful for predicting neurologic involvement in very young patients.

TREATMENT AND PROGNOSIS. Iron therapy may partially correct the anemia, but the persistent use of iron in the presence of adequate iron stores increases the risk of hemochromatosis. Splenectomy is performed for severe and persistent thrombocytopenia or when mechanical factors cause massive swelling, abdominal pain, or gastrointestinal dysfunction. Correction of the thrombocytopenia occurs immediately after the operation, with a less dramatic improvement noted in the anemia. In children, the growth curve usually improves. However, splenectomy may hasten the pace of lipid deposition into the liver and bones, and osteolytic lesions may appear within a few months after the operation. Therefore, the surgeon may elect to leave in place any accessory spleen tissue that is present or to perform a partial splenectomy. Acute lesions in bone and joints are initially treated with immobilization and the prevention of weight bearing. However, as soon as possible, a graduated program of exercises is introduced to maintain joint mobility and prevent further loss of bone. Fractures of the head and neck of the femur are usually treated by prosthetic hip replacement. A few attempts at bone marrow transplantation have been successful, but this procedure is still plagued by a high rate of complications. Enzyme replacement therapy using purified placental enzyme modified by the attachment of mannosyl residues has produced promising results. Weekly infusions of this commercially prepared experimental drug, known as Ceredase, have resulted in a decrease in liver and spleen size and an improvement in hematologic parameters in more than 12 type 1 patients. The prognosis in children with the early onset form of the type 1 disease is poor because of the severe lung, liver, and bone involvement in these cases. In milder cases of later onset, longevity is normal. Children with the infantile neuronopathic form do not survive beyond age 2 to 3 years, whereas those with the juvenile subacute neuronopathic variant may live into their third decade.

Barranger JA, Ginns EI: Glucosylceramide lipidoses: Gaucher disease. In Scriver CR, Beaudet AL, Sly WS, et al. (eds.): The Metabolic Basis of Inherited Disease. 6th ed. New York, McGraw-Hill, 1989. *A comprehensive review of the clinical and metabolic abnormalities in Gaucher disease.*

Eyal N, Wilder S, Horowitz M: Prevalent and rare mutations among Gaucher patients. Gene, in press. *Comprehensive review of mutations and methods for their identification.*

Hobbs JR, Hugh Jones K, Shaw PJ, et al.: Beneficial effect of pre-transplant splenectomy on displacement bone marrow transplantation for Gaucher's syndrome. Lancet 1:1111, 1987. *Result of bone marrow transplantation in six children are discussed.*

Rosenthal DI, Scott JA, Barranger J, et al.: Evaluation of Gaucher disease using magnetic resonance imaging. J Bone Joint Surg 68:802, 1986. *The sensitivity of MRI in detecting bone lesions is documented in this study of 24 patients.*

Rubin M, Yampolski I, Lambrozo R, et al.: Partial splenectomy in Gaucher's disease. J Pediatr Surg 21:125, 1986. *A review of the surgical outcome in 11 children with type 1 Gaucher disease.*

Stowens DW, Teitelbaum SL, Kahn AJ, et al.: Skeletal complications of Gaucher disease. Medicine 64:310, 1985. *Description of bone findings in 327 patients with Gaucher disease.*

175 Niemann-Pick Disease

Edwin H. Kolodny

DEFINITION. The eponym Niemann-Pick disease originally referred to the classic infantile form of lipid storage disease described by Albert Niemann and Ludwig Pick in the first two decades of this century. The lysosomal enzyme sphingomyelinase is absent in this disease; this causes widespread deposition of sphingomyelin, a ceramide phospholipid. Foam cells proliferate within the reticuloendothelial system, and there is nerve cell loss within the central nervous system. This acute neuronopathic form was subsequently designated type A to distinguish it from other variants of sphingomyelin lipidosis that have since been described (Table 175–1).

PATHOLOGY. *Foam Cell.* The cytoplasm of this large histiocyte contains numerous uniform-sized lipid-staining droplets that create a fine reticulated web resembling a honeycomb or mulberry (see Fig. 174–1*B*). Under the electron microscope, these cytosomes consist of both concentrically laminated membranous arrays and dense homogeneous bodies.

Sphingomyelin. The ceramide and phosphorylcholine portions of this lipid are linked by a phosphodiester bond that under normal circumstances is cleaved by sphingomyelinase. Sphingomyelin is increased 15- to 45-fold in the liver and spleen of patients with type A Niemann-Pick disease, and about half as much in type B patients. Sphingomyelin storage occurs in the brain of type A but not type B patients. The organs of type C patients exhibit a threefold to sixfold increase in sphingomyelin. In each variety of Niemann-Pick disease, bis (monoacylglycero) phosphate, unesterified cholesterol, glucosylceramide, and other neutral glycolipids also accumulate.

Sphingomyelinase. Patients with type A and type B Niemann-Pick disease are totally deficient in sphingomyelinase, the acid hydrolase that removes the phosphorylcholine moiety from sphingomyelin. Its complementary DNA (cDNA) has been isolated, and studies have been initiated to find the mutations responsible for types A and B Niemann-Pick disease. In type C patients, sphingomyelinase may be normal or partially deficient, but the principal finding is a defect in esterification and efflux of non-lipoprotein cholesterol from the lysosome. A low molecular weight protein, SAP-2, stimulates sphingomyelinase activity by binding to the enzyme, but no cases of Niemann-Pick disease with SAP-2 deficiency have thus far been reported.

CLINICAL MANIFESTATIONS. *Type A.* Hepatosplenomegaly, diffuse pulmonary infiltration, and developmental delay are noticeable as early as 1 to 2 months of age. Weight gain is poor partly because of vomiting associated with feedings. Lymphadenopathy, opisthotonic posturing, and seizures develop. Eye signs include periorbital puffiness, clouding of the corneas, yellowish discoloration of the lens, and cherry-red maculae. Inter-

mittent jaundice and anemia are present. The affected child becomes emaciated with very thin extremities, a protuberant abdomen, and ascites. Developmental milestones normal for a 1-year-old are never attained, and after the child lingers in a vegetative state for many months, death occurs, usually before the fourth year. Postmortem studies reveal a large yellow liver and atrophic brain with widespread nerve cell loss and gliosis. The cytoplasm of remaining neurons and of the glial cells is ballooned with lipid inclusions. A high percentage of patients with this rare autosomal recessive disorder are of Ashkenazic Jewish ancestry.

Type B. Severe early involvement of the lungs, liver, and spleen also characterizes type B Niemann-Pick disease, but mental development in this variant is normal. The chest radiograph reveals nodular densities throughout the lung fields and thickening of the interlobar fissures. Signs of hypersplenism, such as mild anemia, leukopenia, and thrombocytopenia with easy bruising, often occur. A few patients have been described with a brownish-red spot in the macula, and sea-blue histiocytes are sometimes found in the bone marrow. These cells contain ceroid, which confers on them a bluish cast when stained with Giemsa. Normal longevity is possible but may be limited by chronic pulmonary insufficiency and the mechanical effects of the enlarged spleen and liver on other abdominal organs.

Type C. This diagnosis has been applied to a heterogeneous group of patients with a variable age of onset. In some cases, neonatal jaundice is present during the first 3 months, but this generally subsides despite the progression of the disease. A liver biopsy in these instances may show chronic hepatitis with giant cells. The early-onset group of type C patients develop psychomotor delay during infancy, followed later by a supranuclear gaze palsy, blindness, spasticity, and dementia. The condition of these children deteriorates rapidly over a 2-year period, and they die at age 5 to 6 years. Other type C patients may not develop overt neurologic symptoms until early childhood. These consist of a decline in intellect, progressive impairment of vertical gaze, dysarthria, dysphagia, incoordination, seizures, and involuntary movements. A few have also developed cataplexy. These patients usually survive into adult life. Rarely, there is slower progression with onset in adolescence or adult life.

Type D. This designation is used for cases similar to type C occurring in descendents of an Acadian couple born in Yarmouth, Nova Scotia, in the 1600's.

DIAGNOSIS. Niemann-Pick disease should be suspected whenever vacuolated lymphocytes are present in the peripheral smear and foam cells are present in the bone marrow of a patient with hepatosplenomegaly. The infant of Ashkenazic Jewish heritage who develops slowly would suggest the type A variant. Early jaundice and a subsequent period of normal development might suggest a workup for type C Niemann-Pick disease. The foam cell, a lipid-laden histiocyte, should not be confused with the Gaucher cell, which also contains lipid, but of a different morphologic appearance. Vacuolated leukocytes and foam cells also occur in hypertriglyceridemia and certain other lysosomal storage diseases, such as fucosidosis, mannosidosis, G_{M1} gangliosidosis, Sandhoff disease, Wolman disease, and I-cell disease. In longstanding cases of type B disease, sea-blue histiocytes containing a ceroid-like material are also observed in the bone marrow. The definitive diagnosis of Niemann-Pick disease types A and B is based upon the assay of sphingomyelinase activity. Homogenates of cultured skin fibroblasts or leukocytes from these patients, when incubated with sphingomyelin labeled with ^{14}C in the choline portion of the molecule, have less than 5 per cent of control activity. Intermediate values are obtained for type A and type B heterozygotes. Type C homozygotes may exhibit a partial deficiency, but type C heterozygotes have normal sphingomye-

TABLE 175–1. THE SPHINGOMYELIN LIPIDOSES

Type	Descriptive Name	Racial and/or Geographic Predilection	Affects Brain	Deficiency
A	Acute neuronopathic	Ashkenazic Jewish	Yes	Sphingomyelinase
B	Chronic nonneuronopathic	No	No	Sphingomyelinase
C	Subacute neuronopathic or juvenile dystonic lipidosis	No	Yes	Cholesterol esterification
D	Nova Scotian	Yarmouth County, Nova Scotia	Yes	Unknown

linase activity. The defect in intracellular trafficking and efflux of cholesterol in type C patients and heterozygotes can be demonstrated in fibroblast culture by incubating the cells with low density lipoprotein (LDL) and ^{3}H-labeled oleate and then analyzing their content of unesterified and esterified cholesterol. The ultrastructural examination of skin biopsy specimens from type C patients has demonstrated lysosomes containing loosely arranged, dark, laminated structures within a clear matrix. Prenatal diagnosis of type A and type B Niemann-Pick disease is accomplished by determining the enzyme activity of cultured amniotic fluid cells. Fetuses with type C disease have been identified by studying the intracellular processing of LDL cholesterol in cultured chorionic villus cells.

TREATMENT. No specific treatment is available for any of the sphingomyelin storage diseases. In type B patients, splenectomy may be done to relieve mechanical pressure within the abdomen or to correct a thrombocytopenia with hemorrhagic diathesis. Neither replacement with exogenous enzyme nor organ transplants have been successful, but bone marrow transplanta-

tion has proved beneficial to one 3-year-old type B patient without central nervous system involvement. Type C patients may benefit from attempts to reduce intracellular cholesterol through dietary means and drugs. Animal models of Niemann-Pick disease are available for laboratory trials of these and other potential new therapies.

Fink JK, Filling-Katz MR, Sokol J, et al.: Clinical spectrum of Niemann-Pick disease type C. Neruology 39:1040, 1989. *Analysis of neurologic symptomatology in three phenotypes of Niemann-Pick disease type C.*

Levran O, Desnick RJ, Schuchman EH: Niemann-Pick disease: A frequent missense mutation in the gene encoding acid sphingomyelinase of Ashkenazi Jewish type A and B patients. Proc Natl Acad Sci (USA) 88, in press. *This is the first study to describe a mutation in the sphingomyelinase gene.*

Spence MW, Callahan JW: Sphingomyelin-cholesterol lipidoses: The Niemann-Pick group of diseases. *In* Scriver CR, Beaudet AL, Sly WS, et al. (eds.): The Metabolic Basis of Inherited Disease. 6th ed. New York, McGraw-Hill, 1989. *A comprehensive review of the different clinical forms of sphingomyelin lipidoses. Details of their pathology, metabolic disturbance, and enzymatic aspects are provided, as well as an extensive bibliography.*

Vanier MT, Rousson RM, Mandon G, et al.: Diagnosis of Niemann-Pick disease type C on chorionic villus cells. Lancet 1:1014, 1989. *Techniques for the prenatal diagnosis of Niemann-Pick disease type C are described, and references are provided for the defect in intracellular trafficking of cholesterol in this variant.*

INBORN ERRORS OF AMINO ACID METABOLISM

176 Hyperaminoaciduria (with a Classification of the Inborn and Developmental Errors of Amino Acid Metabolism)

Charles R. Scriver

Study of the appropriate inborn errors has improved our knowledge of amino acid metabolism, as well as the diagnosis and treatment of associated diseases. The inborn errors of renal amino acid transport reveal either a carrier or a metabolic process coupled to the transcellular flux that achieves normal reabsorption.

L-Aminoaciduria, representing less than 2 to 3 per cent of the total urinary nitrogen, is a normal phenomenon. Only 5 per cent

or less of the filtered amino acid load is not reabsorbed by the proximal portion of the renal tubule and is excreted in the urine. Efficiency of renal tubular transport of an amino acid is related to its chemical and steric structure, the amount in the glomerular filtrate, and the sex, age, and physiologic state of the subject. Abnormal aminoaciduria (hyperaminoaciduria) is a result of acquired or hereditary disturbances of cellular metabolism or transport. Table 176–1 shows the known hyperaminoacidurias. (The table includes several disorders of amino acid metabolism that do not show hyperaminoaciduria but affect organic acid and fatty acid derivatives; they can be detected in urine by gas chromatography.)

The hyperaminoacidurias are explained by several mechanisms acting on net reabsorption in the proximal tubule (Fig. 176–1):

1. *Saturation:* The concentration of amino acid in filtrate approaches or exceeds the capacity of the tubular system to reabsorb it (overflow or prerenal aminoaciduria).

2. *Competition:* One amino acid at elevated concentration competes with another sharing the transporter ("combined" aminoaciduria).

Text continued on page 1101

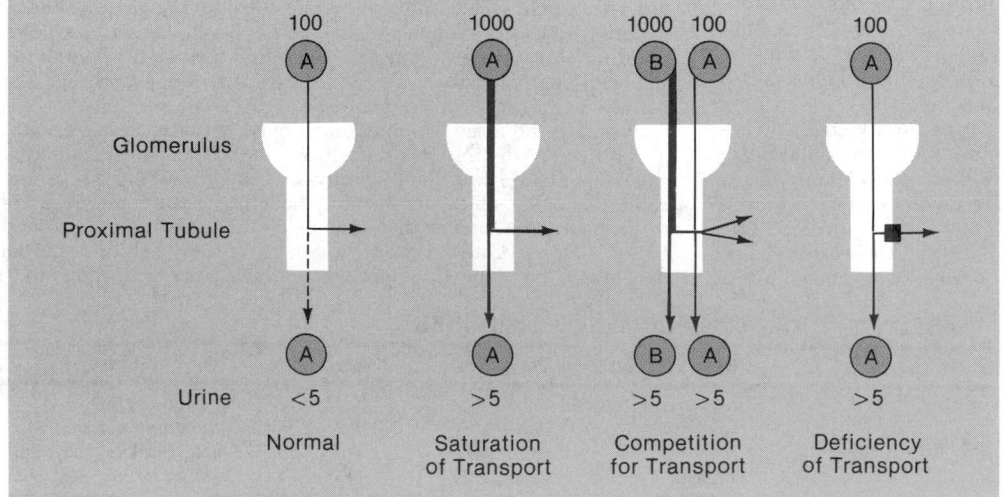

FIGURE 176–1. Mechanism of hyperaminoaciduria. *Panel 1:* Normal reabsorption reclaims more than 95 per cent of filtered amino acid molecules. Hyperaminoaciduria can occur if (*Panel 2*) filtered load increases (10× increase shown) and transport mechanism is saturated or if (*Panel 3*) amino acid (B) (in excess) competes with another (A) on a shared carrier or if (*Panel 4*) carrier is modified or coupling of energy to carrier is impaired.

TABLE 176–1. HEREDITARY AND ACQUIRED AMINOACIDOPATHIES

The aminoacidurias presented in this table are divided into acquired and inherited types. Disturbances related to perinatal adaptive phenomena of multifactorial origin are included. The classification recognizes physiologic factors affecting amino acid distribution between plasma and urine, and whether the disorder primarily affects catabolism or membrane transport of the amino acid(s).

Thus the disorders are grouped according to mechanism and preferred fluid for detection. The data refer to those conditions associated with perturbation of the normal content of ninhydrin-reactive metabolites in plasma or urine; some exceptions have been made to include ninhydrin-negative metabolites.

GROUP IA

The primary defect is in catabolism. There is a low renal clearance of amino acid but a hyperaminoaciduria by saturation of transepithelial transport. Detection in the plasma is preferable unless otherwise indicated, but the use of urine for screening (or diagnosis) is not precluded; assignment to this group implies primarily that diagnosis (or screening) of the condition is feasible by virtue of significant metabolite accumulation in blood (or plasma).

Amino Acid Affected:
↓ = decreased; ↑ = increased. Source of enzyme number is *Enzyme Commission.* IP = apparent inheritance pattern; AR = autosomal recessive; AD = autosomal dominant; (AR) = probably autosomal recessive; XL = X-linked. *Remarks:* CNS = central nervous system; CoA = coenzyme A; CSF = cerebrospinal fluid.

Condition or Disease	Amino Acid Affected	Enzyme Affected (Synonym) In Group A	IP	Remarks
Common Perinatal (Adaptive) Traits*				
Neonatal hyperphenylalani-nemia	Phenylalanine	Phenylalanine 4-mono-oxygenase (phenylalanine-hydroxylating system) [1.14.16.1]	—	Benign; may respond to folic acid; often occurs with tyrosinemia
Neonatal tyrosinemia	Tyrosine	4-Hydroxyphenylpyruvate dioxygenase (p-hydroxyphenyl pyruvic acid hydroxylase) [1.13.11.27]	—	Benign; responds to ascorbic acid and reduced protein intake
Hypermethioninemia	Methionine	? Methionine adenosyltransferase (ATP:L-methionine S-adenosyltransferase) [2.5.1.6]	—	Benign; usually found with high protein intake
Hyperhistidinemia	Histidine	? L-Histidine ammonia-lyase [4.3.1.3]	—	Benign; related to high protein intake
Inherited Traits				
Hyperphenylalaninemia				
Classic phenylketonuria	Phenylalanine	Phenylalanine 4-mono-oxygenase (L-phenylalanine, tetrahydropteridine:oxygen oxidoreductase [4-hydroxylating]) [1.14.16.1]	AR	Plasma phenylalanine >16 mg/100 ml; causes mental retardation; when untreated, L-phenylalanine tolerance in diet is 250–500 mg/day
Atypical phenylketonuria	Phenylalanine	Same	(AR)	Plasma phenylalanine >16 mg/100 ml; similar to entry above, but dietary tolerance for L-phenylalanine is > 500 mg/day
Transient phenylketonuria	Phenylalanine	Same	(AR)	Plasma phenylalanine >16 mg/100 ml; change in status to that of next entry or normal, several months or years after birth
Benign hyperphenylalaninemia	Phenylalanine	Same	AR	Plasma phenylalanine <16 mg/100 ml on normal diet; benign trait
Dihydropteridine reductase deficiency	Phenylalanine	Dihydropteridine reductase [1.6.99.7]	AR	Deficient tetrahydrobiopterin cofactor also impairs biosynthesis of L-dopa and 5-hydroxytryptamine (5-HT) in CNS; low-phenylalanine diet does not correct this
Biopterin synthesis defects	Phenylalanine	Various enzymes in synthesis pathway	AR	See preceding entry
Hypertyrosinemias				
Tyrosinosis (Medes)	Tyrosine	Tyrosine aminotransferase (L-tyrosine:α-ketoglutarate aminotransferase) [2.6.1.5]	(AR)	One case known; myasthenia gravis probably incidental finding
Hypertyrosinemia I	Tyrosine (and methionine in acute stage)	Fumarylacetoacetate hydrolase [3.7.1.2]	AR	Hepatic cirrhosis and renal tubular failure; usually fatal in absence of tyrosine restriction
Hypertyrosinemia II	Tyrosine	Soluble (cytosol) tyrosine aminotransferase [2.6.15]	AR	Associated with developmental retardation; Richner-Hanhart syndrome in some patients
Hawkinsinuria	Tyrosine	4-Hydroxyphenyl pyruvate dioxygenase [1.13.11.27]	AD	Disease signs are variable and include failure to thrive; reflect formation of epoxides and adducts of glutathione

Table continued on following page

TABLE 176–1. HEREDITARY AND ACQUIRED AMINOACIDOPATHIES Continued

Condition or Disease	Amino Acid Affected	Enzyme Affected (Synonym) In Group A	IP	Remarks
Inherited Traits (Continued)				
Hyperhistidinemia†				
Classic form	Histidine (alanine in some cases)	L-Histidine ammonia-lyase [4.3.1.3]; liver, epidermis	AR	Harmless condition in majority
Branched-chain hyperaminoacidemia‡				
Classic maple syrup urine disease	Leucine, isoleucine, valine, alloisoleucine	Branched-chain α-keto acid lipoate oxidoreductase (probably decarboxylase component) [1.2.4.3(4)]	AR	Postnatal collapse; mental retardation in survivors; diet therapy can be effective
Intermittent form	Leucine, isoleucine, valine, alloisoleucine	Branched-chain α-keto acid oxidase(s)§ [1.2.4.3(4)]	(AR)	Intermittent symptoms; development may be otherwise normal
Mild form	Same	Same	(AR)	Unremittent; milder than classic form
Thiamine-responsive form	Same	Same	(AR)	Mild form; responsive to thiamine (vitamin B₁)
Multiple dehydrogenase form	Same (plus pyruvate and α-ketoglutarate)	Dihydrolipoamide dehydrogenase [1.8.1.4]	(AR)	Congenital lactic acidosis plus branched-chain amino-keto acid disorder
Hypervalinemia	Valine	Branched-chain amino-acid aminotransferase (valine aminotransferase) [2.6.1.66]	AR	Retarded development and vomiting; responds to diet
Type I hyperlysinemia	Lysine	Deficient "aminoadipic semialdehyde synthase" (bifunctional enzyme with lysine-ketoglutarate reductase [1.5.1.8] + saccharopine reductase [1.5.1.9] activities)	AR	Associated with mental retardation, hypotonia
Type 2 hyperlysinemia	Lysine, methionine and homocyst(e)ine	Only saccharopine reductase activity of bifunctional enzyme is deficient	AR	Same as above
Homocyst(e)inuria (methylene tetrahydrofolate [THF] reductase deficiency)	Methionine (low) and homocyst(e)ine (high)	5,10-Methylenetetrahydrofolate reductase [1.7.99.5]	AR	Defective remethylation of homocysteine to methionine; neurologic and behavioral symptoms associated
Homocyst(e)inuria (with methylmalonic aciduria)	Homocyst(e)ine (high), methionine (low): plus methylmalonate	Defective cobalamin coenzyme biosynthesis	AR	Defective remethylation of homocysteine and impaired methylmalonyl-CoA mutase (MMA mutase) activity; developmental delay
		Defective cobalamin transport (lysosomal)	(AR)	
Cystathioninuria†	Cystathionine	Cystathionine γ-lyase [4.4.1.1]	AR	Probably benign trait; vitamin B₆ corrects biochemical trait in most patients
Hyperglycinemias				
Ketotic form	Glycine and other glucogenic amino acids	Propionyl-CoA carboxylase (adenosine triphosphate [ATP]–hydrolyzing) propanoyl-CoA:carbon dioxide ligase (adenosine diphosphate [ADP]–forming) [6.4.1.3]	AR	Ketosis, neutropenia, mental retardation; often fatal; detectable in skin fibroblasts
Ibid.	Ibid.	Methylmalonyl-CoA mutase [5.4.99.2]	AR	Symptoms are those of methylmalonic aciduria with acidosis (some mutase-affected patients are responsive to vitamin B₁₂)
Ibid.	Ibid.	Acetyl-CoA acyltransferase (β-ketothiolase) [2.3.1.16] deficiency¶	AR	Signs are those of α-methyl-β-hydroxybutyric aciduria (with or without tiglic aciduria) and acidosis
Nonketotic form	Glycine	Glycine cleavage reaction (CO₂, NH₃, and hydroxymethyltetrahydrofolate formed) [1.4.4.2, 2.1.2.10]	AR	Severe CNS depression soon after birth; high CSF: plasma glycine ratio; benzoate decreases plasma glycine; no effect on CNS prognosis; strychnine improves seizures
Sarcosinemia†	Sarcosine	Sarcosine oxidase (sarcosine:oxygen oxidoreductase [demethylating]) [1.5.3.1]	AR	Benign trait
"Sarcosinemia" (glutaric aciduria, type II)	Sarcosine (glutaric acid and multiple fatty acids)	? Electron transfer flavoprotein (affecting multiple aryl-CoA dehydrogenases) [1.3.99.2–3]	AR	Postnatal lethargy, vomiting, coma, and acidosis; odor; multiple abnormalities of fatty acid oxidation

TABLE 176–1. HEREDITARY AND ACQUIRED AMINOACIDOPATHIES *Continued*

Condition or Disease	Amino Acid Affected	Enzyme Affected (Synonym) *In Group A*	IP	Remarks
		Inherited Traits (Continued)		
Hyperprolinemias				
Type I	Proline	L-Proline dehydrogenase (oxidase) [1.5.99.8]	AR	Benign trait
Type II	Proline	1-Pyrroline dehydrogenase ($\triangle^1$-pyrroline-5-nicotinamide carboxylate: adenine dinucleotide [NAD$^+$] oxidoreductase) [1.5.1.12]	AR	$\triangle^1$-Pyrroline-5-carboxylate and 3-hydroxy-1-pyrroline-5-carboxylate excreted in urine; associated convulsions?
Hyperhydroxyprolinemia	Hydroxyproline	4-Hydroxy-L-proline dehydrogenase (oxidase) [1.1.1.104]	AR	Benign trait
Hyperlysinemias, hypertryptophanemias, and related diseases				
Type I	Lysine (and glutamine)	Saccharopine dehydrogenase (nicotinamide-adenine dinucleotide phosphate [NADP$^+$], lysine-forming) [1.5.1.8]	AR	Associated with mental retardation and hypotonia
Saccharopinuria†	Lysine, saccharopine, citrulline	? Saccharopine dehydrogenase (NADP$^+$, L-glutamate–forming) (saccharopine dehydrogenase) [1.5.1.10]	AR	Associated with mental retardation
Pipecolic acidemia†	Pipecolic acid	L-Pipecolate dehydrogenase (pipecolate oxidase) [1.5.99.3]	AR	Hepatomegaly and mental retardation (peroxisomal disease)
α-Aminoadipic aciduria	α-Aminoadipic acid	?Mitochondrial α-aminoadipate amino transferase [2.6.1.39]	(AR)	Variable clinical features
α-Ketoadipic aciduria	α-Aminoadipic and α-ketoadipic acids	? α-Ketoadipic decarboxylase	(AR)	Mental retardation
Glutaric aciduria type I	Glutaric acid	? Glutaryl-CoA dehydrogenase [1.3.99.7]	(AR)	Mental retardation
Glutaric aciduria type II (multiple acyl-CoA dehydrogenase deficiency)	Glutaric acid, complex organic aciduria, sarcosine	Electron transport flavoprotein [1.3.99.2–3]	AR	Severe form, neonatal metabolic disease; adult form, recurrent hypoglycemia
Hydroxylysinemia	Free hydroxylsine	? Hydroxylysine kinase [2.7.1.81]	(AR)	Mental retardation
Tryptophanemia	Tryptophan (with indoleketonuria)	? Formamidase [3.5.1.9]	(AR)	Variable, probably benign
Hyperammonemias				
Carbamyl phosphate synthetase (CPS) deficiency	Glycine, glutamine	Carbamate kinase (ATP carbamate phosphotransferase) [2.7.2.2]	AR	Group of diseases with ammonia intoxication, protein intolerance, hepatomegaly, vomiting, and so on; argininosuccinicaciduria also has trichorrhexis nodosa
Ornithine transcarbamylase (OTC) deficiency	Glutamine	Ornithine carbamoyltransferase (carbamoylphosphate:L-ornithine carbamoyltransferase) [2.1.3.3]	XL	Same as above
Citrullinemia	Citrulline	Argininosuccinate synthetase (L-citrulline:L-aspartate ligase adenosine monophosphate [AMP]–forming) [6.3.4.5]	AR	Same as above
Argininosuccinicaciduria†	Argininosuccinic acid	Argininosuccinate lyase (L-argininosuccinate arginine-lyase) [4.3.2.1]	AR	Same as above
Hyperargininemia	Arginine	Arginase (L-arginine amidinohydrolase) [3.5.3.1]	AR	Deterioration of CNS function and IQ in childhood; hyperammonemia (inconstant) aggravated by protein
Hyperornithinemia	Ornithine	Unknown (mitochondrial ornithine transport system?)	AR	Associated with hyperammonemia and homocitrullinemia (HHH syndrome)
Hyperornithinemia (without hyperammonemia)	Ornithine	L-Ornithine; 2-oxoacid aminotransferase [2.6.1.13]	AR	Associated with gyrate atrophy of choroid and retina but no hyperammonemia
Hyperalaninemia	Alanine	Pyruvate dehydrogenase (lipoate) (pyruvate dehydrogenase) [1.2.4.1] deficiency	AR	Lactic acidosis
		Pyruvate carboxylase [6.4.1.1] deficiency, and other defects	AR	Intermittent lactic acidosis, intermittent hypoglycemia

Table continued on following page

TABLE 176–1. HEREDITARY AND ACQUIRED AMINOACIDOPATHIES *Continued*

Condition or Disease	Amino Acid Affected	Enzyme Affected (Synonym) *In Group A*	IP	Remarks
Inherited Traits (Continued)				
Aspartylglucosaminuria	Glycoasparagines	Aspartylglucosylaminase (2-acetamido-1[β¹-L-aspartamidol]-1,2-dideoxyglucose amidohydrolase) [3.5.1.26]	AR	Lysosomal disease; mental retardation
Glutathionemia†	Glutathione or related peptides	γ-Glutamyltransferase (γ-glutamyltranspeptidase) [2.3.2.2]	AR	Mental retardation associated with finding
Hyperthreoninemia	Threonine	Unknown	(AR)	Seizures
Other Conditions That May Affect Amino Acids in Plasma				
Protein-calorie malnutrition	Tryptophan/leucine/isoleucine/valine ↓; tyrosine/glycine/proline ↑	—	—	Severity of change related to severity of malnutrition
Prolonged fasting	Alanine ↓; threonine, glycine ↑	—	—	Early fasting does not show same pattern
Obesity	Leucine/isoleucine/valine/phenylalanine/tyrosine ↑; glycine ↓	—	—	Reflects insulin insensitivity
Hepatitis	Methionine/tyrosine ↑	—	—	Reflects severity of liver disease

*These conditions have been detected by screening methods applied in the newborn period of life. They should not be misdiagnosed as permanent disorders of amino acid metabolism also identifiable by screening.

†Urine screening is as efficient as, or even more reliable than, blood screening in these conditions.

‡A number of disorders of branched-chain amino acid catabolism cause accumulation of substances that are Ninhydrin negative. These compounds can usually be detected by gas-liquid chromatographic methods (see Goodman SI: Am J Hum Genet 32:781, 1980).

§Partial activity; more than 2 per cent of normal.

¶Hyperglycemia observed only in some patients with this enzyme deficiency.

GROUP IB

The primary defect is in catabolism. There is a high renal clearance of amino acid and a hyperaminoaciduria by saturation of transeptithelial transport. Detection in the urine is preferable.

Source of enzyme number is *Enzyme Commission*. IP = apparent inheritance pattern; AR = autosomal recessive; (AR) = probably autosomal recessive; AD = autosomal dominant.

Condition or Disease	Substance Affected (Synonym)	Enzyme Affected (Synonym) [Enzyme Commission No.]	IP	Remarks
Hypophosphatasia	Phosphoethanolamine	?Deficiency of ethanolaminephosphate phospho-lyase (O-phosphorylethanolamine phospholyase) [4.2.99.7]	AR	"Rickets" unresponsive to vitamin D; craniosynostosis; hypercalcemia; pyridoxal phosphate accumulation
Pseudohypophosphatasia	Phosphoethanolamine	? Same as above; activity present but altered	(AR)	Same as above
β-Aminoisobutyricaciduria	β-Aminoisobutyric acid	?	AD/AR	Benign polymorphic trait
4-Hydroxybutyricaciduria (γ-amino butyrate pathway)	γ-OH butyrate	Succinic semialdehyde dehydrogenase [1.2.1.24]	AR	Mental retardation, hypotonia; detectable by gas chromatographic analysis of urine, plasma, CSF
Hyper-β-alaninemia	β-Alanine	? β-Alanine-pyruvate aminotransferase (β-alanine transaminase) [2.6.1.18]		Seizures; somnolence; mental retardation
Carnosinemia	Carnosine	Aminoacyl-histidine dipeptidase (carnosinase) [3.4.13.3]	AR	Seizure and mental retardation; or benign possibly
Pyroglutamic aciduria*	L-Pyroglutamic acid (5-oxo-L-proline; pyrrolidone-2-carboxylic acid)	Glutathione synthetase [6.3.2.3]	AR	L-Pyroglutamic acid (5-oxo-L-proline) results from overproduction via modified γ-glutamyl cycle

*Urine screening is as efficient as, or even more reliable than, blood screening in these conditions.

TABLE 176–1. HEREDITARY AND ACQUIRED AMINOACIDOPATHIES *Continued*

GROUP II

There is a primary defect in catabolism and a secondary defect in transport. Hyperaminoaciduria is of combined origin—saturation and competition. Detection is possible in both plasma and urine.

Disease	Amino Acids		Remarks
	Affected in Plasma	*Present in Urine*	
Hyperprolinemia, types I and II	Proline	Proline, + hydroxyproline and glycine	See entries in group 1A; competition occurs on iminoglycine transport system (see group III)
Hyper-β-alaninemia	β-Alanine	β-Alanine, + β-aminoisobutyric acid and taurine	See Hyper-β-alaninemia in group IB; competition occurs on β-amino transport system
Hyperlysinemia	Lysine	Lysine, + ornithine and arginine	See entries in group IA; competition occurs on "dibasic" transport system (see group III)
Hyperargininemia	Arginine	Ornithine and lysine and sometimes generalized hyperaminoaciduria	See Hyperargininemia in group IA; competition occurs on "diabasic" transport system (see group III); pathogenesis of generalized aminoaciduria unknown

GROUP III

The primary defect is in the renal membrane transport site. There is a high renal clearance of amino acid, and detection is possible only in the urine.
Activity Affected: Presumed gene product activity affected by mutant gene. IP = apparent inheritance pattern; AD = autosomal dominant; (AD) = probably autosomal dominant; AR = autosomal recessive; (AR) = probably autosomal recessive; XL = X-linked. *Remarks:* PTH = parathyroid hormone.

Trait	Substance Affected	Activity Affected	Other Tissues Affected	IP	Remarks
Common Perinatal (Adaptive) Traits					
Neonatal iminoglycinuria	Proline, hydroxyproline, glycine	Specific proline and specific glycine transport (probably)	—	—	Benign adaptive trait; prolinuria subsides at ~ 100 days, glycinuria at ~ 200 days after full-term birth
Neonatal cystine-lysinuria	Cystine and dibasic amino acids (lysine, ornithine, and arginine)	Specific dibasic transport system	—	—	Transient; evident in newborn period in some but not all infants
Inherited Hyperaminoacidurias					
Selective					
Hyperdibasic aminoaciduria type 2 (Lysinuric-protein intolerance)	Lysine, ornithine, arginine ("dibasic" group)	Shared "dibasic" amino acid transport system in basolateral membrane	Intestine (basolateral membrane, efflux defect); fibroblasts (plasma membrane; efflux defect on y⁺ system)	AR	Associated with protein intolerance, failure to thrive, hyperammonemia basolateral membrane defect; silent carrier
Hyperdibasic aminoaciduria type I	Lysine, ornithine, arginine	Shared "dibasic" amino acid transport system (brush-border membrane)	Intestine	AR/AD	Associated with mental retardation in one reported patient; carriers have hyperdibasic aminoaciduria
Isolated hyperlysinuria	Lysine	Lysine-specific system (brush border)	Intestine	AR	One proband reported
Classic cystinuria	Lysine, ornithine, arginine, and cystine	Shared system in brush-border membrane	Intestine	AR	"Negative" reabsorption of affected amino acid can occur; three alleles (? same locus), each causing different phenotypes: in type I carrier (vs. types II and III) no excess of amino acids in urine ("silent"); in type III patient, intestinal transport intact (or partial defect)
Hypercystinuria	Cyst(e)ine	Specific system for cyst(e)ine	?	(AR)	One pedigree only
Iminoglycinuria	Proline; hydroxyproline; glycine	Shared system for imino acids, glycine (and sarcosine)	Intestine	AR	Four alleles (? same locus); I and II are silent carriers; III and IV are hyperglycinuric carriers; I associated with intestinal defect; IV with Kₘ mutant
Hartnup disorder	Neutral amino acids (excluding imino acids, glycine, cyst(e)ine, and β-amino acids)	Shared system for large neutral amino acid group (luminal membrane)	Intestine	AR	Three alleles (? same locus); I, intestine affected; II, intestine normal; III, kidney normal; carrier "silent" in all

Table continued on following page

TABLE 176–1. HEREDITARY AND ACQUIRED AMINOACIDOPATHIES Continued

Trait	Substance Affected	Activity Affected	Other Tissues Affected	IP	Remarks
Inherited Hyperaminoacidurias (Continued)					
Hyperhistidinuria	Histidine	Specific sytem for histidine	Intestine	AR	Associated with mental retardation in siblings
Hyperdicarboxylic aminoaciduria (glutamate-aspartate transport defect)	Glutamic acid, aspartic acid	Shared dicarboxylic acid transport system (brush-border membrane)	Intestine ±	AR	Benign
Idiopathic (primary genetic) Fanconi's syndrome	Generalized effect on all solutes and water	? Coupling of energy; ? tight junction integrity	Secondary to renal phenotype	AR (and AD)	Adult-onset and infantile-childhood forms are differentiated; basic defect unknown; probably several alleles
Secondary genetic forms of Fanconi's syndrome					
Cystinosis; type I, type II	Same as above (secondary response)	Cystine storage (lysosomal defect), with secondary damage to tubule and glomerulus (later)	Organ damage from cystine storage (thyroid, retina; CNS, and so on)	AR*	Several alleles; infantile (type I) and adolescent (type II) forms have differing rates for onset of nephropathy; "adult" form (type III) has no nephropathy
Hereditary fructose intolerance	Same as above, + fructose	Fructose-1-phosphate aldolase (fructose bisphosphate aldolase) (with secondary effects on cellular ATP)	Secondary to renal phenotype (hepatic cirrhosis)	AR	Nephropathy dependent on intact PTH-cAMP axis in kidney; responds to fructose withdrawal
Galactosemia	Same as above, + galactose	Galactose-1-phosphate uridyltransferase (with secondary effects on cellular ATP)	Secondary to renal phenotype (cataracts, CNS effects)	AR	Fanconi's syndrome responds to galactose withdrawal; "galactosemia" due to galactokinase deficiency does *not* include Fanconi's syndrome
Hereditary tyrosinemia	Same as above, + tyrosine metabolites	Unknown (with secondary effects on cellular ATP)	Secondary to renal phenotype (hepatic cirrhosis)	AR	Fanconi's syndrome responds to tyrosine restriction
Wilson's disease	Same as above, with proximal and distal renal tubular acidosis	Unknown (? secondary effects on cytochrome oxidase system)	Hepatolenticular degeneration	AR	Fanconi's syndrome responds to depletion of copper storage
Lowe's oculocerebrorenal syndrome	Generalized dysfunction with defective urinary NH₃ production	Unknown	An oculocerebro-intestinal-renal syndrome (? involving tissues with high γ-glutamyl cycle activity)	XL†	Basic defect still unknown: treatment for tubular reclamation defects does not improve mental retardation or the cataracts and hydrophthalmia
Vitamin D dependency (pseudodeficiency rickets)	Generalized defect (secondary response)	Type I: 25-Hydroxyvitamin D-1-α-hydroxylase Type II: defective binding of hormone	Deficiency of synthesis or AR binding affects intestinal absorption of calcium and initiates PTH response	AR	Nephropathy dependent on PTH excess and hypocalcemia (phenocopy occurs in vitamin D deficiency)
Miscellaneous					
Glycoglycinuria	Glucose and glycine	Unknown (the two solutes do *not* share a common carrier)	—	AD	Asymptomatic; normal T_m (maximal tubular reabsorptive capacity of kidneys) (type B) glucosuria; possibility that there is a heterozygous manifestation of a Fanconi-like tubulopathy merits consideration
Luder-Sheldon syndrome	Generalized amino acids, glucose, and phosphate	Unknown	—	AD	Symptoms of Fanconi's syndrome have occurred in probands
Rowley-Rosenberg syndrome	Generalized aminoaciduria	Unknown	—	AR	Associated components of syndrome; growth retardation, muscular hypoplasia, pulmonary involvement, and right ventricular hypertrophy

*For each type.
†Recessive.

Benson PF, Fensom AH: Genetic Biochemical Disorders. Oxford Monographs on the Medical Genetics No. 12. Oxford, Oxford Univesity Press, 1985. A "handbook," leaner than The Metabolic Basis of Inherited Disease (*the standard "encyclopedia"*), *that covers, in short essays, nearly all entries in Table 176–1.*

Scriver CT, Tenenhouse HS: Mendelian phenotypes as "probes" of renal transport systems for amino acids and phosphate. Handbook of Physiology (Renal Section), in press. *A review of the amino acid transport systems (in kidney and other tissues) delineated by mutations in humans and of their relative importance in metabolic homeostasis.*

Wellner D, Meister A: A survey of inborn errors of amino acid metabolism and transport in man. Annu Rev Biochem 50:911, 1981. *A crisp review of events in a field that now moves more slowly than it once did.*

3. Modification of transporter: The amino acid is not transported efficiently because its carrier is altered (renal aminoaciduria).

4. *Inhibition of substrate transfer:* The coupling of energy to the transporter is altered, and flux is impaired (renal aminoaciduria).

Renal transporters show preferences for either single free amino acids or specific groups of them. The transport systems identified in Table 176–1 (group III) were revealed through loss of function in the variant (mutant or developmental) state. Oligopeptides are transported on carriers different from those used by free amino acids.

Scriver CR, Beaudet A, Sly W, Valle D (eds.): The Metabolic Basis of Inherited Disease. 6th ed. New York, McGraw-Hill, 1989. *The Mendelian disorders of amino acid metabolism (catabolism or transport) are described, chapter by chapter, in detail.*

Scriver CR, Tenenhouse HS: Mendelian phenotypes as probes of renal transport systems for amino acids and phosphate. *In* Windhager E (ed.): Handbook of Physiology: Renal Physiology. 2nd ed. New York, Oxford University Press, in press. *An up-to-date review of the inborn errors of renal amino acid transport and associated transport systems.*

177 The Hyperphenylalaninemias

Charles R. Scriver

A widely accepted medical model of disease attributes manifestations (signs and symptoms) to a deviant underlying process (pathogenesis) that has its origins in both proximate and ultimate causes. According to this model, phenylketonuria, the best known form of hyperphenylalaninemia, is no longer a disease, although it continues to be a risk factor, because its principal manifestations (mental retardation, pigment dilution, mousy odor, neurotransmitter deficiency) occur only in rare cases escaping early diagnosis. This satisfactory turn of events came about because the pathogenesis of hyperphenylalaninemia (the risk factor) is offset by treatment. Genetic forms of hyperphenylalaninemia are described here; they are all autosomal recessive disorders. About 0.01 per cent of live births are affected.

PHENYLALANINE METABOLISM. Phenylalanine is an essential amino acid. The normal concentration in plasma is less than 0.1 mmole per liter (0.1 mM, 1.6 mg per deciliter). The balance between intake and utilization is largely controlled by a hydroxylation reaction (Fig. 177–1A). Impaired hydroxylation is the chief explanation for hyperphenylalaninemia. The reaction requires the apoenzyme *phenylalanine hydroxylase,* molecular oxygen, and *tetrahydrobiopterin* cofactor; the last-named is consumed in stoichiometric amounts to form tyrosine, the reaction product. The catalytic property of phenylalanine hydroxylase requires both moment to moment regeneration of tetrahydrobiopterin from dihydrobiopterin, a by-product of the hydroxylating reaction, and long-term renewal of the tetrahydrobiopterin pool by synthesis from precursors. The former is achieved by the enzyme *dihydropteridine reductase,* the latter by a *synthesis pathway* in which several enzymes act in sequence (Fig. 177–1B). Accordingly, there are several ways to impair phenylalanine hydroxylation. Failure to recognize the biologic heterogeneity of hyperphenylalaninemia may lead to erroneous counseling and ineffective (or unnecessary) treatment; all of its forms require special management of women during the reproductive period of life.

DISORDERS OF PHENYLALANINE HYDROXYLASE INTEGRITY. The phenylalanine hydroxylase enzyme is multimeric and homopolymeric. The polypeptide is encoded by a gene on chromosome 12, region q24.1, which is expressed only in liver in humans. Mutations at this locus cause either phenylketonuria (with plasma phenylalanine values above 1 mM on a normal diet) or nonphenylketonuric hyperphenylalaninemia (values below 1 mM, but greater than 0.125 mM). Phenylketonuria is typically associated with mental retardation in the untreated patient; the other form is not. The incidence of the phenylketonuric form varies by population (lower than 1 in 10,000 births in Ashkenazi

Jews, Finns, and Blacks; higher in Scots, Irish, and Yemenite Jews).

The hydroxylation reaction accounts for about three quarters of the moment by moment outflow of phenylalanine; incorporation into protein is the other important route (Fig. 177–1A). If there is deficient hydroxylating activity, and dietary intake is not curtailed, phenylalanine accumulates in body fluids. Overflow into the alternative pathways generates excessive amounts of metabolites derived from phenylalanine, such as the pyruvic (causing phenylketonuria), lactic, and acetic acid derivatives (Fig. 177–1A). Overburden of phenylalanine and its by-products impairs brain development in ways still not fully understood.

Phenylketonuria was first described as a clinical entity in 1934 by Asjborn Fölling, who surmised that the disorder was autosomal recessive and an inborn error of metabolism. In the following three decades, phenylketonuria was seen as a paradigm for the biochemical basis of mental disease, of disease that could be prevented by deliberate restoration of normal metabolism, and of chemical individuality that could be used as the basis for a screening test and early diagnosis. Newborn screening for hyperphenylalaninemia is now one of the most widely applied "genetic" tests. The incidence of the risk factor has not changed, but the frequency of the associated disease is now trivial in screened populations. The practical issues for physicians are interpretation of a positive screening test result, accuracy of the test, and maternal hyperphenylalaninemia (all discussed below).

TETRAHYDROBIOPTERIN-DEFICIENT FORMS OF HYPERPHENYLALANINEMIA. Not every case of persistent hyperphenylalaninemia is explained by a primary hydroxylase deficiency. Tetrahydrobiopterin insufficiency impairs function of three hydroxylases (for phenylalanine, tryptophan and tyrosine) and synthesis of their products, notably 5-hydroxytryptophan (the precursor of serotinin) and L-dopa (the precursor of catecholamines) (Fig. 177–1B). The products function as neurotransmitters in brain, and deficiency of them gives rise to central nervous system disease (including retarded psychomotor development, basal ganglion dysfunction, and instability of body temperature). Regeneration of tetrahydrobiopterin is necessary to maintain catalytic function of the three hydroxylases. *Deficient activity of quininoid dihydropteridine reductase* (encoded by a gene on chromosome 4, region p15.3) blocks the cycle maintaining catalytic amounts of tetrahydrobiopterin. *Deficient activity of guanosine triphosphate, cyclohydrolase I, or 6-pyruvoyl tetrahydropterin synthase and "primapterinuria"* (due to an enzyme deficiency as yet uncharacterized) impair synthesis of tetrahydrobiopterin. The relevant genes have not yet been mapped or cloned in humans.

SCREENING AND DIAGNOSIS. Screening of newborn infants for hyperphenylalaninemia is normal practice. Capillary blood collected on filter paper from heel puncture is analyzed by the bacterial inhibition (Guthrie) assay, fluorimetric analysis, or other quantitative methods. Blood phenylalanine values above 2 mg per deciliter (0.125 mM) on the first day of life or thereafter are considered abnormal and require further investigation. The screening test is not infallible, and false-negative results do occur, some for biologic reasons. Urine screening for "phenylketones" is not reliable.

Every infant with persistent hyperphenylalaninemia is investigated to rule out disorders of tetrahydrobiopterin homeostasis. Urine pterin metabolites or blood cofactor levels are measured under special conditions; there are distinctive urine profiles as well as low blood levels in the disorders of tetrahydrobiopterin synthesis. The tests are done at established centers and require experienced interpretation. Measures of phenylalanine hydroxylase require liver biopsy and are seldom done. Dihydropteridine reductase can be measured in blood spots, fibroblasts, and amniocytes; the cyclohydrolase in phytohemagglutinin-stimulated leukocytes but not in fibroblasts; and the synthase in erythrocytes.

After exclusion of disorders of tetrahydropterin metabolism, hyperphenylalaninemia is classified as follows. About one half of cases with primary phenylalanine hydroxylase deficiency have "phenylketonuria," a generic term for severe hyperphenylalaninemia (>1 mM), low phenylalanine tolerance (<500 mg per day), and high risk of mental retardation in the absence of treatment. The remainder have nonphenylketonuric hyperphenylalaninemia

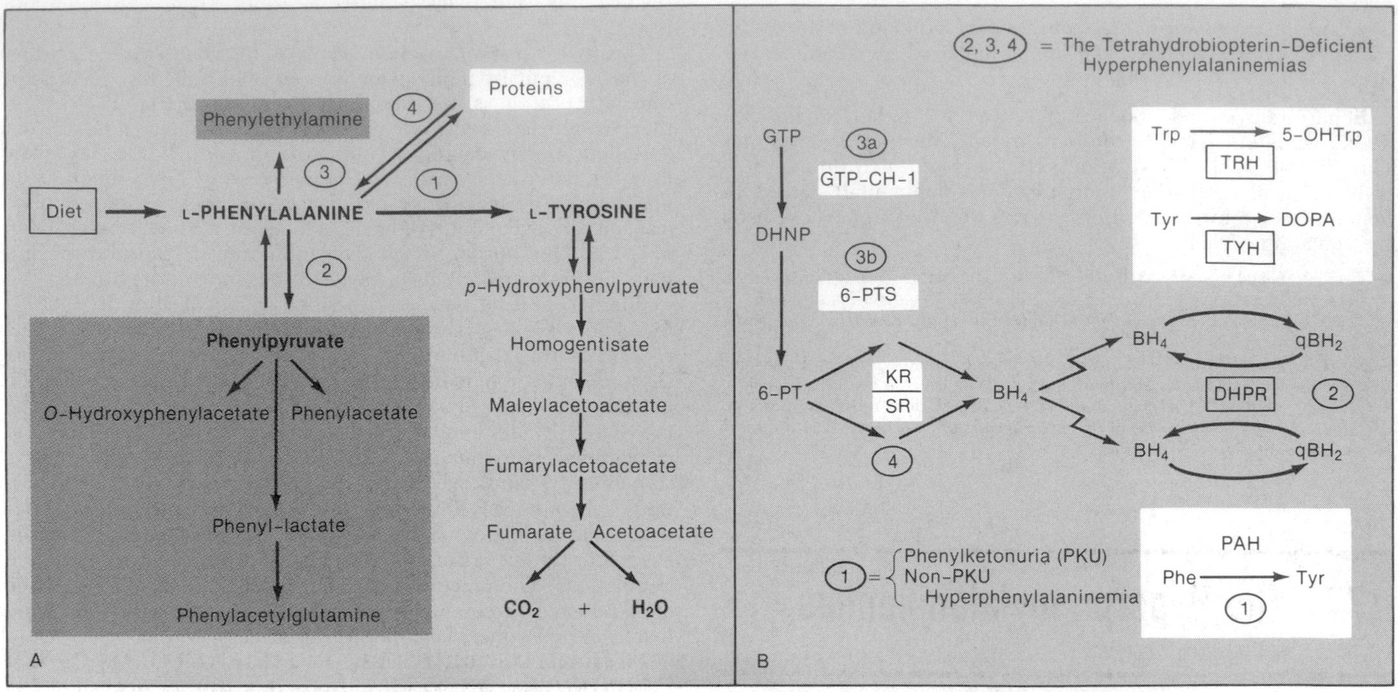

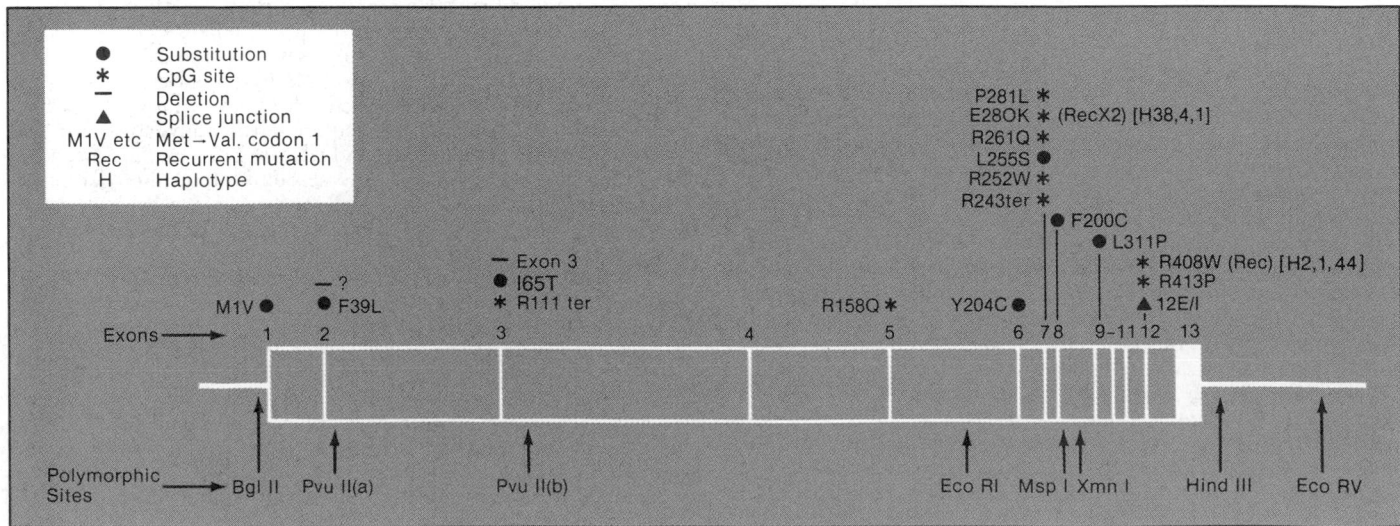

FIGURE 177–1. *A,* Intake of phenylalanine (an essential amino acid supplied only by diet) and its disposal by hydroxylation (1) (representing three quarters of normal runout), transamination (2), decarboxylation (3), and incorporation into proteins (4) (representing under a quarter of runout). *B,* Interrelations between phenylalanine hydroxylase (PAH), dihydropteridine reductase (DHPR), and the tetrahydrobiopterin (BH$_4$) biosynthesis pathway serving aromatic amino acid hydroxylation reactions. Mutations at the relevant chromosomal loci impair the hydroxylation reactions with effects on PAH activity only (1); DHPR activity (2); GTP-cyclohydrolase 1 (GTP-CH-1) activity (3); 6-pyruvoyltetrahydropterin synthase activity (6-PTS) (4); and "primapterin" metabolism (4). Disorders 2, 3a, 3b, and 4 impair function of three hydroxylases: PAH, tyrosine hydroxylase (TYH), and tryptophan hydroxylase (TRH). GTP = guanosine triphosphate; DHNP = dihydroneopterin triphosphate; 6-PT = 6-pyruvoyltetrahydropterin; KR = 2′-ketotetrahydropterin reductase; SR = sepiapterin reductase; qBH$_2$ = quinonoid dihydrobiopterin.

with lower blood phenylalanine values (<1mM), higher tolerance for dietary phenylalanine (>500 mg per day), and no elevated risk for mental retardation if not treated. There is a correlation between level of hepatic hydroxylase activity and clinical form; in broad terms, activity is less than 1 per cent of normal in phenylketonuria and more than 1 per cent of normal in nonphenylketonuric hyperphenylalaninemia.

DNA analysis (by polymerase chain reaction [PCR], nucleotide sequence analysis, Southern blot, and other methods) is useful in identifying mutations at the hydroxylase (Fig. 177–2) and the reductase loci. Interpretation of phenotype by mutation analysis is of increasing clinical relevance. Prenatal diagnosis by analysis of DNA in chorionic villus samples or amniocytes is now feasible for most (≈85 per cent) couples at risk.

FIGURE 177–2. Diagram of the phenylalanine hydroxylase (PAH) gene (≈90 kb, chromosome 12q24.1), showing exons *(vertical bars),* polymorphic restriction sites *(arrows),* and regions of over half the known mutations associated with phenylketonuria. The code (e.g., M1V) indicates normal residue, position in the PAH polypeptide, and replacement residue. One third of mutations involve hypermutable CpG dinucleotides; three mutations are "recurrent."

TREATMENT. The mainstay of treatment for primary phenylalanine hydroxylase deficiency is dietary restriction of the amino acid. There are several semisynthetic diet products ("orphan foods") for this purpose. Phenylketonuric patients can tolerate only 250 to 500 mg of phenylalanine per day to maintain the blood phenylalanine level well below 1 mM. Intake, blood levels of phenylalanine, and growth rate are monitored at frequent intervals to avoid undertreatment or overtreatment. Treatment into adult life is now recommended. Well-treated patients have normal or near-normal intellectual development.

The tetrahydrobiopterin-deficient forms require continuous replacement therapy of cofactor alone or in combination with neurotransmitter precursors and folinic acid is used in dihydropteridine reductase deficiency. Whether effective postnatal treatment of these disorders is feasible remains to be seen.

MATERNAL HYPERPHENYLALANINEMIA. This problem is relevant to all practitioners who counsel women about pregnancy. Intrauterine hyperphenylalaninemia places the fetus at risk of microcephaly, mental retardation, and organ malformations (notably cardiac). Accordingly, all females with hyperphenylalaninemia should be identified, followed (registries exist for this purpose), counselled about risk when they attain reproductive age, and treated with diet to maintain near-normal blood phenylalanine levels before conception and throughout the pregnancy. This treatment prevents harm to the fetus, but it is still under evaluation.

GENETICS. Mutant alleles (at all relevant loci) are recessive. Their aggregate frequency in the population is ≈0.01, meaning that 2 per cent of the population is heterozygous. Explanations for the high frequency of this "rare" phenotype and its genes include founder effects and genetic drift (observed in some populations), selective advantage in the heterozygote (unproved), hypermutability at the locus (observed), reproductive compensation (unlikely), and multiple loci involved in the trait (observed).

Levy HL: Maternal phenylketonuria. Prog Clin Biol 281:227, 1988. *A good up-to-date discussion of a major problem (maternal hyperphenylalaninemia).*

Scriver CR, Kaufman S, Woo SLC: The Hyperphenylalaninemias. *In* Scriver CR, Beaudet AL, Sly WS, et al. (eds.): The Metabolic Basis of Inherited Disease. 6th ed. New York, McGraw-Hill, 1989, pp 495–546. *A reference covering all major issues concerning the hyperphenylalaninemias.*

Trefz FK, Lichter-Konecki U, Konecki D: Phenylketonuria. Curr Opinion Pediatr 1:421, 1989. *A reference covering developments occurring after the preceding reference went to press.*

178 Alcaptonuria

James B. Wyngaarden

DEFINITION. Alcaptonuria is a rare hereditary disease in which homogentisic acid oxidase activity is missing. Homogentisic acid produced during the metabolism of phenylalanine and tyrosine accumulates and is excreted in the urine. It causes pigmentation of cartilage and other connective tissue (ochronosis) and in later years a degenerative arthritis of the spine and the larger peripheral joints. The disease has historical significance, for it was chiefly on the basis of study of families with alcaptonuria that Sir Archibald Garrod developed the concept of inborn errors of metabolism. The disease is inherited as an autosomal recessive trait. No method of detection of heterozygotes has been found.

INCIDENCE AND PREVALENCE. At least 600 cases have been reported, including one in an Egyptian mummy 3500 years old. A prevalence of three to five per million individuals was found in Northern Ireland.

PATHOGENESIS. The activity of homogentisic acid oxidase in the normal adult human liver is sufficient to metabolize over 1600 grams of homogentisic acid per day. Normally, no homogentisic acid can be detected in plasma or urine. In alcaptonuric individuals there is no detectable activity of this enzyme in liver or kidney tissue. Plasma levels of homogentisic acid rise to about 3 mg per deciliter, and the urinary excretion ranges from 4 to 8 grams per day. Mammalian tissue contains an enzyme called homogentisic acid polyphenoloxidase that catalyzes the oxidation of homogentisic acid to an ochronotic pigment, but pigment can also be produced nonenzymatically in the presence of oxygen and alkali, as, for example, in urine. The homogentisic acid polymer has a high affinity for cartilage and connective tissue macromolecules. The stained tissue is fragile and eventually may break down, leading to degenerative intervertebral disc or joint disease. Homogentisic acid may also have a direct effect upon collagen synthesis through inhibition of lysyl hydroxylase.

PATHOLOGY. In an adult alcaptonuric patient, cartilage in many areas, particularly the costal, laryngeal, and tracheal cartilage, is densely pigmented, sometimes being coal-black in appearance. Pigmentation is also present throughout the body in fibrous tissue, fibrocartilage, tendons, and ligaments. To a lesser degree, it is also found in the endocardium, in the intima of larger vessels, in various organs such as kidney and lung, and in the epidermis.

CLINICAL MANIFESTATIONS. Homogentisic acid is present in urine from birth, but urine is colorless when passed. Before the days of disposable diapers, the diagnosis was sometimes made when diapers turned brown in alkaline soaps. Pigment may appear in perspiration and stain clothing in the axillary and genital regions. Generally, the earliest change that can be detected externally is a slight pigmentation of the sclerae or the ears, beginning at 20 or 30 years of age. The cartilage of the ears may be slate blue or gray and feel irregular and thickened. Sometimes dusky discolorations of underlying tendons can be seen through the skin over the hands. In many patients, however, pigment is scarcely evident. The arthritis usually presents with limitation of motion of the hips, knee joints, or shoulders. There may be periods of acute inflammation, and later there is usually rather marked limitation of motion and ankylosis in the lumbosacral region. The arthritic complications are often severe and painful and may lead to extensive crippling. In addition, alcaptonuric patients appear to have a high incidence of cardiovascular disease, including generalized arteriosclerosis and chronic mitral and aortic valvulitis, with calcification of valves and annulus. At least one degenerated pigmented aortic valve has been replaced with a prosthesis. Myocardial infarction is a common cause of death. Other reported complications include ruptured intervertebral discs, prostatitis, and renal stones.

RADIOGRAPHIC CHANGES. These may be almost pathognomonic of alcaptonuria. The vertebral bodies of the lumbar spine show degeneration of the intervertebral discs with narrowing of the space and dense calcification of remaining disc material. There is variable fusion of vertebral bodies, but little osteophyte formation and minimal calcification of intervertebral ligaments. The degenerative changes of ochronotic arthritis are most severe in the hip, shoulder, and knee, and there may be calcific deposits in the tendons. The sacroiliac joints and smaller joints of the extremities usually show little or no abnormality. Ear cartilage may be calcified.

DIAGNOSIS AND DIFFERENTIAL DIAGNOSIS. The diagnosis is suggested by the history of pigmentary changes of urine, the presence of non-glucose reducing substance, the pigmentation of sclerae or cartilage, the arthritic episodes, and especially the typical radiographic changes of the lumbar spine. Specific identification of homogentisic acid in urine can be accomplished by chromatographic or enzymatic assays.

The ochronotic changes of skin and cartilage may be confused with pigmentary changes resulting from prolonged use of quinacrine hydrochloride (Atabrine) or from use of carbolic acid dressings for chronic cutaneous ulcers. The arthritis must be differentiated chiefly from rheumatoid arthritis, osteoarthritis, and gout.

TREATMENT. There is no effective treatment. Dietary restriction of phenylalanine and tyrosine of the degree necessary to reduce homogentisic aciduria is impractical and potentially deleterious. Large amounts of ascorbic acid have been given in an effort to reduce pigment formation. Ascorbic acid protects lysyl hydroxylase from inhibition by homogentisic acid in vitro. It does not alter the metabolic defect.

Justesen P, Anderson PE Jr: Radiologic manifestations in alcaptonuria. Skeletal Radiol 11:204, 1984. *Characteristic radiologic findings are demonstrated.*

La Du BN: Alcaptonuria. *In* Scriver CR, Beaudet AL, Sly WS, et al. (eds.): The Metabolic Basis of Inherited Disease. 6th ed. New York, McGraw-Hill, 1989, p 775. *A detailed discussion of the history, clinical features, and biochemical derangements of alcaptonuria and ochronosis.*

179 The Hyperprolinemias and Hydroxyprolinemia

Lloyd H. Smith, Jr.

The imino acids proline and hydroxyproline are nonessential; proline is readily synthesized in the body from glutamate and ornithine and hydroxyproline from proline. The synthesis of hydroxyproline occurs uniquely in peptide linkage largely as a constituent of collagen. Three rare genetic disorders of the degradative pathways of the acids have been described.

HYPERPROLINEMIAS. Two distinct disorders of proline metabolism, both transmitted as rare autosomal recessive traits, are associated with hyperprolinemia. In type I hyperprolinemia there is a block in the metabolism of proline to Δ'-pyrroline-5-carboxylate because of decreased activity of the enzyme proline oxidase. In type II hyperprolinemia, there is a block at the second step in the degradative pathway, the conversion of Δ'-pyrroline-5-carboxylate to L-glutamate, because of decreased activity of Δ'-pyrroline-5-carboxylate dehydrogenase. In both disorders the accumulation of proline in the blood leads to prolinuria and, through competition for a common renal tubular transport mechanism, to hydroxyprolinuria and glycinuria as well. In the type II disorder, there is also excessive urinary Δ'-pyrroline-5-carboxylate. The disorders can be diagnosed by finding the characteristic changes of hyperprolinemia and iminoaciduria as noted above. Although various forms of renal disease have been described with the type I disorder and neurologic abnormalities and seizures in some patients with either type I or type II hyperprolinemia, these may represent the bias of ascertainment. Since no clinical entity has been clearly established, there is no indicated therapy for either form of hyperprolinemia.

HYDROXYPROLINEMIA. An increased plasma level of free hydroxyproline associated with hydroxyprolinuria has been described in members of several families, but this disorder has not resulted in prolinuria or glycinuria. The disorder is assumed to be an autosomal recessive trait in which the homozygote has deficient activity of hydroxyproline oxidase. There is no associated abnormality of collagen metabolism, and the urinary excretion of peptide-bound hydroxyproline is normal. As in the case of the hyperprolinemias, no clinical entity has been demonstrated and no treatment is indicated.

180 Diseases of the Urea Cycle

Lloyd H. Smith, Jr.

Humans are ureotelic; they depend upon the synthesis of urea for nitrogen excretion. The only source of net urea formation is through the urea cycle (Fig. 180–1), which consists of five enzymes necessary for the sequential synthesis of carbamyl phosphate, citrulline, argininosuccinate, arginine, and urea. The pathway also serves for the de novo synthesis of arginine. When the function of this pathway is impaired, ammonia tends to accumulate. Genetic diseases associated with blocks at each of these five steps have been discovered and are described briefly below. In addition, one patient has been described with deficiency of N-acetylglutamate synthetase, which catalyzes the formation of acetylglutamate, which is required for the activation of carbamyl phosphate synthetase in step 1 (Fig. 180–1).

The associated clinical disorders resulting from the enzymatic defects prior to the synthesis of arginine are similar and can be described under two headings:

1. Neonatal presentation. After a normal pregnancy and delivery, the infant typically becomes symptomatic in 24 to 72 hours, with lethargy, vomiting, hypothermia, and hyperventilation. These symptoms rapidly progress to coma. The plasma ammonia level is high, and the blood urea nitrogen level is markedly reduced. A computed tomographic (CT) scan of the head reveals cerebral edema.

2. Late-onset presentation. These patients may present in later infancy or early childhood with recurrent episodes of hyperammonemia, characterized clinically by vomiting and central nervous system symptoms varying from lethargy, disorientation, and seizures to coma. These episodes may be precipitated by the stress of an infection or a change in diet or may appear with no evident precipitating cause. As in patients with neonatal presentation, respiratory alkalosis is common.

In all of the disorders of the urea cycle associated with hyperammonemia, ammonia itself appears to be the toxic metabolite, since the syndrome can be simulated in experimental animals by the infusion of ammonia. It is speculated that the central nervous system abnormalities can be attributed, at least in part, to the secondary intracellular accumulation of glutamine, with resulting increased osmolarity within the brain, particularly in astrocytes.

CARBAMYL PHOSPHATE SYNTHETASE (CPS) DEFICIENCY. Carbamyl phosphate (CAP) channeled for urea synthesis, in contrast to pyrimidine-channeled CAP, is synthesized in mitochondria from ammonia, bicarbonate, and ATP in a reaction catalyzed by CPS in the presence of N-acetylglutamate as an enzyme activator. Patients with deficiency of CPS usually present with hyperammonemia, protein intolerance, and neurologic symptoms as described above. The diagnosis is established by

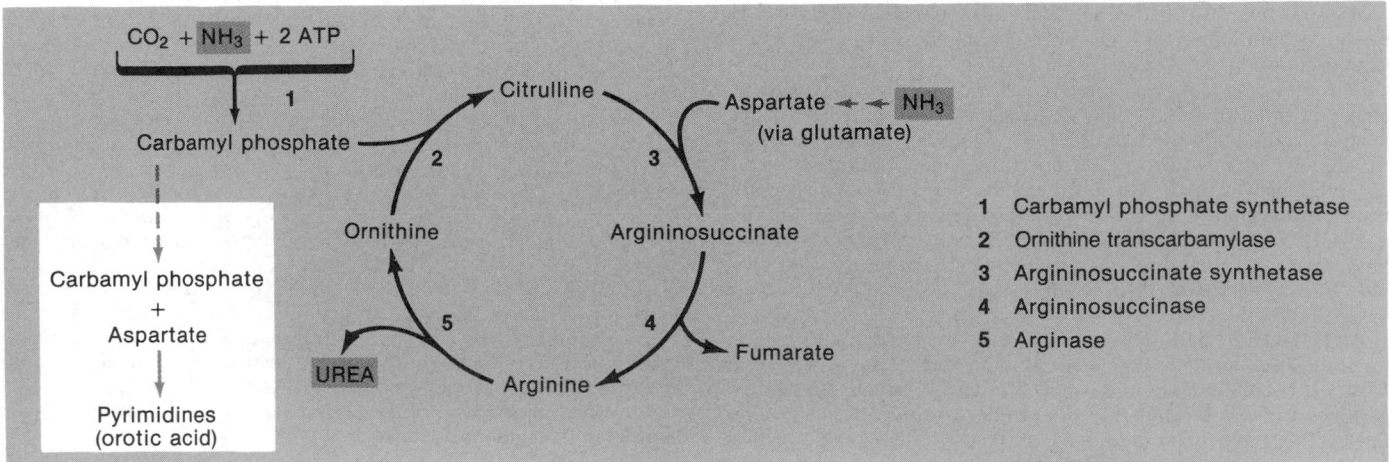

FIGURE 180–1. The urea cycle.

measuring carbamyl phosphate synthetase in a liver biopsy or in peripheral leukocytes. There are no characteristic changes in amino acids in blood or urine. Treatment is by protein restriction, the use of essential amino acids, and the administration of sodium benzoate or phenylacetate to enhance nitrogen excretion as hippurate or phenylacetylglutamine.

ORNITHINE TRANSCARBAMYLASE (OTC) DEFICIENCY. OTC, which catalyzes the mitochondrial carbamylation of ornithine by CAP to form citrulline, is coded for in band p 21.1 of the X chromosome. This most frequent genetic disorder of the urea cycle is therefore transmitted as an X-linked dominant trait, with hemizygous males rarely surviving the neonatal period; females manifest varying degrees of protein intolerance. The clinical onset can be acute and neonatal or late and intermittent, as noted above. As in the case of CPS deficiency, there are no detectable abnormalities of amino acid metabolism. Mitochondrial CAP accumulates, however, and spills over into the cytosol to drive pyrimidine synthesis (Fig. 180–1). This results in orotic aciduria as a constant finding. The enzyme defect can be shown in biopsy specimens from liver or intestinal mucosa or in leukocytes. Prenatal diagnosis of the disease is now possible using a gene-specific probe. The treatment is the same as that described above for CPS deficiency. In both CPS and OTC deficiencies, arginine becomes an essential amino acid. The addition of dietary citrulline as an arginine precursor is therefore recommended.

ARGININOSUCCINATE (ASA) SYNTHETASE DEFICIENCY (CITRULLINEMIA). Citrulline synthesized in mitochondria normally diffuses into the cytosol, where it is condensed with L-aspartic acid in the presence of ATP to form argininosuccinic acid. This reaction is catalyzed by ASA synthetase. Patients with neonatal citrullinemia have exhibited marked heterogeneity in the severity of their clinical and chemical manifestations. The associated hyperammonemia is, in general, less severe than in deficiency of CPS or OCT but does occur after protein ingestion. Citrulline is increased in blood and urine, sometimes more than 100-fold, but there is no evidence that it is toxic per se. Secondary orotic aciduria has been noted, presumably reflecting excess CAP. Patients with a late-onset form of presentation have been described, especially in Japan.

ARGININOSUCCINASE (ASase) DEFICIENCY (ARGININOSUCCINIC ACIDURIA). Cytosolic argininosuccinic acid undergoes reversible cleavage to arginine and fumarate catalyzed by ASase. Approximately 60 patients have been described with argininosuccinic aciduria. Clinical findings, which vary widely in severity, have included mental retardation, seizures, ataxia, hepatomegaly and hepatic fibrosis, and friable hair (trichorrhexis nodosa). In addition to large amounts of ASA in blood, urine, and cerebrospinal fluid (readily demonstrable by chromatography), patients with ASase deficiency may have citrullinemia. As part of dietary therapy, patients should receive supplementary arginine.

ARGINASE DEFICIENCY (HYPERARGININEMIA). Arginine is hydrolyzed to urea and ornithine, catalyzed by arginase, in the last step of the urea cycle. Patients with deficiency of arginase have exhibited mental retardation and spasticity. Arginine is increased in blood and urine and may occasionally cause secondary cystinuria owing to competitive inhibition of the renal tubular transport of dibasic amino acids. Hyperammonemia may be found after protein ingestion. The absence of arginase can be conveniently demonstrated in circulating erythrocytes.

181 Branched-Chain Aminoaciduria

Lloyd H. Smith, Jr.

Leucine, isoleucine, and valine are essential, so-called branched-chain amino acids that have certain structural resemblances and share some common metabolic pathways. Two rare genetic disorders in the degradative pathways of the branched-chain amino acids are described briefly.

MAPLE SYRUP URINE DISEASE. This disorder, also called *branched-chain ketonuria*, derives its name from the character-

istic odor of the urine of affected infants. The disease is transmitted as a rare (1 in 68,000 to 290,000 births in large surveys) autosomal recessive trait in which the affected homozygote exhibits deficient activity in components of the branched-chain keto acid dehydrogenase multienzyme complex, which functions in the oxidative decarboxylation pathway of the keto acids of leucine, isoleucine, and valine. As a consequence, these three amino acids and their corresponding keto acids accumulate in excess in blood and urine and presumably throughout the body. A few patients have a variant disorder that responds in part to treatment with large amounts of thiamine (>150 mg thiamine per day), which may serve to stabilize the dehydrogenase multienzyme complex. The pathogenesis of the deleterious effects in maple syrup urine disease has not been firmly established and may be complex, but probably relates mostly to the accumulation of leucine.

In typical maple syrup urine disease, severe hypotonia, lethargy, feeding difficulties, and hypoglycemia develop in the first week in an infant who seemed normal at birth. Convulsions and decorticate rigidity may develop, and most patients die, commonly of intercurrent infection, within the first year of life (often within the first few weeks). Atypical cases with less severe or even intermittent clinical manifestations have been described. The diagnosis can usually be suspected from the characteristic odor of the urine and is confirmed by the abnormal pattern of amino acids and keto acids in blood and urine. The enzyme defect is demonstrable in leukocytes and fibroblasts.

Treatment—by careful dietary control of leucine, isoleucine, and valine—is simple in theory but difficult in practice because of the necessity to balance three individual essential amino acids that are not easily analyzed. In those few cases in which rigid dietary control with careful monitoring of plasma levels has been instituted early, the results have been gratifying. Thiamine therapy with pharmacological doses should be tried for at least several weeks in addition to dietary restrictions.

ISOVALERIC ACIDEMIA. This rare genetic disorder in the degradative pathway of leucine (>60 cases reported) is due to a block in the conversion of isovaleric acid to beta-methylcrotonic acid, which is catalyzed by isovaleryl-CoA (coenzyme A) dehydrogenase. Isovaleric acid accumulates in blood and urine and gives rise to an odor that has been described as being like sweaty feet. The pathogenesis of the associated clinical features has not been established. Symptoms, which usually begin in the first week of life, consist of attacks of vomiting, acidosis, tremors, lethargy, or even coma. Leukopenia, anemia, thrombocytopenia, and hyperammonemia have been observed during acute attacks. In addition to the acute neonatal form of isovaleric acidemia, a chronic intermittent form of intermediate severity may occur. As in the case of maple syrup urine disease, which it may clinically resemble, isovaleric acidemia may be suspected from the associated odor. The diagnosis is established by the demonstration of excess isovaleric acid in the serum by gas-liquid chromatography or of isovalerylglycine in the urine. Treatment is by strict control of dietary leucine. More recently, therapy with glycine and carnitine has shown promise by enhancing the removal of isovaleric acid as isovalerylglycine and isovalerylcarnitine, respectively.

Hyperprolinemia and Hydroxyprolinemia

Phang JM, Scriver CR: Disorders of proline and hydroxyproline metabolism. *In* Scriver CR, Beaudet A, Sly W, et al. (eds): The Metabolic Basis of Inherited Disease. 6th ed. New York, McGraw-Hill, 1989, pp 577–597. *An extensive analysis of the chemical derangements in these rare disorders.*

Diseases of the Urea Cycle

Beaudet AL, O'Brien WE, Bock H-GO, et al.: The human argininosuccinate synthetase locus and citrullinemia. Adv Hum Genet 15:161, 1986. *An excellent general review of this rare disorder, with particular emphasis on the molecular analysis of the defective gene.*

Brusilow SW, Horwich AL: Urea cycle enzymes. *In* Scriver CR, Beaudet A, Sly W, et al. (eds.): The Metabolic Basis of Inherited Disease. 6th ed. New York, McGraw-Hill, 1989, pp 629–663. *A large number of disorders are associated with derangements in urea synthesis. This chapter gives a lucid summary of the biochemistry of urea synthesis and the pathogenesis of the various disorders associated with that pathway. As always in The Metabolic Basis of Inherited Disease, there is a large and useful bibliography (347 references).*

Rowe PC, Newman SL, Brusilow SW: Natural history of symptomatic partial ornithine transcarbamylase deficiency. N Engl J Med 314:541, 1986. *Studies of the disease in a series of symptomatic female heterozygotes with a description of clinical manifestations, therapy, and outcome.*

Branched-Chain Aminoaciduria

Danner DJ, Elsas LJ: Disorders of branched chain amino acid and keto acid metabolism. *In* Scriver CR, Beaudet A, Sly W, et al. (eds.): The Metabolic Basis of Inherited Disease. 6th ed. New York, McGraw-Hill, 1989, pp 671–692. *This is the most sophisticated general presentation of the pathogenesis of this group of disorders. Although the emphasis is on the biochemical basis, there is a useful clinical discussion and an extensive bibliography (268 references).*

182 Homocystinuria

S. Harvey Mudd

DEFINITION. The term *homocystinuria* designates a biochemical abnormality, not a disease entity. Several known genetic disorders lead to homocystinuria. Most common is cystathionine beta-synthase deficiency. In this condition ectopia lentis, mental retardation, bone abnormalities, osteoporosis, and thromboembolic phenomena are frequent.

PREVALENCE. More than 600 adequately documented cases of cystathionine beta-synthase deficiency have been reported. Screening of newborn infants indicates a *minimal* prevalence of 1 in 300,000 worldwide.

ETIOLOGY AND PATHOGENESIS. Cystathionine beta-synthase deficiency is inherited as an autosomal recessive trait. Deficient activity of this enzyme has been demonstrated in liver extracts, in brain, and in cultured skin fibroblasts and lymphocytes. The enzyme deficiency results in failure of homocysteine to react with serine to form cystathionine on the pathway to cysteine. Homocystine is the disulfide oxidation product formed from two molecules of homocysteine. Homocysteinyl moieties are currently detected in normal human plasma at total concentrations of 6 to 14 μM, depending upon the laboratory and method used. In vivo, some 75 to 80 per cent of these moieties are bound by disulfide linkage to proteins; the remainder are not protein bound. In cystathionine beta-synthase–deficient patients, fasting plasma concentrations up to 200 μM of non–protein-bound homocystine have been reported. The urine may contain up to 1 mmol of homocystine per day. Plasma methionine levels are also raised, and plasma cystine is low. Detailed studies, chiefly of cultured fibroblasts, suggest extensive heterogeneity in the genetic lesions producing deficient activity of cystathionine beta-synthase. An important manifestation of such genetic heterogeneity is pyridoxine responsiveness. In 40 to 50 per cent of cystathionine beta-synthase–deficient patients, administration of relatively large amounts of pyridoxine markedly reduces or eliminates homocystinuria, homocystinemia, hypermethionemia, and hypocystinemia. Within any one sibship, all affected sibs are either B_6 responsive or B_6 nonresponsive.

PATHOLOGY. There is breakage of the zonular fibers of the lens (possibly due to disruption of the highly disulfide-linked proteins of the microfibrillar system), with resulting subluxation. The skeleton is markedly osteoporotic, and the vertebrae show rarefaction with biconcave compression. Thrombi and emboli have been reported in almost every artery or vein. These result in brain infarcts, coronary occlusion and myocardial infarction, pulmonary infarcts, renal infarcts, and thrombophlebitis with pulmonary emboli. The pathogenesis of the thrombotic tendency is not clearly understood, but increase of plasma homocyst(e)ine, rather than plasma methionine, is likely to cause the thrombotic tendency.

CLINICAL MANIFESTATIONS. Among individuals with cystathionine beta-synthase deficiency, there is marked variation with regard to the major clinical features of this condition, their time of onset, and severity. Clinical manifestations tend to be less prevalent, slower in onset, or less marked among B_6-responsive patients than among nonresponsive ones. A survey of 629 patients showed that mental capabilities ranged from severely retarded to IQs as high as 130. Median IQ for B_6-responsive patients was 78; for B_6-nonresponsive patients, 56. Mental retardation, when present, most commonly becomes manifest during the first few years of life.

The incidence of dislocated optic lenses increases with age. By the age of 10 years, 55 per cent of B_6-responsive patients and 82 per cent of B_6-nonresponsive patients have dislocated lenses. Acute glaucoma and reduced visual acuity may result.

Thromboembolism is the life-threatening complication of cystathionine beta-synthase deficiency. By age 15, chances of having had a clinically detected thromboembolic event are 12 per cent among B_6 responders and 27 per cent among B_6 nonresponders. Large and small arteries and veins may be affected. Major cerebrovascular thrombosis may occur. Venous thrombosis with pulmonary emboli is common. By age 30 years, 4 per cent of B_6-responsive patients and 23 per cent of B_6-nonresponsive patients have died.

The spine is the most common site of osteoporosis, followed by the long bones. By age 15, chances of having radiologically detected spinal osteoporosis are 36 per cent among B_6 responders and 65 per cent among B_6 nonresponders. Scoliosis occurs in many individuals, although kyphosis is infrequent. Vertebral collapse and pathologic fractures of long bones may occur. The long bones are generally thin and excessively lengthened. Pectus carinatum or excavatum is common.

DIAGNOSIS AND DIFFERENTIAL DIAGNOSIS. The diagnosis is suggested by ectopia lentis and thromboembolic phenomena, together with other aforementioned features. On occasion, patients present with thrombotic disease and a paucity of other manifestations. The urinary cyanide-nitroprusside reaction is positive. Other disulfidurias—for example, cystinuria—also produce a positive cyanide-nitroprusside reaction, so homocystinemia and homocystinuria distinguish cystathionine beta-synthase deficiency from alternative forms of disulfiduria. Cystathionine beta-synthase deficiency is confirmed by demonstration of markedly reduced enzyme activity with cultured skin fibroblasts or phytohemagglutinin-stimulated lymphocytes or in a liver biopsy specimen.

Heterozygotes may be identified by assay of cystathionine beta-synthase activity in liver biopsy tissue. Cystathionine beta-synthase activities in cultured fibroblasts or phytohemagglutinin-stimulated lymphocytes from most heterozygotes are below the control range, but there is some overlap. For unequivocal identification, such studies are best accompanied by methionine loading tests. In some young adults, premature peripheral or cerebral occlusive arterial disease may be due to heterozygosity for cystathionine beta-synthase deficiency, and there is increasing evidence that mild homocysteinemia, whatever its cause, is an independent risk factor for vascular disease.

Rarer forms of homocystinuria are caused by decreased 5-methyltetrahydrofolate–dependent homocysteine methylation, owing either to decreased 5,10-methylenetetrahydrofolate reductase activity or to a variety of lesions that interfere with the ability to produce methylcobalamin. In all of these, plasma methionine levels are low. The condition is first noted in childhood. Homocystinuria also occurs following 6-azauridine triacetate administration.

TREATMENT. Management is directed toward the biochemical abnormality, with the aim of preventing or ameliorating clinical manifestations, and toward the clinical treatment of complications.

Newborns with cystathionine beta-synthase deficiency have almost always been treated with a low-methionine diet (usually accompanied by cystine supplementation). Such therapy prevents mental retardation and may decrease the rate of lens dislocations and reduce the incidence of seizures. It is too early to assess the effects on thromboembolic events, osteoporosis, or mortality. When the condition is diagnosed at later ages in B_6-responsive patients, pyridoxine treatment (doses up to 500 to 1000 mg per day) accompanied by folate repletion has been shown to produce a statistically significant reduction in the rate of initial thromboembolic events. When diagnosis is made at later ages in B_6-nonresponsive patients, strict methionine limitation, if accepted and carefully adhered to, may be beneficial in preventing thromboembolic events. In early studies of such patients, betaine, which lowers homocysteine by accelerating its methylation, has appeared useful. Antithrombotic therapy with aspirin and dipyridamole has also been advocated.

Cochran FB, Sweetman L, Schmidt K, et al.: Pyridoxine-unresponsive homocystinuria with an unusual clinical course. Am J Med Genet 35:519, 1990. *A patient presenting with asthma, pneumothoraces, and superior sagittal sinus thrombosis.*

Gibson MA, Kumaratilake JS, Cleary EG: The protein components of the 12-nanometer microfibrils of elastic and nonelastic tissues. J Biol Chem 264:4590, 1989. *Studies of the components that may be affected in the connective tissue disorders.*

Malinow MR, Kang SS, Taylor LM, et al.: Prevalence of hyperhomocyst(e)inemia in patients with peripheral arterial occlusive disease. Circulation 79:1180, 1989. *A useful summary of modern methods for analysis of plasma homocyst(e)ine and a review of studies implicating mild homocysteinemia as an independent risk factor for early vascular disease.*

McGill JJ, Mettler G, Rosenblatt DS, et al.: Detection of heterozygotes for recessive alleles. Homocyst(e)inemia: Paradigm of pitfalls in phenotypes. Am J Med Genet 36:45, 1990. *Critical discussion of problems in the identification of heterozygotes.*

Mitchell GA, Watkins D, Melancon SB, et al.: Clinical heterogeneity in cobalamin C variant of combined homocystinuria and methylmalonic aciduria. J Pediatr 108:410, 1986. *Contains a useful brief summary of other causes of homocystinuria.*

Mudd SH, Levy HL, Skovby F: Disorders of transsulfuration. *In* Scriver CS, Beaudet AL, Sly WS, et al. (eds.): The Metabolic Basis of Inherited Disease. 6th ed. New York, McGraw-Hill, 1989. *A detailed review of the clinical features of confirmed cases of cystathionine beta-synthase deficiency, with a discussion of metabolic factors in homocystinuria.*

Mudd SH, Skovby F, Levy HL, et al.: The natural history of homocystinuria due to cystathionine-β-synthase deficiency. Am J Hum Genet 37:1, 1985. *An international questionnaire study covering 629 patients. The natural history of the untreated disease is defined for the major clinical manifestations and the effects of therapies evaluated statistically.*

DISORDERS OF PURINE AND PYRIMIDINE METABOLISM

183 Gout

James B. Wyngaarden

Gout is a term representing a heterogeneous group of genetic and acquired diseases manifested by *hyperuricemia* and a characteristic *acute inflammatory arthritis* induced by *crystals* of monosodium urate monohydrate. Some patients develop aggregated deposits of these crystals (*tophi*) in and around the joints of the extremities that can lead to severe crippling. Many patients develop a *chronic interstitial nephropathy*. In addition, uric acid *urolithiasis* is common in gout.

These manifestations of gout can occur in different combinations. However, essential hyperuricemia alone, even when complicated by uric acid lithiasis, should not be called gout; gout signifies inflammatory arthritis or tophaceous disease.

A classification emphasizing the heterogeneity of gout is presented in Table 183–1.

PREVALENCE AND INCIDENCE. The prevalence of gout varies from about 0.13 to 0.37 per cent in Europe and the United States to 10 per cent in adult male Maori of New Zealand. Exceptionally high prevalences are also found in Filipinos in the United States and in natives of the Mariana Islands. During World Wars I and II, acute gouty arthritis was uncommon in Europe. When dietary protein again became plentiful, its frequency returned to prewar levels. Although formerly rare in Japan, gout has now become common in parallel with the increase in protein consumption in that country.

Primary gout is chiefly a disease of adult men; only about 5 per cent of cases are found in women, largely in the postmenopausal group. The frequency of gout is increased in patients taking diuretics, especially of the thiazide group; in certain nephropathies; and in polycythemia vera, myeloid metaplasia, or chronic hemolysis. Gout in all of its forms makes up about 5 per cent of arthritis cases.

GENETICS OF GOUT. A family history of clinical gout is generally found in 6 to 18 per cent of patients in the United States and Denmark. Figures of 40 to 80 per cent have been reported from England and also from the United States following tenacious family studies. About 25 per cent of first-degree relatives of gouty subjects are hyperuricemic, and about 20 per cent of these have symptomatic gout. Familial hyperuricemia is polygenic and multifactorial. Hyperuricemia is correlated with maleness, surface area, obesity, ponderal index, protein intake, social status, educational level, and alcohol ingestion. In primary gout associated with hypoxanthine-guanine phosphoribosyltransferase

(HPRT) deficiency and phosphoribosylpyrophosphate (PP-ribose-P) synthetase variants, the genetic transmissions are X linked. Glycogen storage disease type I, which is associated with a specific form of secondary gout, is an autosomal recessive trait.

PATHOGENESIS AND PATHOLOGY. The hallmark of gout is hyperuricemia. The risk of gout increases with the degree of hyperuricemia and also with age (Table 183–2). Virtually all patients with gout have serum urate values above 7.0 mg per deciliter. An occasional patient has a lower value at the time of attack, perhaps attributable to the urate diuresis that sometimes accompanies the inflammatory response. Repeat analyses show hyperuricemia during quiescent periods.

In normal prepubertal children, serum urate values average 3.6 mg per deciliter in both sexes. At puberty these levels increase. In the United States, the central 95 per cent segment of the distributions encompasses values of 2.2 to 7.5 mg per deciliter in adult males and 2.1 to 6.6 mg per deciliter in adult premenopausal females. After the menopause, mean values in women increase to approximate levels in men. Definitions of hyperuricemia based on distributions of serum urate are useful for epidemiologic studies. But statistical expressions are not adequate definitions of the pathophysiologic significance of hyperuricemia, for it is the *solubility* of urate in plasma and body fluids that is important. There is no evidence that urate in solution is toxic; all of the features of gout derive from responses to the urate crystal.

The solubility of urate in body fluids is strongly influenced by pH and temperature (Table 183–3). At pH 7.4 and 37°C, the solubility of urate in fluid having the sodium composition of plasma is 6.4 to 6.8 mg per deciliter. An additional 0.4 mg per deciliter is protein bound, chiefly to an alpha$_1$-alpha$_2$ globulin. Thus 7.0 mg per deciliter is about the solubility limit of urate in plasma at normal central body temperature and defines hyperuricemia in a physicochemical sense. But solubility is considerably less at the temperature of peripheral joints, which may be 32°C in the knee and 29°C in the ankle (Hollander, 1949).

Mechanisms of Hyperuricemia. The concentration of urate in plasma is determined by the balance between absorption and production of purines on the one hand and destruction and excretion on the other. Exogenous purines contribute substantially to body uric acid stores. Purine restriction leads to a reduction in the serum urate level of 0.6 to 1.8 mg per deciliter in normal subjects and in patients with idiopathic gout. Abnormalities of purine absorption have not been implicated as a cause of hyperuricemia.

Human beings lack uricase; therefore uric acid is the end-product of purine metabolism. In normal subjects approximately one third of the uric acid disposed of each day is degraded by bacteria in the gut, and two thirds is excreted unchanged by the

TABLE 183–1. CLASSIFICATION OF HYPERURICEMIA AND GOUT

Type	Disturbance in Uric Acid Metabolism	Inheritance
Primary		
I. Idiopathic (>99% of primary gout)		
A. Normal urinary excretion (80–90% of primary gout)	Decreased renal clearance ± overproduction	Polygenic
B. Increased urinary excretion (10–20% of primary gout)	Overproduction ± decreased renal clearance	Polygenic
II. Associated with specific enzyme or metabolic defects (<1% of primary gout)		
A. Increased activity of PP-ribose-P synthetase	Overproduction; increased synthesis of PP-ribose-P	X-linked
B. "Partial" deficiency of hypoxanthine-guanine phosphoribosyltransferase	Overproduction; increased PP-ribose-P concentration	X-linked
Secondary		
I. Associated with increased purine biosynthesis de novo		
A. "Complete" deficiency of hypoxanthine-guanine phosphoribosyltransferase	Overproduction; Lesch-Nyhan syndrome	X-linked
B. Glucose-6-phosphatase deficiency	Overproduction and decreased renal clearance; glycogen storage disease, type I (von Gierke)	Autosomal recessive
II. Associated with increased nucleic acid turnover	Overproduction, e.g., chronic hemolysis; polycythemia; myeloid metaplasia	—
III. Associated with decreased renal clearance of uric acid	Reduced renal functional mass; inhibition of secretion and/or enhanced reabsorption by drugs, toxins, or endogenous metabolic products	—

kidney. Decreased uricolysis has been excluded as a mechanism for hyperuricemia. In fact, with high urate concentrations in body fluids, enteric uricolysis is enhanced; with the onset of renal insufficiency, intestinal uricolysis assumes increased importance and in extreme instances may account for 80 per cent of daily urate disposition. By contrast, both increased purine biosynthesis and decreased renal excretion of uric acid play important roles in the pathogenesis of primary hyperuricemia.

Random urine samples in normal men commonly contain 500

TABLE 183–2. PREVALENCE OF GOUTY ARTHRITIS IN MEN IN RELATION TO SERUM URATE CONCENTRATION AND AGE

Serum Urate Level (mg/dl)	Mean Age 49 Years* (%)	Mean Age 58 Years† (%)
6.0–6.9	2	2
7.0–7.9	4	17
8.0–8.9	11	25
9.0–9.9	30	90
10 +	48	90

*Data from Zalokar et al.: J Chronic Dis 25:305, 1972.
†Data from Hall et al.: Am J Med 42:27, 1967.

TABLE 183–3. SOLUBILITY OF URATE ION AS A FUNCTION OF TEMPERATURE IN THE PRESENCE OF 140 mM Na*

Temperature (° C)	Maximal Equilibrium Concentration of Urate in the Presence of 140 mM Na+ (mg/dl)
37	6.8
35	6.0
30	4.5
25	3.3
20	2.5
15	1.8
10	1.2

*From Loeb: Arthritis Rheum 15:189, 1972. Reprinted from Arthritis and Rheumatism Journal, copyright 1972. Used by permission of the American College of Rheumatology.

to 1000 mg per 24 hours. In men on a purine-restricted diet these values average 418 ± 70 mg per 24 hours. From 10 to 20 per cent of gouty subjects show basal values above the m + 2SD value. However, urinary urate measurements are insensitive in the assessment of purine production. With labeled uric acid, the miscible pool of uric acid in normal humans averages 1200 mg, and the daily rate of production averages 750 mg. One half to three fourths of the pool turns over each day. The difference between the rate of production and the rate of excretion of urate ranges from 100 to 365 mg per day and represents intestinal uricolysis. This method discloses an enlarged urate pool in all gouty subjects studied and increased turnover in most.

A second method of study of uric acid production involves measurement of incorporation of an isotopically labeled purine precursor, usually glycine, into urinary uric acid. The incorporation can be corrected for extrarenal disposal to give total incorporation values. By use of these methods, evidence of some degree of excessive production of uric acid has been obtained in about two thirds of gouty patients studied. The most extreme values are found in subjects with HPRT deficiency or PP-ribose-P synthetase variants, but these represent fewer than 1 per cent of gouty subjects. Many patients whose 24-hour urinary uric acid values fall within the normal range show modest increases in the rate of turnover of an enlarged uric acid pool and/or overincorporation of glycine into urate. Studies of the intramolecular distribution of ^{15}N in uric acid following administration of ^{15}N-glycine show excessive labeling of position 9, which is derived from the amide-N of glutamine and from ammonia. Thus many more gouty subjects show evidence of mild overproduction of purine than would have been deduced from urinary uric acid measurements alone.

The first unique reaction of purine biosynthesis and the site of metabolic regulation by purine ribonucleotide inhibitors is that which synthesizes phosphoribosylamine, catalyzed by amido-phosphoribosyltransferase:

$$\text{Glutamine} + \text{PP-ribose-P} + \text{H}_2\text{O} \xrightarrow{\text{Mg}^{2+}}$$
$$\text{phosphoribosylamine} + \text{glutamic acid} + \text{PPi}$$

There are several possible mechanisms for loss of regulation at this site and acceleration of purine biosynthesis. These include (1) excessive concentrations of the substrates PP-ribose-P, glutamine, or both; (2) a structural alteration or increased amount of the enzyme, rendering it more active or less sensitive to inhibition by purine ribonucleotides; or (3) a reduced concentration of one of the regulatory nucleotides (adenosine monophosphate [AMP] or guanosine monophosphate [GMP]) that exert cooperative allosteric inhibition of enzyme activity. Intracellular levels of PP-ribose-P are strikingly raised in HPRT deficiency and also in PP-ribose-P synthetase overactivity. The increased concentration of PP-ribose-P drives purine biosynthesis both by furnishing more of the rate-limiting substrate and by allosteric activation of amidophosphoribosyltransferase. PP-ribose-P turnover is accelerated in gouty patients in whom uric acid is overproduced. However, erythrocyte PP-ribose-P levels are normal in gouty patients without specific enzyme defects. Plasma glutamate values are slightly raised in gouty subjects, both in the fasting state and after oral glutamate loads, but plasma glutamine levels are normal. Although reduced activities of glutaminase and of glutamic dehydrogenase have been postulated in gout, no direct evidence for such enzyme deficiencies exists. Any process that results in accelerated breakdown of intracellular adenyl nucleotides may lead to hyperuricemia by prompt degradation of daughter purine compounds to uric acid and to secondary acceleration of purine synthesis de novo through release of inhibition of amidophosphoribosyltransferase. This biphasic mechanism has been implicated in glycogen storage disease type I following fructose infusion, following alcohol ingestion, and in a gouty patient with a variant AMP deaminase that showed reduced sensitivity to guanosine triphosphate (GTP), its normal regulator. The last example has been proposed as a possible general mechanism in idiopathic gout. There are no examples of gout attributable to intrinsic alterations of the amidophosphoribosyltransferase itself.

In the normal turnover of nucleic acids and nucleotides, some are degraded to free purine bases, chiefly hypoxanthine and guanine. Nucleotides synthesized de novo in excess of nucleic acid requirements are promptly degraded to hypoxanthine. Guanine is deaminated to xanthine by guanase. Hypoxanthine and xanthine are oxidized to uric acid by xanthine oxidase (Fig. 183–1). Hepatic xanthine oxidase activity is increased in gouty overproducers, but this appears to be an induced rather than a primary change. Nevertheless, this is an additional factor contributing to accelerated uric acid synthesis in these patients.

In a substantial fraction of gouty subjects, the immediate pathogenetic mechanism of hyperuricemia appears to be a decreased renal tubular clearance of urate. Renal excretion of urate is a complex function of glomerular filtration, tubular reabsorption, and tubular secretion. Filtration of plasma urate is assumed to be complete, on the basis of micropuncture studies in animals and ultrafiltration studies of human plasma in vitro. Less than 5 per cent of plasma urate is protein bound in humans under physiologic conditions at 37°C. Filtered urate appears to be almost completely reabsorbed in the proximal tubule (presecretory reabsorption). Some of the secreted urate is also reabsorbed in the distal portion of the proximal tubule and to a lesser extent in the ascending portion of the loop of Henle and in the collecting ducts (postsecretory reabsorption). Excreted urate is thought to arise almost entirely by tubular secretion.

Studies in gouty patients have been interpreted as indicating reduced secretion of urate per nephron, but enhanced postsecretory reabsorption would also explain the data. The renal contribution to hyperuricemia is most marked in patients with normal 24-hour excretion values of urate, normal turnover values of the uric acid pool, and normal values of glycine incorporation into uric acid. But reduced renal urate clearances per nephron are not restricted to this group. With the exception of patients with HPRT deficiency or PP-ribose-P synthetase variants, overproducer gouty subjects as a group also show reduced renal urate clearance (Simkin). Thus, although some investigators have separated the large group of patients with an undefined biochemical lesion, *idiopathic gout*, into two discrete subgroups termed metabolic (overproducer) and renal gout, the evidence does not support such a categoric distinction, inasmuch as many subjects show both defects. Since chronic excessive alcohol consumption is common in gouty subjects and causes excessive turnover of adenine nucleotides and increased urate production and excretion, it is possible that some of the metabolic contributions to hyperuricemia in idiopathic gout are alcohol related.

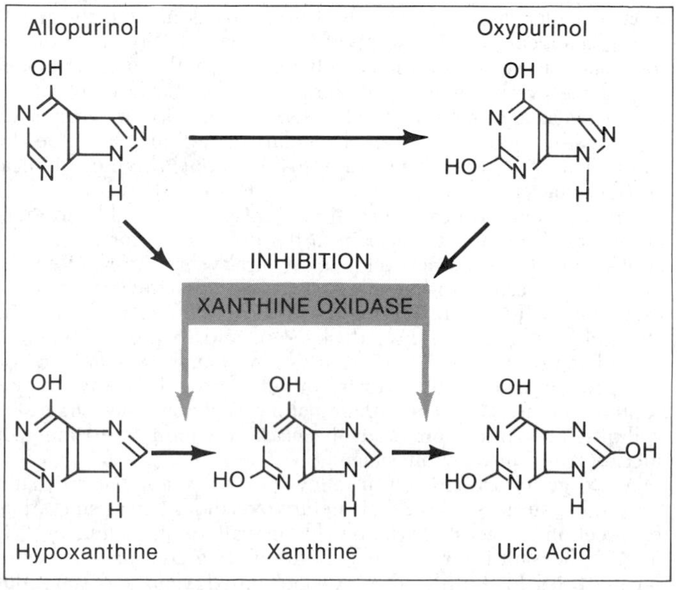

The complexity of the pathogenesis of hyperuricemia is illustrated by two additional observations. The first is that asymptomatic hyperuricemia begins at puberty in the male as an exaggeration of the modest increase in serum urate concentration that normally occurs at that age and at the menopause in the female. Clearly, hormonal factors influence serum urate levels. The second is that both pathogenetic mechanisms may be reversible. Subjects with primary (idiopathic) gout are, on average, 15 to 30 per cent overweight, and 75 per cent or more show fasting hypertriglyceridemia. (Hyperuricemia is present in more than 80 per cent of all patients with hypertriglyceridemia.) In some gouty patients, weight reduction and abstinence from alcohol reverse hypertriglyceridemia, hyperuricemia, excessive urate excretion, and evidence of overproduction by isotopic studies, as well as evidence of impaired renal urate clearance.

The Acute Gouty Attack. In 1859, A. B. Garrod, in the second and fourth of his 10 propositions on the "The True Nature of Essence of Gout," wrote the following: "Investigations recently made in the morbid anatomy of gout, prove incontestably that true gouty inflammation is *always* accompanied with a deposition of urate of soda in the inflamed part. . . . The deposited urate of soda may be looked upon as the cause, and not the effect, of the gouty inflammation." The role of the urate crystal in acute gout was rediscovered in 1961 by McCarty and Hollander. In laboratory animals experimental gouty arthritis requires the presence of leukocytes. However, synovitis can also be produced experimentally by other crystals of similar size and shape, and it occurs in pseudogout caused by calcium pyrophosphate dihydrate crystals.

Although a number of cellular mechanisms are activated by the urate crystal, the exact sequence by which inflammation is initiated is uncertain. Hageman's factor, kallikrein, kinin-like peptides, and the complement system all participate in the response, but each has also been excluded as an obligatory factor. Urate crystals are leukotactic. Leukocytes and synovial lining cells ingest the urate crystals. Within minutes leukocytes release leukotriene B$_4$ (LTB$_4$) and a glycoprotein chemotactic factor (mw = 11,500). Production of these chemoattractants is blocked by colchicine. The acute inflammatory response to injected urate crystals is also blocked by prior treatment with colchicine, but the inflammatory response to purified crystal-induced chemotactic factor is not. Thus this factor and LTB$_4$ may be important mediators of the inflammatory reaction in gout. Monocytes are also stimulated by urate crystals in vitro, with release of interleukin 1. IL-1 may also contribute to initiation and amplification of gouty inflammation.

Crystal-cell interactions may be modulated by proteins adherent to the crystals. Crystals from patients with acute gout have surface coats of IgG and, to a lesser extent, of IgM, IgA, C3, and fibrinogen, but not of albumin. In studies in vitro, IgG coating enhances neutrophil responsiveness to urate crystals, whereas certain other proteins inhibit. Such modulating factors may account for the variable inflammatory responses to urate crystals in gouty subjects.

Phagocytosis of the crystal leads to rapid destruction of the phagolysosome membrane with release of hydrolytic enzymes into the cell. This results in cell necrosis and release of the crystal and lysosomal and cytoplasmic enzymes into the surrounding tissue.

The events leading to the putative burst of microcrystals of urate that initiates the acute attack are largely speculative. Three major theories have been advanced. The first postulates that trauma may result in shedding of crystals from pre-existing cartilaginous tophi into the synovial fluid. The second emphasizes the ability of organized proteoglycans of cartilage to absorb (solubilize) urate. Disruption and increased turnover of proteo-

FIGURE 183–1. Pathway of uric acid synthesis catalyzed by xanthine oxidase and the site of action of allopurinol.

glycans are postulated to occur following trauma, with release of additional urate into the already supersaturated synovial fluid and resulting crystallization. The third postulates a joint effusion with trauma, followed by a more rapid rate of reabsorption of water than of solute, resulting in further supersaturation of synovial fluid with urate and precipitation of crystals. The first metatarsophalangeal joint is exposed to the greatest pressure per unit area of any joint in the body during walking, and it and other lower extremity joints, which are the joints predominantly involved in gout, are especially susceptible to trauma. In addition, the low temperature of peripheral leg joints favors crystallization of urate from supersaturated synovial fluid. Thus each of these theories, which are not mutually exclusive, has merit.

Tophi. The pathognomonic lesion of gout is the *tophus*, a deposit of fine acicular crystals of monosodium urate monohydrate, surrounded by a mononuclear reaction and a foreign body granuloma of epithelial and giant cells, some of which may be multinucleate. Urate crystals are water soluble, but when tissues are treated with nonaqueous fixatives (e.g., absolute alcohol), the crystals are preserved and are brilliantly anisotropic and negatively birefringent in compensated polarized light. Tophi are commonly found in articular and other cartilage, synovia, tendon sheaths and other periarticular structures, epiphyseal bone, the subcutaneous layers of the skin, and the interstitial areas of the kidney. The articular cartilages are the most common and at times the exclusive sites of urate deposition. The deposits, although superficial, are actually embedded in the intercellular matrix. In the joint, cartilaginous degeneration, synovial proliferation and pannus, destruction of subchondral bone, proliferation of marginal bone, and sometimes fibrous or bony ankylosis develop. The punched-out lesions of bone commonly seen on roentgenograms represent marrow tophus deposits, which may communicate with the urate crust on the articular surface through defects in the cartilage. In vertebral bodies, urate deposits involve the marrow spaces adjacent to the intervertebral discs, as well as the discs themselves.

All of these sites of urate deposition are rich in proteoglycans, and the postulated role of these substances in attracting and solubilizing urate when organized, and of releasing urate during metabolic turnover, cited above, may serve to explain both localization and occurrence of tophi. Curiously, the process in the tissues evokes only a minimal inflammatory response in comparison with the violence of the acute gouty attack brought about by crystals within the synovial space. Urate crystals stimulate mesenchymal cells of joints to produce collagenase and prostaglandin E_2, both of which may play roles in articular destruction.

The Gouty Kidney. The only distinctive histologic feature of the gouty kidney is the presence of sodium urate crystals in the medulla or pyramids and surrounding round cell and giant cell reaction. These are found in a high percentage of gouty patients at autopsy and are associated with acute and chronic interstitial inflammatory changes, fibrosis, tubular atrophy, glomerulosclerosis, and arteriolar nephrosclerosis. The earliest change in the kidney is an interstitial reaction, maximal near the loops of Henle, associated with tubular damage. In kidneys without tophi, the interstitial reaction tends to spare the medulla and juxtamedullary cortex. Although renal disease is common in gout, it is generally mild and only slowly progressive. The origin of the interstitial nephropathy is not known. It is not even certain that in the absence of crystalline deposits it is related to hyperuricemia. Other possibilities include nephrosclerosis, uric acid stone disease, urinary infection, aging, and lead poisoning. Crystalline deposits may occur within the distal tubules and collecting ducts and are probably composed of uric acid and related to the intratubular concentration of uric acid and the acid pH of the urine; they lead to dilatation and atrophy of the more proximal tubules. Deposits within the interstitium are composed of sodium urate and are believed to be related to the elevated urate concentration of plasma and interstitial fluid.

Uric Acid Urolithiasis. The overall incidence of renal stones in gout is about 20 per cent, about 200-fold higher than in the general population. In 84 per cent of gouty subjects, the stones are pure uric acid (not sodium urate); in 4 per cent, uric acid and calcium oxalate; and in 12 per cent, calcium oxalate or phosphate

alone. The incidence of stones rises with the degree of hyperuricemia and approximates 50 per cent at serum urate values above 12 mg per deciliter. Marked hyperuricemia probably influences stone formation primarily by increasing uric acid *excretion*. The incidence of stones rises above 20 per cent in gouty subjects when the uric acid excretion exceeds 700 mg per 24 hours, and reaches 50 per cent at values above 1100 mg per 24 hours. Patients with increased uricaciduria also have an increased incidence of calcium oxalate stones. Urate (not uric acid) can participate in "heterogeneous nucleation" with calcium oxalate.

Other factors in the pathogenesis of uric acid stones include the *concentration of uric acid in urine*, the *acidity* of urine, and possibly the availability of stone *matrix* and the level of *solubilizing substances* in the urine. The solubility of urate decreases with fall of pH because of the shift to free uric acid. The pKa of uric acid is 5.75. In plasma at pH 7.4, more than 99 per cent is present in ionized form (urate), whereas in urine at pH 5.0, about 85 per cent is un-ionized (uric acid). At this pH only 15 mg of uric acid per deciliter of urine is soluble at 37°C, so supersaturation is required to excrete an average uric acid load in a normal urine volume. The solubility increases more than 10-fold at pH 7.0 and more than 100-fold at pH 8.0 over pH 5.0.

Both gouty and nongouty uric acid stone formers exhibit unusually low urinary pH values when fasting and throughout the day. The persistently acid urine has been attributed to subnormal ammonium production with a compensatory increase in titratable acidity. There is debate whether these data reflect occult or measurable renal damage (e.g., interstitial nephropathy), aging, or an intrinsic renal defect. Regardless of the explanation, the tendency toward persistently acid urine favors uric acid stone formation.

CLINICAL MANIFESTATIONS. The clinical manifestations of gout are conveniently described in four categories: acute gouty arthritis, tophaceous gout, gouty nephropathy, and uric acid urolithiasis.

Clinical gout is extraordinarily rare before puberty, when males at risk for primary idiopathic gout first develop hyperuricemia. Exceptions occur in the juvenile gout of the Lesch-Nyhan syndrome or glycogen storage disease type I, in which marked hyperuricemia is present from infancy. Only about 20 per cent of hyperuricemic subjects ever develop acute gout, although this figure rises as the degree of hyperuricemia increases (Table 183–2). The peak age of onset of gout is about 45 years in men. Thus the usual gouty male is exposed to 30 years of hyperuricemia before an attack occurs. In women gout usually occurs some years after the menopause, when serum urate values rise to hyperuricemic levels in those genetically at risk for gout.

Acute Gouty Arthritis. When acute gouty arthritis develops, it often appears as a fulminating arthritic attack of incapacitating severity. Acute gout is predominantly a disease of the lower extremity. Seventy-five to 90 per cent of initial attacks are monoarticular, and at least half of first attacks involve the metatarsophalangeal joint of the great toe (podagra). Next in order of frequency as sites of initial involvement are the instep, ankle, heel, knee, wrist, finger, and elbow. Later attacks are more often polyarticular and may include the shoulder or hip, or rarely such joints as the sacroiliac, sternoclavicular, mandibular, or even the spine. The more distal the site of involvement, the more typical are the attacks.

Some patients report short, trivial episodes of "ankle sprains" or sore heels or twinges of pain in the great toe prior to the first attack, sometimes going back over several years. More often the first attack occurs with explosive suddenness during apparent excellent health, often at night. Within minutes to hours the affected joint becomes hot, dusky red, and exquisitely painful. Lymphangitis may be evident. Systemic signs of inflammation may include fever, leukocytosis, and elevation of the erythrocyte sedimentation rate. The inflammatory reaction may suggest a cellulitis or septic joint, and on occasion a joint is erroneously incised by an unwary physician.

Acute gouty arthritis often follows a precipitating event, such as trauma, surgery, alcohol or dietary overindulgence, starvation, or infection. Attacks may follow a long walk, golf, or hunting trip (e.g., "pheasant hunter's toe"). Postoperative gout usually occurs on the third to the fifth day. Alcohol intoxication and starvation increase serum urate levels by inhibition of renal excretion by the accompanying lactic acidosis and ketosis, respectively. Regular ingestion of alcohol also increases urate production by stimulating purine nucleotide catabolism. Thus the legendary association of gout with imbibition has a sound metabolic explanation. Experimentally, urate crystals coated with endotoxins are particularly inflammatory; a subthreshold dose of injected uncoated crystals becomes violently inflammatory when endotoxin is given intravenously. Perhaps these observations bear upon the role of infection in precipitating attacks. It is postulated that uricosuric agents and allopurinol may induce acute attacks by lowering synovial fluid urate levels and favoring shedding of synovial crystals during dissolution.

The course of an untreated attack is highly variable. Initial attacks are usually self-limited. Mild attacks may subside in several hours or a few days. Severe attacks may last many days to several weeks. As the attack subsides, the inflamed skin may desquamate. Once the attack has broken, recovery is generally rapid and complete. The patient then re-enters an asymptomatic phase, often termed *intercritical* gout. The subsequent course is difficult to predict. Some patients never have a second attack. Others never fully recover from the first episode and suffer a series of exacerbations leading directly to chronic gouty arthritis. More commonly, a pattern of recurrences develops. In an extensive series, 62 per cent of patients had recurrences within the first year, 16 per cent in 1 to 2 years, 11 per cent in 2 to 5 years, and 4 per cent in 5 to 10 years; 7 per cent had no recurrence during prolonged follow-up. In the untreated patient, the frequency of attacks often increases, and they may become more severe, last longer, and eventually resolve less completely, leading to permanent disability not responsive to measures usually effective in acute attacks.

Tophaceous Gout. Before effective control of hyperuricemia became possible, more than one half of gouty patients developed visible tophi. The incidence now ranges from 13 to 25 per cent. In noncompliant patients it still exceeds 50 per cent. Development of tophi is correlated with the degree of hyperuricemia, severity of renal involvement, and duration of disease. The time from initial attack to visible tophaceous involvement ranged from 3 to 42 years in one large series, with an average of 11.6 years. In 0.5 per cent of patients, tophi are present at the time of the initial attack; virtually all such patients have gout secondary to a myeloproliferative disease.

Chronic gouty arthritis is a consequence of the progressive inability to dispose of urate as rapidly as it is produced. Crystalline deposits of urate appear in and around joints. Destruction of tissue is particularly evident in cartilage and bone, leading to radiolucent "punched-out" lesions and to cortical erosions with characteristic "overhanging margins" (Fig. 183–2). A frequent site of tophaceous deposits is the external ear, especially the helix and antihelix. Subcutaneous deposits, especially of fingertips, palms, and soles, may be visible as yellowish-white infiltrates. Tophaceous deposits may produce irregular asymmetric tumescences over joints. The classic gout shoe has a window cut to accommodate a tender prominent joint, usually the first metatarsophalangeal. At later stages, fusiform or nodular enlargements of Achilles tendons, or saccular distentions of olecranon bursae, are common and characteristic.

The process of tophaceous deposition advances insidiously, and although the tophi themselves are relatively painless, often progressive stiffness and persistent aching limit the use of affected joints. Eventually, extensive destruction of joints and large subcutaneous tophi may lead to grotesque deformities and progressive crippling (Fig. 183–2). The tense, shiny, thin skin overlying

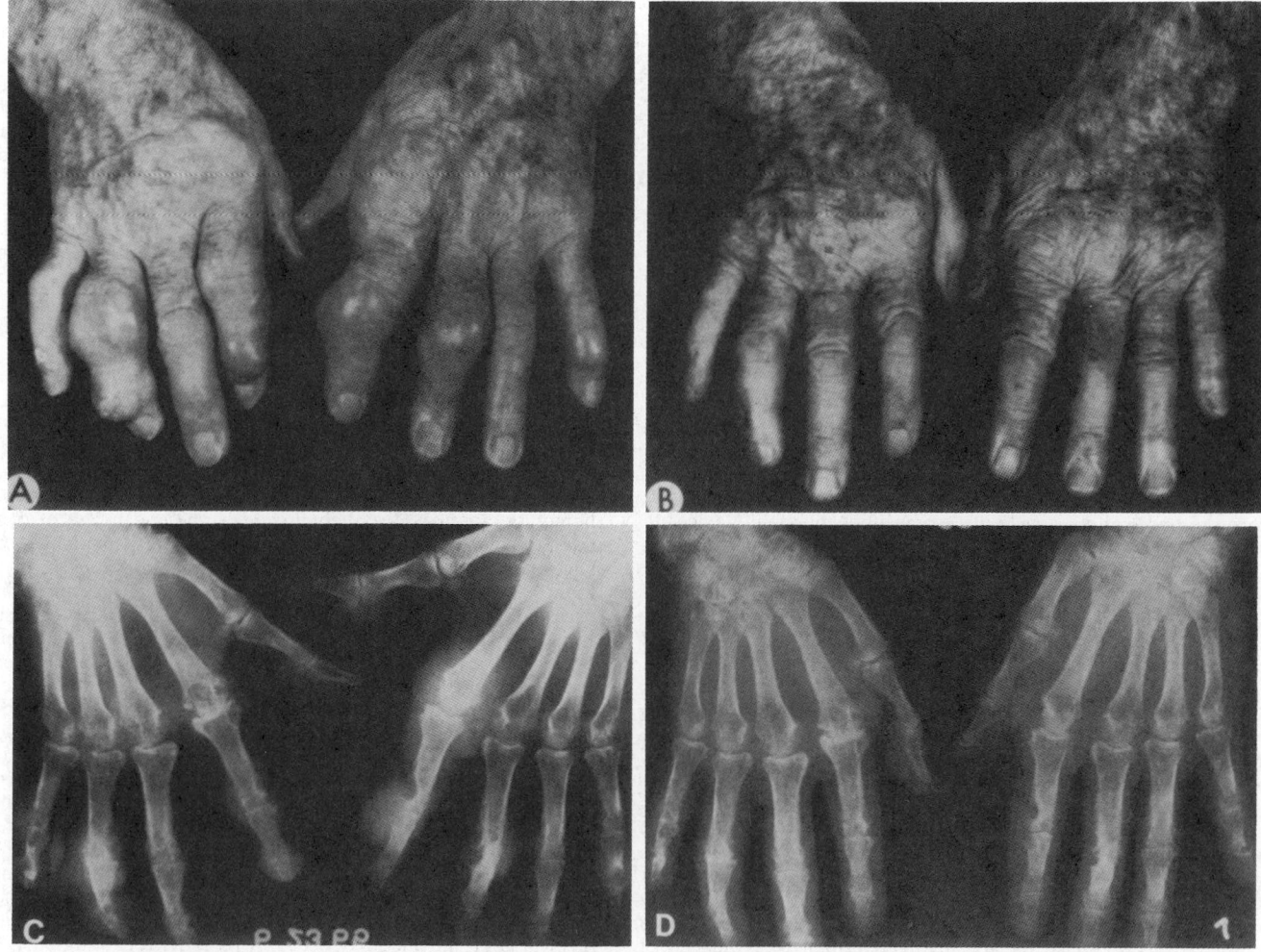

FIGURE 183–2. Chronic gouty arthritis (*A*) with tophaecous destruction of bone and joints (*C*), and improvement after three years of treatment with allopurinol, prophylactic colchicine, and a moderately low purine diet (*B* and *D*). (Courtesy of R. Wayne Rundles, Duke University Medical Center.)

the tophus may ulcerate and extrude white chalky or pasty material composed of myriads of fine, needle-like crystals. The olecranon bursa may be massively distended with "urate milk." Rarely, tophi may involve the tongue, epiglottis, vocal cords, arytenoid cartilage, corpus cavernosum and prepuce of the penis, aorta, aortic or mitral valves, and cardiac conducting system, causing rhythm disturbances. They do not involve the liver, spleen, lungs, or central nervous system.

As chronic gouty changes and renal disease advance, acute attacks occur less frequently and are milder. No joint is exempt from chronic gouty involvement, although those of the lower extremity and hand are most commonly involved. The hip and spinal joints are rarely affected in the absence of extensive disease elsewhere. Radiographic changes of the sacroiliac joint and aseptic necrosis of the hip are sometimes attributable to gout.

Gouty Nephropathy. Renal disease is common in gout. One third of patients show isosthenuria and moderate proteinuria. The glomerular filtration rate is well preserved in many gouty subjects, but in others it gradually falls. Decline in renal function appears to be correlated with aging, renovascular disease and hypertension, renal calculi, pyelonephritis, or independently occurring nephropathy, including that of lead poisoning. Only occasionally is it ascribable to gout alone. Hyperuricemia alone had no deleterious effect upon renal function during follow-up studies of gouty subjects ranging up to 12 years (Berger and Yu). Renal dysfunction does not shorten life expectancy in the average gouty subject, even though uremia is the eventual cause of death in 17 to 25 per cent of subjects. The majority of gouty patients die of cardiac or cerebrovascular disease (60 per cent) or malignant disease, which occur in about the same incidence and at about the same time of life as in nongouty American men.

Hypertension is present in one third to one half of patients and may be severe (diastolic pressure >130 mm Hg) in 10 per cent. Arterial and arteriolar nephrosclerosis are frequently prominent post mortem. There are no characteristic clinical or laboratory features to distinguish gouty kidney from other causes of chronic renal failure. Renal failure from gouty nephropathy in the absence of gouty arthritis, tophi, or stones is extraordinarily rare; indeed, the entity is open to question.

Gouty nephropathy, sometimes referred to as *urate nephropathy* to emphasize the identity of the interstitial crystals, must be distinguished from *uric acid nephropathy*, an entirely different entity leading to acute renal failure from tubular obstruction by uric acid crystals (see Ch. 80).

Urolithiasis. The incidence of urolithiasis in gout is correlated with both the degree of hyperuricemia and the magnitude of the 24-hour uric acid excretion. Above serum levels of 12 to 13 mg per deciliter or excretion values of 1100 mg per 24 hours, the incidence is 50 per cent. Many of these subjects will have secondary gout, with a myeloproliferative disease such as polycythemia vera or myeloid metaplasia. The incidence of stones in such patients is 35 to 40 per cent. Of gouty subjects who pass stones, about one third have their first episode of urolithiasis before the onset of gouty arthritis, sometimes more than a decade earlier. Pure uric acid stones are radiolucent and are demonstrable in the body only by use of contrast media. Renal stones are reduced in frequency in gouty patients given allopurinol.

GOUT ASSOCIATED WITH SPECIFIC ENZYME DEFECTS. Gout occurring on the basis of specific enzyme defects has special clinical features. These forms of gout are rare, accounting for fewer than 1 per cent of cases.

Glycogen Storage Disease Type I (see Ch. 169). Over 50 cases of von Gierke's glycogen storage disease (glucose-6-phosphatase deficiency) and gout have been recorded. Gout does not complicate other forms of glycogen storage disease, although hyperuricemia has been reported in several forms with muscle involvement and attributed to excessive adenosine triphosphate (ATP) degradation following exercise. Subjects with glycogen storage disease type I may develop gouty arthritis by the end of the first decade of life. Chronic tophaceous gout and gouty nephropathy may account for a major portion of morbidity when these patients become adults. The sexes are involved equally. Avoidance of nocturnal hypoglycemia by a diet high in starch or by continuous intragastric feeding may markedly reduce or even correct hyperuricemia and ameliorate gout. The hyperuricemia also responds

to allopurinol, less well to uricosuric agents because of renal disease.

Hypoxanthine-Guanine Phosphoribosyltransferase Deficiency. Deficiency of HPRT gives rise to two different X-linked syndromes. A complete deficiency is associated with the Lesch-Nyhan syndrome (see Ch. 184). There is extreme exaggeration of uric acid production, and the greatly increased excretion leads to crystalluria, renal stones with ureteral colic, and sometimes uric acid nephropathy. Death from renal failure usually occurs by age 10; if allopurinol therapy is begun early, the patients may live into their 20's. A few of the more than 100 reported patients, all males, have had typical attacks of gouty arthritis.

An incomplete deficiency of HPRT is associated with renal stones and recurrent acute gouty arthritis. Erythrocytes show 0.2 to 50 per cent of normal HPRT activity; the disorder is heterogeneous. Fifteen per cent of patients show minimal to moderate neurologic dysfunction resembling spinocerebellar ataxis or cerebral palsy. A few have survived neonatal episodes of uric acid nephropathy. Gout usually begins in the second or third decade; tophi develop early. Three quarters of patients have renal stones, half of these before age 10. These subjects have more marked hyperuricemia (usually >10 mg per deciliter) and uricaciduria (usually >1 gram per 24 hours) than most gouty subjects. More than 100 cases—again, all males—have been described. HPRT normally catalyzes a reaction between hypoxanthine or guanine and PP-ribose-P in reconstituting ribonucleotides, often called a "salvage" reaction. In HPRT deficiency, intracellular PP-ribose-P levels are raised and drive the first reaction of purine biosynthesis to excess. The female heterozygous carriers of complete HPRT deficiency are not hyperuricemic, and their erythrocytes show normal HPRT assay values. Carriers of the partial defect may be hyperuricemic and may show intermediate levels of HPRT activity. Presumably, only cells possessing at least minimal HPRT activity survive lyonization. Heterozygotes for the partial defect may develop uric acid stones or typical gout, which may occur before the menopause. Partial HPRT deficiency should be considered in all women with gout or uric acid stones who exhibit raised urinary uric acid excretion values.

Phosphoribosylpyrophosphate Synthetase Variants. Patients with these variants resemble those with partial HPRT deficiency in showing marked hyperuricemia and uricaciduria and in developing uric acid stones or gout, and sometimes uric acid nephropathy, at an early age. They do not have neurologic abnormalities. Purine overproduction is prodigious. The enzyme abnormalities, of which there are four different types leading to increased activity (see Ch. 177), result in increased intracellular concentrations of PP-ribose-P and excessive purine biosynthesis. This, too, is an X-linked disorder, and all gouty patients are males. Fewer than 20 families with this disorder have been identified.

SECONDARY GOUT. Any acquired hyperuricemic state may be complicated by secondary gout. This disorder occurs in 5 to 10 per cent of patients with polycythemia vera or myeloid metaplasia, occasionally in secondary polycythemia complicating congenital heart disease or chronic pulmonary disease, in chronic myelogenous leukemia, in multiple myeloma, or in chronic hemolytic anemias. In such instances the mean age of onset is later (59 years), women are more commonly involved (16 per cent), and both serum and urinary uric acid values tend to be higher than in idiopathic primary gout. Acute gouty arthritis may occasionally antedate evidence of the myeloproliferative disorder by many months, or even by several years. A syndrome of coexisting sarcoidosis, psoriasis, and gout has been described but may represent fortuitous concurrence of common diseases.

In all the instances mentioned above, hyperuricemia appears to result from an increase in turnover of nucleic acid. Hyperuricemia may also result from reduced renal excretion of urate, either because of drug effects or because of parenchymal disease.

Hyperuricemia frequently follows the use of potent diuretic agents. Mean increases in serum urate concentrations are less than 2 mg per deciliter, but some subjects exhibit rises of 4 to 5 mg per deciliter. The hyperuricemic effect of diuretic agents results from salt and water loss, volume contraction, and avid solute reabsorption (including urate) in the proximal tubule. Typical gouty attacks may occur in patients receiving such drugs as hydrochlorothiazide, ethacrynic acid, or furosemide. In the 14-year study of the adult population of Framingham, Massachusetts, one half of the new cases of gout occurred in subjects taking potent diuretics. Ingestion of many other drugs may also lead to hyperuricemia. For example, patients with chronic renal failure treated with erythropoietin frequently develop hyperuricemia. Three to 5 per cent of patients with gout have diabetes, but this incidence is not far from that of diabetes in the population of equivalent age. In markedly obese patients, total caloric restriction may result in extreme hyperuricemia, which is correlated with serum levels of beta-hydroxybutyric acid and may be associated with severe attacks of acute gouty arthritis, especially of knees and ankles.

Chronic renal disease is a frequent cause of hyperuricemia, but only about 1 patient per 1000 develops gout. Uremia appears to interfere in some way with the inflammatory response to urate crystals. Gout continues to be found in patients who survive lead exposure early in life and go on to develop slowly progressive lead nephropathy. In addition, saturnine gout is particularly prevalent in the southeastern United States, where it is attributed to the chronic ingestion of moonshine whiskey of high lead content with resulting renal tubular damage. Lead nephropathy and polycystic renal disease predispose to gout more often than do other forms of chronic renal disease.

DIAGNOSIS. The diagnosis of acute gouty arthritis is not difficult when there is an explosive onset of a typical inflammatory attack of characteristic severity in a peripheral joint, especially of the lower extremity. The diagnosis is established by the demonstration of typical negatively birefringent needle-shaped crystals of sodium urate in the leukocytes of synovial fluid (Fig. 183–3). With proper technique, including the use of a polarizing microscope, intraleukocytic sodium urate crystals are found in over 95 per cent of aspirates from joints in acute gout. The leukocyte count may range from 1000 to more than 50,000, depending on the acuteness of the inflammation. A Gram stain should always be obtained to evaluate infection, which may coexist. In the rare event of failure to find crystals on the first attempt, a second aspirate obtained some hours later is usually positive. Urate crystals must be distinguished from calcium pyrophosphate dihydrate crystals of pseudogout. The latter are weakly positively birefringent under polarized light and usually more rectangular than urate crystals. A rapid response of pain and inflammation to the administration of colchicine is so characteristic as to be of diagnostic value as well. Responses of rheumatoid arthritis and sarcoid arthritis to colchicine are not so dramatic or complete as those in gout. The finding of hyperuricemia is anticipated and helpful, but since hyperuricemia is common (13 per cent of hospitalized male patients), it may coexist with other acute arthropathies. The presence of tophi or of typical roentgenographic findings of punched-out, destructive bone lesions helps establish the diagnosis of chronic tophaceous gout. In 70 per cent

of patients with crystal-proven gout, extracellular urate crystals are demonstrable in asymptomatic first metatarsophalangeal joints. Such crystals are rare (5 per cent) in hyperuricemic subjects who have never had clinical gout.

Each gouty patient should also have a determination of the 24-hour urinary excretion of uric acid. The sample should be collected after 3 days of moderate purine restriction, during an intercritical period. Values of greater than 600 mg per 1.72 square meters per day under these conditions probably indicate overproduction, and those of over 800 mg per day warrant additional studies for a specific subtype of primary gout, such as HPRT deficiency of PP-ribose-P synthetase overactivity, or of secondary gout, such as a myeloproliferative disorder. Elevated urinary uric acid values also signify that the patient is at higher risk for renal stone and represent an indication for allopurinol rather than uricosuric drug therapy for gout.

Chronic gouty arthritis may be diagnosed by the presence of urate deposits in or near the affected joints or bursae or of soft tissue deposits in the helix of the ear, the fingertips, the Achilles tendon, or other locations. The diagnosis may be confirmed by removal of the chalky contents of a tophus, by microscopic identification of sodium urate crystals by optical means, by chemical identification by the murexide test, or, preferably, by ultraviolet spectrophotometry and degradation by uricase.

DIFFERENTIAL DIAGNOSIS. Acute gout must be differentiated from acute rheumatic fever, rheumatoid arthritis, traumatic arthritis, osteoarthritis, pyogenic arthritis, sarcoid arthritis, cellulitis, bursitis, tendinitis, and thrombophlebitis. Podagra, the most common initial presentation of gout, can be mimicked by trauma, degenerative arthritis, acute sarcoidosis, psoriatic arthritis, pseudogout, palindromic rheumatism, Reiter's syndrome, or infection. Acute monoarticular arthritis of the great toe in the immediate postoperative period following parathyroidectomy can be caused by hydroxyapatite crystals. These various forms of "pseudopodagra" may be suggested by a negative examination of synovial fluid for urate crystals. Pseudogout (see Ch. 271), which is manifested by acute attacks of arthritis of knees and other joints, is usually accompanied by calcification of joint cartilage; the synovial fluid contains nonurate crystals of calcium pyrophosphate. However, gout and pseudogout may coexist, and both types of crystals will then be found in synovial fluid leukocytes.

Chronic gouty arthritis must chiefly be differentiated from rheumatoid arthritis, osteoarthritis, traumatic arthritis, and residua of pyogenic arthritis. The history of onset, progression, response to colchicine, and demonstration of hyperuricemia, asymmetric tumescences, typical roentgenographic changes, and tophi or crystals of urate in synovial fluid and leukocytes should establish the diagnosis.

TREATMENT. The therapeutic aims in gout are (1) to terminate the acute gouty attack as promptly and gently as possible, (2) to prevent recurrences of acute gouty arthritis, (3) to prevent or reverse complications of the disease resulting from deposition of sodium urate in joints and kidneys, and (4) to prevent formation of uric acid kidney stones. The therapeutic program differs according to the stage of the disease and the complications present. In the majority of patients it is possible to abort or prevent acute attacks, to control hyperuricemia, and to prevent chronic gouty arthritis, nephropathy, and stones.

Acute Attack. The affected joint should be placed at rest, and an anti-inflammatory agent administered promptly. Three types of agents are available: colchicine, nonsteroidal anti-inflammatory agents, and glucocorticoids (or adrenocorticotropic hormone [ACTH]). *Colchicine* is the only agent of specific diagnostic value in acute gout. It should be given as soon as the diagnosis is suspected. The initial dose of 0.6 to 1.2 mg of colchicine is followed by 0.6 mg every hour for 8 hours and then every 2 hours until pain is relieved or until nausea, vomiting, cramping, or diarrhea develops. Maximum tolerated doses range from 4 to 8 mg. In many patients dramatic relief of pain and onset of gastrointestinal side effects occur simultaneously. The diarrhea may be treated with paregoric, 4 ml, or Kaopectate, 30 ml, after each loose stool. Colchicine should be discontinued until gastrointestinal symptoms subside. Since the effective dose of colchicine varies, each patient should learn his or her own tolerance dose and stop just short of this in treatment of subsequent attacks. If

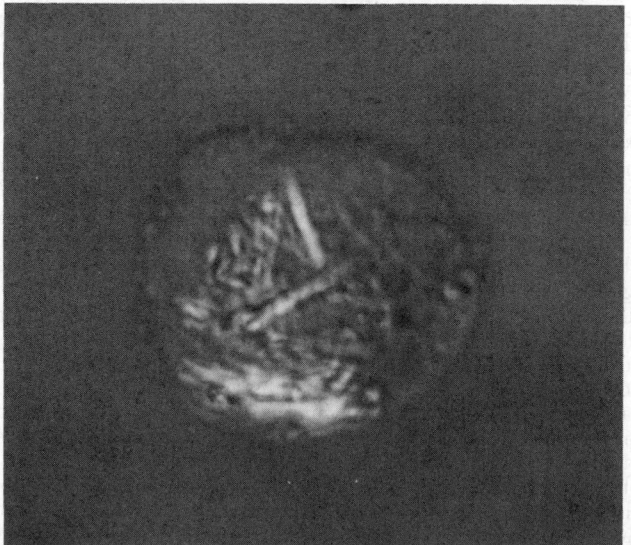

FIGURE 183–3. Sodium urate monohydrate crystals phagocytized by leukocyte in synovial fluid from acute gouty arthritis, examined by polarized light. (Courtesy of Edward W. Holmes, Duke University Medical Center.)

started promptly, colchicine affords relief over 90 per cent of the time; if treatment is delayed beyond 12 hours, only 75 per cent of patients will respond within 24 to 48 hours. Since colchicine is concentrated within cells and turns over with a half-life of about 30 hours, repeated courses of colchicine carry a higher risk of toxicity; treatment failures should be treated with a nonsteroidal anti-inflammatory drug (NSAID).

Colchicine may also be given intravenously (subcutaneous infiltration may result in tissue necrosis). The usual initial dose is 1 to 2 mg in 20 ml of saline solution given slowly, and if a single dose is not effective, the injection may be repeated once in 4 to 5 hours (maximum intravenous dose, 3 to 5 mg). Gastrointestinal symptoms are uncommon with intravenous administration, although occasionally nausea occurs.

Dose-related toxic responses to colchicine include alopecia (reversible), bone marrow suppression (leukopenia, thrombocytopenia, anemia), and hepatocellular damage. The drug should not be used in patients with advanced hepatic or renal disease.

NSAID's are equally effective in acute gout and are usually preferred to colchicine because they are so much milder for the patient. Indomethacin has been most widely used. It is given orally in initial doses of 50 mg three or four times a day. When pain is relieved, doses are tapered over another 48 to 72 hours. Other NSAID's, such as *naproxen* and *ibuprofen*, can also be used. With all NSAID's, renal function should be monitored, especially in hypertensive patients. *Phenylbutazone* and *oxyphenbutazone* (Tandearil) are also effective in acute gouty arthritis and may be preferred when the gouty attack has proceeded for some time or when the attack does not abate completely with colchicine or indomethacin. The initial dose is 400 mg orally, followed by 100 mg every 4 to 8 hours for 2 to 3 days. Bone marrow suppression may rarely occur, even after a short course of either drug.

If full doses of colchicine or NSAID's are contraindicated (e.g., in postoperative gout) or ineffective, *ACTH* may be employed by intravenous drip (40 units per day) or as intramuscular gel (40 to 80 units per day), or systemic glucocorticoids may be given for 2 to 3 days, rarely longer, following which the doses are reduced in stepwise fashion and discontinued. Unfortunately, rebound attacks of gout are rather common after such therapy. *Triamcinolone hexacetonide* in a dose of 5 to 20 mg injected intra-articularly into the involved joint is useful in treating acute gout limited to a single joint or bursa, particularly in patients in whom the standard drugs cannot be used, and relief from pain is usually prompt and complete within 24 to 36 hours. Steroid hormones are not recommended for parenteral use in acute gout, as the effects are inconsistent and rebound attacks frequent.

Uricosuric agents and allopurinol are of no value in treatment of the acute attack.

Interval Phase. The patient with gout should avoid high-purine foods so as to lessen the burden of uric acid excretion. A severe limitation of purine-containing foods is rarely indicated, unless renal function is poor. Gradual weight reduction is indicated if the patient is overweight and may of itself reduce hyperuricemia and the tendency to develop attacks of gout. Sudden weight reduction may precipitate gouty attacks and should be avoided. In general, diets of moderate protein content, somewhat low in fat, are preferred. Hypertension should be treated vigorously, even if antihypertensive agents worsen hyperuricemia; the result can be countered with appropriate antihyperuricemic drug therapy.

A high fluid intake is advisable to maintain a urinary output of 2000 ml per day to promote uric acid excretion. Beer, ale, and wine may precipitate attacks. Distilled alcoholic beverages in moderation generally have little influence on the gouty process. Illicit liquor (moonshine) should be prohibited. Excessive alcohol use in any form should be avoided, as it enhances purine production and also leads to hypertriglyceridemia.

Patients who recognize prodromal symptoms may abort acute attacks by prompt institution of colchicine, phenylbutazone, or indomethacin therapy; they frequently require only a few tablets to achieve success. The daily ingestion of 0.6 to 1.8 mg of colchicine is generally effective in reducing the number of acute gouty attacks in patients who are subject to frequent episodes. Toxicity is rare, but may include alopecia, bone marrow suppres-

sion, and hepatocellular damage. Maintenance colchicine therapy is particularly important during the first months or year after institution of uricosuric drugs or of allopurinol. Daily ingestion of indomethacin, 25 or 50 mg, has also been employed for this purpose and appears to be effective. The risks of renal and gastrointestinal toxicity make use of indomethacin undesirable as a prophylactic agent or as regular therapy for chronic gouty arthritis.

Chronic Gouty Arthritis. Use of a drug to lower the serum level of uric acid to 6 mg per 100 ml or less is indicated in all gouty patients with visible tophi, with roentgenographic evidence of urate deposits, or with a history of two or more major attacks of acute gouty arthritis. Allopurinol is the drug of choice unless the patient is already well managed with a uricosuric agent. With either type of agent the number of acute gouty attacks may be increased during the first few months unless maintenance colchicine therapy is given, whereas after 12 to 18 months the number may be decidedly reduced.

Allopurinol controls serum urate levels by inhibiting xanthine oxidase and thereby regulating production of uric acid (see Fig. 183–1). Allopurinol is converted to oxypurinol in the body, and the latter compound has a longer biologic half-life (28 hours), ultimately being largely excreted in the urine. Inhibition of conversion of hypoxanthine and xanthine to uric acid permits these precursors to be excreted instead. In gouty subjects other than those with HPRT deficiency, the increment in hypoxanthine plus xanthine excretion is only about two thirds of the decrement in uric acid excretion, presumably because of enhanced feedback inhibition of purine synthesis de novo by nucleotides reconstituted from hypoxanthine. The induced xanthinuria has not resulted in xanthine stone formation in the usual gouty subjects but has done so in a rare patient with HPRT deficiency and in patients being treated with antineoplastic agents. Use of allopurinol results in reduction of levels of uric acid in serum *and in urine.* The drug is effective even in the presence of renal failure, when uricosuric agents generally are not. Its action is not blocked by salicylates. The usual dose is 300 mg, given orally once a day. In the presence of moderate nitrogen retention, the dose of allopurinol should be reduced by one half or more (see Ch. 23), as the biologic half-life of the active metabolite, oxypurinol, is prolonged. Allopurinol is usually well tolerated but may cause gastric irritation, diarrhea, or skin rash or induce an attack of gout. Toxic hepatitis, epidermal necrolysis, and vasculitis may occasionally be severe, even fatal. Toxic effects are more frequent and more severe in the presence of renal failure. Intramuscular crystals of xanthine and oxypurinol have been described in patients receiving allopurinol, but their significance in terms of toxicity is not clear. Uricosuric agents may be used concurrently with allopurinol to hasten mobilization of urate deposits, but combined therapy may require larger doses of allopurinol because uricosuric drugs also enhance the excretion of oxypurinol. Since allopurinol decreases uric acid excretion, it is also very useful in controlling uric acid stone formation, especially in patients who are overproducers of uric acid. If the serum urate values can be controlled at levels below saturation of urate in body fluids, extensive resolution of soft tissue tophi and modest reduction in the size of bone erosions may be achieved, together with some recalcification of bone lesions (see Fig. 183–2). Joint mobility and comfort may be greatly improved.

Uricosuric drugs block tubular reabsorption of filtered urate. Those of use in gout are probenecid and sulfinpyrazone. These agents begin to lose effectiveness when the creatinine clearance falls below 80 ml per minute and are ineffective when the clearance falls below 30 ml per minute. *Probenecid* is given in doses of 0.5 gram to 3 grams daily in two or three evenly spaced doses (average dose, 1 to 1.5 grams). This drug may produce gastrointestinal upsets, headaches, or skin rash. *Sulfinpyrazone* may be given in doses of 100 to 600 mg daily in three or four divided doses (average dose, 300 mg). This drug is related to phenylbutazone and may cause untoward reactions but is generally somewhat better tolerated than probenecid. *Salicylates* block the uricosuric action of both probenecid and sulfinpyrazone and must not be used concurrently. Salicylates are uricosuric when given in high doses (4 to 6 grams daily), but few patients can tolerate these quantities.

With all uricosuric agents, the doses should be low initially to avoid sudden excretion of large quantities of urate and should be increased at weekly intervals to maintenance levels. Fluids should be forced to prevent formation of concentrated urine, especially during the late hours of the night. During the first days or weeks of therapy, the urine should be kept at pH 6 or above, by administration of sodium bicarbonate or sodium citrate–citric acid (Shohl's solution); this may be difficult to achieve, as acid urine tends to be produced in gouty patients. In patients in whom urate is being mobilized, and especially those in whom uric acid gravel is formed, alkalinization during the night, when fluid intake is reduced, is important. A single 250-mg tablet of acetazolamide (Diamox) taken at bedtime serves to keep the urine alkaline and dilute throughout the night.

In selected patients surgical removal of large extra-articular urate deposits, such as those in olecranon bursae, may be advisable. Occasionally, amputation of irreparably damaged digits, especially those containing draining sinuses, is indicated. Physical therapy and appropriate self-help devices are valuable in patients who are partially disabled.

Asymptomatic Hyperuricemia. Asymptomatic hyperuricemia is frequent in family members of patients with gout and in the general population. It usually requires no therapy, as only about one fifth of patients ever develop articular attacks, and adequate therapy can be instituted when these supervene. Exceptions may exist in patients with markedly elevated serum levels of uric acid, especially if urinary urate excretion is low and there is a family history of tophaceous disease. In such circumstances the asymptomatic subject should be treated with allopurinol before articular or renal complications develop. It is essential that the physician maintain frequent close observation of the patient.

Berger, L. Yu T-F: Renal function in gout: IV. An analysis of 524 gouty subjects including long-term follow-up studies. Am J Med 59:605, 1975. *An important study showing that deterioration of renal function in gout is largely associated with aging, renovascular disease, hypertension, renal calculi with pyelonephritis, or independently occurring nephropathy. Hyperuricemia alone had no deleterious effect on renal function over periods up to 12 years.*

Cherian PV, Schumacher HR Jr: Immunochemical and ultrastructural characterization of serum proteins associated with monosodium urate crystals (MSU) in synovial fluid cells from patients with gout. Ultrastruct Pathol 10:209, 1986. *Various proteins associated with intracellular urate crystals, IgG > IgM or IgA > C3 or fibrinogen, may influence the inflammatory properties of those crystals.*

Reibman J, Haines KA, Rich AM, et al.: Colchicine inhibits ionophore-induced formation of leukotriene B$_4$ by human neutrophils: The role of microtubules. J Immunol 136:1027, 1986. *The mechanisms of colchicine action in inhibiting production of leukotriene B$_4$ by neutrophils appears to depend upon its effect on the number and integrity of the microtubules.*

Simkin PS: Uric acid excretion in patients with gout. Arthritis Rheum 22:98, 1979. *An analysis of six published studies relating the rate of urate excretion to plasma urate levels in normal and gouty subjects. The kidneys of the average gouty person lag significantly behind the normal in their response to any concentration of plasma urate. The kidneys of overproducers (38 of 73 gouty subjects) were no less handicapped than those of other gouty subjects.*

Spillberg I, Mandell B, Mehta J, et al.: Mechanism of action of colchicine in acute urate crystal–induced arthritis. J Clin Invest 64:775, 1979. *Phagocytosis of urate crystals by neutrophils induces the synthesis and release of a glycoprotein that is chemotactic both in vitro and in vivo. Colchicine decreases production and release of this factor. Colchicine abrogates the acute arthritis produced by urate crystals in rabbits but has no effect upon the arthritis induced by injection of purified cell-derived chemotactic factor.*

Wyngaarden JB, Kelley WN: Gout. In Stanbury JB, Wyngaarden JB, Fredrickson DS, et al. (eds.): The Metabolic Basis of Inherited Disease. 5th ed. New York, McGraw-Hill Book Company, 1983. *A detailed account of purine metabolism and the pathogenesis of primary gout.*

Wyngaarden JB, Kelley WN: Gout and Hyperuricemia. New York, Grune & Stratton, 1976. *Everything you have always wanted to know about gout but never dared to ask, condensed into 500 pages.*

184 Other Disorders of Purine Metabolism

Edward W. Holmes

XANTHINURIA

Classic xanthinuria, which is inherited as an autosomal recessive trait, is the consequence of an isolated deficiency of xanthine oxidase. As a result of this enzyme deficiency, uric acid is replaced by xanthine and hypoxanthine as the end-products of purine metabolism. Serum urate concentrations in these patients range from 0 to 1.4 mg per deciliter, and urinary uric acid excretion ranges from 0 to 8 mg per day; serum oxypurine (xanthine plus hypoxanthine) concentrations and urine oxypurine excretion are increased in this disorder.

More than 50 patients with classic xanthinuria have been described, and the prevalence of this disorder is estimated to be approximately 1 in 45,000. Over 50 per cent of individuals with classic xanthinuria are asymptomatic, the diagnosis being suspected by the incidental finding of a very low serum urate concentration during evaluation of presumably unrelated medical problems. The diagnosis is virtually established by the demonstration of low serum and urinary uric acid levels in association with increased urinary oxypurine excretion, and it is confirmed by assaying liver or intestinal mucosa for xanthine oxidase activity. One third of patients develop radiolucent renal calculi composed of xanthine. Four adult patients have had myopathic symptoms characterized by muscle cramps following exercise, and crystalline deposits of xanthine and hypoxanthine have been found in skeletal muscle. Recurrent polyarthritis has been described in three patients, and it has been suggested, but not established, that this symptom may represent crystal-induced synovitis.

A subtype of xanthinuria has been described in which the deficiency of xanthine oxidase is associated with a deficiency of sulfite oxidase. Both of these enzymes require a molybdenum cofactor for catalytic activity, and absence of this cofactor has been demonstrated in the liver of a patient with this combined enzyme defect. Fifteen patients with an inherited deficiency of these two enzymes have been reported, and all presented in the first weeks of life with a severe neurologic disorder characteristic of isolated sulfite oxidase deficiency. Symptoms include feeding difficulties from birth, tonic-clonic seizures, nystagmus, enophthalmus, ocular lens dislocation, and Brushfield spots. As in isolated sulfite oxidase deficiency, urinary excretion of sulfate is low, while that of sulfite, thiosulfate, S-sulfocysteine, and taurine is increased. Characteristic biochemical findings of xanthinuria are also present.

An acquired phenocopy of the combined defect has been described in a 20-year-old male with short-bowel syndrome maintained for 18 months with total parenteral nutrition. In addition to hypouricemia and hypouricaciduria, urinary excretion of sulfite and thiosulfate was increased while excretion of sulfate was decreased. Following infusion of commercially available amino acid solutions the patient experienced headaches, night blindness, irritability, lethargy, and then coma.

The prognosis in classic xanthinuria is excellent, as shown by the high percentage of patients who are asymptomatic. Therapy for xanthine calculi includes high fluid intake, and on occasion allopurinol has been used in patients with residual xanthine oxidase activity to increase the excretion of hypoxanthine relative to xanthine, the former being more soluble than the latter. In patients with the inherited form of combined xanthine oxidase and sulfite oxidase deficiency, the neurologic symptoms have been refractory to therapy with a number of agents, including oral ammonium molybdate. With the acquired form of this combined disorder, treatment with ammonium molybdate reversed the biochemical abnormalities, and the neurologic symptoms were markedly ameliorated.

Holmes EW, Wyngaarden JB: Hereditary xanthinuria. In Scriver CR, Beaudet AL, Sly WS, et al. (eds.): The Metabolic Basis of Inherited Disease. 6th ed. New York, McGraw-Hill, 1989, pp 1085–1094. *A thorough coverage of the clinical and biochemical abnormalities found in classic xanthinuria.*

Johnson JL, Wadman SK: Molybdenum cofactor deficiency. In Scriver CR, Beaudet AL, Sly WS, et al. (eds.): The Metabolic Basis of Inherited Disease. 6th ed. New York, McGraw-Hill, 1989, pp 1463–1475. *Metabolic and clinical observations on 15 patients with this disorder.*

THE LESCH-NYHAN SYNDROME AND PARTIAL DEFICIENCY OF HYPOXANTHINE-GUANINE PHOSPHORIBOSYLTRANSFERASE

The Lesch-Nyhan syndrome, caused by a virtually complete deficiency of hypoxanthine-guanine phosphoribosyltransferase (HPRT) activity, is manifested clinically by hyperuricemia, excessive production of uric acid, and neurologic features, including self-mutilation, choreoathetosis, spasticity, and mental retardation. Partial deficiency of HPRT activity is associated with uric acid overproduction, severe gout, and occasionally neurologic abnormalities, but self-mutilation is absent. The Lesch-Nyhan syndrome occurs in about 1 in 100,000 births, and partial deficiency of HPRT is noted in less than 1 per cent of the gouty population.

ETIOLOGY AND PATHOGENESIS. The gene for HPRT is located on the X chromosome. Studies employing protein sequencing, RNA mapping, restriction fragment length polymorphism (RFLP), and DNA sequencing techniques have revealed a striking molecular heterogeneity as the basis for this disorder. Failure to reutilize hypoxanthine in the salvage pathway as a result of HPRT deficiency leads to increased oxidation of this purine base to uric acid. An increase in the intracellular concentration of phosphoribosyl-pyrophosphate, which also results from reduction in hypoxanthine reutilization, leads to an increase in the rate of purine biosynthesis de novo. The combined effect of these abnormalities is increased uric acid production resulting in hyperuricaciduria, which predisposes to uric acid crystal and stone formation, and hyperuricemia, which leads to gouty arthritis and tophaceous deposits. The biochemical basis for the unusual and devastating neurologic abnormalities seen in the Lesch-Nyhan syndrome is not clearly understood, but abnormalities in dopamine neuron function have been described. Positron-emission tomography has demonstrated a selective decrease in glucose utilization in the caudate nucleus.

CLINICAL MANIFESTATIONS. The deficiency of HPRT activity is fully expressed only in affected males. Females heterozygous for HPRT deficiency may have subtle abnormalities in purine metabolism, but they are generally asymptomatic.

Infants with the Lesch-Nyhan syndrome are normal at birth, and the earliest consistent abnormality is a delay in motor development noted at 3 to 4 months of age. Between 8 and 12 months, extrapyramidal signs develop, leading to choreoathetosis, and at about 1 year of age signs of pyramidal tract involvement, such as hyperreflexia, clonus, and scissoring of the legs, appear. Compulsive self-destructive behavior appears any time between early childhood and adolescence. This is the most distinctive neurologic feature of the syndrome and is manifested by biting of the fingers, lips, and buccal mucosa. Repeated attempts at self-injury, such as placing extremities in dangerous areas and self-inflicted head trauma, are also common. Sensation is intact in these children. Mental retardation is noted in most cases, but it is unclear whether the enzyme deficiency per se causes this or whether it is the result of poor performance on formal testing in children with dysarthria and choreoathetosis. Growth retardation is also a prominent feature of the syndrome. Uric acid crystalluria may be noted as orange crystals on the diaper during the first weeks of life and in untreated patients progresses to uric acid nephrolithiasis, obstructive uropathy, and azotemia. Hyperuricemia is usually present and may attain levels of 18 mg per deciliter, but the serum urate concentration may be normal, especially before puberty. Gout is unusual in the Lesch-Nyhan syndrome before 12 to 15 years of age. Death usually occurs in the second or third decade from infection or renal failure.

Patients with partial deficiency of HPRT develop uric acid crystalluria and renal calculi in childhood, and gouty arthritis often occurs before 20 years of age. Neurologic manifestations, including mental retardation, mild spastic quadriplegia, dysarthria, cerebellar ataxia, and seizures, are noted in 20 per cent of patients with partial HPRT deficiency, but self-mutilation does not develop. Patients with partial HPRT deficiency may seek medical attention with the only symptom being the passage of a renal calculus or an attack of gouty arthritis. Life expectancy is normal in these patients.

DIAGNOSIS. Self-destructive behavior is the most distinguishing clinical feature of the Lesch-Nyhan syndrome; whereas retarded children with other disorders will bite their fingers, mutilation to the point of tissue destruction is rare in any disorder other than the Lesch-Nyhan syndrome. Severe self-biting in other neurologic disorders is usually associated with a loss of pain sensation. As pointed out, hyperuricemia is usually present, but this is not an invariable finding. The diagnosis is established by demonstrating a virtual absence of HPRT activity in readily accessible tissues such as erythrocytes. Analyses of erythrocyte lysates are not useful in identifying heterozygous female carriers, but this can be accomplished with cell culture of skin fibroblasts or through analysis of hair follicles.

Partial deficiency of HPRT should be suspected in male patients with the onset of gouty arthritis before 20 years of age and in young males with uric acid crystalluria or uric acid nephrolithiasis. Uric acid overexcretion is found invariably in patients with normal renal function, and the diagnosis is confirmed by enzyme assay. Patients with partial HPRT activity have erythrocyte lysate values that are usually in the range of 0.1 to 5 per cent of control values, rarely up 30 to 50 per cent of control values, while patients with the Lesch-Nyhan syndrome have values less than 0.01 per cent of control values.

TREATMENT. Uric acid stone formation, tophi, and gouty arthritis can be controlled in both the Lesch-Nyhan syndrome and partial deficiency of HPRT with drugs that inhibit xanthine oxidase activity. However, a few patients have developed xanthine stones with this therapy. No drugs have been found that correct the neurologic deficits, but supportive measures, such as restraints that reduce the tendency to self-mutilation, are well accepted by the patient. Drugs such as diazepam help control the movement disorder. Given the devastating neurologic complications of the Lesch-Nyhan syndrome, therapeutic abortion has been used as a preventive measure following heterozygote identification and intrauterine diagnosis.

Edwards NL, Recker D, Fox IH: Overproduction of uric acid in hypoxanthine-guanine phosphoribosyltransferase deficiency. J Clin Invest 63:922, 1979. *A careful analysis of the basis for uric acid overproduction in patients with HPRT deficiency.*

Stout JT, Caskey CT: Hypoxanthine phosphoribosyltransferase deficiency: The Lesch-Nyhan syndrome and gouty arthritis. In Scriver CR, Beaudet AL, Sly WS, et al. (eds.): The Metabolic Basis of Inherited Disease. 6th ed. New York, McGraw-Hill, 1989, pp 1007–1029. *A detailed description of the clinical and biochemical consequences of HPRT deficiency.*

Wilson JM, Stout JT, Palella TD, et al.: A molecular survey of hypoxanthine-guanine phosphoribosyltransferase deficiency in man. J Clin Invest 77:188, 1986. *A description of specific mutations at the molecular level in patients with HGPRT deficiency.*

2,8-DIHYDROXYADENINE RENAL STONES

Deficiency of adenine phosphoribosyltransferase (APRT), an enzyme in the salvage pathway of purine nucleotide synthesis, leads to the accumulation and increased urinary excretion of 2,8-dihydroxyadenine, the product of adenine oxidation by xanthine oxidase. Because of the insolubility of this purine, patients with this autosomal recessive disorder are predisposed to development of renal calculi composed of 2,8-dihydroxyadenine. More than 30 individuals homozygous for this enzyme deficiency have been identified; 6 presented with acute renal failure, and 3 of these patients suffered permanent renal damage. Renal colic may occur within the first months of life, as late as 40 years of age, or individuals with this disorder may be asymptomatic. 2,8-Dihydroxyadenine stones are usually radiolucent. The diagnosis is confirmed by analyzing the stone with ultraviolet, infrared, or mass spectrometry or x-ray crystallography or by demonstrating the absence of adenine phosphoribosyltransferase activity in erythrocyte lysates. Except for the excessive excretion of adenine and its metabolites, with the consequent development of renal calculi, no other biochemical or clinical abnormalities have been reported in individuals homozygous for this enzyme deficiency.

The prevalence of the homozygous state is not documented, but it is calculated to occur once in 35,000 to 250,000 births, since the prevalence of heterozygosity for adenine phosphoribosyltransferase deficiency varies from 0.4 to 1.1 per 100. Individuals heterozygous for the enzyme deficiency have no recognized clinical abnormalities.

Prognosis depends on renal function at the time of diagnosis. Therapy with dietary purine restriction, high fluid intake, and allopurinol—to prevent oxidation of adenine to 2,8-dihydroxyadenine—is effective in reducing stone formation and preserving renal function.

Simmonds A, Sahota AS, Van Acker KL: Adenine phosphoribosyltransferase deficiency. In Scriver CR, Beaudet AL, Sly WS, et al. (eds.): The Metabolic Basis of Inherited Disease. 6th ed. New York, McGraw-Hill, 1989, pp 1029–1044. *A detailed review of all known cases of complete APRT deficiency and discussion of the metabolic defect.*

Van Acker KJ, Simmonds A, Potter C, et al.: Complete deficiency of adenine

Adenine, 8-hydroxyadenine, and 2,8-dihydroxyadenine amounted to 25 per cent of urinary purines in two homozygous male children, one of whom had "pure uric acid stones" later correctly identified as 2,8-dihydroxyadenine.

IMMUNE DYSFUNCTION ASSOCIATED WITH PURINE ENZYME DEFICIENCIES

Adenosine deaminase deficiency is an uncommon disorder, approximately 100 to 150 families having been identified, that leads to a clinical syndrome of severe combined immunodeficiency, i.e., a defect in both T cell and B cell function. About one fifth of patients with severe combined immunodeficiency, in which the disorder is inherited as an autosomal recessive condition, or more rarely as an X-linked recessive disorder, have this enzyme deficiency. Approximately 85 per cent of patients with adenosine deaminase (ADA) deficiency come to medical attention at 1 to 2 months of age with recurrent infections of the skin and the gastrointestinal and respiratory systems. Both ordinary and opportunistic pathogens are encountered, and candidiasis is almost invariably present. Diarrhea is common, as well as delayed physical growth and development. Physical findings are for the most part unremarkable except for the absence of lymph nodes and pharyngeal lymphoid tissue. A rachitic rosary, or prominence of the costochondral junctions, has been noted in some patients. Laboratory tests show absence of a thymic shadow, lymphopenia, negative skin test results for delayed hypersensitivity, attenuated lymphocyte responses to lectins and antigens in vitro, and hypogammaglobulinemia. The diagnosis is established by documenting ADA deficiency in erythrocyte lysates or other cell extracts. Approximately 15 per cent of individuals with this disorder have a milder disease with later age of onset and relative sparing of humoral immunity. In the severe form of this disorder, if untreated, overwhelming infection and sepsis lead to death before 2 years of age.

Current mechanisms favored to explain the immune defects observed in ADA deficiency are deoxy–adenosine triphosphate (ATP) accumulation leading to inhibition of ribonucleotide reductase with resultant decrease in DNA replication, and S-adenosylhomocysteine accumulation leading to inhibition of transmethylation reactions. Either or both of these proposed mechanisms could reduce lymphocyte proliferation and function.

Treatment of ADA deficiency by bone marrow transplantation has resulted in virtually complete immune reconstitution in some patients, and at present this is the preferred therapy if compatible donors are available. Enzyme replacement with PEG-ADA* has been documented to improve immune function, and this therapy is effective in long-term trials, i.e., more than 4 years of follow-up. Gene therapy has been approved for this disorder, and trials are under way at the present time.

Purine nucleoside phosphorylase (PNP) deficiency is less common than ADA deficiency, approximately 15 to 20 patients with this disorder having been recognized. PNP deficiency is also inherited as an autosomal recessive disorder, but it leads to a defect in cell-mediated immunity with little, if any, abnormality in humoral immunity. In patients with this disorder, diagnosis has been made as early as 4 months and as late as 9 years of age, with infections involving skin, lung, middle ear, mastoids, and urinary tract. Infections with nonbacterial agents have been most common, reflecting the primary defect in cellular immunity. Laboratory tests show lymphopenia, diminished number of circulating T cells, reduced lymphocyte response to antigens, and negative skin test results for delayed hypersensitivity. Immunoglobulin levels are normal, but several patients have exhibited signs of immunoregulatory abnormalities, as shown by autoimmune hemolytic anemia, antinuclear antibodies, and rheumatoid factor. In addition, patients with PNP deficiency have hypouricemia, a finding of no clinical consequence in itself, but one that suggests the diagnosis of this enzyme deficiency in a child with recurrent infections.

Confirmation of the diagnosis is obtained by assay of erythrocyte lysate or other cell extracts for purine nucleoside phosphorylase activity. It has been proposed that accumulation of deoxyguanosine triphosphate in T cells, with resultant inhibition of ribonucleotide reductase and DNA replication, is responsible for the immune defect in this disorder. The prognosis in purine

*Polyethylene glycol–modified ADA.

nucleoside phosphorylase deficiency is generally better than that for adenosine deaminase deficiency, but therapy with bone marrow transplantation and erythrocyte transfusion has been less successful.

Giblett ER: Adenosine deaminase and purine nucleoside phosphorylase deficiency: How they were discovered and what they may mean. *In* Elliot K, Whelan J (eds.): Enzyme Defects and Immune Dysfunction. Ciba Found Symp 68:3, 1979. *An interesting story about scientific serendipity and discovery of a new group of clinical disorders.*

Hershfield MS, Buckley RH, Greenberg ML, et al.: Treatment of adenosine deaminase deficiency with polyethylene glycol–modified adenosine deaminase. N Engl J Med 316:589, 1987. *Description of a novel form of enzyme replacement therapy that provides active enzyme with a prolonged half-life in the circulation.*

Kredich N, Hershfield MS: Immunodeficiency diseases caused by adenosine deaminase deficiency and purine nucleoside phosphorylase deficiency. *In* Scriver CR, Beaudet AL, Sly WS, et al. (eds.): The Metabolic Basis of Inherited Disease. 6th ed. New York, McGraw-Hill, 1989, pp 1045–1075. *An authoritative review of the clinical, laboratory, and biochemical abnormalities in these disorders. This chapter also includes a detailed discussion of purine nucleoside metabolism in normal and pathologic situations.*

MYOPATHY ASSOCIATED WITH MYOADENYLATE DEAMINASE DEFICIENCY

Deficiency of myoadenylate deaminase has been noted in approximately 2 per cent of muscle biopsies submitted for routine investigation in some centers. This isozyme of adenosine monophosphate (AMP) deaminase is found predominantly in skeletal muscle, and this is the only organ affected by this enzyme deficiency. In approximately half of the cases that have been carefully studied, AMP deaminase deficiency is not associated with other neuromuscular pathology, and in these individuals the enzyme deficiency is marked (<1 per cent of normal). In cases in which the residual enzyme activity is higher (1 to 10 per cent of normal), the patients have a broad spectrum of neuromuscular diseases. Three quarters of patients with primary myoadenylate deaminase deficiency report exercise-related symptoms of easy fatigability, cramps, and myalgias, usually beginning in childhood or young adulthood. Weakness without exercise is noted in fewer than one third of patients. Hypotonia has been described in two patients. Reduced AMP deaminase activity has occasionally been reported in patients with other neuromuscular disorders, but no definite association of this enzyme deficiency has been established with any symptom complex other than easy fatigability, cramps, and myalgias. Since a few individuals with myoadenylate deaminase deficiency have been reported to be asymptomatic, factors in addition to AMP deaminase deficiency may contribute to the exercise-related manifestations described above.

Serum creatine kinase activity is mildly and variably increased in about one half of patients with this disorder, and routine laboratory studies, including electromyography and histochemistry of muscle, are not diagnostic. In the patient with exercise-related symptoms, the specific diagnosis of myoadenylate deaminase deficiency is suggested by the finding of reduced NH_3 production in a forearm ischemic exercise test. Since all patients with reduced NH_3 production following ischemic forearm exercise do not have myoadenylate deaminase deficiency, the diagnosis needs to be confirmed by direct assay of AMP deaminase activity in skeletal muscle.

Adenosine monophosphate deaminase is one of the components of the purine nucleotide cycle, a series of reactions that is potentially important in energy production and utilization in skeletal muscle. Deficiency of myoadenylate deaminase activity may impair energy generation through diminished production of citric acid cycle intermediates, and it may adversely affect energy utilization through a reduction in the rate of adenosine triphosphate (ATP) hydrolysis by myofibrillar adenosine triphosphatase (ATPase).

The prognosis in myoadenylate deaminase deficiency is generally good. Present experience suggests that the symptoms are slowly progressive, and the disorder leads to mild disability in most cases, although there have been exceptions to these generalizations. No effective therapy is available at this time.

Fishbein WN: Myoadenylate deaminase deficiency: Inherited and acquired forms. Biochem Med 33:158, 1985. *Review of biochemical data supporting primary and secondary forms of AMP deaminase deficiency.*

Sabina RL, Swain JL, Holmes EW: Myoadenylate deaminase deficiency. *In* Scriver

CR, Beaudet AL, Sly WS, et al. (eds.): The Metabolic Basis of Inherited Disease. 6th ed. New York, McGraw-Hill, 1989, pp 1077–1084. *Discussion of the clinical and biochemical findings in 130 patients with myoadenylate deaminase deficiency, as well as a review of the role of the purine nucleotide cycle in skeletal muscle function.*

Sabina RL, Swain JL, Olanow CW, et al.: Myoadenylate deaminase deficiency: Functional and metabolic abnormalities associated with disruption of the purine nucleotide cycle. J Clin Invest 73:720, 1984.

185 Disorders of Pyrimidine Metabolism

Lloyd H. Smith, Jr.

Pyrimidine nucleotides share equally with purine nucleotides the chemical chore of transmitting genetic information for reproduction or for phenotypic expression within the cell. They also function in the intermediary metabolism of lipids and carbohydrates. Only a few disorders of pyrimidine metabolism have been recognized.

Hereditary orotic aciduria is a rare genetic disorder of pyrimidine metabolism characterized by megaloblastic anemia resistant to the usual hematinic agents, leukopenia, failure of normal growth and development, and the continued excessive urinary excretion of orotic acid. Patients also have impaired cellular immunity with intact humoral immunity. Orotic acid is highly insoluble and often forms a heavy sediment of urinary crystals that may on occasion result in ureteral or urethral obstruction. The disorder, which is transmitted as an autosomal recessive trait, is usually characterized by a reduction in two consecutive enzymatic activities in pyrimidine biosynthesis, orotate phosphoribosyltransferase (OPRT) and orotidine 5'-phosphate decarboxylase (ODC). Both enzymatic activities reside in a single multifunctional protein, uridine monophosphate (UMP) synthase, for which the gene is located on the long arm of chromosome 3. A single patient has been described with isolated deficiency of ODC. There is a prompt and sustained hematologic and general clinical response to oral uridine (2 to 4 grams per day), which must be continued indefinitely as replacement therapy. The disease has attracted special attention because it represents a block in the de novo pathway of pyrimidine synthesis, is an example of a double defect in enzymatic activity (although now known to be attributable to a single protein), and produces a requirement for replacement of a normal metabolic intermediate, uridine.

Orotic aciduria, without the characteristic hematologic abnormalities, also occurs in *ornithine transcarbamylase deficiency*. It is presumed that this results from the overflow of carbamyl phosphate from urea synthesis (partially blocked in this disease) to pyrimidine synthesis. Orotic aciduria has also been found in purine nucleoside phosphorylase deficiency and in PP-ribose-P synthetase deficiency (see Ch. 184).

Excessive urinary excretion of orotic acid and orotidine occurs during treatment with *allopurinol* or *6-azauridine*.* Metabolic products of both compounds inhibit orotidine 5'-decarboxylase activity.

Pyrimidine 5'-nucleotidase deficiency is a rare form of hereditary hemolytic anemia, transmitted as an autosomal recessive trait. The erythrocytes exhibit prominent basophilic stippling owing to aggregates of undegraded ribosomes and on analysis contain very high concentrations of cytidine and uridine nucleotides. The mechanism by which the nucleotidase deficiency leads to hemolysis is unclear. Lead inhibits pyrimidine 5'-nucleotidase activity and leads to a similar anemia with basophilic stippling, possibly through this mechanism.

Dihydropyrimidine dehydrogenase deficiency is a rare disorder affecting an enzyme in the degradative pathway for the pyrimidine bases uracil and thymine. As a result, uracil and thymine accumulate in plasma and are excreted excessively in the urine. No distinctive clinical picture has been noted, although most cases have been found through screening studies for organic aciduria in patients with a variety of neurologic disorders.

Paglia DE, Fink K, Valentine WN: Additional data from two kindreds with genetically-induced deficiencies of erythrocyte pyrimidine nucleotidase. Acta Hematol 63:262, 1980. *This is the best description of clinical findings and the altered pyrimidine metabolism leading to hemolytic anemia in this rare but interesting genetic disease.*

Suttle DP, Becoft DMO, Webster DR: Orotic aciduria. *In* Scriver CR, Beaudet A, Sly W, et al. (eds.): The Metabolic Basis of Inherited Disease. 6th ed. New York, McGraw-Hill, 1989, pp 1095–1126. *This is the most complete description of normal pyrimidine metabolism in humans and the derangements that occur in hereditary orotic aciduria and in other disorders of pyrimidine metabolism.*

*Investigational drug.

INHERITED DISORDERS OF CONNECTIVE TISSUE

186 The Mucopolysaccharidoses

William S. Sly

The mucopolysaccharidoses (MPS) are a group of lysosomal storage diseases, each of which is produced by an inherited deficiency of an enzyme involved in degradation of acid mucopolysaccharides (now called glycosaminoglycans and abbreviated GAG's). They are clinically progressive and have many common features that result from accumulation of partially degraded GAG's in various tissues. They produce disability primarily from storage-related abnormalities of the connective tissue, the heart, the bony skeleton, and the central nervous system.

Delineation of this group of diseases on the basis of clinical features, radiologic findings, and biochemistry of the urinary GAG's led to the famous classification of McKusick into MPS I to VI in 1966. Over the next 6 years, an exciting series of investigations from the laboratories of Neufeld and co-workers led to the discoveries that fibroblasts from patients with these disorders show storage abnormalities in culture, that fibroblasts from genetically different patients could "cross-correct" each other in culture, and that this "cross-correction" was due to secretion and recapture of lysosomal enzymes by the complementing fibroblast cell lines, each of which could secrete the enzyme the other was missing and take up the "corrective factor" for which it was deficient. These complementation studies served for nearly a decade as means for clinical diagnosis and for segregation of the disease into complementation groups (e.g., segregation of Hurler and Scheie syndromes into one complementation group, and separation of Sanfilippo syndrome into several complementing groups); they also guided the purification of the corrective factors, each of which was eventually identified as a specific GAG degradative enzyme. Although still useful in certain situations, the complementation assays have largely been replaced by direct assays for the enzymes listed in Table 186–1 as deficient for each of the disorders.

ETIOLOGY OF GLYCOSAMINOGLYCAN STORAGE. The GAG's are long linear polysaccharide molecules composed of repeating dimers, each of which contains a hexuronic acid (or galactose in the case of keratan sulfate) and an amino sugar. They are usually found in covalent linkage to a core protein on which they are synthesized and from which they branch like bristles from a brush. The individual GAG's differ from one another in the hexuronic acid-amino sugar combinations in the repeating dimers, in the linkages between these components, in the link-

TABLE 186–1. THE MUCOPOLYSACCHARIDOSES (MPS STORAGE DISEASES I TO VII)

Abbreviation	Eponym	Enzyme Deficiency	Major Storage Product	Urinary GAG's	Clinical Features
MPS U-H	Hurler	α-L-Iduronidase	DS ± HS	↑ 5–25X DS > HS	Onset 6–12 mo, coarse features, rhinorrhea, grunting respiration, corneal clouding, cardiac disease, visceromegaly, dwarfism, dysostosis multiplex, progressive mental retardation after the first year; death by 5–10 yr
MPS I-S (formerly MPS V)	Scheie	α-L-Iduronidase	DS + HS	↑ 5–25X DS > HS	Onset 5–15 yr, corneal clouding, stiff joints, clawhand, genu valgum, dysostosis multiplex, aortic valve disease; however, normal height, normal intelligence, and long survival (difficult to distinguish clinically from mild MPS VI)
MPS I-H/S	Hurler-Scheie	α-L-Iduronidase	DS + HS	↑ 5–25X DS > HS	Onset 2–4 yr, all findings of MPS-H but milder, slower progression, and survival into 20's
MPS II, severe	Hunter, severe form	L-Sulfoiduronate sulfatase	HS + DS	↑ 5–25X DS = HS	Onset 2–4 yr, clear corneas, deafness, all other features of MPS I-H, but milder; mental retardation progresses to profound state; death by 10–15 yr
MPS II, mild	Hunter, mild form	L-Sulfoiduronate sulfatase	HS + DS	↑ 5–25X DS = HS	Onset in first decade, short stature, clear corneas, joint stiffness, dysostosis multiplex, visceromegaly, cardiac disease, nerve entrapments, near-normal intelligence; survival to 30's–60's, depending on heart involvement
MPS III-A	Sanfilippo, type A	Heparan sulfate sulfamidase	HS	↑ 5–20X 85% HS	Onset 2–6 yr, large head, normal height; Hurler-like features, dysostosis multiplex, hepatomegaly are all mild; mental retardation is rapidly progressive and severe; death at end of puberty
MPS III-B	Sanfilippo, type B	N-acetyl-α-D-glucosaminidase	HS	↑ 5–20X 85% HS	Clinically indistinguishable from MPS III, type A
MPS III-C	Sanfilippo, type C	Acetyl CoA: α-glucosamide N-acetyltransferase	HS	↑ 5–20X 85% HS	Clinically indistinguishable from MPS III, type A
MPS III-D	Sanfilippo, type D	N-acetyl-α-D-glucosamine-6-sulfatase	HS	↑ 5–20X 85% HS	Clinically indistinguishable from MPS III, type A
MPS IV-A	Morquio, classic form	N-acetylgalactosamine-6-sulfatase (gal-6-sulfatase)	KS + Ch 6-S	↑ 3–5X KS + Ch-S	Characteristic facies, short-trunk dwarfism, deformed thorax, corneal clouding, hearing deficit, aortic valve disease, unstable neck, spinal cord transection; intelligence is normal; death usually in 20's from cardiorespiratory problems
MPS IV-B	Morquio-like syndrome	β-Galactosidase deficiency	KS + Ch 4-S	↑ 2–5X KS = Ch-S	Short stature, corneal clouding, mild dysostosis multiplex, prominence of lower face, pectus carinatum, hip deformity, normal intelligence
MPS VI	Maroteaux-Lamy, severe	N-acetylgalactosamine-4-sulfatase (arylsulfatase B)	DS + ?Ch 4-S	↑ 4–20X 70–90% DS	Onset 2–4 yr, growth failure from age 4 slowly progressive, joint stiffness, corneal clouding, aortic valve disease, and severe hip deformity; dysostosis multiplex, striking white cell inclusions; intelligence normal; death in 20's
	Maroteaux-Lamy, mild	N-acetylgalactosamine-4-sulfatase (arylsulfatase B)	DS + ?Ch 4-S	↑ 4–20X 70–90% DS	Onset 5–7 yr, short stature, severe osseous changes, especially in the hips; nerve entrapment, corneal clouding, aortic valve disease; normal intelligence, long survival; difficult to distinguish from MPS I-S
MPS VII	Sly	β-Glucuronidase	HS, DS, Ch-S	↑ 6–8X HS, DS Ch 4/6-S	Onset 1–2 yr, mild to moderate Hurler-like features, dysostosis multiplex, pectus carinatum, visceromegaly, cardiac murmurs, short stature, moderate mental retardation; slowly progressive after infancy; striking granulocyte inclusions; milder forms exist, as does a more severe form with neonatal ascites and death within 2 yr

DS = dermatan sulfate; HS = heparan sulfate; Ch-S = chondroitin sulfate; KS = keratan sulfate.

ages between repeating dimers, and in the degree to which individual sugar components are N-acetylated or N-sulfated. The major GAG's and their respective repeating dimers are chondroitin sulfate (glucuronic acid β1-3 N-acetylgalactosamine-4/6-sulfate); dermatan sulfate (iduronic acid α1-3 N-acetylgalactosamine-4-sulfate); heparan sulfate, which has both glucuronic acid and iduronic acid linked β1-4 and α1-3, respectively, to either N-acetylglucosamine or glucosamine N-sulfate; and keratan sulfate (galactose β1-4 N-acetylglucosamine-6-sulfate). The large proteoglycan molecules made up of protein cores and their GAG branches are secreted by cells and constitute a significant fraction of the extracellular matrix of connective tissue. Their turnover depends on their subsequent internalization by endocytosis, their delivery to lysosomes, and their digestion by lysosomal enzymes. Lysosomal proteases digest the core protein, endoglycosidases reduce the size of the GAG's to oligosaccharides of varying length, and many exoglycosidases act sequentially to degrade the GAG's to their monosaccharide components. Each lysosomal enzyme is specific for a specific linkage. An inherited deficiency for any enzyme involved disrupts the sequential degradative process and leads to accumulation in lysosomes of partially degraded GAG. The accumulation is progressive and eventually disrupts cellular architecture and disturbs cell function. The tissues and organs most affected and the severity depend on the degree of enzyme deficiency, i.e., whether partial or complete. Severity also depends on which enzyme is missing, since individual GAG's vary in their tissue distribution and their rate of turnover.

The causative enzyme deficiencies, the major storage products, and the clinical features of the mucopolysaccharidoses are summarized in Table 186–1. There is marked genetic heterogeneity within this group of disorders, with many different clinical phenotypes resulting from the different enzyme deficiencies (see MPS I–VII, Table 186–1). It is now clear also that quite different phenotypes can result from the same enzyme deficiency, depending on whether it is partial or complete (see MPS I-H, MPS I-S, and MPS I-H/S in Table 186–1).

GENETICS OF THE MUCOPOLYSACCHARIDOSES. Except for Hunter syndrome (MPS II), in which the missing enzyme is specified by a gene on the X chromosome and the inheritance is X linked, all of the mucopolysaccharidoses result from deficiencies of enzymes specified by autosomal genes. Thus the inheritance pattern is autosomal recessive. In most cases, affected offspring can be shown to be the products of heterozygous carrier parents, both of whom have about half-normal levels of the enzyme for which the affected patient is deficient. Even though the enzymes can now be measured for most of these disorders, the disorders are too rare to make screening for carriers practical. However, carrier status can be determined by enzyme assays in high-risk individuals, and prenatal diagnosis for most of these disorders is available to high-risk mothers, such as mothers of an affected offspring, who face a 25 per cent chance of another affected offspring in a subsequent pregnancy.

CLINICAL AND PATHOLOGIC CONSEQUENCES OF GLYCOSAMINOGLYCAN STORAGE. Connective tissue storage produces connective tissue laxity in most of these disorders, manifest by inguinal and umbilical hernias. Connective tissue thickening also occurs, owing in part to GAG storage and in part to excessive collagen deposition. This combination leads to coarse facial features, peripheral nerve entrapments, thickened meninges that may lead to cord compression and hydrocephalus, and thickened joint capsules. Connective tissue deposition in valve leaflets, the endocardium, and the myocardium produces symptomatic heart disease, a common cause of death in these patients, to which coronary vascular insufficiency also contributes. Most of these disorders produce short stature, partly because of impaired long-bone growth and partly because of vertebral abnormalities. These and many other changes in the bony skeleton are collectively referred to as *dysostosis multiplex*. Central nervous system storage may produce progressive mental retardation, especially in disorders involving impaired degradation of heparan sulfate (MPS I, II, and III). Corneal clouding and visual handicap result from storage of the partially degraded GAG's in the corneal stroma, especially in disorders involving impaired degradation of dermatan sulfate and keratan sulfate (MPS I, IV, and VI).

Hepatomegaly is common and may be massive but rarely is important clinically. Excessive urinary excretion of incompletely degraded GAG's (mucopolysacchariduria) is a constant finding of considerable diagnostic significance (Table 186–1) but has little pathologic significance.

HURLER SYNDROME (MPS I-H). *Pathology.* The basic defect is a deficiency of alpha-L-iduronidase, an enzyme that participates in degradation of dermatan sulfate and heparan sulfate. Accumulation of membrane-enclosed storage material in parenchymal and mesenchymal cells is the chief pathologic finding. It affects every organ. Vacuolated cells distended with storage material distort normal cell and tissue architecture. In most cells this storage material is granular and composed of GAG's. In neurons, lipids are also present, presumably because stored GAG's inhibit sphingolipid degradation.

Clinical Features. Although patients are thought to be normal until 6 months of age, they develop persistent nasal discharge, noisy breathing, frequent upper respiratory infections, stiff joints, a thoracolumbar gibbus, and some degree of chest deformity in the second half of the first year of life. Over the second year, the classic syndrome develops, with large head, coarse features, corneal clouding, hypertelorism, prominent eyebrows, thick lips, and broad, flat nose with depressed nasal bridge. The hands are short and stubby, and joint limitation produces a clawhand deformity. Abdominal protuberance results from hepatosplenomegaly and lax abdominal musculature, often with inguinal and umbilical hernias. Dwarfism is obvious by the end of the second year, by which time cardiac murmurs are present.

Developmental delay is obvious before 18 months of age, and mental retardation progresses slowly. Limitation of joint movement leads to contractures of the hands, the elbows, and the knees. Death usually occurs by the age of 10 from pneumonia or heart failure, after about 5 years of steady regression and nearly total loss of acquired skills. Hearing loss is usually moderate to severe, and coronary insufficiency and peripheral vascular insufficiency are important late findings.

Radiologic abnormalities of dysostosis multiplex are striking. The skull is large and scaphocephalic, and the calvarium is thickened. The sinuses are poorly developed. The sella is enlarged anteriorly and referred to as **J** shaped. The ribs are oar shaped, being narrow posteriorly and greatly expanded anteriorly. The medial third of the clavicle is thickened. The vertebrae are initially rounded and appear ovoid. One or two lower thoracic and upper lumbar vertebrae are often hypoplastic and wedge shaped, producing the gibbus deformity. The pelvis shows flared iliac wings, a small body of the ilium, and shallow oblique acetabula. The hips show coxa valga deformities. The metatarsals and phalanges are short and wide; the proximal ends of the metacarpals taper sharply, a classic finding called proximal pointing. The long tubular bones have expanded diaphyses. There is loss of normal angulation of the humerus at the shoulder. The radiologic changes are progressive, but the changes vary considerably from patient to patient at a given age. The lower extremities are generally more mildly affected than the upper extremities, except for the hips, which often show changes resembling aseptic necrosis of the femoral heads, changes that correlate with severe hip disability clinically.

Diagnosis. The diagnosis can be suspected on clinical and radiologic grounds, supported by demonstration of mucopolysacchariduria (dermatan sulfate [DS] > heparan sulfate [HS]), and established definitively by demonstration of the enzyme deficiency, using the commercially available phenyl-L-iduronide substrate. Enzyme activity can be measured in extracts of leukocytes or cultured fibroblasts.

Treatment. Only supportive and symptomatic treatment can be offered to patients, as no effective treatment for the storage abnormality is available.

SCHEIE SYNDROME (MPS I-S). This rare disorder is also due to a deficiency of alpha-L-iduronidase and is characterized by severe corneal clouding, deformity of the hands, and aortic valve disease. Symptoms appear between the ages of 5 and 15. The height is normal, as is the intelligence. The striking joint stiffness of the hands is similar to that seen in Hurler syndrome but is complicated by the carpal tunnel syndrome with median nerve entrapment. Aortic stenosis, regurgitation, or both are present but are usually not symptomatic in early life. Life expectancy may be nearly normal. Diagnosis depends on the same criteria as for Hurler syndrome. Corneal transplant and aortic valve replacement are reasonable, since intelligence is normal.

THE HURLER-SCHEIE COMPOUND (MPS I-H/S). Some patients with a phenotype that is intermediate between that of Hurler and that of Scheie syndromes are thought to represent compound heterozygotes, having inherited one Hurler and one Scheie gene from each parent.

HUNTER SYNDROME (MPS II). Hunter syndrome is distinguished from Hurler syndrome by three features: (1) slower progression with longer survival, (2) lack of corneal clouding, and (3) X-linked rather than autosomal recessive inheritance. A severe form and a mild form exist. The severe form has most of the features of Hurler syndrome, but they are slightly milder except for hearing impairment, which is more severe. The patients usually die by age 15. A much milder form has been reported with near-normal intelligence and near-normal survival. Diagnosis is made on the basis of the clinical findings, radiologic evidence of dysostosis multiplex, increased urinary GAG's, and demonstration of sulfoiduronate sulfatase deficiency on serum or on extracts of leukocytes or cultured fibroblasts. Carrier detection is still imperfect, but prenatal diagnostic tests are reliable.

SANFILIPPO SYNDROME (MPS III). This syndrome can be produced by a deficiency of at least four different enzymes, all of which participate in degradation of heparan sulfate (Table 186–1). Early development is normal but slows or halts between the ages of 2 and 6 years, after which mental deterioration is often rapid. Gait becomes unsteady, muscles atrophy, and the patient becomes bedridden. Death usually occurs by puberty. The head is large, the hair coarse, and hirsutism common. Visceromegaly is mild to absent. Cardiac involvement is rare. Height may be normal through the first decade and then falls behind. Skeletal findings of dysostosis multiplex are mild and include thickened calvarium, ovoid vertebral bodies, mild dysplasia of the pelvis, and mild rib changes. The clinical diagnosis may be suspected from the severe mental retardation, which appears disproportionate to relatively mild somatic and radiologic abnormalities, supported by the presence of heparan sulfaturia, and established definitively by demonstration of the specific enzyme deficiency.

MORQUIO SYNDROME, CLASSIC FORM (MPS IV-A). The predominant clinical features relate to skeletal abnormalities and to symptoms of spinal cord compression resulting from instability of the neck. Intelligence is normal. By the age of 2 years, pigeon chest deformity, genu valgum, and gait disturbance appear. Knees and wrists enlarge. The neck appears short, and the head seems to sit on the deformed thorax. Universal platyspondylisis, evident on radiographic examination, kyphoscoliosis, and contractures at the knees and hips all contribute to dwarfism. The face is unusual because of mid-face hypoplasia, depressed nasal bridge, flared nares, and prominence of the lower third of the face on side view. The teeth are widely spaced, and the dental enamel is thin. Corneal clouding is mild but slowly progressive. Long survival is rare, with death occurring between the ages of 20 and 40 from cardiopulmonary complications. The cardiac disease is valvular (aortic regurgitation). The respiratory problems arise from thoracic deformities and from neurotrophic myelopathy caused by atlantoaxial subluxation. Diagnosis depends on the clinical and radiologic features, which are characteristic; the finding of keratan sulfaturia (which may disappear in adolescence); and the deficiency of N-acetylgalactosamine-6-sulfatase, which is active on both GalNAc 6-S in chondroitin sulfate and Gal 6-S in keratan sulfate. The enzymatic assay is available in only a few laboratories. Treatment is symptomatic. Posterior cervical fusion should be done early in the disease to prevent spinal cord damage. Correction of the genu valgum requires a single operation at about 6 years.

THE MORQUIO-LIKE SYNDROME WITH BETA-GALACTOSIDASE DEFICIENCY (MPS IV-B). Short stature, mild pectus carinatum, corneal clouding, odontoid hypoplasia with cervical instability, mild dysostosis multiplex, moderate lumbar kyphosis, and mild genu valgum are all features that are found in this Morquio-like disease resulting from beta-galactosidase deficiency. Absent are hearing deficit, dental abnormalities, cardiac murmurs, hepatomegaly, and joint laxity. Keratan sulfaturia is present. The diagnosis is based on normal N-acetylgalactosamine-6-sulfatase levels and reduced beta-galactosidase levels. Presumably, this disorder reflects a mutation that impairs the

activity of the enzyme on galactose linkages in keratan sulfate but spares its activity on GM_1 ganglioside. Thus the findings of chondrodystrophy predominate, and the neurologic manifestations of GM_1 gangliosidosis are absent.

THE MAROTEAUX-LAMY SYNDROME, SEVERE AND MILD TYPES (MPS VI). Maroteaux and colleagues recognized a new form of mucopolysaccharidosis in 1963 that resembled Hurler syndrome but differed in that intelligence of the dwarfed, deformed patients was spared; the urinary GAG was almost exclusively dermatan sulfate; and the leukocytes exhibited striking metachromatic inclusions. Affected patients often die in their 20's from cardiac failure. Many suffer cervical cord compression and hydrocephalus resulting from thickened meninges. Since specific enzymatic assays have become available both for arylsulfatase B, missing in MPS VI, and alpha-L-iduronidase, missing in MPS I, it has become clear that many patients with milder forms of MPS VI exist who might previously have been thought to have Scheie syndrome. No specific treatment is available for the storage abnormality. However, shunting for hydrocephalus, spinal fusion for atlantoaxial subluxation, corneal transplants for visual handicap, and cardiac valve and hip replacement are all reasonable when required, because intelligence is preserved and patients with milder forms of the abnormality have the potential for long survival.

BETA-GLUCURONIDASE DEFICIENCY MUCOPOLYSACCHARIDOSIS (MPS VII). Most patients present by age 3 with a Hurler-like illness manifested by frequent upper respiratory infections, chest deformities, cardiac murmurs, hepatosplenomegaly, hernias, dysostosis multiplex, and mild to moderate mental retardation. Many develop corneal clouding. About 20 patients, showing a wide range of clinical severity, have been recognized. Most of the patients have shown slow progression in clinical abnormalities after the age of 6. The natural history beyond the teens is yet to be determined. Urinary GAG's have been increased, and heparan sulfate, dermatan sulfate, and chondroitin sulfate have all been reported to be increased in urine. Striking inclusions in leukocytes are typical, as in MPS VI. The diagnosis depends on the demonstration of the enzyme deficiency. Carrier detection and prenatal diagnosis are available.

OTHER DISORDERS RELATED TO THE MUCOPOLYSACCHARIDOSES. Mucolipidosis II (also called I-cell disease) and mucolipidosis III (also called pseudo-Hurler polydystrophy) are severe and milder forms, respectively, of a Hurler-like disease having many features in common with the mucopolysaccharidoses. However, these patients do not have mucopolysacchariduria.

These disorders result not from a deficiency of a single lysosomal enzyme, as do the mucopolysaccharidoses, but from a defect in the processing of N-acetylglucosaminyl phosphotransferase that normally targets acid hydrolases to lysosomes. Failure to add the phosphomannosyl recognition marker that normally directs their segregation into lysosomes allows acid hydrolases to be secreted instead. As a consequence, there is an intracellular deficiency of most of the enzymes involved in the degradation of GAG's (and an extracellular excess), which is part of a general pattern of deficiency involving nearly all lysosomal enzymes. The absence of mucopolysacchariduria, and the 10- to 50-fold elevations of levels of acid hydrolases in serum, distinguish these two disorders from the mucopolysaccharidoses with single-enzyme deficiency.

Another group of disorders, not classified with the mucopolysaccharidoses, may produce a Hurler-like picture, including mental retardation, visceromegaly, and dysostosis multiplex. These disorders result from single-enzyme deficiencies for enzymes involved in the catabolism of the oligosaccharide components of glycoproteins. Included are mannosidosis, fucosidosis, and the more recently delineated group of sialidoses (one of which has been described under the name mucolipidosis I). The sialidoses result from a deficiency of oligosaccharide N-acetylneuraminidase. The primary storage products in these disorders are oligosaccharides derived from glycoproteins. However, there is some storage of keratan sulfate as well. It appears that these enzymes are required for degradation of some oligosaccharide side chains on keratan sulfate. Impaired degradation of keratan sulfate may explain the dysostosis multiplex that mimics the skeletal findings of the mucopolysaccharidoses in these disorders.

Kelly TE: The mucopolysaccharidoses and mucolipidoses. Clin Orthop 114:116, 1976. *A nice summary of clinically relevant information.*

McKusick VA, Neufeld EF, Kelly TE: The mucopolysaccharide storage diseases. *In* Stanbury JB, Wyngaarden JB, Fredrickson DS, et al. (eds.): The Metabolic Basis of Inherited Disease. 5th ed. New York, McGraw-Hill, 1983. *A comprehensive chapter with good historical perspective.*

Neufeld EF, Muenzer J: The mucopolysaccharide storage diseases. *In* Scriver CR, Beaudet AL, Sly WS, et al. (eds.): The Metabolic Basis of Inherited Disease. 6th ed. New York, McGraw-Hill, 1989. *A current, comprehensive treatment of biochemical and genetic information.*

187 The Marfan Syndrome

Peter H. Byers

DEFINITION. The Marfan syndrome is a dominantly inherited connective tissue disorder characterized by musculoskeletal abnormalities (arachnodactyly, tall stature, scoliosis, pectus deformities, and ligamentous laxity), cardiovascular abnormalities (mitral valve prolapse and regurgitation, aortic valve insufficiency, and aortic dilatation, aneurysm, and dissection), lens dislocation, and myopia.

ETIOLOGY AND PATHOGENESIS. For most patients the molecular defect is not known. Recent studies have shown that monoclonal antibodies to fibrillin, a component of microfibrils of elastic fibers and of other microfibrils, stain the matrix of skin and the extracellular matrix of cultured fibroblasts from individuals with the Marfan syndrome poorly when compared with normal persons. Linkage studies using anonymous DNA markers indicate that the gene responsible for the Marfan syndrome is on the long arm of chromosome 15.

PREVALENCE. The Marfan syndrome affects about 1 in 15,000 individuals without racial or ethnic predilection.

PATHOLOGY. The mitral and aortic valves are characterized by "myxomatous degeneration" or the appearance of large pools of nonfibrous material that separate the normal cells of the valves. The valves may be thickened. In the absence of dissection there is accumulation of metachromatic material in the aortic media and disruption of the normal elastic laminae. Aortic dissection characteristically begins in the ascending aorta and may proceed in both directions. Death frequently results from cardiac tamponade due to hemopericardium, coronary occlusion, occlusion of the arteries to the brain, internal hemorrhage, or loss of perfusion of multiple abdominal organs.

CLINICAL MANIFESTIONS. The Marfan syndrome is highly variable in its clinical manifestations, and affected members within the same family may differ in the degree to which they express the mutation; the differences between families may be explained, in part, by different mutations in a single connective tissue gene or mutations in different connective tissue genes. The diagnosis can be made occasionally in newborns because of lens dislocation, mitral valve prolapse, scoliosis, and tall stature with arachnodactyly. More commonly, affected infants may be tall, but cardiac findings are minimal. Many have mild to moderate scoliosis with pectus deformities (excavatum or carinatum); progression of scoliosis or pectus deformities may be rapid during the adolescent growth spurt. About half the patients with the Marfan syndrome have ocular lens dislocation, usually in a superior and nasal direction and generally nonprogressive after adolescence. Cataract formation and glaucoma are occasional complications of ectopia lentis. Mitral valve prolapse is seen in virtually all patients with the Marfan syndrome and in some progresses to symptomatic mitral regurgitation; associated rhythm disturbances may be symptomatic.

The major life-threatening complication of the Marfan syndrome is aortic dissection and rupture, and most deaths result from cardiovascular disease. The risk of dissection is well correlated with aortic diameter. In some children aortic root diameters, measured by echocardiography, are greater than normal, but, more commonly, aortic diameters do not exceed the normal range (20 to 37 mm) until adulthood and usually enlarge gradually,

although the rate may vary. Aortic dissection in the Marfan syndrome is occasionally asymptomatic, but usually there is prolonged, severe substernal chest pain of a tearing or searing quality, often with radiation into the neck, back, and arms. It is often accompanied by diaphoresis, hypotension, and shock. Blood pressure in the two arms may differ. Rarely, pregnancy may be complicated by dissection, even in the presence of a normal aortic diameter.

DIFFERENTIAL DIAGNOSIS. The Marfan syndrome is one of several disorders in which the characteristic habitus is seen. *Contractural arachnodactyly* is a dominantly inherited disorder characterized by arachnodactyly, joint contracture, small, cup-shaped ears, pectus deformity, mild scoliosis, and mitral valve prolapse, but lens dislocation is absent and aortic dilatation is not a complication. *Homocystinuria* (see Ch. 182) is characterized by autosomal recessive inheritance, tight joints, peripheral vascular disease, thrombosis of arterial vessels, lens dislocation, osteoporosis, and, often, mild mental retardation. The diagnosis is confirmed by detection of excessive homocystine in the urine. In the *nonasthenic form* of the Marfan syndrome, body habitus is normal, but lens dislocation and mitral valve prolapse are common, and death from aortic aneurysm and dissection often establishes the diagnosis. Aortic dissection generally occurs in the fifth to seventh decades; the disorder is inherited in an autosomal dominant fashion. The *mitral valve prolapse syndrome* is commonly mistaken for the Marfan syndrome because of the presence of mitral valve prolapse, tall stature, and some of the mild skeletal features of the Marfan syndrome. The disorder is inherited in an autosomal dominant fashion; the absence of lens dislocation and progressive aortic root dilatation distinguishes it from the Marfan syndrome. Patients with the *Stickler syndrome* may have a marfanoid habitus, degenerative arthritis of multiple joints, cleft palate, and, generally, vitreal degeneration. The *marfanoid habitus* may be seen in some patients with sickle cell disease, the Klinefelter syndrome (the 47 XXY karyotype, see Ch. 222), and multiple endocrine adenomatosis type IIB (see Ch. 228).

TREATMENT. Treatment of the Marfan syndrome has several objectives: control of excessive height, prevention of glaucoma, regulation of blood pressure, and prevention of aortic dissection. Excessive height may be controlled by administration of testosterone (to boys) and estrogens (to girls) prior to puberty to hasten epiphyseal closure. Routine ophthalmologic examination is important to assure that dislocation of the lens into the anterior chamber does not occur and to treat any retinal detachment (the consequence of the high myopia that accompanies the syndrome). Rarely, the lenses must be removed because of recurrent anterior chamber displacement or because the lens edge is in the center of the visual field and adequate correction cannot be achieved. Blood pressure should always be maintained in the normal range. There is some indication that treatment with agents that decrease cardiac contractility (beta-adrenergic blockers, for example) may delay the rate of aortic progression, but this is an area of controversy, and appropriate controlled studies have not yet been published; nonetheless, in some centers such treatment is routine.

Recently, the advances in surgical technique have made replacement of diseased portions of the aorta a routine treatment that provides increased life expectancy. Replacement should be considered when aortic root diameter reaches approximately 55 mm and prior to decompensation of the left ventricle as a result of aortic valve insufficiency. A composite graft that includes an aortic valve is now used. In some patients, mitral valve function is compromised and the valve requires replacement or repair. Techniques for replacement of large portions of the aorta have also helped to prolong survival.

PROGNOSIS. The prognosis in the Marfan syndrome depends largely on the vascular complications. In one major study the mean age of death for all affected individuals was in the early 40's, and virtually all died of the cardiovascular complications. The judicious use of surgical replacement of the ascending aorta and, if needed, of additional parts of the aorta appears to prolong survival. If the controlled studies of treatment with beta-adrenergic blockade demonstrate effectiveness, then another treatment of the cardiovascular complications will be available.

Patients with the Marfan syndrome should be observed yearly by an internist, a family physician, or a geneticist. Echocardiography should be performed yearly to follow aortic root diameter and the magnitude of mitral regurgitation and aortic insufficiency. Patients should see an ophthalmologist regularly and should consult with a cardiac surgeon as the aortic root diameter passes 50 to 55 mm.

Pregnancy usually is completed without complication, but women in whom the aortic diameter is greater than 40 mm (above the upper limits of normal) may be at greater risk for complications. All pregnancies should be followed in a high-risk center.

Prenatal diagnosis, the only form of prevention, is not currently available. Genetic counseling is important for all members of the proband's family to identify those who are affected.

Gott VL, Pyeritz RE, Magovern GJ Jr, et al.: Surgical treatment of aneurysms of the ascending aorta in the Marfan syndrome: Results of composite-graft repair in 50 patients. N Engl J Med 314:1070, 1986. *A review of the surgical approach to the patient with the Marfan syndrome: outcome, complications, criteria for selection, and longevity.*

Hollister DW, Godfrey M, Sakai LY, et al.: Immunohistologic abnormalities of the microfibrillar-fiber system in the Marfan syndrome. N Engl J Med 323:152, 1990. *Demonstration of defective staining of fibrillin and discussion of its presumed relevance in the Marfan syndrome.*

Kainulainen K, Pulkkinen L, Savolainen A, et al.: Location on chromosome of the gene defect causing Marfan syndrome. N Engl J Med 323:935, 1990. *Location of the Marfan gene using the techniques of "reverse genetics."*

Maumenee IH: The eye in the Marfan syndrome. Trans Am Ophthalmol Soc 79:684, 1981. *The most comprehensive review of the eye findings in the Marfan syndrome and their differential diagnosis.*

McKusick VA: Heritable Disorders of Connective Tissue. 4th ed. St. Louis, CV Mosby Company, 1972, pp 61–200. *Still the most comprehensive description of patients with the Marfan syndrome. Many case histories, easy and interesting to read; anecdotal.*

Pyeritz RE, McKusick VA: The Marfan syndrome: Diagnosis and management. N Engl J Med 300:772, 1979. *A more formal statistical compilation of the frequency of physical findings and complications in patients with the Marfan syndrome. Recommendations for management and follow-up.*

188 Ehlers-Danlos Syndrome

Peter H. Byers

DEFINITION. Ehlers-Danlos syndrome (EDS) is a group of more than 10 inherited connective tissue disorders characterized by abnormalities of the skin, ligaments, and internal organs. The clinical manifestations include skin fragility, abnormal scar formation, excessive bruising, joint laxity, and, in one variety, rupture of viscera and arteries (Table 188–1).

ETIOLOGY. Some forms of EDS result from defects in the synthesis and processing of types I and III collagens, the major proteins of skin, ligaments, tendons, blood vessels, and viscera. The molecular bases of EDS types I, II, III, V, and VIII are not known. The known defects include mutations affecting the structure, synthesis, processing, or stability of type III collagen (EDS type IV); deficient hydroxylation of lysyl residues in type I and type III collagen (EDS type VI); defective conversion of type I procollagen to collagen (EDS type VII); defective collagen cross-linking and abnormal cellular utilization of copper (EDS type IX); and a functional defect in fibronectin (EDS type X).

PREVALENCE. The prevalence of EDS is about 1 in 5000 births. EDS type III, benign familial hypermobility, accounts for most patients identified as having EDS; some forms are uncommon (EDS types IV, VI, VII, and VIII); others have been found in only a few families (EDS types IX and X). There is no racial or ethnic predisposition for any of the common types of EDS.

PATHOLOGY AND PATHOGENESIS. Dermal collagen fibrils in patients with EDS types I, II, III, and VI are larger than normal and irregular in outline when viewed by electron microscopy. In EDS type IV, skin is thin and collagen fibril diameter is frequently smaller than normal. Arterial wall thickness is usually less than normal, and tensile strength is diminished. Fibroblastic cells in dermis frequently have marked dilatation of the rough endoplasmic reticulum as a result of defective secretion of type III procollagen. There are no specific pathologic features of the other types of EDS.

CLINICAL MANIFESTATIONS. The clinical manifestations of each type of EDS are different (Table 188–1); it is important to identify patients with EDS type IV because of the grave consequences of the disease and to identify those with EDS types VI, V, and IX because of the risk of recurrence in their families.

EDS types I and II are characterized by marked joint laxity; soft, velvety, and hyperextensible skin; easy bruising; and "cigarette-paper" scars in areas of trauma. They differ in severity. Prematurity is common in EDS type I but rare in EDS type II. The major complications of both are recurrent joint dislocations, skin fragility, and early-onset osteoarthritis. The manifestations of joint laxity are more severe in childhood and decrease following puberty. At present the diagnosis depends on recognition of the appropriate clinical findings; electron microscopic studies of dermis may be confirmatory but are not specific. Patients with EDS type III are commonly seen by rheumatologists because of the joint discomfort and early onset of degenerative joint disease.

EDS type IV, the most severe form, usually results from dominant mutations in the genes of type III collagen; autosomal recessive inheritance has been described but is very rare. The diagnosis is confirmed by finding decreased amounts of type III collagen in skin, by identifying a defect in the structure, synthesis, or secretion of type III procollagen by cultured dermal fibroblasts, or by identifying a defect in gene structure. In the newborn

TABLE 188–1. CLINICAL FEATURES, MODE OF INHERITANCE, AND BIOCHEMICAL DISORDERS OF THE EHLERS-DANLOS SYNDROME

Type	Clinical Features	Inheritance*	Biochemical Disorders
I. Gravis	Soft, velvety, hyperextensible skin; easy bruising; "cigarette-paper" scars; hypermobile joints; varicose veins; prematurity	AD	Not known
II. Mitis	Similar to type I, but less severe	AD	Not known
III. Familial hypermobility	Soft skin, no scarring, marked large and small joint hypermobility	AD	Not known
IV. Arterial	Thin, translucent skin with visible veins; marked bruising; skin and joints have normal extensibility; arterial, bowel, and uterine rupture	AD (AR)	Abnormal type III collagen synthesis, secretion, or structure
V. X linked	Similar to type II	XLR	Not known
VI. Ocular	Soft, velvety, hyperextensible skin; hypermobile joints, scoliosis; ocular fragility and keratoconus	AR	Lysyl hydroxylase deficiency
VII. Arthrochalasis multiplex congenita	Congenital hip dislocation, joint hypermobility; soft skin with normal scarring	AD	Abnormal structure of the amino-terminal cleavage site in proα1(I) and proα2(I)
VIII. Periodontal	Generalized periodontitis; skin similar to type II	AD	Not known
IX. Cutis laxa, bladder diverticula	Soft, extensible, lax skin; bladder diverticula and rupture; short arms, limited pronation and supination; broad clavicles; occipital horns	XLR	Abnormal copper utilization with defect in lysyl oxidase
X. Fibronectin defect	Similar to type II	AR	Defect in fibronectin

* AD = Autosomal dominant; AR = autosomal ressessive; XLR = X-linked recessive.

period some infants already have bruising, but most affected infants are difficult to identify. By adolescence the veins are readily visible on the trunk and extremities, and bruising is common. Vascular or bowel rupture is rare during childhood. Arterial fragility may manifest as sudden death, stroke, shock from retroperitoneal or intra-abdominal bleeding, or compartmental syndromes, depending on the site of vessel rupture. Prompt surgical intervention may be lifesaving, although tissue friability may make repairs difficult. Pregnancy may be complicated by arterial or uterine rupture, either of which is often fatal. Recurrent abdominal pain may result from repeated mural hemorrhage in the small intestine. Sigmoid rupture is common. Survival beyond the fifth decade is rare.

EDS type VI is an autosomal recessive disorder characterized by a marfanoid habitus, skin and joint findings similar to those in EDS type II, ocular fragility, and scoliosis. The diagnosis is made by finding decreased amounts of hydroxylysine in skin and confirmed by low levels of lysyl hydroxylase measured in cultured dermal fibroblasts. Late complications may include vascular rupture, as well as blindness from retinal detachment or globe rupture.

EDS type VII is often detected in the newborn period, because of bilateral congenital hip dislocation and marked joint laxity. The hips are often difficult to stabilize, and recurrent dislocation may continue at the hips and other joints. When suspected clinically the diagnosis can be confirmed in some patients by identifying intermediates in the conversion of type I procollagen to collagen in skin and confirming the defect in cultured dermal fibroblasts. The most common defect recognized is an abnormal structure of the proα2(I) chain caused by exon 6 skipping.

EDS type VIII is characterized by the combination of noninflammatory gingival loss (often leading to loss of teeth) and the cutaneous and joint signs of the EDS type II phenotype.

EDS type IX is noted in childhood with skin hyperextensibility and laxity, drooping facies, and minor skeletal anomalies. Evidence of bladder dysfunction may be present by the age of 6 years, and diverticula of the bladder and hydronephrosis may occur. Mild chronic diarrhea, orthostatic hypotension, short upper arms with limited pronation and supination, and the occipital inferior horns become apparent during adolescence. Intelligence is usually in the normal range; inheritance is X-linked recessive. The diagnosis is made by the low serum copper and ceruloplasmin levels and confirmed by low lysyl oxidase levels in cultured dermal fibroblasts. Maintenance of normal urinary drainage is important to prevent renal failure, and continuing bladder drainage may be essential to prevent rupture. There is some variation in severity among families.

DIFFERENTIAL DIAGNOSIS. The differential diagnosis is generally limited to the varieties of EDS, although some patients with the Marfan syndrome have marked joint laxity and others with forms of osteogenesis imperfecta have joint laxity and easy bruising. Patients with EDS type IV and EDS types I and II are often investigated for a bleeding diathesis before the correct diagnosis is made. Because of joint instability and laxity many patients with EDS types I, II, III, VI, and VII are investigated for developmental delay before it is recognized that they have a form of EDS.

TREATMENT. The gaping skin wounds that occur in some forms of EDS should be approximated carefully, and the removable sutures should be left in place for twice the usual time. Recurrent dislocations can often be repaired surgically, although further recurrence is more common than in unaffected individuals. Arterial rupture in patients with EDS type IV needs to be treated surgically unless bleeding is controlled by compartmental limitation (e.g., some retroperitoneal bleeding). The repair of affected arteries is often difficult because of extreme friability. If colon rupture recurs, the colon should be excised to prevent further episodes. Rupture of the small bowel is very rare. Some patients with EDS type VI respond to ascorbic acid (1 to 4 grams per day) with some symptomatic improvement and increased excretion of hydroxylysine in the urine. There is no metabolic treatment for other forms of EDS, and management is largely symptomatic.

PROGNOSIS. The prognosis in EDS depends on the specific type with which the patient is affected. Life expectancy is considerably shortened in EDS type IV because of organ and vessel rupture and may be decreased in EDS type VI; in all others, life expectancy is normal. With the exception of EDS type VI, no specific therapy is available that affects the natural history of the condition.

Prevention by prenatal diagnosis is feasible for some types of EDS. Heterozygosity for the EDS type VI mutation has been recognized by examination of amniotic fluid cells in a family at risk for recurrence. The structural mutations in EDS type VII and in EDS type IV should be recognizable by studies of collagens synthesized by chorionic villus cells in culture, but this approach has not yet been used. Analysis of copper uptake and distribution by amniotic fluid cells should facilitate prenatal diagnosis of EDS type IX. All families should have genetic counseling once a proband is identified.

Byers PH, Holbrook KA: Molecular basis of clinical heterogeneity in the Ehlers-Danlos syndrome. Ann NY Acad Sci 460:298, 1985. *The most comprehensive and up-to-date review of the molecular lesions in EDS.*

McKusick VA: Heritable Disorders of Connective Tissue. 4th ed. St Louis, C. V. Mosby Company, 1972, pp 292–371. *Although the classification is not up to date, the richness of clinical detail is unsurpassed. A delight to read because of the many case histories and the personal touch.*

189 Osteogenesis Imperfecta

David W. Rowe

Osteogenesis imperfecta (OI) is a heritable disorder of connective tissue that results primarily in fragile bones that break with minimal trauma. The disease may be limited to a few fractures in childhood, result in 50 to 100 fractures by adulthood with severe long-bone and chest deformity, or cause death in the newborn. The prevalence is 5 per 100,000 live births, and there is no known racial or ethnic predilection. A sufficiently large number of patients with varying degrees of bone disease have been characterized at the molecular level to develop molecular and clinical correlations. Thus it is now possible to predict with some degree of confidence the relative severity of bone disease that will result from a specific mutation within the type I collagen genes. Not only is it important for the internist to be aware of the genetic basis of classic forms of OI (Table 189–1), it will also be prudent to recognize those individuals with unusual forms of osteoporosis or those with a striking family history of osteopenic bone disease as potential candidates for mild OI due to a recognizable mutation in type I collagen genes.

PATHOGENESIS. The tissues that are abnormal in OI are composed primarily of type I collagen. This collagen type has a triple-helical conformation formed by two genetically distinct but related polypeptide chains in a ratio of two α1(I) and one α2(I) chains. The mildest form of OI (type I) appears to result from underproduction of type I collagen caused by reduced accumulation of α1(I) collagen messenger RNA (mRNA) within the

TABLE 189–1. CLINICAL CLASSIFICATION OF OSTEOGENESIS IMPERFECTA

Type	Description	Inheritance	Suspected Mutation
I	Mild, nondeforming	AD	Deficient amounts of α1(I) mRNA
II	Lethal in the perinatal period	NDM, GM (AR)	Mutations within helical domain of the α1(I) gene
III	Severe long-bone deformity and scoliosis	NDM, GM (AR)	Mutations within helical domain of either the α1(I) or the α2(I) gene
IV	Severity is intermediate between I and III with long-bone deformity	AD	Mutation within helical domain of the α2(I) gene

AD = autosomal dominant; GM (AR) = germinal mosaicism, which can appear as an autosomal recessive; NDM = new dominant mutation.

cytoplasm. In the more severe forms of OI (types II, III, and IV), there are mutations within the helical regions of either the α1(I) or the α2(I) chain. These changes result from either a partial gene deletion or a nucleotide point mutation that alters an amino acid essential to the helical conformation of the α chains. Molecules containing a mutant α chain do not form normal triple-helical molecules. Furthermore, molecules containing a mutant chain interfere with the interactions of adjacent normal molecules, thus weakening the entire structure. Such a mechanism accounts for the dominant inheritance of the disease. The severity of the clinical defect is probably related to the qualitative nature of the mutation and the extent to which the abnormal chains accumulate within specific tissues. Still unanswered is why bone is more severely affected in OI than are other tissues equally rich in type I collagen. Animal models of spontaneous or transgenically induced OI may provide a better understanding of the pathogenesis of bone fragility.

TYPE AND CLINICAL MANIFESTATIONS. The terms OI tarda and OI congenita have been replaced by a classification scheme based on relatively distinct syndromes that reflect fundamentally different defects in type I collagen biosynthesis (Table 189–1). Type I OI is the mildest form and is associated with nondeforming fractures during childhood, which cease after puberty. Fractures can reappear with trauma and in postmenopausal women. In most cases a dominant family history can be elicited, with the associated features of blue sclerae, joint laxity, and thin skin, findings that are less obvious in older affected individuals. More variable are hearing abnormalities, short stature, and dentinogenesis imperfecta. Sporadic cases occur and presumably reflect a new mutation. Fractures heal normally, and osteopenia is appreciated only on quantitative bone densitometry. By contrast, the most severe form of OI (type II) results in infants who do not survive the newborn period. Their bones have a crumpled appearance on roentgenography and are so weak that dismemberment may occur. The disorder is usually acquired as a sporadic new mutation, but recurrences clearly occur secondary to germinal mosaicism of one parent. In OI types III and IV, there are severe deformities of the long bones, marked short stature, and moderate joint laxity. Gray sclerae, impaired hearing, and dentinogenesis imperfecta are frequently present. Fractures and deformity are usually present at birth. A spectrum of severity makes prediction of outcome shortly after birth hazardous. Scoliosis can progress to a point of causing restrictive lung disease, and severe long-bone deformity can preclude ambulation. However, infants born with identical deformities can eventually ambulate with the assistance of external bracing or internal fixation of the long bones. The more severe outcome is classified as type III OI, while the milder form is type IV. Patients with type IV constitute the most heterogeneous group, and any individual case may have features of either type I or type III. Both dominant and recessive modes (germinal mosaicism) of inheritance are observed.

DIAGNOSIS. The diagnosis of each form of OI is based on the history, physical examination, family pedigree, and radiographic features. Only the milder forms of this disease should pose a diagnostic problem with other disorders that cause minimal bone deformity or fractures and osteopenia. The bowing and fractures associated with osteomalacia or rickets are differentiated by roentgenography and the biochemical measures of calcium, phosphorus, parathyroid hormone, and vitamin D. Juvenile, disuse, and steroid-induced osteoporosis can be distinguished by history. Other rare diagnoses to be considered are infantile cortical hyperostosis (Caffey's disease) and hypophosphatasia. Studies of collagen synthesis and collagen mRNA in cultured fibroblasts, plus analysis of restriction fragment length polymorphisms for the type I collagen genes, are beginning to provide the means for a specific diagnosis of the various forms of the disease. However, most of these methods remain experimental. Prenatal diagnosis by ultrasonography continues to be the primary technique for diagnosis of the severer forms (type II and type III) of the disease.

TREATMENT. The use of supplemental calcium, vitamin D, fluoride, anabolic steroids, calcitonin, growth hormone, and pyrophosphate has not been shown to provide a satisfactory response. Since many of these drugs were used in heterogeneous groups of patients with OI, there may be subgroups of patients who could benefit from certain medical regimens. At present, therapy primarily involves orthopedic treatment with external bracing and surgical straightening with intramedullary splinting (rodding) of the long-bone deformities. Use of lightweight plastic bracing will assume a greater role in promoting ambulation. However, attempts to halt the progression of scoliosis in OI, as well as maintenance of good muscle tone and range of motion, are crucial to the optimal use of the extremities. Creative use of physical therapy, especially in the form of swimming, may be the most useful preventive measure in this disorder.

Akeson WH, Bornstein P, Glimcher MJ: Symposium on Heritable Disorders of Connective Tissue. St. Louis, C. V. Mosby Company, 1982. *See Ch. 20 to 23 for a general review of clinical and morphologic aspects of OI.*

Albright JA, Millar EA: Osteogenesis imperfecta. Clin Orthop 159:2, 1981. *A collection of numerous articles on the pathology and treatment of this disease. Unfortunately, treatment strategies have not improved since this article was published.*

Rowe DW, Shapiro JR: Osteogenesis imperfecta. In Avioli L, Krane S (eds.): Metabolic Bone Disease. 2nd ed. Philadelphia, W.B. Saunders Company, 1990. *Contains detailed discussion on the molecular basis of each clinical type of OI. For the latest update of known mutations, see Sykes B: Nature 348:18, 1990.*

Smith R, Francis MJO, Houghton GP: The Brittle Bone Syndrome. London, Butterworth Company, 1982. *A comprehensive clinical review by one group of investigators having a large experience with OI. Chapter 7 contains a thorough differential diagnosis.*

190 Pseudoxanthoma Elasticum

Jouni Uitto

Pseudoxanthoma elasticum (PXE) (synonyms: Grönblad-Strandberg syndrome, systemic elastorrhexis) is a generalized progressive connective tissue disorder primarily affecting the elastic fibers. Clinically, PXE manifests as characteristic cutaneous lesions, ocular changes, and widespread vascular abnormalities. The relative severity of these changes results in a variety of clinical pictures. The onset of the disease may be in early childhood, and in most cases the cutaneous changes are evident before the age of 30 years. The exact incidence of PXE is not known, although estimates are about 1 in 160,000 persons. The male-female ratio is probably 1:1.

CLINICAL MANIFESTATIONS. Skin. The primary cutaneous lesions are relatively small (1 to 3 mm) yellowish papules that give the affected area a pebbly, "plucked chicken skin" appearance. The primary lesions tend to coalesce into larger plaques, and the skin of the involved areas becomes thickened and leathery (Fig. 190–1). Gradually, the affected skin becomes redundant, lax, and inelastic. The predilection sites are the face, neck, axillary folds, lower abdomen, and thighs. The nasolabial folds and chin creases may be strikingly accentuated. Yellowish lesions similar to those noted on the skin can also be seen on the mucous membranes.

Eye. The ocular changes are characterized by angioid streaks, i.e., grayish or brownish-red, poorly defined streaks radiating across the fundus of the eye. Their development usually starts later than that of the cutaneous lesions, often during the third or fourth decade. The ocular changes are commonly bilateral and include hemorrhages and exudates in Bruch's membrane, an elastin-rich structure located between the retina and the choroid. The degenerative changes of the eye frequently lead to impaired vision, and complete blindness, although rare, is one of the major complications of PXE. Angioid streaks may be present without noticeable cutaneous changes, but other accompanying observations, such as vascular changes, may lead to correct diagnosis of PXE. Angioid streaks can also be associated with other diseases—for example, Paget's disease of bone, sickle cell anemia, tumoral calcinosis, lead poisoning, and idiopathic thrombocytopenia.

Vascular Manifestations. The early manifestations of arterial involvement include hypertension, weak peripheral pulses, and, occasionally, intermittent claudication. The most devastating complications develop as a result of coronary occlusion or cerebral

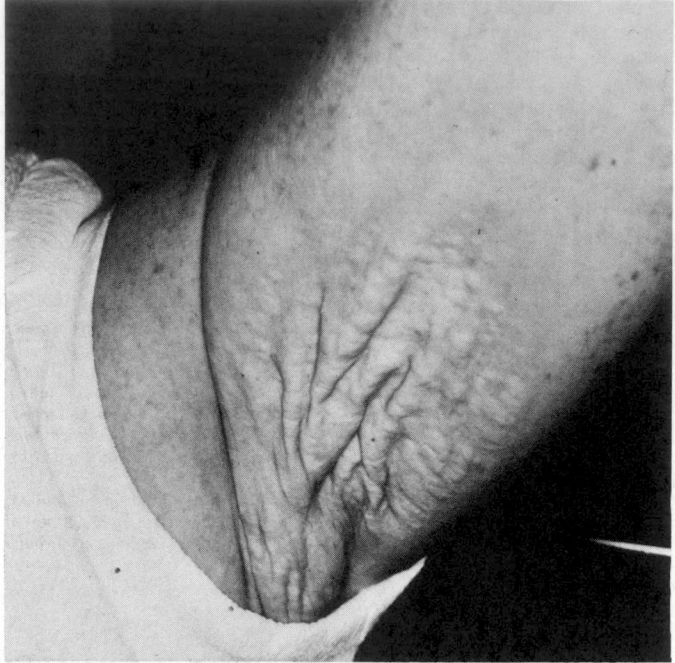

FIGURE 190–1. Typical cutaneous manifestations of pseudoxanthoma elasticum. The lesion demonstrates redundant and inelastic skin in the axillary fold.

hemorrhage; the most frequent complication is recurrent bleeding from the gastrointestinal tract. A common site of the gastrointestinal bleeding is the gastric mucosa, where the elastic fibers of the arteries are particularly affected. Bleeding from the urinary tract can also occur.

INHERITANCE. Most cases of PXE are inherited as an autosomal recessive disease. However, autosomal dominant inheritance has been documented in a few families, although delayed onset, incomplete expression, and lack of carrier detection complicate the genetic analysis.

In addition to the inherited forms, several cases with cutaneous findings consistent with PXE but without family history and without vascular or ocular involvement have been reported. In some of these cases, the development of skin lesions is related

to external trauma, such as exposure to Norwegian saltpeter. Patients with an unusual perforating variant of cutaneous PXE have been described. In these patients the lesions are confined to the abdomen, most often in a periumbilical distribution. Periumbilical perforating PXE appears to be a distinct acquired form of the disease.

PATHOLOGY. Histopathologic examination of the involved skin demonstrates an accumulation of structures in the middle or lower dermis that stain positively with stains specific for elastic fibers, e.g., Verhoeff's stain. In contrast to the elastic fibers in normal skin, the elastic material in PXE appears irregularly clumped and fragmented. The accumulation of elastic fibers has also been quantitated by computerized morphometric analyses and by assay of desmosine, an elastin-specific crosslink compound. Characteristically, the fragmented elastic fibers contain calcium that appears bluish on routine hematoxylin-eosin stain and that can be demonstrated by calcium-specific stains. Electron microscopy of affected skin demonstrates that the amorphous elastin component has been replaced by bundles of granular material with staining properties different from those of normal elastin. Also, foci containing calcium hydroxyapatite crystals can be detected in the elastic fibers. These morphologic findings thus provide evidence for derangement in the organization of the elastic structures in PXE. Biochemical proof of the exact molecular defect in the structure or metabolism of elastin is, however, lacking, and it is unclear whether the calcification of elastic fibers is a primary or secondary event.

THERAPY. No specific treatment is available, and the primary prevention entails genetic counseling. Although treatment with vitamin E, vitamin C, or a low-calcium diet has been advocated in isolated case reports, no clinical proof of the efficacy of any of these therapies is available in the form of controlled clinical trials. In selected cases, plastic surgery may be helpful in improving the cosmetic appearance of the skin.

Neldner KH: Pseudoxanthoma elasticum. Clin Dermatol 6:1, 1988. *Extremely useful clinical account of PXE, based on the author's data on 100 patients followed over a 10-year period.*

Neldner KH, Martinez-Hernandez A: Localized acquired cutaneous pseudoxanthoma elasticum. J Am Acad Dermatol 1:523, 1979. *Clinical description of a distinct acquired form of pseudoxanthoma elasticum.*

Uitto J: Elastic fibers in cutaneous diseases. Curr Concepts Skin Dis 6:19, 1985. *A review of the molecular defects of elastin in heritable connective tissue diseases, including pseudoxanthoma elasticum.*

Uitto J, Paul JL, Brockley K, et al.: Elastic fibers in human skin: Quantitation of elastic fibers by computerized digital image analyses and determination of elastin by a radioimmunoassay of desmosine. Lab Invest 49:499, 1983. *Demonstration of increased elastin concentrations in the lesional skin in pseudoxanthoma elasticum.*

DISORDERS OF PORPHYRINS OR METALS

191 The Porphyrias

Karl E. Anderson

The porphyrias result from deficiencies of specific enzymes of the heme biosynthetic pathway, are usually inherited, and may be associated with striking accumulations of heme pathway intermediates. Porphyrias are more prevalent, and more often manifested in adults, than are most well-characterized inborn errors of major metabolic pathways. Clinical expression is variable and is influenced by factors such as hormones, drugs, and nutrition that have regulatory effects on the heme biosynthetic pathway. Different types of mutations of structural genes for heme pathway enzymes have been found for several types of porphyria. How-

ever, genetic heterogeneity does not explain the variable clinical expression of these diseases.

Two major types of clinical manifestations are characteristic. First, cutaneous photosensitivity occurs in types of porphyria in which porphyrins accumulate. Tissue damage results from excitation of porphyrins by long-wave ultraviolet light. Second, neurologic effects occur in porphyrias characterized by accumulation of the porphyrin precursors δ-aminolevulinic acid (ALA) and porphobilinogen (PBG).

Because the porphyrias are uncommon and their symptoms are nonspecific, the diagnosis depends on a high index of suspicion. Confirmation by appropriate laboratory testing is essential. Porphyria must be differentiated from (1) "porphyrinuria," which can occur in various clinical conditions, and (2) minimal departures from reference ranges, both of which may have no clinical significance.

ENZYMES AND INTERMEDIATES OF THE HEME BIO-SYNTHETIC PATHWAY IN THE PORPHYRIAS.

A type of porphyria has been associated with a deficiency of seven of the eight enzymes of the heme biosynthetic pathway (see Fig. 191–1). Heme is synthesized from glycine and succinyl CoA. Intermediates in the pathway include ALA, an amino acid; PBG, a pyrrole; and hydroxymethylbilane, a linear tetrapyrrole that undergoes spontaneous closure to form uroporphyrinogen I, which is not metabolized beyond coproporphyrinogen I. Uroporphyrinogen III cosynthase catalyzes inversion of one of the pyrroles of hydroxymethylbilane and closure of the molecule to form a porphyrin macrocycle, uroporphyrinogen III. The next two enzymes result in decarboxylation of six of the eight side chains of uroporphyrinogen, with sequential formation of 7-, 6-, and 5-carboxylate porphyrinogens, coproporphyrinogen, 3-carboxylate porphyrinogen, and protoporphyrinogen. The final two enzymes catalyze oxidation of protoporphyrinogen IX to protoporphyrin IX and insertion of ferrous iron in the porphyrin macrocycle to form heme.

Heme is synthesized in largest amounts in bone marrow and liver, where it is used primarily to make hemoglobin and cytochrome P450, respectively. Hepatic heme biosynthesis is regulated primarily by ALA synthase, which is under sensitive feedback control by cellular free heme content. ALA synthase is induced by many of the same drugs and steroids that induce hepatic cytochrome P450. Additional pathway enzymes and cellular uptake of iron are important in the regulation of heme synthesis in erythroid cells. Intracellular concentrations of intermediates, which are generally less than the Michaelis constant (K_m) values for heme pathway enzymes, may greatly influence reaction rates.

Heme pathway intermediates are utilized efficiently and excreted only in small amounts. Normally, ALA and PBG are excreted in much larger amounts than are porphyrins. Porphyrinogens undergo auto-oxidation outside cells and are excreted primarily as porphyrins. ALA, PBG, uroporphyrin, and 7-, 6-, and 5-carboxylate porphyrins are excreted mostly in urine, coproporphyrin in urine and bile, and harderoporphyrin (3-carboxylate porphyrin) and protoporphyrin in bile and feces. ALA, PBG, and porphyrinogens are colorless and nonfluorescent. Porphyrins are reddish and fluoresce when exposed to long-wave ultraviolet light.

CLASSIFICATION. Traditionally, porphyrias have been divided into erythropoietic and hepatic types, based on whether the excess production of intermediates takes place primarily in bone marrow or liver (Table 191–1). Some porphyrias have both erythroid and hepatic features. Porphyrias with neurovisceral symptoms are also termed "acute porphyrias." They share many clinical features and are similarly managed. Several "cutaneous porphyrias" manifest similar skin lesions, but treatment and prognosis differ considerably. Now that these disorders are better characterized, they are best classified in terms of their specific enzyme deficiencies.

PORPHYRIA WITH ALA-DEHYDRATASE DEFICIENCY (ALA-D PORPHYRIA).

In this very rare autosomal recessive disorder, ALA dehydratase is markedly reduced (1 to 2 per cent of normal), and urinary excretion of ALA and coproporphyrin III is increased. In this and other disorders in which ALA accumulates, coproporphyrin III may originate from excess ALA by metabolism to coproporphyrinogen III in tissues other than that in which the excess ALA originates. Symptoms resemble those of acute intermittent porphyria but may begin in childhood. Hemolysis may be present.

Other Conditions Associated with ALA-Dehydratase Deficiency. Lead poisoning and hereditary tyrosinemia can cause increased ALA and symptoms, including abdominal pain, ileus, and motor neuropathy, that are strikingly similar to those of the acute porphyrias. Lead concentrates in erythroid cells and inhibits ALA dehydratase. It also inhibits ferrochelatase, leading to excess erythrocyte protoporphyrin (complexed with zinc). Urinary coproporphyrin is increased.

In hereditary tyrosinemia, a deficiency of fumarylacetoacetase causes accumulation of succinylacetone (2,3-dioxoheptanoic acid), a structural analogue of ALA and a potent inhibitor of ALA dehydratase. Other heavy metals or styrene exposure can also inhibit ALA dehydratase.

ACUTE INTERMITTENT PORPHYRIA (AIP).

This is an autosomal dominant disorder that results from an approximately 50 per cent deficiency of PBG deaminase (formerly known as uroporphyrinogen I synthase). The enzyme is deficient in all individuals who inherit the mutant gene and remains fairly constant over time. Most persons with PBG deaminase deficiency remain asymptomatic.

Prevalence. AIP can occur in all races. Its prevalence in most countries has not been precisely estimated but may be most common (perhaps 5 per 100,000) in northern European populations. Prevalence in a chronic psychiatric population in the United States was estimated to be 210 per 100,000.

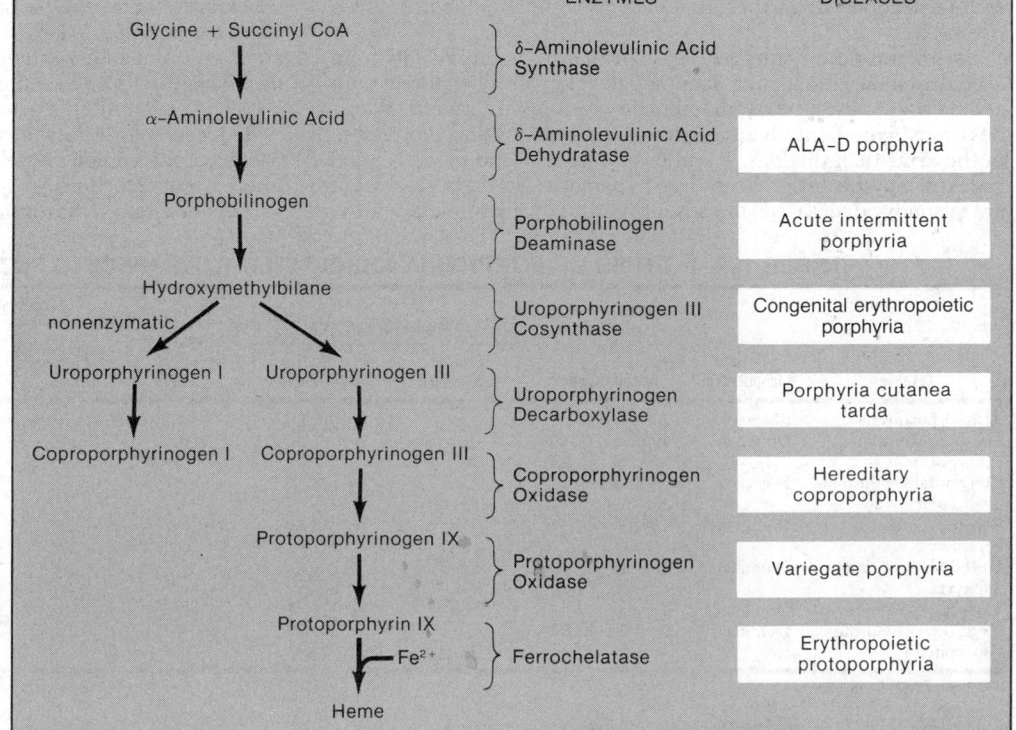

FIGURE 191–1. Intermediates and enzymes of the heme biosynthetic pathway, and diseases of porphyrin metabolism associated with deficiencies of specific enzymes. The initial and last three enzymes (in red) are mitochondrial, and the other four (in black) are cytosolic.

Etiology and Pathogenesis. In most patients with AIP, PBG deaminase is decreased in all tissues. However, the nature of the mutation at the PBG deaminase gene locus varies among AIP lineages. One type of mutation causes the enzyme to be deficient only in nonerythropoietic tissues.

Partial deficiency of PBG deaminase probably does not of itself greatly impair hepatic heme synthesis or induce ALA synthase. This fact is suggested by normal urinary ALA and PBG values and apparently normal cytochrome P450 content in most persons with clinically latent AIP. When the demand for hepatic heme is increased by drugs, hormones, or nutritional factors, induction of ALA synthase is accentuated by the presence of PBG deaminase deficiency. In clinically expressed AIP, hepatic cytochrome P450 may be reduced and can be restored by heme therapy.

Most drugs that are harmful in AIP induce hepatic ALA synthase and cytochrome P450. Sulfonamide antibiotics are not inducers and may inhibit PBG deaminase. Reduced caloric and carbohydrate intakes enhance induction of ALA synthase in animals and increase ALA and PBG levels and precipitate symptoms in AIP. Administration of carbohydrate can reduce hepatic ALA synthase and cytochrome P450.

The mechanism of neural damage in AIP is unknown, but porphyrias and related disorders associated with increased ALA have similar neurologic manifestations. ALA is structurally analogous to γ-aminobutyric acid (GABA) and can interact with GABA receptors. However, ALA and other products of the heme pathway have not been convincingly shown to be neurotoxic. The suggestion that heme deficiency may occur in nervous tissue in these disorders is also unproved.

Clinical Manifestations. Symptoms rarely occur before puberty and seldom, if ever, recur throughout adult life. Symptoms can begin after menopause. Characteristically, attacks last for several days or longer, often require hospitalization, and are followed by complete recovery. Abdominal pain is the most common symptom; it is usually steady and poorly localized but may be cramping. Other manifestations include nausea; vomiting; constipation; tachycardia; hypertension; mental symptoms; pain in the limbs, head, neck, or chest; muscle weakness; and sensory loss. Ileus, with distention and decreased bowel sounds, is common. However, increased bowel sounds and diarrhea may be present. Because the abdominal symptoms are neurologic rather than inflammatory, tenderness, fever, and leukocytosis are generally absent or mild. Tachycardia, hypertension, restlessness, fine tremors, and excess sweating may be due to sympathetic overactivity. Dysuria and bladder dysfunction may occur and require catheterization. Recurrent attacks tend to be similar in a given patient.

Peripheral neuropathy in AIP is primarily motor, results from axonal degeneration, and does not develop in all patients with acute attacks, even when abdominal symptoms are severe. Weakness most commonly begins in proximal muscles and more often in the arms than the legs. It can be asymmetric and focal. Tendon reflexes may be little affected or hyperactive in early stages but are usually decreased or absent with advanced neuropathy.

Cranial and sensory nerves can be affected. Progression to respiratory and bulbar paralysis and death seldom occurs unless porphyria is not recognized, harmful drugs are not discontinued, and appropriate treatment is not instituted. Sudden death, presumably the result of cardiac arrhythmia, may also occur.

The central nervous system can be involved. Anxiety, insomnia, depression, disorientation, hallucinations, and paranoia, which can be especially severe during acute attacks, may suggest a primary mental disorder or hysteria. Depression and other mental symptoms may be chronic. Seizures may occur as an acute neurologic manifestation of AIP itself or as a result of hyponatremia, or they can be due to causes unrelated to porphyria. Treatment of seizures is problematic because virtually all antiseizure drugs (except bromides) can exacerbate AIP. Hyponatremia may be due to hypothalamic involvement and inappropriate antidiuretic hormone (ADH) secretion or to vomiting, diarrhea, poor intake, or excessive renal sodium loss.

After several days, an attack may resolve quite rapidly; abdominal pain may disappear within a few hours and paresis within a few days. Even advanced neuropathy is potentially reversible. Repeated attacks may result in profound malnutrition.

Although liver function is generally well preserved, hepatic abnormalities may be more common in AIP than was previously recognized. AIP may predispose to chronic hypertension and may be associated with impaired renal function.

Precipitating Factors. Recognition of precipitating factors, which as a rule are multiple, is important in management. That endogenous steroid hormones are probably most important is indicated by the rarity of symptoms and excess ALA and PBG before puberty, more frequent clinical expression in women, premenstrual attacks in some women, and exacerbations after administration of sex steroid preparations. Progesterone and progesterone and androgen metabolites with a 5β-H configuration are potent inducers of hepatic ALA synthase. Cyclic attacks usually occur when progesterone levels are highest. Estrogens produce little or no induction of ALA synthase. However, administered estrogens may increase ALA and PBG excretion. Pregnancy is usually well tolerated. Attacks during pregnancy may result from hyperemesis gravidarum and reduced caloric intake.

Drugs remain important as causes of AIP attacks. Hormones and nutrition are often additive. Probably for this reason, (1) drugs may induce attacks in adults but are rarely reported to do so in children with PBG deaminase deficiency, (2) anticonvulsants do not induce attacks in some PBG deaminase–deficient subjects, and (3) barbiturate anesthetics more often exacerbate porphyria if symptoms were present before exposure to anesthetics. The major drugs known to be harmful or safe in the acute porphyrias are listed in Table 191–2. Barbiturates and sulfonamides are most notorious. Benzodiazepines are much less hazardous. There is insufficient published information to allow most drugs to be classified as definitely harmful or safe.

Reduced caloric intake, usually instituted in an effort to lose weight, is a common cause of attacks. They are also provoked by intercurrent infections, major surgery, and other conditions.

Diagnosis and Differential Diagnosis. The diagnosis of AIP is

TABLE 191–1. TYPES OF PORPHYRIA ASSOCIATED WITH SPECIFIC ENZYME DEFICIENCIES

Disease	Autosomal Inheritance	Classification	Presenting Symptoms		Excess Accumulations and Excretions				
			Photo-sensitivity	Neurologic	δ-Amino-levulinic Acid	Porpho-bilinogen	Uro-porphyrin	Copro-porphyrin	Proto-porphyrin
ALA-D porphyria	Recessive	—	–	+	+	–	–	+	+
Acute intermittent porphyria	Dominant	Hepatic	–	+	+	+	+	±	–
Congenital erythropoietic porphyria	Recessive	Erythropoietic	+	–	–	–	+*	+*	±
Porphyria cutanea tarda	Dominant†	Hepatic	+	–	–	–	+‡	+‡	–
Hereditary coproporphyria	Dominant†	Hepatic	+	+	+	+	±	+	–
Variegate porphyria	Dominant†	Hepatic	+	+	+	+	±	+	+
Erythropoietic protoporphyria	Dominant	Erythropoietic	+	–	–	–	–	–	+

*Mostly type I isomers.
†Homozygous forms of these disorders also occur.
‡Accompanied by 7-, 6-, and 5-carboxylate porphyrins and isocoproporphyrins.

TABLE 191–2. SOME SAFE AND UNSAFE DRUGS IN THE ACUTE PORPHYRIAS

Unsafe

Barbiturates	Succinimides
Sulfonamide antibiotics	Carbamazepine
Meprobamate	Valproic acid
Glutethimide	Pyrazolones
Methyprylon	Griseofulvin
Ethchlorvynol	Ergots
Phenytoin	Danazol
Mephenytoin	Alcohol
Chlorpropamide	Estrogens and progestins

Safe

Narcotic analgesics	Digoxin
Aspirin	Bromides
Acetaminophen	Insulin
Phenothiazines	Atropine
Penicillin and derivatives	Diazepam (small doses)
Streptomycin	Dicumarol
Glucocorticoids	Diphenhydramine
Propranolol	Ether
Guanethidine	Nitrous oxide
Neostigmine	Thiazides
Succinylcholine	Heparin

often delayed because symptoms are nonspecific and physical findings minimal. A high index of suspicion and demonstration of a marked increase in PBG are required. Assays for PBG employ Ehrlich's aldehyde (*p*-dimethylaminobenzaldehyde), which forms reddish-purple chromagens with PBG, urobilinogen, and other substances in urine. The Watson-Schwartz test is still widely used to screen for increased PBG but is subject to misinterpretation and false-positive reports, does not quantify PBG, and is less sensitive and only slightly more rapid than quantitative methods such as that Mauzerall and Granick described in 1956. Therefore, qualitative tests for PBG are not recommended. If used for screening, positive samples should be retested by a quantitative method. During an acute attack, PBG excretion generally is in the range of 50 to 200 mg per day (reference range, 0 to 4 mg per day), and ALA excretion is 20 to 100 mg per day (reference range, 0 to 7 mg per day). Such increases virtually assure a diagnosis of AIP, variegate porphyria (VP), or hereditary coproporphyria (HCP).

It is useful to follow ALA and PBG excretion because these values generally decrease with clinical improvement. Such reductions are particularly dramatic after heme therapy. After an attack, it is distinctly unusual for ALA and PBG to decrease to normal levels, except after prolonged periods of latency. In HCP and VP, excretion of ALA and PBG may decrease to normal levels more readily. Fecal porphyrins are usually normal or minimally increased, which distinguishes AIP from HCP and VP.

Decreased levels of PBG deaminase (most conveniently measured in erythrocytes) confirm the diagnosis of AIP. However, in some AIP lineages, the enzyme is deficient only in nonerythropoietic tissues. A wide normal range (up to threefold, which somewhat overlaps the AIP range) and increases in hemolytic disorders also impair interpretation of erythrocyte PBG deaminase results. Measurement of erythrocyte PBG deaminase is highly useful for analyzing pedigrees of known patients with AIP, but not for screening individual acutely ill patients. When family members are screened, the urinary PBG level should also be measured.

No single laboratory test fully excludes AIP, HCP, and VP. However, a normal result of a quantitative test for urinary PBG virtually excludes these disorders as a cause of current symptoms. Efforts to provoke increases in ALA and PBG for diagnostic purposes by glycine loading or administration of phenobarbital or estrogen may be dangerous and are not definitive.

Treatment. Acute attacks usually require hospitalization for treatment of severe pain, nausea, and vomiting and for administration of intravenous glucose and heme. Hospitalization also facilitates observation for neurologic complications, electrolyte imbalances, and nutritional status and investigation of precipitating factors. Narcotic analgesics are usually required for abdominal pain and small to moderate doses of a phenothiazine for nausea, vomiting, anxiety, and restlessness. Chloral hydrate can be employed for insomnia. Diazepam in low doses is probably safe if a minor tranquilizer is required.

Carbohydrate can be given orally as sucrose, glucose polymers, or carbohydrate-rich foods. If oral intake is poorly tolerated or is contraindicated by distention and ileus, intravenous administration of glucose (at least 300 grams daily) is usually indicated. A central venous line facilitates more complete parenteral nutrition support and helps avoid excess fluid volumes.

Heme therapy is more effective than glucose in reducing ALA and PBG. Although glucose infusions may be employed first, heme therapy should probably be initiated early. Its effectiveness is reduced when treatment is delayed. A lyophilized hematin (hydroxy-heme) preparation is available in the United States. It is reconstituted with sterile water but is unstable and must be infused promptly. The usual recommended dosage is 3 to 4 mg per kilogram of body weight infused intravenously once or twice daily, but lower dosages (e.g., 1 to 1.5 mg per kilogram once daily) may be equally effective. More stable preparations of heme (heme arginate and heme albumin) are available in Europe. Heme therapy should be instituted only after the diagnosis of a porphyric attack is confirmed at least by a markedly increased urinary PBG value. Diagnosis is more difficult after heme administration, which can at least transiently normalize porphyrin precursor excretion.

Response to heme therapy depends on the degree of neuronal damage and may not be observed for at least 48 hours. Severe neurologic damage and subacute or chronic symptoms are unlikely to respond. Excessive dosages of hematin may induce acute renal tubular damage. Recommended doses of hematin commonly cause phlebitis at the site of infusion and a transient anticoagulant effect. Heme arginate seldom has these effects.

β-Adrenergic blocking agents may control tachycardia and hypertension in acute attacks of porphyria and are considered by some to hasten recovery. However, these agents may be hazardous in patients with hypovolemia, in whom increased catecholamine secretion may be an important compensatory mechanism. Many other therapies have been tried in this disease, without consistent success.

Treatment is facilitated by identifying and removing inciting factors, such as harmful drugs, and by nutritional restitution. Symptoms during the luteal phase of the menstrual cycle usually resolve with the onset of menses.

Prognosis. The outlook for persons with latent AIP is excellent and is further improved when precautions are taken to avoid attacks. Recurrent attacks of porphyria can be disabling but do not occur throughout adult life and during the past decade have only rarely been fatal. Most patients do well after the diagnosis is established and harmful factors are avoided.

Prevention. The diagnosis of AIP in utero is possible but is seldom indicated in view of the favorable outlook for most PBG deaminase–deficient patients. Although subjects with latent AIP are less sensitive to inducing factors than are patients with prior porphyric symptoms, they are advised to take similar precautions. Latent AIP should never be construed as a health risk that limits availability of health insurance.

Some specific measures help prevent the clinical expression of AIP:

1. Family members should be screened to detect latent cases.
2. Harmful drugs should be avoided.
3. "Crash diets" for weight reduction and even brief periods of starvation (e.g., during postoperative periods or intercurrent illnesses) should be avoided. Regimens for obesity should provide for gradual weight loss during periods of clinical remission of porphyria.
4. Investigational approaches for preventing frequent (especially cyclic) attacks include administration of gonadotropin-releasing hormone analogues or periodic heme infusions. Oophorectomy is an unacceptable option.

CONGENITAL ERYTHROPOIETIC PORPHYRIA (CEP).

This is an autosomal recessive disorder that is caused by a deficiency of uroporphyrinogen III cosynthase, and only about 100 cases have been reported. CEP occurs in several animal species (including all fox squirrels).

Etiology and Pathogenesis. An approximately two-thirds reduction in uroporphyrinogen III cosynthase (intermediate reductions occur in heterozygotes) is found in erythrocytes and other tissues of patients with CEP. Type I porphyrin isomers are produced in greatest excess. Bone marrow production and excretion of type III isomers and formation of heme are also increased, reflecting a hemolytic state. Excess formation of uroporphyrinogen III and heme occurs at the expense of a considerable accumulation in bone marrow of hydroxymethylbilane, which is converted nonenzymatically to uroporphyrinogen I.

Hemolysis varies in degree and is an important influence on disease severity. Excess porphyrins in circulating erythrocytes may predispose to hemolysis. Erythroid cells in marrow are also destroyed and release porphyrins. Splenomegaly, which may be a response to the increased uptake of abnormal erythrocytes, can contribute to anemia and cause leukopenia and thrombocytopenia. Sunlight, other sources of ultraviolet light, and minor trauma to friable skin are other determinants of clinical expression. Drugs, steroids, and nutrition have little influence.

Clinical Manifestations. Reddish urine and severe cutaneous photosensitivity generally are noted in early infancy. However, the clinical expression is variable, and in at least five cases symptoms began in adult life. Bullae and vesicles on sun-exposed skin are prone to rupture and become infected. Areas of skin may be thickened, hypopigmented, or hyperpigmented and may manifest hypertrichosis. Loss of digits and facial features and corneal scarring can be severe. Porphyrins are deposited in the teeth (producing a reddish-brown color termed "erythrodontia") and in bone. Bone demineralization can be substantial. There are no neurologic manifestations. Hemolysis and splenomegaly are almost always present. Life expectancy is often shortened by infections or hematologic complications.

Diagnosis and Differential Diagnosis. Porphyrin excretion and concentrations in red cells and plasma are generally much greater in CEP than in other forms of porphyria. Porphyrins in urine are primarily uroporphyrin and coproporphyrin and in feces are mostly coproporphyrin. ALA and PBG values are normal. In most cases, uroporphyrin I predominates in erythrocytes. A predominance of protoporphyrin in red cells has been described in some cases of CEP and is characteristic of bovine CEP. Stimulation of erythropoiesis increases uroporphyrin and coproporphyrin. CEP is readily distinguished from erythropoietic protoporphyria (EPP) (see further on). *Hepatoerythropoietic porphyria* (homozygous familial porphyria cutanea tarda [PCT]) is clinically similar to CEP but is distinguished by excess isocoproporphyrin in feces and urine and decreased uroporphyrinogen decarboxylase activity in erythrocytes. Very rare homozygous cases of variegate porphyria and hereditary coproporphyria may also be characterized by photosensitivity in childhood and increased erythrocyte porphyrin levels.

Treatment and Prevention. Protection of the skin from sunlight and minor trauma and prompt treatment of secondary bacterial infections help prevent scarring and mutilation. Blood transfusions sufficient to suppress erythropoiesis may be the most effective treatment. Improvement may occur after splenectomy. Oral charcoal may be helpful by increasing fecal excretion of porphyrins. Because homozygotes can be detected in utero, affected families have options for preventing genetic transmission.

PORPHYRIA CUTANEA TARDA (PCT). This is the most common of the porphyrias and is due to a deficiency of uroporphyrinogen decarboxylase in the liver.

Etiology and Pathogenesis. Several forms of this disease have been identified:

1. In the "sporadic" form (type I), which appears to include most adult cases of PCT, the enzyme is deficient in liver but not in erythrocytes and may represent an acquired form of PCT or an underlying genetic trait that remains to be identified.

2. In a familial form (termed type II), uroporphyrinogen decarboxylase is deficient in erythrocytes and other tissues in addition to the liver. This autosomal dominant disorder has a high degree of variation in clinical expression and often no family history of photosensitivity.

3. Recently, a type III has been described, in which the enzyme is deficient in liver but not other tissues, and the deficiency is clearly inherited. Types I to III are clinically similar and difficult to distinguish.

4. Hepatoerythropoietic porphyria, the homozygous form of familial PCT, resembles CEP clinically.

5. Examples of *toxic porphyria* have resembled PCT. Most notably, an extensive outbreak of porphyria occurred in eastern Turkey from 1955 to 1958 after seed wheat containing the fungicide hexachlorobenzene was used for food. Subsequently, hexachlorobenzene and several other chlorinated cyclic hydrocarbons, when administered to animals, caused decreased uroporphyrinogen decarboxylase (only in liver) and a pattern of excess porphyrins resembling that in PCT. Dichlorophenols and trichlorophenols and 2,3,7,8-tetrachlorodibenzo-*p*-dioxin (TCDD, dioxin) have been implicated in smaller outbreaks and single cases in humans. Patients with sporadic PCT seldom have a history of exposure to such chemicals.

6. A severe and intractable form of PCT occurs in some patients with advanced renal disease. Associations of PCT with systemic lupus erythematosus and the acquired immunodeficiency syndrome (AIDS) have also been described.

In liver, a massive accumulation of porphyrins, which may require many months, precedes the appearance of excess porphyrins in plasma and urine. Worsening of PCT by drugs (other than alcohol, estrogens, or iron) or other factors that induce heme synthesis is seldom reported. Hepatic ALA synthase may be little increased because amounts of porphyrins produced are small relative to rates of hepatic heme formation. By contrast, during attacks of the acute porphyrias, much larger amounts of intermediates are excreted (as porphyrin precursors) and ALA synthase is substantially induced.

Ferrous iron can inactivate normal uroporphyrinogen decarboxylase or the half-normal hepatic enzyme activity in familial PCT. Hepatic iron content is important in the clinical expression of PCT. Alcohol intake may promote iron absorption and stimulate hepatic heme and porphyrin synthesis. In some cases of PCT, a heterozygous state for hereditary hemochromatosis contributes to mild hepatic siderosis. Iron removal by therapeutic phlebotomy in PCT restores the enzyme after a prolonged remission, but not immediately.

The complex pattern of porphyrins in PCT is partly due to accumulation of type I and III isomers of uroporphyrin and the 7-, 6-, and 5-carboxylate porphyrins. In addition, 5-carboxylate porphyrinogen can be metabolized by coproporphyrinogen oxidase to a series of 4-carboxylate porphyrins termed isocoproporphyrins.

Biochemical findings in homozygous familial PCT are similar to those in adult heterozygous cases of PCT. Increased erythrocyte protoporphyrin in homozygotes may reflect an earlier accumulation of uroporphyrinogen, which, with cessation of hemoglobin synthesis, is metabolized to protoporphyrin. Similar explanations may account for increased erythrocyte protoporphyrin in other homozygous forms of porphyria.

Clinical Manifestations. PCT is most common in men but has become more frequent in women in association with alcohol and estrogen use. Cutaneous photosensitivity is the major clinical feature. Vesicles and bullae develop on the face, dorsa of the hands and feet, forearms, and legs. Sun-exposed skin also becomes friable. Minor trauma may precede the formation of bullae or cause denudation of the skin. Small white plaques ("milia") may precede or follow vesicle formation. Involved skin tends to heal slowly. Hypertrichosis and hyperpigmentation are sometimes present even in the absence of vesicles. Thickening, scarring, and calcification of affected skin ("pseudoscleroderma") may be striking. Neurologic effects are absent.

Porphyria cutanea tarda develops in some men treated with estrogens for prostate cancer and in some women treated with estrogens or oral contraceptives. Most patients with PCT have a history of moderate or heavy alcohol intake. Liver histopathology is usually nonspecific and not diagnostic of alcoholic liver disease. Cirrhosis and hepatocellular carcinomas are most common in older patients or at autopsy. Very rarely, hepatic tumors themselves contain and presumably produce excess porphyrins. Some of these cases have resembled PCT.

Diagnosis and Differential Diagnosis. Skin lesions in PCT, VP, and HCP are indistinguishable clinically and histologically, but it is important to differentiate these conditions before embarking on therapy. A predominance of uroporphyrin and 7-carboxylate porphyrin in urine and increased isocoproporphyrin in feces are diagnostic of PCT. In PCT, the urinary ALA level may be slightly increased; the PBG level is normal. Total fecal porphyrins are usually less increased in PCT than in other types of porphyria with photosensitivity. Plasma porphyrins are always increased in patients with porphyric skin lesions; their patterns can distinguish VP and EPP from PCT (see further on).

Treatment. PCT is the most readily treated form of porphyria. Patients are advised to discontinue alcohol, estrogens, iron supplements, or other contributing factors. Phlebotomies can gradually reduce hepatic iron stores and almost always produce remissions. Iron stores in PCT are seldom markedly increased and may be normal. Therefore, remission is sometimes achieved after only a few phlebotomies (an average of five to six in one series). About 500 ml of blood can be removed at intervals of 1 to 2 weeks, or longer as iron stores decrease. Ferritin and plasma or urinary porphyrin levels decrease before remission. These should be measured during a course of phlebotomies to avoid unnecessary depletion of iron stores and anemia. With remission, continued phlebotomies may not be needed even if ferritin levels later return to normal. Longstanding remissions may be achieved even after several relapses. Desferrioxamine may be effective in PCT but is much less efficient.

Courses of low-dose chloroquine (e.g., 125 mg twice weekly for several months, or as needed) or hydroxychloroquine are useful when repeated phlebotomies are contraindicated. Chloroquine concentrates in the liver, complexes to excess porphyrins, and promotes their removal. Chloroquine given in usual doses to patients with PCT may cause marked increases in photosensitivity and porphyrin excretion, as well as nausea, malaise, fever, and hepatocellular damage. Although these adverse effects are generally transient and are followed by complete remission, it is prudent to avoid them by using a low-dose regimen.

In patients with PCT and advanced renal disease, phlebotomy is usually contraindicated by anemia, and other treatments are not effective. Recent studies indicate that genetic recombinant erythropoietin can mobilize excess iron, support phlebotomy, and lead to remission of PCT; however, this treatment is still investigational.

HEREDITARY COPROPORPHYRIA (HCP) AND VARIE-GATE PORPHYRIA (VP). These acute porphyrias are due to approximately 50 per cent deficiencies of coproporphyrinogen oxidase and protoporphyrinogen oxidase, respectively, and are autosomal dominant conditions. Both are much less common than AIP in most countries. VP is quite prevalent in South Africa, where most cases have been traced to a couple who emigrated from Holland in the late 1600's.

Etiology and Pathogenesis. Excess ALA and PBG levels during acute attacks of HCP and VP reflect induction of hepatic ALA synthase and the relatively low normal activity of PBG deaminase. Loss of coproporphyrinogen from the liver occurs more readily than loss of other porphyrinogens, and loss is even greater when heme synthesis is stimulated. In VP, protoporphyrinogen accumulates and is auto-oxidized to protoporphyrin. A functional association between protoporphyrinogen oxidase and coproporphyrinogen oxidase in mitochondria may help explain excretion of coproporphyrin in VP.

In *harderoporphyria*, a variant of HCP, a structurally altered enzyme with reduced substrate affinity results in accumulation of harderoporphyrin as well as coproporphyrin. *Dual porphyria* refers to kindreds and individual double heterozygotes with both VP and familial PCT.

Clinical Manifestations. Drugs, steroids, and nutritional factors that are detrimental in AIP provoke exacerbations of HCP and VP. Neurologic manifestations are identical to those in AIP. Skin manifestations are similar to those of PCT and usually occur apart from the neurovisceral symptoms. Impaired biliary excretion by concurrent liver diseases or use of drugs such as contraceptive steroids can cause porphyrin retention and worsen photosensitivity.

Diagnosis and Differential Diagnosis. Urinary levels of ALA, PBG, and uroporphyrin are increased during acute attacks. With resolution of symptoms, these levels normalize more readily than in AIP. The urinary coproporphyrin value is markedly increased in both HCP and VP. A marked, isolated increase in fecal coproporphyrin level is distinctive for HCP. Fecal coproporphy-

rin and protoporphyrin values are about equally increased in VP. The fluorescence spectrum of plasma porphyrins (at neutral pH) is characteristic and very useful for rapidly distinguishing VP from the other porphyrias. A different spectrum distinguishes EPP.

Treatment and Prognosis. Acute attacks of VP are treated like those in AIP. Striking decreases in attacks and deaths from VP in South Africa are attributed to identification of latent cases, avoiding harmful drugs, and better treatment during acute attacks. Measures that protect the skin from sunlight are helpful for photosensitivity. Cholestyramine may decrease photosensitivity occurring with liver dysfunction. Phlebotomies and chloroquine are not effective.

ERYTHROPOIETIC PROTOPORPHYRIA. This is an autosomal dominant condition caused by a deficiency of ferrochelatase. Although EPP was not clearly described until 1961, it is now perhaps the second most common form of porphyria.

Etiology and Pathogenesis. Excess protoporphyrin is found in erythroid cells, plasma, bile, and feces of patients in whom EPP is clinically expressed. Ferrochelatase is probably deficient in all tissues in EPP but becomes rate limiting for protoporphyrin metabolism primarily in bone marrow. Some obligate carriers have little or no increase in red cell protoporphyrin. Increases in plasma and fecal protoporphyrin are also variable. Such variations in clinical expression are not well explained.

Bone marrow reticulocytes are the primary source of protoporphyrin in EPP. Circulating erythrocytes and the liver contribute smaller amounts. In EPP, protoporphyrin in erythrocytes is not complexed with zinc and, compared with zinc protoporphyrin (found in lead poisoning, iron deficiency, and homozygous forms of porphyria), diffuses more readily into plasma. Zinc protoporphyrin dissociates less readily from hemoglobin-binding sites and persists in the red cell as long as it circulates. Disposition of the excess protoporphyrin in EPP depends on hepatic uptake, biliary excretion, and degree of enterohepatic circulation and is impaired by liver damage.

Clinical Manifestations. Cutaneous manifestations in EPP, which usually begin in childhood, are distinct from those of other porphyrias. Burning, itching, erythema, and swelling can occur within minutes of sun exposure. Diffuse edema of sun-exposed areas may resemble angioneurotic edema. Other characteristic skin changes include lichenification, leathery pseudovesicles, labial grooving, and nail changes. Scarring is rarely severe or deforming. Vesicles, pigment changes, friability, and hirsutism are unusual. There is no fluorescence of the teeth, and neuropathic manifestations are absent. Drugs that exacerbate hepatic porphyrias are not known to worsen EPP, although they are generally avoided as a precaution.

Hemolysis is uncommon or very mild in uncomplicated cases. Erythropoiesis and iron metabolism are generally normal. Mild anemia with hypochromia and microcytosis is noted in some cases and is unexplained. Gallstones composed at least partly of protoporphyrin may develop.

Liver function is usually normal in patients with EPP. Liver disease develops in only a minority of cases but can progress rapidly to liver failure and death. Excess protoporphyrin itself may have cholestatic effects and damage hepatocytes. Intercurrent factors such as viral hepatitis, alcohol, iron deficiency, fasting, and oral contraceptive steroids have sometimes contributed.

Diagnosis and Differential Diagnosis. Protoporphyrin is increased in bone marrow, circulating erythrocytes, plasma, bile, and feces. Urinary porphyrins and porphyrin precursors are at normal levels. Hepatic complications of EPP are often preceded by increasing levels of erythrocyte and plasma protoporphyrin, abnormal liver function findings, marked deposition of protoporphyrin in liver cells and bile canaliculi, and increased photosensitivity.

Treatment and Prognosis. β-Carotene has been developed and marketed primarily for treating EPP. Its clinical benefits have been substantiated in large series of patients. No side effects other than a mild and dose-related skin discoloration caused by carotenemia have been noted. Its mechanism of action may involve quenching of singlet oxygen or free radicals. Cholestyramine may reduce protoporphyrin levels by interrupting its enterohepatic circulation. Iron deficiency, caloric restriction, and drugs or hormone preparations that impair hepatic excretory function should be avoided.

Hepatic complications may resolve spontaneously if a reversible cause of liver dysfunction, such as viral hepatitis or alcohol, is contributing. Transfusions or intravenous hematin to suppress erythroid and hepatic protoporphyrin production, splenectomy, correction of iron deficiency, and cholestyramine or activated charcoal may be beneficial. Some patients have undergone liver transplantation. However, similar complications may develop in the transplanted liver.

Anderson KE: The porphyrias. In Williams WJ, Beutler E, Erslev AJ, et al. (eds.): Hematology. New York, McGraw-Hill, 1990, pp 722–742. One of several recent and detailed reviews on the genetic, biochemical, and clinical aspects of the porphyrias.

Anderson KE, Goeger DE, Carson RW, et al.: Erythropoietin for the treatment of porphyria cutanea tarda in a patient on long-term hemodialysis. N Engl J Med 322:315, 1990. Therapeutic approach to a previously intractable form of porphyria cutanea tarda.

Derooij F, Beaumont C, Wilson P, et al.: A point mutation G→A in exon-12 of the porphobilinogen deaminase gene results in exon skipping and is responsible for acute intermittent porphyria. Nucleic Acids Res 17:6637, 1989. Example of the recent advances in characterizing specific gene mutations in the porphyrias.

Held JL, Sassa S, Kappas A, et al.: Erythrocyte uroporphyrinogen decarboxylase activity in porphyria cutanea tarda—a study of 40 consecutive patients. J Invest Dermatol 93:332, 1989. Distinguishing types I to III of porphyria cutanea tarda in part by measuring erythrocyte uroporphyrinogen decarboxylase.

Mustajoki P, Tenhunen R, Pierach C, et al.: Heme in the treatment of porphyrias and hematological disorders. Semin Hematol 26:1, 1989. Review of heme therapy in the acute porphyrias.

Winkler MG, Anderson KE: Vampires, porphyria, and the media: The medicalization of a myth. Perspect Biol Med 33:598, 1990. How scientists and the media have distorted the image of a disease.

192 Wilson's Disease

Andrew Deiss

DEFINITION. Wilson's disease (hepatolenticular degeneration) is a hereditary disorder characterized by the accumulation of copper in the body, especially in the liver, brain, kidneys, and corneas. The excess copper leads to tissue injury and ultimately, if effective treatment is not instituted, to death.

ETIOLOGY AND PREVALENCE. Wilson's disease is inherited as an autosomal recessive trait. The gene responsible for the disturbance in copper metabolism is closely linked to the esterase D and retinoblastoma genes within chromosome 13q14–q21. The prevalence of the disease is approximately 30 per million.

PATHOGENESIS. Normally, loss of copper from the body occurs primarily through the bile. Much of biliary copper is secreted in a poorly absorbable form and thus is lost in the feces. Copper balance is normally maintained by this mechanism. In Wilson's disease biliary excretion of copper is impaired, and as a consequence total body copper is progressively increased. The specific nature of the metabolic abnormality that causes this defect is not known.

Positive copper balance begins in infancy in Wilson's disease and continues thereafter unless appropriate therapy is given. However, the distribution of copper changes as the disease progresses. Liver copper is actually greater in presymptomatic homozygotes than in symptomatic ones. Thus not only does net deposition of liver copper cease, but also a portion of previously deposited copper is lost from the liver and deposited elsewhere. This copper redistribution probably takes place when liver injury occurs. If this injury occurs abruptly in many hepatocytes, liver disease may be clinically manifested, and a large amount of copper may be released over a short period, creating the potential for acute erythrocyte injury and hemolytic anemia as well. However, if hepatocyte injury is more gradual, acute liver disease will not occur, and the patient will remain asymptomatic as the important site of copper deposition shifts to the brain. With the latter course, most patients present at a later time with neurologic or psychiatric symptoms, usually with clinically inapparent cirrhosis.

The serum concentration of the copper-containing protein ceruloplasmin is low in 95 per cent of patients with Wilson's disease. The hypoceruloplasminemia is probably due in part to a decrease in ceruloplasmin gene transcription, but it is not believed to play a pathogenetic role in the disease.

PATHOLOGY. The diagnosis cannot be made on the basis of histologic sections of the liver. Fatty change and glycogen-filled nuclei are present early, followed later by piecemeal necrosis, lymphocytic infiltration, erosion of limiting plates, parenchymal collapse, and fibrosis. Ultimately, these abnormalities evolve into postnecrotic cirrhosis. Stains for copper are unreliable, being negative most frequently during the early stages of the disease, when diagnostic help is most needed.

In the brain, abnormal astrocytes and neuronal necrosis are widely distributed, and there is atrophy or cavitation of the basal ganglia and occasionally the cerebral cortex.

CLINICAL MANIFESTATIONS. Wilson's disease is a disorder of young persons. Although the disease may occur at any time from the age of 5 years into the sixth decade, two thirds of patients seek medical attention between the ages of 8 and 20. The physician should suspect the disorder in young people with signs of chronic or recurrent hepatic dysfunction or with characteristic neurologic abnormalities.

The hepatic symptoms are quite diverse. Commonly, a brief illness characterized by malaise, anorexia, jaundice, and increased aminotransferases is mistaken for viral hepatitis. Similar episodes may recur at intervals of months or years, or a latent period may occur during which the patient is asymptomatic until neurologic symptoms begin. If clinically overt hepatocyte injury persists over a longer period, a syndrome resembling chronic active hepatitis results. Occasionally, liver injury occurs precipitously; without rapid institution of appropriate treatment, death is likely in these patients and the need for prompt diagnosis is urgent. More commonly, however, hepatocyte injury is gradual and is not accompanied by symptoms of liver disease; nevertheless, cirrhosis develops ultimately in all patients. This liver injury may not be recognized until neurologic disease is evaluated.

Episodes of hemolytic anemia occur when massive release of copper from the liver takes place. Thus hemolysis is usually accompanied by overt liver disease; it occurs regularly in patients with fulminant hepatic failure. Hemolysis usually lasts only a short period and disappears spontaneously.

The neurologic signs at onset may take a variety of forms. Patients may start with a slightly dystonic facies in which the upper lip is drawn tightly over the teeth. Shortly afterwards they develop awkward, dystonic postures in the upper extremities and often an unsteady gait. Once recognized by prior experience, these particular neurologic manifestations are seldom mistaken. In other patients, tremor may be the initial sign, often a characteristic "wing-beating" rhythmic oscillating tremor of the upper extremities that in severe cases gradually extends to the trunk. Frequently, loss of coordination of fine movements, such as those required for handwriting, is the earliest neurologic sign. As the disease progresses, patients may develop combinations of these abnormalities. Dysarthria, rigidity, drooling, and titubation are late features. Seizures are infrequent and sensory abnormalities absent. The Kayser-Fleischer (K-F) ring, described below, is definitively diagnostic in the neurologic variety and nearly so in the hepatic form of the disease.

Psychological symptoms of Wilson's disease are prominent and consist of early development of intellectual deterioration, personality changes, and unstable behavior. Children begin to fail at school, and young adults may show difficulty in performing jobs once considered routine. Schizophreniform symptoms and other forms of bizarre behavior may appear, but the mental status examination always shows signs of organic dementia. Effective removal of excess copper often improves but usually fails to eliminate these symptoms completely.

Kayser-Fleischer rings are golden brown or greenish rings or arcs in Descemet's membrane at the limbus of the cornea. They are composed of copper-containing granules and develop primarily after redistribution of liver copper. They may be visible with the unaided eye, but slit-lamp examination should always be performed. K-F rings are present in all or nearly all patients in the neurologic or psychiatric stage of the disease but are not present in about one third of those with hepatic symptoms.

Rare symptoms ascribable to Wilson's disease include cholelithiasis, sunflower cataracts, arthropathy, renal calculi, heart disease, and the Fanconi syndrome.

DIAGNOSIS. The classic diagnostic features of K-F rings, low serum ceruloplasmin concentration (<20 mg per deciliter), and increased amounts of liver and urinary copper (>250 μg per gram of dry weight and >100 μg per 24 hours, respectively) are present in nearly all patients with fully evolved neurologic Wilson's disease, but only in about two thirds of those presenting with liver disease. In these patients, K-F rings often have not yet formed, and the serum ceruloplasmin concentration may be difficult to interpret. Even in Wilson's disease, serum ceruloplasmin increases during inflammation, estrogen administration, and pregnancy and may decrease during liver failure. Measurement of the copper content of the liver should resolve the problem. Hepatic copper is often greater than normal (50 μg per gram of dry weight) in a variety of chronic liver diseases, but it seldom reaches the concentration seen in most patients with Wilson's disease (>250 μg per gram of dry weight). In a patient with a disease clinically suggestive of Wilson's disease, hepatic copper of this magnitude is essentially diagnostic. If the diagnosis is still in doubt, incorporation of radioactive copper into ceruloplasmin can be measured; incorporation is negligible in Wilson's disease, normal in other liver disease, even with copper loading, and intermediate in 75 per cent of heterozygotes. All measurements of copper metabolism should be entrusted only to laboratories experienced with their determination, and the normal values of that laboratory should be used.

In primary biliary cirrhosis and chronic cholestasis, diseases with acquired abnormalities of copper excretion, liver copper may be greatly increased and K-F rings occur rarely. The age, symptoms, and laboratory abnormalities of patients with these diseases help distinguish them from those with Wilson's disease.

Early during the hemolytic anemia the urinary copper excretion is very great. The Coombs test result is negative. When hemolysis and acute liver disease occur concurrently in a young person, Wilson's disease is the most probable cause.

Examination of all siblings of patients with Wilson's disease is mandatory to identify presymptomatic homozygotes. K-F rings are usually absent. Serum ceruloplasmin concentration is reduced in 95 per cent of homozygotes and 20 per cent of heterozygotes. If it is low, liver copper content should be measured. Hepatic copper is slightly increased in most heterozygotes. If the copper is greater than 250 μg per gram of dry weight, Wilson's disease is present, and it should be treated as in symptomatic patients. Heterozygotes never become symptomatic and should not be treated. Some homozygotes will be missed by this evaluation, so continued follow-up is necessary.

TREATMENT. Without effective lifetime therapy, Wilson's disease is inevitably fatal. If treatment is begun early enough, symptomatic recovery usually is complete, and a life of normal length and quality can be expected. If treatment is begun too late, death may not be prevented, or recovery will be only partial.

Effective therapy depends upon establishing negative copper balance, thereby preventing deposition of more copper and mobilizing for excretion excess copper already deposited. Three agents are available that seem to be equally efficacious.

D-Penicillamine remains the drug of choice, at least until there is substantially more experience with the other agents. The usual dosage is 1 gram per day, given in divided doses 1 hour before meals and at bedtime. Response typically is quite slow, occurring over months, but it may occur more rapidly. A year or more is often required to obtain maximum improvement. At least 10 per cent of patients experience a worsening of their neurologic symptoms during the first month or two of treatment, and this phenomenon should not suggest that the diagnosis is in error. Compliance and the effectiveness of therapy must be monitored at 1- to 2-month intervals for the first year and twice yearly thereafter; monitoring consists of measurements of urinary copper, serum ceruloplasmin, and serum nonceruloplasmin copper (total serum copper minus ceruloplasmin copper). Nonceruloplasmin copper should decrease early and ceruloplasmin more gradually if treatment is adequate. Urinary copper levels increase at once to 1 to 5 mg per 24 hours during the first few months and then gradually decline as the excess of copper decreases.

Toxic effects are frequent. Rash, fever, adenopathy, neutropenia, or thrombocytopenia often occurs during the first 2 weeks of treatment. In such circumstances, penicillamine should be discontinued; when the symptoms have cleared, prednisone should be begun at a dose of 40 mg per day and penicillamine resumed at 250 mg per day and gradually increased to full dose over a period of a few weeks. The steroids can then be tapered and stopped. Side effects that occur later after initiation of penicillamine administration include proteinuria, nephrotic syndrome, systemic lupus erythematosus, Goodpasture's syndrome, and a variety of chronic skin diseases. These side effects can often be reversed by temporarily stopping penicillamine and resuming it after the symptoms have abated, sometimes with the addition of steroids. Suspension of treatment should never be permitted for more than a few months.

If penicillamine toxicity is not manageable, either trientine (250 mg 1 hour before meals and at bedtime) or zinc (50 mg of elemental zinc 1 hour before meals, preferably as the acetate) is an effective alternative. Experience is not extensive with either, but side effects have been minimal.

Some patients, especially those with fulminant hepatic failure, are so severely ill that the benefits of medical treatment cannot occur rapidly enough to prevent death. In these patients, liver transplantation, if successful, is curative.

Brewer GJ, Yuzbasiyan-Gurken V, Young AB: Treatment of Wilson's disease. Semin Neurol 7:209, 1987. *A thorough discussion of the details of treatment.*

Cartwright GE: Diagnosis of treatable Wilson's disease. N Engl J Med 298:1347, 1978. *An excellent description of the protean and often confusing clinical presentations of Wilson's disease and a few illustrations of what happens when the diagnosis is missed.*

Scheinberg IH, Sternlieb I: Wilson's Disease. Philadelphia, W. B. Saunders Company, 1984. *The authoritative monograph based on the authors' vast experience with all aspects of Wilson's disease.*

Walshe JM: Diagnosis and treatment of presymptomatic Wilson's disease. Lancet 2:435, 1988. *Criteria for identifying asymptomatic homozygotes in families of patients with Wilson's disease. Liver biopsies should be obtained for confirmation as the author recommends, and therefore more frequently than he has actually done.*

193 Hemochromatosis (Iron Storage Disease)

Arno G. Motulsky

DEFINITION. The most frequent cause of iron overload in persons of European origin is a common genetic disorder known as hemochromatosis. Massive iron deposits may develop after years of increased iron absorption, and functional organ impairment ensues. Secondary hemochromatosis with parenchymal cell involvement also occurs in a variety of anemias associated with ineffective erythropoiesis, increased iron absorption and multiple transfusions—most commonly in homozygous β-thalassemia.

ETIOLOGY, GENETICS, AND PATHOGENESIS. "Idiopathic" hemochromatosis results from an autosomal recessive gene that causes increased iron absorption in the gut. The nature of the basic defect remains unknown. Over many years, the excess iron is deposited in parenchymal cells of the liver and other organs. Clinical signs and symptoms develop when total body iron stores have reached levels of 15 to 40 grams, compared with normal total iron stores of 0.2 to 2.0 grams.

The gene for hemochromatosis is located on the short arm of chromosome 6 and is linked to the human leukocyte antigen (HLA) locus. The hemochromatosis gene is physically close to the HLA-A allele of the HLA complex. Clinically useful DNA markers are not yet available. About 70 per cent of hemochromatosis patients carry the HLA-A$_3$ allele, compared with 25 to 30 per cent of the general population.

Recombination between the hemochromatosis gene and the HLA-A allele is very rare. Since these genes are separate, hemochromatosis is not likely to be a direct effect of HLA-A gene action. An increased frequency of HLA-B$_7$ and HLA-B$_{14}$ is also observed and is caused by "hitchhiking" of each of these determinants with the closely linked hemochromatosis gene (linkage disequilibrium). The development of hemochromatosis requires a "double dose" of the mutant gene, and affected patients are homozygotes. Among sibships that include at least one homozygote whose condition has been definitely diagnosed, additional homozygotes as well as heterozygote carriers can often be defined by HLA testing using the principles of genetic linkage. Thus, the HLA status of the affected patient who has inherited a hemochromatosis gene from each of his or her parents is determined (Fig. 193–1). Sibs with both HLA haplotypes identical to that of the affected patient carry the linked hemochromatosis allele on the maternal as well as the paternal chromosome 6. Such persons are homozygous, are at high risk to develop iron overload, or may already be affected. Sibs who share only one HLA haplotype are heterozygotes, and sibs who share none are normal, not having inherited any hemochromatosis gene. No tests to detect heterozygotes in the general population exist. Detection of homozygotes in the population at large must utilize measures of iron status such as transferrin saturation and serum ferritin levels. HLA testing is of no value for population screening, nor is it useful for diagnosis in the absence of family testing.

The actual amount of stored iron at a given time depends upon factors such as age, sex, iron content of food, caloric intake, degree of alcohol ingestion, and unknown factors such as allelic heterogeneity. The amount of iron absorbed in younger persons is not enough to produce organ damage. Males generally eat larger quantities of food than females and therefore absorb more iron. Females lose iron periodically during menstruation and occasionally during pregnancy. Therefore, while the prevalence of homozygotes for the hemochromatosis gene is identical in both sexes, *clinically* apparent hemochromatosis occurs at least 10 times more frequently in males. Excessive alcohol intake further contributes to liver damage, and many patients give a history of excessive alcohol intake. Alcohol may stimulate iron absorption, and certain alcoholic beverages such as red wines contain increased amounts of iron.

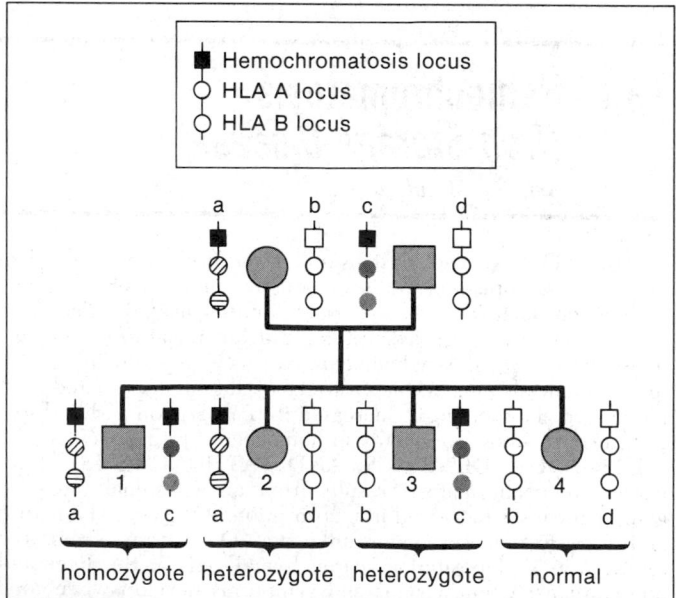

FIGURE 193–1. Hypothetical distribution of iron-loading alleles, each designated by an HLA haplotype, among family members of a patient (1) with fully developed idiopathic hemochromatosis. The "topographic" relationships between the gene (■) and the HLA loci (○) are diagrammatic approximations. The mother of the patient has two number 6 chromosomes, designated a and b, of which chromosome a carries the mutant allele of the hemochromatosis locus. In the father the mutant allele occurs on the sixth chromosome that is designated c. The patient inherited both mutant genes and is a homozygote. (From Bothwell TH, Charlton RW, Motulsky AG: Idiopathic hemochromatosis. *In* Stanbury JB, Wyngaarden JB, Fredrickson DS, et al. [eds.]: The Metabolic Basis of Inherited Disease. 5th ed. New York, McGraw-Hill Book Company, 1983.)

Excessive iron in various parenchymal organs is required before clinical manifestations develop. There is a fairly good correlation between the quantity of iron stored and the development of clinical signs and symptoms. Heterozygotes for the hemochromatosis gene may absorb somewhat increased amounts of iron, and minor, clinically benign iron overload may occur. However, test results of iron status in heterozygotes are closer to those found in normal individuals. It is conceivable that heterozygotes are at higher risk to develop iron overload under conditions in which normal persons would not be affected, as in porphyria cutanea tarda. However, iron overload in alcoholic liver disease appears *not* to be associated with the heterozygote state for hemochromatosis. Not all homozygotes develop clinical disease. In the fraction of those who do so, the development of disease depends upon the various circumstances affecting iron balance already discussed and upon unknown factors. It is clear that full-blown clinical findings are the "tip of the iceberg" and that many homozygotes have no symptoms or exhibit only mild, nonspecific findings.

PATHOLOGY. Although iron in reticuloendothelial cells is relatively harmless, parenchymal cell deposits are noxious. Iron in hemochromatosis is stored mostly in parenchymal cells as insoluble gold-brown aggregates known as hemosiderin. Normally, most iron is stored as ferritin, but with increasing iron overload the proportion of hemosiderin increases. With advancing hemosiderosis, fibrosis increases, and cirrhosis is frequent in fully developed cases.

Skin pigmentation is caused by epidermal melanin, while the slate-gray appearance is caused by hemosiderin. Pancreatic iron deposits are found in acinar cells and are not associated with clinically manifest exocrine deficiency. In the islets, B cells are selectively affected. Iron pigment is deposited in the sarcoplasm of cardiac myocytes and in synovial linings. The gonadotropic cells of the anterior pituitary gland may be heavily infiltrated with hemosiderin, leading to secondary testicular atrophy. Early cases exhibit significantly fewer pathologic findings.

PREVALENCE. Studies in Utah, Brittany (France), and Australia suggest homozygote frequencies varying between 1/200 and 1/600. This implies a high frequency of the heterozygote state for the disease, ranging from 8 to 13 per cent. The reasons for this high frequency are unknown. Hemochromatosis is one of the most common genetic diseases among Caucasoids. Since not all homozygotes develop typical findings, the frequency of the clinical disease is lower and was estimated to be roughly 1/5000 in the Pacific Northwest of the United States and 1/500 and 1/1000 in autopsy series in Scotland and southern Sweden, respectively. The frequency of hemochromatosis is much higher than usually suspected, since the majority of affected homozygotes do not exhibit classic symptoms.

CLINICAL MANIFESTATIONS IN THE FULL-BLOWN DISEASE. Because of the long time required to produce organ damage, the onset of clinical disease is usually, but not always, delayed to the age of 40 to 60. Males are more frequently and earlier affected than menstruating females. The most important clinical signs and symptoms in the fully developed disease include hepatomegaly, skin pigmentation, weakness and lethargy, chronic abdominal pain, diabetes, arthralgia, loss of libido, and impotence. However, more and more patients with few or no clinical findings are being discovered fortuitously.

Skin pigmentation is most pronounced in exposed areas and scars. With increasing hemosiderin deposits, the skin takes on a slate-gray appearance.

Hepatomegaly is the most common physical finding and may occur without symptoms and with normal liver function test results. Episodes of hepatic failure are rare but may be precipitated by blood loss or surgical procedures. *Splenomegaly* occurs. Chronic aching *abdominal pain* is common once cirrhosis has developed and may be the presenting symptom. Carcinoma of the liver is a relatively frequent late complication. Unfortunately, *once cirrhosis has developed, the risk of a malignant hepatoma appears undiminished by iron removal, emphasizing the importance of early case detection and initiation of iron-removing therapy* (see below). Other malignancies do not appear to occur more frequently. Atrial tachyarrhythmias and dilated cardiomyopathy with congestive heart failure are often observed.

Insulin-dependent diabetes is often seen. *Arthralgia* and *arthropathy* different from but often confused with rheumatoid arthritis or osteoarthritis are common. The second and third metacarpophalangeal joints are usually first involved. Knees, hips, shoulders, and lower back may be affected, and acute synovitis with pseudogout of the knees has been observed. Roentgenograms show chondrocalcinosis with small cysts characteristically affecting the second or third metacarpophalangeal joints. Osteoporosis is sometimes observed. *Loss of libido* and sexual impotence with testicular atrophy are common among men. Lethargy, increased sleep requirements, and inability to think clearly are frequent complaints. Infections with unusual organisms that grow better with excess iron may sometimes occur (*Yersinia enterocolitica, Pasteurella pseudotuberculosis,* and *Vibrio vulnificus*).

DIAGNOSIS. The clinical diagnosis of hemochromatosis requires a high index of suspicion and needs to be sought more frequently. Many patients are being detected fortuitously after discovery of abnormally saturated iron-binding capacity and high plasma ferritin levels. Iron overload should be considered among patients who present with any one or a combination of the following: hepatomegaly, weakness and lethargy, abnormal skin pigmentation, atypical arthritis, diabetes, impotence, unexplained chronic abdominal pain, or cardiomyopathy. Excessive alcohol intake increases the diagnostic probability. Diagnostic suspicions should be particularly high when the family history—particularly among sibs—is positive for clinical findings that might suggest hemochromatosis.

The diagnosis requires laboratory testing for iron overload. The most practical screening test is the determination of serum iron, of transferrin saturation, and of plasma ferritin. The serum iron value is elevated in patients with hemochromatosis, and there is increased iron saturation of transferrin, ranging between 60 and 100 per cent (normal is less than 50 per cent). However, abnormally high transferrin saturation can occur as a result of sample contamination, physiologic plasma iron fluctuation, iron therapy, liver disease, and red cell disorders. An abnormal value for transferrin saturation is seen early in the course of the disease and does not reflect the extent of iron storage. In contrast, a valuable noninvasive test to assess iron stores is the measurement of serum ferritin, which correlates reasonably well with the extent of iron storage in the absence of excessive alcohol consumption, inflammation, rheumatoid arthritis, neoplasia, and liver disease such as that induced by drugs or viral hepatitis. Without such complications, a level above 300 μg per liter in males and above 200 μg per liter in females suggests increased iron stores and requires further investigation. Ferritin levels ranging between 700 and several thousand micrograms per liter may be seen. The combination of testing for high transferrin saturation and for an elevated serum ferritin level gives the most reliable results. Rare families with significant iron overload and normal ferritin values have been described. Various imaging techniques such as hepatic computer tomography, magnetic resonance imaging, and magnetic susceptibility measurements promise to become useful for the assessment of hepatic iron stores.

Because of problems with specificity and sensitivity with all laboratory and imaging tests, and the absence of a test for the fundamental genetic defect, the "gold standard" test for hemochromatosis is a *liver biopsy.* Parenchymal hemosiderin deposits can be demonstrated histochemically, and the actual concentration of iron should be estimated biochemically. The extent of liver damage and cirrhosis will be apparent. Phlebotomies can be used as a therapeutic test to establish the diagnosis when a liver biopsy to assess the amount of iron biochemically is not available or not feasible. Weekly venesections of 500 ml (200 to 250 mg of Fe) deplete normal iron stores relatively rapidly. Patients with hemochromatosis require prolonged weekly venesections (2 to 3 years) until they are iron depleted (see below).

DIFFERENTIAL DIAGNOSIS. The most common differential diagnostic problem is raised by alcoholic liver disease not associated with HLA-linked hemochromatosis. Many such patients have an increased amount of stainable liver iron but no increased iron stores (usually less than 3 grams). Unlike genetic hemochromatosis, the iron in this disease is mostly located in reticuloendothelial cells. Liver function abnormalities are more severe than in hemochromatosis. Appropriate tests (including serum ferritin, liver biopsy, and sometimes a trial of phlebotomies—see above) can establish whether there is increased generalized iron storage. Iron overload due to chronic anemias (see below) rarely raises diagnostic problems.

FAMILY DETECTION FOR PREVENTION. Early treatment can remove increased iron stores that ultimately cause disease. Most important, treatment before the onset of cirrhosis appears to prevent the high frequency of hepatoma observed in hemochromatosis. All efforts should therefore be made to detect the disease *as early as possible.* Since the disease is an autosomal recessive trait, there is a 25 per cent chance that sibs of a patient are similarly affected. Testing for iron overload in sibs is therefore imperative. In addition, all family members should have a *single* determination of their HLA status to ascertain which sibs share all HLA determinants with the index case and therefore are homozygotes for the disease. If the characteristic abnormalities in iron metabolism are found, phlebotomies should be initiated after a liver biopsy has assessed the extent of iron storage. Sib testing should be begun at about puberty for males and after the age of 20 years for females. HLA-identical male sibs found to have a normal iron load should be restudied every 2 to 3 years, females somewhat less frequently. Frequent blood donations (three times a year) prevent potentially toxic iron accumulation and are recommended for HLA-identical sibs. Since the heterozygote frequency of hemochromatosis appears to be high among Causasians (~10 per cent), matings of homozygotes with heterozygote carriers are not uncommon, and one half of the offspring of such couples will be homozygotes (pseudodominant vertical transmission). Thus while parents and children of affected patients are usually obligate heterozygote carriers, some of these relatives may also be homozygotes. Family detection therefore should include the entire family.

Differentiation of heterozygotes from homozygotes with early disease may be difficult by serum ferritin and transferrin testing, since heterozygotes often have slightly abnormal values. Determination of HLA status may aid in such cases, since heterozygotes usually share only one-half their HLA haplotypes with their homozygote sibs. Treatment to remove iron is *not* required in heterozygotes.

TREATMENT. Excess iron can be removed by periodic venesections. The removal of one unit (approximately 500 ml) of blood depletes the body of 200 to 250 mg of iron. Weekly venesections are required for about 2 to 3 years to return iron stores to normal levels in patients with the full-blown disease and for lesser periods for those with early disease. Even though there is no medical contraindication to using blood from hemochromatic patients for blood transfusions, many blood banks discard such blood.

Phlebotomies should be monitored by frequent hematocrit determinations and plasma iron and ferritin levels 6 to 10 times per year (Fig. 193–2). After an initial fall, hematocrit levels stabilize at approximately 90 per cent of pretreatment levels. Indicators of iron status do not change until significant depletion of iron stores has occurred. After iron stores have been normalized as shown by ferritin and transferrin tests, venesections are required at 2- to 3-month intervals to prevent reaccumulation of iron. An iron-free diet is not necessary at any time during treatment. Treatment of hepatic, cardiac, endocrinologic, and metabolic complications is along conventional lines. Many manifestations of hemochromatosis *except* arthropathy, cirrhosis, and hepatoma are improved by phlebotomy therapy. Hypogonadism may also be irreversible, and diabetes may become milder but will not disappear.

PROGNOSIS. The 5-year survival rate after diagnosis in untreated patients with the fully developed disease was found to be 18 per cent and the 10-year survival rate, 6 per cent. The principal cause of death in such patients related to liver complications: hepatic failure and portal hypertension (30 per cent) and malignant hepatoma (30 per cent). An additional one third of patients died of cardiac failure.

Recently, 163 treated patients with relatively advanced signs and symptoms were studied in West Germany. There were 53 deaths. Cumulative survival was 92 per cent at 5 years, 76 per cent at 10 years, 59 per cent at 15 years, and 49 per cent at 20 years. Life expectancy was worse in patients who had cirrhosis or diabetes or who required more than 18 months of venesection for iron depletion. Death was due to cirrhosis in 25 per cent and to hepatoma in 25 per cent. By contrast, in *treated patients without cirrhosis, survival expectation was identical to that of*

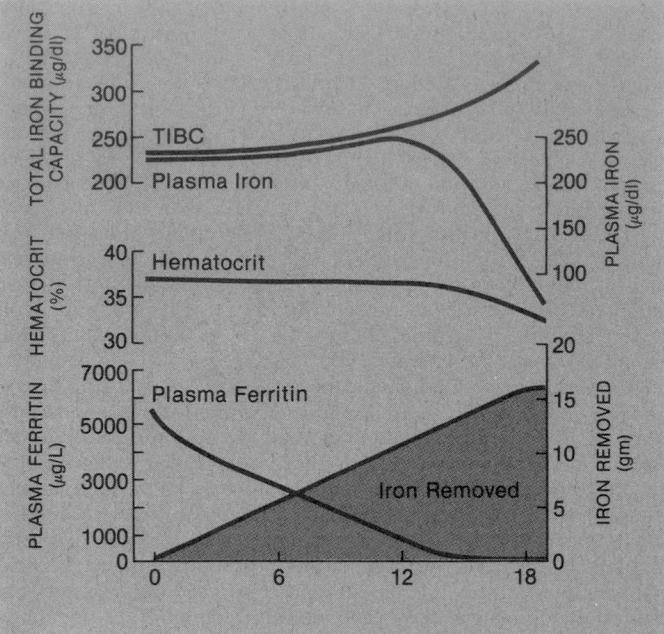

FIGURE 193–2. Serial changes in the hematocrit, plasma iron concentration, total iron-binding capacity, and plasma ferritin concentration in a subject with idiopathic hemochromatosis on repeated venesection therapy. (From Bothwell TH, Charlton RW, Cook JD, et al.: Idiopathic haemochromatosis. *In* Iron Metabolism in Man. Oxford, Blackwell Scientific Publications, 1979.)

the unaffected control population. It is noteworthy that hepatoma has never been reported in hemochromatosis without cirrhosis.

SECONDARY HEMOCHROMATOSIS. Excessive iron deposits in parenchymal cells can be observed in anemias associated with ineffective erythropoiesis, as in β-thalassemia major, in which severe iron loading already occurs before transfusion. Repeated transfusions produce further iron overload, and clinical symptoms of hemochromatosis occur early in life. Hepatic fibrosis is already common in children, as is retarded growth and delayed puberty. Cardiac death usually occurs in adolescence or early adulthood unless iron removal is carried out. Phlebotomies cannot be done, since these patients are severely anemic. Chelation therapy with desferrioxamine, together with frequent transfusions, has improved the prognosis markedly. Death due to complications of iron storage can be prevented if iron removal can be initiated before clinical signs and symptoms of iron overload appear.

Patients with hypoplastic anemias do not absorb increased amounts of iron but often require blood transfusions over prolonged periods. The transfused iron is largely stored in macrophages, and no clinical signs or symptoms are usually seen. Rarely, redistribution to parenchymal cells with development of hepatic cirrhosis or other typical organ involvement occurs.

Bothwell TH, Charlton RW, Motulsky AG: Hemochromatosis. *In* Scriver CR, Beaudet AL, Slye WS, et al. (eds.): The Metabolic Basis of Inherited Disease. 6th ed. New York, McGraw-Hill Book Company, 1989, pp 1433–1462. *A detailed discussion of all aspects of iron metabolism, genetics, and clinical findings in HLA-linked and secondary hemochromatosis.*

Edwards CQ, Griffen LM, Goldgar D, et al.: Prevalence of hemochromatosis among 11,065 presumably healthy blood donors. N Engl J Med 318:1355, 1988. *Attempts at screening for hemochromatosis in a general population.*

Fairbanks VG, Baldus WP: Hemochromatosis: The neglected diagnosis. Mayo Clin Proc 61:296, 1986. *A succinct summary of this underdiagnosed disease and practical advice regarding laboratory tests.*

Simon M, Fauchet R, LeGall JY, et al.: Immunogenetics of idiopathic hemochromatosis and secondary iron overload. *In* Immunogenetics of Endocrine Disorders. New York, Alan R. Liss, 1988. *Extensive discussion of iron overload with emphasis on HLA testing, but covering all aspects.*

Smith LH Jr: Overview of hemochromatosis. *In* Smith LH Jr (ed.): Cecil Textbook of Medicine. Update 1, pp 1–12. Philadelphia, W.B. Saunders Company, 1989. *An excellent referenced review of basic and clinical aspects of hemochromatosis.*

Strohmeyer G, Niederau C, Stremmel W: Survival and causes of death in hemochromatosis: Observations in 163 patients. Ann NY Acad Sci 526:245, 1988.

Recent data on natural history and survival of treated patients with fairly severe disease.

Weintraub LR, Edward CQ, Krikker M (eds.): Hemochromatosis. Proceedings of the First International Conference. Ann NY Acad Sci, Vol. 526, 1988. *The useful proceedings of an international conference on hemochromatosis that covered all basic and clinical aspects.*

194 Phosphorus Deficiency and Hypophosphatemia

Lloyd H. Smith, Jr.

Phosphorus is necessary for the structural and functional integrity of all living things. In hydroxyapatite it is a key constituent of bone; as a part of phospholipids (lecithin, sphingomyelin) it is necessary for the structure of all cell membranes, both external and internal (endoplasmic reticulum, lysosomes, nuclear membranes). It furnishes the backbone of nucleic acids, captures and stores metabolic energy ($\sim$P), serves as a second messenger in endocrinology (cyclic adenosine monophosphate [cAMP], cyclic guanosine monophosphate [cGMP]), regulates the release of O_2 by hemoglobin (2,3-diphosphoglycerate), and buffers urine. Even this partial list indicates that a severe deficiency of phosphorus would lead to widespread and serious consequences.

In an adult of average size there are approximately 700 to 800 grams (25 moles) of phosphorus, of which 80 to 85 per cent is in the skeleton and 10 per cent in muscle. Phosphate is the major anion of intracellular fluid (about 100 mM), where it is found mostly as phosphoproteins, phospholipids, or phosphosugars rather than as free orthophosphate. In extracellular fluid the normal concentration of phosphorus in adults is 2.7 to 4.5 mg per deciliter (0.9 to 1.5 mM), of which most is free; perhaps 10 per cent is protein bound. Serum phosphorus is normally higher in children (4.0 to 7.0 mg per deciliter). (It is conventional to express serum phosphate as the amount of elemental P, since pH influences the relative amounts of $H_2PO_4^-$ and HPO_4^- present.) The average American diet contains about 1000 mg of P, most of which is absorbed by active transport, increased by 1,25-dihydroxycholecalciferol. Approximately 90 per cent of that absorbed from the diet is excreted in the urine by a process involving filtration and partial renal tubular reabsorption. The tubular reabsorption of phosphate is diminished by parathyroid hormone (PTH), acting with cAMP as a second messenger. Through vitamin D, PTH, calcitonin, and the mineralization of osteoid, phosphate metabolism is closely linked with that of calcium. These interrelationships are discussed more completely in Ch. 232.

Hyperphosphatemia that is sustained occurs almost exclusively in three clinical conditions: (1) renal insufficiency (see Ch. 76), (2) hypoparathyroidism (including various types of pseudohypoparathyroidism) (see Ch. 235), and (3) acromegaly or gigantism (see Ch. 213). When severe, hyperphosphatemia may contribute to the acidosis of uremia, further reduce the extracellular fluid concentration of ionized calcium, or lead to metastatic calcification in extraosseous sites. Transient hyperphosphatemia may occur with acute tissue destruction, such as the tumor lysis syndrome or rhabdomyolysis.

CAUSES OF HYPOPHOSPHATEMIA. Hypophosphatemia (serum P < 2.7 mg per deciliter) may be associated with a normal total body phosphate (representing a transient intracellular shift) or with phosphate deficiency. The two most common causes of transient hypophosphatemia are (1) ingestion of carbohydrates, which deplete phosphate in extracellular fluid in the process of their intracellular transport and metabolism, and (2) acute respiratory alkalosis, which leads to an intracellular shift of phosphate through mechanisms not fully explained.

It is convenient to summarize the causes of hypophosphatemia as those that usually result in only moderate reductions in serum P (1.0 to 2.5 mg per deciliter) and those that may result in severe hypophosphatemia (P < 1.0 mg per deciliter) (Table 194–1).

Moderate hypophosphatemia may occur transiently during carbohydrate metabolism or alkalosis, as noted above, in the

TABLE 194–1. CAUSES OF HYPOPHOSPHATEMIA*

I. **Moderate hypophosphatemia (P 1.0 to 2.5 mg per deciliter)**
 Hyperparathyroidism—primary or secondary (in the absence of renal failure)
 Osteomalacia (usually with hyperparathyroidism), malabsorption, deficiency of vitamin D, familial hypophosphatemic rickets, vitamin D–dependent rickets, oncogenic rickets
 Carbohydrate administration or ingestion or enhanced metabolism—glucose, fructose, glycerol, lactate, insulin administration
 Hypomagnesemia
 Extracellular fluid (ECF) volume expansion
 Acute alkalosis—bicarbonate infusion or moderate hyperventilation
 Hemodialysis
II. **Severe hypophosphatemia (P less than 1.0 mg per deciliter)**
 Chronic alcoholism and alcoholic withdrawal
 Diabetic ketoacidosis, recovery phase
 Enteric phosphate binding—excessive use of agents binding phosphate in the gut
 Hyperalimentation
 Nutritional recovery syndrome
 Uptake by rapidly proliferating malignant tumors (rare)

*Modified from Knochel JP: Hypophosphatemia. West J Med 134:15, 1981.

absence of phosphate depletion. Increased PTH, associated with either primary or secondary hyperparathyroidism, reduces the renal tubular reabsorption of phosphate and leads to renal phosphate wasting. In familial hypophosphatemic rickets there may be a primary defect in the renal tubular reabsorption of phosphate. The association of hypophosphatemia with hyperparathyroidism and the various types of osteomalacia or rickets is discussed more fully in Ch. 234 and 235. In the various forms of the Fanconi syndrome, renal tubular dysfunction leads to phosphate wasting (Ch. 82). Hypomagnesemia and extracellular fluid volume expansion may result in reduced renal tubular reabsorption of phosphate and mild hypophosphatemia. Hemodialysis with equilibration against a dialysate deficient in phosphate may lead to overshoot hypophosphatemia. There are no well-defined acute metabolic consequences of moderate hypophosphatemia. Prolonged hypophosphatemia in this range may result in the defective mineralization of bone characteristic of osteomalacia or rickets.

Severe hypophosphatemia may cause serious metabolic consequences as described below. The most frequent cause of severe hypophosphatemia in clinical practice is *alcoholism*, especially during the withdrawal phase. The causes of phosphate depletion in alcoholics are complex and may include (1) poor dietary intake, (2) vomiting, (3) diarrhea, (4) the use of antacids that bind phosphate and reduce its absorption, (5) a possible phosphaturic effect of ethanol itself, (6) magnesium deficiency with phosphaturia, and (7) calcium deficiency with secondary hyperparathyroidism. The serum P level may be further reduced by the hyperventilation characteristic of alcohol withdrawal and by the therapeutic infusion of glucose. Patients with *uncontrolled diabetes mellitus* often become phosphate depleted through catabolism of intracellular organic phosphates and phosphaturia secondary to osmotic diuresis. Initial serum P levels are often normal or even high during diabetic ketoacidosis but rapidly fall to hypophosphatemic levels during the first 6 to 12 hours of treatment with volume expansion, glucose, and insulin. Hyperventilation with *marked respiratory alkalosis* can cause profound hypophosphatemia within minutes; metabolic alkalosis of the same degree causes only moderate hypophosphatemia. Excessive ingestion of *phosphate-binding antacids*, such as aluminum hydroxide, may inhibit phosphate absorption from the intestine sufficiently to cause chronic depletion, especially when combined with reduced dietary ingestion of phosphate. Excessive utilization of phosphate during tissue repletion may occasionally result in severe hypophosphatemia during *hyperalimentation* (without adequate supplementary P) and during the *nutritional recovery syndrome* of refeeding patients with protein-calorie malnutrition or starvation. Whatever its cause, severe hypophosphatemia requires early attention because of its potential consequences.

CONSEQUENCES OF SEVERE HYPOPHOSPHATEMIA

(Table 194–2). The long-term consequences of severe hypophosphatemia are largely structural, those of metabolic bone disease (see Ch. 234). The short-term consequences may be considered to be metabolic, although the distinction is an arbitrary one.

Red cell dysfunction in severe hypophosphatemia may result from two biochemical abnormalities, depletion of intracellular 2,3-diphosphoglycerate (2,3-DPG) and of adenosine triphosphate (ATP). Phosphate is a cofactor for glyceraldehyde-3-phosphate dehydrogenase, an enzyme in the pathway of the synthesis of 2,3-DPG. When intracellular erythrocytic phosphate decreases, a block in the glycolytic pathway results, with accumulation of triose phosphates and depletion of 2,3-DPG. This molecule normally exercises a unique allosteric effect on the dissociation curve of oxyhemoglobin, shifting it "to the right" and thereby enhancing the tissue availability of oxygen (see Ch. 136.2). Reduction of erythrocytic 2,3-DPG, conversely, impairs effective oxygen delivery to the periphery. The same block in the glycolytic pathway reduces ATP synthesis. The degradation of AMP to inosine 5'-phosphate (IMP) by AMP deaminase is enhanced when the restraining influence of phosphate is reduced, further depleting the intracellular concentration of adenine nucleotides. As a result, the concentration of erythrocytic ATP tends to fall in parallel with the reduction of serum phosphorus. At a critical level of ATP (usually with serum $P < 0.5$ mg per deciliter), the energy metabolism of the erythrocyte may become inadequate to maintain the integrity of its membrane, and *hemolysis* may occur.

Leukocyte dysfunction has been demonstrated during phosphate depletion in experimental animals, characterized by impaired chemotaxis, phagocytosis, and bactericidal function. These defects presumably result from inadequate ATP for normal cellular functions, possibly including the synthesis of phospholipids in membranes. Similarly, *platelet dysfunction* occurs in experimental phosphate depletion, but no hemorrhagic diathesis has been attributed to phosphate deficiency in humans.

Many patients with severe hypophosphatemia complain of *weakness*. This is often nonspecific and difficult to delineate from that caused by the associated disorder, but improved diaphragmatic contractility has been noted following the treatment of hypophosphatemia in patients with respiratory failure. *Rhabdomyolysis* is an occasional complication of severe hypophosphatemia, perhaps being somewhat analogous to hemolytic anemia in its pathogenesis, i.e., related to deficiency of ATP. The severity of rhabdomyolysis varies from that manifested solely by an elevated serum level of "muscle enzymes" (aldolase and creatine phosphokinase) to a full-fledged syndrome of muscle weakness, pain, tenderness, and stiffness associated with myoglobinuria. Interestingly, the release of phosphate from the necrosis of muscle may suffice to return the serum P level to normal. A few patients with severe phosphate depletion have exhibited congestive cardiomyopathy, which has seemed to respond to phosphate repletion. These clinical observations are strengthened by the demonstration of decreased myocardial contractility during experimental phosphate depletion in dogs.

Severe hypophosphatemia may result in *central nervous system dysfunction* with a constellation of symptoms and signs designated as metabolic brain disease or metabolic encephalopathy (see Ch. 443). These abnormalities may vary from irritability, weakness, and paresthesias to obtundation, seizures, and coma. It is presumed that this central nervous system dysfunction results from

TABLE 194–2. CONSEQUENCES OF SEVERE HYPOPHOSPHATEMIA

I. **Acute—"metabolic"**
 Hematologic
  Red cell dysfunction and hemolysis
  Leukocyte dysfunction
  Platelet dysfunction
 Muscle
  Weakness
  Rhabdomyolysis
  Myocardial dysfunction
 Central nervous system dysfunction
 Peripheral neuropathy
 Hepatic dysfunction

II. **Chronic—"structural"**
 Osteomalacia or rickets (Ch. 234)

deranged energy metabolism of the brain secondary to ATP depletion. Observations have suggested that hepatic function is further impaired in alcoholics with severe hypophosphatemia, with early improvement during replacement therapy, but a clinical entity of *hypophosphatemic hepatic dysfunction* has not yet been well established.

TREATMENT OF HYPOPHOSPHATEMIA. The treatment of hypophosphatemia depends upon its cause, its acuteness, and its severity. Hypophosphatemia caused by acute respiratory alkalosis or the infusion of carbohydrates does not require replacement therapy. Chronic hypophosphatemia associated with aluminum hydroxide therapy, for example, may require reduction of the antacid and an oral source of supplemental phosphate such as milk (1 gram of P or 30 to 35 mmol per quart) or a balanced solution of phosphate salts (sodium or potassium salts, as in Fleet enema solution or Neutra-Phos). It is rare that hypophosphatemia is so acute and severe as to require parenteral replacement therapy. When such treatment is undertaken, it is well to remember that (1) it is unusual for hypophosphatemia to cause metabolic disturbances at concentrations greater than 1.0 mg per deciliter, so full parenteral replacement is neither necessary nor desirable; and (2) if hyperphosphatemia results, there is a danger of producing a decrease in ionized calcium (with tetany or convulsions) and/or metastatic calcification of soft tissues. It is usually safe and sufficient to administer intravenously 1 mmol of phosphate per kilogram of body weight evenly over a 24-hour period in the treatment of acute, severe hypophosphatemia associated with phosphate depletion. Since potassium depletion is so frequently associated with phosphate depletion both in alcoholics and in patients with diabetic ketoacidosis, it may be useful as a guideline to give half of parenterally administered potassium as its phosphate salt. Obviously, parenteral phosphate should not be given in the face of hyperphosphatemia.

Knochel JP: The clinical status of hypophosphatemia. N Engl J Med 313:447, 1985. *This useful editorial emphasizes the adverse effect of phosphate depletion on muscle function.*

Knochel JP, Jacobson HR: Renal handling of phosphorus, clinical hypophosphatemia, and phosphorus deficiency. *In* Brenner BM, Rector FC Jr (eds.): The Kidney. 3rd ed. Philadelphia, W. B. Saunders Company, 1986, pp 619–662. *This chapter in a major textbook offers an extensive discussion of the normal physiology of phosphate homeostasis and the causes and consequences of hypophosphatemia. There are 459 references.*

Rasmussen H, Tenenhouse HS: Hypophosphatemias. *In* Scriver CR, Beaudet AL, Sly WS, et al. (eds.): *The Metabolic Basis of Inherited Disease.* 6th ed. New York, McGraw-Hill, 1989, pp 2581–2609. *An authoritative discussion of phosphate homeostasis and the inherited syndrome of hypophosphatemic rickets caused by defects in renal tubular phosphate reabsorption.*

Yu GC, Lee DBN: Clinical disorders of phosphorus metabolism. West J Med 147:569, 1987. *This article gives an excellent general review of the clinical and pathophysiologic aspects of phosphate deficiency syndromes in humans.*

195 Disorders of Magnesium Metabolism

Lloyd H. Smith, Jr.

Magnesium is the fourth most common cation in the human body (after sodium, potassium, and calcium) and the cation in second highest concentration intracellularly. The average adult body contains about 25 grams (1000 mmol) of magnesium, of which 50 to 60 per cent is in bone. The normal serum magnesium concentration is 1.6 to 2.1 mEq per liter, approximately one fourth to one third being protein bound. The average American diet contains approximately 500 mg (20 mmol) of magnesium, much of this in chlorophyll. It has been estimated that about 0.15 mmol (3.5 to 4.5 mg) of dietary magnesium per kilogram per day is necessary to maintain a positive balance in adults. More is required in children. Magnesium is actively absorbed in the small intestine by a process that is enhanced by 1,25-dihydroxycholecalciferol, resulting in a net absorption of about 30 to 40 per cent of that ingested. This net absorption is balanced

at equilibrium by renal excretion, which reflects filtration of the 65 to 75 per cent not protein bound followed by net renal tubular reabsorption of approximately 95 per cent. The kidney can control the excretion of magnesium over a wide range—from more than 250 mmol to less than 1 mmol per day. The factors that control the renal tubular reabsorption of magnesium are not completely understood but include sodium excretion, calcium excretion, parathyroid hormone, and extracellular fluid volume. Excretion is also increased by ethanol and by many diuretic agents.

Magnesium has a structural role in bone crystal. It also serves as an activator of a large number of specific enzymes. Of particular importance, it is a cofactor in all transphosphorylation reactions involving adenosine triphosphate (ATP), so that it is intimately involved in energy metabolism and the synthesis of macromolecules, for example. Perhaps even more basic in biology is its obligate role in the function of chlorophyll. By and large it has not been possible to correlate the signs or symptoms of magnesium deficiency or excess with any one of its specific biochemical functions.

HYPERMAGNESEMIA. Because of the ability of the normal kidney to excrete a magnesium load, significant hypermagnesemia is rarely seen in clinical practice. In the past, magnesium ion was occasionally infused as a hypotensive agent in the treatment of acute hypertension with the secondary production of symptomatic hypermagnesemia. In patients with renal insufficiency, the excessive use of magnesium, as in magnesium-containing antacids, may cause hypermagnesemia. The manifestations of hypermagnesemia are largely in the central nervous system and the cardiovascular system. Ionized magnesium is a sedative that depresses the function of the central nervous system and exerts a curare-like effect on the neuromuscular junction at high concentrations (>10 mEq per liter). The cardiovascular effects of hypermagnesemia are those of peripheral vasodilatation, resulting in hypotension, generalized depression of the cardiac conduction system, bradyrhythmias, and asystole with cardiac arrest in diastole. The cardiac effects of Mg^{2+} are usually manifested at serum concentrations greater than 10 mEq per liter, with asystole at levels greater than 25 mEq per liter, but a few patients have exhibited exceptional sensitivity with cardiotoxicity at levels of 4.5 to 5.5 mEq per liter. Factors that augment the cardiotoxicity of Mg^{2+} include hypocalcemia, hyperkalemia, acidosis, digitalis therapy, and renal insufficiency (beyond its effect on the serum Mg^{2+} level). Treatment of hypermagnesemia is usually limited to discontinuing its exogenous source. In severe hypermagnesemia, intravenous treatment with calcium may temporarily reverse many of the toxic effects because of the pharmacologic antagonism of ionized calcium and magnesium in the central nervous system.

HYPOMAGNESEMIA. Hypomagnesemia is a much more frequent metabolic derangement than hypermagnesemia and usually occurs as one component of a complex deficiency state, affecting many minerals, vitamins, and nutrients.

Causes of Hypomagnesemia. Magnesium deficiency and hypomagnesemia result from decreased absorption or from increased excretion (Table 195–1). Very rarely, hypomagnesemia may result from "loss" into bone during excessive osteogenesis, the "hungry bone syndrome," during the repair of osteitis fibrosa generalisata following the removal of a parathyroid tumor (see Ch. 235). Serum levels may also fall, as do those of calcium, during acute pancreatitis. In general, decreased absorption of magnesium occurs in the same circumstances as does decreased calcium absorption, especially that caused by dietary deficiency and malabsorption syndromes of whatever origin. Decreased absorption in uremia may result from deficiency of 1,25-dihydroxycholecalciferol. A few infants have been described with convulsions associated with hypocalcemia and hypomagnesemia in the absence of renal magnesium wasting. They have responded to continued high ingestion of magnesium, but not of calcium, and are thought to have a selective defect in gut absorption of magnesium. It is not clear whether ethanol diminishes magnesium absorption directly or only through diminished ingestion or vitamin D deficiency.

Increased loss of magnesium can occur from excessive vomiting, from diarrhea, or via the kidney. Rarely, patients may exhibit what appears to be an inherited renal tubular defect in magnesium reabsorption. These patients have tended to have potassium wasting as well and to present with hypokalemia, hypomagnesemia, and hypocalcemia (secondary to hypomagnesemia). In general, magnesium clearance tends to parallel that of sodium and calcium and may be increased by diuretics (osmotic, thiazides, ethacrynic acid, furosemide), by ionized calcium, and possibly by ethanol. Renal magnesium wasting also occurs as a result of the renal tubular effect of certain drugs, especially aminoglycosides, amphotericin B, and cisplatin. The magnesium wasting of uncontrolled diabetes mellitus probably results from tissue catabolism and osmotic diuresis. Lactation hypomagnesemia, well described in cattle, has been documented in two women.

Consequences of Hypomagnesemia. Hypomagnesemia rarely occurs as a single deficiency, so that it is not always possible to distinguish its signs and symptoms from those of associated deficiency states. Selective magnesium deficiency has been produced experimentally in humans, however, and it is based on these observations, together with clinical correlations in patients, that the spectrum of manifestations listed in Table 195–2 has been described. Patients with magnesium deficiency are lethargic, weak, and irritable with decreased attention span. They may have tetany with positive Chvostek's and Trousseau's signs because of associated hypocalcemia (see below). In experimental magnesium deficiency, muscles are weak and may show hyaline and vacuolar degeneration of myofibers, sometimes followed by leukocytic infiltration, segmental necrosis, and early calcification. Patients with hypomagnesemia are generally anorectic and may have nausea, vomiting, and poor intestinal motility. Hypomagnesemia may occur in congestive heart failure because of anorexia, malabsorption, and the excessive use of diuretic agents. Magnesium deficiency increases the sensitivity of the heart to digitalis glycosides, so that digitalis toxicity occurs at a lower serum level and also tends to persist longer. Hypomagnesemia has also been associated with cardiac arrhythmias independent of digoxin, including ventricular premature beats, ventricular tachycardia, and ventricular fibrillation. This association is often difficult to establish because other abnormalities generally coexist, especially hypokalemia.

Magnesium metabolism has a number of interesting interrelationships with that of calcium: (1) both are absorbed by the gut through mechanisms enhanced by vitamin D; (2) excess magnesium may inhibit calcium absorption, but not vice versa; (3) calcium and magnesium may compete for renal tubular reabsorption; (4) calcium and magnesium are physiologic antagonists in the central nervous system; and (5) magnesium is necessary for the normal secretion of parathyroid hormone (PTH) in response to hypocalcemia and also for the activity of PTH as a hormone at the site of its target organs. *Hypocalcemia* is one of the most consistent and important findings in magnesium deficiency with

TABLE 195–1. CAUSES OF HYPOMAGNESEMIA (SEEN MOST FREQUENTLY CLINICALLY IN ALCOHOLISM AND MALABSORPTION)

I. **Decreased absorption from dietary sources**
   Diet poor in magnesium
   Parenteral feeding without magnesium
   Ethanol effect on absorption
   Malabsorption syndromes
   Uremia
   Selective intestinal defect for magnesium absorption (rare)
II. **Increased loss of magnesium from the body**
   Gastrointestinal tract—diarrhea, fistulas, suction
   Kidney
      Primary renal tubular defects
      Secondary—diuretics, Ca^{2+}, ethanol, expansion of ECF,
         diabetes mellitus, treatment with gentamicin, cisplatin, or
         amphotericin B
   Breast—lactation hypomagnesemia (mostly in cattle, rarely in
      humans)
III. **Internal redistribution**
   Acute pancreatitis
   Increased loss into bone ("hungry bone syndrome")

TABLE 195–2. CONSEQUENCES OF MAGNESIUM DEFICIENCY

Neuromuscular
   Lethargy, weakness, fatigue, decreased mentation, paresthesias
   Neuromuscular irritability, in part due to associated hypocalcemia
   Hyaline and vacuolar degeneration of myofibers with segmental
      necrosis
Gastrointestinal
   Anorexia, nausea, vomiting
   Paralytic ileus
Cardiovascular
   Increased sensitivity to digitalis glycosides
   Cardiac arrhythmias
Metabolic
   Hypocalcemia—probably due to the combined result of decreased
      PTH secretion and decreased end-organ responsiveness to PTH
   Hypokalemia—tendency toward renal potassium wasting

hypomagnesemia. Hypocalcemia responds promptly to magnesium replacement and is accompanied by a rise in plasma PTH. A burst of PTH secretion occurs within minutes after the infusion of magnesium intravenously into patients with combined hypocalcemia and hypomagnesemia. Many of these patients show evidence of resistance to exogenous PTH as well. Hypomagnesemia therefore results in a complex combination of functional hypoparathyroidism and acquired pseudohypoparathyroidism. This entity should be suspected especially in alcoholics or patients with malabsorption who present with hypocalcemia. *Hypokalemia* is frequently found with hypomagnesemia. Although some of the conditions that cause magnesium depletion also produce potassium depletion, there is evidence that magnesium deficiency itself enhances renal excretion of potassium. This associated hypokalemia is usually resistant to potassium replacement unless magnesium is replaced first.

Treatment of Hypomagnesemia. The treatment of hypomagnesemia is rarely an acute emergency. When rapid replacement therapy is judged to be vital (convulsions, tachyrhythmias), 2 grams of $MgSO_4$ (16.3 mEq) can be given intravenously over several minutes. This can be followed by a constant intravenous infusion of approximately 1 mEq of magnesium per kilogram per 24 hours, which usually suffices for initial replacement therapy. Ampules often contain 1 gram of $MgSO_4 \cdot 7H_2O$, which is 8.1 mEq of Mg, so that initial replacement therapy usually requires 8 to 10 grams of $MgSO_4$ given either intravenously as above or intramuscularly as 2 grams every 4 hours for five doses. After the first day, approximately 0.5 mEq of Mg per kilogram per 24 hours should be given intravenously or intramuscularly for 2 to 5 days, based on the return of the serum magnesium level to normal. Parenteral replacement therapy is often preferable to oral therapy because of the tendency of magnesium salts to cause diarrhea. When renal function is impaired, the aforementioned schedules for magnesium replacement must be followed with extra caution and with careful monitoring of serum levels. When there is chronic loss of magnesium (renal wasting, for example), oral therapy is preferred and can be carried out with various preparations as tolerated without diarrhea—magnesium hydroxide tablets, magnesium acetate solution, or liquid milk of magnesia.

Shils ME: Magnesium in health and disease. Annu Rev Nutr 8:429, 1988. *This is an excellent general review of magnesium metabolism by an author who is an authority in the field. Extensive (203) references.*

Sjögren A, Edvinsson L, Fallgren B: Magnesium deficiency in coronary artery disease and cardiac arrhythmias. J Intern Med 226:213, 1989. *The authors give a useful analytic review of magnesium as a coronary dilator and its role in cardiac arrhythmias and in coronary artery disease.*

Whang R: Magnesium deficiency: Pathogenesis, prevalence, and clinical implications. Am J Med 82(Suppl 3A):24, 1987. *A succinct general review with a useful up-to-date list of 43 references.*

OTHER HEREDITARY DISORDERS

196 Familial Mediterranean Fever

Daniel G. Wright

DEFINITION. Familial Mediterranean fever (FMF) is an inherited, recurrent inflammatory disease of unknown cause. The disease is characterized by acute self-limited attacks of fever and peritonitis, sometimes accompanied by pleuritis, arthritis, and erythematous skin lesions. Among affected individuals in the Middle East and Europe, FMF is frequently complicated by amyloidosis and progressive renal failure. Familial Mediterranean fever has been given a number of other names: familial paroxysmal polyserositis, benign paroxysmal peritonitis, periodic peritonitis, and periodic disease. The first of these is descriptively accurate and an appropriate alternative name for the disease; the other terms, however, are misleading. Familial Mediterranean fever is not a benign condition, given the potentially lethal complication of amyloidosis. Moreover, attacks of acute serositis in FMF affect sites other than the peritoneum, and they recur at irregular, unpredictable intervals that do not reflect true periodicity.

INCIDENCE, PREVALENCE, AND GENETICS. Although FMF has been recognized in many parts of the world, it is largely restricted to ethnic groups originating in the eastern Mediterranean area. It is an uncommon disease, even in Israel, where the largest number of cases is seen. Half the reported cases of FMF are in patients of Sephardic Jewish ancestry; approximately 20 per cent of patients are Armenian, and another 20 per cent are of Turkish or Arabic descent. Most of the remaining patients are of Italian, Greek, or Ashkenazic Jewish ancestry. However, the disease has also been recognized rarely in individuals with Anglo-Saxon or northern European origins. The disease is familial, and in well-studied affected kindreds it appears to be inherited as an autosomal recessive trait. Nonetheless, nearly 50 per cent of patients do not give a positive family history for the disease. Among reported cases males predominate by a ratio of 3:2. Active efforts are under way to identify a genetic abnormality in this disease by genomic linkage studies of DNA from members of affected kindreds.

ETIOLOGY. Although many pathogenetic explanations have been suggested for the acute inflammatory episodes of FMF, the etiology of this disease remains unknown. Extensive studies have failed to establish an infectious or allergic basis for the disease, and no good evidence exists to support suggestions that FMF represents a hormonal or psychosomatic disturbance. Recently, it has been proposed that FMF might be caused by a genetically determined defect in the normal regulation of acute inflammatory responses. Abnormalities of suppressor T lymphocytes, altered metabolism of lipoxygenase products of arachidonic acid, and absence of a normal inhibitor of the complement-derived anaphylatoxin C5a have been described in FMF. However, the possible etiologic significance of these observations remains to be clarified and confirmed.

PATHOLOGY. Pathologic findings in FMF are those of nonspecific, acute inflammation. Neutrophilic infiltration predominates in exudates recovered from peritoneal, pleural, or joint spaces at the time of acute attacks. Serosal thickening and secondary adhesions may occur, which in the abdomen can lead to mechanical bowel obstruction. Amyloidosis is the most serious histopathologic finding in FMF. In affected individuals, amyloid is deposited in the intima and media of arterioles and in the subendothelium of venules in all major organs. There is also parenchymal deposition of amyloid, particularly in the renal glomeruli, adrenals, spleen, and alveolar septa of the lung, while the liver and heart are characteristically spared.

CLINICAL MANIFESTATIONS. In most patients the signs and symptoms of FMF begin during the first two decades of life, usually between the ages of 5 and 15 years. Rarely, however, the onset of the disease may occur in infancy or as late as the fifth or sixth decade. The duration and frequency of attacks vary considerably, even in the same patient. Acute attacks typically last 24 to 48 hours and recur once or twice a month. However, attacks may recur as frequently as several times a week or as infrequently as once a year, and symptoms may persist for as long as a week during individual episodes. Some patients experience spontaneous remission that persists for years, followed by recurrence of frequent attacks. Pregnancy is often associated with remission of attacks, which resume post partum. Some patients relate the occurrence of attacks to cold weather and find that they experience attacks more frequently during winter than summer. Recurrent attacks may also become less severe and/or less frequent as patients age or as they develop amyloidosis. Between attacks, patients typically feel entirely well.

Temperatures as high as 39° to 40°C accompany almost all attacks. Fevers may occur without concomitant evidence of serositis, but this is unusual. The rise in temperature is sometimes preceded by chills and typically peaks by 12 to 24 hours; diaphoresis frequently accompanies defervescence.

More than 95 per cent of patients experience abdominal pain and signs of peritonitis during acute attacks. Pain often begins in one quadrant and then becomes diffuse, sometimes with distention, rigidity, rebound tenderness, and ileus with nausea and vomiting. Pain may radiate to the back or to the shoulders, and upright abdominal roentgenograms may show small air-fluid levels and edema of the bowel. Although these signs and symptoms are self-limited, they can be indistinguishable from those of an acute abdominal emergency, and patients may undergo one or more exploratory laparotomies before the true nature of their disease is recognized. Potential uncertainties about the clinical management of acute abdominal episodes have led to the recommendation that elective appendectomy be carried out during a symptom-free period so that acute appendicitis does not confuse a patient's subsequent care.

Pleuritic pain occurs during acute attacks in 75 per cent of patients. Symptoms of pleuritis may sometimes precede abdominal pain, and a few patients experience pleuritic attacks without abdominal symptoms. Chest pain is usually one sided and may be associated with diminished breath sounds, a friction rub, plate atelectasis, and transient pleural effusion.

Nonspecific, mild arthralgia is a common feature of febrile attacks, and acute, monoarticular, or oligoarticular arthritis may occur. Although arthritis is unusual among patients in the United States, it is a frequently observed manifestation of FMF among Israeli patients. Arthritis usually affects large joints, the knee in particular, and effusions are common. Although arthritic episodes are typically short lived, joint symptoms may also be protracted and follow a course distinct from that of the acute abdominal and/or pleuritic attacks. Roentgenographic findings are nonspecific.

As many as a third of patients experience transient, erysipelas-like skin lesions that appear typically on the lower leg, ankle, or dorsum of the foot. These lesions are well-circumscribed, painful, erythematous areas of swelling, 5 to 20 cm in diameter, that subside spontaneously within 24 to 48 hours.

Self-limited pericarditis, conjunctivitis, aseptic meningitis, and other forms of serositis have been reported as manifestations of this disease but are unusual. Migraine-like headaches and emotional lability have also been observed during acute attacks, but it is unclear whether these are primary or secondary manifestations.

The most serious complication of FMF is systemic amyloidosis of the AA type. The natural history of amyloidosis in this disease is one of relentless progression to renal failure and death, which may occur in adolescence or even earlier. While a substantial proportion of Turkish and Israeli patients develop amyloidosis, this complication has been very unusual among patients in the United States and in several well-studied Armenian and Arabic kindreds. The genetic and/or environmental factors that explain these differences in the incidence of amyloidosis remain unclear.

In Israel, 90 per cent of patients who develop amyloidosis (particularly common in Sephardic Jews) do so after experiencing typical attacks of FMF (phenotype I); however, amyloidosis may occur in asymptomatic siblings of FMF patients, or it may precede the onset of typical FMF attacks (phenotype II).

Laboratory findings in FMF are nonspecific. During acute attacks, a prominent leukocytosis (up to 30,000 per cubic millimeter) is present, and the erythrocyte sedimentation rate and acute phase reactants are increased. These values return to normal between attacks. Elevated plasma dopamine beta-hydroxylase levels (which become normal during colchicine treatment) have been reported in patients with FMF, but confirmatory studies have yet to be done to determine whether this finding represents a specific diagnostic test for FMF. With amyloidosis, laboratory abnormalities reflect the associated nephrotic syndrome and renal failure.

DIAGNOSIS. The diagnosis of FMF is based primarily upon clinical presentation and history. In individuals of appropriate ethnic background with typical recurrent, self-limited attacks, diagnosis should not be difficult; in such individuals, delay in recognizing the disease is usually because the diagnosis is not considered. Nonetheless, when a patient is first seen or when attacks are infrequent, a variety of other acute febrile conditions must be considered and excluded by appropriate diagnostic studies and follow-up—in particular, appendicitis, pancreatitis, cholecystitis, and intestinal obstruction. Familial hyperlipidemia and porphyrias associated with abdominal symptoms must also be considered.

The diagnosis is usually most elusive when patients have a limited or atypical symptom complex. Isolated pleural attacks may closely mimic acute infections or pulmonary emboli. Arthritis, when it is a prominent manifestation, can at first be clinically indistinguishable from various infectious and noninfectious arthritides, and skin lesions on the lower legs may resemble cellulitis or superficial thrombophlebitis. Rare patients have febrile episodes without serositis, and these may require orderly evaluation to determine their origin. Recently, it has been reported that infusion of metaraminol diluted in normal saline provokes acute signs and symptoms of FMF with a high degree of specificity for the disease. However, the appropriate role of such a test in establishing the diagnosis remains unclear. At present, this procedure, which carries intrinsic risks from catecholamine effects and salt load, should be considered experimental and not for use in general practice.

Once FMF is diagnosed, a degree of diagnostic vigilance must be maintained, for patients are not immune to the more common acute illnesses that FMF mimics. Of note, these patients appear to be particularly prone to develop gallbladder disease.

TREATMENT. Colchicine treatment is effective in FMF. Several controlled clinical trials, together with extensive, uncontrolled clinical experience since the mid 1970's, have shown that prophylactic colchicine,* 0.6 mg orally two or three times a day, prevents or substantially reduces the acute attacks of FMF in 75 to 90 per cent of patients. Treatment failures are often associated with noncompliance and/or intolerance to the drug. Some patients can abort attacks with intermittent courses of colchicine, beginning at the onset of attacks (0.6 mg orally every hour for 4 hours, then every 2 hours for 4 hours, and then every 12 hours for 2 days). In general, patients who benefit from intermittent colchicine therapy are those who experience a recognizable prodrome before developing fever and clear-cut acute symptoms. Colchicine does not alter fully developed attacks. Patients who experience gastrointestinal intolerance to colchicine may benefit from reduced doses. Although definite chronic complications from colchicine have not become apparent with its long-term use in FMF, it is still recommended that a trial of intermittent colchicine therapy be attempted, particularly in young patients, before long-term colchicine prophylaxis is used. Azoospermia and chromosomal nondisjunctions have been associated with the use of this drug. This recommendation does not apply to individuals from ethnic groups and in geographic regions associated with a high risk of amyloidosis, for it is now evident that long-term colchicine therapy not only prevents the development of amyloidosis but may also arrest its progression in FMF.

---

* This use of colchicine is not listed in the manufacturer's directive.

Symptomatic and supportive treatment is indicated for patients who do not respond to colchicine. However, every effort should be made to avoid the use of narcotics. In the United States, addiction to narcotics has been a major long-term complication among FMF patients.

It has been estimated that patients with FMF and end-stage renal amyloidosis represent up to 6 per cent of the candidates for renal transplantation in Israel. Many such patients have received successful renal grafts. Of note, it has been suggested recently that these patients may be particularly susceptible to gastrointestinal and other side effects of the immunosuppressive drug cyclosporine.

PROGNOSIS. The prognosis for normal longevity for patients in the United States with FMF is excellent, and since the recognition of colchicine's efficacy in this disease, most patients can be maintained almost entirely symptom free. Except in very rare cases, this disease does not affect the physical growth and development of children. Long-term colchicine therapy has also clearly improved the prognosis of patients in the Middle East who are prone to develop amyloidosis, even those whose symptomatic attacks continue. However, among patients in whom amyloidosis has led to nephrotic syndrome or uremia and who are unable to receive a renal transplant or in whom renal transplantation has failed, the likelihood of eventual death from renal failure remains great.

Barakat MH, Karnik AM, Majeed HWA, et al.: Familial Mediterranean fever (recurrent hereditary polyserositis) in Arabs—a study of 175 patients and review of the literature. Q J Med 60:837, 1986. Meyerhoff J: Familial Mediterranean fever: Report of a large family, review of the literature, and discussion of the frequency of amyloidosis. Medicine 59:66, 1980. *These articles provide extensive reviews of the clinical and pathologic manifestations of FMF and describe differences in the incidence of amyloidosis.*

Dinarello CA, Wolff SM, Goldfinger SE, et al.: Colchicine therapy for familial Mediterranean fever. A double-blind trial. N Engl J Med 291:934, 1974. *One of several controlled trials that clearly established the efficacy of prophylactic colchicine therapy in preventing FMF attacks.*

Wright DG, Wolff SM, Fauci AS, et al.: Efficacy of intermittent colchicine therapy in familial Mediterranean fever. Ann Intern Med 86:162, 1977. *A double-blind study that shows intermittent courses of colchicine can successfully abort attacks in some patients with FMF.*

Zemer D, Pras M, Sohar E, et al.: Colchicine in the prevention and treatment of the amyloidosis of familial Mediterranean fever. N Engl J Med 314:1001, 1986. *A retrospective review of 1070 patients that provides convincing evidence that long-term colchicine therapy arrests the development of amyloidosis.*

---

197 The Amyloid Diseases

Joel N. Buxbaum

DEFINITION. The amyloid diseases constitute a group of conditions of diverse causes characterized by the accumulation of ultrastructurally fibrillar material in various tissues in quantities sufficient to compromise vital organ function. The associated disease states may be inflammatory, hereditary, or neoplastic, and the deposition can be local or systemic. The clinical outcome may be benign or as malignant as the most aggressive of neoplasms. In many senses, amyloid deposition is a symptom of an underlying disorder, much as anemia is a symptom of a variety of pathologic states. The symptoms of the amyloidoses depend upon the amount and localization of the deposits.

In tissue sections, with conventional staining techniques, all amyloid appears homogeneous and eosinophilic. All types bind Congo red and under polarized light emit an apple-green fluorescence when stained with this dye. With the electron microscope, amyloid is seen to contain two discrete structures: a major fibrillar component with a characteristic periodicity and a minor rodlike component that, when extracted and viewed on end, has the appearance of a pentagon with a hollow core (the P-component). The P-component appears to be physically and chemically identical in all amyloids and normally circulates as a soluble serum protein (SAP). Its role in the process of tissue infiltration has not been established.

The deposited fibril, regardless of its chemical nature, when isolated and analyzed has the x-ray diffraction pattern characteristic of a beta-pleated sheet. It is insoluble at physiologic salt concentrations but can be released from tissue deposits by extraction with distilled water. The latter observation, made in the early 1970's, allowed the chemical analysis of fibrils obtained from many preparations of amyloid from the tissues of individuals with different diseases. These studies have, in turn, permitted a more precise, chemically based, classification of the various amyloid syndromes (Table 197–1).

PATHOGENESIS

Amyloid A (AA) Amyloidosis. AA amyloid, so designated because it was the first nonimmunoglobulin amyloid fibril to be characterized chemically, is most frequently found when deposition takes place in the course of chronic inflammatory disease. In the past, chronic infectious processes, such as tuberculosis and osteomyelitis, were the usual precipitating causes. In recent years, the most commonly associated conditions have been the chronic noninfectious inflammatory disorders. Amyloid deposits have been found in up to 20 per cent of autopsies of patients with rheumatoid arthritis, but they are clinically significant in only 3 to 5 per cent of cases. For reasons that are unknown, the prevalence in juvenile rheumatoid disease varies considerably in different countries (e.g., 0.14 per cent in the United States to 10 per cent in Poland). Other inflammatory joint diseases, including the seronegative spondyloarthropathies, gout, and psoriasis, as well as inflammatory bowel disease, even without arthritis, have been associated with amyloid deposition. Some populations of drug abusers, particularly those using the subcutaneous injection route because of depleted vascular access, have been found to have a high frequency of AA disease. The chronic or recurrent skin abscesses found in these patients seem to be particularly effective in the induction of amyloidosis.

Renal deposition of the AA protein has been the ultimately fatal event in the course of some groups of patients with *familial Mediterranean fever* (FMF) (Ch. 196). In the past, 40 per cent or more of North African Sephardic Jews and 20 per cent or more of Turks with this disease succumbed to renal failure secondary to AA amyloid.

AA deposition is also seen in atrial myxomas, a variety of nonlymphoid tumors, and some non–immunoglobulin-producing lymphomas. Renal and gastric carcinomas and Hodgkin's disease have been the tumors most frequently associated with AA amyloid.

Kidneys, liver, and spleen are the most important sites of AA deposition. The nephropathy is characterized initially by proteinuria of the glomerular type. Early in the disease, the kidneys may be enlarged, but with time they shrink, and the course is one of progressive renal failure. A variety of tubular disorders have also been described, including renal tubular acidosis, because of impaired bicarbonate reabsorption, nephrogenic diabetes insipidus, glycosuria, and hyperkalemia produced by decreased renal potassium exchange. The liver disease is relatively nonspecific, usually resulting in only moderate hepatomegaly and liver function test abnormalities.

In the past, when chronic infections were the most frequent stimuli to amyloid deposition, a small number of cases were reported in which eradication of the infection resulted in arrest of progression, or actual regression, of the amyloidosis, as documented by biopsy. In general, even without treatment the course of AA disease is more chronic than that of AL amyloid (see below).

The deposited AA protein appears to be a discrete proteolytic product of its precursor apo-SAA that has a monomer molecular weight of 12,500 but circulates as a molecule of molecular weight 220,000 to 235,000 complexed to high density lipoprotein. It has also been found complexed to albumin. It behaves like an acute phase protein, rising rapidly in the course of inflammation (infectious or noninfectious), peaking, and then falling to normal levels with resolution of the episode. Serum levels are generally higher in the elderly. Its synthesis is stimulated by the monokine interleukin 6 (IL6), which, in turn, can be mediated by interleukin 1 and tumor necrosis factor. It appears that the predisposition to develop AA deposits resides in the production of an amyloidogenic isotypical form of SAA, the inability to degrade SAA completely, or both occurring in the same individual.

AL Amyloidosis. AL (or immunoglobulin [Ig] light chain–related) deposition is the most common form of amyloidosis currently seen in clinical practice. The proportion of the total number of cases that represent multiple myeloma or primary amyloid is difficult to judge, since marrow plasmacytosis may be

TABLE 197–1. CHEMICAL CLASSIFICATION OF THE AMYLOIDOSES

Clinical	Fibril Precursor	Fibril	Common Abbreviation
Systemic			
Primary or myeloma with amyloid	Ig light-chain or light-chain fragment	Light-chain fragment	AL
Secondary*	Serum amyloid A (SAA)	Amyloid A (AA)	AA
Dialysis associated	Beta$_2$-microglobulin (β_2m)	β_2m monomer or dimer	AB
Familial			
Neuropathic	Transthyretin (TTR)†	TTR variants	ATTR
	Apolipoprotein A1 (Apo-A1)	Apo-A1	AApoA1
	Gelsolin‡	Gelsolin peptides	AGel
Cardiomyopathic	TTR	TTR variants	ATTR
Nephropathic	SAA	AA	AA
Vascular			
HCHWA (Iceland)	Cystatin C§	Cystatin variant	ACys
HCHWA (Denmark)	Beta protein precursor	Beta protein	AB
Localized			
Senile			
Cardiac			
Atria	Atrial natriuretic factor (ANF)	ANF	AANF
Ventricles	TTR	TTR normal or variant	ATTR
Brain (Alzheimer's disease)	Beta protein precursor	Beta protein	AB
Pancreas	Islet-associated polypeptide (IAPP)‖	IAPP	AIAPP
Endocrine			
Medullary carcinoma thyroid	Procalcitonin	Procalcitonin, calcitonin	ACal
Islet cell tumor/insulinoma	IAPP	IAPP	AIAPP

*Inflammation associated.
†Transthyretin, formerly known as thyroxine-binding prealbumin, also carries retinol-binding protein.
‡Gelsolin is an actin-binding cytoskeletal protein.
§Cystatin C is a lysomal protease inhibitor also known as gamma trace.
‖The islet-associated polypeptide has also been called amylin.

significant in both and other diagnostic distinctions between the primary disease and myeloma may be blurred (Ch. 151). Functionally, both diseases are malignant. In myeloma, the outcome is related primarily to the proliferative capacity of the neoplastic clone. When AL deposition is present, it contributes to the poor prognosis. In primary amyloid, the growth of the dominant plasma cell clone appears to be limited, but the amyloidogenicity of its homogeneous product results in the ultimately fatal compromise of organ function, most commonly renal or cardiac.

AL deposition is more likely to occur in tongue, heart, lymph nodes, spleen, carpal ligaments, joints, peripheral nerves, and skin than in the AA type. Hence, macroglossia, cardiac failure, arrhythmias, carpal tunnel syndrome, peripheral neuropathy, and ecchymoses are more frequent in AL disease. A deficiency of Factor X has been reported with an attendant bleeding diathesis. There is evidence to suggest that some AL proteins may have affinity for the clotting factor, with resultant lowering of the plasma levels. Removal of an amyloid-laden spleen has reversed the deficiency in some patients. Blood vessels tend to be fragile in AL patients, since the amyloid is deposited in vessel walls. The deposits also decrease vascular compliance, thus contributing to the body's reduced capacity to respond to reflex-mediated changes in body position. The latter may lead to severe orthostatic hypotension as a major clinical problem. Coronary artery amyloid deposition can result in angina pectoris or myocardial infarction. Infiltration of the bowel wall or autonomic nerves may cause diarrhea, with or without malabsorption.

A large number of studies have documented that the deposited fibril protein is related to the excess monoclonal Ig light chain produced by the expanded plasma cell clone and found in the patient's serum, urine, or both. The actual tissue protein may represent the whole light chain or a fragment containing at least the variable region. Most consist of the entire variable and a portion of the light chain constant region. Amino acid sequence analyses of tissue AL protein and the light chain isolated from the same patient have demonstrated chemical identity.

Despite much careful investigation, it is still not clear what makes a given light chain amyloidogenic. Lambda chains are more frequently associated with amyloid deposition than kappa, and the $V\lambda_{VI}$ subgroup is heavily overrepresented. It has been suggested that tissue affinity could be charge related or that the interaction between light chain and tissues could represent that of an incomplete autoantibody with its antigen. Neither of these hypotheses has convincing experimental support. Further, it has not been established whether amyloidogenesis involves only the processing of intact light chains to fragments or whether some of the molecules are of synthetic origin and are predisposed to deposition without further processing. It is possible that both events occur.

Most AL patients, even those with primary amyloid, have a detectable monoclonal Ig (M-protein), usually free light chains of a single class, found in the serum or urine; however, up to 20 per cent have not had such proteins detectable. Analyses of a small number of the latter patients indicated that in short-term tissue culture their bone marrow cells synthesized an excess of free monoclonal light chains. Because of their low concentration in the serum and their presumably high affinity for tissues, they cannot be detected by conventional immunochemical techniques. In only one instance has an Ig heavy chain fragment been found to make up the fibril isolated from human amyloid tissue.

Individuals have been described in whom organ compromise has taken place because of the deposition of monoclonal light chains or light and heavy chain fragments, without discrete fibril formation. Some of the patients had clinical multiple myeloma; others did not. While the proteins have been identified in tissue deposits by immunofluorescence, only a few chemical studies of the tissue forms have been carried out; therefore, formal proof of their identity with a circulating precursor is lacking. The condition appeared to be analogous to AL amyloid, but with the deposited proteins not having the intrinsic properties necessary to form beta-pleated sheets of sufficient size and stability to make fibrils. More recently, individual patients with both fibrillar (amyloid) and nonfibrillar deposits of antigenically similar material have been described, making this simple explanation unlikely.

Senile Amyloidoses. The term *senile amyloid* has been used to describe Congo red–binding material found at autopsy in the tissues of elderly individuals. Such material is most commonly found in the heart but has also been noted in the pancreas, prostate, and brain. Recent data have shown that the fibrils are derived from a variety of tissue-specific proteins.

The cerebral plaques identified in Alzheimer's disease (Ch. 450) are Congophilic and appear to be critical in its pathogenesis. Techniques used to extract and characterize other forms of amyloid have been used to analyze material isolated from the plaques and from amyloid-containing cerebral vessels of these patients. It has been found to consist of a 4200-d polypeptide, the beta protein, which is a portion of a larger protein found in a variety of tissues, including the alpha granules of platelets, where it had previously been identified as a protease inhibitor, nexin 1.

Amyloid material has also been noted in the brain lesions of Creutzfeldt-Jakob patients (Ch. 478.6) and animals suffering from scrapie. Immunohistochemical and nucleotide sequence analyses have indicated that the Alzheimer and Creutzfeldt-Jakob proteins are separate entities.

While many individuals in their eighth and ninth decades have scattered atrial amyloid deposits, clinically significant cardiac disease, characterized by either congestive heart failure or arrhythmia, results from ventricular deposits, which occur less frequently. Once symptoms appear, the prognosis is poor. The presence of a chronic inflammatory disease (e.g., rheumatoid arthritis) or multiple myeloma does not increase the incidence of senile cardiac amyloid deposition, suggesting an independent pathogenesis for each of the three conditions.

The amyloid fibrils isolated from ventricular myocardium have an amino acid sequence identical to that of serum transthyretin (TTR), a normal molecule responsible for the transport of thyroxine and retinol-binding protein. Since TTR is not known to be synthesized by myocardial cells, its cardiac deposition suggests that the precursor is produced at a remote site and localizes at its target by an as yet unknown mechanism. Clinical studies have suggested that pulmonary involvement may be regularly associated with the cardiac deposition, implying that TTR fibrils may be more systemic than previously appreciated and that the disease should be called senile systemic amyloidosis (SSA). It is not yet clear whether the deposited TTR is normal or variant in its primary structure.

AL and AA disease and SSA make up the bulk of the amyloid diseases encountered in clinical practice; however, there are additional forms, the analyses of which have yielded insight into the general process of fibril deposition. One localized form has been found in approximately 40 per cent of medullary carcinomas of the thyroid, in which the fibrillar protein consists of procalcitonin and processed forms of calcitonin.

Structural analyses of the fibrils extracted from the Congo red–binding structures seen in the pancreas of elderly patients with type II diabetes mellitus, and insulinomas have shown that they are derived from a normal peptide product of the beta cell, which probably plays a role in normal glucose metabolism and is now known as islet amyloid polypeptide (IAPP), or amylin.

Hemodialysis-Associated Amyloidosis. During the past decade, a syndrome has been recognized in patients who have been maintained on long-term hemodialysis. It is characterized by carpal tunnel syndrome, i.e., compression of the median nerve by a thickened carpal ligament, and arthropathy, frequently severe enough to require joint replacement. Examination of the surgically excised ligaments and synovial and rectal biopsies from affected individuals have revealed amyloid. Chemical analysis of the fibrils shows that they consist of monomers and dimers of beta$_2$-microglobulin, the light chain of cell-surface major histocompatibility antigens A, B, and C. It has been suggested that the deposition is secondary to the accumulation of the normally totally excreted beta$_2$-microglobulin, which is retained by dialysis membranes with relatively small pore sizes.

Familial Amyloidosis. A growing number of genetically transmitted amyloid deposition diseases with characteristic clinical syndromes have been described; they are summarized in Table 197–2. The majority are primarily neuropathic with autosomal dominant inheritance. Other hereditary forms with nephropathic, cardiopathic, or cutaneous manifestations have also been delineated. Some of these, particularly those involving the heart, appear late in life and may be confused with AL heart disease. The

TABLE 197–2. FAMILIAL AMYLOID SYNDROMES*

Syndrome	Onset (yr)	Clinical Findings	Fibril
Neuropathic			
Portuguese-Japanese (I)†	20–40	Lower limbs, autonomic	ATTR Met 30†
Swedish (I)	30–50	Upper and lower extremities, pupillary abnormalities, renal disease, autonomic and central nervous system dysfunction	ATTR Met 30
Illinois-German (I)	>50	Lower limbs, bowel, renal	ATTR Tyr 77
Swiss-Indiana (II)	>40	Upper extremities, vitreous opacities	ATTR Ser 84
Maryland-German (II)	>40	Upper extremities	ATTR Leu 58
Appalachian	>40	Peripheral neuropathy, autonomic, cardiac	ATTR Ala 60
Israel	20's	Upper and lower extremities, autonomic dysfunction, vitreous opacities	ATTR Ile 33
Iowa (IV)	20–40	Upper and lower extremities, pupillary abnormalities and renal disease	AApoA1 Arg 26
Finland (V)	40's	Facial neuropathy, lattice corneal dystrophy	AGel Asn 187 (15)
Nonneuropathic			
Familial Mediterranean fever (FMF)	10–30	Inflammatory serositis, nephropathy	AA
Derbyshire	10–30	Deafness, urticaria, fever, renal disease	Not known
Polish	40–60	Splenomegaly, hypertension, renal disease	Not known
Irish-American-German (VIII)	40–60	Lung, renal disease	Not known
Iceland (VI)	20–40	Cerebral hemorrhage	ACys Gln 68
Denmark (III)	30–70	Cardiac failure	ATTR Met 111

*All appear to be autosomal dominant diseases except FMF, which is autosomal recessive.
†Roman numerals represent the clinical classification used when these were all called familial amyloidotic polyneuropathy.
‡Thyroxine-binding prealbumin or transthyretin; see Table 197–1.
§Position 49 substitution is not found in fibrils extracted from all tissues.

absence of an M-component and a firm or suggestive family history are more consistent with late-onset familial disease.

CLINICAL MANIFESTATIONS. Regardless of the type of protein, the clinical manifestations of amyloid deposition in a given organ are similar. The renal disease is manifested primarily by proteinuria, reflecting the glomerular localization of the deposition. Renal tubular defects have also been reported. Azotemia and renal failure usually occur late. The latter may be associated with vascular involvement. There is a 5 to 15 per cent incidence of renal vein thrombosis, particularly in patients with AA disease and the nephrotic syndrome. Amyloid renal disease may be associated with hypertension. The kidneys can be small, normal sized, or enlarged. Contraction of the kidneys is generally a late event.

The most characteristic cardiac presentation is that of a restrictive cardiomyopathy with congestive heart failure. Supraventricular arrhythmias are common, as are varying degrees of atrioventricular (AV) block. Echocardiographic studies usually show a thickened interventricular septum and posterior ventricular wall without a dilated ventricle and may reveal a "sparkling" of the myocardial echoes. In vitro studies have demonstrated binding of both calcium channel blocking drugs and digitalis glycosides to amyloid fibrils. It is likely that the sensitivity of some patients with myocardial amyloidosis to digoxin is due to the concentration in the myocardium by this mechanism, and these drugs are generally not used. Pulmonary involvement tends to mirror the cardiac disease both in frequency and in extent, but rarely it becomes the dominant clinical syndrome with impairment of both the mechanics of respiration and gas exchange. Localized upper and lower airway amyloid infiltration can present major mechanical problems requiring surgical intervention.

Gastrointestinal involvement is most frequently manifested by bleeding, although diarrhea and malabsorption due to either submucosal infiltration or autonomic neuropathy have been reported.

DIAGNOSIS. The diagnosis of amyloidosis is made by the demonstration of the typical tissue deposits. Over the years the choice of appropriate tissue for biopsy has widened. In patients in whom the diagnosis is suspected on clinical grounds, recent data suggested that subcutaneous fat aspiration yields Congo red–positive material in up to 85 per cent of cases of AL disease and two thirds of patients with AA deposits. Rectal biopsy in similar patients yields positive results in 70 to 80 per cent if adequate mucosal and submucosal tissue is obtained. Some patients may have a positive rectal biopsy result and a negative subcutaneous fat aspirate, while others may show the reverse. Gingival tissue gives positive results in about one quarter of cases. Bone marrow biopsies have been positive in up to 40 to 50 per cent of patients with AL disease. These sites may be sampled with little chance of serious complications.

When there is evidence of involvement of a particular organ, diagnostic yields improve considerably. Operative specimens from carpal tunnel releases performed on patients with AL or hereditary neuropathic disease may show 95 per cent positivity. Renal biopsies in individuals with proteinuria have been reported to be positive in more than 90 per cent of patients. Liver biopsies also have a high yield; however, as with closed renal biopsies, significant, even fatal, bleeding has occurred. Hence these procedures are performed only after a thorough evaluation of clotting parameters. Liver biopsy is generally not carried out if a coagulopathy is present. Endomyocardial biopsy has become extremely useful in the diagnosis of the cardiac forms of amyloid deposition.

It has now become possible to distinguish the chemical types of amyloid in biopsy material. In the past a diagnosis of AL disease could be inferred by the presence in the serum and urine of monoclonal Ig's or light chains. Now diagnosis is facilitated by the use of antisera to the different light chain classes, AA proteins, beta$_2$-microglobulin, transthyretin, and gelsolin in the immunofluorescent or immunoperoxidase staining of biopsy samples. Since each of the deposited proteins arises from a different precursor, presumably in response to a different stimulus, it is reasonable to assume that these discriminatory methods will eventually have therapeutic implications.

As previously noted, all deposits, regardless of the origin of the fibril, contain P-component and stain with antibodies specific for that protein. Studies in experimental models of amyloid, as well as humans with the disease, have shown that exogenous P-component, administered intravenously, will home to amyloid deposits. Early results indicate that the procedure may be clinically useful in localizing and quantifying the extent of tissue deposition.

TREATMENT AND PROGNOSIS. AL deposition associated with multiple myeloma has been treated in the course of treating the neoplastic process. While 50 to 60 per cent of patients with myeloma respond to treatment with alkylating agents and prednisone with extension of survival, the disease has not yet been cured, nor has the amyloid deposition been reversed.

A number of patients with AL disease, but without overt myeloma, have been reported to show prolonged survival after therapy with protocols like those used for myeloma. As yet, no controlled study has shown enhanced survival with any treatment; nonetheless, it appears that some patients may respond to these regimens. There have also been occasional reports of improvement in AL disease during administration of the organic solvent dimethyl sulfoxide,* usually with concurrent alkylating agent therapy.

The most successful therapy of any form of amyloidosis has been the prophylactic use of colchicine* in patients with FMF (see Ch. 196). As a result of this experience and the observation that colchicine also prevents experimental casein-induced murine AA deposition, several groups have instituted large-scale trials of colchicine in both AA and AL disease. Apart from the FMF experience and the occasional AL patient, no regimen has been uniformly successful in the reversal of any form of amyloid deposition once it has become established; nonetheless, the increased efficacy of supportive care has resulted in longer survival with a better quality of life for many affected individuals. Both cardiac disease and renal disease have been managed more effectively with the judicious use of more potent diuretics. Some patients with AL disease and renal failure, whose monoclonal protein production has been stopped by alkylating agent therapy, have undergone successful renal transplantation. More potent antibiotics have improved the outcome of infectious episodes, and newer agents, such as somatostatin analogues to treat the diarrhea associated with amyloid bowel infiltration and autonomic neuropathy, have had a favorable impact on patient management.

Browning MJ, Banks RA, Tribe CR, et al.: Ten years' experience of an amyloid clinic. Q J Med 54:213, 1985. *The experience of a large British referral clinic, worth comparing with that of the Mayo Clinic (see Kyle reference, below).*

Buxbaum JN, Chuba JV, Hellman GC, et al.: Monoclonal immunoglobulin deposition disease: Light chain and light and heavy chain deposition diseases and their relation to light chain amyloidosis. Ann Intern Med 112:455, 1990. *Comparison of clinical and laboratory features of fibrillar and nonfibrillar Ig deposition (71 references).*

Castano EM, Frangione B: Human amyloidosis, Alzheimer disease and related disorders. Lab Invest 58:122, 1988. *A review of the human amyloidoses with emphasis on pathogenesis as related to the structure of the fibrils and their precursors (141 references).*

Isobe T, Araki S, Uchino F, et al.: Amyloid and Amyloidosis. New York, Plenum Press, 1988. *The proceedings of the Fifth International Symposium, summarizing current work and thinking in the field, including clinical, epidemiologic, and basic science reports covering all forms of amyloidosis.*

Johnson KH, O'Brien TD, Betsholtz C, et al.: Islet amyloid, islet amyloid polypeptide and diabetes mellitus. N Engl J Med 321:513, 1989. *A concise description of the structure of the fibril of pancreatic amyloid and its potential role as a mediator of the pathogenesis of type II diabetes mellitus (46 references).*

Kyle RA, Greipp PR: Amyloidosis (AL), clinical and laboratory features in 229 cases. Mayo Clin Proc 58:665, 1983. *The Mayo Clinic experience, with an excellent description of the relevant features of the most commonly encountered clinical form of amyloid (117 references).*

*This use is not listed in the manufacturer's directive.

198 Hereditary Syndromes Involving Multiple Organ Systems

Arno G. Motulsky

The emergence of clinical genetics as a specialty has led to the definition of a large number of previously undifferentiated birth defects and syndromes. In some of these diseases the origin is monogenic, and multiple organ involvement is caused by the action of the mutant gene in various tissues. In other cases, a detectable chromosomal error or a known teratogen (such as Dilantin) causes multiorgan birth defects. Most frequently, neither a specific genetic nor environmental cause can be identified. Clinical genetics has grown rapidly, and most physicians are unable to keep abreast of the many newly described syndromes.

While most of these conditions become manifest in infancy or childhood, adolescent and adult patients with such conditions often initially come to internists and primary care physicians, who should be aware of the various diagnostic, genetic, and management problems. A vague diagnosis of "multiple birth defects" or "genetic syndrome" usually is not sufficient. Optimal care often requires knowledge of the specific diagnosis and natural history of a given syndrome and appropriate genetic counseling must be based on a definite diagnosis. The reader is referred to various textbooks and compendia for orientation and diagnostic approaches. Because of phenotypic variability in most syndromes, diagnosis may be difficult and new syndromes continue to be described. A significant proportion of such cases remain undiagnosed, even by expert dysmorphologists. In this chapter a few selected syndromes are discussed briefly.

Buyse ML (ed.): Birth Defects Encyclopedia. New York, Mosby, 1990. *A massive multiauthored reference book listing all known birth defects regardless of etiology, with descriptions, illustrations, and references. For on-line search and retrieval, contact Maxwell Online, Inc., 8000 Westpark Drive, McLean, VA 22102 (telephone, 800-055-0906).*

de Grouchy J, Turlean J: Clinical Atlas of Human Chromosomes. 2nd ed. New York, John Wiley & Sons, 1984. *A good general reference volume for standard syndromes associated with cytogenetic abnormalities.*

Emery AEH, Rimoin DL: Principles and Practice of Medical Genetics. Vols. 1 and 2. New York, Churchill Livingstone, 1990. *The standard reference text in clinical genetics with full descriptions of disease entities and their genetics.*

Gorlin RJ, Pindborg JJ, Cohen MM Jr (eds.): Syndromes of the Head and Neck, 3rd ed. New York, Oxford University Press, 1990. *Helpful for reference and differential diagnosis.*

Jones KL: Smith's Recognizable Patterns of Human Malformation. 4th ed. Philadelphia, W. B. Saunders Company, 1988. *The short "bible" for description of malformation syndromes. Many photographs and accounts of many different types of defects. Practically useful.*

McKusick V: Mendelian Inheritance in Man. 9th ed. Baltimore, Johns Hopkins University Press, 1990. *Standard reference source listing definite and possible monogenic diseases, traits, and syndromes with short descriptions and literature citations. Continuously updated and also available with computer access. Contact OMIM User Support, Welch Medical Library, 1830 E. Monument Street, Baltimore, MD 21205 (telephone, 301-955-7058).*

Schinzel A: Catalogue of Unbalanced Chromosome Aberrations in Man. New York, W. de Gruyter, 1984. *The definitive detailed reference for unbalanced chromosomal aberrations.*

WERNER'S SYNDROME

Werner's syndrome is a rare disorder with some clinical features that resemble early aging. Onset of clinical findings is usually in the second or third decade. Affected patients are short because of absence of the adolescent growth spurt and have slender limbs. There is premature graying and then loss of hair. Atrophy and hyperkeratosis of the skin with ulcerations around the feet are often seen. A characteristic squeaky voice and atrophy of muscle, fat, and bone of the extremities are the rule. Soft tissue calcifications usually develop. Atherosclerosis is premature with coronary heart disease and medial calcification of peripheral vessels. Juvenile cataracts and osteoporosis are typical. Hypogonadism occurs in both sexes, and mild diabetes is common. Malignant tumors occur in about 10 per cent of cases, with an unusually high occurrence of meningiomas and sarcomas. Mean age of death is in the early 40's. The phenotype of Werner's syndrome has been considered a "caricature" of senescence rather than a true model of the normal aging process. The condition is inherited as an autosomal recessive trait. Fibroblasts from skin biopsies of patients with Werner's syndrome are difficult to culture. They grow more slowly, assume a senescent morphology more rapidly, and demonstrate a markedly reduced lifespan in vitro. DNA repair is normal. Karyotype preparations show a normal number of chromosomes, but spontaneously increased chromosome breakage and variable stable chromosomal rearrangements such as translocations involving several chromosomes (variegated translocation mosaicism) are seen. Werner's syndrome therefore can be classified among the group of chromosomal instability syndromes. No single enzymatic defect has been discovered yet to explain the multiple clinical, biochemical, and cytogenetic manifestations. Werner's syndrome is sometimes termed adult progeria, but it is entirely unrelated to the pediatric syndrome of progeria (Hutchinson-Gilford), in which death occurs in early adolescence from cardiac or cerebrovascular disease.

Epstein CJ, Martin GM, Schultz AL, et al.: The Werner's syndrome. Medicine 45:177, 1966. *A detailed summary of clinical and laboratory characteristics of 125 cases of Werner's syndrome.*

Salk W, Fujiwara Y, Martin GM (eds.): Werner's Syndrome and Human Aging. New York, Plenum Press, 1985. *Many articles dealing with more recent studies.*

SYNDROMES ASSOCIATED WITH HYPOGONADISM AND VARIOUS CONGENITAL ANOMALIES

LAURENCE-MOON-BARDET-BIEDL SYNDROME AND RELATED DISORDERS. The Laurence-Moon-Bardet-Biedl syndrome exhibits retinal dystrophy (usually pigmentary retinopathy), truncal obesity, hypogonadism, variable mild to severe mental retardation, and polydactyly. Renal structural or functional abnormalities are very common. Total blindness usually occurs after the age of 30 years. Hypogonadism is less frequently found in females, as are mental retardation and polydactyly. Interstitial nephritis may lead to renal failure.

Some investigators (the "splitters") distinguish between the Bardet-Biedl and the Laurence-Moon syndrome by the presence of spastic paraplegia and the absence of polydactyly and obesity in the latter condition. However, others (the "lumpers") believe that these distinctions relate to variable expression of a single disorder.

Alstrom's syndrome appears distinct and is also associated with retinal dystrophy and obesity. Affected patients are usually blind in early childhood and develop moderately severe deafness before age 10. Diabetes mellitus and slowly progressive chronic nephropathy in young adults are seen. Mental retardation and digital anomalies are not encountered.

Carpenter's syndrome (acrocephalopolysyndactyly) is a syndrome characterized by acrocephaly, syndactyly, and a characteristic facial appearance associated with polydactyly of the feet, obesity, mental retardation, and hypogonadism. The various characteristic skeletal findings should cause few diagnostic difficulties.

All these conditions (the syndromes of Laurence-Moon-Bardet-Biedl, Alstrom, Carpenter) are inherited as autosomal recessive traits.

PRADER-WILLI SYNDROME. In this not uncommon condition, infants are born with severe hypotonia and feeding difficulties. Boys exhibit a small penis and cryptorchidism. Thin, turned-down upper lips and up-slanting palpebral fissures are often seen. Skin and hair color tend to be fair and darken with age. Compulsive hyperphagia with development of severe central obesity occurs in later childhood. Hands and feet are characteristically small (acromicria). Young adults may present with pickwickian syndrome manifesting as cardiopulmonary compromise and somnolence. Severe obesity is the major cause of morbidity and mortality in this disorder. This syndrome is the most common syndromal cause of marked obesity. Affected patients are short, and there is hypogonadotrophic hypogonadism with sterility. Menstruation may be delayed or does not occur. Mild to severe mental retardation with behavioral and personality problems are the rule. Mild diabetes mellitus is often seen.

In many cases a chromosome abnormality affecting band q11-12 of the long arm of chromosome 15 has been detected by high-resolution methods. The defect usually is a small deletion in chromosome 15 transmitted from the clinically unaffected father. Although the syndrome usually occurs as a sporadic event, extremely rare familial cases have been reported. Parental chromosomes are usually normal or are balanced translocations. It is likely that an as yet undetectable chromosomal defect exists in those cases in which no visible chromosomal abnormality has been found. The relationship of the unique and specific chromosomal deletion to the pathogenesis of the syndrome remains unknown. An identical chromosome defect (15q11-12), if transmitted from the mother, causes the completely different Angelman (happy puppet) syndrome. These findings illustrate the important role of parental "imprinting" on chromosomal expression during development. The same defect has different effects, depending upon maternal or paternal origin.

NOONAN'S PHENOTYPE. This phenotype is often diagnosed, but its boundaries are not sharply defined because of marked clinical variability. Its frequency has been estimated as 1 in 1000 to 1 in 2500. There are no chromosomal abnormalities, in contrast to the Turner syndrome (XO) that it somewhat resembles ("male" Turner syndrome). However, females can be affected as well. Affected adolescents and adults have a triangular micrognathic facial appearance with frequent hypertelorism, occasional ptosis, and posteriorly angulated low-set ears with a thick helix. A short webbed neck is common. The simultaneous presence of superior pectus carinatum and inferior pectus excavatum is helpful diagnostically. Pulmonary valve stenosis is seen frequently and can be accompanied by other types of congenital heart defects. Mild mental retardation is occasionally found. Lymphatic dysplasia causing lymphedema and a mild bleeding tendency (Factor XI deficiency or von Willebrandt disease or thrombocytopenia) occur sometimes.

Autosomal dominant inheritance can be frequently documented, but many cases are sporadic and presumably caused by new mutations. Careful examination of first-degree relatives often shows minor signs of the condition.

Allanson JE: Noonan syndrome: Am J Med Genet 24:9, 1987. *A useful review.*

Butler MG: Prader-Willi syndrome: Current understanding of cause and diagnosis. Am J Med Genet 35:319, 1990. *Review of all aspects (including detailed cytogenetics) of the syndrome.*

Green JS, Parfrey PS, Harnett JD, et al.: The cardinal manifestations of Bardet-Biedl syndrome—a form of Lawrence-Moon-Biedl syndrome. N Engl J Med 321:1002, 1989. *Clinical findings of the syndrome among 32 patients in Newfoundland.*

Greenswag LR: Adults with Prader-Willi syndrome. A survey of 232 cases. Dev Med Child Neurol 29:145, 1987. *Review with special attention to adults.*

Ranke MB, Heidemann P, Kupfer C, et al.: Noonan syndrome, growth and clinical manifestations in 144 cases. Eur J Pediatr 148:220, 1988. *Review of clinical findings.*

Schachat AP, Maumenee IH: The Bardet-Biedl syndrome and related disorders. Arch Ophthalmol 100:285, 1982. *A critical assessment of these conditions.*

PART XV

NUTRITIONAL DISEASES

199 Nutrient Requirements

Robert M. Russell

Recommended Dietary Allowances

Recommended Dietary Allowances (RDA's) have been established for most essential nutrients by the Food and Nutrition Board of the National Academy of Sciences. A nutrient is defined as essential if its absence from the diet results in a deficiency disease. For certain nutrients, notably some trace elements, essentiality has not been established. The United States RDA's are but one set of many recommendations put out by various countries and organizations (e.g., World Health Organization, Food and Agriculture Organization). In the United States the RDA's are used as a standard upon which several food assistance programs are based. For example, the school lunch program must meet 33 per cent of the RDA's for 12-year-old children in its meal planning. It is necessary in meeting such standards, however, that planners choose foods that will be eaten and enjoyed. The RDA's (Table 199–1) do not represent nutrient requirements for individuals; they are designed as guidelines for the daily intake of nutrients sufficient to ensure that almost all members of the population are not at risk of developing nutrient deficits. Thus, the RDA's exceed the nutrient requirements for most healthy individuals. Recommendations for energy intakes are an exception in that they represent values derived by multiplying resting energy expenditure (REE) by an activity factor for particular age and sex groups.

RDA's have been determined by balance studies, measurement of the amount of a nutrient needed to result in tissue saturation, examination of the food supplies of healthy populations, examination of minimal nutrient intakes required to prevent or correct either a naturally occurring or an experimentally produced deficit, epidemiologic observations, and animal studies. Precise RDA's have not been established for some nutrients (e.g., biotin, manganese) because of limited experimental data. However, ranges of safe intakes of these nutrients have been determined by the National Academy of Sciences and are provided in Table 199–2. Continued consumption of trace minerals above the upper limit of the recommended ranges can lead to toxic effects, as is the case with most individual nutrients.

The RDA's should be met by a variety of foods for two major reasons. First, certain dietary components (e.g., carotene, fiber, and possibly others as yet undefined) that are not considered "required" may nevertheless have a beneficial effect on body functioning. For example, if an individual is limited to a diet containing only preformed vitamin A, he or she could be deprived of the alleged beneficial effects of carotene (a vitamin A precursor). Second, a monotonous diet over a prolonged period may not supply a beneficial ratio of individual nutrients (e.g., a diet of very high carbohydrate content may increase the body's need for thiamine). Although other nutrient interactions have been defined (vitamin B_{12} is necessary for the demethylation of 5-methyl tetrahydrofolate; zinc is needed for the oxidation of retinol to photochemically active retinaldehyde), many such interactions are not fully known at present.

Body growth, body size, pregnancy, and lactation alter the RDA's. Pregnancy increases nutrient needs for the expansion of blood volume and for the growth and development of the fetus, placenta, uterus, and breasts. Similarly, lactation increases nutrient needs in proportion to the quantity of milk produced. Pregnancy and lactation RDA adjustments are provided in Table

199–1. Other factors that result in an alteration of dietary needs include environmental temperature, fever, menstruation (an increased requirement for iron), disease, and medication. Disease and/or drugs may change nutrient requirements by altering nutrient absorption or bioavailability, storage capacity, or excretion or by changing a nutrient's metabolism. For example, kidney disease may result in a decreased ability to change 25-hydroxyvitamin D to its active 1,25-dihydroxylated form (Ch. 233); drugs that stimulate microsomal cytochrome P-450-mediated enzyme activities (e.g., alcohol) cause an increased hepatic metabolism of vitamin A. The physician should remember that the RDA's were not designed for sick or traumatized patients or for individuals with metabolic disorders such as hyperthyroidism. Despite all of these caveats, the RDA's do serve as useful guidelines for the practitioner to judge the adequacy of an individual's diet. Table 199–3 provides a guide to the possible effects of medication on nutrient requirements and the mechanisms by which these interactions occur.

Nutrient requirements and dietary recommendations for adults are defined in broad age classes in Table 199–1, namely 19 to 24 years, 25 to 50 years, and 51 years and older. In the absence of adequate information, the present recommendations for the elderly are the same as for the young adult population. However, old people eat fewer calories than young people, and accompanying this diminished calorie intake is a concomitant reduction in intake of almost all other nutrients. For nutrients whose requirements are fixed (rather than relative to calories), such across-the-board reductions may result in intakes that are insufficient to meet metabolic demands; for example, the amount of dietary protein needed for nitrogen equilibrium is not reduced with age. Age-related changes affect the absorption, metabolism, and excretion of many nutrients, so that age-specific standards for the elderly are needed. In addition, chronic disability, illness, and the increased use of medications in the elderly introduce other variables. Suffice it to say that the elderly person's diet should be of high quality in terms of nutrient density (i.e., quantity of nutrients/calorie).

Since parenteral administration of some nutrients bypasses any problems due to limited absorption, nutrient requirements are generally less when delivered by the parenteral route than by the enteral route. However, the underlying cause (e.g., disease, trauma) that necessitates parenteral delivery in a patient often dictates overall higher nutrient requirements (see Ch. 207).

WATER

Owing to a high ratio of surface area to volume, infants are more prone to dehydration than adults. The average adult needs a minimum of 700 to 1000 ml of water per day in order to survive, but 2000 ml per day (1 ml per Kcal intake) provides a safe and adequate basal maintenance amount. Approximately 100 ml per day of water is lost in feces, 500 to 1000 ml in evaporation and exhalation (insensible loss), and the remainder in urine. Diets providing a high renal solute load (e.g., diets high in protein, sodium, potassium, chloride) will result in higher urinary water losses. In a sick patient additional water must be supplied if body temperature is elevated (each 1°C elevation over normal results in an additional obligatory water loss of 200 ml per day), if diarrhea is present, or if polyuria is present (e.g., from uncontrolled diabetes mellitus or kidney disease). In such cases, measured losses may be added to the maintenance requirements. Elevated environmental temperature and exercise increase insensible losses (for each 2°C rise in temperature above 32°C, 500 ml of extra water should be provided). Acute alterations in water balance can be estimated by rapid changes in body weight.

TABLE 199–1. FOOD AND NUTRITION BOARD, NATIONAL ACADEMY OF SCIENCES—NATIONAL RESEARCH COUNCIL RECOMMENDED DIETARY ALLOWANCES,ᵃ Revised 1989

Designed for the maintenance of good nutrition of practically all healthy people in the United States

Category	Age (years) or Condition	Weightᵇ (kg)	Weightᵇ (lb)	Heightᵇ (cm)	Heightᵇ (in)	Protein (g)	Vitamin A (μg RE)ᶜ	Vitamin D (μg)ᵈ	Vitamin E (mg α-TE)ᵉ	Vitamin K (μg)	Vitamin C (mg)	Thiamine (mg)	Riboflavin (mg)	Niacin (mg NE)ᶠ	Vitamin B6 (mg)	Folate (μg)	Vitamin B12 (μg)	Calcium (mg)	Phosphorus (mg)	Magnesium (mg)	Iron (mg)	Zinc (mg)	Iodine (μg)	Selenium (μg)
Infants	0.0–0.5	6	13	60	24	13	375	7.5	3	5	30	0.3	0.4	5	0.3	25	0.3	400	300	40	6	5	40	10
	0.5–1.0	9	20	71	28	14	375	10	4	10	35	0.4	0.5	6	0.6	35	0.5	600	500	60	10	5	50	15
Children	1–3	13	29	90	35	16	400	10	6	15	40	0.7	0.8	9	1.0	50	0.7	800	800	80	10	10	70	20
	4–7	20	44	112	44	24	500	10	7	20	45	0.9	1.1	12	1.1	75	1.0	800	800	120	10	10	90	20
	7–10	28	62	132	52	28	700	10	7	30	45	1.0	1.2	13	1.4	100	1.4	800	800	170	10	10	120	30
Males	11–14	45	99	157	62	45	1,000	10	10	45	50	1.3	1.5	17	1.7	150	2.0	1,200	1,200	270	12	15	150	40
	15–18	66	145	176	69	59	1,000	10	10	65	60	1.5	1.8	20	2.0	200	2.0	1,200	1,200	400	12	15	150	50
	19–24	72	160	177	70	58	1,000	10	10	70	60	1.5	1.7	19	2.0	200	2.0	1,200	1,200	350	10	15	150	70
	25–50	79	174	176	70	63	1,000	5	10	80	60	1.5	1.7	19	2.0	200	2.0	800	800	350	10	15	150	70
	51+	77	170	173	68	63	1,000	5	10	80	60	1.2	1.4	15	2.0	200	2.0	800	800	350	10	15	150	70
Females	11–14	46	101	157	62	46	800	10	8	45	50	1.1	1.3	15	1.4	150	2.0	1,200	1,200	280	15	12	150	45
	15–18	55	120	163	64	44	800	10	8	55	60	1.1	1.3	15	1.5	180	2.0	1,200	1,200	300	15	12	150	50
	19–24	58	128	164	65	46	800	10	8	60	60	1.1	1.3	15	1.6	180	2.0	1,200	1,200	280	15	12	150	55
	25–50	63	138	163	64	50	800	5	8	65	60	1.1	1.3	15	1.6	180	2.0	800	800	280	15	12	150	55
	51+	65	143	160	63	50	800	5	8	65	60	1.0	1.2	13	1.6	180	2.0	800	800	280	10	12	150	55
Pregnant						60	800	10	10	65	70	1.5	1.6	17	2.2	400	2.2	1,200	1,200	320	30	15	175	65
Lactating	1st 6 months					65	1,300	10	12	65	95	1.6	1.8	20	2.1	280	2.6	1,200	1,200	355	15	19	200	75
	2nd 6 months					62	1,200	10	11	65	90	1.6	1.7	20	2.1	260	2.6	1,200	1,200	340	15	16	200	75

ᵃThe allowances, expressed as average daily intakes over time, are intended to provide for individual variations among most normal persons as they live in the United States under usual environmental stresses. Diets should be based on a variety of common foods in order to provide other nutrients for which human requirements have been less well defined.

ᵇWeights and heights of Reference Adults are actual medians for the designated age, as reported by NHANES II. The use of these figures does not imply that the height-to-weight ratios are ideal.

ᶜRetinol equivalents. 1 retinol equivalent = 1 μg retinol or 6 μg β-carotene.

ᵈAs cholecalciferol. 10 μg cholecalciferol = 400 IU of vitamin D.

ᵉα-Tocopherol equivalents; 1 mg D-α-tocopherol = 1 α-TE.

ᶠ1 NE (niacin equivalent) is equal to 1 mg of niacin or 60 mg of dietary tryptophan.

TABLE 199–2. ESTIMATED SAFE AND ADEQUATE DAILY DIETARY INTAKES OF SELECTED VITAMINS AND MINERALS[a]

Category	Age (years)	Vitamins		Trace Elements[b]				
		Biotin (μg)	Pantothenic Acid (mg)	Copper (mg)	Manganese (mg)	Fluoride (mg)	Chromium (μg)	Molybdenum (μg)
Infants	0–0.5	10	2	0.4–0.6	0.3–0.6	0.1–0.5	10–40	15–30
	0.5–1	15	3	0.6–0.7	0.6–1.0	0.2–1.0	20–60	20–40
Children and adolescents	1–3	20	3	0.7–1.0	1.0–1.5	0.5–1.5	20–80	25–50
	4–6	25	3–4	1.0–1.5	1.5–2.0	1.0–2.5	30–120	30–75
	7–10	30	4–5	1.0–2.0	2.0–3.0	1.5–2.5	50–200	50–150
	11+	30–100	4–7	1.5–2.5	2.0–5.0	1.5–2.5	50–200	75–250
Adults		30–100	4–7	1.5–3.0	2.0–5.0	1.5–4.0	50–200	75–250

[a]Because there is less information on which to base allowances, these figures are not given in Table 199–1 and are provided here in the form of ranges of recommended intakes.

[b]Since the toxic levels for many trace elements may be only several times usual intakes, the upper levels for the trace elements given in this table should not be habitually exceeded.

ENERGY

Energy needs vary with body size, growth phase, age, sex, and activity. Factors that increase energy requirements are cold exposure, pregnancy, lactation, infection, fever, hyperthyroidism, and trauma. Recommended energy allowances for all ages are presented in Table 199–4. A normal variation of ± 20 per cent is accepted for younger adults, the ranges being wider for children. In pregnancy, energy allowances should be increased 300 Kcal per day for the second and third trimesters of pregnancy. Lactation increases energy requirements by 500 Kcal per day. The energy allowances for children from birth through age 10 are World Health Organization figures. The allowances for adults are based on median weights and heights from the second U.S. Health and Nutrition Examination Survey (NHANES II) for moderate work (e.g., walking, shopping, playing golf). In addition to the age groups 19 to 24 and 25 to 50 years, energy recommendations for older people are provided for those over age 50. The aging process normally results in a progressive decrease in energy needs, primarily as a result of a decrease in energy expenditure.

Protein and carbohydrate supply approximately 4 Kcal per gram, alcohol 7 Kcal per gram, and fat 9 Kcal per gram. Resting energy expenditure (REE) is the amount of oxygen consumed under resting conditions extrapolated to 24 hours. A simple rule of thumb to estimate REE is 25 Kcal per kilogram body weight. However, this formula is not useful in overweight people. Since adipose tissue is relatively inert from a metabolic point of view, the relationship between REE and body weight becomes nonlinear in overweightness. A more accurate estimate of REE for healthy individuals is the Harris-Benedict equation:

Men: REE = 66 + (13.7 weight in kg) + (5 × height in cm) − 6.8 (age in years)

Women: REE = 665 + (9.6 × weight in kg) + (1.7 × height in cm) − 4.7 (age in years)

Depending on factors such as activity level and illness, energy needs may be increased many times over the basal level. Ingestion and metabolism of food increase the caloric requirement by about 7 per cent of the REE, provided that a mixed diet is being consumed. Activity increases energy requirements over a wide range (1.1 to 10.3 Kcal per kilogram per hour) depending on the intensity and type of work being done. The number of daily calories that should be provided in addition to the REE are 400 to 800 Kcal for sedentary activity, 800 to 1200 Kcal for light activity (e.g., sewing, desk work), and 1200 to 1800 Kcal for moderate work (e.g., walking). The number of kilocalories to be added for heavy work (e.g., running, swimming) ranges from 1800 to 4500 Kcal per day. Although fasting and malnutrition reduce energy expenditure, the stress of illness increases caloric requirements. For each 1°C of fever, a 13 per cent increase in calories is required. In catabolic patients, 50 to 100 per cent of the REE may be necessary to prevent further tissue breakdown.

PROTEIN

A constant supply of protein (i.e., amino acids) is needed to maintain body function and structure. On a protein-free diet, the average net loss of body protein by males is about 0.34 gram per kilogram of body weight. However, when allowance is made for incomplete utilization of dietary protein and for variability in needs, the allowance recommended for adults rises to 0.75 gram of protein per kilogram. Protein needs are dependent, in part, on energy intake. Increased energy intake results in protein conservation and decreased energy intake results in the diversion of protein to meet energy needs. Pregnancy and lactation increase the body's protein requirement.

There is a continuum of food protein quality depending on the digestibility of the protein and its amino acid composition. Nine essential amino acids must be provided in the diet, since the human body lacks the ability to synthesize them. These are lysine, leucine, isoleucine, valine, methionine, phenylalanine, tryptophan, threonine, and possibly histidine, especially for infants.

High-quality proteins are those that have a high degree of bioavailability (i.e., they are easily digested and absorbed) and have a high biologic value (a measure of the efficiency of utilization of absorbed protein, which in turn is dependent on adequate amounts and proportions of essential amino acids). The highest quality proteins are found in eggs and milk. Seeds and nuts, rice, corn, and grain proteins are of lesser quality. It is recommended that 10 to 15 per cent of caloric intake be derived from protein. Amino acids supplied in excess of the body's requirement are not

TABLE 199–3. EXAMPLES OF DRUG-NUTRIENT INTERACTIONS

Drug	Increased Requirement	Potential Mechanism	Deficiency Symptoms
Antacids (aluminum and magnesium hydroxides)	Phosphate	Formation of insoluble salts	Malaise, paresthesias, anorexia
Anticonvulsants (phenobarbital, phenytoin)	Vitamin D	Induction of hepatic microsomal enzymes resulting in inactive vitamin D metabolites	Rickets, osteomalacia
Oral contraceptives (norethindrone/mestranol)	Folic acid	Inhibition of polyglutamic folate absorption	Megaloblastic anemia
Antituberculous drugs (isoniazid, cycloserine)	Vitamin B$_6$	Excretion of pyridoxal hydrazone complex	Peripheral neuropathy
Anticoagulants (coumarin, warfarin)	Vitamin K	Inhibition of vitamin K recycling	Hypoprothrombinemia
Diuretics (benzothiadiazides)	Potassium	Enhancement of renal excretion	Hypokalemia

TABLE 199–4. MEDIAN REFERENCE HEIGHTS AND WEIGHTS AND RECOMMENDED ENERGY INTAKE

Category	Age (years) or Condition	Weight (kg)	Weight (lb)	Height (cm)	Height (in)	REE[a] (Kcal/day)	Average Energy Allowance (Kcal)[b] Multiples of REE	Average Energy Allowance (Kcal)[b] per Kg per Day[c]	Average Energy Allowance (Kcal)[b]
Infants	0.0–0.5	6	13	60	24	320		108	650
	0.5–1.0	9	20	71	28	500		98	850
Children	1–3	13	29	90	35	740		102	1,300
	4–6	20	44	112	44	950		90	1,800
	7–10	28	62	132	52	1,130		70	2,000
Males	11–14	45	99	157	62	1,440	1.70	55	2,500
	15–18	66	145	176	69	1,760	1.67	45	3,000
	19–24	72	160	177	70	1,780	1.67	40	2,900
	25–50	79	174	176	70	1,800	1.60	37	2,900
	51+	77	170	173	68	1,530	1.50	30	2,300
Females	11–14	46	101	157	62	1,310	1.67	47	2,200
	15–18	55	120	163	64	1,370	1.60	40	2,200
	19–24	58	128	164	65	1,350	1.60	38	2,200
	25–50	63	138	163	64	1,380	1.55	36	2,200
	51+	65	143	160	63	1,280	1.50	30	1,900
Pregnant	1st trimester								+0
	2nd trimester								+300
	3rd trimester								+300
Lactating	1st 6 months								+500
	2nd 6 months								+500

[a]Calculation based on Food and Agricultural Organization equations, then rounded.
[b]In the range of light to moderate activity, the coefficient of variation is ±20%.
[c]Figure is rounded.
Source: Food and Nutrition Board, National Academy of Sciences–National Research Council, Recommended Dietary Allowances, revised 1989.

stored but are degraded to metabolic products (urea, uric acid, etc.), and the carbon skeleton is converted to carbohydrate and fat or oxidized for energy. It is important that a mixed diet be consumed so that adequate amounts of each essential amino acid are received. Some amino acids are complementary; for example, tyrosine may in part meet the body's requirement for phenylalanine, and cystine may in part meet the body's requirement for methionine. The ability of the body to utilize protein is impaired if one essential amino acid is missing, underscoring the need for mixed sources of dietary proteins.

In parenterally fed patients, zero nitrogen balance may be achieved with as little as 0.5 gram per kilogram per day of mixed amino acids (including all essential amino acids). However, patients with abnormal losses or increased demands (burns, trauma, wound repair) may require 1.2 to 1.6 grams per kilogram of desirable body weight per day.

In the clinical setting, the state of nitrogen balance can be crudely estimated by measuring the 24-hour urinary urea nitrogen excretion:

$$\text{Nitrogen balance} = \frac{\text{protein intake (g)}}{6.25} - [\text{urinary urea nitrogen (g)} + 4]$$

CARBOHYDRATE

Carbohydrate supplies 65 per cent of the world's food energy (50 per cent in developed countries, 75 per cent in developing countries), and of this 10 to 50 per cent is from simple sugars. Although a diet low in carbohydrate may result in ketosis, there is no fixed requirement for carbohydrate in the diet. Carbohydrate may be divided into available (i.e., digestible and utilizable as sugars) and unavailable (i.e., dietary fiber). The primary sources of both available and unavailable carbohydrates are of vegetable origin. Dietary fiber reaches the large intestine intact but then may undergo fermentation by bacteria, with the subsequent absorption of breakdown products and some "rescue" of calories. Dietary fiber is made up of crude fiber (cellulose, lignin), mucilages, pectins, hemicellulose, and water-soluble gums. Each type of fiber has different characteristics with regard to water holding, cation exchange, and adsorptive properties (e.g., for bile acids and drugs). For example, mucilages have a high capacity for water holding, and pectins avidly adsorb bile acids. Increases in stool weight and faster intestinal transit result from increases in dietary fiber. Primarily because of epidemiologic disease patterns (e.g., for colon cancer and diverticulitis), an increase of dietary fiber has been suggested. At least 20 to 25 grams of dietary fiber per day are needed for a therapeutic effect in the

irritable bowel syndrome. Gums and pectins have been shown to have a beneficial effect on diabetes by delaying the absorption of glucose. As with most dietary components, too much fiber may be harmful: Large amounts of dietary fiber may contribute to trace metal deficiency in certain parts of the world by adsorbing divalent cations (e.g., zinc) and making them unavailable for gastrointestinal absorption. Carbohydrate intolerance syndromes (e.g., lactose intolerance) are described in Ch. 102.

FAT

Fat, a concentrated source of calories, serves as a carrier for fat-soluble vitamins and as a source of essential fatty acids. All body cells with the exception of the central nervous system and erythrocytes can directly utilize fatty acids as a source of energy. Polyunsaturated essential fatty acids (linoleic, linolenic) and their derivatives serve as precursors for eicosanoids, which include the leukotrienes, prostaglandins, and thromboxanes. They are also needed for membrane structure and integrity. Polyunsaturated fatty acids have been shown to promote carcinogenesis in experimental animals, however, and may reduce circulating HDL cholesterol and promote gallstone formation. Thus, an upper limit of 10 per cent of calories taken in as polyunsaturated fats is advised. Monounsaturated fatty acids are effective for optimizing plasma lipoproteins. There is recent interest in the role of N-3 polyunsaturated fatty acids, derived from linolenic acid or from fish oils, in the prevention of ischemic heart disease. However, more investigation is needed on the interaction between N-6 and N-3 fatty acids in human tissue before sound dietary recommendations can be made. Linoleic acid is a prominent component of dietary fats, but deficiency has been recognized only among patients on prolonged parenteral feedings containing no fat. Two per cent of calories in the form of linoleic acid and 0.5 per cent as linolenic acid are sufficient for preventing essential fatty acid deficiency.

VITAMINS AND MINERALS

Requirements for vitamins and minerals are discussed in Ch. 204 and 205.

NUTRITIONAL RECOMMENDATIONS

The Surgeon General's Report on Nutrition and Health published in 1988 outlines prudent dietary recommendations for the United States population in order to avoid diseases and disabilities that appear to have a relation to diet. Other sets of similar recommendations have been proposed by organizations such as the American Heart Association and the National Cancer Institute. Such dietary goals include a reduction in the percentage of calories ingested as fat by the United States public from 37 per cent to 30 per cent (<10 per cent saturated, <10 per cent polyunsaturated). At least 12 per cent of total calories should be ingested as protein. Further recommendations are that total calories ingested as carbohydrate be increased to approximately 60 per cent, with an increase in complex carbohydrates (e.g., starches, fiber) and naturally occurring sugars to approximately 50 per cent. Refined and processed sugar ingestion should be decreased to about 10 per cent of the total caloric intake. With a view toward reducing coronary artery disease, the American Heart Association recommends, in addition, a restriction of dietary cholesterol to less than 300 mg per day and of sodium to less than 3 grams per day. The judicious diet is outlined in detail in Ch. 12.

Diet and Health. Washington, D.C., National Academy of Sciences, 1989. *A comprehensive analysis of the scientific literature on the role of diet in the etiology and prevention of chronic disease in the United States.*

Energy and Protein Requirements, Report of a Joint FAO/WHO/UNU Expert Consultation. Geneva, WHO, 1985.

National Research Council: Recommended Dietary Allowances, 10th ed. Washington, D.C., National Academy of Sciences, 1989.

Roe DA: Drug Induced Nutritional Deficiencies, 2nd ed. Westport, CT, AVI Publishing Company, Inc., 1985.

The Surgeon General's Report on Nutrition and Health. US Dept of Health and Human Services (DHHS) Publication No 88-50211. Washington, D.C., 1988. *This report's major conclusion is that overconsumption of fat at the expense of foods high in complex carbohydrates is detrimental to health.*

200 Nutritional Assessment

Robert M. Russell

The recognition and treatment of malnutrition that accompanies illness play important roles in optimizing patient care. New modes of delivering nutrients to sick patients by both the parenteral and enteral routes may result in reductions in morbidity and mortality and shorten the length of hospitalization for both medical and surgical patients (Ch. 206 and 207).

Methods of nutritional assessment that have been used for some time to judge the severity of malnutrition among populations in lesser developed countries (e.g., anthropometric measures) are now being applied to hospitalized patients. An unexpectedly high prevalence (up to 40 per cent) of protein-energy malnutrition has been identified among Western patients. Reasons for the lack of recognition of malnutrition in hospitalized patients include preoccupation with the treatment of the disease process, neglect of the overall nutritional status of the patient (e.g., failure to obtain regular weights or to observe a patient's dietary intake), lack of sensitivity of casual observation in the recognition of protein-energy malnutrition, absence of a single indicator for diagnosis of malnutrition, and latent onset of clinical signs of malnutrition and relative lack of specificity of these signs. A single nutrient deficiency rarely occurs in a patient; rather, a complex and confusing array of deficiencies is most often present.

The diagnosis of malnutrition should be made on the basis of several consolidated pieces of information, including dietary history, anthropometric and laboratory measurements, and clinical examination. By using all of this information in a coordinated fashion, a more accurate diagnosis of the malnourished can be achieved, and an effective plan of treatment can be instituted.

DIET

It is not expected that the physician will interpret dietary records of a patient in detail. However, a physician should be able to perform a dietary evaluation by assessing the intakes of major food groups (milk-yogurt-cheese, meat-poultry-fish-eggs, fruits-vegetables, breads-cereals-grains, alcohol, fats such as oil, butter, bacon, and gravy) and the quality of selection within these groups. This is best done by asking the patient to recall all foods eaten within the last 24 hours (including snacks) and the approximate portion sizes. A mixed diet is a desirable goal, when advising patients on healthful diets (Ch. 12). Moreover, the clinician should be aware of the key questions to ask patients, which provide clues about whether or not the patient's dietary intake requires adjustment (Table 200–1). A detailed medical and social history can alert the physician to an existing dietary problem or the likelihood of a dietary problem occurring in the future. For example, poverty, physical or mental disability, complaints of dysphagia, anorexia, nausea, abdominal pain while eating, ill-fitting dentures, and alcoholism may all be factors that prevent adequate dietary intake. Increased nutritional requirements can result from diarrhea, fever, open wounds or burns, malabsorption, diabetes, and hyperthyroidism. The physician should be able to counsel patients regarding general dietary guidelines (Ch. 12) and recognize cases for referral to a dietitian for more detailed counseling.

The elderly are a group with an increased risk of malnutrition. The reasons for this include poverty, the inability to move around easily, the cumulative effects of chronic disease necessitating multiple medications, social isolation, and the lack of knowledge for adequate preparation of meals (particularly among elderly men). Problems often arise when interviewing the elderly person for dietary habits (e.g., by 24-hour dietary recall, food frequency questionnaires) if the individual is senile or has impaired short-term memory. Even a 3- to 7-day dietary record, wherein the patient records everything eaten during that period, has proven difficult for the elderly patient to keep. A family member may therefore be of great assistance when obtaining dietary information. Finally, appropriate standards for judging the elderly person's diet are not currently available. The Recommended Dietary Allowances (see Table 199–1) were developed as population standards (not individual requirements) and are set to meet the needs of most healthy individuals. The standards for adults are based almost exclusively on young adults. As a result, they may not be appropriate for meeting the needs of the elderly patient who has an array of chronic diseases or aging disorders, or both.

ANTHROPOMETRIC MEASUREMENTS

Sophisticated and specialized methods to assess body composition are available, e.g., underwater weighing for body density, CT scanning, neutron activation analysis, and ^{40}K counting. However, none of these methods is available for widespread clinical use. Anthropometric reference values derived from measurements on normal populations provide inexpensive, quick, and convenient estimates of a patient's nutritional status in terms of protein and fat reserves. The most useful anthropometric meas-

TABLE 200–1. KEY QUESTIONS TO ASK AS PART OF THE NUTRITIONAL ASSESSMENT OF THE ADULT

1. Is there recent weight gain or weight loss? How much?
2. Are there alterations in appetite, sense of smell, or taste?
3. Are there problems with chewing or swallowing? Does the patient have poor dentition or poorly fitting dentures?
4. Are there symptoms of gastrointestinal disorders: diarrhea, constipation, nausea, vomiting, early satiety?
5. Does the patient live alone? If not, who prepares meals? Does he/she know how to cook?
6. What type of cooking facilities and refrigeration are in the patient's home?
7. Does the patient purchase a variety of foods? If not, is it due to financial difficulties?
8. How many meals are eaten per day? How many snacks? Are one or more meals eaten outside of the home? If so, where?
9. Is the patient physically or mentally handicapped? Does this prevent the individual from shopping, cooking, or feeding herself or himself?
10. Does the patient take any dietary supplements (e.g., vitamins)?
11. How much alcohol does the patient consume?
12. Does the patient use prescription or nonprescription drugs?
13. Are there any religious or ethnic beliefs or food intolerances that prevent adequate food intake?
14. Does the patient follow a dietary restriction? Is it prescribed or self-imposed?
15. Is the patient depressed?

TABLE 200–2. REFERENCE WEIGHTS FOR VARIOUS HEIGHTS DERIVED FROM ACTUARIAL (MORTALITY EXPERIENCE) DATA OF THE 1979 BUILD AND BLOOD PRESSURE STUDY FOR USE IN AGES 20 TO 55*

Height		Weight			
		Male		Female	
in	cm	lb	kg	lb	kg
58	147.3	—	—	114	51.7
59	149.9	—	—	116.5	52.8
60	152.4	—	—	119	53.9
61	154.9	—	—	122	55.3
62	157.5	133	60.3	125	56.7
63	160.0	135	61.2	128	58.0
64	162.6	137.5	62.4	131	59.4
65	165.1	140	63.5	134	60.8
66	167.6	143	64.9	137	62.1
67	170.2	146	66.2	140	63.5
68	172.7	149	67.6	143	64.9
69	175.3	152	68.9	146	66.2
70	177.8	155	70.3	149	67.6
71	180.3	158.5	71.9	152	69.0
72	182.9	162	73.9	—	—
73	185.4	166	75.3	—	—
74	188.0	169.5	76.9	—	—
75	190.5	174	78.9	—	—

*Weights represent the midpoint of the middle frame for each height. These values correct the 1983 Metropolitan Tables to nude weights and heights.

ures include height, weight, triceps skinfold (actually fatfold) thickness, and midarm muscle area. Accurate measurements require only three simple pieces of equipment: a beam or lever balance scale with a vertical measuring rod and a headpiece, a constant tension skinfold caliper, and a flexible measuring tape, preferably with an insertion.

WEIGHT FOR HEIGHT. Single reference weights for each inch of height have been derived from United States life insurance actuarial data on longevity and have been termed "ideal" or "optimal" by some investigators. However, these single weights should not be interpreted as "ideal," since they represent the midpoint of an acceptable range for a person of medium frame and were derived from the mortality experience of only those men and women between the ages of 20 to 59 years who could afford life insurance. These weights are neither age- nor race-specific and do not represent all cultural groups. Further, these reference weights cannot be applied to patients with peripheral edema or ascites. Despite the recognized flaws in using such

TABLE 200–3. MEDIAN WEIGHT FOR VARIOUS HEIGHTS FOR AGE 55 to 74 FROM COMBINED NHANES I AND II DATA SETS

Height		Weight			
		Male		Female	
in	cm	lb	kg	lb	kg
58	147	—	—	125.4	57
59	150	—	—	136.4	62
60	152	—	—	143.0	65
61	155	—	—	140.8	64
62	157	149.6	68	140.8	64
63	160	154.0	70	143.0	65
64	163	156.2	71	145.2	66
65	165	158.4	72	147.4	67
66	168	162.8	74	145.2	66
67	170	171.6	78	158.4	72
68	173	171.6	78	154.0	70
69	175	169.4	77	158.4	72
70	178	176.0	80	160.6	73
71	180	184.8	84	—	—
72	183	178.2	81	—	—
73	185	193.6	88	—	—
74	188	209.0	95	—	—

Adapted from Frisancho AB: Am J Clin Nutr 40:808, 1984.

single reference weights as standards, clinicians have found the 1983 Metropolitan Life Insurance Reference Weights for Height useful for judging a patient's nutritional status reflecting caloric sufficiency. These reference weights (corrected to the nude state) are provided in Table 200–2 and may be used for judging underweightness or overweightness for the population age group 20 to 55. For people over the age of 55 it is recommended to use age-specific weight-for-height median values (medium frame size) derived from the combined data sets of the National Health and Nutrition Examination Surveys of 1971 to 1974 and 1976 to 1980 (NHANES) (Table 200–3). Body mass index (weight ÷ height squared) is another means of assessing relative body weight which has the advantage of minimizing height as a factor in estimating overweightness and underweightness. Body mass index thus partially compensates for the shrinkage in height which takes place during the adult life span (Ch. 203). A nomogram for determining and interpreting body mass index is provided in Figure 200–1. In children, weight and height are often used as separate measures to indicate malnutrition and are expressed as percentiles of a cross-section of American children. Weight and height tables for children can be found in most pediatric textbooks.

The amount of weight lost and the rate at which it was lost by

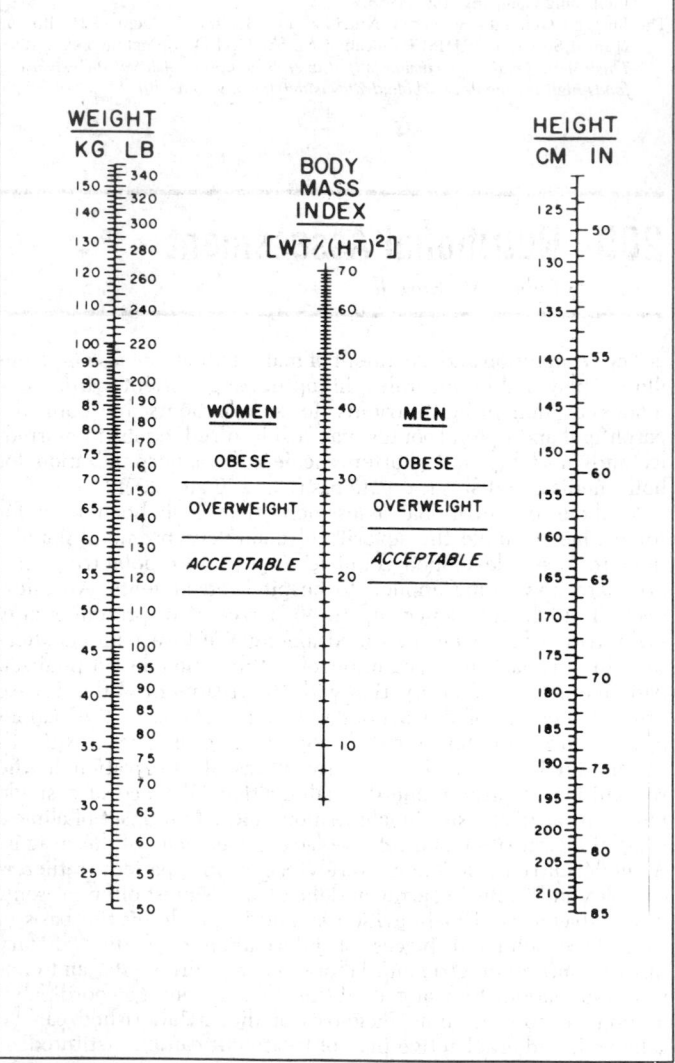

FIGURE 200–1. A nomogram for determining body mass index (BMI). To use this nomogram, place a ruler or other straight edge between the column for height and the column for weight connecting an individual's numbers for those two variables. Read the BMI in kg/m² where the straight line crosses the middle lines when the height and weight are connected. Overweight: BMI of 25–30 kg/m²; obesity: BMI above 30 kg/m². Heights and weights are without shoes or clothes. (From Bray GA: Obesity: definition, diagnoses and disadvantages. Med J Aust 142:S2–S8. Copyright 1985, The Medical Journal of Australia; reprinted with permission.)

TABLE 200-4. SUGGESTED CRITERIA TO JUDGE MALNUTRITION AND OBESITY IN THE UNITED STATES POPULATION

	Standard Male/Female	At Risk for Malnutrition (% of standard)	At Risk for Obesity (% of standard)
Weight/Height			
Age 20–55	Table 200–2	<80	>130
Age >55	Table 200–3	<80	>120
Triceps skinfold (mm)			
Age 25–54	12/23	<50	>170
Age 55–75	12/25	<50	>150
Midarm muscle area (cm²)			
Age 25–54	55/31	<70	NA
Age 55–75	52/35	<65	NA

The percentages below and above the given standards for assessing malnutrition and obesity correspond to less than the 15th percentile and greater than the 85th percentile, respectively, on the combined data sets of NHANES I and II normative values.

a patient are also important for judging an individual's nutritional status. A weight loss of 1 kg represents approximately a 7000-calorie deficit. A history of unintentional weight loss of 10 per cent or greater (6 per cent in an overweight patient) over a 6-month period can be indicative of malnutrition.

TRICEPS SKINFOLD THICKNESS. This measurement provides an estimate of the body's fat reserves. The measurement should be taken at a marked point on the right arm, halfway between the acromial process of the scapula and the olecranon process of the elbow. The patient's arm should be relaxed when the fatfold is grasped posteriorly between the thumb and forefinger of the examiner. The fold should be raised, allowing underlying muscle to fall back to the bone, and the calipers applied. The measurement is useless if arm edema or paralysis is present. Age- and sex-specific standards for triceps skinfold (TSF) thickness for all ages through 75 years are summarized in Table 200–4. A wide range on either side of the standard is considered an acceptable TSF measure, since large variances are found for fatfold thicknesses in the normal population. A patient whose TSF thickness is less than 50 per cent of the NHANES standard is considered to have depleted body fat stores, whereas the patient whose TSF thickness is more than 150 to 170 per cent of standard is considered obese.

MIDARM MUSCLE AREA. This derived value is used to estimate lean body or skeletal muscle mass. To calculate this value, the midarm circumference must first be measured at the same site as for the triceps fatfold, with the patient's right arm in a relaxed posture. The formula to calculate bone-free, upper-arm midarm muscle area (MAMA) is:

$$\frac{\{\text{midarm circumference (cm)} - [0.314 \times \text{TSF (mm)}]\}^2}{4\pi} \begin{array}{l} - 10 \text{ (males)} \\ - 6.5 \text{ (females)} \end{array}$$

Median values are summarized in Table 200–4. Thirty to 35 per cent below this standard (depending upon age) is indicative of a depletion of lean body mass. Neither TSF nor midarm muscle area standards have been derived for the very elderly (i.e., older than 75 years). A summary of criteria to judge malnutrition and obesity by anthropometric measurements is presented in Table 200–4.

CLINICAL ASSESSMENT

By noting certain physical changes in the patient (e.g., temporal muscle wasting, hair depigmentation, edema), the clinician may have the clinical impression of protein-calorie malnutrition, which objective anthropometric and laboratory measurements can confirm. However, early clinical symptoms and signs of malnutrition are rather vague and often include weakness, lethargy, irritability, and lightheadedness. Many of the symptoms and signs are nonspecific for a single nutrient deficit and may be caused by insufficiency of one of several nutrients. For example, flaking dermatitis may accompany deficiencies of protein, riboflavin, or linoleic acid. On the other hand, when certain clinical signs

TABLE 200-5. CLINICAL SIGNS AND SYMPTOMS OF NUTRITIONAL INADEQUACY IN ADULT PATIENTS

	Clinical Sign or Symptom	Nutrient
General	Wasted, skinny	Calorie
	Loss of appetite	Protein-energy
Skin	Psoriasiform rash, eczematous scaling	Zinc
	Pallor	Folate, iron, vitamin B₁₂, copper
	Follicular hyperkeratosis	Vitamin A
	Perifollicular petechiae	Vitamin C
	Flaking dermatitis	Protein-energy, niacin, riboflavin, zinc
	Bruising	Vitamin C, vitamin K
	Pigmentation changes	Niacin, protein-energy
	Scrotal dermatosis	Riboflavin
	Thickening and dryness of skin	Linoleic acid
Head	Temporal muscle wasting	Protein-energy
Hair	Sparse and thin, dyspigmentation	Protein
	Easy to pull out	
Eyes	History of night blindness (also impaired visual recovery after glare)	Vitamin A, zinc
	Photophobia, blurring, conjunctival inflammation	Riboflavin, vitamin A
	Corneal vascularization	Riboflavin
	Xerosis, Bitot spots, keratomalacia	Vitamin A
Mouth	Glossitis	Riboflavin, niacin, folic acid, vitamin B₁₂, pyridoxine
	Bleeding gums	Vitamin C, riboflavin
	Cheilosis	Riboflavin
	Angular stomatitis	Riboflavin, iron
	Hypogeusia	Zinc
	Tongue fissuring	Niacin
	Tongue atrophy	Riboflavin, niacin, iron
	Scarlet and raw tongue	Niacin
	Nasolabial seborrhea	Pyridoxine
Neck	Goiter	Iodine
	Parotid enlargement	Protein
Thorax	Thoracic rosary	Vitamin D
Abdomen	Diarrhea	Niacin, folate, vitamin B₁₂
	Distention	Protein-energy
	Hepatomegaly	Protein-energy
Extremities	Edema	Protein, thiamine
	Softening of bone	Vitamin D, calcium, phosphorus
	Bone tenderness	Vitamin D
	Bone ache, joint pain	Vitamin C
	Muscle wasting and weakness	Protein, calorie, vitamin D, selenium, sodium chloride
	Muscle tenderness, muscle pain	Thiamine
	Hyporeflexia	Thiamine
	Ataxia	Vitamin B₁₂
Nails	Spooning	Iron
	Transverse lines	Protein
Neurologic	Tetany	Calcium, magnesium
	Paresthesias	Thiamine, vitamin B₁₂
	Loss of reflexes, wrist drop, foot drop	Thiamine
	Loss of vibratory and position sense	Vitamin B₁₂
	Dementia, disorientation	Niacin
Blood	Anemia	Vitamins E, B₁₂, folate, iron, pyridoxine
	Hemolysis	Phosphorus

appear, the nutrient deficit may be very severe (e.g., scleromalacia, a leading and rapidly progressive cause of blindness due to vitamin A deficiency). Table 200–5 contains a listing of the most prevalent clinical presentations and the associated nutrient deficits that may cause them.

Functional and end-organ testing has been advocated for diagnosis of specific nutrient deficits (e.g., dark adaptation for vitamin A, taste and smell for zinc, bone density for vitamin D). However, functional tests are not available to assess the status of most nutrients, and, as with clinical signs, the functional tests are often nonspecific. For example, impairment of dark adaptation may be caused by zinc deficiency as well as vitamin A deficiency. Taste and smell may be affected by age, smoking, and drugs as well as by zinc nutriture. Bone density is diminished in both osteoporosis and vitamin D deficiency (osteomalacia).

As with dietary assessment, the elderly present a particular problem when evaluated for the presence or absence of clinical signs or symptoms of malnutrition. Some of the changes associated with malnutrition may also be a function of normal aging (e.g., hypogeusia, dry skin, sparse hair, atrophy of the tongue, bleeding gums from ill-fitting dentures). Nevertheless, as with younger patients, clinical signs should be assessed for dietary, laboratory, and anthropometric correlates vis-à-vis possible nutritional implications.

LABORATORY ASSESSMENT

Laboratory measurements are another tool that can aid the physician in making a diagnosis of malnutrition, although, once again, certain laboratory abnormalities that could reflect malnutrition can also have a non-nutritional cause (e.g., calcium, albumin, hematocrit). Modern analytical instruments (e.g., high-performance liquid chromatography), techniques (e.g., radio or enzyme immunoassays), and computerization have greatly increased the capability of nutritional biochemical testing. Currently available biochemical tests for assessing nutritional status include the direct measurement of a nutrient or nutrient metabolite in blood, other body fluids (e.g., urine, saliva), or tissues (e.g., white blood cells, hair, liver) and the measurement of a biochemical function that is nutrient specific. For example, laboratory tests for pyridoxine status may include the direct measurement of pyridoxal 5'-phosphate in plasma or the enzymatic activity of erythrocyte transaminase, for which pyridoxal 5'-phosphate is a cofactor. The latter test involves the calculation of an activity coefficient whereby red blood cell transaminase activity is determined before and after the addition of pyridoxal 5'-phosphate. An activity coefficient of greater than 2.2 is indicative of pyridoxine deficiency.

The establishment of normal nutrient values in body fluids or tissues for each sex varies from laboratory to laboratory, and the normal range usually represents a mean ± 2 SD of a normal population. Optimally, a low biochemical nutrient value in body fluids or tissue should be coupled with a specific functional abnormality before making the diagnosis of a nutrient deficiency. However, in practice this is rarely done. One guide for interpretation of laboratory values that reflects the status of various nutrients in the blood or serum of adults is presented in Table 200–6. For some nutrients (e.g., vitamin A) children have a different normal range than adults. The reader is referred to a pediatric text for children's normal values. Normal biochemical ranges have not been established for the very old (i.e., over 75 years). The physician must rely upon values derived from younger populations to judge the nutritional biochemical parameters for this group.

Many nutrient biochemical diagnostic tests are not readily available in a hospital clinical chemistry laboratory. Nevertheless, there are several laboratory tests that are routinely performed (e.g., hemoglobin level, serum protein level) that may aid the physician in assessing the nutritional status of his or her patients. In the absence of liver disease, a low serum albumin may be used as an indicator of protein nutriture. In sick patients who are obese, silent kwashiorkor (protein malnutrition) may develop (Ch. 201), as reflected by low serum protein values, although the patient may continue to look overnourished and anthropometric

TABLE 200–6. GUIDE FOR INTERPRETATION OF SERUM AND/OR BLOOD INDICES FOR SELECTED NUTRIENTS

Nutrient	Normal*	Deficient	Marginal
Albumin	3.5–5.5 grams/dl	2.8–3.2	3.2–3.5
Transferrin	200–400 mg/dl	< 200	
Transthyretin	10–40 mg/dl	< 10	
Ferritin	12–300 ng/ml	< 12	
Retinol	30–90 µg/dl	< 15	15–30
Carotene	40–240 µg/dl	< 40	
Vitamin E	0.5–1.8 mg/dl	< 0.5	0.5–0.7
Vitamin D (25-OH-D₃)	15–40 ng/ml		
Thiamine (erythrocyte)	0.9–1.25†	> 1.25	1.25–1.20
Riboflavin	0.9–1.39†	> 1.40	1.30–1.40
Pyridoxine	0.9–2.2†	> 2.2	
Niacin (urine 2-pyridone/N'-methyl nicotinamide—metabolite ratio)	1.0–4.0	< 1.0	
Serum folate	6–20 ng/ml	≤ 3.0	3–6
Red cell folate	150–450 ng/ml	< 150	
Vitamin B₁₂	>200 pg/ml	< 150	150–200
Vitamin C	0.3–2.0 mg/dl	< 0.2	0.2–0.3
Calcium	8.5–10.5 mg/dl	< 8.5	
Phosphorus	2.5–4.5 mg/dl	< 2.5	
Iron	50–170 µg/dl		
Zinc	70–130 µg/dl	≤ 65	65–70
Copper	70–160 µg/dl	< 70	
Magnesium	1.4–2.5 mg/dl	≤ 1.4	

*These normal values will vary with the method used and in different laboratories.
†An enzymatic assay. Values represent an activity coefficient.

measures may be normal or exceed the normal range. Other proteins that are synthesized in the liver and that have a more rapid turnover than albumin (e.g., transferrin, transthyretin) may also be used to diagnose protein malnutrition at an earlier stage, provided that the patient does not have liver damage. The transferrin in serum, if not directly measured, may be estimated from the total iron binding capacity (TIBC) according to the formula: $(0.8 \times TIBC) - 43$. Protein values that are more than 20 per cent below the lower limit of the normal range are generally regarded as severely substandard.

Muscle protein can be estimated from urinary creatinine excretion; this complements the anthropometric indicator MAMA. The amount of creatinine appearing in the urine over 24 hours is proportional to muscle mass. A crude standard for creatinine excretion can be derived by multiplying an individual's reference weight-for-height by 23 or 18 (for males or females, respectively). Twenty per cent below these derived values may represent muscle protein depletion. However, several factors are known to affect creatinine excretion (e.g., kidney disease, diet, fever, strenuous exercise, menstrual cycle), and the interpretation, therefore, must be carried out cautiously.

In protein-energy malnutrition, the number of circulating lymphocytes diminishes, and the patient demonstrates impaired delayed hypersensitivity to common skin antigens (e.g., mumps, Candida, tuberculin). Thus, these tests also may be used in assessing the patient's nutritional status, although anergy may result from many non-nutritional factors as well (e.g., disease, drugs). A lymphocyte count of fewer than 1200 per cubic millimeter is regarded as severely substandard. The effect of advanced age on these parameters is uncertain.

The value of nutritional assessment parameters in predicting patient outcome is unproven. A prognostic nutritional index has been derived from various nutritional assessment indices (e.g., albumin, transferrin, triceps skinfold, delayed hypersensitivity) and applied to surgical patients to predict postoperative complications and mortality. In one study a higher prognostic nutritional index score correlated with greater postoperative problems, but further evaluation is necessary. Moreover, it is not known whether this index has any value in predicting outcomes in medical patients.

Andres A: Mortality and obesity: The rationale for age specific height-weight tables. *In* Andres R, Bierman EL, Hazzard WR (eds.): Principles of Geriatric Medicine. New York, McGraw-Hill, 1985, pp 311–318. *This article discusses the problems with available weight-height standards and describes a U-shaped relationship between body mass index and mortality.*

Frisancho AR: New standards of weight and body composition by frame size and height for assessment of nutritional status of adults and the elderly. Am J Clin Nutr 40:808, 1984. *This article presents American standards for weight and height from ages 1 to 75, derived from the combined data sets of NHANES I (1971–1974) and II (1976–1980).*

201 Protein-Energy Malnutrition

Robert B. Baron

Protein-energy malnutrition (PEM) occurs when inadequate protein and/or calories are ingested to meet an individual's nutritional requirements. PEM may be primary, as a result of inadequate food intake, or secondary, as a result of illness. In developing nations, PEM is most often primary and affects predominantly infants and children. It is the most important nutritional disorder and one of the developing world's most important health problems. In industrialized nations, PEM is most often secondary to other diseases and affects both children and adults. In North America and Europe, 28 to 80 per cent of hospitalized patients have been reported to have secondary PEM. This chapter emphasizes clinical features of secondary PEM as seen in industrialized nations.

Pathogenesis

Secondary PEM is caused by decreased intake of calories and protein, increased nutrient losses, or increased nutrient requirements (Table 201–1). It can develop slowly owing to chronic illness or chronic semistarvation or quite rapidly owing to acute illness.

In uncomplicated starvation and semistarvation, metabolism adapts to reduce the breakdown of lean body mass. Fat and fat-derived fuels gradually replace glucose as the major energy source. During the initial phase of a complete fast, glucose requirements for the brain, bone marrow, renal medulla, and peripheral nerves are provided by glycogen. Glycogen stores, however, last for only 12 to 24 hours. As glucose levels decline, insulin levels also decline and glucagon levels increase. Amino acids, particularly alanine, are released by muscle. Hepatic gluconeogenesis from amino acids provides glucose for the central nervous system and other glycolytic tissues. The changes in insulin and glucagon also favor lipolysis. Mobilized fatty acids provide the fuel for the remaining tissues. By the second week of a complete fast, fatty acids are less completely oxidized and more of them form ketone bodies. Ketones become the primary energy source for the brain and reduce the need for glucose. The muscles catabolize less protein and release less alanine, thus conserving their protein content.

Adaptation also decreases the body's total energy requirement, by as much as 40 per cent in severe chronic undernutrition. Absolute requirements decrease as body weight diminishes owing to a decrease in body mass. More importantly, however, energy

TABLE 201–1. CAUSES OF PROTEIN-ENERGY MALNUTRITION IN HOSPITALIZED PATIENTS

Decreased Oral Intake

Anorexia	Poverty
Nausea	Old age
Dysphagia	Social isolation
Pain	Substance abuse
Gastrointestinal obstruction	Depression
Poor dentition	

Increased Nutrient Losses

Malabsorption	Nephrosis
Diarrhea	Fistula drainage
Bleeding	Protein-losing enteropathy
Glycosuria	

Increased Nutrient Requirements

Fever	Trauma
Infection	Burns
Neoplasms	Medications
Surgery	

requirements also decrease per unit of body mass. Both ingested food and circulating endogenous substrates are utilized more efficiently. More endogenous amino acids, for example, are utilized for protein synthesis than for oxidation. In addition, virtually all of the body's biochemical and physiologic processes are curtailed. Less energy is expended for the sodium potassium pump, protein turnover, temperature regulation, the inflammatory response, and the function of most body organs during chronic undernutrition.

During a severe acute illness, hormonal and inflammatory responses prevent this adaptation to starvation and result in changes in protein and energy metabolism that can rapidly lead to PEM. Circulating levels of the catecholamines, glucocorticoids, glucagon, and growth hormone are all increased. Although necessary to mediate the body's response to physical stress, these hormonal and inflammatory changes result in marked increases in energy expenditure, nitrogen loss, gluconeogenesis, and the failure of ketoadaptation. In this manner, changes in body composition, including depletion of protein and fat stores, may occur rapidly. A number of other compounds may also play important roles in the metabolic response to injury. Of particular interest are the metabolic effects of the cytokines, such as tumor necrosis factor and interleukin 1, and the eicosanoids, such as prostaglandins, thromboxane, prostacyclin, and leukotrienes.

The resting metabolic expenditure (RME) may increase significantly during the response to illness. In burns involving greater than 40 per cent of the body surface area, for example, the RME may double. In other critical illnesses such as trauma or sepsis, the RME typically increases by 20 to 50 per cent. Nitrogen losses also typically increase by 20 to 100 per cent. During the response to illness, amino acids are released by skeletal muscle at a markedly accelerated rate. Released amino acids can then be metabolized for energy or shifted to the liver or other visceral organs, where their need for protein synthesis is more immediate. During prolonged illness and continued energy and protein deficiency, however, depletion of visceral protein also occurs and functional impairment of body organs can result.

Physiologic Consequences

Virtually every organ and organ system of the body can undergo marked morphologic and functional changes during protein-energy malnutrition

BODY WEIGHT. The most obvious manifestation of chronic PEM is loss of body weight. Most patients can tolerate a loss of 5 to 10 per cent of body weight without significant consequences, but losses greater than 40 per cent below ideal weight are almost always fatal. Both adipose tissue and the lean body mass are depleted, but losses of adipose tissue are greater. Extracellular water remains nearly constant, resulting in its relative increase. In severe PEM, the body's organs also decrease in size. In experimental animals, for example, a 7-day fast results in a 40 per cent decrease in liver mass, 28 per cent decrease in the gastrointestinal tract, 20 per cent decrease in the kidneys, and 17 per cent decrease in cardiac mass. During acute PEM caused by critical illness, changes in body weight and adipose stores may be less marked despite changes in organ morphology and function. Many patients may actually gain weight owing to retention of sodium and therefore of body water.

HEART. Severe PEM results in both quantitative and qualitative changes in the heart. In the "Minnesota experiment," for example, in which 32 male volunteers were semistarved for 6 months, a 24 per cent decrease in body weight was associated with an 18 per cent decrease in cardiac stroke volume and a 38 per cent decrease in cardiac index. Animal studies have demonstrated similar findings, as well as decreases in left ventricular contractility and compliance, decreased myocardial glycogen, myofibrillar atrophy, and interstitial edema. These changes are reversed with nutritional repletion.

LUNG. The lung parenchyma is minimally affected during PEM, but marked changes in pulmonary function can occur as a result of the loss of mass and strength of the muscles of respiration. In the "Minnesota experiment," vital capacity, tidal volume, and minute volume were decreased by 8 per cent, 19 per cent, and 30 per cent, respectively, after 24 weeks of semistarvation.

The ventilatory response to hypoxia is also decreased during semistarvation, but the clinical significance of this is unclear.

GASTROINTESTINAL TRACT. During severe PEM, gastric motility is slowed and gastric acid secretion is decreased. The most significant effects of PEM on the luminal gastrointestinal tract are seen in the small intestine. Total small bowel mass is decreased, primarily owing to mucosal atrophy and loss of villi. Lymphocytic infiltration of surface epithelial cells can occur, and epithelial cell renewal is decreased. Both disaccharidase enzyme activity and the rate of absorption of amino acids are decreased. Although pancreatic endocrine activity is spared, exocrine insufficiency can occur in severe PEM. Similar changes in the gastrointestinal tract are observed in individuals fed exclusively with parenteral nutrition, suggesting that stimulation of the gut by intraluminal nutrients is necessary for normal gut structure and function.

LIVER. In typical secondary PEM, liver mass decreases but the liver histology remains normal. Fat, protein, and glycogen are depleted, but the number of hepatocytes is preserved. In contrast, children with severe, primary protein deficiency resulting in kwashiorkor have enlarged livers with fatty infiltration and excess glycogen. In both instances, serum levels of albumin and other serum transport proteins are commonly decreased owing to diminished hepatic synthesis.

KIDNEY. Renal mass is also decreased during PEM, but renal histology remains normal. Renal function is well preserved except for an impaired concentrating ability due to a lowering of the medullary osmotic gradient.

ENDOCRINE. The endocrine response to PEM is complex and greatly affected by the extent of concurrent illnesses, as discussed above. In addition, serum thyroxine is typically at the lower limits of normal or slightly decreased. Peripheral conversion of thyroxine (T_4) to triiodothyronine (T_3) is commonly decreased, favoring the conversion to reverse triiodothyronine (Ch. 216). Serum TSH and the TSH response to TRH, however, are unaltered. Gonadal hormones are also affected. In men, testosterone levels are decreased and LH and FSH levels are appropriately increased. In women, however, gonadotropin release is depressed despite low levels of circulating estrogens.

IMMUNOLOGIC FUNCTION. The effects of severe PEM on the immune system are among its most important consequences. Virtually all components of the immune system are adversely affected in rough proportion to the degree of nutritional impairment. Peripheral blood lymphocyte counts are commonly decreased, with values often less than 1200 per cubic millimeter. Both the percentage of T cells and T-cell function are depressed. Skin tests for delayed hypersensitivity reactions are often nonreactive, and lymphocyte response to phytohemagglutinin and poke weed mitogens is decreased.

Humoral immunity is also affected, but in a more variable fashion. Specific antibody responses are depressed in some instances and preserved in others. For example, antibody production following administration of poliovirus, tetanus, diphtheria, measles, and pneumococcal polysaccharide antigens is normal, whereas impaired responses have been observed after the administration of yellow fever and influenza A vaccines. In some instances, the affinities and binding capacity of antibodies are reduced.

Slight neutropenia may occur during PEM, but the usual concurrent bacterial infections cause leukocytosis. Neutrophils are normal morphologically, but some measures of neutrophil function, including chemotaxis and bacterial killing, are abnormal. Phagocytosis is usually normal.

Levels of individual complement components, other than C4, and total serum hemolytic complement activity are commonly decreased. Other nonspecific host defense mechanisms, including interferon production, opsonization, and plasma lysozyme production, may also be adversely affected by protein-calorie undernutrition. Acute phase reactants such as C-reactive proteins, α_2-macroglobulin, α_1-antitrypsin, and haptoglobin tend to be elevated. Changes in the body's anatomic barriers to infection, including atrophy of the skin and gastrointestinal mucosa, may contribute to an increased risk of infection.

It is not possible to define the exact mechanisms of enhanced susceptibility to infections observed with PEM. Each of the abnormalities of the immune response probably contributes in part. Micronutrient deficiencies may occur concurrently with PEM and can also cause significant abnormalities in the immune response.

WOUND HEALING. Almost all aspects of wound healing are adversely affected in patients with severe PEM. Neovascularization, fibroblast proliferation, collagen synthesis, and wound remodeling are delayed. Local factors, such as edema associated with hypoalbuminemia and micronutrient deficiencies, may contribute to poor wound healing in undernourished patients. In mild PEM, however, wound healing is relatively well-preserved despite negative nitrogen balance. Even during complete starvation, endogenous substrates can be effectively utilized for collagen synthesis during the early phases of wound healing.

Clinical Manifestations

The clinical manifestations of PEM are extremely diverse, ranging from mild growth retardation and weight loss to several distinct clinical syndromes. This diversity is due to differences in the relative degree of protein and energy deficiency, the cause of the deficiency, the severity and duration of the deficiency, the age of the patient, and the association with other illnesses or nutritional deficiencies. In children in the developing world with severe PEM, for example, the classic syndromes of kwashiorkor (predominant protein deficiency) and marasmus (predominant energy deficiency) may develop. Marasmic kwashiorkor, an intermediate syndrome, may be seen when protein deficiency develops in combination with chronic energy deficiency. Although these syndromes are not typically encountered in secondary PEM in industrialized nations, they serve to illustrate the range of manifestations of PEM.

KWASHIORKOR. The child with severe kwashiorkor commonly has a decreased blood pressure, bradycardia, and hypothermia. Body weight is usually low but may be normal owing to edema and anasarca. The child is usually apathetic, lethargic, and anorectic, with decreased spontaneous movement. The skin demonstrates a "flaky paint" dermatitis with dry, hyperpigmented, hyperkeratotic lesions over the face, extremities, and perineum. The hair is typically sparse, dry, and brittle and may be reddish or yellowish. The abdomen is distended owing to hepatomegaly and ascites. The extremities are commonly wasted and edematous. Clinical signs of concurrent micronutrient deficiency may also be present (Ch. 205).

The serum albumin is typically less than 2.8 grams per deciliter and the lymphocyte count less than 1200 cells per cubic millimeter. A mild anemia is common; it is usually normochromic and normocytic unless other deficiencies coexist. The serum transferrin is usually decreased but may be normal or slightly elevated if iron deficiency is also present. Other serum transport proteins, including prealbumin and retinol-binding protein, are decreased. Serum glucose and lipids are decreased. Serum levels of liver enzymes are most often normal and may be low. Blood urea nitrogen and urinary urea nitrogen are low. Fluid and electrolyte disorders are common, particularly hypokalemia, hypophosphatemia, and a hyperchloremic metabolic acidosis.

MARASMUS. Children with marasmus have less characteristic manifestations. Although the pulse, blood pressure, and body temperature may be low, patients tend to be less apathetic and lethargic and to have a good appetite. Growth is retarded and the weight is low. There is obvious muscle wasting and loss of body fat and the patient looks emaciated, but there is no edema. The skin is dry and loose with decreased turgor. The dermatitis of kwashiorkor is usually absent. The hair is thin, dry, and dull. The abdomen is thin without signs of hepatomegaly or edema. Typically, there are fewer laboratory abnormalities than in children with kwashiorkor. Serum albumin and other transport proteins are often normal. A mild anemia is common. Any of the other laboratory abnormalities of kwashiorkor may be present but are usually absent.

SECONDARY PROTEIN-ENERGY MALNUTRITION. Secondary PEM, as seen in industrialized nations, is usually due to a deficiency of both protein and energy. Clinical manifestations vary considerably, in large part reflecting the associated illness that has caused the malnutrition and the nutritional status of the patient prior to the illness. In mild forms of secondary PEM, growth retardation in children and weight loss in adults may be the only manifestation. In more severe cases, depletion of fat stores results in loss of subcutaneous fat in the face and extremities. Reduction of lean body mass is reflected in loss of skeletal muscle, most noticeably in the interosseous and temporal muscles. The skin is often dry with decreased turgor, and the hair may be brittle and thin. Serum proteins are often decreased, and if particularly low, may result in dependent edema or anasarca. Patients with low serum proteins have a poor prognosis.

Obese patients who develop secondary PEM may have persistent fat stores and adequate subcutaneous fat and may demonstrate few of the manifestations of PEM. Although skeletal muscle is usually decreased, evaluation is difficult if large amounts of body fat are present. Serum proteins may be decreased or normal.

Diagnosis

The absence of distinct clinical manifestations can make the diagnosis of PEM quite difficult. A high index of suspicion based on the patient's risk factors for malnutrition, the overall clinical setting, and close observation of the patient are often necessary.

BODY WEIGHT. The most sensitive diagnostic measure is a documented history of weight loss. Weight loss should be quantified as a per cent of original body weight. Significant changes in weight may be obscured by edema. Some patients, particularly those with a severe acute illness such as sepsis, burns, or multiple trauma, can develop severe protein depletion rapidly without significant weight loss. Unfortunately, no standard amount of weight loss occurring over an established period of time clearly indicates clinically significant PEM. Nevertheless, most authors consider a 10 per cent loss of body weight occurring during the present illness to be clinically significant.

LABORATORY TESTS. Each of the clinical abnormalities seen in patients with severe PEM can be used as a diagnostic test to detect undernutrition. Most valuable are the serum albumin, other serum transport proteins such as transferrin, prealbumin, and retinol-binding protein, anergy to skin test antigens, total lymphocyte count, blood urea nitrogen, urinary excretion of creatinine, and anthropomorphic measures of body composition, such as skinfold thickness and mid-arm muscle circumference. Each of these tests when abnormal, like a history of weight loss, has been shown to predict poor clinical outcomes in patients in a wide variety of clinical settings. Combining these tests into indices such as the prognostic nutritional index further improves their predictive accuracy. Unfortunately, it remains unclear whether the poor outcomes predicted by excessive weight loss or by abnormalities in these tests reflect the consequences of PEM or the severity of the underlying illness.

A number of other nutrition assessment methods have been developed to more specifically define abnormalities in body composition. These include isotopic measurement of body composition, densitometry, computed tomography, nuclear magnetic resonance imaging, ultrasonography, whole-body impedance, and measures of muscle function. Although many of these are useful research techniques, their application in clinical practice is limited.

CLINICAL ASSESSMENT. A thorough, nutritionally focused history and physical examination can predict outcomes as well as any of the above tests and indices. The history should emphasize recent reduction in dietary intake, changes in body weight, gastrointestinal symptoms, the underlying illness, and the patient's functional status. The physical examination should emphasize loss of subcutaneous fat, muscle wasting, volume status, and signs of micronutrient deficiencies (Ch. 205). The initial clinical assessment is often equivocal; that is, the presence of clinically significant undernutrition is uncertain. In such cases, serial evaluations of the clinical examination, body weight, and laboratory parameters and close observation of the patient's nutrient intake as a function of estimated requirements is necessary to make the diagnosis of PEM.

Treatment

The goals of treatment of PEM are to provide adequate energy, protein, and micronutrients to restore body composition to normal and to treat the underlying process that caused the deficiency to develop.

STRATEGY. Treatment should proceed in two stages. In severe PEM, the first priority should be correction of fluid and electrolyte abnormalities and treatment of acute medical problems, most commonly infections. Although any combination of electrolyte and acid-base abnormalities can occur, most common are hypokalemia, hypocalcemia, hypophosphatemia, hypomagnesemia, and a hyperchloremic metabolic acidosis.

In the second phase one must provide adequate nutritional substrate to begin repletion. Nutrients should be provided quite slowly to prevent complications of overfeeding. In most adult patients no more than 0.8 gram of protein per kilogram and 30 Kcal per kilogram of actual body weight should be provided per day. As the patient becomes stabilized, protein and energy intake can be increased to 35 to 40 Kcal per kilogram and 1.0 to 1.5 grams of protein per kilogram per day. Adequate micronutrients must also be simultaneously provided. Patients with severe, life-threatening PEM should be fed even more cautiously.

ROUTE OF THERAPY. Nutrients can be provided either enterally or parenterally. Patients whose gastrointestinal tract is functioning and who can protect their airway should be fed enterally, either by mouth, feeding tube, or tube enterostomy (Ch. 206). Patients with contraindications to enteral feeding can be given required nutrients parenterally via either peripheral or central veins (Ch. 207). An algorithm for selecting the most appropriate method of nutritional support is shown in Figure 201–1.

COMPLICATIONS OF THERAPY. Particular care must be taken to avoid complications of refeeding. Many deaths attributable to PEM occur not during starvation but during repletion.

Electrolyte abnormalities, for example, are common during refeeding. The provision of energy and protein to a severely undernourished patient may convert a catabolic state to an anabolic one. As new tissues are synthesized and old tissues replenished, potassium and other electrolytes are transported intracellularly and may precipitate an acute drop in serum levels and result in life-threatening cardiac arrhythmias.

Congestive heart failure and pulmonary edema can be precip-

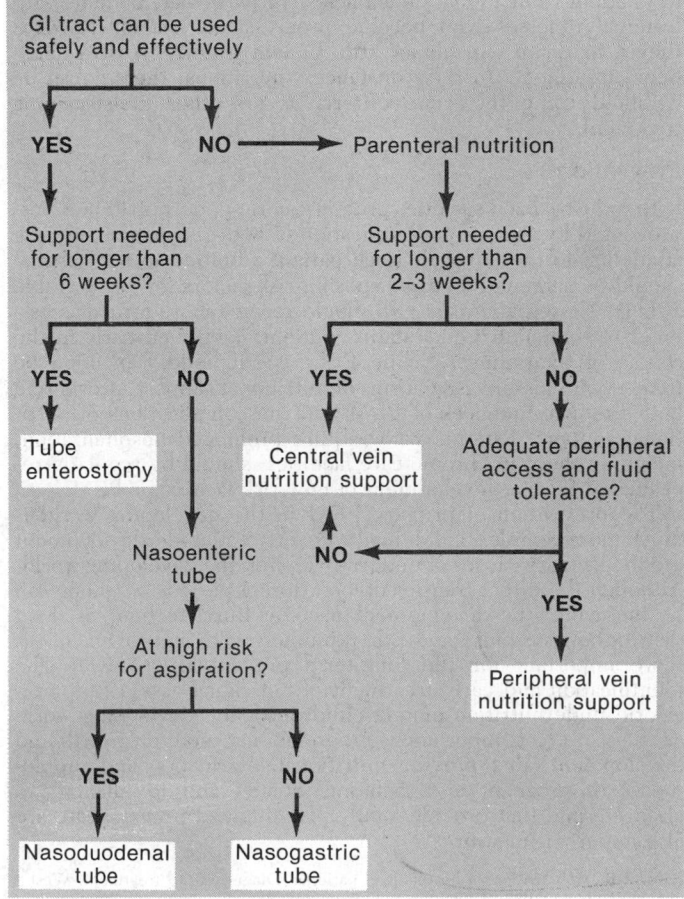

FIGURE 201–1. Decision tree concerning method of nutritional support.

itated by refeeding. As noted above, undernutrition is associated with decreased cardiac mass, decreased cardiac index and stroke volume, a slowing of the metabolic rate, and hypovolemia. The acute provision of carbohydrate, fluid, and sodium may correct the metabolic and volume abnormalities more rapidly than the depressed myocardium can handle and result in fluid overload. Should this complication occur, standard measures for the treatment of congestive heart failure should be used together with a slowing of the rate of nutritional repletion.

Benign refeeding edema must be differentiated from refeeding congestive heart failure. Many severely undernourished patients develop edema in dependent areas during refeeding without an associated increase in left ventricular filling pressures. The cause of refeeding edema is unclear. Changes in renal sodium retention, in part due to increased serum insulin, and poor venous tone have both been implicated. Treatment should include reassurance, elevation of dependent areas, and modest sodium restriction. Diuretics are rarely effective and may result in exacerbation of fluid and electrolyte abnormalities.

Diarrhea may result from enteral refeeding. Severely malnourished patients have atrophy of the gastric mucosa, decreased disaccharidase activity, and a mild deficiency of the exocrine pancreas. The provision of intraluminal nutrients can thus result in malabsorption and diarrhea. Gradual refeeding and restriction of lactose and lipid during the early refeeding phase decrease the risk of diarrhea.

REHABILITATION. Treatment of patients with PEM requires more than the provision of nutrients. Physical therapy and other measures to improve the patient's functional status are effective adjuncts to nutritional treatment. Physical therapy may result in greater repletion of muscle mass and smaller adipose tissue stores than nutritional repletion without muscle contraction.

The most important non-nutritional factor in the treatment of these patients is the resolution of the disease or social process that caused the PEM. In most instances, if the underlying process cannot be effectively treated, little benefit is derived from treating the patient's nutritional deficiencies. In particular, patients with terminal illnesses who become progressively malnourished as they near death will obtain little benefit from aggressive nutritional treatment. In these instances, nutritional therapy can be withheld using the same criteria as for other life-sustaining treatments.

Prevention

In industrialized societies protein-calorie undernutrition is best prevented by the early identification of high-risk patients during admission to the hospital. Each patient admitted to the hospital should be screened for predisposing risk factors for PEM (Table 201–1). Those patients at risk should receive more formal assessment of their nutritional status. Patients identified early in the course of their illness, while PEM is still mild, can often be treated with less invasive forms of nutritional support, preventing both the consequences of PEM and the complications of nutritional support. Patients who require prolonged hospitalization, including those in chronic care facilities, should be regularly re-evaluated for the development of new risk factors for PEM.

The prevention of primary PEM in the developing world is much more complex and difficult. Poverty and underdevelopment are the primary causes of undernutrition in the developing world. Although the direct transfer of food during periods of famine can be lifesaving, the development of agricultural techniques, food distribution systems, and other public health improvements is more important for the long-term prevention of PEM. The identification and early treatment of individual cases of protein-calorie undernutrition among children of the developing world are also of great importance. Programs that monitor growth and development, that provide nutritional information and supplements to pregnant and lactating women and to infants and children, and that provide family planning and prenatal care are also important measures.

Baron RB: Malnutrition in hospitalized patients: Diagnosis and treatment. West J Med 144:63, 1986. *A brief review of current controversies in the diagnosis and treatment of secondary protein-energy malnutrition.*

Goldstein SA, Elwyn DH: The effects of injury and sepsis on fuel utilization. Annu Rev Nutr 9:445, 1989. *A detailed review of the metabolic and hormonal alterations occurring during critical illness and their impact on nutritional status.*

Heymsfield SB, Williams PJ: Nutritional assessment by clinical and biochemical methods. *In* Shils ME, Young VR (eds.): Modern Nutrition in Health and Disease, 7th ed. Philadelphia, Lea & Febiger, 1988. *A comprehensive review of traditional and newer techniques for diagnosing protein-energy malnutrition.*

Silberman H: Parenteral and Enteral Nutrition, 2nd ed. Norwalk, CT, Appleton & Lange, 1988. *An excellent brief textbook covering theoretical and practical aspects of nutrition support of patients with protein-energy malnutrition.*

Torún B, Viteri FE: Protein-energy malnutrition. *In* Shils ME, Young VR (eds.): Modern Nutrition in Health and Disease. 7th ed. Philadelphia, Lea & Febiger, 1988. *A balanced review of the classic syndromes of primary protein-energy malnutrition.*

202 The Eating Disorders
Douglas A. Drossman

The eating disorders—anorexia nervosa, bulimia, and rumination—attract much public attention and scientific inquiry. Diagnosis and treatment require an understanding that these disorders result from a combination of biologic, psychological, and social influences.

ANOREXIA NERVOSA

DEFINITION. Anorexia nervosa is a chronic disorder characterized behaviorally by self-induced weight loss, psychologically by body-image and other perceptual disturbances, and biologically by physiologic alterations (e.g., amenorrhea) that result from nutritional depletion.

HISTORICAL NOTE. The disorder was first reported 300 years ago by Morton in describing an 18-year-old patient as a "skeleton only clad with skin" with "total suppression of her monthly courses." In 1874, Gull first used the term *anorexia nervosa* in reporting a "nervous, morbid disease" associated with loss of appetite and severe wasting. It is now recognized that these patients are not truly anorectic; they are *preoccupied* with food and struggle against hunger to achieve the desired goal of thinness.

EPIDEMIOLOGY. Anorexia nervosa afflicts predominantly young, affluent white females (95 per cent). The incidence may be increasing. In one community study the number of new cases per year over a 10-year period rose from 0.55 per 100,000 to 3.26 per 100,000. The disorder is associated with higher social class, occurring in up to 1 in 250 adolescent students in private school and with a prevalence of 1 per cent.

ETIOLOGY AND PATHOGENESIS. *Sociocultural Factors.* The cultural ideal for women's bodies has shifted in the last century from that of plumpness (formerly representing wealth, abundance, maternalism, and fertility) to a slimmer female image (representing independence, assertiveness, and success). Thinner women predominate on prime-time television and among beauty pageant contestants and high-fashion models. Social pressures from peers, particularly during adolescence, seem to influence young women and girls to engage in anorectic behaviors. These factors are probably not sufficient for the disorder to develop but may create the proper environment for its expression in the predisposed individual. Recent studies also report an association of childhood sexual abuse history among patients with anorexia nervosa. The possible relationship of abuse in the pathogenesis of the disorder needs further study.

Psychological Factors. It is believed that anorectics have an incompletely developed personal identity and struggle to maintain a sense of control over their environment. Psychiatric interviews suggest that the patient develops within a family that values outward appearance, proper behavior, and achievement more than self-actualization. In response to parental expectations, the pre-anorectic child learns to be hard working, eager to please, and attentive to family needs. In turn, the parents support and indulge in the behaviors of their model child ("best little girl in the world"). Therefore, these actions are mutually reinforced, leading to interdependence among the family members (enmeshment). However, the high standards within the family are rarely achieved by the child, who obsessively struggles for parental approval.

It follows that "negative" childhood behaviors (e.g., assertiveness, rebellion) are not permitted. These behaviors are believed necessary for the development of individual identity. As a result, the pre-anorectic child comes to rely on externally imposed ideal values to maintain self-esteem, but at the expense of self-actualization and a sense of autonomy.

It is not surprising that a distressing period for the pre-anorectic child occurs during or soon after puberty, when physical, social, and psychological events (menarche, growth spurt, school, and adolescent peer pressure) encourage separation from the family and individuation. Over 80 per cent of anorectic patients develop the disorder within 7 years of menarche. The compounded life events at this time are experienced with feelings of helplessness and ineffectiveness. The decision to diet, while not fully understood, may be a desperate attempt for control of one's body, at least, in a distressing new environment.

Biologic Factors. There is an increased risk of anorexia nervosa among siblings (6 per cent), with a four- to five-fold difference in concordance rates for monozygotic twins, suggesting a predisposing role for genetic factors. Also, there are more perinatal complications reported among anorexia nervosa patients. The higher birth weight and the increased prevalence of obesity preceding the onset of illness suggest that premorbid obesity is an influencing factor. Abnormalities in satiety, temperature regulation, and endocrine function suggest that a hypothalamic abnormality exists, although no specific lesion has been identified. It is more likely that the hypothalamus serves a modulating role. In the predisposed individual, the biologic and psychosocial events around the time of adolescence may produce neurotransmitter, endocrine, or immune changes via the hypothalamus, leading to the physiologic and behavioral changes characteristic of the disorder. The biologic findings of anorexia nervosa can be viewed as homeostatic adaptations to self-imposed energy depletion.

CLINICAL MANIFESTATIONS. There are no characteristic pathologic or physiologic findings, and no consistent psychiatric diagnosis is found. The consistency of the medical and behavioral features, however, argues for classifying the disorder as a clinical entity.

Psychological and Behavioral Features. Pursuit of Thinness. Patients are not truly anorectic, but struggle against hunger to achieve an unrealistic degree of weight loss. Interestingly, they are preoccupied with food and exhibit bizarre food preferences or elaborately prepare food for others. For most anorectics, weight loss is accomplished through dietary restriction and exercise (restrictor subgroup), although up to 50 per cent will also self-induce vomiting or take purgatives (bulimic subgroup).

Perceptual Disturbances. Anorectics overestimate their body width, insisting they are too fat despite profound weight loss. Their assessment of the body habitus of others is not affected. Anorectics may also exhibit abnormalities in the perception of enteroceptive stimuli. They distort hunger awareness, deny fatigue, and fail to recognize emotional states such as anger and depression.

Sense of Ineffectiveness. Patients feel as though they are controlled by their environment and seem unable to function separately from family or other relationships. They gauge their responses to the expectations of others.

Cognitive Deficits. Patients may exhibit deficits in conceptual thought and abstract reasoning. They may be unable to view situations in anything but extremes, and they interpret events in a rigid and highly personalized form.

Medical Features. Most of the physical, metabolic, and endocrine abnormalities of anorexia nervosa are also seen in starvation secondary to the other conditions. The severity of the findings correlates with the nutritional state.

Physical Signs. Patients may have severe loss of subcutaneous fat and exhibit bony prominences. Core temperature, blood pressure, and pulse are decreased. Examination of the skin may reveal acrocyanosis, downy hair (lanugo), and a yellow discoloration (hypercarotenemia). Elevated serum carotene and vitamin A levels are due either to an excess intake of dietary carotenoids or to an acquired defect in the utilization or metabolism of these compounds. Secondary sexual features are absent in the patient who develops anorexia nervosa before puberty.

Endocrine Abnormalities. *Gonadal.* The endocrine hallmark is gonadal dysfunction, and for women this presents as amenorrhea. Male anorectics lose libido and are infertile. Patients have decreased follicle-stimulating (FSH) and luteinizing hormone (LH) and do not exhibit secretory bursts of LH throughout the day in response to endogenous luteinizing hormone-releasing factor (LHRF), indicating an abnormality in hypothalamic regulation. This "immature" secretory pattern, characteristic of prepubertal girls, may result from the loss of a critical amount of body fat content or from the psychophysiologic effects of stress in the absence of significant weight loss. Normal menses usually recur with weight gain, when body fat content reaches 22 per cent.

Thyroid. Patients may exhibit clinical features suggestive of hypothyroidism, such as decreased vital signs, dry skin, constipation, cold intolerance, and a delayed ankle jerk, although lethargy is not usually observed. T_3 levels tend to be low, with a corresponding increase in reverse T_3, the relatively inactive isomer of T_3 (Ch. 216). Under the stress of malnutrition, the liver preferentially deiodinates T_4 to rT_3. The clinical findings of mild hypothyroidism may arise from a decreased availability of the more active T_3 isomer, which preferentially binds to the thyroid receptor. However, free thyroxine, total T_4 levels, and the TSH response to TRH are normal. Clinically significant hypothyroidism does not occur, and treatment with exogenous thyroid is not indicated.

Adrenal. Anorectic patients usually have normal or slightly elevated plasma cortisol levels with decreased urinary excretion of 17-hydroxycorticosteroids. This is due to a decrease in the metabolic clearance of cortisol from plasma with an increase in cortisol-binding capacity. The 24-hour cortisol production rate and basal ACTH secretion are normal. The response to ACTH stimulation may be increased, and the response to metyrapone stimulation is normal. Decreased libido and delayed virilization in males may be due to a shift of androgen metabolism from the 5α-reductase enzyme system (yielding testosterone and its congeners) to the 5β-reductase system, producing the weaker androgen etiocholanolone (Ch. 222).

Growth Hormone. Human growth hormone (hGH) levels are normal or slightly elevated. Concurrently there is a decrease in somatomedin levels. This growth-promoting peptide is produced by the liver and other tissues under the influence of hGH. Somatomedin mediates the anabolic effects of hGH but not its lipolytic effects. Thus, anorectic patients and other malnourished individuals maintain their adipose tissue breakdown (increased hGH) without growth effects.

Cardiovascular Abnormalities. Patients exhibit depressed cardiovascular function with a decreased cardiac O_2 consumption, left ventricular wall thickness, cardiac chamber size, and blood pressure. These are adaptive responses to malnutrition and decreased catecholamine levels. Electrocardiographic changes include bradycardia, decreased QRS amplitude, prolonged QT interval, nonspecific ST segment changes, and U waves. Patients may also develop arrhythmias (tachycardia, sinus arrest, and ectopic atrial, junctional, or ventricular rhythms) due either to the primary disorder or to metabolic disturbances secondary to purgation. Sudden death has been reported among severely emaciated patients.

Hematologic Findings. Leukopenia and decreased white cell function, anemia, thrombocytopenia, and hypocomplementemia may occur. Anorectic patients do not seem to have a greater susceptibility to infection, however.

Gastrointestinal Findings. Constipation, delayed gastric emptying, pancreatic fibrosis, and jejunal dilatation may occur. Malabsorptive diarrhea and acute gastric dilatation may develop with rapid refeeding.

DIAGNOSIS. It is difficult to know when the diagnosis should be made, since social and cultural factors promote and maintain anorectic behaviors. Five per cent of college women without weight loss display attitudes and behaviors consistent with the diagnosis. Within some population groups (e.g., high-fashion models, ballerinas) low body weight is *de rigueur* and the associated anorectic behaviors are accepted. The diagnosis of anorexia nervosa should be considered when the person voluntarily restricts food intake in the face of hunger to achieve an unrealistic degree of weight loss and becomes psychosocially dysfunctional. The diagnosis is confirmed by identifying the described behavioral features and by excluding any treatable medical disorders.

The use of clinical criteria such as those proposed by the American Psychiatric Association (Table 202–1) is recommended. The differential diagnosis in this young population includes primary endocrine disorders (panhypopituitarism, Addison's disease, hyperthyroidism, diabetes mellitus), gastrointestinal disease (Crohn's disease, celiac sprue), chronic infection (tuberculosis), neoplastic disorders (lymphoma), and, rarely, CNS disorders (hypothalamic tumor, vascular malformation).

All patients should receive a nutritional assessment to determine the severity of the malnutrition and to establish a baseline for follow-up. Height and weight are usually sufficient. Patients with marked weight loss should have other nutritional measures obtained (serum transferrin, albumin, measurement of triceps skin fold thickness, skin test reactivity to *Candida* antigen) in order to gauge the approach to nutritional treatment.

TREATMENT. There are two goals in the treatment of patients with anorexia nervosa: nutritional restitution with alleviation of medical complications, and modification of the psychological and environmental factors that promote anorectic behavior. No single treatment is superior, and a multidisciplinary approach involving medical, psychiatric/psychological, and nutritional (dietitians, pharmacists) personnel is needed.

General Medical Care. The medical physician performs the initial clinical assessment, is responsible for the medical and nutritional care of the patient, and provides psychological support. The general approach should include (1) fostering a sense of autonomy in the patient by encouraging her to take personal responsibility in the treatment plan, (2) remaining objective, consistent, and honest in order to maintain the patient's trust, (3) involving the family as part of the treatment program, (4) serving as liaison and patient advocate with the various consultants and counselors.

Nutritional Care. All anorectic patients require some dietary management, although nutritional supplementation is not needed unless the patient is at risk of medical complications. With mild degrees of weight loss (e.g., weight 80 per cent of ideal or better), nutritional and psychological counseling is sufficient. The physician's role includes personal support, education about adolescent body development and its relationship to diet, and scheduling of periodic visits to observe for clinical deterioration. With moderate malnutrition (weight 65 to 80 per cent of ideal) nutritional supplements may be necessary, but hospitalization usually is not required. Oral replacement with a palatable, nutritionally complete formulation (e.g., Ensure Plus) may help, with the goal being intake of 250 to 500 calories above daily energy requirement. In some cases metoclopramide or bethanechol may be used to improve gastric emptying and the patient's tolerance of larger meals. With severe malnutrition (weight less than 65 per cent of ideal) hospitalization is usually required. Oral replacement

TABLE 202–1. DIAGNOSTIC CRITERIA FOR ANOREXIA NERVOSA*

A. Refusal to maintain body weight over a minimal normal weight for age and height (e.g., weight loss leading to maintenance of body weight 15% below that expected) or failure to make expected weight gain during period of growth, leading to body weight 15% below that expected.

B. Intense fear of gaining weight or becoming fat, even though underweight.

C. Disturbance in the way in which one's body weight, size, or shape is experienced (e.g., claiming to "feel fat" even when emaciated or belief that one area of the body is "too fat" even when obviously underweight).

D. In females, absence of at least three consecutive menstrual cycles when otherwise expected to occur (primary or secondary amenorrhea; a woman is considered to have amenorrhea if her periods occur only following hormone [e.g., estrogen] administration).

*American Psychiatric Association Diagnostic and Statistical Manual of Mental Disorders (DSM-IIIR), 4th ed. Washington, D.C., Copyright APA 1987. Used with permission.

may be attempted, but if the patient is unable or unwilling to comply, tube feeding into the duodenum may be necessary. The patient can receive 400 to 600 calories above daily caloric need, with the goal being no more than 1 to 2 kg weight gain per week.

If the patient is severely malnourished and tolerates a feeding tube poorly or refuses to eat, parenteral nutrition may be considered. The peripheral venous route is preferred, since central hyperalimentation is more expensive and is associated with a greater frequency of complications. If a central venous route is chosen, it should be supervised by an experienced hyperalimentation team. Caloric delivery should begin with one half of the daily requirement, progressing to full requirement by day three or four. Electrolytes, serum chemistries, and hepatic and renal function must be monitored.

The goal of enteral or parenteral supplementation is to *slowly* get the patient to a body weight out of the range of medical risk. Rapid refeeding produces excess water stores and edema, secondary metabolic disturbances, and possibly cardiac failure. Continued nutritional intervention beyond achieving a "dry weight" of 80 per cent of ideal is not recommended. These procedures are psychologically invasive and minimize the patient's involvement in treatment, thereby increasing anxiety and resistance. Furthermore, supplements interfere with appetite and with attempts to re-establish normal eating patterns.

Pharmacotherapy. No pharmacologic agent is of proven value. Chlorpromazine, amitriptyline, lithium carbonate, and cyproheptadine have been reported effective in small, short-term inpatient treatment trials. Their use should be ancillary to the long-term nutritional and behavioral approaches.

Psychotherapy. Psychotherapy is used to help the patient modify the aberrant eating behavior and to improve psychosocial function. Behavior modification is an effective means of achieving short-term weight gain. Family therapy offers the best potential for long-term benefit, since treatment is directed toward modifying the family interactions that maintain the anorectic behavior. Insight therapy may occasionally help the motivated patient.

PROGNOSIS. The short-term prognosis is generally favorable; over 75 per cent of patients will attain a body weight above 75 per cent of ideal. Menses will resume in at least half; however, less than one third of patients will resume normal eating patterns. The long-term prognosis is variable, and relapses requiring hospitalization occur in about half of the patients. The mortality rate among hospitalized patients averages 6 per cent, with the main causes of death being inanition and severe electrolyte disturbances; suicide occurs in 1 per cent. A poorer prognosis is associated with a late age of onset, self-induced vomiting or laxative abuse, long duration of illness, male sex, and the presence of associated psychiatric disturbance. A better prognosis is associated with the patient's ability to achieve a degree of social integration (e.g., with parent, spouse, and friends). It appears that anorexia nervosa is a lifelong behavioral disorder with periodic exacerbations requiring medical, psychological, and nutritional intervention.

BULIMIA

DEFINITION. Bulimia, derived from the Greek meaning "ox-eating," is a behavioral disorder characterized by episodes of overeating (binging), usually followed by acts to "undo" the threatened weight gain with self-induced vomiting, cathartic or diuretic abuse (purging), fasting, or excessive physical activity. Bulimia nervosa is sometimes used to distinguish the behavior of patients who binge and purge from that of other bulimics who binge but do not purge. Compared with anorectics, bulimics have normal body weight and tend to have less distortion of body image. Bulimics are more aware that their behavior, although secretive, is aberrant, and they may therefore be more accepting of treatment.

EPIDEMIOLOGY. Although bulimia was only first reported as a diagnostic entity in 1979, its prevalence is very high and it has probably existed a long time. Binge eating, at least once, occurs in half of the population, and weekly binge eating is reported by up to 15 per cent. Self-induced vomiting or laxative/diuretic abuse associated with binge eating occurs in up to 20 per cent of college students, and 4 per cent report this type of behavior at least weekly. Bulimia is almost exclusively diagnosed in young (<30 years) women (>95 per cent). Most bulimics carry on their activity secretly; less than one third have discussed their behavior with their physician, and in one survey only 2.5 per cent were under medical care.

ETIOLOGY AND PATHOGENESIS. Patients commonly report obesity during childhood or adolescence, and the onset of bulimia is associated with a conscious decision to diet. At some point the patients lose control of their compulsion to eat large amounts of "forbidden foods" and binge. Self-induced vomiting is discovered as a convenient method of re-establishing weight control. Thus, a binge-purge cycle becomes established.

As with anorexia nervosa, societal influences seem to play a prominent role in the desire to be thin. Also, there are historical and social precedents for self-induced vomiting. The ancient Romans ate lavishly and then induced vomiting at feasts. Socialites who must attend many dinner parties sometimes induce vomiting. Bulimics report coming from families that emphasize hearty eating and where food is used to celebrate happy times and to console during sad times. For these patients eating takes on greater meaning than simply to achieve nutritional benefit, and this may help to explain the emotional and behavioral investment present in food and eating.

A possible role for cholecystokinin (a satiety-inducing nerve-gut peptide) has been implicated in bulimia. When compared with healthy subjects, bulimic patients have a blunted meal-induced secretion of cholecystokinin.

CLINICAL MANIFESTATIONS. *Psychological and Behavioral Features.* The characteristic behavioral feature is the binge-purge cycle: an eating compulsion with a failure to achieve or to respond to normal satiety. These episodes occur secretly and are often associated with feelings of frustration, loneliness, or the sight of tempting foods. Binges are usually planned, and the preparation is associated with anxiety and excitement. During the binge, high-calorie "junk" foods are pleasurably consumed. The binge is usually terminated when feelings of guilt or physical discomfort such as nausea, abdominal pain, or headache occurs. At this point the patient self-induces vomiting and/or takes cathartics or laxatives. Bulimics generally look healthy, and their behaviors are unnoticed by friends and family. They are more outgoing than their anorectic counterparts. Some patients may exhibit impulsive or antisocial behaviors such as drug abuse, kleptomania, and sexual promiscuity. The patient who seeks help does so because of feelings of guilt, anxiety, or depression, or she is no longer able to continue the habit and still function in daily activities.

Medical Features. The medical findings of bulimia are consequences of the vomiting and laxative abuse. The physical examination may reveal parotid or salivary gland swelling due to vomiting, bruising of the knuckles from their rubbing against the upper incisors during the induction of vomiting, pharyngitis and dental erosions from reflux of gastric acid, or conjunctival hemorrhages from retching.

Frequent vomiting may also be complicated by esophagitis, Mallory-Weiss tears, or aspiration pneumonitis. Hypokalemic hypochloremic metabolic alkalosis due to loss of H^+, Cl^-, and K^+ is the most common metabolic complication, and this may lead to cardiac arrhythmias or renal injury. Secondary metabolic disturbances may produce weakness, tetany, and seizures. Emetics such as ipecac may produce cardiac conduction defects and arrhythmias. Stimulant laxatives can produce a "cathartic colon" with degeneration of Auerbach's plexus.

The majority of patients are clinically depressed by the time of clinical presentation, and 5 per cent have attempted suicide. It is believed that bulimia may be a manifestation of an underlying depressive disorder, since a large proportion of patients have first-degree relatives with major affective disorders.

DIAGNOSIS. The diagnosis of bulimia is based on recognition of the binge eating pattern and the exclusion of other medical diseases that might explain the behavior. The differential diagnosis, which is limited in this young population group, would include schizophrenia, use of oral contraceptives, seizures, and rare neurologic disorders. The latter may include *Klüver-Bucy syndrome*, a disorder of bilateral temporal lobe damage associated with indiscriminate sexual behavior, hyperphagia, and pica, and *Kleine-Levin syndrome*, a sleep disorder associated with hypersomnia and overeating.

TREATMENT. The goal of treatment is to help the patient overcome the urge to overeat. Bulimic patients recognize their behaviors as maladaptive. Compared with anorectics, they are more aware of associated psychological difficulties and are more willing to work with physicians and counselors in a treatment plan.

The current psychotherapeutic technique is cognitive-behavioral treatment in which the patient identifies the abnormal behaviors and then uses behavioral techniques to extinguish them, thereby accomplishing greater self-control. The treatment is safe and probably effective.

Antidepressants have been reported to be successful in decreasing the binge activity and in increasing the patient's sense of well-being.

RUMINATION SYNDROME

Rumination syndrome, or merycism, is an eating disorder in which the person repetitively regurgitates small amounts of food from the stomach, rechews the food, and then reswallows it. The disorder has been recognized as a medical curiosity for over 300 years, and ruminators have been known for their tendencies to offer public performances.

Infants frequently ruminate, and the disorder is described among institutionalized adults and children with emotional and intellectual deficits. No characteristic psychological profile or psychiatric diagnosis has been reported. There may be two subpopulations with the disorder, those in whom the behavior develops in childhood as a learned maladaptive habit worsening at times of stress, and those in whom rumination is associated with bulimia. A familial association is reported, although the role for genetic factors in the pathogenesis is not established.

The prevalance of rumination in adults is unknown, since generally physicians are unfamiliar with the clinical features. Patients who seek treatment report symptoms of weight loss, regurgitation, or vomiting and may express concern about there being an underlying medical disorder. Parents may bring the adolescent child to the doctor because of halitosis or dental problems.

Rumination in humans is not the same physiologic event as in ruminant animals, since reverse peristalsis does not occur. Radiographic and manometric studies indicate that an episode is initiated by a belch or swallow, at which time the lower esophageal sphincter pressure is lowered, creating a common channel between the stomach and esophagus. At the same time diaphragmatic and rectus muscle contractions raise the intra-abdominal pressure, thereby leading to regurgitation. When the upper esophageal sphincter is relaxed, food is ejected into the mouth, where it is expectorated or reswallowed.

The diagnosis depends on identifying the characteristic clinical features in the absence of other organic or psychiatric disease. Medical conditions such as esophageal stricture, reflux esophagitis, intestinal obstruction, or esophageal motor disorders (achalasia, diffuse esophageal spasm) should be excluded by radiography, video-fluoroscopy, and manometry. Since the disorder appears to be a learned maladaptive habit, behavioral modification and biofeedback techniques are recommended as approaches to treatment. However, cure may be difficult because the act is pleasurable and patients may not be motivated to change.

Balaa MA, Drossman DA: Anorexia nervosa and bulimia: The eating disorders. DM 31:1, 1985. *This monograph comprehensively reviews the epidemiology, pathophysiology, medical and psychosocial characteristics, diagnosis, and treatment of the two major eating disorders.*

Diagnostic and Statistical Manual of Mental Disorders. 4th ed (DSM-IIIR). Washington, DC, American Psychiatric Association, 1987. *This manual provides the standards of nomenclature and diagnostic criteria for anorexia nervosa and bulimia.*

Harris RT: Bulimarexia and related serious eating disorders with medical complications. Ann Intern Med 99:800, 1983. *Provides a good review of the medical complications in bulimia.*

Hsu LKG: The treatment of anorexia nervosa. Am J Psychiatry 143:573, 1986. *A review of treatment, including discussion of the approach to the patient, pharmacotherapy, psychotherapy, and behavior modification.*

Mitchell JE, Seim HC, Colon E, et al.: Medical complications and medical management of bulimia. Ann Intern Med 107:71, 1987. *This is an excellent general review documented with 86 useful references concerning this common disorder.*

Levine DF, Wingate DL, Pfeffer JM, et al.: Habitual rumination: A benign disorder. Br Med J 287:255, 1983. *Presents some of the clinical features of nine patients with rumination syndrome.*

203 Obesity

F. Xavier Pi-Sunyer

Obesity is a frustrating problem for patient and physician alike. Its underlying cause is rarely clear, and its treatment is fraught with difficulty and failure. Management of obesity therefore requires much understanding and persistence.

About 34 million adult Americans (26 per cent of those aged 20 to 75 years) are overweight, 12.4 million severely so. The per cent of adult women who are overweight (27.1 per cent) is somewhat greater than that of men (24.2 per cent).

DEFINITION

Visual inspection of a patient can give a subjective but fairly accurate estimate of the degree of obesity. More objective measures are height-weight tables, weight-related indices, and other anthropometric measurements.

The three most commonly used indices are (1) tables of average weights by height and age; (2) tables of desirable weights for height associated with lowest mortalities in insured populations; and (3) indices derived from height and weight, of which the body mass index is the most useful.

TABLES OF AVERAGE WEIGHTS. National Health and Nutrition Examination Surveys (NHANES) are periodically conducted on a representative United States population and then compiled in percentile tables as weights for height for sex. These cross-sectional data can be used for defining obesity, with a commonly made arbitrary decision that above the 85th percentile is "overweight." This comparison to a reference population makes no statement as to health risk involved at any weight level. The biggest problem is that of finding an appropriate reference population, particularly for minorities.

IDEAL WEIGHT TABLES. The Metropolitan Life Insurance Company Tables of Heights and Weights indicate the weight at which longevity is greatest, based on those insured. The 1983 tables are derived from the pooled data of 25 insurance companies in the United States and Canada, including about 4.2 million policies issued between 1950 and 1971. People with major diseases were screened out. The tables show weights based on lowest mortality for men and women at ages 25 to 59 by height and body frame.

The Metropolitan tables have been criticized as being inaccurate because (1) insured subjects do not represent a random sample of the population; (2) insured subjects are screened for illness and so are healthier than average; (3) no actual body frame measurements were taken when data were gathered so that the division into three frame categories (small, medium, and large) was a post hoc manipulation of the data; (4) about 20 per cent of the subjects used in the tables reported their heights and weights but were not actually measured (the bias being that women tend to under-report their weight and men to over-report their height); (5) the tables do not distinguish between obesity and overweight.

BODY MASS INDEX (BMI). In an effort to clear the confusion about how to classify overweight, the BMI has been computed:

$$BMI = kg/(ht \text{ in meters})^2$$
$$\text{or } BMI = lb/(ht \text{ in inches})^2 \times 703.1$$

This simple measurement correlates quite highly with other estimates of fatness, although some very muscular individuals may be classified as obese when they are not. It is also a somewhat more accurate index of fatness for males than for females.

The mean BMI (weighted for the height distribution of the United States population) taken from the mid-point of the medium frame of the 1983 Metropolitan tables is 22.4 kg/m² for men and 22.5 kg/m² for women. Patients can be divided for degree of obesity as shown in Figure 203–1. Health risks increase as BMI increases above 25.

Aging is a fattening process, so that a young and old person of comparable body weight are not comparably obese (Fig. 203–2). This has led to controversy concerning whether it is the total weight of an individual that should stay constant from 25 years

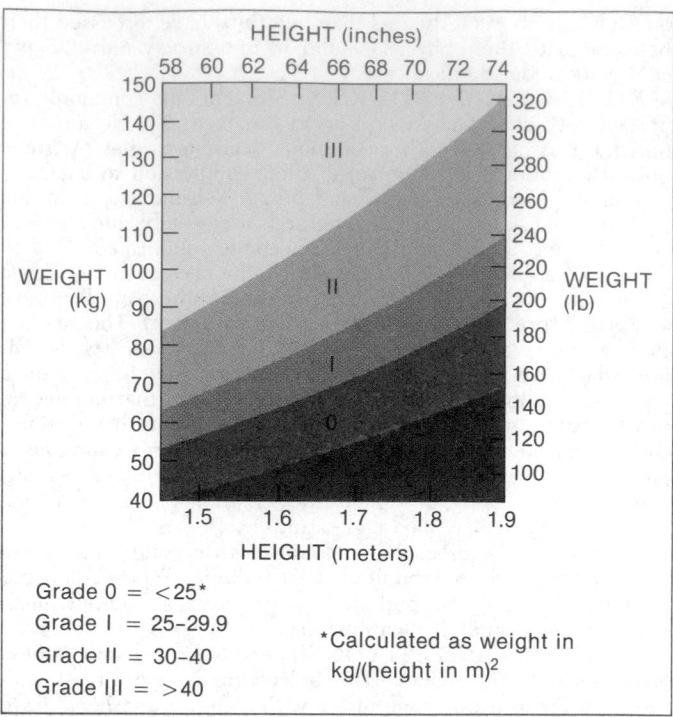

FIGURE 203–1. Grades of obesity as defined by body mass index. (Reproduced with permission from Garrow JS: Treat Obesity Seriously. Edinburgh, Churchill Livingstone, 1981, p 3.)

Grade 0 = <25*
Grade I = 25–29.9
Grade II = 30–40
Grade III = >40

*Calculated as weight in kg/(height in m)²

to 70 years or the fat-free mass, that is, the working cellular mass of the body plus the skeleton. The average weight data from the United States population show a gradually increasing weight with age, more pronounced and sustained for women than for men (Fig. 203–3).

Whereas many studies suggest that an increase from one's weight at 25 years old may increase mortality, a number have suggested that for the lowest mortality, the pattern of body

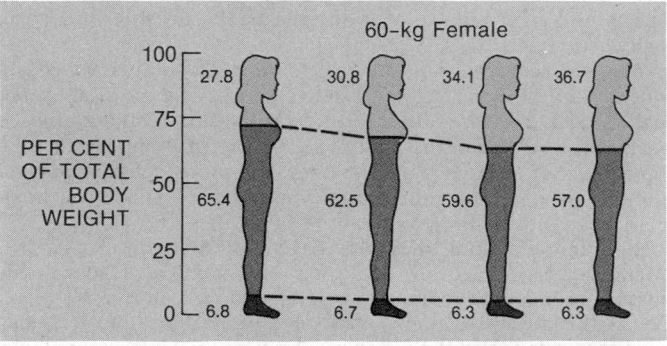

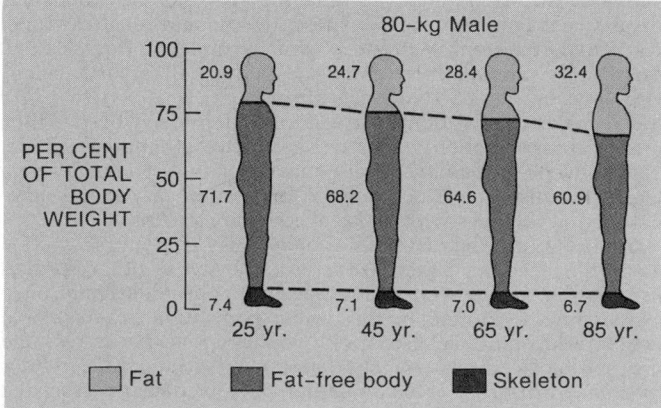

FIGURE 203–2. Body composition change with aging of representative normal adults. (Adapted from Moore FD, Olesen KH, McMurrey JE, et al.: The Body Cell Mass and Its Supporting Environment. Philadelphia, W. B. Saunders Company, 1963.)

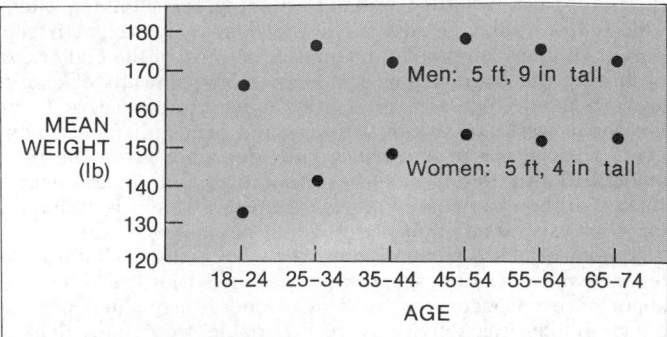

FIGURE 203–3. Weight change with aging for men and women. (Adapted from National Center for Health Statistics: Weight by height and age for adults 18–74 years, United States, 1971–1974. DHEW Publication No. [PHS] 79-1656, Series 11, No. 208, 1979.)

weight should be leanness in the twenties followed by a very moderate weight gain as one gets older. The minimal mortality points in relation to BMI for each age-sex grouping have been calculated. The regression lines, computed separately for men and women, are presented in Figure 203–4. Clearly, age strongly affects the BMI associated with the lowest mortality in this study. Also, the regression lines for men and women are nearly the same. The "best" BMI gradually increases with age in both sexes, with no consistent difference between men and women. As a result, a single set of weight goal tables (Table 203–1) can be constructed which are applicable for both men and women. The goals, which are somewhat more liberal for certain age groups than are the Metropolitan tables, are given by decade of age, with generally higher allowable weights as persons get older. Until the issue is further clarified, these goals seem to be reasonable for a physician to utilize in counseling patients in preventive medicine. Two caveats must be added. First, these tables have been derived from and are applicable primarily to white men and women in the United States. Second, the tables have been derived from populations without known risk factors. Patients with significant risk factors such as coronary artery disease, hypertension, and diabetes mellitus are better counseled

TABLE 203–1. AGE-SPECIFIC WEIGHT-FOR-HEIGHT TABLES* (GERONTOLOGY RESEARCH CENTER)

	Weight Range for Men and Women by Age (Years)†				
Height	25	35	45	55	65
ft–in			lb		
4–10	84–111	92–119	99–127	107–135	115–142
4–11	87–115	95–123	103–131	111–139	119–147
5–0	90–119	98–127	106–135	114–143	123–152
5–1	93–123	101–131	110–140	118–148	127–157
5–2	96–127	105–136	113–144	122–153	131–163
5–3	99–131	108–140	117–149	126–158	135–168
5–4	102–135	112–145	121–154	130–163	140–173
5–5	106–140	115–149	125–159	134–168	144–179
5–6	109–144	119–154	129–164	138–174	148–184
5–7	112–148	122–159	133–169	143–179	153–190
5–8	116–153	126–163	137–174	147–184	158–196
5–9	119–157	130–168	141–179	151–190	162–201
5–10	122–162	134–173	145–184	156–195	167–207
5–11	126–167	137–178	149–190	160–201	172–213
6–0	129–171	141–183	153–195	165–207	177–219
6–1	133–176	145–188	157–200	169–213	182–225
6–2	137–181	149–194	162–206	174–219	187–232
6–3	141–186	153–199	166–212	179–225	192–238
6–4	144–191	157–205	171–218	184–231	197–244

*Values in this table are for height without shoes and weight without clothes. To convert inches to centimeters, multiply by 2.54; to convert pounds to kilograms, multiply by 0.455.

†Data from Andres R: Gerontology Research Center, National Institute of Aging, Baltimore, MD.

on stricter tables, such as the Metropolitan Life Tables of 1983 (Ch. 200).

OTHER METHODS. Over half of the fat in the body is deposited under the skin. Its thickness can be measured at various sites using standard skin calipers. It is not difficult to become adept in the use of the calipers, and a running record of a patient's estimated body fat can be easily kept. The most useful and accurate tables are based on the measurement of four skinfold thicknesses—biceps, triceps, subscapular, and suprailiac. For such tables, see the British Journal of Nutrition 2:77, 1974.

Other methods of defining obesity are more difficult and expensive and therefore are used mostly for research purposes: (1) Total body water can be measured by dilution with tritiated or deuterated water. Water is then assumed to be a fixed proportion of fat-free mass (FFM = water mass/0.73), and FFM is subtracted from total body weight to obtain total body fat. (2) Body density can be measured by underwater weighing (with accurate correction for lung and abdominal air) and the amount of fat-free mass and body fat can be calculated. (3) The amount of body potassium can be estimated by measuring the amount of its naturally radioactive isotope ^{40}K in a whole-body counter. From this figure the lean body mass can be calculated as LBM = total K^+ (mmol)/68.1. Total body fat can be calculated as total weight minus LBM.

ETIOLOGY

Very little is known about the etiology of obesity. There are probably many different causes, and some may even co-exist in one individual. Obviously excess lipid deposition occurs because energy intake exceeds energy expenditure. An obese individual may have increased intake, decreased expenditure, or both.

GENETICS. Recent twin and adoption studies indicate that human fatness is under strong genetic control. From 64 to 88 per cent of the variance in skinfold thickness, body mass index, and relative weight has been attributed to genetic factors. The studies that have shown this degree of variance describe the genetic influences found in persons living under particular environmental conditions, namely those of western society. Since the environment in which heritable characteristics are expressed affects the expression, these variance ranges may not apply to all societies. Not only is there a strong genetic component to fatness, but there is also a similarly strong genetic component to regional

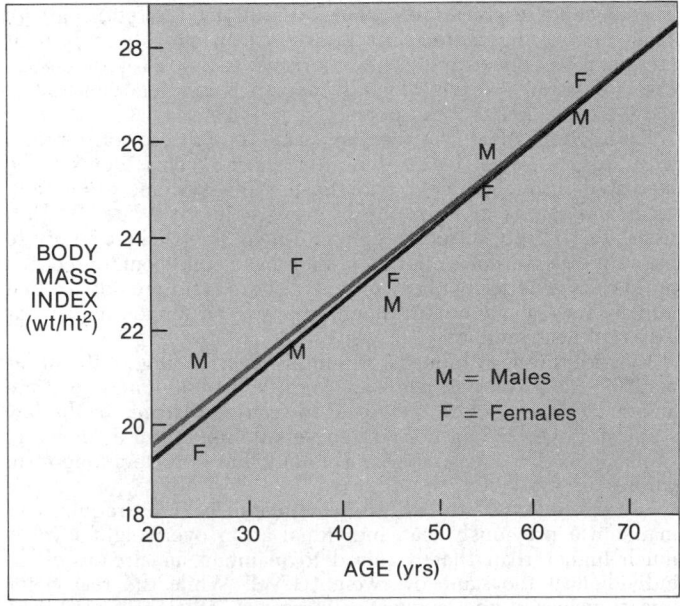

FIGURE 203–4. The effect of age on the body mass index (BMI) associated with lowest mortality. Minimal mortality points were computed for each age-sex group. The regression lines were computed separately for men (dark red line) and for women (light red line). Note that there is a strong effect of age on the BMI associated with lowest mortality and that the regression lines for men and women are nearly identical. (From The Build Study, 1979. Adapted by Andres R: *In* Andres R, Bierman EL, Hazzard WR, Blass JP (eds.): Principles of Geriatric Medicine. Copyright © 1990 by McGraw-Hill, Inc. Used by permission of McGraw-Hill Book Company.)

fat distribution. Thus, a person's genotype is an important determinant of how adaptation to excess energy intake occurs. Environment is also clearly important, and the interrelation of genetics to particular environments needs to be further investigated.

A number of rare genetic diseases are associated with obesity, but through unknown mechanisms: the Prader-Willi syndrome, the Laurence-Moon-Biedl syndrome, the Alstrom syndrome, the Cohen syndrome, the Carpenter syndrome, and Blount's disease. The reader is referred to textbooks on genetic disorders for further descriptions of these entities.

ENERGY INTAKE. Hyperphagia is the striking cause of obesity in a number of animal models (both genetic and brain-lesioned). The cause of human obesity is usually much less straightforward, however. Obesity has been regarded as an eating disorder for centuries, but the presumed eating abnormality has been difficult to document. Measuring food intake in a free-living environment is subject to large errors. It is also difficult to agree on what constitutes abnormal intake, since the range of caloric intake varies greatly even in lean individuals. Most studies have suggested that obese persons do overeat (at least in their weight-gaining phases). There are numerous examples of individuals who categorically deny overeating but who lose weight when brought into a metabolic ward and placed on a calculated weight-maintaining diet for their height and age.

Possibly obese persons are unduly attracted by the hedonic aspects of food, or they have impaired feedback signals registering satiety, or they have insensitive central reception centers for the feedback signals. It has also been suggested that feeding behavior is learned and that satiety is a conditioned response. Maladaptive conditioning is said to occur in obese persons. None of these theories has been scientifically validated.

ENERGY EXPENDITURE. Resting Metabolic Expenditure. Obese individuals may gain weight because they are "thrifty"; i.e., less ingested nutrient is spent as heat and thus more is available for storage. This argument has been put forward by those who contend that obese individuals do not eat more than lean ones and may actually eat less. Impaired thermogenesis exists in certain animal models of obesity. While it has been more difficult to document in humans, recent studies in both adults and infants have reported that a low rate of energy expenditure may predispose to obesity.

Thermogenesis can be divided into three components—resting metabolic rate (RMR), thermic effect of food (TEF), and thermic effect of exercise or activity (TEE).

RMR is the energy expended in the postabsorptive state to drive basic life-supporting processes under thermoneutral conditions. RMR, expressed as total amount of energy spent per unit time, is higher in obese persons than in lean ones. RMR can be well correlated with total weight but can be better correlated with lean body mass (LBM). This explains why men have higher RMR's than women and why RMR's decrease with age.

Obese individuals have a higher LBM than those who are lean, since they require an extra amount of sustaining cell mass to maintain the extra fat. When RMR is expressed as kilocalories per kilogram of LBM, obese persons have values equivalent to the lean. It is only when RMR is expressed as kilocalories per kilogram of body weight that they have values below those who are lean. This is because per unit of weight they have a relatively lower amount of metabolizing cell mass and a larger amount of stored fat, which is relatively inert in energy utilization. In terms of basal or resting energetics, therefore, the obese once they are obese do not have impaired RMR's and are not more "efficient" than lean persons. Some recent studies have reported, however, that in certain individuals a low RMR may predispose them to gain weight.

The RMR varies as much as ±15 per cent from individual to individual, even when they are matched for age, sex, and surface area. If a difference in metabolic rate between individuals can be as great as one third, it is clear that at a given caloric intake one individual may gain weight and another may lose it. Energy balance depends on matching intake to expenditure. It is not surprising that different individuals maintain weight on widely differing caloric intakes.

Expenditure in Activity. The obese expend more energy during physical activity, since an obese person is moving a greater load

through space, whether walking, running, or climbing stairs. This is true, although less so, even when body weight is supported, as in cycle ergometer exercise, because of the higher cost of moving the larger leg mass. Thus, more kilowatts of energy are expended. Increases in energy expenditure relative to increases in work are similar in obese and lean individuals, however. That is, if lean and obese individuals are given the same amount of work to do, once the constant amount of extra energy related to the extra cost of moving the extra weight is accounted for, they expend an equivalent amount of energy.

Studies of obese persons, however, show most of them to be less active, both in engaging in physical activities and in moving about once engaged. The amount of energy expended over 24 hours in physical activity is very variable from individual to individual, however, and it is difficult to generalize.

Expenditure After Food. Food is an important thermogenic stimulant, since it generates heat as it is metabolized. Because of this, a fed person has a higher metabolic rate than a fasting one. This elevation of postcibal metabolic rate above basal has been called the thermic effect of food (TEF). With a mixed diet, about 10 per cent of the metabolizable energy ingested is lost as heat.

Obese persons may have TEF responses equivalent to lean persons, or they may have a somewhat depressed response. The impaired response appears to be related to insulin resistance. Obese persons with insulin resistance have a slower glucose disposal. The impaired utilization of glucose by the cells of the body slows down heat production. Thus, glucose loads in an insulin-resistant obese person can generate lesser amounts of heat per calorie ingested. This impaired thermogenic effect can be normalized by giving insulin, so that an equivalent thermic response to that of insulin-sensitive persons occurs. Thus, it seems likely that a thermogenic defect relating to carbohydrate disposal is found in obese patients who are insulin resistant and not found in those who are equivalently obese but insulin sensitive. Thus, there is evidence for an overall somewhat diminished thermic effect of food in obese as compared to lean individuals. However, even insulin-resistant obese persons with a decreased TEF have an overall energy expenditure greater than do lean persons for the 3- to 4-hour period after the meal, since the slight decrease in TEF is less than the inherent elevation in their RMR.

In summary, although hypometabolism may predispose to obesity in some cases, RMR is higher once obesity is present. Thermogenic responses to ordinary stimuli (food, stress, cold) are small per se, and differences between lean and obese persons are small to nonexistent. The net result is that 24-hour energy expenditure in the typical obese person is greater than that of the typical sedentary lean person.

Expenditure After Overfeeding. Small rodents can waste rather than store much of excess ingested calories. This seems to be mediated through the sympathetic nervous system, which activates and causes hypertrophy of brown adipose tissue (BAT), a tissue that is specialized to generate heat. A deficient ability to burn off excess calories in this fashion has been documented in a number of genetically obese rodents. There is little evidence that humans have an adequate amount of brown fat to mount a similar excess of heat production, however.

In studies in lean humans, significant overfeeding (of the order of 2000 extra calories per day) for a sufficient length of time (about 10 days or more) may lead to energy wastage. In the few studies of overfeeding done in obese volunteers, no evidence of similar energy wastage has been found, but very few long-term studies are available.

In experimental studies, the number of calories required to maintain a previously lean individual at an overweight level is much higher than that required to maintain an already obese individual at the same overweight level. While the reason for this is unclear, it does suggest an increased "efficiency" of at least some obese subjects.

Do obese people lack a protective mechanism, i.e., heat dissipation, that lean people possess if they overeat? There is not much convincing experimental evidence to date, although it is a tempting hypothesis that needs to be further investigated.

PATHOPHYSIOLOGY

FAT CELLS. Fat cells (adipocytes) form a reservoir of energy that expands or contracts according to the energy balance of the organism. Fat cells develop from precursor preadipocytes to accommodate excess nutrient calories. Adipocytes gradually increase in volume to about 1 μg of mass, at which point little further enlargement seems to be possible. With continuing positive energy balance, new adipocytes form from precursor cells and the total cell number increases. Adipocytes can increase their number in an unlimited fashion, so that fat mass can reach huge dimensions through hyperplasia.

Once fat cells are formed, it is difficult to dedifferentiate them. This has been termed the "ratchet effect," because a ratchet turns in only one direction. Even though weight may be lost, fat cell numbers remain fixed. As a result, fat cell size reverts toward normal and with sustained weight loss may actually go below normal (Fig. 203–5).

What the stimulus is for the differentiation of preadipocytes into adipocytes is unknown. Adipose tissue lipoprotein lipase (LPL) may be involved. LPL acts on circulating chylomicrons and very low density lipoproteins (VLDL), activating the breakdown of triglyceride to glycerophosphate and free fatty acids (FFA). The FFA can then enter adipocytes, be re-esterified to triglycerides, and be stored. Adipose tissue LPL activity is high in obesity. Whether it is primary and causative for obesity or is secondary to the obesity is unclear. While LPL activity seems to rise with weight loss and is thought to be important in the accelerated weight regain of many patients, it seems to drop after the maintenance of weight loss for a time, suggesting that its elevation in the obese patient may be secondary rather than primary.

REGIONAL DISTRIBUTION OF ADIPOSE TISSUE. Fat mass is distributed differently in men and women. The android, or male, pattern is characterized by fat distributed predominantly in the upper body above the waist, whereas the gynecoid, or female, pattern shows fat predominantly in the lower body, that is, lower abdomen, buttocks, hips, and thighs. Upper body fat has a significantly worse prognosis for morbidity and mortality than does lower body fat. The regional distribution can be measured in a variety of ways. The easiest, most common, and very useful way is by measuring body circumference at the waist and at the hips and calculating a waist:hip ratio. A ratio of greater than 0.85 in women and greater than 1.0 in males can be considered abnormal.

Fat cells from the upper body seem to be functionally different from fat cells in the lower body. They are more sensitive to catecholamines and insulin. It is likely that the greater lipolytic and lipogenic potential of the upper body cells is related to an underlying difference in sex-hormone response of the two tissues. Thus, testosterone and estrogen influences may be important and may act differently on upper and lower body fat cells.

Abdominal or android fatness carries a greater risk for hypertension, cardiovascular disease, hyperinsulinemia, diabetes mellitus, gallbladder disease, and stroke. It also carries a greater risk of overall mortality. Since more men than women have the android distribution, they are more at risk for these conditions. Also, women who deposit their excess fat in a more android manner have a greater risk than women whose fat distribution is more gynecoid. Upper body fat deposition tends to occur primarily by hypertrophy of the existing cells, whereas lower body fat deposition is by differentiation of new fat cells, i.e., hyperplasia. Reducing a normal number of enlarged fat cells to normal size is easier than reducing large numbers of the cells in the lower body hyperplastic depot to normal or below normal sized cells. This may explain the weight loss difficulties of many women with lower body obesity.

Thus, three components of body fat are associated with health risk: per cent body fat, subcutaneous truncal or abdominal fat, and visceral fat in the abdominal cavity. While partly correlated with each other, they do show independence of expression.

SET POINT. The concept of a "set point" of body weight suggests that each person has a control system that "sets" how much weight, or alternatively how much fat, he or she should have. How the control system is regulated, that is, where the feedback signals from "weight" or "fat" originate and how they might be transmitted (humoral, neural, both?) to the hypothalamic feeding and satiety areas are totally unknown.

This set-point theory suggests that people are at a given weight because they are "set" there. That is, one's set point is the weight one normally maintains. Although this is circular thinking, set-point theory has been used to suggest that weight loss programs are misguided and that the effort to lose weight is inevitably fraught with failure because set point will bring individuals up to their pre-weightloss weight.

Animals with ventromedial hypothalamus (VMH) lesions seem

FIGURE 203–5. Fat cell hypertrophy, proliferation, and shrinkage to and below initial size. (Adapted with permission from Van Itallie TB: The enduring storage capacity of fat. *In* Stunkard AJ, Stellar E (eds.): Eating and Its Disorders. New York, Raven Press, copyright 1984.)

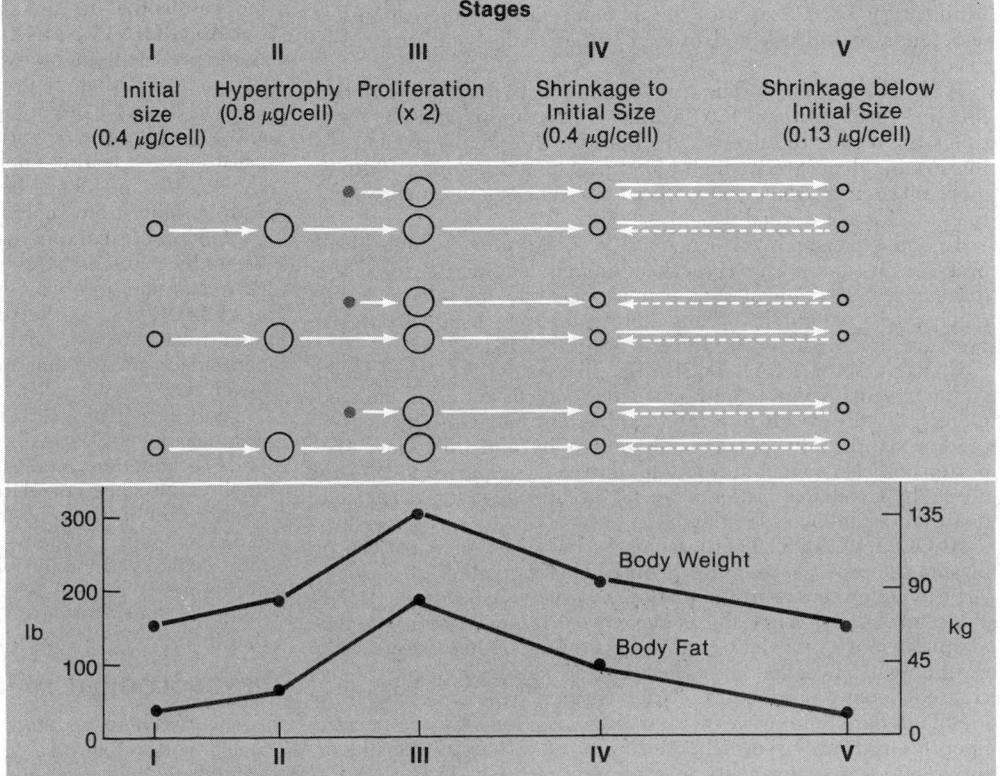

to "set" themselves at a higher prevailing weight, from which they then once more regulate their weight normally. That is, once they have attained their plateau higher weight, they gain more weight if overfed but return to previous weight if they are allowed to eat ad lib; if they are food-deprived, they lose weight and when fed ad lib also return to their previous plateau weight. In a similar manner, animals with lesions in the lateral hypothalamus are hypophagic and lose weight to a new lower weight "set point," which they then return back to from either overweight if they have been overfed or underweight if they have been further underfed. Genetically obese animals, such as the Zucker rat, also seem to defend elevated weights.

If and how these models relate to human obesity is unclear. The set-point theory has been used to suggest that exercise and some drugs lower set point and most palatable foods raise it. Once these statements have been made, however, no closer understanding of the regulation of body weight and of food intake has been attained. Certainly, if there is a "set point," it is a very movable one that seems to change easily under the influence of a number of environmental conditions.

CLINICAL MANIFESTATIONS

INSULIN RESISTANCE. Obesity induces an insulin-resistant state in man, one that is associated with both basal and stimulated hyperinsulinemia. This results from a change in β-cell insulin release rather than in the threshold to glucose stimulation. The enlarged fat cell is less sensitive to the antilipolytic and lipogenic actions of insulin. While a decreased number of insulin receptors contributes to the insulin resistance, the resistance is generally much greater than would be predicted from the magnitude of this decrease. A "postreceptor" defect is therefore presumed to occur as well. This defect in glucose utilization occurs also in other insulin-sensitive tissues, particularly muscle. The liver is also less responsive to insulin. As the insulin resistance becomes more profound, glucose uptake in peripheral tissues is impaired and glucose output by the liver is increased.

DIABETES MELLITUS. In a certain number of obese individuals, diabetes mellitus occurs, as the non-insulin-dependent (NIDDM) type (Ch. 218). The prevalence of diabetes is approximately three times higher in overweight than in nonoverweight persons. In the United States about 85 per cent of patients with NIDDM are obese. Clinically manifest diabetes develops only with the appropriate genetic legacy, but obesity, by enhancing insulin resistance, increases the demand on the pancreatic islets and tends to unmask and exacerbate an underlying propensity for diabetes.

HYPERTENSION. The prevalence of hypertension (blood pressure greater than 160/95 mm Hg) is approximately three times higher for the overweight than for the nonoverweight. In the Framingham Study, high blood pressure developed 10 times more often in persons who were 20 per cent or more overweight than in those of normal weight.

The mechanism by which obesity contributes to high blood pressure is unknown. Hyperinsulinemia leading to increased tubular reabsorption of sodium may be a factor. Whatever the mechanism, weight loss from dieting leads to a fall in arterial pressure, even when salt intake is not restricted.

CARDIOVASCULAR DISEASE. In obesity, increased blood volume, stroke volume, left ventricular end-diastolic volume, and filling pressure result in a high cardiac output. This can lead to predominantly left ventricular hypertrophy and dilatation. Hypertension also contributes to left ventricular hypertrophy. Thus, obese hypertensive patients are at greater risk for congestive heart failure and sudden death.

BLOOD LIPIDS. There seems to be an adverse pattern of plasma lipoproteins in obese people. This is manifested particularly by a low concentration of high density lipoprotein (HDL) cholesterol. LDL cholesterol may be elevated. Hypertriglyceridemia is more prevalent in obese persons, possibly because the insulin resistance and hyperinsulinemia of obesity lead to increased hepatic production of triglycerides. This hypertriglyceridemia generally improves with weight loss, but if a true genetic lipoprotein disorder coexists, more intensive therapy specific for the lipoprotein abnormality may be required (Ch. 172).

RESPIRATORY PROBLEMS. Severe obesity can lead to chronic hypoxia with cyanosis and hypercapnia. Associated with this are an increased demand for ventilation, an increased breathing workload, respiratory muscle inefficiency, and decreased functional reserve capacity and expiratory reserve volume. Peripheral lung units can close, resulting in a ventilation-perfusion mismatch.

The end-stage associated with severe obesity is the pickwickian syndrome, in which hypoventilation is so marked that hypoxia leads to long periods of somnolence. In these patients, pulmonary hypertension occurs and cardiac failure may supervene.

SLEEP APNEA. Sleep apnea is very common in severely obese patients (Ch. 70). The relationship between obesity and sleep apnea is unclear, since the most obese individuals are not necessarily the most severely affected. Apnea can be obstructive or central, and both are more prevalent in obese persons. In obese persons the upper airways may be obstructed by the large local accumulation of fat tissue, often in combination with micrognathia and enlarged tonsils and adenoids. The obstruction leads to hypoventilation and hypoxia, which somehow trigger apneic episodes that then make the hypoxia and hypercapnia worse. These patients benefit from weight loss and sometimes from surgical removal of some of the obstructive tissues. Central apnea is characterized by a cessation of ventilatory drive from brain centers, so that diaphragmatic excursions stop for periods of 10 to 30 seconds. The reason obese persons are prone to this condition is unknown. Pharmacotherapy is sometimes helpful. Daytime somnolence is common in obese patients with apnea, partly from hypoxia and partly from the continual disturbance of sleep at night, since they tend to awake after each apneic episode.

VENOUS CIRCULATORY DISEASE. Severely obese individuals often have varicose veins and venous stasis. Congestive heart failure may add to dependent edema, with the further complications of trophic changes of the skin and an increased propensity for thrombophlebitis and thromboembolism. Pulmonary embolism is much more common in the obese than in those of normal weight (Ch. 65).

CANCER. Endometrial cancer is two to three times more common in obese than in lean women. Risk of breast cancer increases with increasing BMI in postmenopausal women. It has been speculated that this increased risk is due to the stimulatory effect of increased levels of estrogens in the postmenopausal period. Obese women also have a higher incidence of cancer of the gallbladder and of the biliary system. Obese men have a higher mortality from cancer of the colon, rectum, and prostate for reasons that are unknown.

GASTROINTESTINAL DISEASE. Cholesterol gallstones are more prevalent in obesity. The pathogenetic sequence is presumed to be that of greater cholesterol production in the increased body fat depots, greater biliary excretion of cholesterol, and a resulting supersaturation of the cholesterol in bile. The gallstones can lead to cholecystitis (see Ch. 126) and the need for cholecystectomy. The obese carry a greater risk for complications and mortality from such abdominal surgery.

Many obese patients have fatty livers with modest abnormalities of liver function tests, but hepatic diseases in general are not more common in obese than in lean persons.

ARTHRITIS. As the severity of obesity increases, joint symptoms related to osteoarthritis become common. Excess stress is particularly placed on joints of the lower extremities and the lower back.

There is a strong correlation between body weight and serum uric acid level. With obesity, urate clearance is decreased and urate production increased. Since hypertension and diabetes mellitus also are correlated with elevated uric acid levels, the relationship between hyperuricemia and obesity is multifactorial.

SKIN. Skin problems are common in obesity, particularly intertrigo in redundant folds of skin. Fungal and yeast infections of skin are common. Acanthosis nigricans occurs in a minority of morbidly obese patients. These patients can manifest a syndrome that includes severe insulin resistance.

PSYCHOLOGICAL MANIFESTATIONS

The psychological toll of severe obesity is large. Poor self-image and impaired social relationships are common. Obese individuals are often discriminated against in educational and

TABLE 203–2. PATTERN OF EXCESS MORTALITY VARIATION WITH EXCESS WEIGHT (MEN AGES 15–34 YRS AT ENTRY)

Weight Relative to Average Weight (per cent)	Mortality Ratio
105–115	110
115–125	127
125–135	134
135–145	141
145–155	211
155–165	227

Adapted from Build Study 1979. Chicago, Society of Actuaries and Association of Life Insurance Medical Directors of America, 1980.

professional settings, engendering anxiety, anger, and self-doubt. There is no evidence, however, of any particular neurotic or psychotic character in obese individuals. The depression and anxiety seem to be situational rather than endogenous and often improve if the obesity can be ameliorated.

MORTALITY

Obesity is associated with increased mortality. The effect of obesity on cardiovascular mortality generally occurs through linkage with other risk factors such as hypertension, diabetes, and hyperlipidemia. However, obesity can also make independent contribution to mortality. In the Framingham Study, for every 10 per cent rise in relative weight, systolic blood pressure rose 6.5 mm Hg, plasma cholesterol 12 mg per deciliter, and fasting blood glucose 2 mg per deciliter. The causes of increased mortality for those 20 per cent or more overweight include coronary heart disease, cerebral "hemorrhage" (stroke), diabetes, digestive diseases, and cancer (Table 203–2).

OBESITY AND THE ENDOCRINE SYSTEM

Although obesity has often been described as an "endocrine" disease, less than 1 per cent of obese patients have any significant endocrine dysfunction. Hypothalamic, pituitary, thyroid, adrenal, ovarian, and possibly pancreatic endocrine syndromes have been related to obesity.

HYPOTHALAMIC DISEASE. In this type of obesity, the appetite systems or tracts located in the hypothalamus are affected. Bilateral damage in the ventromedial hypothalamus produces obesity in the rat; conversely, bilateral damage in the extreme lateral portion of the hypothalamus causes aphagia. Rather than a single balance of a "feeding center" and a "satiety center," however, it is now clear that diffuse excitatory and inhibitory neuronal systems controlling feeding course through the limbic system and the whole brain. Following trauma, inflammation, or a tumor in the hypothalamus, a few patients develop hyperphagic obesity, most of them after surgery for tumors in the hypothalamic area. Craniopharyngioma has been most commonly associated with rapidly progressive obesity. The diagnosis is usually based on history and physical findings, which may or may not include focal neurologic defects, depending on the nature and extent of the injury.

PITUITARY AND ADRENAL DYSFUNCTION. Cushing's disease is the most common form of pituitary dysfunction leading to obesity (Ch. 217). ACTH is excessively produced either by a pituitary tumor or by hyperactive pituitary cells, which leads to excess production of cortisol by the adrenal cortex. Cushing's syndrome can also have a variety of other causes, including exogenous glucocorticoids, primary disorders of the adrenal, and paraneoplastic syndromes of excess ACTH production. The hypercortisolism causes adipocytes located primarily at the center of the body to expand, while those at the extremities do so much less. With this central obesity comes hypertension and diabetes.

THYROID DISEASE. Obesity is often ascribed to "hypometabolism" caused by underactivity of the thyroid gland, but this is in fact seldom true. Severe hypothyroidism can lead to some increased fat, but most of the excess weight is actually edema, which is lost with the institution of thyroid hormone replacement.

POLYCYSTIC OVARIAN SYNDROME (Ch. 224). Mild hirsutism, irregular menses or amenorrhea, and obesity have been linked in the "polycystic ovarian syndrome." In this syndrome the ovaries have atretic follicles, the patient is anovulatory, and

menstrual disturbance (long-term amenorrhea to oligomenorrhea) is the rule. The ovaries overproduce androgens, some of which are converted to estrogens peripherally, primarily in adipose tissue. Hirsutism is common, but virilization is not. The relation of obesity to the polycystic ovarian syndrome is not clear, but the two conditions often coexist.

ENDOCRINE CONSEQUENCES OF OBESITY. One of the pathophysiologic consequences of obesity may be certain endocrine abnormalities. The sex-hormone abnormalities associated with obesity are different in males and females. While mildly obese men have no detectable abnormalities, severely obese men have mild hypogonadotropic hypogonadism, with less than two thirds the normal mean plasma levels of total testosterone, free testosterone, and follicle-stimulating hormone. Gonadotropic hormones are suppressed by elevated plasma estrogens derived from increased aromatization of adrenal precursors in the excessive body fat. Obesity may be associated with increased metabolic clearance rates of testosterone, caused partly by decreased sex hormone-binding globulin (SHBG). Spermatogenesis, libido, and potency, however, are normal.

Estrogens are not elevated in obese premenopausal women, probably because the amount of estrone conversion by the adipose tissue is small in comparison with regular ovarian estradiol production. Estrogens are elevated, however, in postmenopausal obese women, most likely owing to increased peripheral conversion of the prehormone androstenedione to estrone. This may be a partial explanation as to why there is less osteoporosis in obese women.

There are differences in the androgen-estrogen environment in persons with upper (UBO) and lower (LBO) body obesity. This is more clearly defined in women. Women with UBO have higher androgen production rates and higher concentrations of testosterone and estradiol levels than those with LBO. They also have decreased levels of SHBG, so that free testosterone concentrations are higher. Women with LBO have increased estrone from peripheral aromatization of circulating androgens.

In obesity, insulin resistance develops and hyperinsulinemia results. Whether impaired glucose tolerance or frank diabetes ensues depends on the degree of insulin resistance and the underlying genetic make-up of the individual. Triiodothyronine (T_3) may be elevated to high normal in conditions of high caloric intake with adequate carbohydrate, while thyroxine levels and TSH levels are normal. Slightly low blood cortisol levels may be present in obesity, probably because of enhanced turnover rates of cortisol. The circadian rhythm of cortisol secretion is usually normal in obesity. Urinary free cortisol levels are normal if related to the lean body mass or urinary creatinine. Also, these obese patients usually suppress normally with dexamethasone (Ch. 217).

Pseudotumor cerebri (benign intracranial hypertension) (Ch. 486) occurs most commonly in young women who are frequently obese. No intracranial pathology has been found, although headache and blurred vision occur. Why obesity is common in so many of these patients is unclear. It is possible that altered function of the ventromedial or paraventricular region of the brain occurs owing to the increased intracranial pressure.

Hypothalamic control of prolactin and growth hormone is often defective in obesity, with poor response to insulin hypoglycemia. These abnormalities generally revert to normal with significant weight loss, but not always. Whether these pituitary abnormalities reflect altered hypothalamic control due to obesity or abet the obesity in some way is unclear.

TREATMENT

Obesity is very difficult to treat, because the primary emphasis must be on active patient self-control rather than on passive drug therapy. The responsibility of the physician is to be as supportive and helpful as possible. The three approaches to weight control are diet, exercise, and drugs.

DIET. A truly motivated individual will generally stay on a diet for a long time, initially for weight loss and then for weight maintenance. Crash diets for a few days or weeks generally accomplish little of permanent value. Because of the long-term requirement for a diet, it must be tailored to a person's tastes and habits.

The diet must be nutritionally adequate. It is not possible to calculate a diet under 1100 calories that contains adequate amounts of vitamins and minerals. If the diet is lower in calories than this, vitamin and mineral supplements are necessary. The goal of weight loss is loss of as much fat as possible while losing as little lean body mass as possible. A mixed, balanced diet is a sensible approach to long-term weight reduction. A diet of at least 0.8 to 1.2 grams of protein per kilogram of desirable body weight will minimize nitrogen losses. The protein should be of high quality, so that essential amino acids can be utilized to maintain lean body mass.

It is a common strategy in many popular weight-reduction programs to use very unbalanced diets that focus on particular food groups at the expense of others. The high-fat–low-carbohydrate diets that are low in calories are ketogenic, whereas the low-fat–high-carbohydrate diets are not. These diets have in common a marked imbalance of macronutrients, with a concomitant imbalance of micronutrients. They cannot be recommended. If such diets are used, careful calculations for nutritional adequacy must be made, and appropriate supplements must be taken daily by the patient. These supplements require a number of tablets and capsules each day, so that compliance becomes a greater problem that must be strictly monitored.

VERY LOW CALORIE DIETS. Very low calorie diets (VLCD) severely limit daily intake to 300 to 700 calories. Some diets are strictly limited to protein and have been called protein-supplemented modified fasts (PSMF). Others allow both protein and carbohydrate. The concept of protein-supplemented fasting arose because this regimen improves nitrogen balance over fasting programs. There is little evidence, however, that at equicaloric levels protein alone is better than protein with carbohydrate. The extra weight lost early in the diet when protein alone is given is that of water. With this water diuresis there is electrolyte loss as well. The calories can be given either in liquid formula form or as natural foods. High-quality protein must be given. It is also imperative that adequate supplements of vitamins and minerals be taken. Although these very severe diets have been given for extensive periods of time, it is dangerous to allow them for longer than 12 weeks. The heavier the patient, the safer the diet seems to be. The lighter the patient, the more LBM is lost per unit of weight loss, so that more caution, more liberal calories, and a shorter time period of diet should be followed. These diets, especially those relying on liquid formulas, have been popular because of their relative ease and because, since they are so hypocaloric, the weight loss is more rapid. However, they can have serious side effects.

Side effects of these severe diets include orthostatic hypotension (secondary to both sodium loss and impaired norepinephrine secretion), fatigue, cold intolerance, dry skin, hair loss, and menstrual irregularities. Cholelithiasis, cholecystitis, and rarely pancreatitis occur. Unfortunately, most individuals rapidly regain weight after being on these crash programs, perhaps in large measure because the very low caloric content and the liquid form of the diet do not educate the patient to make the adjustments in lifestyle and eating behavior necessary to maintain the weight loss.

BEHAVIOR MODIFICATION. Psychoanalysis and psychotherapy have not been very helpful in weight control. An extended change in eating behavior requires a great change in life style, however, so behavior modification programs have proliferated. Behavior therapy is a fundamental departure from the traditional "dietary" training of the past, in which a list of foods, the allowable quantities, and specific menus were supplied. In behavior modification the patient is first made aware of what and how much he or she eats as a background for changing that behavior. Many persons eat quite unconsciously, with little thought of how much they eat and with little or no knowledge of its caloric content. Initially, in the education process, careful food intake diaries are kept. Patients record not only what was eaten, but where, with whom, how, their feelings, and their degree of hunger. These diaries are analyzed, and nutrient densities of foods are discussed. New modes of eating are suggested, including not eating between meals, eating always at table, eating only three times per day, watching the portions of food eaten, not doing other activities while eating, and eating slowly with concentration. Behavior modification also strives at stimulus control and environmental management. The aim is to break learned associations between environmental cues and food intake. Particular situations that trigger eating are avoided or controlled. Behavior modification therapy is usually done in groups, with continued dialogue between the trained group leader (psychologist, nutritionist, physician), the other group members, and the patient.

EXERCISE. Obesity is a consequence of greater energy intake than energy expenditure. To lose weight, the imbalance must be tipped the other way, with expenditure becoming greater than intake. This is done not only by hypocaloric dieting, but also by increasing activity. Obese persons tend to be inactive; it is therefore important to increase caloric utilization. The patient should be taught the approximate number of calories being expended over basal level in individual activities. Most patients are surprised at how much exercise it takes to expend just a few calories (Table 203–3).

Moderate exercise only transiently increases the metabolic rate. The calories expended are the calories of work done. In the obese, moderate exercise does not actually lower food intake, but intake does not increase to keep pace with the extra expenditure, as it does in lean persons. This is helpful in inducing weight loss.

DRUG THERAPY. Drugs in weight control have been used as short-term adjunctive therapy to diet and exercise. Over the long term the use of drugs has been disappointing, owing to small effects on weight loss or adverse side effects. In general, drugs affect appetite modestly. The anorectic drugs act centrally through brain catecholamine, dopaminergic, or serotoninergic pathways. For example, amphetamine and its derivatives seem to produce anorexia through stimulating the central hypothalamic neurochemical pathways in which norepinephrine and/or dopamine is the principal neurotransmitter.

Amphetamine not only decreases appetite; it also elevates mood and increases arousal, probably mediated through making norepinephrine and dopamine more abundant at synapses. In

TABLE 203–3. APPROXIMATE ENERGY EXPENDITURE IN SELECTED ACTIVITIES FOR PEOPLE OF DIFFERENT WEIGHTS (CALORIES PER 30 MINUTES)*

Activity	Weight (pounds)					
	110	130	150	170	190	210
Aerobic dancing						
"walking pace"	99	114	132	150	168	186
"jogging pace"	159	186	213	243	270	300
"running pace"	204	240	276	315	351	387
Basketball	207	243	282	318	357	396
Canoeing—leisure	66	78	90	102	114	126
Canoeing—racing	156	183	210	237	267	294
Carpentry	78	93	105	120	135	147
Cycling—5.5 mph	96	114	132	147	165	183
Cycling—9.4 mph	150	177	204	231	258	285
Dancing—ballroom	78	90	105	117	132	144
Dancing—disco	156	183	210	237	267	294
Gardening	150	177	204	231	258	285
Golf	129	150	174	195	219	243
Judo	294	345	399	450	504	558
Lying or sitting down	33	39	45	51	57	63
Mopping floor	96	105	120	138	153	171
Running						
11.5 minutes per mile	204	240	276	315	351	387
9 minutes per mile	291	342	393	447	498	552
7 minutes per mile	366	417	468	522	573	624
5.5 minutes per mile	435	513	591	669	747	828
Skiing, cross-country	216	252	291	330	369	408
Standing quietly	39	45	51	57	66	72
Swimming						
backstroke	255	300	345	390	435	486
crawl	192	228	261	297	330	366
Table tennis	102	120	138	156	174	195
Tennis	165	192	222	252	282	312
Walking						
3 mph	102	114	126	138	153	165
4 mph	120	141	162	186	207	228

*Adapted from The High Energy Factor, by B. Gutin. Copyright © 1983 by B. Gutin. Reprinted by permission of Random House, Inc.

contrast, fenfluramine is thought to increase brain serotonin. Mazindol probably works through a dopaminergic mechanism. It therefore appears that increasing the activity of norepinephrine, dopamine, and/or serotonin at certain central nervous system sites can lead to anorexia and weight loss.

All of the drugs mentioned have a greater effect on appetite control than do placebos. Problems arise, however, from abuse potential and side effects. Amphetamine has clearly addictive properties. Amphetamine and phenmetrazine have disturbing side effects, such as sleep disturbances, agitation, and psychosis. Irritability and insomnia have been reported with diethylpropion, mazindol, and phentermine. Fenfluramine often causes depression, sedation, and diarrhea. Contraindications include severe hypertension, coronary artery disease, glaucoma, and history of drug abuse.

These drugs are generally prescribed for short periods of time, in an effort to help patients over difficult weight "plateaus" or crisis periods. Some experts, however, suggest that certain of the drugs lower "set point" of weight and should be given chronically. This is not, however, generally accepted practice.

GOALS. Very often the patient, and sometimes the physician, has unrealistic goals of what can be accomplished. One pound of fat is equivalent to 4000 kilocalories. With a deficit of 400 kilocalories per day, losing one pound takes 10 days. The more accurate the knowledge of daily energy expenditure and energy intake is, the closer a physician can predict the rate of weight loss. This may prevent unrealistic goals and disappointment by both patient and therapist.

SURGERY. Certain patients have severe obesity (greater than 100 per cent of desirable weight), have tried weight control programs without success, and often have complications like sleep apnea, heart failure, phlebitis, and arthritis. Their life expectancy is much lower than normal. These patients may be candidates for surgery for obesity, since nonoperative management rarely leads to permanent weight reduction.

Surgery for obesity should be considered experimental, as there is no one accepted procedure and all carry significant risks and complications. Short bowel procedures (jejunoileal bypass) generally leave about 50 cm of small bowel between the ligament of Treitz and the ileocecal valve, with the bypassed portion of bowel draining directly into the ileal remnant (end-to-end or end-to-side) or into the colon. Jejunoileal bypass generally produces weight loss but is fraught with complications, including diarrhea, electrolyte losses, vitamin deficiencies, hepatic toxicity, calcium oxalate kidney stones, intestinal pseudo-obstruction, and polyarthritis. As a result, it cannot be recommended.

Because of the severe side effects of intestinal surgery, gastric surgical procedures have become popular. In these operations, no part of the stomach is resected, so that the operation is theoretically reversible. A small fundic pouch or reservoir is created so that the individual is severely limited in the amount of food that he or she can eat. The pouch is generally created by stapling across the stomach, leaving a very small reservoir. The distal stoma created for the pouch has variably been designed to empty into the rest of the stomach or into a loop of jejunum, with the rest of the stomach and duodenum becoming a blind loop. Alternatively, in vertical banded gastroplasty, as opposed to horizontal banding, only a small tubular reservoir remains for food entering from the esophagus. Side effects include gastric distress and vomiting. If vomiting is severe enough, electrolyte disturbances can occur. Also, some patients do not lose much weight, because many eat "around" the small reservoir with frequent servings of liquid or semisolid foods. A mean weight loss of two thirds of excess weight has been reported, but failure is not uncommon. Dilatation of the gastric pouch, stomal dilation, stomal obstruction, and staple line dehiscence can occur as complications.

Surgery is still unsatisfactory and experimental, but it may be advisable in some cases. Because life-long follow-up and vitamin and mineral supplementation are necessary, a responsible and cooperative patient and an experienced surgeon are a requisite duo.

WEIGHT REGAIN

The most difficult problem in the treatment of obesity is the maintenance of a reduced body weight. The ability to maintain weight loss may depend on the severity of obesity and the amount of hypercellularity of the adipocytes in a given individual.

A person who is modestly overweight with enlarged adipocytes but little proliferation of extra adipocytes can more easily maintain weight loss. The adipocyte hyperplasia of greater obesity is likely to create a much greater problem in maintenance of weight loss. The degree of filling of adipocytes is very likely a regulated factor in energy balance. Obese persons with adipocyte hyperplasia begin to decrease the mass of each adipocyte as they lose weight. If the adipocyte mass drops below a normal lower level of about 0.5 µg per cell, individuals seem to have greater difficulty in maintaining weight reduction. Adipocyte mass seems to be a regulated factor with a feedback effect on energy intake, so that the reduced obese seem to experience strong food intake cues that they have trouble resisting.

Lipogenic enzyme activities increase when a hypocaloric diet is liberalized as a patient goes from a weight-loss to a weight-maintenance period. This is consequent to an increase in caloric intake rather than being primarily caused by the reduction in weight. It is not clear whether an increased food efficiency is present, but reduced obese individuals have been reported to require about 25 per cent fewer calories per square meter of surface area to maintain their body weight than do either normal persons or obese individuals who have not dieted and lost weight. Thus, reduced obese persons have energy requirements typical of a semifasted state despite their taking sufficient calories to maintain weight at a level that is still above normal.

PREVENTION

The propensity toward obesity is partially inherited, but a large component is also environmental. Obesity leads to an increased morbidity and mortality from a number of diseases, especially for those who are under 45 years old. Being overweight in early adult life is more dangerous than it is at older ages.

It is incumbent on physicians to make their patients aware of these risks and try to keep patients at a body mass index of grade 0 to grade 1 (see Fig. 203–1). This is particularly true for those patients who already have, or have a family history of, the diseases that are precipitated and abetted by obesity.

Hubert HB, Feinleib M, McNamara PM, et al.: Obesity as an independent risk factor for cardiovascular disease: A 26-year follow-up of participants in the Framingham Heart Study. Circulation 67:968, 1983. *A re-examination of the relationship of the degree of obesity and the incidence of cardiovascular disease over 26 years in more than 5200 men and women indicates that obesity is a significant independent predictor, particularly among women.*

Kissebah AH, Vydelingum N, Murray R, et al.: Relation of body fat distribution to metabolic complications of obesity. J Clin Endocrinol Metab 54:254, 1982. *A study in women of the sites of fat predominance as an important prognostic marker for glucose intolerance, hyperinsulinemia, and hypertriglyceridemia.*

Krotkiewski M, Bjorntorp P, Sjostrom L, et al.: Impact of obesity on metabolism in men and women. Importance of regional adipose tissue distribution. J Clin Invest 72:1150, 1983. *A study of the regional differences between the sexes with regard to adipose tissue distribution and of the differential risk of upper and lower body obesity as it relates to lipid and carbohydrate metabolism.*

Lew EA, Garfinkel L: Variations in mortality by weight among 750,000 men and women. J Chron Dis 32:563, 1979. *A description of the mortality experience of men and women in a long-term prospective study by the American Cancer Society, documenting that individuals 30 to 40 per cent heavier than average had a mortality rate 50 per cent higher than those of average weight. Mortality comparisons as a function of weight for all common diseases are included.*

National Institutes of Health Consensus Development Panel on the Health Implications of Obesity: Health implications of obesity. Ann Intern Med 103:147, 1985. *A statement on the risks of obesity.*

Ravussin E, Lillioja MB, Knowler WC, et al.: Reduced rate of energy expenditure as a risk factor for body-weight gain. N Engl J Med 318(8):467–471, 1988. *A report of hypometabolism as a predisposing cause of obesity.*

Segal KR, Pi-Sunyer FX: Exercise, resting metabolic rate, and thermogenesis. Diabetes/Metab Rev 2:19, 1986. *A review of the differences in thermogenic response to food and to exercise in lean and obese persons.*

Sims EA: Mechanisms of hypertension in the overweight. Hypertension 4:43, 1982. *A review of the pathophysiology of hypertension in the obese.*

Sims EAH, Danforth E: Expenditure and storage of energy in man. J Clin Invest 79:1019, 1987. *An excellent, up-to-date review of energy balance in man with a useful bibliography of 71 references.*

Stunkard AJ, Sorensen TIA, Harris C, et al.: An adoption study of human obesity. N Engl J Med 314:193, 1986. *A study of the contributions of genetic factors and the family environment to human fatness, concluding that genetic influences have an important role in determining human fatness in adults.*

Van Itallie TB, Yang MU: Diet and weight loss. N Engl J Med 297:1158, 1977. *A review and a careful metabolic study of the effects of macronutrient composition of low-calorie reducing diets on body composition.*

Wadden TA, Van Itallie TB, Blackburn GL: Responsible and irresponsible use of very low calorie diets in the treatment of obesity. JAMA 263:83–85, 1990. *A useful and responsible commentary on treatment with very low calorie diets.*

204 Disorders of Vitamin Metabolism: Deficiencies, Metabolic Abnormalities, and Excesses

Richard S. Rivlin

In approaching disorders of vitamin metabolism, several considerations should be kept in mind about the properties of vitamins, their roles in medicine, and the evolving patterns of their deficiency syndromes as commonly encountered.

Although generations of students are familiar with the syndrome of pellagra (niacin deficiency) as involving four D's (dermatitis, diarrhea, dementia, and death), in clinical practice in the United States such a classic syndrome is encountered only rarely. Rather, the typical picture one sees in severely ill patients with protein-calorie malnutrition is that of multiple vitamin deficiencies without manifestations of any single classic deficiency syndrome. Overt vitamin deficiencies caused by diet are seldom isolated for several reasons. First, a diet poor in one vitamin is usually poor in several others. In addition, one vitamin is often required for the metabolism of another. An example is riboflavin, which is involved in the metabolism of folic acid, pyridoxine, vitamin K, and niacin. Thus a vitamin deficiency may develop secondary to the inadequate dietary intake of a related nutrient.

The clinical development of vitamin deficiencies is typically gradual; the physical examination is usually not useful in detecting deficiencies of specific vitamins early in their development. For example, by the time that perifollicular hemorrhages characteristic of scurvy have developed, vitamin C deficiency is already far advanced. Even the abnormalities detected by physical examination late in the course of the deficiency state are often not pathognomonic. Cheilosis and glossitis, typically attributed to deficiency of riboflavin, can be observed with deficiencies of a number of other B vitamins. Finding an abnormality of this kind on physical examination helps to establish the diagnosis of malnutrition but usually does not identify a specific nutrient as missing from the diet.

Increasing attention is now being paid to drugs and alcohol as significant causes of specific vitamin deficiencies. Drug-induced vitamin deficiencies often are poorly recognized and become evident most frequently in chronically ill patients requiring long-term treatment who have a marginally adequate diet. The elderly are particularly vulnerable to the deleterious effects of ethanol. This commonly used and abused substance is now established as the major cause of deficiencies of folate and thiamine among individuals 65 years of age and older, and probably in many younger age groups as well.

In general, most vitamins must be acquired from dietary sources because they cannot be synthesized in the body. There are several exceptions to this rule in that certain vitamins are synthesized in the body but in very small amounts. An example is niacin, which is formed in vivo from an essential amino acid, tryptophan. A tryptophan-poor diet, such as that consumed when corn is the major food staple, cannot provide sufficient precursor to meet the metabolic needs for niacin, and pellagra may develop. Other examples of vitamins synthesized by the body, or more correctly by the intestinal microflora, are vitamin K and biotin. Deficiency of these vitamins often results from long-term antibiotic therapy, which eliminates the bacterial sources. Under the usual circumstances, however, bacterial synthesis of vitamin K and biotin is not sufficient, and some must be obtained from food sources. Vitamin D is synthesized in the skin in considerable amounts after exposure to light (Ch. 233), and constitutes a source of the vitamin which is at least as important as its dietary intake.

The B vitamins as a group function as essential coenzymes required in intermediary metabolism. The dietary form of each vitamin is first converted into its active derivatives before serving as a coenzyme. Examples include dietary thiamine and its coenzyme derivative, thiamine pyrophosphate, pyridoxine and pyridoxal phosphate, and riboflavin and flavin mononucleotide (riboflavin-5'phosphate) and flavin adenine dinucleotide. Vitamin deficiencies may arise not only because of dietary deficiencies but also because conversion of the dietary form of the vitamin to its coenzyme derivatives is diminished by drugs, disease, or other factors. Vitamin deficiencies may also be caused by abnormalities of intestinal absorption, plasma transport, tissue storage, binding to proteins, or excretion. Ensuring adequate vitamin status involves exogenous factors, such as dietary adequacy and food processing, preparation, and storage, as well as endogenous factors, such as hormones, that control vitamin utilization by the body.

The rate at which stores of vitamins are depleted following restriction of their dietary intake varies widely among vitamins. The body stores of vitamin B_{12} may not be depleted for years, whereas folic acid, thiamine, and niacin may be depleted within weeks or months of reduced dietary intake. In general, the body's capacity for storage of water-soluble vitamins is limited, and when the storage capacity is exceeded, the excess is usually excreted rapidly rather than stored; their tissue concentrations often cannot be increased beyond a certain point even by massive doses. By contrast, body stores of fat-soluble vitamins may become very great with prolonged administration of doses greatly exceeding their recommended dietary allowances (RDA).

At present, many individuals are consuming vitamins in doses far in excess of the RDA. More than one third of individuals 65 years of age and older in the United States are estimated to be taking some kind of nutritional supplement. Left to their own judgment, many persons will not select supplements appropriately. Supplement use is greater among females than males, whites than blacks, and well educated than poorly educated; vitamin C is the most commonly consumed individual supplement. Serious toxicity may develop with prolonged use of vitamins A and D at 5 to 10 times the RDA, particularly in children. Individuals vary considerably in the rate at which they develop toxicity with prolonged use of megadoses of vitamins. Certain conditions predispose to early symptoms. For example, individuals who become dehydrated may be at increased risk for developing hypercalcemia from large doses of vitamin D, and the onset of acute liver disease may precipitate vitamin A toxicity in a stable patient who previously had taken megadoses of this vitamin.

Vitamins increasingly may play specific roles in prevention of disease. Examples include vitamin A and β-carotene in possible prevention of certain malignancies and B vitamins and vitamin C in the possible prevention of neural tube defects when consumed during pregnancy. These subjects are under active investigation at the present time and remain controversial. It is still too early to make firm recommendations on either subject.

For certain disorders vitamins may be used quite appropriately as drugs. For example, ascorbic acid is widely employed to acidify the urine in cases of refractory urinary tract infections. Certain derivatives of vitamin A, in particular the 13-*cis* isomer of retinoic acid, have potent antikeratinizing effects that have been applied to the treatment of cystic acne. Nicotinic acid is widely utilized in the management of severe hyperlipoproteinemia. Certain pyridoxine-dependency syndromes require pharmacologic doses of vitamin B_6. In these and other vitamin-responsive inborn errors of metabolism, therapy must be specific and targeted. Thus, the therapeutic applications of vitamins extend far beyond their roles in correcting dietary deficiency. Both the therapeutic role of vitamins and their potential for toxicity should be kept in mind by the practicing physician.

While the emphasis in clinical medicine is appropriately on the correction of vitamin deficiencies, under certain conditions decreased vitamin intake may confer certain advantages. In malaria, vitamin supplementation programs have been observed to worsen parasitemia, and deficiencies of vitamin E and riboflavin appear to have antimalarial actions. Dietary deficiency of riboflavin, as well as of structural analogues, drugs, and diseases that interfere with the metabolism of this vitamin, all exert antimalarial effects.

Elsas LJ, McCormick DB: Genetic defects in vitamin utilization. Part 1: General aspects and fat-soluble vitamins. Vitam Horm 43:103, 1986. *Review of inherited disorders with special vitamin requirements.*

Machlin LJ (ed.): Handbook of Vitamins, 2nd ed. New York, Marcel Dekker, 1990. *Recently updated volume covering new research and therapeutic applications of vitamins.*

Rivlin RS: Vitamin deficiency. *In* Samiy A, Douglas RG Jr, Barondess J (eds.): Therapeutic Medicine for Practicing Physicians. Philadelphia, Lea and Febiger, 1990, in press. *Discussion of vitamin deficiency syndromes and their therapies.*

VITAMIN B₁ (THIAMINE)

Structure and Biochemical Function

The thiamine molecule is shown in Figure 204–1. The principal biochemical role of thiamine is that of precursor of thiamine pyrophosphate, a coenzyme required for oxidative decarboxylation of α-ketoacids to aldehydes. These reactions are widely distributed in intermediary metabolism and are an important source of energy generation. In addition, thiamine pyrophosphate serves as the coenzyme for transketolase, which catalyzes the conversions of the two 5-carbon sugars, xylulose-5-PO₄ and ribose-5-PO₄, to the 7-carbon sugar, sedoheptulose-7-PO₄ and the 3-carbon sugar, glyceraldehyde-3-PO₄. This reaction is used as a functional index of thiamine nutritional status, as discussed later in this chapter.

It has been suggested that thiamine may have an additional role in conduction of impulses in peripheral nerves apart from its function as a coenzyme in intermediary metabolism. The initiation of nerve impulses is associated with hydrolysis of thiamine diphosphate and thiamine triphosphate.

Normal Physiology

Dietary thiamine is absorbed from the intestinal tract both by passive diffusion (at high concentrations) and by active transport (at low concentrations.) The absorptive process is associated with phosphorylation of the thiamine molecule within the mucosal cell. In folate deficiency the absorption of thiamine is diminished. About 30 per cent of thiamine is bound to serum proteins normally. Muscle serves as the major storage organ for thiamine; most of the body stores are in the form of thiamine pyrophosphate, with lesser amounts stored as thiamine triphosphate, thiamine monophosphate, and thiamine itself. The degradation and excretion pathways of thiamine are not known with certainty, and more than 25 metabolites of the vitamin have been recovered from urine.

Requirements and Dietary Sources

The RDA for thiamine in adult males is 1.2 to 1.5 mg per day and in adult women, 1.0 to 1.1 mg per day, depending upon age, with a 50 per cent increase during pregnancy and lactation. The allowance is generally related to caloric intake, expressed as 0.5 mg per 1000 kcal, although it is recommended that thiamine intake not go below 1.0 mg per day even with a caloric intake reduced below 2000 kcal. The best dietary sources of thiamine are beef, pork, whole grains, enriched cereal grains, peas, beans, and nuts. The milling and polishing of rice, unless it is subsequently fortified, greatly reduces the thiamine content. Thiamine is rapidly destroyed at alkaline pH and is also heat sensitive when not under strongly acid conditions. Some food items, particularly raw fish, coffee, tea, betel nuts, and many plants, have been shown to contain thiaminases, enzymes that destroy the dietary supply of thiamine. A number of antithiamine factors have been identified from both plant and animal sources, and their consumption in large amounts has resulted in frank deficiency.

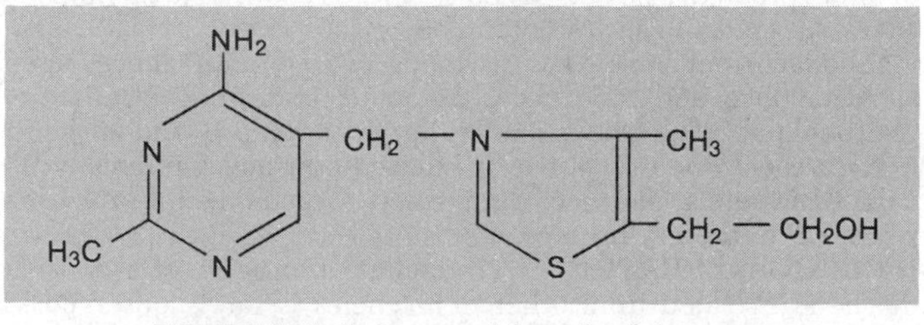

FIGURE 204–1. Structural formula of thiamine.

Deficiency

PATHOGENESIS. In addition to being caused by a poor diet, thiamine deficiency in the United States most commonly occurs as a result of alcoholism. Thiamine absorption is exquisitely sensitive to ingested ethanol, which significantly interferes with thiamine absorption even in healthy individuals. Repeated drinking throughout the day prevents most of the dietary thiamine from being absorbed, particularly in alcoholic patients in whom some degree of malabsorption is quite common. Approximately 25 per cent of alcoholic patients admitted to general hospitals in the United States have some evidence of thiamine deficiency by either clinical or biochemical criteria. Alcoholism is clearly the most important cause of thiamine deficiency in older age groups and probably in younger age groups as well. There is some evidence that alcohol also affects adversely the intermediary metabolism of thiamine, and chronic liver disease secondary to alcoholism may diminish the conversion of thiamine to thiamine pyrophosphate. Refeeding an alcoholic patient without additional thiamine may precipitate thiamine deficiency.

In developing countries that rely on polished rice as a staple in the diet, beriberi prevalence remains very high. It is likely that other factors, such as heavy coffee consumption, possibly may diminish the intestinal absorption of thiamine. Thiamine deficiency is also observed with diabetes, cancer, and other chronic illnesses and with long-term parenteral nutrition or use of intravenous fluids not containing thiamine.

CLINICAL FEATURES. Early thiamine deficiency is characterized by anorexia, irritability, and weight loss. Later, patients experience weakness, peripheral neuropathy, headache, and tachycardia. Advanced thiamine deficiency presents with involvement of two major organ systems predominantly: the cardiovascular system (the syndrome known as "wet beriberi," i.e., beriberi heart disease) and the nervous system, both central and peripheral (known as "dry beriberi").

The following criteria are generally accepted for the diagnosis of beriberi heart disease: absence of other known etiologic factors, history of at least 3 months of documented dietary thiamine deficiency, associated peripheral neuritis, enlarged heart with normal sinus rhythm (usually tachycardia), peripheral edema, nonspecific ST- and T-wave changes, and rapid therapeutic response to thiamine administration. Beriberi heart disease is well recognized as a cause of high-output failure, which is a consequence of the profound peripheral vasodilation. Resting tachycardia, weakness, and weight loss often resemble the clinical features of apathetic hyperthyroidism, with which it is frequently confused.

The central nervous system manifestations of thiamine deficiency consist primarily of the Wernicke-Korsakoff syndrome (Ch. 456). The Wernicke's component is an acute disorder consisting of variable degrees of vomiting, horizontal nystagmus, ophthalmoplegia caused by weakness of the rectus muscles, fever, ataxic gait, and progressive mental impairment. Patients have died when the disease has been unrecognized and allowed to progress. The Korsakoff syndrome typically has loss of memory and confabulation as prominent features.

The peripheral nervous system abnormalities of thiamine deficiency typically consist of a symmetric lesion that involves motor, sensory, and reflex responses. The legs are usually involved earlier and more completely than the arms. Pain and paresthesias may be particularly disabling to afflicted patients. An abnormal transketolase with high Km for thiamine pyrophosphate has been described, which may predispose certain alcohol abusers to severe neurologic impairment when thiamine deficiency develops.

DIAGNOSIS. Thiamine status can be evaluated using bioassays, microbiologic techniques, chemical analyses, and functional enzyme assays. The most sensitive method for analyzing thiamine in small quantities in body fluids, tissues, and foods is high performance liquid chromatography (HPLC). In actual practice, the two most widely used assays are urinary thiamine excretion and the transketolase activity coefficient. Urinary thiamine can be determined accurately, but the results may be misleading if there has been recent thiamine intake in a previously deficient patient or if the patient has recently taken diuretics, which promote thiamine excretion. The results obtained under those circumstances would not yield the expected low value.

Transketolase, as noted above, requires thiamine pyrophosphate as its coenzyme. In thiamine deficiency, the erythrocyte apoenzyme is not fully saturated with its cofactor, and addition of the cofactor in vitro to an erythrocyte hemolysate results in an increase in measured enzyme activity. The degree of increase in the activity coefficient (i.e., enzyme activity after incubation with the coenzyme in vitro compared to that before, expressed as per cent increase) is an indication of the degree of unsaturation of the apoenzyme with thiamine pyrophosphate. The degree of unsaturation, in turn, is indicative of the magnitude of depletion of body stores of thiamine. An activity coefficient of 15 to 20 per cent or greater is generally regarded as reflecting significant thiamine deficiency. If these assays are unavailable, a therapeutic trial of thiamine, which provides rapid improvement (in 12 hours or less) in cardiovascular function and in ophthalmoplegia, may be regarded as supportive evidence for the diagnosis of thiamine deficiency. In a patient with beriberi, cardiac output may diminish and vascular resistance increase within 30 minutes of intravenous administration of a single 100-mg dose of thiamine.

TREATMENT. If thiamine deficiency is suspected, rapid treatment with large doses of the vitamin is essential. Generally, 50 to 100 mg are administered intramuscularly or intravenously every day for the first few days, after which lower doses in the range of 5 to 10 mg may be given orally. Other therapeutic applications for which pharmacologic doses of thiamine are required include several rare inborn errors of metabolism: thiamine-responsive branched-chain ketoaciduria (maple syrup urine disease), as well as subacute necrotizing encephalomyelopathy (Leigh's syndrome), a condition in which thiamine triphosphate is deficient in the brain.

Toxicity

Thiamine can be given safely by mouth in very large amounts without fear of toxicity. When given by the intravenous route, large doses of thiamine on very rare occasions have been associated with poorly understood reactions resembling anaphylactic shock. Fortunately, these reactions occur so rarely that intravenous therapy with thiamine should not be withheld from a seriously ill patient in whom thiamine deficiency is suspected.

Gubler CJ: Thiamin. *In* Machlin LJ (ed.): Handbook of Vitamins, 2nd ed. New York, Marcel Dekker, 1990, p 233. *Comprehensive review of biochemical and nutritional aspects of thiamine.*

Haas RH: Thiamin and the brain. Ann Rev Nutr 8:483, 1988. *Review of effects of thiamine deficiency on brain function.*

Iber FL, Blass JP, Brin M, et al.: Thiamin in the elderly—Relation to alcoholism and to neurological degenerative disease. Am J Clin Nutr 36(Suppl):1067, 1982. *Discussion of prevalence of thiamine deficiency and effects of alcohol and drugs upon thiamine bioavailability.*

Mukherjee AB, Svoronos S, Ghazanfari A, et al.: Transketolase abnormality in cultured fibroblasts from familial chronic alcoholic men and their male offspring. J Clin Invest 79:1039, 1987. *Confirmatory description of an inborn error of transketolase predisposing to severe consequences of thiamine deficiency.*

VITAMIN B₂ (RIBOFLAVIN)

Structure and Biochemical Functions

Riboflavin (Fig. 204–2) must be converted to its coenzyme derivatives, flavin mononucleotide (riboflavin-5'-PO₄, FMN) and flavin adenine dinucleotide (FAD), in order to be metabolically active. These coenzymes are formed sequentially from dietary riboflavin after reacting with ATP and function as cofactors for a wide variety of enzymes in intermediary metabolism, particularly those involving oxidation-reduction reactions. FAD-dependent enzymes include α-glycerophosphate dehydrogenase, xanthine oxidase, and NADPH-cytochrome c reductase. A small fraction of tissue flavins is found in covalent linkage with proteins and includes the enzymes monoamine oxidase (MAO) and succinic dehydrogenase.

Normal Physiology

Riboflavin and FMN are absorbed from the upper gastrointestinal tract by a specific and saturable transport process. FAD, the predominant form in foods such as meat, must first be degraded to riboflavin and FMN prior to being absorbed. Cova-

lently bound flavins are largely unavailable as nutritional sources of riboflavin. A number of metals and drugs form complexes or chelates with dietary riboflavin and may influence the bioavailability of this vitamin. Such agents include copper, zinc, iron, saccharin, tryptophan, ascorbic acid, and dietary fiber. Dietary fiber in the form of psyllium but not wheat bran decreases the apparent intestinal absorption of a single 30-mg dose of riboflavin; effects of fiber on usual amounts of dietary riboflavin are not known.

After absorption, riboflavin is bound loosely to serum albumin and more tightly to immunoglobulins, particularly IgA and IgG. The amount of riboflavin bound to serum proteins varies widely in normal individuals. In pregnancy there are specific riboflavin-binding proteins that appear to be essential to normal fetal development. The renal tubule transports riboflavin in both directions, and in urine the predominant form detected is riboflavin rather than the coenzyme derivatives. There are additional metabolites of riboflavin in human urine including 7-hydroxymethylriboflavin, 8-α-sulfonylriboflavin, and trace amounts of other substances.

Thyroid and adrenal hormones regulate the conversion of riboflavin to FMN, FAD, and covalently bound flavins, and riboflavin metabolism is impaired in adult hypothyroid patients. Analogues of riboflavin interfere with certain actions of aldosterone.

Requirements and Dietary Sources

The RDA for riboflavin in adult males is 1.4 to 1.7 mg per day and in adult females, 1.2 to 1.3 mg per day, depending upon age. Allowances are increased during pregnancy and lactation and probably should be increased with heavy exercise. When riboflavin is consumed in amounts greater than the RDA, increased urinary excretion occurs promptly. In the United States, milk and dairy products supply close to half the daily intake of riboflavin, with meat, fish, poultry, eggs, and legumes providing other important sources; the remainder comes largely from green leafy vegetables, fruits, and grain products. In developing countries, the principal sources are cereals, roots, and tubers. Riboflavin is light-, acid-, and alkali-sensitive and rapidly loses biologic activity when exposed to sunlight or when treated with sodium bicarbonate, a common but unfortunate practice used to retain the color of green vegetables.

Deficiency

PATHOGENESIS. Riboflavin deficiency arises not only because of an inadequate diet but also when hormones, drugs, or disease impair the absorption, utilization, metabolic transformations, binding, or excretion of this vitamin. In experimental animals, the psychotropic drugs chlorpromazine, imipramine, and amitriptyline and the antitumor agent doxorubicin, as well as several antimalarial agents, all diminish the conversion of riboflavin to its active coenzyme derivatives, FMN and FAD. Chlorpromazine treatment greatly accelerates the development of riboflavin deficiency. The underlying mechanism of this effect appears to be inhibition of flavokinase, the enzyme that converts riboflavin to FMN, the first of two steps in the biosynthesis of FAD.

Phototherapy of newborn infants with hyperbilirubinemia leads to some decomposition of riboflavin because of its light sensitivity. Ethanol diminishes both the intestinal absorption of riboflavin and its bioavailability from food sources. Deficiency of riboflavin likely results also after severe trauma, burns, surgery, chronic debilitating diseases, dialysis, and severe and prolonged diarrhea. Increased riboflavin excretion occurs under conditions of negative nitrogen balance, including diabetes, after withdrawal of insulin, or after certain drugs, such as boric acid. Hypothyroidism impairs riboflavin metabolism, as noted above.

Riboflavin deficiency has particularly important effects upon fat metabolism and alters the plasma and tissue concentrations of phospholipids. The conversion of dietary vitamin B₆ and folic acid to their coenzyme derivatives is blocked by riboflavin deficiency. In β-thalassemia, there is diminished formation of FMN from riboflavin in the erythrocyte.

CLINICAL FEATURES. The clinical picture of riboflavin deficiency isolated from other deficiencies is rarely observed as noted above. Early symptoms of riboflavin deficiency include

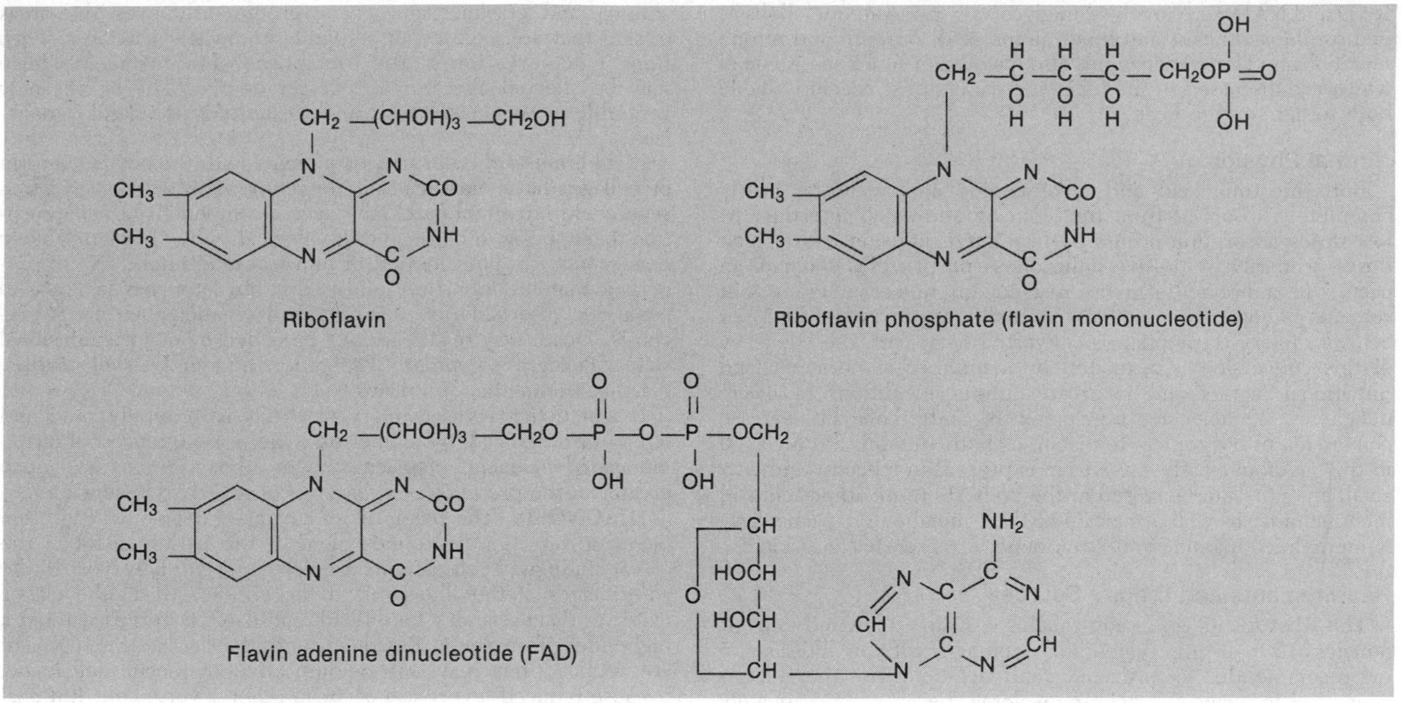

FIGURE 204–2. Structural formulae of riboflavin (vitamin B_2) and its coenzyme derivatives.

soreness of the mouth, burning and itching of the eyes, and personality deterioration. Advanced riboflavin deficiency produces a constellation of findings that include cheilosis, angular stomatitis, seborrheic dermatitis, glossitis, corneal vascularization, reticulocytopenia and anemia, and retarded intellectual development. Cheilosis and angular stomatitis, once thought to be specific for riboflavin deficiency, are now known to occur frequently in other nutritional deficiencies, particularly B_6 deficiency. Riboflavin deficiency is a major cause of congenital malformations in experimental animals, but it is unclear at present whether malformations result from human maternal riboflavin deficiency. The rate of metabolism of a number of drugs is altered in riboflavin deficiency, at least in part because the microsomal hydroxylase system requires flavin coenzymes. There is evidence that riboflavin deficiency antagonizes *Plasmodium* infection in both animals and humans.

DIAGNOSIS. In riboflavin deficiency, there is a reduction in urinary excretion of riboflavin as well as a reduction in the concentrations of various flavins in plasma and in erythrocytes. Assays of urinary excretion of riboflavin in longstanding deficiency may be misleading if there has been some recent intake of this vitamin. A useful functional test of riboflavin status is the activity coefficient of erythrocyte glutathione reductase, an FAD-requiring enzyme. When FAD is added in vitro to an erythrocyte hemolysate, the increase in activity measured is much greater in erythrocytes from riboflavin-deficient than from riboflavin-replete individuals. As with transketolase and thiamine pyrophosphate (referred to above), this assay reflects the lesser degree of saturation of the apoenzyme with its cofactor in deficient compared with normal individuals. Results are expressed as the activity coefficient, i.e., the ratio of enzyme activity after incubation with FAD in vitro to that before incubation. Activity coefficients greater than 1.2 to 1.3 are generally considered to be indicative of a riboflavin-deficient state.

TREATMENT. Riboflavin deficiency can be treated satisfactorily with food sources high in riboflavin, such as milk, liver, meat, eggs, and green, leafy vegetables, or with the vitamin itself. Deficient patients treated with 10 to 15 mg per day of riboflavin undergo healing of skin lesions within days to weeks of initiation of therapy. The intravenous administration of riboflavin, which may be needed in debilitated patients or in those with serious disorders of the gastrointestinal tract, is greatly restricted by its limited solubility in aqueous solution.

Riboflavin in large doses has been utilized to treat several rare inborn errors of metabolism, including congenital methemoglobinemia, pyruvate kinase deficiency, glutaryl-CoA dehydrogenase deficiency, and defects of β-oxidation.

Toxicity

Riboflavin, FMN, and FAD are completely free of any known clinical toxicity. There is a theoretical possibility that the photosensitizing properties of riboflavin may constitute some risk.

Cooperman JM, Lopez R: Riboflavin. *In* Machlin LJ (ed.): Handbook of Vitamins, 2nd ed. New York, Marcel Dekker, 1990, p 283. *Update on riboflavin metabolism, sources, and deficiency.*

McCormick DB: Riboflavin. *In* Brown ML (ed.): Present Knowledge in Nutrition, 6th ed. Washington, D.C., International Life Sciences Institute, The Nutrition Foundation, 1990, p 146. *Discussion of the physiology, sources, functions, and metabolic roles of riboflavin.*

Pinto JT, Huang YP, Rivlin RS: Mechanisms underlying the differential effects of ethanol upon the bioavailability of riboflavin and flavin adenine dinucleotide. J Clin Invest 79:1343, 1987. *Study showing how alcohol causes riboflavin deficiency.*

Rivlin RS: Medical aspects of vitamin B_2. *In* Muller F (ed.): Chemistry and Biochemistry of Flavins. Boca Raton, CRC Press 1990, in press. *Review of diseases that disturb riboflavin metabolism clinically and their treatment.*

NIACIN (UNOFFICIALLY CALLED VITAMIN B_3)

Structure and Biochemical Function

The term "niacin" is used generally to refer to nicotinic acid and nicotinamide and other biologically active pyridine derivatives, as shown in Figure 204–3. The term "niacin" is sometimes used loosely to refer to nicotinic acid only. Niacin is a precursor of two coenzymes, nicotinamide adenine dinucleotide (NAD) and nicotinamide adenine dinucleotide phosphate (NADP), which

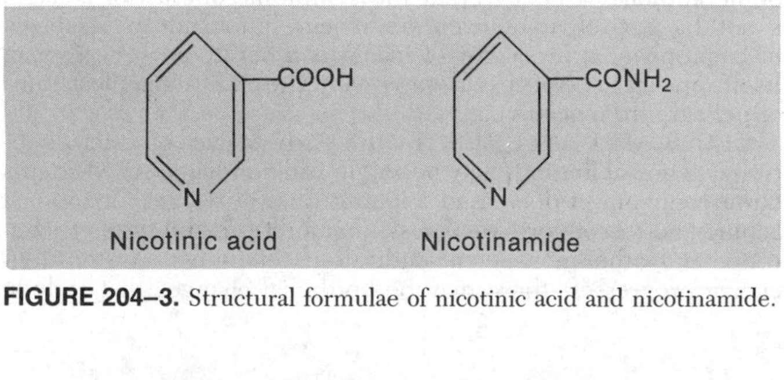

FIGURE 204–3. Structural formulae of nicotinic acid and nicotinamide.

function in a wide number of oxidation and reduction reactions. NAD and NADP are involved in glycolysis, pyruvate metabolism, pentose biosynthesis, and lipid, amino acid, protein, and purine metabolism. These coenzymes also have other functions, some of which are discussed in the following paragraphs. Niacin is stable both to light and to heat.

Normal Physiology

Both nicotinic acid and nicotinamide appear to be nearly completely absorbed from the stomach and small intestine. At low doses absorption occurs by facilitated diffusion and at high doses primarily by passive diffusion. A portion of dietary niacin occurs in a bound form (as niacinogen) in cereal grains but remains biologically available. Normally, approximately 1.5 per cent of dietary tryptophan is converted to niacin. The efficiency of this conversion is regulated by a number of hormonal and nutritional factors and is greater under conditions of niacin deficiency. Deficiencies of vitamin B_6 and riboflavin decrease conversion of tryptophan to niacin, as both vitamins are involved in this metabolic pathway. Niacin is present in all cells, and only small amounts can be stored in the body. Both nicotinic acid and nicotinamide, as well as certain of their metabolites, particularly N-methylnicotinamide and 2-pyridone, are excreted in urine.

Requirements and Dietary Sources

The RDA for niacin in adult males is 15 to 19 mg and in adult females, 13 to 15 mg, depending upon age, with an additional 5 mg recommended for pregnancy and lactation. The allowance is expressed in terms of niacin equivalents, because approximately 60 mg of dietary tryptophan are needed to form 1 mg of niacin. Proteins of animal origin such as meat, milk, and eggs have a relatively high tryptophan content and therefore are good sources of endogenously generated niacin. Vegetable proteins also supply tryptophan, but the concentration is lower than in animal proteins. Diets dependent heavily upon corn are a particular problem because the tryptophan content is low. Niacin from wheat sources has limited bioavailability. Pyridoxine deficiency and riboflavin deficiency increase the dietary requirement for niacin, because they are required for the biosynthesis of niacin from tryptophan, as noted above.

Deficiency

PATHOGENESIS. Niacin deficiency or pellagra may develop because of a number of factors. First, dietary deficiency develops when corn is the major staple of the diet. Pellagra caused by consumption of corn was once very common in the southeastern United States but fortunately has largely disappeared at the present time. Secondly, niacin deficiency may arise as a result of alcoholism, a condition in which diet is often poor and erratic. It is likely that in prolonged alcoholism, particularly in the presence of other nutrient deficiencies, the absorption and metabolism of niacin may be impaired. In addition, certain drugs interfere with niacin metabolism to a clinically significant degree, the best known of which is isonicotinic acid hydrazide (INH). The neurologic symptoms occurring with INH treatment can be ameliorated by administration of pyridoxine. Certain anticancer drugs, particularly 6-mercaptopurine, may produce niacin deficiency. In the rare inborn error of Hartnup's disease, pellagra may develop because of a defect in the intestinal and renal tubular transport of tryptophan and of several other amino acids (Ch. 176). Malnourished patients with the malignant carcinoid syndrome have been known occasionally to exhibit manifestations of pellagra because of diversion of dietary tryptophan to serotonin (Ch. 230). Some authorities believe that the symptom complex of pellagra is not due entirely to deficiency of niacin, but rather to deficiency of tryptophan, a precursor of niacin and serotonin. Tryptophan itself appears to be necessary to prevent the clinical manifestations of pellagra from occurring.

CLINICAL FEATURES. In the early stages of niacin deficiency, clinical findings may be vague and nondiagnostic. Patients often complain of decreased appetite, loss of weight, abdominal aching and discomfort, weakness, irritability, inability to concentrate, and other nonspecific indications of illness. As the deficiency progresses, there may be epithelial changes that include glossitis, stomatitis, soreness and pain in the mouth (particularly the tongue), and eventually development of the characteristic skin lesions. These lesions, when well established, are dark, scaling, and cracking and occur prominently over the areas of skin that are exposed to sunlight, frequently leaving a sharp line of demarcation at the unexposed skin surfaces. These may be affected also but to a lesser degree. The lesions may resemble a necklace and are described as Casal's necklace.

In addition to the dermatitis, patients with the advanced form of pellagra have diarrhea and dementia. The diarrhea is often severe and intractable and may have a component of malabsorption that appears to be related to villous atrophy. The latter likely results from the long period of minimal food intake. Neuropsychiatric manifestations are mild at first but later may progress to confusion, disorientation, seizures, hallucinations, and frank psychosis. Death may result, usually preceded by major confusional states. Pellagra is popularly known for the four D's—dermatitis, diarrhea, dementia, and death.

Niacin deficiency secondary to drugs is generally mild and often unrecognized by clinicians. The consequences of drug-induced deficiencies of niacin and of other vitamins are much greater in the presence of a marginal or frankly deficient diet.

DIAGNOSIS. The diagnosis of advanced deficiency can often be made on clinical grounds alone if the patient exhibits the classic findings. Such patients are very unusual, however. In the early stages of the illness or in the absence of all the classic features, diagnosis may be difficult and is often missed without a high index of suspicion. Blood concentrations of NAD and NADP are reduced but may not be indicative of niacin deficiency, because reduced levels also occur in other severe, constitutional illnesses that are unrelated to niacin intake. Attention has therefore turned to assay of urinary metabolites of niacin as indices of niacin nutriture. The most widely used is N-methylnicotinamide. Low urinary levels are interpreted as indicative of niacin deficiency. The excretion of another metabolite, 2-pyridone, is less widely used and requires a cumbersome assay. Some investigators have considered the ratio of these two metabolites in urine to be the most accurate index of niacin nutriture. Urinary metabolites can now be measured accurately by HPLC.

TREATMENT. The treatment of advanced pellagra can be accomplished satisfactorily by administering large oral doses (approximately 50 to 150 mg) of nicotinamide (the form present in most commercial vitamin formulations). The exact dose given is somewhat empiric. The therapeutic response is often dramatic, and patients may show marked improvement within several days after the start of therapy. Maintenance levels are then given together with dietary repletion. Nicotinamide is usually well tolerated under these conditions. Nicotinic acid is also effective against pellagra.

Other therapeutic applications of niacin include its use as nicotinic acid in the control of an elevated serum cholesterol level in daily doses of 3 grams or more (Ch. 172). Nicotinic acid may be useful in treating patients with types II, IV, and V hyperlipoproteinemia. The mechanism of the therapeutic effect on lipid metabolism is not known with precision, and this property is not shared by nicotinamide. With nicotinic acid treatment, HDL levels tend to rise because of a slight decrease in synthetic rate with a large decrease in degradative rate. Therapy is generally initiated with low doses of nicotinic acid and gradually increased with frequent monitoring of appropriate laboratory tests.

Doses in the range of those used to treat pellagra are also needed to treat niacin deficiency in Hartnup disease and in the carcinoid syndrome. Massive doses of niacin have not proven useful in the treatment of schizophrenia and other psychiatric disorders, despite the claims of food faddists and "orthomolecular" therapists.

Toxicity

At the doses of nicotinamide used to treat niacin deficiency (described previously) there is little if any toxicity. When nicotinic acid in doses of 3 grams or more is used in the treatment of a lipid disorder, the most common side effect observed is flushing of the face due to vascular dilation. Administering one tablet of aspirin prior to the dose of nicotinic acid often ameliorates the flushing. Other common side effects of nicotinic acid may include dryness, itching, and increased pigmentation of the skin and abdominal pain. Rarely, hepatotoxicity, hyperuricemia, and worsening of peptic ulcer and glucose tolerance have been observed. Abnormalities in liver function tests are common toxicities, but both biochemical and histologic findings generally regress with discontinuation of nicotinic acid. There is some evidence that so-called sustained-release capsules of nicotinic acid may be more toxic than crystalline nicotinic acid.

Henderson LaVM: Niacin. In Darby WJ, Broquist HP, Olson RE (eds.): Annual Review of Nutrition. Vol. 3. Palo Alto, Annual Reviews Inc, 1983, p 289. This review covers transport, metabolism, and physiologic and pharmacologic effects of niacin.

Krieger I, Statter M: Tryptophan deficiency and picolinic acid: Effect on zinc metabolism and clinical manifestations of pellagra. Am J Clin Nutr 46:511, 1987. Report providing evidence that pellagra is due to tryptophan deficiency.

Van Eys J: Nicotinic acid. In Machlin LJ (ed.): Handbook of Vitamins, 2nd ed. New York, Marcel Dekker, 1990, p 312. Recent review stressing metabolism, pharmacology, and toxicity of niacin.

VITAMIN B₆ (PYRIDOXINE)

Structure and Biochemical Function

The term "vitamin B_6" or "pyridoxine" is often used to refer to three closely interrelated compounds—pyridoxine, pyridoxamine, and pyridoxal—together with their phosphate derivatives. Of all these compounds, pyridoxal-5'-phosphate (Fig. 204–4) is the most important, because it constitutes the major coenzyme involved in the intermediary metabolism of amino acids, including aminotransferases, decarboxylases, racemases, and synthetases. Pyridoxal phosphate is involved in metabolism of several vitamins and in biosynthesis of heme and sphingosine. It is estimated that more than 100 reactions involve pyridoxal-5'-phosphate as a cofactor. In certain circumstances pyridoxamine phosphate can also fulfill a coenzyme function. Pyridoxine is the major dietary source found in plants, whereas pyridoxal and pyridoxamine constitute the major forms in foods from animal sources. Pyridoxine is stable in acid solutions in the absence of light but is highly light-sensitive in acid or neutral solutions. Pyridoxal and pyridoxamine are destroyed at high temperatures, particularly by autoclaving and in the presence of protein or amino acids.

Normal Physiology

Dietary pyridoxine and related compounds are absorbed from the upper gastrointestinal tract, probably by simple diffusion. The vitamin is widely distributed in the body; muscle constitutes an important storage organ, in which it is bound to phosphorylase a, thus serving to stabilize the enzyme molecule. The various forms of pyridoxine are readily interconverted to one another by the liver and erythrocytes. Under ordinary circumstances only very small amounts of dietary pyridoxine are converted to pyridoxal phosphate. In urine, pyridoxine, pyridoxal, and pyridoxamine can all be detected but at low concentrations; the major metabolite of pyridoxine, 4-pyridoxic acid, is found in urine in high concentrations, particularly in alcoholic patients.

Thyroid hormones reduce the concentrations of vitamin B_6 in various tissues, and increased sensitivity to insulin is demonstrable during B_6 deficiency.

Requirements and Dietary Sources

The RDA for vitamin B_6 is 2.0 mg per day for adult males and 1.6 per day for adult females, regardless of age, with a 0.5 mg

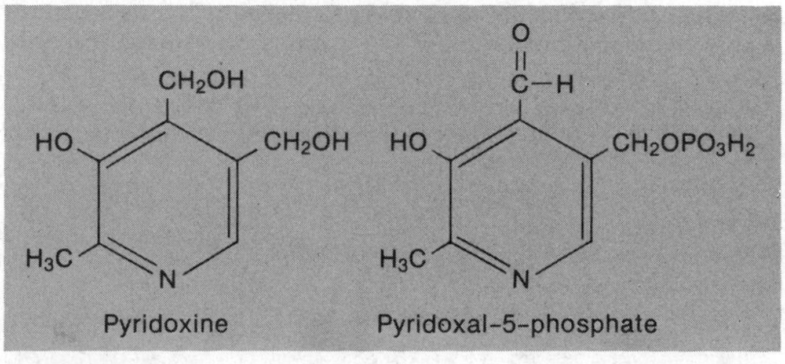

FIGURE 204–4. Structural formulae of pyridoxine and its phosphate derivative.

per day increase during pregnancy and lactation. The requirement for vitamin B_6 is greater with a higher protein intake.

Vitamin B_6 is widely distributed in the food supply and can be derived from both plants and animals. Sources of vitamin B_6 are similar to those of other B vitamins and include liver, meat, wheat, nuts, beans and other vegetables, fruits, and cereals. Considerable losses occur during prolonged cooking, particularly pressure cooking. The bioavailability of vitamin B_6 from dietary sources varies widely, averaging about 70 per cent; bananas and walnuts have nearly 80 per cent B_6 bioavailability, spinach only 22 per cent, and orange juice 9 per cent. Bioavailability is low when there is high glycosylated B_6 in the food item.

Deficiency

PATHOGENESIS. Dietary deficiency of pyridoxine may occur occasionally despite its widespread sources in the food supply. Deficiency of pyridoxine is recognized increasingly as a consequence of prolonged therapy with certain medications. Foremost among these drugs is isoniazid, which complexes with pyridoxal phosphate to a clinically significant degree. Individuals with the genetic trait of inactivating isoniazid at a slow rate are particularly susceptible to B_6 deficiency from this drug. Isoniazid induces peripheral neuritis and diarrhea in adult patients; in children it produces anemia and seizures that can be prevented by coincident administration of pyridoxine. Cycloserine, another drug widely used for tuberculosis, is also a vitamin B_6 antagonist. With the widespread use of penicillamine for the treatment of rheumatoid arthritis, its B_6 antagonistic properties are of increasing clinical importance. Pyridoxine deficiency occurs frequently in alcoholism in association with deficiencies of other vitamins, particularly folic acid. The principal effect of ethanol is to accelerate catabolism of pyridoxal phosphate. The increased urinary excretion of certain tryptophan metabolites, particularly xanthurenic acid, in women treated with oral contraceptives has been interpreted as indicating vitamin B_6 deficiency, because B_6 is needed for conversion of tryptophan to niacin. L-Dopa, used for Parkinson's disease, may also cause B_6 deficiency over a prolonged period of time.

CLINICAL FEATURES. Deficiency of vitamin B_6 is not thought to produce a characteristic syndrome. As with deficiencies of other B vitamins, dermatitis, glossitis, cheilosis, and stomatitis may be manifestations of pyridoxine deficiency. Markedly B_6-deficient patients may have irritability, weakness, depression, dizziness, peripheral neuropathy, and seizures. As noted previously, deficiency in infants and children is typically characterized by diarrhea, anemia, and seizures. The rapidity with which drug-induced deficiency of B_6 occurs depends upon the adequacy of the patient's diet as well as the dosage and duration of drug therapy. Chronic vitamin B_6 deficiency also leads to secondary hyperoxaluria, increasing the risk of kidney stone formation (Ch. 88).

In addition to the deficiency syndromes of vitamin B_6 caused by diet or drugs or both, there is a group of disorders in which the affected patients do not display manifestations of deficiency yet require pharmacologic doses of this vitamin for adequate treatment. These disorders are known as dependency syndromes and include such diverse entities as pyridoxine-dependent convulsions, pyridoxine-responsive anemia, homocystinuria caused by cystathionine synthetase deficiency, cystathioninuria, xanthurenic aciduria, and some cases of primary hyperoxaluria.

Of these dependency syndromes, pyridoxine-responsive anemia requires special mention because it is often confused with iron-deficiency anemia; both disorders are characterized by hypochromic, microcytic red cells. In the pyridoxine-responsive anemia, however, serum iron is generally elevated with an increase in saturation of transferrin and an increase in iron absorption from the intestinal tract. There is evidence of iron overload, with hemosiderin deposits in bone marrow, liver, and other organs. Many patients have hepatosplenomegaly, and a hemolytic component may contribute to the anemia. It is important to differentiate this syndrome from iron-deficient anemia, because inadvertent administration of iron worsens pyridoxine-responsive anemia. The blood count rises satisfactorily in response to pharmacologic doses of vitamin B_6. In patients with cystathionine synthetase deficiency, the greatly elevated serum concentrations of homocysteine and methionine can be normalized with doses of pyridoxine of several hundred milligrams per day.

DIAGNOSIS. The diagnosis of pyridoxine deficiency can be made by direct assay of vitamin B_6 in blood (normal levels generally are greater than 50 ng per milliliter) or by determining the urinary excretion of the main metabolite of pyridoxine, 4-pyridoxic acid. The excretion of less than 1.0 mg per day of this compound is generally considered suggestive of deficiency. Less frequently, the excretion of pyridoxine in urine is also determined. Functional enzyme assays, similar to those in use for diagnosing thiamine and riboflavin deficiencies, have also been developed for vitamin B_6 using aspartate aminotransferase or alanine aminotransferase in erythrocyte hemolysates. Enzyme activity is determined with and without the addition of pyridoxal phosphate in vitro. When activity coefficients (as defined previously) are greater than 1.5 for aspartate aminotransferase and 1.2 for alanine aminotransferase, they are considered indicative of pyridoxine deficiency. These procedures have generally supplanted the tryptophan load test, in which the increased excretion of xanthurenic acid is taken as an index of B_6 nutriture. Probably the most widely accepted index of vitamin B_6 nutriture at present is the direct measurement of pyridoxal phosphate concentrations in blood.

TREATMENT. Dietary deficiency of pyridoxine can be treated satisfactorily with oral doses in the general range of 2 to 10 mg per day; doses of 10 to 20 mg per day may be needed in pregnancy. Pyridoxine deficiency occurring in association with specific drugs that inhibit pyridoxine metabolism, such as isoniazid, cycloserine, and penicillamine, requires higher doses, perhaps up to 100 mg per day, to ameliorate peripheral neuropathy. Rather than administer B_6 when symptoms develop, it may be much more beneficial to attempt to prevent these side effects by administering vitamin B_6 at the time when therapy with a B_6-antagonizing drug is initiated and particularly when a prolonged course of treatment is anticipated. Since iatrogenic vitamin B_6 deficiency is entirely preventable, B_6 is now routinely prescribed for patients receiving INH. Treatment with high doses of vitamin B_6 is contraindicated in patients receiving L-dopa, however, as it may interfere with the efficacy of the drug.

Treatment of a pyridoxine-dependency syndrome requires much higher doses of B_6, and amounts in the range of 300 to 500 mg per day generally have been prescribed. In patients with gyrate atrophy, a rare genetic eye disease in which progressive visual loss develops as a result of chorioretinal degeneration, there is a deficiency of the mitochondrial enzyme ornithine aminotransferase. The elevated serum ornithine in these patients can be corrected by treatment with pyridoxal phosphate, the cofactor of this enzyme. In common with homocystinuria and several other genetic disorders, gyrate atrophy occurs in a vitamin B_6-responsive and vitamin B_6-unresponsive form.

The possible effectiveness of pyridoxine in the management of the carpal tunnel syndrome and premenstrual tension is controversial. In some women on contraceptive steroids, vitamin B_6 has appeared to ameliorate depression. Pyridoxine is regarded as ineffective in treating schizophrenia, autism, and childhood hyperactivity, as well as peripheral neuropathies in which there is no known B_6 deficiency, such as in diabetes.

Toxicity

A sensory neuropathy has been described in a small number of patients receiving 2 grams or more of pyridoxine per day, and some subjects have had symptoms on 500 mg or possibly less per day. This potentially important finding requires confirmation and extension. At the present time, there are probably no indications for treatment of any disorder, even a pyridoxine-dependency syndrome, with doses of this magnitude. Thus, pyridoxine appears to be safe when prescribed in the appropriate milligram amounts needed to correct deficiency and to treat vitamin B_6-dependency states.

McCormick DB: Two interconnected B vitamins: riboflavin and pyridoxine. Physiol Rev 69:1170, 1989. *Review of the interrelations between vitamins B_2 and B_6.*

Ramesh V, McClatchey AI, Ramesh N, et al.: Molecular basis of ornithine aminotransferase deficiency in B_6-responsive and -nonresponsive forms of gyrate atrophy. Proc Natl Acad Sci USA 85:3777, 1988. *Report that pyridoxine-responsive and nonresponsive forms of gyrate atrophy result from mutations in the ornithine aminotransferase structural gene.*

Reynolds RD, Leklem JE: Vitamin B_6: Its Role in Health and Disease. New York, Alan R. Liss, 1986. *Volume covering the proceedings of a conference on this vitamin in nutrition and metabolism.*

Schaumburg H, Kaplan J, Winderbank A, et al.: Sensory neuropathy from pyridoxine abuse. A new megavitamin syndrome. N Engl J Med 309:445, 1983. *Description of B_6 toxicity.*

VITAMIN B₁₂ (COBALAMIN) AND FOLIC ACID

The structure, function, pathophysiology, and therapeutic use of vitamin B_{12} and folic acid are discussed in Ch. 132 in association with the megaloblastic anemias.

VITAMIN C (ASCORBIC ACID)

Structure and Biochemical Function

Ascorbic acid resembles glucose in having several polyhydroxyl groups adjacent to one another (Fig. 204–5). Ascorbic acid can be oxidized to dehydro-L-ascorbic acid, which is also biologically active, and can be generated from the latter by reacting with reduced glutathione. Ascorbic acid is a precursor of oxalate, an important component of kidney stones.

Ascorbic acid participates in oxidation-reduction reactions and in hydrogen ion transfer. This vitamin is a powerful reducing agent or antioxidant, particularly in lipid and vitamin metabolism, and is especially important in preventing oxidation of tetrahydrofolate. In addition, ascorbic acid enhances the intestinal absorption of nonheme iron. This vitamin is involved in collagen metabolism, and defects in collagen biosynthesis are believed to be the basis for many of the symptoms of scurvy. In the absence of vitamin C, dopamine-B-hydroxylase activity is reduced, impairing the biosynthesis of neurotransmitters. Ascorbic acid is also involved in carnitine biosynthesis, tyrosine metabolism, wound healing, and immune function and is a component of drug-metabolizing enzyme systems.

Prolonged storage or excessive cooking diminishes the biologic activity of ascorbic acid. This highly water-soluble vitamin is also destroyed by oxidation, particularly by exposure to air in the presence of copper ion and an alkaline medium.

Normal Physiology

Ascorbic acid is absorbed by a limited-capacity mechanism in the distal small intestine. As dietary intake of ascorbic acid increases, a progressively smaller proportion is absorbed—that is, about 95 per cent at 100 mg, 75 per cent at 1 gram, and 20 per cent at 5 grams. Within the usual range of dietary ascorbic acid intake of 10 to 130 mg per day, the plasma level is proportional to the amount ingested. Because of limited absorptive capacity, ingestion of massive amounts of ascorbic acid has only a small effect upon elevating plasma levels of this vitamin. In addition, as the dietary intake increases further, the low renal threshold for excretion assures that excess plasma levels of ascorbic acid are promptly excreted. Another mechanism protecting against excessive accumulation of ascorbic acid is the microsomal enzyme NADPH monodehydro-ascorbate transhydrogenase, which is induced by its substrate, ascorbic acid; in response to a large dietary load of ascorbic acid, degradative capacity is rapidly and substantially increased.

The body pool of ascorbic acid in adult males consuming about 80 mg per day is estimated to be approximately 1500 mg, and the rate of catabolism is about 3 per cent of the pool size per day. Increasing the dietary intake of ascorbic acid to more than 80 mg per day seems not to increase significantly the tissue stores of this vitamin. Similar to most B vitamins, the storage capacity

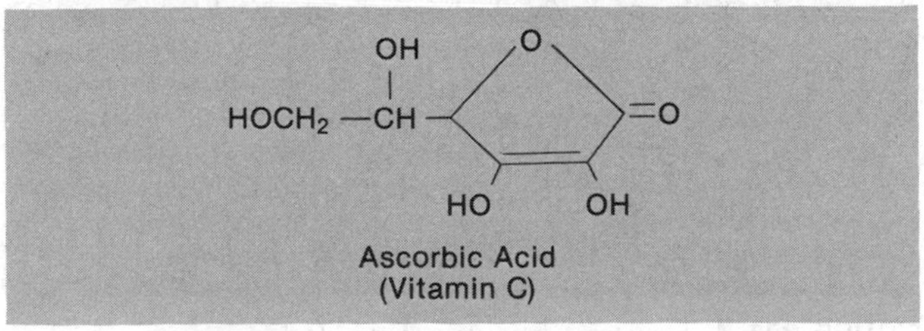

FIGURE 204–5. Structural formula of ascorbic acid.

for vitamin C is limited. Urinary excretion is in the form of ascorbic acid and dehydro-L-ascorbic acid, as well as several metabolites, including a sulfated derivative, ascorbate-2-sulfate, and oxalic acid, as noted above.

Requirements and Dietary Sources

The RDA for ascorbic acid is 60 mg per day for healthy adult males and females regardless of age. This allowance is generally regarded as quite generous inasmuch as amounts as low as 10 mg per day prevent scurvy. Amounts greatly in excess of the RDA have potential for toxicity. The recommended dietary allowance is increased to 70 mg per day during pregnancy and to 90 to 95 mg per day during lactation. Human milk contains about 30 to 55 mg per liter. It is especially important for women to maintain an adequate intake of ascorbic acid during lactation, because the vitamin concentration in milk is closely dependent upon dietary intake.

Serum ascorbic acid levels are lowered in smokers, possibly as a result of accelerated metabolism or diminished intake, and in users of oral contraceptive drugs, but the implications of these findings are unclear. The decreases are quantitatively small and can be corrected with a modest increase in consumption of ascorbic acid from dietary sources (about 40 mg for smokers, the amount contained in a glass of fresh orange juice). Patients who are exposed to cold or heat stress or who are febrile, undergoing surgery, or subjected to trauma may have increased requirements for vitamin C. Patients receiving parenteral nutrition exclusively have higher requirements because of urinary losses.

The best dietary sources of ascorbic acid appear to be citrus fruits and green vegetables, especially broccoli, green peppers, tomatoes, cabbage, oranges, grapefruits, and lemons. Care must be taken during food preparation in order to avoid losses of the vitamin. Much smaller amounts are contained in milk, meats, and cereals. As noted above, ascorbic acid is heat-sensitive and is destroyed by alkali. Some decreased vitamin content is also observed with prolonged storage.

Deficiency

PATHOGENESIS. Urban poor, particularly the elderly, are at increased risk for dietary deficiency of ascorbic acid, in large measure because economic deprivation prevents them from obtaining the richest sources, namely citrus fruits, leafy vegetables, and tomatoes.

An increasingly important cause of ascorbic acid deficiency in the United States today is food faddism and bizarre nutritional practices. The strict macrobiotic diet may lead to scurvy, particularly with pressure cooking of food items that have little ascorbic acid to begin with. Elderly individuals following a "tea and toast" diet are vulnerable to a number of deficiencies, particularly of ascorbic acid, as these sources are grossly inadequate. Children may develop scurvy when fed unsupplemented cow's milk exclusively for the first year of life. Vitamin C deficiency progressing to scurvy is common in chronic alcoholic patients, probably because the diet is notably deficient in vitamin C–containing food items. Vitamin C deficiency, however, is not generally as prevalent as deficiencies of B vitamins in chronic alcoholism. Scurvy was not prominent during the famine in Ireland in the nineteenth century, as people subsisted on raw potatoes, a good source of vitamin C.

CLINICAL FEATURES. In the early stages of deficiency, symptoms and signs may be nonspecific and include general malaise, lethargy, and weakness. As the disease progresses, probably 1 to 3 months after onset, patients may complain of dyspnea and pain in bones and joints, due predominantly to hemorrhages below the periosteum. Perifollicular hemorrhages, particularly about hair follicles, are indicative of advanced deficiency. Petechiae often are prominent and may appear over the arms after application of a sphygmomanometer. This finding is known as the Rumpel-Leed test. With progressive vitamin C depletion, ecchymoses and purpura may develop initially at areas of trauma, irritation, or pressure. Joints, muscles, and subcutaneous tissues may become sites of hemorrhage. Swollen, bleeding gums are characteristic of advanced deficiency. Pallor and anemia may be the result of prolonged bleeding or associated folic acid deficiency, with which scurvy commonly occurs. In children, disturbances of growth occur, and teeth, bones, blood vessels,

and other collagen-rich structures develop abnormally. Preformed teeth may become loose and fall out because of alveolar bone resorption.

Wounds heal poorly, and previously healed wounds may open up again. In very advanced deficiency, edema, oliguria, and neuropathy are prominent. Should intracerebral bleeding occur, serious neurologic sequelae and even death may result.

DIAGNOSIS. The diagnosis of advanced scurvy can be made on clinical grounds alone because the skin changes often are quite characteristic. These classic presentations occur rarely, however. Capillary fragility is commonly abnormal. Radiographs are useful in demonstrating subperiosteal elevation, disturbances of calcification of the cartilage matrix, fractures and dislocations, ground glass appearance of the cortex, alveolar bone resorption, and other findings.

Plasma ascorbic acid levels are greatly reduced in scurvy, usually to 0.1 mg per deciliter or lower. Some depression of plasma ascorbic acid levels occurs, however, in a variety of other conditions, including cigarette smoking, tuberculosis, rheumatic fever, and many chronic disorders and in some women using oral contraceptive drugs. These conditions must be considered when a low ascorbic acid level is detected.

The assay of ascorbic acid in serum or plasma can be accomplished with titrimetric, spectrophotometric, or fluorometric methods. Some laboratories prefer to make the diagnosis of scurvy by assay of platelet or white blood cell ascorbic acid content.

TREATMENT. As little as 10 mg per day of ascorbic acid can completely prevent the clinical manifestations of scurvy. Even far-advanced cases of scurvy respond rapidly to ascorbic acid in the range of 100 to 200 mg per day. Marked improvement is to be expected within several days. Patients should also be instructed in the importance of a proper diet to prevent further recurrences.

Patients with rare inborn errors of metabolism, including tyrosinemia, osteogenesis imperfecta, and Chédiak-Higashi syndrome, have had some apparent benefit from the use of ascorbic acid in the range of 50 to 200 mg per day. Certain forms of the Ehlers-Danlos syndrome are disorders in which pharmacologic doses (4 grams) have been reported to be effective.

Special mention must be made of two conditions in which the use of megadoses of ascorbic acid has attracted wide attention in the popular press: the common cold and advanced cancer. Many studies have been performed on the possible benefits of 2 grams and higher per day of ascorbic acid on the prevention of colds and on the alleviation of symptoms once colds develop. On balance, the predominance of evidence favors the view that while some individuals may receive slight benefit in terms of symptoms, probably as a result of a mild antihistamine action of ascorbic acid, no consistent, reproducible improvements occur in the frequency, duration, or severity of illness in the great majority of cases.

With respect to treatment of cancer, there is some theoretical basis for the view that maintenance of immune function may depend upon the adequacy of vitamin C nutriture, as may wound healing, collagen formation, and cytotoxicity of a number of chemotherapeutic drugs. Nevertheless, treatment of patients with advanced colon cancer with megadoses of vitamin C after chemotherapy and radiation has been ineffective when evaluated in an objective manner. The use of vitamin C under no circumstances should replace established methods of treating cancer with chemotherapy, surgery, or radiation.

Vitamin C at a dose level of approximately 0.5 to 3 grams per day has long been used empirically to acidify the urine in cases of refractory urinary tract infections. Ascorbic acid is only a weak acidifying agent, and its efficacy under these circumstances is difficult to evaluate.

Ascorbic acid in amounts ordinarily contained in food may be useful in facilitating the intestinal absorption of nonheme iron. To be effective, the ascorbic acid and the iron sources must be consumed together. As little as 100 ml of orange juice, which contains 40 to 50 mg of ascorbic acid, has been reported to increase the absorption of iron from vegetable sources more than threefold. Iron from meat is not absorbed more efficiently by ascorbic acid.

A potentially useful application of ascorbic acid lies in its ability to inhibit the conversion of nitrites and secondary amines to the carcinogenic nitrosoamines in vitro, and, under certain circumstances, in vivo. Whether ascorbic acid can achieve this effect in vivo under ordinary circumstances of food consumption is important to determine. It is of interest that consumption of foods high in vitamin C is associated with reduced risk of gastric and esophageal cancer. The antioxidant effect of ascorbic acid may be synergistic with that of vitamin E and β-carotene, and trials of cancer prevention with a combination of antioxidants are now in progress in patients at high risk.

Another potential therapeutic role for vitamin C may lie in diabetes. Doses of 500 to 2000 mg per day of ascorbic acid have been reported to reduce erythrocyte concentrations of sorbitol possibly implicated in the pathogenesis of complications of diabetes. There is recent evidence that ascorbic acid alone or in combination with zinc, iron, calcium, or EDTA may reduce the body burden of lead.

Toxicity

At the dose range of approximately 1 to 2 grams per day and higher there is potential for some adverse side effects. There is great variability among individuals in regard to their susceptibility to the adverse effects of large doses of ascorbic acid. In the intestinal tract, large doses (2 grams and higher) of ascorbic acid may produce pain, discomfort, and an osmotic diarrhea. Doses of ascorbic acid above 1 gram may give a false-negative guaiac test for blood, thereby obscuring recognition of occult bleeding. Urine tests for glucose also may be misleading when very large doses of ascorbic acid are ingested, producing a false-negative glucose oxidase reaction (Tes-Tape) and false-positive copper-reduction reaction (Clinitest) and making urine strips more difficult to read. At daily doses of 3 grams and higher, automated measurements of alanine aminotransferase, lactate dehydrogenase, and uric acid may be affected.

As oxalate is a degradative product of ascorbic acid, large amounts of this vitamin are expected to increase biosynthesis and renal excretion of oxalate, posing the potential risk of formation of oxalate stones in susceptible individuals. The increase in oxalate excretion is small in magnitude, however, and in most cases still falls within the normal range. There is recent evidence that patients with recurrent formation of kidney stones exhibit increased production and urinary excretion of oxalate following a 2-gram load of ascorbic acid. Uricosuria and uric acid stones are also believed to occur with increased frequency after large doses of ascorbic acid. Nevertheless, the real risk of kidney stone formation in users of large doses of ascorbic acid is not known with precision at the present time. Precipitation of calcium oxalate stones is favored by an alkaline urine. With chronic consumption of large doses of ascorbic acid, there is a likelihood of exacerbating systemic acidosis in those disorders with failure of urinary acidification, such as chronic renal disease and renal tubular acidosis. Certain patients with diminished glucose-6-phosphate dehydrogenase activity may be at increased risk for hemolytic episodes with large doses of ascorbic acid therapy. There is some concern that indiscriminate use of ascorbic acid, which increases intestinal absorption of iron, may put patients with hemochromatosis at risk for hyperabsorption of iron. Vitamin C may also increase the risk of iron overload in patients with β-thalassemia and other disorders that require frequent long-term blood transfusions.

Block G, Menkes M: Ascorbic acid in cancer prevention. In Moon TE, Micozzi MC (eds.): Nutrition and Cancer Prevention. Investigating the Role of Micronutrients. New York, Marcel Dekker, 1989, p 341. Current status of epidemiology of vitamin C intake and cancer prevalence.

Burns JJ, Rivers JM, Machlin LJ (eds.): Third conference on vitamin C. NY Acad Sci Vol. 498, 1987. Proceedings of a recent symposium on advances in understanding of vitamin C metabolism.

Hathcock JN, Rader J: Micronutrient safety. In Bendich A, Chandra R (eds.): Micronutrients and Immune Function. New York, Academy of Sciences, 1990, Vol. 587, p 257. Recent review of toxicities of vitamins and minerals.

Levine M: New concepts in the biology and biochemistry of ascorbic acid. N Engl J Med 314:892, 1986. Important update of biochemistry, physiology, and nutritional applications of vitamin C.

VITAMIN A

Structure and Biochemical Function

Vitamin A refers to retinol, although the term is often used loosely to indicate all related compounds (Fig. 204–6). The term "retinoids" has been used to designate all the natural and synthetic isomers and derivatives of vitamin A. Retinol is oxidized to vitamin A aldehyde (retinal), which is critical to vision. Retinoic acid (vitamin A acid) is the major oxidative metabolite of retinol. Retinoic acid can fulfill the growth-promoting and epithelium-differentiating roles of retinol but cannot fully maintain its function in reproduction, nor can retinoic acid fulfill the functions of retinal in vision. Carotenoids are larger precursor molecules that undergo cleavage to yield retinal. The most important of the more than 30 carotenoids with pro-vitamin A activity is β-carotene.

Of the various metabolic roles of vitamin A, the best understood is the visual process. Retinal is the prosthetic group of all the visual pigments that capture light. The human retina contains four kinds of visual pigments: rhodopsin in rods and three iodopsins in cones. In the dark-adapted retina, rhodopsin is activated by photons of light. This event initiates the visual cycle, during which retinal changes its conformation from a cis to a trans isomer and other conformational changes occur in the protein. During dark adaptation, these processes are reversed and rhodopsin is regenerated. In view of the absolute requirement for retinal, it is not surprising that loss of highly sensitive night vision is an early symptom of vitamin A deficiency. Vitamin A probably serves additional roles in the normal functioning of the retina.

The mechanism of action of vitamin A in growth and differentiation is not known. One hypothesis is that vitamin A is similar to steroid hormones in influencing events in the genome following attachment to specific cellular binding proteins. The striking effects of vitamin A upon differentiation, particularly of epithelial tissues, underlie the current concept that this vitamin and its derivatives may have a role in the prevention of certain cancers, particularly of epithelial origin.

Retinol is fat soluble, sensitive to acid and heat, and rapidly oxidized upon exposure to light and oxygen. β-Carotene is relatively less heat-sensitive than retinol. β-Carotene is capable of quenching singlet oxygen and is a powerful antioxidant, protecting cell membranes from damage caused by free radicals.

Normal Physiology

Foods containing vitamin A (largely in the form of retinyl esters) or carotenoids are digested by gastric and intestinal enzymes, and then both forms are absorbed by the intestinal mucosa. About 80 to 90 per cent of dietary vitamin A is absorbed. The rate of absorption of dietary β-carotene is much slower, and only 40 to 60 per cent is absorbed, the percentage decreasing at higher doses. Absorption of β-carotene is more dependent than vitamin A upon interactions with bile salts.

Within the intestinal mucosa, β-carotene is cleaved to two molecules of retinal, which are then reduced to retinol (Fig. 204–6). The retinol generated from β-carotene, as well as that absorbed directly, is esterified subsequently. The retinyl esters formed are incorporated into chylomicrons and transported via lymph to the general circulation, where the triglycerides in the chylomicrons are degraded by lipoprotein lipase. The smaller chylomicron remnants remaining are then cleared by the liver, the major storage organ for vitamin A, which contains approximately 90 per cent of the total body reserves. Retinyl esters, mostly in the form of retinyl palmitate, are stored in the liver, and their hydrolysis generates retinol, which binds to a specific hepatic apo-retinol binding protein (RBP). The holo-RBP is secreted into the plasma, where it forms a 1:1 molar complex with a tetrameric protein, formerly called prealbumin, which also binds thyroxine and triiodothyronine. In recognition of both roles, this protein is now named transthyretin.

Cell surfaces recognize the RBP-retinol complex rather than retinol, and once inside the cell, all trans-retinol binds to a specific protein, cellular retinol binding protein (CRBP). CRBP may deliver retinol to intranuclear binding sites that mediate genomic expression and/or transport retinol across cellular membranes. CRBP concentrations are increased in certain animal and human tumors. A cellular retinoic acid binding protein (CRABP) has also been detected in a number of neonatal tissues and epithelial tumors that are sensitive to retinoic acid therapeutically.

Retinoic acid does not accumulate in liver, and it fulfills some but not all of the physiologic functions of retinol. In vitamin A deficiency, hepatic concentrations of vitamin A are nearly completely depleted before total plasma RBP levels begin to fall. With vitamin A repletion, the liver apo-RBP becomes more saturated, and levels of holo-RBP begin to rise in blood.

The degradative metabolism of retinol and its derivatives proceeds by a series of chain-shortening steps to yield a group of compounds of little if any intrinsic biologic activity.

Requirements and Dietary Sources

The RDA for vitamin A is currently 1000 µg of retinol equivalents (RE) for adult males and 800 µg for adult females. One RE is defined as 1 µg of retinol or 6 µg of β-carotene. The allowances are calculated in this fashion because the overall utilization of β-carotene is only about one sixth that of retinol, as a result of the relative inefficiency with which β-carotene is absorbed and converted to vitamin A.

Vitamin A allowances were formerly expressed in terms of international units (IU), and this nomenclature still appears on most commercial vitamin bottles. One RE is equal to 3.33 IU retinol and 10 IU β-carotene. The RDA for vitamin A expressed in terms of IU is 5000 for adult males and 4000 for adult females. These figures are based upon the estimate that the American diet contains approximately equal amounts of β-carotene (2500 IU = 250 RE, for males) and retinol (2500 IU = 750 RE, for males).

β-Carotene is derived from plant sources, including vegetables such as carrots and sweet potatoes, leafy green vegetables, and some fruits, such as cantaloupe and papaya. Preformed vitamin A is derived almost exclusively from animal sources. Liver obviously is a rich source, followed by kidney, milk and milk products, and fish. Fish liver oils have unusually high concentrations of vitamin A.

Deficiency

PATHOGENESIS. Vitamin A deficiency is a very common problem worldwide, particularly in developing countries, as a consequence of famine or shortages of vitamin A–rich foods. The ocular manifestations of vitamin A deficiency are such a serious problem that half a million preschool children become blind every year as a result. In such situations, a diet high in rice, wheat, maize, and tubers contains little if any β-carotene. Breast and cow's milk do not provide enough vitamin A to meet the needs of the growing child.

In the United States, vitamin A deficiency may be encountered among the urban poor, the elderly, alcohol abusers, patients with malabsorption, and other individuals on a marginal diet. In alcoholism, vitamin A deficiency may develop for several reasons. Zinc deficiency, which frequently coexists in alcoholism, impairs the release of holo-RBP from liver, thereby interfering with vitamin A mobilization from storage sites. Thus, alcohol-associated zinc deficiency may intensify sequelae of dietary vitamin A deficiency. In addition, in alcoholism the degradative enzyme, alcohol dehydrogenase, which also converts retinol to retinal in the retina, may be so saturated with ethanol that retinal production is sharply diminished. Furthermore, as malabsorption develops in chronic alcoholism, dietary carotenes and vitamin A may be lost in increasing amounts in the stool.

Vitamin A deficiency may occur after long-term use of mineral oil, because this fat-soluble vitamin is dissolved in the oil. Other laxatives may result in vitamin A deficiency because of rapid intestinal transit and diminished intestinal absorption. Vitamin A deficiency may result also after prolonged use of certain drugs, such as cholestyramine, colestipol, neomycin, and colchicine.

CLINICAL FEATURES. Night blindness, as noted previously, may be an early manifestation of vitamin A deficiency. It has been suggested that the frequent episodes of falling and of traffic accidents involving chronic alcoholic persons at night may be due to some degree to underlying night blindness. In addition, dryness or xerosis of the conjunctivae and later of the cornea may develop (xerophthalmia), leading to softening and perforation of the cornea and development of Bitot's spots (small, white patches) on the sclerae. Because of the role of vitamin A in maintaining differentiated epithelium, dietary deficiency leads to abnormalities of epithelial tissue and keratinization, particularly in the eye, lung, sweat glands, and gastrointestinal tract. Loss of taste may also occur. Vitamin A deficiency leads to increased frequency, severity, and mortality rate of infectious diseases.

It has been suggested that decreased intake of β-carotene or vitamin A–rich foods or both may be associated with an increased prevalence of epithelial cancers, particularly lung cancers, among smokers. In some studies, intake of β-carotene but not vitamin A has had a strong negative correlation with cancer risk. Also, vitamin A–deficient animals have an increased risk of chemical carcinogenesis; administration of retinoids can prevent chemically induced cancers in animals.

DIAGNOSIS. The demonstration of abnormal dark adaptation is important evidence for the diagnosis of vitamin A deficiency. Techniques are being developed that can be carried out under field conditions without expensive equipment. Retinol can be detected directly in serum by immunoassay. Normal levels are in the range of 30 to 65 µg per deciliter. Serum levels may be increased by hypothyroidism, nephrotic syndrome, oral contraceptives, and disorders of lipid metabolism. By the time serum levels of retinol begin to decrease from dietary deficiency, liver reserves are already nearly completely depleted. A new technique, conjunctival impression cytology, may be useful in detecting early histologic abnormalities in the cornea.

TREATMENT. The extensive eye problems of vitamin A deficiency that are encountered in developing countries are best

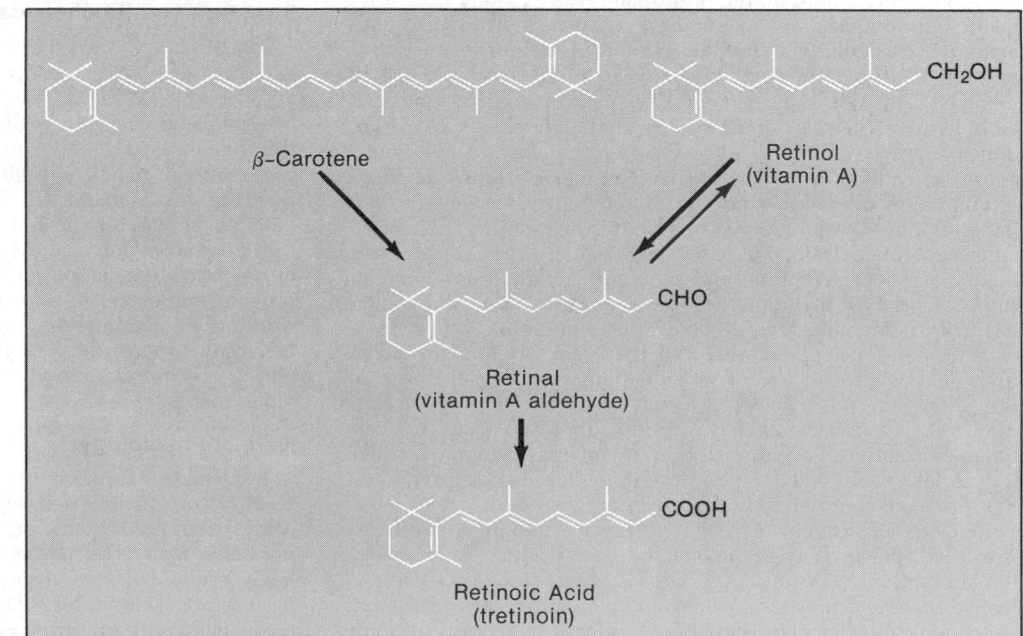

FIGURE 204–6. Structural formulae and interconversions of retinol, retinal, retinoic acid, and β-carotene.

approached through a systematic plan of prevention. Such programs are increasing in scope and magnitude. Injections of vitamin A in large doses (50,000 to 100,000 IU) every 4 to 6 months are highly effective and are tolerated remarkably well. In children from population groups that have a high prevalence of vitamin A deficiency, capsules containing 200,000 IU given every 6 months have reduced mortality markedly, particularly from infectious diseases. In the United States, only when dietary deficiency is far advanced should it be treated with similar doses and for several days only; then maintenance doses should be administered. Water-soluble forms of vitamin A should provide great assistance in patient management.

Derivatives of vitamin A (referred to as retinoids), particularly 13-cis-retinoic acid (isotretinoin), have been used to treat cystic acne with considerable success. Investigations are continuing in other dermatologic disorders, including psoriasis, actinic keratosis, leukoplakia, and pityriasis rosea. The mechanism of action of this derivative may lie in inhibition of keratinization, suppression of sebaceous gland secretion, or possibly a direct anti-inflammatory effect.

The use of β-carotene or retinoids or both, especially the less toxic forms, for the possible prevention of epithelial cancers is under intense study. Smokers should be expected to benefit particularly by increasing their intake of carotenoids, but no amounts of these agents are large enough to protect completely against the harmful effects of smoking. Consumption of foods rich in carotenes and vitamin A is not a substitute for failure to stop smoking. The exact doses necessary to achieve preventive effects are not known at present.

A new therapeutic application for vitamin A is in children with severe measles infection. Measles depresses the serum levels of vitamin A, and vitamin A deficiency greatly increases risk of pneumonia, diarrhea, and death in infected patients. Treatment with large doses of water-miscible retinyl palmitate reduces severity of complications and death rate in severely ill children with malaria.

Toxicity

β-Carotene is entirely without toxicity when consumed in food or as a nutritional supplement. Because only limited amounts of β-carotene can be converted to vitamin A by the body, consumption of β-carotene in amounts several-fold above the RDA does not lead to vitamin A toxicity. Consumption of β-carotene in large amounts from foods such as carrots may stain the skin a yellow-orange color, but this phenomenon is entirely benign and may even be beneficial in providing protection against solar exposure. The sclerae remain white in carotenemia; thus, the condition can easily be differentiated from jaundice.

Vitamin A (retinol), on the other hand, can be quite toxic when taken continuously for a few days to several weeks in large amounts (particularly at 100,000 IU and higher) or for periods of several months or more at lower doses of 25,000 to 50,000 IU per day. The skin may become dry, pruritic, coarse, and scaly with fissures; hair loss may occur. Both vitamin A excess and deficiency have adverse effects upon the skin. Sore mouth, anorexia, and vomiting may ensue. The most serious side effects of vitamin A overdosage pertain to the central nervous system: patients may develop severe headaches, drowsiness, irritability, failure to concentrate, increased intracranial pressure, and papilledema. These symptoms and signs may mimic those of a brain tumor. The liver may enlarge, rarely progressing to fibrosis and cirrhosis. Generalized lymph node enlargement may occur. There may be painful hyperostoses, and there are preliminary indications that long-term use of vitamin A may accelerate the bone loss of aging, possibly by sensitizing vitamin D receptors to calcitriol. Hypercalcemia may develop after large doses. Congenital malformations have occurred in the infants of women consuming 25,000 to 50,000 IU per day or higher during pregnancy. Symptoms of acute vitamin A toxicity are shown in Table 204–1.

In cases of vitamin A toxicity, serum vitamin A levels are increased, particularly in the form of retinyl esters. In an asymptomatic patient consuming megadoses of vitamin A, the onset of liver disease, such as viral or alcoholic hepatitis, may precipitate overt clinical toxicity, presumably by releasing stored retinol into the general circulation. With discontinuation of large doses of vitamin A, the symptoms gradually recede. Low-protein diets enhance hepatic toxicity of vitamin A, and treatment with tetracycline may increase the risk for increased intracranial pressure. Treatment with zinc may facilitate mobilization of vitamin A from the liver, a useful adjunct when there is hepatotoxicity.

The development of synthetic retinoids with lower toxicities and greater uptake in target organs is expected to facilitate the safe application of these agents to the possible chemoprevention of cancer. At present it is essential to realize that derivatives of vitamin A such as 13-cis-retinoic acid may cause birth defects and other manifestations of vitamin A toxicity.

TABLE 204–1. SIGNS AND SYMPTOMS OF ACUTE VITAMIN A TOXICITY

Children	Adults
Anorexia	Abdominal pain
Bulging fontanelles	Anorexia
Drowsiness	Blurred vision
Increased intracranial pressure	Drowsiness
Irritability	Headache
Vomiting	Hypercalcemia
	Irritability
	Muscle weakness
	Nausea, vomiting
	Peripheral neuritis
	Skin desquamation

From Hathcock JN, Hattan DG, Jenkins MY, et al.: Evaluation of vitamin A toxicity. Am J Clin Nutr 52:183, 1990.

Goodman DS: Vitamin A and retinoids in health and disease. N Engl J Med 310:1023, 1984. *This comprehensive review highlights advances relating vitamin A and retinoids to clinical medicine and public health, particularly ophthalmology, nutrition, dermatology, and cancer.*
Hathcock JN, Hattan DG, Jenkins MY, et al: Evaluation of vitamin A toxicity. Am J Clin Nutr 52:183, 1990. *Review of vitamin A toxicity, particularly with respect to causing birth defects.*
Hussey GD, Klein M: A randomized controlled trial of vitamin A in children with severe measles. N Engl J Med 323:160, 1990. *Large doses of vitamin A reduce death rate and severity of complications.*
Olson JA: Vitamin A. *In* Brown ML (ed.): Present Knowledge in Nutrition, 6th ed. Washington, D.C., International Life Sciences Institute, The Nutrition Foundation, 1990, p 96. *Review of physiology, binding proteins, metabolism, and function of vitamin A.*
Ziegler RG: A review of epidemiological evidence that carotenoids reduce the risk of cancer. J Nutr 119:116, 1989. *Documents evidence that low intake of fruits and vegetables is associated with increased risk for certain cancers.*

VITAMIN D

Vitamin D is discussed in Chapter 233 in association with calcium metabolism and metabolic bone diseases.

VITAMIN E

Structure and Biochemical Function

Vitamin E activity is derived from a series of dietary tocopherols and tocotrienols, the most potent of which is D-α-tocopherol (Fig. 204–7). At least eight compounds with vitamin E activity have been isolated from plants. The most widely accepted function of this vitamin is as an antioxidant, protecting polyunsaturated fatty acids in membranes and other cellular structures from attack by free radicals. Vitamin E deficiency in animals increases the likelihood of membrane and cellular damage from ozone, nitrogen dioxide, and hyperbaric oxygen. Dietary selenium is a precursor of selenite, a cofactor for glutathione peroxidase, which also provides important protection against lipid peroxidation in vivo, working in conjunction with vitamin E and other enzymes, including superoxide dismutase and catalase. Dietary selenium under certain circumstances may spare the requirement for vitamin E.

Normal Physiology

Intestinal absorption of dietary vitamin E requires normal mechanisms of digestion and absorption of fat, particularly bile acids. About 20 to 50 per cent of tocopherols are absorbed normally, with lower percentages at higher doses. Medium-chain triglycerides enhance absorption of tocopherols, and polyunsaturated fatty acids inhibit absorption. Tocopherols are absorbed as micelles primarily from the mid-small intestine. Vitamin E in blood is bound to all the lipoproteins, and levels correlate with those of lipoproteins to which they are bound both normally and in various disease states. In contrast to vitamin A, there does not appear to be a specific carrier protein in blood for vitamin E, nor a specific organ in which it is stored. Some vitamin E is also transported in erythrocytes. The most important storage sites of the vitamin are fat, liver, and muscle. Recent reports raise the possibility of specific binding proteins for E in tissues. Vitamin E undergoes little metabolic transformation after absorption. The major excretory route is through the feces.

Since dietary deficiency occurs only under very unusual circumstances, cases of vitamin E deficiency have usually been identified primarily in patients with prolonged and severe fat malabsorption. Vitamin E deficiency has also been detected in patients receiving parenteral nutrition without adequate E replacement.

Requirements and Dietary Sources

The dietary allowance for vitamin E is expressed in terms of milligrams of α-tocopherol equivalents (α-TE) and is 10 mg per day (15 IU) for adult males and 8 mg per day (12 IU) for adult females, with increases of 2 mg per day for pregnancy and 3 to 4 mg per day for lactation. The increased requirement for vitamin E with diets high in polyunsaturated fatty acids is thought not to be clinically relevant, since the items highest in vitamin E content—soybean, corn, cottonseed, wheat germ, and safflower oils and their derivatives—are also high in polyunsaturated fatty acids. As a group, the tocopherols and tocotrienols are widely distributed in the food supply. They are relatively unstable and lose significant activity during storage and cooking.

Deficiency

PATHOGENESIS. Clinical deficiency of vitamin E is generally encountered in the setting of severe malabsorption. The most serious deficiency is associated with a genetic disorder, abetalipoproteinemia, in which there is failure both of intestinal absorption and of serum transport of vitamin E. Vitamin E deficiency occurs in children with biliary atresia, cystic fibrosis, and chronic cholestasis, as well as in adults who survive these diseases or who have celiac disease, Crohn's disease, or other serious forms of malabsorption (Ch. 102).

An apparent inborn error of vitamin E metabolism, named familial isolated vitamin E deficiency, has recently been identified. Affected patients have a common pattern of neurologic abnormalities, are vitamin E deficient despite consuming an adequate diet, have no evidence of vitamin E malabsorption, and can achieve normal serum levels as well as neurologic improvement after treatment with large doses of the vitamin (800 to 1000 mg per day). The defect appears to reside in inability to incorporate dietary vitamin E into VLDL, resulting in very rapid clearance from plasma.

CLINICAL FEATURES. Deficiency of vitamin E has generally not been recognized as a clearly definable syndrome. The red cell half-life may be shortened, although anemia is uncommon in the absence of other causes. Most importantly, clinical and neuropathologic evidence of posterior column and spinocerebellar tract abnormalities have been described, with areflexia, ophthalmoplegia, and disturbances of gait, proprioception, and vibration. In premature infants, vitamin E deficiency is associated with hemolytic anemia, thrombocytosis, edema, intraventricular hemorrhage, and increasing risk of retrolental fibroplasia and bronchopulmonary dysplasia, both of which are related to oxygen toxicity.

DIAGNOSIS. Diagnosis of vitamin E deficiency is usually made by measurement of plasma vitamin E levels; normal levels are generally 0.50 to 0.70 mg per deciliter and higher. In several of the hemolytic anemias, such as sickle cell anemia and G-6-PD deficiency, serum vitamin E levels tend to be low. Serum vitamin E concentration should be expressed in relation to serum lipid levels when vitamin E nutritional status is being evaluated, inasmuch as serum vitamin E levels correlate with those of serum cholesterol and total lipids and may be elevated in diabetes and primary lipid disorders.

TREATMENT. The therapeutic role of vitamin E remains controversial at the present time. Although vitamin E has been advocated by food faddists as an "anti-aging" vitamin, there is no evidence that it prolongs life in man. This vitamin has been claimed to enhance sexual performance, an attribute that also has not been substantiated. Some patients with intermittent claudication appear to have improved after therapy with vitamin E. Hemolytic anemia in the premature newborn is generally benefited by vitamin E therapy, and the severity but not the incidence of retrolental fibroplasia may be reduced. Administration of vitamin E has reduced the incidence of intraventricular hemorrhage in premature infants. Large doses of vitamin E have diminished the neurologic complications in abetalipoproteinemia, cholestatic liver disease, and cystic fibrosis.

There are a number of other effects of vitamin E demonstrable in vitro in experimental animals and in some instances in humans, but their clinical relevance remains unresolved. These effects include reducing platelet aggregation, inhibiting conversion of nitrites to nitrosamines, inhibiting prostaglandin synthesis, improving immune function, protecting against environmental toxicants and pollutants, and diminishing progression of cataracts, among others. There is much interest in the potential therapeutic role of vitamin E as an antioxidant. Vitamins E and C are synergistic in their antioxidant activities in vitro. A number of studies have found that elevated serum levels of vitamin E are associated with lower risk of cancer, as noted above. Such relationships possibly may relate to the antioxidant properties of vitamin E. Current investigations are seeking to determine whether vitamin E delays the emergence of cancer, heart disease, and other major health problems.

Toxicity

Vitamin E is far less toxic than vitamins A and D, and a daily intake in the range of 200 to 800 mg per day (20 to 80 times the RDA) is generally considered safe. Nausea, flatulence, and diarrhea have been reported at doses in excess of 1000 mg. In animals the intestinal absorption of vitamin A and K is reduced at high doses of E, which may be clinically significant in patients on marginal diets. Vitamin E appears to increase the vitamin K requirement, and megadoses of vitamin E administered together with the anticoagulant drug warfarin may result in overt bleeding.

Bieri JG, Corash L, Hubbard VS: Medical uses of vitamin E. N Engl J Med 308:1063, 1983. *This article reviews the rationale for treatment with vitamin E in various clinical disorders, limitations of treatment, and toxicities encountered.*

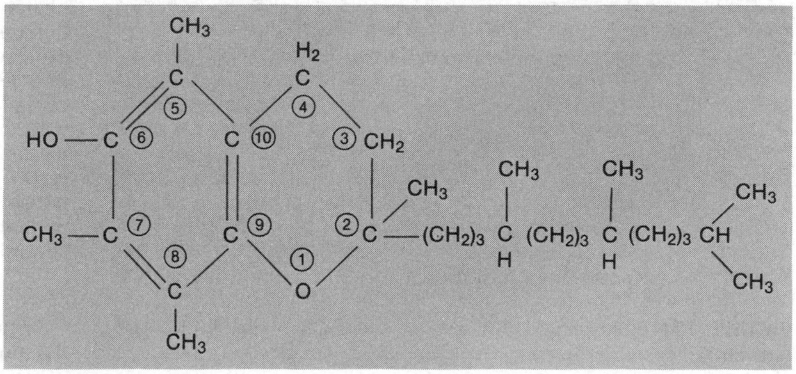

FIGURE 204–7. Structural formula of D-alpha tocopherol (vitamin E).

Machlin LJ: Vitamin E. *In* Machlin LJ (ed.): Handbook of Vitamins, 2nd ed. New York, Marcel Dekker, 1990, p 99. *Up-to-date review of physiology and medical uses of vitamin E.*

Murphy SP, Subar AF, Block G: Vitamin E intakes and sources in the United States. Am J Clin Nutr 52:361, 1990. *Survey identifying sources of dietary intake of E.*

Traber MG, Somol RJ, Burton GW, et al.: Impaired ability of patients with familial isolated vitamin E deficiency to incorporate α-tocopherol into lipoproteins secreted by the liver. J Clin Invest 85:397, 1990. *Research into mechanism of vitamin E deficiency in a familial disorder.*

VITAMIN K

Structure and Biochemical Functions

Vitamin K occurs naturally in two forms, differing from one another only in their side chains. Vitamin K_1 (now called phylloquinone) is made by plant sources; vitamin K_2 (menaquinone) is synthesized by normal intestinal flora. It is also contained in some animal tissues. Vitamin K_3 (menadione) is an artificial provitamin that can be converted to menaquinone by the liver (Fig. 204–8). Compounds with vitamin K activity are sensitive to ultraviolet light and alkali.

It has been proposed that the mechanism of action of vitamin K consists of a post-translational γ-carboxylation of glutamic acid moieties in inactive precursor proteins, which confers calcium-binding properties to the proteins. The most widely known of these proteins are involved in blood coagulation. Four clotting factors are dependent upon vitamin K for this important action: prothrombin (Factor II), proconvertin (Factor VII), Christmas factor (Factor IX), and Stuart-Prower factor (Factor X). Lack of vitamin K may result in death from uncontrolled hemorrhage.

The anticoagulant drugs warfarin and dicoumarol inhibit the vitamin K–dependent γ-carboxylation by interfering with activation of vitamin K to its metabolically active hydroquinone form. As a result of this inhibition, the activation of the four clotting factors is greatly reduced.

Proteins that are involved in the mineralization of bone (osteocalcin) and possibly also in calcium resorption from the renal tubule also require vitamin K for their synthesis. Other vitamin K–dependent proteins have been identified (protein C, protein S). The vitamin K antagonists warfarin and dicoumarol also cause a marked decrease in formation of osteocalcin, presumably by interfering with γ-carboxylation.

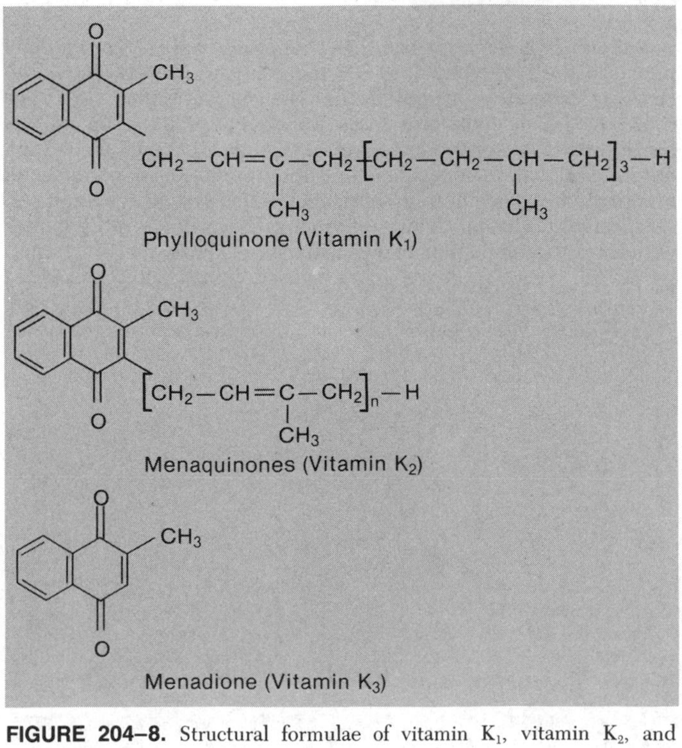

FIGURE 204–8. Structural formulae of vitamin K_1, vitamin K_2, and vitamin K_3.

Normal Physiology

The intestinal absorption of various forms of vitamin K resembles that of vitamin E in requiring bile salts and other normal mechanisms of fat absorption and in being incorporated into micelles. Vitamin K_1 is absorbed principally in the proximal segment via a saturable energy-dependent process, whereas vitamin K_2 is absorbed by the small intestine and by the colon via a non–carrier-mediated, non–energy-dependent process. Liver and other parenchymal organs store vitamin K, but apparently only to a limited degree. The efficiency of absorption varies greatly and is markedly diminished by mineral oil, other fat solvents, and laxatives. In patients who have fat malabsorption that is severe and prolonged, as in sprue, regional ileitis, and other disorders, or in patients with obstruction to bile flow, vitamin K deficiency commonly develops. Deficiency also may occur after prolonged antibiotic therapy, destroying the intestinal synthesis of vitamin K.

After absorption, vitamin K is transported via the lymphatic system in association with chylomicrons. Liver is probably the most important storage site for vitamin K; high concentrations are also found in the adrenal glands, lungs, bone marrow, kidneys, and lymph nodes. The main excretory products of vitamin K in urine are glucuronide derivatives that have undergone chain shortening and beta oxidation.

Requirements and Dietary Sources

The best sources of vitamin K are green leafy vegetables, particularly turnip greens, broccoli, brussels sprouts, spinach, and lettuce. There are moderate amounts in liver, bacon, cheese, butter, coffee, and green tea. Significant amounts are synthesized by intestinal bacteria. There may be discrepancies in the analysis of foods by several different methods. In 1989 for the first time a recommended dietary allowance was made for vitamin K by the National Academy of Sciences. It is recommended that normal adult males consume 70 to 80 μg per day and normal adult females 60 to 65 μg per day. No increase is recommended for either pregnancy or lactation. Dietary deficiency based upon consuming less than this amount is uncommon at the present time in the United States, because the usual diet contains ample amounts of vitamin K.

Deficiency

PATHOGENESIS. Vitamin K deficiency occurs frequently in newborn infants for several reasons. First, fetal stores tend to be low because very little of this vitamin is transported across the placenta. In addition, the fetal gut is sterile, and therefore the newborn lacks the supply of vitamin K that can be provided by normal intestinal flora. As the intestinal tract becomes colonized postnatally, the synthesis of vitamin K becomes appreciable. Deficiency generally does not develop unless there is an abnormality of intestinal function or antibiotic therapy.

CLINICAL FEATURES. Vitamin K deficiency may be manifested clinically as increased tendency to hemorrhage. Such bleeding episodes may be particularly severe in newborn infants.

DIAGNOSIS. The only practical and reliable method for diagnosis of vitamin K deficiency is direct assay of one or more of the four vitamin K–dependent clotting factors. Hypothyroidism inhibits both the synthesis and degradation of these four clotting factors.

TREATMENT. Vitamin K deficiency responds rapidly to the administration of vitamin K, provided that liver function is normal. A number of preparations of vitamin K are available, some of which are water soluble, e.g., menadiol sodium diphosphate. These forms are more toxic than the lipid-soluble phylloquinone form. In patients with advanced liver disease, the serum prothrombin is decreased and responds poorly if at all to administration of vitamin K. Patients with low serum prothrombin caused by vitamin K deficiency can be distinguished from those with low prothrombin caused by liver disease because in vitamin K deficiency the prothrombin precursor in blood is not γ-carboxylated; usually γ-carboxylated prothrombin is found in patients with liver disease. When vitamin K is given orally to patients with malabsorption, bile salts may also need to be administered to achieve optimal results.

Toxicity

Consumption of large quantities of foods rich in vitamin K is not believed to produce clinical toxicity. Certain water-soluble derivatives administered parenterally have caused hemolytic anemia and jaundice.

Olson RE: Vitamin K. *In* Goodhart RS, Shils ME (eds.): Modern Nutrition in Health and Disease, 6th ed. Philadelphia, Lea & Febiger, 1980, pp 170–180. *Thorough discussion of nutritional aspects of vitamin K, with emphasis upon biochemical mechanisms.*

Suttie JW: Current concepts of the mechanism of action of vitamin K and its antagonist. *In* Lindenbaum J (ed.): Nutrition in Hematology. Contemporary Issues in Clinical Nutrition. Vol. 5. New York, Churchill Livingstone, 1983, pp 245–270. *Discussion of the basic biochemistry of vitamin K and its relation to clotting factors.*

Suttie JW: Vitamin K. *In* Machlin LJ (ed.): Handbook of Vitamins, 2nd ed. New York, Marcel Dekker, 1990, p 145. *Comprehensive review of nutritional aspects of vitamin K.*

205 Disturbances of Trace Mineral Metabolism

Clifford Tasman-Jones

The bulk of living material is formed by 11 elements, all of which are from the lower atomic numbers of the periodic table (H, C, N, O, Na, Mg, P, S, Cl, K, and Ca). In addition to these, there are essential minerals that are present in trace amounts. These include F, Si, V, Cr, Mn, Fe, Co, Ni, Cu, Zn, Se, Mo, Sn, and I.

While deficiencies of trace minerals and vitamins are uncommon in humans eating a variety of foods, trace mineral deficiencies can occur in premature infants and in those with disordered eating habits owing to physical or psychological causes and with the use of enteral and parenteral feeding. Deficiencies developing during parenteral nutrition have stimulated interest in trace mineral function in human metabolism.

Trace minerals essential for life act as essential cofactors of enzymes and as organizers of the molecular structures of the cell (e.g., mitochondria) and its membrane. There is an optimal tissue concentration for trace minerals; excess can be toxic and insufficiency leads to metabolic failure.

Trace mineral bioavailability is affected by the physiologic status of the person (intrinsic factors), as well as by dietary availability (extrinsic factors). The absorptive mechanisms in the intestine vary with the trace mineral. Once in the plasma they are bound either to specific proteins or to albumin for transportation. The excretory path varies, but most are excreted into the gastrointestinal tract, many by way of bile; some are excreted into the urine and some by sweat glands. Not all trace minerals have been shown to be clinically important. Some, such as iron and iodine, are so important in specific disorders that they are covered separately in this volume.

ZINC

METABOLISM. Although zinc represents only 0.003 per cent (1.4 to 2.3 grams) of the human body, it is an intrinsic part of at least 110 metalloenzymes and other cellular components and is essential for the synthesis of protein, DNA, and RNA. Zinc is an important stabilizing component of macromolecules and biomembranes. It is required for growth at all stages of life, particularly during fetal growth in pregnancy.

Zinc is widely available from food of both animal and vegetable origin. Zinc from flesh food is generally more available than that from cereals.

Zinc is absorbed from the small intestine, although the exact mechanism for this remains uncertain. Its absorption is influenced by dietary factors and is inhibited by phytate, high dietary fiber, oxalate, iron, copper, and tin but enhanced by animal protein. A low molecular weight zinc-binding ligand, possibly secreted from the pancreas, is a postulated mechanism for absorption.

The highest concentrations of zinc are in the prostate, the skin and its appendages, the brain choroid, liver, pancreas, bone, and blood. In blood approximately 80 per cent of zinc is in erythrocytes, 16 per cent in plasma, 3 per cent in leukocytes, and the remaining 1 per cent in platelets. Plasma zinc is normally 12 to 20 μmol per liter. Zinc is excreted mainly in the feces, but small amounts (between 4.0 and 12.0 μmol per 24 hours) are secreted in the urine.

DEFICIENCY SYNDROMES (Table 205–1). In man zinc deficiency has been described in a chronic and an acute form. In Iran and Egypt hypogonadal dwarfism in males is associated with deficiency of zinc and dietary protein. Additionally, many of these children usually eat clay, which may bind zinc, making it unavailable for absorption.

Acrodermatitis enterohepatica, a rare autosomal recessive inherited disorder of zinc metabolism, represents a chronic form of pure zinc deficiency. This entity is characterized by diarrhea; an unpleasant skin rash of the extremities, face, and perineum; alopecia; mental irritability; muscle wasting; and depression. Although the nature of the disease remains in doubt, it may be caused by an absence of the ligand essential for zinc absorption. This ligand is present in human milk but not in cow's milk.

Acute zinc deficiency has been described in patients receiving parenteral nutrition. This syndrome is characterized by diarrhea; disturbance of the central nervous system with mental irritability and depression; skin lesions of the face, perineum, limbs, and skin folds; alopecia; loss of taste; and defects in the immunologic mechanisms. Treatment with zinc supplementation, usually in the form of zinc sulfate, results in a dramatic response.

The true importance of zinc in premature and young infants has still to be fully evaluated. A scaly erythema of the cheeks and diaper areas can be caused by zinc deficiency and incorrectly diagnosed as an eczematous rash. Many of the artificial milk formulas have added zinc, and it is suggested that zinc in human milk may sometimes be inadequate.

Zinc deficiency may occur in a number of conditions, including AIDS, diabetes, uremia, inflammatory bowel disease, malabsorption, cirrhosis, and alcoholism. The potential causes of zinc deficiency are indicated in Table 205–2.

In Crohn's disease, when there is severe catabolism, zincuria may be severe, depleting body stores that are needed during metabolism.

Individuals with sickle cell anemia may have delayed puberty, decreased hair, poor growth, and roughened skin related to zinc deficiency.

EXCESS. Zinc taken in excess may cause gastrointestinal upset with nausea and vomiting.

COPPER

The best-described function of copper is its effect on erythropoiesis. Ceruloplasmin ferroxidase transports iron essential for hemoglobin formation. Copper-containing monoamine oxidase enzymes explain its role in pigmentation and in central nervous system function. Copper-containing lysyl oxidase is necessary for elastin and collagen cross-linking in connective tissues. Cytochrome c oxidase and superoxide dismutase play key roles in the defenses against free radicals.

TABLE 205–1. CLINICAL FEATURES OF ZINC DEFICIENCY

Symptoms	Signs	Laboratory	Treatment
Growth retardation in adolescent males	Failure to thrive	Low plasma zinc	Oral 1 mg zinc/kg body weight as sulfate or acetate
Reduced taste (hypoguesia)	Hypogonadism in males	Hypercholesterolemia	
Reduced smell (hyposmia)	Skin rash of face, perineum, and extremities		
Irritability and depression, diarrhea	Alopecia		

TABLE 205–2. CAUSES OF ZINC DEFICIENCY

Inadequate dietary intake
  Anorexia
  Total parenteral nutrition
  Eating disorders (e.g., anorexia nervosa)
Increased requirement
  Growth
  Wound healing
  Infection
Decreased absorption
  Inflammatory bowel disease
  Surgical resection
  Intestinal fistulae
  Competing minerals (e.g., iron)
  Reduced availability (e.g., dietary fiber)
Increased loss
  Zincuria
  Fecal loss
  Skin loss

Usually copper is excreted in the bile as a metallocomplex. There is an additional copper loss in the urine (0.16 to 0.95 μmol per day) and saliva (0.006 to 0.008 μmol per day).

The highest concentrations of copper occur in the liver, brain, heart, spleen, kidneys, and blood. The mean daily requirement of copper is estimated to be between 5 and 15 μmol when given intravenously and between 30 and 40 μmol when given orally.

The copper content of plant foods is influenced by the copper content of the soil. Similarly, foods derived from animals vary according to their diet. The richest source of copper is liver, but nuts, peas and beans, soy beans, wheat germ, and bran provide good sources. Milk, both human and cow's milk, is a poor source of copper.

DEFICIENCY SYNDROMES. Hypocupremia occurs in a number of inherited disorders such as Wilson's disease (a disease of copper excess), Menkes' kinky hair syndrome (a syndrome of neurologic disorder with hypocupremia), and familial hypoceruloplasminemia. It may also be found with decreased copper intake, as in parenteral nutrition, or with the poor absorption or increased loss associated with protein-losing enteropathy, the nephrotic syndrome, cystic fibrosis, and other malabsorptive diseases such as celiac disease and sprue. Premature and underweight infants may manifest a deficiency of copper, the importance of which is still undefined.

SELENIUM

METABOLISM. Selenocysteine in the enzyme glutathione peroxidase is important in protecting lipids of cell membranes, proteins, and nucleic acids against oxidant damage.

In the United States, the blood level of selenium is 1.90 to 3.17 μmol per liter. A low blood selenium concentration reflecting a low soil content has been noted in Finland, China, New Zealand, Sweden, and Denmark.

The daily requirement for selenium is estimated to be 0.72 μmol for women and 1.02 μmol for men. It probably depends on the supply of other trace minerals, including zinc, copper, magnesium, and iron and also the supply of other antioxidant substances, such as vitamin E and vitamin C. In the United States the intake is 0.76 to 2.79 μmol per day.

DEFICIENCY (Table 205–3). *Keshan disease* is a syndrome of endemic cardiomyopathy in the People's Republic of China that is alleviated by giving oral sodium selenite. In the areas of China where Keshan disease is prevalent, the dietary intake is estimated to be less than 0.38 μmol.

Selenium deficiency has been associated with intravenous feeding when the patient has developed muscle pain and tenderness associated with a very low blood selenium level. These symptoms are alleviated by giving selenomethionine.

Decreased levels of selenium in patients who have had acute myocardial infarction have been reported, and in Finland a reduced serum selenium concentration has been shown to correlate with cardiovascular death and acute coronary artery disease. The significance and importance of this remain to be confirmed.

A moderate drop in the selenium levels has been reported in patients with diseases of the gastrointestinal tract, particularly celiac disease and ulcerative colitis. Because of the importance of selenium in immune function, such a decrease may have clinical significance.

In newborn infants the level of selenium is about one-half that of the average adult. Because of a reduced selenium level in patients with malignant disease, there is interest in the possibility of a relationship between this trace mineral and cancer.

EXCESS. Selenium is a cell toxin and, as such, should be given with considerable care. Selinosis occurs with daily intake in excess of 6.35 μmol.

FLUORINE

METABOLISM. Fluorine is universally present in body fluids, tissues, and the skeleton. The environmental water and soil content of fluoride is the principal determinant of the fluoride status of the body.

Fluorine is readily absorbed in the intestine after release into its ionic form. It is retained in the body, mainly deposited in bones, and is excreted principally in the urine.

The principal health-related importance of fluorine is its ability to maintain the structure of the teeth. Fluoride, taken regularly throughout life, enhances the resistance of teeth to acidic dental plaque–related caries. Its role in the maintenance of normal bone calcification is not clear but may be important.

As water is a major source of fluoride, beverages provide a major source of fluoride intake. All foods, however, contain traces of fluoride, with plant foods containing more than animal foods.

CLINICAL FEATURES. The principal clinical importance of fluoride deficiency is in dental caries and possibly in the development of osteoporosis. Where the food and water sources of fluoride are deficient, fluoride can be given either by water fluoridation or by use of fluoride tablets, with further supplementation through toothpastes, dentifrices, and mouth rinses.

EXCESS. There is a risk of overexposure, and this manifests itself by fluorosis with defects of the tooth enamel.

TRACE MINERALS OF MINOR CLINICAL IMPORTANCE

Manganese

METABOLISM. Manganese, a trace element essential for life, is present in an amount of approximately 12 to 20 mg in the average adult. Maximally absorbed in the duodenum by an unknown transport mechanism, manganese is bound to transmanganin, a specific β-globulin transport protein. Manganese is concentrated in tissues rich in mitochondria and is widely distributed in the body, with maximal concentrations in the brain, kidneys, pancreas, bone, and liver. The blood and serum levels vary widely. Manganese is excreted principally in bile.

Manganese is an activator of many enzymes, but pyruvate carboxylase is the only manganese metalloenzyme. Manganese appears to be intimately involved in the synthesis of DNA, RNA, and protein.

DEFICIENCY. A syndrome has been described with impaired growth, skeletal abnormalities, abnormal reproductive function, ataxia, convulsions, and anomalies of fat metabolism. This deficiency is very rare.

EXCESS. Manganese poisoning, which usually occurs after industrial exposure, induces a syndrome that closely resembles Parkinson's disease.

Chromium

METABOLISM. Chromium is an essential micronutrient required for the maintenance of normal blood glucose levels. The

TABLE 205–3. CLINICAL FEATURES OF SELENIUM DEFICIENCY

Symptoms	Signs	Diagnosis	Treatment
Heart failure Skeletal muscle weakness	Cardiac dilatation	Selenium levels 0.55 μ mol/L	Oral selomethionine 100–200 g/day

recommended daily intake is 50 to 200 μg, and the normal serum level is 0.5 to 9.0 μg per liter. Chromium is present in yeast, meat, and grain. The chromium glucose tolerance factor is postulated to facilitate insulin receptor activity.

DEFICIENCY. Chromium deficiency is characterized by impaired glucose tolerance, encephalopathy, and neuropathy. Because of impaired insulin activity, patients may develop hyperglycemia with hyperosmolar nonketotic coma. Chromium deficiency may give a confusional state similar to hepatic encephalopathy with ataxia and peripheral neuropathy. A suggested association between chromium deficiency and coronary artery disease awaits confirmation.

EXCESS. If too much chromium is given, symptoms of nausea, vomiting, gastrointestinal ulceration, liver damage, kidney damage, and central nervous system abnormalities with convulsions may occur.

Vanadium

Analysis of vanadium is difficult. The total body vanadium content is about 100 μg. Blood levels are very low, 0.005 to 8.4 μmol per liter.

Vanadium depresses plasma cholesterol levels, Na^+,K^+-ATPase, myosin, Ca^{2+} ATPase, adenylate kinase, and phosphofructokinase and stimulates adenyl cyclase. Vanadium deficiency has been postulated to play a role in nutritional edema, and vanadium excess has been postulated to be a factor in manic-depressive illness. Neither of these suggestions has been confirmed.

Silicon

Silicon is found in high concentrations in tendons, aorta, and eye tissues. It is necessary for mammalian bone growth and calcification. In experimental animals, silicon appears to inhibit atheroma development. Chronic inhalation of silicon as silica (SiO_2) produces lung disease, as described in Ch. 527.

Cousins RJ: Absorption, transport and hepatic metabolism of copper and zinc. Special reference to metallothionein and ceruloplasmin. Physiol Rev 65:238, 1985. *A comprehensive review of copper and zinc metabolism, with particular reference to the key role of the liver.*

Featherstone JDB: The mechanism of dental decay. Nutr Today 22:10–16, 1987. *The role of fluoride in stabilizing enamel.*

Fitzgerald FT, Tierney IM: Trace metals in human disease. Adv Intern Med 30:337, 1984. *An overall introduction to trace metals in human disease.*

Nève J, Vertongen F, Molle L: Selenium deficiency. Clin Endocrinol Metab 14:629, 1985. *A useful review emphasizing the current knowledge and areas of poor understanding.*

O'Dell BL: Bioavailability of trace elements. Nutr Rev 42:301, 1984. *A useful review of problems of determining and understanding trace mineral availability.*

Prasad AS: Clinical manifestations of zinc deficiency. Am Rev Nutr 5:341, 1985. *A full review of the etiological and clinical features of zinc deficiency.*

Robinson MF: Selenium in human nutrition in New Zealand. Nutr Rev 47:99–107, 1989. *Blood selenium concentrations reflect low selenium soil content. Intravenous feeding may also be associated with a low selenium blood level and muscle pain responsive to selenomethionine.*

Wallach S: Clinical and biochemical aspects of chromium deficiency. J Am Coll Nutr 4:107, 1985. *A comprehensive readable review of chromium metabolism indicating its importance in clinical medicine.*

Williams DG: Copper deficiency in humans. Semin Hematol 20:118, 1983. *Major features of normal copper metabolism and copper deficiency are summarized in a very readable form.*

206 Principles of Nutritional Support: Enteral Nutritional Therapy

David H. Alpers

Enteral nutritional therapy implies modification of the usual diet and is used for two major general indications. The first is supplementation of protein and calories in a wide variety of situations with the intention of providing part or all of the daily requirements. This use is not disease-specific. The second and more traditional indication involves the use of diets for specific

TABLE 206–1. STRATEGY FOR CALORIE AND PROTEIN SUPPLEMENTATION

Route of Delivery	Incomplete Provision	Complete Provision
Enteral	Oral supplementation Table foods, e.g., milk, peanut butter, egg	Forced enteral feeding Nutritionally complete commercial diets
	Commercial supplements Individual macronutrients (e.g., protein, fat, carbohydrate)	Blenderized formulas
	Nutritionally complete supplement	
Parenteral	Peripheral (e.g., 3 per cent amino acids, 5 to 10 per cent dextrose, 10 per cent lipid emulsion)	Central (e.g., 4.25 per cent amino acid, 25 per cent dextrose, vitamins, minerals, fatty acids)

diseases or pathophysiologic situations. The diets used involve restricting a particular element of the diet (e.g., fat, lactose), adding a nutrient that may be required in larger amounts than are available from a well-balanced diet (e.g., calcium, potassium), or altering the consistency of the diet (e.g., high-fiber, full-liquid). These two major indications are discussed in this chapter. Also included is a discussion about formulating a plan for calorie and protein supplementation, which places this and the following chapter on parenteral nutrition in proper perspective.

PROTEIN AND CALORIE SUPPLEMENTATION

Initial Decisions: Completeness of Nutrient Provision and Route of Administration

The range of methods for providing protein and calorie supplements has expanded greatly beyond table foods in recent years, and likewise the range of available products for this use is very great. For many patients all that may be needed is a careful history of dietary intake, estimation of protein and caloric requirements, and adjustment of the diet to provide the needed nutrients. Whether table foods or commercial supplements are used, there are two major considerations for the physician to provide the most appropriate therapy for each patient: (1) Is the supplement intended as a partial fulfillment of daily needs (incomplete provision) or a total replacement of calories and protein (complete provision)? (2) Are the nutrients to be delivered by the enteral or the parenteral route? Table 206–1 summarizes these major choices. Forced enteral feeding refers to the delivery of nutrients to the small intestine via a small (7 to 8 French) polyurethane or silicone catheter placed through the nose or percutaneously via the endoscope (percutaneous endoscopic gastrostomy) or by a surgical procedure. Parenteral supplementation by peripheral or central vein will be discussed in Ch. 207. The options listed in Table 206–1 are not mutually exclusive. For example, sometimes forced enteral feeding can be used together with peripheral vein feeding; nutritionally complete commercial supplements can be used orally in some patients to supply total macronutrient requirements; central vein feeding can be supplemented by oral intake.

Formulating a Protein-Calorie Support Plan

Figure 206–1 illustrates a flow diagram used for selecting patients in negative protein and calorie balance for intensive nutritional support. The correct choice for nutritional support (enteral versus parenteral, oral versus forced enteral) depends largely upon the four key questions outlined in the figure. The physician should estimate protein and caloric requirements for the individual patient. Methods for making these estimates are available in a number of handbooks. While the estimates are fairly crude, they are clinically useful, because they provide some quantitative guidelines for deciding the magnitude of supplementation needed. The most commonly used formulas for determining basal requirements are those of Harris and Benedict:

$$BMR_{women} = 655 + (9.6 \times W) + (1.8 \times H) - (4.7 \times A)$$
$$BMR_{men} = 66 + (13.7 \times W) + (5 \times H) - (6.8 \times A)$$

where BMR is basal metabolic requirement in kcal; W is ideal weight in kg; H is height in cm; A is age in years. For ambulatory patients the basal requirements can be estimated at two thirds of their total caloric need. This equation underestimates BMR in malnourished patients by up to 10 per cent and overestimates it in obesity. Most ill hospitalized patients do not require calories in excess of their estimated basal requirement, based on their usual weight. Hospitalized patients receiving protein of high biologic value (egg, milk, meat) need only 0.6 gram per kilogram body weight per day for mild illness if body protein is not depleted by prior chronic or acute illness. For ambulatory patients this figure becomes 0.8 to 0.9 gram per kilogram per day to allow for the protein content of a mixed animal and vegetable diet. For severely ill patients, even if depleted of protein, the requirement rarely exceeds 1.2 grams per kilogram per day. Larger amounts of protein cannot be assimilated by sick patients, largely because of increased catabolism and the high caloric requirement needed to retain amino acids as protein. In general, calorie and protein requirements for ill or hospitalized patients have been overestimated in the past.

If the diet is meeting requirements (question 1), no further therapy is needed. If the diet is inadequate, an assessment of the patient's present nutritional status is then obtained. Caloric reserves are monitored most easily by body weight and protein reserves by serum albumin levels. Other available methods are discussed in Ch. 200. If the degree of depletion (question 2) as assessed by body weight is mild (about 5 per cent decreased) and the gastrointestinal tract is intact, oral supplements may be used. If the degree of depletion is moderate (5 to 10 per cent decreased) to severe (over 10 per cent decreased) and the anticipated duration of support is long (question 3), intensive therapy may be needed. As is apparent in the algorithm in Figure 206–1, the definition of *long* is crucial for decision making. If the patient can be expected to lose up to 10 per cent of body weight during

the illness, the needed duration of treatment is considered to be long. Alternatively, an arbitrary number of days with inadequate intake can be considered "long": 7 to 10 days for normally nourished patients, 3 to 5 days for poorly nourished patients. Whether forced enteral feeding or total parenteral nutrition (TPN) via a central vein is chosen depends on the availability or adequacy of the gastrointestinal tract (question 4). The gastrointestinal tract is usually evaluated by history (the presence or absence of diarrhea or malabsorption), physical examination (normal motility or ileus), and barium radiographs. Some patients are selected for TPN because of the need for complete bowel rest. Data to support the use of this therapy have been obtained in the acute management of Crohn's disease and ulcerative colitis and in the postoperative adaptive period of the short-bowel syndrome, and severe pancreatitis (see Ch. 106). Some patients with these disorders can be treated with forced enteral feeding. Often, however, bowel rest will control symptoms more rapidly. Other considerations (social, economic) may play a role in the final choice of therapy for a given patient. The patient may be unwilling to maintain a nasal or gastric feeding tube, or hospitalization may not be possible because of cost restrictions. Finally, some patients may need to be fed via gastrostomy or jejunostomy.

The percutaneous gastrostomy has allowed relatively simple establishment of this feeding route and has expanded the indications for gastrostomy. Gastrostomy feeding is now used, especially in the United States, when the anticipated time for enteral supplementation is long, and the patient cannot swallow. The tube is placed endoscopically or radiographically if the esophagus is patent (e.g., stroke) or surgically if it is not. Complications include pneumoperitoneum, abdominal and gastric wall hematomas, and subcutaneous emphysema. A more detailed discussion of the indications for TPN can be found in the following chapter (Ch. 207).

The following categories of patients are commonly considered for enteral nutrition therapy: (1) chronically ill patients with anorexia, (2) patients with chronic inflammatory illnesses who

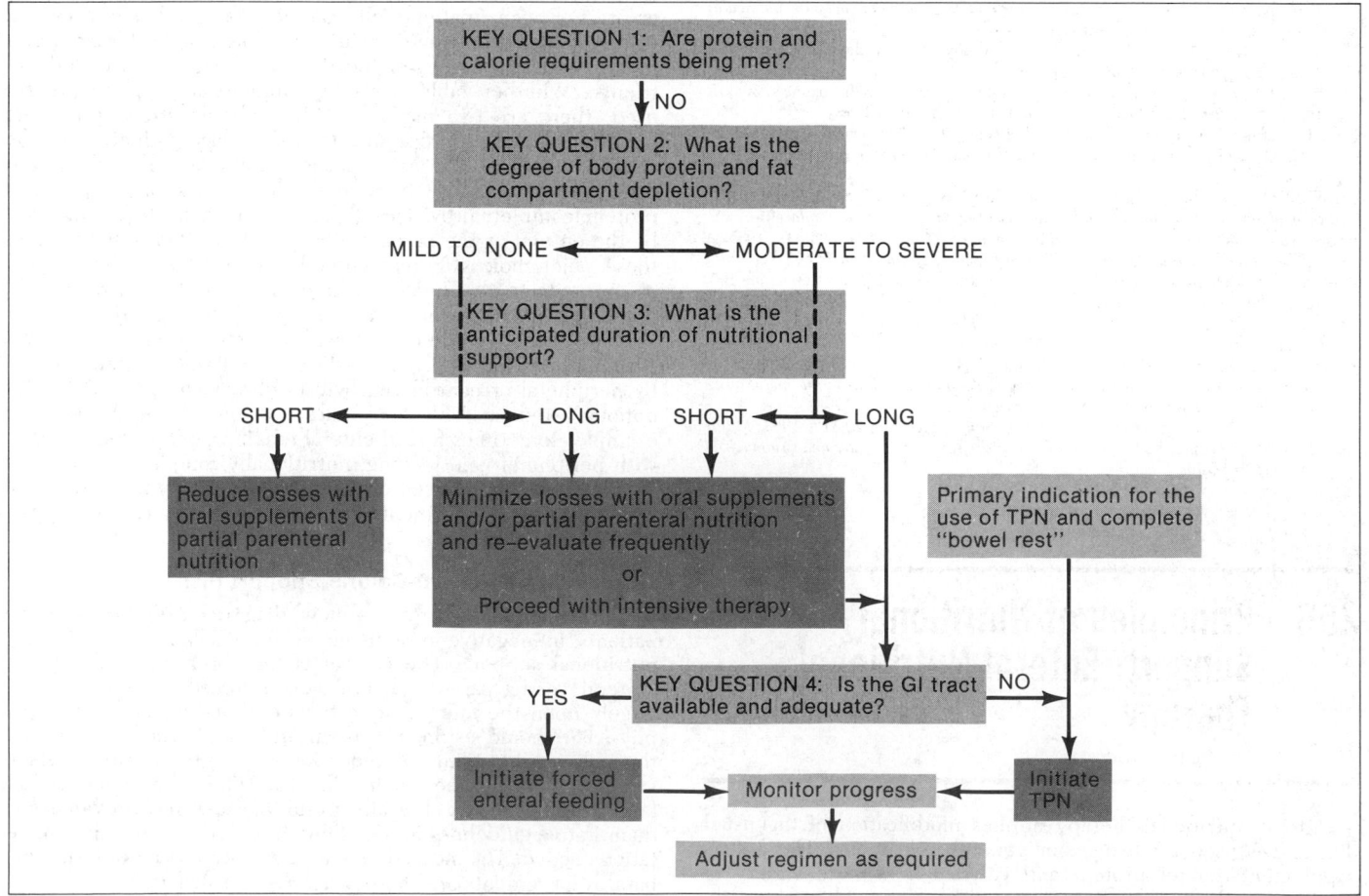

FIGURE 206–1. Flow diagram useful for selecting patients in negative protein and calorie balance for intensive nutritional support. TPN = total parenteral nutrition; GI = gastrointestinal.

have increased requirements but who can tolerate only a usual caloric intake for their size, (3) poor or marginally nourished patients preparing for tests or intestinal surgery, and (4) patients with specific dietary needs that benefit from the special characteristics of some commercial supplements (e.g., low-residue, lactose-free). Forced enteral feeding typically is used for those patients who have moderate to severe anorexia, those who cannot maintain a calorie and protein intake commensurate with their needs (e.g., burn patients), or those whose illnesses prevent them from satisfactory oral feeding (e.g., patients with cervical spine fractures or swallowing disorders).

Delivery of Enteral Supplements

TABLE FOODS

If requirements are not great and appetite is good, table foods can be recommended as protein and calorie supplements. Each ounce of meat, fish, poultry, or cheese contains about 7 grams of protein, an egg 6 to 7 grams, and one cup of milk 8 grams. One-half cup of dried beans, peas, or nuts contains 5 grams or more of protein, but these sources contain protein of a lower biologic value (sustains growth less well) and are not usually recommended for a major role in "catch up" therapy in nutritionally depleted patients. Milk products are very useful, provided that lactose intolerance is not a problem. Meat and fish are helpful if fat is well tolerated. Otherwise, poultry without skin or tuna canned in water should be selected. Peanut butter contains 8 grams of fat and 4.2 grams of protein per tablespoon and is a good source of concentrated calories and protein. Table foods remain an excellent choice for oral supplementation, because they are tasty, esthetically and socially appealing, reasonable in cost, easily obtained, and available in a wide variety of choices. If well tolerated and adequate for the requirements, they should not be supplemented by commercial supplements unless the supplements exhibit specific properties that make them preferable.

COMMERCIAL SUPPLEMENTS

Commercial supplements, like table foods, display a diversity of characteristics that help the physician determine the choice for each patient. They are available as sources of single macronutrients (protein, carbohydrate, or lipid) or as nutritionally complete supplements, containing all necessary macronutrients and micronutrients. These products are of high caloric density and precisely defined nutrient composition but have the disadvantages of limited esthetic and taste appeal, taste fatigue with constant use, frequent occurrence of diarrhea, and higher cost than table foods. The nutritionally incomplete supplements can be used when the deficiency is specific (protein or calorie) or the deficiency is anticipated only for a short time, as in preparation for surgery. Protein is not wisely provided without another source of calories, since about 25 to 40 nonprotein kilocalories are needed per gram of protein to maintain positive nitrogen balance. Otherwise, a portion of the amino acids in the protein is converted to carbohydrate to provide the energy needed for amino acid assimilation.

The nutritionally complete supplements are largely distinguished by four major characteristics: (1) the presence or absence of lactose, (2) the use of intact protein or hydrolyzed protein (or amino acids), (3) the presence of small or large amounts of fat as caloric sources, and (4) isotonic or hypertonic osmolality. Supplements that are isotonic or nearly so contain less available carbohydrate and more lipid, which is osmotically less active. This characteristic is of greatest importance when forced enteral feeding is used, but any of the hypertonic solutions may be diluted or infused at a slower rate. The other three characteristics are more important for patients with abnormal intestinal absorption. Hydrolyzed protein may be useful for patients with pancreatic insufficiency, lactose-free supplements for patients with lactose intolerance, and low-fat supplements for those with limited intestinal fat absorption. The nutritionally complete supplements just described are designed to be the sole source of daily nutrients and thus contain all needed micronutrients in adequate quantities, if deficiencies are not present and if requirements are usual. Nonprescription milk-based products also provide good sources of protein and calories in a wide variety of flavors. If the patient is lactose tolerant, they may be used very successfully.

COMPLICATIONS OF ENTERAL FEEDING USING

COMMERCIAL SUPPLEMENTS. The use of enteral feeding with highly concentrated supplements can be limited by side effects. The most common is diarrhea, which can be due to intolerance to one of the macronutrients (fat, lactose) or intolerance to the osmotic load. Altering the rate of delivery or the concentration of the supplement is often helpful, but may compromise the delivery of adequate calories. Complications of forced enteral feeding alone include esophagitis and tracheobronchial aspiration. Volume or sodium overload can occur, especially in the edema-prone patient.

THERAPEUTIC DIETS FOR SPECIFIC DISORDERS OR PATHOPHYSIOLOGIC STATES

The diets most commonly used to control symptoms are those that restrict one or another element in the diet. Diets restricted for each of the major macronutrients (fat, carbohydrate, and protein) have their individual uses (Table 206–2). As expected, these diets are helpful in altering pathophysiologic states and are not specific for any disease. Any condition causing steatorrhea can be improved symptomatically by limiting fat (triacylglyceride) intake. Care must be taken with any restrictive diet to supplement any nutrients that have been secondarily limited with fat restriction. However, levels of intake that improve symptoms in most cases (40 to 50 grams per day) still supply sufficient fat sources so that deficiency of fat-soluble vitamins does not occur. A fat-restricted diet can be made isocaloric only by increasing carbohydrate intake, because most food sources of fat also contain protein. For this diet to be successful the patient must not have any generalized carbohydrate intolerance. Similarly, the low-lactose or low-available-carbohydrate diet is low in calcium.

Most restrictive diets do not eliminate the nutrient whose content is altered. A low-lactose diet is much easier to achieve than a truly lactose-free one and is usually sufficient to relieve symptoms. Control of symptoms is the usual goal of dietary management, and restriction of the appropriate nutrient to the point at which symptoms are altered is an acceptable goal. Thus, a low-protein diet for hepatic encephalopathy should still deliver the estimated daily protein allowance (0.5 to 0.8 gram per kilogram of body weight) to avoid protein deficiency. This concept is especially important in the management of chronic renal failure, a situation in which the protein requirement may be actually increased. When the glomerular filtration rate (GFR) falls below 25 ml per minute, the protein allowance should not be more than 1.3 grams per kilogram per day (referring to ideal body weight) and falls to 0.6 gram per kilogram per day for a GFR of 4 to 10 ml per minute. Over 50 per cent of the protein intake should be of high biologic value (with high essential amino acid content). Requirements actually increase with dialysis because of the loss of amino acids in the dialysate. The allowance rises with hemodialysis to 1 gram per kilogram per day, and to 1.2 to 1.5 grams per kilogram per day with chronic peritoneal dialysis.

TABLE 206–2. THERAPEUTIC DIETS CHARACTERIZED BY RESTRICTION OF DIETARY COMPONENTS

Diet	Typical Indication
Low fat (60–75 grams/day)	Steatorrhea, mild (see Ch. 102)
Low fat (40–60 grams/day)	Steatorrhea, severe (see Ch. 102)
Low oxalate	Enteric hyperoxaluria (see Ch. 102)
Low lactose	Lactose intolerance (see Ch. 102)
Gluten free	Celiac sprue (see Ch. 102)
Low fiber	Acute diarrhea, bowel preparation (see Ch. 101)
Low protein	Hepatic encephalopathy (see Ch. 123)
	Chronic renal failure (see Ch. 77)
Elimination	Food allergies
Controlled carbohydrate	Diabetes mellitus (see Ch. 218)
Calorie restricted	Obesity (see Ch. 203)
Low sodium	Edematous states (see Ch.75)
Low fat, cholesterol, or carbohydrate according to type	Hyperlipidemia (see Ch. 172)
Low copper	Wilson's disease (see Ch. 121)
Low phosphate	Chronic renal failure (see Ch. 77)

Some of the diets used for therapy control or modify the content of macronutrients rather than restrict them. The diet for diabetes mellitus is a good example of this principle (see Ch. 218). Successful management of the obese diabetic combines a weight reduction diet with regulation of the carbohydrate content. The prudent diet recommended by the American Diabetes Association still contains 40 to 55 per cent of calories as carbohydrates, with relatively less (5 to 15 per cent) as simple sugars (requiring no pancreatic digestion) and more (30 to 45 per cent) as starch. There is also less cholesterol and saturated fats to reduce blood lipids. These latest recommendations contain relaxed restrictions on carbohydrate intake. High-starch diets are well tolerated by diabetics as long as total caloric intake is controlled. Many patients require diets that may utilize elements from diets designed specifically for weight reduction, diabetes mellitus, hyperlipidemias, and chronic renal failure.

Diets That Supplement Dietary Components

Although less commonly required, diets that add a component to the normal diet are often employed (Table 206–3). A high fiber intake has not been clearly shown to have a beneficial effect on the symptoms of all patients with irritable bowel syndrome and on the recurrence of attacks of acute diverticulitis, although supplementation with fiber is now commonly used for these disorders. The reasons for the uncertainty are that (1) these disorders are identified mostly by clinical criteria, (2) the irritable bowel syndrome is probably a heterogeneous group of motility disorders, (3) the definition of fiber and estimation of its intake are imperfectly developed, and (4) many types of fiber supplements are used, containing different components of dietary fiber. Dietary fiber is useful in the prevention and treatment of constipation not associated with laxative abuse. A diet low in fiber (see Table 206–2) is useful in acute diarrheal illness and as a preparation for barium enema, colonoscopy, and intestinal surgery. The diet is then additionally modified in the form of a clear liquid diet for further reduction in ileal residue.

There are limited data on the food content of the major components of dietary fiber, i.e., cellulose, hemicelluloses, pectin, mucilage and gums, and lignins. Thus, it is not always clear when an individual patient is ingesting a low-fiber diet, although total daily average fiber intake in the United States is probably about 12 to 15 grams lower than what is considered ideal. Most often fiber is supplemented by ingestion of commercial preparations containing psyllium seed or by the use of bran. Psyllium is rich in hemicelluloses, while bran contains more cellulose. Present practice recommends the addition of 6 to 10 grams of fiber per day (2 teaspoons of psyllium seed or three-quarters cup of bran) for the irritable bowel syndrome (characterized by alternating diarrhea and constipation) and for recurrent diverticulitis. Benefits of high fiber intake (type and amount variable) have also been reported for diabetes mellitus, maintenance of lower calorie intake, lowering of serum cholesterol, and prevention of colon cancer. At present the data do not clearly support a specific role for a fiber-supplemented diet in any of these disorders.

The best treatment for postmenopausal osteoporosis is still debatable, but it is no longer agreed that increased calcium intake needs to be an important component of the treatment plan (Ch. 238). Published reports show only a modestly positive relationship between dietary calcium and cortical bone mass, but no correla-

TABLE 206–3. THERAPEUTIC DIETS CHARACTERIZED BY SUPPLEMENTATION OF DIETARY COMPONENTS

Diet	Typical Indication
High fiber	Irritable bowel, prevention of recurrent diverticulitis
High calcium (milk products, CaCO₃, or combination)	Postmenopausal osteoporosis
High protein (high biologic value)	Chronic hemodialysis or peritoneal dialysis
High protein	Malabsorption
Supplemental potassium	Diuretic use
High calorie	Weight loss due to illness

TABLE 206–4. SODIUM AND POTASSIUM CONTENT OF COMMON FOODS*

Food	Portion	Sodium Content (mg)	Potassium Content (mg)
Milk	cup	120	350
Meat, fish, poultry	ounce	25	100–180
Most fruits and their juices	cup	4–10	300–490
Most vegetables	½ cup	5–9	300–500

*Content refers to uncooked or unprocessed foods.

tion with trabecular bone where rapid turnover occurs, and which comprises up to 50 per cent of bone in the spine. Calcium supplementation appears to be inferior to estrogen therapy in slowing bone loss in postmenopausal women. The probable long-term effects of calcium, however, are not clear, because most studies have been for 2 years or less.

When diuretics and low-sodium diets are used, potassium is frequently replaced as an inorganic salt, but dietary supplementation can often be used and would be more palatable. For instance, the salt substitutes often used with low-sodium diets contain about 12 mEq of potassium per gram, and potassium is present in fairly high concentration in most fruits and vegetables and their juices (Table 206–4). Eight ounces of frozen orange or tomato juice contains 12 mEq potassium and one medium orange or banana 6 to 8 mEq. Milk is also a good source of potassium, but because of its high sodium content would be an inappropriate supplement for a patient taking diuretics. Only some patients taking diuretics daily in appropriate doses develop hypokalemia. Urinary potassium loss can be measured; if not excessive, it can be matched by table foods. Therefore, for many patients, advice on dietary potassium supplements will be sufficient.

Protein supplements are needed for conditions characterized by excessive protein loss, such as protein-losing enteropathy, dialysis, and burns. These supplements can be supplied as table food or as commercial supplements. For each 10 grams of protein added, another 250 kcal from nonprotein sources must also be ingested to ensure that the amino acids will be converted into body protein.

Diets That Alter the Consistency of Food

One of the most common dietary manipulations used in hospitalized patients is the *liquid diet*. The *clear* liquid diet provides the daily requirement for water mostly in the form of juices, bouillons, and gelatins, and requires minimal digestion and intestinal motility, but it does not provide adequate amounts of protein, calories, vitamins, or minerals. It is also a low-fiber diet. If the patient who requires such a diet is already protein and calorie malnourished, the diet needs to be supplemented with carbohydrate, protein, or both, and with micronutrients. Even so, it is difficult to provide much more than 1000 kcal per day. For long-term use the *full* liquid diet is more often prescribed, including milk and other dairy products, cereals, and eggs. If table foods from all food groups are used or the diet is enriched with commercial supplements, the diet can be nutritionally complete. Care should be given to determining the actual food ingested, however, because a full liquid diet is often used for a patient who has some difficulty in swallowing table food. Thus, the ingested food may not equal what is ordered. This precaution, of course, should be exercised when any diet is used for therapy, but it is particularly important when impairment of food ingestion or anorexia is the reason for the prescribed diet.

The *bland diet* restricts spicy foods and is often combined with a mechanical soft diet for the treatment of peptic ulcer disease. Despite this widespread use, there are no data that clearly support the value of such a diet for any clinical condition, and present practice does not favor its use (see Ch. 98). Restriction of seasonings makes the food less palatable and discourages the successful use of whichever diet is being presented.

Alpers DH, Clouse RE, Stenson WF: Manual of Nutritional Therapeutics, 2nd ed. Boston, Little, Brown and Company, 1988. *A detailed practical account of the use of diets and enteral therapy. Includes nutritional characteristics of most commercial supplements and diets.*

American Dietetic Association: Handbook of Clinical Dietetics. New Haven, Yale University Press, 1982. *A comprehensive and carefully outlined source of obtaining the details of most diets.*

Diet and Health: Implications for reducing chronic disease risk. Committee on Diet and Health, Food and Nutrition Board; Commission on Life Sciences, National Research Council. Washington, D.C., National Academy Press, 1989. *An up-to-date extensive survey of dietary patterns and guidelines pertaining to chronic disease, including suggestions for future research. Its conclusions are general and may not apply in all clinical situations.*

Garrow JS: Treat Obesity Seriously. London, Churchill Livingstone, 1981. *A sensible and multifaceted approach to the therapy of obesity, especially for use of diet.*

Gorlin R. The biological actions and potential clinical significance of dietary ω-3 fatty acids. Arch Intern Med 148:2043, 1988. *A judicious review of the potential uses of fish oil.*

Kabadi UM: Nutritional therapy in diabetics. Postgrad Med 79:145, 1986. *A balanced review of carbohydrate restriction.*

Physiological Effects and Health Consequences of Dietary Fiber. Washington, D.C., Life Sciences Research Office, Federation of American Societies for Experimental Biology, 1987. *Summarizes the evidence for the role of fiber in human disease.*

Report of the National Cholesterol Education Program Expert Panel on Detection, Evaluation, and Treatment of High Blood Cholesterol in Adults. Arch Intern Med 148:36, 1988. *The most definitive statement available on the rationale for and use of altered fat diets for atherosclerosis.*

The Surgeon General's Report on Nutrition and Health. U.S. Dept of Health and Human Services. DHHS (PHS) Publication No. 88–80210, 1988. *Focus is on the relationship of diet to chronic diseases, more from the point of view of nutritional policy makers than individual physicians.*

Taylor TV: Miscellaneous problems in the stomach and duodenum: Percutaneous endoscopic gastrostomy. Curr Opinion Gastroenterol 5:874, 1989. *A brief summary of recent experience with this technique.*

207 Parenteral Nutrition

Ray E. Clouse

Parenteral nutrition includes delivery of micronutrients and macronutrients, and all recognized human nutrients can be provided. Those nutrients that rapidly become depleted in disease, such as water and major minerals, are administered routinely by vein to the hospitalized patient. Concentrated solutions are needed to provide protein and calories, and central venous access is often required. The complications associated with these solutions and with the access catheters become important limiting factors in the routine use of more comprehensive parenteral nutrition for the average patient. Although parenteral nutrition could be utilized in much the same way as enteral supplements or forced enteral feeding when an appropriate nutritional support plan is designed (see Ch. 206), parenteral nutrition is usually reserved for those requiring the total daily administration of protein and calories by the intravenous route.

PARENTERAL ENERGY AND PROTEIN DELIVERY

Protein and calorie requirements are closely linked. Positive nitrogen balance, reflecting net positive endogenous protein synthesis, is most successfully accomplished when positive energy balance has been achieved. If parenteral nonprotein calories are provided for the average hospitalized patient in a ratio of calories to amino acid nitrogen (in grams) of greater than or equal to 150:1, delivered amino acids are likely to be utilized for protein synthesis. The required ratio decreases in more intense catabolic states (e.g., major burns) and increases in less stressed situations.

ENERGY (CALORIE) SOURCES. Both carbohydrate and lipid are used as parenteral calorie sources (Table 207–1). The monohydrate form of dextrose used in most commercial intravenous solutions provides 3.4 kcal per gram, in contrast to 4 kcal per gram for the carbohydrate alone. Dextrose can be used as the sole nonprotein calorie source. Aproximately 50 per cent of patients require insulin supplementation in the parenteral infusion if dextrose is used to meet all daily calorie requirements. Lipid emulsions contain a source of calories in the form of emulsified droplets of soybean or safflower oil, which provide 9 kcal per gram, supplemented slightly by the caloric contribution of the emulsifiers (Table 207–1). Lipid emulsions may be used to supply the essential fatty acid linoleic acid as well as up to 70 per cent of the daily caloric requirement. A contraindication to the use of the emulsions is pre-existing hyperlipidemia. Complications related to the lipids are uncommon but may limit their use (see below).

The preferred parenteral energy source or combination of sources varies with different patient situations. Positive energy balance and nitrogen balance can be achieved if dextrose is used alone to provide daily calories, as long as adequate amino acids are also supplied. This fact is of importance to the patient intolerant to the lipid emulsions. Lipid emulsions reduce the likelihood of hyperglycemia, the volume of fluid needed, and the metabolic response to the infusion. They also are utilized for their essential fatty acid content. Thus, a combination of lipids and dextrose is usually employed as the energy source. Lipids also have theoretical and practical advantages in patients with respiratory compromise because they have a lower respiratory quotient (0.7) than carbohydrates (1.0): Less carbon dioxide is produced from delivery of a lipid-dextrose combination than from an equicaloric dextrose solution.

Lipid emulsions are somewhat more expensive than dextrose and usually necessitate additional intravenous equipment. The use of a combination of lipid and dextrose with other nutrients in a single infusion bag has eliminated some of the cumbersome equipment required for lipid infusion, but not all patients are in stable enough condition to make this technique practical.

PROTEIN DELIVERY. Protein requirements are met in parenteral nutrition by infusion of amino acids. Amino acid profiles in standard commercial products are based largely on normal plasma amino acid concentrations, with modifications to stimulate anabolism. The amino acid content (in grams) is roughly comparable to the dietary protein in the RDA, except for differences due to absorption efficiency and slight differences related to dissimilarities of amino acid profiles in average dietary proteins and in the solutions.

Amino acid ratios in specialized commercial products have been modified for use in renal failure, liver failure, and increased metabolic stress. Relatively reduced concentrations of essential amino acids are found in the plasma profiles of patients with renal failure, possibly as a result of the catabolic state of uremia. Blood urea nitrogen levels are reduced yet positive nitrogen balance is attained if a large percentage of the protein requirement is provided as essential amino acids in these patients. The parenteral formulation employed depends on the conditions of the renal failure. In chronic stable renal failure without dialysis, a modified commercial solution with higher proportions of essential amino acids may prevent worsening of uremia yet accomplish positive nitrogen balance. Once dialysis is employed, a more balanced, standard amino acid solution should be used. Consistent benefit of commercial solutions with increased proportions of essential amino acids has not been demonstrated in acute renal failure, but outcome of these patients depends upon many variables. The use of essential amino acids alone in relatively low quantities in conjunction with concentrated dextrose is being studied. In principle, the dextrose should partially inhibit amino acid use for gluconeogenesis, thereby slowing urea formation and forcing reutilization of nonessential amino acids for protein synthesis. Both essential and nonessential amino acids are ultimately necessary, however, for sustained anabolism.

Parenteral solutions favoring the branched-chain amino acids (isoleucine, leucine, valine) are used in some cases of liver failure and in metabolic stress. Routine use of these formulas remains controversial because of their expense in relation to their documented benefits. In liver failure, blood levels of aromatic amino acids (phenylalanine, tyrosine, tryptophan) are elevated, whereas levels of branched-chain amino acids are decreased; the cause for this alteration is unclear. Aromatic amino acids enter the brain and participate in encephalopathy. In order to meet protein

TABLE 207–1. PROTEIN AND CALORIE SOURCES UTILIZED IN PARENTERAL NUTRITION

Macronutrient Category		Parenteral Form of Macronutrient	Nonprotein Caloric Value
Protein		Crystalline amino acids	
Calories	Carbohydrate	Dextrose monohydrate	3.4 kcal/g
	Fat	Lipid emulsion	10% emulsion—1.1 kcal/ml 20% emulsion—2.0 kcal/ml

requirements without further promoting encephalopathy, parenteral formulations with increased ratios of branched-chain amino acids to aromatic amino acids can be used (branched-chain amino acids increased to 35 to 45 per cent of total from the usual of 20 to 25 per cent in standard solutions). Besides not promoting encephalopathy, the branched-chain amino acids do not require any hepatic processing as metabolic substrates. Best use of modified amino acid solutions in liver disease may be in mildly encephalopathic patients with acute exacerbations of chronic liver failure. The branched-chain amino acids are oxidized extrahepatically in skeletal muscle, heart, and kidney and serve as a fuel source for muscle in the injured state. These amino acids also appear to have a regulatory role in preventing protein degradation and stimulating protein synthesis both in liver and muscle. Because of these observations, parenteral formulas with branched-chain amino acids composing 45 to 50 per cent of total amino acids have been suggested for use in cases of sepsis or extreme metabolic stress, situations of marked catabolism resistant to reversal.

PRACTICAL APPLICATIONS. A combination of dextrose, amino acids, and water provides the base solution to which vitamins and minerals can be added. Parenteral nutrition solutions that provide all energy and protein requirements are administered through a central vein in most cases because they are so hyperosmotic. For example, a formulation made from 500 ml of 50 per cent dextrose (2500 mOsm per liter) and 500 ml of 8.5 per cent amino acids (850 mOsm per liter) would provide 850 kcal (from nonprotein sources) and 42.5 grams of amino acids with a resultant osmolarity of 1675 mOsm per liter. All additives, particularly major minerals (e.g., sodium, potassium), further raise the final osmolarity. Lipid emulsions are infused in parallel with the base solution or are added directly to the solution bag. If lipids, dextrose, and amino acids are combined ("3-in-1" solutions), compatibility restrictions limit the range of formulations. Macronutrient delivery can be shortened for patients in stable condition to a 10- to 12-hour period, e.g., at night. Both methods of calorie and protein delivery are effective in achieving positive energy and nitrogen balance. Gradual conversion over 2 to 3 days is required from a 24-hour schedule to the cyclic schedule. Once conversion is effected, the base solution (and lipid emulsion, if used as a daily energy source) is discontinued each morning by reducing the rate in two or three 30-minute steps. The rate is similarly increased at the reinitiation of infusion in the evening. These precautions are effective in preventing hypoglycemia for most patients. Patients on cyclic regimens are then free from infusion in the daytime.

Macronutrients may also be provided through peripheral veins. Lesser concentrations of dextrose and amino acids are required to keep the final osmolarity less than 600 to 800 mOsm per liter and thereby reduce the likelihood of thrombophlebitis. Continuous coadministration of isotonic lipid emulsion reduces the osmolarity yet allows for the total energy and protein requirement to be infused. For this reason, lipid emulsions are regularly used as daily energy sources in peripheral vein parenteral nutrition. Parenteral prescriptions that provide fewer calories than the daily energy requirement can serve as supplements to an inadequate enteral regimen or can be used alone to reduce negative nitrogen balance. Even with excessive amino acid infusion (greater than 2 grams per kilogram per day), however, sustained positive nitrogen balance is not accomplished without adequate energy supply. Thus this parenteral nutrition practice is not a substitute for more intensive support, if nutritional restoration is the goal.

TOTAL PARENTERAL NUTRITION

Besides amino acids and calorie sources, all other recognized nutrients can be provided by a parenteral route. Total parenteral nutrition (TPN) is required for short or long periods by patients with either temporarily or permanently unusable or inadequate small intestines. In most instances, a central venous access is employed. Detailed techniques of TPN are beyond the scope of this textbook and are described in many monographs and handbooks. The most successful TPN programs involve direction by a knowledgeable physician and the cooperation of informed and interested colleagues in the pharmacy, nursing, and dietetics departments.

INDICATIONS. A small number of patients require lifelong TPN because of extensive resection (e.g., from mesenteric vascular accidents, Crohn's disease, trauma) or advanced small bowel disease (e.g., scleroderma, radiation enteritis). The majority of patients with short-bowel syndrome from resection, however, can eventually be managed with oral feeding after an initial adaptation period. More commonly TPN is indicated as a temporary nutritional therapy for two patient groups: (1) those selected for intensive nutritional support in whom the intestinal tract is not usable for forced enteral feeding (see Ch. 206) and (2) those in whom a nothing-by-mouth regimen ("bowel rest") would be beneficial to a primary gastrointestinal disease. The majority of patients placed on a TPN regimen are those with the first indication. Figure 206–1 gives a flow diagram incorporating the various questions used in deciding which patients are indeed candidates for intensive nutritional support. In general, this group (a) has moderate to severe protein compartment depletion at the initial evaluation and is expected to suffer significant additional losses with the current illness, or (b) will be undergoing a surgical intervention or specialized treatment (e.g., radiation) that will predictably interfere with enteral nutritional support.

Gastrointestinal Diseases. Parenteral nutrition has two potential roles in patients with gastrointestinal diseases: (1) to provide nutritional restoration and (2) to assist disease regression by allowing the bowel to remain in an unstimulated state (bowel rest). The ability of TPN to reverse malnutrition associated with gastrointestinal disease is not disputed, and TPN is indicated for any patient selected for intensive nutritional support by the conventional algorithm. Thus, patients with nutritional deterioration from severe inflammatory bowel disease may well benefit from TPN for nutritional restoration. The value of bowel rest, in contrast, remains controversial, particularly for inflammatory bowel disease. A summary of reported responses to TPN and bowel rest for a variety of gastrointestinal diseases is listed in Table 207–2. In most of these disorders, enteral dietary treatment is also effective, other treatments (such as corticosteroids for inflammatory bowel disease) have influenced the reported results, and overall efficacy of the bowel rest regimen remains unproven. Because of these observations, the primary indication for TPN in gastrointestinal disease is for nutritional support when enteral treatment is not feasible. Bowel rest regimens are generally reserved for patients who fail other conventional treatments. In the case of inflammatory bowel disease, colonic disorders are less likely than small intestinal disorders to respond to bowel rest.

TPN with or without bowel rest is also often indicated in gastrointestinal disorders associated with severe symptoms, especially if the patient would also be selected for intensive nutritional support. Such conditions include severe diarrhea,

TABLE 207–2. SUMMARY OF THE EFFECTS OF TOTAL PARENTERAL NUTRITION (TPN) WITH BOWEL REST IN VARIOUS DISEASES

Disease	Nutritional Maintenance or Repletion Achieved	Short-Term (In-Hospital) Disease Regression	Long-Term Disease Regression
Ulcerative colitis*	Majority	30–50%	20–30%
Crohn's disease*	Yes	60–80%	50–60%
Subgroup with fistulas†	Yes	30–40%	10–30%
Subgroup with colitis†	Yes	60%	NA‡
Enterocutaneous fistulas (not Crohn's disease)	Yes	30–70% closure§	NA
Severe pancreatitis	Yes¶	NA	NA

*Many patients in reported series treated with corticosteroids as well as TPN and bowel rest.

†Small patient series; subgroups not always designated.

‡Adequate data not available.

§Many patients eventually managed with surgical therapy; wide range of reported success rates.

¶Parenteral nutrition is successful and does not contribute to morbidity of pancreatitis despite theoretical concern regarding pancreatic stimulatory effects.

intractable vomiting, and small intestinal disorders that interfere significantly with enteral feeding (e.g., radiation enteritis, obstruction from inflammatory adhesions, following small bowel resection).

Perioperative Management. A strong correlation exists between nutritional status and postoperative morbidity and mortality. Advantages from routine use of preoperative TPN, however, have not been established. One large and well-designed study has demonstrated the value of 10 days of preoperative TPN in malnourished patients undergoing surgery for gastrointestinal tract malignancies. Guidelines for choosing patients for preoperative TPN remain incomplete, but 7 to 10 days of preoperative treatment for malnourished subjects needing a major abdominal or thoracic operation are now recommended. Data are also absent to support the use of TPN in managing postoperative complications. However, TPN prevents nutritional deterioration in subjects with complications that interfere with eating (e.g., prolonged ileus, mechanical obstruction) or that increase metabolic demands (e.g., wound dehiscence, intra-abdominal abscess). In some of these instances, forced enteral feeding may be successful and more cost effective.

Other Diseases. When TPN is utilized in management of patients with disease not involving the gastrointestinal tract, bowel rest is not enforced. Use of TPN with modified amino acid formulas in patients with hepatic and renal disease has been mentioned. Despite intuitive impressions that TPN should reduce mortality and could improve organ function in these disorders, results from clinical studies have not been conclusive. In patients with cancer, nutritional status can be maintained or improved with an adequate TPN program, but this has not proved to be of overall benefit in enhancing tumor responsiveness to antineoplastic agents. The best candidates for intensive nutritional support are those who have tumors potentially responsive to anticancer therapy, but who could not receive optimal management because of the combined detrimental effects of the planned therapy and malnutrition. Patients undergoing allogeneic bone marrow transplantation for leukemia often typify this situation. Some patients can be managed with forced enteral nutrition rather than TPN. Patients who are severely catabolic or who will likely need major surgery may also be candidates for intensive nutritional support. Such candidates would be selected by following the algorithm outlined in Ch. 206.

Home TPN. Home administration should be considered for patients with irreversible gastrointestinal disease or for patients whose conditions are relatively stable and who need TPN for a month or more. The cyclic method of macronutrient delivery and long central catheters burrowed through a subcutaneous tunnel on the anterior chest are employed. Approximately one third of patients requiring home TPN have malignant disease or intestinal complications related to therapy for malignant disease (resection or radiation). One third have inflammatory bowel disease, and the remainder have a variety of intestinal disorders, including severe gastrointestinal motility disturbances (such as scleroderma bowel) and short-bowel syndrome following trauma or ischemic insult.

NUTRIENTS PROVIDED DURING TPN (Table 207–3). Protein requirements (as described in Ch. 199) are met with crystalline amino acids in commercially available solutions. Nonprotein calories are provided by concentrated dextrose and by lipid emulsions. Two liters of a base solution composed of equal amounts of 8.5 per cent amino acids and 50 per cent dextrose in conjunction with 500 ml of a 10 per cent lipid emulsion is a feasible daily protein-calorie prescription. This provides approximately 80 grams of protein as amino acids, 1680 carbohydrate calories, and 550 fat calories. The resultant nonprotein calorie–nitrogen ratio is 170:1, with 25 per cent of the daily calories provided by fat. An alternate regimen would provide all the nonprotein calories as dextrose. The daily protein and calorie prescription should be tailored to a patient's requirements or exceed them by 20 to 40 grams of protein and 500 to 1000 kcal, if restoration of depleted compartments is a goal. Water requirement varies, depending on the capability of the patient to excrete an osmotic load, 30 ml per kilogram (or approximately 1 ml per kilocalorie delivered) being typical. Increased water delivery is necessary for fever (360 ml per day per degree Celsius elevation) and anabolism (300 to 400 ml per day).

Major mineral requirements vary considerably from patient to

TABLE 207–3. TYPICAL DAILY NUTRIENT PROVISIONS DURING TOTAL PARENTERAL NUTRITION (TPN) FOR STABLE ADULT PATIENTS WITHOUT CARDIAC, HEPATIC, OR RENAL FAILURE

Calories	Dextrose	60–80% of requirement (see Ch. 199)
	Lipid emulsion*	20–40% of requirement
Protein	Crystalline amino acids	100% of requirement (see Ch. 199)
Minerals	Sodium	90–120 mEq
	Potassium	90–150 mEq
	Chloride	90–150 mEq
	Calcium	12–16 mEq
	Phosphorus	20–40 mmol
	Magnesium	12–16 mEq
	Iron†	
	Zinc‡	2.5–4 mg
	Copper	300–500 µg
	Chromium	10–20 µg
	Manganese	0.15–4 mg
	Selenium§	40–80 µg
	Iodine§	70–140 µg
	Molybdenum§	100–200 µg
Vitamins	A	3300 IU
	D	200 IU
	E	10 IU
	B_1 (thiamine)	3.0 mg
	B_2 (riboflavin)	3.6 mg
	Pantothenic acid	15.0 mg
	Niacin	40.0 mg
	B_6 (pyridoxine)	4.0 mg
	Biotin	60.0 µg
	Folic acid	400.0 µg
	B_{12} (cobalamin)**	5.0 µg
	C (ascorbic acid)	100.0 mg††
	K	5 mg/wk‡‡
Essential Fatty Acid§§	Linoleic acid	4% of total calories

*See text for a discussion of the use of lipid emulsion as a daily calorie source. May be co-administered with the base sodium.

†The daily requirement (not taking phlebotomy losses into consideration) is about 1.5 mg and can be met by giving 1 ml (50 mg Fe) of iron-dextran solution intramuscularly per month. Replacement is usually dictated by indices of iron stores.

‡Requirements are increased if intestinal fluid losses are great (see Ch. 205).

§Additive usually reserved for patients on long courses of TPN.

**May be given by monthly intramuscular injection.

††Daily provision often increased to 500 mg or more during periods of catabolic stress.

‡‡Not provided by multivitamin preparation; given by separate injection.

§§Provided by lipid emulsions on a biweekly or triweekly basis. Linolenic acid is also present in some emulsions and may be required during long-term TPN (see text).

patient and during any one patient's course of TPN. In particular, potassium requirements may be initially large because of extracellular to intracellular fluxes with glucose (and possibly insulin) infusion and because of reversal of the catabolic state. The ranges of major mineral requirements listed in Table 207–3 are typical for the average adult patient, but careful monitoring of serum levels is always necessary to determine the correct provision, especially in the first few weeks of TPN.

Deficiencies of trace elements are rarely observed in patients receiving oral feedings because these nutrients are widely distributed among foods and the requirements are low. Deficiencies of zinc, chromium, copper, molybdenum, and selenium may occur during long courses of TPN, however. Such deficiencies are now prevented by supplementing TPN fluid with trace elements from the outset. Zinc, copper, chromium, and manganese are commonly provided; selenium and iodine (and occasionally molybdenum) are usually given only to patients receiving long courses of TPN, as during home TPN. Manganese deficiency has not yet been reported in TPN patients. See Ch. 205 for further discussion of the trace elements.

Recommendations for vitamin supplementation are given in

Table 207–3; few detrimental effects have appeared when these guidelines have been followed. More commonly, vitamin deficiency results from the inadvertent omission of folate or cobalamin, which may not be included in the multivitamin preparation used, or from omission of vitamin K, which is not included in any parenteral multivitamin formulation. Less vitamin D than the recommendation is necessary for patients undergoing long-term therapy.

Linoleic, linolenic, and arachidonic acids cannot be synthesized by humans. However, essential fatty acid (EFA) deficiency can usually be prevented by supplying adequate quantities of linoleic acid alone. EFA deficiency is rarely observed as an isolated deficiency except during TPN. A large amount (8 to 10 per cent) of the fat in adipose tissue contains the EFA's. However, the high insulin levels observed during TPN with concentrated dextrose are believed to impair access to this store through inhibition of lipolysis. Manifestations of EFA deficiency include dry, cracked skin, coarsening of the hair, hair loss, and impaired wound healing. It is estimated that 4 to 5 per cent of the daily energy requirement should be provided by linoleic acid to prevent deficiency, and lipid emulsions (500 ml of 10 per cent emulsion triweekly) satisfy this requirement. A report of linolenic acid deficiency in a child receiving a lipid emulsion low in this fatty acid during long-term TPN suggests that linoleic acid alone may not always be adequate to prevent EFA deficiency in humans. Use of a lipid emulsion with both linoleic and linolenic acid is currrently recommended to avoid EFA deficiency during long courses of TPN.

COMPLICATIONS OF PARENTERAL NUTRITION

Both administration-related and metabolic complications may occur with parenteral nutrition (Table 207–4). Several complications can be detected by a chest radiograph (in expiration if pneumothorax is suspected) after central-vein catheter insertion, a practice that should always be followed. Some degree of clinically inapparent catheter-related thrombosis may occur in as many as 50 per cent of patients. At present, only symptomatic patients (certainly less than 5 per cent of those with subclavian vein catheters) are observed and treated for noninfected thrombosis along the catheter path. *Thrombophlebitis* from hyperos-

TABLE 207–4. COMPLICATIONS OF PARENTERAL NUTRITION

Administration-related Complications
Central vein catheter
  Infection
  Inappropriate tip placement
  Pneumothorax
  Venous thrombosis
  Hemothorax
  Air embolus
  Arterial laceration
  Brachial plexus injury
  Catheter fragmentation and embolization
Peripheral vein catheter
  Thrombophlebitis
  Infection

Metabolic Complications
More frequent
  Hyperglycemia and hyperosmolarity
  Hypoglycemia
  Electrolyte disturbances
  BUN elevation
  Liver dysfunction
  Fatty liver
  Hypercapnia
  Cholelithiasis (long-term treatment)
  Hyperlipidemia from lipid emulsion
Rare
  Vitamin and trace mineral deficiency (Fig. 207–1)
  Essential fatty acid deficiency
  Metabolic bone disease
  Other adverse reaction to lipid emulsion
  Hyperammonemia

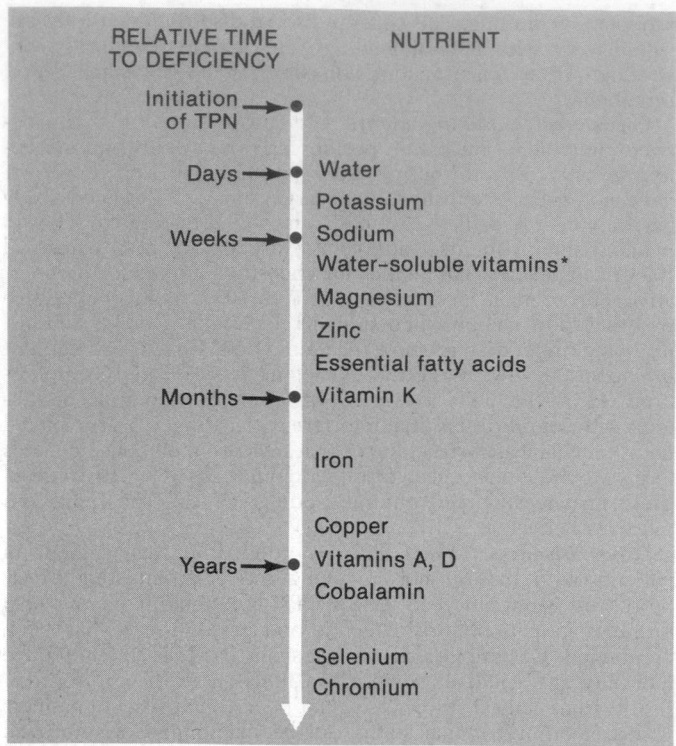

FIGURE 207–1. Relative time to the development of nutrient deficiencies during inadequately supplemented total parenteral nutrition (TPN). The time is proportional to body stores and inversely related to the fractional catabolic rate of the nutrient in an individual patient. Thus, the relative times given are only estimates. (*Excluding cobalamin.)

molar solutions is the most frequent administration-related complication when a peripheral vein is used.

Catheter-related sepsis can be held to no more than 5 per cent of patients treated with TPN of varying course length in a typical hospital-based program if maximal efforts are being made to prevent infection. Contamination from the catheter hub is often responsible for catheter-related infection. Culturing of material from removed catheter tips indicates whether the source of fever was actually an infected catheter.

Metabolic complications include the appearance of nutritional deficiencies resulting from inadequately prescribed TPN. Figure 207–1 shows the relative time to appearance of deficiencies under these circumstances. Each deficiency, of course, becomes more quickly apparent if body stores of that nutrient were originally depleted. Deficiencies are rare if nutrients are attentively prescribed.

Hyperglycemia is common in patients given concentrated dextrose by central vein. Regular insulin should be added to the base solution to keep serum glucose below 200 mg per deciliter. *Hypoglycemia* is not likely to occur if (1) exogenous insulin is added to the base solution rather than given subcutaneously, (2) the base solution is not interrupted abruptly, and (3) parenteral nutrition is terminated slowly over 24 hours or more with a stepwise reduction in the rate of glucose delivery. Incorrect provisions of major minerals can also be detected by regular laboratory monitoring, especially during the first 2 weeks of parenteral nutrition therapy.

Hepatic dysfunction not infrequently occurs. Increases in serum levels of liver enzyme activities are frequently noted following initiation of TPN. Transaminase increases usually do not persist. Delayed or persistent increases (> 20 days) may indicate toxic hepatitis related to the amino acid infusion or, more likely, a process not related to parenteral nutrition. Elevations of alkaline phosphatase values (up to two times normal) are noted in half of patients receiving TPN for more than 20 days. In some patients this represents fat accumulation from excessive carbohydrate feeding. Painful hepatomegaly may occur in these circumstances; fatty liver may be detected by computed tomography. Prevention or correction of increases of liver enzymes has been observed in some patients treated with metronidazole. Reduction in overgrowth of intestinal organisms and their toxic by-products in the portal stream has been speculated as the mechanism of this effect.

Periarticular, long-bone, and back pain, a syndrome that usually appears months into a course of TPN, is of unclear cause, but is likely related to altered vitamin D metabolism. Other factors contributing to bone disease include hypercalciuria observed during the TPN infusion (probably related to glucose loading and/or increased organic sulfate burden) and possibly improper trace mineral administration. Patients respond to discontinuation of TPN and removal of vitamin D from the TPN fluid.

Early or immediate *reactions to lipid emulsions* (dyspnea, cyanosis, cutaneous allergic phenomena, nausea, headache, back pain, autonomic discharge) occur with an incidence of less than 1 per cent. Hyperlipidemia resulting from the infusion should clear within 4 hours after the infusion. Poor lipid clearance is common with renal or hepatic failure. Delayed adverse reactions include hepatomegaly, jaundice, splenomegaly, thrombocytopenia, and leukopenia. Alterations in pulmonary function studies may occur in patients receiving lipid emulsions. A reduction in pulmonary diffusing capacity may be the most significant change, a change that has been seriously detrimental to premature infants with hyaline membrane disease, but less clinically significant to adults with respiratory disease.

As many as one third of patients treated with TPN for a period of 2 years have detectable *gallstones.* The prevalence is even higher (50 per cent) in the subset with ileal disease (Crohn's disease or prior resection or both). Gallbladder stasis and an increase in bile saturation with fasting are possible explanations for these higher than expected prevalences.

Alpers DH, Clouse RE, Stenson WF: Manual of Nutritional Therapeutics, 2nd ed. Boston, Little, Brown and Company, 1988. *This manual outlines parenteral nutrient requirements and describes techniques of parenteral nutrition in a chapter devoted to the subject. It is also a reference source for nutrient composition of proprietary products.*

A.S.P.E.N. Board of Directors: Guidelines for use of local parenteral nutrition in the hospitalized adult patient. J Parent Enteral Nutr 10:441, 1986. *A more comprehensive list of current recommendations for the use of parenteral nutrition in various disease settings.*

Berger R, Adams L: Nutritional support in the critical care setting. Chest 96:139, 1989. *A review of the principles and practical applications of parenteral nutrition in the intensive care unit.*

Detsky AS, Baker JP, O'Rourke K, Goel V: Perioperative parenteral nutrition: A meta-analysis. Ann Intern Med 107:195, 1987. *A comprehensive review of the trials examining TPN in the perioperative setting.*

Seidman EG: Nutritional management of inflammatory bowel disease. Gastroenterol Clin North Am 17:129, 1989. *Comparison of parenteral and enteral nutrition management strategies in patients with inflammatory bowel disease.*

PART XVI
ENDOCRINE AND REPRODUCTIVE DISEASES

208 Principles of Endocrinology

Gordon N. Gill

Communication is essential for all life processes. Accurate sensing of the environment and appropriate coordinated responses depend on the nervous and endocrine systems, which are tightly interwoven. Nervous system functions are mediated by hormones, and the endocrine system is centrally controlled by the nervous system. Communication between cells is necessary for development from a single fertilized egg to a mature adult, for an orderly reproductive cycle, and for homeostatic adjustments to a constantly changing environment. Hormones, distinct chemical messengers, transmit information from one cell to another to coordinate homeostatic adaptations, growth, development, and reproduction. Hormones, a word derived from Greek meaning "excite" or "set in motion," bind with high affinity and specificity to receptors, which are allosteric proteins. Receptor proteins have two essential functional characteristics: a recognition site, which binds hormone with high specificity and affinity, and an activity site, which transduces the information received into a biochemical message. Allosteric receptor proteins adopt various conformational states; binding of the hormone ligand results in the active conformation. The initial event in hormone action is thus a bimolecular reaction dependent on the concentration of hormone, the concentration of receptor, and the affinity of receptor for hormone.

$$[\text{Hormone}] + [\text{Receptor}] \underset{k_{-1}}{\overset{k_1}{\rightleftharpoons}} [\text{Hormone-Receptor}]$$

$$\text{Inactive} \qquad\qquad\qquad \text{Active}$$

Factors that control the concentration of both hormone and receptor determine biologic responses of cells, of organs, and of the whole organism.

Traditional endocrinology dealt with the glands that produce hormones and the concentrations of hormone to which cells expressing receptors are exposed. Biosynthesis, secretion, transport of hormone to target cells, and metabolic inactivation determine the effective hormone concentration. Diseases of endocrine glands that impair hormone production result in deficiency states, while diseases that cause excessive production result in hormone excess states. Expression of receptor is equally important in forming the active hormone-receptor complex. Genetic and acquired diseases that impair receptors result in deficiency states even though hormone concentrations are compensatorily increased. Increased receptor expression results in an excess state, an event that occurs with growth factor receptors in malignant transformation.

Hormones are produced not only by the glands of internal secretion but by a variety of cells throughout the body. Neurohormones, produced in the hypothalamus, are also produced in cells throughout the nervous system to modulate neuronal function. Gastrointestinal hormones are produced within the nervous system. Hormones that regulate production and maturation of cells of the hematopoietic and immune systems are made in cells of these lineages and in endothelial and mesenchymal cells. Growth-promoting and -inhibiting hormones (growth factors and growth inhibitors) are produced by macrophages and mesenchymal cells. Many of these signaling molecules do not travel long distances through the blood to reach target cells as do classic hormones (endocrine), but act on target cells in the vicinity of the producer cell (paracrine) or even on the producer cell itself (autocrine). During development, cell surface hormones may act on the cell surface receptor of a neighbor cell as a cell-cell communication system. Regardless of signaling distance, the same principles of hormone-receptor interactions operate.

HOW HORMONES WORK

Two classes of hormones operate via two types of receptors (Fig. 208–1). Peptide hormones are synthesized as parts of larger protein molecules and are processed as secretory proteins. They act via receptors located in the cell membrane with the recognition/binding site exposed on the cell surface and the activity domain facing the inside of the cell. Activated cell surface receptors use a variety of strategies to transduce signal information, often activating second messengers, which amplify and distribute the molecular information. Many peptide hormones ultimately signal via regulation of protein phosphorylation. In this most common process through which proteins are covalently modified, a phosphate group is donated to the protein by adenosine triphosphate. This allows peptide hormones to change rapidly the conformation and thus the function of existing cell enzymes. It also allows somewhat slower changes in gene tran-

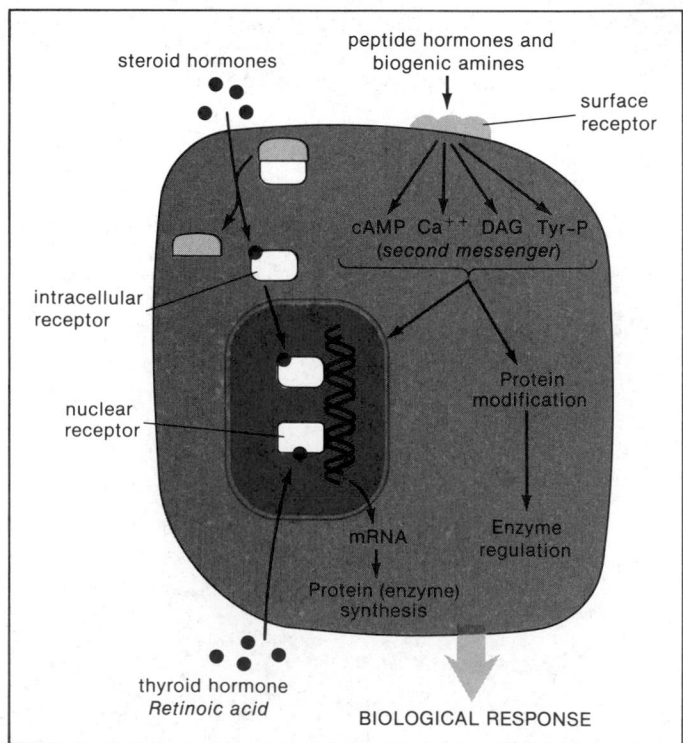

FIGURE 208–1. Mechanisms by which peptide and steroid hormones signal.

scription to regulate the concentration of enzyme proteins. Biogenic amines function like peptide hormones.

Steroid hormones are synthesized from precursor cholesterol. Thyroid hormone, retinoic acid (vitamin A), and vitamin D are synthesized via separate pathways but act through the same family of receptors and mechanisms as do steroid hormones. This group of hormones acts via structurally related receptors that bind to DNA recognition sites to regulate transcription of target genes. They change the concentration of cell proteins, primarily enzymes, and thus the metabolic activity underlying the physiologic response.

Peptide Hormones Act Via Cell Surface Receptors

HORMONE BINDING AND SIGNAL TRANSDUCTION. Peptide hormone receptors have one of three general structures (Fig. 208–2): (1) a seven membrane–spanning structure, in which the recognition site is formed by exterior sequences between membrane-spanning helices and the activity site is formed by interhelical regions inside the cell, (2) a single membrane-spanning helical structure separating the recognition domain from the cytoplasmic domain, which contains an intrinsic enzyme activity, and (3) a single membrane-spanning helix that separates the recognition domain from an intracellular domain that couples to second messenger systems as do the seven member–spanning receptors. The protein coupled may be an intracellular tyrosine kinase or other enzyme.

Hormone ligands and receptors bind with high affinities (equilibrium dissociation constants (K_D) of nM to pM), thus providing the specificity necessary for cells to decode the information provided by the low concentration of hormone present among the many other circulating and extracellular proteins. Measurements of hormone binding to cell surface receptors yield complex functions. These are likely due to interaction of hormone-receptor complexes with cell proteins but may arise from receptor aggregation, receptor modification, or cooperativity in binding.

The conformational change resulting from peptide hormone binding activates receptors to signal from the cell surface. Removal of receptors from the cell surface results in down-regulation and attenuation of the response. Binding affinities and dose-response curves for the initial event in cell signaling are the same. For example, binding of ACTH and production of cAMP occur with similar affinities and saturation; binding of insulin and activation of protein tyrosine kinase also occur with the same affinity and saturation. Biologic responses consequent to these initial events occur via a series of amplifications, each with its own affinity. The result is a dose-response curve for biologic

activities which is more sensitive than that for binding and activation of the initial response. Full biologic responses may thus occur at a low concentration of hormone that results in occupancy of only 10 per cent or less of receptors. This provides high sensitivity to small changes in hormone concentration. It also provides significant reserve. Hormone-induced down-regulation may remove 90 per cent of receptors from the cell surface. This renders the cell refractory to the initial hormone concentration, but if the need is great enough, hormone concentrations can increase 10-fold and fully activate the residual 10 per cent of receptors to give full biologic responses. Such a response system provides high initial sensitivity, buffering via down-regulation against excessive hormone responses, but a reserve that can operate when the signal is strong enough.

Receptors are mobile in the plane of the membrane. Ligand binding not only transduces signals but also induces down-regulation by removing receptors from the cell surface. Ligand binding may induce sequestration of receptors and their retention inside the cell via interactions with cell proteins, as occurs with rhodopsin and adrenergic receptors. Ligand binding may induce endocytosis via clathrin-coated pits with ultimate degradation via lysosomal enzymes, as occurs with insulin and epidermal growth factor receptors. The concentration of cell surface receptors is regulated by interaction with hormone ligand and by other signals that regulate its synthesis and affinity. The concentration of receptors determines the cells' responsiveness. Antagonists occupy receptors but in general do not induce desensitization. When antagonists are removed, receptor concentrations are high and cells are very responsive to hormone exposure. Effects on receptor concentration are seen clinically as up-regulation (e.g., as excessive adrenergic responses when β blockers are rapidly withdrawn) and as down-regulation (e.g., insulin resistance in type II diabetes). Regulation of receptor synthesis is an important mechanism by which one hormone regulates responsiveness to another to coordinate biologic effects.

A class of cell surface receptors serves a nutrient delivery rather than an informational function. These molecules include the low density lipoprotein (LDL) receptor, the transferrin receptor, and the asialoglycoprotein receptor. LDL and transferrin receptors, which are clustered in coated pits, internalize, deliver LDL (cholesterol) and iron to the cell interior, and then recycle to the cell surface. Such receptors do not down-regulate, but undergo recycling to provide the cell with essential nutrients.

INTRACELLULAR SECOND MESSENGERS. cAMP and cGMP. The concept of second messengers was established by

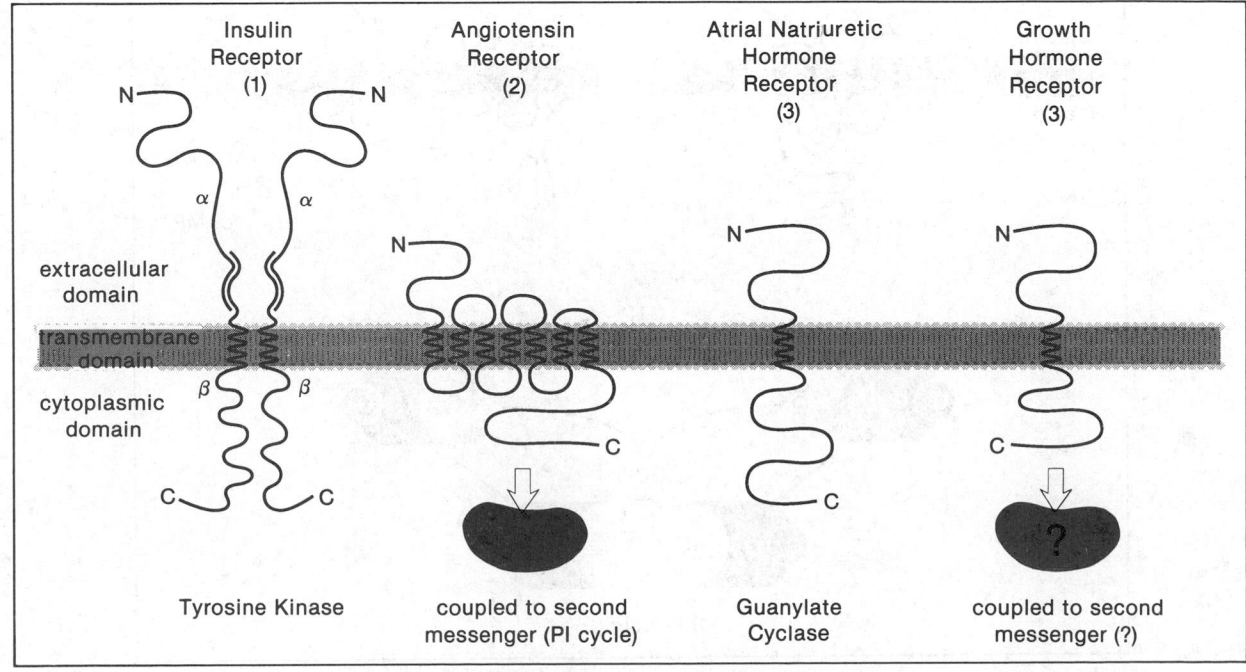

FIGURE 208–2. Structures of peptide hormone receptors.

Earl Sutherland, who discovered cAMP, an intracellular allosteric effector that mediates the action of many peptide hormones. Hormone receptors are coupled to catalytic adenylate cyclase via guanosine nucleotide binding (G) proteins, the β-adrenergic receptor being a paradigm for this signaling pathway (Fig. 208–3). This receptor belongs to the seven membrane–spanning class. On ligand binding, the receptor interacts with a G protein trimer consisting of α, β, and γ subunits. G proteins are ancient signaling molecules involved in regulating many cell processes, including initiation and elongation of protein synthesis, protein transport between membrane compartments, and signal transduction. In all cases binding of GDP results in an inactive conformation, whereas binding of GTP results in an active conformation. The activity of G proteins is thus regulated by the ratio of GTP to GDP, which is, in turn, linked to the energy state of the cell. Because G proteins bind GDP with higher affinity than GTP, guanine nucleotide exchange is triggered by proteins that facilitate exchange of GTP for GDP. Activity is reversed by hydrolysis of GTP to GDP. Binding of hormones to receptors that operate through the cAMP second messenger system results in a conformational change causing receptors to bind to G proteins. Ligand-activated receptors facilitate exchange of GTP for GDP so that the activated $G_{\alpha}s$ (stimulating α GTP-binding subunit) dissociates from the β and γ subunits. The [ligand-hormone receptor]-[$G_{\alpha}s$-GTP] complex activates adenylate cyclase to catalyze formation of cAMP from ATP. Each hormone ligand induces formation of multiple cAMP molecules via this mechanism. Inhibitory G proteins operate in a similar manner to decrease cAMP formation. In both cases ligand-activated receptors act to exchange GTP for GDP, analogous to proteins that catalyze this process to regulate protein synthesis.

Adenylate cyclase is a large complex molecule with a 12 membrane–spanning structure resembling the family of glucose transporters, sodium and calcium channels, and the mutated gene in cystic fibrosis. The two large cytoplasmic domains have internal sequence similarities and are related to sequences in guanylate cyclase. Four adenylate cyclases have been identified, and their channel-like structure suggests that they may function as transporters in addition to catalyzing formation of cAMP.

Activation of adenylate cyclase is buffered and terminated by several mechanisms: (1) Hormone dissociates from receptor. Binding of G_{α}-GTP to the receptor decreases affinity for hormone about one order of magnitude to facilitate this dissociation. (2)

Receptors desensitize and are removed from the cell surface by a process involving phosphorylation and interaction with cell proteins termed "arrestins." (3) Most importantly, G_{α} proteins possess intrinsic GTPase activity so that GTP is hydrolyzed to GDP and, on GDP binding, G_{α} is inactivated and reassociates with the β/γ subunits. If hormone exposure is short, receptors are dephosphorylated and reappear on the cell surface; if exposure is prolonged, receptors are degraded and resensitization requires new receptor synthesis.

There are many consequences when this mechanism of signal transduction is perturbed. Continuous exposure to hormone results in desensitization or tachyphylaxis. Deficiency of G protein, which occurs in certain forms of pseudohypoparathyroidism, results in insensitivity to hormone. Cholera toxin, which activates ADP ribosylation of $G_{\alpha}s$, inhibits GTPase activity, interfering with reversibility so that profound and prolonged elevations in cAMP occur. Mutations in G_{α} proteins that are predicted to impair GTPase activity have been described in tumors. The *ras* family of G proteins is frequently mutated and oncogenic in human tumors. Mutations impair interaction of these proteins with GTPase-activating proteins, so that, by analogy to cholera toxin, the mutant *ras* proteins remain in the GTP-bound active conformation. *ras* proteins are presumed to couple a signaling pathway different from adenylate cyclase because *ras* cannot substitute for mammalian G_{α}.

cAMP, an intracellular allosteric effector, binds to the regulatory subunit of cAMP-dependent protein kinase. A-kinase is a tetrameric protein consisting of two regulatory and two catalytic subunits. Binding of cAMP dissociates the inhibitory regulatory subunits as a dimer from the two catalytic subunits. The latter then catalyze the transfer of the γ phosphate of ATP to serine and threonine residues in proteins. This covalent modification by phosphorylation causes an allosteric conformational change in the substrate protein that results in a change in its activity. The hormonal signal is transduced into an alteration in enzyme activity and thus in cell function.

cAMP actions are reversed by hydrolysis of cAMP by phosphodiesterase to 5′ AMP, and protein phosphorylation is reversed by the action of phosphatases. Phosphodiesterases are regulated and are a frequent target of inhibitor drugs, such as methyl xanthines, which prolong cAMP action by blocking its degradation. Phosphatases are regulated by phosphatase inhibitor proteins, which are fine tuned by phosphorylation of these molecules.

A conceptually similar but structurally distinct system provides

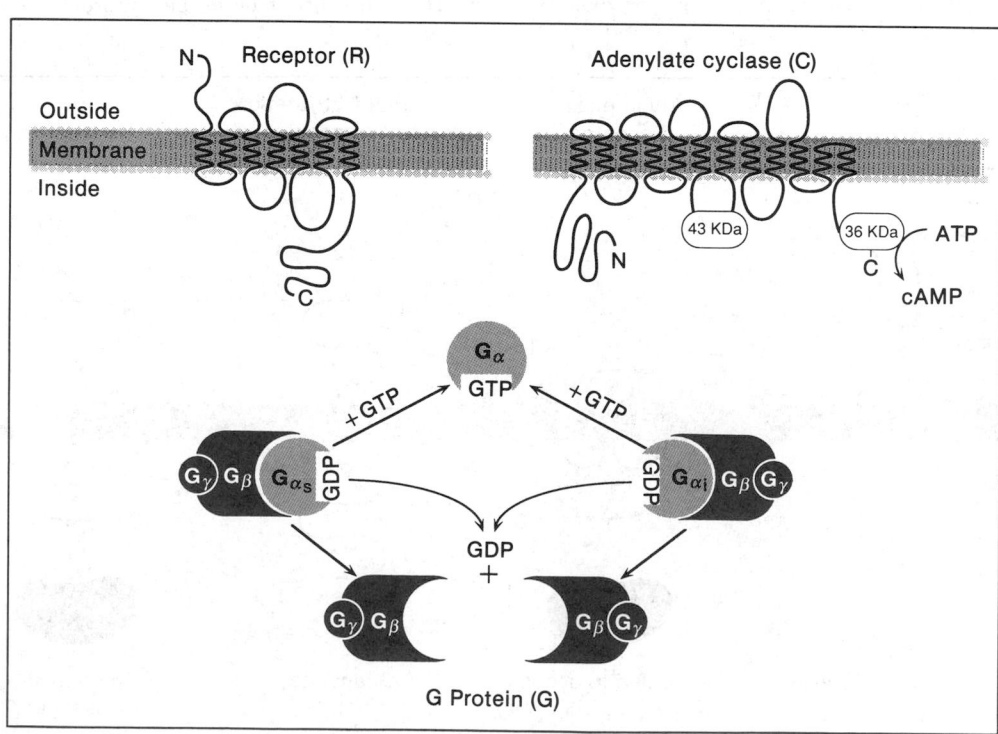

FIGURE 208–3. Hormone-regulated adenylate cyclase.

signal transduction via the second messenger cGMP. Two forms of guanylate cyclase catalyze formation of cGMP from GTP. The best characterized mammalian enzyme is the receptor for atrial natriuretic hormone (ANH) (Ch. 211). The binding site for ANH is located on the extracellular portion of its receptor separated by a single membrane–spanning domain from the cytoplasmic guanylate cyclase (see Fig. 208–2). In contrast to adenylate cyclase, receptor and catalytic activities reside in the same molecule. Activity is regulated primarily by ligand binding but also depends on phosphorylation of the enzyme, with dephosphorylation causing desensitization. A cytoplasmic form of guanylate cyclase contains a heme moiety and is activated by nitrous oxide and free radicals.

cGMP acts by binding to the regulatory domain of cGMP-dependent protein kinase. G-kinase, a dimeric enzyme that is evolutionarily related to A-kinase, is allosterically activated on cGMP binding. Like A-kinase, it catalyzes protein phosphorylation to alter enzyme function and physiologic responses. Reactions are terminated by cGMP phosphodiesterase and protein phosphatases. cGMP phosphodiesterase is activated by binding of calcium-calmodulin, a mechanism providing biochemical communication between two signaling systems.

Calcium and Diacylglycerol. Hormone receptors that activate the phosphatidylinositol (PI) cycle transmit information to the interior of the cell via two second messengers: calcium (Ca^{2+}) and diacylglycerol (DAG) (Fig. 208–4). The cycle of PI metabolism consists of synthesis of this phospholipid, its breakdown, and its resynthesis. PI is composed of a three-carbon glycerol backbone with long-chain fatty acids esterified at carbons 1 and 2 and an inositol ring esterified via a phosphoester bond at carbon 3. Distinct kinase enzymes catalyze phosphorylation of the inositol ring at positions 3, 4, and 5. Quantitatively the principal phosphorylations occur sequentially at position 4 and then 5 (PI 4-kinase and PI 4(P)-5-kinase). Although both kinases are regulated, the principal function of activated hormone receptors is to stimulate phosphoinositidase (phospholipase C), which releases the phosphorylated inositol to generate inositol triphosphate (IP_3, inositol 1,4,5 P_3) and DAG (the glycerol backbone with fatty acids attached at carbons 1 and 2). IP_3 increases the concentration of cytoplasmic [Ca^{2+}]. It mobilizes stored intracellular Ca^{2+} by binding to specific receptors on intracellular membranes and by facilitating opening of calcium channels. The concentration of basal cytoplasmic Ca^{2+} is at least 1000-fold less than that in storage sites and outside the cell. The release from intracellular stores or entry of Ca^{2+} into the cell rapidly increases cytoplasmic [Ca^{2+}].

Ca^{2+} plays a regulatory role in muscle contraction, in neuromuscular transmission, and in hormone signaling. Ca^{2+} binds to calmodulin and alters its conformation, causing the Ca^{2+}-calmodulin complex to bind to a variety of enzymes to regulate their activities. Ca^{2+}-calmodulin regulates protein kinases, including myosin light chain kinase involved in smooth muscle contraction, phosphorylase kinase involved in breakdown of glycogen, and calmodulin-dependent protein kinase important in synaptic transmission. Ca^{2+}-calmodulin regulates cyclic nucleotide phosphodiesterase and adenylate and guanylate cyclases to influence cAMP and cGMP concentrations, and it is involved in microtubule assembly and disassembly. Ca^{2+}-calmodulin is thus able to bind to a variety of other proteins and to alter their activity in response to information provided by the cytoplasmic Ca^{2+} concentration. This provides for diffusion and integration of information received at the cell surface.

DAG acts as a second messenger by binding to protein kinase C to activate this important regulatory enzyme. Protein kinase C also requires Ca^{2+} for activation, so both second messengers of this pathway cooperate to increase the activity of this enzyme. Tumor promoters, such as active phorbol esters, are DAG analogues and act via protein kinase C.

The components of this second messenger system are diverse and complex. There are multiple isoenzyme forms of protein kinase C and of phosphoinositidase. Additional kinases phosphorylate alternate positions on the inositol ring; PI 3-kinase appears to be activated by certain tyrosine kinases to yield unique PI metabolites with functions distinct from Ca^{2+} mobilization. Sphingosine, a component of glycosphingolipid metabolism, inhibits protein kinase C, which provides dual regulation of this protein. Specific phosphatases remove the phosphate groups from the inositol ring to terminate its activity; lithium blocks the activity of one of these phosphatases to enhance accumulation of the biologically active inositol phosphates. Like other information pathways, this one is diffused to generate coordinated cellular responses and is buffered and ultimately turned off when the signal strength decreases.

Protein Tyrosine Kinases. A group of peptide hormone receptors contains intrinsic protein tyrosine kinase activity. Ligand binding to the extracellular domain results in an allosteric change that is

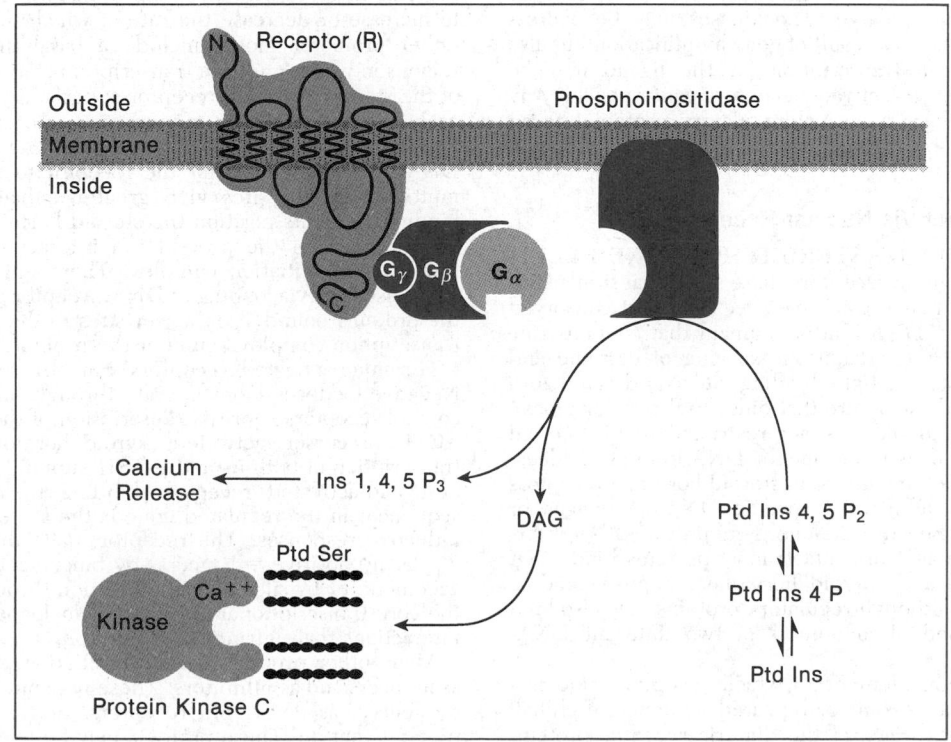

FIGURE 208–4. The phosphatidylinositol signaling pathway.

transmitted across the single membrane-spanning segment to activate the cytoplasmic kinase domain (see Fig. 208–2). In a second structural motif a transmembrane receptor is coupled to a distinct cytoplasmic tyrosine kinase subunit. The lymphocyte receptor CD4 and cellular p56[lck] belong to this second class.

Within the cell the great majority of protein-bound phosphate is attached to serine and threonine residues; only a small fraction (3 to 10 parts per 10,000) is attached to tyrosine. Numerous kinases, however, covalently modify tyrosine residues in proteins as a central regulatory function in cell proliferation, developmental processes, and differentiated function. Historically, this was revealed by the discovery that tyrosine kinase activity is intrinsic to the transforming protein of the Rous sarcoma virus. Several transforming retroviruses presumably "captured" cellular tyrosine kinases in the past and have disarmed their regulatory features or have constitutively expressed them under strong retroviral promoters. When introduced into cells, these retroviruses result in unregulated excessive tyrosine kinase activity and transformation of cells from normal to unrestrained malignant proliferation (Ch. 376).

The extracellular ligand-binding domains of receptors of this class contain cysteine-rich regions that create the binding sites either as monomers (epidermal growth factor [EGF] receptor) or as dimers (insulin receptor), or contain immunoglobulin-like structures (platelet-derived growth factor [PDGF] and fibroblast growth factor [FGF] receptors). The cytoplasmic protein tyrosine kinase domains are highly homologous, containing ATP and substrate-binding sites, but different receptors recognize distinct substrates to give specific biologic responses. For example, insulin stimulates glucose uptake while EGF stimulates cell proliferation. The tyrosine kinases contain variable domains on both sides of the tyrosine kinase core as well as inserts within the kinase domain which provide regulatory sites that modulate ligand-activated tyrosine kinase activity.

Increased tyrosine kinase activity is reversed by three principal mechanisms: (1) by ligand-induced endocytosis and down-regulation of surface receptors, (2) by tyrosine phosphatases, which specifically remove phosphate from tyrosine residues, and (3) by reversal of the kinase reaction to transfer the phosphate from tyrosine residues in protein to ADP.

Regulation and reversibility of ligand-activated tyrosine kinases are very important. Mutations involving these proteins occur frequently in cells transformed from normal to cancerous patterns of growth. Mutations may bypass regulatory features so that the kinases are constitutively active. The kinases may be overexpressed, most frequently as a result of gene amplification but also as a result of enhanced transcription; or the ligand may be constitutively expressed to activate receptors continuously. Any of these changes converts a normal regulatory protein into an oncoprotein, one capable of causing neoplastic transformation (Ch. 157).

Steroid Hormones Act Via Nuclear Receptors

THE SUPERFAMILY OF STEROID HORMONE RECEPTORS. All steroid hormone receptors share structural similarities indicative of a common ancestral molecule. The most conserved structural feature is the DNA-binding domain that contains zinc "fingers" (Fig. 208–5). The diagnostic spacing of cysteine and histidine residues creates a tight binding site coordinated to a Zn^{2+} atom and a peptide structure that binds to the major groove of DNA. This structural motif is not restricted to the steroid receptor gene family nor is it specific for DNA binding. It does, however, create the protein surface in steroid hormone receptors that binds with high affinity to specific DNA sequences or recognition elements. Because the energy of protein-DNA interaction depends on the area of contact, most proteins bind DNA as complexes. Steroid and thyroid hormone receptors bind to DNA as homodimers, although regulatory proteins may also bind as heterodimers formed of monomers of two different DNA-binding proteins.

The DNA recognition element to which receptors bind frequently consists of a palindrome or repeated sequence, each half binding one monomer surface of the dimeric receptor protein. Small variations in the DNA-binding domain and in the DNA

recognition element provide specificity for hormone action. Cortisol receptors bind to glucocorticoid DNA response elements (GRE's) but not to estrogen DNA response elements (ERE's). Specificity is quantitative, not absolute. For example, progesterone receptors bind to GRE's, and retinoic acid receptors bind to thyroid hormone receptor DNA response elements (TRE's). Specificity is sufficient for generating hormone-specific responses but may permit overlapping functions, as in ligand-activated progesterone receptor induction of glucocorticoid-regulated genes. Targeting via DNA-binding domains can be clearly demonstrated by swapping the DNA-binding domain of one receptor for another. Replacing the DNA-binding domain of the estrogen receptor with that of the cortisol receptor targets the hybrid receptor to GRE's, resulting in estrogen-inducing genes normally regulated by cortisol.

Hormone binding activates the biologic function of the receptor. Cortisol receptors exist in inactive complexes with other proteins; cortisol binding induces an allosteric change that facilitates dissociation, allowing the ligand-bound receptor to bind to GRE DNA. Thyroid hormone and retinoic acid receptors exist bound to DNA rather than complexed to protein; hormone binding results in an allosteric change that activates the receptor, so it interacts with other components of the transcription machinery.

The steroid hormone receptor family is a large one, extending to include receptors for $1,25(OH)_2$ vitamin D, thyroid hormone, and retinoic acid. There are also subfamilies of receptors—at least four for retinoic acid, two for thyroid hormone, and a group of "orphans" whose ligands remain to be identified. This structural motif is an important one, which in evolution has diverged to specify responses to many hormonal signals and to control expression of numerous genes. Identifying the orphan receptors will expand understanding of ligand molecules that can signal metabolic and developmental information.

REGULATION OF GENE TRANSCRIPTION. Hormone-activated receptor proteins bound to their DNA response element targets act as *cis*-active enhancers. They act from various positions relative to the start of transcription and in various combinations with other regulatory proteins to control the rate of initiation of gene transcription. Gene promoters lie upstream of the site where eukaryotic RNA polymerase II initiates transcription of messenger RNA. The best-characterized promoter contains a TATA box that binds a protein, transcription factor II D (TFIID), which directs accurate transcription by RNA polymerase II approximately 30 base pairs downstream. A variety of regulatory proteins interact with the basic transcription initiation complex to increase or decrease the rate at which mRNA is synthesized. Other promoter motifs include a basal initiator and GC-rich regions in which multiple transcription start sites exist. Members of the steroid hormone receptor superfamily regulate genes with each of these promoter sequences. Gene expression is induced by increasing the rate of transcription. The gene must contain a DNA binding element for the receptor to generate a response; multiple binding sites give greater enhancement. The DNA binding elements position the steroid hormone receptors so that other regions of the protein can interact with proteins in the transcription initiation complex. These enhancers can act over large distances via looping of DNA. Adaptor proteins may connect the proteins bound at enhancer sites to the proteins of the basal transcription complex bound at the promoter.

Hormone-activated receptors can also repress transcription. Negative feedback loops operate through this process. Activated cortisol receptors repress transcription of the gene encoding the ACTH precursor; activated thyroid hormone receptors inhibit transcription of both α- and β-TSH subunit genes. The principle of ligand-activated receptors binding to specific DNA target sequences in the regulated gene is the same as that required for inductive responses. The receptor may inhibit transcription by displacing positive enhancers, by blocking RNA polymerase engagement, or by silencing transcription through interactions with the core transcriptional machinery, analogous to protein-protein interactions that enhance transcription.

Many other proteins regulate initiation of transcription, both as inducers and as inhibitors. These may bind to DNA via specific sequences, as do steroid receptors, or they may interact with proteins that do. These proteins may be modified in response to hormonal signals initiated at the cell surface. Such alterations account for the changes in gene transcription due to hormones acting via surface receptors. Genes regulated by cAMP contain DNA sequences that specify binding of a specific nuclear transcription regulator, the cAMP response element binding protein (CREB). This protein, which is a member of a family of related transcriptional regulators, is a required final mediator of gene induction by peptide hormones that act at the cell surface to activate adenylate cyclase and cAMP-dependent protein kinase. This chain of effects alters transcription of mRNA's and cell protein concentrations to dictate changes in cell function and organ physiology.

BIOSYNTHESIS OF HORMONES AND RECEPTORS

Synthesis and Delivery of Peptide Hormones

Peptide hormones are small secretory proteins; their biosynthesis and secretion occur via the same processes as other nonhormonal secretory proteins. In general, peptide hormones are synthesized as part of larger precursor proteins that contain additional information. Within the endoplasmic reticulum space, the precursor protein is cleaved, covalently modified, and folded into the form that will ultimately be secreted.

The precursor structure may have a variety of functions. Precursors for antidiuretic hormone and oxytocin contain specific neurophysins that serve as carriers of the peptides from the site of synthesis in the hypothalamus to storage granules in axon terminals in the posterior pituitary (Ch. 214). The ACTH precursor, pro-opiomelanocortin, contains information for several peptides that may be coordinately involved in stress responses (Ch. 209). The precursor for gonadotropin-releasing hormone contains a potent prolactin-inhibitory peptide, a structure that allows reciprocal regulation of lactation and reproductive function. Structures in the precursor protein may serve to fold the peptide correctly. The connecting peptide in the insulin precursor between the β and the α subunits facilitates folding for formation of mature insulin with correctly formed disulfide bonds between and within the two chains (Ch. 218). The connecting peptide is then excised and removed from mature α-β insulin.

Within the endoplasmic reticulum and Golgi apparatus, glycosylation of TSH, LH, FSH, and hCG occurs. Secretory granules containing highly concentrated hormone accumulate in the unstimulated cell. During secretion the membrane of the secretory granule fuses with the plasma membrane and stored hormone is discharged into the circulation, a process termed exocytosis. Rapid release of hormone in response to stimuli reflects discharge of secretory granules, whereas prolonged secretion reflects release of newly synthesized hormone.

Peptide hormones may also be derived from precursors with receptor-like structures or from circulating forms. EGF and transforming growth factor α (TGF-α) are made as a part of the surface domain of a transmembrane protein with a receptor-like structure. These are released by proteolysis, although they may act on adjacent cells without processing to provide cell-to-cell

communication. Renin, an enzyme released from juxtaglomerular cells, acts on angiotensinogen secreted from liver. Active angiotensin is synthesized by progressive extracellular proteolysis of a precursor: renin to yield angiotensin I and angiotensin-converting enzyme to yield angiotensin II.

Secreted peptide hormones have a short half-life of about 3 to 7 minutes in the circulation. Glycoprotein hormones have longer half-lives of 1 to 4 hours. The short circulating half-life and peptide degradation by gastric acid and intestinal enzymes have precluded oral use of this class of hormones. Several attempts to prolong half-lives have met with partial success: Complexing with Zn^{2+} and protamine creates a slowly absorbed and longer-acting form of injectable insulin; removing the amino group from the N′ terminal amino acid and substituting a D-arginine creates a longer-acting ADH which can be absorbed from nasal mucous membranes. At present direct use of peptide hormones is limited to injectable forms. Prolonged action results in receptor desensitization, so recapitulation of normal cyclic secretion typical of endogenous production presents a second difficulty. Use of GnRH must be both by parental routes and pulsatile in nature to induce ovulation and successful pregnancy.

Synthesis and Transport of Steroid Hormones

Steroid hormones are derived from cholesterol provided by de novo cellular synthesis from acetate or by uptake of circulating cholesterol made in the liver and delivered to cells via low density lipoprotein particles. Because synthesized steroid hormones are not stored, secretory rates directly reflect production rates. In adrenal and gonadal tissues the rate-limiting step for increased steroid hormone biosynthesis is transfer of substrate cholesterol to the side chain cleavage enzyme located in the inner mitochondrial membrane. Cleavage of the side chain of cholesterol is catalyzed by a cytochrome P-450 enzyme that resembles other steroid hydroxylases. These enzymes progressively modify the cholesterol nucleus by the sequential addition of hydroxyl groups to specific sites. The rate-limiting step is stimulated in target cells by ACTH, LH, and FSH to result in rapid increases in steroid hormone biosynthesis. The trophic stimulatory hormones also maintain the structure of the target glands and induce each of the enzymes involved in hormone biosynthesis. With hypophysectomy or feedback inhibition of pituitary hormone production, the entire steroid biosynthetic pathway decreases and the adrenal, ovary, and testis atrophy. Addition of trophic hormones induces enzymes and regrowth of target glands. Induction of biosynthetic enzymes appears directly mediated via second messenger pathways, primarily cAMP, but growth requires coordinated provision of growth factors because cAMP, in general, inhibits growth.

The pattern of biosynthetic enzymes expressed during cell differentiation determines which steroid hormone is produced

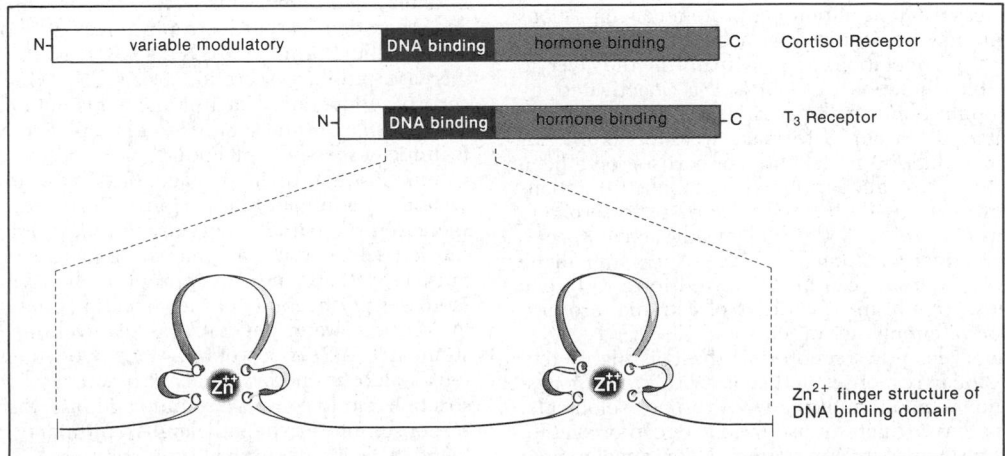

FIGURE 208–5. Structural features of steroid hormone receptors. The cortisol and T_3 receptors have variable modulatory domains but highly conserved DNA-binding domains. The DNA-binding domains contain two Zn^{2+} fingers.

and is the basis of the differentiated function of adrenal and gonads. The fascicularis zones of the adrenal cortex express cytochrome P-450 enzymes that catalyze hydroxylations at carbons 21, 17, and 11. They also express 3β-hydroxysteroid dehydrogenase, $\Delta^{4,5}$ isomerase which forms cortisol. The zona glomerulosa of the adrenal cortex makes aldosterone through a similar series of reactions, but the pathway lacks 17α-hydroxylase and contains an activity that acts at carbon 18. The testis lacks 21- and 11β-hydroxylases, so reactants flow to testosterone. Ovarian synthesis of estradiol requires cooperation between adjacent theca interna and granulosa cells. Granulosa cells express aromatase, the enzyme that catalyzes placement of three double bonds in the A ring of estrogens but cannot provide precursor androstenedione, which is synthesized in the theca interna cell located adjacent to the granulosa cell. Granulosa cells efficiently convert precursor androstenedione provided by the theca interna to estrone and estradiol.

The active form of vitamin D, 1,25(OH)$_2$D, is also made from cholesterol, but the biosynthetic enzymes are located in three separate organs: skin, liver, and kidney (Ch. 233). Vitamin D$_3$ is formed from 7-dehydrocholesterol by ultraviolet irradiation of skin. D$_3$ is then hydroxylated at carbon-25 in the liver to yield 25(OH)D. This is converted by 1α-hydroxylase to 1,25(OH)$_2$D in proximal tubule cells of the kidney. In this unique endocrine system, the major site for regulation is the final 1α-hydroxylation in renal proximal tubule cells, a step controlled by parathyroid hormone and phosphate.

In contrast to peptide hormones, steroid hormones have longer circulating half-lives and may be active when administered orally. Following secretion into the circulation, steroid hormones are bound to transport glycoproteins made in the liver. The transport proteins, which have a binding but not an activity site, provide a reservoir of hormone, protected from metabolism and renal clearance, which can be released to cells. Three transport proteins have been characterized: corticosteroid-binding globulin (CBG) which binds cortisol and progesterone, sex steroid hormone–binding globulin (SHBG) which binds testosterone with greater affinity than estradiol, and vitamin D–binding protein which binds precursor 25(OH)D with greater affinity than 1,25(OH)$_2$D. Thyroid-binding globulin (TBG) binds L-thyroxine to provide its uniquely long half-life of 7 days. Estrogen induces and androgens inhibit synthesis of these transport proteins. Albumin provides a large carrier system that weakly binds hormones.

Free steroid hormone, which is in equilibrium with that bound to transport protein, enters cells to bind intracellular receptors and generate biologic responses. The free fraction is also the active one in feedback regulation, so it is the concentration of free hormone that is altered in homeostatic responses. The free fraction is very small compared to the bound fraction, but total hormone concentrations from both fractions are measured in most clinical assays. Conditions, such as pregnancy, that alter binding protein concentrations alter total measured hormone but not the biologically relevant free hormone concentrations. In special clinical situations measurement of binding protein concentrations and of free hormone may be required for accurate assessment.

Steroid hormones are metabolized principally in the liver to inactive water-soluble metabolites. Cortisol is inactivated by reduction of the double bond in the A ring, and conjugation to glucuronide or sulfate at carbon 3 to make it water-soluble for renal excretion. More than 50 metabolites of cortisol have been identified, all inactive. Not all peripheral metabolic alterations are inactivating, however. 5α-Reductase converts testosterone to 5α-dihydrotestosterone, which is the biologically active species in male reproductive tract and skin (Ch. 222). Androstenedione produced in ovary and adrenal can be converted to testosterone in peripheral tissues. Significant quantities of estradiol are produced by conversion of circulating precursors.

Like their hormonal ligands, receptor synthesis is highly regulated to control cellular responses and sensitivity to hormones. Gene promoter regions contain multiple DNA response elements, which bind proteins that regulate transcription. Receptor synthesis is increased in response to environmental or development need or is repressed in negative feedback loops and during stages of development. Receptor concentration is as important as hormone concentration in determining cell responses. Regulation of receptor synthesis is therefore central to providing coordinated and appropriate endocrine responses.

INTEGRATION OF ENDOCRINE RESPONSES
Feedback Loops

A number of hormones cooperate to coordinate development, reproduction, and homeostasis. When a hormone has elicited an appropriate response, the signal must be terminated. In addition to the buffering that occurs in target cells, feedback control is the principal mechanism through which this occurs (Fig. 208–6). Feedback loops are especially important for communication between organs that are spatially separated. The hormonal products of peripheral endocrine glands, such as thyroid, adrenal cortex, ovary, and testis, exert negative feedback control over the synthesis and secretion of the stimulatory pituitary hormone. Feedback, which occurs at the level of the pituitary cell and in the hypothalamus, operates via control of several essential steps. The neurohormone TRH stimulates thyrotropes of the anterior pituitary to synthesize and secrete TSH, which in turn increases synthesis and secretion of thyroid hormone. Increased production of thyroid hormone induces appropriate metabolic responses in target organs; it also inhibits production of TSH to return the system to baseline. The prohormone L-thyroxine (T$_4$) is converted in the pituitary thyrotrope to active T$_3$, and T$_3$ binds to nuclear T$_3$ receptors to inhibit transcription of both α- and β-TSH subunit genes. T$_3$-bound receptors also decrease synthesis of TRH receptors, rendering cells less responsive to stimulatory TRH. In addition, T$_3$ inhibits hypothalamic production of TRH. Conversely, when thyroid hormone concentrations are low, feedback inhibition is relieved and TRH stimulates increased production of TSH, which increases production of T$_4$ and thus re-establishes homeostasis. Feedback principles provide an exquisitely sensitive system for making appropriate changes and then returning to the homeostatic set-point.

Feedback operates not only via steroid and thyroid hormones but also through peptides and ions. Pituitary FSH production is feedback regulated by the ovarian steroid hormone estrogen and by the ovarian peptide hormone inhibin. Parathyroid hormone regulates serum Ca^{2+} concentrations; with hypocalcemia PTH increases and re-establishes normocalcemia. The increase in serum [Ca^{2+}] feedback inhibits PTH synthesis and secretion to re-establish serum PTH concentrations appropriate to normocalcemia (Ch. 235).

Recruitment of Coordinate Responses

Physiologic responses result from many different cell types and organs acting in concert. The necessary coordination is provided both by a hormone acting at multiple sites and by each hormone eliciting multiple responses, which sum to give the overall effect. Integrated responses require that one hormone regulate the synthesis or action of another; the nervous system is integrated into the overall response. Paradigms of such coordinated responses include stress, fasting, and reproduction.

A major stress, such as trauma with pain and hypovolemia, initiates a central nervous system response that includes synthesis and secretion of corticotropin-releasing hormone (CRH) and antidiuretic hormone (ADH). CRH is the major stimulus to increase pituitary secretion of ACTH, which increases adrenal cortisol production. Cortisol maintains not only blood glucose but also vascular responsiveness to epinephrine and norepinephrine. It limits excessive inflammatory responses to prevent further volume loss and tissue damage. CRH acts, in the central nervous system, to stimulate the peripheral sympathetic nervous system. Increased sympathetic nervous system activity mediates adaptive cardiovascular responses, including increased blood pressure and pulse rate. It also induces appropriate behavioral responses. ADH increases permeability of the collecting duct of the distal nephron to conserve water and intravascular volume. It facilitates CRH-stimulated ACTH secretion. With hypovolemia the renin-angiotensin-aldosterone system is also activated to enhance vasoconstriction and to conserve sodium and intravascular volume. These responses of the hypothalamus, pituitary, and adrenal cortex together facilitate survival from stresses.

With fasting, blood glucose concentrations are maintained for 12 to 24 hours by glucagon- and epinephrine-mediated release of glucose from glycogen stores. With more prolonged fasting cortisol-stimulated gluconeogenesis is the major mechanism that sustains blood glucose. Insulin secretion is suppressed. Metabolic demands are decreased by inhibition of 5' deiodinase to decrease conversion of T_4 to active T_3 in peripheral tissues. Growth-promoting hormones, such as insulin-like growth factor I, are also suppressed under conditions of substrate lack. With starvation gonadotropin secretion decreases and reproductive capacity is diminished.

Female reproductive cycles result from coordinated signaling by hypothalamic, pituitary, and ovarian hormones. Pulsatile secretion of GnRH stimulates pituitary production of LH and FSH. During the follicular phase of the menstrual cycle these peptide hormones regulate ovarian secretion of estrogen and direct maturation of follicles, one of which increases 1000-fold in diameter and becomes dominant for ovulation (Ch. 224). FSH induces LH receptors in ovarian granulosa cells, and both LH and FSH induce aromatase as part of the mechanism that enhances estrogen production. LH and FSH increase during the follicular phase and, with follicle development, estrogen secretion rises. Positive feedback effects of estrogen result in the mid-cycle surge of LH and FSH, which induces ovulation. The remaining granulosa and theca cells reorganize to form the corpus luteum, which produces progesterone as well as estrogen. Concentrations of these hormones negatively inhibit FSH and LH production and induce additional uterine changes necessary for implantation. Ovarian inhibin also feedback inhibits FSH production. If fertilization and implantation occur, the corpus luteum is regulated by hCG until placental steroidogenesis is established. If fertilization does not occur, negative feedback of estrogen and progesterone inhibits LH and FSH, and the luteal phase of the menstrual cycle ends after about 10 days when the corpus luteum, now deprived of trophic stimulation, decreases estrogen and progesterone production. Menstruation occurs and, in the absence of negative feedback, FSH and LH again rise to initiate a subsequent reproductive cycle.

Cycles and Rhythms

Nervous system rhythms are evident within feedback loops and coordinate hormonal responses. Several pituitary hormones are secreted with a frequency of 15 to 60 minutes owing to pulsatile secretion of hypothalamic hormones. Longer rhythms are superimposed on these pulses. Pulsatile secretion of peptide hormones maximizes target cell responses by preventing excessive receptor down-regulation. ACTH and consequently cortisol exhibit a diurnal rhythm with early morning secretion exceeding evening secretion at least twofold. Growth hormone is entrained to deep sleep, with maximal daily production occurring coincident with EEG-defined slow wave sleep. Cycles also occur at different stages of development. At puberty nocturnal increases in gonadotropins occur, a rhythm much less pronounced in adult life. Measured hormone levels must be interpreted relative to these rhythms and cycles, as well as to stages of the menstrual cycle, when assaying reproductive hormones.

ASSESSMENT OF ENDOCRINE FUNCTION

Quantitation of Circulating Hormones and Metabolic Products

Endocrine function is assessed by accurately measuring the concentration of hormones present in blood. Even though circulating concentrations are low (nM to μM for steroid hormones and thyroxine and pM to nM for peptide hormones), precise assays based on competitive protein binding are widely available. Most clinical assays use antibodies that bind the hormone of interest with high affinity and high specificity. Both polyclonal and monoclonal antibodies are used; monoclonal antibodies have the advantage of purity and virtually unlimited supply. As originally developed, radioimmunoassays (RIA) mix radiolabeled hormone with specific antibody in the presence of increasing con-

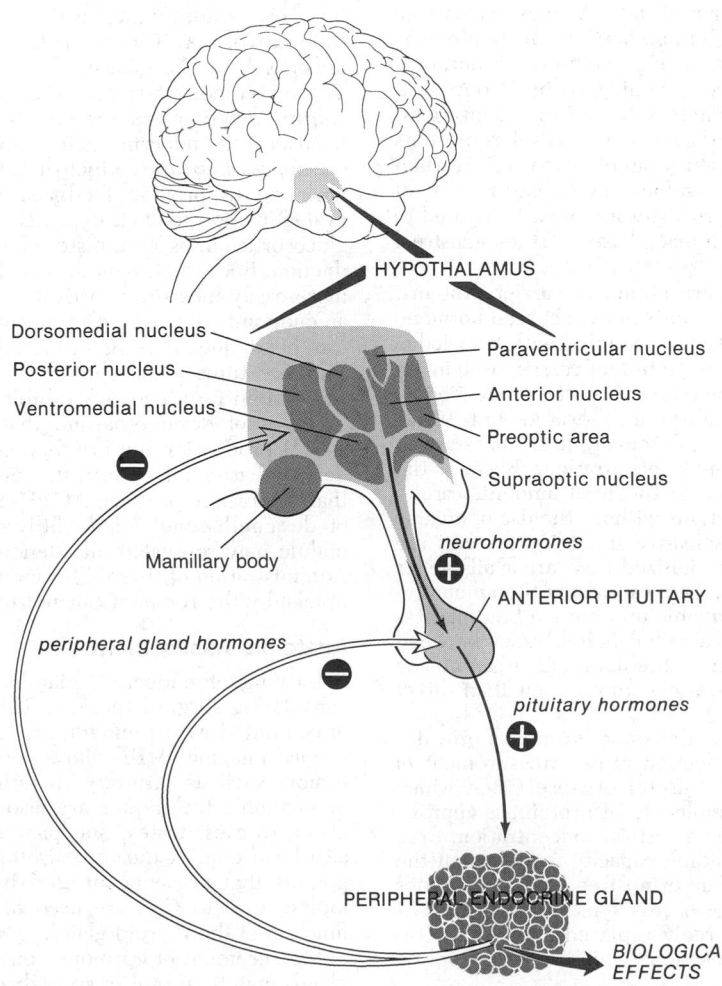

FIGURE 208–6. Forward regulation and negative feedback.

centrations of standard unlabeled hormone. Unlabeled hormone competes with radiolabeled hormone for binding to antibody to generate a standard curve of decreasing radioactive hormone bound to antibody. Samples for assay are mixed with radiolabeled hormone and antibody, and the extent of displacement of radiolabeled hormone from subsequently isolated antibody can be directly compared to displacement by known amounts of hormone. For a sensitive, precise assay a specific high-affinity antibody, a radiolabeling procedure that does not damage the hormone, and unlabeled pure hormone are required. To avoid radioactivity, enzyme-linked immunoabsorbent assays (ELISA) have been increasingly adapted. These assays use enzyme activity to generate a color change that can be quantitated with a spectrophotometer. Two antibodies directed against different epitopes in the same hormone molecule may be used. The first antibody binds hormone and is immobilized; the second antibody with an attached enzyme is then added and the amount of antibody-bound enzyme activity provides a measure of the amount of hormone attached to the first antibody. Other assays use fluorescent dyes attached to either the hormone standard or to a second antibody. Improved sensitivity and accuracy of hormone measurements reduce the need to perform more complex stimulation and suppression tests.

Even with sensitive and precise assays of hormone concentration, clinical assessment is essential. Measured values must be interpreted in relation to clinical signs and symptoms. It is also extremely helpful to measure both arms of a feedback loop. Most hormone concentrations exhibit a gaussian distribution of normal values, so an individual measurement at either end of the normal range may be normal or abnormal for that individual. Coincident measurement of TSH and T_4, LH and testosterone, ACTH and cortisol, PTH and Ca^{2+} gives greater information than either alone. A T_4 at the lower end of the normal range with an elevated TSH indicates thyroid gland failure, whereas the same T_4 with a normal TSH likely indicates a euthyroid state. An elevated cortisol with suppressed ACTH indicates autonomous production of cortisol by an adrenal tumor. Cycles and rhythms of hormone secretion must also be considered. Evening cortisol concentrations are half or less of peak morning values. Coincident measurement of ACTH clarifies whether a low cortisol represents diurnal rhythm or adrenal insufficiency; an elevated ACTH when cortisol is low suggests adrenal insufficiency. Measurement of gonadotropins and estradiol and progesterone must be related to normal values for follicular and luteal phases of the menstrual cycle.

Steroid and thyroid hormones are bound to carrier proteins. Most measurements use organic solvents to extract total hormone for assay. This is usually sufficient when coupled with knowledge of effects of hormones on the concentration of carrier protein. In pregnancy, in which estrogen increases hepatic production of carrier proteins, cortisol and T_4 values are elevated, but ACTH and TSH are normal. On occasion, however, it is necessary to measure the free, active hormone concentration. Because the free fraction is very small relative to the total amount, careful separation of bound from free fractions without the use of organic solvents is necessary, and very sensitive detection systems are required. Assays for free T_4 and for ionized Ca^{2+} are available for specialized clinical circumstances. One can assess the amount of binding globulin by RIA or the available unoccupied binding sites by measuring the distribution of a radiolabeled tracer between soluble binding globulin and an insoluble matrix (T_3 resin uptake tests). These indirect tests provide less information than direct measurements of free hormone.

Measurement of urinary excretion of some hormones provides an integrated value for daily production rates. Measurement of urinary free cortisol is particularly useful because CBG, which binds one cortisol molecule per molecule of protein, is approximately saturated at the peak morning cortisol concentration. Free unbound cortisol that exceeds binding capacity is filtered at the glomerulus, so an elevated 24-hour urine free cortisol provides an accurate assessment of cortisol excess syndromes (Ch. 217). Precise RIA's or ELISA's have largely replaced chemical methods, such as the Porter-Silber reaction, which measure only a fraction of cortisol metabolites.

Measurement of metabolic effects is an essential component of endocrine evaluation. Insulin function is assessed by measuring plasma and urine glucose concentrations, PTH by measuring serum $[Ca^{2+}]$, aldosterone by measuring serum $[K^+]$, and ADH by measuring serum and urine osmolalities.

Stimulation and Suppression Tests

Measurement of both arms of a feedback loop provides sufficient laboratory information in most endocrine deficiency or excess states. Additional diagnostic information can be gained, however, by perturbing the feedback system through administration of hormones.

For *stimulation tests* a hormone is administered and the ability of the target gland to respond is assessed by measuring its product. This provides an estimate of the ability of the target gland to synthesize hormone, of its trophic maintenance, and of its exposure to feedback inhibition. Baseline measurements are made before hormone administration and at the established normal time of peak target gland response. Ranges of normal responses have been established for comparison. Examples include TRH stimulation tests, in which serum levels of pituitary-produced TSH are measured. In hypopituitarism, serum TSH fails to rise in response to a standard intravenous injection of TRH. In primary hypothyroidism, in which feedback inhibition by thyroid hormone is small, TSH rises excessively, whereas in hyperthyroidism excessive feedback inhibition results in minimal or no increases in TSH. For ACTH stimulation tests $ACTH_{1-24}$ is administered as an intravenous injection to assess the ability of the adrenal cortex to produce cortisol. A low baseline cortisol that fails to rise indicates adrenal insufficiency. Interpretation requires integration of clinical information because failure to respond to ACTH may also occur when the adrenal cortex has been suppressed as a result of treatment with synthetic glucocorticoids. A variation of stimulation tests involves interruption of the feedback loop by metabolic inhibitors of hormone biosynthesis. Metyrapone, an inhibitor of 11β-hydroxylase, decreases serum cortisol, relieving feedback suppression of ACTH production. The resulting increase in ACTH can be measured directly. Alternatively, ACTH-stimulated 11-desoxycortisol, the precursor of cortisol, can be measured as an indicator of increased ACTH. The metyrapone test provides an assessment of pituitary corticotrope function and reserve. Stimulation tests are most useful in suspected endocrine deficiency states.

Suppression tests, which measure the ability of administered hormone to provide feedback inhibition, are most useful in evaluating hormone excesses. Dexamethasone, a potent synthetic glucocorticoid, is administered to feedback inhibit ACTH production. Because dexamethasone is not detected in cortisol assays, more easily measured cortisol rather than ACTH can be used as an endpoint. In Cushing's syndrome, the source of cortisol excess can be deduced using dexamethasone suppression (Ch. 217). Pituitary tumors that produce excess ACTH frequently retain susceptibility to feedback inhibition. These tumors are resistant to doses of dexamethasone that suppress normal corticotrope ACTH production but are feedback inhibited by higher doses of dexamethasone. In contrast, adrenal gland tumors and tumors that ectopically produce ACTH are resistant to even high doses of dexamethasone. In a euthyroid patient a hyperfunctioning nodule may represent an adenoma or a thyroid gland remnant. Administration of thyroid hormone suppresses radioactive iodine uptake by the remnant but not by the adenoma.

Anatomic Assessment

Imaging of endocrine glands is important, especially when considering surgical therapy. The high sensitivity and precision of computed axial tomography (CAT) and nuclear magnetic resonance imaging (MRI) allow detection of even small endocrine tumors such as pituitary, parathyroid, and adrenal adenomas. Sonographic techniques are also useful for imaging the thyroid gland, ovaries, testes, and pancreas. Radionuclide imaging may also be useful. Radioactive isotopes of iodine (^{123}I, ^{131}I) or compounds that are concentrated by the thyroid gland similar to iodine, such as ^{99}Tc, are used to determine anatomy and imply function of the thyroid gland.

Measurement of hormone concentrations in venous effluent of glands may be useful in specialized circumstances to localize the source of abnormal production. Measurement of ACTH in petrosal sinus blood may be useful in localizing pituitary tumors, PTH in neck and chest veins in localizing unusually located parathyroid adenomas, and insulin in mesenteric venous drainage in localizing pancreatic insulinomas.

Cytologic and immunocytochemical techniques are important. Fine-needle aspiration of thyroid nodules with cytologic examinations analogous to those used in Papanicolaou smears has become the procedure of choice to distinguish benign and malignant thyroid nodules. Staining of surgical tissues with antihormone antibodies provides proof of hormone production and serves as a guide to future therapy.

Receptors are not routinely measured but can be quantitated using immunologic techniques. Recombinant DNA technologies can be used to define inherited defects in receptors. When oncogenes are identified in specific endocrine neoplasms, these can be measured and mutations identified using DNA hybridization techniques. Autoimmune endocrine diseases can be documented by quantitating antibodies directed against specific organs (thyroid-stimulating immunoglobulin, anti–islet cell antibodies, antiadrenal antibodies).

ABERRATIONS IN DISEASE

Deficiency States

The most prevalent endocrine disorders result from hormone deficiencies. A variety of disease states impair or destroy endocrine glands: defects in organ development, genetic defects in biosynthetic enzymes, immune-mediated destruction, neoplasia, infections, hemorrhage, nutritional deficits, and vascular insufficiency. Endocrine gland failure may be acute with rapid development of symptoms or chronic with slower development of symptoms but more pronounced physical changes. Defects in a gland such as the thyroid may result in a multisystem disorder due to failure to produce a single hormone, whereas defects in the hypothalamus or pituitary may result in a multisystem disorder, including thyroid deficiency, due to failure to produce many hormones. Multiple endocrine gland deficiencies may also result from autoimmune-mediated mechanisms in the polyglandular autoimmune deficiency syndromes (Ch. 228). Because hormones participate in coordinated responses, secondary changes in other endocrine responses often result from deficiency of a single hormone.

Deficiency states also result from defects in hormone receptors and in signaling mechanisms. Defects may be inherited or acquired. Genetic abnormalities in androgen receptors result in unresponsiveness to androgens and an XY male with a female phenotype (Ch. 221); defects in vitamin D receptors result in vitamin D–resistant rickets (Ch. 233); defects in thyroid hormone receptors result in the resistance to thyroid hormone of Refetoff's syndrome (Ch. 216); defects in growth hormone receptors result in ateliotic dwarfism of Laron's syndrome (Ch. 213). Acquired receptor defects most often result from immunologic mechanisms whereby antibodies bind to receptors, blocking ligand access.

Postreceptor defects may occur. A defect in $G_\alpha s$ results in pseudohypoparathyroidism with unresponsiveness to PTH. Such patients fail to respond normally to other hormones whose receptors couple to adenylate cyclase (TSH, glucagon, LH). Type II diabetes mellitus, which is inherited, is characterized by insulin resistance (Ch. 218). The molecular defect has not yet been characterized, but understanding this pathophysiology underlies therapeutic approaches directed at reducing resistance to and augmenting secretion of insulin. Because receptor and postreceptor defects are characterized by hormone resistance, feedback does not occur and producer glands enlarge and circulating hormone concentrations are high despite clinical evidence for deficiency.

Excess States

Excessive production of hormone and clinical evidence of such excess imply failure of normal feedback mechanisms. This occurs most commonly with neoplasia and with autoimmunity, in which antireceptor antibodies act as hormone agonists. Tumors of endocrine glands characteristically produce excessive amounts of the hormone made by the cell of origin but are no longer subject to normal feedback controls. Some tumors, such as pituitary adenomas that produce ACTH, retain feedback but require higher concentrations of cortisol to suppress ACTH. Prolactinomas retain dopamine suppression, and both their function and growth can be inhibited by dopamine agonists. Tumors arising in peripheral endocrine glands that are under pituitary trophic hormone regulation are autonomous because they are not normally subject to negative feedback. More undifferentiated tumors may also be insensitive to feedback regulation.

Hormones may be produced in excess by tumors arising from cells that do not normally produce the hormone (Ch. 161). Ectopic production of peptide hormones is common in a variety of neoplasms, and symptoms due to the hormone excess may contribute significantly to morbidity. Because steroid hormones are made via a multienzyme pathway, excesses of these hormones occur only with tumors arising in the producer gland or when there is excessive production of the trophic peptide hormone. Cortisol excess may result from adrenocortical tumors or from excessive stimulation by ACTH produced by pituitary or ectopic neoplasms.

The most prevalent disease due to agonistic antibodies is Graves' disease, in which antibodies are produced that activate the TSH receptor (Ch. 216). Because many hormones are available as therapeutic agents, some patients take excessive amounts and present with an endocrine excess syndrome.

Genetic Determinants of Disease

Many endocrine diseases result from genetic mutations, although only a minority of these have been characterized. Genetic defects in biosynthetic enzymes may result in deficiency states: Hypothyroidism may result from thyroid peroxidase or deiodinase enzyme defects; adrenal insufficiency may result from 21-hydroxylase deficiency or a defect in other steroid biosynthetic enzymes; a form of male hypogonadism may result from 5α-reductase deficiency. Receptor defects are thought to be uncommon, but methods to define these have only recently become available. Type II diabetes, the most common endocrine abnormality, is inherited but its molecular basis is not yet known. Autoimmune endocrine disease also has a genetic basis involving an inherited defect in immune surveillance. Multiple endocrine neoplasia syndromes are likely due to defects in tumor suppressor genes analogous to that which occurs in retinoblastoma (Ch. 228).

As normal structures become defined, mutations can be identified. Once these are defined, precise diagnostic methods using nucleic acid probes can be used to make precise diagnoses in disease states and to provide predictive information before overt disease develops. Because genetic defects are present in all DNA, peripheral blood cells or skin fibroblasts provide a ready source of material for assay. Development of such assays will improve precision in diagnosis of endocrine disorders.

Alberts B, Bray D, Lewis J, et al. (eds.): Molecular Biology of the Cell. New York, Garland Publishing Inc., 1989. *Chapter 12 gives an excellent overview of hormonal signaling mechanisms.*

Beato M: Gene regulation by steroid hormones. Cell 56:335, 1989. *Concise review of mechanisms of steroid hormone action.*

Berridge MJ, Irvine RF: Inositol phosphates and cell signalling. Nature 341:197, 1989. *Review of this second messenger signaling system.*

Bourne HR, Sanders DA, McCormick F: The GTPase superfamily: A conserved switch for diverse cell functions. Nature 348:125, 1990. *Thoughtful review of how the large number of G proteins work.*

Felig F, Baxter JD, Broadus AE, et al. (eds.): Endocrinology and Metabolism, 2nd ed. New York, McGraw-Hill, 1987. *Textbook of endocrinology containing six introductory chapters on principles of endocrinology and pathophysiology of diseases affecting the endocrine system.*

Gilman AG: G proteins and regulation of adenylyl cyclase. JAMA 262:1819, 1989. *Albert Lasker Award lecture concisely reviewing G protein function.*

Levitzki A: From epinephrine to cyclic AMP. Science 241:800, 1988. *Summary of signaling by β-adrenergic receptors; a good model for receptors that signal via cAMP.*

Weinberg RA (ed.): Oncogenes and the Molecular Origins of Cancer. Cold Spring Harbor, New York, Cold Spring Harbor Laboratory Press, 1989. *Monograph that provides a precise summary of concepts of regulation of growth and how normal control mechanisms are disordered in malignancy.*

West JB (ed.): Best and Taylor's Physiological Basis of Medical Practice, 12th ed. New York, Williams & Wilkins, 1990. *Sections 7 and 8, Metabolism and Endocrine Systems, detail physiologic principles of each of the major endocrine glands and metabolic systems.*

209 The Endorphin Family of Opioid Peptides: Biochemistry, Anatomy, and Physiology

Stanley J. Watson

Many structures throughout the central and peripheral nervous system contain cells that secrete peptides. Major among these is a family of endogenous neuropeptides capable of mimicking many actions of opiate alkaloids, such as morphine and heroin. These peptides have a common pentapeptide sequence at their amino terminus [Tyr-Gly-Gly-Phe-Met (or-Leu)], which is important for their opiate activity. All such *endogenous opioid peptides* carry the generic name of endorphins (*endogenous morphines*). There are actually three main families of endorphins, each with its own separate protein precursor, mRNA, and gene (Fig. 209–1). (1) *Pro-Opio-Melano-Cortin* (or POMC), (2) Pro-Enkephalin, and (3) Pro-Dynorphin/Neo-Endorphin. POMC produces one opiate peptide, β-endorphin, and several nonopioid products, e.g., ACTH and α-, β-, and γ-melanocyte-stimulating hormones (MSH). In contrast, pro-enkephalin has seven repeated opioid sequences, and pro-dynorphin has three.

The discovery of three families of endorphins with their many active peptides grew out of a rich set of pharmacologic tools and behavioral paradigms. Briefly, the structural pharmacology of the opiate alkaloids allowed the description of active and inactive stereoisomers of both opiate agonists and antagonists. The introduction of radiolabeled versions of the active alkaloids made it possible, in the early 1970's, to describe the existence of opiate receptors in brain. A search for their natural ligands followed, and more than 20 active peptide fragments were extracted and sequenced during the next decade—chief among these are β-endorphin, met- and leu-enkephalin, and dynorphin. Gene and mRNA information radically improved our knowledge of the sequences of the endorphins within their precursors and provided better understanding of their relationships with their nonopiate fragments. The availability of peptide and precursor sequences then allowed the production of antibodies and nucleic acid probes

for studying the anatomy, peptide biochemistry, nucleic acid biochemistry, receptors, and physiology of all three endorphin families.

All three members of the endorphin family are widely distributed, including being found in brain, heart, lung, adrenal, ovary, pituitary, testes, and gut. Each endorphin originates in a separate set of cells and rarely coexists in the same neuron or endocrine cell with other endorphins. Specifically, POMC is found in the corticotrophs of the anterior lobe of the pituitary, in the arcuate nucleus in the base of the hypothalamus, and in the nucleus tractus solitarius in the brain stem. POMC fibers project heavily through limbic, autonomic, and pain systems. The dynorphin system, more widespread both within the brain and in the periphery, is found in testes, ovary, gut wall, adrenal cortex, and LH and FSH cells of anterior pituitary. In brain the dynorphin system is linked through a very complex fiber network to sympathetic tone, pain systems, motor systems, endocrine control, limbic system, and cortical functions. The enkephalin system, even more widespread than dynorphin and POMC, is found with the catecholamine cells of the adrenal medulla; it is also in heart, lung, gut wall, sympathetic ganglia, and pituitary and shows many brain fiber systems. In brain it is extremely widespread, so that currently only very few circuits linking enkephalin cells and fibers have been described. The most obvious systems impacted by enkephalin are motor, pain, endocrine, autonomic, limbic (reward), cortex, and hippocampus.

As the structure of the endorphin peptides and precursors became clear, major questions arose concerning the biosynthetic processing of the peptides in different neural and endocrine tissue. The most obvious example of tissue-specific processing of the endorphins is found with POMC in the pituitary of the rat. In the anterior lobe the corticotrophs produce, among other peptides, the stress hormone ACTH (1-39). In contrast, in the intermediate lobe (found in most species, but in humans present only in pregnant women and fetuses) that same molecule is further processed to make α-melanocyte-stimulating hormone [or N-acetyl ACTH 1-13 amide and ACTH (18-39)]. Similar tissue-specific processing patterns are found for other POMC peptides, such as β-endorphin, as well as for pro-dynorphin– and pro-enkephalin–produced peptides. For example, pro-enkephalin in adrenal is cleaved into larger fragments, whereas in brain it is actively processed to much smaller peptides.

Several principles have emerged about the processing of neuropeptides. A given precursor can give rise to one set of products in one tissue and a different set of products in another tissue.

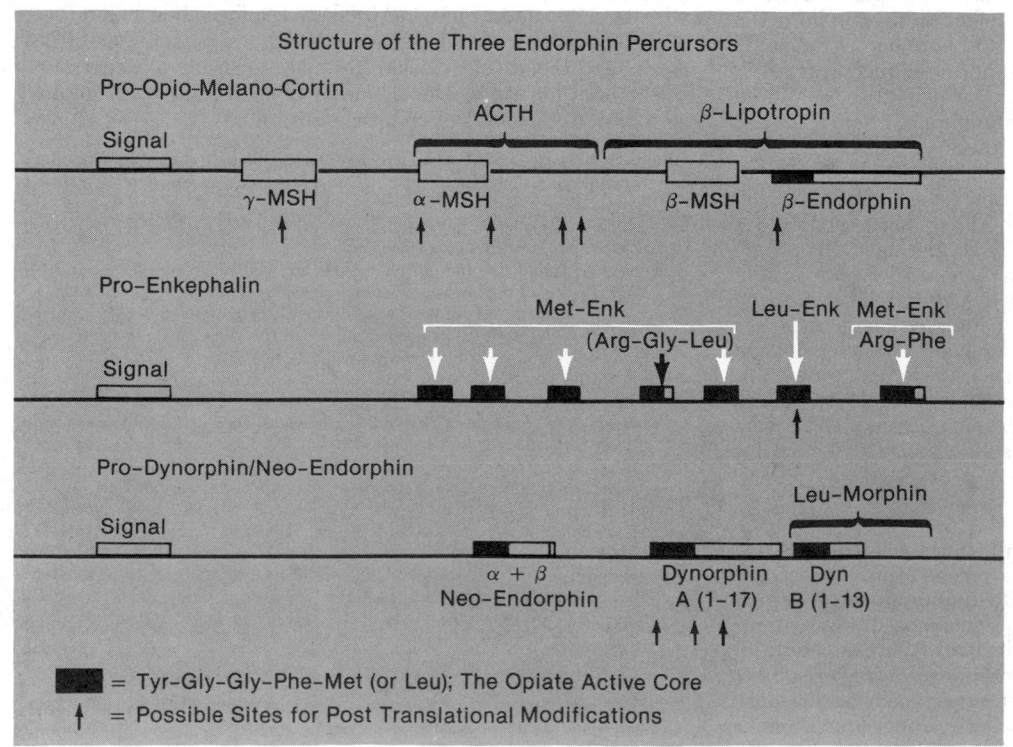

FIGURE 209–1. Simplified schematic of the precursors for all three endorphin families. Note the many peptides produced from each precursor, their similar size, and in the case of pro-enkephalin and pro-dynorphin, the multiple copies of opioid peptides produced by each.

General processing differences are due to the cleavage site chosen, indicated by the presence of a dibasic peptide bond (e.g., lysine-argenine). In a second type of processing variant other chemical moieties are added to a given site in a peptide sequence, e.g., amidation, acetylation, sulfation, or phosphorylation. Both types of processing choices can alter the nature and potency of these molecules. For example, the addition of an acetyl group to the amino terminal tyrosine of β-endorphin decreases its opiate activity by more than 1000-fold. Thus, two of the largest problems in peptidergic systems, especially in brain, are in understanding the precursor-processing pathways and the final structure of the peptides produced by each precursor, in a tissue of interest. Figure 209–1 provides a simplified version of this information for each precursor.

Peptidergic cells have a range of control over the materials that they secrete. To add further complexity, several peptides arise from each of the three endorphin precursors, and nonopioid peptides can be co-produced and co-secreted along with the endorphins (e.g., ACTH and β-endorphin from anterior lobe).

Three main opiate receptor subclasses, each with a different distribution pattern in brain, gut, pituitary, adrenal, and reproductive tissues, have been described (μ, κ, δ).

The μ receptor is very sensitive to morphine; the δ receptor seems to prefer enkephalin-like peptides; the κ receptor was characterized by the action of dynorphin-like peptides. In addition, an ε receptor has been suggested for β-endorphin, although it has been demonstrated only in peripheral tissue. The selectivity of the receptors is not absolute. For example, dynorphin, while κ preferring, is also a potent μ agonist, and enkephalins, while δ preferring, can also interact with the μ site. More accurate characterization of these receptors and their biochemistry, structure, and ligand preferences will depend on the cloning of their respective genes and on study of post-translational modifications of gene products in specific tissues. In addition, there is not a one-to-one anatomic link between κ receptors and dynorphin-producing cells and fibers; nor is there one for the δ receptor and pro-enkephalin systems. Rather, one tends to see two or even three opiate receptor subtypes associated with the terminal systems of the peptidergic neurons. It is conceivable that the processing choices of a cell, by altering the peptide products, can alter the receptor preference of the materials secreted. In effect, it is possible that the cell modulates its products as a function of physiologic or pharmacologic demand, to act on different receptor subtypes at the synapse. Thus, such a system would be extremely flexible in the way it modulates its synaptic transmission.

With a multiplicity of peptides and receptors across a variety of tissues, it is clear that endorphins do not have a single physiologic role. Furthermore, multiple active transmitters and modulators may exist in the same cell. A particularly clear example of "co-transmission" can be found with the pro-dynorphin peptides in the hypothalamus. Pro-dynorphin peptides (and mRNA) are found in the same cells that produce vasopressin. Consistent with this finding, arginine vasopressin (AVP) and dynorphin are co-released from the posterior pituitary with the same stimuli. It is hypothesized that dynorphin provides local feedback inhibition on further AVP secretion. Other examples of co-transmission among the endorphins include enkephalin and catecholamines in the adrenal medulla, enkephalin and catecholamines in the sympathetic nervous system, and dynorphin and LH/FSH in the anterior pituitary.

Table 209–1 summarizes the main physiologic observations associated with the endorphins. The endorphins have been classically associated with modulation of stress and pain. The neuronal and endocrine systems involved in these responses are, in the case of stress, the hypothalamic-pituitary-adrenal system and the limbic system. In fact, each major component of the stress-response system contains endorphins. For example, the hippocampus, a main site of corticosteroid feedback, contains enkephalin and dynorphin neurons; the hypothalamus contains all three opioid families; the anterior pituitary contains POMC and enkephalin; and the adrenal medulla produces enkephalin and the adrenal cortex, dynorphin. A similar pattern is seen in pain-modulatory systems in the spinal cord, periaqueductal central gray, thalamus, and the limbic system. It seems clear that stress and pain responses are, in several ways, dependent on endorphin physiology.

TABLE 209–1. PROPOSED FUNCTIONS AND KNOWN ANATOMIC LOCALIZATIONS OF THE ENDOGENOUS OPIOID SYSTEMS

Function	Anatomic Localization
Appetite modulation and eating behavior	Limbic system, including hypothalamus and amygdala
Cardiovascular regulation	NTS, parabrachial nucleus
Drinking and water balance	Subfornical organ, magnocellular hypothalamic-pituitary system
Endocrine responses	Hypothalamic-pituitary-peripheral axis
Stimulatory effects on Growth hormone Melanocyte-stimulating hormone Prolactin	Hypothalamus and anterior lobe
Inhibitory effects on Follicle-stimulating hormone Luteinizing hormone Thyroid-stimulating hormone	Hypothalamus and anterior lobe
Inhibition of release of vasopressin and oxytocin	Hypothalamus and posterior lobe
Gastrointestinal motility	NTS, area postrema, and GI nervous plexi
Pain inhibition	Thalamus, periaqueductal gray, substantia gelatinosa, NTS, spinal cord
Respiration	Parabrachial nucleus, NTS
Response to stress	Hypothalamic-pituitary-adrenal axis
Sensory-motor integration	Nigrostriatal system, globus pallidus, inferior and superior colliculi
Thermoregulation	Hypothalamus

NTS = Nucleus tractus solitarius.

The physiology of the endorphins presents certain patterns in Table 209–1: (1) These peptides are implicated in a wide variety of physiologic events. (2) Many of these events correlate fairly well with the anatomy of the opioid peptides. For example, all three endorphins are found in the nucleus tractus solitarius and are implicated in cardiovascular regulation; gut motility is controlled from the brain and gut opiatergic loci; respiration is regulated partially by the parabrachial nucleus, an area with both opiate peptides and receptors; and motor integration actively involves the nigrostriatal system, rich in opioid anatomy. (3) The functions associated with the endorphins are basic, homeostatic, limbic, "core" functions; they do not seem to be primarily cognitive but may be more affective or drive related. (4) There are a few "unexpected" physiologic links, such as appetite modulation, drinking, and thermoregulation.

The current state of endorphin biology does not allow precise links between particular peptides, neural circuits or receptors, and specific behaviors. Only a few such inferences can be made. For example, dynorphin in posterior pituitary may play a role in thirst regulation, or anterior pituitary POMC may be involved in stress responses.

Finally, perhaps the most exciting set of advances has come from the study of the regulation of the transcription of pro-enkephalin and POMC genes. Several enhancer and repressor DNA sequences have been identified in the 5' untranslated flanking regions of both genes. Among these are sequences that respond to A and C kinase second messenger systems, and to glucocorticoids. The specific proteins that bind to those sites have been described and in some cases sequenced.

It is clear that the next decade will be one of consolidation and organization of the great wealth of biologic data on these important systems. One of the main foci will be a clearer view of the physiology-peptide-receptor interface; the other will be an increased understanding of the genetic regulation of these systems. With the increasing clarity will come an improved appreciation of the regulation of a whole series of critical basic brain functions.

Akil H, Bronstein D, Mansour A: Overview of the endogenous opioid systems. In Rodgers RJ, Cooper SJ (eds.): Endorphins, Opiates and Behavioral Processes.

Chichester, John Wiley and Sons Limited, 1988, pp 1–23. *A general overview of the biochemistry, anatomy, and physiology of endorphins.*

Herbert E, Seasholtz A, Comb M, et al.: Study of the regulation of expression of neuropeptide genes by gene transfer methods. *In* Psychopharmacology: The Third Generation of Progress. New York, Raven Press, 1987, pp 373–384. *A summary of the gene structure and promoter elements of several peptide genes.*

Holoday JW: Endogenous opioids and their receptors. *In* Current Concepts. Kalamazoo, Mich. Upjohn Company, 1984, pp 4–64. *A summary of some of the physiologic functions attributable to the endogenous opioid systems. It is particularly recommended for the novice who wishes to have a general summary of opioid systems and their possible function.*

Khachaturian H, Lewis ME, Schafer MK, et al.: Anatomy of the CNS opioid systems. Trends Neurosc 8(3):111, 1985. *A summary of the cells and circuits that contain endorphin peptides in brain.*

Mansour A, Khachaturian H, Lewis ME, et al.: Anatomy of CNS opioid receptors. Trends Neurosc 11(7):308, 1988. *A summary of the distribution of the three types of opioid receptors in rat brain.*

Mansour A, Schafer MKH, Newman SW, et al.: Central distribution of opioid receptors: A cross-species comparison of the multiple opioid systems of the basal ganglia. *In* Almeida OFX, Shippenberg TS (eds.): Opioid Peptides and Receptors. Berlin, Springer-Verlag, in press.

Martin WR: Pharmacology of opioids. Pharmacol Rev 32:283, 1984. *An authoritative and comprehensive review of opiate pharmacology. The author presents an in-depth analysis of how different classes of opiates may influence analgesia, respiration, cardiovascular function, pupil dilation, temperature, EEG, and dependence.*

Millan MJ, Herz A: The endocrinology of the opioids. Int Rev Neurobiol 26:1, 1985. *A comprehensive review of the role of the opioid peptides and receptors in neuroendocrine responses. The authors have worked many years in this area and provide a thoughtful review of this field.*

210 Prostaglandins and Related Compounds

Garret A. FitzGerald

Arachidonic acid, derived from dietary sources, is transported in plasma in both esterified and nonesterified forms, primarily bound to lipoproteins and albumin, respectively. The relative importance of these two sources for cellular delivery is poorly understood. Esterified arachidonic acid in low density lipoproteins is taken up by cells by a process dependent on the low density lipoprotein receptor. The fatty acid is compartmentalized in the phospholipid domain of cell membranes. This localization appears relevant to the availability of arachidonate for release (in response to specific stimuli as well as to nonspecific physical and chemical perturbation of membranes) for subsequent oxygenation by either cyclo-oxygenase or lipoxygenase to give rise to biologically active compounds. A third pathway of metabolism via cytochrome P-450 also exists (Fig. 210–1).

All cells can release arachidonic acid, but the predominant enzymatic products that are formed are highly cell specific. Because they are derived from a polyunsaturated eicosanoic (C_{20}) fatty acid, these compounds—thromboxane A_2, the prostaglandins (PG's), epoxygenases, leukotrienes, and lipoxins—are collectively known as eicosanoids. Because of their diverse biologic properties and rapid metabolism to inactive products, the eicosanoids have

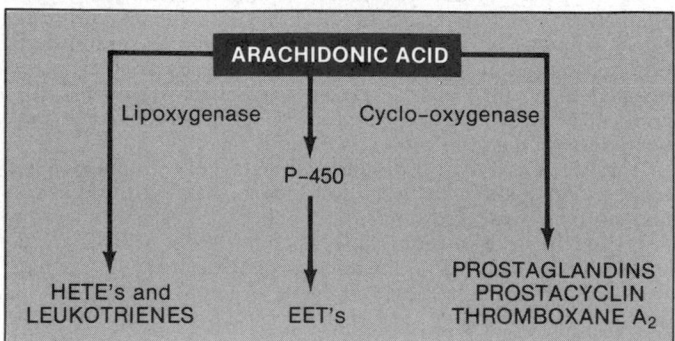

FIGURE 210–1. Major pathways of metabolism of arachidonic acid.

been implicated as local mediators of receptor-dependent events in a range of physiologic processes and in diverse human diseases, including bronchial asthma, inflammation, and unstable coronary disease. Arachidonic acid itself and its metabolites may also function as intracellular second messengers, particularly in the modulation of ion channels.

THE CYCLO-OXYGENASE PATHWAY (Fig. 210–2)

The biotransformation of arachidonic acid into thromboxane (Tx)A_2, prostacyclin (PGI$_2$), PGE$_2$, PGF$_{2\alpha}$, and PGD$_2$ is catalyzed by a common enzyme, the fatty acid cyclo-oxygenase. The product of the cyclo-oxygenase reaction is an unstable endoperoxide, PGG. A second oxygen molecule is then introduced at C_{15}; this results in the 15-hydroperoxy endoperoxide PGH, and liberates a free radical. The cyclo-oxygenase and peroxidase activities reside in a single membrane-associated protein, PGG/H synthase, for which the human gene has been cloned and localized to chromosome 9.

PGH is metabolized by cell-specific enzymes to form either the "classic" prostaglandins of the D, E, and F series, PGI$_2$, or TxA$_2$. Arachidonic acid contains four double bonds ($\Delta^{5,8,11,14}$). It is apparent from the sequence of biosynthesis (Fig. 210–2) that two double bonds remain in its (bisenoic) cyclo-oxygenase products. This is denoted by the subscript 2, as in TxA$_2$ and PGE$_2$. Analogous metabolism of other fatty acid substrates gives rise to monoenoic or trienoic prostaglandins and thromboxanes (Fig. 210–3). For example, metabolites of eicosatrienoic acid ($C_{20:3}$n-6) contain only one (Δ^{13}) double bond. Eicosapentaenoic acid (EPA) ($C_{20:5}$n-3), which is prevalent in certain fish and aquatic mammals, is transformed by cyclo-oxygenase to metabolites with three ($\Delta^{5,13,17}$) double bonds, such as PGI$_3$ and TxA$_3$. Structurally, prostaglandins of the D, E, and F series possess a cyclopentane ring and differ only in their substituent groups. The F series prostaglandins are referred to as PGF$_{1\alpha}$, PGF$_{2\alpha}$, and PGF$_{3\alpha}$. In man, many of the metabolites formed from PGD$_2$ contain an F ring and one of these, $9\alpha,11\beta$-PGF, contracts bronchial and vascular smooth muscle and inhibits platelet aggregation.

THROMBOXANE A$_2$. TxA$_2$, the predominant cyclo-oxygenase product formed by platelets, stimulates aggregation of these cells and constricts vascular and bronchial smooth muscle. These biologic properties are shared by the PG endoperoxides. Use of analogues of PGH$_2$ and/or TxA$_2$ has identified specific binding sites for these eicosanoids on many tissues, including platelets, vascular smooth muscle cells, and glomerular mesangial cells. A cDNA encoding a placental TxA$_2$ receptor has been cloned. The relative rank order potency of different ligands suggests that distinct receptors mediate platelet aggregation and smooth muscle cell contraction. Indeed, it appears that different forms of the receptor (or distinct receptors) transduce the platelet shape change and aggregation responses to these eicosanoids. The relative affinity of these receptors for PGH$_2$ and TxA$_2$ is unknown. Platelet aggregation is induced via receptors linked to a G protein (that is insensitive to pertussis toxin) to activate phospholipase (PL) C. TxA$_2$ is very evanescent at physiologic pH; its half-life has been estimated at 30 seconds.

In addition to initiating aggregation of platelets, TxA$_2$ that is generated by platelets aggregated in response to epinephrine, adenosine diphosphate (ADP), and platelet-activating factor (PAF) is responsible for a "secondary wave" of aggregation. Aspirin inhibits platelet aggregation by preventing the formation of TxA$_2$, although the capacity of platelets to form TxA$_2$ must be inhibited by greater than 95 per cent for even modest inhibition of platelet function.

PROSTACYCLIN. Prostacyclin (PGI$_2$), the predominant cyclo-oxygenase product of arachidonic acid formed by vascular endothelium and also by subendothelium, both inhibits the aggregation of platelets by all recognized agonists and disaggregates previously aggregated platelets. PGI$_2$ inhibits the adherence of platelets and neutrophils to foreign surfaces and damaged endothelium and dilates both bronchial and vascular smooth muscle. PGI$_2$ acts at specific binding sites to activate adenylate cyclase via the stimulatory G protein, G$_s$. Another important property of PGI$_2$ is the modulation of cholesterol efflux from arterial walls. Nanomolar quantities of PGI$_2$ stimulate the activity of both the lysosomal and cytoplasmic cholesterol ester hydrolases when added experimentally to vascular smooth muscle cells but have

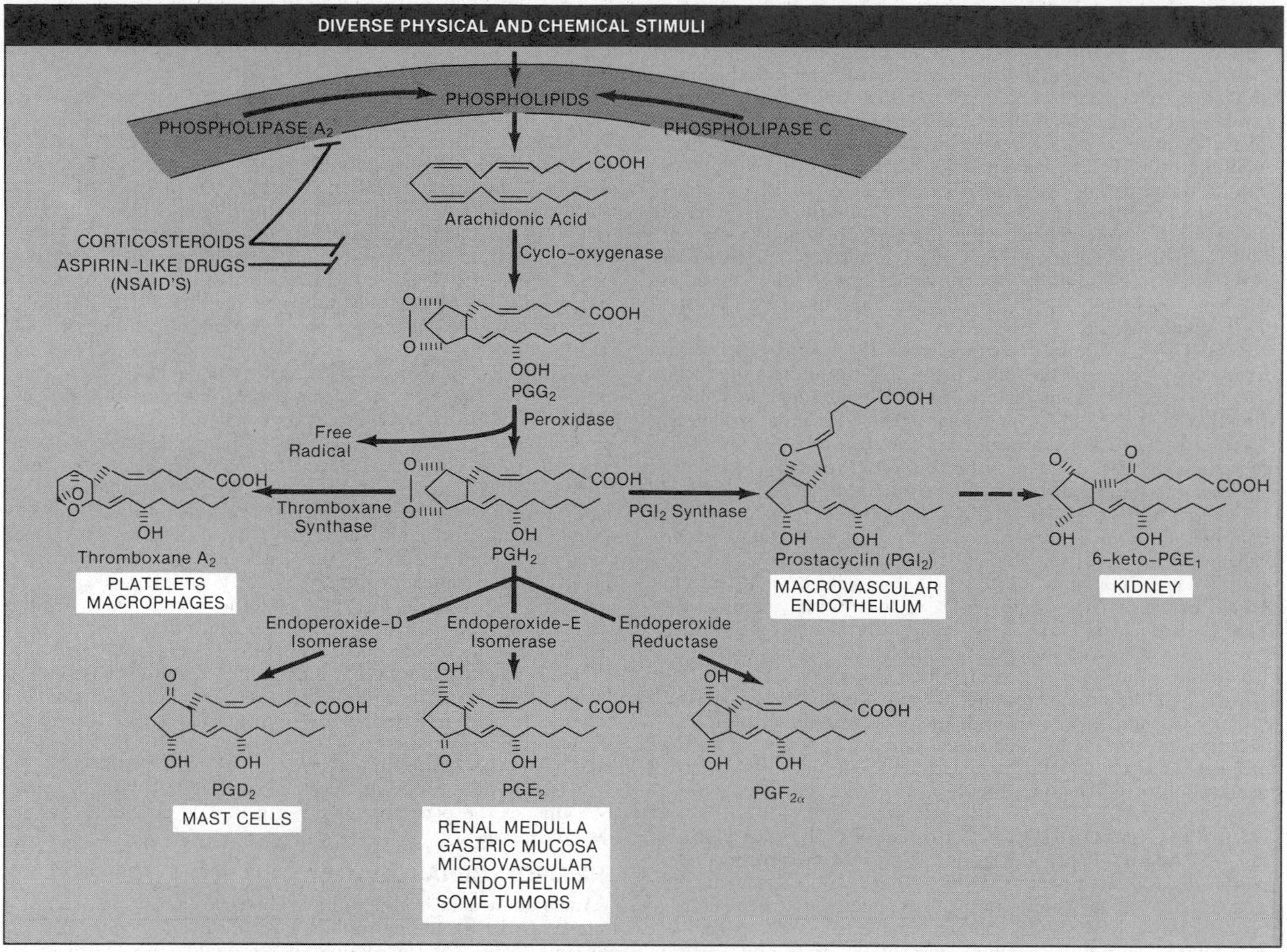

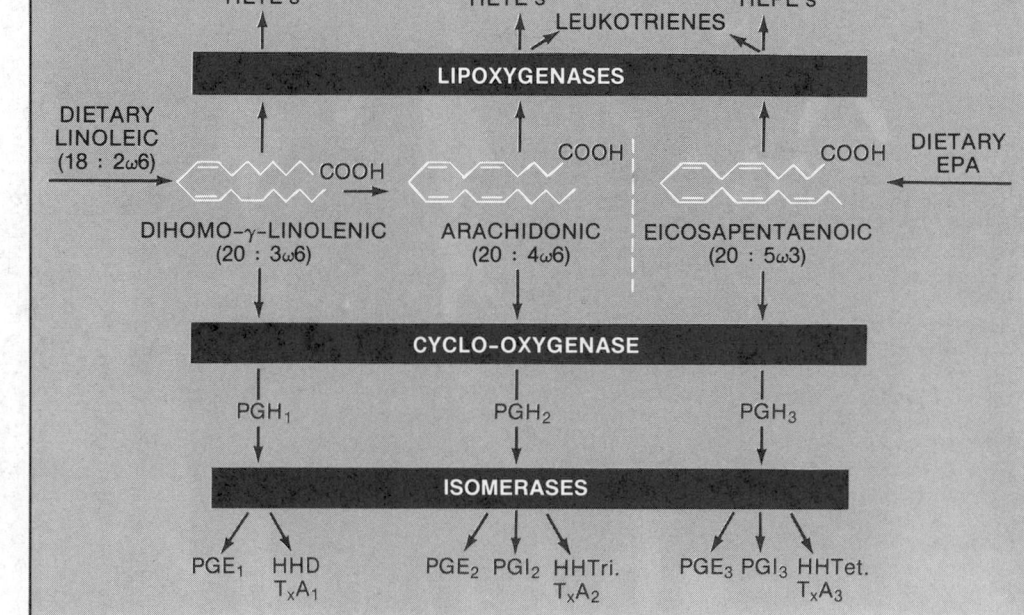

FIGURE 210–2. Metabolism of arachidonic acid by fatty acid cyclo-oxygenase. The major tissues of origin of the eicosanoids are shown.

FIGURE 210–3. Analogous formation of mono-, bis-, and trienoic prostaglandins. (Reproduced with permission from FitzGerald GA, Price P, Knapp HR: Biochemical and functional effects of dietary substrate modification in man. *In* Simopoulos AP, Kifer RR, Martin RE (eds.): Health Effects of Polyunsaturated Fatty Acids in Seafoods. Orlando, FL, Academic Press, 1986, pp 61–80.)

no effect on the microsomal acyl-CoA cholesterol acyl transferase (ACAT), which re-esterifies free cholesterol.

PGI_2, like TxA_2, is evanescent at physiologic pH (half-life of 3 minutes). Although PGI_2 differs from other prostaglandins in undergoing minimal metabolism during transit through the lung, circulating concentrations are rarely, if ever, sufficient to mediate a systemic response. Many factors associated with thrombogenesis and vasoconstriction, such as trauma, thrombin, ADP, PAF, endothelin, PGH_2/TxA_2, and platelet-derived growth factor, stimulate PGI_2 formation by endothelial cells in vitro. This suggests that local formation may serve both to limit the deposition of platelets and leukocytes following vascular injury and to prevent their further recruitment. PGI_2 biosynthesis is increased in several human diseases in which evidence of platelet activation is present, including severe peripheral arterial disease and unstable coronary disease.

PROSTAGLANDIN D_2. Prostaglandin D_2, the principal cyclo-oxygenase product of the mast cell, is released, together with histamine and other mediators, by IgE-dependent and other stimuli. Infusion of PGD_2 in humans results in nasal stuffiness, systemic hypotension, and flushing. These symptoms are characteristic of the syndrome of systemic mastocytosis in which there is diffuse mast cell infiltration of tissues (Ch. 252). A minority of patients with this disorder exhibit a rise in blood pressure, rather than hypotension, in association with flushing. One possible explanation for this observation is preferential conversion of PGD_2 to its $9\alpha,11\beta$-PGF metabolite, which contracts vascular smooth muscle in vitro. The role of PGD_2 in the normal immunologic response is unclear. PGD_2 is increased in bronchoalveolar lavage fluid following antigen challenge in atopic individuals, suggesting that it may contribute to the bronchomotor response in allergic asthma. PGD_2 is a minor product of the platelet cyclo-oxygenase. Both PGD_2 and its $9\alpha,11\beta$-PGF metabolite inhibit platelet aggregation by stimulating adenylate cyclase, thereby increasing intraplatelet cyclic AMP. In experimental animals, central administration of PGD_2 induces sleep, an event that is countered by infusion of PGE_2.

PROSTAGLANDIN E_2. The formation of PGE_2 from PGH_2 is catalyzed by a PGE_2 isomerase that is present in renal medulla, gastric mucosa, and platelets. PGE_2 rather than PGI_2 may be the predominant prostaglandin formed by microvascular endothelium. In the kidney, PGE_2 can act both as a vasodilator and as an inhibitor of tubular sodium absorption. In rabbit cortical collecting tubular cells, PGE_2 acts via distinct receptors to stimulate and inhibit adenylate cyclase via G_s and G_i, respectively. In human platelets, PGE_1 and PGI_2 apparently act at an identical receptor site to stimulate adenylate cyclase via G_s and inhibit aggregation. PGE_2 can also act at this site. There is some evidence that PGE_2 can act at a distinct site to exert negative control of the cyclase via G_i.

PGE_2 is the predominant cyclo-oxygenase product of arachidonic acid formed in gastric mucosa. It participates in the regulation of gastric blood flow and limits the effects of diverse physical and chemical insults to the gastric mucosa. This "cytoprotective" property is shared by PGI_2, but the mechanism by which this protection occurs is unknown. Other biologic properties of PGE_2 include relaxation of bronchial smooth muscle, contraction of uterine smooth muscle (19-hydroxylated E prostaglandins are the major arachidonic acid products in human semen), and modulation of lymphocyte function. PGE_2 modulates neurotransmission via presynaptic receptors on adrenergic neurons in vitro.

In a minority of patients with solid tumors, PGE_2 production by the tumor causes hypercalcemia via stimulation of osteoclast activity (Ch. 161). In such cases, suppression of PGE_2 biosynthesis lowers the level of serum calcium. When metastases to bone occur, however, local mechanisms for hypercalcemia supervene. High concentrations of PGE_2 are found in the joint fluid of patients with rheumatoid arthritis. The role of PGE_2 in this setting is unknown, although the clinical response to cyclo-oxygenase inhibitors suggests that eicosanoids are of relevance to the local inflammatory process.

PROSTAGLANDIN $F_{2\alpha}$. $PGF_{2\alpha}$, formed from PGH_2 by the action of an endoperoxide reductase, contracts bronchial and uterine smooth muscle and vasoconstricts some uterine beds. Although increases in $PGF_{2\alpha}$ metabolites have been described during dysmenorrhea and allergen-evoked bronchospasm, a unique site for formation of this prostaglandin and its role in pathophysiology remain to be determined. Novel PGF isomers have been detected in human plasma and urine that are formed by a free radical–catalyzed, cyclo-oxygenase-independent process. One of these compounds, 8-epi-$PGF_{2\alpha}$, is a potent renal vasoconstrictor.

THE LIPOXYGENASE PATHWAY (Fig. 210–4)

Arachidonic acid is also widely subject to lipoxygenation reactions (Fig. 210–4). In neutrophils, insertion of an oxygen molecule adjacent to one of the double bonds yields the hydroperoxy

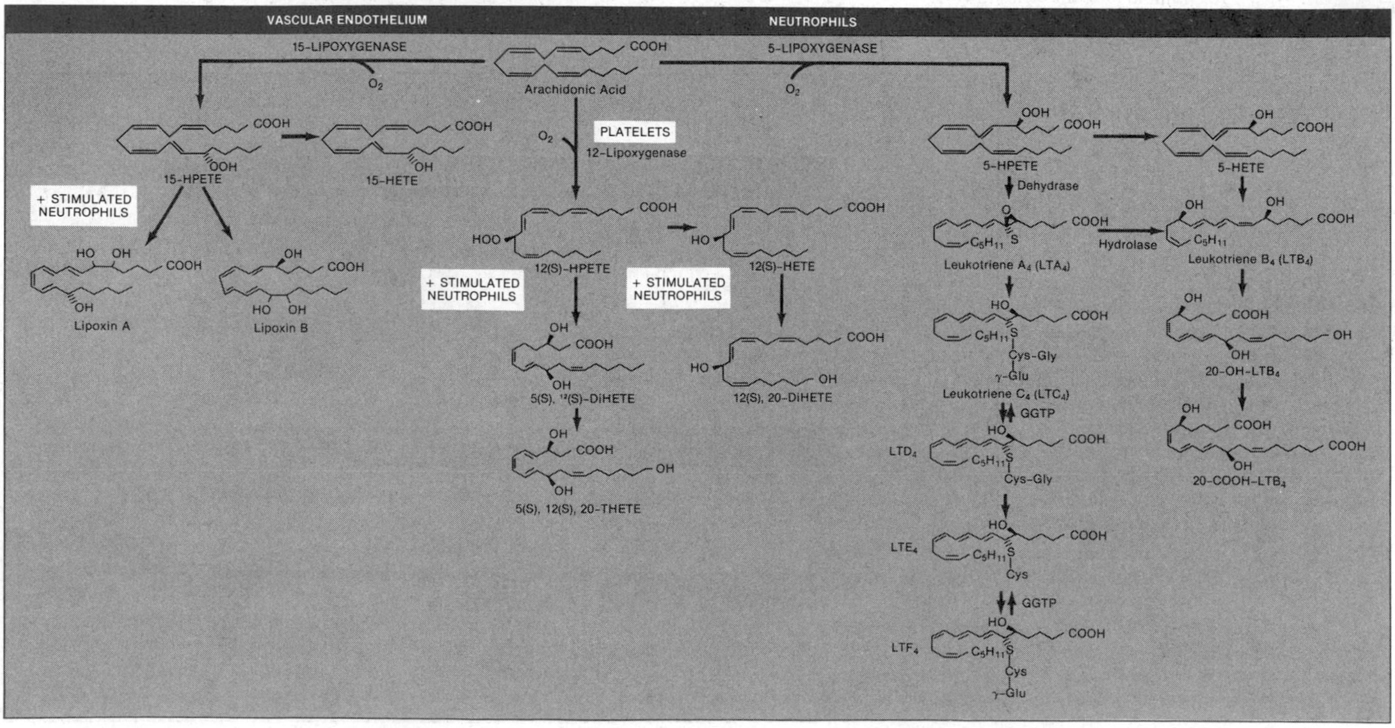

FIGURE 210–4. Metabolism of arachidonic acid by lipoxygenase enzymes.

derivative, 5-hydroperoxyeicosatetraenoic acid (5-HPETE). This can undergo further metabolism to either a 5-hydroxyeicosatetraenoic acid (5-HETE) or to an unstable 5,6-epoxide intermediate, leukotriene (LT)A$_4$. This compound can be hydrolyzed to 5,12-dihydroxyeicosatetraenoic acids, one of which is LTB$_4$. The subscript 4 refers to the number of double bonds. Thus, analogous to the nomenclature for cyclo-oxygenase products, substitution of eicosapentaenoic acid for arachidonic acid as a substrate would result in formation of LTB$_5$. The site of the initial lipoxygenation reaction tends to vary with cell type. Thus, 12-HETE is formed predominantly in platelets, 5-HETE by polymorphonuclear leukocytes, and 5-HETE, 11-HETE, and 15-HETE by endothelial cells as measured in culture.

The 5-lipoxygenase of human neutrophils, a cytosolic enzyme, is translocated to the membrane for metabolism of arachidonic acid. It requires an 18K protein, termed the five lipoxygenase activating protein (FLAP), to achieve full activation. The development of both 5-lipoxygenase inhibitors and of a translocation inhibitor is likely to elucidate the role of the products of this pathway in human physiology and disease. Analogous activating proteins do not appear necessary for expression of 12- and 15-lipoxygenase activity. The primary structures of two distinct 12-lipoxygenases have been reported. One, in porcine leukocytes, is immunologically identical to that in porcine brain and human tracheal cells. It is closely related to the 15-lipoxygenase. The human platelet 12-lipoxygenase is a distinct gene product. The role of 12-HETE in platelets is unknown. Platelet 12-lipoxygenase is translocated from the cytosol to the membrane in a calcium-dependent manner, and 12-HETE inhibits the mobilization of a glycoprotein IIb/IIIa complex in tumor cell lines. This complex is analogous to that which serves as a receptor for adhesive macromolecules, such as fibrinogen, in activated platelets. 12-Lipoxygenase products regulate potassium channel flux in Aplysia. Formation of 15-HETE is reportedly increased in atherosclerotic blood vessels, and recent in situ hybridization studies suggest that expression of the enzyme is increased and colocalized with oxidized low density lipoproteins in human atherosclerotic plaques.

LTA$_4$ is conjugated enzymatically with glutathione to yield LTC$_4$. This compound is metabolized to LTD$_4$ and LTE$_4$ by successive elimination of a γ-glutamyl residue and glycine. The cysteinyl-containing leukotrienes are powerful bronchoconstrictors and vasoconstrictors. In addition, they have been shown to be identical with "slow-reacting substance of anaphylaxis"—a product first identified following immunologic challenge or addition of cobra venom to guinea pig ileum. These compounds also dilate microvessels, increase vascular permeability, and stimulate mucus secretion. LTC$_4$ causes pulmonary bronchoconstriction, an effect that is partially blocked by cyclo-oxygenase inhibitors. This implies that LTC$_4$ may mediate this effect via the release of a bronchoconstrictor prostaglandin, such as thromboxane A$_2$. LTC$_4$ may cooperate with luteinizing hormone–releasing hormone (LHRH) in the control of LH release by cells of the anterior pituitary, judged by in vitro studies.

LTB$_4$ stimulates adhesion, migration, aggregation, enzyme release, and generation of superoxide by polymorphonuclear leukocytes. These biologic properties strongly suggest a role for lipoxygenase products in both inflammation and antigen-evoked bronchoconstriction. DiHETE's can be formed via transcellular metabolism, at least in vitro. Examples include 12,20-DiHETE formed by a mixed suspension of platelets and polymorphonuclear leukocytes. Leukocytes can utilize erythrocyte LTA$_4$ to generate LTB$_4$ and endothelial cells can utilize platelet-derived PGH$_2$ to generate PGI$_2$.

Stimulated human leukocytes can convert 15-HPETE to products termed lipoxins (LX) containing a characteristic tetraenoic structure (Fig. 210–4). The two major products are identified as LXA and LXB. LXA is a potent stimulus to superoxide generation by neutrophils and contracts pulmonary tissue. Both LXA and LXB inhibit natural killer cell cytotoxicity in vitro, by a mechanism distinct from that of PGE$_2$, which decreases the binding between target and effector cells. Another series of compounds with potent biologic properties in vitro are the hepoxilins, formed by an intramolecular rearrangement of 12-HETE. Glutathione conjugates of hepoxilin A$_3$ cause hyperpolarization of rat brain neurons at nanomolar concentrations. Definitive evidence for the formation of either LX's or hepoxilins in vivo has yet to be provided.

THE EPOXYGENASE PATHWAY (Fig. 210–5)

In addition to metabolism by cyclo-oxygenase and lipoxygenase enzymes, arachidonic acid is subject to ω and ω-1 oxidation by cytochrome P-450 enzymes in microsomal preparations. This results in the formation of 19-OH and 19-oxo-eicosatetraenoic acid (by ω-1-oxidation) and 20-OH-eicosatetraenoic and eicosatetraene-1,20-dioic acids (by ω oxidation). In addition, a series of epoxides 14(15)-epoxy-, 11(12)-epoxy-, 8(9)-epoxy-, and 5(6)-epoxy-eicosatrienoic acids (EET's) can be formed by this enzyme from arachidonic acid. These compounds can then be further transformed to vicinyl diols by epoxide hydrolases. One such compound, 11,12-dihydroxyeicosatrienoic acid, inhibits the Na$^+$-K$^+$-ATPase enzyme in vascular smooth muscle. 5(6)-EET inhibits sodium absorption and potassium secretion by the rabbit cortical collecting duct, and synthetic 5(6)-EET stimulates the release of LH and somatostatin by pituitary cells in culture. Interestingly, 8,9-EET and 14,15-EET stereospecifically inhibit human platelet cyclo-oxygenase. By contrast, all EET's studied inhibit platelet aggregation in vitro by a nonspecific mechanism, independent of an effect on thromboxane formation. EET's weakly inhibit monocyte and platelet adherence to endothelial cells. Finally, 5(6)-EET is metabolized to epoxides of PGG$_1$, PGH$_1$, and PGE$_1$ and to the 5S, 6S and 5R, 6R isomers of 5-hydroxy-PGI$_1$. The biosynthesis of EET's has recently been confirmed in vivo. Urinary excretion of their vicinyl diols (DHET's) is increased in normal pregnancy, and further increments, particularly of 14(15)-DHET, are observed in patients with pregnancy-induced hypertension.

PHARMACOLOGIC AND DIETARY REGULATION OF BIOSYNTHESIS

With the exception of P-450–derived metabolites, none of the oxygenated products of arachidonic acid are stored in significant quantities for subsequent release by cells. Release is equivalent to biosynthesis. Arachidonate release may occur by several mechanisms. Phosphatidylinositol (PI) may be hydrolyzed by a PI-specific PLC, yielding diacylglycerol (DAG) and inositol phosphate. DAG is then further hydrolyzed, yielding free arachidonic acid and other fatty acids. Alternatively, phosphatidylcholine (PC) may be hydrolyzed by phospholipase A$_2$(PLA$_2$), yielding arachidonic acid from the sn-2 position. PLA$_2$ may also liberate arachidonic acid from phosphatidylethanolamine. Selectivity of phospholipid compartmentalization and phospholipase action permits some HETE's and EET's to modulate second messenger formation. Thus, 15-HETE incubated with endothelial cells is selectively incorporated into PI, and agonist-evoked activation of PLC results in release of a 1-stearoyl-2(15-HETE)-DAG. Similarly, PLD-catalyzed formation of a modified phosphatidic acid has been demonstrated.

CORTICOSTEROIDS. The effects of steroids on eicosanoid biosynthesis are complex. It is thought that they induce formation of a phospholipase-inhibitory protein, variously named lipocortin, macrocortin, lipomodulin, and renomodulin (see Fig. 210–2). It is hypothesized that initially steroids bind to specific cytosolic receptors and that the complex is then transferred to the nucleus where steroids regulate the expression of genes and subsequently the synthesis of a PLA$_2$-inhibitory protein (Ch. 208). The lipocortin family is derived from a monomeric 40K protein, phosphorylation of which by protein kinases results in its activation as an inhibitor. Interestingly, there is a striking sequence homology between this protein and the 40K protein that is phosphorylated following the binding of epidermal growth factor to its receptor. The amino acid sequence of one member of the family, lipocortin III, is identical to that of inositol 1,2-cyclic phosphate 2 phosphohydrolase. It is possible that other lipocortins are also enzymes that regulate the intracellular levels of inositol phosphate messages during cellular activation. Prevention of protein synthesis blocks the inhibitory effect of steroids on the release of radiolabeled arachidonate by neutrophils with the chemoattractant peptide, f-Met-Leu-Phe. A cDNA has been isolated and cloned that encodes for a 40K protein that inhibits arachidonic acid release from prelabeled cells. Such a role for lipocortin has been disputed, however, especially as lipocortins bind nonspecifically to phospholipids. The effects of steroids on eicosanoid biosynthesis in vivo are complex and appear to exhibit cellular specificity. Although steroids do not affect the activity of constitutively expressed PGG/H synthase, they block its induction in several systems by agents such as interleukin-1, bacterial lipopolysaccharide, and DMSO. There is also some evidence that steroids regulate stimulated increases in phospholipase mRNA. Further studies are necessary to elucidate the contribution of these mechanisms to the therapeutic efficacy of corticosteroids in man.

CYCLO-OXYGENASE INHIBITORS. Nonsteroidal anti-inflammatory drugs (NSAID's) prevent the formation of prostaglandins by inhibiting the enzyme cyclo-oxygenase. This group of drugs includes aspirin, salicylates, indomethacin, ibuprofen, piroxicam, fenoprofen, paracetamol, phenylbutazone, oxyphenbutazone, bolmetin, sulfinpyrazone, and sulindac. Paracetamol (acetaminophen) is a considerably less potent inhibitor than the other compounds, except perhaps in the brain. Aspirin is also unlike the other compounds in that it acetylates a serine residue at position 529, close to the active site of the platelet PGG/H synthase, and inhibits the enzyme irreversibly. This accounts for the unique effects of aspirin on the platelet. While other cells have the capacity for de novo protein synthesis, the anucleate platelet does not; thus inhibition of TxA_2 formation by aspirin persists for the lifetime of the platelet. By contrast, the effects of aspirin on eicosanoid formation by other cells (e.g., prostacyclin biosynthesis by vascular endothelium) are not so prolonged. The irreversible actions of aspirin on platelet cyclo-oxygenase also account for the cumulative inhibition of platelet TxA_2 formation by the repeated administration of low dosages of aspirin (20 to 40 mg per day; a regular aspirin tablet contains 325 mg). This results in partial inhibition of platelet cyclo-oxygenase after single-dose administration. Even though low doses of aspirin tend to depress PGI_2 formation, its effect is more pronounced on platelet TxA_2 biosynthesis during long-term therapy. This relative "biochemical selectivity" for TxA_2 may result from partial recovery of PGI_2 formation or pharmacokinetic properties of the drug. A differential sensitivity of the enzyme in platelets and endothelial cells is a superficially unlikely explanation, given the identity of the deduced primary structures of the PGG/H synthases in the two tissues. Aspirin is subject to extensive first-pass metabolism by the liver, and its deacylated product, salicylic acid, is a weak inhibitor of platelet cyclo-oxygenase. Reduction in the rate of drug delivery in a controlled release preparation permits more efficient hepatic extraction of aspirin. This still permits cumulative inhibition of platelet cyclo-oxygenase in the presystemic circulation, while protecting the cyclo-oxygenase in the systemic vasculature from aspirin exposure.

Tissue-selective inhibition of cyclo-oxygenase may also be possible with sulindac and sulfinpyrazone. These compounds are prodrugs that are converted by the intestinal flora to their sulfide derivatives, which are potent cyclo-oxygenase inhibitors. Renal tissue possesses the capacity to retroconvert these sulfides to their inactive sulfones, and evidence suggests that renal prostaglandin synthesis may be spared by doses of these drugs that completely inhibit TxA_2 formation by platelets.

THROMBOXANE SYNTHASE INHIBITORS AND RECEPTOR ANTAGONISTS. Many imidazole and pyridine analogues selectively inhibit thromboxane synthase. These compounds depress TxA_2 formation without coincidental inhibition of PGI_2 synthesis, as seen with NSAID's. Indeed, following Tx synthase inhibition, accumulated platelet PGH_2 can be utilized by vascular PGI_2 synthase. Tx synthase inhibitors increase the biosynthesis of platelet-inhibitory, vasodilator prostaglandins, such as PGI_2 and PGE_2 at the platelet-vascular interface in man. Although limited clinical trials have failed to demonstrate benefit from these compounds, this may reflect incomplete suppression of TxA_2 biosynthesis throughout the dosing interval with these reversible inhibitors and/or substitution for the action of TxA_2 by accumulated PGH_2. In this regard, antagonists of the shared TxA_2-PGH_2 receptor are currently under study in man. Synergy of these compounds with Tx synthase inhibitors has been demonstrated in animal models of thrombosis, and several drugs that combine both properties are under study in man.

DIETARY SUBSTRATE MODIFICATION. Mortality from coronary heart disease seems to be lower in populations who consume large quantities of n-3 fatty acids, such as EPA, from aquatic mammals or fish. One hypothesis has been that a shift toward the formation of TxA_3 (which is less biologically active than TxA_2) and PGI_3 (which is a platelet-inhibitory, vasodilator compound like PGI_2) may favorably influence platelet–vessel wall interactions (see Fig. 210–3). Although fish oil supplementation of the western diet has only modest effects on platelet function, it has caused apparent regression of atherosclerosis in several animal models. The biologic properties of many eicosanoids suggest their relevance to the evolving atherosclerotic lesion. It is possible that the altered biologic activity of their trienoic analogues, together with other properties of marine oils, such as

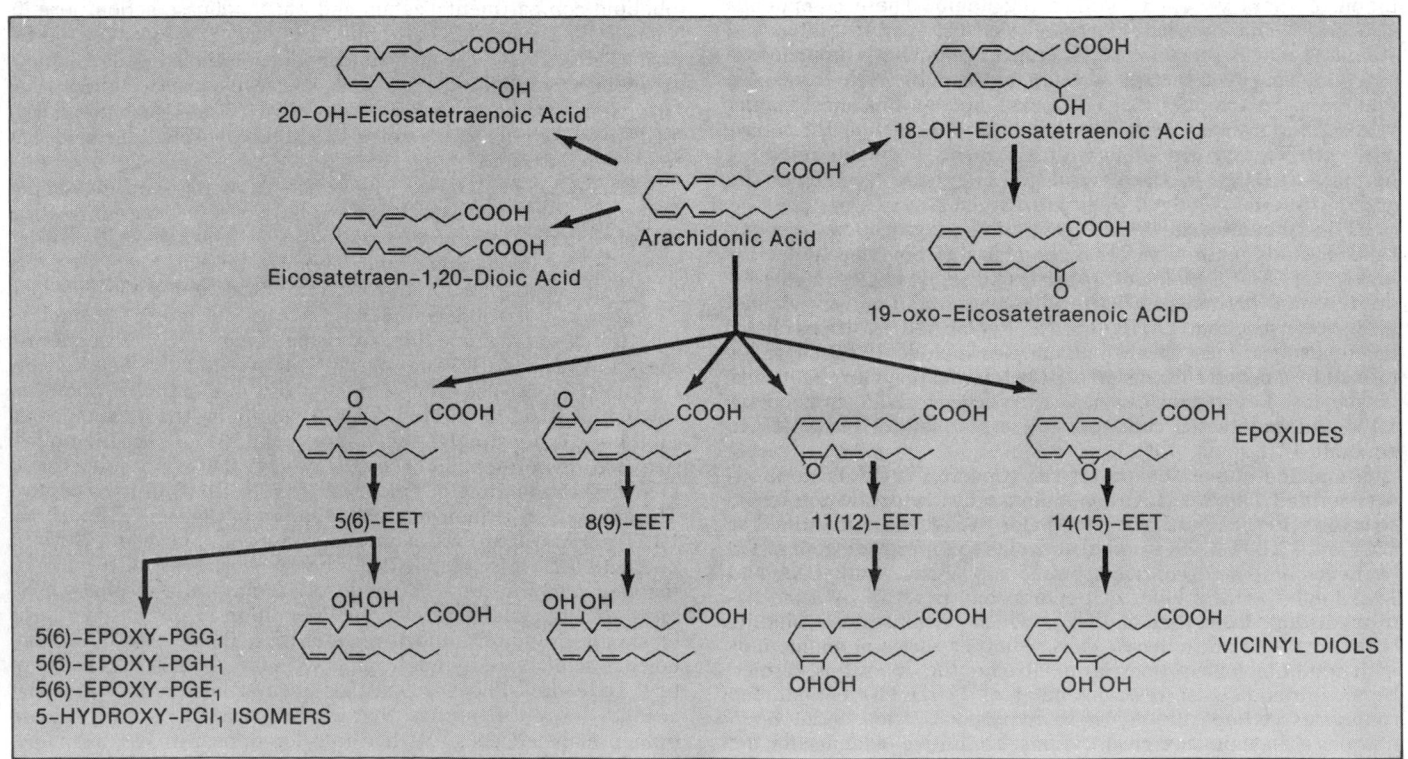

FIGURE 210–5. Metabolism of arachidonic acid by cytochrome P-450.

their ability to influence plasma lipids and cell membrane fluidity, may facilitate plaque regression.

Supplementation of the diet with n-3 fatty acids lowers blood pressure in patients with mild essential hypertension. This effect is not obviously related to altered eicosanoid formation. Similarly, it has been hypothesized that marine oils might modulate inflammatory or immune diseases by altering the profile of lipoxygenase product formation.

LIPOXYGENASE INHIBITORS AND ANTAGONISTS. Several selective 5-lipoxygenase inhibitors are bioavailable and well tolerated in man, and preliminary evidence of efficacy has been obtained using surrogate endpoints in both ulcerative colitis and allergic rhinitis. Prototype sulfidopeptide leukotriene antagonists diminish the early- and late-phase bronchoconstrictor response to allergen challenge in asthmatic patients. No selective inhibitors of epoxygenase product formation are currently available for use in humans.

FUNCTIONS OF ARACHIDONIC ACID METABOLITES IN VIVO

The evidence implicating arachidonate metabolites in mechanisms of some human diseases includes measurements of their biosynthesis and the effects of drugs that prevent their formation or antagonize their actions. Because of the evanescence of the primary compounds, estimates of in vivo synthesis have largely been based upon measurement of long-lived but biologically inactive metabolites. Quantitative assays for the major urinary metabolites of primary prostaglandins, PGI_2 and TxA_2, have been useful in identifying potential targets for drugs designed to modulate their actions. Similar methodology is now available to explore lipoxygenase and epoxygenase product formation in vivo. The capacity of tissues to generate arachidonic acid metabolites greatly exceeds the actual production rates in vivo. Thus, artifacts related to sample collection (for example, platelet activation ex vivo during blood sampling, catheter-induced vascular trauma, or formation of free radical–catalyzed derivatives during sample storage) can seriously confound attempts to measure these compounds in the bloodstream. Measurement of metabolite excretion in urine has been favored as a noninvasive, albeit indirect, approach. The most specific and sensitive method for measurement of eicosanoid metabolites is gas chromatography–mass spectrometry, which has been used to validate radioimmunoassays and enzyme immunoassays for selected compounds.

THE CARDIOVASCULAR SYSTEM. TxA_2 is one of many platelet agonists generated in vivo. While aspirin inhibits Tx-dependent aggregation, other agonists, such as thrombin and high doses of collagen, can induce aggregation in vitro despite the presence of aspirin. In view of these properties, it is superficially surprising that aspirin has been shown to influence clinical outcome in a variety of trials in cardiovascular disease, presumably because of its effects on TxA_2 formation. This may reflect the importance of TxA_2 as an amplifying signal for other platelet agonists.

Aspirin reduces significantly the incidence of stroke in patients suffering transient ischemic attacks and those with nonvalvular atrial fibrillation, the incidence of thrombotic occlusion following coronary artery bypass graft implantation, and the incidence of myocardial infarction and death in patients with unstable coronary disease. The risk of a combined endpoint of myocardial infarction, stroke, and vascular death is reduced by about 25 per cent in aspirin-treated patients. The most convincing evidence that aspirin reduces mortality in patients who have suffered an acute myocardial infarction is provided by the ISIS-2 study of more than 17,000 patients. The reduction in mortality achieved by aspirin and the thrombolytic agent streptokinase were comparable and additive.

Clear-cut evidence of the benefit of aspirin has been obtained in smaller trials of patients with unstable angina. This may reflect the early initiation of aspirin therapy and the more prominent role of thrombosis in determining outcome in these patients. Angioscopic and angiographic evidence of thrombosis is present in unstable angina, and phasic increases of TxA_2 formation coincide with episodes of cardiac ischemia. By contrast, the alteration of TxA_2 formation after myocardial infarction is transient, and there is no evidence of platelet activation in patients with chronic stable angina. Thus, if entry to the trial is delayed after a

myocardial infarction, patients represent a more "dilute" population potentially susceptible to benefit from antiplatelet therapy. Although aspirin has been used in combination with dipyridamole in many of these studies, there is little evidence that this latter drug contributes to the antithrombotic efficacy of aspirin in humans. The lowest dose of aspirin that has been shown to be effective in unstable angina has been 75 mg per day.

The use of PGI_2 and its analogues as a platelet-inhibitory drug has been restricted by the need to administer it as an infusion and its steep dose-response relationship. Doses that inhibit platelet function are close to those that cause side effects, such as gastric cramping and hypotension. Nonetheless, its potential efficacy as a platelet inhibitor is illustrated by its effects on platelet adhesion and aggregation in extracorporeal circuits, such as pump oxygenators and hemodialysis units, a setting in which aspirin is markedly less effective. Attempts to assess the efficacy of PGI_2 in atherosclerotic disease involving major vessels in the lower limb have been confounded by a high placebo response rate, but preliminary results look more convincing in thromboangiitis obliterans (Buerger's disease).

Infusion of PGE_1 may reduce the incidence of reocclusion following coronary thrombolysis. Several prototype, orally available PGI and PGE analogues are under investigation.

THE RESPIRATORY SYSTEM. While preliminary evidence indicates that sulfidopeptide antagonists blunt both the early- and late-phase bronchoconstrictor responses to inhaled allergen, the utility of these compounds in the treatment of asthma remains to be defined. Although TxA_2 as well as LT biosynthesis is increased coincident with the bronchoconstrictor response to inhaled allergen, experiments with aspirin and thromboxane antagonists suggest that its functional importance is marginal. A minority of asthmatics, perhaps 10 per cent, exhibit bronchoconstrictive, hypersensitivity reactions to aspirin. This appears to reflect a role for prostaglandins, TxA_2, or leukotrienes, as these attacks are provoked by a range of structurally distinct inhibitors of cyclo-oxygenase but rarely by salicylate, which resembles aspirin but is a weak inhibitor of that enzyme. No evidence currently supports an allergic basis for this condition. Drug-induced reactions in such patients may be quite severe and often feature profuse rhinorrhea and flushing in addition to bronchospasm. Whether such attacks are mediated by differential inhibition of bronchoconstrictor versus bronchodilator prostaglandins, by a shunting of the arachidonate substrate toward lipoxygenation and the formation of bronchoconstrictor leukotrienes, or by reduced formation of a prostaglandin that normally inhibits release of other mediators of bronchoconstriction is unknown.

Aspirin may also trigger a hypersensitivity response in which alterations in blood pressure, flushing, tachycardia, and diarrhea predominate over bronchospasm. Some of these patients have systemic mastocytosis (Ch. 252).

THE GASTROINTESTINAL SYSTEM. Both PGI_2 and PGE_2 are cytoprotective of gastric mucosa in vitro and are thought to contribute to the regulation of mucosal blood flow. The dose-related gastrointestinal side effects of NSAID's are thought to reflect increased susceptibility to local injury (e.g., H^+ backdiffusion) due to inhibition of these prostaglandins. Oral dimethyl PGE analogues have been approved for use as an adjunct to NSAID therapy. The watery diarrhea associated with multiple endocrine neoplasia often responds to treatment with prostaglandin inhibitors. Excessive formation of LTB_4 has been demonstrated in colonic mucosa and rectal dialysates obtained from patients with inflammatory bowel disease.

RENIN RELEASE AND RENAL FUNCTION. While sympathoadrenal activity is the principal regulator of renin release, it appears to be via a cyclo-oxygenase metabolite of arachidonic acid. PGI_2 is the most potent of the prostaglandins as a renin secretagogue. Inhibition of cyclo-oxygenase by NSAID's has implications for the diagnostic application of renin measurements. The associated reduction in aldosterone production may be deleterious for patients with hyperkalemia.

Metabolites of arachidonic acid contribute little to the regulation of renal blood flow under physiologic circumstances. Under conditions of increased vasoconstrictor tone, however, preservation of renal blood flow becomes increasingly dependent upon the generation of vasodilator prostaglandins. This is particularly so in patients with chronic glomerulonephritis, Bartter's syndrome, the nephropathy of systemic lupus erythematosus, congestive heart failure, or combined hepatic and renal dysfunction. It has been proposed that the decline in renal function in such patients following administration of NSAID's is less likely to occur with sulindac as a result of retroconversion of the sulfide to the sulfone.

The kidney possesses the capacity to generate TxA_2 in addition to vasodilator prostaglandins. Renal biosynthesis of TxA_2 is increased in some patients with severe nephropathy in association with systemic lupus erythematosus, and infusion of a PGH_2-TxA_2 receptor antagonist improves indices of renal function in such patients. Increased TxA_2 biosynthesis by the kidney has been demonstrated in animal models in response to ureteric obstruction, renal vein thrombosis, and development of hypertension following partial renal ablation and coincident with the development of cyclosporine-induced nephrotoxicity. Increased TxA_2 formation during renal allograft rejection has been reported in humans; however, it is unknown whether this is an epiphenomenon or of primary importance in the rejection process. 16,16-Dimethyl PGE_2 delays renal allograft rejection in man, although the mechanism is unknown.

PGE_2 is the major product formed from arachidonic acid in the renal medulla, where it appears to inhibit sodium reabsorption in the distal tubule. The consequent sodium retention caused by administration of a cyclo-oxygenase inhibitor persists only for a day or two, after which sodium balance is reversed despite continued treatment. Prostaglandins may also influence free water clearance. Indomethacin diminishes the excessive water elimination in nephrogenic and lithium-induced diabetes insipidus.

Although P-450–catalyzed metabolism of arachidonate occurs in renal tissue and several of the compounds influence tubular ion flux, glomerular filtration rate, and vascular tone, their precise role in renal physiology and pathology remains to be established.

THE REPRODUCTIVE SYSTEM. Both PGE_2 and $PGF_{2\alpha}$ are potent stimulants of myometrial contraction. Both they and their methylated analogues have been utilized as abortifacients and in the induction of labor, usually as an adjunct to low amniotomy. Cyclo-oxygenase inhibitors are currently being evaluated in the treatment of premature labor. A potential hazard of this approach has been premature closure of the ductus arteriosus, although the incidence of the complication is unknown. Closure of a persistent ductus arteriosus can be achieved with indomethacin in the neonatal period. This implies that a cyclo-oxygenase metabolite contributes to ductal patency. Infusion of PGE_1 has been used to maintain an open ductus in infants with pulmonary atresia until corrective surgery is performed.

Biosynthesis of the prostaglandins increases during pregnancy, particularly during labor. In the case of PGI_2, biosynthesis is increased markedly from as early as the first trimester. Interestingly, this increment is less pronounced in patients with pregnancy-induced hypertension (PIH). Indeed, diminished PGI_2 biosynthesis is apparent prior to the rise in blood pressure. Studies of TxA_2 biosynthesis indicate that platelet activation is present in normal pregnancy and is further increased in patients with severe PIH. TxA_2 is a potent vasoconstrictor in the placental bed and may contribute to the depressed placental blood flow that is a hallmark of PIH. Encouraging results from several small studies have prompted the initiation of multicenter trials to determine if aspirin will reduce the incidence of PIH in women at risk of developing the disease. It has been difficult to document a teratogenic risk from maternal consumption of aspirin in the first trimester.

FEVER AND INFLAMMATION. Cyclo-oxygenase inhibitors share antipyretic, analgesic, and anti-inflammatory actions. Paracetamol differs from the other compounds in being an efficient antipyretic despite weak anti-inflammatory properties in the periphery. The prostaglandins that mediate fever are unknown. Vasodilator prostaglandins seem to act in concert with other mediators to augment the inflammatory response. Among these may be the leukotrienes, which enhance capillary permeability and function as chemoattractants and leukocyte activators. These properties suggest that combined cyclo-oxygenase and lipoxygenase inhibitors may be more effective anti-inflammatory agents than aspirin-like drugs.

Fitzpatrick F, Murphy R: Cytochrome P450 metabolism of arachidonic acid: Formation and biological actions of "epoxygenase" derived eicosanoids. Pharmacol Rev 40:229, 1989. *A comprehensive review of this pathway of arachidonic acid metabolism.*

Hennekens MD, Buring JE, Sandercock P, et al.: Aspirin and other antiplatelet agents in the secondary and primary prevention of cardiovascular disease. Circulation 80:749, 1989. *A comprehensive review of clinical trials of aspirin, including ISIS-2.*

Hirata M, Hayashi Y, Ushikube F, et al.: Cloning and expression of cDNA for a human thromboxane A_2 receptor. Nature 349:617, 1991. *The first cloning of a receptor for an eicosanoid.*

Kerins D, Murray R, FitzGerald GA: Prostacyclin and PGE_1: Molecular mechanisms and therapeutic utility. Prog Hemostasis 10:307, 1991. *A comprehensive review of basic and clinical knowledge about these prostaglandins.*

Leaf A, Weber PC: Cardiovascular effects of n-3 fatty acids. N Engl J Med 318:549, 1988. *A review of the biochemistry and potential benefits of fish oils in cardiovascular disease.*

Samuelsson B: Leukotrienes: Mediators of immediate hypersensitivity and inflammation. Science 220:568, 1983. *A review that concentrates on the biosynthesis and metabolism of these compounds and their role in inflammation.*

Vane JR: The road to prostacyclin. Adv Prostaglandin Thromboxane Leukotriene Res 15:11, 1985. *An account of the discovery and pharmacology of this prostaglandin.*

211 Natriuretic Hormones

Dennis A. Ausiello

In the last decade, considerable interest has focused on endogenous factors that play a role in the regulation of water and electrolyte balance. The isolation and cloning of the cardiac-derived atrial natriuretic peptide (ANP) has led to a rapid definition of its biosynthesis, storage, release response, and action. Although there are still some uncertainties, a picture of its role in physiology and pathophysiology and a possible therapeutic agent have been developed. A second compound (or compounds), called natriuretic hormone (NH), whose presumed structure and function are distinct from those of ANP, has not yet been completely characterized. Therefore, its physiology, pathophysiology, and therapeutic potential are still unclear.

NATRIURETIC HORMONE (NH)

Experimental observations led to the concept of the existence of an endogenous regulator of mammalian Na^+-K^+-ATPase (the Na^+ pump) more than 25 years ago. At that time intravascular expansion with saline in dogs produced a brisk natriuresis with no change in renal perfusion pressure, glomerular filtration rate, or mineralocorticoid activity. The natriuretic effects of extracellular fluid volume expansion in one animal also occurred in a second animal cross-circulated with the blood of the first. The presumption was that the natriuresis was due to a circulating substance that exerted its effects directly on the renal tubular Na^+ reabsorptive process without affecting renal hemodynamics. Further experiments confirmed that active extracts from plasma, urine, and tissue sources that were natriuretic in vivo had a direct effect on transepithelial sodium transport. These substances have digitalis-like characteristics, although there is no reason to assume a structural identity between the postulated endogenous Na^+-K^+-ATPase inhibitor and the cardiac glycosides. Digitalis is a potent inhibitor of Na^+-K^+-ATPase and causes both natriuresis and an increase in vascular resistance, although these are not its major pharmacologic effects. Using the digoxin radioimmunoassay, digitalis-like immunoactivity has been found in the urine and plasma of sodium-loaded normal human subjects and in uremic and hypertensive subjects. Whether NH and digitalis-like compounds are the same endogenous Na^+-K^+-ATPase inhibitors remains to be defined.

BIOLOGIC ACTIVITIES. The biologic effects that have been claimed for the putative NH include (a) natriuresis in vivo, (b) inhibition of sodium transport in vitro, (c) Na^+-K^+-ATPase inhibition, (d) positive cardiac inotropism, and (e) increased vascular reactivity.

BIOCHEMICAL CHARACTERIZATION. Controversy still exists about the chemical nature of the substance. Some maintain that it is a peptide, whereas others have found its properties inconsistent with this class of compounds and propose a steroidal nature.

SITE OF ORIGIN. The site of origin of the NH also remains uncertain, but the brain has been favored, since the natriuretic effects of extracellular fluid volume expansion appear to depend on an intact central nervous system. In addition, Na^+-K^+-ATPase inhibitory activity has been extracted and partially purified from cerebral and hypothalamic tissue. A ouabain-like compound has been isolated from human cerebrospinal fluid. The hypothalamus represents an enriched source of an endogenous inhibitor of Na^+-K^+-ATPase, if not the site of its production.

NH AND THE PATHOPHYSIOLOGY OF ESSENTIAL HYPERTENSION. NH may play a role in normal volume regulation and in the pathophysiology of hypertension and secondary edema states. NH may have an extrarenal action leading to enhanced vascular reactivity. The hypothesis proposed is that in hereditary forms of hypertension, there is a persistent tendency toward renal retention of sodium. This may be due to increased Na^+-K^+ cotransport or Na^+-H^+ exchange in the proximal tubule, occurring as a manifestation of a generalized genetic defect in Na^+-Na^+ (Na^+-Li^+) countertransport. This defect exists in the erythrocytes of some patients with essential hypertension and in their first-degree normotensive relatives. The renal sodium retention leads to a transient increase in extracellular fluid volume, which serves as a stimulus for the release of a Na^+-K^+-ATPase inhibitor. The sodium pump inhibitor acts on the renal tubule to promote sodium excretion, thus restoring extracellular fluid volume to normal levels. It has similar inhibitory effects on the Na^+-K^+-ATPase in vascular smooth muscle cells, resulting in a tonic increase in vascular tone, increased total peripheral resistance, and hypertension. It is assumed that Na^+-K^+-ATPase inhibition in vascular smooth muscle results in an increase in cytosolic free calcium concentration, which must occur to produce the arterial vasoconstriction. How this occurs is unclear. One of the hypotheses is that altered Na^+-Ca^{2+} exchange resulting from partial sodium-pump inhibition may account for an increase in intracellular free Ca^{2+} concentration. At this time, this hypothesis remains attractive but unproven.

ATRIAL NATRIURETIC PEPTIDE (ANP)

ANP, a peptide hormone, is secreted primarily by the cardiac atria and produces natriuresis, diuresis, smooth muscle relaxation, and inhibition of renin and aldosterone secretion. Its major sites of action include the cardiovascular, renal, and endocrine systems. Although the exact mechanisms triggering the release of ANP are not clear, stretch of the atria appears to be the principal stimulus.

It has been known for several decades that membrane-bound secretory granules exist in the cardiac atria. In 1981 in a pioneering report, DeBold and his colleagues observed that bolus injection of crude extracts of rat atria, but not ventricles, produced a rapid, massive, and short-lasting diuresis and natriuresis and a modest kaliuresis. This suggested the existence of a natriuretic hormone in the atrial granules. Subsequently, this unique hormonal system has been thoroughly studied. The amino acid sequence of the active circulating peptide and its prehormone forms have been defined together with their gene structure, target tissue receptors, and signal transduction pathways.

STRUCTURE, BIOSYNTHESIS, AND SECRETION. The atrium first produces a pre-pro ANP (151 amino acids), the final 126 amino acids of which are pro ANP. The pro ANP, the principal storage form of the hormone in the atrial granules, is the immediate precursor of the biologically active 28 amino acid ANP, the predominant circulatory peptide. Circulatory ANP has a cysteine-cysteine disulfide crosslink that is essential for its activity.

The human gene for pre-pro ANP is located on the short arm of chromosome 1. Transcription of the pre-pro ANP gene proceeds at a high rate in the cardiac atria, estimated to be 1 to 3 per cent of all mRNA in the atrial cardiocytes. ANP gene expression is transcriptionally regulated by dexamethasone and thyroid hormone. ANP is also expressed at very low levels in other tissues, such as brain, anterior pituitary, adrenal medulla, lung, kidney, thyroid, and submandibular gland. The major site of ANP synthesis is the myocytes of the right cardiac atrium, with lesser production in the left atrium. Pro ANP is cleaved by a specific atrial protease, probably at the time of exocytotic fusion of atrial granules with the plasma membrane and possibly even soon after secretion from the myocyte, resulting in ANP as the predominant form entering the coronary sinus blood.

STIMULI FOR RELEASE. Atrial stretch, measured as atrial transmural pressure, is the principal stimulus for ANP secretion into the circulation. Atrial pressure is also correlated with release of ANP. During infusion of isotonic saline in humans, plasma ANP increases in parallel with the increase of right atrial pressure. This results from rapid conversion of pro ANP to ANP and/or release of ANP. With cardiovascular or pulmonary disease, a significant correlation exists between circulating ANP levels and the right and left atrial pressures.

Mineralocorticoids, as well as glucocorticoids administered in high doses, increase mRNA encoding for pre-pro ANP and circulating ANP levels, indicating an increase in ANP production and release. In addition, adrenalectomized rats do not respond to increased atrial pressure with increased atrial and circulating ANP levels in the absence of glucocorticoid or mineralocorticoid replacement. Thus these hormones may play a permissive role in the volume response mediating ANP release as well as inducing ANP secretion directly.

BIOLOGIC AND PLASMA HALF-LIFE. A sensitive radioimmunoassay, generally specific for the mid to C-terminal peptides of ANP, will detect levels of 1 to 10 pg of the peptide in plasma. In subjects on varied sodium diets, the plasma ANP levels range from 10 to 40 pg per milliliter.

After release from the atrium or after intravenous administration, ANP is rapidly cleared with a plasma half-life between 2 and 4 minutes in humans. Biologic activity of ANP critically depends on the intact ring structure and carboxy-terminal residues. The rank order of tissue degradative potency appears to be kidney > liver > lung > plasma > heart.

ANP RECEPTORS. ANP receptors are localized on the cell surface of target tissues, including most notably adrenal, kidney, and the vasculature. They are also found, to a lesser extent, in the central nervous system, hepatocytes, colonic smooth muscle, and lung. In kidney, ANP binding sites are most prevalent in large vessels, glomeruli, and the renal medulla. In the adrenal, ANP binding is limited primarily to the zona glomerulosa.

Molecular cloning has defined three ANP receptors: (a) the ANP-C (or ANP-R2) clearance receptor, which is not coupled to cGMP production, the signal transduction pathway involved in ANP action. Clearance receptors do not mediate any known physiologic effect. The receptors for ANP in the kidney and vascular smooth muscle are predominantly clearance receptors. Their abundance accounts for the short half-life of circulatory ANP. It seems probable that the atrial peptide system has a novel receptor-mediated sequestration and clearance mechanism that is responsible, at least in part, for maintaining plasma levels of the hormone. (b) Two structurally similar plasma membrane receptors, ANP-R1 and ANP-R3, are the biologically active receptor forms. ANP binding to the extracellular domain of R1 or R3 activates the cytoplasmic domain of the receptor, which is a guanylate cyclase responsible for the generation of the second messenger, cGMP.

CELLULAR ACTION. The most apparent action of ANP is to increase intracellular cGMP concentration. ANP is a unique peptide hormone in its use of cGMP as a second messenger, which mediates most of the physiologic actions of the hormone. ANP also influences intracellular calcium homeostasis, which may be responsible for some of its biologic effects.

The physiologic responses to ANP include (a) relaxation of vascular and other smooth muscles, (b) increase in glomerular filtration rate and inhibition of tubular water and sodium transport in the kidney, and (c) inhibition of hormone secretion (Fig. 211-1).

KIDNEY ACTION. The kidney is the primary target organ for ANP. ANP causes natriuresis and diuresis by a concerted action at several nephron segments. The primary sites of action of ANP are the glomerulus, the renal vasculature, and the inner medullary collecting duct, although other nephron segments may be involved in the response to ANP. ANP can increase glomerular filtration rate by raising the glomerular hydraulic pressure gradient from capillary lumen to Bowman's space through differential effects on afferent and efferent arteriole tone. By relaxing glomerular mesangial cells, ANP also increases the glomerular ultrafiltration coefficient, Kf. The combined effects result in an increased filtration pressure and thus an increased filtration fraction, with a higher load of salt and water being delivered to the tubules for excretion.

The increased quantity of sodium filtered is not completely reabsorbed. There is an increased delivery of sodium to the distal tubule and collecting duct, where ANP reduces sodium reabsorption and vasopressin-induced water reabsorption, leading to a profound natriuresis. In addition, redistribution of blood flow from the cortex to inner medulla, which dilutes the papillary interstitium, results in an increase in sodium and water excretion.

CARDIOVASCULAR ACTION. ANP directly relaxes arterial vascular smooth muscle through the action of its second messenger, cGMP. This ANP-induced vasorelaxation occurs independent of the presence of endothelium. ANP most effectively relaxes large-caliber arteries, such as the aorta, renal, and iliac arteries. The more peripheral vascular segments of the arterial tree are less sensitive to the hormone. ANP causes vasorelaxation of the aorta constricted with norepinephrine or angiotensin II, compatible with its role as one of the most potent vasodilators known and as a functional antagonist of a variety of vasoconstrictors.

ANP at pharmacologic concentrations reduces mean arterial pressure in man by reducing peripheral vascular resistance and decreasing intravascular volume. This is followed by a decrease in cardiac output attributed to (1) a shift of volume from the intravascular to extravascular space, probably due to alteration in capillary permeability or an increase in resistance to venous return at the site of postcapillary circulation; hemoconcentration, secondary to a decreased plasma volume, may occur in humans in response to ANP; and (2) preload reduction due to relaxation of venous smooth muscle, leading to an augmentation of venous capacitance and a reduction of venous return.

ENDOCRINE ACTION. ANP modulates renin-angiotensin-aldosterone secretion. Administration of ANP causes a prompt decline in circulatory renin and aldosterone levels. ANP blocks both basal and agonist-stimulated (angiotensin II, ACTH, K⁺)

secretion of aldosterone in isolated adrenal zona glomerulosa cells. This appears to be a direct action of ANP on these cells. In addition, ANP decreases the biosynthesis and release of vasopressin. The decrease in vasopressin may potentiate a decrease in vascular tone and augment the diuresis and natriuresis induced by ANP.

SIGNIFICANCE OF ANP IN BODY FLUID HOMEOSTASIS

It is not yet possible to describe definitively the physiologic relevance of ANP. Some evidence suggests that ANP exerts a trivial influence on the normal regulation of body fluid homeostasis: (1) Infusion of ANP into conscious animals and normal human subjects results in plasma concentrations slightly above the physiologic range but produces only a slowly developing and relatively modest natriuresis. (2) Ingestion of food containing salt does not increase plasma ANP, yet a natriuresis routinely occurs postprandially. (3) In a number of common physiologic and experimental conditions, circulating ANP levels do not correlate with renal sodium excretion.

Other evidence suggests that ANP plays a significant role in regulation of body fluid homeostasis: (1) ANP is potent, has a short duration of action, and the hormone responds to physiologically relevant stimuli in a feedback-controlled system. (2) The peptide circulates at nanomolar concentrations, which is consistent with its Kd for receptor binding and second messenger activation in target cells. (3) Long-term, low-dose ANP infusion directly into the renal artery of conscious dogs supports a physiologic action of ANP to promote urinary sodium excretion. (4) The role played by ANP in volume regulation is highly complex and the kidney responds with increased sodium excretion only when a constellation of natriuretic forces is appropriately assayed. Therefore, a rise in ANP levels may be a necessary, but not sufficient, condition to induce natriuresis.

ROLE OF ANP IN PATHOPHYSIOLOGY
Diseases of Disordered Volume Regulation (Edematous States)

CONGESTIVE HEART FAILURE (CHF). CHF is associated with increased atrial pressure and elevated ANP levels. Despite

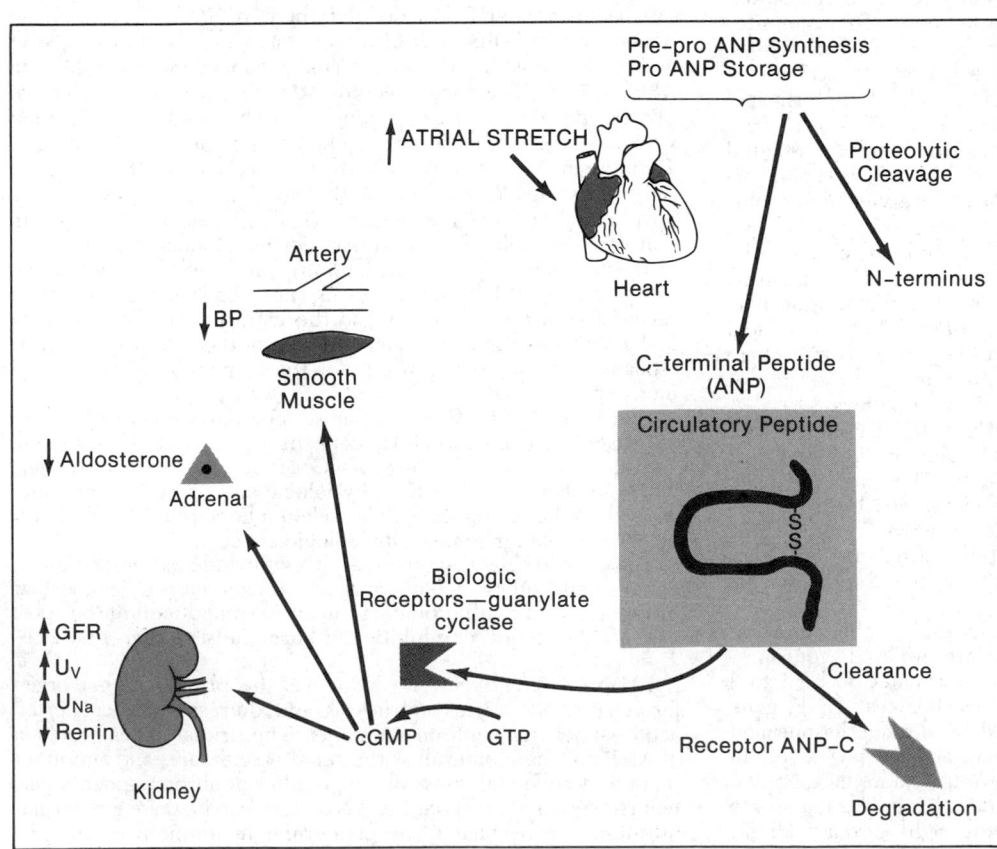

FIGURE 211–1. Major target organs and actions of atrial natriuretic peptide (ANP).

high circulating ANP, however, these patients retain salt and water. CHF is associated with a decreased response of the kidney to ANP, which could result from receptor down-regulation due to high plasma ANP concentrations. These high levels of circulating ANP appear to play a role in the maintenance of sodium excretion by modulating the renal, hemodynamic, and endocrine effects of CHF. The degree of ANP elevation increases with the severity of the clinical disease, as measured by the New York Heart Association functional classification. Class I patients have normal or only moderately elevated levels; class III and IV patients have dramatic elevations. The direct correlation between the severity of the heart failure and plasma ANP has allowed the use of ANP levels to serve as a marker for CHF in adults and children, including those with congenital heart disease. ANP levels correlate directly with right atrial pressure, pulmonary capillary wedge pressure, and pulmonary artery pressure and inversely with cardiac output and cardiac index.

CIRRHOSIS. Progressive cirrhosis of the liver is accompanied by renal sodium and water retention with the development of ascites and edema. This state is usually accompanied by elevated plasma ANP levels, consistent with the "overflow" theory of ascites formation. As in CHF, raised ANP plasma concentrations in the presence of total body volume expansion implies a "refractory" or "reset" response to ANP. This hyporesponsiveness to ANP in cirrhosis is supported by the observation that ANP levels can be stimulated to increase further by water immersion, peritoneovenous shunting, and acute volume expansion with a resultant natriuresis in some patients. It is probable that a complex balance between ANP and antinatriuretic factors is responsible for renal sodium retention in early and late cirrhosis. In the former, hepatic venous outflow obstruction results in renal salt retention and intravascular volume expansion (overflow hypothesis). This in turn leads to an elevation in ANP levels counterbalanced by antinatriuretic factors such that the net effect is ascites formation. In late cirrhosis, with loss of intravascular volume into the peritoneal compartment (underfill hypothesis), there is a reduced stimulus for ANP secretion such that ANP plasma levels no longer offset antinatriuretic processes.

NEPHROTIC SYNDROME. Why edema forms in the nephrotic syndrome is not completely understood. Traditionally it has been suggested that renal sodium and water retention is a consequence of the lower plasma oncotic pressure from hypoalbuminemia and the resultant reduction in plasma volume. Consistent with this hypothesis, nephrotic syndrome is found to be associated with normal or diminished circulatory levels of ANP that can be stimulated to rise after intravascular volume expansion. Head-out water immersion conducted on patients with nephrotic syndrome demonstrated that ANP levels increased, but renal salt and water excretion was blunted. There thus appears to be an impaired renal response to ANP in the nephrotic syndrome.

ESSENTIAL HYPERTENSION. Patients with essential hypertension have a wide range of plasma ANP concentrations, suggesting that the contribution of ANP may vary in the heterogeneous population of patients with this disease. This finding precludes the use of ANP levels to differentiate among the various causes of hypertension.

RENAL DISEASE. Progressive renal disease is frequently associated with plasma volume expansion and elevated ANP levels. In patients undergoing regular dialysis, ANP levels can be used as an indicator of volume status. Decreased levels correlate with the amount of weight loss and fluid removal in dialysis patients.

THERAPEUTIC POTENTIAL

ANP may have a role as a therapeutic agent, especially in critical care situations. Intervention, in general, is limited by a lack of an effective oral agent. ANP must be administered intravenously. Its potency as a pharmacologic agent in altering cardiovascular and renal function makes it potentially attractive in treating patients with diseases associated with edema (CHF, cirrhosis, nephrotic syndrome), hypertension, and ischemic renal injury: (a) In patients with CHF, the natriuretic and diuretic effects of pharmacologic concentrations of ANP are often limited, but the effect on augmenting cardiac output is quite favorable; (b) in cirrhosis, the renal hyporesponsiveness together with a

relative increased sensitivity to hypotension make the therapeutic use of ANP problematic; (c) in patients with nephrotic syndrome, ANP infusion may result in a natriuresis; (d) variable short-term benefits have been reported in patients with hypertension. The use of low-dose ANP with other agents may prove effective if a satisfactory oral agent is developed; and (e) a potentially important therapeutic action of ANP may be the prevention and reversal of acute renal failure (Ch. 76). In various animal models of acute renal failure, ANP given prophylactically or immediately following the hemodynamic insult restores GFR. The therapeutic potential of ANP in human acute renal failure still needs to be assessed.

ANP infusion in all human studies has not exceeded a duration of a few hours. Therefore all reported responses to ANP in humans are acute. Prolonged administration of ANP with a nonparenteral analogue will be necessary to evaluate its therapeutic potential in chronic human diseases.

Blain EH: Atrial natriuretic factor plays a significant role in body fluid homeostasis. Hypertension 15:2, 1990. *Debate on the role ANP plays in body fluid homeostasis.*

Brenner BM, Ballermann BY, Gunning ME, et al.: Diverse biological actions of atrial natriuretic peptide. Physiol Rev 70:665, 1990. *Comprehensive review of the current understanding of the structure of ANP, its synthesis, secretion, cellular and target organ action, and its role in various pathophysiologic states.*

Cogan MG: Atrial natriuretic peptide. Kidney Int 37:1148, 1990. *Comprehensive review of the renal properties of ANP.*

Floras JS: Sympathoinhibitory effects of atrial natriuretic factor in normal humans. Circulation 81:1860, 1990. *Integrative cardiovascular responses to ANP in normal humans.*

Goetz KL: Evidence that atriopeptin is not a physiological regulator of sodium excretion. Hypertension 15:9, 1990. *Debate on the role ANP plays in body fluid homeostasis.*

Haupert GT: Sodium pump regulation by endogenous inhibition. Curr Top Membrane Transport 34:345, 1989. *Review of current knowledge of the hypothalamic ouabain-like factor.*

ACKNOWLEDGMENT: I would like to thank Eliezer Holtzman for his invaluable help in preparing this chapter.

212 Neuroendocrine Regulation and Its Disorders

Lawrence A. Frohman

NEUROENDOCRINE REGULATION

The central nervous system exerts profound regulatory control over hormonal secretion and metabolic processes. The integration of this control is focused in the region of the ventral hypothalamus and consists of three major systems:

1. A neuronal pathway descending through the base of the brain, the autonomic nervous system pathways of the spinal cord, and terminating in the liver, gastrointestinal tract, pancreas, adrenal medullae, and adipose tissue. This pathway, which consists of bidirectional fibers, participates in neurometabolic regulation, and its greatest effects are on blood glucose and fatty acid regulation and on metabolic homeostasis, i.e., appetite control (satiety), temperature control (thermoregulation), and body fat stores (nutrient regulation).

2. A neurosecretory pathway from the anterior hypothalamus that traverses the floor of the ventral hypothalamus and pituitary stalk and terminates in specialized neuronal elements called pituicytes, located in the posterior pituitary. This system is involved in osmoregulation, through the production of vasopressin, and in parturition and nursing, through the secretion of oxytocin. A detailed discussion of this system is provided in Ch. 214.

3. A neuroendocrine system involving clusters of peptide- and monoamine-secreting cells in the anterior and mid-portion of the ventral hypothalamus whose products are transported along nerve fibers to terminals in the outer layer of the median eminence, from which they are released into the capillary vessels of the

hypothalamic-hypophyseal portal system and transported to the pituitary to regulate the secretion of the hormones of the anterior pituitary.

Neuroendocrine Anatomy

The *neurometabolic function* of the hypothalamus can be divided into those components associated with the sympathetic or the parasympathetic branches of the autonomic nervous system. Although medial sympathetic and lateral parasympathetic zones of the hypothalamus can be distinguished, the cellular elements (neuronal perikarya) involved in a particular function cannot be precisely localized to one specific nuclear region. Neurons involved in the inhibitory control of food intake (satiety) are located medially, and those responsible for appetite stimulation are located laterally. This distinction probably explains why destructive lesions of the hypothalamus, which frequently occur in the midline, are more likely to result in obesity than in starvation. A second reason is that fibers from the hypothalamic controlling centers cross the midline, and thus bilateral hypothalamic destruction is necessary for interruption of normal regulatory control.

Neurons of the *neurohypophyseal system* constitute a more anatomically distinct entity with cell bodies located in the paraventricular and supraoptic hypothalamic nuclei. Within these areas are also neurons producing other neuropeptides. The posterior pituitary hormones, oxytocin and vasopressin, along with their specific carrier proteins (neurophysins), are synthesized in the cell bodies as part of a single precursor molecule and transported along axonal fibers through the ventral hypothalamus and pituitary stalk, during which time the hormones are cleaved from the precursor. In the pituicytes of the posterior pituitary they are packaged into storage granules to be released in response to stimulation (e.g., osmotic, barometric) of receptors on the cell bodies in the hypothalamus. The posterior pituitary is therefore functionally an integral part of the brain.

The cell bodies of the neuroendocrine system are diffusely distributed throughout the mediobasal hypothalamus in an area known as the hypophysiotropic region. Although the hypothalamic hormone-secreting neurons receive input from other brain regions in response to changes in the external environment, they continue to function even in the absence of extrahypothalamic input, indicating that their most important homeostatic stimuli are blood borne. Cells secreting thyrotropin releasing hormone (TRH) and somatotropin release inhibiting factor (SRIF) that regulate pituitary function are located in the anterior hypothalamus, while those secreting growth hormone releasing hormone (GRH) are concentrated in the region of the arcuate nuclei. Cells secreting gonadotropin releasing hormone (GnRH) are more widely distributed, with cell bodies in both the anterior hypothalamus and the arcuate nuclei. Cell bodies of corticotropin releasing hormone (CRH) neurons terminating in the median eminence are located predominantly in the paraventricular nucleus. A prolactin inhibiting factor (PIF) exhibits a distribution identical to that of GnRH.

The releasing and inhibiting hormones are stored in nerve terminals in the median eminence. Since the portal blood flow to the pituitary is not compartmentalized, i.e., various cell types in the pituitary are distributed throughout the gland, releasing and inhibiting factors secreted into the portal system have access to all cell types of the anterior pituitary. Specificity of action is achieved by the presence of specific receptors on individual pituitary cell types.

The cells of both the neuroendocrine and neurohypophyseal systems have been called transducer cells, containing both neuronal and endocrine characteristics. They respond to classic neurotransmitter-mediated signals, yet they release peptide hormones into a regional or systemic circulation.

PORTAL VASCULAR SYSTEM. The vascular supply of the anterior pituitary has no direct connections with the arterial system. All of the arterial blood flows through the hypothalamic arteries and forms a capillary plexus within the outer layer of the median eminence in juxtaposition to nerve terminals of the hypophysiotropic neurons. In contrast to most other brain regions, the blood-brain barrier in the area of the median eminence is incomplete, permitting protein and peptide hormones as well as other charged particles access to the intercapillary spaces and the nerve terminals contained therein. These terminals (and/or their perikarya) respond to changes in concentrations of circulating hormones and metabolic signals as well as to neuronal stimuli by secreting releasing and inhibiting factors into the portal system. The portal capillaries coalesce into a series of veins that descend through the pituitary stalk and form a second capillary plexus that bathes the cells of the anterior pituitary. Venous drainage from the anterior pituitary passes through the posterior pituitary and from there into systemic veins.

Releasing and Inhibiting Hormones

The hypothalamic hormones that control the secretion of anterior pituitary hormones and their effects on pituitary hormone secretion are shown in Figure 212–1. Several different patterns of control exist: (1) multiple hypothalamic hormones stimulating release of a single pituitary hormone (CRH and vasopressin [VP]: ACTH), (2) a single hypothalamic hormone stimulating release of several pituitary hormones (GnRH:luteinizing hormone [LH] and follicle-stimulating hormone [FSH], TRH:thyroid-stimulating hormone [TSH] and prolactin), and (3) dual stimulatory/inhibitory influences of hypothalamic hormones on pituitary hormones (GRH and SRIF:growth hormone [GH]).

With one exception, the predominant influence of the hypothalamic hormones on the pituitary is stimulatory. Interference with the integrity of the hypothalamic-pituitary connection results in decreased secretion of all pituitary hormones except for prolactin, the secretion of which is increased when hypothalamic influence is removed.

All of the recognized hypothalamic hormones whose structures have been determined are, with one exception, peptides with sequence length ranging from 3 to 44 amino acids. As the length of the structures increases, both multiple forms of the peptide (see section on somatostatin and GRH) and marked species variation in sequence occur. Whereas the sequences of TRH, GnRH, and SRIF are identical in all mammalian species studied to date, those of GRH and CRH exhibit marked species specificity. The existence of a separate PRF is still controversial, although a candidate for this title is vasoactive intestinal polypeptide (VIP). The one nonpeptide hypophysiotropic hormone is dopamine. In addition to its major role as a neurotransmitter, dopamine is the most important physiologic inhibitor of prolactin. A 56-amino acid prolactin-inhibiting peptide has been identified as a carboxyterminal extension on the GnRH precursor molecule. The physiologic roles of this GnRH-associated peptide (GAP), as well as other less fully characterized prolactin-releasing factors, remain to be confirmed.

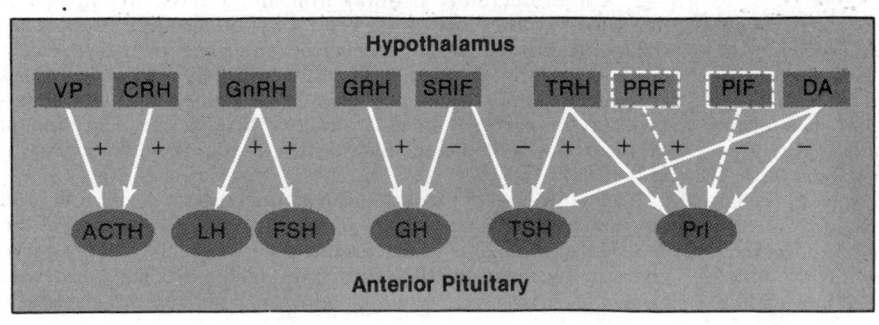

FIGURE 212–1. Interrelationships between hypothalamic and pituitary hormones. Solid lines denote hormones, the structures of which have been determined. Interrupted line indicates factors, the identity of which is still unknown.

ROLE OF BIOGENIC AMINES AND NEUROPEPTIDES IN THE REGULATION OF HYPOTHALAMIC HORMONE SECRETION.

The major neurotransmitter systems utilized for intercellular communication within the central nervous system consist of monoamines and peptides. Neurotransmitters can influence the hypothalamic hormone-secreting neurons at several sites (Fig. 212–2). These include axodendritic connections (site 1) and axoaxonic connections involving presynaptic receptors on the hormone-containing nerve terminals (site 3). Multiple neurotransmitters may also participate in the regulation of hormone secretion through intermediary neurons (site 2), and neurotransmitters may be released directly into the portal system to modify the effect of hypothalamic hormones on the pituitary (site 4). Major advances in the understanding of hypothalamic-pituitary function have occurred as a consequence of the availability of neuropharmacologic compounds that selectively alter neurotransmitter function.

Catecholamines (Dopamine, Norepinephrine, Epinephrine). The common precursor for the catecholamines is tyrosine, which is actively transported from the blood into catecholaminergic neurons in the CNS. Tyrosine is converted to dihydroxyphenylalanine (L-dopa) by tyrosine hydroxylase, which, because of its low concentration, represents the rate-limiting step in catecholamine biosynthesis. It is therefore the enzyme most susceptible to pharmacologic blockage by tyrosine analogues such as α-methylparatyrosine. L-dopa is rapidly decarboxylated by aromatic L-amino acid decarboxylase to dopamine (5-hydroxytryptamine). This enzyme can be inhibited by L-dopa analogues such as α-methyldopa and α-methyldopahydrazine (carbidopa). In dopaminergic neurons, dopamine is stored in secretory granules and released as a neurotransmitter, while in noradrenergic and adrenergic neurons it is further hydroxylated by dopamine β-hydroxylase to form norepinephrine. Copper-chelating agents such as disulfiram are potent inhibitors of this step and impair the conversion of dopamine to norepinephrine. In noradrenergic neurons, this transmitter is packaged similarly to that of dopamine, whereas in selective neurons it is converted to epinephrine by phenylethanolamine-N-methyltransferase. See Ch. 229 also for a discussion of catecholamine metabolism.

In nerve endings, newly synthesized catecholamines are stored in secretory granules that protect them from enzymatic degradation. There are at least two distinct pools of neurotransmitters that are differentially susceptible to releasing stimuli. A long-lasting depletion of catecholamines can be produced by reserpine, which causes a slow but constant release of the monoamines and inhibits reuptake. Catecholamine release occurs in response to nerve stimulation by fusion of the secretion vesicle membrane with the cell membrane and extrusion of the amine directly into the intercellular space. Once released, catecholamines bind to postsynaptic receptors that appear to be similar in the hypophysiotropic neurons to those demonstrated in other neural sites. In addition, they bind to presynaptic receptors on the nerve terminals to effect a feedback regulation. Alterations in presynaptic and postsynaptic receptor activity are accomplished by the use of receptor agonists and antagonists. Catecholamine action terminates primarily by reuptake of the neurotransmitter into the presynaptic neuron, but also by removal into the circulation and metabolic degradation. Drugs such as cocaine, tricyclic antidepressants, or nomifensine inhibit reuptake, resulting in enhancement of catecholamine effects. Metabolic degradation occurs by two enzymes: monoamine oxidase (MAO) and catechol-O-methyltransferase. Catecholamine action is therefore enhanced by MAO inhibitors such as pargyline and tranylcypromine.

Indolamines (Serotonin, Melatonin). Tryptophan, the precursor of serotonin, is actively transported from blood to brain. Since tryptophan hydroxylase activity is not saturated at physiologic concentrations, fluctuations in plasma tryptophan levels determine the rate of brain serotonin synthesis. After hydroxylation, 5-hydroxytryptophan is converted to serotonin by aromatic L-amino acid decarboxylase. Serotonin functions as a neurotransmitter and, in the pineal, also serves as a precursor of melatonin. Serotonin synthesis can be inhibited by p-chlorophenylalanine, which inhibits tryptophan hydroxylase, and by L-dopa, which competes with 5-hydroxytryptophan for decarboxylation. The storage, release, and uptake of serotonin are similar to those of norepinephrine, with many of the same agents (i.e., amphetamine) releasing both compounds. Tricyclic antidepressants inhibit serotonin uptake, although in contrast to norepinephrine, imipramine and amitriptyline are more potent than their desmethyl derivatives (desmethylimipramine and nortriptyline). Alteration of serotonin receptor activity can be produced by agonists such as quipazine and LSD and by antagonists (methysergide and cyproheptadine). Termination of serotonin effects occurs by presynaptic reuptake and metabolic degradation involving MAO. Drugs interfering with MAO activity also enhance serotonin effects.

Acetylcholine. Acetylcholine is synthesized from acetyl-CoA and choline. The source of choline is probably phosphatidylcholine which, after crossing the blood-brain barrier, is partially degraded to choline. Choline is then converted to acetylcholine by choline acetyltransferase. There are two types of acetylcholine receptors, muscarinic and nicotinic, which have different anatomic distribution and physiologic function. Arecoline and atropine, a muscarinic agonist and antagonist, respectively, cross the blood-brain barrier and modify acetylcholine receptor activity. Inhibitors of acetylcholinesterase, such as pyridostigmine, enhance cholinergic tone.

Gamma-Aminobutyric Acid (GABA). In the mammalian hypothalamus GABA is an inhibitory neurotransmitter. It is formed by the decarboxylation of L-glutamate and is metabolized by transamination. Numerous agents inhibit GABA synthesis and metabolism, but only one, valproate, an inhibitor of GABA degradation, has been shown to be useful clinically in altering neuroendocrine function.

Histamine. Histamine is synthesized within the CNS from histidine by a specific decarboxylase and the nonspecific aromatic L-amino acid decarboxylase. Alteration of histamine effects is brought about primarily by histamine receptor antagonists. There are two classes of histamine receptors: H_1 and H_2. Drugs such as diphenhydramine and cyproheptadine inhibit H_1 receptors, while cimetidine and ranitidine inhibit H_2 receptors.

Neuropeptides. A large number of neuropeptides have been

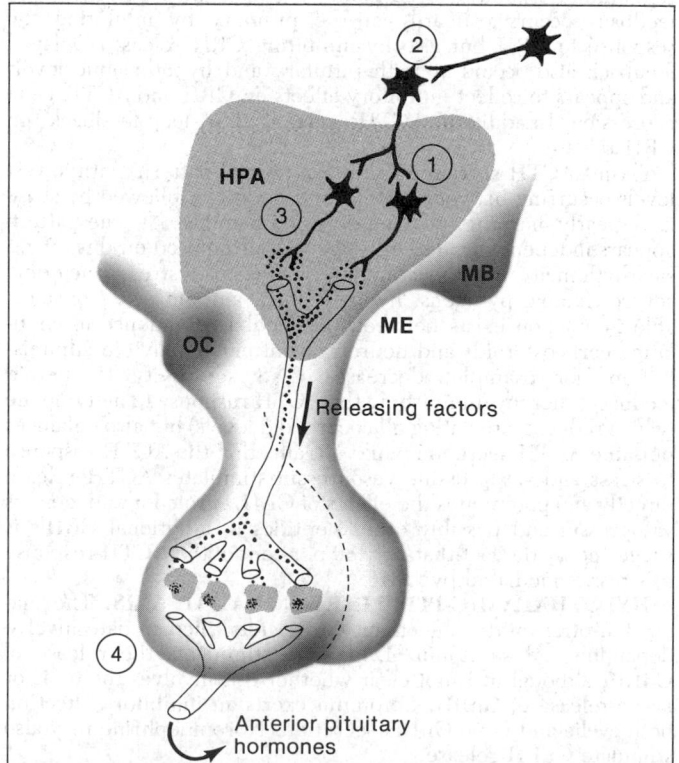

FIGURE 212–2. Sites of potential neurotransmitter effects on hypothalamic releasing and inhibiting hormone secretion and function. HPA = Hypophysiotropic area; OC = optic chiasm; ME = median eminence; MB = mamillary body. Refer to text for description of effects at each site. (From Frohman LA: Clinical neuropharmacology of hypothalamic releasing factors. N Engl J Med 286:1391, 1972. Reprinted by permission of the New England Journal of Medicine.)

identified in the hypothalamus, and their role in the regulation of neuroendocrine function is, at present, only incompletely understood. A list of neuropeptides with potential effects on releasing and inhibiting hormones is provided in Table 212–1. Many of these peptides are widely distributed in extrahypothalamic CNS and function as neurotransmitters or neuromodulators in other pathways. Of particular significance is a group of peptides common to both the CNS and the gastrointestinal tract. Although the function of many of these peptides within the CNS remains to be determined, they appear to have a role in integrative systems relating to homeostatic mechanisms. Their presence throughout evolution and as far back as unicellular organisms underscores their essential role in intercellular communication. With the exception of analogues of enkephalin capable of crossing the blood-brain barrier and of TRH, neuroendocrine effects of peptides other than hypophysiotropic hormones have not been convincingly documented in man. Limited information is available concerning biosynthesis, storage, secretion, and local metabolism of hypothalamic neuropeptides. The hypothalamus also contains numerous lymphokines and monokines, and these immunoregulatory signals are capable of affecting neuroendocrine function. Interleukin (IL)-1, IL-6, and thymic peptides release both hypothalamic and pituitary hormones.

MECHANISM OF ACTION OF HYPOTHALAMIC HORMONES. Hypophysiotropic hormones affect pituitary hormone secretion by several mechanisms. Specific, high-affinity receptors are present on the anterior pituitary target cells, and evidence now points to the participation of several intracellular mediator or second messenger systems, including adenylate cyclase–cyclic AMP, calcium-calmodulin, and phosphatidylinositol–protein kinase C. In addition, at least some releasing hormones stimulate pituitary hormone gene expression and exhibit mitogenic effects, since stimulation can lead to cellular hyperplasia and even tumor formation.

The mechanism of action of the inhibitory hormones somatostatin and dopamine is less well understood. Somatostatin inhibits cyclic AMP formation and enhances phosphodiesterase activity, both of which actions impair hormone release mediated by cyclic AMP. Somatostatin also inhibits transmembrane Ca^{2+} transport and may have other effects on exocytosis. The inhibitory effects of dopamine appear to be independent of cyclic AMP levels, and, like somatostatin, occur at a late stage in the secretory process. Dopamine also exhibits inhibitory effects on gene expression in lactotrophs.

The effects of all the hypophysiotropic hormones studied to date are modified by target gland hormones, i.e., thyroxine, cortisol, estrogens, androgens, inhibin, and insulin-like growth factors. These hormones alter the number of releasing or inhib-

TABLE 212–1. NEUROPEPTIDES WITH POTENTIAL EFFECTS ON HYPOTHALAMIC RELEASING HORMONES

Gastroenteropancreatic peptides
  Cholecystokinin
  Galanin
  Gastrin
  Gastrin-releasing peptide
  Glucagon
  Insulin
  Motilin
  Neuropeptide PHI/PHM
  Neurotensin
  Pancreatic polypeptide
  Secretin
  Substance P
  Vasoactive intestinal peptide

Hypothalamic hormones
  Corticotropin-releasing
    hormone
  Growth hormone–releasing
    hormone
  Somatostatin
  Thyrotropin-releasing hormone
  Vasopressin

Endorphin-enkephalin peptides
  α-Melanocyte stimulating
    hormone
  β-Endorphin
  Dynorphin
  Methionine/leucine enkephalin

Immunomodulators
  Interleukin-1
  Interleukin-6
  Thymosin fraction 5

Others
  Angiotensin
  Bradykinin
  Calcitonin
  Calcitonin gene–related product
  Neuropeptide PYY

iting hormone receptors, but also exhibit effects at postreceptor sites.

Regulation of Hypophysiotropic and Pituitary Hormone Secretion

The control of hypophysiotropic hormone secretion is best appreciated when considered in conjunction with that of the five major pituitary hormone systems they regulate: ACTH, LH and FSH, TSH, GH, and prolactin. Each consists of feedback (closed loop) systems involving primarily blood-borne signals on which are superimposed other neurotransmitter-mediated signals mostly originating within the CNS (open loop) and representing environment (temperature, light-dark), stress (pain, fear, psychic), and intrinsic rhythmicity (ranging from ultradian or short-term to diurnal, monthly, and seasonal). Thus, both internal and external environmental factors are important determinants of the activity of these systems. A summary of neurotransmitter effects on pituitary hormone secretion is provided in Table 212–2.

HYPOTHALAMIC-PITUITARY-ADRENOCORTICAL AXIS. Nearly all of the monoamine neurotransmitters affect CRH release. Acetylcholine stimulates CRH release predominantly through nicotinic receptors and appears to be the primary neurotransmitter mediating stress-induced CRH release. Serotonin also stimulates CRH release, but the effect is likely mediated through a cholinergic interneuron, since it can be blocked by atropine. Norepinephrine inhibits the cholinergic effects on CRH release through an α-adrenergic receptor, and GABA exerts a similar effect. Melatonin inhibits CRH and may be responsible for the circadian pattern of CRH release that is entrained to the light-dark cycle. Enkephalins exert inhibitory effects on the pituitary-adrenal axis. This effect is believed to occur within the hypothalamus at the level of CRH release, although an additional action on the pituitary has not been excluded. Interleukin-1 (IL-1), a neuroimmunomodulator, also stimulates CRH release.

CRH stimulates ACTH release, which in turn stimulates the secretion of glucocorticoids and mineralocorticoids from the adrenal cortex. Glucocorticoids inhibit ACTH secretion by both rapid (minutes) and delayed (hours) feedback mechanisms. Rapid feedback occurs primarily at the pituitary by inhibiting the response to CRH but also by inhibiting CRH release. Delayed feedback also occurs at both pituitary and hypothalamic levels and appears to reflect inhibitory effects on CRH and ACTH gene expression. In addition, ACTH exerts a "short-loop feedback" on CRH release.

Plasma ACTH secretion exhibits a diurnal pattern, with lowest levels occurring between 10 P.M. and midnight followed by a rise in the early morning, peaking between 6 and 8 A.M. The pattern appears independent of sleep stage. Superimposed on this intrinsic rhythmicity are the stimulatory effects of stress, including severe trauma, pyrogens, hypoglycemia, and anxiety. Considerable interaction exists between the feedback influence of circulating corticosteroids and neurotransmitters. Phenytoin administration, for example, decreases CNS sensitivity to steroid feedback, thereby diminishing the ACTH response to metyrapone (which reduces circulating glucocorticoid levels) but also enhances pulsatile ACTH secretion while not affecting the ACTH response to stress and vasopressin. Vasopressin stimulates ACTH release directly and potentiates the effects of CRH. A role for endogenous vasopressin and possibly other peptides as additional CRH's is suggested by the fact that only 80 per cent of the ACTH response to stress is mediated by CRH.

HYPOTHALAMIC-PITUITARY-GONADAL AXIS. The major neurotransmitter effects on GnRH identified to date involve dopamine and serotonin. Dopamine stimulates the release of GnRH, although it is not clear whether this involves the tonic or cyclic release of GnRH. Serotonin exerts an inhibitory effect on both cyclic and tonic GnRH secretion. Norepinephrine may also stimulate GnRH release.

The regulation of the hypothalamic-pituitary-gonadal axis varies with age and sex. LH and FSH are present in circulation from birth, and through the early stages of puberty FSH levels gradually increase to a greater degree than do LH levels. During this period, FSH responses to GnRH are greater than are LH responses, a pattern opposite to that seen after puberty, and the hypothalamus is exceedingly sensitive to the suppressive effects of gonadal steroids. In the later prepubertal period (7 to 9 years) sleep-related pulsatile LH secretion begins, and synchronization occurs between LH and FSH pulses. These pulses stimulate the secretion of testosterone in boys and estradiol in girls that initiates the clinical characteristics of puberty. At the same time, evidence for lessening sensitivity of hypothalamic GnRH secretion in response to steroid feedback can be demonstrated. In females, development of positive feedback on LH and FSH by gonadal steroids generates the cyclic preovulatory gonadotropin surge resulting in the establishment of cyclic ovulation by the mid-teens. In adult males the LH secretory pattern is characterized by eight to ten pulses occurring at regular intervals through the day, and the teenage relationship to the sleep-wake pattern disappears. Similar pulsatile secretion of LH and FSH occurs in mature women, the frequency and magnitude of the pulses varying with the phase of the menstrual cycle. When ovarian follicles disappear at menopause, secretion of the major ovarian hormones decreases, and the loss of negative feedback of these hormones enhances secretion of FSH and, to a lesser extent, LH. A similar increase in LH and FSH is observed in men in the seventh and eighth decades in response to decreasing testicular function.

In men, surgical stress results in a transitory rise in the level of LH followed by a prolonged fall, accompanied by a fall in testosterone levels. No changes have been observed in women, although hypothalamic anovulation is frequently seen during periods of stress. Pheromones or other environmental factors have been implicated as the cause for the synchronization of menstrual cycles seen in women living in close association.

Steroid hormones regulate LH and FSH secretion by two major mechanisms. Gonadal steroids regulate tonic secretion by a negative feedback mechanism. Testosterone appears to be more potent than estrogen in this negative feedback effect, while progesterone has an intermediate effect. Inhibin, a peptide produced by ovarian granulosa cells and testicular Sertoli cells, has a selective action in inhibiting FSH release, possibly by impairing the effects of GnRH. Cyclic release of LH and FSH is stimulated by a positive feedback effect of ovarian steroids during the final phases of follicular growth prior to ovulation. The preovulatory surge of LH is preceded by an increase in circulating estrogen levels in the presence of low or decreasing progesterone levels. The positive effects occur at both the hypothalamic and pituitary levels, although the latter appear to be more important. GnRH is released in a tonic pulsatile manner by the hypothalamus approximately every 90 minutes, and this pattern of secretion is critical for its effects on the pituitary. In an individual deficient in GnRH secretion, pulsatile administration of GnRH allows restoration of normal cyclic ovulation. In contrast, constant infusion of GnRH leads to down-regulation of pituitary GnRH receptors and a suppression of gonadotropin secretion. This phenomenon has resulted in major advances in therapy aimed at enhancing or preventing fertility.

HYPOTHALAMIC-PITUITARY-THYROID AXIS. TSH secretion by the pituitary is regulated by TRH, dopamine, and somatostatin. For a discussion of the control of somatostatin secretion, the reader is referred to the section on the regulation of GH secretion. TRH secretion is stimulated by norepinephrine and dopamine and is inhibited by serotonin. TRH stimulates TSH secretion, which in turn enhances the release of thyroxine and triiodothyronine by the thyroid. The feedback effects of these hormones, primarily triiodothyronine, occur principally in the pituitary, where they inhibit the TSH response to TRH. A reduction in circulating thyroid hormone levels leads to a prompt rise in TSH levels. TRH is not required for this acute response, although it is necessary for the full expression of TSH hypersecretion over a long time. In addition, TRH is required for maintaining basal TSH secretion. In addition to its effects on the pituitary, triiodothyronine exerts an inhibitory effect on TRH gene expression in the hypothalamus.

Acute changes in environmental conditions requiring increased metabolic activity, such as cold exposure, lead to a TRH-mediated increase in TSH secretion. This effect is readily demonstrable in infants but not in adults, in whom other mechanisms of thermogenesis (mediated by the autonomic nervous system and resulting in shivering and free fatty acid mobilization) are more important. Agents inhibiting adrenergic neurotransmission block the TSH response to cold.

Dopaminergic agents exert an inhibitory effect on TSH release by the pituitary which is most pronounced in patients with elevated TSH levels but is also seen in normal individuals. A role of endogenous dopamine in suppressing TSH secretion has also been demonstrated.

Somatostatin inhibition of TSH secretion exerts a relatively minor physiologic role under normal circumstances, but increases in hypothalamic somatostatin release as a result of elevated GH levels can suppress TSH secretion to subnormal levels. Somatostatin, however, is a less potent inhibitor of TSH than of GH.

HYPOTHALAMIC-PITUITARY-SOMATOTROPH AXIS. GH secretion is regulated by releasing and inhibiting hormones: GRH and SRIF (somatostatin). GH is secreted in a pulsatile pattern with basal levels at or beneath the level of detection, superimposed on which are pulses of GH related to an inherent neural rhythmicity resulting in pulsatile release of both GRH and SRIF. The majority of pulsatile GH secretion occurs about 1 hour after the onset of sleep and is associated with sleep stages 3 and 4. With age, GH secretion changes dramatically, both qualitatively and quantitatively. Extremely high levels seen in the first few days of life decrease by 2 weeks of age. During the pubertal period levels comparable to or greater than those of adults are seen, and the GH surges occur more frequently. After the fourth decade, there is a gradual and progressive decrease in spontaneous GH secretion and responses to GH releasing stimuli also decrease. Neurotransmitter regulation of GH secretion has been extensively defined. Dopamine, norepinephrine (through the α receptor), epinephrine, serotonin, GABA, and acetylcholine have all been shown to stimulate GH secretion. Melatonin has both stimulatory and inhibitory effects, TRH and CRH exhibit inhibitory effects (both peptides stimulate SRIF release), and endorphins-enkephalins have stimulatory effects, all mediated within the CNS.

GH secretion is profoundly affected by nutrients. Elevations of amino acid levels, decreases in free fatty acids, and hypoglycemia all stimulate GH secretion, while hyperglycemia inhibits GH release. GH secretion is increased by exercise, anxiety, and emotional or physical stress. Many hormones affect GH secretion. Estrogen administration increases GH responsiveness, while corticosteroid and thyroid hormone deficiency and excess decrease responsiveness. In pubertal and prepubertal males, androgen

TABLE 212–2. EFFECTS OF AMINERGIC AND PEPTIDERGIC NEUROTRANSMITTERS ON ANTERIOR PITUITARY HORMONE SECRETION

	Norepinephrine	Dopamine	Serotonin	Acetylcholine	Histamine	GABA	Other
ACTH	α ↑	−	↑	↑	−	−	Enkephalins ↓
LH and FSH	(↑)	↓	−	−	−	−	−
TSH	↑	↓	↑	−	−	−	Neurotensin ↓
GH	α ↑ β ↓	↑	↑	↑	−	(↑)	Neurotensin ↓ Substance P ↓ Enkephalins ↑
Prolactin	−	↓	↑	−	↑	↑	Neurotensin ↓ Enkephalins ↑ VIP ↑

NOTE: ↑ = stimulates; ↓ = inhibits; − = no effect or insufficient data; ( ) = conflicting data exist. All effects reflect CNS rather than pituitary sites of action (with the exception of dopamine). The data are derived (whenever possible) from studies in humans.

administration also enhances GH responses. GH secretion is sexually dimorphic: Women have higher basal levels and smaller pulses than do men. These differences may, in part, contribute to sex-related differences in growth patterns and selected enzyme activity.

In addition to these "open-loop" stimuli is a closed-loop feedback system. GH stimulates the production of somatomedin C (insulin-like growth factor [IGF-I]) by numerous tissues, and both GH and IGF-I exhibit feedback effects. IGF-I stimulates the release of somatostatin, inhibits that of GH, and also inhibits basal and GRH-stimulated GH synthesis and release by the pituitary. GH itself stimulates SRIF secretion and inhibits GRH gene expression and secretion.

HYPOTHALAMIC-LACTOTROPH-BREAST AXIS. Prolactin secretion is predominantly controlled by inhibitory CNS influences, with dopamine being the major prolactin-inhibiting factor. Two peptides, TRH and vasoactive intestinal polypeptide (VIP), appear to have physiologic prolactin-releasing factor (PRF) activity, although their relative importance is not yet clear. Neurotransmitter influences on prolactin secretion are extensive. Serotonin stimulates prolactin release by effects on PRF. Melatonin and histamine have stimulatory effects within the CNS, as do opioid peptides and GABA. The effect of the latter two agents appears due to their inhibitory effects on the tuberoinfundibular dopaminergic system.

Prolactin secretion is increased by tactile stimulation of the breast via receptors in the nipple and areola that reach the spinal cord by the intercostal nerves. During pregnancy, prolactin levels increase as a result of estrogen stimulation. Following parturition, the rapid decline in estrogen and progesterone levels allows the unopposed action of prolactin to stimulate lactation from the estrogen-primed breast. The suckling stimulation of prolactin secretion is in part controlled by VIP. Prolactin levels return to normal after several months even during continual lactation. Prolactin is a stress-responsive hormone, and increased secretion is observed after surgical stress, exercise, and insulin hypoglycemia. Prolactin secretion is increased in states of thyroid hormone deficiency and decreased in the presence of thyroid hormone excess.

Bateman A, Singh A, Kral T, et al.: The immune-hypothalamic-pituitary-adrenal axis. Endocr Rev 10:92, 1989. *A critical review of the developing field of neuroimmunology. The interaction of cytokines with the neuroendocrine system, while not yet completely understood, is likely to become of major importance.*

Frohman LA, Krieger DT: Neuroendocrine physiology and disease. *In* Felig P, Baxter JD, Broadus AE, et al. (eds.): Endocrinology and Metabolism, 2nd ed. New York, McGraw-Hill Book Company, 1987, pp 185–247. *A systematic in-depth presentation of the anatomy and physiology of human neuroendocrinology, along with the clinical manifestations, diagnosis, and therapy of anatomic and functional disorders. Designed for the medical student, clinical trainee, and practicing physician.*

Krieger DT, Brownstein M, Martin JB (eds.): Brain Peptides. Vol 2. New York, John Wiley & Sons, 1987. *A comprehensive collection of monographs on the role of brain peptides as transmitters, hypophysiotropic hormones, and messengers throughout the nervous system. This is a definitive reference volume. Of interest to the medical student, neurobiologist, and clinical trainee.*

Marshall JC, Kelch RP: Gonadotropin-releasing hormone: Role of pulsatile secretion in the regulation of reproduction. N Engl J Med 315:1215, 1986. *An excellent discussion of the importance of pulsatility in the biologic effects of gonadotropin-releasing hormone on the pituitary.*

Morley JE: Neuropeptide regulation of appetite and weight. Endocr Rev 8:256, 1987. *The regulation of food intake is a complex issue that involves several distinct brain regions and neurochemical mediators. This review provides an up-to-date assessment of the importance of various brain peptides in this activity.*

Muller EE: Neural control of somatotropic function. Physiol Rev 67:962, 1987. *An excellent review of the current knowledge of neuroendocrine regulation of growth hormone secretion.*

Nieman LK, Loriaux DL: Corticotropin-releasing hormone: Clinical applications. Annu Rev Med 40:331, 1989. Taylor AL, Fishman LM: Corticotropin-releasing hormone. N Engl J Med 319:213, 1988. *Two excellent reviews of the physiology, pathology, and clinical utility of the releasing hormone.*

DISEASES OF THE CENTRAL NERVOUS SYSTEM WITH ALTERED NEUROENDOCRINE AND NEUROMETABOLIC FUNCTION

The frequent association of altered hormone secretion with disorders of the CNS has been recognized for many decades. Although attention was initially focused on the hypothalamus

because of its crucial role in neuroendocrine regulation, diseases localized to extrahypothalamic brain regions as well as nonlocalized CNS disorders can also produce disturbances in neuroendocrine function. The clinical and laboratory manifestations of these disorders are frequently indistinguishable from those of hypothalamic origin, since their mediation is usually via the hypothalamus. Similarly, the distinction between hypothalamic and pituitary causes of certain pituitary hormone secretory disorders may be difficult for other reasons.

Because of the reticular organization of the anatomic structure of the hypothalamus, only certain functions can be localized to a precise site. In addition, neurons within a specific hypothalamic locus may be involved in several separate regulatory functions. Consequently the extent of endocrine or metabolic disturbance is more dependent on the location than the size of the hypothalamic lesion. Furthermore, slowly growing lesions tend to be silent until they have reached considerable size, whereas rapidly enlarging lesions, depending on location, can cause dramatic clinical and laboratory manifestations even when quite small.

Acute hypothalamic damage is associated with impairment of consciousness, sustained hyperthermia, and severe disturbances of cardiovascular, gastrointestinal, or respiratory function. In contrast, persistent disease in the hypothalamus results in alterations in cognition and complex homeostatic functions. Although disorders of neuroendocrine regulation can be produced by acute lesions that destroy the median eminence or the pituitary stalk, they generally tend to be seen with chronic disorders and often result in an inability of the endocrine system to adapt to environmental changes rather than in an alteration of basal hormone secretion. Because hypothalamic neuronal projections, in contrast to those involving sensory and motor function, are generally not lateralized, unilateral damage seldom results in significant or prolonged symptoms. Thus disturbances of hypothalamic function are most commonly seen with diffuse infiltrative or inflammatory diseases, with tumors of the midline that expand bilaterally, or with disorders affecting the median eminence, the final common effector pathway to the pituitary.

Etiology of Hypothalamic Disease

Anatomically defined disorders of the hypothalamus vary in frequency with age groups and are summarized in Table 212–3. In addition, disturbances of neuroendocrine or neurometabolic function are frequently unassociated with anatomic evidence of hypothalamic disease using available neuroradiologic techniques. Many have been attributed to disorders of neurochemical function, although precise mechanisms are currently not known.

TUMORS. Hypothalamic tumors are frequently located in the region of the third ventricle. Those tumors located in the inferior portion of the third ventricle or the anterior mediobasal hypothalamus commonly produce disturbances in neuroendocrine and neurometabolic regulation. The most frequent hypothalamic tumors are craniopharyngiomas (see next section) and their variants (ependymomas and epidermoid cysts), followed by astrocytomas and dysgerminomas. Two other tumor types, hypothalamic pinealomas and hamartomas, are considered separately because of their association with specific neuroendocrine disorders. Since they are frequently of developmental origin, the majority of hypothalamic tumors occur in patients under 25 years of age. Endocrine disturbances generally result from destruction of those neuronal elements required for normal pituitary function. The most frequently occurring manifestations are diabetes insipidus, hypogonadism, and growth retardation. Disturbances in thyroid and adrenal function are less common. The diagnosis of a hypothalamic tumor is made by magnetic resonance imaging and visual field measurement. The combination of an atypical visual field defect (i.e., loss of inferior visual fields), normal sellar anatomy, and intact responses to releasing hormones in a patient with hypopituitarism points to primary hypothalamic disease. It is difficult to remove hypothalamic tumors completely without destroying normal tissue critical for maintaining homeostasis. Many of these tumors, because of their developmental origin, tend to be slow growing and may even undergo spontaneous growth arrest or regression. Cystic tumors can be aspirated or marsupialized into the cerebroventricular system. Radiotherapy is also effective in many of these tumors. The loss of endocrine function is, however, rarely reversible, and replacement hormone therapy is required.

Neonates
Intraventricular hemorrhage
Meningitis: bacterial
Tumors: glioma, hemangioma
Trauma
Hydrocephalus, hydranencephaly, kernicterus

1 Month–2 Years
Tumors: glioma, especially optic glioma, histiocytosis X, hemangiomas
Hydrocephalus, meningitis
"Familial" disorders: Laurence-Moon, Bardet-Biedl, Prader-Labhart-Willi

2–10 Years
Tumors: craniopharyngioma, glioma, dysgerminoma, hamartoma, histiocytosis X, leukemia, ganglioneuroma, ependymoma, medulloblastoma
Meningitis: bacterial, tuberculous
Encephalitis: viral and demyelinating, various viral encephalitides and exanthematous demyelinating encephalitides, disseminated encephalomyelitis
"Familial" disorders: diabetes insipidus, etc.
Damage from nasopharyngeal radiation therapy

10–25 Years
Tumors: craniopharyngioma, pituitary tumors, glioma, hamartoma, dysgerminoma, histiocytosis X, leukemia, dermoid, lipoma, neuroblastoma
Trauma
Subarachnoid hemorrhage, vascular aneurysm, arteriovenous malformation
Inflammatory diseases: meningitis, encephalitis, sarcoidosis, tuberculosis
Associated with midline brain defects: agenesis of corpus callosum
Chronic hydrocephalus or increased intracranial pressure

25–50 Years
Nutritional: Wernicke's disease
Tumors: glioma, lymphoma, meningioma, craniopharyngioma, pituitary tumors, angioma, plasmacytoma, colloid cysts, ependymoma, sarcoma, histiocytosis X
Inflammatory: sarcoidosis, tuberculosis, viral encephalitis
Subarachnoid hemorrhage, vascular aneurysms, arteriovenous malformation
Damage from pituitary radiation therapy

50 Years and Older
Nutritional: Wernicke's disease
Tumors: sarcoma, glioblastoma, lymphoma, meningioma, colloid cysts, ependymoma, pituitary tumors
Vascular: infarct, subarachnoid hemorrhage, pituitary apoplexy
Infectious: encephalitis, sarcoidosis, meningitis

Adapted from Plum F, Van Uitert R: Non-endocrine diseases of the hypothalamus. *In* Reichlin S, Baldessarini RJ, Martin JB (eds.): The Hypothalamus. New York, Raven Press, 1978, p 415.

Hamartomas. One type of hypothalamic tumor, the hamartoma, has been associated with increased, rather than decreased, hypothalamic function. Hamartomas consist of masses of redundant, partially disoriented glial and neuronal cells or an abnormally lodged collection of normal nerve tissue. Hamartomas associated with precocious puberty consist of encapsulated nodules in the posterior hypothalamus containing membrane-bound secretion granules similar to those in hypothalamic neurosecretory cells. Vessels in the hamartoma have fenestrations characteristic of those in the median eminence, suggesting a secretory process similar to that in the median eminence. These vessels are presumed to connect to the pituitary portal system. The secretion granules contain GnRH, which is found in high concentrations in CSF from patients with this disorder. Hamartomatous cells are believed to secrete GnRH in a pulsatile manner, but are not under normal prepubertal inhibitory influences. The resultant hormonal effects produce pubertal changes that in girls lead to menarche and cyclic ovulatory menses as early as the second year of life.

Hamartomas are present in one third of all children with this form of precocious puberty. Specific therapy aimed at the hamartoma appears unnecessary, since its course is benign with no other neuroendocrine disturbances and no loss of nonendocrine hypothalamic structure or function. Therapy of the precocious

puberty, however, is of great importance both for psychological reasons and for prevention of premature epiphyseal fusion and stunted growth. Optimal therapy is currently achieved with the use of a GnRH agonist to down-regulate pituitary GnRH receptors, resulting in diminished gonadotropin secretion and suppression of bone growth.

Hypothalamic hamartomas have also been associated with gigantism, acromegaly, and GH-secreting pituitary tumors. They have been shown to contain GRH, which is secreted into the portal system, resulting in GH hypersecretion and somatotroph hyperplasia and tumor formation.

Gangliocytomas. A closely related tumor, the gangliocytoma, consists of randomly oriented large ganglion cells similar to those in the hypothalamic magnocellular (large cell) nuclei. Intrapituitary gangliocytomas are also seen in association with acromegaly and GH-secreting tumors of the pituitary and contain GRH. In contrast to hypothalamic hamartomas, the axons of the intrapituitary tumors directly contact the somatotropic cells. A CRH-containing pituitary gangliocytoma has also been described in association with ACTH hypersecretion and Cushing's disease.

Pineal Tumors. Pineal tumors constitute less than 1 per cent of all intracranial neoplasms and consist of three separate tumor types: pinealomas (pineal parenchymal tumor [20 per cent]), glial tumors (25 per cent), and germinomas (also called ectopic pinealomas or teratomas [55 per cent]). The neuroendocrine effects (precocious puberty) of the first two types are most likely a consequence of destruction of the normal pineal by tumor, leading to loss of pineal secretory products (possibly melatonin, arginine vasotocin, or another factor) that normally inhibit the initiation of sexual maturation. Only a small percentage of pineal tumors cause sexual precocity and usually not until they extend beyond the pineal region. Some pineal tumors are associated with delayed puberty, which may be mediated by production of an antigonadotropic factor. Precocious puberty associated with germinomas, which are similar both histologically and functionally to ovarian and testicular germ cell tumors, is caused by the production of chorionic gonadotropin. Levels as high as those seen during the first month of pregnancy are often present. Many of the "ectopic" pinealomas occur in the midline of the ventral hypothalamus and result in loss of other endocrine functions. Surgical treatment of pinealomas is generally unsatisfactory although the tumors consisting of germinal elements are exquisitely radiosensitive. Many tumors, however, contain nongerminal elements (teratomas) that are relatively radioresistant. See also Ch. 215.

INFILTRATIVE AND INFLAMMATORY DISEASES. Histiocytosis X (see also Ch. 149). This granulomatous disease of the histiocytic type, with eosinophilic elements, involves the ventromedial hypothalamus and is associated with diabetes insipidus, anterior hypopituitarism due to destruction of releasing hormone-secreting neurons, or both. The three clinical subgroups of the disease are Hand-Schüller-Christian disease, the most common type, characterized by polyuria, exophthalmos, and skull defects; Letterer-Siwe disease, a more rapidly progressive form; and eosinophilic granuloma, in which similar pathologic findings are present in bones. The disease may begin with diabetes insipidus, which is present in nearly 50 per cent of patients with Hand-Schüller-Christian disease. Less commonly, growth failure, hypogonadism, and panhypopituitarism are seen. The diagnosis is established by bone or intracranial biopsy. The CNS forms of the disease may respond to high-dose glucocorticoid therapy or chemotherapy, but the impairment in neuroendocrine function appears irreversible.

Sarcoidosis (see Ch. 67). Involvement of the CNS by sarcoidosis is uncommon. When it is present, however, the hypothalamus and pituitary are frequently involved with infiltrating granulomatous nodules. Patients may develop diabetes insipidus, galactorrhea due to hyperprolactinemia, partial or total anterior pituitary insufficiency, and neurometabolic and neurovegetative symptoms such as somnolence or hyperphagia. In general, the usual treatment with glucocorticoids does not improve the endocrine dysfunction. Granulomatous hypothalamic disease, producing the same endocrine disturbances, can also occur in the absence of peripheral manifestations of sarcoidosis.

TRAUMA. Basal skull fractures are frequently accompanied by shearing of the pituitary stalk, leading to panhypopituitarism and diabetes insipidus. In patients who become comatose following skull fractures, impairment in the pituitary-thyroid and pituitary-gonadal axes has been reported in the absence of stalk damage. Gonadal and thyroid hormones generally return to normal upon recovery.

RADIATION-INDUCED HYPOTHALAMIC DYSFUNCTION. Radiation therapy for intracranial neoplasms, including pituitary tumors, and for nasopharyngeal and maxillary sinus carcinomas frequently leads to hypopituitarism. The interval between therapy and appearance of hormone deficiencies ranges from 1 to 10 years or possibly longer. Children appear more susceptible than adults, and the critical dose is believed to be about 4000 rads. In children, growth failure associated with reduced GH secretion, hypogonadotropic hypogonadism, and hypothyroidism is seen. The site of the defect appears to be variable, with some patients exhibiting hypothalamic and others pituitary damage. In some, but not all, patients, pituitary hormone responses to the injection of hypothalamic releasing hormones may distinguish the anatomic site of the defect.

FUNCTIONAL DISEASES OF THE CENTRAL NERVOUS SYSTEM WITH NEUROENDOCRINE DISTURBANCES

Disturbances in neuroendocrine function manifested by both decreased and increased pituitary hormone secretion can occur in the absence of structurally detectable disease in the pituitary or CNS. With the aid of releasing hormones to test specifically the pituitary component and other stimuli to test the hypothalamic-pituitary unit, some degree of discrimination can be made as to the source of the disordered hormone secretion. The following are recognized functional disturbances that have been attributed to hypothalamic (or possibly other CNS) disease. The specific biochemical defect responsible remains to be determined.

HYPOTHALAMIC HYPOGONADISM. This disorder is defined as an impairment in pituitary-gonadal function caused by deficient or disordered secretion of GnRH. The manifestations vary according to the age at presentation (see also Ch. 222 and 224).

Prepubertal. The presence of hypothalamic hypogonadism prior to puberty results in failure of normal sexual maturation. Other pituitary hormone deficiencies, also attributed to hypothalamic dysfunction, may coexist. A major subgroup of this disorder, most frequently seen in boys, includes anosmia or hyposmia (*Kallmann's syndrome* or olfactory-genital dysplasia). This syndrome may be associated with other neurologic defects such as color blindness and nerve deafness. The disorder is frequently familial, although sporadic cases have also been reported. Midline developmental defects occasionally occur, and hypoplasia in the region of the anterior commissure, olfactory bulb, and hypothalamus has been found. In some patients there is an additional defect characterized by decreased testicular response to LH. The gonadotropin responses to a single injection of GnRH are markedly impaired or absent, indicating a lack of prior GnRH function. Repeated administration of GnRH, given to prime the gonadotrophs, eventually produces a normal or supranormal gonadotropin response and serves to differentiate this disorder from that of primary gonadotroph failure. Standard therapy consists of the use of gonadal steroids for the development and maintenance of secondary sexual characteristics. GnRH can produce similar effects and promote fertility if administered by an intermittent infusion pump to simulate endogenous gonadotropin secretion.

Postpubertal. Postpubertal hypothalamic hypogonadism is more frequently seen in women but also affects men. In women, it is manifested clinically by secondary amenorrhea or oligomenorrhea and occasionally by infertility associated with anovulatory cycles. The terms *functional* or *psychogenic amenorrhea* and *infertility* have also been used for this disorder. Patients may exhibit normal basal levels of gonadotropins and estradiol, resulting in maintenance of secondary sexual characteristics, although pulsatile secretion of LH is absent, and the cyclic ovulatory surge of gonadotropins does not occur. The gonadotropin responses to a single injection of GnRH reveal enhancement of the FSH rather than the LH response. These women respond normally to clomiphene, an estrogen receptor antagonist, suggesting that the defect is related to a functional derangement in the positive estrogen feedback mechanism. The disorder is usually self-limited. In men, the presenting symptoms are decreased libido and impotency. Therapy consists of testosterone alone unless there is also a desire for fertility.

Hyperprolactinemia exerts an inhibitory effect on the positive feedback effect of estradiol on GnRH secretion that has been attributed to enhanced tuberoinfundibular dopamine secretion. The negative estrogen feedback mechanism appears intact, since elevated FSH and LH levels are maintained in postmenopausal women with hyperprolactinemia. In men, hyperprolactinemia produces hypogonadism, manifested most frequently by diminished libido and potency and occasionally by gynecomastia.

In severe cases, basal estradiol levels and serum gonadotropin responses to GnRH are reduced, implying a defect in tonic as well as cyclic GnRH secretion. Similar physiologic disturbances are seen in some patients with hyperprolactinemia irrespective of cause. Marked increases and decreases in body weight are often accompanied by amenorrhea, as occurs with severe obesity and in professional ballet dancers, female athletes, and anorexia nervosa (see details later in this section). Evidence for decreased GnRH secretion has also been found in male athletes.

Treatment of this disorder depends on the extent of hypogonadism and the patient's desire for fertility. Restoration of ovulatory menses may be accomplished by cycles of clomiphene administration, cyclic estrogen-progestin (oral contraceptive) therapy, gonadotropin administration, or GnRH infusions, depending on the desired goal. In hypoestrogenemic women, decreased vaginal secretions, leading to dyspareunia and decreased libido, and the long-term consequences of osteopenia and metabolic bone disease warrant replacement therapy. In men, testosterone replacement therapy is indicated if endogenous hormone levels are subnormal.

Polycystic Ovary Syndrome (see also Ch. 224). The polycystic ovary (Stein-Leventhal) syndrome is characterized by amenorrhea, obesity, hirsutism, and consistently elevated LH levels. It is occasionally associated with a history of childhood CNS injury or "encephalitis." The altered hormonal secretory pattern of polycystic ovaries appears to be secondary to the increased LH secretion. This syndrome is occasionally seen in patients with hyperprolactinemia, but the causal relationship remains to be established.

HYPOTHALAMIC HYPOTHYROIDISM. This is an uncommon disorder manifested by hypothyroidism, a low or normal plasma TSH level, and an exaggerated and delayed response of TSH to TRH. In patients with this disorder, peak TSH responses occur at 90 to 120 minutes, in contrast to the 15- to 30-minute peak response time seen in normal subjects. Some patients have elevated basal TSH levels with decreased biologic activity, but in most, basal levels are normal. Hypothalamic hypothyroidism can occur as an isolated defect or, more commonly, is seen in association with deficiencies of gonadotropin, GH, or ACTH secretion. Treatment of this disorder is with thyroxine.

HYPOTHALAMIC-ADRENAL DYSFUNCTION. Decreased ACTH secretion on the basis of hypothalamic or other CNS disorders is relatively rare. It is seen most commonly in association with other pituitary hormone deficiencies during childhood and, by inference, has been attributed to a CNS cause. Disturbances of ACTH diurnal rhythm and suppressibility of ACTH are common in patients with a variety of intracranial diseases and reflect disturbances in neuroendocrine control mechanisms. They do not have major clinical significance, but subtle effects on behavior cannot be excluded. In particular, patients with affective disorders (unipolar depression) or experiencing bereavement exhibit a lack of normal glucocorticoid suppressibility similar to that seen in Cushing's disease.

IDIOPATHIC HYPERPROLACTINEMIA. Idiopathic hyperprolactinemia (IH) is a disorder in which prolactin levels are elevated in the absence of demonstrable pituitary or CNS disease and of any other recognized cause of increased prolactin secretion (see Ch. 226). The clinical manifestations of IH consist of galactorrhea and amenorrhea. In some patients, oligomenorrhea is present, and in a few, sporadic ovulation persists. Prolactin levels are elevated, but rarely exceed 150 ng per milliliter. The disease is confined to women of child-bearing age. The diagnosis remains inferential and based on exclusion of a pituitary microadenoma.

Many patients in whom IH was previously diagnosed have subsequently been found by magnetic resonance imaging to harbor microadenomas. Extensive testing using neuropharmacologic probes has failed to distinguish patients with IH from those with microadenomas, suggesting that the same pathophysiologic mechanism underlies both disorders. IH has been attributed to a CNS neurotransmitter defect related to dopamine metabolism, based on the observations that drugs impairing dopaminergic neurotransmission (i.e., neuroleptic dopamine receptor antagonists) increase prolactin secretion. The major action of these drugs in elevating prolactin levels, however, appears to be at the pituitary rather than within the CNS. IH is a benign condition, since less than 5 per cent of patients observed over a period of years subsequently show evidence of a pituitary tumor.

Therapy depends on the level of symptoms and the degree of inconvenience they produce. Bromocriptine (2.5 mg two or three times a day) is a dopamine receptor agonist that suppresses prolactin levels, eliminates galactorrhea, and restores cyclic menses and fertility. Nearly 80 per cent of patients experience menses within 2 months of initiating therapy, and 65 per cent become fertile. The effect of the drug is of short duration, however, and hyperprolactinemia recurs following its discontinuation. In some patients, hyperprolactinemia may remit spontaneously or following a pregnancy subsequent to bromocriptine administration. There is no evidence that long-term bromocriptine therapy per se restores prolactin secretory dynamics to normal. Even in the absence of a desire for fertility, the increased risk of osteopenia in hyperprolactinemic, hypoestrogenemic women provides the rationale for therapy.

HYPOTHALAMIC DISORDERS OF GROWTH HORMONE SECRETION. Idiopathic Growth Hormone Deficiency. Idiopathic GH deficiency (IGHD) occurs as either an isolated hormone deficiency or in association with other anterior pituitary hormone deficiencies and as both a familial and sporadic disorder. It is a disease of childhood, the diagnosis frequently being made because of impaired linear growth when the child is between 2 and 3 years of age. Impairment in GH secretion may be complete, with basal levels barely detectable, or partial, with subnormal responses to stimuli. The absence of radiologic abnormalities of the pituitary and the frequent coexistence of TRH- and GnRH-responsive deficiencies of TSH and gonadotropins suggest that the defect is located in the hypothalamus. Limited histologic studies of the pituitary or hypothalamus are available because of the generally benign nature of the disease. It is assumed to be due to a deficiency of GRH secretion, most likely on the basis of a neurotransmitter or biosynthetic abnormality, rather than to a structural defect in the hypothalamus. Approximately 75 per cent of patients with IGHD exhibit an intact GH response to GRH, indicating that the disorder has a heterogeneous etiology. Several other subgroups of GH deficiency are now also recognized, including one in which partial deletion of the GH gene results in complete absence of the hormone and another in which there is spontaneous recovery of GH secretion. In addition, other defects may be present in the pituitary, rendering it unresponsive to GRH. Therapy of IGHD should be initiated as soon as the diagnosis is established and consists of administration of biosynthetic human GH. Preliminary results using GRH as therapy indicate that this releasing hormone may effectively substitute for GH in about half of the patients with IGHD. Hypothyroidism, if present, must also be treated. If gonadotropin deficiency is present, therapy with gonadal steroids is postponed as long as possible to avoid accelerating bone growth and producing epiphyseal closure before acceptable linear bone growth is achieved by GH.

Psychosocial Dwarfism. A pattern indistinguishable from IGHD is seen occasionally in children reared in environments with deficient maternal care and affection. Children with this disorder, also termed the emotional deprivation syndrome, exhibit impaired GH responses to stimuli when studied. Within a short time in an improved environment, however, GH secretion returns to normal, and linear growth is restored. It is presumed that the impaired GH secretion is secondary to a behaviorly associated alteration in neurotransmitter metabolism impairing normal GRH-SRIF interrelationships.

Cerebral Gigantism. This childhood disease is characterized by rapid growth, accelerated bone age, and mental retardation. Ventricular enlargement is present, although no focal CNS lesions have been detected. GH secretion has been normal in the few patients described with this disorder. A variant of the syndrome is associated with lipodystrophy, hyperpigmentation, hypertrichosis, hepatosplenomegaly, increased adrenal steroid production, and hyperlipemia.

CENTRAL NERVOUS SYSTEM DISORDERS OF WATER REGULATION. Organic lesions of the CNS and drug therapy can lead to "cerebral hyponatremia" or "cerebral hypernatremia," which are entities distinct from diabetes insipidus (see Ch. 214).

Hyponatremia. The syndrome of inappropriate secretion of antidiuretic hormone (ADH) results from the autonomous secretion of vasopressin, resulting in hyponatremia, renal sodium loss, and inability to excrete dilute urine in the presence of normal renal, pituitary, adrenal, and thyroid function; resistance to correction by hypertonic saline; and reversibility following restriction of water (see Ch. 75). The increased renal sodium excretion occurs secondary to expanded extracellular volume. When measured, plasma vasopressin levels have been increased.

This syndrome has been reported in patients with carcinoma metastatic to the brain, primary brain tumors, cerebral infarction, basal skull fracture, subarachnoid hemorrhage, meningoencephalitis, and acute intermittent porphyria, but it may also occur in the absence of any underlying structural disease. Certain hypoglycemic and antineoplastic drugs can produce the same syndrome. The former, including chlorpropamide and tolbutamide, augment ADH action on the renal tubule and also stimulate ADH release. Vincristine and cyclophosphamide have direct neurotoxic effects on neurohypophyseal tissue. Other agents such as carbamazepine (Tegretol), amitriptyline (Elavil), thioridazine (Mellaril), and clofibrate (Atromid-S) also produce the syndrome, presumably by affecting endogenous vasopressin release.

Hypernatremia. Patients with intracranial lesions with or without disturbances of consciousness may exhibit hypernatremia in the presence of normal renal function, adequate fluid intake, absence of thirst, and failure of forced fluid intake to correct the hyperosmolality. This syndrome has been attributed to impaired regulation of thirst as well as vasopressin secretion and has been described in association with histiocytosis, craniopharyngioma, optic nerve glioma, pineal tumor, encephalitis, and ruptured intracranial aneurysm. The treatment of this disorder, above and beyond that of the specific causative lesion, is similar to that for diabetes insipidus.

DISORDERS OF NEUROMETABOLIC REGULATION. Acute Disorders. Acute disturbances of metabolic regulation occur most commonly in states of stress that activate the sympathetic nervous system. Thus, patients with hyperthermia, trauma, sepsis, and burns, and undergoing general anesthesia, may exhibit hyperglycemia and hyperglucagonemia along with impaired insulin secretion. In most instances these changes represent merely an extension of normal physiologic processes, do not result in significant clinical problems, and resolve spontaneously when the stress disappears. However, when stress is prolonged, as in severe burns, the responses can produce a severe catabolic state that can be life threatening.

Stress diabetes, seen frequently in the same clinical disorders, may have several causes. Some patients may manifest true diabetes mellitus for the first time under circumstances in which there is enhanced secretion of cortisol, glucagon, catecholamines, and GH, but in other patients the marked hyperglycemia may be unrelated to true diabetes. A syndrome indistinguishable from nonketotic hyperglycemia with or without coma is associated with severe head injury, cerebral thrombosis, encephalitis, and heat stroke. The severity of the hyperglycemia and its duration predict the probability of survival following head injury. Treatment consists of hydration and small doses of insulin.

Hypoglycemia is seen only rarely with hypothalamic disease. It has been reported in association with subdural hemorrhage.

Chronic Disorders. Destruction of the ventromedial hypothalamus leads to a syndrome of obesity, while damage to the ventrolateral hypothalamus results in anorexia and inanition. Because bilateral destruction is necessary, inanition is infrequently observed, since the concomitant loss of other important homeostatic mechanisms is usually incompatible with prolonged survival. An anatomically identifiable hypothalamic lesion is present in only a small percentage of patients with extensive obesity or inanition. However, the remarkable similarity of clinical and biochemical features in patients with and without definable lesions suggests that many "functional" disorders of caloric homeostasis ("essential" obesity and anorexia nervosa) are caused by biochemical disturbances in hypothalamic function that are currently undefined.

Hypothalamic Obesity. Ventromedial hypothalamic destruction resulting from encephalitis, infiltrative diseases (leukemia or histiocytosis X), trauma, vascular accidents, and tumors has been associated with obesity. Oxygen consumption, insulin secretion, body composition, and adipose metabolism are similar in patients with hypothalamic obesity and those with essential obesity. Adipose tissue mass increases primarily as the result of hypertrophy rather than hyperplasia. Marked insulin resistance is present, and diabetes may develop in some patients. GH secretion is impaired, and hypogonadism is common.

A number of familial disorders (Laurence-Moon, Bardet-Biedl, Alstrom-Hallgren, Prader-Willi) are associated with extreme obesity and evidence of other hypothalamic disturbances, including hypogonadism, temperature intolerance, and loss of diurnal rhythms; and of extrahypothalamic disturbances, such as deafness, pigmentary retinopathy, hypotonia, and mental retardation.

Therapy of hypothalamic obesity is not very successful. Once true destruction has occurred, the functional alterations are almost always irreversible. In children with hypothalamic leukemic infiltrates, successful chemotherapy can lead to cessation of hyperphagia and reduction of weight to normal. In general, therapeutic measures are aimed at treatment of the morbidly obese patient.

Anorexia Nervosa. This disorder is seen almost exclusively in young women and consists of weight loss, amenorrhea, and behavioral disturbances. Bulimia may also be present (see Ch. 202).

Almost every neuroendocrine system is affected by the disorder. Gonadotropin secretion "regresses" to a prepubertal stage characterized by absence of pulsatile secretion of LH and altered FSH-LH responses to GnRH. GH levels are normal or, at times, elevated, particularly in the presence of severe malnutrition, in which a paradoxic response to glucose may be observed. TSH responses to TRH are reduced, but thyroid function tends to be normal. Plasma cortisol levels are elevated, but diurnal variation is generally preserved. Patients tend to be poikilothermic, exhibiting difficulty in maintaining body temperature in response to changes in the environment. Impaired vasopressin secretion can be demonstrated but is rarely of clinical importance.

Most of the endocrine metabolic disturbances can be attributed to the severe malnutrition, and successful therapy resulting in weight gain is usually accompanied by restoration of normal neuroendocrine responses. One exception is gonadotropin secretion, which frequently remains abnormal and results in persistence of amenorrhea in up to one third of patients. Another is osmoregulation, which is accompanied by dysregulated vasopressin secretion for prolonged periods.

Prognosis for the reversal of cachexia and weight loss is reasonably good. Mortality is currently less than 5 per cent, and the majority of patients return to within 10 per cent of original body weight. Only 40 per cent of patients maintain their weight over a long term; the remainder exhibit moderate to severe weight loss with time.

CENTRAL NERVOUS SYSTEM BEHAVIORAL DISORDERS AFFECTING NEUROENDOCRINE FUNCTION. Disturbances of endocrine function have been observed in patients with a variety of psychiatric illnesses. The association is presumably through disordered neurotransmitter metabolism, although it is still unclear whether the same defect underlies both the behavioral and neuroendocrine dysfunction or whether altered behavior itself secondarily affects neuroendocrine function.

Of all the conditions studied, depressive affective behavior and the manic-depressive state have been most clearly shown to exhibit endocrine changes. Cortisol secretion in depressed patients is enhanced, and they are relatively resistant to dexamethasone suppression. This abnormality reverts to normal with successful treatment. In manic-depressive patients, cortisol secretion tends to be decreased during manic states and elevated during depressive periods.

Brown WA (ed.): Endocrinology of neuropsychiatric disorders. Endocrinol Metab Clin North Am 17:1–239, 1988. *An excellent collection of review articles on the variety of behavioral and other CNS disorders that have effects on neuroendocrine function.*

Goldman MB, Luchins DJ, Robertson GL: Mechanisms of altered water metabolism in psychotic patients with polydipsia and hyponatremia. N Engl J Med 318:397, 1988. *A carefully conducted study of the mechanisms underlying altered water metabolism in association with behavioral disease.*

Kopelman PG: Neuroendocrine function in obesity. Clin Endocrinol (Oxf) 28:675, 1988. *Obesity is associated with a number of neuroendocrine disturbances, some of which appear to be secondary and others primary. This article reviews the most important aspects.*

Lamberts SWJ: The role of somatostatin in the regulation of anterior pituitary hormone secretion and the use of its analogs in the treatment of human pituitary tumors. Endocrinol Rev 9:417, 1988. *This hypothalamic hormone and its superactive analogue have now become important in the suppression of many endocrine and exocrine functions. Its physiology and clinical use are reviewed in relation to pituitary tumors.*

Manasco PK, Pescovitz OH, Hill SC, et al.: Six-year results of luteinizing hormone releasing hormone (LHRH) agonist treatment in children with LHRH-dependent precocious puberty. J Pediatr 115:105, 1989. *The most comprehensive results available demonstrating the efficacy of an analogue in blocking the pituitary responses to endogenous GnRH and markedly affecting outcome of a significant neuroendocrine disorder.*

Sano T, Asa SL, Kovacs K: Growth hormone-releasing hormone–producing tumors: Clinical, biochemical, and morphological manifestations. Endocrinol Rev 9:357, 1988. *A comprehensive review of tumors that secrete a hypothalamic hormone and cause growth hormone hypersecretion and acromegaly. Although uncommon, the disorder requires treatment that is different from that of the typical patient with acromegaly.*

Whitcomb RW, Crowley WF Jr: Clinical review 4: Diagnosis and treatment of isolated gonadotropin-releasing hormone deficiency in men. J Clin Endocrinol Metab 70:3, 1990. *The understanding of the physiology of GnRH secretion has permitted the use of the hormone in treating endogenous GnRH deficiency. The authors review their extensive experience with this agent.*

213 The Anterior Pituitary

Lawrence A. Frohman

ANATOMY

The pituitary is located in a saddle-shaped cavity, the *sella turcica*, which is an integral portion of the sphenoid bone. Its anterior boundary is the midline *tuberculum sellae* and the anterior clinoid processes that project posteriorly from the sphenoid wings. The posterior limit is the *dorsum sellae*, which projects laterally to form the posterior clinoid processes. The lateral boundaries of the sella are nonosseous and consist of the medial wall of the cavernous sinus, in which is contained the internal carotid artery. The *diaphragma sellae*, a thickened reflection of the *dura mater*, forms the roof of the sella and is attached to the clinoid processes. Only the external layer of the dura extends into the sella as a periosteal lining, and thus the pituitary is normally extradural and not in direct communication with cerebrospinal fluid. The pituitary stalk and its blood vessels pass through a foramen in this membrane that may be incomplete or fenestrated.

The shape of the sella varies from ovoid to spheroid, resulting in considerable variation in normal pituitary dimensions. The average dimensions of the pituitary are 10 mm (anterior-posterior) by 13 mm (transverse) by 6 mm (height). Pituitary weight varies from 0.5 to 0.7 gram, being slightly greater in women. The anterior lobe constitutes about 75 per cent of the total pituitary weight and during pregnancy can increase up to twofold in size.

The arterial blood supply of the pituitary originates from the internal carotid artery via branches from the circle of Willis and hypophyseal arteries. Whereas the posterior lobe is supplied directly by the inferior hypophyseal artery, the blood supply of the anterior lobe is derived entirely from the portal vascular system (see Ch. 212). Venous drainage from the anterior lobe enters the posterior pituitary capillary bed and then the cavernous sinus. The nerve supply of the anterior pituitary consists of postganglionic sympathetic fibers that accompany and terminate on arteriolar vessels and nerve fibers connecting the posterior and anterior lobes. Their function is currently unknown.

EMBRYOLOGY

The glandular portion of the pituitary (*adenohypophysis*) is derived from Rathke's pouch, an ectodermal evagination of the oropharynx that fuses with a diencephalic outpouching of the region of the third ventricle in the developing embryo that eventually differentiates into the *neurohypophysis,* or posterior lobe. That portion of Rathke's pouch not in contact with the diencephalon differentiates to form the *pars anterior,* or anterior lobe. Two lateral outgrowths from the anterior lobes fuse in the midline and extend forward along the hypophyseal stalk to form the *pars tuberalis,* which in humans is limited to a small group of cells along the anterior region of the stalk. The portion of Rathke's pouch contiguous with the neurohypophysis develops less extensively and forms the *pars intermedia,* or intermediate lobe. This structure is not well defined in humans and tends to become intermingled with the anterior lobe. This combined structure has been called the *pars distalis.*

Differentiation of the pars anterior results in cells that secrete growth hormone (GH), prolactin, corticotropin (ACTH), thyroid-stimulating hormone (TSH), luteinizing hormone (LH), and follicle-stimulating hormone (FSH) as well as non–hormone-secreting cells. Cells of the pars intermedia secrete ACTH, lipotropin, and endorphins. Pituitary tumors developing in various regions of the pars distalis tend to reflect the predominant cell types in each region.

The lumen of Rathke's pouch is obliterated during development, although remnants may persist at the boundary of the neurohypophysis as either a cleft or small colloid-filled cysts. The connection with the oropharynx disappears early in development, because of growth of the sphenoid bone, although a few cells in the lower portion of the pouch may persist along the tract, occasionally within the sphenoid bone, and are known as the pharyngeal pituitary. These cells contain secretory granules for GH and prolactin, can be a source of "ectopic" pituitary tumor development, and conceivably could exhibit significant endocrine function subsequent to destruction or removal of the pars distalis.

Pituitary hormones are detected immunochemically as early as the seventh week of fetal life, and some CNS control of anterior pituitary hormone secretion occurs early in gestation. In contrast, true functional maturation, including aspects of feedback regulation, do not develop until postnatal life.

CELL TYPES

The anterior pituitary contains many cell types, the predominant function of which is the synthesis, storage, and release of a specific hormone(s). The frequency of heterogeneous cell type clustering suggests the presence of paracrine effects on hormone secretion.

SOMATOTROPHS. Originally identified as acidophilic cells, these cells secrete GH and are located predominantly in the lateral portions of the anterior lobe where they constitute up to 50 per cent of all cells. Tumors derived from this cell type lead to acromegaly.

LACTOTROPHS. Lactotrophs are also acidophilic and secrete prolactin. They are slightly less numerous than somatotrophs, tend to be located more peripherally than somatotrophs, and have smaller secretion granules. During pregnancy and fetal life, lactotrophs are increased in number, reflecting the effects of increased estrogen levels. Virtually all of the increase in pituitary size during pregnancy can be accounted for by lactotroph proliferation. Both lactotrophs and somatotrophs appear to be derived from a common stem cell, the somatomammotroph, tumors of which may secrete both GH and prolactin.

THYROTROPHS. The basophilic staining cells that secrete TSH occur most frequently at the anterior edge of the pituitary near the midline, although they are also present in deeper portions of the gland. Their secretory granules are smaller than GH and prolactin granules. Thyrotrophs normally constitute only about 6 per cent of anterior lobe cells. In primary hypothyroidism they undergo marked hypertrophy.

GONADOTROPHS. These cells are located deep in the lateral portion of the gland in association with lactotrophs and secrete both LH and FSH. Although constituting only 3 to 4 per cent of anterior pituitary cells normally, they increase in number following castration and decrease during pregnancy as a result of placental gonadotropin production.

CORTICOTROPHS. Cells of this type, which can be chromophobic or basophilic, are found in two separate locations. One group of cells resides most commonly in the medial mucoid region of the anterior lobe. A second group migrates during development to the junctional region of the anterior and posterior lobes and also to the pars tuberalis. Anterior lobe corticotrophs exhibit sparse granulation, whereas those in the pars tuberalis–posterior lobe region contain large, electron-dense granules. The same precursor molecule is present in both cell types, although processing enzyme activity varies, resulting in different ratios of hormones derived from the precursor (ACTH, melanocyte-stimulating hormone [MSH], lipotropins, and endorphins) in the two different regions. Anterior lobe corticotrophs increase in number with glucocorticoid deficiency, whereas those in the intermediate-posterior lobe region decrease, suggesting that only the former are physiologically important ACTH-secreting cells.

OTHER CELL TYPES. As many as 15 to 20 per cent of anterior pituitary cells cannot be stained by antibodies to any of the recognized anterior pituitary hormones. Some of these may represent resting degranulated cells or undifferentiated primitive secretory cells. However, others may be responsible for the secretion of as yet uncharacterized pituitary hormones such as tissue-specific growth factors. One such cell type is stellate, with cellular processes extending into the perivascular spaces in a manner suggestive of primitive follicle formation. These *folliculostellate* cells generally do not contain secretory granules but have recently been shown to produce an endothelial cell growth factor.

ANTERIOR PITUITARY HORMONES

The anterior pituitary secretes six well-recognized hormones, all of which are readily measurable in serum. They can be divided into three general categories: corticotropin and related peptides, glycoprotein hormones, and somatomammotropin hormones. The chemical characteristics of these hormones are given in Table 213–1.

CORTICOTROPIN-RELATED PEPTIDES. ACTH and its related family of peptides are synthesized as a single precursor molecule, pro-opiomelanocortin, with a molecular weight of approximately 29,000. Following glycosylation, the molecule is differentially cleaved into an NH_2-terminal fragment of uncertain biologic activity; a midportion, which contains ACTH; and a COOH-terminal portion, β-lipotropin (LPH). Subsequent processing, which varies in the different groups of corticotrophs, may also cleave ACTH into α-MSH and corticotropin-like intermediate lobe peptides. β-LPH is also differentially processed further to β-endorphin and other endorphin-related peptides (see Ch. 212). Although the structures of β-MSH and met-enkephalin are contained within the β-LPH sequence, the former is not synthesized in postnatal human pituitaries, and the biosynthesis of the latter occurs through a separate precursor.

ACTH. The primary effects of ACTH are stimulation of secretion of glucocorticoid, mineralocorticoid, and androgenic steroids by the adrenal cortex. ACTH binds to specific receptors on adrenocortical cell membranes and stimulates steroidogenesis through a cyclic AMP–mediated mechanism by enhancing cholesterol conversion to pregnenolone. ACTH also stimulates adrenal protein synthesis, leading to cellular growth and hyperplasia.

Extra-adrenal effects of ACTH include stimulation of lipolysis in adipose tissue, insulin-releasing effects on the pancreatic B cell, stimulation of GH secretion, and enhancement of glucose and amino acid transport into muscles. Except in patients with ACTH-secreting tumors, it is unlikely that plasma ACTH levels sufficient to produce these effects are ever achieved. Although ACTH has less potent pigmenting effects than α-MSH or β-MSH, it has long been considered the major pigmenting hormone in man. Recent studies, however, have indicated control of pigmentation to be a complex process, and the importance of ACTH has come under question.

Plasma levels of ACTH exhibit great variability, in part because of its episodic secretion. Levels in normal adults range from undetectable to 80 pg per milliliter (the lower limit of detection in most assays is approximately 10 pg per milliliter). In addition to its episodic secretion, a diurnal rhythm can be detected with lowest levels in the evening and peak levels in the early morning. Changes in plasma ACTH levels can be shown to precede those of plasma cortisol with a short lag period. With stress, plasma

ACTH levels can reach several hundred picograms per milliliter. In patients with ectopic ACTH production, immunoreactive ACTH levels may be exceedingly high and consist in part of larger molecular sized forms ("big" ACTH) believed to represent partially processed but biologically inactive precursor molecules. ACTH is rapidly eliminated from plasma; its half-life is 3 to 9 minutes, leading to an estimated secretion rate of 25 μg per day, which represents approximately 5 per cent of pituitary hormone content.

β-LPH, Endorphins, and Related Peptides. β-LPH and β-endorphin are secreted in an equimolar ratio to ACTH in response to all types of stimulation. The presence of both molecules in the same precursor as ACTH provides an explanation for this observation. The plasma levels of β-LPH and β-endorphin, however, do not necessarily parallel those of ACTH because of their slower metabolic clearance rates. β-LPH is cleared primarily by the kidneys, and its levels rise disproportionately to those of ACTH in renal failure. Since ACTH secretion is normal in this disorder, β-LPH must exert relatively little feedback effect on its own secretion or that of ACTH. β-LPH and β-endorphin have not been shown to have any effects peripherally at the levels normally seen in plasma.

GLYCOPROTEIN HORMONES. The pituitary glycoprotein hormones consist of an α and β subunit, each containing a peptide core with branched carbohydrate side chains that are required for biologic activity and for stability in plasma. The α subunits of the glycoprotein hormones are identical, whereas the β subunits vary, thereby providing the biologic specificity of each hormone. There is considerable homology between β subunits of the different hormones as well as cross-species homology of both α and β subunits, which explains why bovine or ovine glycoprotein hormones are active in humans. The isolated subunits have no intrinsic biologic activity. Hormone heterogeneity, related to the degree of glycosylation, has been suggested as the explanation for the reported variations in glycoprotein bioactivity at different times in the menstrual cycle. The genes encoding the individual subunits are located on different chromosomes, and the rate-limiting step in glycoprotein hormone secretion is regulated by β subunit production. Elevations in plasma α subunit levels can be seen after both TRH and GnRH stimulation and occasionally in pituitary tumors.

TSH. TSH effects on the thyroid cells are largely analogous to those of ACTH on the adrenal cortex. High-affinity receptors are present on cell membranes, and TSH binding leads to activation of adenylate cyclase, enhanced iodine transport and binding to protein, increased thyroglobulin and thyroid hormone synthesis, and increased thyroglobulin proteolysis with release of thyroid hormones. RNA and protein synthesis are also stimulated, leading to an increase in thyroid size and vascularity.

TSH is measured by a specific assay utilizing an antibody directed to antigenic determinants on the β subunit that exhibit little or no cross-reactivity with other glycoprotein hormones. Normal levels of plasma TSH are from 0.5 to 5 μU per milliliter, with most assays exhibiting a sensitivity of 0.1 μU per milliliter. In primary hypothyroidism, TSH levels may increase to greater than 100 μU per milliliter and responses to thyrotropin-releasing hormone (TRH) are enhanced. A few patients have been described with hypothyroidism and only slightly elevated TSH levels in whom administration of TRH results in an exaggerated TSH increase and a concomitant increase in thyroxine. Evidence for a biologically less potent TSH due to altered glycosylation has been found in such individuals. TSH is cleared from circulation with a half-life of 75 to 80 minutes, and the secretion rate of the hormone is 100 to 200 mU per day. In hypothyroidism, secretion rates may be increased 10 to 15 times that in normals.

LH and FSH. Gonadal function is regulated by two pituitary hormones: (1) FSH, which stimulates ovarian follicular growth, testicular growth, and spermatogenesis, and (2) LH, which promotes ovulation and follicular luteinization, stimulates testicular interstitial cell function, and enhances production of steroids in both ovary and testis. In the ovary, FSH promotes growth and maturation of the primordial follicle, and LH stimulates progesterone production by the corpus luteum by enhancing the conversion of cholesterol to pregnenolone. In the testis, FSH acts on the Sertoli cell, where, in conjunction with testosterone, the production of an androgen-binding protein is stimulated. The target cell of LH is the Leydig cell, leading to enhanced testosterone production. The androgen binding protein serves to transport testosterone in high concentrations into tubular cells to stimulate spermatogenesis. (See also discussion in Ch. 222.) Inhibin, a glycoprotein produced by ovarian granulosa cells and testicular Sertoli cells in response to both FSH and testosterone, exerts a preferential inhibitory feedback effect on FSH secretion.

The gonadotropin assays exhibit a slight degree of cross-reactivity between the hormone and the subunits, although this is not a practical problem at present. Of importance, however, is the cross-reactivity due to the great similarity between LH and chorionic gonadotropin β subunits. While chorionic gonadotropin assays are quite specific, most LH assays do not discriminate between the two hormones.

Plasma levels of FSH and LH in women vary with the menstrual cycle. FSH levels rise slightly and then decline progressively during the early follicular phase of the cycle, during which time LH levels are generally stable or rise slightly. An abrupt rise in LH at midcycle, initiated by increasing estrogen secretion by the developing follicle and accompanied by an FSH

TABLE 213–1. ANTERIOR PITUITARY HORMONES IN HUMANS

Class	Members	Molecular Weight	Amino Acids	Carbohydrate	Other Features
Corticotropin-lipotropin	ACTH	4,500	39		All members of class derived from a single precursor
	α-MSH	1,800	13		N-terminal 13 amino acids of ACTH. In humans, found only in fetal life and in tumors
	β-Lipotropin	11,200	91		
	β-Endorphin	4,000	31		C-terminal (amino acids 61–91) portion of β-LPH
Glycoprotein	LH	29,000	α subunit: 89 β subunit: 115	1% sialic acid	All have two subunits, with the α subunit being identical or nearly identical and the β subunit conferring biologic specificity
	FSH	29,000	α subunit: 89 β subunit: 115	5% sialic acid	
	TSH	29,000	α subunit: 89 β subunit: 112	1% sialic acid	
	Chorionic gonadotropin*	46,000	α subunit: 92 β subunit: 139	12% sialic acid	
Somatomammotropin	Growth hormone	21,800	191		All single-chain proteins with two or three disulfide bridges
	Prolactin	22,500	198	†	
	Placental lactogen*	21,800	191		

Adapted from Frohman LA: Diseases of the anterior pituitary. *In* Felig P, Baxter JD, Broadus AE, et al. (eds.): Endocrinology and Metabolism, 2nd ed. Copyright © 1987 by McGraw-Hill, Inc. Used by permission of McGraw-Hill Book Company.
*Of placental origin and included for comparison purposes.
†Carbohydrate-containing forms of prolactin have been identified.

rise, triggers ovulation. Both hormone levels decline during the luteal phase. Levels of FSH and LH in males are similar to those in females during the follicular phase. FSH and LH levels increase in response to age-related decreases in gonadal function in both sexes. In women this occurs at menopause, and in men a gradual increase is seen during the sixth to eighth decades. The half-life of LH in circulation is approximately 30 minutes, whereas that of FSH is twice as long, the difference being attributed to the varying sialic acid content of the hormones. This permits clear detection of a pulsatile pattern of LH secretion but less so for FSH.

SOMATOMAMMOTROPIC HORMONES. This hormonal class consists of GH, prolactin, and a structurally similar placental hormone, chorionic somatomammotropin, or placental lactogen. Extensive interspecies homology exists for both GH and prolactin, suggesting relatively limited changes in gene duplication during evolution. Despite the similarity, subprimate growth hormones are biologically inactive in humans. GH and placental lactogen exhibit 83 per cent homology, in contrast to only 16 per cent homology between GH and prolactin. Despite these differences, each hormone has both intrinsic lactogenic and growth-promoting activity. Large-molecular-weight–sized hormones ("big" GH and prolactin) have been identified in both pituitary and plasma. The big hormones appear to be dimers connected by interchain disulfide linkages. They are secreted by the pituitary, bind to the hormone target cell receptors, and exhibit reduced biologic activity as compared to the monomer. Some of the large molecular weight GH is actually GH bound to its binding protein, which represents the extracellular domain of the GH receptor. There are four or five additional GH variants, including proteolytically modified forms, electrophoretic variants, and a smaller molecule ("20K variant") lacking amino acids 32 to 46, which is encoded by a separate mRNA species derived from the authentic GH gene and formed by differential splicing of pre-mRNA to mRNA. This variant, while representing 10 per cent of pituitary GH, constitutes less than 5 per cent of secreted GH, and levels in circulation do not change in response to GH secretagogues. It appears to have the same biologic effects as 22K GH. The GH-placental lactogen family consists of five genes, one of which encodes a GH variant that is secreted by the placenta. It is biologically active and most likely accounts for the suppression of pituitary GH secretion during pregnancy.

Growth Hormone. GH is important for linear growth and regulation of metabolic processes. GH administration results in positive nitrogen balance, decreased urea production, decreased body fat stores, and enhanced carbohydrate utilization. Biphasic effects on circulating glucose, amino acid, and free fatty acid levels occur in response to GH with an initial decrease and subsequent return to normal or an increase. The acute effects of GH in isolated tissues resemble those of insulin and include increased amino acid uptake and incorporation into protein, stimulation of RNA synthesis, and enhanced glucose utilization. GH also antagonizes the lipolytic effect of catecholamines in adipose tissue. These acute effects disappear within 3 to 4 hours, by which time a series of delayed effects appears. These include enhanced triglyceride lipolysis, increased sensitivity to catecholamine-mediated lipolysis, and inhibition of glucose uptake and utilization secondary to impaired pyruvate decarboxylation. These effects form the basis of the diabetogenic action of the hormone. GH also exhibits multiphasic effects on insulin secretion. There is an acute direct stimulatory effect on the β cell, a subsequent inhibitory effect, and a late and persistent stimulation of insulin release that occurs secondary to the impairment of carbohydrate utilization. The last effect has the greatest pathophysiologic significance in the development of diabetes secondary to GH hypersecretion.

Many GH effects cannot be produced by acute exposure of tissues to the hormone and are mediated by a group of GH-dependent growth factors that are synthesized in numerous tissues. GH binds to a specific cell-membrane receptor to stimulate their production. The most important of these factors is somatomedin C or insulin-like growth factor I (IGF-I), a peptide of about 7500 daltons that has many similarities to insulin, including structural resemblance to proinsulin and binding to insulin receptors. Somatomedin C receptors are present in many tissues, including cartilage, where sulfate incorporation into proteoglycan and amino acid uptake and incorporation are stimulated.

The importance of IGF-I in the growth-promoting effects of GH is illustrated by the Laron dwarf, in whom a mutation of the GH receptor impairs GH stimulation of IGF-I production, resulting in severe growth retardation. IGF-I may be synthesized in the same cell in which it acts (autocrine) or in neighboring cells (paracrine). Thus, while circulating IGF-I levels are a measure of GH secretion, they most likely reflect local IGF-I production rather than serving as a source for tissue uptake even though systemically administered IGF-I can enhance growth. It is currently believed that cell differentiation and growth require both GH and IGF-I, with GH serving to commit a precursor cell to a specific pathway of differentiation and IGF-I enhancing growth and replication. Other growth factors, such as IGF-II platelet-derived growth factor and epidermal growth factor, do not appear to be GH dependent although GH does stimulate production of the EGF receptor. GH also stimulates cardiac and renal hypertrophy and production of specific hormones such as renin and aldosterone and conversion of thyroxine to triiodothyronine.

Immunoreactive measurements of GH are valid indicators of GH bioactivity. Mean GH levels during adolescence and adult life are generally less than 3 ng per milliliter, although the spontaneous secretory pulses of GH can produce elevations as great as 30 to 50 ng per milliliter in young adult subjects. Levels in women during the childbearing age are generally greater than in men, particularly in response to exercise or other stimuli. GH is cleared from plasma primarily by the liver and to a lesser extent by the kidney. The half-time of GH disappearance from circulation is 20 minutes, and the overall secretion in normal adults ranges from 300 to 500 µg per square meter per day.

Prolactin. The major effect of prolactin is to stimulate the synthesis of milk constituents, including lactalbumin, casein, lipids, and carbohydrates (see Ch. 226). Prolactin receptors are present on alveolar surfaces of mammary cells and, in addition, have been identified in liver and kidney. Prolactin is not required for normal breast development in humans, and pathologic elevations of the hormone are not generally associated with an increase in breast size. During pregnancy, prolactin, in conjunction with estrogen, progesterone, and placental lactogen, results in further breast development and milk formation. Following parturition, the abrupt decrease in estrogen and progesterone derived from the placenta permits initiation of lactation. This effect underlies the previous use of estrogens to inhibit lactation in the postpartum period and explains the frequent onset of galactorrhea in hyperprolactinemic women after discontinuance of oral contraceptives. Continued prolactin secretion is required to maintain lactation once initiated, and the return of prolactin to normal levels in the postpartum period is delayed in women who nurse for prolonged periods. The actual milk let-down reflex is mediated by the release of oxytocin rather than by prolactin. Oxytocin stimulates contraction of myoepithelial cells surrounding the terminal acinar lobules that expel their milk into the lobular ducts. Although prolactin has numerous effects on behavior and on fluid and electrolyte metabolism in lower species, no such effects have been convincingly demonstrated in humans.

Normal prolactin levels do not exceed 15 ng per milliliter in men or 20 ng per milliliter in women. There are no significant changes during the menstrual cycle, but levels decrease at menopause. During pregnancy, prolactin levels rise continuously from early gestation to values of 150 to 200 ng per milliliter at term. Prolactin is cleared from circulation with a half-time of approximately 50 minutes. The liver and, to a lesser extent, the kidney are the major sites of prolactin removal.

TESTS OF ANTERIOR PITUITARY HORMONE FUNCTION

ACTH. Since ACTH levels in normal subjects may be undetectable at times, random measurements of the hormone are of limited value. In a patient with signs and symptoms of adrenocortical insufficiency and low plasma cortisol levels, a low or even normal ACTH level is suggestive of hypothalamic-pituitary disease. The most useful test at present for evaluating ACTH function is that of insulin hypoglycemia. A dose of insulin, generally 0.1 U per kilogram, to decrease the fasting blood glucose to 40 mg per deciliter is given intravenously, and plasma cortisol levels are measured over a 2-hour period. A rise greater than 10 μg per deciliter or a peak level greater than 20 μg per deciliter is indicative of a normal hypothalamic-pituitary-adrenal axis. The dose of insulin should be decreased by 50 per cent when hypopituitarism is strongly suspected and increased by 50 per cent in patients with anticipated insulin resistance (i.e., obesity). No treatment is necessary for catecholamine-mediated symptoms of hypoglycemia, but those of central glucopenia (impaired mentation or altered states of consciousness) require immediate therapy. This test must not be performed in patients with suspected primary adrenal insufficiency.

Corticotropin-releasing hormone (CRH) is a safe and specific means of assessing ACTH secretory function. Ovine CRH is more potent than human CRH, presumably because of its longer plasma half-life. When given at a dose of 1 μg per kilogram, CRH elicits both an ACTH and cortisol response. A rise in ACTH without a corresponding increase in cortisol suggests a chronically unstimulated adrenal gland and therefore a hypothalamic dysfunction. In contrast, absence of an ACTH response indicates primary pituitary disease. CRH has not yet been approved for use in the United States. When available, it should eliminate the need for the use of insulin hypoglycemia in most cases. Impairment of normal cortisol feedback using metyrapone, an 11β-hydroxylase inhibitor, at a dose of 750 mg orally every 4 hours for six doses, with measurement of plasma 11-desoxycortisol or urinary 17-hydroxycorticoids, is an alternative way to test the entire hypothalamic-pituitary-adrenal axis. This test is less useful than insulin hypoglycemia in predicting normal responsiveness of the axis to stress. ACTH stimulation has also been used as an indirect method of assessing endogenous ACTH secretory activity.

The best test of suspected excessive ACTH and cortisol secretion is by dexamethasone suppression. The rapid dexamethasone suppression test involves administration of 1 mg dexamethasone orally at 11 P.M. and measurement of plasma cortisol at 8 o'clock the following morning. A level of less than 5 μg per deciliter indicates normal suppressibility. In patients in whom normal suppression is not demonstrated, a standard low-dose dexamethasone suppression test (0.5 mg orally every 6 hours for 48 hours) is performed. Plasma cortisol will be suppressed to less than 5 μg per deciliter, and urinary free cortisol levels will be suppressed to less than 20 μg per 24 hours in normal subjects but not in patients with ACTH hypersecretion or primary adrenocortical hypersecretion. In patients in whom suppression fails, a high-dose dexamethasone suppression test (2 mg orally every 6 hours for 48 hours) is then used to distinguish between pituitary and adrenal causes.

TSH. Impaired TSH secretion should be suspected in hypothyroid patients when plasma TSH levels are not elevated. Differentiation of pituitary from hypothalamic causes of TSH deficiency can usually, but not always, be accomplished by administering TRH, 500 μg (intravenously), and measuring plasma TSH levels. In normal persons, plasma TSH increases to at least 8 μU per milliliter after TRH administration, and peak levels usually occur at 15 to 30 minutes. In hypothalamic hypothyroidism, the response may be exaggerated and is frequently prolonged, with peak values at 90 to 180 minutes. Since thyroxine impairs the TSH response to TRH, it is not possible to assess TSH function in patients receiving thyroid hormone replacement therapy until at least a month after discontinuation of medication.

LH AND FSH. LH and FSH deficiency should be suspected in patients with clinical evidence of hypogonadism and subnormal testosterone or estradiol levels in whom gonadotropin levels are not elevated. Administration of gonadotropin-releasing hormone (GnRH) may be useful in distinguishing between hypothalamic and pituitary causes of hypogonadism. In normal subjects, a single GnRH injection increases LH levels three- to fivefold. Multiple injections may be necessary to distinguish between hypothalamic and pituitary causes, since impaired responses may be seen after a single injection in both disorders. Clomiphene, an estrogen antagonist, stimulates gonadotropin levels in some patients with hypothalamic hypogonadism.

GROWTH HORMONE. The most frequently employed stimulus for GH secretion is insulin hypoglycemia. The details of testing and the cautions required are as described under ACTH testing. Peak GH levels usually occur at 60 or 90 minutes, and a

peak level of 9 ng per milliliter or greater is considered normal. Up to 30 per cent of normal subjects may not respond to insulin hypoglycemia. L-Arginine (0.5 gram per kilogram intravenously during a 30-minute period), L-dopa (0.5 gram orally), and clonidine (25 μg orally) are other effective stimuli used to test GH secretory reserve and may be used in series with insulin. The responses are comparable in magnitude to those after insulin. Other stimuli (glucagon plus propranolol, endotoxin, vasopressin, ACTH) have no advantage over those described. Although still investigational, GRH is often useful in distinguishing between hypothalamic and pituitary causes for GH deficiency. Lack of an adequate GH response, however, may also be due to excessive somatostatin secretion.

Suppressibility of GH secretion in patients with elevated GH levels is evaluated with a standard glucose tolerance test. A decrease in GH levels to less than 2 ng per milliliter is seen in normal subjects. TRH is also used in distinguishing between types of suspected GH hypersecretion. TRH has no effect on GH levels in normal subjects, whereas a rapid increase in GH levels occurs in most patients with acromegaly.

PROLACTIN. Impaired prolactin secretion is rarely a clinical problem. It should be suspected in patients with levels of less than 2 ng per milliliter, and the diagnosis is confirmed by the absence of a response to TRH. Elevated prolactin levels in nearly all patients, with the exception of occasional patients with prolactin-secreting tumors and patients with chronic renal failure, can be suppressed by dopamine infusions, L-dopa, or other dopaminergic agents. These tests are not useful in the differential diagnosis of hyperprolactinemia.

Brook CGD, Hindmarsh PC, Stanhope R: Growth and growth hormone secretion. J Endocrinol 119:179, 1988. *A clearly written review of the role of GH secretion in promoting growth.*

Chin WW: Hormonal regulation of thyrotropin and gonadotropin gene expression. Clin Res 36:484, 1988. *An up-to-date review of the hormonal control of TSH and LH using techniques of molecular biology.*

Frohman LA: Diseases of the anterior pituitary. *In* Felig P, Baxter JD, Broadus E, et al. (eds.): Endocrinology and Metabolism, 2nd ed. New York, McGraw-Hill Book Company, 1987, pp 247–338. *A detailed systematic description of the chemistry, physiology, and pathophysiology of the pituitary. Of particular use to the clinical trainee and practicing physician.*

Frohman LA, Jansson J-O: Growth hormone-releasing hormone. Endocrinol Rev 7:223, 1986. *A review of basic and clinical aspects of GRH, its use as a diagnostic and therapeutic agent, and disorders of GRH secretion.*

Gold PW, Kling MA, Whitfield HJ, et al.: The clinical implications of corticotropin-releasing hormone. Adv Exp Med Biol 245:507, 1988. *An excellent review of the recent advances in knowledge of the hypothalamic-pituitary axis resulting from the use of CRH in humans.*

Grave GD, Cassorla FG (eds.): Disorders of Human Growth: Advances in Research and Treatment. Springfield, IL, Charles C Thomas, 1988, pp 1–386. *A review of the therapeutic potentials for treatment of growth hormone deficiency along with an up-to-date review of studies on the physiologic regulation of growth hormone secretion.*

Gross KM, Matsumoto AM, Bremner WJ: Differential control of luteinizing hormone and follicle-stimulating hormone secretion by luteinizing hormone-releasing hormone pulse frequency in man. J Clin Endocrinol Metab 64:675, 1987. Sauder SE, Frager MS, Case GD, et al.: Effects of changing gonadotrophin-releasing hormone pulse frequency on gonadotrophin secretion in men. Clin Endocrinol (Oxf) 28:647, 1988. *Two excellent physiologic studies demonstrating the importance of pulsatile GnRH secretion on pituitary gonadotropin secretion in humans.*

Kovacs K, Horvath E, Ezrin C: Anatomy and histology of the normal and abnormal pituitary gland. *In* Degroot LJ, Besser LJ, Cahill GF Jr, et al. (eds.): Endocrinology, 2nd ed. Philadelphia, W. B. Saunders Company, 1989, pp 264–283. *A well-organized and referenced presentation of pituitary structure with emphasis on changes in human disease.*

Sheldon W Jr, DeBold CR, Evans WS, et al.: Rapid sequential intravenous administration of four hypothalamic releasing hormones as a combined anterior pituitary function test in normal subjects. J Clin Endocrinol Metab 60:623, 1985. *Description of a rapid, simple, and safe method of testing pituitary hormone secretory reserve.*

Spratt DI, O'Dea LSL, Schoenfeld D, et al.: Neuroendocrine-gonadal axis in men: Frequent sampling of LH, FSH, and testosterone. Am J Physiol 254:E658, 1988. *A carefully conducted study of the pulsatile nature of gonadotropin and testosterone secretion in men.*

HYPOPITUITARISM

DISEASE STATES ASSOCIATED WITH HYPOPITUITARISM (Table 213–2). The subject's age, rapidity of onset of the disorder, and the extent of impaired hormone secretion as well as the specific pathologic process all influence the clinical manifestations. When acute and complete, the disease can be life threatening, but in a mild form it can remain undetected for many years. Hypopituitarism can occur as a result of a *primary*

TABLE 213–2. ETIOLOGY OF HYPOPITUITARISM

A. Primary

Pituitary tumors
  Primary intrasellar (chromophobe adenoma, craniopharyngioma)
  Parasellar (meningioma, optic nerve glioma)
Ischemic necrosis of the pituitary
  Postpartum (Sheehan's syndrome)
  Diabetes mellitus
  Other systemic diseases (temporal arteritis, sickle cell disease and trait, arteriosclerosis, eclampsia)
Aneurysm of intracranial internal carotid artery
Pituitary apoplexy (almost always related to a primary pituitary tumor)
Cavernous sinus thrombosis
Infectious disease (tuberculosis, syphilis, malaria, meningitis, fungal disease)
Infiltrative disease (hemochromatosis)
Immunologic (granulomatous or lymphocytic hypophysitis)
Iatrogenic
  Irradiation to nasopharynx
  Irradiation to sella
  Surgical destruction
Primary empty sella syndrome
Metabolic disorders (chronic renal failure)
Idiopathic (frequently monohormonal and occasionally familial)

B. Secondary

Destruction of pituitary stalk
  Trauma
  Compression by tumor or aneurysm
  Iatrogenic (surgical)
Hypothalamic or other central nervous system disease
  Inflammatory (sarcoidosis)
  Infiltrative (lipid storage diseases)
  Trauma
  Toxic (vincristine)
  Hormone induced (glucocorticoids, gonadal steroids)
  Tumors (primary, metastatic, lymphomas, leukemia)
  Idiopathic (frequently congenital or familial, often restricted to one or two hormones, and may be reversible)
  Nutritional (starvation, obesity)
  Anorexia nervosa
  Psychosocial dwarfism

Adapted from Frohman LA: Diseases of the anterior pituitary. *In* Felig P, Baxter JD, Broadus AE, et al. (eds.): Endocrinology and Metabolism, 2nd ed. Copyright © 1987 by McGraw-Hill, Inc. Used by permission of McGraw-Hill Book Company.

pituitary disorder or *secondary* to CNS disease. In the latter, pituitary hormone deficiency occurs because of a lack of appropriate releasing hormones.

The classic example of *primary hypopituitarism* is ischemic postpartum pituitary necrosis, first associated with the clinical features of hypopituitarism by Simmonds and characterized by Sheehan. The mechanism of acute ischemic necrosis is believed to relate to vasospasm of hypophyseal vessels, possibly influenced by estrogen-induced sensitivity to the vasoconstrictive stimulus of hypoxia. This disorder occurs most frequently in the immediate postpartum period associated with severe hemorrhage and hypotension. Some degree of hypopituitarism occurs in up to one third of women experiencing severe hemorrhage during delivery. The disorder is recognized by absence of lactation in the postpartum period and failure of normal cyclic menstruation to resume. Because of the slowly progressive nature of this disease the presence of postpartum lactation does not preclude development of the disorder at a later time. Since complete hypopituitarism requires at least 90 per cent destruction of the pituitary, the diagnosis may never be made in many patients with pituitary necrosis and minimal evidence of hypopituitarism. The disease is currently much less common than previously, because of the marked improvement in obstetric care during the past half century. Ischemic pituitary necrosis can be seen with other disorders, although much less commonly.

The most common cause of hypopituitarism is a pituitary tumor (discussed in the following section). Other parasellar mass lesions, including CNS tumors and internal carotid aneurysms, can also invade the sella and destroy the pituitary. Intrapituitary hemorrhage (*pituitary apoplexy*) associated with pituitary tumors may produce varying degrees of hypopituitarism. If bleeding occurs

gradually, the pituitary is compressed and symptoms of hypopituitarism predominate. If the hemorrhage is sudden, presenting symptoms include headache, visual field defects or blindness, ophthalmoplegia, and subarachnoid irritation. Hemorrhage within a pre-existing pituitary tumor may cause its sudden expansion. Immediate glucocorticoid therapy is essential in such patients. Most recover without the need for surgical intervention, but it may be necessary in some to restore visual function.

Radiation therapy for treatment of malignant tumors of the head and neck frequently causes primary or secondary hypopituitarism. Growth disturbances are the most common manifestations in children, whereas hypogonadism is more common in adults. Hypopituitarism may occur at any time from 6 months to more than 5 years after a dose of 3000 rads or greater, and children appear to be more susceptible than adults. Lymphocytic hypopituitarism, a recently recognized disorder, tends to occur in the postpartum period and may present as an expanding pituitary mass lesion associated with hypopituitarism (and occasionally hyperprolactinemia). Destruction of pituitary tissue with lymphocyte infiltration has been found histologically, but the cause is unknown. Hypopituitarism may occur without detectable underlying disease and may be limited to one or two hormones. Both autosomal and X-linked recessive forms have been reported. Partial hypopituitarism also occurs in patients with chronic renal failure and is reversible after renal transplantation.

Secondary hypopituitarism can be caused by diverse CNS disorders, all of which disrupt the delivery of releasing factors to the pituitary. The distinction between CNS and pituitary causes can frequently, but not always, be made on the basis of responses to the hypothalamic releasing hormones. Diseases of the pituitary stalk are most frequently due to trauma. Basilar skull fractures often shear the stalk, rupturing both neural and vascular connections. Parasellar tumors and aneurysms can compress the stalk sufficiently to impair blood flow to portal vessels. Disorders of the CNS, primarily the hypothalamus, that impair releasing hormone secretion are described in Ch. 212.

CLINICAL FEATURES. In the most dramatic form of hypopituitarism, panhypopituitarism occurring after surgical hypophysectomy, severe pituitary apoplexy, or withdrawal of hormone replacement therapy, clinical features are noted within a few hours (diabetes insipidus) to a few days (adrenal insufficiency). In partial hypopituitarism the signs and symptoms develop slowly and may be vague and nonspecific.

Hormone-specific Features. **ACTH.** Manifestations of ACTH deficiency are similar to those of adrenocortical deficiency. Weakness, postural hypotension, malaise, dehydration, and cold intolerance are common, although a true addisonian crisis is infrequent because some aldosterone secretion is maintained through the renin-angiotensin mechanism, which is independent of ACTH. Nausea, vomiting, and severe hypothermia can occur, and hypoglycemia associated with prolonged fasting or alcohol ingestion may be seen as a result of impaired gluconeogenesis. In contrast to Addison's disease, in which hyperpigmentation occurs, patients with ACTH deficiency frequently exhibit depigmentation and decreased tanning after exposure to sunlight. If ACTH secretion is partially impaired, symptoms may be experienced only during periods of stress. Adrenal androgen deficiency contributes to decreased libido and loss of axillary and pubic hair in women although in men it is of little consequence if testicular function is preserved.

TSH. The features of primary and secondary TSH deficiency are quite similar with the exception of severity. Patients experience cold intolerance, dry skin, pallor, mental slowing, bradycardia, hoarseness, and constipation. True myxedema and hypercholesterolemia are seen only infrequently. Menstrual flow may be increased or more likely decreased because of associated gonadotropin deficiency. During childhood, TSH deficiency results in growth retardation that is unresponsive to GH treatment.

LH and FSH. In women, gonadotropin deficiency results in amenorrhea and signs of estrogen deficiency, including breast atrophy, skin dryness, decreased vaginal secretions, and, occasionally, decreased libido. In males, the testes decrease in size and become softened. Decreased androgen production results in a loss of libido and potency, decreased rate of growth of secondary sexual hair, and reduced muscular strength. If the deficiency occurs prior to puberty there is total or partial impairment of secondary sexual development. If GH secretion is unaltered, failure of sex steroid–induced epiphyseal closure of the long bones produces excessive growth of limbs, leading to a eunuchoid appearance.

Growth Hormone. GH deficiency in the adult is unassociated with clinically recognized symptoms. Carbohydrate tolerance is impaired in GH-deficient subjects, but this disorder is distinct from diabetes mellitus and is not associated with microangiopathy. In children, GH deficiency results in growth retardation. Fasting hypoglycemia is often seen, particularly when ACTH deficiency is also present.

Prolactin. Prolactin deficiency results only in the absence of postpartum lactation.

Vasopressin. Deficiency of vasopressin results in diabetes insipidus, described in detail in Ch. 214. The impairment of water reabsorption by the kidneys results in polyuria and polydipsia, and, if fluid intake is not maintained, severe dehydration. Extreme thirst may be present that is preferentially relieved by ice water. Polyuria may not occur when ACTH deficiency coexists because of the requirement of cortisol for free water excretion. The appearance of polyuria during ACTH or glucocorticoid administration is highly suggestive of combined vasopressin and ACTH deficiency.

Oxytocin. Oxytocin deficiency is unassociated with any clinically apparent disease in humans. In particular, in women with panhypopituitarism who become pregnant, initiation of labor is normal, as is parturition.

General Clinical Features. The skin of hypopituitary patients often exhibits decreased turgor and a waxy character. Perioral and periorbital wrinkling is common, giving the appearance of premature aging. Nutrition, in general, is quite well preserved. Moderate anemia is common; it is usually normochromic and normocytic, but it may be hypochromic or macrocytic and is attributed to a combination of thyroid, testosterone, and erythropoietin deficiencies. Mental slowing and apathy are common, as are other psychiatric symptoms, including delusions and occasionally paranoid psychosis. Carbohydrate metabolism is generally intact in nondiabetics, but in insulin-requiring diabetics, hypopituitarism necessitates reduction of insulin dosage, frequently to less than half of the original level; there is also an increased tendency for hypoglycemic reactions. These changes may persist even with full glucocorticoid replacement therapy.

The sequence of pituitary hormone loss varies among patients with hypopituitarism. In general, deficiencies of GH and gonadotropins are the earliest to occur and thus the most frequently observed. ACTH and TSH deficiencies are less common and are seen at a later stage in the natural history of the disease. The pattern, however, is not predictable in individual patients, thus precluding the usefulness of evaluating pituitary function by measurement of only one or two hormones.

DIFFERENTIAL DIAGNOSIS. The major categories of disease with which hypopituitarism can be confused include (1) disorders of multiple target glands or of the CNS and (2) diseases that share the generalized features of hypopituitarism that are unassociated with endocrine dysfunction.

While measurement of pituitary hormones is indispensable in the differential diagnosis, certain clinical features have discriminatory value. Primary adrenal insufficiency is associated with hyperkalemia, hyperpigmentation, and salt craving, all of which are absent in hypopituitarism. Some patients with primary gonadal failure exhibit a discrepancy between the loss of gonadal steroid production and the loss of spermatogenesis or ovulation. Both components of gonadal function are diminished to the same extent in hypopituitarism. Primary ovarian failure results in characteristic symptoms (hot flashes) that are usually not seen when ovarian failure is secondary to gonadotropin deficiency.

Patients with chronic malnutrition or liver disease exhibit weakness, lethargy, cold intolerance, and decreased libido, frequently raising the possibility of hypopituitarism. The presence of cachexia is important in suggesting a nonpituitary disease. Although anorexia nervosa may often be confused with hypopituitarism, the severe weight loss, psychiatric symptoms, and preservation of axillary and pubic hair are all useful discriminating factors (see Ch. 202).

DIAGNOSIS. The diagnosis of hypopituitarism should be carefully and appropriately established because therapeutic decisions imply lifelong hormonal replacement therapy. In addition, neuroanatomic studies directed at determining the etiology of the hypopituitarism are an integral part of the workup and are discussed in the section on pituitary tumors.

Functional studies of each of the anterior pituitary hormones have been described in the previous section, where the specific testing details are provided. Certain general concepts used in testing are described here.

In evaluation of ACTH secretion, it is important to consider the practical implications. Testing is performed to identify patients with suspected partial adrenal insufficiency in whom an inadequate response to stress may occur. The best stimulus for this purpose is insulin hypoglycemia, in which the response to cortisol correlates well with that to surgical stress. The same test can also be used to evaluate GH responsiveness. Insulin hypoglycemia can be dangerous and should not be used in patients suspected of primary adrenal insufficiency. Recent administration of glucocorticoid therapy can complicate the workup of a patient with suspected hypopituitarism. The suppressive effects of glucocorticoids on the hypothalamic-pituitary-adrenal axis can result in a subnormal response or absence of response to any of the stimuli used. Glucocorticoids should be discontinued for at least 1 month, if possible, prior to definitive testing.

A similar problem occurs in evaluating TSH function in patients who have been receiving long-term thyroid hormone therapy, which can impair the TSH response to TRH for at least 1 month.

In patients with gonadotropin deficiency, a single GnRH challenge is frequently of little help in distinguishing between hypothalamic and pituitary causes and is useful primarily when neuroanatomic evidence of pituitary disease is present and the status of the gonodotrophs is being questioned.

Documentation of GH deficiency is important primarily in children of short stature when therapy with exogenous GH is being considered. The high frequency (> 75 per cent) of GH responses to GRH in children with no anatomic evidence of hypothalamic-pituitary disease argues for a hypothalamic etiology in most GH-deficient children. Decisions concerning GH therapy require careful assessment because of the effort and expense involved. Failure of response to at least two stimuli, usually insulin hypoglycemia and arginine, is generally required before institution of GH therapy. However, the use of exogenous GH in treating partial GH deficiency states is considered by some to be of value. In addition, hypothyroidism, if present, must be corrected prior to GH testing. In adults, GH deficiency serves as a marker for acquired hypopituitarism, particularly for pituitary tumors. In children and adults with obesity, GH responses to all stimuli tested are impaired, even in the presence of seemingly normal growth.

THERAPY. Hormonal replacement therapy must be determined individually and treatment goals specifically defined. The therapeutic use of pituitary hormones is restricted to GH for correcting growth retardation and gonadotropins for inducing fertility. GnRH may be used for introduction of puberty and treatment of infertility and GRH can be substituted for GH when the cause of hormone deficiency is hypothalamic rather than pituitary. For the most part, target organ hormones are used because of their cost advantage, ease of administration, and prolonged action.

ACTH. ACTH deficiency is treated with glucocorticoids. Cortisone (25 mg orally), hydrocortisone (20 mg orally), or prednisone (5 mg orally) given in two divided doses provides adequate therapy for most patients under normal conditions. Supplemental mineralocorticoid therapy is unnecessary because of the partial preservation of aldosterone secretion. The use of prednisone is preferred because of its lower cost. Occasional patients may require full glucocorticoid replacement therapy (a dose 50 per cent greater than those listed), but in most patients this dose is excessive. The clinical assessment of the adequacy of therapy relates to the patient's sense of well-being and the absence of excessive weight gain. During stress, the dose should be increased two- to threefold and then gradually tapered. If oral medication cannot be retained, injectable steroids (hydrocortisone hemisuccinate [Solu-Cortef] for initial emergency use, 100 mg intramuscularly or intravenously), or cortisone acetate for long-term use (50 to 100 mg intramuscularly every 12 hours) is indicated. Treatment of the acutely ill hypopituitary patient requires the same dosage of hydrocortisone (100 to 300 mg per day) as used in primary adrenal insufficiency. Preoperatively, patients should receive hydrocortisone hemisuccinate 50 mg intramuscularly every 6 hours beginning the night prior to surgery and continuing through the immediate postoperative period, followed by gradual tapering to maintenance dosage. Treatment of patients with partial ACTH deficiency without symptoms in the nonstressed state is more controversial. With adequate education, many patients do not need maintenance replacement therapy except in times of stress. Such patients in particular should wear appropriate medical identification bracelets.

TSH. TSH deficiency is treated with L-thyroxine 0.125 mg per day, although a lower dose may suffice in occasional patients. Clinical assessment of the patient and serum thyroxine levels during initiation of therapy are used to establish the appropriate dose. Adrenal insufficiency must be corrected first, although patients with partial adrenal insufficiency may require glucocorticoid replacement only after thyroid hormone replacement is started. The use of triiodothyronine, particularly as long-term therapy, is not recommended, because its shorter biologic half-life results in more rapid appearance of thyroid deficiency in the event therapy is omitted.

LH and FSH. Treatment of gonadotropin deficiency requires consideration of both gonadal steroid replacement and treatment of infertility. The subjects are considered in greater detail in Ch. 222 and 224.

Women. Estrogen replacement therapy is indicated in premenopausal women to maintain secondary sex characteristics and to reduce the risk of osteoporosis and possibly coronary artery disease. This can be accomplished with ethinyl estradiol 5 to 20 μg per day or conjugated estrogens (Premarin) 0.6 to 1.25 mg per day. The lowest possible dose that produces the desired clinical effects should be used. To induce cyclic bleeding, estrogen should be given for 25 days each month, accompanied on the last 5 days by a progestinic agent such as medroxyprogesterone 5 to 10 mg per day. Alternatively, an oral contraceptive preparation containing no more than the equivalent of 25 μg estradiol per day can be used. The advantage of replacement therapy after the menopause is still controversial, and the potential risks and benefits should be discussed with the patient to help make an appropriate decision. Estrogen therapy usually corrects the dyspareunia attributable to local estrogen deficiency in women with hypopituitarism, but decreased libido due to the absence of adrenal androgens often persists. This can be corrected by injection of a small dose of long-acting androgen such as testosterone enanthate 50 mg every 1 to 2 months or by oral administration of fluoxymesterone 5 to 10 mg once or twice weekly.

Restoration of fertility is possible in a large percentage of women with clomiphene or GnRH therapy (the latter given in a pulsatile manner by an intermittent infusion pump) if the cause of the disorder is hypothalamic or with combined FSH-LH preparations if pituitary disease is present. An FSH-rich preparation from postmenopausal urine is used to initiate follicular growth and maturation; it is monitored by measurement of plasma estradiol levels. Human chorionic gonadotropin is then injected to induce ovulation. This therapy is expensive, entails the risk of superovulation and multiple pregnancy, and should be undertaken only under the direction of an experienced physician.

Men. Testosterone replacement therapy in adult males is accomplished by intramuscular injection of a long-acting testosterone preparation (testosterone enanthate or cypionate, 200 mg every 3 weeks). The endpoints are restoration of full androgenization, including beard growth, and improvement in muscular strength, libido, and potency. Androgen therapy should be withheld as long as possible in the adolescent with growth retardation to avoid premature epiphyseal closure, which limits the potential for future linear growth. Testosterone therapy may be required for many months before full restoration of libido and performance. If gonadotropin deficiency has developed before puberty, full androgenization may never occur. In patients with longstanding hypogonadism, psychosocial behavioral changes affecting the patient's entire lifestyle may be disrupted by initiation of testosterone therapy, leading to major adjustment problems with both sexual and nonsexual relationships.

Infertility in men with hypopituitarism can be corrected with a combination of FSH and human chorionic gonadotropin (hCG), although therapy is required for several months, and the success rate is less than 50 per cent. GnRH, given intermittently as in women, is an alternate method of therapy in individuals with hypothalamic hypogonadism.

Growth Hormone. GH therapy is indicated for the correction of impaired linear growth, and its use is thus confined almost exclusively to childhood and adolescent years. Early establishment of the diagnosis is critical, since the probability of successful long-term therapy is inversely related to the extent of growth retardation. Treatment requires the use of human GH, which was originally extracted and purified from human pituitaries obtained at autopsy. The association of pituitary GH therapy with Creutzfeldt-Jakob disease led to a discontinuation in its use in 1985 and substitution of GH produced by recombinant DNA technology. GH is administered intramuscularly or subcutaneously at a dose of 0.1 mg per kilogram three times weekly; its use is continued until the final height is achieved, coincident with long-bone epiphyseal closure. A goal of 5 feet 4 inches is generally pursued but not always achieved. Careful attention must be given to concomitant thyroid hormone deficiency. Glucocorticoids should be used sparingly because of their interference with growth-promoting effects of GH. Small doses of oral androgens may be used simultaneously to increase growth velocity, although this has not gained widespread acceptance. Estrogens are to be avoided because of their greater effect on epiphyseal closure. Gonadal steroid therapy is usually initiated during the years of puberty to avoid psychosocial problems. However, if significant catch-up growth is required, its use should be delayed. GH therapy increases height age more rapidly than bone age, may initially be associated with a decrease in body fat, and also corrects the fasting hypoglycemia of GH-deficient children. GRH, or one of its analogues, may be useful in treatment of at least 50 per cent of children with isolated GH deficiency and in the future may be administered by noninjectable routes. Recent studies have suggested that metabolic disturbances and muscle work performance impairment of adults with GH deficiency can be improved with GH therapy. However, the use of GH in adults must still be considered experimental.

Guay AT, Agnello V, Tronic BC, et al.: Lymphocytic hypophysitis in a man. J Clin Endocrinol Metab 64:631, 1987. Scanarini M, D'Avella D, Rotilio A, et al.: Giant-cell granulomatous hypophysitis: A distinct clinicopathological entity. J Neurosurg 71:681, 1989. *Two unusual forms of hypopituitarism that can mimic a pituitary tumor.*
Komatsu M, Kondo T, Yamauchi K, et al.: Antipituitary antibodies in patients with the primary empty sella syndrome. J Clin Endocrinol Metab 67:633, 1988. Bjerre P, Lindholm J, Videbaek H: The spontaneous course of pituitary adenomas and occurrence of an empty sella in untreated acromegaly. J Clin Endocrinol Metab 63:287, 1986. *The spectrum of the empty sella syndrome is reflected in these two reports of primary and secondary forms of the disease.*
Lam KSL, Tse VKC, Wang C, et al.: Early effects of cranial irradiation on hypothalamic-pituitary function. J Clin Endocrinol Metab 64:418, 1987. Littley MD, Shalet SM, Beardwell CG, et al.: Hypopituitarism following external radiotherapy for pituitary tumours in adults. Q J Med 70:145, 1989. *Hypopituitarism following cranial irradiation for both pituitary and nonpituitary disease is being recognized more frequently in adults as well as children.*
Libber SM, Plotnick LP, Johanson AJ, et al.: Long-term follow-up of hypopituitary patients treated with human growth hormone. Medicine (Baltimore) 69:46, 1990. Binnerts A, Wilson JHP, Lamberts SWJ: The effects of human growth hormone administration in elderly adults with recent weight loss. J Clin Endocrinol Metab 67:1312, 1988. *An excellent review of the long-term effects of GH treatment of hypopituitary children, in which the results are encouraging, if not completely satisfying, contrasted with a report of acute effects in adults, the long-term significance of which is unknown.*
Phillips JA III, Vnencak-Jones CL: Genetics of growth hormone and its disorders. Adv Hum Genet 18:305, 1989. *A current review of genetic aspects of GH deficiency from clinical and molecular levels.*
Sheehan HL, Summers VK: The syndrome of hypopituitarism. Q J Med 42:319, 1949. *The classic monograph describing the clinical-pathologic correlations of hypopituitarism. Its lucid and detailed presentation makes it worthwhile reading even after more than four decades.*
Whitcomb RW, Crowley WF Jr: Diagnosis and treatment of isolated gonadotropin-releasing hormone deficiency in men. J Clin Endocrinol Metab 70:3, 1990. Blunt SM, Butt WR: Pulsatile GnRH therapy for the induction of ovulation in hypogonadotropic hypogonadism. Acta Endocrinol (Copenh) 119:58, 1988. *Pulsatile GnRH therapy is useful in the treatment of both men and women with gonadotropin deficiency, as reviewed in these articles.*

PITUITARY TUMORS

CLASSIFICATION. Pituitary tumors are subdivided by their histologic characteristics and also by their functional activity.

Specific considerations of hormone-secreting pituitary tumors are found in the next section. The two major histologic types of primary pituitary tumors are the adenoma and the craniopharyngioma. In addition, parasellar tumors such as optic nerve glioma, meningioma, chordoma, sphenoid wing sarcoma, as well as metastatic tumors, can also be present within the sella turcica.

Pituitary Adenomas. This cell type constitutes greater than 90 per cent of all pituitary tumors. The classic subdivision into chromophobic and chromophilic tumors has given way to more specific identification on the basis of immunohistochemical stains for individual hormones. Using these techniques, only 10 to 20 per cent of pituitary adenomas appear to be nonfunctioning. Pituitary tumors account for 6 to 18 per cent of all brain tumors, and small adenomas, many of which are functioning, have been detected in up to 30 per cent of unselected autopsy series. The growth pattern of pituitary adenomas appears unrelated to hormone secretion. Rapidly enlarging tumors are often recognized because of their mass effects, whereas slowly growing tumors tend to allow for greater expression of the hormone hypersecretory effects. The peak incidence of nonfunctioning pituitary adenomas is between 40 and 50 years, and the frequency is uninfluenced by sex. Many "nonfunctioning" tumors actually produce portions of hormones (e.g., the glycoprotein α subunit common to TSH, LH, and FSH) or may synthesize but be incapable of releasing the hormone. Although pituitary adenomas are almost always histologically benign, they may exhibit aggressive growth behavior with invasion of surrounding structures, making their total removal impossible. Adenomas are generally solid with a well-defined capsule, although they may on occasion be cystic and hemorrhagic. Calcification, if present, results from organization of a previous hemorrhage.

Craniopharyngiomas. These tumors are of congenital origin, may be partly or entirely cystic, and are always benign. The cyst fluid may be cholesterol rich. Calcification, generally concentric, is present in 50 per cent. The tumors grow at variable rates and may remain dormant for many years. Although half of the tumors are seen during childhood, they may appear at any time during life. The site of origin of most tumors is in the midline at the upper portion of the pituitary stalk, and approximately 15 per cent involve the upper portion of the anterior lobe and are therefore intrasellar. Variations of craniopharyngiomas include ependymomas and epidermoid cysts.

CLINICAL FEATURES. The manifestations of pituitary tumors are neuroanatomic, endocrinologic, and radiologic. Presenting symptoms of pituitary tumors have changed in frequency over the years with refinements in diagnostic procedures. Whereas nearly 90 per cent of patients diagnosed 30 years ago exhibited visual disturbances, only 25 per cent do so at present. In contrast, the most common presentation today relates to impaired gonadal function, frequently associated with prolactin-secreting pituitary tumors. A small percentage of patients (less than 5 per cent) are discovered accidentally on review of head-imaging procedures obtained for other purposes.

Neuroanatomic manifestations occur secondary to tumor growth causing pressure on the overlying dura and the diaphragma sellae. This results in headaches that are variable in nature, imprecisely located, generally of dull quality, unassociated with nausea or visual symptoms, unrelated to position, and inconsistently relieved by analgesics. Disappearance of headache is frequently a sign of rupture of the dura. With continued suprasellar expansion the tumor exerts pressure on the optic chiasm, leading to the classic findings of bitemporal hemianopsia. At early stages the field defects may be asymmetric and involve only the superior temporal fields. Eventually, blindness and optic atrophy occur. Anterior growth of the tumor may cause symptoms limited only to one eye. Papilledema occurs in one fourth of craniopharyngiomas but rarely in pituitary adenomas. Further growth results in hypothalamic compression leading to temperature instability, hyperphagia, altered sleep patterns, and emotional disturbances. Pressure on the third ventricle results in internal hydrocephalus. Rarely, temporal or frontal lobe compression may cause behavioral changes and seizures, and midbrain compression may produce long-tract signs. Lateral extension is more common and leads to compression of the third, fourth, and sixth cranial nerves in the cavernous sinus, resulting

in ophthalmoplegia and diplopia. Expansion inferiorly into the sphenoid sinus may result in cerebrospinal fluid rhinorrhea. Hemorrhage into the tumor, *pituitary apoplexy,* may result in rapid expansion of the tumor and lead to the sudden appearance of headache of varying intensity that subsides after a few days. If the tumor is intrasellar, hypopituitarism often results; if extrasellar, there may be rapid deterioration of vision. "Spontaneous" cures of hormone-secreting pituitary tumors may also occur as the result of hemorrhagic tumor necrosis.

Neuroradiologic presentations consist of a deformed or enlarged sella seen on standard skull roentgenography or a mass lesion seen on computed tomography (CT) or magnetic resonance imaging (MRI).

Endocrine symptoms include diminished function secondary to destruction of normal pituitary tissue by tumor or interference with portal blood supply and hyperfunction due to tumor or hyperplasia. The two may be combined. In addition, diminished function may occur secondary to the effects of hormone hypersecretion (i.e., hypogonadism secondary to hyperprolactinemia). The frequency of presentation and the manifestations are described in the previous section.

DIAGNOSTIC PROCEDURES. Diagnosis of a pituitary tumor necessitates differentiation from other parasellar disorders, determination of the tumor size and extent of extrasellar extension, and assessment of hormone deficiencies and/or hypersecretion. Endocrine evaluation should be performed prior to definitive therapy, if possible, because the extent of hypopituitarism and presence of hormone hypersecretion may influence the type and extent of therapy. Patients with pituitary tumors undergoing stressful procedures must be considered to have panhypopituitarism unless proven otherwise and pretreated with glucocorticoids.

Neuroradiologic procedures have improved remarkably during the past decade, and MRI today constitutes the definitive study. This technique provides exquisite anatomic resolution and, using a combination of coronal and sagittal images, defines the tumor in relation to the sellar contents as well as the extrasellar structures (Fig. 213–1). Precise information concerning displacement of the pituitary stalk (if present) and relationship of the tumor to the optic chiasm and cavernous sinus usually provides sufficient data for deciding on a surgical approach, if indicated, or the need for other procedures. As an alternative, CT performed with contrast media also provides high-quality imaging of the pituitary (Fig. 213–2). Despite its lower cost, CT provides resolution inferior to that of MRI and subjects the patient to radiation exposure. If repeat imaging studies are necessary, the radiation dose may become considerable.

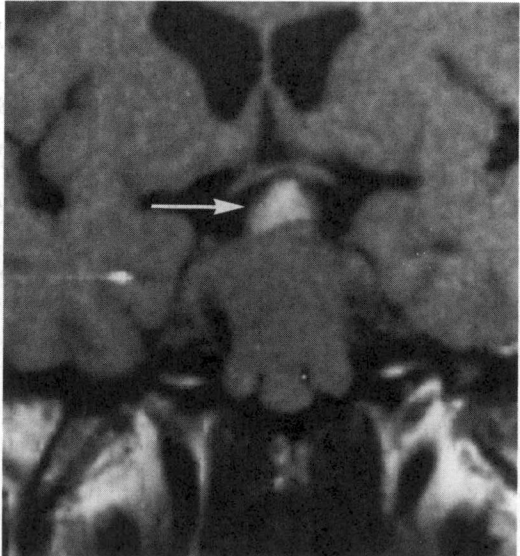

FIGURE 213–1. Magnetic resonance image (MRI) of a pituitary adenoma (coronal view). The large tumor mass extends inferiorly and superiorly. The intense (white) signal (*arrow*) in the dorsal portion of the tumor represents recent hemorrhage. The superiorly displaced optic chiasm is seen just above the tumor.

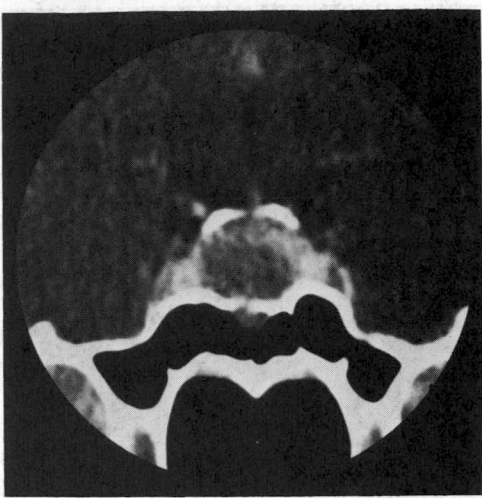

FIGURE 213–2. Computed tomographic (CT) scan of pituitary (coronal view) demonstrating a pituitary tumor with suprasellar extension and erosion of the sellar floor with inferior extension of the tumor into the sphenoid sinus.

The most important neuro-ophthalmologic study is evaluation of visual fields. Test objects of varying sizes and colors can provide an excellent assessment of both central and peripheral fields. The technique is reproducible and sensitive and useful in observing patients for serial changes. Bitemporal field defects are, however, not specific for pituitary tumors; they may occur with parasellar tumors, vascular abnormalities, arachnoiditis, or rarely with chiasmal prolapse into the sella associated with the empty sella syndrome. Atypical field defects may also occur, even those suggesting superior rather than inferior pressure.

DIFFERENTIAL DIAGNOSIS. Disorders that must be differentiated from pituitary tumors include the empty sella syndrome, parasellar diseases, and pituitary enlargement associated with other endocrine disorders.

The *empty sella* is partly or nearly completely filled with CSF and results from extension of the subarachnoid space into the intrasellar region. The pituitary gland is flattened along the posterior portion of the floor and the dorsum. Primary empty sella syndrome is unassociated with prior surgical or irradiation therapy and has been found in up to one quarter of autopsy series, usually unassociated with endocrine disease. The etiology is unknown, but the syndrome has been postulated to be due to incomplete formation of the diaphragma sella, permitting CSF pressure to be transmitted to the sella and gradually leading to herniation of the arachnoid and remodeling of the sella. Nearly all patients are asymptomatic, although some may have nonspecific headaches. The syndrome is seen commonly in obese women and in association with systemic hypertension, benign intracranial hypertension (pseudotumor cerebri), and CSF rhinorrhea. The sella is usually symmetrically enlarged or ballooned and may be deformed. Endocrine function is generally normal, although diminished TSH and gonadotropin secretion, hyperprolactinemia, and rarely panhypopituitarism or diabetes insipidus may be present. The diagnosis is established by CT or MRI. The empty sella may coexist with a pituitary tumor, which is usually hyperfunctional. The secondary empty sella syndrome is seen in patients following pituitary surgery or irradiation or intratumoral bleeding.

The signs and symptoms of parasellar disorders may mimic those of pituitary tumors. Parasellar disorders include inflammatory and granulomatous diseases (sarcoidosis, eosinophilic granuloma), degenerative disorders (aneurysms), and neoplasms (meningiomas, hamartomas, chordomas, and metastatic tumors). Suprasellar tumors usually present with the neurologic manifestations of increased intracranial pressure, hypothalamic symptoms, visual impairment, and internal hydrocephalus. Endocrine manifestations tend to follow rather than precede neurologic symptoms. CT and MRI are extremely valuable in differentiating these disorders from primary pituitary tumors.

Longstanding primary hypothyroidism or hypogonadism can result in sellar enlargement, increased TSH or gonadotropin

secretion, hyperplasia of tropic hormone–producing cells, and in some patients, hormone-secreting tumors. Institution of appropriate replacement hormone therapy can reverse the hypersecretory and hyperplastic (although not neoplastic) changes.

THERAPY. Treatment of nonfunctioning pituitary tumors is indicated to prevent or limit the loss of pituitary function and the consequences of extrasellar extension. The two therapeutic methods are surgery and radiation therapy.

Pituitary surgery is the conventional therapy for pituitary tumors. The transsphenoidal approach is currently used for all tumors except those with extensive suprasellar extension, particularly when separated from the intrasellar portion by a narrow neck. Tumors encircling optic nerves or encasing cerebral vessels can be removed only by a transfrontal approach. Currently the operative mortality is less than 1 per cent. The transsphenoidal approach includes the use of modern fluoroscopic aids and microsurgical techniques. It provides better visualization of the sellar contents and permits selective adenomectomy to be performed. If preoperative evaluation reveals preservation of anterior pituitary function, a conservative approach is indicated to preserve remaining pituitary hormone secretion, since a small rim of adenohypophyseal tissue is often sufficient to maintain adequate pituitary function. Glucocorticoid coverage is essential for the perioperative period even for patients with intact pituitary-adrenal function and is accomplished with parenteral administration of hydrocortisone, 50 mg intramuscularly every 6 hours. Postoperatively the patient must be carefully observed for the development of diabetes insipidus, particularly since an obtunded patient may not perceive thirst. Transient polyuria and increased plasma osmolality commonly occur in the immediate postoperative period as a result of mild trauma to the pituitary stalk. Persistence of these findings beyond the first 48 hours usually indicates significant destruction of the stalk or posterior pituitary and permanent impairment of function. However, fluctuations in posterior pituitary function may occur for a period of several weeks, and recovery has been observed as late as many months postoperatively. Initially the patient should be treated with aqueous vasopressin (5 U subcutaneously) or desmopressin (DDAVP) (1 or 2 µg subcutaneously) rather than with a long-acting preparation so the natural history of the process can be observed.

Radiation therapy can be used as an alternative to surgical excision of the pituitary tumor or as adjunct therapy. Although less popular as primary therapy, because of its delayed effects, radiation therapy using conventional high-energy sources (supravoltage) or heavy-particle (proton beam) sources is an effective method of treatment. Radiation therapy is to be avoided in patients with significant suprasellar extension or in the presence of marked visual field defects.

The recurrence rate of pituitary tumors following surgical treatment alone ranges from 25 to nearly 100 per cent in different series. Since postoperative radiographic and endocrine studies indicate that intraoperative assessment of the extent of pituitary tumor removal is often inaccurate, postoperative irradiation is indicated in all patients with nonfunctioning pituitary adenomas unless specifically contraindicated. The dose currently employed is 4500 to 5000 rads, which can be given with minimal side effects. Some late loss of pituitary function occurs in 15 to 25 per cent of patients. Thus, if preservation of fertility is desired, radiation therapy should be delayed.

Cardoso ER, Peterson EW: Pituitary apoplexy: A review. Neurosurgery 14:363, 1984. *A thorough discussion of the varied manner in which this disorder presents and a rationale for management.*

Davis PC, Hoffman JC Jr, Spencer T, et al.: MR imaging of pituitary adenoma: CT, clinical, and surgical correlation. AJR 148:797, 1987. Peck WW, Dillon WP, Norman D, et al.: High-resolution MR imaging of pituitary microadenomas at 1.5 T: Experience with Cushing disease. AJR 152:145, 1989. L'Huillier F, Combes C, Martin N, et al.: MRI in the diagnosis of so-called pituitary apoplexy: Seven cases. J Neuroradiol 16:221, 1989. *The availability of MRI has markedly improved the diagnostic accuracy in suspected pituitary tumors and increased the likelihood of appropriate therapy.*

Grigsby PW, Simpson JR, Fineberg B: Late regrowth of pituitary adenomas after irradiation and/or surgery: Hazard function analysis. Cancer 63:1308, 1989. Harris PE, Afshar F, Coates P, et al.: The effects of transsphenoidal surgery on endocrine function and visual fields in patients with functionless pituitary tumours. Q J Med 71:417, 1989. *Nonfunctioning tumors of the pituitary continue to remain a vexing therapeutic problem as reflected by these two reports that examine outcome and long-term sequelae.*

Heshmati HM, Turpin G, Kujas M, et al.: The immunocytochemical heterogeneity of silent pituitary adenomas. Acta Endocrinol (Copenh) 118:533, 1988. Kovacs K, Lloyd R, Horvath E, et al.: Silent somatotroph adenomas of the human pituitary: A morphologic study of three cases including immunocytochemistry, electron microscopy, in vitro examination, and in situ hybridization. Am J Pathol 134:345, 1989. *Studies of "nonfunctioning" tumors of the pituitary gland reveal that many exhibit evidence of hormone storage and in vitro secretion. These reports illustrate the variety of such observations.*

Klibanski A, Zervas NT: Diagnosis and management of hormone-secreting pituitary adenomas. N Engl J Med 324:822, 1991. *This is a valuable, succinct general review of pituitary tumors; with 114 up-to-date references.*

PITUITARY HYPERFUNCTION: HORMONE-SECRETING PITUITARY TUMORS

Pituitary hormone hypersecretion generally involves overproduction of only a single hormone except in the case of certain hormone-secreting tumors. Hormone overproduction occurs in response to altered feedback signals (i.e., hyperprolactinemia due to increased estrogen secretion in pregnancy; ACTH, TSH, and gonadotropin hypersecretion in response to diminished target organ feedback in primary hypofunction of the adrenal, thyroid, and gonads; and GH hypersecretion associated with caloric deprivation). Whereas these changes begin as functional alterations, prolonged stimulation can result in hyperplastic as well as hypersecretory changes. Pathologic hyperfunction occurs in association with pituitary hyperplasia or tumor unrelated to regulatory feedback mechanisms. These disorders involve primarily somatotrophic, lactotrophic, and corticotrophic cells, although all cell types may be affected.

Growth Hormone–Secreting Tumors: Acromegaly

GH hypersecretion is most commonly associated with a pituitary somatotroph tumor or rarely somatotroph hyperplasia. These tumors previously were considered eosinophilic (due to GH storage granules) or chromophobic (when little hormone was stored). Tumors with abundant hormone storage tend to be better differentiated and more slowly growing, resulting in more pronounced clinical features of GH hypersecretion, whereas the less differentiated nonhormone–storing tumors tend to grow more rapidly, leading to more pronounced effects of an expanding tumor mass.

CLINICAL FEATURES. The clinical manifestations of GH hypersecretion depend on the age of onset. During childhood and prior to epiphyseal fusion, GH hypersecretion produces proportional skeletal growth leading to gigantism. Hypogonadism is frequently present, leading to delayed epiphyseal closure and thus a more prolonged growth period. The tallest reported patient with gigantism reached a height of nearly 9 feet. It is more common for patients to exhibit features of both gigantism and acromegaly, reflecting persistence of GH hypersecretion into adult life.

Signs and symptoms of GH hypersecretion beginning during adult life develop slowly. Soft tissue swelling and hypertrophy involving the extremities and face are the earliest findings (Fig. 213–3). These changes are usually best documented by comparing photographs taken over a one- to two-decade span. Spadelike changes develop in the fingers, and increased soft tissue volume necessitates ring enlargement and increases in glove and shoe sizes. The skin becomes thickened and leathery, and skin folds increase in prominence. A generalized increase in hair growth and pigmentation often occurs. Fibroma molluscum (pedunculated epithelial tags) and acanthosis nigricans are common. The skin becomes oily, and sebaceous cyst formation is common. Increased sweating occurs in most patients and is a sensitive biologic indicator of disease activity.

Bony changes occur more slowly and include cortical thickening, tufting of terminal phalanges, and osteophyte proliferation. Degenerated articular cartilages and ligamentous hypertrophy produce a hypertrophic arthropathy that eventually leads to deforming and crippling arthritis. Prognathism results from mandibular enlargement and causes a significant overbite of the lower incisors and increased spacing of the teeth. Bony overgrowth of the frontal, malar, and nasal bones occurs; increase in size of the paranasal sinuses together with vocal cord hypertrophy leads to

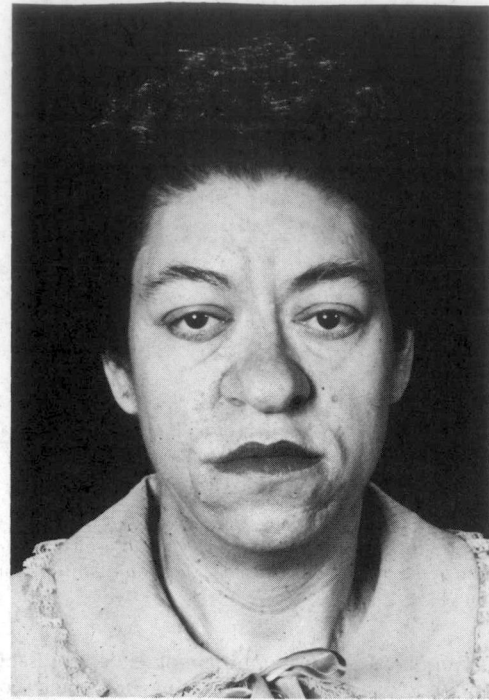

FIGURE 213–3. Clinical features of a 43-year-old patient with acromegaly of 15 years' duration. Coarsened features result from soft tissue overgrowth about the eyes, nose, and mouth. Lacrimal overgrowth, thickening of skin folds, and fibroma molluscum are also present. (From Frohman LA: *In* Felig P, Baxter JD, Broadus AE, et al. (eds.): Endocrinology and Metabolism, 2nd ed., p 302. Copyright © 1987 by McGraw-Hill, Inc. Used by permission of McGraw-Hill Book Company.)

deepening of the voice. Eustachian tube mucosal hypertrophy often produces obstruction and serous otitis media and that of the nasopharynx may lead to sleep apnea.

Peripheral neuropathy commonly occurs because of nerve entrapment by surrounding tissue overgrowth, most commonly affecting the median nerve and producing the carpal tunnel syndrome. Axonal demyelinization of peripheral nerves associated with perineural and subepineural proliferation results in palpable nerve fibers. Paresthesias, sensory losses, and proximal muscle weakness occur frequently.

Prolonged hypersecretion of GH leads to generalized visceromegaly involving salivary glands, liver, spleen, and kidneys. Salivary gland enlargement is detectable clinically whereas that of the other organs is not, and significant hepatosplenomegaly usually implies the presence of a coexisting disease. Both secretory and reabsorptive functions of the kidney are increased in acromegaly.

Thyroid enlargement with nodule formation is common, but true hyperfunction is infrequent. Parathyroid hyperplasia and adenoma may occur, often reflecting the multiple endocrine neoplasia syndrome (Type I), leading to hypercalciuria and nephrolithiasis. Elevations of prolactin levels occur in one third of patients, resulting in galactorrhea, amenorrhea, and decreased libido.

The effects of GH on the cardiovascular system are controversial. Hypertension is common but generally mild and responsive to drug therapy. Cardiomegaly is routinely found, but there is no characteristic form of acromegalic heart disease. Cardiac failure, when it occurs, appears related to hypertension and not to the effects of GH hypersecretion. Yet the incidence of cardiovascular disease is increased in acromegalics, as is mortality. Weight gain is uncommon, but carbohydrate intolerance and diabetes are seen in 25 per cent of acromegalics, primarily in those with a family history of diabetes. Insulin resistance is common and occasionally associated with ketosis. Diabetic microangiopathy, however, is extremely uncommon, even in longstanding disease.

LABORATORY STUDIES. The diagnosis of acromegaly is established by the finding of elevated plasma GH levels that do not respond normally to physiologic suppression and stimulation;

in adults, a GH value greater than 2 ng per milliliter in males or 5 ng per milliliter in females after oral glucose administration is confirmatory. Randomly obtained samples with markedly elevated levels are also diagnostic. However, in normal children and young adults, GH levels as high as 50 ng per milliliter are sporadically exhibited, thereby necessitating dynamic studies of GH secretion in many patients. TRH stimulates GH secretion in 70 to 80 per cent of acromegalics but not in normal subjects, and this procedure is also useful in following patients after therapy. GH secretion in acromegalics differs in other ways from that in normal persons, including absence of a sleep-associated increase in GH and a tendency for wide spontaneous fluctuations in GH levels, indicating intermittent secretory activity. Plasma GH levels increase after GRH in most acromegalics, but the test is not of diagnostic help.

Plasma IGF-I (somatomedin C) levels are also increased in acromegaly and provide good correlation with the clinical manifestations of GH hypersecretion. Determination of IGF-I levels for assessing disease activity after therapy is useful, particularly when GH levels are borderline.

DIFFERENTIAL DIAGNOSIS. The clinical features of acromegaly are not confused with those of other diseases. The question commonly raised is whether features suggestive of the disease are associated with active disease, inactive disease, or no disease. Dynamic studies of GH secretion are required to differentiate these possibilities. Gigantism during childhood occasionally occurs in the absence of GH hypersecretion (cerebral gigantism) through a yet to be determined mechanism. GH levels are elevated in patients with renal failure, cirrhosis, protein-calorie malnutrition, and anorexia nervosa and in the Laron dwarf (growth retardation caused by a genetic defect in the GH receptor), but in these conditions the clinical features of acromegaly are absent.

PATHOGENESIS. Acromegaly occurs nearly always as a primary tumor of somatotrophs within the pituitary, although rarely it may be secondary to excessive somatotroph stimulation by an ectopic GRH-secreting tumor, hypersecretion of GRH from the CNS, or an ectopic GH-secreting tumor. Selective removal of the GH-secreting adenoma is followed in most patients not only by restoration of normal GH values but by normal responses to dynamic testing.

GH-secreting tumors are monoclonal (as judged by X chromosome inactivation analyses). In addition, a genetic point mutation has been found in the guanine nucleotide regulatory protein ($G_s \alpha$) in 40 per cent of GH-secreting pituitary adenomas, the result of which is autonomous GH hypersecretion and cell growth. These studies therefore support the concept of a primary pituitary disease. In some patients, however, GH-secreting tumors have been associated with GRH-secreting carcinoid tumors of the bronchus and foregut, pancreatic islet tumors, and small cell carcinoma of the lung. Removal of the extrapituitary tumor has resulted in a return of GH levels to normal and regression of the pituitary tumor. Pituitary histology in patients with secondary acromegaly ranges from local or generalized somatotroph hyperplasia to actual tumor formation. In addition, neuronal tumors present in the hypothalamus (hamartomas) or in the pituitary, contiguous with the somatotroph adenoma (gangliocytoma or choristoma), may also be the source of GRH production in a few patients with acromegaly. Since excessive stimulation by GRH is capable of inducing adenomas as well as hyperplasia, it is possible that some patients now considered to have primary pituitary disease actually have a hypothalamic disorder characterized by excessive GRH production from nontumorous tissue.

Comparison of the limited numbers of reported patients with secondary acromegaly does not provide any evidence of differences in either clinical manifestations or responses to dynamic studies of GH secretion, with the possible exception of decreased frequency of GH responses to GRH. In patients with ectopic GRH production or even with CNS overproduction, immunoreactive plasma GRH levels are readily detectable, in contrast to patients presumed to have primary pituitary disease in whom levels are near or beneath the limits of detectability.

THERAPY. Therapy for patients with acromegaly involves three potential methods: surgery, irradiation, and medical (pharmacologic). Considerations of the space-occupying mass and of hypopituitarism are similar to those described for nonfunctioning pituitary tumors. Prior to initiation of therapy to the pituitary itself, consideration should be given to the possibility of an extrapituitary tumor, removal of which may reverse the GH hypersecretion.

Surgical treatment of GH-secreting pituitary tumors is currently the treatment of choice. Transsphenoidal or, if necessary, transfrontal adenomectomy is indicated once the presence of the disease has been established, even though the radiologic findings are minimal. The results in published series vary. The described "success" or "cure" rate varies considerably, depending on the criteria used for defining normal GH levels as well as on the initial size of the tumor. Using a criterion of 5 ng per milliliter, success rates of up to 90 per cent have been reported with small tumors. Using a more stringent and widely accepted criterion of 2.5 ng per milliliter, however, the success rate is probably not more than 50 to 60 per cent. Normalization of GH levels is inversely related to the size of the tumor; less favorable results occur with tumors greater than 2 cm in diameter or plasma GH levels greater than 100 ng per milliliter. The clinical features of GH, however, are frequently improved even without complete restoration of GH values to normal. In patients whose GH levels return to the normal range, tumor recurrence is infrequent (approximately 5 per cent), but with incomplete removal the recurrence rate is greater than 50 per cent if no further therapy is administered.

Radiation therapy, using methods similar to those for nonfunctioning tumors, is effective as a primary means of treatment of acromegaly. The reduction in GH hypersecretion is, however, slow, the response is inversely related to the initial GH level, and achievement of normal levels may require 5 or even 10 years, although about half of patients exhibit normal GH levels after 2 to 4 years. Postoperative irradiation is indicated when GH levels remain elevated and, used in conjunction with surgery, offers the best prognosis.

Pharmacologic therapy in acromegaly is of limited value. Bromocriptine, a dopamine receptor agonist, lowers GH levels to normal in only 25 per cent and decreases tumor size in only 5 per cent of patients. Dosages of up to 60 mg per day may be required, and side effects are frequent. Octreotide, a somatostatin analogue, is effective in reducing GH levels to normal in nearly half of acromegalics and in decreasing tumor size in nearly the same percentage. The drug must be injected three to four times daily or given by constant subcutaneous infusion and is associated with a number of side effects (acholic stools, mild carbohydrate intolerance), the most worrisome of which is the development of cholelithiasis in more than 40 per cent of patients. Neither of the drugs is tumoricidal, and each is effective only during continued administration. They should, therefore, be considered only as adjunct therapy or in patients who are not surgical candidates.

Frohman LA: Therapeutic options in acromegaly. J Clin Endocrinol Metab, 1991, in press. *A current review of the relative advantages and limitations of the various forms of therapy of this disorder.*

Frohman LA, Downs TR: Ectopic GRH syndrome. *In* Robbins RJ, Melmed S (eds.): Acromegaly. New York, Plenum Press, 1987, pp 115–125. Sano T, Asa SL, Kovacs K: Growth hormone-releasing hormone-producing tumors: Clinical, biochemical, and morphological manifestations. Endocr Rev 9:357, 1988. *The spectrum of acromegaly secondary to excess secretion of growth hormone–releasing hormone is reviewed from the clinical, laboratory, histologic, and therapeutic aspects in these two reviews.*

Lamberts SWJ: The role of somatostatin in the regulation of anterior pituitary hormone secretion and the use of its analogs in the treatment of human pituitary tumors. Endocrinol Rev 9:417, 1988. Page MD, Millward ME, Taylor A, et al.: Long-term treatment of acromegaly with a long-acting analogue of somatostatin, octreotide. QJ Med 74:189, 1990. Ho KY, Weissberger AJ, Marbach P, et al.: Therapeutic efficacy of the somatostatin analog SMS 201-995 (octreotide) in acromegaly. Ann Intern Med 112:173, 1990. *Three excellent series summarizing the use of octreotide in treatment of acromegaly.*

Macleod AF, Clarke DG, Pambakian H, et al.: Treatment of acromegaly by external irradiation. Clin Endocrinol (Oxf) 30:303, 1989. Littley MD, Shalet SM, Swindell R, et al.: Low-dose pituitary irradiation for acromegaly. Clin Endocrinol (Oxf) 32:261, 1990. *The role of irradiation in therapy of acromegaly is clearly described in these two series.*

Melmed S: Acromegaly. N Engl J Med 322:966, 1990. *An excellent review of current knowledge of acromegaly from the standpoint of pathogenesis and therapy.*

Ross DA, Wilson CB: Results of transsphenoidal microsurgery for growth hormone-secreting pituitary adenoma in a series of 214 patients. J Neurosurg 68:854, 1988. Oyen WJG, Pieters GFFM, Meijer E, et al.: Which factors predict the results of pituitary surgery in acromegaly? Acta Endocrinol (Copenh) 117:491, 1988. *Large surgical series indicating the effectiveness (and limitations) of the surgical treatment of acromegaly and a careful assessment of the predictors of surgical outcome.*

Prolactin-Secreting Tumors: Amenorrhea-Galactorrhea Syndrome

Hyperprolactinemia is the most common form of pituitary hyperfunction. It is present in as many as 25 per cent of infertile women. The incidence in men is much lower. In patients with pituitary tumors the incidence of elevated prolactin levels ranges from 60 to 80 per cent and is greater than that of any other pituitary hormone. The distinction between patients with *idiopathic hyperprolactinemia* and those with *prolactin-secreting tumors* is currently made on the basis of CT or MRI examination of the pituitary. Thus, changes in the relative frequency of the two diagnoses reflect primarily recent improvements in radiologic technology.

CLINICAL FEATURES. In women, hyperprolactinemia causes galactorrhea, oligomenorrhea or amenorrhea, and infertility (see Ch. 226 for a discussion of galactorrhea). Galactorrhea requires near-normal levels of ovarian steroids and is therefore not seen in all patients. It frequently occurs in association with oral contraceptive use, usually following its discontinuation. The reported incidence of galactorrhea in patients with prolactin-secreting tumors varies from 50 to 90 per cent. Oligomenorrhea or amenorrhea occurs in a similar percentage of patients and in nearly all with radiographic evidence of a pituitary tumor. The development of amenorrhea and the development of galactorrhea are not necessarily related to one another and are of no diagnostic importance. The cause of amenorrhea is related to effects of altered CNS neurotransmitters, principally dopamine, as a result of hyperprolactinemia, which interferes with the positive feedback effect of estradiol on GnRH secretion and the self-priming effect of GnRH. The effects of anovulation include hypoestrogenemia, which results in decreased vaginal secretion, and dyspareunia, which may be responsible for diminished libido. Mild hirsutism may also occur in association with increased dehydroepiandrosterone sulfate production by the adrenals. Longstanding hyperprolactinemia has, in some women, been associated with decreased bone density, only part of which may be attributed to the hypoestrogenemia. Whether such women are at increased risk for the development of clinically significant osteoporosis is controversial.

In men, hyperprolactinemia results in impotence and diminished libido and, rarely, gynecomastia and galactorrhea. A defect in endogenous GnRH secretion is present, along with diminished testosterone secretion. The decreased libido is, however, not explained entirely on this basis, since it often persists despite testosterone replacement therapy. In some men oligospermia is also present.

LABORATORY STUDIES. Plasma prolactin levels in patients with prolactin-secreting tumors vary from slightly above normal (15 to 20 ng per milliliter) to values greater than 10,000 ng per milliliter. Levels less than 200 ng per milliliter are of little use in distinguishing between the various causes of the disorder, whereas levels greater than 200 ng per milliliter are invariably associated with prolactin-secreting tumors. Since prolactin is a stress-responsive hormone and levels fluctuate in normal subjects, repeated sampling in patients with moderate degrees of hyperprolactinemia is essential.

A large number of dynamic studies of prolactin secretion reveal differences between normal persons and those with pathologic hyperprolactinemia, but none is reliable in distinguishing between idiopathic hyperprolactinemia and prolactin-secreting tumors. Prolactin responses to submaximally suppressive infusions of dopamine are impaired in such patients, as compared to those with known extrapituitary disorders causing hyperprolactinemia, although the latter can usually be distinguished on clinical grounds. Patients with prolactin-secreting tumors and idiopathic hyperprolactinemia have impaired responses to dopamine receptor–blocking agents, to stimulation with TRH, and to a combination of L-dopa plus the dopa decarboxylase inhibitor, carbidopa.

In some patients with pituitary tumors and mild hyperprolactinemia (i.e., less than 100 ng per milliliter) the tumor may not secrete prolactin, but rather appears to increase prolactin secretion by interruption of hypothalamic-pituitary portal blood flow.

DIFFERENTIAL DIAGNOSIS. Consideration should be given to an extrapituitary cause for hyperprolactinemia in all patients, since subtle changes on CT or MRI studies may not indicate the presence of a pituitary tumor. This is particularly true in patients with prolactin levels less than 200 ng per milliliter. The differential diagnosis of hyperprolactinemia is given in Table 213–3. If none of the disorders listed is present and there is no history of drug ingestion, the patient with a normal radiographic examination is considered to have idiopathic hyperprolactinemia.

The many similarities between patients with idiopathic hyperprolactinemia and those with small prolactin-secreting pituitary tumors (microadenomas) have led to the belief that these entities represent different stages of the same disorder. Follow-up evaluation of idiopathic hyperprolactinemia suggests that only a small percentage of cases (less than 5 per cent) progress to demonstrable pituitary tumor formation and that among cases of microadenoma the vast majority remain stable for years with respect to both prolactin levels and tumor size.

Some patients with galactorrhea have normal or borderline elevation of prolactin levels, normal dynamic studies of prolactin secretion and ovulatory menses, and normal fertility. These patients represent the most common type of nonpuerperal galactorrhea, termed *normoprolactinemic galactorrhea*, which is attributed to enhanced sensitivity of the breast to prolactin. The disorder often presents as persistence of postpartum galactorrhea or following discontinuation of oral contraceptives.

PATHOGENESIS. As with GH-secreting tumors, a controversy currently exists about whether prolactin-secreting tumors represent a primary pituitary disease or are secondary to altered hypothalamic influence. Using X-chromosome inactivation studies, prolactin-secreting adenomas also appear to be monoclonal, favoring a pituitary etiology. Prolactinomas may also occur in association with other tumors, in particular pancreatic islet tumors and parathyroid tumors/hyperplasia as part of the multiple endocrine neoplasia syndrome (Type I) (Ch. 220).

A hypothalamic etiology (or component) is supported by a large number of pharmacologic studies suggesting impaired CNS dopaminergic tone. However, evidence for prolactin resistance to dopamine has also been demonstrated, although this appears to be unrelated to altered dopamine receptors. Oral contraceptives do not exert a pathogenic role, although the possibility of a role for a yet unidentified prolactin-releasing factor still exists.

THERAPY. The treatment of prolactin-secreting tumors has undergone considerable change in the past decade. Although surgery has been the therapy of choice in the past, many prolactinomas can now be treated as effectively by medical

TABLE 213–3. DIFFERENTIAL DIAGNOSIS OF NONPHYSIOLOGIC HYPERPROLACTINEMIA

A. Pharmacologic Agents
  Monoamine synthesis inhibitors (α-methyldopa)
  Monoamine depletors (reserpine)
  Dopamine receptor antagonists (phenothiazines, butyrophenones, thioxanthines)
  Estrogens (oral contraceptives)
  Narcotics (morphine, heroin)

B. Central Nervous System Disorders
  Inflammatory/infiltrative (sarcoidosis, histiocytosis)
  Traumatic (stalk section)
  Neoplastic (hypothalamic or parasellar tumors)

C. Pituitary Disorders
  Prolactin-secreting tumors
    Macroadenomas
    Microadenomas
  Empty sella syndrome

D. Idiopathic Hyperprolactinemia

E. Other
  Hypothyroidism
  Renal failure
  Cirrhosis
  Granulomatous or lymphocytic hypophysitis
  Chest wall/breast disease or surgery
  Thoracic spinal lesions

(pharmacologic) means. Prolactinomas are divided into three subgroups when therapy is considered:

1. *Macroadenomas with only slightly elevated prolactin levels* (i.e., <100 to 150 ng per milliliter). This tumor (also called a *pseudoprolactinoma*) is composed primarily of nonprolactin-secreting cells and should be managed similarly to the nonfunctioning tumor, i.e., surgical removal of tumor mass with preservation of pituitary function.

2. *Microadenomas.* Primary surgical therapy of microadenomas has resulted in up to 90 per cent "cure" rates as judged by restoration of cyclic menses and fertility. However, growth of microadenomas is infrequently observed (5 to 10 per cent become macroadenomas), and this, plus their presence in one third of unselected autopsies, raises the question of whether their removal is indeed necessary in most patients. Furthermore, long-term follow-up of presumably cured patients indicates recurrence of hyperprolactinemia in up to 25 per cent. The most frequent reason for treatment of microadenomas is infertility. The most rapid and effective means of reducing prolactin levels to normal in such patients is by use of the dopamine agonist bromocriptine, which suppresses prolactin secretion in all forms of hyperprolactinemia by an action directly on the lactotroph. Prolactin levels are decreased by more than 90 per cent, and galactorrhea is improved or eliminated in most patients, even if prolactin levels remain slightly elevated. Similarly, cyclic menses and fertility may return without complete normalization of prolactin levels. The dosage required for most patients is 5 to 7.5 mg per day in divided doses although some may require up to 15 mg per day. Side effects consist primarily of nausea and vomiting due to stimulation of the emesis center, occasionally hypotension due to a CNS-mediated mechanism, and mood changes. The side effects may be minimized by initiating therapy with a small dose and gradually increasing it, although 5 to 10 per cent of patients are unable to tolerate the drug. Even when given throughout pregnancy bromocriptine appears to be safe. It is, in fact, the recommended therapy for women who develop signs and symptoms of a prolactin-secreting tumor during pregnancy. Even when fertility is not of concern, reduction of prolactin levels is warranted to restore normal estrogen levels and possibly to correct osteopenia and prevent subsequent symptomatic osteoporosis. The same rationale is used for treating idiopathic hyperprolactinemia.

3. *Macroadenomas with markedly elevated prolactin levels.* This tumor is composed almost exclusively of lactotrophs. In addition to the above considerations, the tumor size can be markedly decreased by bromocriptine, most dramatically when the tumor is very large. In about two thirds of patients, bromocriptine reduces tumor size by 50 to 75 per cent. The effects are usually quite rapid, occurring within days, but in some patients, tumor shrinkage may require several months. The reduction in size continues for as long as therapy is continued, even for more than a decade. Discontinuation of the drug after 1 year or less of therapy may be associated with rapid regrowth of the tumor, and symptoms may recur within days. However, after several years, drug dosage can be markedly reduced and in occasional patients, discontinued without evidence of tumor regrowth. Bromocriptine is useful in reducing the size of very large tumors prior to surgery, in postoperative treatment of patients in whom only partial tumor removal was accomplished, and in patients who are not candidates for surgery.

Bromocriptine is also effective in males with prolactinomas. Restoration of serum testosterone levels and of libido and potency follows institution of therapy and normalization of prolactin levels.

Another dopamine agonist, pergolide, recently approved for treatment of Parkinson's disease, is also useful as a prolactin-suppressive agent.

Kleinberg DL, Boyd AE, Wardlaw S, et al.: Pergolide for the treatment of pituitary tumors secreting prolactin or growth hormone. N Engl J Med 309:704, 1983. *This agent, a dopamine agonist like bromocriptine, is useful in treatment of both prolactin- and growth hormone–secreting tumors.*

Mehta AE, Reyes FI, Faiman C: Primary radiotherapy of prolactinomas. Am J Med 83:49, 1987. *This modality of therapy is effective. Its onset is slow, however, and the long-term risks of hypopituitarism must be considered.*

Molitch ME: Management of prolactinomas. Annu Rev Med 40:225, 1989. Dalkin AC, Marshall JC: Medical therapy of hyperprolactinemia. Endocrinol Metabol Clin North Am 18:259, 1989. *Two excellent reviews that discuss the role of pharmacotherapy in the treatment of prolactinomas.*

Schlechte J, Dolan K, Sherman B, et al.: The natural history of untreated hyperprolactinemia: A prospective analysis. J Clin Endocrinol Metab 68:412, 1989. *This article shows that untreated hyperprolactinemia is generally a stable and minimally progressive disorder.*

Schlechte J, El-Khoury G, Kathol M, et al.: Forearm and vertebral bone mineral in treated and untreated hyperprolactinemic amenorrhea. J Clin Endocrinol Metab 64:1021, 1987. Klibanski A, Biller BMK, Rosenthal DI, et al.: Effects of prolactin and estrogen deficiency in amenorrheic bone loss. J Clin Endocrinol Metab 67:124, 1988. *Patients with prolactinomas have decreased bone mineral density, although controversy exists as to whether the effects are specific to prolactin and the nature of the long-term risk associated with the finding.*

ACTH-Secreting Tumors: Cushing's Disease

Basophilic adenomas of the pituitary associated with bilateral adrenocortical hyperplasia and the features of hypercortisolism constitute a disorder first described by Cushing. The tumors, which tend to be located in the midline or near the anterior-posterior pituitary junction, are usually benign, but in contrast to other pituitary tumors, often exhibit more aggressive growth behavior, may have true malignant potential, and on rare occasions metastasize within and without the CNS. Corticotroph tumors may first become clinically apparent following bilateral adrenalectomy in patients with Cushing's disease (Nelson's syndrome). They may also be chromophobic and are found in 5 to 7 per cent of pituitaries at autopsy in patients without evidence of ACTH hypersecretion during life. Defects in the hormone secretory process may be responsible for these nonfunctioning tumors.

CLINICAL FEATURES. The clinical features of corticotroph tumors consist of those related to hypercortisolism and those caused by hypersecretion of ACTH and related peptides. The signs and symptoms of hypercortisolism are indistinguishable from those associated with adrenocortical adenomas or exogenous hormone administration and include centripetal obesity, hypertension, diabetes, amenorrhea, hirsutism, acne, osteoporosis and compression fractures, muscle atrophy, violaceous striae, capillary fragility, impaired wound healing, decreased resistance to infection, and behavioral changes. These are discussed in greater detail in Ch. 217. Increased secretion of ACTH and β-LPH produces pigmentation similar to that seen in Addison's disease. In addition to generalized pigmentation, the pressure points (knuckles, elbows, knees, belt or brassiere strap regions), areolae, genitalia, mucous membranes, and recently healed scars are particularly affected. Because ACTH production is only partially autonomous in this disease, hyperpigmentation is mild or moderate in the early stages but may be more pronounced after adrenalectomy or in very large tumors.

LABORATORY STUDIES. Randomly obtained plasma cortisol levels are elevated in only about half of the patients with Cushing's disease. The 24-hour urinary free cortisol is the most reliable screening measurement for distinguishing patients with increased adrenocortical function. Normal values are less than 100 μg per 24 hours. Of the dynamic tests, dexamethasone suppressibility is the most reliable and widely used. In normal subjects, low-dosage dexamethasone (0.5 mg every 6 hours for 2 days) decreases urinary free cortisol to less than 20 μg per 24 hours and plasma cortisol to less than 5 μg per deciliter. Patients with corticotroph tumors exhibit impaired suppression with the low dosage but at least 50 per cent suppression with the high dosage (2.0 mg every 6 hours for 2 days). In some patients, however, larger doses may be required to demonstrate suppression. An overnight dexamethasone suppression test (1 mg orally at 11 P.M. with a plasma cortisol measurement at 8 A.M. the next morning) provides comparable screening sensitivity except in obese subjects, in whom false-positive results are more frequent. Dexamethasone at any dose does not suppress cortisol secretion in patients with adrenal adenomas or ectopic ACTH. These conditions can be distinguished by measurement of plasma ACTH levels, which are absent in the former and very high in the latter. Patients with Cushing's disease exhibit ACTH hyperresponsiveness to CRH; those with adrenal adenomas or ectopic ACTH production do not respond to CRH. CT and MRI of the pituitary demonstrate the adenoma in only 60 to 70 per cent of patients with Cushing's disease. If the tumor location is unclear, petrosal sinus catheterization and sampling for ACTH levels, preferably in combination with CRH administration, often provide definitive information.

DIFFERENTIAL DIAGNOSIS. ACTH-secreting tumors are responsible for approximately 80 per cent of cases of endogenous hypercortisolemia. Adrenal tumors are present in about 15 per cent, and the remainder are caused by ectopic ACTH-secreting or, rarely, by CRH-secreting tumors. The differential diagnosis of these disorders is discussed in greater detail in Ch. 217. Ectopic ACTH production can occur in a variety of tumors, most commonly small cell lung carcinomas, carcinoids, and pancreatic islet tumors (see Ch. 161). The disease can mimic that of corticotroph tumors, although in patients with malignant diseases, weight gain is often absent and severe hypokalemia is a prominent feature. Some of these tumors have been shown to secrete CRH alone or in combination with ACTH, explaining the occasional similarity in responses to dynamic hormone testing to those in patients with corticotroph tumors. Ectopic ACTH secretion should be suspected when the clinical and biochemical features of hypercortisolism occur on a periodic or intermittent basis.

Mild elevations of plasma cortisol, loss of diurnal variation, and absence of dexamethasone suppressibility are seen in patients under stress, during periods of bereavement, and in patients with depressive illness. Biochemically it is frequently impossible to distinguish these patients from those with ACTH-secreting tumors, although the clinical features of hypercortisolism are generally absent.

PATHOGENESIS. Arguments have been made for both a hypothalamic and a pituitary cause of ACTH-secreting tumors. Hypothalamic tumors have been identified in association with Cushing's disease, suggesting tumorous overproduction of CRH. Patients with ACTH-secreting tumors generally respond to CRH, as does tumor tissue tested in vitro. Basophilic hyperplasia, rather than tumor, is occasionally found in patients with Cushing's disease. In addition, cyproheptadine, a serotonin-receptor blocker, suppresses ACTH secretion in some patients with the disorder, providing strong support for a primary CNS role. The major argument for a primary pituitary disorder is based on the successful treatment by transsphenoidal adenomectomy, which includes re-establishment not only of normal quantitative cortisol secretion but of diurnal periodicity and glucocorticoid suppressibility. It is possible that two subgroups of the disease exist that are not readily distinguishable by clinical or laboratory methods currently available. Several lines of evidence suggest the presence of two subgroups, including the ultradian pattern of ACTH and cortisol secretion and the biochemical responses of the tumor in vivo and in vitro. In support of this, X-chromosome inactivation studies reveal about half of ACTH-secreting tumors to be monoclonal and the remainder polyclonal. The latter group could represent responses to increased CRH stimulation. Both groups, however, have a common characteristic: diminished sensitivity to feedback inhibition by cortisol.

THERAPY. Definitive treatment of ACTH-secreting pituitary tumors is indicated as soon as the diagnosis has been established. Once ectopic ACTH or CRF production has been excluded, surgical removal of the pituitary ACTH-secreting tumor is indicated. Tumors may be extremely small and difficult to identify. If the tumor cannot be located or if the patient remains hypercortisolemic following surgery, anterior hypophysectomy or bilateral total adrenalectomy is necessary, the decision being influenced by the patient's age, desire for subsequent pregnancy, and overall general health. Following pituitary adenomectomy, adrenocortical hypofunction requiring glucocorticoid replacement therapy may persist for as long as 2 years. A success rate of up to 85 per cent has been reported in patients with small ACTH-secreting tumors, although in those with large tumors this figure is reduced to about 30 per cent.

Radiation is also effective as primary therapy in ACTH-secreting tumors, although its use is generally limited to patients who are not surgical candidates. Cure rates have been reported of 80 per cent in children and 60 per cent in adults with either conventional radiotherapy or proton beam therapy. Some long-term loss of other pituitary function has been noted after radiotherapy.

Pharmacologic therapy of Cushing's disease is directed at suppression of cortisol biosynthesis by the adrenals, using aminoglutethimide, metyrapone, or mitotane (o,p'-DDD) or ketoconazole; at neurotransmitter metabolism within the CNS; or at the pituitary directly. Detailed discussion of drugs acting on the adrenal is provided in Ch. 217. They have been used, together with radiotherapy, as an alternative to surgical treatment in selected patients. The serotonin-receptor blocker cyproheptadine and the GABA agonist sodium valproate have been successful in a small number of patients with Cushing's disease in restoring both ACTH and cortisol secretion to normal. Responses have also been seen in patients with Nelson's disease. A few patients also exhibit decreases in ACTH secretion during bromocriptine therapy. There is no evidence for regression of tumor size by these agents.

Howlett TA, Plowman PN, Wass JAH, et al.: Megavoltage pituitary irradiation in the management of Cushing's disease and Nelson's syndrome: Long-term follow-up. Clin Endocrinol (Oxf) 31:309, 1989. *The use of radiotherapy alone has proven disappointing in terms of its results, although this form of therapy is of value in patients with inadequate responses to pituitary surgery.*

Loli P, Berselli ME, Tagliaferri M: Use of ketoconazole in the treatment of Cushing's syndrome. J Clin Endocrinol Metab 63:1365, 1986. Schteingart DE: Cushing's syndrome. Endocrinol Metabol Clin North Am 18:311, 1989. *The use of pharmacotherapy is discussed in these articles and is most effective when directed at the inhibition of adrenocortical hormone biosynthesis.*

McCance DR, McIlrath E, McNeill A, et al.: Bilateral inferior petrosal sinus sampling as a routine procedure in ACTH-dependent Cushing's syndrome. Clin Endocrinol (Oxf) 30:157, 1989. *Widespread experience with this procedure has made it useful in confirming the pituitary origin of the disease when radiographic imaging studies are nondiagnostic; it is also frequently of help in lateralizing the tumor.*

Nieman LK, Cutler GB Jr, Oldfield EH, et al.: The ovine corticotropin-releasing hormone (CRH) stimulation test is superior to the human CRH stimulation test for the diagnosis of Cushing's disease. J Clin Endocrinol Metab 69:165, 1989. *This procedure is of greatest help in differentiating a pituitary tumor from ectopic production of ACTH.*

Tindall GT, Herring CJ, Clark RV, et al.: Cushing's disease: Results of transsphenoidal microsurgery with emphasis on surgical failures. J Neurosurg 72:363, 1990. Guilhaume B, Bertagna X, Thomsen M, et al.: Transsphenoidal pituitary surgery for the treatment of Cushing's disease: Results in 64 patients and long term follow-up studies. J Clin Endocrinol Metab 66:1056, 1988. *Two surgical series representative of the overall success that has been achieved in treatment of Cushing's disease by selective pituitary adenomectomy.*

Other Hormone-Secreting Tumors

TSH and gonadotropin secretion by pituitary tumors is extremely rare. TSH-secreting tumors are detected during the workup of hyperthyroid patients with elevated rather than suppressed TSH levels. The clinical manifestations consist of hyperthyroidism and a pituitary tumor mass. Occasionally mixed pituitary cell types are present with coexisting GH or prolactin hypersecretion. TSH secretion is not completely autonomous, since suppression of thyroxine production by methimazole frequently results in an increase of TSH secretion. Treatment must be directed to removal of the tumor mass, although medical therapy to suppress the elevated thyroxine levels is required preoperatively. Octreotide also suppresses TSH secretion in these patients, but no reduction in tumor size has been observed.

FSH- and FSH/LH-secreting pituitary tumors are very rare and often associated with longstanding hypogonadism. Many tumors otherwise considered to be nonfunctioning, however, may secrete the isolated glycoprotein α subunit, which lacks any biologic activity and serves primarily as a tumor marker. Some of these tumors may respond to either bromocriptine or octreotide.

Gesundheit N, Petrick PA, Nissim M, et al.: Thyrotropin-secreting pituitary adenomas: Clinical and biochemical heterogeneity: Case reports and follow-up of nine patients. Ann Intern Med 111:827, 1989. *This article illustrates the range of settings in which TSH-secreting tumors are seen and the long-term history of the tumors.*

Heseltine D, White MC, Kendall-Taylor P, et al.: Testicular enlargement and elevated serum inhibin concentrations occur in patients with pituitary macroadenomas secreting follicle stimulating hormone. Clin Endocrinol (Oxf) 31:411, 1989. Klibanski A, Deutsch PJ, Jameson JL, et al.: Luteinizing hormone–secreting pituitary tumor: Biosynthetic characterization and clinical studies. J Clin Endocrinol Metab 64:536, 1987. *Clinical and biochemical characterizations of gonadotropin-secreting tumors emphasize the effect on reproductive hormone physiology.*

Ishibashi M, Yamaji T, Takaku F, et al.: Secretion of glycoprotein hormone alpha-subunit by pituitary tumors. J Clin Endocrinol Metab 64:1187, 1987. Demura R, Jibiki K, Kubo O, et al.: The significance of α-subunit as a tumor marker for gonadotropin-producing pituitary adenomas. J Clin Endocrinol Metab 63:564, 1986. *Glycoprotein α-subunit may be secreted independently of glycoprotein hormones by tumors. Although the monomeric subunit is bioinactive, it defines the tumor cell type as of thyrotroph/gonadotroph origin.*

214 The Posterior Pituitary

Thomas E. Andreoli

ANTIDIURETIC HORMONE

The neurohypophysis of humans elaborates two hormones: *arginine vasopressin* (AVP), which exhibits vasopressor and antidiuretic activity, and *oxytocin*, which is galactobolic and uterotonic. Both hormones are octapeptides of approximately 1100 daltons, with a 20-member ring structure created by disulfide bonds. The antidiuretic and vasopressor activities of AVP are each approximately 100 times as great as those of oxytocin, a difference that is related to the different tertiary conformations of the two peptides.

The posterior pituitary gland contains terminal axons whose cell bodies lie in hypothalamic cell clusters known as the *supraoptic* and *paraventricular nuclei.* Synthesis of posterior pituitary hormones occurs in these hypothalamic nuclei rather than in the posterior pituitary gland: (1) AVP can be demonstrated immunochemically in cells of both the supraoptic and the paraventricular nuclei; and (2) neurosecretory granules accumulate only on the hypothalamic side of a sectioned hypophyseal stalk.

The cardinal steps in the biosynthesis of antidiuretic hormone (ADH) are illustrated in Figure 214–1. Neurohypophyseal hormones, including vasopressin, are synthesized as prohormones in conjunction with specific carrier proteins called neurophysins. Vasopressin, specifically, is synthesized as a prohormone in conjunction with neurophysin II, and the complex is sometimes termed the van Dyke protein. Both vasopressin and neurophysin II come from a common precursor gene, located on human chromosome 20 (Fig. 214–2). The hormone precursor contains three peptide regions: a signal peptide and ADH at the N-terminal, a neurophysin II region, and a C-terminal glycoprotein region of unknown significance. Each region of the precursor protein is, in turn, coded for by one of three different exons on the vasopressin precursor gene. Thus, the main steps in the biosynthesis of ADH are transcription of the vasopressin precursor mRNA; translation of the mRNA to a pre-prohormone; and removal of the signal peptide sequence while the peptide is still attached to the ribosome, yielding the prohormone. The prohormone peptide is transported in neurosecretory granules to the posterior pituitary gland. During transport, the prohormone peptide is cleaved to neurophysin II and ADH. In the posterior pituitary gland, the neurosecretory granules rest in terminal projections of axonal plasma membranes, juxtaposed to systemic circulation capillaries. Other pituicyte nerve fibers terminate in the median eminence and along the third ventricle, thus allowing access of vasopressin to cerebrospinal fluid.

There are two pools of AVP-containing neurosecretory granules in pituicytes: one adjacent to the cell membrane and therefore available for immediate release, and a second storage pool removed from immediate contact with the plasma membrane.

Release of hormone occurs by an exocytotic process involving fusion of neurosecretory granules with pituicyte plasma membranes. In other words, AVP release is quantal. A stimulus to the hypothalamic pituicyte cell body is transmitted to the site of granule storage, where it causes cell membrane depolarization, an associated increase in calcium permeability, and rapid calcium entry into the pituicytes. This influx of calcium activates the exocytosis of AVP-containing neurosecretory granules.

RELEVANT PHYSIOLOGY. Detailed accounts of the renal and pituitary processes resulting in the formation of dilute or concentrated urine are presented in Ch. 73 and 75. ADH exerts major physiologic effects on discrete regions of the nephron and also affects vascular smooth muscle tone. There are two distinct receptors for these ADH effects. Those in smooth muscle, also found on hepatocytes, are denoted V_1 receptors. Those within epithelia, for example, collecting ducts, are designated V_2 receptors. The V_2 receptors have a greater affinity for ADH than do V_1 receptors.

In all epithelia that respond to ADH, the hormone binds to V_2 receptors on the basolateral plasma membrane of the cell and, in so doing, activates the enzyme adenylate cyclase. Adenylate cyclase increases the production of $3',5'$-cyclic adenosine monophosphate (cAMP) from its substrate adenosine triphosphate (ATP). Cyclic AMP then acts as a second messenger to activate a cell-specific protein kinase, protein kinase A, which induces the final cellular response to the hormone (see Ch. 208). ADH-stimulated adenylate cyclase is present in the collecting duct and in the medullary, but not cortical, thick ascending limb of Henle (mTALH) of mammalian kidneys.

The *cardinal* physiologic effect of ADH is to promote the formation of hypertonic urine, which depends particularly on two sets of events operating in parallel within the renal medulla. First, in the thick ascending limb of Henle, approximately 15 to 20 per cent of the filtered load of sodium chloride is absorbed. Since the mTALH is water impermeable, this process contributes simultaneously to the maintenance of a hypertonic medullary interstitium and to the formation of dilute urine. Under normal circumstances, the osmolality of the renal medullary interstitium rises from isotonic, at the corticomedullary junction, to very hypertonic, approximately 1200 mOsm per kilogram of H_2O, at the papillary tip. Since the enrichment of medullary interstitial osmolality and dilution of tubular fluid both depend on sodium chloride absorption by the water-impermeable mTALH, the latter region of the nephron is commonly termed the medullary diluting segment. Approximately 10 per cent of fluid filtered at the glomerulus, or about 18 liters daily, reaches the early distal tubule with an osmolality of approximately 50 mOsm per kilogram of H_2O.

When ADH is absent, the water permeability of collecting ducts is at a minimum. Thus there is reduced osmotic equilibration of fluid passing through collecting ducts with the medullary interstitium, and most of the fluid escapes unchanged as hypotonic urine. Since only 10 per cent of filtered water normally

FIGURE 214–1. Flow diagram for the pathway of posterior pituitary hormone biosynthesis. (From Reeves WB, Andreoli TE: The posterior pituitary and water metabolism. *In* Foster DW, Wilson JD [eds.]: Williams Textbook of Endocrinology, 8th ed. Philadelphia, W.B. Saunders Company, 1991.)

Form	Molecular Weight	Synthetic Step
Preprohormone	$\simeq 21,000$	Protein synthesis; magnocellular neuron ribosomes
Prohormone	$\simeq 23,000$	Glycosylation and membrane packaging; magnocellular neuron; Golgi apparatus
Neurosecretory Granule (NSG)	$(23,000)_n$	Transport down supraopticohyophyseal tract as osmotically inactive granules
Neurophysin + Hormone	$\simeq 10,000$ $\simeq 1,100$	Storage in posterior pituitary; cleavage within NSG

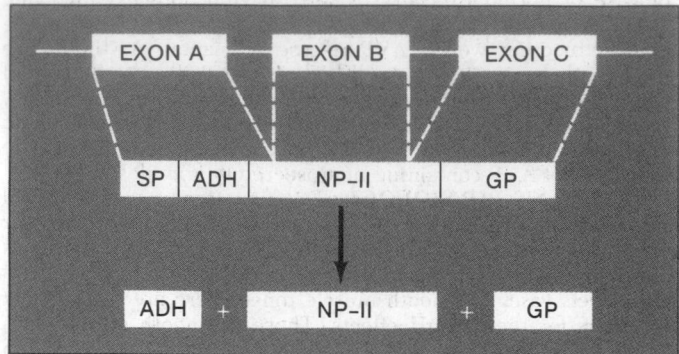

FIGURE 214–2. A schematic representation of the organization of the ADH gene and its relation to the pre-prohormone and final peptide products. SP= Signal peptide; NP-II= neurophysin II; GP= glycoprotein.

reaches the collecting duct system, the maximal degree of polyuria in a patient with complete pituitary diabetes insipidus (or complete nephrogenic diabetes insipidus) is therefore approximately 18 liters daily. During normal antidiuresis, ADH, by way of cAMP, increases the water permeability of luminal (urinary) cell membranes of cortical and outer medullary collecting ducts. Thus in the presence of ADH, there is osmotic equilibration of hypotonic luminal fluid in collecting ducts with the hypertonic medullary interstitium and, consequently, water absorption, a reduction in urine volume, concentration of urine, and conservation of body water.

The ADH-dependent increase in the water permeability of collecting ducts is due to a hormone-dependent increase in the number of water-specific channels available for water transport through luminal membranes. These channels are rather narrow, approximately 2 Å in radius, and therefore exclude urea and NaCl. As a consequence, the luminal fluid concentrations of these two solutes increase when water is abstracted from cortical and outer medullary collecting ducts during antidiuresis. In turn, the increase in luminal urea concentration creates a favorable gradient for passive urea diffusion out of inner medullary (papillary) collecting ducts into the interstitium, thereby maintaining interstitial hypertonicity. ADH also causes a slight increase in papillary duct urea permeability, thus favoring passive movement of urea down its concentration gradient for recirculation through the medullary interstitium.

A *second ADH-mediated* event in the antidiuretic response is to increase the rate of NaCl transport in medullary, but not cortical, mTALH. This process involves a furosemide-sensitive electroneutral cotransport of $Na^+:K^+:2Cl^-$ from luminal fluid into cells; virtually all of the potassium entering cells through this process is recycled back into luminal fluid via potassium-specific channels in luminal membranes. Consequently, ADH increases urinary concentrating power in two ways: by enhancing the water permeability of collecting ducts and by increasing the net rate of salt absorption by the mTALH, thus enriching medullary interstitial osmolality.

This latter effect of ADH on medullary diluting segments is opposed by at least three other factors. (1) As interstitial NaCl concentrations increase, the backleak of NaCl into the tubular lumen of the mTALH also increases and thereby tends to reduce net NaCl absorption by the mTALH. (2) Increases in interstitial osmolality down-regulate the ADH stimulation of NaCl cotransport. (3) Prostaglandins of the E series, which are produced in the renal medullary interstitium in response to increasing interstitial osmolality, inhibit competitively the ADH-mediated increases in the rate of intracellular cAMP formation.

These three processes have a negative feedback on ADH enhancement of active NaCl absorption in the mTALH, so that the diluting power of the mTALH remains constant during either antidiuresis or water diuresis.

Finally, prostaglandins of the E series also antagonize the ADH-dependent enhancement of collecting-duct water permeability. This effect may be produced either by prostaglandins

synthesized endogenously by collecting-duct cells or by prostaglandins synthesized within the medullary interstitium. Thus prostaglandins blunt urinary concentrating power by offsetting ADH effects in at least two loci, the mTALH and the collecting duct.

At levels of hormone that exceed those necessary for antidiuresis, ADH also has pressor activity (this was the first known effect of posterior pituitary extract and provided the basis for the name vasopressin) that is the result of a direct constricting effect on vascular smooth muscle via the V_1 receptors described above. At all but high pharmacologic doses, this pressor effect is easily overcome by compensatory vasodilatory reflexes, so that hypertension is not routinely seen during AVP replacement therapy. Lesser doses may, however, cause significant vasoconstriction of coronary arteries. Another effect of vasopressin, seen at levels that supersede those necessary for antidiuresis, is stimulation of intestinal motility. Finally, AVP released into the CSF and thalamic centers may play a role in such diverse processes as memory and regulation of corticotropin release.

OSMOTIC REGULATION OF ADH RELEASE. Verney's elegant studies demonstrated a strong antidiuretic response to perfusion of carotid vessels with hypertonic solutions of various solutes, including sodium salts and glucose; hypertonic urea solutions elicited no such response. Therefore he concluded that specific cells that acted as osmoreceptors were present within the distribution of the carotid circulation and that the plasma membranes of these cells were impermeable to sodium salts and glucose but permeable to urea. In the presence of extracellular hyperosmolality induced by impermeable species, these osmosensing cells reached osmotic equilibrium by losing water to the hypertonic plasma. In other words, Verney deduced that osmoreceptor shrinkage, produced by raising plasma osmolality with solutes restricted to the extracellular compartment, was the stimulus for ADH release.

When the anterior wall of the third ventricle is exposed to hypertonic saline, neurons in both the anterior hypothalamus and the preoptic area have increased rates of depolarization. Concomitantly, about half of the pituicytes in hypothalamic nuclei show a characteristic depolarization pattern, and plasma antidiuretic activity increases. Therefore it is probable that the neurons in the anterior hypothalamus and preoptic areas, which depolarize in response to hypertonic saline, represent Verney's osmoreceptors.

In normal man, plasma AVP levels are undetectable below a plasma osmolality of 280 mOsm per kilogram of H_2O. Since the usual plasma osmolality in man is approximately 287 mOsm per kilogram of H_2O, secretion of AVP is tonic; the average circulating hormone levels are between 2.0 and 2.5 pg per milliliter. Vasopressin levels increase in a linear fashion with increasing plasma osmolality, such that a rise in plasma osmolality of only 1 per cent (2.9 mOsm per kilogram of H_2O) evokes a 1 pg per milliliter rise in AVP. Parallel examinations of plasma AVP and urine osmolality indicate that each unit increase in AVP allows an increase of 250 mOsm per kilogram of H_2O in urinary concentration. Since the maximal concentrating ability of the human kidney is approximately 1200 mOsm per kilogram of H_2O, maximal water conservation is therefore achieved at a plasma AVP level of 5.0 pg per milliliter.

Combining these relations yields a measure of the efficiency of the water homeostatic mechanism: for each 1 mOsm per kilogram of H_2O change in plasma osmolality there is a change in urinary concentration of 95 mOsm per kilogram of H_2O, which represents a gain of almost 100-fold. The ingestion of water sufficient to decrease plasma osmolality by only 1 mOsm per kilogram of H_2O reduces urinary concentration by 95 mOsm per kilogram of H_2O, thus allowing the water to be excreted and osmotic balance to be restored. The opposite effect, water loss, results in stimulation of ADH release, increase in urinary concentration, and conservation of body water by the same magnification phenomenon.

NONOSMOTIC REGULATION OF ADH RELEASE. Isotonic or hypotonic volume depletion results in an antidiuretic state. Evidence now exists for stretch receptors, or baroreceptors, that sense changes in vascular wall tension in both the venous (low pressure) and arterial (high pressure) circulations. Immersion and negative pressure breathing, i.e., maneuvers that augment intrathoracic blood volume, as well as balloon distension of the left atrium, all produce water diuresis that can be overcome by

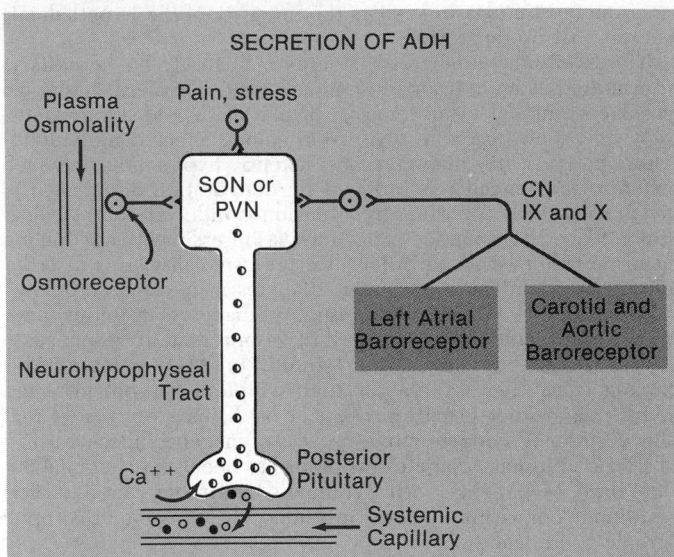

FIGURE 214–3. Secretory stimuli for calcium-dependent ADH release: van Dyke protein (◐), vasopressin (●), neurophysin II (○). SON = Supraoptic neuron, PVN = paraventricular neuron.

TABLE 214–1. CONDITIONS THAT ALTER ANTIDIURETIC HORMONE ACTIVITY

Enhance	Suppress
Drugs and Conditions That Modify Release of ADH	
Surgical stress	Phenytoin
Vincristine	Alcohol
Cyclophosphamide	Narcotic antagonists
Clofibrate	α-Adrenergic agents
Carbamazepine	
Barbiturates	
Morphine and narcotic analogues	
Nicotine	
β-Adrenergic agents	
Hypoxia	
Hypercapnia	
Drugs That Modify the ADH Effect on Collecting Ducts	
Chlorpropamide	Lithium
Biguanides	Methoxyflurane
Indomethacin	Demeclocycline

administering ADH. Conversely, positive pressure breathing and upright posture, which reduce intrathoracic blood volume, or left atrial collapse, produce antidiuresis. These observations indicate that the left atrium and the pulmonary vasculature are the major loci for low pressure baroreceptors that modulate ADH release.

Hypotension, or selective clamping of major systemic arterial vessels, also produces profound antidiuresis. These data indicate the presence of a baroreceptor system in the arterial circulation, localized to the carotid bifurcations and aortic arch, that also modulates ADH release. This type of nonosmotic ADH release is modulated by stimulatory or inhibitory signals arriving from the baroreceptors via parasympathetic pathways in the vagus and glossopharyngeal nerves. The low pressure baroreceptors are more sensitive regulators of ADH release than those in high pressure regions of the circulation. These relations are summarized in Figure 214–3.

Circulating levels of ADH rise with vascular volume depletion. However, volume-mediated, nonosmotic ADH release has a "threshold" requiring more than 7 per cent blood volume depletion, with greater degrees of blood volume contraction eliciting exponential rises in circulating ADH levels. Thus nonosmotic ADH release differs strikingly from osmotically mediated ADH release, which occurs with only a 1 to 2 per cent increase in plasma osmolality and rises linearly with further increases in plasma osmolality. With less than a 7 per cent decrease in blood volume, ADH release is governed wholly by plasma osmolality. At greater reductions in blood volume, ADH release is increasingly dominated by nonosmotic, volume-dependent stimuli. This observation explains the finding of progressive fluid dilution in patients with hypovolemia or states of decreased cardiac output.

Finally, the vasoconstrictor peptide endothelin-1 is also released from the posterior pituitary following water depletion. Since administered endothelin-1 increases plasma ADH levels, endothelin-1 may also play a role in ADH release.

Input from higher cortical functions also appears to influence ADH release. Pain, emotion, stress, and some psychotic states are associated with ADH stimulation or inhibition. Most common is the transient antidiuresis that occurs postoperatively.

PATHOLOGIC ALTERATION OF ADH RELEASE. A wide variety of agents and conditions are known to affect ADH activity (Table 214–1). Nicotine, as a stimulant of ADH release, and acute alcohol ingestion, as an inhibitor of ADH release, have figured prominently in devising means to assess neurohypophyseal integrity. Stimulatory drugs such as clofibrate and chlorpropamide have been utilized to treat states of partial ADH insufficiency. Other drugs, such as lithium and demeclocycline, are prominent for their effect on the renal collecting duct, making it unresponsive to ADH and thereby producing nephrogenic diabetes insipidus.

The syndrome of inappropriate antidiuretic hormone secretion (SIADH) is characterized by persistent hyponatremia, an inappropriately elevated urine osmolality, and no discernible stimulus for ADH release. A common cause for this condition is neoplastic, most notably oat cell carcinoma of lung; SIADH is due to ectopic production of ADH by the tumor, with persistent release of hormone independent of regulatory influences. Inflammatory disorders of the lung, such as pneumonia or cavitary tuberculosis, provide other sites for ectopic ADH production. The syndrome also occurs in patients with head trauma or with other diseases of the central nervous system and often terminates with recovery of neurologic function. The SIADH syndrome is discussed in detail in Ch. 75.

THIRST REGULATION. Body water content is governed not only by ADH modulation of renal water excretion but also by regulation of water intake through thirst. Both systems operate in parallel under the influence of osmotic and volume mediators. Thirst also requires an intact cerebral cortex, which transforms the urge to drink into appropriate behavior to secure water.

Hyperosmolality, and presumably shrinkage of thirst receptors, is the primary stimulus for thirst and requires only a 2 per cent rise in plasma osmolality. The thirst "threshold" in conscious humans is about 294 mOsm per kilogram, the same osmolality at which maximal urinary concentration under ADH is achieved. Hypovolemia also stimulates thirst via an angiotensin II–mediated mechanism. Indeed, hyperreninemic states such as malignant hypertension are often accompanied by pathologic thirst. Phenothiazines enhance thirst and contribute to the hyponatremia seen in some patients treated with these drugs for affective disorders. Finally, prostaglandin E also stimulates thirst. The polydipsia that accompanies hypokalemia probably depends on increased production of prostaglandin E.

WATER REPLETION REACTION. The positive limb of the water repletion reaction has two cardinal features—redundancy and variable gain. Thus two sets of stimuli—osmotic and nonosmotic—stimulate both thirst and antidiuresis. The osmotic stimuli represent, especially for antidiuresis, the system that is activated by 2 per cent changes in effective plasma osmolality and has a linear gain. In contrast, nonosmotic stimuli enhance thirst and antidiuresis only in response to rather large (that is, more than 7 per cent) reductions in effective circulatory volume. Moreover, particularly with respect to antidiuresis, greater degrees of volume contraction provide exponential rather than linear increases in concentrating power.

SUPPRESSION OF WATER REPLETION. At least two separate factors suppress both ADH release and thirst. First, water ingestion, via the *oropharyngeal reflex*, promptly suppresses ADH release, even prior to absorption of the ingested water. Passage of water through the pharynx also suppresses thirst, even when an esophageal fistula prevents net water absorption. These anticipatory responses for both thirst and ADH secretion are accompanied by reduced electrical activity in the hypothalamus and probably involve a neural mechanism.

Second, atrial natriuretic peptide, or atriopeptin, may have a central role in the negative feedback limb of the water repletion reaction. The factors responsible for the biosynthesis and release of atriopeptin are described in detail in Ch. 211. Stated briefly, atriopeptin is released from atrial granules in response to increases in effective circulating volume. Moreover, immunoreactive atriopeptin is produced in the anterolateral periventricular areas of the hypothalamus. In the present context, two actions of either circulating or centrally released atriopeptin have particular relevance: blunting of ADH release in response to osmotic or nonosmotic stimuli and suppression of angiotensin-mediated thirst. These effects suggest a central role for atriopeptin in negative feedback regulation of the water repletion reaction.

Reeves WB, Andreoli TE: The posterior pituitary and water metabolism. *In* Foster DW, Wilson JD: Williams Textbook of Endocrinology, 8th ed. Philadelphia, W. B. Saunders Company, 1990. *A complete analysis of the physiology of the water repletion reaction.*
Schmale H, Fehr S, Richter D: Vasopressin biosynthesis—from gene to peptide hormone. Kidney Int 32:S8, 1987. *A summary of vasopressin biosynthesis.*
Thrasher TN, Keil LC, Ramsay DJ: Drinking, oropharyngeal signals, and inhibition of vasopressin secretion in dogs. Am J Physiol 253:R509, 1987. *The role of the oropharyngeal reflex in modulating thirst and ADH release.*

DIABETES INSIPIDUS

Pituitary Diabetes Insipidus

DEFINITION. Pituitary diabetes insipidus is a polyuric syndrome that results from a lack of sufficient ADH to effect appropriate concentration of the urine or water conservation. The disease is identified by the persistence of an inappropriately dilute urine in the presence of strong osmotic or nonosmotic stimuli to ADH secretion, and in the absence of renal concentrating defects, and a rise in urine osmolality upon the administration of vasopressin. Pituitary diabetes insipidus may result either from destruction of the centers of ADH synthesis or from failure of the mechanisms effecting ADH release.

ETIOLOGY. Trauma to the neurohypophysis, either accidental or as a result of hypophysectomy, is the major identifiable cause of diabetes insipidus. A second major cause for pituitary diabetes insipidus is an intracranial tumor, which may be primary, as in craniopharyngioma, or metastatic, among which breast carcinoma is the most likely cause. Less frequent causes of pituitary diabetes insipidus are granulomatous lesions of the central nervous system, including tuberculosis and sarcoidosis, the histiocytoses, encephalomeningitis, or vascular lesions. There is a rare familial form of pituitary diabetes insipidus which affects either sex, occurs at any age, and is associated with extensive gliosis of neurohypophyseal nuclei. Finally, 30 to 40 per cent of all patients with pituitary diabetes insipidus have no identifiable cause for the disorder.

PATHOGENESIS. Pituitary diabetes insipidus depends on one of at least four different pathogenic mechanisms. Most commonly the disorder occurs when there is atrophy or destruction of the hypothalamic centers responsible for hormone production. In experimental circumstances, preservation of as few as 15 per cent of magnocellular neurons prevents polyuria, whereas evident diabetes insipidus occurs when only 6 to 8 per cent of neurons remain. Neither removal of the posterior pituitary gland alone nor low section of the neurohypophyseal tract with preservation of hypothalamic nuclei is sufficient to produce a permanent polyuric state. Rather, direct trauma to the pituitary gland or low section of the neurohypophyseal tract results in transient diabetes insipidus; for example, the polyuric state following low stalk section lasts for only 1 to 2 weeks postsurgery. Since the anterior and posterior lobes of the pituitary gland have totally separate blood supplies, infarction of the anterior pituitary gland does not disrupt posterior pituitary function.

A second group of cases has been identified, often classed under the heading essential hypernatremia, in which osmotic stimuli fail to elicit ADH release, while nonosmotic stimuli result in antidiuresis. Although euvolemic, these patients are polyuric and excrete hypotonic urine, and water deprivation alone fails to elicit an antidiuretic response. However, when volume contraction occurs in these patients, significant antidiuresis ensues. Thus, in this disorder there is selective failure of osmoreceptors to stimulate ADH release. The intact response of ADH release to nonosmotic stimulation verifies the integrity of the hypothalamic centers that produce ADH.

Third, pituitary diabetes insipidus may rarely be hereditary, transmitted as an autosomal dominant trait. This form has equal occurrence in males and females, displays father-to-son transmission, and shows variable expression among affected individuals. These patients may maintain a persistently hypotonic urine even when hyperosmolality is induced by dehydration or infusion of hypertonic saline, or when hypotension is induced pharmacologically. Since all respond to exogenous vasopressin with a reduction in urine volume and elevation of urine osmolality, this disorder differs from familial nephrogenic diabetes insipidus (see below). Some patients with familial pituitary diabetes insipidus have shown detectable levels of plasma vasopressin in response to strong osmotic or nonosmotic stimuli to ADH release. This finding, plus the observation that symptoms of polyuria and polydipsia are not usually present at birth, have suggested that this disorder is a degenerative process of magnocellular neurons.

Finally, pituitary diabetes insipidus has been reported in about one third of patients with Wolfram's syndrome, an inherited condition comprising diabetes insipidus, diabetes mellitus, optic atrophy, and deafness.

Nephrogenic Diabetes Insipidus

DEFINITION. The term *nephrogenic diabetes insipidus* should be applied to disorders in which renal tubular unresponsiveness to ADH, without disturbances either in solute delivery to the loop of Henle or in countercurrent multiplication or exchange processes, is responsible for polyuria and hyposthenuria. Thus nephrogenic diabetes insipidus may be due to inability of ADH to raise cellular cAMP concentrations, to inability of cAMP to increase the water permeability of luminal membranes of collecting ducts, or to a combination of these two disorders.

FAMILIAL NEPHROGENIC DIABETES INSIPIDUS. This familial disorder occurs primarily in males and exhibits a hereditary pattern of X-linked transmission with variable penetrance in females. In normal individuals or patients with pituitary diabetes insipidus, exogenous ADH can increase the rate of urinary cAMP excretion. In the majority of patients with familial nephrogenic diabetes insipidus, comparable doses of ADH do not increase rates of urinary cAMP excretion. However, in two groups of children with nephrogenic diabetes insipidus, both basal and ADH-stimulated rates of urinary cAMP excretion exceeded those of normal children. These disparate results led to the postulate that familial nephrogenic diabetes insipidus is a heterogeneous disorder produced by either a defect in hormone receptor adenylate cyclase stimulation or a defect beyond the generation of cAMP.

The lack of response to ADH in familial nephrogenic diabetes insipidus is restricted to those responses mediated by the V_2 receptor, since V_1 receptor–mediated effects such as vasoconstriction are normal. The V_2 receptor defect appears to be generalized. For example, extrarenal effects mediated by V_2 receptors include an increase in von Willebrand factor and Factor VIII, a fall in diastolic blood pressure, and stimulation of renin release. In most patients with familial nephrogenic DI, these extrarenal V_2-mediated responses are absent, indicating a generalized defect in the V_2 receptor signal transduction pathway.

ACQUIRED NEPHROGENIC DIABETES INSIPIDUS. Vasopressin-resistant hyposthenuria associated with otherwise normal or nearly normal renal function may occur as a complication of drug therapy or in association with systemic diseases. This acquired nephrogenic diabetes insipidus is to be distinguished from the rare familial disorder described earlier.

Vasopressin-unresponsive hyposthenuria occurs in patients receiving demeclocycline; both the concentrating defect and vasopressin-unresponsiveness are reversible and disappear shortly after discontinuance of antibiotic therapy. The glomerular filtration rate in these patients is generally normal, as is the ability for maximal urinary dilution (positive free water formation), indicating that solute abstraction from the loop of Henle is probably unimpaired.

In human renal medulla, demeclocycline noncompetitively inhibits basal adenylate cyclase activity, ADH-stimulated adenylate cyclase activity, and cAMP-dependent protein kinase activity, but does not affect nucleotide phosphodiesterase activity. These data suggest that demeclocycline may inhibit both cAMP accumulation and cAMP effects on renal tubular membranes.

Nephrogenic diabetes insipidus may also be produced by volatile fluorocarbon anesthetics. Methoxyflurane anesthesia is complicated by a full spectrum of renal injury, ranging from vasopressin-resistant polyuria and hyposthenuria to acute tubular necrosis. Both fluoride and oxalic acid, which are metabolic products of methoxyflurane, contribute to the nephrotoxicity of the anesthetic. However, the polyuric state is related to the markedly increased serum concentration and urinary excretion of inorganic fluoride. Sodium fluoride causes vasopressin-resistant polyuria in dogs, and in rats inorganic fluoride seems to reduce collecting duct water permeability without affecting salt transport in the ascending limb.

Serum lithium concentrations of 0.5 to 1.5 mEq per liter, which are generally regarded as being in the therapeutic range for affective disorders, produce vasopressin-resistant diabetes insipidus. Nephrogenic diabetes insipidus has been observed in 12 to 30 per cent of patients receiving lithium therapy; the defect is usually reversible, and urinary concentrating ability returns toward normal when lithium is discontinued. This defect may be due to a lithium-dependent inhibition of ADH-stimulated cAMP accumulation in collecting ducts. Finally nephrogenic diabetes insipidus characterized by persistent, vasopressin-resistant hyposthenuria and polyuria occurs rarely in certain systemic diseases, including most notably sarcoidosis and Sjögren's syndrome.

ACQUIRED POLYURIC STATES. Other disorders may present with polyuria and relative vasopressin resistance, although not necessarily with profound hyposthenuria. Rather, these polyuric disturbances are generally characterized by inability to concentrate urine maximally in response to vasopressin, either stimulated endogenously or administered exogenously; random urine samples are ordinarily not profoundly hypotonic but are usually only slightly hypotonic or modestly hypertonic.

In general, such polyuric disorders occur most commonly in association with hypokalemic nephropathy (Ch. 75) or hypercalcemic nephropathy (Ch. 235), or as a consequence of diseases that disrupt medullary architecture and consequently impair the generation and maintenance of a hypertonic medullary interstitium. The latter disorders include those diseases that affect particularly the renal interstitium, such as sickle cell disease, pyelonephritis, analgesic nephropathy, and multiple myeloma. These diseases are considered in Ch. 80.

Finally, states characterized by osmotic, or solute, diuresis, for example, in diabetic ketoacidosis and hyperglycemic nonketotic states, may result in polyuria with isotonic urine formation and unresponsiveness to vasopressin. In these disorders, the fraction of isotonic glomerular filtrate delivered to the loop of Henle is greatly increased because of failure to absorb solute, for example, glucose, in the proximal nephron. Thus the amount of solute and water reaching the loop of Henle becomes large with regard to the diluting or concentrating ability of the loop of Henle and collecting ducts, respectively, and vasopressin-resistant polyuria and isosthenuria ensue. Consequently the polyuric state in osmotic diuresis differs from that in nephrogenic diabetes insipidus in two respects; urinary solute excretion is dramatically increased in osmotic diuresis but not in nephrogenic diabetes insipidus; and the urine osmolality is nearly isotonic in solute diuresis but rather hypotonic in nephrogenic diabetes insipidus.

Pituitary or Nephrogenic Diabetes Insipidus

CLINICAL MANIFESTATIONS. The foremost clinical feature of either pituitary or nephrogenic diabetes insipidus is *polyuria*, with urine volumes ranging from 3 to 15 liters per day. Along with polyuria there is near-continuous thirst, often with a preference for ice cold water. The disease is almost always accompanied by *nocturia*, in contrast to persons with primary polydipsia (compulsive water drinking), in whom nocturia is usually absent. The onset of polyuria in pituitary diabetes insipidus is most often abrupt, with peak urine flow reached in 1 or 2 days. Therefore, polyuria developing over weeks or months suggests a disease other than pituitary diabetes insipidus. The polyuria of familial nephrogenic diabetes insipidus is present from birth.

The polyuria in complete diabetes insipidus, either pituitary or nephrogenic, has an upper limit of approximately 18 liters

daily, or about 10 per cent of filtered water, since 90 per cent of the glomerular filtrate is normally absorbed by the nephron prior to reaching the collecting system. In partial pituitary diabetes insipidus, the daily urine volume may be considerably smaller. In contrast, persons afflicted with compulsive water drinking, often referred to as primary or psychogenic polydipsia, not infrequently ingest more than 20 liters of fluid daily. Therefore, the daily urine volume in these patients may also exceed 20 liters.

Modest degrees of volume depletion may curtail polyuria, even in complete diabetes insipidus, for two reasons. First, volume contraction increases the fraction of glomerular filtrate absorbed by the proximal nephron, so that a smaller volume of hypotonic fluid reaches the collecting duct system. Second, even in the absence of ADH, or when collecting ducts are unresponsive to ADH, collecting ducts have a slight permeability to water; consequently, a small fraction of the water reaching the collecting duct system can be absorbed even without ADH. Since the volume of glomerular filtrate reaching the collecting duct system is reduced during volume contraction, the further absorption of relatively small volumes of water by collecting ducts during the volume-contracted state can result in dramatic reductions in polyuria.

Aside from the discomfort and inconvenience of polyuria and polydipsia, patients with pituitary or nephrogenic diabetes insipidus suffer no ill effects unless they are *deprived of access to water*. When this happens, *circulatory collapse* or *hypertonic encephalopathy* may occur. Because of the high rates of urine flow in some patients with diabetes insipidus, these complications may develop in a period of hours. For example, a patient with pituitary diabetes insipidus might excrete 5 per cent of his glomerular filtrate daily, or about 9 liters of urine. In a 70-kg man having 42 kg of body water, this loss, if not continually replenished, would result in a 20 per cent reduction in body water in only 24 hours.

Hypertonic Encephalopathy. Acute increases in intracellular fluid osmolality to levels exceeding 350 mOsm per kilogram of H_2O produced by solutes such as NaCl or glucose (in diabetes), which cross cell membranes poorly, result in central nervous system dysfunction ranging from lethargy to frank coma. Since comparable elevations of plasma osmolality produced by urea, which permeates cell membranes freely, do not produce the disorder, it is evident that hyperosmolality per se is not the basis for the disturbance. Rather, acute hypertonic encephalopathy occurs because cell membranes, being freely permeable to water, are in virtually constant osmotic equilibrium with extracellular fluid. When hypernatremia develops acutely, cellular water loss produces brain shrinkage, and the increase in brain solute content is accounted for entirely by a rise in intracellular Na^+, K^+, and Cl^- concentrations.

In children who develop acute hypernatremia and attain a serum sodium concentration above 160 mEq per liter in 24 hours, the mortality exceeds 40 per cent; about two thirds of the survivors have permanent neurologic sequelae. At autopsy, cerebral vessels are markedly congested and engorged, hemorrhages are evident both in subcortical brain parenchyma and subarachnoid spaces, and venous thrombosis occurs.

When hypernatremia develops gradually, the incidence of hypertonic encephalopathy is greatly reduced, both in man and in experimental animals. This occurs because brain cells adapt to gradually developing hypernatremia by accumulating solutes intracellularly. The sum of brain Na^+, K^+, and Cl^- accounts for approximately 40 to 50 per cent of intracellular solutes; the remaining solutes include amino acids, myoinositol, betaine, and urea. Thus in chronic hypernatremia, the accumulation of idiogenic osmoles in the brain minimizes the extent of water loss and consequently brain shrinkage. This in turn reduces the frequency with which encephalopathy develops.

Posthypophysectomy Course. The acute diabetes insipidus following hypophysectomy has a characteristic triphasic response. For a few hours to days following the insult, there exists a polyuric, hyposthenuric phase that depends on inhibition of ADH release. Next, there follows a period with reduced urine volume and a rise in urine osmolality. During this phase, there is persistent release of ADH from atrophying neurons, an inability to excrete a water load, and the risk of progressive hypotonicity with continued parenteral administration of large volumes of hypotonic fluids. The final phase, if the diabetes insipidus becomes permanent, is marked by recurrence of polyuria and hyposthenuria.

LABORATORY MANIFESTATIONS. Persistent hyposthenuria, with urine specific gravity of 1.005 or less and urine osmolality less than 200 mOsm per kilogram of H_2O, is the hallmark of the diabetes insipidus syndromes. In euvolemic patients, the glomerular filtration rate (GFR) is normal. Since patients with diabetes insipidus ingest water in response to plasma hypertonicity, random plasma osmolality determinations in these patients will be, on the average, above the usual norm of 287 mOsm per kilogram of H_2O. The serum sodium concentrations are also elevated and account quantitatively for the increases in plasma osmolality. In contrast, persons with primary polydipsia have a primary aberration of the thirst mechanism and ingest water independent of physiologic stimuli. These patients often have mild dilutional hyponatremia.

In patients whose diabetes insipidus, either pituitary or nephrogenic in origin, begins in childhood, considerable dilation of the urinary bladder, ureters, and renal pelvis may occur. This dilation has led to a reduction in GFR in some patients.

DIAGNOSIS. Based on the underlying pathophysiology, the polyuric syndromes may be grouped into the following general categories: (1) pituitary diabetes insipidus, in which there is absence or diminished production and secretion of ADH; (2) solute diuresis, in which excessively high rates of solute delivery to the loop of Henle overwhelm quantitatively the ability of distal nephron segments to dissociate solute and water absorption; (3) nephrogenic diabetes insipidus, either familial or acquired, in which collecting duct cells are partially or completely unresponsive to ADH; (4) renal concentrating disorders, in which there is impaired generation of a hypertonic medullary interstitium by renal countercurrent multiplication and exchange processes; and (5) primary polydipsia, in which the ingestion of unusually large volumes of water results in polyuria, the appropriate physiologic response.

Disorders such as diabetes mellitus, which produces solute diuresis, are characterized by isotonic urine and by glycosuria. The history and laboratory data are adequate to identify disorders such as sickle cell disease or interstitial nephritis, both of which impair the ability to generate a hypertonic medullary interstitium. Routine laboratory screening readily identifies the presence of hypercalcemia or hypokalemia. Finally, congenital nephrogenic diabetes insipidus is identified by a history of having been present since birth, generally in males, and by *persistent* unresponsiveness to exogenous ADH. Acquired nephrogenic diabetes insipidus is recognized by ADH unresponsiveness combined with a history of exposure to agents, such as lithium, demeclocycline, or methoxyflurane anesthesia, which antagonize the action of ADH on collecting ducts.

The more difficult diagnostic problem is the differentiation of patients with partial or complete deficiency of ADH from those with primary polydipsia. Certain factors may point toward the most likely diagnosis. For example, a 24-hour urine volume greater than 18 liters, a random plasma osmolality determination below 285 mOsm per kilogram of H_2O, and a history of episodic polyuria all suggest compulsive water drinking as the underlying disorder. A history of head trauma or neoplasm, a history of sudden onset of unrelenting polyuria, and a random plasma osmolality determination greater than 290 mOsm per kilogram of H_2O all suggest pituitary diabetes insipidus.

The basis of all tests for pituitary diabetes insipidus rests on the ability of the kidney to excrete hypertonic urine after an osmotic stimulus. The simplest maneuver is to produce hypertonicity of body fluids by water deprivation. The absolute level of urine concentration achieved with water deprivation is nondiagnostic, since maximal concentrating ability depends on the degree of medullary hypertonicity as well as the presence of adequate amounts of ADH. For example, the maximal urine osmolality produced by water deprivation in a group of randomly selected hospitalized patients was found to be 764 mOsm per kilogram of H_2O as compared with 1067 mOsm per kilogram of H_2O in healthy volunteers. Presumably the lower value for maximal urine concentrating ability in hospitalized patients reflects a reduction in medullary interstitial hypertonicity with respect to that present in normal volunteers.

Even in patients with a reduced medullary interstitial tonicity, the maximal urine osmolality achieved with water deprivation depends on maximal degrees of endogenous ADH release in response to dehydration. Therefore, in those with intact mechanisms for ADH production and release, the administration of exogenous ADH will not produce an increase in the maximal urine osmolality achieved via water deprivation. This rationale forms the framework for a test scheme, illustrated in Figure 214–4, for distinguishing complete or partial pituitary diabetes insipidus from other polyuric syndromes.

In patients with mild polyuria, water deprivation may begin the night preceding the test; patients with severe polyuria should have water restricted during the day, to allow for close observation. The test begins with paired measurements of urine and plasma osmolality. All water intake is then withheld and hourly measurements of urine osmolality and body weight are made. When two sequential urine osmolalities vary by less than 30 mOsm per kilogram of H_2O, or when 3 to 5 per cent body weight is lost, 5 units of aqueous vasopressin is injected subcutaneously. A final urine osmolality is measured 60 minutes later.

The time required to achieve a maximal urine concentration varies from 4 to 18 hours. In normal persons, water deprivation results in urine osmolality two to four times greater than that of plasma. More important, the subsequent administration of ex-

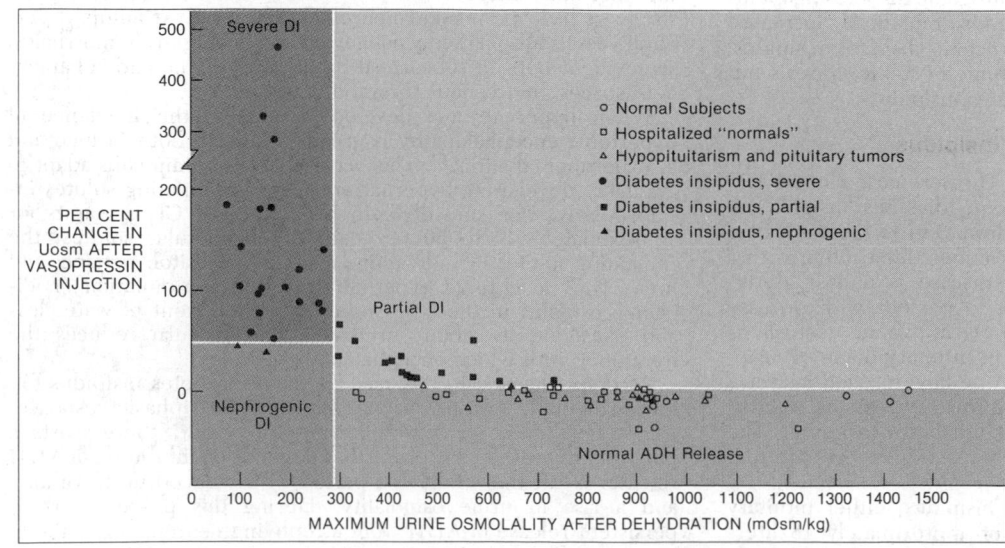

FIGURE 214–4. Maximal urine osmolality after dehydration versus the percentage change in urine osmolality induced by subsequent vasopressin injection. DI = Diabetes insipidus; ADH = antidiuretic hormone. (From Miller M, et al.: Ann Intern Med 73:721, 1970. Reprinted with permission of the publisher.)

ogenous ADH results in a less than 5 per cent further increase in urine osmolality. In patients with primary polydipsia, who have reduced medullary interstitial tonicity as a result of prolonged water diuresis, the urine may concentrate only slightly after water deprivation. However, they too will have stimulated endogenous ADH release maximally and will exhibit a less than 5 per cent rise in urine osmolality with supplemental ADH.

In patients with complete pituitary diabetes insipidus urine osmolality does not rise above that of plasma in response to water deprivation but shows a greater than 50 per cent increase in response to injection of ADH. In patients with partial pituitary diabetes insipidus the urine may concentrate to some degree in response to water deprivation, but urine osmolality also increases by at least 10 per cent after ADH injection. An interesting observation is that patients with partial pituitary diabetes insipidus often show a peak urine osmolality that decreases with further water restriction. This suggests a limited reserve of neurohypophyseal hormone that is depleted after an initial secretory burst. Finally, in patients with nephrogenic diabetes insipidus deprived of water, the urine osmolality fails to rise above that of plasma even when they are given exogenous ADH. When a diagnosis of pituitary diabetes insipidus is made, a careful evaluation for neoplasm involving the hypothalamus or neurohypophyseal tract is mandatory.

Levels of circulating vasopressin measured by radioimmunoassay have heretofore been available only for research purposes. A commercial assay is now marketed for clinical use, but its utility is, as of now, undefined. Hypertonic saline infusions have also been utilized to test for release of ADH. This procedure is hazardous in patients with limited cardiac reserve, in whom volume expansion may precipitate cardiac decompensation. Moreover, the results of the test are uninterpretable if the patient develops salt diuresis, thus fixing urine osmolality near isotonicity.

Nicotine, a nonosmotic stimulus to ADH secretion, has been used to elicit antidiuresis in those patients who have "essential hypernatremia," i.e., ADH release in response to volume contraction but not to hypertonicity. A better diagnostic approach in these patients is to assess the antidiuretic response to mild volume contraction.

TREATMENT. Patients with diabetes insipidus, either pituitary or nephrogenic, may require emergency treatment of hypertonic encephalopathy or maintenance therapy for polyuria.

Hypertonic Encephalopathy. The goal in treating this medical emergency is to replenish body water, thereby restoring osmotic balance and replenishing cell volume, at a rate that avoids significant complications. Since the brain adjusts to hypertonicity, at least in part, by increasing intracellular osmolar content, rapid repletion of body water with extracellular fluid dilution, causes translocation of water into cells to achieve osmotic equilibrium. The result of this water movement is cell swelling and cerebral edema. Seizures occur in up to 40 per cent of patients treated for severe hypernatremia by rapid infusions of hypotonic solutions. If water repletion is undertaken at a slower rate, brain cells lose the accumulated intracellular solutes and osmotic equilibration can occur without cell swelling. Consequently, a good rule of thumb is to administer fluids at a rate that reduces the serum sodium concentration to normal over a 36- to 48-hour period, or to reduce the serum sodium concentration by about 1 mEq per liter every 2 hours.

The choice of fluid to be administered in the diabetes insipidus syndromes depends in large part on three factors: the extent to which circulatory collapse may be present; the rate at which hypernatremia has developed; and the magnitude of hypernatremia. Hypotonic NaCl solutions are best used as initial therapy in patients with modest volume contraction and only modest elevations of serum sodium concentrations, that is, less than 160 mEq per liter. However, in more advanced cases of hypernatremia, particularly if the hypernatremia has developed gradually, that is, over a period greater than 24 hours, and is accompanied by signs of circulatory collapse, more prudent initial therapy is to administer normal saline solutions. The reasons for this choice are twofold: in advanced hypernatremia, a normal saline solution is dilute relative to the patient's body fluid osmolality and thus dilutes the latter while minimizing the risk of iatrogenic cerebral swelling; at the same time, the normal saline solution provides an effective means of volume expansion. Finally, 5 per cent glucose solutions may be used to replenish body water in acute hypernatremia without significant circulatory collapse. However, the glucose infusion rate must be less than the rate of glucose metabolism to avoid glycosuria. Otherwise, the resulting osmotic diuresis will thwart attempts to replenish body free water. The treatment of drug-induced nephrogenic diabetes insipidus consists of removal of the offending agent.

Polyuria. Patients with partial hormonal deficiency and volumes of urine output between 2 and 6 liters daily may require no treatment as long as they are assured access to water. Specific therapy for pituitary diabetes insipidus is some form of ADH replacement. A variety of hormone preparations are available which differ in the ratio of antidiuretic to vasopressor activity and the duration of biologic effect. These relations are depicted in Table 214–2.

Early preparations of dried posterior pituitary extract, termed pituitary snuff, were given by nasal insufflation, had an effective biologic life of only a few hours, and inevitably produced chronic rhinitis, which often led to inadequate absorption of hormone. Aqueous vasopressin injection, having an activity span of only a few hours, is not practical for long-term use. It is useful, however, for diagnostic testing or for acute management of polyuria following central nervous system trauma or surgery.

Nasal sprays of aqueous lysine vasopressin may provide intermittent relief of polyuria. Rhinitis, although not so severe as with dried extract, is also a frequent concomitant to this form of therapy.

The most widely used preparation has been Pitressin Tannate in Oil, which is given intramuscularly, As little as 0.5 ml per day may provide adequate hormone for 24 to 48 hours. Great care must be exercised in preparing the injection by careful warming and mixing of the ampule so as to suspend the pellet of hormone in the oil. Failure to do so may result in injection of the oil vehicle alone and apparent "vasopressin resistance." Pain at injection sites and sterile abscesses are frequent complaints with this preparation. Persistent abdominal pain from the effect of ADH on intestinal motility is a not uncommon problem.

A synthetic analogue of vasopressin, dDAVP (1-deamino,8-D-arginine vasopressin), provides antidiuretic activity for 8 to 20 hours with negligible pressor effect, can be taken as a nasal spray, and is the current drug of choice. The drug is best started at night to find the lowest dose that will prevent nocturia. This dose, usually 5 to 10 µg, can be given twice daily or doubled as a single morning dose. A nasal catheter is provided, which is measured for convenient dosing in the 5 to 24 µg range. Headache

TABLE 214–2. COMPARISON OF NEUROHYPOPHYSEAL HORMONES AND SYNTHETIC ANALOGUES

Preparation	Activity						Duration of Activity	Route of Administration
	Antidiuretic	:	Vasopressor	:	Oxytocic			
8-Arginine vasopressin								
Pitressin, aqueous	100	:	100	:	5		2–6 hours	Intravenous
Pitressin tannate in oil							24–48 hours	Intramuscular
8-Lysine vasopressin								
Lypressin	60	:	70	:	1		2–6 hours	Nasal insufflation
1-Deamino, 8-D-arginine vasopressin								
(dDAVP), desmopressin	290	:	0.14				6–20 hours	Nasal insufflation
Oxytocin	1	:	1	:	100			

may be a troublesome side effect with large doses but usually disappears with a reduction of dosage.

For patients having some residual ADH production, the oral hypoglycemic agent chlorpropamide may provide adequate amelioration of symptoms. This drug stimulates ADH secretion and augments the activity of residual ADH on the collecting duct. Doses of 250 to 500 mg daily are sufficient to reduce polyuria in most patients with partial pituitary diabetes insipidus, but the side effect of hypoglycemia limits the drug's usefulness.

Thiazide diuretics may reduce the volume of urine in patients with all forms of diabetes insipidus, that is, either pituitary or nephrogenic, by causing a state of mild salt depletion. This results in a secondary increase in isotonic proximal tubular fluid absorption and a decrease in the volume of fluid delivered to the collecting duct. The effect is produced by 50 to 100 mg of hydrochlorothiazide daily, is sustained even in the absence of diuretics by salt restriction, and can be abolished by salt loading even with continued diuretic administration.

Vasopressin infusions have also been used to treat bleeding esophageal varices by reducing splanchnic blood flow. Desmopressin, a synthetic analogue of arginine vasopressin, stimulates the production of clotting Factor VIII. These other actions are discussed elsewhere in this textbook.

Nephrogenic Diabetes Insipidus. The therapeutic considerations outlined above, particularly with respect to the treatment of hypertonic encephalopathy and to the value of a chronic mild salt-depleted state in minimizing polyuria, apply equally well to the care of patients with pituitary or nephrogenic diabetes insipidus. In patients with nephrogenic diabetes insipidus acquired as a consequence of drug therapy (for example, lithium or demeclocycline), the offending agent should be discontinued.

Finally, it is important to stress the need to minimize the extent of polyuria in children with congenital nephrogenic diabetes insipidus, since there is a close correlation between repeated bouts of dehydration during childhood and mental dullness in adulthood. Alternatively, in patients in whom episodes of dehydration have been minimal, both mental and physical growth retardation can be avoided.

Barlow ED, DeWardener HE: Compulsive water drinking. Q J Med 28:235, 1959. *A thorough examination of the clinical course and pathophysiology of urinary concentration in a group of patients with primary polydipsia.*

Bichet DG, Razi M, Arthus M-F, et al.: Epinephrine and dDAVP administration in patients with congenital nephrogenic diabetes insipidus. Evidence for a precyclic AMP V_2 receptor defective mechanism. Kidney Int 36:859, 1989. *Analysis of the V_2 receptor defect in familial nephrogenic diabetes insipidus.*

Cunnah D, Ross G, Besser GM: Management of cranial diabetes insipidus with oral desmopressin (dDAVP). Clin Endocrinol 24:253, 1986. *The use of dDAVP in pituitary diabetes insipidus.*

Knoers N, van der Heyden H, van Oost BA, et al.: Three-point linkage analysis using multiple DNA polymorphic markers in families with X-linked nephrogenic diabetes insipidus. Genomics 4:434, 1989. *Linkage analysis in familial nephrogenic diabetes insipidus.*

Miller M, Dalakos T, Moses AM, et al.: Recognition of partial defects in antidiuretic hormone secretion. Ann Intern Med 72:721, 1970. *A concise guide to testing procedures for states of ADH insufficiency and a rational scheme for interpreting the test results.*

Reeves WB, Andreoli TE: The posterior pituitary and water metabolism. In Foster DW, Wilson JD (eds.): Williams Textbook of Endocrinology, 8th ed. Philadelphia, W. B. Saunders Company, 1991. *A full review of the polyuric syndromes, their differential diagnosis and treatment; extensively referenced.*

THE SYNDROME OF INAPPROPRIATE ADH PRODUCTION (SIADH)

For convenience SIADH has been discussed in Ch. 75 as a major disorder producing hyponatremia.

OXYTOCIN

Oxytocin is produced in the same hypothalamic nuclei and by the same synthetic mechanism as vasopressin. AVP and oxytocin are produced in both the paraventricular and the supraoptic nuclei of the hypothalamus. However, a given neuron in these nuclei produces only one hormone. Neurophysin I is the specific carrier protein synthesized with oxytocin and has been used as a marker for oxytocin release.

PHYSIOLOGY. The primary stimuli for oxytocin secretion are nipple stimulation (suckling) and deformation of the reproductive tract (especially the vagina) in females and muscular contraction of the reproductive organs in the male. The neural arcs serving these stimuli are not well defined, but some evidence suggests that the final synaptic transmitter is dopamine. Estrogens appear to influence secretion directly, based on observations of increased neurophysin I in blood during estrogen peaks of the menstrual cycle, or permissively, based on findings of a graded response to vaginal distension over the period of a menstrual cycle and an enhanced response with exogenous estradiol. Progesterones inhibit response to mechanical stimuli. Hypertonicity of body fluids also appears to cause oxytocin secretion. For example, in congenitally vasopressin-deficient Brattleboro rats, hypertonicity causes degranulation of the neurohypophysis, indicating sustained secretion of oxytocin, a relatively weak antidiuretic principle. Finally, relaxin, an ovarian peptide that suppresses uterine contraction and relaxes pelvic connective tissue during parturition, suppresses oxytocin release.

BIOLOGIC ACTIVITY. In females, oxytocin initiates its primary effect by binding to specific myometrial receptors, the affinity of which increases strikingly in the presence of estrogen. Exogenously administered oxytocin elicits contractions of the fundus indistinguishable from those of labor. However, the initiation of labor is apparently oxytocin independent, with increasing secretions seen only with dilation of the birth canal. Oxytocin may play a key role in final expulsion of the fetus and placenta. The total absence of oxytocin does not prevent parturition, although prolonged labor is seen in such women. The cellular events leading to uterine contraction are unknown but parallel an oxytocin-induced increase in ion permeability with depolarization of the myometrial cell membrane.

The milk-ejection reflex is also mediated via oxytocin. Contraction of mammary myoepithelium is stimulated, leading to a rise in intramammary pressure and expulsion of milk from alveolar channels to large sinuses, where it is accessible to the suckling infant. A true galactogenic effect of oxytocin leading to increased milk production has not been convincingly demonstrated. Absence of oxytocin abolishes the milk-ejection reflex.

In the male, oxytocin increases ejection of sperm into the semen in response to stimulation of the reproductive organs. Oxytocin retains some antidiuretic activity, about 1 per cent of AVP, but exerts no significant antidiuretic effect at physiologic levels of secretion. Vascular smooth muscle is relaxed by oxytocin, causing a decrease in blood pressure, cutaneous flushing, and increased limb blood flow. Reflex tachycardia and sympathetic responses quickly restore hemodynamics to normal except when such reflexes are rendered inactive as in deep anesthesia.

THERAPEUTIC USE. The primary use of oxytocin (Pitocin) is to induce or to improve the quality of labor. The uterus is relatively resistant to oxytocin in early pregnancy, but infusions given with hypertonic saline injections may speed abortions of later pregnancy.

With long-term infusion of oxytocin, patients may experience sufficient antidiuretic effects to be at risk of water intoxication. Antidiuresis may be detected at oxytocin infusion rates of 15 mU per minute, and maximal urinary concentration is usually attained at rates of 45 mU per minute. Infusions for delivery and control of postpartum uterine hemorrhage may reach 20 to 40 mU per minute, and infusions for therapeutic abortions range from 20 to 100 mU per minute.

Feeney JG: Water intoxication and oxytocin. Br Med J 285:243, 1982. *An account of water intoxication following oxytocin administration.*

Roberts JS: Oxytocin, Vol I. Montreal, Eden Press, 1977. *This review covers the extensive work in oxytocin physiology and chemistry; very readable and fully referenced.*

215 The Pineal Gland

Alfred J. Lewy

The mammalian pineal is located in the "center" of the brain (above the quadrigeminal plate, just behind the posterior commissure) but is actually outside of the "blood-brain barrier." Postganglionic neurons from the superior cervical ganglia release norepinephrine, which in turn stimulates β_1-adrenergic receptors on the pinealocytes (Fig. 215–1). This results in the synthesis and release into the CSF and venous circulation of melatonin, the principal putative hormone of the pineal gland. The (paired) suprachiasmatic nuclei are the source of an approximately 24-hour rhythm in melatonin production that persists in conditions of constant darkness or blindness. Photic input, conveyed to the suprachiasmatic nuclei (SCN) via the retinohypothalamic tracts, synchronizes (entrains) the SCN and its output circadian rhythms to the 24-hour light-dark cycle. Between the SCN and the cell bodies of the preganglionic sympathetic neurons in the spinal cord, there are synapses in the paraventricular nuclei.

Melatonin production by the human pineal is decreased by β-blockers and α_2 agonists and is increased by certain tricyclic antidepressants that block reuptake of norepinephrine. Melatonin production is also increased by extreme physical exercise, norepinephrine, and psoralen. In general, diet and activity have no effect. Increased melatonin in manic states and decreased melatonin in depression probably occur but most likely represent epiphenomena following changes in adrenergic activity.

FUNCTION OF MELATONIN

The function of melatonin in humans remains elusive. In some fish and reptiles melatonin coalesces melanin-containing melanosomes and in this way causes blanching, but this effect has been lost in most animals. Melatonin may possibly have this effect on the mammalian retinal pigmented epithelium. The association of pineal tumors with disorders of puberty is most likely explained by compression of the hypothalamus, since no

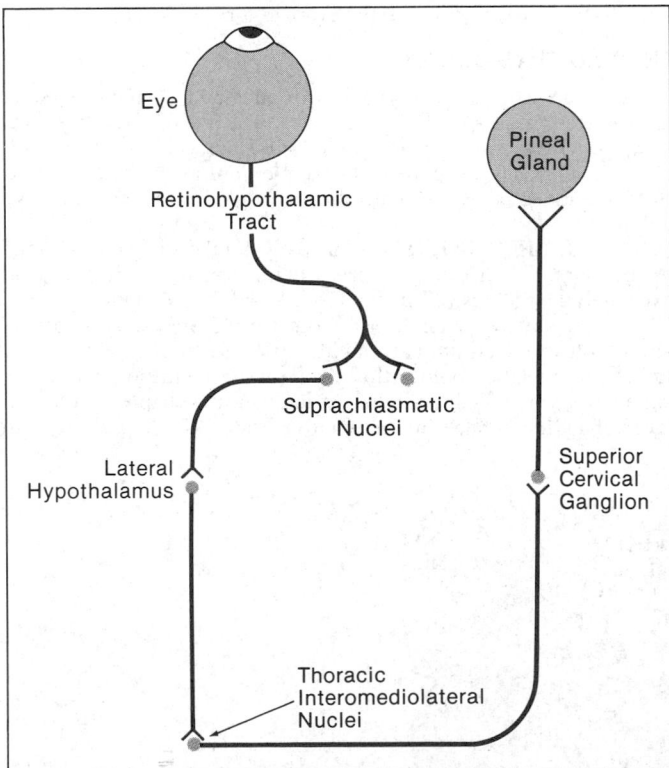

FIGURE 215–1. Schematic diagram for the neuroanatomic regulation of the timing of mammalian melatonin production. Norepinephrine, released by postganglionic sympathetic neurons, stimulates β_1-adrenergic receptors on the pinealocytes, resulting in a sequence of biochemical events which culminates in the synthesis and activation of N-acetyltransferase (the rate-limiting enzymatic step in the synthesis of melatonin and its precursor, N-acetylserotonin) and the release of melatonin into the CSF and venous circulation. The (paired) suprachiasmatic nuclei (SCN) are the source of an approximately 24-hour rhythm in melatonin production that persists in conditions of constant darkness or blindness. Photic input, conveyed to the SCN via the retinohypothalamic tracts, synchronizes (entrains) the SCN and its output circadian rhythms to the 24-hour light-dark cycle. Between the SCN and the cell bodies of the preganglionic sympathetic neurons in the spinal cord, there are synapses located in the paraventricular nuclei of the lateral hypothalamus.

melatonin-secreting tumor has yet been found. Furthermore, it now appears that the main effect of melatonin on the reproductive system lies in its ability to communicate the time of the year to animals that are seasonal breeders. In such animals it can have either anti- or progonadal activity depending on whether the species is a spring or fall breeder, respectively. Reproductive and endocrine effects of exogenous melatonin administration, not to mention endogenous melatonin secretion, have not been well documented in humans.

CHRONOBIOLOGY OF MELATONIN

Melatonin is produced only during nighttime darkness in both diurnal and nocturnal animals with an approximately 12-hour "on" phase and a 12-hour "off" phase. These phases persist even in constant darkness, although several days in constant darkness cause the melatonin rhythm to free run, beating in and out of phase with the sleep-wake cycle. Many blind people with a complete absence of light perception have free-running endogenous circadian rhythms. When these individuals are out of phase with their sleep-wake cycles (which have remained more or less synchronized to clock time), they are symptomatic (nighttime insomnia and daytime sleepiness). A pattern of insomnia that recurs every few weeks is almost pathognomonic for free-running circadian rhythms in totally blind individuals.

Darkness does not induce melatonin production. In sighted people, exposure to sufficiently bright light during the night immediately suppresses melatonin production. Two models have been proposed to explain how the nightly melatonin profile is shaped. In the *two-pacemaker model*, it is hypothesized that separate endogenous pacemakers control the onset and offset of melatonin production, cued primarily to dusk and dawn, respectively. In the *"clock-gate" model*, the suppressant effect of light (probably unique to melatonin) participates in the shortening of the duration of nighttime melatonin production during long photoperiods. Both models attempt to explain the shorter duration of melatonin secretion during the briefer summer nights compared to the longer winter nights.

The changing duration of nighttime melatonin secretion during the calendar year seems to be responsible for the reproductive effects of the light-dark cycle in seasonal breeders. Seasonal rhythms have not been well documented in humans, but it is clear that humans have most, if not all, of the circadian rhythms found in other higher animals. Whereas seasonal rhythms respond to the duration of the photoperiod or scotoperiod, circadian rhythms respond to the 24-hour light-dark cycle. In animals, the light-dark cycle's phase-shifting effects on circadian rhythms can be described by a phase response curve (PRC). This appears to be the case in humans as well. The PRC can be explained in the following way. Delay responses (shifts to a later time) result when exposure to light occurs during the first part of the night; advance responses (shifts to an earlier time) result when the exposure occurs during the latter part of the night. These phase shifts are greatest in magnitude in the middle of the night and are least during the middle of the day.

Although the suppressant effect of light is probably unique to melatonin, phase-shifting by light affects the endogenous circadian pacemaker (SCN) and all of its driven rhythms. In fact, the timing of the SCN's circadian rhythms is best measured by the circulating levels of melatonin. In some species injections of exogenous melatonin are capable of causing phase shifts and/or entrainment. In some instances, a PRC for melatonin has been described that is more or less the opposite of the PRC for light; that is, the melatonin PRC resembles a dark-pulse PRC. In humans, orally administered melatonin appears to have circadian phase-shifting effects, which can be described by a PRC that resembles a dark-pulse PRC. Thus, melatonin—which is produced only during the night—may be the chemical messenger of darkness. Therefore, human melatonin production may normally have a role, however small, in the entrainment of the SCN's circadian rhythms. Not being seasonal breeders, perhaps humans have retained the suppressant effect of light in order to use endogenous melatonin to more effectively augment entrainment and phase-shifting effects of the light-dark cycle. The melatonin PRC may also provide the rationale for precise scheduling of exogenous melatonin administration for therapeutic purposes, such as to treat chronobiologic sleep and mood disorders and to facilitate adaptation to shift work and air travel.

PINEAL TUMORS

Four main types of tumors arise that are usually malignant in the pineal: (1) pineoblastomas or pineocytomas, the term used depending on the degree of differentiation of this tumor of the pineal parenchyma, (2) germinomas, (3) embryonal carcinomas, and (4) glial tumors. Invasion of the pineal by cysts has also been reported. Destruction of pineal tissue can reduce or even ablate melatonin production, but increased circulating levels of melatonin have not been conclusively associated with pineocytomas. Melatonin production decreases with age, but this does not seem to be related to pineal calcification. By occluding the cerebral aqueduct, pineal tumors can produce symptoms associated with increased intracranial pressure, sometimes necessitating a shunt. Through pressure on the quadrigeminal plate, pineal tumors can produce Parinaud's syndrome, which includes paresis of upward conjugate gaze. Some germinomas and embryonal carcinomas secrete human chorionic gonadotropin, which has been implicated in cases of delayed onset of puberty. Treatment modalities include surgical extirpation, radiation, and chemotherapy, depending on tumor type and location and the absence or degree of metastases.

Lewy AJ, Sack RL, Singer CM, et al.: Winter depression and the phase shift hypothesis for bright light's therapeutic effects: History, theory and experimental evidence. J Biol Rhythms 3:121, 1988.

Lewy AJ, Wehr TA, Goodwin FK, et al.: Light suppresses melatonin secretion in humans. Science 210:1267, 1980.

Neuwelt EA (ed.): Diagnosis and Treatment of Pineal Region Tumors. Baltimore, Williams & Wilkins, 1984.

Reiter RJ: The pineal gland. In DeGroot LJ, Besser GM, Cahill GF Jr (eds.): Endocrinology, 2nd ed. Philadelphia, W. B. Saunders Company, 1989, pp 240–253.

Relkin R (ed.): The Pineal Gland. New York, Elsevier Biomedical, 1983.

216 The Thyroid

P. Reed Larsen

The thyroid gland secretes thyroxine, 3,5,3',5'-tetraiodothyronine (abbreviated T_4) and small amounts of 3,5,3'-triiodothyronine (abbreviated T_3). The principal role of these substances is to regulate tissue metabolism. In infants, adequate supplies of thyroid hormone are necessary for the development of the normal central nervous system in the first 1 to 2 years of life. The absence of thyroid hormone during this period results in irreversible mental retardation, a syndrome known as *cretinism*. The hormone is also required for normal growth and bone maturation in children. Despite these important functions, the body can withstand marked reductions in thyroid hormone for long periods, although at the cost of abnormal function of many organ systems.

EMBRYOLOGY AND ANATOMY

The thyroid develops from a combination of pharyngeal midline and bilateral primitive tissues from the fourth branchial pouch. These primitive thyroid cells migrate from the pharyngeal floor, leaving behind a residual thyroglossal duct that normally becomes obliterated. The major portion of the thyroid cell mass is derived from the median mid-pharyngeal tissue. The lateral thyroid anlagen migrate medially to fuse with median-derived thyroid tissue, but primarily contribute the *parafollicular* or *C cells*. The C cells secrete calcitonin, not thyroid hormone, and do not play a role in thyroid physiology (see Ch. 236). The evolution of thyroid function occurs over the first 10 to 12 weeks of fetal life, with definite appearance of T_4 in the gland by 10 to 11 weeks. The placenta is impermeable to T_3 and T_4; the fetus depends on its own thyroid for its supply of these hormones. The adult size (15 to 20 grams) of the thyroid is reached at about age 15. The thyroid gland has the configuration of a butterfly, with the two lobes measuring about 5×2 cm. The lobes are composed of spherical structures called *follicles*, consisting of *colloid* surrounded by a single layer of epithelial cells enclosed by a basement membrane. Colloid consists predominantly of the protein *thyroglobulin*, which is the storage form of T_4 and T_3.

THYROID PHYSIOLOGY

The structures of the thyroid hormones and their precursors, monoiodotyrosine and diiodotyrosine (MIT and DIT), are shown in Figure 216–1. Iodine accounts for 65 per cent of the weight of T_4. Since this is a relatively scarce element in the earth's crust, the thyroid cell has mechanisms to concentrate and conserve iodine.

IODINE METABOLISM. The daily intake of iodine in man varies markedly in different areas of the world. It ranges from extremely low levels (20 μg or less per day) to as high as 600 or 700 μg per day in certain areas of the United States. The optimal iodine intake for adults is thought to be 150 to 300 μg per day. Levels appreciably below this lead to the condition known as *endemic goiter*, which is discussed later in this chapter. The high level of iodine intake in the United States is, in part, due to

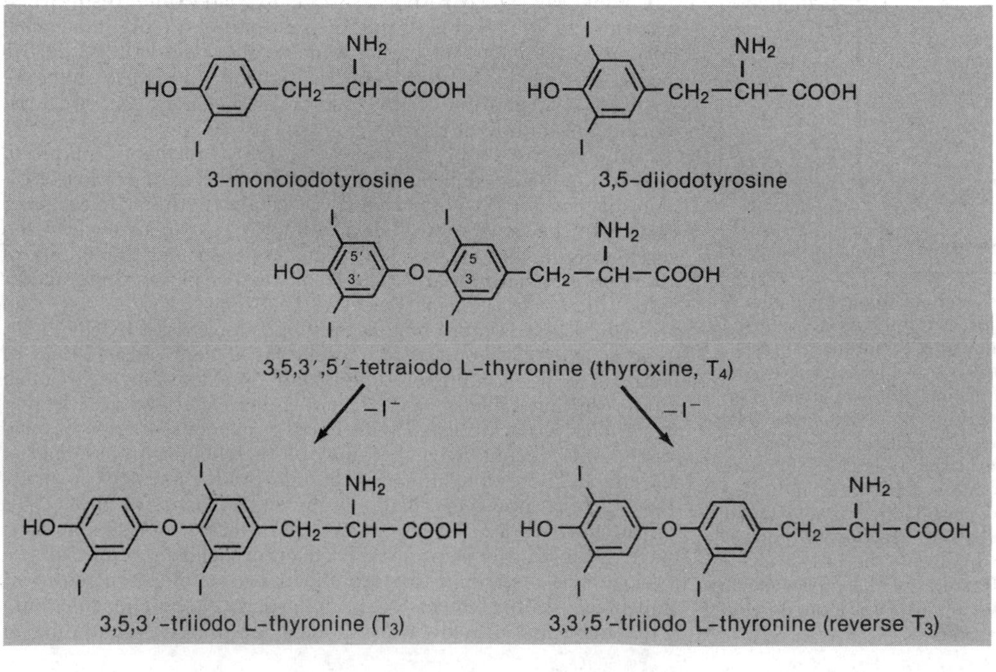

FIGURE 216–1. Structure of the thyroid hormones and their precursors.

iodination of salt. Iodine in all forms is reduced to iodide (I⁻) in the gastrointestinal tract and absorbed within 30 minutes of ingestion. I⁻ leaves the blood via two mechanisms. It is concentrated by the thyroid or excreted in the urine. There is a wide variation in the fraction of I⁻ concentrated by the thyroid per 24 hours, depending on iodine uptake. In the United States, iodine uptake by the thyroid varies from about 5 to 30 per cent.

INTRATHYROIDAL IODIDE METABOLISM. In Figure 216–2 are shown the steps involved in the synthesis of the thyroid hormones. Because the concentrations of I⁻ in the plasma are so low, the thyroid cell concentrates I⁻, the cell-plasma ratio being about 20 to 40:1. The trapped I⁻ is rapidly oxidized and incorporated into protein. As a consequence, there is little I⁻ per se in the thyroid gland. The process of I⁻ oxidation and its incorporation into tyrosine is known as *organification*. The substrate for iodine is the 660,000 molecular weight glycoprotein thyroglobulin. Only about 25 per cent of the tyrosine residues of this specialized protein are available for iodination. Both MIT and DIT are formed. In a typical molecule of fully iodinated human thyroglobulin, there are approximately 6 to 7 residues of MIT, 4 to 5 of DIT, 3 to 4 of T₄, and 0.2 to 0.3 of T₃. The T₄ and T₃ arise from the coupling of either 2 DIT residues or 1 MIT and 1 DIT residue, a reaction that requires thyroid peroxidase. This process is known as *coupling*. Both organification and coupling are inhibited by *thiourea compounds*, which are used in the treatment of patients with hyperthyroidism (see below). The thyroglobulin is iodinated at the apical border of the cell and is then exocytosed into the colloid. Under normal circumstances, T₄ and T₃ secretion occurs from this pool. The thyroid secretory process starts with phagocytosis of thyroglobulin by the apical cell membrane, leading to the formation of a *colloid droplet*. This is combined with a lysosome, and as the colloid droplet traverses the thyroid cell, proteolysis occurs with eventual release of T₄ and T₃ at the basal cell border. Deiodination of T₄ to T₃ also occurs during this process, resulting in a ratio of T₄ to T₃ in thyroid secretion that is somewhat less than the 15:1 value found in the thyroglobulin itself. To conserve iodine for reuse in the thyroid cell, a *deiodinase* is present that removes the iodine from MIT and DIT, allowing it to recycle.

CIRCULATING T₄ AND T₃. Thyroid hormones in plasma exist in two forms, free and protein bound. Although only about 0.02 per cent of total plasma T₄ and 0.3 per cent of plasma T₃ are free, it is the free hormone concentration that is maintained constant by the feedback regulatory system and that appears to parallel the rate of cellular uptake of these hormones. It is, therefore, the free hormone concentration that determines the thyroid status irrespective of the total plasma concentration. In the euthyroid person the total hormone is determined by the quantity and affinity of certain thyroid hormone–binding proteins, which are *thyroxine-binding globulin* (TBG), transthyretin (formerly termed thyroxine-binding prealbumin), and albumin. TBG is by far the most important of these, transporting about 75 per cent of serum T₄ and T₃. It is a glycoprotein, with a molecular weight of 55,000, which is synthesized in the liver. TBG has a high affinity for both T₄ and T₃, although the affinity for T₄ is about 10- to 15-fold higher than that for T₃. There is normally sufficient TBG in serum to bind approximately 20 μg of T₄ per deciliter at a molar ratio of 1:1. The serum TBG concentrations change under many circumstances, which are listed in Table 216–1. It is important to recognize these conditions, since the resultant changes in total T₄ and T₃ may duplicate abnormalities that are found in patients with thyroid dysfunction. For example, during pregnancy, serum total T₄ and T₃ are increased but serum free T₄ and T₃ concentrations remain constant. The relationships are described in the following equation:

$$[\text{TH}] \text{ is proportional to } \frac{[\text{TH-TBG}]}{[\text{TBG}]}$$

where TH = free T₄ or T₃, [TH-TBG] = TBG-bound T₄ or T₃, and TBG = unoccupied TBG. When [TBG] increases, the bound hormone also increases until a new steady state is achieved at which [TH] is again normal. This occurs through both decreased metabolism and increased secretion of T₄ and T₃. To interpret a total serum T₄ or T₃ measurement accurately it is necessary to know the fraction of the hormone that is free; alternatively the free hormone can be measured directly or estimated (see Direct Tests of Thyroid Function later in this chapter). Certain compounds compete with T₄ and T₃ for binding to TBG. Two such drugs are salicylates and phenytoin. About a 20 to 30 per cent reduction in serum T₄ and T₃ is observed when 300 mg of phenytoin or salicylates in excess of 2 grams per day are given.

KINETICS OF T₄ AND T₃. Deiodination of the iodothyronines is the most significant metabolic transformation of the thyroid hormones. In the case of T₄, deiodination of the distal ring, occurring predominantly in liver and kidney, gives rise to T₃, which has approximately three to four times the metabolic potency of the parent hormone (Fig. 216–1). About 30 to 40 per cent of the 80 μg of T₄ produced per day is metabolized via this pathway (Table 216–2), giving rise to about 80 per cent of the T₃ produced daily. Loss of an iodine in the proximal ring of T₄ leads to formation of *reverse T₃* (3,3′,5′-triiodothyronine), a compound that appears to have no metabolic effect. About 40 per cent of T₄

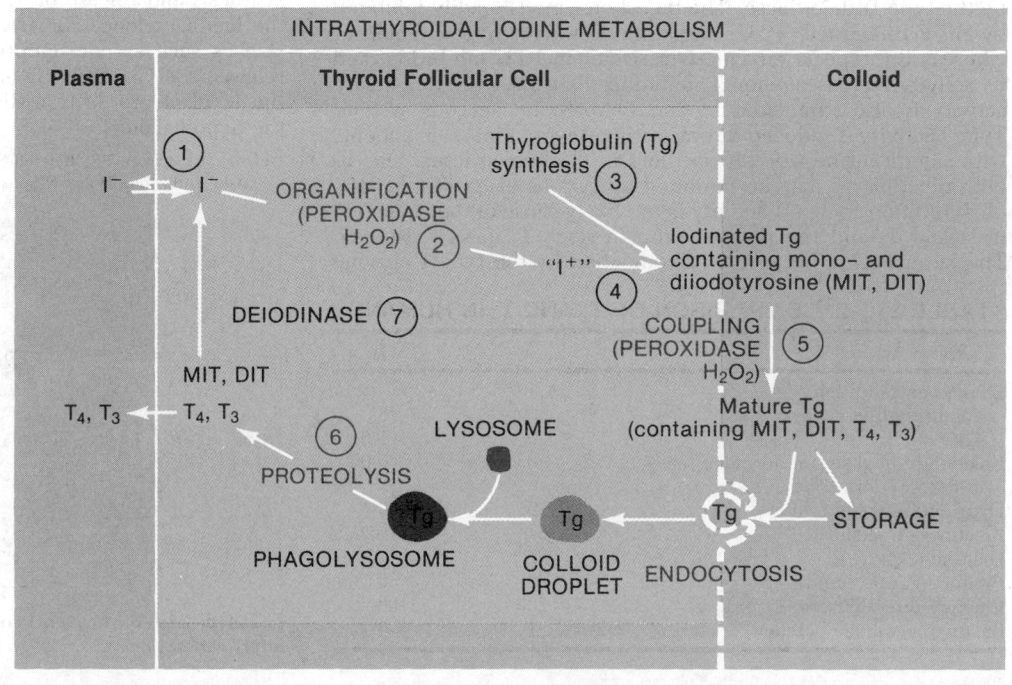

FIGURE 216–2. Principal steps in the synthesis and secretion of thyroid hormones. MIT = Monoiodotyrosine; DIT = diiodotyrosine. The steps denoted by the numbers are those in which defects have been identified in patients with inherited abnormalities in thyroid hormone biosynthesis (see Sporadic and Endemic Goiter, later in this chapter).

TABLE 216-1. CIRCUMSTANCES ASSOCIATED WITH CHANGES IN THE CIRCULATING CONCENTRATION OF THYROXINE-BINDING GLOBULIN (TBG)

Increased TBG
1. Pregnancy
2. Treatment with supraphysiologic amounts of estrogens, including oral contraceptives
3. In some patients with cirrhosis or acute hepatitis
4. As a congenital abnormality
5. In acute intermittent porphyria
6. After administration of heroin, methadone
7. After administration of clofibrate

Decreased TBG
1. Protein malnutrition, hepatic failure, chronic illness
2. Nephrotic syndrome
3. After administration of L-asparaginase
4. As a congenital abnormality (usually X-linked)
5. During treatment with androgenic steroids or pharmacologic doses of glucocorticoids

is metabolized via this pathway, the remainder being excreted via the biliary tract into the feces following conjugation with glucuronide. T_3 and reverse T_3 are, in turn, deiodinated in both proximal and distal rings, giving rise to the predicted monoiodothyronines and diiodothyronines, none of which has physiologic effects. T_4 to T_3 conversion and reverse T_3 deiodination appear to be catalyzed by the same enzyme. If this reaction is inhibited, as it is under diverse circumstances, a reduction in serum T_3 and an increase in the serum reverse T_3 concentrations occur.

The differences between T_3 and T_4 in terms of distribution volume, the intracellular fraction, and half-life can be attributed principally to the differences in the affinities of these two hormones for the plasma-binding proteins (Table 216–2). The higher intracellular T_3 content explains in part its higher potency relative to T_4. Given the 3 to 4:1 ratio of metabolic potency of T_3 and T_4 and the fact that approximately one third of T_4 is converted to T_3, it appears that T_4 has little intrinsic metabolic activity in man.

REGULATION OF T_4 TO T_3 CONVERSION. Two classes of enzymes convert T_4 to T_3 (iodothyronine 5'-deiodinases). One of these (type I), most active in liver and kidney, provides the bulk of the T_3 to the plasma pool. Plasma T_3 is the source of most of the intracellular T_3 for the liver, kidney, heart, and skeletal muscle. A second enzyme (type II), present in the central nervous system, pituitary, brown adipose tissue (BAT), and placenta, selectively provides T_3 to the cells of these tissues. For example, about 80 per cent of intracellular T_3 in cerebral cortex and 50 to 60 per cent of T_3 in the anterior pituitary or BAT are provided by the type II deiodinase. The type I enzyme is readily inhibited by propylthiouracil (PTU) and decreases with hypothyroidism, whereas the type II enzyme is resistant to PTU inhibition, and its activity increases when T_4 is reduced. In BAT the deiodinase activity is also stimulated by the sympathetic nervous system. Type I activity is reduced during fasting, severe illness, in patients with significant hepatic disease, and in the human fetus. One or both deiodinases may be inhibited by various drugs (Table 216–3). Inhibition of type I activity is the likely cause of the reduction in serum T_3 and the rise in serum reverse T_3 in sick patients. The latter occurs because 5'-deiodination by the type I enzyme

TABLE 216-2. COMPARISON OF T_3 AND T_4 IN HUMANS

	T_3	T_4
Serum concentration		
Total (µg/dl)	0.14	8
Free (ng/dl)	0.4	1.6
Fraction of total serum hormone that is in the free form (%)	0.3	0.02
Distribution volume (liters)	35	10
Fraction intracellular (%)	64	10–20
Half-life (days)	1	7
Production rate (µg/day)	33	80
Fraction directly from thyroid (%)	20	100
Relative metabolic potency	1	0.3

TABLE 216-3. DRUGS THAT CAN INFLUENCE THYROID FUNCTION OR ALTER TEST RESULTS

Type of Effect	Common Examples
Suppress TSH secretion	Dopamine, L-dopa, glucocorticoid excess
Inhibit thyroid hormone synthesis or release	Iodide, lithium carbonate, phenylbutazone, sulfonylureas
Decrease hormone-protein binding	Salicylates, phenytoin, fenclofenac, furosemide
Inhibit T_4 to T_3 conversion	
Type I 5'-deiodinase	Propylthiouracil, not methimazole (Tapazole)
	Propranolol (not other β-adrenergic antagonists)
	Glucocorticoid excess
Types I and II 5'-deiodinase	Amiodarone (Cordarone), Iopanoic acid (Telepaque), ipodate (Oragrafin)

is a rate-limiting step in reverse T_3 degradation. The increase in type II activity during hypothyroxinemia acts as a homeostatic mechanism to maintain normal intracellular T_3 concentrations in certain tissues when T_4 production is reduced. The capacity for PTU and glucocorticoid to inhibit type I activity is important in short-term treatment of severe hyperthyroidism.

MECHANISM OF ACTION OF THYROID HORMONE. Thyroid hormone regulation of protein synthesis occurs through effects on gene transcription and messenger RNA stabilization. A DNA- and T_3-binding nucleoprotein, the T_3 receptor, has about tenfold higher affinity for T_3 than for T_4, explaining in part why T_3 is the active hormone. There are two genes coding for similar thyroid hormone receptor proteins, which are both members of the erb A-related hormone receptor superfamily. Effects of thyroid hormone in many tissues can be related to the degree of saturation of these receptors by T_3. Other direct effects of thyroid hormone at the cell membrane or mitochondria may also occur. The regulation of the type II deiodinase by T_4 does not require protein synthesis, but the mechanism for this action is not understood.

REGULATION OF THYROID FUNCTION. The feedback loop for regulation of thyroid function is presented in Figure 216–3. *Thyrotropin-releasing hormone* (TRH) is secreted by hypothalamic cells and stimulates synthesis and release of thyrotropin (TSH, thyroid-stimulating hormone). This hormone in turn stimulates all of the steps involved in thyroid hormone synthesis and release through activation of adenylate cyclase. T_4 and smaller amounts of T_3 are released from the gland with monodeiodination of T_4 to T_3 in liver and kidney. Both serum T_3 and T_4 (via its intrapituitary conversion to T_3) suppress the synthesis and release of TSH competing with TRH to complete the feedback loop. *Somatostatin* (SRIF) and possibly other substances such as neuropeptides and dopamine also inhibit TSH release (see Ch. 212). T_3 also has a direct suppressive effect on the level of pro TRH mRNA in the paraventricular nucleus of the hypothalamus.

DeGroot LJ, Larsen PR, Refetoff S, et al.: The Thyroid and Its Diseases, 5th ed. New York, John Wiley & Sons, 1984. *A basic text.*

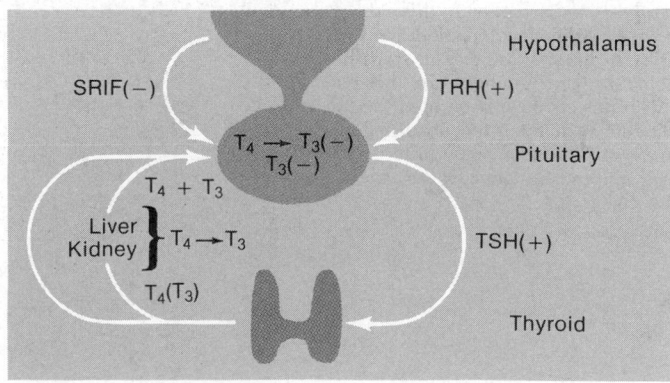

FIGURE 216–3. Current concepts of hypothalamic-pituitary-thyroid interrelationships.

Ingbar SH, Braverman LE: *In* Werner's The Thyroid, 5th ed. Philadelphia, J. B. Lippincott Company, 1986. *A basic text.*

Kaplan MM, Larsen PR (eds.): Symposium on thyroid disease. Med Clin North Am 69:847, 1985. *This issue contains chapters directed at the most important clinical aspects of thyroid disease authored by experts in their respective fields.*

Larsen PR: Feedback regulation of thyrotropin secretion by hormones. N Engl J Med 306:23, 1982. *A detailed, but clinically oriented, discussion of the feedback regulation of TSH secretion by thyroid hormones.*

Sakurai A, Takeda K, Ain K, et al.: Generalized resistance to thyroid hormone associated with a mutation in the ligand-binding domain of the human thyroid hormone receptor β. Proc Natl Acad Sci USA 86:8977, 1989. *Evidence that thyroid hormone resistance is caused by point mutations in the human gene coding for the β form of the thyroid hormone receptor.*

TESTING FOR SUSPECTED THYROID DYSFUNCTION

The thyroid gland is unique among the endocrine organs in that symptoms may arise from two general types of problems. Hyperfunction of the thyroid (*hyperthyroidism* or *thyrotoxicosis*) or decreased secretion of thyroid hormone (*hypothyroidism* or *myxedema*) may cause the patient to seek medical help. Alternatively, physical enlargement of the thyroid (*goiter*) may cause respiratory embarrassment or dysphagia or, more commonly, cosmetic abnormalities. Goiter may exist in the absence of any functional abnormality. Although the most severe forms are dramatic and unmistakable, milder degrees of thyroid dysfunction lead to many symptoms that are nonspecific, requiring biochemical tests for diagnostic confirmation.

PHYSICAL EXAMINATION OF THE THYROID

The high prevalence of thyroid disease, particularly in the female (5 to 10 per cent), makes a careful examination of the thyroid gland an important part of the general physical examination. Thyroid enlargement may be the first clue to thyroid functional abnormalities in a patient with otherwise nonspecific symptoms. A cup of water is a necessity, and the patient should first be asked to swallow with the neck moderately extended while the anterior area of the neck is inspected. Significant thyroid enlargement and thyroid nodules can often be discerned by this maneuver. The position of the trachea should then be determined, followed by palpation of the thyroid. The isthmus of the thyroid is first identified and is usually found just inferior to the cricoid cartilage. The left and right thumbs are then employed in turn to palpate the left and right lobe of the gland as the patient swallows. The normal thyroid gland is palpable in a large proportion of younger persons, although in the elderly patient it is not surprising to find the cricoid cartilage at or below the sternal notch. The pyramidal lobe, a small cylinder of tissue extending vertically from the isthmus to the thyroid cartilage to the left or right of the midline, can often be palpated as well.

DIRECT TESTS OF THYROID FUNCTION

MEASUREMENT OF TOTAL SERUM THYROID HORMONE CONCENTRATIONS. Serum T_4 and T_3 are both readily quantitated by specific radioimmunoassays that require 200 μl or less of serum. Typical normal ranges for the total T_4 and T_3 concentrations are presented in Table 216–4, as well as the values in patients with alterations in TBG and in those with thyroid dysfunction.

SERUM FREE T_4 AND T_3 AND THE FREE T_4 INDEX. Since the concentration of free, rather than total, thyroid hormones parallels the thyroid status, the ideal thyroid function test

TABLE 216–4. SERUM THYROID HORMONE CONCENTRATIONS IN NORMAL PERSONS AND PATIENTS WITH THYROID DISEASE

	Serum T_4 (μg/dl)		Serum T_3 (ng/dl)	
	Mean	*Range*	*Mean*	*Range*
Euthyroid				
Normal TBG	8	5–11	140	80–220
Increased TBG	12	8–20	190	120–320
Reduced TBG	2	<1–5	60	20–100
Infants				
Cord serum	11	8–15	48	20–80
Age 6 weeks	10	7–14	163	120–220
Hyperthyroidism	21	8–35	480	200–1600
Hypothyroidism	2	<1–5	50	<20–150

would be the direct determination of free thyroid hormones. The absolute serum free T_4 and T_3 can be measured either by immunoassay of a dialysate of human serum or by estimating the dialyzable (free) fraction of T_3 and T_4, multiplying this by the total hormone concentration (see Table 216–2). In patients who have abnormal total T_4 and T_3 concentrations caused by changes in serum TBG concentration but who are euthyroid, the free hormone concentrations are normal. Unfortunately, such determinations are time consuming.

An indirect estimate of the free fraction of T_4 and T_3 can be obtained by estimating the thyroid hormone–binding ratio (THBR). These tests, formerly termed T_3 or T_4 uptake tests, are performed by analyzing the distribution of tagged T_3 or T_4 in a sample of dilute serum. A common method has been to add charcoal or resin to this sample and quantitate the fraction of the tagged iodothyronine bound to this matrix. The result should be expressed as the ratio of matrix-bound counts to serum protein-bound counts, with a typical normal range of 33 to 50 per cent. To improve reproducibility, this result should be normalized to that obtained in samples of normal sera assayed simultaneously, such that the normal range is 0.85 to 1.15. The ratio of tracer thyroid hormone bound to the inert matrix to that bound to serum protein is directly proportional to the free fraction of thyroid hormone. While the relative distribution of T_3 on the serum-binding proteins is slightly different from that of T_4 (T_3 is only weakly bound to transthyretin), its distribution is sufficiently similar so that in many laboratories it is used instead of T_4. The similarity between the free fraction of thyroid hormones and the THBR can be formalized by calculating the free T_4 (or T_3) index. This is the product of a normalized THBR value and the total serum T_4 or T_3 concentration. The normal range for these indices in units is approximately the same as that for the total thyroid hormone concentrations. In my laboratory, the normal free T_4 index is 4.7 to 10.5. The free T_4 index is an excellent approximation of the free T_4.

An alternative estimate of the free T_4 may be obtained by using one of several commercial kits. While there are some technical advantages to these tests, they do not measure the free T_4 directly, but provide only an estimate of its concentration, as does the free T_4 index. One notable clinical situation in which both methods often provide falsely high estimates of the free T_4 is in patients with familial dysalbuminemic hyperthyroxinemia. In patients with this syndrome a portion of the serum albumin binds T_4, but not T_3, with abnormally high affinity. The total T_4 value is elevated, but the free fraction of T_4 by dialysis is reduced; therefore the free T_4 concentration is normal. Since T_3 does not bind to the abnormal albumin with increased avidity, estimation of THBR employing T_3 is normal, and therefore a free T_4 index calculated using this value is elevated. Other artifacts in the analogue method kits result in the same falsely high estimate of free T_4. The use of T_4 in estimation of THBR would solve the problem in this syndrome and in other situations such as severe illness in which the changes in the binding of T_3 and T_4 are not identical. The terms T_3 *uptake* and T_3 *resin* are sometimes confused with the direct immunoassay of serum T_3 concentrations, and these terms should be discarded in favor of the THBR.

COMPARISON OF THE UTILITY OF T_4 AND T_3 DETERMINATIONS. The free T_4 index is the best screening test for thyroid dysfunction. It is superior to the free T_3 index by virtue of the fact that the principal thyroid secretory product is T_4. About 80 per cent of circulating T_3 derives from T_4 to T_3 conversion. Therefore, in patients who are sick or who have received any of the drugs listed in Table 216–3, which inhibit T_4 to T_3 conversion, the serum T_3 is invariably reduced relative to the serum T_4, but this does not imply thyroid disease. In hypothyroidism, serum T_3 may be normal despite significant impairment of thyroid function. On the other hand, in hyperthyroidism there is a small fraction of patients in whom serum T_4 is not elevated but the concentration of serum T_3 is. This condition is called T_3 *thyrotoxicosis* (see below).

SERUM REVERSE T_3 AND OTHER IODOTHYRONINES. The normal concentration of reverse T_3 is 15 to 30 ng per deciliter. It derives exclusively from peripheral metabolism of T_4, and its concentration in the blood reflects a combination of that process and the rate of its degradation. Its measurement is not generally useful clinically, although it is an excellent barometer of the rate of T_4 to T_3 conversion. Immunoassays have been developed for both monoiodinated and diiodinated thyronines, but these measurements do not have clinical applicability.

SERUM THYROID HORMONE–BINDING PROTEIN CONCENTRATIONS. The normal concentration of circulating TBG and transthyretin can be measured by immunoassay or by determination of the binding capacity. The normal concentration of TBG is 1.5 mg per deciliter. This quantity of protein binds approximately 20 μg of T_4 (1 mole T_4 per 1 mole TBG). The binding capacity of transthyretin is approximately 250 μg T_4 per deciliter. These measurements are rarely necessary for clinical purposes. Estrogen treatment increases the glycosylation of human TBG. This reduces its metabolic clearance rate and accounts for the two- to threefold increase in the circulating TBG during pregnancy or exogenous hyperestrogenism.

RADIOACTIVE IODINE UPTAKE (RAI UPTAKE). The normal 24-hour thyroidal uptake of radioiodine ranges from 5 to 30 per cent. All the radioiodine in the thyroid at this time is in the organified form. Because of the broad normal range for this test, it is not a reliable method for determining thyroid status. Its major diagnostic use is in separating patients who have hyperthyroidism caused by subacute thyroiditis in whom the uptake is reduced or absent from those with Graves' disease (see next section). It is contraindicated in pregnancy.

TESTS OF THYROID REGULATION

SERUM THYROTROPIN. The normal range for serum TSH is 0.5 to 5.0 μU per milliliter. In patients with thyroid hypofunction, TSH increases, and when thyroid function is autonomous, TSH is reduced, as expected from the normal feedback relationships (Fig. 216–3). Newer TSH assays can discriminate between normal TSH concentrations and those that are reduced. Previously it was necessary to employ the TRH infusion test to make this differentiation. With this immunometric assay (TSH-IMA), so called because a combination of monoclonal antibodies is usually employed, serum TSH values less than 0.1 μU per milliliter correlate well with absence of a TSH increase in response to TRH (see below). The TSH-IMA should prove to be useful in monitoring the status of hypothyroid patients receiving replacement therapy and those patients in whom TSH suppression is desired, such as those with thyroid carcinoma or TSH-dependent nodular goiter. It may also be used as a screening test in patients suspected of thyroid disease as an alternative to the free T_4 index (Fig. 216–4). Virtually all patients with clinical symptoms attributable to primary hypothyroidism have serum TSH concentrations greater than 20 μU per milliliter, and many subjects with minimal symptoms or goiter alone have results between 10 and 20 μU per milliliter. An elevation of the serum TSH concentration almost always indicates that thyroid function is impaired. It is also the critical test for separating patients with primary thyroid disease from those with hypothyroidism resulting from hypothalamic or pituitary dysfunction.

THYROTROPIN-RELEASING HORMONE INFUSION TEST. TRH can be infused intravenously and TSH measured in serum to determine whether TSH is present in the pituitary. Pituitary TSH is reduced in patients with hyperthyroidism and in those with autonomous thyroid hormone production and often in patients with hypothalamic pituitary disease. This test has been superseded by the TSH-IMA described above. Typical normal and pathologic responses are shown in Figure 216–5. In practice, a basal serum sample is obtained, followed by intravenous infusion of 400 μg of TRH over 1 minute. A second serum sample is obtained 30 minutes after the infusion, and both are assayed for TSH. In normal persons the minimal TSH increment is 2 μU per milliliter except in males over the age of 40, in the seriously ill, or in patients with depression or exogenous or endogenous glucocorticoid excess in whom the normal response can be lower. The response is amplified (30-minute value greater than 25 μU per milliliter) in patients with primary hypothyroidism. A significant increment in TSH eliminates the diagnosis of hyperthyroidism except in the extremely rare patient with the TSH-induced form of this disease.

METABOLIC INDICES OF THYROID STATUS

BASAL METABOLIC RATE (BMR). Since thyroid hormone is an important factor in the regulation of the rate of oxygen consumption, this test should theoretically be useful in evaluating thyroid status. However, it has given way to serum measurements, since these are more specific and usually more accurate. The normal range for the BMR is usually from -15 to $+5$ per cent.

DEEP TENDON REFLEX CONTRACTION AND RELAXATION TIMES. Thyroid status is reflected in the rate (not amplitude) of contraction and relaxation of skeletal muscle. These rates are more rapid in hyperthyroidism and slowed in hypothyroidism. Some clinicians have employed a kinemometer tracing to quantitate these events and have observed as high as 70 per cent diagnostic accuracy with this test. Like the BMR, it is less specific than serum hormone measurements, since hypothermia, peripheral neuropathy, gross edema, and many other conditions may slow the rate of relaxation. However, a clinically apparent delay in the relaxation phase of the deep tendon reflexes is almost invariably present in patients with significant hypothyroidism, although the more rapid relaxation in hyperthyroidism is difficult to appreciate visually.

ANATOMIC EVALUATION OF THE THYROID GLAND

THE THYROID SCAN. The capacity of the thyroid gland to trap ions such as I^- or molecules with a similar charge and configuration has provided a useful method for correlating structure and function. Of the iodine isotopes either ^{123}I or ^{131}I can be used. ^{123}I, although more expensive, is preferred for scanning, particularly in younger persons, since the radiation dose to the thyroid is 7.5 mrads per microcurie administered, as opposed to 800 mrads per microcurie for ^{131}I. Another isotope that gives a low radiation dose is $^{99m}TcO_4^-$ (pertechnetate), which is trapped, but not organified, by the thyroid. For this reason, a scan is obtained 30 minutes after intravenous injection of this isotope. The thyroid scan is usually used to determine the functional state

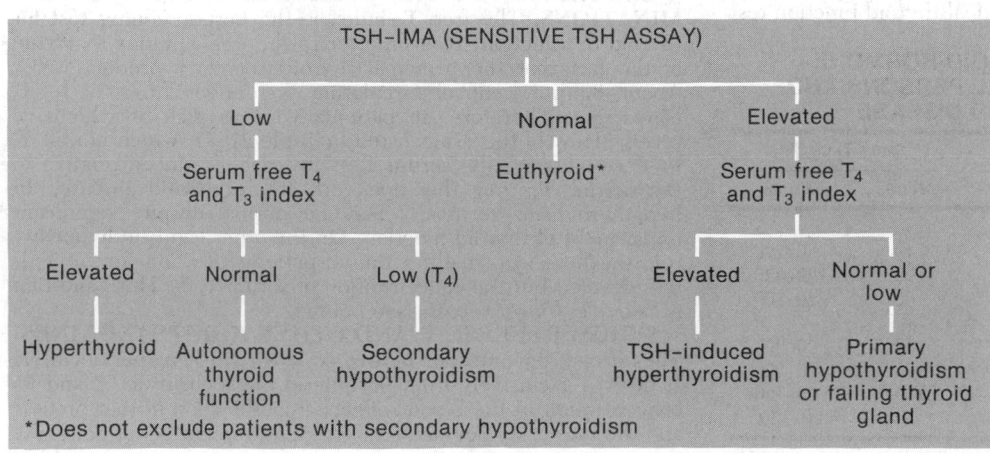

TSH-IMA (SENSITIVE TSH ASSAY)

Low — Normal — Elevated

Serum free T_4 and T_3 index — Euthyroid* — Serum free T_4 and T_3 index

Elevated — Normal — Low (T_4)   Elevated — Normal or low

Hyperthyroid — Autonomous thyroid function — Secondary hypothyroidism   TSH-induced hyperthyroidism — Primary hypothyroidism or failing thyroid gland

*Does not exclude patients with secondary hypothyroidism

FIGURE 216–4. Proposed schema for evaluation of patients based on the TSH-IMA. The TSH-IMA is capable of differentiating the lower limit of normal from the TSH concentration in the sera of patients with autonomous thyroid hyperfunction as well as quantifying elevated levels. The current experience suggests that this approach would not be useful in patients with nonthyroidal illness in whom TSH may be suppressed by factors other than thyroid hyperfunction.

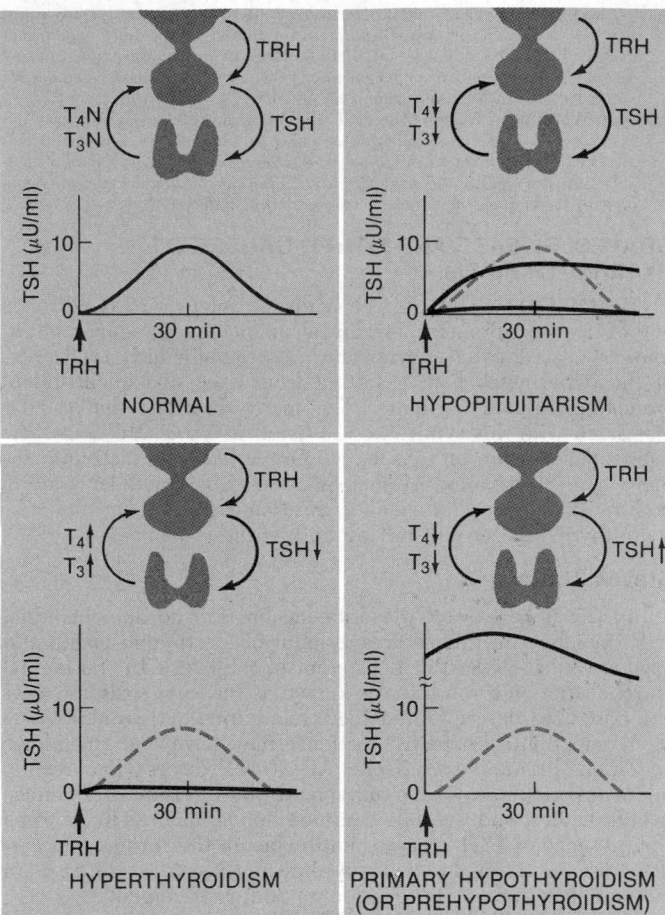

FIGURE 216–5. Typical responses to the infusion of TRH in patients with hyperthyroidism and primary and secondary hypothyroidism. In patients with hypopituitarism or hypothalamic disease virtually any TRH response pattern can be seen. The most pertinent diagnostic information is that serum TSH is not increased in a patient with a reduced serum free T_4 index.

of a palpable thyroid nodule (see later in chapter) or in evaluating masses in the neck or upper part of the chest to see if thyroid tissue is present.

THYROID ULTRASOUND. Whether a given thyroid mass is solid or cystic can be determined by ultrasonography. Ultrasound is now sufficiently sensitive to allow identification of 1- to 3-mm nodules that are too small to be palpated. Such nodules are present in as many as 40 per cent of the population and have unknown clinical significance. Ultrasound may serve as a useful objective method for following the response of a thyroid nodule to TSH suppressive therapy.

NEEDLE BIOPSY OR ASPIRATION. Either a fine (23 to 25 gauge) or cutting needle (Vim-Silverman) can be used to obtain a sample of thyroid cells for histologic examination. These techniques have received increased attention in recent years as a method for evaluation of thyroid nodules. Accurate interpretation of a fine-needle aspirate requires an experienced cytologist.

OTHER TESTS SPECIFICALLY RELATED TO THYROID FUNCTION OR DISEASE

ANTITHYROID ANTIBODIES. In autoimmune thyroid disease (Hashimoto's thyroiditis or Graves' disease), antibodies that bind to various antigens of thyroid tissue are present in the serum. The most important of these is the *thyroid microsomal antibody (TMAb)*. Thyroid peroxidase is the principal antigen in thyroid microsomes. TMAb is found in approximately 95 per cent of patients with Hashimoto's thyroiditis and in only about 10 per cent of adults with no apparent thyroid disease. The test is generally performed by a tanned red cell hemagglutination technique, and the results are reported as the highest titer causing agglutination. Titers in excess of 1:100 are significant. About 55 per cent of patients with Graves' disease also have circulating

TMAb's. *Thyroglobulin antibodies* (TgAb's) are also present in the serum of about 60 per cent of patients with Hashimoto's disease.

Antibodies directed against the thyroid TSH receptor (TRAb's), present in the sera of patients with Graves' disease, can be measured by many techniques that quantitate their interaction with the TSH receptor on thyroid cells. These immunoglobulins are usually stimulatory at the receptor level but may block TSH-TSH receptor interaction without causing stimulation (see Graves' Disease and Other Causes of Hyperthyroidism).

SERUM THYROGLOBULIN. The normal serum thyroglobulin (Tg) concentration is 2 to 20 ng per milliliter. Serum Tg may be increased in any patient with an enlarged thyroid or following acute trauma to the thyroid, whether a consequence of inflammation, surgery, or radiation. Thyroglobulin determinations are most useful in the follow-up of patients with metastatic thyroid carcinoma following thyroidectomy. An increase in serum Tg indicates the presence of tumor tissue, although a normal value does not eliminate this possibility. Serum thyroglobulin concentrations are generally reduced in patients who have *thyrotoxicosis factitia*, and this measurement may be useful in separating this group of patients from those with hyperthyroidism due to thyroid inflammation.

THE EFFECTS OF NONTHYROIDAL ILLNESS AND COMMON DRUGS ON THYROID FUNCTION TESTS

ILLNESS. The physiologic response to illness changes a number of aspects of thyroid function. With moderate to severe illness, T_4 deiodination to T_3 is impaired, leading to a decrease in the serum T_3 concentration. Since the type I deiodinase that converts T_4 to T_3 is also involved in reverse T_3 degradation, the metabolic clearance of reverse T_3 decreases and reverse T_3 concentrations rise, sometimes markedly so. In many patients, the binding of thyroid hormones to the normal serum hormone-binding proteins is reduced, which decreases serum T_4 concentrations and, depending on the degree of illness, increases the free fraction of both T_3 and T_4. It is not certain whether the increase in the free hormone fractions is due to the presence of a binding inhibitor in the serum or an intrinsic change in the binding affinity of the circulating thyroid hormone–binding proteins. Whatever the cause of this decreased thyroid hormone binding, it is not recognized by the simpler techniques used to assess this binding, such as the resin or charcoal T_3 uptake, nor by the current T_4-analogue–based estimates of free T_4. The clinical relevance of this difficulty is that the free thyroxine index may be artifactually low in sick patients. If the free thyroxine is measured by equilibrium dialysis or ultrafiltration, the free thyroxine concentrations are normal. With chronic illness, the serum TBG and albumin concentrations may be lowered and the free fraction of thyroid hormones and the THBR rise. This is especially true in patients with severe hepatic disease or nephrotic syndrome.

Serum TSH concentrations are generally normal in patients with critical illness, although a normal value is not physiologically appropriate for a patient with a substantive reduction in the serum free T_3. This observation has been used as evidence that there is hypothalamic or pituitary suppression of TSH release during illness which contributes to the abnormalities of thyroid function. Paradoxically, in rare patients the TSH may be elevated, although this is more common during recovery from severe illness. Since dopamine or glucocorticoid can directly suppress TSH, individuals receiving these agents may have an additional reason to develop transient pituitary hypothyroidism. Dopamine can suppress the appropriately elevated serum TSH of a patient with primary hypothyroidism, theoretically even into the normal range. Thus, the evaluation of patients receiving dopamine infusions is complex.

The goal of thyroid function testing in ill patients should be to rule out pre-existing hypothyroidism or hyperthyroidism. The sooner after admission estimates of serum thyroid hormone levels and TSH are obtained, the more effective the results are in achieving this goal. Thus, the clinician should have a low threshold for ordering thyroid function tests during the initial evaluation of the sick patient. In the presence of a markedly reduced free thyroxine index in an extremely ill patient, the concentration of serum TSH is very important. If this is not above 5 μU per milliliter, it is quite likely that the apparent thyroid dysfunction is due to the illness and/or its treatment. If TSH is elevated, parenteral replacement therapy with thyroxine should be provided, except for patients with symptomatic coronary artery disease (see below). Since it is usually impossible to evaluate critically ill patients endocrinologically or radiographically for hypothalamic-pituitary disease, it may be necessary to treat some empirically with replacement thyroxine and to provide glucocorticoid as well if the plasma cortisol concentration is not appropriate for the patient's physiologic stress (>15 μg per deciliter). Such patients are then evaluated for underlying thyroid/pituitary disease after recovering from their acute illness.

Occasionally a patient may have severe illness and an elevated level of serum T_4. Such patients should be suspected of having underlying autonomous thyroid function and often must be treated for hyperthyroidism if the serum TSH is less than 0.1 μU per milliliter. This phenomenon may also occur in patients with *acute psychiatric illness* and *hyperemesis gravidarum*. Serum T_3 determinations are usually not useful in patients with systemic illness owing to the impairment of T_4 to T_3 conversion. As with the patient suspected of thyroid hypofunction, definitive evaluation for underlying hyperthyroidism is performed when the patient's clinical condition permits.

DRUGS. Many therapeutic agents interfere (or appear to interfere) with thyroid function. The most commonly used and troublesome agents are listed in Table 216–3. The suppression of TSH secretion by dopamine or pharmacologic administration of glucocorticoids can transiently suppress TSH concentrations and may contribute to the reduced serum T_4 often seen in the seriously ill patient. Lithium carbonate may cause goiter or hypothyroidism, especially in individuals with mild underlying Hashimoto's thyroiditis. Phenylbutazone and sulfonylurea drugs inhibit normal thyroid gland function if given in sufficient dosage. In addition to the agents listed in Table 216–1, salicylates (>2 grams per day), phenytoin, fenclofenac, and furosemide all inhibit thyroid hormone-protein binding. Because these agents are weak binding inhibitors, they do not usually cause an abnormality in the THBR, and therefore the free T_4 index is mildly reduced. Agents that inhibit the type I 5'-deiodinase generally cause a reduction in serum T_3. If this is severe and prolonged enough, a compensatory increase in TSH secretion occurs, and the serum T_4 concentration rises. In patients receiving more than 200 mg propranolol, mild elevations in the serum free T_4 index are not uncommon.

Amiodarone has complex effects on thyroid function. Since this drug is about 30 per cent iodine by weight, it may produce all of the effects of iodide, that is, either hypothyroidism or hyperthyroidism. Even after discontinuation of this agent, tissue stores of iodine are significantly increased for 6 to 9 months. In addition, amiodarone seems to inhibit both pathways for T_4 to T_3 conversion and causes compensatory hyperthyroxinemia. There is some question whether it might also be a peripheral antagonist of thyroid hormone action, a further stimulus to a compensatory increase in TSH secretion. Iopanoic acid and ipodate, radiographic agents used for visualization of the gallbladder, are also effective inhibitors of T_4 to T_3 conversion. Their effect is transient and disappears within 3 to 4 weeks. All agents that inhibit peripheral T_4 to T_3 conversion raise the ratio of serum T_4 to T_3. In a patient receiving these agents, a TSH-IMA or a TRH test may be required to determine if hyperthyroidism is present.

Ain KB, Refetoff S: Relationship of oligosaccharide modification to the cause of serum thyroxine–binding globulin excess. J Clin Endocrinol Metab 66:1037, 1988. *Evidence that changes in serum TBG during pregnancy or estrogen therapy are a consequence of altered glycosylation and the resultant reduced hepatic clearance of this protein.*

Kaplan MM: Clinical and laboratory assessment of thyroid abnormalities. Med Clin North Am 69:863, 1985. *A detailed examination of the clinical application of thyroid function tests and a review of the effects of drugs that can influence these.*

Spencer CA, Lai-Rosenfeld AO, Guttler RB, et al.: Thyrotropin secretion in thyrotoxic and thyroxine-treated patients: Assessment by a sensitive immunoenzymometric assay. J Clin Endocrinol Metab 63:349, 1986. *The performance of a TSH-IMA in monitoring patients undergoing thyroid hormone replacement or with thyrotoxicosis.*

Surks MI, Hupart KH, Pan C, et al.: Normal free thyroxine in critical nonthyroidal illnesses measured by ultrafiltration of undiluted serum and equilibrium dialysis. J Clin Endocrinol Metab 67:1031, 1988. *Evidence showing that during severe illness free thyroxine concentrations are normal or even elevated despite markedly lowered total thyroxine concentrations.*

Wiersinga WM, Endert E, Trip MD, et al.: Immunoradiometric assay of thyrotropin in plasma: Its value in predicting response to thyroliberin stimulation and assessing thyroid function in amiodarone-treated patients. Clin Chem 32:433, 1986. *An example of the utility of the TSH-IMA in that most challenging diagnostic situation, the patient with amiodarone-induced thyroid dysfunction.*

GRAVES' DISEASE AND OTHER CAUSES OF HYPERTHYROIDISM

DEFINITION. The clinical syndrome of hyperthyroidism is one of the most dramatic in clinical medicine. The major symptoms associated with this syndrome are predominantly a reflection of the hypermetabolism resulting from excessive quantities of circulating thyroid hormone. The many disorders that can be associated with this syndrome are listed in Table 216–5 in their approximate order of frequency. Graves' disease accounts for more than 85 per cent of such patients. Toxic nodular goiters, both multinodular *(Plummer's disease)* and uninodular, and subacute thyroiditis account for the bulk of the remainder.

Graves' Disease

In 1835, Robert Graves described a clinical syndrome including hypermetabolism, diffuse enlargement of the thyroid gland, and *exophthalmos* (forward displacement of the eyes). In continental Europe, the same condition is known as Basedow's disease after von Basedow's description in 1840. In addition to thyroid involvement and ophthalmopathy, patients may have a dermatologic condition, *pretibial myxedema*. As Graves' disease is currently defined, patients may have only one of these three major clinical manifestations, and the only common denominator is likely to be the presence of TSH receptor antibodies in the serum. *Jodbasedow* disease refers to hyperthyroidism (Basedow's disease) in iodine-deficient patients after iodine (jod) replacement.

ETIOLOGY AND PATHOGENESIS. The precise etiology of Graves' disease is still not known, but it seems likely that it is an autoimmune disorder. Hyperthyroidism is its principal manifestation, yet TSH is suppressed and no intrinsic regulatory abnormalities in the thyroid have been identified. Thus the thyroid stimulation seems likely to be a consequence of a circulating, non-TSH, thyroid stimulator. This "stimulator" is now thought to be a γ globulin or a family of γ globulins.

It is postulated, with increasing evidence, that in Graves' disease, for reasons as yet unclear, B lymphocytes secrete antibodies directed against the TSH receptor. These antibodies, termed TRAb, are generally polyclonal and may be stimulatory or inhibitory at the receptor, depending on the nature of their interaction with the receptor site. The reason for the appearance of TRAb and their perpetuation in Graves' disease has not been elucidated. Assays for the presence of TRAb depend either on the capacity of the serum to activate adenylate cyclase in thyroid cell membranes or thyroid cell lines or to compete with labeled TSH for binding to the TSH receptor on thyroid cells or on guinea pig adipocyte membranes. TRAb are found in 85 to 90 per cent of patients with clinical evidence of Graves' disease.

The etiology of Graves' exophthalmopathy is not known. Patients with exophthalmos and particularly those with dermopathy almost invariably have high titers of circulating TRAb, suggesting

TABLE 216–5. DISEASES OR CLINICAL SYNDROMES ASSOCIATED WITH THYROTOXICOSIS

Graves' disease
Toxic multinodular goiter
Toxic adenoma
Iodide-induced hyperthyroidism
Subacute thyroiditis
Factitious (exogenous) thyrotoxicosis
Neonatal thyrotoxicosis (mother with Graves' disease)
TSH-secreting pituitary tumor
Nontumorigenic pituitary-induced hyperthyroidism
Choriocarcinoma (uterine or testicular origin) or hydatidiform mole
Struma ovarii
Hyperfunctioning thyroid carcinoma (usually metastatic)

that these two clinical manifestations represent the most severe form of this disease. Antibodies to soluble human eye muscle antigens were found in 17 of 23 patients with Graves' ophthalmopathy, but not in Graves' patients without this manifestation and rarely in those with Hashimoto's thyroiditis. This suggests a similar autoimmune etiology for ophthalmopathy and for hyperthyroidism. It has also been proposed that Tg-anti-Tg circulating immune complexes may bind to eye muscles and play a pathogenic role. Further studies will be required to resolve this question.

Emotional Factors in the Etiology of Hyperthyroidism. The emotional lability of the patient with hyperthyroidism has led many clinicians to question the role of psychologic trauma in the pathogenesis of this disease. Numerous anecdotes have been cited to suggest that emotional trauma may somehow trigger the onset of overt hyperthyroidism. If this is so, it would still appear to require participation of the immune system, since circulating TRAb are such a constant feature of the clinical picture. In my mind, it seems more likely that an episode of physical or emotional trauma brings the patient to medical attention, at which time pre-existing hyperthyroidism is recognized.

INCIDENCE. Graves' disease is common, affecting as many as 1.9 per cent of the female population and about a tenth that number of males, according to a population survey in northern England. It reaches its peak incidence in the third and fourth decades. The reason for the female predominance in this as in all thyroid diseases is not known. There is a strong familial component to Graves' disease with a family history of autoimmune thyroid disease (Graves' disease, Hashimoto's thyroiditis, or "goiter") in a significant fraction of patients. The importance of genetic inheritance in the predisposition to this syndrome has been confirmed by finding a higher relative risk of this condition in patients with the histocompatibility antigens HLA-B8 (Caucasians), HLA-B35 (Japanese), and HLA-Bw46 (Chinese).

PATHOLOGY. The thyroid of the patient with Graves' disease is diffusely enlarged and hypercellular. In patients undergoing thyroidectomy without prior treatment with antithyroid drugs or iodine, a diffusely hyperplastic epithelium is noted with little or no colloid present and often with lymphocytic infiltration, varying from minimal to extensive. In some specimens it is impossible to distinguish the microscopic picture from Hashimoto's thyroiditis (a condition sometimes called hashitoxicosis). If the patient receives iodide preoperatively, the gland contains large amounts of colloid, cells are of normal height, and the vascularity is markedly reduced. Other tissues show no specific changes except in severely hyperthyroid patients. In those situations there may be edema and focal necrosis in the liver with cellular infiltration.

In hyperthyroid patients with mild eye manifestations of Graves' disease such as lid retraction and stare, no significant orbital pathology is found, and these changes probably are due to the hyperthyroidism per se. In more severe cases, edema of the extraocular muscles occurs in association with infiltration with lymphocytes, plasma cells, and neutrophils. In addition, hydrophilic mucopolysaccharide collects in the orbital tissues. The conjunctivae may show perivascular lymphocytic infiltration and edema (*chemosis*). The end stage of these processes is fibrosis, which most often involves the inferior eye muscles, causing restriction of upward globe movement.

CLINICAL PICTURE. The common clinical symptoms of thyrotoxicosis are listed in Table 216–6. These occur in any

TABLE 216–6. COMMON SYMPTOMS AND SIGNS OF HYPERTHYROIDISM (THYROTOXICOSIS)

Symptoms	Signs
Nervousness and/or tremor	Tachycardia or atrial fibrillation
Weight loss (usually with increased appetite)	Widened pulse pressure with increased systolic and decreased diastolic pressures
Palpitations	
Heat intolerance and excessive perspiration	Hyperdynamic precordium and accentuated S1
Emotional lability	Warm, smooth skin
Muscle weakness	Tremor
Hyperdefecation	Proximal muscle weakness
	Thyroid enlargement or abnormality

patient with excessive thyroid hormone secretion whether due to Graves' disease or some other cause. They are a consequence of the stimulatory effect of thyroid hormone on the metabolic rate and on many other tissues, especially the heart and central nervous system. The typical patient with Graves' disease is in her mid-20's with symptoms that can often be dated to 6 to 12 months previously. The patient is nervous, anxious, and fidgeting, and speaks rapidly. She complains of her agitated fatigue, palpitations, and, in warmer climates, heat intolerance. There may be weight loss despite increased appetite, or the patient may merely report success in her efforts at weight control. An increased frequency of bowel movements and, rarely, diarrhea may be noted. Emotional lability is often apparent during the interview, and a history of deteriorating domestic or occupational relationships may be obtained. A history of neck swelling (often not noted first by the patient) may be present. Amenorrhea or oligomenorrhea is not uncommon. Rarer manifestations of hyperthyroidism include pruritus and urticaria. About 5 per cent of males may experience gynecomastia, and even less commonly *hypokalemic periodic paralysis* may occur. For unknown reasons, this condition is much more common in males of Oriental extraction.

Apathetic or Masked Hyperthyroidism. The symptoms given in Table 216–6 are those generally found in the younger patient. The clinician should be aware that in some patients, particularly the elderly, the clinical symptoms and signs of hypermetabolism may not be so dramatic. Rather than appearing agitated, the elderly patient with hyperthyroidism may be depressed. Weight loss and symptoms of congestive heart failure can be the predominant manifestations of the hypermetabolic syndrome. Often this is complicated by atrial fibrillation or other supraventricular tachyarrhythmia, leading to suspicion that the heart, rather than the thyroid, is the source of the problem. Because of the subtlety of this clinical form of hyperthyroidism it is recommended that any patient with the recent onset of atrial fibrillation have tests of thyroid function. In this way a reversible cause of congestive heart failure and/or recurrent arrhythmias may be recognized and appropriate treatment instituted.

Graves' Ophthalmopathy. Eye symptoms are present in more than 50 per cent of patients with Graves' disease but, except for modest lid lag and stare, are rare in patients with other causes of hyperthyroidism. This is a useful point in establishing the diagnosis. Common complaints are protruding eyes; easy tearing, especially on exposure to wind or cold; photophobia; a gritty foreign body sensation in the eyes; and, less commonly, diplopia (Fig. 216–6). The patient with significant *proptosis* (exophthalmos) may complain of irritation, particularly on arising, since the eyelids do not completely cover the sclera when the patient is sleeping (*lagophthalmos*). Rarely, severe chemosis, inflammation, and periorbital edema occur (malignant exophthalmos). Eye complaints are usually bilateral, but may be unilateral, and Graves' disease is one of the most common causes of unilateral exophthalmos.

Pretibial Myxedema. In a few patients with Graves' disease (1 to 2 per cent) a brawny, nonpitting swelling of the pretibial area, ankles, and/or feet is present. This can appear in plaques. It has an orange-skin appearance and is usually not tender. This dermopathy, found exclusively in Graves' disease, is termed *pretibial myxedema*. The name derives from the histologic similarity of the mucopolysaccharide infiltration of the subcutaneous tissues to that found in advanced hypothyroidism (myxedema).

Euthyroid Graves' Disease. In a small fraction of patients with Graves' disease, eye manifestations (unilateral or bilateral) with or without pretibial myxedema appear, but hyperthyroidism is not present. This can arise because of destruction of the thyroid as a result of coexistent Hashimoto's disease, or hyperthyroidism may be delayed in its appearance for months or years after the first eye symptoms. In many such patients, appropriate testing often reveals subtle evidence of thyroid dysfunction.

PHYSICAL SIGNS. In younger patients, tachycardia is almost universal. The systolic blood pressure is elevated primarily because of the increased inotropic effect of thyroid hormone on the heart. The diastolic pressure is reduced owing to a decrease in peripheral vascular resistance associated with increased skin capillary blood flow. Body temperature is usually normal. The

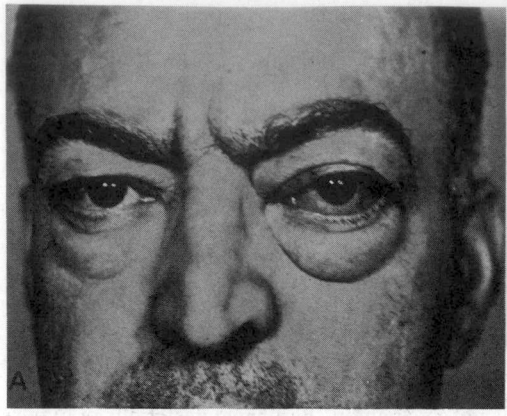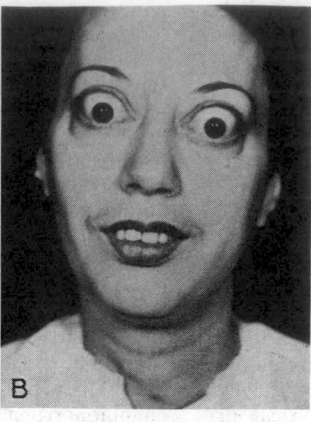

FIGURE 216–6. Two patients showing the typical ophthalmopathy characteristic of Graves' disease. Patient A demonstrates marked periorbital swelling, exophthalmos, chemosis, and conjunctival injection. The proptosis, limitation of extraocular movements, and other manifestations of ophthalmopathy are much more severe in Patient A than in Patient B. Patient B has marked widening of the palpebral fissures owing to lid retraction and also has significant proptosis. Patient A is euthyroid; Patient B is mildly hyperthyroid. (From Williams RH (ed.): Textbook of Endocrinology, 6th ed. Philadelphia, W. B. Saunders Company, 1981, p 189.)

skin is smooth, warm, and moist, and the patient may radiate heat. A fine tremor of the outstretched hands and occasionally *onycholysis* of the fourth and fifth fingers or clubbing (*thyroid acropachy*) are observed. The thyroid is almost always diffusely enlarged from 1.5 to 5 to 6 times normal. One third of elderly patients do not have a detectable goiter. The gland may be soft or firm, depending on the degree of hyperthyroidism and the level of iodine intake. Auscultation of the neck may reveal a multitude of sounds. In the younger patients a *venous hum* may be heard over the external jugular vein, particularly with the patient in the sitting position. Third or fourth heart sounds are heard easily in the neck, and a carotid bruit is not uncommon. In addition, a bruit over the thyroid gland is present in some patients, a manifestation of the high blood flow to this organ. A diffuse lymphadenopathy may be present in hyperthyroidism, and splenomegaly is found in 10 per cent of patients. The liver is not enlarged except in elderly patients with congestive failure. The neurologic examination shows tremor and proximal muscle weakness. Eye signs include lid lag, a failure of the upper lid to cover the upper margin of the iris as the globe traverses from upward to downward gaze, a widened palpebral fissure so that the sclera is visible above and/or below the iris, conjunctival injection and chemosis, periorbital swelling, and proptosis. The last-named finding is determined by measuring the distance from the lateral portion of the bony orbit to the cornea, using the *exophthalmometer*. In the white population this distance is 17 mm or less, with an upper limit of normal of 20 mm (22 mm for the black population). The difference between the two eye measurements should not be more than 3 mm. In addition to these moderate abnormalities, there may be impairment of globe movement. The most common restriction is in upward and/or outward gaze. This is due not to weakness of the superior eye muscles but to swelling and fibrosis of the inferior rectus and inferior oblique muscles beneath the globe. In addition, abduction and convergence may also be affected. Eye signs may be absent or mild, are usually bilateral when present, but may be asymmetric.

Laboratory Diagnosis of Hyperthyroidism

The various steps to be followed in establishing the laboratory diagnosis of hyperthyroidism are outlined in Figure 216–7. The initial screening test is to determine the free T_4 index. In virtually all patients an elevation in the free T_4 index is present. In the hospitalized patient the diagnosis may be somewhat more complicated if the patient is severely ill or has received any of the agents listed in Table 216–3, which cause inhibition of T_4 to T_3 conversion. In these patients an impairment of T_4 clearance or inhibition of T_4 to T_3 conversion may lead to an elevation in the serum free T_4 index without hyperthyroidism. Other causes of an elevated free T_4 index not necessarily indicating hyperthyroidism are familial dysalbuminemia (see Direct Tests of Thyroid Function), hyperemesis gravidarum, and acute psychosis. In the last two conditions the increase in the free T_4 index is usually transient. An alternate approach is to use the strategy depicted in Figure 216–4. Except in seriously ill patients this approach should be equally effective.

In such patients and in patients in whom the clinical suspicion of hyperthyroidism is present but the free T_4 index is normal or equivocal, a serum T_3 measurement is required. The ratio of T_3 to T_4 is increased in the thyroid gland in patients with Graves' disease. As a consequence, the T_3 production rate and the fraction of T_3 coming directly from the thyroid are increased. Thus the serum T_3 is elevated to a greater extent than is the serum T_4 (see Table 216–4). Patients in whom serum T_3 is elevated but the serum free T_4 index is not have *T_3 thyrotoxicosis*, which occurs in 3 to 5 per cent of patients in the United States but is more common in areas where dietary iodine is lower. The diagnosis of hyperthyroidism cannot be eliminated until the free T_3 index (as well as the free T_4 index) has been found to be normal. Even in hyperthyroidism, a substantial fraction of T_3 derives from periph-

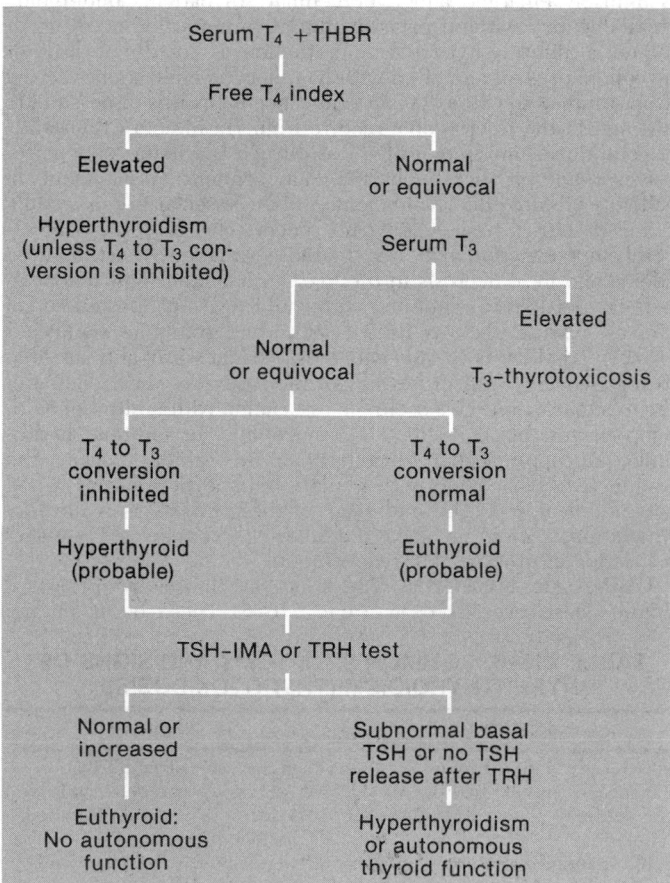

FIGURE 216–7. Laboratory diagnosis of hyperthyroidism. THBR refers to the thyroid hormone–binding ratio (formerly termed T_3 or T_4 uptake). TSH-IMA refers to the serum TSH measured by an immunometric assay that can discriminate between normal and suppressed as well as elevated TSH concentrations.

eral T_4 to T_3 conversion. Impairment of this process from any cause (illness or drugs) can lead to a reduction in serum T_3. However, in hyperthyroidism, even with severe illness, the serum T_3 is rarely depressed to less than 100 ng per deciliter. To eliminate the possibility of a TSH-producing pituitary tumor and to confirm the hyperthyroid state, the serum TSH should be measured. A normal TSH-IMA eliminates all forms of hyperthyroidism except the patient with increased TSH secretion (see Fig. 216–4). Since patients with fixed or autonomous, but not supranormal, thyroid hormone production also have a reduced serum TSH, an abnormal test does not always indicate the presence of hypermetabolism and the need for treatment.

In patients with a classic history and laboratory abnormalities, an RAI uptake and thyroid scan are not necessary to establish the diagnosis. However, if the hyperthyroidism is of brief (less than 3 months') duration, if the thyroid is not enlarged or if it is tender, subacute thyroiditis must be considered, and an uptake and scan should be performed after pregnancy has been excluded. These tests are also required when nodular goiter or factitious thyrotoxicosis is suspected (see Table 216–5).

Unilateral Ophthalmopathy. Since Graves' ophthalmopathy may be unilateral and not associated with frank hyperthyroidism, local pathology such as orbital tumor, pseudotumor of the orbit, cavernous sinus-carotid aneurysm, and sphenoid ridge meningioma must be considered. In addition to the free T_4 index, serum T_3, and TRH test, such patients require orbital radiography, ultrasonography, and computed tomography. In almost all patients with Graves' ophthalmopathy, bilateral involvement of the extraocular muscles is found even though clinically the process appears unilateral. Positive serum tests for TRAb or TMAb provide further support for this diagnosis.

OTHER CHEMICAL ABNORMALITIES ASSOCIATED WITH HYPERTHYROIDISM. In 5 to 20 per cent of patients with hyperthyroidism any of the following may be found: modest hypercalcemia, increased alkaline phosphatase (bone or hepatic isozyme), increased direct bilirubin, and a mild anemia of "chronic disease." Modest neutropenia may occur (1000 to 2000 per cubic millimeter).

Differential Diagnosis of Hyperthyroidism

Few clinical syndromes mimic hyperthyroidism. Pheochromocytoma and neurocirculatory asthenia may cause some clinical confusion, but appropriate laboratory testing eliminates these from consideration. Differentiation of patients with Graves' disease from those with other forms of hyperthyroidism is rarely difficult based solely on the history and physical examination (see Table 216–5). The use of the RAI uptake and scan to identify patients with subacute thyroiditis or nodular disease has been discussed. Iodine-induced hyperthyroidism is due to either multinodular goiter or Graves' disease (jodbasedow). Factitious thyrotoxicosis, the ingestion of excess thyroid hormone, should be considered particularly in paramedical personnel in whom symptoms and laboratory manifestations are associated with a nonpalpable thyroid gland. TSH-induced hyperthyroidism is diagnosed by finding an elevated or normal TSH in the presence of an increased free T_4 or T_3 index. It can be associated with either pituitary resistance to thyroid hormone or a thyrotroph tumor. Chorionic gonadotropin–induced hyperthyroidism is confirmed by the elevation in serum hCG in association with molar pregnancy or choriocarcinoma.

Treatment

TREATMENT OF HYPERTHYROIDISM OF GRAVES' DISEASE. The treatment of patients with Graves' disease must be considered in the context of its natural history. In 10 to 50 per cent of patients, depending on the series, thyroid function returns to normal (remission) in association with (but probably not because of) drug treatment directed at the thyroid, not at the apparent primary defect in the immune system. If the patient destined for remission could be identified, a rational treatment approach for this disease could be developed. At present this is not possible, although a reduction in circulating TRAb titers generally accompanies remission, and it may be possible to employ such assays in the future to guide therapy. Early studies suggested that if patients were given antithyroid drugs for 12 to 18 months, approximately 50 per cent would remain euthyroid

after discontinuation of the drugs. More recently that fraction may have decreased to 10 to 20 per cent. The reason for the apparent change in the natural history of hyperthyroidism in the United States is not clear. One possible explanation is the recent increase in iodine intake. Since antithyroid drugs markedly deplete thyroidal iodine, the capacity to re-establish excessive secretion of thyroid hormone could be influenced by the iodine supply. In patients with Graves' disease who undergo a remission, hypothyroidism may occur some 20 to 30 years later. This is presumably autoimmune in origin, further emphasizing the similarities between Graves' disease and Hashimoto's thyroiditis. Lastly, in patients whose condition is in remission, relapse may occur months to years later.

As the underlying cause for Graves' disease is not known, no specific therapy for this condition is available. There are two phases of the treatment of the hyperthyroidism of Graves' disease. The first is acute therapy with the goal of re-establishing euthyroidism. The second phase is definitive therapy, the induction of a permanent alteration in thyroid function.

Short-Term Treatment of Hyperthyroidism. Antithyroid Drugs. In a typical patient with hyperthyroidism caused by Graves' disease, the first step in management is to suppress the elevated thyroid hormone secretion rate. The drugs of choice for this purpose are derivatives of thiourea. In the United States, propylthiouracil (PTU) and methimazole (Tapazole) are used. Both inhibit the organification of iodine by the thyroid gland as their major mechanism of action. Neither drug affects I^- trapping, nor does either inhibit the release of preformed thyroid hormone. PTU, but not methimazole, is an inhibitor of T_4 to T_3 conversion, giving it a modest therapeutic advantage over the latter agent. This drug has special importance in the short-term treatment of hyperthyroidism. Carbimazole, rapidly converted to methimazole in the body, is used in Europe and is equal in potency to methimazole.

PTU and methimazole are rapidly absorbed and are probably concentrated by the hyperactive thyroid. Although the plasma half-life is relatively short, suggesting the need for frequent dosage, in practice it is often possible to maintain satisfactory suppression of thyroid hormone synthesis by administration of these drugs twice or even only once per day. Methimazole is approximately 15 times as potent as PTU. Initial treatment consists of 300 to 450 mg of PTU per day (or the equivalent of methimazole) divided into three doses. Rarely as much as 1600 mg per day of PTU is required, but problems with compliance are common at such dosages. Since there is a 5- to 10-day half-time for the disappearance of the metabolic effects induced by excess thyroid hormone, it is not unusual for the serum level of T_4 to fall before the patient begins to obtain relief from the symptoms of hyperthyroidism. It is my practice to see the patient 3 to 4 weeks after the initial visit, obtaining a free T_4 index and serum T_3 at that point to ascertain the progress of therapy. If clinical improvement has not occurred, the serum T_4 has not decreased, and compliance has been maintained, the dose of antithyroid drug should be increased. After the first months of treatment, the dose of antithyroid drug can be reduced to a level of 100 to 300 mg per day of PTU, and the patient seen at 2- to 3-month intervals. In patients to be treated for 6 to 18 months, therapy can be monitored by both clinical and laboratory parameters. The serum T_3-T_4 ratio is increased because of intrathyroidal iodine deficiency and the increased thyroidal T_3-T_4 ratio in Graves' disease. Therefore both serum T_3 and the free T_4 index should be monitored. Serum TSH may increase if the serum T_4 falls below normal even if serum T_3 is normal. This is undesirable, since it can lead to further thyroid enlargement and possibly an exacerbation of eye symptoms.

Thiourea derivatives have several side effects. A maculopapular rash occurs in 2 to 8 per cent of patients but does not usually require discontinuation of the drug. Both agents can rarely cause hepatocellular damage, and PTU can cause vasculitis. The most serious side effect of both agents is agranulocytosis. This occurs in 2 to 5 of 1000 patients and can be fatal if not recognized. Since this reaction may be abrupt in onset and is so rare, it is not, in the opinion of many experts, necessary to monitor the white blood count (WBC) at frequent intervals. Instead, a baseline WBC and differential are obtained, and the patient is cautioned on each visit about the symptoms and significance of agranulocytosis. The patient is instructed to report immediately if infection occurs and to stop the medication. The WBC and differential are repeated and the drug discontinued permanently if indicated. The reaction may appear at any time during therapy and does not appear to be dose related (except at extremely high doses). It is seen most commonly in the first few months of therapy. If such a reaction occurs, the drug should be withdrawn and appropriate supportive care provided. Recovery occurs in almost all patients, and an alternative treatment method should then be used. Special precautions about the use of antithyroid drugs in pregnancy are discussed below. Iodide (saturated solution of potassium iodide, 1 gram KI per milliliter) 3 drops twice a day or Lugol's solution (125 mg I⁻ per milliliter) 10 drops three times a day is the most effective antithyroid drug for short-term use, since it inhibits both thyroid hormone release and thyroid hormone synthesis (through the Wolff-Chaikoff effect). Iodide alone can be given to patients with allergies to thiourea drugs to suppress thyroid function for periods of 10 to 28 days. Since the initially depressed hormone release increases gradually during treatment, iodide administration should not be prolonged beyond 2 to 3 weeks. Iodide is often used to decrease the vascularity of the thyroid gland in the preparation of patients who are to have surgery. Since it interferes with the subsequent administration of ¹³¹I, it should not be used in the weeks prior to this treatment.

The benefits of bed rest, adequate diet, and the extrication of the patient from the usual occupational or domestic pressures cannot be overemphasized. Remarkable clinical improvement is often noted within 1 to 2 days simply as a result of hospitalization. The short-term treatment of severe hyperthyroidism is discussed below under Thyroid Storm.

β-Adrenergic Blocking Agents and Other Drugs. The similarity of the symptoms of hyperthyroidism to those of catecholamine excess is striking. The molecular basis for this similarity is not clearly established. Although animal studies have shown thyroid hormone–induced increases in β-adrenergic receptors in cardiac tissue, the receptor number is normal in lymphocytes from patients with thyrotoxicosis. Plasma catecholamine concentrations are normal in hyperthyroidism. Nevertheless, blockade of β-adrenergic receptors by propranolol or other β-receptor antagonists may result in symptomatic improvement prior to a decrease in serum thyroid hormones. A dose of 20 to 40 mg of propranolol every 4 to 6 hours may be used, but patients with congestive heart failure or bronchial asthma should not receive this therapy. In most patients with mild to moderate hyperthyroidism this adjunctive therapy is not necessary and may complicate the therapeutic regimen. In patients with more profound tachycardia or with thyroid storm (see below), it may have an important beneficial effect. Propranolol, although decreasing pulse rate and cardiac output in patients with hyperthyroidism, does not alter the elevated basal metabolic rate. Therefore the tissues continue to consume oxygen at a high rate in the presence of a decrease in cardiac output.

Lithium inhibits release of preformed thyroid hormone from the thyroid gland, probably by inhibiting hydrolysis of thyroglobulin, and may also inhibit peripheral T_4 degradation. In patients with allergies to thiourea drugs and iodide, lithium carbonate 0.9 to 1.5 grams per day (serum lithium concentrations of 0.5 to 1.0 mEq per liter) may be of value in the treatment of acute hyperthyroidism. Serum lithium levels must be closely monitored, as some of the toxic effects of lithium are similar to those of thyrotoxicosis.

Iopanoic acid (Telepaque) and ipodate (Oragrafin) contain iodide and also are potent inhibitors of type I and type II 5'-deiodinase activities. These agents therefore appear to be ideal for short-term treatment of hyperthyroidism. However, both remain in the body for long periods, which may prohibit subsequent ¹³¹I therapy. They can be used in emergency situations, especially if surgery is contemplated as definitive therapy, and might also be as effective as PTU for blocking T_4 to T_3 conversion, such as might be required in the rare patient with severe exogenous thyrotoxicosis.

The Second Phase of Hyperthyroidism Treatment. If the symptoms of hyperthyroidism are not severe or after short-term treatment of symptoms with thiourea drugs, a decision must be made as to long-term therapy. There are three choices: further antithyroid drugs with hopes of a spontaneous remission, surgery, or radioiodine. None of these is ideal, and the choice for each patient must be made individually.

Long-Term Antithyroid Drug Therapy. If long-term antithyroid drug therapy is undertaken in anticipation of a remission, it should be continued for 6 to 18 months. If the quantities of drug required to maintain euthyroidism remain relatively large (e.g., 200 mg of PTU or greater) and serum T_3 and T_4 rise when the dosage is reduced, then a remission has not occurred. If the thyroid becomes smaller and the required amount of antithyroid drug lower, then a remission is probable. Some authorities recommend a TSH assay at this juncture, but I prefer to determine serum T_3 and T_4, to discontinue the treatment, and to repeat these tests in 4 weeks. The serum T_3 is especially important, since it may become elevated prior to the T_4 when a relapse occurs. If thyroid hormones remain normal, the patient should be seen at bimonthly intervals for 1 year, at which time the visits can be reduced in frequency.

Surgery. Surgical removal of a portion of the thyroid gland to regulate hyperthyroidism is a time-honored and effective treatment in the hands of expert surgeons. Hyperthyroidism rarely recurs, although roughly 50 to 60 per cent of patients eventually become hypothyroid. In most patients, hyperthyroidism is controlled by antithyroid drugs for 1 to 2 months prior to surgery. About 7 to 10 days before surgery, saturated solution of potassium iodide or Lugol's solution should be given to reduce the vascularity of the thyroid (see above).

Alternatively, propranolol alone may be used to prepare the patient, or it may be combined with I⁻. One to 2 weeks of pretreatment with 40 mg of propranolol every 6 hours has been given. This approach should not be employed for patients who can undertake standard preoperative therapy with thiourea drugs. Aside from hypothyroidism, other potential complications of surgery include neck hemorrhage, recurrent laryngeal nerve damage, and hypoparathyroidism. In highly experienced clinics, such complications are quite rare (<1 per cent).

Radioiodine. Treatment of hyperthyroidism with ¹³¹I has been used since the late 1940's. The principal complication of this treatment is hypothyroidism, which occurs in about 10 per cent of patients in the first year and increases about 5 per cent per year thereafter over 20 years. Depending on the dose given, about 20 per cent of patients require a second treatment. No increased risk of thyroid carcinoma or leukemia occurs after such treatment. For many years, there was a reluctance to employ ¹³¹I in the treatment of women in the childbearing age group, but the ovarian dose from a typical 10-mCi treatment is approximately 2 to 4 rads, which is in the same range as that from hysterosalpingography or a barium enema. Although any unnecessary radiation is to be avoided, the calculated increase in the gamete mutation rate from exposure in this range is only a small fraction of the spontaneous mutation rate. Thus ¹³¹I therapy does not appear to offer a significant risk of fetal malformation, although it is recommended that pregnancy not be undertaken for 6 months after this therapy to avoid transient radiation-induced changes in the gametes.

I generally pretreat patients who are to have ¹³¹I therapy with thiourea derivatives to provide symptomatic relief and avoid the remote chance of an exacerbation of hyperthyroidism from radiation thyroiditis. These are discontinued 4 days prior to determining the 24-hour ¹³¹I uptake. My practice is to administer orally an amount of ¹³¹I which when multiplied by the RAI uptake will result in thyroidal accumulation of 6 mCi ¹³¹I. This results in an average dose of 80 to 90 μCi per gram, or 6000 to 7000 rads, which is associated with resolution of hyperthyroidism in about 80 per cent of patients within 6 months. Therapy with thiourea drugs may be restarted after 1 week, although it is not usually required. Patients are seen monthly thereafter with appropriate diagnostic and therapeutic measures to maintain the euthyroid state. At least 6 months is allowed to elapse before considering a second treatment. Since radioiodine crosses the placenta and would be concentrated by the thyroid of the fetus at 12 weeks and older, it is imperative that the possibility of pregnancy be eliminated before radioiodine is administered.

The therapist administering radioiodine is committed to the planning of adequate follow-up. This consists of thoroughly informing the patient about the risks of delayed hypothyroidism (occurring in 80 to 100 per cent), providing written documentation of the treatment and its complications, and maintaining proper communication with referring physicians as to the need for indefinite follow-up. Patients are alerted to the symptoms of hypothyroidism and instructed that after the acute phase of treatment they should be seen at least every 4 to 6 months for appropriate thyroid function testing until hypothyroidism appears and treatment is initiated.

Choice of Therapy. None of the three long-term therapies for hyperthyroidism is ideal. Some thyroidologists do not use radioiodine in patients under the age of 35 or 40 because of the fear of long-term complications, whereas others employ radioiodine routinely in the treatment of hyperthyroidism in children. On balance, from the point of view of lack of immediate complications and effectiveness, radioiodine treatment is the most effective approach currently available. My approach is to inform the patient of all treatment options and to recommend antithyroid drugs only to patients who have goiters less than three times normal or in patients who are hesitant regarding radioiodine therapy. In women in whom pregnancy is planned, a requirement for high doses of antithyroid drugs indicates the need for definitive treatment prior to undertaking pregnancy. Surgery is recommended only for patients with extreme thyroid enlargement or those who have coexisting nonfunctioning thyroid nodules. The physician advising patients regarding this decision must consider not only these theoretical arguments and the patient's preferences but also the availability of an experienced surgeon.

Graves' Disease and Pregnancy. The peak incidence of Graves' disease occurs in women during the reproductive period. Therefore, it is not uncommon to find hyperthyroidism in a pregnant patient or for pregnancy to occur during therapy with antithyroid drugs. There is a tendency for Graves' disease to exacerbate during the first trimester of pregnancy and to ameliorate during the third trimester. One to 2 months after delivery, an exacerbation is not uncommon. Since PTU and methimazole cross the placenta, whereas thyroid hormones do not do so in appreciable amounts, minimal quantities of these agents must be used during pregnancy. PTU crosses the placenta less well than does methimazole. While pregnant patients tolerate moderate degrees of hyperthyroidism quite well, uncontrolled thyrotoxicosis is associated with an increased risk of spontaneous abortion and may be associated with thyroid storm at the time of delivery.

With these facts in mind, pregnant patients with hyperthyroidism should be seen at monthly intervals, with careful clinical examination supplemented by measurements of serum T_3, T_4, and THBR. It should be recalled that the normal range for both serum T_4 and T_3 is higher during pregnancy (see Table 216–4). PTU should be given at the lowest dosage that maintains the patient at an acceptable euthyroid state. I do not employ supplemental thyroid hormones in the treatment of most pregnant hyperthyroid patients. An attempt to reduce the antithyroid drug dose should be made as the third trimester approaches. If the patient's hyperthyroid symptoms cannot be controlled on less than 300 to 400 mg of PTU per day, then subtotal thyroidectomy should be considered during the second trimester. Iodides can be given for 7 to 10 days in preparation for surgery but should not be given over a long period during pregnancy, since the fetus may develop hypothyroidism because of transplacental iodide transfer and the Wolff-Chaikoff effect.

The newborn infant of the mother with Graves' disease should be examined carefully for either hypothyroidism as a consequence of excessive antithyroid drug or hyperthyroidism resulting from transplacental passage of TRAb. In either situation goiter may be present, which may lead to respiratory embarrassment. Even the most meticulously managed patients may have infants with modest reductions in serum T_4 that quickly normalize in the first week of life. Neonatal hyperthyroidism is transient but occasionally must be treated with antithyroid drugs and digitalis for tachycardia.

The quantities of PTU in the milk of mothers receiving 200 to 300 mg PTU per day are not great enough to cause impairment of an infant's thyroid function. It seems likely that nursing mothers could take PTU at low doses, although the infant could still be at risk for nonthyroidal complications of this drug. Methimazole (and presumably carbimazole) is present in milk in significant amounts and should not be given to nursing mothers.

Thyroid Storm. Some patients with hyperthyroidism develop severe manifestations that are exaggerations of many of the symptoms listed in Table 216–6. Often these occur because of superimposed stress or infection. The patient may be febrile, have abdominal pain, and become delirious, obtunded, or psychotic. This condition, called *thyroid storm,* has a mortality of 20 to 40 per cent. It should be suspected in any patient with severe hyperpyrexia, or extreme tachycardia, particularly if goiter is present. Patients with suspected thyroid storm should be hospitalized and treated with a protocol such as is outlined in Table 216–7. I⁻ is the most effective agent for inhibiting release of preformed thyroid hormone. If it is thought that the patient has a surgical abdomen, intravenous propranolol may be used intraoperatively to control tachycardia, assuming that there are no contraindications. The line between severe hyperthyroidism and thyroid storm is nebulous. In patients with severe symptoms but without fever, I⁻ should be added to PTU therapy to achieve a more rapid decrease in thyroid hormones. The I⁻ can be discontinued after 1 week.

Treatment of Ophthalmopathy. In most patients with ophthalmopathy no specific therapy is needed. Return of the patient to the euthyroid state often results in amelioration of many of the minor symptoms, including stare and lid lag. It is important to avoid hypothyroidism, as anecdotal data suggest that this may be associated with an exacerbation of eye symptoms. The patient may note periorbital edema, especially on arising in the morning. An extra pillow or elevation of the head of the bed will relieve this. Alternatively, a diuretic can be administered at bedtime. In patients with more severe symptoms, artificial tears or 1 per cent methylcellulose are prescribed.

A small fraction of patients with Graves' disease have more severe problems than can be relieved by these minor therapeutic measures. In patients with severe proptosis, desiccation of the sclera or cornea may occur at night because of lagophthalmos. Taping the lids closed at night may alleviate this symptom, although lateral tarsorrhaphy is a more permanent solution. Diplopia may be treated by prisms or, if permanent, by muscle repositioning or relief of fibrous adhesions. This procedure should not be performed until the eye disease has stabilized, often a matter of 2 to 3 years. In the patient with severe inflammation and chemosis *(malignant exophthalmos),* prednisone is required. Although 15 to 20 mg per day may be sufficient, in many patients

TABLE 216–7. MANAGEMENT OF PATIENTS WITH THYROID STORM

Diagnostic
1. Serum T_3 and T_4 concentrations, resin or charcoal T_3 uptake
2. Appropriate evaluation for underlying precipitating causes such as infection, acute surgical abdomen, central nervous system lesions, or psychological trauma
3. Baseline WBC and differential, electrolytes, Ca, P
4. Plasma cortisol

Therapeutic
1. Intravenous fluids—dextrose with or without electrolytes as indicated, multivitamins
2. Propylthiouracil, 400 mg every 6 hours (by nasogastric tube, if necessary), to inhibit thyroid hormone synthesis and block T_4 to T_3 conversion
3. Sodium iodide, 250 mg every 6 hours (orally or intravenously)
4. Hydrocortisone, 50 to 100 mg every 6 hours intravenously
5. External cooling and acetaminophen (300 to 600 mg) every 4 to 6 hours for severe hyperpyrexia (do not use salicylates, which increase free thyroid hormones and oxygen consumption)
6. Propranolol—in patients without asthma, chronic bronchitis, or nonarrhythmia-related, congestive heart failure, 10 to 40 mg may be given every 4 to 6 hours orally; a slow intravenous infusion of 1 mg per minute for 2 to 10 minutes with careful monitoring of blood pressure and ECG may be used if oral therapy is not feasible; propranolol may precipitate pulmonary edema in a few patients with hyperthyroidism; reserpine or guanethidine do not appear to have any advantages over propranolol in this situation
7. Oxygen may be helpful
8. Digitalis glycosides should be employed for therapy of congestive failure and for blockade of a rapid ventricular response to an atrial tachyrhythmia
9. Appropriate treatment of precipitating event if any

as much as 100 mg per day is necessary with the attendant complications of treatment. Such patients should have frequent measurements of visual acuity and visual fields. Deterioration of either test is an emergency requiring steroid treatment and ophthalmologic consultation. An alternative treatment is orbital irradiation, 2000 rads being given to the retro-orbital region to suppress local lymphocytic infiltration. This is usually used in conjunction with glucocorticoid administration. In the case of optic compression or persistent corneal ulceration, surgical decompression may be required. Fortunately, in most patients the severity of the eye manifestations abates after 12 to 18 months, although in many the proptosis never reverts to normal.

Pretibial Myxedema. The lesions of pretibial myxedema are not generally incapacitating but may be cosmetically disfiguring. They may be treated with topical application of glucocorticoids, with enhancement of absorption by occlusive dressings if necessary.

PROGNOSIS. In most patients, Graves' disease is a benign disorder in which the physician can play an important role in providing considerable relief to the patient. Because of the complications of treatment and the possibility of hypothyroidism even in patients with a spontaneous remission, patients with Graves' disease require lifelong observation.

TREATMENT OF OTHER CAUSES OF HYPERTHYROID-ISM. The short-term treatment of hyperthyroidism associated with toxic multinodular goiter or toxic adenoma does not differ from that of patients with Graves' disease. These entities are discussed in detail later in the chapter. The hyperthyroidism associated with subacute thyroiditis (particularly the lymphocytic variety) is discussed in the section Thyroiditis.

TSH-secreting pituitary tumor must be treated by surgery. Patients with this condition are identified and separated from the group with nontumorigenic TSH-induced hyperthyroidism by finding an elevation of the serum α-TSH subunit as well as of TSH. Nontumorigenic hypersecretion of TSH is thought to be due to a reduction in feedback sensitivity to T_3 and T_4 at the pituitary level. Such patients are treated with antithyroid drugs. In patients with choriocarcinoma or hydatidiform mole, removal of the tumor relieves these symptoms. Extremely rare is the ovarian teratoma containing thyroid tissue, *struma ovarii*. This should be treated surgically. In general, thyroid carcinoma does not function well enough to lead to hyperthyroidism. Hyperthyroidism can occur if extensive metastases that retain a significant degree of function are present, as may be seen occasionally in follicular carcinoma. This condition is readily diagnosed and is treated with [131]I.

Burrow GN: The management of thyrotoxicosis in pregnancy. N Engl J Med 313:562, 1985. *A review of factors to be considered when managing the pregnant patient with active Graves' disease.*

Cohen JH, Ingbar SH, Braverman LE: Thyrotoxicosis due to ingestion of excess thyroid hormone. Endocr Rev 10:113, 1989. *A review of the approach to the patient suspected of ingesting excess thyroid hormone.*

Davis PJ, Davis FB: Hyperthyroidism in patients over the age of 60 years. Medicine 53:161, 1974. *An excellent summary of the clinical syndrome of hyperthyroidism in the elderly patient.*

Gesundheit N, Petrick PA, Nissim M, et al.: Thyrotropin-secreting pituitary adenomas: Clinical and biochemical heterogeneity. Ann Intern Med 111:827, 1989. *Thorough description of a rare but important cause of hyperthyroidism—thyrotropin-secreting pituitary tumors.*

Henneman G, Krenning EP, Sankaranarayanan K: Place of radioactive iodine in treatment of thyrotoxicosis. Lancet 1:1369, 1986. *The author makes a persuasive argument for the use of radioiodine as the first-line treatment for patients with Graves' disease. A brief but thorough review of the pros and cons of this approach to therapy.*

McKenzie JM, Zakarija M: Clinical review 3: The clinical use of thyrotropin receptor antibody measurements. J Clin Endocrinol Metab 69:1093, 1989. *A review of when and when not to request thyrotropin receptor antibody measurements in patients suspected of Graves' disease.*

Silva JE: Effects of iodine and iodine containing compounds on thyroid function. Med Clin North Am 69:881, 1985. *The author reviews all aspects of iodine excess and deficiency. The discussion of iodide-induced hyperthyroidism is particularly relevant for this section.*

Smallridge RC, Parker RA, Wiggs EA, et al.: Thyroid hormone resistance in a large kindred: Physiologic, biochemical, pharmacologic, and neuropsychologic studies. Am J Med 86:289, 1989. *A review of the clinical manifestations of thyroid hormone resistance in a large family.*

Smith BR, McLachlan SM, Furmaniak J: Autoantibodies to the thyrotropin receptor. Endocr Rev 9:106, 1988. *Studies of the etiology of Graves' disease are reviewed.*

HYPOTHYROIDISM AND MYXEDEMA

DEFINITION. *Hypothyroidism* is the clinical syndrome that results from a deficiency of thyroid hormone. In severe hypothyroidism a hydrophilic mucopolysaccharide substance accumulates in subcutaneous tissues, causing a nonpitting edema referred to as *myxedema*. Some authorities use the terms *hypothyroidism* and *myxedema* interchangeably, whereas others reserve the latter term for the severe form of this syndrome.

ETIOLOGY. A list of causes to be considered in patients with hypothyroidism is given in Table 216–8. *Primary hypothyroidism*, that caused by thyroid gland malfunction, accounts for over 95 per cent of such cases, of which Hashimoto's thyroiditis, idiopathic myxedema (probably a variant of Hashimoto's thyroiditis), and thyroid destruction resulting from ^{131}I therapy or surgery for hyperthyroidism account for the greatest proportion. Hashimoto's and subacute thyroiditis are discussed in the next section. Hypothyroidism after therapeutic irradiation to the thyroid area for lymphoma or Hodgkin's disease is found in 10 to 30 per cent of these patients, usually within 1 to 2 years of treatment.

Hypothyroidism can also occur with normal or nearly normal thyroid tissue when there is a superimposed stress on thyroid hormone synthesis. Hypothyroidism may be caused either by severe iodine deficiency (<25 μg iodine per day) or by naturally occurring goitrogens such as have been found in Colombia or are generated by eating the cassava plant in Africa (see Sporadic Goiter and Endemic Goiter). In patients with Graves' disease, especially after RAI treatment, or in those with mild Hashimoto's thyroiditis, iodine excess may cause hypothyroidism through the Wolff-Chaikoff effect (I^--induced inhibition of organification). These glands are unable to reduce I^- uptake in the presence of an elevated plasma I^- as normally occurs. The drugs listed in Table 216–8 inhibit organification of thyroidal I^-. In most cases the hypothyroidism associated with these drugs is mild.

Screening of newborns for hypothyroidism is now widely practiced, and the incidence of this condition is about 1 in 4000 births. About 65 per cent of infants with congenital hypothyroidism in North America have thyroid agenesis or hypoplasia, 25 per cent have ectopic thyroid glands, and about 10 per cent have

TABLE 216–8. CAUSES OF HYPOTHYROIDISM

I. **Primary hypothyroidism**
   A. Acquired
      1. Destructive lesions
         a. Hashimoto's thyroiditis
         b. Idiopathic myxedema (probably the end-stage of Hashimoto's thyroiditis)
         c. [131]I therapy for hyperthyroidism
         d. Subtotal thyroidectomy, especially for Graves' disease
         e. Therapeutic external x-ray treatment to the neck for other diseases
         f. After subacute thyroiditis (may be transient)
         g. Cystinosis
      2. Impaired function of a normal or nearly normal gland
         a. Endemic goiter—iodine deficiency or naturally occurring goitrogens
         b. Iodine excess (>6 mg per day) in patients with underlying thyroid disease
         c. Drug-induced: lithium carbonate, para-aminosalicylic acid, thiourea drugs, sulfonamides, phenylbutazone, and others
   B. Congenital
      1. Defects in enzymes required for thyroid hormone synthesis (congenital goiter)
      2. Thyroid agenesis
      3. Thyroid dysgenesis or ectopy
      4. Maternal iodide or antithyroid drugs
II. **Secondary hypothyroidism**
   A. Hypothalamic dysfunction
      1. Neoplasms
      2. Eosinophilic granuloma
      3. Therapeutic irradiation
   B. Pituitary dysfunction
      1. Neoplasms
      2. Pituitary surgery or irradiation
      3. Idiopathic hypopituitarism
      4. Sheehan's syndrome (postpartum pituitary necrosis)
      5. Dopamine infusion and/or severe illness(?)
III. **Tissue resistance to thyroid hormone**

defects in one of the steps required for thyroid hormone synthesis (see Sporadic Goiter and Endemic Goiter).

Secondary hypothyroidism occurs as a result of hypothalamic or pituitary dysfunction. Dopamine infusion and/or severe illness may suppress TSH release sufficiently to cause a modest, transient hypothyroidism. A rare cause of hypothyroidism is tissue resistance to thyroid hormones, which is usually due to an abnormality in the nuclear receptor for these hormones.

INCIDENCE. Hypothyroidism is common in adults. In one epidemiologic survey, 1.4 per cent of adult females and about 0.1 per cent of adult males were affected. Autoimmune destruction of the thyroid gland is the most common cause of thyroid gland failure in adults. This generally affects women over the age of 40 but can occur at any age. Hypothyroidism is also a common congenital disease, occurring in about 1 of 4000 neonates in North America and Western Europe and more frequently in areas of iodine deficiency.

PATHOLOGY. The pathology of the thyroid gland in hypothyroidism depends on the etiology of the syndrome. In "idiopathic myxedema," the thyroid tissue is generally replaced by fat with few intact follicles and lymphocytic infiltration (see also Thyroiditis). When the thyroid cells remain partly functional, the elevated serum TSH leads to hyperplasia and hypertrophy. In secondary hypothyroidism, the number of follicular cells is low and considerable colloid is present. The gland is small in contrast to the goiter found when thyroid cell dysfunction is present and TSH secretion is increased.

The nonthyroidal pathology of the hypothyroid state is the same regardless of its etiology. The longer the duration and the more severe the deficiency, the greater are the changes. The accumulation of mucopolysaccharide in connective tissues has already been mentioned. This material may also appear in muscle. Effusions, which often have a high protein content, occur in various serous cavities.

CLINICAL MANIFESTATIONS. The common clinical manifestations of this syndrome in the adult are summarized in Table 216–9. These symptoms and signs can be attributed to either deceleration of cellular metabolic processes or the accumulation of the hygroscopic mucopolysaccharide in the vocal cords or oropharynx, as well as the more obvious changes in the subcutaneous tissues. The symptoms are nonspecific, particularly in the early phases, and may either pass unnoticed by the patient or be attributed to advancing age. Characteristically, the patient becomes aware of their multiplicity and severity only after thyroid hormone replacement leads to a return of normal function. This is particularly true of younger patients. In the elderly, hearing impairment, somnolence, and decreased memory and ability to calculate may occur. These may lead to an apparent psychological withdrawal and paranoia at times requiring hospitalization. The term *myxedema madness* has been used to describe this syndrome, which can be mistaken for cerebrovascular insufficiency or senile dementia. Alternatively, the patient may confabulate or respond with humorous non sequiturs to draw the interviewer's attention from his or her limited recall of recent events. This behavior has been termed *myxedema wit*. A variety of menstrual disorders may be present, although menorrhagia is said to be the most common pattern. Pregnancy may occur in patients with hypothyroidism, and the increased hormone requirements of that condition may cause a previously borderline functioning thyroid to decompensate. Despite the developmental abnormalities associated with congenital hypothyroidism, the symptoms of hypothyroidism in infants are few. Severe thyroid hormone deficiency is associated with growth retardation in the older infant

TABLE 216–9. COMMON SYMPTOMS OF HYPOTHYROIDISM

Weakness, fatigue, lethargy
Dry, coarse skin
Swelling of the hands, face, and extremities
Cold intolerance, decreased sweating
Coarsening or huskiness of the voice
Modest weight gain (~10 lbs) with anorexia
Decreased memory, hearing impairment
Arthralgia, paresthesias
Constipation
Muscle cramps

and child. In the adolescent, thyroid enlargement, *adolescent goiter*, may be the only manifestation and is usually seen in the pubertal female. In some patients in whom the hypothyroidism is of rapid onset, cramps in large muscle groups may be a prominent symptom. Such symptoms usually occur after a rapid change from a hyperthyroid to a hypothyroid state, such as after surgery for Graves' disease, a second RAI treatment for hyperthyroidism, or even vigorous antithyroid drug therapy.

Many of the common signs of hypothyroidism are the opposite of those seen in the hyperthyroid patient. Bradycardia is common and is sometimes associated with hypothermia. Systolic pressure is generally reduced and diastolic pressure increased, the latter resulting from increased peripheral vascular resistance. Myxedema is manifested by a puffy, nonpitting swelling of the subcutaneous tissue, which may particularly collect in the periorbital area. Body and scalp hair are reduced; the skin may be coarse, the texture of sandpaper, and is usually cool and sallow. The yellow complexion is due to the accumulation of carotene in the serum in patients with significant hypothyroidism. The thyroid may be enlarged, of normal size, or not palpable, depending on the cause. The heart sounds are distant, and the heart shadow is often enlarged. The latter can be a manifestation of pericardial effusion, which is common but rarely leads to tamponade. In addition to the cortical dysfunction previously mentioned, cerebellar ataxia may be present. Other neurologic signs, including delayed relaxation of the deep tendon reflexes, peripheral neuropathy, and carpal tunnel syndrome, can completely resolve with treatment.

Certain physiologic abnormalities are characteristic of hypothyroidism. Cardiac output is reduced, although not out of proportion to the decrease in O_2 consumption. Glomerular filtration is also subnormal, leading to an impairment of the capacity to excrete free water. In addition, inappropriate antidiuretic hormone (ADH) secretion may lead to hyponatremia. Gastrointestinal motility is reduced, and occasionally the patient may develop an apparent obstruction, *myxedema megacolon*. There are important abnormalities in the respiratory center. The sensitivity to both hypercarbia and hypoxia is reduced, and such patients may readily develop CO_2 narcosis or cardiac arrhythmias associated with hypoxia. This is one of the chief causes of death in the severe form of myxedema, *myxedema coma*. Pituitary function is impaired in severe hypothyroidism even of the primary variety. Hypoglycemic stress does not elicit normal growth hormone or cortisol responses in such patients, so that testing pituitary function must be delayed until the hypothyroid state has been corrected. Serum prolactin is increased in moderate to severe primary hypothyroidism, and this may lead to galactorrhea in a small percentage of patients.

LABORATORY DIAGNOSIS. The diagnosis of hypothyroidism can be easily confirmed by using the scheme outlined in Figures 216–4 and 216–8. When the diagnosis is not made, it is usually because the nonspecificity of signs and symptoms does not immediately suggest this cause. This disease is one of the "great imitators," and a high index of suspicion should be maintained, as the condition is so readily diagnosed and treated. In all patients with hypothyroidism, the free T_4 index is reduced. Serum T_3 concentrations are often in the normal range in hypothyroid patients, and this test is not useful in the diagnosis of this condition. It is unlikely that significant symptoms are present in patients with an equivocal reduction in this hormone. Once a reduced free T_4 index has been found, it is imperative to determine whether the cause of the disease is primary, i.e., owing to thyroid disease, or secondary, involving the hypothalamic-pituitary axis. An increase in serum TSH establishes the diagnosis of primary hypothyroidism. If the serum TSH concentration is normal or borderline, then the diagnosis of pituitary or hypothalamic hypothyroidism is made, and further steps are taken to evaluate the possibility of a deficiency of other pituitary hormones. It is extremely important that this be done prior to the onset of therapy, since thyroid replacement exacerbates mild ACTH insufficiency associated with hypothalamic or pituitary disease. *If unrecognized, such patients may have an addisonian crisis provoked by thyroid hormone replacement.* There are two circumstances in which primary hypothyroidism is not associated with TSH elevation. This may be the case when hypothyroidism follows shortly after a period of hyperthyroidism, since the latter causes suppression of pituitary TSH synthesis lasting 4 to 5 weeks. Dopamine infusion may also cause suppression of an elevated TSH concentration into the normal range.

In the patient whose symptoms are nonspecific or borderline and in whom an equivocally reduced free T_4 index is obtained, the serum TSH may be significantly elevated. Elevated serum TSH is the most sensitive index of impairment of thyroid gland function. Whether or not such patients are actually metabolically hypothyroid cannot be determined by using tests. This condition has been called *subclinical hypothyroidism*.

There are a few clinical situations in which the free T_4 index is reduced but serum TSH is not elevated in the absence of hypothalamic or pituitary disease. This may occur in severely ill patients without thyroid disease, but who presumably have transient hypothalamic-pituitary hypothyroidism. In such patients, a serum cortisol determination is indicated to eliminate the possibility of ACTH deficiency. If clinically indicated, therapy can then be initiated with both thyroxine and glucocorticoid. Patients receiving 2 to 3 grams per day of salicylate or 300 mg per day of phenytoin may have a reduction in the free T_4 index without hypothyroidism (see Table 216–3), and also patients ingesting replacement quantities (25 µg or more) of triiodothyronine (Cytomel) have reduced serum T_4 due to suppression of TSH, even if the thyroid gland is normal. A 24-hour RAI uptake test may not separate hypothyroidism from the euthyroid state and is not useful in diagnosis.

Other Biochemical Abnormalities and Associated Diseases in Patients with Hypothyroidism. Serum cholesterol and triglycerides, creatine phosphokinase (MM isozyme), aldolase, lactic dehydrogenase, and SGOT may all be elevated in the patient with moderate to severe hypothyroidism. Hyponatremia with or without the inappropriate ADH syndrome is seen. There is often a modest anemia of chronic disease that may be macrocytic. Serum vitamin B_{12} should be measured in these patients because of the 3 to 6 per cent coexistence of pernicious anemia with Hashimoto's thyroiditis. Other conditions found with increased frequency in patients with autoimmune thyroid disease include idiopathic adrenocortical deficiency, diabetes mellitus, hypoparathyroidism, myasthenia gravis, vitiligo (Ch. 228), and mitral valve prolapse.

DIFFERENTIAL DIAGNOSIS. There are few conditions that can masquerade as hypothyroidism in its classic form. However, patients with nephrotic syndrome or hypoalbuminemia and associated peripheral edema may be suspected of this diagnosis. Although the serum T_4 in these conditions is reduced because of hypoproteinemia, the THBR is generally quite elevated with a consequent normal free T_4 index. Patients with chronic renal disease may have symptoms entirely similar to those of hypothyroidism (including hypothermia), and laboratory tests are required to evaluate the possible coexistence of these two diseases. In patients with spontaneous primary hypothyroidism, the tests for autoantibodies to either thyroglobulin or microsomal components

of the thyroid cell are generally positive. This is true even if the typical thyroid enlargement of Hashimoto's thyroiditis is not present. The other causes of hypothyroidism have already been discussed (see Table 216–8), and reversible causes should be eliminated.

THERAPY. Hypothyroidism is a readily treatable disease. The preparations available for thyroid replacement are listed in Table 216–10. Levothyroxine is most frequently used as replacement therapy, since it provides stable and easily measureable serum concentrations for use in monitoring therapy and allows physiologic regulation of extrathyroidal T_3 production. Ideally, both serum T_3 and T_4 concentrations should be normalized for satisfactory replacement. Since in the euthyroid individual, 20 per cent of T_3 is derived directly from the thyroid gland (see Table 216–2), one would predict that normalization of serum T_3 in hypothyroid individuals would be associated with a serum free T_4 index that is about 60 per cent above the euthyroid value. Because intrapituitary T_3 is derived independently from both serum T_4 *and* serum T_3, this could well result in a subnormal TSH-IMA. At present the data are too incomplete to allow an informed decision whether serum T_3 or serum TSH concentrations should be normalized, assuming that both goals cannot be achieved simultaneously. It is recognized that excessive thyroid hormone replacement may be deleterious to cardiac function and to bone mineralization. At present, I use a combination of clinical evaluation and the TSH-IMA test as the guidelines for adequate replacement, although serum T_3 is measured periodically. The dose of levothyroxine required to achieve symptomatic and biochemical replacement in most patients is about 1.5 µg T_4 per kilogram (about 0.7 µg T_4 per pound). This is a significantly lower requirement than previously used because of improvements in tablet formulation. In most female patients a dose of 87 to 100 µg is quite adequate. The difference between this amount and the T_4 production rate of 1.1 µg per kilogram per day is due to the incomplete absorption of orally administered levothyroxine. In patients who become hypothyroid after ^{131}I treatment for Graves' disease, the requirement may be lower because of residual, nonsuppressible T_4 or T_3 secretion.

In patients who are in good health otherwise or whose hypothyroidism is very modest, therapy can be initiated with half-replacement doses immediately on establishment of the diagnosis. This can be increased to full replacement after 1 month. In patients with more severe hypothyroidism, elderly patients, or those with a history of cardiovascular disease, I prefer to begin therapy with smaller amounts (25 µg of thyroxine per day) and to increase these by 25-µg increments at 4-week intervals (with due attention to symptoms) until a replacement dose is achieved. In patients with primary hypothyroidism there may rarely be associated primary autoimmune hypoadrenalism (*Schmidt's syndrome*). Such patients require adequate replacement of glucocorticoid prior to institution of thyroid hormone replacement. A similar procedure must be employed in patients in whom hypothalamic-pituitary disease is a cause of hypothyroidism.

Long-term monitoring of thyroid hormone replacement should

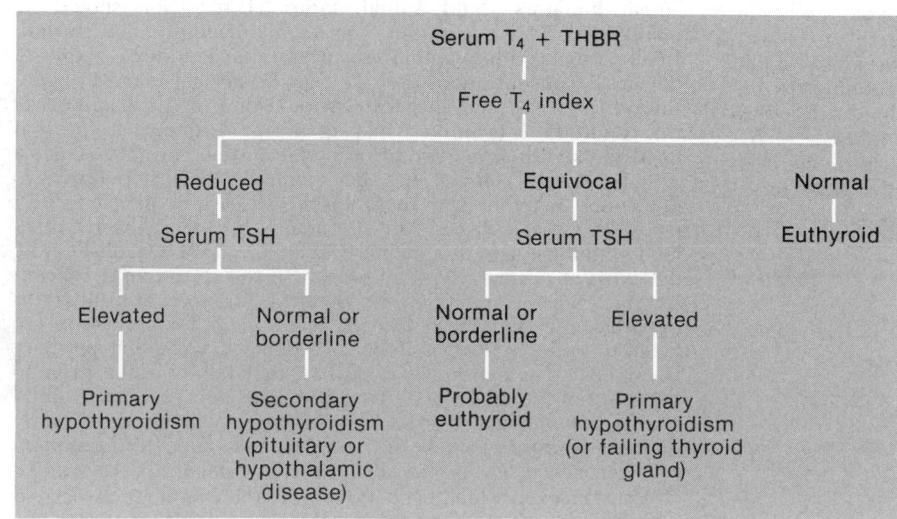

FIGURE 216–8. Laboratory diagnosis of hypothyroidism. THBR refers to the thyroid hormone–binding ratio (formerly termed T_3 or T_4 uptake).

TABLE 216–10. HORMONE CONTENT OF THYROID REPLACEMENT PREPARATIONS
(AMOUNTS APPROXIMATELY EQUIVALENT TO 1 GRAIN [65 mg] OF DESICCATED THYROID)

| | Levothyroxine | Liotrix | | Desiccated Thyroid (1-Grain Tablets) | | Levotriiodothyronine |
		Euthroid-1	Thyrolar-1	Armour	Proloid	
T_4 (μg)	100	60	50	63	55	0
T_3 (μg)	0	15	12.5	12	16	25

include annual measurements of the serum free T_4 index, TSH, and serum T_3. The replacement dose of T_4 may be 20 to 40 per cent lower in elderly patients. Thyroxine requirements increase about 25 to 50 per cent in most pregnant women with primary hypothyroidism, decreasing again immediately after delivery. Serum hormone and TSH concentrations should be monitored at monthly intervals during the first trimester and the dosage of thyroxine adjusted as needed to maintain the serum TSH in the normal range.

Special Problems in Hypothyroid Patients. The patient who presents simultaneously with angina and hypothyroidism poses a serious therapeutic problem. In some patients with coronary artery disease, reintroduction of thyroid hormones results in increased myocardial oxygen demands without an adequate increase in myocardial blood flow. A trial of propranolol with small increments of thyroxine may reduce myocardial oxygen consumption without decreasing the pulse rate to unacceptably low levels. If an exacerbation of angina occurs during thyroxine therapy, T_4 to T_3 conversion may be acutely reduced in peripheral tissues with propylthiouracil (see Graves' Disease and Other Causes of Hyperthyroidism). In patients with localized coronary artery disease in whom bypass graft surgery is indicated, the frequent adverse effects of thyroxine replacement have raised the possibility that surgery should be performed prior to thyroid hormone replacement. The overall morbidity may be lower in patients operated on in the hypothyroid state than in patients in whom replacement is attempted prior to surgery.

Although theoretical considerations suggest that hypothyroidism would impair the physiologic response to surgical stress, patients with mild to moderate hypothyroidism do not appear to have more perioperative complications with major surgery than do euthyroid patients, at least as assessed in retrospective studies. While elective surgery should not be performed in the untreated hypothyroid patient, a moderate degree of hypothyroidism does not preclude carefully managed emergency procedures.

Patients with subclinical hypothyroidism (low-normal free T_4 index and TSH >10 μU per milliliter) may benefit from therapy even though their symptoms are not obvious. This biochemical pattern together with a small goiter and positive antithyroid microsomal antibodies indicates the presence of Hashimoto's thyroiditis (see below), and it is my practice to treat such patients to prevent further thyroid enlargement.

Treatment of Myxedema Coma. In severe myxedema the patient may lapse into coma. This serious complication (mortality, 20 to 50 per cent) occurs most commonly in patients with severe hypothyroidism who are subjected to an additional physiologic stress. This may occur spontaneously, following cold exposure, or during infection, but in all too many instances it is iatrogenic. The administration of sedatives to hypothyroid patients may precipitate coma, as drugs are not metabolized as rapidly in these patients. The reduced sensitivity of the respiratory center to changes in blood gases may lead to inappropriately small ventilatory responses. In other situations, surgery may be performed in a patient who is not recognized to be severely hypothyroid, and postoperative opiates or sedatives lead to clinical deterioration. In Table 216–11 are shown the important steps in management of patients with myxedema coma. In these emergent situations it is important to institute treatment immediately. If the serum free T_4 index is reduced, treatment is begun even if the cause of the hypothyroidism (primary versus secondary) has not been identified. Accordingly, testing for adrenal function is carried out immediately, followed by institution of glucocorticoid replacement. Because of the irregularities of either intramuscular or gastrointestinal absorption in hypothyroidism, medications should be given intravenously. Glucocorticoid replacement

should not be given in pharmacologic quantities, since this impairs T_4 to T_3 conversion.

PROGNOSIS. The prognosis of hypothyroidism is excellent, provided that thyroid hormone replacement is maintained at an appropriate level.

Withdrawal of Thyroid Hormone After Prolonged Replacement. The question sometimes arises whether thyroid hormone therapy is indicated in a patient already receiving it. If, based on the history, the physician is skeptical of the need for replacement, the dosage of thyroxine may be reduced to about 50 per cent of the estimated maintenance dose. Measurements of serum free thyroxine index and TSH are then performed at monthly intervals. If these remain normal for 2 months, the thyroxine may be discontinued and monitoring continued for an additional 2 months. If the free T_4 index and TSH are normal at that time, one can exclude the diagnosis of significant hypothyroidism.

Becker C: Hypothyroidism and atherosclerotic heart disease: Pathogenesis, medical management, and the role of coronary artery bypass surgery. Endocr Rev 6:432, 1985. *A review of clinical experience in treating patients with a combination of hypothyroidism and coronary artery disease.*

Gow SM, Caldwell G, Toft AD, et al.: Relationship between pituitary and other target organ responsiveness in hypothyroid patients receiving thyroxine replacement. J Clin Endocrinol Metab 64:364, 1987. *A correlation of serum TSH-IMA and thyroid hormones with various other markers of thyroid status in hypothyroid patients receiving levothyroxine.*

Mandel SJ, Larsen PR, Seely EW, et al.: Increased need for thyroxine during pregnancy in women with primary hypothyroidism. N Engl J Med 323:91, 1990.

Rees-Jones RW, Rolla AR, Larsen PR: Hormonal content of thyroid replacement preparations. JAMA 243:459, 1980. *Analyses of desiccated thyroid tablets show that some generic preparations have reduced quantities of T_4 and T_3 relative to those contained in brand-name products.*

Vulsma T, Gons MH, de Vijlder JJM: Maternal-fetal transfer of thyroxine in congenital hypothyroidism due to a total organification defect or thyroid agenesis. N Engl J Med 321:13, 1989. *Convincing evidence of transplacental passage of maternal thyroxine to the congenitally hypothyroid fetus.*

THYROIDITIS

Thyroiditis is classified into three types: acute, subacute, and chronic. Despite the common factor of inflammation in all of these entities, there are marked differences in their clinical presentations and etiology.

Acute Thyroiditis

Acute thyroiditis results from a bacterial infection of the thyroid gland with typical symptoms of such involvement, including a

TABLE 216–11. MANAGEMENT OF PATIENTS WITH MYXEDEMA COMA

Diagnostic

1. Serum T_4, T_3 uptake (or equivalent), TSH
2. CBC, glucose, electrolytes, blood gases, BUN, creatinine, CPK
3. Plasma cortisol before and 30 and 60 minutes after cosyntropin (Cortrosyn), 0.25 mg, intravenous bolus
4. Careful evaluation for concomitant disease; continuous ECG and temperature monitoring

Therapeutic

1. Levothyroxine, 2 μg per kilogram intravenously over 5 to 10 minutes initially, and 100 μg intravenously every 24 hours thereafter
2. Cover to conserve body heat; do not rewarm externally
3. Tracheal intubation and mechanical ventilation as required
4. Intravenous fluids as determined by initial blood glucose and electrolytes and by the state of hydration; watch for water retention
5. Hydrocortisone, 100 mg by intravenous bolus, then 25 mg every 6 hours as a continuous intravenous drip
6. Vigorous treatment of associated and precipitating conditions such as infection

fever, local tenderness, and swelling. This condition is quite rare. The infection may involve the whole gland or only a portion of it. Laboratory studies generally show normal thyroid function, but there is an elevated leukocyte count with a polymorphonuclear predominance. The thyroid scan may show an area of decreased uptake corresponding to the involved portion, but the 24-hour RAI uptake is usually normal. Treatment of this condition requires proper identification of the causative agent and appropriate antimicrobial drugs. This may require a needle aspiration. If localized abscess formation occurs, the abscess should be drained. The process usually responds rapidly to these measures.

Subacute (Nonsuppurative) Thyroiditis

This condition is also referred to as *giant cell thyroiditis, granulomatous thyroiditis,* or *de Quervain's thyroiditis.* In the classic form of this disease the patient presents with an exquisitely tender thyroid, which is pathologically characterized by follicular cell destruction and by a lymphocytic and polymorphonuclear leukocyte infiltration, together with multinucleate giant cells. In recent years, a different type of subacute thyroiditis has appeared, which is often painless and associated with hyperthyroidism. It shares some pathologic features with Hashimoto's thyroiditis (see below). This condition, which will be denoted *subacute lymphocytic thyroiditis,* is discussed separately below because of its unique features. The disease described by de Quervain will be referred to as *subacute granulomatous thyroiditis.*

INCIDENCE. The incidence of subacute granulomatous thyroiditis is not known, but it is not rare. It is most common in the third to fifth decades, and females are affected about three to four times more commonly than males. It occurs with increased frequency in HLA-B35–positive individuals.

ETIOLOGY. The granulomatous form of subacute thyroiditis often follows a viral infection by several weeks. At the time of the acute illness, elevated titers of antibody to influenza virus, coxsackievirus, or adenovirus can be found. Over the next few months these fall in many patients, suggesting that an acute infection has recently occurred. In only two cases has a virus been cultured from thyroid tissue, which in both cases was mumps. Some authorities interpret the thyroiditis as being a consequence of a process set in motion by the viral illness but not representing a direct infection of the gland. The precise etiology is unknown.

PATHOLOGY. The classic pathologic picture includes the cellular infiltrate described above, along with severe destruction of the normal follicular architecture. Fibrosis appears in the latter phases. Despite the extensive destruction, complete restoration of the normal thyroid structure generally occurs.

CLINICAL MANIFESTATIONS. Subacute granulomatous thyroiditis is characterized by an often exquisitely painful two- to threefold enlargement of the thyroid gland together with systemic symptoms, including fever, chills, and malaise. Patients often complain of neck or ear pain or dysphagia and may have had evaluation for pharyngeal infection. Symptoms of hyperthyroidism may also be present. The patient may report a prior viral illness. If symptoms of hyperthyroidism are present, they are generally of very short duration (less than 2 months) and are due to the release of thyroid hormones resulting from thyroid destruction. Physical examination may show fever, tachycardia, and exquisite tenderness of the slightly enlarged thyroid gland. This generally involves the whole gland but may be asymmetric.

DIAGNOSIS. The leukocyte count is mildly elevated, but there is characteristically a marked elevation of the erythrocyte sedimentation rate (ESR). This has been one of the hallmarks of this disease. The free T_4 index may be normal or increased. As would be expected from the pathology, the RAI uptake is low and the thyroid is poorly visualized on scan. The RAI uptake is the principal test for separating patients with this disease from those with hyperthyroidism resulting from Graves' disease. There may be an asymmetric involvement of the thyroid with decreased function in that area. Antimicrosomal and antithyroglobulin antibodies are absent or low in titer, although the serum thyroglobulin may be increased, reflecting the destructive process.

TREATMENT. Since this is a self-limited disease, treatment is symptomatic. Mild analgesics such as aspirin (2 to 4 grams per

day) should be given for neck discomfort. In a significant fraction of patients, this is not sufficient, and prednisone, 20 to 40 mg per day, is required. The immediate relief associated with this therapy is almost diagnostic. The glucocorticoid should be continued for 2 to 3 weeks and then tapered over the next 3 weeks. There may be an exacerbation of the original symptoms during discontinuation of glucocorticoid requiring reinstitution of this therapy. Eventually this will not occur. The hyperthyroidism is usually mild but may require propranolol. Antithyroid drugs are of no use, as the serum T_4 and T_3 decrease when the glandular supply is exhausted.

There may be transient hypothyroidism following subacute granulomatous thyroiditis, and this may be severe enough to require treatment in some patients. Therefore it is important for these patients to be followed closely during the recovery period to ascertain whether or not this complication has occurred. Replacement thyroxine can be discontinued after 3 to 6 months with appropriate biochemical monitoring to establish that thyroid function has returned to normal. In 5 to 10 per cent of patients, permanent hypothyroidism supervenes. Occasionally a patient will be seen initially in the hypothyroid phase of this illness. An elevation in serum TSH and low thyroid hormones in the absence of antimicrosomal or antithyroglobulin antibodies should alert the physician to this possibility.

Subacute Lymphocytic Thyroiditis

This disease has been referred to by a variety of descriptive terms, including *painless thyroiditis, lymphocytic thyroiditis, lymphocytic thyroiditis with spontaneously resolving hyperthyroidism, hyperthyroiditis,* and *atypical subacute thyroiditis.* This confused nomenclature reflects the principal clinical and pathologic features of the disease: hyperthyroidism that is self-limited and lymphocytic infiltration of the thyroid.

ETIOLOGY. The etiology of the disease is unknown. There is little suggestion of a prior viral illness in these patients. The pathologic features are much closer to those of Hashimoto's disease than to those of granulomatous thyroiditis, suggesting an autoimmune etiology.

INCIDENCE. The precise incidence is not known, but one suspects that it has been increasing over the last 5 to 10 years. This condition may account for 5 to 20 per cent of patients with hyperthyroidism. About two thirds of reported cases are in women, with patients ranging from 13 to over 80 years of age.

PATHOLOGY. Lymphocytic infiltration is the common feature in all specimens studied. Destruction of follicular architecture and fibrosis similar to that of subacute granulomatous thyroiditis is seen, but foreign body giant cells are rare. Germinal centers characteristic of Hashimoto's disease are rarely seen.

CLINICAL MANIFESTATIONS. The principal symptoms of this form of subacute thyroiditis are those of hyperthyroidism, as described in the section Graves' Disease and Other Causes of Hyperthyroidism. Nonthyroidal stigmata of Graves' disease, exophthalmos and pretibial myxedema, are not present, although a stare and widened palpebral fissure may occur as a consequence of the hyperthyroidism per se. The duration of the hyperthyroid phase is short (usually less than 3 months), and it is generally modest in severity. Physical signs include those typical of hyperthyroidism and a normal or slightly enlarged thyroid gland which is not tender. The gland may be firm.

The natural history of thyroid function in a patient who had a typical episode of this disease is presented in Figure 216–9. The acute phase of hyperthyroidism resolved rapidly and spontaneously and was followed by a period of transient hypothyroidism requiring treatment. This was discontinued after 3 months, and after an initial period of thyroidal resistance to TSH, normal function returned. A phase of significant hypothyroidism such as this follows the hyperthyroidism in about one third of patients. For obscure reasons, this form of thyroiditis occurs with increased frequency in the first few months post partum.

LABORATORY DIAGNOSIS. Serum T_4 and T_3 concentrations are generally elevated, the TSH subnormal, the leukocyte count normal, and the ESR normal or only slightly elevated (<50 mm at 1 hour, Westergren). This is in marked contrast to the results in the granulomatous form of the disease. The 24-hour RAI uptake is reduced and will not increase even after TSH injection. Serum thyroglobulin is increased in the acute phase of the disease, and the titers of TMAb and TgAb may be low or elevated, depending on the clinical pattern. In postpartum thyroiditis, these antibody titers are elevated, and the condition appears to be associated with underlying Hashimoto's thyroiditis. In such patients, repeated episodes of hyperthyroidism followed by transient hypothyroidism should be anticipated with each pregnancy.

This disease must be separated from other causes of hyperthyroidism, notably Graves' disease. The best test for this is the 24-hour RAI uptake. A low uptake may occasionally also be observed in a patient with Graves' disease who has received excess iodide. This may be obvious from the history or can be eliminated by measuring the urinary iodide, which must be considerably elevated (>2 mg per 24 hours) to suppress the uptake in hyperthyroidism associated with thyroid hyperfunction. A needle biopsy will also be diagnostic. In *factitious hyperthyroidism,* the serum thyroglobulin is reduced in the presence of a low serum TSH concentration. This finding distinguishes this condition from subacute lymphocytic thyroiditis.

TREATMENT. As with subacute granulomatous thyroiditis, treatment is symptomatic. β-Adrenergic blockade may be required for the hyperthyroid phase, but propylthiouracil is of no value except to inhibit T_4 to T_3 conversion. Glucocorticoid is not required because there is no tenderness, but more rapid resolution of the hyperthyroidism has been reported in patients given a 4-week course of prednisone starting at 40 mg per day. A hypothyroid phase should be treated for 3 to 6 months, followed by withdrawal of the therapy.

PROGNOSIS. The hyperthyroid phase usually remits within a few months, and the entire history of this disease lasts less than a year. However, the potential for subsequent hypothyroidism indicates the need for annual examination of thyroid function in these patients.

CHRONIC THYROIDITIS

There are two types of chronic thyroiditis: Hashimoto's and Riedel's thyroiditis *(Riedel's struma).*

Hashimoto's Thyroiditis

This is an apparently autoimmune disease of the thyroid gland. It appears to be closely related to Graves' disease. Synonyms for this condition are *chronic lymphocytic thyroiditis* and *lymphadenoid goiter.*

ETIOLOGY. The sera of patients with this condition contain antibodies to one or more thyroid antigens, including thyroid peroxidase (antithyroid microsomal antibodies), thyroglobulin, or a colloid antigen that can be separated from thyroglobulin. At present it is not certain whether these antibodies are the cause or the result of this disease. The pathologic features of the condition can be reproduced in laboratory animals by immunization with thyroid tissue. However, the experimental disease is not sustained once immunizations have been discontinued, nor can the injury be induced by serum from immunized animals. Since the disease can be transferred by sensitized lymphocytes, it has been proposed that the destruction is produced by cell-mediated processes. On exposure to thyroid tissue antigens in vitro, lymphocytes of patients with Hashimoto's thyroiditis (and Graves' disease) produce substances causing inhibition of leukocyte migration. This response is not found in patients with other forms of thyroid disease or by exposure to extracts of other tissues. Similar observations have been made in patients with idiopathic myxedema, suggesting that the atrophic thyroid found in this condition is affected by a similar process. Other evidence supporting the autoimmune hypothesis is the increased prevalence of many of the so-called autoimmune diseases in patients with Hashimoto's thyroiditis. These include Sjögren's syndrome, lupus erythematosus, idiopathic thrombocytopenic purpura, and pernicious anemia. As many as 6 per cent of patients with Hashimoto's disease have been reported to have pernicious anemia. Although rare, involvement of other endocrine glands by this immunopathologic process may occur. Idiopathic Addison's disease and Hashimoto's disease may appear in the same patients. This combination is called Schmidt's syndrome (see Ch. 228). The parathyroids, the β cells of the pancreatic islets, the pituitary, and the gonads may also be involved. There are a few reports of transplacental passage of maternal thyroid antibodies leading to transient impairment of thyroid function in neonates, but such cases are the exception rather than the rule. An increased risk of the atrophic form of Hashimoto's thyroiditis is present in patients who are HLA-DR3 or HLA-B8 positive.

INCIDENCE. Women are affected four to five times more frequently than men. The incidence increases with increasing age. TMAb have been found in about 10 per cent and 3 per cent of asymptomatic adult females and males, respectively. Thyroid peroxidase is now recognized to be the antigen in thyroid microsomes. Ten to 20 per cent of these persons can be expected to have biochemical evidence of thyroid disease. This disease is probably the most common cause of goiter in adolescents, although the incidence is not as high as in older women.

PATHOLOGIC FINDINGS. The thyroid gland is normal or

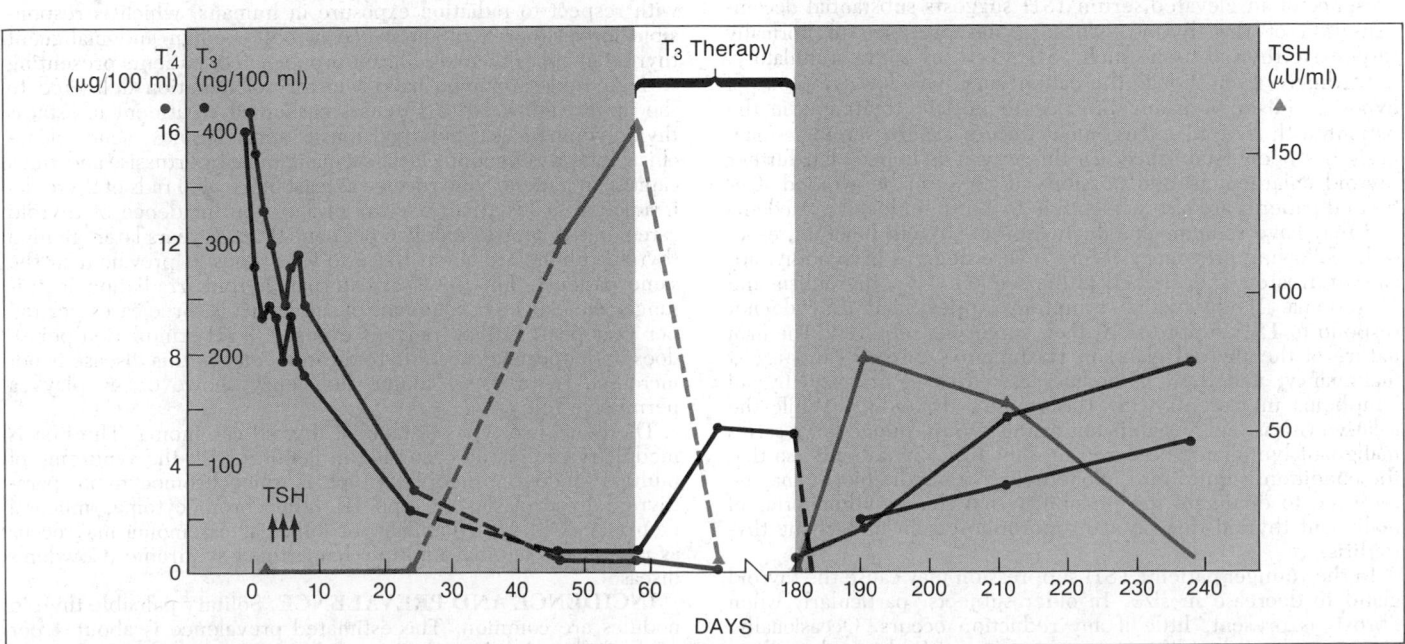

FIGURE 216–9. Changes in serum T_3, T_4, and TSH in a patient with subacute lymphocytic thyroiditis. The rapid decrease in serum T_3 and T_4 in the first 5 days is due to exhaustion of thyroidal stores as a consequence of the destructive process. Transient T_3 replacement was employed because of prolonged hypothyroidism. Normal thyroid function had returned by 8 months after the initial episode. (From Larsen PR: Serum triiodothyronine, thyroxine, and thyrotropin during hyperthyroid, hypothyroid, and recovery phases of subacute nonsuppurative thyroiditis. Metabolism 23:467, 1974. © 1974, The Williams & Wilkins Company, Baltimore.)

may be enlarged two- to fivefold, depending on the degree of fibrosis. Microscopic examination reveals that varying degrees of infiltration with lymphocytes and plasma cells, fibrosis, and, in many cases, germinal centers are present. An oxyphilic change may be present in the cytoplasm of the residual thyroid follicular cells. It may occasionally be difficult to differentiate Hashimoto's disease from primary lymphoma of the thyroid gland.

CLINICAL MANIFESTATIONS. Two clinical forms of thyroid involvement are described. In the so-called atrophic form the gland is normal or reduced in size, and hypothyroidism is the prominent symptom (see Table 216–9). This may well be the same syndrome as idiopathic myxedema. In other patients, variable degrees of thyroid enlargement and hypothyroidism occur, but goiter is the most common chief complaint. The gland is generally symmetrically enlarged, and often the pyramidal lobe is quite prominent, suggesting generalized hypertrophy. The thyroid is firm and may feel lobular or diffusely enlarged. Occasionally Hashimoto's disease presents as a single nodule in the thyroid gland, which represents the residual functioning thyroid tissue in a gland, the remainder of which has been destroyed by this disease. The patient may have a family history of Graves' or Hashimoto's disease, pernicious anemia, or other autoimmune phenomena. As mentioned in the discussion of *lymphocytic thyroiditis,* as many as 5 to 10 per cent of women may have postpartum episodes of transient hyperthyroidism followed by transient hypothyroidism associated with elevated TMAb.

LABORATORY DIAGNOSIS. The serum free T_4 index is reduced and serum TSH increased in many patients with this syndrome. Approximately 95 per cent of patients have positive TMAb tests, and about 50 to 60 per cent have positive TgAb. The RAI uptake may be reduced, normal, or even increased, depending on the residual thyroid cell function and the serum TSH. The thyroid scan generally reveals a heterogeneous uptake of the isotope. Occasionally a single island of functioning tissue remains. This can be differentiated from a functioning adenoma of the thyroid by appropriate tests of thyroid function. If the diagnosis remains in doubt, a needle biopsy can be performed and will reveal the characteristic changes of lymphocytic infiltration in the majority of cases.

TREATMENT. In the early phases of Hashimoto's thyroiditis, goiter may be present and the serum TSH mildly increased, but the free T_4 index is in the lower normal range. Nevertheless, the presence of an elevated serum TSH suggests substantial decompensation of the thyroid, since in the presence of normally responsive thyroid tissue such TSH levels are quite stimulatory. Accordingly, even though the patient may have few symptoms of hypothyroidism, it is my practice to initiate treatment in the patient with thyroid enlargement once a secure serologic diagnosis has been established. In this way it is hoped that further thyroid enlargement and possibly surgery can be avoided. Untreated patients are also susceptible to iodide-induced myxedema and may have spontaneous fluctuation in thyroid function, especially following pregnancy. More severe degrees of hypothyroidism are treated as described in the section, Hypothyroidism and Myxedema. If obstructive symptoms appear and they do not respond to TSH suppression, then surgery is required. The firm nature of the thyroid gland in Hashimoto's disease can suggest malignancy, and there is an increased risk of primary thyroid lymphoma in patients with Hashimoto's thyroiditis. While the relative risk is highly significant in this group, in one large series malignant lymphoma occurred in only 4 of 829 patients, so that the condition is quite rare. Nonetheless, a needle biopsy may be required to eliminate the possibility that this or other forms of malignant thyroid disease are superimposed on underlying thyroiditis.

In the younger patient, TSH suppression may cause the thyroid gland to decrease in size. In older subjects, particularly when fibrosis is present, little if any reduction occurs. Occasionally, Hashimoto's thyroiditis may present with hyperthyroidism ("hashitoxicosis"), which should be treated as is Graves' disease. Appropriate observation of the patient for the involvement of other tissues by autoimmune disease should be carried out as indicated.

PROGNOSIS. The prognosis of this condition is excellent as long as thyroid hormone therapy is provided when indicated. In patients with serologic evidence of Hashimoto's thyroiditis but normal thyroid function, an annual evaluation for hypothyroidism is indicated.

Riedel's Thyroiditis

This is a rare disorder of unknown cause in which a sclerosing fibrous infiltration of the thyroid gland occurs, causing the gland to become extremely firm. As the disease progresses, local muscles in the neck and the trachea are infiltrated and hypothyroidism appears. This condition may be difficult to differentiate from carcinoma of the thyroid. It is clinically associated with both retroperitoneal fibrosis and sclerosing cholangitis. Obstruction of the trachea may occur as the fibrosis proceeds, and a surgical approach is the only satisfactory method of treatment to relieve tracheal obstruction. Glucocorticoid therapy can be beneficial to some patients.

Amino N, Mori H, Iwatani Y, et al.: High prevalence of transient post-partum thyrotoxicosis and hypothyroidism. N Engl J Med 306:14, 849, 1982. *A prospective survey showing a 5.5 per cent incidence of transient thyrotoxicosis or hypothyroidism post partum.*

DeGroot LJ, Quintans J: The causes of autoimmune thyroid disease. Endocr Rev 10:537, 1989. *A review of current concepts regarding the etiology of autoimmune thyroid diseases.*

Holm L-E, Blomgren H, Lowhagen T: Cancer risks in patients with chronic lymphocytic thyroiditis. N Engl J Med 312:601, 1985. *An extensive epidemiologic study showing that while the relative risk of lymphoma is increased in individuals with chronic lymphocytic thyroiditis, the incidence of this complication is extremely low.*

Tunbridge WMG, Evered DC, Hall R, et al.: The spectrum of thyroid disease in a community: The Whickham survey. Clin Endocrinol 7:481, 1977. *The epidemiology of thyroid disease in an English community; this study provides a firm basis for estimates of the prevalence of Hashimoto's and Graves' disease as well as nodular goiter.*

BENIGN AND MALIGNANT TUMORS OF THE THYROID: THE SOLITARY THYROID NODULE

In this section are discussed those benign and malignant tumors that usually present as a solitary thyroid nodule. Multinodular goiter is discussed in the next section, Sporadic and Endemic Goiter. Virtually all tumors of the thyroid arise from glandular cells and are therefore adenomas or carcinomas. A scheme for evaluation of the patient with a solitary thyroid nodule is presented at the end of this chapter.

ETIOLOGY. The fundamental cause of thyroid tumors is unknown. However, two factors, exposure to ionizing radiation and the presence of TSH, have been found to be important for inducing thyroid tumors in animals. Similar data are available with respect to radiation exposure in humans, which is responsible for an increased incidence of both benign and malignant thyroid neoplasms. A significant proportion of patients presenting with thyroid carcinoma have a history of radiation delivered to the upper thorax 10 to 15 years earlier for treatment of "status thymolymphaticus," enlarged tonsils and adenoids, acne, eustachian tube dysfunction, facial hemangiomas, pertussis, and tinea capitis. In patients who receive at least 300 to 400 rads of thyroidal irradiation at less than 5 years of age, the incidence of thyroid carcinoma is approximately 6 per cent 10 to 20 years later. Benign thyroid tumors are about three to four times as prevalent in the same patients. For doses of external thyroid irradiation in this range, the expected incidence of carcinoma is three cases per rad per year per 1 million persons exposed. TSH stimulation per se does not appear to cause thyroid carcinoma, as this disease is not increased in areas of iodine deficiency; however, it plays a permissive role.

There are two types of familial thyroid carcinoma. The first is medullary carcinoma occurring in families with the syndrome of multiple endocrine neoplasia type II (pheochromocytoma, parathyroid hyperplasia) or type III (pheochromocytoma, mucosal neuroma) (Ch. 228). Papillary or follicular carcinoma may occur as part of the familial multiple hamartoma syndrome (Cowden's disease).

INCIDENCE AND PREVALENCE. Solitary palpable thyroid nodules are common. The estimated prevalence is about 4 per cent of the adult population, with a 2 to 1 preponderance of females. There is some difficulty in obtaining precise figures in this area, since a significant number of nodules that seem to be solitary by palpation are found to be dominant nodules in multinodular goiters at surgery or autopsy. This estimate represents a relatively small fraction of the true prevalence of thyroid nodules, which is about 40 to 50 per cent as revealed by autopsy studies or high-resolution ultrasonography. Such nodules are rarely true neoplasms. The estimated incidence of thyroid nodules is 0.1 per cent per year, but since many nodules are found at autopsy that were not suspected clinically the true incidence may be higher. The incidence of thyroid carcinoma is estimated to be 36 new cases per year per 1 million persons. These two estimates suggest that about 3 or 4 per cent of patients who develop solitary thyroid nodules have thyroid carcinoma. Many surgical series report thyroid carcinoma in 10 to 30 per cent of resected solitary nodules, which indicates that the screening procedures employed to identify high-risk patients are effective. Various autopsy series have reported an incidence of thyroid carcinoma ranging from 0.1 to 6 per cent. The higher figures are from studies in which an extremely careful search was made for microscopic carcinomas, virtually all being less than 5 mm in diameter. The clinical significance of such lesions is negligible, and this "background" of asymptomatic microscopic lesions should be kept in mind when evaluating this literature.

Benign Neoplasms

PATHOLOGY. The *follicular adenoma* is by far the most common benign thyroid tumor. It varies from microscopic to 8 to 10 cm in size and is composed of a normal-appearing thyroid epithelium arranged in a follicular structure. An intact capsule surrounds these tumors, and there is often evidence of compression of surrounding normal thyroid tissue. The follicles may range from extremely small with little colloid (*fetal adenoma* or *microfollicular adenoma*) to large distended structures (*macrofollicular adenoma*). The *embryonal* adenoma is an even more primitive-appearing structure possessing very little colloid. On occasion, the tumors may be composed of oxyphils (*oxyphil adenoma* or *Hürthle cell adenoma*). None of these differences in microscopic picture appears to bear on the functional characteristics of these nodules, nor do such nodules appear to become malignant. The hypercellular adenomas may be extremely difficult to differentiate from follicular carcinomas, especially when only a needle biopsy sample is available. Follicular adenomas have specific receptors for TSH, and these cells respond to TSH normally. However, many of these tumors do not possess the capacity for concentrating iodide or other similar substances. Since such nodules do not concentrate isotopes, they are referred to as *nonfunctioning* or *cold*.

CLINICAL MANIFESTATIONS. Thyroid adenomas fall into two categories: those that produce significant quantities of thyroid hormones and those that do not. The latter are the more common (90 to 95 per cent). Patients with these tumors present with an asymptomatic mass in the neck. The patient may be discovered to have this tumor on routine physical examination and often is completely unaware of its existence. The tumor usually becomes palpable by the time it reaches 1 cm in diameter, but it may reach 5 to 10 cm without being noticed by the patient. Thyroid function studies in patients with nonfunctioning follicular adenomas are normal, and the thyroid scan generally reveals an area of decreased or absent uptake of $^{123}I^-$ or $^{99m}TcO_4^-$ (a "cold" nodule). The precise diagnosis can be made only by obtaining a tissue specimen by aspiration biopsy, cutting needle biopsy (Vim-Silverman needle or its equivalent), or excision of the nodule. As these nodules may outgrow their blood supply, cystic degeneration may occur. Ultrasonography of such a lesion reveals a cystic cavity within the nodule.

Functioning follicular adenomas may present with or without symptoms of hyperthyroidism, largely depending on their size. Lesions over 3 cm in diameter tend to cause thyrotoxicity and constitute about 50 per cent of these adenomas in patients 60 years and older. T_3 thyrotoxicosis was found in 46 per cent of such patients in one large series. More commonly the patient is asymptomatic, and a thyroid scan shows that the only area concentrating radioactivity is the nodule itself. Such patients generally have normal or high-normal serum thyroid hormone levels, the serum TSH-IMA is subnormal, and TRH infusion will not cause TSH release. Such nodules are functioning autonomously at a rate sufficient to suppress TSH synthesis in the pituitary (hence the lack of function in the remainder of the thyroid) but not at a sufficiently high level to cause metabolic hyperthyroidism. Functional lesions that have suppressed TSH synthesis but not caused hyperthyroidism are denoted *warm* nodules, whereas those associated with hyperthyroidism are called *hot* nodules. Assessment of the thyroid functional state is necessary for proper evaluation of these lesions, since the thyroid scan is identical. This is especially important, since Hashimoto's disease may present as a solitary focus of functioning thyroid tissue, as may congenital absence of one lobe of the thyroid. The presence of potentially functioning thyroid tissue can be demonstrated by injection of 10 units of bovine TSH, followed in 24 hours by a thyroid scan. Unlike multinodular goiters, follicular adenomas of the thyroid rarely grow large enough to cause significant physical encroachment on the trachea or esophagus.

TREATMENT. The finding of an autonomously functioning nodule virtually eliminates the diagnosis of thyroid carcinoma. Treatment at that point depends on the thyroid status. If the patient is euthyroid (a warm thyroid nodule), nothing more than an annual follow-up with appropriate thyroid function tests (including a serum T_3) is necessary. In the hyperthyroid patient, surgery or ^{131}I is available for definitive treatment, although antithyroid drugs may be necessary to control symptomatic hyperthyroidism prior to definitive therapy. The choice of treatment depends on the age of the patient and the size of the nodule. In patients under the age of 20, surgical resection should be performed, as the radiation delivered to extranodular tissue after radioiodine therapy may reach a level that is considered carcinogenic. In older patients with cosmetically disfiguring lesions or those that are compressing vital structures in the neck, surgery is also preferred. For the rest, ^{131}I is indicated. I attempt to deliver 10 mCi of ^{131}I into the nodule. Following either surgery or radioactive iodine treatment, a period of 4 to 6 weeks is required for re-establishment of pituitary TSH secretion, following which function of the previously suppressed normal thyroid tissue should occur. The patient may need to receive thyroxine supplementation during this interim period but may not require indefinite replacement. The approach to the *nonfunctioning thyroid nodule* is described below under Clinical Manifestations and Diagnosis of Thyroid Carcinoma—The Solitary Nodule.

Malignant Thyroid Tumors

Four types of malignancy are found in the thyroid gland. *Papillary carcinoma* comprises the largest fraction, about two thirds of all cases of thyroid malignancy. *Follicular carcinoma* accounts for another 20 per cent, including the *Hürthle cell* variant with *medullary*, and *poorly differentiated* carcinomas about 5 per cent each. Another 5 per cent is accounted for by *non-Hodgkin's lymphoma*, which has become more common in recent years. Medullary carcinoma is a tumor of calcitonin-producing C cells and has no relationship to the thyroid follicular epithelium.

PATHOLOGY AND NATURAL HISTORY. *Papillary carcinoma* is the most benign and the most common form of thyroid carcinoma. It is two to three times more common in women than in men and occurs with equal frequency in the third to seventh decades. Since the less well-differentiated forms of carcinoma increase with age, papillary carcinoma is the most common malignant thyroid tumor in younger patients. The size of these tumors varies from microscopic to several centimeters in diameter. Of the clinically apparent variety, the *occult* tumors (defined as those less than 1.5 cm in diameter) are differentiated from the *intrathyroidal* tumors, which are larger but do not extend through the thyroid surface. The tumor is classified as *extrathyroidal* if it extends through the thyroid capsule and involves surrounding tissues. Microscopically, papillary carcinoma consists of well-differentiated thyroid epithelium covering papillary fibrovascular stalks. The nuclei are frequently clear, as opposed to the denser appearance of normal nuclei. A virtually pathognomonic feature in about 40 per cent of papillary thyroid carcinomas is the so-called *psammoma body*. These calcific globules are 5 to 100 μ in diameter and are often present in the tips of the papillary projections. Their etiology is unknown, but their presence in the thyroid tumor raises the high likelihood of its carcinomatous nature. Cervical lymphatic involvement even with occult thyroid tumors is common, occurring in as many as 50 per cent. Blood-borne metastases are uncommon. The presence or absence of lymph node metastases does not seem to alter the prognosis. In a large series studied at the Mayo Clinic, the 20-year survival of patients with occult or intrathyroid papillary carcinoma was not significantly different from that of a control group. However, the 20-year survival for patients with extrathyroidal carcinoma was about 40 per cent, and this dropped to 20 per cent over the next 10 years. Many thyroid cancers have areas of follicular as well as papillary structure, and blood-borne metastases may occur that have a follicular pattern even though the primary tumor is papillary. Thus, many predominantly papillary tumors have follicular elements, but the biologic behavior of these lesions seems to be a function of the predominant microscopic appearance.

Follicular carcinomas also are more common in women than in men but tend to increase in incidence with increasing age. The tumors vary from well-differentiated, virtually normal-appearing thyroid tissue to nearly solid sheets of follicular epithelium with little evidence of follicle formation. The former are differentiated from follicular adenomas only by demonstration of capsular and vascular invasion. Such a diagnosis generally cannot be made without the entire nodule for examination, and even at frozen section the carcinomatous nature of the lesion may not be recognized. Cyst formation may occur as it does in benign follicular tumors, and calcification may occur centrally. Follicular carcinomas tend to metastasize via blood vessel invasion and not, in general, via lymphatics. Metastases may not be evident at the time of initial evaluation but may appear years later despite apparent complete excision of the tumor. It is not unusual for the follicular carcinoma to concentrate radioiodine, although it does so considerably less well than does normal thyroid tissue. Thus, it is only in the absence of normal thyroid tissue and in the presence of increased TSH that this potential is appreciated. However, it is useful in treatment in some of these tumors (see below). Patients who have had removal of well-encapsulated, noninvasive follicular carcinomas appear to have a normal lifespan. On the other hand, patients with tumors that show extensive local involvement and angioinvasion at the time of initial surgery have an approximately 30 per cent 10-year survival, which is decreased to less than 20 per cent at 20 years.

The most aggressive form of thyroid epithelial carcinoma, anaplastic or undifferentiated, may appear in *giant* or *spindle cell* forms. The small cell variety of this lesion has proven to be a lymphoma in most cases. Undifferentiated thyroid carcinoma is the most highly malignant tumor of the thyroid gland. It is found almost exclusively in patients over the age of 60. The average prognosis from diagnosis to death in the giant cell tumors is less than 6 months, whereas patients with small cell carcinoma may have 5-year survival of 20 to 25 per cent. Both tend to extend locally and often cause tracheal obstruction. Distant metastases may occur with either type.

Medullary carcinoma of the thyroid is a malignant tumor of the C cell and produces thyrocalcitonin. Its occurrence in association with multiple endocrine neoplasia syndromes has been mentioned. It may also occur spontaneously. These tumors are characterized by sheets of tumor cells separated by a hyaline-amyloid–containing stroma. The amyloid is formed by the tumor cells and deposited in the stroma. The tumors may also produce ACTH, prostaglandin, or carcinoembryonic antigen. In familial syndromes, the penetrance of this tumor is complete, so that screening of family members is indicated by use of calcium and/or pentagastrin infusions to stimulate calcitonin release from pathologic cells (see Ch. 236).

Lymphoma is usually the nodular histiocytic form and generally arises in a gland affected by Hashimoto's thyroiditis. It should be considered diagnostically in patients with Hashimoto's disease who present with a rapidly enlarging mass in the thyroid gland, and a core or aspiration biopsy should be performed with appropriate cytochemical stains. Depending on the clinical stage, these lesions may respond quite well to radiotherapy, with or without chemotherapy. Complete cure by surgical resection of small lesions has also been reported.

CLINICAL MANIFESTATIONS AND DIAGNOSIS OF THYROID CARCINOMA—THE SOLITARY NODULE. The approach to the patient with a solitary thyroid nodule is a matter of considerable disagreement among clinicians. For some, thyroid carcinoma is sufficiently serious to require a surgical approach to

all potentially carcinomatous lesions; others believe that considerable selection should be used prior to surgery. The benign nature of the common forms of thyroid carcinoma and the relatively large number of benign nodules make a conservative approach rational. There are several clinical characteristics that dictate an open surgical approach to a nonfunctioning thyroid nodule. This includes a history of prior irradiation. Nodules in such patients carry a 20 to 25 per cent risk of carcinoma. A history of rapid growth, evidence of recurrent nerve paresis, obvious involvement of lymph nodes, or fixation of the nodule to surrounding tissues should also lead to serious consideration of immediate surgery. Statistically, the risk of a solitary cold nodule being malignant is higher in a male than in a female, since benign disease of the thyroid is much more common in females. Thyroid nodules in children are more likely to be carcinoma than those in adults.

In the absence of specific signs pointing to a diagnosis of thyroid carcinoma, there are two avenues of approach (Fig. 216–10A and B). If there is no obvious thyroid dysfunction (either hyperthyroidism or hypothyroidism) and an experienced cytopathologist is available, a needle aspiration can be performed (Fig. 216–10A). If the lesion is a simple cyst, this will be curative; otherwise the cytologic report guides therapy. If carcinoma is found, surgical exploration is indicated. If a cellular follicular aspirate is obtained that is consistent with a benign or a malignant lesion, a ^{123}I (or ^{131}I) scan is performed. If the lesion is hypofunctional, surgical exploration is advised. If it is warm or hot,

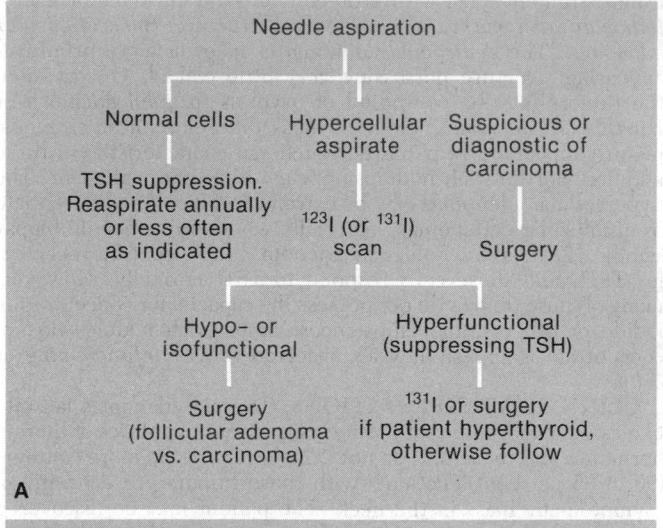

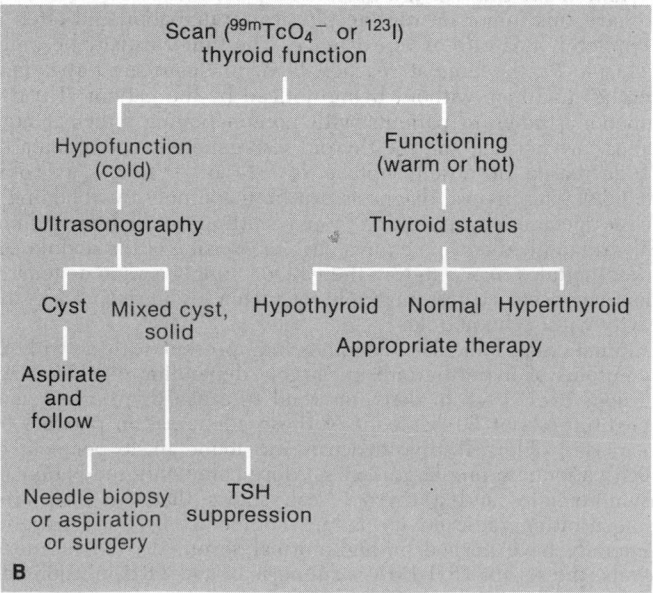

FIGURE 216–10. *A* shows a schema for the diagnostic evaluation of a patient with a solitary thyroid nodule based on aspiration biopsy cytology. *B* presents an alternative solution to the same problem starting with a thyroid scintiscan.

management is as discussed earlier under autonomous nodules. If the cytologic report indicates that the lesion is benign, thyroxine is given to suppress TSH, and this is monitored by TSH-IMA measurement. The need for surgery is then determined by the subsequent course of the individual patient. Aspiration biopsy cytology yields false-positive results (i.e., papillary carcinoma) very rarely, and false-negative results, that is, a benign diagnosis in a patient with a malignant lesion, should occur in only 2 to 3 per cent of patients. This figure, however, may be higher during the early experience with this technique in a given center. A number of patients are referred for surgery because of a cytologic picture that is suspicious but not clearly diagnostic. Nonetheless, in most clinics, aspiration cytology has reduced the apparent need for surgical exploration by 50 to 60 per cent. In other words, approximately 40 per cent of patients with solitary nodules require surgical exploration because of frankly or suspiciously malignant lesions.

If a trained cytopathologist is not available, then thyroid scanning is performed followed by ultrasonography if the nodule is not hyperfunctioning (Fig. 216–10B). Rarely a malignant nodule will be warm by $^{99m}TcO_4^-$ but cold by iodide scan. This should be suspected and tested for when warm lesions do not suppress function in the remainder of the gland. Ultrasonography of hypofunctioning nodules is performed. A cystic lesion can be treated by aspiration and the procedure repeated twice more if the fluid reaccumulates before surgery is indicated. In the nonfunctioning solid nodule, needle aspiration cytology, cutting needle biopsy, or surgical exploration is advised. I recommend surgical excision for patients under 20 and for those high-risk patients with familial carcinoma and radiation exposure. The availability of experienced thyroid surgeons plays an important role in this approach, since serious morbidity attends inadvertent resection of the parathyroid glands or recurrent laryngeal nerve paresis. In the other patients, the approach is dictated by the response to TSH suppression. Most nodules do not change in size, and therapy is individualized, whereas patients with nodules that increase during TSH suppression are referred for surgery, and those patients with nodules that decrease in size are followed with continued suppression. None of these responses clearly differentiates a benign from a malignant lesion.

At the time of initial surgery a frozen section should be obtained from all solitary thyroid nodules and an attempt made to provide definitive treatment. A reasonable approach to intrathyroidal papillary carcinoma is to perform a lobectomy with isthmectomy and explore for and remove any involved lymph nodes. An examination of the other lobe should be made for tumor, but, except in the irradiated patient, bilateral lobectomy is not required. With extrathyroidal extension of papillary carcinoma or bilateral lymph node metastases, a total thyroidectomy is performed with great care to preserve the recurrent laryngeal nerves and parathyroid glands. A follicular carcinoma is approached as are the papillary lesions, except that the presence of distant lymph node metastases or extensive capsular and vascular invasion in the initial frozen section should lead to consideration of bilateral thyroidectomy. This is done to remove residual normal tissue to facilitate radioiodine therapy (see below). Radical neck dissection does not offer any advantage over the less mutilating procedures described above. Medullary carcinoma of the sporadic variety may be treated as papillary carcinoma, but the familial form requires bilateral lobectomy. It is, of course, important to determine that pheochromocytoma and hyperparathyroidism are not present before undertaking surgery. Anaplastic carcinoma is rarely restricted enough to lend itself to surgical therapy, except for palliation to prevent tracheal compression. Lymphoma should be treated by radiotherapy and chemotherapy in consultation with a hematologist.

RADIATION THERAPY. I⁻ may be concentrated to a sufficient degree to be useful by as many as 50 to 60 per cent of well-differentiated thyroid tumors. This can be demonstrated only after the establishment of hypothyroidism with an increase in serum TSH. In general, prophylactic therapy with radioiodine in patients with papillary carcinoma does not appear to be beneficial, although metastases may respond to this method. In follicular carcinoma with evidence of vascular invasion or in patients with follicular metastases, particularly to the lungs, significant amelioration of symptoms and dramatic changes in the radiographic picture may be associated with this therapy. It does not appear

to be as useful for patients with bone metastases. To be weighed against these beneficial effects is the increased incidence of leukemia, which is 2 to 3 per cent in patients treated with large doses of ^{131}I (300 mCi and more).

The usual approach to evaluation of the feasibility of this therapeutic method is to remove residual functioning thyroid tissue surgically or by ^{131}I administration. After this, the patient is switched to triiodothyronine (50 μg per day) for a period of approximately 2 weeks, following which administration of the hormone is discontinued. Within 2 to 3 weeks, most patients show the maximal uptake in metastatic tissue. At that time, a tracer dose of ^{131}I should be given with appropriate dosimetry of the tumor mass, bone marrow, and lungs. Following this, the maximal tolerable ^{131}I dose should be given and the patient started on TSH-suppressive therapy with thyroxine 1 day later. Local recurrences of papillary carcinoma can often be treated surgically by removal of involved lymph nodes. In such patients this is preferable to ^{131}I, which should be reserved for a nonresectable lesion.

Despite the poor function of thyroid tumors in terms of radioiodine trapping, carcinomatous thyroid cells have TSH receptors and respond to TSH in vitro. Accordingly, efforts should be made to suppress TSH below normal, as monitored by TSH-IMA or by demonstrating that TRH does not increase TSH into the measurable range of a conventional assay. In patients who have had total thyroidectomy and radioiodine ablation, serum thyroglobulin concentrations should be monitored, since normal or increased levels of this protein then indicate the presence of residual thyroid tumor.

Hay ID, Grant CS, Taylor WF, et al.: Ipsilateral lobectomy versus bilateral lobar resection in papillary thyroid carcinoma: A retrospective analysis of surgical outcome using a novel prognostic scoring system. Surgery 102:1088, 1987. *An evaluation of the difficult issue of the appropriate surgery for patients with papillary thyroid carcinoma.*
Kaplan MM, Garnick MB, Gelber R, et al.: Risk factors for thyroid abnormalities after neck irradiation for childhood cancer. Am J Med 74:272, 1983. *This study shows that both benign and malignant thyroid nodules, as well as hypothyroidism, may appear 5 to 35 years after therapeutic irradiation to the neck.*
McConahey WM, Hay ID, Woolner LB, et al.: Papillary thyroid cancer treated at the Mayo Clinic 1946 through 1970: Initial manifestations, pathologic findings, therapy, and outcome. Mayo Clin Proc 61:978, 1986. *An update of a large retrospective evaluation of the results of various treatment modalities in patients with well-differentiated thyroid carcinoma.*
Pottern LM, Kaplan MM, Larsen PR, et al.: Thyroid nodularity after childhood irradiation for lymphoid hyperplasia: A comparison of questionnaire and clinical findings. J Clin Epidemiol 43:449, 1990. *An evaluation of the effect of radiation for tonsillar disease on thyroid nodularity in a large group of patients treated at Boston Children's Hospital. There is about a two- to threefold increase in the prevalence of thyroid nodules in the irradiated population compared with a large group of similarly examined controls.*

SPORADIC AND ENDEMIC GOITER

DEFINITION. *Sporadic goiter* refers to thyroid enlargement, which is found in a relatively small fraction of a given population. The cause for the thyroid enlargement may be different from patient to patient. The term *endemic goiter* refers to a condition seen in a much larger fraction of the population, which is presumably a consequence of one or several environmental influences, most commonly iodine deficiency. Although the causes of sporadic and endemic goiter are, by definition, different, the pathophysiology and pathology underlying these conditions are probably quite similar, and they are therefore grouped together.

ETIOLOGY. The common factor that is thought to lead to thyroid enlargement is *hypersecretion of TSH*. TSH increases in response to decreased production of thyroid hormones, especially T_4, as a consequence of an intrinsic abnormality in the process of thyroid hormone synthesis in the case of sporadic goiter, or the lack of adequate quantities of iodine in the diet or the presence of a goitrogen in the environment in endemic goiter. TSH increases as T_4 falls. As a consequence of the increased TSH secretion, iodine turnover by the thyroid is accelerated, the T_3 to T_4 ratio in thyroid secretion is increased, and serum T_3 may remain entirely normal. Such patients appear to be clinically euthyroid at the expense of an elevated serum TSH concentration and an enlarged thyroid gland.

PATHOLOGY. In the early phases, the thyroid gland may be diffusely enlarged with cellular hyperplasia as a result of TSH stimulation. Later, large follicles form with low epithelium. As the process continues, there is further stimulation of some thyroidal areas and atrophy of others with concomitant fibrosis. These multiple nodules have markedly varying activity. The accumulation of thyroglobulin, particularly in the iodine-deficient patients, may occur because poorly iodinated thyroglobulin is relatively resistant to digestion by endogenous proteases. To some extent, the same phenomenon may be occurring in the multinodular goiters which are sporadic and in which a specific cause has not been identified.

Sporadic Goiter

Sporadic goiter affects about 5 per cent of the population in the United States. Females outnumber males by a 3:1 ratio. In some patients an enzymatic defect in one of the steps in thyroid hormone synthesis can be identified (see Fig. 216–2). However, in most patients no specific cause can be isolated, but it is possible that milder forms of similar enzymatic deficiencies may be present.

CONGENITAL GOITER. This condition is sometimes referred to as *sporadic cretinism,* a syndrome of infantile myxedema characterized by growth failure, mental retardation, diffuse myxedema, and many of the signs and symptoms of hypothyroidism outlined in the section Hypothyroidism and Myxedema. Goitrous hypothyroidism can be due to a defect in any of the steps leading to the formation of thyroid hormone synthesis already discussed in the introduction. Defects have been identified in (1) iodide transport; (2) organification of iodide due to reduction in or absence of peroxidase, to an abnormal enzyme, or to diminished peroxide generation; (3) synthesis of an abnormal thyroglobulin molecule; (4) a structural abnormality in peroxidase, impairing its function as an iodine acceptor; (5) abnormal interrelationships of iodotyrosine; (6) impaired thyroglobulin proteolysis; and (7) a defect in iodotyrosine deiodination. The numbers given refer to the specific steps shown in Fig. 216–2. In some disorders of thyroglobulin synthesis the formation of an iodinated albumin-like protein has been described. All of these defects are rare. In North America and Europe they constitute less than 10 per cent of the approximately 1 in 4000 infants with congenital hypothyroidism.

A detailed description of each of these various defects is beyond the scope of this general text. The most common defect is the inability to organify iodine (defects in steps 2, 3, or 4). Such patients accumulate large amounts of I^- in the thyroid. This can be demonstrated by performance of a *perchlorate (CIO_4^-) discharge test.* In some patients this condition has been found in association with eighth nerve deafness and has the eponym *Pendred's syndrome.*

Regardless of the specific defect, these patients present with goiter and hypothyroidism, the serum T_4 index is reduced, and serum TSH is elevated. Further evaluation for the type of biochemical defect requires careful laboratory investigation. The treatment of such patients is with exogenous thyroid hormone. Thyroxine treatment causes regression of the enlarged thyroid, and mental retardation may be ameliorated or prevented if treatment is started before 3 months of age. Genetic counseling is desirable so that these patients are aware of the risk of hypothyroidism in subsequent offspring.

MULTINODULAR GOITER IN THE ADULT. The hypothesis that adults with multinodular goiter have mild defects in thyroid hormone synthesis similar to the more complete forms found in infants remains to be proved. If this is the case, then the goiter could be explained by modest increases in TSH, which is secreted by the pituitary in response to the reduced serum T_4. A significant physiologic increase in TSH may be as little as 2 to 3 μU per milliliter, often below the sensitivity of the TSH immunoassay that is clinically available. The compensatory increase in the size of the thyroid gland under these circumstances results in adequate rates of thyroid hormone formation, so that the vast majority of patients with this abnormality are euthyroid.

CLINICAL MANIFESTATIONS. Patients with multinodular goiter may come to the physician because of respiratory obstruction or dysphagia. More often the patient is asymptomatic and

the enlarged multinodular thyroid is discovered on a routine physical examination. Such patients should be questioned carefully for symptoms of respiratory obstruction. The goiter often extends retrosternally; this may be demonstrated by having the patient extend the arms directly over the head. If a significant substernal goiter is present, jugular venous distention and suffusion of the face occur *(Pemberton's sign).* Aside from physical obstruction, the most significant clinical aspect of the multinodular goiter is the tendency for hyperthyroidism to develop late in life *(Plummer's disease).* It is postulated that after decades of stimulation by TSH one or more of the nodular hyperplastic areas become autonomous. Since this condition generally appears in the elderly patient, the resulting hyperthyroidism may be of the apathetic variety (see the section Graves' Disease and Other Causes of Hyperthyroidism). In one series, administration of 50 to 100 mg of KI per day to eight patients with multinodular goiter resulted in hyperthyroidism in four patients, which required definitive treatment. The etiology of this form of iodide-induced thyrotoxicosis (probably not jodbasedow) is not clear, but caution is needed before the administration of iodide or iodine-containing drugs, such as amiodarone, to patients with multinodular goiter.

LABORATORY DIAGNOSIS. The physician must investigate both the anatomic and the functional nature of the thyroid pathology. Anatomic information is gained by chest or esophageal radiography, from a scintiscan, and when indicated by computed tomography of the neck and upper thorax. ^{131}I is recommended for thyroid scanning of these patients because the γ rays emitted by $^{99m}TcO_4^-$ and $^{123}I^-$ may not be strong enough to penetrate the sternum. The scintiscan image shows patchy focal uptake of radioactivity in an enlarged thyroid gland. The significance of the nonfunctioning areas in such scintiscans is discussed below. Measurements of serum free T_4 index, T_3, TSH, and TMAb and TgAb should be obtained, especially since Hashimoto's thyroiditis may present as a multinodular goiter. A TSH-IMA or a TRH test is especially important if Plummer's disease is suspected.

TREATMENT. The proper treatment depends on the clinical manifestations in the individual patient. Hyperthyroidism associated with multinodular goiter is best treated with radioactive iodine. However, because of the heterogeneity of the tissue uptake of radioiodine, a larger dose of radioiodine is necessary (180 μCi per gram or 10 mCi in a typical gland). The not uncommon coexistence of cardiac or pulmonary disease in this age group, together with the large size of the thyroid gland and the possibility of radiation thyroiditis, has led me to pretreat most elderly hyperthyroid patients with antithyroid drugs prior to radiotherapy. The antithyroid drugs are discontinued approximately 4 to 5 days prior to treatment. If a high plasma I^- (low RAI uptake) does not permit the use of radioiodine, then surgical treatment must be undertaken after appropriate preparation with antithyroid drugs.

Hypothyroid patients require treatment with thyroxine as described in the section Hypothyroidism and Myxedema. Young euthyroid patients with diffuse thyroid enlargement may be started on thyroxine replacement therapy to suppress TSH, particularly if this is slightly elevated. One may block further thyroid enlargement by this treatment as well as cause regression of goiter in some. In patients over the age of 40, it is unlikely that significant amelioration in physical symptoms will occur with TSH suppression, but this hormone may be administered on a trial basis. Great care must be exercised, particularly in the elderly, since one or more of the hyperplastic thyroid nodules may be functioning autonomously. In all patients with multinodular goiter it is suggested that a TSH-IMA or TRH test be performed prior to initiation of therapy with thyroid hormone to avoid iatrogenic hyperthyroidism. When autonomous function is present, well-meaning attempts to suppress TSH can cause iatrogenic hyperthyroidism. If physical symptoms of obstruction are present or there is evidence of recurrent laryngeal nerve dysfunction, surgical treatment is generally in order.

The Multinodular Goiter and Thyroid Carcinoma. Nodular disease of the thyroid is common and thyroid carcinoma is relatively rare. Poorly functioning areas may be present in the thyroid scintiscans of multinodular goiters, but this is not an indication for surgery for malignant disease. As heterogeneity of function is the rule, other criteria must be employed for recognition of malignancy in the multinodular goiter. Factors that raise this possibility include previous exposure to therapeutic thyroidal irradiation in childhood, a family history of thyroid carcinoma or enlargement of cervical lymph nodes, recurrent laryngeal nerve palsy, or the continuing enlargement of a single "cold" nodule in an otherwise stable gland. In situations in which doubt exists, needle biopsy may provide the requisite microscopic diagnosis to reassure the patient and the physician that conservative therapy is the appropriate course of action.

PROGNOSIS. Patients with euthyroid multinodular goiter should have thyroid function and physical findings evaluated at annual intervals. Most do not require surgery.

Endemic Goiter

Iodine deficiency is the most common cause of thyroid disease in the world population, although iodination of salt has eliminated this problem in North America. Areas in which iodine intake remains low include mountainous regions such as the Andes and Himalayas. In addition, there are areas of endemic goiter in central Africa, New Guinea, and Indonesia. Iodine prophylaxis, either in foodstuffs or in the form of iodized oil injection, has been successful in many of these countries, but iodine deficiency remains a considerable public health problem. In a few geographic locations, ingestion of a goitrogen has been implicated in the high incidence of goiter. Examples include a thiocyanate derivative from the cassava, which is eaten in large quantities in central Africa, and a goitrogenic hydrocarbon found in the water supply in parts of Colombia and in Chile.

CLINICAL MANIFESTATIONS IN ADULTS. The minimal quantity of iodine required for normal thyroid function is approximately 100 μg per day. As the level of iodine in the diet decreases below this level, there is a progressive fall in serum T_4 and a progressive rise in serum TSH. Serum T_3 concentrations remain normal or slightly elevated, a persistently elevated TSH being required for this compensation. Serum TSH concentrations may exceed 100 μU per milliliter. In the presence of lifelong stimulation of this degree, enormous hypertrophy and hyperplasia of the thyroid gland can occur. Such glands may weigh 1 to 5 kg, producing considerable physical impairment.

EFFECTS OF IODINE DEFICIENCY IN INFANTS. In areas of endemic goiter, cretinism is not uncommon. Despite the capacity of the placenta to transport I^-, in areas where iodine intake is severely reduced (25 μg per day or less) the 24-hour maternal RAI uptake is virtually 100 per cent. Infants in these areas may be born with congenital hypothyroidism as a consequence of iodine deficiency.

In areas such as the Andes or New Guinea where iodine intake may be less than 20 μg per day, a different form of *endemic cretinism* may be seen. As opposed to dwarfism and mental retardation, some children in these areas have spastic diplegia, squint, and deafness. The etiology of this syndrome is still not clarified. It may be a manifestation of the effect of iodine deficiency per se on the embryologic development of the central nervous system. Fetal or maternal hypothyroidism as a consequence of severe iodine deficiency may also contribute to this problem.

TREATMENT. The treatment of iodine deficiency is to supply this element either as a food additive or by direct injections of iodinated oil. This has often been difficult because of the inaccessibility and restricted governmental resources of those countries in which iodine deficiency is a problem. The *jodbasedow phenomenon* (iodine-induced hyperthyroidism) occurs in some patients receiving iodine supplementation. These presumably are patients with underlying Graves' (Basedow's) disease who are given adequate supplies of the substrate for thyroid hormone synthesis.

Dumont JE, Vassart G, Refetoff S: Thyroid disorders. *In* Scriver CR, Beudet A, Sly WS, et al.: The Metabolic Basis of Inherited Disease, 6th ed. New York, McGraw-Hill Book Company, 1989, pp 1843–1879. *The emphasis is on the emzymology of pathogenesis.*

Lever EG, Medeiros-Neto GA, DeGroot LJ: Inherited disorders of thyroid metabolism. Endocr Rev 4:213, 1983. *A comprehensive review of this topic.*

Studer H, Peter HJ, Gerber H: Natural heterogeneity of thyroid cells: The basis for understanding thyroid function and nodular goiter growth. Endocr Rev 10:125, 1989. *A careful study of the probable cause of hyperthyroidism in nodular goiter.*

Thilly CH, Delange F, Lagasse R, et al.: Fetal hypothyroidism and maternal thyroid status in severe endemic goiter. J Clin Endocrinol Metab 47:354, 1978. *The effects of iodine deficiency on mother and newborn are described, comparing treated and untreated patients.*

Wolff J: Congenital goiter with defective iodide transport. Endocr Rev 4:240, 1983. *The clinical, pathophysiologic, and biochemical findings in patients with this form of sporadic goiter.*

217 Disorders of the Adrenal Cortex
J. Blake Tyrrell and John D. Baxter

217.1 STRUCTURE AND DEVELOPMENT OF THE ADRENAL CORTEX
John D. Baxter

The major function of the adrenal cortex is to produce glucocorticoid and mineralocorticoid hormones, of which cortisol and aldosterone, respectively, are the most important in humans. The glucocorticoids, named for their carbohydrate-regulating properties, are essential for survival, at least in times of stress, and regulate intermediary metabolism, hemodynamic functions, and developmental processes. The mineralocorticoids regulate sodium, potassium, and hydrogen ion balance and secondarily affect the blood pressure. Either an excess or a deficiency of these steroids can have deleterious effects. Glucocorticoid excess is termed Cushing's syndrome. Adrenocortical insufficiency due to destruction of the adrenal gland is called Addison's disease. Aldosterone excess and deficiency are referred to as aldosteronism and hypoaldosteronism, respectively. Whereas diseases of the adrenal cortex are relatively uncommon, their clinical stigmata are part of the differential diagnosis of common problems. In addition, iatrogenic glucocorticoid excess is a common clinical problem due to the widespread usage of glucocorticoids in therapy. Secondary hyperaldosteronism is also a common problem sometimes requiring antimineralocorticoid therapy.

The human adrenal cortex produces at least 50 other steroids. This gland is a major source of androgenic steroids in the female (see Ch. 224) but is a trivial source of these steroids in the male compared to the testes (see Ch. 222). The adrenal production of dehydroepiandrosterone (DHEA) and its sulfate derivative is about half that of cortisol. Although these steroids typically are designated "adrenal androgens," they may have other, as-yet-undefined actions. The adrenal produces only minute quantities of estrogens and progestins. Some other adrenal steroids (e.g., deoxycorticosterone or testosterone) can cause clinical abnormalities when they are produced in excess in certain pathologic states.

STRUCTURE. There are two adrenal glands, located extraperitoneally at the upper poles of each kidney lateral to the eleventh thoracic to first lumbar vertebrae. The right gland tends to be higher and more lateral than the left. The average gland weighs 4 grams and is 2 to 3 cm wide and 4 to 6 cm long. A series of small arteries arising from the abdominal aorta, from renal and phrenic arteries, and occasionally from ovarian or spermatic arteries, feed the gland. Because of this, arterial infarction is unusual. The venous drainage of the gland on the left is ordinarily into the renal vein and on the right into the inferior vena cava. The gland is innervated by autonomic fibers.

The adrenal cortex comprises about 90 per cent of the gland and surrounds the centrally located medulla that produces catecholamines. The cortex has three zones. The ill-defined zona glomerulosa, about 15 per cent of the cortex, is present under the capsule and contains foci of cells, with a small cytoplasmic volume and lipid content, that produce aldosterone. The remainder of the cortex, the zonae reticularis and fasciculata, can be considered a single unit involved predominantly in cortisol and androgen production. Cells of the zona fasciculata, about 75 per cent of the cortex, appear vacuolated or clear on stained sections because of their high cholesterol content. The cells of the inner zona reticularis are more compact with less lipid.

The morphology of the gland is influenced by corticotropin (ACTH), angiotensin II, and potassium. Elevations of ACTH levels increase adrenal blood flow within minutes and adrenal weight within hours; the clear fasciculata cells lose their lipid, attain the compact morphology and ultrastructural features of reticularis cells, and produce cortisol. Prolonged stimulation results in hyperplasia and hypertrophy. Increases in angiotensin II and potassium result in hypertrophy and hyperplasia of the glomerulosa cells and increased aldosterone production. Deficiency of angiotensin II leads to atrophy of the zona glomerulosa, and deficiency of ACTH to atrophy of the zonae fasciculata and reticularis; this is reversible upon restimulation. Occasionally, accessory adrenal glands may be present in a variety of locations in the abdomen or pelvis and can assume significant function in states of ACTH excess.

DEVELOPMENT. The adrenal cortex is derived from mesenchymal tissue. Cortical cells emerge to form a primitive fetal cortex around the sixth week of development. This evolves into a fetal zone involved predominantly in synthesis of androgen and estrogen precursors, and a definitive zone destined to become the adult gland. The fetal zone, the major bulk of the adrenal cortex at birth, begins to recede by the last intrauterine month and disappears around the end of the first year. The permanent cortex is formed from cells of the outer portion of the fetal gland and is not developed completely until around 3 years of age.

217.2 SYNTHESIS, CIRCULATION, AND METABOLISM OF ADRENAL STEROIDS

John D. Baxter

SYNTHESIS

The structures and steps in biosynthesis of a number of steroid hormones are shown in Figure 217–1. The letter designation for the carbon rings and the number designation of the carbon atoms are shown for pregnenolone, a key biosynthetic intermediate. α- and β- designate positions of the side groups above (β) or below (α) the plane of the molecule. The various steroids differ in (1)

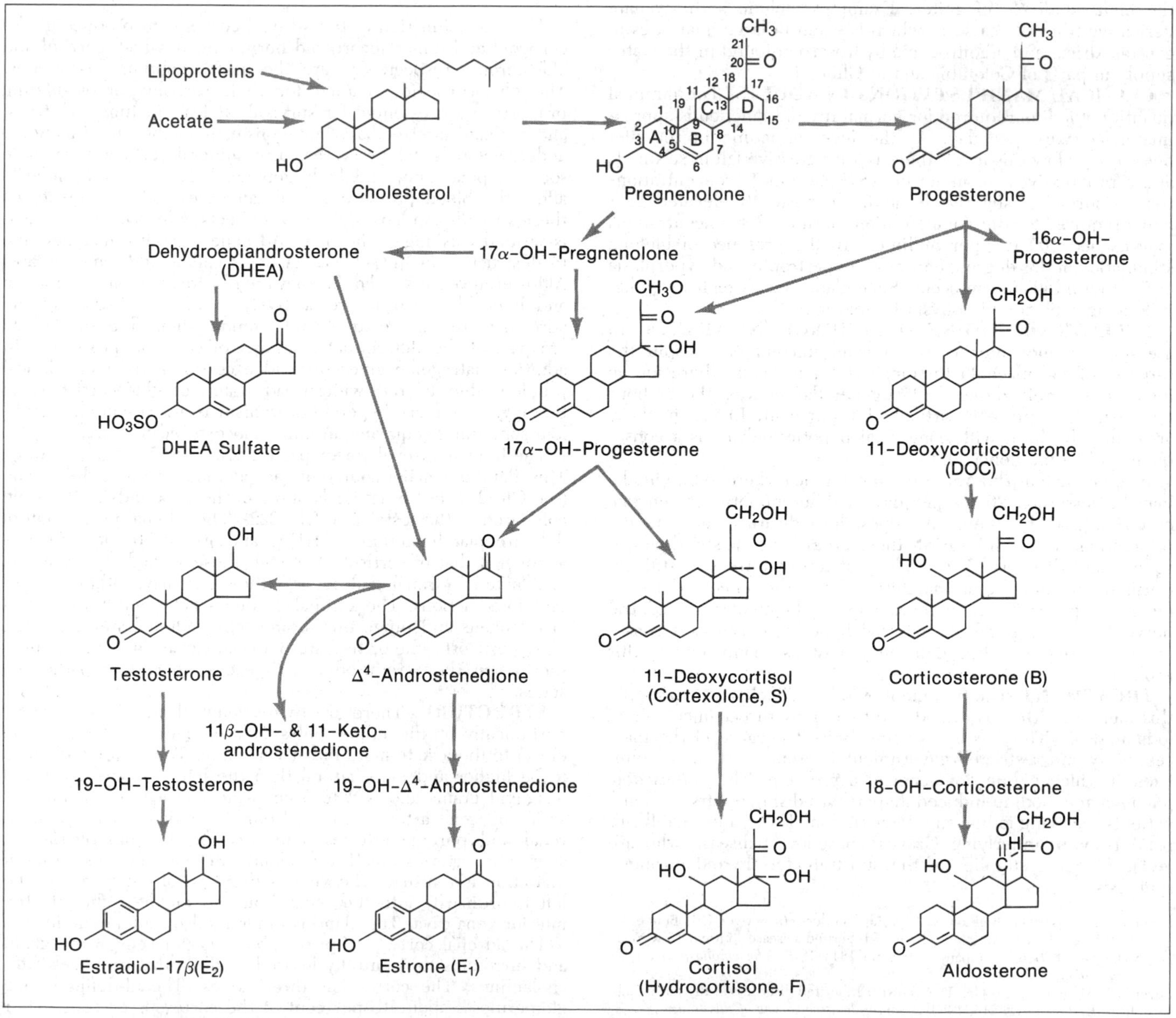

FIGURE 217–1. Steps in adrenal steroid biosynthesis. The numbers for the carbon atoms and the letters designating the rings of the steroid molecule are shown for pregnenolone. Arrows indicate the conversion pathways; the use of two arrows between intermediates indicates that more than one step is involved in the interconversion. (Adapted from Baxter JD, Tyrrell JB: *In* Felig P, Baxter JD, Broadus AE, et al. (eds.): Endocrinology and Metabolism, 2nd ed. New York, McGraw-Hill Book Company, 1987, p 516.)

TABLE 217–1. SECRETION RATES AND PLASMA CONCENTRATIONS OF ADRENAL STEROIDS*

Steroid	24-hr Secretion (mg)	Mean Plasma Concentration (ng/ml)
Aldosterone	0.15	0.16
Androstenedione	2.4	1.5
Corticosterone	2.5	3
Cortisol	16	100
11-Deoxycorticosterone (DOC)	0.6	0.16
11-Deoxycortisol	0.4	1.7
DHEA	0.7(F), 3.0(M)	5.4
DHEA-S	7	1200
Progesterone	nil	0.2(M,F), 12(F)†
17α-Hydroxyprogesterone	nil	0.2(M), 0.6(F), 2.0(F)†
Testosterone	0.2	5.6(M), 0.5(F)

Modified from Baxter JD, Tyrrell JB: The adrenal cortex. In Felig P, Baxter JD, Broadus AH, et al. (eds.): Endocrinology and Metabolism, 2nd ed. New York, McGraw-Hill Book Company, 1987, p 521, where references to primary source material can be found.

*Mean values are reported for adults. Individual female (F) and male (M) values are reported only when these differ by more than twofold.

†Refers to the luteal phase of the menstrual cycle.

the saturation of the A ring (Δ indicates a double bond); (2) hydroxyl and ketone groups at positions 3, 11, 17, and 21; (3) the presence of a three-carbon side chain at position 17; and (4) an aldehyde group at position 18. Since the chemical nomenclature is cumbersome, trivial names for the steroids are used most frequently.

All steroids are derived from cholesterol that is obtained mostly by receptor-mediated internalization of plasma low density lipoproteins and to a lesser extent from synthesis by the gland. This uptake mechanism is increased when the adrenal is stimulated.

Subsequent steps occur in the mitochondrion or endoplasmic reticulum. The first step is the conversion of cholesterol to pregnenolone. This rate-limiting step is regulated by the major factors (ACTH, angiotensin II, and potassium) that stimulate steroid biosynthesis. This conversion involves several steps, catalyzed by the enzyme 20,22-desmolase (cholesterol side chain cleavage enzyme). Pregnenolone is then modified either (1) by converting its 5,6 to a 4,5 double bond with the use of 3β-hydroxysteroid dehydrogenase and Δ⁵-oxysteroid isomerase, resulting in progesterone; or (2) by addition of a 17α-hydroxyl group with the use of 17α-hydroxylase, resulting in 17α-hydroxypregnenolone. The former pathway occurs in the glomerulosa, which lacks 17α-hydroxylase activity; although controversial, the latter pathway probably predominates in the fasciculata-reticularis, with subsequent conversion of 17α-hydroxypregnenolone to 17α-hydroxyprogesterone.

CORTISOL. Cortisol is synthesized by two successive hydroxylations of 17α-hydroxyprogesterone. The first is at the 21 position, catalyzed by 21-hydroxylase, and results in 11-deoxycortisol (also called compound S). The second, at the 11 position of 11-deoxycortisol, is catalyzed by 11β-hydroxylase and yields cortisol (also called hydrocortisone or compound F). These hydroxylations also require a flavoprotein dehydrogenase and a cytochrome P-450.

ALDOSTERONE. Aldosterone is produced by 21-hydroxylation of progesterone to form deoxycorticosterone (DOC); 11β-hydroxylation of DOC to form corticosterone; 18-hydroxylation of the latter to form 18-hydroxycorticosterone (18-OHB); and oxidation of the 18 CH₂OH group to an aldehyde to form aldosterone with the use of 18-hydroxycorticosteroid hydroxylase. This step is unique to the glomerulosa.

ANDROGENS. The adrenal androgens have 19 carbon atoms (C-19 steroids) and serve as precursors for more potent androgens produced in peripheral tissues. These are DHEA and its sulfate (DHEA-S), androstenedione, and testosterone. DHEA is derived from 17α-hydroxypregnenolone by removal of its C-17 side chain, that leaves a keto group, with the use of C-17,20-lyase, and 17β-hydroxysteroid dehydrogenase. The sulfation of DHEA at the 3 position to DHEA-S is catalyzed by a sulfokinase. Androstenedione can be derived from either 17α-hydroxyprogesterone or DHEA, as illustrated. The adrenal synthesizes minute quantities of the C-18 steroids estradiol and estrone (Fig. 217–1). However,

DHEA and DHEA-S synthesized by the fetal adrenal account for substantial amounts of maternal production of estriol, estradiol, estrone, testosterone, and androstenedione.

PRODUCTION RATES. The production rates and the blood levels under basal conditions of the major adrenal steroids are shown in Table 217–1. More cortisol is produced than any other steroid; much less aldosterone is produced. The production of DHEA plus DHEA-S is about half that of cortisol; although the plasma levels of DHEA are only a fraction of those of cortisol, plasma levels of DHEA-S are severalfold higher than those of cortisol because of the slow metabolism of DHEA-S. Corticosterone has substantial glucocorticoid activity but is produced at much lower levels than cortisol. Similarly, DOC has substantial mineralocorticoid activity, and more DOC than aldosterone is produced, but free levels of this steroid in plasma are much lower than those of aldosterone even though total levels are similar. The adrenal production of progesterone and 17α-hydroxyprogesterone is minimal. The production of testosterone is at levels similar to those of aldosterone.

INHIBITORS. Several compounds can inhibit adrenal steroid biosynthesis at various steps. They can be useful for diagnosis and therapy of adrenal disorders (discussed below). Of these, metyrapone (SU-4885), aminoglutethimide, and mitotane (o,p'-DDD) have been used most commonly. Metyrapone predominantly inhibits 11β-hydroxylation and to a lesser extent 21-hydroxylation. Aminoglutethimide blocks the early steps in conversion of cholesterol to pregnenolone (cholesterol to 20α-hydroxycholesterol). Mitotane blocks adrenal mitochondrial functioning and results in generalized inhibition of steroid biosynthesis and adrenal atrophy. Ketoconazole, an antifungal agent, also inhibits steroid biosynthesis by inhibiting the actions of cytochrome P-450 enzymes. Spironolactone can block aldosterone biosynthesis by inhibiting the 11β- and 18-hydroxylation steps; these actions may add to the antimineralocorticoid actions of this compound.

PLASMA BINDING OF ADRENAL STEROIDS

GLUCOCORTICOIDS. Approximately 90 to 93 per cent of the circulating cortisol is bound by plasma proteins. About 80 per cent of this binding is due to specific and high-affinity association of cortisol with corticosteroid-binding globulin (CBG, also termed transcortin). A lesser quantity is bound by albumin and a negligible amount by other plasma proteins. CBG is synthesized in the liver and at its usual concentrations in plasma has a capacity for binding cortisol of around 25 μg per deciliter; thus, when cortisol levels begin to exceed this saturation capacity, the proportion of free cortisol is increased. Although several other steroids (e.g., corticosterone, progesterone) can bind to CBG, under most circumstances such occupancy is minimal.

CBG concentrations in plasma vary on a genetic basis and are also regulated by hormones and other factors. CBG levels are increased in pregnancy (by almost twofold during the third trimester), in hyperthyroidism, in diabetes, and by estrogens and oral contraceptives. Such effects can be maximal in 3 to 5 days and reversed by 2 to 3 weeks after cessation of the stimulus. CBG levels can be low congenitally and in liver disease (decreased protein production), multiple myeloma, obesity, hypothyroidism, and the nephrotic syndrome (through urinary loss).

The physiologic role of the plasma steroid-binding proteins is unknown. CBG is not required to transport cortisol, as it is soluble at physiologically effective concentrations. CBG is also not required for cortisol action. For instance, tissue culture cells respond to cortisol in the absence of detectable CBG. Further, the free rather than the plasma-bound steroid is physiologically active, and physiologic mechanisms that regulate cortisol levels respond to the free rather than the total steroid concentration. Thus, when the CBG levels are primarily elevated or depressed, there are elevations or depressions, respectively, of the total cortisol in plasma, but the free cortisol concentration remains the same. This point is critical for evaluation of states of glucocorticoid excess or deficiency.

That CBG may have some importance is suggested by its ubiquity in mammals, even though plasma levels vary enormously, and by the fact that congenital absence of CBG in humans has never been found. A possible role for CBG is to provide a more even distribution of cortisol within larger organs. The free steroid is immediately available for tissue uptake. Thus, when blood enters a large organ such as the liver, the proximal portions of the tissue (outer hepatocytes in the lobule) could sequester most of the free hormone, making it unavailable for more distal uptake (closer to the central vein). In the presence of CBG-bound cortisol, however, the uptake of free hormone by cells would lead to the release of bound hormone to reestablish the equilibrium. Since the blood is moving, such dissociation would occur more distally, where the newly derived free cortisol would then be available for uptake. Such binding may also slow the degradation of steroids as they pass through the liver by reducing the rate at which they are taken up. In addition, CBG or CBG-like proteins can be located intracellularly, and in the kidney they may sequester cortisol and prevent it from occupying the mineralocorticoid receptors. This would preserve the latter for occupancy by aldosterone as the major salt-regulating hormone. Finally, the protein binding of steroids in the blood may buffer rapid changes in plasma free cortisol levels that would otherwise occur as a result of episodic release of cortisol from the adrenal gland.

MINERALOCORTICOIDS. Under physiologic conditions, about 60 per cent of the total plasma aldosterone is protein bound, largely to albumin. The binding is weaker than that of cortisol with CBG, and the free plasma aldosterone seems to be physiologically active.

DOC has potent mineralocorticoid activity, and its plasma levels are similar to those of aldosterone. However, DOC is not normally a physiologically important mineralocorticoid, since over 95 per cent of it is bound to plasma proteins and thus its free levels are much lower than those of aldosterone.

METABOLISM OF ADRENAL STEROIDS

The hydrophobic steroids, although filtered by the renal glomerulus and excreted into the urine, are mostly reabsorbed. For example, only about 1 per cent of the cortisol produced daily is excreted unchanged in the urine. Nevertheless, the kidneys account for over 90 per cent of the excretion of metabolized steroids (DOC and corticosterone are exceptions); the remainder is lost in the gut. To promote their renal elimination, the steroids are inactivated and made more water soluble through enzymatic modifications. These involve hydroxylation of the keto groups, reduction of the double bond in the A ring, and conjugation at the 3 or 21 positions with glucuronide or sulfate. These conversions occur mostly in liver, although during pregnancy the placenta assumes metabolic importance. The conversions alter the steroids so that the renal clearance of a major cortisol metabolite, tetrahydrocortisone glucuronide, is around 70 per cent that of the creatinine clearance. More than 50 metabolites of cortisol and aldosterone have been detected in humans. The pathways shown in Figure 217–2 appear generally to be dominant.

GLUCOCORTICOIDS. Cortisol is cleared from the plasma with a half-life of 80 to 120 minutes. About 70 per cent of infused cortisol, and presumably of that secreted, is eliminated within 24 hours. The 11β-hydroxyl group of cortisol can be oxidized by the enzyme 11β-hydroxysteroid dehydrogenase to the ketone, forming cortisone, which is devoid of glucocorticoid activity. Cortisone can also be converted to cortisol by 11-oxo-steroid reductase. Thus, administered cortisone is largely converted to active cortisol in the liver. Conversely, however, in parts of the kidney cortisol is predominantly converted to cortisone. This prevents cortisol from binding to the mineralocorticoid receptor, which in turn allows aldosterone to serve as the major mineralocorticoid. In other tissues, such as brain, where cortisol is not efficiently converted to cortisone, cortisol does occupy and act through mineralocorticoid receptors.

Cortisol and cortisone have similar subsequent metabolic fates, and overall roughly equivalent quantities of metabolites of these steroids are produced. Quantitatively the most important subsequent modification involves reduction of the 3-keto moiety to form dihydrocortisol and dihydrocortisone, followed by a reduction of the 4,5 double bond to form tetrahydrocortisol and tetrahydrocortisone. When the 3-hydroxyl group is formed, over 95 per cent of the products are conjugated at this position to form the glucuronide and to a lesser extent the sulfate derivatives. Conjugates of these two steroids make up around 30 per cent of

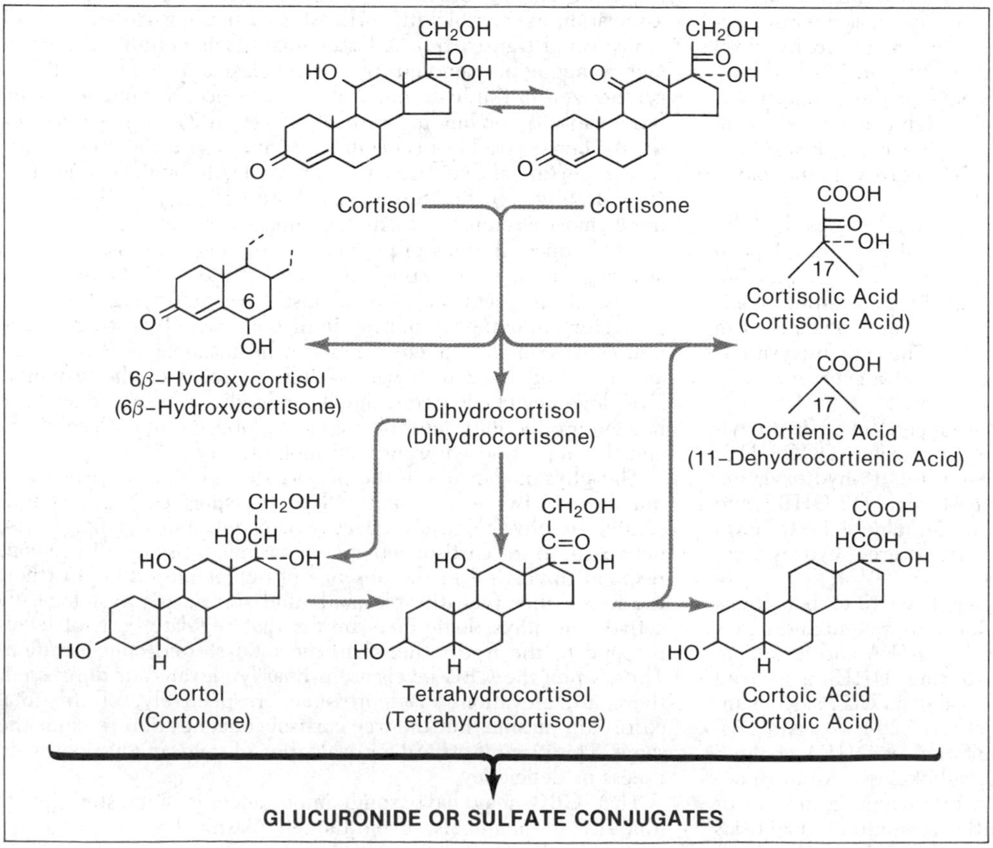

FIGURE 217–2. Metabolism of cortisol. See text. The interconversion of cortisol to cortisone is shown. The other steroid metabolites can be derivatives of either cortisol or cortisone. Structures shown and names are for the cortisol derivatives. The names of the cortisone derivatives are shown in parentheses. In some cases, only part of the steroid molecule is shown; in these cases numbers refer to the steroid carbons for orientation. For tetrahydrocortisol, tetrahydrocortisone, and their derivatives, the 3-hydroxyl and 5-hydrogen are shown in the α and β configurations, respectively, but both α and β orientations occur at both positions. For a more extensive discussion and references, see Baxter JD, Tyrrell JB: In Felig P, Baxter JD, Broadus AE, et al. (eds.): Endocrinology and Metabolism, 2nd ed. New York, McGraw-Hill Book Company, 1987, p 544.

Cortisol — Cortisone

Cortisolic Acid (Cortisonic Acid)

6β-Hydroxycortisol (6β-Hydroxycortisone)

Cortienic Acid (11-Dehydrocortienic Acid)

Dihydrocortisol (Dihydrocortisone)

Cortol (Cortolone)

Tetrahydrocortisol (Tetrahydrocortisone)

Cortoic Acid (Cortolic Acid)

GLUCURONIDE OR SULFATE CONJUGATES

the urinary cortisol metabolites. The second major site for modification involves the reduction of the 20-ketone to a hydroxyl, with subsequent reduction of the A ring, resulting in cortol (11-OH) or cortolone (11-keto). These account for approximately 25 per cent of the cortisol metabolites. Alternatively, there can be conversion of the 21-hydroxyl to a COOH to form cortisolic or cortisonic acid from cortisol and cortisone, respectively. Cortoic (11-hydroxyl) or cortolonic (11-keto) acid results from this modification of tetrahydrocortisone and tetrahydrocortisol, respectively, and these metabolites account for about 10 per cent of the cortisol metabolites. Other minor pathways involve the C-17 modifications discussed above without A-ring reduction, removal of the C-17 side chain with formation of 17-keto or 17-COOH moieties, formation of the C-21 COOH (without C-20-keto) and 6β-hydroxylation. The latter modification constitutes a major pathway in infants in whom the esterification mechanism has not been developed and for the synthetic glucocorticoids used in therapy.

MINERALOCORTICOIDS. Aldosterone is cleared with a half-life of around 15 minutes. Its conversion to metabolites is so effective that very little aldosterone survives passage through the liver. This is in part due to the weak plasma binding of aldosterone which allows it to be taken up by the liver (discussed above). Less than 0.5 per cent of the aldosterone appears in the urine in the free state. The metabolism of aldosterone is similar to that of cortisol. About 35 per cent of the steroid appears as tetrahydroaldosterone glucuronide (3 position). However, two major differences are that there is much less 11β-hydroxy to 11-keto conversion, and 15 to 20 per cent of the aldosterone appears as a C-18 glucuronide that is acid labile; measurements of the urinary "aldosterone" usually reflect this metabolite.

ANDROGENS. The metabolism of androgens is discussed in Ch. 222.

VARIATIONS IN RATES OF METABOLISM. The rate of steroid metabolism can be altered in certain clinical states and by various drugs. Agents that affect plasma steroid-binding proteins secondarily affect metabolism because of inhibitory influences of plasma binding on clearance. In chronic liver disease, hypothyroidism, infancy, very old age, anorexia nervosa, and protein-calorie malnutrition, the rate of steroid metabolism is decreased. The converse occurs in hyperthyroidism. These states are in general not associated with abnormal free steroid levels (anorexia nervosa is an exception) because the regulatory systems tend to compensate by altering steroid production. The conversion of cortisone to cortisol is not substantially impaired in liver disease. The conversion of prednisone to prednisolone may be impaired, however, and prednisolone rather than prednisone is recommended for glucocorticoid therapy in patients with severe liver disease. Also, there is no major effect of renal disease (even though it does affect the clearance of some metabolites) or of most chronic diseases, obesity, and stress.

Drugs that affect steroid metabolism usually increase 6β-hydroxylation. This is a minor pathway in adults, and these drugs do not have a major effect on endogenous cortisol. They have a greater effect on the clearance of synthetic glucocorticoids such as dexamethasone and prednisone, and this is therefore an important consideration with steroid therapy or with the use of glucocorticoids to assess the hypothalamic-pituitary-adrenal axis. These drugs include mitotane, phenytoin, rifampicin, aminoglutethimide, and barbiturates. Glycyrrhetinic acid, present in licorice, and carbenoxolone, used for treatment of peptic ulcer disease, block 11β-hydroxysteroid dehydrogenase and thereby the conversion of cortisol to cortisone. This leads to increased actions of cortisol through mineralocorticoid receptors and a hypermineralocorticoid state.

217.3 REGULATION OF ADRENAL STEROID PRODUCTION

John D. Baxter

Adrenal cortisol and androgen production is regulated by the hypothalamic-pituitary-adrenal axis, whereas aldosterone production is regulated predominantly by the renin-angiotensin system and by potassium (Fig. 217–3). These systems allow for basal and circadian steroid production, regulation of plasma steroid levels in normal circumstances, and increased or decreased steroid production in response to a number of specific stimuli.

REGULATION OF GLUCOCORTICOID PRODUCTION

The hypothalamus, pituitary, and adrenal comprise a neuroendocrine axis concerned with regulation of cortisol production (see

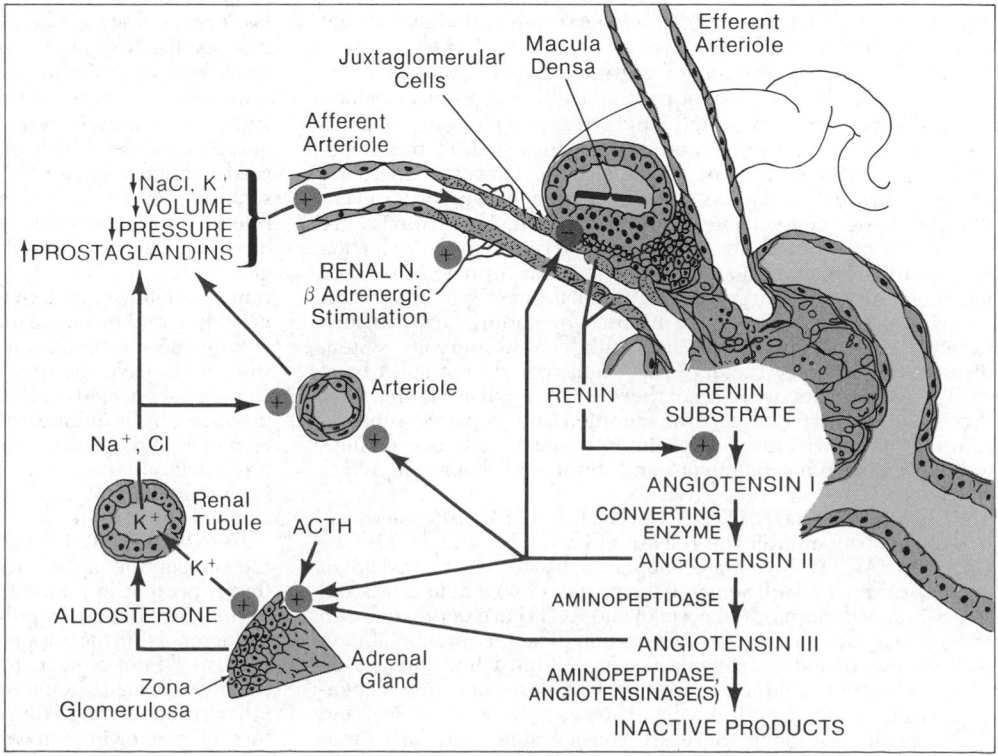

FIGURE 217–3. Renin-angiotensin system. The plus and minus signs indicate stimulation and inhibition, respectively. (Reprinted from Baxter JD, Perloff D, Hsueh W, et al.: *In* Felig P, Baxter JD, Broadus AE, et al. (eds.): Endocrinology and Metabolism, 2nd ed. New York, McGraw-Hill Book Company, 1987, p 701.)

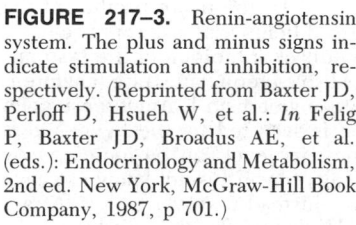

Ch. 212). Corticotropin-releasing factor (CRF) and arginine vasopressin (AVP) are elaborated by the hypothalamus and travel through its portal system to the anterior pituitary where they stimulate the release of ACTH, which in turn increases adrenal cortisol production.

Three major types of mechanisms are involved in regulating cortisol release: (1) circadian rhythms of secretion are established by the brain, (2) a number of types of excitatory factors can increase cortisol production, and (3) production of CRF and ACTH is regulated negatively by glucocorticoids.

ACTH AND RELATED PEPTIDES. ACTH circulates free in the plasma with a half-life of around 10 minutes. It is derived from the proteolysis of pro-opiomelanocortin, a larger precursor pituitary protein of about 290 amino acids that also contains the sequences of several other proteins, including β-endorphin, α-, β-, and γ-melanocyte-stimulating hormones (MSH), β-lipotropin (β-LPH), and an amino-terminal fragment (see Ch. 208). Although MSH itself has the greatest pigment-stimulating activity, this activity in humans is due predominantly to MSH sequences contained within ACTH (α-MSH), β-LPH (β-MSH), and the amino-terminal fragment (γ-MSH), as very little MSH is present in the circulation. ACTH stimulates cortisol release within 2 to 3 minutes. This is due to increased cortisol synthesis primarily through stimulation of cholesterol to pregnenolone conversion, rather than through effects on secretion of stored hormone. More prolonged stimulation results in increased protein, RNA, and DNA synthesis with both hypertrophy and hyperplasia. ACTH binds to surface receptors and activates adenylate cyclase. This results in increased cyclic AMP generation with consequent stimulation of protein phosphorylation and of the production of phospholipids that may be involved in the stimulation of steroidogenesis. The actions of ACTH are also Ca^{2+} dependent. These effects increase cholesterol side chain cleavage and cholesterol esterase and lipoprotein uptake and block cholesterol ester synthesis with a resulting stimulation of the conversion of cholesterol to pregnenolone.

SPONTANEOUS RHYTHMS. The circadian rhythm of ACTH and cortisol results in decreasing release through the afternoon and evening. Secretion begins to increase around 3 to 4 A.M., peaks by around 8 A.M., and then begins to decline. This release occurs in pulses with intervals between them of 40 minutes to hours; the changes in overall cortisol production are due to the number of pulses that occur. These result in cortisol levels that vary enormously within minutes; thus, single plasma cortisol determinations may not give an adequate integrated assessment of overall cortisol production.

The spontaneous rhythm of cortisol secretion can be interrupted acutely by a variety of psychological and physical factors. These can vary from seemingly mild stresses such as the confrontation for venipuncture to more severe ones such as the preparation for cardiac surgery or severe anxiety. However, there are major individual variations. Major trauma or surgery, severe illness, hypoglycemia, fever, burns, and intensive exercise are illustrative of physical stresses that increase cortisol production by up to sixfold. Minor illnesses such as upper respiratory infections or minor surgery have minimal or no influence. Variations in cortisol levels can be blunted by chronic diseases such as congestive heart failure and with central nervous system disease and pituitary tumors even when they do not affect basal ACTH release. In depression there is a circadian rhythm, but there can be increased cortisol secretion and impaired suppression by glucocorticoids. Serotonin antagonists such as cyproheptadine inhibit both spontaneous and stimulated changes in ACTH release.

FEEDBACK INHIBITION OF ACTH RELEASE. Glucocorticoids feedback-inhibit the release of both CRF and ACTH (see Ch. 208). ACTH levels are increased up to 10- to 20-fold in primary adrenal insufficiency. Conversely, endogenous levels and stress-induced increases of cortisol and ACTH are depressed with exogenous glucocorticoid administration. The feedback inhibition in response to glucocorticoids occurs within a few minutes, is progressive with continual exposure in a dose- and time-dependent fashion, affects both basal and stress-stimulated release, and is reversible. Although there are considerable individual variations, administration of a large dose of glucocorticoids for a few

days does not, in general, result in suppression of pituitary function for more than a few hours; more prolonged exposure is accompanied by substantial suppression. Thus after several years of glucocorticoid therapy and then withdrawal of steroid administration or following surgical removal of a tumor causing Cushing's syndrome, a year or more may be required for the hypothalamic-pituitary-adrenal axis to return to normal functioning. Although significant suppression occurs at both the hypothalamic and pituitary levels, the quantitative contribution of each of them has not been clarified.

REGULATION OF MINERALOCORTICOID PRODUCTION

Aldosterone production is controlled predominantly by the renin-angiotensin system and potassium, although other factors such as sodium, ACTH, dopamine, and serotonin also affect aldosterone secretion (Fig. 217–3). The renin-angiotensin system is important for adaptive blood pressure changes and is involved in the pathogenesis of some forms of hypertension.

RENIN. Renin, a glycoprotein of 340 amino acids, is produced in the juxtaglomerular cells of the afferent renal arteriole as a precursor protein (prorenin) that is cleaved to yield active renin. These cells release renin into the circulation where it has a half-life of around 15 minutes. Prorenin is also made in a number of other tissues, and in some of these, including the adrenal, it may be converted to active renin. The role of extrarenal renin-angiotensin systems is currently a subject of intense study. However, extrarenal prorenin does not contribute to the plasma renin, and conditions that result in impaired renal release of renin lead to aldosterone deficiency. The release of renin is stimulated by lowering the blood pressure, assumption of the erect posture, salt depletion, β-adrenergic or central nervous system stimulation, and certain prostaglandins. It is inhibited by increases in blood pressure (except with malignant hypertension), salt loading, angiotensin II, vasopressin, potassium, calcium, β-adrenergic antagonists, α-methyldopa, clonidine, and inhibitors of prostaglandin synthesis such as indomethacin.

Four factors mediate most of the changes in renin release: (1) Changes in renal tubular sodium chloride concentration are detected by the macula densa, a specialized segment of the distal tubule that makes contact with the juxtaglomerular cells of the afferent arteriole just before it enters the glomerulus. This information is transmitted to the juxtaglomerular cells so that factors that reduce volume or lower the plasma sodium and chloride levels (e.g., dehydration, fluid or blood loss) increase renin release. (2) Renal baroreceptors stimulate renin release in response to decreases in renal perfusion pressure as with fluid loss or decreases in blood pressure. These receptors can function independently of innervation and salt delivery and respond more to changes in pressure than to the absolute pressure. (3) Renal sympathetic nerves that terminate in the juxtaglomerular cells and smooth muscle cells of the renal afferent arterioles secrete norepinephrine, which in turn stimulates renin release through β-adrenergic receptors. Blockage of this mechanism by agents such as propranolol probably explains how they decrease renin release. However, catecholamines can have other indirect effects on renin release through influences on renal blood flow and glomerular filtration. (4) Angiotensin II, the major product of the renin-angiotensin system (discussed below), blocks renin release, providing one mechanism for feedback inhibition of the system.

Renin acts in the plasma and cleaves renin substrate (angiotensinogen) to yield the decapeptide angiotensin I. Angiotensinogen contains about 450 amino acids, is secreted by the liver, and is produced by a number of tissues; its level can be increased by estrogens and glucocorticoids. Angiotensin I is not known to have physiologically important actions; instead it serves as a substrate for production of angiotensin II. Normally the production of angiotensin I is rate limiting for angiotensin II generation.

CONVERTING ENZYME. The conversion of angiotensin I to the octapeptide angiotensin II is catalyzed by converting enzyme that is present in a number of tissues and in high concentrations in the lung. In certain pulmonary diseases there can be decreases or increases in the plasma levels of the enzyme, although these changes do not appear to have a physiologically important effect on angiotensin II generation. Converting enzyme also catalyzes other reactions, including the inactivation of bradykinin. Inhibitors of converting enzyme, such as captopril, enalapril, and lisinopril, are widely used to treat hypertension and heart failure.

ANGIOTENSIN II. Angiotensin II is a potent vasoconstrictor with direct effects on arterioles. It inhibits renin release as described above. It is a potent stimulator of aldosterone release, and stimulates both early and late steps in aldosterone biosynthesis, resulting in increased conversion of cholesterol to pregnenolene and of corticosterone to 18-hydroxycorticosterone. Angiotensin II binds to cell surface receptors and stimulates Ca^{2+} influx and phospholipid turnover but does not activate adenylate cyclase. Angiotensin II also has a tropic influence on the adrenal zona glomerulosa, and it may also stimulate the proliferation of smooth muscle and other cells of the body. The hormone also has other complex effects on the kidney that affect salt balance, possibly through influences on kallikreins and prostaglandins. Plasma concentrations of angiotensin II can vary up to 25-fold; the hormone has a half-life of only 1 to 2 minutes. There are several breakdown products of angiotensin II. One of these, angiotensin III, a polypeptide of seven amino acids, has angiotensin II activity, but its biologic importance is probably less than that of angiotensin II.

POTASSIUM. Increased potassium stimulates and decreased potassium inhibits aldosterone production. These effects are elicited by changes in potassium of as little as 0.1 mEq per liter in the physiologic range and are independent of sodium or angiotensin II. Prolonged hyperkalemia, like excess angiotensin II, has a tropic influence on the adrenal.

OTHER FACTORS. Other factors of lesser importance also affect aldosterone release. ACTH has a transient effect, and, rarely, aldosterone production can be blunted with chronic ACTH deficiency. Atrial natriuretic peptide blocks and other pituitary factors may stimulate aldosterone release. Sodium deficiency decreases and sodium loading increases aldosterone release, but these influences are probably mediated through effects on renin. Dopamine agonists can inhibit and dopamine antagonists can increase plasma aldosterone. Aldosterone release is episodic and shows a tendency to a circadian rhythm that is similar to but much less prominent than that of cortisol.

REGULATION OF ADRENAL ANDROGEN PRODUCTION

Adrenal androgen production is regulated by ACTH in a manner similar to that of cortisol. Plasma levels of these hormones also show the same circadian periodicity as cortisol, although this is masked in the case of DHEA-S because of its prolonged plasma half-life. Adrenal androgen release is also altered during prepuberty (adrenarche) by poorly understood mechanisms. Further, it should be remembered that androgens released by the testes and ovaries contribute to plasma androgen levels.

217.4 ACTIONS OF ADRENAL STEROIDS

John D. Baxter

GLUCOCORTICOIDS

Glucocorticoids have diverse actions that affect most mammalian tissues and are also essential for survival, at least in times of stress.

INTERMEDIARY METABOLISM. Glucocorticoids have multiple influences on glucose metabolism with diverse secondary effects (Fig. 217–4). In most tissues these steroids inhibit glucose uptake. Liver, heart, brain, and erythrocytes are exceptions. In many of these tissues the steroids also block protein and nucleic acid synthesis and stimulate turnover of these macromolecules. In adipose tissue the steroids inhibit lipolysis and block lipogenesis. In liver the steroids stimulate glycogen deposition, gluconeogenesis, the ability of other hormones to stimulate gluconeogenesis, and lipoprotein synthesis. Gluconeogenesis is further facilitated because of increased availability of glycerol and amino acid substrate due to the effects in peripheral tissues. The steroids also tend to stimulate the appetite, and in adrenal insufficiency there is anorexia. Finally, glucocorticoids tend to blunt the actions of insulin and decrease the affinity for insulin binding to its receptors.

The net effect of these influences is a glucocorticoid-induced tendency to hyperglycemia, ketosis, and hyperlipidemia. How-

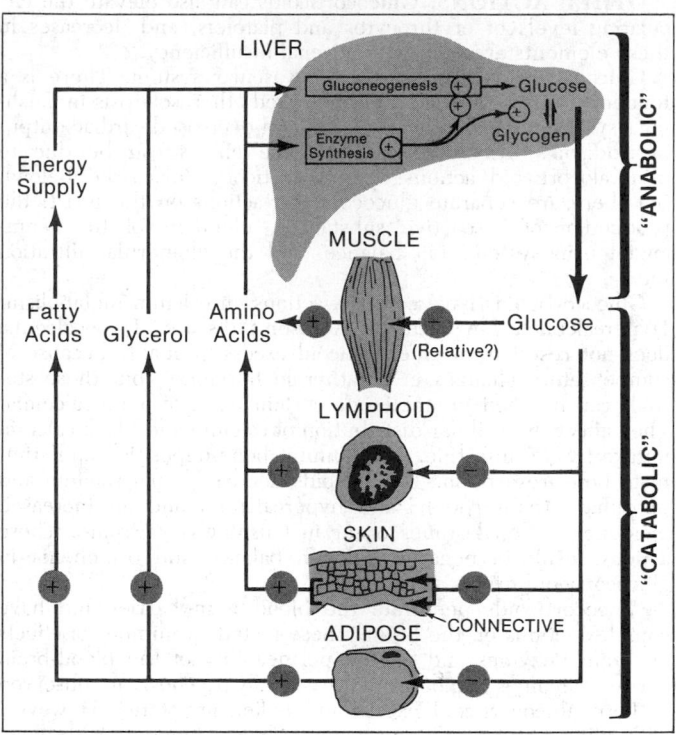

FIGURE 217–4. Glucocorticoid influences on intermediary metabolism. Plus and minus signs refer to stimulation and inhibition, respectively. (Modified from Baxter JD, Forsham PH: Tissue effects of glucocorticoids. Am J Med 53:579, 1972.)

ever, in normal subjects the elevated levels of glucose increase insulin release that in turn blunts the effects of the steroid. However, in diabetes or latent diabetes, significant hyperglycemia and insulin resistance can ensue. Lipogenesis induced by secondary increases in plasma insulin levels along with the increased food intake due to appetite stimulation may explain the truncal and sometimes generalized obesity seen in Cushing's syndrome. Conversely, in adrenal insufficiency there is a tendency to hypoglycemia; usually this is not marked in the adult, but it can be significant if there is concomitant fasting. Many of the actions of glucocorticoids on intermediary metabolism can be perceived as a protection against fasting; there is peripheral catabolism with sparing of essential tissues (heart, brain, blood cells) to make available substrate for maintenance of the blood sugar levels.

These actions of glucocorticoids on intermediary metabolism also explain many other effects of glucocorticoid excess. Thus inhibition of metabolic functions in peripheral tissues may explain glucocorticoid-induced myopathy, inhibition of immunologic and inflammatory responses, poor wound healing, thinning of the skin, striae, and osteoporosis.

INFLAMMATORY AND IMMUNOLOGIC RESPONSES. In excess, glucocorticoids suppress inflammatory and immunologic responses, but it is not clear whether they normally modulate immunologic systems. In excess, glucocorticoids inhibit antigen processing; T cell function; synthesis of cellular mediators of the inflammatory response such as interleukins, plasminogen activator, lymphokines, other active peptides, and prostaglandins and other eicosanoids; cellular migration and action at sites of inflammation; and inflammatory reactions themselves. In general they do not affect most antibody responses, although there are a few exceptions. Some populations of lymphocytes are killed by glucocorticoids; this explains the efficacy of these steroids in treating certain leukemias such as acute lymphoblastic leukemia of childhood. The steroids also affect mononuclear cell trafficking, tend to decrease blood monocyte, lymphocyte, and eosinophil levels, and increase polymorphonuclear leukocytes; there are reciprocal changes during adrenal insufficiency. Interestingly, glucocorticoids do not produce any permanent impairment of the immunologic system.

OTHER ACTIONS. Glucocorticoids can also elevate the circulating levels of erythrocytes and platelets, and decreases in these elements are seen with adrenal insufficiency.

Glucocorticoids affect the cardiovascular system. There is a tendency to hypertension and increased atherosclerosis in Cushing's syndrome and to hypotension and decreased cardiac output in Addison's disease. Some of these effects can be due to mineralocorticoid actions of glucocorticoids (discussed below), but there are separate glucocorticoid actions on the heart, the production of vasoactive substances, elements of the renin-angiotensin system, ion balance, and the glomerular filtration rate.

Glucocorticoids have complex actions on calcium metabolism. Hypercalcemia can occur in Addison's disease. Hypocalcemia does not result from glucocorticoid excess (probably because of compensatory changes in parathyroid hormone), but these steroids can be used to ameliorate certain types of hypercalcemia. They affect the cellular distribution of calcium and block calcium uptake by the intestine. They inhibit bone deposition and stimulate bone resorption. The steroids decrease renal calcium and phosphate reabsorption, and hypercalciuria and an increased incidence of renal stones occur in Cushing's syndrome. These actions result in negative calcium balance and osteopenia in glucocorticoid excess states.

Glucocorticoids penetrate the blood-brain barrier and have complex actions on the brain. These include a number of effects on brain enzymes and on the permeability of the blood-brain barrier. Changes in mood and occasionally psychosis are observed in both glucocorticoid excess and deficiency states. However, with glucocorticoid therapy, euphoria is common. Addisonian subjects commonly have increased sensitivity to a variety of sensory stimuli such as smell or taste. The mechanisms of these influences are poorly understood. Glucocorticoids increase intraocular pressure, probably by blocking fluid uptake by the trabecular meshwork. Glucocorticoid therapy can precipitate glaucoma in susceptible individuals and can enhance cataract formation.

In the gastrointestinal tract glucocorticoids inhibit DNA synthesis and tend to enhance stimuli to gastric acid secretion. They probably also enhance the tendency to form duodenal ulcers and, in high doses, the tendency to develop gastritis.

In excess, glucocorticoids inhibit linear growth, as a result of their inhibitory influences on a number of tissues. However, glucocorticoid action is required for a number of developmental processes. One particularly important process is the synthesis of surfactant in the lung. Lack of glucocorticoid induction of this factor in premature birth contributes to the respiratory distress syndrome of the newborn.

Complex interrelationships exist between glucocorticoids and other hormones. Glucocorticoids inhibit vasopressin release; conversely, ACTH deficiency can lead to hyponatremia with water intoxication. Glucocorticoids secondarily increase insulin and parathyroid hormone (PTH) levels and in some cases blunt the production of growth hormone, prolactin, insulin, glucagon, thyroid-stimulating hormone (TSH), and testosterone. Multiple synergisms and antagonisms between glucocorticoids and other hormones also exist at the cellular level. For example, they are synergistic with epinephrine and glucagon in stimulating hepatic gluconeogenesis. These effects are sometimes termed permissive glucocorticoid actions.

STRESS. Why glucocorticoids are essential for survival in times of stress is poorly understood. Two factors are probably operative. First, stress increases the production of a number of biologically active substances such as catecholamines, prostaglandins and other arachidonic acid metabolites, proteases, and kinins. Glucocorticoids, by contrast, tend to blunt the production and actions of these substances, which, if left unchecked during stress, would lead to shock and vascular decompensation. Second, the stimulation of cardiovascular functions by glucocorticoids may be critical in times of stress when other compensatory systems may be less effective.

MOLECULAR MECHANISMS OF ACTION. Glucocorticoids penetrate cells and bind to intracellular receptors. The receptors that mediate most actions of the glucocorticoids are termed "glucocorticoid" receptors. These bind active glucocorticoids with high affinity and have a much lower affinity for other classes of steroids. Glucocorticoids can also bind to the "mineralocorticoid" receptors that mediate the actions of aldosterone. As mentioned earlier, metabolic conversion of cortisol to cortisone prevents cortisol actions through mineralocorticoid receptors in the kidney, but cortisol does act through receptors in the brain, hypothalamus, heart, and other sites. The complexes of the glucocorticoids with either of these classes of receptors then bind to specific sites on the DNA where they either enhance or inhibit the ability of RNA polymerase to stimulate transcription of glucocorticoid-responsive genes (see Ch. 208). These actions result in changes in the levels of specific mRNA's transcribed by these genes with consequent fluctuations in the levels of their protein products that in turn mediate the glucocorticoid responses. Also, some glucocorticoid effects occur by mechanisms that do not involve stimulation of transcription.

MINERALOCORTICOIDS

Mineralocorticoid hormones act on kidney, gut, salivary glands, and sweat glands to affect the balance of electrolytes. Direct actions on other tissues including brain, mammary gland, placenta, and pituitary can occur, but the physiologic importance of these is unknown. Thus the spectrum of mineralocorticoid action is more restricted than that of glucocorticoid action.

In the kidney, the most important target organ, mineralocorticoids promote the reabsorption of sodium ion and secretion of potassium ion in the cortical collecting tubules, and possibly in the connecting segment of the nephron, and stimulate the secretion of hydrogen ion in the medullary collecting tubules. Thus, with mineralocorticoid excess, there is sodium retention, hypokalemia, and alkalosis. In primary mineralocorticoid excess, hypertension develops with time. With mineralocorticoid deficiency there is sodium ion loss and a tendency to hyperkalemia and acidosis. The overall effects of mineralocorticoids on both sodium and potassium ions also depend on the level of salt intake. Increased sodium intake results in more tubular sodium for reabsorption; this enhances potassium secretion. Conversely, sodium restriction diminishes aldosterone-induced kaliuresis. In most circumstances with persistent mineralocorticoid excess, the sodium retention that occurs reaches a limit such that the body "escapes" from further sodium retention. This is due to secondary increases in the secretion of other factors or hormones such as atrial natriuretic factor (ANF) and changes in renal hemodynamics with compensating influences of sodium excretion. Exceptions are the secondary hyperaldosteronism of heart failure and of cirrhosis with ascites in which sodium retention is progressive. As noted, hyperkalemia directly stimulates aldosterone secretion, which in turn enhances renal potassium excretion. This servomechanism forms an important component of the body's defense against hyperkalemia.

Mineralocorticoid actions are mediated through molecular mechanisms similar to those described above for cortisol and in Ch. 208. The mineralocorticoid receptors bind aldosterone and DOC with high affinity; they also bind cortisol with around 10 per cent of the affinity for aldosterone. Since plasma free cortisol concentrations are around 100-fold higher than those of aldosterone, there is a need to modulate occupancy of mineralocorticoid receptors by cortisol, as mediated through renal conversion of cortisol to cortisone, as discussed above. The synthetic steroid 9α-fluorocortisol binds tightly to mineralocorticoid receptors and is used for mineralocorticoid replacement therapy, since it is more stable than aldosterone after oral administration. Mineralocorticoid antagonists such as spironolactone bind to these receptors and block aldosterone action.

Aldosterone stimulates the synthesis of several renal proteins that result in increases in (1) sodium permeability in the apical membrane exposed to the tubular lumen; (2) various mitochondrial enzymes that increase cellular ATP and thereby enhance the actions of the Na^+-K^+-ATPase; (3) the Na^+-K^+-ATPase; and (4) probably other as yet unidentified factors of the basolateral membrane. These combined actions result in Na^+ reabsorption. Potassium ion secretion increases secondarily to the Na^+-K^+ exchange because of the pumping action of the Na^+-K^+-ATPase; however, other mechanisms must also operate because there can be independent actions of aldosterone on Na^+ and K^+.

Aldosterone-stimulated renal tubular transport of hydrogen ion, about which little is known, can probably occur independently of the effects on Na^+ and K^+. However, potassium ion deficiency decreases Na^+-K^+ exchange, which in turn increases the Na^+-H^+ exchange and hydrogen ion excretion. As in the case of potassium, hydrogen ion loss can be blunted with sodium restriction. The mineralocorticoid-induced alkalosis is also promoted by hydrogen ion movement into cells in exchange for losses in potassium.

The major known extrarenal targets for aldosterone are the sweat and salivary glands, ileum, and colon where the steroid promotes potassium loss and sodium retention. These actions are ordinarily minor in terms of overall salt balance.

217.5 LABORATORY EVALUATION OF ADRENOCORTICAL FUNCTION

J. Blake Tyrrell

The function of the adrenal cortex is best assessed by plasma assays of the major steroids and measurement of their trophic hormones, e.g., ACTH and related peptides or renin and angiotensin. Certain urinary assays remain useful, however, despite the disadvantage of 24-hour collections. The following considerations must be remembered when using these assays: (1) Current assays for plasma steroids measure total hormone concentration, not bioactive free hormone. (2) Plasma levels of cortisol and ACTH vary greatly because of episodic secretion and many other factors (see below); thus single determinations should not in general be relied upon for a definitive diagnosis. (3) In assessing adrenal function, stimulation and suppression testing provide the most definitive information.

GLUCOCORTICOID FUNCTION

ACTH AND RELATED PEPTIDES. Immunoassays for ACTH are extremely useful but are technically difficult. ACTH is unstable in plasma and adheres to glass; specimens should be collected in anticoagulated plastic or silicon-coated tubes on ice, centrifuged in the cold without delay, and frozen until assayed. The normal range of plasma ACTH in the morning (8 to 9 A.M.) is 20 to 100 pg per milliliter in most assays. Values at other times of the day are lower, but marked episodic variation may occur.

Plasma ACTH levels are used primarily to differentiate pituitary, adrenal, and other causes of adrenal dysfunction. Thus, in patients with cortisol deficiency elevated ACTH levels (generally greater than 250 pg per milliliter) confirm the diagnosis of primary adrenal insufficiency (Addison's disease). Conversely, with secondary adrenal insufficiency due to hypothalamic or pituitary disease or steroid therapy, ACTH levels are low normal or subnormal (usually <20 pg per milliliter). In states of cortisol excess (Cushing's syndrome), a suppressed or undetectable ACTH level (<20 pg per milliliter) is diagnostic of an adrenal tumor hypersecreting cortisol or of exogenous glucocorticoid administration. With ACTH-producing pituitary tumors (Cushing's disease), plasma ACTH levels are normal to modestly elevated (40 to 200 pg per milliliter), whereas in the ectopic ACTH syndrome they are usually elevated markedly (100 to >1000 pg per milliliter). ACTH levels in the two latter conditions may overlap, but very high (>300 pg per milliliter) values strongly suggest an ectopic tumor. Plasma ACTH levels are also elevated in congenital adrenal hyperplasia proportional to the extent of cortisol deficiency and are markedly elevated in pituitary tumors that arise following bilateral adrenalectomy (Nelson's syndrome).

Immunoassays for other peptides derived from pro-opiomelanocortin are also available. The antisera usually measure both β-LPH and β-endorphin. Reported normal morning values of immunoreactive β-LPH/β-endorphin are 20 to 200 pg per milliliter. Levels of these peptides vary similarly to those of ACTH, but because of its longer plasma half-life, β-LPH levels show less episodic variability than ACTH, and β-LPH is considerably more stable than ACTH in plasma.

PLASMA CORTISOL AND RELATED STEROIDS. Plasma cortisol is most frequently measured by radioimmunoassay; current antisera show little cross-reactivity with other natural or synthetic steroids. Competitive protein binding and high-performance liquid chromatography assays are also in use. Normal

TABLE 217–2. CONDITIONS CAUSING ELEVATED CORTISOL LEVELS

Increased CBG	Increased Secretion
Estrogen therapy	Spontaneous Cushing's syndrome
Pregnancy	Exercise
Hyperthyroidism	Physical stress
Diabetes mellitus	Anxiety
Hematologic disorders	Depression
Congenital	Starvation
	Anorexia nervosa
	Alcoholism
	Chronic renal failure

values of plasma cortisol vary with the circadian rhythm of ACTH. Mean levels at 8 A.M. are 10 to 12 μg per deciliter with a range of 3 to 20 μg per deciliter. Values at 4 to 6 P.M. are approximately 50 per cent of the morning levels, although there is great variability. Values obtained between 10 P.M. and 2 A.M. are less than 3 μg per deciliter and may be unmeasurable. Episodic variability and the numerous conditions increasing cortisol secretion or CBG concentrations (Table 217–2) limit the utility of single cortisol determinations.

Measurement of plasma 11-deoxycortisol (compound S) by radioimmunoassay is used in metyrapone testing of pituitary-adrenal reserve (see below) and in the assessment of patients with congenital adrenal hyperplasia or adrenal tumors.

URINARY CORTICOSTEROIDS. Measurements of urinary steroids have been traditionally used to evaluate adrenal function and provide an integrated assessment of steroid production and excretion. With the exception of urinary free cortisol, these methods are less advantageous and have been largely supplanted by plasma measurements of cortisol or other steroids.

Urine free cortisol, although less than 1 per cent of total adrenal cortisol secretion, is a useful measurement in the diagnosis of hypercortisolism. The steroid is measured by radioimmunoassay or competitive protein binding. Normal values range from 20 to 100 μg per 24 hours. Elevated levels are almost always present in Cushing's syndrome but not in simple obesity; this ability to separate these conditions is a major advantage. Urinary cortisol excretion is increased by any condition that increases adrenal cortisol secretion (Table 217–2) and is decreased in renal failure.

Urinary 17-hydroxycorticosteroids (17-OHCS) and 17-ketogenic steroids (17-KGS) measure steroid metabolites, predominantly those of cortisol and 11-deoxycortisol. These methods are currently not recommended in most situations, because the methods are not specific, the levels are altered in many disease states, and the assays are subject to interference by many commonly used drugs and medications.

SUPPRESSION TESTS. Suppression tests evaluate the ability of dexamethasone, a potent synthetic glucocorticoid not measured in current cortisol assays, to inhibit ACTH and cortisol secretion. In Cushing's syndrome glucocorticoids do not normally inhibit ACTH release. There are two types of dexamethasone suppression tests: (1) Low-dose tests are used to document the abnormal responsiveness of the hypothalamic-pituitary-adrenal axis that is characteristic of Cushing's syndrome. (2) High-dose tests are used to distinguish the various causes of Cushing's syndrome. The techniques for performing these tests and the expected responses are summarized in Table 217–3.

Low-Dose Dexamethasone Tests. The overnight 1-mg dexamethasone suppression test is an excellent screening procedure for Cushing's syndrome. The test can be used on an ambulatory basis, and in this setting abnormal responses occur in about 95 per cent of patients with Cushing's syndrome. False-positive responses occur in 25 per cent of hospitalized and chronically ill patients, in 15 per cent of obese patients, and in a number of other conditions, including acute illness, anxiety, depression, alcoholism, anorexia nervosa, estrogen therapy, and uremia. Drugs that accelerate dexamethasone metabolism, especially phenytoin and phenobarbital, also cause false-positive results. The 2-day low-dose test provides the same information as the 1-mg

TABLE 217–3. DEXAMETHASONE SUPPRESSION TESTS

Low-Dose Tests

Overnight test
Dexamethasone 1 mg p.o. at 11 P.M.; plasma cortisol at 8 to 9 A.M.
Normal response—plasma cortisol <5 μg/dl

2-day test
Dexamethasone 0.5 mg p.o. q6h for 8 doses; plasma cortisol 1 hr
after last dose and 24-hr urine free cortisol and/or 17-OHCS during
second day of dexamethasone

Normal response—plasma cortisol <5 μg/dl; urine free cortisol <25
μg/24 hr; urine 17-OHCS <4 mg/24 hr or <1 mg/gram urine
creatinine

High-Dose Tests

Overnight test
Dexamethasone 8 mg p.o. at 11 P.M.; plasma cortisol before and at 8
to 9 A.M. after dexamethasone

Response—Cushing's disease; suppression of cortisol to <50% of
baseline; ectopic ACTH/adrenal tumors: no cortisol suppression

2-day test
Dexamethasone 2.0 mg p.o. q6h for 8 doses; plasma cortisol before
dexamethasone and 1 hr after last dose; 24-hr urine free cortisol
and/or 17-OHCS before dexamethasone and during second day
Response—Cushing's disease; suppression of plasma or urine steroids
to <50% of baseline; ectopic ACTH/adrenal tumors: no steroid
suppression

overnight test. It is most useful when the results of other tests are equivocal or inconclusive.

High-Dose Dexamethasone Tests. Glucocorticoids in pharmacologic doses suppress ACTH and cortisol secretion in most patients with ACTH-producing pituitary tumors, but not in patients with adrenal and ectopic tumors. Two tests are available (Table 217–3). The overnight high-dose test is simpler and more accurate than the 2-day high-dose test. Approximately 90 per cent of patients with pituitary ACTH-producing tumors have suppression of cortisol levels to less than 50 per cent of baseline levels, whereas about 95 per cent of those with adrenal tumors or the ectopic ACTH syndrome do not achieve this degree of suppression. With the 2-day high-dose test about 25 per cent of patients with Cushing's disease fail to achieve greater than 50 per cent suppression of urine 17-OHCS, urine free cortisol, or plasma cortisol.

STIMULATION TESTS. These procedures assess the reserve capacity of the hypothalamic-pituitary-adrenal axis and its ability to respond appropriately to stressful situations. These tests act at different sites of the axis and thus can be used to assess its different functions.

CRF Testing. Corticotropin-releasing factor (CRF) testing is utilized in the diagnosis of adrenal insufficiency and Cushing's syndrome. CRF is generally administered intravenously in a dose of 1 μg per kilogram of body weight. ACTH and cortisol secretion peak at 30 to 60 minutes and may be sustained for several hours. Flushing and occasionally hypotension have been observed; thus the test should be performed with the patient supine. Subnormal ACTH and cortisol responses occur in secondary adrenocortical insufficiency due either to hypothalamic-pituitary disorders or to glucocorticoid therapy, and a subnormal cortisol response with high ACTH levels occurs in primary adrenocortical insufficiency. Most but not all patients with pituitary ACTH-producing tumors have supranormal ACTH and cortisol responses, whereas there is no response in patients with cortisol-producing adrenal tumors and in most patients with ectopic ACTH-producing tumors.

ACTH Testing. The administration of ACTH, which allows direct assessment of adrenal glucocorticoid reserve, is useful in the diagnosis of both primary and secondary adrenal insufficiency. The rapid ACTH stimulation test is performed with synthetic human α1-24 ACTH (Cosyntropin [Cortrosyn]), which has full

biologic potency and a lesser incidence of allergic reactions than previously used ACTH preparations. Cortrosyn, 250 μg, is administered intravenously or intramuscularly; plasma cortisol levels are obtained prior to and at 30 or 60 minutes after ACTH administration. Normally the peak plasma cortisol level is greater than 15 to 20 μg per deciliter, depending on the laboratory, and increases by at least 5 μg per deciliter. Subnormal responses to ACTH stimulation establish the diagnosis of adrenal insufficiency. A normal response excludes primary adrenal failure and complete secondary insufficiency, but it does not exclude partial secondary adrenal insufficiency. A normal response to ACTH in the latter case occurs when there is sufficient basal ACTH secretion to prevent adrenal atrophy but not enough pituitary reserve to respond to stress. When this infrequent situation is suspected, the issue can be resolved with the use of metyrapone or insulin hypoglycemia testing.

The rapid ACTH stimulation test gives no information regarding the cause of adrenal dysfunction. This distinction can be made by measuring either the basal plasma ACTH level, which is elevated in primary adrenal insufficiency and is low in secondary adrenal insufficiency, or the aldosterone response to ACTH stimulation (normally an increment in the plasma aldosterone of at least 4 ng per deciliter above baseline). The latter test is based on the fact that the zona glomerulosa responds acutely to ACTH and that this response is preserved in secondary adrenal insufficiency, but is deficient in the primary form in which the entire adrenal cortex is destroyed.

Metyrapone Testing. Metyrapone inhibits the synthesis of cortisol predominantly by blocking 11β-hydroxylation. As a result, ACTH secretion increases and drives the production of steroids proximal to the site of the block. Thus, measurement of plasma 11-deoxycortisol following metyrapone administration can be used to assess the functional reserve of both the adrenal and pituitary. The test is most useful when secondary adrenal insufficiency is suspected in the setting of a normal ACTH stimulation test. The overnight test is most commonly used because of its rapidity and simplicity; because of the short duration of inhibition of cortisol synthesis there is little risk of precipitating acute adrenal insufficiency. Metyrapone is given at midnight with food, and plasma for 11-deoxycortisol and cortisol determinations is obtained at 8 A.M. The dose of metyrapone* is 2 grams for patients less than 70 kg; 2.5 grams for those 70 to 90 kg; and 3 grams for patients weighing more than 90 kg. A plasma cortisol value less than 10 μg per deciliter indicates adequate 11β-hydroxylase inhibition, and in normal persons plasma 11-deoxycortisol increases to greater than 7 μg per deciliter. A normal response to metyrapone indicates adequate function of both the pituitary and adrenals. A subnormal response establishes the diagnosis of adrenal insufficiency and correlates well with deficient responses to stress and hypoglycemia. The test per se does not differentiate primary and secondary causes. However, in the presence of a normal response to the rapid ACTH stimulation test a subnormal response to metyrapone indicates secondary adrenal insufficiency.

Insulin Hypoglycemia Testing (see Ch. 219). Hypoglycemia elicits a stress response that stimulates CRF and ACTH secretion and, as a consequence, cortisol release. A normal cortisol response to hypoglycemia indicates a normal hypothalamic-pituitary-adrenal axis and rules out adrenal insufficiency or decreased pituitary ACTH reserve. This test is most often utilized in the evaluation of suspected hypothalamic or pituitary disorders, since growth hormone reserve can be assessed simultaneously with that of ACTH.

MINERALOCORTICOID FUNCTION

PLASMA RENIN. Assessment of plasma renin is essential in the diagnosis of states of excess and deficient mineralocorticoid secretion; it is also helpful in the evaluation of other types of hypertension (see Ch. 44). Currently used assays do not measure the plasma renin concentration directly, but instead measure the plasma renin activity (PRA) by quantifying the amount of angiotensin I (AI) generated over time in the patient's plasma. The normal values of PRA depend on the salt intake and postural status. In subjects with moderate salt intake (around 110 mEq Na+ per day) and in the supine and standing positions, for 1

*This dose is not listed in the manufacturer's directive.

hour, the plasma renin activity ranges, respectively, from 1 to 3 and 3 to 6 ng of AI generated per milliliter per hour. In individuals in whom salt has been restricted (20 mEq Na^+ per day) for 4 days and who have been in the upright posture for 2 hours the values range from 5 to 10 ng AI per milliliter per hour. In clinical practice, diuretic therapy is the most commonly observed factor that increases the PRA. In patients with primary hyperaldosteronism the PRA is characteristically suppressed. With most aldosterone-producing adenomas and in a small subset of patients with hyperplasia (primary adrenal hyperplasia), the PRA is unresponsive or only weakly responsive to provocative stimuli, whereas in those with primary aldosteronism with bilateral hyperplasia (idiopathic hyperaldosteronism), and in a small subset of patients with adenoma (renin-responsive adenoma), the PRA, although suppressed, usually responds to such stimuli.

In patients with borderline low PRA in whom primary aldosterone excess is suspected, stimulation tests with measurement of PRA may be necessary. Patients can be subjected to salt restriction (10 to 20 mEq of sodium per day for 5 days), given 40 to 60 mg of furosemide intravenously, or given 50 mg of captopril orally; blood samples are then taken after 1 to 4 hours in the upright posture. If the plasma renin does not increase under these conditions and the plasma and/or urinary aldosterone levels are elevated, primary aldosteronism is probable. Caution should be exercised in performing these tests, since severe and life-threatening volume depletion or hypokalemia could ensue; these risks must be weighed before the test is performed.

ALDOSTERONE AND 18-HYDROXYCORTICOSTERONE MEASUREMENTS. These measurements are utilized in the diagnosis of primary aldosteronism and in the differentiation of its subtypes of adenoma and hyperplasia. Plasma measurements ordinarily involve extraction and chromatography of the steroid followed by radioimmunoassay. The urine measurements ordinarily quantify by radioimmunoassay the 18-glucuronide metabolite of aldosterone (about 15 per cent of the total aldosterone production). Less commonly, urinary tetrahydroaldosterone is measured.

Measurements should be made after adequate sodium repletion (a sodium intake of at least 120 mEq per 24 hours for 4 days) and withdrawal of diuretics for at least 2 to 3 weeks, and in the case of plasma measurements after at least 6 hours of recumbency. Normal values for aldosterone excretion are 4 to 17 μg per 24 hours; elevated values are typically seen with both adrenal adenoma and hyperplasia causing primary aldosteronism. Basal plasma values in the supine patient are usually 4 to 12 ng per deciliter. Plasma aldosterone levels are almost always elevated above 20 ng per deciliter in patients with an aldosterone-producing adenoma. By contrast, with primary aldosteronism due to bilateral adrenal hyperplasia, plasma aldosterone levels are usually less than 20 ng per deciliter and are commonly in the normal range. Plasma and urinary aldosterone values must be interpreted with caution in the presence of hypokalemia that results in decreased aldosterone production; normal aldosterone levels may be found in patients with primary aldosteronism and hypokalemia.

Plasma 18-hydroxycorticosterone (18-OHB) measurements (normal range 10 to 30 ng per deciliter) are also especially useful in the differential diagnosis of primary aldosteronism. When sampled at 8 A.M. after overnight recumbency and during a high-salt diet as described above, plasma 18-OHB levels almost always exceed 100 ng per deciliter in patients with an aldosterone-producing adenoma. Levels are less than this with primary aldosteronism due to bilateral hyperplasia.

The use of both aldosterone and 18-OHB measurements has greatly simplified the diagnosis and differential diagnosis of primary aldosteronism. However, in circumstances in which plasma renin values are suppressed and aldosterone values are normal or borderline, suppression tests can be performed. These include (1) high-sodium diet (300 mEq per day for 5 days), (2) fludrocortisone acetate (9α-fluorocortisol) 0.3 mg per day for 3 days, or (3) 2 liters of saline intravenously over 4 hours. These maneuvers reduce plasma aldosterone levels to less than 5 ng per deciliter in normal subjects, but the levels ordinarily exceed 10 ng per deciliter in patients with primary aldosteronism.

Two additional methods for differentiating primary aldosteronism due to an adenoma from that due to hyperplasia take advantage of the fact that plasma aldosterone and 18-OHB levels in hyperplasia, but not adenoma, are under control of the renin-angiotensin system. The first involves postural studies. The plasma aldosterone is initially measured in the supine position at 8 A.M. after 4 days of a sodium intake of at least 120 mEq per 24 hours and then subsequently after 2 to 4 hours in the upright posture. In patients with an adenoma there is generally either no increase or an actual decrease in plasma aldosterone in the upright position, whereas with hyperplasia, there is almost always an increase in plasma aldosterone concentrations after 2 to 4 hours in the upright position. The second test involves a saline infusion. Patients receiving 120 mEq of sodium per day receive an intravenous infusion of 1250 ml of isotonic saline between 8 A.M. and 10 A.M. after overnight recumbency. The ratio of 18-OHB to cortisol is measured in plasma samples taken before and immediately after the infusion. This ratio generally increases in patients with an aldosterone-producing adenoma but decreases in patients with hyperplasia.

ADRENAL ANDROGENS

Plasma levels of the predominant adrenal androgens, DHEA, DHEA-S, and androstenedione, can be measured. These assays plus that of testosterone are most frequently used for the evaluation of hirsutism. Stimulation and suppression tests have not been as useful as in other pituitary and adrenal disorders. Plasma free testosterone measurements usually provide a better index of total androgenicity than total levels of the hormone, since androgen excess decreases sex hormone–binding globulin levels and can result in a normal total level in the presence of an elevated free testosterone concentration. Measurement of androstanediol and its glucuronide, metabolic products of dihydrotestosterone, provides an index of peripheral androgen production and may provide the best index of androgen excess.

Urinary 17-ketosteroid excretion assesses adrenal androgen production and reflects metabolites of DHEA and DHEA-S. However, this test has limited utility, since the more potent androgens such as testosterone and dihydrotestosterone contribute less than 1 per cent of the total urinary 17-ketosteroids. Furthermore, 17-ketosteroids are increased in obesity without androgen excess, and there is interference by multiple drugs and medications.

217.6 ADRENOCORTICAL HYPOFUNCTION
J. Blake Tyrrell

Adrenal insufficiency is defined by deficient production of glucocorticoids or mineralocorticoids or both. Primary adrenocortical insufficiency (Addison's disease) is due to destruction of the adrenal cortex, whereas in secondary adrenocortical insufficiency impaired cortisol production is due to deficient ACTH production. Hyporeninemia causes selective aldosterone deficiency. Selective adrenal defects due to congenital enzyme deficiencies also occur (see Ch. 221).

PRIMARY ADRENOCORTICAL INSUFFICIENCY

ETIOLOGY. Primary adrenocortical insufficiency has multiple causes. In the United States over 80 per cent of the cases are due to autoimmune destruction of the adrenal. Tuberculosis is the second most frequent cause and remains a common cause of the disease in underdeveloped countries. Acquired immunodeficiency syndrome (AIDS) has become a more frequent cause of the disorder. Other rare causes include hemorrhage due to sepsis, anticoagulation, coagulopathies, trauma, surgery, and pregnancy; bilateral infarction, e.g., due to thrombosis or arteritis; fungal infection; invasive disorders such as lymphoma, metastatic tumors, amyloidosis, sarcoidosis, and hemochromatosis; surgery; cytotoxic agents such as mitotane; and congenital hypoplasia and hyporesponsiveness to ACTH. Primary adrenocortical insufficiency due to any cause is a rare disease with an estimated incidence in Western countries of around 50 per million population.

The idiopathic autoimmune form of adrenal insufficiency is two- to threefold more common in females and is usually diagnosed in the third to fifth decades of life. Early in the disease there is lymphocytic infiltration of the glands, and there is a high association (40 to 53 per cent of patients) with disorders of other endocrine glands or with pernicious anemia or vitiligo. Antibodies to the adrenal cortex are commonly present, and there is evidence for abnormal cell-mediated immunity.

The association of Addison's disease with the other disorders has been referred to as *Schmidt's syndrome*, autoimmune endocrine failure, and the polyglandular failure syndromes (Ch. 228). Approximate associations are ovarian failure, 25 per cent of female patients (testicular failure in males is unusual); hyperthyroidism, 7 per cent (mostly female); hypothyroidism or Hashimoto's thyroiditis with goiter, 9 per cent; subclinical thyroiditis, up to 80 per cent; diabetes mellitus (type I), 12 per cent; vitiligo, 9 per cent, presumably due to immunologic destruction of melanocytes; hypoparathyroidism, 6 per cent; and pernicious anemia, 4 per cent. The development of autoimmune adrenocortical insufficiency shows some hereditary predisposition, and an autosomal recessive pattern of inheritance has been suggested. About 40 per cent of patients have first- or second-degree relatives with one of the associated disorders. Further, there is an increased incidence of histocompatibility antigen (HLA) types B8, Dw3 and of the haplotype HLA-A1,B8.

Patients with AIDS commonly have subtle abnormalities of adrenal function which are not clinically significant. However, a small percentage of these patients develop frank adrenocortical insufficiency.

CLINICAL MANIFESTATIONS. The development of clinical manifestations of adrenocortical insufficiency requires loss of more than 90 per cent of the adrenal cortices. The rate of destruction varies, depending on the cause, but with the idiopathic variety this usually requires several months. With gradual destruction, increases in ACTH secondary to the lower cortisol levels tend to stimulate the gland maximally. Thus in the period prior to complete destruction there may be normal plasma cortisol levels but absence of responsiveness to stress. In about 25 per cent of patients symptoms first appear in a crisis or impending crisis. However, in the majority of cases destruction becomes more complete, and the patient experiences symptoms that lead to medical evaluation before a crisis occurs. The destruction of the gland results in loss of both glucocorticoid and mineralocorticoid functions and secondary increases in ACTH and in renin.

The clinical presentation depends on the rate and degree of adrenal destruction, the presence of stressful influences, and the pathology of associated or causative conditions. For these reasons it is convenient to discuss separately the chronic and acute presentations.

Chronic primary adrenocortical insufficiency develops gradually over months to years. The major clinical features (Table 217–4) are generalized weakness and fatigue, weight loss, anorexia, hyperpigmentation, hypotension, gastrointestinal upset (including vague discomfort, nausea, vomiting, and less commonly diarrhea), salt craving, and postural dizziness. Weight loss is due both to dehydration secondary to salt loss and to anorexia. The blood glucose concentration is ordinarily in the low-normal range, although hypoglycemia can occur with fasting, vomiting, or illness and in children. Female patients can also have amenorrhea and loss of axillary hair, the latter due to decrease of adrenal androgens. Although dehydration can be significant, this may be compensated for by increased salt intake. Hyponatremia is present in most patients, although it may be masked somewhat

TABLE 217–4. CLINICAL FEATURES OF CHRONIC PRIMARY ADRENOCORTICAL INSUFFICIENCY

Feature	%	Feature	%
Weakness and fatigue	100	Hypotension	88
Weight loss	100	Gastrointestinal symptoms	56
Anorexia	100	Salt craving	19
Hyperpigmentation	92	Postural symptoms	12

Data from Nerup J: Acta Endocrinol 76:127, 1974 and Thorn GW: The Diagnosis and Treatment of Adrenal Insufficiency. Springfield, IL, Charles C Thomas, 1951, and reprinted in Baxter JD, Tyrrell JB: The adrenal cortex. *In* Felig P, Baxter JD, Broadus AH, et al. (eds.): Endocrinology and Metabolism, 2nd ed. New York, McGraw-Hill Book Company, 1987, p 587.

if there is dehydration. Mild hyperkalemia is also usually present; the presence of severe hyperkalemia should suggest concomitant renal or other disease. A normocytic, normochromic anemia is common but can also be masked by dehydration and hemoconcentration. There tends to be neutropenia, lymphocytosis, and eosinophilia. Dehydration when present leads to increases in blood urea nitrogen and creatinine, and there may be mild acidosis. The heart tends to be small and vertical on radiographic examination; the abdominal radiograph is usually normal but can show adrenal calcification in about 50 per cent of those cases due to tuberculosis. Calcification of the ear lobes sometimes occurs in longstanding cases.

Hyperpigmentation, an important diagnostic feature, may precede other manifestations. It is generalized; but is accentuated in sun-exposed areas; pressure points such as the elbows, knees, knuckles, and toes; and on palmar creases, nail beds, buccal mucosa, tongue, nipples, areolae, and perivaginal or perianal mucosa; and in recent surgical scars. In blacks, pigmentation of the tongue is of diagnostic helpfulness. Hyperpigmentation is commonly misinterpreted as an excessive suntan and the "healthy" appearance of the patient may lead to a dismissal of other symptoms.

Acute adrenocortical insufficiency is seen most commonly in a patient with either undiagnosed or diagnosed adrenocortical insufficiency who is exposed to one of the stresses discussed earlier and who therefore has an increased requirement for glucocorticoids. It can also be seen with acute adrenal destruction secondary to hemorrhage, most commonly associated with septicemia or anticoagulant therapy (adrenal apoplexy). In these cases, anorexia is often profound with nausea and vomiting that exaggerates volume depletion and dehydration. Abdominal pain is frequent and may mimic a surgical condition of the abdomen; however, these symptoms are usually vague. The blood pressure falls, and hypovolemic shock develops that is incompletely responsive to fluid replacement. Fever is common and may or may not be due to the precipitating event. Hyperpigmentation will be present or absent, depending on the duration of the disease; when present it is an important diagnostic sign. The presence of hyperkalemia, lymphocytosis, and eosinophilia should also suggest the diagnosis. Severe hypoglycemia is uncommon and is more likely to occur in children or in adults with secondary adrenal insufficiency (see below). The diagnosis of acute adrenocortical insufficiency should be considered in any patient with unexplained shock, and the consideration of this should not be diverted by the presence of an accompanying disorder such as infection or diabetic ketoacidosis.

SECONDARY ADRENOCORTICAL INSUFFICIENCY. Secondary adrenocortical insufficiency results from inadequate ACTH production. The causes are discussed in Ch. 213. Pituitary and hypothalamic tumors are the most common spontaneous causes. In these cases there is progressive loss of ACTH such that cortisol production and responses to stress are decreased, but mineralocorticoid production is usually normal. Chronic suppression of ACTH production with exogenous glucocorticoids followed by their withdrawal also causes the syndrome and is by far the most frequent cause.

The development of clinical manifestations is usually gradual, but like primary adrenocortical insufficiency can be acute. The presenting features are similar to those of primary adrenocortical insufficiency with four exceptions: (1) Since hypersecretion of ACTH and related peptides is absent, there is no hyperpigmentation; in fact, patients with hypopituitarism commonly exhibit pallor of the skin. (2) The electrolyte abnormalities of hyponatremia, hyperkalemia, and mild acidosis are absent because of preservation of aldosterone secretion. Hyponatremia, if present, is due to decreased glomerular filtration rate, hypothyroidism, or increased vasopressin release and not to dehydration. (3) Other features of hypopituitarism (see Ch. 213) may be present. (4) Hypoglycemia is more common because of the combined ACTH and growth hormone deficiency.

DIAGNOSIS. The clinical suspicion of adrenocortical insufficiency should be confirmed by laboratory testing. Since the rapid ACTH stimulation test (discussed below) requires only 30 minutes, it is unusual that testing cannot be performed before initiating therapy, even in sick patients. However, in seriously ill patients, in whom the diagnosis is suspected, therapy should not be delayed by prolonged diagnostic measures; if means for a rapid diagnosis are unavailable, therapy should be initiated and diagnostic testing performed at a later date. Although an elevated plasma cortisol level (e.g., greater than 20 μg per deciliter) makes the diagnosis unlikely, cortisol levels below 20 μg per deciliter can be present with impaired adrenal responsiveness to stress. Thus, in circumstances when the plasma cortisol is less than 22 μg per deciliter, the adrenal reserve should be tested.

Figure 217–5 shows a diagnostic strategy. If adrenocortical insufficiency is suspected, the rapid ACTH stimulation test should be performed. This test requires only 30 minutes and can be done even in most acute situations. A normal response excludes the diagnosis of primary adrenocortical insufficiency; an abnormal response establishes the presence of adrenocortical insufficiency. Rare patients with secondary adrenocortical insufficiency respond normally. The basal plasma ACTH level, determined prior to ACTH administration, is measured to distinguish between primary and secondary adrenocortical insufficiency. In primary adrenocortical insufficiency, the levels exceed 250 pg per milliliter and usually are greater than 400 pg per milliliter. By contrast, plasma ACTH levels in secondary adrenocortical insufficiency are inappropriately low, ranging from 0 to 20 pg per milliliter. The plasma aldosterone response to ACTH can also be used to differentiate primary from secondary adrenocortical insufficiency, but there is less extensive experience with this procedure.

Further diagnostic procedures are needed only in exceptional cases, for example, in suspected secondary adrenocortical insufficiency with a normal response to ACTH or in cases in which plasma ACTH measurements are unavailable. In these cases the metyrapone or insulin hypoglycemia tests can be helpful. The latter test is usually performed in suspected hypopituitarism, since simultaneous assessment of both growth hormone and ACTH can be carried out (see Ch. 213). The metyrapone test is performed in patients in whom hypoglycemia is contraindicated or in those who have had prior glucocorticoid therapy, since it provides essentially the same information and is of less potential risk to the patient. An abnormal response to metyrapone or insulin hypoglycemia establishes the diagnosis of secondary adre-

nocortical insufficiency when the primary form has been excluded by the ACTH stimulation test. The presence of low-normal or low ACTH levels further confirms this diagnosis.

In spontaneous adrenocortical insufficiency of any type, the clinical evaluation should include an assessment of associated disorders or precipitating factors. In primary adrenocortical insufficiency the laboratory evaluation should include blood glucose and serum calcium and phosphorus; thyroid function tests, including TSH and thyroid antibody determinations; and testing for tuberculosis and HIV infection. If there is oligomenorrhea or amenorrhea, FSH and LH levels should be determined. First- and second-degree relatives should be screened for endocrine deficiency syndromes because of the increased risk in these individuals. In secondary adrenocortical insufficiency, patients should be examined for other pituitary dysfunction, pituitary or hypothalamic tumors, and prior glucocorticoid therapy (see Ch. 213). In acute adrenocortical insufficiency, the precipitating cause should be determined, since this is often infectious.

TREATMENT. *Acute Adrenocortical Insufficiency.* In an acute crisis, therapy should be instituted as soon as the diagnosis is suspected (Table 217–5). A soluble glucocorticoid, such as cortisol hemisuccinate or phosphate, should be given intravenously. Volume depletion, electrolyte abnormalities, and hypoglycemia should be corrected and general supportive measures instituted. Precipitating factors should be assessed and corrected. If recovery is satisfactory, the glucocorticoid dose can be reduced on the second day and then tapered to oral maintenance doses by the fourth to fifth day. Mineralocorticoid replacement is unnecessary when high doses of cortisol are given, but should be given when the cortisol dose has been tapered to near-maintenance levels (40 to 60 mg per 24 hours).

Chronic Adrenocortical Insufficiency. The treatment of the primary form of this condition requires both glucocorticoid and mineralocorticoid replacement, whereas the secondary form usually requires only glucocorticoid replacement (Table 217–5). Patients must be made aware that a lifetime of replacement is necessary and of the need to increase glucocorticoid replacement in times of stress. Each patient should carry an identification bracelet or card. Cortisol at levels similar to physiologic production is given in a way that approximates the circadian rhythm. Thus, for ordinary maintenance, 15 to 20 mg of cortisol are given in the early morning and 5 to 10 mg in the late afternoon. An equivalent amount of prednisolone or prednisone (about 5 mg per day) or cortisone acetate (37.5 mg per day) is also acceptable; however, the potency of dexamethasone has probably been underestimated, and this steroid is not recommended. For mineralocorticoid replacement, 9α-fluorocortisol (fludrocortisone) 0.05 to 0.2 mg orally per day, is recommended. Follow-up is mainly by clinical assessment of a feeling of well-being, examination of signs of glucocorticoid or mineralocorticoid excess or deficiency, and measurements of serum electrolytes. The serum potassium and in some cases the plasma renin levels (evaluated in conjunction with a 24-hour urinary sodium determination) can be particularly helpful for evaluating the adequacy of mineralocorticoid replacement. Measurements of cortisol and ACTH are

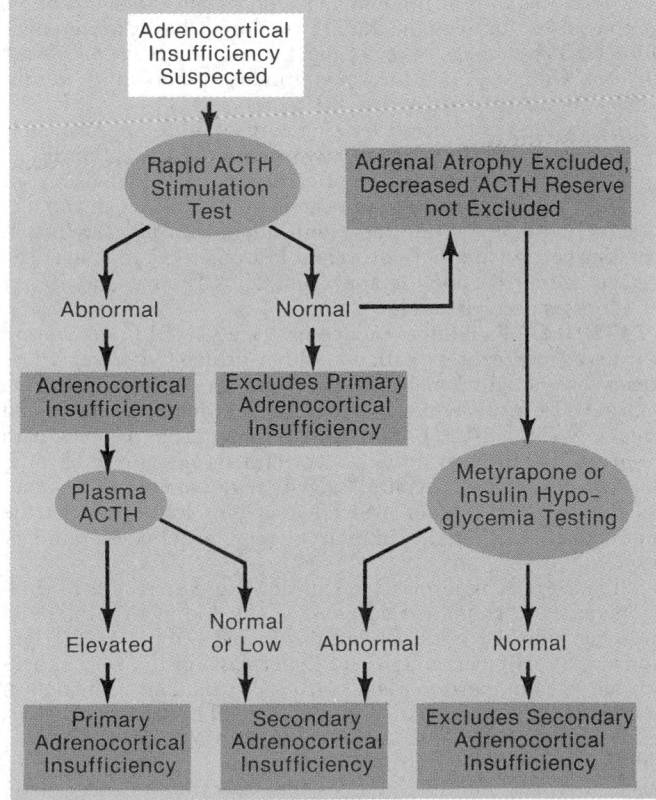

FIGURE 217–5. Evaluation of suspected primary or secondary adrenocortical insufficiency. Boxes enclose clinical decisions and ovals enclose diagnostic tests. (Reprinted from Baxter JD, Tyrrell JB: The adrenal cortex. *In* Felig P, Baxter JD, Broadus AE, et al. (eds.): Endocrinology and Metabolism, 2nd ed. New York, McGraw-Hill Book Company, 1987, p 593.)

TABLE 217–5. THERAPY OF ADRENAL INSUFFICIENCY

Acute Crisis

1. Cortisol (hydrocortisone) 100 mg IV, every 6 hr for 24 hr. If stable, reduce to 50 mg every 6 hr and then taper to oral maintenance in 4 to 5 days. Maintain or increase dose to 200 to 400 mg per 24 hr if complications persist or occur.
2. Correct volume depletion, dehydration, hypotension, and hypoglycemia with intravenous saline and glucose.
3. Correct precipitating factors, especially infection.

Maintenance

1. Cortisol 15 to 20 mg p.o. q. A.M.; 5 to 10 mg at 4 to 6 P.M.
2. 9α-Fluorocortisol 0.05 to 0.1 mg q. A.M. (primary).
3. Follow weight, blood pressure, and electrolytes.
4. Educate patient to increase cortisol dosage during stress.

Modified from Tables 12–17 and 12–18 in Baxter JD, Tyrrell JB: The adrenal cortex. *In* Felig P, Baxter JD, Broadus AH, et al. (eds.): Endocrinology and Metabolism, 2nd ed. New York, McGraw-Hill Book Company, 1987.

usually less helpful. The doses may need to be adjusted somewhat. Many of the subjective complaints of Addison's disease can be reversed within a few days; a somewhat longer time is required before strength returns to normal and hyperpigmentation subsides.

In times of stress, it is sometimes difficult to predict the need for increased glucocorticoid administration. It is best to err on the side of overreplacement rather than underreplacement. For minor illnesses such as significant upper respiratory infections, the cortisol dose should be doubled or tripled and then tapered over a few days. It is not usually necessary to change the 9α-fluorocortisol dose. Patients with vomiting and diarrhea should seek medical attention and receive parenteral cortisol. Patients who may not have early access to medical attention should keep injectable cortisol available and be instructed in its use.

In the event of major trauma or severe illness, treatment should be similar to that for adrenal crisis discussed above. In the case of elective major surgery the protocol described in Table 217–6 has been shown to be effective.

PROGNOSIS. Survival of patients in whom adrenocortical insufficiency is adequately diagnosed and treated now approximates that of the normal population. This is in sharp contrast to the period before steroids were available or when only mineralocorticoid replacement was available, at which time the survival rate was usually 2 years or less.

HYPOALDOSTERONISM

PATHOGENESIS. Hypoaldosteronism can occur in association with hypocortisolism or as an isolated defect. The major cause of isolated hypoaldosteronism is defective renal renin secretion (hyporeninemic hypoaldosteronism) (see Ch. 75). Other rarer causes include isolated adrenal biosynthetic defects (18-hydroxylase syndrome) and focal destruction of the adrenal glomerulosa (hyperreninemic hypoaldosteronism), transient deficiency following removal of an aldosterone-producing tumor, unresponsiveness to aldosterone (pseudohypoaldosteronism) with normal or increased aldosterone production, marked potassium depletion, and heparin administration.

HYPORENINEMIC HYPOALDOSTERONISM. This is seen generally in older patients with renal disease. It is most commonly due to diabetic nephropathy but can also occur with other renal diseases such as interstitial nephritis or multiple myeloma. It has also been observed following removal of an aldosterone-producing tumor or rarely without any apparent cause in association with hypertension. The hyporeninemia leads to decreased aldosterone production and impaired ability of the zona glomerulosa to respond to stimuli. However, the gland usually retains some capacity to secrete aldosterone through stimulation by potassium. Hypoaldosteronism results secondarily in hyperkalemia, which is disproportionate to the extent of renal disease. Chronic renal disease per se ordinarily does not lead to hyperkalemia unless the glomerular filtration rate is severely impaired (e.g., less than 10 ml per minute). In fact, hyporeninemic hypoaldosteronism is the most common cause of hyperkalemia in patients with renal disease and creatinine clearance rates greater than 10 ml per minute. Although these patients can develop hyponatremia, in adults this is less common, probably because of the fact that the primary disease tends to favor sodium retention. These patients

TABLE 217–6. STEROID COVERAGE FOR SURGERY

1. Correct electrolytes, blood pressure, and hydration if necessary.
2. Hydrocortisone phosphate or hemisuccinate, 100 mg IM, on call to operating room.
3. Hydrocortisone phosphate or hemisuccinate, 50 mg IM or IV, in recovery room and every 6 hr for the first 24 hr.
4. If progress is satisfactory, reduce dosage to 25 mg every 6 hr for 24 hr; then taper to maintenance dosage over 3 to 5 days. Resume previous 9α-fluorocortisol dose when patient is taking oral medications.
5. Maintain or increase cortisol dosage to 200 to 400 mg per 24 hr if fever, hypotension, or other complications occur.

Modified from Baxter JD, Tyrrell JB: The adrenal cortex. *In* Felig P, Baxter JD, Broadus AH, et al. (eds.): Endocrinology and Metabolism, 2nd ed. New York, McGraw-Hill Book Company, 1987, p 596.

also tend to develop a metabolic acidosis due to the lack of H^+-secreting actions of aldosterone; this can be accentuated by a decreased glomerular filtration rate. This form of acidosis has been classified as type IV renal tubular acidosis (see Ch. 82).

TREATMENT. The treatment of hypoaldosteronism involves therapy for the primary condition plus mineralocorticoid replacement as described above for primary adrenocortical insufficiency. However, in some patients with hypertension, treatment with 9α-fluorocortisol is not indicated and diuretics are used instead. Conversely, some patients require higher doses of mineralocorticoids, probably because the renal disease renders them more refractory to the steroid. Therapy is monitored by measuring serum potassium levels.

217.7 CUSHING'S SYNDROME

J. Blake Tyrrell

Cushing's syndrome is the result of chronic glucocorticoid excess. It occurs most commonly in patients receiving supraphysiologic doses of glucocorticoids. Spontaneously occurring Cushing's syndrome, a rare disorder, occurs as a result of either primary tumors of the adrenal gland that hypersecrete cortisol or from excess ACTH secretion that may be of pituitary or nonpituitary (ectopic ACTH syndrome) sources. In addition, Cushing's syndrome can be due to excessive CRF secretion from hypothalamic or ectopic tumors.

Cushing's disease (spontaneous hypercortisolism due to excessive pituitary ACTH secretion) accounts for two thirds of reported cases. This disorder is most common in women 20 to 40 years old, with a female-male ratio of 8:1.

Secretion of ACTH from ectopic tumors accounts for about 15 per cent of cases of Cushing's syndrome. The true incidence of this disorder is probably higher, since many patients lack the typical clinical features of cortisol excess because of the dominance of the manifestations of cancer and the rapidity of progression. Because of the current predominance of oat cell carcinoma of the lung in males, the ectopic ACTH syndrome has a female-male ratio of 1:3 and an age of onset most frequently between 40 and 60 years. CRF secretion from nonpituitary tumors rarely results in the stimulation of excess ACTH secretion.

Primary adrenal tumors secreting cortisol cause approximately 15 per cent of cases of Cushing's syndrome. In adults there is an equal frequency of adenoma and carcinoma. In childhood prior to the age of 10 years, adrenal carcinoma is the most frequent cause of Cushing's syndrome. Both adenomas and carcinomas secreting cortisol are more prevalent in women than in men. The average age at diagnosis is approximately 40 years, and 70 per cent of cases occur in adults.

PATHOLOGY. Pituitary adenomas (see Ch. 213) are present in over 90 per cent of patients with Cushing's disease. These tumors are usually small; 50 per cent are 5 mm or less in diameter. They are typically basophilic and unencapsulated and contain ACTH, β-LPH, and β-endorphin. The patients with Cushing's disease who do not have pituitary adenomas have (1) diffuse hyperplasia; (2) hyperplasia with multiple nests of adenomatous cells; (3) an adenoma or adenomatous hyperplasia of the intermediate lobe of the pituitary; or (4) no obvious pituitary disorder.

Adrenocortical hyperplasia in Cushing's disease results in modest increases in combined adrenal weight due to hyperplasia of the zonae reticularis and fasciculata. In the ectopic ACTH syndrome, adrenal enlargement and hyperplasia of the zona reticularis are usually more marked, with a concomitant reduction in the number of zona fasciculata cells. Bilateral nodular hyperplasia occurs in approximately 20 per cent of cases of ACTH excess. In addition to diffuse hyperplasia of the zonae reticularis and fasciculata, there are multiple nodules that vary from microscopic to several centimeters in diameter and that contain clear cells similar to those of the zona fasciculata.

Cortisol-secreting adenomas are usually encapsulated, range from 2 to 6 cm in diameter, typically secrete cortisol alone, and are usually composed of zona fasciculata–like cells. Adrenal carcinomas that secrete cortisol are usually large at the time of diagnosis, may be palpable as abdominal masses, and usually secrete a number of steroids. Histologically these tumors may appear benign or exhibit considerable pleomorphism, and the histologic appearance does not predict benign or malignant behavior. Therefore the diagnosis of adrenal carcinoma is dependent on the demonstration of either local tumor invasiveness or metastatic spread. Extension of these tumors occurs locally, and common sites of metastases are the liver and lung.

ETIOLOGY AND PATHOGENESIS. The etiology of Cushing's disease is unknown. It is possible that primary pituitary tumors arise spontaneously. In the uncommon cases in which diffuse or adenomatous hyperplasia is present, excessive secretion of CRF or some other factor may stimulate the pituitary. Rarely hypothalamic or ectopic CRF-producing tumors have been reported. The ectopic ACTH syndrome occurs in a relatively small number of tumor types. Oat cell carcinoma of the lung accounts for approximately 50 per cent of cases. The greatly increased production of cortisol and 11-deoxycorticosterone (DOC) stimulated by very high ACTH levels commonly results in manifestations of both mineralocorticoid and glucocorticoid excess.

Other ACTH-secreting tumors include thymomas and thymic carcinoids, islet cell tumors of the pancreas, carcinoid tumors, medullary carcinomas of the thyroid, and pheochromocytomas. Many other tumors may secrete ACTH, but this occurs very rarely.

Cortisol-producing adrenal tumors arise spontaneously and are not under normal control by the hypothalamic-pituitary axis; their secretion of cortisol and the other steroids is autonomous, episodic, and random.

Nodular adrenocortical hyperplasia is usually due to ACTH excess, but rare cases have been described with persistently suppressed ACTH levels.

CLINICAL FEATURES. The classic features, most typically seen in Cushing's disease (Fig. 217–6, Table 217–7) usually develop insidiously over several years. The most common mani-

TABLE 217–7. INCIDENCE OF CLINICAL FEATURES OF CUSHING'S SYNDROME

Feature	%
Obesity	94
Facial plethora	84
Hirsutism	82
Menstrual disorders	76
Hypertension	72
Muscular weakness	58
Back pain	58
Striae	52
Acne	40
Psychological symptoms	40
Bruising	36
Congestive heart failure	22
Edema	18
Renal calculi	16
Headache	14
Polyuria/polydipsia	10
Hyperpigmentation	6

Data from Plotz CM, et al.: Am J Med 13:597, 1952, and Ross EJ, et al: Q J Med 35:149, 1966, and reprinted from Baxter JD, Tyrrell JB: The adrenal cortex. *In* Felig P, Baxter JD, Broadus AE, et al. (eds.): Endocrinology and Metabolism, 2nd ed. New York, McGraw-Hill Book Company, 1987, p 606.

festation is central obesity with rounding of the face and fat accumulation around the trunk, supraclavicular areas, and dorsocervical spine. Serial photographs are helpful in recognizing these gradual changes. Classically this pattern of obesity spares the extremities; however, generalized obesity including the extremities occurs in about 50 per cent of patients. Atrophy of the skin and underlying connective tissue is frequent. This leads to facial plethora, easy bruisability, and red to purple depressed striae. The last occur most commonly over the lower abdomen, but can also be more generalized on the trunk and upper legs. Patients also have poor healing of minor or major injuries and abrasions and an increased incidence of superficial fungal infections. Hirsutism is present in approximately 80 per cent of female patients as a result of excessive adrenal androgen secretion. Hypertension is present in the majority of patients; it is rarely accompanied by hypokalemia in Cushing's disease, although this is common in the ectopic ACTH syndrome or adrenal carcinoma. Hypertension contributes greatly to the mortality of untreated Cushing's syndrome.

Additional common manifestations include hypogonadism in both male and female patients, psychological disturbances (usually depression), which occur in the majority, and proximal muscle weakness. Osteopenia is present in virtually all patients and may progress to frank osteoporosis (see Ch. 238). Back pain is common, and compression fractures of the spine occur in approximately 20 per cent. Renal stones, secondary to hypercalciuria, and thirst and polyuria, which may be due to hyperglycemia, can also occur. Routine laboratory abnormalities include high normal or modestly elevated values for the hematocrit, slightly elevated white cell counts, and a depressed percentage of lymphocytes and eosinophils. Electrolyte abnormalities occur only rarely in Cushing's disease, but hypokalemia occurs commonly with the ectopic ACTH syndrome or adrenal carcinoma.

DIAGNOSIS. A suggested plan for the evaluation of suspected Cushing's syndrome is shown in Figure 217–7. If the syndrome is suspected, the 24-hour urine free cortisol should be measured and the overnight 1-mg dexamethasone suppression test performed.

If results of both of these tests are normal, the diagnosis of Cushing's syndrome is excluded, with two exceptions: (1) Rare patients whose disease activity is episodic can have normal tests during periods of inactivity. In these cases, repeated evaluation during periods of disease activity establishes the diagnosis. (2) Rare patients with Cushing's disease have delayed clearance of dexamethasone and therefore have normal responses to low-dose dexamethasone. However, these patients have elevated urine free cortisol levels.

If the 24-hour urine free cortisol level is elevated and the 1-mg overnight dexamethasone suppression test is abnormal, then

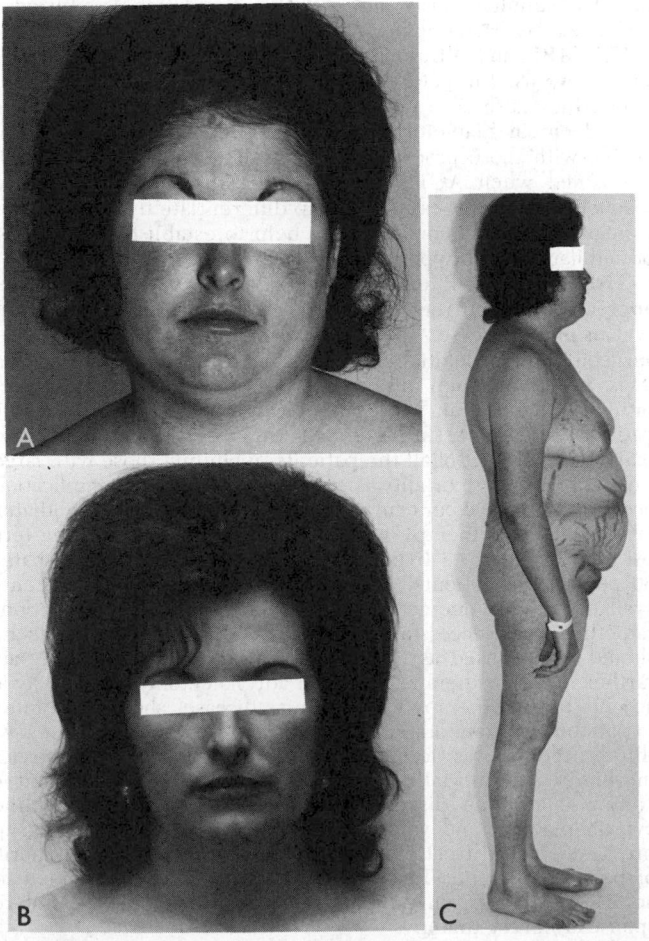

FIGURE 217–6. The appearance of a patient with Cushing's syndrome (*A*) before and (*B*) 1 year after removal of an adrenal adenoma. (*C*) Profile, before treatment.

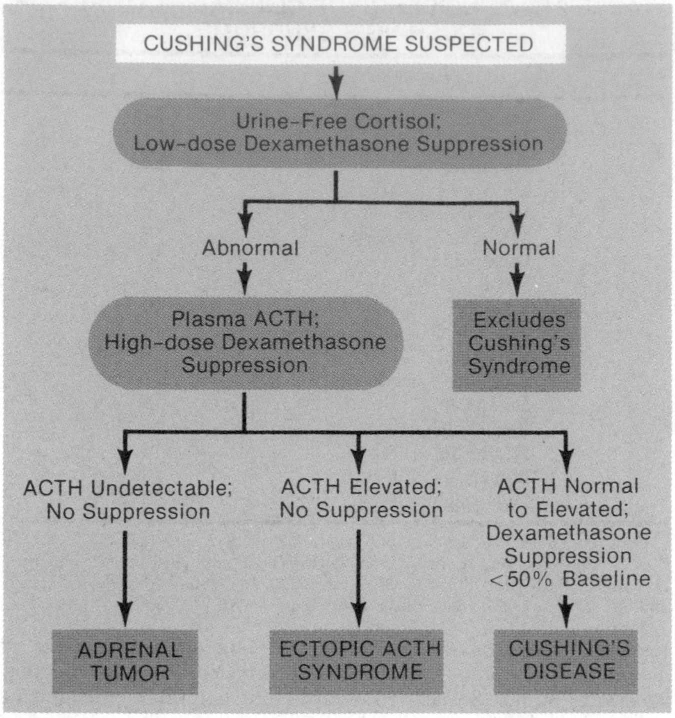

FIGURE 217–7. Evaluation of Cushing's syndrome. Boxes enclose clinical decisions and ovals enclose diagnostic tests. See the text for details and the potential for false-positive and false-negative results. (Reprinted from Baxter JD, Tyrrell JB: The adrenal cortex. *In* Felig P, Baxter JD, Broadus AE, et al. (eds.): Endocrinology and Metabolism, 2nd ed, New York, McGraw-Hill Book Company, 1987, p 609.)

spontaneous Cushing's syndrome is present provided that several abnormalities that lead to false-positive responses can be excluded. Results of the dexamethasone suppression test can be abnormal in obesity, estrogen therapy, drug therapy that increases dexamethasone metabolism (listed in Ch. 27), and chronic renal failure, although the 24-hour urine free cortisol is almost always in the normal range. In the case of obesity or estrogen therapy, the 2-day low-dose dexamethasone test should be performed; the results are almost always normal in the absence of Cushing's syndrome. Response to both the 24-hour urine free cortisol and the 1-mg dexamethasone suppression tests can be abnormal in alcoholism, acute and chronic illness, depression and other states of substantial emotional stress, and anorexia nervosa. In these cases, in the absence of spontaneous Cushing's syndrome the abnormalities subside following cessation of the condition.

ETIOLOGIC DIAGNOSIS. Once the diagnosis of Cushing's syndrome has been established, it is essential to determine its specific cause. The two most useful procedures are (1) the measurement of basal plasma ACTH levels and (2) the high-dose dexamethasone suppression test. In Cushing's disease, ACTH levels are normal to modestly elevated (50 to 200 pg per milliliter), and in 90 per cent of these patients, plasma or urinary steroid levels are suppressed to less than 50 per cent of baseline values in response to the high-dose dexamethasone test. In the ectopic ACTH syndrome, plasma ACTH values are often markedly elevated and are more than 200 pg per milliliter in two thirds of patients. In about 95 per cent of these patients, hypothalamic-pituitary control of ACTH and cortisol secretion is absent, and there is no response to high-dose dexamethasone suppression. Exceptions occur mostly in patients with relatively benign tumors, especially carcinoids, in whom ACTH levels may be only modestly elevated and in whom the high dose of dexamethasone may suppress ACTH release. With glucocorticoid-secreting adrenal tumors, plasma ACTH levels are suppressed to either low normal or undetectable levels, and dexamethasone suppression testing produces no reduction in cortisol levels.

Two major problems are encountered in determining the cause: (1) In approximately 10 per cent of patients with Cushing's disease

the cortisol levels are not suppressed adequately in response to dexamethasone, and (2) approximately 5 per cent of patients with ectopic tumors have suppression in response to high-dose dexamethasone and thus may appear to have Cushing's disease. In some cases, lack of suppression with pituitary adenomas occurs with larger tumors that are apparent when computed tomographic (CT) or magnetic resonance imaging (MRI) is performed. Also, this problem is more frequent when there is nodular adrenal hyperplasia. With these cases it is necessary to use additional procedures to establish the diagnosis. These include the use of head and body imaging studies to search for an ectopic tumor, selective venous sampling of the petrosal sinuses that drain the anterior pituitary and of other suspected regions with plasma ACTH determinations to identify the site of increased ACTH release, and utilization of higher doses of dexamethasone to suppress the activity of the pituitary tumor.

Tumor Localization. In Cushing's disease MRI is the current procedure of choice and allows excellent resolution of the hypothalamus and pituitary with better definition of parasellar structures (cavernous sinuses, pituitary stalk, and optic chiasm) than does CT (Fig. 217–8). However, the ability of MRI to detect the 50 per cent of tumors that are less than 5 mm in diameter is still limited even with gadolinium enhancement. In the absence of a radiologically evident lesion consistent with an adenoma it is recommended that selective venous sampling for ACTH be performed prior to surgical intervention. This technique is very useful in establishing a pituitary cause of Cushing's syndrome in those patients with normal neuroradiologic studies and in those with dexamethasone-nonsuppressible Cushing's disease. This procedure also excludes a pituitary etiology of ACTH excess when an occult ectopic ACTH-secreting tumor is present. The technique requires an experienced radiologist, since sampling from the inferior petrosal sinuses is required to assess pituitary ACTH secretion adequately. A gradient of 2:1 of central to peripheral ACTH levels establishes the presence of Cushing's disease. The most accurate results are obtained if the petrosal sinuses are sampled simultaneously and if CRF stimulation is utilized to maximize ACTH secretion.

CT, MRI, and ultrasonographic imaging of the adrenal (Fig. 217–9) are used in patients with suspected adrenal tumors or in whom the cause is in doubt. Adrenal tumors are usually larger than 2 cm in diameter when diagnosed and thus are readily visible with those procedures. Adrenal scanning should also be performed when ACTH levels or dexamethasone studies are inconclusive. In this case they help differentiate hyperplasia from primary adrenal tumors and may help to establish the diagnosis of nodular adrenal hyperplasia.

TREATMENT. Pituitary microsurgery with a transsphenoidal approach is the current method of choice for the initial therapy of Cushing's disease. It is critical that it be performed by a surgeon with substantial experience with the technique because it is not a common procedure. Under ideal circumstances, pituitary tumors can be located at surgery in 90 per cent of patients, and successful responses to surgery occur in approximately 80 per cent of all the patients, including those with larger tumors. Surgical mortality is rare, and significant complications occur in less than 2 per cent of patients. Heavy-particle irradiation is also effective therapy for Cushing's disease, with long-term correction of cortisol hypersecretion occurring in approximately 80 per cent of patients. Unfortunately this therapy is currently available in only one center in the United States. Conventional radiotherapy is successful in only 15 to 25 per cent of adults and should not be used as initial therapy because it precludes any further radiation therapy. Bilateral adrenalectomy, previously an accepted initial therapy for Cushing's disease, should be limited to patients in whom other therapies are unsuccessful. In the past, this procedure was accompanied by a high degree of surgical morbidity and mortality and the subsequent development of Nelson's syndrome (discussed below). Reserpine, bromocriptine, cyproheptadine, and valproate sodium have been used to suppress ACTH and treat Cushing's syndrome, but only a minority of patients respond. In general their use is recommended for adjunctive therapy in patients who have had unsuccessful responses to other therapy.

Drugs that inhibit adrenal cortisol secretion can also be used as adjunctive therapy or in patients in whom more definitive treatments have been unsuccessful. Ketoconazole, the current drug of choice, is effective in most patients, has a gradual onset of action, and has relatively few side effects. The effective dosage is 400 to 500 mg given twice daily, and cortisol levels gradually decline over 1 to 2 weeks. The major adverse effect is hepatic toxicity, which is only rarely severe. Alternatively, metyrapone* (ordinarily 2 grams per day) and aminoglutethimide (1 gram per day) are given simultaneously in four divided doses. These drugs are expensive, have frequent side effects (predominantly gastrointestinal), and result in secondary increases in ACTH levels that sometimes are sufficient to overcome the enzyme inhibition. They are not usually used for long-term therapy of Cushing's disease. Mitotane, 3 to 6 grams per day in divided doses, can be used if tolerated. Although remission rates with the drug in Cushing's disease are approximately 80 per cent, relapse occurs following discontinuation of therapy. In addition, the response to mitotane is slow, requiring weeks to months to control cortisol excess, and side effects that include nausea, vomiting, diarrhea, somnolence, and skin rash occur in the majority of patients. Since the use of these drugs may produce hypoadrenalism, careful monitoring of steroid levels and glucocorticoid replacement are required.

In the ectopic ACTH syndrome the tumor hypersecreting ACTH should be removed. This may be possible in the minority of patients with the more benign tumors such as thymoma, bronchial carcinoid, or pheochromocytoma. Unfortunately in the majority of patients the tumors are malignant and metastasize prior to the diagnosis of cortisol excess. In such patients, drug therapy as discussed above is used to control cortisol excess. Ketoconazole, metyrapone, and aminoglutethimide are preferred to mitotane because of their more rapid onset of action; multiple drugs may be required if the hypercortisolism is severe. Hypokalemia should be corrected, and spironolactone therapy may be useful in blocking the mineralocorticoid effects of cortisol and 11-deoxycorticosterone. Bilateral adrenalectomy may be considered in a rare patient in whom drug therapy is inadequate and the cortisol excess rather than the tumor is life threatening.

The treatment of adrenal tumors is primarily surgical. Patients

*This use is not listed in the manufacturer's directive.

with unilateral adrenal adenoma should undergo resection of the affected adrenal. Although surgical cure of adrenocortical carcinoma is unusual, surgical removal of the primary tumor is indicated to reduce cortisol secretion even when metastases are present. Mitotane, 6 to 12 grams per day in divided doses, if tolerated, is recommended for patients with residual or nonresectable carcinoma, and approximately 75 per cent of patients achieve reduced steroid secretion. Only about one third of patients undergo reduction in tumor bulk, however, and it is not clear whether the drug prolongs survival. Ketoconazole, metyrapone, and aminoglutethimide can be used in patients who do not respond to or tolerate mitotane. The prognosis is poor with adrenal carcinoma; most patients survive less than 5 years following the onset of symptoms.

The normal hypothalamic-pituitary-adrenal axis is suppressed in Cushing's syndrome of all causes, and months to sometimes 2 years are required for it to recover following removal of an adrenal, pituitary, or ectopic tumor. Thus, following the resection of a cortisol- or ACTH-producing tumor, glucocorticoid replacement therapy, as described above for secondary adrenocortical insufficiency, is required until normal pituitary and adrenal function recovers.

NELSON'S SYNDROME. Defined as the clinical progression of an ACTH-secreting pituitary adenoma following bilateral adrenalectomy for Cushing's disease, this syndrome appears to occur in at least one third of such patients. Fortunately the incidence of this disorder has dropped dramatically because of the decreased use of bilateral adrenalectomy for treatment of Cushing's disease.

The syndrome probably results when cortisol feedback inhibition is removed by bilateral adrenalectomy, thus allowing progression of the adenoma. Nelson's syndrome is characterized by increasing hyperpigmentation, usually within 1 to 2 years following adrenalectomy. In addition, these patients frequently exhibit local manifestations, including hypopituitarism, visual loss, headache, cavernous sinus invasion with extraocular muscle palsies, and rarely malignant changes with metastatic spread. Plasma ACTH levels are dramatically elevated and usually range from 1000 to 10,000 pg per milliliter. The majority of these tumors

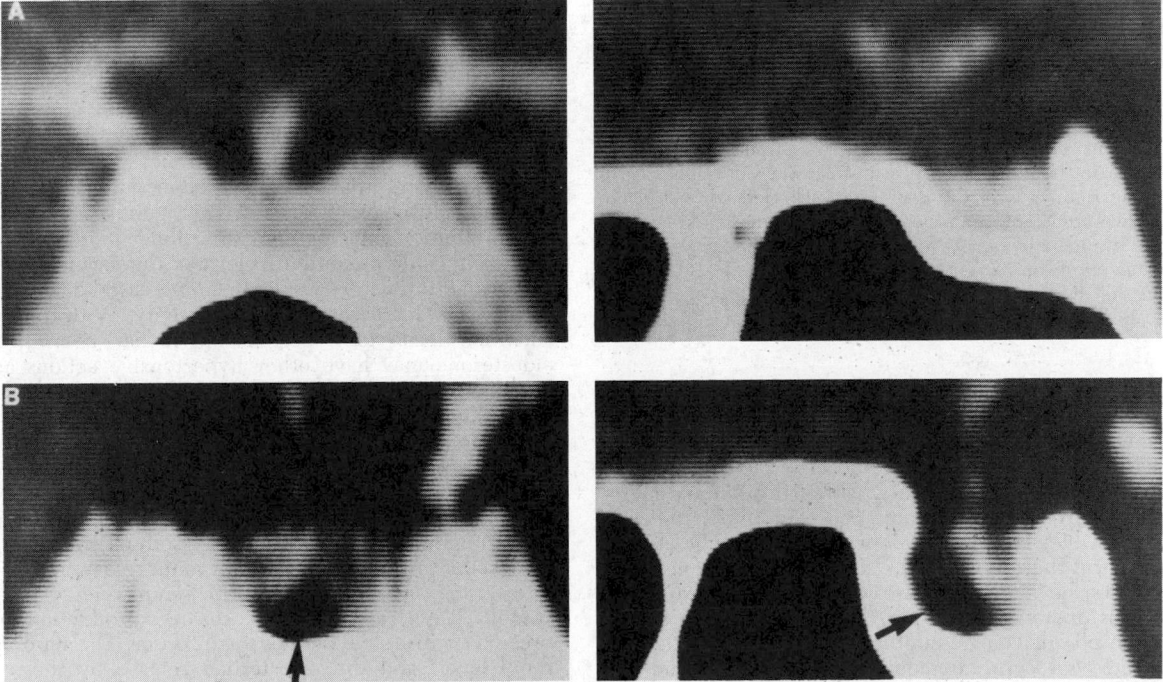

FIGURE 217–8. CT scans of normal and abnormal pituitary glands. The sections shown are computer re-formations derived from 1.5-mm axial sections through the sella turcica. Coronal re-formations are shown on the left and sagittal ones on the right. *A*, Normal pituitary gland. The upper border is flat; the pituitary stalk (seen on the coronal section) is midline; and the gland is relatively homogeneous in density. The lateral margins of the sella turcica (see coronal section) are formed by the contrast-enhancing cavernous sinuses. *B*, In a patient with Cushing's disease, a 3- to 4-mm pituitary adenoma is visualized as a low-density lesion in the anterior inferior portion of the anterior lobe (*arrows*). (Reprinted from Findling JW, Tyrrell JB: *In* Greenspan FS, Forsham PH (eds.): Basic and Clinical Endocrinology, 2nd ed. Los Altos, Calif., Lange Medical Publications, 1986, p 65.)

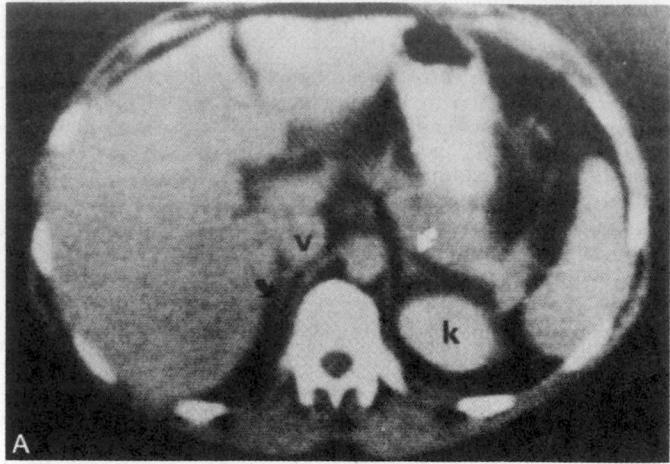

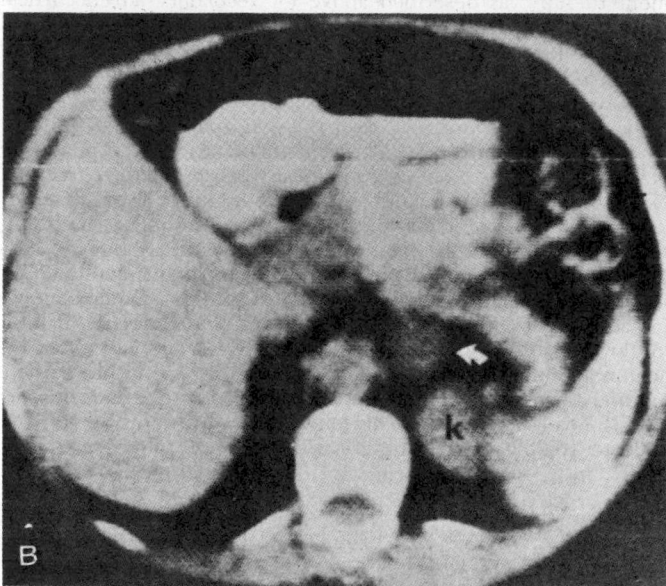

FIGURE 217–9. CT scans in Cushing's syndrome. *A*, Patient with ACTH-dependent Cushing's syndrome. The adrenal glands are not detectably abnormal by this procedure. The curvilinear right adrenal (*black arrow*) is shown posterior to the inferior vena cava (v) between the right lobe of the liver and the right crus of the diaphragm. The left adrenal (*white arrow*) has an inverted **Y** appearance anteromedial to the left kidney (k). *B*, A 3-cm left adrenal adenoma (*white arrow*) anteromedial to the left kidney (k). (From Korobkin M, White EA, Kressel HY, et al.: Computed tomographs in the diagnosis of adrenal disease. AJR 132:231, 1979. © 1979, American Journal of Roentgenology, The Williams & Wilkins Company.)

are greater than 1 cm in diameter and are readily localized by MRI or CT of the sella turcica.

The treatment of Nelson's syndrome is considerably less successful than that of Cushing's disease because of the large size and aggressive nature of these tumors. Although pituitary microsurgery is the preferred initial therapy, complete tumor resection is usually not possible. Heavy-particle irradiation may be utilized either as primary therapy or after surgery in patients with intrasellar tumors; however, in those with extrasellar extension, conventional postoperative radiation therapy should be undertaken. Although pharmacologic inhibition of ACTH secretion has been attempted with cyproheptadine, bromocriptine, and valproic acid, it appears that only a minority of patients respond. Nevertheless, trials of these medications are indicated if surgical treatment and radiotherapy are unsuccessful.

INCIDENTAL ADRENAL MASSES

The routine use of CT, MRI, and ultrasonography for the evaluation of intra-abdominal conditions has led not infrequently to the incidental detection of unilateral adrenal masses or less

commonly of bilateral adrenal enlargement. The great majority of such patients with unilateral lesions have benign nonfunctional adrenocortical adenomas or cysts; a few patients have functioning adenomas or rarely carcinomas of the adrenal cortex or medulla. When such lesions are identified, the patient should undergo screening tests for pheochromocytoma, Cushing's syndrome, aldosterone excess, and adrenal carcinoma. If a functioning tumor is present, it should be resected regardless of its size. Nonfunctioning lesions less than 6 cm in diameter should be re-imaged in 6 and 18 months; if growth occurs, resection is recommended. Nonfunctioning lesions greater than 6 cm should be resected because adrenal carcinoma is more common with larger lesions. The incidental discovery of bilateral adrenal enlargement is very unusual and presents a difficult diagnostic challenge. These patients may have a variety of infectious, metastatic, invasive, or hemorrhagic lesions that may ultimately lead to adrenal insufficiency (Ch. 217.6). Rare lesions are bilateral adrenal carcinomas, bilateral pheochromocytomas, and congenital adrenal hyperplasia. In such cases, if screening tests for adrenal hyper- and hypofunction are negative, needle biopsy of the adrenal should be considered to establish a histologic diagnosis and direct appropriate therapy.

217.8 MINERALOCORTICOID EXCESS STATES

John D. Baxter

PRIMARY ALDOSTERONISM

Increased and inappropriate production of aldosterone from the adrenal is known as primary aldosteronism and leads to sodium retention with hypertension, suppression of plasma renin, and hypokalemia and its manifestations. It is due mainly to an adrenocortical adenoma, bilateral adrenocortical hyperplasia, or rarely to an adrenal carcinoma. The disease occurs in all age groups, with a peak incidence during the third and fourth decades. About 70 per cent of the adenomas occur in women. Although primary aldosteronism almost always results in hypertension (normotensive primary hyperaldosteronism is extremely rare), the syndrome is present in less than 2 per cent of patients with hypertension. Nevertheless, this largely reversible form of hypertension should be considered in all hypertensive patients.

ALDOSTERONE-PRODUCING ADENOMAS. With an aldosterone-producing adenoma (Conn's syndrome), aldosterone excess leads to sodium retention and potassium and hydrogen loss. Other steroids that are normally synthesized in the zona glomerulosa (i.e., deoxycorticosterone, corticosterone, and 18-hydroxycorticosterone) are also produced in excess, although they are probably not important in the overall pathophysiology. Sodium retention expands the extracellular fluid volume, increases total body sodium content, elevates the serum sodium concentration and ultimately results in an increased intracellular sodium content that increases vascular reactivity. With time, the sodium retention leads to hypertension. It has been proposed that aldosterone may have other hypertensive actions as well. The hypokalemia results in muscular weakness, a tendency to cardiac irritability and arrhythmia, carbohydrate intolerance, resistance to vasopressin (nephrogenic diabetes insipidus), and abnormalities in baroreceptor function. The latter results in a more volume-dependent hypertension. The expansion of the extracellular fluid and plasma volume is registered by the stretch receptors at the juxtaglomerular apparatus and by sodium chloride flux at the macula densa with suppression of renin release, low plasma renin levels, and unresponsiveness of renin release to provocative stimuli. Thus, increased aldosterone production with a suppressed renin system defines the disorder. The suppressed plasma renin levels and the aldosterone release by these tumors are generally unresponsive to the usual stimuli such as posture or diuresis, although they are responsive in a small subset of patients (renin-responsive adenoma).

The sustained hypertension leads to compensatory effects that act to decrease the plasma volume, which can be normal or increased. However, an increased sodium and extracellular fluid volume persists, and the hypertension continues to be aldosterone dependent. The hypertension can also lead to many complications, such as renal damage, stroke, and myocardial infarction.

BILATERAL ADRENAL HYPERPLASIA. Bilateral adrenal hyperplasia can be diffuse or nodular, and selectively involves the glomerulosa cells. It accounts for perhaps 30 per cent of the patients in whom primary aldosteronism is diagnosed; however, its precise incidence is not known, since there is a gradient between what is termed low-renin essential hypertension without frank aldosterone excess and this syndrome. Adrenal hyperplasia does not in general precede development of an adenoma.

The pathophysiology of the most common form of hyperplasia (idiopathic hyperaldosteronism) shows several differences from that of adenoma: (1) Although the plasma renin is suppressed, it does respond to postural and other stimuli. (2) The adrenal is hypersensitive to angiotensin II, exhibiting a marked increase in aldosterone production rather than insensitivity. (3) The aldosterone hypersecretion is less than with the adenoma, a feature that is useful in the differential diagnosis. By contrast, the blood pressure in the two groups tends to be similar. (4) The hypertension in most patients does not respond to adrenalectomy, implying that common factors produce both hypertension and enhanced adrenal sensitivity to angiotensin II. The mechanisms for the development of hyperplasia are unknown. There is active inquiry whether there is abnormal production (or loss) of factor(s) that enhance adrenal and vascular sensitivity to angiotensin II.

There are also subgroups of hyperplasia. A few per cent of patients have what has been termed primary adrenal hyperplasia. In these patients the plasma aldosterone and 18-OHB levels tend to be higher; the aldosterone and renin responses to provocative stimuli resemble those with aldosterone-producing adenomas; the hypertension commonly responds to adrenalectomy; and the hyperplasia is typically nodular, being either unilateral or bilateral. In rare patients the hypertension and aldosterone excess respond to glucocorticoid therapy.

CLINICAL PRESENTATION. Patients present with elevated blood pressure detected on routine screening or, less commonly, because of hypokalemia. The blood pressure elevations range from mild to severe, with mean presenting pressures in the range of 200 mm Hg systolic and 120 mm Hg diastolic. Malignant hypertension is rare. A history of hypertension in pregnancy is common with female patients who develop the disorder. When present, symptoms of hypokalemia include tiredness, loss of stamina, weakness, nocturia, and lassitude. Symptoms of more severe depletion include alkalosis; rarely tetany with a positive Trousseau or Chvostek sign; increased thirst and polyuria with low urine specific gravity and unresponsiveness to vasopressin; paresthesias; cardiac arrhythmias such as ventricular tachycardia; and postural hypotension with dizziness. Headache is a frequent incidental complaint. There are no characteristic physical findings. In spite of fluid overload, edema is only rarely present. The heart is usually only mildly enlarged, if at all, and electrocardiographic changes are usually those of moderate left ventricular hypertrophy and potassium depletion. There tend to be fewer funduscopic changes than in other forms of hypertension of comparable severity. These patients are particularly sensitive to the potassium-wasting effects of diuretics.

DIAGNOSIS. The hallmarks of the disorder are hypertension with hypokalemia, suppression of the renin-angiotensin system, and increased aldosterone production. The serum sodium is rarely less than 139 mEq per liter in the absence of diuretic therapy. A suggested evaluation plan is shown in Figure 217–10. The initial step is to determine whether hypokalemia is present, since this is the primary clue to mineralocorticoid excess. All patients with hypertension should be screened, especially those with spontaneous hypokalemia, after diuretics have been withheld for at least 3 weeks.

The evaluation of hypokalemia requires control of the sodium balance, since sodium depletion from decreased intake or diuretics can decrease urinary potassium excretion and thus mask hypokalemia. Random serum potassium levels may be normal in up to 20 per cent of patients with primary aldosteronism, but salt loading unmasks hypokalemia in virtually all patients with adenoma and in most patients with hyperplasia. In the latter group the serum potassium levels are almost always below 4 mEq per liter. If according to the dietary history the patient's usual sodium intake is 120 mEq or greater per 24 hours, measurement of normal potassium levels on three occasions obviates the need

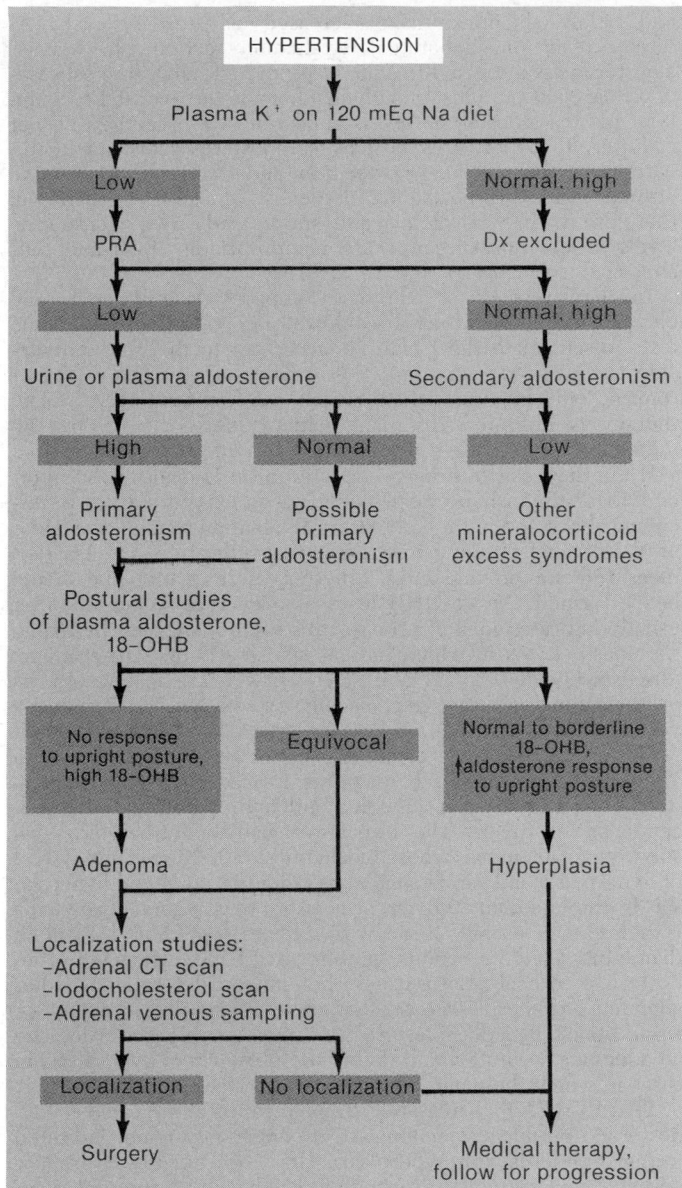

FIGURE 217–10. Flow diagram for diagnosis of primary aldosteronism and differentiation of adrenal adenoma from hyperplasia. (Adapted from Baxter JD, Perloff D, Hsueh W, et al.: *In* Felig P, Baxter JD, Broadus AE, et al. (eds.): Endocrinology and Metabolism, 2nd ed. New York, McGraw-Hill Book Company, 1987, p 756.)

for further evaluation. If dietary intake is inadequate or unclear, the patient is instructed to consume a normal diet supplemented with 1 gram of NaCl with each meal for 4 days, and the serum potassium is then measured.

If the plasma potassium value is low, other causes of hypokalemia should be ruled out: diuretic therapy, gastrointestinal loss due to vomiting or diarrhea, other mineralocorticoid excess syndromes (discussed below), starvation, insulin and glucose therapy, metabolic acidosis, renal disease, and renovascular and accelerated hypertension.

Random unstimulated plasma renin activity (PRA) or plasma renin concentration (PRC) should be determined as the next step in diagnosis. In primary aldosteronism this is suppressed even after short-term diuretic therapy, salt restriction, assumption of erect posture, or exercise, although other causes of low renin must be excluded. If PRA is normal or high, primary aldosteronism is unlikely.

If the plasma renin value is low or marginally low, 24-hour urinary aldosterone and plasma aldosterone levels should be measured. It is critical to monitor the salt intake and posture, as discussed earlier, because patients with essential hypertension and a low-salt intake have increased aldosterone levels. As discussed in the Laboratory Evaluation section, the urinary aldosterone is increased to over 17 µg per 24 hours in most cases of primary aldosteronism. With an adenoma the overnight recumbent plasma aldosterone levels almost always exceed 20 ng per deciliter. In hyperplasia the plasma aldosterone levels are ordinarily less than 20 ng per deciliter and frequently are in the normal range. Hypokalemia decreases aldosterone secretion; therefore with hypokalemia and suppressed PRA, aldosterone levels in the normal range are inappropriately high and thus abnormal.

In the presence of marginally suppressed PRC and mild elevation of plasma or urinary aldosterone, one of the stimulation tests (discussed earlier) may be necessary to diagnose primary aldosteronism. Marginal cases are usually due to primary aldosteronism with hyperplasia, in which case antimineralocorticoid therapy is indicated. In many patients such therapy can be initiated and the patient re-evaluated at a later time.

If the diagnosis of primary aldosteronism is made, it is important to distinguish between adenoma and hyperplasia. As discussed above and in the Laboratory Evaluation section, the levels of plasma aldosterone provide an initial indication, but 18-OHB measurements provide an even better discrimination and should be performed. An 18-OHB level of over 100 ng per milliliter usually indicates adenoma; below this value it suggests hyperplasia. In situations in which these tests, or CT or MRI scanning (discussed below), do not give a clear answer, the postural studies or the saline infusion tests usually are helpful in reaching a decision.

CT or MRI scanning of the adrenals should be performed in all patients in whom the diagnosis is made; this can help in distinguishing between adenoma and hyperplasia and in localization of the tumor. The scan also usually identifies the small subgroup of adenomas whose biochemical indices are more typical of hyperplasia and can in some cases identify unilateral hyperplasia. In the less than 20 per cent of patients in whom an adenoma is not found, usually those with tumors less than 1.4 cm in diameter, selective venous sampling with measurements of aldosterone-cortisol ratios is usually helpful, can determine whether adenoma or hyperplasia is present, and can lateralize an adenoma. In addition, an iodocholesterol scanning technique can localize an adenoma accurately and detect the presence of hyperplasia in cases in which the diagnosis remains uncertain.

TREATMENT. Unilateral adrenalectomy is indicated for aldosterone-producing adenomas. Adrenalectomy is not indicated for most patients with hyperplasia. However, in cases of primary adrenal hyperplasia with biochemical indices that resemble adenoma, removal of a unilaterally hyperplastic gland or of one gland (preferably the left because of surgical considerations) in patients with bilateral hyperplasia is frequently effective. However, these patients also respond to antimineralocorticoid therapy. Prior to surgery the blood pressure and serum potassium should be normalized by treatment with the mineralocorticoid antagonist spironolactone (200 to 400 mg per day) or the potassium-sparing diuretic amiloride (20 to 40 mg per day). These dosages of spironolactone can be reduced to around 100 to 150 mg per day once normalization of blood pressure and hypokalemia has occurred. Medical therapy can be continued in the rare patient in whom surgery is contraindicated or in patients in whom the etiologic diagnosis is uncertain. This form of treatment also tends to reactivate the suppressed renin-angiotensin system so that the incidence of postoperative hypoaldosteronism is reduced. Also the response of the blood pressure to this therapy provides an excellent indication of the anticipated response to surgery.

Following surgery the blood pressure returns to normal in around 50 per cent of patients, with reduction of hypertension in another 25 per cent. However, hypertension, but not hyperaldosteronism, returns in about 40 per cent by 10 years postoperatively.

Medical therapy is recommended for most patients with bilateral hyperplasia. Spironolactone in doses described above or amiloride corrects the hypokalemia but not the hypertension in most cases. Additional antihypertensive medications are usually necessary. Although treatment with a glucocorticoid is effective in the rare subgroup of patients with glucocorticoid-hyperplasia,

it is debatable whether patients should be screened for this responsiveness.

OTHER FORMS OF HYPERTENSION ASSOCIATED WITH MINERALOCORTICOID EXCESS

There are several other mineralocorticoid-excess conditions. DOC excess can occur in the 11β- and 17α-hydroxylase syndromes (see Ch. 221), in patients with Cushing's syndrome, especially with ectopic ACTH-producing carcinoma, and with adrenal adenomas and carcinoma. In these cases the PRC is suppressed as it is in primary aldosteronism; however, plasma aldosterone levels are usually suppressed as well. Rarely mineralocorticoid-excess hypertension results from excessive ingestion of licorice or carbenoxolone (discussed in Ch. 217.2), 9α-fluorocortisol used for treating postural hypotension, or mineralocorticoid-containing nasal sprays. It can be present in rare cases of insensitivity to glucocorticoids when elevated cortisol levels have mineralocorticoid actions. There are rare syndromes (predominantly observed in children) in which there are hypertension, hypokalemia, and suppressed PRC with no detectable elevations of known mineralocorticoids; in some instances these syndromes are due to 11β-hydroxysteroid dehydrogenase deficiency, which impairs renal cortisol to cortisone conversion with a consequent cortisol-induced mineralocorticoid excess state. In all of these conditions there are hypertension, hypokalemia, and suppression of PRC without an associated increase of aldosterone.

SECONDARY HYPERALDOSTERONISM

Secondary hyperaldosteronism results from stimulation of the adrenal glomerulosa by extra-adrenal factors, usually the renin-angiotensin system. It can be physiologic or contribute to the pathology of disease states. A physiologic increase occurs during excessive potassium intake as part of the body's defense against hyperkalemia. Secondary hyperaldosteronism can occur during the luteal phase of the menstrual cycle and occasionally during oral contraceptive use. Aldosterone secretion increases progressively during normal pregnancy; levels reach 10 times those of nonpregnant women by the third trimester. This is presumably due to an increase in renin and angiotensin, possibly due to a decrease in blood pressure. Interestingly, renin levels are more elevated during the first trimester, whereas plasma aldosterone levels are highest during the third trimester. This may be due to a progressive increase in sensitivity of the adrenal glomerulosa to angiotensin II. Aldosterone secretion increases when there is excessive sodium loss and when there is dietary restriction of sodium. Aldosterone increases in some patients with congestive heart failure and with significant hypoalbuminemia such as with nephrotic syndrome. In heart failure the aldosterone levels result from counterbalancing influences of decreased renal perfusion secondary to reduced cardiac output that increases renin and aldosterone release, and of sodium retention that suppresses renin and aldosterone levels. Renin and aldosterone levels are commonly elevated in cirrhosis when ascites is present; this is accentuated by decreased clearance of aldosterone. The increased aldosterone further promotes sodium retention and potassium loss. Elevated aldosterone levels are found in Bartter's syndrome (see Ch. 82). Finally, secondary hyperaldosteronism and hypertension can occur with renal artery stenosis, unilateral renal ischemia, accelerated hypertension, and renin-secreting tumors. Since secondary aldosteronism occurs in response to other primary processes and is an adaptive response, treatment is usually not indicated. However, in certain situations such as heart failure or cirrhosis, in which the excessive sodium retention and potassium loss are deleterious, antimineralocorticoid therapy, such as spironolactone, can be helpful.

Baxter JD, Tyrrell JB: The adrenal cortex. *In* Felig P, Baxter JD, Broadus AE, et al. (eds.): Endocrinology and Metabolism, 2nd ed. New York, McGraw-Hill Book Company, 1987, pp 511–650. *An extensive review of the physiology and pathology of the adrenal cortex.*

Baxter JD, Perloff D, Hsueh W, et al.: The endocrinology of hypertension. *In* Felig P, Baxter JD, Broadus AE, et al. (eds.): Endocrinology and Metabolism, 2nd ed. New York, McGraw-Hill Book Company, 1987, pp 693–788. *A description of the renin-angiotensin system and an analysis of the pathophysiology and approaches to diagnosis and treatment not only of primary aldosteronism but also of other types of endocrine hypertension.*

Crapo L: Cushing's syndrome: A review of diagnostic tests. Metabolism 28:955, 1979. *This paper, although published over a decade ago, still provides an excellent overview of the approaches to the diagnosis of Cushing's syndrome.*

Dluhy RG: The growing spectrum of HIV-related endocrine abnormalities. J Clin Endocrinol Metab 70:563, 1990. *An overview of adrenal and other abnormalities in AIDS.*

Findling JW: The Cushing syndromes: An enlarging clinical spectrum. N Engl J Med 321:1677, 1989. *An overview of causes of and diagnostic approaches to Cushing's syndrome.*

Funder JW, Pearce PT, Smith R, et al.: Mineralocorticoid action: Target tissue specificity is enzyme, not receptor, mediated. Science 242: 583, 1988. *An examination of the role of cortisol-to-cortisone conversion in the actions of cortisol and aldosterone.*

Hall PF: Tropic stimulation of steroidogenesis: In search of the elusive trigger. Recent Prog Horm Res 41:1, 1985. *A review of the mechanisms regulating steroid biosynthesis.*

Irony I, Kater CE, Biglieri EF, et al.: Correctable subsets of primary aldosteronism: Primary adrenal hyperplasia and renin responsive adenoma. Am J Hypertens 3:576, 1990. *An analysis of the types of primary aldosteronism and how to manage them.*

Kaye TB, Crapo L: The Cushing syndrome. An update in diagnostic tests. Ann Intern Med 112:434, 1990. *This updates and complements the 1979 paper by Dr. Crapo listed above.*

Keller-Wood ME, Dallman M: Corticosteroid inhibition of ACTH secretion. Endocr Rev 5:1, 1984. *A review of the kinetics and mechanisms whereby glucocorticoids block both CRF and ACTH release.*

Marver D, Kokko JP: Renal target sites and the mechanism of action of aldosterone. Miner Electrolyte Metab 9:1, 1983. *A review of the actions of aldosterone.*

May RE, Carey RM: Rapid adrenocorticotrophic test in practice. Am J Med 79:679, 1985. *An assessment of the usefulness of this test.*

Melby JC: Primary aldosteronism. Kidney Int 26:769, 1984. *An overview of mineralocorticoid-excess syndromes.*

Munck A, Guyre P, Holbrook NJ: Physiological functions of glucocorticoids in stress and their relation to pharmacological actions. Endocr Rev 5:25, 1984. *A proposal that explains how glucocorticoids are useful in the body's response to stress.*

Parker LN, Odell WD: Control of adrenal androgen secretion. Endocr Rev 1:392, 1980. *An excellent examination of the factors that regulate adrenal androgen production.*

Re NJ: Cellular biology of the renin-angiotensin systems. Arch Intern Med 144:2037, 1984. *An excellent overview of the renin-angiotensin system.*

218 Diabetes Mellitus

Jerrold M. Olefsky

DEFINITION. Diabetes mellitus is a heterogeneous primary disorder of carbohydrate metabolism with multiple etiologic factors that generally involve absolute or relative insulin deficiency or insulin resistance or both. All causes of diabetes ultimately lead to hyperglycemia, which is the hallmark of this disease syndrome.

CLASSIFICATION AND DIAGNOSIS

The currently accepted classification and the criteria for the diagnosis of diabetes mellitus are summarized in Table 218–1. Diabetes can be separated into two general disease syndromes: (1) *Type 1*, or *insulin-dependent diabetes mellitus* (IDDM), is present in patients with little or no endogenous insulin secretory capacity. These patients develop extreme hyperglycemia, ketosis, and the associated symptomatology unless treated with insulin, and they are therefore entirely dependent on exogenous insulin

TABLE 218–1. CLASSIFICATION OF DIABETES

1. Insulin-dependent, or type I diabetes (IDDM). Formerly called juvenile-onset or ketosis-prone diabetes.
2. Non–insulin-dependent, or type II diabetes (NIDDM). Formerly called adult-onset, maturity-onset, or nonketotic diabetes.
   A. Obese (~80%)
   B. Nonobese (~20%)
3. Secondary diabetes
   A. Pancreatic disease (e.g., pancreatectomy, pancreatic insufficiency, hemochromatosis)
   B. Hormonal (excess counterinsulin hormones, e.g., Cushing's syndrome, acromegaly, pheochromocytoma)
   C. Drug-induced (e.g., thiazide diuretics, steroids, phenytoin)
   D. Associated with specific genetic syndromes (e.g., lipodystrophy, myotonic dystrophy, ataxia-telangiectasia)
4. Impaired glucose tolerance (IGT). Formerly called chemical, latent, borderline, or subclinical diabetes.
5. Gestational diabetes: glucose intolerance with onset during pregnancy.

therapy for immediate survival. This form of the disease usually, but not always, develops prior to early adulthood. Older terms for this syndrome are juvenile onset, ketosis prone, or brittle diabetes. (2) *Type II*, or *non–insulin-dependent diabetes mellitus* (NIDDM), occurs in patients who retain significant endogenous insulin secretory capacity. Although treatment with insulin may be necessary for control of hyperglycemia, these patients do not develop ketosis in the absence of insulin therapy and are not dependent on exogenous insulin for immediate survival. Previous terms for this form of the disease are maturity or adult onset, nonketotic, and stable diabetes. The diagnosis of diabetes in patients with the insulin-dependent form of the disease is usually unequivocal, and the distinction between type I and type II diabetes can usually be made on clinical grounds. However, there are occasional patients with minimal, but clearly detectable, endogenous insulin secretion in whom the disease is difficult to categorize initially. Usually these are lean adult, sometimes elderly, patients who at the time of initial diagnosis retain sufficient insulin secretory function so that the disease meets the classification of type II diabetes; with time, insulin secretion diminishes to the point that the disease merges into the category of type I diabetes.

The diagnosis of NIDDM is based on a distinction between normal and abnormal levels of glycemia and therefore is less precise. Prior to the report of the National Diabetes Data Group, oral glucose tolerance tests were commonly used to establish this diagnosis. This approach is fraught with difficulties because oral glucose tolerance is affected by numerous other variables that can cause mild abnormalities of glucose metabolism independent of diabetes. Concomitant illness, stress, physical inactivity, hypocaloric or low carbohydrate intake, various drugs, and aging are among those factors that can adversely influence glucose tolerance. Therefore, when employed, glucose tolerance testing must be rigorously controlled by administering a standard oral glucose load (75 grams), ensuring an appropriate antecedent diet (eucaloric with at least 200 grams of carbohydrate per day), adequate physical activity, and the absence of drugs affecting carbohydrate metabolism. Even with these precautions, only a minority (15 to 25 per cent) of individuals who have normal fasting plasma glucose levels with abnormal glucose tolerance tests go on to develop overt diabetes. In recognition of the above facts, relatively stringent criteria for establishing the diagnosis of NIDDM have been recommended: (1) fasting venous plasma glucose concentration greater than 140 mg per deciliter on at least two separate occasions, or (2) in the absence of fasting hyperglycemia, a diagnosis of NIDDM can be made following ingestion of the standard 75-gram oral glucose tolerance test if the 2-hour venous plasma glucose and one other sample (the 30-, 60-, or 90-minute sample) exceed 200 mg per deciliter.

Impaired glucose tolerance exists if the fasting plasma glucose level is less than 140 mg per deciliter and if the 30-, 60-, or 90-minute plasma glucose concentration exceeds 200 mg per deciliter along with a 2-hour plasma glucose level between 140 and 200 mg per deciliter. Microvascular complications of diabetes rarely occur in individuals with impaired glucose tolerance, and the great majority of these cases do not deteriorate to overt diabetes in long-term follow-up. Most instances of impaired glucose tolerance, therefore, are probably unrelated to the disease syndrome of NIDDM. Almost all patients who meet the criteria for NIDDM during oral glucose tolerance testing show fasting hyperglycemia (greater than 140 mg per deciliter) when evaluations are repeated. Furthermore, in those few patients who meet the criteria for NIDDM in the absence of fasting hyperglycemia, many do not develop fasting hyperglycemia during prolonged follow-up, and clinical symptoms of diabetes are unusual. Thus, the clinical significance of impaired glucose tolerance is unclear. As previously mentioned, only a minority (2 to 35 per cent, depending on the population examined) of these patients go on to develop overt NIDDM when followed for up to 20 years. The real challenge is to develop markers to detect which patients with impaired glucose tolerance have a benign nonprogressive abnormality of glucose intolerance and which have a prediabetic state. Patients with impaired glucose tolerance who secrete low amounts of insulin, compared to normal individuals, have a much higher risk of developing overt diabetes (perhaps up to 40 per cent), whereas those who secrete high amounts of insulin seldom (about 5 per cent) progress to frank diabetes. In brief, glucose tolerance testing is unnecessary for patient management in the absence of clinical signs and symptoms of diabetes, although this is still a highly useful procedure for epidemiologic or research purposes. An exception to this would be in a pregnant subject suspected of having gestational diabetes, since criteria for this diagnosis are less stringent and vigorous management of minimal degrees of hyperglycemia is important.

Glucose tolerance declines with age. Insulin secretion is not decreased in aging, whereas insulin resistance due to a postreceptor defect in insulin action is a common finding in aged populations. Age-related variables such as inadequate diet, increasing adiposity with decreased lean body mass, and physical inactivity can contribute to this insulin-resistant state, but the aging process itself also plays a significant role. The glucose intolerance of aging tends to be mild and is most easily detected following an oral glucose challenge. When mild abnormalities of oral glucose tolerance tests were used to diagnose diabetes, age-adjusted criteria for these tests had to be employed. However, with the current more stringent criteria noted above, this problem is largely obviated, since the glucose intolerance of aging does not cause significant fasting hyperglycemia (more than 140 mg per deciliter) and only rarely would cause glucose intolerance severe enough to meet the new criteria in the absence of hyperglycemia.

EPIDEMIOLOGY AND CLINICAL PRESENTATION

Overall, in the United States the prevalence of diabetes is probably between 2 and 4 per cent, with IDDM comprising 7 to 10 per cent of all cases. The prevalence of IDDM (0.2 to 0.3 per cent) is probably more accurate than the estimates for NIDDM, because of the relative ease of ascertainment and the fact that many patients with NIDDM are asymptomatic and the disease is undiagnosed.

The prevalence of diabetes has been difficult to quantitate accurately because the criteria for the diagnosis of NIDDM have varied from survey to survey over the years; the less stringent the criteria the greater the prevalence and vice versa. Furthermore, the prevalence of diabetes differs widely among different populations, depending on ethnic group constituents, age, economic conditions, and probably other environmental factors. For example, the prevalence of diabetes is extremely high among Pima Indians (about 35 per cent) and certain Micronesian cultures (about 35 per cent). Indians, particularly after emigrating from their country, have a higher rate of diabetes than other ethnic groups. Thus, Indians living in South Africa, Trinidad, Singapore, Malayasia, and Fiji exhibit a higher prevalence of diabetes than the local population and than those living on the Indian subcontinent. A low prevalence of diabetes has been noted in Eskimos, Athabascan Indians (Alaska), and Chinese (although prevalence increases in Chinese populations living in Western countries). The proportion of IDDM to NIDDM also differs widely among different populations; IDDM is extremely rare in Pima Indians, Micronesians, and Eskimos, but is more common in Caucasian populations.

A few facts concerning the prevalence of major diabetes-related complications serve to underscore the enormous impact of this disease. Approximately 25 per cent of all new cases of end-stage renal failure occur in patients with diabetes. About 20,000 amputations (primarily of toes, feet, and legs) are carried out in patients with diabetes, representing approximately half of the nontraumatic amputations performed in the United States. Furthermore, diabetes is the leading cause of new cases of blindness, with approximately 5000 new cases occurring each year.

INSULIN-DEPENDENT DIABETES MELLITUS (IDDM, TYPE I). These patients have little or no endogenous insulin and usually present with relatively abrupt clinical symptoms of *polyuria, polydipsia,* and *polyphagia. Weight loss,* fatigue, and infection can often accompany the initial presentation. Because of the extreme hypoinsulinemia and hyperglucagonemia, these patients readily develop *ketosis,* and the initial onset of this disease may be clinically evident as full-blown ketoacidosis. At the time of the first clinical presentation, symptoms can usually be traced back for several days to a few weeks; however, in most cases β cell destruction began months and usually years prior to the onset of clinical symptoms. In some cases, detection of this preclinical state may be possible by assessing the presence of circulating antibodies to islet cells or insulin. Unfortunately, proven methods to delay or prevent the full-blown disease are not available. The peak age of onset of IDDM is 11 to 13 years, coinciding with early adolescence and puberty. A secondary peak is noted at age 6 to 8 years, and by the third decade of life the incidence falls to a steady but still substantial level. It is unusual for IDDM to begin past age 40. Once IDDM is diagnosed, insulin therapy is required to achieve initial metabolic control. In many patients a "honeymoon" period follows initial treatment in which the disease remits and little or no insulin is required. This remission is due to a partial return of endogenous insulin secretion, which may last for several weeks or months and occasionally 1 to 2 years; ultimately, however, the disease recurs, and insulin therapy is required permanently.

NON–INSULIN-DEPENDENT DIABETES MELLITUS (NIDDM, TYPE II). Patients with NIDDM typically present with polyuria and polydipsia of several weeks' to months' duration. Polyphagia can occur but is less common, whereas weight loss, weakness, and fatigue are frequent. Dizziness, headaches, and blurry vision are common accompanying complaints. In many patients no symptoms are apparent and the disease is diagnosed by routine blood or urine testing. In others, diabetes is advanced, and the presenting complaints are related to neuropathic, retinopathic, or vascular complications. NIDDM patients are usually but not always older than 40 at presentation. Obesity is a frequent feature of NIDDM, at least in Western cultures; in the United States 80 to 90 per cent of NIDDM patients are obese. Obesity by itself leads to insulin resistance and predisposes or exacerbates the NIDDM state. The mechanisms of obesity-induced insulin resistance are unclear, but the linkage between obesity and NIDDM is indisputable. Certain patterns of distribution of excess adipose tissue may be metabolically more deleterious. Abdominal, or upper body, obesity is more closely associated with NIDDM than is lower body obesity (adipose tissue deposits mainly around the hips and thighs). Endogenous insulin secretion is relatively preserved and may even be excessive; thus, ketosis is rare, explaining why NIDDM is categorized as nonketotic or ketosis resistant.

SECONDARY DIABETIC STATES. In addition to the major categories of diabetes (IDDM and NIDDM), many secondary forms of diabetes exist when some other readily identifiable primary disease entity or pathophysiologic state causes or is strongly associated with the diabetic state (Table 218–1). These cases comprise only a small proportion of the total cases of diabetes. Any disease process that limits insulin secretion or impairs insulin action can cause secondary diabetes. Disorders that lead to pancreatic destruction such as chronic pancreatitis, cystic fibrosis, or hemochromatosis can reduce insulin secretion enough to cause diabetes. Conditions in which excess amounts of counterinsulin hormones are secreted, such as Cushing's disease, acromegaly, pheochromocytoma, and glucagonoma, can also produce diabetes. A number of drugs such as thiazide diuretics, glucocorticoids, and adrenergic agents can lead to, or at least exacerbate, diabetes. Many unusual genetic diseases are associated with a higher than normal incidence of diabetes through unknown mechanisms; these include muscular dystrophy, myotonic dystrophy, Friedreich's ataxia, Turner's syndrome, and others.

Finally, several rare syndromes have been identified, the biochemical mechanisms of which are well described and which primarily involve abnormalities of insulin-glucose physiology. Certain patients with extreme insulin resistance, acanthosis nigricans, and diabetes have circulating anti-insulin receptor antibodies. These antibodies are part of a more generalized autoimmune process, since proteinuria, leukopenia, and antinuclear and anti-DNA antibodies also exist. Other patients with the triad of acanthosis nigricans, insulin resistance, and diabetes do not have antireceptor antibodies, but instead have a profound decrease in cellular insulin receptors. Typically these are young females with hirsutism and polycystic ovaries. In some of these patients, family members also have decreased insulin receptors and insulin resistance, suggesting that this disorder is due to a genetically mediated decrease in insulin receptors. In a few subjects, molecular cloning has revealed mutations in insulin receptor gene alleles, demonstrating the genetic nature of these unusual cases. In some patients, abnormal insulin products are synthesized and secreted. For example, familial hyperproinsulinemia involves a defect in the proinsulin molecule that prevents normal cleavage of proinsulin to insulin in the pancreatic β cell. This leads to the secretion of large amounts of proinsulin (which is biologically less active than insulin) instead of insulin. This disorder can lead to impaired glucose tolerance, but has not yet been associated with overt fasting hyperglycemia. Rarely patients carry mutations in the insulin structural gene itself that lead to the secretion of insulin species with single amino acid substitutions resulting in markedly reduced biologic activity. These patients have a clinical picture of typical NIDDM. These mutant insulins are immunologically reactive and are secreted in large quantities in response to the hyperglycemic state. The clinical hallmark of this condition is the presence of hyperglycemia and marked hyperinsulinemia in a patient with normal sensitivity to exogenous insulin.

GENETICS

Diabetes has long been termed a geneticist's nightmare. The disease clearly aggregates in families and has a strong familial component. However, the precise genetic contribution to diabetes has been difficult to ascertain for at least four reasons: (1) No specific genetic marker has been identified. Glucose tolerance is the currently used method of diagnosis, but because of differences in the way tests are performed and the criteria used, it is difficult to compare one study to another. (2) There is a great deal of etiologic heterogeneity between IDDM and NIDDM and within these categories. This indicates genetic heterogeneity even though the phenotype (hyperglycemia) is comparable. It is also possible that, depending on environmental factors, there can be variable phenotypic expression of a common genotype. (3) It is likely that "diabetogenic genes" interact with external factors as well as with other genetic components, making the specific genetic influences underlying the final phenotypic expression of the diabetes hard to detect. (4) Actual transmission rates of diabetes from generation to generation are low.

Genetic factors are clearly important in the etiology of diabetes. This is demonstrated by classic twin studies. When twins below the age of 40 years are studied, if one twin has diabetes (mostly IDDM based on age) then the other twin develops diabetes only 30 to 50 per cent of the time. If the two pairs are concordant, the second twin usually develops diabetes within a couple of years of the first. For a purely genetic disease, concordance should be 100 per cent. This suggests that while genetic factors are important in IDDM, they are only predisposing and must interact with environmental influences if diabetes is to develop. This does not exclude the possibility that in some patients IDDM occurs entirely because of genetic or environmental factors. In twins over 40 years the concordance rate for diabetes (almost all NIDDM based on age) approaches 100 per cent. This suggests that genetic factors are more important in this form of diabetes and may be causal or closely associated with causal mechanisms.

Despite the contribution of genetic factors, direct transmission of diabetes from parent to offspring is surprisingly low. If one parent has IDDM, the risk to the offspring of developing IDDM is on the order of 2 to 5 per cent. If one child has IDDM, the average risk for another sibling is 5 to 10 per cent. However, the risk is much greater if the second sibling is HLA (human leukocyte antigen)-identical to the first, intermediate if HLA-haploidentical, and very low if HLA-nonidentical. The risk for developing diabetes in a monozygotic twin of an IDDM patient is 30 to 50 per cent. Not only does this indicate the importance of nongenetic "triggering" factors in the etiology of IDDM but it also defines the maximal predictive value that could be achieved by tests based on genetic characteristics. The risk for IDDM is less in HLA-identical siblings than in monozygotic twins: This indicates that genes outside of, or not linked to, the HLA region contribute to the etiology of IDDM, pointing to the multigenic nature of this disease. The type of diabetes tends to run true in families, and the incidence of NIDDM in the offspring of an IDDM parent is probably not greater than normal. If one parent has NIDDM, the risk is 10 to 15 per cent for offspring developing the disease. When both parents have NIDDM, the transmission risk increases, but adequate data are not available to quantitate the

increase in risk. If one sibling has NIDDM, the risk for another sibling is 10 to 15 per cent. These low rates of transmission make it difficult to trace models of inheritance in family studies, but the facts are clinically important in counseling and reassuring diabetic patients who wish to have children.

Strong associations have been identified between IDDM and specific HLA's encoded by the major histocompatibility complex region located on the short arm of the sixth chromosome (see Ch. 250) At each of these loci numerous alleles (genes) exist, some of which confer increased risk for the development of IDDM. These high-risk alleles include: HLA-DR3, HLA-DR4, HLA-B8, and HLA-B15. The HLA-A, B, and C antigens are present on virtually all nucleated cell types, whereas the HLA-DR antigens show tissue restriction and are predominantly expressed on B lymphocytes and macrophages. It is possible that DR antigens are also expressed on islet cells, but this is unproven at the current time.

An HLA haplotype refers to a particular set of alleles at the four closely linked HLA loci A, B, C, and D, on one of the sixth chromosomes (each person inherits two haplotypes, one from each parent). In this system, some of the alleles are in linkage disequilibrium. This means that certain HLA antigens encoded by alleles at the different HLA loci occur together more frequently within the same haplotype than would be predicted by random statistical chance, taking gene (allele) frequency into account. The antigens encoded by the HLA alleles associated with higher risk for IDDM do not directly cause or predispose to the disease. Rather, these alleles are believed to be in linkage disequilibrium with genes in the HLA region (possibly certain immune response genes) that are directly related to the etiology of IDDM. In other words, through linkage disequilibrium one "looks" at the "diabetogenic gene" via the more easily measured HLA antigens.

The D locus appears to be more important than the B locus because it is more closely linked to the etiologically important genes. The increased risk for IDDM development imparted by inheritance of HLA-B8 and B15 is most likely a result of linkage disequilibrium between these HLA B locus alleles and the HLA alleles DR3 and DR4, respectively. Likewise, the risk imparted by HLA-DR4 is probably due to linkage disequilibrium with HLA-DQ B. HLA-DR and DQ molecules are heterodimers composed of α and β subunits. Both subunits are transmembrane molecules and are associated with each other in a noncovalent manner. Specific alleles at the DQ B locus may define at least one proximate diabetes risk gene encoding an immune system antigen that directly participates in IDDM etiology. A specific DQ B allele, missing the aspartic acid codon at position 57 of the B chain, can be detected by direct DNA analysis, and this allele is in linkage disequilibrium to the DR4 allele and directly predisposes to IDDM. The DR3 association with IDDM is linked to some other gene not associated with the DQ locus, and this gives evidence for the multigenic etiology of this disease. Interestingly, homozygosity at any of these alleles (i.e., DR3/DR3) does not lead to greater risk than when the allele occurs on only one haplotype. However, if both sixth chromosomes bear two different diabetes-associated alleles at a particular locus (i.e., DR3/DR4), the increase in risk is more than additive. The diabetes-associated HLA antigens are quite frequent in the nondiabetic population (although clearly less frequent than in IDDM). For example, 30 to 35 per cent of normal persons are positive for DR3 or DR4. Thus, far more people who are positive for these antigens are normal than have IDDM (e.g., if the average risk for IDDM in a population is 0.2 per cent, and if a particular HLA haplotype confers a 10-fold increase in risk, then the risk would still be only 2 per cent for those with this haplotype). This is an important point to realize in thinking about HLA typing for screening or predictive value in a practical or clinical sense.

Despite all this information, the model of inheritance for IDDM is obscure, although it is clearly not autosomal dominant. The low penetrance of the diabetes-associated genes combined with the relative degrees of HLA associations suggests that the genetic predisposition must interact with specific environmental factors for IDDM to occur. Additionally, the disease could be multigenic, with at least two genes necessary for IDDM to develop. With this model, environmental factors would still be necessary.

In NIDDM no HLA associations have been identified, demonstrating the differences in etiology between the two major forms of diabetes. Although the location of the genetic component for NIDDM is not known, possible changes have been noted on the eleventh chromosome, which contains the insulin gene. A 1.5 to 3.4 kilobase insertion of extra DNA, about 500 base pairs upstream from the 5′ flanking end of the insulin gene, has been described by some workers as a polymorphism more frequent in patients with NIDDM than in normal persons or patients with IDDM. However, the association is slight and has not been found by all workers. Restriction fragment length polymorphisms have also been observed in the insulin receptor as well as glucose transporter genes, some of which have a statistically significant association with the NIDDM phenotype. However, the potential importance of any of these associations is unknown at present. Identification of the NIDDM gene(s) is of major interest, with enormous diagnostic and therapeutic potential. Since this is most likely a heterogeneous multigenic disease, the search will be a most difficult task.

PATHOGENESIS

Before discussion of the pathogenetic aspects of diabetes it is important to review briefly some of the essential features of insulin and glucose physiology. Insulin is produced in the pancreatic B cell as the primary biosynthetic product preproinsulin containing 109 amino acid residues (MW ~ 11,500). This peptide is rapidly converted to proinsulin (86 amino acid residues, MW ~ 9000) by cleavage of the amino terminal 23 amino acid "pre" sequence. Within the B cell secretory granules, proinsulin is converted by proteolytic cleavage to insulin (51 amino acids, MW ~ 6000) and C peptide (31 amino acids, MW ~ 3000). Thus, the final B cell secretory product is 95 per cent insulin and C peptide in equimolar amounts and 5 per cent unconverted proinsulin. In familial hyperproinsulinemia, mutations in the proinsulin sequence prevent proteolytic conversion within the secretory granule, leading to release of large amounts of proinsulin having only 7 to 10 per cent of insulin's biologic activity. The regulation of insulin release is extremely complex, being influenced by glucose, amino acids, gut insulinogenic hormones, glucagon, neural influences, and other factors. However, glucose is the most important stimulus for insulin secretion.

After a brief circulating time ($t_{1/2}$ 4 to 8 minutes) insulin interacts with target tissues to exert its biologic effects. At the target cell, insulin action is initiated by binding of the hormone to specific cell surface insulin receptors. The complete amino acid structure of the insulin receptor has been elucidated. Following formation of the insulin receptor complex one or more signals are propagated (second messengers) that interact with a variety of cellular effector systems such as enzymes and glucose transport proteins to produce insulin's ultimate biologic effects. Insulin exerts its major effects on carbohydrate homeostasis by stimulating peripheral glucose disposal and inhibiting hepatic glucose production. A variety of abnormalities in insulin biosynthesis, secretion, and action can lead to diabetes.

A number of other hormones, termed anti-insulin or counter-regulatory hormones (glucagon, growth hormone, cortisol, and catecholamines), affect carbohydrate homeostasis. Among these, glucagon is probably most important in terms of the pathophysiology of diabetes. Glucagon is 29 amino acids (MW ~ 3000) in length and is synthesized in the pancreatic α cells as proglucagon (MW ~ 9000 to 11,000). Its release is stimulated by hypoglycemia, amino acids, neural influences, and stress. Its major effect on glucose metabolism is exerted at the liver where it binds to surface receptors, stimulates cyclic AMP generation, and promotes glycogenolysis, gluconeogenesis, and ketogenesis. Its lipolytic effects are minimal in man, and glucagon has little if any effect on peripheral glucose uptake. Thus, glucagon affects glucose metabolism by influencing hepatic glucose production, and glucagon levels are absolutely or relatively increased in both IDDM and NIDDM.

NIDDM. Abnormalities of insulin and, to a lesser extent, glucagon secretion and action are central to the pathogenesis of NIDDM. Syndromes involving abnormalities of insulin biosynthesis have already been discussed. These include familial hyperproinsulinemia and mutations in the structural gene for insulin leading to secretion of a biologically defective insulin molecule. These rare syndromes lead to mild degrees of glucose intolerance or a clinical picture indistinguishable from NIDDM. Beyond these unusual syndromes, however, insulin biosynthesis is qualitatively normal in NIDDM.

Secretion of insulin is not normal in NIDDM. In some patients with impaired glucose tolerance, substantially reduced amounts of insulin are secreted in response to a glucose load. These subjects are not insulin resistant and the defect in insulin secretion appears adequately to account for their abnormal glucose metabolism. These patients have a relatively high propensity to develop overt NIDDM (up to 50 per cent) and should be followed for progression. Other patients with impaired glucose tolerance secrete normal or increased amounts of insulin, although in some cases the dynamics of secretion may be altered with a delay in release of insulin following a glucose stimulus. These patients are insulin resistant primarily because of decreased insulin receptors. This is true in both the obese and nonobese categories of this classification. In relatively few (about 5 per cent) of the hyperinsulinemic insulin-resistant patients with impaired glucose tolerance is there progression to fasting hyperglycemia.

The great majority of patients with NIDDM are both insulin deficient and insulin resistant. The decrease in insulin action exists whether they are obese or nonobese (although approximately 80 per cent are obese). Patients with NIDDM may have normal or elevated fasting insulin levels, but they almost always secrete decreased amounts of insulin following oral glucose or meals. Other functional abnormalities that have been identified include a marked decrease in early release of insulin (first phase) after intravenous administration of glucose, and much greater blunting of the insulin response to glucose compared to other insulin stimuli (amino acids, sulfonylureas, glucagon, or β agonists). These latter findings have given rise to the idea that β cell dysfunction in NIDDM may be characterized by a defect in glucose recognition by islet cells. Insulin deficiency tends to be more severe in patients with longstanding disease. Interestingly, amyloid-like proteinaceous deposits are found in the islet interstitium of many such patients. A peptide termed "islet amyloid polypeptide (IAPP)," or amylin, has been isolated from this islet amyloid material. IAPP is cosecreted with insulin from β cells, but its physiologic function is unknown. Possibly, deposition of IAPP to form these amyloid deposits has a deleterious impact on β cell function in longstanding NIDDM.

In addition to these abnormalities of insulin secretion, patients with NIDDM are also insulin resistant. Insulin action is a complex sequence of events beginning with binding to surface receptors; insulin resistance can be due to any abnormality at any step along the insulin action pathway. For convenience, the cellular causes of insulin resistance can be broadly divided into binding and postbinding defects (Fig. 218–1). A binding defect involves a decrease in insulin binding due to a decrease in either receptor number or affinity or to both. A postbinding defect refers to any biologically significant abnormality in the activity of effector proteins (such as insulin sensitive enzymes or transport proteins) or an impairment in the coupling or transducing mechanisms between insulin receptor complexes and effector units. In subjects with impaired glucose tolerance who are insulin resistant, binding defects exist (decreased receptor number), but postbinding function is normal. In NIDDM, insulin resistance exists in the great majority of patients. Although a receptor defect (decreased number) is present in most insulin-resistant NIDDM patients, this does not appear to be the major abnormality. Postbinding defects also exist, and these appear to play the predominant role in causing the insulin-resistant state. As far as glucose homeostasis is concerned, several postbinding defects have been described in NIDDM; e.g., these patients exhibit decreased β subunit tyrosine kinase activity, decreased rates of cellular glucose transport, and diminished glycogen synthase activity.

Insulin deficiency and insulin resistance both contribute to the hyperglycemia of NIDDM. In addition, another abnormality also contributes to the hyperglycemia. Hepatic glucose production rates are increased in NIDDM, and the magnitude of this increase is proportional to the level of fasting hyperglycemia. This hepatic abnormality is, at least partially, due to resistance to insulin's normal restraining effect on liver glucose production. Additionally, glucagon levels are often elevated, either absolutely or

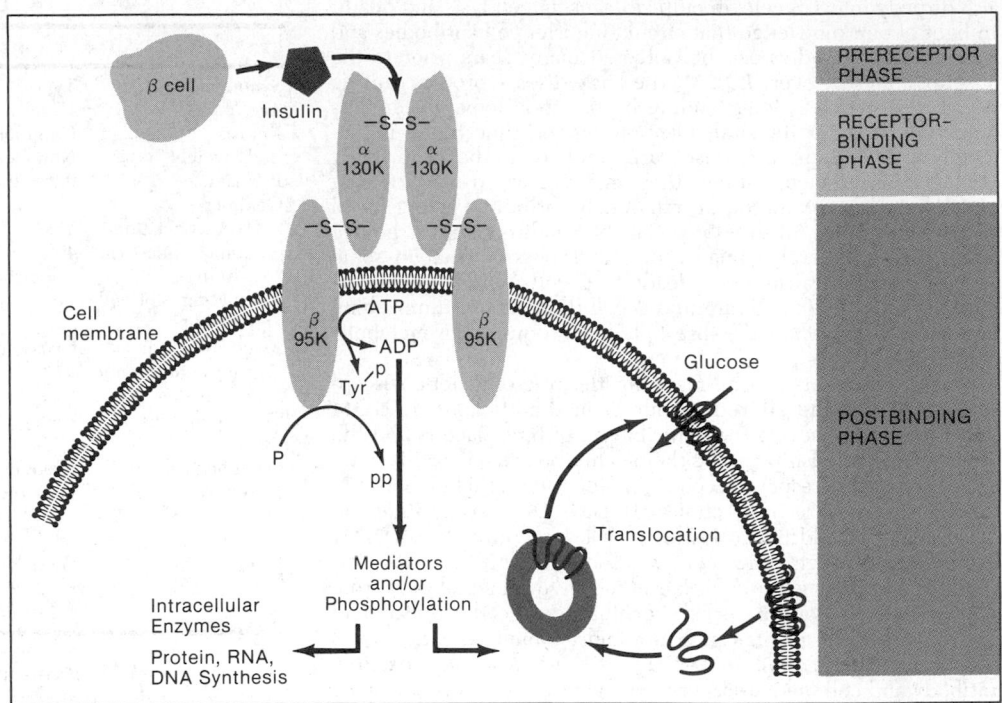

FIGURE 218–1. Model of insulin action and categories of insulin resistance. Insulin binds to the extracellular α-subunits of its receptor, stimulating tyrosine autophosphorylation of the transmembrane β subunits. This is followed by mediation of insulin's pleiotropic biologic effects, including recruitment of intracellular glucose transport proteins to the cell surface to facilitate glucose uptake. Abnormalities can occur at the prereceptor phase, involving biosynthesis and secretion of abnormal β cell products; at the receptor binding phase, involving decreased insulin binding to receptors due to decreased receptor number or affinity; or at the postbinding phase, involving any defect in the insulin action cascade distal to the initial binding event.

relatively, in NIDDM, and it is possible that excess glucagon stimulation also contributes to the increase in glucose production.

Thus, insulin deficiency, insulin resistance, and accelerated hepatic glucose production all exist in NIDDM, and all contribute to the hyperglycemia (Fig. 218–2). It is tempting to suggest a unifying pathogenetic hypothesis in which one metabolic lesion is primary and the others are secondary. Unfortunately it is not possible to choose any particular sequence at this time. All three abnormalities can be generated in animal models by inducing hyperglycemia and hypoinsulinemia, and all three are at least partially reversible with weight loss, oral sulfonylureas, or insulin therapy.

IDDM. *Autoimmunity* plays a major role in the etiology of IDDM. Circulating antibodies to thyroid, gastric mucosa, and the adrenal are far more common in patients with IDDM than in normal persons. More importantly, up to 90 per cent of patients with new-onset IDDM have demonstrable serum titers of islet cell antibodies. These antibodies are heterogeneous, some binding to cytoplasmic antigens common to all islet cells and others directed against the β cell surface. The latter lyse β cells

in culture in the presence of complement, consistent with a pathophysiologic role in vivo. These islet cell antibodies are also observed in BB rats, an animal model that spontaneously develops an IDDM-like syndrome. Anti-insulin antibodies are also present with high frequency in IDDM sera. In humans, islet cell and anti-insulin antibodies can be detected at least several years prior to IDDM onset. Titers of these antibodies fall after the onset of clinical disease; by 5 years only 20 per cent of patients have demonstrable titers, and by 10 to 20 years the prevalence falls to 5 to 10 per cent. Patients who continue to demonstrate antibodies after several years may be examples of heterogeneity within IDDM. In these patients IDDM may represent a primary autoimmune disease, since they are largely female, show a great prevalence of other organ-specific antibodies, and have a strong family history of autoimmune disease. Patients with onset of IDDM at an older age tend to fall into this group. Genetically, they may also be different, since they have a greater prevalence of HLA-B8 and DR3. In cases of IDDM in which islet cell antibodies are cleared within 1 year of the disease's onset, patients are more often male, do not typically show signs of other autoimmune phenomena, experience onset of disease at a younger age, and have a higher association with HLA-B15 and HLA-DR4. Circulating antibodies may not be the only component of the immune response associated with IDDM; a cell-mediated immune response may also be involved. Increased K cells (killer lymphocytes) have been reported in IDDM along with alterations in T lymphocyte subpopulations. Both antibody-induced and cell-mediated immune phenomena may be involved in the pathogenesis of IDDM.

A strong genetic component is involved in the etiology of IDDM, but extragenetic factors must also contribute, at least in most patients. Several lines of evidence suggest a role for viruses in IDDM: (1) Autopsies of IDDM patients dying within a few months of the disease's onset have revealed an "insulitis" consisting of round cell infiltration of islet tissue. (2) A modest seasonal variation to the incidence of IDDM has been noted in some studies. (3) A clinical history of preceding viral-type illness, particularly coxsackie B and mumps, is often reported at the onset of IDDM. (4) Increased viral titers, including coxsackievirus B4, have been reported in IDDM patients at or near the time of the disease's onset. (5) Certain diabetogenic viruses (encephalomyocarditis M, coxsackievirus B, and rheovirus) can cause diabetes when inoculated into rodents. Further, the susceptibility of different rodent strains to develop virus-induced diabetes appears to be under genetic control. (6) Diabetogenic viruses can

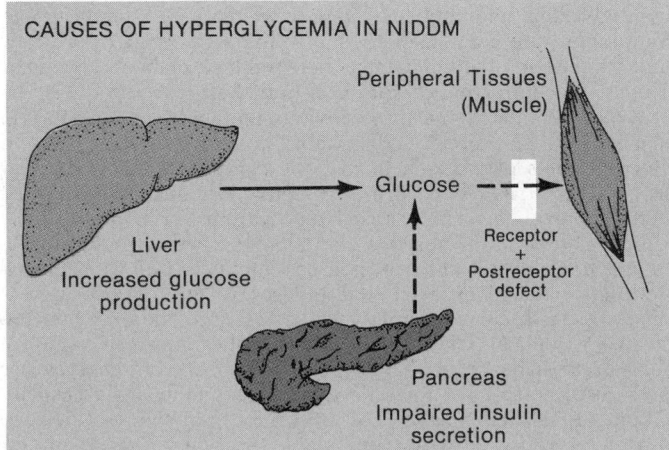

FIGURE 218–2. Summary of the metabolic abnormalities in NIDDM which contribute to the hyperglycemia. Increased hepatic glucose production, impaired insulin secretion, and insulin resistance due to receptor and postreceptor defects all combine to generate the hyperglycemic state.

also directly infect β cells in culture, causing cell lysis and death. In light of our knowledge that circulating islet cell antibodies and anti-insulin antibodies can be detected many years prior to the onset of clinically overt IDDM, the basic disease process causing β cell destruction is longstanding by the time hyperglycemia is detected. Thus, acute viral infections in the time frame immediately prior to disease onset are unlikely to be of primary etiologic importance; rather, they may act as stresses causing metabolic decompensation in individuals with pre-existing β cell destruction. Since 80 to 90 per cent of β cell mass must be lost before overt hyperglycemia occurs, it is possible that in some cases an acute viral infection leads to β cell dysfunction superimposed on chronic autoimmune β cell destruction, diminishing insulin secretion below the threshold level required for metabolic homeostasis.

Strong arguments can be made for the role of genetic susceptibility viruses, and altered immunity in the etiology of IDDM (Fig. 218–3). However, the contribution of these factors and the sequential relationship among them cannot be stated at this time. Clearly, immune responses could provide the causal link between the HLA associations and clinical IDDM. One way to integrate these factors would be to postulate that susceptibility to IDDM is inherited through genes closely associated with the HLA loci. Given this proper genetic background, environmental triggering agents such as certain viruses exhibiting β cell tropism and possibly chemical agents can injure and in some cases destroy β cells. Following β cell injury, an immune response (possibly antibody and cell mediated) directed against β cells occurs owing to release of β cell antigens into the circulation, alteration of β cell antigens, cross-reactivity with viral antigens, or primary modulation of the immune response. In any event, the immune response would then exacerbate or complete the initial viral or chemical β cell injury. Of course this is only one of several sequences that can be proposed. IDDM is probably heterogeneous, and no single sequence of pathogenetic events necessarily explains all cases. For example, IDDM patients who are HLA-B8/DR3 display other organ-specific autoantibodies and probably have a primary autoimmune disease and do not need an environmental factor to trigger the disease. Regardless of the exact nature of the intertwining of genetic, viral, and immune influences, it is clear that β cell destruction is gradual, even though the clinical onset of metabolic decompensation is usually abrupt when destruction of β cell mass reaches a critical point or an intercurrent illness occurs. This raises the possibility of intervention therapies following the onset of β cell injury but prior to clinical manifestations of IDDM, since by the time IDDM appears β cell destruction may be too far advanced for effective preventive therapy. Such an approach would require a method to detect preclinical IDDM. Using a combination of autoantibody measurements and tests of insulin secretion, prediction of IDDM development is now possible in certain first-degree relatives of IDDM patients. This has allowed investigators to initiate clinical trials aimed at IDDM prevention in these selected individuals.

C peptide is secreted in equimolar amounts compared to insulin. Since C peptide has a much longer half-life than insulin, it provides an excellent measure of insulin secretory capacity, especially in those patients with circulating anti-insulin antibodies that interfere with usual insulin radioimmunoassays. In patients with IDDM who have been treated with insulin for longer than

TABLE 218–2. SOME FEATURES DISTINGUISHING INSULIN-DEPENDENT FROM NON–INSULIN-DEPENDENT DIABETES

	IDDM	NIDDM
Synonym	Type I	Type II
Age of onset	Usually <30	Usually >40
Ketosis	Common	Rare
Body weight	Nonobese	Obese (80%)
Prevalence	0.2%–0.3%	2%–4%
Genetics		
HLA association	Yes	No
Monozygotic twin studies	40%–50% concordance rate	Concordance rate near 100%
Circulating islet cell antibodies	Yes	No
Associated with other autoimmune phenomena	Occasional	No
Treatment with insulin	Always necessary	Usually not required
Complications	Frequent	Frequent
Insulin secretion	Severe deficiency	Variable: moderate deficiency to hyperinsulinemia
Insulin resistance	Occasional: with poor control or excessive insulin antibodies	Usual: due to receptor and postreceptor defects

5 years, C peptide levels are usually undetectable. However, C peptide may be measured in many of these patients during the first years of their disease. This shows that complete loss of β cell secretion in IDDM is not abrupt, but progresses for several years after the diabetes becomes clinically apparent. For the most part, ease of diabetic management and stability of metabolic control in IDDM are correlated with the degree of residual insulin secretion. Those patients with the highest levels of circulating C peptide are easier to treat, and in those with undetectable levels the disease is more unstable. Some of the major clinical and pathophysiologic distinctions between IDDM and NIDDM are listed in Table 218–2.

TREATMENT

In this section, details concerning the various methods of diabetic management are discussed. However, since the severity and clinical picture of diabetes are quite variable, therapeutic methods are also varied. In particular, major differences exist in the approach to NIDDM versus IDDM, and whenever possible therapeutic distinctions for these two forms of diabetes will be made.

RELATIONSHIP BETWEEN HYPERGLYCEMIA AND COMPLICATIONS. It is important to start with more general principles and to identify overall therapeutic goals. A consideration of therapeutic goals involves one of the most important questions in the field, that is, what is the relationship between hyperglycemia and the development of diabetic complications? Simply put, are complications due to hyperglycemia or are they due to genetic or other factors independent of hyperglycemia? This is the central clinical question in diabetes.

Hyperglycemia is the most obvious metabolic abnormality in diabetes. It is therefore reasonable to suspect that elevated glucose levels play a role in diabetic complications. Consistent with this is a large body of retrospective evidence showing that better control is usually associated with fewer complications. Unfortunately, in the absence of randomized, prospective studies in which significant differences in glycemic control are achieved between matched experimental and control groups over an extended period, current clinical studies can provide only nonconclusive evidence. Classic diabetic complications can occur in secondary diabetes (in which genetic aspects of diabetes are presumably missing) and in normal kidneys following transplantation into diabetic patients. Furthermore, in twin studies the degree of retinopathy is comparable in twins concordant for IDDM, whereas in discordant pairs the nondiabetic twin does not have retinopathy. Certain abnormalities seen in diabetes, such as retinal capillary leakage (as demonstrated by fluorescein angiography), slowed motor nerve conductive velocity, and mi-

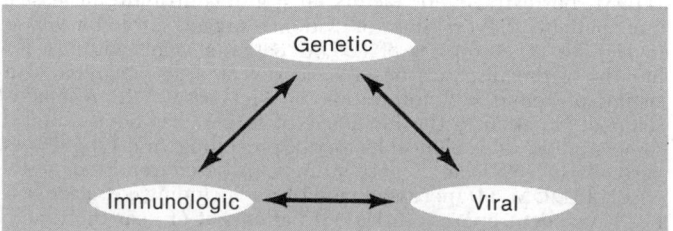

FIGURE 218–3. An interplay of genetic, immunologic, and viral etiologies contributes to the pathogenesis of NIDDM. The importance of each factor probably differs in subpopulations of IDDM, demonstrating the heterogeneity of this disease.

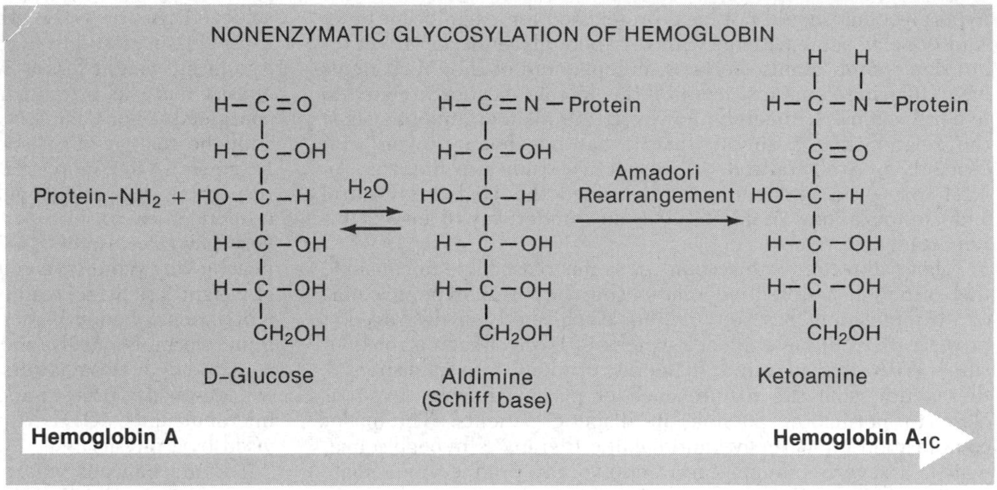

NONENZYMATIC GLYCOSYLATION OF HEMOGLOBIN

FIGURE 218–4. Chemical reactions underlying the nonenzymatic glycosylation of hemoglobin A to hemoglobin A_{1C}.

$$\text{Protein-NH}_2 + \begin{array}{c} \text{H–C}=\text{O} \\ | \\ \text{H–C–OH} \\ | \\ \text{HO–C–H} \\ | \\ \text{H–C–OH} \\ | \\ \text{H–C–OH} \\ | \\ \text{CH}_2\text{OH} \end{array} \underset{\text{H}_2\text{O}}{\rightleftarrows} \begin{array}{c} \text{H–C}=\text{N–Protein} \\ | \\ \text{H–C–OH} \\ | \\ \text{HO–C–H} \\ | \\ \text{H–C–OH} \\ | \\ \text{H–C–OH} \\ | \\ \text{CH}_2\text{OH} \end{array} \xrightarrow[\text{Rearrangement}]{\text{Amadori}} \begin{array}{c} \text{H} \quad \text{H} \\ | \quad | \\ \text{H–C–N–Protein} \\ | \\ \text{C}=\text{O} \\ | \\ \text{HO–C–H} \\ | \\ \text{H–C–OH} \\ | \\ \text{H–C–OH} \\ | \\ \text{CH}_2\text{OH} \end{array}$$

D-Glucose   Aldimine   Ketoamine
(Schiff base)

Hemoglobin A   **Hemoglobin A_{1C}**

croalbuminuria, can be reversed by intensive insulin therapy, but the relationship between these physiologic abnormalities and clinically significant complications has not been demonstrated. In animal experiments a number of studies have shown good correlation between the level of hyperglycemia and microvascular complications similar (but perhaps not identical) to those seen in human diabetes. In animals, these complications can also be prevented or reversed with insulin therapy.

Several biochemical mechanisms have been proposed that may link hyperglycemia to complications. Proteins can be nonenzymatically glycosylated in vivo, and the degree of this glycosylation is directly related to the degree of hyperglycemia. Chromatography of red blood cell hemolysates shows four minor components (HbA_{1a1}, HbA_{1a2}, HbA_{1b1}, HbA_{1c}) of HbA, referred to as the HbA_1 fraction or "fast" hemoglobins (because of their more rapid elution from columns). HbA_1 is due to post-translational, nonenzymatic modification of HbA and comprises about 6 per cent of total hemoglobin in normal persons. HbA_{1c} comprises approximately two thirds of these minor components and is increased in the presence of hyperglycemia. To form HBA_{1c}, glucose combines with the N terminal valine of β chains to form a Schiff base aldimine (Fig. 218–4). This compound is relatively unstable, and the reaction is readily reversible. The aldimine undergoes an Amadori rearrangement to form the more stable ketoamine. HbA can also be glycosylated through the same chemical reaction at the N terminus of the α chain and ε amino groups of lysines. HbA_{1c} can be measured by various chromatographic techniques, and total glycosylated hemoglobin can be measured chemically. Glycosylation occurs continuously within the red cell and is a direct reflection of the average glucose concentration to which the cell is exposed throughout its 120-day lifespan. Measurement of glycosylated hemoglobin content therefore provides a useful means to assess the chronic degree of hyperglycemia that existed in a given patient over the preceding several weeks and is not affected by acute changes in plasma glucose level. Additionally, the nonspecific and nonenzymatic nature of hemoglobin glycosylation raises the possibility that glycosylation of other body proteins can occur, leading to structural or functional changes that may be related to chronic diabetic complications. Increased amounts of glycosylated low-density lipoprotein (LDL) molecules, for example, circulate in hyperglycemic diabetic patients and do not bind normally to LDL receptors. Since abnormal glycosylation may affect all tissues, this mechanism could be related to a variety of diabetic complications.

Additional biochemical lesions related to hyperglycemia have been proposed for nervous tissue. *Sorbitol* is a polyhydroxyl alcohol (polyol) produced from glucose by aldose reductase in nerve tissue; once formed, sorbitol can be converted to fructose (Fig. 218–5). It is theorized that this polyol pathway is particularly active in diabetes because of the hyperglycemia. This could lead to increased intracellular osmolarity (due to accumulation of sorbitol and fructose) with water influx, swelling of Schwann cells, anoxia, and demyelination. Consistent with this, an increase

in sorbitol content has been found in nerve tissue of diabetic rats, and it is reversible with insulin therapy. However, Schwann cell swelling and increased water content have not yet been demonstrated, and further testing of the polyol pathway hypothesis is necessary. Another hyperglycemia-related metabolic lesion in nervous tissue has been proposed involving *myoinositol*. Concentrations of this compound are decreased in peripheral nerves of diabetic rats, and this is associated with a decrease in nerve conduction velocity. These abnormalities can be prevented by insulin or oral myoinositol supplements. It is possible that uptake of myoinositol by nerves is inhibited by hyperglycemia, leading to depletion and pathologic sequelae. A link may exist between polyol and myoinositol metabolism in that increased activity of the polyol pathway contributes to the reduction in nerve myoinositol content.

The above discussion cites clinical and biochemical evidence supporting the relationship between hyperglycemia and complications. On the other hand, there is evidence against this relationship. For example, patients have been reported with diabetic complications at the time of onset of IDDM, when

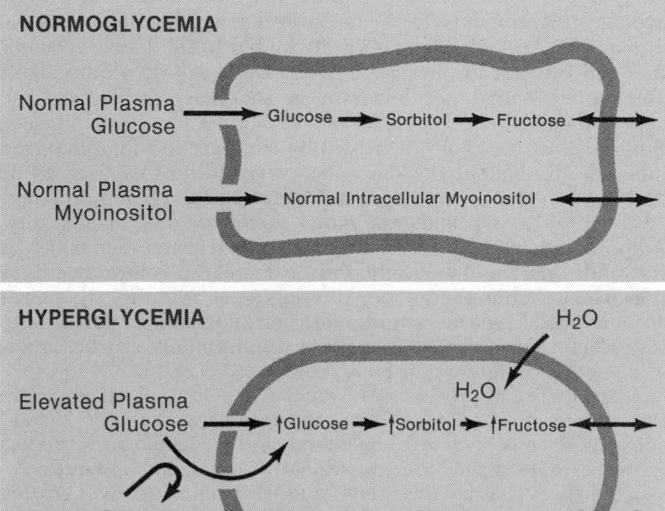

FIGURE 218–5. Metabolic theories for the pathogenesis of diabetic neuropathy secondary to hyperglycemia. This demonstrates the suggested effects of hyperglycemia to increase intracellular sorbitol and fructose concentrations, leading to an osmotic increase in intracellular water content. In addition, it has been suggested that hyperglycemia depletes intracellular myoinositol content by competitively inhibiting the uptake of myoinositol from the extracellular space.

hyperglycemia should not have pre-existed for a significant time. Additionally, some patients with very poor glycemic control never develop complications. Perhaps, independent of IDDM, patients have differing genetic susceptibilities to complications related to hyperglycemia. Ultimately, however, the main argument against the relationship is simply that it has not been proven with certainty by well-controlled, prospective studies in humans. An NIH-sponsored multicenter study called the Diabetes Control and Complications Trial (DCCT) is now under way to answer this important question.

Taking all factors into account, it seems reasonable to conclude that although a definitive relationship between hyperglycemia and complications has been neither established nor disproved at present, the bulk of evidence weighs in favor of such a relationship. With this in mind it seems prudent to establish as a therapeutic goal the maintenance of plasma glucose levels as close to normal as possible in diabetic patients. The major complication of aggressive antidiabetic therapy is hypoglycemia, which, if severe enough, can unequivocally produce immediate and irreversible CNS damage. Therefore, diabetic management should be pushed until glucose levels are normal or near normal, unless recurrent, overt episodes of hypoglycemia develop. If this occurs, then compromises are necessary in the degree of glycemic control achieved. Other therapeutic goals include (1) normal growth and development in children, (2) normal pregnancy and childbirth in females, (3) reduction of diabetes-related atherosclerosis risk factors, especially in adult diabetic patients, and (4) minimal interference with normal lifestyle in all diabetics.

DIETARY TREATMENT. Dietary treatment is an integral part of the overall therapeutic plan in all diabetic patients. In many NIDDM patients dietary therapy can be the predominant method of treatment. Dietary therapy is concerned with the total number of calories ingested, the distribution of calories throughout the day, the individual food sources that make up these calories, and maintenance of proper nutrition. Dietary therapy is much different in NIDDM and IDDM, because patients in the former are usually obese, whereas in the latter they are not, and NIDDM patients retain endogenous insulin secretion while IDDM patients do not.

Total Caloric Intake. Since most NIDDM patients are overweight, caloric restriction is advisable and can be of great benefit. The essential tenet of weight reduction is straightforward: If caloric expenditure exceeds intake, weight will be lost. There are many ways to calculate daily caloric expenditure, but on the average this amounts to 30 to 35 kcal per kilogram in normal humans; 25 kcal per kilogram is attributed to the basal metabolic rate and the rest to physical activity. Daily caloric requirements are about 30 kcal per kilogram in sedentary individuals and approximately 35 kcal per kilogram in moderately active subjects. For those who engage in brisk physical exertion for prolonged intervals throughout the day caloric expenditure can exceed 35 kcal per kilogram. Another factor affecting caloric requirements (at least on a per kilogram basis) is the degree of adiposity. Adipose tissue is predominantly storage triglyceride, which is relatively inert metabolically with a decreased caloric need per unit weight. Thus the greater the degree of adiposity, the lower an individual's caloric requirement per kilogram. In very obese, sedentary individuals, daily caloric requirements can be as low as 25 kcal per kilogram of body weight.

A number of approaches to weight reduction exist that vary in the degree of caloric restriction and rate of weight loss, dietary constituents, as well as behavioral and psychological support measures. These include nutritionally sound and modestly restricted diets that achieve slow gradual weight loss over several months, nutritionally balanced very low calorie diets for rapid weight loss, behavior modification, pharmacologic aids, and even surgical procedures (i.e., gastric plication) in the morbidly obese patient in whom medical therapy fails. These approaches are discussed in detail in Ch. 203.

For all these methods, inducing the initial period of weight loss is not the major problem in weight reduction, but, rather, the major problem is weight regain or recidivism. Motivated patients can usually successfully lose weight over the initial dietary period, but it is the unusual patient who successfully keeps the pounds off. The major challenge in weight reduction

therapy is to develop a proper supportive environment and patient motivation to maintain weight loss after it has been achieved. In the NIDDM patient, significant caloric restriction is usually successful in lowering plasma glucose levels even before significant weight loss is achieved. Depending on the degree of obesity that was present initially and the amount of weight loss, continued beneficial effects on glycemic control can be maintained after the goal weight is achieved and a eucaloric diet is initiated. In general, the more recent the onset of NIDDM, the more responsive the patient will be to the beneficial effects of weight reduction. In patients with pronounced fasting hyperglycemia, very low calorie diets (300 to 600 kcal per day) are often useful in achieving rapid glycemic control as well as an initial rapid rate of weight loss (which can often be of important psychological and motivational benefit). Very low calorie diets usually consist of liquid formula meals and should not be utilized unless they contain adequate amounts (a minimum 30 to 40 grams per day) of high-quality protein and are supplemented with vitamins and micronutrients. NIDDM patients on such diets should be supervised by a physician.

The mechanisms whereby weight reduction improves hyperglycemia in NIDDM are not completely clear. Weight loss leads to a reduction in the accelerated rates of hepatic glucose production, ameliorates the degree of insulin resistance by increasing insulin receptors and reducing the magnitude of the postreceptor defect in insulin action, and possibly improves β cell secretion. However, the precise cellular mechanisms leading to these effects are not known. Patients with IDDM are seldom obese, and an important nutritional goal is maintenance of adequate nutrition, particularly to assure normal growth and development in children and pregnant women.

Distribution of Calories. In addition to total caloric consumption, attention should also be paid to the distribution of calories throughout the day in any dietary prescription. Two principles should be kept in mind: (1) calories should be spread as evenly as possible throughout the major daily meals to avoid a large concentration of calories at any one meal and not to overwhelm the diabetic patient's impaired capacity to metabolize food; and (2) in those patients receiving exogenous insulin, caloric intake should be temporally adjusted to coincide with the time course of action of the administered insulin. The latter point highlights a major difference in dietary consideration between patients with IDDM and those with NIDDM. In NIDDM, endogenous insulin secretion is still present and the β cell can respond at the appropriate times (albeit to a limited degree) to food ingestion, regardless of when it occurs throughout the day. This is even true, although to a lesser extent, in NIDDM subjects who are treated with insulin. Thus, in these patients it is sufficient to balance calories throughout the day, but the patient has a good deal of leeway to determine the timing of specific meals as long as calories are ingested at times of peak exogenous insulin action. For practical purposes, the only insulin present in patients with IDDM is that which is administered exogenously. Therefore, patients must pay close attention to the timing of meals and must be certain that there is reasonable concordance between meal ingestion and the time course of action of the insulin they have taken. To a certain extent the patient can elect a temporal pattern suitable to his lifestyle and preference and the insulin therapy regimen can then be tailored appropriately. In this way greater flexibility is allowed that improves overall patient compliance and quality of life.

Nutrient Content of Diet. A great deal of attention is currently being paid to the individual components comprising the diabetic diet. When patients consume eucaloric diets, it is important that they be properly balanced and nutritionally sound. A generally accepted protein requirement is 0.8 gram per kilogram per day for adults, but larger amounts are usually consumed in Western diets. Thus, protein usually comprises about 15 per cent of total caloric consumption. With this as a base, the proportions of fat and carbohydrate (CHO) are inversely related. Previous attempts to restrict total CHO intake are no longer deemed advisable, and most authorities now advocate liberalization of CHO intake to 50 to 55 per cent of total calories. This means that total fat intake should not exceed 30 to 35 per cent, and because diabetic patients are predisposed to macrovascular disease, saturated fat (primarily animal fat) intake should be reduced so that the polyunsaturated-saturated fat ratio is equivalent to 1:0. Ideally, cholesterol intake should not exceed 450 mg per day, and even lower levels of intake are advisable. The recommendation of a low saturated fat, low cholesterol diet is particularly important in NIDDM patients because of the high prevalence of concomitant hyperlipidemias. The makeup of the CHO portion of the diet also requires attention. In the past it was believed that diabetics should rigorously avoid sucrose because it is rapidly absorbed and raises the blood glucose level inordinately. Although this may be true when sucrose is consumed as the sole nutritive component, as in soft drinks or certain candies, it is less of a problem when modest amounts of sucrose are eaten in a mixed meal setting. Because of this, up to 5 per cent of total CHO can be consumed as added sucrose, as long as it is taken in the context of a mixed meal and spaced out through the day. This allows the diabetic a wider variety of food choices, making the diet more palatable; a side benefit of this approach is that it improves patient adherence to the dietary prescription and to the other elements of the overall therapeutic plan. The remainder of the CHO should consist predominantly of starches. All complex CHO cannot be lumped together as a single food group because the glycemic response to different starches differs widely, being lowest for lentils and pasta and highest for wheat and potatoes. More work needs to be done to determine the glycemic potency of a large number of foods, singly and together, in diabetic patients before the precise composition of the CHO in the diet can be recommended with certainty. At this stage it is advisable for the diabetic to consume 50 to 55 per cent of calories as CHO with a modest restriction in sucrose intake and emphasis on ingestion of those complex CHOs with low glycemic potency.

Fructose is a nutritive sweetener that may also have a place in the diabetic diet. This simple CHO is somewhat sweeter than sucrose and has similar properties when prepared in foods. Thus, fructose can be substituted for sucrose in most foods with little change in taste or texture. The advantage is that fructose is absorbed from the gastrointestinal tract more slowly than sucrose and is predominantly taken up and metabolized by the liver through non–insulin-dependent mechanisms. Within the liver, fructose is phosphorylated and eventually converted to glycogen or triglyceride through the triose phosphate intermediates. Thus, little fructose escapes hepatic uptake to enter the peripheral circulation, and only a small amount of fructose is converted to glucose for release from the liver. Ingestion of fructose leads to a minimal postprandial rise in plasma glucose or insulin levels in normal persons and in diabetics when taken alone or as part of a mixed meal. For these reasons, fructose offers some advantage in the diabetic diet, and amounts up to 75 grams per day can be safely consumed. The major exception occurs in patients with severely uncontrolled NIDDM or in poorly insulinized IDDM patients. In these conditions glycogen production is inhibited and fructose enters the gluconeogenic pathway and is ultimately released as glucose, causing hyperglycemia.

Dietary fiber can also influence CHO absorption. Glycemic excursions are reduced and insulin secretion diminished when normal persons and subjects with NIDDM consume fiber-enriched diets. This effect is mediated through delayed gastric emptying and overall slowing of the rate of CHO digestion and absorption. Since large amounts of fiber (10 to 15 grams per meal) are needed to observe these effects, major changes in dietary patterns would be necessary to achieve beneficial results. Nevertheless, when fiber is consumed as natural foods, there do not seem to be any untoward effects of increased fiber ingestion, and some studies indicate that increased fiber intake can lower serum triglyceride levels. The only potential caveat to this statement involves growing children and pregnant women, since subtle undesirable changes in micronutrient absorption due to high fiber ingestion have not been ruled out.

A minority of diabetic patients adhere to the recommended dietary regimens. To a large extent this is due to inadequate understanding on the part of the patient as well as the physician regarding dietary goals and methods. An additional factor is that dietary therapy must be individualized, taking into account each patient's lifestyle, economic status, food preferences, and social needs. This can be a time-consuming process, and few physicians have the time or training to participate with patients in this type of detailed dietary management. For this reason it is critical to incorporate a dietitian or nutritionist trained in the principles of dietary therapy of diabetes as part of the health care team. One cannot simply give pamphlets, instructional aids, and meal plans and expect even motivated patients to adhere to the necessary regimens. Detailed instruction by a nutrition counselor is necessary to tailor the diet to each patient's special needs. Dietary therapy is a means of long-term treatment, and therefore the longer view is important. Occasional deviations from recommended meal plans for special occasions are acceptable, provided that the patient has a clear understanding of how this should be managed. Often this allows for better patient compliance with the overall diet plan. Periodic meetings with a nutrition counselor are necessary to implement and maintain individualized dietary regimens.

ORAL HYPOGLYCEMIC AGENTS. Oral hypoglycemic agents are often therapeutically effective in NIDDM patients. In patients who do not respond satisfactorily to diet and do not have severe hyperglycemia (i.e., plasma glucose levels consistently greater than 250 mg per deciliter), oral agents are an appropriate therapeutic choice. In patients with severe hyperglycemia, insulin therapy is preferable, at least initially, to gain more rapid control of clinical symptoms and to prevent hyperosmolarity. While sulfonylureas are effective in patients with NIDDM, they are ineffective in IDDM. Some have suggested that combinations of oral agents with insulin can reduce insulin requirements of IDDM; however, this has not been proven, and would be of minor clinical importance anyway.

The mechanism of action of sulfonylureas is complex. In the short term, they augment β cell insulin secretion. However, after several months of therapy, insulin levels return to pretreatment values while glucose levels remain improved. These findings led to the demonstration that sulfonylureas exert extrapancreatic effects on glucose metabolism: (1) They reduce the accelerated rates of hepatic glucose production in NIDDM; (2) they partially reverse the postbinding defect in insulin action; and (3) they increase the number of cellular insulin receptors. These all represent significant components of the insulin resistance of NIDDM, so sulfonylureas can improve glycemia by improving insulin's effectiveness at target cells. The relative importance of each of these actions in ameliorating hyperglycemia is unclear, but it is likely that the pancreatic and extrapancreatic effects of these agents combine to produce the hypoglycemic action of these drugs.

There are several different kinds of sulfonylureas, differing primarily in potency, pharmacokinetics, and modes of metabolism as outlined in Table 218–3. *Tolbutamide* is metabolized to inert products by the liver and has a relatively short half-life, necessi-

TABLE 218–3. CHARACTERISTICS OF SULFONYLUREAS

Generic Name	Brand Name	Dosage Range (mg)	Duration of Action (hr)	Comments
Tolbutamide	Orinase	500–3000	6–12	Metabolized by liver to inert products, given 2–3 ×/day
Chlorpropamide	Diabinese	100–500	60	Metabolized by liver (~70%) to less active metabolite, and excreted intact (~30%) by kidneys; can potentiate ADH action, given 1×/day
Acetohexamide	Dymelor	250–1500	12–24	Metabolized by liver to active metabolite, given 1–2 ×/day
Tolazamide	Tolinase	100–1000	10–18	Metabolized by liver to active product, given 1–2 ×/day
Glyburide	Micronase	2.5–30	10–30	Metabolized by liver to inert products, given 1×/day
Glipizide	Glucotrol	5–40	18–30	Metabolized by liver to inert products, given 1×/day

tating administration two to three times a day. Although it is the least potent of the available sulfonylureas on a weight basis, it has not been clearly demonstrated that any sulfonylurea produces greater hypoglycemic potency at maximal doses in diabetic patients. Therefore, for practical purposes, the differences in relative potency of the different drugs simply mean that more or less of a given agent should be used. *Tolazamide* and especially *acetohexamide* are metabolized by the liver to biologically active products that are then excreted by the kidneys. These drugs have intermediate half-lives and are usually given twice (but sometimes once) a day. *Chlorpropamide* also undergoes considerable hepatic degradation into less active metabolites excreted in the urine. This compound can cause significant water retention and hyponatremia by potentiating ADH action on the kidney. Chlorpropamide has the longest circulating half-life and duration of action (about 60 hours) and is given only once a day. Hypoglycemia is the major complication of sulfonylureas, and this can be particularly severe with chlorpropamide because of its long duration of action. Elderly NIDDM subjects are more susceptible to hypoglycemia, especially those prone to skip meals. The route of metabolism of the different compounds may influence the choice of agent. One should be cautious about the use of chlorpropamide, acetohexamide, and, to a lesser extent, tolazamide in patients with compromised renal function because of the route of excretion. Second-generation sulfonylureas, such as *glibenclamide* (or glyburide) and *glipizide*, have rapidly assumed a major share of the market, largely displacing the first-generation agents. These compounds are metabolized by the liver and have a relatively long duration of action. They can often be given once a day, although twice a day dosing is usually required in patients with initial fasting glucose levels greater than 220 mg per deciliter. A general guideline would be to progress up to 10 mg per day in the A.M. for either drug and if satisfactory control is not achieved then add a P.M. dose. It is claimed, but not rigorously demonstrated, that the second-generation sulfonylureas are more effective than the first-generation drugs.

The other major category of oral hypoglycemic agents consists of the biguanides, such as *phenformin*. The exact mechanism of action of these drugs is not clear, although they may interfere with hepatic gluconeogenesis. However, these drugs were strongly implicated in the development of lactic acidosis and have been prohibited from clinical use in the United States by the Food and Drug Administration.

In NIDDM, the usual practice is to begin with a low dose of a given sulfonylurea, advancing the dose until the therapeutic response is satisfactory or a maximal dose is reached. Occasionally patients who do not respond to one drug can be switched to another with beneficial effect. Most patients who do not achieve a therapeutic response with a given sulfonylurea will not respond satisfactorily by switching to another. Enough patients do respond to this approach, however, so that it is an appropriate tactic before it is concluded that oral hypoglycemic drugs are not effective in a specific patient. Certain drug interactions occur with sulfonylureas, that is, phenylbutazone and anticoagulants compete for hepatic removal mechanisms with sulfonylureas. A disulfiram (Antabuse)-like reaction can occasionally occur following alcohol consumption by patients taking sulfonylureas. This is most frequently reported with chlorpropamide and has not yet been noted with the second-generation agents. Potential interactions of this sort should always be kept in mind in the appropriate clinical context.

Approximately 10 to 20 per cent of NIDDM patients do not respond to oral agents, and treatment is termed primary failure. Secondary failure occurs when a patient responds initially to an oral agent, but then ceases to respond in the next year or two. This occurs in 5 to 20 per cent of patients, but these proportions obviously depend on the particular NIDDM population studied. For example, patients with new-onset diabetes respond better than those with longstanding disease. In some cases, secondary failure is due to dietary noncompliance in a patient who previously successfully adhered to a dietary regimen. However, this is often not the case, and the mechanisms of secondary failure in many patients with NIDDM remain unknown.

Debate exists as to which patients with NIDDM are appropriate candidates for oral sulfonylurea therapy. In view of the evidence implicating hyperglycemia with diabetic complications, the therapeutic goal with oral agents should be the maintenance of glucose levels as near to normal as possible. In patients with mild to moderate fasting hyperglycemia (140 to 230 mg per deciliter), dietary therapy should be tried first; if the above therapeutic goals are not achieved with this approach, then a sulfonylurea can be added. The problem arises in patients with more severe fasting hyperglycemia (more than 230 mg per deciliter) who have pronounced clinical symptoms despite dietary treatment. In these patients, some would advise an initial period of sulfonylurea therapy, and if satisfactory control is not achieved, then insulin treatment should be substituted. Others would suggest an initial period of insulin therapy following which the patient is switched to sulfonylureas; if satisfactory control is achieved, the drug is continued. Alternatively, insulin can be used indefinitely in these patients. Clearly this is a gray area, and the particular approach should be individualized to each patient, taking into account the total clinical context of the patient's disease, acceptance of the various therapeutic methods, level of diabetes education, and motivation. In a patient in whom severe fasting hyperglycemia is maintained, with marked clinical symptoms and incipient hyperosmolarity, oral agents are probably not appropriate, at least initially. In these patients insulin therapy should be the primary mode of treatment and can be continued indefinitely, or a therapeutic trial of sulfonylureas can be substituted once the hyperglycemia has been brought under control by the initial period of insulin treatment. In general, response to sulfonylurea therapy is best if the onset of diabetes is recent and the patient is over 40 years of age and not thin.

INSULIN TREATMENT. Insulin is the primary mode of therapy in all patients with IDDM and in many with NIDDM (see above). The goals of therapy include (1) normal growth and development in children, (2) normal pregnancy, delivery, and conceptus in women, (3) minimal interference with psychosocial adjustment, (4) acceptable glycemic control, with minimal hypoglycemia, and (5) prevention of complications. Little disagreement exists concerning goals 1 to 3; however, different views exist of how best to achieve goals 4 and 5. There are many different methods of insulin therapy, and the method chosen is highly dependent on one's views of goals 4 and 5. If a physician holds closely to the important relationship between control and complications, then "acceptable control" will be much more rigorously defined and a method of insulin treatment that is designed to produce the desired response will be chosen. On the other hand, those who question the link between hyperglycemia and complications are advocates of looser control and utilize a less intensive method of insulin delivery. In general, it is quite easy to eliminate overt symptoms of hyperglycemia with any method of insulin therapy, but it is extremely difficult, and probably impossible, to achieve euglycemia on a 24-hour basis. How close one comes to this ideal depends on the method of insulin delivery chosen, which in turn depends on one's philosophy of diabetic management.

At this time, the prevailing opinion among diabetologists is that hyperglycemia contributes substantially to complications. With this view, treatment of hyperglycemia (with any therapeutic modality) should be undertaken with specific glycemic target ranges in mind in order to bring the plasma glucose as close to normal as possible without unacceptable hypoglycemia. Target glucose levels recommended by the American Diabetes Association for NIDDM management are: fasting blood glucose less than 140 mg per deciliter and 2-hour postprandial blood glucose less than 200 mg per deciliter.

Insulin Preparations. To begin a discussion of the methods of insulin treatment, let us first consider the many different kinds of insulin available. Commercial insulin comes in concentrations of 100 units per milliliter (U-100) and 500 units per milliliter (U-500). The various insulin preparations differ in their time course of action (rapid, intermediate, and long acting), degree of purity, and source (beef, pork, beef-pork, or human synthetic insulin); these properties are outlined in Table 218–4. By adjustment of pH during preparation, the size of the zinc-insulin crystal can be modified; the larger the crystals, the slower the release after subcutaneous injection, and this accounts for the differences in time of action between semilente (rapid-acting) and ultralente (long-acting) insulin. Lente (intermediate-acting) insulin is simply a 30:70 mixture of semilente and ultralente, respectively. The

Class	Type	Peak Effect (hr)	Duration of Action (hr)
Rapid	Regular crystalline insulin (CZI)	2–4	6–8
	Semilente	2–6	10–12
Intermediate	Neutral protamine (NPH)	6–12	18–24
	Lente	6–12	18–24
Long Acting	Protamine zinc (PZI)	14–24	36
	Ultralente	18–24	36

other method to delay the onset of action of injected insulin is to mix it with a protein (protamine) and adjust the pH. This results in NPH (intermediate-acting) and PZI (long-acting) preparations. It should be cautioned that the values for peak onset and duration of action listed in Table 218–4 are simply estimates. There is a great deal of variability in these values from patient to patient as a result of circulating anti-insulin antibodies that alter the pharmacokinetics of insulin, variation in subcutaneous absorption, individual responses, and other factors. Additionally, absorption of insulin may be quite variable within a single patient from day to day, since absorption of subcutaneous insulin is markedly increased by vigorous exercise of the injected extremity, or by heating or massage of the injection site. Differences in purity also exist. Conventional insulin preparations contain less than 10,000 parts per million (ppm) of impurities; improved single peak insulin, less than 50 ppm; and "purified" insulin, 1 to 10 ppm. The impurities mentioned are predominantly proinsulin, with smaller amounts of insulin dimers, proinsulin-like products, glucagon, pancreatic polypeptide, somatostatin, and vasoactive polypeptide. For practical purposes, commercially available insulin preparations are labeled as purified (1 to 10 ppm); if they are not specifically labeled, they contain 20 to 50 ppm. The older, less pure forms are no longer widely distributed. Essentially all preparations can be obtained as purified pork, beef, or beef-pork mixtures. Finally, highly purified human insulin is now available as a product of recombinant DNA biosynthesis or chemical conversion of pork to human insulin.

Methods of Treatment. The insulin regimen can be more or less intensive, depending on the number of injections per day, types of insulin used, and frequency and method of assessing control. Many NIDDM patients, and occasional IDDM patients, can achieve excellent glycemic control with a single daily (morning) injection of an intermediate-acting insulin. Because of post-breakfast hyperglycemia, it is often necessary to mix a short-acting preparation with this single dose. In most patients who realize excellent control with this regimen, endogenous insulin secretion is retained. A somewhat more intensive method to regulate glycemia involves a split-dosage regimen. This includes morning (before breakfast) and evening (before dinner) injection of mixtures of intermediate- and rapid-acting insulin. About two thirds of the total daily dose is usually given in the morning and about one third in the evening; the proportion of intermediate- to rapid-acting insulin at each injection is usually two thirds to one third. In patients receiving single-dose therapy who require more than 50 to 60 units per day a split-dose regimen should usually be tried. In a 70-kg man, normal 24-hour insulin output has been estimated at 25 units per day. Therefore, in normal-sized diabetic subjects starting insulin therapy, it is reasonable to begin with a total daily dose of about 20 units per day with upward adjustments every several days based on the level of blood glucose. In mildly obese IDDM patients, starting doses can be 5 to 10 units per day higher. Because of insulin resistance, obese NIDDM patients requiring insulin often need 60 to 90 units per day. With the availability of highly purified insulins (both human and animal) that are less antigenic, it is probably advisable to start all new patients with one of these insulin preparations. With the above methods of insulin delivery, assessment of glycemic control can be carried out in several ways. Measurements of urinary glucose and ketones can be obtained before breakfast and once or twice throughout the day. Patients should be instructed to void 30 minutes before obtaining urine for glucose determination (double voiding), particularly for the morning sample, so that the urinary glucose is more representative of the corresponding blood glucose. Regardless of how carefully urinary glucose is determined, it provides only a rough approximation of blood glucose levels. Factors such as renal threshold, renal blood flow, and urine volume greatly affect the meaning of urine glucose measurements (i.e., a 4+ reaction in a concentrated urine sample is of little significance compared to a 4+ reaction in a dilute sample). For these reasons, urinary glucose is a poor way to monitor diabetic control and if at all possible should not be relied upon as the sole guide on which to base the insulin regimen. Twenty-four-hour urinary glucose excretion can be periodically assessed to provide a better estimate of daylong control (less than 5 grams per day is excellent control). Glycosylated hemoglobin can be measured and provides an excellent assessment of the overall state of glycemic control during the preceding few weeks. The best current method to assess glycemic control is home-, or self-, monitoring of glucose (see below). This requires the patient to assess his own blood glucose level daily and to make appropriate adjustments in insulin dosage. This approach places a large part of the management responsibility in the hands of the patient and emphasizes the need for a continuous outpatient education program.

When patients with new-onset IDDM are started on insulin therapy, after an initial period of stabilization, insulin requirements frequently decrease dramatically over the ensuing few weeks. This is the so-called honeymoon phenomenon, and it is sometimes possible to maintain nearly normal levels of glycemia without administering any insulin. This honeymoon phase may last for a few weeks and sometimes as long as 1 to 2 years. It is invariably followed by worsening of metabolic control with permanent recrudescence of the insulin-dependent state. Some experts have recommended that during this honeymoon period insulin administration should never be completely stopped, even if dosages have to be reduced to homeopathic levels. The reason for this is the fear that if there is a prolonged period in which insulin is not administered, once insulin therapy is reinstituted an anamnestic response with rising titers of anti-insulin antibodies might occur. However, with use of the highly purified insulin preparations now available, or with biosynthetic human insulin, this may be less of a problem.

If more intensive insulin management is required to achieve closer to normal glycemic control, then multiple daily injections of insulin or continuous subcutaneous insulin infusion (CSII) are used. At the current time these approaches are generally limited to patients with IDDM. However, if ideal control of glycemia is the therapeutic goal, there is no reason these methods could not be used in patients with NIDDM whose disease cannot be satisfactorily controlled by other means. Multiple injections involve administration of regular insulin before each meal, with the dose adjusted to the anticipated meal size. This is usually combined with either a long-acting or an intermediate-acting preparation in the evening.

The most intensive method of insulin delivery is CSII. This consists of constant insulin delivery into a subcutaneous site in the abdominal wall via an open loop delivery device consisting of a small insulin pump that must be worn by the patient essentially 24 hours a day. The key to this method of therapy is the constant delivery of basal insulin. The basal insulin infusion is supplemented by a preprandial bolus of insulin given 15 minutes prior to meal ingestion. This gives the patient a fair degree of flexibility in the timing and content of meals, since the preprandial bolus is given at the patient's discretion in an amount picked to match meal size. In general, the basal insulin infusion accounts for about 50 per cent of the total daily insulin dose and usually averages 0.5 to 1 unit per hour. Typically, preprandial boluses are 5 to 10 units, depending on meal size, time of day, and proximity to time of exercise. To be successful, intensive insulin therapy regimens must be combined with home- (or self-) monitoring of glucose. This requires the patient to obtain capillary blood by finger prick for glucose measurement, using a reflectance meter. There are numerous devices and algorithms for constant insulin delivery and various approaches to the frequency and method of glucose self-measurements. A detailed discussion of these issues is beyond the scope of this chapter. With properly motivated and educated patients and physicians, excellent control can be achieved in nearly all subjects. Patients generally accept this mode of therapy quite well and report an increased feeling of well-being. However, CSII should not be used indiscriminately, since pump dysfunction does occur, and hypoglycemia is a real problem, especially nocturnally. Additionally, a great deal is asked of patients when they participate in these programs in terms of dedication, education, and changes in lifestyle.

Many other insulin treatment schedules have been proposed, all of which represent variations on the above common themes. Some of these are listed in Table 218–5. No single method is inherently superior to any other, and it is probably best for a physician to become accustomed to one or two methods and use them more or less exclusively so that he will be familiar with problems associated with insulin therapy and its individualization. All of these approaches are meant as guidelines rather than rigid algorithms.

Regardless of the insulin regimen employed, an established daily dose in a given patient must not be considered to be fixed. Even long-established insulin dosages may need to be increased because of changes in growth status, subtle intercurrent illness or stress, or development of anti-insulin antibodies. Dosages may need to be decreased because of consistent increases in physical activity, dietary changes, or changes in concomitant drug therapy (e.g., stopping steroids). Additionally, absorption may vary from one anatomic site to another, and the rate of absorption of insulin can be augmented by exercise involving a particular injection site. This simply means that the physician and the patient must constantly review the treatment program and be prepared to make changes when indicated.

Complications of Insulin Therapy. The most significant complication of insulin treatment is *hypoglycemia*. This is because even the best mode of insulin delivery is still an imperfect method to mimic the homeostatic mechanisms in normal subjects. Normal persons respond to food ingestion, exercise, and stress in such a way as to keep the blood glucose level within narrowly defined limits. One can hope to approach this, but not match it, with the methods used for delivery of exogenous insulin. For example, when normal individuals exercise, peripheral glucose uptake increases, and this is matched by a corresponding increase in hepatic glucose production. A decrease in insulin secretion allows the increase in hepatic glucose production to occur. Obviously this degree of fine tuning is difficult to achieve with exogenous insulin administration. Consequently hypoglycemia is a common complication of insulin therapy as the result of overzealous insulin administration or inappropriate timing. Most often this occurs in a situation in which tight control is attempted. Occasional mild episodes of hypoglycemia are probably acceptable if they appear in a patient in whom excellent control is generally achieved and who is fully aware of their occurrence and of methods to abort

TABLE 218–5. DIFFERENT INSULIN REGIMENS

Split dose intermediate (NPH or lente) + regular insulin
   A.M. dose: ⅔ TDD
               ~70% intermediate
               ~30% regular
   P.M. dose: ⅓ TDD
               50%–70% intermediate
               30%–50% regular

Intermediate + preprandial regular insulin
   Breakfast: Regular, 25%–40% TDD
   Lunch: Regular, 25%–30% TDD
   Dinner: Regular, 25%–30% TDD
   Night: NPH or lente, 15%–25% TDD

Ultralente + preprandial regular insulin
   Breakfast: Regular, 15%–25% TDD
   Lunch: Regular, 15%–25% TDD
   Dinner: Regular, 15%–25% TDD
               Ultralente, 40%–60% TDD

Triple A.M. mixture: regular, lente + ultralente insulin

Double A.M. mixture: regular + NPH (or lente) insulin

TDD = total daily dose

them. However, frequent and severe hypoglycemic reactions are unacceptable. These are serious and occasionally can be fatal. Furthermore, the long-term effects on the central nervous system of frequent hypoglycemic episodes have not been determined. If satisfactory control cannot be achieved without recurrence of such reactions, then compromises in the overall therapeutic plan must be made. It would seem imprudent to expose patients to known complications of hypoglycemia in the hope that superior control will prevent chronic diabetic complications in the future. Some IDDM patients are particularly susceptible to hypoglycemia, seemingly because of impaired secretion of counter-regulatory hormones, particularly glucagon.

An interesting aspect of hypoglycemic episodes is the so-called *Somogyi phenomenon*. This involves rebound hyperglycemia due to excessive secretion of counter-regulatory hormones following a previous episode of hypoglycemia. The classic situation involves nocturnal hypoglycemia followed by marked hyperglycemia prior to breakfast. This can induce a self-defeating cycle in which the insulin dose is progressively raised in response to the fasting hyperglycemia when a reduction in insulin dose, to prevent the nocturnal hypoglycemia, would be more appropriate.

A minority of patients beginning insulin therapy experience a variety of local allergic reactions at the injection site. Manifestations include local itching; erythematous, indurated lesions; and occasional small, discrete subcutaneous nodules. These local reactions are usually self-limited and eventually disappear with continued insulin treatment. Antihistamines may be used for symptomatic relief if necessary. The frequency of these problems has decreased significantly with the use of the newer more highly purified insulins. Rare patients may develop systemic reactions, including generalized urticaria and even anaphylactic reactions. This usually occurs when insulin therapy has been stopped for a time and then reinstituted. If these symptoms cannot be controlled by antihistamines, and if insulin treatment is mandatory for the patient's well-being, then formal desensitization regimens are necessary. Other local reactions at the injection site include lipoatrophy and hypertrophy. Lipoatrophy at the injection site is a benign condition usually due to impurities in the insulin preparation. It can usually be corrected by changing to a highly purified pork insulin and injecting this into the lipoatrophic areas, which then fill in with subcutaneous fat in a normal fashion. Most likely the new highly purified human insulin preparations will also be suitable for this purpose. Insulin hypertrophy is attributed to the local lipogenic effects of the injected insulin. In advanced cases the underlying tissue can be fibrous and less vascular, making the overlying skin anesthetic. This explains why many patients prefer these areas as sites of injection. This problem can usually be corrected by carefully rotating injection sites.

FUTURE MODES OF THERAPY

Even with the most meticulous mode of insulin therapy in the most motivated patients, euglycemic control is difficult to achieve for prolonged periods. Thus the search for better, more effective, and, in some cases, curative forms of therapy continues. Transplantation of the pancreas or islet cells continues to receive extensive study. Numerous logistic, immunologic, and technical problems need to be overcome before such therapies become available for routine clinical purposes, but there are signs that some positive results might be seen in the next several years. This is the one mode of therapy that might actually be considered curative.

Efforts continue to be expended in developing newer and better external or implantable insulin-delivery devices. Unquestionably the mechanical and engineering aspects of insulin-delivery devices will continue to improve dramatically over the next several years, and pumps that are smaller, safer, and more flexible will be produced. It also seems likely that reliable implantable devices are in the offing. However, unless such devices can be used to administer insulin via the portal route, the advantage of implantable pumps appears to be mostly aesthetic. An additional hope for internal devices is that a closed-loop system can be designed. This would require development of a reliable, fail-safe glucose sensor integrated into the appropriate algorithms for insulin delivery. If such artificial pancreases become readily available, they would obviously have wide applicability. Finally, since hyperglucagonemia has been implicated in the pathogenesis of the hyperglycemia in diabetes, agents that specifically suppress glucagon secretion have been sought. Attempts to develop a glucagon-specific somatostatin derivative continue; such a compound might be a useful adjunctive therapy in the management of diabetes.

ACUTE COMPLICATIONS

The acute metabolic complications of diabetes are diabetic ketoacidosis, hyperosmolar nonketotic coma, lactic acidosis, and hypoglycemia.

Diabetic Ketoacidosis (DKA)

DKA is due to insulin deficiency. Before consideration of the pathogenesis of the metabolic derangement, it is important to review the normal physiologic effects of insulin on carbohydrate, protein, and fat metabolism, since DKA simply represents a reversal of these normal insulin-stimulated processes.

PHYSIOLOGY OF FED AND FASTED STATE. When food is ingested, insulin functions as the major anabolic hormone facilitating the disposition of carbohydrate, protein, and fat and their synthesis into macromolecules for storage (Fig. 218–6A). Glucose is absorbed into the portal vein, and approximately 60 per cent of the ingested glucose-derived carbons end up in liver glycogen in the postprandial period. A significant portion of this is probably not a result of direct hepatic glucose uptake, but is due to peripheral metabolism of glucose to three-carbon fragments (lactate, pyruvate) that are then recycled to the liver where they enter the gluconeogenic pathway and are synthesized into glycogen. Glycogen then serves as the storage form of carbohydrate for later release. When glucose is metabolized via the glycolytic (anaerobic) pathway, 2 moles of ATP are generated per mole of glucose. Aerobic, or oxidative, metabolism (Krebs' cycle) is far more efficient as an energy-producing process and generates 12 moles of ATP per mole of glucose. Insulin exerts multiple anabolic effects on this process. It stimulates glucose uptake and glycogen synthesis by muscle and inhibits glycogenolysis. In liver, insulin does not directly stimulate glucose uptake, but it does actively promote glycogenesis and inhibit glycogenolysis. Although most of the ingested glucose, or glucose-derived carbon, ends up in the liver in the postprandial period, over a 24-hour day the central nervous system (CNS) (primarily brain) is the predominant tissue of glucose consumption, accounting for about 70 per cent of total glucose utilization. Glucose is the primary source of energy for brain, and glucose uptake and metabolism in this tissue are independent of insulin. A major purpose of glucose homeostasis is to store glucose as liver glycogen postprandially when glucose and insulin levels are high, so that it can be released in the interprandial period for CNS consumption. Protein digestion and absorption lead to a postprandial rise in circulating amino acid levels. Insulin plays a dominant role in converting amino acids to protein by stimulating amino acid uptake in muscle and liver and by augmenting protein synthesis and inhibiting proteolysis. Fat is absorbed as chylomicrons that enter the circulation via the lymphatic system. Insulin affects fat assimilation in a number of ways. Lipoprotein lipase, an enzyme synthesized primarily by fat and muscle tissue, is secreted into the extracellular space and incorporated into the surface of nearby endothelial cells. In this location, lipoprotein lipase hydrolyzes fatty acids from triglyceride-rich lipoproteins (chylomicrons and very low density lipoproteins). These fatty acids are then taken up, predominantly by adipose tissue, where they are esterified into triglyceride for storage in the fat droplets of adipocytes. Insulin stimulates the synthesis and secretion of lipoprotein lipase and also strongly inhibits lipolysis of triglycerides stored in adipose tissue. Additionally, by promoting glucose uptake, insulin increases the supply of glycerol within adipocytes for esterification of fatty acids. Insulin is also lipogenic and stimulates the synthesis of fatty acids from glucose or other substrates that form pyruvate.

Many of these insulin effects are antagonized by the counter-regulatory hormones, glucagon, epinephrine, cortisol, and growth hormone. When mild (fasting) or severe (DKA) insulin deficiency exists, the processes outlined in Figure 218–6A are reversed, and characteristic metabolic derangements occur. This is illustrated in Figure 218–6B. A 24-hour fast causes mild insulin deficiency, and this results in a marked decrease in peripheral glucose uptake. This is accompanied by a decrease in synthesis of

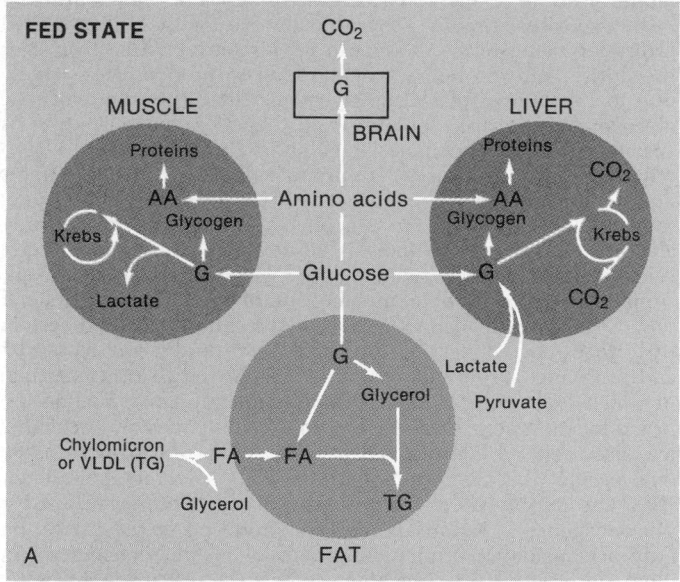

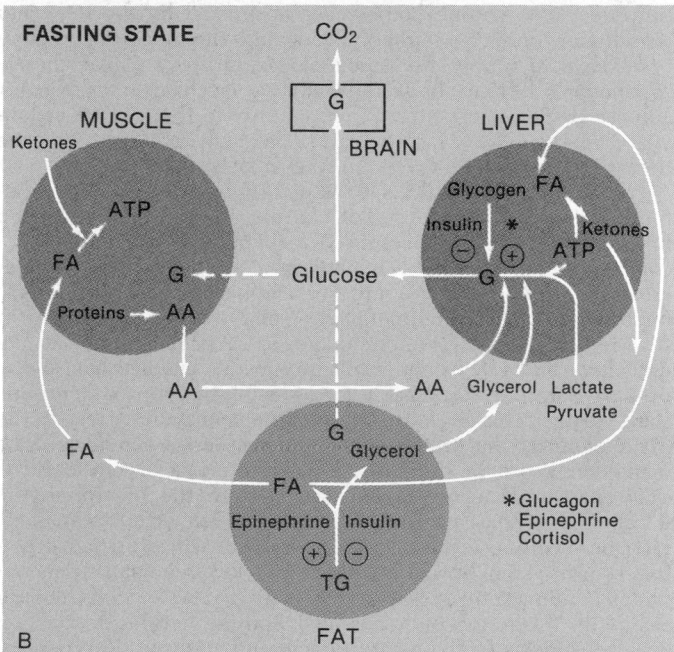

FIGURE 218–6. *A,* Fuel homeostasis during the immediate postprandial fed state. The key features of this diagram are the storage of glucose (G), amino acids (AA), and fatty acids (FA) as the macromolecules glycogen, protein, and triglyceride (TG) in tissue depots; each of these processes is facilitated by the anabolic effects of insulin. *B,* Reversal of the anabolic effects of insulin during the insulinopenic fasting state. The major purpose of these homeostatic responses is to maintain a supply of glucose for obligate glucose uptake by the CNS while other tissues cease their consumption of glucose in favor of fatty acids from adipose tissue depots.

glycogen, protein, and triglyceride, along with increased breakdown of these storage macromolecules by accelerated glycogenolysis, proteolysis, and lipolysis. These catabolic processes increase as a result of the lack of insulin effect, but breakdown of macromolecules is also augmented by increased concentrations of counter-regulatory hormones. Thus, glucagon stimulates glycogen breakdown and is also strongly ketogenic, but has no in vivo effect on glucose uptake, lipolysis, or proteolysis. Epinephrine promotes glycogenolysis and lipolysis and also inhibits peripheral glucose uptake. Cortisol probably has effects that are additive or possibly synergistic with the other counter-regulatory hormones and may independently stimulate proteolysis. Growth hormone probably plays a minor role in these events mediated through inhibition of glucose uptake. Taken together, fasting-induced insulin deficiency plus increased counter-regulatory hormones lead to a marked decrease in glucose metabolism by insulin-sensitive tissues, "sparing" glucose for the obligate CNS utilization. The source of glucose in this setting is the liver. For the initial 12 to 24 hours, hepatic glucose production is largely due to breakdown of stored glycogen. After this time, hepatic glycogen stores are depleted and hepatic glucose output is sustained by gluconeogenesis. Hepatic gluconeogenesis is supported by the increased supply of gluconeogenic substrates flowing from the periphery, that is, muscle proteolysis, leading to an increased supply of gluconeogenic amino acids (mainly alanine) and increased lipolysis resulting in enhanced glycerol release from adipose tissue. Some lactate and pyruvate are supplied from anaerobic metabolism of glucose in peripheral tissues (Cori cycle). Thus the liver is the central clearinghouse in this process by converting the breakdown products of stored fat and protein to supply glucose for the CNS in a setting (fasting) in which exogenous glucose is unavailable. In this situation the predominant energy source for non-CNS tissues is circulating free fatty acids (FFA) derived from breakdown of adipose tissue triglyceride (the CNS cannot utilize FFA as a metabolic fuel). FFA also supply the liver with the energy necessary to drive gluconeogenesis. Ketone bodies are produced in the liver from fatty acid oxidation under conditions of insulin deficiency and glucagon excess. In fasting this serves an important homeostatic purpose, since ketone bodies can be utilized by the CNS and muscle for energy, markedly reducing the need for protein breakdown to supply gluconeogenic percursors for liver glucose production. Ketone bodies provide a mechanism to convert adipose tissue energy stores into a substrate that can be metabolized in the CNS; this spares critical body proteins, allowing humans to survive relatively long-term fasts.

PATHOPHYSIOLOGY OF DKA. In DKA, all of these homeostatic processes are out of control, leading to pronounced hyperglycemia and ketonemia. The hyperglycemia is due to a combination of increased hepatic glucose production and decreased peripheral glucose uptake. The biochemical mechanisms underlying the hyperketonemia are somewhat more complex, as seen in Figure 218–7. Ketone bodies are produced in hepatocyte mitochondria by β oxidation of fatty acids, and glucagon is the primary hormone responsible for inducing the hepatic ketogenic state. It does this by lowering malonyl coenzyme A levels, the first committed substrate in fatty acid synthesis, which leads to a marked increase in the activity of carnitine acyl transferase I. This enzyme translocates fatty acids from the cytosol to the intramitochondrial space, where they are converted to ketones. Hepatic carnitine levels are also increased, which further drives this transfer step by mass action. The key regulatory point in understanding ketogenesis is that in the fed state, entry of fatty acids into the mitochondria is low, limiting fatty acid oxidation and ketogenesis in favor of fatty acid and triglyceride synthesis; thus the liver is rate limiting in ketone body formation. When the level of insulin is low and glucagon high (as in starvation or DKA), fatty acids freely enter mitochondria to be converted to ketones, and therefore the supply of fatty acids to the liver is rate limiting for ketogenesis. Fatty acids are freely permeable across the hepatocyte plasma membrane, and thus the plasma concentration of FFA drives ketogenesis. In starvation, fatty acid levels are only moderately increased, leading to enhanced, but controlled, ketogenesis; in DKA, FFA levels are much higher, leading to uncontrolled ketogenesis. Another factor enhancing ketonemia in DKA is related to ketone body utilization. Insulin normally stimulates ketoacid uptake by peripheral tissues, and this is inhibited in DKA; additionally, very high levels of ketones may saturate the uptake mechanisms, further limiting utilization.

All of the pathophysiologic sequelae of DKA follow from hyperglycemia and hyperketonemia (Fig. 218–8). Thus, acidosis and ketonuria are directly due to the buildup of the ketoacids β-hydroxybutyrate and acetoacetate. The hyperglycemia and hyperketonemia produce an osmotic diuresis that causes intravascular volume depletion and dehydration and urinary electrolyte loss. The hyperosmolarity further exaggerates intracellular dehydration.

CLINICAL PICTURE. Diabetic ketoacidosis can be a life-threatening situation, and the clinical presentation is often dramatic. An antecedent history of polyuria and polydipsia for one

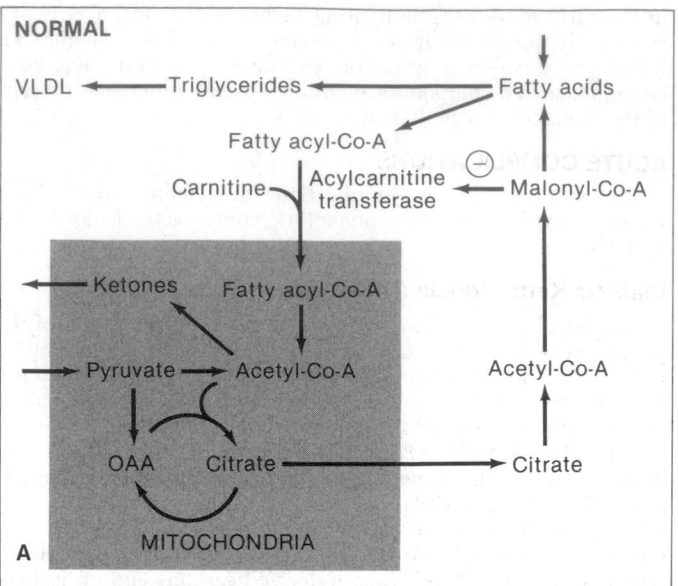

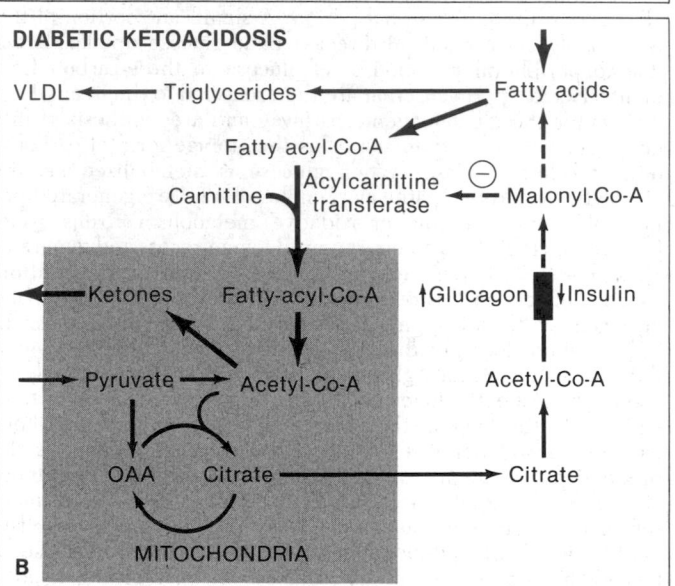

FIGURE 218–7. Hepatic fatty acid and ketoacid metabolism in the normal state *(upper panel)* and insulinopenic diabetic ketoacidotic state *(lower panel)*. Malonyl-Co-A is a key regulatory intermediate in this scheme, competitively inhibiting the ability of acyl carnitine transferase to translocate fatty acyl-Co-A molecules from the cytosol to the intramitochondrial space in the normal state. In diabetic ketoacidosis, glucagon excess and insulin deficiency inhibit the generation of malonyl-Co-A, releasing the inhibition of acyl carnitine transferase. See text for further details. VLDL = Very low density lipoproteins; OAA = oxaloacetic acid.

to several days is typical, and nausea, vomiting, and anorexia are frequent accompanying symptoms. Occasionally, abdominal pain is a predominant feature, sometimes mimicking an acute abdominal condition. Often this is due to gastric stasis and distention. In the obtunded patient with gastric distention, nasogastric suction should be considered to avoid vomiting with aspiration. Physical findings include tachypnea, dehydration, and disorientation, or even coma. If systemic acidosis is severe, Kussmaul respirations are present. Precipitating causes of DKA include failure of the patient to take insulin, infection, intercurrent illness, trauma, or emotional stress. When a known diabetic presents with signs and symptoms of DKA, the diagnosis is usually straightforward. However, DKA can also be the initial presenting episode of diabetes. DKA is a disease of IDDM, only rarely occurring in NIDDM, and only when precipitating causes are extreme.

Although the diagnosis of DKA can be strongly suspected on a clinical basis, confirmation is based on laboratory analyses. The diagnosis is made by demonstrating hyperglycemia and hyper-

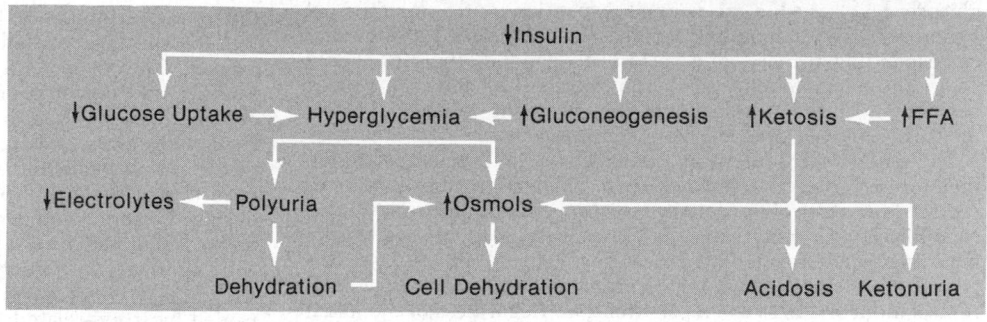

FIGURE 218–8. Pathophysiology of diabetic ketoacidosis. Severe insulin deficiency leads to hyperglycemia and ketonemia, and from this all of the other pathophysiologic sequelae result. FFA = free fatty acids.

ketonemia in the presence of acidosis. However, the severity of these abnormalities can vary over a wide range. Occasionally the presenting episode may be severe ketonemia and acidosis and only mild hyperglycemia (200 to 400 mg per deciliter). Other patients may have severe hyperglycemia and only mild ketonemia and acidosis. Occasionally, alcoholic patients have ketonemia and hyperglycemia, and this condition, termed alcoholic ketoacidosis, must be differentiated from DKA (see next section). Direct quantitative measurements of acetoacetate and β-hydroxybutyrate are not usually readily available, and most physicians rely on reagent strips (Ketostix) or tablets (Acetest) for measurements. With this method, a nitroprusside reaction is the indicator; nitroprusside reacts mainly with acetoacetate, to a lesser extent with acetone, and not at all with β-hydroxybutyrate. Since β-hydroxybutyrate levels are much higher than acetoacetate levels in DKA, this method can sometimes be confusing. For example, when concomitant lactic acidosis exists, acetoacetate production may be inhibited in the presence of very high levels of β-hydroxybutyrate. In this setting the nitroprusside reaction may not be strongly positive. During the course of insulin therapy for DKA, β-hydroxybutyrate levels may fall out of proportion to acetoacetate levels, giving the impression that therapy is less effective than it actually is. Serum sodium levels are usually mildly decreased. This is due to the hyperglycemia- and hyperketonemia-induced hyperosmolarity, which attracts extracellular water from the intracellular space, leading to dilution of serum sodium. It should be kept in mind that the osmolar contribution of the hyperketonemia can often approach the contribution of the hyperglycemia. Serum bicarbonate levels are depressed, and the magnitude of decrease is in proportion to the degree of acidosis. BUN levels are usually modestly elevated as a result of dehydration and a component of prerenal azotemia. Serum potassium levels can be high, low, or normal, depending on the degree of dehydration and acidosis. In all cases, severe total body and intracellular potassium depletion exists. Because of cellular buffering mechanisms, which exchange intracellular potassium for extracellular hydrogen ion, extracellular potassium levels are often maintained in acidotic states. Nevertheless, greater than 95 per cent of total body potassium is intracellular, so in the presence of acidosis, extracellular potassium levels do not reflect total body potassium stores unless the potassium concentration is plotted on a nomogram related to serum pH (Fig. 218–9).

TREATMENT OF DKA. The treatment of DKA should be started as soon as it is diagnosed. The goals of therapy are to increase the rate of glucose utilization by insulin-dependent tissues, to reverse ketonemia and acidosis, and to correct the depletion of water and electrolytes. To accomplish this, treatment can be divided into four general areas: (1) insulin administration, (2) replacement of fluid and electrolytes, (3) treatment of any precipitating problems, and (4) avoidance of complications.

A variety of *insulin* regimens are possible, ranging from constant intravenous infusion to intermittent administration of intravenous, subcutaneous, or intramuscular boluses. The aim of all forms of insulin administration is to achieve a rapid and maximal insulin effect. In vivo insulin action is near maximal at an insulin concentration of about 200 μU per milliliter, and achieving higher levels has little further benefit. Since insulin is rapidly cleared from the circulation ($t_{1/2}$ = 7 minutes), boluses must be given frequently (every 30 to 60 minutes) to maintain maximally effec-

tive insulin levels. With constant intravenous administration, serum insulin levels are maintained at a steady state throughout the infusion. In normal subjects, an infusion rate of 10 units per hour results in an insulin level of approximately 200 μU per milliliter by 30 minutes, and if this mode of treatment is chosen a priming dose (10 to 20 units) should be given initially. Advocates of constant intravenous infusion maintain that the rate of metabolic improvement is smoother and more predictable and hypoglycemia is less common. Additionally, problems of variable or inadequate absorption from subcutaneous or intramuscular sites are avoided. One difficulty with this method occurs in the occasional patient with severe insulin resistance due to sepsis or high titers of insulin antibodies. If clear-cut metabolic improvement is not seen within the first few hours of constant insulin infusion, a bolus of insulin (20 to 30 units) should be given and the rate of insulin infusion increased.

Fluid replacement should also be started immediately. Patients with DKA are dehydrated and hypovolemic and usually have fluid deficits of 5 to 8 liters or more. Thus, rapid expansion of intravascular volume is essential, and this is achieved by an initial infusion of 1 to 2 liters of normal saline, or equivalent, over the first 1 to 2 hours. Of course, caution should be used in those patients with underlying cardiovascular or oliguric renal disease. Following initial rapid fluid administration, the rate of replacement can be slowed to restore estimated losses by 16 to 24 hours, depending on the patient's degree of dehydration and underlying cardiovascular-renal status. Much of the initial decline in plasma

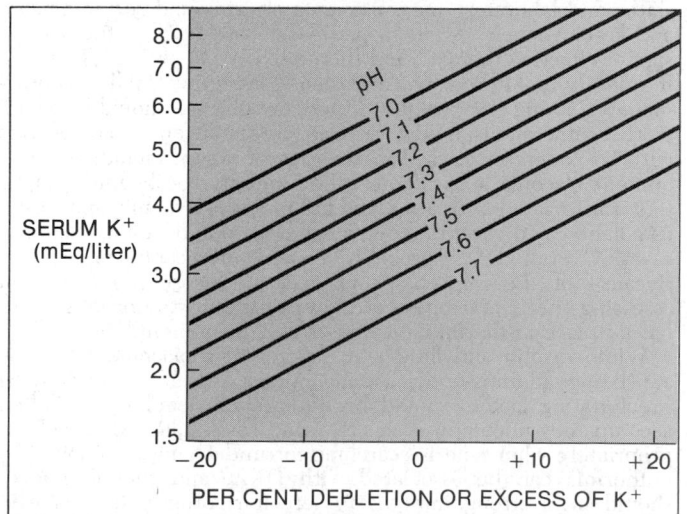

FIGURE 218–9. Nomogram depicting the relationship between total body potassium depletion, serum potassium, and serum pH. Per cent potassium depletion or excess is calculated by drawing a horizontal line from the ordinate intercept of the serum potassium concentration to the intersection of the diagonal line corresponding to the coexisting serum pH. From this intersection a vertical line is dropped to the abscissa and per cent potassium depletion or excess is read from the abscissal intercept. For example, at a serum potassium concentration of 4.0, at a concomitant serum pH of 7.2, an approximate 10 per cent depletion of total body potassium stores exists.

glucose level is due to volume expansion with reduction of hyperosmolarity, along with increased glomerular filtration and corresponding urinary glucose loss. In general, the aim should be to initiate metabolic correction rapidly, but once the patient has shown clear-cut substantial improvement, further replacement therapy can proceed more cautiously.

The electrolyte content of administered fluids must be closely monitored. Over the entire course of therapy the goal is to replace the electrolyte deficit, which averages 200 to 400 mEq each for sodium, potassium, and phosphate. Patients are usually ingesting some form of calories by 16 to 24 hours, and this provides the most physiologic replacement method. Potassium replacement requires the most attention. Regardless of the initial serum potassium level, total body reserves are depleted and serum levels fall dramatically as acidosis and hyperglycemia are corrected. As glucose is taken up by cells under the influence of insulin, potassium is also transported intracellularly, and as acidosis is reversed the cellular buffering process exchanging intracellular potassium for extracellular hydrogen ion diminishes. To prevent hypokalemia, potassium should be included in the intravenous fluids once it is established that renal perfusion and urine flow are adequate following initial intravascular fluid expansion. To accomplish this, 40 mEq of potassium can be added to each liter of intravenous fluids as the phosphate salt. Phosphate depletion is also uniform in DKA, and some replacement is advisable, particularly if serum phosphate levels are low. This can be accomplished by administering 10 to 20 mmol per hour and can be accomplished along with potassium replacement by giving potassium phosphate. Since excessive phosphate repletion can cause hypocalcemia, ongoing phosphate administration should be guided by the serum phosphorus and calcium levels. Bicarbonate replacement should be initiated in patients with severe acidosis (pH < 7.0). This can be administered at the rate of 44 mEq per liter with appropriate monitoring of pH until it rises above 7.0. Three to four ampules of bicarbonate (44 mEq per ampule) usually suffice to achieve this goal. Excessive bicarbonate replacement is contraindicated because it exacerbates the tendency toward hypokalemia and may also result in rebound CNS acidosis. The latter occurs because carbon dioxide is more rapidly diffusible across the blood-brain barrier than is bicarbonate ion, causing CNS pH to fall at a time when peripheral pH is rising. This can lead to stupor and worsening of CNS status at a time when metabolic improvement is occurring.

Therapy should be monitored by frequent assessment of clinical status and laboratory measurements of urine and serum glucose and ketone levels. A fall in plasma glucose level is the earliest sign of effective therapy, and therefore plasma glucose should be frequently monitored. Once plasma glucose levels fall to approximately 250 mg per deciliter, 5 per cent glucose should be added to the intravenous fluids. Occasionally children or adolescents with DKA exhibit marked mental deterioration, including development of coma 4 to 6 hours after therapy has begun. Usually this is associated with a marked fall in hyperglycemia and serum osmolality, and cerebral edema has been noted in a few autopsy cases. Overall this is probably a rare complication of therapy. Because of the importance of plasma glucose monitoring in assessing the effectiveness of therapy, administration of glucose has no place in the initial stages of DKA treatment.

While insulin and fluid and electrolyte replacement therapy are being administered, a concomitant search for underlying precipitating factors should be undertaken. Leukocytosis often accompanies uncomplicated DKA and so should be viewed appropriately when one is searching for underlying infection. Hypothermia can be associated with DKA, and therefore fever should be a strong impetus to screen rigorously for a site of infection.

The major complications of DKA are mostly the result of treatment and include *hypokalemia, late hypoglycemia, rebound CNS acidosis,* and *CNS deterioration* (possibly due to cerebral edema). However, with proper attention to therapeutic details the former two can always be avoided, and the latter are fortunately rare. Recurrence of DKA can occur in the hospital if the vigorous phase of therapy is relaxed too soon. Maintenance of a flow chart with all therapies and laboratory tests recorded is an important means of coordination so that unexpected results do not go undetected and inappropriate therapies are not given.

Alcoholic Ketoacidosis

Alcoholic ketoacidosis can sometimes present a problem in the differential diagnosis of DKA when the patient is not a known diabetic or when a diabetic patient ingests large amounts of alcohol. This syndrome is characterized by hyperketonemia, acidosis, and dehydration. Serum glucose levels can be normal or sometimes elevated to the lower range of values seen in DKA. In the latter case a diagnostic problem can occur. The clinical picture of alcoholic ketoacidosis occurs in alcoholics following a recent, and sometimes prolonged alcoholic debauch; abstinence during the immediately preceding 12 to 24 hours is a common finding. The patient is usually anorexic, sometimes with nausea and vomiting, and some degree of starvation over the preceding 1 to 3 days is always present. The starvation, perhaps accompanied by stress-related hyperglucagonemia, creates a ketogenic state in the liver. This is accompanied by elevated FFA levels similar to those seen in starvation, which are perhaps augmented by adrenergic activation related to alcohol withdrawal, creating the metabolic environment for ketoacidosis. It is unusual for these patients to have hyperglycemia, but it can occur. When it does, the pathogenesis is unclear. In some patients, abnormalities of glucose tolerance exist after therapy, and thus the hyperglycemia may be stress related in previously glucose-intolerant patients. Alternatively, adrenergic mechanisms related to alcohol withdrawal could suppress residual endogenous insulin secretion, facilitating mild hyperglycemia. Regardless of the underlying mechanisms, the metabolic abnormalities are rapidly reversed by intravenous administration of fluids and glucose. Only occasionally is insulin needed in the early stages of treatment.

Nonketotic Hyperosmolar Syndrome

The term *nonketotic hyperosmolar coma* has frequently been applied to this syndrome, but by no means do all patients display coma or even mental obtundity. Rather, this syndrome comprises a spectrum ranging from mild degrees of hyperosmolarity with minimal CNS symptoms to severe hyperosmolarity with minimal CNS symptoms to severe hyperosmolarity with accompanying coma. The biochemical hallmarks are extreme hyperglycemia (mean 1000 mg per deciliter, range 600 to 2400 mg per deciliter) in the absence of overt ketoacidosis. Dehydration, hypovolemia, and disorientation are accompanying features. This syndrome usually develops over a much longer interval than DKA, with symptoms of polyuria antedating clinical presentation by several days and sometimes weeks. This syndrome usually occurs in elderly patients with NIDDM (often not previously diagnosed) who for some reason are unable to keep up with the osmotic diuresis by adequate water ingestion and this results in severe dehydration. The severe hyperglycemia is at least partly caused by decreased renal glucose excretion due either to intrinsic underlying renal disease or to decreased glomerular filtration and prerenal azotemia secondary to the marked hypovolemia and dehydration. Frequently this condition is associated with steroid, diuretic, or phenytoin therapy as a precipitating cause. Other precipitating factors include infections, cerebrovascular events, or therapeutic maneuvers such as hypertonic peritoneal dialysis or parenteral nutrition.

Serum sodium and potassium levels are usually normal while serum bicarbonate levels are often somewhat depressed. This is usually not associated with significant ketonemia and probably reflects an underlying component of lactic acidosis due to hypovolemia. The BUN is uniformly elevated because of hypovolemia and prerenal azotemia. In these cases, however, acidosis is mild, and serum osmolality can be approximated by the formula:

$$\text{serum osmolality (mOsm/L)} = 2 \times [\text{Na}^+ + \text{K}^+ \text{ (mEq/L)}] + \frac{\text{plasma glucose (mg/dl)}}{18} + \frac{\text{BUN (mg/dl)}}{2.8}$$

Since urea is freely diffusible across cell membranes, it does not alter the effective serum osmolality, which is the clinically important factor to consider in this hyperosmolar condition. Most experts do not consider BUN levels in this calculation and prefer to estimate effective serum osmolarity as:

$$\text{Osm}_E = 2 \times [\text{Na}^+ + \text{K}^+ \text{ (mEq/L)}] + \frac{\text{plasma glucose (mg/dl)}}{18}$$

Values above 300 mOsm per liter are abnormal and above 320 mOsm per liter are indicative of clinically significant hyperosmolarity.

The reason ketosis is not a feature of this condition has not been satisfactorily explained. FFA levels are not as high in this syndrome as they are in DKA, and most investigators attribute the relatively lower FFA levels and decreased rates of ketogenesis to higher residual insulin levels in patients with the hyperosmolar syndrome. This answer is not entirely satisfactory, however, since measured peripheral insulin levels overlap with those reported in DKA. On the other hand, peripheral insulin levels do not always reflect portal insulin concentrations, and significant differences in portal insulin levels may exist in DKA versus hyperosmolar syndrome, with the higher levels in hyperosmolar syndrome restraining hepatic ketogenesis.

In some series, the mortality has ranged up to 50 per cent. However, the relatively high mortality reflects selection criteria because mortality tends to be higher with greater severity of the hyperosmolality. The first priority of treatment should be intravascular volume expansion to restore circulatory integrity. This is accomplished by infusion of 1 to 2 liters of normal saline, or equivalent, over 1 to 2 hours, provided that absolute cardiovascular contraindications do not exist. Even normal saline is hypotonic relative to serum in these patients, and therefore this therapy initiates the correction of the hyperosmolality. As in DKA, insulin can be administered by constant intravenous infusions or bolus therapy. Since absorption of insulin administered subcutaneously or intramuscularly is variable because of dehydration and hypovolemia, and since late hypoglycemia is a more common complication of the hyperosmolar syndrome, constant intravenous administration of insulin can be very effective in this condition, leading to a predictable and fairly constant, smooth decline in plasma glucose levels. Once plasma glucose begins to decrease, and provided that acceptable volume expansion and urine flow have been established, potassium phosphate salts should be added to the intravenous fluids. Subsequent to the initial volume expansion, intravenous fluids can consist of 0.5 normal saline with added potassium phosphate. Once plasma glucose levels decline to approximately 250 mg per deciliter, 5 per cent glucose should be added to the intravenous fluids. The above comments are meant more as guidelines than hard and fast rules, since, as in DKA, therapy must be individualized as far as replacement of fluids and electrolytes is concerned. This is best done by maintaining an organized flow chart with frequent measurements of plasma glucose, electrolytes, blood pressure, and urine volume. Despite even the best therapy, morbidity and mortality are high in this condition. Thrombosis and embolic events as well as infections, particularly pneumonia with accompanying adult respiratory distress syndrome, contribute significantly to adverse outcomes. In summary, rigorous but carefully monitored hydration and re-establishment of circulatory integrity are critical for successful therapy. These goals should be pursued while hyperosmolarity is corrected by administration of relatively hypotonic fluids with adequate free water along with insulin to reduce the hyperglycemia. Concomitantly a careful workup should be instituted to uncover precipitating factors with appropriate therapy when necessary.

CHRONIC OR LATE COMPLICATIONS OF DIABETES

Retinopathy (See Color Plate 14E)

Eye disease is common in diabetes, and permanent loss of vision is one of the most striking and feared complications. Approximately 25 per cent of all newly reported cases of blindness are attributed to diabetes. When diabetics of all ages and types are considered together, the incidence of blindness from diabetic retinopathy is 0.2 per cent per year in all diabetics and 0.6 per cent per year in diabetics with retinopathy. This is 11 and 29 times greater, respectively, than the incidence of blindness from all other causes combined in the general population.

The major form of diabetic eye disease is diabetic retinopathy. Two general categories exist: nonproliferative or background retinopathy and proliferative retinopathy. Nonproliferative retinopathy can include venous abnormalities, microaneurysms, retinal hemorrhages, retinal edema, and exudates. This may progress to proliferative retinopathy, characterized by neovascularization, glial proliferation, and vitreoretinal traction. In general, diabetic retinopathy is progressive and tends to worsen with the duration of disease. However, most diabetics do not develop proliferative retinopathy. The incidence of this complication is substantially lower in NIDDM then in IDDM, even when corrected for duration of disease. However, since there are many more patients with NIDDM than IDDM, the absolute numbers of NIDDM and IDDM patients with proliferative retinopathy are roughly comparable.

NONPROLIFERATIVE RETINOPATHY. Probably the earliest retinal change is increased capillary permeability seen on fluorescein angiography. This abnormality can be readily reversed by effective glycemic control, but the relationship of this form of capillary permeability to retinopathy is unknown. Nonperfusion of retinal capillaries occurs early in diabetic retinopathy (so-called capillary dropout), and this leads to areas of retinal ischemia and infarction. Microaneurysms are small (15 to 50 µm diameter) excrescences along capillaries and are particularly prominent along the edges of areas of capillary nonperfusion. Fusiform aneurysms, or general dilatation of capillary loops, can also occur. Retinal veins are often tortuous and dilated; dilatation can be segmental, giving rise to a beaded or "sausage string" appearance. Exudates can be of two types: (1) *Hard, waxy exudates* are white to yellowish, shiny, with defined borders but without surrounding pigmentation. These exudates are due to lipid- and protein-containing fluid that has leaked from surrounding capillaries. (2) *Cotton-wool, or soft, exudates* are really areas of nonperfusion representing retinal microinfarcts and are often surrounded by microaneurysms. Clinically, an increase in cotton-wool areas indicates progressive capillary dropout and is a poor prognostic sign. Subretinal hemorrhages tend to be small and dot shaped and may resorb within a few weeks. Larger, flame-shaped hemorrhages occur in the superficial retinal layers and resorb more slowly. Preretinal hemorrhages are more serious and can impair vision if they are large or if they impinge on the macula. Following resorption, scarring and vitreous retraction or retinal detachment can occur. Edema of the retina is due to abnormal capillary permeability and ischemia. When persistent macular edema exists, vision is seriously impaired, and usual forms of therapy (photocoagulation) may not be effective. The primary pathogenetic events underlying these changes of nonproliferative background retinopathy are unclear, but loss of supporting capillary pericytes, endothelial proliferation, and hyperviscosity with red cell aggregation, together or alone, have all been proposed.

PROLIFERATIVE RETINOPATHY. The hallmark of proliferative retinopathy is new vessel formation or neovascularization. These capillary fronds or loops can grow on the surface of the retina or extend into the vitreous. Often this is accompanied by proliferation of glial elements in the region of the optic disc or along the new vessel arcades. Traction between the vitreous and the neovascular and glial elements can ultimately develop, leading to retinal detachment or large-scale hemorrhage into the vitreous. These events lead to serious loss of vision or blindness. It has been suggested that the stimulus for neovascularization is retinal ischemia with local release of growth-promoting factors.

Photocoagulation is the therapy of choice for proliferative diabetic retinopathy. With this therapy, a light beam is focused on the retina to produce a burn or coagulum in a precisely defined area. By this means, one can selectively destroy microaneurysms, leaky vessels, neovascular elements, and areas of microinfarction or edema. Destruction of vessels prone to hemorrhage or causing traction directly prevents further deterioration. Destroying areas of retina that are poorly perfused and hypoxic may curtail the ischemic stimulus for neovascularization, preventing further proliferative changes. Regardless of the mechanism, the cooperative trial of the Diabetic Retinopathy Study Research Group clearly showed that photocoagulation decreases the incidence of retinal detachment, hemorrhage, and loss of vision. Thus, photocoagulation involves selective treatment of new vessels as well as panretinal treatment to destroy 20 to 30 per cent of the remaining retinal tissue. Photocoagulation therapy may also be useful for proliferative retinopathy as indicated by results from the Early Treatment Diabetic Retinopathy Study. All patients with significant diabetic retinopathy should be followed by an ophthalmologist and photocoagulation considered when new vessel formation or preretinal hemorrhage occurs.

Photocoagulation early in the course of diabetic retinopathy can also be advisable. In the past, hypophysectomy was used as treatment for proliferative retinopathy. However, the therapeutic responses to this maneuver are quite variable, and significant complications exist. With the advent of photocoagulation, use of hypophysectomy has been largely abandoned. In patients with severe vitreal involvement, total vitrectomy may offer some possibility of improvement and preservation of vision.

Other Complications of Diabetes Affecting Vision

In addition to retinopathy, the eyes are affected in other ways by diabetes mellitus. Diabetics may experience temporary blurring of vision and *changes in refraction*, most likely due to osmotic changes in lens shape as a result of fluctuations in hyperglycemia. These changes can be disconcerting, but patients should be advised not to seek new refractions until a stable period of metabolic control is produced. It may take 6 to 8 weeks before the hyperglycemia-induced changes in visual acuity subside. *Glaucoma* is also more frequent in diabetics. Rubeosis iridis is due to capillary neovascularization of the iris, which can produce closed-angle glaucoma. Usually occurring when diabetic retinopathy is advanced, this form of glaucoma is generally refractory to treatment. Open-angle glaucoma is also more frequent in diabetics, and this may relate to fibrosis or scarring of the canals of Schlemm, which drain the anterior chamber. Although *cataracts* are common in diabetics, it has not been rigorously demonstrated that the incidence of cataracts is increased in this condition. For the most part, cataracts in diabetics are indistinguishable from senile cataracts in nondiabetic patients, and the indications for surgery are the same as in nondiabetics. It is possible that the presence of diabetes accelerates the development of senile cataracts so that they occur at an earlier age than in nondiabetics. It has been postulated that hyperglycemia leads to increased sorbitol production in the lens, resulting in osmotic changes that accelerate cataract formation. While evidence in favor of this theory exists, it still remains to be proved. Opacities in the lens termed snowflake cataracts are occasionally noted in young patients whose diabetes is in poor control. This form of cataract is more specific for diabetes but can occur in other conditions and, unlike the senile cataract, can regress when glycemic control is achieved.

Nephropathy

Kidney disease is common in diabetes (see also Ch. 83 for an extensive discussion of the kidney in diabetes), and renal failure is one of the major causes of death.

PATHOLOGY. The dominant form of diabetic nephropathy is microvascular disease affecting the renal glomerulus. A number of distinct morphologic and functional abnormalities characterize diabetic glomerulopathy. Early in diabetes the kidney increases in size, and the associated glomerular hypertrophy leads to an increased glomerular filtration rate with hyperfiltration and microalbuminuria in up to 50 per cent of patients with new-onset IDDM. The hyperfiltration and increased kidney size revert to normal following effective insulin therapy and are unassociated with other glomerular lesions. Later in the disease, diffuse thickening of the glomerular basement membrane is noted along with increased mesangial volume. Patients with substantial histologic changes can exhibit normal renal function; however, impaired renal function probably does not occur in the absence of morphologic changes. Later in the disease, when decreased renal function is evident, the mesangium further expands and occupies a greater proportion of the glomerular volume while the thickness of the glomerular basement membrane is not necessarily increased. Glomerular occlusion accompanies this picture. Often characteristic nodular hyaline-like deposits, termed nodular glomerulocapillary sclerosis or Kimmelstiel-Wilson lesions, are evident in the center of peripheral glomerular capillary lobules.

CLINICAL AND FUNCTIONAL ASPECTS. The manifestations of diabetic nephropathy are quite heterogeneous. Asymptomatic, mild proteinuria can remain constant for many years. In other patients proteinuria may increase and be followed by progressive reduction in glomerular filtration and renal function. Persistent proteinuria (3 to 5 grams per day or greater) is a poor prognostic sign, usually heralding renal failure within 5 years. However, exceptions exist. The proteinuria may progress to include all of the classic features of the nephrotic syndrome. Once azotemia develops, progression to renal failure and uremia is inevitable within a few months to 2 to 3 years.

The diagnosis of diabetic nephropathy is usually made on clinical grounds, and renal biopsy is rarely indicated. Invasive diagnostic procedures should be aimed at detection of reversible features such as infection or obstruction. Contrast studies should not be conducted without clear indications, since rapid deterioration of renal function with acute renal failure sometimes follows intravenous pyelography or angiography in azotemic diabetic patients. When the study is performed, patients should be well hydrated before testing.

If renal failure develops in a diabetic, dialysis or transplantation must be considered. As recently as 10 to 15 years ago, uremic diabetics were thought to be extremely poor risks for dialysis, with very low survival rates and high rates of complications, particularly infections and deterioration of vision. However, in recent years, results have been much better with a first-year survival of over 80 per cent and 3-year survival of over 60 per cent. Additionally, far fewer cases of progressive visual impairment and blindness occur. Thus, in the absence of other negative factors, the presence of diabetes should not be considered a contraindication to dialysis, and decisions to initiate this form of therapy should generally proceed as in nondiabetic uremic patients. Chronic ambulatory peritoneal dialysis (CAPD) has been tried in some patients, but overall experience is still limited. Indications for CAPD vary widely among treatment centers, as does enthusiasm for this mode of therapy. Recent experience with renal transplantation has also been encouraging. Regardless of donor source (cadaver or related donor), survival rates after renal transplantation in diabetics approach those in nondiabetics. Interestingly, diabetic-type glomerular changes have been noted in biopsy specimens from the transplanted kidney in many of these patients.

Neuropathy (See also Ch. 498)

Diabetic neuropathy is perhaps the most common disabling chronic complication of diabetes. Although death seldom results from neuropathic changes alone, a great deal of morbidity and reduced quality of life can be attributed to diabetic neuropathy. The incidence and severity of neuropathy generally progress with duration of diabetes, and severe neuropathy can often exist in the absence of other chronic diabetic complications. A number of different classification schemes have been proposed, but none is entirely satisfactory, primarily because the causes of diabetic neuropathy are not known, and therefore classification must be descriptive in nature rather than based on pathogenetic mechanisms. Table 218–6 provides a simplified method of classification that may prove useful. Polyneuropathy is a diffuse symmetric disorder of peripheral nerve function. Asymmetric neuropathy implies a cluster of signs and symptoms that can be anatomically related to dysfunction of a single nerve trunk (mononeuropathy) or to more than one nerve trunk (mononeuropathy multiplex) either simultaneously or successively. It has been proposed that the symmetric or diffuse neuropathies are due to "metabolic" abnormalities of the neurons or the Schwann cells, whereas the asymmetric or focal neuropathies are due to vascular occlusion and ischemia. Diabetic neuropathy is very common in both IDDM and NIDDM, and mild to severe disease can exist in up to 50 per cent of patients. The incidence of symmetric neuropathy is comparable in IDDM and NIDDM when corrected for duration of disease, but focal neuropathies are more common in older NIDDM patients, suggesting a vascular contribution to the etiology.

TABLE 218–6. CLASSIFICATION OF DIABETIC NEUROPATHY

1. Symmetric distal polyneuropathy
2. Asymmetric neuropathy
   A. Cranial mononeuropathy and mononeuropathy multiplex
   B. Peripheral mononeuropathy and mononeuropathy multiplex
   C. Neuromuscular syndromes
3. Autonomic neuropathy

NEUROPATHIC LESIONS AND THE DIABETIC FOOT.

Loss of sensation can lead to the development of a Charcot joint as a result of repeated undetected trauma. More commonly, neuropathic ulcers develop, particularly on the plantar aspect of the foot. This can be due to weakness of the intrinsic muscles of the foot secondary to neuropathy, leading to abnormal pressure distribution. Weight bearing is then accentuated on the metatarsal heads, causing degeneration of the underlying fat pads and eventually leading to the typical open, draining neuropathic ulcer. Ulcers can also result from penetrating wounds caused by stepping on tacks or other sharp objects the patient does not feel. The best therapy is preventive. All diabetics should be trained to examine their feet daily for callous formation, blisters, or trauma. Shoes should be properly fitted; orthotic or other devices to aid in proper weight distribution are sometimes helpful. Patients should be advised never to walk barefoot. In all cases the feet should be kept clean and dry, and professional trimming of toenails and callosities is often advisable. Neuropathic foot ulcers can lead to gangrene and the requirement for amputation. Meticulous foot care substantially decreases the incidence of these ulcers and is a major form of preventive therapy that all diabetics should receive. Once open ulcers develop, healing can still occur if peripheral circulation is adequate. A high index of suspicion should be maintained for underlying osteomyelitis. Treatment is supportive with bed rest, elevation of the foot, warm (but not hot) foot soaks, debridement, and in some cases antibiotics. Protective plaster casts are sometimes advised. If these therapies fail and gangrene develops, amputation is the only recourse.

SYMMETRIC DISTAL POLYNEUROPATHY. This form of diabetic neuropathy can be divided into two types: (1) relatively asymptomatic and (2) painful. The first form is diffuse, distal, usually in the lower extremities with a stocking type of distribution. It is characterized by numbness, tingling, or pins-and-needles sensation, often worse at night. Although the course may wax and wane, it is generally progressive and irreversible. Symptoms of the painful form can range from burning or dull aching sensations to cramping or excruciating, lancinating pain. The pain is often worse at night and partially relieved by movement. Hyperesthesia can be so marked that even light touch is so painful that the patient cannot tolerate bed covers. Physical examination is similar in both types and is often rather unremarkable. The single most common finding is absence of deep tendon reflexes in the lower extremities (i.e., loss of knee and ankle jerks).

ASYMMETRIC NEUROPATHY. Diabetic mononeuropathies of the cranial nerves usually involve the third, sixth, or fourth cranial nerve in order of frequency. This gives rise to extraocular muscle paralysis with diplopia. The most common syndrome is isolated third nerve palsy accompanied in 80 per cent of cases by sparing of the pupillary reflex. Mononeuropathies of peripheral nerves most frequently occur at sites of external pressure or entrapment (i.e., carpal tunnel). Manifestations include footdrop, wristdrop, or other symptoms related to the particular nerve involved.

Another diabetic neuropathic syndrome involves *radiculopathy*. This syndrome is characterized by dysesthesias and painful hyperesthesia localized to the anatomic distribution of one or more spinal nerves. Symptoms can resemble herpes zoster, although skin lesions are seldom noted.

Diabetic neuropathic cachexia is a syndrome of elderly male diabetics characterized by marked weight loss, painful peripheral polyneuropathy, and depression. The weight loss is so marked that patients appear cachectic, leading to a diagnosis of suspected underlying malignant disease. Other complications of diabetes are typically absent, and patients spontaneously recover in about 1 year.

For a thorough discussion of diabetic symmetric distal polyneuropathy, asymmetric neuropathy, and autonomic neuropathy, see Ch. 498.

Cardiovascular Disease

Cardiovascular disease is the major cause of death in diabetic patients and is far more prevalent than in the nondiabetic population because of accelerated atherogenesis. Not only is cardiovascular disease more frequent, but onset is at an earlier age, and manifestations are more severe. The etiology of the accelerated atherosclerosis in diabetes is incompletely understood, but the causes are probably multifactorial. Most forms of hyperlipoproteinemia are more common in diabetic subjects, and high-density lipoprotein levels tend to be decreased in patients with uncontrolled diabetes. Furthermore, in patients with chronic hyperglycemia, circulating lipoproteins become glycosylated, adversely altering their turnover and sites of tissue deposition. This phenomenon might contribute to the increased risk of atherosclerosis in the absence of grossly elevated circulating lipid levels. Abnormalities of endothelial cell function have also been proposed that would enhance the susceptibility of arterial walls to injury. Increased platelet aggregation and hyperviscosity have also been proposed. Medical management of these risk factors is similar to that in nondiabetic subjects. Thus, specific diet and drug therapy for the various hyperlipoproteinemias should be used when indicated (Ch. 172). On occasion, lipid-lowering drugs such as nicotinic acid may accentuate glucose intolerance. Because of the high risk for atherogenesis, diabetics should be strongly encouraged to abstain from cigarette smoking. Arterial hypertension is a frequent concomitant of diabetes and should be treated promptly. Interestingly, epidemiologic studies have suggested that the existence of hypertension causes little in the way of additive risk for atherosclerosis in diabetics. The diabetic has a substantially greater risk for the development of all forms of cardiovascular disease even when hypertension and hyperlipoproteinemia are taken into account.

The pattern of coronary artery disease (CAD) has been reported to be different in diabetics and nondiabetics, exhibiting in diabetics a greater tendency toward diffuse distal lesions in addition to the usual proximal lesions. However, systematic studies have not uniformly confirmed this notion, suggesting that if this is a feature of CAD in diabetes, then only a minority of patients show diffuse distal occlusive disease. This is important, since one would expect coronary artery bypass surgery to be less successful in patients with distal disease and poor runoff. Overall the indications for myocardial revascularization are probably no different in diabetics and nondiabetics, although a greater incidence of postoperative complications is seen in diabetics. The presence of diabetes substantially eliminates the sex differences in CAD, since the incidence of CAD is roughly comparable in premenopausal diabetic women and age-matched diabetic men. Complications of myocardial infarction are more frequent in diabetics, and postinfarction survival is less. Although angina pectoris is common in diabetic patients, atypical anginal syndromes are seen more frequently than in nondiabetics. Various atypical pain patterns have been described. Painless myocardial infarction has been described in diabetics, probably due to disturbance of afferent nerve fibers. The diagnosis should be suspected in diabetic patients with the sudden onset of left ventricular failure. A syndrome of diabetic cardiomyopathy has been described and is characterized by congestive heart failure in the absence of proximal CAD. It is thought that this syndrome is due to small-vessel occlusive disease. Whether a distinct cardiomyopathy exists in diabetes in the absence of any CAD is still being debated.

Peripheral vascular disease is far more frequent in the diabetic than in the nondiabetic population, and this is particularly so for distal vascular insufficiency of the lower limbs. When combined with the neuropathic complications of diabetes, this unfortunately presents an ideal setting for the development of ischemia and gangrene, necessitating amputation. Because of the marked distal small-vessel disease, vascular bypass surgery is often satisfactory. Most forms of cerebrovascular disease and stroke are also seen more frequently in diabetes.

Dermatologic Lesions

Dermatologic abnormalities are common in diabetes. For example, these patients are more prone to various skin infections such as carbuncles and furuncles. These can often be extensive and difficult to treat. Vaginal candidiasis is frequent in hyperglycemic glycosuric women. Antifungal agents are effective in treating this disorder, but recurrences are common until glycosuria is effectively controlled. Necrobiosis lipoidica diabeticorum consists of round or oval, sharply defined, plaque-like lesions on the anterior surface of the lower legs. The borders of these lesions are frequently elevated, and the center may be depressed. The centers tend to be yellowish, while the borders are hyperpigmented. Although this lesion is uncommon in diabetics, when it does occur, the plaques can ulcerate upon minimal trauma. Diabetic dermopathy (shin spots) is the most frequent dermatologic lesion seen in diabetic patients, occurring in 60 per cent of males and 30 per cent of females. These lesions are common over the tibial area, but also can be observed on forearms and thighs. They begin as small reddish papules that gradually heal, leaving thin hyperpigmented atrophic areas behind. Typical xanthomatoses can occur secondary to hyperlipoproteinemia. In insulin-dependent diabetic subjects, tight waxy skin over the dorsum of the hands in conjunction with joint contractions has been observed. This may be an important clinical observation, since these patients appear to have accelerated development of other microangiopathic complications.

SUMMARY

Diabetes mellitus is a chronic disease and therefore the approach to the patient and methods of management must encompass a long-term view. Patients with diabetes will be interacting with health care providers for the remainder of their lives. The patient must become well educated concerning the disease and eventually learn to individualize all the various components of therapy to his or her own personal circumstances. Ultimately many of the day-to-day therapy and management decisions rest in the hands of the patient. Since much of the treatment of diabetes involves intensive self-care, in a very real sense the patient may be his or her own most important physician. This requires education, motivation, and psychological adjustment.

Brand PW: The diabetic foot. In Ellenberg M, Rifkin H (eds.): Diabetes Mellitus. Theory and Practice, 3rd ed. New Hyde Park, NY, Medical Examination Publishing Co., 1983, pp 829–849. An in-depth review of the clinical manifestations and management of diabetic foot problems.

Bunn HF: Evaluation of glycosylated hemoglobin in diabetic patients. Diabetes 30:613, 1981. A review of the biochemistry, clinical significance, and use of glycosylated hemoglobin in diabetes.

Early Treatment Diabetic Retinopathy Study Research Group: Photocoagulation for diabetic macular edema. Arch Ophthalmol 103:1796, 1985. A report of the multicenter study designed to determine at what point photocoagulation is appropriate therapy for diabetic retinopathy.

Feingold KR: Hypoglycemia: A pitfall of insulin therapy. West J Med 139:688, 1983. An excellent clinical discussion of this important complication of the therapy of diabetes, with 56 references.

Felig PU, McCurdy DK: The hypertonic state. N Engl J Med 297:1444, 1977. A discussion of the pathophysiology and clinical treatment of the hyperosmolar syndrome.

Geffner ME, Lippe BM: The role of immunotherapy in Type I diabetes mellitus. West J Med 146:337, 1987. A recent review covering the pros and cons of the various forms of immunotherapy which have been used or considered for the early treatment of IDDM.

Given BD, Mako ME, Tager H, et al.: Circulating insulin with reduced biological activity in a patient with diabetes. N Engl J Med 302:129, 1980. The first description of a patient producing a biologically defective insulin molecule.

Goetz FC: Recent progress in the management of end-stage diabetic nephropathy. Clin Endocrinol Metab 11:579, 1982. A good discussion of the relative success rates of dialysis and transplantation in end-stage diabetic neuropathy.

Greene DA, Lattimer S, Ulbrecht J, Carroll P: Glucose-induced alterations in nerve metabolism: Current perspective on the pathogenesis of diabetic neuropathy and future directions for research and therapy. Diabetes Care 9:290, 1985. A comprehensive review article discussing current concepts about the pathogenesis of diabetic neuropathy with a view toward therapy.

Kreisberg RA: Diabetic ketoacidosis. In Rifkin H, Porte D Jr (eds.): Ellenberg and Rifkin's Diabetes Mellitus, 4th ed. New York, Elsevier Science Publishing Co., 1990, pp 591–603. A thorough and current review of the pathogenesis and treatment of this disorder.

Kroc Collaborative Study Group: Blood glucose control and the evolution of diabetic retinopathy and albuminuria. N Engl J Med 311:365, 1984. A report of a well-designed multicenter clinical trial to examine the effect of intensive diabetic control on diabetic complications.

Lernmark A, Baekkeskov S: Islet cell antibodies—Theoretical and practical implications. Diabetologia 21:431, 1981. A discussion of the potential role of autoantibodies directed against β cells in the pathogenesis of diabetes.

L'Esperance FA Jr, James SA Jr: The eye and diabetes mellitus. In Ellenberg M, Rifkin H (eds.): Diabetes Mellitus. Theory and Practice, 3rd ed. New Hyde Park, NY, Medical Examination Publishing Co., 1983, pp 727–757. A general review of the ocular complications of diabetes mellitus with particular emphasis on retinopathy.

McGarry JD, Foster DW: Regulation of hepatic fatty acid oxidation and ketone body production. Ann Rev Biochem 49:395, 1980. Detailed review of the intermediary metabolism of ketogenesis and the pathogenesis of diabetic ketoacidosis.

National Diabetes Data Group: Classification and diagnosis of diabetes mellitus and other categories of glucose intolerance. Diabetes 63:843, 1977. A description of the unified classification system and methods and criteria for diagnosis of diabetes mellitus.

Olefsky JM, Molina JM: Insulin resistance. In Rifkin H, Porte D Jr (eds.): Ellenberg and Rifkin's Diabetes Mellitus, 4th ed. New York, Elsevier Science Publishing Co., Inc., 1990, pp 121–153. A review of the pathogenesis and mechanisms of insulin resistance in NIDDM and their contribution to the overall diabetic state.

Peacock I, Tattersall R: Methods of self monitoring of diabetic control. Clin Endocrinol Metab 11:485, 1982. A review of the rationale and technique of self-monitoring of glucose in diabetes mellitus.

Rotter JI, Rimoin DL: The genetics of diabetes. Hosp Pract 22:79, 1987. A useful general discussion of the genetics of the various types of diabetes mellitus, with a tabular summary of a large number of genetic syndromes associated with it.

Rotter JI, Anderson CE, Rimoin DL: Genetics of diabetes mellitus. In Ellenberg M, Rifkin H (eds.): Diabetes Mellitus. Theory and Practice, 3rd ed. New Hyde Park, NY, Medical Examination Publishing Co., 1983, pp 481–503. A review of the inheritance patterns and the genetic contributions to the etiology of type I and type II diabetes mellitus.

Schade DS, Santiago JV, Skyler JS, et al.: Intensive Insulin Therapy. Princeton, Excerpta Medica, 1983. A monograph outlining the physiologic principles and methods of administering intensive therapy by multiple injections as well as CSII.

Segall M: HLA and genetics of IDDM. Holism vs. reductionism? Diabetes 37:1005, 1988. A review of the interrelationships between the genetic predisposition to IDDM, immunologic abnormalities, and their relationship to the HLA system.

Unger RH, Orci L: Glucagon and the A cell. Physiology and pathophysiology. N Engl J Med 304:1518, 1575, 1981. A review of the physiology of glucagon secretion and action as well as its role in the pathophysiology of diabetes.

Zata R, Brenner BM: Pathogenesis of diabetic microangiopathy. Am J Med 80:443, 1986. A discussion of the role of hemodynamic abnormalities in the pathogenesis of diabetic microangiopathy.

Ziegler AG, Herskowitz RD, Jackson RA, et al.: Predicting Type I diabetes. Diabetes Care 13:762, 1990. A state-of-the-art summary of the current methods that might be useful in predicting the eventual development of type I diabetes. This is particularly important in view of the emergency concepts concerning new therapies that might be useful early in the course of this disease, before clinical manifestations appear.

219 Hypoglycemic Disorders
F. John Service

Hypoglycemia is a pathophysiologic state and not a disease. Just as pain, fever, or vomiting requires identification of the underlying condition, hypoglycemia warrants diagnosis of the primary disorder causing the low plasma glucose concentration.

Hypoglycemia could be considered to be present at glucose concentrations below the lower limit of normal fasting plasma glucose, e.g., below 70 mg per deciliter. However, because hypoglycemic disorders are usually symptomatic clinical syndromes, hypoglycemia is usually defined as a glucose concentration below the level at which symptoms are expected to occur, e.g., below 45 mg per deciliter.

PHYSIOLOGY

Plasma glucose is maintained within narrow bounds, in spite of intermittent food ingestion and periods of fasting, as the net balance between the rates of glucose production and utilization. Following food ingestion, the increase in plasma glucose, in concert with an incretion effect from enteric factors, results in an increase in plasma insulin, which accelerates glucose utilization and suppresses hepatic glucose production. As the plasma glucose concentration falls early in the postabsorptive state, plasma insulin decreases, which restores glucose utilization and production to the preprandial rates. There is then a transition from a state of glucose storage to one of carefully husbanded glucose production at rates designed to satisfy the obligatory needs of the body (see Fig. 218–6). A more extensive discussion of glucose homeostasis is given in Ch. 218.

Glycogenolysis

In the postabsorptive period 4 to 6 hours after food ingestion, plasma glucose concentrations are generally 80 to 90 mg per deciliter, and glucose is produced and utilized at a rate of approximately 2 mg per kilogram per minute. About half of the glucose produced is metabolized by the central nervous system. At this time most glucose (70 to 80 per cent) is produced from hepatic glycogenolysis, with a small contribution (20 to 25 per cent) from gluconeogenesis. Hepatic glycogen stores become exhausted after 24 to 36 hours of fasting.

Glycogenolysis is stimulated by epinephrine and glucagon and inhibited by insulin. Several enzymes are involved in the cleavage of glucose moieties from glycogen and the final appearance of free glucose in the circulation. Abnormalities of these enzymes may result in hypoglycemia. For example, deficient activity of glucose-6-phosphatase (von Gierke's disease) may cause severe hypoglycemia, whereas deficient activities of glycogen phosphorylase and debrancher enzyme cause milder degrees of hypoglycemia (Ch. 169). Deficiency of glycogen synthetase results in severe hypoglycemia in newborns.

Gluconeogenesis

Gluconeogenesis is the generation of new glucose from non-carbohydrate substrates. Defects in this process result in hypoglycemia after prolonged fasting when glycogen stores have been depleted. Lactate and pyruvate, glycerol, and amino acids account for approximately 58 per cent, 13 per cent, and 29 per cent, respectively, of the glucose produced via gluconeogenesis. Defects in gluconeogenesis may arise from (1) diminished substrate availability, e.g., hypoglycemia in renal failure; (2) altered redox state, which inhibits several important gluconeogenic enzymes, e.g., alcohol hypoglycemia; and (3) inhibition of fatty acid oxidation, which diminishes the energy source for gluconeogenesis, e.g., poisoning from the unripe ackee fruit.

Alanine and glutamine are the most important amino acids that act as glucose precursors. The carbon source of alanine is muscle-derived pyruvate, and the nitrogen source for the transamination of pyruvate to alanine is thought to be branched-chain amino acids. Impaired metabolism of leucine, a branched-chain amino acid, observed in maple syrup urine disease, is associated with reduced alanine production and sometimes with hypoglycemia (Ch. 181). After 3 days of fasting, glucose production is derived primarily from hepatic gluconeogenesis. During starvation, renal gluconeogenesis may account for approximately 50 per cent of glucose production.

Hormonal Control of Glucose Homeostasis

The effects of insulin, glucagon, catecholamines, cortisol, and growth hormone on glucose homeostasis and recovery from hypoglycemia are shown in Table 219-1. Insulin is the primary hypoglycemic hormone; the others act by a variety of mechanisms to elevate glucose concentrations. Although glucagon, catecholamines, cortisol, and growth hormone increase in response to insulin-induced hypoglycemia, glucagon makes the major contribution to the acute recovery from hypoglycemia. Catecholamines can modestly elevate glucose concentration in the presence of glucagon deficiency or severe hypoglycemia.

CLINICAL EVALUATION

Defects of many of the mechanisms that maintain plasma glucose in the normal range are associated with readily recognizable clinical syndromes. In some instances the symptoms and signs of the primary disorder predominate over those of hypoglycemia, or at least point to the existence of the primary disorder causing hypoglycemia. In some patients with multisystem disease, poor nutrition, or multiple drug use, the causes of hypoglycemia may be uncertain and the patient too ill to undergo extensive evaluation.

When a patient is observed with symptoms of hypoglycemia, 10 to 20 ml of blood should be drawn in addition to that for glucose determination. Additional analyses (which should include measurement of sulfonylurea if plasma glucose proves to be low) can be determined by the clues generated from the history and physical examination. Such an opportunity may provide sufficient data to establish the cause of the hypoglycemic disorder or to narrow the diagnostic possibilities. Glucose or glucagon should be administered, following blood withdrawal, to any patient suspected of being hypoglycemic. Prompt treatment shortens the duration of hypoglycemia, and, if the patient is not hypoglycemic, no harm is done.

In patients with asymptomatic hypoglycemia one must be alert to artifactual hypoglycemia. Whole blood glucose values may be spuriously low in polycythemia vera because of the unequal distribution of glucose between erythyrocyte and plasma and excessive glycolysis by erythrocytes and in leukemia from excessive glycolysis by leukocytes. Prompt measurement of glucose in plasma in these conditions should provide accurate results.

An uncommon and challenging problem is the low plasma glucose concentration in an asymptomatic patient in whom laboratory error and spurious result have been ruled out. Such patients may have adapted to longstanding hypoglycemia or have mild symptoms that have been completely unrecognized.

A flow diagram of a clinical approach to the evaluation of a suspected hypoglycemic disorder is presented in Figure 219-1. Note that the evaluation is directed to patients who appear healthy. For those who do not appear healthy, the results of the history and physical examination determine the direction of the investigation.

Hypoglycemic disorders cause a constellation of symptoms that usually recur as discrete episodes at irregular intervals. A useful but not infallible historical aid is the timing of symptoms in relation to food intake: Those occurring within 5 hours of food intake are the food-stimulated hypoglycemias and those occurring 5 or more hours after food intake are the food-deprived hypoglycemias (Fig. 219-2).

Considerable effort should be expended to obtain from the patient and family members a detailed description of symptoms, and careful attention should be paid to their occurrence in relation to food intake. The food-stimulated hypoglycemias usually cause symptoms mediated by the autonomic nervous system—sweating, shakiness, anxiety, palpitations, and weakness—and rarely those of impairment of central nervous system function. The food-deprived hypoglycemias, on the other hand, usually result in impairment of central nervous system function—reduced intellectual capacity, confusion, irritability, abnormal behavior, convulsions, and coma. Hypothermia may be observed. Often the autonomic symptoms that precede the central nervous system symptoms go unrecognized. Symptoms of hypoglycemia usually occur at plasma glucose concentrations of about 45 mg per deciliter or less. They are not related to the rate of fall in glucose concentration. The symptoms of hypoglycemia are nonspecific. For this reason it is necessary to demonstrate a low plasma glucose concentration concomitant with symptoms and subsequent relief of symptoms by correction of the hypoglycemia, i.e., *Whipple's triad*. This triad should be demonstrated before hypoglycemia can be considered to be the basis for a patient's symptoms, regardless of the cause of the hypoglycemia. Since persons without a hypoglycemic disorder may feel better after eating, it is imperative to confirm that symptoms are due to hypoglycemia. Every medication used by the patient, including nonprescription drugs, must be examined.

TABLE 219-1. HORMONAL CONTROL OF GLUCOSE HOMEOSTASIS

Hormone	Hepatic Glucose Production	Extrahepatic Glucose Utilization	Basal Glucose Production	Relative Importance to Recovery from Insulin-induced Hypoglycemia
Insulin	↓	↑	↓	+ + +
Glucagon	↑	—	↑	+
Catecholamine*	↑	↓	—	—
Cortisol	↑	↓	↑	—
Growth hormone†	↑	↓	—	

↑ = increase; ↓ = decrease; — = no effect.
*Epinephrine is approximately 10 times more potent than norepinephrine. Its action is primarily through a β-adrenergic mechanism. In the presence of glucagon deficiency, catecholamines make a modest contribution to the recovery from hypoglycemia.
†Has an acute and transient hypoglycemic effect.

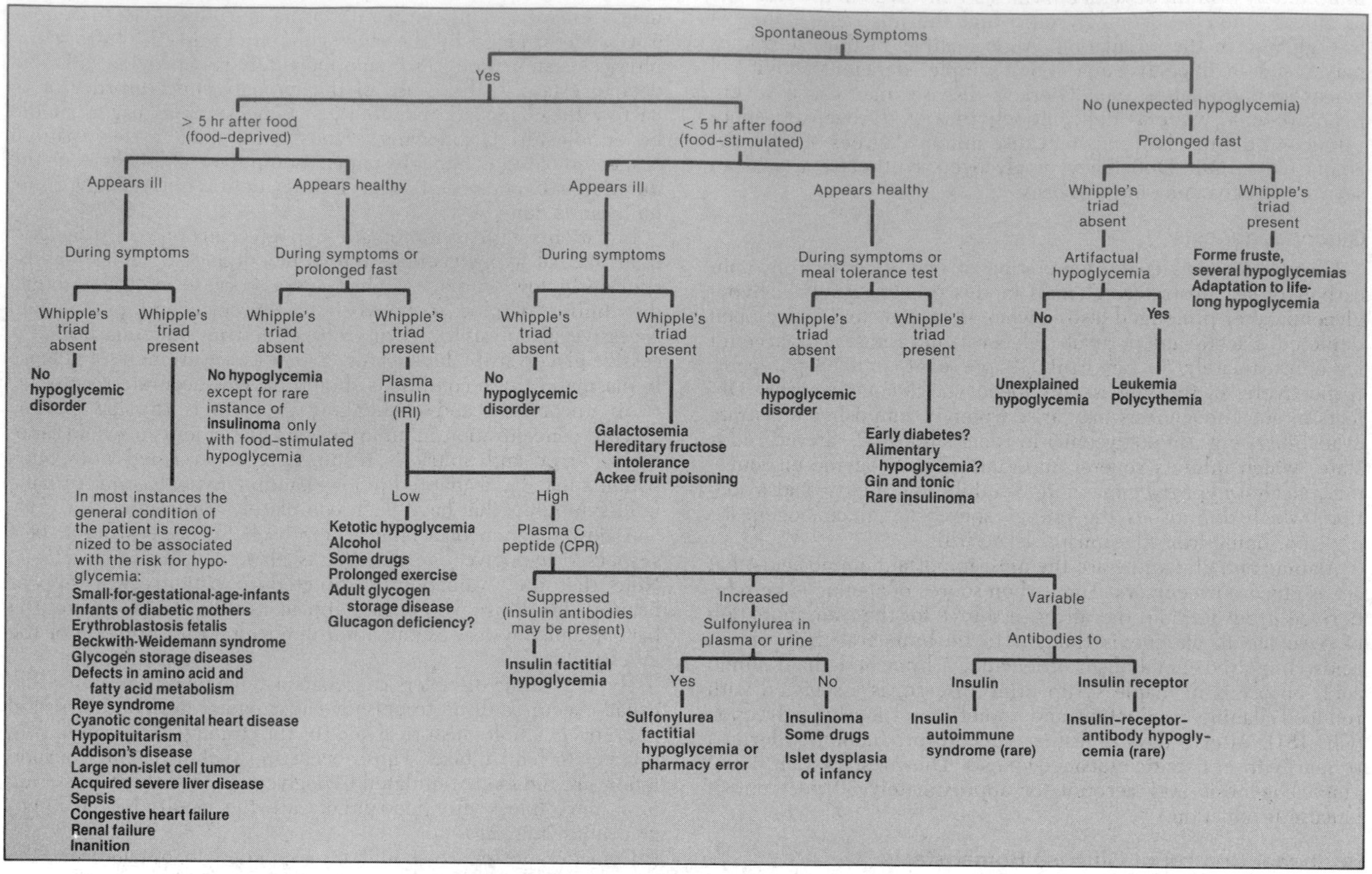

Spontaneous Symptoms

Yes — No (unexpected hypoglycemia)

Yes branch:

> 5 hr after food (food-deprived) — < 5 hr after food (food-stimulated)

> 5 hr after food (food-deprived):

Appears ill — Appears healthy

- Appears ill → During symptoms
  - Whipple's triad absent → **No hypoglycemic disorder**
  - Whipple's triad present → In most instances the general condition of the patient is recognized to be associated with the risk for hypoglycemia:
    **Small-for-gestational-age-infants
    Infants of diabetic mothers
    Erythroblastosis fetalis
    Beckwith-Weidemann syndrome
    Glycogen storage diseases
    Defects in amino acid and fatty acid metabolism
    Reye syndrome
    Cyanotic congenital heart disease
    Hypopituitarism
    Addison's disease
    Large non-islet cell tumor
    Acquired severe liver disease
    Sepsis
    Congestive heart failure
    Renal failure
    Inanition**

- Appears healthy → During symptoms or prolonged fast
  - Whipple's triad absent → **No hypoglycemia except for rare instance of insulinoma only with food-stimulated hypoglycemia**
  - Whipple's triad present → Plasma insulin (IRI)
    - Low → **Ketotic hypoglycemia
      Alcohol
      Some drugs
      Prolonged exercise
      Adult glycogen storage disease
      Glucagon deficiency?**
    - High → Plasma C peptide (CPR)
      - Suppressed (insulin antibodies may be present) → **Insulin factitial hypoglycemia**
        - Yes → **Sulfonylurea factitial hypoglycemia or pharmacy error**
        - No → **Insulinoma Some drugs Islet dysplasia of infancy**
      - Increased → Sulfonylurea in plasma or urine
        - Yes → (Sulfonylurea factitial hypoglycemia or pharmacy error)
        - No → (Insulinoma, Some drugs, Islet dysplasia of infancy)
      - Variable → Antibodies to
        - Insulin → **Insulin autoimmune syndrome (rare)**
        - Insulin receptor → **Insulin-receptor-antibody hypoglycemia (rare)**

< 5 hr after food (food-stimulated):

Appears ill — Appears healthy

- Appears ill → During symptoms
  - Whipple's triad absent → **No hypoglycemic disorder**
  - Whipple's triad present → **Galactosemia Hereditary fructose intolerance Ackee fruit poisoning**

- Appears healthy → During symptoms or meal tolerance test
  - Whipple's triad absent → **No hypoglycemic disorder**
  - Whipple's triad present → **Early diabetes? Alimentary hypoglycemia? Gin and tonic Rare insulinoma**

No (unexpected hypoglycemia):

Prolonged fast

- Whipple's triad absent → Artifactual hypoglycemia
  - No → **Unexplained hypoglycemia**
  - Yes → **Leukemia Polycythemia**
- Whipple's triad present → **Forme fruste, several hypoglycemias Adaptation to life-long hypoglycemia**

FIGURE 219–1. Evaluation of hypoglycemic disorders.

Because of the erratic occurrence of symptoms of hypoglycemia, glucose determination from a venipuncture specimen may not be feasible. Prompt provision by the patient of a capillary blood sample from a lancet puncture of a fingertip during the occurrence of spontaneous symptoms may be useful. Such a sample may be placed on filter paper or into a capillary tube for subsequent measurement of glucose in a laboratory. Reflectance meter measurement of glucose may be inaccurate in the hypoglycemic range.

FOOD-STIMULATED (POSTPRANDIAL) HYPOGLYCEMIAS

Many patients with postprandial symptoms suggestive of hypoglycemia have normal concomitant blood glucose concentra-

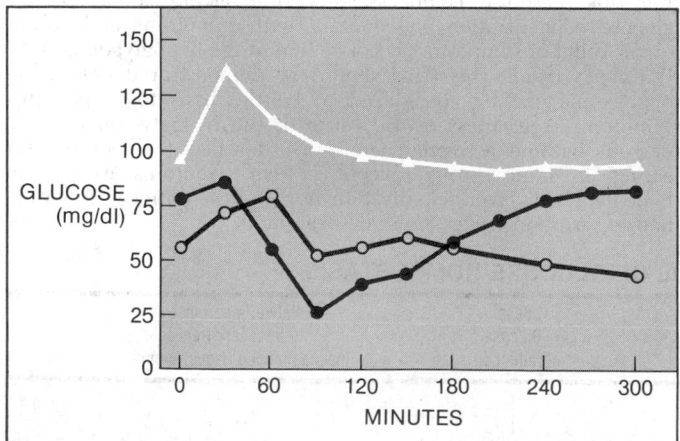

FIGURE 219–2. Differential plasma glucose responses to a mixed meal between patients with food-stimulated hypoglycemia (*closed circles*) and food-deprived hypoglycemia (*open circles*) in contrast to healthy subjects (*triangles*). (Modified from Service FJ: Hypoglycemias. *In* Smith LH Jr (ed): Cecil Textbook of Medicine Update. Philadelphia, WB Saunders Company, 1990.)

tions. For such cases the term "functional hypoglycemia" was coined. Eventually reliance on Whipple's triad was replaced by use of the oral glucose tolerance test (OGTT). If the symptoms experienced during ordinary daily activities were reproduced and a glucose nadir of 50 mg per deciliter or less was documented during the OGTT, the presence of a food-stimulated hypoglycemic disorder was considered to have been confirmed. Use of the OGTT is often misleading, however, since (1) in at least 10 per cent of healthy persons the plasma glucose nadir is less than 50 mg per deciliter; (2) there is no correlation between the nadir of plasma glucose concentrations and the occurrence of symptoms of hypoglycemia in patients with symptoms suggestive of food-stimulated hypoglycemia; (3) the results of OGTT are variable upon repeated testing; (4) subjects with symptoms during an OGTT may have similar symptoms during a placebo OGTT; and (5) glycemia less than 50 mg per deciliter after oral glucose cannot usually be reproduced after a mixed meal despite the presence of symptoms during both. Measurement of plasma cortisol responses, calculation of rates of glucose descent, and hypoglycemic indices have not improved the accuracy of the OGTT.

Unfortunately, reliance on the OGTT for the diagnosis of food-stimulated hypoglycemia has led to extensive literature, not on disorders of hypoglycemia but on the test itself. Although there undoubtedly are patients with true postprandial hypoglycemia, most persons with symptoms following meals have psychoneurosis. Low carbohydrate–high protein diets, sulfonylureas, biguanides, and anticholinergic agents have not been shown to be effective treatment for such patients.

Hypoglycemia following the ingestion of substances that are toxic to susceptible persons may be considered in the category of postprandial hypoglycemias. The ingestion of large amounts (equivalent of three highballs) of ethanol and carbohydrate (gin and tonic) may cause hypoglycemia within 3 to 4 hours in some healthy persons. The unripe ackee fruit may result in hypoglycemia in children or adults with chronic malnutrition by inhibiting the transport of long-chain fatty acids into mitochondria, thereby suppressing their oxidation and depressing gluconeogenesis. Postprandial hypoglycemia occurs in children with galactosemia (Ch.

TABLE 219–2. SYMPTOMS OF HYPOGLYCEMIA

Autonomic nervous system dysfunction
  Sweating
  Shakiness
  Anxiety
  Palpitations
  Weakness

Central nervous system dysfunction
  Diplopia
  Blurred vision
  Confusion
  Abnormal behavior
  Amnesia
  Unconsciousness
  Seizures

168) and hereditary fructose intolerance (Ch. 170) should the relevant offending hexose be eaten.

FOOD-DEPRIVED (FASTING) HYPOGLYCEMIAS

Drug-Induced Hypoglycemias

Drugs constitute the most common cause of hypoglycemia, when treatment of diabetic persons with insulin and sulfonylureas is included. Errors in filling prescriptions by substitution of a sulfonylurea for the intended medication and drug administration errors by hospital staff or the patient are increasingly common causes of hypoglycemia. Factors increasing the risk of drug-induced hypoglycemia are extremes of age, antecedent food deprivation, and impaired renal and hepatic function. Other drugs implicated as the cause of hypoglycemia are salicylates (in children), propranolol (in patients with other conditions having the potential to cause hypoglycemia), ethanol, disopyramide (Norpace), sulfamethoxazole and trimethoprim (Bactrim, Septra) (in the presence of renal failure), pentamidine (Lomidine), and quinine (when used for cerebral malaria). Since a wide variety of drugs has been implicated as the cause of hypoglycemia, the reader is referred to review articles on this subject.

Ethanol-induced hypoglycemia arises from inhibition of gluconeogenesis as a result of the increase in the NADH-NAD ratio in instances of depleted hepatic glycogen. The increased NADH-NAD ratio suppresses the conversions of lactate to pyruvate, glycerophosphate to dihydroxyacetone phosphate, and glutamate to ketoglutarate and several tricarboxylic cycle reactions. Infusion of ethanol into healthy subjects for 4 hours results in hypoglycemia, reduced rates of hepatic glucose production, suppressed plasma insulin concentrations, increased plasma lactate, β-hydroxybutyrate, glycerol, and free fatty acid concentrations, and increased lactate-pyruvate and β-hydroxybutyrate-acetoacetate ratios. Hypoglycemia usually develops within 6 to 36 hours of the ingestion of even moderate amounts of ethanol by persons chronically malnourished or by healthy persons who have missed one or two meals. Healthy children are especially susceptible to ethanol hypoglycemia. Blood ethanol levels may not be elevated when the patient is hypoglycemic.

INSULINOMA

Insulinoma is a rare disorder; its incidence is approximately 1 patient per 250,000 person-years. Insulinoma may occur slightly more commonly in women. It is uncommon in persons less than 20 years of age and rare in those less than 5 years of age. The median age at diagnosis is about 50 years, except in patients with the multiple endocrine neoplasia syndrome type 1 (MEN 1), in which it is in the mid 20's.

Of patients with insulinoma, approximately 87 per cent have single benign tumors, approximately 7 per cent have multiple benign tumors, and approximately 6 per cent have malignant tumors. Eight per cent of insulinoma patients have MEN 1 (Ch. 228). Sixty per cent of patients with MEN 1 have multiple tumors. Fifty per cent of patients with multiple insulinomas have MEN 1.

Some tumors secrete hormones in addition to insulin: gastrin, 5-hydroxyindoles, ACTH, glucagon, and somatostatin. In rare instances, insulinomas have occurred in non–insulin-dependent diabetic persons but have never been documented in an insulin-dependent patient.

Clinical Picture

Symptoms may be present for many years prior to the diagnosis. In one series 85 per cent of patients had various combinations of diplopia, blurred vision, sweating, palpitations, and weakness; 80 per cent had confusion or abnormal behavior; 53 per cent had unconsciousness or amnesia; and 12 per cent had grand mal seizures (Table 219–2). Twenty per cent of cases may be misdiagnosed, the belief being that the patient has a neurologic or psychiatric disorder.

Hypoglycemia usually occurs 5 or more hours after any meal. In rare instances, symptoms may occur solely in the postprandial period (2 to 4 hours after eating) and never during fasting. Symptoms may be aggravated by exercise, alcohol use, a high protein–low carbohydrate diet, treatment with sulfonylureas, and fasts. Less than 20 per cent of patients with insulinoma gain weight.

Diagnosis

The diagnosis of insulinoma is based on the demonstration of Whipple's triad and nonsuppressed plasma insulin and C-peptide levels, either with spontaneous hypoglycemia or with that induced by a prolonged fast. A simplified diagnostic scheme is shown in Figure 219–3. Insulin antibodies are usually undetectable but may be present in low titers. In lieu of demonstrating Whipple's triad during the spontaneous occurrence of symptoms, useful diagnostic tests are the prolonged supervised fast, the intravenous tolbutamide test, and the C-peptide suppression test.

SUPERVISED FAST. The prolonged supervised fast is the classic test for the diagnosis of insulinoma. During the fast the patient should be active during the day. Noncaloric beverages may be consumed. The frequency of blood sampling should be guided by the patient's history of tolerance to food withdrawal

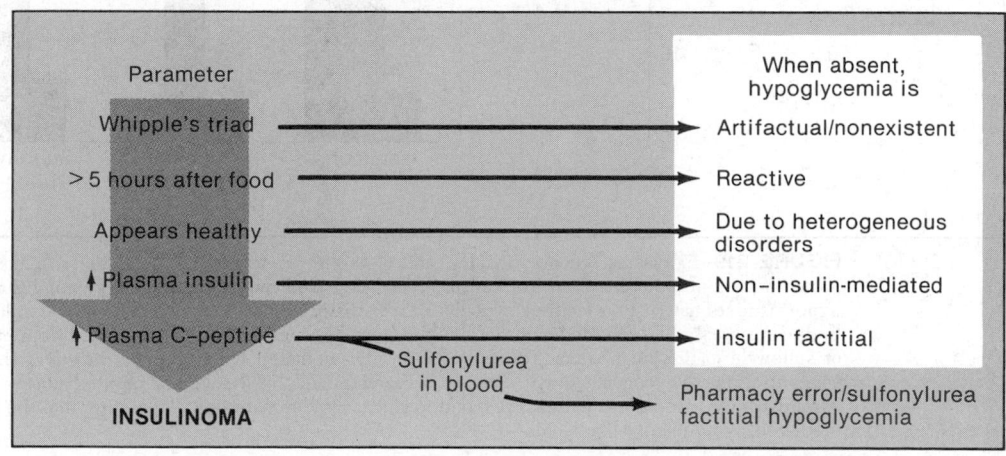

FIGURE 219–3. Important parameters for the diagnosis of insulinoma.

Parameter	When absent, hypoglycemia is
Whipple's triad	Artifactual/nonexistent
>5 hours after food	Reactive
Appears healthy	Due to heterogeneous disorders
↑ Plasma insulin	Non–insulin-mediated
↑ Plasma C-peptide	Insulin factitial
Sulfonylurea in blood	Pharmacy error/sulfonylurea factitial hypoglycemia
INSULINOMA	

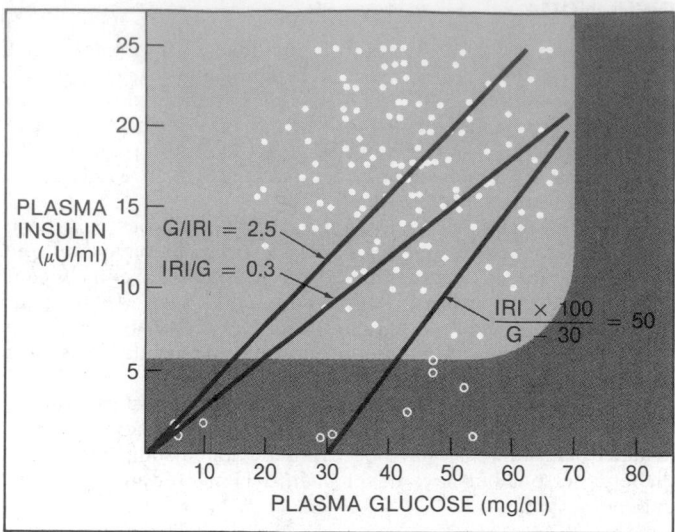

FIGURE 219–4. Simultaneously measured plasma glucose and insulin concentrations in patients with histologically confirmed insulinoma (*closed circles*) and in patients with non–insulin-mediated hypoglycemia (*open circles*). Various ratios: Glucose/insulin = 2.5, insulin/glucose = 0.3, and insulin × 100/glucose − 30 = 50, designed to establish relative hyperinsulinemia, are much less useful than using a value of plasma insulin of 6 μU per milliliter as a discriminator. (Reprinted with permission from Service FJ: Clinical presentation and laboratory evaluation of hypoglycemic disorders in adults. *In* Service FJ (ed.): Hypoglycemic Disorders. Boston, GK Hall, 1983, pp 73–95.)

and be increased as the plasma glucose approaches the hypoglycemic range. Whenever blood is withdrawn for glucose determination, plasma insulin and C-peptide should be measured. Plasma should also be submitted for detection of sulfonylurea, especially if accidental or surreptitious ingestion of this drug is suspected. The patient's mental status should be checked regularly. During prolonged fasting healthy women experience lower plasma glucose concentrations than do healthy men: Values as low as 42 mg per deciliter in men and 34 mg per deciliter in women may be unaccompanied by symptoms. Therefore, it is essential to continue the fast to the point at which symptoms develop, or to 72 hours. Upon demonstration of Whipple's triad, either during the prolonged fast or spontaneously, glucagon, 1 mg, should be injected intravenously. Whereas a prompt increase in glucose concentration indicates an insulin-mediated hypoglycemic disorder such as insulinoma, a blunted glucose response indicates glycogen storage disease or a disorder that impairs glycogenesis or glycogenolysis.

Plasma insulin concentrations frequently are "normal" when the plasma glucose is in the hypoglycemic range (Fig. 219–4). Since patients with insulinoma have been observed to have plasma insulin levels as low as 6 μU per milliliter during hypoglycemia, relative hyperinsulinemia (nonsuppressed insulin levels) may be considered as values of 6 μU per milliliter or more. Glucose-insulin ratios are less helpful in confirming relative hyperinsulinemia (Fig. 219–4). The patterns of plasma glucose, insulin, and C-peptide during hypoglycemia and the plasma glucose response to intravenous glucagon, 1 mg, are shown in Figure 219–5 for insulinoma and other causes of food-deprived hypoglycemia.

In a large series, Whipple's triad was demonstrated within 12 hours of the last meal in 29 per cent of patients, within 24 hours in 71 per cent, within 36 hours in 79 per cent, within 48 hours in 92 per cent, within 60 hours in 97 per cent, and within 72 hours in 98 per cent. In rare instances, patients with insulinoma may not develop hypoglycemia during prolonged fasting of even up to 96 hours. At the time of hypoglycemic symptoms, plasma glucose concentrations were 46 mg per deciliter or less in 100 per cent of patients, 39 mg per deciliter or less in 75 per cent, 35 mg per deciliter or less in 50 per cent, and 28 mg per deciliter or less in 25 per cent.

THE INTRAVENOUS TOLBUTAMIDE TEST. This test (tolbutamide, 1 gram intravenously over 3 minutes) should be performed only in persons for whom the fasting plasma glucose is known to exceed 50 mg per deciliter immediately prior to the test and who have not been food deprived for several days preceding the test. The best criterion for the interpretation of the tolbutamide test is the mean of the values at 120, 150, and 180 minutes (Fig. 219–6). The criterion of 55 mg per deciliter for lean persons and 62 mg per deciliter for obese persons provides 95 per cent and 100 per cent sensitivity, respectively,

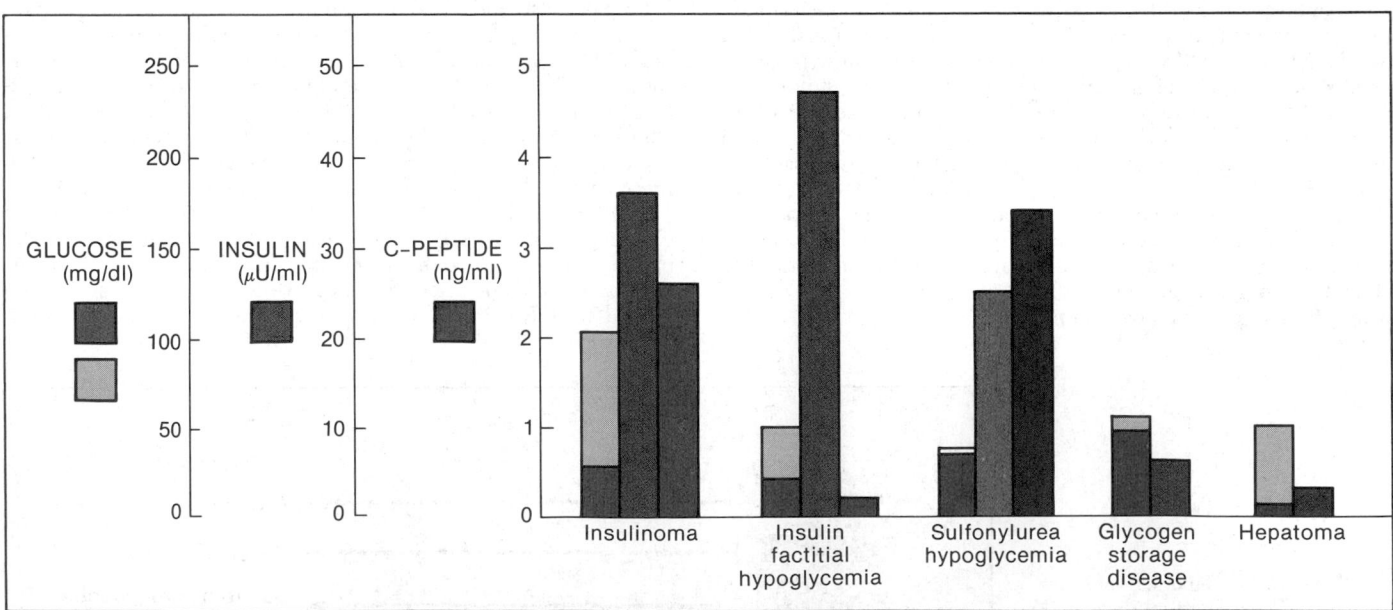

FIGURE 219–5. Plasma glucose, insulin, and C-peptide concentrations and the response of plasma glucose to intravenous glucagon (1 mg) in five causes of food-deprived hypoglycemia. Three conditions are characterized by hyperinsulinemia: Insulin factitial hypoglycemia is distinguished from insulinoma and sulfonylurea hypoglycemia by the suppressed C-peptide level. Sulfonylurea hypoglycemia can be distinguished from insulin only by detection of sulfonylurea in the plasma. The two non–insulin-mediated hypoglycemic disorders show low plasma insulin concentrations. Glycogen storage disease is characterized by a severely blunted glucose response to glucagon administration. Hepatoma patients respond to glucagon administration, suggesting that the hypoglycemia is in part mediated by an insulin-like factor—IGF II?

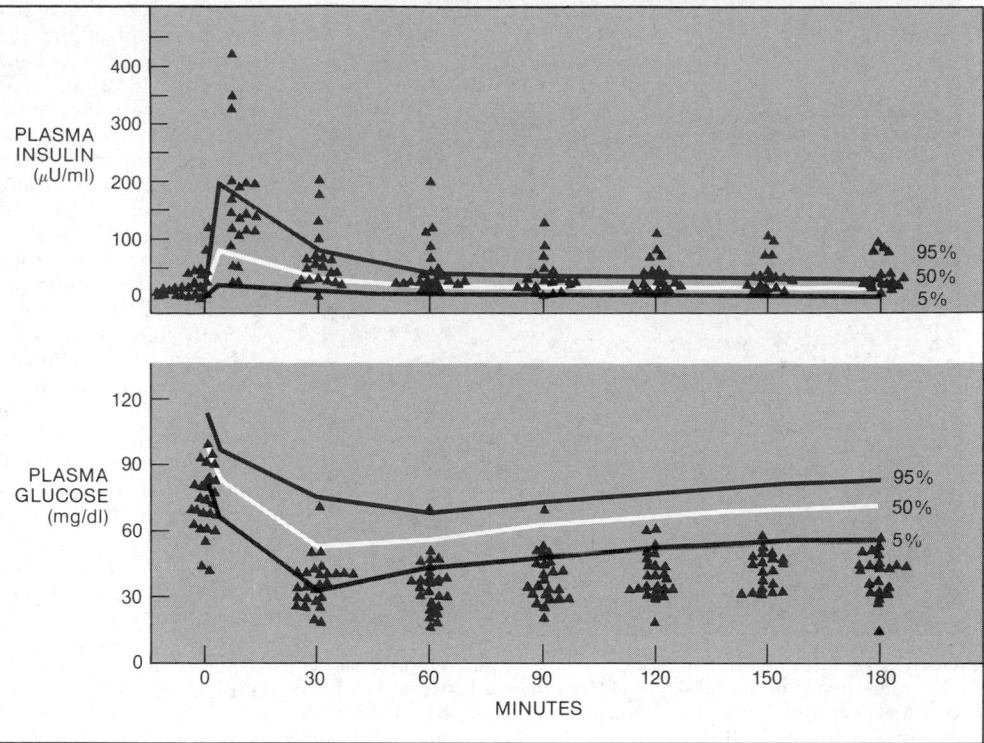

FIGURE 219-6. Plasma glucose and insulin responses to the intravenous tolbutamide test in 261 lean, healthy persons shown as the 5th, 50th, and 95th percentiles and 27 lean patients with insulinoma shown as triangles. (Modified from McMahon MM, et al.: Diagnostic interpretation of the intravenous tolbutamide test for insulinoma. Mayo Clin Proc 64:1481, 1989.)

at 95 per cent specificity. Plasma insulin responses are less sensitive diagnostic discriminators. If the plasma glucose responses to intravenous tolbutamide are normal, the insulin values should be ignored.

THE C-PEPTIDE SUPPRESSION TEST. This test (insulin 0.125 unit per kilogram over 60 minutes or an equivalent total dose given at a slower rate over 3 hours) is based on the observation that hypoglycemia induced by exogenous insulin fails to suppress C-peptide concentration normally in those with insulinomas (Fig. 219-7). The criteria for normal C-peptide suppression are influenced by age and body mass index. The euglycemic C-peptide suppression test involves maintenance of euglycemia during insulin infusion. This approach relies on inhibition of insulin release by insulin itself and has the advantage of avoiding hypoglycemia. It is difficult to know how useful this approach to C-peptide suppression is because it has been used in only a few patients. Furthermore, if the patient is hypoglycemic prior to the test, the test is virtually in process: Measurement of plasma glucose, insulin, and C-peptide will provide a diagnosis. If the patient is not hypoglycemic, the standard test (insulin infusion without maintaining euglycemia) can be conducted.

THE INTRAVENOUS GLUCAGON TEST. This test (glucagon, 1 mg intravenously) has an accuracy of 50 to 80 per cent using criteria of peak insulin of 130 μU per milliliter or more or an increase above basal level of 100 μU per milliliter or more when conducted after an overnight fast. Unfortunately, many medications influence the response to glucagon.

OTHER TESTS. The utility of other tests such as glycosylated hemoglobin, human pancreatic polypeptide, and infusions of alcohol, calcium, epinephrine and propranolol, diazoxide, and somatostatin-tolbutamide in the diagnosis of insulinoma is unproven or inadequate. Human chorionic gonadotropin or one of its subunits may be a marker for functioning malignant insulinomas. Eighty per cent of patients with insulinoma may have elevated proinsulin concentrations (>20 per cent of total immunoreactive insulin). Recently improved assays for proinsulin may enhance its diagnostic accuracy.

Localization

Only after the diagnosis of insulinoma has been confirmed biochemically should a localization procedure be done. Pancreatic

angiography has been reported to have a high rate of success if stereoscopy, magnification, and subtraction are used. Insulinomas appear as homogeneous, intensely vascular, sharply circumscribed masses within the substance of the pancreas.

Computed tomography has had limited success in localization. Real-time high-resolution ultrasonography performed by a skilled operator is the preferred localization procedure. Success at finding the tumor is 68 per cent for preoperative ultrasonography and 86 per cent for intraoperative ultrasonography (Fig. 219-8). Percutaneous transhepatic portal venous sampling for insulin has the disadvantage of being highly invasive. It is usually unnecessary if a skilled ultrasonographer is available. Failure to localize an insulinoma preoperatively should not deter pancreatic exploration in a patient for whom the diagnosis has been firmly established, because the combination of a skilled surgeon and an ultrasonographer experienced with insulinomas is highly successful in finding the tumor.

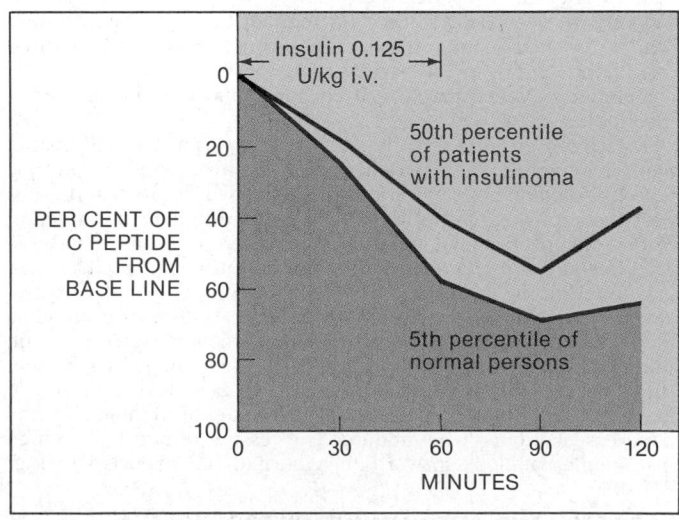

FIGURE 219-7. C-peptide suppression test shows less suppression of C-peptide in a typical patient with insulinoma in contrast to normal persons.

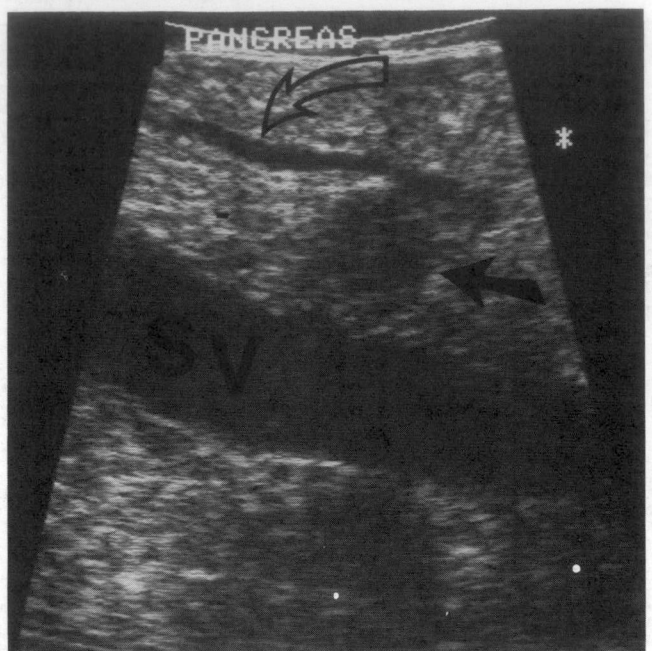

FIGURE 219–8. Intraoperative sonogram showing discrete hypoechoic lesion (*solid arrow*) in the substance of the pancreas between the main pancreatic duct (*open arrow*) and splenic vein (SV). (Reprinted with permission from Gorman B, Charbonneau JW, et al.: Benign pancreatic insulinoma: Preoperative and intraoperative sonographic localization. AJR 147:929, 1986. © 1986, American Roentgen Ray Society.)

Treatment

Surgical removal is the preferred treatment for insulinoma. In a large series, 58 per cent of subjects underwent successful enucleation of the tumor; 33 per cent, partial pancreatectomy; and the remainder, a variety of other procedures. In the series, 88 per cent were cured, 2 per cent had diabetes, and the remainder required medical treatment to control persistent hypoglycemia from malignant insulinoma, islet hyperplasia, or a tumor missed during surgery. Operative mortality has not been observed for many decades. The postoperative complication rate is about 10 per cent. The risk of recurrence is 8 per cent at 20 years following initial successful resection.

Intraoperative glucose monitoring should not be relied upon for surgical management, since there is a high (23 per cent) incidence of failure of plasma glucose to increase after successful insulinoma removal.

The median diameter of benign tumors is 1.5 cm. Malignant tumors (identified on the basis of metastases) are usually larger. Tumors are evenly distributed throughout the pancreas, whether benign or malignant, single or multiple. Ectopically located insulinoma and islet hyperplasia are very rare. There is no correlation between the severity of symptoms and the size of the insulinoma.

Treatment of persistent hypoglycemia in a patient with malignant insulinoma, in a patient in whom insulinoma cannot be found at pancreatic exploration, or in one who refuses surgery is best accomplished with diazoxide, which inhibits insulin release. Phenytoin, propranolol, and verapamil have been used successfully in some cases. A long-acting somatostatin analogue has been disappointing in the lack of effective control of hypoglycemia in several patients with malignant insulinoma. Malignant insulinoma metastasizes primarily to local structures such as regional lymph nodes and liver; distant metastases are uncommon. The chemotherapeutic regimen of choice consists of streptozotocin and 5-fluorouracil. Survival exceeds that in adenocarcinoma of the pancreas. Patients who undergo successful removal of benign insulinoma can look forward to a normal life expectancy (Fig. 219–9).

FACTITIAL AND AUTOIMMUNE HYPOGLYCEMIA

Nondiabetic persons who secretly take insulin or sulfonylureas are predominantly women in the third and fourth decades of life who are employed in health-related occupations. Patients with factitial hypoglycemia have an erratic pattern in the occurrence of symptoms and may tolerate prolonged periods of fasting. With the exception of the rare instance of the insulin autoimmune syndrome and occasional insulinomas, the presence of insulin antibodies is strong evidence of repeated injection of insulin. In addition, the presence of low plasma concentrations of C-peptide concomitant with elevated insulin levels and hypoglycemia indicates an exogenous source of insulin (see Fig. 219–5). Insulin antibodies cause spurious radioimmunoassayable plasma insulin concentrations: very high if the double-antibody assay is used and undetectable if the charcoal-coated dextran assay is used. Results of tests for insulinoma (including the C-peptide suppression test if the patient is taking a sulfonylurea) may be indistinguishable between an insulinoma patient and a patient who secretly took the hypoglycemic agent prior to the test (see Fig. 219–5). Concentrations of sulfonylurea should be measured in the plasma or urine if it is suspected of being the hypoglycemic agent. The clinical pattern in diabetic subjects consists of increased frequency of hypoglycemia during treatment and persistence of hypoglycemic episodes after complete cessation of use of the agent. The presence of insulin antibodies is of no help in the diagnosis in the insulin-treated patient. An inverse relation between C-peptide and insulin levels during hypoglycemia is diagnostic of surreptitious insulin administration. Insulin has been used for suicide, homicide, and child abuse.

Autoimmune hypoglycemia comprises two classes of patients, those with insulin antibodies who have apparently never been exposed to exogenous insulin and those with insulin receptor antibodies. The patients with spontaneous generation of insulin antibodies have ranged in age from a few days old to elderly. Hypoglycemia may be severe, may occur during fasting or postprandially, and is often self-limited. During episodes of hypoglycemia, plasma free insulin levels have been found to be elevated and plasma C-peptide concentrations have varied from elevated to suppressed. Distinguishing between insulin antibody autoimmune hypoglycemia and factitial hypoglycemia may be very difficult. The observation of intermittent production of an abnormal insulin that is immunogenic has not been supported by other studies. Species specificity, association constants, and binding capacities for human, porcine, and bovine insulins of the antibodies from patients with autoimmune hypoglycemia are not different from those of antibodies from insulin-treated diabetics. However, there are sufficient differences in the frequency and duration of insulin administration between patients with factitial hypoglycemia and insulin-treated diabetics to require full characterization of the insulin, proinsulin, and C-peptide antibodies in proved factitial hypoglycemia for comparison with those of the autoimmune hypoglycemic syndrome. Distinction between autoimmune and factitial hypoglycemia by antibody characteristics may become even more difficult now that human insulin has come into common use. Neither the biochemical characteristics of this syndrome nor the mechanism of the hypoglycemia has been fully elucidated.

Hypoglycemia has been observed in persons with insulin receptor antibodies. During hypoglycemia, plasma insulin levels have been found to be elevated and C-peptide levels have been suppressed. Most of the patients with hypoglycemia had preexisting insulin-resistant diabetes and evidence for autoimmune disease prior to the development of hypoglycemia. Antagonist and agonist action of insulin receptor antibodies may be due to different populations of insulin receptor antibodies which recognize different antigenic sites. This syndrome may respond to glucocorticoid therapy or methylpalmoxinate, an inhibitor of free fatty acid oxidation, but is not improved by immunosuppressive agents or plasmapheresis.

NON–BETA CELL TUMOR HYPOGLYCEMIA

A wide variety of tumors of mesenchymal or epithelial origin and some malignant hematologic diseases have been associated with hypoglycemia.

Mesenchymal tumors account for 45 to 64 per cent of the reported cases. Approximately one third of the tumors are located in the chest and two thirds are in the abdomen, usually in the retroperitoneum. They usually are large and therefore readily detectable. Hepatomas account for 22 per cent of cases.

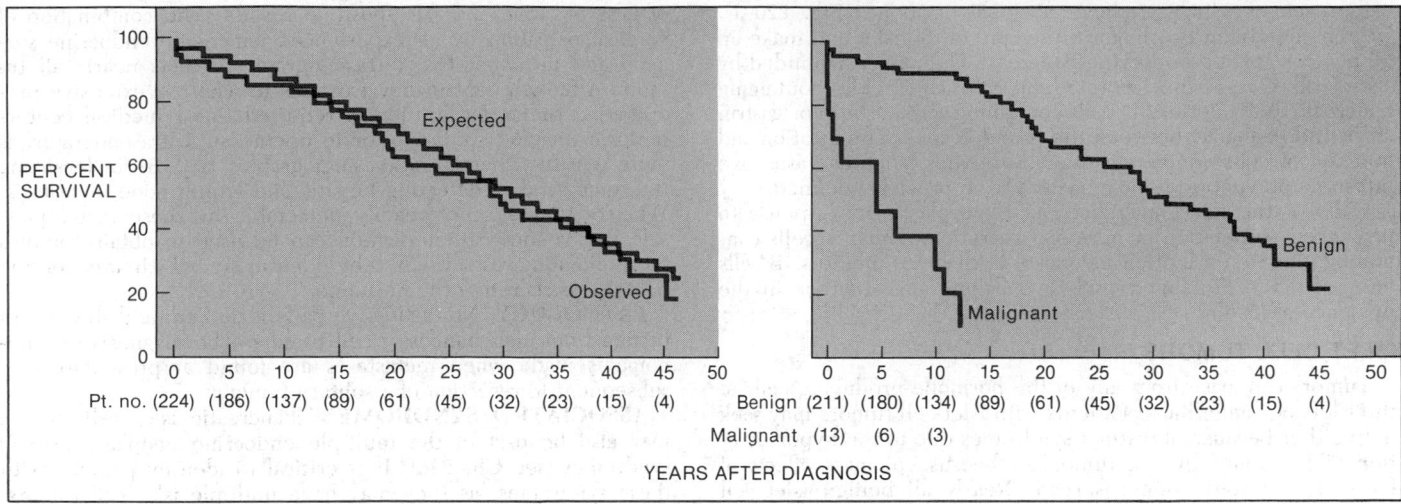

FIGURE 219–9. Survival (%) after histologic confirmation of insulinoma observed in 224 patients over 45 years in contrast to expected survival, and in benign versus malignant insulinoma. (Reprinted with permission from Service FJ, Nelson RL: Insulinoma. Compr Ther 6:70–74, 1980.)

No single pathogenetic mechanism satisfactorily explains all cases of tumor-related hypoglycemia. In some, more than one mechanism may be involved. Metastatic destruction of the adrenals or pituitary and extensive metastatic involvement of the liver can impair glucoregulatory mechanisms. Some tumors evince a high rate of glucose utilization. In others, substances such as tryptophan metabolites may impair gluconeogenesis. There has not been convincing documentation of insulin secretion by a non–islet cell tumor, although hyperinsulinism resolved following tumor removal in one patient. Although elevated levels of insulin-like growth factor II (IGF II) and IGF II mRNA have been observed in some patients with non–islet cell tumor hypoglycemia, there is controversy regarding the role of the polypeptide in the genesis of hypoglycemia. Total or partial surgical removal of the tumor usually results in amelioration of the hypoglycemia.

HYPOGLYCEMIA IN HEPATIC, RENAL, AND ENDOCRINE DISORDERS AND MISCELLANEOUS CONDITIONS

Symptomatic hypoglycemia is uncommon in liver disease because glucose homeostasis can be maintained with as little as 20 per cent of healthy parenchymal cells, but biochemical hypoglycemia has been reported in a wide variety of acquired hepatic diseases. The hypoglycemia of congestive heart failure, sepsis, and Reye's syndrome is considered to be due to hepatic mechanisms. During hypoglycemia, plasma insulin and C-peptide concentrations are suppressed.

Hypoglycemia is uncommon in adrenocortical insufficiency. Hypoglycemia in hypopituitarism is common in children under 6 years of age but less so beyond that age. Asymptomatic hypoglycemia has been observed in isolated growth hormone deficiency after prolonged fasting. Spontaneous hypoglycemia has been reported to be a frequent finding in isolated ACTH deficiency. Adults surgically deprived of epinephrine are not subject to hypoglycemia.

Hypoglycemia in nondiabetic persons with renal failure may be due to inadequate gluconeogenic substrate availability. Glucagon deficiency is a theoretic mechanism for hypoglycemia, but the existence of this disorder has not been confirmed.

Hypoglycemia is a concomitant of starvation. It has been observed in persons with protein-calorie malnutrition as a result of anorexia nervosa or extreme food faddism. Inanition may be one of several factors in the genesis of hypoglycemia in patients with multisystem disease and prolonged intravenous fluid therapy. Prolonged, severe exercise may provoke hypoglycemia in untrained persons but is less likely to do so in athletes.

Garber AJ, Bier DM, Cryer PE, et al.: Hypoglycemia in compensated chronic renal insufficiency. Substrate limitation of gluconeogenesis. Diabetes 23:982, 1974. *Data are presented indicating that hypoglycemia in chronic renal failure may be due to inadequate availability of alanine.*

Hogan MJ, Service FJ, Sharbrough F, et al.: Oral glucose tolerance test compared with a mixed meal in the diagnosis of reactive hypoglycemia. A caveat on stimulation. Mayo Clin Proc 58:491, 1983. *The authors demonstrated the inadequacy of the oral glucose tolerance test for the diagnosis of postprandial symptoms. Patients considered to have food-stimulated hypoglycemia after oral glucose tolerance testing had no hypoglycemia after a mixed meal despite the presence of postprandial symptoms. In addition, EEG monitoring during postprandial symptoms showed no changes.*

Lowe WL, Roberts CT Jr, LeRoith D, et al.: Insulin-like growth factor-II in nonislet cell tumors associated with hypoglycemia: Increased levels of messenger ribonucleic acid. J Clin Endocrinol Metab 69:1153, 1989. *Nonislet cell tumors associated with hypoglycemia were found to produce large amounts of IGF-II mRNA.*

Marks V: Hypoglycemia. Oxford, Blackwell Scientific Publications, Ltd., 1981. *An authoritative reference work on hypoglycemic disorders.*

Palardy J, Havrankova J, Lepage R, et al.: Blood glucose measurements during symptomatic episodes in patients with suspected postprandial hypoglycemia. N Engl J Med 321:1421, 1989. *The importance of measuring glucose during the occurrence of spontaneous symptoms of hypoglycemia is clearly demonstrated by the data in this paper. When self-collected capillary blood specimens on filter paper were analyzed for glucose, only 5 per cent had values less than 2.8 mM per liter (50 mg per deciliter).*

Scarlett JA, Mako ME, Rubenstein AH, et al.: Factitious hypoglycemia. Diagnosis and measurement of serum C-peptide immunoreactivity and insulin-binding antibodies. N Engl J Med 297:1029, 1977. *Seven cases of surreptitious injection of insulin are described. The authors emphasize the importance of the triad of low plasma glucose and high plasma insulin levels and suppression of plasma C-peptide for diagnosis of this condition. In addition, there is a useful discussion of characteristics of antibodies to insulin, proinsulin, and C-peptide of human, porcine, and bovine origin for the distinction between factitial and autoimmune hypoglycemia.*

Seltzer HS: Severe drug-induced hypoglycemia: A review. Comp Ther 5:21, 1979. *An excellent reference source regarding the drugs implicated and the conditions conducive to drug-induced hypoglycemia.*

Service FJ, McMahon MM, O'Brien PC, et al.: Incidence, recurrence and survival of insulinoma. A sixty-year study. In preparation. *This paper provides new information on the natural history of insulinoma generated from experience over a 60-year period with 224 patients with insulinoma.*

Taylor SI, Greenberger G, Marcus-Samuels B, et al.: Hypoglycemia associated with antibodies to the insulin receptor. N Engl J Med 307:1422, 1982. *The authors report a nondiabetic patient with fasting hypoglycemia ascribed to the action of autoantibodies to the insulin receptor. Although the few other patients with this syndrome had a history of prior diabetes, evidence for coexistent autoimmune disease is a clue to the presence of antireceptor antibodies.*

220 Pancreatic Islet Cell Tumors

Carl Grunfeld

THE ISLETS OF LANGERHANS

Dispersed throughout the exocrine pancreas are nests of endocrine cells, the islets of Langerhans. The islet itself is a miniature organ with a distinctive organization of individualized cells, each of which produces a single hormone (Fig. 220–1). Insulin-containing B cells form the core of the islet and make up 60 per cent of the endocrine pancreas. They are surrounded by a rim of A cells that secrete glucagon or F cells containing pancreatic polypeptide. D cells containing somatostatin or gastrin are found primarily between the A and B cells. The location and function of cells containing other hormones, such as vasoactive intestinal polypeptide, have not yet been precisely defined.

Cells of the islets may become hyperplastic in response to prolonged stimulation of hormone secretion. Thus, A cells containing glucagon are often increased in diabetes mellitus. B cells increase after prolonged excessive caloric ingestion or in the presence of insulin resistance.

ISLET CELL TUMORS

Tumors can arise from any of the hormone-producing cells of the islets of Langerhans. Patients with islet cell tumors may seek help either because of distinct syndromes due to the hypersecretion of hormones by the tumors or because of mass effects of local or metastatic tumor spread. Nearly all benign islet cell tumors and more than 80 per cent of carcinomas secrete clinically significant amounts of hormone; some secrete multiple hormones. Clinical presentation usually reflects the dominance of one hormone (Table 220–1).

The tumor is named after the hormone responsible for the syndrome or, in asymptomatic patients, the hormone found in highest concentration in the circulation or in the tumor. For example, a tumor producing insulin is known as an insulinoma, and one producing glucagon is a glucagonoma. Tumors may also secrete human chorionic gonadotropin or chromogranin A and B.

DIAGNOSIS. Diagnosis of islet cell tumors is usually made by detecting elevated basal or fasting levels of the suspected hormone in the presence of the characteristic syndrome. Provocative tests have also been developed that use pharmacologic agents to discriminate between secretion from a tumor and from normal pancreas. In addition, tumors usually secrete a larger proportion of prohormone or other species of high molecular weight than do normal islet cells.

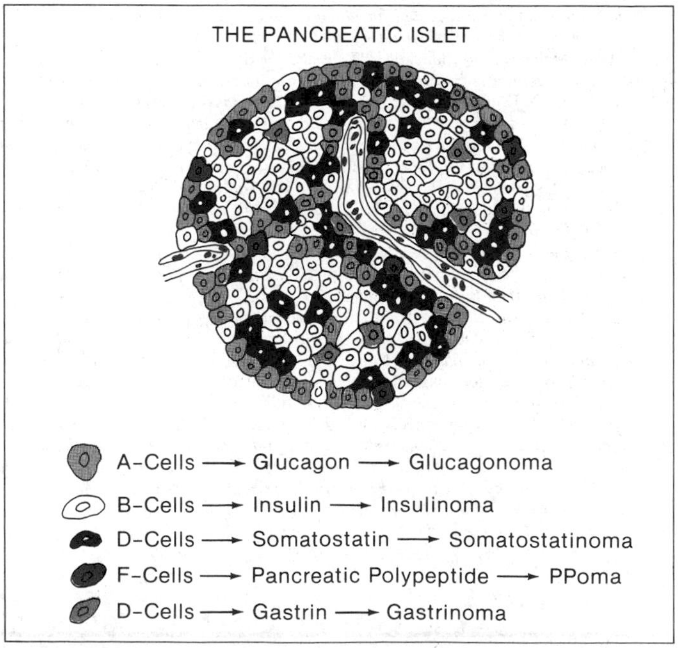

THE PANCREATIC ISLET

A–Cells ——→ Glucagon ——→ Glucagonoma

B–Cells ——→ Insulin ——→ Insulinoma

D–Cells ——→ Somatostatin ——→ Somatostatinoma

F–Cells ——→ Pancreatic Polypeptide ——→ PPoma

D–Cells ——→ Gastrin ——→ Gastrinoma

FIGURE 220–1. Morphology of the islets of Langerhans. This schematic representation of a typical islet demonstrates the distinctive distribution of hormone-secreting cells within the islet. Insulin-containing B cells, forming the core of the islet, are surrounded by glucagon-containing A cells. D cells are interspersed. In the posterior portion of the head of the pancreas, the proportion of cells containing pancreatic polypeptide is increased and the number of glucagon-secreting cells is strikingly decreased. (Modified from Unger RH, Orci L: Glucagon and the A cell: Physiology and pathophysiology. N Engl J Med 304:1518, 1981. Reprinted by permission of the New England Journal of Medicine.)

Imaging techniques should not be relied upon to make the diagnosis of an islet cell tumor, as there are a significant number of false-negative and false-positive results. The combination of surgical palpation by an experienced pancreatic endocrine surgeon and intraoperative ultrasonography detects nearly all tumors. Although controversy exists as to whether extensive preoperative tumor localization is required, most medical centers perform imaging studies prior to operation. Ultrasonography is more sensitive than CT scan, angiography, or MRI for localizing the tumor and in detecting hepatic and lymph node metastasis. When a tumor is not readily detectable by these techniques, selective venous catheterization can be used to obtain samples for radioimmunoassay, thereby identifying which area of the pancreas is secreting the hormone.

PATHOLOGY. No distinctive pathologic finding distinguishes benign from malignant islet cell tumors. The diagnosis of carcinoma is made when metastases are found at presentation or subsequent to resection of a solitary tumor.

ASSOCIATED SYNDROMES. Pancreatic islet cell tumors may also be part of the multiple endocrine neoplasia (MEN) syndromes (see Ch. 228). It is critical to identify patients with these syndromes, as they may have multiple islet cell tumors. Identification of the tumor or area of the pancreas responsible for excess secretion is essential to allow limited pancreatic resection. Unfortunately in patients with an MEN syndrome, tumors may recur, necessitating total pancreatectomy. The presence of hypercalcemia in patients with islet cell tumors is suggestive of the MEN 1 syndrome, as 85 per cent of patients with MEN type 1 have hyperparathyroidism at some time.

THERAPY. The primary therapy of solitary islet cell tumors is surgical resection. Therapy for islet cell carcinoma with metastasis is directed toward ameliorating the symptoms of the presenting syndrome and may include pharmacologic inhibitors of hormone secretion and action, chemotherapeutic agents, radiotherapy, or surgical debulking. Octreotide, a long-acting analogue of somatostatin approved for treatment of VIP (vasoactive intestinal polypeptide)-omas and carcinoids, is effective at reversing the symptoms of most islet cell tumors. Symptomatic relief may occur without complete suppression of circulating hormone levels. Although octreotide has become the mainstay for treating the hormone-produced syndromes, symptoms eventually recur with growth of tumor. Specific agents are discussed under each tumor.

Similar syndromes resulting from hypersecretion of pancreatic hormones occasionally occur secondary to diffuse hyperplasia of islet cells. The treatment of hyperplastic syndromes is partial or near-total pancreatectomy.

Insulinoma

The most common islet cell tumor is the insulinoma, which may produce life-threatening hypoglycemia. Insulinoma is reviewed in Ch. 219.

Gastrinoma

The second most common islet cell tumor is the gastrinoma associated with Zollinger-Ellison syndrome, producing recurrent peptic ulcers due to hypersecretion of gastric acid. This syndrome is discussed in Ch. 98.

VIPoma or the Diarrheogenic Syndrome

CLINICAL PRESENTATION. VIPoma or the diarrheogenic syndrome, associated with islet cell tumors, severe watery diarrhea, and hypokalemia, is also called pancreatic cholera, Verner-Morrison syndrome, WDHA (water diarrhea, hypokalemia, achlorhydria) syndrome, or WDHH (water diarrhea, hypokalemia, hypochlorhydria) syndrome. Patients have profound but intermittent secretory diarrhea; peak diarrhea output exceeds 3 liters per day in 80 per cent. A more general discussion of secretory diarrhea is contained in Ch. 101. Unlike the diarrheal discharge of long-term laxative abuse, the discharge in VIPoma is rich in electrolytes; fecal potassium loss can reach 300 mEq per day. Serum potassium is usually less than 3 mEq per liter and is accompanied by acidosis due to severe loss of bicarbonate.

The severe hypokalemia may lead to profound weakness, to flaccid paralysis, and to renal failure due to hypokalemic nephropathy. More than half of the patients have frank diabetes or glucose intolerance, which is probably secondary to hypokalemia, a known inhibitor of insulin secretion (see Ch. 75 for a discussion of hypokalemia). Hypercalcemia is found in half of the patients during attacks and is not usually indicative of hyperparathyroidism (and the MEN 1 syndrome), as parathyroid hormone levels are suppressed and the hypercalcemia remits with resection of the primary islet cell tumor. Despite hypercalcemia, tetany due to hypomagnesemia has been described. Flushing of the skin has been reported.

DIFFERENTIAL DIAGNOSIS. Secretory diarrhea may result from three other endocrine tumors (gastrinoma, carcinoid, and somatostatinoma), but peak volume of diarrhea rarely exceeds 3 liters per day in these syndromes. Further, the diarrhea in Zollinger-Ellison syndrome is caused by hypersecretion of gastric acid and can be reversed by gastric suction or with cimetidine. The diarrheogenic syndrome is almost always accompanied by achlorhydria or hypochlorhydria; decreased gastric acid secretion persists when the diarrhea is in remission and the serum potassium is normal.

PATHOLOGY. Eighty per cent of the patients with the diarrheogenic syndrome have islet cell tumors. Nearly half are malignant. Patients without islet cell tumors often have diffuse islet cell hyperplasia. The diarrheogenic syndrome has also been reported with bronchial tumor, pheochromocytoma, and ganglioneuroblastoma.

The diarrhea probably results from excess secretion of VIP. Infusion of VIP into laboratory animals and humans results in secretory diarrhea, hypokalemia, inhibition of gastric acid secretion, and hypercalcemia. Increased plasma VIP levels have been found in patients in whom islet cell tumor, islet cell hyperplasia, bronchogenic carcinoma, ganglioneuroblastoma, or pheochromocytoma was found to be the cause of the syndrome. VIP is difficult to detect in the circulation of normal humans; therefore the absence of VIP does not rule out the diagnosis. VIPomas also synthesize and secrete peptide histidine methionine (PHM), a peptide produced by the same mRNA as VIP that also enhances intestinal fluid secretion. Islet cell tumors producing only pancreatic polypeptide (another presumed hormone of unknown normal function) or prostaglandin E_2 have also been reported to be associated with this syndrome.

THERAPY. Treatment of the diarrheogenic syndrome is primarily by surgery. Because of the profound systemic effects of this tumor, resection is considered even in the presence of metastases. When no tumor is found, subtotal pancreatectomy is usually attempted. If hyperplasia is then identified on histopathologic examination and symptoms persist, total pancreatectomy should be considered. Octreotide is useful in preparing patients for surgery or as a palliative for metastatic disease. The tumors may also be transiently responsive to steroids, indomethacin, metoclopramide, lithium carbonate, or trifluoperazine. Radiotherapy, streptozotocin and interferon-α have been reported to reduce the size of metastases and volume of diarrhea.

Glucagonoma

CLINICAL PRESENTATION. The glucagonoma syndrome is characterized by a waxing and waning skin rash (necrolytic migratory erythema), diabetes, hypoaminoacidemia, weight loss, and anemia. The classic cutaneous lesion begins as an erythematous base, becomes indurated, and develops superficial central blistering. The blisters then erode and crust over. Healing may be accompanied by hyperpigmentation. This process takes 7 to 14 days, with lesions developing in one area while others are resolving. The rash is most prominent on the perineum, along intertriginous folds, and around the mouth and nose. Glossitis, stomatitis, and cheilitis are common. Onycholysis and brittle nails may be present.

Although cutaneous lesions were the hallmark of the first reported cases, the rash is actually present in only two thirds of patients with glucagonoma. The remainder usually present because of widespread metastatic disease.

Frank diabetes occurs in 60 per cent of patients with glucagonoma, and an additional 30 per cent have glucose intolerance. Even in patients with severe hyperglycemia, diabetic ketoacidosis is rarely observed in the glucagonoma syndrome, despite the known ability of glucagon to stimulate hepatic ketogenesis. There appear to be adequate levels of insulin to suppress lipolysis, limiting the free fatty acid substrates for hepatic ketone production.

Weight loss and anemia are found at the time of diagnosis in half of the patients with glucagonoma. Gastrointestinal symptoms include diarrhea, abdominal pain, and nausea and vomiting. Thromboembolic disease has also been described.

Glucagonoma is infrequently found in the MEN 1 syndrome. However, rare MEN 1 kindreds have been reported in which some members have glucagonoma and others have hyperglucagonemia without clinically detectable tumors. In addition, a familial glucagonoma syndrome has been reported in the absence of other endocrine tumors.

DIAGNOSIS. The diagnosis of glucagonoma is made by detecting elevated levels of glucagon and excluding other conditions associated with hyperglucagonemia, including diabetic ketoacidosis and hyperosmolar syndromes, chronic renal failure, cardiovascular collapse, and cirrhosis of the liver. Normal circulating levels of glucagon are 50 to 150 pg per milliliter. Most patients with glucagonoma have levels in excess of 500 pg per milliliter (occasionally as high as 10,000 pg per milliliter), while glucagon levels in the previously mentioned syndromes average 200 to 500 pg per milliliter. At the time of presentation 60 per cent of glucagonomas have metastasized, most commonly to the liver and local lymph nodes.

THERAPY. Surgery is the treatment of choice for glucagonoma confined to the pancreas. Surgery may also be indicated with

TABLE 220–1. SYNDROMES ASSOCIATED WITH ISLET CELL TUMORS

Tumor	Major Findings	Minor Findings	Other Hormones in Tumor or Plasma	Per Cent Malignancy	Hyperplasia	MEN Syndrome
Insulinoma	Adrenergic: palpitations, tremor, hunger, sweating Neuroglycopenic: confusion, seizures, transient focal deficit, coma	Ischemic cardiovascular disease, permanent neurologic deficits	Gastrin, glucagon, pancreatic polypeptide, somatostatin, GRF*	10	Occasional	10%
Gastrinoma	Peptic ulcers, enhanced acid secretion	Diarrhea, malabsorption, weight loss, dumping	ACTH, insulin, glucagon, VIP, 5-HIAA, MSH, somatostatin, calcitonin, pancreatic polypeptide	40–60	10%	25%
VIPoma	Watery diarrhea, hypokalemia, hypochlorhydria	Hypercalcemia, hyperglycemia, weakness, hypomagnesemia	PHM, pancreatic polypeptide, prostaglandins (?), GRF, gastrin	40	20%	Rare
Glucagonoma	Rash, diabetes, weight loss, anemia	Diarrhea, abdominal pain, thromboembolic disease	Pancreatic polypeptide, VIP, 5-HIAA, gastrin, insulin	60	Occasional	Occasional
Somatostatinoma	Diabetes, cholelithiasis, steatorrhea, malabsorption, weight loss	Indigestion, abdominal pain, anemia, diarrhea, ductal obstruction, hypoglycemia	ACTH, gastrin, calcitonin, PGE₂, glucagon, GRF, pancreatic polypeptide, VIP, 5-HIAA, substance P	66	None reported	One case (MEN 3)
PPoma	None	Watery diarrhea, hypokalemia, achlorhydria; abdominal pain, weight loss	Glucagon, insulin, somatostatin, VIP	40	Occasional	25%

*GRF = growth hormone–releasing factor; 5-HIAA = 5-hydroxyindoleacetic acid; MSH = melanocyte-stimulating hormone; PGE₂ = prostaglandin E₂; PHM = peptide histidine methionine.

metastatic disease, as debulking of the tumor mass may ameliorate the glucagonoma syndrome. Octreotide usually decreases glucagon secretion from glucagonomas and improves symptoms. It can be used to prepare patients for surgery or to ameliorate symptoms from metastatic disease. Streptozotocin, with or without 5-fluorouracil and dacarbazine (DTIC), may induce significant remission. Phenoxybenzamine may also inhibit glucagon secretion from tumors. The skin rash often resolves within a few days of successful surgery or octreotide therapy.

Somatostatinoma

CLINICAL PRESENTATION. Somatostatinomas are not common; most are found incidentally during laparotomy or during the workup of obstructive jaundice or abdominal pain, with identification made retrospectively on the basis of elevated concentrations of somatostatin in the tumor or in the patient's plasma. The tumors contain granules characteristic of D cells. The primary tumor is located in the duodenum or jejunum in 40 per cent of cases.

A syndrome associated with hypersomatostinemia includes diabetes mellitus, cholelithiasis, steatorrhea with malabsorption, dyspepsia, and significant weight loss. Patients may also have hypochlorhydria, watery diarrhea, anemia, and flushing. The diabetes is usually mild.

The pathophysiology of the syndrome is consistent with the known effects of somatostatin. Infusion of somatostatin in humans inhibits the release of multiple hormones, including insulin, glucagon, secretin, gastrin, and motilin. Hyperglycemia results from suppression of insulin secretion, but ketosis is infrequent, presumably because of the concomitant inhibition of glucagon secretion. Suppression of secretin, motilin, and gastrin, which decreases hydrochloric acid secretion, gastric emptying, and duodenal motility, may cause indigestion and abdominal pain. Inhibition of gallbladder contraction may predispose to cholelithiasis. Malabsorption is produced by inhibition of pancreatic exocrine function.

It is difficult to make the prospective diagnosis of somatostatinoma, as all of these symptoms are nonspecific and are found more commonly in other disorders. The incidence of cholelithiasis is increased in patients with diabetes. Malabsorption may occur in diabetics with chronic pancreatitis. This diagnostic difficulty is further compounded, as many patients with documented somatostatinoma have none of the components of the proposed syndrome. Some patients had severe hypoglycemia and were suspected to have insulinomas. Their tumors also contained insulin, and secretion of small amounts of insulin from the tumors with concomitant suppression of compensatory release of glucagon from the normal pancreas may have resulted in hypoglycemia.

Somatostatinomas may secrete additional hormones that modify the clinical syndrome. Striking elevations of serum calcitonin can cause watery diarrhea due to the effects of calcitonin on water and electrolyte transport in the gut. Somatostatinomas can produce ACTH, causing Cushing's syndrome, or prostaglandin E_2, causing flushing. Hyperplasia of cells containing pancreatic polypeptide (resulting in excess secretion of this hormone) has been reported in the presence of somatostatinoma.

DIAGNOSIS. The diagnosis of somatostatinoma is made by detecting elevated basal or stimulated levels of circulating somatostatin. Tolbutamide or calcium-pentagastrin infusion results in marked elevation of somatostatin in patients with somatostatinoma and normal basal somatostatin levels but not in controls.

THERAPY. Two thirds of patients with somatostatinoma have metastases at presentation; this may reflect the difficulty in the clinical diagnosis of this syndrome. Surgical resection should be performed if possible. Streptozotocin therapy reduces tumor size and plasma somatostatin levels.

Other Hormones Produced by Islet Cell Tumors

PANCREATIC POLYPEPTIDE. Many endocrine tumors of the pancreas and gut produce pancreatic polypeptide (PP) as a secondary hormone, allowing it to serve as a marker for islet cell tumors. Increasing numbers of islet cell tumors that produce PP as their major hormone are being identified; these may account for some of the tumors previously identified as "nonfunctional."

The role of PP in normal islet physiology is not apparent, and no clinical syndrome has been definitively associated with PPomas. A few cases of islet cell tumors associated with watery diarrhea, hypokalemia, and achlorhydria have been accompanied by elevated serum levels of PP with normal VIP levels.

ACTH. Pancreatic islet cell tumors producing ACTH account for nearly 10 per cent of cases of Cushing's syndrome due to ectopic ACTH production. Such tumors are usually found to secrete multiple hormones, including insulin, gastrin, serotonin, or somatostatin. However, it is more common to find Cushing's *disease* due to a pituitary adenoma associated with other islet cell tumors in patients with MEN type 1.

GROWTH HORMONE–RELEASING FACTOR. Acromegaly has been reported in patients with islet cell tumors secreting growth hormone–releasing factor. Although these patients often have hyperplasia of the growth hormone–secreting cells of the pituitary, it is very difficult to distinguish them from patients with classic acromegaly due to a pituitary adenoma (see Ch. 213). In either case the sella may be normal or enlarged, and growth hormone levels may show paradoxic responses to provocative testing.

Bloom SR, Polak JM: Glucagonoma syndrome. Am J Med 82(5B):25, 1987. *A comprehensive and useful general review, with 44 references.*

Berelowitz M: Somatostatin-producing tumors. Adv Exp Med Biol 188:475, 1985. *Only 6 of 21 patients with pancreatic somatostatinoma and none of 13 patients with a small intestine primary tumor showed clinical symptoms of the proposed somatostatinoma syndrome.*

Jensen RT (ed.): Gastrointestinal endocrinology. Gastroenterol Clin North Am 18(4): December, 1989. *This volume has eight articles covering the clinical presentation, localization, and treatment of islet cell tumors as well as four articles on the properties of the hormones.*

Krejs GJ: VIPoma syndrome. Am J Med 82(5B):37, 1987. *An excellent general review of this interesting entity, with 120 references. A good place to start.*

221 Disorders of Sexual Differentiation

Julianne Imperato-McGinley

NORMAL SEXUAL DIFFERENTIATION

The fetus is bipotential for sexual differentiation. The bipotentiality includes the gonad, the internal sex structures, and the external genitalia.

Development of the Bipotential Gonad

In fetuses of both sexes an undifferentiated gonad develops during the fifth week of fetal life. A thickened area of coelomic or germinal epithelium on the medial aspect of the mesonephros proliferates and with the underlying mesenchyme produces a prominence designated the gonadal ridge. Then cords of cells known as primary sex cords proliferate from the epithelium into the mesenchyme. The primordial germ cells are visible early in the third week among the endodermal cells of the wall of the yolk sac. During folding of the embryo, they multiply and migrate by a combination of ameboid movement and passive transfer along the dorsal mesentery to the gonadal ridges and later into the underlying mesenchyme. By the end of the sixth week the bipotential gonad is formed (Fig. 221–1). The primordial germ cells develop into spermatogonia in the male and ova in the female, the sex cords become either seminiferous tubules or primary ovarian follicles, and the mesenchymal cells form either the Leydig cells or the theca and stromal cells in the female.

Gonadal Differentiation—Development of the Testes and Ovaries

Testicular differentiation begins with the evolution of the *testicular or seminiferous cords* from primary sex cords of the indifferent gonad at approximately the seventh week of gestation (Fig. 221–1). The Sertoli cells differentiate within each cord, enlarge, aggregate, and engulf the germ cells. The distal ends of the cords interconnect to form the rete testes, which is in contact with the wolffian (mesonephric) ducts. By the sixth month the

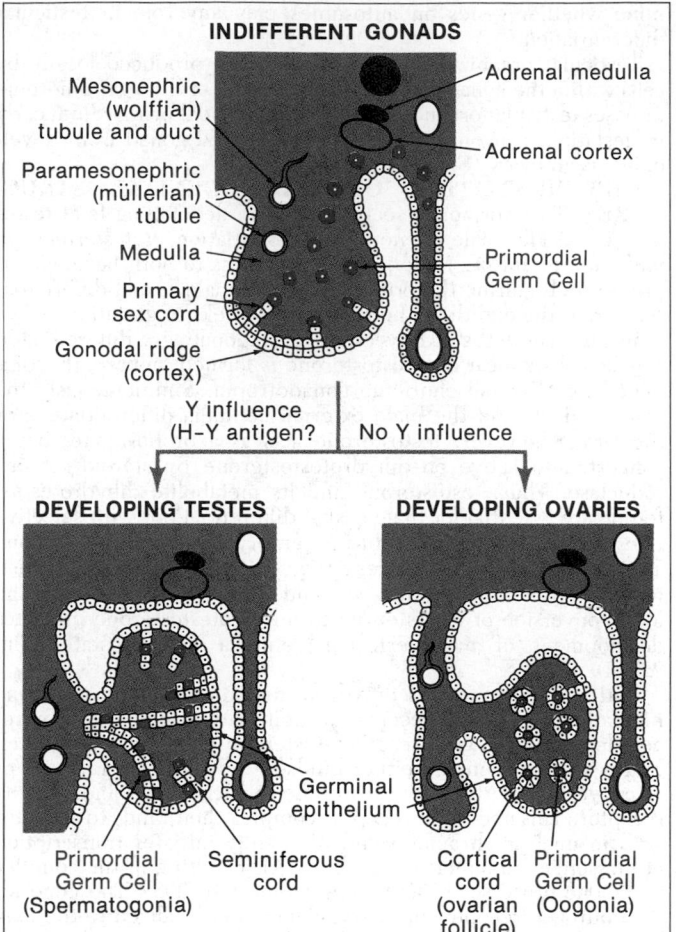

FIGURE 221–1. Development of the bipotential gonad from coelomic epithelium (primary sex cords) underlying mesenchymal tissue and primordial germ cells and its differentiation to either a testis or an ovary.

ends of the rete testes develop a lumen continuous with the mesonephric tubules, which develop into the ductuli efferentia. The fetal Leydig cells, apparent by 8 weeks of fetal life, fill the interstitial spaces at 3 months of gestation.

Ovarian differentiation from the indifferent gonad begins at approximately 50 days of gestation (Fig. 221–1). The primary sex cords form irregular groups of cells called medullary cords containing primitive granulosa cells that engulf primordial oogonia. As the oogonia differentiate, the primitive granulosa cells organize around them and form a single layer constituting the primordial follicle. At 18 to 20 weeks of gestation, there are approximately 7 million oogonia and oocytes, whereas by birth the number decreases to approximately 2 million.

Phenotypic Differentiation

DUCTAL DEVELOPMENT

Every fetus has both *wolffian (mesonephric) ducts,* which develop into epididymis, vas deferens, and seminal vesicles in the male, and *müllerian (paramesonephric) ducts,* which develop into fallopian tubes, uterus, and upper third of the vagina in the female (Fig. 221–2). In the male as the initial event the müllerian ducts regress by about 7½ weeks of gestation, following which the mesonephric wolffian ducts differentiate to form the epididymis, vas deferens, seminal vesicles, and ejaculatory ducts. In the female the wolffian ducts regress at approximately 10½ weeks, and the müllerian ducts differentiate to form the fallopian tubes, uterus, and upper portion of the vagina.

DEVELOPMENT OF THE EXTERNAL GENITALIA

The external genitalia of both sexes (like the gonad) develop from common primordia, the urogenital tubercle, urogenital folds, and urogenital swellings (Fig. 221–2). In the male, external genital masculinization begins shortly after wolffian ductal differ-

entiation and is completed by 14 weeks of gestation. The urogenital tubercle elongates to become the glans penis, the urogenital folds fuse to become the shaft of the penis, and the urogenital swellings become the scrotum. The prostate arises from endodermal buds in the urethral lining at 10 weeks and grows into the mesenchyme, which forms the muscular and connective tissue components. Descent of the testes and growth of the penis occur between 20 weeks of gestation and term. In the female the urogenital tubule becomes the clitoris, the urogenital swellings, the labia majora, and the urogenital folds the labia minora. Female differentiation occurs after the embryo has reached 10½ weeks.

Determinants of Phenotypic Differentiation

Since the fetus is bipotential, what are the determinants of the male or female phenotype?

FEMALE PHENOTYPIC DIFFERENTIATION

Ovarian tissue containing primary follicles is found in human abortuses with a 45 XO complement. Thus, ovarian differentiation

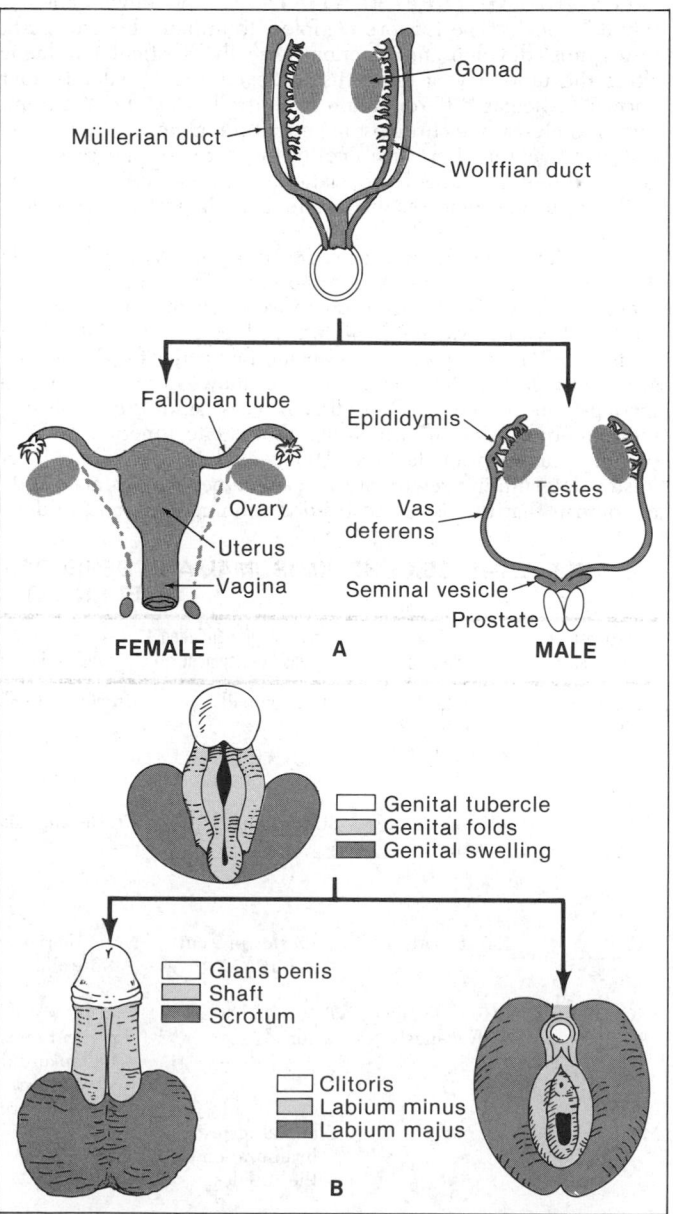

FIGURE 221–2. Summary of male and female sexual differentiation. *A,* Internal sexual differentiation from wolffian and müllerian ducts. *B,* Development of male and female external genitalia from common primordia.

does not appear to require a 46 XX chromosomal complement. Adults, however, with a 45 XO complement have only streak gonads made of whorls of connective tissue. A complete 46 XX complement, therefore, although not necessary for ovarian differentiation, is essential for maintenance of normal ovarian follicular development. Deletion of either the long or short arm of the X chromosome results in streak gonads. Deletion of the short arm of the X chromosome (XXp-) is associated with streak gonads and the skeletal and somatic anomalies of subjects with 45 XO Turner's syndrome. In contrast, long arm deletions (XXq-) are usually associated with streak gonads and none of the stigmata of Turner's syndrome (Table 221–1). See Ch. 224 for a complete discussion of XO and XX gonadal dysgenesis.

In the absence of gonads, either ovaries or testes, the wolffian anlagen regress and the müllerian ducts differentiate to form fallopian tubes, uterus, and upper portion of the vagina, and the external genital primordia differentiate as female (Fig. 221–2). Thus, femaleness is the innate tendency of every fetus and does not require gonadal influence.

MALE PHENOTYPIC DIFFERENTIATION

TESTICULAR DIFFERENTIATION. The development of the male phenotype is more complex; to initiate the process the testes must develop and function normally. Testicular influence alters the tendency of the fetus to develop as female. In man, normal testicular differentiation is controlled by the Y chromosome. Analysis of Y chromosome structural abnormalities in man suggests that the short arm (Yp) of the chromosome carries the gene(s) directing testicular formation. Simple absence of the (Yp) of the Y chromosome results in a female phenotype, with streak gonads.

Testicular differentiation occurred in an XX male who carried 60 kilobase pairs of the Y chromosome. Thus, 60 kilobases of segment 1A1 of the Y chromosome were left to search. As DNA markers became available, this was reduced to 35 kilobases and from this a single copy gene was made that codes for an 80 amino acid motif that is highly conserved. It shows homologies for the mating-type protein MC of fission yeast and the nonhistone nuclear HmG protein, which are thought to function as DNA-binding transcription factors. The gene has been named SRY (testes determining region of the Y). Further studies are needed to confirm that this is the testes-determining gene and to determine whether genes on autosomes play any role in testicular differentiation.

Testicular organizing factor or substance produced locally by cells within the gonad and under the control of the Y chromosome imposes testicular organogenesis on the gonadal primordium early in gestation, preventing the undifferentiated gonad from developing as an ovary (Fig. 221–3).

DIFFERENTIATION OF MALE GENITAL STRUCTURES. Two hormones secreted by the developing fetal testes are essential for male phenotypic differentiation, *testosterone* and *müllerian inhibiting factor*. Responsiveness to both hormones is present only during the critical period of male sexual differentiation, from the eighth to the fourteenth weeks of gestation.

In the male fetus at 8 weeks of gestational age, differentiated Leydig cells appear and testosterone is formed, apparently stimulated by placental chorionic gonadotropin. Simultaneously the wolffian ducts and the male external genitalia differentiate. For the latter, however, testosterone acts as a prohormone, being converted to active 5α-dihydrotestosterone by steroid Δ^4 5α-reductase. Thus, testosterone and its metabolite dihydrotestosterone are essential for male sexual differentiation, with selective roles for each hormone during embryogenesis. Testosterone acting locally mediates differentiation of the wolffian ductal system to the vas deferens, epididymis, and seminal vesicles, while the local conversion of testosterone to dihydrotestosterone mediates development of male external genitalia and prostate (Fig. 221–4).

Both testosterone and dihydrotestosterone bind to the same high-affinity androgen receptor protein within the cells of androgen-dependent target areas. Testosterone enters the target cell by passive diffusion and either binds to the androgen receptor or is converted to dihydrotestosterone, which then binds to the receptor. This androgen receptor complex then binds to acceptor sites in nuclear chromatin and ultimately initiates transcription of messenger ribonucleic acid (mRNA), resulting in the complex metabolic processes of androgen action (Ch. 208). The gene for the androgen receptor has been cloned and localized to the long arm of the X chromosome near the centromere.

The inhibition of the müllerian anlage is under the control of müllerian inhibiting factor, a high-molecular-weight glycoprotein, a product of the Sertoli cells of the seminiferous tubules. The human gene for müllerian inhibiting factors has been cloned and localized to the tip of the short arm of chromosome 19. Its secretion begins shortly after the initiation of seminiferous tubular differentiation. The müllerian ducts are receptive to this hormone

TABLE 221–1. SEX CHROMOSOMAL AND DEVELOPMENTAL ABNORMALITIES LEADING TO ABNORMAL SEXUAL DIFFERENTIATION AND DEVELOPMENT

Chromosomal Complement	Disorder	Gonadal Differentiation and Development	Internal Sex Structures	External Genitalia	Pubertal Development	Comments
XO, XXp-, XXq-	Gonadal dysgenesis	Streak gonads	Uterus and fallopian tubes	Female	None	XO to XXp- associated with short stature. Can be XX with abnormal X chromosome at the molecular level.
XY	XY gonadal dysgenesis	Streak gonads	Uterus and fallopian tubes	Female	None	A spectrum. See Table 221–3. Abnormality at the molecular level affecting testes determining gene.
XY	XY agonadism	No testes present at birth	No müllerian structures. No wolffian structures.	Female		Part of a spectrum. Mildest form normal male without testes.
XO/XY	Mixed gonadal dysgenesis	Testes and streak gonads	Uterus, vas deferens, if present on side of testes. Fallopian tube on side of streak, occasionally next to vas deferens.	Most commonly ambiguous (range— female to normal male)	Male	Most common cause of ambiguity in the newborn after congenital adrenal hyperplasia.
XX	XX males	Bilateral testes; hyalinization of the tubules	Normal	Usually normal. Can have ambiguous genitalia.	Male	X chromosome contains testes determining region of the Y chromosome.
XX, XX/XY, XY	True hermaphroditism	Ovary and testes; ovotestis	Uterus almost invariably present. Vas deferens on side of testes. Fallopian tube on side of ovary.	Most commonly ambiguous		May be familial. XX male in same family.

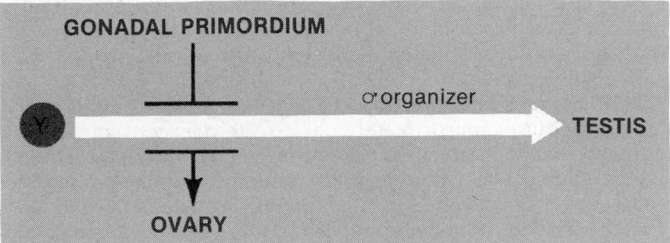

GONADAL PRIMORDIUM

♂organizer → **TESTIS**

↓ **OVARY**

FIGURE 221–3. Testicular organizing substance under Y chromosome control imposing testicular organogenesis on the indifferent gonad.

before 8 weeks of gestation. Postnatally, the levels are high in normal boys prior to 2 years of age. They fall progressively in older boys and decrease sharply at puberty.

In summary, male phenotypic development requires normal testicular differentiation and function, so that at a critically isensitive period in utero (8 to 14 weeks) müllerian inhibiting factor, secreted by the Sertoli cells, and testosterone, secreted by the Leydig cells, are produced in sufficient amounts. Müllerian inhibiting factor, acting locally, suppresses the müllerian anlage, and testosterone, also acting locally, causes differentiation of the wolffian anlage to cpididymis, vas deferens, and seminal vesicles. Testosterone is converted by the enzyme 5α-reductase to dihydrotestosterone in the anlage of the external genitalia, resulting in male external genital differentiation (Fig. 221–4). Depending upon specific target tissue, either testosterone or dihydrotestosterone complexes with the androgen receptor, to initiate androgen action at the nuclear level.

Genetic Control of Male Sexual Differentiation

Male sexual differentiation is under complex genetic control. Testicular differentiation requires gene(s) normally found on the Y chromosome. The enzymes involved in testosterone biosynthesis, as well as the enzyme 5α-reductase converting testosterone to dihydrotestosterone, are regulated by genes located on the autosomes. A gene located on the X chromosome codes for the androgen receptor at the androgen-dependent target areas. Inherited forms of müllerian inhibiting factor deficiency are transmitted as a recessive trait, either autosomal or X linked.

Thus, male phenotypic development is regulated by multiple genes located on the autosomes as well as on both X and Y chromosomes.

Byskov AG: Differentiation of mammalian embryonic gonad. Physiol Rev 66:71, 1986. *All aspects of gonadal differentiation are covered, from formation of the gonadal primordium to theories of gonadal differentiation. Excellent bibliography.*

ABNORMALITIES OF SEXUAL DIFFERENTIATION

Male Pseudohermaphroditism

The known etiologic factors in male pseudohermaphroditism or incomplete masculinization can be divided into three categories: (1) disorders of testicular differentiation; (2) disorders of testicular function; and (3) disorders of function at the androgen-dependent target areas. Table 221–2 lists the specific clinical entities within each category.

DISORDERS OF TESTICULAR DIFFERENTIATION AND DEVELOPMENT

XY GONADAL DYSGENESIS. Clinical Presentation. Subjects with pure gonadal dysgenesis have a 46 XY chromosomal complement but are phenotypic females with primary amenorrhea, tall stature, eunuchoidal proportions, and scant axillary and pubic hair. The uterus and fallopian tubes are present, and streak gonads are found. The incomplete forms of this condition have variable amounts of functional testicular tissue, and consequently at birth the subjects frequently have clitoromegaly, ambiguous genitalia, or, rarely, a penile urethra. The degree of virilization at puberty is also variable. In pure gonadal dysgenesis, postpubertal gonadotropins are increased to the castrate range with castrate levels of testosterone. However, when functioning testicular tissue is present, testosterone can vary from castrate levels to low-normal male levels. Additionally, if müllerian inhibiting factor is produced there may be partial or complete absence of müllerian structures (Table 221–1; Fig. 221–5).

Pathophysiology. In pure gonadal dysgenesis the testes do not

FIGURE 221–4. Schematic representation of the factors involved in male and female sexual differentiation.

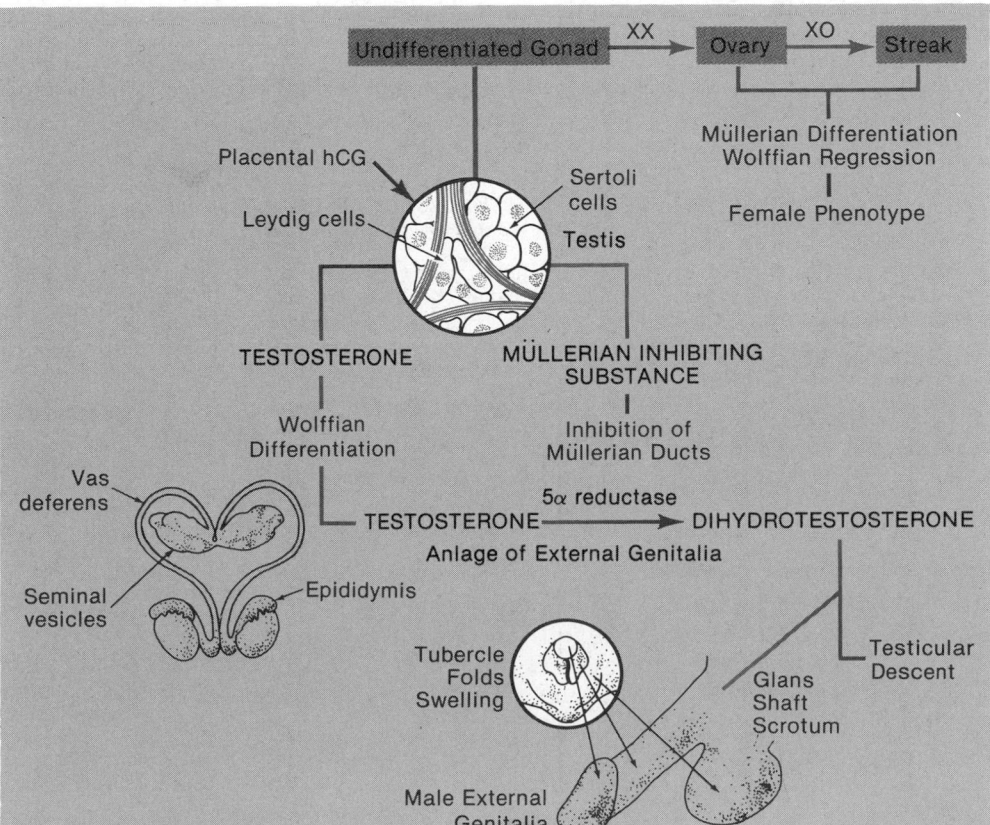

TABLE 221–2. CLASSIFICATION OF THE CAUSES OF MALE PSEUDOHERMAPHRODITISM

I. Disorders of testicular differentiation and development
  A. Testicular dysgenesis, affecting both Leydig cell and seminiferous tubule development
    1. Y chromosomal abnormalities
    2. XY gonadal dysgenesis
    3. XO/XY gonadal dysgenesis
    4. Testicular regression syndrome
  B. Leydig cell agenesis or dysgenesis—selective absence or decrease in Leydig cell differentiation and function—seminiferous tubule embryogenesis occurring normally
    1. Abnormality of the hCG-LH receptor: absence of precursor Leydig cell

II. Disorders of testicular function
  A. Abnormalities of müllerian inhibiting factor synthesis or action—persistent müllerian duct syndrome
  B. Enzyme deficiencies affecting testosterone biosynthesis
    1. Cholesterol 20,22-desmolase
    2. 17α-Hydroxylase
    3. 17,20-Desmolase
    4. 3β-Hydroxysteroid dehydrogenase:Δ^{5-4} isomerase
    5. 17β-Hydroxysteroid dehydrogenase

III. Disorders of function at the androgen-dependent target areas
  A. Disorders of androgen action (complete and partial androgen insensitivity)
    1. Cytosol androgen-receptor binding abnormalities
    2. Post cytosol androgen-receptor binding abnormalities
  B. Disorders of testosterone metabolism
    1. 5α-Reductase deficiency

differentiate at all, and in the absence of a functional testis phenotypic development is female, with wolffian duct regression and müllerian differentiation. In the incomplete forms there are varying degrees of testicular development and of fetal masculinization. The etiology of this condition could be due to a number of theoretical causes involving testicular organizing substance. Deletion of gene (SRY) on the Y chromosome near the centromere results in streak gonads. Thus, this gene is purported to code for the testicular organizing substance. There could also be abnormalities in its structure, due to deletions or point mutations of the testes determining gene or lack or decrease in binding of the gonadal specific receptor. Neither the receptor nor its gene has yet been identified.

Familial cases of pure gonadal dysgenesis occur, transmitted by either X-linked recessive or autosomal dominant-sex limited inheritance with variable expressivity. Some sibs may have the pure form and a female phenotype and others present with ambiguous genitalia.

Management and Therapy. The streak gonads should be removed because approximately 20 to 30 per cent of subjects develop gonadoblastomas or dysgerminomas within the streaks. Dysgerminomas may be malignant, and approximately 5 to 8 per cent of gonadoblastomas contain malignant elements. In pure gonadal dysgenesis, infants are invariably reared as female and come to the attention of the physician at puberty because of lack of secondary sexual development. Estrogen and progesterone replacement therapy should be instituted at the time of puberty and after prophylactic removal of the streak gonads. In incomplete forms of testicular dysgenesis, the child should be reared in the sex that will be more functional, and appropriate surgical correction of the genitalia carried out. Intra-abdominal testicular tissue should always be removed because of the increased risk of malignancy. This necessitates the use of testosterone replacement therapy at puberty, if the child is being reared as a male.

MIXED GONADAL DYSGENESIS. ***Clinical Presentation.*** Subjects with mixed gonadal dysgenesis usually have a streak gonad on one side, a testis on the contralateral side, and XO/XY mosaicism on chromosomal analysis. The phenotypic spectrum ranges from phenotypic females, with or without the clinical characteristics of Turner's syndrome, to subjects with ambiguous genitalia, to normal phenotypic males. The genitalia are sufficiently ambiguous that approximately two thirds are raised as girls, with the stigmata of Turner's syndrome occurring in one third. Affected subjects have a uterus, and most have bilateral fallopian tubes. The vas deferens, if present, is on the side of the testis, and frequently a fallopian tube also exists adjacent to the vas deferens. Virilization generally occurs at puberty. The testes appear histologically normal before puberty. However, after puberty the seminiferous tubules demonstrate thickened walls with few if any germ cells. Consequently, affected subjects are infertile. If pubertal gynecomastia occurs, a gonadal tumor should be suspected.

Pathogenesis. XO/XY mosaicism in subjects with this condition can be best explained as resulting from mitotic nondisjunction or anaphase lag, resulting in loss of the Y chromosome. Perhaps the lack of testicular differentiation of the streak gonad is related to the preponderance of the XO cell line in that gonad. Despite good Leydig cell function with virilization at puberty, the testis must have been functionally dysgenetic (between the eighth and fourteenth weeks of gestation—the critically responsive period), as evidenced by absence of or incomplete virilization of the

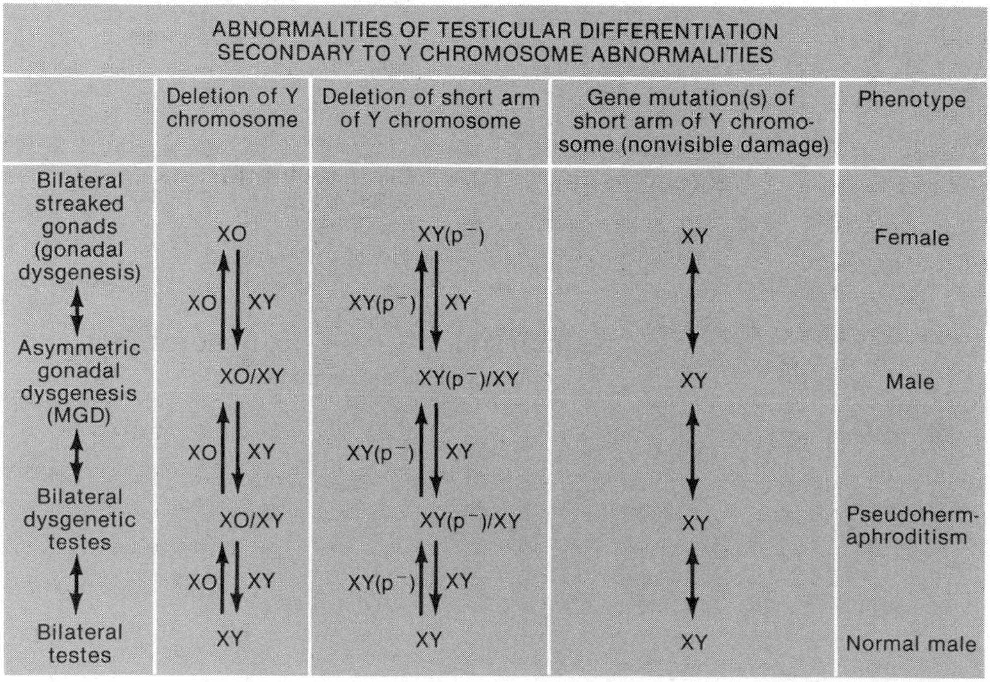

ABNORMALITIES OF TESTICULAR DIFFERENTIATION SECONDARY TO Y CHROMOSOME ABNORMALITIES

	Deletion of Y chromosome	Deletion of short arm of Y chromosome	Gene mutation(s) of short arm of Y chromosome (nonvisible damage)	Phenotype
Bilateral streaked gonads (gonadal dysgenesis)	XO	XY(p⁻)	XY	Female
↕	XO ↕ XY	XY(p⁻) ↕ XY	↕	
Asymmetric gonadal dysgenesis (MGD)	XO/XY	XY(p⁻)/XY	XY	Male
↕	XO ↕ XY	XY(p⁻) ↕ XY	↕	
Bilateral dysgenetic testes	XO/XY	XY(p⁻)/XY	XY	Pseudohermaphroditism
↕	XO ↕ XY	XY(p⁻) ↕ XY	↕	
Bilateral testes	XY	XY	XY	Normal male

FIGURE 221–5. The abnormalities of testicular differentiation may be thought of as a spectrum of disorders that can be produced by more than one genotype.

external genitalia. Theoretically a delay in testicular differentiation and function in utero could result in delayed secretion of testosterone and müllerian inhibiting factor, completely or partially missing the critically responsive period and resulting in the presence of female or ambiguous genitalia and müllerian structures.

There are subjects with an XO/XY chromosomal complement and bilateral streak gonads as well as XO/XY subjects with bilateral testes. Thus the classic clinical syndrome of mixed gonadal dysgenesis may be one clinical entity in a spectrum ranging from streak gonads and a female phenotype to varied abnormalities of testicular development (symmetric or asymmetric) and genital ambiguity, possibly depending upon the preponderance of a particular cell line, either XO or XY, within the gonad at the time of differentiation (Table 221–1; Fig. 221–5).

Management and Therapy. Owing to the increased incidence of tumor formation, an intra-abdominal testis that cannot be brought into the scrotum should be removed as well as the streak gonad. A scrotal testis should be preserved. In infants, when the testes cannot be brought to the scrotum and must be removed, and the external genitalia are severely ambiguous, the sex of rearing should be female and appropriate genital surgery performed. At the time of puberty, estrogen and progesterone therapy should be given to induce and maintain feminization. If the child is to be raised as a male, testosterone replacement therapy will be needed at the time of puberty.

XY AGONADISM, TESTICULAR REGRESSION, OR VANISHING TESTES SYNDROME. *Clinical Presentation.* Typically these subjects are 46 XY phenotypic females with absent gonads and no müllerian or wolffian internal structures. The lack of müllerian structures and gonadal remnants separates this entity from pure XY gonadal dysgenesis. The condition appears to be secondary to regression of the differentiating testis before the onset of androgen secretion, resulting in lack of wolffian differentiation, but after the onset of secretion of müllerian inhibiting factor, resulting in inhibition of female internal structures. There is, however, a phenotypic spectrum of agonadal subjects perhaps related to the time of testicular regression, during or after the critical period of male sexual differentiation. Affected subjects therefore vary widely in phenotypes: from those with total absence of internal sex structures and female external genitalia, to subjects with ambiguous genitalia, to normal males with absent testes.

Pathophysiology. The etiology of the testicular regression is unknown. These subjects are unequivocally 46 XY, and chromosomal abnormalities have never been demonstrated. Familial cases of agonadism in XY subjects occur, however, suggesting that in some cases it may be an inherited condition. Variable phenotypic expression in agonadal siblings from the same kindred also occurs, suggesting that this condition is a clinical spectrum due to the time of regression of the embryonic testes.

Management and Therapy. Sex hormone therapy should be instituted at puberty in accordance with the sex of rearing.

LEYDIG CELL AGENESIS OR DYSGENESIS, GONADOTROPIN UNRESPONSIVENESS. *Clinical Characteristics.* Adult subjects with Leydig cell agenesis or dysgenesis have either normal female external genitalia or slight posterior fusion of the labia majora and have been raised as females. An epididymis and vas deferens are present in affected subjects, indicating that little testosterone is needed at a critical period to initiate wolffian differentiation. No müllerian structures are found, confirming that müllerian inhibiting factor is secreted by the Sertoli cells of the seminiferous tubules. In the adults, normal-appearing Sertoli cells with few spermatogonia and few or no Leydig cells are present in the testis.

Pathophysiology. Plasma androgen levels do not significantly change with administration of human chorionic gonadotropin (hCG). Luteinizing hormone (LH) levels are elevated in adulthood.

Theoretically the absence or decrease in Leydig cells can result from (1) an absence of or decrease in precursor cells destined to become functioning Leydig cells under hCG-LH stimulation or (2) a decrease in the hCG-LH receptor or receptor response of the precursor Leydig cells. It can be theorized that the hCG-LH receptor mediates Leydig cell differentiation, and without these receptors, precursor Leydig cells are not formed. A complete phenotypic spectrum of subjects with this disorder can be anticipated, dependent upon the severity of the developmental defect.

Management and Therapy. Affected subjects should be raised in the sex in which they will be more apt to function normally. In most instances because of the severe genital ambiguity this would be female. Thus the testes should be removed and corrective genital surgery performed. At puberty appropriate sex hormone therapy should be instituted concordant with the individual's gender.

DISORDERS OF TESTICULAR FUNCTION

In disorders of testicular function, the testes have differentiated normally, but the secretion of either müllerian inhibiting factor or testosterone is abnormal.

MÜLLERIAN INHIBITING FACTOR DEFICIENCY. *Clinical Presentation.* Males with this condition have a uterus and bilateral fallopian tubes. They have bilateral testes with normal male differentiation of wolffian structures and external genitalia and undergo normal male puberty. This entity most frequently occurs as unilateral cryptorchidism with a contralateral inguinal hernia containing müllerian structures, "uteri inguinale," and a testis. The incidence of testicular tumors is approximately 13 per cent, similar to the incidence in cryptorchidism. An inguinal hernia most often brings affected males to a physician's attention. Although fertility has been described, azoospermia is frequently noted. More than 80 cases have been reported, including at least eight families with two affected sibs. Pedigree analysis suggests an X-linked or autosomal recessive inheritance. In 5 per cent of affected patients, either seminomas or other germ cell tumors occur.

Pathogenesis. Theoretically this entity could be due to a number of abnormalities affecting the synthesis, structure, timing of secretion, or action of müllerian inhibiting factor. Some children with this condition possess no müllerian inhibiting factor and others possess normal amounts, suggesting genetic heterogeneity. Documentation of the precise biochemical abnormalities will have to await further studies of the MIF gene and its receptor. The ultimate effect is lack of suppression of the müllerian anlage, resulting in the presence of a uterus. Androgen secretion is adequate during the critical period of sexual differentiation, and the wolffian ducts and external genitalia differentiate normally.

Management and Therapy. The müllerian structures should be surgically removed if they are in the inguinal canal. Since malignant change in müllerian structures has never been reported, surgical removal is not necessary if they are located in the abdomen. The cryptorchid testes should be brought into the scrotal sac and the patient examined frequently for the development of testicular tumors.

Imperato-McGinley J: Sexual differentiation—Normal and abnormal. Curr Top Exp Endocrinol 5:231, 1983. *Of particular interest in this review is the section on male pseudohermaphroditism, including an extensive bibliography for each clinical entity described.*

DEFICIENCIES OF TESTOSTERONE BIOSYNTHESIS.
Clinical Features. Five enzymatic steps involving four genes are required to convert cholesterol to testosterone; deficiencies of these enzymatic steps constitute the nonvirilizing forms of the adrenogenital syndrome. The five enzymatic steps are (1) cholesterol 20,22-desmolase, (2) 3β-hydroxysteroid dehydrogenase:Δ^{5-4} isomerase, (3) 17α-hydroxylase, (4) 17,20-desmolase, and (5) 17β-hydroxysteroid dehydrogenase (Fig. 221–6). The enzymatic activities 17α-hydroxylase and 17,20-desmolase reside in the same enzyme. Deficiencies of the enzymes cholesterol 20,22-desmolase and 3β-hydroxysteroid dehydrogenase:Δ^{5-4} isomerase impair production of aldosterone and cortisol. 17α-Hydroxylase deficiency impairs cortisol production, while 17,20-desmolase and 17β-hydroxysteroid dehydrogenase deficiencies affect only androgen biosynthesis. Since androgens are the precursors of estrogens, it follows that estrogen production is also low in all of the enzyme deficiencies except 17β-hydroxysteroid dehydrogenase (Table 221–3). These disorders are inherited as autosomal recessive traits. Genotypic females are phenotypically normal at birth, with the exception of females with 3β-hydroxysteroid dehydrogenase deficiency, who may be mildly virilized.

The testes differentiate normally, and normal amounts of müllerian inhibiting factor are secreted, so müllerian structures

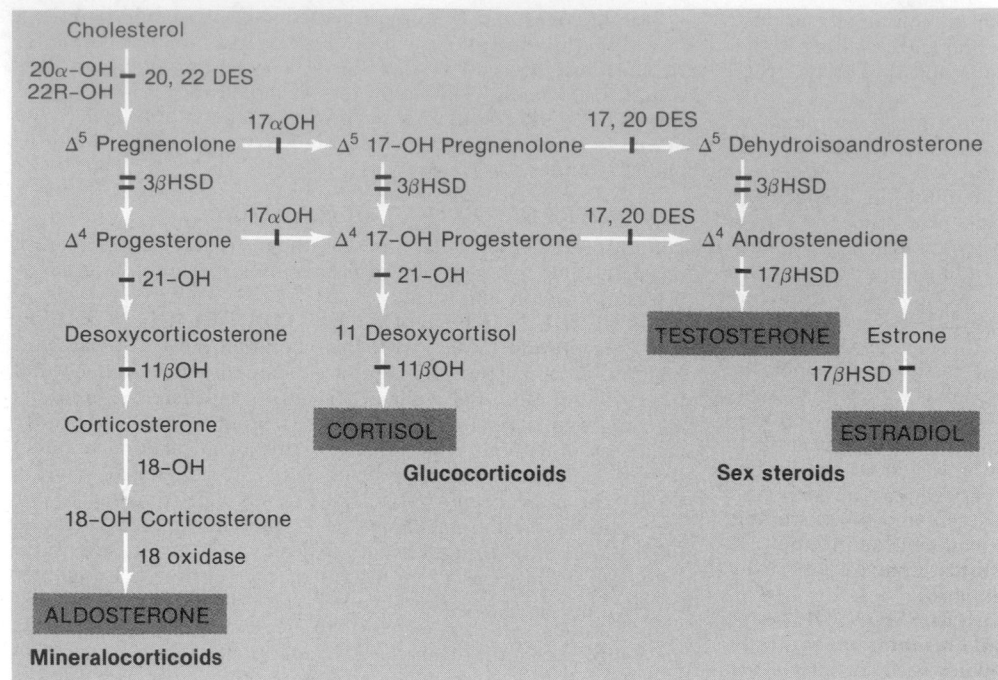

Cholesterol

20α-OH
22R-OH — 20, 22 DES

Δ⁵ Pregnenolone —I→ Δ⁵ 17-OH Pregnenolone —I→ Δ⁵ Dehydroisoandrosterone
   3βHSD   3βHSD   3βHSD
Δ⁴ Progesterone —I→ Δ⁴ 17-OH Progesterone —I→ Δ⁴ Androstenedione
   21-OH   21-OH   17βHSD
Desoxycorticosterone 11 Desoxycortisol   TESTOSTERONE   Estrone
   11βOH   11βOH   17βHSD
Corticosterone   CORTISOL   ESTRADIOL
   18-OH   Glucocorticoids   Sex steroids
18-OH Corticosterone
   18 oxidase
ALDOSTERONE
Mineralocorticoids

FIGURE 221–6. Congenital adrenal hyperplasia. *Left,* Enzyme deficiencies resulting in male pseudohermaphroditism. Cholesterol 20,22-desmolase, 17α-hydroxylase, 3β-hydroxysteroid dehydrogenase:Δ⁵⁻⁴ isomerase, 17,20-desmolase, 17β-hydroxysteroid dehydrogenase. *Center* and *right,* Enzyme deficiencies resulting in female pseudohermaphroditism. 21-Hydroxylase, 11β-hydroxylase, 3β-hydroxysteroid dehydrogenase:Δ⁵⁻⁴ isomerase. (DES = desmolase; OH = hydroxylase; HSD = hydroxysteroid dehydrogenase.)

are absent. However, the impaired secretion of testosterone by Leydig cells at the critical period of sexual differentiation in utero causes ambiguity of the external genitalia. Wolffian differentiation is normal. In general, the severity of the enzyme defect is reflected in the degree of external genital ambiguity at birth and the amount of virilization at puberty. Each specific enzyme deficiency, however, may show considerable variation in clinical presentation from totally female external genitalia to males with mild hypospadias and cryptorchidism.

The causes for the enzymatic abnormalities include deletions or mutations at structural gene loci coding for the amino acid sequences of the enzymes. Mutations at sites other than structural loci can be classified as *regulatory,* altering the rate of synthesis or degradation of the enzyme; *architectural,* affecting incorporation of enzyme molecules into active sites in the cell; or *temporal,* affecting the development of the tissue or the time of activation of regulatory systems.

Congenital Lipoid Adrenal Hyperplasia (Cholesterol 20,22-Desmolase Deficiency). A genetic male from a consanguineous marriage exhibited wolffian differentiation but with female external genitalia. The infant died in adrenal crisis at 6 days of age. At autopsy the adrenals were large and yellowish and contained cortical cells with foamy, spongy cytoplasm that stained positively for lipids. Approximately 32 cases have been subsequently described with equal numbers of both sexes affected. Most died in adrenal crisis in infancy, owing to severe deficiencies of glucocorticoid and mineralocorticoid production and with similar pathologic findings.

The affected genotypic males have abdominal or inguinal testes with wolffian differentiation, and no müllerian structures. The external genitalia are either female or severely ambiguous. As would be expected, genotypic females have normal female genitalia.

Pathogenesis. A deficiency in the conversion of cholesterol to pregnenolone results in decreased glucocorticoid, mineralocorticoid, and sex steroid production (Fig. 221–6). All plasma steroid values are low to unmeasurable, and little or no urinary 17-ketosteroids, 17-hydroxysteroids, or aldosterone is found (Table 221–3). cDNA clones that encode the gene responsible for the cleavage of the side chain of cholesterol (P-H50 SCC) have been isolated and the corresponding gene located on chromosome 15. The gene defects in this condition will be forthcoming.

Management and Therapy. Signs of adrenal insufficiency with hyperkalemia and hyponatremia usually occur within the first 2 weeks of life. The condition must be distinguished from 3β-hydroxysteroid dehydrogenase deficiency or congenital adrenal hypoplasia. In a phenotypic female or a patient with ambiguous genitalia and adrenal insufficiency, demonstration of a 46 XY karyotype distinguishes this condition from congenital adrenal hypoplasia. Low urinary 17-ketosteroid and low plasma dehydroepiandrosterone levels distinguish it from 3β-hydroxysteroid dehydrogenase deficiency. Once the diagnosis is established, glucocorticoid and mineralocorticoid therapy should be immediately instituted and is essential for survival. In genotypic males, sex hormone therapy should be instituted at puberty in accordance with the sex of rearing. In most instances, because of the severity of the genital defect, the sex of rearing should be female. Genotypic females also require appropriate female sex hormone therapy at puberty.

3β-Hydroxysteroid Dehydrogenase:Δ⁵⁻⁴ Isomerase Deficiency. Clinical Presentation. Affected 46 XY subjects with 3β-hydroxysteroid dehydrogenase:Δ⁵⁻⁴ isomerase deficiency have genital ambiguity, although mild to moderate hypospadias is more common than severe perineoscrotal hypospadias. Internal male sexual differentiation is normal, with wolffian differentiation and müllerian ductal inhibition. Curiously, genetic males who reach puberty develop gynecomastia, the etiology of which is not known. At birth genotypic females have normal or slightly virilized external genitalia, with clitoral hypertrophy and slight labial fusion.

Severely affected children have adrenal insufficiency and die in infancy as a result of salt-losing crisis if not adequately treated. In the milder cases sufficient cortisol and aldosterone are synthesized to avoid this complication.

Pathogenesis. The enzyme deficiency results in decreased cortisol production, increased ACTH secretion, and increased production of Δ⁵,3β-hydroxysteroids (Fig. 221–6). Plasma levels of pregnenolone, 17α-hydroxypregnenolone, and dehydroepiandrosterone and their sulfate conjugates are increased, with decreased levels of aldosterone and cortisol. The slight virilization of the external genitalia in the female is due to the mild androgenic effect of excess plasma dehydroepiandrosterone and its subsequent peripheral conversion to Δ⁵-androstenediol and other androgens (Table 221–4). Surprisingly, plasma Δ⁴ steroids, i.e., progesterone, 17α-hydroxyprogesterone, androstenedione, and occasionally testosterone, may be normal or even increased. This may reflect intact hepatic and peripheral 3β-hydroxysteroid dehydrogenase:Δ⁵⁻⁴ isomerase enzyme activity. Also in some

TABLE 221–3. XY MALE PSEUDOHERMAPHRODITISM WITH AN ENZYMATIC DEFECT IN TESTOSTERONE BIOSYNTHESIS

| Enzyme Deficiency | External Genitalia | | Secretion | | | Puberty | Comments |
	Female or Urogenital Sinus	Ambiguous	Cortisol	Aldosterone	Androgens		
Cholesterol 20,22-desmolase	+ + + +	+	↓	↓	↓	↓	
3β-Hydroxysteroid dehydrogenase:Δ$^{5-4}$ isomerase	+	+ + + +	− ↓	− ↓	↑ DHEA ↑ 17OH preg	Gynecomastia despite low estrogens	Intact peripheral 3βHSD with conversion of Δ^5 to Δ^4 steroids
17α-Hydroxylase	+ + + +	+ +	− ↓	B ↑ DOC ↑	↓	Gynecomastia despite low estrogens	Hypertension due to ↑ DOC with ↓ renin and aldosterone
17,20-Desmolase	+ + + +	+	−	−	↓		
17β-Hydroxysteroid dehydrogenase	+ + + +	+ +	−	−	↓ T ↑ Δ^4	Gynecomastia due to increased estrogen and decreased T	Peripheral conversion of androstenedione to E$_1$

↑ = elevated; ↓ = decreased; − = normal; + = relative frequency of occurrence; B = corticosterone; DOC = desoxycorticosterone; DHEA = dehydroepiandrosterone; 17OH Preg = 17α-hydroxypregnenolone; T = testosterone; Δ^4 = androstenedione; 3βHSD = 3β-hydroxysteroid dehydrogenase; E$_1$ = estrone.

affected subjects, the gonadal defect is not as severe as the adrenal defect, suggesting that the same enzyme may be under different regulatory control in different areas. The 3-BHSD gene has been cloned and localized to chromosome 1. In both gonadal and adrenal tissue it appears to be encoded by the same structural gene, but under separate regulatory control.

Management and Therapy. In infancy the diagnosis is suggested in a 46 XY male with ambiguous genitalia and adrenal insufficiency. In contrast to an infant with cholesterol 20,22-desmolase deficiency, urinary 17-ketosteroid values are normal to high with increased plasma dehydroepiandrosterone. Treatment involves mineralocorticoid and glucocorticoid replacement therapy. If needed, sex steroid therapy should be instituted at puberty to induce sexual development in accordance with the sex of rearing.

17α-Hydroxylase Deficiency. **Clinical Presentation.** Many cases of 17α-hydroxylase deficiency have been reported in both genetic males and females. In 46 XY subjects the defect of the external genitalia is usually severe, resulting in completely female external genitalia at birth. Müllerian structures are absent, and wolffian structures are either developed or hypoplastic. Often gynecomastia develops at puberty with little or no virilization. Thus, males with this enzyme deficiency can have the same phenotype in adulthood as subjects with the complete androgen insensitivity syndrome. In 46 XX females with this condition secondary sexual development is absent at puberty and there is primary amenorrhea. Classically the affected subjects also have hypertension and hypokalemia.

Pathogenesis. 17α-Hydroxylase activity resides in the same P-450 enzyme as 17,20-desmolase activity (see section below), coded for by a gene located on chromosome 10. 17α-Hydroxylase deficiency can be characterized by partial or complete defects in either or both 17α-hydroxylase/17,20-desmolase activities. Some of the mutations that have been found include (1) a seven base pair (bp) duplication in the N-terminal region XYP17 (P-450 17α), producing a premature stop codon, (2) a triplet deletion of the

TABLE 221–4. CLASSIFICATION OF CAUSES OF FEMALE PSEUDOHERMAPHRODITISM

I. Androgenic influences
  A. Fetal
    1. Congenital adrenogenital syndrome
      a. 21-Hydroxylase deficiency
      b. 11β-Hydroxylase deficiency
      c. 3β-Hydroxysteroid dehydrogenase:Δ$^{5-4}$ isomerase deficiency
  B. Maternal
    1. Excess maternal androgen production
    2. Maternal ingestion of virilizing substances
II. Idiopathic

N-terminal of the CYP-17 gene, (3) a four-base duplication on exon 8, and (4) a stop codon in place of tryptophan at amino acid 17, leading to the formation of a truncated protein.

17α-Hydroxylase activity converts pregnenolone and progesterone to 17α-hydroxypregnenolone and 17α-hydroxyprogesterone, respectively (Fig. 221–6). These steps are necessary for the ultimate formation of cortisol and C19 androgens, including testosterone. Thus a deficiency results in decreased plasma cortisol, an increase in ACTH, and hypersecretion of the plasma precursor 17-deoxysteroids (pregnenolone, progesterone, desoxycorticosterone, corticosterone, 18-hydroxycorticosterone) and their urinary metabolites. Excess circulating desoxycorticosterone increases sodium retention and plasma volume, resulting in hypertension, hypokalemia, and suppression of plasma renin. The plasma aldosterone value is also low secondary to a low level of plasma renin (see Table 221–3). 17α-Hydroxylated steroids are decreased, i.e., plasma 17α-hydroxypregnenolone, 17α-hydroxyprogesterone, 11-deoxycortisol, cortisol, androstenedione, dehydroepiandrosterone, testosterone, and estrogen. Consequently, urinary levels of 17-hydroxysteroids and 17-ketosteroids are low. Despite markedly impaired cortisol production, signs of glucocorticoid deficiency do not generally occur, due to the inherent glucocorticoid activity in the high levels of circulating corticosterone.

In affected adults, gonadotropin values are elevated, sex steroid levels are low, and in the male there is little or no testicular 17α-hydroxyprogesterone and testosterone response to hCG administration. Consanguinity has been documented in some cases, as has an occurrence of the disorder in siblings of both the same and opposite sex.

Management and Therapy. Hypertension associated with hypokalemic alkalosis in an XY individual with female external genitalia or ambiguous genitalia should suggest the diagnosis. It should also be suspected in any XX female with the same symptom complex who has primary amenorrhea and lack of secondary sexual development. Glucocorticoid replacement therapy reverses the metabolic abnormality and lowers the blood pressure. Appropriate sex steroid therapy concordant with the sex of rearing should be administered at puberty.

17,20-Desmolase Deficiency. **Clinical Presentation.** In 1972 a child with male ambiguous genitalia was described with a defect postulated to be secondary to 17,20-desmolase deficiency. A male pseudohermaphroditic cousin and maternal 46 XY "aunt" were included in the report. Since then other cases of the enzyme deficiency in 46 XY males have been reported, all phenotypic females or subjects with severely ambiguous genitalia. A genetic female with primary amenorrhea and lack of secondary sexual development has also been reported.

Pathogenesis. 17,20-Desmolase activity resides in the same P-450 enzyme as 17α-hydroxylase. Partial or complete lack of this activity in the adrenal and gonads results in decreased cleavage of the two-carbon side chain from either 17α-hydroxyprogesterone or 17α-hydroxypregnenolone with a resultant decrease in androstenedione and dehydroepiandrosterone production, respectively (Fig. 221–6). This step is essential for the ultimate formation of testosterone and estrogens. A deficiency in 17,20-desmolase activity can also be associated with a deficiency of 17α-hydroxylase activity (see above).

It is not known why the basal plasma levels of progesterone, pregnenolone, 17α-hydroxyprogesterone, and 17α-hydroxypregnenolone are elevated, particularly in prepubertal subjects with this enzyme deficiency. Since the enzyme 17,20-desmolase is not involved in cortisol biosynthesis, ACTH levels should be normal with subsequent normal amounts of the C21 precursor steroids mentioned above (Fig. 221–6).

Management and Therapy. In genotypic males the sex of rearing depends upon the degree of ambiguity of the external genitalia. In more severe cases, patients should be raised as females, with castration carried out in early childhood. Sex hormone therapy at puberty is invariably necessary. In genotypic females, estrogen and progesterone supplementation is invariably needed at the time of puberty.

17β-Hydroxysteroid Dehydrogenase Deficiency. Clinical Presentation. This condition, described only in 46 XY males, is characterized by either female external genitalia or mild ambiguity of the genitalia. With few exceptions, those affected have been raised as girls. In subjects with totally female-appearing external genitalia at birth, the abnormality is not noted until puberty, when virilization frequently occurs with clitoral enlargement. At puberty there are two distinct clinical presentations. Some subjects develop gynecomastia in addition to virilization, while others undergo strong virilization with a male pattern of body hair, deep voice, android build, and no gynecomastia. All subjects raised as females throughout childhood who were castrated prior to or during their teenage years have maintained a female gender identity.

Pathogenesis. 17β-Hydroxysteroid dehydrogenase catalyzes the conversion of androstenedione to testosterone, the final step in the synthesis of testosterone (Fig. 221–6), and the oxidation-reduction of estrone and estradiol, dehydroepiandrosterone, and Δ^5-androstenediol. In affected 46 XY subjects, the enzyme deficiency results in increased circulating plasma levels of androstenedione, while plasma levels of testosterone are low to low normal (Table 221–3). Plasma luteinizing hormone (LH) is increased, while plasma follicle-stimulating hormone (FSH) is normal to increased. Approximately 90 per cent of circulating testosterone arises from the extragonadal conversion of androstenedione. Thus in the adult the defect appears to affect the testes while peripheral enzyme activity appears to be intact. However, for masculinization of the external genitalia to be minimal or absent in the fetus, peripheral conversion of androstenedione to testosterone and dihydrotestosterone in the anlage of the external genitalia must be insignificant or absent during early gestation. Thus, peripheral as well as testicular 17β-hydroxysteroid dehydrogenase activity appears deficient in utero, whereas peripheral enzyme activity appears to be intact in the adult. The elevated plasma levels of androstenedione result in increased peripheral conversion to estrone (Table 221–3). In some subjects the conversion of estrone to estradiol also appears to be as severely impaired as the conversion of androstenedione to testosterone, while in others it is impaired to a lesser degree or not at all, suggesting that the 17β-hydroxysteroid dehydrogenase enzyme(s) converting estrone to estradiol and androstenedione to testosterone may be under different regulatory control. The lower the plasma testosterone-estradiol ratio, the greater the likelihood of gynecomastia developing in an affected subject at the time of puberty.

Management and Therapy. 46 XY affected subjects with female external genitalia should be raised as females and castration carried out either before or during early puberty to avoid significant virilization. Female sex hormone therapy should be instituted at puberty. In those subjects with ambiguous genitalia that can be surgically corrected, a male sex of rearing should be considered. If the diagnosis is made peripubertally or postpubertally, careful psychosexual evaluation should be performed to determine the gender identity before any therapy is instituted. If a gender change from female to male has occurred with puberty, corrective male genital surgery is needed.

New MI, White P, Pang S, et al.: The adrenal hyperplasias. *In* Scriver C, Baudet A, Sly W, et al. (eds.): *The Metabolic Basis of Inherited Disease*, 6th ed. New York, McGraw Hill, 1989, pp 1881–1918. *A review of the biochemical aspects of nonvirilizing and virilizing forms of congenital adrenal hyperplasia.*

Peterson RE, Imperato-McGinley J: Male pseudohermaphroditism due to inherited deficiencies of testosterone biosynthesis. *In* Serio M, Motta M, Zanisi M, et al. (eds.): *Sexual Differentiation: Basic and Clinical Aspects*. Vol. 2. New York, Raven Press, 1984, pp 301–319. *A detailed study of the clinical characteristics and the biochemistry of male pseudohermaphroditism due to deficiencies in testosterone biosynthesis.*

DISORDERS OF FUNCTION AT ANDROGEN-DEPENDENT TARGET AREAS

COMPLETE ANDROGEN INSENSITIVITY—TESTICULAR FEMINIZATION. Clinical Presentation. In this inherited form of male pseudohermaphroditism, genetic and gonadal males have a female phenotype and totally female psychosexual orientation. The testes differentiate and secrete müllerian inhibiting factor, resulting in absent fallopian tubes, uterus, and upper portion of the vagina. Despite normal to high-normal plasma levels of testosterone, wolffian structures are absent or rudimentary, and the external genitalia are totally female. Affected subjects are raised as girls, and the condition is rarely suspected prior to puberty. A prepubertal diagnosis is made when inguinal or labial masses are palpated in a phenotypic female child and are found to be testes.

Adequate breast development occurs at puberty, but pubic and axillary hair is scant to absent. Medical attention is usually sought because of primary amenorrhea. Rarely, patients with 17α-hydroxylase deficiency have the same phenotypic presentation at puberty.

Pathogenesis. In patients with complete androgen insensitivity, absence of high-affinity binding to the androgen receptor (receptor-negative) has been demonstrated in cultured fibroblasts from genital skin. A variety of qualitative abnormalities of the androgen receptor have also been described, suggesting different structural changes of the receptor protein. Deletions and point mutations of the DNA and steroid-binding domains of the androgen receptor have been described in this condition. Postreceptor variants with normal androgen receptor binding have also been demonstrated. In the latter individuals, the mutation may affect the steps in the initiation of androgen action subsequent to nuclear binding, i.e., failure of RNA synthesis or an abnormality in its processing (Fig. 221–7).

The receptor-negative form of complete androgen insensitivity is maternally transmitted with only males expressing the condition, suggesting inheritance as X-linked recessive or autosomal dominant-sex limited (males). The gene for the androgen receptor is on the long arm of the X chromosome near the centromere.

Plasma testosterone levels are normal to high with mild to moderately elevated plasma levels of LH. FSH levels are normal to elevated. Urinary estrogens and plasma estradiol levels are generally in the low female range with increased production rates for estrone and estradiol, which are mainly testicular in origin. The elevated circulating estrogens together with the androgen unresponsiveness result in an unopposed estrogen effect resulting in breast development at puberty.

The histology of the testes resembles that of normal prepubertal males. Postpubertally, Sertoli cells and spermatogonia are present, but no evidence of spermatogenesis exists. The Leydig cells are hyperplastic, correlating with the elevated plasma testosterone levels.

Management and Therapy. Testicular neoplasms occur in approximately 2 to 5 per cent of patients with complete androgen insensitivity, but rarely before the age of 25 to 30 years. For this reason the testes should be removed following puberty to allow complete breast development. Following castration, cyclic estrogen replacement therapy is necessary to maintain adequate breast turgor. In general, the vagina is adequate for normal coital function. Occasionally it is too shallow, but can frequently be enlarged with vaginal dilators, thereby avoiding reconstructive surgery.

PARTIAL ANDROGEN INSENSITIVITY. Clinical Presentation. Partial forms of androgen insensitivity occur. Affected subjects range from XY subjects with genital ambiguity and minimal to moderate pubertal virilization and gynecomastia, to normal males with gynecomastia or infertility. Several pedigrees compatible with X linkage have been reported. Studies of genital

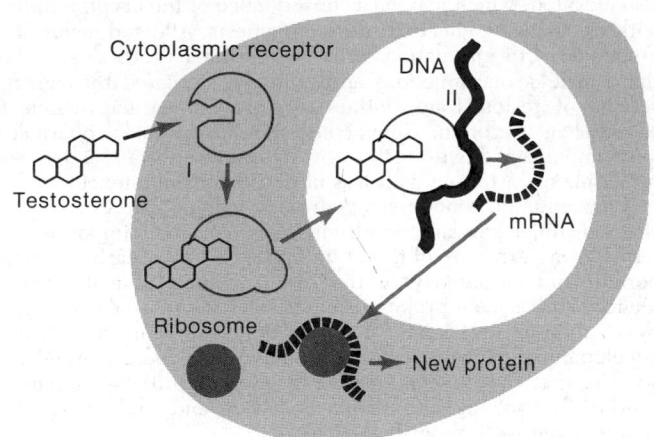

I. Abnormalities affecting binding to the cytosol receptor

  A. Quantitative

    1. Absent binding to cytosol receptor

  B. Qualitative

    1. Thermolability
    2. Failure of stabilization with sodium molybdate
    3. Altered binding affinity
    4. Lability of cytosolic receptor under conditions that normally promote transformation to the DNA–binding state

II. Nuclear or postnuclear receptor binding defect

    1. Impaired nuclear retention
    2. Impaired augmentation of receptor binding following incubation with androgen

FIGURE 221–7. Illustration of the abnormalities of androgen action resulting in androgen insensitivity.

skin fibroblasts from a mother of affected subjects demonstrate two clonal populations, one with normal dihydrotestosterone binding and one with a qualitative abnormality altering binding to the cytosol receptor, confirming X linkage in this form of androgen insensitivity. Affected subjects within the same pedigree may exhibit the variable phenotypes described. Thus these syndromes may represent variable phenotypic expressions of the same gene mutation.

Pathogenesis. In general, the endocrine profile is similar to that demonstrated in subjects with complete androgen insensitivity. Plasma LH and testosterone levels are generally elevated. The total amount of 17β-estradiol produced and the quantity secreted by the testes can be greater than those found in patients with complete androgen insensitivity. However, despite increased estrogen production, the degree of feminization at puberty is not as marked as in complete androgen insensitivity, which may be a consequence of the incomplete androgen resistance with a less severe androgen and estrogen imbalance at the cellular level.

In some affected males with incomplete androgen insensitivity, the binding capacity and affinity of the androgen receptor for dihydrotestosterone are normal. Thus this condition may be a variant of complete androgen insensitivity with normal cytosol-binding activity. Other affected males, however, have a reduced number of binding sites for dihydrotestosterone; this may represent a variant of complete androgen insensitivity with absence of androgen-binding activity. Qualitative defects in the receptor have also been demonstrated.

A form of incomplete androgen insensitivity is infertility in phenotypically normal men with either azoospermia or severe oligospermia. The mean plasma levels of LH and testosterone can be normal or elevated. The most frequent finding in cultured genital skin fibroblasts is a decrease in androgen-binding capacity of the androgen receptor. How frequently this is a cause of infertility is unknown.

Management and Therapy. Subjects with incomplete androgen insensitivity can be distinguished biochemically from male pseu-

dohermaphroditism with defects in testosterone biosynthesis. Following puberty, a normal to elevated plasma testosterone level with a normal androstenedione-testosterone ratio as well as normal plasma progesterone and dehydroepiandrosterone levels distinguishes subjects with this condition from subjects with 17β-hydroxysteroid dehydrogenase deficiency, 17α-hydroxylase deficiency, and 3β-hydroxysteroid dehydrogenase deficiency, who can have the same appearance. True hermaphrodites most commonly have an XX karyotype and can often be distinguished on that basis. Incomplete androgen insensitivity in puberty commonly results in gynecomastia and varying degrees of virilization.

Subjects with moderate to severe defects in masculinization of the external genitalia should be raised as females and castrated before puberty to prevent virilization. Estrogen therapy should be added at puberty. Those with mild hypospadias can be raised as males but require surgery for correction of both the hypospadias and the gynecomastia, if present.

Griffen JD, Wilson JD: The androgen resistance syndromes: 5α reductase deficiency, testicular feminization, and related disorders. *In* Scriver C, Baudet A, Sly W, et al. (eds.): The Metabolic Basis of Inherited Disease, 6th ed. New York, McGraw-Hill, 1989, pp 1919–1944. *A comprehensive review of the biochemical abnormalities in complete and partial androgen insensitivity.*

5α-REDUCTASE DEFICIENCY. *Clinical Presentation.*

Most patients with this condition have pseudovaginal perineal hypospadias with separate urethral and vaginal openings within a urogenital sinus. Rarely a blind vaginal pouch opens into the urethra. All patients have epididymides, vas deferens, and seminal vesicles. The incidence of cryptorchidism is significantly higher in childhood than adulthood, suggesting that occasionally the testes descend during puberty.

The pubertal events include deepening of the voice, development of a muscular habitus, growth of the phallus, rugation and hyperpigmentation of the scrotum, and testicular descent. The prostate is small or absent, even in elderly subjects. Subjects have erections with ejaculation from the perineal urethra. Facial hair is decreased or absent and body hair is decreased.

Pathogenesis. The enzyme Δ^4,5α-reductase catalyzes the reduction of the double bond at the 4–5 position of both C19 steroids, such as testosterone, and C21 steroids. It is present in high quantities in the liver and peripheral tissues, particularly the sebaceous glands, hair follicles, and skin of the external genitalia, where it converts testosterone to dihydrotestosterone (Fig. 221–8). When the enzyme is deficient, plasma testosterone is normal to elevated and dihydrotestosterone is decreased. The urinary 5α-reduced metabolites of testosterone, i.e., androsterone and androstanediol, and of C21 and C19 steroids other than testosterone, i.e., cortisol, corticosterone, 11β-hydroxyandrostenedione, and androstenedione, are decreased. Diminished 5α-reductase activity has been demonstrated both in skin slices and in fibroblasts cultured from genital skin. An autosomal recessive inheritance has been demonstrated.

Male pseudohermaphrodites with 5α-reductase deficiency represent a unique clinical model, defining major actions for testosterone and dihydrotestosterone in male sexual differentiation and development. Since the developmental defect is limited to the external genitalia and prostate, their development appears to be effected through the actions of dihydrotestosterone. In contrast,

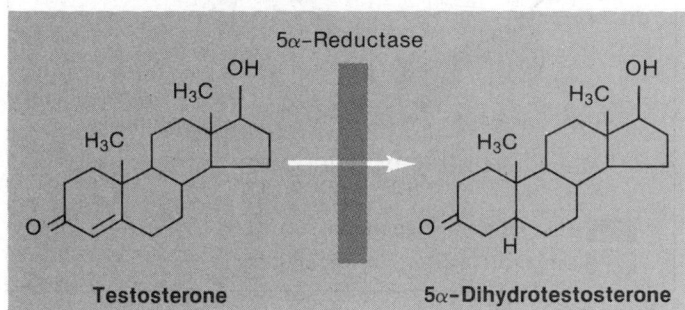

FIGURE 221–8. The conversion of testosterone to dihydrotestosterone by the enzyme 5α-reductase.

wolffian differentiation develops normally and appears to be a testosterone-mediated function (Fig. 221–9). At puberty the affected males develop rugation and hyperpigmentation of the scrotum, growth of the phallus, an increase in muscle mass, and deepening of the voice (Fig. 221–10). Their ultimate height is similar to that of their fathers and normal male sibs. Thus these pubertal events are mainly effected through the actions of testosterone. In contrast, prostatic development or enlargement, acne, normal male facial and body hair, and temporal recession of the hairline do not occur in affected males and appear to be effected mainly through the actions of dihydrotestosterone.

It is puzzling that the effects of dihydrotestosterone in dihydrotestosterone-dependent areas are not mimicked by testosterone, since both androgens share a common cytosol receptor. Two possible explanations can be submitted: (1) the cytosol receptor at certain target sites is modified so that it favors 5α-dihydrotestosterone over testosterone or (2) the 5α-dihydrotestosterone receptor complex has a higher affinity for the acceptor sites in chromatin.

In a few affected subjects with descended testes, testicular biopsy has demonstrated complete spermatogenesis; thus testosterone may be more important than dihydrotestosterone in the process of spermatogenesis. The question of fertility, however, remains unanswered. The cryptorchid testes of most subjects demonstrate seminiferous tubular damage with either Sertoli cells only or aberrant spermatogenesis. Plasma LH is increased despite normal to high plasma levels of testosterone, suggesting a role for dihydrotestosterone in the negative feedback control of LH. The elevated plasma LH levels correlate with the microscopic findings of Leydig cell hyperplasia. Plasma FSH levels are also elevated, which may be a consequence of the cryptorchidism with its damaging effect on spermatogenesis. Affected males have erections, with ejaculation from the perineal urethra, and thus these male sexual functions appear to be mediated through the actions of testosterone, either directly or via conversion to estradiol in the brain. Conversely, administration of pharmacologic amounts of dihydrotestosterone causes a substantial decrease in plasma testosterone with loss of libido and impotence.

A documented gender change from female to male in untreated affected subjects in large kindreds underscores the importance of testosterone exposure of the brain in utero, in the early postnatal period, and at puberty in the determination of male gender identity. It has been proposed that gender identity becomes fixed by 18 months to 4 years of age, around the time of language development. However, from studies with these patients, it appears that the development of gender identity in humans is continually evolving throughout childhood and adolescence, becoming fixed with puberty.

Management and Therapy. Subjects who have been diagnosed in infancy and in early childhood should be raised as males and their sex changed. Dihydrotestosterone cream should be administered to increase phallic size to facilitate surgical correction.

The most serious debate involves how to manage subjects who were raised as females but were diagnosed as having 5α-reductase deficiency in the peripubertal and postpubertal period. After careful psychiatric evaluation some subjects are found to have a male gender identity and should be helped to take their place as males in society. Other subjects who are not able consciously or subconsciously to admit the fact of maleness cannot and should not be encouraged to change gender roles. All these factors must be considered by the physician and a psychiatrist working in concert with the patient and the family before a final decision concerning the sex of rearing is made.

Imperato-McGinley J, Gautier T: Inherited 5α-reductase deficiency. Trends Genet 2(5):130, 1986. *A review of the inheritance and clinical and biochemical findings of this unusual experiment of nature.*

Imperato-McGinley J: 5α Reductase deficiency. *In* Bardin CW (ed.): Current Therapy in Endocrinology and Metabolism—4. Philadelphia, B. C. Decker, 1991. *A review of the condition with a comprehensive discussion of management and therapy.*

XX Males and True Hermaphroditism

XX MALES

Clinical Presentation. Approximately 50 cases of XX males have been reported, including members within the same family. The incidence in newborn males is estimated to be 1 in 20,000. Classically XX adult males have short stature, a normal-sized penis, small firm testes generally less than 2 cm, and infertility. One third have gynecomastia. The phenotypic appearance resembles that of males with Klinefelter's syndrome (XXY) with the notable exception that XX males are shorter in stature than the average male. The histologic features of the testes also resemble those of subjects with Klinefelter's syndrome. The seminiferous tubules are hyalinized and contain only Sertoli cells or a few immature spermatogonia, correlating clinically with azoospermia or oligospermia. The Leydig cells are hyperplastic. Levels of FSH and LH are elevated, with decreased plasma testosterone and increased plasma estradiol levels. XX children with bilateral testes and ambiguous genitalia have been reported, suggesting a phenotypic spectrum of this condition (Table 221–1).

Pathogenesis. Three possible mechanisms for the expression of masculinity in XX individuals have been proposed—(1) translocation of part of the Y chromosome to the X chromosome or to an autosome, (2) undetected mosaicism XX/XY or XXY, and (3) a mutant autosomal gene determining maleness in an XX individual. DNA digests from the nuclei of cells from testes of an XX male have demonstrated Y-specific DNA fragments. Studies using Y-specific DNA probes have demonstrated the presence of Y chromosomal material in the genome of some XX males. Thus, most 46 XX males appear to be a consequence of a paternal X-Y interchange containing the testes-determining gene on the Y chromosome.

TRUE HERMAPHRODITISM

Clinical Presentation. In true hermaphroditism both ovarian and testicular tissue is present with each gonad containing its

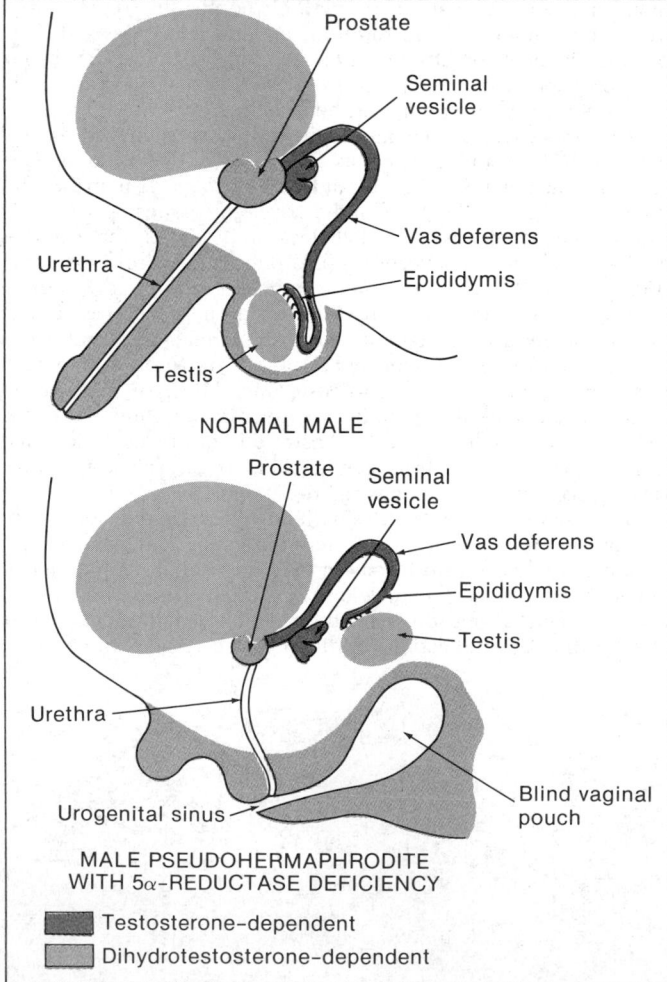

Prostate

Seminal vesicle

Vas deferens

Epididymis

Urethra

Testis

NORMAL MALE

Prostate

Seminal vesicle

Vas deferens

Epididymis

Testis

Urethra

Urogenital sinus

Blind vaginal pouch

MALE PSEUDOHERMAPHRODITE WITH 5α-REDUCTASE DEFICIENCY

■ Testosterone-dependent

■ Dihydrotestosterone-dependent

FIGURE 221–9. Illustration of the hypothesis for the specific actions of testosterone and dihydrotestosterone in male sexual differentiation in utero.

corresponding gamete. Most subjects have ambiguous genitalia, although approximately 7 per cent of true hermaphrodites have normal female external genitalia; 75 per cent of affected subjects are raised as males. The most common gonadal associations are an ovary and testis or an ovotestis and ovary. Gonadal tumors occur in approximately 2 per cent.

A fallopian tube is always found adjacent to an ovary and also most commonly adjacent to an ovotestis. An epididymis is present in approximately one third and a uterus in approximately 90 per cent of affected subjects.

With puberty, variable virilization and feminization occur. About half of affected subjects menstruate; in those raised as males with mild or moderate hypospadias or a penile urethra, menstruation can present as cyclic hematuria. Gynecomastia develops in 80 per cent of subjects. Pregnancy and childbirth have been reported in true hermaphrodites following removal of testicular tissue and correction of the external genitalia. A few subjects with functional testicular tissue are fertile (Table 221–1).

Pathogenesis. A 46 XX complement is present in approximately two thirds of cases, XX/XY mosaicism in one third of cases, and 46 XY complement in one tenth of the cases. A reported case of true hermaphroditism in a subject whose brother and paternal uncle were XX males suggests that XX males and XX true hermaphrodites may be variants of the same condition. Interestingly, Y-specific DNA has been found in some XX true hermaphrodites. The pathogenesis of the presence of both ovarian and testicular tissue is unknown.

Management and Therapy. The sex assignment in true hermaphroditism diagnosed in infancy and childhood is best determined by the appearance of the external genitalia, together with the gonadal tissue and internal structures. If an ovary-ovotestis and a uterus are present, the ovotestis and any male internal structures should be removed and feminizing surgery of the external genitalia performed. If bilateral ovotestes are present, and if a good line of demarcation is seen between ovarian and testicular tissue, the testicular portion should be removed, the genitalia surgically feminized, and the child raised as female. If a testis is present on one side and an ovotestis on the contralateral side, the testis should be brought into the scrotum and the child raised as male if the external genitalia can be surgically corrected. If an ovary is present on one side and a testis on the contralateral side, the sex of rearing should be decided by evaluation of the appearance of the external and internal sex structures, and appropriate surgical correction should be performed. Peripubertal or postpubertal surgical correction of the internal and external sex structures should depend exclusively upon the gender identity of the affected individual. Although testicular tumor formation is rare, if the individual is to be raised as male the testis should be brought into the scrotum, so that periodic examination can be accomplished.

McLaren A: What makes a man a man? Nature 346:216, 1990. *Discussion on the latest development in the quest for the testes determining gene.*

Female Pseudohermaphroditism

Female pseudohermaphroditism can result from either fetal or maternal androgenic influences (Table 221–4). Cases of undetermined etiology have also been described.

CONGENITAL ADRENAL HYPERPLASIA— VIRILIZING FORMS

Three adrenal enzyme defects, 21-hydroxylase deficiency, 11β-hydroxylase deficiency, and 3β-hydroxysteroid dehydrogenase deficiency, can result in increased androgen production in utero with virilization of the female fetus (Table 221–5). They are the virilizing forms of congenital adrenal hyperplasia (Fig. 221–6). 21-Hydroxylase and 11β-hydroxylase deficiency can result in severe virilization of the female fetus. The virilization with 3β-hydroxysteroid dehydrogenase deficiency is mild; it is also a cause of male pseudohermaphroditism, and is discussed in the section Male Pseudohermaphroditism. The adrenal enzyme defects decrease cortisol production; pituitary ACTH secretion therefore increases and drives adrenal androgen overproduction. In the genotypic female, since ovaries and not testes are present, müllerian inhibiting factor is not produced, and the internal structures are female, i.e., uterus and fallopian tubes. Despite the masculinization of the external genitalia, wolffian differentiation does not occur. Affected 46 XY males with either 21-hydroxylase or 11β-hydroxylase deficiency appear phenotypically normal at birth.

21-HYDROXYLASE DEFICIENCY. Clinical Features. 21-Hydroxylase deficiency is the most common cause of ambiguous genitalia in 46 XX infants. Its incidence varies from approximately 1 in 300 births in Alaskan Eskimos to 1 in 15,000 births in Caucasians in Wisconsin. In the classic form of the disease, the spectrum of masculinization varies at birth from female infants with minimal clitoromegaly and fusion of the labioscrotal folds to infants with a penile urethra and the appearance of a cryptorchid

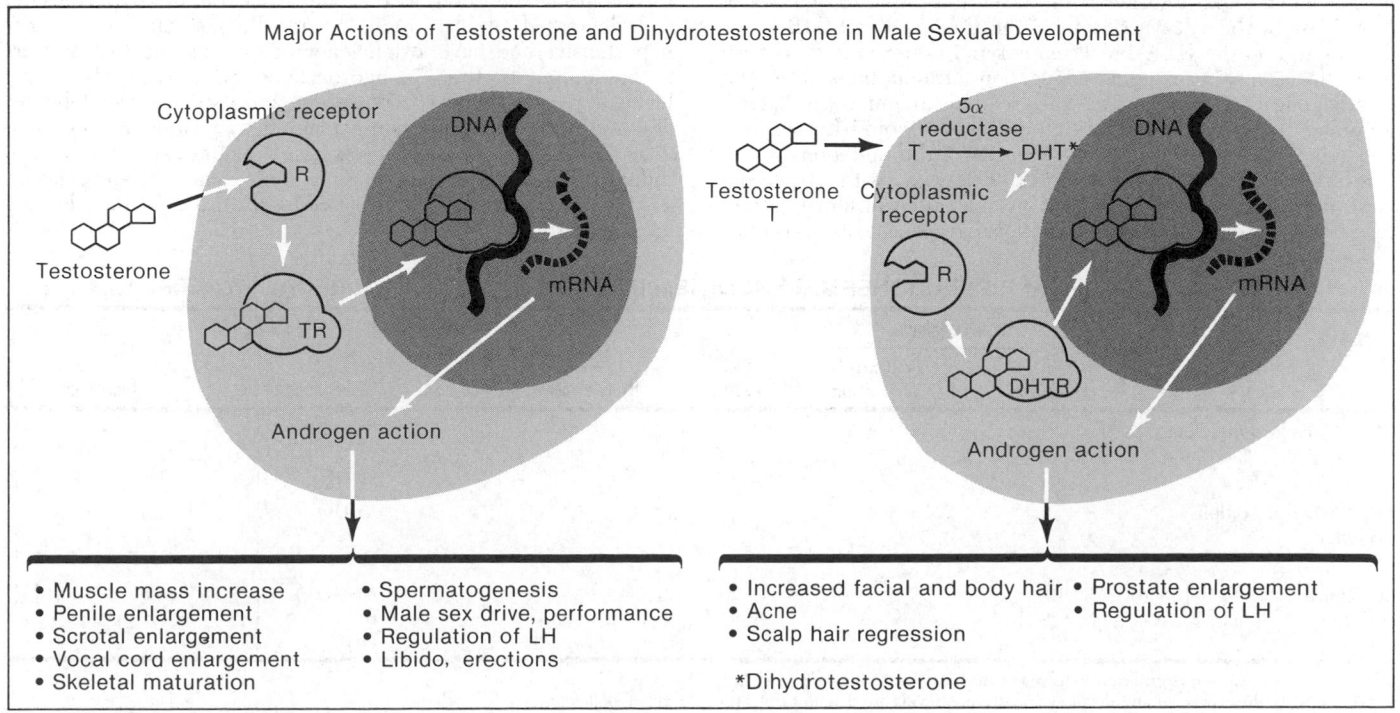

Major Actions of Testosterone and Dihydrotestosterone in Male Sexual Development

• Muscle mass increase	• Spermatogenesis
• Penile enlargement	• Male sex drive, performance
• Scrotal enlargement	• Regulation of LH
• Vocal cord enlargement	• Libido, erections
• Skeletal maturation	

• Increased facial and body hair	• Prostate enlargement
• Acne	• Regulation of LH
• Scalp hair regression	

*Dihydrotestosterone

FIGURE 221–10. Illustration of the major actions of testosterone and dihydrotestosterone at puberty.

male. Some infants also have salt wasting and may die in infancy. If affected XX children are untreated in infancy, there is rapid acceleration of growth; enlargement of the clitoris; increase in muscle mass; precocious development of pubic, axillary, and body hair; and advancement of bone age. Although they are tall in childhood, premature closure of the epiphyses eventually results in short stature in adulthood. At the time of expected puberty, there is absence of breast development and menstruation. Untreated males with this condition also show precocious maturation with short stature in adulthood. The excessive androgen production can inhibit gonadotropin secretion, so that untreated adult males, although strongly virilized, can have small soft testes and azoospermia. However, because of the adrenal androgen excess, they are capable of having erections. Frequently, however, true puberty occurs in untreated males with normal FSH and LH secretion, testicular enlargement, and spermatogenesis. ACTH-dependent testicular "tumors," most probably of adrenal origin, have been described and can occur either unilaterally or bilaterally.

Females with a nonclassic or late-onset form of the disease are born with normal female genitalia but may develop hirsutism, acne, and menstrual irregularities at puberty.

Pathogenesis. 21-Hydroxylase deficiency results in decreased synthesis of cortisol with consequent increase in ACTH and increase in plasma progesterone, 17α-hydroxyprogesterone, and C19 androgens (dehydroepiandrosterone, androstenedione, and testosterone; Figure 221–6; Table 221–5). In the newborn, determination of plasma 17α-hydroxyprogesterone is the test most diagnostic for this condition. The increased adrenal androgen production in the female fetus in utero virilizes the external genitalia. In the salt-losing form, aldosterone production is deficient, but the salt loss may also be due to increased production of progesterone and 17α-hydroxyprogesterone, which act as aldosterone antagonists. Obligate carrier parents and sibs frequently demonstrate increased 17α-hydroxyprogesterone levels in response to a 1-hour ACTH stimulation test.

The gene for 21-hydroxylase deficiency is closely linked to the HLA locus of chromosome 6. HLA-A3, BW47, DR7, and BW60 are associated with the salt-wasting form, HLA-B5 with the simple virilizing form, and HLA-B14, DR1 with the nonclassic or late-onset form of this condition.

There are two 21-hydroxylase genes, CYP-21A (a pseudogene) and CYP-21B, located adjacent to C4A and C4B genes that encode the fourth component of serum complement. About one quarter of the classic forms of the disease are due to deletion of CYP-21B. In the salt-wasting form the CYP-21B and C4B genes are deleted on the HLA-BW47 haplotype. Other mutations arise from the transfer or gene conversion of mutations from the pseudogene CYP-21A to CYP-21B, leading to amino acid alterations and aberrant splicing. The clinical severity of 21-hydroxylase deficiency is correlated with the severity of the mutation.

Management and Therapy. Affected females with 21-hydroxylase deficiency have ovaries and normal internal female structures with potential for fertility. Therefore, diagnosis and treatment should be carried out early and the child appropriately treated and raised as a female. Surgical correction of the masculinized external genitalia should be performed early so that gender confusion does not occur later on in childhood and adolescence. Medical therapy involves adequate glucocorticoid replacement therapy to lower ACTH secretion and to suppress adrenal androgen excess. Overtreatment should be avoided to prevent the signs and symptoms of glucocorticoid excess, which can lead to growth retardation.

Overt salt losers must be given mineralocorticoid as well as glucocorticoid replacement therapy. Many affected subjects without overt signs of adrenal crisis have impaired mineralocorticoid production, characterized by decreased sodium content and plasma volume with resultant increase in plasma renin, and may benefit from mineralocorticoid supplementation.

The nonclassic or late-onset form of the disease can be treated with a single low dose of a glucocorticoid administered in the late evening. This blunts the rise of ACTH in the morning hours and decreases adrenal androgen production. The treatment results in regulation of menses and improvement in fertility, as well as in hirsutism and acne.

11β-HYDROXYLASE DEFICIENCY. Clinical Features. Females with this disorder can have mild to severe masculinization of the external genitalia. A late-onset form results in mild hirsutism, clitoral hypertrophy, and irregular menses to severe virilization. Males with this condition show precocious male sexual maturation but develop gynecomastia at puberty. The cause of the gynecomastia is unknown, but it has been postulated to be secondary to elevated plasma desoxycorticosterone levels. Patients usually have hyporeninemic hypertension due to elevated desoxycorticosterone levels.

Pathogenesis. 11β-Hydroxylase deficiency results in decreased cortisol production, which causes an increase in ACTH, in C19 androgen secretion, and in desoxycorticosterone production (Fig. 221–6). Elevation of the plasma 11-desoxycortisol level is diagnostic of this enzyme deficiency and distinguishes it from 21-hydroxylase deficiency. Plasma cortisol as well as the urinary cortisol metabolites tetrahydrocortisone and tetrahydrocortisol can be normal to low. Urinary 17-ketosteroids, reflecting adrenal androgen overproduction, and urinary 17-hydroxysteroids, reflecting elevated levels of plasma 11-desoxycortisol, are increased. Excretion of pregnanetriol, a metabolite of 17α-hydroxyprogesterone, is usually normal or slightly increased. Plasma desoxycorticosterone is increased, as is its urinary metabolite tetrahydrodesoxycorticosterone, while corticosterone and aldosterone are decreased. The increased production of desoxycorticosterone results in salt retention, increased plasma volume, hypertension, and decreased plasma renin. Some affected subjects are not hypertensive and have a deficiency of the enzyme that appears to be limited to the 17α-hydroxylated pathway, with normal levels of plasma desoxycorticosterone and its urinary metabolites (Table 221–5). This has been explained by postulating the presence of either two 11β-hydroxylase enzyme systems or two different regulatory systems for 17α-hydroxylase steroids and for 17-desoxysteroids. The gene that codes for this enzyme is located on chromosome 8.

TABLE 221–5. XX FEMALE PSEUDOHERMAPHRODITISM DUE TO CONGENITAL ADRENAL HYPERPLASIA

| Enzyme Deficiency | External Genitalia | | Salt-wasting | Hypertension | Cortisol | Mineralocorticoids | | Androgens | |
	Ambiguous	Postnatal Virilization							
21-Hydroxylase deficiency	+ + + +	+ + + +	50–80%	−	− ↓	*ALDO ↓ *B ↓ *DOC ↓		T ↑ Δ4 ↑ ↑ ↑ 17OHP ↑ ↑ ↑ ↑	
11β-Hydroxylase deficiency†	+ + +	+ + + +	−	+ +	− ↓	ALDO ↓ B ↓ DOC ↑		T ↑ Δ4 ↑ ↑ 17OHP ↑ ↑	
3β-Hydroxysteroid dehydrogenase deficiency	+ +	+ +	±	−	− ↓	ALDO ↓ − B ↓ − DOC ↓		DHEA ↑ ↑ ↑ 17OH preg ↑	

*Mineralocorticoids are significantly decreased in the salt-wasting form of 21 O-hydroxylase deficiency.
†Elevated 11-desoxycortisol and desoxycorticosterone levels are diagnostic of 11β-hydroxylase deficiency.
↑ = elevated; ↓ = decreased; − = normal; + = relative frequency of occurrence; ALDO = aldosterone; B = corticosterone; DOC = desoxycorticosterone; T = testosterone; Δ4 = 4-androstenedione; 17OHP = 17-hydroxyprogesterone; DHEA = dehydroepiandrosterone; 17OH preg = 17α-hydroxypregnenolone.

Management and Therapy. Glucocorticoid replacement therapy effects biochemical normalization, decreases blood pressure, and arrests precocious development. In females, surgical correction of the external genitalia should be carried out as in females with 21-hydroxylase deficiency.

VIRILIZATION OF THE FEMALE FETUS SECONDARY TO EXCESS MATERNAL ANDROGEN PRODUCTION OR EXOGENOUS MATERNAL ADMINISTRATION OF VIRILIZING HORMONES

Masculinization of the female infant may occur in mothers with ovarian luteomas, virilizing adrenal tumors, and untreated maternal congenital adrenal hyperplasia. Why virilization of the female fetus does not occur in all states of maternal hyperandrogenicity may be related to the onset and the degree of hyperandrogenicity and the potency of the androgens secreted. The placenta may also offer some protection for the fetus by aromatization of the maternal androgens to estrogens.

Administration of testosterone or its derivatives to pregnant women may virilize a female fetus but with no effect on differentiation of the wolffian ductal system. Paradoxic masculinization of the female fetus associated with maternal administration of diethylstilbestrol early in pregnancy has been reported rarely.

Cutler GB Jr, Laue L: Seminars in Medicine of the Beth Israel Hospital, Boston: Congenital adrenal hyperplasia due to 21-hydroxylase deficiency. N Engl J Med 323:1806, 1990. *A concise, up-to-date review of this most common form of the virilizing forms of congenital adrenal hyperplasia.*

Miller WL: Molecular biology of steroid hormone synthesis. Endocr Rev 9(3):295, 1988. *An inclusive review and bibliography at the molecular level of the enzymes involved in steroid hormone biosynthesis.*

White PC, New MI, Dupont B: Congenital adrenal hyperplasia. N Engl J Med 316:1519, 1580, 1987. *An excellent review and extensive bibliography of the enzyme deficiencies resulting in adrenal hyperplasia, with particular emphasis on 21-hydroxylase deficiency; 107 references.*

222 The Testis and Male Sexual Function

Alvin M. Matsumoto

The testis has three major physiologic functions: (1) During embryogenesis, the testis plays a vital role in normal male sexual differentiation. Production of testosterone by the fetal testis stimulates the development and growth of male internal and external genitalia. The fetal testis also produces müllerian inhibitory factor, which prevents the differentiation of female internal genitalia (see Ch. 221). (2) Beginning at the time of puberty and continuing into adulthood, testosterone produced by the testis is necessary for the development and maintenance of secondary sexual characteristics (virilization) and sexual functioning (libido and potency). (3) Spermatozoa produced by the testis are necessary for fertility.

Disorders of the testis are common and have profound effects on patients. Infertility affects approximately 14 per cent of all married couples in the reproductive age group. Disorders of sperm production cause or contribute to the infertility in 40 per cent of these couples; therefore, 5 to 6 per cent of all men wishing to father children are unable to do so because of a disorder of testicular function. Klinefelter's syndrome, which results in permanent androgen deficiency and infertility, affects approximately one in 400 to 500 males. Impotence and gynecomastia, which often result from testicular dysfunction, are very common complaints for which men seek medical attention. High doses of androgenic steroids are widely used by competitive athletes, often with serious side effects. Finally, cancer of the testis remains one of the most common fatal neoplasms of young men.

Many disorders of the testis can be treated effectively. Testosterone replacement therapy in androgen-deficient men results in the development or restoration of secondary sexual characteristics and normal sexual functioning. Gonadotropin treatment of hypogonadotropic men often stimulates spermatogenesis and induces fertility in addition to restoring androgen secretion. Finally,

seminomas are exquisitely responsive to radiation therapy, and the treatment of nonseminomatous testicular cancers with multidrug chemotherapy has markedly improved survival.

TESTICULAR STRUCTURE AND PHYSIOLOGY

Functional Anatomy

The normal adult testis weighs approximately 20 grams and normally measures 3.5 to 5.5 cm in length and 2.0 to 3.0 cm in width. Normal testis volume is between 15 and 30 ml. About 90 per cent of the volume of the testis is composed of seminiferous tubules, where spermatozoa are produced. Therefore, any significant reduction in testicular size is likely to be reflected in a decrease in total sperm production.

During fetal development, the testes descend from an intra-abdominal position into the scrotum. The scrotal location of the testes allows them to function at a temperature approximately 2°C lower than that of the abdomen. The pampiniform plexus of veins that drains the testes surrounds the testicular artery and cools the arterial blood supply to the testes by a countercurrent heat-exchange mechanism. The lower testicular temperature is necessary for normal spermatogenesis in man. Failure of the testes to descend into the scrotum (cryptorchidism) or an abnormality in the cooling mechanism (varicocele) impairs sperm production.

The testis is composed of two structurally distinct compartments: the *interstitial* or *Leydig cell compartment* and the *seminiferous tubule compartment* (Fig. 222–1). These compartments are responsible for the two major physiologic roles of the testis, namely production of testosterone and spermatozoa, respectively.

The interstitial compartment is composed of *Leydig cells*, which produce sex steroid hormones, primarily testosterone. Leydig cells are nestled between seminiferous tubules, in close proximity to blood vessels. This location is important, since it facilitates delivery of high concentrations of testosterone to the seminiferous tubule compartment (intratesticular testosterone levels being approximately 100 times those found in peripheral blood) and the diffusion of testosterone into the blood vessels, for delivery to the rest of the body. The high intratesticular concentration of testosterone is important in stimulating normal spermatogenesis.

The seminiferous tubule compartment is composed of developing *germ cells* and *Sertoli cells*. Spermatogenesis involves the differentiation and maturation of spermatogonia, the most primitive germ cell, into spermatozoa. In humans, spermatogenesis takes approximately 74 days. Sperm transport through the epi-

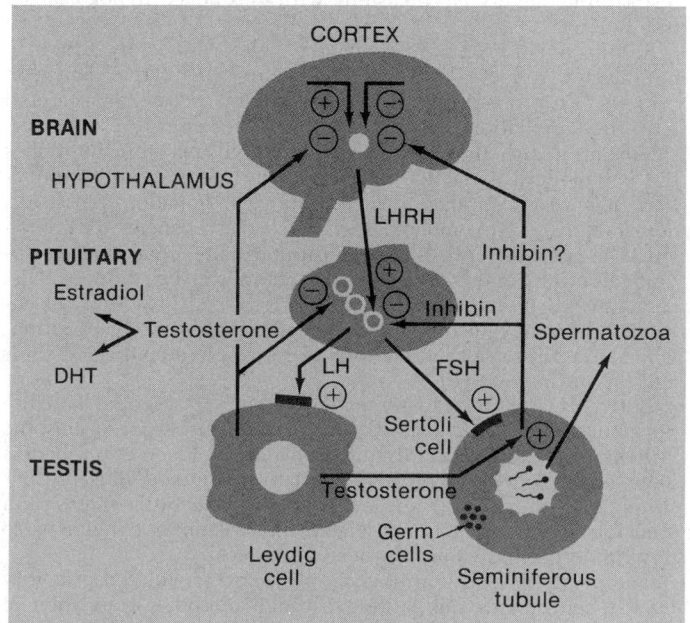

FIGURE 222–1. Diagram of the normal physiology of the hypothalamic-pituitary-testicular axis. (Adapted from Matsumoto AM, Bremner WJ: Bailliere's Clin Endocrinol Metab 1:71, 1987.)

didymis and vas deferens takes another 12 days. Therefore, processes that adversely affect early spermatogenesis may not be manifest by reduced sperm counts in the ejaculate until 2 to 3 months after the insult.

Sertoli cells perform many varied functions. By forming tight junctions at the basal portion of the seminiferous tubules, they maintain a barrier to the passage of macromolecules from the blood and interstitial compartment into the seminiferous tubules (the blood-testis barrier). Sertoli cells support spermatogenesis by synthesizing and secreting androgen-binding protein (ABP) and other protein products, by phagocytosing cellular remnants, and by participating in the movement and release of the maturing sperm and the secretion of fluid into the seminiferous tubule lumen. Sertoli cells produce *inhibin*, a glycoprotein that inhibits follicle-stimulating hormone secretion from the pituitary gland, but whose physiologic role remains unclear. They also produce another glycoprotein, *müllerian inhibitory factor (MIF)*, which is responsible, in the fetus, for causing the regression of the müllerian ducts (which normally develop into the female internal genitalia) during male sexual differentiation (see Ch. 221). Finally, Sertoli cells are capable of aromatizing testosterone to estradiol and producing paracrine factors that modulate Leydig cell function.

Central Nervous System Regulation of Gonadotropin Secretion

Normal testicular function depends on adequate stimulation by the gonadotropins, *luteinizing hormone (LH)*, and *follicle-stimulating hormone (FSH)*, which are secreted by the anterior pituitary gland (Fig. 222–1). Like thyroid-stimulating hormone and human chorionic gonadotropin (hCG), both LH and FSH are glycoprotein hormones composed of an α and a β subunit. These subunits are encoded on different genes, synthesized separately, glycosylated, and noncovalently assembled prior to secretion from the pituitary. The α subunits of all four glycoprotein hormones are identical and biologically inactive, whereas the β subunits are unique for each hormone and determine their biologic activity.

Measurements of serum gonadotropin levels are usually performed by radioimmunoassay (RIA). In normal young men, LH and FSH levels range from 5 to 20 mIU per milliliter (normal ranges vary according to the reference preparations used). Most gonadotropin assays are not sufficiently sensitive to distinguish between low and low-normal gonadotropin levels. Therefore, a hormonal profile of low-normal gonadotropin levels and low testosterone levels is consistent with secondary hypogonadism (see below).

Serum gonadotropin measurements determined by RIA may not always reflect the levels of biologically active hormone present. Free α subunit is synthesized in excess and secreted into the circulation by the pituitary. Because it cross-reacts significantly with the RIA for the intact glycoprotein hormones but is biologically inactive, alterations in free α subunit production may result in discrepancies between gonadotropin levels determined by RIA and bioassay. Such discrepancies have been found in gonadotropin-secreting pituitary adenomas and α subunit-secreting tumors, such as pancreatic islet cell tumors. Discrepancies between the immunoreactivity and bioactivity of gonadotropins may also result from alterations in glycosylation, which can affect both their intrinsic biologic activity and their half-life in the circulation.

Both LH and, to a lesser extent, FSH are secreted into the peripheral circulation from the anterior pituitary in an episodic fashion (Fig. 222–2). Pulsatile gonadotropin secretion begins during sleep in early puberty, and by adulthood it is present throughout the day. Knowledge of the fluctuations of serum gonadotropin levels has influenced blood sampling regimens to determine normal values of these hormones.

The pulsatile secretion of gonadotropins is regulated primarily by the central nervous system through episodic stimulation of the pituitary by *LH-releasing hormone (LHRH)*. LHRH, a decapeptide synthesized by hypothalamic neurons, stimulates release of both LH and FSH from the pituitary gland (see Fig. 222–1). Low-dose pulsatile LHRH administration has been used successfully to induce normal testicular function in patients with hypogonadotropic eunuchoidism, who presumably lack endogenous LHRH. By contrast, administration of high-dose, continuous LHRH or potent, long-acting LHRH agonists results in marked suppression of gonadotropin and testicular function. This paradoxic action of superactive LHRH agonists has been used clinically in the treatment of androgen-dependent tumors, such as prostate cancer.

The hypothalamic LHRH neuronal system plays an important integrative role in the regulation of testicular function (see Fig. 222–1). It receives input both from higher neural centers, such as the cerebral cortex and limbic system, through numerous stimulatory and inhibitory neurotransmitter (e.g., catecholamine and serotonin) and neuropeptide (e.g., opioid) systems and from testicular feedback signals, primarily sex steroid hormones. The input from these sources alters LHRH output, which, in turn, regulates pituitary gonadotropin secretion and testicular function. Increasing knowledge of how the central nervous system regulates LHRH secretion has helped to further our understanding of the mechanisms by which stress, malnutrition, and certain pharmacologic agents (such as catecholaminergic and opiate drugs) affect testicular function (Ch. 212).

Gonadotropin Regulation of Testicular Function

LH REGULATION OF TESTOSTERONE PRODUCTION. LH binds to specific membrane receptors on Leydig cells of the interstitial compartment of the testis and stimulates testicular steroidogenesis and secretion of *testosterone*, the major steroid product of the testis (see Fig. 222–1). LH increases the conversion of cholesterol to pregnenolone by the cholesterol side chain cleavage enzyme complex (20,22-desmolase), the rate-limiting step in testosterone biosynthesis.

Testosterone is secreted both locally within the testes and into the peripheral circulation (see Fig. 222–1). Healthy young men secrete approximately 5 to 7 mg of testosterone daily, essentially all from the Leydig cells. Total testosterone concentrations in plasma, as determined by RIA, range from 3 to 10 ng per milliliter (300 to 1000 ng per deciliter). Like gonadotropins, testosterone is secreted in a pulsatile fashion (Fig. 222–2).

In early puberty, testosterone secretion increases from very low to near adult levels during sleep in response to sleep-associated rises in LH levels. In adults, testosterone secretion occurs throughout the entire day. In young healthy men testosterone levels exhibit a circadian variation of about 1.5 ng per milliliter, with maximal levels occurring at 8 A.M. and minimal levels occurring at 9 P.M.

Under the influence of LH stimulation, Leydig cells also convert testosterone to *estradiol*. However, secretion of estradiol by the testis accounts for only about 15 per cent of the daily production of estradiol. The remainder of estradiol in blood is produced from testosterone and androstenedione (an adrenal androgen) by the enzyme aromatase in peripheral tissues, mostly adipose tissue.

TESTOSTERONE TRANSPORT. Like other steroid hormones, the majority of testosterone secreted into the circulation is bound to plasma proteins, primarily albumin and *sex hormone–binding globulin (SHBG)*. Approximately 30 to 40 per cent of total testosterone is bound to SHBG and is not biologically available. Only 1 to 2 per cent is free (i.e., unbound to plasma proteins) and physiologically active. Albumin-bound testosterone seems also to be available to act on many target organs. Therefore, measurement of non-SHBG-bound testosterone may provide the best estimate of biologically available testosterone. In certain clinical situations, alterations in SHBG levels result in total testosterone measurements that do not reflect bioavailable testosterone levels. SHBG (and total testosterone) levels are decreased with obesity, hypothyroidism, androgens, nephrotic syndrome, Cushing's disease, and acromegaly and increased with hepatic cirrhosis, hyperthyroidism, and estrogens. In these situations, free or non-SHBG-bound testosterone levels should be obtained.

PERIPHERAL METABOLISM OF TESTOSTERONE. The metabolism of circulating testosterone plays a very important role in its biologic actions on target tissues. Testosterone may be converted in peripheral tissues to either *dihydrotestosterone (DHT)* or *estradiol*, which mediates many of the physiologic actions of testosterone (see Fig. 222-1). These active metabolites of testosterone can be formed and act locally on androgen target tissues or circulate in blood and act on distant target tissues.

In many androgen-dependent target tissues, testosterone is converted intracellularly to a more potent androgen, DHT, by the enzyme 5 α-reductase. This conversion is required for normal male sexual differentiation. Males with 5 α-reductase deficiency, who cannot form DHT from testosterone in utero, fail to develop normal male external genitalia and as a result are born and raised as phenotypic females (Ch. 221). DHT is also thought to be important in mediating the androgenic effects of testosterone on skin and accessory sexual organs (i.e., prostate, seminal vesicles, and epididymis). In many peripheral tissues, especially in adipose tissue, testosterone is aromatized to estradiol, a potent estrogen. Obesity therefore results in increased peripheral estrogen formation. In men estrogens have diverse physiologic actions that may be agonistic or antagonistic to those of androgens. Therefore, the physiologic effects of testosterone result from the actions of testosterone itself in combination with those of its active metabolites, DHT and estradiol. Finally, 5β-reduced metabolites of androgens may be important mediators of androgen action on bone marrow.

Circulating testosterone and its active metabolites are metabolized to inactive metabolites mostly in the liver, and these inactive metabolites are excreted primarily in the urine. In sexual tissue (including skin and prostate), DHT is efficiently metabolized to 3 α-androstanediol and then to 3 α-*androstanediol glucuronide (3 α-diol G)*. Blood and urine measurements of 3 α-diol G are useful markers of peripheral androgen action. In disorders in which DHT formation is reduced (such as 5 α-reductase deficiency), 3 α-diol G levels are reduced (Ch. 221).

ANDROGEN ACTION AND FUNCTIONS. At the target cell, testosterone and DHT bind to intracellular androgen receptors, which interact with specific chromosomal sites to alter gene transcription and protein synthesis, resulting in expression of androgen action (Ch. 208). Quantitative or qualitative abnormalities of the androgen receptor, resulting in impaired androgen action, cause varying degrees of male pseudohermaphroditism (Ch. 221).

The major functions of androgens are the differentiation of male internal and external genitalia (primary sexual characteristics) during embryogenesis; the development and maintenance of secondary sexual characteristics, sexual functioning (libido and potency), certain behavioral characteristics (such as aggression), and feedback regulation of gonadotropins; and the initiation and maintenance of spermatogenesis.

FSH REGULATION OF SERTOLI CELL FUNCTION. FSH binds to specific membrane receptors on Sertoli cells of the seminiferous tubule compartment of the testis and stimulates the production of seminiferous tubule fluid and a variety of proteins thought to be important in regulating spermatogenesis (e.g., ABP, transferrin, plasminogen activator), in feedback control of pituitary FSH secretion (inhibin and activin), and possibly in intratesticular paracrine modulation of Leydig cell function (see Fig. 222-1). Testosterone produced by adjacent Leydig cells also regulates these Sertoli cell functions through androgen receptors. The relative roles of FSH and testosterone in the regulation of Sertoli cell function are poorly understood. Developing germ cells are enveloped in the cytoplasmic processes of the Sertoli cells, which nurture and coordinate the completion of sperm maturation in the seminiferous tubule.

HORMONAL CONTROL OF SPERMATOGENESIS. Both FSH and LH stimulation are required for the initiation of spermatogenesis at the time of puberty. At this time, LH causes the differentiation of Leydig cells from interstitial connective tissue precursors and stimulates them to produce high intratesticular levels of testosterone, which are essential for the initial phases of sperm production. By stimulating Sertoli cell function, FSH plays an important role in the later stages of spermatid maturation (spermiogenesis) during this initial wave of spermatogenesis.

Normal levels of either FSH or LH do not appear to be absolute requirements for the maintenance of spermatogenesis in adult men. Selective gonadotropin replacement in adult men with experimentally induced gonadotropin deficiency results in stimulation of qualitatively normal sperm production with either FSH or LH treatment alone. However, replacement of both LH and FSH is necessary to maintain quantitatively normal spermatogenesis in these hypogonadotropic men.

Clinically, replacement of both FSH and LH activity is generally required to initiate sperm production in prepubertal hypogonadotropic hypogonadal patients. In contrast, initiation and maintenance of spermatogenesis in postpubertal men with acquired hypogonadotropic hypogonadism can usually be achieved with replacement of LH activity alone.

Seminal fluid analysis is used to evaluate the function of the seminiferous tubules. It is performed on seminal fluid samples obtained by masturbation, usually after 48 hours of abstinence from ejaculation. Normal ejaculate volume ranges from 2 to 6 ml. Although the normal range of sperm concentration is gener-

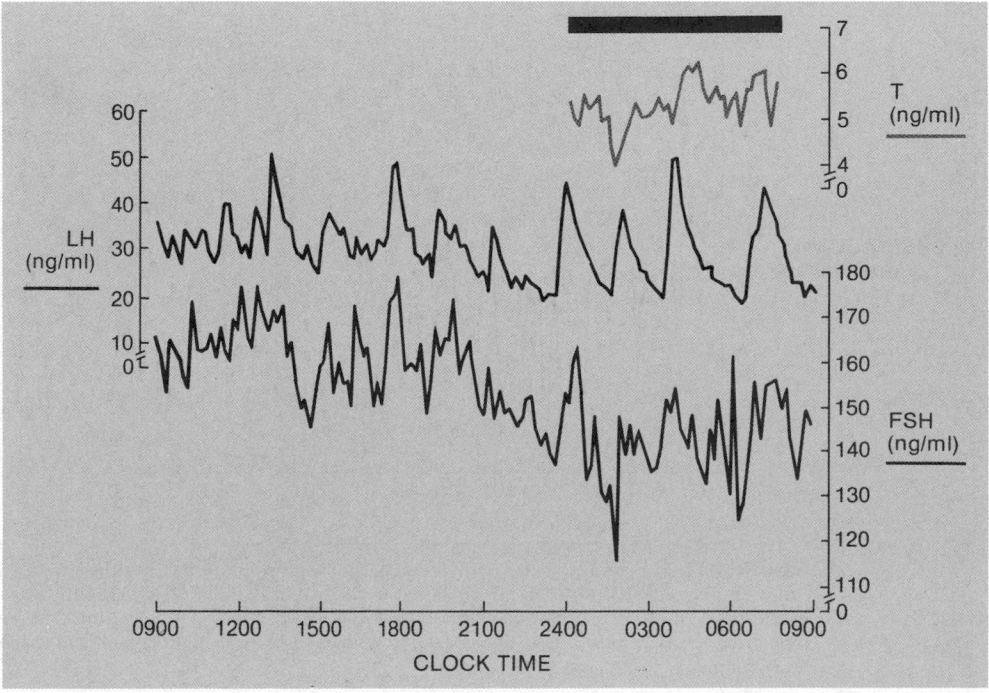

FIGURE 222–2. Example of pulsatile LH and FSH secretion throughout a 24-hour day and episodic testosterone secretion at night in a healthy young man. Blood samples were drawn at 10-minute intervals. Black bar denotes sleep, as documented by electroencephalogram.

ally considered to be 20 to 200 million per milliliter, sperm concentrations below 20 million per milliliter may be sufficient for fertility. In addition to determining sperm count, a careful microscopic examination of the seminal fluid is usually performed to assess sperm motility and morphology. Normally, greater than 60 per cent of sperm examined within 1 hour after ejaculation are motile, and greater than 60 per cent have a normal oval head morphology.

The minimal levels of sperm concentration, per cent motility, and per cent oval forms compatible with fertility are not clearly defined. In any individual, sperm counts normally exhibit extreme variability (Fig. 222-3) and are often temporarily suppressed by factors such as fever. Therefore, a reasonable estimate of mean sperm production requires at least three seminal fluid analyses over a 2-month period. Functional tests of sperm penetration into cervical mucus of various mammalian species or zona pellucida–free hamster ova may be helpful in assessing fertilizing capability of spermatozoa.

Testicular Feedback Regulation of Gonadotropin Secretion

Both steroid and nonsteroidal products of the testis are involved in negative feedback control of pituitary gonadotropin secretion. Increased production of these testicular products results in suppression, whereas decreased production of these factors results in stimulation of gonadotropin secretion (see Fig. 222-1). Testosterone and its active metabolites, DHT and estradiol, exert profound inhibitory effects on both LH and FSH secretion, although the relative roles of these steroids are not clearly defined. Testosterone may affect both the hypothalamic release of LHRH and the pituitary sensitivity to LHRH stimulation. Inhibin, a glycoprotein product of the Sertoli cell, selectively inhibits FSH secretion at the pituitary gland. At present, the physiologic significance of inhibin is unclear.

Knowledge of these negative feedback relationships has proved to be clinically useful in the diagnosis of hypogonadal states (see below). In addition, the potent negative feedback effect of administering exogenous testosterone has been utilized to suppress endogenous gonadotropin and sperm production in the development of male contraceptives.

Matsumoto AM, Bremner WJ: Endocrinology of the hypothalamic-pituitary-testicular axis with particular reference to the hormonal control of spermatogenesis. Bailliere's Clin Endocrinol Metab 1:71, 1987. *This paper reviews the normal physiologic regulation of testicular function, which forms the basis for understanding the pathophysiology and treatment of testicular disorders. An up-to-date discussion of the hormonal regulation of human spermatogenesis is also provided.*

Steiner RA, Cameron JL: Endocrine control of reproduction. *In* Patton HD, Fuchs AF, Hille B, et al. (eds.): Textbook of Physiology: Circulation, Respiration, Body Fluids, Metabolism and Endocrinology, 21st ed. Philadelphia, W. B. Saunders Company, 1989, p 1289. *This chapter contains an excellent, concise, and up-to-date general discussion of the physiology and pathophysiology of the male reproductive axis.*

PHYSIOLOGY OF MALE SEXUAL FUNCTION

Normal male sexual function requires coordinated regulation of the following physiologic events: *libido* or sexual desire, sustained penile tumescence or *erection, ejaculation, orgasm,* and *detumescence.*

Libido

Libido is generated in the central nervous system and stimulated by a variety of visual, tactile, imaginative, auditory, and gustatory stimuli. These stimuli are received in a number of cortical and subcortical regions of the brain, including the limbic system, and relayed via the preoptic–anterior hypothalamic area to spinal cord centers that control penile erection. Therefore, disturbances in libido are nearly always accompanied by disturbed erectile function or impotence.

Libido is regulated primarily by psychic factors and the sex steroid milieu, in particular serum testosterone concentrations. Thus, psychological disturbances of all degrees (from stress to major psychiatric illnesses), central nervous system lesions, drugs that alter brain function, and androgen deficiency may disturb normal libido and potency. Occasionally, castrated males maintain sexual desire and erectile function for long periods, suggesting that the requirement for androgens may be quite variable.

Erection

Erections are generated by two separate but synergistic mechanisms, one involving sensory stimulation of the genitalia, mediated through a spinal reflex arc (reflexogenic erections), and another involving psychogenic stimuli from higher brain centers (psychogenic erections). In reflexogenic erections, afferent sensory fibers from the penis travel in the pudendal nerve to the sacral spinal erection center (S2 to S4). Efferent parasympathetic fibers arising from this center travel in the nervi erigentes and innervate the blood vessels of the corpora cavernosa of the penis; efferent somatic fibers traveling in the pudendal nerve innervate the pelvic floor (ischiocavernosus and bulbocavernosus) muscles. Sympathetic fibers originating in the thoracolumbar spinal erection center (T12 to L1) innervate the muscles of the vas deferens, accessory sex glands, and internal sphincter of the bladder. In psychogenic erections, projections from higher brain centers descend in the lateral spinal columns and regulate both the thoracolumbar and sacral spinal erection centers.

Penile erectile tissue consists of paired corpora cavernosa on

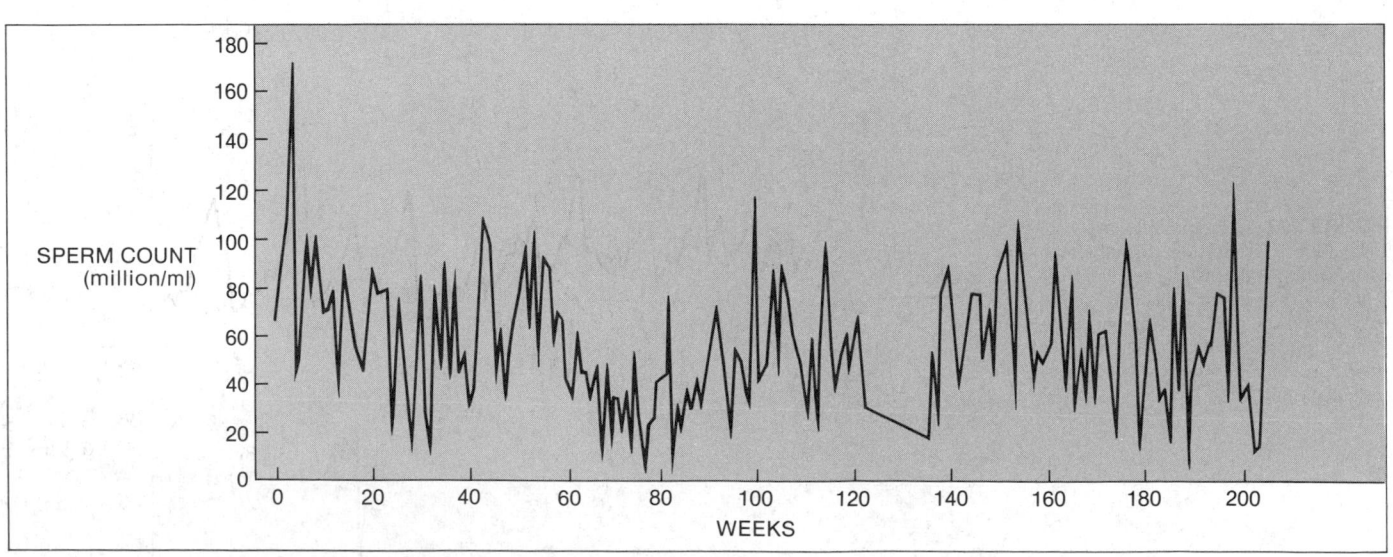

FIGURE 222–3. Example of the normal variations in sperm count in a healthy young man. Normal range of sperm count is generally considered to be between 20 and 200 million per milliliter. Despite good health and no medications, the sperm count may occasionally fall below the normal range, into the oligospermic range. (Adapted from Bardin CW, Paulsen CA: The testes. *In* Williams RH (ed.): Textbook of Endocrinology, 6th ed. Philadelphia, W.B. Saunders Company, 1981.)

the dorsum of the penis and the corpus spongiosum that surrounds the urethra and forms the glans penis. The corpora are composed of spongelike, interconnected trabecular spaces lined by vascular epithelium and smooth muscle and are surrounded by a thick fibrous sheath, the tunica albuginea. Activation of the spinal erection centers results in relaxation of the penile smooth muscle and vasodilation of the cavernosal arteries (branches of the internal pudendal arteries). These actions are mediated by cholinergic, β-adrenergic, and peptidergic (e.g., vasoactive intestinal peptide) receptors. As a result, blood flow into the trabecular spaces of the corpora is increased, causing engorgement of the penis (tumescence). Expansion of the trabecular walls against the tunica albuginea compresses subtunical venules and impedes venous outflow, resulting in sustained tumescence, i.e., an erection.

Failure to achieve an adequate erection or impotence has many potential etiologies, including androgen deficiency, central and peripheral nervous system diseases, vascular disorders, and penile abnormalities. Impotence as it relates to the differential diagnosis of hypogonadism is discussed in a subsequent section of this chapter.

Ejaculation

Ejaculation is stimulated by sympathetic nervous system activation, which results in contractions of the vas deferens and accessory sex glands and emission of seminal fluid into the urethra. Emission is followed by reflex rhythmic contractions of the ischiocavernosus and bulbocavernosus muscles and expulsion of semen from the urethra, i.e., ejaculation. Like erection, the ejaculatory reflex is under considerable control by higher cerebral centers. Sympathetic activation also stimulates closure of the internal urethral sphincter, thereby preventing retrograde ejaculation.

Premature ejaculation is usually due to performance anxiety or an emotional disorder and rarely has an organic etiology. Retrograde ejaculation into the bladder usually occurs in patients with sympathetic neuropathy (e.g., with diabetes) or after bladder neck surgery. Reduced or absent ejaculation may occur with androgen deficiency, sympatholytic drugs, sympathectomy, or extensive retroperitoneal/pelvic surgery.

Orgasm

Orgasm, the pleasurable sensation that usually accompanies ejaculation, is primarily a central nervous system–mediated phenomenon that, under normal circumstances, is influenced by ascending pathways associated with ejaculation. However, orgasm can occur in the absence of erection or ejaculation (e.g., with temporal lobe lesions). Conversely, normal libido, erection, and ejaculation can occur without orgasm; this is nearly always due to a psychological disorder.

Detumescence

Detumescence results from contraction of the penile smooth muscle and α-adrenergic vasoconstriction of the cavernosal arteries, which reduce arterial blood flow into the penis. As a result, the trabecular spaces of the corpora collapse, subtunical venules are decompressed, venous outflow is increased, and the penis becomes flaccid. In many cases, premature detumescence may contribute to the pathophysiology of impotence (e.g., venous leak or incompetence). Failure of detumescence, priapism, is often painful and unrelated to sexual intercourse. It is commonly idiopathic in etiology but may be associated with spinal cord injury, sickle cell disease, chronic myelogenous leukemia, and intracorporal injection of vasodilatory substances used in the treatment of impotence.

Meyer JK: Disorders of sexual function. *In* Wilson JD, Foster DW (eds.): Williams' Textbook of Endocrinology. Philadelphia, WB Saunders Company, 1985, p 476. *This chapter contains a well-organized, clear, and comprehensive discussion of the physiologic and anatomic basis of male sexual function and dysfunction.*

HYPOGONADISM

Hypogonadism is the most common disorder of testicular function encountered in clinical practice. The clinical manifestations of male hypogonadism differ depending on (1) whether there is *impairment of testosterone production,* which is nearly always accompanied by impairment of sperm production, or

isolated impairment of sperm production, with normal testosterone production; (2) whether androgen deficiency occurs *during embryogenesis, before puberty,* or *after puberty;* and (3) whether testicular hypofunction is the result of a *primary* defect in the testis or is *secondary* to hypothalamic-pituitary dysfunction.

Androgen Deficiency

The clinical presentation of androgen deficiency depends on the stage of sexual development in which it occurs.

During early fetal development, testosterone and its active metabolite, DHT, mediate the differentiation of male internal and external genitalia from the wolffian duct system and the indifferent anlage of external genitalia, respectively. Androgen deficiency (e.g., as a result of a genetic androgen biosynthetic enzyme defect) or impaired androgen action (androgen resistance) occurring during this period of development results in varying degrees of ambiguous genital development, or *male pseudohermaphroditism.* These disorders are discussed in greater detail in Ch. 221.

During puberty, testosterone is responsible for the development of male secondary sexual characteristics, such as (1) the growth of the penis and scrotum, (2) the development of accessory sexual organs (prostate and seminal vesicles) necessary to produce an ejaculate, (3) a male pattern of hair growth (face, external ear canals, chest, lower abdomen, pubis, perianal area, legs, and inner thighs) and frontal scalp regression, (4) the enlargement of the larynx and thickening of the vocal cords with consequent deepening of the voice, (5) the development of skeletal musculature and increase in strength (especially in the shoulder and pectoral muscles), (6) a redistribution of body fat, and (7) stimulation of erythropoiesis. Testosterone also stimulates the pubertal spurt of long bone growth and, eventually, the closure of long bone epiphyses, which results in cessation of bone growth. Finally androgens stimulate libido (sexual drive), potency (erectile function), and aggressive behavior and play an important role in initiation of spermatogenesis, which determines the development of fertility.

Patients who develop androgen deficiency before the onset of puberty usually present to physicians as adolescents or young adults with delayed puberty or poor male sexual development. Prepubertal testosterone deficiency results in *eunuchoidism* (Fig. 222–4), which is characterized by infantile development of genital and accessory sexual organs, failure to develop an ejaculate (aspermia), lack of male hair pattern, high-pitched voice, poor muscular development and strength, lower abdominal-pelvic girdle fat distribution, and excessive long bone growth (due to lack of closure of long bone epiphyses). The testes are small, usually less than 2 cm in length or 2 ml in volume. A eunuchoidal body habitus is characterized by excessively long arms and legs in proportion to height. Although there are racial differences in body proportions, eunuchoidal body measurements consist of an arm span that exceeds height by greater than 5 cm or a distance from the floor to the symphysis pubis that is 5 cm greater than that from the symphysis to the crown of the head. Patients with prepubertal androgen deficiency fail to develop normal sexual functioning (libido and potency) and are infertile. Testosterone deficiency before puberty may occasionally result in gynecomastia (benign enlargement of breast tissue).

In the adult, testosterone is responsible for the maintenance of libido, potency, and secondary sexual characteristics and participates in the maintenance of spermatogenesis. The major complaints of men with adult-onset androgen deficiency are poor sexual performance, as a result of diminished libido and/or impotence; infertility, as a result of impaired spermatogenesis; and gynecomastia. Rapid development of severe androgen deficiency (such as surgical castration) may also result in vasomotor instability or hot flushes, similar to those that many women develop at the time of menopause. Androgen deficiency may also result in behavioral changes, such as passivity, lack of motivation, and irritability.

Secondary sexual characteristics do not regress to the prepubertal state in men who develop testosterone deficiency as adults. However, with longstanding androgen deficiency, there may be significant loss of hair in androgen-dependent areas of the body, fine wrinkling of skin (most noticeable around the eyes and mouth), diminished muscle strength and mass, osteoporosis, and altered fat distribution. In hypogonadal men, pubic hair may assume a female type, inverted triangle pattern (female escutcheon), in contrast to the male type, diamond-shaped distribution, with hair extending to the umbilicus (male escutcheon). The amount and distribution of facial and body hair vary considerably, depending on an individual's ethnic and genetic background. The testes are usually small in hypogonadal states that result in androgen deficiency. However, depending on the specific cause and severity of the disorder, testis size may be normal. For example, men with recent onset of gonadotropin deficiency from a destructive pituitary tumor may have normal size testes, despite severe testosterone deficiency.

Serum testosterone levels are low in states of androgen deficiency. Very sensitive and specific RIA's for serum testosterone are generally available and are relatively inexpensive. Routinely available assays measure total testosterone and may give falsely low values in clinical states in which sex hormone–binding globulin is reduced (such as protein deficiency states and obesity). In these instances serum free or non-SHBG-bound testosterone levels should be measured.

Testosterone helps to maintain quantitatively normal spermatogenesis in man; androgen deficiency, therefore, almost always results in abnormalities in sperm production. Impaired spermatogenesis is usually confirmed by a low sperm count on seminal fluid analysis. Sperm counts are highly variable in any individual and are often suppressed by illness (e.g., fever). At least three sperm counts should be obtained over a period of 2 months, while patients are well, before diagnosing low sperm counts (oligospermia).

Isolated Deficiency in Sperm Production

In contrast to patients with androgen deficiency, men with an isolated deficiency of sperm production present postpubertally with infertility as their major complaint, without symptoms of testosterone deficiency. Testis size may be reduced or normal and an undescended testis or *varicocele* (varicose dilatation of the pampiniform venous plexus of the testis) may be found. The remainder of the physical examination is usually unremarkable. Sperm counts are usually low (less than 20 million per milliliter) or zero (*azoospermia*), and there may be isolated or associated abnormalities of sperm motility and/or morphology on seminal fluid analysis. Serum testosterone levels are normal in disorders causing isolated impairment of sperm production.

Differential Diagnosis

The major manifestations of androgen deficiency in adults are impotence, infertility, and gynecomastia. Although hypogonadism resulting in testosterone deficiency is a major cause of these clinical manifestations, there are many other causes.

IMPOTENCE. Impotence is defined as a consistent inability to achieve or maintain penile erection that is adequate for completion of sexual intercourse. It is a commonly encountered complaint in medical practice, occurring in 10 to 35 per cent of adult men with medical problems and increasing in prevalence with advancing age. Impotence is often underdiagnosed because of reluctance of patients and physicians to discuss sexual dysfunction as a medical problem. Although psychogenic impotence is common, the majority of men with impotence who are followed in a general medical clinic have one or more organic causes of erectile dysfunction. Furthermore, organic causes of impotence often result in performance anxiety and secondary psychogenic sexual dysfunction.

Penile erection sufficient to complete intercourse requires (1) normal *central nervous system* and thoracolumbar sympathetic and sacral parasympathetic *spinal cord* outputs to the penis; (2) an intact *arterial supply* and *venous drainage* of the penis; and (3) an *anatomically normal penis*. Dysfunction of any of these components interferes with normal initiation and maintenance of penile erection (Table 222–1).

Normal central nervous system function is necessary to produce adequate penile erections. *Libido* or sexual desire, mediated by the cerebral cortex and limbic system, has a profound influence on erectile function. In most central nervous system disorders that cause sexual dysfunction, reduced libido is usually associated with impotence. All degrees of *psychiatric disturbance*, from minor stress and performance anxiety to major psychiatric illness, such as depression and schizophrenia; *chronic debilitating illness*, such as cardiac, respiratory, renal, or liver disease or malignancy; and *drugs* that affect central nervous system function (sedatives, antipsychotics, antidepressants, centrally acting antihypertensive agents, and alcohol), are central nervous system causes of impotence and generally reduce libido as well as erectile function. *Androgen deficiency, hyperprolactinemia,* and *thyroid dysfunction* (hyperthyroidism and hypothyroidism) also impair libido and potency. Elevated prolactin levels may cause impotence by inducing secondary hypogonadism and androgen deficiency. However, impotence may not resolve with androgen replacement therapy alone and may require, in addition, therapy aimed at reducing the elevated prolactin levels (e.g., bromocriptine). In contrast to these disorders, *destructive or infiltrative diseases* of certain regions of the *brain* (such as tumor or infarction of the

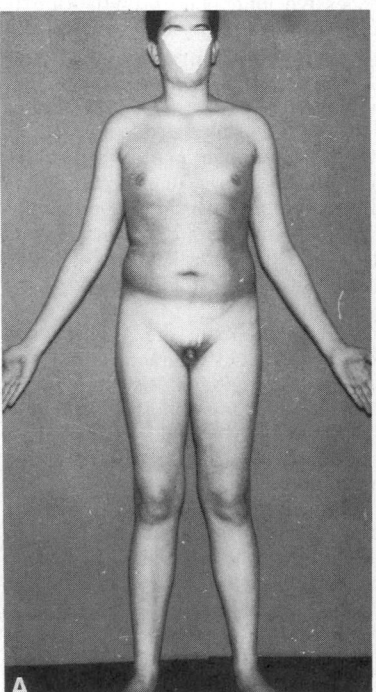
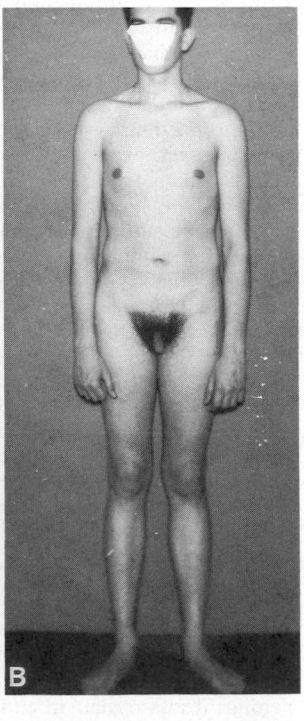
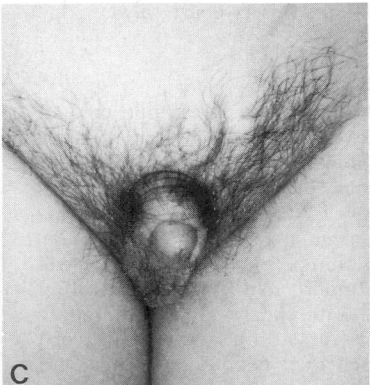
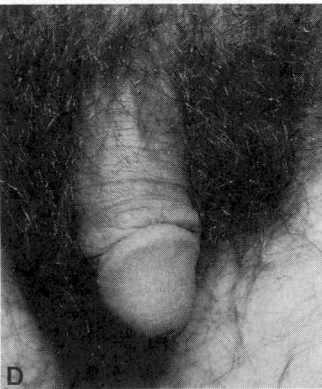

FIGURE 222–4. Example of eunuchoidism as a result of prepubertal androgen deficiency due to functional prepubertal castrate syndrome. *A* and *C*, Before androgen therapy, note the eunuchoidal features of infantile genital development, lack of male hair pattern, poor muscular development, pelvic girdle and lower abdominal fat distribution, and disproportionately long arms and legs. No testicular tissue was identified at the time of surgical exploration. *B* and *D*, After 18 months of testosterone treatment, scalp hair recession, penile development, and pubic hair growth have occurred. A masculine body habitus has developed, with an increase in pectoral and shoulder muscle development and loss of pelvic girdle and lower abdominal fat. (From Bardin CW, Paulsen CA: The testes. *In* Williams RH (ed.): Textbook of Endocrinology, 6th ed. Philadelphia, W.B. Saunders Company, 1981.)

TABLE 222–1. CAUSES OF IMPOTENCE

I. Disorders of Central Nervous System Control	II. Disorders of Peripheral Erectile Response
Psychiatric Illness	Drugs
Stress	Anticholinergic drugs
Performance anxiety	Antidepressants
Depression	Antihistamines
Major psychiatric illness	β-Adrenergic
Chronic Illness	blockers
Cardiac disease	Sympathomimetic
Respiratory disease	drugs
Renal disease	α-Adrenergic agonists
Liver disease	Antihypertensive
Malignancy	agents
Central Nervous System–	Autonomic Neuropathy
Active Drugs	Pelvic surgery
Sedatives	Diabetes
Antipsychotics	Other peripheral
Antidepressants	neuropathies
Central antihypertensives	Vascular Disease
Alcohol	Distal aortoiliac
Endocrine Disorders	atherosclerosis
Hypogonadism (androgen	Diabetes
deficiency)	Trauma
Hyperprolactinemia	Venous incompetence
Thyroid disease	Penile Abnormalities
Central Nervous System	Peyronie's disease
Disease	Chordee
Temporal lobe disorders	Priapism
Limbic system disorders	Trauma
Spinal Cord Disease	Microphallus or
Trauma	micropenis
Multiple sclerosis	
Syphilis	
Other spinal cord lesions	

temporal lobe or limbic system) or *spinal cord diseases* (such as injury, tumor, multiple sclerosis, or syphilis) may cause impotence without associated loss of libido. Patients with high spinal cord lesions (above T11) usually retain the ability to have reflexogenic erections.

In addition to intact central nervous system functioning, normal penile erection requires intact peripheral nervous system function, adequate blood flow to the penis, and normal erectile structures within the penis. *Disorders of peripheral autonomic nerve function* which cause impotence include extensive pelvic surgery, such as aortoiliac bypass, pelvic lymph node dissection, abdominoperineal resection of the rectum, lumbar sympathectomy, and prostatectomy; diabetes; and other conditions causing peripheral autonomic and sensory neuropathy. Atherosclerotic *peripheral vascular disease* involving the distal aortoiliac arteries and *trauma* to these vessels are the most common causes of vascular impotence. These patients usually have diminished or absent femoral pulses and may present with *Leriche's syndrome,* although claudication may be absent in some cases. In addition, autonomic neuropathy and atherosclerotic macro- and microvascular disease are major etiologic factors contributing to erectile dysfunction in the 30 to 50 per cent of diabetic men who develop impotence. Penile venous incompetence (venous leak) resulting in inadequate veno-occlusion to sustain an erection is an uncommon cause of impotence. *Penile abnormalities,* such as Peyronie's disease, chordee, priapism, and microphallus, may also cause erectile dysfunction. *Drugs* may cause erectile dysfunction by inhibiting penile smooth muscle relaxation and arterial vasodilation (anticholinergic drugs, antidepressants, antihistamines, β-adrenergic blockers) or by inducing premature detumescence (sympathomimetic drugs, α-adrenergic agonists). The mechanism of impotence associated with certain antihypertensive agents (e.g., diuretics, vasodilators, sympatholytic agents) is unclear.

Normal testosterone levels are necessary for maintenance of libido and potency. Hypogonadism resulting in androgen deficiency is a cause of impotence in approximately 15 to 20 per cent of men complaining of sexual dysfunction in a general medical clinic. Therefore, all impotent patients should have serum testosterone and gonadotropin levels measured as part of their diagnostic workup.

A thorough history and physical examination provide invaluable clues to the etiology of impotence. Erectile dysfunction that occurs abruptly and is transient, intermittent, or temporally associated with stress is usually psychogenic in origin. Men with psychogenic impotence often have spontaneous nocturnal or morning erections and are able to achieve normal erections with some partners but not with others or with masturbation but not during sexual intercourse. Patients with impotence related to central or peripheral nervous system or vascular disease or penile abnormalities usually demonstrate clinical manifestations of the underlying disorder. A careful drug history may reveal offending medications that cause impotence.

Measurement of nocturnal penile tumescence (NPT) and buckling pressure may be used to differentiate psychogenic from organic impotence. NPT is usually present in psychogenic impotence but absent if there is an organic cause of erectile dysfunction. Formal evaluation is done in a sleep laboratory with EEG monitoring to detect sleep disturbances that may disturb NPT. Resistance of the penis to buckling is also measured; this measurement correlates better than NPT alone with ability to have sexual intercourse. A simpler assessment of NPT can be made by wrapping the penis with perforated paper (e.g., stamps) or a snap gauge; NPT is detected by breaking of the perforations or wires of different tensile strength.

Doppler determination of the ratio of supine penile systolic blood pressure to brachial systolic blood pressure (penile/brachial index) may be useful in diagnosing patients with penile arterial vascular insufficiency. An index greater than 0.75 is normal; one between 0.75 and 0.60 is indeterminate; and one less than 0.6 is suggestive of arteriovascular impotence, which may be confirmed by arteriography. Recently, intracavernosal injection of vasodilatory agents (e.g., papaverine) with and without duplex ultrasonography or direct pressure monitoring has been used in the evaluation of impotence. Development of a sustained erectile response implies normal vascular status, whereas a short-lived, partial, or absent response suggests a hemodynamic abnormality. Corporal veno-occlusion is usually evaluated by cavernosometry and cavernosography following intracavernosal injection of a vasodilating drug. In the absence of neurogenic bladder dysfunction, electromyographic determination of the bulbocavernosus reflex latency and somatosensory evoked response of the dorsal nerve may be useful in detecting peripheral and sacral spinal abnormalities contributing to impotence.

Treatment of impotence is directed at the underlying causes of erectile dysfunction. Psychosexual education, counseling, and therapy are very successful in restoring sexual function in many men with psychogenic impotence. Testosterone therapy should be reserved for hypogonadal men with androgen deficiency in whom libido and potency are restored with adequate androgen replacement. Men with impotence and hypogonadism due to hyperprolactinemia may require agents to lower prolactin levels (e.g., bromocriptine) in addition to testosterone replacement to improve potency. Self-administration of intracavernosal injections of vasodilatory drugs (e.g., papaverine and/or phentolamine) induces penile erections sufficient for sexual intercourse in many patients with impotence. In general, it is very effective and well tolerated. Patients with severe arterial insufficiency or venous leaks are least likely to respond to this therapy. Select patients with vascular impotence are candidates for corrective surgical procedures.

In patients for whom effective therapy is not available, surgical implantation of a penile prosthesis offers rigidity sufficient for sexual intercourse without interfering with ejaculation or orgasm. Recently, vacuum-constriction devices have been introduced as a nonsurgical alternative to penile prostheses for the treatment of impotence. A condom-like cylinder is placed over the flaccid penis; a vacuum is applied to generate negative pressure, drawing blood into the penis and resulting in an erection. A constrictive band is then placed around the base of the penis to prevent the drainage of blood from the penis, maintaining tumescence for the duration of intercourse.

INFERTILITY. Infertility is defined as the inability of a couple to achieve a pregnancy after 1 year of unprotected intercourse. An estimated 5 to 6 per cent of men in the reproductive age group are infertile. Most causes of male infertility result in abnormal sperm count or semen quality, as reflected by an abnormal seminal fluid analysis. About 90 per cent of male infertility is caused by hypogonadism resulting in impaired spermatogenesis; and 80 to 90 per cent of these men have isolated deficiency of sperm production with normal androgen production of unclear etiology, i.e., *idiopathic oligospermia or azoospermia* (see below). Other causes of male infertility include *coital disorders, ductal obstruction, ejaculatory dysfunction,* and *disorders of accessory sexual organs* (Table 222–2). Even if a cause of male infertility is diagnosed, the female partner should undergo diagnostic evaluation, since a concomitant female factor causing infertility is found in 30 per cent of infertile couples.

Although uncommon, *defects* in the *coital technique,* such as timing of intercourse during menses, rather than at the time of ovulation near mid-cycle, premature withdrawal of the penis, prior ejaculation, and infrequent intercourse are causes of male infertility. They are important to remember because they are potentially reversible with proper patient education. Basal body temperature measurements or rapid RIA kits measuring urinary LH levels are commercially available methods often used to estimate the timing of ovulation in the partner's menstrual cycle. *Erectile dysfunction* from any cause may result in unsuccessful intercourse and infertility.

Impediment of sperm transport from the testis to the urethra results in azoospermia and infertility. Causes of *ductal obstruction* include congenital absence of the vas deferens or seminal vesicles; congenital defects of the epididymis or vas, e.g., as a consequence of diethylstilbestrol exposure in utero; fibrosis as a complication of genitourinary infection, especially epididymitis; cystic fibrosis or Young's syndrome, in which thickened, inspissated mucous secretions lead to blockage of the epididymis and vas deferens; and vasectomy.

Obstructive azoospermia must be differentiated from a severe defect in spermatogenesis. Measurement of a serum FSH level is often helpful, since elevated levels generally indicate disordered seminiferous tubular function. Normal FSH levels may occur in either obstructive azoospermia or seminiferous tubule dysfunction. In obstructive azoospermia, radiologic examination, i.e., a vasogram, will demonstrate the ductal obstruction, and a testicular biopsy will reveal normal spermatogenesis. Evaluation of azoospermia is one of the few indications for performing a testicular biopsy. Vasectomy has been used widely and successfully to induce infertility in men who desire fertility control, without any deleterious effects on the hypothalamic-pituitary-testicular axis or general health. Using microsurgical techniques, vasovasostomy has been used successfully to restore fertility in vasectomized men. Despite return of sperm in the ejaculate in 80 to 90 per cent, fertility is restored in only 30 to 50 per cent of men after vasovasostomy.

Ejaculatory dysfunction, such as premature or retrograde ejaculation, can cause infertility by preventing the normal deposition of sperm into the female genital tract. Premature ejaculation is often successfully treated by sex therapy techniques. Retro-

TABLE 222–2. CAUSES OF MALE INFERTILITY

Coital Disorders
  Defects in Technique
    Poor timing with menses
    Premature withdrawal
    Infrequent intercourse
  Impotence
Hypogonadism (Deficiency of Sperm Production)
Ductal Obstruction
  Congenital Defects of Vas Deferens, Epididymides, or Seminal
    Vesicles
  Postinfectious Obstruction
  Cystic Fibrosis/Young's Syndrome
  Vasectomy
Ejaculatory Dysfunction
  Premature Ejaculation
  Retrograde Ejaculation
Disorders of Accessory Glands
  Epididymitis/Seminal Vesiculitis/Prostatitis
  Immunologic

grade ejaculation most commonly results from diabetic autonomic neuropathy, prostatic resection, pelvic surgery, or administration of sympatholytic drugs. It is suspected if orgasm produces little or no ejaculate and is confirmed by the presence of large numbers of sperm in a postejaculation urine sample. Sympathomimetic drugs, imipramine, and harvesting and concentrating of sperm from the urine for artificial insemination have been used to treat retrograde ejaculation.

Disorders of the *accessory sexual organs* result in infertility by a number of mechanisms. Infections of the epididymis, seminal vesicles, and/or prostate have been reported to cause infertility by affecting sperm maturation or function directly or by inducing antisperm antibodies that, in turn, affect sperm function. Offending organisms include *Neisseria gonorrhoea, Chlamydia trachomatis,* coliforms, *Ureaplasma urealyticum,* and *Mycobacterium tuberculosis.* Antisperm antibodies present in the semen may cause sperm agglutination and reduce sperm motility. Induction of these antibodies after vasectomy may be responsible for the discrepancy between the success rate for return of sperm in the ejaculate and restoration of fertility after vasectomy reversal. High-dose glucocorticoid therapy can lower antisperm antibody titers and improve fertility in some patients.

GYNECOMASTIA. Gynecomastia, a benign glandular enlargement of the male breast, is usually asymptomatic, but its rapid development may cause pain and tenderness. It is often very difficult to distinguish between true gynecomastia and an increase in adipose tissue in obese boys or men. The technique used to examine the female breast, namely palpation with the flat of the hand against the chest wall, often misses significant amounts of breast tissue in the male. In order to adequately detect gynecomastia, fingers should be used to grasp the tissue surrounding the areola in a pinching action.

Although usually bilateral, gynecomastia may be markedly asymmetric or rarely unilateral. In these instances, gynecomastia must be distinguished from other benign chest wall tumors (such as lipomas, neurofibromas, and lymphomas) and male breast cancer. In contrast to benign breast conditions, breast carcinoma is usually eccentric in location, hard, and associated with skin or nipple retraction and bloody discharge; lymphadenopathy due to metastatic disease may also be found.

Gynecomastia usually occurs when the breast is exposed to a hormonal milieu of increased estrogen concentration relative to testosterone concentration, i.e., an increased estrogen/testosterone ratio. An increased ratio may result from pathologic conditions or drugs that either increase estrogen or reduce testosterone levels or action of these hormones. Since both of these hormonal alterations commonly result in primary or secondary hypogonadism, hypogonadal states are major causes of gynecomastia. Unless hyperprolactinemia induces androgen deficiency by inhibiting gonadotropin secretion, elevated prolactin levels do not usually cause gynecomastia. Hyperprolactinemia may, however, contribute to the development of *galactorrhea* (milky breast discharge) in patients with gynecomastia. The clinical causes of gynecomastia are summarized in Table 222–3.

Gynecomastia may sometimes be *physiologic* rather than pathologic. Transient gynecomastia is usually seen in neonatal boys, as a result of exposure in utero to high maternal estrogen concentrations. At the time of puberty, gynecomastia is observed in 60 to 70 per cent of boys. This pubertal gynecomastia usually lasts for months to years and does not persist into adulthood. Although there is a transient rise in the estrogen/testosterone ratio during puberty, the pathogenesis of pubertal gynecomastia is unclear. Finally, small amounts of palpable breast tissue (2 to 3 cm in diameter) can be detected by careful examination in 40 per cent of healthy normal adult men, increasing in prevalence with advancing age. This mild gynecomastia is always asymptomatic and generally goes unnoticed.

Most of the pathologic causes of gynecomastia are associated with alterations in the hypothalamic-pituitary-testicular axis, resulting in a hypogonadal hormonal profile. Gynecomastia may occur with any of the causes of hypogonadism that result in *androgen deficiency,* including both primary testicular disorders and those secondary to gonadotropin deficiency.

In addition to androgen deficiency or *disorders of androgen action,* gynecomastia may be caused by a number of *drugs.* Gynecomastia may result from exposure to exogenous estrogen, e.g., from administration of diethylstilbestrol for metastatic pros-

TABLE 222–3. CAUSES OF GYNECOMASTIA

222 THE TESTIS / 1341

TABLE 222–3. CAUSES OF GYNECOMASTIA

I. **Physiologic Gynecomastia**
  Neonatal
  Pubertal
  Adult
II. **Hypogonadism (Deficiency of Androgen Production)**
III. **Androgen Resistance Syndromes**
IV. **Drug-Induced Gynecomastia**
  Hormones
    Estrogens
    Aromatizable androgens hCG
  Drugs Interacting with Estrogen Receptor
    Marijuana
    Digitalis
  Drugs Altering Androgen Production or Action
    Spironolactone
    Cimetidine
    Ketoconazole
    Cytotoxic agents
  Central Nervous System–Active Drugs
    Antihypertensive agents
    Tranquilizers
    Sedatives
    Antidepressants
    Amphetamines

V. **Tumors**
  Estrogen-Secreting Tumors
    Adrenal carcinoma
    Leydig cell or Sertoli cell tumor of testis
  Gonadotropin-Secreting Tumors
    Testicular carcinoma
    Lung carcinoma
    Liver carcinoma
VI. **Systemic Disorders**
  Hepatic Cirrhosis
  Renal Failure
  Thyrotoxicosis
VII. **Miscellaneous**
  Refeeding Gynecomastia
  Familial
  Increased Peripheral Aromatization
  Local Chest Trauma

tate cancer, ingestion of estrogen-treated animal foodstuffs, use of or contact with estrogen-containing creams, and accidental occupational exposure. Excessive circulating estrogens inhibit endogenous gonadotropin secretion, which results, in turn, in reduced testosterone production. Secondary hypogonadism induced by estrogens may contribute to the development of gynecomastia. Administration of high doses of aromatizable androgens, especially to prepubertal boys or severely hypogonadal men, may induce gynecomastia analogous to that which occurs at puberty. hCG binds to the LH receptor on the Leydig cell of the testis and has biologic activities identical to those of LH. By stimulating relatively greater testicular production of estradiol compared to testosterone, hCG treatment of hypogonadotropic hypogonadal men may cause gynecomastia. Certain drugs result in breast enlargement by interacting with the estrogen receptor (marijuana, digitalis) or by interfering with androgen production or action (spironolactone, cimetidine, ketoconazole, certain chemotherapeutic agents). Finally, many central nervous system–active drugs, such as certain antihypertensives, sedatives, tranquilizers, antidepressants, and amphetamines, are associated with gynecomastia.

Although very uncommon, gynecomastia may be the initial manifestation of an *estrogen-secreting tumor* of the adrenal gland or testis. Feminizing adrenal tumors are usually malignant and present with a palpable abdominal mass. In contrast, estrogen-secreting tumors of the testis are often small and benign. Unlike many exogenous estrogen preparations, which do not cross-react with the RIA for estradiol, these tumors secrete large amounts of estradiol, which are detected in blood by clinically available estrogen assays. *hCG-secreting tumors*, such as testicular, lung, and hepatic carcinoma, may cause gynecomastia by stimulating excessive estrogen relative to testosterone secretion by Leydig cells. hCG cross-reacts with most routinely available LH assays; patients with hCG-secreting tumors may therefore have elevated LH levels. Also, since LH cross-reacts with most intact hCG assays, a specific β-hCG assay should be used to confirm the diagnosis of an hCG-secreting tumor.

Certain *systemic disorders* are associated with gynecomastia. In hepatic cirrhosis, gynecomastia is associated with increased estrogen production, primarily by accelerated peripheral conversion of adrenal androgens (androstenedione) to estrone. In addition, serum SHBG levels are elevated, and total and bioavailable serum testosterone levels are low, which also favor an increased estrogen/testosterone ratio. The gynecomastia observed in patients with renal failure is associated with androgen deficiency resulting from primary testicular failure, and estrogen production is not increased. High estradiol levels and relatively reduced

bioavailable testosterone levels (as a result of increased SHBG levels) are commonly found in patients with thyrotoxicosis and contribute to the development of gynecomastia in this condition.

Gynecomastia is often associated with nutritional repletion and weight gain after a period of starvation and weight loss. This *refeeding gynecomastia* was originally described in former prisoners of World War II who developed tender gynecomastia following their liberation and resumption of a normal diet. A similar condition may occur upon recovery from any prolonged, severe illness associated with malnutrition and weight loss. Refeeding gynecomastia may contribute to the gynecomastia associated with hemodialysis in chronic renal failure patients and to that related to isoniazid treatment in men with tuberculosis. Malnutrition results in severe suppression of the hypothalamic-pituitary-testicular axis. Refeeding and restoration of nutrition and body weight result in resumption of normal gonadal function, a dynamic hormonal situation similar to the onset of puberty. The rapid restoration of gonadal function ("second puberty") may explain the gynecomastia associated with refeeding. *Familial gynecomastia* and *idiopathic increase in peripheral aromatase activity* are very rare causes of gynecomastia.

Treatment of gynecomastia should focus on the correction of the underlying disorder or withdrawal of the offending drug. Prophylactic low-dose irradiation of the breast prior to the institution of diethylstilbestrol treatment in men with prostatic carcinoma prevents gynecomastia. Testosterone treatment of androgen deficiency may occasionally result in resolution of gynecomastia. Experience with the estrogen antagonists (such as tamoxifen), nonaromatizable androgens (such as dihydrotestosterone), and aromatase inhibitors in treating gynecomastia has been limited and variably effective. Severe, longstanding gynecomastia of any cause is usually associated with increased fibrous tissue stroma and requires surgical reduction mammoplasty.

Dial LK (ed.): Geriatric sexuality. Clin Geriatr Med 7:1, 1991. *The entire issue is devoted to sexuality in older adults, with very good chapters on sexuality and impotence in aging men, urologic and endocrine considerations in geriatric sexual dysfunction, and the impact of medications and chronic diseases on sexual function in the elderly.*

Glass AR: Gynecomastia. *In* Becker KL (ed.): Principles and Practice of Endocrinology and Metabolism. Philadelphia, JB Lippincott Company, 1990, p 1000. *This is a well-organized chapter that provides a very good review of the causes and treatment of gynecomastia.*

Howards SS, Lipshultz LI (eds.): Male infertility. Urol Clin North Am 14:1, 1987. *An excellent, comprehensive discussion of the evaluation and treatment of male infertility by several authors.*

Krane RJ (ed.): Impotence. Urol Clin North Am 15:1, 1988. *The entire issue is devoted to a comprehensive overview of the pathophysiology, evaluation, and treatment of impotence. Chapters on the surgical and nonsurgical treatment of impotence are particularly clear and contain excellent figures.*

Krane RJ, Goldstein I, Saenz de Tejada I: Impotence. N Engl J Med 321:1648, 1989. *An excellent, concise, recent review of the anatomy, physiology, pathophysiology, diagnosis, and treatment of impotence.*

Mahoney CP: Adolescent gynecomastia. Differential diagnosis and management. Pediatr Clin North Am 37:1389, 1990. *An excellent review of pubertal and pathologic gynecomastia in adolescents.*

Stine CC, Collins M: Male sexual dysfunction. Prim Care 16:1031, 1989. *A very good review of the causes and treatment of impotence and premature ejaculation from the standpoint of a primary care physician.*

Swerdloff RS: Infertility in the male. Ann Intern Med 103:906, 1985. *This is an extensive review of the diagnostic evaluation and treatment of male infertility (over 100 references).*

CAUSES OF MALE HYPOGONADISM

Once the diagnosis of male hypogonadism is suspected from the clinical manifestations described above, the diagnosis is confirmed by measurement of serum testosterone level and sperm count. A low serum testosterone concentration confirms androgen deficiency, and reduced sperm counts confirm a deficiency in sperm production.

The majority of hypogonadal men with *androgen deficiency* also have impairment in sperm production. Once androgen deficiency is diagnosed (low serum testosterone and sperm count), an effort should be made to distinguish between disorders that result from primary testicular disease (*primary hypogonadism*) and those that are secondary to inadequate gonadotropin stimulation of the testis (*secondary hypogonadism*), as a result of either pituitary or hypothalamic disease.

In addition to helping to define the specific etiology of androgen deficiency, the distinction between primary and secondary hypogonadism may have practical therapeutic implications. For example, regardless of the specific etiology, primary hypogonadism is usually treated with androgen replacement. In the majority of cases, the infertility in primary hypogonadism is not treatable. However, secondary hypogonadism may result from destruction of pituitary gonadotropin-secreting cells, for example by a pituitary tumor. In this instance, in addition to androgen deficiency, the space-occupying effects of the tumor mass on brain function (such as visual fields and cerebroventricular flow) and alterations (both increase and decrease) in the secretion of other anterior pituitary hormones (such as ACTH, thyroid-stimulating hormone [TSH], growth hormone, and prolactin) need to be considered in formulating a therapeutic plan (Ch. 213). Furthermore, since the testes usually function normally in response to adequate gonadotropin stimulation in patients with secondary hypogonadism, gonadotropins or LHRH may be administered in these patients to stimulate spermatogenesis and induce fertility.

The negative feedback relationship between gonadotropin secretion and circulating testosterone levels (see Fig. 222–1) provides the physiologic basis and rationale for the use of serum gonadotropin levels to distinguish between primary and secondary testicular disorders that result in androgen deficiency. Because the negative feedback effect of testosterone on gonadotropin secretion is reduced, men with primary hypogonadism have reduced serum testosterone and elevated serum LH and FSH levels; i.e., they have hypergonadotropic hypogonadism. Not uncommonly, serum FSH levels may be disproportionately elevated compared to LH levels, especially with severe seminiferous tubule dysfunction. However, selective elevation of serum LH levels is distinctly unusual and suggests the presence of a substance, such as hCG or α subunit, that cross-reacts in the RIA for LH.

In contrast to primary testicular dysfunction, men with secondary hypogonadism are not able to increase gonadotropin secretion appropriately in the presence of reduced testosterone negative feedback and have inadequate gonadotropin stimulation of the testis. These men have a hormonal pattern of reduced serum testosterone and low to low normal serum LH and FSH levels; i.e., they have hypogonadotropic hypogonadism. Gonadotropin levels are often in the low normal range in men with secondary hypogonadism because most clinically available gonadotropin assays lack sufficient sensitivity to distinguish low from low normal values.

The majority of hypogonadal patients with isolated impairment of sperm production have primary testicular disease. These patients generally present with infertility and have no clinical manifestations of androgen deficiency. Serum testosterone and gonadotropin levels are usually normal. Therefore, hormone determinations are not routinely obtained as part of an infertility workup unless clinical androgen deficiency is also present. Infertile patients who present with no sperm in their ejaculate, i.e., azoospermia, may have either severe seminiferous tubule failure or obstruction of the genital tract. Measurement of serum FSH level may be helpful in evaluation of an azoospermic patient. A selective elevation of serum FSH levels with normal LH levels in a patient with azoospermia implies severe germ cell dysfunction with loss of negative feedback influences (such as inhibin) on the pituitary gland and poor prognosis for fertility. No further workup is usually necessary. A normal serum FSH level in an azoospermic patient leaves open the possibility of a surgically correctable ductal obstruction, and a vasogram and testicular biopsy are usually performed. In addition to severe seminiferous tubule dysfunction, selective elevation in serum FSH levels may be observed in patients with gonadotropin-secreting pituitary adenomas. Uncommonly, isolated deficiency of sperm production results from inadequate gonadotropin stimulation of the testis. In these instances, serum gonadotropin levels are generally reduced, and very rarely selective FSH deficiency may occur.

The vast majority of adults with male hypogonadism have either primary or secondary testicular failure. Very rarely, disorders of androgen action may present in adults with a clinical picture of hypogonadism. Unlike the severe androgen resistance syndromes, which present at birth with male pseudohermaphroditism (Ch. 221), these disorders are characterized by mild defects in androgen action, resulting in a nearly normal male phenotype (frequently with varying degrees of hypospadias). Both serum testosterone and gonadotropin levels are usually elevated.

In summary, clinical manifestations combined with measurements of serum testosterone, sperm count, and basal serum gonadotropin levels permit a physiologic classification of the causes of male hypogonadism into primary and secondary hypogonadism and subclassification into disorders that result in deficiency of both sperm and androgen production and those with isolated deficiency in sperm production with normal androgen production (Table 222–4).

Primary Hypogonadism

DEFICIENCY OF SPERM AND ANDROGEN PRODUCTION. *Congenital or Developmental Disorders.* Klinefelter's syndrome is the most common cause of primary testicular failure resulting in impairment of both spermatogenesis and testosterone production. The syndrome is characterized by small, firm testes, azoospermia, gynecomastia, varying degrees of eunuchoidism and testosterone deficiency, and elevated gonadotropin levels. Klinefelter's syndrome is a very common disorder, affecting 1 in every 400 to 500 men. The incidence of Klinefelter's syndrome increases to 5 per cent when maternal age is over 45 years. The incidence of this syndrome, in particular of its variants, is significantly increased in mentally retarded individuals. The fundamental defect in Klinefelter's syndrome and its variants is the presence of one or a number of extra X chromosomes.

Classically, the karyotype in Klinefelter's syndrome is 47 XXY, resulting from meiotic nondisjunction in either the maternal or paternal gamete. Variants of the syndrome demonstrate a variety of karyotypes, including XXYY, more than two X (poly X) plus Y, and mosaicism. The karyotypes in mosaic Klinefelter's syndrome are a combination of the normal, classic, and variant karyotypes and may vary among different tissues within the same individual. In classic Klinefelter's syndrome (47 XXY), the presence of an extra X chromosome is responsible for the presence of a sex chromatin or Barr body in the nucleus of epithelial cells obtained on buccal smear, a normal finding in females, who carry two X chromosomes. Variant syndromes characterized by more than two X chromosomes may exhibit more than one Barr body per nucleus, the number of sex chromatin bodies always being one less than the number of X chromosomes. Confirmation of the presumptive diagnosis of Klinefelter's syndrome made on buccal smear examination is accomplished by karyotyping of blood lymphocytes or testicular tissue.

Although Klinefelter's disease is a congenital disorder, clinical features are not evident prior to puberty. At the time of puberty, the testes fail to increase in size and become firmer in consistency. This is a result of fibrosis and hyalinization of the seminiferous tubules. The most remarkable clinical feature of Klinefelter's syndrome is the very small size of the testes, rarely exceeding 2 cm in length, in contrast to a lower limit of 3.5 cm in the normal adult. Clinical androgen deficiency is usually present, but the degree of androgen deficiency is variable, resulting in varying degrees of eunuchoidism (Fig. 222–5). In contrast to other conditions that result in prepubertal androgen deficiency and classic eunuchoidism (see above), Klinefelter's syndrome often results in a disproportionate increase in lower extremity compared to upper extremity long bone growth. Careful palpation usually reveals bilateral gynecomastia in about 80 to 90 per cent of patients. Although the incidence of mental retardation is greater, the majority of patients with Klinefelter's syndrome have normal intelligence. Most patients exhibit character and personality disorders, which may be related, in part, to the psychosocial consequences of androgen deficiency. There is a slightly increased incidence of certain systemic diseases in Klinefelter's syndrome. These include diabetes, chronic obstructive pulmonary disease, autoimmune disorders (e.g., systemic lupus erythematosus, Hashimoto's thyroiditis), malignancy (breast cancer, lymphoma, germ cell neoplasms), and varicose veins.

The clinical manifestations of Klinefelter's syndrome variants differ from those of the classic 47 XXY syndrome. In general, the presence of more than two extra X chromosomes results in a much higher incidence of mental retardation and somatic abnormalities, such as hypospadias, cryptorchidism, and bony abnormalities of the radius and ulna. The majority of patients with mosaic Klinefelter's syndrome exhibit less severe clinical manifestations, particularly if a normal XY cell line is present. Indeed, fertility in patients with mosaic Klinefelter's syndrome (XXY/XY) has been documented. Patients with an additional Y chromosome tend to be tall and have extremely aggressive, antisocial behavioral abnormalities. Very rarely, a patient exhibits the classic features of Klinefelter's syndrome with a normal (46 XY) karyotype, a so-called mutant or phenocopy. Finally, phenotypic males with a 46 XX karyotype may demonstrate the typical clinical manifestations of classic Klinefelter's syndrome, except for having shorter stature and a higher incidence of hypospadias. The mechanism by which these individuals develop a male phenotype in the apparent absence of a Y chromosome is unclear (Ch. 221). In some patients with this condition, Y chromosomal material is translocated onto the X chromosome.

Azoospermia is present in over 95 per cent of patients with classic Klinefelter's syndrome. Serum testosterone levels are usually low but may be in the low normal adult range. However, free testosterone levels are reduced in most patients with Klinefelter's syndrome. Serum estradiol levels are often elevated, which results in elevated SHBG concentrations (and total testosterone levels within the normal range) and contributes to the development of gynecomastia. Serum gonadotropin levels, especially serum FSH levels, are uniformly elevated. Occasionally, serum LH levels may fall in the high normal adult range.

Treatment of Klinefelter's syndrome is aimed primarily at correction of the androgen deficiency with testosterone replacement therapy (see below). The infertility is irreversible. Gynecomastia may be a source of great social embarrassment, in which case reduction mammoplasty should be performed.

The *functional prepubertal castrate syndrome (congenital anorchia)* is characterized by bilateral absence of functioning testicular tissue, occasionally associated with absent epididymides, in a genotypic and phenotypic man. The presence of otherwise normal male internal and external genitalia, without müllerian duct derivatives, and descent of the vas and testicular blood vessels into the scrotum imply that a normally functioning testis was present during fetal and prepubertal life. It is hypothesized that testicular damage during the fetal or prepubertal period results in atrophy of the gonads. Patients with this syndrome usually present with delayed puberty, eunuchoidal features with sexual infantilism, absence of palpable testes ("empty scrotum"), and, unlike other conditions associated with eunuchoidism, short stature (see Fig. 222–4). Congenital anorchia must be distinguished from bilateral abdominal cryptorchidism, which also presents with absent scrotal testes. Because of the increased risk of malignancy, intra-abdominal testes require orchiectomy or orchiopexy. The absence of a testosterone response to exogenous hCG (e.g., 2000 IU three times weekly for 3 to 4 weeks) in patients with congenital anorchia may be helpful in distinguishing it from bilateral abdominal testes. However, there have been reports of responses to hCG stimulation in patients with congenital anorchia and absent responses in patients with bilateral cryptorchidism. Laparoscopy or surgical exploration is often necessary to confirm the diagnosis. Treatment of this syndrome consists of androgen replacement therapy to induce full sexual maturation. Insertion of testicular prostheses may be of psychological value.

Noonan (Bonnevie-Ullrich) syndrome, an autosomal recessive disorder, occurs in karyotypically normal males and females. It is characterized by a number of clinical features similar to those of females with Turner's syndrome. Characteristic findings include short stature, typical facies (hypertelorism, antimongoloid eye slant, ptosis, low-set ears, micrognathia, high-arched palate, and dental malocclusions), webbed neck, shield-like chest, pectus excavatum, cubitus valgus, mental retardation, cardiovascular

TABLE 222–4. CAUSES OF MALE HYPOGONADISM

I. Primary Hypogonadism
   Deficiency of Sperm and Androgen Production
      Congenital or Developmental Disorders
         Klinefelter's syndrome and variants
         Functional prepubertal castrate syndrome
         Noonan (Bonnevie-Ullrich) syndrome
         Myotonic dystrophy
         Polyglandular autoimmune disease
         Complex genetic disorders
         ? Normal aging
      Acquired Disorders
         Orchitis (mumps, leprosy, etc.)
         Surgical or traumatic castration
         Drugs (spironolactone, ketoconazole, H_2 receptor blockers,
            alcohol, marijuana, digitalis, cytotoxic drugs)
         Irradiation
      Systemic Disorders
         Chronic liver disease
         Chronic renal failure
         Malignancy (Hodgkin's, testicular)
         Sickle cell disease
         Paraplegia
         Vasculitis (periarteritis)
         Infiltrative disease (amyloidosis)
   Isolated Deficiency of Sperm Production
      Congenital or Developmental Disorders
         Germinal cell aplasia (Sertoli cell–only syndrome)
         Cryptorchidism
         Varicocele
         Immotile cilia syndrome (Kartagener's syndrome)
         Myotonic dystrophy
      Acquired Disorders
         Orchitis (mumps, leprosy, etc.)
         Thermal trauma
         Irradiation
         Cytotoxic drugs
         Environmental toxins
      Systemic Disorders
         Acute febrile illness
         Paraplegia
         Idiopathic Oligospermia or Azoospermia

II. Secondary Hypogonadism
   Deficiency of Sperm and Androgen Production
      Congenital or Developmental Disorders
         Hypogonadotropic eunuchoidism (Kallmann's syndrome)
         Hemochromatosis
         Complex genetic syndromes
      Acquired Disorders
         Hypopituitarism
         Hyperprolactinemia
         Estrogen excess
         Progestins
         Opiate-like drugs
      Systemic Disorders
         Glucocorticoid excess (Cushing's syndrome)
         Acute stress or illness
         Nutritional deficiency (protein-calorie malnutrition,
            anorexia nervosa)
         Chronic illness
         Massive obesity
   Isolated Deficiency of Sperm Production
      Androgen Excess
         Congenital adrenal hyperplasia (21- and 11β-hydroxylase
            deficiency)
         Androgenic anabolic steroids
         Androgen-secreting tumors
      Hyperprolactinemia
      Isolated FSH Deficiency

   Androgen Resistance Syndromes
      Reifenstein's Syndrome
      Idiopathic Oligospermia or Azoospermia
      ? Celiac Disease

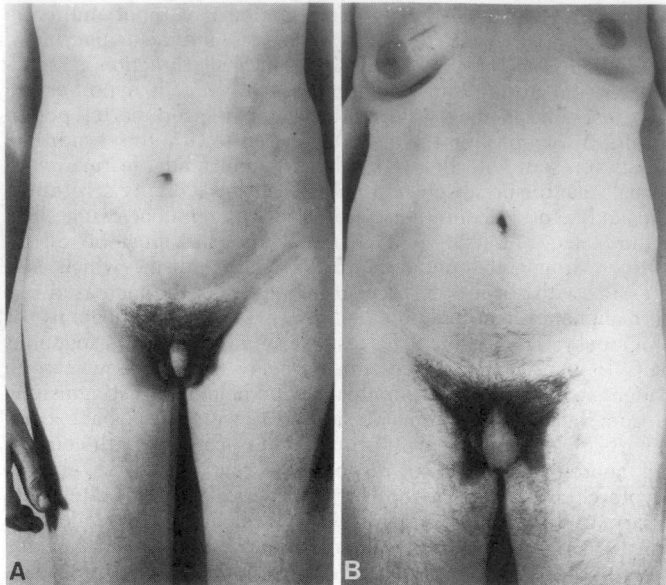

FIGURE 222–5. Two patients with untreated Klinefelter's syndrome, demonstrating the variability in degree of androgenization in this disorder. *A*, The small penis, diminished pubic hair with a female escutcheon, and sparse body hair indicate severe androgen deficiency. *B*, Normal penile development and adequate pubic and body hair indicate nearly normal androgen production by the testes. Gynecomastia is present in both patients, although only visible in the patient shown in *B*. The testes in both subjects were less than 2 cm in length. (From Bardin CW, Paulsen CA: The testes. *In* Williams RH (ed.): Textbook of Endocrinology, 6th ed. Philadelphia, W.B. Saunders Company, 1981.)

anomalies (pulmonic stenosis and atrial septal defects), and lymphedema. Males with Noonan syndrome (also called male Turner's syndrome) exhibit primary testicular dysfunction with impairment of both sperm and androgen production and elevated serum gonadotropin levels. Cryptorchidism is frequently present. Treatment of this disorder consists of testosterone replacement to correct the androgen deficiency and orchiopexy for associated cryptorchidism, both for psychological reasons and to monitor the testes for malignancy.

Myotonic dystrophy (see also Ch. 504) is an autosomal dominant disorder characterized by progressive weakness and atrophy of muscles, especially those of the face, neck, and distal extremities. An important diagnostic feature in this disorder is the presence of myotonia, or prolonged contraction of muscles. Other characteristic findings include cataracts, cardiac arrhythmias, dysphagia, premature frontal balding, mild intellectual deterioration, and gonadal atrophy. Testicular atrophy, which occurs in middle age, is found in about 80 per cent of men affected by myotonic dystrophy. The majority of these men have isolated impairment of spermatogenesis with normal androgen production. However, approximately 20 per cent of men with myotonic dystrophy have manifestations of androgen deficiency as a result of primary testicular failure. In addition to treating the androgen deficiency, testosterone replacement therapy may help to maintain or improve muscle function in these men.

Polyglandular autoimmune disease (see also Ch. 228) is a disorder in which there is concurrence of organ-specific autoimmune disease involving several endocrine and nonendocrine organs, associated with the presence of circulating autoantibodies to these organs. Specific conditions that occur in association with each other in this disorder are Addison's disease, hypothyroidism, insulin-dependent diabetes, pernicious anemia, ovarian failure, hypoparathyroidism, vitiligo, mucocutaneous candidiasis, Graves' disease, hypopituitarism, and alopecia. Although much less common than primary ovarian failure, primary testicular failure, associated with antitesticular antibodies and resulting in androgen deficiency, may occur in males with polyglandular autoimmune disease.

Normal aging in healthy men significantly reduces levels of total, free, and non-SHBG-bound testosterone and diminishes

spermatogenesis compared to that in young men. In addition, the normal circadian variation in testosterone levels is markedly attenuated in old compared to young men. Both LH and FSH levels are significantly elevated in healthy old men, suggesting that the reduction in testosterone levels which occurs with normal aging is mostly the result of primary testicular dysfunction. Indeed, elderly men exhibit reduced testosterone responses to stimulation by exogenous hCG administration. The physiologic significance of reduced testosterone levels in aging men is unknown. Normal aging in men is also accompanied by an increased incidence of sexual dysfunction, as well as decreased muscle and bone mass. Whether these changes in body function with aging are related to the reduction in androgen production remains to be investigated.

Primary hypogonadism may present in a number of *complex genetic disorders*, such as *Alstrom, ataxia telangiectasia, Sohval-Soffer, Weinstein,* and *Werner* syndromes. Rarely, patients with *Prader-Labhart-Willi* and *Laurence-Moon-Biedl* syndromes demonstrate primary, rather than the more commonly associated secondary, hypogonadism.

Acquired Disorders. In general, seminiferous tubule function and spermatogenesis are much more sensitive to external or environmental influences (such as irradiation, cytotoxic agents, or heat) than is Leydig cell production of testosterone. This greater sensitivity is due, in large part, to the fact that spermatogenesis involves active and coordinated cellular division and differentiation, requiring complex regulation. As a result, most acquired primary testicular disorders causing hypogonadism result more commonly in isolated impairment of spermatogenesis with normal androgen production (see below) than in androgen deficiency.

Viral orchitis, most frequently due to *mumps,* is a very common cause of acquired primary testicular failure. Approximately 15 to 25 per cent of males with mumps develop acute orchitis. The few boys who develop mumps orchitis before puberty usually recover completely without subsequent testicular dysfunction. However, acute mumps infection of pubertal or adult testes usually results in permanent seminiferous tubule damage and, in severe cases, Leydig cell dysfunction with androgen deficiency. Although clinical mumps orchitis is unilateral in the majority of cases, degenerative changes have been observed in the clinically uninvolved testis. During the acute phase of orchitis, which usually develops within a few days of parotitis, there is interstitial edema and sloughing of the germinal epithelium. This may be followed by progressive tubular sclerosis and testicular atrophy over the next several months. The availability and use of mumps vaccine have significantly reduced the incidence of mumps orchitis. Orchitis may also complicate infections with viruses such as *echoviruses* and *arboviruses.* Uncommon causes of orchitis include *gonorrhea, leprosy, tuberculosis, brucellosis, glanders, syphilis,* and certain parasitic diseases such as *filariasis* and *bilharziasis.* As in mumps, orchitis complicating these disorders results more commonly in isolated impairment of sperm production, although in severe cases androgen production is also affected.

Bilateral surgical or traumatic castration results in acute androgen deficiency, and castration after puberty often causes hot flushes and irritability, similar to that of women at the time of menopause.

Certain *drugs* may produce androgen deficiency by inhibiting testosterone biosynthesis and/or by blocking androgen action. The aldosterone antagonist *spironolactone* inhibits testosterone synthesis, as well as interfering with androgen action by competitively binding to the androgen receptor. *Ketoconazole,* an antifungal agent, inhibits testosterone synthesis and in high doses may also inhibit adrenal steroidogenesis. H_2 *receptor blockers* (e.g., cimetidine) also block androgen receptors and act as weak androgen antagonists. *Alcohol* has direct toxic effects on both spermatogenesis and steroidogenesis in the testis in the absence of alcoholic cirrhosis. *Marijuana* (tetrahydrocannabinol) has direct inhibitory effects on testicular function in addition to its central nervous system effects. *Digitalis* has been reported to elevate serum estradiol levels and reduce serum testosterone levels, perhaps through its interaction with both the estrogen and androgen receptors. A number of *cytotoxic drugs* used in cancer chemotherapy interfere with spermatogenesis and, more rarely, with androgen production. In some *malignancies,* androgen deficiency may also be present in the absence of exposure to chemotherapeutic agents (e.g., Hodgkin's disease or testicular cancer). Androgen deficiency may be the result of general debilitation and malnutrition associated with some malignancies. *Irradiation* of the testes rarely causes permanent androgen deficiency. However, exposure of the testes to very large doses (over 600 to 800 rads) may compromise Leydig cell function.

Systemic Disorders. A number of systemic diseases cause deficiencies in sperm and androgen production, primarily by affecting testicular function directly, although gonadotropin secretion may also be affected in many of these conditions. In patients with *chronic liver disease* (cirrhosis), gynecomastia and testicular atrophy are commonly present (in 50 to 75 per cent). Total serum testosterone levels are low or low normal. Because SHBG levels are elevated, free or non-SHBG-bound testosterone levels are low. Serum LH levels are usually elevated but may fall in the high normal range. LH secretion may be partially suppressed by the high circulating levels of estrogens found in cirrhotic patients. Increased estrogen concentrations result from impaired hepatic clearance of adrenal androgens (androstenedione), leading to an increased substrate for peripheral aromatization to estrone and estradiol. The increased estrogen/testosterone ratio may contribute to the formation of gynecomastia. Treatment of androgen deficiency in patients with cirrhosis with an aromatizable androgen may result in worsening of gynecomastia.

Chronic renal failure usually causes reductions in both sperm and androgen production. LH and FSH levels are elevated, as a result of increased production as well as reduced renal clearance. The response of testosterone levels to hCG stimulation is impaired. Elevated serum prolactin levels and zinc deficiency may also contribute to testicular dysfunction in uremia. Hemodialysis does not significantly improve testosterone production. However, successful renal transplantation may result in some return of testicular function, which may be tempered by the drugs used for chronic immunosuppressive therapy to prevent graft rejection. In addition to treating androgen deficiency, testosterone replacement therapy may also improve the anemia of renal failure.

Sickle cell disease often results in low serum testosterone and elevated serum gonadotropin levels, implying primary testicular failure. *Paraplegia* may result in a transient reduction in serum testosterone levels that return to normal in the chronic paraplegic state unless chronic malnutrition occurs. *Vasculitis* involving the testis (e.g., periarteritis nodosa) or *infiltrative diseases* (e.g., amyloidosis, leukemia) may also result in primary testicular failure.

ISOLATED DEFICIENCY OF SPERM PRODUCTION.

Congenital or Developmental Disorders. *Germinal cell aplasia, or Sertoli cell–only syndrome,* is an uncommon condition characterized on testicular biopsy by seminiferous tubules of moderately reduced size, lined with Sertoli cells but devoid of germ cells and having little or no tubular fibrosis. Patients with this syndrome are normally androgenized but infertile. They have slightly smaller than normal testes, azoospermia, and elevated serum FSH levels, indicative of severe seminiferous tubule dysfunction. Serum testosterone levels are normal, and LH levels are normal or slightly elevated. Testosterone response to hCG stimulation may be reduced. These findings suggest that mild, subclinical Leydig cell dysfunction may also be present. It is hypothesized that congenital absence of germ cells is the basis for this syndrome. However, in some familial cases of germinal cell aplasia, germ cells have been found on testicular biopsy prior to puberty but are lost during and after puberty. The karyotype is usually 46 XY, although 47 XYY and 47 XXY karyotypes have also been found. Other gonadal disorders causing severe seminiferous tubule damage (such as mumps orchitis, cryptorchidism, irradiation, or cytotoxic drugs) may result in seminiferous tubules lined only with Sertoli cells. In these acquired causes of Sertoli cell–only syndrome, however, the tubules are usually extensively sclerosed and hyalinized and the testes are much smaller. Infertility in congenital germinal cell aplasia is irreversible but may be reversible with time in some acquired cases of severe germ cell damage.

In *cryptorchidism* the testes fail to descend normally into the scrotum. Cryptorchid testes are usually located in the abdomen or inguinal canal. *Ectopic testes* are located outside the normal pathway of testicular descent and may be found in the perineal, femoral, or superficial inguinal areas. To avoid unnecessary treatment, cryptorchid testes must be distinguished from *retractile testes,* which are located in the scrotum, but are withdrawn into the inguinal canal or abdomen with minimal stimulation.

The testes usually descend into the scrotum about the eighth month of fetal life. Undescended testes are found in approximately 3 to 4 per cent of full-term newborn males, but the testes descend during the first year in all but 0.7 to 0.8 per cent. The prevalence of cryptorchidism in adult males is about 0.3 to 0.4 per cent. Inguinal hernia is associated with cryptorchidism in 50 to 80 per cent of cases.

Bilateral cryptorchidism may be the presenting complaint in a number of hypogonadal disorders, such as the functional prepubertal castrate, the Noonan syndrome, and Reifenstein's syndrome. It may also be variably associated with many other causes of hypogonadism, such as Klinefelter's syndrome and hypogonadotropic eunuchoidism. In these disorders, cryptorchidism is usually associated with androgen deficiency. In contrast, when cryptorchidism is not associated with other hypogonadal disorders, it rarely affects Leydig cell function and usually causes isolated impairment of spermatogenesis.

Even when cryptorchidism is unilateral, testicular dysfunction is very common, suggesting that both testes have altered function. Abnormal testicular function may contribute to the failure of the testes to descend properly. In rare instances, normal testicular descent may be impeded by anatomic abnormalities along the pathway of descent, e.g., external inguinal hernias. In these instances, both testes function normally, and orchiopexy before puberty usually results in preservation of normal testicular function.

Careful physical examination of the scrotum should be performed to distinguish cryptorchidism from retractile testes, which is a more common condition. The diagnosis is particularly difficult in obese patients, and repeated examinations may be necessary. Examination should be performed in the standing, squatting, and recumbent positions, and observation in warm water may be helpful. The Valsalva maneuver and applied pressure to the lower abdomen are useful procedures to detect a mobile testis, which does not require therapy. In patients with retractile testes, elicitation of a cremasteric reflex may result in a localized puckering of the scrotal skin. Failure to palpate a testis after repeated examinations suggests that the testis is intra-abdominal, severely atrophic, or absent. Ultrasonography or CT scan may be helpful in localizing nonpalpable testes.

As a result of exposure of the seminiferous tubules to higher extrascrotal temperatures at the time of puberty, the germinal epithelium of cryptorchid testes shows severe degeneration, eventually resulting in tubular fibrosis. Bilateral cryptorchidism causes infertility. Sperm counts are low, and serum FSH levels are usually elevated. Leydig cell function is usually preserved, and serum testosterone and LH concentrations remain normal. The risk of malignancy in undescended testes is five to nine times greater than in scrotal testes, and the risk remains increased even after orchiopexy. Previous reports, based on retrospective studies, markedly overestimated this risk.

Therapy for cryptorchidism should be instituted before puberty, when the degenerative changes of the germinal epithelium occur. The exact age at which treatment should be instituted is controversial. Administration of hCG (1000 IU three times weekly) or LHRH to prepubertal boys with cryptorchidism may cause testicular descent in some patients. When such therapy is successful, it is probable that the testis would have descended spontaneously at puberty. Reports of the efficacy of hormonal therapy are widely discrepant, probably as a result of inclusion of variable proportions of patients with retractile testes. If hormonal therapy is unsuccessful in causing testicular descent, orchiopexy is performed in an attempt to preserve testicular function, to allow easier examination of the testis for malignant degeneration, and for cosmetic reasons. Despite orchiopexy, fertility rates in patients with cryptorchidism are usually reduced, particularly in patients with bilateral undescended testes. Often, bilateral testicular biopsies are performed at the time of orchiopexy to determine the degree of testicular abnormality. If a unilateral cryptorchid testis is atrophic and shows extensive tubular fibrosis, an orchiectomy is usually performed, provided that the contralateral testis is in the scrotum.

A *varicocele* is an abnormal dilatation of the pampiniform plexus of veins surrounding the spermatic cord, caused by retrograde blood flow into the internal spermatic vein. Palpable varicocele occurs in about 10 per cent of the general population and in 30 per cent of men with infertility. Varicocele is clearly associated with infertility. However, approximately 50 per cent of men with varicoceles have normal seminal fluid analyses, and some men with varicocele and abnormal seminal fluid parameters are fertile. About 90 per cent of varicoceles occur on the left side, as a result of valvular incompetence between the left internal spermatic vein and the renal vein. Occurrence of an isolated right-sided varicocele may be an early clue to venous obstruction by malignancy or to situs inversus. Varicoceles may affect testicular function by a variety of mechanisms, including increasing testicular temperature and blood flow. Seminal fluid analysis usually shows low sperm concentration with reduced motility and increased numbers of sperm with abnormal morphology (e.g., increased tapered and amorphous forms). Testicular size and serum testosterone, LH, and FSH levels are usually normal. Surgical repair of varicoceles in infertile men has been reported to improve semen quality and fertility, although well-controlled clinical studies have not been performed.

Immotile cilia syndrome, or *Kartagener's syndrome*, is characterized by sinusitis, bronchiectasis, and situs inversus. Patients usually suffer from chronic respiratory infections because of impaired mucociliary clearance in the respiratory tract. In addition, these patients produce nonmotile spermatozoa. Cilia in the respiratory tract and the sperm tail are immotile in Kartagener's syndrome because of an abnormality in *dynein*, a protein that is important in microtubular filament movement. Other patients have a *deficiency of protein carboxyl methylase*, an enzyme that is important in sperm motility. Infertility in this disorder is not treatable.

The majority of patients with *myotonic dystrophy* (see above) may have isolated impairment of spermatogenesis with normal androgen production.

Acquired Disorders. The majority of adults who develop mumps *orchitis* and orchitis due to other infectious agents sustain severe germ cell damage and isolated impairment of spermatogenesis with normal Leydig cell function (see above). Seminiferous tubule function is much more sensitive to damage from external or environmental agents than is Leydig cell function. Therefore, exposure of the testis to *thermal trauma, irradiation, cytotoxic drugs,* and *environmental toxins* often results in deficiency of sperm production without androgen deficiency. Even relatively minor thermal trauma, such as that induced by tight underwear or hot tubs, may result in suppression of sperm production.

The human testis is very sensitive to irradiation. Only 15 rads of x-irradiation may suppress spermatogenesis temporarily; more than 600 rads usually produces permanent infertility. Doses of radiation used in therapy of malignant lymphoma have been reported to result in permanent germ cell damage and infertility, despite shielding of the testis. Spermatogenesis is also very sensitive to damage by cytotoxic cancer chemotherapeutic agents, especially to alkylating agents. The likelihood of severe seminiferous tubule damage and permanent infertility is greater with combination chemotherapy regimens, such as MOPP for Hodgkin's disease. Despite being very sensitive to radiation and cytotoxic drugs, the germinal epithelium has remarkable regenerative properties, and recovery of spermatogenesis may occur despite very severe germ cell loss associated with high doses of these cytotoxic agents. Both irradiation (over 800 rads) and cytotoxic agents occasionally produce androgen deficiency. Sperm banking offers some hope of fertility for patients who will develop permanent infertility as a result of irradiation or chemotherapy for malignant disease. Sulfasalazine has been associated with oligospermia, reduced sperm motility, and infertility, but these findings may also be related to the underlying inflammatory bowel disease and catabolic state.

Damage to the germinal epithelium has been reported in workers exposed to carbon disulfide, a solvent used in production of rayon, and to dibromochloropropane, an insecticide. A number of other chemical agents used in industry and laboratories have been implicated as direct testicular toxins (e.g., lead, deuterium oxide, cadmium, fluoroacetamide, nitrofurans, dinitropyrroles, diamines, α-chlorhydrin, other insecticides, and rodenticides).

Systemic Disorders. A number of relatively minor *acute febrile illnesses* may result in temporary suppression of sperm production (e.g., minor viral infections). Over 50 per cent of men with spinal cord lesions resulting in *paraplegia* exhibit diminished testicular function, the majority demonstrating impaired sperm production with normal androgen production. Reduced spermatogenesis may be a result of elevated testicular temperature, caused by increased scrotal skin temperature (from loss of lumbar sympathetic innervation) and loss of the cremasteric reflex.

Idiopathic Oligospermia or Azoospermia. In most men who present with infertility and isolated impairment of spermatogenesis, no apparent cause can be found, leading to the diagnosis of *idiopathic oligospermia or azoospermia.* Because of the high prevalence of male infertility (5 to 6 per cent of reproductive age men), idiopathic oligospermia or azoospermia is the most common cause of male hypogonadism. Since the pathogenesis of impaired sperm production is not known, therapy for this disorder has been largely empiric and unsatisfactory. Trials of treatment with large doses of testosterone, gonadotropins, clomiphene citrate, testolactone, cortisone, thyroid hormone, caffeine, and vitamins have generally been unsuccessful in improving fertility rates over those achieved by placebo treatment or untreated patients, who have a 20 per cent fertility rate in 1 year. At present, infertility in these patients should be considered irreversible and couples should be offered artificial insemination, using donor semen, or adoption as alternatives.

Secondary Hypogonadism

Secondary hypogonadism is testicular failure due to inadequate gonadotropin secretion as a result of either hypothalamic or pituitary dysfunction. In the majority of cases, both LH and FSH secretion are diminished, resulting in impairment of both sperm and androgen production. Rarely, there may be isolated deficiency of sperm production.

DEFICIENCY OF SPERM AND ANDROGEN PRODUCTION. Congenital or Developmental Disorders. *Hypogonadotropic eunuchoidism,* or *Kallmann's syndrome,* is a congenital and often familial disorder, characterized by isolated hypogonadotropic hypogonadism (resulting in eunuchoidal features) and anosmia or hyposmia. Gonadotropin deficiency in this disorder is caused by a defect in synthesis and/or release of LHRH from the hypothalamus; chronic exogenous LHRH administration results in stimulation of normal testicular function. A developmental failure of the olfactory lobes is responsible for absent or reduced sense of smell. There is considerable genetic heterogeneity in this disorder. Kallmann's syndrome may be inherited as an autosomal dominant with variable (male-predominant) expression, an autosomal recessive, or an X-linked recessive condition.

Usually, patients with Kallmann's syndrome present with delayed puberty. They exhibit eunuchoidal features and prepubertal size testes. An early prepubertal manifestation of Kallmann's syndrome is micropenis. In addition to anosmia or hyposmia (present in approximately 80 per cent of cases), these patients may also exhibit other mid-line defects (e.g., cleft-lip or -palate, color blindness, renal agenesis, nerve deafness), cryptorchidism, and skeletal abnormalities (e.g., syndactyly, short fourth metacarpals, craniofacial asymmetry). Patients with Kallmann's syndrome are often aspermic (i.e., have no ejaculate). Serum testosterone, LH, and FSH levels are low, while other anterior pituitary functions are normal. The degree of gonadotropin deficiency is highly variable. A single dose LHRH test may not result in stimulation of gonadotropin secretion, but repeated LHRH administration will increase LH and FSH levels. Clomiphene citrate is an antiestrogen that stimulates hypothalamic release of LHRH and as a result increases gonadotropin secretion. In men with Kallmann's syndrome gonadotropins are paradoxically suppressed by clomiphene citrate.

The differentiation between Kallmann's syndrome and constitutional delayed puberty is very difficult (especially in the absence of anosmia or hyposmia) and cannot be reliably made in the prepubertal age range. Usually, androgen therapy is initiated to induce sexual maturation in both of these conditions. It is intermittently stopped to determine whether spontaneous onset of puberty occurs. Patients with Kallmann's syndrome continue to require androgen therapy to achieve and maintain sexual maturation, whereas patients with constitutional delayed puberty do not require treatment after spontaneous endogenous gonadotropin and testosterone secretion begin. When fertility is desired, androgen replacement treatment is discontinued, and spermatogenesis may be induced with gonadotropin or LHRH therapy. Previous androgen therapy does not alter the subsequent testicular response to gonadotropin therapy. However, gonadotropin therapy is much less successful in patients who have associated cryptorchidism, particularly if it is bilateral.

A variant form of Kallmann's syndrome is *isolated LH deficiency*, which is also called the *"fertile" eunuch syndrome*. This syndrome is characterized by a selective deficiency in LH secretion, which results in prepubertal androgen deficiency and eunuchoidism. FSH secretion is preserved, resulting in testes of nearly normal size in which well-advanced spermatogenesis is present. Spermatogenesis is not normal in these patients, however, and they are not fertile, as the name of the syndrome would imply. Treatment with hCG, which contains predominantly LH-like hormonal activity, stimulates Leydig cell production of testosterone, ameliorates androgen deficiency, and increases spermatogenesis.

Hemochromatosis is an autosomal recessive disorder in which there is parenchymal iron deposition in a variety of tissues, most prominently in the liver, skin, pancreas, and heart (Ch. 193). Iron deposition in the pituitary gland selectively inhibits gonadotropin production without significantly affecting other anterior pituitary hormone secretion. The resulting hypogonadotropic hypogonadism and androgen deficiency are responsible for the common complaint of impotence in this disorder. Frequent phlebotomies or treatment with desferrioxamine to decrease iron overload may restore gonadotropin secretion in some patients. Even in the presence of significant iron overload, administration of gonadotropins can stimulate testicular function, including induction of spermatogenesis. Parenchymal iron deposition resulting in hypogonadotropic hypogonadism may also occur in patients with conditions that require frequent blood transfusions, such as thalassemia.

Secondary hypogonadism may be present in a number of *complex genetic syndromes*, such as *Prader-Labhart-Willi, Laurence-Moon-Biedl, Biemond, Carpenter, familial cerebellar ataxia, dyskeratosis congenita, familial ichthyosis, Borjeson, Kraus-Rupert, Lowe, steroid sulfatase deficiency, RUD, CHARGE, LEOPARD, Martsolf, Rothmund-Thompson,* and *Richards-Rundle* syndromes.

Acquired Disorders. Hypopituitarism. Any destructive or infiltrative lesion of the hypothalamus and/or pituitary may cause impairment of gonadotropin secretion, either selectively or in conjunction with deficiency of other anterior pituitary hormones (Ch. 213). Specific pathologic conditions include functioning and nonfunctioning pituitary adenomas; suprasellar tumors, such as craniopharyngioma, meningioma, optic glioma, or astrocytoma; metastatic neoplasms; lymphoma; surgical ablation or irradiation of the pituitary; infarction; vasculitis; apoplexy; hypophysitis; aneurysm; abscess; trauma; granulomatous disease, such as tuberculosis, sarcoidosis, fungal disease, and histiocytosis X; and transfusional iron overload.

Usually, destructive processes involving the pituitary gland result in progressive loss of anterior pituitary function in the following order: Gonadotropin and growth hormone secretion are the first to be affected, followed by TSH production, and finally ACTH secretion. The combination of gonadotropin and growth hormone deficiency is most important to recognize in prepubertal children with growth retardation. In adults, clinical secondary hypogonadism, in the absence of other anterior pituitary dysfunction, may be the initial manifestation of a hypothalamic or pituitary process. Because loss of TSH and ACTH secretion is associated with greater degrees of pituitary destruction, secondary hypothyroidism and hypoadrenalism usually do not occur without concurrent secondary hypogonadism.

Patients with prepubertal gonadotropin deficiency present with delayed puberty and have eunuchoidal features and small testes, usually less than 2 cm. Children with associated growth hormone deficiency also demonstrate short stature (dwarfism). Men with postpubertal gonadotropin deficiency usually present with diminished libido and potency. Initially, testicular size may be normal, but with longstanding gonadotropin deficiency the testes become small. In addition to hypogonadism, patients with hypopituitarism may have findings of deficiency or excess of other anterior pituitary hormones or tumor mass effects.

Serum testosterone levels and sperm counts are low. Serum LH and FSH levels are low or in the low normal adult range. The gonadotropin response to single dose LHRH administration does not reliably differentiate hypothalamic and pituitary causes of gonadotropin deficiency. In many instances, LHRH administration fails to stimulate gonadotropin secretion in patients with hypothalamic disease; alternatively, it may stimulate gonadotropin levels in men with pituitary disease. Clinical evaluation of patients with secondary hypogonadism should include anatomic studies (such as CT scan and visual field examination) to determine the presence and effects of a hypothalamic or pituitary tumor and investigation of other anterior pituitary hormone functions.

Treatment is aimed at the process causing hypopituitarism and correction of androgen deficiency with testosterone replacement therapy. If fertility is desired, androgens are discontinued and gonadotropin therapy is instituted.

Hyperprolactinemia. This condition, resulting from a pituitary adenoma, central nervous system–active drugs (such as phenothiazines and other antipsychotics, opiates, sedatives, antidepressants, stimulants), or adrenergic dopaminergic antagonist drugs (antihypertensives, metoclopramide) may cause secondary testicular failure (Ch. 226). In men, prolactin-secreting adenomas are usually large (macroadenomas), and gonadotropin deficiency may be caused primarily by destruction of pituitary gonadotrophs. Even in the absence of a tumor, prolactin has an inhibitory effect on gonadotropin secretion, resulting in secondary hypogonadism. In some men with hyperprolactinemia, correction of androgen deficiency with testosterone replacement therapy does not correct impotence. The addition of bromocriptine, a dopamine agonist that decreases pituitary prolactin secretion, may be useful in these situations.

The negative feedback effects of *estrogen excess* in men causes inhibition of gonadotropin secretion and secondary hypogonadism. Estrogen excess may result from either exogenous administration of estrogens or estrogenic substances (e.g., diethylstilbestrol administration in men with prostate cancer) or endogenous secretion from an estrogen-producing neoplasm (e.g., feminizing adrenal carcinoma). Patients with estrogen excess usually manifest varying degrees of gynecomastia. *Progestins* (e.g., medroxyprogesterone acetate) and *opiate-like drugs* (e.g., morphine, methadone, and heroin) also inhibit gonadotropin production and may cause secondary hypogonadism.

Systemic Disorders. *Glucocorticoid excess*, as a result of either Cushing's syndrome or high-dosage glucocorticoid administration, suppresses gonadotropin secretion, resulting in secondary testicular failure with loss of libido, impotence, and oligospermia. Activation of the hypothalamic-adrenal axis resulting in stimulation of corticotropin-releasing factor (which is thought to inhibit LHRH secretion) and high circulating levels of endogenous glucocorticoids may contribute to the reduction in serum testosterone, LH, and FSH levels observed with *acute stress or illness*, such as emotional stress, vigorous physical exercise, trauma, myocardial infarction, surgery, burns, sepsis, etc. *Nutritional deficiency*, such as that associated with protein-calorie malnutrition or anorexia nervosa, inhibits gonadotropin production and may cause secondary hypogonadism. Concurrent primary testicular dysfunction may also be associated with inadequate nutrition. Malnutrition may contribute to the secondary testicular failure associated with a number of *chronic illnesses*, such as malignancy and chronic heart, respiratory, liver, and kidney disease. Moderate obesity results in reduction in SHBG and total testosterone levels, with normal free testosterone levels. Some men with *massive obesity* demonstrate clinical androgen deficiency with low free testosterone concentrations and reduced gonadotropin levels.

ISOLATED DEFICIENCY OF SPERM PRODUCTION. *Congenital adrenal hyperplasia* caused by either 21-hydroxylase or 11β-hydroxylase deficiency results in excessive production of adrenal androgens. Androgen excess suppresses gonadotropin secretion, resulting in secondary hypogonadism. Testicular androgen and sperm production are suppressed. Excessive adrenal androgen production causes premature virilization and precocious pseudopuberty, rather than androgen deficiency. Secondary hypogonadism is therefore manifested by isolated impairment of spermatogenesis. Glucocorticoid treatment of some patients with congenital adrenal hyperplasia may result in true precocious puberty, with premature activation of the hypothalamic-pituitary-gonadal axis. These patients demonstrate premature induction of spermatogenesis and normal gonadotropin levels. Androgen excess caused by administration of *testosterone* or *androgenic anabolic steroids* or *androgen-secreting tumors* (e.g., testicular Leydig cell tumors) also result in secondary hypogonadism presenting with isolated deficiency in sperm production with normal androgenization. High doses of testosterone have been used in normal men to suppress sperm production in trials to develop male contraceptives.

Rarely, *hyperprolactinemia* impairs sperm production despite normal gonadotropin and testosterone levels. *Isolated FSH deficiency,* an extremely rare condition, results in normal virilization in males, with normal serum testosterone and LH levels. Spermatogenesis and fertility have not been well characterized in this disorder, although testicular biopsy in one man revealed arrest of sperm maturation at the spermatid stage.

Androgen Resistance Syndromes

Androgen resistance syndromes are caused by defects in androgen action (Ch. 221). The severity of androgen insensitivity determines the clinical presentation of these disorders. Most androgen resistance syndromes result in severely defective androgen action, and patients with these syndromes present at birth as either phenotypic females (testicular feminization) or with ambiguous genitalia (male pseudohermaphroditism). However, some men with mild, incomplete androgen insensitivity or *Reifenstein's syndrome* may present as adults with a clinical picture of mild androgen deficiency with a nearly normal male phenotype. Patients with Reifenstein's syndrome may have hypospadias, gynecomastia, varying degrees of virilization, a small prostate gland, impaired spermatogenesis, and cryptorchidism. They may be distinguished from patients with true hypogonadism by having elevated serum testosterone, LH, and FSH levels. Some men with very mild androgen insensitivity may present with only oligospermia or azoospermia and no other phenotypic abnormalities. Some men with celiac disease are infertile and have elevated serum testosterone and LH levels, suggesting androgen resistance.

Delayed Puberty

Puberty in boys usually begins between the ages of 9 and 14 years. With the maturation of the central nervous system mechanism that regulates LHRH production, pulsatile gonadotropin and testosterone secretions begin, initially during sleep and then throughout the day. The first clinical indications of the onset of puberty are an increase in the testicular size (above 3 cm) and a wrinkling and pigmentation of the scrotal skin. Subsequently, there are increase in penile length and appearance of pubic hair, followed by increasing long bone growth and development of other secondary sexual characteristics, such as hair growth in other androgen-dependent areas, increase in muscle mass, enlargement of the larynx, and growth of the prostate. The increase in testicular size precedes the appearance of pubic hair by about 2 years and the peak velocity in growth of height by 3 years. The onset and duration of puberty and the degree to which secondary sexual characteristics develop vary considerably, largely attributable to the genetic background of an individual.

Delayed puberty is the lack of sexual maturation before the age of 15 years. A number of the disorders discussed above that cause *hypogonadism,* including those causing primary and secondary testicular failure and androgen resistance, may result in delayed sexual maturation. *Severe systemic illnesses* (such as malabsorption, asthma, diabetes, malignancy) that also cause growth retardation and *thyroid hormone deficiency* may also cause delayed puberty. The great majority of boys with delayed puberty, however, have physiologic or *constitutional delayed puberty.* This is a benign form of delayed adolescence which represents a normal variation in the onset of puberty. It is frequently familial. These boys eventually undergo a delayed but normal puberty and attain normal sexual maturation and height.

The diagnosis of constitutional delayed puberty can be strongly suspected in a healthy boy with retardation of growth and bone age, normal growth velocity in relation to bone age, a family history of delayed adolescence, a testicular volume above 2 ml, and a bone age between 12 and 13 years. These clinical features are often not present and the diagnosis can be very difficult. Diagnostic evaluation should be undertaken to exclude organic causes of delayed puberty, i.e., hypogonadism, systemic illness, and hypothyroidism. In the absence of anosmia or other morphologic manifestations, constitutional delayed puberty cannot be distinguished from hypogonadotropic eunuchoidism or Kallmann's syndrome (see above).

Delayed sexual maturation often results in severe psychosocial distress to both the patient and his parents. Therefore, after systemic and endocrine disorders are excluded, patients with delayed puberty are usually treated with androgen replacement therapy to induce sexual maturation. It is generally recommended that patients not be treated with androgens until after 15 years of age. The emotional stress and trauma of delayed puberty often result in treatment beginning at about 13 to 14 years of age, however, so that the onset of sexual maturation coincides with those of his contemporaries. Androgen treatment is intermittently stopped to determine if spontaneous onset of puberty has occurred.

TREATMENT OF HYPOGONADISM
Androgen Therapy

Androgens are principally used to treat testosterone deficiency in hypogonadal men; the therapeutic goal of androgen therapy is to restore the normal physiologic effects of testosterone. In prepubertal androgen-deficient boys, the aim of androgen replacement is to stimulate and maintain male secondary sexual characteristics, somatic development, and sexual function without compromising adult height by premature closure of long bone epiphyses. In adult androgen deficiency, the objective of therapy is to restore and maintain libido, potency, and secondary sexual characteristics. Androgen treatment is very successful in accomplishing these goals. However, testosterone cannot be administered in sufficiently high doses to achieve the high intratesticular levels required to stimulate spermatogenesis.

The long-acting 17β-hydroxyl esters of testosterone, *testosterone enanthate* and *cypionate,* are the most effective, safest, and most practical preparations currently available to treat androgen deficiency. Intramuscular injection of 200 mg of either preparation results in peak serum testosterone levels at the upper limits of the normal adult range in 1 to 2 days. Testosterone levels remain in the normal range for about 2 weeks. Therefore, in adults with androgen deficiency, replacement therapy is usually initiated with either testosterone enanthate or cypionate at a dose of 200 mg intramuscularly every 2 weeks. In these men, testosterone administration generally results in stimulation of libido and potency, improvement in energy level, increase in physical and social drive, and increase in hemoglobin concentration.

In an elderly androgen-deficient man with symptoms of bladder neck obstruction secondary to an enlarged prostate gland, it is wise to begin testosterone therapy gradually with a short-acting testosterone preparation. *Testosterone propionate,* a short-acting 17β-hydroxyl ester of testosterone, given in doses of 25 to 50 mg intramuscularly three times weekly, is useful in this situation. The shorter duration of action of this preparation permits rapid withdrawal if androgen stimulation results in prostatic growth or urinary obstruction.

Androgen replacement therapy is much more complicated in prepubertal boys with delayed puberty. Although testosterone is very effective in inducing secondary sexual characteristics and stimulating long bone growth, overly aggressive androgen therapy can result in premature closure of long bone epiphyses and compromise final adult height. Furthermore, it is often not possible to differentiate patients with constitutional delayed puberty, who require only temporary androgen replacement, from those with permanent hypogonadotropic hypogonadism. Therefore, in boys with delayed puberty whose height is far below the expected adult height, androgen therapy is begun with testosterone enanthate or cypionate, 50 to 100 mg intramuscularly every 2 weeks, and gradually increased to full replacement doses. Androgen therapy is intermittently stopped for 3 to 4 months to determine whether spontaneous pubertal development will occur.

Currently, all oral androgen preparations available in the

United States are 17α-alkylated derivatives of testosterone, which have the potential for serious hepatotoxicity. When used for the treatment of androgen deficiency, parenteral 17β-hydroxyl esters of testosterone do not cause hepatotoxicity. Because of the greater risk of oral androgen preparations, as well as their increased cost and reduced efficacy, they should be avoided in the treatment of androgen deficiency. In the very rare circumstance of a patient who will not or cannot take parenteral androgens, *methyltestosterone*, 25 to 50 mg orally or 10 to 25 mg buccally, or *fluoxymesterone*, 5 to 10 mg orally daily, may be used.

Androgen therapy is absolutely contraindicated in men with androgen-sensitive cancers, i.e., prostatic carcinoma and male breast carcinoma. Full replacement doses of androgens may be inappropriate for hypogonadal men with mental retardation or severe psychopathology and for elderly androgen-deficient men with severe bladder neck obstruction from prostatic hyperplasia, who are not good surgical candidates.

Excessive stimulation of libido and erections by androgens is very uncommon, usually occurring in prepubertal boys or in men with longstanding androgen deficiency given large doses of testosterone. These symptoms usually resolve with time or reduction in dosage. Androgen administration causing acute urinary retention is very uncommon in the absence of underlying prostatic carcinoma. Patients given testosterone to induce puberty may develop acne or gynecomastia, similar to that observed in normal puberty. Adult hypogonadal men less commonly develop acne and rarely develop gynecomastia, except when a predisposing condition such as hepatic cirrhosis exists. Androgens may cause mild weight gain as a result of sodium retention and protein anabolic effects, and patients with underlying edematous states may develop worsening edema during therapy.

Erythropoiesis is stimulated by androgen administration. Occasionally, significant erythrocytosis requiring phlebotomy and reduced testosterone dosage occurs. Testosterone has also been reported to worsen or induce obstructive sleep apnea. All oral 17α-alkylated androgens have been reported to cause hepatic cholestasis and occasionally clinical jaundice. Although rare, more serious and potentially life-threatening complications of oral androgens are the development of peliosis hepatis (blood-filled cysts in the liver), hepatic adenoma, hepatoma, or hepatic angiosarcoma. Hepatotoxicity does not result from replacement dosages of parenteral 17β-hydroxyl esters of testosterone. Depending on the androgen preparation, dose, duration of therapy, and individual susceptibility, androgen administration may induce virilization in women, manifested by acne, hirsutism, and menstrual dysfunction, and in severe cases frontal balding, voice changes, breast atrophy, and clitoral hypertrophy.

Androgens have also been used in the treatment of anemias related to renal and bone marrow failure, micropenis and microphallus, hereditary angioneurotic edema, female breast cancer, lichen sclerosus, endometriosis, and senile osteoporosis. The use of androgenic steroids has not been demonstrated to be of long-term value in promoting protein anabolism in catabolic states associated with a variety of acute and chronic illnesses. However, in many illnesses (such as burns, chronic liver disease, and illnesses requiring chronic glucocorticoid therapy), serum testosterone levels are often low. The efficacy of androgen therapy in this subset of catabolic diseases has not been examined.

Androgenic anabolic steroids are commonly used by competitive athletes with the hope of improving endurance, strength, and performance. Numerous studies have demonstrated that androgens are of dubious value in increasing strength and performance, in the absence of intensive training and high-protein diets. Many athletes often take multiple androgenic anabolic agents (including 17α-alkylated agents) in very high doses, with little regard for potentially serious side effects. Hepatotoxicity (including hepatoma) and impaired spermatogenesis resulting in infertility have been reported in athletes taking these androgenic steroids. Furthermore, the long-term sequelae of taking massive doses of 17β-hydroxyl ester preparations are unknown. The potential risks of high-dose anabolic steroid use far outweigh the potential benefits to athletic performance, and the use of these agents for this purpose should be strongly discouraged.

Gonadotropin and LHRH Therapy

The aim of gonadotropin therapy is to stimulate spermatogenesis and to establish or restore fertility in gonadotropin-deficient hypogonadal patients. The gonadotropin preparations usually used for this purpose are *hCG*, which is purified from the urine of pregnant women and contains LH-like biologic activity almost exclusively; and *human menopausal gonadotropin* (*hMG*, Pergonal), which is purified from the urine of postmenopausal women and contains both FSH and LH activity. A more purified preparation of *human FSH* (*hFSH*, Metrodin) is now available for clinical use; it has been used primarily to induce ovulation so far. Both hCG and hMG are expensive and require multiple injections per week. Therefore, testosterone, rather than gonadotropin therapy, is used to induce and maintain androgenization in patients with hypogonadotropic hypogonadism.

Initiation of spermatogenesis in prepubertal patients with hypogonadotropic hypogonadism usually requires treatment with both hCG and hMG. Because of the relative ineffectiveness of hMG to stimulate the immature testis and the greater expense, treatment is initiated with hCG alone, at a dosage of 2000 IU subcutaneously or intramuscularly two to three times weekly for 6 to 12 months. Clinical evidence of sexual maturation and the increase in serum testosterone levels are monitored to determine the need for adjustments in dose. During hCG treatment, testosterone produced by the Leydig cells causes the Sertoli cells to mature and spermatogenesis to be initiated to varying degrees of completeness. Occasionally, hCG alone stimulates spermatogenesis sufficiently for sperm to appear in the ejaculate. However, the majority of prepubertal patients with hypogonadotropic hypogonadism require FSH activity, in the form of hMG, in addition to hCG to complete spermatogenesis and induce fertility. Therefore, hMG, at a dosage of 75 IU subcutaneously or intramuscularly three times weekly, is usually added to hCG if there is no evidence of sperm in the ejaculate with hCG alone. Gonadotropin induction of sperm production may take as long as 1 year. Even with combined hCG and hMG treatment, sperm output in the ejaculate may not be normal. Despite very low sperm counts, fertility may be induced, however.

Once initiated, spermatogenesis may be maintained with hCG treatment alone. In adults with acquired hypogonadotropic hypogonadism, sperm production may also be restored with hCG treatment alone. Previous androgen treatment does not alter testicular responsiveness to subsequent gonadotropin therapy. The presence of primary testicular disease, such as cryptorchidism, worsens the prognosis for induction of sperm production and fertility by gonadotropin treatment.

In patients with Kallmann's syndrome, pulsatile administration of low doses of LHRH has been used successfully to stimulate endogenous gonadotropin secretion and to initiate and maintain spermatogenesis to induce fertility. Pulsatile administration more closely mimics the normal physiologic situation; however, a portable infusion pump must be used to deliver small doses of LHRH every few hours (e.g., 5 to 20 μg subcutaneously every 2 hours) throughout the day, making LHRH therapy a much more complex management problem than gonadotropin therapy. LHRH and gonadotropin therapy are probably similar in their ability to stimulate spermatogenesis in men with Kallmann's syndrome.

Castro-Magaña M, Bronsther B, Angulo MA: Genetic forms of male hypogonadism. Urology 35:195, 1990. *This is an excellent review article on the pathophysiology, clinical manifestations, and treatment of genetic causes of primary and secondary hypogonadism in men.*

Handelsman DJ, Swerdloff RS: Male gonadal dysfunction. Clin Endocrinol Metab 14:89, 1985. *A very complete review of clinical and laboratory evaluation of male gonadal disorders.*

Hopwood NJ: Pathogenesis and management of abnormal puberty. Spec Topics Endocrinol Metab 7:175, 1985. *An excellent review of pubertal disorders.*

Lee PA, St L O'dea L: Primary and secondary testicular insufficiency. Pediatr Clin North Am 37:1359, 1990. *This is a well-organized and well-written review of the diagnosis and treatment of primary and secondary testicular failure in the pediatric age group.*

Matsumoto AM: Clinical use and abuse of androgens and antiandrogens. *In* Becker KL (ed.): Principles and Practice of Endocrinology and Metabolism. Philadelphia, JB Lippincott Company, 1990, p 991. *This chapter reviews the pharmacology of androgen preparations, their clinical use in treatment of male hypogonadism and other conditions, the inappropriate use of androgens, and their potential side effects.*

Plymate SR, Paulsen CA: Male hypogonadism. *In* Becker KL (ed.): Principles and Practice of Endocrinology and Metabolism. Philadelphia, JB Lippincott Company, 1990, p 948. *This chapter contains an excellent comprehensive discussion of disorders causing primary and secondary hypogonadism, with 181 references.*

Rosenfeld RL: Diagnosis and management of delayed puberty. J Clin Endocrin

Metab 70:559, 1990. *A concise, up-to-date review of the diagnosis and treatment of delayed sexual development.*

PRECOCIOUS PUBERTY

Isosexual precocity is defined as the development of sexual maturation before the age of 9 years. In boys, premature development of secondary sexual characteristics results in virilization. This is accompanied by accelerated skeletal maturation and linear growth and premature closure of long bone epiphyses, resulting in short stature as an adult. *True precocious puberty* is caused by premature secretion of gonadotropins. Testicular androgen and sperm production is stimulated by gonadotropins and results in virilization and increased testis size. *Precocious pseudopuberty* results from secretion of androgens from the adrenal gland or testis. Androgen excess results in virilization, but normal sperm production is not stimulated and the testes remain small. Occasionally, high local testosterone concentrations within the testis can stimulate some degree of spermatogenesis.

True Precocious Puberty

In the majority of cases of true precocious puberty no identifiable cause for premature activation of gonadotropin secretion is found. This condition is called *idiopathic precocious puberty.* It is often inherited as a male-limited autosomal dominant or X-linked recessive trait. Patients have an increased incidence of seizure disorders and abnormal electroencephalograms. The remaining cases of true precocious puberty are primarily caused by *central nervous system lesions* involving the posterior hypothalamus. Lesions include hypothalamic and pineal tumors, craniopharyngioma, hamartomas, hydrocephalus, postencephalitic lesions, congenital brain defects, neurofibromatosis, and tuberous sclerosis. Central nervous system lesions may also result in disturbances of other hypothalamic functions, causing diabetes insipidus, eating disorders, somnolence, emotional lability, and altered temperature regulation, as well as mental and psychomotor retardation and seizures. Precocious puberty may precede the onset of a clinically detectable neurologic lesion. Therefore, a prolonged period of follow-up observation with repeated neurologic evaluation is necessary to exclude central nervous system lesions. Rarely, an *hCG-secreting tumor* (e.g., hepatoblastoma) or *hCG administration* for cryptorchidism (iatrogenic precocious puberty) causes true precocious puberty.

Precocious Pseudopuberty (Ch. 221)

Adrenocortical hyperfunction, either from congenital adrenal hyperplasia (21-hydroxylase or 11β-hydroxylase deficiency) or a virilizing adrenocortical tumor, is the most common condition causing precocious pseudopuberty in boys. Patients with congenital adrenal hyperplasia caused by 21-hydroxylase deficiency usually have markedly elevated serum 17-hydroxyprogesterone and urinary pregnanetriol levels. Rarely, *Leydig cell tumor* of the testis, autonomous Leydig cell function (*testotoxicosis*), and administration of *androgenic steroids* may cause precocious pseudopuberty.

Treatment of these conditions is directed at the underlying cause. For idiopathic precocious puberty, drugs to inhibit pituitary gonadotropin secretion (medroxyprogesterone acetate, LHRH analogues) or androgen synthesis (ketoconazole), or to block androgen action (flutamide, cyproterone acetate) have been used with varying success to prevent further sexual maturation. With the exception of LHRH analogues, these treatments do not usually prevent premature closure of long bone epiphyses.

Kaplan SL, Grumbach MM: Pathophysiology and treatment of sexual precocity. J Clin Endocrinol Metab 71:785, 1990. *A concise and up-to-date review of the pathophysiology and management of precocious pubertal development.*

Wheeler MD, Styne DM: Diagnosis and management of precocious puberty. Pediatr Clin North Am 37:1255, 1990. *This is an excellent, comprehensive review of the diagnosis and treatment of sexual precocity.*

TUMORS OF THE TESTIS

Tumors of the testis are uncommon, representing about 1 per cent of all cancers in men. They occur more commonly in white than in black males. The annual incidence of testicular tumors is 6 per 100,000 males. About 95 per cent of testicular tumors are malignant and derive from the germ cells. The remaining 5 per cent are non–germ cell or stromal tumors derived mostly from Leydig and Sertoli cells of the gonadal stroma and are usually benign. Gonadoblastoma is a rare testicular neoplasm containing both germ cell and stromal elements, arising in dysgenetic testes containing a Y chromosome. The peak age of incidence of testicular cancer is 20 to 35 years. It is the most common malignancy in this age group. Advances in treatment have transformed testicular cancer from the most common cause of cancer death in this age group 20 years ago into one of the most curable of all cancers today. A testicular mass in a patient over 50 years is more likely to be a lymphoma than a germ cell tumor.

The most significant risk factor for developing testicular cancer is cryptorchidism. In unilateral cryptorchidism, the contralateral, normally descended testis also carries an increased risk of malignant degeneration. Orchiopexy at an early age (2 to 3 years) permits easier palpation and detection of testicular cancer and may reduce the risk of neoplasm. Carcinoma in situ has been found in men with oligoazoospermia presenting with infertility and in the contralateral testes of patients with presumed unilateral testicular cancer, suggesting that these conditions may also carry an increased risk for testicular neoplasm.

Germ Cell Tumors

Germ cell cancers may be classified according to their pathologic characteristics into *seminoma* and *nonseminoma. Nonseminomatous cancers* include *embryonal cell carcinomas, choriocarcinomas,* and *teratomas.* Forty per cent of germ cell cancers contain a mixture of seminomatous and nonseminomatous elements. The presence of any nonseminomatous element in a tumor that is predominantly seminoma dictates its classification as a nonseminoma. The distinction between seminoma and nonseminoma is important to plan for staging and subsequent therapy. Seminomas usually metastasize via regional lymph nodes to retroperitoneal, mediastinal, and supraclavicular lymph nodes and are very sensitive to radiation therapy. On the other hand, nonseminomas metastasize by both lymphatic and hematogenous routes (especially to liver and lungs) and are radioresistant.

Most patients with germ cell tumors present with a painless mass in the testis. Rapid onset of a painful testicular mass is usually caused by bleeding into the neoplasm. Back or abdominal pain (from retroperitoneal lymphadenopathy), shortness of breath (from diffuse pulmonary metastases), gynecomastia (from hCG secretion), supraclavicular lymphadenopathy, or ureteral obstruction may also be present.

Germ cell tumors, especially nonseminomatous cancers, often secrete biologic markers (Ch. 160). Embryonal cell cancers may secrete α-*fetoprotein.* Pure seminomas never elaborate α-fetoprotein, and its presence in serum implies the presence of nonseminomatous elements in the tumor or metastases. *hCG* is secreted by nearly all choriocarcinomas, a third of embryonal cell carcinomas and teratocarcinomas and, rarely, by pure seminomas. This marker may be detected and differentiated from cross-reacting LH in serum with a specific β-hCG assay. Both of these tumor markers may be used to monitor response to therapy. They may precede clinically detectable disease by weeks to months.

In seminoma, orchiectomy and radiotherapy to the periaortic and iliac lymph nodes have resulted in cure rates of 80 to 95 per cent. In nonseminomatous testicular cancer, the addition of cisplatin to aggressive, multiple-drug chemotherapeutic regimens has resulted in response rates of over 90 per cent and long-term remission in 50 to 90 per cent of patients.

Non–Germ Cell Tumors

Non–germ cell tumors are rare tumors that develop from the two major elements of testicular stroma, the *Leydig* and *Sertoli cells.* They are usually benign, but about 10 per cent are malignant and metastasize via regional lymphatics. Both Leydig and Sertoli cell tumors may secrete a variety of steroid hormones, primarily androgens or estrogens, that may result in virilization or feminization, respectively. These tumors are usually small and difficult to diagnose; selective venous catheterization and sampling to determine the site of increased steroid production are often helpful. Gynecomastia is present in about 30 per cent of patients with non–germ cell tumors. Children may present with either isosexual (virilizing) or heterosexual (feminizing) precocious pseudopuberty. Treatment consists primarily of orchiectomy.

Ozols RF, Williams SD: Testicular cancer. Curr Probl Cancer 13:285, 1989. *An excellent comprehensive review of the classification, epidemiology, staging, treatment, and prognosis of testicular cancer (98 references).*

223 Diseases of the Prostate

Charles B. Brendler

This chapter discusses three common disorders of the prostate: prostatitis, benign prostatic hyperplasia, and adenocarcinoma of the prostate. A brief review of the normal anatomy, physiology, and biochemistry of the prostate is provided first.

THE NORMAL PROSTATE

ANATOMY. The normal adult prostate, a firm, elastic organ weighing about 20 grams, is located caudad to the base of the bladder and is traversed by the first portion of the urethra. It is bordered anteriorly by the symphysis pubis and posteriorly by the rectum. The paired seminal vesicles are attached to the prostate and are located posterior to the bladder (Fig. 223–1).

The human prostate has two concentric anatomic regions: an inner periurethral zone composed of short glands and an outer peripheral zone composed of longer, branched glands. These regions are separated by a thin layer of fibroelastic tissue, the so-called surgical capsule (Fig. 223–2). Benign prostatic hyperplasia (BPH) arises within the inner periurethral zone in a specific region near the verumontanum, called the transition zone. In contrast, prostatic carcinoma usually arises in the outer peripheral zone.

PHYSIOLOGY. The secretions of the prostate and other sex accessory organs presumably protect or enhance the functional properties of the spermatozoa. Of the total average human ejaculate volume of 3.5 ml, the prostate secretes 0.5 ml and the seminal vesicles secrete 2.0 to 2.5 ml.

Two specific components of prostatic secretion, zinc and acid phosphatase, have aroused interest because of their high concentrations in seminal fluid. Zinc is higher in concentration in the prostate than in any other organ in the body, but its function is unknown. The biologic function of acid phosphatase is also unknown. Prostate cancer cells often continue to secrete acid phosphatase after they have metastasized, and the measurement of prostatic acid phosphatase in the serum is used both as a screening test for prostatic carcinoma and to follow the response to therapy in patients with metastatic disease.

BIOCHEMISTRY. The growth and secretory function of the prostate depend on functioning testes; prostatic maturation does not occur in a male castrated before puberty. Testosterone, the major circulating androgen, is converted to dihydrotestosterone (DHT) by the enzyme 5α-reductase in prostatic epithelial cells. DHT, the major active androgenic metabolite within the prostate,

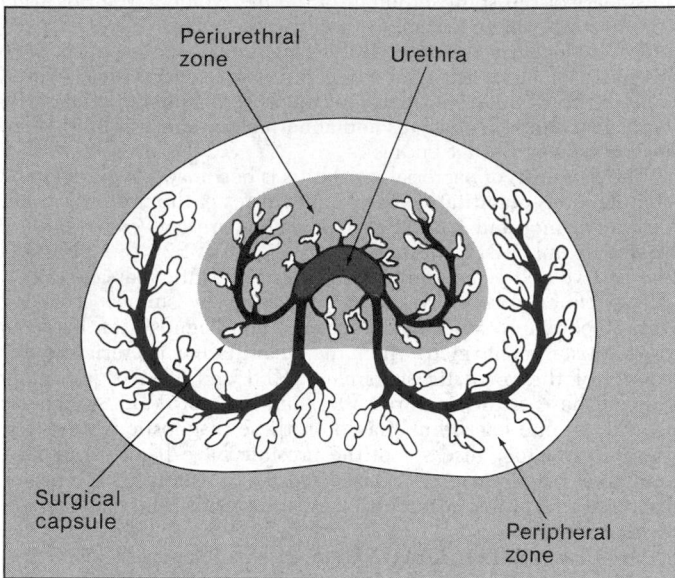

FIGURE 223–2. A coronal section through the prostate demonstrating the anatomic relationships between the urethra, periurethral tissue, surgical capsule, and peripheral tissue. (After Brendler H. *In* Glenn JF (ed.): Urologic Surgery, 3rd ed. Philadelphia, J. B. Lippincott Comany, 1983.)

binds to a cytoplasmic receptor, is transported to the nucleus, and there initiates RNA synthesis, protein synthesis, and cell replication.

Estrogens inhibit prostatic growth, largely by blocking the release of luteinizing hormone from the pituitary, thus inhibiting testicular synthesis of testosterone. If castrated animals are given both estrogens and androgens, normal prostate growth occurs, indicating that estrogens do not block androgen-induced growth in the prostate itself.

PROSTATITIS

INCIDENCE AND ETIOLOGY. About 50 per cent of men experience symptoms of prostatic inflammation during adult life. Only about 5 per cent of these cases are due to bacterial infection of the prostate. The etiology of these symptoms in the remaining 95 per cent of patients is unclear.

Most bacterial infections of the prostate are caused by gram-negative organisms, most commonly *Escherichia coli*. Enterococci, staphylococci, and streptococci are rare causes of prostatic infection. *Chlamydia trachomatis* and *Ureaplasma urealyticum* probably cause prostatitis infrequently, but this topic remains controversial.

PATHOGENESIS. Most episodes of bacterial prostatic infection are due to a previous urethral infection with direct ascent of bacteria from the urethra through the prostatic ducts into the prostate. The organisms that cause bacterial prostatitis are the same as those that produce bacteriuria, and chlamydial and gonococcal infections of the urethra may involve the prostate.

Prostatic infection may also result from impairment of host defense mechanisms. The concentrations of prostatic antibacterial factor and magnesium, zinc, calcium, citric acid, spermine, cholesterol, and lysozyme are decreased in the prostatic fluid of men with chronic bacterial prostatitis. Whether these alterations contribute to or result from prostatic infection is unknown. About 10 per cent of men with chronic bacterial prostatitis have more than one organism, and many after cure develop reinfection of the prostate by a different organism, further suggesting impaired host defense function.

DIAGNOSIS. The diagnosis of prostatitis is based on examination of expressed prostatic secretions (EPS) and quantitative bacterial localization cultures. Although microscopic examination of the EPS is important, it can be misleading. The clinician should always compare the microscopic appearance of the EPS

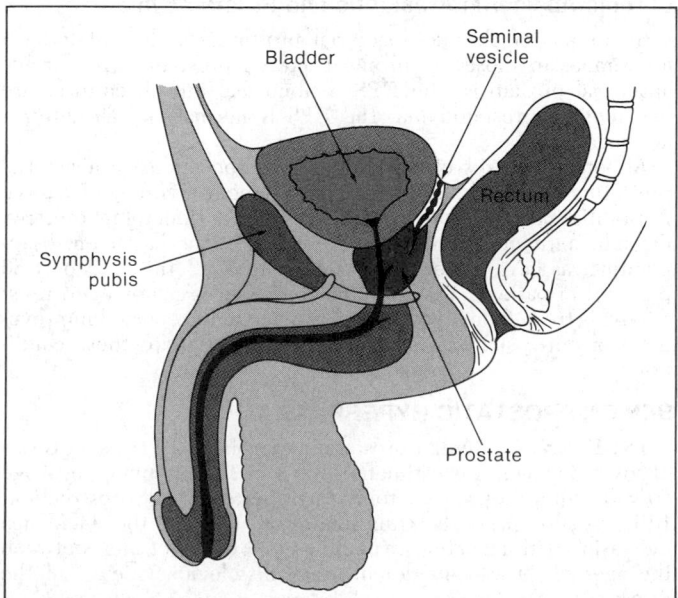

FIGURE 223–1. The anatomic relationship of the prostate to adjacent structures. (After Brendler H. *In* Glenn JF (ed.): Urologic Surgery, 3rd ed. Philadelphia, J. B. Lippincott Company, 1983.)

to smears of the spun sediment of the first voided 10 ml of urine (the urethral specimen) and the midstream urine (bladder specimen) to localize the site of the inflammatory response. The presence of more than 20 white blood cells per high-powered field in the EPS is abnormal. During prostatic inflammation, EPS typically contain leukocytes and abnormal numbers of lipid-laden macrophages (oval fat bodies).

The diagnosis of bacterial prostatitis is best made by performing simultaneous quantitative bacterial cultures of the urethral urine, bladder urine, and EPS. Four specimens are collected: the first voided 10 ml (VB1), the midstream aliquot (VB2), the EPS, and the first voided 10 ml immediately after prostatic massage (VB3). All specimens are cultured quantitatively by surface streaking onto blood and MacConkey agar. The diagnosis of bacterial prostatitis is confirmed when the quantitative bacterial colony counts of the prostatic specimens (EPS and VB3) significantly exceed those of the urethral (VB1) and bladder (VB2) specimens by at least one logarithm. Based on these diagnostic maneuvers, the inflammatory diseases of the prostate have been subdivided into four categories: (1) acute bacterial prostatitis, (2) chronic bacterial prostatitis, (3) nonbacterial prostatitis, and (4) prostatodynia.

DIFFERENTIAL DIAGNOSIS. All patients with lower urinary tract complaints require a full urologic evaluation. The differential diagnosis of patients with lower urinary tract irritative symptoms should include upper urinary tract infection with secondary colonization of the bladder, carcinoma of the bladder, neurogenic bladder, prostatic obstruction, and urethral stricture. Because the irritative urinary symptoms in men with prostatitis are identical to those of patients with flat in situ carcinoma of the bladder, a urinary cytology and cystoscopy should be performed in these patients to exclude the presence of bladder malignancy.

Acute Bacterial Prostatitis

Acute bacterial prostatitis is a fulminant condition that occurs mainly between the ages of 20 and 40. Patients present with the acute onset of fever, chills, and malaise associated with marked urinary irritative and obstructive symptoms. Pain may be experienced in the suprapubic region, lumbar spine, and perineum.

On physical examination, patients frequently have a fever as high as 39 to 40°C. Patients may have marked suprapubic tenderness if prostatic infection results in urinary retention. Rectal examination to rule out a prostatic abscess should be done very carefully, as it is extremely uncomfortable for the patient and may result in septicemia or secondary epididymitis if the prostate is massaged too vigorously. The prostate is variably enlarged, markedly tender, and hot to palpation. A prostatic abscess should be suspected if an abnormally fluctuant area is palpated within the prostate.

Patients with acute bacterial prostatitis almost always have associated bacteriuria, and, therefore, a urinalysis and urine culture are helpful in establishing the diagnosis and identifying appropriate antibiotic therapy. With recurrent bacterial prostatitis, intravenous pyelography or abdominal ultrasonography should be done to rule out upper urinary tract pathology. A pelvic ultrasound or computed tomography scan may be helpful in diagnosing a prostatic abscess.

Patients with acute bacterial prostatitis are frequently quite ill and need to be hospitalized for their initial treatment. Urinary retention may necessitate placement of a temporary suprapubic cystostomy or urethral catheter. Intravenous antibiotics are usually given; a combination of gentamicin to cover gram-negative organisms and ampicillin to cover enterococci should be used. Supportive measures include hydration, analgesics, and stool softeners. Following initial intravenous therapy, the patient should be placed on an antibiotic with broad gram-negative coverage that diffuses readily into the prostatic fluid. Trimethoprim, trimethoprim-sulfamethoxazole, and the new quinolone derivatives are the usual choices. Since bacterial infections may be difficult to eradicate, oral antibiotics should be continued for 4 to 6 weeks after the acute episode. It is worthwhile to examine the EPS and VB3 6 to 12 weeks after starting therapy to be sure that the infection has resolved.

Granulomatous lesions of the prostate, observed in about 1 per

cent of tissue specimens obtained either by biopsy or by partial prostatectomy, usually result from previous bacterial infection or prior transurethral resection of the prostate. Systemic diseases commonly associated with granuloma formation, such as tuberculosis, account for only a small minority of cases. Granulomatous prostatitis may cause induration that mimics prostatic carcinoma, requiring a biopsy to distinguish the two conditions. Granulomatous prostatitis may result in irritative and obstructive urinary symptoms that usually resolve spontaneously. The value of antibiotics in this condition is controversial.

Chronic Bacterial Prostatitis

Chronic bacterial prostatitis is one of the most common causes of recurrent urinary tract infection in men. The symptoms, similar to but milder than those of acute bacterial prostatitis, include urinary frequency and dysuria along with vague lower abdominal, lumbar, and perineal pain. Fever and urethral discharge are uncommon. The diagnosis is made by examination of the EPS and quantitative bacterial cultures. The EPS should be considered abnormal if there are greater than 10 leukocytes per high power field (hPF) and more than one or two lipid-laden macrophages per hPF. Men with chronic bacterial prostatitis may have a normal EPS while on antibiotic therapy but may continue to have recurrent infections once antibiotics have been discontinued. Furthermore, 5 to 10 per cent of men with no symptoms of prostatic inflammation have more than 10 leukocytes per hPF in their EPS.

An alternative approach to quantitative bacterial cultures, which are expensive and time consuming, is to obtain a quantitative culture of the bladder urine (VB2) and a nonquantitative culture of the EPS on the first office visit. If these cultures are both negative, the prostate is probably not infected. Recovery of gram-negative bacteria from either of these specimens identifies patients who might have chronic bacterial prostatitis and provides a rationale for conventional bacterial localization cultures on the second office visit.

Chronic bacterial prostatitis is frequently difficult to treat. Antibiotic therapy alone eradicates only about 30 to 50 per cent of the infections, but suppressive antimicrobial therapy usually results in complete symptomatic relief and reduces the risks of serious illness. The usual antibiotics used in this condition are trimethoprim-sulfamethoxazole, carbenicillin, or one of the new quinolones, such as ciprofloxacin or norfloxacin, in a 4- to 12-week course of therapy. Suppressive antibiotic therapy with trimethoprim, trimethoprim-sulfamethoxazole, and nitrofurantoin is effective. Experimentally, direct injection of antibiotics, such as thiamphenicol and aminoglycosides, has given promise in patients who failed previous oral antibiotic therapy.

Chronic Abacterial Prostatitis and Prostatodynia

Symptoms of chronic abacterial prostatitis and prostatodynia are similar to those of chronic bacterial prostatitis. In chronic abacterial prostatitis, the EPS is abnormal but all cultures are negative. In prostatodynia, the EPS is normal and all cultures are negative.

Although cultures of prostatic biopsy specimens in abacterial prostatitis are rarely positive, some patients with nonbacterial prostatitis and prostatodynia improve with antimicrobial therapy. Overall, antibiotic therapy in these conditions has been disappointing, as have all forms of therapy to date. In one report 86 per cent of patients with chronic abacterial prostatitis and prostatodynia treated only with stress management reported improvement or cure, suggesting a psychological basis for these conditions.

BENIGN PROSTATIC HYPERPLASIA

INCIDENCE. Benign prostatic hyperplasia (BPH) is a disease of advancing age; it is estimated that 1 in 10 men living until age 80 will require a prostatectomy for relief of urinary obstruction. BPH usually presents clinically after age 50, the incidence increasing with age, but as many as two thirds of men between the ages of 40 and 49 demonstrate histologic evidence of the disease.

ETIOLOGY. BPH is closely related to both aging and age-associated changes in circulating hormones. Circulating androgens clearly play a role; BPH does not develop in men who are castrated or lose testicular function before puberty. Castration causes atrophy of prostatic epithelium.

With aging, serum testosterone levels decline while serum estrogen levels increase, resulting in an increase in the ratio of plasma estrogens to plasma testosterone. It is unclear, however, whether these shifts in circulating hormone levels are directly involved in the pathogenesis of BPH. Androgens and estrogens seem to act synergistically in the development of BPH in the dog, estrogens increasing prostatic androgen receptors by two-fold. Levels of DHT are not actually elevated in BPH tissue, but enzymatic changes occur within the hyperplastic gland that would tend to favor the accumulation of DHT.

PATHOGENESIS. As the hyperplastic prostate enlarges, it compresses the urethra, producing symptoms of urethral obstruction that ultimately may progress to urinary retention. Urethral obstruction may cause incomplete emptying of the bladder, giving rise to urinary stasis, urinary tract infection, and bladder calculi. Furthermore, hypertrophy of the bladder muscle may cause hydronephrosis and bladder diverticula. Bladder neoplasms are more likely to arise in bladder diverticula, especially if the diverticula drain poorly and are chronically infected.

SYMPTOMS. Symptoms due to BPH are either obstructive or irritative. *Obstructive symptoms* include hesitancy to initiate voiding, straining to void, decreased force and caliber of the urinary stream, prolonged dribbling after micturition, a sensation of incomplete bladder emptying, and urinary retention. These symptoms result directly from narrowing of the bladder neck and prostatic urethra by the hyperplastic prostate.

Irritative symptoms include urinary frequency, nocturia, dysuria, urgency, and urge incontinence. These symptoms may result from incomplete emptying of the bladder with voiding or may be due to urinary tract infection secondary to prostatic obstruction. More commonly, irritative symptoms result from reduced bladder compliance as a result of prostatic obstruction. It is important to recognize that irritative symptoms may be caused by other conditions such as bladder carcinoma, neurogenic bladder, and urinary tract infection unrelated to prostatic obstruction. All too frequently, patients with irritative urinary tract symptoms are presumed to have prostatic obstruction without an adequate diagnostic evaluation, resulting in delayed and sometimes inappropriate therapy.

PHYSICAL EXAMINATION. Other than a distended bladder, the usual physical findings in BPH are confined to the prostate. Examination of the prostate should be performed with the patient in either the knee-chest position or bent over the bed with his chest touching his elbows. The examining glove should be well lubricated, and the index finger should be inserted slowly into the rectum to allow the anal sphincter time to relax.

The normal prostate, the size of a walnut, has the consistency of a pencil eraser. The hyperplastic prostate is variably enlarged, usually no more than two or three times normal, but occasionally exceeding the size of a lemon. The consistency remains rubbery but is somewhat more fleshy, particularly in the larger glands. Rectal examination affords only a rough estimate of prostatic size and should never be relied upon to rule out prostatic obstruction. A much more accurate anatomic appraisal of the prostate can be obtained with transrectal ultrasonography and cystourethroscopy. The rectal examination is, however, the single most valuable screening test for prostatic carcinoma. The entire posterior surface of the gland should be examined for areas of induration suggestive of malignancy.

DIAGNOSTIC TESTS. The most valuable test for documenting urinary obstruction is measurement of the urinary flow rate. Inexpensive flowmeters allow an accurate determination of the patient's voided volume and peak urinary flow rate, which can be plotted against the patient's age on a nomogram. A decreased flow rate per se is never an indication for prostatectomy, but, when used and interpreted correctly, uroflowmetry is an excellent physiologic test for prostatic obstruction.

An abdominal ultrasound examination is useful to rule out associated upper tract pathology, such as hydronephrosis, as well as to detect renal masses. Furthermore, ultrasound measurement of postvoid residual urine volumes and prostatic size is extremely accurate.

Cystourethroscopy, although often employed, may be misleading as a screening test for prostatic obstruction. An anatomically small prostate may produce significant obstruction during voiding, while an anatomically large prostate may produce little or no obstruction at all. The place for cystourethroscopy is in making the decision about whether the prostate is small enough to be resected transurethrally or sufficiently large to require open surgical removal. Before proceeding to prostatectomy, a careful inspection of the bladder is made to rule out bladder diverticula, stones, and, most importantly, tumors.

A retrograde urethrogram may be helpful in evaluating patients with symptoms of BPH when a urethral stricture is suspected. Formal urodynamic testing including a cystometrogram may be indicated in patients with complex voiding symptomatology or a suspected neurogenic bladder.

TREATMENT. The most common treatment for BPH is partial prostatectomy. The indications for prostatectomy are (1) voiding symptoms that are troublesome to the patient; (2) urinary retention; (3) recurrent urinary tract infections caused by postvoid residual urine; (4) compromised renal function due to hydronephrosis from prostatic obstruction; (5) recurrent gross hematuria with no other explanation; and (6) urge incontinence due to prostatic obstruction.

A partial prostatectomy done for BPH attempts to re-establish a wide-open bladder neck and prostatic urethra by selectively removing all of the hyperplastic prostatic tissue down to the so-called surgical capsule, leaving the peripheral prostate intact (Fig. 223–2). This is accomplished either by transurethral resection or by open surgical enucleation of the adenoma, depending usually on the size of the gland. Adenomas less than 70 grams are usually approached transurethrally.

Transurethral prostatectomy (TURP) is generally regarded as a safe and effective procedure, but recent evidence suggests that it may be less effective than open prostatectomy in overcoming urinary obstruction and that TURP may be associated with higher long-term mortality. Alternatives to transurethral prostatectomy include (1) transurethral incision of the bladder neck, (2) balloon dilatation of the prostate, (3) treatment with sympathetic α-adrenergic inhibitors, and (4) antiandrogen therapy.

Transurethral incision is done by making one or two longitudinal incisions with an endoscope through the muscular fibers of the bladder neck and prostatic urethra to spring open the prostate and thus enlarge the caliber of the prostatic urethra. Transurethral incision can be performed as an outpatient procedure under local anesthesia, and operative time and blood loss are greatly reduced. Transurethral incision is probably as effective as transurethral resection in treating small prostates (< 20 grams) but appears less effective for larger, bulkier glands.

Balloon dilatation is done by inflating a balloon endoscopically within the prostatic urethra to a diameter of 90 French for 10 minutes at 4 atm. The pressure from the balloon compresses and may rupture the prostatic tissue, reducing urethral obstruction. Significant hemorrhage may occur infrequently, but morbidity is otherwise minimal. About 70 per cent of patients are improved symptomatically at 6 months; further follow-up is necessary to determine the long-term value of this procedure.

Sympathetic blockade relieves prostatic obstruction by inhibiting α-adrenoceptor–mediated contractions of the prostatic capsule, prostate adenoma, and bladder neck. Selective α_1 blockers, such as terazosin and prazosin, have fewer side effects than nonselective α blockers. Terazosin has the additional advantage of once-daily dosing. The response rate to these agents appears to be about 70 per cent.

Antiandrogen therapy relieves prostatic obstruction by causing atrophy of the prostatic epithelium. Prostate size decreases an average of 30 per cent after 3 to 6 months of therapy, but the prostate quickly regrows after cessation of therapy. Although there is a significant placebo effect on clinical symptoms, urodynamic improvement has been marginal in most studies.

CARCINOMA OF THE PROSTATE

INCIDENCE. Carcinoma of the prostate is rare before age 50, but the incidence subsequently increases steadily with age. Overall, it is the second most common malignancy in American men and the third most common cause of cancer deaths in men over 55 (behind lung and colorectal cancer). Carcinoma of the prostate is more common among black American men (22 deaths per 100,000 men) than white American men (14 deaths per 100,000 men).

ETIOLOGY. The etiology of prostatic carcinoma is unknown. The disease does not occur in men castrated before puberty and regresses following castration or estrogen therapy, but a hormonal etiology has not been established. BPH does not appear to be causally related. Environmental factors may be involved, since men migrating from areas where prostatic cancer is uncommon to areas where it is more common develop the disease with increased frequency. Oncogenic viruses have been detected within prostatic cancer cells, but a direct etiologic relationship has not been established.

PATHOGENESIS. Ninety-five per cent of prostatic cancers are adenocarcinomas, with the remainder being transitional cell carcinomas, squamous cell carcinomas, and sarcomas. Adenocarcinoma of the prostate usually arises in the peripheral region of the prostate (Fig. 223–2), although it commonly invades the periurethral tissue where BPH orginates, subsequently producing urethral obstruction. Prostate cancer may produce ureteral obstruction either by direct extension into the bladder or by spreading behind the bladder through the seminal vesicles. Distant spread occurs through lymphatic and hematogenous routes. Prostatic cancer most commonly metastasizes to the pelvic lymph nodes and skeleton, especially the pelvis and lumbar spine. Visceral metastases, which occur later and less commonly, most frequently involve the lungs, liver, and adrenals.

In its unpredictable natural history, prostatic cancer progresses very slowly in some men, who may do well for many years without treatment. In others the disease exhibits rapid metastatic spread leading to early death. In the absence of the ability to predict which patients can be followed conservatively and which require prompt treatment, we are obliged to treat patients with prostatic cancer aggressively, to the extent that an individual's age and general health permit.

SYMPTOMS. Early carcinoma of the prostate is asymptomatic. As the disease spreads into the urethra, it may cause symptoms of urinary obstruction indistinguishable from those produced by BPH. If the tumor has progressed to obstruct the ureters, the patient may present with uremia. Skeletal pain and pathologic fractures caused by metastatic disease may be the initial symptoms of advanced disease.

PHYSICAL EXAMINATION. The patient may present with lymphadenopathy, signs of uremia, and congestive heart failure, or in urinary retention with a distended bladder. More commonly, the pathologic physical findings are confined to the prostate. On rectal examination the prostate feels harder than the normal or hyperplastic prostate, and the normal boundaries of the gland may be obscured. Approximately 50 per cent of localized indurated areas within the prostate are malignant, with the remainder due to prostatic calculi, inflammation, prostatic infarction, or postsurgical change in a patient having previously undergone a partial prostatectomy for BPH. If induration is detected that is suggestive of carcinoma, the examiner should determine whether it is focal or diffuse in nature and whether it seems to extend beyond the border of the prostate.

DIAGNOSIS. The diagnosis of prostatic cancer is made with an accuracy rate of greater than 90 per cent by a transperineal or transrectal needle biopsy of the prostate. Alternatively, a transrectal fine-needle aspiration of the prostate may be performed for a cytologic diagnosis, although there is less experience with this technique in the United States.

Transrectal ultrasonography is also capable of demonstrating prostate cancers, which typically appear as hypoechoic lesions within the prostate (although some may appear hyperechoic or have mixed echogenicity). Although more sensitive than digital examination, transrectal ultrasonography is not sufficiently specific at present to be used as a screening test for prostate cancer. Overall, only 30 to 40 per cent of the abnormal lesions detected on sonography are malignant. Similarly, measurements of serum prostate specific antigen (PSA) are not sufficiently accurate to diagnose men with early prostate cancer. For example, 15 to 20 per cent of men with BPH have PSA values greater than 10 ng per milliliter (normal, <4.0 ng per milliliter).

STAGING CLASSIFICATION. The treatment of prostatic carcinoma depends primarily on the stage of the disease, as illustrated in the Whitmore staging system (Fig. 223–3).

Stage A prostatic carcinoma refers to tumors that are discovered incidentally on histologic examination of prostatic tissue that has been removed for presumed BPH. Stage A tumors are subdivided into stage A1 lesions, which are well- or moderately well-differentiated tumors involving less than 5 per cent of the removed tissue, and stage A2 lesions, which are either poorly differentiated or involve more than 5 per cent of the removed tissue.

Stage B tumors are palpable on rectal examination and are confined within the boundaries of the prostate. Stage B1 includes tumors involving less than one posterior lobe, and stage B2 includes tumors that involve one whole or both posterior lobes.

Stage C tumors extend beyond the boundaries of the prostate but are confined within the pelvis. These tumors have penetrated the peripheral capsule of the prostate and may extend cephalad into the seminal vesicles or laterally toward the bony pelvic sidewalls.

Stage D tumors are metastatic. Stage D1 tumors have spread to the pelvic lymph nodes, and stage D2 tumors have distant metastases.

STAGING EVALUATION. The treatment of prostatic carcinoma is predicated largely on the stage of the tumor; accurate staging is therefore essential. The digital rectal examination is valuable in assessing the local extent of tumor, but transrectal ultrasonography and magnetic resonance imaging of the prostate may be useful when the findings on physical examination are not definitive.

Enzymatic determination of serum acid phosphatase remains a basic screening test for metastatic prostatic cancer, with an elevated value being about 70 per cent sensitive and virtually 100 per cent specific for metastatic disease. Measurement of serum PSA appears of limited value in the staging of prostate cancer. Ninety per cent of men with prostate cancer have PSA values between 10 and 50 ng per milliliter, but values within this range do not distinguish organ-confined from more advanced disease. Conversely, PSA is extremely helpful in evaluating patients after radical prostatectomy. Since PSA is made only by the prostate, serum levels following surgery should be undetectable. A measurable level of PSA postoperatively is thus highly suggestive of residual disease.

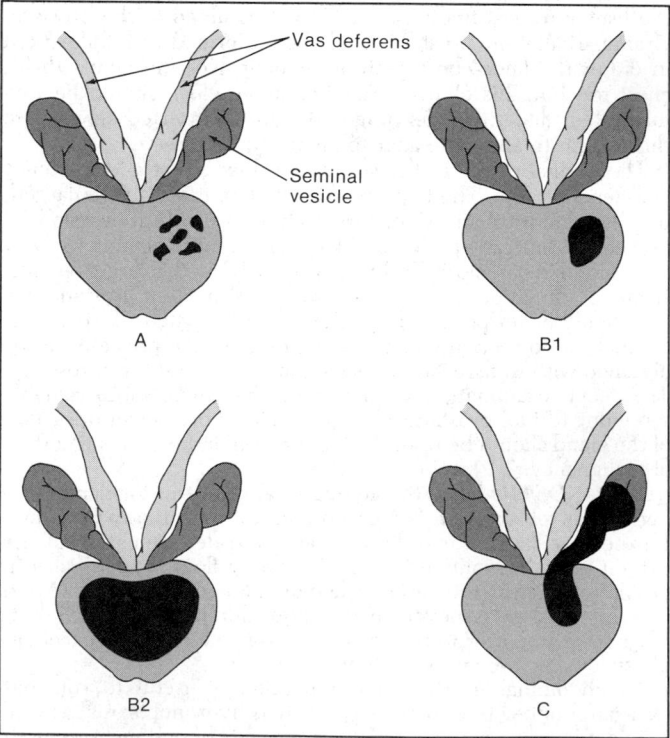

FIGURE 223–3. Whitmore staging classification of prostatic carcinoma. A = Microscopic disease in a clinically benign gland. B1 = Nodule involving less than one posterior lobe. B2 = Nodule involving one entire lobe or both posterior lobes. C = Extension beyond the peripheral capsule of the prostate. D (not pictured) = Metastatic disease.

The radionuclide bone scan is highly accurate and far more sensitive than conventional skeletal radiography in detecting osseous metastases. Pelvic lymph node metastases in prostatic carcinoma are more difficult to detect. Pedal lymphangiography does not consistently demonstrate the primary sites of lymphatic drainage from the prostate, which are the obturator and hypogastric lymphatic chains. Pelvic computed tomography scan has proved similarly unreliable. In patients with otherwise localized disease, a staging pelvic lymphadenectomy is usually done prior to performing a radical prostatectomy, either in conjunction with the operation, relying on a frozen-section evaluation of the lymph nodes, or several days earlier to allow a full histologic evaluation of the nodal tissue. Pelvic lymphadenectomy has a low morbidity and seems justified as a staging procedure to spare those patients with positive lymph nodes from a radical prostatectomy.

TREATMENT. Surgery. Patients with stage A1 disease have traditionally been treated conservatively, since the disease was thought to be latent and of no clinical significance. More recently it has been learned that approximately 16 per cent of untreated patients with A1 disease develop metastatic carcinoma of the prostate within 10 years. Thus, it may be advisable to treat healthy men under age 65 with stage A1 disease aggressively.

Patients with stages A2 and B disease require further therapy, since, untreated, many develop metastatic disease. The treatment options for these clinical stages include radical prostatectomy and radiation therapy. In radical prostatectomy the entire prostate and seminal vesicles are removed through either a perineal or a retropubic approach. The cure rate for patients undergoing radical prostatectomy for localized disease is excellent, with the 15-year survival rate for patients with pathologically confined disease equalling that of age-matched men without prostatic cancer. The major complications of radical prostatectomy are urinary incontinence and impotence. Recent advances in surgical technique, however, have reduced the risk of significant urinary incontinence to less than 5 per cent and have allowed preservation of potency in over 70 per cent of patients.

Radiation. Radiation therapy is administered either via external beam or via interstitial radioactive seeds that are implanted surgically into the prostate. Although the issue remains controversial, radiation therapy seems most appropriate in patients with localized disease who either are unwilling to undergo radical prostatectomy or are not surgical candidates for reasons of age and health. Radiation therapy also is the treatment of choice for patients with clinical stage C disease that has extended beyond the borders of the prostate and is therefore not curable surgically.

Endocrine. Hormonal therapy, the mainstay of treatment for patients with stage D disease, attempts to deprive prostatic tumors of circulating androgens and thereby produce regression of both primary and metastatic lesions. Hormonal ablation can be achieved either by castration or by administration of exogenous estrogens. Diethylstilbestrol (DES), administered at a dose of 3 mg per day, lowers plasma testosterone to castrate levels. Lower doses of DES may produce incomplete suppression of testosterone, whereas doses higher than 3 mg produce no further suppression and are associated with an increased incidence of cardiovascular complications.

Androgen ablation can also be achieved with luteinizing hormone–releasing hormone analogues that inhibit testosterone synthesis, used either alone or in combination with antiandrogens that block androgen action in the prostate itself. In the United States, the most commonly used analogue is leuprolide acetate (Lupron) administered in a depot form intramuscularly, 1 mg monthly. The most commonly used antiandrogen is flutamide (Eulexin), administered in a dose of 250 mg orally three times daily. These agents appear as effective as conventional hormonal therapy with estrogens or orchiectomy, but they seem to provide minimal if any survival advantage. Prostatic cancer is presumably composed of a heterogeneous cell population, some cells being hormone sensitive and others hormone resistant. Relapse following hormonal therapy is due to continued growth of hormone-resistant cells, and further attempts to lower serum testosterone provide no additional palliation.

Patient response to hormonal therapy varies considerably: 10 per cent of patients live less than 6 months, 50 per cent survive less than 3 years, and only 10 per cent live longer than 10 years. The timing of endocrine therapy also appears to make little difference in the course of the disease. Initiation of treatment at the time of diagnosis may provide a longer symptom-free interval but little in the way of effective palliation once relapse has occurred. For this reason, it may be preferable to delay hormonal therapy until the patient has become symptomatic in the hope of providing increased long-term palliation.

Chemotherapy. Cytotoxic chemotherapy for carcinoma of the prostate has so far yielded discouraging results. A major goal for the future is to develop new forms of therapy that will be effective against the hormone-resistant cell population. The discovery of such agents will represent a major advance in the treatment of this disease.

Blaivas JG: Pathophysiology and differential diagnosis of benign prostatic hypertrophy. Urology 32(6 Suppl):5, 1988. *An excellent review of the physiology and diagnosis of BPH.*

Catalona WJ, Scott WW: Carcinoma of the prostate. *In* Walsh PC, Gittes RF, Perlmutter AD, et al. (eds.): Campbell's Urology, 5th ed. Philadelphia, W. B. Saunders Company, 1986, pp 1463–1543. *This chapter provides a comprehensive review of all aspects relative to the diagnosis and treatment of carcinoma of the prostate.*

Catalona WJ, Smith DS, Ratliff TL, et al.: Measurement of prostate-specific antigen in serum as a screening test for prostate cancer. N Engl J Med 324:1156, 1991. *This large study concluded that measurement of serum PSA levels is a useful addition to screening by rectal examination alone.*

Coffey DS: The biochemistry and physiology of the prostate and seminal vesicles. *In* Walsh PC, Gittes RF, Perlmutter AD, et al. (eds.): Campbell's Urology, 5th ed. Philadelphia, W. B. Saunders Company, 1986, pp 233–274. *An excellent review of prostate biochemistry and physiology.*

Fair WR: Managing prostatitis: Practical aspects of antibiotic therapy. Urology 24:1, 1984. *A symposium on etiology, diagnosis, and treatment of prostatitis.*

Fowler JE Jr: Bacteriuria and associated infections of the reproductive system in men. *In* Urinary Tract Infection and Inflammation. Chicago, Year Book Medical Publishers, 1989, pp 92–123. *An updated review of the etiology, diagnosis, and treatment of male genital tract infections.*

Gittes RF: Medical progress: Carcinoma of the prostate. N Engl J Med 324:236, 1991. *An excellent recent review.*

New approaches in the treatment of benign prostatic hyperplasia. Prostate (Suppl) 3:23, 1990. *A multiauthored review of alternative treatments for BPH.*

Walsh PC: Benign prostatic hyperplasia. *In* Walsh PC, Gittes RF, Perlmutter AD, et al. (eds.): Campbell's Urology, 5th ed. Philadelphia, W. B. Saunders Company, 1986, pp 1248–1265. *A comprehensive review of all aspects relative to the diagnosis and treatment of benign prostatic hyperplasia.*

224 THE OVARIES

Robert W. Rebar

The ovaries episodically release female gametes (oocytes or eggs) and secrete sex steroid hormones, principally androstenedione, estradiol, and progesterone. Oocytes are released only during the adult reproductive years when sex steroid secretion is also greatest, but the ovaries are physiologically active throughout life.

Sex steroids affect the growth, differentiation, and function of a variety of tissues and organs throughout the body; therefore abnormalities of the ovaries and of sex steroid secretion should be recognized by all physicians. A rational approach to the diagnosis and treatment of reproductive disorders in women requires an understanding of the functions of the ovaries and of their most important unit, the follicle, throughout life.

EMBRYOLOGY AND ANATOMY OF THE OVARIES

EMBRYOGENESIS AND DIFFERENTIATION. Prior to 6 to 7 weeks of fetal age the gonads are paired, undifferentiated gonadal ridges overlying the mesonephros. By the sixth week of gestation, the primordial germ cells have migrated from their site of origin in the yolk sac to the gonadal ridges. Beginning during the sixth to eighth weeks the ovaries rapidly differentiate, and the number of germ cells, now called oogonia, increases by mitosis to 6 to 7 million. The germ cells next undergo meiosis such that all germ cells (now called oocytes) are arrested in meiotic prophase by the seventh month of gestation. From midgestation onward the number of germ cells progressively decreases until the menopause, by which time virtually no oocytes

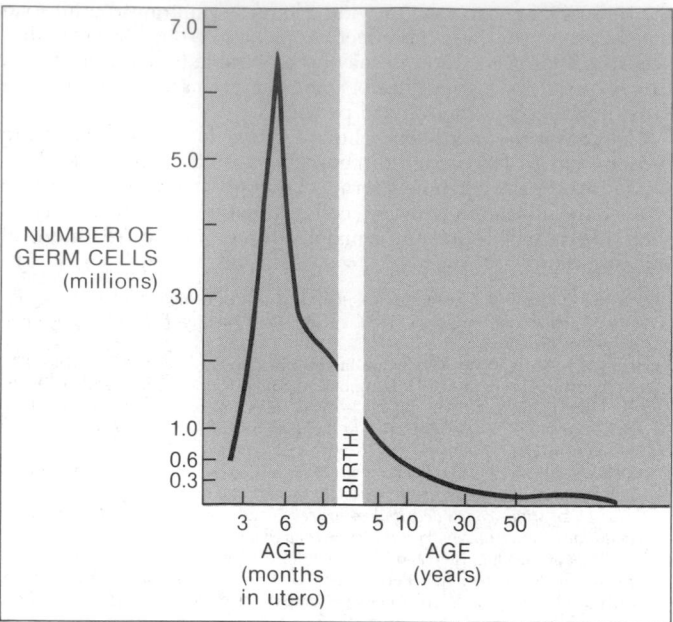

FIGURE 224–1. The number of oocytes present in both ovaries at different ages. (Adapted from Baker TG: *In* Austin CR, Short RJ (eds.): Reproduction in Mammals. I. Germ Cells and Fertilization. London, Cambridge University Press, 1972, pp 14–45. Reproduced from Rebar RW: Semin Reproduct Endocrinol 1:169–176, 1983.)

remain (Fig. 224–1). Thus the human female is born with a finite and decreasing number of germ cells. The germ cells are eliminated from ovaries by *ovulation* and by *atresia* (degeneration), which accounts for the elimination of 99.9 per cent of all germ cells. The development of the ovaries is described in greater detail in Ch. 221.

THE ADULT OVARY. The adult ovary consists of two principal parts: a central medulla surrounded by the predominant outer cortex (Fig. 224–2). The entire ovary is limited by a single cell layer termed the germinal epithelium. The medulla contains the blood vessels and nerves as well as nests of steroid-secreting hilus or ovarian Leydig cells. The cortex contains the *follicle complexes*, composed of the *oocyte*, *granulosa cells*, and *theca*

cells. Characteristic changes occur in each component during follicle growth and differentiation. Interactions among the follicular components give rise to the gamete (ovum) and to sex steroid hormones necessary for establishing and maintaining early pregnancy following fertilization of the ovum.

Follicles can be divided into two major classes, nongrowing and growing. The nongrowing or *primordial* follicles comprise 90 to 95 per cent of the ovarian follicles throughout reproductive life of the female. The ability of a woman to menstruate and reproduce depends totally upon the pool of primordial follicles. Each primordial follicle contains a small oocyte arrested in meiotic prophase, surrounded by a layer of squamous cells from which granulosa cells originate. These cells are bounded by the basal lamina, which is selectively permeable to solutes in plasma. This complex is surrounded in turn by stroma, which consists of supporting connective tissue cells, contractile cells, and steroid-secreting thecal interstitial cells. Primordial follicles are recruited sequentially to become growing follicles, which then pass through primary, secondary, and tertiary (or graafian) phases. Atresia may occur in any phase.

Erickson GF, Schreiber JR: Morphology and physiology of the ovary. *In* Becker KL, et al. (ed.): Principles and Practice of Endocrinology and Metabolism. Philadelphia, J. B. Lippincott, 1990, pp 776–788. *A treatise on follicular growth and development.*

OVARIAN FUNCTION IN CHILDHOOD AND PUBERTY

PHYSICAL CHANGES AT PUBERTY. Puberty extends from the earliest signs of sexual maturation until the attainment of physical, mental, and emotional maturity. Pubertal changes in girls result directly or indirectly from maturation of the hypothalamic-pituitary-ovarian unit. Hormonally, human puberty is characterized by a resetting of the negative gonadal steroid feedback loop, the establishment of new circadian and ultradian (frequent) gonadotropin rhythms, and the acquisition in the female of a positive estrogen feedback loop controlling the menstrual cycle as interdependent expressions of the gonadotropins and ovarian steroids. In girls, pubertal development generally occurs between 8 and 14 years of age. The age of onset and the rate of progress through puberty are variable and depend upon genetic, socioeconomic, nutritional, physical, and psychological factors.

Physical changes occur in an orderly sequence over a definite time frame during puberty (Fig. 224–3). Breast budding in girls is usually the first pubertal change, followed shortly by the appearance of pubic hair, with menarche occurring late in pu-

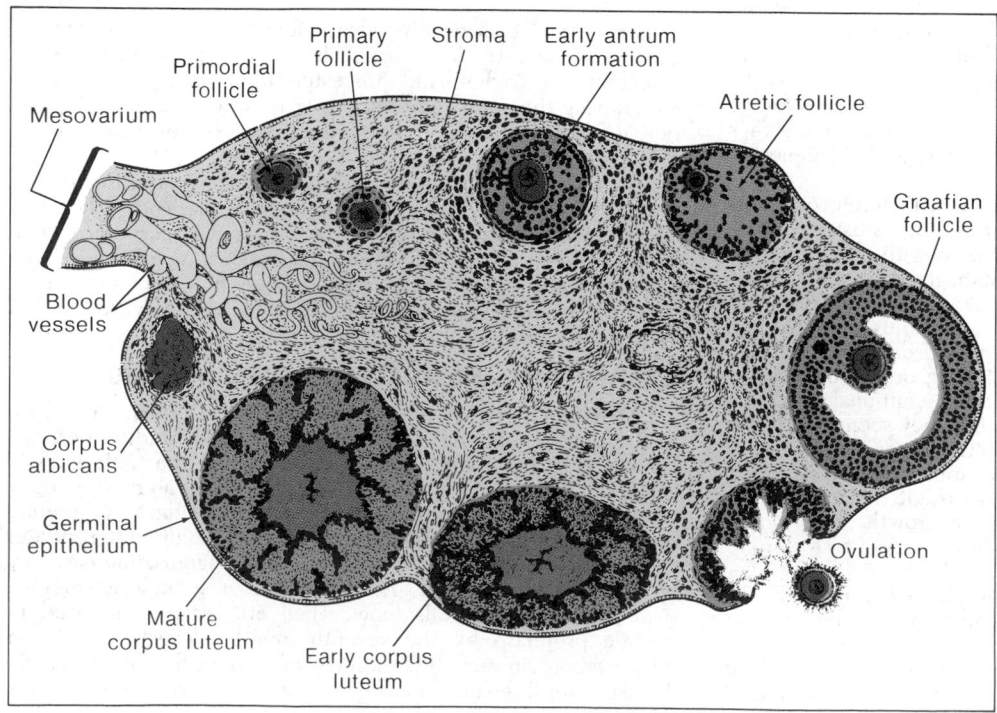

FIGURE 224–2. Diagrammatic illustration of the microscopic anatomy of the ovary. Changes in the components of the follicular complex occurring during atresia and ovulation are shown, progressing clockwise, from a primordial follicle (*upper left*) to a corpus albicans (*lower left*). (Adapted from Ross GT, Schreiber JR: *In* Yen SSC, Jaffe RB (eds.): Reproductive Endocrinology—Physiology, Pathophysiology and Clinical Management, 2nd ed. Philadelphia, W.B. Saunders Company, 1986, pp 115–139.)

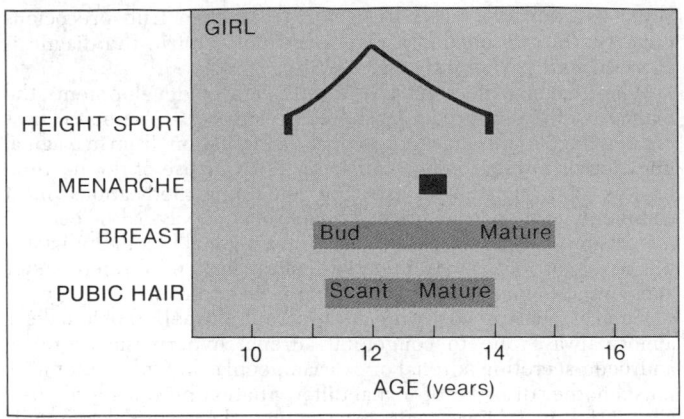

FIGURE 224–3. Temporal sequence of events for the "average" girl during puberty. (Reproduced from Rebar RW: *In* Yen SSC, Jaffe RB (eds.): Reproductive Endocrinology—Physiology, Pathophysiology and Clinical Management, 2nd ed. Philadelphia, W. B. Saunders Company, 1986, pp 683–733.)

bertal development. The time from breast budding (median age of onset 9.8 years) to menarche approximates 2 years. Breast development results from increasing ovarian estrogen production; pubic and axillary hair, from increasing ovarian androgen production. Estrogens are required for growth of pubic hair as well.

The ovarian sex steroids join with growth hormone and adrenal androgens to produce the adolescent growth spurt. Peak growth velocity is achieved relatively early with little growth observed following menarche. Lean body mass, skeletal mass, and body fat are equal in prepubertal boys and girls, but by maturity women have twice as much body fat and less lean body mass and skeletal mass as men, as a result of differences in sex steroid secretion beginning at puberty. Estrogens are necessary for normal formation, mineralization, and maturation of bones. Well-established standards exist for determining radiographically, typically by examining radiographs of the bones of the wrist, whether bone age is appropriate for chronologic age. Estrogen deficiencies retard and excesses advance bone age in relation to chronologic age.

HORMONAL CHANGES. The ovaries function even in early childhood. The low levels of luteinizing hormone (LH) and follicle-stimulating hormone (FSH), which are normally present, increase if the ovaries are removed prior to puberty, just as they do later in life, indicating exquisite sensitivity of the hypothalamic-pituitary unit to extremely low circulating sex steroid levels. As puberty nears there is a progressive decrease in sensitivity of the hypothalamic-pituitary unit to sex steroids, leading to increased secretion of pituitary gonadotropins, stimulation of sex steroid output, and the development of secondary sex characteristics. Increased secretion of both LH and FSH initially occurs at night with sleep and is associated with increased estradiol secretion the following morning (Fig. 224–4). As is true for most hormones, both LH and FSH are secreted in an episodic or pulsatile rather than a continuous fashion. It is possible that the sleep-entrained pulsatile secretion of gonadotropins commences in response to increased pulsatile secretion of gonadotropin releasing hormone (GnRH). Later in puberty, secretion of LH and FSH is increased, relative to childhood, throughout the 24-hour period, except during the early follicular phase when nighttime increases still occur. Basal levels of estradiol, the major estrogen secreted by the ovaries, increase throughout puberty. A "critical body mass" may be required for positive estrogen feedback and ovulation. During the first 2 years after menarche, up to 90 per cent of menstrual cycles may be anovulatory because of a delay in the synchronization of the hypothalamic-pituitary-ovarian axis.

ABERRATIONS OF PUBERTAL DEVELOPMENT

DEFINITION. Abnormalities of pubertal development can be divided into four major categories (Table 224–1):

1. *Precocious puberty* represents any pubertal changes before the age of 8 years. The precocious development is *isosexual* when the development is common to the phenotypic sex of the individual and *heterosexual* when the development is characteristic of the opposite sex. *True precocious puberty* is due to premature maturation of the hypothalamic-pituitary axis. In the absence of increased hypothalamic-pituitary activity, *precocious pseudopuberty* exists.

2. *Delayed (or interrupted) puberty* is defined as the absence of any secondary sex characteristics by the age of 13 years or of menarche by age 16 or by passage of 5 or more years from breast budding to menarche.

3. *Asynchronous pubertal development* occurs when there is deviation from the normal pattern of pubertal development.

4. *Heterosexual pubertal development* is development occurring at the appropriate time, but with some features characteristic of the opposite sex.

PRECOCIOUS PUBERTY. Differential Diagnosis. The temporal sequence in which the signs and symptoms of sex steroid hormone excess appear is most important. *Incomplete isosexual precocious puberty* indicates premature development of only a single pubertal feature. If breast budding occurs prior to the age of 8 years in the absence of any other development, the diagnosis may be *premature thelarche*. Premature thelarche is believed due to transient increases in estrogen secretion or increased breast sensitivity to the small quantities of circulating estrogens present prior to puberty. If pubic and/or axillary hair develops alone and persists, *premature pubarche* and *adrenarche* must be considered. These abnormalities are associated with slight increases in adrenal androgen secretion, but not with clitoromegaly or other signs of virilization. These syndromes require no treatment, and affected girls typically begin true puberty at the usual age.

When precocious development is isosexual, the purpose of evaluation is to determine if the cause is central (true precocious puberty) or not. Careful questioning of the patient and her parents may indicate inadvertent ingestion or absorption of sex steroids (iatrogenic or factitious). About 10 per cent of individuals with true precocious puberty have one of several organic brain diseases, including neoplasms, tuberous sclerosis, neurofibromatosis, encephalitis, meningitis, and hydrocephalus. The seriousness of intracranial lesions mandates that girls with precocious

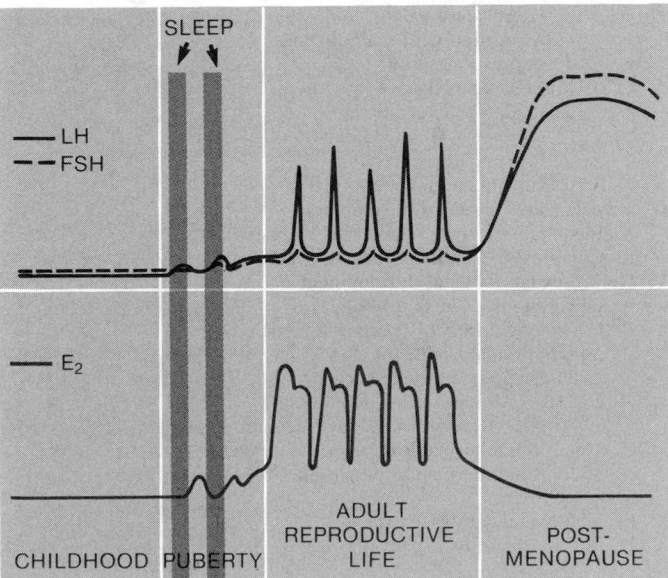

FIGURE 224–4. The changing patterns of LH, FSH, and estradiol (E$_2$) concentrations in peripheral blood throughout the life of a woman. The elevated levels of LH and FSH present in the first several weeks of life are not shown, nor is the fact that both LH and FSH are secreted in a pulsatile fashion. The pubertal period has been expanded to illustrate the sleep-associated increases in LH and FSH followed by morning increases in E$_2$ that are observed during puberty. (Reprinted with permission from *Endocrine and Metabolism Continuing Education Quality Control Program*, 1982. Copyright American Association for Clinical Chemistry, Inc.)

puberty have skull films and/or computed tomography (CT) of the brain. In almost 90 per cent of girls with true precocious puberty, however, no cause is identified (idiopathic or constitutional).

The physical examination may also provide critical information about the etiology of the precocious development. Cutaneous café au lait spots, facial asymmetry, polyostotic fibrous dysplasia, and other skeletal abnormalities, cranial nerve deficits, and multiple ovarian follicular cysts suggest *McCune-Albright syndrome* in a girl with precocious puberty. (At present it is uncertain whether the McCune-Albright syndrome produces precocious puberty through a central or a peripheral mechanism stimulating ovarian estrogen secretion.) Precocious development associated with short stature, congenital bodily asymmetry, a triangular facies, and clinodactyly suggests the *Silver-Russell syndrome*. Characteristic signs and symptoms may suggest the coexistence of primary hypothyroidism and precocious puberty, especially if galactorrhea is also present. In these patients, thyroid hormone replacement therapy will halt progression of pubertal development until the expected age of puberty. (Engimatically, primary hypothyroidism may also lead to delayed pubertal development. Thyroid hormone replacement will permit the onset of puberty.)

Abdominal and rectal examination may reveal a mass and suggest an adrenal or ovarian tumor. Because palpable ovarian cysts may develop rarely prior to ovulation in true precocious puberty, the presence of a mass need not confirm the diagnosis of precocious pseudopuberty.

When vaginal bleeding is the only sign of development, the diagnosis of sexual precocity should be suspect. Common causes of bleeding in this age group include irritation from a vaginal infection or foreign body, sexual assault, prolapse of the urethral meatus, and ingestion of estrogen-containing medications (most commonly oral contraceptive preparations). A vaginal or cervical neoplasm is also a rare possibility. Thus, vaginal bleeding dictates the need for vaginal examination, often best performed under anesthesia, before further evaluation is undertaken.

Heterosexual precocity in an apparent prepubertal female is almost always due to congenital adrenal hyperplasia or to an androgen-secreting adrenal or ovarian neoplasm. Only very rarely must another disorder of sexual differentiation be considered (see Ch. 221). It is important to examine the external genitalia carefully because congenital adrenal hyperplasia is usually associated with some degree of sexual ambiguity.

Excessive androgens produced endogenously by abnormal fetal adrenal glands in utero or diffusing across the placenta to the fetus from the mother can virilize the external genitalia and result in female pseudohermaphroditism. The extent of virilization varies from an enlarged clitoris only to sexual ambiguity sufficient to make gender assignment difficult.

Excessive maternal androgen secretion, typically from an ovar-

---

TABLE 224–1. ABERRATIONS OF PUBERTAL DEVELOPMENT

I. **Precocious development (before age 8)**
  A. Isosexual precocity
    1. Incomplete sexual precocity
      a. Premature thelarche
      b. Premature pubarche
      c. Premature adrenarche
    2. True precocious puberty
      a. Idiopathic (constitutional)
      b. Due to CNS lesions
      c. McCune-Albright syndrome
      d. Primary hypothyroidism
      e. Silver-Russell syndrome
    3. Precocious pseudopuberty
      a. Ovarian neoplasms
      b. Adrenal neoplasms
      c. Iatrogenic (estrogen-containing preparations)
      d. hCG-secreting neoplasms distinct from CNS and ovarian tumors
  B. Heterosexual precocity
    1. Ovarian neoplasms
    2. Adrenal neoplasms
    3. Congenital adrenal hyperplasia
    4. Other rare disorders of sexual differentiation
II. **Delayed pubertal development**
  (no development by age 13; absence of menarche by age 16; passage of 5 years or more from breast budding without menarche)
  A. Anatomic abnormalities
    1. Müllerian agenesis or dysgenesis (Rokitansky-Küster-Hauser syndrome)
    2. Distal genital tract obstruction
      a. Transverse vaginal septum
      b. Imperforate hymen
      c. Vaginal agenesis
  B. Hypergonadotropic hypogonadism (FSH > 40 mIU per milliliter)
    1. Gonadal dysgenesis
      a. With stigmata of Turner's syndrome
      b. Pure (46,XX or 46,XY)
      c. Mixed
    2. Ovarian failure with normal ovarian development
      a. Autoimmune disorders
      b. Gonadotropin receptor and/or postreceptor defects (?Resistant ovary or Savage syndrome)
      c. Enzymatic defects (17α-hydroxylase deficiency, galactosemia)
      d. Physical causes
        i. Irradiation
        ii. Chemotherapeutic agents
        iii. Viral agents
      e. Idiopathic
  C. Hypogonadotropic or normogonadotropic hypogonadism (LH and FSH < 10 mIU per milliliter or LH and FSH 6–25 mIU per milliliter with at least one being greater than 10 mIU per milliliter)
    1. Isolated gonadotropin deficiency
      a. In association with midline defects (Kallmann's syndrome)
      b. Independent of associated disorders
    2. Neoplasms of the hypothalamic-pituitary axis
      a. Craniopharyngiomas
      b. Pituitary tumors
      c. Others
    3. Hand-Schüller-Christian disease (eosinophilic granuloma; histiocytosis X)
    4. Idiopathic hypopituitarism
    5. "Hypothalamic" forms of amenorrhea
      a. Psychogenic
      b. Exercise associated
      c. Associated with malnutrition
      d. Anorexia nervosa
    6. Miscellaneous disorders
      a. Prader-Willi syndrome
      b. Lawrence-Moon-Bardot-Biedl syndrome
      c. Primary hypothyroidism
    7. Constitutional delayed puberty
III. **Asynchronous pubertal development**
  A. Incomplete forms of androgen insensitivity
  B. Complete forms of androgen insensitivity
IV. **Heterosexual pubertal development**
  A. Polycystic ovarian syndrome
  B. Congenital adrenal hyperplasia (female pseudohermaphroditism)
    1. 21-Hydroxylase deficiency
    2. 11β-Hydroxylase deficiency
    3. 3β-ol-Hydroxysteroid dehydrogenase deficiency
  C. Male pseudohermaphroditism due to 5α-reductase deficiency
  D. Male pseudohermaphroditism due to partial androgen insensitivity
  E. Mixed gonadal dysgenesis
  F. Androgen-producing neoplasms
    1. Ovarian
    2. Adrenal
  G. Cushing's syndrome

ian or adrenal neoplasm, can lead to virilization of a female fetus. This occurs very rarely, because of the great capacity of the placenta to aromatize naturally occurring androgens to estrogens. Virilization of a female fetus is much more apt to occur if a pregnant woman has ingested a synthetic steroid preparation with androgenic properties, because available synthetic compounds generally cannot be aromatized.

Excessive androgen secretion beginning in utero is usually associated with defective cortisol synthesis. As a consequence, ACTH secretion is increased, resulting in congenital adrenal hyperplasia and excessive androgen secretion. The three different enzyme defects in the steroidogenic pathway that can lead to virilization of the female fetus are described in Ch. 221. 21-Hydroxylase deficiency is the most common form of congenital adrenal hyperplasia, accounting for more than 90 per cent of affected individuals. The defect may vary from partial to complete deficiency of the enzyme.

Diagnostic Tests. MEASUREMENT OF PEPTIDE AND STEROID HORMONES. Increased levels of immunoreactive human chorionic gonadotropin (hCG) may suggest a chorionic gonadotropin (hCG)-secreting neoplasm, most commonly an ovarian teratoma or dysgerminoma. In such cases, the hCG, which is antigenically and biologically similar to LH, stimulates ovarian steroid secretion and pseudopubertal development. Because even specific LH immunoassays show some cross-reactivity with hCG, values for serum LH may be elevated in individuals with hCG-secreting tumors. Immunoreactive hCG is always elevated in the presence of such tumors. Levels and ratios of FSH and LH typical of pubertal as opposed to prepubertal girls help in diagnosing true precocious puberty. Timed urine collections rather than blood samples can be used to measure gonadotropin secretion if necessary. Excessively high circulating levels of estrogen suggest an estrogen-producing neoplasm. High levels of serum testosterone suggest an ovarian source of excess androgen in girls with heterosexual development, while increased levels of dehydroepiandrosterone (DHEA) or its sulfate (DHEA-S) (the principal precursors of 17-ketosteroids) suggest an adrenal source. High levels of serum 17-hydroxyprogesterone imply congenital adrenal hyperplasia (CAH) secondary to 21-hydroxylase deficiency, whereas high levels of serum 11-deoxycortisol imply an 11β-hydroxylase deficiency. In CAH these hormone levels should decrease promptly following oral administration of suppressive doses of dexamethasone. Suppression in response to exogenous corticoids occurs much less consistently in individuals with adrenal cortical adenomas and carcinomas and rarely in those with ovarian androgen-secreting neoplasms (see Ch. 217, 221).

ADDITIONAL STUDIES. Ultrasonic scanning of the adrenals and ovaries and CT of the adrenals may be indicated to confirm clinical suspicions. In girls with ovarian or adrenal neoplasms the tumor can almost always be localized radiographically. Catheterization of the ovarian and adrenal veins and measurements of the effluent steroids from each gland should be pursued only when CT, ultrasonography, or magnetic resonance imaging fails to identify what is suspected to be a neoplasm. Although plain skull films are of use in screening for pituitary and parapituitary tumors, CT or MRI of the skull is indicated in the presence of definite neurologic deficits or if true precocious puberty is suspected. Radiographic estimation of bone age is indicated in all cases and serves as a useful tool to follow the results of treatment.

Treatment. Treatment for precocious puberty should be initiated promptly so that: (1) The patient's ultimate height is not compromised as a result of sex steroid–induced premature epiphyseal closure. (2) Emotional disturbances in the patient and her parents are prevented or attenuated.

Gonadotropin-releasing hormone analogues are now the preferred therapy for suppressing gonadotropin secretion and also may prevent bone maturation. The analogues are not effective in children with McCune-Albright syndrome. Medroxyprogesterone acetate (100 to 200 mg intramuscularly every 2 to 4 weeks) also may be used to suppress gonadotropin secretion. Medroxyprogesterone acetate, however, does not always prevent premature epiphyseal closure and the resultant short stature.

Individuals with CNS or steroid-secreting neoplasms must undergo therapy appropriate for the particular lesion. Girls with congenital adrenal hyperplasia are appropriately managed with glucocorticoids (plus mineralocorticoids when indicated) as outlined in Ch. 221.

DELAYED PUBERTY. Typically girls with delayed puberty present at the age of 16 years or later because of primary amenorrhea, but younger girls may present because of failure to initiate pubertal development. Because of the anxiety generated by delayed puberty, some evaluation is always indicated regardless of the age of the patient.

When pubertal development progresses normally but menstruation does not begin, an abnormality in the genital tract should be considered. Congenital malformations of the müllerian ducts are uncommon, occurring in 0.02 per cent of all women. Most do not cause amenorrhea, and many do not impair reproduction. The anomalies associated with amenorrhea vary in severity from an imperforate hymen to complete aplasia of all müllerian duct derivatives with vaginal atresia. Although aplasia generally involves all of the müllerian duct derivatives, defects may involve only a single part of the distal genital tract.

A müllerian duct anomaly is suggested by (1) normal levels of serum gonadotropins and steroids, (2) an abnormal outflow tract, (3) a history of cyclic abdominal pain with or without a palpable mass, and (4) normal development of secondary sex characteristics. Normal ovarian function still induces endometrial growth and shedding after menarche if the uterus is normal. In the absence of a normal outflow tract, however, the menstrual effluent is retained and may or may not be able to escape into the abdominal cavity. Free in the abdominal cavity, the effluent may cause endometriosis. Constrained to the uterine cavity, the effluent causes hematometra and a large abdominal mass. In the absence of a mass or cyclic pain, a karyotype is indicated in girls with evidence of an abnormal genital tract to rule out any of several disorders of sexual differentiation (see Ch. 221). Such disorders, however, almost never occur together with completely normal pubertal development. In girls with a normal karyotype and a genital tract anomaly, examination under anesthesia and diagnostic laparoscopy should be undertaken to delineate the extent of the defect. When the abnormality consists of an imperforate hymen or transverse vaginal septum only, surgical restoration can be accomplished relatively simply. Attempts to provide an outflow tract for the uterus should not be undertaken if there is no cervix because of the high risk of recurrent pelvic infection. Even with a functional cervix, the creation of an outflow tract that will permit successful pregnancy is unlikely. A functional vagina can be created surgically or by the daily use of ever larger dilators. To prevent shrinkage and scarring, surgery should be deferred until the patient is willing to use dilators postoperatively on a daily basis or she is about to become sexually active.

Other causes of delayed puberty and primary amenorrhea are the same as those that may cause amenorrhea in older women (see below). When no apparent cause for delayed development is found, constitutional delayed puberty must be entertained as a diagnosis of exclusion. A strong family history of delayed maturation adds support to this presumption. Small doses of estrogen may be administered to induce some pubertal development but may obscure a pathologic cause for the delay and may compromise linear growth and ultimate height.

ASYNCHRONOUS PUBERTAL DEVELOPMENT. Asynchronous pubertal development is characteristic of male pseudohermaphroditism due to androgen insensitivity, especially complete testicular feminization. This syndrome of androgen insensitivity is inherited either as an X-linked recessive or as a sex-limited autosomal dominant trait. Despite the presence of intra-abdominal or inguinal testes, there is complete failure of virilization. Affected individuals develop breasts (but only to Tanner stage 3) and a typical female habitus with unambiguous female external genitalia but with absence of internal female structures, generally having only a foreshortened blind-ending vagina. Little or no pubic and axillary hair develops. The karyotype is obviously 46,XY in these individuals. Circulating testosterone levels are equivalent to or higher than those found in normal men, and LH levels are elevated while FSH levels are normal compared to menstruating women. This syndrome is further discussed in Ch. 221.

HETEROSEXUAL PUBERTAL DEVELOPMENT. *Polycystic ovarian (PCO) syndrome,* by far the most common cause of heterosexual pubertal development, is associated with the development of some secondary sex features characteristic of males at the normal age of puberty. Feminization occurs in affected girls, and they develop normal breasts and a typical female habitus, but masculinization also occurs. (In contrast, girls with congenital adrenal hyperplasia generally show little if any female development at puberty.) A heterogeneous syndrome, PCO syndrome most typically begins at or near puberty with hirsutism and irregular menses from the time of menarche. Menarche may be delayed as well, so that young women may present with primary amenorrhea. Basal LH levels tend to be somewhat elevated in perhaps 80 per cent of cases, and circulating levels of all androgens are elevated moderately.

Congenital adrenal hyperplasia is generally diagnosed prior to puberty, and heterosexual precocious pseudopuberty is typical. However, if the defect is mild and changes to the external genitalia are minimal, masculinization may occur at the expected age of puberty. This attenuated or nonclassic form of 21-hydroxylase deficiency seems to occur in families with a strong family history of hirsutism. Affected girls generally have some defeminization with flattening of the breasts, severe hirsutism, relatively short stature, and obesity.

Mixed gonadal dysgenesis designates asymmetric gonadal development, with a germ cell tumor or a testis on one side and an undifferentiated streak, rudimentary gonad, or no gonad on the other. The extent of genital virilization prior to puberty is variable in this rare disorder. The vast majority are reared as girls in whom virilization occurs at puberty; some may note breast development as well. Affected individuals generally have a mosaic karyotype, with 45,X/46,XY being most common. Short stature and other stigmata associated with a 45,X karyotype in Turner's syndrome are less common in patients with tumors than in patients with testes. Gonadectomy is indicated in all individuals with a Y chromosome to eliminate the increased neoplastic potential of such dysgenetic gonads and in all patients in whom virilization occurs at puberty to remove the source of androgen. Estrogen replacement therapy is warranted following gonadectomy. Other causes of male pseudohermaphroditism associated with heterosexual pubertal development are described in Ch. 221.

An androgen-producing neoplasm or Cushing's syndrome may occur rarely during the pubertal years and lead to heterosexual development.

Marshall WA, Tanner JM: Variations in the pattern of pubertal changes in girls. Arch Dis Child 44:291, 1969. *A classic paper that is required reading for all serious students.*

Simpson JL, Rebar RW: Normal and abnormal sexual differentiation and development. *In* Becker KL (ed.): Principles and Practice of Endocrinology and Metabolism. Philadelphia, J. B. Lippincott Company, 1990, pp 710–739. *A detailed discussion of the disorders of sexual differentiation organized similarly to the discussion in this chapter.*

Styne DM, Grumbach MM: Puberty in the male and female. Its physiology and disorders. *In* Yen SSC, Jaffe RB (eds.): Reproductive Endocrinology, 2nd ed. Philadelphia, W. B. Saunders Company, 1986, pp 313–384. *A detailed and excellently referenced discussion of normal and abnormal pubertal development.*

THE NORMAL MENSTRUAL CYCLE

CHARACTERISTICS OF THE MENSTRUAL CYCLE. Between menarche at approximately age 12 years and the menopause at about age 51 years, the reproductive organs of normal women undergo a series of closely coordinated changes at approximately monthly intervals that together comprise the normal menstrual cycle. The menstrual cycle is the expression of the coordinated interaction of the hypothalamic-pituitary-ovarian axis with associated changes in the target tissues (endometrium, cervix, vagina) of the reproductive tract.

A menstrual cycle begins with the first day of genital bleeding (day 1; menses) and ends just prior to the next menstrual period. The median menstrual cycle length is 28 days, but normal ovulatory menstrual cycles may range from about 21 to 40 days in length. Menstrual cycles vary most greatly in length in the years immediately following menarche and in the years immediately preceding menopause, largely because of an increased incidence of anovulatory cycles. Irregularities in menstrual cycle length also may be caused by abrupt changes in diet, exercise, or environment; serious emotional disturbances; and following

parturition or abortion. The menstrual cycle can be divided into three distinct phases: *follicular, ovulatory,* and *luteal.*

The Follicular or Preovulatory Phase. Variable in length, the follicular phase begins with the first day of menstrual bleeding and extends to the day prior to the preovulatory LH surge. A rise in serum FSH begins in the late luteal phase of the previous menstrual cycle, continues into the early follicular phase, and initiates growth and development of a group of follicles (Fig. 224–5). The preovulatory follicle destined for ovulation is selected from this cohort in a manner that is not yet understood. Circulating LH levels rise slowly throughout the follicular phase, but FSH levels fall after the early follicular phase increase. Approximately 7 to 8 days before the preovulatory LH surge, estradiol (E_2) and estrone (E_1) begin to increase, generally reaching a maximum on the day before or the day of the LH surge. The divergence in LH and FSH levels may be related to the follicular secretion of *inhibin* (folliculostatin), a hormone that specifically inhibits the release of FSH. Several days before the LH surge, plasma androgens (androstenedione and testosterone) and some progestins (17α-hydroxyprogesterone and 20α-dihydroprogesterone) begin to increase. They peak on the day of the LH surge. Progesterone itself does not increase until just prior to the onset of the LH surge.

The Ovulatory Phase. During this phase the ovum is released from the mature graafian follicle 16 to 32 hours after the onset of the preovulatory surge of LH by the pituitary gland. The ovulatory phase extends from 1 day prior to the LH surge to 1 day following the LH surge. Some women experience brief (a few minutes to a few hours in length), dull, unilateral pelvic pain near the time of ovulation, termed mittelschmerz. The association of this pain to ovulation is unknown, but it may be due to leakage of follicular fluid into the abdominal cavity at ovulation. Mittelschmerz may occur before or after actual ovulation or not at all

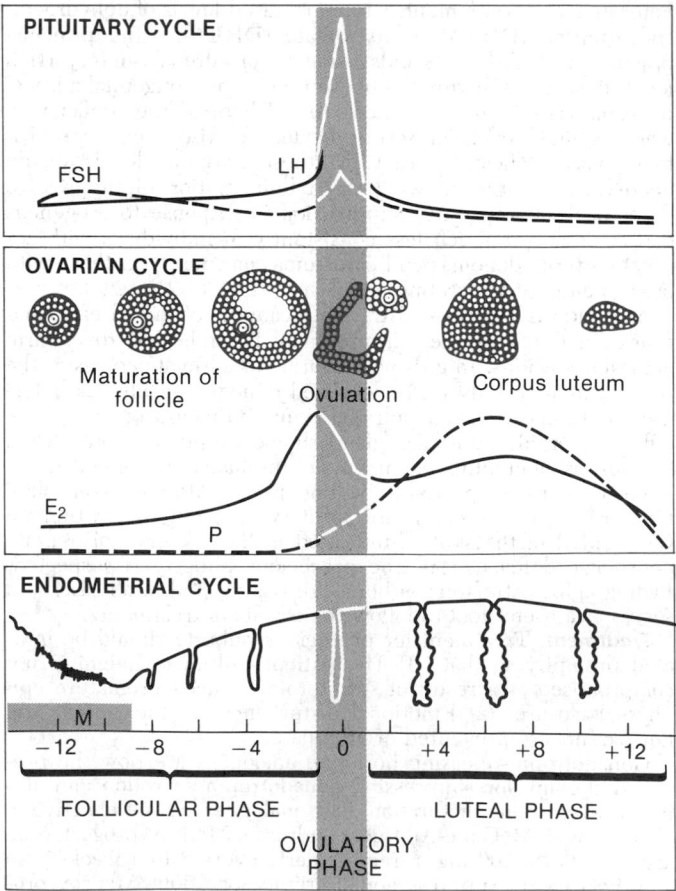

FIGURE 224–5. The idealized cyclic changes observed in gonadotropins, estradiol (E_2), progesterone (P), and uterine endometrium during the normal menstrual cycle. The data are centered about the day of the LH surge (day 0). Days of menstrual bleeding are indicated by M. (Reprinted with permission from *Endocrine and Metabolism Continuing Education Quality Control Program,* 1982. Copyright American Association for Clinical Chemistry, Inc.)

in ovulatory women. During the ovulatory phase a rapid rise in plasma LH results in response to positive estrogen feedback, leading to final maturation of the follicle and to ovulation. As peak LH levels are reached, E_2 levels drop, but progesterone levels continue to increase.

The Luteal or Postovulatory Phase. The more constant half of the menstrual cycle, the luteal phase, is approximately 14 days in length and ends with the onset of menses. This phase represents the functional lifespan of the corpus luteum ("yellow body") of the ovary, which supports the released ovum by secreting progesterone. In the luteal phase, progesterone secretion increases to peak 6 to 8 days after the LH surge. Parallel but smaller increases in 17α-hydroxyprogesterone, E_2, and E_1 levels also occur. Progesterone levels decrease toward menses unless the ovum is fertilized and pregnancy results. The finding of serum progesterone levels greater than 10 ng per milliliter 1 week prior to menses is probably diagnostic of normal ovulation. Progestins increase basal morning body temperature so that a "thermogenic shift" of more than 0.3°C occurring after a nadir is a presumptive sign of ovulation and progesterone secretion. Unfortunately, taking basal temperatures on a daily basis is tedious, subject to error, and not very reliable.

CYCLIC CHANGES IN TARGET ORGANS. Endometrium. During the menstrual cycle the endometrium undergoes remarkable histologic and cytologic changes, which culminate with menstrual bleeding when the corpus luteum ceases to secrete progesterone. The *basal layer of the endometrium*, which is not lost during menses, then regenerates the *superficial layer* of compact epithelial cells lining the uterine cavity and an *intermediate layer of spongiosa*, both of which are shed at each menstruation. Endometrial glands in these layers proliferate under the influence of estrogen in the follicular phase so that the mucosa thickens. In the luteal phase, under the influence of progesterone, the glands become coiled and secretory, with increased vascularity and edema of the stroma. As both E_2 and progesterone decline in the late luteal phase, the stroma becomes increasingly edematous, endometrial and blood vessel necrosis occurs, and endometrial bleeding ensues. Local release of prostaglandins may initiate vasospasm and ischemic necrosis in the endometrium as well as the uterine contractions accompanying menstrual flow. Thus prostaglandin synthetase inhibitors can relieve dysmenorrhea (menstrual cramping). Fibrinolytic activity in the endometrium also peaks at the time of menstruation, accounting for the noncoagulability of menstrual blood. Because the histologic changes during the menstrual cycle are so characteristic, endometrial biopsies are used to date the stage of the cycle and to assess the tissue response to gonadal steroids.

Cervix and Cervical Mucus. During the follicular phase, cervical vascularity, congestion, and edema increase progressively under the influence of estrogen. The external cervical os opens to a diameter of 3 mm at ovulation and then decreases to 1 mm. Cervical mucus increases in quantity (10- to 30-fold) and in elasticity (spinnbarkheit). "Palm leaf" arborization (ferning) becomes prominent just prior to ovulation (if cervical mucus is allowed to dry on a glass slide and examined microscopically). Under the influence of progesterone during the luteal phase, cervical mucus thickens, becomes less watery, and loses its elasticity and ability to fern. The characteristics of cervical mucus are useful clinically to evaluate the stage of the cycle and the amount of estrogen present.

Vagina. When ovarian estrogen secretion is low, as in the early follicular phase, vaginal epithelium is pale and thin. In the follicular phase under the influence of estrogens the epithelium thickens, and the number of mature cornified epithelial cells increases. During the luteal phase, progesterone causes a decrease in the percentage of cornified cells and an increase in the number of precornified intermediate cells and polymorphonuclear leukocytes. There is also increased cellular debris and clumping of shed desquamated cells. Histologic changes in the vaginal epithelium and in the cervical mucus are the most sensitive indicators of estrogen status in the body. However, the reliability of vaginal smears depends upon the absence of infection or exogenously administered steroid hormones that have antiestrogenic effects. Steroid hormones also facilitate progression of spermatozoa toward the ovaries and of ova toward the uterine cavity through effects on the fallopian tubes.

Ovary. A small primordial follicle with a diameter of 50 μm

transforms and grows into a mature graafian follicle 1 to 2 cm in diameter in two distinct phases: (1) The oocyte and follicle grow to form a *primary follicle*, apparently independent of gonadotropin control. The oocyte increases tenfold in diameter (from 15 to 150 μm) and becomes surrounded by a zona pellucida, a translucent "shell" of glycoproteins. In addition, the single layer of cells surrounding the oocyte becomes cuboidal and takes on the characteristics of granulosa cells. (2) In a second phase completely dependent upon gonadotropin and steroid hormones, the follicular unit develops into a *mature graafian follicle*, which is capable of being released in response to the midcycle surge of LH and FSH. Under the influence of FSH, granulosa cells acquire specific receptors for FSH, undergo mitosis, multiply to form secondary follicles consisting of several granulosa cell layers, and also acquire the ability to aromatize androgens to estrogens. Simultaneously, thecal interstitial cells begin to develop around the basement membrane surrounding the granulosa cells, develop specific cell membrane receptors for LH, and synthesize and secrete androgens, primarily Δ⁴-androstenedione and testosterone, in response to LH. The androgens can diffuse across the basement lamina where they are aromatized to estrogens. The rising E_2 in the follicular phase then feeds back on the hypothalamic-pituitary unit via the systemic circulation (Fig. 224–6). Just described is the so-called *two-cell theory*, which holds that both granulosa and theca are required for estrogen biosynthesis and maturation of the follicle.

A tertiary graafian follicle that contains an antrum or fluid-filled cavity increases from 200 μm to 1 to 2 cm in diameter, primarily because of accumulation of follicular fluid, again under the direct control of FSH. In tertiary follicles, FSH induces the appearance of specific LH receptors on granulosa cell membranes. These LH receptors are responsible for the stimulation of progesterone secretion prior to ovulation (luteinization) and for continued production of progesterone in the luteal phase.

Approximately 2 weeks are required for the presumptive preovulatory follicle to complete its growth and expel a mature oocyte. The oocyte is inhibited from resuming meiotic maturation by granulosa cell–oocyte interaction and an oocyte maturation

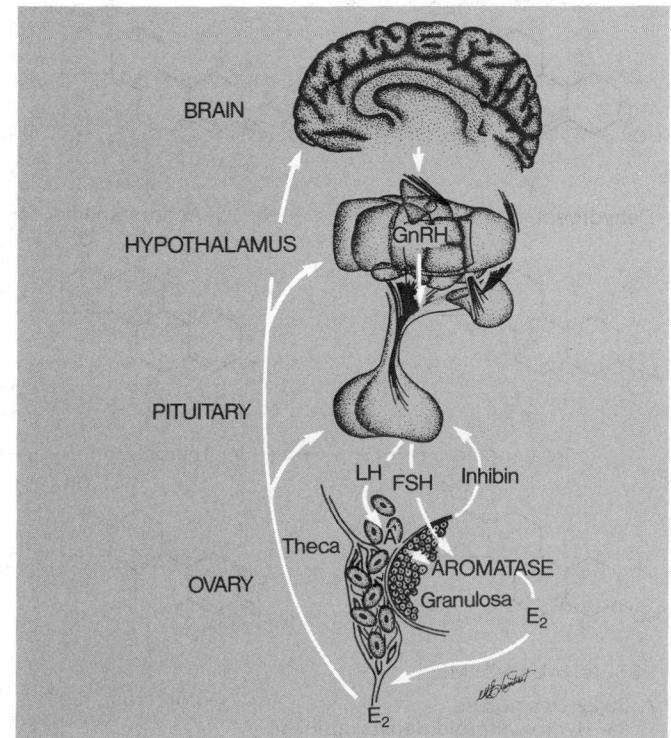

FIGURE 224–6. The hypothalamic-pituitary-ovarian axis in the regulation of follicular maturation and steroidogenesis. A = Androgens; E_2 = estradiol. (Modified from *Endocrine and Metabolism Continuing Education Quality Control Program,* 1982. Copyright American Association for Clinical Chemistry, Inc.)

inhibitor (OMI) until following the LH-FSH surge. Within 36 hours of the onset of the surge the oocyte completes the first meiotic division (reduction to 22 + X chromosomes) and a first polar body is extruded. The second meiotic division is completed only if the oocyte is fertilized by a spermatozoon. During the LH-FSH surge the preovulatory follicle bulges above the surface of the ovary. A stigma or avascular area develops on the follicle surface. Under the influence of local prostaglandins, plasminogen activator, and other hormones, a cluster of granulosa cells surrounding the oocyte and the oocyte itself (together known as the cumulus oophorus) are extruded.

The corpus luteum is formed from the granulosa and theca cells of the former preovulatory follicle following ovulation and secretes progesterone and E₂ for approximately 14 days. It then degenerates unless fertilization occurs. The lifespan of the corpus luteum may depend in part upon prostaglandins and prolactin as well as upon progestin. If fertilization occurs, chorionic gonadotropin (hCG), which is similar to LH, is secreted by the developing blastocyst and helps to support the corpus luteum until the fetoplacental unit can support itself. Pregnancy tests in common use have been developed utilizing antibodies to the specific β subunit of hCG and have little if any cross-reactivity with LH.

OVARIAN STEROIDOGENESIS. The ovaries and the developing follicles synthesize sex steroid hormones (estrogens, androgens, and progestins), which play important roles in ovulation and in preparing the uterus to accept a fertilized ovum via two separate pathways: (1) the so-called Δ^5 pathway, in which 17α-hydroxypregnenolone and DHEA with double bonds between carbons 5 and 6 are intermediates, and (2) the Δ^4 pathway, in which pregnenolone is converted to progesterone and in which 17α-hydroxyprogesterone and androstenedione with double bonds between carbons 4 and 5 are the alternative intermediates (Fig. 224–7).

Although cholesterol as substrate for steroid synthesis is obtained normally from circulating low-density lipoproteins (LDL), it can be synthesized de novo from two-carbon fragments (acetate). Different structures and cells within the ovary synthesize different steroids, in part because of stimulation by the gonadotropins. Gonadotropin binding to its receptor activates adenylate cyclase and stimulates cyclic AMP production. The cAMP in turn activates protein kinases that catalyze phosphorylation of proteins to mediate the cellular effects of each gonadotropin (see Ch. 208). LH also increases phosphatidylinositides within the ovary. LH

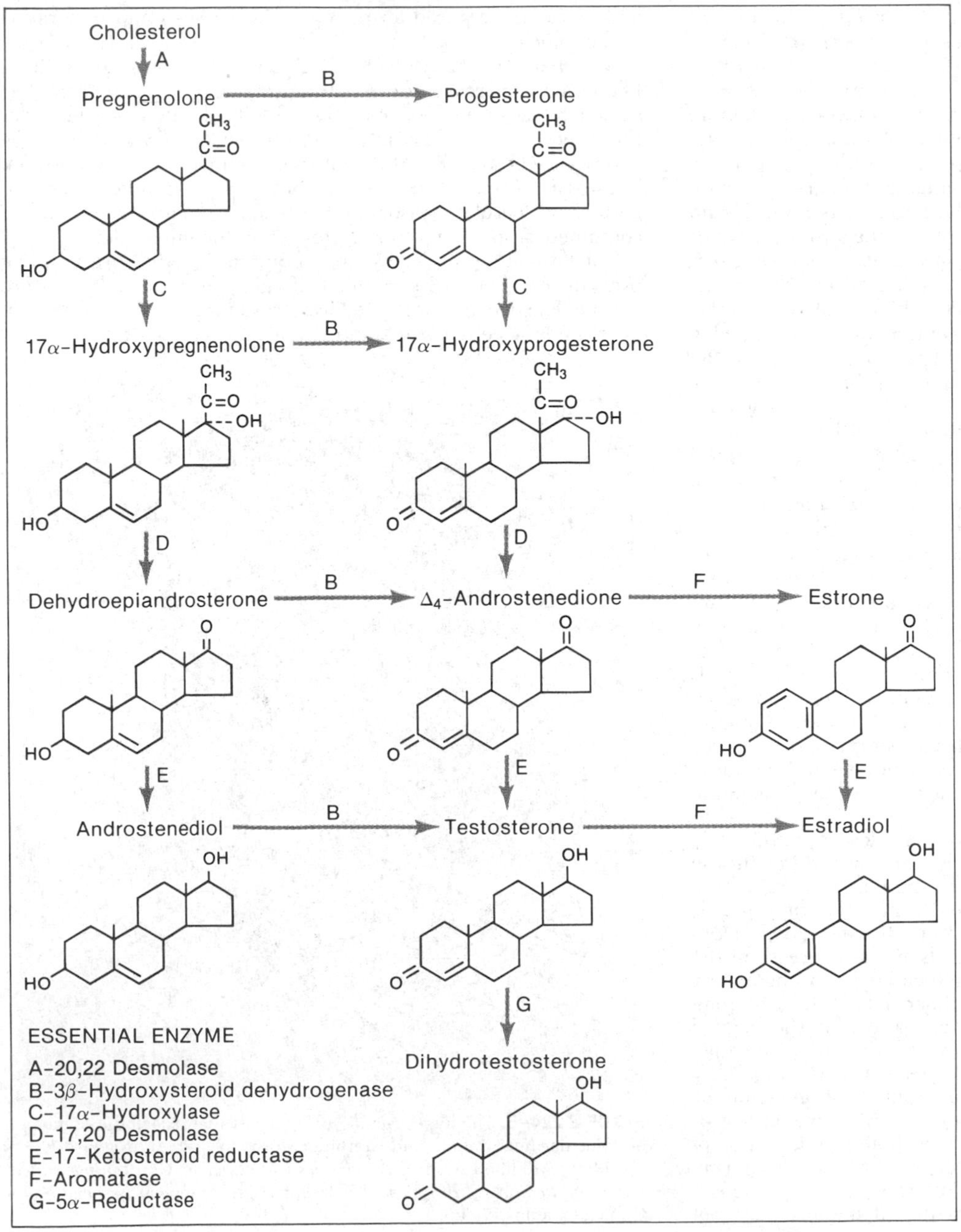

FIGURE 224–7. Steps in ovarian biosynthesis of steroid hormones. (Modified from data of Ross GT: *In* Rudolph AM (ed.): Pediatrics 16:1726, 1977. Copyright American Academy of Pediatrics 1977.)

ESSENTIAL ENZYME

A–20,22 Desmolase
B–3β–Hydroxysteroid dehydrogenase
C–17α–Hydroxylase
D–17,20 Desmolase
E–17-Ketosteroid reductase
F–Aromatase
G–5α–Reductase

acts primarily to regulate the first step in steroid hormone biosynthesis, that is, the conversion of cholesterol to pregnenolone. FSH acts to aromatize androgens to estrogens. Thus, LH acts to enhance substrate flow and the synthesis of androgens and/or progesterone. In the absence of LH, FSH action is reduced because of diminished substrate for aromatization.

Androgens, primarily androstenedione and testosterone, are secreted by interstitial and theca cells and serve as the substrate for the granulosa cell aromatase enzyme for synthesis of estrogens. Androstenedione, the major ovarian androgen, can also be converted to testosterone and estrogens in peripheral tissues. When ovarian androgen synthesis is excessive, as in ovarian androgen-producing tumors, or when conversion of androgen to estrogen in the ovary is reduced, as in PCO syndrome, hirsutism and even virilism can result. Testosterone, the most biologically potent androgen, is bound tightly to sex hormone–binding globulin (SHBG; also known as testosterone-estradiol–binding globulin, TeBG) so that only about 1 per cent of circulating testosterone is biologically free and active. Secretion rates and circulating concentrations in normal adult premenopausal women are given in Table 224–2.

Estrogens are produced predominantly in ovarian follicles by granulosa cell aromatization of the A ring of theca cell androgens. Naturally occurring estrogens are 18-carbon steroids, which by definition stimulate proliferation of the endometrium and bind to specific, saturable cytosolic receptors. The amount of estrogen secretion depends on the phase of the menstrual cycle (Table 224–2). In the early follicular phase the secretion rates of E_2 and E_1 are almost equal (60 to 170 μg per day). As the dominant follicle is selected, E_2 secretion increases to as much as 800 μg per day, with almost all the E_2 synthesized by the dominant follicle. The corpus luteum also produces significant quantities of E_2 (250 μg per day). In the late follicular and luteal phases, E_1 secretion is about one-fourth that of estradiol. The dominant follicle and corpus luteum synthesize about 95 per cent of circulating E_2; E_1 is of little significance in the ovulating woman. In the postmenopausal years, however, E_1 becomes the predominant estrogen in the absence of functioning follicles. E_1 is synthesized by peripheral conversion of adrenal androgens, especially androstenedione. As much estrogen is synthesized during the 9 months of pregnancy as would be synthesized during 100 years of normal menstrual cycles.

Progesterone synthesis is low in the follicular phase, but increases to 10 to 40 mg per day during the luteal phase (Table 224–2). Should pregnancy occur, progesterone production increases to as much as 300 mg per day at term. Why the corpus luteum atrophies at about 14 days is not known, but may be due to the effects of intraovarian estrogen and/or prostaglandins. However, LH stimulation is required for progesterone production by the corpus luteum. Progesterone induces secretory changes in the endometrium in preparation for implantation of the fertilized ovum.

NEUROENDOCRINE REGULATION OF THE OVARIES.

Neurons containing various peptide hormones that can release or inhibit secretion of the gonadotropins are found in the hypothalamus (see Ch. 212). Specifically, cells containing gonadotropin-releasing hormone (GnRH) occur in the area including the arcuate nucleus and median eminence and the preoptic area. Axons from these neurons run in the tuberoinfundibular tract and terminate on capillaries within the median eminence; this allows for delivery of their products through the portal vascular system to the anterior pituitary gland. It appears that classic neurotransmitters, including norepinephrine, dopamine, and serotonin, as well as neuromodulators, such as endogenous opiates and prostaglandins, influence secretion of GnRH by the hypothalamus. In addition, estrogens and androgens bind to cells in the hypothalamus and the anterior pituitary, and progestins bind to cells in the hypothalamus to influence hypothalamic-pituitary regulation of ovarian function.

GnRH is secreted in a pulsatile fashion (perhaps because of an inherent oscillator within the arcuate nucleus) and is responsible for pulsatile release of gonadotropins. Pulsatile gonadotropin release in turn appears to account for the pulsatile secretion of sex steroids from the ovaries. The ovarian sex steroids then feed back on the hypothalamic-pituitary unit to modulate both the frequency and amplitude of the gonadotropin pulse (see Fig. 224–6). Thus, gonadotropin pulses vary throughout the menstrual cycle. Pulses occur at approximately 60- to 90-minute intervals in the follicular phase and at intervals of greater than 180 minutes in the luteal phase.

Gonadal steroids can exert both negative and positive feedback effects on gonadotropin secretion. Among ovarian steroids, 17β-estradiol is the most potent inhibitor of gonadotropin secretion, acting on both the hypothalamus and pituitary. For women to ovulate, E_2 must also elicit a positive feedback effect on gonadotropin release. The feedback effects are both time and dose dependent. In the normal menstrual cycle the positive feedback action of E_2 leading to the LH surge is preceded by a period when lower E_2 levels are present with their negative feedback effects.

It appears that the ovary is the "clock" for the timing of ovulation, with the hypothalamus stimulating pulsatile release of the gonadotropins. The follicle complex and corpus luteum develop in response to gonadotropin stimulation. For appropriate ovarian regulation of reproductive function in women, three biologic characteristics are necessary: (1) an appropriate balance and sequence of negative and positive feedback actions; (2) differential feedback effects on the release of LH and FSH; (3) local intraovarian controls on follicular growth and maturation, separate from but interrelated to the effects of gonadotropins on the ovaries.

di Zerega GS, Hodgen GD: Folliculogenesis in the primate ovarian cycle. Endocr Rev 2:27, 1981. *A detailed discussion of recruitment and selection of the dominant follicle, summarizing a series of elegant studies.*

TABLE 224–2. CONCENTRATIONS, METABOLIC CLEARANCE RATES, PRODUCTION RATES, AND OVARIAN SECRETION RATES OF SEX STEROID HORMONES IN BLOOD

Steroid	Plasma MCR (liters/day)	Binding	Phase of Menstrual Cycle or Stage of Life	Plasma Concentration (ng/dl)	Plasma Production Rate (μg/day)	Ovarian Secretion Rate (μg/day)
Androstenedione	2000	Albumin	Premenopausal	40–240	3200	800–1600
			Postmenopausal	30–120	1600	
Testosterone	700	TeBG, albumin	Premenopausal	19–70	260	
			Postmenopausal	15–70	150	
Estradiol	1350	TeBG, albumin	Early follicular	2.5–6	70–200	60–170
			Late follicular	20–40	445–945	400–800
			Midluteal	15–25	270	250
			Postmenopausal	<1.0–2.5		
Estrone	2200	Albumin	Early follicular	2–6	70–200	60–170
			Late follicular	10–20	300–600	250–500
			Midluteal	10–15	240	160
			Postmenopausal	1.5–5.0	55	
Progesterone	2200	CBG, albumin	Follicular	3–10	700–2500	1500
			Luteal	10–25	3000–30,000	24,000

CBG = Cortisol-binding globulin; MCR = metabolic clearing rate; TeBG = testosterone-estradiol–binding globulin.

Erickson GF, Schreiber JR: Morphology and physiology of the ovary. *In* Becker KL (ed.): Principles and Practice of Endocrinology and Metabolism. Philadelphia, J. B. Lippincott Company, 1990, pp 776–788. *A detailed discussion of ovarian function.*

Rebar RW, Kenigsberg D, Hodgen GD: The normal menstrual cycle and the control of ovulation. *In* Becker KL (ed.): Principles and Practice of Endocrinology and Metabolism. Philadelphia, J. B. Lippincott Company, 1990, pp 788–797. *A more detailed discussion of the control of ovulation than is described here.*

Richardson GS: Steroidogenesis. *In* Sciarra JJ (ed.): Gynecology and Obstetrics. Vol. 5. Philadelphia, Harper and Row, 1986 (rev. ed.), pp 1–17. *A detailed summary of the steroidogenic pathway.*

ABNORMALITIES OF THE REPRODUCTIVE YEARS

DYSMENORRHEA AND ENDOMETRIOSIS. Dysmenorrhea, perhaps the most common of all gynecologic disorders, affects about 50 per cent of postpubertal women. Dysmenorrhea can be classified as primary or secondary.

Primary dysmenorrhea occurs only in ovulatory cycles. Prostaglandins that are released from the endometrium just prior to and during menstruation cause contraction of uterine smooth muscle and produce dysmenorrhea by initiating painful, exaggerated uterine contractions and myometrial ischemia. Associated systemic symptoms include nausea, diarrhea, headache, and emotional changes. Primary dysmenorrhea is much more common than is secondary dysmenorrhea.

In *secondary dysmenorrhea* there is a pathologic cause for the dysmenorrhea. Endometriosis, the ectopic occurrence of endometrial tissue generally within the abdominal cavity, is the most common cause in severe cases. Other possible causes include pelvic inflammatory disease, congenital abnormalities such as atresia of a portion of the distal genital tract and cystic duplication of the paramesonephric ducts, and cervical stenosis.

Prostaglandin synthetase inhibitors such as naproxen, ibuprofen, mefenamic acid, and indomethacin are the mainstays of treatment. If the dysmenorrhea is still severe, addition of an oral contraceptive preparation to inhibit ovulation and limit prostaglandin release is generally effective. In cases in which the pelvic pain still remains intractable, additional evaluation is warranted. If thorough evaluation of the gastrointestinal and urinary tracts fails to reveal a definitive cause, examination under anesthesia and diagnostic laparoscopy may be indicated.

If endometriosis is diagnosed at laparoscopy, treatment varies, depending on the severity of the disease and the goals of the patient regarding fertility. It may be possible to fulgurate implants or lyse adhesions through the laparoscope. In general, endometriosis should be treated medically, with additional surgery deferred until infertility (if present) becomes manifest. Medical therapy can consist of continuous suppression with GnRH analogues, progestins, oral contraceptive agents, or danazol for 3 to 6 months. GnRH analogues are rapidly becoming the most frequent form of medical suppressive therapy. After a course of therapy, use of oral contraceptive agents probably should be continued until fertility is desired. Conservative surgical resection of endometriosis at laparotomy should almost always be deferred until it is established as the cause of infertility. Surgery may be required, however, for continuing severe pain, severe endometriosis, or large ovarian cysts containing endometriosis (endometriomas). If symptoms continue despite adequate treatment or if psychological overlay is suspected, psychiatric evaluation may be indicated. Medical causes of dysmenorrhea, however, should be eliminated first.

PREMENSTRUAL SYNDROME. Premenstrual syndrome (PMS), also known as premenstrual tension (PMT), is a complex of physical and/or emotional symptoms that occur repetitively in a cyclic fashion before menstruation and that diminish or disappear with menstruation. Typically these cyclic symptoms are sufficiently severe to interfere with some aspects of life. Women with definitive psychiatric disturbances probably should not be included among those with PMS. More than 150 different symptoms are now thought to vary with the menstrual cycle (Table 224–3). Estimates of the prevalence of PMS range from 25 to 100 per cent. For most women the syndrome is merely annoying; it is likely that PMS causes serious difficulties for no more than 5 to 10 per cent. The diagnosis is best established by requiring patients to keep prospective daily records of symptoms over a 2- to 3-month period. Less than 50 per cent of women presenting with PMS are found to have the syndrome when such records are examined.

Most women seek help for PMS in their 30's after 10 or more years of symptoms. Many report that their symptoms began at menarche; approximately half state that symptoms began following childbirth. Severity and duration of symptoms are often reported to increase following each successive pregnancy, to become more severe with advancing age. Women with severe longstanding PMS almost always experience secondary psychological reactions, including social difficulties, such as marital discord, difficulty relating to their children, difficulty maintaining friendships, and withdrawal from social activities.

The etiology of PMS is unknown, but theories abound: alterations in the ratio of estrogen to progesterone in the luteal phase, alterations in α-melanocyte stimulating hormone (MSH) or β-endorphin activity, alterations in monoamine neurotransmitters, alterations in prolactin activity, increase in vasopressin secretion, alterations in mineralocorticoid secretion, alterations in prostaglandins, endogenous allergies to steroids (especially progesterone), reactive hypoglycemia, and many others.

Patients should be informed that no one therapy has been effective in all women and that none of the currently popular therapies has proved consistently effective. Still, women with mild premenstrual symptoms often benefit from simple changes in lifestyle, including addition of mild aerobic exercise each day; reduction in intake of xanthine-containing beverages, salt, and refined sugar in the day, particularly in the luteal phase; stress reduction; and adequate rest. Women with more severe PMS may benefit from treating predominant complaints symptomatically. Thus bromocriptine* (generally 2.5 mg twice a day) or danazol (100 to 400 mg daily in two divided doses) may be given continuously for relief of mastalgia, with the understanding that both may have unpleasant side effects. Prostaglandin synthetase inhibitors may help reduce dysmenorrhea and may benefit headaches. Mild sedatives and tranquilizers may help reduce insomnia and anxiety. Mild diuretics (especially spironolactone at doses up to 100 mg each morning) may be of benefit if cyclic edema can be documented by the presence of substantial weight gain in the luteal phase and by signs of dependent edema. The administration of 50 mg of pyridoxine per day has been urged by many as at least a harmless placebo, since it is a required cofactor in several enzymatic reactions, but, rarely, vitamin toxicity can develop when doses as low as 250 mg per day are given for a protracted time.

Since PMS requires the occurrence of cyclic ovulation, oophorectomy is sometimes considered for patients with particularly intractable symptomatology. Because GnRH analogues that induce a "medical castration" appear to have some effectiveness in PMS, the rationale seems valid. However, oophorectomy may create new problems related to estrogen deficiency for women with PMS treated in this permanent fashion.

Natural progesterone, particularly in the form of vaginal suppositories given at doses of up to 800 mg per day, has been used

TABLE 224–3. COMMON SYMPTOMS OF CYCLIC PREMENSTRUAL SYNDROME

Somatic Symptoms

Abdominal bloating	Constipation or diarrhea
Acne	Headache
Alcohol intolerance	Peripheral edema
Breast engorgement and tenderness	Weight gain
Clumsiness	

Emotional and Mental Symptoms

Anxiety	Insomnia
Change in libido	Irritability
Depression	Lethargy
Fatigue	Mood swings
Food cravings (especially salt and sugar)	Panic attacks
	Paranoia
Hostility	Violence toward self and others
Inability to concentrate	Withdrawal from others
Increased appetite	

---

*This use is not listed in the manufacturer's directive.

enthusiastically by many clinicians, but results of double-blind placebo-controlled trials have generally provided no evidence of efficacy. Likewise, the use of large quantities of multiple vitamins or of oil of evening primrose, containing the essential fatty acid γ-linolenic acid, a precursor of prostaglandins, is unsubstantiated.

Keye WR Jr (ed.): The Premenstrual Syndrome. Philadelphia, W. B. Saunders Company, 1988. *A simple multiauthored text detailing what is known about this disorder.*

Stillman R: Endometriosis. *In* Becker KL (ed.): Principles and Practice of Endocrinology and Metabolism. Philadelphia, J. B. Lippincott Company, 1990. *A succinct summary of this enigmatic disorder.*

ABNORMAL UTERINE BLEEDING. **Differential Diagnosis.**

The causes of abnormal uterine bleeding in the reproductive years include complications from the use of oral contraceptive preparations; complications of pregnancy (especially threatened, incomplete, or missed abortion and ectopic pregnancy); coagulation disorders (most commonly idiopathic thrombocytopenic purpura and von Willebrand's disease); and pelvic disease such as intrauterine polyps, leiomyomas, and tumors of the vagina and cervix. Clear-cell adenocarcinoma of the vagina or cervix may occur in women exposed to diethylstilbestrol (DES) during fetal life as a result of maternal ingestion. Affected women also may have congenital abnormalities of the upper vagina, cervix, and uterus. Because a history of DES exposure is not always obtained and because this malignant tumor may be fatal, clinical suspicion should remain high. Women with a history of DES exposure should be reassured, however, that the incidence of malignancy is extremely low. Trauma (postcoital or otherwise), foreign bodies, systemic illnesses including various endocrinopathies (such as diabetes mellitus, hypothyroidism and hyperthyroidism, Cushing's syndrome, and Addison's disease), leukemia, and renal disease may also present with abnormal bleeding.

Dysfunctional uterine bleeding (DUB), abnormal uterine bleeding with no demonstrable organic genital or extragenital cause (75 per cent of cases), is most frequently associated with anovulation. Postmenarchal bleeding in adolescents secondary to immaturity of the hypothalamic-pituitary-ovarian axis accounts for about 20 per cent of all cases, and premenopausal bleeding consequent to incipient ovarian failure constitutes more than half of the cases. Most anovulatory bleeding is due to either estrogen withdrawal or estrogen breakthrough bleeding. In anovulatory women, estrogen stimulates the endometrium unopposed by progesterone. As a consequence, the endometrium proliferates, becomes thicker, and may shed irregularly, especially if estrogen levels drop. Anovulatory bleeding tends to occur at less frequent intervals, while organic lesions tend to cause bleeding more frequently than cyclic menses.

Evaluation and Treatment. All cases of abnormal bleeding should be evaluated, including obtaining a thorough history with special emphasis on the amount and duration of blood loss. Prospective charting of the days that the patient bleeds may be required to evaluate the bleeding pattern. Complications of pregnancy or a bleeding diathesis must always be ruled out.

The physical examination (including the Papanicolaou smear) is normal in dysfunctional bleeding except for signs of anemia in the more severe cases. Laboratory tests should include a complete blood count, platelet count, coagulation studies, thyroid function tests, and fasting blood glucose. DUB must be a diagnosis of exclusion. Management of DUB depends upon the age of the patient and the extent of the bleeding. A sample of the endometrium should be obtained by biopsy or by dilatation and curettage from all women over age 35 and from those at increased risk of developing endometrial carcinoma because of prolonged anovulatory bleeding.

Even profuse bleeding in anovulatory women can almost always be successfully treated by administering one combination oral contraceptive pill every 6 hours for 5 to 7 days. Bleeding should cease within 24 hours, but patients should be warned to expect heavy bleeding 2 to 4 days after stopping therapy. If anemia and signs of acute blood loss are profound, blood transfusion may be necessary. If the bleeding continues despite therapy, curettage can be carried out. Recurrence can be prevented by giving the patient combination oral contraceptive agents cyclically for 3 or more months. If spontaneous cyclic menses do not resume and pregnancy is not desired, the patient can be treated with cyclic progestin (medroxyprogesterone acetate 5 to 10 mg for 10 to 14

days each month) or oral contraceptive agents. If pregnancy is desired, ovulation can be induced, as discussed subsequently.

Acute episodes of anovulatory bleeding also can be treated with conjugated estrogens administered intravenously (25 mg every 4 hours for up to three doses) until bleeding ceases. Progestin therapy (medroxyprogesterone acetate 5 to 10 mg orally for 10 days) should be started simultaneously. Withdrawal bleeding will occur after cessation of therapy, and the patient can then be treated with oral contraceptive agents for at least three cycles.

For individuals with anovulatory bleeding without an episode of profuse bleeding, treatment with cyclic oral contraceptive agents or progestin can be provided unless pregnancy is desired, in which case ovulation must be induced.

Speroff L, Glass RH, Kase NG: Dysfunctional uterine bleeding. *In* Speroff L, Glass RH, Kase NG: Clinical Gynecologic Endocrinology and Infertility, 4th ed. Baltimore, Williams & Wilkins Company, 1989, pp 265–282. *A detailed and logical approach to the treatment of abnormal uterine bleeding.*

AMENORRHEA. **Definition and Etiology.**

Amenorrhea is the absence of menstruation for 3 or more months in women with past menses (*secondary amenorrhea*) or the absence of menarche by the age of 16 years regardless of the absence or presence of secondary sex characteristics (*primary amenorrhea*). If an intact genital outflow tract exists and there is no primary disease of the uterus, amenorrhea is a sign of failure of the hypothalamic-pituitary-ovarian axis to produce cyclically the hormones necessary for menses. Amenorrhea is a sign of any of several disorders involving different organ systems. Amenorrhea is physiologic in the prepubertal girl, during pregnancy and early in lactation, and after the menopause. At any other time it is pathologic and demands evaluation. Use of the term *post-pill amenorrhea* to refer to women who fail to resume menses within 3 months of discontinuing oral contraceptives is inappropriate. Such individuals should be evaluated in the same manner as any woman with amenorrhea. Similarly, individuals with menses occurring at infrequent intervals of greater than 40 days, termed oligomenorrhea, should be evaluated identically to women with amenorrhea.

Clinical Evaluation. The patient with amenorrhea should be viewed as a bioassay subject in whom even subtle hormonal abnormalities may be manifested by obvious signs and symptoms. For example, breast development indicates exposure to estrogens, while the presence of pubic and axillary hair indicates androgenic stimulation.

Patients should be questioned especially closely for evidence of psychological disturbances, dietary and exercise habits, lifestyle, environmental stresses, a family history of genetic anomalies, and abnormal growth and development. Patients should also be asked about and examined for the presence of any signs of hyperandrogenism, including hirsutism, temporal balding, deepening of the voice, increased muscle mass, clitoromegaly, and increased libido, as well as for any signs of defeminization, including decreasing breast size and vaginal atrophy. Any history of galactorrhea, the nonpuerperal secretion of milk from the breasts, should be determined (see Ch. 226). A history of symptoms related to thyroid and adrenal dysfunction should also be sought.

The physical examination should focus on evaluating (1) body dimensions and habitus, (2) the extent and distribution of body hair, (3) breast development and secretions, and (4) the genitalia.

In normal adult women the arm span is similar to the height, while in hypogonadal women the span is generally more than 5 cm greater than the height. The general appearance of the patient should be evaluated to determine if the habitus is that of an adult female. The distribution and quantity of body hair should be considered in view of the family history. The extent of any hirsutism (increased sexually stimulated terminal hair; see Ch. 225) should be recorded, preferably by photographs. Other signs of virilization should be sought carefully. Breast development should be graded according to the method of Tanner (Table 224–4). Breast secretion should be sought by applying pressure to the breasts while the patient is seated. Any secretion should be examined microscopically for the presence of perfectly round fat globules of varying size, which are always present in milk and indicate galactorrhea. Finally, the female genitalia should be examined carefully because they are such sensitive indicators of

TABLE 224-4. CRITERIA FOR DISTINGUISHING TANNER STAGES 1 TO 5 DURING PUBERTAL MATURATION

Tanner Stage	Breast	Pubic Hair
1 (Prepubertal)	No palpable glandular tissue or pigmentation of areola; elevation of areola only	No pubic hair; short, fine vellous hair only
2	Glandular tissue palpable with elevation of breast and areola together as a small mound; areolar diameter increased	Sparse, long, pigmented terminal hair chiefly along the labia majora
3	Further enlargement without separation of breast and areola; although more darkly pigmented, areola still pale and immature; nipple generally at or above midplane of breast tissue when individual is seated upright	Dark, coarse, curly hair extending sparsely over mons
4	Secondary mound of areola and papilla above breast	Adult-type hair, abundant but limited to mons and labia
5 (Adult)	Recession of areola to contour of breast; development of Montgomery's glands and ducts on areola; further pigmentation of areola; nipple generally below midplane of breast tissue when individual is seated upright; maturation independent of breast size	Adult-type hair in quantity and distribution; spread to inner aspects of the thighs in most racial groups

Data from Ross GT: Disorders of the ovary and female reproductive tract. In Wilson JD, Foster DW (eds.): Textbook of Endocrinology, 7th ed. Philadelphia, W. B. Saunders Company, 1985, pp 206–258; Speroff L, Glass RH, Kase N: Clinical Gynecologic Endocrinology and Infertility, 3rd ed. Baltimore, Williams & Wilkins Company, 1983, p 377; and Kustin J, Rebar RW: Menstrual disorders in the adolescent age group. Primary Care 14:139–166, 1987.

hormonal milieu. The Tanner stage of pubic hair development should be noted (Table 224–4). Since the sensitivity of the genitalia to androgens decreases onward from early in fetal development, the extent of any virilization is important. Fusion of the labia and enlargement of the clitoris with or without formation of a penile urethra are observed in women exposed to androgens during the first 3 months of fetal development (see Ch. 221). Significant clitoromegaly in the absence of other signs of sexual ambiguity and in the presence of other signs of virilization requires marked androgenic stimulation and strongly implicates an androgen-secreting neoplasm in the absence of a history of ingestion of exogenous steroids. The development of the labia minora in postpubertal women indicates the influence of estrogens. Overt anomalies of the distal genital tract and especially any evidence of obstruction to the escape of menstrual blood should be sought in the remainder of the pelvic examination. The vaginal mucosa and the cervical mucus are exquisitely sensitive to estrogen. Under the influence of estrogen the vaginal mucosa changes during sexual maturation from a tissue with a shiny, bright red appearance with sparse, thin secretions to a dull, gray-pink rugated surface with copious, thick secretions.

The history and physical examination quickly differentiate among several causes of amenorrhea, regardless of the age of the patient (Table 224–5). The various disorders of sexual differentiation and the other peripheral causes are often apparent on inspection. Distal genital tract obstruction should be identified at the time of pelvic examination even if the specific abnormality is not obvious. The physical stigmata of Turner's syndrome, discussed subsequently, generally make the diagnosis simple. Any sexual ambiguity indicates the need for chromosomal analysis and the measurement of 17-α-hydroxyprogesterone to rule out congenital adrenal hyperplasia. Pregnancy and gestational trophoblastic disease may be suspected and confirmed by measuring circulating concentrations of hCG. The possibility of intrauterine

TABLE 224-5. CAUSES OF AMENORRHEA

Disorders of sexual differentiation
Distal genital tract obstruction (müllerian agenesis and dysgenesis)
Gonadal dysgenesis
Ambiguity of external genitalia (male and female pseudohermaphroditism)

Other peripheral causes
Pregnancy
Gestational trophoblastic disease
Amenorrhea traumatica (Asherman's syndrome)

Chronic anovulation or ovarian failure
Degree of sexual development
Galactorrhea
Evidence of androgen excess
Evidence suggestive of adrenal or thyroid dysfunction

synechiae or adhesions (Asherman's syndrome) must be considered in individuals developing amenorrhea following curettage or endometritis. Tuberculous endometritis, especially in younger women, may also lead to this disorder. Without hormonal measurements it may be impossible to distinguish among individuals with chronic anovulation, in whom hypothalamic-pituitary-ovarian function is insufficiently coordinated to produce cyclic ovulation, and those with ovarian failure, in whom in most cases the ovaries are devoid of oocytes. Still, it is generally possible to form some strong clinical impressions about the etiology of the amenorrhea. It can be noted if the patient has absence of, incomplete, or complete development of secondary sex characteristics. The presence of excess body hair or galactorrhea may provide clinical evidence of the pathogenesis of the amenorrhea. Signs and symptoms of adrenal or thyroid dysfunction may be important as well.

The administration of a progestin has been advocated to assess the level of endogenous estrogen. This test is of limited value, however, because almost half the young women with premature ovarian failure experience withdrawal bleeding in response to progestin.

To ascertain if the outflow tract is intact, an orally active estrogen, such as 2.5 mg conjugated estrogen daily for 21 days with 5 to 10 mg of oral medroxyprogesterone acetate for the last 5 to 10 days, may be administered. Withdrawal bleeding should occur if the endometrium is normal. Still, hysterosalpingography and hysteroscopy may be required to diagnose Asherman's syndrome because some patients do continue to have some withdrawal bleeding.

Laboratory Evaluation. Basal levels of FSH, prolactin, and TSH should be measured in all amenorrheic and oligomenorrheic women to confirm the clinical impression (Fig. 224–8).

Increased TSH levels with or without increased levels of prolactin imply primary hypothyroidism, and further evaluation for this disorder is indicated (see Ch. 216). Although hypothyroidism commonly results in anovulation, amenorrhea occurs in only some hypothyroid women. Menorrhagia and oligomenorrhea may occur as well. The newly available very sensitive immunoassays for TSH permit identification of women with hyperthyroidism as well because TSH levels are suppressed in those individuals.

If the prolactin concentration is increased (typically greater than 20 to 30 ng per milliliter) and the TSH level is normal (generally less than 5 μU per milliliter), measurement of the prolactin concentration in the basal state should be repeated before more extensive evaluation is undertaken. This is the case because prolactin levels are increased by nonspecific stressful stimuli, sleep, and food ingestion. Prolactin levels may be elevated in as many as one third of women with amenorrhea. Evaluation of galactorrhea and hyperprolactinemia is detailed in Ch. 226.

Increased FSH levels (generally greater than 40 milli International Units [mIU] per milliliter) imply ovarian failure and require further evaluation. Chromosomal evaluation is indicated in all individuals with elevated FSH levels who are under the age of 30 years at the time the amenorrhea begins.

If prolactin and TSH concentrations are within normal ranges and FSH levels are low or normal, the measurement of total testosterone levels is indicated whether or not there is any evidence of hirsutism or virilization. Hyperandrogenic women need not be hirsute because some have relative insensitivity of the hair follicles to androgens. Mildly increased levels of testosterone (and perhaps DHEA-S as well) suggest PCO syndrome. However, total circulating androgen levels are rarely not elevated because of the alterations in metabolic clearance rate and SHBG that are present in PCO syndrome. Circulating levels of LH and FSH may aid in differentiating PCO syndrome from hypothalamic-pituitary dysfunction. LH levels are frequently elevated in PCO syndrome such that the ratio of LH to FSH is increased; however, LH levels may be identical to those observed in normal women in the follicular phase. In contrast, levels of LH and FSH are normal or slightly reduced in hypothalamic-pituitary dysfunction. There is some overlap between women with "PCO-like" disorders and those with hypothalamic-pituitary dysfunction. Radiographic assessment of the sella turcica is indicated in all amenorrheic women in whom both LH and FSH levels are very low (both less than 10 mIU per milliliter) to exclude a pituitary or parapituitary neoplasm. Other pituitary functions should be evaluated in any individual with significantly impaired LH and FSH secretion, as detailed subsequently. Both total testosterone and DHEA-S levels should be measured in hirsute or virilized women. Testosterone levels of greater than 200 ng per deciliter should lead to investigation for an androgen-producing neoplasm, most likely of ovarian origin. DHEA-S levels greater than 7.0 μg per milliliter should lead to evaluation for an adrenal neoplasm, and DHEA-S levels between 5.0 and 7.0 μg per milliliter should lead to evaluation for "adult-onset" congenital adrenal hyperplasia (see Ch. 221).

Hypergonadotropic Amenorrhea (Presumptive Ovarian Failure). DIFFERENTIAL DIAGNOSIS. Gonadal failure may begin at any time during embryonic or postnatal development and may result from many causes (Table 224–6). Normally the ovaries fail at menopause when virtually no functioning follicles remain. However, premature loss of oocytes prior to age 40 may occur and lead to premature ovarian failure, possibly from abnormalities in the recruitment and selection of oocytes. Since FSH is the principal regulator of folliculogenesis, it would seem that most causes of premature ovarian failure may somehow involve FSH secretion or action. Circulating gonadotropin levels increase whenever ovarian failure occurs, because of decreased negative estrogen feedback to the hypothalamic-pituitary unit.

Genetic Abnormalities. Several pathologic conditions with dys-

genetic gonads have elevated gonadotropin levels and amenorrhea. The term *gonadal dysgenesis* refers to individuals with undifferentiated streak gonads without any association with either extragonadal stigmata or sex chromosomal aberrations. Because individuals with gonadal dysgenesis have the normal complement of oocytes at 20 weeks of fetal age but virtually none by birth, this disorder is a form of premature ovarian failure.

Turner's syndrome describes patients with streak gonads composed of fibrous stroma and four cardinal features: (1) a female phenotype, (2) sexual infantilism, (3) short stature, and (4) several physical abnormalities, sometimes including a webbed neck, low-set ears, multiple pigmented nevi, double eyelashes, micrognathia, epicanthal folds, shieldlike chest with microthelia, short fourth metacarpals, an increased carrying angle to the arms, and certain renal and cardiovascular defects (most commonly coarctation of the aorta and aortic stenosis). The diagnosis can sometimes be made at birth because of unexplained lymphedema of the hands and feet. The syndrome is associated with an abnormality of sex chromosome number, morphology, or both. Most commonly the second sex chromosome is absent (45,X). This is the single most common chromosomal disorder in humans, but more than 95 per cent of such fetuses are aborted so that the incidence in newborns is approximately 1 in 3000 to 5000. Chromosomal breakage and mosaicism occur frequently as well. In mosaic individuals with a normal 46,XX cell line, sufficient follicles may persist postnatally to initiate pubertal changes and to cause ovulation so that pregnancy is possible.

Pure gonadal dysgenesis is the term given to phenotypically female individuals with streak gonads who are of normal stature and have none of the physical stigmata associated with Turner's syndrome. Such individuals have either a 46,XX or 46,XY karyotype. The 46,XX defect may be inherited as an autosomal recessive, with 10 per cent having associated nerve deafness. The 46,XY defect may be inherited as an X-linked recessive, with clitoromegaly occurring in 10 to 15 per cent and gonadal tumors developing in 25 per cent if the gonads are not removed.

Trisomy X (46,XXX karyotype) is also associated with premature menopause, while many such individuals actually have normal reproductive lives. Premature menopause can also occur in mosaic individuals with cell lines with excess X chromosomes. When gonadal abnormalities occur in women with excess X chromosomes, they seem to occur after ovarian differentiation so that some ovarian function is possible. Only later in life do such women develop secondary amenorrhea and premature ovarian failure.

OTHER CAUSES. *Physical, Chemical, and Infectious Causes.* Irradiation and chemotherapeutic agents, especially alkylating

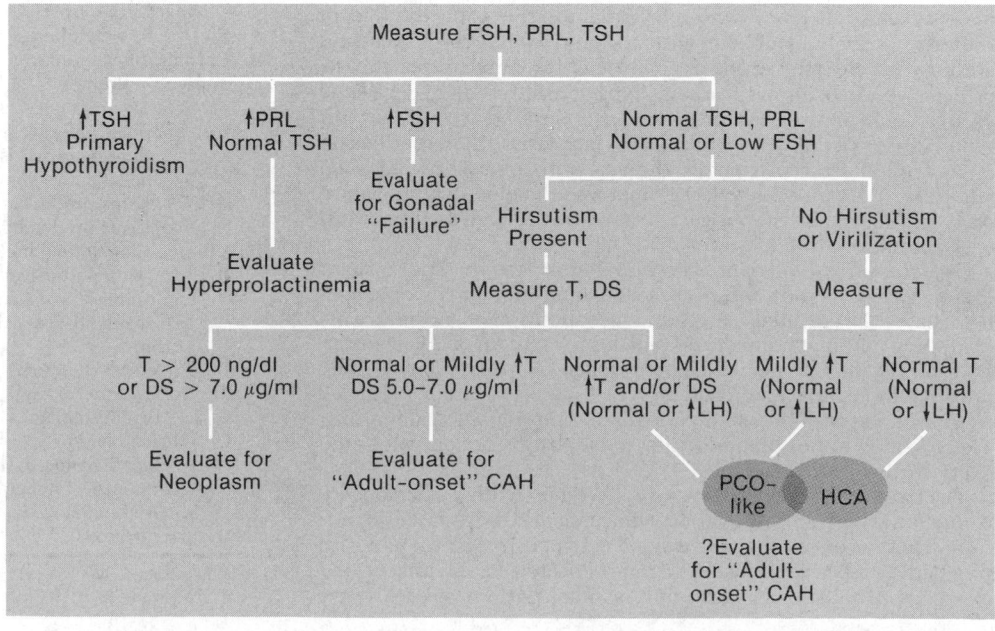

FIGURE 224–8. Biochemical evaluation of amenorrhea. This schema must be considered as an adjunct to the clinical evaluation of the patient. See text for details. **Abbreviations:** FSH = follicle-stimulating hormone; PRL = prolactin; TSH = thyroid-stimulating hormone; T = testosterone; DS = dehydroepiandrosterone sulfate; LH = luteinizing hormone; PCO-like = polycystic ovarian–like; HCA = hypothalamic chronic anovulation; CAH = congenital adrenal hyperplasia.

TABLE 224–6. CLASSIFICATION OF HYPERGONADOTROPIC AMENORRHEA (FSH > 40 mIU PER MILLILITER)

I. Menopause
II. Genetic abnormalities
  A. Genetically reduced cell endowment
  B. Accelerated atresia
  C. Gonadal dysgenesis
    1. With stigmata of Turner's syndrome (45,X)
    2. Pure (46,XX or 46,XY)
    3. Mixed
  D. Trisomy X with or without chromosomal mosaicism
  E. In association with myotonia dystrophica
III. Physical causes
  A. Gonadal irradiation
  B. Chemotherapeutic (especially alkylating) agents
  C. Viral agents
  D. Surgical extirpation
IV. Autoimmune disorders
  A. Polyglandular, involving ovarian failure and any combination of thyroiditis, hypoadrenalism, hypoparathyroidism, diabetes mellitus, myasthenia gravis, vitiligo, mucocutaneous candidiasis, and pernicious anemia
  B. Isolated ovarian failure
V. Enzymatic defects
  A. 17α-Hydroxylase deficiency
  B. Galactosemia
VI. Defective gonadotropin secretion and/or action
  A. Resistant ovary or Savage syndrome
  B. Secretion of biologically inactive forms
  C. α or β subunit defects
VII. Congenital thymic aplasia
VIII. Circulating gonadotropin antibodies
IX. Idiopathic premature ovarian failure

agents, utilized to treat various malignant diseases also may cause premature ovarian failure. Ovulation and cyclic menses return in some of these patients even after prolonged intervals of hypergonadotropic amenorrhea associated with signs and symptoms of profound hypoestrogenism. Rarely, mumps affects the ovaries and causes ovarian failure.

Autoimmune Disorders. Premature ovarian failure may occur in conjunction with a variety of autoimmune disorders. The most well known syndrome involves hypoadrenalism, hypoparathyroidism, and mucocutaneous candidiasis together with ovarian failure (see Ch. 228). Thyroiditis is the most commonly associated abnormality. Antibodies to the FSH receptor have been identified in a very few cases. These associations make it mandatory to rule out other potentially life-threatening endocrinopathies in young women with hypergonadotropic amenorrhea.

Enzymatic Defects. In girls with the rare syndrome of 17α-hydroxylase deficiency who survive until the expected age of puberty, sexual infantilism and primary amenorrhea occur together with elevated levels of gonadotropins. Increased synthesis of desoxycorticosterone leads to hypertension with hypokalemic alkalosis; serum progesterone levels are elevated as well. As with other causes of congenital adrenal hyperplasia, the hypertension is controlled by replacement therapy with glucocorticoids (see Ch. 221). Women with galactosemia also develop ovarian failure early in life, even when a galactose-restricted diet is introduced early in infancy (see Ch. 168).

Defective Gonadotropin Secretion and/or Action. The resistant ovary (Savage) syndrome occurs in young amenorrheic women who have (1) elevated peripheral gonadotropin concentrations, (2) normal (although immature) follicles present on ovarian biopsy, (3) a 46,XX karyotype with no evidence of mosaicism, (4) fully developed secondary sex characteristics, and (5) ovarian resistance to stimulation with human menopausal or pituitary gonadotropins. There seems to be some block to gonadotropin action within the ovary in this syndrome.

THERAPEUTIC CONSIDERATIONS. Women with hypergonadotropic amenorrhea and ovarian failure should be treated identically whether or not they have signs of hypoestrogenism or desire pregnancy. Ovarian biopsy is not indicated to document the existence of follicles because only a small portion of each ovary can be sampled and because pregnancies have resulted in patients who had biopsies devoid of follicles. Estrogen replacement is warranted to prevent the accelerated bone loss known to occur in affected women (see Ch. 238). The estrogen should be given sequentially with a progestin to prevent endometrial hyperplasia. Young women with ovarian failure may require twice as much estrogen as postmenopausal women for relief of signs and symptoms of hypoestrogenism.

Women with hypergonadotropic amenorrhea are rarely able to become pregnant. Pregnancy is more likely to occur with estrogen replacement therapy than with any other therapy. It is not clear why pregnancy is rarely possible in such women. Even with estrogen replacement the pregnancy rate is less than 10 per cent. The most successful treatment of young women with hypergonadotropic amenorrhea involves hormone replacement to mimic the normal menstrual cycle and embryo transfer utilizing donor oocytes. Pregnancy rates are higher than in other women undergoing in vitro fertilization and typically exceed 30 per cent per cycle.

Differential Diagnosis and Treatment of Chronic Anovulation. Chronic anovulation, the most frequent form of amenorrhea encountered in women of reproductive age, implies that functional ovarian follicles remain and that cyclic ovulation can be induced or reinitiated with appropriate therapy (Table 224–7). Appropriate management requires that the etiology of the anovulation be determined. The pathophysiologic bases for several forms of anovulation are unknown, but the anovulation can be interrupted transiently by nonspecific induction of ovulation in the majority of affected women. It is important to recognize that anovulation can result in either amenorrhea or irregular (generally less frequent) menses.

TABLE 224–7. CAUSES OF CHRONIC ANOVULATION

I. Chronic anovulation of hypothalamic-pituitary origin
  A. Hypothalamic chronic anovulation
    1. Psychogenic
    2. Exercise associated
    3. Associated with diet, weight loss, and/or malnutrition
    4. Anorexia nervosa and bulimia
    5. Pseudocyesis
  B. Forms of isolated gonadotropin deficiency (including Kallmann's syndrome)
  C. Due to hypothalamic-pituitary damage
    1. Pituitary and parapituitary tumors
    2. Empty-sella syndrome
    3. Following surgery
    4. Following radiation
    5. Following trauma
    6. Following infection
    7. Following infarction
  D. Idiopathic hypopituitarism
  E. Hypothalamic-pituitary dysfunction or failure with hyperprolactinemia (multiple causes)
  F. Due to systemic diseases
II. Chronic anovulation due to inappropriate feedback (i.e., polycystic ovarian syndrome)
  A. Excessive extraglandular estrogen production (i.e., obesity)
  B. Abnormal buffering involving sex hormone–binding globulin (including liver disease)
  C. Functional androgen excess (adrenal or ovarian)
  D. Neoplasms producing androgens or estrogens
  E. Neoplasms producing chorionic gonadotropin
III. Chronic anovulation due to other endocrine and metabolic disorders
  A. Adrenal hyperfunction
    1. Cushing's syndrome
    2. Congenital adrenal hyperplasia (female pseudohermaphroditism)
  B. Thyroid dysfunction
    1. Hyperthyroidism
    2. Hypothyroidism
  C. Prolactin and/or growth hormone excess
    1. Hypothalamic dysfunction
    2. Pituitary dysfunction (microadenomas and macroadenomas)
    3. Drug induced
  D. Malnutrition

Modified from Rebar RW: Chronic anovulation. *In* Serra GB (ed.): The Ovary. New York, Raven Press, 1983, pp 217–240.

HYPOTHALAMIC CHRONIC ANOVULATION (HCA).

HCA is a heterogeneous group of disorders with similar manifestations. Emotional and physical stress, exercise, diet, weight loss, body composition, malnutrition, environment, and other unrecognized factors may contribute in varying proportions to the anovulation. Abrupt cessation of menses in women under 30 years of age who have no anatomic abnormalities of the hypothalamic-pituitary-ovarian axis and no other endocrine disturbances suggests a diagnosis of HCA. Affected individuals tend to be bright, educated, and engaged in intellectual occupations and may well give a history of psychosexual problems and socioenvironmental trauma. HCA is characterized by low to normal levels of gonadotropins and relative hypoestrogenism. Rarely, however, do affected women present with signs and symptoms of estrogen deficiency. Psychological counseling and/or a change in lifestyle, especially for those women engaged in strenuous exercise programs, may be effective in inducing cyclic ovulation and menses. For women desiring pregnancy, ovulation can also be induced with clomiphene citrate (50 to 100 mg per day for 5 days beginning on the fifth day of withdrawal bleeding). Treatment with human menopausal gonadotropin and human chorionic gonadotropin (hMG-hCG) or with GnRH administered in a pulsatile fashion may be effective in women who do not ovulate in response to clomiphene. Most physicians advocate the use of exogenous steroids to prevent osteoporosis. A regimen can be used consisting of oral conjugated estrogens (0.625 to 1.25 mg), ethinyl estradiol (20 μg), or micronized estradiol-17β (1 to 2 mg) or of transdermal estradiol-17β (0.05 to 0.10 mg) daily with oral medroxyprogesterone acetate (5 to 10 mg) added for the first 12 to 14 days of each month. Sexually active women can be given oral contraceptive agents as an alternative. If steroid therapy is administered, patients must be informed that the amenorrhea probably will be present when therapy is discontinued. Other physicians believe only periodic observation is indicated, with barrier methods of contraception recommended for fertility control. Adequate ingestion of calcium should be ensured regardless of therapy. Contraception is needed for sexually active women with HCA, because the functional defect is mild in these disorders and may resolve spontaneously at any time, with ovulation occurring prior to any episode of menstruation.

Individuals with amenorrhea and significant weight loss should be examined for the possibility of *anorexia nervosa* (see Ch. 202). This disorder may be the most severe form of functional HCA, or it may be a distinct entity.

Kallmann's syndrome (isolated gonadotropin deficiency or familial hypogonadotropic hypogonadism) is a familial disorder consisting of gonadotropin deficiency, anosmia or hyposmia, and color blindness in men or, more rarely, in women. Other midline defects such as cleft lip and palate can occur in the affected individual or in family members. The trait is transmitted as an X-linked recessive or a male-limited autosomal dominant trait, but genetic heterogeneity may occur. Partial or complete agenesis of the olfactory bulb is present on autopsy, accounting for use of the term *olfactogenital dysplasia*. The disorder affects only gonadotropin secretion, and all other pituitary hormones are secreted normally. Isolated gonadotropin deficiency in the absence of anosmia occurs as well. Sexual infantilism with a eunuchoidal habitus is the clinical hallmark of this disorder, but moderate breast development may occur. Circulating LH and FSH levels are quite low, but almost always detectable. Ovulation induction requires use of hMG-hCG or pulsatile GnRH. Estrogen replacement therapy is indicated in these women until such time as pregnancy is desired. It may not be possible to distinguish between partial isolated gonadotropin deficiency and functional HCA in all cases.

Hypopituitarism may be obvious upon cursory inspection or sufficiently subtle to require endocrine testing (see Ch. 213). The clinical presentation depends on the age of onset, the etiology, and the nutritional status of the individual. Failure of development of secondary sex characteristics or for development to progress once puberty is initiated must always raise the question of hypopituitarism. Ovulation can be induced successfully with exogenous gonadotropins when pregnancy is desired and after the hypopituitarism is treated appropriately. Replacement therapy with estrogen is indicated to prevent signs and symptoms of estrogen deficiency.

Galactorrhea associated with hyperprolactinemia, whatever the

etiology, almost always occurs together with amenorrhea caused by hypothalamic-pituitary dysfunction or failure. Many conditions can cause excess prolactin secretion (see Ch. 226). It is unclear if all individuals with chronic anovulation associated with hyperprolactinemia and no other cause have pituitary microadenomas, even in the absence of identifiable radiographic changes of the sella turcica. Hirsutism may be observed occasionally in association with amenorrhea-galactorrhea and hyperprolactinemia. Elevated levels of the adrenal androgens DHEA and DHEA-S may be observed and may account for the polycystic-like ovaries present in some hyperprolactinemic women.

The hypothalamic-pituitary unit also may fail to function normally in a number of stressful, debilitating, systemic illnesses that interfere with somatic growth and development. Chronic renal failure, liver disease, and diabetes mellitus are the most prominent examples.

CHRONIC ANOVULATION DUE TO INAPPROPRIATE FEEDBACK.

PCO syndrome, which causes anovulation because of inappropriate feedback signals to the hypothalamic-pituitary unit, is a heterogeneous disorder in which there is considerable clinical and biochemical variability among affected individuals. Although patients usually present with amenorrhea, hirsutism, and obesity, affected women may instead complain of irregular and profuse uterine bleeding, may not have hirsutism, and may be of normal weight. Excess androgen from any source or increased extraglandular conversion of androgens to estrogens can lead to the typical findings of PCO syndrome. Included are such diverse disorders as Cushing's syndrome, mild congenital adrenal hyperplasia, virilizing tumors of adrenal or ovarian origin, hyperthyroidism and hypothyroidism, obesity, and primary PCO syndrome with no other recognizable etiology. In the primary syndrome the irregular menses, mild obesity, and hirsutism begin during puberty and typically become more severe with time. Obesity alone can lead to a PCO-like syndrome, with the degree of obesity required to cause anovulation varying widely from individual to individual. All such patients are well estrogenized regardless of whether they present with primary or secondary amenorrhea or dysfunctional bleeding. As noted, LH concentrations tend to be elevated, with relatively low and constant FSH levels, but both may be in the normal range compared to levels in women in the follicular phase of the menstrual cycle. Levels of most circulating androgens, especially testosterone, tend to be mildly elevated. The etiology of PCO syndrome is unknown, but current evidence suggests that the hypothalamic-pituitary unit is intact and that a functional derangement, perhaps involving insulin-like growth factors such as somatomedin C within the ovary, results in abnormal gonadotropin secretion.

The aim of the diagnostic evaluation is to rule out any causes (such as neoplasms) that require definitive therapy. Hirsutism should be evaluated as detailed in Ch. 225. PCO syndrome itself is a benign disorder. Patients generally require therapy for hirsutism, for induction of ovulation if pregnancy is desired, and for prevention of estrogen-induced endometrial hyperplasia and cancer. No ideal therapy exists, but rather the therapeutic approach must be individualized to the needs of each patient.

In the anovulatory woman not desiring pregnancy who is not hirsute, therapy with intermittent progestin administration (such as medroxyprogesterone acetate 5 to 10 mg orally for 10 to 14 days each month) or oral contraceptives can be provided to reduce the increased risk of endometrial carcinoma that is present in such a woman with unopposed estrogen. All women utilizing intermittent progestin administration should be cautioned about the need for effective contraception if they are sexually active, because these agents will not inhibit ovulation when administered intermittently.

The approach to the hirsute anovulatory woman not desiring pregnancy is detailed in Ch. 225. Oral contraceptive agents are the first line of therapy for such women with mild hirsutism and offer protection from endometrial hyperplasia.

In women with PCO syndrome desiring pregnancy, clomiphene citrate is the first approach to inducing ovulation because of its simplicity and high success rate. Approximately 75 to 80 per cent conceive with such therapy. Other possible methods of inducing ovulation include use of hMG-hCG, purified FSH, pulsatile GnRH, wedge resection of the ovaries at laparotomy, and laser or cautery destruction of follicles at laparoscopy. Surgical treatment is warranted only rarely and only in women in whom all other methods fail, in whom there is a question of an ovarian tumor because of ovarian size or circulating androgen levels, and in whom fertility is not an issue (because of the risk of pelvic adhesions from the surgery leading to infertility).

A particularly severe subset of affected women present with marked obesity, anovulation, mild glucose intolerance and high levels of circulating insulin with insulin resistance, acanthosis nigricans, hyperuricemia, and severe hirsutism with markedly elevated circulating androgen levels. These women have *hyperthecosis of the ovaries* in which the androgen-producing cells in the stromal, hilar, and thecal components of the ovaries are increased greatly in number. Although considered a separate entity by some clinicians, hyperthecosis probably should be viewed as a part of the spectrum comprising PCO syndrome.

Chronic Anovulation Due to Other Endocrine and Metabolic Disorders. Adrenal hyperfunction appears to cause chronic anovulation by inducing a PCO-like syndrome secondary to increased adrenal androgen secretion, but other possible mechanisms also exist.

Both hyperthyroidism and hypothyroidism are associated with a variety of menstrual disturbances, including dysfunctional uterine bleeding and amenorrhea as a result of alterations in the metabolism of androgens and estrogens. These metabolic changes in turn result in inappropriate steroid feedback and chronic anovulation.

Rebar RW: Exercise and the menstrual cycle. Exercise-related factors can lead to hypothalamic dysfunction. *In* Soules MR (ed.): Controversies in Reproductive Endocrinology and Infertility. New York, Elsevier, 1989, pp 41–58. *A detailed discussion of the effects of exercise on reproduction in women.*

Rebar RW: Practical evaluation of hormonal status. *In* Yen SSC, Jaffe RB (eds.): Reproductive Endocrinology, 2nd ed. Philadelphia, W. B. Saunders Company, 1986, pp 683–733. *A clinician describes a systematic approach to assessing ovarian function and clinical diagnosis. Bibliography is exhaustive.*

Rebar RW, Erickson GF, Coulam CB: Premature ovarian failure. *In* Gondos B, Riddick D (eds.): Pathology of Infertility. New York, Thieme Medical Publishers, Inc., 1987, pp 123–141. *A detailed discussion of the diagnosis and treatment of premature ovarian failure.*

Yen SSC: Chronic anovulation caused by peripheral endocrine disorders. *In* Yen SSC, Jaffe RB (eds.): Reproductive Endocrinology, 2nd ed. Philadelphia, W. B. Saunders Company, 1986, pp 441–499. *A detailed discussion of many of the causes of anovulation with an exhaustive bibliography.*

Yen SSC: Chronic anovulation due to CNS-hypothalamic-pituitary dysfunction. *In* Yen SSC, Jaffe RB (eds.): Reproductive Endocrinology, 2nd ed. Philadelphia, W. B. Saunders Company, 1986, pp 500–545. *A complete discussion of hypothalamic amenorrhea with an extensive bibliography.*

DISORDERS OF FOLLICULOGENESIS.

The recognized disorders of folliculogenesis are not identified until at or following ovulation, but they are believed to be manifestations of abnormalities in follicular development.

Luteinized Unruptured Follicle (LUF) Syndrome. The LUF syndrome describes development of a dominant follicle without its subsequent disruption and release of the ovum. The abnormality can be diagnosed by ultrasonography or by the absence of evidence of ovulation when the ovary is viewed at laparoscopy. The disorder is believed to occur infrequently and sporadically and is probably not a significant cause of infertility. Menstrual cycles in which no ovum is released are characterized by presumptive evidence of ovulation, including biphasic basal body temperatures, secretory endometrium, a normal LH surge, and normal progesterone production in the luteal phase. In fact, although the syndrome is believed to occur, data to substantiate its existence are only circumstantial (although strongly so) at present.

Luteal Phase Dysfunction. Progesterone secretion in the luteal phase may be reduced in duration (termed luteal phase insufficiency) or in amount (termed luteal phase inadequacy). More rarely the endometrium may be unable to respond to secreted progesterone because of the absence of progesterone receptors. These disorders are believed to represent causes for infertility (because of inability of fertilized ova to implant) in approximately 5 per cent of infertile couples. Abnormalities of the follicular phase, especially in the frequency of gonadotropin pulses, may account for most luteal phase dysfunction. Luteal phase defects also may occur sporadically in normally ovulating women approximately once each year.

Luteal phase dysfunction may be associated with several clinical entities, including mild or intermittent hyperprolactinemia (of any etiology), strenuous physical exercise, inadequately treated 21-hydroxylase deficiency, and habitual abortion. Luteal dysfunction occurs more commonly at the extremes of reproductive life and in the first menstrual cycles following full-term delivery, abortion, or discontinuation of oral contraceptives. It also may occur during ovulatory cycles induced with clomiphene citrate or hMG-hCG.

The diagnosis of luteal phase dysfunction can be made either by endometrial biopsy or by serial progesterone determinations. Endometrial biopsies obtained from the uterine fundus in the late luteal phases of two different cycles must be at least 2 days out of phase from the expected date of bleeding, as judged from the subsequent menstrual cycle, for the diagnosis to be made. The absolute concentration that progesterone must achieve and the length of time progesterone must be increased in the luteal phase to exclude luteal dysfunction are unclear. Luteal dysfunction is extremely rare in women with menstrual cycles greater than 25 days in length in whom a single random progesterone determination is greater than 15 ng per milliliter.

Treatment of luteal dysfunction is controversial. Any underlying defect should be treated. If subsequent luteal function depends on prior follicular development, modification of follicular development with either clomiphene citrate (25 to 100 mg daily by mouth for 5 days beginning on cycle day 3 to 5) or FSH (75 to 300 IU intramuscularly for 3 to 5 days beginning on cycle day 3 to 5) is reasonable. hCG (2500 to 5000 IU intramuscularly at 2- to 3-day intervals beginning with the shift in basal body temperature) or progesterone (12.5 mg intramuscularly in oil daily or 25 mg twice a day as rectal or vaginal suppositories) can be utilized as well. Bromocriptine may correct the abnormality in individuals with hyperprolactinemia. Synthetic progestational agents should not be used to treat luteal phase defects because of their possible (although unproven) association with congenital anomalies. Furthermore, the synthetic progestins produce an abnormal endometrium. None of these agents has been shown to increase the pregnancy rate.

Daly DC: Luteal phase defects. *In* Gondos B, Riddick DH (eds.): Pathology of Infertility. New York, Thieme Medical Publishers, Inc., 1987, pp 169–184. *A complete review of what is known about luteal dysfunction.*

McNeely MJ, Soules MR: The diagnosis of luteal phase deficiency: A critical review. Fertil Steril 50:1, 1988. *A consideration of the difficulties involved in diagnosing luteal dysfunction.*

INFERTILITY. *Infertility* may be defined as involuntary inability to conceive. *Sterility* is total inability to reproduce. In either case the situation may or may not be correctable, especially for each particular couple. Failure to reproduce thwarts a basic human instinct and causes anger, guilt, and depression. More than 10 per cent of couples in the United States seek medical assistance for infertility.

The requirements for pregnancy to occur are several:

1. The male must produce adequate numbers of normal, motile spermatozoa.
2. The male must be capable of ejaculating the sperm through a patent ductal system.
3. The sperm must be able to traverse an unobstructed female reproductive tract.
4. The female must ovulate and release an ovum.
5. The sperm must be able to fertilize the ovum.
6. The fertilized ovum must be capable of developing and implanting in appropriately prepared endometrium.

Infertility is too frequently viewed primarily as a problem of the female. In fact, in approximately 40 per cent of cases, infertility is caused by the male (Table 224–8). In perhaps one third of couples more than one cause contributes to the infertility.

Peak age of fertility in the female is 25 years. For nulliparous women of this age the average time during which unprotected intercourse occurs until conception is 5.3 months. For parous women the average duration of intercourse until conception is 2.7 months. The reproductive performance of couples is influenced by the ages of the female and male partners, the frequency of intercourse, and the length of time the couple has been attempting to conceive. There is a decline in both female and male reproductive performance after age 25.

TABLE 224–8. CAUSES OF INFERTILITY AND THEIR APPROXIMATE INCIDENCE (%)

I. **Male factors (40%)**
  A. Decreased production of spermatozoa
    1. Varicocele
    2. Testicular failure
    3. Endocrine disorders
    4. Cryptorchidism
    5. Stress, smoking, caffeine, nicotine, recreational drugs
  B. Ductal obstruction
    1. Epididymal (postinfection)
    2. Congenital absence of vas deferens
    3. Ejaculatory duct (postinfection)
    4. Postvasectomy
  C. Inability to deliver sperm into vagina
    1. Ejaculatory disturbances
    2. Hypospadias
    3. Sexual problems (i.e., impotence), medical or psychological
  D. Abnormal semen
    1. Infection
    2. Abnormal volume
    3. Abnormal viscosity
  E. Immunologic factors
    1. Sperm-immobilizing antibodies
    2. Sperm-agglutinating antibodies
II. **Female factors**
  A. Fallopian tube pathology (20 to 30%)
    1. Pelvic inflammatory disease or puerperal infection
    2. Congenital anomalies
    3. Endometriosis
    4. Secondary to past peritonitis of nongenital origin
  B. Amenorrhea and anovulation (15%)
  C. Minor ovulatory disturbances (<5%?)
  D. Cervical and uterine factors (10%)
    1. Leiomyomas and polyps
    2. Uterine anomalies
    3. Intrauterine synechiae (Asherman's syndrome)
    4. Destroyed endocervical glands (postsurgery or postinfection)
  E. Vaginal factors (<5%)
    1. Congenital absence of vagina
    2. Imperforate hymen
    3. Vaginismus
    4. Vaginitis
  F. Immunologic factors (<5%)
    1. Sperm-immobilizing antibodies
    2. Sperm-agglutinating antibodies
  G. Nutritional and metabolic factors (5%)
    1. Thyroid disorders
    2. Diabetes mellitus
    3. Severe nutritional disturbances
III. **Idiopathic or unexplained (< 10%)**

Couples who complain of infertility merit evaluation regardless of the length of infertility. If the couple believes there is a problem, it is the physician's responsibility to reassure them by appropriate evaluation and subsequent explanation of all findings and the prognosis.

The evaluation begins with a detailed history obtained from both partners and physical examinations of both individuals. The couple should be seen together for the first visit. Each couple should be questioned together and separately, since separate interviews may uncover information that would not be imparted in the presence of the partner.

Initial evaluation of infertility generally includes (1) assessment of semen, (2) documentation of ovulation by basal body temperature, serum progesterone determination approximately 6 to 8 days before menses, or endometrial biopsy less than 3 days before onset of menses, and (3) evaluation of the female genital tract by hysterosalpingography. Basal serum levels of prolactin and thyroid hormones should be measured. Diagnostic laparoscopy with tubal dye instillation should be performed if all previous tests are normal, since 30 to 50 per cent of women are found to have endometriosis or tubal disease on surgical evaluation. Treatment must be predicated on the findings of the infertility evaluation.

Glass RH: Infertility. *In* Yen SSC, Jaffe RB (eds.): Reproductive Endocrinology, 2nd ed. Philadelphia, W. B. Saunders Company, 1986, pp 571–613. *A summary of the approach to the infertile couple.*

SEXUAL FUNCTION AND DYSFUNCTION. Although sexual responses begin following puberty, they can continue for the duration of a woman's life. Sexual responses generally are divided into four phases: excitement, plateau, orgasm, and resolution.

With sexual arousal and excitement, vasocongestion and muscular tension increase progressively, primarily in the genitals, manifested by vaginal lubrication in the female. The lubrication is due to formation of a transudate in the vagina. Sexual excitement is initiated by any of a variety of psychogenic or somatogenic sexual stimuli and must be reinforced to result in orgasm. With continued stimulation, the excitement phase increases in intensity into a plateau phase during which a high state of sexual interest is maintained. The plateau phase may be short or long, and it is from this phase that an individual can shift to orgasm. The orgasmic phase tends to be brief and is characterized by rapid release from the developed vasocongestion and muscular tension. The orgasmic release is also known as the climax because peak psychological and physical intensity is achieved and there is an attendant feeling of satisfaction. Copious secretions and transudate may flow during orgasm in women. While women may resolve toward sleep following orgasm, many remain responsive to sexual stimulation and may return to plateau and subsequent orgasm.

Characteristic genital and extragenital responses occur during these phases. Estrogens magnify the sexual responses, but responses may occur in estrogen-deficient women. For women these changes occur in the breasts and in the pudendal region and are variable from one response cycle to another. For some women, excitement proceeds quickly through plateau to orgasm, and orgasm is explosive and accompanied by vocalization and involuntary contractions of the pelvic skeletal muscles. For other women, the responses are slow in building, controlled in amplitude, and long lasting. For a few women orgasm never occurs; for many it is intermittently absent.

The somatic sensate focus enabling orgasmic release is variable and may include stimulation of the breast, vagina, or clitoris. The psychological aspect of coitus may involve concentration on the current partner or act or fantasies about other times and persons. While orgasms may vary in physiologic intensity, what is important is psychological satisfaction. Satisfaction for both men and women may be had without orgasm.

Women may seek consultation because of disturbances in normal sexual arousal or orgasm. Such sexual dysfunction may be due to either organic or functional disturbances.

A variety of diseases affecting neurologic function, including diabetes mellitus and multiple sclerosis, may prevent sexual arousal. So, too, may local pelvic disorders, such as endometriosis and vaginitis, which cause dyspareunia and lead to sexual avoidance. Estrogen deficiency causing vaginal atrophy and dyspareunia is a relatively common cause of sexual dysfunction. Debilitating systemic diseases such as malignant disease may also affect sexual function indirectly.

In most cases the cause of sexual dysfunction is psychological. For instance, vaginismus involves involuntary contractions of the muscles surrounding the introitus and leads to dyspareunia. It is a conditioned response engendered by a previous imagined or real traumatic sexual experience. Feelings of guilt, caused by incest or rape as examples; of inadequacy, caused by hysterectomy or mastectomy; or of depression or anxiety may lead to failure to be aroused. Failure to achieve orgasm may be viewed as a dysfunction if the woman is frustrated or dissatisfied.

Treatment of sexual dysfunction is best accomplished by eliminating functional causes and providing the patient, often together with her partner, with appropriate psychological counseling. Behavioral modification is effective in treating many women with psychological sexual dysfunction.

Kaplan HS: The Evaluation of Sexual Disorders: Psychological and Medical Aspects. New York, Brunner-Mazel, 1983. *A good general text detailing sexual disorders.*
Kaplan HS: The Illustrated Manual of Sex Therapy, 2nd ed. New York, Brunner-Mazel, 1987. *A simple text graphically detailing the therapeutic techniques first introduced by Masters and Johnson.*
Kolodny RC, Masters WH, Johnson VE: Textbook of Sexual Medicine. Boston, Little, Brown and Company, 1979. *A widely used text detailing sexual problems and their therapy.*
Masters W, Johnson V: Human Sexual Response. Boston, Little, Brown and

Company, 1966. *The classic work detailing human sexual response. Required reading for all individuals seriously interested in this field.*

Nadelson CC, Marcotte DB (eds.): Treatment Interventions in Human Sexuality. New York, Plenum Press, 1983. *A multiauthored text that considers sexual problems in detail.*

HORMONAL THERAPY DURING THE REPRODUCTIVE YEARS

INDUCTION OF OVULATION. Induction of ovulation should never be attempted until serious disorders precluding pregnancy are ruled out or treated. Furthermore, ovulation induction should be utilized only in women with chronic anovulation, because women with ovarian failure are unresponsive to any form of ovulation induction. In general, the use of pharmaceutical agents does not improve the quality of an ovum, and thus the chance of pregnancy is not improved in women who ovulate regularly.

Clomiphene citrate is the agent that usually induces ovulation most easily. Clomiphene should be utilized in individuals without hyperprolactinemia who have the ability to release LH and FSH. A typical course of clomiphene therapy is begun on the fifth day following either spontaneous or induced uterine bleeding. The initial dosage is 50 mg daily for 5 days. Clomiphene appears to act as an anti-estrogen and stimulates gonadotropin secretion by the pituitary gland to initiate follicular development. If ovulation is not achieved in the very first cycle of treatment, the daily dosage is increased to 100 mg. If ovulation is still not achieved, dosage is increased in a stepwise fashion by 50 mg increments to a maximum of 200 to 250 mg daily for 5 days. The highest dose should be continued for 3 to 6 months before the patient is regarded as a clomiphene failure. The quantity of drug and the length of time that it can be used, as suggested here, are greater than those recommended by the manufacturers, but conform with published series.

The ovulatory surge of LH may occur 5 to 12 days (average, 7 days) after the completion of the last day of clomiphene treatment in each course. Couples are advised to have intercourse every other day during this time interval. Ovulation can be documented by monitoring changes in basal body temperature or preferably by measuring serum progesterone approximately 14 days after the last clomiphene tablet is taken. In addition, menses should occur about 3 weeks after the last day of therapy. Withdrawal bleeding with progestin can be induced if the patient fails to bleed within 4 weeks of therapy and if a serum hCG level documents that the patient is not pregnant.

Some clinicians give 5000 to 10,000 IU of hCG intramuscularly 7 days after the last day of clomiphene therapy to trigger ovulation, but this approach has not been established to increase effectiveness. The administration of hCG, however, does serve to time ovulation and may be helpful in selected couples. Ovulation can be expected to occur approximately 36 hours after hCG administration.

In appropriately selected patients, 75 to 80 per cent will ovulate and 40 to 50 per cent can be expected to become pregnant. About 15 per cent of pregnancies can be expected with each ovulatory cycle. The multiple pregnancy rate is about 8 per cent, with almost all being twins. The incidence of congenital anomalies is not increased.

Side effects of clomiphene are uncommon and very rarely serious. The most serious side effects include vasomotor flushes (10 per cent), abdominal discomfort (5 per cent), breast tenderness (2 per cent), nausea and vomiting (2 per cent), visual symptoms (1.5 per cent), and headache (1 per cent). Significant ovarian enlargement may occur but is rare (5 per cent).

The addition of dexamethasone, 0.5 mg orally at bedtime to blunt the nighttime secretion of ACTH, may be useful in hyperandrogenic women with an adrenal component who fail to ovulate in response to clomiphene. Other individuals failing to respond to clomiphene typically require hMG-hCG or perhaps pulsatile GnRH to induce ovulation.

Bromocriptine, a dopamine agonist, is effective in inducing ovulation in hyperprolactinemic women (see Ch. 226). The drug should be stopped once pregnancy is confirmed. Ovulatory menses and pregnancy are achieved in about 80 per cent of patients with galactorrhea and hyperprolactinemia. The majority of women with prolactin-secreting pituitary tumors remain asymptomatic during pregnancy. It is extremely rare for a patient with either a microadenoma or a macroadenoma to develop a problem related to the tumor that affects either the mother or the fetus during pregnancy. Monitoring during pregnancy need consist only of questioning the patient about the development of visual symptoms and headaches. Formal assessment of visual fields and CT or MRI should be carried out in any patient developing suspicious symptoms. Symptoms generally abate with institution of bromocriptine therapy. No adverse effects of bromocriptine on fetuses or pregnancies have been reported.

hMG, a purified preparation of gonadotropins extracted from the urine of postmenopausal women, must be administered intramuscularly. Each vial contains 75 units of FSH and 75 units of LH. Purified FSH has become available for use recently. Biochemically engineered preparations of both products will become available in the future. hMG is administered at doses of two to four vials for 5 to 12 days to achieve follicular development as monitored by ultrasound and serum or urinary E_2 concentrations. hCG, 5000 to 10,000 IU, is administered as a single intramuscular dose when follicular maturation is apparent. The hCG should be withheld if more than three follicles mature together. GnRH analogues are now being utilized to suppress endogenous follicular activity before initiating therapy with hMG and continued until hCG is given in older women and those with poor responses to hMG alone. Use of the analogues necessitates administration of larger quantities of hMG. Success rates, however, seem to be somewhat improved with this combined therapy.

Because of the expense and the complication rate, thorough evaluation should be carried out to exclude other causes of infertility before hMG-hCG is used. Ovulation can be induced in almost 100 per cent of patients, but pregnancy will occur in only 50 to 70 per cent. There is no increased risk of congenital anomalies with hMG-hCG.

The rate of multiple pregnancies with hMG-hCG may approach 30 per cent, with 5 per cent being triplets or more. Ovarian hyperstimulation is the major side effect and may be life threatening. The ovaries enlarge remarkably in this treatment-induced syndrome, and multiple follicle cysts, stromal edema, and multiple corpora lutea are present. There is a shift of fluid from the intravascular space into the abdominal cavity with resultant hypovolemia and hemoconcentration. The cause of the ascites is unknown. Treatment is conservative, with monitoring of fluid and electrolyte status. Pelvic examinations should not be performed for fear of rupturing the ovaries. The hyperstimulation generally will resolve slowly over about 7 days.

GnRH, administered intravenously or less effectively subcutaneously at doses of 5 to 20 μg every 60 to 120 minutes, also can be used to induce ovulation in women with an intact pituitary gland. It is most effective in individuals with hypothalamic chronic anovulation. hCG can be administered to support the corpus luteum after ovulation at a dose of 1500 IU intramuscularly every 3 days for three to four doses. The advantage of GnRH rests in the fact that hyperstimulation is extremely unlikely. However, reported pregnancy rates have been no greater than those achieved with hMG-hCG. Furthermore, some patients do not tolerate wearing the infusion pump that must be utilized.

Speroff L, Glass RH, Kase NG: Induction of ovulation. *In* Speroff L, Glass RH, Kase NG: Clinical Gynecologic Endocrinology and Infertility, 4th ed. Baltimore, Williams & Wilkins Company, 1989, pp 583–609. *A detailed and practical survey of how to induce ovulation.*

STEROIDAL CONTRACEPTION. *Physiologic Actions and Metabolic Effects.* Oral contraceptive pills are the most widely used contraceptives worldwide, with more than 50 million users. Combination (estrogen-progestin) and progestin only preparations are available. The estrogen may be either mestranol or ethinyl estradiol, while the progestin is usually one of six derivatives of 19-nor-testosterone: norethindrone, norethindrone acetate, norethynodrel, ethynodiol diacetate, norgestrel, and levonorgestrel. New progestins will soon be widely available.

The low-dose combination pills currently in use (containing 30 to 35 μg of estrogen with reduced amounts of progestin) were developed to reduce the biochemical changes produced by contraceptive steroids, but the majority of studies were conducted with the older high-dose preparations. It is known that virtually all biochemical changes are dose related.

Combination oral contraceptives inhibit the midcycle gonadotropin surge by inhibiting GnRH release from the hypothalamus. Cervical mucus becomes thick, viscid, and scanty in amount, thus retarding sperm penetration. Fallopian tube motility and secretion are altered as well, and the endometrial glands produce less glycogen. Efficacy is substantiated by a failure rate of 0.1 per cent during the first year of combination oral contraceptive use, lower than with any other reversible form of contraception.

Oral contraceptives decrease maturation of the vaginal epithelium and somehow render the vagina more susceptible to candidiasis. The endometrium becomes atrophic with variable degrees of decidual change, leading to diminished menstrual flow. Follicular development is arrested with low estrogen and progesterone secretion. Both circulating LH and FSH levels are reduced and constant.

The general metabolic effects of oral contraceptives resemble those of pregnancy. Glucose tolerance is impaired, with an increase in plasma insulin levels. The "mini-pill" containing progestin only in low dosage may cause no changes in glucose metabolism. Levels of circulating triglycerides and of very low density lipoproteins (VLDL) are often increased, almost entirely because of the estrogenic component (see Ch. 172). Only slight changes are seen with the low-dose combination preparations. Only very high estrogenic formulations will increase mean serum cholesterol levels. Because of a direct effect of estrogens on the endoplasmic reticulum in the liver, α_2 globulins, including angiotensinogen, and β globulins are increased, while serum albumin levels are decreased somewhat. A number of blood coagulation factors and carrier proteins (including thyroid-binding globulin, transferrin, ceruloplasmin, SHBG, and corticosteroid-binding globulin) are also increased.

Interactions with Other Drugs. Oral contraceptive steroids interact with several other drugs, leading to reduced effectiveness of the contraceptives or of the other drug. Such interactions occur because of altered drug absorption or metabolism. The majority of these interactions occur only with long-term use of the pharmacologic agent. By inducing hepatic microsomal enzymes, long-term administration of antibiotics may reduce the contraceptive efficacy of the steroids. The short-term use of antibiotics is probably of little concern. Anticonvulsants also sharply reduce the efficacy of contraceptive steroids, as do antacids, which may decrease the absorption of steroids. Conversely, contraceptive steroids oppose the therapeutic effects of anticoagulants, antidiabetic agents, and certain antihypertensive agents, such as guanethidine and α-methyldopa, because of their metabolic effects. Because of the impaired elimination of certain drugs, such as phenothiazines, oral contraceptive users may require lower doses.

Complications, Side Effects, and Benefits. Although the complications and side effects of combination oral contraceptives have been widely reported, the low-dose formulations currently available have minimized the side effects compared to the older, high-dose preparations without sacrificing contraceptive efficacy or reducing the substantial health benefits associated with oral contraceptive use.

The use of oral contraceptives increases the risk of *thromboembolism*, possibly as much as 4- to 13-fold with the doses of estrogens used in early preparations. The estrogen content of oral contraceptives appears to be correlated roughly with the risk of venous thromboembolic disease. Lower dosages of estrogen than were used initially in oral contraceptive preparations may not significantly increase the risk of any cardiovascular complications. Advanced maternal age and smoking seem to be the major risk factors for the use of oral contraceptives. In the absence of smoking and in women under the age of 45 years who do not suffer from obesity, hypertension, diabetes mellitus, or inherited lipoprotein abnormalities, there is little, if any, increased risk to low-dose combination oral contraceptive users for cardiovascular disease, including myocardial infarction. Some clinicians believe that these preparations may be used safely in normal women until the menopause.

In the absence of smoking and hypertension, it appears unlikely that there is an increased risk of fatal and nonfatal stroke from the use of low-dose oral contraceptives, in contrast to the enhanced risk of both thrombotic and hemorrhagic stroke reported earlier from the use of preparations containing larger amounts of estrogens. Some but not all women with migraine headaches may note increasingly frequent headaches with oral contraceptive use. Women with migraine headaches do not seem to be at increased risk of stroke.

Women using oral contraceptives are more likely to become hypertensive, especially if over the age of 35 years. Smoking may contribute to the incidence of hypertension. Increases in blood pressure are generally reversible shortly after oral contraceptives are discontinued. Failure of the blood pressure to return to normal when oral contraceptives are discontinued suggests underlying disease.

Contraceptive steroids do not appear to be teratogenic. Derivatives of 19-nor-testosterone can virilize female fetuses when administered in large doses to women early in pregnancy, but the doses required are far in excess of those contained in oral contraceptives.

Use of oral contraceptives reduces the risk of benign breast neoplasia, including fibrocystic disease and fibroadenoma. Since benign breast disease is a significant risk factor for the subsequent development of breast cancer, oral contraceptives may afford protection against breast cancer in this manner. Indeed, the incidence of breast cancer does not seem to be increased by use of oral contraceptives. Furthermore, oral contraceptives reduce the risk of developing endometrial carcinoma by about half and of developing ovarian carcinoma by about 40 per cent. In the cases of both endometrial and ovarian cancers, the protection is related to duration of use and persists for at least 10 years after stopping oral contraceptives.

Use of combined oral contraceptives may result in an increased risk for the development of *hepatocellular adenoma*, and this risk may increase with increased duration of contraceptive use. Rarely in patients with such adenomas the liver may rupture, and death may even occur because of hemorrhage. There is no evidence of any increased risk of developing liver cancer.

The relationships of oral contraceptive use to cervical carcinoma, pituitary tumors, and melanoma are unclear. Some studies show positive relationships between cervical dysplasia and oral contraceptive use, while other studies do not. Cervical dysplasia is increased in women with first coitus at an early age and those who have multiple sexual partners. Since oral contraceptive use may encourage such sexual behavior, any such relationship is difficult to interpret. In addition, Pap smear screening is much more common among oral contraceptive users so that cervical neoplasia may be detected more frequently in these women. There is some evidence that the incidence of prolactinomas may be increasing in women, but the use of contraceptive steroids has not been shown to increase this risk.

So-called *post-pill amenorrhea* is sometimes regarded as a side effect of oral contraceptive use. The return to ovulation following discontinuation of contraceptive use is variable but occurs within 4 to 8 weeks in most patients. Approximately 1 in 500 patients will have amenorrhea for 6 months or longer, with 15 per cent of these having associated galactorrhea. This prolonged amenorrhea is probably caused by underlying disorders unrelated to oral contraceptive use. In normal women subsequent fertility is unimpaired.

Nausea and vomiting occur occasionally when use begins, but generally abate with continued use. Mastalgia and increased breast size may occur, but also tend to subside in several cycles. Chloasma (hyperpigmentation of the face) is a leading cause of pill discontinuation. Acne is usually improved, but occasionally may be exacerbated. Dizziness, headaches, visual disturbances, depression, and increased or decreased libido have been reported. Easy bruisability due to increased capillary fragility and edema also may occur.

Other therapeutic benefits exist with oral contraceptive use as well. The risk of pelvic inflammatory disease appears reduced by half. Decreased menstrual blood loss results in a lower incidence of iron deficiency anemia. Acne frequently improves and dysmenorrhea decreases in the majority of patients. Symptomatic relief of endometriosis occurs in some patients. The risk of functional ovarian cysts is decreased, as are the incidences of ectopic pregnancies and uterine fibroids. Women with PCO syndrome treated with oral contraceptives are afforded protection from endometrial carcinoma. Oral contraceptives may possibly afford protection against development of rheumatoid arthritis as well.

Absolute contraindications to the use of oral contraceptives include thrombophlebitis, thromboembolic disorders, cardiovascular disease, or a history of these conditions; markedly impaired liver function; known or suspected estrogen-dependent neoplasia; undiagnosed abnormal genital bleeding; known or suspected pregnancy; and congenital hyperlipidemia. Oral contraceptives generally should be administered with caution to smokers, women who are obese, and those with varicose veins. If headaches develop or become more frequent with pill use, oral contraceptives should be discontinued. Because of a possible increase in postsurgical thromboembolic complications in women using oral contraceptives, use of oral contraceptives should be discontinued 2 weeks prior to surgery and begun again 2 weeks postoperatively.

Low-dose combination oral contraceptive pills offer superb protection for sexually active women not desiring pregnancy. For most such individuals the benefits of the low-dose preparations clearly outweigh the adverse effects, but possible side effects and complications must be considered in treating individual patients.

Henzl MR: Contraceptive hormones and their clinical use. In Yen SSC, Jaffe RB (eds.): Reproductive Endocrinology, 2nd ed. Philadelphia, W. B. Saunders Company, 1986, pp 643–682. A detailed discussion of steroidal contraception.

Zatuchni GI: Known and potential complications of steroidal contraception. In Becker KL (ed.): Principles and Practice of Endocrinology and Metabolism. Philadelphia, J. B. Lippincott Company, 1990, pp 868–872. A detailed consideration of the risks of oral contraceptives.

THE MENOPAUSE AND POSTMENOPAUSAL YEARS

DEFINITIONS AND EPIDEMIOLOGY. The *menopause* is the final menstrual period denoting the cessation of cyclic ovarian function as manifested by cyclic menstruation. The *climacteric* is the physiologic period during which regression of ovarian function occurs. Its onset generally is signalled by alterations in the menstrual cycle or vasomotor symptomatology. Menopause occurs at a mean age of approximately 51 years. Today's average woman in the Western world can expect to live one third of her life in the postmenopausal phase.

SYMPTOMATOLOGY AND SIGNS. Most signs and symptoms associated with the postmenopausal years result from decreased circulating estrogen. Common symptoms include hot flushes, paresthesias, palpitations, cold hands and feet, headaches, vertigo, irritability, anxiety, nervousness, depression, fatigue, weight gain, insomnia, night sweats, forgetfulness, and inability to concentrate.

Vasomotor instability is perhaps the most common complaint. Over 75 per cent of women experience hot flushes with decreasing estrogen levels, and these may persist for years. In a typical hot flush, the skin, especially of the head and neck, becomes red and warm for a few seconds to 2 minutes with cold chills thereafter. Accompanying physiologic changes include a rise in skin temperature, peripheral vasodilatation, increased heart rate, decreased skin resistance, and concomitant LH pulses. The mechanism for hot flushes is unknown but must involve thermoregulatory centers in the hypothalamus.

Any increase in bleeding or bleeding after 6 months of amenorrhea demands examination and sampling of the endometrium to exclude carcinoma. Women note relocation of fat deposits, with increased fat in the lower abdomen, hips, and breasts. The genital skin becomes thin and pale, with a decrease in the size of the labia minora, clitoris, uterus, and ovaries, and the women often complain of dyspareunia. Decreased elastic tissue of skin is noted, and osteoporosis may occur in about 25 per cent of postmenopausal women (see Ch. 238).

Menopausal signs and symptoms may begin long before menses have ceased. Symptoms may be difficult to diagnose in women with previous hysterectomies. Following bilateral oophorectomy young women develop identical signs and symptoms.

ENDOCRINOLOGIC CHANGES. During the menopausal transition regular menstrual cycles may continue up to the menopause. The cycles may become shorter, due to shortened follicular phases, with increased FSH, normal LH, and decreased E_2 and progesterone levels in comparison to normal ovulatory cycles. Variable cycles also may occur prior to the menopause, with some being ovulatory and others being anovulatory. Waning ovarian follicular activity with decreasing E_2 production must be central to these changes, and yet some follicles have been found on occasion in ovaries of postmenopausal women.

In postmenopausal women, circulating FSH and LH concentrations are greatly increased. Estrogen levels are decreased markedly, but androgen levels are decreased only slightly. The postmenopausal ovaries continue to secrete substantial amounts of androgen (androstenedione and testosterone), which together with adrenal androgens are converted to estrogens by extraglandular conversion in the periphery. The peripheral conversion of androgens accounts for most circulating estrogen in postmenopausal women.

CLINICAL MANAGEMENT. Treatment of postmenopausal women must be individualized and based on a personal dialogue with each patient. Exogenous estrogen replacement will stop or diminish hot flushes, reverse atrophic genital changes, decrease osteoporotic fractures (see Ch. 238), and may decrease the incidence of atherosclerotic coronary artery disease.

Estrogen replacement therapy is absolutely contraindicated in postmenopausal women with estrogen-dependent tumors of the breast, uterus, or kidney; acute liver disease; cerebrovascular disease; deep-vein thrombosis and embolism; malignant melanoma; and undiagnosed genital bleeding. Replacement therapy must be considered carefully and other therapy may require modification in women with estrogen-associated hypertension, diabetes mellitus, cholecystitis and cholelithiasis, pancreatitis, congestive heart failure, past endometriosis, and neuro-ophthalmologic vascular disease. Individual exceptions to even the absolute contraindications exist.

Many treatment regimens are currently being utilized. Estrogen should be administered together with a progestin in a cyclic fashion to women with a uterus to prevent an increased risk of endometrial hyperplasia and carcinoma. Oral estrone sulfate (0.625 to 1.25 mg), micronized estradiol-17β (1 mg), or transdermal estradiol (0.05 mg) may be given daily. To this should be added a progestin such as medroxyprogesterone acetate (5 to 10 mg orally for 12 to 14 days each month, beginning on the first day of the month). Menstrual bleeding will occur in more than half of the women. As a consequence, continuous daily administration of a combination of an estrogen and a progestin has been advocated. The ratios of estrogen to progestin utilized are empiric. Unfortunately, irregular breakthrough bleeding occurs frequently in the first several months of therapy, even though the majority of women eventually become amenorrheic. Although continuous combined therapy is an option, it cannot be advocated strongly until more data accumulate regarding its safety and efficacy. Still another regimen provides estrogen and progestin Monday through Friday of each week, with no medication given on the weekends. Similar dosages of estrogen alone may be administered continuously to women who have undergone hysterectomy, particularly because progestins may impact negatively on several beneficial metabolic effects of estrogen. Younger women may require twice as much estrogen as older women to alleviate symptoms.

Even the continuous combined replacement therapy differs from oral contraceptive preparations in that the doses of estrogen and progestin are lower. Moreover, the estrogens utilized in replacement therapy have fewer metabolic effects than do the synthetic estrogens used in oral contraceptives. There is no evidence that postmenopausal estrogen administration increases the risk of thromboembolic phenomena.

Before beginning estrogen replacement therapy, patients should have a complete history and physical examination. A pretreatment mammogram is indicated because estrogens stimulate glandular tissue and may make diagnosis of breast masses more difficult. Periodic Papanicolaou smears should be obtained, and patients should undergo endometrial biopsy for any breakthrough bleeding and perhaps at intervals of 1 to 2 years while receiving estrogen replacement therapy. Some clinicians believe endometrial biopsies are not needed so long as there is no abnormal bleeding and withdrawal bleeding does not begin until at least 11 days after beginning progestin.

Side effects of therapy are common and may require modifications of therapy. Breast tenderness occurs frequently if too much estrogen is given. The dose of progestin should be reduced in the woman who complains of depression and/or bloating.

Medroxyprogesterone acetate (20 to 40 mg) or megestrol acetate (40 to 80 mg) orally each day may be utilized to treat hot flushes in women who cannot or will not take estrogens. Clonidine skin patches programmed to deliver 0.1 mg per day may also reduce the intensity and frequency of hot flushes in individuals who cannot take estrogens. Postural hypotension, however, is a common side effect with this therapy. Vaginal lubricants may be used for symptomatic treatment of dyspareunia in such individuals.

EFFECTS OF ESTROGEN ON LIPIDS AND CARCINOMA.
Unlike the effects of oral contraceptives in younger women, estrogen replacement in postmenopausal women does not raise blood pressure. This may be true because some estrogens, particularly those synthetic ones used in oral contraceptives, increase hepatic synthesis of renin substrate (angiotensinogen). The naturally occurring estrogens E_2 and E_1, however, do not increase renin substrate.

Estrogen administration tends to lower total cholesterol levels, although the degree of reduction varies with the dose and potency of the estrogen used. More importantly, estrogen decreases the LDL-cholesterol and increases the HDL-cholesterol fraction. Increased levels of the subfraction HDL_2 are most strongly associated with both estrogen ingestion and diminished cardiovascular risk. Thus the net effect of estrogen administration is to shift the HDL-LDL ratio to one associated with a decreased risk of cardiovascular disease. Overall, the risk of cardiovascular disease appears reduced by half in postmenopausal users of estrogen, but this reduced risk has not yet been confirmed by prospective studies. Estrogen administration to postmenopausal women may increase plasma triglycerides slightly, but these increases are generally of no significance except in some individuals with genetic disorders of triglyceride metabolism in whom marked elevations in triglycerides may occur.

Progestins, especially those derived from 19-nor-testosterone (such as norethindrone and norgestrel), oppose the effects of estrogens on plasma lipid and lipoprotein fractions. Even orally administered medroxyprogesterone, which is relatively neutral when given alone, appears to cancel the favorable changes induced by estrogens when given in combination with estrogen.

Estrogen-containing oral contraceptive preparations have not been linked conclusively to increased risks of endometrial or breast cancer. However, as noted, estrogen given alone to postmenopausal women greatly increases the risk of endometrial cancer over those never given estrogen. The risk of endometrial carcinoma is reduced markedly, if not abolished, by the cyclic addition of a progestin. Whether estrogen therapy increases the risk of breast cancer is not clear, but the majority of studies have not shown such a relationship. If there is any increased risk of breast cancer, the increase in risk appears modest. Because the likelihood of death from cardiovascular disease is far greater than that from breast cancer, it appears that the benefits of estrogen replacement therapy outweigh the risks in most postmenopausal women.

Korenman SG (ed.): The Menopause. Norwell, Mass, Serono Symposia, USA, 1990. *A review by leading authorities on the physiologic changes and therapeutic approaches to the menopause.*

Mezrow G, Rebar RW: The Menopause. *In* Sciarra JJ (ed.): Gynecology and Obstetrics, Vol. 4. Revised edition—1990. Philadelphia, J. B. Lippincott Company, pp 1-22. *An up-to-date summary of the management of the menopause.*

OVARIAN TUMORS

Ovarian tumors may cause ovarian dysfunction, either by secreting hormones or by stimulating adjacent non-neoplastic stromal cells. Only perhaps 5 per cent of ovarian tumors, however, show functional activity. Most nonfunctional tumors are asymptomatic until late in their evolution; more than three fourths are diagnosed only in advanced stages. In contrast, women with functioning neoplasms commonly present with altered sexual development or reproductive abnormalities, and thus diagnosis is made much earlier. Ovarian tumors may occur in all age groups but are less common in younger women, especially before puberty.

Ovarian tumors generally are classified as (1) common epithelial tumors derived from coelomic epithelial cells; (2) sex cord stromal tumors composed of granulosa cells, theca cells, Sertoli-Leydig cells, or their progenitors; (3) lipid or lipoid cell tumors; (4) germ cell tumors, including teratomas, dysgerminomas, and choriocarcinomas; (5) gonadoblastomas; (6) soft tissue tumors not specific to the ovary; and (7) secondary metastatic tumors. Each of these major classes of tumors includes several different histologic types. Sex cord stromal tumors are most apt to be functioning.

Ovarian neoplasms must be distinguished from tumor-like conditions of the ovary, which include luteomas of pregnancy (nodular theca-lutein hyperplasia) that may result in virilization of the mother but regress spontaneously post partum; hyperplasia of ovarian stroma (hyperthecosis), frequently associated with severe hirsutism; functional follicle and corpus luteum cysts; germinal inclusion cysts lined by surface epithelium; simple cysts; paraovarian cysts; inflammatory lesions; and endometrial cysts or endometriomas.

Ovarian neoplasms are diagnosed most commonly at the time of routine pelvic examination. Even most functioning neoplasms are palpable; those that are not may be identified by ultrasonography. As an ovarian tumor grows, it distends the abdomen, leading to pressure on the bladder or rectum and a sensation of pelvic fullness and discomfort. Ascites may develop if the neoplasm is malignant or sometimes when it is not (Meigs' syndrome).

TABLE 224–9. CLINICAL FEATURES OF HORMONE-PRODUCING OVARIAN TUMORS

Tumor	Hormones Produced*	Incidence Age in Years Peak	Range	Malignancy	Bilaterality	Size Range in cm (per cent Palpable)	Miscellaneous
Androblastoma (arrhenoblastoma)	*Androgens*, estrogens	20–40	4–69	20%	Rare	<5–>25 (85)	Most common virilizing ovarian neoplasm
Dysgerminoma	Androgens, *chorionic gonadotropin*	10–30	6–76	100%	15%	3–50 (60)	May be "mixed" with other tumors originating from germ cells
Gonadoblastoma	*Androgens*, estrogens	10–30	6–38	50%	40%	<1–>30 (?)	Usually occur in genetic males with female external genitalia
Granulosa-theca cell	*Estrogens*, androgens, progestogens	30–70	<1–92	5–20%	10–15%	<1–>30 (80–90)	Most common functioning ovarian neoplasm
Hilar cell	*Androgens*, estrogens	45–75	4–86	Rare	Rare	1–9 (50)	Hypertension in 50%, diabetes in 50%
Lipoid cell (adrenal-like)	*Androgens*, estrogens	20–50	6–78	20%	Rare	0.5–30	Diabetes associated with lesion in 50%
Teratomas, benign	Serotonin, thyroxine	10–40	<1–78	Rare	10%	2–45 (90)	Carcinoid syndrome only in patients with large carcinoid tumors
Teratomas, malignant	Chorionic gonadotropin	6–15	6–42	100%	Rare	>5 (100)	Not all secrete chorionic gonadotropin

Modified from data of Rose GI, Vande Wiele RL: *In* Williams RH (ed.): Textbook of Endocrinology, 5th ed. Philadelphia, W. B. Saunders Company, 1974, pp 368–422.
*When more than one hormone is secreted, the major one is *italicized.*

Abdominal and pelvic pain may occur with torsion, hemorrhage, or rupture of the tumor.

Functioning ovarian tumors can produce other clinical manifestations as well (Table 224–9). Some tumors are associated with clinical manifestations of decreased hormone production. Intervals of amenorrhea caused by steroid suppression of gonadotropins may alternate with excessive vaginal bleeding produced by steroid stimulation of the endometrium during the reproductive years. In some young girls, steroid-secreting ovarian tumors may cause pseudopubertal development. In postmenopausal women, increased estrogens, secreted by the tumor itself or from peripheral aromatization of androgens secreted by the tumor, may stimulate the endometrium and result in bleeding.

Any pelvic mass identified on examination must be investigated. What constitutes such a "mass" and what evaluation is indicated depend on the age of the individual. Adnexal masses less than 5 cm in diameter may well be due to normal follicular development in women of reproductive age and may resolve with observation over 2 to 8 weeks. Even cystic masses greater than 5 cm in diameter, as documented by ultrasound examination, may resolve over a few weeks. Those that do not resolve require surgical removal. Any palpable adnexal mass in a postmenopausal woman, in whom the ovaries normally atrophy and cannot be detected during examination, should be removed.

Yeh I-T, Zaloudek C, Kurman RJ: Functioning tumors and tumor-like conditions of the ovary. *In* Becker KL (ed): Principles and Practice of Endocrinology and Metabolism. Philadelphia, J. B. Lippincott Company, 1990, pp 848–854. *An excellent discussion of the clinical manifestations of ovarian tumors for any physician who undertakes the medical care of women.*

225 Hirsutism
Roger S. Rittmaster

DEFINITION. Normal Hair Growth. Most body hair can be classified as vellus or terminal. Vellus hairs are fine and unpigmented, such as those that cover the face of children. Terminal hairs, pigmented and coarser, may be sex hormone–dependent (such as those over the chin and abdomen of men) or sex hormone–independent (such as eyebrows and eyelashes) (Fig.

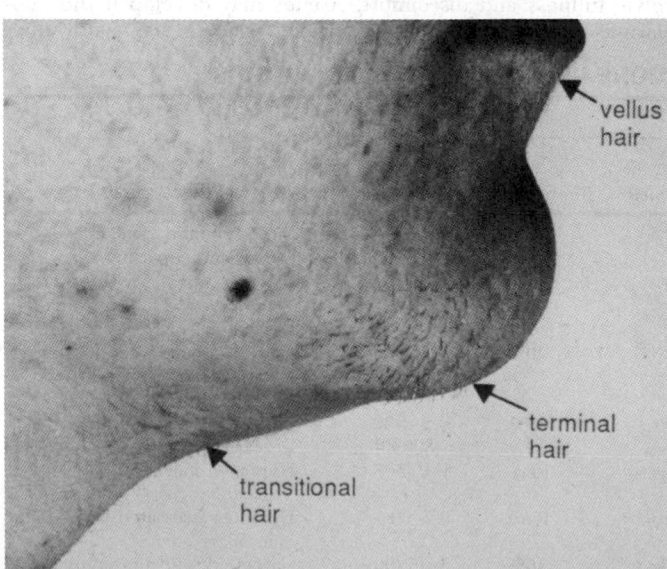

FIGURE 225–1. Facial hair growth in a hirsute woman. Vellus hair is fine, unpigmented hair. Terminal hair is coarse and pigmented. Transitional hair is intermediate between vellus and terminal. This woman also has mild acne, another androgen-dependent process. (Reprinted with permission from Rittmaster RS: Hirsutism. Med North Am 14:2686–2695, 1987.)

225–1). Androgens convert vellus hair to terminal hair in sex hormone–dependent areas.

Hirsutism. Hirsutism is the presence of excess hair in women. This is usually an androgen-dependent process. Twenty-five to thirty-five per cent of young women have terminal hair over the lower abdomen, around the nipples, or over the upper lip. Most women gradually develop more androgen-dependent body hair with age. Nevertheless, "normal" patterns of female hair growth are unacceptable to many women. At the other extreme, severe hirsutism may rarely be the earliest sign of masculinizing diseases. More often, however, severe hirsutism reflects only increased androgen production in women with no serious underlying disorder.

ETIOLOGY. Hirsutism may be divided into androgen-dependent and androgen-independent etiologies. Androgen-dependent hirsutism is restricted to areas where men typically become hirsute and often begins with adolescence. In women, androgens arise from the ovaries, the adrenal glands, or exogenous sources such as anabolic steroids (Table 225–1). Often, no definite abnormality exists; the hirsutism simply results from modestly increased androgen production and/or increased skin sensitivity to androgens.

Androgen-independent hirsutism is caused by drugs (cyclosporine, glucocorticoids, minoxidil, diazoxide, and possibly phenytoin) or starvation (anorexia nervosa); it may be associated with the skin lesions of porphyria; or it may be an inherited condition. Androgen-independent hirsutism is characterized by long, fine hairs occurring over much of the body, including such areas as the forehead and flanks. Androgens may exacerbate androgen-independent hirsutism, giving rise to a clinically confusing presentation. The pathophysiology of androgen-independent hirsutism is unknown.

PATHOPHYSIOLOGY OF ANDROGEN-DEPENDENT HIRSUTISM. To be active in skin, testosterone, the major circulating androgen, must first be converted to dihydrotestosterone by the enzyme 5α-reductase. Hirsute women have elevated skin 5α-reductase compared to nonhirsute women. Nevertheless, increased 5α-reductase alone is usually insufficient to induce hirsutism.

Hirsute women as a group also have increased androgen production from the adrenal glands, the ovaries, or both. Either testosterone itself is secreted, or androgen precursors such as androstenedione are secreted, which are then converted in the liver or skin to active androgens. Most hirsute women do not have an underlying disease, but simply fall at one end of the spectrum of androgen production and skin 5α-reductase activity.

The ovarian and adrenal causes of hirsutism listed in Table 225–1 lead to increased androgen production. Virilizing tumors secrete androgens directly. The pituitary adenomas in Cushing's disease release ACTH, which stimulates the adrenals to secrete both cortisol and androgens (Ch. 217). The virilizing forms of congenital adrenal hyperplasia involve enzyme defects that impair cortisol synthesis, leading to increased ACTH secretion (Ch. 217). The enzyme block causes shunting of cortisol precursors to

TABLE 225–1. CAUSES OF ANDROGEN-DEPENDENT HIRSUTISM

Ovarian causes
  Polycystic ovarian syndrome
  Severe insulin resistance
  Virilizing ovarian tumors
Adrenal causes
  Congenital adrenal hyperplasia
    21-Hydroxylase deficiency
    3β-Hydroxysteroid dehydrogenase deficiency
    11-Hydroxylase deficiency
  Cushing's disease
  Ectopic ACTH-producing tumors
  Virilizing adrenal tumors
Combined ovarian and adrenal causes
  "Idiopathic" hirsutism
Exogenous androgens
  "Anabolic" steroids
  Danazol
  Postmenopausal hormone replacement formulations containing androgens

androgens. The most common form, 21-hydroxylase deficiency, leads to an overproduction of 17-hydroxyprogesterone. While severe forms of 21-hydroxylase deficiency cause ambiguous genitalia in female infants, milder forms may lead only to hirsutism and/or irregular menses. This "attenuated" form of 21-hydroxylase deficiency is present in about 1 per cent of hirsute women.

In the polycystic ovarian syndrome, both the ovaries and adrenals secrete excess androgens, although the majority of the androgens are usually of ovarian origin (Ch. 224). Obesity is an important predisposing factor to the development of polycystic ovarian syndrome and, as such, can indirectly cause hirsutism.

CLINICAL MANIFESTATIONS. Androgen-induced hirsutism of benign origin usually begins in adolescence and becomes gradually worse with time. Family history is often positive. The hirsutism may vary from mild to severe. Usually hair growth begins over the lower abdomen, on the breasts, and over the upper lip. Hirsutism over the chin, above the umbilicus, and over the central chest requires somewhat greater androgenicity. Widespread hirsutism over the upper back, upper abdomen, and upper chest implies severe hyperandrogenism. Some women may have only facial hair or other unusual patterns of hirsutism, probably due to local variation in skin 5α-reductase activity.

Severe, rapidly progressive hirsutism, beginning in childhood or beyond adolescence, suggests an androgen-secreting tumor. Such tumors can cause signs of virilization: deepening of the voice, excess muscle development, and marked clitoral enlargement. Signs of virilization, however, simply imply severe hyperandrogenism and can occasionally be seen with all causes of hirsutism. Androgen-secreting tumors are rare, and most severely hirsute women have either polycystic ovarian syndrome or hirsutism alone.

Attenuated congenital adrenal hyperplasia is clinically indistinguishable from simple hirsutism or polycystic ovarian syndrome, and the diagnosis must be made biochemically. Cushing's disease may be suspected when the patient presents with central obesity, hypertension, diabetes, and/or thinning of the skin (see Ch. 217).

DIAGNOSIS. The diagnostic evaluation of hirsutism is directed at ruling out a significant underlying cause. Important historical points include a drug history (including use of oral contraceptives), age of onset and rate of progression of hirsutism, presence of thinning of scalp hair or deepening of the voice, menstrual history, history of obesity, and family history of hirsutism. The physical examination should include an assessment of the quality and distribution of hair growth, signs of virilization or Cushing's syndrome, and presence of abdominal or pelvic masses.

Laboratory Evaluation. In women with androgen-dependent hirsutism, regular ovulatory menses, and no physical signs of Cushing's syndrome, hormonal evaluation is usually unnecessary. Virilizing tumors have not been reported in such patients, and hirsutism associated with attenuated congenital adrenal hyperplasia need not be treated differently from other benign forms of hirsutism (see Treatment section).

In hirsute women with irregular menses, a reasonable laboratory evaluation includes measurement of serum testosterone, 17-hydroxyprogesterone, prolactin, LH, and FSH. A testosterone level less than 170 mg per deciliter (6 nmol per liter) rules out an androgen-secreting tumor, although re-evaluation may be necessary if the hirsutism continues to progress or signs of virilization appear. Testosterone levels above 170 mg per deciliter may also be seen with polycystic ovarian syndrome. To rule out attenuated 21-hydroxylase deficiency, serum 17-hydroxyprogesterone should be measured between 7 and 9 A.M. during the first week of the menstrual cycle (values may be elevated during the luteal phase). Values less than 200 mg per deciliter (6 nmol per liter) rule out this diagnosis. Mildly elevated values (less than 1000 mg per deciliter) (30 nmol per liter) may be seen in both heterozygous and homozygous 21-hydroxylase deficiency (the heterozygous disorder is not associated with hirsutism) and in polycystic ovarian syndrome. To distinguish between these conditions, 17-hydroxyprogesterone should be measured 30 to 60 minutes after the intravenous administration of 250 μg synthetic ACTH. Levels are greater than 1500 ng per deciliter (45 nmol per liter) in homozygous 21-hydroxylase deficiency. Other forms of attenuated congenital adrenal hyperplasia are too rare to justify routine hormonal screening. Serum prolactin, LH, and FSH are used to evaluate the possibility that a prolactinoma, ovarian failure, or polycystic ovarian syndrome is contributing to the irregular menses. These tests are not directly relevant to the evaluation of hirsutism itself. Measurement of dehydroepiandrosterone sulfate (DHEAS) as an index of adrenal androgen production is generally unhelpful.

TREATMENT. Hirsutism is a cosmetic problem that may have severe psychosocial consequences. Because it is not a disease in itself, the benefits and risks of any therapy should be carefully weighed and the treatment individualized.

Mechanical Hair Removal. For mild hirsutism, bleaching and mechanical hair removal are adequate and safe. Shaving is the easiest method of temporarily removing visible hair. While shaving does not increase hair growth rates, it may leave a stubble and is unacceptable to many women. Plucking and waxing may control mild hirsutism, but they also do not resolve the problem and may lead to scarring. Electrolysis can provide a safe, effective alternative for localized mild to moderate hirsutism and is a useful adjunct to medical therapy in more severe cases. Electrolysis is expensive, however, and long-term treatment may be necessary.

Drug Treatment. Successful medical therapy results in a gradual return of terminal hair to finer, less pigmented vellus hair. Younger women with mild hirsutism of brief duration respond best to medical therapy. More severe hair growth can be prevented, and resolution of the hirsutism is possible. Nevertheless, drug treatment is not a cure, and lifelong therapy may be necessary to prevent recurrence. Generally, 6 months is needed to judge the efficacy of a given therapy, although improvement may continue indefinitely. No drug is currently approved by the Food and Drug Administration for treatment of hirsutism.

Antiandrogens. Antiandrogens (spironolactone, cyproterone acetate), which block the androgen receptor, are the drug treatment of choice for hirsutism. They are effective in reducing hair growth in at least 70 per cent of women, and hirsutism in the remaining women stabilizes. Spironolactone is usually given in a starting dose of 50 mg twice daily. Although higher doses (up to 200 mg daily) may improve efficacy, side effects are dose related. The most common side effect is increased frequency of menses, which can be controlled by combining spironolactone with an oral contraceptive. Spironolactone should not be given to pregnant women or to women with renal insufficiency. Cyproterone acetate, a potent antiandrogen and progestin, is often given as 50 to 100 mg daily on days 5 to 15 of the menstrual cycle, combined with 35 to 50 μg of ethinyl estradiol on days 5 to 26. Alternatively, it may be given with an oral contraceptive, at a starting dose of 50 mg daily from days 1 to 10 of the birth control pill cycle. Side effects are similar to those of the oral contraceptive alone. Although widely used in Europe and Canada, cyproterone acetate has not been approved by the Food and Drug Administration at the time of publication.

Ovarian Suppression. Although oral contraceptives are often used to control menstrual cycles in women given antiandrogens, they are usually ineffective for treating hirsutism when used alone (although they may prevent the hirsutism from becoming worse). Birth control pills differ in the androgenicity of the progestational component, but this difference has never been shown to have clinical significance in the treatment of hirsutism. Gonadotropin-releasing hormone analogues suppress the ovary by suppressing LH and FSH secretion. They are effective in treating hirsutism associated with polycystic ovarian syndrome but are expensive and lead to menopausal symptoms unless estrogens are given concurrently.

Glucocorticoids. Glucocorticoids suppress adrenal cortisol and androgen secretion. They are frequently ineffective in low doses, and higher doses can cause Cushing's syndrome. They also can cause a drug-induced hirsutism in some women and cannot be recommended as a routine treatment. While glucocorticoids have traditionally been used to treat congenital adrenal hyperplasia, antiandrogens are more effective in treating the hirsutism associated with this disorder.

PROGNOSIS. Untreated, hirsutism usually becomes gradually worse with time, and most therapies need to be continued indefinitely. However, worsening hirsutism is easily prevented with antiandrogen therapy, and most women experience a satisfactory improvement with the judicious use of mechanical and medical therapies.

Horton R, Lobo RA (eds.): Androgen metabolism in hirsute and normal females. Clin Endocrinol Metab 15(2):213, 1986. *An excellent collection of reviews on aspects of the pathophysiology and treatment of hirsutism.*

Mahajan DK (ed.): Polycystic ovarian disease. Endocrinol Metab Clin North Am 17(4):621, 1988. *A series of well-written reviews on the pathophysiology and clinical approach to polycystic ovarian syndrome.*

Rittmaster RS, Loriaux DL: Hirsutism. Ann Intern Med 106:95, 1987. *A detailed review of the pathophysiology, evaluation, and treatment of hirsutism.*

Spritzer P, Billaud L, Thalabard J, et al.: Cyproterone acetate versus hydrocortisone treatment in late-onset adrenal hyperplasia. J Clin Endocrinol Metab 70:642, 1990. *Another example of the excellent clinical results with antiandrogens.*

226 Nonmalignant Diseases of the Breast

Douglas J. Marchant

Approximately one in every four women in the United States requires medical attention for breast symptomatology. More than half of all women have some degree of fibrocystic changes during their lifetime, and most have histologic changes that could be described as "fibrocystic disease." It is recommended, however, that the term *fibrocystic disease* be abandoned and the term *fibrocystic change* or *condition* be substituted because it is more descriptive of the clinical entity.

The physician should be knowledgeable about these common benign conditions and provide treatment or referral when indicated. This chapter discusses growth and development of the breasts, puberty, pregnancy and lactation, and the common benign conditions for which consultation is requested. Diagnostic studies, including examination of the breast, aspiration, and indications for surgical biopsy and referral, are emphasized. Gynecomastia, the main nonmalignant abnormality of the male breast, is described in Ch. 222.

GROWTH AND DEVELOPMENT OF THE BREAST

The functional units of the breast are of ectodermal origin. The epithelial ridge that eventually forms the breast tissue, recognizable by the thirty-fifth day of embryonic life, undergoes a series of alterations to form the lactiferous ducts and alveolae. At 15 weeks, mesenchymal cells differentiate into the smooth muscle of the nipple and the areola. The breast unit is complete at birth, as demonstrated by the occasional appearance of "witch's milk" caused by high levels of maternal hormones. During the third trimester of pregnancy, placental hormones in the fetal circulation stimulate further development of the functional units. This colostral secretion declines within 3 to 4 weeks, the breast tissue involutes, and no additional differentiation occurs until puberty.

Development of the mature breast begins with the onset of puberty and continues for several years. Estrogen levels increase, and the areolae become enlarged and pigmented. Adipose tissue is deposited to form and shape the breast and to provide a steroidogenic milieu for the conversion of hormones directly in the breast. In addition to estrogen and progesterone, insulin, cortisol, thyroxin, growth hormone, and prolactin are required for complete functional development.

The mature breast consists of the functional units—the alveolae, lactiferous ducts, and their supporting tissues. The alveolae are inconspicuous in the nonpregnant, nonlactating breast. The much larger ducts lie embedded in a stromal network consisting of fibrous tissue, fat, blood vessels, and lymphatics.

ABNORMALITIES OF GROWTH AND DEVELOPMENT

A number of congenital anomalies may be referred to the clinician for evaluation and treatment. The most frequently observed is the accessory nipple, or polythelia. This tissue, which may be mistaken for a pigmented nevus, lies along the milk line extending from the axilla to the groin. Rarely, functioning breast tissue is found along this milk line. Most commonly this ectopic breast tissue is located in the axilla, where it may enlarge and become quite painful during pregnancy and lactation.

Patients may be referred for failure of breast development, premature development, and breast hypertrophy. Normal sexual development and puberty are discussed in Ch. 224. Complete absence of the breast is rare and usually is associated with defects in the chest wall and muscles. Premature development is usually associated with the appearance of a mass beneath the nipple-areola complex. Other manifestations of sexual maturation are absent and hormonal studies are normal. A vaginal smear reveals little or no estrogen effect, consistent with the prepubertal state. No treatment is required; in particular to be avoided is surgical removal of the mass in the mistaken belief that it represents a tumor. If this area is removed, breast tissue will not develop on the affected side. Asymmetric breast development is common and requires no further treatment. Breast hypertrophy, on the other hand, is often uncomfortable and disturbing both to the patient and to the parents. These patients require considerable counseling because if reduction mammoplasty is recommended too early, a repeat operation will be necessary. A reduction mammoplasty, if required, should be performed only after completion of breast development, which may take several years.

THE BREAST DURING PREGNANCY AND THE PUERPERIUM

With the completion of breast development during and following puberty, the breasts are quiescent until pregnancy. During pregnancy the breast grows and develops due to lobular alveolar growth, the formation of secretory cells, and changes in the supporting tissues. Insulin responsiveness also is acquired during pregnancy. Further growth requires estrogen, progesterone, prolactin, and human placental lactogen. During pregnancy, serum prolactin increases from a nonpregnant level of approximately 10 ng to 200 ng per milliliter or more at term. Human placental lactogen reaches serum concentrations of approximately 6000 ng per milliliter at term. Lactation is suppressed by estrogen and progesterone, which inhibit prolactin action at the receptor level. With the rapid drop in estrogen and progesterone levels following delivery, this inhibition is removed and milk production begins. A decrease in the prolactin-inhibiting factor (PIF) by suckling increases prolactin and further promotes lactation. In the final event oxytocin is released and acts on the myoepithelial cells to contract the duct system for the delivery of the milk. By the end of the third or fourth month, suckling is the only stimulus required for continued lactation. If breast feeding does not occur, prolactin rapidly returns to nonpregnant levels.

Mastitis occasionally complicates lactation, usually following the first pregnancy. There is a localized area of inflammation and tenderness and slight elevation of temperature. Treatment includes continuation of breast feeding and the use of appropriate antibiotics. Since the most common organism is *Staphylococcus aureus*, penicillin or one of its derivatives is the treatment of choice. If the patient does not respond and if the tenderness and fever persist, a breast abscess should be suspected, for which the treatment is adequate drainage under general anesthesia in an operating room setting. Antibiotics should be continued in full therapeutic doses for 7 to 10 days following adequate drainage. The breast rapidly returns to normal and the cosmetic result is excellent.

The discovery of a dominant mass during pregnancy or lactation requires careful consideration. Early in pregnancy, a dominant mass is easily distinguished from fibrocystic changes. Often the patient gives a history of a mass first discovered many years before and followed in the belief that it represented a benign fibroadenoma. With rare exception, the cause of all dominant masses discovered during pregnancy or the puerperium should be resolved. This requires an open biopsy using a local anesthesia. Biopsy can be safely performed during lactation. The patient is requested to empty the breast early on the day of the operation. The mass is removed with careful approximation of the breast tissues and a pressure dressing temporarily applied. This can be removed later in the day and often the patient can breast feed on the operated side.

FIBROCYSTIC CHANGES

Fibrocystic changes, which represent an exaggerated physiologic response to a changing hormonal environment, include painful lumpy breasts (mastodynia, mastalgia), a dominant mass, and nipple discharge.

The peak incidence of fibrocystic changes occurs between the ages of 30 and 50. Breast tenderness often occurs premenstrually, which suggests that progesterone may play an important role in the development and symptomatology of these changes. In the resting breast there is minimal epithelial proliferation in the proliferative phase of the menstrual cycle and maximal proliferation in the secretory phase, a pattern quite different from that of the endometrium. Whether this dissimilarity between breast and endometrial epithelium reflects receptor content or some more indirect effect on proliferation is unclear. Estrogen is a mitogen for the endometrium but not for the breast, and the idea, derived largely from endometrial studies, that progestins are protective for the breast is difficult to sustain. The relative contributions of estrogen and progesterone to the etiology of benign breast conditions require further investigation.

Most, if not all, women experience these fibrocystic changes, and to label this condition a "disease" is inappropriate. Physical examination usually reveals irregular thickening, particularly in the upper outer quadrants. The changes associated with this process and its symptomatology constitute one of the most difficult challenges in the office practice of the physician.

MASTODYNIA (MASTALGIA)

Breast pain is common; it may occur in as many as 50 per cent of women. Usually the etiology is unclear, and relief of symptoms often is proportional to the time that the physician spends with the patient. The discomfort generally is classified as (1) cyclic mastalgia or mastodynia occurring immediately prior to the menses; (2) fibrocystic changes, including duct ectasia and sclerosing adenosis; or (3) referred pain such as costochondritis.

Almost all women complain of occasional breast discomfort for the first few days preceding the onset of menses, and most do not seek medical attention. It is the discomfort occurring at other times during the menstrual cycle, or throughout the cycle, that brings the patient to the physician.

Perimenopausal patients not infrequently note breast discomfort. The cause is unknown. Postmenopausal patients should be carefully evaluated for referred pain. They often perceive the discomfort to be in the breast when in reality it is related to the pectoral muscles, the chest wall, or even the cardiovascular system. Trauma is not an infrequent cause of breast discomfort. The usual presentation is a tender erythematous or ecchymotic area. In some cases open biopsy must be performed to rule out carcinoma.

NIPPLE DISCHARGE

Nipple discharge may be physiologic or pathologic, provoked or spontaneous. In most cases the patient can be immediately reassured that cancer is unlikely, since 10 per cent or fewer of breast cancers present with nipple discharge. A careful and detailed history is essential. Is the discharge produced only at the time of breast self-examination when the nipple is squeezed? Does it occur only with sexual stimulation? What type of physical exercise does the patient do? Does she wear a sport brassiere? Does she take any medication? Has she ever been pregnant? What is the menstrual history? Most patients can describe the character of the discharge, although not necessarily in a reliable fashion. For example, many patients complain of bloody nipple discharge, but when the secretions are examined on a gauze or by cytology, the color is blackish green and no blood cells are found.

Three types of discharge deserve further comment: galactorrhea, serosanguinous or bloody discharge, and discharge from the postmenopausal breast.

GALACTORRHEA. Galactorrhea is the spontaneous secretion of a milky discharge not immediately associated with a pregnancy. Usually it is persistent and occasionally it is voluminous. Elevated prolactin levels may be associated with galactorrhea. Physiologic causes of hyperprolactinemia include breast stimulation, coitus, eating, exercise, pregnancy, sleep, and stress. Hyperprolactinemia may also be due to pathologic factors, including brain and pituitary disorders, encephalitis, and pituitary microadenomas or macroadenomas. In addition, a number of pharmacologic agents may produce hyperprolactinemia, as noted in Table 226–1.

TABLE 226–1. CAUSES OF NONPUERPERAL GALACTORRHEA

I. **Central origin**
A. Organic
1. Suprahypophyseal lesions
a. Hypothalamic disorders—infiltrative processes (histiocytosis, metastatic diseases); masses (craniopharyngioma, meningioma); infarction; embolism
b. Pituitary stalk lesions—section; impingement by tumors (all types with suprasellar extension); vascular insult
2. Hypophyseal tumors
a. Prolactin secreting* (solitary; part of multiple endocrine adenomatosis syndrome mixed with GH, TSH, ACTH)
B. Functional
1. Drug related
a. Psychotropic (butyrophenones, phenothiazines)*
b. Antihypertensive (reserpine, α-methyldopa)
c. Cannabinoids (morphine, heroin)
d. Contraceptives
e. Antigastroplegics (metoclopramide)*
2. Unclassified (idiopathic, stress, empty sella syndrome)
II. **Peripheral origin**
A. Due to pituitary prolactin
1. Due to primary failure of target endocrine gland
a. Hypothyroidism
b. Addison's disease
2. Due to excess estrogen formation from target endocrine glands
a. Feminizing adrenal carcinoma
b. Polycystic ovarian syndrome
3. Due to decreased metabolic clearance of prolactin
a. Renal failure
b. Liver failure
c. Hypothyroidism
4. Due to local breast conditions
a. Mechanical stimulation or suckling
b. Thoracic and/or breast trauma, burn
c. Inflammation, i.e., mastitis, herpes zoster
B. Due to ectopic prolactin production
1. Renal neoplasia
2. Bronchogenic neoplasia

*Most common causes of highest serum prolactin levels.

Prolactin is secreted in a sleep-related circadian rhythm with maximal release between 3:00 A.M. and 5:00 A.M. Serum samples, therefore, should be obtained in a fasting state between 8:00 A.M. and 12:00 noon. Prolactin levels do not change during the menstrual cycle. A serum level of prolactin of greater than 20 ng per milliliter may be abnormal and should be further evaluated. Other diagnostic studies include microscopic evaluation of the breast discharge, which may reveal refractile fat globules, confirming the diagnosis. A thorough history should be taken to rule out physiologic or pharmacologic causes, and the menstrual history should focus on amenorrhea, oligomenorrhea, infertility, or a short luteal phase.

Prolactinomas, or prolactin-secreting pituitary adenomas, are common causes for hyperprolactinemia in women. Prolactinomas may be microadenomas (< 1 cm in diameter) or macroadenomas (> 1 cm). The diagnosis usually is made by computed tomography (CT) scan using contrast media. Modern CT or magnetic resonance imaging has replaced older methods of diagnosing pituitary tumors, such as the cone view tomogram or plain skull film.

SEROUS OR BLOODY BREAST DISCHARGE. This type of nipple discharge must be investigated. Usually it is caused by a benign intraductal papilloma, but carcinoma occurs in 10 to 15 per cent of these patients. Often it is difficult to demonstrate the exact quadrant of the breast from which the discharge appears at the nipple. A microscopic examination of the fluid may identify red blood cells, confirming the clinical impression and the need for open biopsy.

POSTMENOPAUSAL NIPPLE DISCHARGE. Any nipple discharge that occurs during the postmenopausal period must be viewed as suggestive of carcinoma of the breast. Careful examination of the breast may reveal a mass or other findings consistent with carcinoma, which must be followed up, as described in Ch. 227.

DETECTION AND DIAGNOSIS

HISTORY. The diagnostic evaluation begins with a careful history, noting the age of the patient, the date of the last menstrual period, family history of breast disease, use of medication, the date of birth of the first child, and any surgery related to previous breast disease. Inquiry should be made concerning the use of oral contraceptives, including the type of medication and for how long it has been taken. If the patient has received estrogen replacement therapy, the type of medication and the length of time that the medication has been used should be noted. Pelvic surgery, including oophorectomy and a history of pelvic malignancy, particularly ovarian carcinoma and endometrial carcinoma, should be recorded. Did the patient notice the symptom casually or by employing deliberate breast self-examination, or was it first noted by another health care provider? Does the patient wear a brassiere? What type of medication has the patient used to provide relief? Are there any emotional factors that should be considered? The history should be recorded with particular emphasis on the date of onset of the symptom, the exact location in the breast and, finally, the disposition.

PHYSICAL EXAMINATION. For careful evaluation the breasts are first examined in the sitting or standing position. Contour, symmetry, and skin changes are noted. The vascular pattern is observed and the condition of the areola and nipple recorded. These changes may be exaggerated by asking the patient to elevate the arm or to place her hands on the hips, thus contracting the pectoralis major muscles and exaggerating any small change noted on routine observation. While the patient is in this position, the axilla is palpated, being careful to support the arm with the opposite hand. This relaxes the pectoralis muscle and permits careful evaluation of the axilla. While the patient is in the sitting or standing position, the supraclavicular area should be checked for a cervical rib or other unexpected finding. Examination of the neck may reveal thyroid enlargement.

Following these maneuvers, the patient is placed in the supine position. The breast is palpated in a systematic manner with the flat of the hand. The use of Phisohex or talcum powder permits the identification of even minor alterations. Approximately 80 per cent of American women discover their own lesions, often while taking a shower. The use of this so-called "wet technique" permits the identification of very subtle changes in breast texture. Following the careful evaluation of all quadrants, the areola and nipple should be carefully examined and the nipple gently squeezed. Any discharge is evaluated for location, consistency, and color.

The patient often presents with a chief complaint of a lump. This may or may not be confirmed by careful examination. The usual finding is a vague thickening, particularly in the upper outer quadrant.

The physician must carefully evaluate the chief complaint and then, on the basis of a thorough examination, decide whether the findings represent a dominant mass or an exaggeration of normal breast tissue associated with fibrocystic changes. In the obese patient with very large breasts, it is unlikely that any but the most obvious lesion will be discovered by routine examination. The large breast, therefore, is an indication for mammography to augment what in most cases is an inadequate physical examination.

Once a lesion has been characterized as a mass, a lump, or a dominant mass and has been measured or drawn, its cause must be established. There are no obviously benign lesions. The only exception is a mass in the teenager for whom elective treatment of an obvious fibroadenoma may be recommended.

CYST ASPIRATION

A mass may be cystic, solid, benign, or malignant. Attempts should be made to aspirate the mass with a fine (23 or 24) gauge needle. Local anesthesia is not required. The mass is immobilized with the fingers, the needle inserted, and the fluid withdrawn. If the fluid is clear or cloudy and no residual mass is palpated immediately following the aspiration, it is sufficient to arrange a follow-up examination in 1 month with reassurance and monthly self-examination of the breast. If the mass remains immediately following the aspiration, if the fluid is bloody, or if there is a residual mass on the first follow-up visit, open biopsy is mandatory. If the mass is solid, open biopsy is recommended except for a teenager, for whom excision biopsy can be performed on an elective basis.

Cytologic evaluation of nipple discharge or cyst fluid is seldom rewarding. On the other hand, it is probably advisable to examine spontaneous nipple discharge microscopically, particularly if it is unilateral and serosanguinous or bloody. A positive cytologic examination of cyst fluid in the absence of other indications for biopsy is exceedingly rare. Cytology is not, therefore, recommended as a routine examination.

FINE-NEEDLE ASPIRATION (FNA)

The accurate use of fine-needle aspiration requires an understanding of the techniques involved and a cytopathologist capable of interpreting the smear. A standard disposable syringe can be used with a 23- to 25-gauge needle. Local anesthesia is helpful because several "passes" may be required to obtain an adequate sample of "tissue juice" for appropriate evaluation. The material should not enter the syringe and should be placed directly on the slide and fixed with an appropriate spray. The technique is most useful for the obvious dominant mass. Fine-needle aspiration is useful only if positive; a negative finding is unreliable. Some radiologists prefer that a mammogram be performed prior to fine-needle aspiration because the procedure may distort the anatomy of the breast.

OTHER DIAGNOSTIC STUDIES

Ultrasonography is useful to confirm the presence or absence of macrocysts, particularly when these lesions are discovered by mammography and are nonpalpable. The procedure should not be performed on a routine basis, since it is unsuitable for screening and is an extra expense to the patient. It is much simpler to immediately attempt aspiration with a fine-gauge needle. Thermography and diaphonography are experimental procedures and should not be employed, except with evaluative protocols.

Mammography may be used as a screening examination in the asymptomatic patient or to confirm the findings noted on physical examination. The accuracy of mammography depends upon a number of factors, including the size and density of the breast and the location of the lesion. False-negative results, which occur even in the best institutions, may reach 10 per cent and in some centers approach 25 per cent. The presence of a dominant mass and a negative mammogram clearly do not preclude the recommendation for referral and an open biopsy.

BREAST BIOPSY

Certain features of the breast biopsy are important when discussing such a recommendation with the patient. In the past, open biopsy was performed solely as a diagnostic procedure to determine the presence or absence of cancer. Currently, the biopsy often becomes part of conservative treatment, and therefore it must be executed by surgeons familiar with contemporary treatment for breast cancer (Ch. 227). It is essential that the biopsy be performed in an operating room setting with trained personnel familiar with the biopsy technique and the use of local anesthesia.

MANAGEMENT OF BENIGN BREAST DISORDERS

The medical management of benign breast conditions often challenges even the most well-informed physician. For patients with mild fibrocystic changes and minimal symptomatology, reassurance only is indicated. Occasionally, a well-fitting brassiere, salt restriction, and a mild analgesic to control discomfort are all that is required.

For patients with greater discomfort, a detailed history is often the key to appropriate diagnosis and therapy. Mammography may be helpful in ruling out significant breast pathology and in reassuring the patient. Treatment strategy often depends upon the "complaint threshold of the patient and the safety threshold of the physician." In the absence of highly effective specific therapy, a number of treatment regimens have been proposed:

the topical use of progestational agents, tamoxifen, bromocriptine, various vitamin formulations, and primrose oil. For most patients treatment is directed toward a reasonable and rational explanation rather than any specific medication.

Danazol is effective but for most patients the cost and the side effects are prohibitive. Moderate doses of danazol decrease follicular maturation and increase anovulatory periods. Danazol has intrinsic androgenic activity and also decreases sex hormone–binding globulin, which increases free testosterone levels. Estradiol secretion is reduced because of the lack of follicular maturation. For some patients who have been incapacitated by breast discomfort and nodularity, a short course of danazol (400 to 600 mg daily for 6 months) may provide symptomatic relief and a marked change in the physical examination. The use of danazol should be restricted to those patients who have failed more conservative measures to control their symptomatology.

The treatment of patients with galactorrhea varies according to its etiology and the patient's desires. For patients with a pituitary microadenoma, bromocriptine, 5 mg daily, is usually effective. Unfortunately, if bromocriptine is discontinued, hyperprolactinemia usually returns, leading to galactorrhea and amenorrhea. Therapy therefore must be continued indefinitely.

The objectives for therapy of prolactinomas are to normalize the prolactin levels and menstrual function, to preserve function of the anterior pituitary, and to reduce the tumor mass. Patients with macroadenomas or with extrasellar extension of the tumor should be treated first with bromocriptine, followed by surgery when maximal reduction of the tumor size has been obtained. Surgery should be performed without discontinuing bromocriptine, since the adenoma may rapidly regrow.

Women with no evidence of pituitary adenoma but with unacceptable rates of galactorrhea may benefit from bromocriptine even if the serum prolactin level is normal. If galactorrhea is not symptomatic in such patients, however, treatment is not necessary. It is appropriate to refer most of these patients for further endocrine evaluation and to a reproductive endocrinologist if fertility is desired.

Occasional patients present with nonlactational mastitis, i.e., periodic drainage of purulent material from the nipple-areola complex in spite of previous attempts at drainage. In this condition, known as squamous metaplasia, it is not clear whether infection occurs initially followed by squamous metaplasia and intermittent discharge or whether squamous metaplasia occurs first followed by infection. The treatment, however, is complete excision of the involved duct system. Antibiotics are seldom helpful.

The most common benign neoplasm of the breast is the fibroadenoma, usually first presenting in the teenager but occasionally discovered on routine examination during the early reproductive years. Most of these lesions should be removed. In the occasional young patient with more than one mass, it is appropriate to use ultrasonography to document the actual number of lesions. Most surgeons prefer to remove the palpable lesion, usually as day surgery under local anesthesia, a procedure that is easy to do when the lesion is small. Patients who have discovered these lesions almost invariably request removal. The role of the primary care physician is to document the finding and then arrange for appropriate referral.

SUMMARY

The diagnosis and treatment of nonmalignant diseases of the breast constitute one of the most difficult challenges facing the primary care physician. The symptomatology is extremely subjective, and conclusions based even upon the most careful examination are subject to error.

Even specific complaints, such as nipple discharge, require considerable judgment when recommending treatment or referral. No lesion is obviously benign. Since 80 per cent of women with breast cancer have no identifiable risk factors, careful breast examination must be included as part of every physical examination.

Brookshaw JD: Danazol treatment of benign breast disease: A survey of U.S.A. multi center studies. Postgrad Med J 55:52, 1979. *Danazol has been approved by the FDA for the treatment of fibrocystic changes. It is costly, however, and there are a number of side effects. This article describes the results of a multicenter study in the United States.*

Feig SA: Decreased breast cancer mortality through mammographic screening: Results of clinical trials. State Art Radiol 167:659, 1988. *Although mammography screening can lead to a remarkable improvement in breast cancer survival, the degree to which any program achieves potential gain depends upon the technical quality of the study, the interpretive expertise of the radiologist, the screening facility, and the number of projections.*

Hindle WH: Fine needle aspiration. *In* Hindle WH (ed.): *Breast Disease for Gynecologists*, Norwalk, CT, Appleton and Lange, 1990, pp 67–118. *This chapter covers the history and evolution of the fine-needle aspiration technique, including recommendations and contraindications for its use.*

Kleinberg DL, Noel GH, Frantz AG: Galactorrhea: A study of 235 cases including 48 with pituitary tumors. N Engl J Med 296:589, 1977. *This classic article is perhaps the most comprehensive report on the clinical entities associated with galactorrhea.*

Leis HP Jr: Management of nipple discharge. World J Surg 13:736, 1989. *This report of a series of over 8000 breast operations discusses the incidence of breast cancer in patients presenting with nipple discharge and the management of significant discharges.*

Love SM, Gelman SR, Silen W: Fibrocystic disease of the breast, a non disease. N Engl J Med 307:1010, 1983. *This article traces the history of fibrocystic "disease." Since most, if not all, women have these changes, the condition should not be called a disease. In most cases there is no relationship between fibrocystic changes and the later development of breast cancer.*

Yen SSC: Prolactin in human reproduction. *In* Yen SSC, Jaffe RB (eds.): *Reproductive Endocrinology*. Philadelphia, W. B. Saunders Company, 1986, pp 237–263. *This chapter describes abnormalities in prolactin secretion and the treatment of the clinical sequelae.*

227 Breast Cancer

Brian J. Lewis

EPIDEMIOLOGY AND PATHOGENESIS

In 1990, 150,000 new cases of female breast cancer and 900 new cases of male breast cancer were projected for the United States. In terms of annual mortality, 49,000 women and 350 men die of breast cancer. These figures and the 1 in 12 lifetime risk that a woman in the United States has for developing breast cancer make this disease a significant health problem.

The cause of breast cancer is unknown, but there are several factors that correlate with its occurrence: age, family history, ethnic influences, and hormonal effects.

AGE. Only about 15 per cent of cases of breast cancer occur before the age of 40. The age-adjusted incidence steadily increases thereafter, with two thirds of cases occurring in postmenopausal women.

FAMILY HISTORY. Daughters or sisters of breast cancer patients have a two- to three-fold greater risk of developing breast cancer than do women without an affected first-degree relative. More specifically, this relative risk can range from 1.5 if the mother or sister was postmenopausal at diagnosis to 8.8 if she was premenopausal and had bilateral disease. Unlike patients in the general population, women with the highest relative risk among those with a positive family history have a greater tendency to have their disease before the age of 40. Careful counseling, screening, and tracking of high-risk patients are essential. Increased monitoring should be given to patients with prior curative treatment for breast cancer, since they have a 10 to 15 per cent lifetime chance of developing a second primary breast cancer.

ETHNIC INFLUENCES. Ninety per cent of breast cancer patients lack a positive family history. While ethnic background has a role, it is necessary to control for the influences of allied cultural and nongenetic factors. Oriental women have a much lower risk of breast cancer than women in western countries. Women of Japanese descent who reside in the United States have a higher risk than women in Japan. Within the United States itself, the probability of developing breast cancer by age 75 shows considerable variation: for white women, it is 8.2 per cent; for black women, 7.0 per cent; for Hispanic women, 4.8 per cent; for native American women, 2.5 per cent; for Japanese-American women, 5.4 per cent; and for Chinese-American women, 6.1 per cent.

HORMONAL EFFECTS. Estrogens have an impact on the development of breast cancer. Early menarche, late menopause, and late or no pregnancy correlate with a higher risk (relative

TABLE 227–1. RISK FACTORS FOR BREAST CANCER IN WOMEN WITH PROLIFERATIVE BREAST DISEASE

Diagnosis	Relative Risk of Breast Cancer (95% Confidence Interval)
Nonproliferative lesions	1.0
Proliferative disease without atypical hyperplasia	1.9 (1.2 to 2.9)
Atypical hyperplasia	5.3 (3.1 to 8.8)
Atypical hyperplasia + family history of breast cancer	11.0 (5.5 to 24)

Data from DuPont WD, Page DL: Risk factors for breast cancer in women with proliferative breast disease. N Engl J Med 312:146, 1985.

risk of 1.3, 1.5 and 2 to 3, respectively). Conversely, premature loss of ovarian function, late menarche, early menopause, and early or more numerous pregnancies correlate with a decreased risk. The chance for developing breast cancer is increased in men with Klinefelter's syndrome or with other disturbances of estrogen metabolism.

Oral contraceptives seem not to increase the risk of breast cancer, and they may ameliorate the symptoms of fibrocystic disease. There is some concern that the use of exogenous estrogens in postmenopausal patients can increase the risk, but this may correlate with higher doses and more prolonged treatment. There is very little evidence that the replacement doses used for the treatment of osteoporosis increase the risk of carcinoma of the breast (Ch. 239).

Historically, there has been a linkage between fibrocystic disease of the breast and an increased risk for breast cancer. A host of terms has been lumped under "fibrocystic disease" (i.e., macrocysts, microcysts, adenosis, apocrine change, fibrosis, fibroadenoma, and ductal hyperplasia). We now know that the majority of women (70 per cent) who have a biopsy for benign disease are not at increased risk for cancer, but the presence of atypical hyperplasia and a family history of breast cancer greatly increase the probability of developing breast carcinoma (Table 227–1).

OTHER RISK FACTORS. Other risk factors include ionizing radiation and possibly diet. Surprisingly, consumption of even moderate amounts of alcohol may increase risk appreciably. Repeated chest fluoroscopy for tuberculosis, therapeutic radiation of mastitis, and exposure of Japanese women to the atomic bomb blast have been linked to increased rates of breast cancer. Animal models and geographic-ethnic differences in incidence suggest that dietary factors, in particular fat (increased in the western diet), may contribute to the development of breast cancer.

DIAGNOSIS

Clinical Presentation

Breast cancer is usually noted as a painless lump and discovered incidentally by the patient, by routine physical examination, or by mammography. Pain and tenderness are nonspecific findings and herald cancer less than 10 per cent of the time. Physical findings suggestive of a malignancy include a hard, irregular mass and skin dimpling or nipple retraction. Nonbloody nipple discharges are rarely associated with cancer. Bloody discharges correlate with intraductal papillomas in about 30 per cent of cases and with invasive cancer in about one third of cases.

Pertinent history includes a family history of breast cancer on the maternal side, especially in first-degree relatives, prior breast biopsies, whether the lump is new or old, and whether it fluctuates in size, consistency, and tenderness with the menstrual cycle. Such cycling is more suggestive of a benign process but by no means rules out cancer. Physical examination should include careful inspection and palpation of both breasts and assessment of the axillary, supraclavicular, and infraclavicular node areas.

Evaluation of a Breast Mass

A suspicious breast mass requires systematic evaluation and follow-up. A negative mammogram or needle aspiration does not ensure that a mass is benign, and if it remains of concern, it must be excised. To avoid distortion of breast anatomy, a mam-

mogram should precede any biopsy procedure. Breast imaging rules out contralateral lesions and multiple foci in the ipsilateral breast, and it is sometimes redone after biopsy to confirm that the area of interest was in fact removed.

Formerly, diagnosis and treatment were a one-step procedure. A woman with a suspicious lesion had an excision under general anesthesia with frozen section analysis of the tumor. If cancer was found, mastectomy immediately followed, and the woman awoke to confront both the diagnosis of cancer and the loss of her breast. A two-step procedure is now used. Fine-needle aspiration cytology or excisional biopsy under local anesthesia allows an outpatient diagnosis. If cancer is found, the patient and surgeon can then review treatment options.

Screening and Detection

Early detection of a tumor improves the chances for cure. Efforts to screen for and detect early breast cancer have centered on self-examination, physician examination, and techniques for imaging the breast.

Self-examination is simple, without cost, and free of risk. It has been shown to result in earlier detection of tumors, and every adult woman should be instructed in its use. Any mass that is new and persists for more than a few weeks, is rapidly enlarging, or changes from a previously stable lump requires a physician's examination.

Examination by a physician as a screening tool is more costly and is applied less frequently than self-examination. Discovery of an unsuspected mass during a periodic examination by a physician leads to detection of tumors at an earlier stage than in patients who do not have periodic breast examinations. The American Cancer Society recommends that every woman have a routine breast examination at least every 3 years.

Breast imaging techniques include thermography, sonography, and radiographic mammography. Thermography has yet to prove sufficiently sensitive for widespread use. Sonography can help distinguish cystic from solid lesions initially found on radiography. Radiographic mammography is a well-studied and standardized methodology. Annual mammography lowers the mortality from breast cancer in screened populations compared with unscreened control groups. It detects smaller lesions with fewer nodal metastases. Current technology allows a lower dose of radiation per examination. Table 227–2 shows guidelines for screening. Annual examinations are also recommended for women with a prior breast cancer regardless of age.

Breast cancer incidence rose gradually over the first half of the century and turned more sharply upward in the 1960's, concomitant with and possibly as a result of increased attention to education and screening. The mortality (deaths per 100,000), however, has remained constant. It may be that tumors are being found earlier and cured more readily, since more of the tumors found are smaller. Alternatively, a proportion of the early asymptomatic (subclinical) cancers being discovered may have a lower malignant potential than tumors that grow faster and more rapidly become clinically apparent. Thus, screening may appear more efficacious than it really is, since some of the patients discovered to have an "early" cancer may represent a subpopulation with indolent disease who would not otherwise have had clinical expression of the tumor. Nonetheless, there has been a definite reduction in mortality from breast cancer in women who are screened with mammography.

TUMOR BIOLOGY

Breast cancer is more than just a local process; local control of tumor is necessary but not by itself sufficient to address the

TABLE 227–2. GUIDELINES FOR MAMMOGRAPHIC SCREENING OF ASYMPTOMATIC WOMEN

1. Baseline mammogram for all women aged 35 to 40
2. Mammography every one to two years from age 40 to 49
3. Mammography annually for women aged 50 or older
4. Mammography annually for women at any age with a personal history of breast cancer
5. Mammography annually for women aged 40 and over who have a family history of breast cancer or who are otherwise at increased risk

TABLE 227–3. STAGING OF CARCINOMA OF THE BREAST

Stage I	Tumor < 2 cm without skin involvement and with no clinically suspicious axillary nodes.
Stage II	Tumor < 2 cm with clinically suspicious nodes; any tumor 2 to 5 cm with or without clinically suspicious nodes.
Stage III	Any tumor > 5 cm; skin involvement or chest wall attachment; any size tumor with clinically fixed axillary nodes; arm edema; supraclavicular nodes.
Stage IV	Metastatic disease.

threat of distant metastases. Breast cancer is also a chronic illness with a potential for recurrence 10 to 15 years after removal of the primary tumor. While one can extirpate apparent disease in the breast and in the axillary nodes in the majority of cases, at least 50 to 80 per cent of women found to have tumor in the axillary nodes and 30 per cent of those without axillary node metastases will have metastatic disease.

STAGING. The system for clinically staging breast cancer reflects the anatomic extent of tumor (Table 227–3). It allows consistent and comparable description and reporting of cases. The stages correlate with survival and are important in planning treatment, but they do not totally predict the clinical behavior of the tumor. A more complete classification scheme would ideally measure the balance between the inherent virulence of the cancer and the intrinsic antitumor defenses of the host. In addition to tumor size and nodal status, hormone receptor content and nuclear grade reproducibly correlate with prognosis. The infrequent histologic subtypes of papillary, colloid (mucinous), and tubular carcinoma are associated with a more favorable outcome. Other variables such as the percentage of cells in S-phase, oncogene expression, epidermal growth factor receptors, cathepsin-D, and stress response (heat shock) proteins may each provide a means for better predicting who will have metastatic disease (Table 227–4).

METHOD OF SPREAD. Breast cancer spreads directly to the bloodstream as well as to the draining lymphatics. Tumor emboli can traverse the lymph nodes and enter the venous system; and tumor cells can presumably reach lymph nodes by way of the bloodstream. In addition, upon discovery, a breast cancer mass usually contains 10^9 or more cells. Given what is known of doubling times, the cell number at diagnosis implies that the cancer may have been growing for a number of years. It seems logical that there will be shedding of the tumor cells into the venous and lymphatic circulation throughout the life of the tumor, especially early, when tumor growth rate is highest.

Accordingly, it is likely that many more patients with breast cancer have micrometastases than we see with clinical recurrence. Negative axillary nodes may not mean that the tumor was never present in the lymphatic system but rather that it had been there and was unable to flourish. Positive lymph nodes do correlate with subsequent metastases and poor survival. This could reflect simple anatomic spread of cancer past the last "line of defense" imposed by the lymph nodes (Halsted). More probably it implies that because the tumor persisted in the nodes, however it arrived there, it will also persist and grow in other organs.

TABLE 227–4. PROGNOSTIC FACTORS IN BREAST CANCER

Factor	Influence on Risk of Metastases
Tumor size	Risk increases with size
Nodal status	Risk increases with presence and number of nodal metastases
Hormone receptor status	Risk increased if receptors not present
Nuclear grade	Risk increased with high grade
Favorable histology	Risk decreases with favorable subtypes
Per cent S-phase	Risk increases with per cent S-phase
Oncogene expression	Risk appears to increase with increased oncogene expression
Cathepsin-D levels	Risk appears to increase with levels
Epidermal growth factor receptor levels	Risk appears to increase with levels
Stress response process levels	Risk appears to increase with levels

CELL ORIGIN. Most breast tumors derive from mammary epithelium. Eighty per cent of these are infiltrating ductal carcinomas. Less common are infiltrating lobular carcinoma, medullary carcinoma, comedocarcinoma, and tubular, papillary, and colloid carcinoma. Lobular and comedocarcinoma can be bilateral and require increased surveillance of the unaffected breast. Lobular carcinoma in situ poses a special problem. Although it is not an invasive lesion, it is associated with a 1 per cent annual risk for the development of an invasive lesion in either breast. Some surgeons have therefore advocated prophylactic mastectomy. A more conservative approach is to do a "mirror image" biopsy of the contralateral breast to rule out invasive tumor and then to track the patient closely with periodic examinations and prompt biopsy of any suspicious lesions. Ductal carcinoma in situ carries a higher risk for evolving into invasive cancer and requires surgery. Inflammatory breast cancer represents a highly virulent pathologic variant. Clinically, the patient has a red, swollen, warm breast with a characteristic peau d'orange appearance. Microscopically, this is associated with involvement of dermal lymphatics by tumor. It has proven difficult to achieve long-term survival in patients with this diagnosis.

HORMONE RECEPTOR PROTEINS. Estrogen and progesterone receptor proteins (ERP and PRP) are present in normal mammary epithelium and in a proportion of breast cancers. After binding to the steroid, the activated hormone-receptor complex interacts with specific sites on DNA, and this results in the initiation of steroid-specific protein synthesis. One product of estrogen stimulation is PRP, and the presence of PRP signifies functionally intact ERP. A tumor is considered ERP-positive when it contains more than 10 femtomoles of receptor per milligram of protein, as measured using a radioligand binding assay. Monoclonal antibodies against ERP are now available and permit microscopic visualization and enumeration of ERP-positive tumor cells.

ERP is found more frequently and in higher titer in tumors from postmenopausal patients (60 per cent or more versus 30 to 40 per cent positive in premenopausal women). ERP-positive tumors tend to be less virulent and are more likely to respond to hormonal therapy (see below). Tumors that contain both ERP and PRP have the greatest likelihood of regressing after an endocrine maneuver, and the probability of a response increases directly with the titer of the RP. Given the therapeutic and prognostic implications of hormone receptor levels, it is mandatory that all primary breast cancers be submitted for receptor analysis at the time of removal. There is an 80 per cent concordance between the hormone receptor profile of a primary tumor and its metastases, in the absence of intervening hormone treatment. Breast cancers are heterogeneous in the sense that in RP-positive specimens, the majority but not necessarily all of the cells contain RP. When metastatic disease becomes refractory to hormonal therapy after initially responding, the progression reflects the outgrowth of hormone-independent cells that are usually RP-negative.

PRIMARY MANAGEMENT OF BREAST CANCER

Stage I and Stage II Disease

Since Halsted's time, almost three generations ago, the view of breast cancer as a local or regional process has made radical mastectomy or one of its variants the standard approach to the management of resectable tumor confined to the breast and the axillary lymph nodes. Patients often received postoperative radiation therapy to the chest wall and the draining lymph node areas. These treatments have produced a local control rate of 95 per cent, but variations in locoregional therapy have not differed significantly in their impact upon distant recurrence or overall survival. Furthermore, more extensive surgery or surgery followed by radiation increases the risk of arm edema.

These approaches entered general use without the testing of alternative approaches, but recently local tumor excision with breast irradiation has been gaining a wider acceptance. Older, largely uncontrolled studies seemed to indicate similar outcomes either with tumor excision and breast irradiation or with traditional mastectomy. While one cannot refer to the decades of observation on local tumor control and side effects that exist for standard surgical approaches, recent controlled trials show that the techniques are equivalent in terms of tumor recurrence and overall survival.

Public interest in alternatives to mastectomy has increased, and patients are more informed and expect their physicians to provide a comprehensive overview of treatment possibilities, especially ones that would spare them the disfigurement and distress imposed by mastectomy. Likewise, the growing application of plastic surgery for breast reconstruction after mastectomy has lessened the emotional trauma of the operation.

Breast conservation is appropriate therapy for Stage I or Stage II disease. Table 227–5 lists the requirements for its use. Mammography is essential to exclude patients with multifocal disease or with diffuse microcalcifications. (Even if the latter prove benign on biopsy, they will interfere with the subsequent mammographic follow-up used to screen for recurrent cancer.) An adequate surgical resection of the tumor with negative resection margins is essential and is facilitated by inking the margins of the specimen and orienting it for the pathologist. Axillary node dissection determines whether the patient requires adjuvant systemic treatment because of nodal metastasis. Extensive intraductal carcinoma in situ may be a contraindication to breast conservation because of a higher risk of recurrence in the treated breast.

The most common but not necessarily the preferred approach to the primary management of a Stage I or Stage II breast cancer is total mastectomy and axillary lymph node dissection. Postoperative radiotherapy is an individualized rather than "standard" therapy. It is employed when narrow resection margins, extensive nodal disease, the presence of residual tumor, or other high-risk factors for local recurrence are present. With the advent of adjuvant chemotherapy for Stage II disease (see below), there may be even fewer indications for adjuvant radiation therapy, since drug treatment alone may decrease the local failure rate. However, this supposition has yet to be adequately tested in clinical trials.

Clinically suspicious nodes are pathologically negative for tumor 25 to 30 per cent of the time, and, conversely, clinically negative nodes are positive histologically with an equal frequency. With a proper axillary dissection, radiation to the axilla is not usually necessary (and increases the risk for arm edema). While positive axillary nodes increase the likelihood of subclinical supraclavicular and internal mammary node metastases, there is no evidence that adjuvant radiation to those areas will improve survival.

Standard pretreatment evaluation for any of these techniques includes a complete blood count, a profile of serum chemistries with particular reference to studies suggestive of liver or bone

TABLE 227–5. REQUIREMENT FOR LIMITED SURGERY AND RADIOTHERAPY FOR EARLY BREAST CANCER

Patient Selection	Comments
Adequate resection of tumor without major cosmetic deformity	This requires a single discrete tumor, moderate sized breast, tumor diameter < 4–5 cm.
Surgical Criteria	
Wide resection with specimen orientation	Grossly negative surgical margins are essential—re-resection may be required if margins are microscopically involved.
Hormone receptor analysis	
Separate axillary incision	
Radiation Therapy	
4500–5000 rad to entire breast + boost to tumor bed	
Treatment of the Axilla	
Level I and Level II axillary dissection* (not an informal "sampling")	Permits adequate node sampling, controls local tumor, and obviates the need for axillary radiation. Does not impose a major risk for arm edema.

Sources: Harris et al., 1985; Danoff et al., 1985.
*Level I = Complete removal of nodes lateral to the pectoralis minor muscle.
Level II = Removal of nodes beneath the pectoralis minor.

involvement, and a chest radiograph. Many feel that routine bone scans or liver scans are not indicated in patients with clinical Stage I or II disease, although some advocate a baseline bone scan to be used as a reference if the patient should develop skeletal metastases in the future. The yield of positives is extremely low in the absence of symptoms or signs suggesting visceral disease. On the other hand, with locally advanced tumor (Stage III), the yield of screening bone scans is sufficiently high to warrant their use. Likewise, with abnormal blood chemistries suggestive of liver involvement or with symptoms such as bone pain, scans would be required to avoid inappropriate use of a curative procedure in a patient with advanced, incurable disease.

Stage III Disease and Inflammatory Breast Cancer

If a patient's disease is Stage III solely on the basis of tumor size (tumor > 5 cm), but the tumor appears to be as resectable as that of a Stage I or II patient, mastectomy is the primary treatment. For patients with locally advanced but unresectable disease (i.e., invasion of chest wall, fixation of axillary nodes, or positive supraclavicular nodes), control of persistent or recurrent regional disease as well as latent distant metastases is the dominant problem. Inflammatory breast cancer is aggressive locally as well as metastatically. It is properly considered a systemic disease from the outset, even though it appears to be confined to the breast. The treatment plan for the latter two presentations involves an individualized approach using chemotherapy to reduce the tumor volume, followed by radiation therapy and possibly resection of the breast and draining nodes. This strategy requires close consultation from the outset between surgeons, radiation oncologists, and medical oncologists. Prolonged remissions and perhaps cures can be obtained in a fraction of patients.

Metastatic Breast Cancer

CLINICAL FEATURES. Breast cancer most frequently metastasizes to lymph nodes, skin, lung, pleura, bone, liver, brain, and pericardium. In autopsy series, the adrenals are involved in up to half the patients, but adrenal insufficiency is rarely seen. Likewise, the ovaries contain tumor in up to one quarter of patients at autopsy. Rarely metastatic breast cancer may be found incidentally at oophorectomy in a patient whose first sign of breast cancer is an involved ovary presenting as a pelvic mass. Breast cancer is the most common source of metastases to the eye in women.

PATIENT ASSESSMENT. Once a metastatic focus is found, routine studies to map tumor extent include a complete blood count (which can reflect myelophthisis secondary to marrow metastases) and the measurement of serum levels of liver enzymes, bilirubin, and calcium. The carcinoembryonic antigen titer and the CA 15-3 antigen titer can be useful markers for following response to therapy. A chest radiograph is indicated and can reveal lung nodules, mediastinal or hilar node involvement, or a pleural effusion. A bone scan is also mandatory, and positive areas, especially those that are symptomatic or in weight-bearing bones, require follow-up radiographs to determine whether radiation is needed to prevent collapse or pathologic fracture. If physical findings or laboratory studies suggest hepatic involvement, a radionuclide liver scan, a sonogram of the liver, or a liver CT scan confirms the presence of metastatic disease, gauges its extent, and allows comparison with follow-up studies during treatment. "Routine" liver imaging is widely employed, but its yield and cost-effectiveness in the absence of signs suggesting liver metastasis are open to question. The same statement applies to "routine" studies of the brain, although they are clearly indicated in the presence of neurologic symptoms or signs.

COMPLICATIONS. Certain complications occur with some frequency and require urgent attention in patients with metastatic breast cancer: hypercalcemia, metastases to weight-bearing bones, and metastases to the nervous system (the epidural space, the leptomeninges, or the brain).

Hypercalcemia requires standard methods of therapy, such as saline, furosemide, and mithramycin therapy along with treatment of the breast cancer itself (Ch. 235). A positive bone scan, especially in the femur or vertebral column, or bone pain in these areas requires radiographic analysis of the extent of structural damage. Femoral lesions may necessitate orthopedic stabilization and radiation therapy to prevent pathologic fractures.

Vertebral body lesions may require radiation to diminish pain and avoid further collapse.

Patients with persistent back pain are at greater risk for *epidural metastases* and possibly cord compression. Motor or sensory changes in a segmental distribution greatly increase the possibility of an epidural lesion. However, in the presence of back pain, their absence does not exclude an epidural lesion. Pain without a neurologic deficit means that there is still time to treat an epidural lesion with radiation before the cord becomes ischemic and permanently damaged.

Leptomeningeal metastases present with headache and focal sensory or motor changes suggestive of single or multiple nerve root involvement. The diagnosis depends upon the demonstration of breast cancer cells in the cerebrospinal fluid and may require multiple spinal taps to yield a diagnosis (with appropriate studies beforehand, if indicated, to rule out a mass lesion in the brain). Since systemically administered drugs penetrate the blood-brain barrier poorly, intrathecal or intraventricular chemotherapy is necessary.

TREATMENT. The two major types of therapy for disseminated breast cancer are hormonal and cytotoxic. Hormonal therapy is less toxic but can require as long as 8 to 12 weeks to produce maximal benefit. The impact of chemotherapy is more rapid. Responses to all these treatments last a median of 6 to 18 months, and responders have a significantly prolonged survival compared with nonresponders.

The menopausal status of the patient and the hormone receptor profile of the tumor are the major determinants of whether to employ an endocrine maneuver and which particular therapy to use. Other important considerations are the tempo of the disease, the performance status of the patient, and the sites of metastases. A long interval between mastectomy and recurrence suggests indolent disease and would, along with a good performance status, permit the longer observation period needed to gauge response to an endocrine therapy. Bone, soft tissue, and limited pulmonary metastases may respond to hormonal therapy, whereas liver, brain, and extensive lung metastases greatly decrease the probability of a response and therefore require chemotherapy.

Premenopausal Patients. For premenopausal patients with ER-positive tumors, hormonal therapy is first-line treatment in the absence of the contraindications mentioned above. Oophorectomy is the initial choice and causes tumor regression in 30 to 80 per cent of RP-positive patients. If a patient progresses after initial response, then progestins, adrenalectomy (rarely hypophysectomy), and androgens can be used in sequence until there is no longer a response. At that point, the patient should receive chemotherapy.

Some advocate initial endocrine treatment with the antiestrogen tamoxifen, followed later by oophorectomy once the tamoxifen is ineffective. The experience is more limited with this approach. Some women continue to menstruate while receiving tamoxifen, so its exact mechanism of action and the certainty of adequate estrogen blockade are less well established (in premenopausal women). LHRH agonists are being studied and may become the treatment of choice in the next several years.

Adrenal influences can be removed either by surgical adrenalectomy or by use of medical methods to inhibit adrenal function. Surgical ablation requires permanent replacement therapy in addition to the morbidity of surgery. Medical inhibition with aminoglutethimide, by contrast, is reversible once the drug is stopped. Patients receiving aminoglutethimide experience rash and somnolence 10 to 40 per cent of the time, although these side effects wane after several weeks of treatment. The drug blocks adrenal steroidogenesis by inhibiting conversion of cholesterol to pregnenolone. In peripheral tissue, it also blocks the conversion of androstenedione to estrone, a precursor of estradiol. This latter reaction accounts for the bulk of estrogen production in postmenopausal women. In patients who have RP-positive tumors and responded to prior endocrine therapy, responses to aminoglutethimide occur 30 to 60 per cent of the time. Aminoglutethimide therapy requires replacement corticosteroid treatment with hydrocortisone, which also suppresses the increase in pituitary ACTH secretion produced by aminoglutethimide inhibition of cortisol production, an increase that could otherwise override the blockade. A periodic check of plasma dehydroepiandrosterone levels confirms the adequacy of adrenal suppression. Adrenalectomy is usually chosen over hypophysectomy. The two are roughly equal in therapeutic effect. Hypophysectomy requires a neurosurgeon highly skilled in the transsphenoidal approach (less morbid than the transfrontal route), and complications of the surgery range from incomplete pituitary ablation to cerebrospinal fluid leak and infection. Hypophysectomy also requires permanent thyroid *and* adrenal hormone replacement.

Premenopausal patients with RP-negative tumors, or those originally RP-positive who have become refractory to endocrine treatment, require chemotherapy. Drug classes active against breast cancer include alkylating agents (typically cyclophosphamide), antimetabolites (5-fluorouracil, methotrexate), vinca alkaloids (vincristine, vinblastine), anthracyclines (doxorubicin), and mitomycin-C. In various combinations, these agents effect responses in 60 to 70 per cent of patients, with 10 to 15 per cent achieving a complete remission. These responses have a median duration of only 6 to 9 months, however, and studies are in progress using high-dose chemotherapy and autologous bone marrow rescue to see if selected patients can achieve permanent ablation of metastatic disease.

Postmenopausal Patients. For RP-positive tumors in postmenopausal patients who are candidates for endocrine therapy, the antiestrogen tamoxifen has replaced estrogen therapy (diethylstilbestrol, DES) as initial treatment. Tamoxifen has few side effects, in contrast to DES, which much more frequently produces nausea, anorexia, and salt retention. Both drugs have been associated with a tumor "flare" consisting of increased bone pain and hypercalcemia. This occurs in patients with skeletal metastases during the initial weeks of treatment, more commonly with DES. These reactions usually herald an antitumor effect and do not necessitate cessation of therapy as long as symptoms and calcium levels are controlled by standard supportive treatments. Withdrawal of DES, once the tumor progresses, produces further regression of tumor in 20 to 30 per cent of patients (withdrawal effect is less common with tamoxifen). Once the disease progresses after this initial therapy, serial endocrine maneuvers are employed, as discussed for premenopausal patients, until the tumor becomes refractory to hormonal therapy. Oophorectomy has no role in the treatment of postmenopausal patients. Again, for RP-negative tumors or for tumors resistant to endocrine treatment, chemotherapy becomes the treatment of choice.

Adjuvant Drug Therapy

The goal of prophylactic therapy after mastectomy is to eliminate any micrometastases present. Since eradication of tumor cells is more probable when their number is small, the treatment should be applied as soon after primary treatment as possible. Furthermore, because systemic therapy is quite active against metastatic breast cancer in women who have a high tumor burden, it should be all the more effective against microscopic disease. Table 227–6 summarizes the present indications for adjuvant systemic therapy. Ongoing clinical trials are likely to modify these guidelines in the near future.

The following points should be kept firmly in mind: (1) *optimal* treatment for any subset of patients has yet to be defined; (2) physicians should continue to enroll their patients in controlled trials; and (3) the studies to date in axillary lymph node–negative patients show a statistically significant improvement in relapse-free survival with adjuvant drug therapy. Although not yet demonstrated, there is a strong supposition that overall survival will be increased as well. Since 70 per cent of node-negative

TABLE 227–6. INDICATIONS FOR ADJUVANT SYSTEMIC THERAPY

Axillary lymph node metastases not present
1. Tumors ≤ 1 cm—no adjuvant therapy (risk of relapse less than 10%)
2. Tumors >1 cm and especially with adverse prognostic features (see Table 227–4)—consider adjuvant tamoxifen or chemotherapy

Axillary lymph node metastases present
1. Premenopausal, receptor positive or negative—combination chemotherapy
2. Postmenopausal, receptor positive—tamoxifen
3. Postmenopausal, receptor negative—consider chemotherapy, but this cannot be recommended yet as standard practice

women are cured by primary treatment, the challenge remains to identify and treat only the subset at high risk.

The best choice of drugs, dose, schedule, and duration for adjuvant treatment is unresolved. To date, no severe long-term sequelae of chemotherapy have appeared in patients who have received adjuvant therapy.

SPECIAL CONSIDERATIONS

Male Breast Cancer

Carcinoma of the male breast occurs with 1 per cent the frequency of female breast cancer. Its clinical presentation and primary therapy are similar to those in women. Abnormalities of estrogen metabolism are cited as a possible causative factor. The vast majority of tumors that have been examined are estrogen RP-positive. Castration is the treatment of choice for the initial management of metastatic disease. Antiestrogen therapy, adrenalectomy, and hypophysectomy may offer some palliation, and the effects of additive hormonal therapy are less certain than in female breast cancer.

Breast Cancer and Pregnancy

Breast cancer complicates approximately one of every 3000 pregnancies. It has been held for some time that pregnancy adversely affects the outcome of breast cancer, with studies citing a high frequency of axillary lymph node metastases and shortened survival when the diagnosis is made during pregnancy. To some extent, these poor results may have related to a delay in diagnosis and in the initiation of treatment rather than inherently different biologic factors. The treatment considerations are the same as for the nonpregnant patients, and a standard surgical approach poses a 1 per cent or less risk to the developing fetus. When patients present with disseminated disease in the first or second trimester, cytotoxic drug treatment is a significant risk to the fetus and usually requires termination of pregnancy. If clinical considerations permit, treatment can be delayed to the third trimester to permit delivery of a viable fetus.

Patients who develop cancer during pregnancy tend to present with more advanced stages of disease than nonpregnant patients. However, when compared stage for stage, pregnant women have only a slightly less favorable prognosis than nonpregnant women. In a woman who has had an apparent cure of a breast cancer, subsequent pregnancy is not associated with an excessive risk of recurrence. Patients with early stage breast cancer who bear children appear to have a survival equal to that of women who do not become pregnant. A 3-year interval between primary treatment of early breast cancer and a subsequent pregnancy has been advocated.

Brinton LA, Hoover R, Fraumeni JF Jr: Interaction of familial and hormonal risk factors for breast cancer. J Natl Cancer Inst 69:817, 1982. *An evaluation of family history of breast cancer as a risk indicator in relation to hormonal factors. A large, case-controlled study.*

Danoff BF, Haller DG, Glick JH, et al.: Conservative surgery and irradiation in the treatment of early breast cancer. Ann Intern Med 102:634, 1985. *A detailed review of the literature on breast conservation in primary breast cancer management.*

Donegan WL: Cancer and pregnancy. CA 33:194, 1983. *An overview of the issues surrounding breast cancer (and other cancers) and pregnancy.*

Dupont WD, Page DL: Menopausal replacement therapy and breast cancer. Arch Intern Med 151:67, 1991. *This important, authoritative review of a large number of studies concludes that menopausal therapy consisting of 0.625 mg or less of conjugated estrogens daily does not increase the risk of breast cancer.*

Fisher B: Laboratory and clinical research in breast cancer—a personal adventure. Cancer Res 40:3863, 1980. *This article, plus the following references by Fisher et al. and the reference by Veronesi et al., details a shift in thinking about the biology of breast cancer and update clinical trials of primary management designed to test specific hypotheses about the nature of breast cancer.*

Fisher B, Redmond C, Poisson R, et al.: Eight year results of a randomized clinical trial comparing total mastectomy and lumpectomy with or without irradiation in the treatment of breast cancer. N Engl J Med 320:822, 1989.

Fisher B, Redmond C, Fisher ER, et al.: Ten year results of a randomized clinical trial comparing radical mastectomy and total mastectomy with or without radiation. N Engl J Med 312:674, 1985.

Glick JH, Abeloff MD, Brown BW, et al.: National Institutes of Health Consensus Development Conference Statement: Adjuvant chemotherapy for breast cancer. September 9–11, 1985. CA 36:42, 1986. *A summary statement of the conclusions and recommendations reached in the 1985 conference on adjuvant therapy for node-positive patients.*

Harris JR, Hellman S, Canellos GP, et al: Cancer of the breast. In De Vita VT,

Hellman S, Rosenberg SA (eds.): Cancer. Principles and Practice of Oncology. Philadelphia, J. B. Lippincott, 1985. *A comprehensive treatise detailing areas such as surgical technique, pathology, and chemotherapy.*

Harris JR, Hellman S, Kinne DW: Special report. Limited surgery and radiotherapy for early breast cancer. N Engl J Med 313:1365, 1985. *Summary statement of a workshop held to define surgical procedures, patient selection and criteria, and areas of controversy in the use of more conservative surgery plus radiotherapy for the primary management of breast cancer.*

Kopans DP, Meyer JE, Sadowsky N: Breast imaging. N Engl J Med 310:960, 1984. *A review of mammography and other breast imaging methods which includes a critique of the utility and limitations of each technique.*

McGuire WL, Tandon AK, Allred DC, et al.: How to use prognostic factors in axillary node–negative breast cancer patients. J Natl Cancer Inst 82:1006, 1990. *A summary of the utility of prognostic factors in estimating recurrence risk in node-negative patients.*

Petrakis NL, Ernster VL, King M-C: Breast. In Schottenfeld D, Fraumeni JF Jr (eds.): Cancer Epidemiology and Prevention. Philadelphia, W. B. Saunders Company, 1982. *A review of the range of associated risk factors for breast cancer.*

Relman AS: Adjuvant treatment of early breast cancer. N Engl J Med 320:525, 1989. *Two editorials and four articles in this issue show the implications of controlled trials of recent adjuvant treatment in node-negative breast cancer.*

Schatzkin A, Jones DY, Hoover RN, et al.: Alcohol consumption and breast cancer in the epidemiologic follow-up study of the first national health and nutrition examination survey. N Engl J Med 316:1169, 1987. *This article and its accompanying editorial review the increasing evidence that even modest consumption of alcohol increases the risk of breast cancer by 50 to 100 per cent.*

Veronesi U, Del Vecchio M, Greco M, et al.: Results of quadrantectomy, axillary dissection and radiotherapy (QUART) in T_1N_0 patients. In Harris JR, Hellman S, Silen W (eds.): Conservative Management of Breast Cancer. Philadelphia, J. B. Lippincott Company, 1983.

Wood WC: National Institutes of Health Consensus Development Conference Statement: Treatment of early stage breast cancer. June 18–21, 1990. *A summary statement of conclusions and recommendations concerning primary treatment of early breast cancer and adjuvant therapy for node-negative patients.*

228 Polyglandular Disorders

John N. Loeb

A number of different syndromes are characterized by autonomous hyperfunction or hypofunction of more than one endocrine gland. Although the majority of these syndromes are clearly of genetic origin, the fundamental mechanisms leading to hyperfunction or hypofunction thus far remain unknown in any instance. The syndromes to be considered in this chapter are those in which dysfunction appears to be autonomous within the affected endocrine glands themselves; multiple glandular abnormalities resulting from primary abnormalities in the hypothalamic-pituitary axis or ascribable to various locally infiltrative processes are discussed elsewhere.

SYNDROMES CHARACTERIZED BY MULTIPLE ENDOCRINE GLAND HYPERFUNCTION OR NEOPLASIA

The major syndromes characterized by multiple endocrine hyperfunction are those of multiple endocrine adenomatosis (MEA) or multiple endocrine neoplasia (MEN). A number of these syndromes are inherited as autosomal dominant traits and are clinically distinct. The term MEN is now generally preferred because it is more inclusive, comprising both hyperplastic and carcinomatous as well as adenomatous abnormalities. Table 228–1 compares the clinical features of some of these syndromes.

MULTIPLE ENDOCRINE NEOPLASIA, TYPE 1 (WERMER'S SYNDROME). In 1954 Wermer reported the familial occurrence of *multiple tumors of the anterior pituitary, parathyroid glands, and pancreatic islet cells* in association with a high incidence of peptic ulcer. This complex of abnormalities is now most commonly referred to as multiple endocrine neoplasia, type 1 (MEN 1). The syndrome may also include tumor or hyperfunction of the adrenal and thyroid glands, but the relation of these latter endocrinopathies to the underlying genetic abnormality is less well defined. Although it has been proposed that the fundamental defect in MEN 1 is an abnormal differentiation of neural crest tissue, current evidence in support of this hypothesis is by no means conclusive (see also below, under MEN 2a). A circu-

TABLE 228–1. COMPARISON OF THE CLINICAL FEATURES OF THE MAJOR SYNDROMES CHARACTERIZED BY MULTIPLE ENDOCRINE GLAND HYPERFUNCTION

Endocrine Abnormality	MEN 1*	MEN 2a*	MEN 2b*
Hyperparathyroidism [Hyperplasia or multiple adenomas]	90–95%, with high incidence of hypercalcemia and nephrolithiasis	20–30%, but only 10% with frank hypercalcemia or nephrolithiasis	Rare
Pancreatic islet cell hyperfunction [Hyperplasia, adenomas, or carcinoma, with hypersecretion (e.g., of gastrin or insulin)]	30–35%	—†	—
Pituitary adenomas ["Nonfunctioning" or with hypersecretion of prolactin (common) or growth hormone (rare)]	20–30%	—	—
Multiple cutaneous lipomas	20%	—	—
Thyroid adenomas, adrenal cortical adenomas, carcinoid tumors	Rare	—	—
Thyroid C-cell hyperplasia with hypersecretion of calcitonin ± medullary carcinoma	—	"100%"‡	"100%"‡
Pheochromocytoma	—	Probably >20%	Probably >20%
Multiple mucosal neuromas; marfanoid habitus	—	—	Characteristic
Inheritance	Autosomal dominant	Autosomal dominant	Autosomal dominant, but frequently "sporadic"
Chromosomal linkage	Chromosome 11	Chromosome 10	—

*Percentages indicate approximate frequencies among affected individuals manifesting hyperfunction of at least one endocrine gland.

†— = *not part of the syndrome.*

‡Generally taken to be an essential component of the syndrome.

lating factor that is mitogenic for parathyroid cells in culture and similar if not identical to basic fibroblast growth factor has recently been found in the plasma of patients with MEN 1 (but not of patients with MEN 2a). The mutant gene for MEN 1 is on chromosome 11.

More than half of patients with MEN 1 have adenomas of two or more different endocrine glands, and involvement of three or more different glands is seen in up to 20 per cent of affected individuals. The approximate frequencies of glandular involvement in patients exhibiting any manifestation of endocrine hyperfunction are, in descending order, parathyroids (90 to 95 per cent), pancreatic islet cells (30 to 35 per cent), and anterior pituitary (20 to 30 per cent). Less commonly there may be hyperfunction (adenomas) of the adrenal cortex and thyroid gland; carcinoid tumors have been reported occasionally. Initial manifestations are most commonly detected in middle age, and many years may elapse between the manifestation of the first endocrine abnormality and ensuing ones. The clinical course is highly variable, depending in part upon which glands are affected and whether the neoplasm results in hypersecretion or instead in compression of surrounding normal glandular tissue with concomitant loss of function. By far the greatest majority of patients

(over 90 per cent) have problems related to hypercalcemia, peptic ulcer, hypoglycemia, or pituitary dysfunction. In patients with pituitary neoplasms symptoms are most commonly attributable to pituitary enlargement, with headache or visual-field abnormalities, or to hypopituitarism. Acromegaly, the galactorrhea-amenorrhea syndrome with hyperprolactinemia, and, considerably more rarely, Cushing's disease, may also be seen.

Parathyroid gland involvement is by far the most common manifestation of MEN 1 but may be clinically "silent" for many years. Patients may have a history of kidney stones or progressive renal failure as the first manifestation of hyperparathyroidism, or, much more commonly, hypercalcemia may be detected incidentally upon routine screening. All four parathyroid glands are usually abnormal, and pathologic study may reveal either hyperplasia or multiple adenomas. Parathyroid carcinoma is rare.

Islet cell tumors of the pancreas can be either adenomas (generally multiple) or carcinomas; they may be preceded by diffuse hyperplasia of islet tissue and most typically secrete excess gastrin. Hypersecretion of gastrin may give rise to the *Zollinger-Ellison syndrome* (see Ch. 98) characterized by marked hypersecretion of hydrochloric acid, peptic ulceration (sometimes involving esophageal, distal duodenal, or jejunal sites), and, often, diarrhea. Abdominal pain, bleeding, and perforation are more common than in ordinary instances of peptic ulcer, and radiographic signs consistent with hypersecretion of gastric acid (e.g., hypertrophied gastric rugae) are frequently seen. Many patients in whom the Zollinger-Ellison syndrome initially appears in isolation represent a subset of individuals with MEN 1 and ultimately develop manifestations of additional endocrine neoplasms. *Duodenal* gastrinomas occur in high incidence in patients with MEN 1 and hypergastrinemia.

Hypersecretion of insulin by islet cell neoplasms (usually nonmetastasizing) may produce hypoglycemia as an initial manifestation, whereas the elaboration of other substances may, considerably more rarely, result in a variety of other syndromes. Vasoactive intestinal peptide and prostaglandins have been proposed as agents possibly responsible for the intractable watery diarrhea that can be seen even in the absence of hypersecretion of gastrin and the Zollinger-Ellison syndrome, and hypersecretion of glucagon with hyperglycemia, weight loss, and a characteristic skin rash ("necrotizing migratory erythema") has been reported. Islet cell tumors may also secrete pancreatic polypeptide or, rarely, ACTH, serotonin, or somatostatin.

Symptoms caused by *pituitary adenomas* in MEN 1 are most commonly due to local encroachment of tumor upon other structures, with headache or visual-field abnormalities, or to deficiency of one or more of the tropic hormones. Many of these tumors secrete prolactin and may give rise to the galactorrhea-amenorrhea syndrome. More rarely there is hypersecretion of growth hormone with resulting acromegaly. Hypersecretion of ACTH in MEN 1 is almost always attributable to an ectopic (pancreatic) site.

Adrenocortical hyperfunction may be due to ectopic production of ACTH or to independently functioning adrenal adenomas or carcinomas. Functioning adenomas most commonly elaborate hydrocortisone, giving rise to signs of glucocorticoid excess, but predominant secretion of aldosterone has been reported in rare instances. Hyperfunction of the *thyroid* gland has been reported least frequently of all, and, in part owing to the high incidence of thyroid abnormalities in the population at large, it is possible that sporadic instances of thyroid hyperfunction in MEN 1 represent incidental occurrences unrelated to the underlying genetic abnormality. Adenomas, thyroiditis, and rarely papillary and follicular cell carcinomas have all been reported in association with MEN 1; medullary carcinomas are *not* a part of this syndrome (cf. MEN 2a and 2b, below). *Other tumors* that can form a part of the clinical picture of MEN 1 include schwannomas, multiple cutaneous lipomas, thymomas, and both bronchial and small intestinal carcinoids.

Management of the various manifestations of MEN 1 is, for the most part, similar to management of the identical manifestations when they occur in sporadic form and hence is considered elsewhere in this textbook. As indicated above, parathyroid involvement, when it occurs, frequently involves more than one gland, and histopathology far more commonly reveals diffuse hyperplasia than a single adenoma. In such instances a number of surgeons now advocate total parathyroidectomy with reimplantation of a glandular fragment in a location conveniently accessible to subsequent exploration if necessary (e.g., the muscle of the forearm). Management of severe peptic ulceration in MEN 1 has usually required either long-term cimetidine or ranitidine therapy or near-total gastrectomy—rather than an attempt to eliminate the source of excess gastrin—since hypersecretion of gastrin by islet-cell tissue in this syndrome is almost always attributable to either multiple tumors or diffuse hyperplasia. A substantial proportion of patients with MEN 1 and the Zollinger-Ellison syndrome have hypergastrinemia on the basis of duodenal rather than pancreatic gastrinomas. The hypergastrinemia can often be cured or markedly ameliorated when these tumors (frequently small) are removed, so the duodenum should be examined first in patients who have MEN 1 and symptomatic hypergastrinemia.

The sporadic nature of the sequential manifestations of this syndrome makes it important to follow affected individuals with particular attention to the development of new abnormalities. Once the diagnosis has been established in a given patient and baseline films of the sella turcica and prolactin levels have proved to be normal, the major requisite is a careful interval history and a periodic (e.g., yearly) determination of the serum calcium and phosphorus.

Because of the high incidence of the syndrome in first-degree relatives, all such family members should be carefully evaluated, as well as any second-degree relatives who have suggestive histories elicited through questioning of the propositus. Determination of fasting blood sugar, serum calcium, and prolactin levels is generally sufficient if menses or sexual potency is present and if the history and physical examination are negative. Films of the sella turcica are usually unrevealing, and CT scanning is too expensive for use as a routine screen.

MULTIPLE ENDOCRINE NEOPLASIA, TYPE 2a (SIPPLE'S SYNDROME). A second and entirely distinct syndrome, multiple endocrine neoplasia, type 2a (MEN 2a), is characterized by *medullary carcinoma of the thyroid, pheochromocytoma, and parathyroid hyperplasia.* First partially described by Sipple in 1961, this syndrome, like MEN 1, is inherited as an autosomal dominant trait. The pheochromocytomas are frequently bilateral, although rarely extra-adrenal, and the medullary carcinoma of the thyroid generally appears to be multifocal in origin. A particularly convenient and virtually constant feature of the medullary thyroid carcinomas is the hypersecretion of calcitonin, which serves as a useful marker for the presence of this neoplasm. Elevated levels of calcitonin, either under basal conditions or in response to the provocative stimuli of calcium and pentagastrin infusions, are an indication of parafollicular C-cell hyperplasia in the thyroid gland and may herald the presence of the genetic abnormality well before pathologic changes appear that are unequivocally malignant. As in the instance of the pancreatic adenomas in MEN 1, the medullary carcinomas of the thyroid in MEN 2a may secrete a variety of hormones and other biologically active substances that are not secreted by the corresponding normal tissue. These include ACTH, prolactin, histaminase, vasoactive intestinal peptide, serotonin, and a number of prostaglandins. Only rarely does medullary carcinoma of the thyroid present as a palpable mass. Pheochromocytoma is observed in about one half of affected individuals, and hyperparathyroidism in about one quarter. Only about 10 per cent of individuals with MEN 2a exhibit hypercalcemia or nephrolithiasis (cf. the much higher incidence of overt hyperparathyroidism in MEN 1). Glial tumors and meningiomas may also be seen in MEN 2a but occur far less frequently.

It has been suggested that MEN 2a represents a form of neuroectodermal dysplasia in which so-called APUD cells (cells capable of *a*mine *p*recursor *u*ptake and *d*ecarboxylation and possessing rather characteristic histologic staining properties)—following their embryonic migration to the foregut and subsequent localization in a variety of endocrine tissues—later become neoplastic and secrete excessive amounts of hormone in response to a specific genetic defect. Although the evidence for a common APUD cell origin is somewhat better in MEN 2a than it is in MEN 1, it is still by no means wholly convincing. In particular, the high incidence of parathyroid involvement is

difficult to reconcile with this theory, since the bulk of present evidence suggests an epithelial rather than a neural crest origin for this tissue. The medullary thyroid carcinomas in MEN 2a may begin as polyclonal hyperplasia followed by clonal carcinomas; that is, these carcinomas may arise as independent clonal "expansions" on a background of initial hyperplasia. The mutant gene for MEN 2a is on the short arm of chromosome 10.

The pheochromocytomas of MEN 2a are generally benign and are treated surgically. Because they are frequently bilateral, an anterior surgical approach is often recommended; CT scanning, multiple-site venous sampling for catecholamines, and angiography can all be helpful in planning surgery. Medullary carcinoma of the thyroid, on the other hand, runs a typically malignant course, and, because of its multifocal nature, requires total thyroidectomy. Elevated levels of calcitonin per se constitute a sufficient indication for total thyroidectomy, even when the tumor is otherwise clinically silent. The tumor is frequently slow growing, and limited node dissection is thus justified; completeness of tumor removal and the possibility of subsequent recurrence are both conveniently monitored by serum calcitonin levels. The isolated finding of medullary carcinoma of the thyroid should prompt a particularly careful inquiry into the family history, since it is likely that at least 10 per cent of such tumors are familial.

Screening of first-degree relatives of patients with MEN 2a is indicated and should include a 24-hour urine collection for vanillylmandelic acid, metanephrines, and catecholamines (even when the blood pressure is normal) as well as calcium and basal calcitonin determinations. If a thyroid mass is present, a fuller workup is indicated, including measurement of calcium-pentagastrin–stimulated calcitonin levels. Restriction-fragment analysis of DNA from peripheral blood lymphocytes can be employed to identify carriers of the MEN 2a gene.

MULTIPLE ENDOCRINE NEOPLASIA, TYPE 2b (MUCOSAL NEUROMA SYNDROME). This syndrome (MEN 2b) resembles MEN 2a but differs in four important respects: (1) The medullary carcinoma of the thyroid and the pheochromocytomas may be accompanied by striking and often disfiguring neuromas of the lips, buccal mucosa, and tongue, as well as by ganglioneuromas of the gastrointestinal tract, thickened corneal nerves visible upon slit-lamp examination, and café-au-lait spots, neuromas, or neurofibromas of the skin; (2) the body habitus may somewhat resemble that seen in patients with the Marfan syndrome; (3) parathyroid hyperplasia sufficient to result in frank hypercalcemia is rare; and (4) mean survival time in MEN 2b is considerably shorter than that in MEN 2a (30 versus 60 years). In contrast to MEN 1 and MEN 2a, MEN 2b is frequently sporadic, a history of affected family members being obtainable in not more than half of the cases.

McCUNE-ALBRIGHT SYNDROME. In 1937 McCune and Albright and their associates both described a syndrome characterized by a triad of *polyostotic fibrous dysplasia, café-au-lait pigmentation of the skin* (typically over the forehead, nuchal or sacral areas, or buttocks), and *precocious puberty in the female.* The precocious puberty, although predominantly seen in the female, may occur in males as well. This syndrome may be accompanied by a variety of other endocrine abnormalities, including pituitary hyperfunction (with Cushing's syndrome, acromegaly, or gigantism), bilateral pheochromocytomas, hyperthyroidism, and hypercorticism resulting from adrenal adenoma. Frank malignant disease has not been described. Although the sexual precocity appears to be hypothalamic in origin, patients with adrenal adenomas and hyperthyroidism can have low plasma levels of ACTH and TSH, respectively. The cause of the bone lesions is unknown. The disease appears to be sporadic.

SYNDROMES CHARACTERIZED BY MULTIPLE ENDOCRINE GLAND HYPOFUNCTION

Syndromes characterized by hypofunction of multiple endocrine organs are discussed under the separate headings of Schmidt's syndrome and the syndrome of polyglandular deficiency associated with mucocutaneous candidiasis. As noted below, however, evidence that the two syndromes actually represent different entities is incomplete. Table 228–2 compares the clinical features of these syndromes.

MULTIPLE ENDOCRINE DEFICIENCY SYNDROME (SCHMIDT'S SYNDROME). In 1926 Schmidt described two

TABLE 228–2. COMPARISON OF THE CLINICAL FEATURES OF THE MAJOR SYNDROMES CHARACTERIZED BY MULTIPLE ENDOCRINE GLAND HYPOFUNCTION

	Multiple Endocrine Deficiency Syndrome (Schmidt's Syndrome)	Polyglandular Deficiency with Mucocutaneous Candidiasis
Hypoadrenalism	Common	Common
Hypothyroidism	Common	Rare
Diabetes mellitus (Type I)	Common	Rare
Gonadal failure	Less common	Less common
Hypoparathyroidism	Rare	Common
Pituitary insufficiency	Rare	Rare
Autoantibodies to endocrine tissues and gastric parietal cells	Often present	Often present
Sex distribution	Strong female predominance	Female preponderance about 4:1
Inheritance	Usually "sporadic," but susceptibility related to HLA haplotype and may be inherited as autosomal dominant	Generally inherited as autosomal recessive; no apparent HLA association; siblings characteristically affected
Time of onset	Usually becomes evident during adult life	Typically becomes evident during childhood preceded by chronic mucocutaneous moniliasis
Other associated "autoimmune" diseases and characteristics	Pernicious anemia; hyperthyroidism; celiac disease; alopecia; vitiligo; myasthenia gravis; isolated red-cell aplasia	Pernicious anemia; malabsorption; alopecia; vitiligo; IgA deficiency; hypergammaglobulinemia; chronic active hepatitis; proliferative glomerulonephritis

patients with biglandular failure characterized by *idiopathic Addison's disease and lymphocytic thyroiditis.* This syndrome has subsequently been expanded to include "primary" failure of other endocrine glands, including the gonads, endocrine pancreas, and rarely the parathyroids, as well as a number of nonendocrine abnormalities of presumed autoimmune origin (see below). Virtually any combination of the foregoing endocrine deficiencies may appear in a single individual. The order of appearance is extremely variable, and a lag of as much as 17 years has been observed in the manifestation of sequential deficiencies. Hypothyroidism and hypoadrenalism are common; diabetes mellitus (Type 1) and gonadal failure are somewhat less so. The frequencies of the different glandular failures probably vary greatly with ascertainment; if one considers Type 1 diabetes mellitus as part of the syndrome, the association of this with autoimmune thyroid disease may be the most commonly encountered combination.

Characteristic of this syndrome is the presence of autoantibodies to endocrine tissue and at times to gastric parietal cells as well. Such antibodies are often detectable before the appearance of clinical glandular insufficiency and are a hallmark of syndromes of "idiopathic" endocrine failure. Their presence has been implicated in the pathogenesis of the glandular destruction itself rather than merely as reflecting an immune response to tissue antigens released during antecedent glandular degeneration. Thus, for example, approximately two thirds of patients with idiopathic Addison's disease are reported to have autoantibodies to adrenal tissue, whereas such antibodies are generally absent in patients whose adrenal insufficiency is secondary to tuberculous destruction. About twice as many females are affected with idiopathic adrenal insufficiency as males. Although most cases of multiple

deficiency syndromes are sporadic, their occasional appearance in kindreds, as well as the relatively high gene frequency of the HLA-B8 and HLA-DR3 alleles in affected persons, provides strong evidence for a dominantly inherited susceptibility to the development of this type of polyglandular failure. Other "autoimmune" diseases that may accompany the aforementioned endocrine deficiencies include pernicious anemia, celiac disease, myasthenia gravis, alopecia, vitiligo, and isolated red-cell aplasia. Because it occurs in the same families and has the same HLA associations, Graves' disease is considered by many to be another facet of the syndrome.

Although the constellation of adrenal, thyroid, and gonadal failure in a single patient can easily be confused with primary pituitary insufficiency, measurement of the appropriate tropic hormones permits a ready differentiation of the two syndromes. Occasionally the simultaneous presence of hyperpigmentation in such an individual suggests a diagnosis of primary adrenal failure on "clinical" grounds alone. Because of the sporadic appearance and variable sequence of subsequent endocrine deficiencies, patients with a proven idiopathic endocrine deficiency should be periodically screened for evidence of additional endocrine involvement.

POLYGLANDULAR DEFICIENCY ASSOCIATED WITH MUCOCUTANEOUS CANDIDIASIS. A clinical picture somewhat different from that of Schmidt's syndrome is presented by patients with the so-called candidiasis-endocrinopathy syndrome. Characteristically this syndrome is dominated by the presence of extensive mucocutaneous candidiasis that appears in early childhood and is followed by the development of idiopathic adrenal insufficiency or hypoparathyroidism or both. Most typically, but not invariably, the appearance of these endocrinopathies postdates the acquisition of chronic monilial infection (mean age of onset, 13 versus 3 years, respectively). As in Schmidt's syndrome, antibodies against endocrine tissues are frequently demonstrable, and pernicious anemia with antibodies against gastric parietal cells may also be present. Diabetes mellitus, in contrast, is relatively rare. Also contrasting with Schmidt's syndrome, which most typically becomes evident in adult life, is the fact that there is no apparent association with the presence of specific HLA alleles, and the apparent inheritance of the syndrome as an autosomal recessive trait within a single generation of siblings. Chronic active hepatitis and proliferative glomerulonephritis have also been reported. The mucocutaneous candidiasis is associated with hypergammaglobulinemia, IgA deficiency, and anergy to *Candida albicans.* Treatment with oral ketoconazole can produce a striking remission of the mucocutaneous candidiasis, although the latter generally recurs upon discontinuation of therapy. No evidence for disseminated candidiasis has been found in autopsied individuals, nor has *Candida* yet been cultured from an affected endocrine gland.

Albright F, Butler AM, Hampton AO, et al.: Syndrome characterized by osteitis fibrosa disseminata, areas of pigmentation and endocrine dysfunction, with precocious puberty in females. N Engl J Med 216:727, 1937. *One of the two classic descriptions of the McCune-Albright syndrome. Excellent figures.*

Gagel RF, Tashjian AF Jr, Cummings TW, et al.: The clinical outcome of prospective screening for multiple endocrine neoplasia type 2a: An 18-year experience. N Engl J Med 318:478, 1988. *A recent review showing that prospective screening and early treatment of the manifestations of MEN 2a can prevent metastasis of medullary thyroid carcinoma as well as the morbidity and mortality associated with pheochromocytoma.*

Deftos LJ, Catherwood BD, Bone HG III: Multiglandular endocrine disorders. *In* Felig P, Baxter JD, Broadus AE, et al. (eds.): Endocrinology and Metabolism, 2nd ed. New York, McGraw-Hill Book Company, 1987, pp 1662–1691. *Excellent general review with 198 references.*

Pipeleers-Marichal M, Somers G, Willems G, et al.: Gastrinomas in the duodenums of patients with multiple endocrine neoplasia type 1 and the Zollinger-Ellison syndrome. N Engl J Med 322:723, 1990. *Multicenter report of a high incidence of resectable duodenal gastrinomas as a cause of symptomatic hypergastrinemia in patients with MEN 1.*

Rabinowe SL, Eisenbarth GS: Polyglandular autoimmunity. Adv Intern Med 31:293, 1986. *An excellent review of these syndromes with an up-to-date list of 60 references.*

Sobol H, Narod SA, Nakamura Y, et al.: Screening for multiple endocrine neoplasia type 2a with DNA-polymorphism analysis. N Engl J Med 321:996, 1989. *Genetic screening permits identification of individuals at risk for MEN 2a with a high level of certainty.*

Trence DL, Morley JE, Handwerger BS: Polyglandular autoimmune syndromes. Am J Med 77:107, 1984. *A comprehensive review of these interesting disorders supplemented by 110 references.*

Wilkin TJ: Mechanisms of disease: Receptor autoimmunity in endocrine disorders. N Engl J Med 323:1318, 1990. *The best recent article on this topic.*

Zimering MB, Brandi ML, deGrange DA, et al.: Circulating fibroblast growth factor–like substance in familial multiple endocrine neoplasia type I. J Clin Endocrinol Metab 70:149, 1990. *Evidence that the parathyroid hyperplasia characteristic of MEN 1 is attributable to a circulating growth factor similar if not identical to basic fibroblast growth factor.*

229 The Adrenal Medullae

Philip E. Cryer

The sympathochromaffin (sympathoadrenal) system consists of two components: (1) the sympathetic nervous system and (2) the chromaffin tissues, including the adrenal medullae. The primary endocrine, neurotransmitter, and perhaps paracrine products of the sympathochromaffin system are the catecholamines—epinephrine (adrenaline), norepinephrine (noradrenaline), and dopamine. Cells of the sympathochromaffin system also contain a variety of peptides of potential biologic importance. Their pathophysiologic roles, if any, are unknown.

Catecholamine excess commonly results in hypertension along with typical symptoms. It has long been suspected, but is still not proven, that increased sympathetic nervous system activity is the cause of primary (essential) hypertension. Catecholamine overproduction from chromaffin cell tumors—pheochromocytomas—is an uncommon, but often curable, cause of hypertension. Deficient sympathetic neuronal norepinephrine release results in postural (orthostatic) hypotension, a sharp decrease in blood pressure when a person stands. Under certain conditions, deficient adrenomedullary epinephrine secretion results in hypoglycemia. Two of these prominent examples of sympathochromaffin pathophysiology are discussed in the paragraphs that follow. Disorders of the sympathetic nervous system are discussed in Ch. 452.

PHYSIOLOGY OF THE SYMPATHOCHROMAFFIN SYSTEM

CATECHOLAMINE BIOSYNTHESIS. The term *catecholamines* is often used to refer to epinephrine and norepinephrine, although dopamine is also a catecholamine, i.e., has the dihydroxyphenyl ("catechol") ring structure and an amine side chain (Fig. 229–1). The catecholamines are synthesized from the amino acid tyrosine, which is derived from the diet or formed by hydroxylation of the essential amino acid phenylalanine. Tyrosine hydroxylase, the enzyme that converts tyrosine to dihydroxyphenylalanine (dopa), is the rate-limiting enzyme in catecholamine biosynthesis. In the presence of a nonspecific decarboxylase, dopa is converted to dopamine, which is the final product in some systems (e.g., interneurons in the sympathetic ganglia). After transport into cytoplasmic vesicles (storage granules), dopamine can be converted to norepinephrine in the presence of dopamine β-hydroxylase. Norepinephrine is the final product in sympathetic postganglionic neurons. Other tissues, such as the adrenal medullae, have cells that also contain phenylethanolamine-N-methyltransferase, the enzyme that converts norepinephrine to epinephrine, the final product of those cells.

Catecholamines are stored in cytoplasmic granules and released from the cell by exocytosis in response to neural stimulation.

CATECHOLAMINE DEGRADATION AND ELIMINATION. Catecholamines are degraded by two principal enzyme systems, catechol-O-methyltransferase (COMT) and monoamine oxidase (MAO) (Fig. 229–1). COMT converts norepinephrine and epinephrine to their respective O-methyl derivatives, the metanephrines (normetanephrine and metanephrine). MAO converts norepinephrine and epinephrine to dihydroxymandelic acid. These intermediates, the metanephrines and dihydroxymandelic acid, can then serve as substrates for MAO and COMT, respectively, resulting in their conversion to the major end product of extra-CNS catecholamine metabolism, vanillylmandelic acid (VMA). Dopamine metabolism (not shown in Figure 229–1) by MAO and COMT leads to the formation of homovanillic acid (HVA).

In general, catecholamine degradation within the sympathochromaffin cells is via MAO, whereas that of released catecholamines is via COMT. Released catecholamines are also conjugated, largely to sulfate in humans, and this may be another important route of inactivation. Sixty to 80 per cent of plasma epinephrine and norepinephrine and roughly half of the catecholamines excreted in the urine are conjugated.

Catecholamines are cleared rapidly from the circulation. Plasma half-times are 1 to 2 minutes. Clearance is largely extrarenal; less than 5 per cent appears in the urine unaltered.

BIOLOGIC ROLES OF THE CATECHOLAMINES. Epinephrine, norepinephrine, and dopamine are neurotransmitters in the CNS. Outside of the CNS, epinephrine is a hormone of the adrenal medullae, and norepinephrine is primarily the neurotransmitter of sympathetic postganglionic neurons. Dopamine is probably also a neurotransmitter, although its physiologic role has not been defined clearly.

Neurally regulated secretion of epinephrine from extra-adrenal chromaffin tissue (not sympathetic neurons) occurs, but in the absence of the adrenal medullae even stimulated plasma epinephrine levels in adults are not high enough to produce measurable biologic effects. Biologic actions of extra-adrenal epinephrine, if any, must be paracrine/neurotransmitter, not hormonal, in nature, at least in adults. Thus, epinephrine functions primarily as a hormone of the adrenal medulla and its plasma concentration is a valid index of its secretion.

Norepinephrine is released from axon terminals of sympathetic postganglionic neurons in direct relation to adrenergic receptors on innervated target cells. Most released norepinephrine is dissipated locally by reuptake into an axon terminal (uptake$_1$), where it is either stored in vesicles or metabolized, or by uptake into other cells adjacent to the synaptic cleft (uptake$_2$), where it is metabolized. Only a small fraction escapes into the circulation. The plasma norepinephrine concentration is a reasonable index of sympathetic neural activity under common physiologic conditions, at least in the basal state and during upright activity in humans. However, under some conditions, such as hypoglycemia, substantial amounts of norepinephrine (along with large amounts of epinephrine) are released from chromaffin tissues, specifically the adrenal medullae. Under such conditions the plasma norepinephrine concentration is clearly not an index of sympathetic neural activity. During vigorous physical activity and in a variety of pathologic states such as surgery, acute myocardial infarction, and diabetic ketoacidosis, circulating norepinephrine is probably derived from both the sympathetic nerves and the adrenal medullae, and its concentrations can be high enough to produce measurable effects. Under these conditions norepinephrine may function as a hormone as well as a neurotransmitter.

This physiology is relevant to the clinical use of plasma catecholamine measurements. Norepinephrine release from sympathetic neurons in amounts sufficient to produce biologically active norepinephrine concentrations in the synaptic cleft can be associated with very small, even undetectable, increments in its plasma concentration. On the other hand, if norepinephrine is released directly into the circulation (as from a pheochromocytoma) substantial increments in its plasma concentration are required to produce biologically active synaptic cleft concentrations.

BIOLOGIC ACTIONS OF THE CATECHOLAMINES. Catecholamines produce a variety of hemodynamic and metabolic effects. These are the result of catecholamine occupancy of adrenergic receptors (adrenoceptors) on the surface of target cells and a consequent series of intramembrane and intracellular biochemical events. Adrenergic receptors are divided into α- and β-adrenergic receptors, which are subdivided into α$_1$- and α$_2$- adrenergic receptors and β$_1$- and β$_2$-adrenergic receptors on the basis of measurements of the responses to various agonists and antagonists and the binding of a variety of ligands (generally antagonists) and competition for binding of these ligands by agonists and antagonists in vitro. In general, β-adrenergic receptors are linked through a stimulatory guanine nucleotide regulatory protein to adenylate cyclase, and α$_2$- (but not α$_1$-) adrenergic receptors are linked through an inhibitory protein to adenylate cyclase. A discussion of adrenergic receptors is beyond the scope of this chapter, although selected examples are given.

Catecholamines increase the rate and force of myocardial contraction (β_1) and produce vasoconstriction (α) in most vascular beds, although vasodilatation (β_2) occurs in some vascular beds, e.g., those of skeletal muscle. Norepinephrine produces increased vascular resistance and blood pressure (systolic and diastolic); the increased blood pressure reflexively limits the increase in heart rate. Probably because it has a higher affinity than norepinephrine for β_2-adrenergic receptors, epinephrine normally produces a somewhat different pattern: increased systolic, but not diastolic, blood pressure and increased heart rate.

Catecholamines increase the plasma glucose concentration through complex actions. These involve both stimulation of hepatic glucose production and limitation of glucose utilization and are mediated by both direct and indirect mechanisms. Foremost among the indirect mechanisms is limitation of insulin secretion (α_2). The direct actions are largely β mediated. Catecholamines also stimulate lipolysis, ketogenesis, glycolysis, and mobilization of amino acids such as alanine. They also increase thermogenesis.

Symptoms that occur when the sympathochromaffin system is activated include palpitations, anxiety, headache, and diaphoresis. All but the last are attributable to released catecholamines; diaphoresis has been attributed to a sympathetic cholinergic mechanism.

PHEOCHROMOCYTOMA

Pheochromocytomas are catecholamine-releasing tumors that typically produce hypertension. They are an uncommon cause of hypertension; perhaps 1 in 1000 hypertensive patients harbors a pheochromocytoma. Yet it is important to detect a pheochromocytoma for several reasons: (1) Hypertension due to a pheochromocytoma is usually curable by surgical removal of the tumor. (2) Patients with a pheochromocytoma are at risk for a lethal hypertensive paroxysm. (3) Some pheochromocytomas are malignant; early detection and removal would be expected to reduce the frequency of metastatic disease. Parenthetically, malignancy is established convincingly only by proven metastases; histologic criteria in the primary tumor are not reliable. (4) The presence of pheochromocytomas can be a clue to the presence of associated endocrine and nonendocrine familial disorders (Ch. 228). Pheochromocytomas are components of the multiple endocrine neoplasia, type 2 (MEN 2a) and type 3 (MEN 2b) syndromes. These familial disorders are inherited as autosomal dominant traits. MEN 2a includes medullary carcinoma of the thyroid, primary hyperparathyroidism, and pheochromocytoma. MEN 2b includes medullary carcinoma of the thyroid, multiple mucosal neuromas, and pheochromocytoma. Pheochromocytomas are not a component of the MEN 1 syndrome (pituitary and pancreatic adenomas and hyperparathyroidism). Familial pheochromocytomas also occur as an isolated disorder, in neurofibromatosis, and in the von Hippel-Lindau syndrome.

PATHOLOGY. Pheochromocytomas arise from chromaffin cells. Chromaffin cells are widespread and associated with sympathetic ganglia during fetal life. Postnatally most chromaffin cells degenerate; the major residual clusters of chromaffin cells comprise the adrenal medullae. Approximately 90 per cent of pheochromocytomas arise from the adrenal medullae. Extra-adrenal pheochromocytomas (paragangliomas) have been found in sites ranging from the carotid body to the pelvic floor. However, the majority are associated with sympathetic ganglia in the abdomen and most of the others with ganglia in the posterior mediastinum. Multiple pheochromocytomas, including bilateral adrenomedullary tumors, occur in up to 10 per cent of apparently sporadic cases. Bilateral adrenomedullary pheochromocytomas, with or without extra-adrenal tumors, are the rule in familial pheochro-

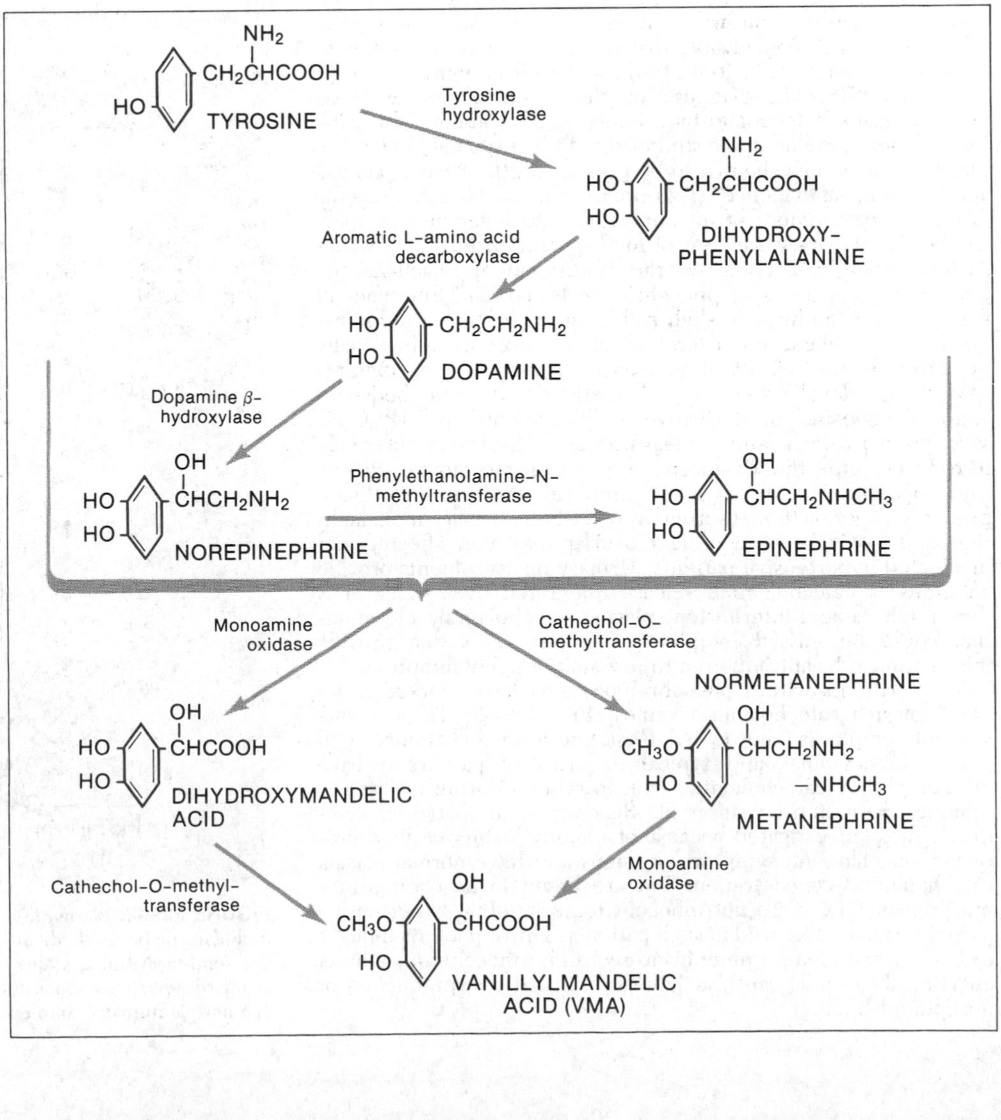

FIGURE 229–1. Catecholamine biosynthesis and metabolic degradation.

mocytoma. Bilateral adrenomedullary hyperplasia, thought to be a precursor to pheochromocytoma, has been found in members of affected families.

The vast majority of pheochromocytomas release norepinephrine, and most also release some epinephrine. Rarely, a pheochromocytoma releases epinephrine predominantly or even exclusively.

CLINICAL MANIFESTATIONS. The clinical manifestations of pheochromocytomas are commonly due to the effects of released catecholamines and only rarely to the mass effect of the tumor. Common symptoms are *headache, palpitations,* and *diaphoresis.* Less common symptoms include abdominal or chest pain, gastrointestinal symptoms, weakness, or visual symptoms. Symptoms are typically paroxysmal and associated with increments in blood pressure. Hypertension is sometimes truly intermittent. In many cases, hypertension is sustained but exhibits marked fluctuations with peak values occurring during symptomatic episodes. In general, plasma catecholamine levels are higher during symptomatic, hypertensive episodes than during asymptomatic, less hypertensive, or even normotensive intervals. The event(s) that precipitates episodic catecholamine release is usually not identifiable. However, the relationship between plasma catecholamine concentrations and blood pressure is not tight. This may reflect contrasting effects of norepinephrine and epinephrine but raises the possibility that hypertension in a patient with a pheochromocytoma may not be exclusively the result of direct effects of circulating norepinephrine on the cardiovascular system. Metabolic features of pheochromocytoma include an increased metabolic rate (some patients complain of heat intolerance, weight loss, or both) and an insulin-resistant state. Glucose intolerance and fasting hyperglycemia occur, but overt diabetes is unusual and probably reflects a coexistent defect in insulin secretion, i.e., genetic diabetes mellitus.

The rare epinephrine-releasing pheochromocytomas can produce different paroxysms. These may include hypotension, prominent tachycardia, noncardiac pulmonary edema, and cardiac arrhythmias. It is conceivable that tumor products in addition to epinephrine might contribute to these manifestations.

DIAGNOSIS. The diagnosis of pheochromocytoma is based upon clinical suspicion and biochemical confirmation (Table 229–1). In general, radiographic studies should be used only to localize pheochromocytomas known to be present on the basis of clinical and biochemical evidence. High-pressure liquid chromatographic (HPLC) measurement of unconjugated catecholamines or spectrophotometric measurement of total metanephrines or VMA in 24-hour urine collections is the traditional approach to the biochemical diagnosis of pheochromocytoma. The frequency of false-negative findings is slightly higher with VMA determinations. Nonetheless, the excretion of all three is substantially increased in the majority of patients with pheochromocytomas.

With the development of sufficiently sensitive methods, including single isotope derivative (radioenzymatic) or HPLC assays, plasma catecholamine measurements have been effectively introduced into the diagnosis of pheochromocytoma. Plasma catecholamine or urinary norepinephrine measurements are probably superior to measurement of 24-hour urinary metanephrine and VMA because of less overlap between affected and unaffected hypertensive patients. Urinary measurements provide an index of catecholamine release integrated over time. Thus they might reflect intermittent plasma catecholamine elevations that could be missed by plasma measurements that provide information relevant only to a time frame of a few minutes.

Most patients with a pheochromocytoma have markedly elevated plasma catecholamine values (Fig. 229–2). Three points warrant emphasis, however. First, occasional patients with pheochromocytomas and typical histories of paroxysms have normal plasma catecholamine concentrations during an asymptomatic, normotensive interval. Second, some patients, commonly those investigated because of a family history of pheochromocytoma, have no symptoms or signs and have normal plasma catecholamine concentrations but are found to have pheochromocytomas. These are not innocent tumors; lethal hypertensive paroxysms have occurred in such patients. Third, patients thought to have predominant epinephrine-secreting pheochromocytomas on clinical grounds can also have substantial overproduction of norepinephrine.

TABLE 229–1. DIAGNOSIS OF PHEOCHROMOCYTOMA

Clinical Suspicion
1. Paroxysmal symptoms (especially headache, palpitations, and diaphoresis)
2. Intermittent or unusually labile hypertension or hypertension refractory to therapy
3. Incidental adrenal mass (rarely a pheochromocytoma in the absence of one or more of the above)
4. Family history of pheochromocytoma, MEN 2, or MEN 3

Biochemical Confirmation
1. Plasma norepinephrine and epinephrine (± dopamine)
   Patient sampled in the basal state (and supine position) and, if possible, during a paroxysm
   Radioenzymatic or HPLC method
   Note blood pressure, heart rate, and any symptoms
2. Urinary catecholamines or metanephrines (or VMA)
   If plasma values are normal or equivocal but clinical suspicion is high, repeated plasma measurements are an alternative
   Can be used as the initial test

Anatomic Localization
1. Computed tomography
   Of the abdomen, including the adrenals, initially; of the pelvis and thorax if the abdomen is negative
   Indicated in the absence of biochemical evidence only if clinical suspicion is very high (e.g., positive family history)
2. Magnetic resonance imaging
3. Iodobenzylguanidine scan

Strict attention to the details of sample collection, handling and storage, the sources of possible biologic variation, and the effects of drugs is critical if diagnostic error is to be avoided in the biochemical assessment of patients with suspected pheochromocytomas. Patients should be studied in the drug-free state if at all possible. Most antihypertensive drugs (other than clonidine) and many other drugs can elevate plasma and/or urine catecholamine levels. Elevated plasma catecholamine concentrations are to be expected during physical or mental stress and in any acute

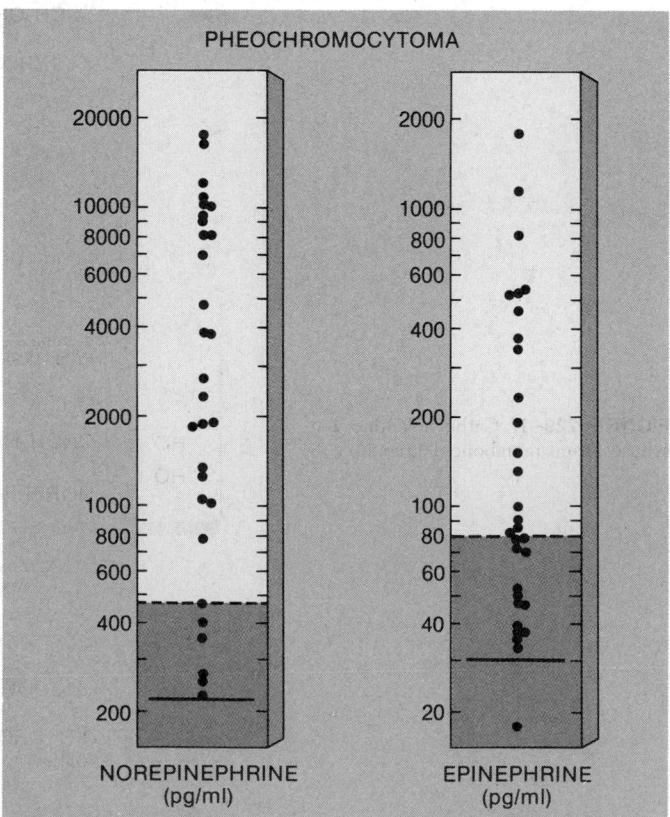

FIGURE 229–2. Plasma norepinephrine and epinephrine concentrations (radioenzymatic method) in 30 patients with pheochromocytomas. Note the semi-logarithmic scales. The interrupted horizontal lines are three standard deviations above the means (solid horizontal lines) of data from 165 normal humans sampled in the supine position.

illness. Elevations, at times marked, have been well documented in patients with acute myocardial infarction, shock, burns, diabetic ketoacidosis, and cerebrovascular accidents, as well as during and immediately after surgery. Stable plasma catecholamine elevations also occur in patients with chronic disorders—for example, hypothyroidism, congestive heart failure, chronic obstructive pulmonary disease, anemia, duodenal ulcer, and depression. Lastly, elevated plasma catecholamine concentrations have been found in some, but certainly not all, patients thought to have essential hypertension.

It is my practice to obtain samples for determination of plasma norepinephrine and epinephrine in the basal state, with the patient supine, when pheochromocytoma is suspected. Substantial elevations over reference values provide strong support for the diagnosis of pheochromocytoma and are commonly found in affected patients. Samples are also obtained during symptomatic paroxysms. However, the interpretation of such values is more judgmental, since reference values cannot be defined precisely. Thus the biochemical diagnosis of pheochromocytoma is more convincingly supported if plasma catecholamine levels are elevated in the basal state and rise further during symptomatic episodes.

It is useful to record the blood pressure and whether or not symptoms are present when plasma samples for catecholamine measurements are drawn from a patient suspected of having a pheochromocytoma. Clearly, normal plasma (or urinary) catecholamine values obtained when the patient is normotensive and free of symptoms do not exclude the presence of a pheochromocytoma. Theoretically, 24-hour urinary catecholamine or metabolite measurements might detect intermittent catecholamine release missed by plasma sampling. These measurements should be obtained if plasma catecholamine levels are normal but clinical suspicion is high.

Substantial plasma norepinephrine elevations are required to produce hypertension in normal humans. Plasma epinephrine elevations within the physiologic range do not raise the diastolic blood pressure. It is reasonable, therefore, to consider normal or even moderately elevated plasma catecholamine levels obtained when the patient is hypertensive to be strong evidence against the diagnosis of pheochromocytoma.

Most patients ultimately found to have pheochromocytomas have distinctly elevated plasma and urinary catecholamine levels. The considerations raised in the preceding paragraphs apply to patients in whom the diagnosis is less clear cut and to the always difficult problem of the degree of certainty of a negative conclusion. Obviously one can never be absolutely certain during life that a given patient does not have a pheochromocytoma. As in many other areas of medicine, clinical judgment must be based upon probability.

Oral clonidine (0.3 mg) suppresses plasma catecholamine levels in hypertensive patients without pheochromocytoma but not in patients with pheochromocytoma. Thus the clonidine suppression test has been suggested to distinguish patients with primary hypertension with elevated basal plasma norepinephrine levels from those with hypertension due to a pheochromocytoma. Definition of the utility of this test awaits further experience. False negatives and false positives have been reported.

LOCALIZATION. Given biochemical confirmation of pheochromocytoma, anatomic localization is desirable. Normal adrenal glands can usually be imaged with modern computed tomography (CT), and the majority of adrenomedullary pheochromocytomas can be seen with this technique. CT is the recommended initial localizing procedure. Magnetic resonance imaging is also useful, and might be more specific. External scanning after the injection of radioactive agents that localize in pheochromocytomas has the conceptual advantage of measuring function rather than anatomy and the practical advantage of permitting scanning of the entire trunk of the body and might, therefore, be expected to localize extra-adrenal pheochromocytomas better than CT scans. The initial experience with [131I]-m-iodobenzylguanidine (MIBG) scans has been encouraging in this regard.

TREATMENT. Treatment is surgical removal of the pheochromocytoma. Patients are usually prepared for surgery by administration of an α-adrenergic antagonist, such as phenoxybenzamine or prazosin, in doses sufficient to produce normal blood pressure and to prevent paroxysms. Treatment for 7 to 10 days prior to surgery is often recommended on the premise that this permits expansion of the blood volume. These drugs can also be used to treat chronic catecholamine excess in patients with metastatic tumor, although they do not influence the growth of a malignant pheochromocytoma. A β-adrenergic antagonist, such as propranolol, can be added to the preoperative regimen if arrhythmias are, or become, a problem.

Most patients are cured by surgery. The differential diagnosis of persistent hypertension includes a missed pheochromocytoma, a surgical complication resulting in renal ischemia, and underlying primary hypertension. Long-term follow-up is important, since late recurrences, including metastatic lesions, are being recognized with increasing frequency.

OTHER NEURAL CREST TUMORS. Pheochromocytomas are tumors of differentiated neural crest cells, the chromaffin cells. Tumors of more primitive cells also occur. These include neuroblastoma, a rather common malignant tumor of infancy and early childhood, usually arising in the adrenal medullae, and ganglioneuroma, a generally benign tumor often arising in sympathetic ganglia. These tumors commonly synthesize catecholamines but usually do not release catecholamines in sufficient quantities to produce clinical manifestations. Presumably the catecholamines are largely inactivated within the tumor. Nonetheless, measurements of catecholamine metabolites such as HVA and VMA are useful, particularly in assessing the response to therapy.

EPINEPHRINE DEFICIENCY

The prevention or correction of hypoglycemia involves both dissipation of insulin and activation of glucose counter-regulatory systems. Whereas insulin is the dominant glucose-lowering factor, there are redundant glucose counter-regulatory factors, and a hierarchy among these. In defense against decrements in plasma glucose, dissipation of insulin is likely most important. Glucagon plays a primary counter-regulatory role. Epinephrine is not normally critical, but it compensates and becomes critical when glucagon is deficient. Hypoglycemia develops or progresses when both glucagon and epinephrine are deficient and insulin is present. Other hormones, neurotransmitters, or substrate effects may be involved, but they are neither critical nor potent.

Selective deficiency of the glucagon response to decrements in plasma glucose is the rule in patients with insulin-dependent diabetes mellitus (IDDM). To the extent that they have deficient glucagon responses, patients with IDDM are largely dependent upon epinephrine to prevent or correct hypoglycemia. Deficient epinephrine responses develop typically later in the course of the disease. Patients with combined deficiencies of the glucagon and epinephrine responses are virtually defenseless against iatrogenic hypoglycemia. They have defective glucose counter-regulation and are at substantially increased risk (25-fold in our experience) for severe hypoglycemia, at least during intensive therapy of IDDM.

Patients with defective glucose counter-regulation often have a history of hypoglycemia unawareness but some do not. They can be identified prospectively with an insulin infusion test. Clearly, euglycemia is not an appropriate therapeutic goal in patients with IDDM and defective glucose counter-regulation, whether the latter is demonstrated with an insulin infusion test or is apparent from recurrent severe hypoglycemia during an attempt at intensive therapy. Administration of a β-adrenergic antagonist such as propranolol impairs recovery from experimental hypoglycemia in most patients with IDDM. Long-term administration of β-adrenergic antagonists has not been shown to increase the frequency of severe hypoglycemia in patients with IDDM, but this has not been examined in the context of intensive therapy.

Bravo EL, Gifford RW Jr: Pheochromocytoma: Diagnosis, localization and management. N Engl J Med 311:1298, 1984. *An extensive experience, including plasma catecholamine data.*

Cryer PE: Pheochromocytoma. West J Med, in press. *A more detailed review of the subject, including discussion of the effects of drugs on catecholamine measurements and other details of diagnostic testing.*

Cryer PE: Diseases of the sympathochromaffin system. *In* Felig P, Baxter JD, Broadus AE, et al. (eds.): Endocrinology and Metabolism, 2nd ed. New York, McGraw-Hill Book Company, 1987, pp 651–692. *A detailed discussion of sympathochromaffin physiology and pathophysiology.*

Cryer PE, Binder C, Bolli GB, et al.: Hypoglycemia in insulin dependent diabetes mellitus. Diabetes 38:1193, 1989. *A review of the physiology and pathophysiology of glucose counter-regulation.*

Duncan MW, Compton P, Lazarus L, et al.: Measurement of norepinephrine and 3,4-dihydroxyphenylglycol in urine and plasma for the diagnosis of pheochromocytoma. N Engl J Med 319:136, 1988. *Includes data comparing plasma and urinary norepinephrine measurements.*

The French MIBG Study Group: Comparison of iodobenzylguanidine imaging with computed tomography in locating pheochromocytoma. J Clin Endocrinol Metab 61:769, 1985. *A large experience demonstrating the strengths and weaknesses of the two approaches.*

230 The Carcinoid Syndrome

Philip E. Cryer

Carcinoid tumors arise from enterochromaffin (Kulchitsky) cells that are located predominantly in the gastrointestinal mucosa. Enterochromaffin cells have the potential to produce a variety of biologically active amines and peptides, including serotonin, bradykinin, histamine, and tachykinins, as well as prostaglandins. Carcinoid tumors are relatively common. Those that release sufficient quantities of mediators into the systemic circulation to produce the clinical carcinoid syndrome—flushing often with diarrhea and sometimes with wheezing or cardiac failure—are rare. Carcinoid tumors are most commonly found in the appendix or rectum, but these rarely produce the carcinoid syndrome. The tumors that produce the syndrome typically arise in the ileum, although the carcinoid syndrome can also result from tumors of the stomach, bile duct, duodenum, pancreas, lung, or even the gonads. Despite the release of a variety of mediators, the biochemical common denominator of the carcinoid syndrome is the overproduction of serotonin and the excretion of its major metabolite, 5-hydroxyindoleacetic acid (5-HIAA).

A variety of ectopic humoral syndromes have been associated with histologic carcinoid tumors. These include Cushing's syndrome (ACTH) and dilutional hyponatremia (vasopressin) with bronchial carcinoids, gynecomastia (chorionic gonadotropin) with gastric carcinoids, acromegaly (growth hormone–releasing hormone) with foregut carcinoids, and hypoglycemia (insulin) with pancreatic carcinoids. Typically, such patients do not have the carcinoid syndrome.

BIOSYNTHESIS AND DEGRADATION OF SEROTONIN. Serotonin is synthesized from dietary tryptophan and later is converted to 5-hydroxyindoleacetic acid through the reactions shown in Figure 230–1.

Approximately 90 per cent of serotonin in the body is normally found in the gut. Serotonin synthesis accounts for only 1 per cent of the metabolism of tryptophan in normal individuals. This may be as high as 60 per cent in patients with the carcinoid syndrome. Indeed, a pellagra-like skin rash has been attributed to diversion of tryptophan from nicotinic acid synthesis in such patients. Normal individuals excrete less than 10 mg of 5-HIAA per 24 hours. Patients with the carcinoid syndrome commonly excrete 50 to 100 mg per 24 hours.

CLINICAL MANIFESTATIONS. Clinical carcinoid syndrome is usually associated with an ileal carcinoid tumor that has metastasized to the liver. Carcinoids in sites, such as those in the lung or ovary, that do not drain into the portal circulation can rarely produce the carcinoid syndrome without evident hepatic metastases. Carcinoid syndrome due to an ileal carcinoid, however, is almost invariably associated with overt hepatic metastases. Presumably the liver clears mediators released from the tumor, and this clearance is impaired by metastatic tumor, resulting in the clinical syndrome.

More than 90 per cent of patients with the carcinoid syndrome have episodes of *cutaneous flushing*. The flush usually begins in the face and may spread to the trunk or even the extremities. It is red initially and then becomes purple; it commonly lasts only a few minutes, but may continue for hours. *Telangiectasias* of the face can result from frequent flushing. The heart rate increases

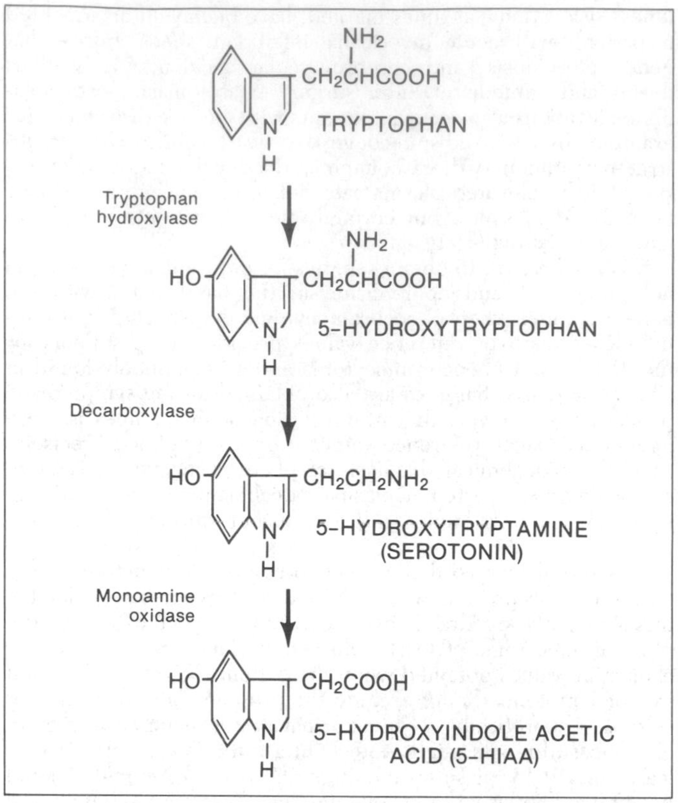

FIGURE 230–1. Synthesis and degradation of serotonin.

and the blood pressure tends to decrease during a flush. This is in contrast to patients with pheochromocytomas who typically have episodes of pallor with hypertension. Bronchial carcinoids may be associated with more intense and long-lasting flushing episodes. In patients with gastric carcinoids, flushing tends to be patchy initially and may be anywhere on the body. Headache commonly follows the flush.

Flushing can be precipitated by alcohol, food, stress, or palpation of the liver, or it may follow the administration of catecholamines, pentagastrin, or reserpine. A single mediator that causes the carcinoid flush has not been identified. It is not serotonin, since inhibition of serotonin synthesis does not prevent flushing. Candidate mediators include bradykinin, histamine, prostaglandins, and tachykinins including substance P.

More than three quarters of patients with the carcinoid syndrome have *diarrhea*, typically exacerbated during episodes of flushing. Serotonin most likely mediates the diarrhea, since it can be reduced by inhibition of serotonin synthesis in most patients. Intestinal symptoms can also result from mesenteric fibrosis. Pleural, peritoneal, and retroperitoneal fibroses also occur. Serotonin may also cause the fibrotic lesions.

Right-sided endocardial fibrosis, perhaps the result of chronic serotonin excess, is found in more than one third of patients with the carcinoid syndrome. Cardiac failure due to pulmonic stenosis or tricuspid insufficiency or both is less common but implies a poor prognosis. Involvement of the left side of the heart is uncommon. It does occur in patients with bronchial carcinoids, which implies that the responsible mediator(s) is ordinarily cleared during passage through pulmonary capillaries.

Bronchoconstriction with wheezing during an episode of flushing is less common, occurring in about 20 per cent of patients. Like flushing, but unlike diarrhea, bronchoconstriction is not prevented by inhibition of serotonin synthesis.

Somatostatin has been reported to decrease flushing, diarrhea, and bronchoconstriction in patients with the carcinoid syndrome. The mechanism(s) of this effect is not known.

DIAGNOSIS. Diagnosis is based upon clinical suspicion—usually a history of flushing and diarrhea—associated with markedly increased urinary 5-hydroxyindoleacetic acid excretion. Metastatic hepatomegaly is common. Since carcinoid tumors produce the carcinoid syndrome rarely, the histologic diagnosis of a carcinoid tumor does not establish the presence of the carcinoid syndrome. Platelet serotonin levels are elevated in most patients with the carcinoid syndrome. Gastric carcinoids appear to have low decarboxylase activity, since 5-hydroxytryptophan, rather than serotonin, is the major product of indole metabolism in some such patients.

Provocative tests, such as the precipitation of episodes with intravenous administration of epinephrine, are seldom necessary and potentially dangerous, since severe hypotension and bronchoconstriction can occur.

False-positive urinary 5-HIAA determinations are common and should be suspected particularly when the values are minimally elevated, e.g., 10 to 20 mg per 24 hours. Increased 5-HIAA excretion can follow the ingestion of chocolate, bananas, tomatoes, pineapples, walnuts, and avocados and the use of drugs, including mephenesin, methamphetamine, methysergide, methocarbamol, reserpine, acetaminophen, and glyceryl guaiacolate (the last in some cough syrups). Increased values have also been reported in Whipple's disease and nontropical sprue.

Computed tomography, radionuclide scans, ultrasonography, and conventional barium-contrast radiographic studies can be used to define tumor anatomy. Despite widespread metastases, the primary tumor can be small and difficult to demonstrate.

TREATMENT. In the presence of documented metastases, resection of a primary ileal carcinoid tumor is not indicated. It may become necessary because of intestinal obstruction or because of intussusception. Rarely, surgical removal of an isolated tumor (e.g., a bronchial or ovarian carcinoid) is curative. Devascularization of metastatic tumor by percutaneous arterial embolization has been reported to produce symptomatic relief in some patients. Resection of localized hepatic metastases and hepatic artery ligation have also been reported to ameliorate symptoms of the carcinoid syndrome temporarily.

Survival of less than 5 years after the onset of the carcinoid syndrome is the rule, but survival for more than 20 years is well documented. Thus, high-risk attempts at curative therapy are generally not indicated. Carcinoid tumors are not radiosensitive. Low-risk chemotherapy has not been very effective.

Symptomatic therapy includes nutritional support plus the provision of nicotinamide to prevent pellagra. Diarrhea has been treated with serotonin antagonists such as methysergide or cyproheptadine as well as with loperamide or even opiates. The drug parachlorophenylalanine, a tryptophan hydroxylase inhibitor, reduces diarrhea. However, allergic reactions and CNS side effects have occurred, and the drug remains experimental. No drug is consistently effective in preventing flushing; H_1 and H_2 histamine antagonists, including cimetidine, are often tried. Phenothiazines and the α-adrenergic antagonist phenoxybenzamine have also been used, as have glucocorticoids. Treatment with leukocyte interferon has been reported to decrease flushing and diarrhea in patients with the carcinoid syndrome. Long-term symptomatic therapy with a somatostatin analogue is promising.

Kvols LK: Metastatic carcinoid tumors and the carcinoid syndrome. Am J Med 81:49, 1986. *A review of chemotherapy and hormonal therapy.*

Norheim I, Theodorsson-Norheim E, Brodin E, et al.: Tachykinins in carcinoid tumors: Their use as a tumor marker and possible role in the carcinoid flush. J Clin Endocrinol Metab 63:605, 1986. *Plasma tachykinin levels often increase during induced flushing and decrease during effective therapy.*

Öberg K, Norheim I, Theodorsson E, et al.: The effects of octreotide on basal and stimulated hormone levels in patients with carcinoid syndrome. J Clin Endocrinol Metab 68:796, 1989. *The somatostatin analogue was shown to block tachykinin release.*

Roberts LJ II: Carcinoid syndrome and disorders of systemic mast-cell activation including systemic mastocytosis. Endocrinol Metab Clin North Am 17:415, 1988. *A more detailed discussion of the carcinoid syndrome.*

231 Ovarian Carcinoma

Howard W. Jones, III

Ovarian carcinoma is the most deadly of the gynecologic malignancies. The age-specific incidence gradually rises, reaching a peak at about age 70, at which time it is 55 per 100,000 among white women. The rate is somewhat lower among black women.

The etiology of ovarian cancer is unknown; except for some relatively rare familial groups, it has not been possible to identify any clinically useful high-risk groups for increased surveillance. Multiple pregnancies and the use of oral contraceptives may be protective because of decreased ovulation and hormonal influences.

Pathology

Four types of ovarian tumors require separate consideration because of their clinical characteristics and prognoses: (1) The common *epithelial tumors* of the ovary include the serous, mucinous, endometrioid, clear cell, and otherwise unspecified adenocarcinomas. These tumors account for almost 90 per cent of ovarian cancers and are most commonly found in postmenopausal women. (2) *Germ cell tumors*, which arise from the totipotent oocytes, are usually benign ("dermoid cysts"). They often occur in young women and are almost always unilateral. When malignant (e.g., dysgerminoma, teratoma), they are highly aggressive but respond very well to combination chemotherapy. (3) *Stromal tumors* are generally low grade, and since they arise from the granulosa, theca, and Sertoli-Leydig cells of the ovary, they may be hormonally functional. They are usually unilateral and may occur in any age group, but most typically in the fourth and fifth decades. Surgical excision alone may be all the therapy required, but combination chemotherapy is effective for metastatic or recurrent disease. (4) Malignancies of other sites that are metastatic to the ovary must always be considered in the evaluation of patients with a pelvic mass. In some cases a pelvic mass is the first indication of a primary gastrointestinal or endometrial carcinoma. Breast cancer also commonly metastasizes to the ovary.

DIAGNOSIS

Clinical Presentation

Early ovarian cancer is usually asymptomatic. Occasionally, ovarian enlargement is found on routine examination and cancer may be discovered incidentally at the time of abdominal or pelvic surgery for other indications. In most cases, however, widespread intra-abdominal metastases are present by the time the diagnosis is made. Symptoms of abdominal swelling, bloating, and pelvic fullness or pressure are common. It is not unusual for the patient to have had vague abdominal complaints or nonspecific gastrointestinal symptoms. Ascites or a palpable abdominopelvic mass may be found on examination. The presence of an irregular mass in the pelvis or cul-de-sac nodularity accompanied by ascites is often diagnostic. Some patients develop malignant pleural effusions and present with shortness of breath.

SCREENING TESTS. Screening tests for ovarian cancer are still controversial. Transvaginal ultrasonography, although quite effective for diagnosing ovarian cysts and tumors, is nonspecific and its use for screening results in surgical exploration of a large number of women with benign ovarian cysts. Even when a cancer is diagnosed by ultrasound screening in an asymptomatic patient, there is still no evidence that survival is improved. Serum levels of the tumor-associated antigen CA-125 above 35 μ per milliliter are highly correlated with serous or endometrioid ovarian cancer in postmenopausal women. Unfortunately, many ovarian tumors (e.g., mucinous, nonepithelial, and about 20 per cent of serous ovarian cancers) do not cause elevated levels of CA-125, while endometriosis, pelvic inflammatory disease, and some benign ovarian tumors may do so. The relative rarity of ovarian cancer, combined with the nonspecific nature of currently available tests, makes ovarian cancer screening unsatisfactory.

DIFFERENTIAL DIAGNOSIS. A pelvic mass can be caused by either a benign or a malignant tumor of the ovary as well as by inflammatory conditions, physiologic cysts, and malignancies of other pelvic organs and structures. Initially, a careful history and physical examination are most helpful in suggesting possible primary sites. Pelvic ultrasonography may allow the dimensions and character of the mass to be determined. Smooth-walled, unilocular ovarian cysts are almost always benign, whereas malignancies are most commonly described as echogenically "complex" with both cystic and solid components. The possibility of ectopic pregnancy must always be considered when a pelvic mass is present. A pregnancy test is, therefore, normally the first laboratory study done in women in the reproductive age group. A careful contraceptive history is important, since functional ovarian cysts, including both follicle cysts and corpus luteum cysts, are common in ovulating women. Inflammatory masses and endometriosis can be confused with ovarian cancer and can cause an elevated CA-125 in addition to a complex adnexal mass. In the older age group, diverticular abscesses and carcinoma of the colon must be considered within the differential diagnosis.

Once a complete history and physical have been done and the size and character of the mass have been confirmed by ultrasonography, several additional studies may be helpful. A barium enema or colonoscopy is almost always indicated prior to surgery to rule out a primary lesion or secondary involvement of the colon. An abdominal and pelvic computerized tomography scan identifies any ureteral obstruction or displacement that may be present and further characterizes the mass. This study may also provide additional information about upper abdominal disease, including aortic lymph node enlargement, omental or liver metastases, and the rare primary carcinoma of the pancreas that mimics ovarian cancer.

Additional studies (e.g., brain scans, bone scans) should generally be reserved for patients whose symptoms or physical findings suggest involvement of the areas to be studied.

TREATMENT

Surgery

In almost all cases of suspected ovarian carcinoma, an exploratory laparotomy is the ultimate diagnostic procedure. If the diagnosis is sustained, tumor debulking, including total abdominal hysterectomy and bilateral salpingo-oophorectomy, if possible, should be done. At this point a definitive diagnosis can be made

TABLE 231–1. DEFINITIONS OF THE STAGES IN PRIMARY CARCINOMA OF THE OVARY*

Stage I	Growth limited to the ovaries
Stage Ia	Growth limited to one ovary; no ascites. No tumor on the external surface; capsule intact.
Stage Ib	Growth limited to both ovaries; no ascites. No tumor on the external surfaces; capsules intact.
Stage Ic	Tumor either Stage Ia or Ib, but with tumor on surface of one or both ovaries; or with capsule ruptured; or with ascites present containing malignant cells or with positive peritoneal washings.
Stage II	Growth involving one or both ovaries with pelvic extension
Stage IIa	Extension and/or metastases to the uterus and/or tubes.
Stage IIb	Extension to other pelvic tissues.
Stage IIc	Tumor either Stage IIa or IIb, but with tumor on surface of one or both ovaries; or with capsule(s) ruptured; or with ascites present containing malignant cells or with positive peritoneal washings.
Stage III	Tumor involving one or both ovaries with peritoneal implants outside the pelvis and/or positive retroperitoneal or inguinal nodes. Superficial liver metastases equal Stage III. Tumor is limited to the true pelvis but with histologically proven malignant extension to small bowel or omentum.
Stage IIIa	Tumor grossly limited to the true pelvis with negative nodes but with histologically confirmed microscopic seeding of abdominal peritoneal surfaces.
Stage IIIb	Tumor involving one or both ovaries with histologically confirmed implants of abdominal peritoneal surfaces, none exceeding 2 cm in diameter. Nodes are negative.
Stage IIIc	Abdominal implants greater than 2 cm in diameter and/or positive retroperitoneal or inguinal nodes.
Stage IV	Growth involving one or both ovaries with distant metastases. If pleural effusion is present, there must be positive cytology to allot a case to Stage IV. Parenchymal liver metastasis equals Stage IV.

*Nomenclature of the International Federation of Gynecology and Obstetrics (FIGO). Staging is based on findings at clinical examination and surgical exploration.

and the extent of the disease accurately staged. Aggressive tumor debulking, even when all cancer cannot be removed, improves the length and quality of survival. If possible, this initial surgery should be done by a gynecologic oncologist whose special training and experience should provide the optimal surgical and postoperative management.

The goal of the initial operation for ovarian cancer is twofold. First, all tumor should be removed if possible to provide the greatest possibility of cure. In approximately two thirds of patients, however, widespread intra-abdominal metastases prevent complete surgical debulking. The second goal of surgery is accurate staging (Table 231–1). In addition to the stage of disease, the volume of residual tumor following initial surgery, the histologic type and grade of the tumor, and the age of the patient have important prognostic significance. Women with minimal residual disease and well-differentiated tumors have the most favorable outcome. Those under age 50 and those with tumors exhibiting mucinous and endometrioid histology also seem to do better.

Careful staging evaluation with peritoneal cytology and multiple biopsies of the upper abdomen (the omentum, diaphragm, and retroperitoneal nodes) is especially important in early stage disease, since microscopic metastases often escape clinical detection. Accurate staging guides the most appropriate postoperative management. Patients with Stage Ia well-differentiated epithelial ovarian cancers do not need additional therapy (Table 231–1).

In patients with advanced disease, aggressive surgical debulking includes bowel resection or colostomy in as many as 25 per cent of patients. Whether such extensive surgical resection actually improves 5- and 10-year survival rates is still controversial. It is agreed, however, that optimal tumor debulking (<1 cm residual) results in prolongation of good-quality survival. This is where the skills and experienced judgment of the gynecologic oncologist are most important.

Chemotherapy

Most patients with ovarian cancer require postoperative chemotherapy. Cisplatin, the cornerstone of most regimens, is usually given in combination with other agents, such as cyclophosphamide, doxorubicin, hexamethylmelamine, or etoposide. Carboplatin, which has fewer renal and neurologic side effects, and ifosfamide are now under investigation. Most patients are treated with intermittent intravenous therapy at 4-week intervals for six monthly cycles, but some centers use intraperitoneal chemotherapy instead. Response rates of 60 to 80 per cent are generally seen, but only about 30 per cent of the treatment group experiences a complete response. Some debilitated patients are still treated with a single alkylating agent, such as oral melphalan, but this therapy is probably not as effective as cisplatin alone or in combination with other cytotoxic drugs. Carboplatin is almost as well tolerated as oral melphalan.

Radiation Therapy

Postoperative external radiation therapy to the whole abdomen is probably as effective as chemotherapy for patients with minimal residual tumor. The toxicity of such therapy, especially that of gastrointestinal obstruction, has usually been greater than that associated with chemotherapy.

Intraperitoneal radioactive colloidal chromic phosphate is also used to treat some women with Stage I or II disease with no gross residual tumor. Only patients with very early disease are good candidates for this therapy, which requires a complete and uniform intraperitoneal distribution of the radioactive suspension.

"Second-look" Surgery

A planned re-exploration in order to evaluate the extent of disease following a course of therapy and to resect any residual malignancy has been called "second-look" surgery. This approach allows an excellent research evaluation of the effect of the primary therapy, but it has not proven to be of significant clinical benefit to patients with ovarian cancer. Measurements of tumor-associated antigens, such as CA-125, used in conjunction with periodic physical examinations and selected radiographic studies, have been helpful in monitoring the disease status of treated patients. Until more effective salvage therapy is available, second-look

TABLE 231–2. CARCINOMA OF THE OVARY: DISTRIBUTION BY STAGE AND 3- AND 5-YEAR SURVIVAL IN THE DIFFERENT STAGES*

Stage	Patients Treated		3-Year Survival (%)	5-Year Survival (%)
	Number	(%)		
I	2230	26.1	79.8	72.8
II	1313	15.4	60.5	46.3
III	3339	39.1	27.1	18.6
IV	1391	16.3	10.1	4.8
Unstaged	268	3.1	31.7	21.6
TOTAL	8541	100.0	43.4	34.9

*Data from Carcinoma of the ovary. In Pettersson F (ed.): Annual Report on the Results of Treatment in Gynecological Cancer, Vol. 20. Stockholm, Panorama Press AB, 1988. The "Annual Report" is published at regular intervals by the International Federation for Gynecology and Obstetrics and contains vast quantities of statistics generated from institutions which submit their treatment results from throughout the world.

surgery in the asymptomatic patient with a normal physical examination is probably not indicated.

Treatment of Recurrent, Metastatic Disease

The overall survival of patients treated for ovarian cancer is only 30 to 40 per cent; many women develop progressive disease despite appropriate primary therapy. Salvage chemotherapy protocols for recurrent disease lead to only a 10 per cent response rate, which is usually partial and short term. Widespread intra-abdominal metastases with bowel obstruction are frequent, but reoperation with resection, bypass, or enterostomy may provide significant palliation. Pleural effusion may require thoracentesis and pleural sclerosis. With the relative effectiveness of current primary chemotherapy, patients may survive to develop late metastases to the liver, brain, and meninges. Localized radiation has been helpful in some of these patients.

PROGNOSIS

The long-term survival rate of patients treated for epithelial ovarian cancer is still disappointing (Table 231–2). Almost 60 per cent of patients have Stage III or IV disease at the time of diagnosis. Although the majority of women with advanced disease live 2 years with a reasonable quality of life, recurrent cancer eventually becomes symptomatic in most, and by 5 years only about 15 per cent still survive. The results are much better for patients diagnosed at an earlier stage. Almost three fourths of women with Stage I ovarian cancer survive 5 years.

Heintz APM, Hacker NF, Lagasse LD: Epidemiology and etiology of ovarian cancer: A review. Obstet Gynecol 66:127, 1985. *This is an excellent review of the many different factors that might be related to the etiology of ovarian cancer. The authors emphasize the significance of family history.*

Jacobs I, Stabile I, Bridges J, et al.: Multimodal approach to screening for ovarian cancer. Lancet 1:268, 1988. *This study describes the use of pelvic examination, CA-125, and ultrasonography to screen patients for ovarian cancer. There is an excellent discussion with good references.*

Sutton GP, Stehman FB, Einhorn LH, et al.: Ten-year follow-up of patients receiving cisplatin, doxorubicin, and cyclophosphamide chemotherapy for advanced epithelial ovarian carcinoma. J Clin Oncol 7:223, 1989. *This is an excellent review of long-term follow-up of patients treated with platinum-based combination chemotherapy. This group has one of the world's largest experiences, and the discussion and references are superb.*

Williams L, Hoskins WJ: Can cytoreductive surgery aid ovarian cancer survival? Contemp Gynecol Obstet 35:13, 1990. *This recent review examines the role of initial cytoreductive surgery as well as second-look operation for ovarian cancer. An excellent review of the literature.*

Williams SD, Blessing JA, Moore DH, et al.: Cisplatin, vinblastine, and bleomycin in advanced and recurrent ovarian germ-cell tumors. Ann Intern Med 3:22, 1989. *This is a report of a gynecologic oncology group study using new chemotherapy approaches for germ cell tumors of the ovary. The results with platinum-based combination therapy are excellent.*

PART XVII

DISEASES OF BONE AND BONE MINERAL METABOLISM

232 Mineral and Bone Homeostasis

Stephen J. Marx

Calcium, phosphorus, and magnesium, three of the principal body elements, have diverse roles. The calcium ion is particularly versatile. In the crystalline phase, it contributes to the varied structural roles of bone. In a supersaturated solution in blood, it contributes to plasma membrane excitability, plasma enzyme activities, and accretion of all minerals in extracellular matrix of bone. In the cytoplasmic fluid, its extraordinarily low concentrations allow rapid rises of its local concentrations to transmit information among cell compartments via its interactions with high-affinity calcium-binding proteins, such as calmodulin or protein kinase C. Phosphate is the principal intracellular anion, with central roles in cytoplasm as a buffer, energy carrier (mainly via the high-energy phosphate bonds of adenosine triphosphate [ATP]), and molecular switch (through phosphorylation and dephosphorylation). Magnesium is the principal cation in cytoplasm, functioning as a cofactor in many chemical reactions (for example, as an Mg-ATP complex or as a cofactor in many steps of DNA or RNA metabolism).

MINERALS IN BLOOD

The State of Calcium, Phosphate, and Magnesium in Blood

Total calcium concentration is tightly regulated, so that typical diurnal fluctuations are not more than 5 per cent from the mean value. Calcium in blood is divided among protein-bound, complexed, and ionized or free fractions (Table 232–1). Protein binding of calcium in blood is principally to albumin, and this binding is decreased by acid pH. The ionized calcium fraction is the focus for metabolic control by the parathyroid gland, and measurements of ionized calcium in blood give the most valid index of pathologic disruptions of calcium homeostasis.

Phosphate and magnesium in blood are principally unbound (Table 232–1), and the concentration of each is regulated over a broader relative variation from its mean than that for calcium. Neither phosphate nor magnesium has a unique endocrine system dedicated to its control. Rather, their blood concentrations are

sustained indirectly by the hormones directed at calcium control and directly by poorly understood local processes in bone, kidney, and other organs.

Steady-State Flow of Minerals to and from Blood

Only 0.1 per cent of the total body calcium is in blood and extracellular fluid (Table 232–2). This calcium pool is in a rapidly exchanging equilibrium with large calcium pools controlled by three organs (bone, intestine, and kidney), each of which is an important site for the regulation of mineral metabolism. The rate of these daily fluxes (Fig. 232–1) is sufficiently large that disturbance of mineral flux to or from any of these organs can result in abnormally high or low concentrations of one of these minerals in blood.

ORGANS EXCHANGING MUCH MINERAL WITH BLOOD

Bone

BONE FUNCTION AND ARCHITECTURE. Major functions of bone include support, locomotion, encasement of hematopoietic tissue, and reservoir for calcium, phosphate, and magnesium. The architecture of bone responds dynamically to changes in mechanical load. The mechanisms whereby the signals from altered load are transduced are poorly understood. Mature bone adopts one of two macroscopic organizations (Fig. 232–2). The cortices of all bones and the interior of certain bones have a continuous structure termed cortical or lamellar bone. Lamellar bone, which is predominant in the long bones, is characterized by little metabolic activity and few cells. It has a highly organized extracellular matrix of mineral and parallel bundles of type I collagen. During embryonic development or in states with pathologic increase of bone turnover, bone assumes a less organized "woven" architecture. Within the vertebral bodies and in portions of the interior of other bones, bone is organized as a series of thin, interdigitating plates; this is termed trabecular, cancellous, or spongy bone. Its ratio of surface to volume is higher than that found in cortical bone and is thus better suited to rapid turnover.

EXTRACELLULAR MATRIX. Newly deposited osteoid must undergo a poorly understood maturation process for 1 to 3 weeks until it becomes competent for mineral accumulation. The mineral phase of bone extracellular matrix is a mixture of multiple amorphous and crystalline states, the latter principally as hydroxyapatite crystals ($Ca_{10}(PO_4)_6OH_2$). Ninety to 95 per cent of osteoid, the organic component of the extracellular matrix, is

TABLE 232–1. CONCENTRATIONS AND STATES OF CALCIUM, MAGNESIUM, AND PHOSPHATE IN NORMAL HUMAN PLASMA OR SERUM*

State	Calcium (mM)	Magnesium (mM)	Phosphate (mM)
Protein bound	1.15 (47)	0.26 (31)	0.15 (13)
Filterable or free†			
Complexed	0.25 (10)	0.06 (7)	0.40 (35)
Ionized	1.06 (43)	0.52 (62)	0.60 (52)

*Number in parentheses indicates percentage of total for that mineral.
†Filterable or free = complexed + ionized.

TABLE 232–2. DISTRIBUTION OF CALCIUM, MAGNESIUM, AND PHOSPHATE IN THE BODY OF A 70-KG ADULT*

Compartment	Calcium (g)	Magnesium (g)	Phosphate (g)
Bones and teeth	1300 (99)	14.0 (54)	600.0 (86)
Extracellular fluid	1 (0.1)	0.3 (1)	0.2 (0.03)
Cells	7 (1.0)	12.0 (46)	100.0 (14)

*Most of calcium is in bone; almost half of magnesium is in cells. Phosphate, as the principal counterion to calcium and magnesium in their dominant pools, has an intermediate proportional distribution. Number in parentheses is the percentage of total for that mineral.

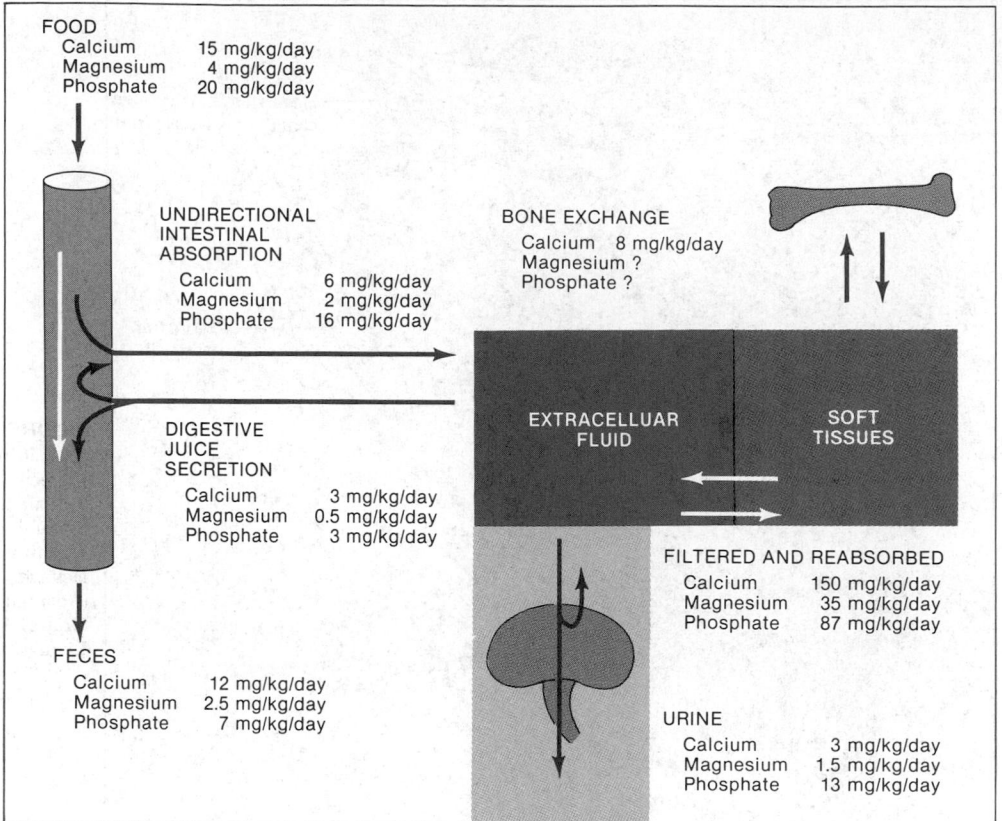

FIGURE 232–1. Typical mineral fluxes in adults. (Modified from Aurbach GD, Marx SJ, Spiegel AM: Parathyroid hormone, calcitonin, and the calciferols. *In* Wilson JD, Foster DW [eds.]: Williams Textbook of Endocrinology. 7th ed. Philadelphia, W.B. Saunders Company, 1985, p 1144.)

composed of bundles of type I collagen, a long triple helix of two alpha$_1$ (type I) chains and one alpha$_2$ (type I) chain. The principal collagen of cartilage matrix is type II as a homotrimer of three alpha$_1$ (type II) chains. Fibrils of collagen play a major role in the strength of bone (type I collagen), cartilage (type II collagen), and elastic tissues (type III collagen). Their disruption results in characteristic disturbances (osteogenesis imperfecta [type I collagen], chondrodysplasia [type II collagen], Ehlers-Danlos syndrome or arterial aneurysms [type III collagen], and even certain variants of familial osteoarthritis [type II collagen]). The second most prominent protein in bone matrix is osteocalcin (or bone gla-protein); it has a molar content of three residues of gamma-carboxyglutamic acid, an unusual amino acid that confers to the molecule high affinity for calcium on bone crystals. The roles of osteocalcin are unknown, but its concentration in blood is a potential index of osteoblast activity. Several other proteins, phosphoproteins, glycoproteins, and so on, in bone matrix have been identified in the search for molecules regulating bone mineral accumulation and bone growth.

BONE CELLS. Several cells are highly characteristic of bone. A flat bone-lining cell (perhaps derived from marrow stroma) with few organelles covers many bone surfaces thought not to be undergoing modification. This cell is perhaps one precursor of the osteoblast. The osteoblast is a cuboidal bone matrix–synthesizing cell. It lines any periosteal, endosteal, or trabecular surface at which bone formation takes place. Its plasma membrane is highly enriched with a bone-specific isoform of the alkaline phosphatase enzyme. This enzyme is believed to promote bone mineralization by catalyzing in supersaturated extracellular fluid of bone the hydrolysis of pyrophosphate and other inhibitors of calcium-phosphate crystallization. The osteocyte is the principal stable cell inside mature bone. It is probably derived from an osteoblast that has encased itself in bone. Osteocytes are interconnected with one another via long processes that traverse bone canaliculi. The role of the osteocyte is unknown, but it is appropriately located to modulate mineral fluxes. The chondrocyte is the dominant cell of cartilage; it releases to the extracellular matrix vesicles that are rich in alkaline phosphatase and that may be a central organelle for calcium accumulation in preparation

for cartilage mineralization. The osteoclast is the main bone-resorbing cell. It is derived from precursors of the premonocyte lineage. It is a highly motile, multinucleated giant cell, with several specialized features for bone. These include organelles that mediate cell attachment to bone surface (podosomes), a strikingly redundant ruffled border at the bone face for ion transport, many enzymes that can function in bone resorption, and a high concentration of carbonic anhydrase II, which participates in acidification of the extracellular pocket between the osteoclast ruffled border and the skeletal resorption surface.

LOCAL REGULATORS OF BONE CELLS. Bone cells are under systemic and local regulation. Known systemic regulators include parathyroid hormone, calcitonin, and calcitriol, which are considered later in this chapter. There is also a highly complex network of local controls. The term "osteoclast-activating factors" was applied in the 1980's to components in incompletely characterized fluids that could activate bone resorption in vitro. Some of their active components have been identified. For example, interleukin 1 and lymphotoxin/tumor necrosis factor–beta are potential stimulators of bone resorption that seem to be released locally by some tumors in bone. They cannot act directly on mature osteoclasts but can act, rather, through nearby cells, such as osteoblasts or marrow stromal cells, that communicate with osteoclasts. Like the activators of bone resorption, the activators of bone formation are poorly understood, particularly since this process involves a complex interplay of osteoblast proliferation and differentiation. Some contributors to this process include type 1 insulin-like growth factor and transforming growth factor–beta; the latter is present selectively and at high concentrations in osteoblasts and osteocytes. In addition, several newly identified proteins (osteogenesis-inducing factor, bone morphogenetic proteins [some of which are homologues of the beta-type transforming growth factor], and so forth) can induce bone formation in soft tissue sites. Prostaglandins can stimulate bone formation or bone resorption, and they may be important mediators in inflammatory processes of the skeletal system.

BONE REMODELING. Bone growth or modeling occurs initially within a membrane or along the edge of cartilage (e.g., periosteum or epiphyseal growth plate). Though it contains few

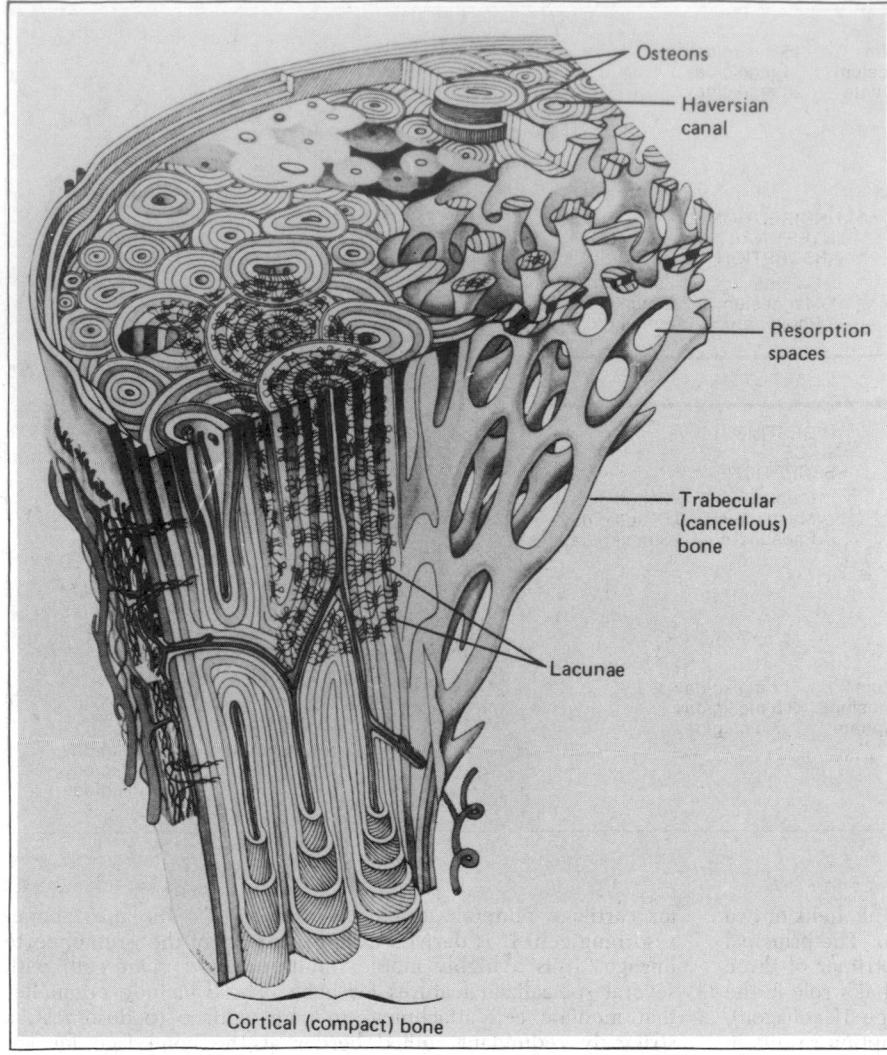

Osteons

Haversian
canal

Resorption
spaces

Trabecular
(cancellous)
bone

Lacunae

Cortical (compact) bone

FIGURE 232–2. Bone organization. Microstructure of mature bone; areas of cortical (lamellar) and trabecular (cancellous) bone are shown. The central area in the transverse section shows differences in mineral density as degrees of shading. Note the organization of osteons, the distribution of osteocyte lacunae, and the organization of bone lamellae. (Adapted from Warwick R, Williams PL [eds.]: Gray's Anatomy. 35th ed. Edinburgh, Churchill Livingstone, 1973, p 217.)

cells, cortical bone is constantly going through slow and orderly cycles of localized resorption and then rebuilding. This process is mediated by the local remodeling unit (alternately termed osteon or basic multicellular unit). Remodeling begins with excavation of a cavity by osteoclasts; as the resorption front advances, osteoclasts are replaced by other cells. Over an interval of several months, new bone is deposited in cylindrical lamellae about the rim of the cavity until it is refilled to complete this cycle. This cycle is an important example of the normal, coordinated relation between the bone resorption and bone formation processes. Most perturbations that modify one component of these two processes also modify the other in the same direction. The determinants of this coupling between bone resorption and formation are not known, but they probably include a host of growth factors present at high local concentrations in bone extracellular matrix and exposed or released by the skeletal resorption process.

Intestines

MINERAL ABSORPTION. The intestinal absorption of magnesium and phosphate is not subject to fine regulation and has not been studied intensively. By contrast, intestinal absorption of calcium is tightly regulated, and its quantitation has been analyzed in detail. Most calcium absorption is accomplished in the small bowel. Over a wide range of intakes, approximately one tenth of dietary calcium is absorbed passively; the remainder of net intestinal absorption of calcium is regulated by active vitamin D metabolites, especially $1\alpha,25(OH)_2D$, in blood. With a normal diet, approximately 30 per cent of calcium is absorbed. With low dietary calcium, the secondarily high blood $1\alpha,25(OH)_2D$ level can drive fractional calcium absorption to approach 90 per cent.

Kidney

ION FILTRATION AND REABSORPTION. The non–protein-bound fractions of calcium, magnesium, and phosphate from plasma cross the glomerulus. The distal portions of the nephron have efficient and selective systems capable of completing the reabsorption from tubular fluid of more than 99 per cent of any one of these minerals. Tubular calcium reabsorption is stimulated principally by parathyroid hormone (PTH); thiazides or lithium can also increase tubular calcium reabsorption. Saline loading with or without loop diuretics can inhibit this. Tubular phosphate reabsorption is mainly under negative influence by PTH. The determinants of tubular reabsorption of magnesium are incompletely understood.

Integrated Fluxes: Mineral Balance and Nutrition

Skeletal growth is maximal throughout childhood, nearing completion during adolescence. Until this time, the rate of skeletal calcium accretion is typically 200 to 400 mg (5 to 10 mmole) per day. Fetal mineralization during the last trimester or milk secretion during lactation imposes similar daily increments on calcium efflux from maternal blood. The skeleton remains in a state of approximate zero mineral balance between ages 20 and 35, after which it slowly loses mass. This loss is greatest in the trabecular bone of the vertebrae, attaining peak rates about the menopause (3 to 10 per cent per year during the first 1 to 4 years after surgically induced menopause).

Normal adults can sustain zero calcium balance with daily

TABLE 232–3. EFFECTS OF PRINCIPAL CALCIOTROPIC HORMONES

Hormone	Principal Target Tissues	Action
Parathyroid hormone	Renal proximal convoluted tubule	Increase serum $1,25(OH)_2D$
	Renal distal convoluted tubule	Increase calcium reabsorption
	Renal proximal and distal convoluted tubules	Decrease phosphate reabsorption
	Bone	Increase calcium and phosphate resorption
Calcitonin	Bone	Decrease calcium and phosphate resorption
$1,25(OH)_2D$	Small bowel	Increase calcium absorption
	Bone	Increase calcium and phosphate resorption
	Parathyroid gland	Decrease release of PTH

calcium intakes between 400 and 1500 mg (10 to 37.5 mmole), mainly as dairy products. Typical daily calcium intakes in the United States are 500 to 800 mg (12.5 to 20 mmole), and there is uncertainty over the minimal level for optimal skeletal health. With a typical daily calcium intake of 700 mg (17.5 mmole), one fourth, or 175 mg (43.7 mmole), is absorbed; during skeletal balance, this amount must equal the amount lost in urinary excretion (disregarding the small amount of calcium lost from skin).

Because of the large mineral fluxes between blood and three principal pools (bone, renal tubular lumen, and intestinal lumen), it is often difficult to assign mild disruptions to one pool. For example, there is uncertainty whether the slow bone losses with idiopathic age-associated osteoporosis reflect primary disturbances of calcium flux in bone, the intestine, or combinations of these.

HORMONAL REGULATORS OF MINERAL HOMEOSTASIS

Parathyroid Hormone

SYNTHESIS, SECRETION, AND METABOLISM. Parathyroid hormone is a rapidly regulated hormone that sustains calcium and $1,25(OH)_2D$ in blood and depresses phosphate in blood (Table 232–3). Parathyroid hormone is stored in the parathyroid cell mainly as a peptide of 84 amino acids. The parathyroid cell secretes PTH as the native molecule or as fragments, only some of which are biologically active. Fragments of PTH are also generated from its metabolism after secretion into blood. The amino-terminus of PTH (residues 1 to 34) contains the requirements for receptor binding and biologic activity. Biologically active forms of PTH are cleared rapidly from blood, perhaps by their receptors, while inactive fragments are cleared more slowly, rendering them likely to be measured in immunoassays not specially designed to measure the intact molecule.

BLOOD CALCIUM EFFECT ON THE PARATHYROID GLAND. The parathyroid gland, as the coordinator of blood levels of PTH and $1,25(OH)_2D$, is exquisitely sensitive to changes of ionized calcium in extracellular fluid. The parathyroid cell responds to calcium in at least three different ways. First, low calcium concentration is a direct stimulus for the gradual increase in size and numbers of parathyroid cells (secondary hypertrophy and hyperplasia). Second, low calcium stimulates the biosynthesis of PTH over 1 to 2 days. Third, depression of the calcium level stimulates within seconds the secretion of preformed PTH. The parathyroid cell differs strikingly from most other hormone secretory cells, which exhibit accelerated secretion in response to increases of extracellular calcium.

PARATHYROID HORMONE MECHANISMS OF ACTION. Parathyroid hormone binds to a plasma membrane receptor; the PTH receptor then causes a rise of cyclic $3',5'$-adenosine monophosphate (cAMP) and perhaps other second messengers in the cytoplasm of its target cells. The consequence is rapid effects of PTH on the target cells in bone and kidney. A different peptide, termed "parathyroid hormone–related peptide," with homology to PTH at the amino-terminus, is secreted by many cancers, causing hypercalcemia through its interactions with PTH receptors.

PARATHYROID HORMONE ACTION IN BONE. Parathyroid hormone in bone stimulates osteoblasts and osteoclasts. The effects on osteoclasts are indirect, since these cells lack receptors for PTH. Very high PTH levels result in clear excess of bone

resorption over bone formation. Controversy exists over whether mild PTH excess might have a net anabolic effect selectively in trabecular bone.

PARATHYROID HORMONE ACTION IN KIDNEY. Parathyroid hormone acts in the kidney to stimulate the synthesis of $1,25(OH)_2D$ by increasing the activity of $25OHD_3$ 1α-hydroxylase in the proximal tubules. Parathyroid hormone acts in the distal portions of the nephron to increase tubular reabsorption of calcium. In addition, PTH inhibits phosphate reabsorption in the distal, and perhaps also the proximal, tubules. Parathyroid hormone also inhibits bicarbonate reabsorption.

PARATHYROID HORMONE ACTION ON INTESTINE. Parathyroid hormone has no important direct action on the intestine. However, the direct renal effect of PTH to increase serum $1,25(OH)_2D$ causes highly important secondary effects in the intestine (see Intestinal Actions of Calcitriol, further on).

Calcitonin

CALCITONIN SYNTHESIS AND SECRETION. Calcitonin is a peptide of 32 amino acids that is normally synthesized and secreted by the parafollicular or C cells, which are neuroectodermal cells within the thyroid gland. Its secretion is stimulated by calcium and also by certain intestinal peptides (gastrin and glucagon) (see Ch. 236).

CALCITONIN ACTIONS. Calcitonin, at high concentrations, can directly inhibit osteoclast function. Calcitonin also can act in the kidney to cause mild natriuresis. These calcitonin actions have not been shown to be important in normal physiology. For the present, the principal interests in calcitonin are as a tumor marker, particularly for familial C cell neoplasia, or as a pharmacologic agent to treat bone disorders, such as Paget's disease.

Vitamin D and Its Metabolites

SYNTHESIS OF VITAMIN D. Vitamin D_3 is a seco-steroid (i.e., a steroid with one ring opened) synthesized from 7-dehydrocholesterol in the skin (Fig. 232–3), in a reaction catalyzed by ultraviolet light derived from the sun. Vitamin D_2, produced synthetically from the plant sterol ergosterol, is a vitamin D_3 analogue used as a dietary supplement or drug. The metabolism of vitamin D_3 and vitamin D_2 is similar in humans (see Ch. 233).

HYDROXYLATIONS OF VITAMIN D METABOLITES. Vitamin D ("D" refers to combinations of the D_3 and D_2 isoforms) is converted to 25OHD in hepatocytes. This reaction is not under metabolic control and is determined principally by the serum levels of its substrate, vitamin D. 25OHD is normally converted to $1,25(OH)_2D$ only in the renal proximal tubule by an enzyme system stimulated by PTH. A similar PTH-independent 1α-hydroxylation occurs in the normal placenta and abnormally in granuloma tissues, as in sarcoidosis. 25OHD and $1,25(OH)_2D$ can also be hydroxylated at other residues (C-23, C-24, C-26), but these and other conversions probably serve mainly to inactivate vitamin D metabolites.

ABSORPTION AND TRANSPORT OF VITAMIN D METABOLITES. Vitamin D metabolites enter the bloodstream like other sterols, and a small fraction of all vitamin D metabolites undergo an enterohepatic recirculation. When cutaneous synthesis of vitamin D is marginal, any cause of intestinal malabsorption can result in vitamin D deficiency. Vitamin D metabolites are lipid soluble; they circulate in plasma bound to a specific 25OHD binding protein and, to a lesser degree, to other carriers.

MECHANISM OF ACTIONS OF VITAMIN D METABOLITES. Vitamin D is an inactive precursor; 25OHD and

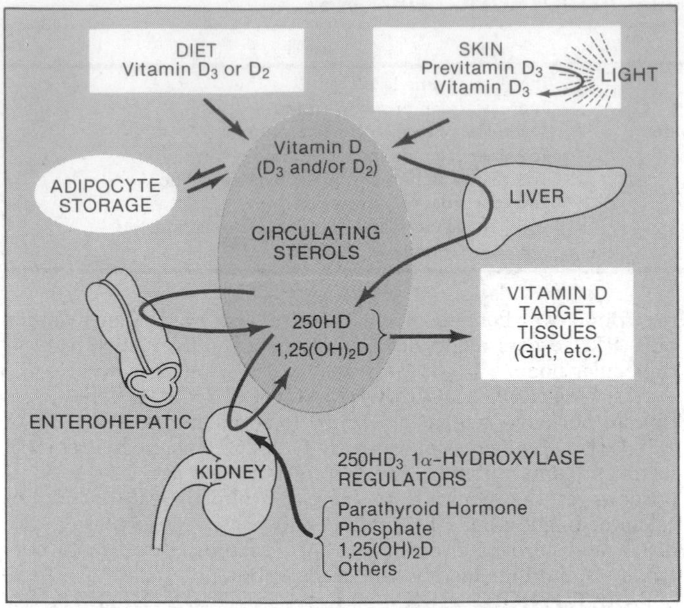

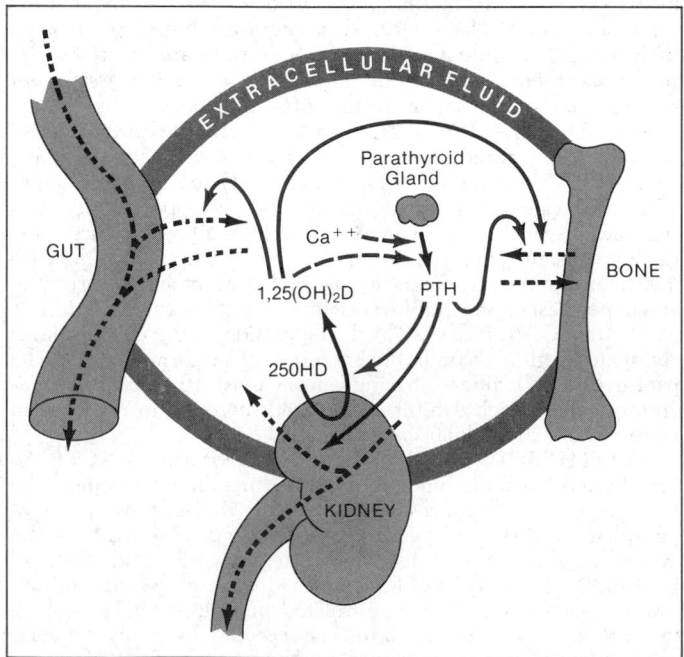

FIGURE 232–3. The vitamin D activation pathway. This involves steps in many different organs. Dysfunction at any step can have clinically important consequences.

1,25(OH)$_2$D are both active. Though the concentration of 25OHD is about 1000-fold higher than that of 1,25(OH)$_2$D in blood, the latter has far higher affinity for the vitamin D receptor and normally determines the degree of vitamin D receptor activation. Calcitriol binds to intracellular receptors in target cells and causes gradual changes in the nuclei of those cells. The vitamin D receptor is highly homologous to the receptors for other steroids and to those for thyroid hormone and retinoic acid. Though vitamin D receptors are present in many organs, only those in duodenal mucosa have been established as important in normal physiology.

INTESTINAL ACTIONS OF CALCITRIOL. Calcitriol (1,25(OH)$_2$D) increases the flux of calcium from the intestinal lumen to blood. Calcitriol, to a much lesser extent, increases the flux of phosphate and magnesium from intestinal lumen to blood. Calcium, magnesium, and phosphate ions have specific processes for their intestinal transport. Calcitriol induces in duodenal mucosa high concentrations of an intracellular calcium-binding protein, termed calbindin. Calbindin belongs to the calmodulin protein family, but its role, if any, in intestinal calcium transport is unknown.

SKELETAL EFFECTS OF CALCITRIOL. The principal effects of calcitriol on bone (antirachitic effects) are indirect results of its action to promote calcium influx from intestinal lumen to blood. The deficient mineralization in vitamin D deficiency states is the consequence of the combination of low calcium in blood and low phosphate in blood, the latter resulting from the renal phosphate-wasting effects from secondary hyperparathyroidism.

The supraphysiologic concentrations of vitamin D metabolites sometimes reached during pharmacotherapy can raise blood calcium in part by increasing osteoclast numbers and activity.

OTHER EFFECTS OF CALCITRIOL. Calcitriol can inhibit PTH biosynthesis and secretion; the direct negative effects of calcitriol might contribute a form of short-loop negative feedback to parathyroid function. Calcitriol exerts direct effects on the renal enzymes that hydroxylate 25OHD; calcitriol inhibits the 25OHD$_3$ 1α-hydroxylase and stimulates the other hydroxylases that catabolize 25OHD in the renal tubule and in other tissues. Possibly important effects of calcitriol in skin and hair are suggested by its protective effect on psoriatic skin at pharmacologic doses and by the striking association of total alopecia with the rare syndrome of severely defective vitamin D receptors. Vitamin D receptors are present in many additional organs, but no role for them has been identified in normal physiology.

Other Hormones

SEX STEROIDS. Sex steroids, particularly estrogens, have slow but extremely important anabolic effects on bone. The effects are exerted directly on the bone organ, perhaps through receptors in the osteoblast. Estrogen deficiency results in accelerated bone remodeling with disproportionate bone resorption, particularly in trabecular bone.

GLUCOCORTICOIDS. Glucocorticoids affect many of the cells that contribute to mineral metabolism. The most striking effect is bone thinning that results from high glucocorticoid concentrations. This thinning is probably a consequence mainly of inhibition of osteoblasts. In addition, glucocorticoids antagonize the actions of vitamin D metabolites by unknown mechanisms.

THYROID HORMONE. Thyroid hormones also have direct effects on bone cells. Excess of thyroid hormones causes increased release of calcium from bone. The skeletal consequences of deficient thyroid hormone are most evident in the disordered growth of cartilaginous epiphyses associated with congenital hypothyroidism.

GROWTH HORMONE. Growth hormone stimulates the growth of bone and cartilage, in part by stimulating local production of type 1 insulin-like growth factor by osteoblasts and chondrocytes.

ADAPTATIONS TO DISRUPTIONS OF MINERAL METABOLISM

Two principal calciotropic hormones, PTH and 1,25(OH)$_2$D, interact with each other and with multiple target tissues to control the metabolism of calcium, phosphate, and, to a lesser degree, magnesium (Fig. 232–4 and Table 232–3). These hormones allow for adaptations over time intervals that are short (minutes) or long (months).

Blood levels of ionized calcium are sustained at nearly invariant levels, with minimal diurnal changes reflecting mainly the sudden rises of calcium influx with meals. Serum levels of PTH and 1,25(OH)$_2$D also show only modest diurnal changes under normal conditions. Serum phosphate typically has broad diurnal fluctuations, with a nadir around 9:00 AM and peaks at around 6:00 PM and 4:00 AM.

Calcium Excess States

States with long-term excess or deficiency of calcium are associated with deviations at multiple steps of the integrated

FIGURE 232–4. Integrated control of secretion and actions of parathyroid hormone (PTH) and calcitriol (1,25(OH)$_2$ vitamin D = 1,25(OH)$_2$D) with emphasis on calcium fluxes. Unfilled arrows show secretion of PTH and calcitriol. Stippled arrows are calcium fluxes. Solid black arrows show stimulatory effects; interrupted black arrows show inhibitory effects.

mineral homeostasis system. The most common calcium excess state in adults is primary overfunction of the parathyroid gland. Of course, this has the potential to distort most of the normal calcium regulatory processes. Primary hyperparathyroidism results in high blood levels of PTH and often of $1,25(OH)_2D$ as well. The results are combinations of increased calcium influx to blood dependent upon the evoked dysfunctions in intestinal, skeletal, and renal pools of calcium. A very different integrated metabolic pattern results when calcium excess is caused by dysfunction outside the parathyroid—for example, with osteolytic metastases, skeletal immobilization, or dietary calcium overload (milk-alkali syndrome). In the latter disturbances, the parathyroid gland reacts appropriately and becomes suppressed by the increase of ionized calcium in blood; blood concentrations of PTH and $1,25(OH)_2D$ become low. The abnormally high filtered load of calcium without the anticalciuric effects of PTH results in severe hypercalciuria; irreversible renal damage can occur over a period of only a few weeks.

Calcium Deficiency States

Calcium deficiency states generally result in the parathyroid gland's recognizing the signal of a low ionized calcium level in blood. Increased PTH secretion (within seconds), increased PTH biosynthesis (within days), or parathyroid cell hyperplasia (within weeks) activates the response pathway. The consequences of this secondary hyperparathyroidism are increased renal tubular secretion of $1,25(OH)_2D$ (if there is not underlying deficiency of 25OHD or 1α-hydroxylase) and increased net calcium flux into blood from the intestinal lumen, from bone, and from the renal tubular lumen. The relative contribution of each calcium pool to this integrated response depends in part on the chromic state of that pool and on the relative levels of PTH and calcitriol. Serum calcium typically begins to fall below normal only when the osteolytic response to PTH or $1,25(OH)_2D$ becomes weakened (from depletion of readily exchangeable calcium pools or other types of tachyphylaxis). Secondary hyperparathyroidism has important effects on phosphate homeostasis through direct effects on bone and kidney, increasing phosphate influx from bone and causing a similar increase in phosphate efflux into urine. With forms of hypoparathyroidism, some residual components of mineral homeostasis can be sustained in the face of deficiency of PTH and secondarily of $1,25(OH)_2D$.

Metabolic Bone Diseases

Certain forms of metabolic bone disease are associated with dramatic imbalances in mineral flux to or from blood; these include increased calcium influx with aggressive osteolytic processes and decreased calcium influx with many forms of osteomalacia. Others, because they do not dramatically compromise the readily exchangeable pools of bone mineral, may have little or no long-term impact on the blood homeostatic system. For example, idiopathic osteoporosis has been categorized into two major forms (perimenopausal and aging associated), but no clearcut changes in blood PTH or $1,25(OH)_2D$ as adaptations to altered serum calcium levels have been identified in either form.

USES OF LABORATORY TESTING
Electrolytes in Blood

CALCIUM IN BLOOD. To stabilize protein concentration, total calcium should be measured in the fasting patient who is seated or recumbent. Most laboratories measure it inexpensively and with high precision. A high or low calcium value during multichannel screening is often the first indication of a treatable disorder. Serum calcium has traditionally been expressed in the United States in units of milligrams per deciliter, with a typical normal range being 8.8 to 10.2 mg per deciliter. Because calcium has a molecular weight of 40 and is divalent, this can be easily converted into milliequivalents per liter (divide milligrams per deciliter by 2.0) or into millimolar units (SI units); divide milligrams per deciliter by 4.0). Simple equations allow measurements of total calcium in serum to be "corrected" for distortions by deviation of albumin concentration (for example, total calcium can be adjusted upward by 1 mg/dl [0.25 mM] for each gram per deciliter that serum albumin is below the normal mean and vice versa). When uncertainty exists with regard to the direction or severity of an abnormality of blood calcium, the ionized calcium fraction should be evaluated, as it is a more valid and direct reflection of pathophysiology. This is a more demanding laboratory procedure than is total calcium, and the reproducibility is generally worse. An abnormality of blood calcium can arise from an abnormal flux to or from the major sites of calcium turnover—in bone, gut, and renal tubular fluid.

PHOSPHATE IN BLOOD. Phosphate measurements in serum represent only the 30 per cent that is in inorganic compounds. By convention, phosphate is reported in units of elemental phosphorus. These conventions avoid some of the confusion that would result from efforts to consider molar anion content (phosphate in serum is in a variable equilibrium between its monobasic and dibasic states). Its principal determinants are PTH, age, sex, food ingestion, and diurnal rhythm. Serum phosphate is only a weak index of intracellular phosphate stores. Its normal range is far wider than that for calcium.

MAGNESIUM IN BLOOD. Serum magnesium, like phosphate, is determined by its threshold for renal excretion and by total body pools. Primary disturbance of magnesium in blood is unusual, but important abnormalities can occur during major illnesses; for example, in association with chemotherapy or with extensive burns, tissue necrosis may increase blood magnesium levels, or large fluid losses could depress it.

Hormones in Blood

PARATHYROID HORMONE. Parathyroid hormone is often the first regulator that should be examined in an evaluation of a possible disturbance of mineral homeostasis. Two types of immunoassay are in widespread use. Radioimmunoassay (RIA) directed at the mid-region or carboxy-terminus of PTH can provide excellent clinical correlations; this assay is an index equally of PTH secretion rate and of renal clearance of inactive PTH fragments. Therefore, with mild to severe renal failure, the values must be interpreted with caution. A two-site immunoradiometric assay (IRMA) can give a result that is a more valid indicator of intact, biologically active PTH. Clinical correlations are excellent with this assay, and no adjustment is generally needed for renal compromise. Because the intact PTH molecule has a much shorter half-time than do its inactive fragments, normal PTH concentrations with the "intact" IRMA are far lower than with the mid-region or carboxy-terminus RIA (typically, 10 to 60 pg per milliliter versus 100 to 400 pg per milliliter, the latter normal range being especially dependent upon what is selected as the laboratory standard).

CALCITONIN. Calcitonin is measured by RIA. Clinical uses are limited. When the RIA is used in family screening for early stages of C cell neoplasia, it is particularly important that the laboratory provide normal ranges adjusted for the selected C cell challenge protocol and the patient's age.

25-HYDROXYVITAMIN D. Vitamin D itself is rarely measured in clinical settings. Two different vitamin D metabolites can be measured by most laboratories. It is essential to understand that these two metabolites, 25OHD and $1,25(OH)_2D$, are usually indicators of two entirely different types of process. Serum 25OHD is a useful index of vitamin D nutritional status. It is also a good index of sterol absorption. Low levels can arise from deficiency of sunlight, from deficiency of vitamin D nutritional supplementation, from fat malabsorption, and from accelerated hepatic catabolism of vitamin D metabolites. Since the body easily compensates for concentrations above normal, dangerously high levels occur only during consumption of pharmacologic doses of vitamin D or of 25OHD.

1,25-DIHYDROXYVITAMIN D. $1,25(OH)_2D$ measurement in serum gives an index of the steroid hormone whose renal production is usually finely regulated by blood PTH. Even with vitamin D intoxication, the serum levels of $1,25(OH)_2D$ may be appropriately low because of this regulatory system. Serum $1,25(OH)_2D$ has only limited diagnostic use. However, certain states can be associated with otherwise unexplainable mineral disturbances that reflect high levels of $1,25(OH)_2D$ (sarcoidosis and other granulomas) or low levels (certain renal tubular disorders, such as X-linked hypophosphatemia).

Blood Indices of Bone Disturbance

Alkaline phosphatase enzyme in serum is an index of its sources in bone, liver, and placenta and of its excretion by the biliary tree. With increased osteoblastic activity, the amount of skeletal alkaline phosphatase enzyme in serum can rise dramatically. Skeletal alkaline phosphatase can be measured selectively through its physicochemical properties (it is the heat-labile component of total alkaline phosphatase) or otherwise (e.g., by RIA, a topic for research in several centers). High skeletal alkaline phosphatase levels can point to high bone turnover (hyperparathyroidism, Paget's disease). Other bone-specific proteins are also under investigation as possible specific indicators of skeletal processes. Osteocalcin (sometimes called bone gla-protein) is another osteoblast-specific protein that has been useful in some long-term studies of bone turnover, but its insensitivity to diffuse bone pathology has compromised its broad clinical use.

Measurements on the Skeleton

BONE RADIOGRAPHS AND SCANS. Standard radiography is often the starting point in the evaluation of bone disorders. Images can be specific for numerous conditions or can direct further diagnostic procedures (i.e., bone biopsy) to sites of focal disturbance. A bone scan with technetium-99m diphosphonate may identify a local disturbance that is not accompanied by radiographic change; the label adsorbs to bone mineral, and increased local blood flow without fracture is sufficient to give a positive signal.

BONE MASS INDICES. Bone mass can be measured noninvasively with a wide variety of techniques. These include dual-channel radiographs, single- and dual-channel photon absorptiometry, radiographs with computed tomography (CT), and other methods under development. Selection among these possibilities should depend largely on local expertise. For sequential studies in a patient, these methods are compromised, to varying degrees, by high cost and lack of precision.

BONE BIOPSY. Bone biopsy can be the final diagnostic tool in identifying local or generalized disturbances of bone. It can be particularly useful in distinguishing osteomalacia from osteoporosis. Maximal information about the bone formation process can be obtained by prior administration of two pulses of tetracyclines 14 days apart (tetracyclines selectively adsorb to the mineralization front of osteoid and provide a fluorescent signal in the biopsy). This test should be considered in consultation with persons knowledgeable about its indications and the details of its processing.

Analyses of the Intestines in Mineral Metabolism

Specific tests of intestinal function are rarely used in current clinical practice. Metabolic balance studies are time consuming and expensive. Calcium absorption studies with radioactive or stable isotopes are not applied outside research settings. General indices of intestinal function are considered in other chapters.

Analyses of the Kidney and Urine

Renal biopsy should be done only for the standard indications related to intrinsic or systemic diseases in the kidney. Urinary excretion of hydroxyproline and other collagen metabolites is a useful index of bone resorption rates because 60 per cent of urinary hydroxyproline is normally derived from collagen in bone.

Urinary excretion of calcium, magnesium, or phosphate is useful in screening for total body excess or deficiency of any of these minerals. Urinary excretion of calcium is central in the evaluation of urolithiasis. More detailed discussion of the workup of urolithiasis is presented elsewhere (see Ch. 88).

Aurbach GD, Marx SJ, Spiegel AM: Parathyroid hormone, calcitonin, and the calciferols. Metabolic bone disease. *In* Wilson JD, Foster DW (eds.): Williams Textbook of Endocrinology. 8th ed. Philadelphia, W.B. Saunders Company, 1991. *Detailed review of mineral metabolism with emphasis on calciotropic hormones. Other major textbooks of endocrinology have similar chapters.*

Avioli LV, Krane SM (eds.): Metabolic Bone Diseases and Clinically Related Disorders. 2nd ed. Philadelphia, W.B. Saunders Company, 1990. *A detailed review of the entire field from multiple authors.*

DeGroot LJ, Besser GM, Cahill GF, et al. (eds.): Endocrinology. 2nd ed. Philadelphia, W.B. Saunders Company, 1989. *Volume 2 of this three-volume encyclopedic text contains 22 chapters by many authors covering the field of mineral metabolism. Controversial areas are treated in depth, but coverage of some topics may be outdated.*

Favus MJ (ed.): Primer on Metabolic Bone Diseases and Disorders of Mineral Metabolism. Kelseyville, Calif., American Society for Bone and Mineral Research, 1990. *Concise chapters that quickly advance the reader to the current frontiers of research on a topic.*

Peck WE (ed.): Bone and Mineral Research. Vols. 1–6, 1983–1989. New York, Elsevier. *An annual volume with authoritative reviews of basic and clinical topics in this area.*

233 Vitamin D
Daniel D. Bikle

Vitamin D is a steroid hormone with two molecular forms: vitamin D_3 (cholecalciferol), which is produced in the skin, and vitamin D_2 (ergocalciferol), which is derived from the plant sterol ergosterol. Vitamin D_2 is the usual form of vitamin D available for pharmaceutical use, although both vitamin D_2 and D_3 are used as food supplements. Despite subtle differences in physiology and biochemistry, vitamin D_2 and D_3 have equivalent potency and mechanisms of action in humans. In the ensuing discussion, lack of a subscript after the D indicates that both forms of vitamin D are implied.

To achieve biologic potency, vitamin D must be further metabolized. Two of these metabolites, 25-hydroxyvitamin D (25OHD) and 1,25-dihydroxyvitamin D (1,25(OH)$_2$D), are produced by successive hydroxylations; the hepatic enzyme vitamin D 25-hydroxylase catalyzes the formation of 25OHD, and the renal enzyme 25OHD 1-hydroxylase catalyzes the formation of 1,25(OH)$_2$D. Both 25OHD (calcifediol) and 1,25(OH)$_2$D (calcitriol) are available to treat disorders of calcium homeostasis. A third metabolite, 24,25-dihydroxyvitamin D (24,25(OH)$_2$D), also shows promise as a therapeutic agent but as yet is available only for investigational purposes. 24,25(OH)$_2$D, like 1,25(OH)$_2$D, is produced from 25OHD, principally in the kidney.

VITAMIN D ENDOCRINE SYSTEM

The vitamin D endocrine system can be divided into three levels (Fig. 233–1): bioavailability of vitamin D from skin and gut; metabolism of vitamin D to its active forms, principally by the liver and kidney; and the action of these metabolites on target tissues.

BIOAVAILABILITY. Vitamin D_3 is produced in the skin by a multistep process. Irradiation of 7-dehydrocholesterol by ultraviolet (UV) light converts it to previtamin D_3, which then undergoes thermal isomerization to vitamin D_3. No clear regulation of vitamin D_3 production has been observed other than by the amount of UV irradiation that reaches the 7-dehydrocholesterol in the epidermis. Increased melanin in the epidermis reduces the effect of UV irradiation. Aging also appears to result in decreased vitamin D production.

Vitamin D is also available from the diet, as it is commonly used as a food supplement in dairy products. Vitamin D is absorbed principally in the jejunum by a process (chylomicron formation) that is facilitated by bile salts, fatty acids, and monoglycerides. Most of the vitamin D absorbed passes through the lymphatic system before entering the bloodstream. The hydroxylated metabolites of vitamin D (i.e., 25OHD and 1,25(OH)$_2$D) depend less on chylomicron formation for their absorption.

Vitamin D and its metabolites are transported in blood bound mainly to an alpha globulin called vitamin D–binding protein (DBP). This protein has a higher affinity for 25OHD and 24,25(OH)$_2$D than for vitamin D and 1,25(OH)$_2$D. Since the amount of DBP in blood (5×10^{-6} M) far exceeds that of vitamin D and its metabolites (Table 233–1), 1 per cent or less of the total amount of these metabolites is actually free to diffuse into cells. It is unclear whether DBP serves principally as a circulating reservoir for the vitamin D metabolites in blood or facilitates the transport of these metabolites into target tissues. Changes in DBP levels affect total concentrations of vitamin D metabolites without necessarily affecting the free concentrations. Pregnancy and estrogen increase DBP; liver disease and proteinuria decrease DBP. The relative importance of free versus total concentration of the vitamin D metabolites has not been established with certainty, although evidence suggesting that the free concentration is the biologically active concentration is accumulating.

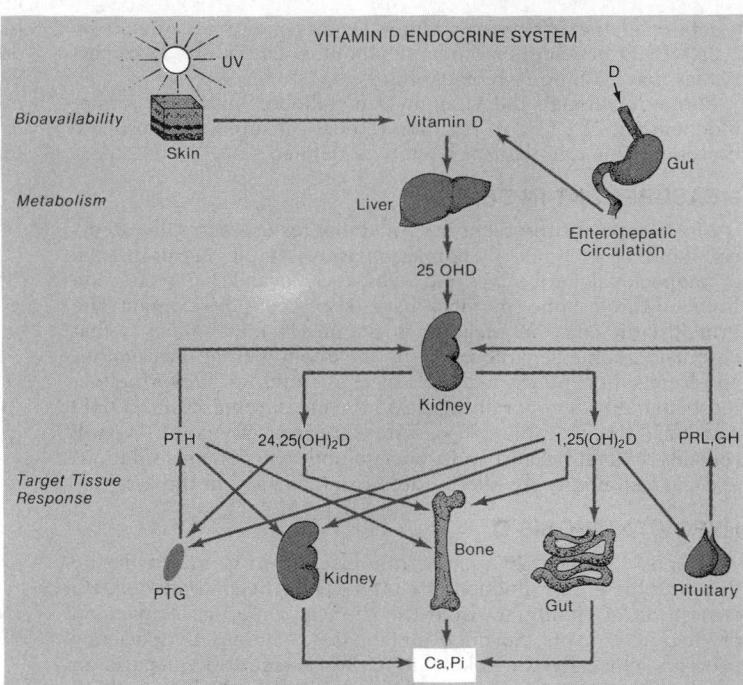

FIGURE 233–1. The vitamin D endocrine system. Vitamin D is made available to the body by photogenesis in the skin and absorption from the intestine. Vitamin D is then hydroxylated in the liver to 25OHD, then in the kidney to $1,25(OH)_2D$ and $24,25(OH)_2D$. The active vitamin D metabolites act on different tissues to produce a variety of responses. The three target tissues principally responsible for calcium (Ca) and phosphate (Pi) homeostasis are kidney, bone, and intestine. Endocrine tissues such as the parathyroid gland (PTG) and anterior pituitary are also target tissues. Their hormones, parathyroid hormone (PTH), prolactin (PRL), and growth hormone (GH), help regulate vitamin D metabolism in the kidney. In addition, PTH has a direct effect on bone and kidney regulation of calcium and phosphate homeostasis. (Reproduced with permission from Bikle DD: The vitamin D endocrine system. *In* Stollerman GH, et al. [eds.]: Advances in Internal Medicine. Vol. 27. Copyright © 1982 by Year Book Medical Publishers, Inc., Chicago.)

METABOLISM. Liver. The first step in the bioactivation of vitamin D occurs in the liver, where vitamin D 25-hydroxylase converts vitamin D to 25OHD. Since 25OHD production by this cytochrome P450 mixed-function oxidase is governed principally by the supply of substrate (i.e., vitamin D), circulating 25OHD levels are a good indicator of vitamin D bioavailability. Hepatic production of 25OHD appears to be well preserved in all but the most severe cases of liver disease unless the vitamin D stores are depleted. Compounds such as phenytoin and phenobarbital, however, which induce drug-metabolizing enzymes in the liver, alter the hepatic metabolism of vitamin D in a manner that may lead to clinical bone disease in subjects with marginal vitamin D stores.

Kidney. The 25OHD produced by the liver is further metabolized to $1,25(OH)_2D$ and $24,25(OH)_2D$, principally in the kidney. Little, if any, $1,25(OH)_2D$ is produced outside the kidney (except by the placenta) under normal circumstances, although other tissues, such as bone, cartilage, skin, and macrophages may produce $24,25(OH)_2D$ and $1,25(OH)_2D$ in limited amounts. Lymphomatous and sarcoid tissue may also contain 1-hydroxylase activity. Both the 1-hydroxylase and the 24-hydroxylase in the kidney are cytochrome P450 mixed-function oxidases located exclusively in the mitochondria of the proximal renal tubule.

TABLE 233–1. VITAMIN D AND ITS METABOLITES

Name	Abbreviation	Generic Name	Serum Concentration*
Vitamin D	D	Calciferol	1.6 ± 0.4 ng/ml
Vitamin D_3	D_3	a. Cholecalciferol	
Vitamin D_2	D_2	b. Ergocalciferol	
25 hydroxy-vitamin D	25OHD	Calcifediol	26.5 ± 5.3 ng/ml
1,25 dihydroxy-vitamin D	$1,25(OH)_2D$	Calcitriol	34.1 ± 9.8 pg/ml
24,25 dihydroxy-vitamin D	$24,25(OH)_2D$		1.3 ± 0.4 ng/ml
25,26 dihydroxy-vitamin D	$25,26(OH)_2D$		0.5 ± 0.1 ng/ml

*Values differ somewhat from laboratory to laboratory, depending on the methodology used and the sunlight exposure and dietary intake of vitamin D in the population studied. Children tend to have higher $1,25(OH)_2D$ levels than do adults. Data are derived from Lambert PW, Fu IY, Kaetzel DM, et al.: Assay for multiple vitamin D metabolites. *In* Bikle DD (ed.): Assay of Calcium Regulating Hormones. New York, Springer-Verlag, 1983, pp 99–124.

Their activities are closely regulated by a variety of ions and hormones, the most important of which are calcium, phosphate, $1,25(OH)_2D$ itself, and parathyroid hormone (PTH). Low serum calcium and phosphate levels and elevated PTH levels stimulate $1,25(OH)_2D$ production. High $1,25(OH)_2D$ levels inhibit $1,25(OH)_2D$ production but increase $24,25(OH)_2D$ production. Other hormones such as prolactin and growth hormone may also stimulate $1,25(OH)_2D$ production, but whether these hormones are important in the control of $1,25(OH)_2D$ production under normal physiologic conditions is not known.

TARGET TISSUE RESPONSE. Bone, gut, and kidney are the primary target tissues for vitamin D, but many other tissues, including the pituitary, parathyroid glands, pancreas, brain, activated lymphocytes, thymocytes, skin, and a variety of tumors, contain a specific receptor for $1,25(OH)_2D$ and respond to it by a change in function. Muscle contains no receptors for $1,25(OH)_2D$ but appears to be a target tissue for 25OHD. These observations suggest that vitamin D influences a much greater range of biologic phenomena than previously appreciated, such as immunoregulation, cellular differentiation, and neural transmission. Whether all tissues that contain receptors for the vitamin D metabolites have a physiologically important response to normal circulating concentrations of the metabolites has not been established.

Intestine. $1,25(OH)_2D$ regulates calcium transport across the intestine in a highly integrated sequence of events. First, $1,25(OH)_2D$ appears to increase the permeability of the brush-border membrane to calcium, permitting calcium to enter from the lumen into the intestinal epithelial cell down a steep electrochemical gradient. The calcium that enters the cell must be accumulated by subcellular organelles, such as the mitochondria, to prevent cytosolic calcium concentrations from reaching toxic levels. $1,25(OH)_2D$ stimulates this accumulation. The calcium must then be transported through the cell and pumped across the basolateral membrane into the bloodstream. A unique calcium-binding protein (CaBP), induced by $1,25(OH)_2D$ in the intestine as well as in a number of other target tissues, appears to modulate intracellular calcium concentrations, perhaps by facilitating the removal of calcium from the cell.

Bone. The role of the vitamin D metabolites in calcium movement in and out of bone is less clear. $1,25(OH)_2D$ is a potent stimulator of bone resorption and inhibitor of collagen production (bone formation) in vitro. On the other hand, $24,25(OH)_2D$ may stimulate bone and cartilage formation without stimulating bone resorption. These results have engendered a controversy over whether all the effects of vitamin D on bone are mediated by 1,25(OH)$_2$D or whether other metabolites, 24,25(OH)$_2$D in particular, have a unique biologic role.

Kidney. Although the vitamin D metabolites may play a role, independent of PTH, in regulating renal calcium and phosphate excretion, this role has not been well defined.

MEASUREMENT IN SERUM

Most assays for the vitamin D metabolites use naturally occurring binding proteins. Radioimmunoassays employing polyclonal or monoclonal antibodies and a bioassay evaluating resorption from cultured bone in vitro have also been developed. The principal difficulty in measuring vitamin D metabolites is that chromatographic separation of the metabolites from one another and from other interfering substances is required. Nevertheless, most laboratories generally agree on the measurements of 25OHD and 1,25(OH)$_2$D (Table 233–1). Measurement of vitamin D itself remains difficult because of its poor solubility in aqueous solutions and modest affinity for the binding proteins used in the assays.

HYPOVITAMINOSIS D

Vitamin D deficiency results from insufficient vitamin D in the diet, insufficient production of vitamin D in the skin, inadequate absorption of vitamin D from the diet, or abnormal conversion of vitamin D to its bioactive metabolites. Vitamin D deficiency presents clinically as rickets in children and osteomalacia in adults. This subject is discussed in detail in Ch. 234.

HYPERVITAMINOSIS D

Hypervitaminosis D may occur in three general settings: (1) excessive consumption, usually for therapeutic purposes, of vitamin D, vitamin D analogues (such as dihydrotachysterol), or vitamin D metabolites; (2) the abnormal conversion of vitamin D to its biologically active metabolites, as occurs in sarcoidosis and possibly other granulomatous diseases; or (3) a change in the sensitivity of the target tissue to vitamin D, as can occur with the remission of a variety of gastrointestinal diseases associated with calcium malabsorption. The initial signs and symptoms of vitamin D intoxication include weakness, lethargy, headaches, nausea, and polyuria and are attributable to the hypercalcemia and hypercalciuria. Ectopic calcification may occur, particularly in the kidneys, resulting in nephrolithiasis or nephrocalcinosis; other sites include blood vessels, heart, lungs, and skin. Infants appear to be quite susceptible to vitamin D intoxication and may develop disseminated arteriosclerosis, supravalvular aortic stenosis, and renal acidosis.

The dose of vitamin D required to produce toxicity varies among patients, reflecting differences in absorption, storage, and subsequent metabolism of the vitamin as well as in target tissue response to the active metabolites. For example, an elderly patient with senile osteoporosis and a low turnover rate of bone also tends to have a reduced ability to absorb calcium in the intestine and a reduced ability to produce 1,25(OH)$_2$D in the kidney. Such a patient can usually ingest 50,000 to 100,000 IU of vitamin D per day without developing hypercalcemia or hypercalciuria. In contrast, a patient of similar age with a similar degree of osteoporosis but in whom the osteoporosis develops as a result of primary hyperparathyroidism would almost certainly be harmed by this amount of vitamin D. In the latter patient, the ability of vitamin D to stimulate bone resorption and intestinal calcium absorption is enhanced in part because of the greater rates of 1,25(OH)$_2$D production and bone turnover observed in primary hyperparathyroidism. Patients with sarcoidosis appear to develop vitamin D intoxication because 1,25(OH)$_2$D production in the abnormal tissue is not subject to the normal feedback mechanisms that regulate renal production of 1,25(OH)$_2$D. Analogues of vitamin D, such as dihydrotachysterol, or the renal metabolite of vitamin D, 1,25(OH)$_2$D, which bypass the normal rate-limiting step of vitamin D bioactivation (the renal 1α-hydroxylase reaction), are more likely than vitamin D or 25OHD to result in hypercalcemia if used in excess.

Hypervitaminosis D is treated by stopping the administration of vitamin D or its analogues or metabolites. If the hypercalcemia is severe, the patient should be placed on a low-calcium diet and given glucocorticoids (e.g., 60 mg of prednisone every day) and generous amounts of fluids. Acute hypercalcemia, when symptomatic, can be treated with saline and furosemide diuresis, as described under the general management of hypercalcemia (Ch. 235). Hypercalcemia lasts for only a few days when caused by excess 1,25(OH)$_2$D, but it may persist for weeks or months when caused by excess vitamin D. The hypercalcemia of sarcoidosis tends to respond within days to glucocorticoid therapy.

Adams JS, Singer FR, Gacad MA, et al.: Isolation and structural identification of 1,25-dihydroxyvitamin D$_3$ produced by cultured alveolar macrophages in sarcoidosis. J Clin Endocrinol Metab 60:960, 1985. *Provides direct evidence that sarcoid macrophages make 1,25(OH)$_2$D.*

Bikle DD: Regulation of intestinal calcium transport by vitamin D: Role of membrane structure. In Aloia RC, Curtain CC, Gordon LM (eds.): Membrane Transport and Information Storage. New York, Wiley-Riss, 1990, pp 191–219. *A comprehensive discussion of the mechanisms by which 1,25(OH)$_2$D regulates intestinal calcium transport.*

Fraser DR: Regulation of the metabolism of vitamin D. Physiol Rev 60:551, 1980. *A thorough, well-balanced review of vitamin D metabolism in the liver and kidney.*

Holick MF: Capacity of human skin to produce vitamin D$_3$. In Kligman A, Takase Y (eds.): Cutaneous Aging. Tokyo, University of Tokyo Press, 1988, pp 223–246. *A thorough discussion of the biochemistry of vitamin D production in the skin, including the environmental variables that limit this process.*

Lambert PW, Stern PH, Avioli RC, et al.: Evidence for extrarenal production of 1α,25-dihydroxyvitamin D in man. J Clin Invest 69:722, 1982. *The demonstration of 1,25(OH)$_2$D levels in anephric humans and the suggestion that vitamin D treatment increases these levels.*

Lee DBN, Zawada ET, Kleeman CR: The pathophysiology and clinical aspects of hypercalcemic disorders. West J Med 129:278, 1978. *This article discusses all the major hypercalcemic disorders, including the diagnosis and treatment of hypervitaminosis D.*

Pillai S, Bikle DD, Elias PM: Vitamin D and epidermal differentiation. Evidence for a role of endogenously produced vitamin D metabolites in keratinocytic differentiation. Skin Pharmacol 1:149, 1988. *Describes both the production of 1,25(OH)$_2$D by epidermal cells and the role of 1,25(OH)$_2$D in modulating the differentiation of these cells.*

Reichel H, Koeffler HP, Norman AW: The role of the vitamin D endocrine system in health and disease. N Engl J Med 320:980, 1989. *A good overview emphasizing recent concepts regarding the role of 1,25(OH)$_2$D in cellular growth and differentiation.*

234 Osteomalacia and Rickets

Daniel D. Bikle

DEFINITIONS

Osteomalacia and rickets are caused by the abnormal mineralization of bone and cartilage. Osteomalacia refers to the defect that occurs in bone in which the epiphyseal plates have closed (i.e., in adults), whereas rickets refers to the defect that occurs in growing bone (i.e., in children). Abnormal mineralization in growing bone affects the transformation of cartilage into bone at the zone of provisional calcification. As a result, an enormous profusion of disorganized, nonmineralized, degenerating cartilage appears in this region, leading to widening of the epiphyseal plate (observed radiologically as a widened radiolucent zone) with flaring or cupping and irregularity of the epiphyseal-metaphyseal junctions. This latter problem gives rise to the clinically obvious beaded swellings along the costochondral junctions (rachitic rosary) and the swelling at the ends of the long bones. Growth is retarded by the failure to make new bone. Once bone growth has ceased (i.e., after closure of the epiphyseal plates), the clinical evidence for defective mineralization becomes more subtle, and special diagnostic procedures may be required for its detection.

PATHOGENESIS—OVERVIEW

The best known cause of abnormal bone mineralization is vitamin D deficiency. Vitamin D, through its biologically active metabolites, ensures that the calcium and phosphate concentrations in the extracellular milieu are adequate for mineralization to occur. Vitamin D may also permit osteoblasts to produce a bone matrix that can be mineralized and then allows them to mineralize that matrix in a normal fashion. Phosphate deficiency can also cause defective mineralization. It may act independently or in conjunction with other predisposing abnormalities, since most hypophosphatemic disorders associated with osteomalacia or rickets also affect the vitamin D endocrine system. Dietary calcium deficiency has been implicated as a cause of rickets and may contribute to the osteomalacia and osteoporosis found in elderly patients. Osteomalacia or rickets may develop despite adequate levels of calcium, phosphate, and vitamin D if the bone matrix cannot undergo normal mineralization. For example, the deficiency in alkaline phosphatase in patients with hypophosphatasia can cause a defect in mineralization. This enzyme cleaves pyrophosphate, an inhibitor of bone mineralization, and a deficiency results in reduced removal of this inhibitor. Finally, drugs such as etidronate and heavy metals such as aluminum can interfere with mineralization and lead to osteomalacia or rickets.

Table 234–1 lists diseases associated with osteomalacia and

TABLE 234–1. THE OSTEOMALACIC SYNDROMES*

A. Disorders in the vitamin D endocrine system
  1. Decreased bioavailability
    Insufficient sunlight exposure
    Nutritional vitamin D deficiency
    Nephrotic syndrome (urinary loss)
    Malabsorption (fecal loss)
      Billroth type II gastrectomy
      Sprue
      Regional enteritis
      Jejunoileal bypass
      Pancreatic insufficiency
      Cholestatic disorders
      Cholestyramine
  2. Abnormal metabolism
    Liver disease
    Chronic renal failure
    Vitamin D–dependent rickets type I
    Tumoral hypophosphatemic osteomalacia
    X-linked hypophosphatemia
    Hypoparathyroidism (?)
    Chronic acidosis (?)
    Anticonvulsants
  3. Abnormal target tissue response
    Vitamin D–dependent rickets type II
    Gastrointestinal disorders
B. Disorders of phosphate homeostasis
  1. Decreased intestinal absorption
    Malnutrition
    Malabsorption
    Antacids containing aluminum hydroxide
  2. Increased renal loss
    X-linked hypophosphatemic rickets
    Tumoral hypophosphatemic osteomalacia
    De Toni-Debré-Fanconi (phosphaturia, aminoaciduria, glycosuria, bicarbonaturia)
    Cystinosis
    Oculocerebrorenal syndrome (Lowe's syndrome)
    Paraproteinemias
    Wilson's disease
    Glycogen storage diseases
    Galactosemia
    Tyrosinemia
    Cadmium poisoning
    Neurofibromatosis
C. Calcium deficiency
  1. Dietary insufficiency
  2. Excessive renal loss (?)
  3. Malabsorption of calcium (?)
D. Primary disorders of bone matrix
  1. Hypophosphatasia
  2. Fibrogenesis imperfecta ossium
  3. Axial osteomalacia
E. Inhibitors of mineralization
  1. Aluminum
    Chronic renal failure
    Total parenteral nutrition
  2. Etidronate
  3. Phenytoin (?)
  4. Fluoride (?)

*This table categorizes diseases that produce osteomalacia according to the presumed mechanism (or mechanisms) by which bone mineralization is inhibited. A question mark indicates that the association of the disease with osteomalacia or the mechanism by which it produces osteomalacia is not established.

rickets according to the presumed mechanism responsible for the mineralization defect. Diseases that appear under multiple headings affect bone mineralization via multiple mechanisms. It is important to understand the mechanism by which a particular disease interferes with bone mineralization in order to choose appropriate diagnostic procedures and therapy.

VITAMIN D DEFICIENCY
Pathogenesis

Vitamin D deficiency results from one, or more often a combination, of the following three causes.

REDUCED SUNLIGHT EXPOSURE. The human skin can generate adequate amounts of vitamin D if exposed to sufficient ultraviolet radiation. In countries with limited sunlight, however, or where the population dresses in a fashion that reduces exposure to sunlight, circulating levels of vitamin D metabolites are often low. These low levels may help explain why the incidence of osteomalacia is higher in Great Britain, the Scandinavian countries, the Middle East, and India than in the United States.

NUTRITIONAL VITAMIN D DEFICIENCY. The fortification of dairy products with vitamin D has made nutritional vitamin D–deficient rickets uncommon in the United States, although it is still prevalent in other parts of the world. Even in the United States, vitamin D deficiency may occur in children of vegetarian mothers who avoid milk products (and presumably have reduced vitamin D stores) and in children who are not weaned to vitamin D–supplemented milk by age 2. The contribution of nutritional vitamin D deficiency to osteomalacia in elderly people is also suspected. Osteomalacia has been observed in 25 to 30 per cent of bone biopsies from elderly patients who have suffered hip fractures in Scandinavia and Great Britain. Most likely, both reduced vitamin D intake and reduced exposure to sunlight contribute to the development of osteomalacia in the elderly.

MALABSORPTION. Fecal loss of vitamin D and its metabolites occurs in patients with malabsorption for several reasons (Fig. 234–1). Ingested vitamin D is absorbed primarily in chylomicrons; disorders that involve the biliary tract, pancreas, or mid to distal portions of the small intestine reduce the efficiency of this process (Ch. 233). Endogenous vitamin D and its metabolites undergo enterohepatic circulation; disorders of the distal small bowel disrupt this circulation. In cholestatic disorders, urinary excretion of vitamin D metabolites is increased, and intestinal absorption is decreased. Drugs, such as cholestyramine, that are used in the treatment of cholestatic disorders may compound the problem by binding to the bile salts required for the absorption of the vitamin D metabolites, thus enhancing their fecal excretion. The resulting bone disease is often a combination of osteomalacia and osteoporosis. The prevalence of osteomalacia in patients with cholestatic and gastrointestinal disorders varies from country to country. It appears to be higher in Great Britain and Northern Europe than in the United States. Fully 25 to 50 per cent of British and European patients who have undergone Billroth type II gastrectomy or jejunoileal bypass or who have cholestatic liver disease or inflammatory bowel disease have osteomalacia when evaluated by bone biopsy.

Diagnosis

In children, the presentation of rickets is generally obvious from a combination of clinical and radiologic evidence. The diagnostic challenge is to determine the etiology. In adults the clinical, radiologic, and biochemical evidence for osteomalacia is often subtle. In situations in which osteomalacia should be suspected (malnutrition, liver disease, malabsorption, and unexplained osteopenia), the clinician must decide whether to obtain a biopsy of bone for histomorphometric examination. This decision must rest on the availability of resources to perform the biopsy and to evaluate the specimen, the index of suspicion coupled with the lack of certainty from other diagnostic procedures, and the degree to which the therapeutic approach will be altered by the additional information.

CLINICAL FEATURES. The clinical presentation of rickets depends on the age of the patient and, to some extent, the etiology of the syndrome (Fig. 234–2). The affected infant or young child may be apathetic, listless, weak, hypotonic, and

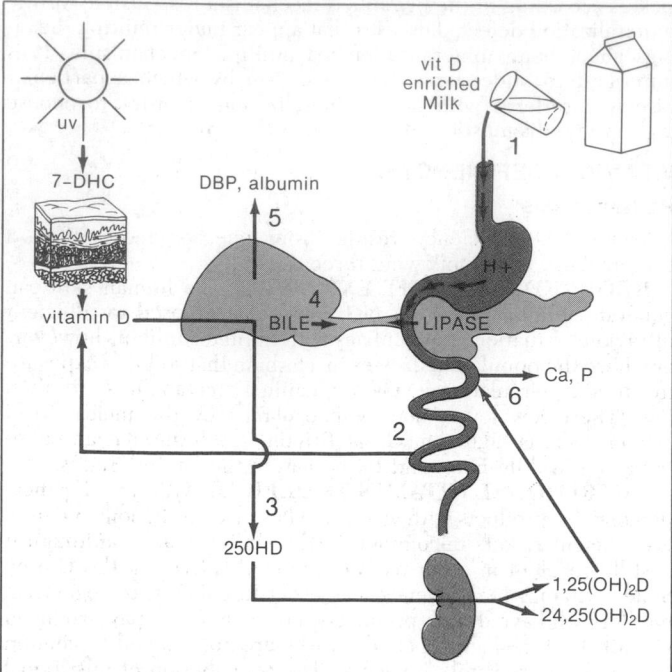

FIGURE 234–1. Six steps in vitamin D absorption and handling that may be altered by hepatogastrointestinal disorders and lead to bone disease. 1, Decreased intake of vitamin D. 2, Decreased absorption of vitamin D secondary to disorders in biliary secretion, pancreatic enzymes, enterocyte function, or intestinal anatomy. 3, Abnormal production of 25OHD by the liver secondary to hepatic parenchymal disease or anticonvulsants. 4, Disruption in the enterohepatic circulation of vitamin D metabolites and conjugates secondary to disorders in biliary secretion. 5, Reduced delivery of vitamin D metabolites to target tissues secondary to decreased vitamin D–binding protein (DBP) and albumin synthesis. 6, Decreased response of the diseased intestine to 1,25(OH)$_2$D with respect to calcium and phosphorus absorption.

growing poorly. A soft, somewhat misshapen head with widened sutures and frontal bossing may be observed. Eruption of teeth may be delayed, and teeth that do appear may be pitted and poorly mineralized. The enlargement and cupping of the costochondral junctions produce the "rachitic rosary" on the thorax. The tug of the diaphragm against the softened lower ribs may produce an indentation at the point of insertion of the diaphragm (Harrison's groove). Muscle hypotonia can result in a pronounced pot belly and a waddling gait. The limbs may become bowed, and joints may swell because of flaring at the ends of the long bones (including phalanges and metacarpals). Pathologic fractures may occur in patients with florid rickets.

After the epiphyses have closed, the clinical signs of rickets or osteomalacia are subtle and cannot be relied upon to make the diagnosis. Patients with severe osteomalacia complain of bone pain and muscle weakness. Difficulty climbing stairs or rising from chairs may be reported. Such individuals may have a history of multiple fractures. However, osteomalacia is often diagnosed by bone histomorphometry in patients who lack obvious symptoms in their musculoskeletal system.

RADIOLOGIC FEATURES. The radiologic features of rickets, like the clinical manifestations, can be quite striking, especially in the young child. In growing bone, the radiolucent epiphyses are wide and flared, with irregular epiphyseal-metaphyseal junctions. Long bones may be bowed. The cortices of the long bones are often indistinct. Occasionally, evidence of secondary hyperparathyroidism—subperiosteal resorption in the phalanges and metacarpals and erosion of the distal ends of the clavicles—is observed.

Pseudofractures (also known as Looser's zones or Milkman's fractures) are an uncommon but nearly pathognomonic feature of rickets and osteomalacia (Fig. 234–3). These radiolucent lines are most often found along the concave side of the femoral neck, the pubic rami, the ribs, the clavicles, and the lateral aspects of the

scapulae. Pseudofractures may result from unhealed microfractures at points of stress or at the entry point of blood vessels into bone. They may progress to complete fractures that go unrecognized and thereby lead to substantial deformity and disability. Bone density is not a reliable indicator of osteomalacia, since bone density can be decreased in patients with vitamin D deficiency or increased in patients with chronic renal failure. In adults with normal renal function, radiologic evidence of a mineralization defect is often subtle and not readily distinguishable from osteoporosis.

BIOCHEMICAL FEATURES. Vitamin D deficiency results in decreased intestinal absorption of calcium and phosphate. In conjunction with the resulting secondary hyperparathyroidism, vitamin D deficiency leads to an increase in bone resorption, increased excretion of urinary phosphate, and increased renal tubular reabsorption of calcium. The net result tends to be a low normal serum calcium level, low serum phosphorus level, elevated serum alkaline phosphatase level, increased parathyroid hormone (PTH) level, decreased urinary calcium level, and increased urinary phosphate level. Finding a low 25OHD level in combination with these other biochemical alterations strengthens the diagnosis of vitamin D deficiency. The 1,25(OH)$_2$D level may be normal, making this determination less useful for the diagnosis of osteomalacia. Both 25OHD and 1,25(OH)$_2$D levels may be reduced in patients with liver disease or nephrotic syndrome, who nevertheless have normal free concentrations of these metabolites and who may not be vitamin D deficient. Other factors, such as age and diet, must be considered. For example, serum phosphorus values are normally lower in adults than in children. Dietary history is important, since urinary phosphate excretion and, to a lesser degree, urinary calcium excretion reflect dietary phosphate and calcium content. Since phosphate excretion depends on the filtered load (the product of the glomerular filtration rate [GFR] and plasma phosphate), urinary phosphate levels may be normal if either the GFR or the plasma phosphate levels are reduced, despite the presence of hyperparathyroidism. Expressions of renal phosphate clearance that account for these variables (e.g., renal threshold for phosphate, or TmP/GFR; TmP = maximal tubular reabsorption of phosphate) are a better indicator of renal phosphate handling than is total phosphate excretion. The TmP/GFR can be calculated from a nomogram using measurements of a fasting serum and urine phosphorus concentration.

HISTOLOGIC FEATURES. Because of the difficulty in di-

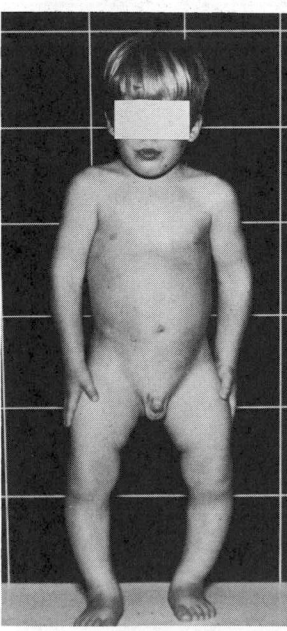
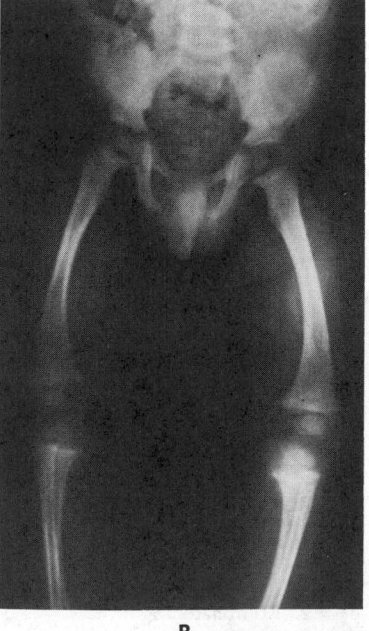

FIGURE 234–2. The clinical (A) and radiologic (B) appearance of a young boy with X-linked hypophosphatemic rickets. The most striking abnormalities are the bowing of the legs, apparent in both femora and tibiae, with flaring of the ends of these bones at the knee. (Photographs courtesy of Dr. Sara B. Arnaud.)

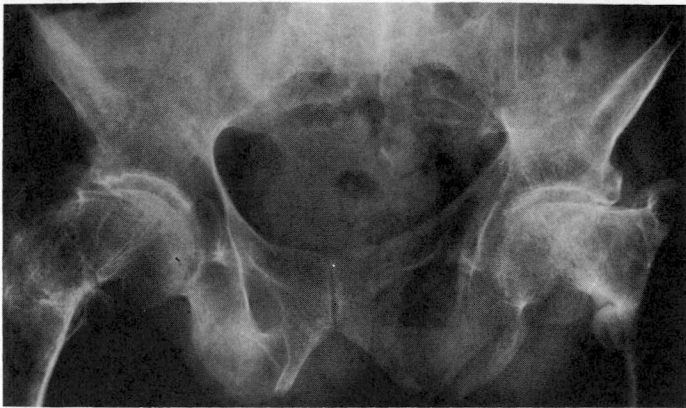

FIGURE 234–3. Roentgenogram of the pelvis of an elderly female with severe osteomalacia. This film reveals marked bowing (varus deformity) of both femoral necks, with pseudofractures of the medial aspect of the femoral necks and the superior aspect of the left pubic ramus. (Photograph courtesy of Dr. Harry K. Genant.)

agnosing osteomalacia in adults by clinical and radiologic means, transcortical bone biopsy may be necessary. A rib or the iliac crest is the site at which a biopsy is generally performed. To assess osteoid content and mineral appositional rate, the bone biopsy specimen is processed without decalcification. This requires special equipment.

In osteomalacia, bone is mineralized poorly and slowly, resulting in wide osteoid seams (>12 μm) and a large fraction of bone covered by unmineralized osteoid. States of high bone turnover (increased bone formation and resorption), such as hyperparathyroidism, can also cause wide osteoid seams and increased osteoid surface, producing a superficial resemblance to osteomalacia. Therefore, the rate of bone turnover should be determined by labeling bone with tetracycline, which provides a fluorescent marker of the calcification front. When two doses of tetracycline are given at different times, the distance between the two labels divided by the time interval between the two doses equals the mineral appositional rate. The normal appositional rate is approximately 0.74 μm per day. Mineralization lag time, the time required for newly formed osteoid to be mineralized, can be calculated by dividing osteoid seam width by the appositional rate corrected by the linear extent of mineralization or calcification front (a measure of the bone surface that is undergoing active mineralization as measured by tetracycline incorporation). It is normally about 20 to 25 days. Depressed appositional rate, increased mineralization lag time, and reduced calcification front clearly distinguish osteomalacia from high turnover states such as hyperparathyroidism. Low turnover states, such as senile osteoporosis, can also have low appositional rates and reduced calcification fronts, but these are distinguished from osteomalacia by normal or reduced osteoid surface and volume.

Treatment

The goal in treating osteomalacia and rickets is to normalize the clinical, biochemical, and radiologic abnormalities without producing hypercalcemia, hyperphosphatemia, hypercalciuria, nephrolithiasis, or ectopic calcification (especially nephrocalcinosis). To realize this goal, patients must be followed carefully, and as the bone lesions heal or the underlying disease improves, the dose of vitamin D, calcium, or phosphate needs to be adjusted to avoid such complications. Table 234–2 lists the available vitamin D metabolites and analogues, including dose range, duration of action, cost, and clinical applications.

Simple nutritional vitamin D deficiency responds to oral doses of 2000 to 4000 IU of vitamin D per day, taken for several months, followed by replacement doses of 200 to 400 IU per day. Radiologic and biochemical evidence of healing requires several months. If the patient fails to respond to treatment, the physician should consider other possible causes of the bone disease.

Patients with malabsorption may respond to large doses of oral vitamin D (25,000 to 100,000 IU per day), or they may require parenteral administration of the vitamin. Since patients with steatorrhea absorb 25OHD (calcifediol) better than they do

vitamin D, 50 to 100 μg of calcifediol per day or every other day should be tried if large doses of vitamin D fail to raise circulating levels of 25OHD into the high normal range. Vitamin D therapy should be supplemented with 1 to 3 grams of calcium per day. Only the osteomalacic component of the bone disease associated with these conditions responds to vitamin D; the osteoporotic component does not. Consequently, patients must be carefully selected for vitamin D treatment and carefully followed. Histomorphometric evaluation of bone biopsies is particularly useful in this regard.

CHRONIC RENAL FAILURE (see also Ch. 77 and 237)
Pathogenesis of Renal Osteodystrophy

Metabolism of 25OHD to 1,25-dihydroxyvitamin D (1,25(OH)$_2$D) and 24,25-dihydroxyvitamin D (24,25(OH)$_2$D) in the kidney is tightly regulated. Renal disease results in reduced circulating levels of both these metabolites. With the reduction in 1,25(OH)$_2$D levels, intestinal calcium absorption falls, and bone resorption appears to become less sensitive to PTH—a result that leads to hypocalcemia. Phosphate excretion by the diseased kidney is decreased, resulting in hyperphosphatemia and aggravation of the hypocalcemia. As a consequence, hyperparathyroidism develops, facilitated by the fact that the levels of the vitamin D metabolites are too low to inhibit PTH secretion. The net effect of deficient 1,25(OH)$_2$D and 24,25(OH)$_2$D and excessive PTH on bone is complex. Patients may have osteitis fibrosa (reflecting excessive PTH), osteomalacia (in part reflecting vitamin D deficiency), or a combination of the two. One particularly debilitating form of renal osteodystrophy is found in a small percentage of patients on hemodialysis in whom only osteomalacia occurs. Such patients have increased aluminum content in their bones, particularly in the zone where mineralization is occurring (calcification front). The aluminum is thought to block mineralization. These patients are particularly debilitated by bone pain, fractures, and muscle weakness.

Diagnosis

Most patients with chronic renal failure and renal osteodystrophy have osteitis fibrosa alone or in combination with osteomalacia (see Ch. 237). If not well controlled, these patients will have a low serum level of calcium and high serum levels of phosphorus, alkaline phosphatase, and PTH. A few patients develop severe secondary hyperparathyroidism in which the PTH level increases dramatically, with restoration of the serum calcium to normal or even elevated levels (sometimes called tertiary hyperparathyroidism). Another small subset of patients with renal osteodystrophy present with normal or low serum levels of PTH and alkaline phosphatase. Their serum calcium levels are often elevated after treatment with small doses of 1,25(OH)$_2$D. These patients have pure osteomalacia on bone biopsy and are thought to suffer from aluminum intoxication (see Ch. 237). Regardless of the type of bone disease, most patients with chronic renal disease have low 1,25(OH)$_2$D and 24,25(OH)$_2$D levels and, unless treated with vitamin D, tend to have low 25OHD levels as well.

Treatment

Patients with renal osteodystrophy generally respond to 1,25(OH)$_2$D (calcitriol, 0.5 to 1.0 μg per day) or dihydrotachysterol (DHT, 0.25 to 0.5 mg per day), calcium supplementation (1 to 3 grams per day), and phosphate restriction (dietary restriction supplemented with phosphate binders such as aluminum hydroxide). The goal is to achieve and maintain normal serum levels of calcium, phosphorus, PTH, and alkaline phosphatase. This regimen treats osteitis fibrosa more effectively than osteomalacia. Some authorities recommend the use of calcifediol rather than calcitriol or DHT, since calcifediol may treat the osteomalacia more effectively. This issue is unresolved. Patients with only osteomalacia usually fail to respond to 1,25(OH)$_2$D alone, but they have responded to 1,25(OH)$_2$D in combination with 24,25(OH)$_2$D, a metabolite not yet available for clinical use. The osteomalacia in renal osteodystrophy also appears to respond to the removal of aluminum with deferoxamine, a drug approved for the treatment of iron overload. Neither 24,25(OH)$_2$D nor deferoxamine has been approved by the United States Food and

TABLE 234–2. AVAILABLE VITAMIN D METABOLITES AND ANALOGUES

	Ergocalciferol	Dihydrotachysterol	Calcifediol	Calcitriol
Abbreviation	D_2	DHT	$25OHD_3$	$1,25(OH)_2D_3$
Physiologic dose	2.5–10 μg (1 μg = 40 units)	25–100 μg	1–5 μg	0.25–0.5 μg
Pharmacologic dose	0.625–5.0 mg	0.2–1.0 mg	20–200 μg	0.25–2.0 μg
Duration of action	1–3 months	1–4 weeks	2–6 weeks	2–5 days
Cost	$0.11/1.25 mg	$0.42/0.4 mg	$0.51/50 μg	$1.50/0.5 μg
Clinical applications	Vitamin D deficiency	Chronic renal failure	Vitamin D malabsorption	Chronic renal failure
	Vitamin D malabsorption	Hypoparathyroidism	Chronic renal failure	Hypoparathyroidism
	Hypoparathyroidism			Hypophosphatemic rickets
	Hypophosphatemic rickets			Acute hypocalcemia
	Anticonvulsant therapy in institutionalized patients			Vitamin D–dependent rickets types I and II

Drug Administration for the treatment of renal osteodystrophy, and both must currently be considered investigational drugs for this purpose.

NEPHROTIC SYNDROME

Even when vitamin D intake is adequate, vitamin D and its metabolites can be lost in the urine. The vitamin D metabolites in serum are tightly bound to an alpha globulin called vitamin D–binding protein (DBP). Patients with the nephrotic syndrome may lose substantial amounts of DBP into their urine and consequently have very low circulating levels of the vitamin D metabolites. Although the total concentration of all the vitamin D metabolites is reduced in this situation, the free (or unbound) concentration may be normal. Thus, the measurement of the total concentration may be misleading as to the severity of the vitamin D deficiency. The incidence of osteomalacia in patients with the nephrotic syndrome is unknown; osteomalacia has only recently been recognized as a complication of this renal disease.

LIVER DISEASE

The hepatic production of 25-hydroxyvitamin D (25OHD) is not tightly controlled. Neither cholestatic nor parenchymal liver disease has much effect on 25OHD production. The low levels of circulating 25OHD found in patients with liver disease can usually be attributed to reduced hepatic synthesis of DBP, poor nutrition, or malabsorption rather than to failure by the liver to metabolize vitamin D. As in patients with the nephrotic syndrome, the low total concentrations of the vitamin D metabolites in patients with liver disease may reflect the low levels of DBP and not a true state of vitamin D deficiency.

ANTICONVULSANTS

Phenytoin and phenobarbital induce drug-metabolizing enzymes in the liver that alter the hepatic metabolism of vitamin D. This effect may account for the lower circulating levels of 25OHD found in patients treated with anticonvulsants. Surprisingly, these drugs do not lead to a reduction in $1,25(OH)_2D$ levels. Chronic anticonvulsant therapy does not seem to lead to clinically significant osteomalacia unless accompanied by other predisposing factors, such as inadequate sunlight exposure or poor nutrition. However, some authorities have raised the possibility that phenytoin may exert a direct inhibitory effect on bone formation. Treatment is generally not required unless serum 25OHD levels are low, in which case modest vitamin D supplementation (400 to 2000 IU per day) may be advised.

HYPOPARATHYROIDISM

Parathyroid hormone is a major stimulator of $1,25(OH)_2D$ production. One would expect osteomalacia to develop when the hormone is absent, because of the reduction in $1,25(OH)_2D$ production. However, osteomalacia appears to be a rare complication of hypoparathyroidism.

VITAMIN D–DEPENDENT RICKETS TYPE I

Vitamin D–dependent rickets type I, or pseudo–vitamin D deficiency, is a rare autosomal recessive disease in which there is a low level of $1,25(OH)_2D$ resulting from a selective deficiency in the renal production of $1,25(OH)_2D$. Although affected patients do not respond to doses of vitamin D that are adequate to treat vitamin D deficiency (i.e., 400 to 4000 IU per day), they do respond to moderate doses (4000 to 40,000 IU per day) of vitamin D or physiologic doses (0.5 to 1.0 μg per day) of $1,25(OH)_2D$.

VITAMIN D–DEPENDENT RICKETS TYPE II

Vitamin D–dependent rickets type II (hereditary $1,25(OH)_2D$–resistant rickets) is a rare condition that occurs in childhood and is not responsive to even huge doses of vitamin D. Many children also present with alopecia. Unlike patients with vitamin D–dependent rickets type I (see above), children with type II disease have high circulating levels of $1,25(OH)_2D$. Their problem involves an abnormality in the number, affinity, or functions of the intracellular $1,25(OH)_2D$ receptor. Recently, the gene for the vitamin D receptor from several affected families has been sequenced, and point mutations in the zinc fingers of the DNA binding domain or in the steroid binding domain (resulting in a premature termination codon) have been identified. Just as the genetic defect in this syndrome varies from family to family, so, too, does the clinical response to $1,25(OH)_2D_3$ (calcitriol), which is generally used in large doses (2 to 6 μg per day).

PHOSPHATE DEFICIENCY

Chronic hypophosphatemia may lead to rickets or osteomalacia independently of other predisposing abnormalities. The principal diseases in which hypophosphatemia is associated with osteomalacia or rickets, however, also include other abnormalities that can interfere with bone mineralization. Chronic phosphate depletion is caused by decreased intestinal absorption or increased renal clearance. Acute hypophosphatemia can result from movement of phosphate into cells (e.g., after infusion of insulin and glucose), but this condition is transient and does not result in bone disease (see Ch. 194).

Seventy to 90 per cent of dietary phosphate is absorbed, primarily in the jejunum. This process is not tightly regulated, although vitamin D, at least in animal models, stimulates phosphate absorption. Meat and dairy products are the principal dietary sources of phosphate, and vegetarian diets that exclude them can cause phosphate deficiency. The incidence of osteomalacia in vegetarians who avoid all meat and dairy products is unknown, but its occurrence has been reported. Since these dietary practices also lead to decreased vitamin D intake, such individuals may be predisposed to bone disease.

Intrinsic small bowel disease and surgical rearrangement of the small bowel interfere with phosphate absorption and, if coupled with diarrhea or steatorrhea, can result in phosphate depletion. The hypophosphatemia may contribute to the osteomalacia seen in such patients, especially when vitamin D levels are reduced.

Eighty-five to 90 per cent of the phosphate filtered by the glomerulus is reabsorbed, primarily in the proximal tubule. This process is regulated by PTH, which reduces renal tubular phosphate reabsorption, and probably also by vitamin D, which appears to increase renal tubular phosphate reabsorption. Many diseases that affect renal handling of phosphate are associated with osteomalacia.

Treatment of phosphate deficiency is generally geared to correction of the primary problem. Oral preparations of phosphate (and the amounts required to provide 1 gram of elemental phosphorus) include Fleet Phospho-Soda (6.12 ml), Neutra-Phos (300 ml), and Phos-Tab (6 tablets). These preparations are usually given in amounts that provide 1 to 3 grams of phosphorus, although diarrhea may limit the dose. Careful attention to both serum calcium and serum phosphate concentrations is required to avoid hypocalcemia or ectopic calcification (should the calcium-phosphate product become too high).

ALUMINUM HYDROXIDE ANTACIDS

A number of widely used antacids (e.g., Mylanta, Maalox, Basaljel, and Amphojel) contain aluminum hydroxide, which binds phosphate and prevents its absorption. Patients who ingest large amounts of these antacids may become depleted in phosphate. This mechanism may contribute to the severity of the osteomalacia observed in patients with chronic renal failure and in those who have undergone partial gastrectomy but who continue to ingest large quantities of antacids (see Ch. 237).

DE TONI-DEBRÉ-FANCONI SYNDROME

The de Toni-Debré-Fanconi syndrome includes a heterogeneous group of disorders characterized by phosphaturia, aminoaciduria, glycosuria, and bicarbonaturia, and frequently mild acidosis and hypercalciuria. In general, the osteomalacia or rickets associated with these proximal tubular disorders responds only to large doses of vitamin D, with correction of the acidosis and hypophosphatemia as needed. The associated bone disease is most likely the result of a combination of systemic acidosis, hypophosphatemia, and abnormal vitamin D metabolism.

X-LINKED HYPOPHOSPHATEMIA

X-linked hypophosphatemia (vitamin D–resistant rickets, or VDRR) is characterized by renal phosphate wasting, hypophosphatemia, and a subtle decrease in $1,25(OH)_2D$ production. Children often present with florid rickets. Although most cases are diagnosed in childhood and have an X-linked dominant form of inheritance, sporadic adult cases and autosomal transmission occur. Most patients have $1,25(OH)_2D$ levels that are inappropriately low for the degree of hypophosphatemia, which ordinarily increases $1,25(OH)_2D$ production. Treatment with oral phosphate and vitamin D suppresses $1,25(OH)_2D$ to even lower levels. The primary abnormality in these patients is thought to be a defect in renal tubular phosphate transport, resulting in renal phosphate wasting. This defect may secondarily alter vitamin D metabolism. X-linked hypophosphatemia is a fairly common form of metabolic bone disease that should be suspected in all individuals who have low levels of serum phosphorus and evidence of bone disease.

The bone disease in patients with X-linked hypophosphatemia responds to the combination of phosphate (1 to 3 grams per day) and either large doses (25,000 to 100,000 IU) of vitamin D or more physiologic doses (0.25 to 1.0 μg per day) of $1,25(OH)_2D$. Neither phosphate nor vitamin D alone is as effective. Unfortunately, oral phosphate preparations also act as laxatives, and tolerance of full doses is sometimes difficult to achieve. A recently recognized complication of such treatment is the development of hyperparathyroidism later in life, thought to be phosphate induced.

TUMOR-INDUCED HYPOPHOSPHATEMIC OSTEOMALACIA

Certain unusual tumors (usually mesenchymal) produce osteomalacia associated with low serum levels of phosphorus and $1,25(OH)_2D$ and increased phosphaturia. The cause of this syndrome is unknown, but it is presumed that a humoral product of the tumor suppresses both $1,25(OH)_2D$ production and phosphate reabsorption in the kidney. Removal of the tumor reverses the abnormalities.

CHRONIC METABOLIC ACIDOSIS

Acute metabolic acidosis results in reduced $1,25(OH)_2D$ production. Although chronic metabolic acidosis is associated with osteomalacia, especially when accompanied by renal loss of phosphate and bicarbonate (as in proximal renal tubular acidosis), it is unclear whether chronic metabolic acidosis has a direct effect on the renal metabolism of vitamin D. Bicarbonate therapy alone is effective in treating the osteomalacia associated with renal tubular acidosis and ureterosigmoidostomy, although the addition of 0.25 to 1 mg of vitamin D per day may facilitate healing.

CALCIUM DEFICIENCY

Calcium deficiency may contribute to the mineralization defect that complicates gastrointestinal disease and proximal tubular disorders, but it is less well established as a cause of osteomalacia than is vitamin D or phosphate deficiency. In one carefully performed study of children who ingested a low-calcium diet, there was clinical, biochemical, and histologic evidence of osteomalacia. The serum phosphorus and 25OHD levels were normal, the serum alkaline phosphatase level was elevated, and the serum and urine calcium levels were low. Since intestinal absorption of calcium decreases with age, the daily requirement for calcium increases from approximately 800 mg in young adults to 1400 mg in the elderly. Calcium deficiency can result not only from inadequate dietary intake but also from excessive fecal and urinary losses. Except in cases in which a renal leak of calcium plays an important role in the etiology of calcium deficiency (certain forms of idiopathic hypercalciuria or following glucorticoid therapy for inflammatory diseases), urinary calcium excretion provides a useful means to determine the appropriate level of oral calcium replacement. Because of its low cost and high percentage of elemental calcium, calcium carbonate is the formulation of choice.

PRIMARY DISORDERS OF THE BONE MATRIX

Intrinsic disorders of bone in which matrix is produced but not normally mineralized are rare. Three diseases appear to fit this category, but none is well understood.

Hypophosphatasia

Hypophosphatasia, transmitted in an autosomal recessive pattern, usually manifests as a severe form of rickets in children, or merely as a predisposition to fractures in adults. The biochemical hallmarks are low serum (and tissue) levels of alkaline phosphatase and increased urinary levels of phosphocthanolamine. The reason these patients develop osteomalacia or rickets is unclear, but the following mechanism has been suggested. Skeletal alkaline phosphatase cleaves pyrophosphate, an inhibitor of bone mineralization; patients deficient in alkaline phosphatase may be unable to hydrolyze this inhibitor and so develop a mineralization defect.

Fibrogenesis Imperfecta Ossium

Fibrogenesis imperfecta ossium is a rare, painful disorder that affects middle-aged men in what appears to be a sporadic fashion. Serum alkaline phosphatase activity is increased. The bones have a dense, amorphous, mottled appearance radiologically and a disorganized arrangement of collagen with decreased birefringence histologically. Presumably, the disorganized collagen matrix retards normal bone mineralization.

Axial Osteomalacia

Unlike fibrogenesis imperfecta ossium, axial osteomalacia is not painful, involves only the axial skeleton, shows no disorganization of collagen on bone biopsy, and is not associated with increased serum alkaline phosphatase activity. The reason for the mineralization disorder in this rare disease is uncertain.

INHIBITORS OF MINERALIZATION

Several drugs are known to cause osteomalacia or rickets by inhibiting mineralization, but in no case is the mechanism fully understood.

Aluminum

Patients on hemodialysis are exposed to aluminum in the dialysate if tap water is used and through the antacid preparations used to control serum phosphorus levels. Most develop bone disease. Bone biopsies show a correlation between the extent of osteomalacia in these patients and the amount of aluminum deposited in bone. It is likely that the aluminum blocks normal mineralization. Severely affected patients respond to a reduction in their exposure to or body stores of the metal.

Many patients who are treated by total parenteral nutrition for extended periods develop bone disease characterized by osteomalacia. In some cases the aluminum content of the casein hydrolysate used to provide amino acids is high. Replacement of casein hydrolysate with purified amino acids may correct or prevent this complication.

Etidronate

Etidronate, the only diphosphonate available for clinical use in the United States, produces osteomalacia at doses greater than 5 to 10 mg per kilogram of body weight. Therefore, the dose must be limited. Etidronate affects osteoblast function and inhibits calcium phosphate crystallization. It is unclear why this drug and not other diphosphonates results in osteomalacia.

Phenytoin

As discussed previously (see Anticonvulsants), phenytoin therapy may cause osteomalacia by inducing enzymes that alter the hepatic metabolism of vitamin D. In addition, phenytoin directly and adversely affects bone mineral metabolism in animals. This effect may also contribute to bone disease.

Fluoride

Fluoride stimulates bone formation, but if it is administered in high doses without adequate calcium supplementation, the bone is poorly mineralized. The mechanism (or mechanisms) by which fluoride alters osteoblast function and bone mineralization is unknown.

Bikle DD: Calcium absorption and vitamin D metabolism. Clin Gastroenterol 12:379, 1983. *A review of the effect of vitamin D on the intestine and the gastrointestinal diseases that lead to osteomalacia.*

Bikle DD, Halloran BP, Gee E, et al.: Free 25-hydroxyvitamin D levels are normal in subjects with liver disease and reduced total 25-hydroxyvitamin D levels. J Clin Invest 78:748, 1986. *This article points out that total vitamin D metabolite concentrations may be reduced in patients with reduced DBP levels without a reduction in the free (and, possibly, the more physiologically relevant) vitamin D metabolite concentrations.*

Brenner RJ, Spring DB, Sebastion A, et al.: Incidence of radiologically evident bone disease, nephrocalcinosis, and nephrolithiasis in various types of renal tubular acidosis. N Engl J Med 307:217, 1982. *The authors point out that bone disease (osteomalacia) is much more common in proximal renal tubular acidosis than in distal renal tubular acidosis.*

Chesney RW, Mazess RB, Rose P, et al.: Long-term influence of calcitriol (1,25-dihydroxyvitamin D) and supplemental phosphate in X-linked hypophosphatemic rickets. Pediatrics 71:559, 1983. *This article discusses the modern therapy for this disease.*

Colussi G, de Ferrari ME, Surian M, et al.: Vitamin D metabolites and osteomalacia in the human Fanconi syndrome. Proc Eur Dial Transplant Assoc 21:756, 1984. *Five patients were evaluated; three had bone disease and low 1,25(OH)₂D levels.*

Curtis JA, Kooh SW, Fraser D, et al.: Nutritional rickets in vegetarian children. Can Med Assoc J 128:150, 1983. *Nutritional vitamin D deficiency continues to be a problem in those who omit milk and dairy products from their diet.*

Dibble JB, Sheridan P, Losowsky MS: A survey of vitamin D deficiency in gastrointestinal and liver disorders. Q J Med 209:119, 1984. *This article reports the results of a survey of 152 patients with gastrointestinal disease and 104 patients with chronic liver disease in whom 25OHD levels were assessed. Low levels of 25OHD were found in many patients, but osteomalacia was detected almost exclusively in patients with 25OHD levels below 2 per milliliter.*

Goldstein DA, Haldimann B, Sherman D, et al.: Vitamin D metabolites and calcium metabolism in patients with nephrotic syndrome and normal renal function. J Clin Endocrinol Metab 52:116, 1981. *This article describes the pathogenesis of osteomalacia in the nephrotic syndrome.*

Hahn TJ, Hendin BA, Scharp CR, et al.: Serum 25 hydroxycalciferol levels and bone mass in children on chronic anticonvulsant therapy. N Engl J Med 292:550, 1975. *The demonstration that chronic anticonvulsant therapy can lead to reduced 25OHD levels and bone mass in children. Vitamin D supplementation increased 25OHD levels.*

Hodsman AB, Iherrard DJ, Wong EGC, et al.: Vitamin D resistant osteomalacia in hemodialysis patients lacking secondary hyperparathyroidism. Ann Intern Med 94:629, 1981. *An early but thorough clinical description of patients with aluminum-associated osteomalacia occurring during hemodialysis.*

Mankin HJ: Rickets, osteomalacia, and renal osteodystrophy. Parts I and II. Am Bone Joint Surg 56A:101, 352, 1974. *A thorough review with an accounting of the history of the subject, a description of the clinical presentation of rickets, and a complete list of the etiologies of bone mineralization disorders.*

Marel GM, McKenna MJ, Frame B: Osteomalacia. Bone Mineral Res 4:335, 1986. *This is an excellent, complete, and up-to-date review of the subject.*

Marie PJ, Pettifor JM, Ross FP, et al.: Histological osteomalacia due to dietary calcium deficiency in children. N Engl J Med 307:584, 1982. *This study indicates that calcium deficiency alone may be sufficient to cause osteomalacia.*

Parfitt AM, Gallagher JC, Heaney RP, et al.: Vitamin D and bone health in the elderly. Am J Clin Nutr 36:1014, 1982. *A review of the importance of adequate vitamin D intake in adults, discussing, among other issues, the high incidence of osteomalacia found in patients with hip fractures.*

Ritchie HH, Hughes MR, Thompson ET, et al.: An ochre mutation in the vitamin D receptor gene causes hereditary 1,25-dihydroxy vitamin D₃-resistant rickets in three families. Proc Natl Acad Sci USA 86:9783, 1989. *Describes a point mutation leading to a premature termination codon in the steroid binding domain. This same group demonstrated other point mutations in the DNA binding domain of the receptor gene from other families with this syndrome.*

Voights AL, Felsenfeld AJ, Flach F: The effects of calciferol and its metabolites on patients with chronic renal failure. Arch Intern Med 143:960, 1205, 1983. *In this two-part review, the authors evaluate the data concerning the most appropriate vitamin D metabolite (or analogue) to use in the treatment of the various types of renal osteodystrophy.*

Weider N, Cruz DS: Phosphaturic mesenchymal tumors: A polymorphous group causing osteomalacia or rickets. Cancer 59:1442, 1987. *An excellent review of 17 cases of this syndrome of reversible bone disease caused by tumors.*

235 The Parathyroid Glands, Hypercalcemia, and Hypocalcemia

Allen M. Spiegel

THE PARATHYROID GLANDS

EMBRYOLOGY AND ANATOMY. Normally, there are four parathyroids, averaging 120 mg in total weight, but as many as 5 per cent of normal individuals may have more than four glands. The superior parathyroids are derived from the fourth (more caudal) branchial pouches and remain almost stationary during embryologic development. Their typical final location is near the upper poles of the thyroid. Aberrant locations include the tracheoesophageal groove and the retroesophageal space. The inferior parathyroids develop (in association with the thymus) from the third branchial pouches. During normal development, they migrate caudally, assuming a final position near the lower poles of the thyroid. The inferior parathyroids may fail to descend, remaining near the angle of the jaw, or, at the other extreme, may descend into the anterior mediastinum in association with the thymus.

SYNTHESIS AND SECRETION OF PARATHYROID HORMONE (PTH). Parathyroid hormone, together with vitamin D (Ch. 233), is the principal regulator of ionized calcium in extracellular fluid. Parathyroid hormone is synthesized in the parathyroid glands as "preproparathyroid hormone," a precursor composed of 115 amino acids. A hydrophobic "leader" peptide of 25 amino acids is first cleaved from the amino-terminus to yield the prohormone, followed by cleavage of a basic, amino-terminal hexapeptide to yield the mature 84-amino-acid hormone. The latter is the principal secreted form of the hormone. There is no evidence for secretion of either the preprohormone or the prohormone. The prohormone possesses less than 0.2 per cent of the biologic activity of the native, 84-amino-acid hormone. The full biologic activity of the intact hormone resides within the amino-terminal 1–34 fragment, whereas fragments from the midregion and carboxy-terminal regions lack biologic activity (Fig. 235–1).

Secretion of PTH is regulated primarily by the concentration of ionized calcium in the extracellular fluid. Normally, PTH secretion is regulated at a "setpoint" that maintains serum ionized calcium within a relatively narrow range. Deviations below the setpoint stimulate, and deviations above the setpoint inhibit, hormone secretion. Effects of calcium on hormone secretion occur acutely (within minutes); low calcium levels have a slower stimulatory action on hormone synthesis. At high calcium concentrations, there is evidence for intracellular degradation of synthesized hormone and possible release of biologically inactive fragments. High magnesium ion concentrations in extracellular fluid, like high calcium concentrations, inhibit PTH secretion, but hypomagnesemia, unlike hypocalcemia, may inhibit hormone

FIGURE 235–1. Secretion, metabolism, and clearance of parathyroid hormone. *Top,* Parathyroid hormone (PTH) is synthesized as a preprohormone and undergoes successive cleavages within the parathyroid to the mature (1–84), major secreted form of the hormone. Under certain conditions (e.g., hypercalcemia), some of the hormone is cleaved intracellularly into biologically inactive, carboxy-terminal fragments, which are also secreted. *Middle,* The major circulating forms of the hormone are the intact 1–84 species (the shaded region corresponds to the amino-terminal 1–34 portion possessing full biologic activity) and biologically inactive carboxy-terminal fragments. The presence of amino-terminal fragments in the circulation is unclear (indicated by "?"). *Bottom,* Peripheral metabolism of the hormone occurs in liver and kidney. The kidney also clears intact hormone and carboxy-terminal fragments from the circulation. (From Endres DE, Villanueva R, Sharp CF Jr, et al.: Measurement of parathyroid hormone. Endocrinol Metab Clin North Am 18:611, 1989.)

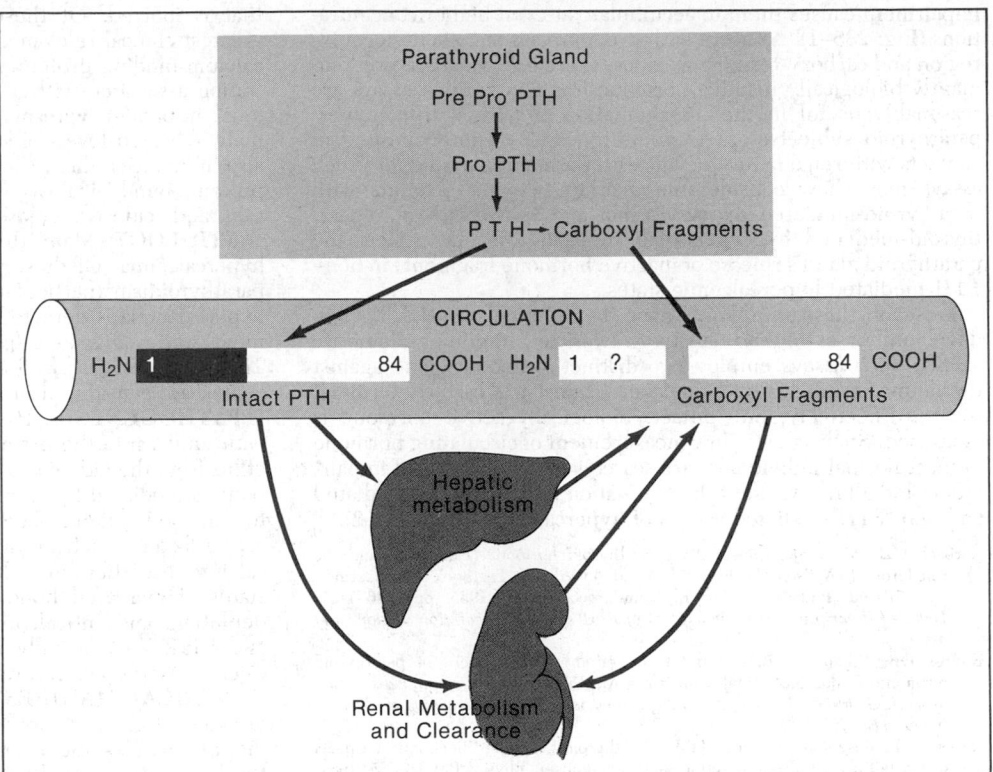

secretion and action. The active metabolite of vitamin D, $1,25(OH)_2D$ (dihydroxycholecalciferol), suppresses both secretion and synthesis of PTH. Reduction in $1,25(OH)_2D$ is a major factor contributing to increased PTH secretion in renal failure.

FORMS OF PARATHYROID HORMONE IN PLASMA. Parathyroid hormone circulates in plasma as the intact hormone secreted from the gland and as fragments derived either from glandular secretion (particularly in hypercalcemic states) or from peripheral metabolism of the intact hormone. Most, if not all, of these fragments lack biologic activity but may, depending on antibody specificity, contribute to immunoreactivity in plasma (Fig. 235–1).

PARATHYROID HORMONE ACTION. Parathyroid hormone acts directly on kidney and bone, and indirectly on the gut, to maintain the normal concentration of serum ionized calcium (see Ch. 232 for a complete discussion of mineral homeostasis). In the kidney, PTH (1) enhances reabsorption of calcium, and also magnesium, from the glomerular filtrate; (2) increases excretion of phosphate and of bicarbonate; (3) activates the enzyme (1-α-hydroxylase) that forms the active metabolite, $1,25(OH)_2D$, of vitamin D. In bone, PTH causes the release of calcium and phosphate into the extracellular fluid. The hormone acts directly on osteoblasts, which secondarily affect osteoclast activity. The hypercalcemic action on bone and the anticalciuric action on kidney combine to raise the serum calcium level. The phosphatemic action on bone would tend to blunt the hypercalcemic effect of the hormone owing to formation of calcium phosphate complexes, but the phosphaturic action counteracts the tendency to hyperphosphatemia. Stimulation of $1,25(OH)_2D$ formation promotes enhanced intestinal absorption of calcium, which also serves to maintain a normal serum calcium level (see Ch. 233). The clinical consequences of PTH excess (or in the opposite directions, hormone deficiency) follow directly from the actions of the hormone: (1) hypercalcemia; (2) a tendency to hypophosphatemia; (3) a tendency to reduced serum bicarbonate levels and hyperchloremia; (4) increased serum levels of $1,25(OH)_2D$; and (5) relative reduction in urinary calcium excretion and increase in urinary phosphate excretion for a given filtered load.

MECHANISM OF PARATHYROID HORMONE ACTION. The first step in PTH action is binding to specific plasma membrane–bound receptors on target cells in bone and kidney. Such receptors are coupled to guanosine triphosphate (GTP)–binding proteins—in particular, the Gs protein that links receptors to stimulation of adenylyl cyclase (for a more general description of the mechanism of polypeptide hormone action, see Ch. 208). Adenylyl cyclase catalyzes the formation of the "second messenger," cyclic adenosine monophosphate (AMP), which mediates hormone action by stimulating the phosphorylation of critical intracellular proteins. A clinically useful peculiarity of PTH action on proximal renal tubular cells is that not only are cyclic AMP levels increased intracellularly but, because of overflow into the extracellular fluid, urinary cyclic AMP excretion is also increased. "Second messengers" other than cyclic AMP may also mediate certain actions of PTH.

ASSAY OF PARATHYROID HORMONE IN PLASMA. Normally, the concentration of biologically active PTH circulating in plasma is quite low (<50 pg per milliliter). Bioassays sensitive enough to detect such low levels include a renal cytochemical assay and several assays based on stimulation of cyclic AMP formation in bone or kidney cells. Unfortunately, such assays are too cumbersome for routine clinical use. Total urinary cyclic AMP excretion (normalized to creatinine clearance by simultaneous measurement of serum and urinary creatinine) is an easily measured and sensitive index of circulating PTH bioactivity. It is elevated in primary hyperparathyroidism, is low in hypoparathyroidism, and falls within 1 hour of successful parathyroidectomy in patients with hyperparathyroidism. Increased urinary cyclic AMP excretion, however, is not absolutely specific for PTH hypersecretion; parathyroid hormone–related peptide, secreted by many malignancies, similarly increases urinary cyclic AMP excretion, and this must be taken into account in the interpretation of urinary cyclic AMP measurements in subjects with hypercalcemia (see Hypercalcemia Associated with Malignancy, below).

Radioimmunoassays are sufficiently sensitive and practial for the routine measurement of circulating PTH. Interpretation of assay results requires an understanding of what a particular antiserum is measuring. Immunoreactivity need not correlate with biologic activity. Indeed, the bulk of circulating PTH consists of biologically inactive mid-region and carboxy-terminal fragments. Since such fragments are cleared by the kidney, renal impairment causes them to accumulate at even higher concentrations (Fig. 235–1). Antisera with predominant specificity for mid-region and carboxy-terminal regions, therefore, measure predominantly biologically inactive hormone fragments. Such assays are reasonably useful in the discrimination of normal from hyperparathyroid subjects, but their utility is much more limited in subjects with renal failure. Even with normal renal function, such assays may show considerable overlap between patients with parathyroid-mediated hypercalcemia and those with non–parathyroid-mediated hypercalcemia. In part, this may reflect the parathyroid gland's release of inactive hormone fragments in non–PTH-mediated hypercalcemic states.

Most of these problems have been circumvented by the development of highly sensitive "two-site" immunoradiometric assays. Such assays employ two distinct antibodies, one against the amino-terminal region and one against the carboxy-terminal region. Effectively, only intact, biologically active hormone is measured. Such assays allow measurement of circulating hormone in most normal individuals, are scarcely affected by renal impairment, and allow excellent discrimination between PTH-mediated and non–PTH-mediated causes of hypercalcemia (Fig. 235–2).

Aurbach GD, Marx SJ, Spiegel AM: Parathyroid hormone, calcitonin, and the calciferols. *In* Wilson JD, Foster DW (eds.): Williams Textbook of Endocrinology. 7th ed. Philadelphia, W.B. Saunders Company, 1985, pp 1146–1157. *Detailed description of basic aspects of PTH synthesis, secretion, action, and assay.*

Endres DB, Villanueva R, Sharp CF Jr, et al.: Measurement of parathyroid hormone. Endocrinol Metab Clin North Am 18:611, 1989. *Complete discussion of methods for PTH assay, including comparison of two-site versus mid-region immunoassays.*

Habener JF, Rosenblatt M, Potts JT Jr: Parathyroid hormone: Biochemical aspects of biosynthesis, secretion, action, and metabolism. Physiol Rev 64:985, 1984. *Extensive review of basic aspects of PTH synthesis and action, together with relevant clinical implications.*

Nussbaum SR, Zahradnik RJ, Lavigne RJ, et al.: A highly sensitive two site immunoradiometric assay of parathyrin (PTH) and its clinical utility in evaluating patients with hypercalcemia. Clin Chem 33:1364, 1987. *Description of prototype of most clinically useful assay for PTH.*

HYPERCALCEMIA

DEFINITION. Hypercalcemia is defined as an abnormal elevation in serum ionized calcium concentration.* Since total,

---

*See Ch. 232 and Part XXVII for calcium and phosphorus reference range values in serum and urine.

rather than ionized, calcium is generally measured, one must be aware of factors that influence the fraction of total serum calcium that is ionized. Of these, serum albumin concentration is of greatest clinical relevance, since albumin is the chief circulating calcium-binding protein. "Normal" total serum calcium concentration associated with a significant reduction in serum albumin (e.g., in patients with malignancy) may actually represent abnormally elevated levels of serum ionized calcium. Acid-base status also influences the proportion of total serum calcium that is protein bound (alkalosis decreases the ionized calcium concentration, and acidosis increases it).

ETIOLOGY. Many different diseases are potential causes of hypercalcemia. Of these, the most common are primary hyperparathyroidism (particularly in asymptomatic individuals whose hypercalcemia is detected by routine serum chemistry measurement) and malignancy (particularly in hospitalized individuals). These disorders, as well as some of the rarer causes of hypercalcemia, are considered in separate sections below.

PATHOGENESIS. Hypercalcemia results from excessive calcium influx into the extracellular fluid from bone and decreased efflux from the kidneys into the urine. Calcium mobilization from bone is mediated by activators of bone resorption. These activators include systemic factors (e.g., PTH, $1,25(OH)_2D$) and locally acting factors, such as various lymphokines. Reduction in renal calcium excretion may lead to hypercalcemia, particularly in states of increased bone turnover. Renal impairment, volume depletion, and anticalciuretic agents, such as thiazide diuretics and PTH, are clinically relevant factors that can reduce renal calcium excretion and provoke hypercalcemia.

CLINICAL MANIFESTATIONS. Many of the manifestations of hypercalcemia are not specific to the underlying cause (specific disease manifestations are discussed under individual disease headings). Extreme hypercalcemia leads to coma and death. Neurologic manifestations in less severe cases may include confusion, lethargy, weakness, and hyporeflexia. Hypercalcemia may be detected by shortening of the QT interval on the electrocardiogram. Arrhythmias are rare, but bradycardia and first-degree heart block have been reported. Acute hypercalcemia may be associated with significant hypertension. Gastrointestinal manifestations include constipation and anorexia; in severe cases, there may be nausea and vomiting. Acute pancreatitis has been reported in association with hypercalcemia of various causes. Hypercalcemia interferes with antidiuretic hormone action, thereby leading to polyuria and polydipsia. Reversible reduction in renal function associated with significant hypercalcemia is

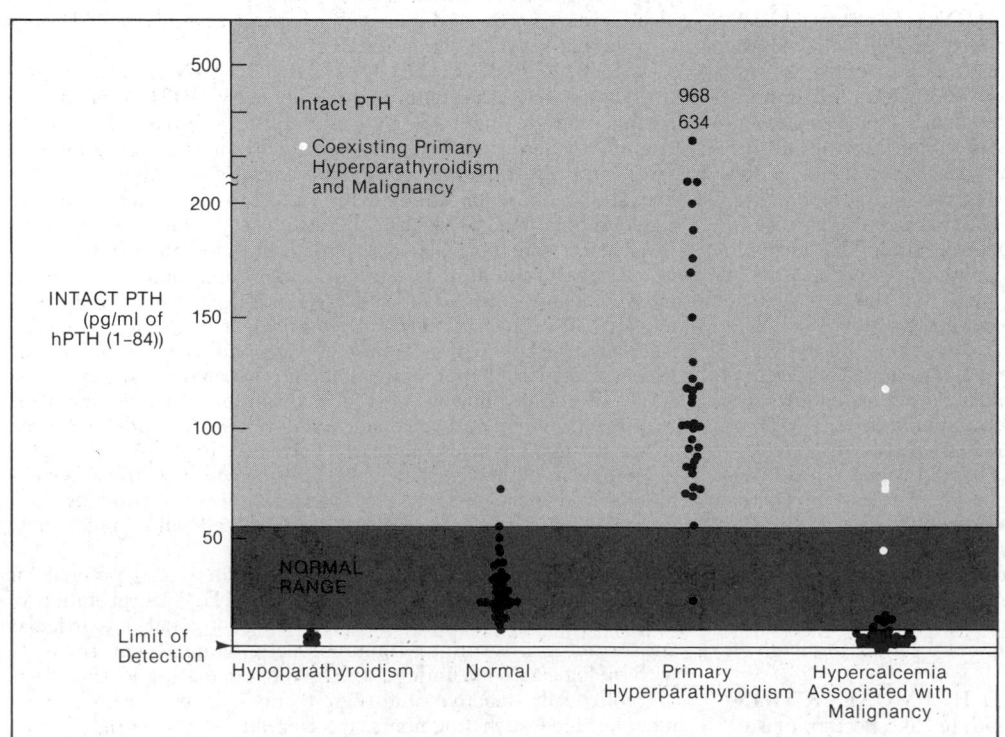

FIGURE 235–2. Two-site immunoassay for PTH in serum. The two-site method measures exclusively intact PTH. The hormone is detectable in the majority of normal subjects and undetectable in patients with various forms of hypoparathyroidism. Almost all patients with primary hyperparathyroidism show values outside the normal range. In contrast, values are low to undetectable in patients with malignancy-associated hypercalcemia, except for four individuals with coexistent primary hyperparathyroidism. (From Endres DB, Villanueva R, Sharp CF Jr, et al.: Measurement of parathyroid hormone. Endocrinol Metab Clin North Am 18:611, 1989.)

TABLE 235–1. CAUSES OF HYPERCALCEMIA

Parathyroid Hormone–Mediated Causes
  Primary hyperparathyroidism
    Sporadic, familial (multiple endocrine neoplasia types I and II)
  Familial hypocalciuric hypercalcemia*
  Ectopic secretion of parathyroid hormone by tumors (very rare)
Non–Parathyroid Hormone–Mediated Causes
  Malignancy associated
    Local osteolytic hypercalcemia
    Humoral hypercalcemia of malignancy
  Vitamin D mediated
    Vitamin D intoxication
    Excessive production of 1,25(OH)$_2$D in granulomatous disorders
  Other endocrinopathies
    Thyrotoxicosis
    Hypoadrenalism
Immobilization with increased bone turnover, e.g., Paget's disease
Acute renal failure with rhabdomyolysis
Calcium carbonate ingestion (milk-alkali syndrome)

*Parathyroid hormone secretion is necessary for hypercalcemia but is not the primary defect.

followed by more permanent damage if hypercalcemia persists. Particularly if serum phosphorus is also increased, hypercalcemia can lead to nephrocalcinosis and interstitial nephritis. Hypercalciuria and nephrolithiasis may also occur. Deposition of calcium in other soft tissues, including skin and cornea, is most likely to occur in patients with associated hyperphosphatemia.

DIFFERENTIAL DIAGNOSIS. Potential causes of hypercalcemia are listed in Table 235–1. These may be divided into PTH-mediated (primary hyperparathyroidism) and non–PTH-mediated diseases (all others). Although ectopic secretion of PTH by tumors was long considered a potential cause of PTH-mediated hypercalcemia, there is now general agreement that ectopic secretion of authentic PTH (as opposed to parathyroid hormone–related peptides; see below) by tumors is extremely rare. The first step in the differential diagnosis of hypercalcemia is to establish whether or not PTH hypersecretion is present, since subsequent diagnostic maneuvers and definitive therapy critically depend on this distinction.

Readily measured blood and urine chemistries may offer some clues to diagnosis. In theory, PTH hypersecretion should be reflected by hypophosphatemia, hyperchloremia, hypobicarbonatemia, increased urinary phosphate excretion, and urinary calcium excretion that is relatively low for the filtered load. Suppression of PTH secretion by hypercalcemia of non-parathyroid etiology should, in theory, change these parameters to the opposite direction. In practice, there is often considerable overlap in each of these parameters between patients with parathyroid-mediated forms of hypercalcemia and those with non–parathyroid–mediated forms. This situation may reflect confounding variables, such as vomiting, diuretic treatment, and renal failure, as well as the ability of certain hypercalcemic agents to mimic many actions of PTH. Most important in this respect is parathyroid hormone–related peptide, first isolated from tumors associated with the syndrome of humoral hypercalcemia. This peptide mimics all of the known actions of PTH on kidney and bone, including increasing urinary cyclic AMP excretion and stimulating renal formation of 1,25(OH)$_2$D. Decreased urinary cyclic AMP excretion (with normal renal function) strongly suggests non–PTH-mediated hypercalcemia, but increased urinary cyclic AMP excretion is compatible with both primary hyperparathyroidism and tumor secretion of parathyroid hormone–related peptide. Serum 1,25(OH)$_2$D concentration also does not allow definitive diagnosis. It may be elevated in primary hyperparathyroidism and vitamin D–related causes of hypercalcemia and may be reduced in other non–parathyroid-mediated causes of hypercalcemia. For reasons that are not entirely clear, the serum 1,25(OH)$_2$D level is often low in patients with malignancies secreting parathyroid hormone–related peptide, despite the ability of the peptide to stimulate 1,25(OH)$_2$D formation.

Definitive distinction between parathyroid- and non–parathyroid-mediated causes of hypercalcemia relies primarily on PTH immunoassay. As discussed earlier, this distinction is best made with the two-site type of assay that measures intact PTH and is unaffected by renal function (Fig. 235–2). An elevated PTH level

secures the diagnosis of primary hyperparathyroidism. In selected cases with coexistent malignancy, the unlikely possibility of ectopic PTH secretion may be excluded by selective venous sampling and assay of PTH, but generally this testing is unnecessary. Hormone levels in the normal range suggest the possibility of familial hypocalciuric hypercalcemia. This entity is discussed further in the section on hyperparathyroidism. Low to undetectable values for PTH place the patient in the non–parathyroid-mediated category. Additional testing is necessary to establish a specific diagnosis within this group. Immunoassays for parathyroid hormone–related peptide have been developed, and these may allow the diagnosis of hypercalcemia caused by tumor secretion of this agent. Complete clinical evaluation, including history (e.g., vitamin ingestion, chronicity of symptoms), physical examination (masses, lymphadenopathy), radiologic studies, and other blood tests (e.g., thyroid and adrenal function), may point to a diagnosis. The diagnostic approach to hypercalcemia is summarized in Table 235–2.

TREATMENT. The definitive treatment of hypercalcemia depends on the specific diagnosis and treatment of the underlying disease, e.g., parathyroidectomy for primary hyperparathyroidism, chemotherapy for a malignancy. The initial treatment of hypercalcemia can be instituted (and in acute hypercalcemic crisis, often *must* be instituted) without a specific diagnosis, but cumulative toxicity and loss of efficacy preclude long-term non-specific treatment. Measures aimed at reducing the serum calcium level act by increasing urinary calcium excretion and by decreasing bone resorption. General measures applicable to every patient include mobilization as soon as feasible (since immobility increases bone resorption) and hydration (since significant hypercalcemia causes dehydration). Volume depletion, by limiting renal calcium excretion, perpetuates a vicious circle that can lead to acute hypercalcemic crisis. Volume expansion with isotonic saline often significantly reduces the serum calcium level by enhancing renal calcium excretion. Only after volume repletion should diuretics be employed to enhance sodium and thereby calcium excretion. With a vigorous saline diuresis, calcium excretion in the range of 1 to 2 grams per day can be achieved as a temporary measure to reduce the serum calcium level. In patients with renal failure, dialysis can be employed almost as effectively to remove calcium from extracellular fluid. Careful monitoring of cardiac function and serum electrolytes is necessary with both saline diuresis and dialysis treatment.

Since increased bone resorption is the principal factor causing hypercalcemia in most patients, measures aimed at inhibiting bone resorption are generally most effective. Agents that inhibit osteoclast function (the "final common pathway" of bone resorption) are effective irrespective of the specific factor causing

TABLE 235–2. DIAGNOSTIC APPROACH TO HYPERCALCEMIA

1. Distinguish parathyroid hormone–mediated forms of hypercalcemia from non–parathyroid hormone–mediated forms: *Parathyroid hormone immunoassay (preferably two-site type) is the definitive test.*
2. If the parathyroid hormone level is elevated, primary hyperparathyroidism is the most likely diagnosis: *Family history for hypercalcemia should be checked to distinguish sporadic from familial (multiple endocrine neoplasia syndromes and hypocalciuric hypercalcemia) disease. Marginal elevation in parathyroid hormone levels, particularly in young, asymptomatic individuals, should prompt urine calcium measurement to exclude familial hypocalciuric hypercalcemia. In patients with coexisting malignancy, selective venous sampling can be done to exclude ectopic parathyroid hormone secretion, but the latter is extremely rare.*
3. If parathyroid hormone is low or undetectable, further laboratory tests (in addition to complete history, physical, and radiologic studies) are needed to distinguish among the various forms of non–parathyroid hormone–mediated forms of hypercalcemia: *Increased urinary cyclic AMP excretion suggests tumor secretion of parathyroid hormone–related peptide (direct radioimmunoassays for this peptide should shortly become widely available). Increased 1,25(OH)$_2$D suggests granulomatous disease (including some types of lymphoma).*

increased bone resorption. Available agents include calcitonin, plicamycin (mithramycin), and biphosphonates (diphosphonates). Calcitonin should theoretically be the ideal agent, given its low toxicity and specific action in inhibiting osteoclast function. In practice, the effectiveness of calcitonin is often limited and transient. Dosages of up to 32 MRC units per kilogram per day have been given by intravenous infusion. Plicamycin, in doses of 25 μg per kilogram as an intravenous bolus, is generally quite effective in lowering the serum calcium level within 24 to 48 hours. Depending on the underlying process, the effect may last for several days. Unfortunately, repeated treatment causes cumulative liver and renal toxicity, as well as thrombocytopenia. Biphosphonates, effective both orally and parenterally, have been used extensively in Europe but are not available in the United States. Only etidronate is available here, and it must be given intravenously in dosages of 7.5 mg per kilogram per day to treat hypercalcemia effectively.

Inorganic phosphate salts lower the serum calcium level when given intravenously but pose a serious danger of metastatic calcification in the hypercalcemic patient. Sudden hypotension, renal failure, and death have been reported after phosphate infusion treatment. Doses of up to 50 mmole (about 1.5 grams of elemental phosphorus) infused over 6 to 8 hours can be given if the serum calcium level must be lowered and all other measures fail. Oral phosphate is considerably safer. It is useful in patients with significant hypercalcemia who are awaiting definitive treatment and in whom one wishes to prevent development of hypercalcemic crisis. Dosages in the range of 2 grams of elemental phosphorus (10 grams of phosphate salts) per day in divided doses can be given. The serum phosphate level and renal function must be carefully monitored.

Glucocorticoids are highly effective in treating hypercalcemia caused by vitamin D–related mechanisms (vitamin D intoxication, overproduction of $1,25(OH)_2D$ in granulomatous disorders) and by certain malignancies (cytokine release associated with myeloma) but are ineffective in most other forms of hypercalcemia, including hyperparathyroidism and most malignancies. Forty to 100 mg per day of prednisone or the equivalent is the usual dose range. Indomethacin was reported to lower the serum calcium level in prostaglandin-mediated hypercalcemia but has proved generally ineffective. Novel agents under study that may become available in the future include gallium nitrate, shown to be effective in the hypercalcemia of malignancy, and WR-2721, reportedly effective in some cases of parathyroid carcinoma.

PRIMARY HYPERPARATHYROIDISM

DEFINITION. Primary hyperparathyroidism is a disorder in which hypercalcemia is due to hypersecretion of PTH.

ETIOLOGY. In most cases (about 85 per cent), hyperparathyroidism is caused by sporadic, solitary adenomas. Hyperplasia of all four glands occurs in about 10 per cent of cases, and these are most often familial, in the context of three distinct autosomal dominant inherited diseases: multiple endocrine neoplasia types I and II and familial hypocalciuric hypercalcemia. Carcinoma occurs rarely (<5 per cent of cases). The genes for multiple endocrine neoplasia types I and II have been linked to chromosomes 11 (q13) and 10, respectively. In no case has the etiology been clearly defined, but molecular genetic evidence indicates that almost all sporadic adenomas, as well as enlarged glands in multiple endocrine neoplasia type I, are monoclonal tumors. A high percentage of such tumors show loss of alleles at 11q13. This finding suggests that loss of a "tumor suppressor gene" from this locus may be instrumental in tumorigenesis. Epidemiologic evidence demonstrates a higher incidence of parathyroid tumors in subjects receiving neck irradiation in the past. Specific mutations associated with such tumors have not been defined. Finally, it has long been postulated that longstanding secondary hyperparathyroidism (e.g., in response to hypocalcemia of renal failure) may evolve into autonomous hypersecretion, "tertiary hyperparathyroidism." If such a transition occurs, its molecular basis has yet to be identified.

INCIDENCE. The incidence of hyperparathyroidism has increased substantially, largely as a result of routine blood calcium measurement. Age-adjusted incidence rates are between 25 and 50 per 100,000, based on recent surveys. A prevalence between 0.1 and 0.5 per cent has been estimated, with females affected about twice as commonly as males. The incidence rises sharply after age 40.

PATHOLOGY. Microscopic distinction between adenoma and hyperplasia is difficult, if not impossible. The distinction between single-gland and multigland disease relies on gross surgical identification of more than one enlarged gland. In multiple endocrine neoplasia types I and II, there is always multigland involvement, although asymmetric gland enlargement is often present. The chief cell generally predominates in parathyroid tumors; oxyphil cell tumors are much rarer.

PATHOPHYSIOLOGY. The primary disturbance is inappropriate secretion of PTH for the level of serum calcium. Studies in vitro with isolated parathyroid cells show that most adenomas either fail to suppress secretion at high calcium levels or show an altered setpoint, i.e., a higher calcium level is required to suppress secretion than for normal cells. Cells from hyperplastic glands may show a normal calcium setpoint for secretion. Hypersecretion of PTH in such cases may be due to a primary defect causing cellular proliferation and to an inability to suppress hormone secretion completely because of increased cell mass.

Slight increases in PTH secretion act on bone to increase turnover and may cause a reduction in cortical rather than trabecular bone density. At very high levels, PTH causes radiographically detectable subperiosteal bone resorption and, eventually, marrow fibrosis and cystic, reparative bone lesions termed "brown tumors." This is the classic form of the disease called "osteitis fibrosa cystica." Parathyroid hormone increases renal calcium reabsorption, but at high filtered loads of calcium, hypercalciuria, nonetheless, develops. Enhanced $1,25(OH)_2D$ formation by the kidneys is prominent in some patients and is associated with increased intestinal calcium absorption. Such patients may be at particular risk for renal stone formation.

CLINICAL MANIFESTATIONS. Most patients today either are asymptomatic at presentation (discovered through incidental blood calcium measurement) or present with vague, nonspecific symptoms, such as fatigue, weakness, and mental disturbance. Patients with significant hypercalcemia show many of the signs and symptoms of hypercalcemia discussed above. Nephrolithiasis, with or without renal colic, is not specifically associated with hyperparathyroidism but is most commonly seen in this setting. Subperiosteal bone resorption is rarely seen today, and osteitis fibrosa cystica even less commonly. Neuromuscular abnormalities, particularly proximal muscle weakness affecting the lower limbs, may be prominent. Joint manifestations include chondrocalcinosis that may lead to pseudogout. It has been claimed that hypertension, peptic ulcer disease, and osteoporosis are manifestations of hyperparathyroidism, but these are all common, and there is no firm evidence for a causal relationship between hyperparathyroidism and any of these disorders. There are no specific physical findings in hyperparathyroidism. A neck mass, if present, most commonly represents a coincidental thyroid nodule, less commonly a benign or malignant parathyroid tumor. "Band keratopathy," calcification at "3 and 9 o'clock" of the cornea, is best seen by slit-lamp examination and occurs most often when hypercalcemia is accompanied by hyperphosphatemia—thus less commonly in hyperparathyroidism than in other hypercalcemic disorders. Radiologic findings include subperiosteal resorption, which, when present, is best seen at the radial sides of the phalanges, distal phalangeal tufts, and distal clavicles. Lucent bone lesions, representing brown tumors, are seen in rare, severely affected patients. Soft tissue calcification may be evident in the joints, kidneys, and lungs. The calcification is best appreciated on bone scans.

DIAGNOSIS. The differential diagnosis of hypercalcemia is discussed above. Parathyroid hormone immunoassay, preferably one of the newer two-site assays, is the key to diagnosis. In making the distinction between hyperparathyroid and normal states (e.g., in patients presenting with nephrolithiasis), repeated careful serum calcium and PTH (including the mid-region type of assay) measurements are most useful. Hypercalcemic subjects taking lithium or thiazides should be retested for hyperparathyroidism after discontinuation of the drug (this may not be feasible in some patients on lithium), since both drugs may alter serum calcium and parathyroid hormone secretion. In relatively young, asymptomatic individuals, or if the serum PTH level is marginally elevated, hypercalcemia may be due to familial hypocalciuric hypercalcemia rather than hyperparathyroidism (see discussion below under Familial Hypocalciuric Hypercalcemia).

PROGNOSIS AND TREATMENT. Surgical parathyroidectomy is the only definitive treatment for hyperparathyroidism. Oral phosphate treatment can lower the serum calcium level, but the long-term safety and efficacy of this approach are unclear. In mildly affected, older women, estrogen treatment has been advocated, particularly to blunt bone resorption, but, again, long-term efficacy is unknown. Thus, the only alternative to surgery at present is conservative medical follow-up. Most experts recommend surgery for all patients with symptomatic disease and even for asymptomatic patients meeting other, somewhat arbitrary, criteria, such as age below 40 or a serum calcium level higher than 11.5 mg per deciliter. The appropriate management of patients not fitting any of these criteria is controversial, with some advocating surgery for all, and others conservative follow-up. The long-term course of untreated hyperparathyroidism is unknown. Controlled studies comparing surgery versus medical follow-up have not been performed. Small series of patients followed conservatively for several years suggest that mild biochemical disease rarely progresses to severe symptomatic disease, but it is difficult to exclude subtle abnormalities, such as reduced bone density. Since definitive treatment recommendations are not possible, therapy must be individualized. The author personally follows a policy of recommending surgery for all but older patients with only mild, biochemical disease.

If the decision is to perform surgery, the crucial issue is to find a highly experienced parathyroid surgeon. A success rate as high as 95 per cent can be expected for initial neck exploration by a skilled surgeon. The success rate is substantially lower with inexperienced surgeons. Preoperative localization is not needed by the skilled surgeon performing initial exploration. Neither localization studies nor neck exploration itself should serve as *diagnostic* maneuvers. Only after the diagnosis has been established biochemically (by PTH assay) should one recommend surgery. In patients undergoing repeat neck exploration for recurrent or persistent disease, localization studies are extremely helpful. Noninvasive studies include ultrasound, technetium-thallium scanning, computed tomography (CT), and magnetic resonance imaging. Invasive techniques include fine-needle aspiration of imaged lesions for PTH assay, selective arteriography, and selective venous catheterization for hormone assay. The latter techniques are best performed by radiologists with specialized experience.

After successful surgery, hypocalcemia is generally mild and transient and rarely requires treatment. In the rare case of subjects with extensive bone disease, severe, prolonged hypocalcemia secondary to "bone hunger" occurs. Persistent relative hypophosphatemia suggests that bone hunger, rather than hypoparathyroidism, is the cause of hypocalcemia in this setting. Acute treatment with calcium infusions and long-term treatment with vitamin D and oral calcium may be needed. Eventually, treatment can be discontinued if normal parathyroid tissue remains. In patients without residual normal parathyroid tissue, lifelong vitamin D therapy is necessary. Autotransplantation of parathyroid tissue in the forearm is an experimental alternative in such cases. Successful surgery generally halts formation of renal stones in patients with nephrolithiasis and allows skeletal remineralization in patients with bone disease. There is no definitive evidence that surgery corrects hypertension or other nonspecific manifestations of hyperparathyroidism.

FAMILIAL HYPOCALCIURIC HYPERCALCEMIA

DEFINITION. This is an autosomal dominant genetic disease with essentially complete penetrance that causes hypercalcemia and relatively low urinary calcium excretion for the filtered load.

ETIOLOGY. The etiology is unknown, and the chromosomal localization of the "disease gene" has yet to be identified.

INCIDENCE. The disorder is relatively rare, but it is overrepresented among patients presenting with unsuccessful neck exploration because of the difficulty in achieving normocalcemia by surgery.

PATHOPHYSIOLOGY. The primary disturbance appears to be in divalent cation transport and/or "sensing" in at least the kidneys and parathyroids. The kidneys show an exaggerated reabsorption of filtered calcium (and magnesium) that leads to hypercalcemia. The parathyroids, however, fail to suppress fully hormone secretion despite hypercalcemia. The process is PTH dependent, since totally parathyroidectomized subjects become hypocalcemic, but even small amounts of parathyroid tissue are sufficient to maintain hypercalcemia. Parathyroid gland mass is generally only mildly increased.

CLINICAL MANIFESTATIONS. The disease leads to few, if any, clinical manifestations—hence its other name, "familial benign hypercalcemia." Nephrolithiasis and bone disease are, in general, not seen. Pancreatitis has been reported, but the specificity of this association is unclear. Hypercalcemia is present at birth. In some neonates, a clinically severe form of the disease is present. This severe form may be due to inheritance of a double dose of the abnormal gene. Otherwise, the main morbidity is that resulting from unsuccessful neck exploration prompted by failure to distinguish this disorder from conventional hyperparathyroidism. There is no evidence of associated endocrinopathies, as in the multiple endocrine neoplasia syndromes.

DIAGNOSIS. A high index of suspicion is needed to recognize this disease. Hypercalcemia associated with relatively young age, with only slight elevation in the serum PTH level, or with a family history of unsuccessful neck exploration should trigger further evaluation. Hypermagnesemia is suggestive; urinary calcium-creatinine ratios less than 0.01:1 strongly support the diagnosis. Screening of first-degree relatives for hypercalcemia may also be helpful. Until specific genetic probes become available, definitive diagnosis is not possible.

PROGNOSIS AND TREATMENT. Since the disease is compatible with normal life expectancy and is associated with little, if any, morbidity, neck exploration would appear to be contraindicated. Successful surgical treatment, moreover, is quite difficult, with permanent hypoparathyroidism or, more commonly, recurrent hypercalcemia, the usual result.

HYPERCALCEMIA ASSOCIATED WITH MALIGNANCY

ETIOLOGY AND PATHOGENESIS. Malignancies can cause hypercalcemia through two non–mutually exclusive mechanisms. First, local osteolytic hypercalcemia is caused by tumor metastatic to bone. Tumor cells may release bone-resorbing factors or so-called "osteoclast-activating factors," which indirectly lead to bone resorption. Cytokines such as lymphotoxin and interleukin 1 are potent osteoclast-activating factors. Second, humoral hypercalcemia of malignancy is caused by tumor secretion of factors into the circulation that act systemically to increase bone resorption. Such factors may show other PTH-like actions, including increasing urinary cyclic AMP and phosphate excretion and decreasing renal calcium excretion. This condition leads to a syndrome with biochemical features closely resembling those of primary hyperparathyroidism. One such factor commonly associated with many tumors has recently been identified as a polypeptide roughly twice as large as PTH and homologous in amino acid sequence to the biologically active, amino-terminus of PTH. This so-called parathyroid hormone–related peptide may also be secreted by tumors metastatic to bone, so that humoral and local osteolytic mechanisms may combine to cause hypercalcemia. Some tumors cause hypercalcemia through excessive synthesis of $1,25(OH)_2D$, in a manner analogous to that seen in sarcoidosis (see below). A role for additional, as yet unidentified, bone-resorbing agents secreted by tumors has not been excluded.

INCIDENCE. Malignancy-associated hypercalcemia occurs most commonly in patients with bone metastases. Breast carcinoma is one of the most frequent causes. Most subjects with bone metastases are not hypercalcemic because of adequate renal compensatory mechanisms. Slight renal impairment may then provoke hypercalcemia. Treatment of women with breast cancer metastatic to bone with tamoxifen has been associated with acute sharp increases in the serum calcium level. Certain hematogenous neoplasms, such as myeloma and human lymphotropic virus type I–associated leukemia/lymphoma, are frequently associated with hypercalcemia. Humoral hypercalcemia of malignancy is much rarer. It is seen most frequently with squamous carcinomas, but biochemical evidence indicates that almost any tumor type, including breast carcinoma, can produce parathyroid hormone–related peptide.

CLINICAL MANIFESTATIONS. Malignancy-associated hypercalcemia often develops acutely, may be quite severe (hypercalcemic crisis), and is frequently a grave prognostic sign. In most cases, particularly of the local osteolytic hypercalcemia variety, the underlying neoplasm is clinically evident. An otherwise occult neoplasm may occasionally manifest with humoral hypercalcemia of malignancy. Accurate and rapid diagnosis is critical in such cases, since successful tumor removal may be feasible.

DIAGNOSIS. As discussed earlier, PTH radioimmunoassay is the critical test for excluding coexistent primary hyperparathyroidism. Parathyroid hormone–related peptide fails to cross-react in such assays. Recently, specific immunoassays for this peptide have been developed, and these facilitate diagnosis of tumor secretion of the peptide. Increased urinary cyclic AMP excretion (coupled with low or undetectable PTH measurement) also favors tumor secretion of parathyroid hormone–related peptide. If both PTH and urinary cyclic AMP levels are low, one is dealing with a vitamin D–mediated or local osteolytic hypercalcemia.

TREATMENT AND PROGNOSIS. Acute, nonspecific treatment of hypercalcemia is instituted if the diagnosis is unclear (see Ch. 165). Definitive treatment must be directed at the underlying neoplasm, if feasible. When tumor treatment is not possible, vigorous treatment of hypercalcemia may be irrelevant. In those cases mediated by vitamin D or lymphokine release, glucocorticoids are often uniquely effective in lowering the serum calcium level.

HYPERCALCEMIA DUE TO GRANULOMATOUS DISEASES

ETIOLOGY AND PATHOGENESIS. Hypercalcemia is caused by unregulated formation of $1,25(OH)_2D$ in granuloma-associated macrophages. Normally, 1-hydroxylation takes place in the kidney and is sensitive to feedback suppression by high serum calcium levels. Unregulated synthesis of $1,25(OH)_2D$ in patients with granulomatous diseases renders them hypersensitive to vitamin D (from the diet or through sun exposure).

INCIDENCE AND PREVALENCE. This form of hypercalcemia has been observed in almost any disease capable of causing granuloma formation. These diseases include sarcoidosis, tuberculosis and fungal infections, berylliosis, and some lymphomas, such as Hodgkin's disease. Overt hypercalcemia may be seen in only about 10 per cent of patients with sarcoidosis, but hypercalciuria and intestinal hyperabsorption of calcium may occur in almost half of such individuals.

CLINICAL FEATURES. Manifestations are those of the underlying disease, as well as the superimposed effects of hypercalcemia. Because this form of hypercalcemia often coexists with relatively higher serum phosphorus levels than those seen in hyperparathyroidism, soft tissue calcification, nephrocalcinosis, and renal impairment are more common. Patients may present with hypercalcemia and relatively few other findings (e.g., subtle hilar adenopathy in sarcoidosis).

DIAGNOSIS. Parathyroid hormone and urinary cyclic AMP are suppressed. The serum level of $1,25(OH)_2D$ is elevated (in cases of vitamin D intoxication, the serum $1,25(OH)_2D$ level may be normal and only serum $25(OH)D$ is increased).

TREATMENT AND PROGNOSIS. The prognosis depends on that of the underlying disease. Glucocorticoids are extremely effective in lowering the serum calcium level in such cases. Chloroquine has been used effectively in subjects who cannot tolerate glucocorticoid treatment.

Attie MF: Treatment of hypercalcemia. Endocrinol Metab Clin North Am 18:807, 1989. *Complete discussion of treatment options and their pathophysiologic basis.*

Aurbach GD, Marx SJ, Spiegel AM. Parathyroid hormone, calcitonin, and the calciferols, *In* Wilson JD, Foster DW (eds.): Williams Textbook of Endocrinology. 7th ed. Philadelphia, W.B. Saunders Company, 1985, pp 1170–1198. *Detailed description of primary hyperparathyroidism and malignancy-associated and other forms of hypercalcemia, including differential diagnosis and treatment.*

Broadus AE, Mangin M, Ikeda K, et al.: Humoral hypercalcemia of cancer. N Engl J Med 319:556, 1988. *Review of pathogenesis of this syndrome and discovery of parathyroid hormone–related peptide.*

Brown EM, LeBoff MS, Oetting M, et al.: Secretory control in normal and abnormal parathyroid tissue. Recent Prog Horm Res 43:337, 1987. *Detailed review of control of normal parathyroid hormone secretion and of abnormal secretion in hyperparathyroidism.*

Friedman E, Sakaguchi K, Bale AE, et al.: Clonality of parathyroid tumors in familial endocrine neoplasia type I. N Engl J Med 321:213, 1989. *Description of molecular genetic abnormalities in familial and sporadic forms of parathyroid neoplasia.*

Heath DA: Primary hyperparathyroidism: Clinical presentation and factors influencing clinical management. Endocrinol Metab Clin North Am 18:631, 1989. *Thorough review of clinical features of hyperparathyroidism and arguments for and against surgery.*

Marx SJ, Spiegel AM, Levine MA, et al.: Familial hypocalciuric hypercalcemia. N Engl J Med 307:679, 1982. *Review of clinical and pathophysiologic features of this disease.*

Singer FR, Adams JS: Abnormal calcium homeostasis in sarcoidosis. N Engl J Med 315:755, 1986. *Review of derangements in vitamin D metabolism causing hypercalcemia and hypercalciuria in granulomatous disorders.*

HYPOCALCEMIA

DEFINITION. Hypocalcemia is an abnormal reduction in serum ionized calcium concentration.* Reduction in total serum calcium, as may occur in patients with hypoalbuminemia, does not necessarily reflect a reduction in ionized calcium. Ionized, not total, serum calcium affects neuromuscular function and is therefore the clinically relevant parameter.

ETIOLOGY AND PATHOGENESIS. Normal serum ionized calcium concentration is maintained by the direct actions of PTH on kidney and bone and by the indirect actions (through $1,25(OH)_2D$) on the intestine (see Ch. 232). Hypocalcemic disorders can be divided according to pathogenesis into two broad categories: (1) primary hypoparathyroidism, in which hypocalcemia is due to deficient secretion and/or action of PTH (specific subtypes are discussed under individual headings below); and (2) hypocalcemia due to target organ malfunction (e.g., renal failure, intestinal malabsorption, vitamin D deficiency). Hypocalcemia occurs in this category despite normal or even increased PTH secretion (secondary hyperparathyroidism). In hypoparathyroidism, there is reduced mobilization of calcium from bone, reduced renal reabsorption of calcium, lowered phosphaturia, and reduced $1,25(OH)_2D$ formation with a resultant decrease in intestinal calcium absorption. The end results are hypocalcemia and hyperphosphatemia. Renal failure (see Ch. 237) and acute phosphate loads (as may occur with chemotherapy of certain tumors such as Burkitt's lymphoma) are other causes of hypocalcemia with hyperphosphatemia. With vitamin D deficiency or malabsorption, hypocalcemia occurs with normal or low serum phosphorus levels (the latter reflecting secondary hyperparathyroidism). Hypocalcemia with low or normal serum phosphorus levels is also seen in acute pancreatitis (attributed to calcium soap formation, but this is unproved) and in some patients with osteoblastic tumor metastases. Table 235–3 summarizes the causes of hypocalcemia.

CLINICAL MANIFESTATIONS. Hypocalcemia of any cause is associated with certain typical signs and symptoms. Most prominent among these is increased neuromuscular excitability. Paresthesias of the fingers, toes, and circumoral region are mild manifestations; in more extreme cases there may be muscle cramping, carpopedal spasm, laryngeal stridor, and convulsions.

---

*See Ch. 232 and Part XXVII for calcium and phosphorus reference range values.

TABLE 235–3. CAUSES OF HYPOCALCEMIA

Hypoparathyroidism
  Deficient parathyroid hormone secretion
    Idiopathic (autoimmune)
    Parathyroid hormone gene mutation
    Surgical
    Infiltrative (iron overload, Wilson's disease)
    Functional
      Hypomagnesemia
      Transient postoperative
  Deficient parathyroid hormone action (hormone resistance)
    Pseudohypoparathyroidism types Ia and Ib
Normal or Increased Parathyroid Hormone Function
  Renal failure
  Intestinal malabsorption
  Acute pancreatitis
  Osteoblastic metastases
  Vitamin D deficiency or resistance

Symptoms reflect not only the degree of hypocalcemia but also the acuteness of the fall in serum calcium concentration. Patients with longstanding severe hypocalcemia may show surprisingly few symptoms. Factors that acutely alter the balance between ionized and protein-bound calcium may precipitate symptoms. For example, alkalosis lowers ionized calcium; thus hyperventilation may provoke symptoms of tetany. Signs of latent tetany include Chvostek's sign (twitching of the upper lip after tapping on the facial nerve below the zygomatic arch) and Trousseau's sign (carpal spasm after inflating a cuff on the upper arm above systolic blood pressure for 2 to 3 minutes).

Various mental disturbances, such as irritability, depression, and even psychosis, have been attributed to hypocalcemia. Papilledema and other signs of increased intracranial pressure have been reported. Intracranial calcifications, particularly of the basal ganglia, may be seen on plain radiographs and even more frequently on CT. Increased sensitivity to the dystonic effects of phenothiazines has been attributed to basal ganglia calcification. Longstanding hypocalcemia may lead to cataract formation. Cardiac effects of hypocalcemia include prolongation of the QT interval and, rarely, congestive heart failure. Dental anomalies depend on age of onset; in children hypocalcemia can cause enamel hypoplasia and failure of the adult teeth to erupt.

DIFFERENTIAL DIAGNOSIS. Measurement of serum calcium, phosphorus, and creatinine levels allows one to categorize the form of hypocalcemia. Hypocalcemia and hyperphosphatemia with normal renal function are pathognomonic of hypoparathyroidism. Low or undetectable PTH by immunoassay despite hypocalcemia confirms the diagnosis. (Rare forms of PTH-resistant hypoparathyroidism show elevated levels of PTH and are discussed further below.) Hypocalcemia and hyperphosphatemia caused by renal failure pose no diagnostic problem. Hypocalcemia with normal or low serum phosphorus levels should prompt measurement of vitamin D metabolites and assessment of gastrointestinal function to check for vitamin D deficiency and malabsorption, respectively. Measurements of PTH should show increased values in such patients, as the normal parathyroids attempt to compensate for hypocalcemia.

TREATMENT. Acute, symptomatic hypocalcemia requires emergency treatment in the form of intravenous calcium infusion. Ten to 20 ml of 10 per cent calcium gluconate solution (contains 10 mg of elemental calcium per milliliter) may be given over 10 to 20 minutes (this may be hazardous in patients taking cardiac glycosides). In less urgent settings, a slow intravenous infusion (over 4 to 8 hours) of 20 mg of elemental calcium per kilogram of body weight may be given. As with hypercalcemic disorders, definitive resolution of hypocalcemia requires treatment of the underlying disease. In patients with hypoparathyroidism, lifelong therapy with vitamin D (with or without oral calcium) is required. This is discussed further under treatment of hypoparathyroidism, below.

HYPOPARATHYROIDISM

DEFINITION. Hypoparathyroidism is defined as deficient PTH secretion and/or action. This condition may lead to overt hypocalcemia and hyperphosphatemia, as discussed above, or may only predispose to hypocalcemia (decreased parathyroid reserve) in times of increased calcium demand, such as pregnancy.

ETIOLOGY AND PATHOGENESIS. *Permanent Deficiency in Parathyroid Hormone Secretion.* This deficiency may result from surgical removal of the parathyroids, from glandular destruction by iron overload (e.g., transfusions in thalassemia) or copper overload (Wilson's disease), and from glandular destruction through a presumed autoimmune mechanism. The latter often has a genetic basis. The parathyroids may fail to develop as part of the DiGeorge syndrome. Some cases termed "idiopathic hypoparathyroidism" may be due to inherited mutations in the PTH gene that prevent synthesis and secretion of PTH.

Transient Deficiency in Parathyroid Hormone Secretion. Reversible hypoparathyroidism can be caused by hypomagnesemia. The latter may compromise both PTH secretion and action. Magnesium replacement corrects the defect. Transient hypoparathyroidism may also result from suppression of normal parathyroids by parathyroid adenomas or other causes of hypercalcemia. This condition rarely lasts more than 1 week. Surgical injury to

the parathyroids is another postulated cause of transiently reduced hormone secretion.

Deficiency in Parathyroid Hormone Action. Secretion of a biologically inactive form of PTH is a theoretical, but unproven, cause of deficient PTH action. Target organ resistance to PTH appears to be the major cause of this form of hypoparathyroidism, which was termed "pseudohypoparathyroidism" by Albright, who described it as the first example of a hormone-resistance disorder. Subsequent studies indicated that the defect in this disease occurs proximal to formation of cyclic AMP (a second messenger of PTH action), since affected subjects lack the normal brisk increase in urinary cyclic AMP excretion observed following infusion of PTH in normal individuals. There are at least two forms of pseudohypoparathyroidism. In type Ia disease, a 50 per cent deficiency has been found in the Gs protein that couples PTH (and many other) receptors to the enzyme that forms cyclic AMP, adenylyl cyclase. This deficiency may limit normal cyclic AMP production in response to PTH as well as to other hormones, such as thyroid-stimulating hormone. As a result, patients with this form of the disease show many abnormalities (e.g., hypothyroidism, hypogonadism) in addition to hypoparathyroidism. In affected subjects from several families with type Ia disease, distinct mutations that prevent synthesis of normal Gs protein have been found in the gene encoding the Gs protein. Inheritance of the mutation is autosomal dominant. In subjects with type Ib disease, the Gs protein is normal, and resistance is limited to PTH. A defective PTH receptor is a likely, but unproven, basis for this disease. In some subjects, hypocalcemia and hyperphosphatemia are associated with radiographically evident osteitis fibrosa cystica. This finding suggests selective renal, as opposed to skeletal, resistance to PTH action. The pathogenesis is unclear.

INCIDENCE. All forms of hypoparathyroidism are relatively rare. The incidence of surgical hypoparathyroidism varies widely as a function of the skill of the surgeon.

CLINICAL MANIFESTATIONS. The manifestations generally associated with hypocalcemia have been discussed above. The clinical features unique to each form of hypoparathyroidism reflect the underlying disease. In autoimmune forms, there may be associated endocrine deficiency, most frequently Addison's disease, as well as a T cell defect predisposing to mucocutaneous candidiasis. Alopecia and vitiligo may also be seen. In pseudohypoparathyroidism type Ib, the appearance is normal, but in type Ia disease, affected individuals show a constellation of abnormal physical findings termed Albright's hereditary osteodystrophy (Fig. 235–3). These findings include obesity; short stature; round face and short neck; metacarpal and metatarsal shortening (most often fourth and fifth), as well as shortening and broadening of the distal phalanges; and subcutaneous calcifications. Such individuals often show slight mental retardation and associated endocrine abnormalities, most commonly hypothyroidism (without goiter) and hypogonadism. First-degree relatives of patients with pseudohypoparathyroidism type Ia may show the physical features of Albright's osteodystrophy without evidence of hormone resistance. This condition has been termed "pseudopseudohypoparathyroidism." Rarely, individuals with pseudohypoparathyroidism (more often of the Ib type) may show radiographic evidence of osteitis fibrosa cystica and elevated serum levels of bone-derived alkaline phosphatase.

DIFFERENTIAL DIAGNOSIS. Low or undetectable serum PTH in the face of hypocalcemia, hyperphosphatemia, and normal renal function establishes the diagnosis of hormone-deficient hypoparathyroidism. Diagnosis of the underlying disease depends on history (e.g., neck surgery), physical findings (e.g., candidiasis, alopecia), and additional laboratory tests (e.g., evidence for hypoadrenalism). Antibodies to parathyroid antigens have been detected in the autoimmune form of the disease, but this test is not available for routine clinical use. If an elevated level of serum PTH is measured by immunoassay in a subject with hypocalcemia, hyperphosphatemia, and normal renal function, this suggests hormone-resistant hypoparathyroidism. Parathyroid hormone infusion (at present with commercially available synthetic 1–34 peptide) and measurement of urinary cyclic AMP excretion can be performed to confirm PTH resistance. Physical appearance can help distinguish type Ia from type Ib pseudohypoparathyroidism, as can testing for other endocrinopathies, such as hy-

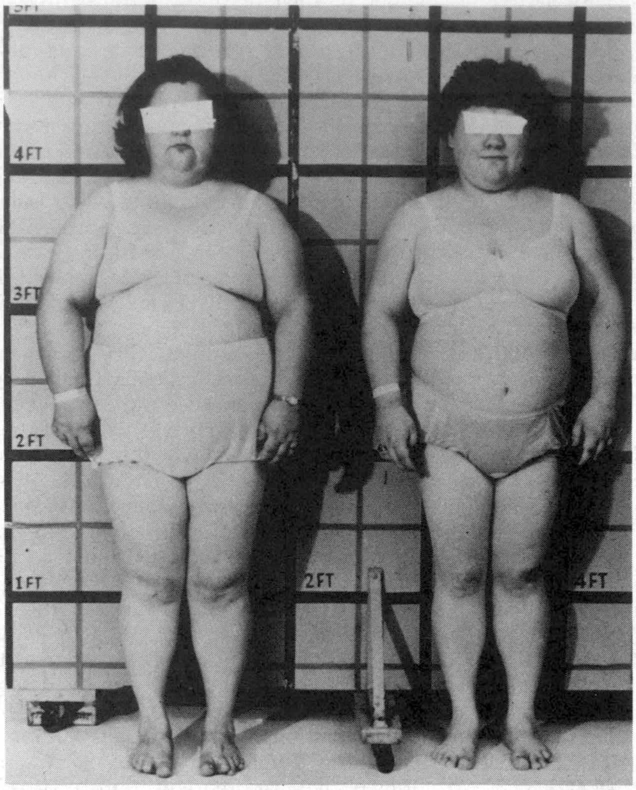

FIGURE 235–3. Phenotypic features of Albright's hereditary osteodystrophy. A mother *(left)* and daughter display many of the features of Albright's osteodystrophy, including obesity, short stature, round face, and short neck. Metacarpal and metatarsal shortening manifest as shortened fourth and fifth fingers (right hands of both subjects) and shortened fourth toes (left feet of both subjects), respectively. Both subjects show resistance to PTH and thyroid-stimulating hormone, as well as deficient Gs protein activity, characteristic of pseudohypoparathyroidism type Ia. (From Spiegel AM: Pseudohypoparathyroidism. *In* Scriver CR, Beaudet AL, Sly WS, Valle D [eds.]: The Metabolic Basis of Inherited Disease. 6th ed. New York, McGraw-Hill, 1989, pp 2013–2027; with permission.)

pothyroidism. Measurement of Gs protein and detection of mutations in the corresponding gene are not routinely available tests.

TREATMENT. Transient forms of hypoparathyroidism may not require treatment. Reversible forms should be treated appropriately, i.e., magnesium replacement for hypomagnesemia. In permanent, hormone-deficient hypoparathyroidism, hormone replacement therapy is not practical. Parathyroid autografting is effective in some patients with surgical hypoparathyroidism. When this is not feasible, and also in subjects with pseudohypoparathyroidism, lifelong treatment with oral vitamin D is required. Vitamin D_2, ergocalciferol (generally 50,000 units per day), is inexpensive by comparison with the active metabolite, $1,25(OH)_2D$ (generally 0.25 μg per day). The latter has the theoretical advantage of more rapid onset (and in case of toxicity, offset) of action, but with appropriate monitoring, vitamin D_2 can be used very effectively. Oral calcium salts (1 to 2 grams of elemental calcium per day in divided doses) may be added for individuals whose dietary calcium intake is highly variable or inadequate. The goal of treatment is the lowest serum calcium concentration compatible with avoidance of symptoms, since without PTH, urinary calcium excretion (and the possibility of nephrolithiasis) will be increased at any filtered load of calcium. Both serum and urine calcium levels, as well as renal function, must be monitored. In forms of hypoparathyroidism that have associated endocrinopathies, appropriate hormone replacement therapy should be instituted.

Ahn TG, Antonorakis SE, Kronenberg HM, et al.: Familial isolated hypoparathyroidism: A molecular genetic analysis of 8 families with 23 affected persons. Medicine 65:73, 1986. *Review of studies of PTH gene as locus of defect in this disease.*

Aurbach GD, Marx SJ, Spiegel AM: Parathyroid hormone, calcitonin, and the calciferols. *In* Wilson JD, Foster DW (eds.): Williams Textbook of Endocrinology. 7th ed. Philadelphia, W.B. Saunders Company, 1985, pp 1199–1207. *Detailed description of clinical and pathophysiologic features of hypocalcemic disorders and the multiple forms of hypoparathyroidism.*

Mallette L: Synthetic human parathyroid hormone 1–34 fragment for diagnostic testing. Ann Intern Med 109:800, 1988. *Description of use of this commercially available peptide in the differential diagnosis of hypoparathyroidism.*

Spiegel AM: Pseudohypoparathyroidism. *In* Scriver CR, Beaudet AL, Sly WS, et al. (eds.): The Metabolic Basis of Inherited Disease. 6th ed. New York, McGraw-Hill, 1989, pp 2013–2027. *Extensive discussion of clinical features and pathogenesis of hormone-resistant forms of hypoparathyroidism.*

236 Calcitonin and Medullary Thyroid Carcinoma

Leonard J. Deftos

Calcitonin (CT) is a 32-residue peptide secreted primarily by the thyroidal C-cells in mammals and by the embryologically related ultimobranchial gland in submammals. The main biologic effect of CT is to decrease bone resorption by inhibiting the osteoclast. This effect results in a decrease in the concentration of blood calcium, with a nadir directly related to bone turnover; thus, the hypocalcemia may be slight in normal adults but considerable when bone resorption is increased pathologically in disease states or physiologically during bone growth. This property of CT makes it an effective drug for hyperresorptive diseases, such as Paget's disease, osteoporosis, and hypercalcemia. The physiologic significance of other reported effects of CT is not well established. The calciuric effect of CT is seen only with pharmacologic doses of the hormone. A variety of gastrointestinal effects are only inconsistently observed. A stimulatory effect on bone formation may be attributable to a CT precursor molecule rather than to CT itself. However, an analgesic effect of CT continues to receive considerable attention and may be related to neuroendocrine features of the hormone. In addition to its role in skeletal physiology and treatment, CT is a serum and tumor marker for medullary thyroid carcinoma (MTC) and is the signal tumor of multiple endocrine neoplasia (MEN) type II.

CALCITONIN

Biochemistry

The 32-residue structure of CT, determined for eight species, reveals a common 1,7 amino-terminal disulfide bridge and carboxy-terminal proline. Seven of the nine amino-terminal residues are identical in all CT molecules. The interspecies structural differences in the rest of the molecule cause the submammalian (ultimobranchial) CT molecules to have a greater potency in mammals than the mammalian CT molecules. Thus, the salmon form of the hormone is widely used for treatment in humans. The greater chemical basicity of these submammalian CT species probably accounts for their increased potency. In contrast to the other major skeletal peptide hormone, parathyroid hormone (PTH), a biologically active fragment of CT has not been identified, and the entire molecule seems to be necessary for biologic activity.

Secretion and Production

The most important secretory regulation of CT is mediated by ambient calcium. An acute increase in blood calcium concentration increases the secretion of CT, and an acute decrease in blood calcium level decreases the secretion of CT. The effects of chronic changes in blood calcium concentration on secretion have not been as well defined. Chronic hypercalcemia may stimulate CT production, but this compensatory response may be limited. Chronic hypocalcemia seems to increase CT storage in C-cells. Although a variety of other factors have been reported to stimulate CT secretion, only pentagastrin and its related peptides are consistent additional secretagogues. The high concentration of pentagastrin necessary to stimulate secretion does not support the presence of a normal entero–C-cell secretory pathway. Nevertheless, pentagastrin and calcium are clinically important agents for the evaluation of CT secretion by both normal and malignant C-cells.

The effect of gonadal steroids and age on CT production remains controversial. It is well established that blood concentrations of CT are higher in males than females and in children than adults. Some studies report a decline in CT secretion during adulthood and a stimulation of CT secretion by estrogens and testosterone. These observations have led to the hypothesis that age- and menopause-related declines in CT production contribute to the corresponding declines in bone mass seen in the elderly, especially postmenopausal women. These observations support the use of CT in the treatment of osteoporosis, but more complex hormonal abnormalities underlie this skeletal disorder.

MEDULLARY THYROID CARCINOMA

Medullary thyroid carcinoma is a tumor of the CT-producing C-cells of the thyroid gland. These cells migrate from the neural crest to the thyroid gland and to other sites of the diffuse neuroendocrine system during embryogenesis in mammals. In submammals, these cells form their own distinct organ, the ultimobranchial gland. The neural crest origin of C-cells accounts for their production of a variety of biologically active substances. This embryologic origin may also explain the common association of MTC with other neuroendocrine tumors. Thus, MTC can occur as part of a multiple endocrine disorder, MEN type II, or sporadically.

Pathology

A palpable tumor is the most common physical finding in the patient with MTC. The tumor is usually firm and located in the middle or upper lobes of the gland. Bilateral tumors are common in MEN. Calcification can be present in the tumor, and this may result in a radiographic pattern that is sufficiently characteristic to assist in clinical diagnosis. Similarly, the presence of amyloid in the tumor can assist in histologic diagnosis. However, cytologic diagnosis is made difficult by the fact that the cells of MTC can be arranged in a variety of patterns. Therefore, the diagnosis of MTC is conclusively made by the demonstration of CT in the tumor by immunohistology. Hyperplasia of the C-cells antedates the frank malignancy of MTC, especially in the familial forms of the tumor. C-cell hyperplasia is often too subtle to be appreciated by light microscopy, and immunohistology for CT is necessary to make this diagnosis.

Tumor Behavior

The clinical behavior of MTC is usually intermediate between that of aggressive anaplastic thyroid cancer and that of indolent papillary and follicular thyroid cancer. Local lymph node spread is common, and metastases to lung and bone can occur. Medullary thyroid carcinoma in which all or most of the cells produce CT may have a better prognosis than a more heterogeneous tumor in which CT production is not uniform. Even in the most aggressive tumors, CT production is usually sufficient to serve as a specific marker for this thyroid cancer. However, there may be rare instances in which CT production has ceased. The 5-year survival of those with MTC approximates 50 per cent. Survival can vary from several months to three decades after diagnosis. Patients under 2 years of age with metastatic disease and over 50 years of age with only localized disease have been reported. C-cell hyperplasia can occur in those as young as 2 years and as old as 45 years of age. Therefore, the tumor can be rapidly aggressive, leading to death within months after diagnosis, or it can be indolent and compatible with survival for decades.

Pathogenesis

Medullary thyroid carcinoma is preceded by C-cell hyperplasia, especially in the familial form of the disease. This progression from hyperplasia to cancer is best documented for MTC in the clinical setting of MEN type II. C-cell adenomas have also been observed. The progression of unregulated growth from hyperplasia to malignancy is similar to that seen in the progression of mucosal cells to a frankly malignant state in colon cancer. In colon cancer, this development is accompanied by a sequential expression of oncogenes. It is thus interesting to speculate that an oncogene cascade is responsible for the progression of normal C-cells through hyperplasia to cancer in MTC. In the familial form of the tumor, an oncogene abnormality may be related to the chromosome 10 site, to which MEN type IIA has been mapped. Abnormalities in oncogene expression have been observed in MTC, but their role in pathogenesis has not yet been defined. It is notable that this same progression of normal cells to hyperplastic and then neoplastic cells is also observed for the other two endocrine components of heritable MTC, pheochromocytoma and parathyroid neoplasia. Thus, the genetic abnormality on chromosome 10 may result in the overexpression (or undersuppression) of an endocrine cell growth factor.

Diagnosis

Overexpression of the CT gene is the molecular hallmark of MTC. This overexpression results in the increased production of CT by the tumor and increased secretion of the hormone into blood. As a result, most patients with MTC have an increased circulating concentration of CT that can be detected by radioimmunoassay and increased tumor concentrations that can be demonstrated directly by immunohistology or through increased messenger RNA (mRNA) expression by in situ hybridization. Usually, the basal blood concentration of CT is sufficiently elevated to be diagnostic of the presence of the tumor. In the early stages of the diseases, however, the basal concentrations of CT cannot be readily distinguished from normal. In these circumstances, provocative testing of CT secretion can reveal the presence of the abnormal C-cells. Such testing is also clinically indicated for the relative of a patient with familial MTC when early diagnosis is sought. The two most commonly used provocative agents for CT secretion are calcium and the synthetic gastrin analogue pentagastrin, alone or in combination. Most tumors respond to either agent with a diagnostic increase in CT secretion. CT blood measurements can also be used to evaluate therapy and monitor tumor recurrence. Interpretation must be made according to the specific parameters of the procedure utilized.

The primary genetic abnormality in MEN type IIA has been localized to chromosome 10. Molecular genetic techniques allow the assignment of gene carrier status with considerable certainty in a patient at risk and with a well-documented pedigree. However, confounding factors such as mistaken diagnoses and nonpaternity can complicate genetic analysis. The ethical considerations that surround all of genetic screening should be considered in the light of the effective and curative treatment that is available for the components of MEN type IIA.

CT Gene Expression

A wide variety of bioactive substances are overproduced by MTC. Some can be attributed to the neural crest origin of the C-cells and some to deregulated CT gene expression. This gene encodes peptides in addition to CT. The CT gene consists of six exons that generate, through differential mRNA splicing, two distinct mRNA's, one of them the CT precursor and the other a precursor for calcitonin gene–related peptide (CGRP). The CT precursor is processed into three peptides: CT; its amino-terminal flanking peptide, N-pro CT; and its carboxy-terminal flanking peptide, C-pro CT. The CGRP precursor is similarly processed. Thus, the CT gene encodes at least six peptides. The peptides derived from the CT precursor, including CT, act on the skeletal system, and the peptide derived from the CGRP precursor acts as a neurotransmitter. This remarkable genetic economy produces two CT precursor–derived peptides that have opposite skeletal effects, with CT inhibiting bone resorption and N-pro CT, its amino-terminal relative, promoting bone cell mitogenesis. Human CT gene expression is summarized in Figure 236–1.

MULTIPLE ENDOCRINE NEOPLASIA (MEN)

Medullary thyroid carcinoma can occur in association with other endocrine tumors as part of a multiple endocrine neoplasia, designated MEN type II, to distinguish it from MEN type I, which consists of parathyroid, pancreatic, and pituitary tumors. MEN type II is an autosomal dominant syndrome that can be clinically classified into two subtypes, type IIA and IIB (Table 236–1).

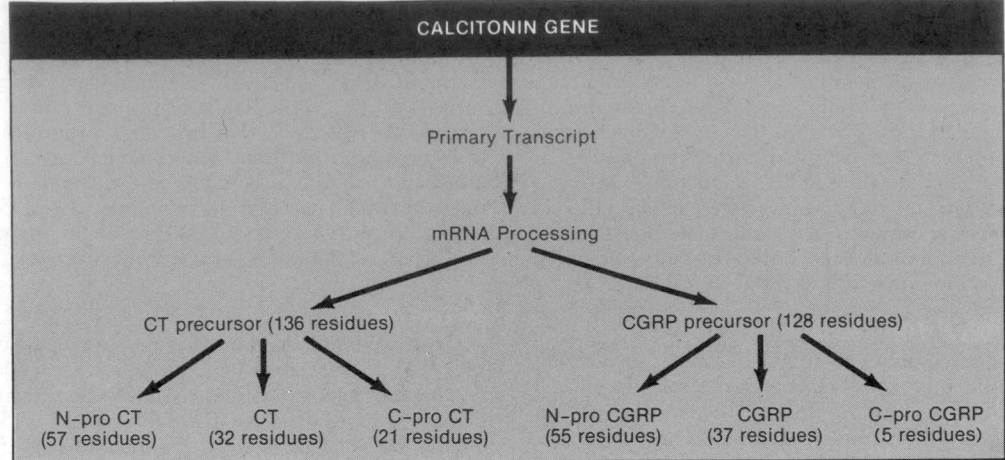

FIGURE 236–1. Summary of human calcitonin (CT) gene expression. The CT pathway occurs primarily in endocrine tissue (e.g., C-cells) and the calcitonin gene–related peptide (CGRP) pathway primarily in neural tissue. The gene has six exons whose primary RNA transcript is differentially spliced into an mRNA for the CT precursor and one for the CGRP precursor. A common 25-residue leader sequence is removed, and these two polypeptide precursors are each processed into their three respective peptide products. (Alternative designations for some of these peptides are as follows: for N-pro CT, PAS-57; for C-pro CT, PDN-21 and katacalcin; for N-pro CGRP, PAS-55). The function of these other peptides is not firmly established.

Pheochromocytoma

Pheochromocytoma is a component of MEN type IIA and IIB. Bilateral and multifocal pheochromocytomas are very common in this clinical setting, with an incidence of over 70 per cent. This figure contrasts with a bilateral incidence of usually less than 10 per cent for sporadic pheochromocytomas and only 20 to 50 per cent for familial pheochromocytomas. Adrenal medullary hyperplasia is a predecessor of the pheochromocytomas seen with MTC. The increase in adrenal medullary mass results from diffuse or multifocal proliferation of adrenal medullary cells, primarily those found within the head and body of the glands. The biochemical as well as clinical manifestations of this tumor may be subtle, so diagnostic tests for pheochromocytoma should be pursued vigorously in MEN type II.

Hyperparathyroidism

Hyperparathyroidism is much more common in MEN type IIA than in MEN type IIB (and it also occurs in MEN type I). The presence of hyperparathyroidism thus should always make one consider the possibility of MEN. Parathyroid hyperplasia is more common than adenoma, an important consideration for surgical treatment. Although a calcium-mediated functional relationship between hyperparathyroidism and MTC has been suggested, the two neoplasias are probably related to the same gene.

Multiple Mucosal Neuromas

The presence of neuromas with a centrofacial distribution is the most consistent component of MEN type IIB. The most common location of neuromas is the oral cavity. The oral lesions are almost invariably present by the first decade and in some cases even at birth. Mucosal neuromas can also be present in the eyelid, conjunctiva, and cornea. The most prominent microscopic feature of neuromas is an increase in the size and number of nerves. These hypertrophied nerve fibers are readily seen with a slit lamp and occasionally by direct ophthalmologic examination.

Gastrointestinal tract abnormalities are part of the multiple mucosal neuroma syndrome. The most common of these is gastrointestinal ganglioneuromatosis, which usually occurs in the small and large intestines but has also been noted in the esophagus and stomach. The lesions are sometimes associated with swallowing abnormalities, megacolon, diarrhea, and constipation. The diarrhea may also be due to excess production of bioactive substances by the MTC. In any case, diarrhea is the most common symptom of MTC.

Marfanoid Habitus

Patients with this component have a tall, slender body with long arms and legs, an abnormal ratio of upper to lower body segments, and poor muscle development. Other features associated with the marfanoid habitus may include dorsal kyphosis, pectus excavatum or pectus carinatum, pes cavus, and high-arched palate. In contrast to patients with true Marfan's syndrome, these patients do not have aortic arch abnormalities, ectopia lentis, homocystinuria, or mucopolysaccharide abnormalities.

Treatment and Clinical Management

Surgery is the treatment of choice for the three neoplasias in MEN type II. All are potentially lethal—especially MTC and pheochromocytoma—but all can be cured in their early stages by surgery. Aggressive therapy is thus warranted. Management of the individual components of MEN syndromes generally follows the accepted procedures for each of the neoplasias. However, the sequence of treatment is guided by the presence of multiple endocrine tumors. Pheochromocytomas, which are commonly bilateral, should be treated first because they can be life threatening and pose risks for surgery of the other tumors. Thyroid and parathyroid surgery must be aggressive because all glandular tissue may be involved.

An essential feature of appropriate clinical management in MEN type II is evaluation of family members, since these tumors are transmitted in an autosomal dominant pattern. Family members must be re-evaluated periodically because of the varying penetrance of the component tumors. Calcitonin measurement remains the diagnostic procedure of choice. Genetic linkage techniques utilizing restriction fragment length polymorphism (RFLP) are increasingly used to identify individuals at risk for the syndrome.

CALCITONIN AS A DRUG

Calcitonin's primary biologic effect of inhibiting osteoclastic bone resorption makes it useful in treating disorders characterized by increased bone resorption and certain forms of hypercalcemia.

TABLE 236–1. COMPONENTS OF MULTIPLE ENDOCRINE NEOPLASIA TYPE II AND THEIR FREQUENCY BASED ON AVERAGE FIGURES FROM THE LITERATURE

Component	MEN Type IIA (%)	MEN Type IIB (%)
Medullary thyroid carcinoma	97	90
Pheochromocytoma	30	45
Hyperparathyroidism	50	Rare
Mucosal neuroma syndrome	—	100

Thus, CT can be prescribed for treating Paget's disease, osteoporosis, and the hypercalcemia associated with malignancy. Both salmon CT and human CT are available, the former being more potent and the latter being less antigenic. Calcitonin is safer than most treatment alternatives, but its effects can be transient. The inconvenience of repeated parenteral administration may be avoided by newer preparations of the peptide.

Burns DM, Birnbaum RS, Roos BA: A neuroendocrine peptide derived from the amino terminal half of rat procalcitonin. Mol Endocrinol 3:140, 1989. *An exposition of the complexities of CT gene expression.*

Deftos LJ: Radioimmunoassay for calcitonin in medullary thyroid carcinoma. JAMA 227:403, 1974. *Early study of the application of CT radioimmunoassay to the diagnosis of MTC.*

Deftos LJ, Roos BA: Medullary thyroid carcinoma and calcitonin gene expression. Bone Miner Res 6:267, 1989. *A detailed exposition of multiple endocrine neoplasia and the regulation of calcitonin-gene products.*

Grauer A, Raue F, Gagel RF: Changing concepts in the management of hereditary and sporadic medullary thyroid carcinoma. Endocrinol Metab Clin North Am 19:613, 1990. *A review of current management approaches.*

Kramer JB, Wells SA Jr: Thyroid carcinoma. Adv Surg 22:195, 1989. *A review of surgical management of medullary thyroid carcinoma.*

Melvin KEW, Tashjian AH Jr, Miller HH: Studies in familial medullary carcinoma. Rec Prog Horm Res 28:399, 1972. *Classic study of MTC.*

Sobol H, Narod SA, Nakamura Y, et al.: Screening for MEN Type IIA with DNA-polymorphism analyses. N Engl J Med 321:996, 1989. *The application of RFLP to genetic analyses in MEN.*

237 Renal Osteodystrophy

Eduardo Slatopolsky

Renal osteodystrophy refers to the complex lesions of bone that are present in the majority of patients with advanced renal failure. The main components of renal osteodystrophy are osteitis fibrosa and osteomalacia (Table 237–1). A lesser role is played by osteosclerosis and osteoporosis. Osteitis fibrosa, a consequence of an increased level of parathyroid hormone (PTH), is characterized by an increase in the number of osteoclasts and an increase in bone resorption and marrow fibrosis. Osteomalacia, a condition secondary in part to alterations in vitamin D metabolism, results from a decreased mineralization of osteoid tissue (shown histologically by an abnormal calcification front in bone). Osteosclerosis is due to localized areas of mineralized woven bone which appear as increased bone density on radiographic studies. Osteoporosis, defined as a decrease in the mass of normally mineralized bone, is an infrequent and minor component of renal osteodystrophy.

OSTEITIS FIBROSA

Secondary hyperparathyroidism occurs universally in chronic renal disease. Chief cell hyperplasia of the parathyroid glands and high levels of immunoreactive parathyroid hormone (i-PTH) are among the earliest findings affecting mineral metabolism in patients with chronic renal failure. Several factors contribute to the development of secondary hyperparathyroidism in renal insufficiency (Table 237–1 and Fig. 237–1).

TABLE 237–1. FOUR COMPONENTS OF RENAL OSTEODYSTROPHY

1. Osteitis fibrosa (secondary hyperparathyroidism)
   a. Phosphate retention
   b. Altered metabolism of vitamin D
   c. Skeletal resistance to PTH
   d. Impaired degradation of PTH
   e. Altered feedback regulation of PTH by Ca^{2+}
2. Osteomalacia
   a. Altered metabolism of vitamin D
   b. Altered synthesis and maturation of collagen
   c. Acidosis
   d. Increased bone magnesium
   e. Increased pyrophosphate
   f. Retention of aluminum
   g. Retention of iron
3. Osteosclerosis ⎫
4. Osteoporosis   ⎬ of lesser quantitative importance

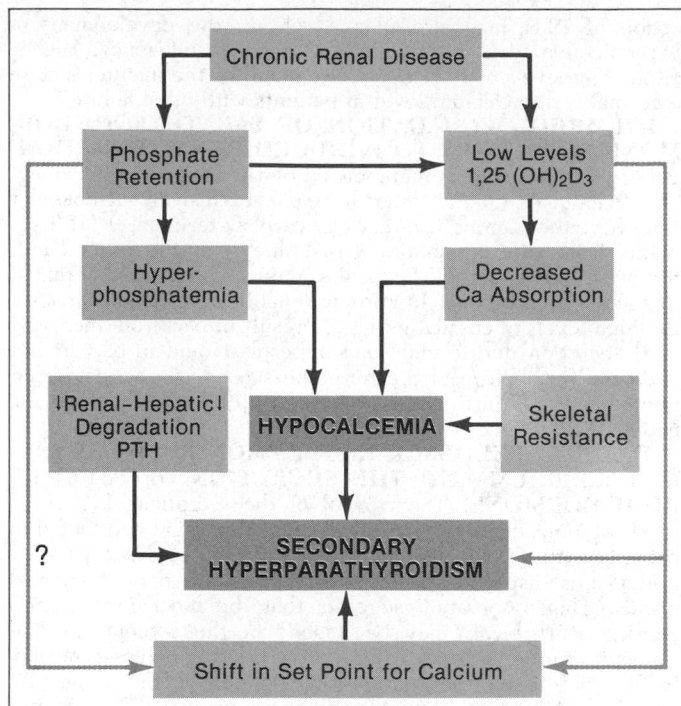

FIGURE 237–1. Diagrammatic representation of the factors involved in the pathogenesis of secondary hyperparathyroidism.

PHOSPHATE RETENTION. An important role of phosphate retention in producing secondary hyperparathyroidism is firmly established. Long-term feeding of a diet high in phosphate to animals with normal renal function can produce secondary hyperparathyroidism. Conversely, restriction of dietary phosphate can prevent the development of secondary hyperparathyroidism in chronic renal failure. The effect of phosphate retention on the parathyroid glands is mediated by lowering the concentration of ionized calcium in extracellular fluid, which in turn results from (1) the complexing of ionized calcium by phosphate; (2) a decreased renal production of calcitriol ($1,25(OH)_2D_3$), the active metabolite of vitamin D; and (3) a direct effect of phosphate on bone, decreasing calcium mobilization from the skeleton. In patients with far-advanced renal failure (a glomerular filtration rate [GFR] less than 20 ml per minute), correction of hyperphosphatemia alone does not completely reverse secondary hyperparathyroidism, since many other factors also contribute to the increased PTH levels in blood.

ALTERATIONS IN VITAMIN D METABOLISM (see also Ch. 233). Renal osteodystrophy may arise in part because of defective renal production of the active form of vitamin D in advanced renal failure. The liver hydroxylates vitamin D_3 to 25-hydroxycholecalciferol ($25(OH)D_3$), the predominant form of vitamin D_3 present in plasma. The $25(OH)D_3$ is further hydroxylated to $1,25(OH)_2D_3$, also termed calcitriol, by a specific hydroxylase enzyme found in the mitochondrial fraction of the renal proximal tubular cells. Parathyroid hormone and low-phosphate diets stimulate the activity of this hydroxylase; lack of PTH, hyperphosphatemia, or hypercalcemia decreases the activity of the hydroxylase. Intestinal absorption of calcium is reduced in patients with far-advanced renal insufficiency, and low levels of calcitriol are found in serum as the probable cause. Calcium malabsorption is usually present in patients with GFR's less than 40 ml per minute. In addition, it is now well accepted that calcitriol has a direct effect on the synthesis and secretion of PTH. The main action is inhibition of PTH gene transcription and synthesis of Pre-pro PTH messenger RNA (mRNA). Low levels of calcitriol observed in patients with chronic renal failure could potentially play a role in the development of secondary hyperparathyroidism.

SKELETAL RESISTANCE TO THE ACTION OF PARATHYROID HORMONE. Skeletal resistance to the calcemic action of PTH may also play a role in the development of hypocalcemia seen in patients with renal insufficiency. Higher circulating levels of PTH may be needed for the maintenance of a normal serum calcium level in patients with renal failure.

IMPAIRED DEGRADATION OF PARATHYROID HORMONE SECONDARY TO REDUCED RENAL FUNCTION. Parathyroid hormone is metabolized by the liver and the kidney. The liver takes up the intact hormone exclusively; it does not remove either amino-terminal or carboxy-terminal PTH fragments from the circulation. The kidney, on the other hand, removes both intact PTH and the amino- and carboxy-terminal fragments from plasma. In chronic renal insufficiency, therefore, the high levels of circulating i-PTH result in part from increased PTH secretion due to chief cell hyperplasia and in part from a decreased catabolism of the hormone secondary to a decreased number of nephrons. There also seems to be decreased hepatic metabolism of intact PTH.

ALTERED FEEDBACK REGULATION BETWEEN IONIZED CALCIUM AND THE SECRETION OF PARATHYROID HORMONE. The control of the secretion of PTH by levels of ionized calcium in extracellular fluid may be blunted in patients with chronic renal insufficiency. Hyperplastic parathyroid glands display less sensitivity to calcium than do normal glands. This observation suggests that the mechanism for increased PTH levels may be a shift in the setpoint for the concentration of ionized calcium as well as the increased mass of parathyroid tissue. The setpoint is defined as the amount of calcium necessary to suppress the secretion of PTH by 50 per cent. Thus, normal concentrations of ionized calcium may not suffice to suppress the release of PTH by the hyperplastic glands of patients with secondary hyperparathyroidism. Low levels of calcitriol play a role in this abnormal setpoint for calcium-regulated PTH secretion.

OSTEOMALACIA

Osteomalacia is defined as an increase in the osteoid seam width accompanied by a decrease in the mineralization front. The presence of excess osteoid per se does not necessarily indicate osteomalacia. An increase in osteoid tissue may be secondary to the abnormal mineralization of osteomalacia, or it may be due to an increased rate of synthesis of bone collagen that is normally mineralized. The use of double tetracycline labeling of the calcification front in vivo can differentiate between these two possibilities. The use of this technique and quantitative bone histology is critical to the diagnosis of osteomalacia. The mechanisms by which deficiency of vitamin D leads to impaired mineralization of bone are poorly understood. Whether vitamin D or calcitriol can directly stimulate bone mineralization or whether it leads to mineralization only by increasing the levels of calcium and phosphate in the extracellular fluid surrounding bone is uncertain. Although the plasma levels of calcitriol are reduced in patients with far-advanced renal insufficiency, overt osteomalacia is found in only a small fraction of such patients and may be absent even in anephric patients. Thus, other factors could also participate in the pathogenesis of osteomalacia in uremic patients—for example, the plasma level of phosphate. Hypophosphatemia per se can produce severe osteomalacia even in patients with normal renal function. Additional factors include alterations in collagen synthesis and maturation, defective bone crystal maturation, increased bone magnesium concentrations, elevated levels of pyrophosphate, and diminished calcium carbonate levels. The combination of these factors may influence the maturation of bone and potentially contribute to the development of osteomalacia. Acidosis also contributes to the skeletal disease. In chronic renal insufficiency the skeleton assists in buffering the retained acids. Administration of bicarbonate and correction of the acidosis in azotemic patients can reduce fecal calcium excretion.

Another type of osteomalacia in renal insufficiency, one that is resistant to vitamin D therapy, is caused by an excess of aluminum. Patients with osteomalacia secondary to aluminum have pathologic fractures, complain of severe bone pain, and characteristically have low levels of PTH. The source may be a high aluminum content in the water and/or the ingestion of phosphate binders containing aluminum. The aluminum is deposited in the interface between the osteoid tissue and the calcification front and has a toxic effect on the osteoblast. Severe iron retention can induce a similar form of osteomalacia.

Finally, after total parathyroidectomy the lack of PTH in patients results in low bone turnover and may sometimes precipitate the development of osteomalacia.

CLINICAL MANIFESTATIONS

The symptoms related to renal osteodystrophy usually appear only when renal failure is advanced. On the other hand, certain biochemical alterations may appear early in the course of renal insufficiency. Knowledge of the presence of these alterations may help the physician to introduce treatment early in the course of renal failure and in this way to prevent severe complications in bone and mineral metabolism.

Bone pain can develop and progress slowly to a point where the patient is bedridden, without regard to whether the bone disease is predominantly osteitis fibrosa or osteomalacia. The bone pain is generally vague and commonly located in the lower back, hips, knees, and legs. Low back pain may result from the collapse of a vertebral body, and sharp chest pain may indicate spontaneous rib fracture. Physical findings are frequently lacking.

Muscular weakness, when present, is usually proximal, appears slowly, and progresses with time. Plasma levels of muscle enzymes, creatine phosphokinase, and transaminases are usually normal, and the electron micrographic changes are nonspecific. The pathogenesis of such muscular weakness is uncertain. In patients with myopathy, the myofibrils are disorganized in a patchy fashion and the Z-band material may be dispersed. These changes revert to normal following treatment with $25(OH)D_3$. *Pruritus* due to calcium deposition in skin is a common symptom in uremic patients, particularly with severe secondary hyperparathyroidism.

Vascular calcification and peripheral ischemic necrosis may occur, producing lesions of the tips of the toes and fingers and violaceous discoloration of the skin. Ulcerations and scar formation may occur, with clear demarcation of the lesions from the surrounding skin. Acute pain and swelling around one or more joints may also develop in uremic patients. The syndrome of *calcific periarthritis*, which may be caused by deposition of hydroxyapatite crystals, is accompanied by marked hyperphosphatemia.

Skeletal deformities are common in azotemic children who are growing. Bowing of the tibia and femur and deformities from slipped epiphyses are not uncommon. Children with renal rickets sometimes exhibit typical radiographic findings of vitamin D deficiency. In adults with renal failure, particularly those with osteomalacia, marked skeletal deformities with lumbar scoliosis, thoracic kyphosis, and deformity of the thoracic cage may be observed. Growth retardation is usually seen in young children before and during maintenance hemodialysis. See Chapter 234 for a further discussion of osteomalacia and rickets.

Another clinical manifestation of renal osteodystrophy that occurs in some patients after renal transplantation is aseptic necrosis of the head of the femur. This condition is more frequently seen in patients with severe bone disease (osteitis fibrosa) before renal transplantation and in those who receive very large doses of glucocorticoids.

BIOCHEMICAL FEATURES

Circulating i-PTH is elevated early in the course of renal insufficiency (a GFR of 60 to 80 ml per minute). As the disease progresses (a GFR less than 40 ml per minute), hypocalcemia and low levels of calcitriol appear. With advanced renal insufficiency, however, the serum calcium level may remain close to normal and values below 7.5 mg per deciliter are infrequent. Usually, hypocalcemia is more marked in severe osteomalacia or with profound metabolic acidosis. Occasionally, hypercalcemia may be observed in uremic patients, particularly in those undergoing long-term dialysis. This complication can arise from (1) severe hyperparathyroidism, (2) the ingestion of large amounts of calcium and vitamin D, (3) the presence of unrelated diseases, such as sarcoidosis or malignancies, or (4) a "pure" mineralizing defect, as may occur in osteomalacia secondary to aluminum retention. Hyperphosphatemia is usually present in patients with a GFR less than 25 ml per minute. The degree of hyperphosphatemia depends on the amount of phosphate ingested, the fraction absorbed in the intestine, and that excreted into the urine. If the patient ingests phosphate binders, the serum phosphate level may remain normal despite advanced renal insufficiency. Patients with severe hyperparathyroidism and advanced renal insufficiency usually have higher concentrations of serum phosphate in plasma.

Advanced renal insufficiency (a GFR less than 15 ml per minute) may be associated with hypermagnesemia and an increased content of magnesium in bone. This may adversely affect crystal formation.

Total serum alkaline phosphatase levels are commonly higher in uremic patients with osteitis fibrosa than in those with osteomalacia. Coexistent liver disease should be excluded as a cause of an elevated alkaline phosphatase level.

RADIOGRAPHIC FEATURES

Secondary hyperparathyroidism increases bone resorption, most commonly evident on the subperiosteal surfaces of bone. Erosions that occur in conjunction with formation of new bone may appear as cysts or osteoclastomas (brown tumors). The presence of subperiosteal erosion correlates with serum i-PTH and with the histomorphometric features of osteitis fibrosa on bone biopsy. Subperiosteal resorption of the phalanges may be the most sensitive radiographic sign of secondary hyperparathyroidism. The tuft of the terminal phalanx or the second or third digit commonly shows resorption. With severe tuft erosion there may be a collapse of the soft tissue and change in the contour of the tuft, so that the finger appears to show clubbing. Bone erosions may also occur at the upper end of the tibia, the neck of the femur or the humerus, and the lower surface of the medial end of the clavicle. In the skull, resorption leads to the mottled and granular appearance commonly associated with altering areas of osteosclerosis.

Osteosclerosis is thought to be another feature of osteitis fibrosa arising from an increase in the thickness and number of trabeculae in spongy bone. Osteosclerosis can lead to a typical "rugger jersey" appearance of the spine.

Osteomalacia is far less distinctive radiographically than is secondary hyperparathyroidism. The Looser zone or pseudofracture is the only pathognomonic radiographic finding of osteomalacia in the adult (Fig. 234–2). Rickets, i.e., widening of the epiphyseal growth plate, cannot develop after epiphyseal closure and hence is limited to children. With mechanical stress following severe prolonged deficiency of vitamin D, a Looser zone may extend across the full width of the bone and produce a true fracture with displacement of fragments. In uremia, osteomalacia is commonly associated with secondary hyperparathyroidism, with concomitant radiographic features of both. The diagnosis of osteomalacia rests on histologic examinations and can be established with certainty only by bone biopsy.

Soft tissue calcification is presumed to be influenced by an increase in the calcium phosphate product in plasma, the degree of secondary hyperparathyroidism, the magnitude of alkalosis, and local tissue injury. Three major varieties include (1) calcification of the medium-sized arteries, (2) articular or tumoral calcifications, and (3) visceral calcifications affecting the heart, lung, and kidney.

TREATMENT

The objectives of the treatment of patients with renal osteodystrophy are (1) to return the blood levels of calcium and phosphate to normal; (2) to suppress secondary hyperparathyroidism; (3) to reverse the histologic abnormalities in the skeleton; and (4) to prevent and reverse extraskeletal deposits of calcium and phosphate. Guidelines for the management of renal osteodystrophy are summarized in Table 237–2.

CONTROL OF PHOSPHATE AND CALCIUM. To control phosphate, dietary phosphate intake should be reduced to 700 to 800 mg per day (determined as phosphorus) by restricting the ingestion of dairy products and by decreasing the amount of protein in the diet. In advanced renal failure, in addition to dietary control, phosphate binders are usually required to reduce its intestinal absorption. Phosphate binders should be ingested along with the meal to increase their efficiency. The use of aluminum-containing gels carries the potential of excessive alu-

---

TABLE 237–2. GUIDELINES FOR MANAGEMENT OF RENAL OSTEODYSTROPHY

Early Treatment
It is important to begin treatment early, i.e., when the GFR is 30 to 40 ml/min, especially for the control of serum phosphate.

Control of Serum Phosphate (P) (3.5 to 4.5 mg/dl)
Restrict phosphorus intake in diet to 600 to 800 mg/day
Phosphate-binding antacids: aluminum carbonate or hydroxide; individualize dosage: Basaljel, Dialume, Alucap, Amphogel, 1–4 capsules with each meal; minimize the use of aluminum binders
Calcium carbonate: 1–3 grams with each meal
Hypophosphatemia should be avoided
Predialysis phosphorus: 4.5–5.5 mg/dl

Adequate Calcium Intake
Oral calcium supplements providing 1–2 grams/day when serum P is controlled: Os-Cal, Titralac
Dialysate calcium, 6.0–6.5 mg per dl (3.0–3.25 mEq/liter)

Use of Vitamin D Sterols
Vitamin D_2 or D_3, 50,000 to 250,000 IU (1.25 to 6.25 mg)/day
Dihydrotachysterol, 0.25–2.0 mg/day
25-Hydroxyvitamin D_3 (calcifediol), 20–100 μg/day (Calderol)
1,25-Dihydroxyvitamin D_3 (calcitriol), 0.5–1.0 μg/day (Rocaltrol)
1,25-Dihydroxyvitamin D_3 (calcitriol) IV, 1.0–3.0 μg 3 times/wk (Calcijex)

Parathyroidectomy: Severe secondary hyperparathyroidism (bone erosions and increased i-PTH) plus any of the following:
Persistent hypercalcemia (serum calcium > 11.5 to 12.0 mg/dl)
Progressive or symptomatic extraskeletal calcification
Persistently elevated serum calcium-phosphorus product
Pruritus not responsive to medical treatment
Calciphylaxis (ischemic ulcers and necrosis)
Symptomatic hypercalcemia after renal transplantation

---

minum absorption and accumulation. They should, therefore, be used with caution. If the patient develops symptoms and signs suggesting aluminum-induced osteomalacia, this drug should be discounted. If phosphate is not controlled, the patient will develop severe secondary hyperparathyroidism and extraskeletal calcification. Calcium carbonate (1 to 3 grams with each meal) helps to bind phosphate and thereby reduces the amount of aluminum binders needed for the treatment of hyperphosphatemia. During treatment with oral calcium carbonate, it is important to determine the total amount of phosphate ingested during 24 hours and during each meal. In this way the relative amount of calcium carbonate given can be adjusted to the phosphate-binding requirements of specific meals. Calcium carbonate also provides a calcium supplement that helps correct the negative calcium balance secondary to the calcium malabsorption of advanced renal insufficiency. The serum phosphorus level should be maintained at normal or nearly normal levels, between 3.5 and 4.5 mg per deciliter, if the patient is not yet on dialysis. The serum calcium concentration should be maintained in the upper limits of normal. Severe hyperphosphatemia should be corrected before the administration of calcium to reduce the risk of metastatic calcification. Supplemental calcium should be discontinued if the serum calcium level increases above 11.0 mg per deciliter. The concentration of calcium in the dialysate affects serum calcium levels during maintenance hemodialysis. In patients ingesting large amounts of calcium carbonate, the ideal calcium concentration in the dialysate is between 5.0 and 5.5 mg per deciliter.

USE OF VITAMIN D AND ITS METABOLITES. Despite dietary control of phosphate, the use of phosphate binders, an adequate dietary calcium intake, and appropriate levels of calcium in the dialysate, uremic patients may still develop skeletal disease. Thus, vitamin D and its metabolites are important and effective agents in the treatment of renal osteodystrophy. Calcitriol, the most active metabolite of vitamin D, is the drug of choice in the treatment of hypocalcemia and secondary hyperparathyroidism (see Ch. 235). The usual dose is 0.5 to 1 μg per day. Calcitriol, given intravenously during dialysis, at the dosage of 1 to 3 μg three times per week, is the best approach to suppress secondary hyperparathyroidism. If osteomalacia predominates on bone biopsy, excellent results have been obtained with the use of $25(OH)D_3$ (20 to 100 μg per day) in addition to calcitriol. With the use of vitamin D or its metabolites, hypercalcemia and, less frequently, hyperphosphatemia may occur as side effects.

PARATHYROIDECTOMY. The regimen outlined above can lead to improved homeostasis of calcium and phosphorus and reverse the symptoms of bone disease and suppression of PTH secretion. Such measures may not be entirely successful, however, and parathyroidectomy may be required. Indications for parathyroid surgery include severe secondary hyperparathyroidism (bone erosions and high levels of i-PTH) in the presence of any of the following: (1) persistent hypercalcemia, particularly when symptomatic; (2) intractable pruritus that does not respond to dialysis or other medical treatment; (3) progressive extraskeletal calcification in conjunction with a high calcium-phosphorus product that is consistently about 75 to 80 despite appropriate phosphate restriction; and (4) the appearance of ischemic lesions of soft tissues. Because of lack of compliance, many patients are unable to control their serum phosphorus levels. In these cases neither calcium supplements nor vitamin D or its metabolites can be recommended safely. Such patients are more likely to develop severe secondary hyperparathyroidism and require parathyroidectomy. Postoperative hypocalcemia may pose a problem if the remaining parathyroid tissue is inadequate and if severe osteitis fibrosa is present preoperatively. Preoperative treatment of such patients with calcitriol (1 to 2 μg per day) may prevent such problems. Serum levels of phosphorus and magnesium sometimes decrease after parathyroidectomy. Aluminum-containing phosphate binders should be withheld if the serum phosphorus level falls below 3.0 mg per deciliter. Rapid remineralization of the skeleton occurs during this period, but once the "hungry bones" have been mineralized, serum calcium levels will rise. A fall in a previously elevated serum alkaline phosphatase toward normal may indicate that rapid skeletal remineralization is nearly complete and that calcium supplements and vitamin D therapy may be reduced or discontinued. In the past, the removal of 3½ parathyroid glands was the procedure of choice. More recently, total parathyroidectomy followed by autotransplantation of some of the parathyroid tissue into the patient's forearm has been utilized. The transplanted tissue is more accessible if subsequent surgical removal is necessary. Total parathyroidectomy without autotransplantation has no place in the management of renal osteodystrophy, since it may predispose to the development of an isolated mineralization defect or osteomalacia in uremic patients. Cryopreservation of removed parathyroid tissue is a useful precaution so that hypoparathyroidism may be treated by reimplantation of parathyroid tissue.

Occasionally after a successful renal transplantation, the patient may develop hypercalcemia. Usually this is due to persistent hyperparathyroidism and increased renal production of calcitriol. In the majority of cases, the hypercalcemia subsides several months after renal transplantation. In some patients, however, severe hypercalcemia (a calcium level of 12 to 13 mg per deciliter) may persist for several months and may affect renal function. In these patients a subtotal parathyroidectomy is recommended.

TREATMENT OF ALUMINUM TOXICITY. If the patient has aluminum-induced osteomalacia, phosphate binders containing aluminum should be discontinued at once. Phosphate should be controlled by using a diet more restrictive in phosphate, and the serum phosphorus level may be allowed to increase to 6 mg per deciliter. Desferoxamine, a drug used for the treatment of iron excess, also chelates aluminum, and its use may relieve aluminum-induced osteomalacia.

Coburn JW, Slatopolsky E: Vitamin D, parathyroid hormone and renal osteodystrophy. *In* Brenner BM, Rector FC (eds.): The Kidney. 4th ed. Philadelphia, W.B. Saunders Company, 1990, pp 2036–2120.

Massry SG: Divalent ion metabolism and renal osteodystrophy. *In* Massry SG, Glassock RJ (eds.): Textbook of Nephrology. Baltimore, The Williams & Wilkins Company, 1983, pp 7.104–7.148.

Slatopolsky E, Weerts C, Norwood K, et al.: Long-term effects of calcium carbonate and 2.5 mEq/liter calcium dialysate on mineral metabolism. Kidney Int 36:897, 1989.

238 Osteoporosis

B. Lawrence Riggs

GENERAL CONSIDERATIONS

Osteoporosis is defined pathologically as an absolute decrease in the amount of bone, leading to fractures after minimal trauma. The disease causes 1.5 million fractures and costs $10 billion in the United States each year. The most common sites of fracture are the vertebrae, distal radius (Colles' fracture), and hip. One third of women over age 65 will have vertebral fractures. By extreme old age, one in every three women and one in every six men will have had a hip fracture; of these, 20 per cent die and another 30 per cent require long-term domiciliary care.

After maximal skeletal mass is achieved in young adulthood, there is a period of stability before bone loss begins. Two distinct phases of bone loss can be recognized: a slow, age-related phase that occurs in both sexes and an accelerated phase that occurs in postmenopausal women. The slow phase begins at about age 35 and continues well into old age, has a similar rate in both sexes, and results in losses of similar amounts of cortical and cancellous bone. Cortical bone predominates in the appendicular skeleton, whereas cancellous bone is concentrated in the axial skeleton, particularly in the vertebrae, and in the ends of the long bones. A transient accelerated postmenopausal phase, caused by estrogen deficiency, is superimposed in women and results in a loss of disproportionately more cancellous than cortical bone. The bone loss declines exponentially with time, and most of the bone is lost during the first 4 to 8 years after menopause.

ETIOLOGY

General

The main underlying cause of fractures in osteoporosis is increased bone fragility as a result of bone loss. Fracture risk is determined by absolute bone density, regardless of age. In the absence of severe trauma, fractures do not occur until bone density has fallen below the values found in young adults (about 1.0 gram per square centimeter for both vertebrae and femur). With further decreases in bone density below the fracture threshold, the incidence of fractures increases. In addition, the increased propensity of the elderly to fall is an independent cause of fractures.

The main factors contributing to osteoporosis are shown in Figure 238–1 and are discussed below.

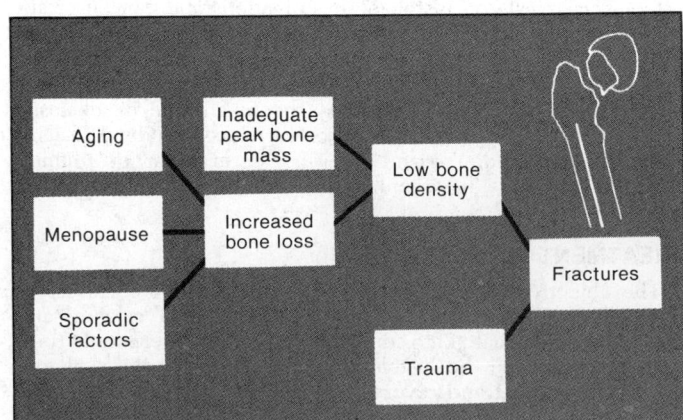

FIGURE 238–1. Model for the pathogenesis of osteoporosis. The major cause of fractures in osteoporosis is a decrease in absolute bone density. In the elderly, trauma due to an increased propensity to fall and an impaired ability to break the fall further increases the incidence of fractures. Low bone density can occur later in life because the amount of bone formed by the completion of growth in young adulthood was inadequate or the rate of bone loss was increased. The latter is a result of the cumulative effect of factors related to aging (that are universally present), of the menopause (in women), and of various sporadic factors (that are present in some but not in other individuals).

Initial Bone Density

Insufficient accumulation of bone mass during skeletal growth predisposes to fractures later in life as age-related bone loss ensues. Differences in bone density at skeletal maturity explain, in part, the racial and sexual differences in the incidence of osteoporosis that have been observed. White women have the lightest skeletons, and black men have the heaviest; white men and black women have skeletons of intermediate density. This rank order corresponds to the rank order for the occurrence of fractures. Women of short stature and of northern European extraction tend to have a more gracile skeleton and also to have an increased incidence of osteoporosis later in life. Moreover, if the rate of bone loss with age is constant, those white women with the lowest bone density values at skeletal maturity are at the greatest risk for fracture in later life. The amount of bone present in young adulthood has been shown to have strong genetic determinants, and the premenopausal daughters of osteoporotic women have lower bone density than do age-matched control women.

Age-Related Factors

Age-related factors are responsible for the slow phase of bone loss. Three age-related factors seem particularly important. First, from the fourth decade onward bone formation is decreased at the cellular level (each osteoblast does less work), and this abnormality becomes more severe with age. Second, as a consequence of impaired calcium absorption, concentrations of serum intact parathyroid hormone increase with aging by about 30 per cent. Impaired calcium absorption is most prominent after age 70 and appears to be caused by impaired metabolism of vitamin D or decreased tissue responsiveness to its active metabolites. The secondary hyperparathyroidism increases overall skeletal turnover (more bone remodeling units are formed), but because of the impairment in osteoblast function, this exacerbates the bone loss. Finally, nutritional vitamin D deficiency may contribute to bone loss in some elderly persons.

Menopause

The excess loss attributable to menopause may be 10 to 15 per cent for the appendicular skeleton and 15 to 20 per cent for the vertebrae. A form of functional hypogonadism associated with decreased vertebral density has been described in female long-distance runners. Postmenopausal administration of estrogen decreases the occurrence of fractures associated with osteoporosis by about one half. Men do not undergo the equivalent of menopause, but gonadal function does decline in some elderly men, and overt hypogonadism is often associated with vertebral fractures.

Sporadic Factors

When present, these sporadic factors increase the rate of bone loss. Smoking and high alcohol consumption increase the risk of developing osteoporosis twofold. Ethanol is toxic to osteoblasts. Obesity is protective, possibly because of increased loading stress to the spine and, in postmenopausal women, because of increased conversion (in fat tissue) of adrenal androgens to estrogens. Nutritional factors may also be important, although this is controversial. Some data suggest that premenopausal women require a calcium intake of 1000 mg per day and postmenopausal women require 1500 mg per day to maintain calcium balance. These levels are well above the average intake—550 mg per day—in middle-aged and elderly women. A high protein intake may decrease retention of dietary calcium, possibly because acid radicals increase urinary calcium excretion.

OSTEOPOROSIS SYNDROMES

Osteoporosis can be classified as primary or secondary, depending on the absence or presence of an associated medical condition known to cause bone loss (Table 238–1). Secondary causes of osteoporosis can be identified in 20 per cent of women and 40 per cent of men presenting with vertebral fractures and should always be sought. Primary osteoporosis may occur, although rarely, in prepubertal boys and girls (juvenile osteoporosis) and characteristically runs an acute clinical course for 2 to 4 years. A spontaneous remission then ensues, followed by resumption of bone growth. An uncommon primary form of

TABLE 238–1. CLASSIFICATION OF CAUSES OF OSTEOPOROSIS

Primary osteoporosis	**Bone marrow disorders**
Juvenile	Multiple myeloma and related
Idiopathic (young adults)	disorders
Involutional osteoporosis	Systemic mastocytosis
Endocrine diseases	Disseminated carcinoma
Hypogonadism	**Connective tissue diseases**
Ovarian agenesis	Osteogenesis imperfecta
Glucocorticoid excess	Homocystinuria
Hyperthyroidism	Ehlers-Danlos syndrome
Hyperparathyroidism	Marfan's syndrome
Diabetes mellitus (?)	**Miscellaneous causes**
Gastrointestinal diseases	Immobilization
Subtotal gastrectomy	Chronic obstructive pulmonary
Malabsorption syndromes	disease
Chronic obstructive jaundice	Chronic alcoholism
Primary biliary cirrhosis	Rheumatoid arthritis (?)
Severe malnutrition	Chronic heparin administration
Alactasia	Chronic administration of
	anticonvulsant drugs (?)

osteoporosis occurs in young adults of either sex (idiopathic osteoporosis) and undoubtedly is heterogeneous etiologically. The main manifestation is vertebral fracture, although fractures of the ribs and appendicular skeleton may also occur. The clinical course may be mild but more often is severe, progressive, and relatively refractory to standard therapy.

The common primary form of osteoporosis, termed "involutional osteoporosis," begins in middle life and becomes increasingly more common with advancing age. Involutional osteoporosis can be separated into two major types based on differences in clinical presentation, in densitometric and hormonal changes, and in the relationship of disease patterns to menopause and aging.

TYPE I ("POSTMENOPAUSAL") OSTEOPOROSIS

This form of the disease typically affects women within 15 to 20 years after menopause. Vertebral fractures and Colles' fractures are the main clinical manifestations. The vertebral fractures are often of the "crush type" and are associated with large deformation and pain. The skeletal sites of these manifestations—vertebral body and the ultradistal radius—contain large amounts of trabecular bone. In patients with type I osteoporosis, the rate of trabecular bone loss is usually two to three times the normal rate, but the rate of cortical bone loss is only slightly above normal. During this accelerated phase, trabecular plate perforation with loss of structural trabeculae weakens the vertebrae and predisposes to acute collapse. Bone turnover is usually high; bone resorption is increased, with inadequate compensatory bone formation. Some osteoporotic women have low bone turnover; these women may have reached a "burned-out" stage and will have little further loss of cancellous bone.

Type I osteoporosis appears to be caused by factors closely related to or exacerbated by menopause. This situation leads to the following cascade: accelerated bone loss, decreased secretion of parathyroid hormone and increased secretion of calcitonin, and functional impairment in 25OHD 1α-hydroxylase activity with decreased production of $1,25(OH)_2D$, therefore leading to decreased calcium absorption. The defect in calcium absorption may further aggravate bone loss. All women are estrogen deficient after menopause, however, and serum levels of sex steroids are similar in postmenopausal women with and without type I osteoporosis. Thus, other factors must augment the rate or duration of the accelerated phase of bone loss; these factors interact with estrogen deficiency to determine individual susceptibility.

TYPE II ("AGE-RELATED") OSTEOPOROSIS

This syndrome occurs in men and women age 70 or older and results from the slow phase of bone loss. It is manifested mainly by hip and vertebral fractures, although fractures of the proximal humerus, proximal tibia, and pelvis are common. The vertebral fractures are often of the multiple-wedge type, leading to dorsal

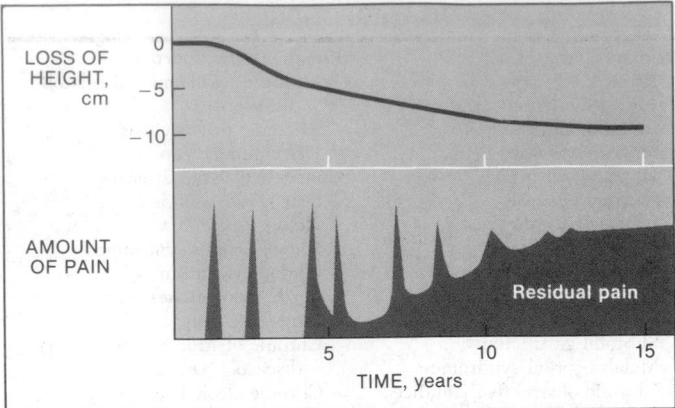

FIGURE 238–2. Clinical course of an untreated or unsuccessfully treated patient with osteoporosis. Upper panel shows continued loss of height. Lower panel shows occurrence of back pain, which is at first acute and intermittent but later chronic.

kyphosis ("dowager's hump"). Thinning of trabeculae associated with the slow phase of bone loss is responsible for gradual and usually painless vertebral deformation. In type II osteoporosis, bone density values for the proximal femur, vertebrae, and sites in the appendicular skeleton are usually in the lower part of the normal range (adjusted for age and sex). This finding suggests proportionate losses of cortical and trabecular bone and a rate of loss that is only slightly higher than the mean for age-matched peers. The age-related processes causing type II osteoporosis affect virtually the entire population of aging men and women, and as the slow phase of bone loss progresses, an increasing number of them have bone density values below the fracture threshold. The two most important of these age-related factors are decreased osteoblast function and secondary hyperparathyroidism. The effects of all risk factors for bone loss encountered over a lifetime, however, are cumulative. Thus, the residual effects of accelerated bone loss after menopause many years before may explain why the incidence of hip fractures is twofold greater in elderly women than in elderly men, although rates of slow bone loss are similar in the two sexes. Conversely, the necessary contribution of age-related slow bone loss accounts for

the absence of an acute increase in the incidence of hip fractures in the immediate postmenopausal period.

CLINICAL CONSIDERATIONS

Clinical Presentation

Osteoporosis is manifested by back pain, loss of height, spinal deformity (especially kyphosis), and fractures of the vertebrae, hips, wrists, and, less frequently, other bones. The most characteristic symptom of osteoporosis is back pain caused by vertebral compression. Typically, a woman within 20 years after menopause develops acute lumbar or thoracic back pain after some ordinary activity, such as raising a window or lifting a sack of groceries. The pain may be mild or severe, and it may be localized or may radiate to the flank. It remits in days or weeks but then recurs with the occurrence of new fractures. After several episodes of acute intermittent pain, a chronic mechanical backache may develop as a result of spinal deformity (Fig. 238–2). In untreated or unsuccessfully treated patients, severe kyphosis may develop, with a loss of 4 to 8 inches of height. In severe cases, the ribcage comes to rest on the pelvic brim. The frequency of occurrence of vertebral fractures and the number of fractures that eventually occur vary widely among patients, but the average is one per year in the initial phase of the disease. In general, progression is slower in elderly women, and substantial dorsal kyphosis and cervical lordosis—the so-called dowager's hump—commonly develop in the absence of significant pain.

Radiologic Findings

Radiographs of the spinal column (Fig. 238–3) show accentuation of the vertebral end-plates, prominence of the weight-bearing vertical trabeculae (caused by disappearance of the horizontal trabeculae), and loss of contrast in radiodensity between the interior of the vertebral body and the adjacent soft tissue. Vertebral deformity may take the form of collapse (reduction of anterior and posterior height), anterior wedging (reduction in anterior height, usually occurring in the thoracic spinal column), or "ballooning" (biconcave compression of the end-plates by pressure of the intervertebral discs, usually occurring in the lumbar spinal column). In addition, the nucleus pulposus may herniate locally into the vertebral body (Schmorl's nodes). Osteoporosis caused by glucocorticoid excess should be considered when there is associated osteoporosis of the skull, fractures of the ribs and pelvic rami, and prominent partially mineralized callus at the site of fracture. In the absence of pseudofractures, osteomalacia may be difficult to distinguish from osteoporosis,

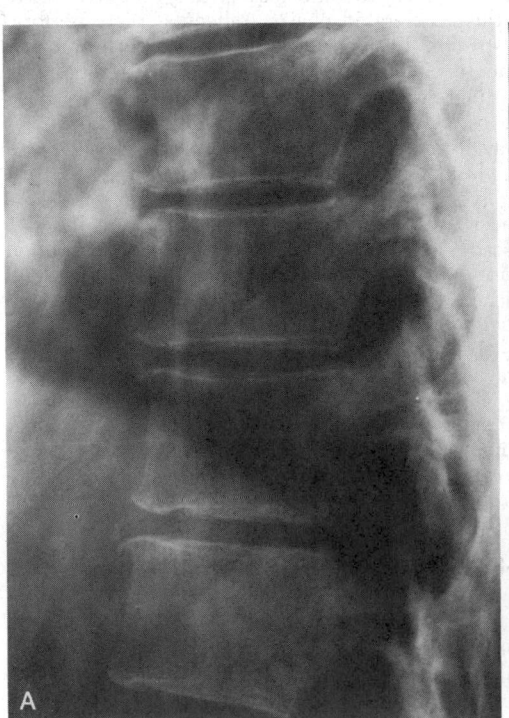

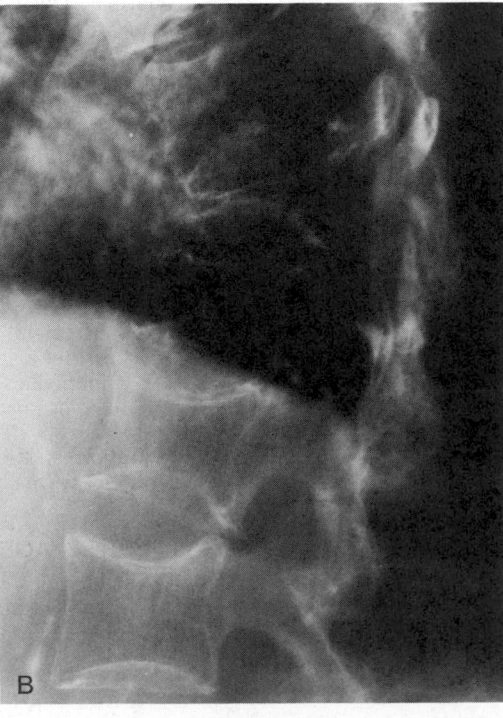

FIGURE 238–3. Radiographs of the spinal column. *A*, Normal bone in a 60-year-old woman. *B*, Vertebral osteoporosis in a 62-year-old woman. There is a decrease in bone density with high-grade collapse fractures of T12 and L1 and ballooning (expansion of the intervertebral discs) of L2 and L3.

but osteomalacia often has a ground glass appearance rather than the characteristic clear glass appearance of osteoporosis. Posterior wedging of a vertebra suggests a destructive lesion rather than osteoporosis.

Diagnostic Evaluation

All patients with newly discovered osteoporosis should have a general medical evaluation to assess severity and exclude secondary diseases that may cause the osteoporosis (Fig. 238–4). Systemic symptoms or abnormal physical findings suggest the presence of an underlying disease. Serum calcium and phosphorus levels are normal in primary osteoporosis. Serum alkaline phosphatase levels also are normal except for transient elevations during healing of vertebral fractures. Sustained elevation of the alkaline phosphatase level, in the absence of liver disease, suggests osteomalacia or skeletal metastasis.

Multiple myeloma may be present without symptoms and with a normal hematogram and erythrocyte sedimentation rate. Although most cases can be diagnosed by serum and urine protein electrophoresis, bone marrow examination may be required to establish its presence (Ch. 151). Sometimes bone marrow examination is also necessary to diagnose disseminated carcinoma.

The severity and the response to treatment can now be assessed directly by measurement of bone density. Three techniques are generally available—dual-photon absorptiometry (DPA), dual-energy x-ray absorptiometry (DEXA), and quantitative computed tomography (QCT)—all of which produce satisfactory clinical results (Table 238–2). Both DPA and DEXA utilize transmission scanning: The photons are generated with a ^{153}Gd source in DPA and an x-ray tube in DEXA. With DPA and DEXA, bone density can be measured at both the lumbar spine and the proximal femur. With QCT, only vertebral density can be assessed. However, unlike the other two methods, QCT can measure cancellous bone in the center of the vertebral body exclusively,

TABLE 238–2. MAJOR METHODS FOR MEASURING BONE MINERAL DENSITY OF THE AXIAL SKELETON

Feature	DPA	DEXA	QCT
Reproducibility (%)	2–4	1–2	3–5
Accuracy (%)	4	4	5–10
Radiation (mrem)	5–10	<5	200–500
Scan time (min)	30	10	10–20

DPA = dual-photon absorptiometry; DEXA = dual-energy x-ray absorptiometry; QCT = quantitative computed tomography.

and it is unaffected by artifacts such as vertebral osteophytes and aortic calcification. In assessing whether therapy has effectively arrested bone loss, measurements should be made at baseline and at yearly intervals during treatment.

Iliac trephine biopsy after double tetracycline labeling may be useful in selected patients to exclude osteomalacia and to assess bone turnover. The biopsy specimen should be processed by an experienced laboratory that will provide quantitative information. Recently, methods have been developed to assess bone turnover noninvasively. Serum osteocalcin, also called bone gla-protein, and serum bone isoenzyme of alkaline phosphatase are specific markers for bone formation. Urine deoxypyridinium reflects the excretion of unique crosslinks of collagen in bone and thus is a specific marker for bone resorption.

TREATMENT

General Therapeutic Measures

Acute back pain responds to analgesics, heat, and gentle massage to alleviate muscle spasm. Sometimes a brief period of bed rest is required. Chronic back pain often is caused by spinal deformity and thus is difficult to relieve completely. Instruction in posture and gait training and institution of regular back extension exercises to strengthen the flabby paravertebral muscles are usually beneficial. Occasionally, use of an orthopedic back brace is required. All patients with osteoporosis should have a diet adequate in calcium, proteins, and vitamins; should be reasonably active physically; and should take precautions to prevent falls.

Drug Therapy

Drugs used in the treatment of osteoporosis can be classified as antiresorptive or formation stimulating (Fig. 238–5). The drugs currently approved by the Food and Drug Administration for the treatment of osteoporosis—calcium, estrogen, and calcitonin—act by decreasing bone resorption. Antiresorptive drugs are most effective when bone turnover is high and have little effect when it is low.

Calcium, which may act by decreasing parathyroid hormone secretion, is safe, well tolerated, and inexpensive. *Vitamin D or its active metabolite, 1,25-dihydroxyvitamin D,* must be used judiciously, if at all, because the dosage that increases calcium absorption is not much smaller than the dosage that increases bone resorption.

Estrogen effectively reduces bone resorption but has significant untoward effects. These commonly include induction of menstruation, mastodynia, and fluid retention. Less common but more serious side effects are endometrial carcinoma, venous thrombosis and pulmonary embolism, aggravation of hypertension, and cholelithiasis. Some evidence suggests that long-term estrogen therapy increases the risk of breast cancer. Beneficial effects include relief of symptoms due to atrophy of estrogen-sensitive tissues and reduction in the risk of coronary artery disease. Estrogen acts directly on bone cells to decrease bone turnover; estrogen receptors have recently been demonstrated in both osteoblasts and osteoclasts. Androgens and synthetic anabolic agents probably are also antiresorptive but may have weak formation-stimulating activity.

Calcitonin is an effective antiresorptive agent, but calcium supplements must be given concurrently to prevent secondary hyperparathyroidism; disadvantages include the requirement for parenteral administration, a relatively high cost, and the development of neutralizing antibodies in some patients. Preparations

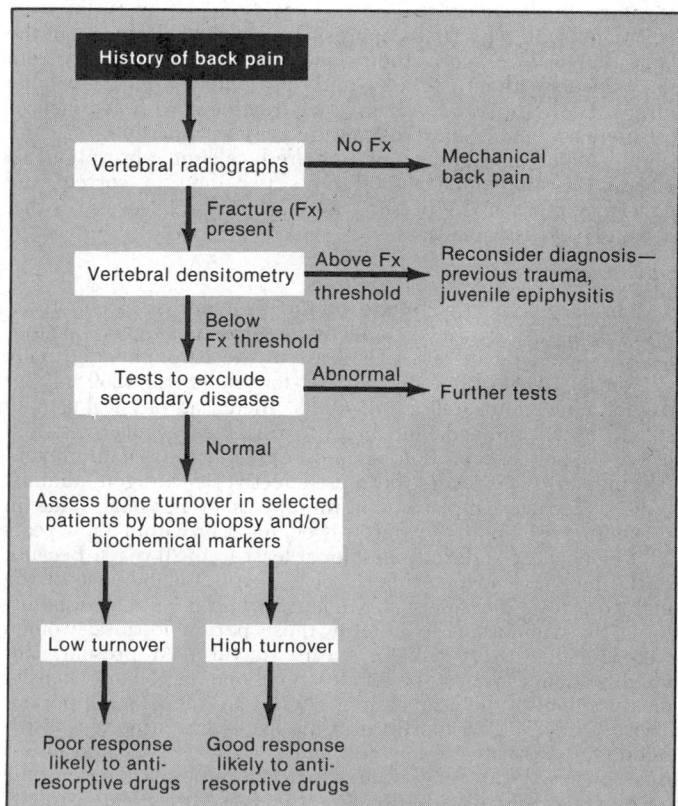

FIGURE 238–4. Diagnostic algorithm for investigation of the patient with osteoporosis. Studies for assessing bone turnover are more important when an effective formation-stimulating regimen becomes available. Nonetheless, it is still important to know whether bone turnover is low, as such patients should be given supplementary calcium and should be saved the expense and side effects of potent antiresorptive drugs, such as estrogen or calcitonin. (Modified from Eastell R, Riggs BL: Diagnostic evaluation of osteoporosis. Endocrinol Metab Clin North Am 17:547, 1988.)

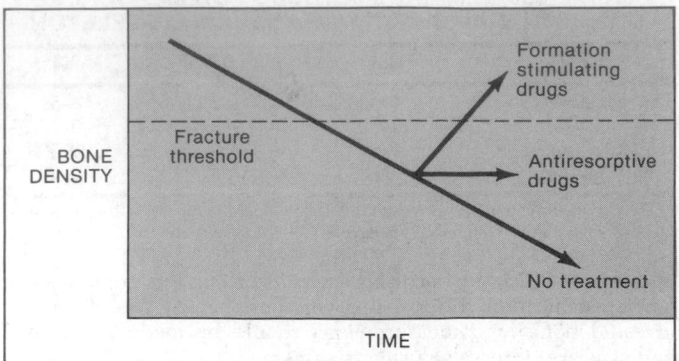

FIGURE 238–5. As bone is lost through the osteoporotic process, the bone density falls below the fracture threshold. As more bone is lost in the untreated patient, progressively more fractures occur. Antiresorptive drug therapy decreases the bone resorption that is responsible for continued bone loss. When a new steady state is attained, after 3 to 6 months of treatment, there is also a decrease in bone formation that approximates the decrease in bone resorption. Thus, the best result that can be obtained with this class of therapeutic agents is maintenance of the existing skeletal mass or slowing of its rate of loss. Regimens that stimulate bone formation have the theoretical potential of increasing bone mass substantially and thus of eliminating the risk of new fractures.

that can be administered transnasally are undergoing clinical trials.

Bisphosphonates are antiresorptive drugs that are adsorbed to bone crystals. When osteoclasts phagocytose bone crystals containing the drug, their metabolic activity is inhibited. The bisphosphonate most widely used in the United States is etidronate. Because this drug also impairs mineralization after long use, it must be administered cyclically. Newer and more potent bisphosphonates are undergoing clinical trials.

Therapy for patients with involutional osteoporosis should be individualized. Calcium supplements (1.0 to 1.5 grams per day) should be given to all patients. Those with more mild disease, especially women within 15 years of menopause, usually receive low-dose estrogen therapy (such as cyclic doses of 0.625 mg of conjugated estrogen or 0.025 mg of ethinyl estradiol daily). Because the risk of endometrial hyperplasia (and therefore carcinoma) is decreased or eliminated by concomitant progestin therapy, 5 mg of medroxyprogesterone acetate should be given daily during the last 10 to 14 days of the cycle. Abnormal menstrual bleeding should be promptly investigated. Continuous estrogen can be given with 2.5 mg of medroxyprogesterone acetate daily without inducing menstrual bleeding in some, but not all, women. The excessive hepatic production of coagulation factors, renin substrate, and bile cholesterol (accounting for an increased risk of venous thrombosis, hypertension, and cholelithiasis) is due to the liver's being exposed to increased estrogen concentration in the first pass after oral administration. These problems can be reduced or eliminated by giving cyclic estrogen as a transdermal patch (0.1 mg of estradiol-17β per day). Annual breast examination and mammograms are mandatory. If bone loss or fractures continue while the patient is receiving hormone treatment, the dosage of both estrogen and progestin should be doubled.

Treatment with vitamin D and its active metabolites should probably be reserved for patients with a documented or suspected impairment in calcium absorption. This impairment can be inferred from a relatively low urinary calcium excretion rate (<75 mg per day), especially if this rate does not increase significantly with calcium supplementation. Calcitonin is an appropriate alternative for women who do not wish to take estrogen or in whom it is contraindicated. The recommended dosage is 50 to 100 units per day accompanied by at least 1.0 gram of supplementary calcium daily.

Regimens that stimulate bone formation have the potential of increasing bone mass substantially and thus of eliminating the risk of new fractures. Sodium fluoride, the synthetic 1–34 fragment of parathyroid hormone in low dosage, and combined therapy with calcitonin and phosphate given orally have been reported to stimulate bone formation, and other regimens are being investigated. Only therapy with sodium fluoride, however, has been widely evaluated. Although fluoride therapy results in large increases in cancellous bone mass, the newly formed bone is qualitatively abnormal. A recent randomized clinical trial showed that it did not decrease the occurrence of vertebral fractures and did increase the occurrence of appendicular fractures.

The same therapeutic approach, with modifications, can be used for other types of osteoporosis. Idiopathic osteoporosis in young adult women often is relatively refractory to therapy. Because the women are premenopausal, there is no reason to prescribe sex steroids. Some of these patients have impaired calcium absorption that is correctable with vitamin D therapy. The mainstay of treatment, therefore, is calcium supplementation with or without pharmacologic doses of vitamin D. Calcitonin can be added to decrease the increased level of bone resorption that may be present.

Although most men with osteoporosis do not have a deficiency of sex steroids, 10 to 20 per cent have partial or complete hypogonadism from various causes. Patients with documented low plasma testosterone levels should receive replacement therapy—for example, with testosterone enanthate in a dose of 200 to 400 mg given intramuscularly every 3 weeks. Calcium supplements with or without pharmacologic doses of vitamin D should also be given.

The most common cause of secondary osteoporosis is chronic use of pharmacologic dosages of glucocorticoids. The single most effective measure is reduction of dosage or, if possible, complete discontinuation of the glucocorticoid. Administering the glucocorticoid once daily or on alternate days may maintain a more favorable balance between its anti-inflammatory and immunosuppressive effects and the osteopenic effect. All patients should be given calcium supplements, and postmenopausal women should be given estrogens. Preliminary data suggest that bisphosphonates may be effective.

Patients with type II osteoporosis have already lost most of the bone they will ever lose, their bone differs little in density from that of peers without fractures, and they generally have low bone turnover. There is no evidence that treatment with estrogen or calcitonin is beneficial. Treatment consists primarily of calcium supplementation (because of impaired calcium absorption), a vitamin D supplement (1000 units per day) to correct any deficiency that may be present, and instruction in measures that decrease the risk of falls.

PREVENTION

Considering the magnitude of the problem of osteoporosis, prevention is the only cost-effective approach. Dietary calcium, if low, should be increased at least to the recommended daily allowance (RDA) of 800 mg per day for adults and 1200 mg per day for adolescents and young adults. Increased physical activity should be encouraged, and bone toxins, such as cigarettes and heavy alcohol consumption, should be eliminated. Of all preventive measures, however, the most effective is estrogen administration. Estrogen replacement therapy is of maximal value in preventing osteoporosis when it is begun at or within a few years after menopause and continued for at least 15 to 20 years. Because of the potential adverse effects of estrogen and because of the high cost of the necessary surveillance while it is being administered, it is important to identify those perimenopausal women who are at greatest risk for future fracture. At present, this identification can best be made by obtaining a bone density measurement of the lumbar spine in the perimenopausal period. Those women in the top third of the age-adjusted normal distribution are at relatively low risk and need not be treated unless this is necessary for relief of menopausal symptoms. Those in the lower third of the distribution are at increased risk, and estrogen replacement therapy should be strongly considered for them. Those in the middle one third of the distribution should have a repeat bone density measurement made after 2 to 3 years and, if substantial bone loss has occurred, should be reconsidered for treatment. In the future, it is possible that bisphosphonate drugs may be substituted for estrogen in some women.

Jackson JA, Kleerekoper M: Osteoporosis in men: Diagnosis, pathophysiology, and prevention. Medicine 69:137, 1990. *Useful review of etiology, presentation, and management of osteoporosis in men.*

Melton LJ III, Eddy DM, Johnston CC: Screening for osteoporosis. Ann Intern Med 112:516, 1990. *Position paper on clinical indications for bone densitometry and the present status of cost-effectiveness of screening. Good discussion on various methods of measurement.*

Riggs BL, Melton LJ III: Medical progress: Involutional osteoporosis. N Engl J Med 314:1676, 1986. *Review of etiology and treatment of osteoporosis and a summary of the evidence that supports the concept of two distinct syndromes of involutional osteoporosis.*

Riggs BL, Hodgson SF, O'Fallon WM, et al.: Effect of fluoride treatment on the fracture rate in postmenopausal women with osteoporosis. N Engl J Med 322:802, 1990. *Results of prospective randomized clinical trial of fluoride therapy in 202 women with type I osteoporosis, using fracture frequency as the end-point. Despite dramatic increases in vertebral bone density, the fracture rate did not change significantly, suggesting that bone strength was decreased.*

Watts NB, Harris ST, Genant HK, et al.: Intermittent cyclical etidronate treatment of postmenopausal osteoporosis. N Engl J Med 323:73, 1990. *Prospective randomized clinical trial in 429 women with type I osteoporosis, showing that this new regimen increases bone mass modestly and reduces the vertebral fracture rate.*

239 Paget's Disease of Bone (Osteitis Deformans)

Frederick R. Singer

INCIDENCE AND EPIDEMIOLOGY

Paget's disease is a common bone disorder second in frequency to osteoporosis. In areas of prevalence, it affects approximately 3 per cent of the population over age 40. The disease is common in the United Kingdom and in the countries to which its inhabitants have migrated, including the United States, Canada, South Africa, Australia, and New Zealand. The disease also is common in France, Germany, and Italy but is rarely found in China, Japan, India, or Scandinavia. There is no major predilection for either sex.

There is evidence of an autosomal dominant transmission that is linked to histocompatibility leukocyte antigens. As many as 25 per cent of patients have been reported to have at least one relative with the disease.

PATHOLOGY

Paget's disease may affect one or many bones, but in the majority of patients most of the skeleton is uninvolved. The earliest phase is characterized by a localized osteolytic process in which proliferation of multinucleated osteoclasts is the dominant lesion. The osteoclasts of Paget's disease may be occasionally quite large and may exhibit more than 100 nuclei in a cross-section of one cell. Adjacent to the advancing osteolytic front, the pathology is characterized by a mixed osteolytic and osteoblastic process of great intensity. Numerous plump osteoblasts line bony trabeculae that have previously been partially resorbed by osteoclasts. The marrow spaces may be devoid of hematopoietic cells and instead are filled with fibroblasts, connective tissue, and blood vessels. The resultant architecture of the bone takes on a "mosaic" pattern in which the cement lines are arranged in a haphazard pattern instead of the normal symmetry of parallel collagen fibers in both cortical and trabecular bone. Occasionally, this abnormal mosaic pattern is present with little or no cellular activity. Osteolytic, mixed osteolytic and osteoblastic, and "burned-out" Paget's disease may be present in a single bone. Paget's disease can usually be readily distinguished from primary hyperparathyroidism, osteomyelitis, and osteomalacia by light microscopy, but electron microscopy studies have provided evidence of a characteristic lesion. The nuclei, and at times the cytoplasm, of the osteoclasts frequently contain abnormal inclusions that resemble the nucleocapsids of viruses of the Paramyxoviridae family. Respiratory syncytial virus and measles virus antigens have been demonstrated in the osteoclasts of Paget's disease by immunohistologic techniques.

ETIOLOGY

Sir James Paget, in his original description of the disease, proposed that the entity was inflammatory in nature. The recent ultrastructural and immunohistologic studies support the concept of a "slow" virus infection, although definitive proof is still to be obtained. No other hypotheses have generated supporting evidence.

CLINICAL FEATURES

In many patients, Paget's disease is not appreciated until an abnormal radiograph or laboratory test is encountered either in the course of a routine evaluation or during assessment of an unrelated complaint. The most common complaints of symptomatic patients are *skeletal deformity* and *musculoskeletal pain*. The bones most likely to be abnormal on physical examination are the cranium, the clavicles, and the long bones, particularly of the lower extremities. The complications associated with skull lesions include hearing loss, vertigo, tinnitus, and, less commonly, headaches. Severe enlargement of the base of the skull may lead to basilar impression and compression of the spinal cord, the brain stem, the cerebellum, and the basilar and vertebral arteries. Slurred speech, impaired swallowing, diplopia, and urinary incontinence may result. Deformity of the facial bones (leontiasis ossea) is much less common in patients with Paget's disease than in patients with fibrous dysplasia, a disease that usually is diagnosed several decades earlier in life. The spine may be involved at any level, but lumbar and thoracic vertebrae are most commonly affected. One or more vertebrae, consecutive or not, can manifest the disease. Back pain may be severe and of complex origin, since degenerative arthritis is common in this age group, and impingement of skeletal tissue on nerve roots or the spinal cord can occur. The sudden onset of intolerable pain suggests that a compression fracture has occurred. Disease affecting the pelvis and proximal femur produces a common severe pain syndrome, weight-bearing pain from degenerative arthritis of the hip. Ambulation may also be impaired when significant lateral or anterior bowing of the femur or tibia develops. These bones are also prone to pathologic fracture. Evidence of disease activity in long bones is manifested by increased skin temperature over the affected bone. This results from the increased cutaneous blood flow associated with the hypervascular bone beneath.

Defects in Bruch's membrane of the retina, termed angioid streaks, may be observed in about 10 per cent of patients and seldom are associated with impaired vision. Cardiac enlargement and frank congestive heart failure may be manifestations of prior increased cardiac output, which is thought to be a consequence of increased vascularity of affected bones. This usually occurs in patients with more than 20 per cent of the skeleton affected by Paget's disease or when the skull is severely involved. Bone tumors such as osteosarcoma and giant cell tumor may develop in lesions of Paget's disease (Ch. 241). A rapid worsening of bone pain or the relatively sudden development of a mass or both are the common modes of presentation.

RADIOLOGY. The radiologic features of Paget's disease are so characteristic that it is seldom necessary to obtain a bone biopsy for diagnosis. The earliest manifestation is a localized osteolytic lesion most readily detected in the skull and at either end of a long bone. In the skull, the circumscribed radiolucent area has been termed osteoporosis circumscripta (Fig. 239–1). The osteolytic lesion in an extremity bone usually progresses with a sharply defined **V** shape at an average rate of progression of 1 cm per year. Linear cortical radiolucencies may develop in the femur or tibia on the convex surface of a curved bone and may be precursors of fractures. An uncommon variant of the osteolytic lesion may occur at the distal end of the tibia, in which a cystlike expansion of the bone is seen. Osteolytic disease of the vertebral bodies is often associated with sclerotic margins, giving a "picture frame" appearance. These vertebrae are prone to compression fractures.

The radiographic manifestations of osteoblastic activity generally appear years or even decades after the onset of osteolysis. In the skull a "honeycomb" appearance of patchy new bone may fill in the underlying osteoporosis circumscripta, and subsequently the classic "cotton-wool" lesions of exuberant chaotic bone formation appear with a strikingly thickened calvarium (Fig. 239–2). In the long bones, the osteolytic lesions evolve into thickened bone with irregular trabeculation. In the pelvis, thickening of the

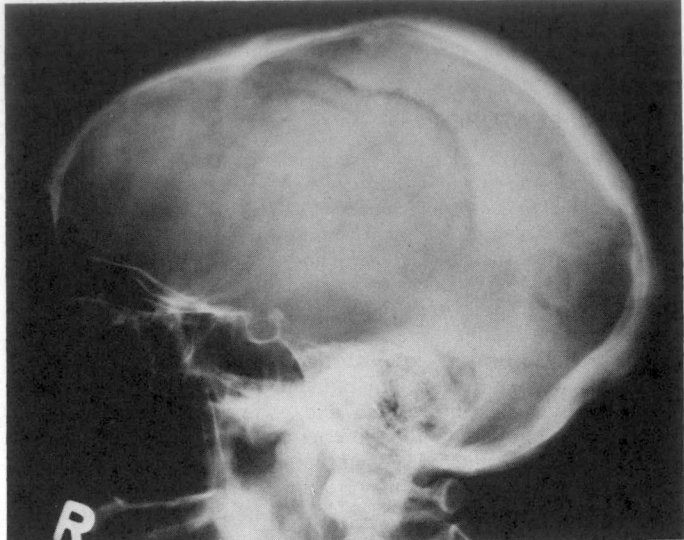

FIGURE 239–1. Osteoporosis circumscripta of the skull, involving the frontal, parietal, and temporal bones.

iliopectineal line, the "brim sign," is nearly pathognomonic of Paget's disease. It is also found in patients with osteopetrosis but rarely in patients with osteoblastic metastases. Enlargement of the ischial and pubic bones is also typical of Paget's disease. Sclerosis of the pagetic vertebral body may be difficult to distinguish from malignant bone involvement, but if the vertebral body is clearly larger than adjacent vertebral bodies, Paget's disease is likely. Computed tomography (CT) of the spine is a useful means of evaluating the detailed anatomy of the spine and is particularly helpful in defining arthritic and neurologic complications in the patient with back pain.

The bone scan is the most sensitive means to detect active lesions of Paget's disease, although it is not a specific diagnostic test. The earliest lesions may not be discernible roentgenographically at the same time an area of increased uptake of the radiolabeled scanning agent is obvious.

BIOCHEMICAL FEATURES

The extent and activity of Paget's disease have been found to correlate reasonably well with serum alkaline phosphatase activity (an index of osteoblastic activity) and urinary hydroxyproline excretion (an index of bone matrix resorption). Patients with very limited active disease have normal biochemical parameters,

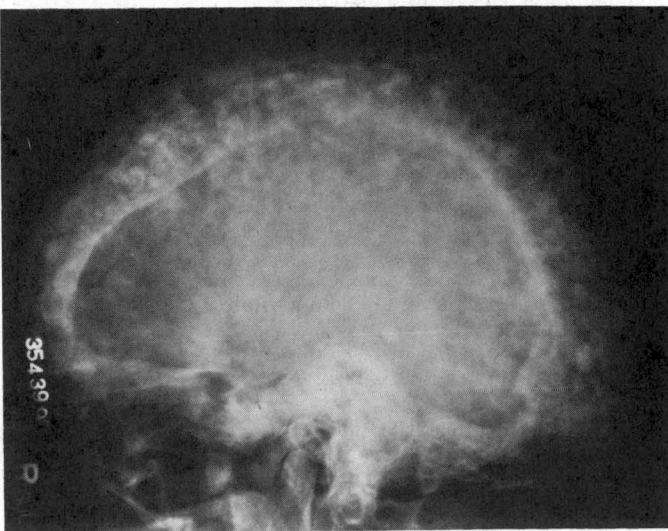

FIGURE 239–2. Advanced involvement of the skull with marked thickening of the entire cranial vault, areas of osteolysis, and patchy new bone formation resulting in a "cotton-wool" appearance.

whereas increases of 50-fold greater than normal sometimes occur in patients with polyostotic disease of greatest extent. The serum calcium concentration is normal except in patients who are immobilized or in whom malignancy or primary hyperparathyroidism develops. Hypercalciuria precedes hypercalcemia in these patients. Hyperuricemia, with or without clinical gout, is sometimes found and may reflect an increased turnover of purines.

MEDICAL AND SURGICAL THERAPY

Most patients with Paget's disease do not require any therapy or may require only analgesic agents, such as aspirin or indomethacin. The leading indications for medical therapy are bone pain and preparation for orthopedic surgery. Prevention of future complications in patients with osteolytic lesions of the skull and weight-bearing bones may be a reasonable objective.

CALCITONIN. Effective and safe therapy of Paget's disease became possible with the availability of salmon calcitonin. Subcutaneous injections of 50 to 100 MRC units daily or on alternate days produce an average decrease of 50 per cent in biochemical parameters and improve many of the manifestations of the disease. Relief of bone pain, healing of osteolytic lesions, reduction of increased cardiac output and elevated skin temperature, stabilization of auditory acuity, and reversal of various neurologic deficits have all been convincingly documented during chronic therapy. Treatment may be necessary for years in patients with active osteolytic lesions. Side effects include nausea, facial flushing, and polyuria, but they seldom require interruption of therapy. Salmon calcitonin elicits an antibody response in more than 50 per cent of patients, since its amino acid sequence differs considerably from that of human calcitonin. Approximately 25 per cent of patients acquire high enough antibody titers to become resistant to hormone action. These patients respond to human calcitonin or to other forms of therapy.

BISPHOSPHONATES. An alternate form of therapy is disodium etidronate, whose main advantage is its oral mode of administration. At a dosage of 5 mg per kilogram of body weight daily for an initial treatment period of 6 months, this drug produces benefits similar to those of calcitonin and can be used in repeated 6-month courses after symptoms return. However, healing of osteolytic lesions has seldom been documented. Long-term use of higher doses should be avoided because of impairment of bone mineralization and resulting susceptibility to fracture. More potent bisphosphonates, which are less likely to impair mineralization, are undergoing clinical trials.

MITHRAMYCIN. Mithramycin is a cytotoxic antibiotic that has not been approved for the treatment of Paget's disease by the Food and Drug Administration (FDA) but has been used in selected patients because of its great potency. The platelet, renal, and hepatic toxicity of this agent warrants great caution in its use. It should be reserved for patients with marked symptomatology in whom other agents fail.

The effectiveness of medical therapy can usually be objectively assessed by measurement of serum alkaline phosphatase activity alone at intervals of 2 to 4 months. Radiographs of osteolytic lesions should be obtained at least annually.

SURGERY. Surgery is an important adjunct to medical therapy in selected patients. Occipital craniectomy may be necessary in patients with basilar impression, and decompression of neurologic structures affected by vertebral lesions is another procedure of critical importance. More commonly, orthopedic procedures are required to enable more normal ambulation in patients with pelvic and lower extremity disease. Degenerative arthritis of the hip is a common complication that can produce severe pain and limit ambulation. Results of total hip replacement are excellent. Deformity of the tibia may also limit ambulation because of knee and ankle pain. Tibial osteotomy leading to restoration of a more normal knee-ankle alignment can also markedly alleviate joint pain and restore a near-normal gait. If possible, 1 to 3 months of medical therapy should be administered prior to surgery to reduce the amount of intraoperative and postoperative bleeding and to prevent immobilization hypercalcemia postoperatively.

Altman RD, Singer FR: Proceedings of the Kroc Foundation conference on Paget's disease of bone. Arthritis Rheum 23:1073, 1980. *A comprehensive coverage of etiologic, metabolic, and therapeutic aspects of the disease.*

Mills BG, Singer FR, Weiner LP, et al.: Evidence for both respiratory syncytial virus and measles virus antigens in the osteoclasts of patients with Paget's disease of bone. Clin Orthop Rel Res 183:303, 1984. *A study documenting antigens of two Paramyxoviridae viruses in osteoclasts of Paget's disease.*

Rebel A: Symposium: Paget's disease. Clin Orthop Rel Res 217:2, 1987.

Singer FR, Krane SM: Paget's disease of bone. *In* Avioli LV, Krane SM (eds.): Metabolic Bone Disease and Clinically Related Disorders. Philadelphia, W.B. Saunders Company, 1990. *A comprehensive review of clinical features, pathology, biochemistry, and treatment of Paget's disease.*

240 Osteonecrosis, Osteosclerosis, and Other Disorders of Bone

Gordon J. Strewler

OSTEONECROSIS

Osteonecrosis is synonymous with aseptic or avascular necrosis of bone; these terms describe infarction of bone. Bone infarcts may be asymptomatic or associated with self-limited pain if they occur in the shaft, as in sickle cell disease or hyperbaric injury (caisson disease). Syndromes with greater morbidity occur with necrosis of subarticular bone, especially in the femoral head.

ETIOLOGY. The most common cause of osteonecrosis is vascular compromise from fracture or dislocation of the femoral neck. Other bones susceptible to posttraumatic osteonecrosis are the carpal scaphoid, the body of the talus, the humeral head, and the lunate. Nontraumatic vascular compromise, usually of the femoral head, is the likely cause of osteonecrosis in sickle cell disease (sludging of sickled erythrocytes), caisson disease (gas bubble emboli), Gaucher's disease (obstruction by histiocytes), hemophilia, and polycythemia vera. Other important causes are glucocorticoid therapy, cytotoxic chemotherapy, radiation injury, and renal transplantation. The prevalence of osteonecrosis after renal transplantation ranges from 3 to 41 per cent in various reports. In addition to corticosteroid therapy, precedent renal osteodystrophy and persistent secondary hyperparathyroidism may be etiologic factors. Osteonecrosis is associated with alcoholism and diabetes mellitus, but diabetics seem to be relatively protected against its development after renal transplantation. The ossification centers of growing bone in children are susceptible to growth disturbances and sometimes to osteonecrosis; here the relative roles of constitutional factors and trauma are poorly defined. Over 50 eponymic syndromes, collectively called osteochondroses, are associated with growth disturbances at various epiphyseal sites. The most common site of true osteonecrosis is the femoral head (Perthes' disease).

PATHOGENESIS. While in some disorders (e.g., sickle cell disease), osteonecrosis can readily be ascribed to vascular obstruction, in others, such as glucocorticoid excess, its cause is unknown. Better understood are the mechanisms by which infarction of bone leads to its eventual collapse. Dead bone does not lose mechanical stability. Bone resorption occurring as part of the reparative process weakens the infarcted area, predisposing to fractures and fragmentation.

CLINICAL MANIFESTATIONS. Besides the femoral head, common sites of nontraumatic osteonecrosis include the femoral condyles, distal tibia, humeral head, and talus. The presenting symptom is pain, often of acute onset. Radiologic diagnosis may be delayed for weeks or months because dead bone and living bone are radiologically indistinguishable. Magnetic resonance imaging or radionuclide scanning may show abnormalities earlier than the radiograph. It is mostly slow reparative processes that are visualized radiographically. A linear subchondral lucency, the "crescent sign," indicates collapse of subchondral bone. Patchy lucencies reflect resorption; patchy sclerosis indicates growth of new bone over the scaffolding of dead trabeculae. These reparative processes may lead to healing if fragmentation or collapse of weakened bone does not supervene. Initial therapy consists of avoidance of weight bearing, but surgery, such as transpositional osteotomy, arthrotomy with removal of fragments, or arthroplasty, is frequently required.

Kenzora JE (ed.): Symposium on idiopathic osteonecrosis. Orthop Clin North Am 16:593, 1985. *Articles on pathogenesis, diagnosis, and therapy of osteonecrosis.*

DISORDERS OF INCREASED BONE DENSITY

Radiographic evidence of increased bone density (osteosclerosis) usually reflects increased bone mass per unit of volume, rather than increased mineral per unit of bone mass. This increase can result from accelerated synthesis and mineralization of the bone matrix or from decreased bone resorption. The pathogenesis of such disorders is rarely known, and their histologic characteristics are often indistinguishable; hence, they are classified on the basis of their radiographic appearance. Sclerosis of the cortex can produce increased width as the result of new bone formation, and this is sometimes referred to as hyperostosis. Bone shape can also be altered by disorders of modeling, the process by which bones assume their adult shape during development.

Trabecular Osteosclerosis

This form of osteosclerosis is the most frequently encountered. Its causes can be categorized as neoplastic, hematologic, or metabolic.

Neoplastic. Prostatic and breast carcinoma, as well as other neoplasms with osteoblastic metastases, can present on occasion as diffuse osteosclerosis; however, localized blastic or lytic areas are generally also present and permit radiologic diagnosis of malignancy. Generalized osteosclerosis is a rare presentation of myeloma and other hematologic malignancies.

Hematologic. In 40 per cent of cases of agnogenic myeloid metaplasia with myelofibrosis, diffuse skeletal sclerosis is seen. Osteosclerosis is also preceded by myelofibrosis when it occurs in mastocytosis and polycythemia vera. Sickle cell disease is manifested in bone by sclerosis, medullary bone infarcts, and subchondral osteonecrosis.

Metabolic. Renal osteodystrophy characteristically gives rise to sclerosis of the vertebral end-plates—the "rugger-jersey" spine—and to trabecular sclerosis in the metaphyses of long bones and the skull (Ch. 237). Cortical erosions of secondary hyperparathyroidism are also typically present. Diffuse osteosclerosis is an unusual presentation of Paget's disease (Ch. 239) and is rare in primary hyperparathyroidism. Fluorosis occurs endemically in areas of India and Africa where the fluoride content of water is high, following industrial exposure in aluminum and fertilizer plants, and, increasingly, in individuals treated for osteoporosis (see Ch. 238). Uniform sclerosis of bone is accompanied by exostoses and roughened cortical calcifications at muscle and ligamentous insertions, which suggest the diagnosis. Periarticular pain and limitation of motion are common. Histologically, thick trabeculae are covered by wide osteoid seams, which indicate the presence of osteomalacia.

Cortical and Trabecular Osteosclerosis

OSTEOPETROSIS

Osteopetrosis (Albers-Schönberg disease, or marble bone disease), a rare disorder of greatly increased bone density, occurs in several distinct forms. The malignant, autosomal recessive form (osteopetrosis congenita) results in replacement of the marrow space with bone, which causes anemia, infection, and early death. The benign, autosomal dominant form (osteopetrosis tarda) may be asymptomatic and rarely limits survival. A mild form with autosomal recessive rather than dominant inheritance is characterized by renal tubular acidosis and absence of the isozyme carbonic anhydrase II. In obligate heterozygotes for this disorder, carbonic anhydrase II activity is one half of normal. This is undoubtedly an important clue to the nature of osteoclast dysfunction in these individuals.

PATHOLOGY. Osteosclerosis results from defective osteoclast function with a failure of normal bone resorption. The medullary cavity is occupied by thickened bone trabeculae with central zones of entrapped calcified cartilage, which indicates a failure to resorb the primary spongiosa. Osteoclasts are abundant. In some cases, defective osteoclast function is suggested by the absence of a ruffled border, the redundantly invaginated membrane structure normally adjacent to bone in actively resorbing osteoblasts.

MALIGNANT OSTEOPETROSIS. The malignant, autosomal recessive form of osteopetrosis presents in infancy with failure to thrive and delayed development. Proptosis, blindness, and frequently deafness and hydrocephalus ensue before age 2, as bone encroaches upon the cranial foramina. Despite its solid appearance, osteopetrotic bone is fragile, and fractures are frequent. Osteomyelitis is common. Obliteration of the marrow space causes extramedullary hematopoiesis, with hepatosplenomegaly and hypersplenism. Leukoerythroblastic anemia and thrombocytopenia are accompanied by elevated acid and alkaline phosphatase levels and, on occasion, hypocalcemia. Radiologically, the bone is everywhere sclerotic, often with metaphyseal bands of increased density. The long bones are poorly modeled and clublike; ragged metaphyseal-epiphyseal junctions may suggest rickets. Untreated, malignant osteopetrosis results in death from infection, bleeding, or anemia.

BENIGN OSTEOPETROSIS. This autosomal dominant variant is asymptomatic in about half of cases and is usually detected in family studies or as an incidental radiologic finding. The remainder of patients present with fractures of brittle osteopetrotic bone (about 40 per cent) or with osteomyelitis, usually of the mandible. Radiographically, the picture resembles that in the malignant form, but bones are well modeled (Fig. 240–1). The only laboratory abnormality is an increased acid phosphatase level in some patients.

TREATMENT. Bone marrow transplantation from human leukocyte antigen (HLA)–identical sibs has been used successfully for treatment of malignant, autosomal recessive osteopetrosis. Establishment of a chimeric state is accompanied by remarkable regression of osteosclerosis and the reversal of anemia and incomplete nerve deficits. A conceptual by-product of these experiments has been the demonstration that the osteoclast originates from hematopoietic elements.

PYKNODYSOSTOSIS

This disease has only recently been distinguished from osteopetrosis. Inherited as an autosomal recessive trait, it is characterized by short stature and generalized osteosclerosis and is distinguished from osteopetrosis by several additional features: an obtuse mandibular angle with receding chin, multiple wormian bones with persistently open cranial fontanelles, and hypoplasia of terminal phalanges and clavicles. Fractures are common. Toulouse-Lautrec is thought to have suffered from pyknodysostosis.

Cortical Osteosclerosis

HYPERTROPHIC OSTEOARTHROPATHY

The term hypertrophic osteoarthropathy describes subperiosteal formation of new bone in the long bones, secondary to some other condition. It often occurs in conjunction with digital clubbing and arthritis (see Ch. 277). The etiologies include pulmonary, hepatic, and intestinal disease. Bronchogenic carcinoma

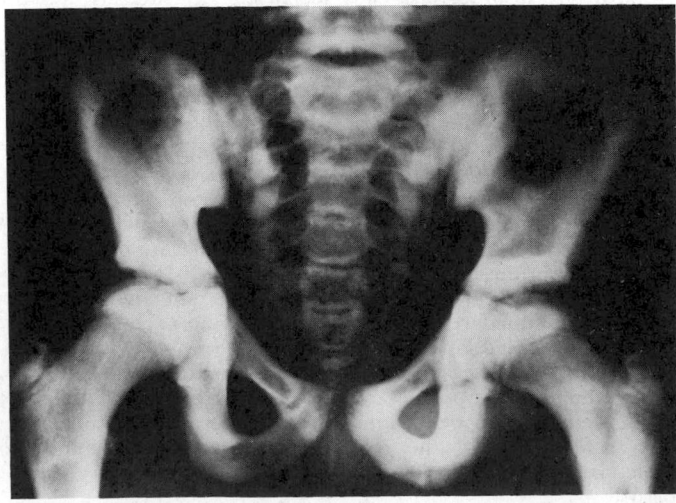

FIGURE 240–1. Roentgenogram of the pelvis of a teenager with the benign, autosomal recessive form of osteopetrosis.

(except small cell carcinoma) is the most common cause of hypertrophic osteoarthropathy and of clubbing; other causes of hypertrophic pulmonary osteoarthropathy are pleural tumors, lung abscesses, and empyema. Hypertrophic osteoarthropathy occurs in as many as 30 per cent of patients with chronic liver disease, often without clubbing. It is occasionally seen in ulcerative colitis and regional enteritis. Hypertrophic osteoarthropathy is unusual in cyanotic congenital heart disease, although clubbing is typically observed.

Hypertrophic osteoarthropathy is usually confined to the distal tibia and fibula and the distal radius and ulna. When advanced, it may involve other bones. However, it rarely involves the distal phalanges, even in the presence of clubbing. Bone pain, tenderness, and soft tissue swelling may be present, but the condition is sometimes asymptomatic. The periosteum is thickened, and subperiosteal formation of new bone is radiographically evident. Initially present as a separate stripe, new bone may eventually fuse with the cortex. The differential diagnosis includes pachydermoperiostosis, thyroid achropachy, hypervitaminosis A, syphilis, and polyarteritis nodosa. The pathogenesis is unknown. However, blood flow to affected extremities is increased, and the condition sometimes responds to vagotomy; these findings suggest that central reflex changes may be operative.

PACHYDERMOPERIOSTOSIS

In pachydermoperiostosis, an autosomal dominant condition, periosteal formation of new bone occurs from puberty in the same distribution as in secondary hypertrophic osteoarthropathy. Also classically present are marked clubbing and thickened, oily skin. Facial features are coarse, and the thickened forehead and scalp are often marked by transverse folds (cutis verticis gyrata). The appearance may superficially resemble that of acromegaly. Pachydermoperiostosis is differentiated from secondary hypertrophic osteoarthropathy by the family history and lack of an antecedent cause.

VITAMIN A INTOXICATION (Ch. 204)

Previously witnessed mostly in abusers of vitamins, this disorder is being seen more often, sometimes with hypercalcemia, in those treated with 13-*cis*-retinoic acid (isotretinoin) for cystic acne, ichthyosis, or malignancy. The characteristic periosteal new bone is often seen as a fusiform excrescence on the mid-shaft or as anterior spurs on vertebral bodies.

PROGRESSIVE DIAPHYSEAL DYSPLASIA

This rare disorder, also known as Camurati-Engelmann disease, is inherited as an autosomal trait. Classically, it is manifest in childhood by a thin body habitus, muscle wasting and weakness with a waddling gait, and bone pain. The serum biochemistry is usually normal, but the alkaline phosphatase level may be increased; the erythrocyte sedimentation rate is also elevated. Radiographs show characteristic hyperostosis of the diaphyseal cortices with symmetric fusiform enlargement of the long bones. The skull is sometimes involved. These changes progress with time, at a pace that slows in adulthood. Bone pain and muscle weakness sometimes respond to corticosteroids, but the changes in bone do not. Progressive diaphyseal dysplasia exhibits considerable phenotypic variation; asymptomatic individuals and a mild adult variant (Ribbing's disease) are common.

HEREDITARY HYPERPHOSPHATASIA

Hereditary hyperphosphatasia has also been called congenital hyperphosphatasia, osteoectasia with hyperphosphatasia, and juvenile Paget's disease. Children affected by this rare, crippling, autosomal recessive condition present before age 2 with an enlarging skull, bowing of the extremities, bone pain, and fractures. Alkaline and acid phosphatase levels and the urinary hydroxyproline level are greatly increased. The calvaria is thickened, with focal densities that resemble cotton-wool balls. Elsewhere, bones are thickened symmetrically and may be demineralized, sometimes with loss of the normal cortex. Several patients have responded dramatically to calcitonin.

Focal Osteosclerosis

Osteopoikilosis is an asymptomatic, autosomal dominant trait. Pea-sized sclerotic spots, prominent in the metaphyseal area, are accompanied in some kindreds by unique cutaneous lesions (dermatofibrosis lenticularis disseminata). These are yellowish papules or plaques with increased elastin. The combination is known as the Buschke-Ollendorff syndrome. *Osteopathia striata*, another autosomal dominant disorder of the sclerosing type, is usually asymptomatic and is characterized by symmetric, parallel arrays of fine streaks in the long bones and pelvis. *Melorheostosis* is a progressive, painful disorder in which discrete hyperostotic areas appear to flow down the long bones like dripping wax. No hereditary predisposition is evident.

Frame B, Honasoge M, Kottamasu SR: Osteosclerosis, Hyperostosis and Related Disorders. New York, Elsevier, 1987. *A comprehensive, readable, profusely illustrated treatise.*
Hansen-Flaschen J, Nordberg J: Clubbing and hypertrophic osteoarthropathy. Clin Chest Med 8:287, 1987. *A good clinical review.*
Sly WS, Whyte MP, Sundaram V, et al.: Carbonic anhydrase II deficiency in 12 families with the autosomal recessive syndrome of osteopetrosis with renal tubular acidosis and cerebral calcification. N Engl J Med 313:139, 1985.

OTHER DISORDERS OF BONE

Fibrous Dysplasia

Fibrous dysplasia occurs in both monostotic and polyostotic forms. The latter is often associated with cutaneous café au lait spots and precocious pseudopuberty in females, and this triad is called the McCune-Albright syndrome.

The etiology of fibrous dysplasia is unknown. It is not heritable. Individual lesions are composed of dense fibrous tissue in medullary bone, interspersed with thin bone trabeculae (often covered by wide osteoid seams) and sometimes islands of cartilage. Radiographically, the lesions have a multilocular appearance beneath a thinned cortex (Fig. 240–2). Within, they have the appearance of ground glass, owing to their fine trabeculations. Although monostotic and polyostotic forms are histologically indistinguishable, monostotic lesions are not associated with an endocrinopathy. They commonly involve the proximal femur, tibia, or ribs, may occur at any age, and can cause bone pain, fractures, or deformity. Malignant transformation occurs in about 1 per cent of lesions.

Polyostotic fibrous dysplasia usually presents in those between the ages of 3 and 10. It may involve over 50 per cent of the skeleton and frequently produces "shepherd's-crook" deformity of the femur and discrepancies in leg length; skull involvement may cause gross facial disfigurement (leontiasis ossea). Fractures are common. Serum biochemistry is frequently normal except for elevation of the alkaline phosphatase level. The café au lait spots sometimes seen in polyostotic fibrous dysplasia have jagged borders that Albright likened to the coast of Maine, to distinguish them from those in neurofibromatosis, which have smooth borders like the coast of California.

About half of girls with polyostotic fibrous dysplasia undergo precocious puberty, which may precede detection of the bone abnormality. Precocious puberty has also been reported in a few boys with this syndrome. Sexual maturation in both sexes is associated with low gonadotropin levels, and fertility does not

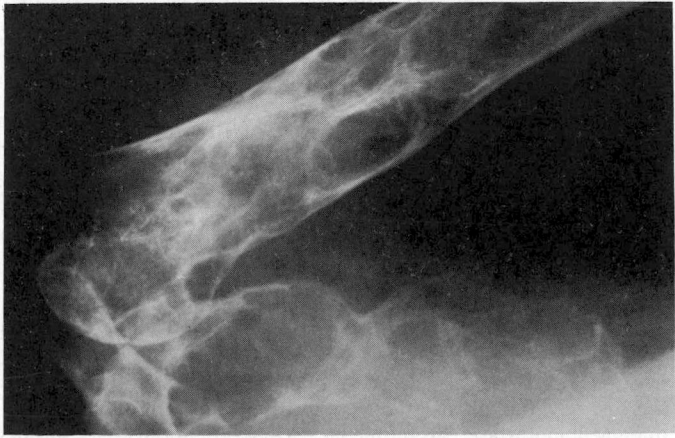

FIGURE 240–2. Roentgenogram of the humerus and scapula of a patient with extensive polyostotic fibrous dysplasia. Both bones are extensively involved with typical lesions.

occur. Histologically, the ovaries display multiple follicular cysts. Several other endocrinopathies have been described in the McCune-Albright syndrome; these include hyperthyroidism (in about 20 per cent), gigantism with acromegaly, and Cushing's syndrome. Levels of thyroid-stimulating hormone (TSH) are suppressed in hyperthyroidism associated with the McCune-Albright syndrome. In these glands, which thus function autonomously, receptors for the respective tropic hormone–luteinizing hormone (LH), follicle-stimulating hormone (FSH), and TSH—are coupled to adenylate cyclase. However, the nature of the regulatory defect remains to be defined and may be unrelated to the receptor–adenylate cyclase system.

Hereditary Multiple Exostoses

This relatively common disorder (also called diaphyseal aclasis) is inherited as an autosomal dominant trait with high penetrance. Irregular bony excrescences protrude from the expanded metaphyses of the long bones. These osteocartilaginous exostoses arise from the growth plate and grow as the bone does. They may subsequently become isolated from the epiphysis or remain in continuity, but they reproduce normal structure, with an outer cortex and an inner spongiosa continuous with that of the bone of origin. Growth ceases in adulthood. Disability results principally from limb-length discrepancies: Linear bone growth decreases as the bone grows transversely. Less common are syndromes of nerve, spinal cord, and vascular compression. The exostoses undergo sarcomatous degeneration in 3 to 10 per cent of affected individuals, and this must be suspected when a lesion enlarges rapidly, especially during adulthood.

Enchondromatosis *(Dyschondroplasia, Ollier's Disease)*

A sporadic condition, enchondromatosis becomes symptomatic in childhood as multiple, growing, cartilaginous masses within the trabecular bone, which produce swelling and interfere with linear bone growth. As with cartilaginous exostoses, these arise from the growth plate, growth ceases at puberty, and replacement of cartilage by mature bone may follow. Enchondromas appear radiologically as radiolucent defects in the metaphyseal area of the tubular and flat bones, often with central calcific stippling. Enchondromatosis must be distinguished from hereditary exostoses and from fibrous dysplasia. Malignant degeneration is uncommon. When enchondromatosis is associated with multiple hemangiomas (Maffucci's syndrome), the enchondromas or hemangiomas undergo malignant transformation in 15 per cent of cases.

Achondroplasia

Chondrodystrophies are disorders of cartilaginous growth that typically eventuate in disproportionate short stature. The most common of them is achondroplasia. Affected individuals are easily recognizable: The limbs are short; the trunk is of relatively normal length; and the head is large, with a bulging forehead and scooped-out nose. Achondroplasia is inherited as an autosomal dominant trait. About 80 per cent of cases represent new mutations; the mutation rate increases with paternal age. To account for short bones and a shortened cranial base but a normal cranial vault, the mutation must affect endochondral ossification, as in the limbs and chondrocranium, but not membranous ossification, as in the vault. Surprisingly, the growth plate is not grossly disorganized histologically, and chondrocytes are normal ultrastructurally. The pathogenesis of achondroplasia remains an enigma. Radiographically, the cranial base and foramen magnum are small, lumbar lordosis is greatly exaggerated, and the lumbar spinal canal narrows from the upper to lower lumbar spine, as indicated by a decreasing interpeduncular distance. The long bones appear massive, owing to their disproportionately normal width. Complications can include hydrocephalus, presumably related to the small size of the foramen magnum, and spinal cord and root compression, a potential consequence of even minimal impingement by a disc or osteophyte upon the small spinal canal. Despite its problems, achondroplasia is compatible with good health and a normal lifespan.

Beighton P: Inherited Disorders of the Skeleton. Edinburgh, Churchill Livingstone, 1988. *A comprehensive monograph that includes inherited osteosclerotic disorders as well as bone dysplasias.*

Nicoletti B, Kopits SE, Ascani E, et al. (eds.): Human Achondroplasia: A Multidisciplinary Approach. New York, Plenum Press, 1988. *Diagnostic, orthopedic, and social aspects.*

241 Bone Tumors

Henry J. Mankin

PRIMARY TUMORS OF BONE

Primary bone tumors are uncommon, but they are important, since they are most frequent in the young (the second to the fourth decades) and they tend to be extraordinarily malignant. Beyond their random occurrence, bone tumors have been associated with (1) genetic disorders of preosseous cartilage (hereditary multiple osteocartilaginous exostoses and enchondromatosis), (2) radiation injury, (3) Paget's disease, (4) bone infarcts, (5) chronic osteomyelitis, and, most recently, (6) specific genetic errors.

CLASSIFICATION AND STAGING

Any connective tissue element that exists in the osseous or preosseous skeleton can be the cell of origin of a neoplastic process; both benign and malignant tumors may be classified according to cell type as osseous, cartilaginous, fibrous, and "other" (including vascular, neural, marrow, lipid, and tumors of unspecified origin). Furthermore, within each broad category, several radiologically, histologically, and biologically distinct types of tumors exist, providing a sometimes puzzling array of diagnoses from which to choose for a patient who presents with an obvious radiographic lesion.

Prior to treatment, all primary bone tumors must be staged to assess the anatomic extent of the lesion (T), the grade of the tumor (G), and the presence or absence of distant metastases (M). The determination of T is best done by physical examination, radiographs, and special imaging studies, including angiography, computed and planar tomography, magnetic resonance imaging, and ^{99m}Tc bone scanning. The grade of the tumor can be determined only by study of biopsy material using both standard and specialized techniques, including, most recently, flow cytometry of DNA kinetics. Since most bone tumors metastasize to the lungs and occasionally other bones, computed tomography of the chest and a bone scan are required to establish "M."

BENIGN BONE TUMORS

Most benign tumors of bone present as a mass or deformity detectable on physical examination, as an incidental finding on a radiograph, or occasionally as a result of a pathologic fracture through a weakened area of the bone. With few exceptions, benign lesions are small and painless. For some, the radiographic features are so characteristic as to be easily recognizable. Benign bone tumors show well-defined cortical margins, absence of a soft tissue mass, and sclerotic bony margination separating the lesion from the normal tissues. Some lesions may require biopsy for definition, and some, particularly those that threaten the integrity of the skeleton, require treatment, which, for most of these lesions, is "intralesional" (such as simple excision or curettage and packing of the defect with methylmethacrylate or autograft or allograft bone), although for some benign lesions the recurrence rate may be high and may necessitate subsequent surgery. An ultimate cure may be anticipated in a high percentage of the cases.

MALIGNANT PRIMARY TUMORS OF BONE

Multiple myeloma, the most common "primary" malignancy of bone, is discussed in Ch. 151. Other primary malignant tumors of bone are considerably less common in frequency than carcinomas or blood element neoplasms. The most frequently encountered bone sarcomas are osteosarcoma and (depending on the age group studied) chondrosarcoma; round cell tumors (Ewing's sarcoma and primary lymphoma of bone), giant cell tumors, and malignant fibrous tumors follow in order of diminishing frequency.

OSTEOSARCOMA. The peak age of incidence for osteosarcoma is in the second decade, with a second, lesser peak occurring in later years (often in association with Paget's disease). The tumor has a predilection for the distal femur or proximal tibia of the rapidly growing child and occurs more frequently in males. Osteosarcoma in later life usually occurs as a complication of Paget's disease, radiation injury of bone, or a bone infarct. Pain, limitation of movement, and swelling are the principal complaints, and even at earliest observation, the radiographic findings show obvious destruction and a soft tissue mass outside the bone. Productive changes within and without the bone suggest the presence of the osteosarcoma. Typically, the serum alkaline phosphatase level is moderately elevated. About 10 per cent of patients have metastases to the lungs at the time of the initial examination or shortly after. If left untreated, the course is fulminant, with a rapid progression of the tumor, widespread metastases, and death in less than a year.

Current treatment consists of preliminary chemotherapy with doxorubicin, methotrexate, and *cis*-platinum, followed by usually limb-sparing surgery using an allograft or metallic implant. Chemotherapy is continued for up to 1 year and has led to survival figures ranging up to 85 to 90 per cent. Even in patients who develop metastases, resection of pulmonary nodules in conjunction with aggressive chemotherapy appears to be successful in effecting cure in over 20 per cent.

ROUND CELL SARCOMA. *Ewing's sarcoma* is a highly malignant tumor of unknown cytogenesis, which primarily affects teenage children and produces a very destructive, lytic tumor often of the pelvis, shaft of the femur, or other long bones. Symptoms and signs include not only local pain, swelling, and a palpable mass, but at times systemic findings, such as fever, malaise, chills, and a rapid erythrocyte sedimentation rate. The prognosis for this tumor is particularly poor without treatment, but the lesions, like the lymphomas of bone, are remarkably chemosensitive and radiosensitive. The combination of chemotherapy and local irradiation or, more recently, of chemotherapy and surgical resection provides a long survival rate exceeding 60 per cent. *Non-Hodgkin's lymphoma* and, less frequently, *Hodgkin's lymphoma* may make their appearance as a bony focus difficult to distinguish radiographically and sometimes histologically from Ewing's sarcoma. Staging of these individuals is essential to be certain that the bone tumor is solitary rather than an osseous focus of diffuse disease. The treatment is similar to that of lymphoma of other sites, depending principally on the radiosensitivity of the primary site and the response of the tumor to chemotherapeutic drugs.

CHONDROSARCOMA. The chondrosarcomas are extraordinarily variable in clinical presentation, degree of malignancy, and biologic behavior. Central chondrosarcomas, most prevalent in middle age, occur most frequently in the pelvis and proximal portions of the appendicular skeleton. Neither radiation nor chemotherapy has proved to be very effective in the treatment of chondrosarcomas, particularly for large tumors. With accurate staging, however, surgery with appropriately wide margins may produce a cure in up to 85 per cent of patients, depending on the stage of the disease.

METASTATIC TUMORS OF BONE

Certain of the malignant neoplasms and tumors of the hematopoietic system have a propensity for metastasis to the skeleton. At times, the presenting complaint for a patient with a primary breast, lung, prostatic, renal, or thyroid carcinoma may be pain in the spine, ribs, or long bones or a pathologic fracture through a metastatic focus. In men, the most frequent source of metastatic carcinoma is carcinoma of the prostate, followed closely by carcinoma of the lung and, with lesser frequency, tumors originating in the genitourinary or gastrointestinal tracts or thyroid gland. In women, carcinoma of the breast is by far the most frequent cause of metastatic bone disease, but the lung is increasingly the primary site in women who smoke. The frequency of metastatic carcinoma far exceeds that of primary tumors of bone, especially in later life, so that staging of any individual with a bone tumor should include a careful clinical, imaging, and laboratory evaluation of the more frequent sites of origin. Conversely, patients who are under treatment for primary tumors of the organs just cited should have frequent bone scans, which are far more sensitive than radiographs in revealing the presence of distant metastases.

Radiographic findings in metastatic bone disease vary with the type of primary tumor and the bony site involved, but almost always the tumorous deposits are in the axial and proximal appendicular skeleton, are centrally placed within the bone, and are quite destructive in appearance. About 90 per cent of prostatic, 50 per cent of breast, and 25 per cent of lung carcinomatous metastases evoke a sclerotic response in the affected bone, producing a mottled increase in osseous density on the radiograph. The treatment of skeletal metastases from a primary carcinoma depends on the patient's general condition, the radiosensitivity of the lesion, the site and extent of involvement, and the proximity of the tumor to vital structures such as the spinal cord. Most skeletal metastases are radiosensitive, and regression and long-term remission can be achieved in some patients with carcinoma of the prostate and breast simply with the use of hormones and radiation (see Ch. 223 and 227). When the integrity of the skeletal system is threatened or a pathologic fracture of a long bone has occurred, prophylactic or therapeutic open reduction and internal fixation are clearly indicated and frequently provide the patient with considerable relief of pain and restoration of function.

Heare TC, Enneking WF, Heare MM: Staging techniques and biopsy of bone tumors. Orthop Clin North Am 20:273, 1989. *Techniques of staging and pitfall of the biopsy.*

Jaffe N: Chemotherapy for malignant bone tumors. Orthop Clin North Am 20: 487, 1989. *A review of current methods of chemotherapy.*

Mankin HJ, Gebhardt MC: Advances in the management of bone tumors. Clin Orthop 200:73, 1985. *An extensive review of this general topic.*

Sweetnam R: Malignant bone tumor management: 30 years of achievement. Clin Orthop 247:67, 1989. *A comprehensive review of progress in the field of bone tumors.*

PART XVIII
DISEASES OF THE IMMUNE SYSTEM

242 Introduction

J. Claude Bennett

The immune system consists of an integrated constellation of various cell types, each with a specifically designated functional role (Fig. 242–1). In addition, secreted molecules (cytokines) are responsible for interactions, modulations, and regulation of the system. Antibody molecules and cells participate in specific interactions with immunogenic epitopes present on foreign materials, i.e., antigens introduced from the exterior world and foreign to the host. Recognition events are the beginning of the physiologic steps identified with the immune response; they initiate a series of processes causing a wide range of effects within the host. These include the pathways through which inflammation takes place, the killing of invading microbial agents, and the disposal of foreign toxic compounds.

Events leading to specific molecular interactions depend upon the differentiation and expansion of the cell clones that are involved. These include production of specific cell-bound receptor molecules (TCR, T-cell receptors) and secreted or cell-bound immunoglobulins (antibodies). The cellular network (Fig. 242–1) results in the elaboration of an enormous array of specific molec-

ular events. Abnormal regulation of the immune system may cause the host to be unable to handle antigenic stimuli, resulting in a state of immune deficiency (see Ch. 244). At the other extreme it may allow the host to react to its own tissues, resulting in an autoimmune process (see Ch. 261).

In an immunocompetent individual, the immune response is initiated by the introduction of an external agent that possesses an immunogenic structural epitope. The appropriate response depends upon the recognition by surface receptors of B and T lymphocytes of the foreignness of the introduced agent. These interactions lead to events that allow proliferation and differentiation of the antigen-stimulated cells. In order to appreciate the exquisite degree of specificity expressed by this remarkable system, one must understand the molecular interactions that result in antigen processing, presentation, and cellular proliferation. B lymphocytes differentiate to produce specifically directed immunoglobulins (antibodies). All such immunoglobulins share an overall structure, but each contains its own antigen-binding area (Fab region) and within any class (e.g., IgG, IgM) a similar constant region (Fc) (Fig. 242–2). Therefore, the product of any given clone of B cells has a unique specificity distinct from that of all other clonal lines of B cells. This provides the enormous diversity in the recognition properties of the immune system. Furthermore, each of the classes of immunoglobulins is imbued with structural elements that set it apart

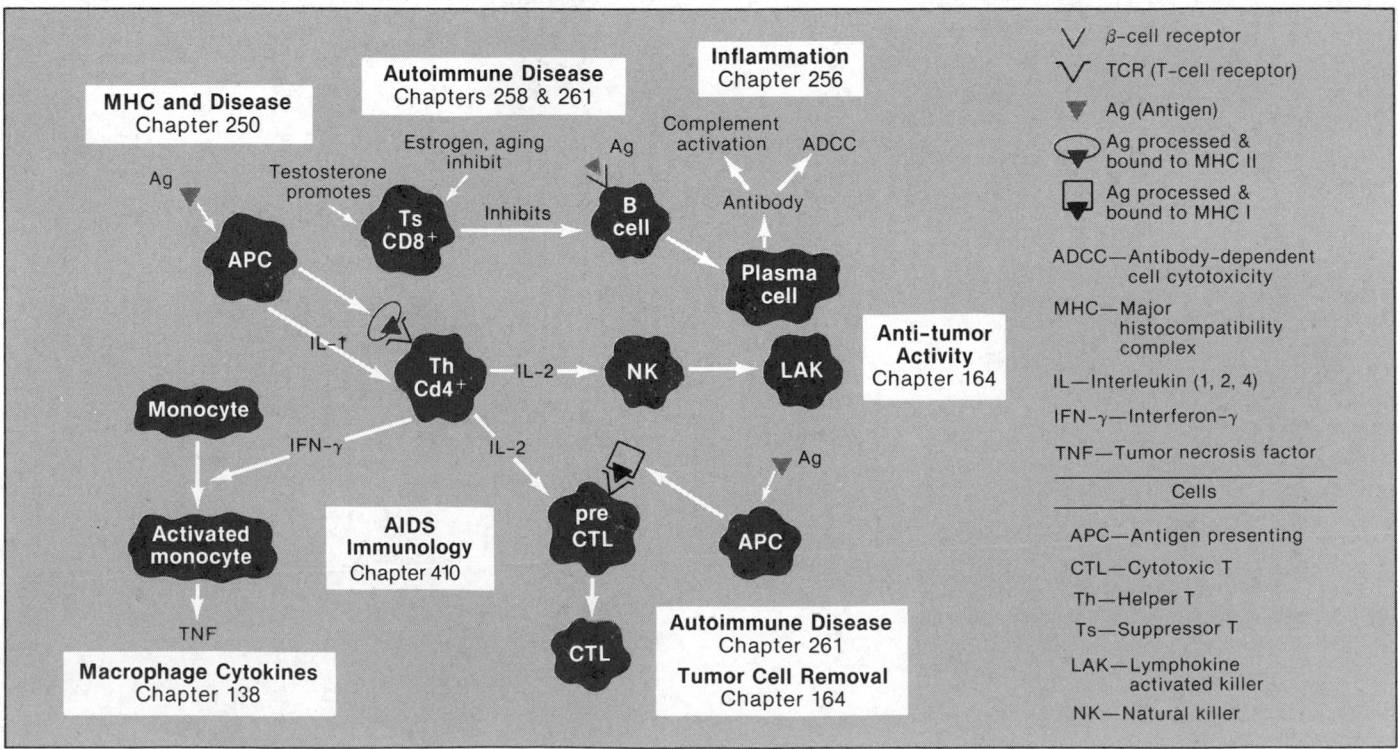

FIGURE 242–1. Schematic diagram of some of the major interactions among the various cell types and secreted molecules of the immune system. Definitions of symbols are given on the right-hand side of the figure. The blocks at various stages in the pathways and at their outcomes indicate their potential significance and refer to chapters elsewhere in this textbook for further reading and in-depth study.

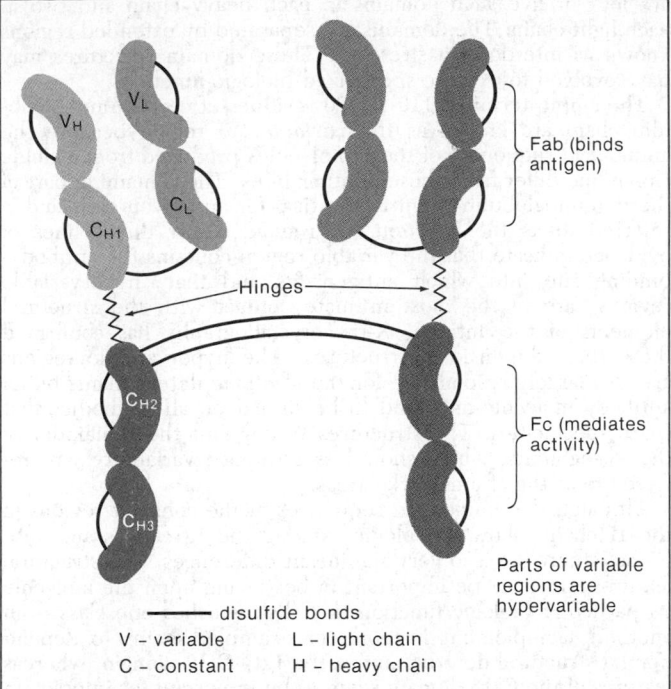

FIGURE 242–2. Diagram of the overall structure of immunoglobulin G, which is the basic structural pattern for all immunoglobulins (see text), drawn to highlight the various reactive areas and to emphasize the globular domain features of the immunoglobulin molecule.

Legend within figure:
Fab (binds antigen)
Fc (mediates activity)
Parts of variable regions are hypervariable
disulfide bonds
V – variable   L – light chain
C – constant   H – heavy chain
Hinges

and define its distinct function in biologic effector mechanisms Table 242–1).

During the initiation of the immune process, T lymphocytes respond to antigen on the surface of macrophages or other specialized antigen-presenting cells (APC) (Figs. 242–1 and 242–3). T cells then differentiate as they express various functions, such as cytotoxic potential, enhanced expression of immunity (helper T cells), or down-modulation of the immune response. Therefore, the T lymphocyte becomes pivotal in the development of both *humoral immunity* by way of its stimulation of B lymphocytes and the development of *cellular immunity* and regulation by virtue of its own intrinsic properties and its role in elaboration of cytokines for cellular communication processes.

Reactions of the immune system may stimulate activation of the complement cascade (Ch. 243) and the production of arachidonic acid derivatives such as prostaglandins and leukotrienes (Ch. 256), which play key roles in the expression of inflammation. Both lymphocytes and macrophages secrete a variety of cytokines, which modulate the immune response and the induction of inflammation (Table 242–2).

Immunologic events can be regulated through networks of antibody-forming cells, helper/suppressor mechanisms, and cytokine mediation or through specific mechanisms of immunologic tolerance. Immunodeficiency states and autoimmune diseases represent the endpoints of either a genetically incompetent or a poorly regulated immune system.

B LYMPHOCYTE LINEAGE AND ANTIBODY PRODUCTION

Secreted antibodies are the products of plasma cells, which represent the terminal phase of differentiation of B lymphocytes. The latter are found in all peripheral lymphoid tissues and also in the circulating pool of lymphocytes. Within their surface membranes, B cells have receptors that allow them to recognize foreign antigenic determinants. These receptors are immunoglobulin molecules, and in the initial stages of differentiation are generally of the IgM and IgD classes. Stimulation by a specific antigen in conjunction with appropriate cytokines results in proliferation of these B cells and the production of secreted antibody (see Fig. 242–1).

In the earliest stages of differentiation (Fig. 242–4), B lymphocytes lack membrane immunoglobulin (mIg). However, these cells begin to express in their cytoplasm the μ chain, which is the heavy (H) chain of IgM. Later they produce the light (L) chain (either kappa [κ] or lambda [λ]) which allows IgM molecules to be expressed on the surface. The binding region on the mIg of each cell line is unique in its specificity and is identical to that of the antibody molecule that is to be secreted. This means that at a very early developmental stage, a given cell is locked into its own specificity. This process involves several gene rearrangements (see below).

B-cell activation, proliferation, and differentiation require a variety of cytokines. Perhaps the most important in man is interleukin 2 (IL-2), which seems to play a central role in these events and thus facilitates the production of immunoglobulins of all isotypes. Although other cytokines (e.g., IL-4 and TGF-β) are identified as being able to amplify and modify antibody production, generally they are unable to do this except in the presence of IL-2 (Table 242–2).

IMMUNOGLOBULIN FUNCTION AND STRUCTURE

The basic structure of all immunoglobulin molecules (see Fig. 242–2) is similar among the various classes. Essentially they consist of two types of polypeptide chains—the larger called the heavy (H) chain, the smaller known as the light (L) chain. Each immunoglobulin subunit consists of two identical H and two identical L chains and would therefore have the molecular formula H_2L_2. The heavy and light chains are connected to each other by disulfide bonds, and similarly there are disulfide bridges between the two heavy chains which vary in number for the different classes and subclasses. They are generally located in the center of the heavy chain region, known as the "hinge" region, which

TABLE 242–1. PROPERTIES OF IMMUNOGLOBULINS BY CLASS AND SUBCLASS

Class	IgG	IgA	IgM	IgD	IgE
Molecular weight	160,000	170,000 or polymer	900,000	180,000	190,000
Sedimentation constant	7S	7S (9, 11, 13)	19S	7S	8S
Serum concentration (mg/dl)	1000–1500	250–300	100–150	0.3–30	0.0015–0.2
Valence	2	2 (monomer)	10	2	2
Molecular formula	$\gamma_2 L_2$	$(\alpha_2 L_2)_n$	$(\mu_2 L_2)_5$	$\delta_2 L_2$	$\epsilon_2 L_2$

Subclass	IgG1	IgG2	IgG3	IgG4	IgA1	IgA2	IgM	IgD	IgE
Subclass per cent of class, in serum	65	20	10	5	90	10			
Complement fixation	+ +	+	+ +	–	–	–	+ +	–	–
Alternative complement fixation					+	+		±	±
Placental passage	+	+	+	+	–	–	–	–	–
Fixing to mast cells or basophils	–	–	–	–	–	–	–	–	+
Binding to									
Macrophages	+	±	+	±	–	–	–	–	–
Neutrophils	+	+	+	+	+	+	–	–	–
Platelets	+	+	+	+	–	–	–	–	–
Lymphocytes	+	+	+	+	–	–	+	–	–
Half-life (days)	23	23	8–9	23	6	6	5	3	2.5
Synthesis rate (mg/kg/day)	25	?	3.5	?	44	22	7	0.4	0.02

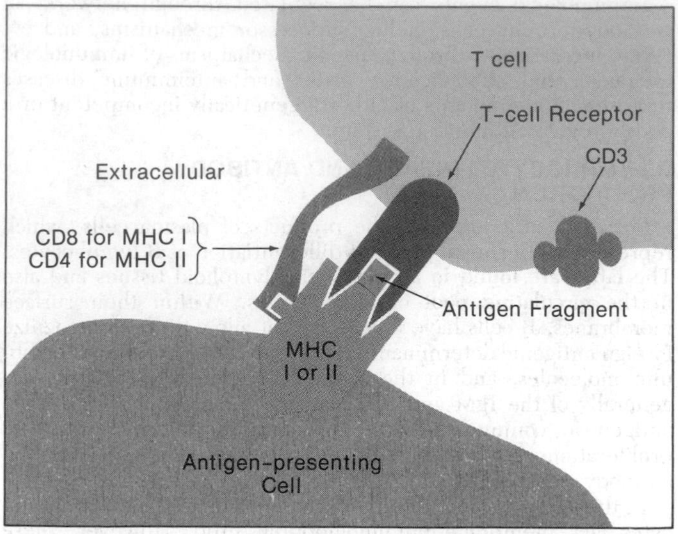

FIGURE 242–3. The molecular events involved in antigen presentation to the T cell. Shown are the interactions among the various molecules, including the major histocompatibility complex (MHC), the T-cell receptor, the CD8 or CD4 molecules, and the CD3 complex. See text for description of the polypeptide chain composition of the various molecules.

is unusually rich in cysteine and proline. Molecular weight of the light chain is about 25,000 daltons, and that of the heavy chain varies between 50,000 and 65,000 daltons. The differences in size of the heavy chains are related to differences in the structure of the hinge region or to the presence of an extra globular domain, as in the case of the μ and ε heavy chains (in IgM and IgE, respectively). Globular domains, formed by intrachain disulfide bonds, each consist of about 110 amino acid residues; and there

are four or five such domains in each heavy chain and two in each light chain. The domains are separated by extended regions known as interdomain stretches. These domain structures may have evolved to execute specialized biologic functions.

The amino terminal 110 to 120 residues of each immunoglobulin chain are known as the *variable* (V) region because the amino acid sequences of those molecules produced from a single clonal line differ from those of other lines. The remaining part of the immunoglobulin chain is identical for any given class and is referred to as the *constant* (C) region. Many direct lines of evidence indicate that the variable region contains the antibody-binding site into which antigen fits and that "hypervariable regions" are in the most intimate contact with the structural elements of the antigen. X-ray crystallography has confirmed these three-dimensional structures. The hypervariable regions are also largely responsible for the *idiotypic* determinants on an antibody molecule and tend to be similar on all antibodies that share specificities. The structures throughout the remainder of the V segments, which show less sequence variability, are referred to as the "framework" areas.

Although the amino acid sequences of the constant regions of the H chains show homologies among the Ig classes and subclasses, there are also very significant differences. The structural features appear to be important in bestowing upon the molecule its particular biologic function that distinguishes one class from another. Complement fixation, for example, seems to depend upon a structural determinant in the IgG CH2 domain, whereas features of the CH3 domain seem to be important for interaction with a variety of cells by way of the Fc receptors. More than one domain in the Fc region of the IgG heavy chain is required for reaction with the binding sites on rheumatoid factors (Ch. 258).

Since Porter's original work on the structure of antibodies, much has been learned about their molecular structure by the use of proteolytic enzymes. For example, papain cleaves IgG into an Fc fragment and two Fab fragments, whereas pepsin degrades the Fc fragment and yields the two Fab fragments still joined by a disulfide bridge (Fab)₂ (see Fig. 242–2). Different enzymes cleave the various classes in different ways, and this approach

TABLE 242–2. CYTOKINES AND THEIR BIOLOGIC ACTIVITIES

Cytokines	Cell Source			Major Activities
	T	Macrophages	Other	
Interleukin-1α and β (IL-1α and β)		+	+	Fever; bone resorption; prostaglandin release; stimulate cytokine production by macrophages and T cells; proliferation of B and T cells.
Interleukin-2 (IL-2)	+			Activates cytotoxic T cells and NK cells. Stimulates proliferation of T cells and NK cells. Stimulates differentiation of T cells and LAK cells. Costimulates proliferation of B cells and antibody secretion.
Interleukin-3 (IL-3)	+			Supports proliferation of mast cells and pre-B cells. Supports differentiation of stem cells.
Interleukin-4 (IL-4)	+		+	Activates resting B cells and macrophages. Induces IgG and IgE secretion in LPS-activated B cells. Stimulates proliferation of T cells and mast cells. Suppresses TNF-α, IL-1, IL-6 in monocytes.
Interleukin-5 (IL-5)	+			Induces IgA production and IgM secretion from LPS-activated B cells. Proliferation of eosinophils; supports differentiation of cytotoxic T cells.
Interleukin-6 (IL-6)	+	+	+	Induces antibody secretion; differentiation of cytotoxic T cells; proliferation of megakaryocytes. Promotes myeloma cell growth.
Interleukin-7 (IL-7)			Thymic strand cells	Proliferation and differentiation of pre-B cells. Proliferation of thymocytes.
Interleukin-8 (IL-8)		+		Neutrophil and T-cell chemotaxis.
Interleukin-9 (IL-9)	+			Growth of T-helper cell clones.
Interleukin-10 (IL-10)	+			Inhibits production of certain cytokines by selected T-helper cell clones.
Tumor necrosis factor-α (TNF-α) (cachectin)	+	+		Fever; shock; activates macrophages; stimulates PMN chemotoxin; angiogenesis, bone resorption; cytotoxic to many cells.
Tumor necrosis factor-β (TNF-β) (lymphotoxin)	+			Activates endothelial cells, granulocytes, and B cells. Inhibits angiogenesis; cytotoxic to many cells.
Interferon-γ (IFN-γ)	+		NK cells	Activates NK cells, cytotoxic T cells, endothelial cells, and macrophages. Has antitumor activity. Stimulates LAK activity; costimulates B-cell proliferation; inhibits T-cell proliferation.

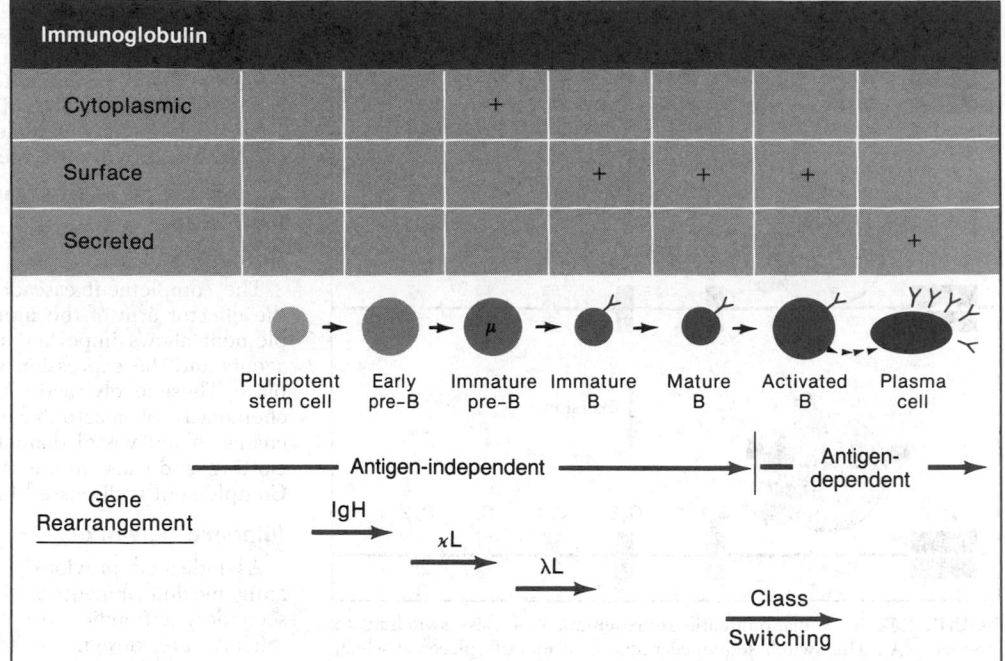

FIGURE 242–4. Presentation of B-cell pathway development in a sequential form showing when immunoglobulin appears in the cytoplasm or on the surface or is secreted. The gene rearrangements that take place at various stages of the differentiation pathway are indicated.

has been important in defining structural corollaries to biologic properties.

Comparisons among the various classes of immunoglobulin are shown in Table 242–1. Certain immunoglobulins appear very different from IgG. For example, IgM is a large molecule but consists of five subunits of the same basic immunoglobulin pattern. It has 10 heavy and 10 light chains and, therefore, 10 antibody-binding sites per molecule. However, because of steric factors, when IgM reacts with large protein antigens, it tends to bind with a valence of five. This can best be seen in the case of IgM rheumatoid factor binding to IgG, which yields a 22 S complex with a formula $(\mu_2L_2)5\text{-}(IgG)5$.

IMMUNOGLOBULIN GENETICS AND GENE ORGANIZATION

Human immunoglobulin genes are contained on chromosomes 2, 14, and 22 (Table 242–3). Several sequences of events must take place for immunoglobulin genes to be expressed. This requires a random process of gene reorganization. As shown in Figure 242–5, each C region is coded by a single gene, but many gene segments are necessary to form the repertoire of V genes. The latter are formed by rearrangement of DNA to bring one V gene into proximity with a J (junction) gene in the case of the L chains; and in the case of the heavy chains, the V must be brought into proximity with a D (diversity) region and a J region. For any given heavy-chain gene, the total V region is formed from a single V region, a single D, and a single J (Fig. 242–5). Combination with a given constant region would determine the Ig class. Recombination activating genes (RAG) activate the V-D-J recombination, and this suggests that they may encode enzymes that have the properties of being V-D-J recombinases.

TABLE 242–3. CHROMOSOMAL LOCATIONS OF THE HUMAN IMMUNOGLOBULIN AND T-CELL RECEPTOR GENES

Chain	Symbol	Locus
Immunoglobulin		
Heavy chain	H	14q32
Kappa light chain	κ	2p12
Lambda light chain	λ	22q11
T-cell receptor		
Alpha and delta chains	α, δ	14q11–12
Beta chain	β	7q32–35
Gamma chain	γ	7p15

The C region genes are located in tandem, so a switching process must occur in order to allow a given assembled V-D-J region to attach to any constant region. This process results in deletion of all intervening genes from that particular clone (Fig. 242–6). In some B lymphocytes both IgD and IgM are present on the cell membrane at the same time, and this occurs through alternative RNA splicing.

There are several mechanisms for generation of antibody diversity which are inherent in the somatic process of Ig gene formation.

1. *Combinatorial diversity*, which results from the combination of various gene segments as described above

2. *Junctional diversity*, which results at the joining site because of some imprecision in codon formation

3. *Junctional insertion*, by which diversity may arise because of insertion of extra nucleotides

4. *Somatic mutational events*

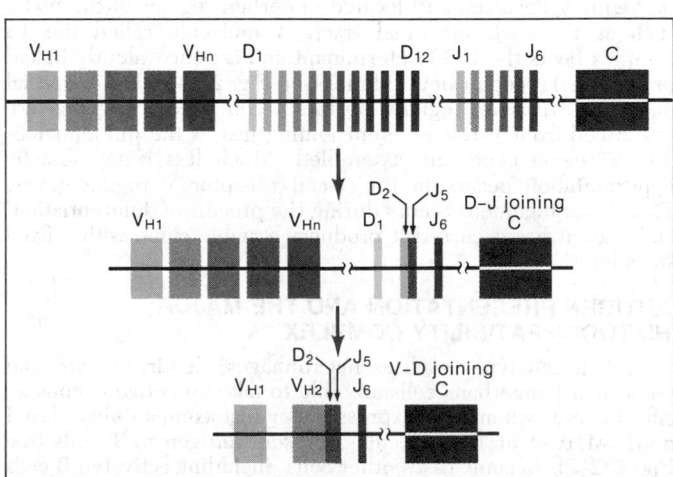

FIGURE 242–5. The mechanisms for DJ and VD joining to form the entire variable region of the heavy chain. Note that intervening gene sequences at each step of joining are deleted, giving rise to the final finished product of an entire V region with the constant region at some distance. This event would be followed by the development of messenger RNA and its splicing to form the entire translatable message sequence (see text for details).

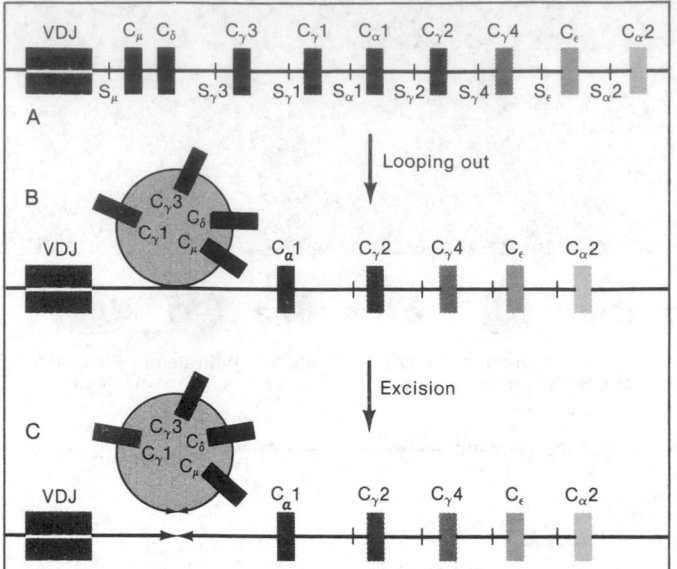

FIGURE 242–6. A diagrammatic representation of class switching to produce IgA₁. The switch sequence regions (S) identify places at which looping can occur. This results ultimately in excision of the loop containing $C\mu$, $C\delta$, $C\gamma_1$, and $C\gamma_3$ and brings $C\alpha_1$ into close juxtaposition to the rearranged VDJ regions. (Adapted with permission from von Schwedler et al.: Nature 345:452–454, 1990. Copyright © 1990 Macmillan Magazines Limited.)

5. *Exchange rearrangement* of the H segments
6. The *combination of associated heavy and light chains*

This process allows an essentially random extrapolation of combinations into the millions of possibilities; i.e., it *generates* antibody diversity.

T LYMPHOCYTES

T-Cell Receptors

The most common form of T-cell receptor consists of a disulfide-linked heterodimer of α and β chains. Both of these chains contain amino-terminal *variable* regions and carboxy-terminal *constant* regions, just as occur in immunoglobulins. These chains contain carbohydrate and are bound within the surface of the T cell with membrane-spanning regions. A subset of T cells possesses similar receptors made up of γ and δ chains that seem to be highly specialized and located in certain regions of the body, such as the gastrointestinal tract. A molecule called the T3 complex bears the CD3 determinant and is noncovalently linked to the T-cell receptor heterodimer (see Fig. 242–3). It is of special note that variable regions of the T-cell receptor genes are assembled from V-D-J segment joining just as the immunoglobulin V region genes are assembled. Much less if any somatic hypermutation occurs in the T-cell receptor V region genes. Thus, rearrangement occurs during the process of differentiation, and once it has occurred it produces a stable clone with a fixed specificity.

ANTIGEN PRESENTATION AND THE MAJOR HISTOCOMPATIBILITY COMPLEX

Certain cell types such as macrophages, dendritic cells, and epidermal Langerhans cells are able to take up antigens nonspecifically and, when they express major histocompatibility class I or II (MHC I or II) molecules, present antigen to T cells (see Fig. 242–3). In some cases other cells, including activated B cells that may express class II MHC molecules, may also act as antigen-presenting cells. The antigen presented has often been processed so that only a relatively small peptide determinant is bound to the MHC for presentation. The presentation event appears to involve the MHC molecule in conjunction with the processed antigen peptide on the surface of the antigen-presenting cell so that it can react with the T-cell receptor, the T3 complex, and

the CD4 molecule in the case of MHC-II, or with CD8 in the case of MHC-I, on the membrane of the T cell (Ch. 250).

Similar membrane recognition events take place when cytotoxic T cells recognize and interact with cells bearing specific foreign antigens. In this case, the cytotoxic T cell may recognize the foreign antigen in conjunction with a class I MHC molecule, and it does so by virtue of its T-cell receptor in the presence of the T3 complex and a CD8 molecule. Such activated cytotoxic T cells can then destroy their target cells by a lytic process.

REGULATION AND MODULATION OF THE IMMUNE PROCESS

Complement

The complement cascade is important in the modification of the effector arm of the immune system. The activation of complement allows important events such as removal of infectious agents and the expression of the inflammatory response to take place. These involve active fragments of the pathway that enhance chemotaxis of macrophages, alter blood vessel permeability, change blood vessel diameters, cause lysis to cells, alter blood clotting, and cause numerous other subtle points of modification. Complement is discussed in greater detail in Ch. 243.

Idiotypic Networks

As indicated previously, antibody molecules express unique antigenic determinants on their variable regions, thereby allowing secondary antibodies to be produced against them. Such determinants are designated *idiotopes*. Therefore, an idiotope of immunoglobulin is functionally equivalent to the *clonotypic* antigenic determinant of a clonal line of T cells. The idiotypic network concept (Fig. 242–7) holds that the immune system is in a dynamic regulatory equilibrium so that members of each clone within the system are recognized by members of other clones through these anti-idiotope interactions. Conceptually, this interrelated system provides mechanisms for regulation based on recognition of receptors without need for exogenous antigen. This method of regulation may allow certain idiotopes to become dominantly expressed and may be operative with unique *clonal markers*, such as those that are observed due to clonal expansion in malignant lymphoid diseases.

Suppression

Regulation of responses to antigenic stimulation and also control of potential immune responses against self components are essential ingredients of a smoothly operating immune system. Suppressor T cells and the suppressor system represent a series of cell types that act in a highly complex fashion. Several distinct types of suppressor systems have been described, and their sequential action appears to have an amplification effect so that direct and graded regulation can take place. Suppressor effector cells can act on antibody-secreting cells and on T cells to downregulate their expression. Although the mechanism of suppression exists, the T-suppressor cell has yet to be isolated.

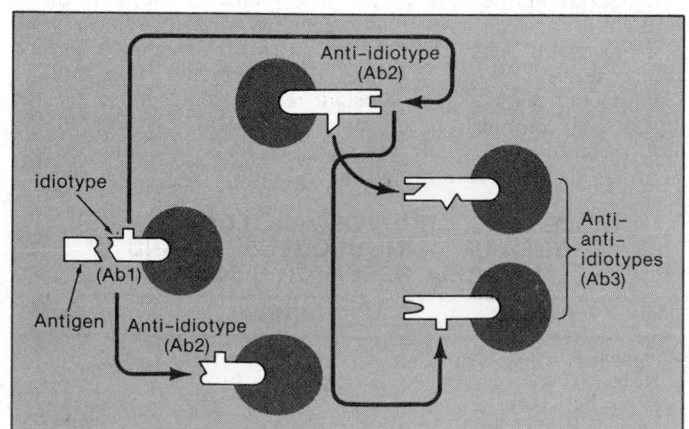

FIGURE 242–7. Diagrammatic representation of the idiotypic network showing the development of anti-idiotypes and anti-anti-idiotypes in sequential processes. This complementary fit mechanism provides the structural basis for the feedback network.

Cytokines

A growing array of molecules have been identified as products of cells that serve to regulate the immune system and to evoke responses in other cells, such as blood vessel endothelial cells and precursor cells in the bone marrow. Cytokines can regulate levels of response or induce differentiation and proliferation of cells. Table 242–2 summarizes the properties of some of these molecules which may be encountered in immune regulation (see also Ch. 256 and 285).

SUMMARY

The immune system is a highly orchestrated and coordinated system that allows a rapid response to foreign substances in a highly specific manner. The organization occurs at the level of the gene, the cell, and the mediator. Therefore, any qualitative or quantitative change in this system can produce profound effects. This is evident as one examines diseases of the immune system, such as those that occur as the result of alteration in immune regulation (see Ch. 258 and 261).

Inflammation, often immunologically mediated and often resulting in tissue damage, is a key feature of diseases of virtually any organ system. Therefore, a knowledge of basic immunology is critical to a clear understanding of the nature of these abnormalities. A student of medicine must be prepared for application of immunology to every branch of internal medicine and for recognizing its importance to an understanding of disease and, hence, the care of the patient.

Balkwill FR, Burke F: The cytokine network. Immunol Today 10:299, 1989. *An excellent integration of cytokine functions.*

Benjamini E, Leskowitz S: Immunology: A Short Course. New York, Alan R. Liss, 1988. *An excellent, manageable general text for the novice.*

Krensky AM, Weiss A, Crabtree G, et al: T-lymphocyte–antigen interactions in transplant rejection. N Engl J Med 322:510, 1990. *Description of T-cell pathways and functional interactions.*

Lai E, Wilson RK, Hood LE: Physical maps of the mouse and human immunoglobulin-like loci. Adv Immunol 46:1, 1989. *Description of the genetic relationships and the methods for generating physical gene maps for this group of structures.*

Maizels N: To understand function, study structure. Cell 60:887, 1990. *A brief discussion of the T-cell receptor structure and its relationship to the structure of immunoglobulins.*

Oettinger MA, Schatz DG, Gorka C, Baltimore D: RAG-1 and RAG-2, adjacent genes that synergistically activate V(D)J recombination. Science 248:1517, 1990. *A detailed description of the mechanisms of Ig class switching.*

Smith KA: Interleukin-2. Sci Am, March 1990, p. 50. *A superb and easy-to-read discussion of the pivotal cytokines in regulation of the immune system.*

243 Complement

John E. Volanakis

Complement is a major effector system of host defense against invading pathogens. It comprises more than 30 proteins that upon activation elaborate protein fragments and protein-protein complexes that interact with specific cellular receptors or directly with cell membranes to mediate acute inflammatory reactions, clearance of foreign cells and molecules, and killing of pathogenic microorganisms. In their native state, complement proteins are either serum soluble or associated with cell membranes (Table 243–1). Most of the serum-soluble proteins are synthesized in the liver. However, a number of other cells—including blood monocytes, tissue macrophages, fibroblasts, epithelial cells of the gastrointestinal and genitourinary tracts, adipocytes, and glial cells—can also produce these proteins. Complement proteins exhibit extensive structural homologies among themselves with remarkable conservation of a small number of repeated structural motifs, indicating that multiple gene duplication events marked the evolution of the system. Functionally, complement proteins are categorized as those participating in the activation sequences, those regulating the activation and activities of the system, and those serving as receptors for biologically active fragments. Some complement proteins overlap these functional categories.

NOMENCLATURE

Eleven of the proteins participating in complement activation are termed complement components and are designated by the letter C and a number from 1 to 9. C1 is a Ca^{2+}-dependent complex of three distinct proteins, C1q, C1r, and C1s. Two additional proteins in this group are designated by the letters B and D. An overbar indicates the enzymatically active form of a complement protein or protein complex, as in C1. Proteolytic cleavage fragments of complement proteins are symbolized by lower case letters, as in C2a and C2b, and inactive fragments by the letter i, e.g., C2ai. Regulatory proteins are designated by capital letters, as in H and I, or by their abbreviated descriptive names, as in DAF for decay-accelerating factor. Five of the complement receptors are symbolized by the letters CR, for complement receptor, and a number from 1 to 5. The remaining receptors are denoted by the symbol of the protein or protein fragment they bind followed by the letter R, as in C5aR.

COMPLEMENT ACTIVATION

Activation of the complement system is necessary for expression of biologic activity and is characterized by operational simplicity and economy of design. The most important host defense activities are derived from two proteins, C3 and C5, that are structurally homologous and probably represent gene duplication products. Additional biologically active products are derived from C4, another structural homologue of C3. Expression of activity requires cleavage of C3 and C5 by highly specific proteases, termed *convertases* (Fig. 243–1). There are two C3 and two C5 convertases. One of each is assembled during activation of the two pathways of complement, which are termed *classic* and *alternative*. C3 convertases are bimolecular, whereas C5 convertases are trimolecular protein complexes. The two activation pathways utilize different proteins to form these enzymes. In addition, the assembly of the convertases is initiated by different activators in the two pathways. However, the resulting enzymes have identical substrate and peptide bond specificity, giving rise to identical biologically active fragments. Characteristic of the simplicity and economy of design of complement activation is the fact that C5 convertases are derivatives of C3 convertases (Fig. 243–1). In each case, a C3b fragment, produced by the action of C3

TABLE 243–1. PROTEINS OF THE COMPLEMENT SYSTEM*

| Prevalent Form in Native State | Functional Group | | |
	Participating in Activation Sequences	*Regulatory*	*Receptors*
Serum soluble	C1q, C1r, C1s, D C4, C3, C2, B C5, C6, C7, C8, C9	C1 INH C4bp, H, I, P C3a/C5a INA S protein	
Membrane associated		CR1, CR2 DAF, MCP HRF, CD59	C1qR, C3aR, C5aR CR1, CR2, CR3 CR4, CR5

*Established symbols have been used for most complement proteins. In addition, the following generally accepted abbreviations have been used: INH, inhibitor; C4bp, C4b-binding protein; INA, inactivator; R, receptor, e.g., CR1, complement receptor type 1; DAF, decay-accelerating factor; MCP, membrane cofactor protein; HRF, homologous restriction factor.

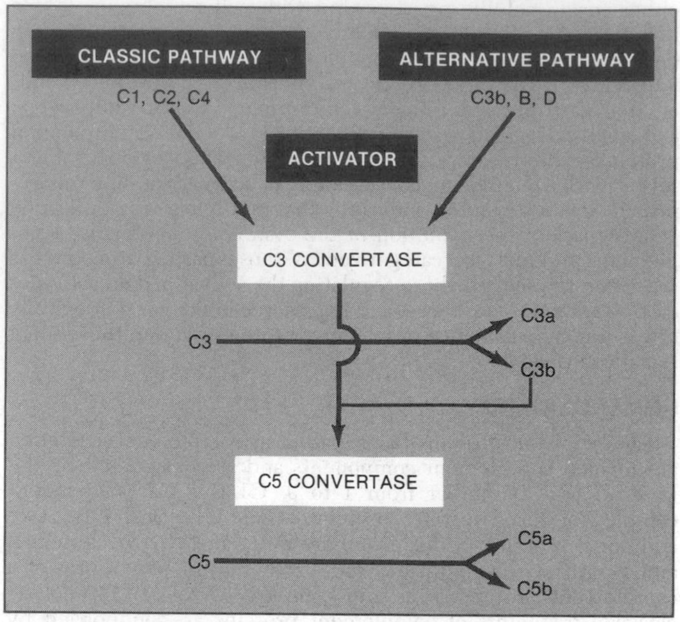

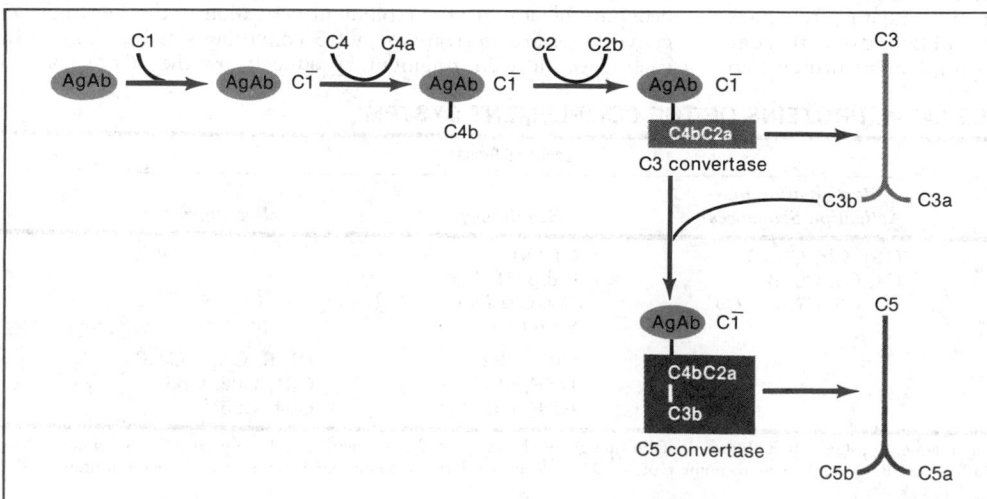

FIGURE 243–1. Activation of the complement system.

completing the assembly of the $\overline{C4b2a}$ complex, which is the C3 convertase of the classic pathway. Cleavage of C3 by the C3 convertase results in the covalent binding of many C3b fragments to the surface of the immune complex and the eventual binding of one C3b to the C4b subunit of the C3 convertase. This leads to the formation of the C3b4b2a complex, which is the C5 convertase of the classic pathway.

ALTERNATIVE PATHWAY. Activation of the alternative pathway is initiated by a variety of cellular surfaces, including those of certain bacteria, parasites, viruses, and fungi. Antibodies can also activate this pathway, but they are not usually required. Assembly of the convertases is intimately related to certain structural features of the multifunctional protein C3. C3 is the most abundant complement protein in blood and is characterized by the presence on its α-chain of an unusual, for blood proteins, thioester bond. Under physiologic conditions, this bond is relatively stable, being hydrolyzed at very slow rates to give rise to $C3_{H_2O}$, which is endowed with the ability to initiate the formation of the short-lived *initiation* C3 convertase. This is accomplished by the formation of a complex between $C3_{H_2O}$ and B and the subsequent cleavage of B by D to generate the $C3_{H_2O}Bb$ complex, the initiation C3 convertase (Fig. 243–3). This series of reactions, starting with the hydrolysis of the thioester bond in native C3 and concluding with the cleavage of C3 into C3a and C3b by the initiation C3 convertase, is considered to occur in the blood continuously at slow rates. Thus, a constant supply of small amounts of freshly generated C3b is available at all times. The initiation C3 convertase is quickly inactivated by the control proteins H and I.

Cleavage of C3 by a C3 convertase induces a pronounced change in the conformation of C3b associated with an extremely labile (metastable) thioester bond that reacts either with water or with hydroxyl or amino groups on the surface of cells or proteins. Thus, C3b becomes covalently attached via an ester or amide bond to surfaces in the immediate vicinity of its generation. The fate of surface-bound C3b depends entirely on the chemical nature of the surface. C3b bound to a nonactivator of the alternative pathway, e.g., host's red cells, is quickly inactivated by the action of control proteins. In contrast, C3b bound to an activator, e.g., *Escherichia coli* cells, preferentially binds B, which is then cleaved by D, generating the $\overline{C3bBb}$ complex, which is the C3 convertase of the alternative pathway. This enzyme is stabilized by the binding of P and is termed the *amplification* C3 convertase because it generates many C3b fragments and thus additional molecules of C3 convertase. Binding of a single C3b molecule to the C3 convertase gives rise to the $\overline{(C3b)_2Bb}$ complex, which is the C5 convertase of the alternative pathway (Fig. 243–3). A biochemical feature determining whether a cell surface can function as an activator of the alternative pathway is the relative amount of sialic acid that is present in membrane-associated glycoproteins and glycolipids. Sialic acid increases the affinity of C3b for the control protein H which prevents the formation of a C3 convertase. Conversely, the absence of cell surface sialic acid favors the binding of B to C3b and the formation of the amplification convertase.

convertase on C3, binds covalently to the C3 convertase and results in the generation of a C5 convertase. Furthermore, C3 and C5 are activated by their respective convertases in similar fashion: A single peptide bond near the NH_2 terminus of the α polypeptide chain of either C3 or C5 is cleaved to generate a small peptide, C3a or C5a, and a large two-polypeptide fragment, C3b or C5b. Each of these four fragments, as well as further cleavage fragments of C3b, express at least one activity important to host defense.

ASSEMBLY OF COMPLEMENT CONVERTASES

CLASSIC PATHWAY. In the classic pathway, assembly of the convertases is initiated by antibodies of the IgG or IgM class complexed with antigen. C1q, one of the three proteins in the C1 complex, binds to two or more Fc regions of antibody molecules within the immune complex. This binding induces a change in the conformation of C1q that causes the autoactivation of C1r, which in turn activates proenzyme C1s to enzymatically active $\overline{C1s}$ (Fig. 243–2). In the next step, $\overline{C1s}$ cleaves C4, resulting in the covalent attachment of its major fragment, C4b, to the surface of the immune complex. Attachment of C4b is accomplished through a transacylation reaction similar to that leading to covalent binding of C3b to activating surfaces (see below). C2 binds to C4b and is also cleaved by $\overline{C1s}$ into two fragments, the larger of which, C2a, remains bound to C4b,

FIGURE 243–2. Formation of complement convertases in the classic pathway of activation.

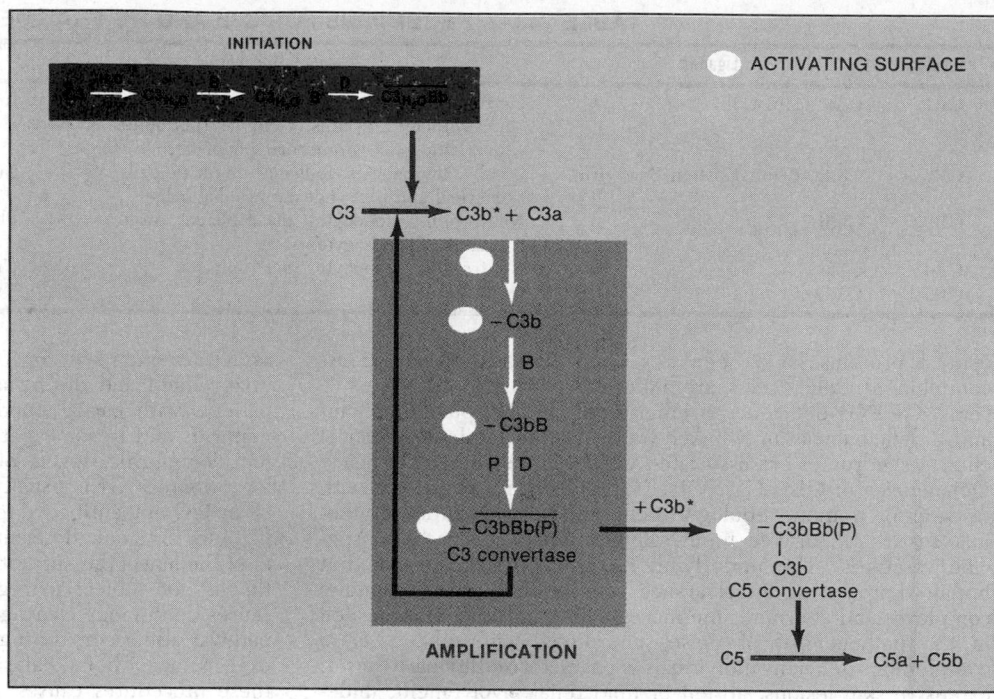

FIGURE 243–3. Formation of complement convertases in the alternative pathway of activation. Assembly of the *initiation* C3 convertase occurs at low levels continuously. When an activator is present, metastable C3b (C3b*) binds covalently to the activating surface and, because it is protected from the action of the regulatory proteins, initiates the assembly of the stable, *amplification* C3 convertase, which forms additional C3 convertase complexes and also the C5 convertase.

BIOLOGIC ACTIVITIES OF COMPLEMENT

With the exception of C5b, the fragments produced by the action of the convertases carry out their biologic functions by interacting with specific cellular receptors (Fig. 243–4). The three complement *anaphylatoxins*, C3a, C5a, and C4a, react with specific receptors to stimulate the release of histamine from mast cells mediating smooth muscle contraction and increased vascular permeability. In addition, C5a evokes neutrophil and monocyte responses, including adherence to vascular endothelia, chemotaxis, release of lysosomal enzymes, and generation of oxygen free radicals. Collectively, the anaphylatoxins allow for the recruitment of host defense molecules and cells to tissue sites invaded by pathogens. C3b and its further cleavage fragments, C3bi and C3dg, react with multiple receptors distributed in a variety of cells (Table 243–2). C3b covalently attached to immune complexes binds to CR1 receptors on erythrocytes, which transport the complexes to the liver, where they are taken up by Kupffer cells and cleared from the circulation. C3b and C3bi interact with CR1 and CR3, respectively, on phagocytic cells to promote ingestion of foreign cells and particles. Reaction of C3bi and C3dg with CR2 on B lymphocytes plays a role in regulating immune responses. C5b initiates the assembly of a large protein-protein complex, termed membrane attack complex (MAC), by interacting sequentially with a single molecule each of C6, C7, and C8 and with 1 to 12 molecules of C9. The MAC interacts directly with the lipid bilayer of biologic membranes through hydrophobic domains of the participating proteins and eventually forms a transmembrane channel that leads to killing of susceptible cells.

CONTROL OF COMPLEMENT ACTIVATION

The multiplicity and potency of the biologic activities generated during complement activation and particularly the ability of complement to mediate acute inflammatory reactions and to produce lethal lesions in cell membranes present a threat not only to invading pathogens but also to the cells and tissues of the host. This self-damaging potential of complement activation is normally kept under effective control by a number of inhibitors and inactivators that act at points of enzymatic amplification and also at the level of effector molecules. C1 INH binds to and inhibits C1r and C1s, regulating the activation and action of C1. A number of plasma and membrane-associated proteins, including C4bp, H, DAF, MCP, CR1, and CR2, control the rate of formation and the activity of complement convertases. Certain of these proteins act as obligatory cofactors for the proteolytic

enzyme I which cleaves C4b and C3b into smaller fragments. The serum S protein, also termed vitronectin, and two cell-associated proteins, HRF and CD59, inhibit the formation of the MAC. HRF and CD59 exhibit species specificity in their action. Finally, C3a/C5a INA, a carboxypeptidase, inactivates the complement anaphylatoxins. Collectively, the complement control proteins perform two important functions: They ensure that complement activation is proportional to the amount and duration of presence of complement activators and protect the cells of the host from the harmful potential of complement activation products.

INHERITED DEFICIENCIES OF COMPLEMENT PROTEINS (Table 243–3)

Hereditary deficiencies of almost all complement proteins participating in the activation sequences and of several of the

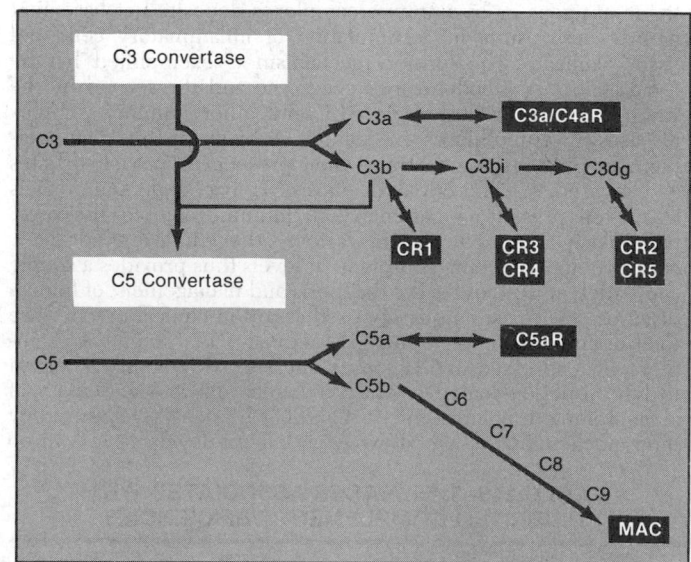

FIGURE 243–4. Interactions of complement fragments with cellular receptors that mediate biologic activities. The complex formed from the binding to C5b of one molecule of C6, C7, and C8 and of 1 to 12 molecules of C9 is termed MAC (membrane attack complex). It forms transmembrane pores by interacting directly with the lipid bilayer of biologic membranes.

TABLE 243–2. RECEPTORS FOR C3b AND ITS FRAGMENTS

Receptor	Ligands	Cellular Distribution	Functions
CR1	C3b, C4b, C3bi	Erythrocytes, neutrophils, eosinophils, monocytes, macrophages, B cells, T-cell subsets, follicular dendritic cells, glomerular podocytes	Immune complex clearance, endocytosis, phagocytosis, immunoregulation
CR2	C3dg, C3bi, Epstein-Barr virus	B cells, thymocytes, follicular dendritic cells, cervical and pharyngeal epithelial cells	Immunoregulation
CR3	C3bi	Neutrophils, monocytes, macrophages, large granular lymphocytes	Phagocytosis, leukocyte adhesion, enhanced cytotoxicity
CR4	C3bi	Neutrophils, monocytes, macrophages	Unknown
CR5	C3dg	Neutrophils	Unknown

control proteins have been described. With two exceptions, complement deficiencies are inherited as autosomal recessive traits. C1 INH deficiency is inherited as an autosomal dominant and P deficiency as an X-linked trait. A rather limited number of clinical syndromes are associated with complement deficiencies. Deficiencies of C1q, C1r, C1s, C4, and C2 are associated with diseases of immune etiology, including systemic lupus erythematosus (SLE), discoid lupus, glomerulonephritis, and nonspecific vasculitis. The underlying mechanisms are unclear, but impaired processing and clearance from the circulation of immune complexes and aberrant immunoregulation have been implicated in the pathogenesis of these syndromes. Clinically, SLE in complement-deficient individuals is characterized by early onset, extensive skin lesions, absent or mild renal involvement, undetectable anti-DNA, and low levels of antinuclear antibodies. Deficiencies of C3, H, I, or P predispose to severe recurrent infections with encapsulated pyogenic bacteria. Lack of or inefficient opsonization of the bacteria by C3b/C3bi apparently causes the susceptibility to infection. Individuals deficient in C5, C6, C7, or C8 are susceptible to disseminated neisserial infections. Direct lysis by complement is probably required for effective defense against gonococci and meningococci. Curiously, individuals with C9 deficiency are usually asymptomatic. Heterozygous deficiency of C1 INH results in hereditary angioedema (Ch. 245), characterized by episodic attacks of circumscribed, nonpruritic edema of the skin or the mucosa of the respiratory or gastrointestinal tract.

Pathophysiology

In certain human diseases, uncontrolled or aberrant activation of complement plays an important pathogenetic role. Activation of the classic pathway at tissue sites by autoantibodies against tissue antigens or by immune complexes deposited at basement membranes results in accumulation of inflammatory cells and tissue damage. The former mechanism is exemplified by the renal lesions of Goodpasture's syndrome and the second by the vascular and renal lesions in SLE and other immune complex diseases. Immunofluorescent staining of biopsy material for complement proteins demonstrates their presence at pathologic sites and is used in differential diagnosis. Hypocomplementemia is also often present in patients with immune complex diseases, particularly SLE, but also in various other clinical syndromes. Measurement of serum complement levels thus provides a simple and widely used tool for the diagnosis and management of human diseases. The most commonly used assays in clinical practice are total hemolytic complement, C4, and C3. Total hemolytic complement, expressed in CH_{50} units, measures the ability of serum to lyse antibody-coated erythrocytes and reflects the activity of all complement components. C4 and C3 are usually measured by immunochemical assays. Low complement levels by all three

TABLE 243–3. DISEASES ASSOCIATED WITH INHERITED COMPLEMENT DEFICIENCIES

Deficient Protein	Diseases
C1q, C1r, C1s, C4, C2	SLE, SLE-like syndrome, discoid lupus, glomerulonephritis, vasculitis
C3, H, I, P	Recurrent pyogenic infections
C5, C6, C7, C8	Recurrent disseminated neisserial infections
C1 INH	Hereditary angioedema

assays are often seen in SLE, particularly in patients with renal involvement and during acute exacerbations of the disease. In patients with partial lipodystrophy with or without glomerulonephritis and in some patients with membranoproliferative glomerulonephritis, levels of total complement and C3 are very low, whereas C4 is usually normal. This is due to the presence of an IgG autoantibody, termed C3 nephritic factor, with specificity for antigenic determinants on the amplification C3 convertase. Binding of this autoantibody to C3bBb creates a stable complex that is not subject to regulation by control proteins and thus causes continuous cleavage of C3. Activation of the alternative pathway also occurs during circulation of the blood through pump oxygenators or hemodialysis machines. The C5a generated during these procedures causes aggregation of neutrophils, leading to their sequestration in the pulmonary vasculature. In some patients this is manifested by symptoms of pulmonary dysfunction and hypoxemia. Complement activation in these cases can best be evaluated by measuring the serum concentration of C3a by radioimmunoassay.

Ahearn JM, Fearon DT: Structure and function of the complement receptors CR1 (CD35) and CR2 (CD21). Adv Immunol 46:183, 1989. *Molecular biology, structure, and function of two important cellular receptors for C3 fragments.*

Campbell RD, Law SKA, Reid KBM, Sim RB: Structure, organization, and regulation of the complement genes. Annu Rev Immunol 6:161, 1988. *An up-to-date review of the genetics and structure of complement proteins.*

Muller-Eberhard HJ: Molecular organization and function of the complement system. Annu Rev Biochem 57:321, 1988. *A comprehensive description of the structure and activation of complement proteins.*

Schifferli JA, Ng YC, Peters DK: The role of complement and its receptor in the elimination of immune complexes. N Engl J Med 325:488, 1986. *Discusses immune complex regulation and disposal.*

Winkelstein JA, Colten HR: Genetically determined disorders of the complement system. *In* Scriver CR, Beaudet AL, Sly WS, Valle DL (eds.): The Metabolic Basis of Inherited Disease. 6th ed. New York, McGraw-Hill, 1989, pp 2711–2737. *An excellent review of heritable disorders of the complement system.*

244 Primary Immunodeficiency Diseases

Rebecca H. Buckley

Since the first genetic defect in immunity was described in 1952, more than four dozen different primary immunodeficiency syndromes have been reported. Such diseases may involve all components of the immune system, including lymphocytes, phagocytic cells, and the complement proteins. This chapter focuses on abnormalities of lymphocytes. Deficiencies of the complement system (see Ch. 243) are mentioned briefly. A review of neutrophil dysfunction syndromes is presented in Ch. 139 and an overall review of the compromised host is given in Ch. 287. The acquired immunodeficiency syndrome (AIDS) is described in Part XXI.

Despite the large body of knowledge gained regarding functional derangements and cellular abnormalities in the various primary disorders of lymphocytes, the fundamental biologic errors for most of them remain unknown. Exceptions include two defects accompanied by purine salvage pathway enzyme deficiencies—adenosine deaminase (ADA) in some cases of autosomal-recessive severe combined immunodeficiency and purine nucleoside phosphorylase (PNP) in some patients with Nezelof's syndrome. In addition, the absence of three different leukocyte surface glycoproteins due to genetic abnormalities in a common 95 Kd β chain (CD18) is the basis of a condition characterized by defective cytolytic lymphocyte and phagocytic cell functions. The genetic errors in many other immunodeficiencies are known to be on the X chromosome, and the abnormal regions for X-linked agammaglobulinemia, X-linked severe combined immunodeficiency, the Wiskott-Aldrich syndrome, X-linked lymphoproliferative syndrome, properdin deficiency, and chronic granulomatous disease (CGD) have been localized. Immune deficiency can also be associated with broad deficiencies of HLA class I and II antigens and these have been shown to be due to different mutations in transacting factors governing the surface expression of these molecules.

Various classifications of immunodeficiency disorders involving lymphocytes have attempted to postulate the cellular levels at which the defects occur. Cells with mature differentiation markers of both T and B lymphocytes, however, have been found in most of the known defects, despite profound deficiencies of T- and/or B-cell function. Thus, in most cases the suspect cell lineage is not missing but malfunctional. Table 244–1 lists the most prominent functional abnormalities and the presumed cellular level of the defect in 19 primary immunodeficiency syndromes.

In contrast to the acquired immunodeficiency syndrome (AIDS), which has a new case acquisition rate of more than 250 per week, primary immunodeficiency diseases are rare. The incidence of agammaglobulinemia is estimated at 1 in 50,000. Selective absence of serum and secretory IgA, the most common, has a reported prevalence of 1 in 333 to 1 in 700.

APPROACHES TO THE PATIENT WITH SUSPECTED IMMUNODEFICIENCY

The number of patients suspected of having primary immunodeficiency will far exceed the incidences of these diseases. So it is important that the tests selected for immunologic assessment be broadly informative, reliable, and cost effective. Familiarity with certain clinical guidelines aids in the initial selection. Patients with antibody, phagocytic-cell, or complement deficiencies have recurrent infections with high-grade encapsulated bacteria. Therefore, those with only repeated viral respiratory infections are not likely to have any of these disorders. By contrast, patients with deficiencies in T-cell function usually manifest

opportunistic infections. Most defects can be ruled out at little cost to the patient if the proper choice of screening tests is made (Table 244–2). Among the most informative are the complete and differential blood counts and the sedimentation rate. Examination of red cells for Howell-Jolly bodies helps exclude asplenia. A normal platelet count rules out Wiskott-Aldrich syndrome. If the sedimentation rate is normal, chronic bacterial infection is unlikely. If the absolute neutrophil count is normal, congenital and acquired neutropenia and severe chemotactic defects are eliminated. If the absolute lymphocyte count is normal, a severe T-cell defect is unlikely. Beyond this, it is well to keep in mind that tests of immune function are far more informative and cost effective than those measuring immunoglobulin concentrations or enumerating lymphocyte subpopulations.

In assessing B cell function, determinations of antibody titers to protein (such as tetanus and diphtheria toxoids) and polysaccharide (such as pneumococcal and *Haemophilus influenzae*) antigens following immunization are the most useful tests. As a rule, patients with B-cell defects for which there is an effective or indicated treatment do not produce antibodies normally. However, the presence of such antibodies does not exclude IgA deficiency, which would also be missed on a serum electrophoretic analysis. Immunoelectrophoresis is not quantitative and, for that reason, is not useful in evaluating immune competence. The quantification of serum IgA is particularly cost effective. If the IgA concentration is normal, this rules out not only IgA deficiency but all of the permanent types of agammaglobulinemia, since IgA is usually very low or absent in those conditions as well. A particularly uneconomical study is IgG-subclass measurement. It is far more helpful to know the results of the above-mentioned antibody studies, since there are well-documented cases of antibody deficiency despite normal concentrations of all immunoglobulin classes and subclasses.

The most cost-effective test for assessing T-cell function is an intradermal skin test with 0.1 ml of a 1:1000 dilution of a known potent *Candida albicans* extract. If the test is positive, as defined by erythema and induration of 10 mm or more at 48 hours, virtually all primary T-cell defects are excluded and the need for more expensive in vitro tests, such as lymphocyte enumeration on a cell sorter or assessments of responses to mitogens, is obviated. Killing defects of phagocytic cells, which should be suspected if the patient has problems with staphylococcal or gram-negative infections, can be screened for in the office by a

TABLE 244–1. CLASSIFICATION OF PRIMARY IMMUNODEFICIENCY DISORDERS

Disorder	Functional Deficiencies	Presumed Cellular Level of Defect
X-linked agammaglobulinemia	Antibody	Pre–B cell
Common variable ("acquired hypogammaglobulinemia")	Antibody	B lymphocyte
Selective IgA deficiency	IgA antibody	IgA B lymphocyte
Secretory component deficiency	Secretory IgA	Mucosal epithelium
Selective IgM deficiency	IgM antibody	T helper cells
Immunodeficiency with elevated IgM	IgG and IgA antibodies	IgG, IgA B lymphocytes; switch T cell
Transient hypogammaglobulinemia of infancy	None; immunoglobulins low, but antibodies present	Unknown
Antibody deficiency with near-normal immunoglobulins	Antibody	Unknown; ?B cell
X-linked lymphoproliferative disease	Anti-EBV nuclear antigen antibody	B cell; ?also T cell
DiGeorge's syndrome	T cellular; some antibody	Dysmorphogenesis of 3rd and 4th branchial pouches
Nezelof's syndrome (including with PNP deficiency)	T cellular; some antibody	Unknown; ?thymus; ?T cell; metabolic defects
Severe combined immunodeficiency syndromes (autosomal recessive; ADA deficiency; X-linked recessive; defective expression of HLA antigens; reticular dysgenesis)	Antibody and T cellular; phagocytic in reticular dysgenesis	Unknown; metabolic defect(s); ?T cell; ?stem cell; ?thymus
Wiskott-Aldrich syndrome	Antibody; T cellular	Unknown
Ataxia-telangiectasia	Antibody; T cellular	B lymphocyte; helper T lymphocyte
Cartilage-hair hypoplasia	T cellular	G1 cycle of many cells
Immunodeficiency with thymoma	Antibody; some T cellular	B lymphocyte; excessive T suppressor cells
Hyperimmunoglobulinemia E syndrome	Specific immune responses; excessive IgE	Unknown
Chronic mucocutaneous candidiasis	Variable cellular	?Antigen overload
Leukocyte adhesion deficiency	Cytotoxic lymphocytes; phagocytic cells	95 Kd β chain of LFA-1, CR3, and p150, 95

TABLE 244–2. APPROACHES TO THE PATIENT WITH SUSPECTED IMMUNODEFICIENCY

Suspected Deficiency	Tests
All immunodeficiency	Complete and differential blood counts; platelet count; examination of red cells for Howell-Jolly bodies
Antibody deficiency	Immunoglobulin quantification; antibody titers to blood group antigens, protein antigens (tetanus, diphtheria), and polysaccharide antigens (*H. influenzae,* pneumococcal)
T-cell deficiency	Absolute lymphocyte count; intradermal skin test with *Candida albicans* 1:1000
Phagocytic cell deficiency	Absolute neutrophil count; nitroblue tetrazolium assay
Complement deficiency	Freeze serum at −70° C immediately for CH50

nitroblue tetrazolium assay. Complement defects can be most effectively screened for in a CH50 assay, which measures the intactness of the entire complement pathway. If these tests are abnormal, or even if they are normal and clinical features of the patient still strongly suggest a host defect, the patient should be evaluated at a center where more definitive immunologic studies can be done before any type of immunologic treatment is begun.

ANTIBODY DEFICIENCY DISORDERS

Antibody deficiency may occur either as a congenital or an "acquired" abnormality, although in both situations it appears to be genetically determined. Most patients are recognized because they have recurrent infections, but some individuals with selective IgA deficiency or infants with transient hypogammaglobulinemia may have few or no infections. Table 244–3 lists some of the general features of these disorders.

X-LINKED AGAMMAGLOBULINEMIA (XAγ). A majority of boys afflicted with this malady remain well during the first 6 to 9 months of life, presumably by virtue of maternally transmitted immunoglobulin. Thereafter they repeatedly acquire infections with high-grade extracellular pyogenic organisms such as pneumococci, streptococci, and *Haemophilus* unless given prophylactic antibiotics or gammaglobulin therapy. The most common types of infections include sinusitis, pneumonia, otitis, septic arthritis, meningitis, and septicemia. Chronic fungal infections are usually not present, and *Pneumocystis carinii* pneumonia rarely occurs unless there is an associated neutropenia. Viral infections and live virus vaccines are also usually handled normally, with the notable exceptions of hepatitis and enterovirus infections. Several examples of paralysis after polio vaccine administration have occurred, presumably because of mutation of persistent vaccine virus to a more neurotropic form. In addition, a dermatomyositis-like syndrome accompanied by chronic, eventually fatal central nervous system disease caused by various echoviruses has occurred in more than 40 patients. Approximately 20 per cent of patients have an arthritis resembling juvenile rheumatoid arthritis.

TABLE 244–3. CLINICAL CHARACTERISTICS OF ANTIBODY DEFICIENCY DISORDERS

1. Recurrent infections with high-grade extracellular encapsulated pathogens
2. Few problems with fungal or viral (except enterovirus) infections
3. Chronic sinopulmonary disease
4. Growth retardation not striking
5. Antibody deficiency in serum and secretions
6. May or may not lack B lymphocytes with surface immunoglobulins or complement receptors
7. Absence of cortical follicles in lymph node and spleen in X-linked agammaglobulinemia
8. Paucity of palpable lymphoid and nasopharyngeal tissue in X-linked agammaglobulinemia
9. Compatible with survival to adulthood or for several years after onset except for those with persistent enterovirus infections, autoimmune disorders, or malignancy

The diagnosis of XAγ is suspected if serum concentrations of IgG, IgA, and IgM are below the 95-per-cent confidence limits for appropriate age- and race-matched controls (usually there is <100 mg per deciliter total immunoglobulin). The demonstration of antibody deficiency in serum and in external secretions is of great importance in distinguishing this disorder from transient hypogammaglobulinemia of infancy. Tests for natural antibodies to blood group substances, for antibodies to antigens given during standard courses of immunization, and for antibodies to and ability to clear bacteriophage φ × 174 are markedly abnormal. Polymorphonuclear functions are usually normal, but some patients with this condition have had transient, persistent, or cyclic neutropenia.

Lymphopenia is uncommon, and the percentages of T cells and T-cell subsets have been found to be normal or elevated in most instances. In contrast, blood lymphocytes bearing surface immunoglobulin, "Ia-like" antigens, or the EBV receptor, or reacting with a specific anti-B-cell serum, are absent or present in very low numbers. Hypoplasia of adenoids, tonsils, and peripheral lymph nodes is the rule; germinal centers are not present, and plasma cells are rarely found. Conversely, normal numbers of pre–B cells are found in the bone marrow. Mixed lymphocyte responsiveness and lymphocyte responses to antigens and mitogens are normal. Cell-mediated immune responses can be detected in vivo, and the capacity to reject allografts is intact. The thymus has appeared normal in all autopsied cases, and lymphoid cells are abundant in thymus-dependent areas of peripheral lymphoid tissues.

Except in those unfortunate patients who develop polio, persistent echovirus infection, or lymphoreticular malignancy, the overall prognosis is reasonably good if humoral replacement therapy is instituted early. Systemic infection can be prevented by administration of intravenous immune serum globulin (ISG, primarily IgG) at a dose of 400 mg per kilogram every 3 to 4 weeks. Such preparations are known to be free of hepatitis and AIDS viruses. Many patients go on to develop crippling sinopulmonary disease despite this therapy, since no effective means exist for replacing secretory IgA at the mucosal surface. Chronic antibiotic therapy is usually necessary in addition for the management of such patients.

COMMON VARIABLE IMMUNODEFICIENCY (CVID). Patients with this condition (formerly known as acquired hypogammaglobulinemia) may appear similar clinically in many respects to those with XAγ. Although this disorder may occur in infants and young children, most patients present with a history of recurrent infection beginning several years after birth. CVID is distinguished from XAγ by later age of onset, somewhat less severe susceptibility to infections, and almost equal sex distribution. In contrast to patients with the X-linked form, patients with CVID may have normal-sized or enlarged tonsils and lymph nodes, and the latter may have cortical follicles. Additionally, such patients often have normal or nearly normal numbers of circulating immunoglobulin-bearing B lymphocytes. Nevertheless, the serum immunoglobulin and antibody deficiencies are usually just as profound by measurement, and the bacterial etiologic agents are the same as in the X-linked disorder. Echovirus meningoencephalitis is rare in patients with CVID.

This condition has been variably associated with a spruelike syndrome, with or without nodular follicular lymphoid hyperplasia of the intestine; thymoma; alopecia areata; and autoantibody formation leading to hemolytic anemia, gastric atrophy, achlorhydria, and pernicious anemia. Frequent complications include giardiasis (seen far more often here than in XAγ), bronchiectasis, gastric carcinoma, lymphoreticular malignancy, and cholelithiasis. Lymphoid interstitial pneumonia, pseudolymphoma, amyloidosis, and noncaseating granulomas of the lungs, spleen, skin, and liver have also been seen.

Despite normal numbers of circulating immunoglobulin-bearing B lymphocytes and the presence of lymphoid cortical follicles, the lymphocytes do not differentiate in vivo or in vitro into immunoglobulin-producing plasma cells, even in the presence of the polyclonal B-cell activator, pokeweed mitogen. Although the primary biologic error responsible for this defect is unknown, in most patients it appears to be due to abnormal terminal differentiation of the B-cell line. Because this disorder occurs in first-degree relatives of patients with selective IgA deficiency (A Def) and some patients with A Def later become panhypogammaglobulinemic, it is possible that these diseases have a common genetic basis. This concept is supported by the recent finding of rare alleles or deletions of Class III major histocompatibility complex (MHC) genes in individuals with either A Def or CVID, suggesting that the susceptibility gene(s) is in this region on chromosome 6. The treatment of CVID is the same as that for the X-linked disorder.

SELECTIVE IgA DEFICIENCY (A Def). An isolated near-absence (i.e., <10 mg per deciliter) of serum and secretory IgA is the most common primary immunodeficiency disorder, a frequency of 1:333 being reported among some blood donors. Although A Def has been observed in apparently healthy individuals, it is commonly associated with ill health. The kinds of health problems experienced often reflect the type of clinic from which the patients are drawn. Among 75 from an allergy-immunology clinic, there were high frequencies of chronic or recurrent respiratory tract infection and atopic diseases. In contrast, 30 A Def patients drawn from a rheumatology clinic had a high frequency of autoimmune and/or collagen vascular disease.

IgA is the major immunoglobulin of external secretions. As would be expected, its deficiency is associated with infections occurring predominantly in the respiratory, gastrointestinal, and urogenital tracts. Bacterial agents responsible are essentially the same as in other types of antibody deficiency syndromes. A high incidence of viral hepatitis was noted in one group of A Def patients, but there is no clear evidence that patients with this disorder have an undue susceptibility to other viral agents. Children with A Def produce local IgM and IgG antipolio antibodies to killed vaccine given intranasally and IgM and IgG antirubella antibodies during convalescence from natural rubella. Serum concentrations of other immunoglobulins are usually normal in patients with A Def, although an IgG_2 subclass deficiency has been reported in some, and IgM (usually increased) may be of the low-molecular-weight variety.

In addition to limiting the attachment of infectious agents to mucosal surfaces, secretory IgA antibodies probably act to prevent absorption of other foreign antigens, such as those in the diet. There is a high incidence of allergy and of IgG antibodies against cow's milk and ruminant serum proteins in patients with IgA deficiency. The antiruminant antibodies often falsely detect "IgA" in immunoassays which employ goat (but not rabbit) antisera. Intestinal nodular hyperplasia has been seen in a few such patients. A spruelike syndrome may occur in adults with selective IgA deficiency and sometimes responds to a gluten-free diet.

The basic defect leading to A Def is unknown. IgA-bearing blood B cells from most such patients also coexpress surface IgM and IgD, similar to cord blood B cells, suggesting maturation arrest. In addition, the B lymphocytes fail to secrete IgA in vitro. Studies of T-cell function have been normal in most patients. The defect may not always be permanent. The occurrence of IgA deficiency in both males and females and in families suggests autosomal inheritance.

Serum antibodies to IgA are found in as many as 44 per cent of such patients. This observation is of possible etiologic and great clinical significance. At least seven IgA-deficient patients have had severe or fatal anaphylactic reactions after intravenous administration of blood products. For this reason, only multiply washed erythrocytes or blood products from other A Def individuals should be administered to these patients; both intramuscular and intravenous ISG (which contain varying amounts of IgA) are contraindicated.

Currently the only treatment for A Def is vigorous treatment of specific infections with appropriate antimicrobial agents. Even if serum IgA could be replaced (in the face of anti-IgA antibodies), it would not be transported into the external secretions, since the latter is an active process involving only locally produced IgA.

SECRETORY COMPONENT DEFICIENCY. A patient with chronic intestinal candidiasis and diarrhea was found to lack IgA in his external secretions, despite having a normal serum IgA concentration. This was traced to a lack of secretory piece, which prevented the normal secretion of locally produced IgA.

SELECTIVE IgM DEFICIENCY. There are very few well-documented cases of this entity (IgM < 10 mg/ml). Fatal septicemia caused by meningococci and other gram-negative organisms, pneumococcal meningitis, tuberculosis, recurrent staphylococcal pyoderma, periorbital cellulitis, bronchiectasis, and

recurrent otitis have all been reported. There is no specific therapy; early and vigorous treatment with antibiotics is recommended.

IMMUNODEFICIENCY WITH ELEVATED IgM (Hypm). This disorder is characterized by very low serum IgG and IgA but markedly elevated polyclonal IgM. Some patients have low-molecular-weight IgM molecules. Like patients with XAγ, those with this defect commonly become symptomatic during infancy with recurrent pyogenic infections, including otitis media, sinusitis, pneumonia, and tonsillitis. In contrast to patients with XAγ, however, the frequent presence of lymphoid hyperplasia often leads away from a diagnosis of immunodeficiency. There is an increased frequency of autoimmune disorders, such as hemolytic anemia and thrombocytopenia, and transient, persistent, or cyclic neutropenia is common. Thymic-dependent lymphoid tissues and T-cell functions are usually normal, but several patients have had partial T-cell deficiencies. A sex-linked mode of inheritance has been proposed, but several examples of the disorder in females now seem to make this less certain.

Normal or only slightly reduced numbers of Ig-bearing B lymphocytes have been found in the blood; however, cultured B-cell lines from most such patients have shown the capacity to synthesize only IgM, suggesting a B-cell maturation defect. Some patients with this condition have, however, been characterized as having normal B cells but a deficiency of "switch" T cells. Plasma cells in lymph nodes contain only IgM.

Because these patients are unable to make IgG antibodies, the treatment is the same as for agammaglobulinemia.

TRANSIENT HYPOGAMMAGLOBULINEMIA OF INFANCY. Unlike patients with XAγ or common variable agammaglobulinemia, those with this condition can synthesize antibodies to human type A and B erythrocytes and to diphtheria and tetanus toxoids, usually by 6 to 11 months of age, well before immunoglobulin concentrations become normal. The finding of only 11 cases of transient hypogammaglobulinemia of infancy among over 10,000 sera tested by the author over a 12-year period suggests that this is not a common entity.

Gammaglobulin replacement therapy is not indicated in this condition. In addition to the known risks of inducing anti-IgG allotype antibodies, passively administered antibodies could block endogenous primary antibody formation in the same manner that RhoGAM suppresses anti-D antibodies in Rh-negative mothers delivering Rh-positive infants.

ANTIBODY DEFICIENCY WITH NEAR-NORMAL IMMUNOGLOBULINS. The author and her associates have studied the antibody-forming capacities of 12 patients with deficient antibody responses despite apparently normal T-cell function and normal or nearly normal immunoglobulin concentrations. Blood group antibody titers were absent in all but 2, diphtheria titers were low in all, and tetanus titers were low in 10. Geometric mean antibody titers to 13 pneumococcal serotypes were significantly lower than those of normal controls before and after immunization with tridecavalent pneumococcal polysaccharide vaccine. All patients cleared bacteriophage φ × 174 normally, but all primary immune responses were far below the normal range. Secondary responses to φ × 174 were also below the normal range in all but two, but, in both cases, most of the secondary response was IgM rather than IgG. This problem will not be detected unless functional tests of antibody-forming capacity are conducted. It may represent an early stage of "acquired" agammaglobulinemia (or CVID). Patients with this disorder are candidates for immunoglobulin replacement therapy.

X-LINKED LYMPHOPROLIFERATIVE DISEASE. This disorder, also referred to as *Duncan's disease* (after the original kindred in which it was described), is characterized by an impaired immune response to Epstein-Barr virus (EBV). Affected persons are apparently healthy until they experience infectious mononucleosis. Two thirds of the more than 100 patients studied thus far died of overwhelming EBV-induced B-cell proliferation during mononucleosis. A majority of the survivors developed hypogammaglobulinemia or B-cell lymphomas or both. Such individuals have marked impairment in production of antibodies to the EBV nuclear antigen, whereas titers of antibodies to the viral capsid antigen have ranged from zero to markedly elevated. Antibody-dependent cell-mediated cytotoxicity against EBV-infected cells and natural killer function are depressed, and there is a deficiency in long-lived T-cell immunity to EBV. Despite normal numbers of B and T cells, there is an elevated percentage of lymphocytes of the suppressor (CD8) phenotype. In addition, lymphocyte immunoglobulin synthesis in response to polyclonal B-cell mitogen stimulation in vitro is markedly depressed. Thus, both EBV-specific and nonspecific immunologic abnormalities occur in these patients.

CELLULAR IMMUNODEFICIENCY DISORDERS

Some important clinical characteristics of cellular immunodeficiency disorders are listed in Table 244–4. In general, patients with partial or absolute defects in T-cell function have infections or other clinical problems for which there is no effective treatment or which are often of a more severe nature than in those with antibody deficiency disorders. It is therefore rare that such individuals survive beyond infancy or childhood.

THYMIC HYPOPLASIA (DiGEORGE'S SYNDROME). This condition results from dysmorphogenesis of the third and fourth pharyngeal pouches, leading to hypoplasia or aplasia of the thymus and parathyroid glands. Other structures forming at the same age are also frequently affected, resulting in anomalies of the great vessels (right-sided aortic arch), esophageal atresia, bifid uvula, congenital heart disease (atrial and ventricular septal defects), a short philtrum of the upper lip, hypertelorism, an antimongoloid slant to the eyes, mandibular hypoplasia, and low-set (often notched) ears. The diagnosis is usually first suggested by the presence of hypocalcemic seizures during the neonatal period. DiGeorge's syndrome has occurred in both males and females, and chromosomal abnormalities (monosomy 22q11 and 10p13) have been noted in approximately 18 per cent. Familial occurrence is rare.

A variable degree of hypoplasia is more frequent than total aplasia of the thymus and parathyroid glands. Some children with the features of this syndrome have little trouble with infections and show evidence of some cell-mediated immunity. They are often referred to as having partial DiGeorge's syndrome. Those with marked thymic hypoplasia may resemble infants with severe combined immunodeficiency in their susceptibility to infection with low-grade or opportunistic pathogens (i.e., fungi, viruses, and Pneumocystis carinii) and to graft-versus-host (GVH) disease from nonirradiated blood transfusions.

Serum immunoglobulins are usually normal for age, but some fractions, particularly IgA, may be diminished and IgE may be elevated. T-cell numbers are decreased, and there is an increased number of B cells. Responses of peripheral blood lymphocytes following mitogen stimulation, like the intradermal delayed hypersensitivity response, have been absent, reduced, or normal. Careful postmortem studies have sometimes revealed tiny nests of thymic tissue containing Hassall's corpuscles and a normal density of thymocytes. Lymphoid follicles usually appear normal, but lymph node paracortical areas and thymus-dependent regions of the spleen show variable degrees of depletion, depending upon the degree of thymic hypoplasia. Because of variability in the severity of the immunodeficiency, it is difficult to evaluate claimed benefits of fetal thymus transplantation.

CELLULAR IMMUNODEFICIENCY WITH IMMUNOGLOBULINS (NEZELOF'S SYNDROME). This syndrome is characterized by lymphopenia, diminished lymphoid tissue, abnormal thymus architecture, and the presence of normal or increased immunoglobulins. Children with this condition may

TABLE 244–4. CLINICAL CHARACTERISTICS OF CELLULAR IMMUNODEFICIENCY DISORDERS

1. Recurrent infections with low-grade or opportunistic infectious agents such as fungi, viruses, or Pneumocystis carinii
2. Delayed cutaneous anergy
3. Accompanied by growth retardation, short life span, wasting, and diarrhea
4. Susceptible to graft-versus-host (GVH) disease if given fresh blood, plasma, or unmatched allogeneic bone marrow
5. Fatal reactions from live virus or BCG vaccination
6. High incidence of malignancy

have recurrent or chronic pulmonary infections, failure to thrive, oral or cutaneous candidiasis, chronic diarrhea, recurrent skin infections, gram-negative sepsis, urinary tract infections, severe varicella, or combinations of these. An autosomal recessive pattern of inheritance has been suggested in some cases, but an X-linked mode seemed more likely in others. Other findings include neutropenia and eosinophilia.

Studies of cellular immune function have shown delayed cutaneous anergy to ubiquitous antigens and low to absent in vitro lymphocyte responses to mitogens and allogeneic cells. Such patients have profound deficiencies of total T cells and T-cell subsets, with usually a normal helper (CD4+) to suppressor (CD8+) cell ratio, in contrast to patients with AIDS, who characteristically have marked inversion of the CD4:CD8 ratio owing to selective deficiency of CD4+ cells. Peripheral lymphoid tissues demonstrate paracortical lymphocyte depletion. The thymuses are very small and have a paucity of thymocytes and usually no Hassall's corpuscles; however, again in contrast to AIDS, thymic epithelium is present. These could all be useful in distinguishing Nezelof's syndrome from pediatric AIDS, since it is the primary immunodeficiency disorder most likely to be confused with it. Fatal or serious infections have included varicella, vaccinia, rubeola, and those due to Pneumocystis carinii, cytomegalovirus, Pseudomonas, and Mycobacterium kansasii. Antibody-forming capacity has been apparently normal in roughly one third of the reported cases. Plasma cells are usually abundant in the lamina propria and lymph nodes. Although very few patients have been reconstituted by bone marrow transplantation, most other forms of therapy have also been unsuccessful.

With Purine Nucleoside Phosphorylase Deficiency. More than 16 patients with Nezelof's syndrome have been found to have purine nucleoside phosphorylase (PNP) deficiency. In contrast to patients with adenosine deaminase (ADA) deficiency, serum and urinary uric acid are markedly deficient, and no characteristic physical or skeletal abnormalities have been noted. Three patients have suffered from a progressive neurologic disorder with spastic tetraplegia, two developed an autoimmune hemolytic anemia, and one, idiopathic thrombocytopenic purpura. Deaths have occurred from generalized vaccinia, varicella, lymphosarcoma, and GVH disease following blood transfusions. In contrast to a majority of patients with Nezelof's syndrome, the thymuses of PNP-deficient patients have had some Hassall's corpuscles, reminiscent of some patients with ADA deficiency. Analyses of lymphocyte subpopulations with monoclonal antibodies in two such patients revealed marked deficiencies of T cells and T-cell subsets but increased numbers of cells with natural killer (NK) phenotype and function. Attempts to correct the immunologic and enzymatic deficiencies of PNP-deficient patients by enzyme replacement or deoxycytidine therapy have not been successful.

SEVERE COMBINED IMMUNODEFICIENCY (SCID) DISORDERS

The syndromes of SCID are characterized by their apparent congenital absence of all adaptive immune function and a great diversity of genetic, enzymatic, hematologic, and immunologic features. Unless immunologic reconstitution can be achieved through immunocompetent tissue transplants or enzyme replacement therapy or unless gnotobiotic isolation can be carried out, death usually occurs before the patient's first birthday. The major subcategories of this disorder are discussed below.

AUTOSOMAL RECESSIVE SEVERE COMBINED IMMUNODEFICIENCY DISEASE. Within the first few months of life, infants affected with this first-described SCID syndrome have frequent episodes of otitis, pneumonia, sepsis, diarrhea, and cutaneous infections. Growth may appear normal initially, but extreme wasting soon develops. Persistent infections with opportunistic organisms such as Candida albicans, Pneumocystis carinii, varicella, measles, parainfluenza 3, cytomegalovirus, and BCG frequently lead to death. These infants also lack the ability to reject foreign tissue and are therefore at risk for GVH disease. GVH reactions can result from maternal immunocompetent cells crossing the placenta or from the administration of blood products containing viable histoincompatible lymphocytes.

Immunologic evaluation reveals serum immunoglobulin concentrations to be diminished, and no antibody formation occurs following immunization. There is a lack of cellular immune function, with lymphopenia and absence of lymphocyte responses to mitogens or allogeneic cells, delayed cutaneous anergy, and inability to reject foreign tissues. Marked heterogeneity of lymphocyte subpopulations exists among SCID patients, even among those with similar inheritance patterns. Despite the uniformly profound lack of T- or B-cell function, some patients have had low numbers of both B and T lymphocytes, whereas others have had elevated numbers of B cells. Cytofluorographic studies with monoclonal antibodies to mature T cells and subsets have generally revealed very small numbers of cells reacting with such reagents; however, there is no increase in cells bearing the CD1 antigen present on immature cortical thymocytes. Thus the lymphocytes present appear to have acquired surface markers characteristic of mature T cells. A new phenotype of SCID was characterized in which virtually all of the lymphocytes of some infants with SCID are large granular lymphocytes with NK cell phenotype and function. NK function has been totally lacking in other SCID patients, again illustrating the striking heterogeneity at a cellular level. Typically, these patients have very small thymuses (less than 1 gram), which usually fail to descend from the neck, contain few thymic lymphocytes, lack corticomedullary distinction, and usually lack Hassall's corpuscles (see exception below). Despite the profound thymocyte depletion in SCID patients, thymic epithelium is present—in contrast to the situation in AIDS in which there is marked epithelial atrophy. Both the follicular and paracortical areas of the peripheral lymph nodes are depleted of lymphocytes. Tonsils, adenoids, and Peyer's patches are absent or extremely underdeveloped.

ISG fails to halt the progressively downhill course of SCID. Transplantation of bone marrow cells from HLA genotypically identical or D locus–compatible donors has resulted in apparent complete correction of the immunologic defect in a number of these patients, with some 50 known long-term survivors since 1968. More recently, techniques to deplete all post-thymic T cells from donor marrow have also allowed the use of haploidentical (half-matched) bone marrow cells for correction of SCID. These employ either a combination of soy lectin agglutination and sheep erythrocyte rosetting (the most successful method) or incubation with monoclonal antibodies to human T cells and complement. Both methods leave the stem cells intact. To date, over 100 infants with SCID who would have otherwise died because of lack of an HLA-identical donor have been treated successfully with T-cell–depleted haploidentical bone marrow with few signs of GVH reaction.

With Adenosine Deaminase (ADA) Deficiency. Absence of the enzyme ADA has been observed in approximately 40 per cent of patients with the autosomal recessive form of SCID. Marked accumulations of adenosine, 2'-deoxyadenosine and 2'-O-methyladenosine directly or indirectly lead to lymphocyte toxicity, which causes the immunodeficiency. Adenosine and deoxyadenosine are apparent suicide inactivators of the enzyme S-adenosylhomocysteine (SAH) hydrolase, resulting in the accumulation of SAH. SAH is a potent inhibitor of virtually all cellular methylation reactions. Although most such patients have had profound lymphopenia from the earliest age studied, a few have had early normal or fluctuating lymphocyte counts that declined by 6 weeks to 2 years of life. In marked contrast to "classic" SCID, some ADA–deficient patients have been found to have a few Hassall's corpuscles in their thymuses and changes suggestive of early differentiation. Other distinguishing features of ADA-deficient SCID patients have included the presence of rib cage abnormalities similar to a rachitic rosary and multiple skeletal abnormalities of chondro-osseous dysplasia on radiographic examination.

Both matched sibling and haploidentical post-thymic T cell–depleted bone marrow transplants have resulted in lymphocyte chimerism and partial or complete correction of the immunologic defect in ADA-deficient SCID. Enzyme replacement therapy with irradiated packed normal erythrocytes or polyethyleneglycol–modified bovine adenosine deaminase on a continuing basis has resulted in improvement in some patients. Recently, this condition became the first in which gene insertion therapy was attempted, as the entire ADA gene has been cloned and sequenced.

X-LINKED RECESSIVE SEVERE COMBINED IMMUNODEFICIENCY DISEASE. This is thought to be the most common form of SCID in the United States. Clinically, immu-

nologically, and histopathologically, these patients appear similar to those with the autosomal recessive form.

DEFECTIVE EXPRESSION OF MAJOR HISTOCOMPATIBILITY COMPLEX (MHC) ANTIGENS. There are two main forms: MHC class I antigen deficiency ("bare lymphocyte syndrome") and MHC class I antigen deficiency plus absence of MHC class II antigens. These autosomal recessive conditions are thought to be due to mutations in X-box binding proteins that result in failure of surface membrane expression of the HLA antigens. Sera from affected individuals contain normal quantities of MHC class I antigens and β_2 microglobulin. Patients (usually of North African descent) present with persistent diarrhea in early infancy and have oral candidiasis, bacterial pneumonia, *Pneumocystis* infection, septicemia, and undue susceptibility to enteroviruses, herpes, and other viral agents. Those with both class I and II antigen deficiencies also have malabsorption. There is variable hypogammaglobulinemia with decreased serum IgM and IgA and poor to absent antibody production. B-cell percentages are usually normal, but plasma cells are absent in tissues. Lymphopenia is only moderate; T-cell functions in vivo and in vitro are decreased but not absent. The thymus and other lymphoid organs are severely hypoplastic. A majority of affected infants die in the first 3 years of life. The associated defects of both B- and T-cell immunity and HLA expression reinforce the important biologic role for HLA determinants in effective immune cell cooperation.

SEVERE COMBINED IMMUNODEFICIENCY WITH LEUKOPENIA (RETICULAR DYSGENESIS). In 1959, identical twin male infants were described who exhibited a total lack of both lymphocytes and granulocytes in their peripheral blood and bone marrow. Seven of eight infants reported died between 3 and 119 days of age from overwhelming infections; the eighth underwent complete immunologic reconstitution from a bone marrow transplant. Autosomal inheritance seems likely from reports of familial occurrences.

PARTIAL COMBINED IMMUNODEFICIENCY DISORDERS

IMMUNODEFICIENCY WITH THROMBOCYTOPENIA AND ECZEMA (WISKOTT-ALDRICH SYNDROME). This X-linked recessive syndrome is characterized clinically by the triad of eczema, thrombocytopenic purpura, and undue susceptibility to infection. Often there is prolonged oozing from the circumcision site or bloody diarrhea during infancy. Atopic dermatitis and recurrent infections usually develop during the first year of life. Infections are caused by pneumococci and other bacteria with polysaccharide capsules, resulting in episodes of otitis media, pneumonia, meningitis, and sepsis. Later, infections with *Pneumocystis carinii* and the herpesviruses become more frequent. Survival beyond the teens is rare; major causes of death are infections and bleeding, but a 12 per cent incidence of fatal malignancy also occurs in this condition. A papovavirus has been recovered from a reticulum cell sarcoma of the brain and from the urine of patients with this syndrome.

The earliest evidence of immunodeficiency is an impaired humoral immune response to polysaccharide antigens. Absent or markedly diminished isohemagglutinin titers are uniformly found, and poor or no responses are seen following immunization with polysaccharide antigens. Antibody titers to protein antigens also fall with time, and anamnestic responses are often poor or absent. Studies of immunoglobulin metabolism have shown an accelerated rate of synthesis—as well as hypercatabolism—of albumin, IgG, IgA, and IgM, resulting in highly variable immunoglobulin concentrations. The predominant dysgammaglobulinemia is a low IgM, elevated IgA and IgE, and a normal or slightly low IgG concentration. Lymphocyte responses are moderately depressed, and cutaneous anergy is a frequent finding. Analyses of blood lymphocytes with monoclonal reagents have revealed moderately reduced percentages of cells reacting with antibodies to all T cells and to the helper (CD4 +) and suppressor (CD8 +) subsets. In addition, the T lymphocytes have deficient or defective cell surface expressions of the sialoglycoprotein CD43.

The thrombocytopenia appears to be due to an intrinsic platelet abnormality, since antiplatelet antibodies are not usually demonstrated and survival times of allogeneic but not autologous ^{51}Cr-labeled platelets have been normal. Megakaryocytes are present in normal number in the bone marrow, but platelet size is small.

Treatment has been directed primarily toward control of bleeding with platelet transfusions, splenectomy, or both and of infections by intravenous administration of ISG. Several patients have had complete corrections of both the platelet and immunologic abnormalities by HLA-matched sibling bone marrow transplants after being conditioned with irradiation or busulfan and cyclophosphamide.

ATAXIA-TELANGIECTASIA. This is a complex syndrome with neurologic, immunologic, endocrinologic, hepatic, and cutaneous abnormalities. The most prominent clinical features are progressive cerebellar ataxia, oculocutaneous telangiectasias, chronic sinopulmonary disease, a high incidence of malignancy, and variable humoral and cellular immunodeficiency. Ataxia typically becomes evident soon after the child begins to walk. Telangiectasias usually develop by 3 to 6 years of age. Recurrent, usually bacterial, sinopulmonary infections occur in roughly 80 per cent of these patients; common viral exanthems have not usually resulted in untoward sequelae, but varicella was fatal in one of the author's patients.

The malignant tumors reported have usually been of the lymphoreticular type, but others have been seen. Cells from patients and heterozygous carriers have increased sensitivity to ionizing radiation, defective DNA repair, and frequent chromosomal abnormalities. The abnormal gene has been mapped to the long arm of chromosome 11 (11q22-23). An autosomal recessive mode of inheritance seems operative.

The most frequent immunologic abnormality is selective absence of IgA, found in 50 to 80 per cent of these patients. IgG_2 or total IgG may also be decreased. IgE concentrations are usually low, and the IgM may be of the low-molecular-weight variety. Specific antibody levels may be decreased or normal. In vivo, there is impaired but not absent cell-mediated immunity, as evidenced by delayed cutaneous anergy and prolonged allograft survival. Death from GVH disease has not been reported. Enumeration of blood T cells and subsets reveals reduced percentages of total T cells and T cells of the helper (CD4) phenotype, with normal or increased percentages of cells of the suppressor (CD8) phenotype. In vitro studies of lymphocyte function have shown moderately depressed proliferative responses to mitogens, decreased T-helper cell function, and an intrinsic defect in B-cell IgA synthesis. The thymus is very hypoplastic and lacks Hassall's corpuscles. No satisfactory treatment has been found.

CARTILAGE-HAIR HYPOPLASIA. An unusual form of short-limbed dwarfism with frequent and severe infections has been reported among the Amish. Features include short and pudgy hands; redundant skin; hyperextensible joints of hands and feet but an inability to completely extend the elbows; and fine, sparse light hair and eyebrows. Severe and often fatal varicella infections appear to be a particular hazard. Progressive vaccinia and vaccine-associated poliomyelitis have also been observed.

The severity of the immunodeficiency varies; in one series, 11 of 77 patients died before age 20, but two were still alive at age 76. Three patterns of immune dysfunction have emerged: defective antibody-mediated immunity, defective cellular immunity, and severe combined immunodeficiency. The most striking abnormality appears to be one of defective cell proliferation due to an intrinsic defect related to the G1 phase, resulting in a longer cell cycle for individual cells. The trait appears to be autosomal recessive with variable penetrance.

IMMUNODEFICIENCY WITH THYMOMA. These patients are adults who almost simultaneously develop hypogammaglobulinemia, deficits in cell-mediated immunity, and benign thymoma (see Ch. 253). The thymomas are predominantly of the spindle cell variety. Eosinophilia or eosinopenia, aregenerative or hemolytic anemia, thrombocytopenia, or pancytopenia may also occur. Antibody formation is poor, although percentages of immunoglobulin-bearing B lymphocytes are normal, and progressive lymphopenia develops. Several patients with this disorder have been shown to have excessive suppressor T-cell activity.

HYPERIMMUNOGLOBULINEMIA E SYNDROME. The hyper-IgE syndrome is a primary immunodeficiency characterized by recurrent staphylococcal abscesses and markedly elevated serum IgE concentrations. The disorder was first reported by the author and her coworkers in two young boys in 1972. These patients all have lifelong histories of severe recurrent staphylococcal abscesses involving the skin, lungs, joints, and other sites. Persistent pneumatoceles develop as a result of their recurrent pneumonias. The pruritic dermatitis that occurs is not typical atopic eczema and does not always persist; respiratory allergic symptoms are usually absent. An autosomal dominant form of inheritance with incomplete penetrance seems possible. Laboratory features include exceptionally high serum IgE concentrations but usually normal IgG, IgA, and IgM concentrations; pronounced blood and sputum eosinophilia; abnormally low anamnestic antibody responses; and poor antibody and cell-mediated responses to neoantigens. In vitro studies have shown normal percentages of CD2-, CD3-, CD4-, and CD8-positive lymphocytes, and there is no increase in the percentage of IgE-bearing B lymphocytes. Lymphocyte responses to mitogens are normal, but responses to antigens or to related allogeneic cells have been absent or very low. Histologic sections of lymph nodes, spleen, and lung cysts show striking eosinophilia.

Phagocytic cell ingestion, metabolism, and killing mechanisms and total hemolytic complement have been normal in all patients. Defects of mononuclear and/or polymorphonuclear chemotaxis are present in some but not most patients and thus are not the basic problem in this syndrome.

The most effective therapy is chronic administration of therapeutic doses of a penicillinase-resistant penicillin, with the addition of other antibiotic or antifungal agents as required for specific infections.

CHRONIC MUCOCUTANEOUS CANDIDIASIS. This clinical syndrome, probably of multiple causes, is associated with chronic candidal infection of the skin and mucous membranes but only rarely life-threatening systemic infections of the types seen in patients with severe T-cell dysfunction. Some patients have endocrinopathies involving the parathyroid, thyroid, adrenal, and/or pancreatic glands (see Ch. 228); however, many have neither associated endocrinopathy nor any demonstrable immunologic abnormality. Ketoconazole (Nizoral) has been found to be the single most effective form of therapy.

LEUKOCYTE ADHESION DEFICIENCY (LAD OR CD11/CD18 DEFICIENCY). This condition is due to an autosomal recessive inherited mutation in the gene encoding the 95 Kd MW β subunit (CD18) shared by three adhesive heterodimers: LFA-1 on B, T, and NK lymphocytes; complement receptor type 3 (CR3) on neutrophils, monocytes, macrophages, eosinophils, and NK cells; and p150,95 (function unknown). Patients have histories of delayed separation of the umbilical cord, omphalitis, gingivitis, recurrent skin infections, repeated otitis media, pneumonia, peritonitis, perianal abscesses, and impaired wound healing. Severe widespread and life-threatening bacterial and fungal infections account for the high mortality. All cytotoxic lymphocyte functions are markedly impaired owing to a lack of the adhesion protein LFA-1; deficiency of LFA-1 also interferes with immune cell interaction and immune recognition. CR3 binds fixed iC3b fragments of C3 and β glucans; its absence causes abnormal phagocytic cell adherence and chemotaxis and a reduced respiratory burst with phagocytosis. Blood neutrophil counts are usually elevated. Deficiencies of these glycoproteins can be screened for by cytofluorography of blood leukocytes with appropriate monoclonal antibodies to CR3 (OKM1, MO1, MAC-1). The disease can be corrected by bone marrow transplantation.

T-CELL ACTIVATION DEFECTS. These conditions are characterized by the presence of T cells that appear phenotypically normal by many criteria but fail to proliferate or produce cytokines in response to stimulation with mitogens, antigens, or other signals delivered to the T-cell antigen receptor (TCR). Recently a number of these have been characterized at the molecular level, including patients who had either (1) defective surface expression of the TCR, (2) defective signal transduction from the TCR to intracellular metabolic pathways, and (3) a pretranslational defect in interleukin-2 (T-cell growth factor) production. These patients have clinical problems similar to those of other severely T-cell–deficient individuals.

PRIMARY DEFICIENCIES OF THE COMPLEMENT SYSTEM

In addition to congenital or hereditary disorders of lymphoid cells, there are several well-defined primary immune defects involving the complement system. Genetically determined deficiencies have been described for all of the components of complement, and undue susceptibility to infection is a characteristic of deficiencies of C2, C3, C5, C6, and C7. The types of infections experienced in C2, C3, and in some with C5 deficiency are with gram-positive encapsulated organisms, whereas those in patients with deficiencies of the terminal components are usually meningococcal or gonococcal. A normal CH50 would exclude all heritable complement deficiencies. The complement system is discussed in detail in Ch. 243.

Alarcon B, Regueiro JR, Arnaiz-Villena A, Terhorst C: Familial defect in the surface expression of the T-cell receptor-CD3 complex. N Engl J Med 319:1203, 1988. *An excellent introduction to the concept of T-cell activation defects.*

Buckley RH: Normal and abnormal development of the immune system. In Joklik WK, Willett HP, Amos DB (eds.): Zinsser Textbook of Microbiology and Immunology. 19th ed. New York, Appleton-Century-Crofts, 1988. *A concise review of ontogeny of the normal human immune system as well as the primary immunodeficiency disorders.*

Buckley RH, Schiff SE, Sampson HA, et al.: Development of immunity in human severe primary T cell deficiency following haploidentical bone marrow stem cell transplantation. J Immunol 136:2398, 1986. *A review of the time course and extent of immune reconstitution in 17 patients with severe T cell defects given haploidentical stem cell transplants.*

Chatila T, Wong R, Young M, et al: An immunodeficiency characterized by defective signal transduction in T lymphocytes. N Engl J Med 320:696, 1989. *An example of a signal transduction defect.*

Fischer A, Lisowska-Grospierre B, Anderson DC, Springer TA: Leukocyte adhesion deficiency: Molecular basis and functional consequences. Immunodef Rev 1:39, 1988. *An excellent review of leukocyte adhesion (CD11/18) deficiency.*

Schaffer FM, Palermos J, Zhu ZB, et al.: Individuals with IgA deficiency and common variable immunodeficiency share polymorphisms of major histocompatibility complex class II genes. Proc Natl Acad Sci USA 86:8015, 1989. *New information concerning the genetic localization of susceptibility genes for selective IgA deficiency and common variable immunodeficiency.*

245 Urticaria and Angioedema

Michael M. Frank

DEFINITION

Urticaria (Table 245–1) is defined as the transient appearance of elevated, erythematous pruritic wheals (hives) or serpiginous exanthem, usually surrounded by an area of erythema. It commonly involves the trunk and extremities, sparing palms and soles, but may involve any epidermal or mucosal surface. The wheals are thought to result from local subcutaneous and intradermal leakage of plasma filtrate from postcapillary venules. In most cases there is associated increased blood flow to the localized area of swelling, resulting in a surrounding erythema. The lesions blanch on pressure, reflecting this pathogenetic process. The appearance of urticaria is thought to reflect an ongoing immediate hypersensitivity reaction.

Angioedema is formed by a similar extravasation of fluid, but in this case the leakage of fluid involves deeper structures, including dermal and subdermal sites. Because of its location in deeper cutaneous structures, it appears as brawny nonpitting edema, usually without well-defined margins. Although urticaria is almost always pruritic, indicating stimulation of nociceptive nerves supplying deeper cutaneous structures, angioedema may be unassociated with itching. Unlike other forms of edema, angioedema is not commonly distributed in dependent areas of the body. Angioedema often involves the lips, tongue, eyelids, genitalia, or dorsum of the hands or feet but also may involve any epidermal or mucosal surface. The transient nature of involvement is important in definition of both urticaria and angioedema; these manifestations appear and peak in minutes to hours and disappear over hours to days.

INCIDENCE AND PREVALENCE

Acute episodes of urticaria/angioedema are arbitrarily defined as those lasting less than 6 weeks. More prolonged episodes are defined as chronic. Acute urticaria and angioedema are very common clinical problems occurring in as many as 20 to 30 per cent of the population at one time or another. They may occur at any age and are the most common form seen in childhood.

TABLE 245–1. CLASSIFICATION OF URTICARIA/ANGIOEDEMA

I. Manifestation of hypersensitivity to a defined agent
   A. Drug reactions
   B. Foods and food additives
   C. Inhaled and contact allergens
II. Presumed immune complex–induced
   A. Collagen disease
   B. Endocrine disease (thyroid disorders)
   C. Serum sickness
   D. Transfusion-induced
   E. Malignancy (tumor antigen–induced)
   F. Infectious agents
III. Physical urticarias
   A. Dermatographism
   B. Familial and acquired cold urticaria
   C. Localized heat urticaria
   D. Cholinergic urticaria
   E. Exercise-induced anaphylaxis/urticaria
   F. Delayed pressure urticaria/angioedema
   G. Familial and acquired vibratory angioedema
   H. Solar urticaria
   I. Aquagenic urticaria
IV. Urticaria pigmentosa and systemic mastocytosis
V. Chronic urticaria and angioedema
VI. Defined complement-related disorders
   A. Hereditary angioedema
   B. Acquired Cl inhibitor deficiency
   C. Complement Factor I deficiency

They occur in persons of all sexes, races, and occupations and at all seasons of the year. Chronic urticaria/angioedema also can occur in individuals of any age, but the peak incidence is noted in young adults. In general, symptoms of urticaria are more striking and are more easily recognized than those of angioedema, and these symptoms are often the presenting complaint. At presentation about 50 per cent of patients are found to have both urticaria and angioedema, approximately 40 per cent have urticaria alone, and about 10 per cent only angioedema. Although the majority of patients clear their lesions spontaneously or respond rapidly to treatment with H_1 antihistamines, a minority of patients continue to have lesions over a period that may last years. It has been reported that of patients with chronic urticaria and angioedema, 75 per cent have symptoms for longer than 1 year, 50 per cent symptoms for longer than 5 years, and 20 per cent symptoms for decades. At times these can be quite debilitating. This clinical syndrome represents a final common pathway of multiple initiating stimuli, and the natural course of disease undoubtedly reflects these multiple initiating factors.

PATHOGENESIS AND PATHOLOGY

Urticaria/angioedema appears to result from dilatation of local small vessels with associated leakage of plasma from local postcapillary venules. Experimentally such leakage can be induced by multiple stimuli. Degranulation of cutaneous mast cells is thought to be the most frequent cause of disease. Mast cells are found in high frequency within the subcutaneous tissues and dermis. Their distribution is particularly rich around blood vessels. These cells stain poorly with the commonly used histopathologic stains and often must be visualized by specific staining techniques. Upon being activated by any of a number of stimuli, these cells degranulate, releasing preformed mediators like histamine present in the granules that can induce capillary permeability and also synthesize various mediators that induce capillary permeability in response to the activation signal, including prostaglandins, HETEs, leukotrienes C, D, and E, and platelet-activating factor (PAF). Recent evidence suggests that with appropriate stimuli, cellular regulatory factors like cytokines can be released without degranulation and release of preformed mediators; these may control the function of other cells within the lesion. Under controlled conditions, the triggering of cutaneous mast cells in normal volunteers induces a typical pruritic hive, lending support to the suggestion that these cells are of critical importance in urticarial reactions in man.

Many stimuli can induce mast cells to degranulate. Probably most important is the interaction of mast cell membrane–bound IgE antibody with specific antigen. Mast cells have on their surface a high-affinity receptor for IgE and in tissues are found coated with IgE antibody derived from plasma or interstitial fluid. Interaction of IgE antibody with its antigen cross-links IgE receptors, a required step in initiating the degranulation process by antigen-mediated cell activation. However, not only IgE meeting its antigen, but also a series of peptides derived from various plasma mediator molecules, can trigger degranulation. For example, peptides derived from activated complement proteins including C3a, C4a, and C5a and small fragments of C2 can induce mast cell degranulation. Similarly, peptides like bradykinin, derived from activation and cleavage of proteins of the kinin-generating system, and neuropeptides like substance P can induce mast cell degranulation. Incompletely defined cellular products derived from circulating mononuclear cells and neutrophils can cause mast cell degranulation as well. Moreover, toxic products from neutrophils and monocytes, whose release is induced by many factors including mast cell products, can on injection induce a typical hive.

Induction of an immediate hypersensitivity response in an allergic individual by the intradermal injection of a sensitizing antigen leads to rapid mast cell degranulation and the immediate appearance of a wheal and flare response that gradually fades. In many individuals 4 to 6 hours later a "late-phase" response is noted with an increase in local inflammation and swelling. Biopsy of such a late-phase reaction reveals the accumulation of neutrophils and eosinophils in the inflamed area and later their gradual replacement by mononuclear cells. The factors that induce the late-phase reaction are not completely defined, but the recent demonstration of the production of chemotactic cytokines some hours after mast cell triggering suggests that these factors may contribute to late-phase inflammation.

An understanding of these experimental findings helps explain biopsy findings in patients with acute and chronic urticaria/angioedema. It should be emphasized that although the disease may be chronic, individual lesions may be quite evanescent, lasting hours to days. On biopsy, subcutaneous edema is prominent with flattened rete pegs, widened dermal papillae, and swollen collagen fibers. There is an increase in the number of cutaneous mast cells noted when compared with normal individuals. Even uninvolved skin from a patient with urticaria shows increased mast cell number when compared with skin of normals. Some mast cell degranulation is seen on biopsy of lesions, and in chronic urticaria a modest mononuclear cell infiltrate containing lymphocytes (predominantly CD4+ helper T cells) and a relatively few monocyte/macrophages is noted. An increase in eosinophils may be seen. Patients with the physical urticaria tend to have more neutrophils and eosinophils on biopsy than are observed in chronic urticaria/angioedema. In a minority of cases with typical urticarial lesions a typical leukocytoclastic vasculitis is observed. This latter finding indicates that the underlying diagnosis is vasculitis and places the patient in a different diagnostic and therapeutic group.

A list of common causes of urticaria/angioedema is provided in Table 245–1. However, it must be emphasized that in most cases the cause of urticaria/angioedema is never found. In one large series 70 per cent of all cases remained in the idiopathic group after all other urticarial syndrome complexes were eliminated. These cutaneous manifestations appear, often are treated, and disappear with no etiologic diagnosis ever made. It is believed that most urticaria/angioedema cases represent hypersensitivity reactions to drugs, foods, or less commonly inhalants, because when a cause is defined it commonly involves one of these sensitizing agents. Penicillin is the drug still most commonly associated with acute urticaria, but aspirin and other nonsteroidal anti-inflammatory agents may exacerbate urticaria, possibly through their inhibition of prostaglandin synthesis, and diuretics, radiocontrast dyes, sulfonamides, and muscle relaxants all are associated with acute urticaria. Opioids can trigger direct mast cell release of histamine and cause urticarial lesions. Among foods, nuts, milk, eggs, chocolate, citrus fruits, tomatoes, fish, shellfish, and food dyes have all been associated with onset of urticaria in some individuals. Nevertheless, so many different antigens, including food additives, drugs, foods, and food contaminants, have been defined as causative in individual cases, and so little antigen may be required to precipitate attacks, that it may be difficult or impossible to define the causative agent. In many patients in whom the disease becomes chronic (defined as lasting longer than 6 weeks) the patient is asked to keep a diary to determine whether a particular food or commercial product is involved with an attack. If it proves impossible to define the precipitating agent by this means, a severely restricted elimination diet, limiting food ingestion to boiled rice and lamb, may be tried to see if elimination of an offending ingested agent will terminate attacks. Too often these attempts are unsuccessful.

There are defined clinical situations in which urticaria and/or angioedema is a common presenting problem: Patients undergoing immune complex–mediated reactions such as occur in active systemic lupus erythematosus and serum sickness may experience waves of urticarial lesions, in this case thought to be due to activation of the various mediatory pathways by circulating immune complexes with generation of kinins and complement-derived anaphylatoxins.

Autoantibodies of various sorts interacting with antigen may induce urticarial reactions. Indeed IgG anti-IgE autoantibodies have been suggested as a major cause of chronic urticaria, and there is some preliminary evidence to suggest that this might be so. Thyroid autoantibodies have been singled out as a cause of urticaria; in one study 90 of 624 patients with chronic urticaria were found to have thyroid autoimmunity, being either hyper- or hypothyroid. Similarly, blood transfusions and infusions of fresh frozen plasma are often associated with hives caused by antibodies in the infused materials encountering host antigen or circulating host antibodies binding antigens in the blood products. One study suggests that as many as 25 per cent of patients receiving fresh frozen plasma (FFP) experience transient urticaria, and some may have anaphylactic symptomatology during the infusion. Similarly, some cancers, for example lymphomas, may be associated with urticarial lesions, thought to be due to an immunologic response to tumor antigens. A similar mechanism is clearly responsible for the hives that may be associated with many infectious agents, particularly viral agents. Here antigens on or released from the infectious agent are bound to antibodies induced in the patient and hives result. Hives are a frequent response to the antibodies formed in the early response to hepatitis A and Epstein-Barr virus infection. Rarely fungal antigens like those derived from *Candida albicans* may precipitate hives or angioedema. Nevertheless, given the rarity of this observation, it is inappropriate to treat patients with chronic urticaria/angioedema with nystatin unless a clear association with a hypersensitivity response to candidal antigens can be demonstrated. Although rare in the United States, many parasitic diseases can at times be associated with urticaria/angioedema with or without hypereosinophilia. Presumably the presence of the urticaria/angioedema reflects an ongoing immediate hypersensitivity reaction to parasite antigens.

Physical Urticarias and Angioedemas

It is important to consider the physical urticaria/angioedema complex when evaluating patients with chronic recurrent urticaria or angioedema, since in one large series these represent 16 per cent of all chronic urticaria/angioedema patients seen. In some patients a highly specific diagnosis can be made, a clear precipitating factor can be defined, and the patient can learn to avoid attacks. Moreover, specific therapy may be available. When one lists these causes of urticaria/angioedema, they appear to be so easily defined that it appears unlikely that they could be missed. However, in practice this is not the case; a detailed history is required to identify these factors. Indeed it is common for these patients to go years before a correct diagnosis is made. The physical urticarias have in common urticaria/angioedema precipitated by a known physical cause. This response may follow exposure to cold, heat, elevated body temperature, pressure, vibration, specific-wavelength ultraviolet rays, or rarely even application of water to the skin. In some cases these reactions are thought to be IgE mediated, as they can be passively transferred with serum of an affected donor to the skin of an unaffected recipient. In other cases the cause is unknown.

Symptomatic Dermatographism

As many as 2 to 5 per cent of the general population may be dermatographic, with the appearance of blanching followed by a linear streak of edema and erythema within 2 to 5 minutes of stroking of the skin. A small proportion of such individuals have sufficiently severe dermatographism that they become symptomatic. In some cases the symptoms can be transferred to a normal recipient by passive transfer of plasma, suggesting that in some way IgE antibody plays a role. In general these individuals can be treated successfully with H_1 and H_2 antihistamines.

Cold Urticaria

These patients experience urticaria/angioedema on exposure to cold and may become hypotensive on diving into a cold swimming pool. Careful studies have shown that mast cell degranulation with histamine release occurs in these patients on cold exposure. Degranulation may be even more extensive when the patient's tissues are warmed following cold exposure. Placing an ice cube on the skin for 5 minutes and then removing it reveals an area of blanching in the shape of the cube followed by edema formation in the same area surrounded by an erythematous flare caused by local hyperemia. In a percentage of these patients passive transfer to the skin of normals has been demonstrated. It has been suggested that upon cold exposure, certain dermal antigens undergo a conformational change that allows specific IgE autoantibody to bind and initiate mast cell degranulation. These patients are typically treated with cyproheptadine, sometimes with the addition of hydroxyzine. Cold urticaria may occur in some systemic diseases as well. In rare cases this may be associated with the presence of cryoglobulin or cryofibrinogen. The symptom complex, however, is not associated with the presence of cold agglutinins. When cold urticaria is associated with underlying disease, treatment of that disease is an essential part of therapy.

In some patients the disease is atypical in that the patient gives a history of typical urticarial symptoms but the ice cube test is negative. In occasional patients dermatographism is brought out by cold exposure; in others exercise-induced urticaria is noted only in the cold. There is a rare familial type of cold urticaria inherited as an autosomal dominant trait in which patients develop urticarial lesions 9 to 18 hours after cold exposure. This cannot be passively transferred with plasma and the cause is unknown.

In a similar fashion, localized heat urticaria has been described, with a wheal and flare response noted 2 to 5 minutes after application of localized heat to the skin.

Cholinergic or Generalized Heat Urticaria

Typically these patients, representing about 4 per cent of all patients with chronic urticaria, develop small (several millimeters), intensely pruritic wheals on an erythematous base on their upper trunk and arms following exercise with sweating or following hot showers. Essential to the development of lesions is a rise in core body temperature. It is generally believed that the parasympathetic nervous system supply to the neuromuscular junction of cutaneous vessels releases acetylcholine as well as neuropeptide, such as vasoactive intestinal peptide, which in an unknown way causes mediator release. In support of this hypothesis is the fact that a proportion of these patients (30 to 50 per cent) develop typical lesions as well as a series of local satellite lesions upon intracutaneous injection of Mecholyl. Atropine may inhibit the skin test but does not successfully treat the disease. These patients are typically highly responsive to hydroxyzine therapy. There is a subset of patients who respond to heat exposure with the development of large urticarial lesions rather than with the typical lesions of cholinergic urticaria. These patients tend not to develop their hives with exercise and are less responsive to hydroxyzine therapy.

Exercise-Induced Urticaria/Anaphylaxis

These patients note urticarial lesions appearing 5 to 30 minutes after the onset of exercise. They last for 1 to 3 hours. In severe cases anaphylactic reactions may be noted. This is an illness generally of young adults. At times symptoms are difficult to distinguish from those of cholinergic urticaria; however, these patients do not develop urticaria on raising core body temperature as in a hot bath.

Pressure-Induced Urticaria

For unknown reasons, in almost all cases urticarial lesions are common at pressure points on the body, e.g., where clothing is tight. Some patients note the development of marked urticarial lesions 4 to 6 hours after pressure is applied to the body. For example, these individuals may note urticarial lesions on buttocks following a long period of sitting on a hard chair or angioedema or urticaria on their feet after prolonged standing in one place. The lesions may be provoked by placing over the shoulders for 20 minutes a 1-inch strap weighted at the ends with 15-pound weights. A systemic response with malaise and even fever is often noted. The response to antihistamines is often poor. The urticaria but not the systemic toxicity may respond to antihistamine therapy. The most severely affected of these patients may require every-other-day glucocorticoid administration for partial relief. They are reported to be unresponsive to nonsteroidal anti-inflammatory agents.

In a similar way, some patients respond to local vibration with the development of urticarial lesions. Typically symptoms are induced by placing a vibrator or vortex mixer on the arm for 5 minutes. Urticaria appears in 1 to 5 minutes.

Solar Urticaria

In general these patients develop urticarial responses to exposure to sunlight; the patients are divided into groups by the wavelength of light that provokes attacks. Patients whose attacks are provoked by light at 280 to 320 nm (type 1) and 400 to 500 nm (type 4) typically have disease that can be passively transferred with serum to nonaffected recipients. This observation suggests the presence of an IgE-dependent mechanism in these cases. Glass absorbs light with wavelength below 320 nm, and patients with urticaria in response to light wavelengths below 320 nm can be protected easily. The erythema-causing band of the solar spectrum, UVB, is at wavelength 290 to 320 nm, and these patients can sometimes be helped considerably by PABA-containing sunscreens, which absorb light in this range. However, many are not protected by the PABA sunscreens. A newly available sunscreen preparation, butyl methoxydibenzoyl methane, absorbs light in the UVA range and may be more useful for this patient group. There are many types of light sensitivity, and sorting these out may be confusing. They range from metabolic abnormalities (erythrogenic porphyria), in which products of metabolism absorb light energy and undergo chemical alteration with the development of toxic products, to photoallergic reactions, in which skin-sensitizing drugs induce allergic reactions when acted upon by sunlight, to phototoxic reactions, in which drugs localized in cutaneous tissues directly cause tissue-damaging reactions when exposed to light of the proper wavelength. In many of these cases the light energy is absorbed by a complex ring structure in the drug with subsequent release of photons and electrons that lead to local generation of toxic products such as singlet oxygen, hydrogen peroxide, and chloramines. Obviously in each case one attempts to identify the cause of the urticaria and eliminate the offending agent if it can be defined.

Aquagenic Urticaria

These patients respond with urticaria within 2 to 30 minutes to application of water to the skin. Typically this is noted in the course of baths or showers, even with water at tepid temperature. In many cases these individuals are probably exquisitely sensitive to additives in the water, e.g., chlorine, but it is reported that rare individuals develop urticaria in response to distilled water.

Chronic Urticaria/Angioedema

It should be clear from the material presented that chronic urticaria/angioedema can be caused by many agents, and identifying the agent may be difficult or impossible. Often after attempts at identifying the etiology of the urticaria have failed, we are left with a patient who requires treatment. H_1 antihistamines are usually the agents of first choice. Some examples of therapeutic agents are listed earlier in the chapter; in patients with chronic disease, high-dose hydroxyzine and cyproheptadine are often effective. These agents make patients drowsy and may not be well tolerated initially, but drowsiness may pass if the drug is continued. Frequently the dose is increased until drowsiness persists and then the dosage is reduced slightly. It is common to find patients who claim to have been unresponsive to these agents because the drugs have not been used properly. Many more conveniently used and less sedating antihistamines have become available in the last few years and have been shown in controlled studies to be effective in chronic angioedema/urticaria. These include terfenadine, astemizol, loratidine, and cetirizine. H_2 inhibitory drugs are often added to H_1 inhibitors if the clinical response is not adequate. Other agents have also proven to be beneficial, including doxipen, a tricyclic antidepressant with anti-H_1 and anti-H_2 properties; nifedipine, a calcium channel blocker; and ketotifin, a drug shown to be efficacious in the physical urticarias. If these agents fail, a course of glucocorticoids may be required. In general one begins with 40 to 60 mg of prednisone per day in divided doses for 1 week. The dosage is then consolidated to a single dose a day, and then the drug is rapidly tapered on an every-other-day schedule until the patient is receiving glucocorticoids once every other day. The dose of glucocorticoids should be tapered to the lowest dose that will maintain the patient with minimal symptoms. Following a course of glucocorticoid therapy, patients often remain in remission for a prolonged time. The illness may recur at a later time or when glucocorticoids are tapered.

DIFFERENTIAL DIAGNOSIS

The etiology of the disorder is multifactorial. Usually the diagnosis of urticaria/angioedema does not present a problem in the patient with clear episodes of pruritic wheals or localized brawny edema. Since many agents can cause these lesions, considerable detective work is required to define these diseases and to develop a suitable specific therapy. During the initial evaluation a number of points must be explored. A history of a fixed rather than evanescent eruption, burning, bruising, or vesiculating lesions must lead one to early biopsy. Similarly, fever or systemic signs and symptoms suggest that further exploration is needed. Patients with idiopathic chronic urticaria typically have a normal sedimentation rate, white count, and differential and these should be examined. In appropriate cases, ANA, heterophile, STS, rheumatoid factor level, cryoglobulins and cryofibrinogen, cold hemolysin, C4, and C1 inhibitor levels should be studied for further clues to the underlying diagnosis. In the patient who responds poorly to therapy or who has atypical disease, a biopsy is clearly indicated. Patients with urticarial vasculitis are treated for the underlying vasculitis.

THERAPY

The use of antihistamines is discussed under each of the various entities and in the section on chronic urticaria/angioedema. The use of glucocorticoids has been discussed in that section as well. Epinephrine is of clinical usefulness in acute management of urticaria/angioedema. In this case the drug is administered as a series of injections (0.2 to 0.3 ml) of 1:1000 dilution subcutaneously, repeated at half-hour intervals two or three times until symptoms are controlled. Obviously the use of epinephrine is contraindicated in certain patient groups such as patients with severe cardiovascular disease. Longer-acting epinephrine preparations such as epinephrine in oil (Sus-Phrine) may be useful.

URTICARIA PIGMENTOSA AND SYSTEMIC MASTOCYTOSIS

Urticaria pigmentosa is characterized by the local accumulation of intradermal masses of infiltrating mast cells (Ch. 252). The lesions may resemble freckles superficially but are raised, as might be expected of infiltrative lesions, and may be somewhat erythematous. They may urticate when stroked (Darier's sign). Systemic mastocytosis is associated with massive accumulation of mast cells in other organs, particularly the bone marrow and gastrointestinal tract. Although some of these patients may present to the physician with acute or chronic urticaria, that presentation is quite rare; systemic signs of histamine toxicity, gastrointestinal disorders, or disorders consequent to destruction of bone marrow or bone are more common.

HEREDITARY ANGIOEDEMA

Hereditary angioedema (HAE) presents clinically as episodic attacks of brawny nonpitting edema that usually involve the extremities but may affect any external body surface including the genitalia. Mucosal surfaces are affected as well and patients frequently have attacks of severe abdominal pain due to swelling of the submucosa of the gastrointestinal tract. On rare occasions attacks may affect the airway, where they can cause respiratory obstruction and asphyxiation. Although attacks are sporadic, about half of the patients note that trauma, particularly associated with local pressure, precipitates an attack, and half the patients note a marked increase in attack frequency at times of emotional stress. About one third of patients note an erythema marginatum–like rash at the onset of attacks which they often describe as nonraised, nonpruritic circles on the skin. In general, attacks become progressively more severe over about 1.5 days and then regress over a similar time period. Swelling of the gastrointestinal mucosa may be associated with exquisite abdominal pain.

Although relatively rare (incidence about 1:10,000), this disease has received a great deal of attention because of the high incidence of lethal complications, because its pathophysiologic basis is best understood of all of the angioedemas, and because adequate therapy is available for most patients. Presence of this disease is associated with either low levels or abnormal function of a plasma regulatory protein, the C1 inhibitor (Ch. 243). This protein functions to control activation of the complement, kiningenerating, fibrinolytic, and intrinsic clotting pathways. Although the precise cause of the capillary leakage is unknown, it is believed that a peptide formed during activation of either the complement or the kinin-generating mediator pathway is the responsible factor. HAE has an autosomal dominant inheritance pattern, affecting 50 per cent of the offspring of a patient and occurring with equal frequency in males and females. This autosomal dominant inheritance reflects the presence of one abnormal gene for C1 inhibitor on chromosome 11. This gene may yield no gene product or may code for a nonfunctional protein.

HAE tends to be mild in childhood, becoming more severe at the time of puberty. The factors that initiate attacks are unknown. There is no relationship between the level or activity of C1 inhibitor and the severity of disease. Patients are described who presumably had the defect from birth but whose attacks began at age 70. Diagnosis is established by demonstration of low levels of C1 inhibitor antigen or function and low levels of the complement protein C4 and/or C2. C1 inhibitor inhibits the function of activated C1 of the classic complement pathway. C1 INH acts by binding to the substrate to be inhibited, and the product of one normal gene is insufficient to control mediator activation. C1 when activated cleaves the next two proteins in the cascade, C4 and C2. Since the function of activated C1 is unregulated in the presence of a relative C1 inhibitor deficiency, C1 continues to cleave C4 and C2. Patients have low levels of circulating C4 and C2 during attacks and usually have low levels between attacks. Interestingly, because of the presence of other control proteins, the levels of C3, the most commonly measured complement protein, are almost always normal. Presumably because of the constant complement activation present in these patients, they have an immune dysregulation, as shown by the higher-than-normal incidence of autoimmune diseases. These include endocrinopathies, granulomatous bowel disorders, arthritides, and SLE.

Patients' angioedema attacks respond poorly to epinephrine, antihistamines, and glucocorticoids, the mainstays of treatment of urticaria and angioedema caused by immediate hypersensitivity reactions. Nevertheless, acute attacks are treated with epinephrine, both nebulized racemic epinephrine in the airway (1:1000 given by nebulization) and subcutaneous injections (0.2 to 0.3 ml 1:1000 SQ repeated q 20–30 min × 3). Epinephrine administered very early in an attack often produces some improvement. Patients also receive antihistamines for sedation. Patients often relate that intravenous administration of FFP to supply the missing inhibitor protein terminates attacks. Nevertheless, a rare patient becomes more edematous following FFP, presumably reflecting increased availability of mediator substrates, and FFP therefore is not recommended for treatment of life-threatening laryngeal edema. In this circumstance endotracheal intubation in the operating room under conditions where tracheostomy can be performed is indicated. FFP can be given in nonemergency situations such as in preoperative patients to prevent attacks. The usual dose of FFP is 2 units, an arbitrary amount that has been used extensively and has proven to be effective. Evidence suggests that infusions of purified C1 inhibitor reliably terminate attacks, but this protein has not yet been made available in the United States. Although short-term therapy and therapy of acute attacks of HAE have not been generally satisfactory, long-term therapy has been quite successful. Patients respond to all of the acetylated artificial androgens with increased C1 INH levels that in some cases approach normal values, a correction of serum C4 and C2, and a marked amelioration of symptoms. In the rare patient in whom the drug is ineffective or in whom drug toxicity is a problem, the plasmin inhibitor ϵ-aminocaproic acid has also been found to be effective. Its mechanism of action is unknown, and there is no change in the amount of C activation reflected in the persistent reduction in the serum level of C4 and C2. With all of these agents there is a high degree of patient-to-patient variation in dosage, and the lowest dose that controls symptoms is chosen. Women are often treated with danazol, an impeded androgen that has few masculinizing side effects. The usual dosage of danazol is 200 to 400 mg per day. Men are often treated with the less expensive but more androgenic agent methyltestosterone in a dose of 10 to 30 mg per day orally.

ACQUIRED C1 INHIBITOR DEFICIENCY

A number of syndromes have been recognized that are associated with a typical hereditary angioedema symptom complex but are a reflection of acquired disease. A decade ago it was recognized that certain patients with malignancies, including lymphosarcoma, leukemia, lymphoma, and paraproteinemia, developed circulating or cellular factors capable of activating C1 and depleting all the C1 inhibitor activity in serum. Later it was noted that rare patients with autoimmune disease also induced massive activation of the complement cascade, with C1 inhibitor utilization and a hereditary angioedema–like clinical picture. More recently, patients have been described with multiple myeloma and anti-idiotypic antibody causing the same symptom complex. Perhaps the most common of these rare individuals are recently described patients who form monoclonal or polyclonal autoantibodies to the C1 inhibitor which destroy its activity. Clinically these patients cannot be distinguished from patients with hereditary angioedema. However, their laboratory tests are unique. All of these patients have profound depressions in functional C1, C4, and C2. Patients with HAE commonly have normal C1 levels. Although their plasma C1 inhibitor antigen level may be normal, these patients have marked depression of C1 INH function. Their treatment involves treating the underlying disease where possible. Some of these patients do respond to danazol or other anabolic steroids. One of the patients with the anti–C1 INH autoantibody has responded to glucocorticoid therapy, and at least one of these patients has responded to cytotoxic therapy.

FACTOR I DEFICIENCY WITH CHRONIC URTICARIA

Factor I is one of the control proteins of the complement activation pathway. The rare individuals with an inherited deficiency of this protein have continuous activation and cleavage of C3 with generation of the anaphylatoxins C3a and perhaps C5a. In vitro these cleavage peptides induce mast cell degranulation and cause chronic urticaria that disappears when the patient is infused with Factor I. In general, this form of urticaria is relatively mild and is treated symptomatically with antihistamines.

Bressler RB, Sowell K, Huston DP: Therapy of chronic idiopathic urticaria with nifedipine: Demonstration of a beneficial effect in a double blinded, placebo controlled, crossover trial. J Allergy Clin Immunol 83:756, 1989. *Seven patients completed this trial. All improved.*
Casale TB, Sampson HA, Harrifin J, et al.: Guide to physical urticarias. J Allergy Clin Immunol 82:758, 1988. *Tables of information on the physical urticarias.*
Champion RH: Urticaria: Then and now. Br J Dermatol 119:427, 1988. *A report of the evaluation of 2300 cases and comments on the literature.*
Champion RH, Greaves MW, Kobza A, et al.: The Urticarias. Edinburgh, Churchill Livingstone, 1985. *The proceedings of a symposium on urticaria-angioedema.*
Frank MM: Hereditary angioedema. In Bayless TM, Brain MC, Cherniack RM (eds.): Current Therapy in Internal Medicine 2. Philadelphia, B. C. Decker, 1987, p 42. *Complete discussion of treatment.*
Frank MM, Gelfand JA, Atkinson JP: Hereditary angioedema: The clinical syndrome and its management. Ann Intern Med 84:580, 1976. *Although old, this represents the classic clinical review of this syndrome.*
Leznoff A, Sussman GL: Syndrome of idiopathic chronic urticaria and angioedema with thyroid autoimmunity. A study of 90 patients. J Allergy Clin Immunol 84:66, 1989. *The best review of this patient group.*
Monroe EN: Chronic urticaria. Review of nonsedating H_1 antihistamines in treatment. J Am Acad Dermatol 19:842, 1988. *Comparison of various H_1 agents and review of published studies.*
Wanderer AA: Cold urticaria syndromes. Historical background, diagnostic classification, clinical and laboratory characteristics, pathogenesis and management. J Allergy Clin Immunol 88:965, 1990. *A thorough review of this syndrome.*

246 Allergic Rhinitis

John E. Salvaggio

DEFINITION. Allergic rhinitis is an IgE-mediated inflammatory disease of the nasal mucous membranes characterized by paroxysms of sneezing; itching of the nose, eyes, palate, and pharynx; nasal stuffiness with partial or total obstruction of air flow; and mucous secretion often accompanied by postnasal drainage. The disease is often seasonal, depending on the pollination patterns of inhalant allergens that have direct impact on the respiratory mucosa. The condition may be perennial when due to nonseasonal allergens.

Patients with allergic rhinitis have an increased number of mast cells in nasal secretions. When appropriately sensitized with specific IgE molecules, mucosal mast cells can interact with allergenic airborne particles that initially affect the respiratory mucosa and release water-soluble allergens during inhalation. Mast cells and basophils concentrate IgE on their surface, which fixes to a glycoprotein receptor site on the membrane by its Fc fragment, resulting in an arrangement that permits exposure of the antibody-combining sites (or Fab) to the surrounding milieu. Cross-linking of two IgE antibody molecules by specific antigen aggregates the corresponding receptor sites and results in initiation of a series of cellular biochemical events that culminate in the expulsion of secretory granule contents with release of pharmacologic mediators. The consequences of mediator release may be apparent within minutes or may require hours to develop (late-phase allergic reactions). They are summarized in Figure 246–1. Among the mast cell–derived mediators, either preformed within their granules or generated from precursor molecules, are

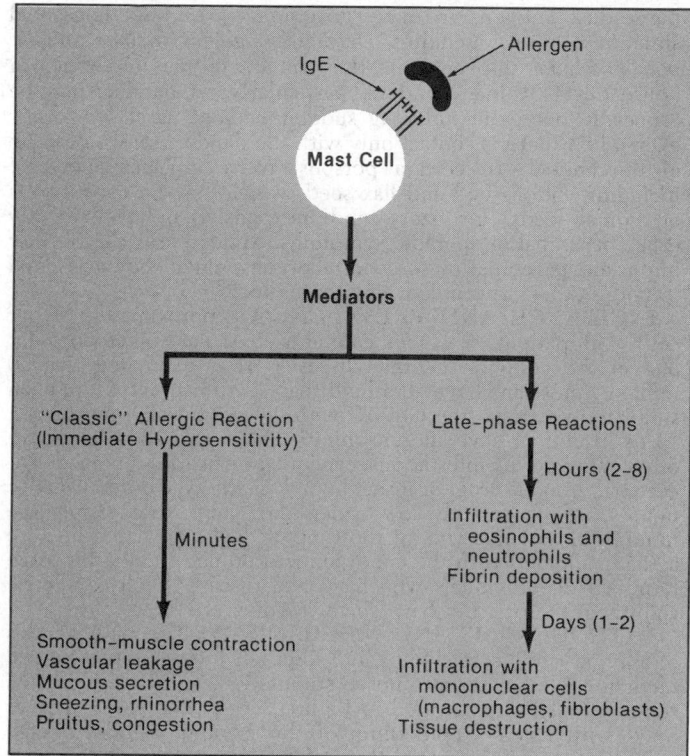

FIGURE 246–1. Mast cell mediator/effector pathways.

histamine; kinins and kininogen; thromboxanes; leukotrienes C_4, D_4, and E_4, which are derived from arachidonic acid released during the allergic reaction; eosinophil chemotactic factors of anaphylaxis (ECF-A), which are derived from the mast cell granule; heparin, which makes up 30 per cent of the dry weight of mast cell granules; superoxide dismutase (SOD), which is formed by the univalent reduction of oxygen; prostaglandins, which are C20 unsaturated fatty acid derivatives of arachidonic acid; platelet-activating factor (PAF), a small phospholipid derivative of phosphoryl choline released from rabbit basophils; neutrophil chemotactic factor of anaphylaxis (NCF-A); inflammatory factors of anaphylaxis, which are constituents of the mast cell granules that can induce a late-phase allergic inflammatory reaction; and a number of enzymes that are found in mast cell granules, such as chymotrypsin, trypsin, and tosyl-arginine-methyl-ester (TAME)-esterase. These enzymes may contribute to the tissue destruction accompanying various late-phase allergic reactions. Both immediate- and late-phase nasal reactions, which occur hours after challenge, have been produced in vivo following nasal challenge with ragweed pollen or other allergens. Histamine; kinins; TAME-esterase; leukotrienes C_4, D_4, and E_4; and prostaglandin D_2 have been directly demonstrated in nasal secretions during the immediate response. With the exception of prostaglandin D_2, these mediators have also been demonstrable in late-phase responses. Since prostaglandin D_2 is released by mast cells but not basophils, this observation suggests an important role for basophils in late-phase reactions. Nasal mucosal biopsy specimens may also reveal increased numbers of ciliated cells, goblet cells, and eosinophils in the epithelium, plus edema and vascular dilation in the submucosa. The inflammation that follows immediate-phase reactions likely results in a primary effect, accounting for much of the hyperreactivity of the allergic nose to a variety of nonspecific stimuli such as strong odors, insecticides, and cigarette smoke.

ETIOLOGY. The most apparent seasonal allergens acting as etiologic agents in allergic rhinitis are pollens such as ragweed. Tree pollens are usually released during the spring, and in most parts of the country the peak of the grass pollen season is late spring to midsummer. Much of the nasal symptoms caused by airborne weed pollens occurs in late summer and early fall. Ragweed pollen is by far the worst offender in the eastern, midwestern, and southern United States. Many individuals with perennial allergic rhinitis have an IgE-mediated response to crude house-dust antigen. In many geographic areas and household situations, mites, including *Dermatophagoides farinae* and *D. petronyssimus*, appear to be the primary sources of antigen in house dusts. Animal danders, particularly cat dander, may be especially potent in inducing sudden, violent nasal symptoms, even when there is contact only with the dander, saliva, or urine of the animal. In certain persons, other inhalant allergens, including cotton seed and flax seed, which may be constituents of animal feeds, fertilizers, and inexpensive upholstery, may cause perennial or sporadic symptoms. Mold spores can be very important perennial or seasonal allergens, since they are found in both outdoor and indoor environments.

INCIDENCE AND PREVALENCE. Approximately 9 per cent of all patients who seek care at a physician's office do so for one of the common allergic diseases. It is estimated that 50 million Americans have allergic diseases: An estimated 9 million suffer from asthma (see Ch. 57) with or without allergic rhinitis; 25 to 30 million have allergic rhinitis alone; and 12 million have other allergic manifestations, such as urticaria, angioedema, eczema, or food, drug, or insect hypersensitivity. These incidence figures are deceptively low, since they approximate only the number of patients who, at the time of the particular study, are actually afflicted with the condition and do not include the large numbers of individuals who have had diseases such as allergic rhinitis in the past but have since "recovered."

PATHOGENESIS AND MECHANISMS. The pathogenesis of allergic rhinitis, including IgE-allergen interaction, mast cell mediator release, sensory nerve stimulation, and CNS-mediated reflex activity, is illustrated in Figure 246–2. The nasal cavity is lined with airways epithelium of the ciliated pseudostratified type. The lamina propria in the anterior part of the nose contains large numbers of seromucous and serous glands. Postganglionic

sympathetic nerves emerge from the stellate ganglion in the neck and reach the nose along arteries. Most of the parasympathetic fibers to the nose travel via the vidian nerve. The parasympathetic fibers are part of a reflex arc with sensory fibers in the trigeminal nerve. The nasal sensory nerves are exposed to stimulation from unconditioned and polluted inhaled air, and there is constant reflex activity in the nerves.

There are immunologic as well as nonimmunologic triggers of this mast cell degranulation process. Histamine sprayed into the nose causes itching, sneezing, discharge, and blockage and directly increases endothelial- and epithelial-cell permeability. This facilitates further allergen penetration into the submucosal areas. Histamine also has a direct effect on vascular H_1 and H_2 receptors, resulting in edema formation. In addition, when released from epithelial basophils, histamine indirectly stimulates sensory nerve H_1 receptors, resulting in a CNS-mediated parasympathetic reflex in the trigeminal and vidian nerves with subsequent itching, sneezing, and increased nasal discharge.

CLINICAL MANIFESTATIONS. Common symptoms include nasal stuffiness, paroxysms of sneezing, profuse mucous secretion, and frequent itching of the nose, eyes, posterior pharynx, or conjunctivae. Soreness or inflammation of the conjunctivae with excessive tearing and mucoid conjunctival discharge may be present in severe cases, and it is not uncommon for patients with recurrent symptoms to note a certain degree of fatigue, malaise, anorexia, and irritability. Many offending plants pollinate during the early morning hours. Thus, morning symptoms may be followed by improvement during the day as exposure lessens. Repeated upward rubbing of the nose to relieve itching may cause a crease to develop across the nose, especially in children. Mouth breathing is common, as are typical dark, discolored infraorbital "shiners" (Fig. 246–3).

Examination of the nasal mucous membranes characteristically reveals bluish, edematous, boggy, pale nasal turbinates, often coated with clear secretion, but many persons with allergic rhinitis have an erythematous, boggy nasal mucosa that can easily be confused with that seen in infectious rhinitis. At times, the nasal airways may be completely obstructed as a result of accumulation of mucus and turbinate swelling. Scleral and conjunctival injection and edema plus periorbital swelling and tearing may be noted. Nasal polyps are relatively uncommonly associated with uncomplicated rhinitis. They may, however, be associated with aspirin intolerance. Since asthmatics with aspirin intolerance often have severe disease, visualization of even small polyps in patients with rhinitis and asthma may provide important diagnostic leads.

In seasonal rhinitis, symptoms recur each year with regularity during the pollination season characteristic for a given area. IgE-mediated perennial rhinitis presents with continuous low-grade symptoms that may improve only if the patient leaves the region of the inciting causes. Perennial rhinitis of unknown cause (also called vasomotor rhinitis) also produces persistent symptoms without correlation to any specific allergen exposure. This type of perennial rhinitis is often worsened by changes in temperature or humidity or with exposure to irritants or other types of air pollutants. It is also often associated with profuse nasal discharge after the patient eats chilled, highly spiced, or very hot foods.

Serous otitis media may be superimposed upon other symptoms of seasonal or perennial allergic rhinitis. In many instances of serous otitis media, however, allergic factors cannot be identified. Serous otitis, which can be an important complication in children, may result from nasal obstruction or obstructive dysfunction of the eustachian tube as a result of mucosal edema and secretions. It can also lead to hearing loss with adverse effects on cognition or speech development in the young child. The tympanic membrane on physical examination is frequently amber colored and retracted and shows decreased motion if there is negative middle-ear pressure or no motion at all if there is a severe effusion.

Chronic sinusitis may be another complication, often manifested by the presence of chronic nasal discharge, nocturnal cough associated with postnasal discharge, pain, fever, headache, and recurrent otitis media. In adults, however, pain, headache, and low-grade fever are the most common signs. Chronic sinusitis as a complication of seasonal allergic rhinitis should be considered whenever symptoms of allergic rhinitis are more protracted than expected, when the patient has severe dull-to-intense throbbing pain over the involved sinus area, or when prolonged or persistent

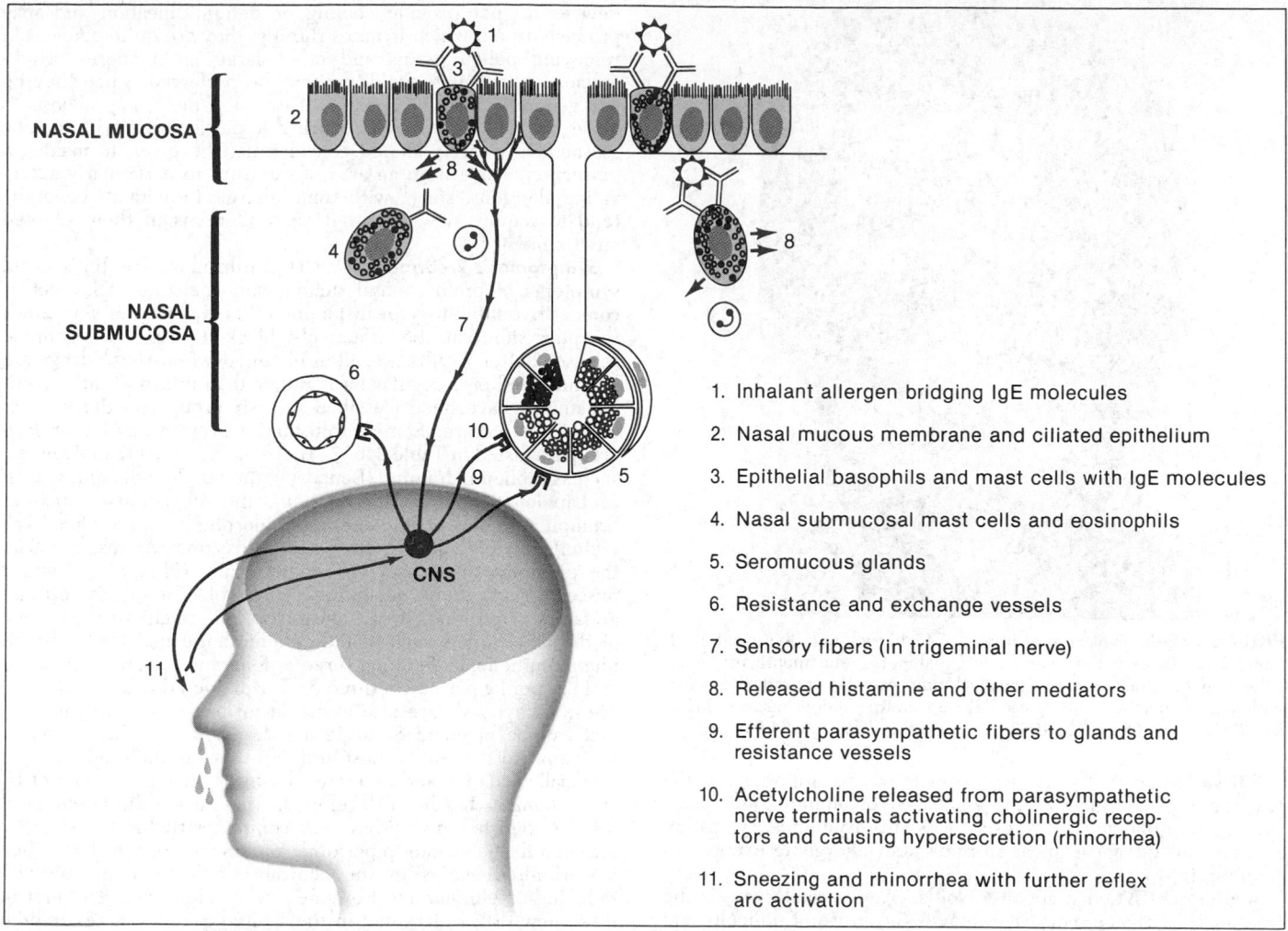

NASAL MUCOSA

NASAL SUBMUCOSA

CNS

1. Inhalant allergen bridging IgE molecules

2. Nasal mucous membrane and ciliated epithelium

3. Epithelial basophils and mast cells with IgE molecules

4. Nasal submucosal mast cells and eosinophils

5. Seromucous glands

6. Resistance and exchange vessels

7. Sensory fibers (in trigeminal nerve)

8. Released histamine and other mediators

9. Efferent parasympathetic fibers to glands and resistance vessels

10. Acetylcholine released from parasympathetic nerve terminals activating cholinergic receptors and causing hypersecretion (rhinorrhea)

11. Sneezing and rhinorrhea with further reflex arc activation

FIGURE 246–2. Pathogenesis of allergic rhinitis; antigen-antibody interaction and mediator release.

cough develops which is suggestive of bronchitis that has failed to respond to appropriate therapy. Transillumination may be helpful in detecting chronic sinusitis, and equipment for ultrasonic evaluation of the sinuses in the office is also available. Roentgenograms often detect opacification, membrane thickening, or an air-fluid level in one or more sinuses.

DIAGNOSIS (WITH DIFFERENTIAL DIAGNOSIS). A good history is most important in correctly diagnosing rhinitis. In addition to the history of classic symptoms, nasal examination should be performed utilizing a nasal speculum along with high-powered illumination. If nasopharyngeal obstruction is present and its cause has not been detected by simpler means, nasopharyngoscopy should be considered. Careful skin testing with common inhalant preparations together with positive and negative control substances is a mandatory procedure in diagnosing specific allergic factors associated with rhinitis. Direct skin tests of the scratch, prick, and intradermal variety are the least expensive and time consuming. The intradermal test should never be performed without prior performance of negative scratch or prick tests. In general, negative skin test responses with common inhalant allergens indicate that rhinitis is of nonallergic origin. Methods of detecting IgE antibodies in vitro have now been available for several years. In patients who are receiving medications that might prevent skin reactivity or in those with extensive eczema or dermatographia that negates the use of skin tests, these in vitro assays for serum IgE antibodies, such as the radioallergosorbent test (RAST), fluorescent allergosorbent test (FAST), multiple thread allergosorbent test, or enzyme-linked immunosorbent assay (ELISA), may be substituted for direct skin testing. Total serum IgE levels are elevated in only 30 to 40 per cent of patients with allergic rhinitis. They may also be elevated

in many nonallergic conditions. Although frequently elevated in allergic rhinitis, the peripheral blood eosinophil count may be normal. A high peripheral eosinophil count may also be seen in nonallergic perennial rhinitis associated with nasal polyps, hyperplastic sinusitis, and idiopathic asthma. Of more significance is a smear of nasal secretions for eosinophils.

Conditions to be considered in the differential diagnosis of rhinitis are listed in Table 246–1. Clear-cut allergic rhinitis due to inhalant allergens seldom presents a differential diagnostic problem. Symptoms of the common cold may, however, be quite similar, although they usually last less than a week and are often associated with fever, pain, and the presence of considerable numbers of neutrophils in nasal secretions. Symptoms associated with structural abnormalities of the nasal area, such as polyps, deviated nasal septum, enlarged tonsils, or foreign bodies, are often unilateral and relatively constant rather than episodic in classic seasonal allergic rhinitis. A suspected diagnosis of so-called rhinitis medicamentosa due to the rebound effects of nose drops, sprays, ovarian hormonal agents (such as oral contraceptives), reserpine derivatives, or hydralazine can often be confirmed when symptoms gradually improve following avoidance of the suspected agent. Nasal symptoms may accompany metabolic disorders such as hyperthyroidism or emotional states, but the relationship is unclear. During pregnancy and the premenstrual period, hormonally related rhinitis may occur. Eosinophilic nonallergic rhinitis resembles allergic rhinitis but is associated with negative skin test reactions and normal IgE levels and tends to respond well only to topical corticosteroid therapy. A condition known as nasal mastocytosis is associated with symptoms of perennial allergic rhinitis; the diagnosis can be made by nasal mucosal biopsy.

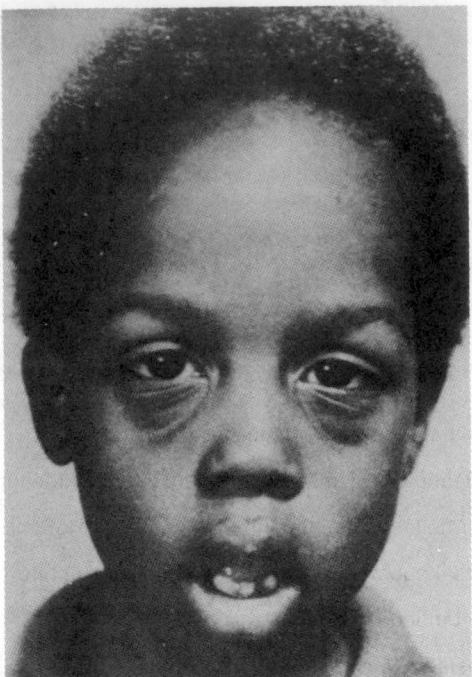

FIGURE 246–3. Typical appearance of highly allergic 6-year-old child. Note dark circles under eyes ("allergic shiners") and mouth breathing. Allergic nasal crease from constant "saluting" was also present. (Reprinted with permission from Mathews KP: Respiratory atopic disease. JAMA 248:2588, 1982. Copyright 1982, American Medical Association.)

TREATMENT. Three basic principles are important in the treatment of allergic rhinitis: avoidance of offending allergens; use of symptomatic treatment such as antihistamines, sympathomimetic drugs, and topical steroids; and allergenic extract immunotherapy.

Avoidance. When practical, avoidance of aeroallergens is the treatment of choice, since it removes the cause of difficulty and prevents symptoms. When a specific food, drug, occupational allergen, or animal dander is involved, avoidance is the only measure that serves both to prevent and to treat disease. All physicians should be familiar, for example, with standard antidust regimens for use in home environments. Although avoidance of outdoor exposure to ubiquitous seasonal and perennial pollens is virtually impossible, common-sense measures to avoid heavy exposure often help to prevent severe exacerbations of symptoms. For example, mold-sensitive patients should avoid barns, working with hay, raking leaves, and mowing grass. Simply keeping doors

TABLE 246–1. DIFFERENTIAL DIAGNOSIS OF RHINITIS

Infections
Allergic
  Seasonal (hay fever)
  Perennial
Eosinophilic nonallergic rhinitis
Rhinitis medicamentosa
Vasomotor rhinitis of pregnancy
"Vasomotor" rhinitis
Disturbed nasal function associated with
  Ciliary dyskinesia
  Hypothyroidism
  Horner's syndrome
  Foreign body
  Nasal polyps
  Nasal septal deviation
  Enlarged tonsils and adenoids
  Nasal mastocytosis
  Sinus disease
  Tumors or granulomas
  Cerebrospinal fluid rhinorrhea
  Aspirin intolerance

and windows closed significantly decreases indoor pollen and mold spore concentrations, and air conditioning makes a closed environment more tolerable. Although electrostatic air-purifying devices do not provide cooling or dehumidification and may produce ozone, which irritates rhinitis, they are quite efficient in removing pollen grains and other large mold spores. High-efficiency particulate air filters may be preferred, since they do not generate ozone. In certain cases a patient may choose to leave an area of exposure during a particularly symptomatic season. Only rarely should consideration be given to making a permanent move from an area of exposure to particularly aggravating allergens, since, with time, allergic individuals generally tend to acquire new sensitivities to allergens in their adopted environment.

Symptomatic Treatment. The H_1 antihistamines often control symptoms of profuse nasal itching and sneezing. They act as competitive inhibitors for histamine at its H_1 receptor site. Since receptor sites can be effectively blocked prior to histamine release, better results are often obtained when these drugs are administered on a regular basis rather than intermittently. Antihistamines have been classified into six groups on the basis of chemical structure. Some antihistamines representative of each group are listed in Table 246–2. These include the ethanolamines, such as diphenhydramine (Benadryl); the ethylenediamines, such as tripelennamine (Pyribenzamine); the alkylamines, such as brompheniramine (Dimetane) and chlorpheniramine (Chlor-Trimeton); the piperazines, such as hydroxyzine (Atarax, Vistaril); the phenothiazines, such as promethazine (Phenergan); and a miscellaneous group, including cyproheptadine (Periactin) and azatadine (Optimine). In a typical case, one might start with one of the alkylamines such as chlorpheniramine maleate or brompheniramine maleate, 4 mg three or four times a day in the adult (0.4 mg per kg per day in three or four divided doses in children). These compounds are also available in long-acting preparations that can be given in 8- to 12-mg doses twice a day. A major limitation to the use of most antihistamines is their side effects, especially sedation and excessive drying. A new generation of H_1 antihistamines has been developed. They lack a direct chemical relation to histamine but have as a common structure an aromatic nitrogen in the form of piperidine, piperazine, or pyridine. They have limited access to the central nervous system, thereby reducing or eliminating drowsiness as a side effect. The first of these new drugs marketed in the United States was terfenidine (Seldane). Another example of these new drugs is astemizole (Hismanil). Several other similar new-generation H_1 antihistamines are under development. Available data have failed to indicate a major enhancement of therapeutic benefit for allergic rhinitis using combined H_1 and H_2 antihistamines.

The most commonly employed sympathomimetic nasal sprays and drops that contain α-adrenergic agonists are phenylephrine hydrochloride, a short-acting agent, and longer-acting preparations such as oxymetazoline hydrochloride. In most cases, use of these compounds for more than a few days results in progressively severe nasal obstruction secondary to rebound swelling of the nasal mucosa that may be a self-perpetuating process (known as rhinitis medicamentosa). Thus these agents are not recommended for long-term use in allergic rhinitis. Sympathomimetic agents administered orally, such as pseudoepinephrine and phenylpropanolamine, may also reduce nasal congestion, although when used alone they may have significant central nervous system effects, often leading to insomnia and nervousness. A 4 per cent solution of cromolyn sodium (Nasalcrom and Opticrom) applied topically can also be beneficial in the treatment and prevention of allergic rhinitis and conjunctivitis if administered frequently. The effect of treatment with Nasalcrom in typical dosage of one spray per nostril four times per day may not be noted until 2 to 4 weeks after initiation of treatment. Thus, there may be an initial need for an antihistamine or decongestant before cromolyn's preventive effect becomes apparent. It is also marketed as a 4 per cent ophthalmic solution that may be employed in treating allergic conjunctivitis. A newer and considerably more potent cromolyn derivative (nedacromil sodium) is currently available in the United Kingdom and Europe but has not yet been approved for marketing in the United States.

Topical corticosteroids are widely used and highly successful in the symptomatic treatment and prevention of allergic rhinitis. These usually include the highly potent and rapidly metabolized

TABLE 246–2. H₁ ANTIHISTAMINE CLASSIFICATIONS

Class (Nonproprietary Name)	Trade Name	Dosage Adult	Child
Ethanolamines			
Diphenydramine hydrochloride	Benadryl	25–50 mg, 3 or 4 times daily	5 mg/kg/day in 3 or 4 divided doses
Carbinoxamine maleate	Clisten	4 mg, 3 or 4 times daily	0.4 mg/kg/day in 3 or 4 divided doses
Ethylenediamine			
Tripelennamine	PBZ	25–50 mg, 3 or 4 times daily	5 mg/kg/day in 3 or 4 divided doses
Methapyrilene hydrochloride	Histadyl	25–50 mg, 4 or 5 times daily	5 mg/kg/day in 3 or 4 divided doses
Alkylamines			
Chlorpheniramine maleate	Chlor-Trimeton, Teldrin, CTM (delayed action), Cosea, Histadur, Rhinihist	4 mg, 3 or 4 times daily 12 mg, 2 times daily	0.4 mg/kg/day in 3 or 4 divided doses
Brompheniramine maleate	Dimetane	4 mg, 3 or 4 times daily	0.4 mg/kg/day in 3 or 4 divided doses
	Dimetane (delayed action) Extentabs	12 mg, 2 times daily	
Piperazines			
Hydroxyzine	Atarax, Vistaril	25–100 mg, 3 or 4 times daily	2 mg/kg/day in 4 divided doses
Phenothiazines			
Promethazine hydrochloride	Phenergan	12.5–25 mg, 2 or 3 times daily	1 mg/kg/day divided into half dose at bedtime and quarter dose every 6 hours in daytime
Trimeprazine tartrate	Temaril	2.5 mg, 4 times daily	2.5 mg in 3 divided doses (3 year olds only) 1.5 mg in 3 divided doses (6 mo to 3 yr)
Miscellaneous			
Terfenadine	Seldane	60 mg, 2 times daily	No recommendation
Astemizole	Hismanil	10 mg, 1 time daily	No recommendation
Cyproheptadine hydrochloride	Periactin	4 mg, 3 or 4 times daily	0.25 mg/kg/day in 3 or 4 divided doses
Azatadine maleate	Optimine	1–2 mg, 2 times daily	No recommendation
Clemastine fumarate	Tavist	2.68 mg, 2 times daily	No recommendation

corticosteroids such as beclomethasone dipropionate (Vancenase and Beconase), flunisolide acetate (Nasilide), budesonide, triamcinolone acetonide, and fluocortin butyl. These agents act primarily topically. Their relatively few side effects may include local burning, irritation, and occasional epistaxis or mild nasopharyngeal candidiasis. Although of substantial value in treating seasonal allergic rhinitis, these may not work well with acute, severe cases associated with considerable nasal mucosal edema and obstruction. They also do not relieve ocular symptoms. If used intermittently on a regular basis, they can help in perennial allergic rhinitis and vasomotor rhinitis. In addition, they may be of some help in weaning patients from excessive use of vasoconstrictor nasal sprays.

Each puff of beclomethasone dipropionate from a nasal inhaler is equal to approximately 42 μg of beclomethasone dipropionate, USP. Seasonal treatment on a daily basis with 400 μg per day is recommended and is considered to be quite harmless. Thus one puff per nostril four times per day from the nasal inhaler would be a typical dosage. In all cases, clinical improvement is usually apparent within several days, but symptomatic relief may not occur in some patients for as long as 2 weeks. There is substantial evidence that no systemic steroid effects occur in adults who use up to 800 μg daily (approximately 16 inhalations). In addition, cushingoid changes probably do not occur until the very large dose of approximately 1 mg* (20 inhalations or more) is reached. When the drug is used, it should be remembered that, in regard to therapeutic potency, eight inhalations is roughly equivalent to 7.5 mg of oral prednisone. These drugs should be used with caution in the presence of viral and fungal nasal diseases such as ocular herpes or related diseases in which there appears to be an associated defect in cell-mediated immunity.

Inhalant Allergen Immunotherapy (Desensitization or Hyposensitization). With this form of therapy, one attempts to alter the immunologic reactivity of an allergic individual so that there is less response upon natural re-exposure to the offending allergen. The clinical decision to use immunotherapy in the patient with allergic rhinitis depends on several factors: (1) the existence of clinically important rhinitis should be confirmed; (2) maximal environmental control procedures should be utilized; and (3) the

response to medication should be well defined. Immunotherapy is usually employed in patients who have substantial allergic components to their illness and who are attaining satisfactory clinical improvement with environmental control and symptomatic treatment. The technique involves injecting increasing amounts of allergen subcutaneously, usually at weekly intervals, starting with a very low dose and gradually increasing (usually a double dose) at each subsequent injection. A satisfactory response to immunotherapy requires achieving an adequate dose with treatment. This can best be achieved using high-quality, well-characterized extracts. The Food and Drug Administration has adopted modern methods of immunologic standardization of allergenic extracts which are significantly improving their quality. After incremental increases in the amount of injected allergen, a maintenance dose is achieved, which is injected at intervals of 2 to 6 weeks, depending upon individual patient activity and requirements. One should always carefully monitor for the development of untoward reactions. In most cases a decrease in nasal symptoms following immunotherapy is obvious during the first 6 months to 1 year and is maximal by 3 years of therapy. Results of a typical controlled clinical study are illustrated in Figure 246–4, which illustrates significant improvement in clinical symptom scores as measured by patient diaries in two groups of patients with ragweed-induced allergic rhinitis who underwent maintenance immunotherapy with aqueous extracts of ragweed prepared by two different methods. There are no universally accepted guidelines for the duration of therapy, and many physicians attempt trials of discontinuation after approximately 4 years of a successful program.

Symptomatic improvement with immunotherapy has been clearly shown in hay fever due to ragweed, grass, mountain cedar pollen, birch pollen, and *Alternaria* sp., and in asthma due to house dust mite, ragweed pollen, grass pollen, and cat dander. Beneficial results depend on a sufficiently high dose of antigen; relapse may occur once continuing maintenance injections are abandoned. Results are specific for particular antigens employed. A variety of immunologic changes have been demonstrated following immunotherapy. Among these changes are a rise in serum IgG-blocking antibodies against the allergens employed; suppression in the usual seasonal rise in IgE antibodies which normally follows environmental seasonal exposure followed by a slow decline in the level of specific IgE antibodies during the

---

*Exceeds dosage recommended by manufacturer.

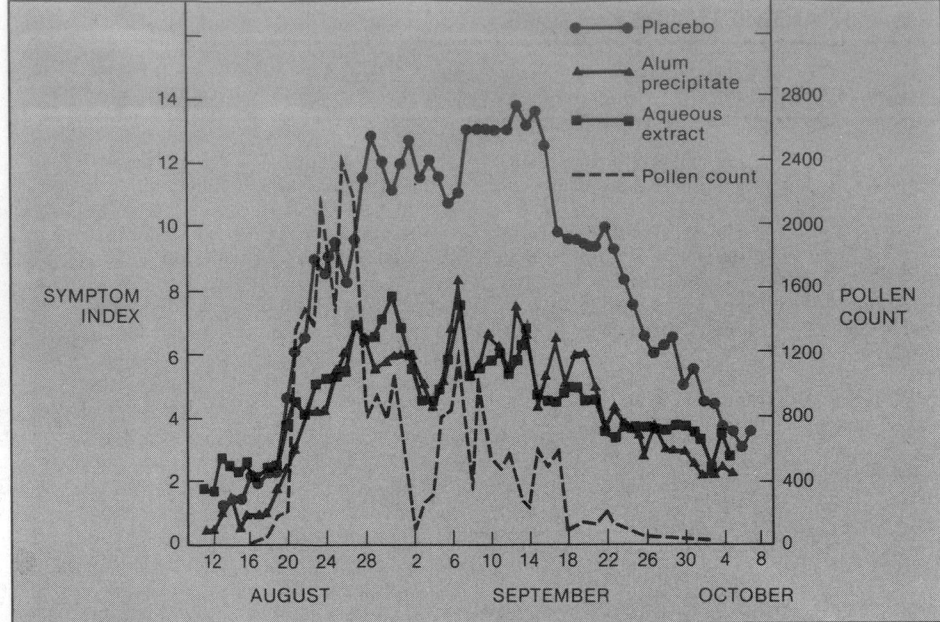

FIGURE 246–4. Daily average symptom scores in three groups of patients. (See text for explanation.) (Reprinted with permission from Norman PS: Trials of alum-precipitated pollen extracts in the treatment of hay fever. J Allergy Clin Immunol 50:31–44, 1972.)

ensuing several years of immunotherapy; increase of blocking IgA and IgG antibodies in secretions; reduced basophil reactivity and sensitivity to allergens; reduced in vitro lymphocyte responsiveness to allergens; and an increase in specific T-suppressor cells following immunotherapy. It is not known which are responsible for clinical improvement, but the serum titer of IgG "blocking" antibodies usually significantly correlates with clinical improvement. In addition, as immunotherapy progresses, the IgG antibodies become largely those of the IgG4 subclass, which are distinguished from antibodies of other IgG subclasses by their inability to cross-link antigen.

New experimental approaches to the therapy of allergic rhinitis include the use of altered antigens (such as allergoids and polymerized forms of antigen) that ultimately result in a heightened degree of immunization, with considerably less chance to trigger sensitized mast cells and produce local or systemic reactions. The use of other routes of antigen administration (e.g., intranasal and oral) has also been attempted, as have efforts to depress specific IgE antibody synthesis, with or without effects on suppressor T cells, by linking allergens to certain agents such as polyethylene glycol, with subsequent production of tolerance. Still other efforts are directed toward such novel ideas as inhibition of IgE receptors on mast cells, basophils, and other IgE receptor–bearing cells.

Therapy of Rhinitis Complications. In treatment of serous otitis media, appropriate medications to keep the nasal airway patent should be used, especially during airplane flights. When fluid and hearing loss persist despite medical treatment, a myringotomy with insertion of a tympanostomy tube usually restores hearing while treatment is continued.

Therapy of chronic sinusitis is based on duration and severity of disease. Since pneumococci, *Haemophilis influenzae*, and β-hemolytic streptococci are frequently offending agents, a broad-spectrum antibiotic such as amoxicillin trihydrate is recommended along with measures to keep the nasal airway patent. Failure to respond to several months of intense therapy may require surgical intervention.

Gershwin ME (ed.): Clinical Reviews in Allergy, Vol. 2, No. 3. New York, Elsevier Scientific Publishing Company, 1984. *A 250-page review of nasal physiology, acute and chronic rhinitis, clinical evaluation, rhinitis therapy, and diagnostic tests.*

Kaplan AP (ed.): Allergy. New York, Churchill Livingstone, 1985. *A comprehensive practical text stressing diagnosis and therapy of common allergic diseases. Diseases based on immediate hypersensitivity are stressed. Chapter on allergic and nonallergic rhinitis by K. P. Mathews is practical and well illustrated.*

Lichtenstein L, Fauci A: Current Therapy in Allergy, Immunology and Rheumatology. Toronto, B. C. Decker, Inc., 1985. *A concise text devoted entirely to the therapy and diagnosis of a wide range of immunologically mediated diseases. Three excellent sections are devoted to allergic rhinitis.*

Lockey RJ, Bukantz SC (eds.): Primer on allergic and immunologic diseases. JAMA 258(20):2581, 1987. *Contains an article by M. Kaliner, P. Eggleston, and K. Mathews on the essentials of respiratory atopic diseases in a setting of other articles that stress the clinical implications of immunology for the medical student and resident.*

Middleton E Jr, Reed CE, Ellis EF: Allergy: Principles and Practice, 3rd ed. St. Louis, C. V. Mosby Company, 1988. *A multiauthored, two-volume reference work, stressing immunologic, pharmacologic, and clinical aspects of the common allergic diseases. A series of pamphlets are sent at intervals to update readers on various chapters as new findings become available.*

Mygind M (ed.): Nasal Allergy. Oxford, Blackwell Scientific Publications, 1978. *A complete text devoted entirely to the structure, function, immunology, diagnosis, and therapy of rhinitis.*

Samter M (ed.): Immunological Diseases. Boston, Little Brown & Co, 1988. *A comprehensive text with in-depth sections on basic immunology, the nonatopic immunologic disorders, the atopic diseases, allergic reaction patterns of the skin, and diseases with prominent immunologic features. The chapter by P. Norman and L. Lichtenstein on allergic rhinitis is particularly thorough in discussing allergenic extract immunotherapy.*

247 Anaphylaxis

Allen P. Kaplan

The term *anaphylaxis* arose from the experiments of Richet and Portier in the early 1900's which showed that dogs who survived a large dose of sea anemone toxin would die within a few minutes after administration of a minute dose a few weeks later. The term meant the opposite of prophylaxis, i.e., a lack of protection rather than the expected immunity. Nevertheless, the reaction is indeed immune in nature and depends upon formation of IgE antibody, the immunoglobulin responsible for typical allergic reactions. The initial sensitization step induces formation of IgE specifically directed to the initiating substance. The IgE binds to high-affinity receptors on basophils and mast cells, and the subsequent combination of antigen with that IgE causes degranulation of basophils and mast cells (see Fig. 246–1). The secretory products of these cells are responsible for the symptoms of allergic reactions (Fig. 247–1). In anaphylaxis, the reaction is systemic in nature, occurs rapidly upon administration of minute concentrations of the offending material, and is potentially fatal. The route of administration of allergen can dictate the manifestations and magnitude of the ensuing allergic reaction; although all routes can lead to anaphylaxis, parenteral administration is more likely than inhaled or ingested allergens to cause elevated circulating levels of unaltered allergen and a systemic reaction. Thus, parenteral administration of medication and insect sting reactions (injected into cutaneous vessels) are among the most common causes of anaphylaxis. Anaphylactoid reactions are de-

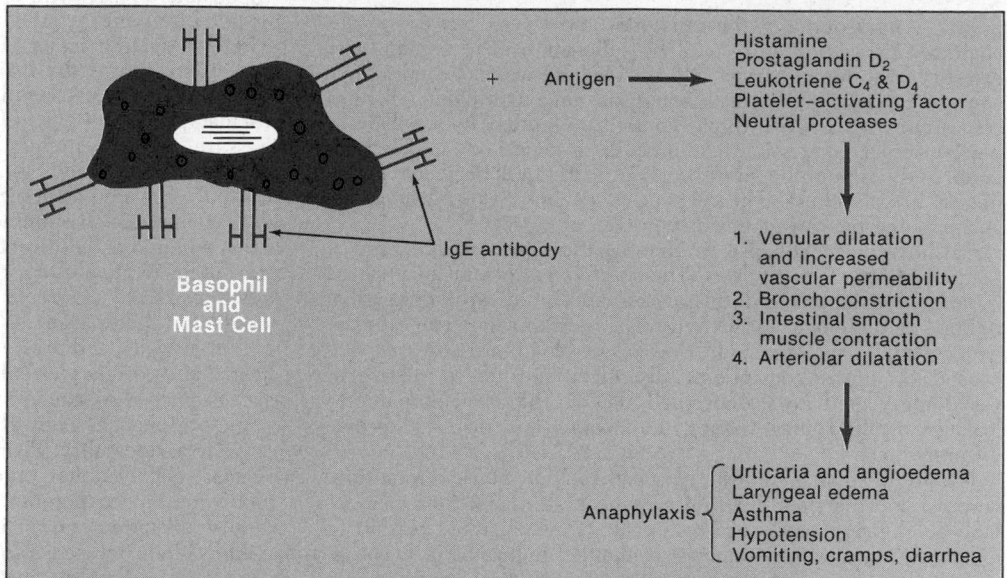

FIGURE 247–1. Acute anaphylaxis.

fined as systemic reactions that have the same symptoms as anaphylaxis but are not due to an IgE-dependent mechanism and are usually not immune. Examples include reactions to radiographic contrast agents and nonsteroidal anti-inflammatory drugs (e.g., acetylsalicylic acid, indomethacin, ibuprofen).

EPIDEMIOLOGY AND ETIOLOGY. The occurrence of anaphylaxis in the early 1900's was largely due to the use of serum from animals immunized with various toxins or bacteria to treat human illness. Between 1895 and 1923, of 41 reported cases of lethal anaphylaxis, 38 were due to serum therapy. Most were due to diphtheria antitoxin injection, and others were due to administration of tetanus antitoxin or antisera to gram-positive bacteria. In the antibiotic era, antibiotics in general and penicillin and sulfa drugs in particular have become the leading causes of fatal anaphylaxis. In recent years, there have been between 100 and 500 deaths per year in the United States due to the administration of penicillin. As new medications and chemicals are produced in a modern society, an ever-expanding number of substances are found capable of causing anaphylaxis. The insect order Hymenoptera is responsible for about 40 deaths each year and is estimated to cause one significant reaction per 10,000 individuals per year, with a mortality of 0.2 per million in the United States. Estimates of penicillin-induced anaphylaxis are 10 to 40 per 100,000 injections.

Although a history of atopy (allergic rhinitis, extrinsic asthma, atopic dermatitis) might be expected to be associated with an increased likelihood of anaphylactic reactions or reactions to antibiotics or insect stings in general, it appears that atopic individuals have, at worst, only a slightly greater risk than nonatopics. Thus, anyone can manifest an IgE response, with clinical symptoms, to the agents responsible for anaphylaxis. There is also no evidence that race, sex, age, occupation, or season intrinsically predisposes an individual to anaphylaxis.

Proteins, polysaccharides, and haptens are capable of eliciting systemic reactions in man (Table 247–1). Proteins are the largest and most diverse group and include antiserum, hormones, seminal plasma, enzymes, Hymenoptera venom (e.g., phospholipase A₂), pollen allergens administered for immunotherapy ("allergy shots"), and foods such as shellfish, eggs, nuts, and wheat products. Polysaccharides such as dextrans are rarer causes. The most common etiologic agents are drugs, low molecular weight substances that are not antigenic themselves but act as haptens and become antigenic upon reaction with host proteins. These include antibiotics, local anesthetics, vitamins, and diagnostic reagents. Although the most common anaphylactic reactions are due to parenteral administration, food-induced anaphylaxis and anaphylactic reactions to an orally administered drug can occur in very sensitive individuals.

CLINICAL MANIFESTATIONS. IgE-mediated reactions can cause symptoms that include the cutaneous, respiratory, cardio-vascular, gastrointestinal, and hematologic systems (Fig. 247–1). In anaphylaxis, there may be manifestations involving multiple organ systems. The onset and manifestations vary depending on route of administration, dose, the release of and sensitivity to vasoactive substances, and differing sensitivities of the responsive organs. These parameters can vary from person to person, and individuals tend to react in a characteristic pattern. The initial manifestations can begin in seconds or take as long as an hour to develop; in severe reactions the onset is usually within 5 to 10 minutes. Initial manifestations often include skin erythema, pruritus, a generalized feeling of warmth and/or impending doom, light-headedness, shortness of breath, nausea, vomiting, or a lump in the throat. Urticaria is the most common manifestation of anaphylaxis. The rash is generalized and intensely pruritic, and consists of well-circumscribed, erythematous, raised wheals with serpiginous borders and blanched centers. Angiocdema may accompany urticaria and typically manifests as swelling of face, eyes, lips, tongue, pharynx, or extremities. The respiratory tract is commonly involved in fatal anaphylaxis. For example, in a study of deaths due to Hymenoptera stings, 70 per cent of victims had involvement of upper or lower airways. The early stages of upper airway edema consist of hoarseness, stridor, and/or dys-

TABLE 247–1. AGENTS CAUSING ANAPHYLAXIS

Type	Common	Rare
Proteins	Venoms (Hymenoptera)	Hormones (insulin, ACTH, vasopressin, parathormone)
	Pollens (ragweed, grass, etc.)	Enzymes (trypsin, penicillinase)
	Foods (eggs, seafood, nuts, grains, beans, cottonseed oil, chocolate)	Human proteins (serum proteins, seminal fluid)
	Horse and rabbit serum (antilymphocyte globulin)	
Haptens and other low molecular weight substances	Antibiotics (pencillins, sulfonamides, cephalosporins, tetracyclines, amphotericin B, nitrofurantoin, aminoglycosides)	Vitamins (thiamine, folic acid)
	Local anesthetics (lidocaine, procaine, etc.)	
Polysaccharides		Dextrans, iron-dextran

phoria. Angioedema of the epiglottis and larynx can cause mechanical obstruction and death by suffocation. The swelling can extend to the hypopharynx and trachea. Between 25 and 50 per cent of patients dying of anaphylaxis have pathologic changes consistent with severe asthma. There is pulmonary hyperinflation, peribronchial congestion, submucosal edema, edema-filled alveoli, and eosinophilic infiltration. The patient experiences shortness of breath, chest tightness, and wheezing. Severe hypoxemia and hypercarbia can manifest rapidly.

Cardiovascular collapse is among the most severe clinical manifestations of anaphylaxis. The exact extent of fatal anaphylaxis is unknown, as anaphylaxis can be associated with myocardial ischemia and ventricular arrhythmias, each of which can cause or be caused by hypotension. Decreased blood pressure may be caused by diffuse peripheral vasodilatation due to release of vasodilatory mediators, decreased effective blood volume due to leakage of fluid into tissues, hypoxemia, or primary cardiac dysfunction.

Gastrointestinal manifestations can include nausea, vomiting, cramps, and diarrhea. Central nervous system abnormalities can include delirium and seizures, each of which may be due to hypoxemia and/or hypotension. Prolonged hypoxia and hypotension can, of course, lead to a variety of secondary, more permanent changes.

DIFFERENTIAL DIAGNOSIS. The diagnosis of systemic anaphylaxis may be obvious when there is a typical history of antecedent exposure to foreign antigenic material and a sequence of events consistent with the syndrome. Confirmation usually requires demonstration of IgE antibody to the substance by skin testing or by RAST (radioallergosorbent test). When the history is absent or when only a portion of the full syndrome is present, it may be difficult to exclude a vascular, cardiac, or neurologic disorder. Possibilities to be considered include acute myocardial infarction, pulmonary embolism, acute asthma, hereditary angioedema, cold urticaria, a seizure disorder, an anaphylactoid or idiosyncratic reaction, transfusion reaction, or a vasovagal reaction. Vasovagal reactions may occur after an injection (e.g., penicillin, xylocaine) and include symptoms such as pallor, sweating, bradycardia, nausea, and hypotension, which can be confused with anaphylaxis. There is absence of any cutaneous manifestations or evidence of respiratory difficulty, and the diagnosis hinges on the cause of the hypotension. In such instances, skin testing is negative. When positive, an elevated plasma histamine (from basophils or mast cells) or tryptase level (mast cell product) suggests anaphylaxis or anaphylactoid reactions that are mast cell–dependent. Hereditary angioedema is due to absence or dysfunction of C1 inhibitor and is associated with laryngeal edema, peripheral angioedema, and acute abdominal pain. It is typically an autosomal dominant disorder with a family history or prior history of typical episodes. Trauma and infections may precipitate attacks of swelling. Patients with cold urticaria may have systemic symptoms due to water immersion such as while swimming; diffuse urticaria, angioedema, and hypotension may ensue. Anaphylactoid reactions can occur by substances causing direct nonimmune release of mast cell products (opiates, tubocurare, dextrans, sulfobromophthalein), which can cause urticaria, angioedema, chest tightness, wheezing, and hypotension. Aspirin and other nonsteroidal agents can cause upper and lower airway obstruction, urticaria, and/or angioedema with no IgE involvement. These agents have in common the property of inhibition of prostaglandin synthetase (cyclo-oxygenase). IgG–anti-IgA immune complexes may cause anaphylaxis-like symptoms when IgA-deficient patients receive blood. Complement activation appears to have a major role in such instances. Finally, radiocontrast media reactions occur in about 1 per cent of studies that employ them. The mechanism is unknown but may relate to their osmolarity. Newer agents seem to markedly diminish the incidence.

PATHOGENESIS. Antigenic induction of IgE formation requires antigenic processing (see Ch. 242) by dendrite cells or macrophages, T-cell help, and switching of B lymphocytes from IgG synthesis to IgE synthesis. Interleukin 4 may be critical for the latter switch and functions as a T-cell helper factor for IgE formation. Subsequent combination of antigen with IgE bound to high-affinity receptors on mast cells and basophils causes

secretion of a variety of vasoactive substances that may be responsible for the symptoms of anaphylaxis (Fig. 247–1). These include histamine, prostaglandin D_2, leukotrienes C_4 and D_4, and platelet-activating factor (PAF) (1-0-alkyl-2-sn-3 phosphorylcholine). Histamine is the major secretory product of basophils and mast cells. It causes venular and arterial vasodilation, increases vascular permeability, and causes a decrease in diastolic blood pressure when systemic levels of approximately 2.5 ng per milliliter are reached. In studies of insect sting anaphylaxis, markedly elevated arterial levels were documented which lasted up to 90 minutes. Histamine has direct inotropic and chronotropic action when injected directly into cardiac muscle, effects that are prevented by H_1 plus H_2 receptor antagonists. Prostaglandin D_2 is synthesized by mast cells but not by basophils. It is a peripheral vasodilator. Leukotrienes C_4 and D_4 are produced by basophils and mast cells and cause profound constriction of peripheral arterial and coronary circulation and may have a role in bronchospasm, since they cause bronchoconstriction and decreased dynamic compliance. They also cause venular dilation and increase vascular permeability. PAF, like prostaglandin D_2, is synthesized by mast cells but not basophils. On a molar basis, it is about 1000 times more potent than histamine in its ability to cause venular dilatation and an increase in cutaneous vascular permeability. When infused into rabbits, it causes profound hypotension, increased pulmonary resistance, pulmonary hypertension, cardiac arrhythmias, and decreased lung compliance, all manifestations of anaphylaxis. It is also a potent chemotactic factor for eosinophils and may account for much of the eosinophilia seen when allergic reactions persist (see Ch. 246).

Bradykinin is a nine–amino acid peptide that may also contribute to the symptoms of anaphylaxis and is generated by cleavage of kininogen by enzymes known as kallikreins. Kinins are peripheral vasodilators, cause systemic hypotension, and constrict coronary vessels. Basophils and mast cells have a kallikrein-like enzyme; organs containing glands (lung, nasal mucosa) secrete a tissue kallikrein that digests low molecular weight kininogen to release bradykinin. Plasma kinin formation is associated with contact activation of Hageman factor, conversion of plasma prekallikrein to kallikrein, and digestion of high molecular weight (HMW) kininogen.

Anaphylaxis is associated with depletion of clotting factors V, VII, and fibrinogen, activation of complement, and depletion of HMW kininogen consistent with acute intravascular coagulation. Clotting defects such as a prolonged partial thromboplastin time are commonly seen. Activation or depletion of these proteins is likely caused by enzymes released from cells that include not only mast cells and basophils but also monocyte/macrophages, eosinophils, and platelets. The latter group of cells possess low-affinity receptors for IgE (CD23) which may mediate cell secretion upon contact with antigen. The participation of these cells in allergic reactions is an area of current investigation.

PREVENTION AND TREATMENT. Patients who have previously experienced anaphylactic episodes should wear a Medic-Alert bracelet and be instructed regarding the importance of relating details of their specific drug reactions before taking medications. The medical history and medical record must include not only the allergic history but a description of the associated symptoms. The physician must be aware of drugs containing cross-reacting antigens. For example, patients with allergy to sulfa-containing antibiotics should avoid other sulfa-containing substances such as chlorthiazide diuretics, furosemide, sulfonylureas, and dapsone.

There is a 15 per cent incidence of a reaction if a cephalosporin is substituted for penicillin because they share the presence of a β-lactam ring. Reactions with second- and third-generation cephalosporins may also occur, but aztreonam is an exception.

When the patient has a history of drug allergy or of taking a drug suspected of causing a reaction, it is appropriate to substitute another non–crossing-reacting therapeutic agent whenever possible. Penicillin causes more anaphylactic reactions than any other drug, yet the history of "allergy" is unreliable, since close to 80 per cent of patients with such a history have negative skin tests to the major determinant (penicillin polylysine) or a minor determinant mixture (penicillin, penicilloic acid, penicillioylamine) and can tolerate the drug with impunity. Anaphylaxis is highly associated with IgE antibody directed to these minor determinants. Thus, a negative skin test to the commercially available major determinant is insufficient testing to administer the drug given a positive history. The addition of testing for minor determinants with negative results renders anaphylaxis or even any allergic reaction rare indeed. The number of alternative antibiotics that can be used in place of penicillin is ever increasing, and avoidance, in the sensitive patient, is the best approach. Nevertheless, there are circumstances in which administration of penicillin or other agents to a known or suspected sensitive patient is necessary. In this circumstance, the patient can be desensitized by gradual administration of increasing concentration of the drug—first intradermally, then subcutaneously, and finally parenterally. Such a procedure should be carried out by experienced personnel in an intensive care unit setting in which anaphylactic reactions can be effectively treated.

When an anaphylactic reaction is encountered, epinephrine given early quickly reverses most manifestations. Administered at a 1:1000 dilution (0.01 ml per kilogram with a maximum dose of 0.5 ml subcutaneously repeated every 20 minutes as necessary), it is initial treatment once an adequate airway is in place. Further exposure to the inducing substance should be limited. When an anaphylactic reaction is initiated by an injection into the arm or leg, a tourniquet may be applied to limit antigen absorption. In the case of a honeybee sting, care should be taken to remove the stinger without compressing the venom sac. Upper airway obstruction must be differentiated from asthma, since laryngeal and epiglottic edema may require endotracheal intubation or emergency tracheostomy to provide an airway. Asthma can be treated with epinephrine, administration of an inhaled β_2 sympathomimetic, and/or intravenous aminophylline at a 6 mg per kilogram loading dose over 20 to 30 minutes, followed by 0.5 to 1 mg per kilogram per hour.

If any respiratory, vascular, or cardiac complications occur, an intravenous line should be placed promptly and a sample of arterial blood obtained for pH, Po_2, and Pco_2 determinations. Supplemental oxygen should be given to reduce hypoxemia. Pulse, blood pressure, and respiratory rate are monitored, and an electrocardiogram is obtained. Hypovolemic shock requires rapid intravenous fluid administration. Additionally, 5 ml of a 1:10,000 solution of epinephrine repeated every 5 to 10 minutes can be given intravenously in severe shock. A vasopressor such as dopamine (2 to 20 μg per kilogram per minute) is indicated to manage hypotension unresponsive to volume expansion. This may increase cardiac output and improve blood flow to coronary, cerebral, renal, and mesenteric vascular beds. Higher doses of dopamine or norepinephrine yield significant α receptor stimulation, which may increase blood pressure but constrict distal vascular beds. In case of significant cardiac dysfunction, an arterial line and a Swan-Ganz catheter should be placed.

Administration of antihistamines at the onset of the acute episode may relieve pruritus, urticaria, and angioedema. Once an intravenous line is placed, 50 to 100 mg of diphenhydramine can be given slowly as a bolus. An H_2-receptor blocker may aid in the therapy of hypotension. Corticosteroids have no value during the acute episode, yet steroids are often also administered intravenously. It takes many hours before their first effect is seen. Thus, administration of steroids helps treat protracted asthma and late reactions that can ensue many hours after the initial episode appears controlled or even 1 to 2 days beyond the initial insult. Thus, observation for at least 24 hours after an anaphylactic event is important.

Dattwyler R, Kaplan AP, Austen KF: Human anaphylaxis. *In* Kaplan AP (ed.): Allergy. New York, Churchill Livingstone, 1985, pp 559–607. *A textbook review of etiology, pathogenesis, and therapy.*

Peters SP: Systemic anaphylaxis. *In* Lichtenstein LM, Fauci AS (eds.): Current Therapy in Allergy, Immunology, and Rheumatology, 1985–1986. Toronto, B. C. Decker, Inc., 1985, pp 75–80. *A detailed description of how to treat anaphylaxis.*

Smith PL, Sobotka AK, Blocker ER, et al.: Physiologic manifestations of human anaphylaxis. J Clin Invest 66:1072, 1980. *Physiologic and biochemical changes monitored in human anaphylaxis occurring during a trial of therapy for insect sting allergy. Includes comments and cautions regarding therapy.*

248 Insect Sting Allergy

Lawrence M. Lichtenstein

The stings of insects of the order Hymenoptera have long been recognized as a potential cause of severe, often life-threatening reactions in susceptible individuals. These reactions are unrelated to the toxic chemicals in the venoms, being due to allergic sensitization. Insect sting allergy has recently become the most intensely studied model of anaphylaxis in man, resulting in important advances that have had rapid clinical application.

EPIDEMIOLOGY. The incidence of immediate hypersensitivity to insect stings based on history is 3 per cent; more than 20 per cent of the population, however, has positive skin test reactions to insect venoms without having had a reaction. Other allergies do not seem to predispose to insect sting sensitivity. The frequency varies with exposure and is therefore greater in children and males as well as those inclined to outdoor activities or beekeeping. Systemic reactions to insect stings cause few fatalities, but the morbidity, fear, and change in life style caused by these reactions is significant. A larger number of people suffer prolonged and unusually severe local inflammatory reactions to insect stings, which are allergic in nature. As with other allergies, there appears to be an inherited predisposition, since multiple family members are often affected.

ETIOLOGY. The only insects possessing true stingers are those of the order Hymenoptera. There are two families of importance, the bees (honeybees, bumblebees) and the vespids (yellow jackets, hornets, wasps). The bees have barbed stingers that remain in the skin after a sting. Yellow jackets are the most common culprits, but honeybees are more commonly implicated in the western United States. Wasps are more common in the south central United States (especially Texas). Sensitivity develops to antigens in the insect venom, most of which have enzymatic activity. A major allergen in both insect families is phospholipase A, but they do not cross-react with one another.

PATHOGENESIS. The injection of foreign proteins commonly causes the production of specific antibodies of the IgE and IgG classes. Individuals may develop venom-specific IgE antibodies after any sting, this response sometimes persisting for less than 3 months and in other instances persisting for more than 25 years. Tissue mast cells and circulating basophils bind IgE antibody, thereby becoming sensitized so that a repeat encounter with the offending allergen triggers release of the mediators of anaphylaxis (see Ch. 57). The initiation and persistence of this sensitization are related to inheritable and other unknown determinants. Sensitization may occur at any time in life, even after many uneventful stings. The sensitizing sting itself causes no unusual reaction and is often so remote as to evade recollection.

Generalized mediator release from sensitized basophils and mast cells causes the many manifestations of anaphylaxis (see Table 252–2). Localization of symptoms to specific target tissues is not well understood. The pathology observed in fatal cases includes upper airway edema and obstruction, the visceral consequences of hypotension, or occasionally no discernible abnormality (see Ch. 247 for a discussion of anaphylaxis).

Large local reactions are IgE dependent; their prolonged time-course is characteristic of the so-called late phase response to antigen which has recently been under intense investigation. These reactions involve a cascade of events beginning with mediator release from mast cells and culminating with local inflammation involving many cell types and numerous mechanisms. The potential roles of eosinophils, neutrophils, basophils, lymphocytes and lymphokines, complement, and mediators with prolonged release or activity are being elucidated.

The venom-specific IgG antibody response to a sting is usually short lived, lasting only a few months. Repeated stings (as in beekeepers) are associated with high titers of IgG antibodies, which protect against allergic reactions. Beekeepers who do not have anaphylactic reactions have high IgG titers, as do affected individuals immunized with venoms. Passive transfer of these IgG antibodies protects sensitive patients from a sting. These protective antibodies are thought to block the allergic reaction by competing with IgE for the allergenic venom proteins and have therefore been termed "blocking" antibodies.

CLINICAL MANIFESTATIONS. Allergic reactions to insect stings are either generalized (systemic) or large local reactions. *Systemic sting reactions* present the classic manifestations of anaphylaxis described in Ch. 247. The observed frequency of the most common symptoms in adult patients is presented in Table 248–1. The risk of a fatal outcome increases, as might be expected, with age and certain drugs, especially antagonists of β-adrenergic receptors. Fatal anaphylaxis may occur without a history of sting allergy.

The onset of systemic symptoms is rapid, within 2 to 3 minutes, and rarely occurs more than 30 minutes after a sting. Symptoms presenting hours later (except large local reactions) are not usually associated with immediate hypersensitivity or IgE antibodies. Unusual reactions such as vasculitis, nephropathies, encephalitis, and other neurologic manifestations have been reported, but no causal relationship has been established. Allergic respiratory symptoms may occur in beekeepers and their families owing to sensitization to the dust in the hives that contain bee body proteins. This sensitivity is unrelated to sting reactions.

Large local reactions are slow in onset and occur with or without concomitant early systemic reaction. The area of induration increases in size progressively for the first 24 to 48 hours and then resolves gradually over several days. These reactions may be so large as to immobilize an entire limb and are a significant cause of morbidity in sensitive individuals. Red streaks resembling lymphangitis may be observed and are often treated with antibiotics despite a lack of evidence for true cellulitis. Some individuals develop large local sting reactions in the absence of allergic sensitivity. These are exaggerated reactions to the toxic and inflammatory venom components and often occur in persons who report similar large swellings after mosquito or fly bites, or who have cutaneous sensitivity to many irritants.

NATURAL HISTORY. The natural history of insect sting allergy has been incompletely documented. The prevalence of venom sensitization in the general population was noted above. It is estimated that about 20 per cent of those at risk by virtue of positive skin tests (but with no history of a systemic reaction) will react on sting. There is considerable variability in the reaction to a sting among those who are clearly allergic as demonstrated by positive skin tests and a history of a previous reaction. In a small study 60 per cent of such adults had a systemic reaction when stung by the appropriate insect. In children, on the other hand, a repeat sting causes a reaction in only 8 per cent. The incidence in adolescents and young adults must lie between these extremes. This variability confounds the prediction of risk associated with sensitization.

Many patients and physicians believe that allergic sting reactions become progressively more severe with every sting. Although some patients progress from large local through mild systemic reactions to life-threatening anaphylaxis, most of those affected maintain a similar pattern of symptoms with every sting. Less than 10 per cent of those experiencing large local reactions subsequently have systemic reactions. Factors favoring a systemic reaction include multiple stings, or stings in close temporal proximity (only weeks apart).

Sensitization generally decreases or disappears in time. This is far more common in children than in adults. However, resensitization has been observed upon re-sting.

DIAGNOSIS. The acute presentation of anaphylaxis is easily diagnosed by the presence of classic symptoms and signs. The insect sting may be inapparent. Differential diagnosis is more difficult in localized reactions such as acute chest pain and dyspnea or syncope without urticaria.

The diagnosis of insect sting allergy currently rests on a convincing history and positive skin tests. Demonstration in vitro of venom-specific IgE by the radioallergosorbent test (RAST) is less sensitive than skin tests but is equally accurate when positive.

Skin tests are performed intradermally with venoms diluted to concentrations in the range of 1 to 1000 ng per milliliter. Five venoms are used: honeybee (HB), yellow jacket (YJ), yellow hornet (YH), white-faced hornet (WH), and *Polistes* wasp (POL). Positive intradermal skin tests develop, within 20 minutes, a wheal greater than 5 mm in diameter with at least 20 mm of erythema. The degree of skin test sensitivity does not correlate with clinical sensitivity. Within a few months after a systemic sting reaction, skin tests are almost uniformly positive. Stings more remote in time are more commonly associated with an apparent loss of sensitivity (similar to the situation in penicillin-related anaphylaxis).

Honeybee venom sensitivity occurs independent of other venom allergies, but about 10 per cent of patients are sensitive to both bee and vespid venoms. The vespid venoms are highly cross-reactive, so that almost all vespid-sensitive patients have positive YJ, YH, and WH skin tests even though most have been stung only by YJs. Half of these patients are also sensitive to POL venom. Very few individuals are allergic to only one or two of the vespid venoms. In vitro RAST inhibition techniques are useful to distinguish cross-reactivity from specific sensitivity. This is clinically relevant in patients with a positive skin test to *Polistes*. This is usually due to cross-reactivity, and the patient may be spared considerable expense and unnecessary immunization by RAST inhibition analysis.

TREATMENT. The treatment of choice for anaphylactic reactions is subcutaneous epinephrine 1:1000, 0.5 ml initially and repeated twice at 10-minute intervals, if necessary, to reverse the progression of symptoms. Sublingual isoproterenol is probably ineffective. Antihistamines and glucocorticoids do not contribute to the management of life-threatening symptoms but may reduce the duration and severity of cutaneous manifestations. Their use should not be considered until the termination of the acute episode. Intravenous volume expansion or airway maintenance may be necessary. In a few individuals, the process is resistant to epinephrine; in such instances an α-adrenergic agent (i.e., norepinephrine) may be tried. Affected persons not yet protected by immunotherapy are advised to carry, and are instructed in the use of, a kit containing a syringe device preloaded with one or two recommended doses of epinephrine.

Venom immunotherapy is successful in virtually all patients. Less than 2 per cent of those immunized have any systemic symptoms after a challenge sting, and these are uniformly less severe than their previous reactions. The indications for venom immunotherapy are now based on an improved understanding of the natural history of the disease. Those with a history of life-threatening reactions should be treated. The risk of progression from strictly cutaneous to life-threatening respiratory or vascular reactions is uncertain in adults but is rare (<1 per cent) in children. Cutaneous reactors who are more likely to be stung in their daily activities or who for a variety of reasons (location, age, cardiovascular disease) can ill afford a more severe reaction should be treated. The cost and inconvenience of treatment may deter other cutaneous reactors from undergoing immunotherapy. Children, much more commonly than adults, have cutaneous symptoms only. These children may be left untreated. Venom immunotherapy is contraindicated in the absence of positive venom skin tests or RAST. Treatment is currently recommended using all venoms causing a positive skin test (for *Polistes*, see above). While other mechanisms may contribute, the induction of increased serum levels of venom-specific IgG antibodies is the most apparent mechanism of protection for venom immunotherapy; less than 3 μg per milliliter is associated with increased risk of sting anaphylaxis.

Rapid immunization in six to eight weekly visits is recommended, since it is associated with a significantly greater and more rapid immune response and with fewer adverse reactions than a slower (more than 20 weeks) regimen. The maintenance dose of 100 μg of each venom is repeated monthly for at least 6 months, and is then continued at 6- to 8-week intervals for 5 years. If treatment is interrupted for more than 3 months, it is

TABLE 248–1. SYMPTOMS REPORTED BY 245 PATIENTS

Symptom	Per Cent
Cutaneous only	14
Urticaria-angioedema	78
Dizziness-hypotension	61
Dyspnea-wheezing	53
Throat tightness-hoarseness	40
Loss of consciousness	33

likely that protection will diminish to inadequate levels. Loss of venom sensitivity during maintenance immunotherapy occurs in only 10 to 20 per cent of patients during 3 to 5 years of treatment. Skin tests should, therefore, be repeated every 2 years. After 5 years it appears that patients can stop therapy and suffer a sting without serious sequelae. Possible exceptions include patients in whom skin test sensitivity has not diminished in 5 years, those who have had systemic reactions during venom immunotherapy, and those with complicating medical conditions. After stopping venom immunotherapy, venom sensitivity continues to decline and is not increased even after stings.

Adverse reactions to venom immunotherapy may be early or late. Immediate reactions include all the manifestations of anaphylaxis. During the initial course of treatment, 10 to 15 per cent of patients report systemic complaints, only half of which require epinephrine. At maintenance doses, systemic reactions occur rarely. After a systemic reaction, the dose should be reduced by up to 50 per cent on the subsequent visit and then increased gradually toward 100 μg again.

Large local reactions occur frequently. Fifty per cent of treated patients experience at least one such reaction. These occur after 10 of every 100 injections in the induction phase, most commonly in the midrange of doses (10 to 50 μg) and much less often at maintenance doses. Large local reactions do not presage systemic reactions and require a reduction of dose only for the most severe reactions. Long-term side effects have not been observed with venom immunotherapy or in beekeepers stung frequently for over 30 years.

Golden DBK, Addison BI, Gadde J, et al.: Prospective observations on patients who discontinue Hymenoptera venom immunotherapy. J Allerg Clin Immunol 88:162, 1989. *Studies of when and how to discontinue venom immunotherapy.*

Golden DBK, Marsh DG, Kagey-Sobotka A, et al.: Epidemiology of insect sting allergy. JAMA 262:240, 1989. *A review of diagnostic and therapeutic problems in insect allergy.*

Hunt KJ, Valentine MD, Sobotka AK, et al.: A controlled trial of immunotherapy in insect hypersensitivity. N Engl J Med 299:157, 1978. *A comparison of venom immunotherapy with whole body extract and placebo. Demonstrates efficacy of venom therapy and the clinical consequences of challenge stings.*

Valentine MD, Golden DBK: Insect venom allergy. In Samter M (ed.): Immunological Diseases. 4th ed. Boston, Little, Brown & Company, 1988, pp 1173–1184. *A general review.*

Valentine MD, Schuberth KC, Kagey-Sobotka A, et al.: The value of immunotherapy with venom in children with allergy to insect stings. N Engl J Med 323:1601, 1990. *A prospective study of the epidemiology and immunotherapy of insect sting allergy in children, indicating that repeat reactions are rare and virtually never of increased severity.*

249 Immune Complex Diseases

Robert R. Rich

DEFINITION. The formation of immune complexes is an invariable consequence of the interaction of antigens with specific antibodies. The inflammatory response that ensues is an important element of normal host defenses, leading to complex clearance and antigen destruction by phagocytic cells. In contrast, immune complex diseases are reflections of excess complex formation or retarded clearance, usually under conditions of exceptional antigen challenge or immunologic dysregulation. Under such circumstances, complexes are deposited or formed at specific tissue sites; the inflammatory response then leads to localized or systemic tissue damage. Clinical manifestations of immune complex disease are protean, with the development of signs and symptoms appropriate to the particular organs involved. This may include virtually any organ, but for reasons described below, sites of predilection include the kidney, lung, skin, joints, and central nervous system. Although immune complex disease may accompany an extraordinary range of pathologic processes, in practice it is encountered most commonly in the course of infectious diseases, in autoimmunity, and as a consequence of therapy for some other primary process.

PATHOGENESIS. Understanding the pathogenesis of immune complex disease requires attention to each of its constituents, i.e., antigen, antibody, the factors that regulate immune complex deposition and clearance, and the inflammatory processes that ensue following their deposition.

Antigens Inducing Immune Complex Diseases. Antigens involved in the development of immune complex diseases can be broadly classified as endogenous, infectious, environmental, and iatrogenic. In many cases the specific antigen is unknown, although the general class can usually be identified. The most familiar example of endogenous immune complexes is the DNA–anti-DNA complexes important to the pathogenesis of systemic lupus erythematosus (SLE). Many other autoimmune diseases are also associated with immune complex formation, but the pathogenetic relevance of the complexes is not always clear. Among autoimmune diseases in which immune complexes are considered important mediators of the inflammatory process are rheumatoid arthritis, cryoglobulinemia, mixed connective tissue disease, polyarteritis nodosa, and other autoimmune vasculitides. Other important sources of endogenous antigens include malignancies in which immune complex formation may contribute to the development of paraneoplastic syndromes.

Infections with organisms of many types, particularly chronic infections, are associated with the development of immune complex disease. Examples among bacterial infections include glomerulonephritis following infection with nephritogenic strains of streptococci, disseminated gonococcal infection, lepromatous leprosy, subacute bacterial endocarditis, allergic bronchopulmonary aspergillosis, secondary syphilis, and chronic *Pseudomonas* infection in patients with cystic fibrosis. Viral diseases in which immune complex deposition may be a prominent feature include hepatitis B infection, dengue, infectious mononucleosis, and subacute sclerosing panencephalitis. Immune complex–mediated disease is also a prominent feature of many parasitic infestations. Particularly noteworthy is the nephrotic syndrome in children with quartan malaria; others include toxoplasmosis, trypanosomiasis, and schistosomiasis.

Extrinsic allergic alveolitis (hypersensitivity pneumonitis) is a frequently encountered immune complex disease associated with exposure to exogenous antigens in the environment. This is usually associated with extraordinary exposure to a particular antigen that is characteristic of certain occupations or hobbies, e.g., the antigens of thermophilic actinomycetes responsible for farmer's lung and bagassosis, and the exposure to avian proteins in patients with pigeon fancier's disease.

A special class of exogenous antigens comprises those encountered as a consequence of medical practice. This includes the prototype of the immune complex diseases, serum sickness, which follows deposition of immune complexes of heterologous serum constituents with autologous antibodies. Serum sickness was regularly seen during the pre-antibiotic decades of the twentieth century when infectious diseases were frequently treated with heterologous antisera. With antibiotic availability, classic serum sickness has been uncommonly encountered. However, as mouse monoclonal antibodies are introduced for treatment of immunologic reactions such as organ transplant rejection, the re-emergence of serum sickness may be anticipated. An iatrogenic disease essentially indistinguishable from classic serum sickness did emerge as a consequence of high-dose antibiotic therapy. The serum sickness–like manifestations of immune responses to drugs reflect the fact that certain drugs, particularly the β-lactam antibiotics and sulfonamides, are effective haptens that are capable of inducing antibody responses upon spontaneous conjugation to autologous proteins. Reactions to tissue allografts following bone marrow or solid organ transplantation are another instance of contemporary practice that may be associated with pathologic immune complex deposition. In the case of solid organ transplants, deposition of complexes within the vasculature of the transplanted organ may contribute importantly to graft rejection.

Factors Affecting Immune Complex Formation and Deposition. Features of both antigen and antibody determine the likelihood of pathologic immune complex formation and deposition. Chief among these are the absolute concentrations of the reactants and their relative molar ration. Most antigens are multivalent for a polyclonal antibody response; antibody molecules are at least bivalent. This theoretically allows for the formation of an extensive antigen-antibody lattice, the size of which is determined largely by the affinity of the antibodies and the molar ration of antigen

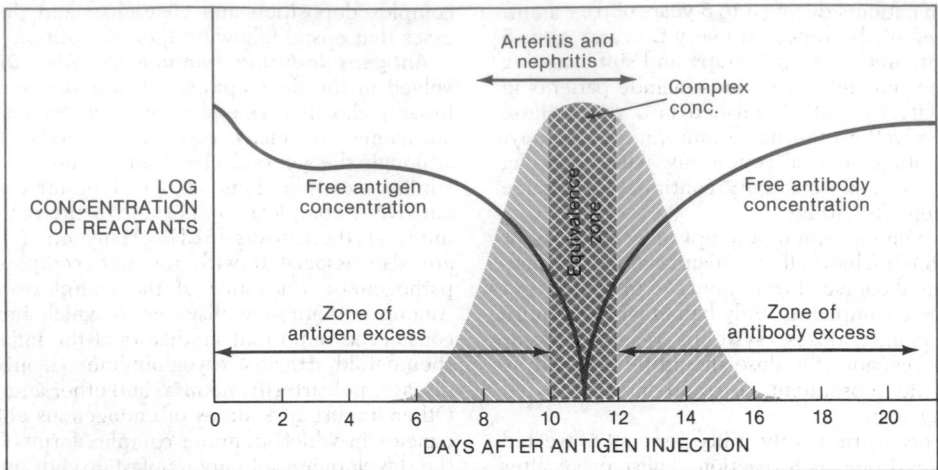

FIGURE 249–1. Development of experimental serum sickness following injection of rabbits with radiolabeled xenogeneic serum. Antibody formation begins after a lag of approximately 5 days. Signs of pathogenic immune complex deposition appear at approximately 8 days and gradually subside with the appearance in the serum of free antibody after the zone of equivalence is passed. Pathogenic complexes are of intermediate size, with a buoyant density of $\geq$ 19S.

to antibody. As illustrated for an experimental model of serum sickness in Figure 249–1, antibody responses begin under conditions in which antigen is present in excess relative to antibody. After a lag of several days, complexes formed initially are small and exhibit little or no pathogenic activity. In contrast, very large complexes are formed as the amount of antigen becomes limiting late in the course of an antibody response under conditions of antibody excess. Because these large complexes are readily cleared by the reticuloendothelial system, they are also relatively nonpathogenic. Immune complex diseases are usually manifest during conditions of slight antigen excess or near the point of equivalence, where lattice formation is maximal and little if any noncomplexed antigen or antibody is detected in the serum. An additional feature of lattice formation important to rapid precipitation of complexes is interaction between Fc portions of antibody molecules (Fig. 249–2) (see Ch. 242). For example, although the valence of F(ab')$_2$ antibodies does not differ from that of whole immunoglobulins, F(ab')$_2$ antibodies form precipitates more slowly. As noted below, such Fc-Fc interactions are important in complement-mediated regulation of immune complex deposition. Antigen charge also plays a role in determining sites of tissue localization; complexes with a substantial positive charge are preferentially attracted to the strong negative charge of basement membranes, particularly in the renal glomerulus.

Localized presence of antigen may largely account for organ-specific immune complex deposition. Diseases such as Goodpasture's syndrome and myasthenia gravis are generally not classified as immune complex diseases because the complexes are formed in situ rather than being preformed in the circulation and then deposited. Nevertheless, the inflammatory process at the site of antigen-specific antibody deposition is essentially the same as that seen following deposition of preformed complexes. Lupus nephritis is an interesting special case in which the disease develops as a consequence of glomerular deposition of DNA–anti-DNA complexes. It has been demonstrated in experimental animals, however, that single-stranded DNA binds avidly to the glomerular basement membrane, presumably attracted by its cationic nature. Thus, DNA–anti-DNA complexes may be formed at the glomerular basement membrane in addition to the localization of preformed complexes at that site.

Features of blood flow and vascular structure are also important in determining the localization of immune complexes. Chief among these is capillary permeability. Because the capillary endothelium is fenestrated in renal glomeruli, pulmonary alveoli, synovia, the choroid plexus of the brain, and the uveal tract of the eye, complexes preferentially deposit in these sites. Hemodynamic variables enhancing immune complex localization include turbulence of flow and increased blood pressure; both of these conditions promote complex deposition in glomeruli and at artery bifurcations.

Immune Complex–mediated Inflammation. Capillary permeability is markedly increased by the action of vasoactive amines such as histamine and platelet-activating factor, which are elaborated at the site of a nascent inflammatory lesion. Consequently, mast cells, basophils, and platelets are important in the initiation of immune complex–mediated inflammatory responses. Mast cell and basophil degranulation may reflect the effects of IgE antibodies specific for the inducing antigen bound to specific Fcε receptors on their surfaces, as well as the elaboration of the anaphylatoxin components of complement, C3a and C5a, as a consequence of complement activation (Ch. 243). Studies in experimental animals have shown that the deposition of circulating immune complexes is promoted by administration of agents

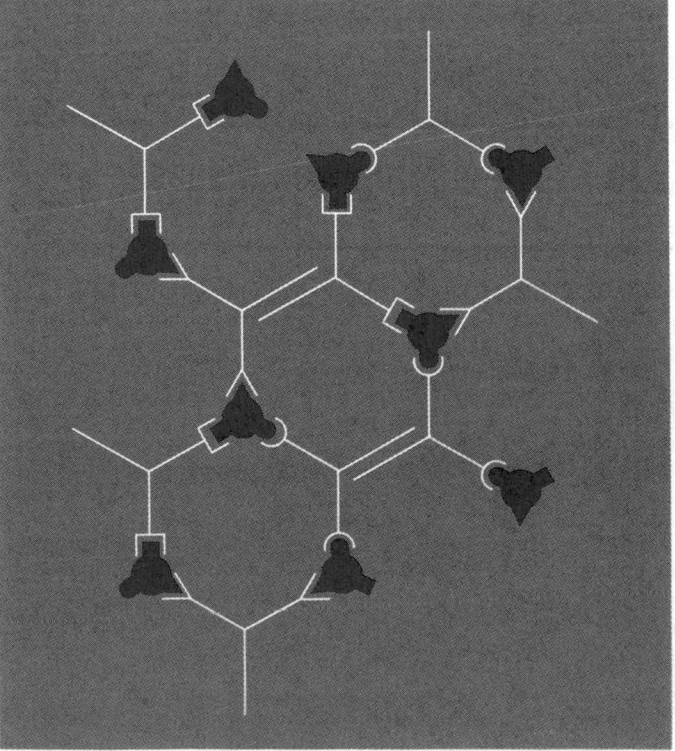

FIGURE 249–2. Immune complex lattice formation near the equivalence point. Neither free antigen nor free antibody is detected. Note that the lattice is formed by noncovalent bonds between antigen and antibody and between Fc portions of adjacent antibody molecules.

that induce mast cell degranulation and is ameliorated by pretreatment with antihistamines. Vascular permeability is also promoted by aggregation of platelets at sites of an inflammatory lesion, with the release of platelet-activating factor and the formation of microthrombi.

The primary cellular effectors of immune complex–mediated inflammation are polymorphonuclear leukocytes in the case of acute immune complex deposition and monocytes and macrophages at sites of chronic deposition. Neutrophils accumulate at the site of immune complex deposition as a consequence of complement activation and production of the chemotactic factor C5a. Their activation and degranulation are promoted by surface binding of complexes to C3b and Fcγ receptors. Tissue damage results from the release of hydrolytic lysosomal enzymes and the formation of toxic oxidants such as superoxide anion (O_2^-) and H_2O_2. Experimental studies of acute immune complex–mediated injury have demonstrated the importance of complement and neutrophils in this process; agents such as cobra venom factor or antineutrophil serum prevent accumulation of neutrophils at the site of complex deposition and consequently prevent injury. Tissue injury at sites of chronic immune complex deposition, for example, in chronic membranous glomerulonephritis and hypersensitivity pneumonitis, is due predominantly to the inflammatory activity of monocytes and macrophages. In experimental models of chronic immune complex deposition, evolution of inflammatory lesions may be inhibited by antimacrophage serum but not by depletion of neutrophils. Mechanisms of monocyte/macrophage-mediated tissue injury are probably similar to those of neutrophils, predominantly the release of hydrolytic enzymes and tissue-reactive oxidants. However, the details of macrophage-mediated inflammation have not been as thoroughly demonstrated experimentally.

Complement and Complement Receptors as Regulators of Immune Complex Deposition. The importance of complement in antibody-mediated inflammation has been appreciated for many years. Consequently, the observation that immune complex diseases, particularly systemic lupus erythematosus, are a prominent feature of genetic deficiencies of complement components presented a difficult paradox. This paradox has been resolved with the more recent realization that complement components can also inhibit immune complex deposition and resolubilize them from sites of deposition. In addition, it is now known that erythrocyte receptors for C3b are important for reticuloendothelial clearance of circulating immune complexes. Analysis of the clinical pattern of immune complex disease in patients with complement deficiencies provides clues to the role of these components in normal prevention of complex deposition. The incidence of immune complex disease in patients with deficiencies of C1q, C1r, C1s, C4, C2, and C3 varies from 60 to 90 per cent, with the majority of these patients exhibiting a lupus-like syndrome. On the other hand, immune complex disease is only occasionally associated with deficiencies of late-acting or alternative pathway components.

The CR1 complement receptors are particularly important to clearance of circulating complexes. Because approximately 90 per cent of blood CR1 molecules are represented on the surfaces of red blood cells, these cells function as efficient scavengers of C3b-containing immune complexes. Studies in baboons revealed that C3b-coated complexes are cleared from erythrocyte surfaces by transfer to the fixed phagocytic cells of the reticuloendothelial system within the liver. Patients with defects in CR1 might be predicted to have deficient complex clearance and an increased predisposition to immune complex disease, a prediction consistent with clinical observations. In patients with SLE but without deficiencies of complement constituents, a significant reduction in the number of erythrocyte CR1 receptors for C3b is frequently observed. The frequent observation of IgA-containing immune complexes and the distinct syndrome of an IgA nephropathy may, at least in part, represent a corollary of these observations. Because IgA does not fix complement via the classic pathway, IgA complexes are less efficiently cleared and are thus more likely to be deposited in capillary beds such as renal glomeruli. At least 60 per cent of patients with focal glomerulonephritis and hematuria following an infectious episode exhibit circulating IgA complexes and complex deposition typical of IgA nephropathy. Whether this represents poor clearance of such complexes, a predisposing defect in IgA regulation, or both requires additional study.

The binding of complement components to immune complexes (Fig. 249–3) prevents the formation of large antigen-antibody lattices and inhibits immune precipitation. This process requires activation via the classic pathway; serum that is deficient in C1q, C4, or C2 does not effectively inhibit lattice formation and complex precipitation. Classic pathway dependence may reflect the initial binding of C1 components, impeding the Fc-Fc interactions between IgG molecules that contribute to immune precipitation. This is followed by covalent bonding of C3b to the complexes, which further inhibits immune precipitation and leads to solubilization of previously deposited complexes. The solubilization process also depends upon activation of components of the alternative pathway, including properdin. Consequently, by promoting clearance of immune complexes and inhibiting their deposition at sites of inflammation, complement components and their receptors should be seen not only as important mediators of immune complex diseases but also as negative regulators that may retard disease development.

EVALUATION OF PATIENTS WITH IMMUNE COMPLEX DISEASES. Because the development of an immune complex disease often represents a secondary immunologic consequence of some other primary process, evaluation of patients with symp-

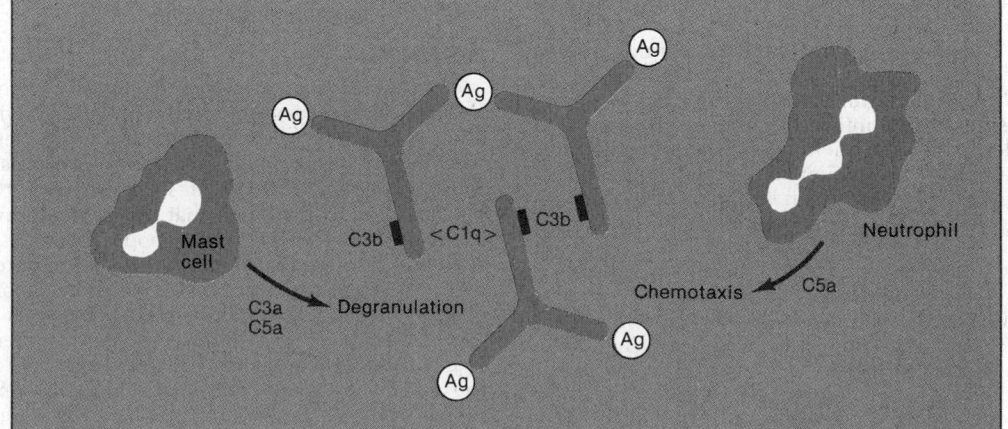

FIGURE 249–3. Positive and negative regulation of immune complex–mediated inflammation by complement components. The anaphylatoxins C3a and C5a, along with antigen binding by surface IgE molecules, promote degranulation of mast cells and basophils and the release of vasoactive amines. C5a also acts as a chemotactic factor attracting polymorphonuclear leukocytes to the site of immune complex deposition. C1q fixation inhibits Fc-Fc interactions between IgG molecules, thereby retarding complex precipitation. Complex formation is inhibited and deposited complexes are solubilized by the covalent attachment of C3b to antibody-antigen complexes; complex solubilization also requires activation of the alternate complement pathway.

toms of immune complex deposition begins with a thorough evaluation of possible sources for high-level antigen exposure. In many instances, such as immune complex disease during a course of antibiotic therapy or as a consequence of chronic infection, the antigen source is obvious. In others, such as hypersensitivity pneumonitis or occasionally in patients with malignancy, an extensive evaluation is required. In cases involving an autoimmune process, the diagnostic process may require extensive serologic investigation. The search for specific antigen within immune complexes is not usually productive. A notable exception is the identification of HBsAg in circulating immune complexes of patients with polyarteritis nodosa, in whom the search provides important insight into the pathogenetic process. More often the actual structure of the antigen is unknown even when its source is identified. A major difficulty is that specific antigen may represent a minor component, particularly with maturation of the antibody response and the development of complexes that form on the basis of immunoglobulin–anti-immunoglobulin interactions.

Many techniques are available for nonspecific detection of immune complexes. The most useful clinically is biopsy with fluorescent or electron microscopic analysis for deposition of various immunoglobulin classes and complement components at the site of a suspected immune complex–mediated inflammatory lesion. Results of such biopsies must be interpreted with caution because complexes may be present at sites not apparently involved in acute inflammation, for example, in apparently normal skin of patients with SLE. Conversely, complexes may have been removed from the site of an ongoing inflammatory process, particularly during its chronic phase. Thus, renal biopsies in acute glomerulonephritis are more likely to reveal immune complex deposition than are biopsies in chronic disease.

Many laboratory methods have been developed for detection of circulating immune complexes based on their physical, chemical, or biologic properties. Among others these include ultracentrifugation, nephelometry, C1q binding, and binding to C3b receptors on a human B-cell line. In all cases, interpretation of the results requires careful attention to conditions of specimen collection and laboratory controls, including appropriate positive and negative standards. Despite the feasibility of quantifying circulating immune complexes, however, the usefulness of such tests has been widely questioned. When appropriately performed, they are often indicative of an ongoing inflammatory process. Nevertheless, a finding of circulating immune complexes is very nonspecific and hence of limited diagnostic usefulness. In addition, the absolute levels do not correlate with disease activity with sufficient predictability to make single determinations helpful in predicting and assessing severity or prognosis. Although serial determinations during the course of disease may correlate roughly with waxing and waning of the inflammatory process, it is only in the unusual patient that such information is particularly helpful in management.

TREATMENT. The therapy of an immune complex disease depends upon its severity and chronicity, the site of inflammatory lesions, and the nature of the primary pathologic process. A first principle when feasible is to eliminate or reduce the source of antigen, for example by effective therapy of an underlying infection, change in an antibiotic, or manipulation of the environment. It should be recognized, however, that if reduction of the antigen load alters the molar ratio of antigen to antibody in complexes, shifting the balance from antigen excess to equivalence, the result may be temporary exacerbation of the inflammatory process. Available alternatives for treatment of the inflammatory process are familiar, including antihistamines, nonsteroidal anti-inflammatory agents, corticosteroids, and cytotoxic agents. When long-term therapy with corticosteroids is anticipated, management with alternate-day therapy is recommended if possible. Cytotoxic agents such as cyclophosphamide have proved to be effective in treatment of systemic vasculitides and severe SLE; a monthly intravenous bolus of cyclophosphamide may prove effective, with reduced toxicity compared to daily therapy. The newer immunosuppressive agents such as cyclosporine are being evaluated for efficacy with chronic immune complex disease developing as a consequence of T-cell dysregulation. Finally, plasmapheresis can dramatically reduce high levels of circulating immune com-

plexes when acute intervention in the inflammatory process is indicated. Such treatment may prove life-saving in patients with severe autoimmune diseases.

Høiby N, Döring G, Schiøtz PO: The role of immune complexes in the pathogenesis of bacterial infections. Annu Rev Microbiol 40:29, 1986.

McDougal JS, McDuffie FC: Immune complexes in man: Detection and clinical significance. Adv Clin Chem 24:1, 1985.

Schifferli JA, Ng YC, Peters DK: The role of complement and its receptor in the elimination of immune complexes. N Engl J Med 315:488, 1986.

Theofilopoulos AN, Dixon FJ: The biology and detection of immune complexes. Adv Immunol 28:89, 1979.

Walport MJ, Lachmann PJ: Erythrocyte complement receptor type I, immune complexes, and rheumatic diseases. Arthritis Rheum 31:153, 1988.

Wilson JG, Fearon DT: Altered expression of complement receptors as a pathogenetic factor in systemic lupus erythematosus. Arthritis Rheum 27:1321, 1984.

250 The Major Histocompatibility Complex and Disease Susceptibility

Benjamin D. Schwartz

The proper functioning of the immune system depends on its ability to distinguish "self" from "nonself." This crucial distinction is achieved via the molecules determined by the major histocompatibility complex, or HLA complex as it is known in humans. It now appears that both foreign and self antigens are recognized by the T lymphocytes of the immune system only in conjunction with HLA molecules. During embryogenesis, a process of T-cell "education" takes place in the thymus whereby T cells recognizing self antigens (in the context of HLA molecules) are normally eliminated and T cells potentially recognizing foreign antigens in the context of self HLA molecules are selected.

For a protein antigen to be recognized by the T lymphocytes of the immune system, it must undergo "processing." During processing, the protein is partially degraded into peptides, some of which are bound by HLA molecules. The peptide and HLA molecule form a complex that is the ligand recognized by the receptor on the T lymphocyte. There appear to be two processing pathways used by the immune system. Intracellular antigens, such as viruses, are processed through the endogenous pathway and are presented by HLA class I molecules to CD8+ (generally cytotoxic) T lymphocytes. In contrast, extracellular antigens are processed through the exogenous pathway and are presented by HLA class II molecules to CD4+ (generally helper) T lymphocytes. Thus, HLA molecules are critical in the recognition of antigen by the immune system.

HISTORY

The existence of a human major histocompatibility complex (MHC) was first suggested in the mid 1950's when leukoagglutinating antibodies were discovered in the sera of multiparous women and multiply transfused leukopenic patients. Analysis of these sera indicated that each serum reacts with the cells of some but not all individuals and that different sera react with the cells of different but overlapping populations of individuals. This pattern suggested that these antisera were detecting alloantigens (i.e., antigens that were present on the cells of some individuals of a given species) which were the products of a polymorphic genetic locus. It was discovered shortly thereafter that these human leukocyte antigens (HLA) had a major role in determining the success of organ transplants, and this finding spurred the initial study of these antigens. Over the ensuing years, the reaction patterns of literally thousands of anti-HLA alloantisera have been codified by computer and have made possible the delineation of the HLA system. In 1973, certain HLA antigens were found to be associated with specific diseases. In addition, at around the same time it was appreciated that the HLA complex regulates several aspects of the human immune response. These findings provided a second impetus for the study of the HLA

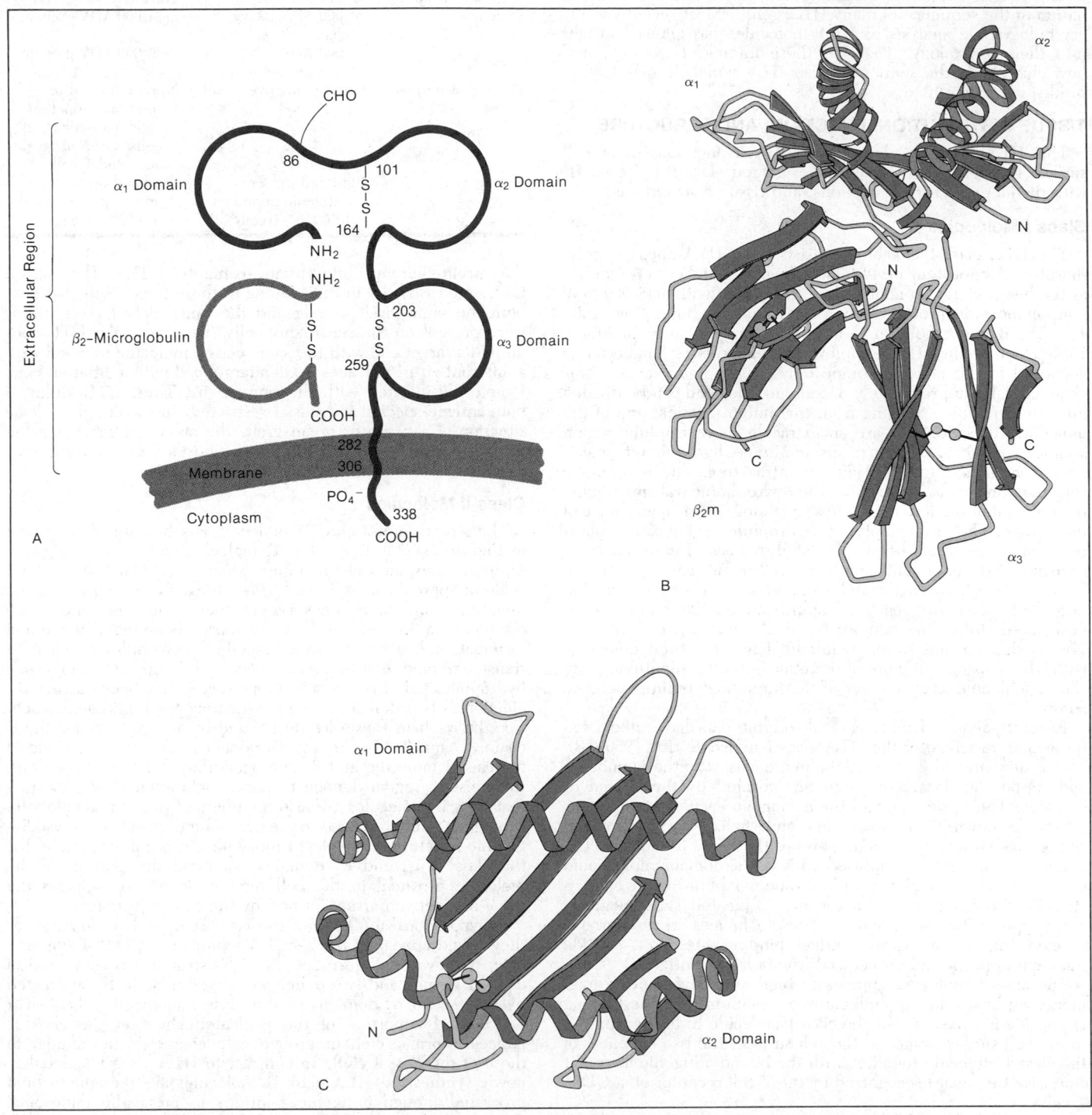

FIGURE 250–1. The HLA class I molecule. *A,* A schematic representation. The molecule consists of a heavy chain, which anchors the molecule in the membrane, noncovalently associated with β₂-microglobulin. Numbers indicate amino acid residues where certain features are found. NH₂ = amino terminus; COOH = carboxy terminus; CHO = carbohydrate; PO₄⁻ = phosphate. α₁, α₂, and α₃ are the three extracellular domains. *B* and *C,* The crystallographic structure. β strands are depicted as thick arrows in the amino to carboxy direction, and α helices are represented as helical ribbons. Connecting loops are shown as thin lines. Disulfide bonds are two connected spheres. *B,* Side view. The molecule is shown with the α₃ domain and β₂-microglobulin at the bottom, and the α₁ and α₂ domains at the top. The β-pleated sheet is seen edge on. The α helices form the cleft into which peptide can fit. *C,* Top view. The α₁ and α₂ domains are seen from above. The β-pleated sheet platform and the cleft formed by the α helices are again visible. (*B* and *C* reprinted by permission from *Nature,* Vol. 329, p. 506. Copyright © 1987 Macmillan Magazines Limited.)

complex. The application of molecular biology technology to the study of the HLA complex over the past 10 years has allowed delineation of additional HLA loci and alleles and the determination of the sequence of many HLA genes. Most recently, x-ray crystallographic analysis of HLA molecules has allowed insight into their physiology. Together these findings have suggested how changes in the sequence of an HLA molecule may lead to predisposition to disease.

TISSUE DISTRIBUTION, FUNCTION, AND STRUCTURE

The HLA complex determines two distinct classes of cell surface glycoprotein molecules, designated class I and class II, with distinct structures, functions, and tissue distributions.

Class I Molecules

The HLA class I molecule consists of an HLA-encoded polymorphic glycoprotein of 44,000 molecular weight (MW) known as the heavy chain, in noncovalent association with a 12,000 MW nonpolymorphic protein known as β_2-microglobulin (Fig. 250–1A). The β_2-microglobulin is encoded by a gene on chromosome 15 and not by the HLA complex. The entire class I molecule is anchored in the cell membrane only by the heavy chain. This chain contains approximately 338 amino acids and can be divided into three regions. Starting from the amino terminal end of the molecule, these regions are an extracellular hydrophilic region (amino acids 1 to 281), a transmembrane hydrophobic region (amino acids 282 to 306), and an intracytoplasmic hydrophilic region (amino acids 307 to 338). The hydrophobic transmembrane region contains 24 amino acids, enabling it to span the cell membrane. The intracytoplasmic hydrophilic region can be phosphorylated, and it has been speculated that class I molecules may transduce external events across the cell membrane.

The extracellular hydrophilic region in turn can be divided into three domains, each of approximately 90 amino acids, designated from the amino terminal end α_1, α_2, and α_3. The α_3 domain and β_2-microglobulin have structural homology with the constant region of immunoglobulin, identifying the class I molecule as a member of the immunoglobulin supergene family.

Recently acquired x-ray crystallographic data have elucidated the actual structure of the HLA class I molecule (Fig. 250–1B). The α_3 domain and β_2-microglobulin are closest to the membrane and support an interactive structure formed by the α_1 and α_2 domains. The α_1 domain and the α_2 domain each consists of four β strands shown as flat arrows and an α helix shown as a coiled ribbon-like structure projecting toward the top of the figure. (The α helix should not be confused with the α domain, nor should the β strand be confused with β_2-microglobulin.) The eight β strands of these two domains form a β-pleated sheet platform that supports the two α helices. These α helices create a groove or cleft that serves as the antigen-binding site for a peptide fragment appropriately processed from a larger antigen.

The class I molecule appears to bind antigenic peptide fragments while still in the endoplasmic reticulum, and the binding of peptide is necessary for the class I molecule to be transported to the cell surface. Once at the cell surface, the two α helices of the class I molecule together with the bound antigenic fragment comprise the ligand recognized by the T-cell receptor on a CD8$^+$ T cell.

A top view of the class I molecule as it would appear to the T-cell receptor of a CD8$^+$ T lymphocyte is shown in Figure 250–1C. The β strands of the α_1 and α_2 domains form the floor of the cleft, and the α helices of the same domains form the sides of the cleft. The majority of alloantigenic determinants recognized both by antibodies and by T cells have been shown to be located in the α_1 and α_2 domains.

The class I antigens are found on virtually every human cell (Table 250–1). This tissue distribution is well suited to the physiologic role of the class I antigens to present foreign antigenic peptides such as viral antigenic peptides to cytotoxic T lymphocytes (CTL's). Precursors of CTL's are specific for a particular viral antigenic peptide in the context of a particular class I molecule. When the precursors encounter this particular combination of the viral antigenic peptide and the class I molecule,

TABLE 250–1. COMPARISON OF HLA CLASS I AND CLASS II MOLECULES

	Class I	Class II
Molecules included	HLA-A, -B, -C	HLA-DR, -DQ, -DP
Structure	44,000 MW heavy chain	~34,000 MW α chain
	12,000 MW β_2-microglobulin	~29,000 MW β chain
Tissue distribution	On virtually every cell	Normal limited to immunocompetent cells, particularly B cells, macrophages, activated T cells
Function	Bind and present antigenic peptides to CD8$^+$ T cells	Bind and present antigenic peptides to CD4$^+$ T cells

they proliferate and differentiate to mature CTL's. The mature CTL's are restricted in their killing to those target cells that bear both the same viral peptide and the same class I molecule as were present on the sensitizing cells. That particular CTL does not kill a target cell with the same class I molecule infected with a different virus, nor does it kill a target cell with a different class I molecule infected with the same virus. Thus, CTL killing is both antigen-specific and class I restricted. In the nonphysiologic situation of a tissue or organ graft, the class I antigens are the principal antigens recognized by the host's CTL's during graft rejection.

Class II Molecules

The structure of a class II molecule is schematically depicted in Figure 250–2A. Each class II molecule consists of two glycoprotein chains, an α chain of approximately 34,000 MW, and a β chain of approximately 29,000 MW. Both of the chains span the membrane and therefore serve to anchor the molecule. Each chain can be divided into three regions. Beginning at the amino terminal end, there is an extracellular hydrophilic region, a transmembrane hydrophobic region, and an intracytoplasmic hydrophilic tail. Each extracellular region has been further divided into two domains of approximately 90 amino acids each. For the α chain these are designated α_1 and α_2, and for the β chain, β_1 and β_2. The α_2 and β_2 domains, like the α_3 domain of the class I molecule and β_2-microglobulin, show homology with the constant region domain of immunoglobulin, thus indicating that class II molecules are also members of the immunoglobulin supergene family. Based on extrapolation from the crystallographic structure of the class I molecules, it is almost certain that the class II α_2 and β_2 domains comprise the portion of the molecule proximal to the cell membrane which supports the distal interactive portion formed by the α_1 and β_1 domains.

A hypothetical top view of the class II α_1 and β_1 domains, as they would appear to the T-cell receptor on a CD4$^+$ T lymphocyte, is shown in Figure 250–2B. The structure is composed of eight β strands and two α helices very similar to those created by the α_1 and α_2 domains of the class I molecule. The two α helices and a portion of the β-pleated sheet of the class II molecule form a cleft or groove with characteristics similar to those of the class I cleft. In contrast to HLA class I molecules, newly synthesized HLA class II molecules are thought to bind processed foreign antigenic peptides in an acidic endosomal compartment during their transport to the cell surface. On the cell surface, the α helices of the class II molecule together with the bound peptide constitute the ligand for the receptor on a CD4$^+$ T cell.

In contrast to the HLA class I molecules, the HLA class II molecules have a limited distribution (Table 250–1). They are found predominantly on immunocompetent cells, including B cells, monocytes, dendritic cells, and activated T cells. Interferon-γ can induce increased expression on macrophages and has also been shown to induce expression of class II molecules on cells where they are not normally expressed, e.g., endothelial cells, thyroid cells, epidermal cells, and renal cells.

The physiologic role of the class II molecules parallels that of the class I molecules. Just as CD8$^+$ T cells recognize foreign antigenic peptide in the context of a class I molecule, CD4$^+$

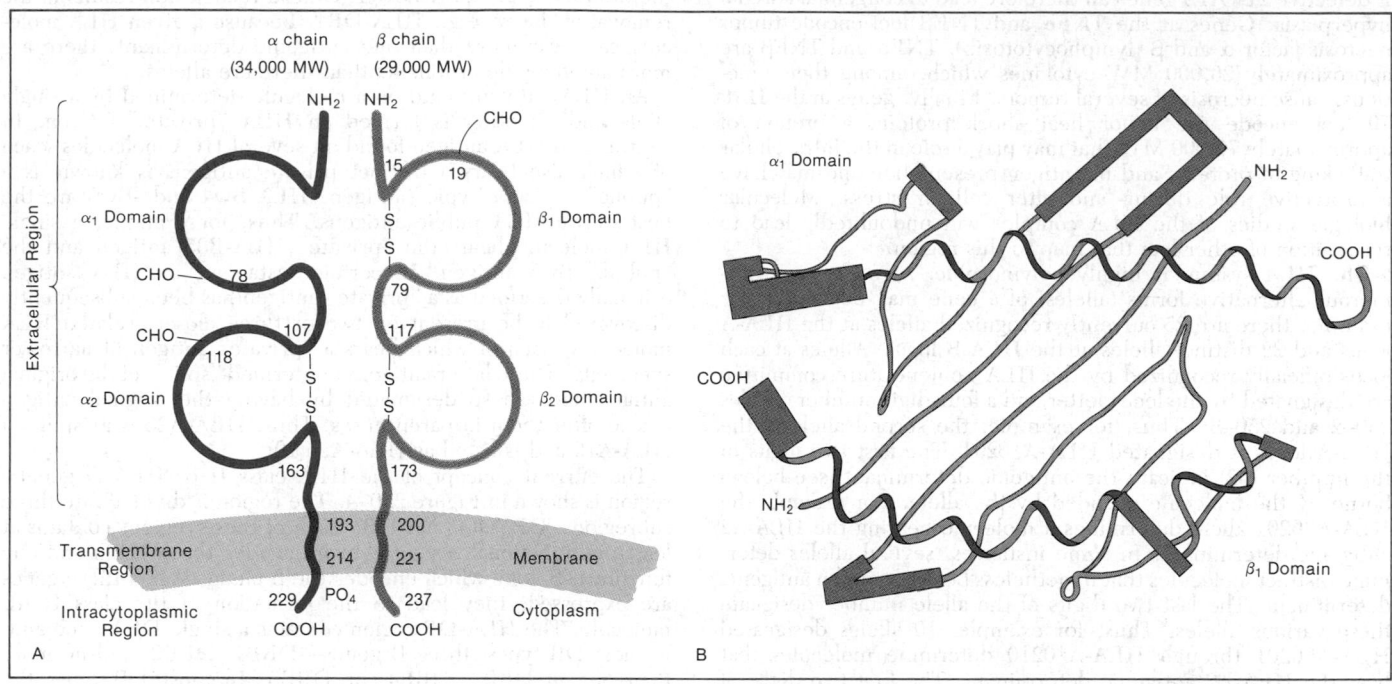

FIGURE 250–2. The HLA class II molecule. *A,* Schematic representation. The molecule consists of an α chain transmembrane glycoprotein noncovalently associated with a β chain transmembrane glycoprotein. The α_1, α_2, β_1, and β_2 domains are indicated. *B,* The postulated crystallographic structure of a class II molecule as seen from above. The antigen-binding cleft is formed by the α_1 and β_1 domains. β strands are depicted as flat thin lines and the α helices as ribbons. The cleft is very similar to that of the class I molecule. For explanation of symbols see Figure 250–1. (*B* reprinted by permission from Nature, Vol. 332, p. 845. Copyright © 1988 Macmillan Magazines Limited.)

(generally helper) T cells recognize foreign antigenic peptide in the context of a class II molecule. In nonphysiologic states such as graft transplantation, the class II molecules present on donor cells can initiate an immune response in the host by stimulating the host's helper T cells.

NOMENCLATURE AND GENETIC ORGANIZATION OF THE HLA COMPLEX

The HLA complex is located on the short arm of chromosome 6. Figure 250–3 schematically depicts the genetic loci currently located within the HLA complex. There are three groups or classes of HLA genes and molecules. Genes at the HLA-A, -B,

and -C loci encode the class I or classic histocompatibility molecules, whereas genes at the HLA-DR, -DQ, and -DP loci determine the class II molecules. As noted above, both class I and class II molecules are cell surface bound.

The HLA complex also contains a series of genes that encode soluble proteins. This set of genes is broadly termed the class III genes. Genes at the Bf, C2, C4A, and C4B loci encode properdin factor B and the second and fourth components of the complement system. Genes at the 21-OHA and -OHB loci encode 21-hydroxylase, an enzyme in the adrenal steroid synthetic pathway. The C4B-linked 21-OHB gene is functional, whereas the C4A-linked 21-OHA appears to be a pseudogene; that is, it is not expressed.

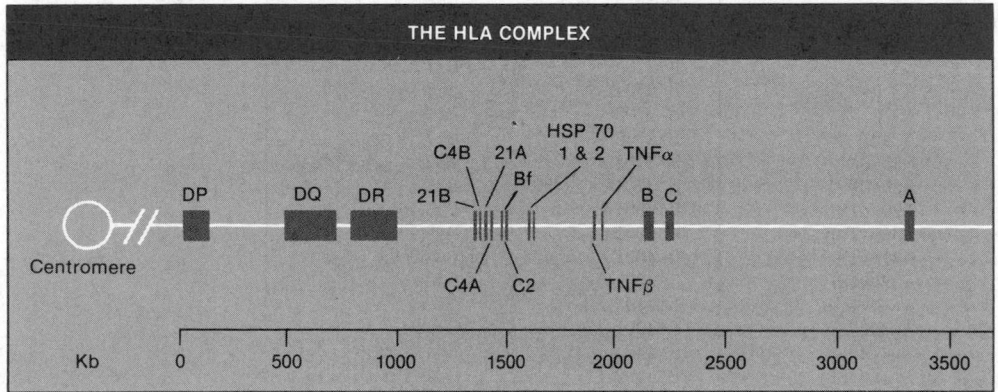

FIGURE 250–3. The current concept of the HLA complex. The class I loci, the class II subregions, and the class III loci are indicated. Distances are given in kilobases (Kb). A, B, and C denote the HLA-A, HLA-B, and HLA-C loci; DP, DQ, and DR designate the HLA-DP, -DQ, and -DR subregions; C2, C4A, C4B, and Bf denote the loci encoding the second, duplicated fourth, and properdin factor B components of the complement system; 21A and 21B designate the 21-hydroxylase A and B loci; TNFα and TNFβ indicate the tumor necrosis factor loci, and HSP 1 and 2 indicate the major heat shock protein 70 loci. Class I loci are shown as thin red blocks, class II loci as thick red blocks, and the complement class III loci as thin vertical bars.

A defective 21-OHB gene can therefore lead to congenital adrenal hyperplasia. Genes at the TNFα and TNFβ loci encode tumor necrosis factor α and β (lymphocytotoxin). TNFα and TNFβ are approximately 20,000 MW cytokines which, among their functions, cause necrosis of several tumors. Finally, genes at the HSP 70 loci encode the major heat shock protein, a protein of approximately 70,000 MW that may play a role in the intracellular trafficking of proteins and in antigen presentation and may have a protective role during and after cellular stress. Molecular biologic studies of the HLA complex will undoubtedly lead to recognition of other loci that map to this region.

The HLA system is highly polymorphic. At each locus, numerous alternative forms (alleles) of a gene may be found. For example, there are 25 currently recognized alleles at the HLA-A locus and 32 distinct alleles at the HLA-B locus. Alleles at each locus officially recognized by the HLA nomenclature committee are designated by the locus letter and a four-digit number (Tables 250–2 and 250–3). Thus, for example, the second allele at the HLA-A locus is designated HLA-A*0201. The first two digits in the number (02) indicate the antigenic determinant (see below) borne by the molecule encoded by the allele. For example the HLA-A*0201 allele determines a molecule bearing the HLA-A2 antigenic determinant. In some instances, several alleles determine distinct molecules that nonetheless bear a common antigenic determinant. The last two digits of the allele number designate these various alleles. Thus, for example, 10 alleles designated HLA-A*0201 through HLA-A*0210 determine molecules that bear the HLA-A2 antigenic determinant. The first two digits of the allele number (02) indicate the HLA-A2 determinant, and the last two digits (01 through 10) designate the 10 distinct alleles, each of which encodes a molecule bearing HLA-A2.

As alluded to above, each functional allele determines a glycoprotein product, the HLA molecule. Each HLA molecule bears antigenic determinants recognized by antibodies. These antigenic determinants are designated by a letter and a number, for example HLA-A1 (Table 250–4). The letter indicates the locus at which the allele encoding the molecule bearing the antigenic determinant is found; the number indicates the number of the antigenic determinant determined by that allele. Antigenic de-

terminants that have been assigned but are not yet officially recognized are signified by a w (for "workshop") placed before the number, e.g., HLA-DRw1. Official recognition results in the removal of the w, e.g., HLA-DR1. Because a given HLA molecule can bear more than one antigenic determinant, there are more antigenic determinants than there are alleles.

An HLA antigen found on a molecule determined by a single allele and no other is termed an HLA "private" antigen. In contrast, an HLA antigen found on several HLA molecules, each of which also bears a distinct private antigen, is known as a "public" or "supertypic" antigen. HLA-Bw4 and -Bw6 are the best-known HLA public antigens. Thus, for example, a single HLA molecule bears the "private" HLA-B35 antigen and the "public" Bw6 antigen. In certain instances, an HLA antigen originally described as a "private" antigen has been subsequently discovered to be present on two or three closely related HLA molecules, each of which bears a "private" antigen of narrower specificity. These latter antigens are termed "splits" of the original antigen and are so designated by having the original antigen placed after them in parentheses. Thus, HLA-A25 is a "split" of HLA-A10 and is listed as HLA-A25(10).

The current concept of the HLA class II or HLA-D genetic region is shown in Figure 250–4. The region is divided into three subregions: DP, DQ, and DR. Each of these regions contains at least one functional A gene which encodes the α chain and one functional -B gene which encodes the β chain. When these genes are expressed, they lead to the formation of the class II αβ molecule. The HLA-DR region contains a single DRA gene and, in most DR types, three B genes—DRB1, DRB2, and no more than one of DRB3, DRB4, or DRB5. In most DR types the DRB2 gene is a pseudogene; that is, it is not expressed. However, the DRB1 and one of the DRB3, DRB4, or DRB5 genes are expressed. The DRα chain can combine with either the DRβ1 chain or the DRβ3 (or DRβ4 or DRβ5) chain to produce the DRαβ1 and DRαβ3 (or DRαβ4 or DRαβ5) molecules. The DRαβ1 molecule bears DR antigens 1 through 18, while the DRαβ3 molecule bears DRw52, the DRαβ4 molecule bears DRw53, and the DRαβ5 molecule is associated with DRαβ1 molecules bearing DRw15 and DRw16 and may itself also bear these determinants.

Certain of the HLA-DR B1 allele types have been organized

TABLE 250–2. DESIGNATIONS OF HLA-A, -B, AND -C ALLELES

HLA Alleles	HLA Antigenic Determinant	HLA Alleles	HLA Antigenic Determinant	HLA Alleles	HLA Antigenic Determinant
A*0101	A1	B*0701	B7	Cw*0101	Cw1
A*0201	A2	B*0702	B7	Cw*0201	Cw2
A*0202	A2	B*0801	B8	Cw*0202	Cw2
A*0203	A2	B*1301	B13	Cw*0301	Cw3
A*0204	A2	B*1302	B13	Cw*0501	Cw5
A*0205	A2	B*1401	B14	Cw*0601	Cw6
A*0206	A2	B*1402	Bw65(14)	Cw*0701	Cw7
A*0207	A2	B*1501	Bw62(15)	Cw*1101	Cw11
A*0208	A2	B*1801	B18	Cw*1201	—
A*0209	A2	B*2701	B27	Cw*1301	—
A*0210	A2	B*2702	B27	Cw*1401	—
A*0301	A3	B*2703	B27		
A*0302	A3	B*2704	B27		
A*1101	A11	B*2705	B27		
A*2401	A24(9)	B*2706	B27		
A*2501	A25(10)	B*3501	B35		
A*2601	A26(10)	B*3701	B37		
A*2901	A29(w19)	B*3801	B38(16)		
A*3001	A30(w19)	B*3901	B39(16)		
A*3101	A31(w19)	B*4001	Bw60(40)		
A*3201	A32(w19)	B*4002	B40		
A*3301	Aw33(w19)	B*4101	Bw41		
A*6801	Aw68(28)	B*4201	Bw42		
A*6802	Aw68(28)	B*4401	B44 (12)		
A*6901	Aw69(28)	B*4402	B44 (12)		
		B*4601	Bw46		
		B*4701	Bw47		
		B*4901	B49 (21)		
		B*5101	B51(5)		
		B*5201	Bw52(5)		
		B*5701	Bw57(17)		
		B*5801	Bw58(17)		

into groups based on their occurrence with DRB3, DRB4, or DRB5 alleles. Thus, for example, the DRB1 alleles determining DR3, DR5, DRw6, and DRw8 have been grouped together because they are in linkage disequilibrium (see below) with DRB3 alleles that determine DRw52 (Table 250–5), and are thought to be evolutionarily related. Similarly, the DRB1 alleles encoding DR4, DR7, and DR9 are grouped together because they are in linkage disequilibrium with DRB4, which encodes HLA-DRw53, and are also evolutionarily related. Finally, the DRB1 alleles determining DR2 all are in linkage disequilibrium with DRB5. Linkage disequilibrium is also responsible for the association of particular DR antigens with particular DQ antigens (Table 250–6).

The DQ subregion contains two pairs of A and B genes. One pair, designated DQA2 and DQB2, are pseudogenes and are not expressed. The other pair, designated DQA1 and DQB1, are expressed and result in the formation of the DQαβ molecule. Likewise, the DP subregion contains two pairs of A and B genes. One pair, designated DPA2 and DPB2, contain pseudogenes. The other pair, designated DPA1 and DPB1, encode the DPα and β chains that form the DPαβ molecule.

The polymorphism of the class II molecules (DR, DQ, and DP) varies somewhat for each set. For the DR molecules, the DRα chain is essentially nonpolymorphic between different DR types, while the DRβ chains are highly polymorphic. For the DQ molecules, both the DQα and DQβ chains demonstrate a high degree of polymorphism. For the DP molecules, the DPα chain shows relatively limited polymorphism, while the DPβ chains are again highly polymorphic.

Two additional class II genes have been mapped to the HLA-D region. One has been designated DNA and the second DOB. Neither of these genes has yet been found to be expressed in vivo, although expression has been induced in in vitro systems. The function of these genes is at present unknown.

It should be noted that there is no HLA-D locus or HLA-D molecule per se. The HLA-D antigens are defined and detected solely by a cellular reaction known as the mixed leukocyte reaction (MLR). Responder cells in the MLR appear to be detecting an array of antigenic determinants present on the HLA-DR, -DQ, and/or -DP molecules. In most cases, it is thought that antigenic determinants on HLA-DR molecules contribute most significantly to the MLR. As a result, HLA-D types tend to be most highly correlated with HLA-DR types (see Table 250–3).

The products of the C2, C4, and Bf loci are complement proteins that can be detected serologically and functionally and also display polymorphism (Table 250–7). Alleles determining properdin factor B can be distinguished by their electrophoretic mobility: a common fast form Bf*F, a common slow form Bf*S, a rare fast form Bf*F1, and a rare slow form Bf*SO.7. There are C2 alleles determining two common forms of C2, C2*C and C2*A, and a rare deficiency allele C2*QO. The C4 locus has been duplicated so that there are two distinct C4 loci designated

TABLE 250–3. DESIGNATIONS OF HLA-DR, -DQ, AND -DP ALLELES

HLA-DR Alleles	HLA-DR Determinants	HLA-D–Associated (T-cell–Defined) Determinants	HLA-DQ Alleles	HLA-DQ Determinants	HLA-D–Associated (T-cell–Defined) Determinants	HLA-DP Alleles	Associated HLA-DP Determinants
DRB1*0101	DR1	Dw1	DQA1*0101	—	Dw1,w9	DPA1*0101	—
DRB1*0102	DR1	DW20	DQA1*0102	—	Dw2,w21,w19	DPA1*0102	—
DRB1*0103	DR'BR'	DW'BON'	DQA1*0103	—	Dw18,w12,28,	DPA1*0103	—
DRB1*1501	DRw15(2)	Dw2			Dw'FS'	DPA1*0201	—
DRB1*1502	DRw15(2)	Dw12	DQA1*0201	—	Dw7,w11	DPB1*0101	DPw1
DRB1*1601	DRw16(2)	Dw21	DQA1*0301	—	Dw4,w10,w13,	DPB1*0201	DPw2
DRB1*1602	DRw16(2)	Dw22			w14, w15,w23	DPB1*0202	DPw2
DRB1*0301	DRw17(3)	Dw3	DQA1*0401	—	Dw8,Dw'RSH'	DPB1*0301	DPw3
DRB1*0302	DRw18(3)	DW'RSH'	DQA1*0501	—	Dw3,w5,w22	DPB1*0401	DPw4
DRB1*0401	DR4	Dw4	DQA1*0601	—	Dw8	DPB1*0402	DPw4
DRB1*0402	DR4	Dw10	DQB1*0501	DQw5(w1)	Dw1	DPB1*0501	DPw5
DRB1*0403	DR4	Dw13	DQB1*0502	DQw5(w1)	Dw21	DPB1*0601	DPw6
DRB1*0404	DR4	Dw14	DQB1*0503	DQw5(w1)	Dw9	DPB1*0801	—
DRB1*0405	DR4	Dw15	DQB1*0601	DQw6(w1)	Dw12,w8	DPB1*0901	DP'Cp63'
DRB1*0406	DR4	Dw'KT2'	DQB1*0602	DQw6(w1)	Dw2	DPB1*1001	—
DRB1*0407	DR4	Dw13	DQB1*0603	DQw6(w1)	Dw18,Dw'FS'	DPB1*1101	—
DRB1*0408	DR4	Dw14	DQB1*0604	DQw6(w1)	Dw19	DPB1*1301	—
DRB1*1101	DRw11(5)	Dw5	DQB1*0201	DQw2	Dw3,w7	DPB1*1401	—
DRB1*1102	DRw11(5)	Dw'JVM'	DQB1*0301	DQw7(w3)	Dw4,w5,w8,	DPB1*1501	—
DRB1*1103	DRw11(5)	—			w13	DPB1*1601	—
DRB1*1104	DRw11(5)	Dw'FS'	DQB1*0302	DQw8(w3)	Dw4,w10,w13,	DPB1*1701	—
DRB1*1201	DRw12(5)	Dw'DB6'			w14	DPB1*1801	—
DRB1*1301	DRw13(w6)	Dw18	DQB1*0303	DQw9 (w3)	Dw23,w11	DPB1*1901	—
DRB1*1302	DRw13(w6)	Dw19	DQB1*0401	DQw4	Dw15		
DRB1*1303	DRw13(w6)	Dw'HAG'	DQB1*0402	DQw4	Dw8,Dw'RSH'		
DRB1*1401	DRw14(w6)	Dw9					
DRB1*1402	DRw14(w6)	Dw16					
DRB1*0701	DR7	Dw17					
DRB1*0702	DR7	Dw'DB1'					
DRB1*0801	DRw8	Dw8.1					
DRB1*0802	DRw8	Dw8.2					
DRB1*0803	DRw8	Dw8.3					
DRB1*0901	DR9	Dw23					
DRB1*1001	DRw10	—					
DRB3*0101	DRw52a	Dw24					
DRB3*0201	DRw52b	Dw25					
DRB3*0202	DRw52b	Dw25					
DRB3*0301	DRw52c	Dw26					
DRB4*0101	DRw53	Dw4,Dw10,Dw13,Dw14, Dw15,Dw17,Dw23					
DRB5*0101	DRw15(2)	Dw2					
DRB5*0102	DRw15(2)	Dw12					
DRB5*0201	DRw16(2)	Dw21					
DRB5*0202	DRw16(2)	Dw22					

TABLE 250–4. CURRENT LISTING OF RECOGNIZED HLA ANTIGENS

HLA-A	HLA-B		HLA-C	HLA-D	HLA-DR	HLA-DQ	HLA-DP
A1	B5	B51(5)	Cw1	Dw1	DR1	DQw1	DPw1
A2	B7	Bw52(5)	Cw2	Dw2	DR2	DQw2	DPw2
A3	B8	Bw53	Cw3	Dw3	DR3	DQw3	DPw3
A9	B12	Bw54(w22)	Cw4	Dw4	DR4	DQw4	DPw4
A10	B13	Bw55(w22)	Cw5	Dw5	DR5	DQw5(w1)	DPw5
A11	B14	Bw56(w22)	Cw6	Dw6	DRw6	DQw6(w1)	DPw6
Aw19	B15	Bw57(17)	Cw7	Dw7	DR7	DQw7(w3)	
A23(9)	B16	Bw58(17)	Cw8	Dw8	DRw8	DQw8(w3)	
A24(9)	B17	Bw59	Cw9(w3)	Dw9	DR9	DQw9(w3)	
A25(10)	B18	Bw60(40)	Cw10(w3)	Dw10	DRw10		
A26(10)	B21	Bw61(40)	Cw11	Dw11(w7)	DRw11(5)		
A28	Bw22	Bw62(15)		Dw12	DRw12(5)		
A29 (w19)	B27	Bw63(15)		Dw13	DRw13(w6)		
A30 (w19)	B35	Bw64(14)		Dw14	DRw14(w6)		
A31(w19)	B37	Bw65(14)		Dw15	DRw15(2)		
A32(w19)	B38(16)	Bw67		Dw16	DRw16(2)		
Aw33(w19)	B39(16)	Bw71(w70)		Dw17(w7)	DRw17(3)		
Aw34(10)	B40	Bw70		Dw18(w6)	DRw18(3)		
Aw36	Bw41	Bw72(w70)		Dw19(w6)			
Aw43	Bw42	Bw73		Dw20	DRw52		
Aw66(10)	B44(12)	Bw75(15)		Dw21	DRw53		
Aw68(28)	B45(12)	Bw76(15)		Dw22			
Aw69(28)	Bw46	Bw77(15)		Dw23			
Aw74(w19)	Bw47			Dw24			
	Bw48	Bw4		Dw25			
	B49(21)	Bw6		Dw26			
	Bw50(21)						

C4A (formerly Rogers), which determines the electrophoretically more acidic group of C4 components, and C4B (formerly Chido), which determines the electrophoretically more basic group of C4 components. There are four well-defined common structural alleles and one deficiency allele at the C4A locus and three well-defined common structural alleles and one deficiency allele at the C4B locus.

HAPLOTYPE

Because of their close linkage, the alleles at each locus on a single chromosome are usually inherited in combination as a unit. This combination is referred to as the haplotype. Because each individual inherits one set of chromosomes from each parent, each individual has two HLA haplotypes. HLA genes are codominant; therefore, both alleles at a given HLA locus are expressed, and two complete sets of HLA antigens can be detected on cells. By simple mendelian genetics, there is a 25 per cent chance that two siblings will share both haplotypes and be fully HLA compatible, a 50 per cent chance that they will share one haplotype, and a 25 per cent chance that they will share no haplotype and thus will be completely HLA incompatible (Fig. 250–5).

LINKAGE DISEQUILIBRIUM

Because of random matings, the frequency of finding a given allele at one HLA locus associated with a given allele at a second HLA locus should simply be the product of the frequencies of each allele in the population. However, certain combinations of alleles are found with a frequency greater than expected. This phenomenon is termed "linkage disequilibrium" and is quantitated as the difference (Δ) between the observed and expected frequencies. For example, the HLA-A*0101 allele, which determines HLA-A1, and the HLA-B*0801 allele, which determines HLA-B8, are found in the Caucasian population with frequencies of 0.161 and 0.104, respectively. Thus, the expected frequency with which the HLA-A*0101, B*0101 haplotype should be found is 0.161×0.104, or 0.0167. However, this haplotype is found with a frequency of approximately 0.0592, almost four times the expected frequency, for a $\Delta = 0.0592 - 0.0167 = 0.0425$. Table 250–8 lists some common examples of linkage disequilibrium. Several hypotheses have been put forth to explain linkage disequilibrium: (1) a selective advantage of a given haplotype, and (2) recent admixture of two inbred populations.

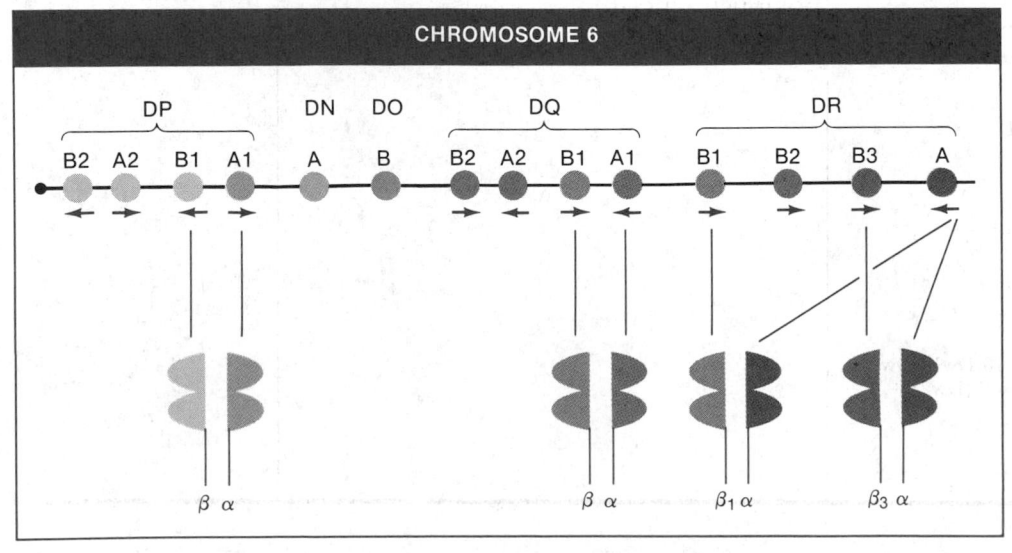

CHROMOSOME 6

FIGURE 250–4. The current concept of the HLA-D region, showing the organization of the three subregions, DP, DQ, and DR. DPA2, DPB2, DQA2, DQB2, and DRB2 are pseudogenes and are not expressed. Pairs of expressed genes (DPA1 and DPB1; DQA1 and DQB1; DRA and DRB1; and DRA and DRB3) which encode class II molecules are indicated. (In other haplotypes, DRA and DRB4 or DRA and DRB5 would be the pair expressed in place of DRA and DRB3.) DNA and DOB are not currently known to be transcribed in vivo. Arrows under genes give the direction of transcription (5' to 3').

TABLE 250–5. ASSOCIATIONS OF DRB1-ENCODED ANTIGENS WITH MOLECULES ENCODED BY DRB3, DRB4, OR DRB5 ALLELES

DRB3	DRB4	DRB5
DR3	DR4	DRw15
DR5	DR7	DRw16
DRw6	DR9	
DRw8		
DRw11 (5)		
DRw12 (5)		
DRw13 (w6)		
DRw14 (w6)		
DRw17 (3)		
DRw18 (3)		

TABLE 250–6. DQ-ASSOCIATED HLA-DR ANTIGENS

HLA-DQ Antigens	Associated HLA-DR Antigens
DQw1	DR1, DRw10, DRw13(w6), DRw14(w6), DRw15(2), DRw16(2)
DQw2	DR3, DR7
DQw3	DR4, DR7, DR9, DRw11(5), DRw12(5)
DQw4	DRw8, DRw15
DQw5	DR1, DRw10, DRw14(w6), DRw16(2)
DQw6	DRw15(2), DRw13(w6)
DQw7	DRw11(5), DRw12(5), DR4
DQw8	DR4
DQw9	DR7, DR9

HLA TYPING

All HLA class I and class II antigens are present on the class I and class II molecules but are defined and detected by different methods. The HLA-A, -B, -C, -DR, and -DQ antigens are defined, detected, and typed serologically by the microlymphocytotoxicity assay. Although some monoclonal antibodies are available for particular HLA antigens, the majority of serologic typing is still done with sera obtained from multiparous women. Typing for the HLA class I antigens is done on purified populations of lymphocytes. Typing of the HLA-DR and -DQ class II antigens is performed on purified populations of B lymphocytes. Alternatively, a two-color dye procedure is used which allows B cells to be distinguished from T cells. HLA-DP antigens are defined and typed by a cellular reaction known as the primed lymphocyte test (PLT), but DP molecules can be detected by monoclonal antibodies. As noted above, HLA-D antigens are defined and typed by the mixed leukocyte reaction (MLR).

The application of molecular biologic techniques to HLA typing has made possible new and more precise methods. The most promising technique is the polymerase chain reaction combined

TABLE 250–7. WELL-DEFINED ALLELES AT THE HLA-LINKED COMPLEMENT LOCI

C2	Bf	C4A	C4B
C2*C	Bf*F	C4A*2	C4B*1
C2*A	Bf*S	C4A*3	C4B*2
C2*Q0	Bf*F1	C4A*4	C4B*3
	Bf*S0.7	C4A*6	C4B*Q0
		C4A*Q0	

with oligonucleotide typing. The polymerase chain reaction is used to amplify the HLA gene(s) to be typed. Because each HLA allele has a unique nucleotide sequence that differentiates it from every other allele, it is possible to synthesize an oligonucleotide (or in some cases, a pair of oligonucleotides) which will hybridize only to this unique sequence. A set of tagged oligonucleotides corresponding to various alleles can therefore be used for HLA typing at the DNA level. Oligonucleotide typing is still in its infancy, and the vast majority of clinical HLA typing is currently done by conventional methodologies.

HLA typing is used primarily for determination of HLA compatibility prior to transplantation and platelet transfusion, for paternity testing, for forensic medicine, and for establishing HLA disease associations.

HLA AND DISEASE

The discovery in 1973 that ankylosing spondylitis (see Ch. 259) is highly associated with HLA-B27 stimulated an intense search for other HLA-disease associations. Well over 100 diseases from virtually all fields of medicine have now been associated with HLA. Despite this broad range of diseases, HLA-associated diseases for the most part share certain common characteristics. In general, these diseases have an hereditary tendency but weak penetrance and do not follow simple mendelian segregation. They lack a known etiologic agent and have an unknown pathophysiology. They are associated with immunologic abnormalities, and many of them are characterized as autoimmune. They follow subacute or chronic courses. Finally, they usually do not affect an individual's ability to bear offspring, thus allowing the HLA-associated diseases to persist in the species.

The association of HLA and disease has been demonstrated by both population and family studies. These two types of studies provide different information. Population studies allow a statistically significant correlation to be established between a particular HLA marker gene and a particular disease state. They do not constitute proof of genetic linkage between a disease susceptibility gene and the HLA marker gene because correlation does not necessarily imply genetic linkage. For example, if a disease susceptibility gene were not linked to HLA but required the presence of a particular HLA antigen for its expression, then an HLA-disease association would be demonstrated in population studies. In contrast, family studies provide an opportunity to determine linkage between a disease susceptibility gene and the HLA marker gene. Because population studies are easier to conduct, the majority of data on HLA and disease derive from this type of study.

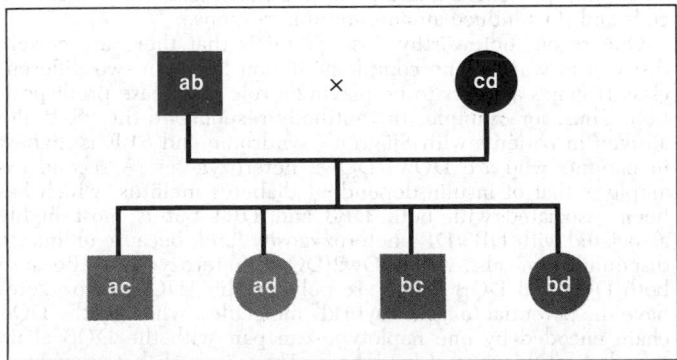

FIGURE 250–5. Inheritance of HLA haplotypes. A haplotype is the combination of alleles at each locus on a single chromosome and is almost always inherited as a unit. Haplotype designations are given by a, b, c, and d. Paternal haplotypes are a and b, and maternal haplotypes are c and d. The mating ab × cd can yield four possible combinations of haplotypes—ac, ad, bc, and bd. Statistically, 25 per cent of the offspring will be HLA identical (e.g., ac and ac), 25 per cent will be total HLA nonidentical (e.g., ac and bd), and 50 per cent will be HLA-haploidentical (e.g., ac and ad).

TABLE 250–8. EXAMPLES OF LINKAGE DISEQUILIBRIUM IN CAUCASIANS

Haplotypes (listed as antigen phenotypes)	$\Delta \, (\times 10^{-3})$
HLA-A1, B8	53.2
HLA-A2, B44 (12)	14.8
HLA-A3, B7	32.4
HLA-B8, DR3	61.3
HLA-B7, DR2	36.8
HLA-DR2, DQw1	93.6
HLA-DR3, DQw2	37.4
HLA-DR7, DQw2	96.7
HLA-DR4, DQw3	87.5
HLA-A1, B8, DR3	28.0
HLA-A3, B7, DR2	11.5

It should be noted that no HLA-disease association is absolute. The majority of individuals with a given disease-associated HLA antigen do not contract the disease, and a given HLA-associated disease can occur in individuals who lack the usual disease-associated HLA antigen. It is now widely accepted that a combination of a particular HLA antigen, other genetic influences, and environmental agents is necessary for the disease to be manifest.

The strength of the association of a particular disease with a particular HLA antigen is quantitated by calculating the relative risk (Table 250–9). The relative risk (RR) is defined by the formula $RR = (P^+ \times C^-)/(P^- \times C^+)$, where P^+ is the number of patients possessing the disease-associated HLA antigen, C^- is the number of controls lacking that particular HLA antigen, P^- is the number of patients lacking that HLA antigen, and C^+ is the number of controls possessing that HLA antigen. The higher the relative risk above 1, the stronger the association between the HLA antigen and the disease. The relative risk can be stated as the chance of developing the HLA-associated disease for an individual with the disease-associated HLA antigen compared to an individual without that HLA antigen. Because there is usually a significant difference in the frequency of a given antigen among different racial groups, it is mandatory to compare a patient group with a control population of the same race. Thus, for example, HLA-B27 is found in 88 per cent of American white patients with ankylosing spondylitis and approximately 8 per cent of American white controls, yielding a relative risk of approximately 85. In contrast, HLA-B27 is found in 48 per cent of American black patients with ankylosing spondylitis but in only 2 per cent of American black controls, giving a relative risk of 45. Table 250–9 gives the relative risks for selected significant HLA-disease associations.

Because of the phenomenon of linkage disequilibrium and the order in which the HLA class I and class II antigens were defined, a particular disease may have appeared to be associated with a particular antigen at a given HLA locus when in actuality it is more highly associated with a particular antigen at a different HLA locus. Thus, for example, the alleles encoding HLA-DQw2, -DR3, and -B8 are known to be in linkage disequilibrium. Before

TABLE 250–9. SELECTED HLA AND DISEASE ASSOCIATIONS IN WHITE PATIENTS

Disease	Antigen	Approximate Relative Risk
Ankylosing spondylitis	B27	81.8
Reiter's syndrome	B27	40.4
Acute anterior uveitis	B27	7.98
Reactive arthritis (*Yersinia*)	B27	17.6
Rheumatoid arthritis	DR4	6.4
Juvenile rheumatoid arthritis		
Seropositive	DR4	7.2
	Dw4	25.8
	Dw14	47
	Dw4/Dw14	116
Pauciarticular	DR5	2.9
	DPw2	3.9
Systemic lupus erythematosus	DR3	2.7
Behçet's disease	B5	3.3
Sjögren's syndrome	DR3	5.6
High-titer anti-SS-A antibody	DQw1/DQw2	—
Graves' disease	DR3	3.8
Insulin-dependent diabetes mellitus	DR3	3.0
Celiac disease	DR3	13.3
Psoriasis vulgaris	B13	4.5
	B17	3.1
	Cw6	7.2
Pemphigus vulgaris	DR4	21.4
Dermatitis herpetiformis	DR3	18.2
Idiopathic hemochromatosis	A3	6.6
	B14	3.7
Goodpasture's syndrome	DR2	19.8
Multiple sclerosis	DR2	2.8
Myasthenia gravis (without thymoma)	B8	3.3
Narcolepsy	DR2	129

any of the HLA class II antigens were well defined, celiac disease was associated with HLA-B8. The definition of the DR antigens allowed a stronger association to be established between celiac disease and HLA-DR3. The subsequent definition of the HLA-DQ antigens suggested an even more significant association between celiac disease and HLA-DQw2. With the application of molecular biology techniques to the study of HLA and disease associations, restriction endonuclease fragments have been identified in the HLA-DP region which yield even more significant associations. Thus, for example, it has recently been reported that 90 per cent of patients with celiac disease have a genomic DNA fragment that can be detected using a DP β chain cDNA probe. Individuals with this fragment have a relative risk of 46 for contracting celiac disease.

In addition, because of linkage disequilibrium, a number of diseases have been associated with what has been termed extended haplotypes. Two such examples are the association of C2 deficiency with the haplotype A*2501, B*1801, C2*QO, BF*S, C4A*4, C4B*2, DRB1*1501, and systemic lupus with the haplotype A*0101, B*0801, BF*S, C2*C, C4A*QO, C4B*1, DRB1*0301.

Several hypotheses have been suggested to explain HLA-disease associations. Four of these apply to diseases associated with both class I and class II antigens. First, HLA molecules may act as receptors for etiologic agents. If only particular HLA molecules can act as receptors for agents that cause particular diseases, then the HLA-disease association would result. The second hypothesis suggests that the antigen-binding cleft of only a particular HLA molecule can accept the processed antigenic peptide fragment that is ultimately responsible for causing disease. The third hypothesis holds that the actual disease susceptibility genes are not the HLA genes themselves but rather T-cell receptor α and β chain genes. This hypothesis suggests that because a particular T-cell receptor α and β chain combination which predisposes to disease recognizes only a particular antigenic peptide fragment in the context of a particular HLA antigen, an *apparent* association with that HLA antigen is seen. The fourth hypothesis, termed the molecular mimicry hypothesis, states that the disease-associated HLA antigen is immunologically similar to the etiologic agent for the disease and then postulates one of two alternatives. The first alternative suggests that because of the similarity of the etiologic agent and the HLA antigen, no immune response is mounted and therefore the etiologic agent can cause disease unabated. The second alternative suggests that a vigorous immune response is mounted against the etiologic agent, but because of the similarity of the etiologic agent and the HLA antigen, the immune response is turned against the HLA antigen and the resulting autoimmune response produces disease.

The majority of HLA-associated diseases have been associated with the class II antigens. The last hypothesis relates only to class II–associated diseases and suggests that class II molecules aberrantly expressed by cells which normally lack class II molecules may present self-antigenic peptide fragments to CD4+ T cells and thus induce an autoimmune response.

One recent noteworthy observation is that there are certain diseases in which gene complementation between two different class II genes appears to be playing a role in disease predisposition. Thus, for example, the antibody response to the SS-A (Ro) antigen in patients with Sjögren's syndrome and SLE is highest in patients who are DQw1/DQw2 heterozygotes. A second example is that of insulin-dependent diabetes mellitus, which has been associated with both DR3 and DR4 but is most highly associated with DR3/DR4 heterozygosity, and, because of linkage disequilibrium, also with DQw2/DQw8 heterozygosity. Because both DQα and DQβ chains are polymorphic, DQ heterozygotes have the potential to form "hybrid" molecules, whereby the DQα chain encoded by one haplotype can pair with the DQβ chain encoded by the second haplotype. Thus, in such heterozygotes, it is possible to form DQw2α/DQw8β and DQw8α/DQw2β molecules. It is postulated that this "hybrid" molecule can present antigenic peptide fragments better than either "parental" molecule to the appropriate CD4+ T cell.

Recently, it has been found that individuals who are predisposed to insulin-dependent diabetes mellitus lack an aspartic acid residue at position 57 of the DQβ chain (i.e., the DQw8 β chain), whereas individuals who are protected from this disease possess an aspartic acid residue at this position (i.e., the DQw7 β chain).

(It should be noted that DQw7 and DQw8 are both splits of DQw3 and have very similar sequences.) Position 57 is found in the α helical portion of the class II peptide-binding cleft. Thus, a single amino acid change in a crucial portion of a class II molecule can dramatically alter disease predisposition.

Finally, it has become apparent that certain regions of the class II molecule, rather than the entire class II molecule, may actually be the elements that confer disease predisposition. These regions have been termed *epitopes*. It has been found that certain DR4 and DR1 class II molecules predispose an individual to rheumatoid arthritis (see Ch. 258). On further analysis, these predisposing DR4 and DR1 molecules were found to share a common amino acid sequence in the α helix of the β chain, and it is thought that this amino acid sequence confers predisposition to rheumatoid arthritis. The fact that two different types of DR molecules share this common disease-predisposing epitope partially explains the lack of absolute HLA-disease associations.

Other mechanisms besides those noted above have also been suggested. It should be emphasized that different mechanisms may be operating to predispose to different diseases and that more than one mechanism may be operating concurrently to produce disease.

McDevitt HO: The HLA system and its relation to disease. Hosp Practice 20:57, 1985. *A clearly written introduction for the neophyte.*
Moller G (ed.): Molecular genetics of class I and II MHC antigens. Parts I and II. Immunol Rev, Vol. 84 & 85. Copenhagen, Munksgaard, 1985. *An in-depth discussion of the organization and basis for polymorphism of the HLA genes.*
Schwartz BD: Infectious agents, immunity, and rheumatic diseases. Arthritis Rheum 33:457, 1990. *A clear discussion of the role of HLA molecules in antigen presentation and the models for HLA-disease associations.*
Tiwari JL, Terasaki PI (eds.): HLA and Disease Associations. New York, Springer-Verlag, 1985. *A comprehensive volume describing virtually all known HLA-disease associations. An excellent referral source.*

251 Drug Allergy

Charles E. Reed

An allergic cause of a drug reaction is suspected when an inflammatory lesion characteristic of those provoked by immunologic mechanisms follows administration of the drug. The variety of drug allergies gives the initial impression that any drug can cause any reaction; in fact, distinct patterns are the rule. Any particular drug tends to cause a similar reaction in different subjects. Typical examples include urticaria after penicillin, lymphocytic pneumonitis after nitrofurantoin, or contact dermatitis from an ointment containing ethylenediamine. Allergic drug reactions need to be distinguished from expected side effects, idiosyncratic reactions of unknown cause, toxic reactions, psychophysiologic reactions, and also from immunologic manifestations of the underlying disease. A further distinction is made between allergic inflammation initiated by a ligand reacting with an antibody or a specifically reacting lymphocyte and similar inflammation initiated by a pharmacologic reaction. Unfortunately these distinctions are not always easily made at the bedside, and there are few reliable clinical or laboratory tests.

Many patients relate a history of allergy to one or more drugs, often without an objective basis. Usually this history can be accepted and serves as a deterrent to excessive drug therapy. Sometimes, however, it is important to evaluate the possibility of allergy to a potentially life-saving drug for which there is no substitute, since many patients with a history of a reaction will tolerate the drug, particularly if several years have passed. If the allergy is still present, taking the drug can be disastrous with fatality from anaphylaxis, Stevens-Johnson syndrome, exfoliative dermatitis, interstitial pneumonitis, or vasculitis. A decision for a particular course of action often rests on judicious weighing of the potential benefits and risks rather than on a definitive diagnosis.

INCIDENCE AND PREDISPOSING FACTORS. Allergic reactions constituted about 6 per cent of all adverse drug reactions in 1968. The frequency is less today because drugs associated with a high frequency of reaction have been displaced by safer ones.

Several predisposing factors exist. Previous drug allergy to the same or a related drug is most important, and the frequency of allergy increases with multiple courses of treatment. Topical administration is the route most likely to sensitize; oral administration, least; and parenteral, intermediate. Parenteral administration provokes more severe reactions, especially anaphylaxis. Children are less likely than adults to react, and men less than women. Persons with history of atopic allergy may be at increased risk of anaphylaxis or urticaria but not of other kinds of allergic drug reactions. Toxic epidermal necrolysis from sulfonamides and several other serious drug allergies are associated with particular HLA phenotypes. The antigenic determinant in drug allergy is often a metabolite rather than the drug itself; genetic differences in drug metabolism therefore influence allergic reactions. For example, persons with reduced acetyltransferase activity were found to be more likely to develop drug-induced systemic lupus erythematosus from procainamide.

MECHANISMS. Foreign macromolecules acting as complete antigens are the most likely to sensitize, eliciting an IgE or IgG antibody response that on a subsequent administration causes anaphylaxis, serum sickness, or vasculitis. Classic serum sickness after injections of large amounts of rabbit or horse serum required large amounts of antigen and relatively high concentrations of circulating immune complexes. Most episodes of urticaria, fever, and arthralgia after relatively small doses involve a combination of IgE- and IgG-initiated events.

Low molecular weight drugs elicit an immune response only after reacting covalently with proteins. This hapten may be the drug itself or a metabolite. The hapten-protein carrier then functions as the complete antigen, both initiating sensitization and eliciting the reaction. An allergic reaction requires a multivalent ligand to cross-link antibody molecules either in fluid phase or bound to cell surface receptors. Univalent haptens actually inhibit cross-linking by occupying the antigen-binding sites. Some chemicals may react with host proteins in such a way that the tertiary structure is altered and the new antigenic determinant is not the hapten itself but the altered structure of the host protein. Drug allergy may take any of the forms of allergic reaction described in Part XVIII. The mechanisms of immune defense and hypersensitivity, like many other biologic functions, exhibit redundancy such that a drug reaction may involve more than one allergic mechanism at the same time. The fact that the hapten often is a drug metabolite may explain the characteristic involvement of some particular organ where the metabolism occurs; alternatively, the hapten may react with a specific organ protein to account for the location of the reaction.

PREVENTION. Avoiding drugs with high sensitizing potential reduces frequency of drug allergy. Interrupted treatment is more likely to sensitize than is continuous treatment, especially with insulin. Beef insulin is more allergenic than pork or human insulin. Recurrence of drug allergy can be reduced by taking a careful history; by exercising a high index of suspicion when fever, rash, or organ damage occurs during treatment; by careful recording of manifestations of drug reactions and diagnosis in the chart when they do occur; and by proper instruction of the patient.

DIAGNOSIS. The history and physical examination provide the essential information for pattern recognition. A key point of the history is the time course of the reaction. Anaphylactic reactions follow within minutes; drug fever, within an hour or two; contact dermatitis, in a day or two; but cholestatic jaundice requires several days or a week. The character of the lesion is also important. Ampicillin characteristically causes a morbilliform rash that may be delayed for 2 days after the drug is stopped. All penicillins may cause urticaria within 10 minutes, but the urticaria may not occur for several days. This distinction is important because the immediate reactions are more likely to be associated with anaphylaxis. A physician observing a drug reaction should record the physical findings for future use. For example, by history alone it is difficult to distinguish between laryngeal edema from anaphylaxis and the hyperventilation syndrome, but the presence of stridor and swelling of pharyngeal or laryngeal

TABLE 251–1. ALLERGIC DRUG REACTIONS

I. Systemic

A. Anaphylaxis

1. Macromolecules
   Allergenic extracts
   Dextrans (including iron dextran)
   Enzymes
   Asparaginase
   Chymopapain
   Trypsin
   Heparin
   Hormones (ACTH, insulin, etc.)
   Human gamma globulin
   Protamine
   Vaccines
   Antisera
2. Diagnostic agents
   Fluorescein
   Iodinated contrast media
3. Antimicrobials
   5-Aminosalicylic acid
   Amphotericin B
   Cephalosporins
   Cinoxacin
   Clindamycin
   Ethambutol
   Kanamycin
   Lincomycin
   Nalidixic acid
   Penicillins
   Streptomycin
   Sulfonamides
   Tetracyclines
   Vancomycin
4. Other drugs and other nonsteroidal anti-inflammatory drugs
   Aspirin
   Benzyl alcohol
   Bleomycin
   Cisplatin
   Colchicine
   Cromolyn
   Cytarabine
   Dantrolene
   Ethylenediamine
   Etoposide
   Flucytosine
   Glucocorticoids
   Indomethacin
   Local anesthetics
   Mephyton
   Meprobamate
   Niacin
   Opiates
   Pentamidine
   Probenecid
   Procainamide
   Sulfite
   Thiopental
   Tolmetin
   Triamterene
   Tubocurarine and other muscle-relaxing agents
   Vitamin B_{12}

B. Serum sickness

1. Macromolecules
   Dextrans
   Heparin
   Hormones (insulin, ACTH, etc.)
   Vaccines
   Antisera
2. Antimicrobials
   Cephalosporins
   Griseofulvin
   Lincomycin
   Minocycline
   Penicillins
   Streptomycin
   Sulfonamides
3. Other Drugs
   Barbiturates
   Hydantoins
   Hydralazine
   Phenylbutazone
   Procarbazine
   Propylthiouracil

C. Drug fever

1. Antimicrobials
   5-Aminosalicylic acid
   Cephalosporins
   Chloramphenicol
   Erythromycin
   Isoniazid
   Kanamycin
   Nitrofurantoin
   Norfloxacin
   Penicillins
   Pyrazinamide
   Quinine
   Streptomycin
   Sulfonamides
   Tetracyclines
2. Other drugs
   Allopurinol
   Captopril
   Heparin
   Hydantoins
   Hydralazine
   Hydrochlorothiazide
   Methyldopa
   Penicillamine
   Phenobarbital
   Pneumococcal vaccine
   Procainamide
   Propylthiouracil
   Quinidine

D. Vasculitis

   Allopurinol
   Atenolol
   Busulfan
   Carbamazepine
   Colchicine
   Diphenhydramine
   Ethionamide
   Furosemide
   Hydantoins
   Hydroxyurea
   Ibuprofen
   Indomethacin
   Isoniazid
   Meprobamate
   Methamphetamine
   Naproxen
   Penicillins
   Phenothiazines
   Phenylbutazone
   Propranolol
   Propylthiouracil
   Streptokinase
   Sulfonamides
   Tetracyclines
   Thiazide diuretics
   Vaccines

E. Systemic lupus erythematosus syndrome

   5-Aminosalicylic acid
   Chloroquine
   Chlorpromazine
   Ethosuximide
   Griseofulvin
   Hydralazine
   Isoniazid
   Methyldopa
   Nitrofurantoin
   Penicillins
   Penicillamine
   Phenytoin
   Procainamide
   Propylthiouracil
   Quinidine
   Tetracycline
   Tocainide
   Trimethadione

II. Skin

A. Urticaria and angioedema

1. Antimicrobials
   5-Aminosalicylic acid
   Aminoglycosides
   Cephalosporins
   Ethambutol
   Isoniazid
   Metronidazole
   Miconazole
   Nalidixic acid
   Penicillins
   Quinine
   Rifampin
   Spectinomycin
   Sulfonamides
2. Other drugs
   Asparaginase
   Aspirin and other nonsteroidal anti-inflammatory drugs
   Calcitonin
   Chloral hydrate
   Chlorambucil
   Cimetidine
   Cyclophosphamide
   Daunorubicin
   Doxorubicin
   Ergotamine
   Ethchlorvynol
   Ethosuximide
   Ethylenediamine
   Glucocorticoids
   Melphalan
   Penicillamine
   Phenothiazines
   Procainamide
   Procarbazine
   Quinidine
   Tartrazine
   Thiazide diuretics
   Thiotepa

B. Morbilliform-maculopapular rash

1. Antimicrobials
   5-Aminosalicylic acid
   Cephalosporins
   Erythromycin
   Gentamicin
   Penicillins
   Streptomycin
   Sulfonamides
2. Other drugs
   Allopurinol
   Barbiturates
   Captopril
   Coumarin
   Gold salts
   Hydantoins
   Thiazide diuretics

C. Toxic epidermal necrolysis and erythroderma and exfoliative dermatitis

   Allopurinol
   Amikacin
   Captopril
   Carbamazepine
   Chloral hydrate
   Chlorambucil
   Chloroquine
   Chlorpromazine
   Cyclosporine
   Diltiazem
   Ethambutol
   Ethylenediamine
   Glutethimide
   Gold salts
   Griseofulvin
   Hydantoins
   Hydroxychloroquine
   Minoxidil
   Nifedipine
   Nonsteroidal anti-inflammatory agents
   Penicillin
   Phenobarbital
   Rifampin
   Spironolactone
   Streptomycin
   Sulfonamides
   Trimethadione
   Trimethoprim
   Tocainide
   Vancomycin
   Verapamil

D. Erythema multiforme

   Acetaminophen
   Barbiturates
   Carbamazepine
   Chloroquine
   Chlorpropamide
   Clindamycin
   Ethambutol
   Ethosuximide
   Gold salts
   Hydantoins
   Hydralazine
   Hydroxyurea
   Mechlorethamine
   Meclofenamate
   Penicillins
   Phenolphthalein
   Phenylbutazone
   Rifampin
   Streptomycin
   Sulfonamides
   Sulfonylureas
   Sulindac
   Vaccines

E. Photosensitive

1. Topical
   Fluorouracil
   Hexachlorophene
   Para-aminobenzoic acid esters
   Promethazine
   Sulfanilamide
2. Systemic
   Carbamazepine
   Chlorpromazine
   Griseofulvin
   Imipramine
   Lincomycin
   Nalidixic acid
   Naproxen
   Norfloxacin
   Phenothiazines
   Piroxicam

TABLE 251–1. ALLERGIC DRUG REACTIONS *Continued*

2. Systemic *Continued*
  Quinethazone
  Sulfonamides
  Sulfonylureas
  Thiazide diuretics
  Triamterene
F. *Fixed drug eruptions*
  Acetaminophen
  5-Aminosalicylic acid
  Aspirin
  Barbiturates
  Benzodiazepines
  Chloroquine
  Dapsone
  Dimenhydrinate
  Diphenhydramine
  Gold salts
  Hydralazine
  Hyoscine
  Ibuprofen
  Iodides
  Meprobamate
  Methanamine
  Metronidazole
  Penicillins
  Phenobarbital
  Phenolphthalein
  Phenothiazines
  Phenylbutazone
  Procarbazine
  Pseudoephedrine
  Quinine
  Saccharin
  Streptomycin
  Sulfonamides
  Tetracyclines
G. *Erythema nodosum*
  Bromides
  Oral contraceptives
  Penicillin
  Sulfonamides
H. *Contact dermatitis*
  Ambroxol
  Amikacin
  Antihistamines
  Bacitracin
  Benzalkonium chloride
  Benzocaine
  Benzyl alcohol
  Cetyl alcohol
  Chloramphenicol
  Chlorpromazine
  Clioquinol
  Colophony
  Ethylenediamine
  Fluorouracil
  Formaldehyde
  Gentamycin
  Glucocorticoids
  Glutaraldehyde
  Heparin
  Hexachlorophene
  Iodochlorhydroxyquin
  Lanolin
  Local anesthetics
  Minoxidil
  Naftin
  Neomycin
  Nitrofurazone

  Opiates
  Para-aminobenzoic
    acid
  Parabens
  Penicillins
  Phenothiazines
  Proflavine
  Propylene glycol
  Streptomycin
  Sulfonamides
  Thimerosal
  Timolol
III. **Lung**
  A. *Asthma*
    Aspirin and other
      nonsteroidal anti-
      inflammatory drugs
    Cromolyn
    Sulfite
    Tartrazine
    Occupational expo-
      sures to:
      Cephalosporins
      Glutaraldehyde
      Pancreatic enzymes
      Papain
      Penicillins
      Psyllium
      Thimerosal
  B. *Eosinophilic*
    pneumonitis
    5-Aminosalicylic acid
    Azathioprine
    Captopril
    Carbamazepine
    Chlorpropamide
    Cromolyn
    Desipramine
    Gold salts
    Imipramine
    Nitrofurantoin
    Penicillins
    Phenytoin
    Sulfonamides
    L-Tryptophan
  C. *Fibrotic and pleural*
    reactions
    Bleomycin
    Busulfan
    Cyclophosphamide
    Gold salts
    Hydralazine
    Hydrochlorothiazide
    Melphalan
    Methotrexate
    Methysergide
    Mitomycin
    Nitrofurantoin
    Procarbazine
IV. **Liver**
  A. *Cholestatic*
    Chlorzoxazone
    Erythromycin estolate
    Ethchlorvynol
    Imipramine
    Nalidixic acid
    Nitrofurantoin
    Phenothiazines
    Sulfamethoxazole

  Sulfonylureas
  Troleandomycin
  B. *Hepatocellular*
    5-Aminosalicylic acid
    Amphotericin B
    Azapropazone
    Ethacrynic acid
    Furosemide
    Gold salts
    Griseofulvin
    Halothane
    Hydantoins
    Isoniazid
    Methyldopa
    Monoamine oxidase
      inhibitors
    Nitrofurantoin
    Propylthiouracil
    Pyrazinamide
    Quinidine
    Rifampin
    Sulfonamides
    Trimethadione
  C. *Chronic active hepatitis*
    Methyldopa
    Nitrofurantoin
V. **Kidney**
  A. *Glomerulitis*
    Allopurinol
    Captopril
    Gold salts
    Nonsteroidal anti-
      inflammatory agents
    Penicillamine
    Penicillins
    Phenytoin
    Probenecid
    Sulfonamides
    Thiazide diuretics
  B. *Interstitial nephritis*
    Allopurinol
    Aztreonam
    Captopril
    Carbamazepine
    Cephalosporins
    Chloramphenicol
    Cimetidine
    Ciprofloxacin
    Colistin
    Furosemide
    Minocycline
    Nonsteroidal anti-
      inflammatory drugs
    Penicillins, especially
      methicillin
    Phenytoin
    Polymyxin B
    Rifampin
    Sulfonamides
    Tetracycline
    Thiazide diuretics
VI. **Bone Marrow and Blood Cells**
  A. *Bone marrow aplasia*
    Chloramphenicol
    Gold salts
    Mephenytoin
    Penicillamine
    Phenylbutazone
    Trimethadione

  B. *Anemia*
    Acetaminophen
    5-Aminosalicylic acid
    Captopril
    Cephalosporins
    Chlorpromazine
    Cisplatin
    Hydantoins
    Ibuprofen
    Insulin
    Isoniazid
    Levodopa
    Mefenamic acid
    Melphalan
    Methyldopa
    Methysergide
    Penicillins
    Quinidine
    Quinine
    Rifampin
    Sulfonamides
    Sulfonylureas
  C. *Thrombocytopenia*
    Acetaminophen
    Acetazolamide
    Acetylsalicylic acid
    5-Aminosalicylic acid
    Carbamazepine
    Chloramphenicol
    Chlorpheniramine
    Cimetidine
    Digitoxin
    Diltiazem
    Ethchlorvynol
    Gold salts
    Heparin
    Hydantoins
    Isoniazid
    Levodopa
    Meprobamate
    Methyldopa
    Penicillamine
    Phenylbutazone
    Procainamide
    Quinidine
    Quinine
    Ranitidine
    Rauwolfia alkaloids
    Rifampin
    Sulfonamides
    Sulfonylureas
    Thiazide diuretics
  D. *Granulocytopenia*
    Captopril
    Cephalosporins
    Chloral hydrate
    Chlorpropamide
    Penicillins (semisyn-
      thetic)
    Phenothiazines
    Phenylbutazone
    Phenytoin
    Procainamide
    Propranolol
    Tolbutamide
  E. *Lymphoid hyperplasia*
    Phenytoin
    Mephenytoin

mucosa makes the distinction clear. Distinction between a drug reaction and an immunologic event from the underlying disease is important. For instance, many children with viral respiratory infections have transient urticaria that can be mistaken for a penicillin rash. Or, on the first or second day of penicillin treatment a patient with endocarditis may have a macular hem-

orrhagic rash and fever, reflecting a reaction to antigens released from the bacteria rather than drug allergy.

Some of the most important patterns of drug reactions are summarized in Table 251–1. For some of the drugs on this list there is no proof that the drug actually caused the reaction. The association is plausible but not certain.

Skin tests may be helpful in predicting anaphylaxis from macromolecules and are usually positive in patients with allergy to foreign serum proteins, insulin, vaccines, and similar materials. With the important exception of penicillin, skin or in vitro allergy tests with low molecular weight drugs are not reliable for detecting anaphylactic (IgE-mediated) drug allergy, although positive skin tests occur after anaphylaxis from muscle-relaxing agents, thiopental, cisplatin, and a few other drugs. Patch tests with single components are useful for identifying contact allergens. Ethylenediamine, one of the ingredients of many creams and ointments, is currently the most frequently encountered contactant. Attempts to adapt lymphocyte transformation tests for diagnosis of drug allergy have been unsuccessful. Eosinophilia, when otherwise unexplained, provides evidence of allergy. Deliberate trial of small doses of the drug strictly for diagnostic purposes is unwise and unnecessary. It may be indicated as a precaution in situations in which the diagnosis of drug allergy is uncertain and no chemically unrelated substitute is available for an urgently needed drug.

MANAGEMENT. In addition to stopping use of the offending drug, symptomatic or supportive treatment of the reaction may be indicated. As a rule it is unwise to attempt to continue using the offending drug under a protective shield of antihistamines or glucocorticoids, although occasional desperate situations may justify an exception. The emergency treatment of anaphylaxis is described in Ch. 247.

SPECIFIC DRUG ALLERGIES. Penicillin. Penicillin is one of the most common drugs causing allergy, and being the most fully understood it serves as a model for other drugs. Penicillin reactions include anaphylaxis, urticaria, vasculitis, dermatomyositis, maculopapular rashes, hemolytic anemia, drug fever, interstitial nephritis, pneumonitis, and contact dermatitis. Airborne penicillin can cause asthma in workers who produce or use it. The nature of the reaction is determined not only by the specific metabolite that becomes the hapten but also by the carrier molecule. For example, the penicilloyl determinant commonly evokes IgE antibody in cases of urticaria, but it also evokes IgG, and after complexing with red cell–membrane protein, it may be responsible for hemolytic anemia during intravenous penicillin treatment. Many patients who claim to be allergic to penicillin tolerate it without adverse effect. In such patients, treatment with more expensive or toxic antibiotics would be unnecessary. Reliable tests are available for predicting which patients with a history of penicillin allergy are at risk of immediate allergic reactions. Cautious skin testing with dilute solutions of the antibiotic itself and with commercially available benzylpenicilloyl-polylysine (Pre-Pen) will provide guidance. If skin test reactions are negative to these reagents and to the "minor" determinants (the plain drug, penicilloate, and penilloate), the probability of a mild allergic reaction is about 2 per cent, no higher than in subjects receiving penicillin for the first time. The minor determinants are as yet available only in research settings, but only about 7 per cent of patients react to this reagent alone. Therefore, for patients who give a history of a penicillin reaction and need a penicillin drug for a serious infection, tests with the available reagents interpreted in the light of the history will allow appropriate treatment to proceed. The skin test with penicilloyl-polylysine begins with a prick of the 6.0×10^{-5} M solution, and, if negative in 20 minutes, one proceeds to intradermal testing. Skin testing with the penicillin solution starts with a prick test with a solution containing 6000 units per milliliter of penicillin G or 4 mg per milliliter of other penicillins. Similar testing with cephalosporin is feasible. The frequency of reactions to cephalosporins in patients allergic to penicillin is controversial.

Desensitization can be undertaken when skin test reactions are positive or when there are other reasons for suspecting an appreciable risk of anaphylaxis but the patient has life-threatening infection with an organism for which no alternative antibiotic is available. Oral desensitization is preferred, except in comatose patients when the same principle can be followed parenterally (Table 251–2).

Radiographic Contrast Agents. Iodinated contrast agents injected for radiographic examination are the most common cause of anaphylactic drug reactions. These reactions are not truly anaphylactic, for these materials do not combine with proteins to act as haptens but rather appear to act pharmacologically. As yet these reactions are not fully understood, but it is known that these drugs activate complement and release histamine, probably because they are hyperosmolar. Skin tests or small test doses do not predict reactivity. Persons who have had a previous reaction are at increased risk of a similar reaction from a subsequent injection. When a second examination is necessary, the patient should be given prednisone 50 mg every 6 hours for three doses, ending 1 hour before the procedure, and an antihistamine shortly before. Alternatively, one of the non-ionic agents with low osmolality can be used.

Local Anesthetics. Most adverse reactions to local anesthetics are either toxic or psychophysiologic, but allergic reactions can occur. The most frequent is contact dermatitis; anaphylaxis is more serious although quite rare. It has not yet been determined that skin testing with local anesthetics is useful in predicting anaphylaxis in patients with a history of reactions to local anesthetic. When local anesthesia is needed, an anesthetic as unrelated as possible to the one suspected of causing the reaction should be chosen, and a small test dose should be given first. Lidocaine seems to carry a low risk of allergy.

Aspirin and Other Nonsteroidal Anti-inflammatory Drugs. Shortly after its introduction in the late nineteenth century, aspirin was observed to provoke severe asthma in some asthmatic patients. Such patients react in the same way to other nonsteroidal anti-inflammatory agents. The typical reaction consists of acute bronchospasm, rhinorrhea, and occasionally urticaria. Most of the asthmatic patients who react to these agents also have nasal polyps and lack IgE-mediated allergy to common airborne allergens. In some patients with chronic urticaria but no respiratory disease, urticaria is the only manifestation of the reaction. The mechanism of this adverse response to aspirin is not allergic; extensive search for IgE antibodies has been unrewarding. Rather, it is presumably due to the inhibition of cyclo-oxygenase, but the molecular mechanism is still undefined. Patients who have reacted to aspirin need not avoid other salicylates (except methylsalicylate), and salicylate-free diets are unnecessary. A very few aspirin-reactive subjects react similarly to tartrazine (FD&C yellow No. 5) added to foods or drugs. Skin tests to aspirin and similar agents are not useful and may be dangerous. No biochemical tests are available for diagnosis.

Angiotensin-Converting Enzyme Inhibitors. These drugs may provoke cough and increase the severity and frequency of episodes of angioedema and asthma, presumably by prolonging the action of bradykinin or other vasoactive peptides.

EOSINOPHILIC SYNDROMES. Adulterated cooking oil and contaminated L-tryptophane capsules have been associated with a multisystem systemic inflammatory illness involving skin, muscle, and lung and characterized by eosinophilia of 1000 to 10,000 cells per 10^{-6} liter. Neither the specific causative agent nor the mechanism of the allergic inflammation has yet been identified.

TABLE 251–2. ORAL DESENSITIZATION PROTOCOL FOR PENICILLIN

Dose*	Units	Route†
1	100	P.O.
2	200	P.O.
3	400	P.O.
4	800	P.O.
5	1,600	P.O.
6	3,200	P.O.
7	6,400	P.O.
8	12,800	P.O.
9	25,000	P.O.
10	50,000	P.O.
11	100,000	P.O.
12	200,000	P.O.
13	400,000	P.O.
14	200,000	S.C.
15	400,000	S.C.
16	800,000	S.C.
17	1,000,000	I.M.

*Interval between doses, 15 min.

†P.O. = oral; S.C. = subcutaneous; I.M. = intramuscular.

From Sullivan TJ, Yecies LD, Shaty GS, et al.: Desensitization of patients allergic to penicillin using orally administered β-lactam antibiotics. J Allergy Clin Immunol 69:276, 1982.

American Academy of Pediatrics Committee on Drugs: "Inactive" ingredients in pharmaceutical products. Pediatrics 76:635, 1985. *A useful source of information about allergic reactions to drugs caused by ingredients other than the active drug itself.*

DeSwait RD: Drug allergy. *In* Patterson R (ed.): Allergic Diseases, Diagnosis and Management, 3rd ed. Philadelphia, J. B. Lippincott Company, 1985. *Detailed, well-referenced review of the subject.*

Moscicki RA, Sockin SM, Corsello BF, et al.: Anaphylaxis during induction of general anesthesia: Subsequent evaluation. J Allergy Clin Immunol 86:325–332, 1990. *Description of procedure for diagnosis and management of this life-threatening reaction.*

Rieder MJ, Uetrecht J, Shear NH, et al.: Diagnosis of sulfonamide hypersensitivity reactions by in-vitro "rechallenge" with hydroxylamine metabolites. Ann Intern Med 110(4):286–289, 1989. *An excellent illustration of the direction of contemporary research in drug allergy.*

Sullivan TJ: Drug allergy. *In* Middleton EJ, Ellis EF, Reed CE, et al. (eds.): Allergy Principles and Practice, 3rd ed. St. Louis, C. V. Mosby Company, 1988.

Weist ME, Adkinson NF: Immediate hypersensitivity reactions to penicillins and related antibiotics. Clin Allergy 18:15–40, 1988. *Review of information about the new antibiotics.*

252 Mastocytosis

Dean D. Metcalfe

Mastocytosis is a rare disease characterized by an abnormal increase in mast cells in the bone marrow, liver, spleen, lymph nodes, gastrointestinal tract, and skin. Mastocytosis can present in any age group and demonstrates a slight male predominance (1.5:1.0). The prevalence of the disease is unknown. Familial occurrence is unusual.

The disease is divided into four distinct clinicopathologic entities on the basis of clinical presentation, pathologic findings, and prognosis (Table 252–1). Patients in the first category have a good prognosis, whereas patients in the other three groups do poorly. Indolent mastocytosis is divided into two subgroups: those with isolated skin involvement and those with systemic disease. In most cases such patients gradually accrue more mast cells with progression of symptoms but can be managed successfully for decades using medications that provide symptomatic relief. The second most common form of mastocytosis is that associated with a hematologic disorder. In this group, examination of the bone marrow and peripheral blood reveals the hematologic abnormality. The prognosis in these patients is determined by the prognosis of the associated hematologic disorder. The third category of mast cell disease is mast cell leukemia; it is the rarest form and has the most fulminant behavior. Mast cell leukemia is distinguished from the other categories by its unique pathologic and clinical picture. The peripheral blood smear shows immature mast cells. The fourth category of patients has an aggressive form of mastocytosis; these individuals have poor prognostic features but do not have a distinctive hematologic disorder or mast cell leukemia. A subset of patients with aggressive mastocytosis have a distinct syndrome that has been termed lymphadenopathic mastocytosis with eosinophilia because of the pronounced eosin-

TABLE 252–1. CLASSIFICATION OF MASTOCYTOSIS

I. Indolent mastocytosis
  A. Skin only
    1. Urticaria pigmentosa
    2. Diffuse cutaneous mastocytosis
  B. Systemic
    1. Marrow
    2. Gastrointestinal
    3. ± Urticaria pigmentosa
II. Mastocytosis with associated hematologic disorder (± urticaria pigmentosa)
  A. Dysmyelopoietic syndrome
  B. Myeloproliferative disorders
  C. Acute nonlymphocytic leukemia
  D. Malignant lymphoma
  E. Chronic neutropenia
III. Mast cell leukemia
IV. Aggressive mastocytosis

TABLE 252–2. REPRESENTATIVE MAST CELL PRODUCTS AND THEIR BIOLOGIC EFFECTS

Granule-associated	
Histamine	Pruritus, increased vasopermeability, gastric hypersecretion, bronchoconstriction
Heparin	Local anticoagulation
Tryptase, chymotryptic proteases	Degradation of local connective tissues
Lipid-derived	
Sulfidopeptide leukotrienes	Increased vasopermeability, bronchoconstriction, vasoconstriction (LTC_4); increased vasopermeability, bronchoconstriction, vasodilation (LTD_4 and LTE_4)
Prostaglandin D_2	Vasodilation, bronchoconstriction
Platelet-activating factor	Increased vasopermeability, vasodilation, bronchoconstriction
Cytokines	
Proinflammatory factors	Fibrosis (TGFβ); activation of vascular endothelial cells, cachexia (TNFα)
Growth enhancing	Colony-stimulating factor (IL-3); eosinophilia (IL-5)

ophilia, hepatosplenomegaly, and lymphadenopathy. Patients with aggressive disease rapidly increase mast cell numbers and are difficult to manage. Prognosis is less optimistic than in patients with indolent mastocytosis.

ETIOLOGY AND PATHOGENESIS. Mast cells originate from pluripotent bone marrow stem cells and migrate through the blood stream and lymphatics to specific sites within the body, where they mature into a fully granulated cell. The targeting of mast cells to defined locations appears to be determined by the sequential expression of cell surface adhesion molecules, including a laminin-binding protein. Thus, mast cells are often found along endothelial and epithelial basement membrane, along nerves, and around glandular structures rich in laminin. Tissues at interfaces between the external and internal environment, i.e., the skin and gastrointestinal tract, are particularly rich in mast cells. In these sites mast cells are believed to contribute to host defense against parasites.

The regulation of mast cell number and mast cell differentiation is under the control of factors produced both in the hematopoietic marrow and by cells in the tissues in which mast cells finally reside. For example, early mast cell differentiation depends on the colony-stimulating factor interleukin 3 (IL-3) and is inhibited by granulocyte-macrophage colony-stimulating factor (GM-CSF). Final maturation and granule composition may depend upon the production of specific mast cell growth factors by fibroblasts and stromal cells.

Regardless of the etiology of the increased burden of mast cells in patients with mastocytosis, the pathogenesis of the disease is largely the result of the increased production of mast cell mediators, which can have effects either at the site of their production or remote from their origin. Mast cell mediators are of three categories, all of which may distribute through the blood stream and lymphatics and produce biologic effects typical of those observed in patients with mastocytosis (Table 252–2).

CLINICAL FEATURES. The various categories of mastocytosis in general share similar clinical features, which are in turn due to the overproduction of mast cell mediators, although some patterns of disease may predominate in a specific category. The skin, gastrointestinal tract, liver, spleen, lymph nodes, bone marrow, and skeletal system yield the most significant management problems. The respiratory tract and endocrine system are generally spared. Also, although mast cells contain mediators that can inhibit immune responses, patients with mastocytosis do not suffer from recurrent infections.

The most common skin manifestation of mastocytosis is urticaria pigmentosa (Fig. 252–1). It is seen in over 90 per cent of patients with indolent mastocytosis and in less than 50 per cent of patients with mastocytosis with an associated hematologic disorder or those with lymphadenopathic mastocytosis with eosinophilia. The lesions of urticaria pigmentosa appear as small, reddish brown macules or slightly raised papules scattered over the body. Mild trauma, including scratching or rubbing of the lesions, usually

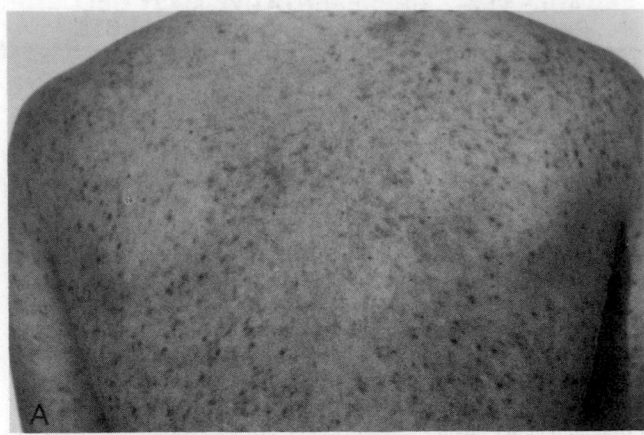

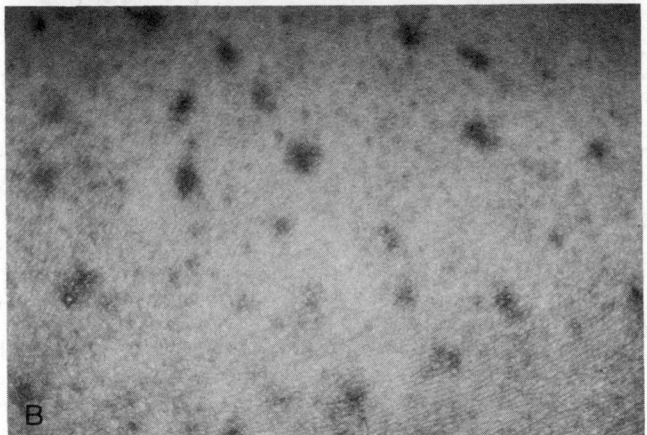

FIGURE 252–1. *A*, Urticaria pigmentosa in a patient with indolent systemic mastocytosis. *B*, Close-up view of urticaria pigmentosa.

causes urtication and erythema around the macules; this is known as Darier's sign. Urticaria pigmentosa is associated with a variable amount of pruritus, which may be exacerbated by changes in climatic temperature, skin friction, ingestion of hot beverages or spicy foods, ethanol, and certain drugs. The diagnosis is confirmed by characteristic skin histopathology. Diffuse cutaneous mastocytosis consists of a diffuse mast cell infiltration of the skin that can occur without discrete lesions. Solitary lesions called mastocytomas do occur but are quite rare. Young children with urticaria pigmentosa or diffuse cutaneous mastocytosis may have bullous eruptions.

Gastrointestinal disease often develops in patients with mastocytosis. The most common problem is gastric hypersecretion due to elevated plasma histamine with resultant gastritis and peptic ulcer disease. Diarrhea and abdominal pain are common and are followed by the onset of malabsorption in approximately one in three patients. Roentgenographic abnormalities fall into three major categories: peptic ulcers; abnormal mucosal patterns such as mucosal edema, multiple nodular lesions, coarsened mucosal folds, or multiple polyps; and motility disturbances. Histopathology of jejunal biopsies has shown moderate blunting of the villi; however, significant mast cell hyperplasia is uncommon.

Hepatic and splenic involvement in indolent systemic mastocytosis is relatively common, although liver function tests are usually normal. The most common chemical abnormality is an elevated alkaline phosphatase; this must be distinguished from bone-derived alkaline phosphatase, which may also be elevated. The most serious manifestation of hepatic and splenic involvement is portal hypertension and ascites associated with fibrosis of the liver and spleen. These conditions appear most commonly in patients who have mastocytosis with an associated hematologic disorder or in those with aggressive mastocytosis.

Bone marrow lesions consist of focal aggregates of spindle-shaped mast cells, often mixed with eosinophils, lymphocytes, and occasional plasma cells, histiocytes, and fibroblasts (Fig. 252–

2). These lesions are rarely seen in children. Anemia, leukopenia, thrombocytopenia, and eosinophilia may occur in association with systemic disease. Bone marrow infiltration with mast cells may induce bone changes that cause radiographically detectable lesions in up to 70 per cent of patients. The proximal long bones are most often affected, followed by the pelvis, ribs, and skull. Bone pain is the most common symptom and is present in 19 to 28 per cent of patients. Skeletal scintigraphy (bone scans) is more sensitive than radiographic surveys in detecting and locating active lesions. In severe or advanced disease, pathologic fractures do occur.

Patients in every category of mastocytosis sometimes experience flushing or frank anaphylaxis. In occasional patients, anaphylaxis may be provoked by alcohol, aspirin, exercise, or infections.

Neuropsychiatric abnormalities have been reported. Problems include a decreased attention span, memory impairment, and irritability. Depression as a consequence of chronic disease or possibly mediated by mast cell products is a possibility.

DIAGNOSIS. The diagnosis of mastocytosis rests on histology, supported by clinical, biochemical, and radiographic data. Mast cells may be overlooked on histologic sections depending on the fixation and/or stain employed. The most useful stains for mast cells include metachromatic stains, such as toluidine blue and Giemsa, and enzymatic stains, such as chloroacetate esterase and aminocaproate esterase. These procedures highlight the granules in the cytoplasm of the mast cell, thereby facilitating identification. In trephine core bone marrow biopsies, decalcification interferes with subsequent attempts to visualize mast cell granules, making their identification more difficult.

Fortunately, the majority of patients with mastocytosis have either urticaria pigmentosa or diffuse cutaneous mastocytosis, which can be recognized on physical examination. These diagnoses should be confirmed by skin biopsy. Blind skin biopsies are not recommended, as other skin conditions including eczema are associated with an increase in dermal mast cells.

In the absence of skin lesions, mastocytosis may be suspected in patients with one or several of the following: unexplained ulcer disease or malabsorption, radiographic or ^{99m}Tc bone scan abnormalities, hepatomegaly, splenomegaly, lymphadenopathy, peripheral blood abnormalities, and unexplained flushing or anaphylaxis. Elevated levels of plasma or urinary histamine or histamine metabolites, prostaglandin D_2 metabolites in the urine, or plasma mast cell tryptase are not diagnostic but do raise the

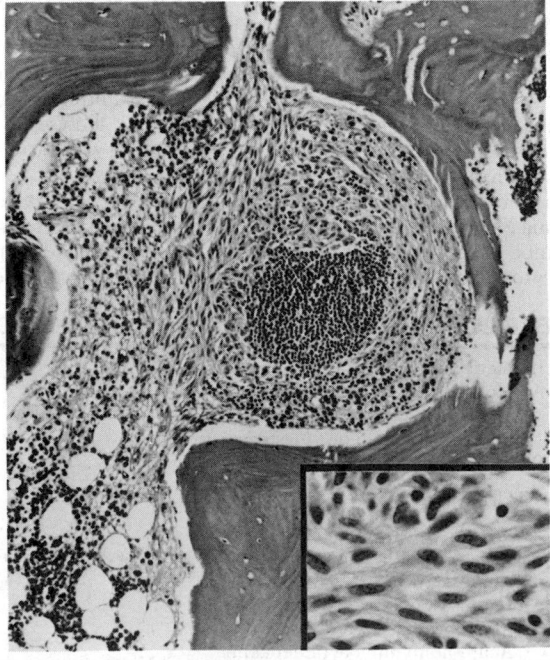

FIGURE 252–2. Bone marrow biopsy shows a characteristic lesion of systemic mastocytosis with nodular, paratrabecular infiltrate of mast cells surrounding a lymphoid aggregate. *Inset:* The mast cells are spindle-shaped, resembling fibroblasts or histiocytes. (Courtesy of W. D. Travis, Bethesda, MD.)

index of suspicion of mastocytosis. Reliable tests for these substances, however, are not generally available except in research laboratories.

Patients suspected of having mastocytosis in the absence of skin lesions should have a bone marrow biopsy and aspirate for diagnosis and categorization of the mastocytosis. Patients with urticaria pigmentosa or diffuse cutaneous mastocytosis should also have this procedure if they have peripheral blood abnormalities, hepatomegaly, splenomegaly, or lymphadenopathy, to determine if they have an associated hematologic disorder. Other tissue specimens, such as lymph nodes, spleen, liver, and gastrointestinal mucosa, define the extent of mast cell involvement but are usually obtained only as dictated by necessity. For example, gastrointestinal biopsies are obtained only if a gastrointestinal workup is indicated, and lymph nodes are biopsied only if lymphoma is considered.

Patients suspected of having mastocytosis should have 24-hour urine 5-hydroxyindoleacetic acid (5-HIAA) and urinary metanephrines measured to help eliminate the possibility of a carcinoid tumor or pheochromocytoma. It should be noted that patients with mastocytosis do not excrete increased amounts of 5-HIAA, suggesting that serotonin, reported in the mast cells of some species, is not synthesized by human mast cells. Idiopathic anaphylaxis and flushing must also be ruled out. Patients with these disorders do not have histologic evidence of significant mast cell proliferation.

TREATMENT. In all categories of mastocytosis, a primary objective of treatment is the control of mast cell mediator–induced signs and symptoms such as anaphylaxis, gastrointestinal cramping, and pruritus. H_1-receptor antagonists such as hydroxyzine and doxepin are helpful in reducing pruritus, flushing, and tachycardia. If insufficient relief occurs, the addition of an H_2 antagonist such as ranitidine or cimetidine may be beneficial. However, many patients continue to complain of bone pain, headaches, and flushing, resulting in part from the inability to block the effects of high levels of histamine with histamine antagonists and the presence of other mast cell mediators. Disodium cromoglycate (cromolyn sodium) is known to inhibit degranulation of mast cells and may have some efficacy in the treatment of mastocytosis. Epinephrine is used to treat episodes of anaphylaxis. Patients should be prepared to self-administer this drug. If subcutaneous epinephrine is insufficient, intensive therapy for anaphylaxis should be instituted. Patients with recurrent episodes of anaphylaxis may be placed on H_1 and H_2 antihistamines to lessen the severity of attacks. Episodes of profound anaphylaxis may be spontaneous but have also been observed following stings from insects.

Methoxsalen with long-wave ultraviolet radiation (PUVA) has been shown to relieve pruritus and whealing after 1 to 2 months of treatment. Relapse of pruritus occurs within 3 to 6 months after stopping treatment. Topical steroids can be used to treat extensive urticaria pigmentosa or diffuse cutaneous mastocytosis, although these lesions eventually recur after discontinuation of therapy.

Treatment of gastrointestinal disease is directed at controlling peptic symptoms, diarrhea, and malabsorption. Gastric acid hypersecretion leading to peptic symptoms and ulcerations is controlled with H_2 antagonists. Diarrhea is difficult to control, and H_2 antagonists are generally not effective. Anticholinergics may give partial relief. Malabsorption, if present, is difficult to manage. In patients with severe malabsorption, systemic steroids have been shown to be effective. Ascites is also difficult to manage. One patient with portal hypertension was successfully managed with a portacaval shunt. Another patient with an exudative ascites was treated successfully with systemic steroid therapy.

Patients with mastocytosis and an associated hematologic disorder are treated as dictated by the specific hematologic abnormality. In mast cell leukemia, chemotherapy has not yet been shown to produce remission or to prolong survival. Chemotherapy has no place in the treatment of indolent mastocytosis. A recent study suggested that splenectomy may improve survival in patients with poor prognostic forms of mastocytosis.

PROGNOSIS. Prognosis must be addressed separately for each category of mastocytosis. One study found seven variables that were strongly associated with poor survival. These included constitutional symptoms, anemia, thrombocytopenia, abnormal liver function tests, lobated mast cell nucleus, a low percentage of fat cells in the bone marrow biopsy, and an associated hematologic disorder. Other poor prognostic variables include absence of urticaria pigmentosa, male sex, absence of skin and bone symptoms, hepatomegaly, splenomegaly, and normal bone radiographic findings.

As a group, patients with indolent mastocytosis and skin involvement alone have the best prognosis. Among children with isolated urticaria pigmentosa, at least 50 per cent of cases resolve by adulthood. Adults with urticaria pigmentosa usually progress gradually to systemic disease and rarely may convert to type II disease. Diffuse cutaneous mastocytosis is usually associated with indolent systemic disease. Patients with mastocytosis with an associated hematologic disorder have a variable course dependent on the prognosis of their hematologic disorder. With mast cell leukemia, mean survival is less than 6 months. Survival with lymphadenopathic mastocytosis with eosinophilia is 1 to 2 years without therapy. The prognosis appears to improve with aggressive symptomatic management.

Cherner JA, Jensen RT, Dubois A, et al.: Gastrointestinal dysfunction in systemic mastocytosis: A prospective study. Gastroenterology 95:657, 1988. *This study describes patterns of gastrointestinal disease in mastocytosis and the implications for clinical management.*

Garriga MM, Friedman MM, Metcalfe DD: A survey of the number and distribution of mast cells in the skin of patients with mast cell disorders. J Allergy Clin Immunol 82:425, 1988. *A study of the value of determination of mast cell numbers in skin biopsies.*

Horny H-P, Kaiserling E, Campbell M, et al.: Liver findings in generalized mastocytosis: A clinicopathologic study. Cancer 63:532, 1989. *A survey of liver histopathology in mastocytosis.*

Schwartz LD, Metcalfe DD, Miller JS, et al.: Tryptase levels as an indicator of mast cell activation in systemic anaphylaxis and mastocytosis. N Engl J Med 316:1622, 1987. *Demonstration of mast cell tryptase in the serum of mastocytosis patients.*

Travis WD, Li C-Y, Bergstralh EJ, et al.: Systemic mast cell disease: Analysis of 58 cases and literature review. Medicine 67:345, 1988. *An excellent review of the histopathologic and clinical features of mastocytosis.*

253 Diseases of the Thymus

Daniel P. Stites

DEVELOPMENT, STRUCTURE, AND FUNCTION. The thymus, a central lymphoid organ, functions in the development and maintenance of immunologic competence. Arising embryologically from the third and fourth branchial clefts, it migrates caudad, as a bilobed organ, to the anterior mediastinum. Ectopic thoracic and cervical thymic rests are present in 30 per cent of normal individuals. The thymus enlarges until late puberty and then involutes, the lymphocytes and epithelial cells being nearly completely replaced with fat by the fifth or sixth decade. The normal thymus varies greatly in size. It is uniquely susceptible to marked involution within hours owing to the stress of serious illness or to treatment with glucocorticoids. The thymus is composed primarily of lymphocytes encased in a lattice of epithelial cells. It also contains a few myoid cells, macrophages, and plasma cells. The thymus is arranged into discrete lobules containing a cortex and medulla. Hassall's corpuscles are specialized aggregates of epithelial cells whose function is unknown.

The thymus begins to function by about 10 to 12 weeks of gestation when immunocompetent T cells can first be detected. Undifferentiated stem cells migrate to the thymus from fetal liver and bone marrow prenatally and from the bone marrow postnatally. Local influences, probably from epithelial cells, induce maturation of thymic lymphocytes, which then divide in the cortex, migrate to the medulla, and emigrate to the peripheral lymphoid tissue as mature T cells. The capacity for self- and nonself-recognition of antigens is conferred upon T cells at this phase within the thymus. The cortex is also the site of intense lymphopoiesis. The thymus secretes a variety of incompletely defined hormones that maintain T-cell competence in peripheral lymphoid organs. The immunosuppressive effects of thymectomy vary with age, being most pronounced at younger ages (see below). The thymus also appears to play an important role in maintenance of tolerance to various antigens, in immune surveillance, and possibly in leukemogenesis (as judged by animal experiments).

THYMIC HYPOPLASIA. Hypoplastic thymus may be either congenital or acquired. In neonates and infants, *congenital thymic hypoplasia* is expressed as marked T-cell and variable B-cell immunodeficiency. Resulting diseases include reticular dysgenesis, severe combined immunodeficiency disease, DiGeorge's and Nezelof's syndromes, and ataxia-telangiectasia (see Ch. 244). Essentially all of these patients are diagnosed in childhood; the severity of the thymic lesion, if untreated, rarely allows survival beyond age 10 or 12 years. Congenital thymic hypoplasia has been treated by thymic or bone marrow transplantation and by thymic hormone injections with variable success. *Acquired hypoplasia* or thymic involution occurs normally with age or results from stress (within hours or days), malnutrition, pregnancy, x-rays, glucocorticoids, or cytotoxic drugs. AIDS and graft-versus-host disease commonly produce severe thymic dysplasia.

THYMIC HYPERPLASIA. An enlarged thymus is very difficult to evaluate accurately because of its large normal variability in size. In the past, so-called status thymolymphaticus, a condition diagnosed with respiratory distress and large thymic shadow on chest roentgenogram, frequently led to unnecessary removal or radiation of normal thymuses. Individuals who received thymic irradiation for "enlarged thymus" have had significant increases in the incidence of thyroid cancer or adenoma. Extrathyroid tumors, particularly breast cancer, also increased slightly but there have been no increases in lymphoreticular malignancy, suggestive of immunodeficiency. The concept of status thymolymphaticus has been abandoned. The thymus may rarely enlarge in thyrotoxicosis, Addison's disease, anencephaly, acromegaly, castration, or tumors (see below). Thymic cysts are usually asymptomatic and the occasional association with neoplasia warrants resection.

THYMUS AND MYASTHENIA GRAVIS. Myasthenia gravis is an autoimmune disease caused by the presence of antiacetylcholine receptor (AchR) antibodies (see Ch. 509). In myasthenia gravis there is a 10 per cent incidence of thymoma. In fact detectable enlargement of the thymus in myasthenia gravis usually heralds the presence of a thymoma. In 65 per cent of cases the thymus is hyperplastic with increased numbers of germinal centers but not clinically enlarged. In the remaining 25 per cent of patients the thymus is normal. In large series of thymomas, 30 to 60 per cent of patients have myasthenia gravis. Rarely myasthenia gravis develops years after total thymectomy for thymoma, which militates against an absolute requirement for thymoma in the pathogenesis of this disorder. Neonatal myasthenia gravis occurs without any thymic abnormality, presumably owing to transplacental transfer of maternal antibody. There is little correlation with serum levels of anti-AchR antibody and clinical improvement in myasthenia following thymectomy. Damage to AchR antigen shared between muscles and thymic epithelial or myoid cells may explain the rather obscure relationship of the thymus to this autoantibody disorder.

EFFECTS OF THYMECTOMY. Total removal of the thymus during the neonatal period in rodents results in severe immunodeficiency, loss of T cells, and a wasting disease, a result of chronic unopposed infection. Thymectomy in adult animals, however, is associated with much subtler changes in T-cell function. What is the effect of thymectomy in humans? Because of the high incidence of extramediastinal thymic rests (30 per cent), thymectomy can rarely be considered total. Total thymectomy intentionally done during cardiothoracic surgery in children does not appear to result in compromised transplantation immunity. In patients with thymoma, a transient decrease in circulating lymphocytes and T-cell functions is noted. Following thymectomy for myasthenia gravis, functional loss in some T-cell populations occurs. However, the long-term effects of thymectomy, either in immunologically normal patients during cardiac surgery or in cancer patients with thymomas, are not known. These individuals should be carefully observed for development of autoimmune disease, infection, certain malignancies, or other signs of T-cell deficiency.

THYMOMA. *Definition.* A thymoma is a neoplasm of thymic epithelial cells. This definition excludes other tumors that may affect the thymus such as lymphoma, germ cell tumors, and carcinoid. Thymomas are rare; fewer than 1000 cases have been reported. Nevertheless, it is the most common tumor of the anterior superior mediastinum (see Ch. 69).

Pathology. Thymomas contain various proportions of epithelial cells and lymphocytes. The latter are T cells and may constitute a large proportion of cellular content of the tumor; hence the term *lymphoepithelioma.* Although their significance is unknown, the activated appearance of these lymphocytes suggests a host reaction to neoplastic epithelial cells. These T cells express surface markers such as CD1a and often such CD4 and CD8 which is characteristic of thymocytes rather than peripheral blood T cells. Various histologic degrees of malignancy from minimal cytologic atypia to undifferentiated carcinoma exist. However, correlation of microscopic appearance with clinical malignancy is notoriously poor. In fact, local invasion of pleura, pericardium, vessels, and nerves is the major criterion for determining clinical malignancy of the tumor.

Clinical Manifestations. Median age of patients with thymoma is about 50 years, and no sex predominance is noted. About 30 per cent of patients present with myasthenia gravis; another 30 per cent are asymptomatic, and the diagnosis is suggested by an anterior mediastinal mass on chest roentgenogram. The remaining 30 to 40 per cent of patients have a variety of symptoms and medical syndromes associated with the tumor (Table 253–1). Symptoms and signs include cough, chest pain, dysphagia, dyspnea, hoarseness, neck mass, and superior vena cava syndrome.

A few patients with spindle cell thymomas have marked *hypogammaglobulinemia.* Whether the relationship is causal is not established. The rare occurrence of red cell aplasia with or without immunodeficiency and thymoma raises the possibility of T cell–mediated suppression of erythropoiesis or immunoglobulin synthesis. Direct evidence to support these notions is only fragmentary.

Diagnosis. The presence of a round or oval anterior mediastinal mass visualized in posteroanterior and lateral chest roentgenograms in the presence of myasthenia gravis or of some other known systemic manifestations is suggestive of thymoma. Computed tomographic (CT) imaging with enhancing contrast media injection is useful in defining the size and location of thymomas and is occasionally useful in differentiating various thymic lesions. Thymic biopsy has no place in evaluation of anterior mediastinal masses, and mediastinoscopy is of little or no value. Some centers claim success with fine needle aspiration and cytology. Thoracotomy with adequate exposure to determine whether capsular invasion has occurred is needed for diagnosis of any thymic tumor. Differential diagnosis includes other primary or secondary thymic tumors (see below), cysts, posttraumatic hemorrhage, aneurysm, or other abnormalities of the anterior mediastinal contents including metastatic tumors, giant lymph node hyperplasia, mesothelioma, thyroid and parathyroid tumors, and paragangliomas (see Ch. 69).

Treatment. Surgical removal of tumor followed by local irradiation if extracapsular extension has occurred is the treatment of choice. Distant metastases are rare; the tumor spreads mainly by local invasion of adjacent structures.

Prognosis. The prognosis is nearly entirely dependent on presence of local invasion and cannot be predicted by histologic appearance of the tumor. Noninvasive thymomas are usually cured by excision. Patients with invasive thymoma have about 50 per cent 5-year survival.

TABLE 253–1. DISEASES ASSOCIATED WITH THYMIC TUMORS

I. Thymoma
    Myasthenia gravis
    Red cell aplasia
    Hemolytic anemia
    Neutrophil agranulocytosis
    Hypogammaglobulinemia (Good's syndrome)
    Systemic lupus erythematosus
    Polymyositis
    Pemphigus vulgaris
    Chronic mucocutaneous candidiasis
II. Carcinoid
    Cushing's syndrome
    Multiple endocrine neoplasia syndromes
      (see Ch. 228)

OTHER TUMORS OF THE THYMUS. *Thymolipoma* probably represents a lipoma arising within normal thymus. This tumor is usually radiolucent and asymptomatic and has not been associated with myasthenia gravis. *Carcinoid tumor* of the thymus arises from neuroendocrine cells within the thymus (see Ch. 230). Fifty per cent produce ACTH-like molecules and cause Cushing's syndrome or hyperparathyroidism, or are associated with multiple endocrine adenomatosis; 30 per cent are malignant and metastasize. Surgery and radiotherapy are indicated. *Carcinomas*, particularly squamous cell types, may rarely occur. *Germ cell tumors* rarely occur: seminoma, teratoma, teratocarcinoma, choriocarcinoma, embryonal cell carcinoma, and yolk sac tumors. The thymus may be involved by *malignant lymphomas*. T-cell lymphomas with acute lymphoblastic leukemia occur in the second decade. Cells from these tumors may have C receptors and are positive for terminal deoxynucleotidyl transferase. Hodgkin's disease usually is of the nodular sclerosing type (see Ch. 147 and 148).

Day DL, Gedgudas E: The thymus. Radiol Clin North Am 22:519, 1984. *A thorough review of thymic anatomy and function. Special emphasis on use of imaging techniques such as CT scans, sonography, and NMR is presented.*

Kornstein MJ, Hoxie JA, Levinson AI: Immunohistology of human thymomas. Arch Pathol Lab Med 109:460, 1985. *Careful phenotypic analysis with monoclonal antibodies of the surface phenotype of various thymomas.*

Namba T, Brunner NG, Grob D: Myasthenia gravis in patients with thymoma with particular reference to onset after thymectomy. Medicine 57:411, 1978. *Excellent review of literature on relationship of thymoma to myasthenia gravis with 72 locally studied cases.*

Salyer W, Eggleston JC: Thymoma. A clinical and pathological study of 65 cases. Cancer 37:229, 1976. *Clinicopathologic description of a large series of thymoma patients, annotating association with other medical syndromes.*

Shore RE, Woodard E, Hildreth N: Thyroid tumor following thymus irradiation. JNCI 74:1177, 1985. *Case control study of 2650 individuals who received thymic irradiation in infancy shows 30 cancers and 59 benign thyroid adenomas in an average of a 29-year follow-up period. No evidence for compromised imune function was detected based on absence of lymphoreticular malignancy.*

PART XIX

MUSCULOSKELETAL AND CONNECTIVE TISSUE DISEASES

254 Approach to the Patient with Musculoskeletal Disease

James F. Fries

The rheumatic diseases present a major challenge to clinical judgment. The chronicity, variability, tendency to exacerbate and remit, biochemical and immunologic complexity, unknown pathogenesis, variable response to specific treatment, and myriad effects upon the patient's lifestyle, family relationships, self-image, and employability combine to complicate the therapeutic equation. Difficult therapeutic decisions must often be made without adequate experimental justification and evaluated against a poorly understood natural history.

In the face of these tremendous uncertainties, contemporary management is relatively straightforward but has recently changed substantially. The therapeutic strategy has shifted from dogma to flexibility. Good management now requires that therapeutic decisions be based upon individual pathophysiology rather than upon diagnosis per se. Further, decisions are never final but are modified in a continuing feedback between application of treatment and observation of response. Decisions change over time as appropriate to the trends, tempo, and previous response of the particular patient. The art of medicine is reborn in the approach to a patient with a chronic disease. The principles underlying contemporary management strategy are set forth in this chapter and are divided into six major topics. The medical history, the physical examination, and the laboratory data, which are discussed in following chapters, are factors in decisions involving these six areas.

DETERMINING THE PATHOPHYSIOLOGY

Diagnosis is *not* the most important factor in selecting management of rheumatic disease. Modern management individualizes therapy within diagnostic categories, based upon subgroups of patients with differing prognoses and different therapeutic requirements. Patients with the same diagnosis often should be managed very differently. Patients with rheumatic disease frequently have features of several diagnostic entities at the same time.

Management in musculoskeletal disease is more closely linked to the underlying pathophysiologic process than to the diagnostic entity. Reversal of the pathophysiologic process (or negation of its impact) requires a clear visualization of that process. Even such a basic pathophysiologic concept as "inflammation" has different therapeutic implications. The inflamed synovial membrane (synovitis) typical of rheumatoid arthritis responds to a different spectrum of anti-inflammatory agents than does the inflammation of ligamentous insertions (enthesitis) typical of ankylosing spondylitis or the inflammation within the joint space induced by microscopic crystals.

Eight specific types of musculoskeletal problems can be readily distinguished by history and physical examination in most patients

and can provide a framework for pathophysiologic categorization. Identification of the predominant pathophysiology in a given patient is usually straightforward. The eight categories are discussed in the following paragraphs and are listed in Table 254–1, together with the prototype disease of the category, examples of the most useful laboratory tests for that category, and the typical treatments required. Management implications for each category are surprisingly distinct and provide guidelines for laboratory investigation and initial treatment. Location of the process is shown in Figure 254–1.

SYNOVITIS. Inflammation of the synovial membrane, with gradual damage to surrounding joint structures, is most strikingly manifested in rheumatoid arthritis. The synovium is tender, thickened, and palpable and may demonstrate warmth and, less often, redness. Joint destruction is caused by the enzymatic products of inflammation and develops slowly over many years. Management is based upon reducing the *rate* of damage to joint structures, and agents directed at retardation of progression (disease-modifying antirheumatic drugs, or DMARD's) should

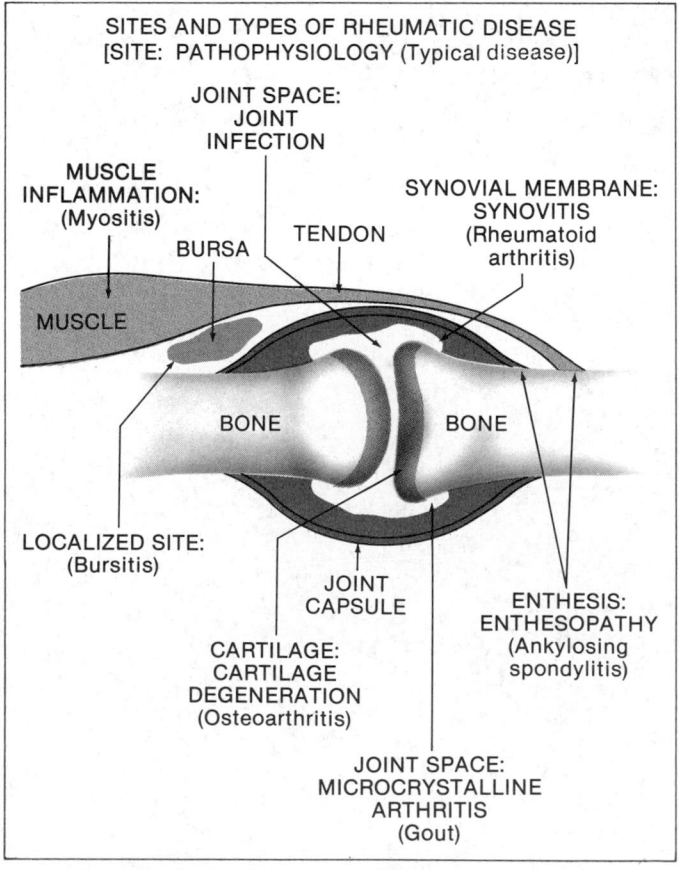

FIGURE 254–1. Location of musculoskeletal disease processes.

usually be employed early in the course and continually throughout. The sedimentation rate is consistently elevated with significant synovitis, and the latex fixation or other tests for rheumatoid arthritis are often useful for further categorization. A wide range of pharmacologic and other treatments may be required, and many patients require sequential trials with a variety of agents. Some useful drugs for synovitis, such as gold, penicillamine, and hydroxychloroquine, have not been proved therapeutically effective in any other category.

ENTHESOPATHY. Inflammation in these diseases is most marked at the enthesis, that transition region where ligament attaches to bone. Such inflammation is the hallmark of a family of rheumatic diseases typified by ankylosing spondylitis and linked to the human leukocyte antigen (HLA)–B27. The distribution of involvement follows the location of regions of enthesis throughout the body. The marked predilection for the sacroiliac joints, heels, and spine identifies a process affecting areas characterized by ligament and tendon attachment. This specific pathophysiology provides a unifying basis for the clinical features of the diseases and their typical response to specific therapy. Rheumatoid factor is predictably absent from the serum. Nonsteroidal anti-inflammatory drugs (NSAID's)—in particular, indomethacin, phenylbutazone, and naproxen—are therapeutically effective and usually are well tolerated over the long term. The spectrum of effective anti-inflammatory drugs used for enthesopathy is different from that in synovitis. Prednisone, for example, is neither indicated nor effective in most patients.

CARTILAGE DEGENERATION. Degenerative and other processes can cause fraying and destruction of the articular cartilage, with subsequent injury to the underlying subchondral bone. This occurrence is usually termed osteoarthritis (or osteoarthrosis), and a group of specific syndromes is recognized within this category. Narrowing of the apparent joint space and development of bone spurs make radiography the most useful investigative procedure; other ancillary tests are usually negative. Few patients have significant inflammation, and it is not surprising that anti-inflammatory treatment is not of great use. The analgesic effects of aspirin or NSAID's may be helpful; doses required for optimal pain relief are often considerably less than doses required for anti-inflammatory effects. Medical treatment is symptomatic and is seldom dramatically effective.

CRYSTAL-INDUCED SYNOVITIS. Microcrystalline arthritis occurs when crystals forming in the synovial fluid (or injected therein) induce an acute inflammatory reaction in the joint fluid and the surrounding synovium. Gout is the prototype disease, with the inflammation induced by crystals of monosodium urate. Similar syndromes may occur with crystals of several other types. The syndrome increases to very intense inflammation within a period of hours and spontaneously resolves without treatment over a period of a few days to a few weeks; this resolution can be markedly accelerated with treatment. The physical factors underlying crystal formation determine that only one or, at most, a few joints are involved at a time. The crucial laboratory observation is inspection of the aspirated joint fluid for crystals under polarized light microscopy. Drugs inhibiting polymorphonuclear leukocytes are particularly effective, as exemplified by colchicine, a drug with little effect in any other rheumatic disease category.

JOINT INFECTION. The synovium encloses a body space that can be the site of direct infection by microorganisms. Critical to investigation of the patient with suspected joint infection is aspiration and culture of the joint fluid and, in many instances, culture of other body fluids as well. Treatment consists principally of prescribing an antibiotic specific for the microorganism involved. Drainage may be required.

MYOSITIS. Inflammation of muscle occurs in two closely related diseases, dermatomyositis and polymyositis, and in an unrelated condition, polymyalgia rheumatica. Determination of muscle enzyme levels and histologic examination of involved muscle may be the critical laboratory observations. In polymyalgia, the sedimentation rate is greatly elevated and is often the sole objective finding. Temporal artery biopsy may be useful when giant cell arteritis is demonstrated. Corticosteroids are almost always required in inflammatory muscle disease and, in contrast to every other rheumatic disease category, are usually required from the outset.

FOCAL CONDITIONS. A wide variety of conditions affecting the musculoskeletal system do not truly warrant the term "disease." Tendinitis, bursitis, low back strain, calcific tendinitis, and other entities can affect almost any area of the body and are the most common of all medical problems. Laboratory aids are few, although radiography may occasionally be useful in locating calcium deposits or spurs or in ruling out fracture. The therapeutic imperative in localized problems (unfortunately often neglected) is to emphasize localized rather than general treatment measures. Treatment of the entire organism for a problem in one local area is seldom rewarding. The use of splints, slings, heat, and local injection is usually the most reasonable initial approach.

GENERALIZED CONDITIONS. A variety of poorly defined entities fall into this category. Terms such as "fibromyalgia" and the "chronic muscle contraction syndrome" are sometimes used to indicate the likelihood of organic disease characterized by sleep disturbance and tender points. The terms "psychogenic rheumatism," "nonarticular rheumatism," and "depressive equivalent" are frequently used to suggest a psychological etiology. These patients are rich in symptoms but poor in objective evidence of pathology. The conditions may be extremely troublesome for the individual but are not progressive and do not result in physical crippling. Laboratory tests, such as the sedimentation rate, give normal results and are employed only to rule out other categories of illness. Treatment is best termed "conservative." The therapeutic approaches to other categories are unlikely to be beneficial, and the physician who attempts pharmacologic intervention rather than reassurance, lifestyle counseling, and support often ends with a drug-dependent patient who gets no better.

These eight categories and the brief descriptions presented are supported by generalizations to which there are some exceptions. However, Table 254–1 summarizes quite specific starting points at which the laboratory investigation and therapeutic approach should begin. The experienced physician soon moves far beyond this table, but it provides a particularly useful framework upon which to place the more detailed clinical knowledge found in the following chapters.

USING THE LABORATORY SELECTIVELY

Laboratory tests in patients with the rheumatic diseases usually provide confirmatory data rather than conclusive evidence. After the three exceptions of (1) the sacroiliac radiograph in ankylosing spondylitis, (2) the identification of specific crystals within the joint fluid, and (3) a positive bacteriologic culture from joint fluid, laboratory tests have varying degrees of lack of sensitivity and lack of specificity and, except in the unusual case, add relatively little to clinical assessment. As a result, the majority of patients presenting with musculoskeletal problems do not require a great amount of laboratory evaluation. The key to appropriate use of the laboratory is selective use. Every test should have a specific indication, and blind "surveys" or "panels" should not be used.

TABLE 254–1. CATEGORIES OF RHEUMATIC DISEASE

Pathology	Prototype	Most Useful Tests	Typical Treatment
Synovitis	Rheumatoid arthritis	Latex, erythrocyte sedimentation rate	Gold
Enthesopathy	Ankylosing spondylitis	Sacroiliac radiographs, HLA-B27	Indomethacin
Cartilage degeneration	Osteoarthritis	Radiographs of affected area	Analgesic
Crystal-induced synovitis	Gout	Joint fluid crystal examination	Colchicine
Joint infection	Staphylococcal	Joint fluid culture	Antibiotics
Myositis	Dermatomyositis	Muscle enzymes, muscle biopsy	Corticosteroids
Focal conditions	Tennis elbow	None, radiographs of affected area	Localized
Generalized conditions	Fibrositis	Erythrocyte sedimentation rate	Conservative

One in six visits by a patient to a health professional is for a musculoskeletal complaint. The great majority of such visits to physicians occur for the common "focal conditions" of life. Low back pain, sprained ankles, tennis elbows, and other common musculoskeletal complaints account for most initial visits. Most such problems are easily identified as self-limited. Optimal management includes ruling out more significant illness, advice about activity or rest, reassurance, occasionally symptomatic medication, and transmission of the expectation that the natural healing process will resolve the difficulty. The usual healing period for local musculoskeletal problems ranges from 2 to 6 weeks, depending upon the magnitude of the often inapparent injury, with the healing process beginning again from the start if there is reinjury during this period. Healing cannot be pharmacologically accelerated. Thus, optimal treatment usually requires "masterly inactivity," with confident reliance upon the natural healing process. Inappropriate vigor with testing or treatment can lead to investigative mishaps, therapeutic side reactions, and an intensity of focus upon the problem inappropriate to its magnitude. The careful clinician uses time to establish the trends and tempo of the condition; time is used to demonstrate the self-limited native condition while avoiding the hazards of inappropriate response.

The critical initial decision, therefore, is whether the problem requires immediate action or whether the decision to investigate or treat can be postponed until the course of the disease and the magnitude of the appropriate response may be better estimated. A 6-week "rule of thumb" is appropriate. In the absence of specific indication or immediate threat, a waiting period of 6 weeks from onset of symptoms serves to minimize inappropriate use of laboratory tests or treatment. Four major exceptions to the 6-week rule obtain. First, a condition that is severe and involves a single joint (or, at most, a few joints) is much more likely, paradoxically, to require immediate attention than is a widespread polyarthritis. Acute gouty arthritis and infections, the usual causes of the "single hot joint," require immediate attention. By contrast, in rheumatoid arthritis, a period of 6 weeks is required even before the criteria for diagnosis can be met, and management in the first days of disease is most appropriately conservative. Many "probable rheumatoid arthritis" patients actually have minor problems that disappear as the viral or minor hypersensitivity reaction subsides. These patients need not be given the emotional burden of a "serious" diagnosis.

Second, a patient who is febrile, systemically ill, and otherwise showing signs of major disease deserves immediate attention. Endocarditis, neoplasm, tuberculosis, and other illnesses are frequently identified through musculoskeletal clues, and a connective tissue disease with systemic manifestations deserves immediate attention.

Third, if the problem is associated with significant trauma, the possible need for immediate orthopedic management should be considered. Fourth, an associated neurologic problem, such as carpal tunnel syndrome, sciatic nerve compression, or cervical nerve root compression may be benefited by immediate attention.

In practice, these four indications for immediate action are relatively unusual. The large majority of patients with initial complaints involving the musculoskeletal system are not found to have conditions requiring either intensive efforts at diagnosis or employment of hazardous therapy.

ESTABLISHING MANAGEMENT GOALS

The impact of disease has too often been defined in terms of numerically expressed test results. The level of autoantibodies, titer of rheumatoid factor, number of radiographic erosions, and sedimentation rate too often become the criteria for therapeutic success. The patient and family are more directly interested in a different list of disease endpoints: in survival, in normal mobility and function, in absence of pain and other symptoms, and in the ability to remain solvent through the duration of a chronic illness. These five "D's" (death, disability, discomfort, drug toxicity, and dollar cost) are the major dimensions of the patient's outcome in the patient's own terms.

In the rheumatic diseases the frequent "trade-offs" among several outcomes must be based upon the values perceived by the particular patient. For example, pain may be reduced by narcotics but disability increased; disability may be reduced by cyclophosphamide but a risk of death incurred; or short-term symptomatic relief by plasmapheresis may be obtained at very high cost.

Establishment of goals must precede development of the individual management strategy. In some instances, a limited goal, such as regaining the ability to walk, may be dramatically useful to the patient and far more valuable than a modest reduction in the general severity of the disease. Some worthy goals may not be achievable in a particular instance, and their pursuit may only increase therapeutic toxicity. The question of what is desirable is subordinate to the question of what is achievable.

PLANNING FOR OPTIMAL LONG-TERM OUTCOME

Hospital-based training tends to focus attention on improving the patient's status by the time of discharge. In chronic illness, such short-term benefits may be desirable but illusory. Corticosteroids, narcotic analgesics, and intra-articular injections often provide obvious short-term benefit. Unfortunately, the agent that provides the best initial response sometimes may lead to iatrogenic disaster over the longer term.

The therapeutic strategy for synovitis has held that simple and less toxic measures should be used first, and hazardous medications withheld unless the simpler approaches fail. Recently, however, it has become recognized that because of severe and prevalent gastric damage, aspirin and NSAID's are more toxic than previously thought and that some DMARD's are relatively well tolerated. As a result, management of synovitis has tended toward earlier and more consistent reliance upon DMARD's, which have a far superior toxic-therapeutic ratio. The old "pyramidal" strategy is being abandoned in favor of a serial DMARD strategy designed to reduce the rate of joint damage.

The inexperienced clinician is often trapped by taking the short view of a chronic illness. A chronic disease cannot be managed by short-term tactics; it requires a long-term strategy, shared and negotiated with the patient.

Such a strategy requires tactical modification at nearly every physician-patient encounter. At each visit, new information is always present, even if only the information about what transpired in response to the last set of decisions. A decision is thus followed by observation, then by further decision, then by another period of observation. The decision strategy is flexible and, in the final analysis, frequently empiric.

USING A COMPLETE CLINICAL REPERTOIRE

Treatment of musculoskeletal disease is frequently discussed in terms of pharmacologic agents. This myopic view neglects the dominant contributions often afforded by reconstructive surgical procedures, by the use of appliances and devices to allow handicapped individuals to function more normally, by exercise to strengthen bones and tissues, or by personal interaction to increase the motivation and improve the self-image of the patient.

A drug-based strategy tends to find its greatest use in early, systemic, inflammatory disease processes. Orthopedic approaches tend to have the greatest utility if the number of joints or regions involved is small, if major problems are concentrated in a single anatomic region, or after an inflammatory process has "burned out." Improvement after occupational therapy is often seen in patients with moderate to major disability who require adaptive devices to render the environment more friendly. Confidence in the ability to live an independent life sometimes can be more important than any specific therapy, and patient confidence (personal efficacy) is a useful therapeutic adjunct. Medical therapy that interferes with mental or emotional adaptation frequently makes things worse.

The novice at managing rheumatic diseases employs only a limited therapeutic repertoire. Typically, the patient requires a diverse program individualized to specific needs and making use of a variety of different disciplines. Development of rational strategies requires intimate knowledge of the strengths and weaknesses of all therapeutic modalities. The physician cannot manage chronic musculoskeletal diseases effectively without knowledge of the techniques of complementary disciplines or a good working relationship with individuals who possess these skills.

ACHIEVING UNDERSTANDING BY THE PATIENT

The informed patient is the physician's greatest single asset in managing chronic illness. Consider even the recommendation that a patient should take aspirin. The lay media describe the hazards of aspirin, colloquialisms associate aspirin with neglect by the physician, and the over-the-counter availability suggests a minor remedy. Yet, for anti-inflammatory treatment with aspirin, the physician may aim for a narrow therapeutic range far above the dose the patient expects. While establishing dosage, the patient is almost certain to encounter one or another side effect, even though the aspirin later may be well tolerated. The informed patient must know that anti-inflammatory and analgesic activities of aspirin are different, that a particular therapeutic range is important, that the drug is active against the inflammatory process itself, and that several weeks may be required to see the full effects of the drug. In the absence of such understanding, it is unusual for a patient to do well on aspirin; education of the patient is a prerequisite for therapeutic success.

Most clinicians believe that patients with positive expectations have better outcomes. While causality is not established by this belief, it is reasonable to assume that restoration of hope and a positive self-image are beneficial parts of treatment. The patient with arthritis is under intense psychological pressures. Self-image is threatened by diseases that may cripple and prevent remunerative employment. The fear of dependence upon others is often present. Yet prognosis is generally better than that anticipated by the patient. The physician who is unaware that every patient with arthritis has significant fears may do great harm by inadvertently increasing those fears.

In addition, the informed patient is more likely to comply with a particular therapeutic regimen. The patient's report of success or failure with previous recommendations is essential for the next clinical decision and must be as accurate as possible, again emphasizing the need for direct patient-physician communication. Unrealistic expectations followed by perceived therapeutic failures are a major cause of a burgeoning business in quack treatment. The patient must be educated to recognize the falsity of overstated claims and the losses in courage, independence, and money that may result. The obscenity of the quack who makes a living by defrauding patients focuses the attention upon the outrage. At the more important level, however, the patient susceptible to the claims of the quack does not have a confident and informed relationship with his or her personal physician.

The management of musculoskeletal disease is directed in large part at maintenance of the independence of the individual. Most persons with arthritis can be independent and healthy individuals despite their musculoskeletal condition. This independence is the final goal of the individualized management strategy.

Fries JF: Toward an understanding of patient outcome measurement. Arthritis Rheum 26:697, 1983. *Review of the concepts and practice of assessment of long-term outcome and the clinical implications thereof.*

Fries JF, Holman HR: Estimating prognosis in systemic lupus erythematosus. Am J Med 57:561, 1974. *Introduction to the concepts of subsets of disease and individualization of prognosis and treatment choice.*

Fries JF, Miller SR, Spitz PW, et al.: Toward an epidemiology of gastropathy associated with non-steroidal anti-inflammatory drug use. Gastroenterology 96:647, 1989. *Review of drug side effect frequency and prevalence, with emphasis upon common, severe, and largely preventable complications.*

Kelley WN, Harris ED, Ruddy S, et al.: Textbook of Rheumatology. 3rd ed. Philadelphia, W.B. Saunders Company, 1989. *Definitive textbook of 2000 pages and many thousand references covering all aspects of rheumatology.*

Schumacher HR (ed.): Primer on the Rheumatic Diseases. 9th ed. Atlanta, Arthritis Foundation, 1988. *Classic, authoritative, current descriptions of all rheumatic diseases and indeed of all rheumatology, available as a public service at nominal cost.*

255 Connective Tissue Structure and Function

Steffen Gay and Renate E. Gay

One of the fundamental characteristics of all connective tissues is the relatively large proportion of extracellular matrix in relation to cells. Until recently, the extracellular matrix was viewed as a passive framework serving mainly as an inert scaffolding for stabilization of the physical structure of tissues. In addition to maintaining this three-dimensional form during morphogenesis and tissue repair, it is now recognized as a dynamic milieu in which cells become organized, exchange signals, and differentiate. Study of these processes has led to discovery of a plethora of new matrix components, matrix receptors, and cell-matrix interactions. The extracellular matrix is composed of multidomain macromolecules that are linked together by covalent and noncovalent bonds to form a highly intricate composite. Two major types of matrices exist: the *interstitium*, which is synthesized by mesenchymal cells and forms the stroma of organs, and the *basement membranes*, which are produced by epithelial and endothelial cells. These matrices comprise four major classes of extracellular macromolecules: (1) the collagens, (2) elastin, (3) noncollagenous glycoproteins, and (4) glycosaminoglycans, which are usually covalently linked to proteins to form proteoglycans.

COLLAGENS. The collagens are the most abundant class of proteins in the human organism, constituting almost 30 per cent of its total protein. The central feature of all collagen molecules is the stiff structure resulting from lengthy domains of triple-helical conformation. Three polypeptide chains, called α chains, are wound around one another to generate a ropelike fold. An absolute requirement for the formation of this triple helix, as well as the most distinctive feature of the α chains, is the presence of lengthy sequences of repeating Gly-X-Y triplets in which the X and Y positions are frequently occupied by prolyl and hydroxyprolyl residues.

Studies based on protein chemistry and complementary DNA (cDNA) sequencing have revealed a genetically determined heterogeneity with as many as 18 homopolymeric or heteropolymeric collagen types. As of this writing, 13 distinct collagen types collectively composed of 25 unique polypeptide chains have been identified. It is of interest that genes coding for the different chains are distributed among several chromosomes in the human genome (Table 255–1). Even simultaneously expressed genes, such as those coding for the two α_1 (I) and one α_2(I) chains of the heteropolymeric type I molecule, are located on different chromosomes. The diversity of the well-defined collagens is reflected by the existence of three distinct forms of general molecular structure. The first of these is represented by the lengthy and essentially linear structure assumed by the triple-helical molecules of the fiber-forming collagens. In contrast, basement membrane collagen type IV molecules contain numerous interruptions of helical conformation within the triple-helical domain, which result in highly flexible molecules. The third molecular form is exemplified by cartilage type IX molecules. These molecules contain three collagenous and four interspersed noncollagenous domains. Most remarkable is the presence of a single chondroitin sulfate chain linked to the noncollagenous domain (NC3) of the α2(IX) chain.

Functional diversity of the various collagen types is accomplished by formation of distinct extracellular aggregates. The most obvious are the interstitial linear polymers of fibrils, derived from collagen types I, II, and III. These fibrils with characteristic banding patterns can be readily visualized by electron microscopy. Type I collagen fibers are found in supporting elements of high tensile strength (e.g., tendon and cornea), whereas fibers formed from type II collagen molecules are restricted to cartilaginous structures. The fibrils derived from type III collagen are prevalent in more distensible tissues, such as blood vessels and parenchymal organs. In addition, collagen types V, VI, IX, and XII are also involved in fiber formation, but largely as adducts. This finding is illustrated by the association of collagen types IX, X, and XI with type II collagen in hyaline cartilage. Adaptation for a special function is shown by type VII collagen molecules, which aggregate as antiparallel overlapping dimers to form the anchoring fibrils required to stabilize the dermoepithelial junction of the skin. In contrast to the interstitial types of collagen, type IV molecules form large polygonal aggregates fulfilling the structural and support requirements of basement membranes.

ELASTIN. Elastic fibers are composed of two morphologically and structurally distinct components: elastin and the microfibrils. Elastin, whose gene has now been characterized, is an insoluble protein polymer. The biosynthetic precursor of elastin, tropo-

TABLE 255–1. POLYMORPHISM OF THE COLLAGEN TYPES

Type	Chain(s)	Locus on Chromosome	Major Molecular Species	Major Distribution
I	α1(I)	17q21.3–q22.05	[α1(I)]₂α2(I)	Skin, tendon, bone, organ capsules
	α2(I)	7q21.3–q22.1		
II	α1(II)	12q13.1–q13.3	[α1(II)]₃	Hyaline cartilage
III	α1(III)	2q31	[α1(III)]₃	Blood vessels, parenchymal organs
IV	α1(IV)	13q34	[α1(IV)]₂α2(IV)	Basement membranes
	α2(IV)	13q34		
	α3(IV)	—		
	α4(IV)	—		
	α5(IV)	—		
V	α1(V)	—	[α1(V)]₂α2(V)	Smooth muscle
	α2(V)	2q31		
	α3(V)	—		
VI	α1(VI)	21q223	[α1(VI),α2(VI),α3(VI)]	Minor collagen of stoma matrices
	α2(VI)	21q223		
	α3(VI)	2q37		
VII	α1(VII)	—	[α1(VII)]₃	Anchoring fibrils of the dermoepidermal junction
VIII	α1(VIII)	—	[α1(VIII)]₃	Descemet's membrane, sclera, dura mater
IX	α1(IX)	6	[α1(IX),α2(IX),α3(IX)]	Hyaline cartilage
	α2(IX)	—		
	α3(IX)	—		
X	α1(X)	—	[α1(X)]₃	Hypertrophic cartilage
XI	α1(XI)	1p21	[α1(XI),α2(XI),α3(XI)]	Hyaline cartilage
	α2(XI)	6p212		
	α1(II)	12q13.1–q13.3		
XII	α1(XII)	—	—	Tendons, ligaments, periosteum
XIII	α1(XIII)	10q11	—	Skin, gut

elastin, is a linear polypeptide composed of about 700 amino acids and is rich in nonpolar amino acids: glycine (>30 per cent), valine, leucine, isoleucine, and alanine. Tropoelastin is synthesized by vascular smooth muscle cells and skin fibroblasts and subsequently incorporated into elastic fibers. Elastic fiber formation involves lysyloxidase-mediated formation of intermolecular crosslinks, called desmosine and isodesmosine. Since these crosslinks do not exist in other proteins and therefore are elastin specific, determination of these two amino acid derivatives in tissue sample reflects the amount of elastin present. The microfibrillar component of interstitial elastic fibers is not fully characterized. However, disulfide-rich glycoproteins, such as *fibrillin*, have been identified and may serve as a scaffold onto which tropoelastin is deposited.

STRUCTURAL GLYCOPROTEINS. The major noncollagenous glycoprotein present in the extracellular matrix is *fibronectin*. Fibronectins are dimeric cell adhesion glycoproteins, composed of two disulfide-bonded subunits and found in rather large quantities in blood plasma (~0.3 mg per milliliter). The diverse functions of fibronectin in cell adhesion are illustrated in Figure 255–1. Some of these functions can be mimicked by synthetic peptides that contain the sequence Arg-Gly-Asp (RGD sequence). Similar sequences are found in other cell adhesion proteins, such as vitronectin, laminin, and collagen type VI. Since fibronectin plays a major role in morphogenesis and tissue remodeling, the regulation of fibronectin biosynthesis by growth factors and cytokines has been a focus of study. For example, it is now established that γ-interferon and transforming growth factor–β

(TGF-β) stimulate fibronectin synthesis, whereas tumor necrosis factor (TNF) and interleukin 1 (IL1) inhibit synthesis.

Vitronectin is a 75-kD protein, which is considerably smaller than the 250-kD fibronectin polypeptide present in plasma and tissue. Vitronectin, also termed serum spreading factor and complement S-protein, promotes cell attachment and spreading, inhibits cytolysis by the complement C5b–9 complex, and modulates antithrombin III–thrombin action in blood coagulation.

Tenascin/hexabrachion is another large glycoprotein of the extracellular matrix. The name hexabrachion refers to the disulfide-linked six-armed structure. Tenascin mediates cell attachment through an RGD-dependent receptor and is expressed in association with mesenchymal-epithelial interactions during morphogenesis and development of undifferentiated tumors. The same protein has also been referred to as myotendinous antigen, GP 250 protein, glial mesenchymal extracellular matrix protein, cytotactin, J1-protein, and brachionectin. As the names suggest, tenascin has been identified in tendons, developing smooth muscle, cartilage, and gut and in neuromuscular and neuronal-glial interactions.

Cartilage Glycoproteins. Several structural glycoproteins have been isolated from various cartilages. They include a 148-kD protein prominent in adult tracheal cartilage, but not present in articular cartilage. On the other hand, articular cartilage contains a 116-kD protein as well as two distinct proteins of 58 kD and 59 kD, which are all localized throughout the interstitial matrix.

PROTEOGLYCANS. Proteoglycans are proteins that carry one or more glycosaminoglycan side chains. Glycosaminoglycans

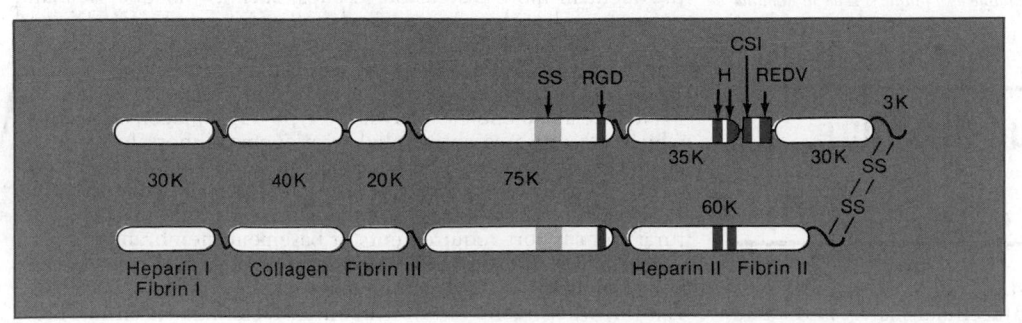

FIGURE 255–1. Multiple cell recognition sites in fibronectin. The fibronectin molecule contains a series of functional domains that bind the indicated ligands. The thick vertical bars indicate cell adhesive recognition sequences. SS = putative synergistic second site; RGD = Gly-Arg-Gly-Asp-Ser site; H = putative sites in the heparin-binding domain; CS1 = the CS1 site in the alternatively spliced IIICS region; REDV = the Arg-Glu-Asp-Val site. (Reprinted with permission from Yamada KM: Fibronectins: Structure, functions and receptors. Curr Opin Cell Biol 1:956–963, 1989. Copyright 1989 by Current Science.)

are long, unbranched polysaccharide chains composed of repeating disaccharide units. One of the two sugar residues in the repeating disaccharide is always an amino sugar (N-acetylglucosamine or N-acetylgalactosamine). Glycosaminoglycans are highly negatively charged owing to the presence of sulfate and carboxyl groups on multiple sugar residues. In contrast, hyaluronic acid, also called *hyaluronan*, is a polymer of glucuronic acid and glucosamine that is not sulfated and not attached covalently to a protein core connected via a link protein. Proteoglycans of almost all sizes and shapes have been biochemically identified. Nevertheless, since cloning and sequence analysis have often identified the same core proteins, the number of distinct proteoglycans is limited (Table 255–2). With respect to their function, they have been referred to as a "multipurpose glue." Proteoglycans not only bind extracellular matrix components together and mediate cell binding to the matrix but also restrain soluble molecules such as growth factors in the matrix and at cell surfaces. Heparan sulfate proteoglycan, for example, binds basic fibroblast growth factor released from injured endothelial cells. The role of proteoglycans in cell adhesion is best exhibited by a membrane-intercalated proteoglycan termed *syndecan*. This molecule binds to collagen and fibronectin through its heparan sulfate chains and mediates cell adhesion.

BASEMENT MEMBRANES. Basement membranes are thin, sheetlike structures deposited by endothelial and epithelial cells but also found surrounding nerve and muscle cells. They provide mechanical support for resident cells, function as a semipermeable filtration barrier for macromolecules in organs such as the kidney and the placenta, and act as regulators of cell attachment, migration, and differentiation. The major constituents are collagen type IV, laminin, entactin (nidogen), and heparan sulfate proteoglycans. Collagen type IV molecules are $[\alpha 1(IV)]_2 \, \alpha 2(IV)$ heterotrimers comprising an N-terminal rod 30 μm long (7S), a linear triple helix containing over 20 noncollagenous sequences, and a C-terminal globular domain (NC1). These molecules can spontaneously aggregate into a network consisting of N-terminal tetramers (7S), lateral associations between the triple-helical rods, and C-terminal dimers (NC1). The network is eventually stabilized by disulfide- and lysyloxidase-derived intramolecular and intermolecular crosslinks, which may provide the scaffold for basement membrane formation. Self-assembly has also been observed with *laminin*, a major basement membrane–associated glycoprotein. The typical features of the laminin molecule are a threadlike long arm terminating in a globular domain and three short arms, each consisting of two globular domains separated by short linear segments. Collagen type IV and laminin appear highly integrated in the basement membrane matrix and are closely associated with a 150-kD, sulfated glycoprotein called

TABLE 255–2. PROTEOGLYCANS (PG) CHARACTERIZED BY SEQUENCING OF THE CORE PROTEIN

Proteoglycan	Glycosaminoglycan
Secreted/extracellular matrix PG	
Large aggregating PG	CS/KS*
Versican	CS/DS
Decorin (PG-40, PGII)	CS/DS
Biglycan (PGI)	CS/DS
Basement membrane PG	HS
Type IX collagen	CS
Intracellular granule PG	
Serglycin (PG19)	CS/DS
Membrane-intercalated PG$_S$	
Syndecan	HS/CS
Invariant chain†	CS
Transferrin receptor†	HS
Thrombomodulin†	HS
Lymphocyte-homing receptor†	CS

*CS = chondroitin sulfate; DS = dermatan sulfate; HS = heparan sulfate; KS = karatan sulfate. These glycosaminoglycans are polymers consisting of the repeating disaccharides: glucuronic acid–N-acetylgalactosamine (CS), iduronic acid–N-acetylgalactosamine (DS), iduronic acid–N-acetylglucosamine (HS and heparin), and galactose-N-acetylglucosamine (KS). DS, HS, and heparin also contain some disaccharide units in which the uronic acid is glucuronic acid instead of iduronic acid.

†These are so-called "part-time proteoglycans"; only some of the molecules are substituted with glycosaminoglycan, and the rest are free protein molecules.

Reprinted with permission from Ruoslahti J: Proteoglycans in cell regulation. J Biol Chem 264:13369–13372, 1989.

entactin (nidogen) in a stable noncovalent complex. Amino acid sequence data of entactin have revealed epidermal growth factor (EGF)–like cysteine-rich motifs, segments showing homology to the EGF precursor, the low density lipoprotein (LDL) receptor, and thyroglobulin. *Heparan sulfate proteoglycans* occur as an integral component in all basement membranes but play different roles in specific tissues. They control permeability of the glomerular basement membranes and have also been implicated in the anchorage of acetylcholinesterase to the neuromuscular junction.

CONNECTIVE TISSUE MATRIX IN CELL REGULATION

It is now well established that matrix components influence the maintenance of cellular phenotypes mediated through matrix receptors.

RECEPTORS FOR EXTRACELLULAR MATRIX COMPONENTS. Adhesive interactions between cells and their surrounding extracellular matrix are not only important in most developmental events but also essential for maintaining the fundamental life processes. Cell proliferation, polarization, migration, differentiation, and protein synthesis depend on interactions between cells and supporting matrix. Diverse families of structurally similar receptors for matrix components have been identified. They include the transmembrane integrin superfamily, peripheral membrane glycoproteins, glycosyltransferases, and proteoglycans. *Integrins* are a group of α/β heterodimers involved in cell binding, some of which involve recognition of an Arg-Gly-Asp (RGD) sequence present in their ligands. The integrins consist of an α-subunit with a molecular mass of 130 to 210 kD and noncovalently associated β-subunits (95 to 130 kD). The cytoplasmic domain of the β-subunit reveals homologies to the EGF, the insulin receptor, and the *neu* oncogene protein. Both subunits define the integrin subfamilies described in Table 255–3.

Since integrins localize in known junctional regions where actin bundles and myofibrils terminate at the cell surface, the major function of integrin receptors appears to be the linkage of extracellular matrix molecules with the intracellular cytoskeletal network. The connection is thereby mediated through the cytoplasmic domain of the β-subunit. That extracellular matrix components may influence gene expression by signal transduction is shown by the finding that fibronectin degradation products induce, via the fibronectin receptor, collagenase and stromelysin gene expression. The latter pathway may play a major role in inflammatory tissue destruction. The pivotal role of these receptors related to infectious diseases is further illustrated by the observation that bacteria use specific receptors to adhere to host connective tissue. For example, it has been shown that certain strains of *Escherichia coli* express a fibronectin receptor that is involved in colonization.

Nonintegrin peripheral membrane glycoproteins serve as matrix receptors in cell binding to laminin and elastin. Whereas integrin laminin receptors bind to the globular end of the long arm of the molecule, a nonintegrin 67-kD receptor binds to a site in the laminin β1 chain. Other nonintegrin matrix receptors have been shown to be restricted to cells of neural origin or chondrocytes. In this regard, a 34-kD protein that binds to cartilage type II collagen has been isolated and termed *anchorin II*. Anchorin II contains segments that are related to a family of Ca^{2+}- and phospholipid-binding proteins, including calpactin, lipocortin, and endonexin. A 90-kD transmembrane glycoprotein, also known as gp90 Hermes or Hermes antigen, mediates lymphocyte binding to the high endothelium of venules during their movement into lymphoid organs. These observations stress that cell-cell and cell-matrix interactions involve multiple types of receptors.

The most provoking question remains: how do matrix receptors transmit information from the extracellular structure to affect gene expression? Figure 255–2 illustrates a model of "dynamic reciprocity," in which the extracellular matrix is postulated to influence gene expression at all levels, including transcription, messenger RNA (mRNA) processing, and translation, via transmembrane and cytoskeletal components. Elucidating the molec-

TABLE 255–3. THE INTEGRIN FAMILY OF CELL RECEPTORS*

Subunits	Designation	Ligands	Distribution
α1β1	VLA-1; CD-/CD29	Collagens I and IV, laminin	F, BM, aT
α2β1	VLA-2; CD49b/CD29	Collagens I, III, IV, V, and VI	F, En, Ep, aT, Pl
α3β1	VLA-3; CD-/CD29	Collagens I and IV, laminin, fibronectin	F, Ep
α4β1	VLA-4; CD49d/CD29	Fibronectin	F, Nc, T, B, M
α5β1	VLA-5; CD-/CD29	Fibronectin	F, En, Ep, aT, Th
α6β1	VLA-6; CD49f/CD29	Laminin	En
αLβ2	LFA-1; CD11a/CD18	Cell adhesion molecules (ICAM-1, 2)	T, B, M, G
αMβ2	Mac-1; CR3; CD11b/CD18	Fibrinogen, Factor X, C3bi	M, G
αXβ2	p150,95; CD11c/CD18	C3bi	M, G
αIIbβ3	gpIIb, IIIa; CD41/CD61	Fibronectin, fibrinogen, von Willebrand factor	Pl
αVβ3	VNR; CD51/CD61	Fibrinogen, von Willebrand factor, vitronectin (VN)	En
αEβ4	—	—	Ec
αVβ5	CD51/CD-	Fibronectin, vitronectin	Ca

*Cloning of the α- and β-subunits has revealed cell-surface proteins on other cells. These include the very late activation (VLA) antigens and the lymphocyte function–associated antigen 1 (LFA-1)/Mac-1/p 150.95 on leukocytes and the platelet IIb/IIIa glycoprotein.

F = fibroblasts; BM = basement membrane associated; aT = activated T lymphocytes only; En = endothelial cells; Ep = epithelial cells; Pl = platelets; Nc = neural crest melanocytes; T = T lymphocytes; B = B lymphocytes; M = monocytes; Th = thymocytes; G = granulocytes; Ca = UCLA-P3 lung adenocarcinoma cells.

Adapted from Springer TA: Adhesion receptors regulate antigen-specific interactions, localization, and differentiation in the immune system. Prog Immunol Springer 7:121–130, 1989.

ular mechanisms of this message system remains one of the key challenges in cell biology.

PATHOPHYSIOLOGY OF CONNECTIVE TISSUE

Some confusion remains about the role of collagen in a wide variety of diseases involving the connective tissues. Historically, the term "collagen disease"—describing a heterogeneous group of acute and chronic diseases, including rheumatoid arthritis, systemic lupus erythematosus, progressive systemic sclerosis, polymyositis, dermatomyositis, Sjögren's syndrome, arteritis, rheumatic fever, ankylosing spondylitis, and amyloidosis—was based on the erroneous notion that "collagen" was equivalent to "connective tissue." However, as outlined above, the different types of collagen and the macromolecular aggregates derived from them are now recognized as distinct structural and histologic entities that exist within a meticulously intercalated connective tissue matrix along with structural glycoproteins and proteoglycans. Consequently, no justification exists for use of the anachronistic term "collagen disease" to encompass a group of such diseases initiated by vastly different pathomechanisms and affecting distinct connective tissue entities. The term "collagen diseases" now exclusively pertains to those inherited conditions in which the primary defect has been demonstrated to be at the gene level and to affect collagen biosynthesis, posttranslational modification, or extracellular processing directly. Recent technologies of gene cloning and gene analysis have led to the delineation of mutations in the fibrillar collagen genes. Collagen type I is the target of certain genetic mutations associated with classic clinical variants of dwarfing syndromes, osteogenesis imperfecta, and Ehlers-Danlos syndrome (types IV and VII) (see Ch. 186, 188, and 189). Moreover, polymerase chain reaction amplification of a series of overlapping segments encoding for the entire helical and telepeptide regions of the human α1(I) collagen cDNA is expected to identify potentially all mutations and polymorphisms.

The acquired disorders of connective tissue involving collagen include conditions that result in repair from overt trauma; in diseases characterized by an excessive deposition of collagenous

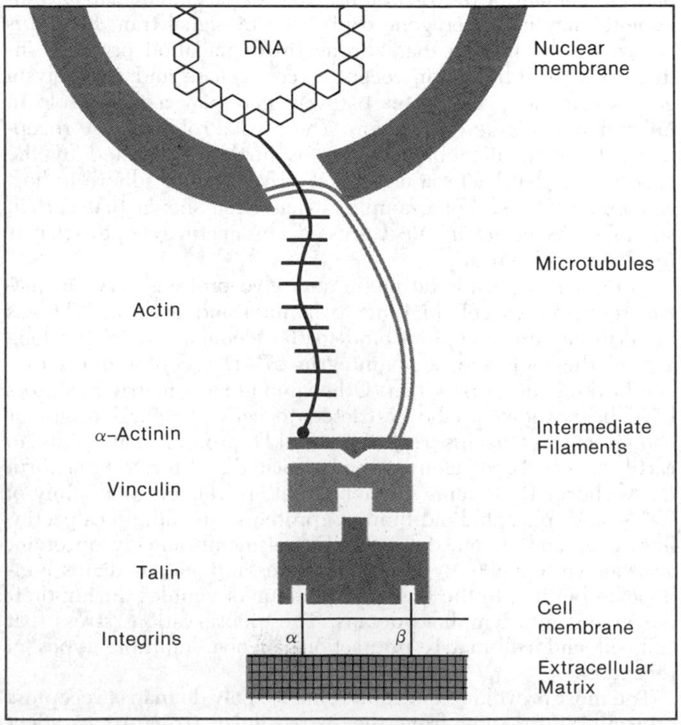

FIGURE 255–2. This refined model for the ultrastructural interaction of cells with extracellular matrix is based on a model of "dynamic reciprocity" whereby the extracellular matrix is postulated to exert an influence on gene expression via transmembrane proteins and cytoskeletal components, proposed originally by Bissell and Carcellos-Hoff (J Cell Sci [Suppl] 8:327, 1987).

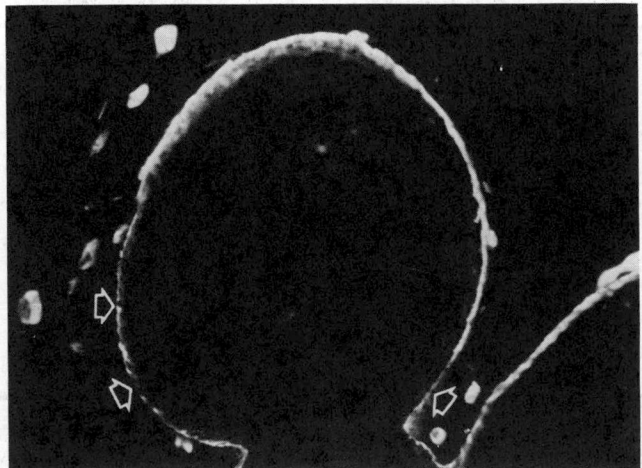

FIGURE 255–3. Frozen section of carcinoma in situ of the breast stained with monoclonal antibodies against human collagen type IV and fluorescence-labeled immunoglobulin antimouse G (IgG). In contrast to other atypical hyperplastic lesions, a thinning and focal loss of basement membrane integrity (arrows) is frequently observed in carcinoma in situ and suggests foci of preceding microinvasion.

FIGURE 255–4. Distribution of collagen types in a normal and rheumatoid joint. The normal synovial lining cell layer is supported by a loose fibrillar network composed of interstitial collagen types I and III, but lacking a continuous basement membrane. Basement membrane collagen type IV is restricted to the vascular endothelium. Vascular smooth muscle cells and pericytes are surrounded with fine, filamentous collagen type V, which is further associated with the interstitial fibers. The vast majority of the interstitial cartilaginous matrix is derived from type II collagen. Collagen types V, IX, and XI are distinctly associated with the hyaline articular interstitium. Synovial fluid normally does not contain collagen. Therefore, detection of collagen in synovial fluid and phagocytes indicates erosive and/or inflammatory joint disease. Detection of type IV collagen suggests endothelial damage and, if found concomitantly with type V collagen, implicates actual necrosis of the vessel walls, i.e., vasculitis. The detection of type I collagen indicates a high level of proteolytic breakdown of synovial stroma and/or bone matrix. Since type II collagen is restricted to the cartilage, the appearance of type II collagen epitopes in synovial fluid and serum represents a sensitive indicator of cartilage destruction and may serve as a tool for monitoring the effects and side effects of antirheumatoid drug therapy. (Reprinted with permission from Gay S, Gay RE: Cellular basis and oncogene expression of rheumatoid joint destruction. Rheumatol Int 9:105–113, 1989.)

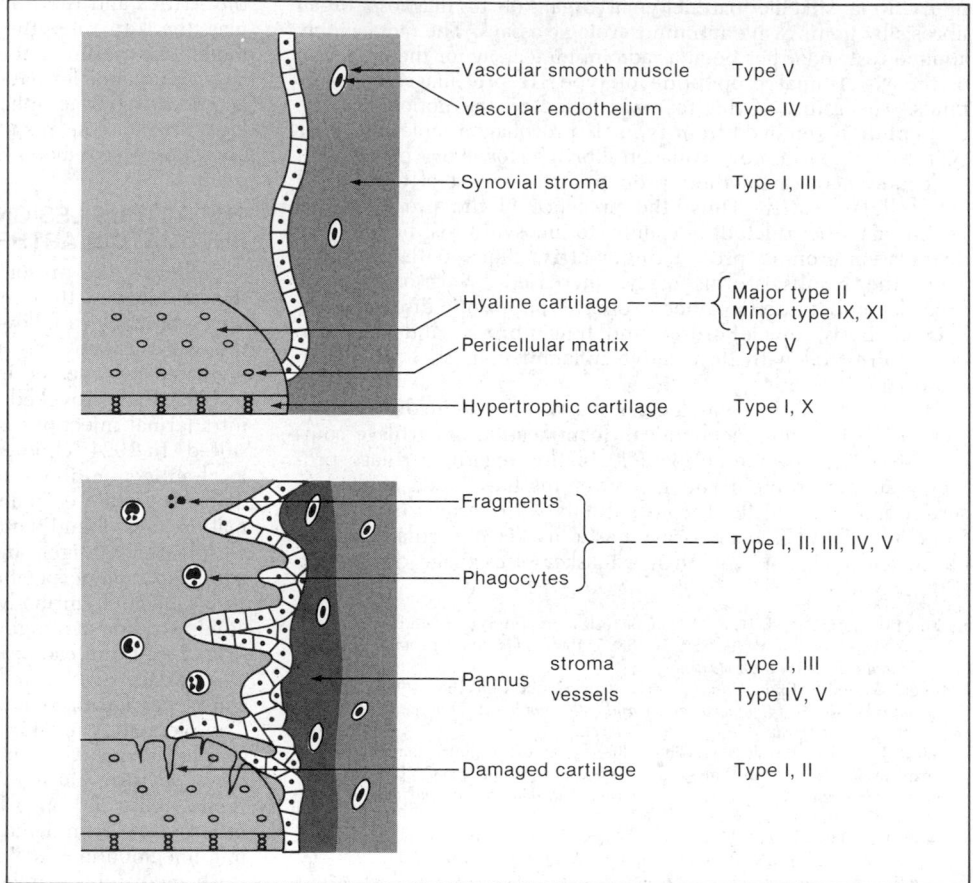

matrix, i.e., fibroproliferative disorders; or in pathologic loss of tissue matrix, including the breakdown of basement membranes in tumor invasion and rheumatoid joint destruction.

Although connective tissue repair after trauma is largely dependent on the type of injury and is, therefore, quite variable, the repair of various connective tissue lesions in wound healing follows a characteristic sequence of events. The initial events involve the synthesis of pericellular and basement membrane collagens in the proliferating epithelial and/or endothelial cells. Subsequently, a loose fibrillar network largely comprising fibronectin and collagen types III and V and single interspersed fibers derived from type I collagen are deposited. Finally, with the formation of scar tissue, the lesions become more fibrous and dense owing to a deposition of collagen fiber bundles derived largely from type I molecules. It is striking that the patterns of collagen deposition in fibroproliferative diseases show certain similarities. For example, damage to the liver is characterized by an initial accumulation of basement membrane collagens in the sinusoidal space of Disse, followed by a fine fibrillar material composed largely of type III collagen and, subsequently, in the case of the development of hepatic fibrosis (cirrhosis, Ch. 122), by an augmented deposition of type I collagen. A similar pattern appears in the development of fibrotic plaques in atherosclerosis (Ch. 47) or the development of cyclosporine-induced myocardial fibrosis in the transplanted human heart.

The major disease affecting almost exclusively the matrix of basement membranes is diabetes mellitus (Ch. 218). The histopathologic hallmark of diabetic microvascular disease is generalized basement membrane thickening. In the kidney, these changes include an increase in glomerular basement membrane permeability followed by decreased glomerular filtration. Evidence exists that accelerated nonenzymatic glycosylation (glycation) plays an important role in the development of diabetic microangiopathy.

The loss of a specialized connective tissue matrix plays a pivotal role in tumor progression and metastasis. With proliferation, malignant tumor cells acquire the capability to invade basement membranes actively and to migrate through the interstitial stroma. Despite the fact that tumor invasion requires a complex sequence of steps, such as the expression of receptors for basement membrane components by the malignant cells, invasion ultimately results in a loss of basement membrane integrity (Fig. 255–3). Severe recessive dystrophic epidermolysis bullosa features a loss of collagen type VII anchoring filaments, which normally connect the epidermal basement membrane to the interstitial matrix of the dermis. In Goodpasture's syndrome, basement membranes are damaged by circulating autoantibodies against basement membrane collagen (Ch. 79). The Goodpasture antigen has been mapped to the C-terminal globular domain of type IV collagen, which explains the high cross-reactivity of the anti–glomerular basement membrane antibodies with alveolar basement membranes.

CONNECTIVE TISSUE MARKERS. The enormous progress in our knowledge of the structure and biology of the connective tissue matrix has caused considerable interest in the development of assays for diagnosis and monitoring therapy in diseases involving connective tissue. Historically, the determination of hydroxyproline as a measure of total collagen content or turnover has been a useful technique in connective tissue research. However, with the discovery of collagen polymorphism and a variety of molecules containing collagenous sequences, the measurement of hydroxyproline now appears to be of only limited value. This observation is based on the fact that there are varying levels of hydroxylation of the different collagens. For example, the type III collagen molecule contains about 30 per cent more hydroxyproline than does type I, and other proteins such as C1q, acetylcholinesterase, and elastin also contain hydroxyproline. Specific immunohistologic and immunoserologic assays have been employed to evaluate the complexity of collagenous proteins in normal and pathologic samples. As illustrated in Figure 255–3, the use of a monoclonal antibody specific for collagen type IV has been advantageous in studies assessing the integrity of basement membranes in neoplastic lesions. Several markers of collagen assembly and turnover have been employed to detect injury to a specific parenchymal organ or to diagnose organ fibrosis by noninvasive immunoserologic assays. The most widely applied test so far has been a radioimmunoassay for the detection of the N-terminal propeptide of type III procollagen in body fluids. The utility of this test was based on the notion that the propeptide is removed from type III procollagen molecules after synthesis to form new collagen fibrils. However, procollagen molecules may retain their propeptide as a part of the normal extracellular matrix. Thus, the presence of the propeptide in serum may be related not only to neosynthesis but also to degradation from a pre-existing matrix. Since both processes affect the results of this assay, increased levels of type III procollagen peptide have been reported in fibrotic diseases, i.e., liver cirrhosis, myelofibrosis, and lung fibrosis, and have also been correlated with destructive inflammation, such as that in acute viral hepatitis.

The development of molecular markers for joint diseases has focused on the immunochemical quantification of cartilage components using specific antibodies. In this regard, cartilage proteoglycan core protein and glycoproteins have been studied in serum and synovial fluid from patients with various arthritides. Keratan sulfate has been assayed as a marker of cartilage metabolism, and collagen type II as a marker of cartilage destruction (Fig. 255–4).

Bashir MM, Indik Z, Yeh H, et al.: Characterization of the complete human elastin gene. Proc Natl Acad Sci USA 264:8887, 1989. *This paper provides the most updated information on elastin.*

Bernfield M (ed.): Extracellular matrix. Curr Opin Cell Biol 1:953, 1989. *A comprehensive and balanced review and collection of expert opinions by leaders in the field of extracellular matrix research.*

Bissell MJ, Carcellos-Hoff MH: The influence of extracellular matrix on gene expression: Is structure message? J Cell Sci (Suppl) 8:327, 1987. *A most interesting hypothesis of how the extracellular matrix may participate in the regulation of gene expression.*

Erickson HP, Bourdon MA: Tenascin: An extracellular matrix protein prominent in specialized embryonic tissues and tumors. Annu Rev Cell Biol 5:71, 1989. *This review article on a specialized structural glycoprotein supplements the articles edited by Bernfield.*

Labhard ME, Hollister DW: Segmental amplification of the entire helical and telopeptide regions of the cDNA for human alpha 1(I) collagen. Matrix 10:124, 1990. *An example of the kind of experimental techniques that are currently applied in hereditary disorders of connective tissue using polymerase chain reaction amplification.*

Lindh E, Thorell JI (eds.): Clinical Impact of Tissue and Connective Tissue Markers. London, Academic Press, 1989. *This book is the proceedings of a recent conference on the use of connective tissue markers.*

McDonald JA: Receptors for extracellular matrix components. Am J Physiol 257:L331, 1989. *A review on how cells interact with matrix via specialized integrin and nonintegrin receptors.*

Miller EJ, Gay S: Collagen structure and function. *In* Cohen IK, Diegelmann RF (eds.): Wound Healing: Biochemical and Clinical Aspects. Philadelphia, W. B. Saunders, 1991. *A complete review on the biochemistry of collagens.*

Rojkind M: Connective Tissue in Health and Disease. Boca Raton, Fla. CRC Press, 1990. *A review on animal models of human connective tissue diseases and methodologies that are applied in current research of organ fibrosis.*

Ruoslahti J: Proteoglycans in cell regulation. J Biol Chem 264:13369, 1989. *A most concise review of the complex roles different proteoglycans play in cellular regulation.*

Sanderson RD, Lalor P, Bernfield H: B lymphocytes express and lose syndecan at specific stages of differentiation. Cell Regul 1:27, 1989. *An example of the role of a most recent proteoglycan named syndecan in the differentiation of B lymphocytes.*

256 Mechanisms of Tissue Injury in Rheumatic Diseases

Gerald Weissmann

Acute inflammation and tissue injury in the rheumatic diseases are caused by host defense mechanisms that have been designed to attack bacteria or viruses but are instead diverted into an attack on the tissues of the host. The two major inflammatory diseases of rheumatology are rheumatoid arthritis (RA) and systemic lupus erythematosus (SLE), and we understand their pathophysiology thanks to three well-studied models of experimental pathology. Whereas some of their *acute* lesions resemble the Arthus and the Shwartzman reactions, in which neutrophils play the key role, the *chronic* features of RA mimic another model of experimental pathology, the tuberculin reaction and its late granuloma formation, in which cytokines, growth factors, and activated macrophages predominate. Joint injury and cartilage degradation result when synovial cells in which proto-oncogenes have been activated form an invasive lesion called *pannus.*

THE ARTHUS LESION AS A MODEL FOR RHEUMATOID ARTHRITIS

Following the prescient observation of Magendie in 1839 that the second and third intravenous injections of foreign proteins into rabbits were followed by increasing distress, Richet coined the word anaphylaxis in 1902 to describe acute catastrophes mediated by repeated intravenous injections of antigens. Arthus, in 1903, then provoked "local anaphylaxis" in rabbits by repeated intradermal injections of antigen; inflammation and necrosis resulted. In 1924, Opie confirmed that the lesions of Arthus were local antigen-antibody reactions in which inflammation was mediated by white cells and that proteolysis was critical. In confirmation it was found that the Arthus lesions could also be provoked by planting antigen in the skin followed by the intravenous administration of specific antibody (the "passive Arthus" reaction) or by injecting antibody in the skin followed by the intravenous administration of antigen (the "reversed passive Arthus" reaction) (Fig. 256–1). In each case, one was dealing with the interactions at a surface of neutrophils that had been attracted by immune complexes localized beneath the endothelium of blood vessels. Complement (Ch. 243), activated by immune complexes, releases anaphylatoxins (C5a and C3a), which liberate histamine. Histamine, in turn, causes reversible gaps to appear between endothelial cells, and once breached, the junctions permit egress of neutrophils. Stimulated by discrete receptors for C5a, C3a, and immunoglobulin G's (IgG's) (FcγRII, FcγRIII), neutrophils release mediators of inflammation: reactive oxygen-derived products (O_2^-, H_2O_2), eicosanoids (see below and Ch. 29), and lysosomal enzymes. These products—especially O_2^-, H_2O_2, and proteases—cause irreversible tissue injury. Predictably, Arthus reactions can be abolished by rendering animals deficient in complement or in neutrophils. Antiproteases or antihistamines are somewhat less effective inhibitors of the Arthus lesion; antiplatelet agents or anticoagulants are useless. It is generally agreed that the local Arthus lesion is one model for immune complex vasculitis in humans, which is also due to interactions of neutrophils with immune complexes and complement. In generalized vasculitis of the Arthus type, the *homotypic* clumping of neutrophils to one another and their *heterotypic* sticking to endothelial cells are mediated by receptors for iC3b (CD11b/CD18), whereas the secretory responses of neutrophils are triggered by receptors for C5a and FcγRII.

The central role of neutrophils in this lesion is mirrored by their abundance in the synovial fluid of patients with RA. Their role in *periarteritis nodosa, leukocytoclastic vasculitis,* some of the *vasculitis of SLE,* and *allergic angiitis* is equally important. Although the *raison d'être* for the preponderance of neutrophils in rheumatoid synovial fluid is not yet clear, their sheer number is impressive. Neutrophils constitute more than 90 per cent of cells found in the synovial fluid of patients with RA, and it has been estimated that the turnover of neutrophils in 30 ml of a rheumatoid joint effusion is greater than a billion. The cells take up self-associating complexes of IgG-IgG rheumatoid factor as well as the more common immunoglobulin M (IgM)–IgG complexes; complement is, predictably, activated. *Rheumatoid vasculitis* is another extra-articular problem mediated by neutrophils in seropositive RA patients. Histologic study of the blood vessels of patients with rheumatoid vasculitis associated with hypocomplementemia has shown a predominantly neutrophilic infiltrate, in response to antigen-antibody complexes and depositions of complement in vessel walls.

THE SHWARTZMAN PHENOMENON AS ANOTHER MODEL OF VASCULITIS

Culture filtrates of gram-negative bacteria injected into the skin of rabbits prepare the site for hemorrhagic necrosis when

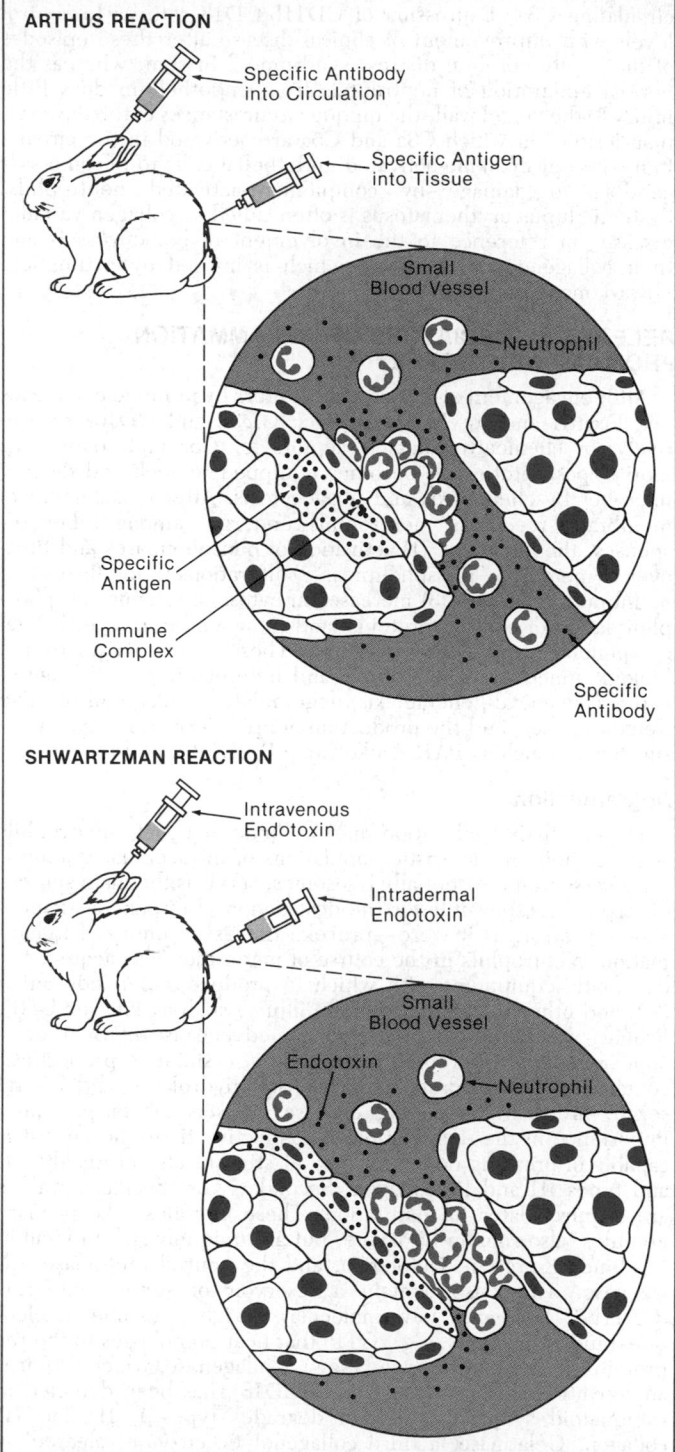

ARTHUS REACTION

- Specific Antibody into Circulation
- Specific Antigen into Tissue
- Small Blood Vessel
- Neutrophil
- Specific Antigen
- Immune Complex
- Specific Antibody

SHWARTZMAN REACTION

- Intravenous Endotoxin
- Intradermal Endotoxin
- Small Blood Vessel
- Endotoxin
- Neutrophil

FIGURE 256–1. In the Arthus model of vascular injury in systemic lupus erythematosus (SLE) (top), intradermal injection of an antigen following intravenous injection of specific antibody leads to immune complex (IC) deposition in vessel walls at the intradermal injection site, which triggers local complement activation, inflammation, neutrophil infiltration, and tissue destruction. In the Shwartzman model (bottom), an intradermal injection of the antigen leads to intravascular alternate pathway complement activation. Antibody is not required, and no IC's are formed. Instead, neutrophils, primed by endotoxin and activated by complement, aggregate within small blood vessels at the intradermal injection, plugging them and causing distal ischemia.

similar filtrates are injected intravenously, a finding first made by Gregory Shwartzman in 1937. The two lesions require a latent, or "preparatory," period of 6 to 24 hours, and the second injection need not be of the same filtrate (Fig. 256–1). The systemic reaction, or "generalized Shwartzman phenomenon," provokes variable degrees of pulmonary or systemic vasculitis and bilateral

renal cortical necrosis as its signature. Like the local lesion, it can be faithfully reproduced by purified endotoxins. Locally or systemically, the *preparatory* injection of endotoxin promotes modest adhesion of neutrophils to postcapillary venules, with escape of some of the white cells from the vessels. The second, or *provocative*, injection leads to microclumps of platelets and leukocytes within the circulation, and these tend to be sequestered in peripheral capillary beds or to attach to the sticky endothelium of venules of the prepared skin site.

The Shwartzman phenomenon can be elicited by second injections not only of endotoxin but also of various polyanions, glycogen, or antigen-antibody complexes, all of which share with endotoxin the capacity to activate complement via the alternate pathway. Moreover, local and systemic Shwartzman reactions can be prevented by rendering animals deficient in complement or neutrophils. In contrast to their inefficacy in the Arthus lesion, anticoagulants and antiplatelet drugs block the local and systemic Shwartzman phenomena. The final Shwartzman lesion is an intravascular insult with secondary damage to endothelial cells. It should be emphasized that the Shwartzman lesion is therefore an exception to the usual circumstances, in which neutrophils fail to injure the endothelial cell layer from which they escape in response to chemoattractants.

Our modern interpretation of the Shwartzman phenomenon is based on recent studies with endotoxin-induced tumor necrosis factor-α (TNF-α) and cellular adhesive molecules displayed by activated endothelial cells and neutrophils. In both the local and the systemic lesions, endotoxin elicits the formation of interleukin 1 (IL1) by Langerhans cells, endothelial cells, or tissue histiocytes and of IL1 and TNF-α from macrophages. These cytokines render venous endothelium sticky—"prepared" in Shwartzman's terms—by inducing the display of adhesive, ligand-like molecules, such as endothelium-leukocyte adhesion molecule 1 (ELAM-1), and by enhancing the procoagulant activity of endothelial surfaces (see below). The enhanced stickiness of endothelial cells induced by endotoxin, TNF, or IL1 leads to *heterotypic* cell-cell adhesion of neutrophils via activation and upregulation of the adhesive integrin CR3 (CD11b/CD18) on the neutrophil surface. The local sites, or small venules in the systemic Shwartzman reaction, have thus been prepared with adherent neutrophils. Some of the neutrophils will already have emigrated to the subendothelium (a noncytotoxic event).

The second, provocative, injection of endotoxin, glycogen, or immune complexes now causes massive *homotypic* neutrophil clumping. With C5a as the major culprit, neutrophils release inflammatory mediators, such as OH_2^-, H_2O_2, eicosanoids, platelet activating factor (PAF), and lysosomal enzymes. As when complement is activated in experimental and clinical examples of the adult respiratory distress syndrome (ARDS; see Ch. 71), leukoaggregates become enmeshed in small capillaries, where the procoagulant effects of endotoxin (via platelets and Factor X) contribute to plugging of the vessels (Fig. 256–2). Tissue injury has been chiefly attributed to H_2O_2 and elastase. Adhesion of neutrophils to endothelial cells—as provoked by TNF, for example—is antagonized by another cytokine: transforming growth factor-β (TGF-β), which in turn is the most potent chemoattractant yet described.

It has now been appreciated that complement-mediated neutrophil aggregation may contribute not only to tissue injury in such diverse conditions as ARDS, acute pancreatitis, Purtscher's retinopathy, acute thermal injury, and the extension of myocardial infarction but also—especially in SLE—to florid vascular crises. Sera from patients with active SLE contain several factors (among them C5a) that cause normal neutrophils to aggregate. Neutrophil-aggregating activity correlates with the activity of the disease and is most pronounced in patients with central nervous system involvement. The availability of radioimmunoassays specific for complement split products permitted documentation of elevated levels of circulating C3a, C5a, and the C5b–9 membrane attack complex in patients with active SLE. Indeed, elevated C3a levels may predict flares of SLE, rising 2 months before disease becomes clinically apparent. Moreover, complement split products Ba and Bb (generated exclusively by the alternate pathway) are also elevated in active SLE; elevated levels of Ba and Bb are better predictors of clinical disease than are conven-

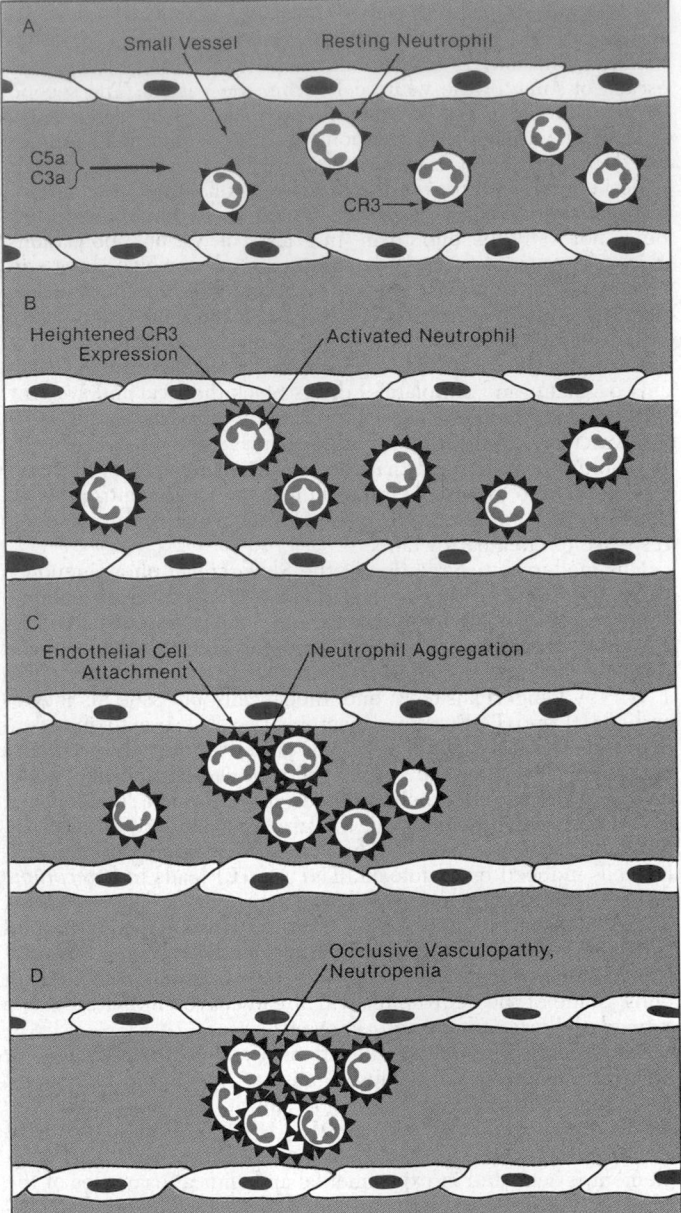

FIGURE 256–2. In active SLE, the process of intravascular complement activation, complement split product (CSP) release, and neutrophil activation may critically involve C5a stimulation of neutrophil CR3 expression (*A* and *B*). A hallmark of the activated neutrophil is heightened expression of surface CR3, which makes the cell stickier; that change can be induced in vitro by C5a. Neutrophils with increased numbers of surface CR3 would then aggregate and adhere to the vascular endothelium (*C*), leading to neutropenia and occlusive vasculopathy (*D*). The role of cytokines (interleukin 1 and tumor necrosis factor) in the interaction of neutrophils and endothelium in SLE is as yet unclear.

tional assays of total C3 and C4 or CH_{50}. In the course of SLE, microthrombosis without inflammation of the vessel wall (i.e., "vasculitis") has been described in lung, kidney, and brain, and histologic evidence has been found of intravascular leukoaggregation associated with elevated levels of circulating complement split products.

With C5a and C3a active in plasma, it is not surprising that cell receptors for complement become activated and upregulated: CR3 (CD11/CD18; see below) has been best studied. As expected, increases in CD11b/CD18 correlate with increased levels of circulating C5a and C3a. Increased expression of CD11b/CD18 on neutrophils has, again, been demonstrated in patients with active, but not inactive, SLE. The highest levels of neutrophil CD11b/CD18 are found in patients with the most severe disease,

especially *cerebritis*, a group that had the highest levels of circulating C3a. Expression of CD11b/CD18 returns to control levels with improvement of clinical disease after these episodes of the "acute cerebral distress syndrome." In sum, whereas the normal emigration of neutrophils from endothelium does little injury to the vessel wall, the unique circumstances of the Shwartzman lesion—in which C3a and C5a are activated in the circulation—permit cytokine-activated endothelial cells to become susceptible to damage by complement-activated neutrophils. Systemic lupus erythematosus is often called a "collagen vascular disease" in reference to the involvement of blood vessels and their collagenous wickerwork, which is injured by Arthus and Shwartzman reactions.

RELEASE OF MEDIATORS OF INFLAMMATION FROM THE NEUTROPHIL

After engagement of its surface receptors by immune complexes (via FcγRII and FcγRIII receptors; CD32 and CD16, respectively) or chemoattractants (receptors for C5a and so on) this motile, postmitotic cell becomes equipped to seek and destroy microbes by chemotaxis and phagocytosis. After engagement of membrane receptors, neutrophils undergo, among other responses, the following: (1) activation of phospholipases and turnover of membrane phospholipids; (2) alterations in ion fluxes and membrane potential; (3) increases in cytosolic calcium; (4) phosphorylation of cellular proteins; and (5) assembly of cytoskeletal components (actin, microtubules). These events regulate the biologic functions of homotypic and heterotypic cell-cell aggregation (see above), chemotaxis, degranulation, release of reactive oxygen species, and the production of lipid-derived inflammatory substances, such as PAF, leukotriene B_4 (LTB_4), and lipoxin A.

Degranulation

During their maturation in the bone marrow, neutrophils acquire their characteristic populations of intracellular granules. These reservoirs, essentially lysosomes, serve as the main sources of enzymes responsible for the destruction of foreign substances and—by error, as it were—provoke the tissue injury of inflammation. Neutrophils in the course of maturation also acquire the enzymatic equipment with which to produce superoxide anion (O_2^-) and other mediators of tissue injury, such as PAF or LTB_4. Primary (azurophil) granules, so named because of their early appearance in neutrophil maturation (or staining properties), contain myeloperoxidase, lysozyme, acid hydrolases, and several serine proteases, including elastase. Elastase is of particular importance in the degradation of connective tissue because it is capable of breaking down not only elastin but also proteoglycans and types III and IV collagen. Secondary, or specific, granules are acquired later in maturation. These granules, like primary granules, also contain lysozyme, but are uniquely rich in vitamin B_{12}–binding protein, lactoferrin, and the neutral proteinase collagenase. They also contain a reservoir of surface integrins (CD11b/CD18) and low molecular weight guanine nucleotide–binding proteins (e.g., GTP) that bear homologies to the *ras* proteins of oncogenesis (see below). Collagenase, which requires an activation step (as does CD11b/CD18), has been detected in rheumatoid synovial fluid and degrades types I, II, and III collagen. Gelatinase, a third collagenolytic enzyme released by the neutrophil, has been localized to the "C" particle compartment, an additional granule subclass. Gelatinase can degrade types IV, V, and 1α2α3α collagen as well as denatured collagen. Thus, neutrophil granules contain three enzymes—elastase, collagenase, and gelatinase—each with different substrate specificity and intracellular origin, which are capable of destroying collagen. These enzymes are differentially released in response to various stimuli.

Neutrophils can discharge the contents of their intracellular granules either *overtly* or *covertly*. During uptake of particles, the neutrophil plasma membrane first invaginates to engulf particles such as immune complexes into a phagocytic vacuole. The vacuole then fuses with lysosomal granules to form a chamber called the phagolysosome, and the granule contents are released into this chamber in the process called *covert degranulation*. Sometimes, however, if the particle is too large, or if the opening of the chamber has not yet closed, lysosomal enzymes are freely discharged into the extracellular milieu, where they may attack host tissues. This *overt degranulation*, a mechanism for extracellular secretion, has been termed "regurgitation during feeding" or, when the material is too large to be ingested (e.g., immune complexes trapped in the matrix of cartilage), has been given the picturesque name of "frustrated phagocytosis" (Fig. 256–3).

Antiproteases, such as alpha₂-macroglobulin and alpha₁-antitrypsin, may prevent tissue damage caused by degradative proteases released inappropriately during overt degranulation. However, the effect of these antiproteases is readily overcome when they are exposed to hypochlorous acid (HOCl), which inactivates them. Since HOCl is formed in the neutrophil after the interaction of myeloperoxidase, chloride anion, and H_2O_2 derived from O_2^- via the NADPH (nicotinamide-adenine dinucleotide phosphate, reduced form) oxidase of the cell, HOCl is important in the mediation not only of bacterial killing (see Ch. 138) but also of tissue injury. Indeed, this HOCl inactivates antiproteases, while simultaneously activating latent collagenase and gelatinase. The identification of destructive enzymes such as myeloperoxidase, collagenase, and elastase at extracellular inflammatory sites in RA patients is consistent with this suggestion. Indeed, the unfortunate interaction of granule enzymes and oxygen metabolites released by neutrophils permits proteases to act unopposed and to elicit the inadvertent tissue injury that accompanies brisk phagocytosis.

Release of Toxic Oxygen Products and Lipid Mediators

The H_2O_2 utilized in the reaction described above is one of several oxygen metabolites, including superoxide anion and hydroxyl radical, that are released during neutrophil activation. The generation of these toxic compounds is governed by the membrane-associated NADPH oxidase system. In addition to contributing to the formation of $HClO^-$, oxygen metabolites can also damage connective tissue directly. For example, superoxide anion is capable of degrading bovine synovial fluid and depolymerizing purified hyaluronic acid.

Neutrophils respond to the engagement of receptors for chemoattractants or immune complexes by mobilizing arachidonate from the sn-2 position of phospholipids. Arachidonate—a fatty acid abbreviated as 20:4 because of its 20 carbons and 4 unsaturated double bonds—is mobilized from membrane stores: directly via a phospholipase A_2 (PLA_2) or indirectly via a phospholipase C (PLC) and followed by the action of a diacylglycerol lipase on diacylglycerol (DAG). Phospholipases A_2, which are associated both with neutrophil granules and with the plasma membrane, have two pH optima (5.5 and 7.5). Purified preparations of PLA_2's require high concentrations of calcium for activity. Neutrophils appear to contain at least two PLC's—one that acts specifically

on phosphatidylinositol (PI) and a second that acts on phosphatidylcholine (PC) to yield DAG. Data on the remodeling of lipids show that not only PLA_2 activity but also the activity of PLC and phospholipase D (PLD) can explain these changes (see below). After treatment with calcium ionophore or with zymosan particles opsonized by C3b, neutrophils release 20:4 from PI and PC to an almost equivalent extent.

Once released from neutrophil phospholipids, 20:4 is transformed to *eicosanoid* metabolites (eicosa = 20), such as 5-hydroperoxyeicosatetraenoic acid (5-HPETE) by 5-lipoxygenase; the peroxide of 5-HPETE spontaneously forms 5-hydroxyeicosatetraenoic acid (5-HETE) or reacts further with the 5-lipoxygenase to form LTA_4, which has an epoxide at the 5,6 position. The 5-lipoxygenase has been purified, sequenced, and cloned. It is a complex enzyme assembly that requires an activation step. Leukotriene A_4 is then acted upon by LTA_4 hydrolase (LTB_4 synthetase) to form 5S, 12R,6, 14-*cis*,8,10-*trans*-dihydroxyeicosatetraenoic acid, or LTB_4. Alternatively, LTA_4 made by the neutrophil can be processed by other cells as well; transcellular metabolism is a rule with eicosanoids (see Ch. 29). Leokotriene A_4 can break down nonenzymatically to 5S,6S or 5S,6R,6,8,10-*trans*,14-*cis*-dihydroxyeicosatetraenoic acid. These nonenzymatic metabolites have, at best, one-tenth the activity of LTB_4 in activating neutrophils. In the presence of exogenous arachidonic acid, neutrophils also show 15-lipoxygenase activity, which, in a parallel manner, produces 15-HPETE and 15-HETE. These products, in turn, are acted upon by an LTA_4 synthetase–like enzyme to make a 14,15-dihydroxy product and finally, in concert with 5-lipoxygenase, can yield the trihydroxy compounds: lipoxins A and B. Mononuclear cells, in contrast, produce stable prostaglandins (PGE_2) and the sulfidopeptides leukotrienes LTC_4, LTD_4, and LTE_4.

Two major candidates for inflammatory mediators made from neutrophils are LTB_4 and lipoxin A. Leukotriene B_4 is a potent chemoattractant and promotes adhesion of neutrophils to endothelial cells from a variety of arterial and venous sites of several species—an effect not shared with other eicosanoids. Prostacyclin from endothelial cells (PGI_2) does not inhibit LTB_4-stimulated adhesion. Finally, lipoxin A has potent vasodilating effects in vivo (but not in vitro) and does not mimic the action of endothelium-derived relaxation factor (EDRF) (nitric oxide). Lipoxin A has only modest effects on neutrophil chemokinesis; since its major biologic action appears to be the inhibition of natural killer (NK) cell activity, lipoxin A may chiefly regulate IgG receptor (Fcγ-RIII)–mediated signal transduction.

STIMULUS-RESPONSE COUPLING: THE BASIS OF CELL ACTIVATION IN INFLAMMATION

Phospholipids and Intracellular Calcium

When chemoattractants such as formyl-methionyl-leucyl phenylalanine (fMLP), C5a, C3a, or LTB_4 engage their receptors, neutrophils respond by generating inositol trisphosphate (IP_3) and DAG. Although signaling via Fc receptors and signaling via receptors for chemoattractants (Fig. 256–4) differ with respect to some details, the general outline of stimulus-response coupling is similar, and neutrophils do not differ in these general pathways from other cells of inflammation.

Cellular IP_3 and DAG concentrations substantially increase within seconds after engagement of the fMLP receptor. By 5 seconds, IP_3 levels begin to decline. In contrast, both DAG and phosphatidic acid (PA) continue to increase over the course of the next 120 to 300 seconds. Although the exact sequence of enzyme reactions whereby the neutrophil generates these elevated levels of DAG and PA is not yet understood, it is likely that both PA and diglycerides play a critical role in maintaining activation of the neutrophil. Indeed, intracellular signaling in neutrophils or macrophages is more complex than that in "suicide" cells like the platelet. In order for neutrophils or macrophages to respond, over time and in space, two signals must be generated: a short "triggering" signal, with an immediate increase in intracellular messengers (e.g., IP_3), and sustained "activation" signals (e.g., DAG or PA) required for the longer processes of chemotaxis and phagocytosis.

But lipid remodeling provides only *some* of the messengers needed for signal transduction. Calcium plays another key role.

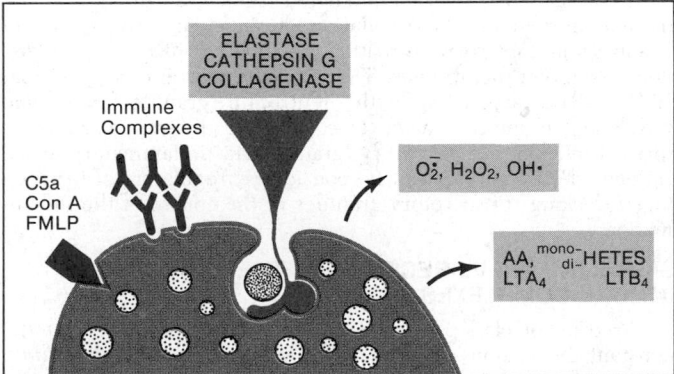

FIGURE 256–3. Release of the mediators of inflammation by the human neutrophil. When neutrophils are engaged by chemoattractants such as formyl-methionyl-leucyl phenylalanine (fMLP, a bacterial peptide analogue), from the complement sequence (C5a), or by lectins (Con A = concanavalin A)—or by immune complexes—they release lysosomal enzymes from intracellular granules to the outside (overt degranulation), assemble and activate the NADPH (nicotinamide-adenine dinucleotide phosphate, reduced form) oxidase that forms toxic oxygen species (O_2^-, H_2O_2, and so on), and turn over membrane phospholipids. These are the precursors for arachidonic acid (AA), which is transformed by an activated 5-lipoxygenase to the intermediate LTA_4, which can be used by neutrophils or other cells to form potent mediators: the leukotrienes (e.g., LTB_4). HETE = hydroxyeicosatetraenoic acid.

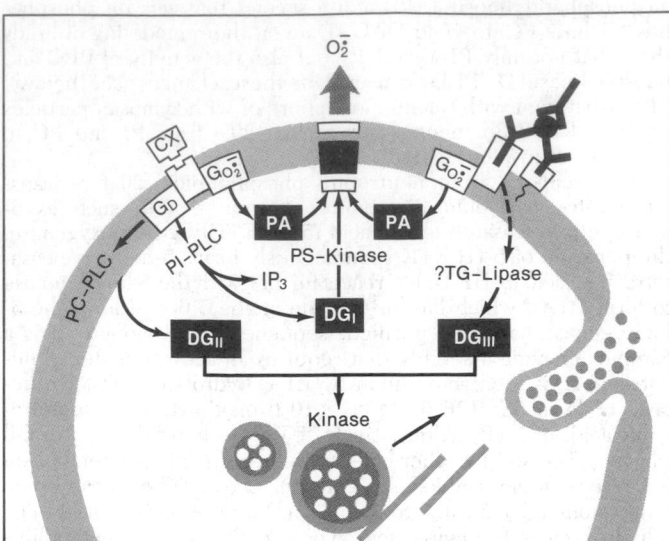

FIGURE 256–4. Stimulus-response coupling in the human neutrophil. Pathways for release of mediators of inflammation by chemoattractants (CX), on the left-hand side of the diagram, differ from those launched by immune complexes (YY), on the right-hand side of the diagram. Three pools of diglyceride (DG) are mobilized, only one of which (DG_{III}) is critical for secretion of lysosomal enzymes. Whereas CX-mediated generation of O_2^- is completely inhibited by pertussis toxin–sensitive G-proteins, only some of the O_2^- assembly in response to immune complex requires this intermediate. Phosphatidic acid (PA) seems to be the main intracellular messenger for assembly of the NADPH oxidase. TG = triglyceride; PI-PLC = phosphatidylinositol–phospholipase C; PC-PLC = phosphatidylcholine–phospholipase C; PS = phosphatidylserine; G_D = the G protein of degranulation; G_{O2^-} = the G protein of superoxide generation.

After treatment with chemoattractants such as C5a or fMLP, neutrophils increase their levels of cytosolic calcium $[Ca]_i$, reaching a peak by 2 to 5 seconds. Over the next 2 minutes, $[Ca]_i$ slowly decreases and then returns *toward*—but not *to*—baseline. The peak levels (300 to 500 nM) are achieved primarily by IP_3-induced mobilization from intracellular stores, since similar levels are achieved in the absence of extracellular calcium. The influx of extracellular calcium begins approximately 5 seconds after calcium has been released from intracellular sites and while IP_3 levels are still dropping. Although IP_4 may in part regulate calcium channels, it is also possible that PA functions in the maintenance of calcium-dependent calcium influx.

Neutrophils break down PI to form DAG and PA within the first 5 seconds of the engagement of receptors by chemoattractants or immune complexes. Suggestions that one or another molecule in the PI-PA cycle mediates these changes in calcium permeability include—among others—the influx via PA-activated "calcium gates" or formation of IP_4 from IP_3 by specific kinases. However, the turnover of IP_3 and IP_4 in consequence of specific phosphatases is extremely rapid (5 to 15 seconds), while DAG and PA continue to accumulate (30 to 120 seconds) after treatment of neutrophils with chemoattractants. In contrast, the formation of DAG proceeds in a biphasic fashion. The first peak is at 2 to 5 seconds, consistent with release of the "triggering" messengers, IP_3 and DAG, by the hydrolysis of polyphosphoinositides. Before this first wave is completed—by 15 to 30 seconds after treatment with fMLP—a second, more sustained wave of DAG formation commences. In contrast, PA rises throughout the time course of activation. There is general agreement that both PLC and PLD are involved in PA function. The concentrations of DAG and PA remain elevated, compared with those of resting neutrophils, for more than 300 seconds, in what has been called the "activation" phase of neutrophil responses. Although the evidence is by no means complete, it appears likely that the second wave of DAG is important in degranulation, whereas the increased levels of PA are important for assembly of the NADPH oxidase that is responsible for generating O_2^-.

GTP-Binding Proteins and Signal Transduction

The superfamily of GTP-binding proteins includes (1) the heterotrimeric proteins which transduce hormonal and sensory signals across the plasma membrane; (2) tubulin (each dimer binds 1 mole of GTP strongly and 1 mole loosely); (3) the elongation and initiation factors of protein synthesis; (4) products of the *ras* oncogene; and (5) putative GTP-binding proteins of cellular secretion. Whereas neutrophils clearly have GTP-binding proteins at their plasmalemma, the protein is neither a classic-G_s- or G_i-protein and appears instead to be at least one novel G-protein: G_n. In turn, at least one function of G_n is to couple receptors for chemoattractants to PLC. Composed of typical β/γ membrane components and an α-subunit of the cytosol, 33 to 50 per cent of the G_n-protein is complexed to the β/γ dimer in the membrane, while the remainder is free in the cytosol. Pertussis toxin (PT) binds to the α-subunit at sites distinct from the GTP site; ribosylation by PT of the soluble α-subunit is enhanced 12-fold by the addition of β/γ-subunits, whereas PT ribosylation of membrane G_n is only modestly enhanced. G_n comprises 1 to 3 per cent of membrane proteins; no great excess of these molecules (10^6 per cell) is present over possible receptors (e.g., receptors for IgG and C5a). The neutrophil G-protein (α-subunit) is a substrate for adenosine diphosphate (ADP) ribosylation both by pertussis and by cholera toxins (CT); both toxins inhibit high-affinity fMLP binding, and the protein is antigenically distinct not only from G_s- or G_i-proteins of other sources, but from the common G_o-protein of brain. Predictably, for G-protein–mediated functions, treatment of intact neutrophils with PT inhibits ligand-mediated O_2^- generation, degranulation, chemotaxis, phospholipid turnover, high-affinity fMLP binding, release of eicosanoids, calcium fluxes, and so on.

But the G-proteins of signal transduction are not the only G-proteins of inflammatory cells; a rapidly growing family of low molecular weight GTP-binding proteins (LMW-GBP's), with a molecular weight in the range of 20 to 30 kD are also present. These proteins are characterized by marked sequence homology to the *ras* oncogene product (*ras* p21). In contrast to their high molecular weight counterparts, no clear function has been attributed to any mammalian *ras*-related protein. Microinjection of human *ras* p21, however, causes degranulation of mast cells, suggesting that LMW-GBP's may play a role in exocytosis. Futhermore, recent evidence implicating *ras* p21 in the activation of a PC-specific PLC suggests that this phospholipase is critical for neutrophil secretion. To date, the strongest evidence for the involvement of *ras*-related proteins in the secretory pathway comes from studies of the yeast *Saccharomyces cerevisiae*, in which these proteins regulate vectorial traffic of vesicles within cells.

In contrast to G-protein–mediated signal transduction at the plasma membrane, the regulation of vesicular movement and fusion seems not to require the transduction of a signal across donor or target membranes. There is good reason to suspect that LMW-GBP's associated with neutrophil granule membrane GBP's are uniquely situated to control the differential and vectorial trafficking of secretory granules in inflammatory cells. Indeed, these proteins can be considered regulators of intracellular "docking" of secretory granules in the course of the inflammation.

SIGNALING VIA Fc RECEPTORS: THE RESPONSE TO IMMUNE COMPLEXES

Three major classes of receptors have been described for the constant Fc region of human IgG's. FcγRI is a *high-affinity receptor* for monomeric IgG (K_a = approximately 10^{-8}M, molecular weight = 72 kD) found mainly on mononuclear cells; recognized by monoclonal antibody 32, it is upregulated in response to interferon (IFN). Neutrophils also have two *low-affinity receptors* (K_a = approximately 10^{-6}M), which bind aggregated IgG's or immune complexes much more avidly than monomeric IgG. FcγRII (or CD32), of approximately 40 kD, is present at 15,000 sites per cell (as recognized by monoclonal antibody IV-3) and is also present on B cells, macrophages, and platelets. FcγRII (1) is resistant to elastase, (2) is not linked to the plasmalemma via PI, (3) is present on neutrophils from patients with paroxysmal nocturnal hemoglobinuria (PNH), (4) appears to mediate O_2^- generation and degranulation, and (5) transduces all of the signal for O_2^- generation and some of the signal for degranulation by means of a PT-sensitive G-protein.

FcγRIII (or CD16) also prefers multimeric IgG and is expressed in heterogeneous fashion on neutrophils, macrophages, and NK cells. FcγRIII has a broad range of molecular weight of 50 to 70 kD, is present at approximately 120,000 sites per neutrophil, and is recognized by monoclonal antibody 3G8. The FcγRIII's on neutrophils and NK cells differ with respect to mass and are products of different but very homologous genes. FcγRIII's of the neutrophil are (1) elastase sensitive, (2) linked to the external plasmalemma via PI, (3) reduced to 90 per cent of controls at the plasmalemma—but not the Golgi region—of cells from patients with PNH, (4) an ineffective trigger of cells for O_2^- or enzyme release, and (5) polymorphic with respect to structure and antigenicity because there are two alleles (CNA1 and NA2). FcγRIII's are shed into the supernatant of neutrophils exposed to fMLP, whereas macrophages and NK cells—in which FcγRIII is a transmembrane structure—do not shed this receptor.

Since cells from patients with PNH respond as well as normal cells to IgG-opsonized particles by O_2^- generation, and all O_2^--generating activity in response to IgG is PT sensitive, we must conclude that the FcγRII is linked to GTP-binding proteins, whereas FcγRIII is not (Fig. 256–4). Recent evidence shows that whereas stimulus-response coupling induced by immune complexes in the bulk phase is largely sensitive to PT, degranulation and O_2^- generation induced by immune complexes on a surface are relatively insensitive to PT. From these observations, it appears that FcγRIII may accumulate at the interface between neutrophils and the immune complexes trapped in the subendothelium. Moreover, signaling via Fc receptors differs from signaling via chemoattractant receptors in that the former is dependent on the integrity of cytoplasmic microtubules, whereas chemoattractant-induced signaling is independent of microtubules. *Colchicine therefore inhibits FcγR signaling.* FcγRIII receptors may serve to cluster Fc receptors in the service of "frustrated phagocytosis" when the discharge of neutrophil contents is launched by an IgG-opsonized particulate too large to digest. Therefore, of the two neutrophil Fc receptors for IgG, it appears that FcγRII triggers cells via classic G-protein–mediated signal transduction, as in synovial fluid. In contrast, FcγRIII receptors unlinked to G-proteins mediate neutrophil discharge in vascular lesions where IgG's are trapped at subendothelial sites, as in vasculitis when the release of mediators of inflammation is by "frustrated phagocytosis."

THE INTEGRINS AND INFLAMMATION

The adhesion of formed elements of the blood to endothelium and to one another is mediated by a superfamily of membrane proteins called "integrins." Three major families of mammalian integrins have been described: (1) receptors for extracellular matrix molecules, such as fibronectin and T lymphocyte receptors, known as very late-appearing antigens (VLA); (2) platelet-surface glycoprotein IIb/IIIa and the vitronectin receptor; and (3) the leukocyte function–associated antigen 1 (LFA-1) family of leukocyte adhesion molecules. The most striking characteristic shared by these molecules is their noncovalently linked α/β heterodimer configuration in which the same β-subunit is shared by all members of a family. In addition, many, but not all, integrins contain a domain that recognizes an Arg-Gly-Asp (RGD) sequence present in their respective ligands.

The LFA-1 family of leukocyte adhesion molecules includes three heterodimeric glycoproteins that share a common 95-kD β chain (CD18): LFA-1, Mac-1 (also called Mo1, gp165/95, and CR3), and gp 150/90, whose α chains have been designated CD11a, 11b, and 11c, respectively. The expression of these three molecules varies according to lineage and stage of maturation of various hematopoietic cells. In addition to mediating cell-cell adhesion, CD11b/CD18 functions as a receptor for iC3b (CR3) and thereby mediates phagocytosis of opsonized particles.

CD11b/CD18 is probably the major neutrophil adhesion molecule involved in *heterotypic* (neutrophil/endothelium) and *homotypic* (neutrophil-neutrophil) adhesion. Children genetically deficient in all three LFA-1 family adhesion molecules suffer from recurrent bacterial infections, impaired pus formation, delayed wound healing, and poor separation of the umbilical cord. Neutrophils from these patients are defective in functions related

to adhesion, such as aggregation, spreading on surfaces, directed migration, and attachment to endothelial monolayers. Normal human neutrophils treated in vitro with a subset of available anti-CD11b/CD18 monoclonal antibodies exhibit defects indistinguishable from those of neutrophils from patients with deficiency.

Although CD11b/CD18 is clearly implicated in the events of neutrophil adhesion, the molecular mechanisms are unclear. Under normal circumstances, neutrophil sticking must be suppressed to permit cells to circulate. Once neutrophils encounter ligands, cell activation is required to render them sticky. In heterotypic adhesion, the other agonist is the endothelial cell. The endothelial cell plays an active role in adhesion and displays to inflammatory cells an inducible, endothelial surface glycoprotein designated ELAM-1, which partially mediates the adhesion of leukocytes, including neutrophils. Interleukin 1, TNF, lymphotoxin (LT), and endotoxin induce the expression of ELAM-1 on endothelial cells. Intercellular adhesion molecule 1 (ICAM-1), a similar but distinct antigen found on a variety of cells, including endothelial cells, is the ligand for LFA-1 and is therefore one of several molecules that direct lymphocyte binding to high endothelial cells, especially those of the chronically inflamed rheumatoid joint. On the other hand, the endothelial side of the equation can be modified by TGF-β. This factor inhibits the adherence of human neutrophils not only to normal endothelium but also to endothelial cells rendered sticky by ELAM-1 as induced by TNF-α.

In homotypic adhesion (neutrophil-neutrophil), the CD11b/CD18 heterodimer receptor engages an as yet unknown ligand on an adherent neutrophil. The putative ligand is unlikely to be adsorbed iC3b, nor is the adhesive ligand likely to be CD11b/CD18 itself because normal neutrophils are capable of aggregating with neutrophils from CD11b/CD18-deficient patients.

CD11b/CD18 is constitutively expressed on the surface of resting neutrophils at a density of 10,000 to 20,000 molecules per cell. Upon activation by a number of stimuli, including especially chemoattractants, neutrophils "upregulate" their surface expression 5- to 10-fold. Since mature neutrophils synthesize little new protein, it is not surprising that upregulation of CD11b/CD18 is due to the translocation of preformed receptor to the plasma membrane from an intracellular source that cosediments with specific granules.

Because each stimulus that enhances neutrophil adhesion also induces Mac-1 upregulation, it was widely believed that these two phenomena were causally related, but recent studies have dissociated neutrophil-neutrophil aggregation from upregulation of CD11b/CD18. Indeed, whereas the constitutive presence on the cell surface of CD11b/CD18 is *required* for neutrophil adhesion, regulation of cell-cell adhesion appears to involve a structural change in each receptor molecule rather than a quantitative change in the number of receptors.

RHEUMATOID ARTHRITIS AS A FORM OF THE TUBERCULIN REACTION

The histopathology of RA can be divided into two phases: (1) the acute inflammatory lesion, the Arthus-type lesion discussed above; and (2) the more chronic, mononuclear cell–mediated, granulomatous disease proceeding in the deeper layers. This lesion—called pannus—is marked by (1) focal collections of β lymphocytes and plasma cells, which synthesize rheumatoid factors locally, (2) various subsets of T lymphocytes, (3) activated macrophages (Fig. 256–5), and (4) the proliferation of other mesenchymal cells of the synovium in which genes for proto-oncogenes have been activated. The two types of activated cells—macrophages and synoviocytes—generate cytokines that cause chondrocytes to participate in their own destruction by releasing proteases and specific collagenase.

The lesions resemble those found in the tuberculin reaction, save for the clusters of B lymphocytes and plasma cells with rheumatoid factor. Indeed, for many years, RA was thought to be a form of tuberculosis, and the gold salts used to treat tuberculosis in the 1920's were first used for RA on the basis of this fuzzy association. We may note that the earliest editions of this text classified RA as a form of "infectious arthritis."

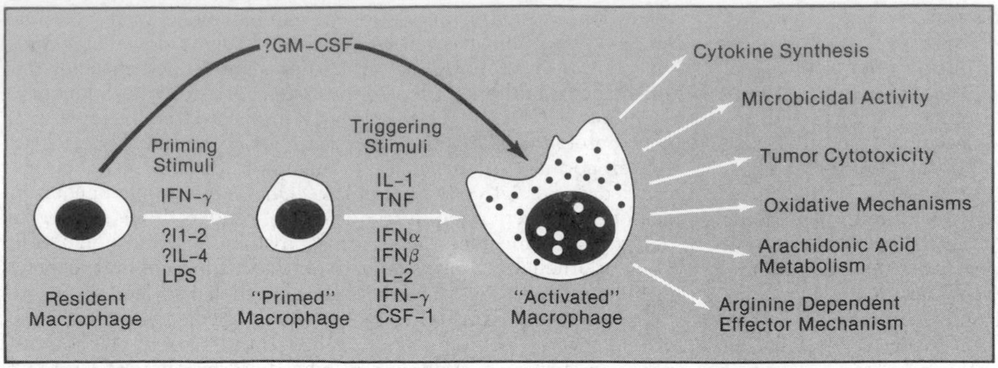

FIGURE 256–5. Schematic depiction of the role of cytokines in the two-stage hypothesis of macrophage activation. Unstimulated cells are primed by treatment with low-dose lipopolysaccharides (LPS), interferon-γ (IFN-γ), and possibly interleukin 2 (IL2). Primed macrophages can be triggered to an activated state by many other cytokines. Activation of the macrophages has classically been defined by demonstrating augmented effector functions as shown.

Although the offending agent of RA is unknown, most modern speculation centers on the likelihood that one or another self-antigen looks very much like the product of a bacterium or virus. The major candidates have been (1) the Epstein-Barr (EB) virus, (2) type II collagen, (3) cartilage proteoglycan, and (4) heat shock (stress) proteins, especially a 65-kD species against which many patients with RA mount a humoral and cellular immune attack. Indeed, there is good evidence that stress proteins are present at the surface of antigen-presenting cells, and recently it was found that a helper T cell clone derived from a patient with tuberculous leprosy reacted with a synthetic peptide found in the third type of variable region of the MLA-DR2 β chain (Ch. 250). The observation that cartilage proteoglycans share epitopes with acetone-extracted fractions of the tubercle bacillus suggests that when humans get RA, they respond to their own tissues as if these were products of the tubercle bacillus or EB virus.

Whatever the offending antigen or antigens prove to be, the mediators released by T and B lymphocytes, by activated macrophages, and by activated synovial cells are the usual battery of cytokines found in chronic inflammation (Table 256–1). These cytokines in turn influence neutrophil function. Indeed, IL1, a proinflammatory cytokine produced chiefly by mononuclear cells, but also by neutrophils, is capable of promoting thymocyte proliferation and synovial fibroblast activation and proliferation. Neutrophils display enhanced adherence to endothelial cells treated with IL1. Among its many other properties, IL1 also induces production of PGE_2 and type II collagenase production by chondrocytes. These actions are regulated by an IL1 inhibitor, which appears to be constitutively present in cartilage cells and in the neutrophil.

Treatment of neutrophils with lymphokine IFN-γ or TNF-β augments neutrophil phagocytic capacity, especially when polymorphonuclear neutrophils are at the surface of cartilage. TNF-β, the most potent chemoattractant, also promotes neutrophil adherence to endothelial cells and stimulates H_2O release and degranulation. Granulocyte-macrophage colony-stimulating factor (GM-CSF), produced largely by fibroblasts, facilitates phagocytosis by neutrophils, possibly by increasing Fc receptor expression. Although many cytokines have no effect on neutrophil chemotaxis, *interleukin 8* (IL8), a macrophage-derived neutrophil chemotactic factor, is one of the most potent neutrophil activators yet found.

Abramson SB, Weissmann G: Complement split products and the pathogenesis of SLE. Hosp Pract 23:45, 1988. *How the Arthus phenomenon and the Shwartzman reaction apply to vasculitis in SLE.*

Bevilaqua MD, Stengelin S, Gimbrone MA, et al.: Endothelial leukocyte adhesion molecule 1: An inducible receptor for neutrophils related to complement regulatory proteins and lectins. Science 243:11, 1989. *Delineation of the critical molecules of endothelial "stickiness."*

Bokoch GM: Signal transduction by GTP-binding proteins during leukocyte activation: Phagocytic cells. In Grinstein S, Rotstein OD (eds.): Mechanisms of Leukocyte Activation. New York, Academic Press, 1990, pp 65–101. *A modern discussion of how the molecular biology of G-proteins has permitted an understanding of the control of signal transduction.*

Haines KA, Reibman J, Weissmann G: Triggering and activation of human neutrophils: Two aspects of the response to transmembrane signals. In Poste G, Crooke ST (eds.): Cellular and Molecular Aspects of Inflammation. New York, Plenum Press, 1988, pp 31–40. *A detailed analysis of the differences between immediate and prolonged responses to signals at the surface of inflammatory cells.*

Harris ED Jr: Pathogenesis of rheumatoid arthritis: A disorder associated with dysfunctional immunoregulation. In Gallin JI, Goldstein IM, Snyderman R (eds.): Inflammation. New York, Raven Press, 1985, pp 751–774. *A review of rheumatoid inflammation with an emphasis on cell-cell interaction in chronic inflammation and cartilage destruction.*

Krane SM, Amento EP, Goldring SR, Stephenson ML: Modulation of matrix synthesis and degradation in joint inflammation. In Glauert AM (ed.): The Control of Tissue Damage. Amsterdam, Elsevier, 1990, pp 179–195. *How IL1 appears to be critical for the self-induced destruction in RA as mediated by PGE_2 and collagenase.*

Nathan CF: Secretory products of macrophages. J Clin Invest 79:319, 1987. *The products of macrophages that provoke tissue injury and constitute cell-cell crosstalk are listed here.*

Pike MC: Chemoattractant receptors as regulators of phagocytic cell functions. In Grinstein S, Rotstein OD (eds.): Mechanisms of Leukocyte Activators. New York, Academic Press, 1990, pp 19–43. *An overview of how neutrophils escape from the capillaries to produce tissue injury.*

TABLE 256–1. CELLULAR SOURCES AND TARGETS OF MAJOR CYTOKINES

Cytokine	Source	Target
IL1-α	Mφ, EC, fibroblasts	Lymphocytes, EC, HCMφ, fibroblasts, others
IL1-β	Mφ	Lymphocytes, EC, HCMφ, fibroblasts, others
IL2	T cells	Lymphocytes, Mφ, others
IL4	T cells	B cells, T cells, others
IL8	Macrophages	PMN
IFN-α	Lymphocytes	Multiple nucleated cells
IFN-β₁	Mφ	Multiple nucleated cells
IFN-β₂ (IL6)	Fibroblasts, Mφ	HC, lymphocytes, others
IFN-γ	T lymphocytes	Mφ, lymphocytes, others
M-CSF, CSF-1	Mφ	Bone marrow, Mφ fibroblasts
GM-CSF	Fibroblasts	Mφ, PMN
TNF-α	Mφ, fibroblasts	PMN, Mφ, others
TNF-β	Lymphocytes, Mφ	Multiple cells
TGF-β	T lymphocytes	PMN, fibroblasts, Mφ
MDNCF	Mφ	PMN

IFN = interferon; TNF = tumor necrosis factor; IL = interleukin; CSF = colony-stimulating factor; M-CSF = macrophage colony-stimulating factor; GM-CSF = granulocyte-macrophage colony-stimulating factor; TGF-β = transforming growth factor–β; Mφ = macrophage; PMN = polymorphonuclear neutrophil; EC = endothelial cell; HC = hepatocytes.

Ritchlin CT, Winchester RJ: Potential for coordinate gene activation in the rheumatoid synoviocyte: Implications and hypotheses. Springer Semin Immunopathol 11:219, 1989. *A discussion at the molecular level of how proto-oncogenes may mediate the cellular phenotypic changes in synoviocytes from RA.*

Smolen JE: Characteristics and mechanisms of secretion by neutrophils. *In* Mallett MB (ed.): The Neutrophil: Cellular Biochemistry and Physiology. Boca Raton, Fla., CRC Press, 1989, pp 24–61. *The mechanisms whereby neutrophils release their inflammatory contents.*

Spaethe SM, Needleman P: Biosynthesis and release of lipid mediate of inflammation. *In* Poste G, Crooke ST (eds.): Cellular and Molecular Aspects of Inflammation. New York, Plenum Press, 1988, pp 153–170. *A review of the cyclo-oxygenase and lipoxygenase pathways in inflammation, with a discussion of the role of essential fatty acid.*

Thomas L: The Youngest Science. New York, Viking Press, 1983, 270 pp. *Read especially Chapters 14 and 15, in which he describes the early days of endotoxin and the Shwartzman reaction.*

Weissmann G: The role of neutrophils in vascular injury. Signal transduction mechanisms in cell/cell interactions. Springer Semin Immunopathol 11:235, 1989. *A review of the Arthus and Shwartzman models and how they relate to the vascular lesions of rheumatic diseases.*

West MA: Role of cytokines in leukocyte activation: Phagocytic cells. *In* Grinstein S, Rotstein OD (eds.): Mechanisms of Leukocyte Activation. New York, Academic Press, 1990, pp 537–570. *A summary of the effects of cytokines, which are released in rheumatoid inflammation, on the activation of neutrophils and macrophages.*

Winfield JB: Stress proteins and autoimmunity. Arthritis Rheum 32:1497, 1989. *How heat shock proteins may be the link between autoantigens and microbial products in the perpetuation of RA.*

Ziff M: Role of the endothelium in chronic inflammation. Springer Semin Immunopathol 11:199, 1989. *How clusters of lymphocytes arrive in the synovial tissues and what the propulsive and adhesive forces are.*

Zvaifler NJ: Pathogenesis of the joint disease of rheumatoid arthritis. Am J Med 75:3, 1983. *A review of chronic inflammation in the joint, with emphasis on classic pathways of tissue injury.*

257 Specialized Procedures in the Management of Patients with Rheumatic Diseases

William J. Arnold and Robert W. Ike

Since rheumatic diseases may be systemic or localized, patients can present with an array of signs and symptoms reflecting multiorgan involvement or pain with limitation of function in a single anatomic area. Optimal management of these patients relies on a thorough history and physical examination, with appropriate laboratory, imaging, and invasive procedures, to arrive at a correct diagnosis and specific therapy. New, exciting, and highly specialized procedures, such as arthroscopy and magnetic resonance imaging (MRI), provide direct and specific information of particular use in the management of patients with localized rheumatic diseases. New serologic testing for Lyme disease and antiphospholipid antibodies can provide important diagnostic information about puzzling new systemic rheumatic disease. The temptation is to rely heavily on the results of these new tests. However, they and the other procedures discussed below must always be interpreted only in the context of a thorough, comprehensive, multifaceted evaluation.

ASPIRATION OF SYNOVIAL JOINTS AND BURSAE

In any patient with undiagnosed arthritis and an associated joint effusion, examination of the synovial fluid is mandatory. Particularly for patients with infectious and crystal-induced inflammation, aspiration and evaluation of synovial fluid are critical elements in the management. Successful joint or bursal aspiration depends on a thorough familiarity with certain principles.

Successful synovial fluid aspiration begins with a well-informed physician. Although most general internists are able to aspirate the knee or olecranon bursa readily, other commonly inflamed structures, such as the shoulder, ankle, elbow, first metatarsophalangeal joint, and subdeltoid bursa, require special expertise for successful aspiration. If the physician is unsure, the advice of a more experienced physician should be sought. Similarly, a well-informed patient is a prerequisite for success. Before the procedure begins, the physician should inform the patient about the

risks and benefits, and the physician should continue to communicate during the procedure. This is also the time to note possible allergies to lidocaine or iodine.

Next, the appropriate supplies and equipment must be made readily available (Table 257–1). The patient must be comfortably positioned to allow muscle relaxation, which will permit full access through the extensor surface to the joint space. For example, when the knee is being aspirated, the patient should be supine with the knee positioned in 10 degrees of flexion, accomplished by resting it on a pillow. The patient should let the leg fall into external rotation, thereby allowing the quadriceps musculature to relax completely. The best evidence for proper positioning and the patient's comfort is a readily movable patella (side to side). If the patient maintains quadriceps contraction, as evidenced by a relatively immobile patella, aspiration will be difficult and painful, if not impossible.

Following skin preparation with iodine and alcohol, the point of entry is determined with the sterile-gloved, nonaspirating hand. In the case of the knee, this entry is located at the midpoint of the patella on the medial aspect of the knee. Local infiltration of the skin and subcutaneous tissue with 1 per cent lidocaine or topical ethyl chloride to reduce the pain of needle entry is optional. The joint space is then entered with an 18-gauge (1½-inch) needle, with a syringe of up to 20 ml attached, depending on the size of the effusion. Larger syringes are too cumbersome to handle. The knee joint capsule is just below the surface of the skin; however, deeper penetration may be required to access sequestered fluid or to penetrate thickened synovium lining the joint capsule. If fluid is not immediately obtained, the syringe should be rotated while the plunger remains retracted. For diagnostic purposes, a 5-ml sample of synovial fluid is more than adequate for all routine studies, including cultures. However, if additional fluid can be obtained without discomfort to the patient, the Kelly clamp can be used to assist in changing syringes.

Following aspiration, the needle should be removed from the joint with one quick motion and hemostasis ensured by applying pressure at the aspiration site for 1 to 2 minutes. An adhesive bandage dressing is then applied, and the patient can be immediately ambulatory. The synovial fluid specimen can be processed efficiently and accurately by immediately placing a single drop on a clean slide with a coverslip (for microscopy) and then putting one half of the specimen in a heparinized tube (for white blood cell [WBC] count and glucose determination) and transporting the other half in the syringe directly to the bacteriology laboratory for culture.

Analysis of the synovial fluid is undertaken as soon as possible after the aspiration to determine if the fluid is inflammatory or noninflammatory (Table 257–2). Synovial fluid from patients with osteoarthritis is characteristically translucent and noninflammatory, with an average synovial fluid WBC count of 600 per cubic millimeter. In contrast, inflammatory synovial fluid, such as that found in patients with rheumatoid arthritis, has a WBC count of

TABLE 257–1. COMPONENTS OF THE ARTHROCENTESIS TRAY

Skin Preparation
Alcohol sponges, iodine swabs
Sterile gauze (2 × 2)
Adhesive bandages
Sterile disposable gloves
Local Anesthetic
1% Lidocaine
Ethyl chloride spray
Aspirating Equipment
Disposable syringes (5, 10, and 20 ml)
18- and 20-gauge aspirating needles
25-Gauge infiltrating needles
Sterile Kelly clamp
Transporting/Analyzing Equipment
Plain and heparinized test tubes
Clean microscope slides with coverslips
Chocolate agar plates
Aerobic/anaerobic bacteria culture media

TABLE 257–2. SYNOVIAL FLUID ANALYSIS

Diagnosis	Appearance	Total White Cell Count per mm³*	Polymorphonuclear cells	Miscellaneous
Normal	Clear, pale yellow	0–200	Less than 10%	—
Group I (Noninflammatory)				
Osteoarthritis	Clear to slightly turbid	50–2000 (600)	Less than 30%	Cartilage fragments
Group II (Mildly inflammatory)				
Systemic lupus erythematosus (SLE)	Clear to slightly turbid	0–9000 (3000)	Less than 20%	—
Scleroderma				
Group III (Severely inflammatory)				
Gout	Turbid	100–160,000 (21,000)	Approximately 70%	Monosodium urate crystals
Pseudogout	Turbid	50–75,000 (14,000)	Approximately 70%	Calcium pyrophosphate dihydrate crystals
Rheumatoid arthritis	Turbid	250–80,000 (19,000)	Approximately 70%	—
Group IV (Infectious)				
Acute bacterial	Very turbid	150–250,000 (80,000)	Approximately 90%	Culture positive
Tuberculosis	Turbid	2500–100,000 (20,000)	Approximately 60%	Culture often negative

*Averages in parentheses.

greater than 2000 per cubic millimeter and may be either translucent or opaque. A rapid determination of opacity can be made by trying to read newsprint placed behind the synovial fluid in a glass tube. Gross tests of inflammation in synovial fluid, such as the mucin clot and string test, can provide additional information about the inflammatory nature of the fluid. Analysis of bursal fluid has shown that bursae react less intensely than synovial joints to specific disease stimuli. A relatively low bursal fluid leukocyte count is often present in patients with septic and gouty bursitis. For instance, in gouty bursitis, an average bursal fluid leukocyte count is 2800 per cubic millimeter, compared with an average of 21,000 per cubic millimeter in synovial fluid.

Every synovial fluid analysis must include a polarizing microscopic evaluation for crystals (see Color Plate 4C). Needle-shaped, intracellular, negatively birefringent crystals of monosodium urate are characteristically seen in patients with gouty arthritis. Rhomboidal, positively birefringent intracellular crystals of calcium pyrophosphate dihydrate are found in patients with the pseudogout syndrome. In both patients with gout and those with pseudogout, a careful, thorough examination of synovial fluid is often necessary to find the pathognomonic crystals. In some patients, both types of crystals may be found. Other crystals found in synovial fluid include calcium oxalate (dialysis-associated arthritis) and calcium hydroxyapatite (Milwaukee shoulder). Occasionally, in patients with chronic effusions accompanied by bleeding (e.g., hemophilia or rheumatoid arthritis), cholesterol crystals may be found. These are platelike and brilliantly birefringent under polarizing microscopy.

The highest synovial fluid WBC counts (15,000 per cubic millimeter or greater) are found in patients with septic arthritis. The most common pathogen is *Staphylococcus aureus*. While a synovial fluid Gram stain revealing gram-positive cocci can be helpful in guiding initial antibiotic therapy, a negative Gram stain does not rule out infection as a cause of the inflammatory arthritis. In these situations, i.e., a negative Gram stain, but with strong suspicion of infectious arthritis, empiric antibiotic therapy must be used until culture results are available.

Neisseria gonorrhoeae is the most frequently found gram-negative organism associated with infectious arthritis. Although gonococcal arthritis may be monoarticular, a polyarticular presentation with fever and skin lesions is characteristic. Gram-negative intracellular diplococci are characteristically seen on a Gram stain of synovial fluid from patients with monoarticular gonococcal arthritis and occasionally (20 per cent) are found in skin lesions of patients with polyarticular gonococcal arthritis.

The clinical course of tuberculous arthritis is usually indolent and monoarticular. The synovial fluid is intensely inflammatory with a high percentage of mononuclear cells. Synovial fluid cultures are usually negative, and signs of active extra-articular disease are minimal. A prompt, accurate diagnosis of tuberculous arthritis requires a high degree of suspicion and culture of synovial biopsy specimens. Often extensive joint destruction is present before a diagnosis of tuberculous arthritis is made.

Determination of the glucose content of synovial fluid is the most valuable chemical assessment performed. When the synovial fluid glucose content is less than 50 per cent of a simultaneously determined serum level, the diagnosis of infectious arthritis should be suspected. In patients with infectious arthritis, serial determinations of synovial fluid glucose level, along with decreasing synovial fluid WBC count and serologic markers of inflammation, such as C-reactive protein level, can be used to follow the efficacy of therapy.

RHEUMATOID FACTOR

Rheumatoid factor is an immunoglobulin M (IgM) antibody directed against normal human immunoglobulin G (IgG). It is usually measured by agglutination tests (agglutination of IgG-coated latex particles) and reported as either negative or positive with a titer. Rheumatoid factor positivity with titers up to 1:320 may be found in otherwise normal people over 70 years old. Rheumatoid factor can be found in 70 to 80 per cent of patients with rheumatoid arthritis but also in patients with other rheumatic diseases (Sjögren's syndrome) and nonrheumatic diseases, such as chronic infections (hepatitis, subacute bacterial endocarditis). In patients with rheumatoid arthritis, the presence of rheumatoid factor is associated with more severe disease, manifested by rheumatoid nodules, rheumatoid vasculitis, and bone erosions. Rheumatoid factor is characteristically absent in patients with the seronegative spondyloarthropathies, such as psoriatic arthritis and ankylosing spondylitis.

ANTINUCLEAR ANTIBODIES

Testing of serum for the presence of antibodies directed against both nuclear and cytoplasmic antigens has contributed greatly to the diagnosis and management of patients with rheumatic diseases. Beginning with Hargraves' description of the LE cell in 1948, subsequent work has refined our knowledge of these antibodies and their clinical associations (Table 257–3).

Routine determination of the presence of antinuclear antibodies is best performed by the indirect immunofluorescent technique

TABLE 257–3. ASSOCIATION BETWEEN RHEUMATIC DISEASES AND ANTINUCLEAR ANTIBODIES

Rheumatic Disease	Antibody Reactive with: (Autoantibody Frequency, %)
Systemic lupus erythematosus	Native DNA (40%), denatured DNA (70%), Sm (30%), nuclear RNP (30%), SSA/Ro (30%), SSB/La (15%)
Drug-induced lupus	Denatured DNA (80%), Histones (> 95%)
Mixed connective tissue disease	Nuclear RNP (> 95%)
Sjögren's syndrome	SSA/Ro (60%), SSB/La (40%)
Dermatopolymyositis	Jo-1 (25%)
Scleroderma	Scl-70 (70% in diffuse scleroderma), centromere (75% in CREST)

Data from Tan EM: Antinuclear antibodies: Diagnostic markers for autoimmune diseases and probes for cell biology. Adv Immunol 44:93–151, 1989.

RNP = ribonucleoprotein; CREST = calcinosis, Raynaud's phenomenon, esophageal dysmotility, sclerodactyly, and telangiectasia.

using Hep-2 cells. The result must be reported as either negative or positive with a titer and pattern. While certain patterns of antinuclear fluorescence correlate loosely with the presence of specific antibodies (e.g., rim pattern with antibodies to native DNA), the presence of specific antibodies can be confirmed only by testing with specific antigens (often referred to as an ANA [antinuclear antibody] profile). Depending on the rheumatic disease, the presence of specific antibodies can be of critical diagnostic significance. For instance, antibody to the Sm antigen is found in only 30 per cent of patients with systemic lupus erythematosus (SLE) but is not found in patients with other rheumatic diseases. The same significance exists for the relationship between antibodies to the Scl-70 antigen and diffuse scleroderma and antibodies to the Jo-1 antigen and polymyositis. Other associations may be of primary therapeutic importance, as in patients with SLE and antibodies to native DNA, in whom there is a higher incidence of renal disease than if these antibodies were absent. There is also a high incidence of complete congenital heart block in infants of normal or SLE mothers who have SSA/anti-Ro antibodies.

SEDIMENTATION RATE

Determination of the sedimentation rate of red blood cells in anticoagulated blood by the Westergren method is a sensitive indicator of the presence of systemic or locally severe inflammation. Characteristically, patients with inflammatory arthritides, such as rheumatoid arthritis and the seronegative spondyloarthropathies, have elevated sedimentation rates, which vary with clinical disease activity. Thus, in this group of patients, determination of the sedimentation rate can assist in following the activity of the disease, but it is of little help diagnostically. In contrast, patients with temporal arteritis and polymyalgia rheumatica frequently have nonspecific symptoms and a negative laboratory serologic evaluation except for an elevated sedimentation rate. In untreated temporal arteritis and polymyalgia rheumatica, a normal Westergren sedimentation rate virtually eliminates the diagnosis. In addition, in these patients, the Westergren sedimentation rate is used together with clinical symptoms to monitor disease activity as a guide to glucocorticoid therapy. Occasionally, as the glucocorticoid dose is tapered, the sedimentation rate rises before symptoms reappear. In patients with the fibromyalgia syndrome, all tests of inflammation are negative or normal, including the sedimentation rate.

C-REACTIVE PROTEIN (CRP)

C-reactive protein is produced in the liver and is normally found in serum in minute amounts (less than 0.6 mg per deciliter). In conditions characterized by inflammation with tissue destruction, particularly bacterial infections, the CRP level may increase 1000-fold in less than 24 hours. Although CRP has been shown to have many effects in the immune system, including complement activation, its specific primary role is still unclear. In the management of patients with rheumatic diseases, serial determinations of the CRP level have certain advantages over following the sedimentation rate. Since numerous serum proteins can influence the sedimentation rate (fibrinogen, haptoglobin, immunoglobulin, ceruloplasmin), changes in the sedimentation rate often do not accurately reflect improvement or deterioration in the clinical condition. Owing to its rapid synthesis and degradation, CRP is a sensitive indicator of therapeutic efficacy in situations in which it is elevated. For example, in patients with septic arthritis, serial serum CRP determinations can provide accurate additional information on the efficacy of antibiotic administration.

ANTIPHOSPHOLIPID ANTIBODY SYNDROME

Antiphospholipid antibodies, including the lupus anticoagulant (LA) and anticardiolipin (ACL), have been reported to be associated with thrombosis, central nervous system disease, and multiple spontaneous abortions in patients with SLE. In addition, in patients without SLE or other obvious connective tissue disease, an increased incidence of arterial and venous thrombosis and loss of fetuses has been suggested to be associated with LA and ACL. Determination of ACL levels is done best by enzyme-linked immunosorbent assay (ELISA). However, this method has been shown to have a high degree of variability and often poor reproducibility even in the best laboratories. The LA is determined by prolongation of the partial thromboplastin time (PTT) when normal plasma is mixed with plasma containing LA. Although LA and ACL are distinct antibodies, they are present together in approximately 70 per cent of patients. LA and ACL are found in approximately 34 per cent and 44 per cent of patients with SLE, respectively.

Although this information engenders a great degree of interest, the lack of prospective study of a group of asymptomatic normal or SLE patients with LA or ACL and a matched population without LA or ACL makes uncertain the exact relationship between antiphospholipid antibodies and disease, particularly in normal subjects. However, since the association of LA and ACL with certain syndromes has been so strong, particularly in patients with multiple spontaneous abortions, clinical trials have been instituted. Oral glucocorticoid or heparin and aspirin therapy of LA-positive, clinically normal women with multiple spontaneous abortions has resulted in successful conception and delivery. Glucocorticoid therapy can alter LA levels but has little effect on ACL levels. An increased incidence of thrombosis, fetal loss, thrombocytopenia, and central nervous system disease has been found in ACL-positive patients with SLE, with no relationship to age, duration of disease, disease severity, or other organ involvement.

LYME DISEASE (see Ch. 343)

A virtual epidemic of testing for Lyme antibodies is sweeping the country. In Wisconsin, where the incidence of Lyme disease is 7.5 per 100,000 population, approximately 1200 per 100,000 Lyme antibody titers were performed in 1988. Since Lyme antibody is frequently absent (50 to 70 per cent) early in the disease, when symptoms and signs are characteristically present, an overreliance on such testing can be very misleading. Newer methodologies, including the Western blot analysis for *Borrelia burgdorferi* antigen, are expensive but promise to add specificity and sensitivity. A PCR (polymerase chain reaction) test for *B. burgdorferi* DNA has been devised, but the sensitivity and specificity have yet to be determined.

Particularly in an endemic area, the decision to treat with antibiotics for Lyme disease must be made more on the basis of clinical suspicion than with reliance on serologic results. Patients with fever and erythema chronicum migrans or polyarthritis, with or without Bell's palsy and cardiac abnormalities (particularly congestive heart failure), should receive antibiotic therapy even if the Lyme antibodies are not present. The presence of Lyme antibodies is most useful diagnostically in patients with an atypical clinical presentation or in late disease (monoarticular arthritis or oligoarthritis and isolated central nervous system disease or psychiatric disorder).

BONE DENSITY MEASUREMENTS

The single most important determinant of hip or vertebral fracture in postmenopausal women is bone density. Therefore, detection and treatment of diminished bone density before menopause should reduce the incidence of fracture in later life. There are certain characteristics in perimenopausal women that, when present, have been thought to predict low bone density (Table 257–4). For the most part, when present, these are reliable indicators of low bone density; however, recent studies have shown bone density to be low in some patients without risk factors. While routine screening of every perimenopausal woman for decreased bone density is not recommended, an accurate determination of bone density can be very useful in determining the need for estrogen therapy and in following the efficacy of therapy for established osteoporosis (see Ch. 238).

Noninvasive techniques for assessing bone density include single- and dual-photon analysis, quantitative computed tomography (CT), and dual-energy x-ray absorptiometry (DEXA). The last-named (DEXA) is now the most accurate method, and dual- and single-photon analyses are the most commonly available. Single-photon analysis is used to assess bone density in the distal radius, while dual-photon analysis accurately assesses bone density in the lumbar spine and proximal femur. Changes in bone density of 1 per cent per year can be accurately assessed with dual-photon analysis. With the use of estrogens and salmon calcitonin, the therapy of osteoporosis can be directed at preventing reabsorption of bone, and fluoride and calcium can stimulate calcified matrix formation. Weight-bearing exercise is the only therapy proven to build bone mass; early results of therapy with Didronel (disodium etidronate) to increase bone mass are encouraging.

IMAGING TECHNIQUES

Plain radiographs of the joints are the least expensive and most readily accessible joint imaging technique. They constitute the gold standard for the diagnosis of osteoarthritis and are the most commonly used means to assess the presence and progression of bone erosions in rheumatoid arthritis. Single anteropostererior radiographs of the hands, feet, pelvis, and knees (weight-bearing joints) are most often used to screen patients with signs or symptoms in these areas. In rheumatoid arthritis, the earliest findings are periarticular osteopenia and soft tissue swelling, particularly evident in the hands. In patients with osteoarthritis, joint space narrowing seen in the medial compartment of the knee on weight-bearing views often precedes the other characteristic features, i.e., subchondral sclerosis, marginal osteophyte formation, subchondral cysts, and varus deformity. A lateral view of the cervical spine in flexion and extension is useful to detect vertebral subluxation (particularly C-1–C-2) in patients with rheumatoid arthritis. A single 20-degree anteroposterior tilt of the pelvis gives excellent visualization of the sacroiliac joints. The limitations of plain radiography in correlating patients' symptoms with intra-articular abnormalities have become evident as more sophisticated imaging techniques have become available. By using both arthroscopic inspection and the newer imaging techniques (MRI), cartilage damage and intra-articular soft tissue abnormalities, such as meniscal tears, have been documented to occur in the presence of normal plain joint radiographs. These observations help to explain the lack of concordance between symptoms and radiographic findings often seen in patients with early osteoarthritis.

Of the new imaging techniques, MRI has had the most dramatic impact on the anatomic assessment of the musculoskeletal system. In a patient with a painful shoulder, the MRI shows rotator cuff inflammation and partial tears with much more sensitivity than does arthography and with more specificity than does ultrasound.

TABLE 257–4. RISK FACTORS FOR OSTEOPOROSIS

Female
Caucasian/Asian
Menopausal
Elderly
Petite female body
Positive family history
Diet deficient in calcium
Alcohol or tobacco consumption
Physical inactivity

In the knee, MRI is extremely sensitive in detecting degenerative changes in menisci and cartilage. Intrameniscal degeneration (grades I and II) unaccompanied by arthroscopically detectable tears is commonly seen on MRI examination in patients with osteoarthritis of the knee. Even meniscal degenerative lesions that appear to be full thickness on MRI (grade III) can occur in the absence of a tear. A similar situation occurs in the lumbosacral spine, where MRI-demonstrable disc degeneration occurs in advance of disc space narrowing on plain radiographs. Thinning and ulceration of hyaline articular cartilage can also be seen before any changes are evident on the plain radiographs. This superior visualization of intra-articular structures holds great promise for the early detection of joint destruction and in guiding specific protective therapy. However, MRI cannot be used to plan or as an indication for arthroscopic interventions in patients with osteoarthritis, since the relationships between the patient's symptoms, the MRI findings, and the response to therapy have not yet been demonstrated.

ARTHROSCOPY

Endoscopic inspection of the joint with therapeutic intra-articular interventions has gone from being "the professor's toy" in the 1970's to being the most commonly performed invasive procedure in the 1990's for patients with arthritis. Fueled by rapid technologic advances, coupled with heightened awareness and expectations on the part of the patient, the dramatic increase in the number of arthroscopies has not yet been accompanied by a clear delineation of the risks and benefits. In addition, the tremendous potential of arthroscopy for research purposes in arthritis to help visually delineate intra-articular abnormalities and obtain synovial biopsy specimens under direct visualization has only just recently begun to be explored.

At present, arthroscopy is performed in an operating room setting, most frequently with the patient under general anesthesia. Sterile conditions are used throughout the procedure. Available instruments include a standard 30-degree rigid operating arthroscope (4 mm in external diameter, fiberoptic light source) in the presence of continuous pressure-controlled saline irrigation. The arthroscope is attached to a television camera, and the image is projected on a screen either in front of or to the side of the arthroscopist. This practice allows accurate visualization as well as the recording of the entire arthroscopic procedure on videotape. Equipment available for arthroscopic intervention includes a variety of motorized and hand-operated instruments. Biopsy forceps and basket forceps for debriding cartilage and menisci come in various sizes and angulations. Motorized equipment includes articular shavers for cartilage and synovial debridement. The basic technique of arthroscopy is triangulation. The arthroscopist must be able to perform diagnostic and therapeutic maneuvers through triangulation while looking at the television screen and not the knee. This is a skill acquired by training on arthroscopic simulators as well as with time and practice. With the use of a standard arthroscope, all compartments of the knee, both weight bearing and non weight bearing, can be inspected, including the posterior compartments and the popliteal space. All intra-articular structures, cruciates, and menisci can be thoroughly inspected and probed to detect defects or laxity. Arthroscopic visualization is now possible for virtually all major joints, including, in order of frequency, the knee, shoulder, ankle, elbow, wrist, and hip. New technologic advances have produced arthroscopes that can be placed in the joint through a 14-gauge needle and now suggest a role for laser therapy in synovial, cartilage, and meniscal debridement.

The most frequent serious complications of arthroscopy at the present time are septic arthritis and hemarthrosis, which occur in fewer than 0.1 per cent of patients. Although no specific series has addressed the complication rate in patients with arthritis, use of local or regional anesthesia rather than general, use of a pressure infusion pump to control bleeding rather than occlusion of blood flow to the leg by thigh tourniquet, and attention to aggressive postoperative rehabilitation should help to lower even further the 1 to 2 per cent overall complication rate for patients with arthritis.

While the role for arthroscopy in the management of patients with arthritis continues to evolve, conceptually, the availability of arthroscopy has already altered the approach to the manage-

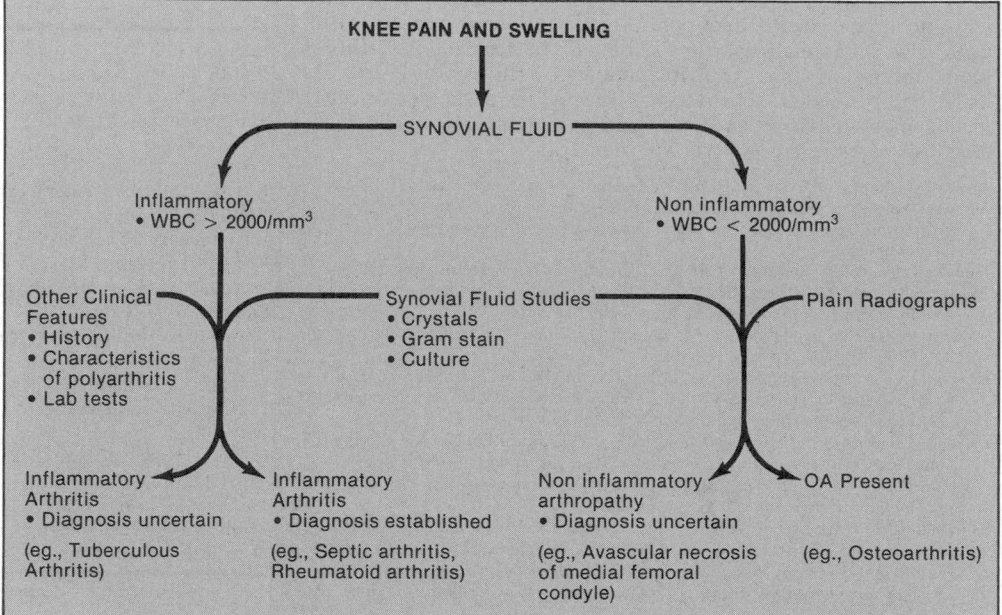

FIGURE 257–1. An arthroscopist's approach to the management of knee arthritis. See text for discussion. WBC = white blood cells; OA = osteoarthritis.

ment of these patients, particularly those with knee arthritis (Fig. 257–1). Clinically, a frequently encountered situation for the rheumatologist is a patient who presents with knee pain and swelling in the absence of trauma. From the arthroscopist's viewpoint, the evaluation of such a patient must be comprehensive and include, in all cases, a complete synovial fluid analysis. If the patient has inflammatory synovial fluid with a positive synovial fluid culture, then immediate management of infectious arthritis will at least involve parenteral administration of antibiotics and repeated needle drainage of the knee. Arthroscopic irrigation and debridement can be used if the infectious arthritis fails to respond. Similarly, if intracellular crystals of monosodium urate are found, then the management should be directed at acute gouty arthritis.

In other patients with knee arthritis and inflammatory synovial fluid, the correct diagnosis of the inflammatory arthritis becomes apparent with time (e.g., rheumatoid arthritis, psoriatic arthritis) and without the need for arthroscopy. More helpful diagnostic information can usually be gained from a thorough history and physical examination that seeks additional articular involvement (e.g., sacroileitis) as well as extra-articular involvement (conjunctivitis, skin rash, digital ulcerations, oral or genital lesions, olecranon nodules, and so on) than from an arthroscopic inspection of an inflamed knee!

However, arthroscopy can be useful at a later time in patients with rheumatoid arthritis, if their comprehensive management program fails to relieve knee pain and disability. These patients usually demonstrate knee inflammation with proliferative synovitis, but at times synovitis can be minimal while the patient notes typical symptoms of internal derangement, such as "locking" and "giving way." Arthroscopic examination might then reveal proliferative synovitis, in which the synovium is capable of being trapped between articular surfaces (synovial impingement syndrome), or actual meniscal tears due to chronic synovitis and loose bodies. These findings can be treated by resection or removal under arthroscopic guidance. Most commonly, a complete, multicompartmental arthroscopic synovectomy will also be performed while addressing any internal derangements present at this time. Patients undergoing complete arthroscopic synovectomy have a much shorter period of rehabilitation and markedly reduced morbidity compared with those who have undergone the previously performed open synovectomy, which is now of historical significance only.

Arthroscopy with synovial biopsy is of greatest value in patients with undiagnosed inflammatory arthritis, particularly if the involvement remains monoarticular. In the past, closed-needle synovial biopsy has been used; however, recent information has documented the dramatic intra-articular variability of synovial

inflammation, requiring biopsy under direct visualization for optimal results. Cultures of synovial biopsy specimens may reveal tuberculous or chronic fungal arthritis, such as blastomycosis or sporotrichosis, while noncaseating granulomas are the characteristic synovial histologic finding in patients with chronic sarcoid arthritis. Pigmented villonodular synovitis, ochronosis, and the arthritis of hemochromatosis also have characteristic synovial histologic findings best obtained with arthroscopic guidance.

In patients with a noninflammatory synovial effusion and a negative synovial fluid analysis, plain radiographs and the physical signs of grating of cartilage surfaces with joint motion and varus deformity will allow the diagnosis of osteoarthritis to be made with certainty. Management to reduce pain and disability then follows a standard comprehensive regimen of exercise, use of heat and cold, nonsteroidal anti-inflammatory drugs, intra-articular glucocorticoid injections, gait-assistive devices, orthoses, and special footwear. Only after failure of this program to relieve pain and disability should arthroscopy be considered to document and treat intra-articular abnormalities. Arthroscopic evaluation of patients with early to moderate radiographic changes of osteoarthritis often reveals significant cartilage defects, torn menisci, and localized areas of inflamed synovial tissue. In these patients, arthroscopic debridement of inflamed or damaged tissue, as well as removal of loose intra-articular debris by saline irrigation, has provided pain relief and improved function. In fact, removal of intra-articular debris with closed tidal saline irrigation, even without arthroscopy, has also produced similar improvement in some patients.

It is in those with the noninflammatory synovial fluid and normal radiographs that the most careful evaluation must be performed prior to arthroscopic intervention. Major diagnostic considerations in this group of patients include avascular necrosis of the medial femoral condyle, malignancy, and osteomyelitis in the femur or tibia abutting the joint. In each of these situations, imaging with MRI can identify characteristic abnormalities, thereby avoiding a potentially unnecessary arthroscopic intervention. In the presence of a normal MRI, arthroscopy contributes little and most frequently reveals degenerative cartilage lesions associated with localized synovial inflammation. Classification of these patients as having early osteoarthritis in the absence of characteristic radiographic and physical findings is tempting but clearly beyond the limits of our present understanding of osteoarthritis.

The full promise of arthroscopy as a research tool in patients with arthritis will be realized as technology improves with the development of smaller arthroscopes and the use of lasers. Serial diagnostic arthroscopy with biopsy as an office procedure may be used to document abnormalities and guide therapy. Lower morbidity with use of the laser compared with motorized instruments will encourage earlier therapeutic intervention in patients with aggressive inflammatory arthritis. Finally, performance of arthroscopic interventions for arthritis patients by rheumatologists will bring badly needed new perspectives to the pathogenesis and management of articular disease and may open new avenues of diagnosis and therapy not yet envisioned.

Arnold WJ, Kalunian K: Arthroscopic synovectomy by rheumatologists: Time for a new look. Arthritis Rheum 32:108, 1989. *A modern perspective on the role of arthroscopic synovectomy and the rheumatologist in the management of rheumatoid arthritis.*

Canoso JJ, Yood RA: Reaction of superficial bursae in response to specific disease stimuli. Arthritis Rheum 22:1361, 1979. *First study to delineate clearly the response of superficial bursae to inflammatory stimuli.*

Goldenberg DL: Synovial fluid analysis in current practice. Postgrad Adv Rheumatol 2:3, 1987. *An updated look at synovial fluid analysis.*

Johnson LL: Arthroscopic Surgery—Principles and Practice. 3rd ed. St. Louis, C. V. Mosby Company, 1986. *Arthroscopy is depicted with excellent photographs and clear textual description.*

Love PE, Santoro SA: Antiphospholipid antibodies: Anticardiolipin and the lupus anticoagulant in systemic lupus erythematosus (SLE) and in non-SLE disorders. Ann Intern Med 112:682, 1990. *Thorough, critical review of all available information on this important association.*

Slemenda CW, Hui SL, Longcope C, et al.: Predictors of bone mass in perimenopausal women. Ann Intern Med 112:96, 1990. *An important study demonstrating the weaknesses of risk factor analysis compared with bone density measurement in identifying women with low bone mass around the time of menopause.*

Sox HC Jr, Liang MH: The erythrocyte sedimentation rate. Guidelines for rational use. Ann Intern Med 104:515, 1986. *Defines the role of the erythrocyte sedimentation rate in the diagnosis and management of patients with rheumatic diseases.*

Steere AC: Lyme disease. N Engl J Med 321:586, 1989. *Complete discussion of clinical, laboratory, and therapeutic aspects of Lyme disease.*

Stoller DW, Genant HK, Helms CA, et al.: Magnetic Resonance Imaging in Orthopedics and Rheumatology. Philadelphia, J. B. Lippincott Company, 1989. *An excellent text devoted to a careful depiction of the MRI findings in the musculoskeletal system.*

Tan EM: Antinuclear antibodies: Diagnostic markers for autoimmune diseases and probes for cell biology. Adv Immunol 44:93, 1989. *Exhaustive, referenced review of the clinical and laboratory significance of antinuclear antibodies.*

258 Rheumatoid Arthritis

Frank C. Arnett

Rheumatoid arthritis (RA) is a chronic systemic inflammatory disease predominantly affecting diarthrodial joints and frequently a variety of other organs. The cause (causes) of RA is (are) unknown, and there is no specific diagnostic test. Therefore, the American College of Rheumatology (ACR) has recently revised classification criteria for RA to guarantee uniformity in investigative and epidemiologic studies (Table 258–1). Although these seven items include the most characteristic clinical features of RA, a variety of other disorders may mimic the disease (see Differential Diagnosis and Table 258–2). It is not recommended that these criteria be relied upon for definitive diagnosis in clinical practice.

Rheumatoid arthritis occurs worldwide in all ethnic groups.

TABLE 258–1. CLASSIFICATION CRITERIA FOR RHEUMATOID ARTHRITIS*

1. Morning stiffness (≥ 1 hr)
2. Swelling (soft tissue) of three or more joints
3. Swelling (soft tissue) of hand joints (PIP, MCP, or wrist)
4. Symmetric swelling (soft tissue)
5. Subcutaneous nodules
6. Serum rheumatoid factor
7. Erosions and/or periarticular osteopenia, in hand or wrist joints, seen on radiograph

*Criteria 1 to 4 must have been continuous for 6 weeks or longer and must be observed by a physician. A diagnosis of rheumatoid arthritis requires that four of the seven criteria be fulfilled.

PIP = proximal interphalangeal; MCP = metacarpophalangeal.

TABLE 258–2. DIFFERENTIAL DIAGNOSIS OF RA

	Subcutaneous Nodules	Rheumatoid Factor (RF)
Acute viral arthritis (rubella, hepatitis B, parvovirus)	−	−
Bacterial endocarditis	+/−	+
Acute rheumatic fever	+	−
Serum sickness	−	−
Sarcoidosis	+	+
Reactive arthritis (Reiter's disease)	−	−
Psoriatic arthritis	−	−
Inflammatory bowel disease	−	−
Whipple's disease	−	−
Systemic lupus erythematosus	+	+
Sjögren's syndrome	−	+
Systemic sclerosis (scleroderma)	−	+/−
Polymyositis	−	+/−
Vasculitis syndromes	−	+
Polymyalgia rheumatica	−	−
Polyarticular gout	+ (tophi)	−
Calcium pyrophosphate disease	−	−
Amyloidosis	+/−	−
Paraneoplastic syndromes	−	−
Multicentric reticulohistiocytosis	+	−
Osteoarthritis (erosive)	−	−

− = not present; + = frequently present; +/− = occasionally present.

Prevalence rates range from 0.3 to 1.5 per cent in most populations, but frequencies of 3.5 to 5.3 per cent have been found in several Native American tribes (Yakima and Chippewa). The peak incidence of onset is between the fourth and sixth decades, but RA may begin at any time from childhood (see Juvenile Chronic Arthritis) to later life. Females are two to three times more likely to be affected than males.

No definitive description of RA exists before the early nineteenth century, and anthropologic evidence of the disease has been found in New World, but not Old World, skeletons. Thus, it has been proposed, but not proved, that an etiologic agent was carried to Europe by early explorers of the Americas. A.B. Garrod first proposed the term "rheumatoid arthritis" in 1858.

ETIOLOGY

Despite intensive research over many decades, the etiology of RA remains unknown. Three areas of interrelated research are currently most promising: (1) host genetic factors, (2) immunoregulatory abnormalities and autoimmunity, and (3) a triggering or persisting microbial infection.

Genetic susceptibility to RA has been clearly demonstrated. The disease clusters in families and occurs more frequently in monozygotic than in dizygotic twins. The major histocompatibility complex (MHC) allele (and encoded antigen) HLA-DR4 (HLA, human leukocyte antigen) is significantly increased in RA patients in most populations (see Ch. 250). Among Caucasians of western European origin, HLA-DR4 occurs in 60 to 70 per cent of seropositive individuals with RA compared with approximately 30 per cent of normal individuals. The presence of this tissue type correlates even more strongly with rheumatoid factor (RF) titer, severe joint destruction on radiographs, rheumatoid lung disease, and Felty's syndrome. HLA-DR1 is found in the majority of HLA-DR4–negative patients and is most strongly associated with the disease in other ethnic groups (Israelis, Asian Indians). Several subtypes of HLA-DR4 were initially defined by mixed lymphocyte cultures (MLC). The HLA-Dw4, HLA-Dw14, and HLA-Dw15 subtypes predispose to RA, while HLA-Dw10 and HLA-Dw13 do not. Molecular genetic studies have recently demonstrated that these HLA-DR4 subtypes result from only a few amino acid differences in the third hypervariable region of the HLA-DR beta chain. HLA-DR1 shares the same amino acid sequence as the HLA-Dw14 subtype of HLA-DR4. Thus, a "shared epitope" among several MHC class II molecules appears to predispose to RA. The critical region on these molecules appears to be a combining site for the T cell antigen receptor (TCR). Since MHC class II molecules present processed antigen to the TCR on helper (CD4+) T lymphocytes (see Ch. 242), it appears likely that an abnormal antigen-specific cellular and/or humoral immune response is inherent to the etiology of RA. The nature of the antigen, whether self or foreign, remains unknown.

Rheumatoid arthritis appears to be an "autoimmune" disease, similar to other MHC class II–associated disorders (see Ch. 250). Autoantibodies to the Fc portion of immunoglobulin G (IgG) molecules, or RF's, are produced by B lymphocytes in the blood and synovial tissues of 80 per cent of RA patients. Such cases are termed seropositive. High titers of serum RF are associated with more severe joint disease and with extra-articular manifestations, especially subcutaneous nodules. Rheumatoid factor detected by the usual clinical methods (latex fixation or sensitized sheep cell agglutination) are immunoglobulin M (IgM) antibodies. IgG, immunoglobulin A (IgA), immunoglobulin E (IgE), and immunoglobulin D (IgD) RF's have also been described. IgM RF can react with five IgG molecules to produce very large complexes (sedimentation coefficient of 22S), and they appear to participate in the pathogenesis of rheumatoid synovitis. Intermediate-sized complexes (between 7S and 19S) containing only IgG molecules, some of which have RF activity against self, have been found and may occur to a greater extent in individuals with widespread systemic disease and vasculitis.

Despite the extremely strong association of RF's with RA, they clearly do not cause the disease. Production of RF occurs commonly in other diseases or disorders in which there is chronic antigenic stimulation, such as bacterial endocarditis, tuberculosis, syphilis, kala-azar, viral infections, intravenous drug abuse, and cirrhosis. Normal individuals occasionally produce RF, especially with increasing age. In none of these situations is RF associated with HLA-DR4.

An infectious origin for RA has been a continuing hypothesis. Streptococci, diphtheroids, mycoplasmas, and *Clostridium perfringens* have all been proposed and later discarded because of lack of definitive evidence. Viral infections such as rubella, Ross River virus, and, more recently, parvovirus B19 have been shown to produce an acute polyarthritis, but no evidence exists that they initiate chronic RA. The Epstein-Barr virus (EBV) remains a viable but unproven candidate for a pathogenetic role. The EBV is a polyclonal B cell activator capable of stimulating autoantibody production, including RF. Increased numbers of EBV-infected B cells have been found in the blood but not the

synovial tissue of RA patients. Antibodies against a nuclear antigen (EBNA) expressed in EBV-infected cells occur in the majority of RA patients, and a variety of other unusual immune responses to EBV are found in RA patients. More recently, an EBV protein has been shown to share the same five amino acids as the HLA-DR4 (Dw4) molecule, which is implicated in susceptibility to RA, thus raising the possibility of "molecular mimicry" as a mechanism. Nonetheless, EBV is highly ubiquitous, and there is no *direct* evidence that this virus initiates the disease.

PATHOLOGY AND PATHOGENESIS

The pathologic hallmark of RA is synovial membrane proliferation and outgrowth associated with erosion of articular cartilage and subchondral bone. Often likened to a malignant tumor, proliferating inflammatory tissue (pannus) may lead subsequently to destruction of intra-articular and periarticular structures and may result in the joint deformities and dysfunction seen clinically.

The events initiating the process are unknown (Fig. 258–1). The earliest findings include microvascular injury and moderate proliferation of synovial cells accompanied by interstitial edema and perivascular infiltration by mononuclear cells, predominantly T lymphocytes. Polymorphonuclear leukocytes and plasma cells are infrequent. With continuation of the process, there is further hyperplasia of lining cells, both DR-positive type A (macrophage-like) and DR-negative type B (fibroblast-like), and the normally acellular subsynovial stroma becomes engorged with mononuclear inflammatory cells, which may collect into aggregates or follicles, especially around postcapillary venules. The composition of cellular infiltrates varies, with some being predominantly T cells, usually CD4 +, others being plasma cell rich, and some having a mixed population of lymphocytes (often CD8 +), plasma cells, macrophages, and interdigitating (dendritic) cells. Mast cells are also commonly present. Occasionally, germinal centers rich in B lymphocytes can be seen. The proliferating synovium (pannus) becomes villous and is vascularized by arterioles, capillaries, and venules.

Roles for both *cellular* and *humoral* immune mechanisms in the rheumatoid synovium have been proposed, and both are

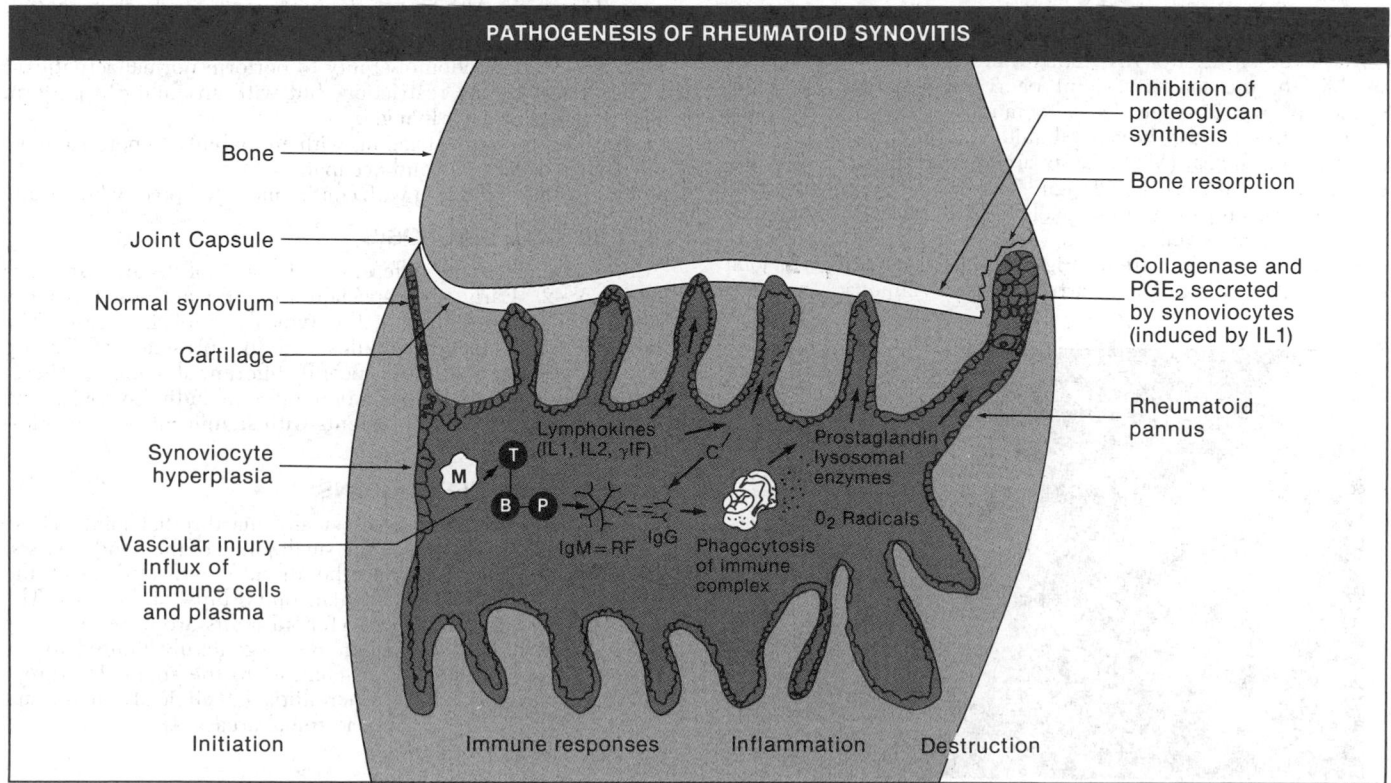

FIGURE 258–1. Events involved in the pathogenesis of rheumatoid synovitis progress from left to right. M = macrophage; T = T lymphocyte; B = B lymphocyte; P = plasma cell; IL1 = interleukin 1; IL2 = interleukin 2; γIF = gamma-interferon; RF = rheumatoid factor; PGE$_2$ = prostaglandin E$_2$; IgM = immunoglobulin M; IgG = immunoglobulin G; C = complement.

supported by immunopathologic findings. A cellular mechanism would involve activation of infiltrating T lymphocytes by some unknown antigen (or antigens) presented by DR-positive cells (type A synoviocytes, macrophages, dendritic cells). A release of a variety of soluble mediators would follow, which would then promote further synovial proliferation and inflammation. Indeed, T cells appear to be activated, and T cell–derived lymphokines (such as interleukin 2 and gamma-interferon) probably play important roles in the inflammatory process. Moreover, interleukin 1, produced by the interaction of monocytes and/or macrophages with activated T cells, induces collagenase and prostaglandin E_2 production by synoviocytes. This monokine also promotes degradation and inhibits synthesis of proteoglycan by chondrocytes, as well as enhances resorption of calcium from bone.

Humoral mechanisms are supported by the demonstration of local RF production within the synovium, the formation of IgM-IgG immune complexes, and activation and consumption of complement via the classic pathway. The sequelae of complement activation include increased vascular permeability and phagocytosis of the immune complexes by phagocytic cells. Aggregates of immune complexes within polymorphonuclear leukocytes are often seen in rheumatoid synovial fluid and have been termed "RA cells" or "ragocytes."

Antigen-antibody complexes formed within the joint cavity can become trapped in hyaline cartilage and fibrocartilage, where they cause changes in matrix macromolecules. Within the synovial fluid, immune complexes activate the complement system, kinins, phagocytic cells, and lysosomal enzyme release. Mediators produced in this process stimulate synovial cells to proliferate and to produce proteinases and prostaglandins. These products cause dissolution of the connective tissue macromolecules, as well as articular cartilage. They may also activate fibroblasts to produce a denser connective tissue matrix (fibrosis).

The ultimate destruction of cartilage, bone, tendons, and ligaments probably results from a variety of proteolytic enzymes, metalloproteinases, and soluble mediators. Collagenase, produced at the interface of pannus and cartilage, is probably largely responsible for the typical erosions after its activation by plasmin.

CLINICAL FEATURES

The mode of onset of RA among different individuals is highly variable. In the majority, joint pain and/or stiffness develops insidiously over several weeks to months. One or more small joints of the hands, wrists, shoulders, or knees and/or the metatarsophalangeal (MTP) joints are frequently the first symptomatic areas. Malaise and fatigue, occasionally with low-grade fever, may accompany musculoskeletal discomfort. As the disease progresses, joint swelling, tenderness, and a red or bluish discoloration become apparent (Fig. 258–2). The pattern of joint involvement is typically polyarticular and symmetric, involving

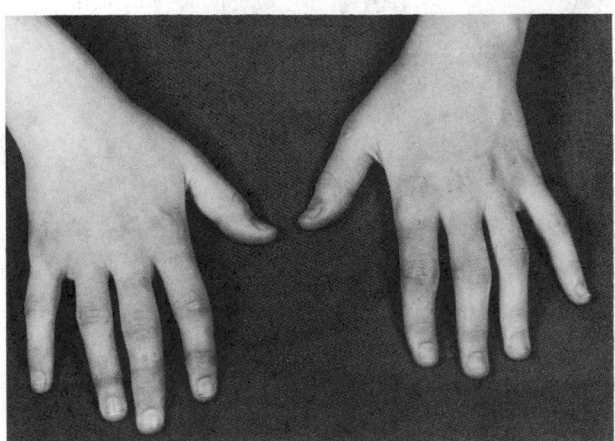

FIGURE 258–2. Early rheumatoid arthritis manifests as symmetric swelling and slight flexion deformities of proximal interphalangeal joints of the hands. Roentgenograms were normal except for evidence of soft tissue swelling.

the proximal interphalangeal (PIP), metacarpophalangeal (MCP), wrist, elbow, shoulder, knee, ankle, and MTP joints. Distal interphalangeal (DIP) joints of the fingers are usually spared. Joint stiffness, especially if lasting more than 1 hour in the morning and after inactivity, is a prominent complaint in RA. So characteristic is this symptom that the duration of morning stiffness is often used as a quantitative guide to the activity of the inflammatory process in both clinical practice and research studies. As the disease process evolves, the patient may experience increasing difficulty with pain and stiffness, as well as impairment of joint function. The simple activities of daily living may be severely compromised, and the ability to continue a productive occupation is threatened. Sleep habits become disturbed, and the patient may experience an associated depression and weight loss.

An "acute" onset occurring over 1 or several days is seen in about 20 per cent of patients. Occasionally, an individual retires in the evening with no symptoms and awakens with acute, generalized RA. Such a rapid onset of pain involving joints, surrounding soft tissues, and muscle can mimic and must be differentiated from acute myositis, viral syndromes, or, if focal, even septic or crystal-induced arthritides. Rare patients experience recurrent (palindromic) episodes of acute monoarthritis, often so severe as to mimic gout, yet lasting only 24 to 48 hours. Such patients, especially if seropositive, eventually develop the typical chronic, symmetric polyarthritis of RA.

The course of RA, like its onset, varies widely. Fluctuating disease activity early in the disease process is usual. Ultimately, joint deformities and variable degrees of disability occur in the majority of patients (Fig. 258–3). Some patients have a relentlessly progressive course leading to early disability or even death, but repeated periods of some degree of remission are the rule. The ACR has proposed criteria for clinical remission in RA. At least five of the following requirements must be fulfilled for at least 2 consecutive months: (1) duration of morning stiffness not exceeding 15 minutes; (2) no fatigue; (3) no joint pain (by history); (4) no joint tenderness or pain on motion; (5) no soft tissue swelling in joints or tendon sheaths; (6) an erythrocyte sedimentation rate (Westergren) less than 30 mm per hour for females or 20 mm per hour for males.

The assessment of functional capacity is frequently necessary in the RA patient. Although various schemes have been proposed, the simple classification that follows serves well in most situations.

Class I: No restriction of ability to perform normal activities.
Class II: Moderate restriction, but with an ability to perform most activities of daily living.
Class III: Marked restriction, with an inability to perform most activities of daily living and occupation.
Class IV: Incapacitation with confinement to bed or wheelchair.

DIFFERENTIAL DIAGNOSIS

Considerations in the differential diagnosis of RA are numerous (Table 258–2). Early RA, especially that of acute onset, is more difficult to diagnose than is the typical established case. The finding of subcutaneous nodules and the presence of RF are useful but are not absolutely specific differential features. Therefore, a complete medical evaluation, often including synovial fluid analysis, is indicated in all patients with significant joint manifestations.

ARTICULAR MANIFESTATIONS

Rheumatoid arthritis can affect any diarthrodial joint. Those most commonly involved are the small joints of the hands, wrists, knees, and feet. With time, the disease may also affect the elbows, shoulders, sternoclavicular joints, hips, and ankles. The temporomandibular and cricoarytenoid joints are less frequently involved. Spinal involvement in RA is generally limited to the upper cervical articulations. In contrast to the spondyloarthropathies, RA does not cause sacroiliitis or clinically significant disease in the lumbar or thoracic spinal areas.

Hands

Swelling of the PIP joints, giving a fusiform or spindle-shaped appearance to the fingers, is one of the most common early signs. Bilateral and symmetric swelling of the MCP joints is also frequent (Fig. 258–2). The DIP joints are usually spared, which

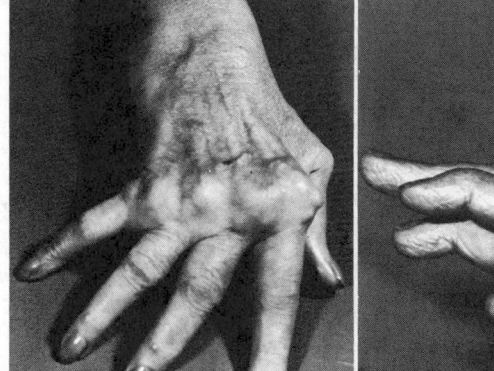

FIGURE 258–3. Hand deformities characteristic of chronic rheumatoid arthritis. *A*, Subluxation of metacarpophalangeal joints with ulnar deviation of digits. *B*, Hyperextension ("swan neck") deformities of proximal interphalangeal joints.

is a useful sign in discriminating RA from osteoarthritis and psoriatic arthritis. Soft tissue laxity gives rise to ulnar deviation of the fingers at the MCP joints (Fig. 258–3A). Swan-neck deformities develop from hypertension of the PIP joints in conjunction with flexion of the DIP joints (Fig. 258–3B). Boutonnière (buttonhole) deformities result from flexion contractures of the PIP joints associated with hyperextension of the DIP joints. These changes result in a loss of strength and dexterity in the hands, as well as the ability to maintain a good pinch. Synovial erosions of extensor tendons, usually at the dorsum of the wrist, may lead to sudden rupture and loss of the ability to extend one or more fingers.

Wrists

The wrists are almost invariably involved in RA and frequently demonstrate easily palpable, boggy synovium, especially over the ulnar styloid. Loss of wrist motion, both flexion and extension,

usually occurs to some degree. The median nerve on the volar side often becomes compressed by proliferating synovium, resulting in a carpal tunnel syndrome (Fig. 258–4). The patient notes paresthesias or pain in the thumb, second and third digits, and radial side of the fourth digit. Symptoms are typically worse at night or with other activities associated with sustained flexion of the wrist. *Tinel's* (Fig. 258–4) and *Phalen's* (Fig. 258–5) signs can usually be elicited, and thenar muscle wasting may be evident.

Knees

Synovial proliferation and effusion are common in these weight-bearing joints. Effusions may be detected by performing ballottement on the patella or by observing a "bulge sign" along the medial aspect of the patella when fluid is pushed into the suprapatellar pouch and then expressed back into the joint. Quadriceps atrophy may occur, and a flexion contracture of the knee may compromise walking. Eventually, destruction of soft tissue around the knee can produce marked joint instability. Popliteal (Baker's) cysts may form owing to effusion or synovial proliferation into the semimembranous bursa (Fig. 258–6). Such synovial cysts may dissect or rupture into the calf, producing symptoms and signs mimicking those of thrombophlebitis. Sonograms are useful in confirming the diagnosis. Venograms may also be necessary because venous occlusion by the cyst can occur.

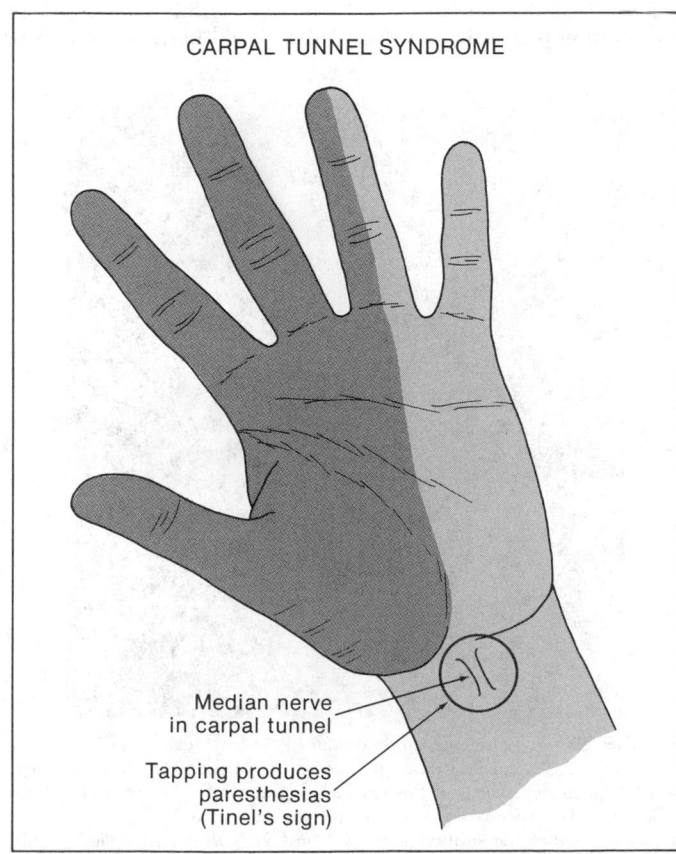

CARPAL TUNNEL SYNDROME

Median nerve
in carpal tunnel

Tapping produces
paresthesias
(Tinel's sign)

FIGURE 258–4. Distribution of pain and/or paresthesias *(shaded area)* when the median nerve is compressed by swelling in the wrist (carpal tunnel).

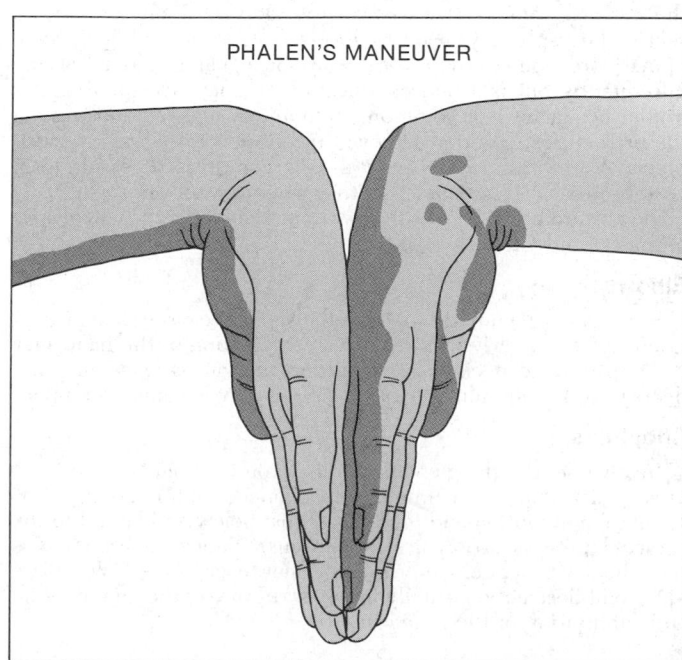

PHALEN'S MANEUVER

FIGURE 258–5. Pain and/or paresthesias are produced in the distribution of the median nerve (Fig. 258–4) when hands are held in forced flexion for 30 to 60 seconds (Phalen's maneuver).

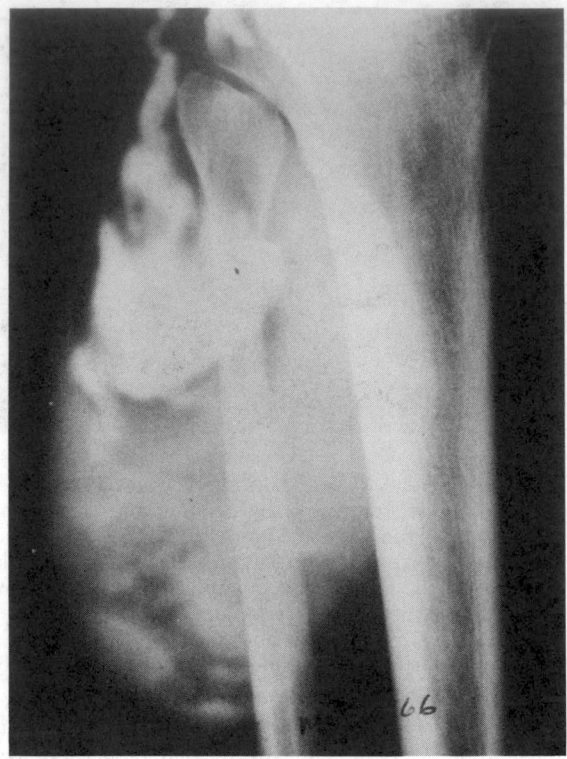

FIGURE 258–6. Arthrogram using a radiocontrast agent injected into the knee. The dye flows into the popliteal space and through a narrow channel into a large synovial cyst (Baker's cyst), which has dissected into the soft tissues of the calf.

Feet and Ankles

The MTP joints are the most commonly involved sites. Subluxation of the metatarsal heads into the soles, often with cock-up and valgus deformities of the toes, results in painful walking and difficulty with footwear.

Neck

Neck pain and stiffness are common. As in other joints, the rheumatoid process can lead to erosion of bone and ligaments in the cervical spine. Atlantoaxial subluxation (C1 on C2) can be seen radiographically in up to 30 per cent of cases (Fig. 258–7). Spinal cord compression with neurologic manifestations occurs infrequently but is a neurosurgical emergency. Occipital and/or frontal headache is a common premonitory sign of weakness in the extremities, bladder or bowel incontinence, or frank quadriplegia. Vertebral arteries may also be compressed, resulting in vertebrobasilar insufficiency with vertigo or syncope, especially on downward gaze. Head tilt may occur from lateral mass collapse of the C1 and C2 vertebrae.

Elbows

Proliferative synovitis in the elbow often causes flexion contractures, even early in the disease. Supination of the hand may be impaired, especially if shoulder motion is concomitantly decreased. Rarely, ulnar or radial nerves may become entrapped.

Shoulders

Involvement of the glenohumeral, acromioclavicular, and thoracoscapular joints is common in advanced but not early RA. Limitation of motion and tenderness just below and lateral to the coracoid process are typical symptoms. Noticeable swelling is rare; however, large synovial cysts may occur (see Color Plate 4D). Joint destruction usually involves rupture of the joint capsule and subluxation of the humerus.

Hips

Pain in the groin, lateral buttock, or lower back may be indicative of hip involvement. Because the hip joint capsule has poor distensibility, severe pain can result if a large effusion occurs. Arthrocentesis should be done to relieve pain and to exclude infection in such cases. Rarely, extreme hip destruction results in protrusion of the femur into the pelvis.

Cricoarytenoid Joints

Synovitis of the cricoarytenoid joints may result in dysphagia, hoarseness, or anterior neck pain. The sudden onset of stridor and dyspnea in a patient with RA is an emergency. Prompt administration of intra-articular or parenteral corticosteroids and/or tracheostomy may be necessary.

EXTRA-ARTICULAR MANIFESTATIONS

Constitutional symptoms, including malaise, fatigue, weakness, low-grade fever and mild lymphadenopathy, are common in RA. All of the extra-articular complications occur almost exclusively in seropositive patients.

Skin

Subcutaneous nodules occur in 20 to 25 per cent of RA patients and are almost always associated with serum RF and more severe articular disease. They occur most commonly in periarticular structures and areas subject to pressure, such as the elbows, extensor and flexor tendons of the hands and feet, Achilles tendons, and, less commonly, occipital and sacral areas. They may occasionally become infected but are usually asymptomatic.

Palmar erythema and fragility of the skin, resulting in easy bruising, are common manifestations. Rheumatoid vasculitis occurs in two major forms. The first is manifested by small, splinter-shaped brown infarcts in the nail folds and digital pulp, often also present over subcutaneous nodules (see Color Plate 4E). Histologic examination may reveal leukocytoclastic vasculitis or a mild venulitis. This is a benign process in most patients and does not indicate serious systemic vasculitis. The second form is a severe necrotizing vasculitis of small and medium arteries indistinguishable from periarteritis nodosa. Digital infarcts, mononeuritis multiplex, fever, and other manifestations of systemic disease should prompt aggressive therapy.

Cardiac Manifestations

Pericardial disease is the most common cardiac feature of RA. Evidence of pericardial involvement with old fibrinous lesions is

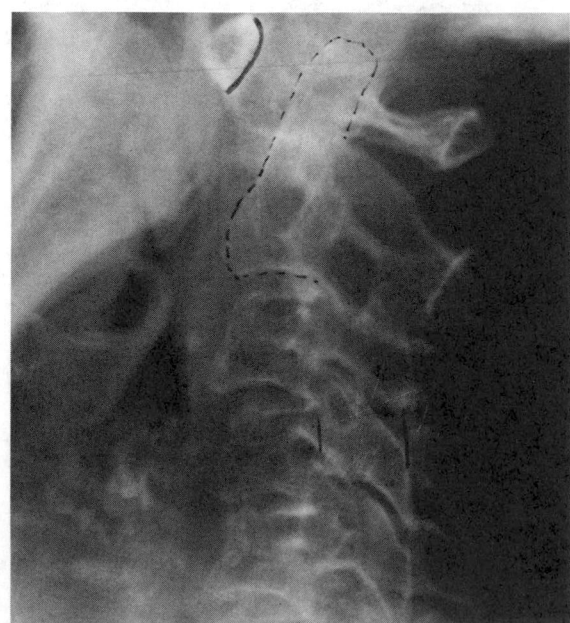

FIGURE 258–7. Lateral roentgenogram of the cervical spine in flexion. The body of C2 and its odontoid process are outlined by broken lines, and the posterior aspect of the anterior segment of C1 is indicated by a solid line. The space between C1 and the odontoid of C2 is markedly increased, indicating subluxation of C1 on C2. Normally, a space of only 2 to 3 mm separates C1 from C2. At a lower level, C3 is also displaced anteriorly owing to rheumatoid erosion of articular and ligamentous structures.

found in approximately 40 per cent of patients at autopsy. A similar frequency of pericardial abnormalities can be detected by echocardiography in asymptomatic RA patients. Clinically evident pericarditis in RA, however, is infrequent. Large pericardial effusions with cardiac tamponade and death are rare. Constrictive pericarditis is somewhat more common and typically presents as dyspnea, right-sided heart failure, and peripheral edema. The pericardial fluid characteristics include a low glucose concentration, increased level of lactate dehydrogenase (LDH), elevated immunoglobulin levels, and low complement activity.

Rheumatoid nodules may develop occasionally in the myocardium or heart valves, and vasculitis may involve the coronary arteries. Conduction abnormalities, valvular incompetence or stenosis, and myocardial infarction are all rare clinical sequelae of rheumatoid heart disease.

Pulmonary Manifestations

Rheumatoid pleural disease, although frequently found at autopsy, is most commonly asymptomatic. Occasionally, a pleural effusion may be of sufficient size to cause respiratory limitation. Neoplasm and infection should be ruled out on the basis of a pleural tap. Typically, the pleural fluid is exudative, and white cell counts vary greatly but generally are less than 5000 per microliter. Glucose levels tend to be low, and the LDH enzyme level is high. Total hemolytic complement, C3, and C4 levels are low. Immune complexes and RF are frequently found in the pleural fluid.

Intrapulmonary nodules may also be seen (Fig. 258–8). Although they are usually asymptomatic, they may become infected and cavitate or rupture into the pleural space, producing a pneumothorax. Malignancy must be excluded in the RA patient, as in any other patient, with a solitary lung nodule. Similar but distinct nodular infiltrates may also be seen in rheumatoid lungs in association with pneumoconiosis (Caplan's syndrome).

Finally, one may see a diffuse interstitial fibrosis with pneumonitis. This may progress to a honeycomb appearance on the roentgenogram, bronchiectasis, chronic cough, and progressive dyspnea. Pulmonary function tests show a diminished compliance and a restrictive ventilatory pattern. Large airways are not involved. An irreversible combination of respiratory insufficiency and resultant right-sided cardiac failure is possible. Rarely, small airway obstruction may develop into a necrotizing bronchiolitis. This complication may also result from therapies with gold and D-penicillamine.

Neurologic Manifestations

Peripheral neuropathies can be produced by proliferating synovium causing compression of nerves. Carpal tunnel syndrome (median neuropathy) (see under Articular Manifestations) is common, and a similar entrapment of the anterior tibial nerve (tarsal

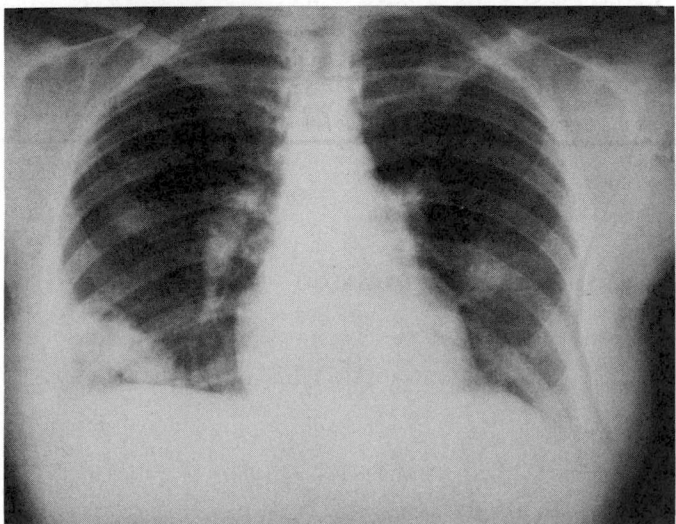

FIGURE 258–8. Chest roentgenogram demonstrating discrete rheumatoid nodules in both right and left lower lobes of the lungs. (Courtesy of Dr. Martin Lidsky, Houston, Texas.)

tunnel syndrome) can result in paresthesias with a foot drop. Rheumatoid vasculitis may cause a mononeuritis multiplex condition with patchy sensory loss in one or more extremities, often in association with a wrist or foot drop. A cervical myelopathy can result from atlantoaxial subluxation (see under Articular Manifestations). The central nervous system is usually spared, although cerebral vasculitis and rheumatoid nodules in the meninges have been described.

Ophthalmologic Manifestations

Sjögren's syndrome is the most frequent ocular complication and may cause corneal damage associated with dryness of the eyes. Xerostomia and/or parotid gland enlargement may accompany ocular dryness. Episcleritis is a self-limited condition associated with redness of the eye and only mild pain. Scleritis is more painful and may result in visual impairment. If this condition progresses to thinning of the tissue, allowing the dark blue color of the choroid below to show through, it is termed scleromalacia perforans. The histologic picture is similar to that of a rheumatoid nodule.

FELTY'S SYNDROME

This triad of chronic RA, splenomegaly, and neutropenia is often accompanied by lymphadenopathy, hepatomegaly, fever, weight loss, anemia, and thrombocytopenia. Hyperpigmentation and leg ulcers may also occur. The syndrome typically appears late in the course of a seropositive, destructive arthritis, often after joint disease is felt to be "burnt out." Recurrent infections with gram-positive organisms constitute the most serious clinical problems and do not correlate with the severity of neutropenia. The bone marrow is typically hyperplastic. Hypersplenism and immune-mediated destruction of white blood cells are believed to cause the neutropenia. Splenectomy may correct the neutropenia and prevent further infections in some patients, but many do not improve. The "large granular lymphocyte syndrome," which is probably a premalignant disorder of T lymphocytes, may mimic Felty's syndrome in RA patients.

LABORATORY FEATURES

A chronic normocytic, normochromic anemia with hematocrit values from 30 to 35 per cent is usual. Typically, both serum iron levels and iron-binding capacity are low. The anemia does not respond to administration of iron, but erythropoietin may be effective when anemia is more severe. The white blood cell count and differential are typically normal, but eosinophilia may occur in severe systemic disease. The platelet count may be moderately elevated owing to chronic inflammation. The erythrocyte sedimentation rate is elevated in most patients but only roughly parallels disease activity. The presence of RF is detected by agglutination methods in more than 80 per cent of cases and is useful in clinical diagnosis. Antinuclear antibodies detected by immunofluorescence, usually in low titer, can be found in 30 to 40 per cent of cases. Although HLA-DR4 can be determined by B cell typing in 60 to 70 per cent of cases, it is not generally useful in diagnosis because it occurs in nearly 30 per cent of normal individuals.

Synovial fluid analysis usually shows a poor mucin clot test and white cell counts in the range of 5000 to 20,000 per cubic millimeter, with 50 to 70 per cent as polymorphonuclear leukocytes (Table 258–3). The synovial fluid glucose concentration is usually normal, but very low values occur occasionally, even in the absence of a superimposed infectious arthritis. Complement levels are typically low.

THERAPEUTIC MANAGEMENT

The prolonged and uncertain course of RA calls for special emphasis on the fact that most patients can continue their accustomed activities, with restrictions tailored to individual cases. Undue or excessive drug therapy, especially adrenocorticosteroids and immunosuppressive agents, can cause greater morbidity than the disease itself. Objectives of management include (1) relief of pain, (2) reduction of inflammation, (3) minimizing undesirable side effects, (4) preservation of muscle strength and joint function, and (5) the return as rapidly as possible to a normal lifestyle. The basic initial program that achieves these objectives for the great majority of patients consists of (1) adequate rest, (2) adequate anti-inflammatory therapy, and (3) physical measures to maintain joint function.

Any confusion arising from the complementary requirements of rest and exercise should be promptly dispelled. As has been noted for many years, it is only a rare patient with RA who does not improve significantly upon being hospitalized. From this we have learned that bed rest tends to decrease the general systemic inflammatory response. Most patients soon learn that their midafternoon fatigue is significantly reduced by a period of rest. During acute attacks, longer rests and perhaps even remaining in bed for the duration of the attack may be required to treat the inflammation.

At the same time, the full range of joint motion should be maintained. This can usually be accomplished by the patient through graded exercise programs. However, during acute attacks, passive range-of-motion exercises by a physical therapist or instructed layperson may be indicated. Physical overexertion increases synovitis and inflammation in the joint affected by RA, but this does not contradict the usefulness of appropriate exercise. Exercise, as well as heat treatments such as showers, baths, warm pools, paraffin baths, or hot packs, should be used to loosen the joints and relieve stiffness. Exercise following the heat treatment maintains the motion of affected joints and prevents muscle atrophy. These goals can generally be achieved without aggressive overactivity and can usually keep a patient fully mobile. Acutely inflamed joints may dictate total body rest or splinting.

NONSTEROIDAL ANTI-INFLAMMATORY DRUGS (NSAID's)

Anti-inflammatory therapy is critical to the basic program. Salicylates are inexpensive, generally well tolerated, and demonstrably effective in controlling RA inflammation. The patient needs to understand that this requires a larger dose than would be used for analgesia alone. A constant blood level of 20 to 30 mg per deciliter is required. For most patients this requires between 3 and 6 grams of aspirin per day. All patients should be monitored for toxic levels by blood tests and should be alerted to report deafness, ringing in the ears, or gastrointestinal intolerance. With the availability of buffered and coated aspirin, a suitable salicylate preparation can be found for almost any patient.

Many other NSAID's that are effective against pain, fever, and inflammation in RA are available. These include derivatives of phenylacetic acid (ibuprofen, ketoprofen, fenoprofen, flurbiprofen), naphthalene acetic acids (naproxen), pyrrolealkanoic acid (tolmetin), indoleacetic acid (indomethacin, sulindac), a halogenated anthranilic acid (meclofenamate sodium), piroxicam, diclofenac, and diflunisal. Most of these drugs are beneficial in RA. They are generally no more effective than aspirin but may be

tolerated in cases in which aspirin is not. Their major problem is high cost. Clinical experience suggests an occasional need to change from one to another of these drugs to minimize side effects and to give maximal benefit to the individual patient.

The NSAID's often cause silent gastrointestinal bleeding. Fortunately, this is usually minimal and tolerable. Overt gastrointestinal tract hemorrhage or ulceration is rare, but if this occurs or gastrointestinal bleeding is contributing to a constant anemia, the therapeutic regimen should be modified. NSAID's should be used cautiously or avoided in patients with impaired renal function.

OTHER THERAPIES

If salicylates and NSAID's fail to control the inflammation or are not tolerated, then one must consider the more slowly acting drugs, including antimalarials, gold, penicillamine, and methotrexate. Antimalarials are usually given as hydroxychloroquine (Plaquenil), 200 mg once or twice daily. This, or chloroquine, may cause retinal lesions and loss of vision; therefore, the patient should be examined by an ophthalmologist at least twice a year.

Gold salts produce remission in many cases. Because of the potential toxicity to kidneys and bone marrow, frequent urinalysis and blood counts must be done, especially during early phases of treatment. An oral gold salt, auranofin, appears to be therapeutically effective and to have less toxicity than do intramuscular injections. A dose of 3 mg two to three times per day is recommended. A therapeutic effect should not be expected before 4 to 6 months. Many patients have been on oral or intramuscular gold therapy for a number of years. Common side effects include pruritic skin rashes and painful mouth ulcers. Severe manifestations include bone marrow suppression, usually leukopenia or thrombocytopenia, renal damage with proteinuria, and rarely a nephrotic syndrome.

Penicillamine may be used in the treatment of RA and is also effective in inducing improvements and sometimes even remissions. Like gold, however, its effects are slow in coming, and it may affect both the bone marrow and the kidneys, so that careful monitoring for toxicity is required. In addition, it may induce other autoimmune diseases, such as myasthenia gravis, Goodpasture's syndrome, or lupus erythematosus.

Immunosuppressive agents such as azathioprine, cyclophosphamide, chlorambucil, and methotrexate have been used to treat especially severe, unremitting RA. Currently, the most widely used and effective form of immunosuppressive therapy for RA appears to be methotrexate. An oral dosage of 7.5 to 15 mg one time per week seems efficacious, and a therapeutic response can be anticipated in several weeks. Side effects include hepatotoxicity and possibly cirrhosis, bone marrow suppression, oral ulcers, and a potential life-threatening pneumonitis. Methotrexate may also cause a leukocytoclastic vasculitis and may promote the formation of rheumatoid nodules.

Because of its side effects, long-term corticosteroid therapy should be reserved for patients with unresponsive and aggressive

TABLE 258-3. SYNOVIAL FLUID FINDINGS IN RHEUMATOID ARTHRITIS AND OTHER FORMS OF ARTHRITIS

Synovial Characteristics	Rheumatoid Arthritis	Gout/Pseudogout	Reiter's/Psoriatic Arthritis	Septic Arthritis	Osteoarthritis, Traumatic Arthritis
Color	Yellow	Yellow-white	Yellow	White	Clear, pale yellow, or bloody
Clarity	Cloudy	Cloudy-opaque	Cloudy	Opaque	Transparent
Viscosity	Poor	Poor	Poor	Poor	Good
Mucin clot	Poor	Poor	Poor	Poor	Good
White blood cell count/mm³	3000–50,000	3000–50,000 or higher	3000–50,000 or higher	50,000–300,000	<3000
% Polymorphonuclear leukocytes	>70	>70	>70	>90	<25
Glucose levels	10–25% less than serum*	10–25% less than serum	10–25% less than serum	70–90% less than serum	5–10% less than serum
Total protein	>3.0 grams/dl	>3.0 grams/dl	>3.0 grams/dl	>3.0 grams/dl	1.8–3.0 grams/dl
Complement	Low	Normal	High	High	Normal
Microscopic features	"RA cells"†	MSU and CPPD crystals	"Reiter's cells"†	Microbes (Gram stain)	Cartilage fibrils†
Culture	Negative	Negative	Negative	Positive	Negative

*Rarely, glucose levels are very low, as in rheumatoid pleural effusions.
†These are not disease specific or diagnostic.
MSU = monosodium urate; CPPD = calcium pyrophosphate dihydrate.

joint disease whose ability to function is threatened. When necessary, the smallest possible dose should be used, i.e., prednisone, 5 mg to 10 mg every other day or daily. Higher doses are necessary for patients with neuropathy, vasculitis, pleuritis, pericarditis, scleritis, and related conditions. Local steroid injections can sometimes be helpful for the relief of persistent effusions and are the treatment of choice for a Baker's cyst of the knee.

Finally, reconstructive orthopedic surgery is of very great importance. Perhaps the greatest contribution of the past two decades to the management of RA has been the development of superb techniques for joint replacement. The use of prosthetic devices for hip and knee joints has given excellent results, and devices for ankle, elbow, and shoulder replacement are improving.

JUVENILE CHRONIC ARTHRITIS

A chronic arthritis beginning in childhood and for which no underlying cause is apparent has been termed *juvenile rheumatoid arthritis*. Because the majority of these cases do not resemble adult RA, the term *juvenile chronic arthritis* (JCA) is a more appropriate designation. Several subgroups of JCA are recognized on the basis of modes of onset, other clinical features, and immunogenetic differences.

Arthritis of systemic onset, or Still's disease, accounts for about 20 per cent of patients. It can begin at any age. Rheumatoid factor and antinuclear antibodies are generally not found. Clinical characteristics include high, spiking daily fevers; an evanescent, salmon-colored rash usually appearing with fever; lymphadenopathy; hepatosplenomegaly; polyserositis; leukocytosis; thrombocytosis; and anemia. Although the disease is rarely life threatening, it can be confused with leukemia or infection. It tends to run a self-limited course in the majority of patients but may recur. Chronic polyarthritis and joint deformities occur in only about 10 per cent of patients.

Disease with a polyarticular onset occurs in approximately 40 per cent of patients. There is a female predominance. The majority of patients are seronegative. Seropositive patients have the worst prognosis, and the disease usually follows a chronic course similar to that in adult RA. HLA-DR4 is strongly associated with seropositive but not seronegative disease. No HLA associations have been found for the seronegative group, except for a small subset with HLA-B27 who develop cervical spine fusion, notably at the C2–C3 apophyseal joints, and, less often, sacroiliitis or ankylosing spondylitis.

Disease with a pauciarticular onset accounts for the remaining 40 per cent of JCA patients. There are at least two subgroups within this group. One is characterized by early age of onset and female predominance. The serum is usually positive for antinuclear antibodies but not RF. Patients in this subgroup are at risk for chronic iridocyclitis, which may progress to blindness. Therefore, frequent ophthalmologic evaluations should be performed. The arthritis usually resolves without deformity. HLA-DR5 and HLA-DRw8 are significantly increased in this subgroup. A second subgroup with pauciarticular onset has a strong male predominance and later age of onset. HLA-B27 occurs in the majority of these patients. The disease in these children follows a course consistent with spondyloarthropathy.

Treatment must be determined on the basis of disease severity. Aspirin is a basic standby, but tolmetin and naproxen can be used safely in children. Physical therapy and psychosocial support are also indicated.

ADULT-ONSET STILL'S DISEASE

Still's disease is one form of juvenile-onset chronic arthritis that may begin in adulthood. Cases have been recognized that span the entire adult age spectrum, including elderly patients. The clinical features are the same as described above. Acute symptoms often respond to salicylates or other NSAID's, but prednisone may be necessary for short periods. The prognosis for complete recovery is good in the majority of patients.

Aptekar RG, Decker JL, Bujak JS, et al.: Adult onset juvenile rheumatoid arthritis. Arthritis Rheum 16:715, 1973. *An excellent clinical discussion of the adult-onset form of Still's disease.*

Arnett FC, Edworthy SM, Bloch DA, et al.: The American Rheumatism Association 1987 revised criteria for the classification of rheumatoid arthritis. Arthritis Rheum 31:315, 1988. *A more in-depth discussion of the development, recommended uses, and potential pitfalls of criteria for RA.*

Fassbender HG: Normal and pathologic synovial tissue with emphasis on rheumatoid arthritis. *In* Cohen AS, Bennett JC (eds.): Rheumatology and Immunology. 2nd ed. Orlando, Fla., Grune & Stratton, 1986. *Comprehensive discussion with excellent illustrations of the course of synovitis.*

Gregersen PK, Silver J, Winchester RJ: The shared epitope hypothesis. An approach to understanding the molecular genetics of susceptibility to rheumatoid arthritis. Arthritis Rheum 30:1205, 1987. *A discussion of how genetic polymorphism may lead to susceptibility to RA.*

Harris ED Jr: Rheumatoid arthritis: Pathophysiology and implications for therapy. N Engl J Med 322:1277, 1990. *A recent comprehensive review of the pathobiology of RA and theoretical basis for rational therapy.*

Olsen NJ, Callahan LF, Brooks RH, et al.: Associations of HLA-DR4 with rheumatoid factor and radiographic severity in rheumatoid arthritis. Am J Med 84:257, 1988. *A large, well-conducted study of the relation of HLA-DR4 to clinical features of RA.*

Southern P, Oldstone MBA: Medical consequences of persistent viral infection. N Engl J Med 314:359, 1986. *Considerations relating to possible infectious origin of RA.*

Strominger JL: Biology of the human histocompatibility leukocyte antigen (HLA) system and a hypothesis regarding the generation of autoimmune disease. J Clin Invest 77:1411, 1986. *Excellent review of concepts relating to autoimmune features of RA.*

Tugwell P, Bennett K, Gent M: Methotrexate in rheumatoid arthritis. Indications, contraindications, efficacy, and safety. Ann Intern Med 107:358, 1987. *An excellent review of efficacy and safety studies of methotrexate therapy in RA.*

Wees SJ, Sunwoo IN, Oh SJ: Sural nerve biopsy in systemic necrotizing vasculitis. Am J Med 71:525, 1981. *Description of a useful diagnostic procedure for vasculitis and peripheral neuropathy.*

Ziff M: Systemic rheumatoid disease: Immunological aspects. Adv Inflam Res 3:123, 1982. *A comprehensive review of the immunologic mechanisms involving the pathogenesis of RA.*

259 The Spondylarthropathies

Andrei Calin

The seronegative spondylarthritides are characterized by involvement of the sacroiliac joints, by peripheral inflammatory arthropathy, and by the absence of rheumatoid factor. Other features include the following:

1. Pathologic changes concentrated around the enthesis (i.e., the site of ligamentous insertion into bone) rather than the synovium. Nonenthesopathic changes may also develop in the eye, the aortic valve, the lung parenchyma, and the skin.

2. Clinical evidence of overlap among the various seronegative spondylarthritides. Thus, a patient with psoriatic arthropathy may well develop uveitis or sacroiliitis, and a patient with inflammatory bowel disease may develop ankylosing spondylitis or mouth ulcers.

3. A tendency toward familial aggregation, with the suggestion that these entities "breed true" within families.

Types

The spondylarthropathies include ankylosing spondylitis, Reiter's syndrome (both the postvenereal, or endemic, and the postinfective, or epidemic, forms), the reactive arthritides (caused by *Yersinia, Salmonella, Helicobacter, Campylobacter,* and other infections), certain subsets of juvenile arthropathy (juvenile ankylosing spondylitis and the seronegative enthesopathic arthropathy syndrome), enteropathic sacroiliitis (ulcerative colitis and Crohn's disease), psoriatic arthropathy, and perhaps a group of rarer disorders (Whipple's disease, Behçet's syndrome, and pustulotic arthro-osteitis) (Fig. 259–1).

These disorders can be categorized according to the specific periarticular or articular involvement. The various spondylarthropathies can be distinguished from one another according to the particular peripheral joints involved, the associated clinical features (i.e., urethritis, conjunctivitis, skin involvement), and the manner in which the disease progresses (i.e., remission or relapse) (Table 259–1).

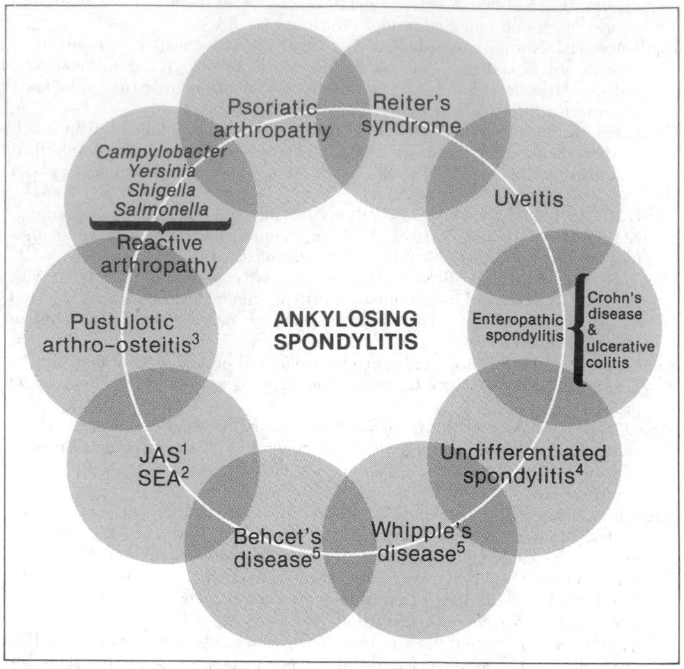

FIGURE 259–1. Individual conditions that overlap to form the spondylarthritides. (1) Juvenile ankylosing spondylitis. (2) Seronegative enthesopathic arthropathy syndrome. (3) Considered by Japanese to be part of spondylarthropathy spectrum (rare in United States and Europe). (4) Undifferentiated spondylitis (i.e., subset of patients who have spondylarthropathic features but who fail to meet criteria for ankylosing spondylitis, Reiter's syndrome, or other condition, e.g., dactylitis, uveitis, plus unilateral sacroiliitis). (5) Not universally accepted as members of the spondylarthropathy group.

Hereditary Factors

Hereditary factors play an important role in the development of spondylarthropathies. Some 5 to 20 per cent of individuals positive for HLA-B27 (HLA, human leukocyte antigen) develop ankylosing spondylitis following an unknown environmental event, while 20 per cent develop Reiter's syndrome after exposure to *Shigella* or other environmental trigger.

The explanation for the link between HLA-B27 and the spondylarthropathies remains unknown. Hypotheses include the following: (1) B27 acts as a receptor site for an infective agent; (2) B27 is a marker for an immune response gene that determines susceptibility to an environmental trigger; or (3) B27 may induce tolerance to foreign antigens with which it cross-reacts.

We now know that the risk of developing ankylosing spondylitis for a B27-positive relative of a B27-positive patient is 25 to 50 per cent compared with about 5 per cent for a random B27-positive subject. This argues for genetic differences between the two B27 groups. Splitting of B27 by monoclonal antibodies and cytotoxic T cells has not provided an explanation for these differences, so there must be an additional susceptibility (and perhaps severity) gene or genes (Fig. 259–2). Chromosomes 2, 14, and 19 may also be operative. The extent to which additional environmental triggers modify disease remains unknown. More than 95 per cent of patients with ankylosing spondylitis are HLA-B27 positive, while 80 per cent of those with Reiter's syndrome carry this antigen, as do only 50 per cent of those with psoriatic or enteropathic spondylitis. A new animal model (transgenic B27+ rat) may help elucidate the nature of the link between B27 and disease.

Etiologic Factors

Numerous infective triggers are recognized for the reactive arthropathies (*Shigella, Salmonella, Chlamydia*, and so forth). By contrast, the arthritogenic environmental event in ankylosing spondylitis has not been adequately defined. However, much interest has focused on *Klebsiella*, plasmids, or other extrachromosomal genetic material emanating from gram-negative enteric bacilli, and heat shock or stress protein.

ANKYLOSING SPONDYLITIS

Criteria for Diagnosis

The criteria for diagnosing ankylosing spondylitis have been evolving in recent years. The newly defined European Seronegative Study Group (ESSG) criteria include all spondylarthropathy patients. A simple approach defines ankylosing spondylitis as the presence of symptomatic sacroiliitis. The condition in a patient with back discomfort and radiologic evidence of sacroiliitis would be diagnosed as ankylosing spondylitis.

Prevalence

Once considered a rare disease, the illness is now known to have a prevalence comparable to that of rheumatoid arthritis. The distribution of ankylosing spondylitis follows the population frequency of HLA-B27 and is more common in whites than in blacks.

Ankylosing spondylitis has often gone undiagnosed; inappropriate diagnostic procedures lead to erroneous diagnoses (e.g., mechanical back disease). Such patients often receive incorrect therapy.

Although ankylosing spondylitis was formerly believed to occur predominantly in men, several studies now suggest that there may be a more uniform sex distribution. Most large series report a 2.5:1 ratio in favor of men. The condition in female patients is less frequently diagnosed, perhaps because physicians and radiologists may be reluctant to diagnose a disease that they consider to be rare in women. In women, the disease may be milder and may present with a greater number of peripheral joint manifestations. In the past, many cases of ankylosing spondylitis in women were inappropriately diagnosed as seronegative rheumatoid arthritis.

Clinical Presentation

A history of several of the following five features is suggestive of inflammatory spinal disease: insidious onset of discomfort, age less than 40 years, persistence for more than 3 months, association with morning stiffness, and improvement with exercise.

If this simple screening test is positive, radiologic evidence of sacroiliitis confirms ankylosing spondylitis. Many radiologists have been unfamiliar with rheumatologic joint disease and have diagnosed ankylosing spondylitis only when evidence of major ankylosis of the sacroiliac joints and spine was present. Ankylosing spondylitis can be diagnosed, however, in the presence of only minimal sacroiliitis. What determines whether a patient will have only a mild pelvic disease, ascending spinal disease, extraspinal articular disease, or extra-articular symptoms remains unknown. Presumably, phenotypic expression depends on numerous interrelating genes. The age at onset is of paramount importance. Some 15 per cent of teenagers (at onset) will require a total hip replacement within 20 years, while those with onset in their 20's are much less at risk for major hip or neck involvement.

Early change in the lumbar spine is manifested as squaring of the superior and inferior margins of the vertebral body. This phenomenon is caused by inflammatory disease at the site of insertion of the outer fibers of the annulus fibrosus, i.e., enthesopathy. Later changes result in the classic, though rare, bamboo spine. Comparable spinal changes are seen in primary ankylosing spondylitis and in the spondylitis associated with inflammatory bowel disease. In spondylitis associated with Reiter's syndrome and psoriatic arthropathy, however, the changes tend to be asymmetric and random.

Radionuclide scans, computed tomography, and other advanced radiologic techniques are usually unnecessary. A simple anteroposterior radiograph suffices.

Physical Examination

Examination of the spine may reveal muscle spasm and loss of the normal lordosis. The degree of restriction of forward flexion can be documented by measuring the distraction, on flexion, of two points—the lower point at the level of the lumbosacral junction and the upper point 10 cm above this level. In a normal individual, the distraction of this 10-cm line is 5 to 8 cm, compared with 0 to 6 cm in an untreated patient with spondylitis. Lateral spinal flexion is measured by the distraction, on contralateral flexion, of a 20-cm line drawn in the mid-axillary plane.

TABLE 259–1. COMPARISON OF SERONEGATIVE SPONDYLARTHROPATHIES

	Ankylosing Spondylitis	Reiter's Syndrome	Psoriatic Arthropathy	Enteropathic Spondylitis	Juvenile Arthropathy (JAS* subset)	Reactive Arthropathy
Sex	Male ≥ female	Male ≥ female	Female ≥ male	Female = male	Male > female	Male = female
Age at onset	20	Any age	Any age	Any age	<16	Any age
Uveitis	+ +	+ +	+	+	+	+
Conjunctivitis	–	+	–	–	–	+
Peripheral joints	Lower > upper: often	Lower usually	Upper > lower	Lower > upper	Lower > upper	Lower > upper
Sex differences	Yes	No	No	No	No	No
Sacroiliitis	Always	Often	Often	Often	Often	Often
HLA-B27	95%	80%	20% (50% with sacroiliitis)	50%	90%	80%
Enthesopathy	+	+	+	+	+	+
Aortic regurgitation	+	+	? +	?	?	+
Familial aggregation	+	+	+	+	+	+
Risk for HLA-B27–positive individual	± 20%	20%	?	?	?	20%
Onset	Gradual	Sudden	Variable	Gradual	Variable	Sudden
Urethritis	–	+	–	–	–	+/–
Skin involvement	–	+	+ +	–	–	–
Mucous membrane involvement	–	+	–	+	–	+
Symmetry (spinal)	+	–	–	+	+	–
Self-limiting	–	+/–	+/–	+/–	+/–	+/–
Remission, relapses	–	+/–	+/–	–	+/–	+/–

*JAS = Juvenile ankylosing spondylitis.

In this case, normal distraction varies from 5 to 12 cm, compared with 0 to 7 cm in patients with spondylitis.

Peripheral joint involvement, especially in the lower limb, occurs at some stage in approximately 20 to 30 per cent of cases. Inflammatory disease of the hip and shoulder may produce progressive disability. Enthesopathic features include plantar fasciitis, costochondritis, and Achilles tendinitis.

Laboratory Findings

HLA-B27 testing should not be used as a routine screening procedure; it is expensive and usually unnecessary. Elevation of the erythrocyte sedimentation rate occurs in most patients but may be normal despite severe disease. Elevation of immunoglobulin A (IgA) levels and the presence of immune complexes suggest aberrant immunity. Serum creatine kinase and alkaline phosphatase levels may be elevated. Lymphocytes predominate in the synovial fluid, and synovial histologic findings are nonspecific.

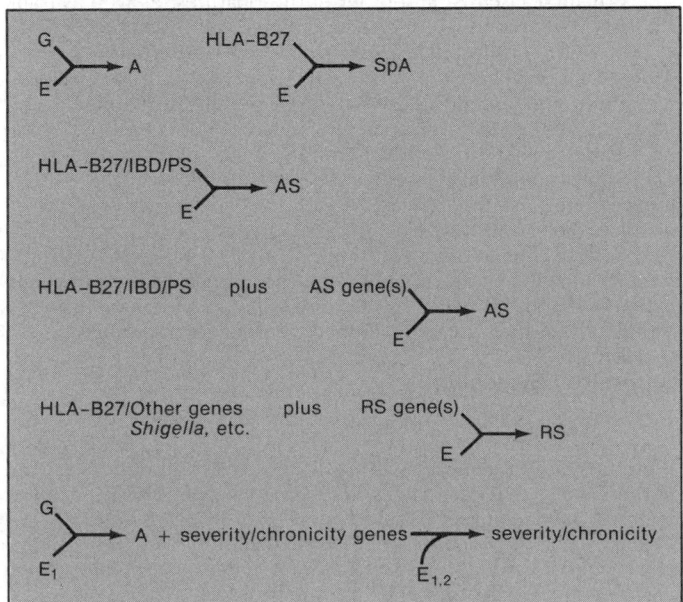

FIGURE 259–2. Relationship between environmental and genetic factors in susceptibility, severity, and natural history of reactive arthropathies and spondylarthritides. G = genetics; E = environment; A = arthritis; SpA = spondylarthropathy; IBD = inflammatory bowel disease; PS = psoriasis; AS = ankylosing spondylitis; E_1 and E_2 = environmental factors; RS = Reiter's syndrome.

Pathology

The synovial lesions of ankylosing spondylitis and rheumatoid arthritis share identical histopathologic characteristics: intimal cell hyperplasia and a diffuse lymphocyte and plasma cell infiltrate. Formation of lymphoid follicles is found less frequently in ankylosing spondylitis than in rheumatoid disease. Synovitis per se, however, does not explain the propensity toward ligamentous ossification and widespread new bone formation observed in ankylosing spondylitis. Inflammation at the enthesis accounts for the unique pathology, or enthesopathy, of ankylosing spondylitis; new bone formation appears to be a specific reparative process occurring at the enthesopathic site. Complications of severe spinal disease include fractures and spondylodiscitis after minimal trauma.

A striking degree of spinal osteoporosis in patients with early and mild disease has been demonstrated, suggesting that bone pathology could be a primary event in disease pathogenesis.

Extraskeletal Involvement

Extra-articular features include fatigue, weight loss, and low-grade fever. Cord compression resulting from spinal fractures or the cauda equina syndrome may cause neurologic symptoms. The negative effects of systemic involvement and of radiotherapy on the survival of patients with ankylosing spondylitis are well recognized.

EYE INVOLVEMENT. Uveitis develops in up to 40 per cent of patients during their illness. It occurs most often in HLA-B27–positive patients. There is no correlation with the severity of the spondylitis, and onset appears to be a random environmental event. The episodes of uveitis are usually self-limited, but may require local steroid therapy.

PULMONARY DISEASE. Patients with severe disease may exhibit chronic infiltrative and fibrotic changes in the upper lung fields that mimic tuberculosis. Pulmonary ventilation is usually well maintained by the diaphragm, despite the chest wall rigidity. The pulmonary fibrosis is occasionally clinically silent, but most affected patients present with cough, sputum, and dyspnea. Cyst formation and subsequent *Aspergillus* invasion may cause hemoptysis.

CARDIOVASCULAR DISEASE. Aortic incompetence, cardiomegaly, and persistent conduction defects occur in 3.5 to 10.0 per cent of patients with severe spondylitic disease. Cardiac involvement may be clinically silent or may dominate the clinical picture. Thickened aortic valve cusps and scar tissue in the root of the aorta represent the major histologic changes.

AMYLOIDOSIS. Amyloid deposition is an occasional complication of ankylosing spondylitis, particularly in Europe.

KIDNEY. In contrast to patients with rheumatoid arthritis, who may show renal impairment as an expression of disease, renal glomerular function is apparently unimpaired in patients with ankylosing spondylitis, despite recognized pathologic changes. An IgA nephropathy, however, has been described in patients with seronegative spondylarthropathy.

Treatment and Prognosis

Ankylosing spondylitis may be a mild or severe disease. As discussed, the younger the age at onset, the more severe the outcome. For example, in an analysis of 1500 cases, 15 per cent of those who were between 15 and 16 years of age at the time of onset needed a total hip replacement within 15 years, compared with 10 per cent of those who were between 19 and 20 years and fewer than 1 per cent of those who were more than 40 years of age (all cohorts were followed for a similar period).

Ankylosing spondylitis is a gratifying condition to recognize and treat early: Much can be accomplished toward ameliorating symptoms and, perhaps, preventing spinal deformity. The primary objectives are to relieve pain, decrease inflammation, begin remedial strengthening exercises, and maintain good posture and function.

Anti-inflammatory agents relieve inflammation, pain, and spasm and permit patients to follow an adequate exercise program. There is some evidence that phenylbutazone decreases the rate of spinal fusion. Nevertheless, indomethacin is the drug of choice. Phenylbutazone, although more efficacious, may be more toxic (in Britain, it can be used only by hospital rheumatologists). Indomethacin, started at a dosage of 25 mg three times a day (or 75 mg slow release at night), may be increased to a maximum of 150 mg daily. The dose should be titrated against response and side effects. Possible side effects include headache, vertigo, and depression, especially in older patients, and nausea, gastric discomfort, and diarrhea in all age groups. Phenylbutazone (100 mg three or four times per day) is remarkably effective but must be used with caution. Dangerous side effects include agranulocytosis and aplastic anemia. Agranulocytosis is an idiosyncratic response, developing chiefly in young individuals within 3 to 6 weeks of the start of therapy. Aplastic anemia appears to be dose-related and occurs primarily in individuals more than 60 years of age.

Nonsteroidal anti-inflammatory drugs (NSAID's) include ibuprofen, naproxen, fenoprofen, tolmetin, sulindac, meclofenamate sodium, piroxicam, diclofenac, and, depending on the country, flurbiprofen, ketoprofen, tiaprofenic acid, etodolac, and others. If indomethacin is efficacious but not tolerated, one of these NSAID's may be given. In general, these agents play a minor role in the management of the spondylarthritides. Phenylbutazone should be tried when indomethacin is ineffective.

Gold and penicillamine have no role to play, but sulfasalazine may be effective. Radiotherapy, once the treatment of choice, is virtually no longer practiced in view of the high risk of inducing leukemia. Azathioprine and methotrexate appear to have no effect on the spinal disease.

The patient also needs remedial strengthening exercises and postural training. A firm mattress and small pillow are ideal when the patient is resting; attention to posture while at work and at rest must be stressed. The best exercise regimen includes extension exercises and hydrotherapy; swimming is highly recommended.

In those few patients who, despite optimal management, develop an irreversible deformity, wedge osteotomy may be indicated. For those with destructive arthropathy of the hip, arthroplasty is a must. The long-term outcome of this procedure is gratifying.

REITER'S SYNDROME

The most common cause of an inflammatory oligoarthropathy in a young man is Reiter's syndrome. This classic triad of urethritis, conjunctivitis, and arthritis represents the one chronic rheumatic disorder related to both a specific genetic background (HLA-B27) and a specific infection. Reiter's syndrome is often not self-limited. Progressive disease may result in major disability. The disease may be defined as an episode of arthropathy within 1 month of urethritis or cervicitis.

Whether a dysenteric (epidemic) or a venereal (endemic) infection is the most common precipitating event is unclear. In young children, the former is the rule. In many cases, the distinction between urethritis as a precipitating factor and urethritis as an integral manifestation of the syndrome remains unclear. In postvenereal Reiter's syndrome, both *Chlamydia* and *Mycoplasma* have been implicated. In a patient with a specific predisposing genetic background, a variety of different organisms may be responsible. *Chlamydia* and *Yersinia* antigenic material has been demonstrated within the synovium, but the "reactive" nature (see below) of Reiter's disease is not in doubt.

Prevalence

Reiter's syndrome develops in at least 1 per cent of patients with nonspecific urethritis. *Shigella* dysentery is followed by Reiter's syndrome in 1 to 2 per cent of cases (i.e., 20 per cent of B27-positive patients). B27 is present in 6 to 14 per cent of whites and 0 to 4 per cent of blacks.

The sex distribution of Reiter's syndrome is difficult to define because the syndrome is diagnosed only with difficulty in women, in whom urethritis and cervicitis are often clinically inapparent. Formes frustes of the syndrome are now being recognized. A woman presenting with or without uveitis and an inflammatory arthropathy of the knee in association with HLA-B27 antigen may have Reiter's syndrome. Similarly, the disorder is difficult to recognize in children; a diagnosis is usually made only if an epidemic of dysentery is present and Reiter's syndrome has been recognized in other family members. Postdysenteric Reiter's syndrome almost certainly has an equal sex distribution.

Clinical Features

Reiter's syndrome should be considered a symptom complex rather than the association of three specific features. The syndrome may manifest as a tetrad (i.e., with the addition of buccal ulceration or balanitis to the classic triad); alternatively, only two of the three cardinal features may be present. Several of the classic features may appear insignificant and be overlooked. For example, the urethritis may be mild, perhaps forgotten; the discharge may be minimal and remembered by the patient only after direct questioning. Balanitis may not be evident unless the prepuce is retracted and the glans penis closely inspected. A red eye may be forgotten or considered irrelevant, and the various skin lesions typified by keratoderma blennorrhagicum may be misdiagnosed.

Rheumatologic features include arthralgias, tenosynovitic episodes, plantar fasciitis, and other enthesopathies, as well as frank arthritis. The typical sausage-shaped digit is a frequent occurrence related to the enthesopathic nature of the disorder.

Some 20 per cent of patients with Reiter's syndrome develop sacroiliitis and ascending spinal disease. Other radiologic evidence of Reiter's syndrome includes plantar spurs and periosteal new bone formation. Cardiac complications similar to those in ankylosing spondylitis occur late in Reiter's syndrome. The hyperkeratotic skin lesions seen in Reiter's syndrome cannot be distinguished from those in psoriasis.

Formerly considered a self-limited process, Reiter's syndrome is now known to be a more or less persistent disease in many patients. About 80 per cent of patients have evidence of disease activity when they are re-examined after a 5-year period.

Laboratory Evaluation

It is unclear whether the presence of HLA-B27 correlates with increased severity of Reiter's syndrome. A patient with severe Reiter's syndrome may have an erythrocyte sedimentation rate in the normal range or one as high as 100 mm per hour or more. Synovial fluid analysis is rarely diagnostic, apart from the fact that it reveals a relatively high complement level (reflecting a nonspecific inflammatory reaction), rather than the low level seen in rheumatoid arthritis (reflecting immune complex disease).

Occasionally, the diagnosis of ankylosing spondylitis and Reiter's syndrome may prove difficult to disentangle. Some patients whose disorder is diagnosed as ankylosing spondylitis may have presented originally with Reiter's syndrome, but the episodes of urethritis have subsequently been forgotten by the physician and patient. Similarly, patients whose disease is diagnosed as Reiter's syndrome may actually have ankylosing spondylitis with peripheral joint disease and a chance of the occurrence of urethritis.

Management

No cure exists for Reiter's syndrome. The patient's feelings of guilt and anxiety about sexual misconduct must be allayed. Although anecdotal evidence suggests that individuals with postvenereal Reiter's syndrome may develop a relapse following sexual activity, many individuals have spontaneous exacerbations. An explanation of allergic response may help the patient: Asthma may develop on exposure to a known or unknown allergen in sensitive individuals; in the same way, Reiter's syndrome may flare up following an unknown allergic event.

Symptomatic management includes the use of indomethacin, phenylbutazone, or other NSAID's. Antibiotic therapy is too late and unnecessary. Patients with severe, recurrent uveitis may require steroid eye drops or subconjunctival preparations. The syndrome may remit, recur, or continue unabated despite steroid or even cytotoxic therapy. For patients with progressive disease, azathioprine or methotrexate may be effective.

THE REACTIVE ARTHROPATHIES

Reactive arthropathy refers to an inflammatory arthritis that follows an infection in which no microbial invasion of the synovial space occurs. The B27-linked arthropathies following *Shigella*, *Salmonella*, *Yersinia*, *Helicobacter*, and *Campylobacter jejuni* infections are in this group. Why some patients develop only an arthropathy whereas others have the full spectrum of Reiter's disease after exposure to one of these agents is unknown.

Yersinia Infection

Yersinia enterocolitica infection may produce the following: fever, mild gastrointestinal illness, and, after a latent period, polyarthropathy and erythema nodosum, especially in B27-positive individuals. The symptom complex may mimic acute rheumatic fever. The arthropathy may last for weeks or months, and in HLA-B27–positive individuals, sacroiliitis may occur.

Salmonellosis

An arthropathy associated with *Salmonella* infections mimics that caused by *Yersinia*. Treatment of these disorders is the same as that of Reiter's syndrome.

JUVENILE CHRONIC ARTHROPATHY

Chronic arthritis in a child or teenager often persists into adulthood; therefore, an awareness of juvenile chronic arthropathy is relevant when attending adult patients. Until recently, the term juvenile rheumatoid arthritis was used, inappropriately, to describe all forms of childhood arthritis. As in adults, arthritis in children may be associated with psoriasis, inflammatory bowel disease, and other conditions. The acute systemic form, Still's disease, manifests with fever, rash, and toxicity in young children who are negative for B27 and rheumatoid factor (IgM anti-IgG). Still's disease is also recognized in adults. Another subset (in the spondylarthropathy group) consists largely of adolescent boys who predominantly exhibit oligoarthropathy affecting the large joints of the lower limbs; such individuals are frequently positive for HLA-B27. This group may develop sacroiliitis or ankylosing spondylitis; the presence of B27 is associated with spinal disease involvement. Another group includes B27-negative individuals (usually girls less than 5 years of age) presenting with an oligoarthropathy characterized by a positive fluorescent antinuclear antibody (FANA) test. These subjects are at risk for developing asymptomatic chronic iridocyclitis, in contrast to FANA-negative and B27-positive patients, who develop clinically obvious acute uveitis. A few older children (preponderantly girls) develop a seropositive, nodular, and erosive disease that resembles adult rheumatoid arthritis. A B27-related syndrome known as seronegative enthesopathy and arthropathy (SEA syndrome) is now also recognized in children. Such individuals often develop sacroiliitis at a later stage.

THE ENTEROPATHIC ARTHROPATHIES

Two major clinical patterns of arthropathy associated with inflammatory bowel disease (ulcerative colitis and Crohn's disease) are peripheral arthropathy and spondylarthropathy.

Peripheral Arthropathy

Approximately 20 per cent of individuals with severe Crohn's disease or ulcerative colitis develop an acute migratory inflammatory polyarthritis, often of abrupt onset and involving the larger joints of the lower extremities. The arthritis resolves in weeks or months. Arthritis flare-ups usually parallel exacerbations of the underlying disorder. The pathogenesis of the joint complication is unknown. The B27 antigen is not present. Treatment is directed at the primary disorder and is more effective in ulcerative colitis than in Crohn's disease.

Spondylarthropathy

About one patient in five with inflammatory bowel disease develops sacroiliitis and, occasionally, severe ankylosing spondylitis. Men and women are equally affected. The spinal disease may precede the bowel disease or follow it. There is no correlation between the severity of the bowel disorder and the spondylitis. Therapy is the same as for classic ankylosing spondylitis. Despite the bowel disease, the NSAID's are usually well tolerated.

A post–intestinal bypass syndrome consisting of arthropathy and occasionally dermatitis is well recognized. Immune alterations have been described in these patients, and B27 is occasionally associated with this syndrome.

PSORIATIC ARTHROPATHY

Different subsets of psoriatic arthropathy are recognized, several forms of which appear to be enthesopathic rather than purely synovitic. Uveitis, sacroiliitis, and ascending spinal disease occur in up to 20 per cent of cases. Patients are seronegative for rheumatoid factor and exhibit sausage digits and characteristic radiologic changes. The disease may be markedly destructive.

Psoriasis itself is a genetically determined disease, associated with HLA-B13, HLA-Bw17, and HLA-Cw6. Moreover, HLA-B27 is present in approximately 20 per cent of individuals with psoriatic arthropathy, even in the absence of sacroiliitis. HLA-Bw38, HLA-DR4, and HLA-DR7 appear to be genetic markers for patients with peripheral arthropathy. About 50 per cent of patients with psoriatic spondylitis are B27 negative; thus, as with inflammatory bowel disease, other genetic or environmental factors are relevant.

Psoriatic arthropathy is a common disease, occurring in about 20 per cent of individuals with psoriasis, particularly in those patients with psoriatic nail disease. Women are affected only slightly more commonly than men, in contrast to the more marked sex distribution in rheumatoid disease. Several forms of psoriatic arthropathy, the separation of which is not entirely distinct, have been described.

1. *Asymmetric oligoarthropathy.* In general, little relationship exists between joint and skin activity. Asymmetric involvement of both large and small joints is seen; the sausage-shaped digit is common. Any patient presenting with this form of arthropathy should be carefully examined for signs of psoriasis (scalp, umbilicus, gluteal region, and nails). In the past, many such individuals were considered to have seronegative rheumatoid arthritis.

2. *Symmetric polyarthropathy resembling rheumatoid arthritis.* Rarely, the pattern of arthritis may be indistinguishable from that seen in rheumatoid disease. This form may represent coincidental rheumatoid arthritis in a patient with psoriasis.

3. *Arthritis mutilans.* A resorptive arthropathy, arthritis mutilans is the severest form of destructive arthritis. The telescoping digits appear as the so-called opera-glass hand.

4. *Psoriatic spondylitis.* Approximately 20 per cent of subjects with psoriatic arthropathy have radiologic sacroiliitis (ankylosing spondylitis). Men predominate, with a sex ratio of 3.5:1.

5. *Psoriatic nail disease and distal interphalangeal joint involvement.* Nail pitting, transverse depressions, and subungual hyperkeratosis often occur in association with distal interphalangeal joint disease. The relationship between the psoriasis and the arthritis remains unclear.

Laboratory Features

An elevated erythrocyte sedimentation rate, anemia, and, rarely, hyperuricemia may occur. The frequency of positive tests for rheumatoid factor is the same as that found in the general population. The synovial tissue and fluid changes are nonspecific.

Radiologic Findings

Characteristic changes in this sometimes highly destructive disease include whittling of the distal ends of the phalanges, giving the joints a "pencil-and-cup" appearance; extensive bone resorption can result in an opera-glass hand. Erosions, ankylosis, periostitis, sacroiliitis, and ankylosing spondylitis are other typical radiologic findings.

Therapy

The skin and joints are treated separately. Improvement of the skin disease may be associated with amelioration of the joint inflammation. For mild arthropathy, indomethacin (25 to 50 mg three times per day) is the drug of choice. If this fails, phenylbutazone may be given. Gold and penicillamine may be useful, but few controlled studies have been done. Methotrexate is helpful in resistant cases.

Human Immunodeficiency Virus (HIV) and Spondylarthropathy

It is well recognized that a patient with rheumatoid arthritis who develops HIV disease may enter remission, at least from the point of view of the rheumatologic event. By contrast, patients with Reiter's syndrome or psoriatic arthropathy experience a dramatic exacerbation of the underlying disorder. Presumably, rheumatoid disease requires CD4+ lymphocytes, while the immunologic nature of spondylarthritis is distinct. Any patient who presents with severe Reiter's syndrome or psoriatic arthropathy, particularly when unresponsive to treatment, should be assessed for HIV disease. Methotrexate can have catastrophic effects on the patient with this infection.

Arnett F: The seronegative spondylarthropathies. *In* McCarty D (ed.): Current Opinion in Rheumatology, Vol. 2, No. 4, 1990. *A series of up-to-date review articles on research and clinical subjects in the spondylarthropathy field.*

Calin A (ed.): Spondylarthropathy. New York, Grune and Stratton, 1984, pp 1–427. *A multiauthored international text on spondylarthropathy, including discussions on immunogenetics, the environment, and ethnic differences.*

Feltkamp TEW (ed.): The pathogenetic role of HLA-B27. Scand J Rheumatol Suppl 87:1–163, 1990. *An excellent recent review of current understanding of B27.*

Will R, Palmer R, Bhalla A, et al.: Marked osteoporosis is present in early ankylosing spondylitis and may be a primary pathological event. Lancet 2:1483, 1989. *A study of the spine in early disease, with striking findings.*

260 Infectious Arthritis

Stephen E. Malawista

BACTERIAL ARTHRITIS

Bacterial arthritis usually results from bloodborne infection and much less commonly from direct penetration (e.g., needle aspiration) or contiguous osteomyelitis. Acute bacterial joint infections may be divided into two general groups, nongonococcal and gonococcal, based on their typically differing target populations, clinical characteristics, and ease of treatment. Differential features of these two classes of bacterial arthritis are presented in Table 260–1.

Nongonococcal Arthritis

Staphylococcus aureus heads the list of common infecting organisms in this group, followed by other gram-positive cocci (*Streptococcus pyogenes, pneumoniae, viridans*) and gram-negative bacilli (*Escherichia coli, Salmonella* sp., *Pseudomonas*, etc.); *Haemophilus influenzae* is unusual except in children under 4 years of age, before protective immunity develops. Patients are often very young, elderly, immunocompromised, or users of intravenous drugs. Risk factors for bacterial arthritis during septicemia include debilitating chronic disease, immunosuppressive therapy, previous joint damage (e.g., rheumatoid arthritis,

TABLE 260–1. DIFFERENTIAL FEATURES OF DISSEMINATED GONOCOCCAL INFECTION AND NONGONOCOCCAL BACTERIAL ARTHRITIS*

Disseminated Gonococcal Infection	Nongonococcal Bacterial Arthritis
Generally in young, healthy adults	Often in very young, elderly, or immunocompromised persons
Initial migratory polyarthralgias common	Polyarthralgias rare
Tenosynovitis in majority	Tenosynovitis rare
Dermatitis in majority	Dermatitis rare
>50% polyarthritis	>85% monoarthritis
Positive blood culture in <10%	Positive blood culture in 50%
Positive joint-fluid culture in 25%	Positive joint-fluid culture in 85–95%

*From Goldenberg DL, Reed JI: Bacterial arthritis. N Engl J Med 312:764–771, 1985. Reprinted by permission of The New England Journal of Medicine.

neuropathic arthropathy, joint surgery), sickle cell anemia, hypogammaglobulinemia, and intra-articular corticosteroid injections. After prosthetic joint replacement, an increasing problem has been late infection by organisms of low virulence, such as *Staphylococcus epidermidis*.

CLINICAL MANIFESTATIONS. A patient may present typically with the abrupt onset of a single, severely tender, red-hot swollen joint, especially the knee or another weight-bearing joint; shaking chills and fever may occur. However, signs of inflammation may be masked in severely debilitated patients or in those receiving adrenocorticosteroids or immunosuppressive agents. Bacterial arthritis superimposed on a noninfectious inflammatory joint disease may also be easily overlooked. For example, infection in one or a few joints of a patient with rheumatoid arthritis may be mistaken for a flare in the chronic disease. An infected joint in a gouty individual may go unrecognized for too long, even when the patient does not respond to his usual regimen for acute gouty arthritis (a good clue that something else is going on). A high index of suspicion is essential in these circumstances, because delay can lead rapidly to destruction of cartilage and bone and eventual fibrous or bony ankylosis.

DIAGNOSIS. When bacterial arthritis is suspected, prompt joint aspiration and both Gram stain and culture of synovial fluid are imperative; most nongonococcal bacteria will be recovered. Cultures for both aerobic and anaerobic organisms should be made. Synovial fluid leukocyte counts are frequently greater than 50,000 per cubic millimeter, and the glucose level is low and lactate level is high compared with those of serum, but these findings are not specific for infection. Bacteriologic studies should of course be extended to blood and other material (sputum, urine, and so forth) from which the infection may have disseminated. On radiograph, only soft tissue swelling is likely to be seen during the first week, but evidence of loss of articular cartilage and erosion of bone may appear rather soon thereafter in untreated patients.

MANAGEMENT. Successful management of bacterial arthritis depends primarily on early institution of appropriate antimicrobial therapy and effective drainage of the joint space. The selection of antimicrobial agents and recommendations regarding dose and duration of therapy are discussed in other areas of the text (Part XX). Antibiotics are given parenterally, often in high doses, for 2 to 4 weeks or more, depending on the clinical situation and the patient's response. They generally attain adequate levels in joint fluid and need not be given intra-articularly; indeed, the latter procedure may induce a chemical synovitis. For drainage, daily (or even more frequent) closed joint aspiration through a large-bore needle is carried out until fluid no longer accumulates. Open surgical drainage can usually be avoided except when the hip or the shoulder is infected (difficult to evacuate completely by needle); when tissue debris or fibrin interferes with closed aspiration; or when loculations, gross joint destruction, or contiguous osteomyelitis is present. The affected joint should be at rest while inflamed and should be mobilized to prevent atrophy when signs of acute inflammation have subsided.

Gonococcal Arthritis

Gonococcal infection is discussed in Ch. 336. The associated arthritis is by far the most common bacterial joint problem in generally healthy, sexually active teenagers and young adults, especially in urban populations. Gonorrhea is more likely to disseminate in women. The risk of dissemination is particularly high during menses and pregnancy, in the postpartum period, and in individuals with genetic deficiency in the terminal components of serum complement (C5, C6, C7, or C8). Additional features that help to distinguish gonococcal from other bacterial arthritides include a high frequency of associated tenosynovitis and rash and of multiple joint involvement, especially in the wrists and hands. Diagnosis is frequently presumptive because synovial fluid smear and culture are often negative, and corroborating cultural evidence from urethra, cervix, throat, rectum, blood, or skin may be lacking. Highly suggestive diagnostically is a history of fever and migratory polyarthralgias that progress to frank oligoarticular arthritis and are associated with tenosynovitis and skin lesions. The latter are either vesiculopustular on an erythematous base, often with necrotic centers, or hemorrhagic. Similar lesions are seen with arthritis caused by the meningococcus. Response to (even oral) antibiotic therapy (Ch. 336) and drainage is usually dramatic. Resistance to penicillin of gonococci that disseminate is uncommon.

Tuberculous Arthritis

The general decline in the frequency of pulmonary tuberculosis in the Western world is reflected in the relative rarity of tuberculous bone and joint disease. Infection usually reaches the joint from hematogenous dissemination to bone and direct extension from an osteomyelitic focus. Formerly, the classic presentation was chronic low back pain in a child because of involvement of lower thoracic or lumbar vertebrae, leading to collapse and sharp-angle kyphosis (Pott's disease). Currently, the typical target is a tuberculin-positive adult, often without evidence of pulmonary disease, who presents with chronic, insidious pain and swelling, usually in a single joint, especially the hip, knee, or wrist; this presentation is often mistaken for monoarticular rheumatoid arthritis. Tenosynovitis is common. Diagnosis depends upon culture of *Mycobacterium tuberculosis* from synovial fluid (positive in 80 per cent) or synovial biopsy (positive in 90 per cent). Sensitivities to chemotherapeutic agents must be determined; caseating granulomas and acid-fast bacilli are sometimes due to atypical mycobacteria resistant to the usual antituberculous drugs. Usual therapy for uncomplicated infections consists of long-term isoniazid and ethambutol or rifampin.

Goldenberg DL: Infectious arthritis complicating rheumatoid arthritis and other chronic rheumatic disorders. Arthritis Rheum 32:496, 1989. *Problems and recommendations in the diagnosis of infection in joints that have other reasons for being inflamed.*
Goldenberg DL, Reed JI: Bacterial arthritis. N Engl J Med 312:764, 1985. *A compact, well-referenced review of the pathophysiology of bacterial arthritis, clinical and microbiologic characteristics of its common forms, and current approaches to diagnosis and therapy.*

VIRAL ARTHRITIS

Many specific viral infections are associated with polyarthritis, notably hepatitis B, rubella, and parvovirus, but also mumps and vaccinia (and formerly, smallpox) and occasionally adenovirus type 7, Epstein-Barr virus (EBV) (in infectious mononucleosis) and other herpesviruses, and certain enteroviruses. Polyarthritis may dominate the picture of various mosquito-transmitted arbovirus infections, especially epidemic polyarthritis of Australia (Ross River virus) and the denguelike illnesses, chikungunya and o'nyongnyong.

In general, diagnosis is suggested by the exposure history (drug abuse for hepatitis B, immunization for rubella, epidemiologic considerations for arboviruses or enteroviruses); recognition of the associated viral syndrome, which often includes fever, rash, and regional lymphadenopathy; brevity of the joint involvement (days to weeks); and changing antibody titers against specific antigens. Routine laboratory tests are nonspecific, and except for rubella, virus has rarely been recovered from synovial fluid. Little is known about pathogenesis, but studies of hepatitis B and rubella provide some clues.

Transient, often symmetric polyarthritis or arthralgias resembling acute rheumatoid arthritis may be associated with hepatitis B, rubella, or parvovirus infection. In the case of *hepatitis B*, 10 to 30 per cent of patients have arthritis, often accompanied by urticaria, fever, and lymphadenopathy, all occurring days to weeks before the onset of frank hepatitis. This prodromal syndrome typically occurs when hepatitis B surface antigen (HBsAg) is in excess over antibody, hypocomplementemia is present, and serum contains immune complexes composed of HBsAg and anti-HB, other immunoglobulins, and complement components. Similar material has been found in affected dermal blood vessels, and the antigen has been seen in synovial tissue. With the development of antibody excess, complexes disappear, the arthritis and rash resolve, and frank hepatitis may supervene. The process resembles experimental serum sickness and suggests an inflammatory pathogenetic mechanism driven by deposition of immune complexes. Joint symptoms may respond dramatically to salicylates.

Rubella arthritis is primarily a disease of adult women. It usually follows onset of the characteristic rash by a few days, but the rash may be absent and rheumatoid factor present, inviting diagnostic confusion. Arthritis is usually sudden in onset, symmetric and polyarticular in distribution (fingers, knees, wrists), brief in duration (less than a month), and without residua. Salicylates are useful for pain and stiffness.

Arthritis may also occur within a few weeks of vaccination by attenuated rubella virus. Again, attacks are brief but may recur periodically for a few years without permanent joint damage. Rubella virus has been recovered from synovial fluid in both the natural and the vaccine-induced disease and more recently in a few patients with various chronic joint syndromes. It seems capable of replicating in synovium; whether its new association with chronic disease is critical or coincidental remains to be determined.

Human parvovirus B19 causes the highly contagious childhood exanthem fifth disease (*erythema infectiosum;* Ch. 365). In infected adults (especially women), a syndrome of short-lived (weeks) inflammatory joint involvement closely resembles that seen in rubella. As in rubella, the characteristic rash is often absent, and the history (of a sick child) is therefore critical for indicating the correct diagnosis; an elevated titer of specific IgM antibody confirms it. Again, treatment is symptomatic; prognosis, excellent.

Schnitzer TJ: Viral arthritis. *In* Kelley WN, Harris ED, Ruddy S, et al. (eds.): Textbook of Rheumatology. 3rd ed. Philadelphia, W.B. Saunders Company, 1989, pp 1611–1628. *Survey of common and uncommon arthritides associated with specific viral illnesses.*
Wands JR, Mann E, Alpert E, et al.: The pathogenesis of arthritis associated with acute hepatitis B surface antigen–positive hepatitis. Complement activation and characterization of circulating immune complexes. J Clin Invest 55:930, 1975. *Clinical description and characterization of immunologic aspects of the syndrome.*

OTHER FORMS OF INFECTIOUS ARTHRITIS

Lyme Disease (See Ch. 343)

Syphilitic Arthritis

Syphilis is discussed in Ch. 340. Joint disease associated with congenital and acquired syphilitic infections is now rare. In infants with congenital disease, musculoskeletal complaints are related to periostitis and osteochondritis. About the time of puberty, painless knee effusions (Clutton's joints) may be confused with rheumatoid or pyogenic arthritis. With acquired infection, arthralgias, arthritis, or tenosynovitis may accompany classic signs of secondary syphilis: rash, mucous plaques, alopecia, or lymphadenopathy. In tertiary lues, gummatous arthritis or periostitis (tibia, clavicles) may occur. Neuropathic arthropathy (Charcot's joint) is reviewed in Ch. 472.

Fungal Arthritis

Any of the invasive mycoses can affect joints, usually by direct extension from bone. Frequent infectious agents include coccidioidomycosis and histoplasmosis—both of which may also be accompanied by erythema nodosum with joint involvement, sporotrichosis (often by direct penetration: rose thorns), blastomycosis, actinomycosis, and candidiasis. Clinically, the affected joint or joints resemble those in other forms of granulomatous arthritis (e.g., tuberculous). For diagnosis, the causative agent must be seen in appropriately stained synovial biopsy material or grown from synovial tissue or fluid.

261 Systemic Lupus Erythematosus

Alfred D. Steinberg

Systemic lupus erythematosus (SLE) is a disease of unknown etiology characterized by inflammation in many different organ systems associated with the production of antibodies reactive with nuclear, cytoplasmic, and cell membrane antigens. Individual patients may have some, but not necessarily all, of the following: fatigue, anemia, fever, rashes, sun sensitivity, alopecia, arthritis, pericarditis, pleurisy, vasculitis, nephritis, and central nervous system disease. The course is often unpredictable, with variable periods of exacerbations and remissions. There is no one clinical abnormality that definitely establishes the diagnosis, nor is there a single test for the disorder. As a result, criteria have been developed and modified in an attempt to include patients with SLE and to exclude patients with other disorders (Table 261–1). Although these criteria were developed for epidemiologic and research purposes, they are helpful in diagnosis as well. Nevertheless, it is possible to fulfill these criteria and not have SLE, and it is possible to fail to fulfill the criteria and still have SLE. Thus, a teenage girl with a "butterfly" rash of the face, pleurisy, and large amounts of serum antibodies reactive with native DNA undoubtedly has SLE even if she does not yet manifest any other criteria.

INCIDENCE. Although SLE can occur at any age (it has been diagnosed at birth and in individuals in the tenth decade of life), more than 60 per cent of patients experience the onset of disease between ages 13 and 40 years. Among children, SLE occurs three times more commonly in girls than in boys. In patients in their teens, twenties, and thirties, 90 to 95 per cent are female. Thereafter, the female predominance again falls to that observed before puberty.

The disorder is approximately three times more common among American blacks than American caucasians. Certain North American Indian tribes (Sioux, Crow, Arapahoe) have an even greater predisposition toward SLE. Asians are affected to approximately the same extent as American blacks. The overall annual incidence of SLE is about 6 new cases per 100,000 population per year for relatively low-risk populations and approximately 35 per 100,000 for relatively high-risk populations. The chance that a black female will develop SLE in her lifetime is approximately 1 in 250.

These data suggest that both genetic factors and sex hormones may affect the probability of developing SLE. If a family member has SLE, the likelihood of SLE increases (approximately 30 per cent for identical twins and 5 per cent for other first-degree relatives). Although males develop SLE less frequently than do females, their illness is not milder.

ETIOLOGY. The etiology of SLE is unknown. The immune hyperactivity that characterizes SLE appears to derive from abnormal immune activation and loss of self-tolerance (Fig. 261–1). An inherited defect in immune regulation may underlie the disorder in many individuals. Environmental agents that trigger disease include foods, drugs, ultraviolet (UV) light, and microorganisms (bacteria, viruses, parasites) (Fig. 261–2). Inherited complement deficiency and other deficiencies (see Ch. 243) may predispose to infections that induce disease activity.

The combination of immune stimulation and impaired regulation leads to a loss of self-tolerance and expansion of B cells able to produce a variety of autoantibodies. Androgens protect against both the polyclonal activation and the loss of self-tolerance, whereas estrogens have the opposite effect. Early in life, idiotopes (unique structures expressed on immunoglobulin molecules) stimulate expansion of T cells with receptors that are able to recognize

TABLE 261–1. CRITERIA FOR CLASSIFICATION OF SYSTEMIC LUPUS ERYTHEMATOSUS*

Criterion		Definition
1. Malar rash		Fixed erythema, flat or raised, over the malar eminences, tending to spare the nasolabial folds
2. Discoid rash		Erythematous raised patches with adherent keratotic scaling and follicular plugging; atrophic scarring may occur in older lesions
3. Photosensitivity		Skin rash as a result of unusual reaction to sunlight, by patient history or physician observation
4. Oral ulcers		Oral or nasopharyngeal ulceration, usually painless, observed by a physician
5. Arthritis		Nonerosive arthritis involving two or more peripheral joints, characterized by tenderness, swelling, or effusion
6. Serositis	a.	Pleuritis—convincing history of pleuritic pain or rub heard by a physician or evidence of pleural effusion
		OR
	b.	Pericarditis—documented by electrocardiogram or rub or evidence of pericardial effusion
7. Renal disorder	a.	Persistent proteinuria greater than 0.5 gram per day or greater than 3+ if quantitation not performed
		OR
	b.	Cellular casts—may be red cell, hemoglobin, granular, tubular, or mixed
8. Neurologic disorder	a.	Seizures—in the absence of offending drugs or known metabolic derangements, e.g., uremia, ketoacidosis, or electrolyte imbalance
		OR
	b.	Psychosis—in the absence of offending drugs or known metabolic derangements, e.g., uremia, ketoacidosis, or electrolyte imbalance
9. Hematologic disorder	a.	Hemolytic anemia—with reticulocytosis
		OR
	b.	Leukopenia—less than 4000/mm³ total on two or more occasions
	c.	Lymphopenia—less than 1500/mm³ on two or more occasions
		OR
	d.	Thrombocytopenia—less than 100,000/mm³ in the absence of offending drugs
10. Immunologic disorder	a.	Positive LE cell preparation
		OR
	b.	Anti-DNA: antibody to native DNA in abnormal titer
		OR
	c.	Anti-Sm: presence of antibody to Sm nuclear antigen
		OR
	d.	False-positive serologic test for syphilis known to be positive for at least 6 months and confirmed by *Treponema pallidum* immobilization or fluorescent treponemal antibody absorption test
11. Antinuclear antibody		An abnormal titer of antinuclear antibody by immunofluorescence or an equivalent assay at any point in time and in the absence of drugs known to be associated with "drug-induced lupus" syndrome

*The classification is based on 11 criteria. For the purpose of identifying patients in clinical studies, a person shall be said to have systemic lupus erythematosus if any 4 or more of the 11 criteria are present, serially or simultaneously, during any interval of observation.

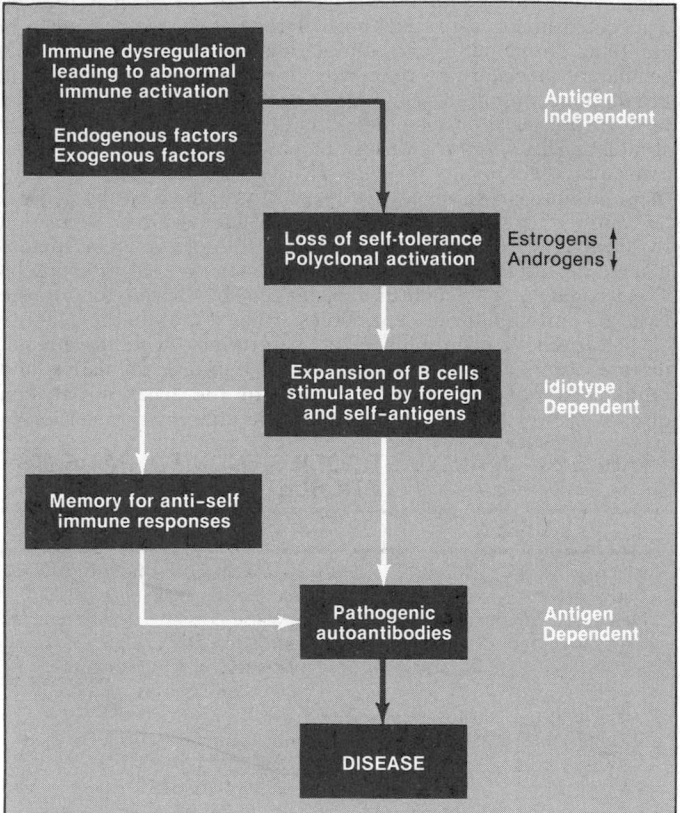

FIGURE 261–1. Flow chart of possible pathogenetic events in systemic lupus erythematosus. A stimulus to humoral immune hyperactivity can result from an endogenous (genetic) predisposition or from environmental triggers, or both. It does not necessarily depend upon stimulation by a specific self-antigen. The immune hyperactivity may lead to a loss of self-tolerance and polyclonal B cell activation. Androgens protect against such effects, whereas estrogens facilitate them. Idiotype stimulation may also contribute to expansion of B cells stimulated by foreign antigens and self-antigens (or antigens cross-reactive with self). Ultimately, selection by self-antigens leads to high-affinity autoantibodies, some of which are pathogenic. Even after the disease is treated, the prior generation of memory B cells allows the autoantibody response to be triggered anew, potentially leading to disease flares.

specific idiotopes but that simultaneously may recognize a self-antigen. In addition, later in life, similar idiotypic stimulation of T cells may provide help for B cells able to produce autoantibodies. For example, an immune complex of antibody and self-antigen (or an antigen cross-reactive with self) may be recognized in such a manner that the idiotype-specific T cell is stimulated by the idiotope on the antibody molecule. This interaction provides help for the B cell, which recognizes the self-antigen and is triggered to produce autoantibodies.

The stimulation of autoreactive B cells leads to both autoantibody-producing cells and memory B cells. The autoreactive B cells are subject to selective pressures by self-antigen, resulting in emergence of clones of B cells able to make antibody of progressively higher affinity for the self-antigen. Some such antibodies are pathogenic and contribute to disease. However, even after treatment, memory B cells may persist. Subsequent stimulation of such B cells may trigger a new disease flare.

Very early in the disease process, autoantibodies may have relatively low affinities for a given self-antigen and may be capable of binding to more than one self-antigen. With time, the selection processes frequently lead to antibodies with high affinity for a given self-determinant and less cross-reactivity with other self-antigens. Therefore, late in disease, the autoantibody "repertoire" becomes relatively fixed.

In some individuals, the inherited predisposition to SLE may be very important, the environmental triggers playing secondary roles. In contrast, other patients may have minimal genetic predispositions and may require very strong environmental triggers for disease expression (Fig. 261–2).

The signs and symptoms are thought to be caused by the

autoantibodies that react with self constituents and initiate inflammatory responses. The more severe the inflammatory response to a given initiator, the more severe the disease. The initiation of this process may be multifactorial and may be different in different individuals. Therefore, several genetic factors may be important in many individuals. These may be genes that allow augmented antibody responses following a variety of stimuli as well as genes that predispose to particular autoantibodies. In addition, hormonal, metabolic, and environmental factors appear to act on the genetically conditioned immune substratum to predispose to or protect against disease expression. Males are protected against SLE by their androgens except in a subgroup of males who inherit a Y chromosome accelerating factor from their fathers. In general, factors that augment humoral immunity favor disease expression, whereas those that retard antibody production tend to protect.

Some patients may have a primary abnormality in the ability of their immune systems to perform normal self-regulatory functions. It is probably best to consider abnormal immune regulation as one of several factors that may contribute to illness. If any one is very abnormal, disease may occur. Under most circumstances, several defects probably combine to incite disease. However, once the process is initiated, impaired self-regulation would favor perpetuation of the disease-inducing abnormalities.

It has long been known that some individuals with SLE have disease exacerbations following exposure to UV light. Several different mechanisms are likely: UV light induces keratinocytes to secrete interleukin 1, which, in turn, stimulates B cells and induces T cells to produce B cell growth and differentiation factors, which stimulate the immune system; UV light impairs processing of antigen and immune complexes, thereby increasing the load of pathogenic complexes on target organs; UV light induces cytosine and thymine dimer formation, which stimulates immune responses.

Certain drugs can cause an SLE-like illness in apparently healthy individuals. The drugs (Table 261–2) do not share common structural or chemical properties. The mechanisms of disease induction probably vary. Even chemicals in foods may induce

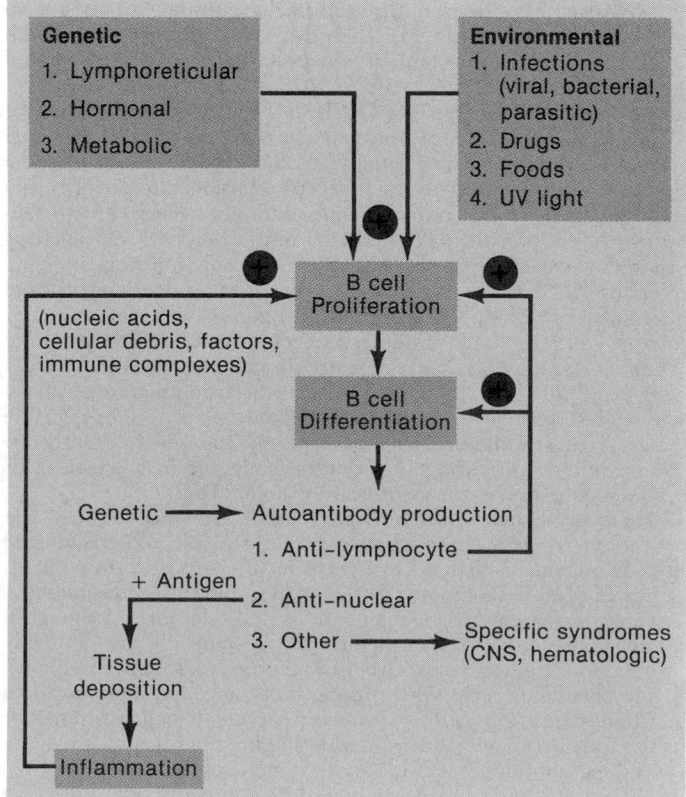

FIGURE 261–2. Initiation and perpetuation of systemic lupus erythematosus.

TABLE 261–2. SOME DRUGS ABLE TO INDUCE FEATURES OF SLE

Related to Dose-Time Administration	More Idiosyncratic
Hydralazine	Aminosalicylic acid
Procainamide	D-Penicillamine
Alpha-methyldopa	Griseofulvin
Isoniazid	Penicillin
Chlorpromazine	Ampicillin
Chlorthalidone	Streptomycin
Phenytoin	Sulfonamides
Mephenytoin	Tetracycline
Trimethadione	Methylthiouracil
Primidone	Propylthiouracil
Ethosuximide	Phenylbutazone
Carbamazepine	Oxyphenisatin
Phenylethylacetylurea	Practolol
	Tolazamide
	Methysergide
	Reserpine
	Quinidine
	Isoquinazepan
	Guanoxan

SLE. For example, alfalfa sprouts contain L-canavanine, which can induce an SLE-like illness. The extent to which "idiopathic" SLE is triggered by such specific environmental factors is unknown.

A variety of complement deficiencies have been associated with SLE. The most common is C2 deficiency. It is not clear whether the association is one of genetic linkage or predisposition because of the deficiency itself. The latter might occur if the deficiency led to increased susceptibility to infections that trigger illness.

For many years it has been thought that there might be a "lupus virus," a particular virus that induces disease. Patients with SLE have, in the endothelial cells of their kidneys and in their lymphocytes, structures that resemble viral nucleocapsids but that are not related to or caused by viruses. In addition, retroviruses have been implicated in the immune complex renal disease of animals with SLE-like disorders. Nevertheless, even if such a virus is important, it is only one of many factors critical to the development of disease.

AUTOIMMUNITY AND DISEASE IN SLE. In past years it was believed that an anti-self response was harmful and that such responses did not occur normally. We now appreciate that normal immune responses involve self-self recognition. Moreover, many individuals produce nonpathogenic antibodies reactive with self-antigens. As a result, disease occurs only when anti-self reactions are either excessive or productive of especially injurious immune responses. SLE is characterized by the production of large amounts of antibodies reactive with antigens having a great variety of specificities. Some antibody molecules cross-react with more than one antigen (DNA and cardiolipin or immunoglobulin G [IgG] and nucleoprotein). As a result, the true range of antibody molecules reactive with self-determinants may be less than the number of specificities as measured by the reactive antigens. Nevertheless, the range of determinants against which SLE antibodies may react is impressive (Table 261–3).

How could such self-reactivity come about? It is believed that self-tolerance is a complex state brought about and maintained by several mechanisms. Very early in life, exposure to antigens tends to produce tolerance rather than immunity. Subsequently, several immune mechanisms maintain self-tolerance. Although B lymphocytes and their progeny are responsible for antibody production, under most circumstances they require helper T lymphocytes for activation, proliferation, and differentiation into antibody-secreting cells. Moreover, some T cells (suppressor cells) appear capable of downregulating immune responses. If the T cell population is self-tolerant, it may prevent B cells from proliferating and differentiating into autoantibody-producing cells. A defect in self-tolerance mechanisms could occur at any of several steps in the immune pathway. Stimulation by a foreign antigen that induces idiotype-specific helper T cells may provide a mechanism for bypassing normal regulatory mechanisms. In addition, strong antigenic stimulation can overwhelm normal regulatory mechanisms, rendering them incapable of regulating the immune stimuli. Strong immune stimuli such as graft-versus-host disease (as after allogeneic bone marrow transplantation) or stimulation by any of a variety of powerful polyclonal immune activators (endotoxin) or even viruses that stimulate B cells (Epstein-Barr virus), may drive B cells to produce antibodies and autoantibodies without the usual requirements for or regulation by T cells. Individuals with B cells capable of producing pathogenic autoantibodies that had been previously held in check by T cells may, under such circumstances, be driven to produce large amounts of injurious antibodies. Since it is often the quantity of pathogenic autoantibody that determines whether or not disease occurs, quantitative aspects of immune regulation and immune stimulation may be critical to the balance between disease and relative health with minor immune abnormalities.

TABLE 261–3. AUTOANTIBODIES FOUND IN PATIENTS WITH SLE

Specificity	Comments
Nuclear	Present in most but not all patients
Native DNA	Essentially restricted to SLE
Denatured (single-stranded) DNA	May also cross-react with double-stranded DNA; high titers in SLE; lower titers in other diseases
Histones H1, H3-H4	SLE
Histones H2A-H2B	More common in drug-induced SLE
Sm	In 25–60% of SLE patients, but not found in other diseases
Nuclear ribonucleoprotein	Found in SLE, but highest titers in "mixed connective tissue disease"; multiple small proteins and combined RNA have been discovered
Nucleolar antigens	Scleroderma, SLE, Sjögren's syndrome
SS-B (La, Ha)	Sjögren's syndrome, SLE
SS-A (Ro)	Sjögren's syndrome, SLE
Proliferating cell nuclear antigen	SLE
RANA	Especially in rheumatoid arthritis (Epstein-Barr virus)
DNA-RNA hybrids, double-stranded RNA	SLE
Cytoplasmic	Less information available on these
Ribosomal ribonucleoprotein	SLE
Mitochondria	Primary biliary cirrhosis, SLE
Microsomal antigens	Chronic active hepatitis, malignancies
Lysosomes	SLE
Single-stranded RNA, tRNA	SLE
SS-B and SS-A	Sjögren's syndrome, SLE
Cell membrane determinants	Common in SLE
Red cells	May occur without important hemolysis
White cells	Granulocytes, T cells, B cells
Platelets	Common without thrombocytopenia
Lipomodulin	SLE, RA, others ?
Receptors	Insulin, IL2, others
MHC Class II	Interferes with immune functions
Others	
Mitotic spindle and intracellular supporting proteins	SLE and other rheumatic diseases
Immunoglobulins	JRA, RA, SLE, Sjögren's syndrome, others
Clotting factors	SLE and other diseases
Phospholipids (e.g., cardiolipin)	SLE, others, without other disease
Thyroid antigens	Thyroid diseases, SLE, Sjögren's syndrome

RANA = RA nuclear antigen; RA = rheumatoid arthritis; JRA = juvenile rheumatoid arthritis; IL2 = interleukin 2.

PATHOGENESIS. Systemic lupus is often classified as an immune complex type of disorder. This designation is, at best, an oversimplification. SLE is a disease primarily mediated by antibodies; however, the details of pathogenesis are not proved for many of the clinical and pathologic findings. It is clear that patients with SLE produce autoantibodies and that many of these are injurious. This has been well demonstrated for the renal disease associated with SLE. Antibody reacts with antigen either in the circulation or in the glomerulus, and complement is fixed, leading to release of chemotactic factors, attraction of leukocytes, and release of their injurious mediators of inflammation. The degree of pathology is determined, to a large extent, by the magnitude of the antibody deposition and the intensity of the inflammatory process initiated. Continued deposition of antibody and continued induction of inflammation ultimately lead to irreversible renal damage. Similar processes occur in other organs. However, antibody and complement may be deposited in the skin or in the choroid plexus with or without an attendant inflammatory response. The qualitative character of the antibody molecules (affinity, isotype, charge), the nature of the antigen or their combined properties (size, molecular configuration), or additional factors may be critical to pathogenesis.

Antibody plays a role in SLE not only by depositing in vessels but also by binding to the surfaces of cells. Patients with SLE produce antibodies to erythrocytes, granulocytes, lymphocytes, and macrophages. These antibodies can cause such cells to be removed from the circulation by the reticuloendothelial system or to be killed by complement-mediated cytotoxicity or, more likely, by the mechanisms of antibody-dependent cellular cytotoxicity (ADCC). In this non–complement-mediated killing, leukocytes recognize antibody-coated target cells and kill them. ADCC may be responsible for some of the pathology initiated in the kidneys and other organs by other antibody-mediated mechanisms. In addition, antibody directed against renal antigens, e.g., renal tubular or glomerular basement membrane, may be generated as a result of immunization by fragments released from the inflammatory process. Such antibody induces additional renal pathology and may account for much of the disease in some patients.

It appears that many of the inflammatory lesions that occur in SLE are initiated by antibody and that the injury occurs in small vessels. Thus, any organ so affected could be a site of inflammation, with the possibility of scarring, dysfunction, or both. Many of the central nervous system problems of patients (seizures, psychoses), as well as hematologic (anemia, thrombocytopenia, leukopenia), cardiac (coronary artery disease), dermal (alopecia, sun sensitivity), and other clinical and laboratory abnormalities, have additional pathogenetic mechanisms. The hematologic abnormalities could all be explained by antibodies specifically reactive with the formed elements of the blood; however, many relate to suppression at the level of the bone marrow. The central nervous system disorders are multiple, and each may have its own pathogenetic mechanism. Because central nervous system involvement in SLE is not a single entity, individual patients may require different approaches to understanding and therapy.

PATHOLOGY. The pathologic abnormalities of SLE follow directly from the pathogenetic mechanisms; moreover, the same degree of variability is encountered. In organs affected by small vessel vasculitis, the first lesions are usually characterized by granulocytic infiltration and periarteriolar edema. This is usually followed by round cell infiltration and ultimately a relatively acellular eosinophilic material composed of fibrin, immunoglobulins, and complement (fibrinoid) containing scattered hematoxylin bodies. These basophilic-staining bodies are nuclear debris, often associated with antinuclear antibody, and represent a correlate of the LE cell in vivo. Immunofluorescence analysis demonstrates immunoglobulin and complement in the vessels in the affected areas. Arterioles, venules, and sometimes arteries and veins are involved.

Individual organs often have their peculiar abnormalities. The spleen has "onion skin lesions," concentric fibrosis of the walls and surrounding tissues of the central and penicilliary arteries. These lesions are thought to be diagnostic of SLE in patients with "idiopathic" thrombocytopenia. Nonbacterial verrucous endocarditis (Libman-Sacks) consists of vegetations on the heart valves or chordae tendineae; they can extend along the endocardium and become quite large.

The renal pathology varies from mild to severe glomerular inflammation and variable interstitial involvement. Most patients have relatively normal kidneys or a renal lesion consisting of minimal focal hypercellularity, thickening of the capillary basement membrane, and fibrinoid change. In clinically important glomerulonephritis, these lesions are more generalized and are usually a mixture of proliferative and membranous changes, with increases in endothelial, mesangial, epithelial, and inflammatory cells, capsular inflammation leading to crescent formation, and focal thickening of the basement membrane and mesangial hypercellularity. Some kidneys have membranous glomerulonephritis with considerable thickening of the basement membrane. Basement membrane thickening, when associated with fibrinoid changes, results in the so-called wire loop lesions. There may also be hyaline thrombi in glomeruli, focal necrosis, hematoxylin bodies, and sclerosis in healed lesions. Tubular degenerative changes and mixed inflammatory interstitial inflammation are common. Some patients have primarily mesangial disease; this carries a better prognosis than does capillary loop involvement. Extensive crescent formation and substantial glomerular or interstitial scarring are unfavorable prognostic signs.

CLINICAL MANIFESTATIONS. SLE is a highly variable disease in onset and course. A young woman may present with a butterfly rash, a history of recent sun sensitivity, pleuropericarditis, arthritis, fever, extreme fatigue, seizures, and nephrotic syndrome. This "typical" presentation, which is easily recognized as SLE, occurs in only a minority of patients. More commonly, patients may have only one or two signs or symptoms of SLE, such as arthritis and fatigue. Only later do additional features of SLE occur. As a result, the initial presentation may allow neither a definitive diagnosis nor insight into the organ systems that may become involved in the future. Many patients never develop major organ involvement. Some have kidney but not central nervous system involvement or vice versa. Thus, the clinical manifestations of one patient may be very different from those of another. Some associations between serologic findings and clinical features are valid on a statistical basis but may not hold for a given individual. Thus, patients with large amounts of anti-DNA, especially precipitating antibodies, are more likely to have renal disease. Those with antibodies to Ro (SS-A) and La (SS-B, Ha) are most likely to have sicca syndrome, muscle disease, lung disease, and inconsequential or no renal disease. In the paragraphs that follow, individual clinical features of patients with SLE are described (see also Table 261–4). Patients vary greatly in organ system involvement and also in the severity of disease when a given organ system is affected. Thus, most patients do not have many of the abnormalities described. In addition, SLE is characterized by periods of active disease followed by periods of less intense disease or even remission. In rare cases the patient has a rapidly progressive disease, but the majority can look forward to the time when the disease no longer interferes with their lives.

Constitutional Problems. The majority of patients have fatigue, fever, and weight loss at the time of diagnosis. However, before attributing these to SLE, a diligent search is necessary to rule out infection. Later in the illness, the recurrence of one or more of these findings often indicates an increase in disease activity. Fatigue, difficult as it may be to evaluate, often is the first sign that a flare is imminent.

Musculoskeletal Problems. Arthralgias are the single most common manifestation in SLE. They characteristically are much more transitory than in patients with rheumatoid arthritis (RA), lasting minutes to days in a given joint. With more longstanding or more severe disease, the pain may be constant and frank arthritis is observed. It is often symmetric, the proximal interphalangeal joints of the hands, metacarpophalangeal joints, wrists, and knees being most commonly affected. Morning stiffness is reported by many patients with SLE and joint disease. Although the bony erosions characteristic of RA do not occur, deformities similar to those in RA develop in 10 to 15 per cent of patients and are thought to result from tendon disease. Occasionally, patients experience rupture of the Achilles or quadriceps tendon. Myalgias occur in approximately 30 per cent of patients; only a portion of these have muscle tenderness. Many patients with SLE and muscle disease do not have elevations of creatine kinase activity; some of these patients have an elevated aldolase value.

TABLE 261–4. COMMON CLINICAL ABNORMALITIES IN PATIENTS WITH SLE

Abnormality	Approximate Frequency (%)*
Constitutional	
Fatigue	90
Fever	80
Weight loss, anorexia	60
Musculoskeletal	
Arthritis, arthralgia	90
Myalgia, myositis	30
Skin and mucous membranes	
Butterfly rash	60
Alopecia	50
Photosensitivity	50
Raynaud's phenomenon	30
Mucosal ulcers	30
Discoid lupus	20
Urticaria	10
Edema or bullae	10
Eye (conjunctivitis/episcleritis/sicca syndrome)	20
Gastrointestinal	30
Serosal (pleurisy, pericarditis, peritonitis)	50
Lymphoreticular	
Lymphadenopathy	50
Splenomegaly	30
Hepatomegaly	30
Hypertension	30
Bacterial infections	40
Pneumonitis (all)	30
"lupus"	10
Renal (all)	50
severe	20
Central nervous system	
Personality disorders	50
Seizures	20
Psychoses	20
Stroke or long tract signs	10
Migraine headaches	10
Cardiac	
Myocarditis	30
Murmurs and valvular disease	30
Coronary artery disease	20
Hematologic	
Anemia (all)	70
Hemolytic	10
Purpura (all)	50
Thrombocytopenia	10
Peripheral neuropathy	10

*Frequencies are compiled from a number of series and are rounded off to the nearest 10 per cent. There was some variation from series to series depending upon patient population, non-SLE therapy, and therapy for SLE. Some abnormalities are more common in younger patients than in older patients (e.g., splenomegaly and lymphadenopathy) and vice versa (e.g., muscle disease and sicca syndrome).

Skin and Mucous Membranes. The typical butterfly rash varies from a slight blush to a clear-cut and somewhat edematous, nonpapular erythematous covering of both cheeks and the bridge of the nose. Patients with a butterfly rash often look as though they have applied too much rouge. This lesion may occur in the absence of sun exposure but may be exacerbated by the sun. It often precedes other manifestations of disease. A maculopapular erythematous eruption is also common. Indistinguishable from a drug-produced eruption, it is often induced or exacerbated by sunlight and sometimes by a drug (sulfisoxazole [Gantrisin] and ampicillin are common offenders). The palms and soles are not always spared. Healing usually occurs without scarring. Urticaria and angioedema are more common than subepidermal bullae, which occur in only a few per cent of patients. Discoid lupus in

SLE is indistinguishable from discoid lupus without systemic involvement; however, systemic disease may develop in patients with longstanding discoid lesions. In this rash, central atrophy, hyperpigmentation and hypopigmentation, telangiectasia, and follicular plugging accompany the usual stages of erythema followed by hyperkeratosis and then by atrophy. The hypopigmentation may be extensive and particularly disturbing to blacks.

Livedo reticularis occurs commonly in patients with SLE, but only rarely is it severe. Splinter hemorrhages, tender fingertip pulp lesions, and palmar erythema are sometimes remarkable. Purpura is more often secondary to vasculitis or capillary fragility (corticosteroid therapy is often responsible) than to thrombocytopenia.

Lupus profundus (relapsing nodular nonsuppurative panniculitis) occurs rarely in SLE patients. It may be limited to superficial panniculitis or may extend deeply into the thighs or buttocks. The overlying skin may ulcerate, and the deeper lesions often calcify.

One fifth of patients demonstrate vasculitic lesions of the skin. These can occur on the fingertips, forearms, lips, or lower leg (the last-named may ulcerate). Although they are signs of disease activity, they do not usually imply impending disaster. The related mucosal ulcers are often painless and occur on the hard and soft palate, the nasal septum, other parts of the upper respiratory tract, and even the vagina. They are usually harmless, but occasional patients with involvement of the upper airway may require emergency tracheotomy.

Alopecia is usually diffuse; patients report increased hair on comb or brush or pillow. The hair will regrow in areas not scarred by discoid lesions.

Raynaud's phenomenon may be severe enough to cause digital gangrene and spontaneous amputation of the distal parts of the digits. More often it follows a more benign and variable course. Thrombophlebitis occurs in approximately 10 per cent of patients and may be accompanied by pulmonary emboli.

Eyes. Conjunctivitis or episcleritis or both are usually observed in younger patients at times of disease activity. Cytoid bodies (white exudates next to retinal vessels) are associated with active central nervous system involvement. Spasm of the retinal vessels may lead to transient or permanent blindness. Keratoconjunctivitis sicca occurs in 10 per cent of patients and is usually slowly progressive, but it often improves temporarily with therapy for other symptoms.

Gastrointestinal System. Anorexia, nausea, vomiting, and abdominal pain are observed in a minority of patients. Diffuse abdominal pain with or without rebound tenderness may be a manifestation of serositis or mesenteric arteritis. The latter can be complicated by intestinal infarct, which may lead to perforation and death. Corticosteroid therapy often improves symptoms in both situations; however, if perforation has already occurred, the symptoms may be blunted and therapy inappropriately delayed. Pancreatitis is occasionally due to SLE.

Dysphagia may be associated with reduced peristalsis or ulcerations of the esophagus caused by arteritis, or, more commonly *Candida albicans* infection.

Liver. Liver enlargement is common but usually inconsequential. Fatty infiltration may rarely be associated with hepatic insufficiency. Liver enzyme elevations often occur early in the illness in the absence of therapy. Aspirin treatment may induce such enzyme elevations. Chronic hepatitis is only occasionally observed in patients with SLE.

Heart. Pericarditis is usually symptomatic but without consequence; however, an occasional patient may experience tamponade. The most common electrocardiographic abnormality is nonspecific T wave changes. A prolonged PR interval or evidence of ischemia or infarction may be found. Myocarditis may be manifested by unexplained tachycardia or dyspnea on exertion. More severe involvement is associated with frank heart failure. Coronary artery disease, most often atherosclerotic but occasionally arteritic, can lead to myocardial infarction, even in women in their early twenties.

Lung. Pleuritic chest pain occurs more commonly than does radiographic evidence of effusion; however, massive effusions may occur. Pneumonitis in patients with SLE is often infectious; however, a noninfectious syndrome that varies from fleeting infiltrates (usually hemorrhagic) to marked consolidation and hypoxia occurs in SLE patients. Diffuse interstitial pneumonitis has also been found in SLE.

Hematologic and Lymphoreticular Problems. Lymphadenopathy and splenomegaly with polyclonal immune hyperactivity may be sufficiently marked to suggest a lymphoproliferative disorder. Hematologic abnormalities are almost invariably present in patients with active disease. The most common is a normocytic anemia caused by impaired erythropoiesis. Hemolysis may occur in patients with or without a positive Coombs test result, but significant hemolysis occurs in fewer than 10 per cent of patients. Iron deficiency often contributes to anemia. Many patients with lupus bruise easily; therapy and capillary fragility are more often the cause than is a bleeding disorder. Mild thrombocytopenia occurs in a substantial proportion of patients; however, serious thrombocytopenia occurs in fewer than 10 per cent. Two types of "anticoagulants" occur. In the first, antibodies may react with clotting factors (VIII, IX, XII, and others) and may be responsible for clinically important bleeding. The other is a laboratory finding caused by antibodies reactive with the phospholipids used in the partial thromboplastin time (PTT) test. This abnormality is not associated with prolonged bleeding and is not a cause of concern with regard to surgery or biopsies. However, patients with antibodies reactive with phospholipids often manifest a syndrome characterized by thromboses, repeated abortions, and lung disease. The thromboses may lead to severe central nervous system dysfunction.

Nervous System. Peripheral neuropathies have been observed in about 15 per cent of patients with SLE, sometimes in the absence of other nervous system involvement. In addition to a sensory neuropathy, a mononeuritis multiplex picture (e.g., foot drop) is notable. Central nervous system involvement is quite variable. Psychological problems include personality disorders of every variety and numerous forms of frank psychosis (depression, paranoia, mania, schizophrenia). Differentiating that caused by lupus and that caused by corticosteroids is often a challenge.

Seizures, often grand mal, are common, especially in younger patients. Migraine headaches and cytoid bodies may be indications of disease activity. An organic brain syndrome with impaired mentation can progress to coma. Recovery may be complete, or there may be residual impairment. Movement disorders are more common in younger patients: chorea, athetosis, and hemiballismus are observed. Cerebellar abnormalities may occur independently or with other defects.

Transverse myelitis occurs in patients with SLE. Paralysis may also develop following intracerebral hemorrhage or thrombosis. Sterile meningitis may be observed. Despite the large variety of lupus-related nervous system problems, bacterial and other non-lupus causes must be sought and treated. In addition, the nonsteroidal anti-inflammatory drugs (NSAID's) used in therapy may induce central nervous system signs or symptoms in patients with SLE.

Kidney Disease. The great majority of patients have some degree of renal involvement. In many, the degree of abnormality is mild enough to escape clinical detection. In others, it is clinically detectable but does not progress to functional impairment. Only a minority of patients have renal involvement that is threatening to the function of the organ. Hypertension and lupus renal involvement synergize in bringing about destructive changes. As a result, the presence of untreated hypertension poses a threat in patients with renal abnormalities.

The renal disease of SLE is of several types: rapidly progressive disease (a subacute glomerulonephritis picture), membranous involvement (usually with some mesangial hypertrophy) with nephrotic syndrome, a nephritic picture (mild to severe), and minimal abnormalities. Most patients have mesangial involvement. The progression to capillary loop pathology carries a worse prognosis. The biopsy features can change from one form to another; as a result, the degree of active disease (e.g., necrosis) and scarring (glomerular hyalinization, interstitial) offers a much more useful measure than do precise histologic classifications. The less scarring, the more there is to treat and preserve. Low-grade activity may be associated with slow progression to renal failure. If renal failure occurs, chronic dialysis and renal transplantation are well tolerated. With modern therapy, most patients avoid renal failure. Complete remissions of renal disease occur.

Menses and Pregnancy. Among outpatients with relatively mild SLE, menstruating women tend to be most symptomatic in the period between ovulation and menses. Menses are frequently irregular during active disease. Bleeding may be increased in patients with antibodies to clotting factors or with thrombocytopenia. Repeated spontaneous abortions are common in some women. Others, especially when in remission, carry to term without difficulty. Patients in remission at the time of conception tend to have relatively normal pregnancies. Advanced cardiac, central nervous system, or renal disease is a contraindication to pregnancy. The risk of a disease flare after induced abortion is the same as after delivery. Patients with active renal disease often experience exacerbation during pregnancy and may develop preeclampsia. Patients without renal involvement tend to have calmer pregnancies, but the disease often flares following delivery or abortion. Increased dosage of corticosteroids during the time of delivery and for several weeks thereafter tends to reduce the likelihood of a disease flare. Babies of mothers with antibodies to SS-A may have congenital cardiac problems, including heart block.

LABORATORY FINDINGS. Specific tests for SLE are not available. The presence of large amounts of antibodies to native DNA is the single most useful diagnostic laboratory finding. The LE cell consists of a nucleus that has been phagocytized. The phagocytosis requires antibodies reactive with DNA-histone and complement. In patients with extremely low complement, LE material that has not been phagocytized may be noted. About 80 per cent of patients with SLE are positive for LE cells. A small percentage of patients with related disorders are also positive: rheumatoid arthritis, especially with Felty's syndrome; Sjögren's syndrome; polymyositis-dermatomyositis. The fluorescent antinuclear antibody test (FANA or ANA) has been used as a screening test; however, many patients with related and unrelated diseases may also have positive tests. It is now possible to measure antibodies specifically reactive with various antigens (native DNA, Sm, various low molecular weight RNA species, SS-A, SS-B, and so on). These are much more informative than the FANA despite the improvement in usefulness of the FANA by virtue of analysis of patterns of staining.

Most patients with active SLE have impaired skin tests. Especially important is the common failure to respond to tuberculin in inactive patients as well.

Hematologic. Anemia usually is present in patients with active disease. Although leukopenia occurs in half of the patients, others may manifest leukocytosis. Corticosteroids may increase the white count. Infection in patients with SLE is to be suspected if there is an increase in percentages of granulocytes or immature granulocytes or both, even in the absence of leukocytosis. Thrombocytopenia may precede other features of SLE. Antibodies to coagulation factors may be measured in coagulation abnormalities. Antibodies to phospholipids, which prolong the PTT, do not cause bleeding. A false-positive serologic test for syphilis is also observed in 15 per cent of patients.

Immune. The erythrocyte sedimentation rate (ESR) is usually but not invariably elevated in patients with active disease. Serum albumin levels are usually near normal except in patients with renal disease. Hypergammaglobulinemia may be marked in an untreated patient. Cryoglobulins may be increased. Rheumatoid factor occurs in low titer in patients with SLE. Reduced hemolytic complement levels (CH_{50}) are common in active disease, especially with renal involvement. Some patients have specific congenital complement deficiencies. Immune complexes may be found in the serum or plasma. Antibodies reactive with leukocytes (granulocytes, B cells, T cells) are found in the majority of patients. Platelet-bound immunoglobulin often occurs in the absence of thrombocytopenia, as does a positive Coombs test result in the absence of hemolysis. Antibodies are found that react with DNA, RNA, histones, nuclear ribonucleoprotein, and cytoplasmic antigenic determinants (see Table 261–3). Rarely, antibodies react with heparin (inducing chylomicronemia), insulin receptors (exacerbating difficulties in sugar regulation), and other functional molecules.

Renal. Proteinuria, granular or cellular casts, and cells (red blood cells [RBC], white blood cells [WBC]) are found in the urine of patients with active kidney disease. Elevated serum creatinine levels may be reversible or fixed. Hypertension is common, even in the absence of renal failure. Renal biopsies are best used to determine therapy rather than to confirm the diagnosis.

Cardiac. Abnormal T waves are the most common electrocardiographic abnormality; evidence of coronary artery or hypertensive disease may be noted. Valvular abnormalities and pericardial fluid may be detected with echocardiograms.

Pulmonary. Pleural fluid may be seen on the x-ray film. It is usually an exudate; however, the protein content may not be very high in patients with hypoalbuminemia. The glucose level is usually much higher than that observed in rheumatoid effusions. LE cells may be seen in the fluid. Pleural biopsies can show varying degrees of fibrosis and infiltration. Lung biopsies may show alveolar hemorrhage only, alveolar damage with interstitial edema and hyaline membranes, hypertrophy with or without vasculitis, or acute alveolitis. There is mild to severe hypoxemia. Patients with interstitial fibrosis show decreased vital capacity; others have disproportionately impaired diffusing capacities.

Nervous System. The electroencephalogram most commonly shows diffuse slowing. Seizures often occur in the absence of the typical patterns observed in patients with foci. The cerebrospinal fluid (CSF) may be normal or may have moderately elevated protein levels. The gamma globulin levels usually are not increased. High levels of protein, including high gamma globulins, in the CSF often accompany inflammation of the spinal cord. Granulocytes are indicative of infection; some patients have small numbers of round cells. Aseptic meningitis with numerous lymphocytes in the CSF occurs occasionally. A loss of brain substance may be noted in patients with chronic disease. Isolated loss of cortical or cerebellar neurons occurs.

DIAGNOSIS. SLE should be suspected in any person with a multisystem disease including joint pain. For epidemiologic and study purposes, 4 of the 11 criteria listed in Table 261-1 are required; however, the diagnosis may be made for other purposes with fewer criteria. SLE should be suspected if any of the criteria shown in Table 261-1 are present and unexplained. The disorder should be considered if any of the following are present: unexplained fever, purpura, splenomegaly, adenopathy, pneumonitis, myocarditis, or aseptic meningitis. The presence of a single symptom, such as serositis, along with antibodies to native DNA in a young woman is highly suggestive of SLE.

The condition in children is frequently misdiagnosed as rheumatic fever or juvenile rheumatoid arthritis. The disease in adults is most commonly misdiagnosed as rheumatoid arthritis. Other diagnoses often applied to patients with SLE include Raynaud's disease, hemolytic anemia, idiopathic thrombocytopenia, thrombotic thrombocytopenic purpura, psychosis, vasculitis, progressive systemic sclerosis, lymphoma, autoimmune neutropenia, secondary syphilis, drug reaction, porphyria, multiple sclerosis, myasthenia gravis, polymyositis, glomerulonephritis, Henoch-Schönlein purpura, personality disorder, stroke, and seizure disorder.

In addition to those just listed, other diseases should be considered in patients suspected of having SLE: subacute bacterial endocarditis, bacterial peritonitis, gonococcal septicemia, meningococcal septicemia, tuberculosis, sarcoidosis, serum sickness, leukemia, leprosy, angioimmunoblastic lymphadenopathy, Wegener's granulomatosis, leptospirosis, Lyme arthritis, Rocky Mountain spotted fever, and acquired immunodeficiency syndrome (AIDS).

Overlaps occur between SLE and other diseases such as progressive systemic sclerosis, polymyositis, and Sjögren's syndrome. Some have defined these as "mixed connective tissue disease" or the "overlap syndrome"; others prefer less rigid categorizations.

THERAPY. The management of patients with SLE is often problematic and fraught with difficulties (Table 261-5). The diagnosis of SLE often induces an emotional reaction. In addition, many patients with SLE have psychological problems that may be a result of the disease. Therefore it is necessary to provide effective emotional support. This includes an honest but optimistic assessment. Most patients with SLE can look forward to a normal lifespan, but with the requirement for periodic visits to the physician and treatment with various drugs. Many of the more serious problems do not affect most people. Thus, although the patient must realize the presence of a serious and chronic disease, a dire prognosis usually should not be issued. Early

TABLE 261-5. SOME SUBOPTIMAL PRACTICES FOR PATIENTS WITH SLE

1. All patients*:
   a. Inappropriate view of severity of disease. An excessively pessimistic view that may lead to overtreatment and unnecessary worry on the part of patient and family. On the contrary, an overly optimistic approach may lead to inappropriate reassurance of the patient and inadequate therapy.
   b. Prolonged (>6 weeks) use of high dosages (1 mg/kg/day of prednisone) of daily corticosteroids, which predisposes to toxicities and especially to infections. [If disease becomes controlled, taper dose and move expeditiously to corticosteroid treatment given every other day—aim for 15–20 mg once every 48 hours in the morning. If disease is inadequately controlled, add an antimalarial and/or introduce a cytotoxic drug.]
2. Patients with moderately severe glomerulonephritis:
   a. Treat with daily corticosteroids, and if proteinuria and nephritic sediment persist add azathioprine. [In many individuals this approach may be more likely to lead to renal failure than if the initial therapy were more vigorous.]
   b. Treat a second renal flare with corticosteroids because there was benefit the first time. [The flare usually is more difficult to treat than the initial nephritis.]
   c. Treat either initial disease or a flare with daily corticosteroids, and if the serum creatinine level rises to approximately 2.5 mg/dl give intravenous cyclophosphamide. [It would be desirable to begin cyclophosphamide much earlier. The better the renal function at the initiation of cyclophosphamide therapy, the higher the probability of preventing renal failure.]
   d. Failure to maintain blood pressure control. [Hypertension and nephritis synergize in causing loss of renal function. A blood pressure kept in the middle of the normal range (110–120/70–80 mm Hg) is not as likely to allow progression to renal failure as is one of 140–155/90–100 mm Hg.]
3. Patients with central nervous system involvement:
   a. Failure to distinguish different central nervous system (CNS) syndromes. [Antiphospholipid syndrome with thrombosis may need primarily anticoagulation rather than strong immunosuppression. Guillain-Barré syndrome in a patient with SLE may be due to vasculitis and may require vigorous therapy.]
   b. Failure to utilize diagnostic approaches. [Infection must be ruled out. Magnetic resonance imaging (MRI) and computed tomographic (CT) scan may suggest particular pathologies. A high CSF protein in the absence of infection should suggest vigorous (bolus cyclophosphamide) therapy.]
   c. Use of prolonged high-dose corticosteroid therapy. [This is associated with increased morbidity and mortality because of infections.]
   d. Failure to use intravenous cyclophosphamide early enough. [For many patients with CNS inflammation secondary to SLE, this therapy can be very rapidly effective.]
   e. Inadequate adjunctive therapy. [Repetitive or continuous seizure activity due to SLE may require, on an acute basis, intravenous corticosteroids in addition to anticonvulsant for control. Phenothiazines may be needed in patients with psychiatric manifestations of SLE until immunosuppression is effective.]
   f. Failure to appreciate impending transverse myelitis. [A high CSF protein level and high gamma globulin percentage are suggestive. An MRI study of the spinal cord may be quite helpful.]

*Comments are provided in brackets.

involvement in educational programs and with physical therapists, dieticians, and occupational therapists may be helpful.

Patients with SLE usually need more than normal rest. Ten hours of sleep at night plus an afternoon nap would not be inappropriate. The more active the disease, the more rest needed. Ultraviolet light should be avoided: outdoor swimming should be limited to periods of reduced exposure (not at noon to 1:00 PM ± 4 hours), and sunscreen should be used even for trips to the store. Drugs that augment the effects of UV light, such as tetracyclines and psoralens, should be avoided. The same is true of foods containing large amounts of psoralens (celery, parsnips, figs, and parsley). Exercise should be appropriate to the clinical situation, but exhaustion should be avoided. Stresses, including surgery, infections, childbirth, abortions, and psychological pressures, may exacerbate the process and dictate additional treatment.

Although certain drugs can induce a lupus-like syndrome,

there is little evidence that those drugs are detrimental to patients with SLE. Therefore, such drugs as alpha-methyldopa and phenytoin (Dilantin) may be used without undue concern. However, sulfonamides are often poorly tolerated; patients with active disease often experience a rash. Estrogens may worsen disease. Since hypertension is synergistic with immune complex disease in bringing about pathology, the blood pressure should be kept in the middle of the normal range for age and sex.

Corticosteroids are frequently given. Short-acting drugs such as prednisone or methylprednisolone are preferred so that therapy every other day can be attempted (see Ch. 27) and the hypothalamic-pituitary-adrenal axis not disrupted. The side effects of steroids given every other day are much less than those of daily therapy. Low doses are less than 30 mg per 1.7 square meters per day of prednisone, and every attempt should be made to maintain patients on less than 25 mg per 1.7 square meters every other day. Moderate doses are 30 to 50 mg per 1.7 square meters per day. Higher doses may be necessary for brief periods. Patients with marked multisystem involvement may temporarily require corticosteroids in divided doses. Azathioprine has long been used to treat patients with SLE; its usefulness may be limited to a subset of patients with moderate kidney disease or those with intractable skin disease or arthritis. Vigorous therapy includes boluses of very large doses of corticosteroids (1 gram or more of methylprednisolone) or of cyclophosphamide (0.85 to 2.0 grams per 1.7 square meters) and plasmapheresis.

A major problem in SLE is long-term management. The clinical picture (history plus physical examination) is usually a very good guide to therapy of nonrenal and nonhematologic problems. In the latter two situations, the laboratory measures are helpful. Anemia, fatigue, and hypergammaglobulinemia tend to weigh in favor of more therapy. The long-term toxicities of corticosteroids (cataracts, aseptic necrosis of bone, infections) must always be balanced against the benefits of continued vigorous therapy. The toxicities of immunosuppressive drugs are less than those of prolonged high-dose corticosteroid therapy. Therefore, it is often prudent to initiate immunosuppressive therapy early for serious disease to minimize the toxicities of corticosteroids. In tapering corticosteroids, it is generally advisable to drop rapidly to 30 mg per 1.7 square meters per day and then to reduce dosage more slowly. The lower the dose, the slower the tapering process should be. Rapid tapering can cause a disease flare, which requires re-institution of high doses.

The variable severity and extent of involvement in SLE dictate individualized treatment. It is helpful to divide problems into those of major organs, which therefore are life threatening, and those that are unpleasant but not life threatening (Table 261–6). The major exception to this division is a syndrome of acute toxic

TABLE 261–6. MAJOR VERSUS NON–MAJOR ORGAN INVOLVEMENT IN SLE

Non–Major Organ SLE*	Major Organ SLE†
Alopecia	Glomerulonephritis
Fever	Central nervous system disease
Fatigue	Myocarditis
Anorexia	Pneumonitis
Arthritis	Thrombocytopenic purpura
Myalgia	Hemolytic anemia (marked)
Pleurisy	Severe granulocytopenia (rare)
Pericarditis	Mesenteric vasculitis
Peritonitis	
Rash	
Skin vasculitis	
Raynaud's phenomenon	
Mucosal ulcers	
Splenomegaly	
Lymphadenopathy	
Peripheral neuropathy	
Episcleritis	
Hepatitis	

*Usually does not require high-dose corticosteroids or other vigorous treatment. In all cases, a careful search for infection is carried out.

†Usually requires high-dose corticosteroids or other vigorous treatment. Individual patients vary greatly and some do not require vigorous therapy. Since prolonged high-dose corticosteroid therapy is very toxic, consideration should be given to immunosuppressive drug therapy.

lupus observed primarily in precorticosteroid times: A young woman with high fever, serositis, rash, and arthritis might succumb to SLE in the absence of major organ involvement. This syndrome is usually responsive to therapy with corticosteroids in modest doses.

Non–major organ involvements are best handled with symptomatic therapy: the less medicine the better. Hydroxychloroquine (200 to 600 mg per day) is effective for skin involvement; it also may help treat arthritis and other manifestations. Nonsteroidal anti-inflammatory drugs, such as aspirin and ibuprofen, are useful for arthritis, serositis, and fever. Some patients tolerate one NSAID better than another—bizarre neurologic reactions may occur in SLE patients receiving ibuprofen or other NSAID's; liver enzyme abnormalities may follow aspirin treatment; gastrointestinal tolerance varies. The combination of hydroxychloroquine and NSAID may be sufficient. The addition of low doses of corticosteroids may be necessary. Initial therapy given every other day may not be possible; however, a subsequent switch to alternate-day treatment reduces steroid-induced side effects. In patients with continued disease activity, symptoms may be prominent every other day, necessitating return to daily steroids. Even in the face of corticosteroid therapy, a NSAID and hydroxychloroquine may add substantial benefit and allow a lower steroid dosage. Fevers occurring in spite of daily corticosteroids may respond to NSAID's. Indomethacin may be especially effective in pericarditis.

The management of major organ involvement is usually directed at preservation of function and prevention of organ failure and disability or death. Myocarditis usually responds to the symptomatic treatment of SLE, but occasional patients may require specific treatment; moderate doses of corticosteroids are usually adequate. Thrombocytopenia and hemolytic anemia are treated more or less as they are in the absence of SLE. Both danazol and intravenous gamma globulin have been given for thrombocytopenia in SLE patients. Administration of plasma or plasma exchange may be helpful in patients with features of thrombotic thrombocytopenia (one should look for fragmented RBC's on the peripheral smear). Patients with Factor VIII deficiency caused by specific antibodies are treated with plasmapheresis and immunosuppression. Mild pneumonitis usually responds to moderate doses of corticosteroids; severe disease requires heroic measures. Central nervous system inflammation may require moderate to high corticosteroid dosages; however, since prolonged therapy with high doses of corticosteroids is inappropriate, a switch to cytotoxic therapy should be considered within 2 weeks. In patients with severe involvement, intravenous cyclophosphamide* (0.85 to 2.0 grams per 1.7 square meters) can be life saving. Seizures require treatment with both corticosteroids and anticonvulsants (Table 261–5). The antiphospholipid antibody syndrome is treated with long-term anticoagulation. Warfarin therapy may be effective with minimal toxicity by keeping the prothrombin time at about 15 seconds.

The most studied and controversial area is the treatment of SLE kidney disease. If there is active disease on biopsy and no scarring, high-dose corticosteroids or corticosteroids plus an oral immunosuppressive drug (e.g., azathioprine*) may be sufficient. If there is active disease and any scarring, vigorous therapy must be considered. The currently available data suggest that renal function can be preserved for long periods with cyclophosphamide therapy. Intermittent boluses are safer than daily oral therapy. Despite substantial loss of renal function, a patient with quiescent disease and moderate scarring usually does not benefit from aggressive and potentially toxic therapy (see Table 261–5).

Alarcon-Segovia D: Anti-phospholipid antibodies and the antiphospholipid syndrome in systemic lupus erythematosus. Medicine 68:353, 1989.

Balow JE: Lupus nephritis. Ann Intern Med 106:79, 1987. *A symposium devoted to pathogenesis and therapy.*

Boey ML (ed.): Proceedings of the Second International Conference on Systemic Lupus Erythematosus, November 26–30, 1989. Singapore, Professional Postgraduate Services International, 1989. *Up-to-date coverage of pathogenesis and patient management.*

DuBois EL: Lupus Erythematosus. Los Angeles, University of Southern California

*This use is not listed in the manufacturer's directive.

Press, 1978. *A lengthy monograph citing many case reports. Extensively referenced.*

Harris EN, Asherson RA, Hughes GRV: Antiphospholipid antibodies—autoantibodies with a difference. Annu Rev Med 39:261, 1988.

Ropes MW: Systemic Lupus Erythematosus. Cambridge, Mass., Harvard University Press, 1976. *Observations of a physician with over 40 years' experience with SLE patients.*

Sibbitt WL Jr: Magnetic resonance and computed tomographic imaging in the evaluation of acute neuropsychiatric disease in systemic lupus erythematosus. Ann Rheum Dis 48:1014, 1989.

Smith HR, Steinberg AD: Autoimmunity—a perspective. Annu Rev Immunol 1:175, 1983. *Discussion of theoretical aspects of autoimmune diseases as well as their classification and pathogeneses.*

Steinberg AD: Therapy of lupus nephritis. Kidney Int 30:769, 1986. *A completely referenced discussion and thorough analysis of difficult problems.*

262 Systemic Sclerosis (Scleroderma)

E. Carwile LeRoy

Scleroderma (hard skin) is an uncommon disease marked by fibrotic increases in the connective tissue of skin and often of visceral organs as well. It varies widely in extent and severity from isolated hardened skin patches of largely cosmetic importance to a life-threatening, generalized condition that can restrict movement "by an ever-tightening case of steel" (Osler) and lead to insufficiency of the peripheral circulation, the lungs, the gut, the heart, and/or the kidneys. Fortunately, most persons with scleroderma are not at risk for the most severe of its consequences. Since the cause is unknown and no cure is available, the physician must distinguish as early as possible the attendant risks for each patient and manage these prospectively.

Distinctions between localized (skin only) and generalized scleroderma and the conditions that mimic each are shown in Table 262–1. Subsets of generalized scleroderma (systemic sclerosis, SSc) are outlined in Table 262–2. It is on occasion difficult to classify the individual patient in this multisystem, multistage disorder in which each target organ independently progresses through stages of inflammation, induration (fibrosis), and atrophy.

DEFINITION. Systemic sclerosis (SSc) is a generalized disorder of small arteries, microvessels, and the diffuse connective tissue characterized by scarring (fibrosis) and vascular obliteration in the skin, gastrointestinal tract, lungs, heart, and kidneys; hidebound skin is the clinical hallmark and organ compromise the prognostic keystone.

PATHOGENESIS AND PATHOLOGY. The mechanism or mechanisms of fibrosis in SSc is not understood. Mesenchymal cells (fibroblasts, smooth muscle cells, and endothelial cells) become activated by unknown stimuli, resulting in the deposition of increased amounts of the usual components of connective tissue (types I and III collagen, proteoglycan, fibronectin) in the interstitium and in the intima of small arteries. Endothelial cell changes, vasomotor and permeability changes, platelet activation, and perivascular mononuclear cell infiltrates are present in target tissues before fibrosis is prominent.

In SSc scar tissue, lesional fibroblasts produce increased quantities of these connective tissue components on a per cell basis even after removal from the patient and propagation in vitro. These same cells show a growth regulatory abnormality characterized by insensitive responses to growth factors and a persistent state of competence (the state of a cell prepared to divide but not yet triggered to proceed), something of a persistently activated state. Interactions, both autocrine (a factor acting on the cell that produced it) and paracrine (a factor acting on an adjacent cell), between two cytokines, transforming growth factor–beta and platelet-derived growth factor, may begin to explain the state of fibroblast activation in SSc. Gene expression in these cells is unusual and as yet incompletely characterized. Understanding the regulatory defect of fibroblast growth may be a key to understanding the unregulated fibrosis in SSc, and perhaps also

TABLE 262–1. DIFFERENTIAL DIAGNOSIS OF SYSTEMIC SCLEROSIS

Vascular Changes
Peripheral vasospasm
  Idiopathic Raynaud's phenomenon (Raynaud's disease)
  Occupational Raynaud's phenomenon
    Vibration and physical trauma (e.g., jackhammer operator)
  Chemical exposure
    Vinyl chloride (plastics industry)
    Mining exposure (coal, silicates, gold, heavy metals)
    Organic solvents (trichloroethylene, others)
  Environmental and drug-associated Raynaud's phenomenon
    Toxic oil syndrome
    Arsenic
    Bleomycin
    Cisplatin
    Ergotamine
    Beta blockers (high dose)
    5-Hydroxytryptophan and carbidopa
  Reflex sympathetic dystrophy (shoulder-hand, thoracic outlet)
  Other diffuse connective tissue diseases (systemic lupus erythematosus, polyarteritis nodosa, dermatomyositis/polymyositis)
  Intravascular causes (cryoglobulinemia, cold agglutinins, nondistensible RBC's, intravascular coagulation)
Telangiectasia
  Hereditary telangiectasia (Osler-Weber-Rendu syndrome)
  Hepatic and hormonal spiders (cirrhosis, contraceptives)

Skin Changes
Localized scleroderma
  Morphea (circumscribed, guttate)
  Generalized morphea
  Linear (with hemiatrophy)
  Other localized hamartomas (collagenoma, tuberous sclerosis, keloids, hypertrophic scars)
  En coup de sabre (with or without facial hemiatrophy)
  Tryptophan-eosinophilia-myalgia-fasciitis syndrome
Scleroderma-like skin changes
  Inflammatory-immunologic
    Undifferentiated connective tissue syndromes (mixed)
    Eosinophilic fasciitis
    Overlap syndromes (SSc with SLE, RA, DM/PM, Sjögren's syndrome [sicca complex and its overlaps])
    Chronic graft-vs.-host disease (CGVHD)
  Occupational, environmental, and drug-associated (see Vascular Changes above)
  Metabolic-genetic (pseudosclerodermas)
    Porphyrias
    Phenylketonuria
    Carcinoid syndrome
    Scleredema with or without paraproteinemia
    Scleromyxedema with or without paraproteinemia
    Lichen sclerosus et atrophicus
    Insulin-dependent diabetes mellitus (digital sclerosis)
    Acromegaly
    Amyloidosis
    Heritable premature aging syndromes (Werner's syndrome, progeria, Rothmund's syndrome)

Visceral Disease
Esophageal hypomotility (diabetes mellitus, aging)
Idiopathic pulmonary fibrosis
Sarcoidosis
Amyloidosis
Infiltrative cardiomyopathies
Intestinal hypomotility syndromes
Malignant hypertension (hyperreninemic, accelerated)
Occupational, environmental, and drug-associated interstitial pulmonary disease (see Vascular Changes above)

RBC's = red blood cells; SLE = systemic lupus erythematosus; RA = rheumatoid arthritis; DM = dermatomyositis; PM = polymyositis.

in liver cirrhosis, atherosclerosis, and other examples of unregulated fibrosis.

Prominent vascular and microvascular lesions dominate the early stages of both limited cutaneous and diffuse forms of SSc (Table 262–2). The unusual cyclic vasoconstrictive-vasodilatory features of Raynaud's phenomenon are present in more than 90 per cent of all SSc patients (Table 262–3). Edema is prominent,

TABLE 262–2. SUBSETS OF SYSTEMIC SCLEROSIS (SSc)

Diffuse Cutaneous SSc (dSSc)
Onset of Raynaud's phenomenon within 1 year of onset of skin changes (puffy or hidebound)
Truncal and acral skin involvement
Presence of tendon friction rubs
Early and significant incidence of interstitial lung disease, oliguric renal failure, diffuse gastrointestinal disease, and myocardial involvement
Absence of anticentromere antibodies (ACA)
Presence of anti-topoisomerase I antibodies (variable)
Nailfold capillary dilatation and dropout

Limited Cutaneous SSc (lSSc)*
Isolated Raynaud's phenomenon for years (occasionally decades)
Skin involvement limited to hands, face, feet (acral)
A significant late incidence of pulmonary hypertension, trigeminal neuralgia, skin calcifications, telangiectasia
A high incidence of anticentromere antibodies (ACA, 70–80%)
Dilated nailfold capillary loops without capillary dropout

Systemic Sclerosis *sine* Scleroderma (ssSSc)
Visceral disease without cutaneous involvement
Examples: (1) esophageal hypomotility, duodenal dilatation with malabsorption, wide-mouthed colonic sacculations; (2) Raynaud's phenomenon, dilated nailfold capillary loops, esophageal hypomotility, oliguric renal failure; (3) Raynaud's phenomenon, dilated nailfold capillary loops, esophageal hypomotility, pulmonary hypertension, and/or interstitial lung disease

*Also termed CREST syndrome, i.e., calcinosis, Raynaud's phenomenon, esophageal hypomotility, sclerodactyly, and telangiectasia.

often occurring episodically, especially in the diffusely involved patient. Circulating evidence of endothelial cell perturbation (elevated plasma levels of Factor VIII–von Willebrand factor) and of platelet activation (elevated serum levels of factors released from platelet alpha-granules) is present in many, but not all, patients. Histologically, vascular lesions are widespread. The small artery lesion in SSc, similar to the lesions seen in chronic homograft rejection, in hemolytic-uremic syndrome, and in thrombotic thrombocytopenic purpura, has three major characteristics: (1) intimal proliferation with smooth muscle cell migration occurring centripetally and the deposition of a mixed mucoid and fibrous connective tissue matrix, (2) medial thinning, and (3) an adventitial cuff of primarily type I collagen, a virtually unique characteristic of the SSc lesion. Cellular proliferation and matrix deposition are prominent in the small arteries of all target organs; when renal involvement, hyperreninemia, and hypertension characterize the clinical course, fibrinoid necrosis is also present. In the nutrient microvascular beds, capillaries are sparse (up to 70 per cent absent), their endothelium is swollen and disrupted, and endothelial basement membranes may be frayed and separated from their cell attachment. Although the endothelial cells bear the brunt of the injury pattern, the basis of this all-out attack on vascular structures in SSc is not known.

Selected immune events point also to the vascular structures. Three of the five defined antigens to which SSc patients show enhanced immune responsiveness are type I collagen, type IV collagen, and laminin (the other two being topoisomerase I and centromere protein), all three components of blood vessels and the second and third being specific for basal lamina, of which the endothelial basement membrane is a prototype. It is possible that a heightened immune response to basement membrane antigens perpetuates the disease in certain immunogenetically selected persons. As in the other rheumatic or diffuse connective tissue disorders that show manifestations of autoimmunity, anti-

TABLE 262–3. RAYNAUD'S PHENOMENON IN MUSCULOSKELETAL DISEASE*

Systemic sclerosis	>90%
Overlap, mixed, undifferentiated	80%
Systemic lupus erythematosus	30%
Dermatomyositis, polymyositis	20%
Rheumatoid arthritis	10%

*From Black CM: Scleroderma, dermatomyositis, and polymyositis. In Dieppe PA, et al.: Atlas of Clinical Rheumatology. Philadelphia, Lea and Febiger, 1986; with permission.

nuclear antibodies are prominent in SSc. With the recent introduction of rapidly proliferating human cell substrates (particularly the human laryngeal carcinoma cell line, HEp-2), greater than 90 per cent of SSc patients have circulating antinuclear antibodies in significant titer. The most sensitive and specific of these is the anticentromere antibody (ACA) pattern, a B cell immune response to a major organizing structure of the chromosome called the centromere. ACA patterns are clinically useful in detecting the limited cutaneous type of SSc. Antibodies to a soluble nuclear isomerase, topoisomerase I, are currently emerging as the newest autoimmune serologic "find" in SSc; both clinical and biologic relevance remains to be determined. Recent studies have demonstrated T cell activation in SSC. The data have been interpreted both as increased T helper function and as decreased T suppressor function. One must remember that circulating differences (increases) may indicate reciprocal changes (decreases) in vascular and interstitial lesions. Thus, a T cell component in SSc seems likely; its cause, possibly viral or chemical, remains unclear.

THE PATIENT. *Diffuse SSc.* The usual age of onset is the fourth decade but may range from the first to the eighth. There is no racial or geographic predilection. There are almost as many men as there are women, in contrast to the female preponderance in limited SSc. The onset may be abrupt and may present as swollen hands, face, and feet associated with Raynaud's phenomenon (episodic pallor of the digits, nose, or ears following cold exposure or stress associated with cyanosis and followed by erythema, suffusion, tingling, and pain). Fatigue is common; overt weakness may be present. The skin reveals a nonpitting fullness, an inability to pinch skin folds, and the loss of skin lines and creases in involved areas. These changes may evolve over 12 to 18 months to include the fingers, hands, forearms, arms, face, thorax, and abdomen, as well as the toes, feet, legs, and thighs. The fingers and toes may be dusky or overtly cyanotic and are usually cool to the touch. Blood pressure and pulse may be elevated, and evaluation of swallowing, breathing, urinary excretory, and cardiac functions may reveal abnormalities. Patients with diffuse SSc should be followed closely for visceral involvement (see Table 262–2 and Fig. 262–1). The cumulative survival rate is reduced in diffuse SSc compared with limited SSc (Fig. 262–2).

Limited Cutaneous SSc. The typical patient with limited cutaneous SSc is a female (or a male who has worked with vibrating machines or plastics or in mining), aged 30 to 50, who presents with a 10- to 15-year history of numbness and a "dead" or "wooden" sensation associated with color changes (often pallor only) of, at first, the second and third fingers of the dominant hand. Full-fledged Raynaud's phenomenon usually develops symmetrically in both hands, fingers 2 through 5, with increasing

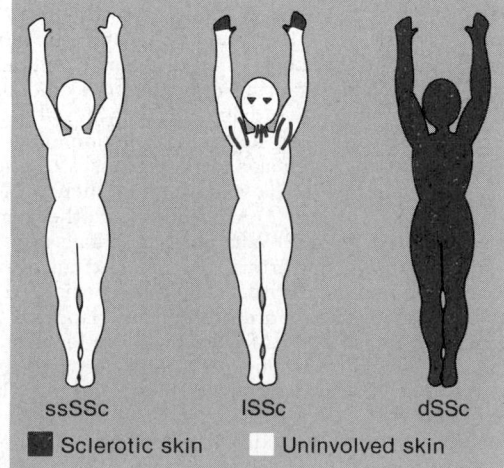

FIGURE 262–1. A pictorial representation of skin involvement in systemic sclerosis. Note that the limited cutaneous SSc patient (Table 262–2) may have subtle thickening of eyelid, neck fold, and armpit skin. Abbreviations: ssSSc = systemic sclerosis *sine* scleroderma; lSSc = limited cutaneous systemic sclerosis; dSSc = diffuse cutaneous systemic sclerosis. (Adapted from Giordano M, et al.: J Rheumatol 13:911, 1986.)

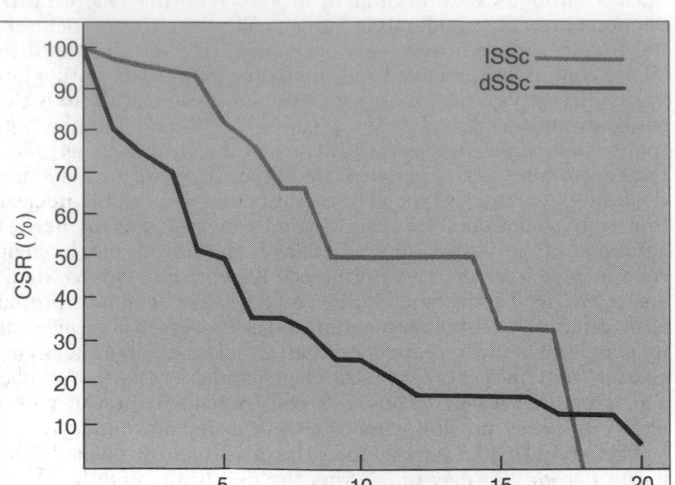

FIGURE 262–2. The cumulative survival rate (CSR, age-adjusted survival) in per cent plotted against time in years for diffuse cutaneous SSc and limited cutaneous SSc (CREST [calcinosis, Raynaud's phenomenon, esophageal dysmotility, sclerodactyly, and telangiectasia] syndrome) patients, showing the substantially reduced survival of diffuse cutaneous SSc patients (Table 262–2). An intermediate group with both intermediate survival and extent of skin involvement has been identified by Giordano et al. Some investigators feel that the intermediate group is not a clearly definable subset as yet. For abbreviations, see Figure 262–1. (Adapted from Giordano M, et al.: J Rheumatol 13:911, 1986.)

frequency, especially in winter; there may be a history of hard, crusting lesions on the fingertips, initially healing in warm weather. General stamina may be decreased, and there may be breathlessness with minimal exertion (see Table 262–2).

DIAGNOSIS. The annual incidence of Raynaud's phenomenon is substantially greater than the incidence of all diffuse connective tissue syndromes combined (Table 262–4). To select those patients with Raynaud's phenomenon who are destined to develop scleroderma and related disorders when a careful history and physical examination reveal no features of connective tissue disease, including no signs of peripheral ischemia, the single best test is wide-field nailfold capillaroscopy—a noninvasive, reproducible, cost-effective, permanent identification of the connective tissue disease–prone patient. Coupled with autoimmune serology and possibly a test of vascular injury or platelet activation/release (such as plasma Factor VIII–von Willebrand factor levels), capillary examination is an important procedure in the early detection of connective tissue disease.

The diagnosis of diffuse SSc is straightforward. A previously well person is now sick with the triad of Raynaud's phenomenon, nonpitting edema, and hidebound skin that may eventually cover virtually the entire body, sparing only the back and buttocks. There are very few alternative diagnoses that must be seriously entertained. Other causes of Raynaud's phenomenon are not usually accompanied by edema, and other causes of edema are not usually associated with Raynaud's phenomenon. The key questions in such patients are (1) Are features of other connective tissue diseases present? and (2) What internal organs are affected?

If symmetric, erosive polyarthritis is present, an overlap between SSc and rheumatoid arthritis should be considered; if fever and a characteristic malar rash are present, overlap with systemic lupus erythematosus is likely. Most often these features are not present, and the second question represents the primary focus. Each visceral target organ (esophagus, lungs, kidneys, heart) of SSc deserves screening.

Abnormal skin texture provides the definitive diagnostic criterion of SSc in over 90 per cent of patients. When distal to the metacarpophalangeal (MCP) joints only, it is called sclerodactyly and is *not* diagnostic of SSc. Firm, taut, hidebound skin proximal to the MCP joints represents the major diagnostic criterion. Skin biopsy is usually *not* more sensitive diagnostically than the experienced touch. Skin changes also distinguish the two prognostically different subsets. If truncal skin changes are present,

TABLE 262–4. POPULATION INCIDENCE OF MUSCULOSKELETAL DISEASE*

Raynaud's phenomenon	1000†
Rheumatoid arthritis	750
Systemic lupus erythematosus	75
Dermatomyositis, polymyositis	10
Systemic sclerosis	10

*From Kammer G: Raynaud's phenomenon. *In* Andreoli TE, et al.: Cecil Essentials of Medicine. Philadelphia, W. B. Saunders Company, 1986; with permission.
†New cases per million adults per year.

the patient has diffuse cutaneous SSc, and close surveillance of visceral function is indicated. If skin changes are limited to the hands, fingers, and face, limited cutaneous SSc is present, yearly evaluation is adequate, and management should focus on the Raynaud's phenomenon. If the skin is of normal texture, two possibilities are suggested: The patient formerly had abnormal skin changes—either diffuse or limited cutaneous—which have subsided; or the patient has visceral disease in the absence of skin changes, which occurs in at least 5 per cent of SSc patients (Table 262–2, SSc *sine* scleroderma).

DIFFERENTIAL DIAGNOSIS. Connective tissue disorders are constellations of organ system involvements (skin, lungs, intestinal tract, serosal surfaces, joints, skeletal muscle, heart, central nervous system); each system involved can show immune-inflammatory, proliferative, or fibrotic-atrophic changes at different stages of the disorder. Virtually none of the systems involved or the stages of involvement of those systems are entirely specific for the particular syndrome or disorder. It is not surprising, therefore, that the nomenclature is confusing. Terms such as mixed connective tissue disease (MCTD), undifferentiated connective tissue syndromes (UCTS), and overlap syndromes have emerged to describe the same patients.

MCTD was introduced to describe anew the already well-known overlap patient with features of myositis, lupus, and scleroderma. The early features of such patients were largely inflammatory and therefore briefly responsive to glucocorticoid therapy; proliferative and fibrotic features were not responsive to treatment. Neither the clinical syndromes, the laboratory tests proposed (extractable nuclear antigen [ENA], antibodies to ribonucleoprotein [RNP]), nor the response to therapy was specific. Therefore, the introduction of MCTD provided no new understanding beyond the time-honored overlap syndrome, which remains the preferred term for established, stable connective tissue disorders with features of more than one traditional disorder (such as rheumatoid arthritis–lupus overlap). In the early patient with inflammatory or edematous features that are insufficient for an established diagnosis, the term undifferentiated connective tissue syndrome (UCTS) is preferred. Some use UCTD here as a hybrid acronym.

Eosinophilic fasciitis is a syndrome that, when acute, is distinct from scleroderma and that blends into the scleroderma spectrum of disorders in its chronic form. Young, vigorous persons note, often after strenuous exertion, the onset of swelling and tautness of the skin of the trunk and proximal extremities with a brawny texture that may be tender. Raynaud's phenomenon is usually absent, and the hands and feet are usually spared. Initially, visceral disease is absent. Deep skin and subcutaneous biopsies show inflammatory changes including the deep fascia, the subcutis, and the dermis. Eosinophilia is present and eosinophils may or may not be present in the skin lesions. Symptoms subside with glucocorticoid therapy and also with no therapy over time. Eosinophilic fasciitis has been associated with aplastic anemia. In a substantial proportion of chronic patients, the visceral involvement of systemic sclerosis has been documented. Several outbreaks of fasciitis-like syndromes, with the added feature of peripheral neuropathy, have recently been documented: the toxic oil syndrome of Spain in 1981–1982 and the L-tryptophan–eosinophilia–myalgia–fasciitis syndrome in the United States in 1989–1990. These events increase the interest in and need for surveillance of environmental triggers in SSc.

CLINICAL MANIFESTATIONS. Peripheral Vascular System. Pallor is the most definitive of the triphasic responses of Raynaud's phenomenon. In the presence of constant or episodic cyanosis alone, the diagnosis should be suspect. The circumstances that provoke pallor and the "dead" sensation of the fingers are usually reproducible in the individual patient (handling cold or frozen items, emotional disturbances). Persistent Raynaud's attacks may lead to a webbing phenomenon (like the frenulum of the tongue) binding the fingernail to the fingertip skin of involved fingers. This is evidence of structural vascular and persistent ischemic disease, as are the more obvious fingertip calluses, digital ulcerations (of fingertips or over dorsal proximal interphalangeal joints), overt ischemic tissue, or calcification; the toes, the nose, and the ears may be affected in Raynaud's attacks as well. The more widespread the areas involved, the more likely is systemic disease.

The Skin. The skin is the most distinctive diagnostic feature of SSc; the diagnosis can be made unequivocally by the texture and location of hidebound skin. In patients with diffuse SSc, skin tautness can limit movement at the wrists, elbows, shoulders, mouth, and thorax (less frequently the hips, knees, and ankles). When fully hidebound, the skin appears to become paper thin over points of bony protrusion, such as the proximal interphalangeal joints, the ulnar styloid process, the olecranon process, the bridge of the nose, and the cheekbones. Gentle pressure over these areas removes all blood from the capillaries; the refilling time can be used as a rough approximation of the degree of ischemia and the propensity to ulcerate.

Gastrointestinal System. If sensitive diagnostic techniques are used, esophageal hypomotility, by far the most common manifestation of gastrointestinal SSc, can be documented in over 90 per cent of patients with both diffuse and limited cutaneous SSc. Many patients do not notice the subtle symptoms of esophageal SSc, which include a vertical substernal burning pain particularly at night, the occasional sense that a pill or large bit of meat "has not gone all the way down," or "heartburn" on lying down soon after a full meal. The single best screening test for esophageal hypomotility is the radionuclide esophageal transit time; it is noninvasive, is safe, and can be relied upon when negative. Because severe esophageal complications, including stricture, can be prevented by early management and because intestinal involvement with SSc does not occur without esophageal involvement, the esophagus of all patients suspected of SSc should be examined for hypomotility. Patients with slow transit times should be further studied both with barium swallow (using light barium and the recumbent position) to detect structural abnormalities (hiatus hernia) and with esophageal motility studies, the definitive procedure for esophageal SSc. The earliest detectable abnormality is a reduction in resting lower esophageal sphincter (LES) pressure, which may be an isolated early finding or may be associated with reduced smooth muscle contraction (secondary and tertiary waves) of the distal two thirds of the esophagus. Upper third, striated muscle dysfunction suggests an overlap syndrome with dermatomyositis. If peptic esophagitis with mucosal ulceration is well established, LES pressure may be increased and the diagnosis of achalasia could be incorrectly entertained. The presence of other features of SSc and reduced LES pressure after treatment are helpful in diagnosis.

Gastric hypomotility may be present but is not often of clinical significance. Small intestinal hypomotility, determined by an upper gastrointestinal (GI) series with small bowel follow-through, occurs in 10 to 20 per cent of patients, all of whom have esophageal hypomotility; this diffuse hypomotility may occur in the absence of cutaneous scleroderma. It need not be searched for in the asymptomatic patient because it consistently declares its presence by postprandial bloating, abdominal distention with diffuse pain, intermittent diarrhea with or without steatorrhea, and weight loss from malabsorption. Abdominal attacks with adynamic ileus may mimic mechanical obstruction and lead to surgical intervention, from which some patients recover poorly and slowly, if at all.

Pulmonary System. Although renal failure was formerly the major threat to life in SSc, the combined impact of several pulmonary abnormalities now seems to be the number one cause of fatal involvement in this disease. Pleurisy and pleural effusions, pulmonary hypertension, interstitial lung disease with fibrosis, and ultimately restrictive pulmonary disease all may be a part of pulmonary SSc. Because the patient is often sedentary from skin or joint restrictions, shortness of breath or dyspnea on exertion is a surprisingly late complaint. Standard chest roentgenography is not a sensitive screening procedure. More than half of SSc

patients selected for the absence of pulmonary symptoms and for a normal chest radiograph show reproducible abnormalities on pulmonary function tests. Patients who smoke show a much higher positive proportion. The single-breath diffusion capacity, which measures the balance between ventilation and perfusion, is a sensitive pulmonary screening tool. Mild reductions in vital capacity are common as well. In smokers, there may be evidence of small airway obstruction. The presence of alveolitis, detected by alveolar thickening on thin-section computed tomography (CT) and/or by the presence of inflammatory cells on bronchoalveolar lavage, is predictive of future pulmonary fibrosis and functional insufficiency. Whether therapeutic intervention at the prefibrotic alveolitis stage can prevent pulmonary functional deterioration is currently under study.

Pleural effusions are usually silent and bland. They take on clinical significance primarily in the patient with established restrictive lung disease (decreased vital capacity) in whom the aspiration of an effusion may improve ventilation. They are present in two thirds of patients at postmortem examination. In the immunosuppressed patient, infection may present with "silent" empyema.

Pulmonary hypertension may be sudden in onset and constitutes a medical emergency. All patients with SSc should be followed closely for changes in the second heart sound over the pulmonic area and for the pulmonic valve closure component of that second sound, detected by the splitting of S2 on deep inspiration. The appearance of tricuspid regurgitation or right ventricular enlargement is evidence of established pulmonary hypertension. The chest radiograph may provide evidence of enlarged pulmonary arteries but often does not; the unassisted echocardiogram, while key in detecting cardiac SSc, has been disappointing in detecting pulmonary hypertension. Combined Doppler/echo techniques measuring tricuspid insufficiency (present in most patients with increased right ventricular pressures) are promising in the early detection of pulmonary hypertension. Aggressive attempts to lower pulmonary artery pressure should be instituted (see Ch. 45).

Renal System. At one time, the abrupt onset of accelerated hypertension and oliguria ("scleroderma renal crisis") accounted for the majority of deaths in SSc. Fortunately, with early identification and treatment with inhibitors of angiotensin-converting enzymes (captopril, enalapril, lisinopril), the consequences of renal involvement have been significantly reduced. All patients fulfilling the criteria for diffuse SSc should be suspect for renal involvement and should be followed with 24-hour urine collections for protein excretion and creatinine clearance three to four times a year. Excretion of greater than 750 mg of protein per 24 hours or clearances of less than 60 ml per minute, or distinct changes in either proteinuria or glomerular filtration rate (GFR), should initiate measurements of resting renin levels and, if elevated, treatment. Increases in blood pressure and pulse rate, accelerated increases in edematous skin tightening (rapidly increasing skin score), or the appearance of microangiopathic hemolytic anemia or disseminated intravascular coagulation (see Ch. 155) may also herald the onset of renal involvement.

The sudden appearance of renal SSc when other features of the disease appear more indolent is a characteristic of the kidney's unique ability to autoregulate its own blood flow. The typical small artery lesion of intimal proliferation develops slowly in the kidney of SSc patients, with gradual reduction in renal blood flow, until both renal flow and glomerular flow drop abruptly and renal failure ensues. A rapid acceleration of these changes is associated with the onset of hyperreninemia. It is during this accelerated phase that hypertension, funduscopic vascular changes (hemorrhages and exudates), and microangiopathic hemolytic anemia appear. The key to successful management of renal SSc is to identify the population at risk (those with diffuse SSc), to detect declining GFR early, and to treat expectantly.

One remarkable feature of renal SSc is the ability of some patients to regain renal function after months to years (up to 4 years) of end-stage renal disease and hemodialysis. Very little is known of the mechanisms of this slow reparative process. The aggressive management of renal SSc with captopril and its converting enzyme inhibitor analogues has improved the 1-year survival from 20 per cent to 80 per cent, with current 5-year survival of about 70 per cent, the first dramatic improvement in the natural history of SSc.

Cardiac System. More than 90 per cent of patients with diffuse SSc (truncal skin involvement) have some form of cardiac involvement. Rarely, acute pericarditis with a friction rub is present; more frequently, a silent pericardial effusion appears slowly, with ankle edema and shortness of breath as the presenting features. Echocardiography is the diagnostic procedure of choice. Pericardial effusions may predispose to renal failure by unknown mechanisms. By electrocardiographic monitoring and electrophysiologic studies, 80 per cent of diffuse SSc patients *without* cardiovascular symptoms have evidence of cardiac involvement; in more recent studies, 95 per cent show abnormalities of thallium reperfusion. Intermittent myocardial ischemia with the acute pathologic concomitant of contraction band necrosis seems to precede fibrosis, suggesting that spasm of the intramyocardial vessels plays a role in cardiac SSc. Most, but not all, of these patients have normal coronary arteries by coronary angiography.

Articular and Musculoskeletal System. Approximately 10 per cent of SSc patients present with a symmetric small joint polyarticular synovitis indistinguishable from rheumatoid arthritis. Within a year, the pattern changes abruptly, with subsidence of joint complaints and the appearance of Raynaud's phenomenon, edema, and diffuse cutaneous SSc. The presence of scleroderma-pattern nailfold capillary changes and a positive antinuclear antibody pattern can identify these patients during their polyarticular phase, prior to the development of cutaneous changes, as destined to develop SSc.

About one half of SSc patients develop stiffness and swelling of the fingers, wrists, knees, and ankles, concomitant with cutaneous changes. Morning stiffness may be present. Signs of inflammation are usually mild. Polymorphonuclear leukocytes are usually present in synovial fluid. On biopsy, the synovium is mildly inflamed, with a distinctive deposition of fibrin throughout the synovium. Obliterative microvascular disease and diffuse fibrotic changes occur at a later stage.

Indolent myopathy is common in SSc. It is difficult to distinguish from atrophy caused by taut skin. Most patients show diffuse atrophy of the extremities with slight elevations of muscle enzyme levels (creatine kinase CK and aldolase); these features are refractory to glucocorticoids or to immunosuppressive therapy. Mild myositis of SSc is best left untreated. Less frequently, abrupt proximal muscle weakness develops and is associated with 10- to 50-fold increases in muscle enzymes, electromyographic features of acute myositis, and lymphoid cell infiltration with muscle fiber necrosis on biopsy. These patients generated the initial confusion regarding mixed, overlap, or undifferentiated connective tissue syndromes; they usually respond to glucocorticoid therapy.

Other. In the second and third decades following the onset of Raynaud's phenomenon, a small but significant proportion of patients with limited cutaneous SSc develop unilateral or bilateral trigeminal neuralgia, which can be disabling.

An increasing number of male SSc patients, especially those with diffuse disease, experience impotence after 1 or 2 years of the onset of symptoms. Impotence is thought to have an organic neurovascular cause, because of diminished or absent nocturnal tumescence. It is refractory to treatment.

Dry eyes (keratoconjunctivitis sicca), dry mouth (xerostomia), or both occur in approximately one fourth of SSc patients. Salivary gland biopsies may show mononuclear cell infiltrates or replacement fibrosis. Supportive care with secretion substitution (artificial tears) and stimulation (lemon candy) provides some relief.

TREATMENT. No therapy has been shown to halt the progression of cutaneous or visceral SSc in a controlled, prospective study. A major source of confusion in assessing therapy is the dependence on softening skin as a key outcome measurement and the natural tendency for hidebound skin to soften after several years (dubbed regressive systemic sclerosis). Skin changes should not be taken as indications of the lessening of the vascular and microvascular disease.

The most distinctive change in the natural history of diffuse cutaneous SSc in the past decade has been the reduction in the proportion of patients who develop renal failure. This change has occurred with the advent of more powerful agents to control the accelerated hypertensive phase of renal failure. Indications for immediate treatment are hypertension (an increase of 30 mm Hg systolic or 15 mm Hg diastolic blood pressure, no matter what the absolute level); a reduction in creatinine clearance of 30 ml per minute or to a clearance below 60 ml per minute; and microangiopathic anemia. If the serum creatinine value is less than 4.0 mg per deciliter, the crisis of renal scleroderma can often, but not always, be averted. Continued intensive treatment is indicated even if hemodialysis is instituted, since some patients can regain function sufficient to obviate dialysis after as long as 4 to 5 years.

D-Penicillamine* has been strongly advocated on the basis of retrospective studies that showed skin softening after 2 years. The proportion of patients who develop significant side effects is 30 to 40 per cent. It is a difficult drug to tolerate. Colchicine* has also been proposed as being capable of influencing cutaneous changes in SSc. Brief crossover studies were inconclusive, and longer open studies were promising but uncontrolled. Colchicine is better tolerated than D-penicillamine.

Glucocorticoids in moderate doses (30 to 40 mg per day in divided daily doses) effectively reduce the inflammatory and edematous changes in SSc but have no effect on the fibrotic features. When pulmonary SSc can be shown to have an active inflammatory component by bronchoalveolar lavage, gallium/indium scans, or high-resolution CT, a brief trial of high-dose (60 to 80 mg in divided daily doses) glucocorticoids is indicated. Also, it may help to reduce pulmonary hypertension if used early in the course of its development, usually in conjunction with calcium channel blockers.

The management of Raynaud's phenomenon has improved in recent years (see Ch. 54); nonetheless, even the most successful management of the vasoactive features of SSc does not appear to slow or stop the continuing appearance of new fibrotic or visceral manifestations. Sometimes a change in lifestyle is sufficient. Clothing should protect the trunk to encourage heat dissipation via peripheral vasodilatation. Extremes of cold, exhaustion, or stress should be avoided. Nitroglycerin ointment applied locally along the course of the digital arteries to those fingers showing severe ischemia is helpful. Selective sympathetic blockade, especially postganglionic alpha blockade with prazosin, usually reduces symptoms but may be difficult to tolerate owing to palpitation and orthostatic hypotension. Inhibitors of the slow calcium channels of cell membranes have been a significant advance in the management of Raynaud's phenomenon. At present, nifedipine in gradually increasing doses is popular, but verapamil, diltiazem, and nicardipine have their proponents as well. When tissue necrosis is present (gangrene), prompt hospital admission for stellate ganglion blockade or epidural blocks is indicated.

As an example of how therapeutic trials in SSc must be conducted to provide meaningful results in this indolent, variable disorder, the negative trial of chlorambucil by Furst and colleagues is cited. The agent was not better than placebo. Fifty-two patients, with a mean of 7.2 years of symptoms, were treated for 3 years each. Extensive inpatient evaluation was carried out at 6, 12, 24, and 36 months, looking for skin, skeletal, pulmonary, cardiac (left and right sides of the heart), renal, upper and lower gastrointestinal, muscular, and global involvement. "Slope estimates" for each patient and each organ system were constructed and compared. Never mind that chlorambucil did not change the course of SSc; the study is a prototype of drug trials until we have a much better understanding of the mechanisms involved.

Jimenez SA, Bashley RI, Rosenbloom J: Regulation of macromolecular biosynthesis in cultured dermal fibroblasts of patients with progressive systemic sclerosis. *In* Black CM, Myers AR (eds.): Current Topics in Rheumatology: Systemic Sclerosis (Scleroderma). New York, Gower Medical Publishing, 1985, pp. 220–225. *A concise review of the data demonstrating that the regulatory defect in the scleroderma fibroblast is at the level of transcription (gene expression).*

Kahaleh MB, LeRoy EC: Vascular factors in the pathogenesis of systemic sclerosis. *In* Jayson MD, Black CM (eds.): Systemic Sclerosis: Scleroderma. Great Britain, Chichester, John Wiley & Sons, 1988, pp 107–118. *A review of the vascular hypothesis in systemic sclerosis.*

Kahaleh MB, LeRoy EC: Interleukin-2 in scleroderma. Correlation of serum level with extent of skin involvement and disease duration. Ann Intern Med 110:446, 1989. *Clinical-biological correlations between disease progression and exaggerated T helper cell function.*

---

*This use is not listed in the manufacturer's directive.

Kallenberg CGM: Early detection of connective tissue disease in patients with Raynaud's phenomenon. Rheumatic Dis Clin North Am 16:11, 1990. *A review of the important hypothesis that virtually all future SSc patients can be detected by capillary and serology examinations, when definitive therapy becomes available.*

Korn JH: Immunologic aspects of scleroderma. Curr Opin Rheumatol 2:922, 1990. *A critical appraisal of genetic associations, T cell subsets (lesional and circulatory), in vivo measures of helper T cell function, and the possibility of retroviral molecular mimicry in the immune events of scleroderma.*

LeRoy EC (ed.): Scleroderma. Rheum Dis Clin North Am 16:1–249, 1990. *A multiauthor discussion of the natural history; early detection; cellular, microvascular, and extracellular matrix; immune; and organ-specific characteristics of systemic sclerosis. A useful reference source.*

LeRoy EC, Black C, Fleischmajer R, et al.: Scleroderma (systemic sclerosis). Classification, subsets and pathogenesis. J Rheumatol 15:202, 1988. *The basis for classifying systemic sclerosis into two subsets based on prognosis.*

LeRoy EC, Smith EA, Kahaleh MB, et al.: A strategy for determining the pathogenesis of systemic sclerosis. Is transforming growth factor β the answer? Arthritis Rheum 32:817, 1989. *The hypothesis that wound healing growth factors are involved in the unregulated scarring of systemic sclerosis.*

Silver RM, Heyes MP, Maize JC, et al.: Scleroderma, fasciitis and eosinophilia associated with ingestion of L-tryptophan. N Engl J Med 322:874, 1990. *A newly recognized syndrome in the scleroderma spectrum of disease.*

Steen VD, Shapiro AP, Medsger TA: Outcome of renal crisis in systemic sclerosis. Ann Intern Med 113:352, 1990. *Documentation of the remarkable efficacy of converting enzyme inhibitors in systemic scleroderma renal crisis.*

Tan EM: Antinuclear antibodies: Diagnostic markers for autoimmune diseases and probes for cell biology. Adv Immunol 44:93, 1989. *A thorough review of humoral autoimmunity in scleroderma in the broader context of human autoimmunity in general by an experienced investigator.*

263 Sjögren's Syndrome

Norman Talal

DEFINITION. Sjögren's syndrome (SS) is a chronic inflammatory and autoimmune disease in which the salivary and lacrimal glands undergo progressive destruction by lymphocytes and plasma cells, resulting in decreased production of saliva and tears. The term autoimmune exocrinopathy has been introduced. The spectrum of this illness includes a primary form (sicca complex), a secondary form accompanying rheumatoid arthritis (or occasionally another connective tissue disease), and a form characterized mainly by lymphoproliferation of either a benign infiltrative or a malignant nature. Females are affected 10 times more frequently than males. The typical appearance of a patient with Sjögren's syndrome who has bilateral parotid swelling is shown in Figure 263–1.

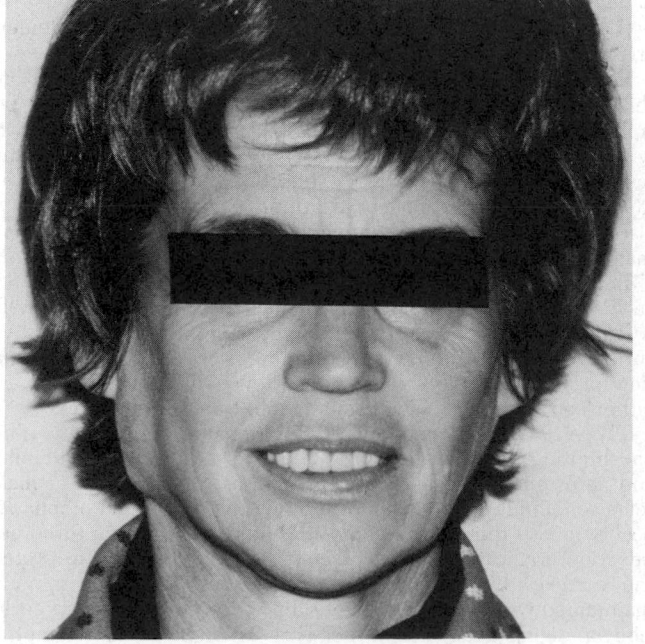

FIGURE 263–1. The characteristic appearance of bilateral parotid swelling has been called the "chipmunk facies" of SS.

A viral etiology for the autoimmune rheumatic diseases has long been suspected but never proved. This possibility has become even more likely because of reports that salivary gland infiltrates and parotid swelling resembling that in SS develop in patients infected with human immunodeficiency virus (HIV). HIV-associated salivary gland disease can occur in adults, children, or after transfusion and may be seen with either AIDS-related complex or AIDS (acquired immunodeficiency syndrome) itself. HIV-related disease must now be added to the differential diagnosis of any patient presenting with parotid swelling. Xerostomia is present in almost all of these patients. Salivary flow rates may be reduced. Dry eyes and arthralgias may also be present. Generalized lymphadenopathy, lymphocytic pulmonary infiltrates, and central nervous system symptoms can occur as well as antinuclear or rheumatoid factor. Anti-Ro/SSA or anti-La/SSB antibodies do not occur. The proper diagnosis can be made by screening for antibodies to HIV with Western blot analysis.

PATHOGENESIS. The several factors involved in the etiology of autoimmune diseases such as SS include genetic, immunologic, hormonal, and probably infectious (? viral) (see also Ch. 261). The discovery of the immune response (IR) genes, which exist in linkage dysequilibrium with other genes in the major histocompatibility complex (see also Ch. 250), has helped distinguish primary from secondary SS. The former is associated with HLA B8, DR3, whereas the latter is associated with DR4 (when rheumatoid arthritis is the accompanying illness). The human leukocyte antigen (HLA) cell-surface antigens, the presumed products of the IR genes, mediate the lymphocyte-lymphocyte and lymphocyte-macrophage interactions necessary for proper immune regulation. Autoimmune diseases probably arise as a consequence of disordered immunologic regulation. Although just how immune regulation becomes disturbed is not yet known, it seems likely that internal factors (such as sex hormones and latent viruses) as well as external factors (drugs or infectious agents) play a role. For example, the predominant female incidence of SS may relate to an ability of androgen to suppress and estrogens to accelerate autoimmune disease, as in the NZB/NZW F_1 mouse model.

CLINICAL MANIFESTATIONS. The symptoms of SS may be subtle and brought out only by careful and persistent questioning.

Ophthalmologic (Keratoconjunctivitis Sicca). The patient may notice accumulation of thick, ropy secretions along the inner canthus caused by a decreased tear film and an abnormal mucous component. Related complaints include erythema, photosensitivity, eye fatigue, decreased visual acuity, and the sensation of a "film" across the field of vision. Desiccation can cause small, superficial erosions of the corneal epithelium. Slit-lamp examination may reveal filamentary keratitis (filaments of corneal epithelium and debris) in severe cases. Conjunctivitis caused by *Staphylococcus aureus* is a complication.

Salivary. Complaints resulting from dryness of the mouth are varied. The "cracker sign" describes the difficulties encountered by trying to eat dry foods without sufficient lubrication. Many subjects require frequent ingestion of liquids. They may resort to carrying water bottles or candy in the purse or pocket. Additional features include oral soreness, adherence of food to buccal surfaces, fissuring of the tongue, and dysphagia. Angular cheilitis resulting from superimposed candidiasis may occur. Patients may lose the ability to discriminate foods on the basis of taste and smell. Dental caries are accelerated. The parotid gland enlarges in many patients (Fig. 263–1) secondary to cellular infiltration and ductal obstruction. Usually asymptomatic and self-limited, the enlargement can be recurrent and associated with pain or erythema. Focal infiltrates of lymphocytes are also found in the minor salivary glands of the lower lip. A biopsy of these lesions provides histologic confirmation and quantification of the degree of infiltration.

Other Symptoms. Dryness may also involve the nasal mucosa, leading to recurrent epistaxis, and may extend throughout the upper respiratory tract, causing hoarseness, recurrent bronchitis, and pneumonitis. Eustachian tube blockage can result in conduction deafness and chronic otitis. Dysphagia may be ascribed to several causes: decreased saliva, infiltration of the glands of the esophageal mucosa, esophageal webbing, and abnormal motility.

Other exocrine gland functions may be affected, leading to loss of pancreatic secretions, hypochlorhydria or achlorhydria, dermal dryness, and lack of vaginal secretions.

Extraglandular Involvement. Extraglandular involvement occurs more frequently in patients with primary than secondary SS. Dependent nonthrombocytopenic purpura is generally associated with hyperglobulinemia. Raynaud's phenomenon is present in 20 per cent of patients. A diffuse interstitial pneumonitis resulting from lymphocytic infiltration may cause dyspnea. Obstructive disease (in the absence of smoking) may result from lymphocytic infiltration surrounding small airways. The most common renal abnormalities involve the tubules, particularly overt or latent renal tubular acidosis and hyposthenuria. The presence of glomerulonephritis should suggest coexisting systemic lupus erythematosus, cryoglobulinemia, or immune complex deposition. Peripheral and cranial neuropathy has been associated with vasculitis involving the vasa nervorum.

Lymphoproliferation and Lymphoma. The incidence of lymphoma is increased 44-fold in SS. Pseudomalignant or malignant lymphoproliferation may be present initially or may develop later in the illness. Most lymphomas belong to the B cell lineage, although the histologic appearance is variable. Many cases previously described as histiocytic lymphoma represent B cell lymphomas and remain sufficiently differentiated to synthesize monoclonal immunoglobulins. Other monoclonal immunoglobulin B cell proliferations in patients with SS include Waldenström's macroglobulinemia, light-chain myeloma, and non–immunoglobulin M (IgM) monoclonal gammopathies (immunoglobulin G [IgG] κ and immunoglobulin A [IgA] λ). A diminution of a previously elevated Ig class may signify malignant transformation. Pseudolymphoma is an intermediate stage in this transition from benign to malignant lymphoproliferation.

Other clinical indications of an increased risk of malignancy include persistent or greatly increased parotid swelling, generalized lymphadenopathy, and splenomegaly. Serial measurement of serum β_2-microglobulin offers another clue to the clinical subset or course. β_2-Microglobulin is elevated in the saliva of patients with SS and in the synovial fluid of patients with rheumatoid arthritis. Salivary levels correspond to the degree of lymphocytic infiltration, and serum levels may be elevated in patients with renal and lymphoproliferative complications.

DIAGNOSIS. Clinical. The presence of dry eyes is suggested by a positive Schirmer test (less than 5 mm of wetting per 5 minutes, with the patient unanesthetized), but the frequency of both false-negative and false-positive results is high. The pattern and intensity of staining with rose bengal dye and slit-lamp examination are more reliable in diagnosis. The presence of filamentary keratitis and corneal ulcerations indicates advanced keratoconjunctivitis sicca.

Diminution in stimulated parotid flow rate (PFR) (<5 ml per gland in 10 minutes) is a sensitive indicator of xerostomia. Salivary scintigraphy, which measures the uptake, concentration, and excretion of ^{99m}Tc-pertechnetate by the major salivary glands, is a sensitive index of glandular function. Scintigraphy is expensive, however, and offers no advantage in diagnostic sensitivity over minor salivary gland biopsy. Lip biopsy is a sensitive and specific diagnostic procedure, is well tolerated by the patient, and causes no disfigurement. Further, biopsy offers more information; in addition to confirming the diagnosis, it allows quantification of the degree of lymphocytic infiltration and tissue damage. Aggregates of lymphocytes within the acinar tissue are scored, each aggregate of 50 or more cells representing a focus. The number of foci within 4 sq mm of glandular tissue is determined and constitutes the focus score. A focus score of more than 1 is characteristic of SS and is seen in fewer than 1 per cent of both normal and autopsy controls. Figure 263–2 demonstrates a strongly positive lip biopsy specimen with a focus score of 8. The diagnosis of SS is based upon the presence of two of the following three criteria: (1) focus score of more than 1 in the labial salivary gland biopsy, (2) keratoconjunctivitis sicca, and (3) an associated connective tissue or lymphoproliferative disorder.

Clinically, a "sicca-like" syndrome may be caused by a number of other disease processes, including hyperlipoproteinemias IV and V, hemochromatosis, sarcoidosis, and amyloidosis. Use of anticholinergic drugs as well as a number of other medications

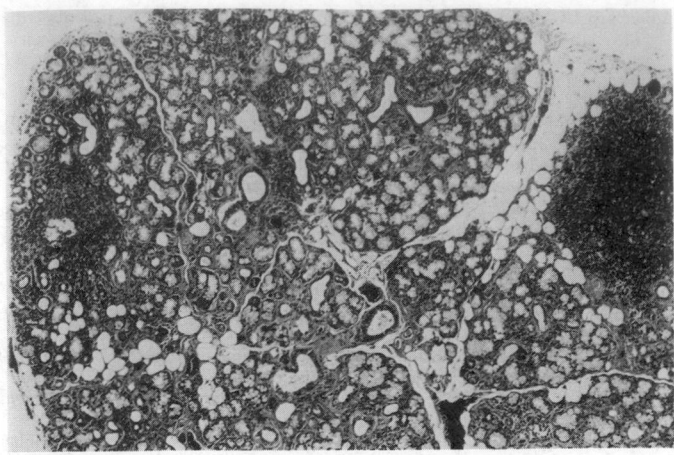

FIGURE 263–2. Several large lymphoid aggregates are seen in this minor salivary gland biopsy from a patient with SS.

may be the single most frequent cause of xerostomia. Thus, it is essential to establish the presence of focal lymphoid infiltrates and autoimmunity in a patient suspected of having SS.

Laboratory. Autoantibodies are common in SS. Rheumatoid factor may be found in 75 to 90 per cent; antinuclear antibodies may be positive in 50 to 80 per cent. Multiple organ-specific antibodies are noted, including antibodies directed against gastric parietal, thyroid microsomal, thyroglobulin, mitochondrial, smooth muscle, and salivary duct antigens.

An autoantibody to a nucleoprotein antigen called SS-B (also termed La) occurs in approximately 50 to 70 per cent of patients with primary SS and, to a lesser extent, in SS accompanied by systemic lupus erythematosus. Antibodies to a related nucleoprotein SS-A (also termed Ro) are less specific for SS, also occur in SLE, and are associated with vasculitis. An antibody (RAP) to an Epstein-Barr (EB) virus–related nuclear antigen (RANA) occurs in secondary SS with rheumatoid arthritis.

Persons with SS manifest B cell hyperactivity. Evidence for this includes the polyclonal hyperglobulinemia seen in more than 50 per cent of patients and the presence of numerous autoantibodies and circulating immune complexes. The lymphoid infiltrates in the salivary glands synthesize immunoglobulins locally. Serum hyperviscosity may result from either macroglobulinemia or polymerizing IgG with rheumatoid factor activity, which forms intermediate complexes. Cryoglobulinemia may be present, as well as vasculitis and glomerulonephritis. A high proportion of patients with SS have circulating immune complexes, as measured by Clq binding and Raji cell assays. Serum levels of complement are only infrequently low.

Peripheral blood T lymphocytes are decreased in about one third of patients. Immunoglobulin-positive lymphocytes in peripheral blood may be increased, particularly in patients with lymphoproliferative or other systemic features. These patients tend to have alterations in T cell subsets and decreased autologous mixed lymphocyte responses. Natural killer (NK) cell activity is also diminished as a consequence of immunoregulatory abnormalities rather than intrinsic deficits.

Reticuloendothelial clearance is defective in patients with SS. In 12 of 19 patients, labeled IgG sensitized autologous red cells, which are usually cleared rapidly by splenic macrophages via surface membrane Fc receptor binding, persisted in the circulation for an abnormally long period. Eleven of the 12 patients had either extraglandular manifestations of SS or secondary SS.

TREATMENT. Treatment of SS is aimed at symptomatic relief and limiting the damaging local effects of chronic xerophthalmia and xerostomia. Ocular dryness responds to the use of artificial tears containing methylcellulose. Since staphylococcal blepharitis occurs in two thirds of patients, the lids should be cultured and infection eradicated. Soft contact lenses may be used to protect the cornea; this practice is controversial. Moisture may be maintained with frequent use of saline drops. Plastic wrap occlusion or diving goggles may be worn at night in an attempt to prevent tear evaporation. Topical steroid use should be avoided unless specifically indicated, because corneal thinning and subsequent perforation may occur. The use of diuretics, many antihypertensive drugs, and antidepressants may further diminish lacrimal and salivary gland function. Xerostomia may respond to an increased fluid intake, use of a 2 per cent solution of methylcellulose, and sour sugar-free candies given as sialagogues. Scrupulous care of teeth is imperative; patients should avoid a high sucrose intake or the frequent use of sugar-containing candies. Vigorous dental plaque control and topical application of fluoride should be used regularly. Oral candidiasis may be treated with nystatin tablets for a prolonged course, with separate treatment of dentures. Vaginal dryness can be treated with propionic acid gels.

Only those patients with severe functional disability or life-threatening complications warrant corticosteroid or immunosuppressive therapy. Prednisone may suppress parotid swelling and improve the restrictive component of pulmonary disease. Immunosuppressive agents have decreased extraglandular lymphoid infiltrates and improved exocrine gland function in some individuals. Their use has been restricted to those patients with severe renal and pulmonary manifestations.

Talal N (ed.): 2nd International Symposium: Sjögren's Syndrome: A Model for Understanding Autoimmunity. London, Academic Press, 1989.
Talal N: Sjögren's syndrome and connective tissue disease with other immunologic disorders. *In* McCarty D (ed.): Arthritis and Allied Conditions. 11th ed. Philadelphia, Lea & Febiger, pp 1197–1213, 1989.

264 The Vasculitic Syndromes

Sheldon M. Wolff

Vasculitis is a clinicopathologic process characterized by inflammation of the blood vessel wall. Associated with this inflammation may be compromise of the vessel lumen with resulting ischemic changes in the tissues supplied by the vessel. Any size, location, and type of blood vessel may be involved, including large muscular arteries, medium-sized and small arteries, arterioles, capillaries, postcapillary venules, and veins. This heterogeneous category of diseases comprises unique syndromes as well as diseases with overlapping clinical and pathologic features. The vasculitis may be the primary process, or it may be a component of another underlying disease. Furthermore, vasculitis varies considerably in its clinicopathologic manifestations. Certain of the vasculitic disorders are rarely life threatening (e.g., the hypersensitivity vasculitic syndromes in which cutaneous involvement usually predominates). Other vasculitic syndromes may be fulminant and, if untreated, rapidly fatal diseases (e.g., Wegener's granulomatosis and polyarteritis nodosa).

The vasculitic syndromes are generally thought to result from immunopathogenic mechanisms; however, the evidence for this varies among the different syndromes. Among these mechanisms, the deposition of circulating immune complexes with subsequent vessel damage has emerged as the major immunopathologic event associated with most of the vasculitic syndromes. The presence of circulating immune complexes does not prove that the associated vasculitis is caused by them, and complexes per se need not result in vasculitis, even in diseases in which vasculitis is present. In only a few diseases has the actual antigen involved in the immune complex been identified. The most noted of these is the hepatitis B surface antigen that has been demonstrated in the circulating immune complexes, cryoprecipitable serum components, and involved tissues of certain patients with hepatitis B antigenemia–associated vasculitis.

The mechanism of tissue damage from immune complexes is thought to be similar to serum sickness. In this model, soluble immune complexes are formed in antigen excess and deposited in blood vessel walls in areas of increased vascular permeability. The increased permeability is attributed to release of vasoactive amines from platelets or mast cells under the influence of specific immunoglobulin E (IgE). Following deposition of complexes, various components of complement are activated, particularly C5a, which is strongly chemotactic for neutrophils. The neutrophils infiltrate the vessel wall at the site of immune complex deposition and release intracytoplasmic enzymes such as collagenase and elastase that directly damage the vessel wall. Compromise of the lumen occurs with resulting ischemic changes.

Certain of the vasculitides are characterized by granulomatous inflammation in and around the blood vessels. Although granulomatous responses are generally of the delayed hypersensitivity type, immune complexes themselves can trigger granuloma formation and thereby produce granulomatous vasculitis.

Why certain persons develop vasculitis and others do not is unknown and likely involves a number of host factors, such as genetic predisposition, immunoregulatory mechanisms, and the integrity of the reticuloendothelial system, which clears the complexes from the circulation. In addition, the reasons that certain complexes cause vasculitis and that certain types of vessels and not others are involved probably relate to the size and physicochemical properties of the immune complex and to other physical factors, such as turbulence of blood flow, hydrostatic pressure within vessels, and previously damaged vessel endothelium.

CLASSIFICATION OF THE VASCULITIC SYNDROMES

The heterogeneity and the obvious overlap among the vasculitis syndromes have led to difficulties in classification of this group of diseases. The first report of a vasculitic syndrome was in 1866 by Kussmaul and Maier, who described the clinicopathologic features in a patient with what is now recognized as classic polyarteritis nodosa. It became evident that there were numerous vasculitic syndromes with diverse clinical and pathologic manifestations, but diagnostic criteria were controversial. More precise and accurate classification schemes now have emerged, based upon re-examination of clinical, pathologic, and immunologic features as well as responses to certain therapeutic regimens. Table 264–1 illustrates one such classification scheme.

The first group of vasculitides is the polyarteritis nodosa group. This syndrome is described in detail in Ch. 265. It is the prototype of the serious systemic necrotizing vasculitides and manifests features such as small and medium-sized muscular artery involvement, hypertension, visceral vessel involvement, and a noticeable lack of lung involvement. Eventually physicians recognized a systemic vasculitis that resembled classic polyarteritis nodosa except that lung involvement was a prominent feature and the patients generally manifested eosinophilia, granulomatous reactions, and a strong allergic diathesis, usually severe asthma. Most of these patients had what is now referred to as allergic angiitis and granulomatosis of the Churg-Strauss type. This disease is quite similar to classic polyarteritis nodosa except for the divergent features mentioned above. Many systemic necrotizing vasculitides manifest clinicopathologic characteristics that overlap

TABLE 264–1. THE CLINICAL SPECTRUM OF VASCULITIS

1. Polyarteritis nodosa group
   Classic polyarteritis nodosa
   Allergic angiitis and granulomatosis (Churg-Strauss disease)
   Overlap syndrome
2. Hypersensitivity vasculitis
   Henoch-Schönlein purpura
   Serum sickness and serum sickness–like reactions
   Vasculitis associated with infectious diseases
   Vasculitis associated with neoplasms
   Vasculitis associated with connective tissue diseases
   Vasculitis associated with other underlying diseases
   Congenital deficiencies of the complement system
   Erythema elevatum diutinum
3. Wegener's granulomatosis
4. Giant cell arteritides
   Cranial or temporal arteritis
   Takayasu's arteritis
5. Other vasculitic syndromes
   Angiocentric immunoproliferative lesions
   Mucocutaneous lymph node syndrome (Kawasaki's disease)
   Behçet's disease
   Vasculitis isolated to the central nervous system
   Thromboangiitis obliterans (Buerger's disease)
   Miscellaneous vasculitides

these two syndromes as well as the hypersensitivity group of vasculitides (discussed below). This subgroup has been referred to as the "overlap syndrome" of systemic necrotizing vasculitis.

In addition to the polyarteritis nodosa group of systemic necrotizing vasculitides, certain other vasculitides are systemic and involve multiple organ systems. However, they are referred to by different names, since they possess characteristic clinical and/or pathologic features. This is true of diseases such as Wegener's granulomatosis (see Ch. 266) and the giant cell arteritides. In the latter group, the two major subcategories—cranial or temporal arteritis (see Ch. 267) and Takayasu's arteritis (see Ch. 53)—are systemic diseases involving large muscular arteries with mononuclear cell and often giant cell infiltration within the walls of the involved arteries. Despite the predisposition for certain vessels in these diseases (temporal artery in cranial arteritis and subclavian artery in Takayasu's arteritis), these are systemic diseases that involve multiple arteries. Lymphomatoid granulomatosis (see Ch. 266) is generally considered in the differential diagnosis of systemic necrotizing vasculitis with lung involvement such as Wegener's granulomatosis. However, it is not, strictly speaking, an inflammatory response in vessels but an infiltration of blood vessel walls with atypical and often neoplastic-looking lymphoid cells. Lymphomatoid granulomatosis will often evolve into a lymphoma, and it has been suggested that these patients should be classified as having an "angiocentric immunoproliferative lesion."

The hypersensitivity vasculitides include a broad and heterogeneous group of disorders that have often caused confusion in categorization. These are discussed in detail in this chapter.

Other vasculitic syndromes can be considered under the category of "miscellaneous" for want of a better term. These include Behçet's disease, the major pathologic feature of which is a true vasculitis (see Ch. 269), and thromboangiitis obliterans, which is an inflammatory and occlusive disease of arteries and veins, although its true vasculitic character has been questioned. In addition to the granulomatous vasculitis of the central nervous system, which is seen in association with certain lymphoproliferative malignancies, there is also a rare syndrome of isolated vasculitis of the central nervous system that occurs in the apparent absence of systemic vasculitis or other systemic disease.

HYPERSENSITIVITY VASCULITIS

Hypersensitivity vasculitis is a term applied to a heterogeneous group of disorders that are thought to represent a hypersensitivity reaction to an antigenic stimulus such as a drug or an infectious agent; hence the word "hypersensitivity." Although the antigenic stimuli associated with this group are heterogeneous, these disorders generally share the characteristic of involvement of small vessels. They can be subdivided into two basic groups. The vast majority of the patients manifest involvement of the postcapillary venules, and hence have a venulitis. A smaller group of patients falls into the second category, in which arterioles are predominantly involved (arteriolitis). Most important, there is a predominant and often exclusive involvement of the vessels of the skin. Confusion in the literature generally resulted from grouping this category of vasculitis with the more serious systemic varieties, such as classic polyarteritis nodosa and related diseases. It is true that the hypersensitivity vasculitides may have variable degrees of organ system involvement other than of the skin. However, this is usually less severe than that of typical systemic vasculitis of polyarteritis nodosa and Wegener's granulomatosis. Most frequently, the skin is exclusively involved, or if other organ systems are involved, the cutaneous disease still dominates the clinical picture.

ETIOLOGY. As indicated by the terminology, the etiology is usually a recognizable antigenic stimulus, such as a drug, microbe, toxin, or foreign or endogenous protein. From an etiologic standpoint the hypersensitivity vasculitides segregate into two distinct groups, depending on the source of the sensitizing antigen. In the classic original group, the antigen is foreign to the host. In the second group the antigen is endogenous. For example, certain connective tissue diseases may manifest a typical hypersensitivity small vessel vasculitis. These diseases are generally characterized by circulating immune complexes in which one of the components is an endogenous protein to which antibody is directed. This is true of patients with systemic lupus erythematosus who develop immune complexes composed of endogenous DNA and anti-DNA antibodies; in addition, patients with rheumatoid arthritis may develop immune complexes of rheumatoid factor with antibody activity against endogenous immunoglobulin. Thus, in most of the hypersensitivity vasculitides, the identity of the etiologic agent that triggers the formation of immune complexes is at least strongly suspected.

INCIDENCE AND PREVALENCE. It is difficult to determine an accurate incidence for the hypersensitivity group of vasculitides owing to the marked heterogeneity among these diverse syndromes. However, the hypersensitivity group of vasculitides is much more common than the polyarteritis group and other syndromes such as Wegener's granulomatosis and Takayasu's arteritis. The disease can be seen at any age and in both sexes; however, this varies considerably with the particular subgroup in question.

PATHOLOGY AND PATHOGENESIS. The histopathologic hallmark of the hypersensitivity vasculitides is a leukocytoclastic venulitis. The term leukocytoclasis refers to nuclear debris derived from the neutrophils that have infiltrated in and around the involved vessels. In skin biopsies, this type of involvement is most common in the postcapillary venules just beneath the epidermis. When biopsies are obtained in the acute phase of active disease, the typical pattern of neutrophil infiltration is readily observed. In the subacute or chronic stages, biopsies often reveal mononuclear cell infiltration. In the second and smaller category of hypersensitivity vasculitis, arterioles and capillaries are predominantly involved. In the typical case of hypersensitivity vasculitis with a predominance of cutaneous involvement, the lesions are usually found in the lower extremities or in the dependent areas such as the sacrum in supine patients. This is most likely due to the increase in hydrostatic pressure within the postcapillary venules in these areas.

Although immune complex deposition is widely considered to be the pathogenic mechanism of this group of vasculitis, not every case of hypersensitivity vasculitis has had immune complexes demonstrated, even when carefully sought, as mentioned above.

CLINICAL MANIFESTATIONS. Just as the broad group is etiologically heterogeneous, so too are the clinical manifestations. However, the hallmark of the group is the predominance of cutaneous involvement. The skin lesions may appear as the classic palpable purpura, which results from the extravasation of erythrocytes into the tissue surrounding the involved venules. In addition, one may see macules, papules, vesicles, bullae, subcutaneous nodules, ulcers, and even recurrent or chronic urticaria.

Even though skin lesions generally dominate, various organ system involvements can be seen. Certain constellations of clinicopathologic findings define relatively distinct syndromes. For example, in *Henoch-Schönlein purpura* the typical syndrome consists of palpable purpura (usually over the buttocks), arthralgias, gastrointestinal symptoms, and glomerulonephritis. Henoch-Schönlein purpura is usually seen in children; however, adults of any age may be affected. The disease usually remits spontaneously after 1 week. However, the disease is remarkable for its tendency to recur a number of times over weeks to months before remission is complete. The characteristic skin lesions are present in virtually all patients. The majority of patients also have arthralgias involving multiple joints, but frank arthritis is rare. The gastrointestinal involvement is usually manifested as colicky abdominal pain which may mimic an acute surgical abdomen. Patients may experience nausea, vomiting, diarrhea, constipation, and occasionally the passage of blood and mucus per rectum. In the more severe and rare case, bowel intussusception may occur. Renal disease is a glomerulitis (see Ch. 79), which is usually expressed as microscopic hematuria without significant renal functional impairment. However, in rare cases renal failure can occur. Most frequently, patients recover spontaneously and completely.

Other groups within the hypersensitivity category include *serum sickness and serum sickness–like reactions*. The classic manifestations are fever, urticaria, arthralgias, and lymphadenopathy occurring 7 to 10 days after primary exposure to the antigen in question, which for serum sickness is usually a heterologous serum protein and for serum sickness–like reactions is usually a drug such as penicillin. Most of the manifestations of this disorder are not the result of vasculitis. However, in some cases cutaneous vasculitis typical of the hypersensitivity group is documented. In addition, patients may rarely progress to a typical systemic necrotizing vasculitis involving multiple organ systems.

A number of disorders have vasculitis as a manifestation of an underlying primary disease. Included in these diseases are *systemic lupus erythematosus, rheumatoid arthritis, mixed cryoglobulinemia*, and *other connective tissue diseases*. In these disorders, the manifestations of the underlying disease usually predominate. When vasculitis is observed, it is generally of the small vessel cutaneous type, which is virtually indistinguishable from the vasculitis seen in the hypersensitivity group with recognized exogenous antigens. However, patients with these disorders, particularly systemic lupus erythematosus and rheumatoid arthritis, may also develop a systemic necrotizing vasculitis that closely resembles the polyarteritis nodosa group in manifestations and severity. Nevertheless, in the typical case, the cutaneous vasculitis usually dominates the clinical picture with respect to the vasculitic process.

Other diseases that may fall into this category of small vessel hypersensitivity vasculitis are the *vasculitis associated with congenital deficiencies of various complement components*, such as Clr, Cls, and C2; *erythema elevatum diutinum; hypocomplementemic vasculitis*; the *vasculitis associated with certain neoplasms, particularly of the lymphoid type;* and the *vasculitis associated with other primary disorders such as ulcerative colitis, Crohn's disease, biliary cirrhosis*, and *retroperitoneal fibrosis*.

DIAGNOSIS. The diagnosis of hypersensitivity vasculitis rests on the demonstration of vasculitis on biopsy. Since the predominant organ involved is the skin, histopathologic material is usually readily available. Because cutaneous involvement is often present in severe systemic vasculitides, one should undertake a systematic workup of other organ systems in patients who present with apparently isolated cutaneous vasculitis. Recently, it has been suggested that the presence of antibiotics against the cytoplasm of neutrophils (ANCA) is supportive evidence for a diagnosis of Wegener's granulomatosis (Ch. 266).

TREATMENT AND PROGNOSIS. Therapy of the hypersensitivity group of vasculitides has in general been unsatisfactory. Since most cases resolve spontaneously, the lack of response to therapeutic regimens is of less importance. However, in those patients who go on to develop persistent cutaneous disease or serious organ system involvement, several regimens have been tried with variable results. In cases in which a recognized antigenic stimulus is present, the first order of therapy is to remove the antigen, e.g., to remove sensitizing drugs or responsible organisms by appropriate antibiotic therapy when possible. In situations in which disease appears to be self-limited, no specific therapy is indicated. However, when disease persists or results in organ system dysfunction, a glucocorticosteroid is the drug of choice. Prednisone is usually administered in doses of 1 mg per kilogram per day with rapid tapering when possible, in some instances directly to discontinuation or initially to an alternate-day regimen followed by ultimate discontinuation (see Ch. 27). In cases that prove refractory to corticosteroid therapy, cytotoxic agents such as cyclophosphamide have been used. The efficacy of these regimens has not yet been fully evaluated in hypersensitivity vasculitis. Thus, one should be reluctant to institute cytotoxic agents in persons with disease limited to the skin, particularly since the response of the cutaneous variety of hypersensitivity vasculitis to cytotoxic agents has not been as dramatic as the response of the systemic vasculitides, such as Wegener's granulomatosis (see Ch. 266) and the polyarteritis nodosa group.

The prognosis of most of the diseases in this category is generally excellent, with spontaneous and complete remissions in most patients. However, certain patients may develop persistent and debilitating cutaneous disease, and others may evolve a typical systemic vasculitis with a serious prognosis.

Christian CL, Sergent JS: Vasculitic syndromes: Clinical and experimental models. Am J Med 61:385, 1976. *Excellent review of the vasculitic syndromes with emphasis on the pathophysiologic mechanisms in several of the human diseases as well as in animal models of vasculitis.*
Cupps TR, Fauci AS: The Vasculitides. Philadelphia, W. B. Saunders Company, 1981, pp 1–21. *Comprehensive treatise on the entire spectrum of the vasculitic syndromes. Pathogenesis, clinicopathologic manifestations, and updated therapeutic approaches are discussed in detail.*

Fauci AS, Katz P, Haynes BF, et al.: Cyclophosphamide therapy of severe systemic necrotizing vasculitis. N Engl J Med 301:235, 1979. *One of the first papers to show that aggressive therapy could lead to dramatic and long-term remissions in these diseases.*
Lipford EH Jr, Margolick JB, Longo DL, et al.: Angiocentric immunoproliferative lesions: A clinicopathologic spectrum of post-thymic T-cell proliferations. Blood 72:1674, 1988. *Detailed description of various stages of lymphomatoid granulomatosis.*
Zeek PM: Periarteritis nodosa and other forms of necrotizing angiitis. N Engl J Med 18:764, 1953. *Classic article that represents the first well-organized approach to the rational classification of the vasculitic syndromes. It is still employed as the backbone of most classification schemes.*

265 Polyarteritis Nodosa Group
Sheldon M. Wolff

DEFINITION. In 1866 Kussmaul and Maier described a patient with polyarteritis nodosa. They introduced the term *periarteritis nodosa* to describe segmental nodules of medium-sized muscular arteries. Because the swelling of the arterial walls often led to occlusion, many of the clinical manifestations were secondary to necrosis. Hence, polyarteritis nodosa is often classified as one of the systemic necrotizing vasculitides. Classic polyarteritis does not involve the lung, as do allergic angiitis and granulomatosis of Churg-Strauss.

Polyarteritis associated with hepatitis B antigenemia was described in 1970 by Gocke and colleagues. The association of hepatitis B antigen-antibody complexes and polyarteritis provides strong support for the hypothesis that the vasculitides in general are secondary to the deposition of soluble immune complexes.

In some patients there are manifestations of both classic polyarteritis nodosa and allergic angiitis and granulomatosis of Churg-Strauss. Such patients are classified as being in the group with the so-called overlap syndrome. Their diagnosis, workup, and management are no different from those of other patients in the polyarteritis nodosa group.

Polyarteritis nodosa occurs from infancy to old age, with a peak incidence in the fifth and sixth decades of life, and the male-female ratio has been estimated at 2 to 3:1.

PATHOLOGY. The lesions of polyarteritis involve arteries of medium and small caliber, especially at bifurcations and branchings. The segmental process involves the media, with edema, fibrinous exudation, fibrinoid necrosis, and infiltration of polymorphonuclear neutrophils, and extends to the adventitia and intima. Thrombosis and infarction or hemorrhage occur at this stage. Subsequently, the regions of fibrinoid necrosis are replaced by granulation tissue, and the intima proliferates. Finally the involved segment is replaced by scar tissue with associated intimal thickening and periarterial fibrosis. These changes produce partial occlusion, thrombosis and infarction, and palpable or visible aneurysms with occasional rupture.

In allergic angiitis and granulomatosis the acute fibrinoid necrosis with cellular infiltration involves arterioles and venules as well as medium-sized muscular arteries. It is characteristic of the polyarteritis nodosa group for the vascular lesions to be in different stages of evolution, i.e., acute, subacute, and healed. In allergic angiitis and granulomatosis, the pulmonary granulomatous lesions in vascular and extravascular sites are accompanied by an intense eosinophilic infiltration.

In patients with polyarteritis associated with hepatitis B antigenemia, the specific antigen has been recognized in immune complexes present in the circulation and deposited in affected vessels along with complement proteins. It is presumed that this pathogenetic mechanism prevails in the entire polyarteritis nodosa group, but the basis for arterial deposition is unknown. The deposition of immune complexes in venules and glomeruli is attributed to changes in permeability and to physical trapping.

CLINICAL MANIFESTATIONS AND DIAGNOSIS. The widespread distribution of the arterial lesions produces diverse clinical manifestations, which reflect the particular organ systems in which the arterial supply has been impaired. Among the early symptoms and signs of polyarteritis nodosa are fever, weight loss, and pain in viscera and/or the musculoskeletal system. Striking and specific presenting signs may relate to abdominal pain, acute glomerulitis, polyneuritis, and, on occasion, myocardial infarction. Pulmonary manifestations, especially intractable bronchial asthma, would indicate allergic angiitis and granulomatosis rather than classic polyarteritis nodosa.

Renal. Renal involvement in two forms, renal polyarteritis and a glomerulitis, may occur separately or together. Approximately 70 per cent of patients with polyarteritis nodosa and renal disease have renal vasculitis, whereas the other 30 per cent have glomerulitis. Renal polyarteritis is the most common lesion seen at postmortem examination. Manifestations of the renal involvement include intermittent proteinuria and microscopic hematuria with occasional hyaline and granular casts. The glomerulitis is manifested by microscopic and even macroscopic hematuria, proteinuria, cellular casts, and progressive renal failure. Hypertension is common. Renal involvement is the cause of death in about two thirds of patients with classic polyarteritis nodosa and about one third of those with allergic angiitis and granulomatosis.

Gastrointestinal. Arterial lesions are commonly found in one or more abdominal viscera. The principal manifestation is pain; anorexia, nausea, and vomiting are less prominent. Impaired arterial blood supply to the bowel can produce mucosal ulcerations, perforation, or infarction with melena or bloody diarrhea. Involvement of appendix, gallbladder, or pancreas can simulate appendicitis, cholecystitis, or hemorrhagic pancreatitis. Liver involvement can range from hepatomegaly with or without jaundice to the signs of extensive hepatic necrosis. Splenomegaly is uncommon. There has been no consistent relationship between the development of necrotizing vasculitis and the appearance of liver disease in patients with hepatitis B antigenemia. Some of the observed combinations include necrotizing vasculitis as the initial clinical finding, superimposed upon chronic active hepatitis, or appearing simultaneously with an acute hepatitis.

Central and Peripheral Nervous System. Central nervous system manifestations are generally late occurrences in the course of polyarteritis nodosa, and their particular presentation reflects the specific area of the brain that is compromised. Headache, seizures, and retinal hemorrhages and exudates occur with or without localizing signs referable to the cerebrum, cerebellum, or brain stem; meningeal irritation may occur as a result of subarachnoid hemorrhage. Multiple mononeuropathy, i.e., involvement of several or even many individual nerves at the same or different times, is a common finding and is attributed to arteritis of the vasa nervorum. The peripheral neuropathy is usually asymmetric, with both sensory and motor distribution. The former can be extremely painful, but the latter has attendant muscular degeneration, which can be severe.

Articular and Muscular. Arthralgias and myalgias are frequent in polyarteritis nodosa. Arthralgias are migratory, generally without swelling, and thought to be due to small, localized arterial lesions. Muscle pain or weakness reflects either direct involvement of the arterial supply or a peripheral neuropathy.

Cardiac. Polyarteritis of the coronary arteries and their branches has a frequency approaching that of renal polyarteritis, and heart failure is responsible for or contributes to death in one sixth to one half of the cases. The clinical manifestations of cardiac involvement are those of partial or complete arterial occlusion, as modified by the superimposition of renal hypertension and an appreciable incidence of acute pericarditis without effusion. Whereas the combination of infarction and hypertension commonly leads to left-sided failure, an occasional patient with allergic angiitis and granulomatosis presents with predominantly right-sided decompensation.

Genitourinary. Involvement of the ovaries, testes, and epididymis is frequent, though usually asymptomatic. Mucosal ulceration in the bladder can occasionally precipitate gross hematuria with dysuria.

Cutaneous. Cutaneous involvement of some form is believed to occur in over 25 per cent of those affected with polyarteritis nodosa. The acute cutaneous manifestations include polymorphic exanthemas—purpuric, urticarial, and multiform in character—and severe subcutaneous hemorrhage, resulting from necrotizing arteritis, with secondary gangrene. Ulcerations and a

persistent livedo reticularis are associated with the more chronic stage of the disease. A most characteristic but uncommon finding is cutaneous and subcutaneous nodules; these occur at any time in the disease course. The nodules tend to group, appear in crops, are usually movable, may regress in days or persist for months, range in size from a pea to a walnut, and may cause the overlying skin to become reddened or to ulcerate.

Pulmonary. Although the bronchial arteries can be involved in classic polyarteritis, only allergic angiitis and granulomatosis that involves the pulmonary arteries and parenchyma with granulomatous lesions give rise to clinical manifestations. Asthma, when present, is intractable and associated with a marked peripheral eosinophilia. Pneumonic episodes are transient or progressive and may be accompanied by hemoptysis and/or pleuritic pain. Respiratory involvement accounts for about one half of the mortality, with the remainder being attributable to the arteritis of other organs.

COURSE UNTREATED. The course of polyarteritis nodosa is progressive with destruction of vital organs. Intermittent acute episodes resulting from thrombosis of vital or nonvital structures are prominent. Death is most frequently attributed to renal involvement in cases of classic polyarteritis nodosa and to pulmonary lesions in those cases classified as allergic angiitis with granulomatosis. Cardiac failure caused by a combination of infarction and renal hypertension is an additional frequent cause of death in both groups, and acute vascular accidents of the gastrointestinal tract or central nervous system account for much of the remaining mortality. In the retrospective postmortem study of Rose and Spencer, the 5-year survival rate was about 10 per cent in classic polyarteritis nodosa and about 25 per cent in allergic angiitis and granulomatosis if onset was dated from the start of respiratory symptoms. The report of the British Medical Research Council in 1960 placed the 54 months' survival rate in polyarteritis nodosa at nearly 50 per cent. Rare patients with polyarteritis limited to nonvital sites have been reported to experience an unusually long course or even a lasting remission.

LABORATORY FINDINGS. Leukocytosis, predominantly polymorphonuclear, is apparent in over 75 per cent of the cases of polyarteritis nodosa or allergic angiitis and granulomatosis, eosinophilia often being marked in the latter group. Hypocomplementemia, which has not been observed in classic polyarteritis nodosa, has been present in patients with hepatitis B antigenemia. The erythrocyte sedimentation rate is customarily elevated. Abnormalities in the urine sediment, especially hematuria and proteinuria, reflect renal involvement. Abnormalities of the electrocardiogram and electroencephalogram are those expected on the basis of arterial occlusive disease or those secondary to the metabolic disturbances of uremia. Lesions apparent on chest roentgenograms are the rule in patients with allergic angiitis and granulomatosis. The findings range from transient or progressive infiltration to consolidation, cavitation, or scarring; upper and lower lobes are involved with equal frequency. As none of these findings are specific, antemortem diagnosis of polyarteritis depends upon biopsy. Since the arterial involvement is segmental and spotty in distribution, it is advisable to obtain tissue from a symptomatic site, and it is essential to section completely the entire specimen. A deep, open surgical biopsy, including subcutaneous tissue and underlying muscle, should be obtained whenever possible from a skeletal muscle exhibiting pain and tenderness. Involvement of the epididymis and testes is sufficiently common to make this a useful biopsy site if palpation reveals the typical nodularity of segmental vascular lesions. Needle and surgical biopsies of internal organs with clinical involvement, such as liver or kidney, are gaining in favor. As an alternative or additional procedure, angiography to detect aneurysms of medium-sized muscular arteries in renal, hepatic, or intestinal sites may be helpful.

DIFFERENTIAL DIAGNOSIS. The differential diagnosis of the polyarteritis group includes not only the constituent syndromes but also all those conditions associated with systemic necrotizing vasculitis. The key differences between classic polyarteritis nodosa and other causes of necrotizing vasculitis include the absence of extravascular granulomas, sparing of the pulmonary arteries, failure of venous involvement except by contiguous spread, and predilection for medium-sized arteries. For allergic angiitis and granulomatosis the striking granulomatous response excludes all but Wegener's granulomatosis. The prominence of bronchial asthma, peripheral eosinophilia, and the usual absence of necrotizing lesions in the upper respiratory tract permit a tentative clinical distinction between allergic angiitis and granulomatosis and Wegener's granulomatosis. Underlying connective tissue diseases are still recognized by their clinical characteristics even when necrotizing arteritis becomes prominent. For example, cases of rheumatoid arthritis with ulcerating cutaneous lesions and peripheral neuropathy often exhibit prominent rheumatoid nodules and a high titer of rheumatoid factor. The specificities of the immunoglobulins that accompany active systemic lupus erythematosus or mixed cryoglobulinemia are distinctive; in addition, in the presence of active renal disease both entities manifest a reduced serum complement level not generally observed in classic polyarteritis nodosa. The giant cell arteritides (i.e., temporal arteritis, Takayasu's arteritis) lack the glomerulitis, peripheral neuropathy, and cutaneous manifestations notable in polyarteritis nodosa. The combination of progressive nephritis and pulmonary hemorrhage seen in Goodpasture's syndrome is unlike polyarteritis nodosa. The drug-induced hypersensitivity vasculitis group may be difficult to separate on purely clinical grounds, although the history of antecedent drug administration, infrequency of gastrointestinal manifestations, and absence of nodules along arteries are useful points. The clinical presentation in Henoch-Schönlein purpura is distinctive.

TREATMENT. The commonly employed nonsteroidal anti-inflammatory agents have no specific therapeutic role in polyarteritis nodosa; thus, corticosteroids have been employed most widely. Large doses, in the range of 40 to 60 mg of prednisone per day, afford symptomatic relief but probably have little effect on the 1-year survival statistics. In our series of 17 patients falling within the polyarteritis group, including 2 with allergic angiitis and granulomatosis and 6 with hepatitis B–associated polyarteritis, 14 experienced dramatic remission with the introduction of cyclophosphamide at a dose of 2 mg per kilogram per day. It was subsequently possible to reduce the cyclophosphamide and to taper the steroids to every other day and yet maintain a remission, and in some instances resolution of microaneurysms on repeat celiac axis angiography was noted.

Churg J, Strauss L: Allergic granulomatosis, allergic angiitis, and periarteritis nodosa. Am J Pathol 27:277, 1951. *This is the classic reference to the polyarteritis nodosa subgroup termed allergic angiitis and granulomatosis; it describes the cardinal clinical and pathologic manifestations.*

Collagen Diseases and Hypersensitivity Panel: Report to Medical Research Council. Br Med J 1:1399, 1960. *This is the classic reference on the natural history of the polyarteritis nodosa group, untreated and with steroid intervention.*

Fauci AS, Katz P, Haynes BF, et al.: Cyclophosphamide therapy of severe systemic necrotizing vasculitis. N Engl J Med 301:235, 1979. *A most important contribution dealing with the effectiveness of cyclophosphamide therapy in the management of a series of patients falling within the polyarteritis group and including such subgroups as allergic angiitis and granulomatosis and hepatitis B–associated polyangiitis.*

Leavitt RY, Fauci AS: Polyangiitis overlap syndrome. Am J Med 81:79, 1986. *Patients are being seen with increasing frequency who do not fit into one of the well-defined vasculitic entities. This is a useful paper that describes 10 such patients.*

Rose GA, Spencer H: Polyarteritis nodosa. Q J Med 26:43, 1957. *This classic article argued most effectively that allergic angiitis and granulomatosis was not a distinct entity from classic polyarteritis nodosa but could most easily be considered polyarteritis nodosa with pulmonary involvement.*

266 Wegener's Granulomatosis and Midline Granuloma

Barton F. Haynes

DEFINITION. Wegener's granulomatosis is a distinct clinical form of systemic necrotizing vasculitis consisting of (1) necrotizing granulomatous vasculitis of the upper and lower respiratory tracts, (2) focal necrotizing glomerulonephritis, and (3) systemic small vessel vasculitis involving numerous organ systems.

ETIOLOGY. The cause of the disease is unknown. It is thought to be a hypersensitivity reaction to unknown inhaled antigen or antigens leading to respiratory tract involvement with granulomatous inflammation, vasculitis, elevated serum immunoglob-

ulin A (IgA) and immunoglobulin G (IgG) levels, and systemic vessel and organ involvement. Although there have been no familial, geographic, or occupational exposure factors associated with the disease, one study has suggested an increased incidence of HLA-B8 antigen in patients with the disease.

INCIDENCE AND PREVALENCE. Originally described in the 1930's, Wegener's granulomatosis is an uncommon, but not rare, disease that is being increasingly recognized in clinical practice. The disease can affect any age group. The mean age at onset is 40 years with a male-female ratio of 3:2.

PATHOLOGY AND PATHOGENESIS. The typical histopathologic lesion seen in the disease is necrotizing vasculitis of small arteries and veins, usually with granuloma formation in the surrounding cellular infiltrates.

In the upper respiratory tract, biopsy of paranasal sinus, nasopharyngeal, or tracheal lesions may show changes of acute or chronic inflammation or may reveal frank vasculitis with or without granulomas. Pansinusitis, nasal crusting with drainage, and serous otitis may result, as well as nasal septal perforation and saddle nose deformity.

Pulmonary lesions are present in 95 per cent of patients, with granulomas and vasculitis the common findings in biopsy material. Lung infiltrates are typically multiple, nodular, bilateral lesions that frequently cavitate. Less frequently, obstructive endobronchial lesions that lead to airway obstruction and atelectasis, or pleural lesions leading to pleural effusions are found. Renal involvement is due to focal segmental glomerulonephritis that can lead to glomerular necrosis, crescent formation, and rapidly progressive renal failure. Any other organ system, most commonly skin and eyes, can be involved with small vessel vasculitis with or without granuloma formation. Although the specific mechanisms that lead to granulomatous vasculitic lesions in Wegener's granulomatosis are poorly understood, considerable evidence suggests that disordered immunity with both antibody- and cell-mediated tissue damage occurs (see Ch. 256). Approximately 50 per cent of patients have elevated levels of circulating immune complexes and test positive for rheumatoid factor, and hypergammaglobulinemia with elevations of serum IgA and IgG levels is common. Deposition of IgG and complement components as well as fibrin can be found in some renal biopsy specimens. Evaluation of pulmonary infiltrates has demonstrated predominantly T cells and macrophages in the granulomatous lesions as well as polymorphonuclear neutrophils (PMN's) in and around inflamed vessels. Some studies have suggested an abnormality of PMN's in this disease, with chemotactic defects, the presence of antineutrophil antibodies, and intravascular lysis of leukocytes reported as early events in the inflammatory process.

It is likely that more than one immunologic mechanism occurs, such that an abnormal or exaggerated antibody response to an inhaled antigen could lead to an immune complex–triggered macrophage–T cell granulomatous response centered in and around vessels.

CLINICAL MANIFESTATIONS. Although Wegener's granulomatosis most commonly presents with upper and lower airway illnesses, it is important to remember that any of the manifestations of the disease can be presenting signs and symptoms (Table 266–1). Organ systems involved during the course of the disease are multiple, with upper and lower respiratory tract, kidney, joint, ear, and eye involvement occurring in 58 to 94 per cent of patients (Table 266–2). Common upper respiratory signs and symptoms include purulent nasal discharge, fever, cough, paranasal sinus pain, nasal mucosal ulceration, and saddle nose deformity. Lung involvement can manifest as cough, hemoptysis, or shortness of breath or can be asymptomatic, with nodular infiltrates seen on routine radiographs.

Renal disease is seen in 85 per cent of patients and is a critical determinant of the clinical outcome. Wegener's granulomatosis of the respiratory tract without renal disease has been termed *limited Wegener's granulomatosis* and was initially thought to be a more benign disease than *generalized Wegener's granulomatosis* with renal and other extrapulmonary system involvement. However, most agree that the limited form constitutes an early form of the generalized disease. Renal manifestations include hematuria, azotemia, proteinuria, and pedal edema. Renal disease can be smoldering but more often, when untreated, rapidly progresses to irreversible renal failure.

TABLE 266-1. PRESENTING SIGNS AND SYMPTOMS IN WEGENER'S GRANULOMATOSIS

Sign or Symptom	%
Pulmonary infiltrates	71
Sinusitis	67
Joint (arthralgia or arthritis)	44
Fever	34
Otitis	25
Cough	34
Rhinitis or nasal symptoms	22
Hemoptysis	18
Ocular inflammation (conjunctivitis, uveitis, episcleritis, and scleritis)	16
Weight loss	16
Skin rash	13
Epistaxis	11
Renal failure	11
Chest discomfort	8
Anorexia or malaise	8
Proptosis	7
Shortness of breath or dyspnea	7
Oral ulcers	6
Hearing loss	6
Pleuritis or effusion	6
Headache	6

Reprinted with permission from Fauci AS, Haynes BF, Katz P, et al.: Wegener's granulomatosis: Prospective clinical and therapeutic experience with 85 patients for 21 years. Ann Intern Med 98:76–85, 1983.

Nearly 70 per cent of patients have some form of joint involvement during the course of the disease. Of those with joint symptoms, one third have an arthritis that is nondeforming and is usually seen in large joints, particularly ankles and knees. The remaining two thirds of patients with joint symptoms have symmetric polyarticular arthralgias without frank arthritis. Eye involvement occurs in 60 per cent of patients and is manifested as proptosis, scleritis, conjunctivitis, uveitis, dacryocystitis, and retinal or optic nerve vasculitis. Scleritis may be in the form of a corneoscleral ring ulcer and in some patients progresses to scleral perforation. Proptosis is usually due to contiguous sinus involvement, with extension of granulomatous inflammation across the lateral wall of the ethmoid sinus into the orbit. Rarely, granulomatous masses can occur in the orbits, causing proptosis in the absence of sinusitis.

Nervous system disease occurs in 20 per cent of patients, involving the peripheral nerves, with mononeuritis multiplex the most common manifestation. Central nervous system involvement can be in the form of cranial nerve dysfunction, diffuse cerebral vasculitis, or hypothalamic granulomas with clinical diabetes insipidus.

Heart involvement is manifested by pericarditis or coronary vasculitis. Less common manifestations of the disease include thyroiditis, mastoiditis, parotid masses, nasolacrimal duct obstruction, pinna and tympanic membrane granulomas, ulcerating breast masses, and anosmia.

Although no laboratory test is diagnostic of the disease, certain laboratory abnormalities are characteristic. These include ele-

TABLE 266-2. ORGAN SYSTEM INVOLVEMENT IN WEGENER'S GRANULOMATOSIS

Organ System	%
Lung	94
Paranasal sinuses	91
Kidney	85
Joints	67
Nose or naospharynx	64
Ear	61
Eye	58
Skin	45
Nervous system	22
Heart	12

Reprinted with permission from Fauci AS, Haynes BF, Katz P, et al.: Ann Intern Med 98:76–85, 1983.

vated erythrocyte sedimentation rate, neutrophilic leukocytosis, anemia, and positive test for serum rheumatoid factor. In addition, the presence of serum antineutrophil antibodies against a cytoplasmic antigen has been reported to be useful for diagnosis.

DIAGNOSIS. The diagnosis of Wegener's granulomatosis should be strongly considered when findings of upper or lower respiratory tract disease, renal disease, and vasculitis involving other organ systems are present. Since early diagnosis and institution of appropriate therapy are essential to preserve renal function and prolong survival, the disease should be considered when any of the typical disease manifestations occurs as an isolated finding (such as proptosis due to granulomatous inflammation and vasculitis) in an otherwise well patient.

To establish a definitive diagnosis of Wegener's granulomatosis, a patient should have evidence of clinical disease in at least two of the following three areas: upper airways, lung, and kidney. Biopsy results should show disease in at least one and preferably two of these organ systems, with lung tissue providing the source of highest diagnostic yield. Open lung biopsy is the procedure of choice to obtain adequate lung tissue for diagnosis. Percutaneous renal biopsy is important early in the evaluation of patients for the disease for both diagnosis and documentation of the extent of renal disease.

Recent studies have shown that serum antibodies against a phorbol myristate acetate–inducible antigen from the cytoplasm of polymorphonuclear leukocytes are specific for Wegener's granulomatosis, and the level of such antibodies correlates with disease activity in Wegener's granulomatosis. Because these antibodies can be found in the serum of patients with vasculitides that do not otherwise fulfill the criteria for Wegener's granulomatosis, at the present time, a positive test for anticytoplasmic antibodies cannot replace a histologic diagnosis.

When the classic triad of Wegener's granulomatosis occurs, the diagnosis, with differentiation from other diseases, is straightforward. However, the diagnosis may be difficult when only isolated features of the disease are present or when less commonly affected organ systems are involved. Thus, the differential diagnosis should include those diseases that can cause pulmonary-renal syndromes, such as Goodpasture's syndrome (see Ch. 79). Idiopathic midline granuloma, also called idiopathic midline destructive disease (see below), is a local disease that destroys facial and palate bones and cartilage, often eroding through maxillary and sphenoidal bones and facial cutaneous tissue. It is not a systemic vasculitis and does not involve lungs or kidneys, but because of the presence of upper airway lesions, it has been confused with Wegener's granulomatosis. Unlike midline granuloma, the lesions of Wegener's granulomatosis do not perforate the palate or erode through major bony structures of the face and upper airway. The only bone commonly destroyed in Wegener's granulomatosis is the medial wall of the orbit, called the *lamina papyracea*.

Another disease frequently confused with Wegener's granulomatosis is *lymphomatoid granulomatosis*. This is a disease characterized by infiltration of various organs with a polymorphic cellular infiltrate consisting of atypical lymphoid and plasmacytoid cells together with granulomatous inflammation in an angiocentric pattern. The disease primarily involves lungs, skin, kidneys, and central nervous system, but not upper airways. Renal involvement is not a glomerulonephritis but rather is an interstitial infiltration with masses of atypical lymphoid cells. Lymphomatoid granulomatosis, unlike Wegener's granulomatosis, is not an inflammatory vasculitis but more likely represents invasion of vessels with premalignant T cells. Up to one half of cases of lymphomatoid granulomatosis evolve into a frank T cell lymphoma that responds poorly even to combined chemotherapy regimens for non-Hodgkin's lymphoma.

TREATMENT AND PROGNOSIS. The treatment of choice for Wegener's granulomatosis is a combination of corticosteroids and a cytotoxic agent. The most efficacious cytotoxic agent in this disease is cyclophosphamide. Irreversible organ system dysfunction can occur if conservative therapy (such as corticosteroids alone) is attempted. In patients with active but stable multisystem disease, oral cyclophosphamide in a dosage of 1 to 2 mg per kilogram per day should be given, with the dosage adjusted to maintain the total leukocyte count above 3000 per cubic millimeter and the PMN count above 1000 to 1500 per cubic millimeter. Close monitoring of the white blood cell count is essential, with weekly assessments necessary to avoid severe leukopenia and infectious complications. In patients with fulminant disease, such as central nervous system vasculitis, severe pulmonary involvement with hypoxemia, rapidly progressive peripheral neuropathy, or rapidly progressive renal failure, cyclophosphamide, in a dosage of 4 mg per kilogram per day, may be given intravenously for 3 days, with a change to the lower oral dosage regimen (1 to 2 mg per kilogram per day) thereafter. Patients should be treated for 1 year after remission has been achieved, and then cytotoxic drug therapy should be stopped and the patient re-evaluated periodically for disease relapse. Complications of cyclophosphamide therapy include hemorrhagic cystitis, bone marrow suppression or failure, opportunistic infections, hair loss, gonadal dysfunction, and rarely bladder carcinoma, leukemia, or lymphoma. Because of the risk of serious complications with cytotoxic therapy, as well as the frequent symptomatic infection of previously damaged upper and lower respiratory tracts with microorganisms such as *Staphylococcus aureus,* the presence of persistent vasculitis should be well documented prior to continuation of long-term cytotoxic therapy (greater than 1 year) for presumed active disease.

Corticosteroids should be administered in an oral daily dose regimen (usually prednisone, 1 mg per kilogram per day) or in divided doses (every 6 hours) for fulminant cases for an initial period (usually 1 to 2 weeks), followed by tapering of the drug to an alternate-day regimen (see Ch. 27). After 3 to 6 months, corticosteroids can usually be discontinued altogether. With this regimen, remissions can be obtained in 90 per cent of patients with Wegener's granulomatosis, once an invariably fatal disease. Those patients who have progressed to end-stage renal failure have had successful renal transplantations while being maintained on this regimen. Patients who relapse while not taking medications or while taking low doses of medication require documentation of disease activity and diagnosis of the disease process present. It is particularly critical in the patient with a new pulmonary infiltrate who has been treated with immunosuppressive therapy to distinguish between a lung infection and a recurrence of pulmonary vasculitis. The use of trimethoprim-sulfamethoxazole oral therapy has been reported to decrease relapses in selected patients with Wegener's granulomatosis, although its use as a first-line drug for the disease remains unproved and cannot be recommended at this time.

Fauci AS, Haynes BF, Katz P, et al.: Wegener's granulomatosis: Prospective clinical and therapeutic experience with 85 patients for 21 years. Ann Intern Med 98:76, 1983. *Long-term follow-up is presented for a large group of patients, detailing presentation, clinical course, and treatment strategy.*
Fauci AS, Haynes BF, Costa, J, et al.: Lymphomatoid granulomatosis. Prospective clinical and therapeutic experience over 10 years. N Engl J Med 306:68, 1982. *Report differentiating lymphomatoid granulomatosis from Wegener's granulomatosis and describing the treatment regimen and outcome for lymphomatoid granulomatosis.*
Haynes BF, Allen NB, Fauci AS: Diagnostic and therapeutic approach to the patient with vasculitis. Med Clin North Am 70:355, 1986. *A concise review that summarizes in detailed tabular form for easy reference the diagnostic and therapeutic approach to patients suspected of having a vasculitic syndrome such as Wegener's granulomatosis.*
Kallenberg CGM, Cohen Tervaert JW, van der Woude FJ, et al.: Autoimmunity to lysosomal enzymes: New clues to vasculitis and glomerulonephritis? Immunol Today 12:61, 1991. *A recent review of the latest theories regarding the pathophysiology of Wegener's granulomatosis.*
Nolle B, Specks U, Ludemann J, et al.: Anticytoplasmic autoantibodies: Their immunodiagnostic value in Wegener granulomatosis. Ann Intern Med 111:28, 1989. *This report shows that if performed using the appropriate techniques, measurement of serum anticytoplasmic antibodies may be an adjunct to the diagnosis of Wegener's granulomatosis and may be of use in monitoring patients with Wegener's granulomatosis for disease activity.*

MIDLINE GRANULOMA

DEFINITION. Idiopathic midline granuloma, also known as idiopathic midline destructive disease, is a progressive, localized destructive process that predominantly involves the nose, paranasal sinuses, and palate, with erosion through bone and soft tissues, frequently involving the face.

ETIOLOGY. The cause of idiopathic midline granuloma is unknown. It has been suggested that the upper respiratory tract and midline facial tissues have an extraordinary capacity to react to antigenic stimulation. In true idiopathic midline granuloma, no primary infectious cause or neoplastic cells are found in involved tissue. Rather, the histologic findings of acute and chronic inflammation with widespread necrosis, with or without granuloma formation, have led to the postulate that this disease is caused by a hypersensitivity reaction to unknown inhaled antigens.

PATHOLOGY. Biopsy of the affected sites demonstrates necrosis and acute and chronic inflammation. Mucosal surfaces of the nose and paranasal sinuses are frequently ulcerated, and inflammation invades and destroys adjacent cartilage and bone. The cellular infiltrate is composed of polymorphonuclear leukocytes, lymphocytes, macrophages, plasma cells, and, less frequently, multinucleated giant cells with well-formed epithelial granulomas. Although perivascular infiltrations and vessel destruction caused by widespread inflammation are common, a primary vasculitis, as a rule, is generally not seen. If foci of atypical lymphocytes or histiocytes are seen, then the presence of an underlying lymphoma or other midline neoplasm should be suspected. Thus, the evaluation of midline granuloma should include a careful search for disseminated lymphoma and other malignancies.

CLINICAL MANIFESTATIONS. Most patients with idiopathic midline granuloma have active sinusitis with superimposed bacterial infections. Symptoms begin with nasal stuffiness and crusting and progress to purulent nasal discharge and nasal bleeding. Ulcerations may appear on the nasal septum, palate, or nose. Progressive perforation and destruction of the nasal septum can occur, resulting in a saddle nose deformity. Destruction of the soft and hard palate can take place, with reflux of food into the upper airway during eating. Paranasal inflammation with swelling is frequently present, resulting in nasolacrimal duct obstruction and dacryocystitis. Relentless midline inflammation

TABLE 266–3. COMPARISON OF CLINICAL FEATURES OF IDIOPATHIC MIDLINE GRANULOMA WITH WEGENER'S GRANULOMATOSIS AND MALIGNANT MIDLINE RETICULOSIS

Feature	Idiopathic Midline Granuloma	Wegener's Granulomatosis	Malignant Midline Reticulosis
Types of upper airway disease	Destructive lesions of sinuses, palate, nose, and facial bones with soft tissue erosions—progesses over months to years	Inflammatory upper airway disease of sinuses and nasal mucosa; palate ulcerations occur without perforation; erosion of medial wall of orbit frequent; otherwise facial bone and soft tissue erosion does not occur	Destructive lesions of sinuses, palate, nose, and facial bones with soft tissue erosion—progresses over weeks to months
Systemic involvment	Disease localized only to upper airway	Systemic involvement of multiple organs characteristic	Destructive lesion local; systemic disease related to disseminated lymphoma
Association with malignancy	None	None	Likely a midline T cell or histiocytic lymphoma
Pathology	Acute and chronic inflammation, with or without granuloma	Necrotizing granulomatous vasculitis	Atypical and pleomorphic cells or frank lymphoma
Treatment	Radiation therapy	Cyclophosphamide and corticosteroids	Radiation therapy and/or combination chemotherapy

Data from Batsakis JG: Ann Otol Rhinol Laryngol 91:541, 1982; Fauci AS, et al.: Ann Intern Med 84:104, 1976.

with necrosis can result in widespread and mutilating destruction of facial bones and tissues, with erosion into the central nervous system, leading to meningitis, or into major blood vessels, leading to life-threatening hemorrhage. Erosion into the orbit can cause retro-orbital masses and lead to orbit destruction and blindness. Loss of smell is common, and recurrent sinus infection with *Staphylococcus aureus* is routine. Most patients are free of systemic signs and symptoms, such as fever, malaise, and arthalgias, except when superimposed bacterial infections are present. There are no characteristic laboratory findings except those related to chronic inflammation and secondary bacterial infections (elevated leukocyte count, erythrocyte sedimentation rate). Computed tomograms and radiographs of the midline structures often show dramatic destruction of facial bones with evidence of widespread sinus inflammation.

DIAGNOSIS. The diagnosis of idiopathic midline granuloma is made by the characteristic clinical presentation of locally destructive lesions restricted exclusively to the upper respiratory tract and the absence of histologic evidence of Wegener's granulomatosis, infections, or lymphoma. Although midline granuloma is a distinct disease, the diagnosis is made by excluding other diseases with similar findings.

While a large number of infectious, collagen vascular, and inflammatory diseases can cause ulcerations of the nose and midline structures, the three entities that are most often confused in the differential diagnosis of idiopathic midline granuloma are presented in Table 266–3. By definition, midline granuloma is a locally destructive disease of the midline facial structures that is relentlessly progressive over months to years. It is not a primary vasculitis and thus is clearly distinct from *Wegener's granulomatosis*. Wegener's granulomatosis is a systemic primary vasculitis that can manifest sinus, nose, and palate lesions. However, the lesions are not progressive; erode only cartilage and thin facial bones, such as the medial wall of the orbit; and frequently heal spontaneously. Erosion of facial bones and tissues in the setting of Wegener's granulomatosis suggests an underlying infection or neoplasm. *Malignant midline reticulosis* is a pleomorphic lymphoma, frequently of the T cell type, that presents with extensive mucosal ulceration, tissue necrosis, bone destruction, and fistula formation in facial midline tissues. Although the clinical picture is similar to that of midline granuloma, the tempo of disease progression is more rapid, and on repeat biopsy, atypical lymphoid cells or frank lymphoma is found. The diagnosis is a difficult one, however, since the clinical picture may suggest an inflammatory process rather than tumor, and on biopsy, the malignant nature of the process may be obscured by an intense inflammatory infiltrate, presumably in response to tumor antigens.

Rarely, other lymphomas, mycosis fungoides, and nonkeratinizing squamous cell carcinomas can produce midfacial destructive lesions. Other less destructive diseases that should be considered in the differential diagnosis of idiopathic midline granuloma are *sarcoidosis* (see Ch. 67), relapsing polychondritis (see Ch. 272), and *necrotizing sialometaplasia*, a self-healing process of 6 to 8 weeks' duration that manifests with large ulcerations of the hard palate and a necrotizing process in minor salivary glands. Infectious diseases that should be ruled out include *chronic bacterial infections, tuberculosis, syphilis, rhinoscleroma* (due to *Klebsiella rhinoscleromatis*), *actinomycosis, leprosy, phycomycosis, blastomycosis, candidiasis, histoplasmosis, coccidioidomycosis,* and *leishmaniasis.* Frequently, there is evidence of secondary bacterial infection in idiopathic midline granuloma. However, for a diagnosis of midline granuloma to be made, there should be no evidence of local or disseminated neoplastic disease.

TREATMENT AND PROGNOSIS. Radiation therapy, approximately 5000 rads, to the midfacial area is the treatment of choice for idiopathic midline granuloma. Prednisone and various types of cytotoxic drug regimens have generally not been successful. Surgical procedures on involved tissues can precipitate acceleration of the destructive process. However, once the disease has been treated with radiation therapy, surgical debridement and aggressive local care measures, such as routine upper airway irrigation and treatment of bacterial superinfections, can aid the healing process. Reconstructive plastic surgery and prosthesis placement for patients with extensive facial disfigurement are often of benefit. In long-term survivors of the disease following

radiation therapy, close monitoring for radiation-induced upper airway neoplasia is essential.

Batsakis JG: Midfacial necrotizing diseases. Ann Otol Rhinol Laryngol 91:541, 1982. *A concise paper summarizing the distinguishing features of idiopathic midline granuloma compared with other syndromes.*

Fauci AS, Johnson RE, Wolff SM: Radiation therapy of midline granuloma. Ann Intern Med 84:104, 1976. *Classic paper describing the distinct clinical features of idiopathic midline granuloma and outlining successful management strategies.*

Fechner RE, Lamppier DW: Malignant midline reticulosis. A clinicopathologic entity. Arch Otolaryngol 95:467, 1972. *Detailed report characterizing this midfacial neoplasm and outlining diagnostic and histopathologic criteria.*

Fu YS, Perzin KH: Non-epithelial tumors of the nasal cavity, paranasal sinuses, and nasopharynx: A clinicopathologic study. X. Malignant lymphomas. Cancer 43:611, 1979. *An important study comparing the features of malignant midline reticulosis with other lymphomas of the head and neck.*

Tsokos M, Fauci AS, Costa J: Idiopathic midline destructive disease (IMDD): A subgroup of patients with the midline granuloma syndrome. Am J Clin Pathol 77:162, 1982. *Paper in which clear diagnostic guidelines are emphasized and a more precise term for idiopathic midline granuloma is proposed.*

267 Polymyalgia Rheumatica and Giant Cell Arteritis

Gene Hunder

Polymyalgia rheumatica and giant cell arteritis are common rheumatic diseases of middle-aged and older persons. Although the etiology of these conditions is unknown and their pathogenesis is poorly understood, it is clear that they are closely related. Some believe that a single etiology causes both conditions and that host and other unknown factors determine whether a patient will develop one or both processes. Another theory is that polymyalgia rheumatica and giant cell arteritis are a single disease but that the arteritis is clinically inapparent in many cases of polymyalgia rheumatica.

POLYMYALGIA RHEUMATICA

Polymyalgia rheumatica is characterized by aching and morning stiffness in the shoulder and hip girdles, the proximal extremities, the neck, and the torso. Usually, it is accompanied by evidence of an inflammatory reaction. The mean age at onset is about 70 years, and it nearly always occurs after the age of 50, with women affected twice as commonly as men.

CLINICAL FINDINGS. Polymyalgia rheumatica may begin abruptly but usually develops in a gradual manner over a number of weeks. In mild or early cases, the symptoms may subside 1 to 2 hours after the patient arises in the morning, only to return later after a period of inactivity. Generally, the discomfort becomes severe enough to interfere with usual activities and may confine the patient to bed. Fatigue, sense of weakness, loss of weight, and a low-grade fever may be present. Joint inflammation has been demonstrated in some cases, which supports the contention that polymyalgia rheumatica is a form of synovitis of the proximal joints and periarticular structures. Upon careful testing, muscle strength is found to be normal or nearly normal. Atrophy of the shoulder girdle muscles and restriction of motion compatible with "frozen shoulder" may evolve later. Tenderness of the painful regions is present in half the number of patients or less.

LABORATORY TESTS. A moderate normochromic normocytic anemia is typical. Usually, the erythrocyte sedimentation rate is markedly elevated, averaging 70 mm to 80 mm in 1 hour (Westergren). Other acute phase protein levels may also be elevated. The leukocyte count, the immunoglobulins, and complement all tend to be normal. About one fourth of patients have mild hepatic dysfunction that reverts to normal with treatment. Tests for rheumatoid factor and antinuclear antibodies in the serum are usually negative.

INCIDENCE. Caucasians appear to be affected more frequently than other groups. The highest recorded incidence rates are from northern Europe and the northern United States. In

TABLE 267–1. POLYMYALGIA RHEUMATICA: DIAGNOSTIC CRITERIA

>50 yr of age
Aching and morning stiffness in at least two of the following areas:
  Neck
  Shoulder girdle
  Pelvic girdle
Erythrocyte sedimentation rate (ESR) >40 mm in 1 hr
Duration of symptoms for 1 mo
No other disease present

one population study, 96 patients were identified in a Minnesota community over a 10-year period, producing an average annual incidence rate of 53.7 per 100,000 persons in those 50 years of age and older (the group at risk). The prevalence was approximately 1 in 200 persons in the population 50 years of age or older. Recent reports on incidence rates in Europe show similar findings.

DIAGNOSIS. Several criteria sets for diagnosing polymyalgia rheumatica have been suggested. Most are similar, and that set shown in Table 267–1 is useful. The morning stiffness should last at least one-half hour. The erythrocyte sedimentation rate is an indicator of systemic inflammation. An additional criterion of rapid response to 10 to 20 mg of prednisone per day is suggested by some. These criteria are only guidelines, since patients occasionally have normal sedimentation rates at onset, and a small number may develop symptoms slightly before the age of 50.

DIFFERENTIAL DIAGNOSIS (Table 267–2). A number of other illnesses may manifest similar findings. Some patients with early rheumatoid arthritis lack the more characteristic distal joint involvement and serum rheumatoid factor and have prominent proximal symptoms. A period of observation may be necessary to determine the ultimate course of the patient's illness in such cases.

Polymyositis and polymyalgia rheumatica both limit physical activity. In the former, the limitation is due to a lack of muscle strength without much discomfort on movement; in polymyalgia rheumatica, however, the limitation is associated with pain. Furthermore, in polymyositis, muscle enzymes are elevated, the electromyograms show distinctive changes, and a muscle biopsy shows an inflammatory myopathy; in polymyalgia rheumatica, these tests are normal.

The fibrositis syndrome or fibromyalgia usually affects younger individuals and tends to be associated with more tender spots on physical examination; laboratory tests are normal. When encouraged to do so, patients with fibromyalgia can move the joints through a full range of motion without great difficulty. Both conditions disturb sleep. The wakefulness in polymyalgia rheumatica is due to discomfort caused by movement in bed. In fibromyalgia, however, there is a more generalized, persistent discomfort that is less tangible. In polymyalgia rheumatica, the sounder the sleep at night, the more intense the morning stiffness. In the case of fibromyalgia, the opposite tends to be true.

Other conditions that occasionally need to be distinguished from polymyalgia rheumatica include chronic infections, such as subacute bacterial endocarditis or viral infections, malignancies, hypothyroidism, and other connective tissue diseases.

GIANT CELL ARTERITIS

Giant cell arteritis (temporal arteritis) affects large and medium-sized arteries, especially those branching from the proximal aorta that supply the neck and the extracranial structure of the head and arms. The lesions tend to be scattered irregularly along the involved vessels, but longer, continuously involved segments also occur. Upon histologic examination, a focal or diffuse granulomatous inflammatory infiltration is present with multinucleated histiocytic and foreign body giant cells, histiocytes, lymphocytes, and fibroblasts. Lymphocytes tend to be predominantly helper T cells.

CLINICAL FINDINGS. This disease affects the same population as polymyalgia rheumatica. The manifestations of giant cell arteritis are diverse, and many presentations have been described.

In most patients, symptoms or signs related to the vascular system develop at some time during the course of the disease (Table 267–3). Headache may be focal or generalized, mild or severe, transient or prolonged. Scalp tenderness may be over the arteries of the head or at other sites.

Visual symptoms are present in about one third of patients; half are transient, and half are permanent. The former includes brief visual blurring, amaurosis fugax, or diplopia. Permanent visual loss may be partial or complete and may occur without warning; about half are unilateral, and half are bilateral. The vision loss is due to narrowing or occlusion of the ophthalmic or posterior ciliary arteries. Ocular symptoms become less common a year or more after onset.

Intermittent claudication occurs in about one half of patients, with the jaw muscles most frequently involved. During mastication of firm foods such as meat, fatigue or discomfort is noted. In a small percentage of patients, claudication of the tongue or throat develops with eating and repeated swallowing. Nervous system alterations are found in up to 30 per cent; 14 per cent were found to have either mononeuritis or polyneuropathy, and 7 per cent were found to have transient ischemic attacks or strokes.

Polymyalgia rheumatica occurs in about 40 per cent of patients with giant cell arteritis. It may precede other symptoms or become manifest only during the withdrawal of corticosteroid therapy given for the arteritis. Diffuse or asymmetric myalgias, arthralgias, or joint swelling may be present in other patients with giant cell arteritis.

PHYSICAL EXAMINATION. The temporal, occipital, or other scalp or cervical arteries may be enlarged, tender, and erythematous. Bruits or pulse deficits may be present over the carotid, subclavian, or brachial arteries. Large artery involvement may be present initially or later, as part of an exacerbation. Findings in the eyes of patients with recent visual loss include

TABLE 267–2. DIFFERENTIAL FEATURES IN POLYMYALGIA RHEUMATICA AND SIMILAR DISORDERS

	Polymyalgia Rheumatica	Giant Cell Arteritis	Rheumatoid Arthritis	Dermatomyositis	Fibromyalgia
Morning stiffness > 30 minutes	+	±	+*	±	Variable
Headache and/or scalp tenderness	0	+	0	0	Variable
Pain with active joint movement	+	0	+*	0	Inconstant
Tender joints	±	0	+*	0	Tender spots
Swollen joints	±	±	+	0	0
Muscle weakness	±†	0	+*	+	0
Normochromic anemia	+	+	+	0	0
Elevated ESR	+	+	+	±	0
Elevated serum creatine kinase	0	0	0	+	0
Serum rheumatoid factor	0	0	70%	0	0
Distinct electromyographic abnormality	0	0	0	+	0
Response to nonsteroidal anti-inflammatory drug (NSAID)	±	0	+	0	0

0 = absent, + = present, ± = present in minority of cases.
* = Associated with affected joints.
† = Pain inhibits movement. Disuse atrophy may occur.

TABLE 267–3. GIANT CELL ARTERITIS: CLINICAL FINDINGS IN 94 PATIENTS*

Clinical Manifestation	Frequency (%)
Headache	77
Abnormal temporal artery	53
Jaw claudication	51
Scalp tenderness	47
Constitutional symptoms	48
Polymyalgia rheumatica	34
Fever	27
Respiratory symptoms	23
Facial pain	14
Diplopia/blurred vision	12
Transient vision loss	5
Blindness (partial or complete)	13
Hemoglobin <11.0 gm/dl	24
Erythrocyte sedimentation rate >40 mm/hr	97

*After Machado EBV, Michet CJ, Ballard DJ, et al.: Trends in incidence and clinical presentation of temporal arteritis in Olmsted County, Minnesota, 1950–1985. Arthritis Rheum 31:745–749, 1988. Adapted from Arthritis and Rheumatism Journal, copyright 1988. Used by permission of the American College of Rheumatology.

papilledema, hemorrhages, and exudates; later, optic atrophy develops.

LABORATORY TESTS. Blood tests are similar to those seen in polymyalgia rheumatica. The platelet count is generally increased. The erythrocyte sedimentation rate averages 80 mm to 100 mm in 1 hour (Westergren), but in 1 to 2 per cent of patients with active arteritis, it is normal or nearly normal. Laboratory tests in patients with visual loss or large artery involvement are not different from tests in patients without these more serious manifestations.

INCIDENCE. Reported incidence rates have varied considerably, from less than 1 per 100,000 persons 50 years of age and older in Israel to about 20 per 100,000 persons 50 years of age and older in northern Europe and the United States. Although the reasons for the variable rates are unknown, ethnic and geographic factors have been suggested. Familial cases of giant cell arteritis and polymyalgia rheumatica have been reported. Giant cell arteritis appears to be one-third as common as polymyalgia rheumatica.

DIAGNOSIS. Giant cell arteritis should be considered in any older person who has developed transient or sudden visual changes, unexplained fever, polymyalgia rheumatica or new headaches, and an elevated erythrocyte sedimentation rate. The arteries of the head, neck, and extremities should be examined carefully. Whereas the significance of slight pulse reductions or minimal degrees of thickness of a temporal artery is difficult to judge, distinct tenderness, redness, and a palpable but nonpulsatile temporal artery are more important clues to the presence of arteritis. In the absence of similar changes in the lower extremities, pulse changes or bruits over the axillary and brachial arteries are more likely to be caused by vasculitis than by arteriosclerosis.

A temporal artery biopsy is recommended for all patients suspected of having giant cell arteritis. A biopsy should be performed on the most clinically abnormal artery segment. When the arteries appear normal on examination, a segment several centimeters long should be removed from one temporal artery, and histologic sections should be examined at multiple levels in an effort to find an involved area. In our experience, if the first temporal artery biopsy is normal, the second site will yield approximately 10 to 15 per cent additional positive cases.

Some patients with polymyalgia rheumatica may be followed carefully without a temporal artery biopsy. If polymyalgia rheumatica is of recurrent onset or has been present for a year or more in the absence of signs or symptoms of vasculitis, biopsy may be deferred and the patient should be followed closely.

DIFFERENTIAL DIAGNOSIS. Conditions that have been confused with giant cell arteritis include systemic infections, amyloidosis with prominent vascular involvement, neoplasms, arteriosclerotic vascular disease in patients with an elevated erythrocyte sedimentation rate that is due to some other cause, arteriovenous fistulas, and other forms of vasculitis.

Follow-up studies of patients who have had a negative temporal artery biopsy have shown that only approximately 10 per cent develop findings of giant cell arteritis and require long-term corticosteroid therapy.

MANAGEMENT

Therapy for polymyalgia rheumatica is aimed at alleviating systemic symptoms and musculoskeletal discomfort. Patients with early or mild polymyalgia rheumatica may try taking nonsteroidal anti-inflammatory drugs. Those not improving with these drugs or those with severe symptoms should be started on 10 mg to 20 mg of prednisone (or the equivalent dose of another corticosteroid). Prednisone acts rapidly, and the patient should notice significant improvement within 24 hours. The corticosteroid dose can be reduced as tolerated after 1 month or earlier. Nonsteroidal anti-inflammatory drugs may be added to control mild discomfort that may occur while corticosteroids are being withdrawn and discontinued.

In giant cell arteritis, the recommended dosage of prednisone is 40 mg to 60 mg per day. Vascular complications seldom occur after corticosteroids have been started. If the response to the initial dose of prednisone is incomplete, the dosage should be increased by 20 mg to 30 mg per day. Usually, if symptoms subside and laboratory values return to normal with a given dose, the disease process is adequately suppressed. Prednisone for both conditions may be administered as a single morning dose or in two to three divided doses per day.

The overall goal of therapy is to administer the lowest dose of corticosteroid that adequately controls the arteritis and prescribe it for the shortest necessary time. The dose needed to achieve control varies among patients and must be determined empirically. There is no evidence that corticosteroid therapy alters the natural course of the disease.

In a small proportion of cases, the corticosteroid dose cannot be reduced without an exacerbation of the disease. Cyclophosphamide, azathioprine, dapsone, and cyclosporine have been reported as steroid-sparing drugs in some instances. However, no controlled studies of these drugs have been done. The average duration of both polymyalgia rheumatica and giant cell arteritis is about 2 years, during which time the intensity of the process may flare up at times but appears to resolve slowly. The course in individual patients, however, varies considerably, and some may continue with active symptoms for several years.

Caselli RJ, Hunder GG, Whisnant JP: Neurologic disease in biopsy-proven giant cell (temporal) arteritis. Neurology 38:352, 1988. *This is a review of the types of neurologic symptoms in 166 consecutive patients with biopsy-proven giant cell arteritis.*

Chuang TY, Hunder GG, Ilstrup DM, et al.: Polymyalgia rheumatica: A 10-year epidemiologic and clinical study. Ann Intern Med 97:672, 1982. *The incidence, manifestations, treatment, course, and outcome of polymyalgia rheumatica in a well-defined population. The relative incidence of giant cell arteritis is also discussed.*

Hunder GG: Giant cell arteritis. Clin Rheum Dis 16:399, 1990. *A discussion on pathogenesis, pathology, diagnosis, and treatment.*

Machado EBV, Michet CJ, Ballard DJ, et al.: Trends in incidence and clinical presentation of temporal arteritis in Olmsted County, Minnesota, 1950–1985. Arthritis Rheum 31:745, 1988. *The incidence and prevalence of giant cell arteritis are determined. Changes in clinical manifestations over a 35-year period are described.*

268 Polymyositis

Robert L. Wortmann

DEFINITION

Polymyositis, an inflammatory disease of skeletal muscle of unknown cause, is characterized by symmetric weakness of limb girdles, neck, and pharynx. The term polymyositis has also been used interchangeably for a group of conditions in which skeletal muscle is damaged by nonsuppurative inflammation; these conditions are more appropriately considered under the classification of idiopathic inflammatory myopathy. These disorders include the traditional diagnosis of adult polymyositis and dermatomyositis (polymyositis with characteristic skin rash) as well as childhood dermatomyositis, cancer-associated myositis, myositis associated with other connective tissue diseases (overlap syndromes), and inclusion body myositis. In this chapter the term idiopathic inflammatory myopathy is used to include all patients with these conditions, and polymyositis is used to denote the adult and prototypic category of inflammatory muscle disease.

INCIDENCE

Idiopathic inflammatory myopathy is a rare condition with an annual incidence ranging between 0.5 and 8.4 cases per million population. The incidence is highest in blacks and lowest in Japanese. Women are more affected than men by a ratio of 2:1. Female predominance is even more pronounced between ages 15 and 44 and in myositis associated with other connective tissue diseases. The sex ratio is equal in older age groups and in myositis associated with malignancy but is reversed in inclusion body myositis. Overall, the age of onset has a bimodal distribution, with peaks in children between 10 and 14 and in adults between 45 and 54. The mean age of onset for the subset of myositis with other connective tissue diseases is similar to that for the associated condition. Individuals with myositis associated with malignancy or inclusion body myositis have a mean age over 60.

PATHOLOGY AND PATHOGENESIS

Abnormalities in skeletal muscle indicative of idiopathic myopathy include muscle fiber degeneration, regeneration, necrosis, phagocytosis, and mononuclear cell infiltration. In polymyositis, necrosis of a single muscle fiber is common, and some nonnecrotic fibers are invaded by T cells and macrophages. Collections of lymphocytes, plasma cells, and histiocytes are found primarily in the endomysium. Inflammatory aggregates contain a high percentage of T cells and few B cells. Over time, fiber diameter variation increases and interstitial fibrosis develops. Although abnormalities in muscle from patients with dermatomyositis may be similar to those in polymyositis, the inflammatory cells tend to be grouped in a perivascular distribution in the perimysium and include a higher percentage of B cells. In the childhood variety of dermatomyositis, vasculopathy, including vascular endothelial hyperplasia, areas of infarction, and perifascicular atrophy, is common, and deposition of immunoglobulin G (IgG), immunoglobulin M (IgM), and C_3 is observed, particularly within the walls of intramuscular arteries and veins. In inclusion body myositis, light microscopy reveals inflammatory changes and characteristic intracellular vacuoles, which are lined with basophilic granules on cryostat sections and eosinophilic material on paraffin sections. Electron microscopy reveals either intracytoplasmic or intranuclear filamentous inclusions. The inclusions are straight and rigid and have periodic striations resembling paramyxoviruses.

The various inflammatory myopathies are believed to be immune-mediated processes that are triggered by environmental factors in genetically susceptible individuals. This theory is in part based on the prevalence of autoantibodies, inflammatory pathology, association with other autoimmune diseases, and response to corticosteroid therapy.

Many patients with polymyositis and dermatomyositis have circulating autoantibodies (Table 268–1). Some are those common in other connective tissue disease (anti-RNP, anti-SSA, anti-SSB), while others occur primarily or exclusively in myositis. The myositis-specific antibodies are directed at cytoplasmic antigens, especially aminoacyl-tRNA (transfer RNA) synthetases. Common antibodies of this type are anti–Jo-1, which is directed at histidyl-tRNA synthetase, and anti-PL7, which is directed at threonyl-tRNA synthetase. These antibodies inhibit the activity of the respective antigenic enzyme protein. Certain picornaviruses can substitute for tRNA and interact with aminoacyl-tRNA synthetase enzymes. It is interesting that some homology exists between amino acid sequences near the active site of histidyl-tRNA synthetase (Jo-1) and some capsid proteins in encephalomyocarditis virus, a *picornavirus* that induces a mouse model of polymyositis. Thus, antibodies initially directed against virus or virus-enzyme complexes could cross-react with homologous areas of host proteins or the enzyme itself. This process is termed molecular mimicry and could explain the autoantibody production.

TABLE 268–1. AUTOANTIBODIES FOUND IN PATIENTS WITH IDIOPATHIC INFLAMMATORY MYOPATHY

Autoantibody	Associated Condition
Anti-SM	SLE
Anti-RNP	SLE, MCTD
Anti-SSA (anti-Ro)	SLE, Sjögren's syndrome
Anti-SSE (anti-La)	SLE, Sjögren's syndrome
Anticentromere	CREST syndrome
Anti-SCL70	Scleroderma
Anti-PM-1	Scleroderma
Anti-Ku	Scleroderma
Anti-Jo-1	PM with interstitial lung disease
Anti-PL-7	PM with interstitial lung disease
Anti-PL-12	PM with interstitial lung disease
Anti-Mi-2	Dermatomyositis

SLE = systemic lupus erythematosus; MCTD = mixed (undifferentiated) connective tissue disease; CREST = calcinosis, Raynaud's phenomenon, esophageal dysmotility, sclerodactyly, telangiectasia; PM = polymyositis.

Several observations emphasize the importance of genetic factors in general and class II antigens (see Ch. 250) in particular in the pathogenesis of inflammatory myopathy. Almost 50 per cent of white patients with polymyositis and dermatomyositis have the HLA-DR3 (HLA, human leukocyte antigen) phenotype. This phenotype is almost always linked with HLA-B8 and is most common in patients with anti–Jo-1 antibodies. HLA-DR52 is found in all patients, black and white, who have myositis and anti–Jo-1 antibodies. The prevalence of the DR1 phenotype is increased threefold in those with inclusion body myositis compared with controls.

Viruses, particularly picornaviruses, are likely causes of myositis. Several viruses, especially coxsackievirus A9, have been associated with myositis in individual cases; elevated titers to coxsackievirus have been found in childhood dermatomyositis; mumps virus antigen has been demonstrated in inclusions in inclusion body myositis; and certain viral infections can induce inflammatory myositis in mice, with inflammation persisting long after virus can be detected. Other infectious agents such as *Toxoplasma gondii* have also been implicated in the pathogenesis of polymyositis.

The pathologic changes in polymyositis and inclusion body myositis appear to result from cell-mediated, antigen-specific cytotoxicity. In these disorders, nonnecrotic muscle fibers are found surrounded by and invaded by CD8+ mononuclear cells, with cytotoxic cells outnumbering suppressor cells by a ratio of 4:1. Studies of circulating mononuclear cells reveal decreased percentages of cells expressing CD8 and increases in those expressing the class II HLA antigen DR, as well as other T cell activation antigens (interleukin 2 receptors; Ta-1, an activation marker also associated with anamnestic responses; and TLiSA-1, a late marker associated with cytotoxic T cell differentiation).

Different immune mechanisms are evident in dermatomyositis. Mononuclear cell invasion of nonnecrotic fibers is rare, cellular infiltration is predominantly perivascular, B cells outnumber T cells, and the CD4-CD8 ratio is higher. In the circulation, DR+ cells and B cells (CD20+ cells) are increased, whereas T cells (CD3+ cells) are decreased. These findings indicate that humoral mechanisms play a significant role in the pathogenesis of dermatomyositis.

Patients with any idiopathic inflammatory myopathy can fulfill the criteria originally developed in 1975 by Bohan and Peter to define polymyositis (Table 268–2).

CLINICAL MANIFESTATIONS

Symptoms usually begin insidiously with no identifiable precipitating event. The cardinal feature of an inflammatory myopathy is symmetric muscle weakness of shoulder and pelvic girdles, at times accompanied by mild pain and tenderness. Weakness of proximal leg and arm muscles, neck flexors, respiratory muscles, and pharyngeal muscles may follow. Early symptoms include difficulty getting up from a chair, climbing stairs, and using hands above the shoulder level. Dysphagia, dysphonia, and dysarthria may develop when the disease affects the pharynx. Morning stiffness, fatigue, and other systemic symptoms are common.

TABLE 268–2. CRITERIA USED TO DEFINE IDIOPATHIC INFLAMMATORY MYOPATHY

1. Symmetric weakness of limb girdle muscles and anterior neck flexors with or without dysphagia
2. Elevation in serum of skeletal muscle enzymes, especially the creatine phosphokinase (CPK)
3. Electromyographic changes consistent with inflammatory myopathy: short, small, polyphasic motor units; fibrillations; positive waves; and bizarre, high-frequency, repetitive discharges
4. Muscle biopsy evidence of fiber necrosis, phagocytosis, and regeneration; variation in fiber size; and inflammatory exudate

Arthralgias are noted with active disease, but frank synovitis is rare. With progression, weakness can become so severe that patients cannot lift their extremities against gravity, involved muscles become atrophic, and contractures develop. An explosive onset with rhabdomyolysis, myoglobinuria, and renal failure is rare. Typically, the neurologic examination is normal except for the motor component of the examination. Deep tendon reflexes are normal or appear slightly decreased because of muscle weakness. Cranial nerve function is normal. Dysphagia is primarily due to weakness of striated musculature in the posterior pharynx and is often associated with a poor prognosis. Patients may have difficulty swallowing liquids, are prone to aspiration, and may have nasal speech. These symptoms may be accentuated by spasm or fibrosis of cricopharyngeal muscles and may require surgical treatment. Esophageal dysfunction may occur but is not often clinically significant.

Pulmonary manifestations develop in some patients because of hypoventilation secondary to muscle weakness, swallowing abnormalities with aspiration, and infection. Approximately 5 to 10 per cent develop interstitial lung disease. Some patients with interstitial pneumonitis have no respiratory symptoms. Others experience nonproductive cough and dyspnea, which may precede the onset of muscle weakness. This restrictive lung disease is associated with bibasilar fine crackles on chest auscultation and reduced diffusing capacity. Symptomatic cardiac problems are unusual, although conduction abnormalities and tachyarrhythmias may be seen on electrocardiograms. Congestive heart failure can result from hypoxemia, pulmonary hypertension, or cardiomyopathy. Raynaud's phenomenon is reported in a small percentage of patients.

Patients with polymyositis may develop periorbital edema. When other cutaneous manifestations are seen, the disease is termed dermatomyositis. Typically, the rash is erythematous and appears on the face, neck, chest, and extensor surfaces of the extremities. The name Gottron's patches is given to raised, red to violet, scaly patches seen over the knuckles, elbows, and knees. A heliotrope rash on the upper eyelids is very characteristic. Capillary nailfold changes are present in some individuals, especially those with Raynaud's phenomenon. These include dilated or distorted capillary loops, sometimes alternating with avascular areas. Childhood dermatomyositis is similar to dermatomyositis in adults except vascular involvement is more prominent. Fever, weight loss, and subcutaneous calcifications are more common, and gastrointestinal tract hemorrhage or perforation may occur.

When myositis occurs in association with another connective tissue or autoimmune disease, the associated conditions may dominate the clinical picture. The most frequently associated disease is systemic lupus erythematosus, but others include scleroderma, rheumatoid arthritis, periarteritis nodosa, giant cell arteritis, autoimmune thyroid disease, insulin-dependent diabetes mellitus, dermatitis herpetiformis, myasthenia gravis, and primary biliary cirrhosis.

Approximately 20 per cent of adults with polymyositis or dermatomyositis also have cancer. Although this may seem higher than expected for the general population, there appears to be no significant difference in the frequency of malignancy when compared with appropriate age-matched control populations. Most often the myositis and malignancy are diagnosed within a year of each other. In general, the location of the neoplasm is as would be expected for the patient's age. Overall, the most commonly associated tumors are of breast and lung. Ovarian and stomach cancers occur more frequently than in the general population; rectal and colon cancers are less frequent. Neoplastic disease is less common in patients with interstitial lung disease or in those with an associated connective tissue disease.

Inclusion body myositis occurs most commonly in older men and can differ from polymyositis by the additional features of distal muscle weakness, asymmetric muscle involvement, and neuropathic findings on physical examination.

CLINICAL COURSE AND PROGNOSIS

The overall 5-year survival rate is approximately 80 per cent, with children having the best prognosis. About half of surviving patients with polymyositis or dermatomyositis essentially recover completely. Older patients, those with associated neoplasms, or those with significant pulmonary, cardiac, and gastrointestinal involvement have a poorer prognosis. Patients with antibodies to aminoacyl-tRNA synthetases (Jo-1) or to signal recognition particles (SRP) do not respond as well to therapy. Patients with inclusion body myositis rarely improve, and they develop fixed or slowly progressive weakness.

LABORATORY DATA

Serum levels of muscle-derived enzymes are elevated at some time during the course of the disease in 99 per cent of patients. Creatine phosphokinase (CPK) levels are the most sensitive, but aldolase, transaminase (serum glutamic-oxaloacetic transaminase [SGOT] and serum glutamic-pyruvic transaminase [SGPT]), and lactate dehydrogenase (LDH) levels are also useful. CPK levels can be used as an index of disease activity or therapeutic response in some but not all patients. When normal CPK values are encountered in the presence of active disease, possible explanations include circulating enzyme inhibitors, a possible associated malignancy, or longstanding disease with severe atrophy. The MB isoenzyme of CPK may be increased in the absence of cardiac involvement owing to its presence in regenerating muscle fibers.

The erythrocyte sedimentation rate remains normal in over half the patients and, when elevated, does not correlate with the degree of weakness. Complete blood count, urinalysis, and other chemistries are usually normal unless an associated connective tissue disease or neoplasm is present.

Antinuclear antibodies are found in low titers in some patients with polymyositis. Certain antibodies (see Table 268–1) may indicate an associated connective tissue disease: anti-SM for systemic lupus erythematosus; anti-SSA and anti-SSB for Sjögren's syndrome; anticentromere for CREST syndrome (calcinosis, Raynaud's phenomenon, esophageal dysmotility, sclerodactyly, and telangiectasia); and anti–PM-1, anti-Ku, and anti-SCL70 for scleroderma. The most common specific autoantibody is to Jo-1. This is found in 10 per cent of patients with dermatomyositis and up to 50 per cent with polymyositis. The majority of patients with anti–Jo-1 antibodies have interstitial lung disease.

The electromyogram (EMG) is abnormal in almost all patients. Classic changes include the triad of (1) small-amplitude, short-duration, polyphasic motor unit potentials; (2) fibrillations, positive waves, and increased insertional irritability; and (3) spontaneous, bizarre, high-frequency discharges. In 10 per cent of patients, the EMG is entirely normal, and in some patients changes are restricted to paraspinal muscles.

DIAGNOSIS AND DIFFERENTIAL DIAGNOSIS

Criteria (see Table 268–2) are useful in establishing the diagnosis of polymyositis. Patients are classified as having definite disease with four, probable disease with three, and possible disease with two. These criteria can be employed only after excluding other causes because no change or test is specific for the diagnosis. Elevation of CPK can occur in a wide number of conditions, as well as with blunt or sharp trauma, aerobic exercise, EMG studies, muscle biopsies, or drugs (such as barbiturate or narcotics) that retard excretion of CPK in the urine. Normal blacks have higher levels of CPK than do whites, frequently with values above the normal ones established for large populations. The EMG changes seen in polymyositis are not specific. Even in the classic case, the change can be considered only myopathic and consistent with inflammation. The EMG is useful in identi-

TABLE 268–3. DIFFERENTIAL DIAGNOSIS OF MUSCLE WEAKNESS

Collagen Vascular
Polymyositis
Dermatomyositis
Polymyalgia rheumatica
Temporal arteritis
Rheumatoid arthritis
Systemic lupus erythematosus
Polyarteritis nodosa
Scleroderma

Endocrine
Hypothyroidism
Hyperthyroidism
Hyperparathyroidism
Hypocalcemia
Cushing's disease
Addison's disease
Hyperaldosteronism

Infectious
Influenza, coxsackie, human
    immunodeficiency virus
    (HIV), and other viruses
Infectious mononucleosis
Rickettsia
Toxoplasmosis
Trichinella
Schistosomiasis
Bacterial toxins:
    Staphylococcal
    Streptococcal
    Clostridial

Toxic (Drug Related)
Alcohol
Clofibrate
Cocaine
Colchicine
Cromolyn
Cyclosporine
Emetine
Gemfibrozil
Hydroxychloroquine
L-Tryptophan
Lovastatin
Penicillamine
Zidovudine (AZT)

Psychosomatic
Hysterical (?)

Idiopathic
Rhabdomyolysis
Inclusion body myositis

Neurologic
Denervating disorders
    Amyotrophic lateral sclerosis
Neuromuscular junction disor-
    ders
    Myasthenia gravis
    Eaton-Lambert syndrome
Muscular dystrophies
    Limb-girdle
    Becker's syndrome
Neuropathies
    Guillain-Barré syndrome
    Diabetes mellitus
    Porphyria

Metabolic-Nutritional
Uremia
Hepatic failure
Malabsorption
Hypercalcemia
Hypocalcemia
Hyperkalemia
Hypokalemia
Hypernatremia
Hyponatremia
Hypomagnesemia
Hypophosphatemia
Periodic paralysis
Vitamin E deficiency
Vitamin D deficiency

Carcinomatous
Neuropathy
Neuromyopathy
Myositis
Microembolization
Eaton-Lambert syndrome

Storage Diseases
    (enzyme-deficiency states)
Glycogen
    McArdle's syndrome (myo-
        phosphorylase)
    Phosphofructokinase
    Debrancher enzyme
    Brancher enzyme
    Phosphoglycerate kinase
    Phosphoglycerate mutase
    Lactate dehydrogenase
Lipid
    Carnitine (primary and
        secondary)
    Carnitine palmitoyltransferase
Purine
    Myoadenylate deaminase

muscle involvement helps differentiate myasthenia gravis, and EMG changes identify Eaton-Lambert syndrome.

Hyperthyroidism can cause proximal muscle weakness. Hypothyroidism and hyperparathyroidism (or any cause of hypercalcemia) can cause proximal weakness, elevated CPK levels, and myopathic EMG changes. Addison's disease, Cushing's disease, primary aldosteronism, and hypokalemia of any cause may lead to muscle weakness. Steroid myopathy usually begins slowly and is accompanied by other signs of glucocorticoid excess. Other drugs may cause myopathy, including alcohol, chloroquine, cimetidine, clofibrate, colchicine, emetine, heroin, lovastatin, penicillamine, phenytoin, and zidovudine.

Several metabolic myopathies can cause proximal muscle weakness, elevated CPK levels, and myopathic EMG abnormalities. These include carnitine deficiency states, myoadenylate deaminase deficiency, and McArdle's disease in some patients. Other patients with McArdle's disease and those with carnitine palmitoyltransferase deficiency develop rhabdomyolysis and symptoms after strenuous exercise. Muscles become swollen and tender and cramp. Serum CPK and urine myoglobin levels increase dramatically.

Infectious causes of chronic myositis include toxoplasmosis, trichinosis, tropical polymyositis, and several viruses, especially coxsackie and influenza. Polymyositis or a polymyositis-like syndrome can develop in some patients with acquired immunodeficiency syndrome (AIDS). Other causes of myopathic clinical presentations include eosinophilic fasciitis, hypereosinophilic syndromes, sarcoidosis, microembolization of atheromas, diabetic amyotrophy, hepatic failure, and uremia.

TREATMENT

During the active stage of the disease, bed rest is essential, and physical therapy with passive range-of-motion exercise should be performed to maintain function and avoid contractures. Smoking is prohibited, and the head of the bed should be elevated in patients at risk for aspiration. Antacids or H_2 (histamine) antagonists may also be useful to raise the pH of gastric fluids.

Treatment with corticosteroids is empiric but standard. Initially, prednisone is used in single daily doses of 1 to 2 mg per kilogram. In responsive patients, muscle strength usually improves in 1 to 2 months, and the CPK level normalizes in these months. Daily high-dose prednisone should be continued until strength has remained normal for 3 to 6 weeks. Once remission is attained, steroids are tapered very gradually, a process that may require up to 2 years. Alternate-day steroid use is recommended only when the disease is under excellent control.

Steroid failures may be attributed to inadequate initial dosage, tapering too quickly, inaccurate diagnosis, an associated malignancy, refractory disease, or coincident steroid myopathy. An improvement in muscle strength when the steroid dose is raised indicates active disease; improved strength with a lower dose of steroid signifies steroid myopathy. Immunosuppressive agents are used in refractory cases and in patients who continue to require high-dose steroid therapy. Daily oral azathioprine, weekly intravenous or oral methotrexate, or pulses of intravenous cyclophosphamide every 1 to 4 weeks may be used.

Only a small percentage of patients with inclusion body myositis respond to steroid or other immunosuppressive therapy. A therapeutic trial is indicated in this disease, but if improvement is not observed soon, drug therapy should be discontinued to avoid side effects and toxicity.

Bohan A, Peter JB, Bowman RL, et al.: A computer-assisted analysis of 153 patients with polymyositis and dermatomyositis. Medicine 56:255, 1977. *Classic paper in the field that first described the clinical spectrum of inflammatory muscle disease using a rational classification scheme.*

Kagen LJ (ed.): Myositis and myopathies. Curr Opin Rheumatol 1:415, 1989. *Includes up-to-date, expert reviews and annotated bibliographies on topics including immunologic aspects of myositis, treatment, the relationship to malignancy, and inclusion body myositis.*

Plotz PH, Dalakas M, Leff RL, et al.: Current concepts in the idiopathic inflammatory myopathies: Polymyositis, dermatomyositis, and related disorders. Ann Intern Med 111:143, 1989. *Review of present classification scheme as well as clinical features, etiology, pathogenesis, and treatment.*

fying areas of abnormality to undergo biopsy, but biopsy should not include the actual site of EMG needle insertion. Because of the symmetric nature of this disease, it is best to limit the EMG to one side of the body and take the biopsy from the other side. Although the possibility of malignancy should be considered in each patient with myositis, extensive undirected testing is not advised. Clues to the coexistence of neoplastic disease are almost always apparent on history, physical examination, or routine laboratory tests.

A variety of other diseases may cause muscle weakness (Table 268–3), and patients with these may actually fulfill some or all four criteria for polymyositis (see Table 268–2); thus, these disorders must be excluded before the diagnosis can be made. Asymmetric weakness and distal extremity involvement, as well as abnormal reflexes, altered sensation, or cranial nerve abnormalities, should suggest a neurologic disease. Patients with inclusion body myositis may be difficult to distinguish from some patients with muscular dystrophy, but in the latter family history is usually present, symptoms begin earlier in life and progress over years, and the muscles involved vary. Ocular and facial

269 Behçet's Disease

Eugene V. Ball

Although there is no invariable feature of Behçet's disease (BD), certain features occur often enough to constitute a definable syndrome and serve as the basis for diagnostic criteria. One set in common use requires the presence of recurrent oral ulcers and any two of the following: genital ulcers; uveitis; cutaneous or large vessel vasculitis; arthritis; and meningoencephalitis. An "incomplete" form has been defined as recurrent aphthous ulcers and any one of the other features. Although oral ulcers are the linchpin of diagnostic criteria, a diagnosis of probable BD is tenable when several of these features occur together in the absence of aphthous ulcers and other known causes can be excluded. Diagnosis has been possible in some patients only after as many as 20 years of minor symptoms.

CLINICAL MANIFESTATIONS

An ascertainment bias is present in reported frequencies of signs as well as differences in reported frequencies of signs between patients in Europe and America and those of the Middle and Far East. Table 269–1 lists manifestations of the disease in one group of 60 patients. Constitutional signs such as fever and weight loss were noted in 63 per cent. Other significant manifestations include meningoencephalitis and abdominal pain. At least 24 patients from Mediterranean areas have had both BD and secondary (AA) amyloidosis.

Oral ulcers are painful, are round or oval, are usually multiple, and may be the only sign of BD; on the other hand, isolated genital ulcers are seldom indicative of BD. Ulcers occur elsewhere, as in the gut and skin, and there is an assortment of nonulcerative skin lesions, such as erythema, erythema nodosum, photosensitivity, and spontaneous pustules. The pustular reaction of the skin to intradermal needle prick (sometimes referred to as pathergy) was once thought to be pathognomonic of BD, but this reaction occurs in no more than 70 per cent of patients, usually in those with extensive disease. Furthermore, it is nonspecific, occurring in 7 per cent of one group of healthy control subjects.

Ten to 15 per cent of acquired blindness among Japanese is thought to be due to the uveoretinitis of BD. Decreased visual acuity results from inflammation, secondary glaucoma, cataracts, or vitreous hemorrhage; and retinal vein thrombosis leading to sudden blindness is not rare.

Phlebitis or arteritis occur in as many as a quarter of all patients and predisposes to thrombosis or aneurysms. For example, 10 per cent of a group of 450 Tunisians had aneurysms, large artery occlusions, or both. Aneurysms are particularly common in pulmonary arteries and are most often single; as many as 14 have occurred in one patient in less than 1 year. Pulmonary vasculitis produces dyspnea, chest pain, cough, or hemoptysis and is a significant cause of death. Its radiographic signs include scattered infiltrates and pleural effusions.

The arthritis of BD is usually intermittent, self-limited, and localized to the knees and ankles; however, erosive changes have been observed in hip, heel, wrist, knee, ankle, and foot radiographs.

Aseptic meningitis occurs in almost all cases of neurologic BD; other manifestations include encephalopathy, seizures, corticospinal abnormalities, bulbar palsy, ataxia, transient ischemic attacks, strokes, and pseudotumor cerebri. These may be acute or gradual in onset, and they may resolve completely or cause death. Focal intracranial abnormalities are detected by imaging studies.

Small and large ulcers in the gut produce symptoms of inflammatory bowel disease and perforation and are more common in Japanese than in Turkish patients.

PREVALENCE

Behçet's disease is rare in the Americas and Europe. It is more prevalent, as well as virulent, in Turkey and the Middle and Far East. Evidence of BD was found in 19 of 1531 persons aged 10 or older in a field survey conducted in rural Turkey; in Hokkaido, Japan, its estimated prevalence was 1 in 1000 persons, but BD is less common in ethnic Japanese living in Hawaii. Its prevalence was estimated at 1 in 25,000 in Olmsted County, Minnesota.

TABLE 269–1. MAJOR MANIFESTATIONS OF BEHÇET'S DISEASE

Manifestation	Prevalence (%)
Mouth ulcers	97
Genital ulcers	83
Cutaneous lesions	75
Uveitis	48
Joint pain	48
Phlebitis	17

GENETICS AND PATHOLOGY

Although not considered hereditary, BD was present in members of four HLA (human leukocyte antigen)-B51–positive families. HLA-B51 has been detected in 51 per cent of BD patients versus 16 per cent of control subjects in Japan and in 62 per cent with BD versus 29 per cent of control subjects in Iraq. Histopathologic characteristics of BD are nonspecific. Despite its classification as vasculitis, fibrinoid necrosis of vessels is not usually found. Mononuclear cells, found in the epidermis and around small vessels in early lesions, are later replaced by neutrophils and plasma cells. Arteritis, which may be catastrophic, is due to inflammation of the vasa vasorum. Abnormalities of the immune system are inconstant, providing no clues to the cause and pathogenesis of BD, which remain unknown.

TREATMENT

Numerous medications have been tried for symptomatic treatment as well as for prevention. Corticosteroids are given in doses up to 1000 mg per day for serious problems, such as central nervous system disease. Colchicine has been the drug of choice for suppression of uveitis in Japan; however, cyclosporine appears to be superior to colchicine in reducing the frequency and severity of ocular attacks. Other immunosuppressive drugs have been used with variable effectiveness and toxicity. Chlorambucil (0.1 mg per kilogram per day) moderates disease expression; however, long-term use is worrisome with respect to oncogenesis. Azathioprine (2.5 mg per kilogram per day) is superior to placebo in preserving visual acuity in patients with eye disease and in reducing the frequency of oral and genital ulcers and arthritis. Acyclovir has failed to alter the course of BD.

Dilsen N, Konice M, Aral O, et al.: Behçet's disease associated with amyloidosis in Turkey and in the world. Ann Rheum Dis 47:157, 1988. *The features of 8 Turkish and 16 other patients with BD and amyloidosis are described.*

Hamza M: Large artery involvement in Behçet's disease. J Rheumatol 14:554, 1987. *Clinical descriptions of 10 of 450 patients evaluated over a 20-year period who were found to have arterial aneurysms (7) and occlusion (3).*

Lee RG: The colitis of Behçet's syndrome. Am J Surg Pathol 10:888, 1986. *A report of severe colitis requiring colectomy and a review of 29 other published cases.*

Masuda K, Urayama A, Kogure M, et al.: Double-masked trial of cyclosporine versus colchicine and long-term open study of cyclosporin in Behçet's disease. Lancet 1:1093, 1989. *A randomized, 16-week, double-blind study comparing colchicine and cyclosporine in 49 and 47 patients, respectively. Thirty-six patients were enrolled in a long-term study of mean duration of 44 weeks.*

Raz I, Okon E, Chajek-Shaul T: Pulmonary manifestations in Behçet's syndrome. Chest 95:585, 1989. *Seven of 72 patients had pulmonary vascular disease manifested as dyspnea, cough, chest pain, and hemoptysis. The clinical and radiographic data of these and 42 other patients were reviewed.*

Yazici H, Pazarli H, Barnes CG, et al.: A controlled trial of azathioprine in Behçet's syndrome. N Engl J Med 322:281, 1990.

270 Panniculitis and Disorders of the Subcutaneous Fat

Gerald S. Lazarus

The subcutaneous tissue is a fibrofatty layer spread between skin and muscles. It functions not only as a thermal and mechanical insulator but also as an active metabolic organ. The characteristic signet ring lipocytes are organized into lobules by fibrous septa, which are continuous with the dermis and contain the blood and lymph vessels and reticuloendothelial cells.

The diagnosis of panniculitis frequently requires deep skin biopsy. The most important histologic characteristic is the location of the inflammatory process. Inflammation primarily in the septa is designated *septal panniculitis,* whereas inflammatory cells primarily in the fat lobules are called *lobular panniculitis.* The presence or absence of vasculitis further differentiates panniculitis into four major groups.

LOBULAR PANNICULITIS WITHOUT VASCULITIS. Nodular Panniculitis—Weber-Christian Disease. Nodular panniculitis describes a group of syndromes or diseases characterized by subcutaneous nodules and inflammatory cells in the fat lobules. The term Weber-Christian disease is applied when cutaneous lesions are associated with systemic complaints; this eponym should be abandoned because lobular panniculitis includes a variety of distinctive disease entities.

The etiology of this group of diseases is unknown. In the early stages, the fat lobules are infiltrated with polymorphonuclear leukocytes. Later, macrophages appear and ingest fat, producing the characteristic lipophagic granuloma. The lesions heal with lobular fibrosis. Modest septal vasculitis may be observed.

Lobular panniculitis most commonly occurs in women between the ages of 30 and 60, although cases have been reported in all age groups. The lesions begin as red, slightly tender nodules deep in the skin. They appear more or less in symmetric crops on thighs and lower legs, but lesions may also occur on arms, trunk, and face. The number of lesions may vary enormously. The lesions become firmer, less red, and less tender over a period of weeks. They heal, leaving a depressed, hyperpigmented scar. *Liquefying panniculitis* is a variant in which the lesions become necrotic and drain an oily, yellow-brown fluid. A substantial number of patients with this clinical picture may have α_1 proteinase deficiency. Biopsy reveals polymorphonuclear leukocytes in the deep reticular dermis as well as in the fat. *Rothmann-Makai syndrome,* a very rare variant of lobular panniculitis, affects children, in whom numerous large lesions develop; the lesions do not liquefy, and healing usually occurs within 12 months.

Systemic nodular panniculitis is a widespread process affecting cutaneous and visceral fat. Patients usually present with unequivocal cutaneous nodules and arthralgias, malaise, fatigue, weight loss, and abdominal pain. Involvement of the bone marrow may produce anemia, leukocytosis or leukopenia, and bone pain. Hepatomegaly, steatorrhea, and intestinal perforation have also been reported. Inflammation may occur in other internal organs, such as lungs, pleura, pericardium, spleen, kidney, and adrenal glands. Visceral involvement may be confined to the retroperitoneal space, producing abdominal pain, nausea, and vomiting. Mesenteric panniculitis resulting in abdominal pain, diarrhea, constipation, and occasional mass lesions may occur without cutaneous findings. Histiocytic cytophagic panniculitis is a disease characterized by panniculitis, fever, serositis, reticuloendotheliomegaly, and a poor prognosis; it is diagnosed by the presence of T lymphocytes and histiocytosis with phagocytosis of erythrocytes, leukocytes, and platelets.

The prognosis of nodular panniculitis is good in patients with only cutaneous involvement. Remissions and exacerbations of the lesions are frequent. Some patients recover after a few months, and permanent remission is usual after several years. On rare occasions, visceral involvement may be fatal.

No specific therapy exists for this disease. Saturated potassium iodide, increasing from five drops three times per day by one drop per day to 30 drops three times per day, has been suggested. Hydroxychloroquine,* 200 mg two times per day, has also been advocated as treatment. High-dose prednisone, 40 to 60 mg for 1 to 2 weeks, with gradual tapering over 6 to 8 weeks, has also been reported to be of value in patients with severe disease; steroids should be used *only for acute* attacks and for limited periods. There are anecdotal reports that cyclosporine may be of value in patients with severe panniculitis.

Lobular Panniculitis Associated with Pancreatic Disease. The diagnosis is made by skin biopsy, which discloses acute fat

---

* This use is not listed in the manufacturer's directive.

necrosis with characteristic ghost cells. These patients often have associated arthritis, ascites, and eosinophilia. Acute pancreatitis, trauma to the pancreas, chronic pancreatitis, pancreatic cysts, and pancreatic carcinoma have been reported to be associated with this syndrome. Diagnosis depends upon the histologic findings at skin biopsy and documentation of a specific pancreatic abnormality. Therapy is directed at the underlying pancreatic disease.

Poststeroid Lobular Panniculitis. Children who receive large doses of steroid for a short period, followed by abrupt discontinuance, may develop lobular panniculitis. Lesions may occur in the viscera, and a fatal case has been reported.

Physical Lobular Panniculitis. Physical trauma of any kind and cold injury, especially in children, can produce lobular panniculitis. A unique traumatic panniculitis occurs in the breasts of obese women in their 50's. Injection of silicones or other foreign materials into female breasts or buttocks and into the male genitalia may induce a granulomatous foreign body nodular panniculitis. Similar inflammatory lesions may be seen following injection of pentazocine (Talwin).

Lobular Panniculitis Associated with Systemic Disease. Lupus erythematosus, sarcoidosis, granuloma annulare, Sweet's disease, acute sudden weight loss from gastrointestinal surgery, and infections, including those caused by deep fungi, mycobacteria, and pyogens, may present as lobular panniculitis. Any patient with acquired immunodeficiency syndrome (AIDS) who has panniculitis must have a biopsy performed and the tissue sent for histologic study and culture to rule out infectious agents. Lymphoma or leukemia may also present as panniculitis; histologically, these lesions demonstrate malignant cells in the fat lobules. Lupus erythematosus confined primarily to the fat is known as lupus profundus. The skin may be exclusively involved, or the panniculitis may be associated with systemic disease.

Lobular Panniculitis with Vasculitis. This category of disease includes *nodular vasculitis* and *erythema induratum.* The eruption consists of recurring, tender, painful nodules on the calves, which often ulcerate and heal with scarring. It is much more common in females than in males. Increased erythrocyte sedimentation rate and hypertension have been associated with this syndrome. Bazin gave the name erythema induratum to this disease when histologic examination revealed caseation necrosis, and the lesions were associated with tuberculosis.

There is no specific therapy. Most patients experience remission of lesions with bed rest. Severe cases have been successfully treated with nonsteroidal anti-inflammatory drugs, dapsone, and prednisone. In the very rare case of nodular vasculitis associated with tuberculosis, appropriate antituberculous therapy is indicated.

SEPTAL PANNICULITIS WITHOUT VASCULITIS. This histologic picture in a patient with nodular, painful, tender lesions, especially on the anterior leg, is diagnostic of *erythema nodosum,* which is discussed in Ch. 525. A chronic disease similar to erythema nodosum clinically and histologically except that the lesions spread peripherally over months, forming rings, is called *subacute migratory panniculitis.* This disease responds to therapy with increasing doses of saturated potassium iodide as described for nodular panniculitis. Septal panniculitis without vasculitis can also be seen in scleroderma, dermatomyositis, and necrobiosis lipoidica diabeticorum. Eosinophilic fasciitis can mimic septal panniculitis. Ingestion of pharmacologic doses of tryptophan for pain or depression has produced a syndrome mimicking acute scleroderma or eosinophilic fasciitis. These diagnostic possibilities should be investigated in all patients.

SEPTAL PANNICULITIS WITH VASCULITIS. *Thrombophlebitis* may present with subcutaneous nodules. Histology reveals inflammation of veins with adjacent panniculitis (see Ch. 54).

Cutaneous polyarteritis is a chronic, recurring, painful nodular eruption, primarily of the legs. An associated mottled livedo vascular pattern is often present. Cutaneous polyarteritis is associated with myalgias, arthralgias, and increased erythrocyte sedimentation rate. Histologic examination demonstrates leukocytoclastic vasculitis of medium-sized arterioles. This disease is not usually associated with systemic involvement. It has a benign course, but lesions may recur for years.

Therapy includes nonsteroidal anti-inflammatory agents and short courses of corticosteroids. Cutaneous polyarteritis associated with granulomatous bowel disease has responded to short courses of cyclophosphamide (Cytoxan).

LIPOATROPHY. Loss of subcutaneous tissue can occur as a consequence of healing in almost any of the panniculitides described previously. The most common diagnosable cause of lipoatrophy is recurrent insulin injection. Insulin lipoatrophy is usually associated with repetitive injections of high doses of insulin in exactly the same location in females. Injections of pentazocine (Talwin) may also produce panniculitis and severe lipoatrophy.

Total lipoatrophy associated with diabetes may occur in children and adults. The clinical picture is dramatic, and there is almost complete loss of subcutaneous fat. Partial lipoatrophy usually begins in children or young adults. It is five times more common in females than in males. Patients often lose the fat in the face and the upper half of the body. In some cases, there is hypertrophy of the fat on the lower half of the body. Patients with partial lipodystrophy often develop progressive mesangiocapillary glomerulonephritis and hypocomplementemia. Diabetes develops in one third of these patients. Retinitis pigmentosum has also been reported with this disease. The prognosis depends upon the severity of the renal disease.

Ackerman AB: Panniculitis. In Ackerman AB: Histologic Diagnosis of Inflammatory Skin Diseases. Philadelphia, Lea & Febiger, 1978, pp 779–826. An outstanding review of the classification and histopathology of panniculitis.

Alegre VA, Winkelmann RK: Clinical and laboratory studies. Histiocytic cytophagic panniculitis. J Am Acad Dermatol 20:177, 1989.

Bondi EE, Lazarus GS: Panniculitis. In Fitzpatrick TB, Eisen AZ, Wolff K, et al. (eds.): Dermatology in General Medicine. 3rd ed. New York, McGraw-Hill Book Company, 1986, pp 1131–1148. A complete overview of panniculitis, emphasizing clinical description, mechanisms, and treatment.

Hendrick SJ, Silverman AK, Solomon AR, et al.: Alpha 1–antitrypsin deficiency associated with panniculitis. J Am Acad Dermatol 18:684, 1988.

Panush RS, Yonker RA, Dlesk A, et al.: Weber-Christian disease. Medicine 64:181, 1985. Excellent review of 15 patients and the world literature.

Wexner SD, Attiyeh FF: Mesenteric panniculitis of the sigmoid colon. Report of two cases. Dis Colon Rectum 30:812, 1987.

271 Crystal Deposition Arthropathies

H. Ralph Schumacher, Jr.

At least three different calcium-containing crystals are now known to deposit in joints and to be associated with a variety of patterns of arthritis in much the same way as urate crystals cause the various features of gouty arthritis. Calcium pyrophosphate and occasionally calcium oxalate produce linear or punctate calcifications in menisci and articular cartilage that can be readily seen on roentgenograms (Figs. 271–1 and 271–2). These calcifications are termed chondrocalcinosis. Both these crystals and calcium apatite can also deposit diffusely in synovium and periarticular tissues, giving a soft tissue pattern on roentgenograms. Radiographs may not show obvious calcifications when crystals are relatively few. Definitive diagnosis is made only by aspiration of synovial fluid for identification of the crystal type.

CALCIUM PYROPHOSPHATE DIHYDRATE (CPPD) CRYSTAL DEPOSITION DISEASE (Pseudogout Syndrome)

This disease is defined by the identification of rod- or rhombus-shaped 2- to 20-μm long, weakly birefringent crystals with positive elongation in synovial fluid or articular tissue. This is a common cause of arthritis; it is most frequent in the elderly. Up to 27 per cent of nursing home patients in their 80's have radiographic evidence of chondrocalcinosis on this basis. Familial cases have been described in populations of various ethnic origins. Both sexes are affected.

The cause of CPPD crystal deposition is not established but

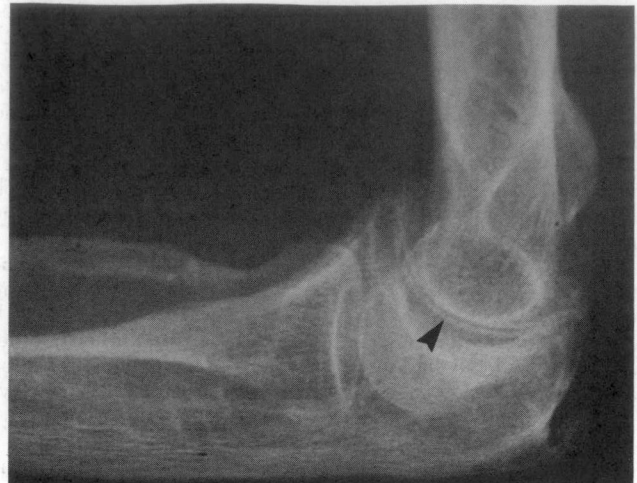

FIGURE 271–1. Chondrocalcinosis (*arrow*) at the elbow joint.

local overproduction of pyrophosphate related to excessive activity of nucleoside triphosphate pyrophosphohydrolase, deficiency of phosphatases, and local changes in proteoglycans are probably important. CPPD crystals deposit only in joints and adjacent tendons or bursae, where they produce hematoxyphilic clumps replacing the normal tissue. Virtually any joint can be involved, but knees, wrists, and second and third metacarpophalangeal joints are most common, so that chronic cases can be confused with rheumatoid arthritis. Acute bouts of crystal-induced arthritis at one or more joints can mimic gout and lead to "pseudogout." Fever with bouts can mimic infection. CPPD crystal deposition often complicates osteoarthritis; this association is more prominent at knees than at hips. Whether crystals contribute to cartilage degeneration in osteoarthritis is not yet clear. Occasional severe arthritis mimics the destruction seen in neuropathic joints. Radiographic evidence of calcification can be present in some cases for years without inducing any symptoms. Others may have crystals in joint fluid with osteoarthritis-like radiographic changes but no visible chondrocalcinosis.

Synovial effusions may have leukocyte counts up to 100,000 per cubic millimeter and with 80 to 90 per cent neutrophils during acute attacks. Between attacks crystals can be seen in clear, noninflammatory joint effusions.

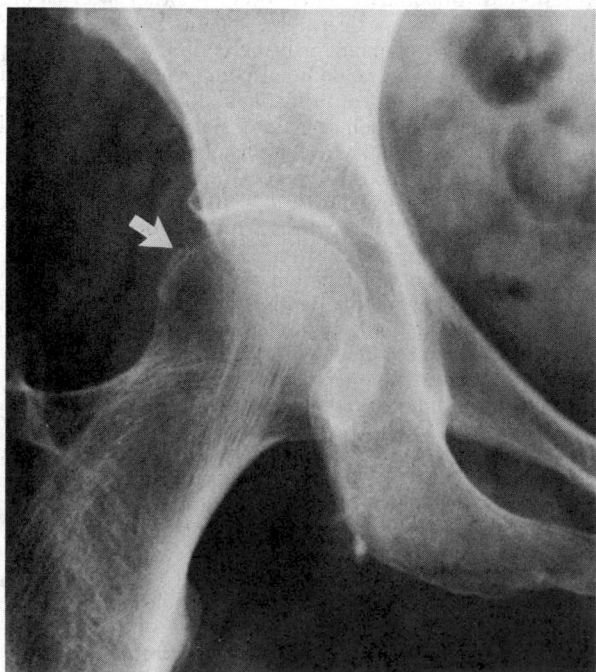

FIGURE 271–2. Chondrocalcinosis in the articular cartilage of the femoral head.

TABLE 271–1. SYSTEMIC CONDITIONS ASSOCIATED WITH CPPD DEPOSITION DISEASE

Hyperparathyroidism
Hemochromatosis
Hypophosphatasia
Hypomagnesemia
Myxedematous hypothyroidism
Ochronosis

CPPD crystal deposition can be an important clue to a number of associated diseases, many of which have specific treatments that can control systemic features if not the arthropathy. Some clearly associated diseases are shown in Table 271–1. CPPD crystal deposition is increased in knees after meniscectomy and may complicate advanced arthritides, such as gout and rheumatoid arthritis.

Treatment of inflammatory episodes with thorough joint aspiration and use of nonsteroidal anti-inflammatory drugs (NSAID's) is generally successful. Intra-articular steroid injections may provide relief in refractory involvement of individual joints. Intravenous colchicine may also be helpful. Chronic therapy with 0.6 to 1.2 mg of colchicine per day can greatly decrease the frequency of acute attacks. Otherwise the prognosis is for slow progression. Joint replacement has been successful when needed.

Alvarellos A, Spilberg I: Colchicine prophylaxis in pseudogout. J Rheum 13:804, 1986. *Colchicine seems well worth trying to prevent acute exacerbations.*
Rachow JW, Ryan LM: Partial characterization of synovial fluid nucleotide pyrophosphohydrolase. Arthritis Rheum 28:1377, 1985. *Overproduction of pyrophosphate by this soluble extracellular enzyme is one possible factor in CPPD crystal deposition.*
Rahman MU, Shenberger KN, Schumacher HR: Initially unrecognized calcium pyrophosphate dihydrate deposition disease as a cause of fever. Am J Med 89:115, 1990. *Even mild crystal-induced joint findings can cause potentially confusing fever.*
Sokoloff L, Varma AA: Chondrocalcinosis in surgically resected joints. Arthritis Rheum 31:750, 1988. *Association of crystals and osteoarthritis is reviewed. CPPD occurs more often in knees than in hips involved with osteoarthritis.*

APATITE CRYSTAL DEPOSITION DISEASE

Individual apatite crystals can be seen only by electron microscopy, but clumps of these crystals appear as 2- to 25-μm shiny (but not generally birefringent) globules that can suggest the diagnosis. Apatite crystal deposition and crystal-induced inflammation are common factors in bursitis and periarthritis. Apatites also occur in some otherwise unexplained acute arthritis, and as with CPPD crystals are common in osteoarthritic joint effusions. Most joints or bursae can be involved, with more common sites including shoulders, hips, knees, and digits. Joint or periarticular inflammation can be acute or chronic. An extremely destructive arthritis has been noted especially at shoulders ("Milwaukee shoulder"), hips, and knees. Radiographs can show soft tissue calcifications with or without bone erosions. Definitive diagnosis of the crystal type is only by electron microscopy with electron probe elemental analysis, x-ray diffraction, or infrared spectroscopy. Other basic calcium phosphates, such as octacalcium phosphate, can be seen along with the apatite. Synovial or bursal effusions can have many or few leukocytes. Serum studies are generally normal except that phosphate levels are often elevated in renal dialysis patients, who are at high risk of apatite deposition.

Apatite deposition can also be associated with scleroderma and the other connective tissue diseases, with repeated depot corticosteroid injections, with tumoral calcinosis due to renal phosphate retention, with central nervous system injury, and with high-dose vitamin D therapy. In most instances the cause of soft tissue apatite deposition is not known. Treatment for acute arthritis or periarthritis is with NSAID's or colchicine. Aspiration of crystals and local injection with depot corticosteroids can also be effective.

Doherty M, Holt M, MacMillan P, et al.: A reappraisal of "analgesic" hip. Ann Rheum Dis 45:272, 1986. *Destructive hip arthritis like the "Milwaukee shoulder" is felt to be related to apatite crystal deposition.*
Paul H, Reginato AJ, Schumacher HR: Alizarin red S staining as a screening test to detect calcium compounds in synovial fluid. Arthritis Rheum 26:191, 1983. *This describes a simple office screening test for apatite and other calcium-containing crystals.*
Pinals RS, Short CL: Calcific periarthritis involving multiple sites. Arthritis Rheum 9:566, 1966. *This recurrent calcific periarthritis is related to apatite crystals.*

Schumacher HR, Somlyo AP, Tse RL, et al.: Arthritis associated with apatite crystals. Ann Intern Med 87:411, 1977. *Clinical picture, diagnostic evaluation, and review.*

OXALATE CRYSTAL DEPOSITION DISEASE

Calcium oxalate deposition can occur in joints along with other tissues of patients with renal failure who are on chronic hemodialysis or peritoneal dialysis, producing radiographic evidence of soft tissue calcification or chondrocalcinosis. Acute or chronic joint effusions with intracellular crystals can be seen. Masses of vertebral oxalates can cause spinal cord compression. Diagnosis is made by identification of typical bipyramidal crystals in joint fluid or biopsy specimens. When less characteristic crystals are seen, other techniques as described under apatite deposition can be used. Vitamin C may potentiate oxalate deposition, so this might be avoided.

Hoffman EC, Schumacher HR, Paul H, et al.: Calcium oxalate microcrystalline-associated arthritis in end stage renal disease. Ann Intern Med 97:36, 1982. *Three cases with oxalosis and arthritis are described. Methods to identify oxalate crystals are included.*
Reginato AJ, Kurnik BRC: Calcium oxalate and other crystals associated with kidney disease and arthritis. Semin Arthritis Rheum 18:198, 1989. *Extensive oxalosis can involve skin, bursae, tendon sheaths, and joints, as well as kidneys and various viscera.*

GOUT

Monosodium urate (MSU) crystal deposition (see Color Plate 4C) in joints and other connective tissues accounts for the most frequent clinical manifestations of gout. The complex genetic, metabolic, and renal factors that interact to produce hyperuricemia and eventually gout are described in detail in Ch. 183. Gouty arthropathy and the gross tophaceous deposits in chronic gout are also described in Ch. 183 but are summarized here, as gout is the most common and prototypical of the crystal deposition diseases.

MSU crystals are rods or needles up to 15 to 20 μm in length and are brightly birefringent with negative elongation when viewed with compensated polarized light. Those from visible tophi or synovial microtophi tend to be more often needle-like. At least some crystals are intracellular during gouty arthritis. Leukocyte counts during attacks usually range from 10,000 to 50,000 per cubic millimeter, with 80 to 90 per cent neutrophils. Gout is most common in middle-aged men but is increasingly seen in women after the menopause and is very rarely noted in premenopausal women but may occur with chronic renal failure. A variety of lower extremity joints are commonly involved, in addition to the classic first metatarsophalangeal joint, but any joint or bursa, including those in the upper extremities, can be affected by either acute or chronic arthritis. Chronic or recurrent acute gout can be polyarticular, can mimic rheumatoid arthritis, and may be misdiagnosed, especially if the typical dramatic early short-lived attacks are not appreciated and synovial fluid is not examined. Tophaceous gout can slowly destroy joints. Crystals are often present in joint fluids even between attacks and may contribute to low-grade inflammation and joint damage.

Radiographs show only soft tissue swelling early in gout but later can reveal cystic erosions with thin, overhanging edges of bone suggestive of gout. Soft tissue tophi are common around joints, in bursae, in Achilles tendons, and at the extensor surface of the forearm; ear tophi appear to be less common than in the past. Gout should be recognized as a syndrome resulting from the many possible causes noted in Ch. 183.

Treatment of acute gouty arthritis can be with NSAID's (although relatively high doses are needed), oral or intravenous colchicine, adrenocorticotropic hormone (ACTH), or prednisone. The last two agents may be needed in complicated patients with renal failure, liver disease, or gastrointestinal disease. Joint aspiration with instillation of depot corticosteroids may also be used if a single joint is involved and infection is excluded. If recurrent attacks develop, chronic low doses of NSAID's or colchicine can suppress inflammation, but crystal accumulation will often continue. Thus, with more frequent attacks or visible tophi, patients should be considered for long-term lowering of urate levels with a uricosuric agent such as probenecid (if renal function is good and the patient is not overexcreting uric acid) or, in other cases, allopurinol, a xanthine oxidase inhibitor.

Lawry GV, Fan PT, Bluestone R: Polyarticular versus monoarticular gout. A prospective, comparative analysis of clinical features. Medicine 67:335, 1988. *Polyarticular gout and other crystal-associated diseases continue to be misdiagnosed without synovial fluid analysis. Fever and other constitutional symptoms are common.*

Wallace SL, Singer JZ: Therapy in gout. Rheum Dis Clin North Am 14:441, 1988. *Some of the complex situations involved in therapy of acute and chronic gout are reviewed. There are risks both from disease progression and from drug toxicities. Colchicine, NSAID'S and allopurinol all require care in appropriate use.*

272 Relapsing Polychondritis

H. Ralph Schumacher, Jr.

This uncommon disease is characterized by recurrent inflammation and destruction of cartilaginous and other connective tissue structures. Frequently involved cartilages are the pinnae of the ears, nasal cartilages, and tracheal rings. Polychondritis occurs nearly equally in both sexes and at any age, but with a peak of onset between the ages of 40 and 60.

The pathologic lesion seen by light microscopy consists of loss of matrix staining, predominantly superficial infiltration with polymorphonuclear neutrophils or lymphocytes, and eventual destruction of normal structures followed by fibrosis. Electron microscopy in addition shows alterations of superficial chondrocytes, matrix, and elastic fibers. The cause of polychondritis is unknown, but the location of lesions and frequency of associated systemic diseases suggest the importance of systemic factors. Antibodies to type II collagen and the presence of cell-mediated immunity to proteoglycan and type II collagen are evidence of immunologic aberrations.

Inflammation of the cartilaginous structures of the ears is the most common initial finding (see Color Plate 10*B*). There may be acute onset of pain and tenderness with erythema and swelling of one or both helices. The lobe is spared. Inner and middle ear involvement can occur, causing hearing loss or vertigo. Nasal cartilage involvement can produce a saddle nose. Laryngeal and tracheal disease can cause hoarseness or life-threatening upper respiratory obstruction. Ocular manifestations are common and include conjunctivitis, episcleritis, iridocyclitis, proptosis, and rarely other problems, such as optic neuritis. Antigens in the eye that are cross reactive with cartilage proteoglycans and their link protein have been identified.

Cardiac involvement, especially of the aortic root with aortic insufficiency, is seen in up to one fourth of cases. There may also be aortic aneurysms. Arthritis is reported in about three fourths of cases. This is generally nondestructive. Fever, rashes, oral or genital ulcers, and neurologic and renal disease can occur. Renal involvement can include glomerulonephritis and immunoglobulin A (IgA) nephropathy.

There are no diagnostic laboratory tests, although the erythrocyte sedimentation rate is often elevated. There may be anemia and leukocytosis. Roentgenograms can detect advanced tracheal narrowing. Cine computed tomographic (CT) scans and pulmonary function tests can detect more subtle airway obstruction.

Relapsing polychondritis is associated with other diseases in one third or more of cases. These include rheumatoid arthritis, systemic lupus erythematosus, Sjögren's syndrome, thyroid disease, ulcerative colitis, psoriasis, spondylarthropathies, Behçet's disease, vasculitis of various types, cryoglobulinemia, diabetes mellitus, biliary cirrhosis, panniculitis, malignancies, sinusitis, and mastoiditis. Lesions of Wegener's granulomatosis can mimic polychondritis.

In mild cases nonsteroidal anti-inflammatory agents can be used for symptomatic treatment, although adrenocorticosteroids in the range of 30 to 60 mg of prednisone per day are generally needed for acute inflammatory episodes and severe respiratory involvement. There is no evidence that steroids alter the long-term course of the disease. Immunosuppressives and cyclosporin A have been used with apparent benefit. Dapsone has been used with variable results in several series.

The course is unpredictable, with about 55 per cent of subjects surviving for 10 years. Infection and systemic vasculitis caused more deaths than did airway obstruction in a recent series. Remissions do occur. Aortic valve disease has required surgery.

Chang-Miller A, Okamura M, Torres VE, et al.: Renal involvement in relapsing polychondritis. Medicine 66:202, 1987. *Glomerulonephritis often responds to corticosteroids or cytotoxic agents.*

Ebringer B, Rook G, Swana T, et al.: Autoantibodies to cartilage and type II collagen in relapsing polychondritis and other rheumatic diseases. Ann Rheum Dis 40:473, 1981. *Immune mechanisms are described and discussed.*

Govet D, Marechaud R, Neu JPH, et al.: Relapsing polychondritis. A critical analysis of the therapeutic effectiveness of dapsone. Presse Med 13:723, 1984. *This interesting agent is not invariably effective.*

Michet CJ, McKenna CH, Luthra HS, et al.: Relapsing polychondritis. Survival and predictive role of early disease manifestations. Ann Intern Med 104:74, 1986. *Anemia, saddle nose deformity, and vasculitis appear to be poor prognostic signs.*

Pazirandeh M, Ziran BH, Khandelwal BK: Relapsing polychondritis and spondylarthropathies. J Rheum 15:630, 1988. *In addition to the many associated autoimmune diseases, one must also consider a possible relationship to psoriasis and spondylarthropathy.*

273 Osteoarthritis (Degenerative Joint Disease)

David S. Howell

Osteoarthritis is a complex response of joint tissues to aging and to genetic and environmental factors, characterized by degeneration of cartilage, bone remodeling, and overgrowth of bone. *Idiopathic osteoarthritis* refers to the common variety encountered during aging that is unrelated to known systemic or local diseases and includes certain hereditary and erosive subsets. *Secondary* osteoarthritis refers to the form that is indistinguishable from the idiopathic (primary) type on a pathologic basis but that is clearly provoked by antecedent events, such as an inflammatory, metabolic, endocrine, developmental, or heritable connective tissue disorder (Table 273–1). Effects of a macrotrauma, repeated microtrauma, or prolonged immobilization on normal joints may predispose the joints to secondary osteoarthritis.

When bone hypertrophy estimated by roentgenographic changes is used as a criterion, the majority of the population over 50 years of age is afflicted with osteoarthritis. By the eighth decade there is evidence of disease in 90 per cent of persons. It is the leading cause of joint pain and related disablements in middle-aged and elderly patients.

PATHOLOGY. Minor cartilage softening in non–weight-bearing sites and hypertrophic bone changes may persist a lifetime without producing symptoms. Osteoarthritis depends on development of progressively deepening clefts and erosions, typically in weight-bearing sites. The disease advances over a period of years but rarely reaches the level of severity seen in rheumatoid arthritis; i.e., there is rarely joint fusion or pannus formation, and major subluxations are uncommon.

The earliest histologic changes may be documented in the surface, subsurface, and deep zones of articular cartilage. These changes include loss of staining reactions for proteoglycans, with areas of cell injury, or loss followed by proliferation. Clefts, microcysts, and erosions arise at the site of these changes. Aggressive lesions consist usually of vertical clefts in cartilage, which progress to deep erosions and exposure of subchondral bone. Bone thickening, eburnation, cysts, and bone-on-bone contact across the joint surface typify end-stage disease.

ETIOLOGY. The most accepted premise is that primary changes in articular cartilage underlie development of osteoarthritis. Nevertheless, in a substantial subset of patients, biomechanical deficiencies arising from dysplasias of major or minor nature are causative. Similar biomechanical deficiencies may arise that are related to adolescent and adult remodeling of bones and abnormal distribution of weight-bearing forces (Table 273–1).

Repeated industrial or sports-invoked macrotraumatic and microtraumatic events may produce excessive wear and hypertrophic remodeling responses. Evidence has been obtained for

TABLE 273–1. ETIOLOGIC CLASSIFICATION OF OSTEOARTHRITIS*

Idiopathic (primary)
Localized
  Hands: Heberden's nodes, erosive interphalangeal
    arthropathy
  Feet: hallux valgus, hammer toes; talonavicular osteoarthritis
  Knees: medial, lateral, patellofemoral compartments
  Hips: sites of cartilage loss—eccentric (superior), concentric (axial,
    medial), diffuse
  Spine: zygoapophyseal joints, osteophytes, intervertebral discs
    (spondylosis); ligaments, e.g., disseminated idiopathic skeletal
    hyperostosis
  Other single sites: shoulder, temporomandibular, carpometacarpal
    joints
Generalized—Includes three or more areas listed above
Mineral deposition diseases
  Calcium pyrophosphate deposition disease
  Hydroxyapatite arthropathy
  Destructive disease (e.g., Milwaukee shoulder)

Secondary
Post-traumatic
Congenital or developmental
  Legg-Calvé-Perthes hip dislocation
  Epiphyseal dysplasias
  Articular cartilage disorders associated with a gene deficiency (e.g.,
    association with type II procollagen gene mutation)
Disturbed local tissue structure by primary disease, e.g., ischemic
  necrosis, tophaceous gout, hyperparathyroid cysts, Paget's disease,
  rheumatoid arthritis, osteopetrosis, osteochondritis
Miscellaneous additional diseases
  Endocrine: diabetes mellitus, acromegaly, hypothyroidism
  Metabolic: hemochromatosis, ochronosis, Gaucher's
    disease
  Neuropathic arthropathies
  Miscellaneous: frostbite, Kashin-Beck disease, caisson
    disease
  Mechanical: obesity, unequal lower extremity length;
    valgus/varus deformities, ligamentous laxity (including
    associations with type I procollagen gene mutations of
    Ehlers-Danlos syndrome).

*Compiled, in part, by Osteoarthritis Diagnostic Criteria Committee. American Rheumatism Association, 1983.

reduced biomaterial properties of cartilage as a function of aging and for possible metabolic disturbances in cartilage metabolism, as in diabetes mellitus, acromegaly, and ochronosis.

The subchondral bone table is disturbed by tissue remodeling early in the disease or by such afflictions as Paget's disease or hyperparathyroidism with subchondral cysts. Hyperlaxity of ligaments per se or as part of certain overt (heritable) disorders of connective tissue can lead to osteoarthritis.

PATHOGENESIS. As a result of a multiplicity of etiologic factors, an apparent final common pathway of disease expression involves breakdown of cartilage both directly by physical injury and by enzymatic degradation resulting from injury to chondrocytes and indirectly by subchondral bone stiffening from remodeling. Most important in this context is injury of the collagen network or framework that holds articular cartilage together. This network retains in a semidehydrated conformed state the abundant, intensely hydrophilic, charged, proteoglycan macromolecules. The latter exert an osmotic pressure of several atmospheres against the network. Ungluing or cleavage of the collagen network by maldistributed or excessive weight-bearing forces or degradation of the network by enzymes elaborated by injured cartilage cells may occur. This response to various precipitating events leads to loss of essential elastic properties.

In early osteoarthritis, repair responses by local chondrocytes are usually of poor quality, leading to almost no replacement of lost tissue. From advanced erosions penetrating the marrow, tissue repair is more effective and consists of mixtures of fibrocartilage and hyaline cartilage. Normal rugged biomaterial properties are never recovered by the repair cartilage. As degeneration proceeds, wear particles and matrix degradation products are released from both original and repair cartilages. These fragments are carried to the synovial lining membrane, where a phagocytic response engenders low-grade inflammation and synovial effusion, proliferation of synovial cells, and thickening of the synovial membranes. Much evidence has accumulated that membrane-engendered inflammatory factors amplify cartilage breakdown.

Several biochemical abnormalities have been noted in osteoarthritic cartilage: increased water content, decreased aggregation and content of proteoglycans, decreased chain length and altered profiles of glycosaminoglycans, exposure of collagen epitopes indicative of enzymatic cleavage, and increased proteolytic enzyme levels.

CLINICAL MANIFESTATIONS. The clinical presentation may be divided into early and late stages. Throughout these stages, there is deep, aching pain in the afflicted joints, morning stiffness of short duration, and variable joint thickening and effusion. Early stages are dominated by pain on motion with stiffness, night pain, and responsiveness to anti-inflammatory medication. The late stages are dominated by joint instability, predominance of pain at rest that is accentuated on weight bearing, and failure to respond to anti-inflammatory agents. The present description of clinical features is developed largely on an anatomic basis inasmuch as signs and symptoms reflect regional patterns of involvement. Roentgenographic and laboratory workup and treatment are discussed later.

Hands. Heberden's nodes refer to the osteoarthritic disfigurements of distal interphalangeal joints, and Bouchard's nodes signify equivalent lesions of the proximal interphalangeal joints of the hands (Fig. 273–1). Early Heberden's nodes have a soft consistency and may be associated with prominent inflammatory signs. In the chronic stage, they are characterized by bony enlargement and angular deformities with variable symptoms.

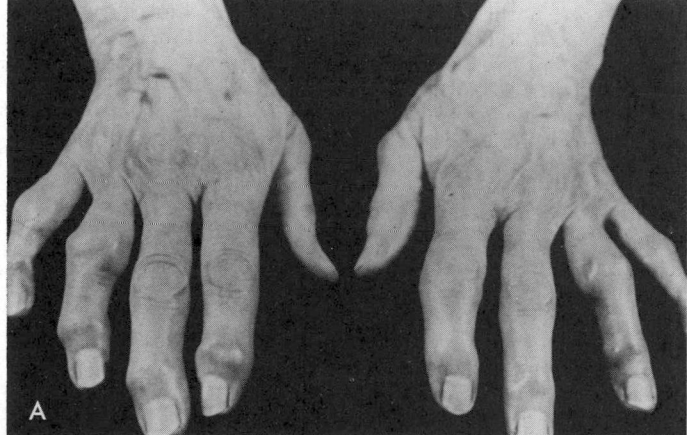
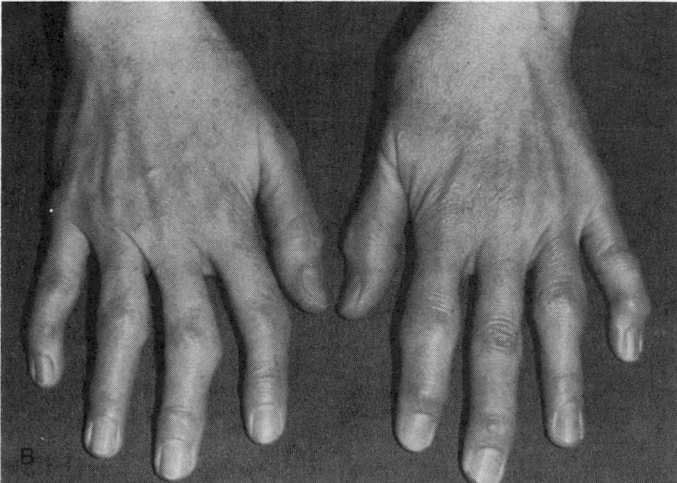

FIGURE 273–1. Typical hand deformities in osteoarthritis. *A*, Typical Heberden's and Bouchard's nodes comprise hypertrophic joint capsular and bony enlargement of the distal and proximal interphalangeal joints, respectively. *B*, Prominent Bouchard's nodes and minor subluxations may cause misdiagnosis of rheumatoid arthritis.

Heredity and sex, in addition to microtrauma, are prominently involved in the development of Heberden's nodes, which are more common in women at menopause or late middle age. The only other common hand lesion involves the first carpometacarpal joint. Such lesions are associated with pain in the radial side of the wrist, pain that is intensified by physical activities such as golf, tennis, and gardening.

Knees. The most common source of major disability in osteoarthritis is knee involvement. At any one time, heat, synovial thickening, or effusions have been documented in at least 50 per cent of cases. Elicitation of crepitus, which persists on repeated flexion and extension of the knee, bony marginal overgrowth, mediolateral instability (in the late stages), and synovial effusion are important diagnostic aids. Degenerative changes are usually more prominent in the medial compartment of the knee, leading to varus (bowleg) deformities. Developmental defects, i.e., knock-knee or bowleg deformity, predispose to osteoarthritis.

Degenerative alteration of the patellofemoral joint is termed chondromalacia patellae. This syndrome of mild effusion and knee pain is usually associated with trauma and occurs predominantly in young adults. It is usually preceded by developmental biomechanical disturbances influencing knee flexion. There is often spontaneous remission of symptoms, but some cases progress to irreversible patellofemoral osteoarthritis.

Hips. Clinical manifestations of primary hip joint disease appear usually in late middle or old age. Perhaps one third or more of cases arise from acetabular dysplasia, as well as growth or maturational disturbances in the femoral neck and head. Altered bone growth as well as developmental thickening at the zenith of the acetabulum may be causative in fewer than 5 per cent of cases. Beyond these factors, there is a background of adult bone remodeling and altered joint incongruity, which may further compromise normal weight-bearing patterns and chondrocyte nutrition. In addition, a variety of acquired disorders, such as rheumatoid arthritis and ischemic necrosis of the femoral head, are important etiologically.

Groin pain on weight bearing or motion is a dominant symptom and is usually referred to the anterior aspect of the thigh above the knee. Over a period of months or a few years, invalidism from severely restricted mobility and pain is a common outcome of untreated disease.

Spinal Osteoarthritis (Including Herniated Disc Syndrome). Throughout the spine, weight-bearing compressive forces are largely supported by one set of articulations—the intervertebral discs. These are elastic organs similar to articular cartilage in respect to the fact that they depend on properties of the semidehydrated proteoglycan molecules. A high osmotic pressure at rest results from proteoglycan confinement by cartilage endplates in two dimensions and the annulus fibrosus in the third. An additional important elastic component is provided by the annulus fibrosus. Rotary motions in the back and neck depend upon the zygoapophyseal joints. All of these joints undergo osteoarthritic changes almost identical in nature to those of the peripheral joints (see Ch. 275 for specific clinical features). Ordinarily, the former joints protect the latter against severe torsional trauma; under certain conditions, especially flexion of the lumbosacral spine, the rotary joints are of much less protectional value, and annular tears may occur under these (and several other) conditions. Resultant displacement of discal products into the spinal foramen adjacent to nerve rootlets and/or spinal canal occurs, depending on the conditions of damage. Injury of these structures both by mechanical trauma and by activated inflammatory pathways believed to involve neural peptides constitutes one of several causes of neural dysfunction leading to symptoms. The relationship of the posterior zygoapophyseal joints in the cervical, thoracic, and lumbar spines to their respective nerve roots as they traverse the intervertebral foramina, and the proximity of an additional set of *joints of Luschka* in the cervical spine (segments C2 to C7), have similar importance because of potential damage to nerves by inflammation secondary to mechanical irritation.

Notably, symptoms of osteoarthritis in the cervical spine depend upon the neural segment involved. Pain, aggravated by motion, often radiates into the supraclavicular and upper trapezius regions, as well as the occiput and distal upper extremities.

Overgrowth of bone in either the cervical or the lumbar spine can cause narrowing of the spinal canal and encroachment on the spinal cord rather than the nerve roots. In the neck, a myelopathy of a painless nature may result. Constriction of the spinal cord by surrounding bone, disc, or ligamentous thickening leads to the syndrome of spinal stenosis most common in the lumbosacral spine. Neurogenic claudication pain (resembling vascular claudication) is an important symptom in this condition and must be differentiated from vascular insufficiency (see Ch. 275 for management of discogenic claudication).

Diffuse Idiopathic Skeletal Hyperostosis. This is characterized by a flowing ligamentous calcification along the anterolateral aspects of vertebral bodies. Symptomatology is variable and focused in the spine or multiple tendon osseous junctions (e.g., at the heel); ankylosis of apophyseal and sacroiliac joints is absent. The thoracic spine is most often affected without intervertebral disc narrowing.

LABORATORY FINDINGS. There are no specific clinical tests for osteoarthritis despite recent evidence for the elevation of levels of soluble cartilage-specific breakdown products in synovial fluid and serum. The sedimentation rate is usually within normal limits, synovial fluid is clear and exhibits a normal range of viscosity, and there is a negative mucin clot test result. Leukocyte counts in synovial fluid generally vary from 150 to 1500 per cubic millimeter; wear particles including whole fragments containing proteoglycans and collagen fibers as well as mineral particles are often identified in the fluid.

ROENTGENOGRAPHIC FEATURES. There is usually narrowing of the radiolucent interosseous joint space resulting from destruction of articular cartilage. Bony cysts varying in size may be seen in subchondral or denuded bone, which may be densely sclerotic. Osteophyte formation at the margins of affected joints is the basis for the most striking roentgenographic findings. Degeneration of lumbar and cervical intervertebral discs results in narrowing of the interspaces. A vacuum sign or marked translucency in the disc may be seen. High-resolution computed tomography (CT) and magnetic resonance imaging (MRI) are important steps in the assessment of spinal lesions and occasionally of osteoarthritis in shoulder, hips, and knees. Oblique views are also valuable for defining bony sclerosis and joint space narrowing of the zygoapophyseal joints of the lumbar spine.

DIFFERENTIAL DIAGNOSIS. Osteoarthritis and rheumatoid arthritis are readily distinguished in terms of their usual clinical presentation. The latter is generally associated with prominent signs of joint inflammation, characteristically afflicting the hands and wrists symmetrically, especially the metacarpophalangeal joints. These joints almost never are affected in osteoarthritis.

Differentiation of these disorders is more complicated when seronegative rheumatoid arthritis involves only (or predominantly) the lower extremities. The presence of a normal erythrocyte sedimentation rate, negative serum rheumatoid factor test result, and minimal synovial fluid change supports the diagnosis of osteoarthritis. Despite severe deformities, occasionally seen with Heberden's and Bouchard's nodes, the lack of ulnar drift and metacarpophalangeal and diffuse wrist involvement help to rule out rheumatoid arthritis. Erosive osteoarthritis characteristically shows bone destruction and inflammatory changes in the proximal and distal interphalangeal joints but not in the metacarpophalangeal joints.

Secondary osteoarthritis must be considered in the presence of joint hypermobility, chondrocalcinosis, heritable disorders such as the Ehlers-Danlos syndrome, mechanical derangements of the joints, metabolic bone disorders, ochronosis, neuropathies, and hemochromatosis. Spinal involvement in osteoarthritis is distinctly different from that in ankylosing spondylitis; the latter predominantly afflicts young men and has characteristic and distinctive roentgenographic features involving sacroiliac sclerosis and fusion, calcification and ossification of the annulus fibrosus and adjacent paravertebral ligaments, and formation of bridging syndesmophytes (bamboo spine).

TREATMENT. Although treatment depends in large measure on the site and severity of joint involvement, the outlook with a multidisciplinary long-term management program is relatively optimistic for functional restoration and symptomatic improvement.

Early disease with signs of mild to moderate inflammation but without joint instability can usually be managed successfully with a combination of measures: (1) Pain may be relieved with mild analgesics (e.g., acetaminophen, 500 mg three or four times a day) or nonsteroidal anti-inflammatory drugs (NSAID's) (e.g., aspirin, 2400 to 3600 mg daily) or both. Indomethacin, ibuprofen, naproxen, fenoprofen, piroxicam, sulindac diclofenac, and tolmetin are alternative agents, advantageous as substitutes for aspirin. Where possible, intermittent rather than continuous usage is encouraged to avoid gastrointestinal side effects, especially acid peptic disease. There is a well-documented substantial morbidity in respect to gastrointestinal intolerance to NSAID's, especially during prolonged usage. Use of gastric protective agents is advised almost routinely (e.g., antacids, histamine-2 receptor blockers, and hydrogen ion pump inhibitors (see Ch. 98). (2) Revision of daily schedule of activities, increased joint rest, and selected avoidance of activities unfavorable to the symptomatic joints must be practiced. (3) The joints must be protected with relevant devices, i.e., splints, crutches, walkers, canes, and so on. (4) Weight-reducing diets must be used. (5) Application of moist heat or cold packs may help. (6) Symptomatic response, in refractory cases, to intra-articular or para-articular injections of small amounts of corticosteroid at infrequent intervals is useful. (7) Once pain and muscle spasm have been relieved, a formalized program of physical therapy followed by a prolonged home exercise program is often recommended in the hope of retarding further joint deterioration.

In the case of cervical osteoarthritis, hyperextension and hyperflexion should be avoided. The patient should sleep flat on one pillow. A cervical collar restricts motion and minimizes pain. (See Ch. 275 for treatment of osteoarthritis in the lumbar spine.)

The principal anatomic regions that are most benefited by orthopedic surgery are the knee, hip, and spine. Several surgical procedures are appropriate for patients with severe hip involvement—wedge osteotomy, various arthroplastics, including total joint replacement, and arthrodesis. For the knee, debridement, either through an arthroscope or via open surgery, osteotomy, and a variety of partial or complete arthroplasties are used for treatment. Tibial or femoral osteotomies may be of long-term benefit by realigning weight-bearing forces, but considerable follow-up rehabilitation is required. Otherwise, joint replacement is the treatment of choice for many cases of advanced osteoarthritis of the knees characterized by intractable pain, loss of function, instability, or all three. Some indications for spinal surgery are: (1) advancing intractable nerve deficits, (2) spinal instability, and (3) spinal stenosis affecting bladder or rectal function because of autonomic nerve involvement.

Altman RD (ed): Pain in osteoarthritis (symposium). Semin Arthritis Rheum 18(S2):1, 1989. *A review of recent progress in research on pain production in various forms of osteoarthritis, presented, for the most part, in terms understandable to practicing physicians.*

McCarty DJ (ed.): Arthritis and Allied Disorders. Philadelphia, Lea & Febiger, 1989, pp 1571–1641. *A comprehensive coverage of multiple important topics, well illustrated with radiographs and clarifying tables.*

Moskowitz RW, Howell DS, Goldberg VM, et al. (eds.): Osteoarthritis: Diagnosis and Management. 2nd ed. Philadelphia, W.B. Saunders Company, in press. *Detailed reference emphasizing both medical and surgical approaches of regional and general importance, readily individualized to the patient.*

274 The Painful Shoulder

David S. Howell

Shoulder pain is a common source of incapacitation and can result from numerous causes. Intrathoracic, diaphragmatic, and cervical pathologic lesions all can cause pain referred to the shoulder, a fact that deserves early consideration and strong emphasis. A characteristic of intrinsic painful disorders is that they often originate in periarticular soft structures—synovial membranes, tendons, and associated muscles. These structures have a unique role in joint stabilization. Loading forces are attenuated by the action of muscles across the coordinated bearings—glenohumeral, acromioclavicular, and sternoclavicular

joints—as well as across the scapulothoracic surfaces. Multiple bursae and tendons near their attachment sites, particularly the rotator cuff tendons, are subject to microinjury and inflammation. Secondary recurrent pain and muscle spasm occur, followed by atrophic or reflex dystrophic responses or both. The most common disorders afflicting these structures are briefly reviewed in this chapter.

CALCIFIC TENDINITIS. A frequently encountered cause of painful shoulder is focal injury or degeneration of the rotator cuff tendons. Roentgenograms reveal calcium-containing minerals in the tendons of the rotator cuff in roughly 3 per cent of middle-aged persons, usually from prior insults. Mineral deposits in tendinous sites may engender bursal inflammation of variable intensity. Acute shoulder pain with radiation into the upper arm and neck is common. Associated muscle hypertonicity with limitation of shoulder motion and guarding, exquisite local tenderness over the inflamed site, and pain on motion or during prolonged rest are prominent. Most often, roentgenograms show linear densities in the supraspinatus, infraspinatus, or subscapularis tendons. Occasionally, a diffuse calcific pattern in the subacromial bursa is seen. Evidence of acute inflammation usually subsides within 1 week, but subacute rotator cuff tendinitis may persist or recur for months to years.

Management is conditioned by the duration and intensity of attacks. Adequate early pain relief is of paramount importance and is usually attainable by use of moist heat or ice compresses; rest, including arm support; analgesics; and a nonsteroidal anti-inflammatory drug (NSAID). Newer agents are discussed in Ch. 258. In most patients, pain and muscle spasm subside with variable reduction of mineral deposits. Injection of an adrenocorticosteroid derivative commonly hastens symptomatic recovery.

Follow-up evaluation is important to assess completeness of recovery. Residual loss of strength or joint motion or chronic pain deserves a conscientious program of active exercises, including both supervised therapy in a physical medicine facility and a home program of daily exercise. Long-term physical therapy or surgical excision of mineral deposits is seldom necessary.

BICIPITAL TENDINITIS. Inflammation of this tendon and synovial sheath is a frequent cause of shoulder pain. The tendon through attrition may subluxate from the bicipital groove or rupture. Localized tenderness on palpation with accentuation of pain by flexion or extension of the elbow against resistance or by internal rotation and abduction distinguishes the diagnosis clinically.

Treatment includes moist heat or ice compresses, rest, and NSAID's in the acute stages, and frequently the instillation of corticosteroids. Chronic recurrent disease is suggestive of the aforementioned mechanical derangements or an additional rotator cuff tear. Surgical transfer of the tendon may lead to satisfactory recovery.

ROTATOR CUFF TEARS. After heavy work, sports, or accidental injury, degenerative lesions in the rotator cuff often engender breakdown with moderate to major tendinous and ligamentous tears, predominantly in middle-aged persons. Complete rupture of the rotator cuff renders the arm incapable of abduction to 90 degrees. With mild tears, there is pain between 60 and 90 degrees of abduction. Either preceding or following these tears, an impingement syndrome frequently occurs at the coracoacromial arch. Often this is associated radiographically with cysts or sclerosis of the greater tuberosity of the humerus, osteophytes at the anterior margin of the acromion, and narrowing of the distance between the humeral head and acromion. These changes are related to trauma from impingement of the aforementioned bones. Since the rotator cuff forms, in part, the roof of the glenohumeral joint and floor of the subacromial and subdeltoid bursae, tears in the cuff permit synovial joint fluid extrusion into these bursae—demonstrable by arthrogram.

Primary treatment of rotator cuff tears consists of heat and aspirin, 2.4 to 3.6 gm per day, or other NSAID's, such as ibuprofen, 1200 to 2400 mg per day. Partial immobilization and exercise programs are indicated for incomplete tears. When these measures fail, surgical repair is often required.

ADHESIVE CAPSULITIS. This (frozen shoulder) disability of middle-aged persons develops more commonly in women than in men and is of unknown etiology. The diagnosis is suspected when persons with no primary shoulder disease develop active and passive restricted motion of the glenohumeral joint attended by increasing pain in the shoulder over a period of weeks to months, and it is more certain when an arthrogram shows a contracted joint capsule. Fibrosis is seen on pathologic study. Rotator cuff tears, hemarthroses, anterior shoulder capsule tear, psychophysiologic shoulder dysfunction, and shoulder-hand syndrome can all cause immobile painful shoulders and may be confused with adhesive capsulitis.

The key feature of management is prevention of severe pain through early use of heat, analgesics, range-of-motion exercises, and, if these are unsuccessful, the judicious use of intra-articular or systemic corticosteroids.

Manipulation mobilization under general anesthesia followed by a course of intensive physical therapy rarely is required for advanced disease.

SHOULDER-HAND SYNDROME. Shoulder pain and stiffness concurrent with pain, swelling, and vasomotor changes in the hands, wrists, and arms of various intensity and duration characterize this syndrome. Thickening of the skin and edema may follow, resembling Sudeck's atrophy. A small percentage of patients eventually develop adhesive capsulitis and sclerodactyly. This syndrome, which affects patients over age 50 years and follows acute severe illness, such as cerebrovascular accident, myocardial infarction, and trauma to the distal upper extremity, is believed to be caused by reflex sympathetic stimulation. Associated changes of cervical osteoarthritis probably have a minor role if any. When the disease is bilateral, the differentiation from acute rheumatoid arthritis or polymyalgia rheumatica may be difficult. The most important feature of treatment is aggressive physical therapy assisted by analgesics and prednisone in a short, moderate-dosage trial of 20 to 30 mg per day for 3 weeks, tapered at the end of the course. Stellate ganglion blocks and local corticosteroid injections are sometimes employed.

AMYLOID ARTHROPATHY. In two thirds of patients, shoulder involvement is present, usually secondary to myeloma. There is para-articular infiltration with amorphous amyloid fibers, causing the "shoulder pad sign." Acute inflammatory signs are usually absent (see Ch. 197).

ISCHEMIC NECROSIS. This disease is half as common in the humeral head as in the hip. Diffuse shoulder pain precedes conventional radiologic changes, the most helpful of which is an irregular translucent band localized in subchondral bone.

POLYMYALGIA RHEUMATICA. This syndrome is often characterized by severely painful shoulders and upper arms in aged persons with anemia, high sedimentation rates, and a negative rheumatoid factor test, and in a small percentage of cases, temporal arteritis and retinal ischemia threatening to vision (see Ch. 518). The dramatic response of shoulder pain to low-dose corticosteroid administration (prednisone, 10 mg per day) is characteristic.

MILWAUKEE SHOULDER. This syndrome consists of a painful, destructive, bilateral arthropathy in middle-aged and elderly patients with capsular calcification, joint effusions, and a high frequency of eroded rotator cuff tendons. Synovial fluids are virtually free of inflammatory cells despite a reported high collagenase activity.

Kozin F: Painful shoulder and the reflex sympathetic dystrophy syndrome. In McCarty DJ (ed.): Arthritis and Allied Conditions. Philadelphia, Lea & Febiger, 1989, pp 1509–1544. *Detailed coverage of etiopathogenesis, differential diagnosis and management; 301 references.*

Post M: The painful shoulder. Clin Orthop 173:2, 1983. *A symposium by multiple authors on various clinically important syndromes and discussion of current management.*

275 The Painful Back

David S. Howell

The back is a complex structure serving weight-bearing and locomotor functions. It provides for major support of body structures and transmission of loading forces through the sacroiliac joints to the lower limbs. The fundamental functioning unit is an articular triad composed of two zygoapophyseal joints posteriorly and the intervertebral disc anteriorly. The disc is composed of a nucleus pulposus encompassed by the annulus fibrosus. These structures are arranged in a series and stabilized throughout the spine by ligaments. The spinal bones also encase the spinal cord and the cauda equina and through successive foramina rootlets connect the spinal cord with peripheral neural pathways. (See Ch. 273 for detailed discussion of the cervical spine, Ch. 259 for the spondyloarthropathies, and Ch. 490 for intervertebral disc disease.)

ETIOLOGY OF BACK PAIN. In Table 275–1, the numerous causes of back pain are displayed according to disease subgroups. Although all vertebral levels can be affected, pain in the low back is most prevalent. The majority of patients present with problems relating to functional or mechanical disturbances, and these must be distinguished from a wide variety of diseases either of focal origin or referred from multiple organ systems. Among degenerative diseases, low back pain is a leading cause of industrial absenteeism and chronic disablement.

MEDICAL HISTORY. *Sex.* Compression vertebral fractures from osteoporosis have their highest prevalence in postmenopausal women. Gynecologic pathology, such as endometriosis, is the basis for some referred patterns of back pain. Reiter's disease, ankylosing spondylitis, and back injuries are found more commonly in males.

Age. Young people with back pain most commonly suffer from muscle or ligament strains, congenital abnormalities, injury, spondyloarthropathies, and herniated disc syndromes. In middle and old age, osteoporosis, vertebral collapse, degenerative states, including spinal stenosis, and malignant lesions are common.

Family History. Familial patterns of segregation are often detected in respect to spondyloarthropathies and uncommonly in respect to spinal degenerative conditions.

Nature of Pain. Events or conditions that accelerate or retard symptoms should be explored. The chronic inflammatory diseases

TABLE 275–1. ETIOLOGY OF BACK PAIN

Mechanical or Traumatic
  Paraspinal ligaments and musculature
    Myofascial syndrome, sacroiliac strain
  Spondylogenic
    Osteoarthritis-related lesions—zygoapophyseal joints
    Degenerative lesions—intervertebral discs
    Mechanical insufficiency, congenital and acquired, of ligaments and bones
    Spondylolisthesis
    Spinal stenosis
    Fractures
Metabolic
  Vertebral bodies, partial collapse and distortion—osteoporosis; osteomalacia—Paget's disease—often with secondary osteoarthritis
Tumors
  Neural tumors, osteosarcoma, metastatic tumors, e.g., from breast, thyroid, kidney
  Myeloma, lymphoma, leukemia
Systemic Inflammatory Disease
  Spondylitis (ankylosing)—Reiter's disease; psoriatic or enteropathic arthropathy
  Disseminated ankylosing skeletal hyperostosis
Infections
  Pyogenic, fungal, tuberculous disc infection, herpes zoster infection, paraspinal abscesses
Referred Pain
  Vascular—aneurysms, sclerosis of aorta and branches
  Tumors or inflammation of pleural, pulmonary, pericardial, cardiac, or neck origin
  Viscerogenic disease of gallbladder, pancreas, stomach, intestines, kidneys, ureters, bladder, prostate, uterus
  Pelvic or retroperitoneal tumors or inflammation
Nonorganic Components
  Hysterical conversion
  Learned painful behavior
  Psychosis
  Litigation neurosis, malingering
  Chronic pain syndrome
  Substance abuse

(spondyloarthropathies) are associated with increased pain and stiffness on inactivity. Patients with lumbar disc protrusion and radicular pain generally are relieved by lying flat with the knees flexed and are uncomfortable sitting. Sudden or acute onset of symptoms is suggestive of a mechanical or infectious origin of symptoms, respectively. Constitutional symptoms such as fever, weight loss, and fatigue are important clues to infectious, inflammatory, or neoplastic disorders.

In regard to localization, the dorsal segment suggests osteoarthritis, vertebral fracture, neoplasm, herpetic radiculitis, or referred pain from the viscera (see later paragraph). Localization of pain in the low back is usually of little help in regard to differential diagnosis.

Claudication-type pain, with onset after sustained walking, suggests either spinal stenosis or arterial insufficiency. The former condition often refers pain to the thigh and is poorly relieved by standing still. Usually neurogenic claudication is relieved by sitting, whereas vascular claudication is reduced by standing.

Referred Pain. A deep aching pain referred to various sites in the upper and midback may be engendered by lesions in the upper gastrointestinal tract. Pain of malignancy (whether local or referred) is typically severe and unrelieved by change of position or mild analgesics.

In respect to neuropathic symptoms, alteration of the structure of the vertebral foramina may lead to radicular dissemination of pain. In such instances, compression or traction of nerve rootlets or extension of inflammation to them can lead to sensory and motor nerve symptoms and signs, i.e., paresthesias, hypoesthesias, and muscle weakness.

Symptomatology. Discogenic pain is characteristically aggravated by cough or sneeze. Rarely, loss of bowel or urinary sphincter function can result from cord compression or bilateral involvement of sacral nerve roots from spinal stenosis, tumors, or infectious lesions.

PHYSICAL EXAMINATION. General examination of the back is discussed in Ch. 254. Descriptions here are confined to vertebral compression fractures, degenerative disc disease, and lumbosacral strains and sprains.

Lumbosacral Strain. This and related myofascial syndromes are the most common ailments seen in the office practice of rheumatology. A history of injury is often followed by prompt or delayed low back pain. Transient disc prolapse, subluxation of facet joints, and injury to muscles or ligaments are diagnostic considerations. Physical signs are usually limited to paravertebral muscle spasm, tenderness, and restricted lower back motion without evidence of nerve root involvement.

Vertebral Compression Fractures. These are the most common complication of osteoporosis, with the resultant traction or compression of rootlets adjacent to collapsed vertebrae. Severe pain may begin suddenly, associated with the postural strain of lifting heavy objects or hyperflexing the trunk. Major physical findings consist of localized tenderness and muscle spasm related to the level of the nerve roots affected. Poorly localized back pain may be associated with osteoporosis in the absence of vertebral collapse. Metastatic tumor, myeloma, and metabolic bone disease, especially osteopenia of aging, are common underlying conditions.

Discogenic Disease. The most common form of low back pain with radiculitis is associated with prolapse, protrusion, or extrusion of intervertebral disc substance (see Ch. 490). Usually the onset of acute symptoms is preceded by chronic intermittent low back pain, although a discrete injury may precipitate an attack. Ninety per cent of disc herniations are localized at L4–L5 or L5–S1 levels. Discs involving the L4 nerve root may cause pain referred along the course of the femoral nerve upon hip extension and knee flexion. Knee extension may be weak and the patellar reflex reduced or absent. Patients with L5 nerve root disturbance complain of classic sciatic distribution of pain, i.e., radiating to the posterior thigh and the anteromedial leg and foot, in association with weakness of the toe extensors. First sacral radiculopathy is associated with pain over the posterior thigh, calf, and heel, weakness of the ankle and toe flexors, and reduced or absent Achilles tendon reflex. Frequently, loss of neurologic function is subtle and requires repeated testing to document. A positive response to straight-leg raising is most frequently indicative of L4–L5 or L5–S1 disc protrusion. Usually there is pain on hip flexion with the knee extended and absence of pain on repetition of hip flexion with the knee flexed (Lasègue's sign). The cauda equina syndrome is a form of spinal stenosis and is an uncommon but important complication of massive disc prolapse. In the cauda equina syndrome, central midline disc displacement causes paralysis of the sacral root with bladder and bowel dysfunction. It is characterized by severe bilateral leg pain, urinary retention, weakness of the anal sphincter, and bilateral nerve root abnormalities. Once complete neurologic block has occurred, deceptively pain is often alleviated, and the patient will require a neurologic examination to verify the need for emergency surgery.

Spondylolisthesis. This condition, which refers to forward displacement of one vertebra on another, commonly involves the L4–L5 and L5–S1 levels. Bursts of segmental severe girdle pain are typical, often worse on activity and relieved by rest.

LABORATORY PROCEDURES. These are dictated by the results of medical history and physical examination. Simple radiographs of the back may suffice if a traumatic injury is causative. In instances of suspected metabolic disturbance, appropriate screening tests, such as serum calcium, phosphorus, and alkaline phosphatase measurements, should be obtained. Complete blood counts, sedimentation rate, urinalysis, and automated serum chemical profiles are sometimes justified to clarify the diagnosis. Anemia and an elevated sedimentation rate should prompt a more extensive search for infectious, inflammatory, and neoplastic diseases.

RADIOGRAPHIC STUDIES. *Routine Radiographic Studies.* These include frontal, lateral, and oblique films of the lumbosacral spine, which can demonstrate foraminal encroachment, compression fractures, degenerative changes, and subluxation of zygoapophyseal joints, as well as interspace narrowing (see Ch. 272). There may be severe degenerative changes on the radiographs, with few or no relevant symptoms, and severe back pain may occur in the absence of significant radiographic signs and be of discogenic origin.

Additional Imaging Procedures. When surgical intervention is planned or a diagnosis remains questionable and requires an imperative answer and high resolution, computed tomography (CT) and magnetic resonance (MRI) imaging (noninvasive) are increasingly preferred to myelography. It is not usually necessary to perform a discogram (injection of radiopaque dye directly into the disc). When osteomyelitis or neoplastic involvement is likely, radionuclide bone scans are helpful. A percutaneous vertebral biopsy under fluoroscopic guidance may be performed to establish histopathologic diagnosis or bacteriologic diagnosis at highly suspicious sites obvious from scans or radiographs. Electromyography can confirm the presence of nerve root deficits.

MANAGEMENT. Conservative therapy for mechanical disorders of the spine and disc herniation focuses on bed rest, analgesics, and anti-inflammatory medication. Use of long-term anti-inflammatory agents should be accompanied by prophylactic protection against peptic ulceration. Application of moist heat, e.g., hydrocollator packs wrapped with a wet towel, may relieve pain and muscle spasm. The amount of bed rest is dependent on the severity of symptoms. After bed rest, gradual ambulation and a program of exercises, together with back protection including a lumbosacral support, are recommended. Most cases of disc herniation respond to conservative therapy; those unresponsive require further measures, including epidural steroids and nerve root or sleeve infiltrations with steroids. Before surgery is indicated, a psychological assessment and exercises emphasizing back stretching and abdominal strengthening should be attempted.

Progressive muscular weakness and progressive neurologic deficit despite bed rest and other aforementioned measures, as well as the cauda equina syndrome, are indications for surgery. Relative indications for laminectomy are severe pain, unrelieved by bed rest, and recurrent episodes of incapacitating pain. Ninety to 95 per cent improvement following surgery is anticipated, although 70 per cent of patients experience relief of pain whether or not the disc is removed.

Following either conservative therapy or surgery, a program of prophylactic management includes postural education, performance of a daily exercise program to strengthen the lumbar and abdominal muscles, and avoidance of lower spine stress. Besides laminectomy, joint fusion for spondylolisthesis and discogenic disease or unroofing procedures for spinal stenosis are sometimes necessary. Myelography, CT scans, or MRI is indicated preoperatively to establish definitively the nature and extent of disease as well as the level of vertebral involvement.

Acute symptoms from compression fractures require appropriate rest and relief of pain with analgesics. Activities must be selected to avoid additional compression fractures. (See Ch. 238 for management of osteoporosis.)

Brown MD, Rydevik B: Advances in the understanding and treatment of low back pain and sciatica. Orthop Clin North Am 22: April, 1991. *An overview of the present management of low back pain, with emphasis on controlled trials and newer diagnostic techniques.*

Manmiche C, Hessels EG, Bentzen L, et al.: Clinical trials of intensive muscle training for chronic low back pain. Lancet 2:862, 1988. *An appropriate program is described for motivated patients with pain refractory to conventional measures.*

Weber H: Lumbar disc herniation: A controlled prospective study with 10 years of observation. Spine 8:131, 1983. *A classic set of observations on the natural history of the disease and discussion of management.*

276 Systemic Diseases in Which Arthritis Is a Feature

Eugene V. Ball

Eleven per cent of adult Americans interviewed in the National Health Survey claimed to have had one or more episodes of painful joints over a period of 6 weeks. Much of this pain was probably due to soft tissue rheumatism and common rheumatic diseases, such as osteoarthritis and rheumatoid arthritis, that are defined by their own attributes and not by associated signs. The arthralgias of a fraction of these persons might have represented early symptoms of systemic diseases diagnosable only by the later appearance of other clinical signs or by laboratory testing. Table 276–1 illustrates the applicability of general medical laboratory tests to the evaluation of nonspecific joint symptoms. The tests afford significant diagnostic clues for certain systemic diseases in which arthralgias can be the earliest and only symptoms. Brief descriptions of musculoskeletal manifestations of a few systemic disorders follow.

PRIMARY BILIARY CIRRHOSIS (see Ch. 122)

More than half of women with primary biliary cirrhosis (PBC) may have serologic abnormalities, such as rheumatoid factors and antinuclear antibodies, in addition to antimitochondrial antibodies. A large number, primarily in this group, have joint pains or

TABLE 276–1. LABORATORY TESTS IN THE EVALUATION OF NONSPECIFIC JOINT SYMPTOMS

Test	Disease
Liver function tests	Primary biliary cirrhosis; chronic active hepatitis
Calcium and phosphorus	Hyperparathyroidism
Serum protein electrophoresis	Hypogammaglobulinemic arthritis; primary amyloidosis
Serum iron and total iron-binding capacity; ferritin	Hemochromatosis
Lipase or amylase	Pancreatic-arthritis syndrome
Thyroxine (T₄), thyroid-stimulating hormone (TSH)	Thyroid myopathy or arthritis
Complete blood count	Leukemia; sickle cell disease
Lipid analysis	Hyperlipidemia-associated arthritis
Partial thromboplastin time	Vasculopathy; hemophilia
Rapid plasma reagin (RPR) or VDRL	Vasculopathy; syphilis
Anti-HIV (human immunodeficiency virus) antibody	HIV arthritis
Antiparvovirus antibody	Parvovirus arthritis

outright rheumatic disease, mainly rheumatoid arthritis, Sjögren's syndrome, or limited scleroderma (CREST syndrome: calcinosis, Raynaud's phenomenon, esophageal dysmotility, sclerodactyly, and telangiectasia). Other defined causes for bone or joint pains in PBC include osteomalacia and hypertrophic osteoarthropathy.

HEMOCHROMATOSIS (see Ch. 193)

Arthritis is frequently the first sign of hemochromatosis and eventually develops in as many as half of all persons with the disease. Typically occurring between the ages of 40 and 50, the arthritis of hemochromatosis has been reported in persons younger than 30 and is easily overlooked or confused with primary osteoarthritis, even though their distributions often differ. It may also be dismissed as idiopathic tendinitis or bursitis. Pain and stiffness frequently appear first in the metacarpophalangeal joints; other joints involved commonly include the wrists, hips, and knees. Signs of inflammation are negligible except during episodes of pseudogout. Chondrocalcinosis is common on radiographs, as are subchondral cysts, sclerosis, and joint space narrowing. The arthritis is not altered by phlebotomy; treatment is symptomatic and may necessitate arthroplasties, particularly in the hips.

SICKLE CELL DISEASE AND OTHER HEMOGLOBINOPATHIES (see Ch. 136)

Almost all persons with sickle cell disease experience musculoskeletal symptoms. Large joint arthritis lasting a few days to a few weeks results from small vessel occlusion caused by local sickling. The aseptic bone infarcts of SC (or less often SS) disease resemble osteomyelitis, which is far more common in persons with sickle cell disease than in normal persons and is often caused by *Salmonella*. Osteonecrosis occurs in both SS and SC disease, often in the head of the femur; however, multiple areas may be infarcted. Hyperuricemia attributable to SS disease has culminated in gout in older patients. Pain due to microfractures in the lower leg, ankle, or foot, lasting up to 1 to 2 years, has been described in almost one half of a group of 50 patients with beta-thalassemia.

HYPOGAMMAGLOBULINEMIA (see Ch. 244 and 287)

Arthritis as a complication of hypogammaglobulinemia is most typical of the X-linked variety (Bruton's disease) in children; however, it also occurs in other types of primary hypogammaglobulinemia. Septic arthritis is caused by common pathogens or by mycoplasmal organisms such as *Ureaplasma urealyticum*. Nonerosive arthritis, without evidence of infection or other demonstrable cause, often resolves following institution of immunoglobulin therapy. Its resolution with treatment does not necessarily constitute *a priori* evidence of an infectious etiology. Intravenous gamma globulin treatment might suppress arthritis through its complex modulating effect on the immune system (for example, it has been shown to increase suppressor T cell functional activity).

WHIPPLE'S DISEASE (see Ch. 102)

The arthritis of Whipple's disease mimics that of rheumatic fever in some respects. It is painful; there is often warmth, redness, and swelling; it favors large joints; subcutaneous nodules have been noted in a few patients; recurrences are common; and it can be migratory. Less often, small joints of the hands and feet are inflamed, and the arthritis becomes chronic and resembles rheumatoid arthritis. The synovial fluid white cell count is sometimes elevated to 50,000 per cubic millimeter, and rod-shaped bacilli may be identified, usually by electron microscopy, in synovial biopsies. Rheumatoid factors and antinuclear antibody are not features of Whipple's disease. The arthritis may antedate gastrointestinal symptoms by years, making diagnosis difficult.

HYPERLIPOPROTEINEMIA (see Ch. 172)

An association exists between type II familial hypercholesterolemia (both homozygous and heterozygous forms) and musculoskeletal symptoms such as Achilles tendinitis, oligoarthritis, and polyarthritis. Transient pain in the Achilles tendon appears to be more common than frank inflammatory tendinitis, which can last a few days and recur two or three times yearly. A few patients have acute painful monoarthritis or pauciarthritis of the knees, ankles, or small joints that lasts a week or more and recurs frequently. Less common is an incapacitating polyarthritis resembling rheumatic fever, persisting a month or more. In one study, 40 per cent of 73 heterozygous patients were symptomatic; articular manifestations appeared at times before the xanthomas that are the major diagnostic sign of familial hypercholesterolemia. Arthritis may also be a feature of type IV hyperlipoproteinemia.

ENDOCRINE DISORDERS (see Ch. 213, 216, and 235)

Aches and stiffness simulating fibrositis may appear early in hypothyroidism; untreated, this may progress to proximal myopathy with elevated creatine kinase levels, simulating polymyositis, or to a syndrome of synovial thickening and joint effusions, simulating rheumatoid arthritis. There also appears to be an association of hypothyroidism with calcium pyrophosphate deposition disease. Unlike myopathy and arthritis, carpal tunnel syndrome is a common manifestation of hypothyroidism. Hyperthyroidism may cause myopathy without elevations of the creatine kinase level but with muscle wasting, which may be severe. Thyroid acropachy, seen rarely in association with pretibial myxedema and Graves' disease, is characterized by diffuse swelling of the fingers and clubbing.

Hyperparathyroidism is another cause of diffuse, vague musculoskeletal pains resembling those of fibrositis. The other musculoskeletal complications of hyperparathyroidism include back pain due to vertebral body fractures; an erosive arthritis predominantly in the hands and wrists; and chondrocalcinosis (with pseudogout occurring most often after parathyroidectomy).

Carpal tunnel syndrome has been reported in almost one half of persons with acromegaly. Raynaud's phenomenon is rare. The arthritis of acromegaly is clinically indistinguishable from osteoarthritis.

SARCOIDOSIS (see Ch. 67)

Joint or juxta-articular pains are experienced by as many as one third of patients with acute sarcoidosis and may be the only symptom of the disease; however, erythema nodosum often accompanies the arthritis and, together with hilar adenopathy, suggests the diagnosis (one should be aware that arthritis may accompany erythema nodosum of any cause). Arthritis often begins in the ankles and spreads symmetrically. The distal interphalangeal joints are typically spared, but any of the other peripheral joints, as well as the heels, may be painful out of proportion to signs of inflammation, which are meager. Episodes last a few days to a few months, and the arthritis usually resolves completely. The erythrocyte sedimentation rate is often elevated; antinuclear antibodies and rheumatoid factors may be present. Treatment with salicylates, nonsteroidal anti-inflammatory drugs (NSAID's), or prednisone is based on the severity of the arthritis. Progressive, deforming arthritis is a feature of chronic sarcoidosis, as are bone lesions, both lytic and sclerotic. Clinically significant sarcoid myopathy is rare.

FAMILIAL MEDITERRANEAN FEVER (see Ch. 196)

Serositis, fever, and arthritis are the major signs of familial Mediterranean fever (FMF). Arthritis occurs in as many as one half of patients; it is usually monoarticular and confined to large joints in the lower extremities. Although it usually lasts less than 1 week, arthritis has been reported to persist for several months. Synovial fluid contains large numbers of granulocytes, and there is intense infiltration of granulocytes and hyperemia in synovial tissue. Diagnosis is suggested by demographic and other clinical features of the disease. In the absence of these, FMF can be easily confused with juvenile rheumatoid arthritis. Colchicine most often prevents recurrent arthritis as well as amyloidosis.

277 Miscellaneous Forms of Arthritis

Eugene V. Ball

NEUROPATHIC JOINT DISEASE (CHARCOT'S JOINTS)

Recognition of neuropathic joint disease and its association with syphilis preceded reports of its association with diabetes mellitus by 64 years, but syphilis has been superseded by the latter as the leading cause of this disorder. Weakness, decreased pain sensation, and impaired position sense contribute to the massive destruction of the knee (or less often the hip or ankle) seen in syphilis, subacute combined degeneration of the spinal cord, paraplegia, and Charcot-Marie-Tooth disease. In syringomyelia, upper limb involvement is typical. Neuropathic disease of the knee or ankle is suggested by effusions, crepitus, enlargement, and relatively little pain, although pain may be severe late in the disease. Neuropathic joint disease in diabetes mellitus (Fig. 277-1) is more likely to cause painless swelling of one or both feet in a patient with longstanding disease and sensory neuropathy. For mechanical reasons, the joints most frequently involved are the tarsometatarsals and the metatarsophalangeals. Destruction also occurs in the talus, the calcaneus, the ankle joints, and the distal tibia. Radiographs characteristically show loss of joint space, sclerosis, multiple irregular bodies representing chip fractures, and new bone formation; analogous changes are seen in osteomyelitis and malignancy. Less severe, but similar, changes have been reported in calcium pyrophosphate deposition disease. Attempts at stabilizing the involved joint with various orthotic devices are often unsatisfactory, and surgical fusion is difficult.

HEMARTHROSIS

Hemophilia (see Ch. 155) is the major medical cause of hemarthrosis, which (with muscle bleeding) accounts for more than 90 per cent of all bleeding episodes in patients with hemophilia. The severity of hemarthrosis is related directly to the levels of clotting factors. For example, infants with severe factor deficiencies often experience hemarthrosis before the age of 1 year. By the age of 15, virtually all persons with severe, inadequately treated factor deficiencies have some form of chronic joint impairment.

Acute bleeding into a joint (most often the knees, elbows, or ankles) is frequently signified by stiffness or discomfort, followed by pain, swelling, and redness. The joint should be immobilized, and adequate factor replacement should be started as early as possible, preferably during the prodromal phase. The joint changes induced by repeated intra-articular bleeding resemble those of rheumatoid arthritis. Hyperplastic synovium appears to be the source of proteases and other enzymes that destroy cartilage and bone, culminating in the absence of articular carti-

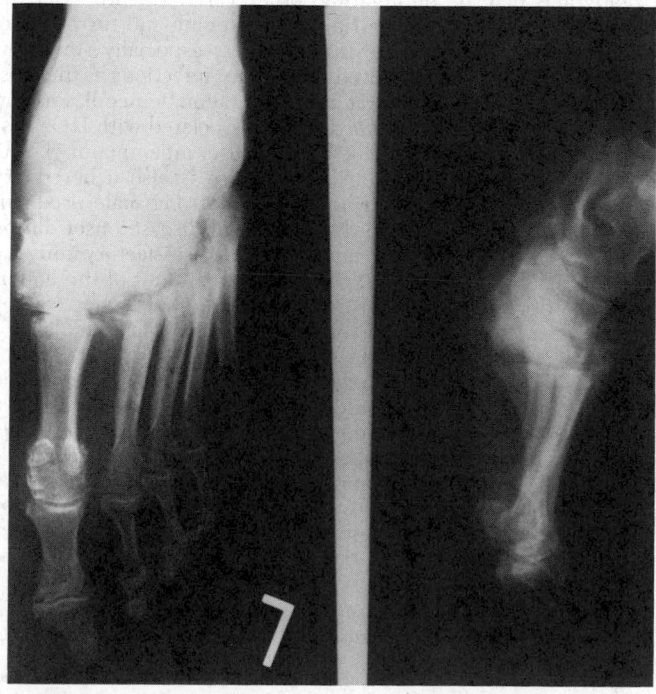

FIGURE 277-1. Diabetes mellitus and neuropathic arthritis. Note lateral displacement of metatarsals (*left*) and fragmentation and osseous debris (*right*).

lage, joint disorganization, and fibrous contractures. Education of the patient and family, as well as home treatment, prevents or attenuates chronic, destructive arthritis. Joint replacements have been done successfully to relieve pain and restore function.

Bleeding into a muscle, which should also be treated with replacement factor, can lead to necrosis and fibrotic scarring. Pseudotumors are cystic bone swellings resulting from intraosseous bleeding and necrosis.

Von Willebrand's disease can produce hemarthrosis and joint destruction comparable to that of hemophilia.

Painful but nondestructive intra-articular bleeding is a common feature of scurvy, and intra-articular tumors such as pigmented villonodular synovitis frequently cause monoarticular bleeding.

MULTICENTRIC RETICULOHISTIOCYTOSIS

The chief manifestations of multicentric reticulohistiocytosis are arthritis and red to purple skin nodules varying in size from 1 to 10 mm. The nodules are found in any part of the skin but tend to concentrate on the face and hands and uncommonly coalesce. The arthritis is most often symmetric and polyarticular. Unlike adult rheumatoid arthritis, it does not spare the distal interphalangeal joints. It can be severely destructive and, in one third of cases, progresses to arthritis mutilans. Systemic signs include fever and weight loss; less often, pericarditis and myositis are present, and it is frequently associated with a malignancy.

The disorder has also been termed lipoid dermatoarthritis because of the lipids contained within the histiocytes and granulomas that constitute the basic lesion. In the absence of a serum or lesional lipid abnormality, lipid deposition is now thought to be nonspecific. Improvement has been reported more consistently with alkylating agents than with prednisone.

HYPERTROPHIC OSTEOARTHROPATHY AND CARCINOMATOUS POLYARTHRITIS

Hypertrophic osteoarthropathy (HO) is a systemic disorder distinguished by periostitis of the distal ends of tubular bones. The lesions presumably begin with increased blood flow and periosteal edema, followed by new bone formation. Isotopic bone scans are positive at an early stage, often preceding radiographic evidence of periosteal new bone. Hypertrophic osteoarthropathy is often manifested as digital clubbing and frequently involves the tibiae, ulnae, radii, femora, metatarsals, and metacarpals. Painful articular swelling appears in approximately 30 per cent of patients and may be debilitating; other variable features of the syndrome include gynecomastia and thickening and furrowing of the facial skin. Intrathoracic malignancies, especially squamous cell carcinoma, have supplanted pulmonary infections as the most common cause of HO. Pleural and diaphragmatic neoplasms and nasopharyngeal carcinomas are strongly associated with HO. Less common causes include chronic liver disease, inflammatory bowel disease, and cyanotic heart disease. There is also a hereditary form termed pachydermoperiostosis, with strong male predominance and a curious bimodal distribution of disease onset during the first year of life or the mid-teens. No satisfactory unifying theory of pathogenesis exists. Successful treatment of the underlying disorder results in regression of HO. In fact, thoracotomy for pulmonary hypertrophic osteoarthropathy may result in a marked decrease in pain and swelling within 24 hours.

The "sudden" onset of polyarthritis resembling rheumatoid arthritis in an older adult should prompt suspicion of an associated malignancy. Carcinomatous polyarthritis may appear months before, or after, detection of malignancy of many types. Its incidence is unknown; in one small series it was almost as common as carcinomatous hypertrophic osteoarthropathy and more common than cancer-related dermatomyositis. Palmar fasciitis has been noted in association with ovarian cancer.

Ginsburg, WW, O'Duffy JD, Morris JL, et al.: Multicentric reticulohistiocytosis: Response to alkylating in six patients. Ann Intern Med 111:384, 1989. *Five of six patients with multicentric reticulohistiocytosis manifesting as skin nodules and polyarthritis were treated with cyclophosphamide. The sixth patient was given chlorambucil. All responded with complete or near-complete remissions lasting as long as 32 months after cessation of treatment.*

Luck JV, Jr, Kasper CKL: General orthopedics: A tribute to J. Vernon Luck Sr.—Symposium: Surgical Management of Advanced Hemophilic Arthropathy: An Overview of 20 Years' Experience. Clin Orthop 242:60, 1989. *A review from a*

large multidisciplinary hemophilia center of the clinical manifestations of hemophilic arthritis and its management, which included 67 prosthetic arthroplasties.

Slowman-Kovacs SD, Braunstein EM, Brandt KD: Rapidly progressive Charcot arthropathy following minor joint trauma in patients with diabetic neuropathy. Arthritis Rheum 33:412, 1990. *This report of neuropathic arthropathy progressing rapidly after minor trauma in three patients is based on the authors' research in experimental arthritis.*

278 Nonarticular Rheumatism

Eugene V. Ball

FIBROSITIS

Primary fibrositis has been defined as a chronic pain syndrome with tender points in predictable sites and disturbed sleep. In the absence of diagnostic laboratory tests or objective physical signs, the syndrome is somewhat controversial, and its existence as a distinct entity has been questioned. The pain of fibrositis is often described as muscular or as deep aching or burning. It is generalized but more severe in the trunk and hands and in proximity to tender "trigger" points. These areas are painful to firm palpation in normal persons but are more tender in persons with fibrositis. Some 14 locations have been identified, e.g., in the second costochondral junction and in the periscapular muscles along the medial border of the scapula, and over the medial collateral ligament of the knee.

Patients may have sleep disturbances of possible pathogenetic significance. Fatigue is virtually universal as a component of this syndrome; headaches and heightened anxiety are common. In these respects, the fibrositis syndrome has a close resemblance to the syndrome of mitral valve prolapse, and it too is more common in women past the age of 20 (although it has been diagnosed in children). There are no confirmed biochemical, immunologic, or anatomic abnormalities in patients with fibrositis. Treatment should emphasize its benign nature. The physician should be wary of overuse of drugs to allay anxiety or induce sleep. In limited studies, amitriptyline and cyclobenzaprine have been found to be superior to placebo in decreasing pain and improving sleep.

BURSITIS

Bursae are small, synovial-lined, fluid-filled sacs located between tendons and bones, which serve to reduce friction between opposing muscles or tendons. Most bursae are present from birth; however, others form in response to repeated pressure.

Of the approximately 80 bursae located on each side of the body, only a few are common sources of pain. The subdeltoid is the largest of the bursae around the shoulder; it is located between the deltoid muscle and the shoulder capsule and extends under the acromion. Acute inflammation of this or nearby bursae and tendons is apt to be exceedingly painful, resulting in restriction of the shoulder movement and tenderness over the rotator cuff. Intrabursal injection of lidocaine is diagnostic and often curative; however, recurrences are common. Bursal calcification predisposes to more frequent attacks.

Trochanteric bursitis is thought to occur as a result of chronic strain on weak quadriceps muscles or overuse of hip and thigh muscles. Pain is often perceived in the lateral aspect of the thigh and the low back and is aggravated by abducting the affected leg and by lying on the affected side. Tenderness is present at the edge of the greater trochanter. Injections of lidocaine often abolish the pain.

TENDINOUS LESIONS

Tendinous lesions include tenosynovitis, a lesion of the gliding surfaces of a tendon and its sheath; tendinitis, painful scarring within a tendon; and trigger lesions, which are localized enlargements of the tendon that engage a constricted part of the sheath (as in "trigger finger"). Tendinous lesions are common, occurring in many areas of the musculoskeletal system. An example is de Quervain's disease, which is stenosing tenosynovitis of the abductor pollicis longus and extensor pollicis brevis at the medial

TABLE 278–1. CONDITIONS CAUSING CARPAL TUNNEL SYNDROME

1. Trauma
2. Occupation
3. Infections: for example, Lyme disease and rubella
4. Rheumatoid arthritis and gout
5. Pregnancy
6. Hypothyroidism and acromegaly
7. Amyloidosis
8. Median artery aneurysm
9. Ganglion cyst, increased fat, hypertrophy of abductor pollicis muscle

styloid. Pain can be localized or can radiate into the hand or back to the shoulder. This and carpal tunnel syndrome occur frequently during pregnancy.

CARPAL TUNNEL SYNDROME

The symptoms of carpal tunnel syndrome are paresthesias and pain in the palmar side of the first three fingers and at times the radial half of the fourth finger; the pain may radiate proximally to the shoulder, creating confusion with a cervical disc syndrome. Physical findings include sensory loss, weakness on abduction and opposition of the thumb, and atrophy of the thenar eminence. Carpal tunnel syndrome is caused by an array of conditions that result in pressure on the median nerve as it passes through the bony flexor compartment of the wrist. Some of these causes are listed in Table 278–1.

Diagnosis is confirmed by electrophysiologic nerve tests. (The clinical tests commonly used are of questionable value.) Magnetic resonance imaging may be useful in defining the cause and thus directing treatment, which might include splinting of the wrist, corticosteroid injections, and surgical release of the transverse carpal ligament. Oral pyridoxine is of questionable value.

TENNIS ELBOW

"Tennis elbow" refers to a lesion of the wrist extensor muscles causing pain at the outer elbow, along the back of the forearm or, less commonly, into the shoulder. The burning or aching pain is produced by resisted extension of the wrist, as in grasping and lifting, and rarely is felt as sudden, searing twinges of intensity sufficient to cause momentary grip paralysis. Tennis elbow usually results from repeated forceful extension of the wrist. The tear most often occurs at the origin of the common extensor tendon from the lateral humoral epicondyle; much less frequently, the tear is in the muscle belly. Treatment includes injection of triamcinolone into the painful scar, manipulation, or tenotomy.

Like tennis elbow, "golfer's elbow" is a misnomer in that both conditions occur frequently in people who play neither sport. Golfer's elbow is less painful than tennis elbow; it represents a lesion of the common flexor tendon at the medial epicondyle. Pain is usually localized to the inner side of the elbow and is produced by resisted flexion of the wrist. Treatment includes triamcinolone injection or massage.

TIETZE'S SYNDROME

Tietze's syndrome is a common cause of chest pain that can be mistaken for visceral pain. There is tender, most often unilateral, swelling at one or more costosternal junctions. Biopsy samples of involved areas have revealed chronic inflammatory fibrosis. The syndrome may result from prolonged coughing or hyperventilation, but it is often idiopathic. Injections into the painful area with triamcinolone are sometimes curative.

Goldenberg DL, Simms RW, Geiger A, et al.: High frequency of fibromyalgia in patients with chronic fatigue seen in a primary care practice. Arthritis Rheum 33:381, 1990. *Of 27 patients with chronic fatigue syndrome seen in a primary care practice, 19 had symptoms and signs of fibromyalgia.*

Sheon RP, Moskowitz RW, Goldberg VM: Soft Tissue Rheumatic Pain: Recognition, Management, Prevention. 2nd ed. Philadelphia, Lea & Febiger, 1987.

279 Articular Tumors

Eugene V. Ball

Articular tumors can be classified as those that arise within the synovium; those that arise from cartilage, bone, or contiguous structures; and neoplasms that are nonarticular in origin but that may metastasize to joints or develop in multiple areas, including joints.

The most common of these are probably synovial chondromatosis and osteochondromatosis, which develop as cartilaginous synovial plaques that sometimes ossify. These cause episodic pain or swelling in a knee, hip, elbow, or shoulder. The joint may lock if the plaques become detached, forming loose bodies. Radiographs reveal multiple opacities if ossification has occurred; arthroscopy may be useful for both diagnosis and treatment.

Pigmented villonodular synovitis (PVNS) is a nonmalignant proliferative disorder of unknown etiology that usually affects the entire synovium of a single joint. This condition occurs most often in early middle age and in the knee in 80 per cent of cases. Uncommonly, two or more joints are involved; similar lesions occur in tendons and bursae. Pain and swelling are characteristic, as is serosanguineous synovial fluid. Radiographic signs include soft tissue swelling, subchondral cysts (particularly in the hip), and pressure erosions. Treatment is synovectomy. Hemangiomas, lipomas, and xanthomas may simulate PVNS.

Synoviomas (synovial sarcomas) are rare, aggressive tumors of young adults. They usually originate in the extremities adjacent to, but not within, a joint. Primary tumors histologically identical to synoviomas have been found in the head and neck, abdominal wall, retroperitoneum, heart, and mediastinum, supporting the view that the tumor originates from mesenchyme rather than synovium. Detection within tumor cells of both cytokeratin (an epithelial intermediate filament) and vimentin (a mesenchymal intermediate filament) has led to the suggestion that the synovioma is a carcinosarcoma. Synoviomas are usually discovered as deep swellings within a tendon sheath, a bursa, or a joint capsule. Pain and tenderness are variable, as are effusions. They metastasize early to lungs, bone, and lymph nodes. Tumor size greater than 4 cm, a high mitotic rate, and local recurrence after excision convey a poor prognosis.

Chondrosarcomas and fibrosarcomas are other malignancies arising within or near joints, and intrasynovial myeloma and lymphoma are rare causes of a swollen or painful joint.

Thorough investigation is required for unexplained pain or swelling within or adjacent to a single joint.

280 Erythromelalgia

Eugene V. Ball

Erythromelalgia (see Ch. 54) is a syndrome of episodic burning pain and redness in the extremities. Attacks may be confined to feet and, if severe and prolonged, may spread to the hands, or they may begin simultaneously in hands and feet. They are most often provoked by increasing environmental temperatures, although a few persons experience attacks only with febrile illnesses. The combination of increasing ambient temperatures and exercise often induces symptoms. Some persons maintain environmental temperatures at levels that are uncomfortably low for themselves, as well as others, to avoid attacks of erythromelalgia. Some sleep bundled up against the cold of an unheated room but with feet protruding uncovered from the blankets. Relief may require immersion of the feet in ice water. The feet appear normal between attacks except in those persons who habitually walk barefoot to avoid attacks provoked by wearing shoes.

Erythromelalgia is sometimes familial. In one remarkable kindred, the disorder is autosomal dominant, afflicting 32 of 66 members. Most often beginning between ages 2 and 8, it has been responsible for severe adjustment problems in youth, engendered in part by an inability to sit comfortably in a heated classroom or to participate in physical activities. In this kindred, the disorder has been frequently misdiagnosed as arthritis, reflex sympathetic dystrophy, or Raynaud's phenomenon; its pathogenesis is unknown, but it is not related to thrombocythemia.

By far the most common recognized cause of nonfamilial erythromelalgia is thrombocythemia, usually a feature of a myeloproliferative disorder. Erythromelalgia was the presenting symptom in 26 of 40 patients with platelet counts in excess of 500×10^9 per liter. Arteriolar inflammation and thrombotic occlusions were found on skin punch biopsy samples. Erythromelalgia disappeared for 3 or 4 days after a single dose of aspirin, which is the duration of its inhibition of platelet aggregation. In the absence of thrombocythemia, aspirins are likely to be ineffective for the treatment or prevention of erythromelalgia.

Other reported associations with erythromelalgia include diabetes mellitus. In addition, nifedipine and bromocriptine can cause an erythromelalgia-like disorder.

Michiels JJ, van Joost T, Vuzevski VD: Idiopathic erythromelalgia: A congenital disorder. J Am Acad Dermatol 21(S Pt. 2): 1128, 1989. *A brief report of idiopathic erythromelalgia in a female whose symptoms began at 2 years of age and increased in severity until age 14, by which time she was sleeping with her feet immersed in ice water.*

Millard FE, Hunter CS, Anderson M, et al.: Clinical manifestations of essential thrombocythemia in young adults. Am J Hematol 33:27, 1990. *Essential thrombocythemia was identified in 13 patients whose median age was 26. Erythromelalgia was the most common complication, occurring in 7 of the 13, of whom 7 were males.*

281 Multifocal Fibrosclerosis

H. Ralph Schumacher, Jr.

In rare instances the delicate fibrous areolar tissue in a certain anatomic region becomes the site of a chronic low-grade inflammatory process, leading to deposition of dense sclerotic plaques, which may obstruct or limit the movement of adjacent viscera. When the process is in the active phase, there are characteristic findings of chronic or granulomatous inflammation, featured by mononuclear cell infiltration, plasma cells, and occasional giant cells. In the end stages the pathologic lesion is simply that of scar tissue, so that by the time this process causes clinical manifestations there may be little evidence of the initial inflammatory reaction. In at least some cases there is an accompanying vasculitis. As a general rule the process tends to originate in the midline, around the great vessels, and then to spread laterally. In most cases a clue to the inciting mechanism is lacking.

Syndromes that have been considered as manifestations of multifocal fibrosclerosis include retroperitoneal fibrosis, mediastinal fibrosis, sclerosing cholangitis (see Ch. 126), Riedel's thyroiditis (see Ch. 216), pseudotumor of the orbit, Peyronie's disease (a sclerotic induration of the corpora cavernosa of the penis), and sclerosing peritonitis. Other sites of a similar fibrosis, such as the testes, vagina, and suprasellar area, have also been reported. Pulmonary and myocardial fibrosis syndromes have generally not been seen as related to multifocal fibrosclerosis, although pleural fibrosis along with retroperitoneal fibrosis can be seen with ergotamine use.

Although most of these syndromes have been described as separate entities, several anatomic areas may become affected in one person. For example, retroperitoneal fibrosis and sclerosing mediastinitis may be present at the same time along with varying combinations of sclerosing cholangitis, Riedel's thyroiditis, and pseudotumor of the orbit. A possible genetic predisposition is suggested by familial cases and by an association between fibrosing syndromes and alpha₁-antitrypsin deficiency. Recent reports have also described familial mediastinal or retroperitoneal fibrosis associated with HLA (human leukocyte antigen)-B27 and seronegative spondyloarthropathies; relations to aortic inflammation with a possible element of reaction to atheromatous components has been described.

Comings DE, Skubi KB, Van Eyes J, et al.: Familial multifocal sclerosis. Ann Intern Med 66:884, 1967. *Description of multiple sites of fibrosis in two brothers.*

Goldbach P, Mohsenifar Z, Salick AI: Familial mediastinal fibrosis associated with seronegative spondyloarthropathy. Arthritis Rheum 26:221, 1983. *Two siblings with both diseases.*

RETROPERITONEAL FIBROSIS

In retroperitoneal fibrosis the process usually begins over the promontory of the sacrum and extends laterally across the ureters and as high as the second or third lumbar vertebra. Less commonly, the lesion develops in other extraperitoneal areas, for example, contiguous with the kidneys, duodenum, descending colon, or urinary bladder. In some cases there has been an associated vasculitis in the skin and subcutaneous tissue, manifested by the formation of nodules, erythematous discolorations, and ulcerations. Similarly, inflammatory changes in small vessels at the sites of the sclerosis have been noted. Glomerulonephritis has been seen in a few patients.

The occurrence of retroperitoneal fibrosis in patients taking methysergide for migraine has been reported with greater frequency than could be due to chance. Occasional cases have been reported after use of other drugs such as ergotamine, various beta-adrenergic blocking agents, hydralazine, or methyldopa. Associated diseases in patients with retroperitoneal fibrosis have included systemic lupus erythematosus, vasculitis, scleroderma, eosinophilic fasciitis, biliary cirrhosis, rubella-associated arthritis, and carcinoid. Retroperitoneal tumors, trauma, or surgery may be a factor in some cases. One patient with associated periarticular fibrosis had elevated plasma levels of a platelet-derived growth factor.

The disorder is about twice as common in males as in females, and the peak incidence is in the fifth and sixth decades. Cases have been reported in children. The manifestations are variable, depending on the anatomic location of the process. Pain is the most common symptom; it is vague, tends to be located in the low back, and may be accompanied by symptoms referable to the gastrointestinal tract. The patient is likely to lose weight and have low-grade fever. There may be some anemia and elevation of the erythrocyte sedimentation rate. Although the ureter is the structure most often affected, symptoms referable to the urinary tract are uncommon until obstructive uropathy has led to azotemia and other clinical manifestations of renal insufficiency. The fibrosing process may surround the inferior vena cava, but obstruction of that vessel is uncommon. Thromboembolism and hypertension can be complications. Arterial invasion has been described. Retroperitoneal fibrosis occasionally develops in association with abdominal aortic aneurysm or aortitis.

Diagnosis of retroperitoneal fibrosis has been most often suggested by the findings at intravenous pyelography: displacement of the ureters toward the midline and evidence of obstruction, usually at the level of the pelvic brim. One or both ureters may be affected. In rare instances a mass can be palpated in the pelvis or on the posterior abdominal wall. Ultrasonography, computed tomographic (CT) scanning, and magnetic resonance imaging (MRI) can also identify the fibrosing masses. Once a mass has been disclosed, the main problem in differential diagnosis lies in distinguishing retroperitoneal fibrosis from retroperitoneal tumor. Multiple deep biopsies should be made at the time of laparotomy.

Surgical treatment, if employed before there has been severe renal damage, is often highly successful. Inasmuch as the fibrosing process is seldom invasive, the constricted organ can usually be freed by blunt dissection so that normal movement or flow is restored. Relief of ureteral obstruction is usually achieved by bringing the ureter out on the anterior surface of the sclerotic mass. Occasionally, however, the obstruction recurs months or years after such treatment. Some surgeons wrap the ureters in omentum to try to decrease recurrent obstruction. Steroid therapy may be helpful in the rare case detected early or may be employed as an adjunct to surgical measures. Azathioprine has been used successfully in a few cases. Other drugs such as penicillamine, colchicine, and gamma-interferon, with theoretical ability to limit clinical fibrosis, have not been studied in this disease. Progesterone has been used with some apparent success in Latin America. When the inferior vena cava is obstructed, surgical relief is technically difficult and risky; here it may be preferable to temporize in the hope that development of collateral pathways may alleviate the circulatory block.

The long-term outlook is fairly good if the disease is recognized and if its obstructive consequences can be treated by surgical means. The disease often tends to run its course and subside. Most deaths have been caused by renal failure.

Cohle SD, Leil JT: Inflammatory aneurism of the aorta, aortitis and coronary arteritis. Arch Pathol Lab Med 112:1121, 1988. *Inflammatory aneurisms of the aorta and other vasculitis may be associated with retroperitoneal fibrosis.*

Ewald EA, Gikas PW, Castor CW: Periarticular fibrosis associated with idiopathic retroperitoneal fibrosis. J Rheum 15: 1443, 1988. *Elevated plasma platelet-derived growth factor is proposed as a possible pathogenetic mechanism.*

MEDIASTINAL FIBROSIS

Taut bundles of collagenous tissue form in the superior and anterior mediastinum, with impingement on the aorta, trachea, bronchi, esophagus, and pericardium, but the predominant manifestations are those caused by obstruction of the superior vena cava: puffy, suffused appearance of the face and conjunctivae; nonpitting edema of the face, neck, and upper extremities; and distended veins in the neck and upper extremities. Rarely the principal vessels affected are the pulmonary arteries, causing pulmonary hypertension. More frequently, the pulmonary veins are involved, and here severe hemoptysis may be the most prominent manifestation. Pericardial fibrosis can lead to constrictive pericarditis. The main task in differential diagnosis is to distinguish this relatively benign condition from obstruction caused by tumor. Roentgenographic examination of the chest may reveal little or no abnormality, but angiographic studies show obstruction of the affected vessels. Thoracotomy may be required for histologic diagnosis.

Histoplasmosis and possibly tuberculosis may cause some mediastinal fibrosis. Mediastinal hemorrhage can lead to fibrosis, and cases have been associated with methysergide use. Some patients with this syndrome have shown gradual improvement over months or years, presumably because of development of collateral circulation. Successful superior vena cava bypass surgery has been described. Steroid and other drug therapy as used with retroperitoneal fibrosis seems reasonable if infection is excluded, but such treatment has not been studied.

Dye TE, Saab SB, Almond MD, et al.: Sclerosing mediastinitis with occlusion of pulmonary veins. J Thorac Cardiovasc Surg 74:137, 1977. *An unusual but serious and treatable cause of hemoptysis.*

Goodwin RA, Nickell JA, Dez Pres RM: Mediastinal fibrosis complicating healed primary histoplasmosis and tuberculosis. Medicine 51:227, 1972. *Excellent review, certainly implicating histoplasmosis.*

SCLEROSING PERITONITIS

A fibrotic syndrome has been observed in patients treated for prolonged periods with the now withdrawn beta-adrenergic blocking drug practolol. Only a few cases have been reported with propranolol or other beta blockers. Some cases have developed a year or longer after cessation of therapy. The peritonitis consists of a thick fibrous encasement of the small intestine, and the symptoms include abdominal fullness, back pain, ascites, weight loss, and signs of subacute obstruction. It has usually been possible to relieve the symptoms by surgery, with blunt dissection to peel away the fibrous tissue. Some improvement occurs with time. A few patients treated with practolol have developed apparently related pericardial or lung disease, conjunctivitis, and dermatitis. Sclerosing peritonitis with many similarities has also been seen in patients treated with chronic ambulatory peritoneal dialysis, in drug abusers, and in an idiopathic form. Silica from talc is a possible factor in some cases. Antibiotics or other agents used in dialysis may also contribute.

Castelli MJ, Armin A-R, Husain A, et al.: Fibrosing peritonitis in a drug abuser. Arch Pathol Lab Med 109:767, 1985. *Perhaps this will become a more common problem.*

Pusateri R, Ross R, Marshall R, et al.: Sclerosing encapsulating peritonitis; report of a case with small bowel obstruction managed by long term hyperalimentation, and a review of the literature. Am J Kidney Dis 8:56, 1986. *This is a serious complication of peritoneal dialysis. Improvement in this patient occurred during parenteral nutrition.*

PART XX
INFECTIOUS DISEASES

SECTION ONE / INTRODUCTION

282 Introduction to Microbial Disease

Gerald L. Mandell

Infectious diseases have profoundly influenced the course of human history. The black plague (caused by *Yersinia pestis*) changed the social structure of medieval Europe. Military campaigns have been profoundly affected by outbreaks of diseases such as dysentery and typhus. Malaria has altered the geographic and racial pattern of distribution of hemogloblins and erythrocyte antigens. The development of *Plasmodium falciparum* is inhibited by the presence of hemoglobin S, and Duffy blood group–negative erythrocytes are resistant to infection with *Plasmodium vivax*. Infections are the major cause of morbidity and mortality in the developing world. AIDS threatens to disrupt the social fabric in some countries of Africa and is severely stressing the health care system in the United States and other parts of the world.

Infection may be defined as multiplication of microbes (viruses, bacteria, fungi, protozoa, or multicellular parasites) in the tissues of the host. The host may or may not be symptomatic. For example, infection with the human immunodeficiency virus may cause no signs or symptoms of illness or tissue damage for years. The definition of infection should also include instances of multiplication of microbes on the surface or in a lumen of the host, causing signs and symptoms of illness or disease. Certain strains of *Escherichia coli* may multiply in the gut and cause a diarrheal illness without invading tissues. This is also considered an infection. Microbes can cause diseases by virtue of toxin production without actually infecting the host. *Clostridium botulinum* can grow in certain improperly processed foods and produce a toxin that can be lethal upon ingestion. At no time does the microbe grow in or on the host. A relatively trivial infection such as that caused by *Clostridium tetani* in a small puncture wound can cause devastating illness because of a toxin released from the organism growing in the tissues.

We live in a virtual sea of microorganisms, and all our body surfaces have an indigenous bacterial flora. This normal flora actually protects us from infection. Reduction of gut colonization increases susceptibility to infection by pathogens such as *Salmonella typhimurium*. The normal flora is thought to exert its protective effect by several mechanisms: (1) utilizing nutrients and occupying an ecologic niche, thus competing with pathogens; (2) production of antibacterial substances that inhibit the growth of pathogens; and (3) induction of host immunity that is cross-reactive and effective against pathogens. In addition to the normal flora, transient colonization may be seen with known or potential pathogens. This may be a special problem in hospitalized patients (see Ch. 289).

Only a very small proportion of microbes may be considered to be principal or professional pathogens, and even among these species only a relatively small number of clones have been shown to cause disease. This supports the concept that pathogenic organisms are highly adapted to the pathogenic state and have developed a set of characteristics which enables them to be transmitted, to attach to surfaces, to invade tissue, and to cause disease. In contrast, opportunistic pathogens cause disease principally in impaired hosts. Organisms that may be harmless members of the normal flora in healthy people may act as virulent invaders in patients with severe defects in host defense mechanisms. Pathogenic organisms may be acquired by several routes. Direct contact has been implicated in the acquisition of staphylococcal disease. Airborne spread, usually by droplet nuclei, is seen in respiratory diseases such as influenza. Contaminated water may be implicated in *Giardia* infection and typhoid fever. Food-borne toxin illnesses may be caused by extracellular toxins produced by *Clostridium perfringens* and *Staphylococcus aureus*. Blood and blood products may be vectors for transmitting hepatitis B virus and the human immunodeficiency virus. Sexual transmission is important for these latter two agents and for a variety of pathogens including *Treponema pallidum* (syphilis), *Neisseria gonorrhoeae*, (gonorrhea), and *Chlamydia trachomatis* (nonspecific urethritis). The fetus may be infected in utero, and this has been seen with rubella virus and cytomegalovirus. Insect vectors may be important, as illustrated by mosquitoes for malaria, ticks for Lyme disease, and lice for typhus.

Pathogens are able to cause disease because of a finely tuned array of adaptations. These include the ability to attach to appropriate cells, often mediated by specialized structures such as the pili on gram-negative rods. Microbes such as *Shigella* species have the ability to invade cells and cause damage in that way. Toxins may act at a distance or may intoxicate infected cells. Pathogens have the ability to thwart host defenses by a variety of ingenious maneuvers. The antiphagocytic capsular coat of the pneumococcus is an example. Organisms may change their surface antigen display so as to outmaneuver the host immune system. This can be seen with influenza virus and trypanosomes. Certain pathogens have the ability to inhibit the respiratory burst of phagocytes (*Toxoplasma gondii*), and others can destroy phagocytic cells that have engulfed them (*Streptococcus pyogenes*). The environment plays an important role in infection, both in transmission and in ability of the host to combat the invader. The humidity and temperature of air may affect the infectivity of airborne pathogens. The sanitary state of food and water is an important factor for the acquisition of enteric pathogens. The "bad air" of swamps associated with malaria turned out to be due to the mosquitoes, but the environmental association was appropriate. The nutritional status of the host clearly is a significant factor in certain infectious diseases. The establishment of infection is a complicated interplay of factors involving the microbe, the host, and the environment.

With rare exceptions, infections are treatable and often curable diseases. Thus it is important to make an accurate etiologic diagnosis and promptly institute appropriate therapy. In acute infections such as pneumonia, meningitis, or gram-negative sepsis, rapid institution of therapy may be life-saving and thus a *presumptive* etiologic diagnosis should be established prior to a *definitive* diagnosis. This presumptive diagnosis can be based on the history, physical examination, epidemiology of illness in the community, and rapid techniques such as microscopic examination of appropriate Gram-stained specimens. Antimicrobial therapy can then be instituted for the presumptive etiologic agents but must be re-evaluated as more definitive diagnostic information becomes available.

1566

283 Introduction to Bacterial Disease

Gerald L. Mandell

Bacteria are classified in the kingdom Procaryotae and contain DNA in a double-stranded loop not bounded by a membrane. The success of bacteria as life forms can be illustrated by the fact that fossils of bacteria 3.5 billion years old have been found. Bacteria are ubiquitous and can grow at temperatures as low as 0°C and as high as 110°C. All bacteria have a bilayered cytoplasmic membrane, and most bacteria (mycoplasma are exceptions) have an outer cell wall containing muramic acid. Morphologic features are often used to categorize bacteria. Bacilli are rods or cylinders with about half the species being motile, while cocci are spherical and nonmotile. It is useful to distinguish bacteria by their ability to retain a basic dye (crystal violet) after iodine fixation and alcohol decolorization (the Gram reaction). Gram-positive organisms retain the dye and contain techoic acids in their cell walls, whereas gram-negative bacteria have an additional outer membrane containing lipopolysaccharide (endotoxin). Capsules may serve as major virulence factors by interfering with the ability of phagocytes to ingest the encapsulated organisms. The capsules of the pneumococcus and *Haemophilus influenzae* are important factors for the virulence of the organisms. Pili or fimbriae are smaller hairlike structures that mediate bacterial attachment to various tissues and body surfaces. Only a very small proportion of species are pathogenic for humans, and new data suggest that even among those pathogenic species only certain clones are true pathogens.

Bacteria may be separated by their ability to reside and replicate intracellularly. Examples of intracellular bacteria include *Salmonella typhi*, *Legionella* species, mycobacteria, and chlamydiae. Extracellular pathogens include streptococci (including pneumococci), staphylococci, and most gram-negative enteric rods such as *Escherichia coli*, *Klebsiella* species, and *Pseudomonas* species. The main technique used for identification of bacteria in patient specimens is culture on artificial media. The ability to grow on the surface of such media in air defines aerobic organisms. Anaerobes cannot grow under such conditions, and facultative organisms can grow either aerobically or anaerobically. Microscopy can be a very useful technique, especially when combined with appropriate staining procedures such as acid-fast stains for mycobacteria or Gram's stain to differentiate grampositive from gram-negative organisms. Newer techniques utilize direct immunofluorescence (e.g., for *Chlamydia trachomatis*), DNA probes (e.g., for *Legionella* species), and latex agglutination tests to detect antigen (e.g., for pneumococcal capsular antigen in spinal fluid). Assays using the polymerase chain reaction are being studied. Tests for antibodies are less useful but may be helpful in some diseases (e.g., Lyme disease).

284 The Febrile Patient

David C. Dale

Fever or *pyrexia* is an elevation of body temperature to a level above normal, i.e., to more than 37.5°C (99.5°F). It is a useful marker of inflammation; usually the height of the fever reflects the severity of the inflammatory process. Anorexia, malaise, myalgias, headache, and other constitutional symptoms often occur concomitantly. When the body temperature changes rapidly, chills and sweats are also observed. Fever with night sweats is a feature of many chronic inflammatory conditions. *Hyperthermia* is a term for fever due to a disturbance of thermal regulatory control: excessive heat production (e.g., with vigorous exercise or as a reaction to some anesthetics), decreased dissipation (e.g., with dehydration), or loss of regulation (e.g., due to injury to the hypothalamic regulatory center).

Most febrile patients have pain, tenderness, redness, and swelling at the site of inflammation, and the cause of the fever is readily identified. In a general medical practice, the most common causes of fever are respiratory illnesses, urinary tract infections, cellulitis, and superficial abscesses. In hospital patients, pneumonia is the most common cause. In otherwise healthy individuals, fever alone is not a cause for hospitalization unless it is quite high (greater than 39°C, or 102°F) or accompanied by shaking chills, hypotension, a change in the sensorium, or other symptoms suggesting bacteremia. However, in immunosuppressed individuals, the elderly, and patients with recent surgery, greater caution is indicated.

FEVER OF UNKNOWN ORIGIN (FUO)

An FUO is usually defined as an illness lasting more than 3 weeks with temperatures greater than 101°F (38.3°C) in which a diagnosis has not been made despite a good hospital or office evaluation. Ordinarily by this time the workup has included a history, physical examination, routine blood and urine tests and cultures, radiographs, and some specialized serologic tests. With careful further evaluation a diagnosis can be made in 70 to 90 per cent of these cases.

Diagnoses for FUO's fall into six general categories: infections, noninfectious inflammatory conditions, neoplastic diseases, drug fevers, factitious illnesses, and a group of less common causes (Table 284–1). The pattern of fever is only occasionally helpful in pointing to a specific diagnosis, e.g., the alternate-day fever in established *Plasmodium vivax* infections, the sustained fever in untreated *Salmonella typhi* infections and other continuous bacteremias, and the relapsing (Pel-Ebstein) fever in Hodgkin's disease and other lymphomas.

Evaluation of the FUO Patient

In patients with persisting fevers, it is important first to carefully review the medical history and repeat the physical examination. New clues may be found in the social, occupational, travel, and medication history. Previous medical and surgical

TABLE 284–1. CAUSES OF FEVER OF UNKNOWN ORIGIN

Infections
Abscesses—hepatic, subhepatic, gallbladder, subphrenic, splenic, periappendiceal, perinephric, pelvic, and other sites
Granulomatous—extrapulmonary and miliary tuberculosis, atypical *Mycobacteria*, fungal infection
Intravascular—endocarditis, meningococcemia, gonococcemia, *Listeria*, *Brucella*, rat-bite fever, relapsing fever
Viral, rickettsial, and chlamydial—infectious mononucleosis, cytomegalovirus (CMV), human immunodeficiency virus (HIV), hepatitis, Q fever, psittacosis
Parasitic—extraintestinal amebiasis, malaria, toxoplasmosis

Noninfectious inflammatory disorders
Collagen-vascular diseases—rheumatic fever, systemic lupus erythematosus, rheumatoid arthritis (particularly Still's disease), vasculitis (all types)
Granulomatous—sarcoidosis, granulomatous hepatitis, Crohn's disease
Tissue injury—pulmonary emboli, sickle cell disease, hemolytic anemia

Neoplastic diseases
Lymphoma/leukemia—Hodgkin's and non-Hodgkin's lymphoma, acute leukemias
Carcinoma—kidney, pancreas, liver, gastrointestinal tract, lung, especially when metastatic
Atrial myxomas

Drug fevers
Sulfonamides, penicillins, thiouracils, barbiturates, quinidine, laxatives (especially with phenolphthalein)

Factitious illnesses
Injections of toxic materials, manipulation or exchange of thermometers

Other causes
Familial Mediterranean fever, Fabry's disease, cyclic neutropenia

illnesses, alcohol intake, and animal contacts are important. On physical examination, special attention should be given to the skin, lymph nodes (including epitrochlear, postauricular, axillary), mucous membranes (including the conjunctivae), and abdominal region (masses, tenderness, and size of the liver and spleen). Usually the basic laboratory tests—CBC, differential, sedimentation rate, urinalysis, liver function tests, skin tests for delayed hypersensitivity (e.g., PPD, mumps), and stool for occult blood—should be repeated. Most patients with active inflammation are anemic, and the leukocyte differential can provide valuable clues. Neutrophilia suggests an occult bacterial infection. Monocytosis suggests tuberculosis, brucellosis, inflammatory bowel disease, or other chronic inflammatory conditions. Severe lymphopenia suggests immunodeficiency or a malignancy. A very elevated sedimentation rate suggests giant cell/temporal arteritis, polymyalgia rheumatica, Still's disease, bacterial endocarditis, or other occult infections, and a normal test rarely occurs with any of these illnesses. If the alkaline phosphatase is elevated, obstructive or infiltrative disease of the liver is the most likely cause, although nonspecific elevation is not uncommon. Other tests, e.g., antinuclear antibodies, febrile agglutinins, complement assays, may be positive but are rarely helpful in the FUO evaluation.

A definitive diagnosis is usually made through a combination of imaging studies, microbiologic tests, and/or biopsies. Previous radiographs should be reviewed carefully for evidence of sinusitis, apical inflammation or small nodules in the lungs, hilar adenopathy, or an intra-abdominal mass. Abdominal ultrasonography, computed tomography (CT), or magnetic resonance imaging (MRI) is very helpful to examine the liver, gallbladder, spleen, and pelvic areas for tumors and abscesses. These tests have reduced, but not completely eliminated, the need for exploratory laparotomies.

Cultures of blood (including for *Mycobacterium avium* in HIV patients), urine (including mycobacterial cultures if tuberculosis is suspected), and other bodily fluids (e.g., cerebrospinal, peritoneal, pleural) should be obtained if at all suggested by the clinical examination. It is useful to do anaerobic cultures of materials from suspected abscess cavities and to examine blood cultures for fastidious bacteria, yeast, and fungi in difficult cases. A tissue diagnosis often can be made from a biopsy of abnormal skin or lymph nodes or the bone marrow. Biopsies or needle aspirations of liver, lung, bone, or other deep tissue sites are also valuable when abscesses or tumors are suspected.

THERAPY

Therapeutic trials with antibiotics, corticosteroids, or antipyretics before the diagnosis is clear can confuse the evaluation. In some instances a trial may be justified but should be time limited, i.e., about 2 weeks. In patients with deep tissue abscesses, fever usually persists despite antibiotics. In patients with noninfectious inflammatory diseases, e.g., sarcoidosis, Still's disease, or vasculitis, a good clinical diagnosis usually can be made before such therapies are begun. In patients with malignancies, rational therapy depends upon a tissue diagnosis. Patients with factitious illness often have serious underlying psychiatric disorders. Care in confrontation is essential to prevent desperate acts including suicide.

Extensive workups of FUO's can be very expensive. In every patient the need for hospital care and testing should be continuously reassessed. When the patient is not severely ill, it is frequently worthwhile to use observation alone as a diagnostic tool. Sometimes even a short period of observation allows an obscure diagnosis to become obvious. In other cases, the fever disappears without the necessity for further diagnostic tests.

Aduan RP, Fauci AS, Dale DC, et al.: Factitious fever and self-induced infection: A report of 32 cases and a review of the literature. Ann Intern Med 90:230, 1979. *A comprehensive review of a large series of patients.*

Bor DH, Makadon HJ, Friedland G, et al.: Fever in hospitalized medical patients: Characteristics and significance. J Gen Intern Med 3:119, 1988. *A careful review of the frequency and outcome of illnesses with fever in an acute care hospital.*

Dinarello CA, Wolff SM: Fever of unknown origin. *In* Principles and Practice of Infectious Diseases. New York, Churchill, Livingstone, 1990, pp 468–478. *A comprehensive discussion of the diagnosis of FUO.*

Larson EB, Featherstone HJ, Petersdorf RG: Fever of undetermined origin: Diagnosis and follow-up of 105 cases 1970–1980. Medicine 61:269, 1982. *A comparison of a series of cases from the 1970's with the series studied by Petersdorf and Beeson in the 1950's.*

Mackowiak PA, LeMaistre CF: Drug fever: A critical appraisal of conventional concepts: An analysis of 51 episodes in two Dallas hospitals and 97 episodes reported in the English literature. Ann Intern Med 106:728, 1987. *Illustrates the causes and courses of drug fevers in 51 cases, with a review of the literature.*

Rowland MD, Del Bene VE: Use of body computed tomography to evaluate fever of unknown origin. J Infect Dis 156:408, 1987. *Outlines the usefulness of CT for FUO patients.*

285 The Pathogenesis of Fever
Bruce Beutler and Steven M. Beutler

FEVER: DEFINITION

Fever (pyrexia) entails an elevation of core body temperature above the level that is normally maintained by the individual. Under normal circumstances, core body temperature (the temperature of blood in the right atrium) is tightly regulated, exhibiting circadian variations over a range that usually does not exceed 0.6°C (1°F), with a mean value of 37°C (98.6°F) (the normal "set point"). An array of thermoregulatory mechanisms, described in detail below, ensures that this temperature is maintained. During episodes of fever, the thermoregulatory set point is shifted, such that the same thermoregulatory mechanisms are employed to maintain an abnormally elevated temperature.

It is important to realize that fever is not equivalent to an elevated core temperature, but to an elevated set point. Under many circumstances, ranging from intense physical exertion to immersion in hot liquids, core temperature may be elevated yet fever does not exist, since an attempt to cope with the departure from homeostasis is in progress. Failure of thermoregulation may also be associated with elevated core temperature; this problem (which obtains in malignant hyperthermia) is also distinct from fever.

THERMOREGULATORY MECHANISMS

Central to any consideration of fever is an understanding of the larger issue of thermoregulation. Core body temperature is determined by two opposing processes, each of which is regulated by the central nervous system. On the one hand, energy in the form of heat is generated by living tissues through a process termed *thermogenesis*. Energy may be passively absorbed from the environment as well. On the other hand, energy is inevitably lost to the environment, chiefly through the emission of infrared radiation and through transfer of energy to a surrounding medium, or to water, which is then volatilized. The temperature at which tissues are maintained is related to heat capacity (i.e., to the amount of energy required to elevate temperature by a defined increment) and to the quantity of energy lost or gained by the system.

Heat is liberated as a product of exothermic chemical reactions, which occur in both anabolic and catabolic pathways. Several "futile cycles" have been defined in which the energy stored in phosphate bonds is liberated in the absence of other net chemical transformation. Such cycles may supply a substantial fraction of the heat produced in thermogenesis. A second thermogenic mechanism consists in the utilization of ATP for the directional transport of ions across biologic membranes. Uncoupling agents, which disrupt the proton gradient so generated in mitochondria, stimulate thermogenesis by increasing the number of chemical transformations performed to achieve a given quantity of work. In humans, liver and muscle tissue are capable of liberating the major portion of energy in the form of heat, although all cells participate to some degree. In other species and in human infants, brown adipose tissue is also an important source of heat.

Metabolic reactions proceed more rapidly at an elevated temperature. Therefore, the passive warming effect of a febrile state leads to accelerated production of energy in the form of heat: For each temperature increment of 0.6°C (1°F), basal metabolic rate increases by approximately 10 per cent. This may, at times, be quite significant from a nutritional point of view. While the resting energy output of an average 70-kg man might approximate 60 watts, it would be expected that the same individual would exhibit an energy output of at least 100 watts when febrile to a temperature of 40.6°C (105°F), based solely upon the accelerated rate of exothermic reactions. Of course, a still greater expenditure of energy might be required to maintain the fever itself.

Muscle is a particularly flexible transducer of chemical energy, since its metabolic activity is largely controlled by the central nervous system. *Shivering thermogenesis* refers to the involuntary process whereby muscles are recruited to produce energy through the exercise of activity, leading to an enhanced metabolic demand. This is one mechanism responsible for the rise in body temperature witnessed in fever. Hence, a sharp "chill" often heralds the onset of fever.

Conservation of energy is effected through piloerection in mammals other than humans. In humans, the development of "gooseflesh" is the equivalent response. Other dermal reactions are also involved: "Flushing" represents a redistribution of circulation to dermal vessels and facilitates heat loss; a blanched appearance of the skin indicates an attempt to conserve heat. Fever is frequently accompanied by a perception of "coldness," prompting efforts to seek warmth.

INITIATION OF FEVER

The neural pathways responsible for thermoregulation originate in the hypothalamus. The exact location of thermoregulatory centers in man remains unknown, although preoptic, supraoptic, anterior, ventromedial, paraventricular, and suprachiasmatic areas have been implicated in animals. A local sensing mechanism exists, wherein the temperature of blood is coupled to the development of autonomic discharge. Elevation of body temperature depends primarily upon sympathetic outflow, leading to shivering thermogenesis and dermal vasoconstriction, whereas cooling mechanisms (sweating and dermal vasodilation) involve a mixture of sympathetic and parasympathetic pathways.

Certain neurotropic drugs are capable of disrupting the hypothalamic thermosensory mechanism or blunting the hypothalamic response and so may interfere with the development of fever. Among these, phenothiazines are the best known for their "poikilothermic" effect. These agents are not specifically active in febrile states; rather, they act to disable thermoregulatory mechanisms at all times following their administration.

CLINICAL ASPECTS OF FEVER

Although fever patterns tend to be nonspecific, they may sometimes provide diagnostic clues. Well known is the alternate-day fever pattern often seen with *Plasmodium vivax* and *Plasmodium ovale* infection. *Plasmodium malariae*, on the other hand, results in fever occurring every third day. A relapsing fever pattern is seen with *Borrelia* infection. Fevers occur daily for 3 to 6 days; a fever-free interval of about 1 week's duration then supervenes. A similar phenomenon is seen in rat-bite fever. Cases of brucellosis and typhoid may be characterized by a continuous "undulating fever." Hodgkin's disease is sometimes accompanied by periodic pyrexia (Pel-Ebstein phenomenon) with cycles lasting variable periods.

Intermittent fevers are seen in many conditions and are therefore of little help in discriminating between various disorders. Intermittent fever may also be caused by the interruption of a continuous fever with antipyretics or cooling measures; such interventions must be taken into account when attempting to analyze a temperature curve.

In addition to considering patterns of pyrexia, it is worthwhile to note the relationship between core temperature and other vital signs. For example, a dissociation between temperature and pulse is sometimes seen in cases of typhoid fever, Legionnaires' disease, psittacosis, and brucellosis. Factitious fever is also accompanied by an inappropriately low pulse. In addition, the respiratory rate may remain unchanged, and normal superimposed diurnal variations in temperature may be absent in factitious fever.

Drug fever may occur in association with nearly any medication. Antibiotics, particularly β-lactam agents, sulfonamides, and nitrofurantoin, are most frequently responsible. Drug fever usually develops within 5 to 10 days following initiation of therapy but can develop after a single dose or after months of administration. Drug fever may persist for several days after withdrawal of the offending agent and occasionally begins after the drug has been withdrawn. There is no characteristic fever pattern. Fevers due to drug allergy tend to be well tolerated but may be accompanied by other allergic phenomena such as nephritis or neutropenia. These, along with rash, may occur in 20 to 60 per cent of patients with drug fever. In the remaining cases, fever may be the sole manifestation. On occasion, drugs appear to induce fever by behaving as exogenous pyrogens (see below).

The response to antipyretics or antibiotics may shed light on the etiology of the fever. For example, fever due to malignancy uncomplicated by infection sometimes responds dramatically to low doses of nonsteroidal anti-inflammatory drugs. Such therapy usually proves ineffective in eliminating fever due to an unremitting infection. Fever caused by pneumococcal pneumonia characteristically resolves promptly upon administration of penicillin; similarly, administration of appropriate antimalarial drugs may result in rapid cessation of fever caused by malaria. Resolution of fever following withdrawal of a medication is characteristic of a drug fever.

Extreme pyrexia (characterized by a core temperature exceeding 41°C, or 106°F) often indicates failure of a distal mechanism of thermoregulation, occurring alone or in combination with infection. Examples of noninfectious causes of such extreme pyrexia include heat stroke, neuroleptic malignant syndrome, and malignant hyperthermia associated with succinylcholine.

CYTOKINES AND FEVER

Hypothalamic dysregulation and fever are triggered by proteins released from cells of the immune system (Fig. 285–1). This communication between the immune system and the nervous system is perhaps the most thoroughly studied "neuroimmunoendocrine" link. In response to invasive stimuli, including components of various microorganisms (e.g., lipoteichoic acid, lipopolysaccharides, and other constituents [collectively termed *exogenous pyrogens*]) or certain chemical agents (e.g., amphotericin and perhaps other drugs), cells of the immune system (principally macrophages and, to a lesser extent, lymphocytes) produce proteins that behave as *endogenous pyrogens*. These proteins are designated "monokines" and "lymphokines," respectively, and are often denoted under the more general heading of "cytokines." During the past decade, several of the cytokines active in the pathogenesis of fever have been isolated, and their structures have been determined by molecular cloning. At present, 11 proteins with pyrogenic activity have been identified (Table 285–1), and it is likely that many others exist. Although mononuclear phagocytes are the principal source of pyrogenic cytokines, the same proteins may sometimes originate from nonimmune cells of neoplastic tissue, in which autonomous production and secretion may occur.

The pyrogenic cytokines are structurally diverse proteins with well-established effects in hematopoiesis, inflammation, and the regulation of cell metabolism. Individual agents are often markedly pleiotropic in their actions. In addition to their involvement in the mediation of fever, cytokines mediate the "acute phase response," which is characterized by increased production of "acute phase reactants" in the liver (fibrinogen, C-reactive protein, complement proteins B, C3, C4, α_2-acid glycoprotein, serum amyloid A, and a variety of proteinase inhibitors among them), decreased production of albumin and transferrin, hypoferremia, hypertriglyceridemia, and other metabolic changes.

Pyrogenic cytokines are presumed to bind to receptors present on vascular endothelial cells that lie within the hypothalamus. They act to reset the hypothalamic thermoregulatory center, prompting an elevation of core body temperature. The resetting is believed to depend largely upon endothelial cell production of prostaglandins (PGE_2 and perhaps $PGF_{2\alpha}$). Thromboxanes and lipoxygenase products may also affect the set point. Cytokines may also interact directly with neural tissues; there is evidence to suggest that the release of corticotropin-releasing factor (CRF) may trigger thermogenesis in response to at least one cytokine (interleukin 1β).

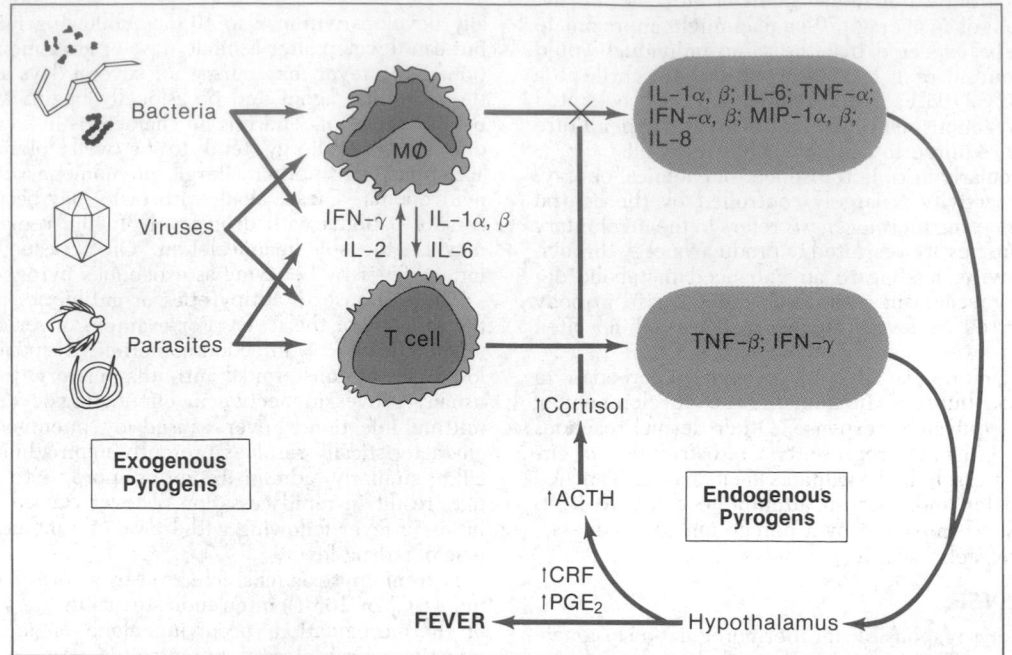

FIGURE 285–1. Production of endogenous pyrogens by macrophages and T lymphocytes. A variety of microbial pathogens produce molecules that function as exogenous pyrogens, triggering the release of endogenous pyrogens from mononuclear cells. ACTH = Adrenocorticotropic hormone; CRF = corticotropin-releasing factor; PGE$_2$ = prostaglandin E$_2$; other abbreviations are defined in the text and Table 285–1.

TABLE 285–1. PROTEINS WITH PYROGENIC ACTIVITY

Endogenous Pyrogen	Other Names/ Abbreviations	Principal Source	Induced by	Principal Effects in Addition to Pyrogenesis	Physical Characteristics
Cachectin/tumor necrosis factor-α	TNF-α	Macrophages	LPS, other microbial products	Fever, shock, anorexia, wasting, tumor necrosis, bone resorption, ↓ adipocyte lipoprotein lipase, neutrophil activation, ↑ endothelial cell adhesiveness/procoagulant effect	Homotrimer; 17 kDa subunit size (nonglycosylated) ↕ 26% identity
Lymphotoxin/tumor necrosis factor-β	TNF-β; LT	Lymphocytes (T & B)	Antigenic/mitogenic stimulation		Homotrimer; 20–25 KDa subunit size (glycosylated)
Interleukin-1α (IL-1α)	Leukocyte ativity factor (LAF), leukocyte endogenous mediator (LEM), mononuclear cell factor (MCF), endogeneous pyrogen (EP)	Macrophages and many other cell types	LPS, other microbial products, TNF	Fever, IL-2 production, bone resorption, pannus formation, neutrophil activation, ↑ endothelial cell adhesiveness/procoagulant effect	Monomer; 17 KDa (glycosylated) ↕ 26% identity
Interleukin-1β (IL-1β)					Monomer; 17 KDa (glycosylated)
Interferon-α	IFN-α; leukocyte interferon	Leukocytes (esp. monocyte-macrophages)		Induction of antiviral state	22 KDa (glycosylated) ↕ 23% identity
Interferon-β	IFN-β; fibroblast interferon	Fibroblasts	LPS, viral infection, double-stranded RNA		22 KDa (glycosylated)
Interferon-γ	IFN-γ; immune interferon; type 2 interferon	T lymphocytes		Macrophage activation Upregulation of Class I and Class II MHC molecules	20–25 KDa (glycosylated)
Interleukin-6 (IL-6)	Interferon-β$_2$, hepatocyte-stimulating factor (HSF), B-cell stimulating factor-2 (BSF-2), B-cell differentiation factor (BCDF)	Many cell types	LPS, TNF	↑ Synthesis of acute phase reactants Weak antiviral effect Terminal differentiation of B cells; T-cell activation	21–26 KDa (glycosylated)
Macrophage inflammatory protein 1α	MIP 1α		LPS		7.9 KDa (nonglycosylated) ↕ 57% identity
Macrophage inflammatory protein 1β	MIP 1β	Macrophages		Neutrophil chemotaxis	7.8 KDa (nonglycosylated)
Interleukin-8 (IL-8)	Monocyte-derived neutrophil chemotactic factor (MDNCF)		LPS, TNF, IL-1		8.0 KDa (nonglycosylated)

No single cytokine is capable of provoking fever of a magnitude equivalent to that elicited by endotoxin, for example. However, it is probable that combined production of several cytokines, as may occur in an inflammatory state, is sufficient to explain most fevers.

One monokine known as cachectin (also referred to as tumor necrosis factor-α) seems capable of reproducing many of the physiologic derangements observed in septic shock and thus appears to mediate most of the deleterious effects of bacterial endotoxin, including fever. A lymphokine known as lymphotoxin (also referred to as tumor necrosis factor-β) is homologous to cachectin, binds to the same receptor as cachectin, and elicits many of the same effects. Two other cytokines (interleukin 1α and interleukin 1β), while incapable of causing shock by themselves, produce many effects similar to those of cachectin, and in some instances synergistic responses have been noted.

Many of the cytokines are mutually inducing, and the concept of a "cytokine cascade" has been offered to describe the production of several factors occurring in response to the elaboration of one member of the group. The temporal sequence of induction may be reflected in the course of fever in vivo. For example, injection of a bolus of cachectin into a rabbit causes an immediate rise in body temperature, as well as a delayed rise, apparently related to secondary production of interleukin 1.

The production of certain cytokines is augmented by the presence of others: For example, cachectin biosynthesis is enhanced by interferon-γ, which also potentiates many of the effects of cachectin. Inhibitory feedback, from the production of glucocorticoid hormones, for example, may block further cytokine synthesis (see below). Thus, a complex relationship exists through which the release of one cytokine may augment (or at times inhibit) the production and effects of a second agent.

MECHANISMS OF ANTIPYRESIS

Nonsteroidal antipyretic agents inhibit fever by blocking the synthesis of prostaglandins within the endothelium of the hypothalamic vasculature, which is accomplished through inhibition of cyclo-oxygenase. However, they do not diminish the elaboration of endogenous pyrogens and may actually increase the production of some of these proteins (notably cachectin). Nonsteroidal antipyretics do not produce poikilothermic effects: They are capable of reducing fever but cannot lower body temperature beneath its normal set point.

Glucocorticoid hormones directly impede the production of endogenous pyrogens by mononuclear phagocytic cells. This is their mechanism of antipyresis and likely explains much of the total anti-inflammatory effect that they exhibit. Inhibition of cytokine synthesis is achieved at more than one level and has been studied most thoroughly in the case of cachectin biosynthesis. Both transcription of the cachectin gene and translation of the cachectin mRNA are downregulated by glucocorticoid agonists. The latter effect seems to depend upon the presence of a sequence motif that is commonly observed in the 3'-untranslated region of mRNA molecules specifying inflammatory mediators; however, the exact means by which glucocorticoid hormones prevent effective translation have not yet been elucidated.

The cyclic (often circadian) course followed in many febrile illnesses has not been fully explained. In some instances (e.g., in malaria), a clear relationship to the life cycle of the pathogen has been demonstrated. Cyclicity may, in other cases, follow from the fact that cells comprising the chief source of endogenous pyrogens are rendered refractory by continued exposure to the stimulatory agent and must recover or be replaced.

THE EVOLUTIONARY BENEFITS OF FEVER

It has been argued that the febrile response would not exist if it did not promote survival. By inference, it has been suggested that antipyretic therapy is best avoided in all but life-threatening circumstances. Modulation of various immune functions has been reported at elevated temperatures in vitro. Moreover, in specific instances, elevation of core temperature has been correlated with a beneficial effect on the course of disease. Most notably, the progression of tertiary syphilis in man is retarded by fever. In an experiment involving rabbits, spirochetal lesions of the skin have

been shown to develop more rapidly in those regions of the skin that have been shaved of fur to allow for local cooling.

Failure to develop a fever in the course of a severe infection foretells a poor outcome. A causal effect has been suggested by studies performed with the lizard *Dipsosaurus dorsalis*. Poikilotherms that are capable of elevating their body temperature only by passive absorption of heat, these animals have been shown to resist lethal infection more effectively at warm temperatures than at cool temperatures.

Contrary to these arguments in support of a beneficial effect, it may be noted that tertiary syphilis is not characterized by fever; hence the causative agent appears to have evolved so as to avoid triggering a febrile response. Indeed, by virtue of their short generation time, microorganisms are generally capable of evading defense mechanisms of the host when compelled to do so in an evolutionary context. Thus, those pathogens that elicit fever may well be impervious to the effects that fever produces. The absence of a pyrogenic response during sepsis could, of course, simply reflect failure of thermoregulatory systems as a result of overwhelming infection.

Ultimately, it must be acknowledged that the immune response is imperfect in that many aspects of immune function may actually injure the host. Fever, like many phenomena associated with inflammation, might sometimes serve no useful function.

TREATMENT OF FEVER

In the absence of specific knowledge concerning the benefits of fever, a conservative approach to the treatment of fever is advisable. Core temperatures beneath 40.6°C (105°F) are well tolerated by most individuals. Moreover, when its source has been defined, fever often serves as an important indicator of therapeutic effect.

Under certain circumstances, aggressive treatment of fever is warranted. Patients with myocardial ischemia, patients predisposed to seizures, and pregnant women may require treatment with antipyretics, since elevation of core temperature increases cardiac output and myocardial oxygen demand, increases the likelihood of seizures, and may exert a teratogenic effect. Acetaminophen or nonsteroidal anti-inflammatory agents are adequate for this purpose in the majority of cases. Physical methods for increasing heat dissipation may also be employed.

Temperatures that exceed 41.1°C (106°F) are life-threatening and must be lowered immediately. Antipyretics are often ineffective in such instances, since pyrexia of this degree does not result from an aberrant hypothalamic set point. It is advisable, in such cases, to lower temperature by any means possible; the most effective action is to immerse the patient in ice water while monitoring core temperature to be certain that a state of hypothermia is not induced.

---

286 The Acute Phase Response

Charles A. Dinarello

ACUTE PHASE CHANGES. Infections, trauma, inflammatory processes, and some malignant diseases induce a constellation of host responses that are collectively referred to as the "acute phase response." The response is associated with characteristic metabolic changes in liver protein synthesis, but, on closer examination, changes also occur in several other systems that include hematologic, endocrinologic, neurologic, and immunologic dysfunctions. These changes are called acute because most are observed within hours or days following the onset of infection or injury, although some acute phase changes also indicate chronic disease. The full spectrum of the response includes dramatic increases in the synthesis of several unique hepatic proteins that are not produced in health. One of these, C-reactive protein, is a marker of the acute phase response and can be used as an indicator of disease. The increased plasma concentrations of acute phase hepatic proteins, glycoproteins, and globulins are responsible for elevated erythrocyte sedimentation rates. Although the liver is producing increasing amounts of a variety of proteins, hepatic albumin synthesis is decreased. Increases in gluconeogenesis, energy expenditure, and muscle proteolysis occur and contribute to weight loss. However, anorexia is often present and may account for most of the weight loss. Fever may be present, and increased sleep and lethargy are frequent clinical complaints. Leukocytosis with increased numbers of circulating immature neutrophils is common, and serum iron and zinc levels are depressed while increased ceruloplasmin levels result in elevated serum copper. Thyroid dysfunction can be present, and there is often abnormal glucose tolerance and lipid metabolism. In addition, anemia develops despite adequate stores of iron, and hypergammaglobulinemia often occurs.

Although the most florid presentation of the acute phase response is observed in patients with bacterial infections, burns, or multiple injuries, clinicians also encounter acute phase changes in patients with occult infections or chronic illnesses such as rheumatoid arthritis, Crohn's disease, and several autoimmune diseases. The presence of acute phase changes can also serve as an indicator of silent disease and some cancers, particularly renal cell carcinoma and Hodgkin's disease. The acute phase response has the outstanding characteristic of being a generalized host reaction irrespective of the localized or systemic nature of the inciting disease. The various components of the response are remarkably consistent despite the considerable variety of pathologic processes that induce it. For example, plasma levels of several acute phase proteins are elevated following myocardial infarction, fracture of a bone, or bacterial pneumonia.

INDUCTION OF ACUTE PHASE CHANGES. How are infections, injuries, and immunologic and inflammatory reactions able to elicit acute phase changes in the host? Moreover, does the acute phase response serve any purpose, and can its presence be used for diagnosing or monitoring the progression of disease? The initiation of the acute phase response is linked to the production of hormone-like polypeptide mediators, now called cytokines. Several cytokines induce acute phase changes: interleukin 1, tumor necrosis factor, interferon-γ, interleukin 6, and leukemia inhibitory factor. Interleukin 1 and tumor necrosis factor induce the production of interleukin 6 from a variety of cells. Interleukin 1 and tumor necrosis factor are produced from phagocytic mononuclear cells, enter the circulation, and affect distant organ systems. Although the primary sources of interleukin 1 and tumor necrosis factor are blood monocytes, phagocytic lining cells of the liver and spleen, and other tissue macrophages, specialized cells such as keratinocytes, gingival and corneal epithelial cells, renal mesangial cells, and brain microglial and astroglial cells also produce these molecules. Interleukin 1 and tumor necrosis factor produced by these latter cell types exert their primary effects within these tissues. In fact, the ability of microbial and inflammatory substances to stimulate the production of these mediators in these strategically located, specialized cells appears to be part of local pathologic changes in many diseases.

Interferon is produced primarily during viral infections. Although it shares with interleukin 1 and tumor necrosis factor the ability to produce fever, sleep, and lethargy, interferon does not induce certain other acute phase changes, and, hence, elevated erythrocyte sedimentation rates and neutrophilia are not commonly observed during viral infections.

The patient with a localized bacterial infection represents an excellent example of the development of the acute phase response. At the onset of the infection, blood monocytes and tissue macrophages become activated either by phagocytosis of the invading microbe or by exposure to its products or toxins; the process results in the synthesis and release of various cytokines within 1 to 2 hours. These mediators enter the circulation and reach the brain where they initiate fever. Fever is the result of prostaglandin E_2 synthesis induced by pyrogenic cytokines in the thermoregulatory center of the brain. Whereas fever is clearly one of the most obvious signs of the acute phase response, other components of the response can be present without apparent clinical manifestations. One of the most sensitive measures of the acute phase response is an increase in the number and immaturity of circulating neutrophils. The release of neutrophils is due to

the direct action of interleukin 1 on the bone marrow. In human subjects injected with small doses of endotoxin or interleukin 1, marked neutrophilia can be measured in the absence of fever. Although not routinely measured, serum zinc and iron levels are depressed. Low serum iron associated with anemia in the face of adequate iron stores is characteristic of the acute phase response. There is a large body of evidence that decreased serum iron probably plays an important role in protecting the host against various bacteria. For example, the reduction in serum iron can suppress the growth rate of several microorganisms and certain tumor cells that have a strict requirement for iron as a growth factor.

Within 8 to 12 hours after the onset of infection or trauma, the liver increases the synthetic rate of the so-called acute phase proteins. The response includes increases in proteins normally found in health as well as the appearance of new proteins that serve as markers of a pathologic event. Several normal plasma proteins increase several-fold during the acute phase response. These include haptoglobin, certain protease inhibitors, complement components, ceruloplasmin, and fibrinogen. However, true acute phase reactants increase several hundredfold. These include serum amyloid A protein, a precursor of the amyloid fibril in secondary amyloidosis, and C-reactive protein. C-reactive protein was named for its ability to interact with the C-polysaccharide of pneumococci and was the first acute phase protein described. Table 286–1 lists the characteristic pattern of increased plasma proteins observed during the acute phase response. Note one exception: The plasma concentration of albumin is decreased.

Of all the acute phase proteins, C-reactive protein and serum amyloid A protein are clinically the most important because their presence serves as an indicator of disease. These proteins are structurally related. C-reactive protein is particularly useful as a marker of the hepatic acute phase protein response and can be measured easily in most hospital clinical laboratories.

Despite the anabolic processes of the liver, the acute phase response is accompanied by a pronounced catabolism of muscle protein associated with loss of body weight and overall negative nitrogen balance. Fever increases oxygen and caloric demands (usually 7 per cent per degree F), and most of the negative nitrogen balance results from oxidation of amino acids from skeletal muscle, which contributes to wasting. These amino acids are largely used for gluconeogenesis. In addition, there can be demineralization of bone. Although the metabolic demands of elevated temperature contribute to the increased need for energy substrates, the host also requires a large supply of amino acids for synthesis of new protein at a time when food intake may be severely impaired or appetite reduced. Amino acids are required for immunologic and reparative processes such as the clonal expansion of lymphocytes and the proliferation of fibroblasts. Also, they are needed for synthesis of hepatic acute phase proteins, immunoglobulins, and collagen. The mechanism of providing ample amino acids for these cellular functions seems to be well orchestrated during the acute phase response. The catabolism during infection and inflammation differs from that of starvation. Unlike starvation, in which large amounts of ketones

TABLE 286–1. PLASMA PROTEINS THAT INCREASE DURING THE ACUTE PHASE RESPONSE

C-reactive protein
Serum amyloid A protein
Alpha-1-acid glycoprotein
Ceruloplasmin
Alpha-macroglobulins

Complement components (C1-C4, factor B, C9, C11)

Alpha-1-antitrypsin
Alpha-1-antichymotrypsin

Fibrinogen
Prothrombin
Factor VIII
Plasminogen

Haptoglobin
Ferritin
Immunoglobulins

Lipoproteins

are spilled into the urine, a septic individual excretes protein with small amounts of ketones. Interleukin 1 and tumor necrosis factor, the primary mediators of acute phase changes, inhibit lipoprotein lipase and hence interfere with lipid metabolism. In addition, these cytokines directly stimulate hepatic lipogenesis, and this mechanism likely accounts for the hypertriglyceridemia observed in patients with acute phase responses, in association with either acute or chronic disease.

MEASUREMENT OF ACUTE PHASE CHANGES IN CLINICAL MEDICINE.
The acute phase response is nonspecific. However, the presence of certain acute phase changes in an otherwise healthy individual can alert the physician to hidden disease. Measuring the levels of ACTH, cortisol, growth hormone, and vasopressin is not particularly useful, although they are elevated during acute phase responses. Increased peripheral neutrophils and erythrocyte sedimentation rate are often used to detect an acute phase response. Measurement of C-reactive protein can assist the physician in determining the presence of disease in patients with vague, constitutional complaints. C-reactive protein levels are usually less than 100 μg per liter but increase within hours 10- to 1000-fold. In severe bacterial infections, the serum level can rise from undetectable to over 100 mg per liter in 48 hours. The presence of elevated levels of C-reactive protein or serum amyloid A protein, even in the absence of fever or neutrophilia, may indicate occult infection or malignant change. Increases in C-reactive protein and serum amyloid A protein occur in patients of any age and also in immunocompromised patients with opportunistic infections.

Not all inflammatory diseases are associated with elevated C-reactive protein. A refractory state can develop in certain diseases such as scleroderma, ulcerative colitis, and lupus erythematosus. Failure to develop hepatic protein changes and the neutrophilia of the acute phase response seems to be related to the presence of circulating inhibitors of cytokines.

TREATMENT OF ACUTE PHASE RESPONSES.
Measurements of fever, acute phase plasma proteins, and peripheral leukocyte numbers are well-established procedures for monitoring many disease states. Although nonsteroidal anti-inflammatory agents are used to treat the fever and associated myalgias of acute phase responses, these drugs do not affect other acute phase changes in the liver, various endocrinologic parameters, or the bone marrow response. Antipyretic blood levels of aspirin and therapeutic concentrations of drugs such as indomethacin or ibuprofen do not reduce production of interleukin 1, tumor necrosis factor, or interleukin 6. On the other hand, corticosteroids are highly effective in reducing cytokine synthesis as well as the effect of these mediators on various tissue targets. Patients receiving therapeutic doses of corticosteroids have blunted acute phase responses with ongoing infections, inflammatory processes, or immunologic reactions.

Most clinicians would agree that alleviation of fever is indicated in many situations, such as in patients with seizure or cardiovascular disorders, in patients with joint destruction, and in patients with debilitating muscle wasting. Treating fever with antipyretics reduces the metabolic and caloric demands of elevated temperature and at the same time ameliorates many of the symptoms of the acute phase response such as headache and myalgias.

The role of acute phase proteins in host defense and repair is not entirely clear. Studies suggest that the major role of C-reactive protein is to bind serum lipids or opsonize pneumococci, whereas serum amyloid A is thought to be immunosuppressive. Ceruloplasmin scavenges toxic free oxygen radicals that are injurious to many tissues. What is clear, however, is that the production and physical structure of these acute phase proteins have been conserved through 400 million years of evolution, and therefore they have presumably been useful to the host. The Limulus crab and fish make C-reactive protein that is nearly identical to human C-reactive protein. This argues that the acute phase response plays a role in survival.

Beisel WR: Magnitude of the host nutritional responses to infection. Am J Clin Nutr 30:1236–1247, 1977. *Discussion of the metabolic imbalances seen in patients with infection and injury.*

Dinarello CA: Interleukin-1 and its biologically related cytokines. Adv Immunol. 44:153–205, 1989. *A comprehensive review of the biologic activities of interleukin 1, interleukin 6, and tumor necrosis factor.*

Feingold KR, Soued M, Serio MK: Multiple cytokines stimulate hepatic lipid synthesis in vivo. Endocrinology 125:267–274, 1989. *Evidence that interleukin*

1, tumor necrosis factor, and interferon may account for the hyperlipidemias observed in patients with acute or chronic inflammatory disease.

Kushner I, Gewurz H, Benson MD: C-reactive protein and the acute-phase response. J Lab Clin Med 97:739–749, 1981. *A brief discussion of the usefulness of measuring C-reactive protein levels in clinical practice.*

Pepys MB, Baltz ML: Acute phase proteins with special reference to C-reactive protein and related proteins (pentaxins) and serum amyloid A protein. *In* Dixon FJ, Kunkel HG (eds.): Advances in Immunology, Vol 34. New York, Academic Press, 1983, pp 141–211. *A comprehensive discussion of the hepatic acute phase protein pattern observed during the acute phase response, with special attention to the acute phase response in various autoimmune diseases.*

287 The Compromised Host

Philip A. Pizzo

Compromised host is a term used to describe patients who have an increased risk for infectious complications as a consequence of a congenital or acquired qualitative or quantitative abnormality of one or more components of the host defense matrix (Table 287–1). Until the early 1980's, this term was largely restricted to patients with congenital immunodeficiencies (Ch. 244) or to those who became immunocompromised as a consequence of cancer or its treatment, bone marrow failure, or treatment with immunosuppressive therapy. The advent of the acquired immunodeficiency syndrome (AIDS) has given the term *compromised host* a new meaning and relevance. The compromised host with AIDS is discussed in detail in Part XXI. In this chapter, the focus is on non-AIDS patients with altered immune defenses. However, many of the complications and approaches to diagnosis and management are generic.

PHYSICAL DEFENSE BARRIERS

The skin and mucosal surfaces represent the primary defense against both endogenous and exogenous sources of infection. Disruption of skin and mucosa may result from trauma, tumor invasion, the cytotoxic effects of chemotherapy or radiotherapy, the use of invasive diagnostic or therapeutic procedures (e.g., intravenous catheters), and effects of locally destructive infections such as oral herpes simplex. Such mucosal alterations provide a nidus for microbial colonization, a focus for localized infection, and a portal of entry for systemic invasion.

The skin and various mucosal surfaces are normally colonized by aerobic and anaerobic bacteria. However, in patients who have been hospitalized, who are neutropenic, or who have received prior broad-spectrum antibiotics, the normal gram-positive flora of the skin can be replaced by other gram-positive organisms such as CDC group JK *Corynebacterium* or *Bacillus* species or by gram-negative organisms (e.g., pseudomonads, enteric gram-negative rods), fungi (e.g., *Candida albicans* or *Aspergillus* species), and atypical *Mycobacterium* species such as *M. chelonei* or *M. fortuitum.*

Similarly, the gastrointestinal tract is normally colonized by an array of aerobic and anaerobic bacteria as well as some fungi, and disruption of its mucosa may lead to infections by a variety of pathogens including polymicrobial infections. A common cause for disruption of the gastrointestinal mucosal integrity is cytotoxic chemotherapy to patients with malignancy, particularly cytarabine (ara-C), the anthracyclines (daunorubicin and doxorubicin), methotrexate, 6-mercaptopurine, and 5-fluorouracil. Although stomatitis is usually the most clinically recognizable manifestation of gastrointestinal toxicity, diffuse gastrointestinal involvement is also likely. Frequently, the differentiation between chemotherapy-induced stomatotoxicity and localized infection (e.g., necrotizing gingivitis due to anaerobic bacteria or mucosal lesions due to herpes simplex virus) can be difficult, particularly in the neutropenic patient.

In addition to mucosal breakdown, mechanical obstruction of body passages can also increase the risk of serious localized infection due to stasis of local body fluids and resultant overgrowth of potentially pathogenic colonizing organisms. Common sites of secondary infection due to obstruction include the lung, urinary tract, biliary tract, or eustachian tube. One should consider an obstructive process when infection at any of these sites fails to respond to appropriate antibiotics.

Anatomic changes can also contribute to the risk of infection. For example, in patients with sickle cell disease, macrophage and splenic dysfunction predisposes to the development of certain bacteremias, especially by *Streptococcus pneumoniae* and *Salmonella* species. Anatomic abnormalities of bones and joints as a result of vaso-occlusive crises caused by infarction of bone marrow, bony cortex, or synovium in patients with sickle cell disease can also predispose to development of infections such as osteomyelitis or arthritis caused by these organisms.

PHAGOCYTE DEFECTS

The polymorphonuclear leukocyte (PMN) and the monocyte are the two most important components of cellular host defense that protect against invasive bacteria and fungi. Both quantitative and qualitative defects affecting PMN and monocytes may occur in compromised patients.

Quantitative Abnormalities of Phagocytes

Granulocytopenia is among the most important risk factors for serious infection in the compromised host. However, it is impor-

TABLE 287–1. PREDOMINANT PATHOGENS IN COMPROMISED PATIENTS: ASSOCIATION WITH SELECTED DEFECTS IN HOST DEFENSE

Host Defense Impairment	Bacteria	Fungi	Viruses	Other
Neutropenia	Gram-negative Enteric organisms (*E. coli, K. pneumoniae, Enterobacter* spp., *Citrobacter* spp.) *Pseudomonas aeruginosa* Gram-positive Staphylococci (coagulase negative, coagulase positive) Streptococci (enterococci α-hemolytic) Anaerobes (anaerobic streptococci, *Clostridia* spp., *Bacteroides* spp.)	*Candida* species (*C. albicans* > *C. tropicalis* > other species) *Aspergillus* species (*A. fumigatus, A. flavus*)		
Abnormal cell-mediated immunity	*Legionella* *Nocardia asteroides* *Salmonella* spp. Mycobacteria (*M. tuberculosis* and atypical mycobacteria) Disseminated infection from live bacteria vaccine (BCG)	*Cryptococcus neoformans* *Histoplasma capsulatum* *Coccidioides immitis* *Candida*	Varicella-zoster virus Herpes simplex virus Cytomegalovirus Epstein-Barr virus Herpes virus 6 Disseminated infection from live virus vaccines (vaccinia, measles, rubella, mumps, yellow fever, live polio)	*Pneumocystis carinii* *Toxoplasma gondii* *Cryptosporidium* *Strongyloides stercoralis*
Immunoglobulin abnormalities	Gram-positive *Streptococcus pneumoniae, S. aureus* Gram-negative *Haemophilus influenzae* *Neisseria* spp., enteric organisms		Enteroviruses Disseminated infection from live virus vaccines (vaccinia, measles, rubella, mumps, yellow fever, polio)	*Giardia lamblia*
Complement abnormalities				
C3, C5	Gram-positive *S. pneumoniae*, staphylococci Gram-negative *H. influenzae, Neisseria* spp., Enteric organisms			
C5-C9	*Neisseria* species (*N. gonorrhoeae, N. meningitidis*)			
Anatomic disruption				
Oral cavity	α-Hemolytic streptococci, oral anaerobes (*Peptococcus, Peptostreptococcus*)	*Candida*	Herpes simplex virus	
Esophagus	Staphylococci, other colonizing organisms	*Candida*	Herpes simplex virus Cytomegalovirus	
Lower gastrointestinal tract	Gram-positive Enterococci Gram-negative Enteric organisms Anaerobes (*B. fragilis, C. perfringens*)	*Candida*		*Strongyloides stercoralis*
Skin (IV catheter)	Gram-positive Staphylococci, streptococci *Corynebacterium, Bacillus* spp. Gram-negative *P. aeruginosa*, enteric organisms Mycobacteria *M. fortuitum, M. chelonei*	*Candida* *Aspergillus*		
Urinary tract	Gram-positive Group D streptococci Gram-negative Enteric organisms *P. aeruginosa*	*Candida*		
Splenectomy	Gram-positive *S. pneumoniae* Gram-negative DFZ bacillus *H. influenzae* *Salmonella* (sickle cell disease)			Babesiosis

From Rubin M, Walsh TJ, Pizzo PA: Clinical approach to the compromised host. *In* Hoffman R, Benz EJ Jr, Shattil SJ, et al. (eds.): Hematology: Basic Principles and Practices. New York, Churchill Livingstone, 1991.

tant to keep in mind that except for congenital neutropenias, there are often other alterations of the host defense matrix that occur in concert with granulocytopenia and can further alter the risk for infection as well as the types of infectious complications that occur.

Granulocytopenia is most commonly associated with malignant disease and its treatment with cytotoxic therapy. This includes patients with hematologic malignancies and lymphomas as well as the increasing number of patients with solid tumors who receive cytotoxic chemotherapy. Patients with primary or secondary bone marrow failure also have neutropenia as their predominant risk for infection. In addition to the neutropenia per se, the patterns of infection are also influenced by the other disease- or treatment-related immune abnormalities. For example, despite equivalent degrees of granulocytopenia, the patient with acute myelogenous leukemia (AML) may present with a different pattern of infection than the patient with aplastic anemia. The disruption of a mucosal defense barrier which occurs in the patient with AML who is receiving cytotoxic therapy appears to increase the risk for infection with enteric gram-negative bacteria, α-streptococci, or anaerobes. In contrast, the patient with aplastic anemia who does not have impaired mucosal integrity may be able to sustain longer periods of granulocytopenia without developing a systemic bacterial infection. On the other hand, if the patient with aplastic anemia is treated with steroids or cyclosporine, the risk for viral or fungal infection may be increased.

Regardless of these modifying factors, the relationship between granulocytopenia and serious infection has been established unequivocally by the classic study of Bodey and colleagues (Table 287–2). This study demonstrated that the risk of infection begins to increase significantly when granulocyte counts fall below 1000 per microliter and is most marked when the counts are 100 per microliter or less. In addition to the absolute granulocyte count, the duration of granulocytopenia is also directly related to the direction of granulocytopenia as well as to whether the counts are rising or falling.

For practical purposes, granulocytopenia is usually defined as a count of 500 or fewer PMN's and band forms per microliter. However, a patient with an absolute granulocyte count of 500 to 1000 per microliter that is rapidly falling is probably at greater risk for infection than a patient with a count of 200 per microliter that is rising. Thus, the absolute granulocyte count, the duration of granulocytopenia, and whether the neutrophil count is falling or rising must all be considered when assessing the risk to any individual patient. Some clinicians also include the monocyte count in this equation to generate an absolute phagocyte index.

Granulocytopenia primarily predisposes patients to bacterial and fungal infection and does not of itself appear to increase the incidence of severity of viral and parasitic infections. In the 1950's and 1960's, when cytotoxic therapy was first being developed, gram-positive bacteria (especially *Staphylococcus aureus*) predominated. In the early 1970's, with the availability of antibiotics to control gram-positive bacteria (e.g., methicillin), gram-negative organisms (e.g., *Escherichia coli*, *Klebsiella*, *Pseudomonas aeruginosa*) emerged as the predominant pathogens in neutropenic patients, perhaps because of the increasing use of more aggressive chemotherapy regimens for the treatment of patients and the use of broader-spectrum antibiotics. During the 1980's, gram-positive organisms re-emerged as common bacterial isolates, and at many centers they now represent the most frequently encountered organisms.

TABLE 287–2. ASSOCIATION OF GRANULOCYTE LEVEL AND CHANCE OF DEVELOPING SIGNIFICANT INFECTION

Granulocyte Level (per cu mm)		Percentage of Serious Infections (Duration of Granulocytopenia in Weeks)							
Initial	Change	1	2	3	4	6	10	12	14
Any level	Any fall	12							
Any level	Fall to 2000	2							
Any level	Fall to 1500	5							
Any level	Fall to 1000	10	30	45	50	65	70	85	100
Any level	Fall to 500	19							
Any level	Fall to <100	28	50	72	85	100			

Adapted from Bodey GP, Buckley M, Sathe YS, et al.: Quantitative relationships between circulatory leukocytes and infection in patients with acute leukemia. Ann Intern Med 61:328–340, 1966.

In addition to these changes in the pattern of infection, institutional variations in the causes of infection and the antibiotic sensitivity patterns of isolates cannot be overemphasized, making it imperative for the physician to have a working knowledge of the specific isolates encountered at his or her own clinical setting.

The gram-negative organisms encountered most commonly in granulocytopenic patients are *E. coli*, *K. pneumoniae*, and *P. aeruginosa*. Together, these have generally accounted for approximately 90 per cent of the gram-negative isolates at most centers. A precise source for gram-negative bacteremia is identified in only a minority of cases, but the gastrointestinal tract, respiratory tract soft tissue, and urinary tract are the most probable sources for infection. Of these three organisms, *P. aeruginosa* is often the most virulent in neutropenic hosts, although in most developed countries the incidence of infection due to *Pseudomonas* declined in neutropenic patients during the 1980's. But as a general rule, virtually any organism can be pathogenic if the host defenses are severely impaired. *Enterobacter* species, *Citrobacter* species, and *Serratia marcescens* are less frequently encountered but are notable because they rapidly become resistant to β-lactam antibiotics through the induction of chromosomally mediated β-lactamases. Other less common gram-negative isolates include *Acinetobacter* species, *Haemophilus* species (usually nontypable *H. influenzae*), and non-*aeruginosa* pseudomonads (often catheter-related and antibiotic-resistant).

The gram-positive organisms most frequently encountered are the coagulase-negative staphylococci (most commonly *S. epidermidis*), coagulase-positive staphylococci (*S. aureus*), enterococci, and α-hemolytic streptococci (e.g., *S. mutans* or viridans group streptococci). Both coagulase-positive and -negative staphylococci are most commonly isolated from the blood, often from patients with indwelling intravenous catheters, or from foreign bodies such as prosthetic heart valves or orthopedic implants. *S. aureus* tends to be significantly more virulent and its sensitivity to β-lactam antibiotics (e.g., methicillin, oxacillin, or nafcillin) can vary from center to center, making it imperative for the physician to be aware of the frequency of methicillin-resistant *S. aureus* (MRSA) at his or her institution. In contrast, the coagulase-negative staphylococci tend to be relatively indolent. During the last decade, the coagulase-negative staphylococci have become increasingly resistant to β-lactam antibiotics, and the majority (50 to 80 per cent) are methicillin-resistant and generally require treatment with vancomycin. Notable are the recent reports of α-hemolytic viridans streptococci that have been associated with septic shock and the adult respiratory distress syndrome (ARDS) in patients who are receiving high-dose cytosine arabinoside and who develop oral mucosal disruption. Other gram-positive bacteria that may be encountered in neutropenic patients include *Bacillus* species (often catheter-related), group CDC-JK *Corynebacterium* (often catheter-related and relatively antibiotic-resistant), *Enterococcus faecium* (may be resistant to vancomycin), and *Lactobacillus* (may also be resistant to vancomycin).

Infections due solely to anaerobic bacteria are less common and are usually associated with a concomitant abnormality in gastrointestinal mucosal integrity. While *Bacillus fragilis* and *Clostridium perfringens* are the most common organisms, other *Bacteroides* species, as well as other *Clostridium* species (e.g., *C. tertium*, *C. septicum*), which are often clindamycin-resistant, can be clinically important. Anaerobes are frequent components of intra-abdominal infections, including peritonitis, intra-abdominal abscesses, and perirectal cellulitis or abscesses. *C. difficile* is a common cause of colitis in neutropenic patients who are treated with antibiotics or cytotoxic agents.

Infections due to *Mycobacterium* species are not increased in frequency in neutropenic patients, although patients with hairy cell leukemia (HCL), who have profound monocytopenia in addition to neutropenia, appear to have an increased risk for developing atypical mycobacterial infection (e.g., *M. kansasii*, *M. fortuitum*, *M. chelonei*, and *M. avium-intracellulare* complex). Rapidly growing mycobacteria (*M. fortuitum* and *M. chelonei*) may also cause exit site infections in patients with indwelling intravenous catheters, or wound infections following surgery.

In contrast to the bacterial infections, which are often associated with the onset of fever in neutropenic patients, fungal infections only rarely cause primary infection (i.e., initial infection in patients not yet receiving antibiotics). More commonly, fungal infections occur as a secondary process in patients receiving antibacterial agents. Although a variety of fungal infections may be encountered in the neutropenic host, *Candida* and *Aspergillus* species predominate.

The vast majority of infections due to *Candida* species are caused by *C. albicans*, with other potential pathogens including *C. tropicalis*, *C. parapsilosis*, *C. krusei*, and *C. glabrata* (also known as *Torulopsis glabrata*). In neutropenic patients, *Candida* infections may include candidemia, catheter-related infections, invasive mucosal infections (e.g., oral, esophageal, or lower gastrointestinal), and disseminated disease, in which the most commonly affected organs are the liver and spleen (so called hepatosplenic candidiasis), the eye (endophthalmitis), and the skin.

Aspergillosis is usually due to *A. fumigatus* and *A. flavus*, although *A. niger* and *A. terreus* can also result in infection. The upper airways (e.g., oral cavity, nasal cavity, or sinuses) and lung are the primary sites involved with *Aspergillus*, and spread is usually by direct invasion into contiguous areas, although widespread dissemination has been described to sites including brain, liver and spleen, gastrointestinal tract, heart, and kidneys. However, positive blood cultures virtually never occur.

Other fungal pathogens that may occur in neutropenic patients include the Mucoraceae species (*Mucor, Rhizopus, Absidia*, and *Cunninghamella*—often clinically resembling *Aspergillus* species infections), *Trichosporon beigelii* (which may cause disseminated visceral and cutaneous disease), *Fusarium* species, *Drechslera*, *Pseudallescheria boydii*, and *Malassezia furfur*.

Qualitative Abnormalities of Phagocytes

The microbicidal activity of granulocytes and monocytes involves complex interactions between the cell and the organism or inflammatory site. Some of the major functions important for microbicidal activity include migration of the cell to the inflammatory site (or chemotaxis), cell activation, phagocytosis, and intra- and extracellular killing via both oxygen-dependent and -independent pathways. These qualitative abnormalities can be operationally divided into the following categories: (1) those associated with malignant or myeloproliferative disease itself, (2) those associated with diseases that do not primarily affect the leukocytes, (3) iatrogenic causes (such as administration of pharmacologic agents or radiation), and (4) primary disorders of phagocytes.

PATIENTS WITH MALIGNANT DISORDERS AND MYELODYSPLASIA. Significant functional defects in mature PMN's can occur in patients with AML and acute lymphoblastic leukemia prior to therapy. Although it has been largely assumed that granulocytes from patients with chronic myelogenous leukemia (CML) have normal microbicidal activity, some studies have documented significant impairment in neutrophil function of morphologically mature PMN's from patients with CML, including abnormalities in phagocytosis, random migration, chemotaxis, and bactericidal activity. Nevertheless, during the stable chronic phase of the disease, infectious complications are rarely seen in these patients.

In addition to immunoglobulin deficiencies that impair opsonization, patients with chronic lymphocytic leukemia (CLL) and multiple myeloma may also have such abnormalities as defective granulocyte adherence, decreased granulocyte migration, a decrease in the number of granulocyte receptors for C3b and IgG, and decreased chemotaxis of monocytes.

Significant defects in granulocyte function have also been found in PMN's from patients with myelodysplastic syndromes and preleukemic states. The clinician should probably assume that neutrophils from patients with myelodysplastic syndromes or preleukemia are functionally defective, and thus patients with "borderline" granulocyte counts should be approached as if they had an absolute neutropenia.

NONMALIGNANT HEMATOLOGIC DISEASE. Although the predominant defect in host defense in most patients with aplastic anemia is neutropenia, followed by immune suppression as a result of therapy (e.g., steroids, antithymocyte globulin, or cyclosporine), deficient production of superoxide and a deficiency of myeloperoxidase can sometimes be observed. Patients with

paroxysmal nocturnal hemoglobinuria (PNH) appear to have an increased susceptibility to bacterial infection. Impaired chemotaxis despite normal phagocytosis and bacterial killing has been described in PNH, and the Fc receptor type III (the major Fc receptor in blood and on neutrophils) has also been shown to be deficient in PNH.

In addition to splenic dysfunction, abnormal complement activation, and defective serum opsonizing capacity, defective phagocytic function has been described in patients with sickle cell anemia, although the significance of this is unclear. Neutrophils from infection-prone children with sickle cell disease have been shown to have defective bactericidal activity, perhaps secondary to zinc deficiency.

Some patients with severe G6PD deficiency appear to have an increased susceptibility to infections caused by catalase-positive bacteria. The clinical picture resembles that of chronic granulomatous disease of childhood, although only rarely are infections reported in the first decade of life. The granulocytes show normal phagocytosis and chemotaxis but defective bactericidal activity.

Although most studies address disseminated intravascular coagulation (DIC) secondary to overwhelming bacterial infection, the potential role of fibrinogen degradation products (FDP's) in modifying PMN function has been suggested by the finding that two FDP's (FDP D and FDP E) can cause substantial in vitro inhibition of PMN chemotaxis, oxidative metabolism, and killing of *E. coli*. DIC associated with infection, then, may represent a vicious circle in which the organism triggers the coagulation abnormalities, which in turn may result in neutropenia and defective PMN function, thus worsening the infection.

PHARMACOLOGIC AGENTS AND RADIOTHERAPY. Most cytotoxic drugs used for treatment of malignant and autoimmune diseases or transplantation have antiproliferative effects, resulting in neutropenia and monocytopenia. Among the antineoplastics, the most commonly implicated agents include methotrexate, 6-mercaptopurine, vincristine, vinblastine, anthracyclines, cyclophosphamide, carmustine, and platinum compounds.

Glucocorticoids are associated with increased susceptibility to infection. As a general rule, the signs and symptoms of even severe infections may be masked or greatly reduced in patients receiving steroids. Steroids impair neutrophil chemotaxis, and at high dosages PMN phagocytosis, microbicidal activity, and antibody-dependent cytotoxicity may also be altered. In addition, steroids may cause monocytopenia as well as defects in monocyte chemotaxis, phagocytosis, and killing of bacteria and fungi. In addition to their action on granulocytes and monocytes, steroids may enhance susceptibility to infection by impairing wound healing, increasing skin fragility, and depressing lymphocyte function, the production of cytokines, and humoral immune responses.

Biologic agents (e.g., colony-stimulating factors [CSF], interleukins, interferons) are being employed increasingly in clinical medicine, and their impact on the host defense matrix must be assessed. Studies to date suggest that granulocyte-macrophage (GM)-CSF or granulocyte (G)-CSF not only may increase cell number but also may enhance a number of neutrophil functions, including oxidative metabolism, phagocytosis, microbicidal activity, and antibody-dependent cytotoxicity. At the same time, in adults undergoing autologous bone marrow transplantation, there appears to be the unanticipated finding of a marked decrease in migration of PMN's toward a sterile, artificially created inflammatory site on the skin during periods of GM-CSF administration. Although the clinical significance of any of these effects has not yet been established, these data underscore the importance of carefully evaluating biologics as they are introduced into the therapeutic armamentarium. For example, although interleukin 2 (IL2) appears promising in mediating tumor lysis (with either lymphokine-activated killer [LAK] cells, tumor infiltrating lymphocytes [TIL], or interferon-α), impaired granulocyte function, decreased chemotaxis, and decreased Fc receptor γ-III expression have been noted in some patients receiving high doses of IL2 and may be associated with an increased incidence of significant infections due to *S. aureus*. In contrast, other biologic agents such as interferon-γ may increase phagocyte function and decrease the risk for infection (e.g., in patients with chronic granulomatous disease).

PRIMARY DISORDERS OF PHAGOCYTE FUNCTION. Chronic granulomatous disease (CGD) has served as a prototype for diseases characterized by defective oxidative metabolism of phagocytes. Although CGD represents a heterogeneous group of disorders from a molecular and genetic perspective, the common denominator is that phagocytes lack essential components of oxidative metabolism and fail to generate the respiratory burst in response to various stimuli, including certain pathogenic organisms. The organisms that cause serious infections in patients with CGD are most often those that contain the enzyme catalase. In the absence of cellular production of H_2O_2, the peroxide generated by non–catalase-containing organisms is enough to ameliorate the neutrophil deficiency and allow microbicidal activity. However, if the organism also contains catalase, the H_2O_2 it produces is rapidly degraded and is not available for participation in oxidative-based killing. The majority of infections in patients with CGD are caused by *S. aureus*, although serious infections can also result from enteric gram-negative bacilli (e.g., *E. coli, K. pneumoniae,* or *Serratia* species), *P. cepacia, Nocardia asteroides,* and *Aspergillus* species.

Serious recurrent infections usually begin in the first year of life in children with CGD. The lung is the most common site of infection (pneumonias and abscesses), with other common infections including skin and soft tissue abscesses, visceral abscesses (particularly hepatic), osteomyelitis (especially of the small bones in the hands and feet), and suppurative lymphadenopathy. Uncommonly, CGD can present in adolescence or adulthood, although with careful history, infectious complications often date back to childhood.

Prophylactic antibiotics, with trimethoprim-sulfamethoxazole, have been advocated by many investigators. Recently, interferon-γ has been shown to reduce the incidence of serious infection and hospital days for patients with CGD.

Myeloperoxidase (MPO) deficiency is perhaps the most common of all granulocyte disorders, with an estimated frequency ranging from 1 in 2000 to 1 in 4000. MPO is a lysosomal enzyme that catalyzes the formation of hypochlorous acid from H_2O_2 produced in the respiratory burst. Interestingly, the majority of individuals identified with MPO deficiency are healthy, and infectious complications are exceedingly rare. Systemic *Candida* infections have occurred in a small number of MPO-deficient patients who also had diabetes mellitus.

Chédiak-Higashi syndrome (CHS) is a rare disorder characterized by autosomal recessive inheritance, recurrent infections, partial oculocutaneous albinism, central and peripheral neuropathy, and increased bleeding time. Neutropenia can also be present. Infections result from combined effects of neutropenia and functional defects in phagocytes, which include impaired degranulation and defective chemotaxis. Infections frequently involve the skin, respiratory tract, and mucous membranes and are most commonly caused by *S. aureus* or gram-negative bacilli. Deficiency of the iC3b receptor (also known as CR3, Mo1, and MAC-1), which is important for adherence and phagocytosis, is a rare disorder. Accordingly, neutrophils demonstrate defects in aggregation, margination, chemotaxis, and phagocytosis. The most common infections are skin and subcutaneous tissue infections, otitis, mucositis, gingivitis, and periodontitis.

A number of disorders have been described which are characterized by defects in chemotaxis of granulocytes and/or monocytes. Infections in these patients tend to be cutaneous, and the most common pathogens are *S. aureus,* streptococci, *C. albicans, E. coli,* and *Trichophyton rubrum.* Depending on the specific syndrome, deep-seated infections may also occur. The "lazy leukocyte" syndrome may also be associated with neutropenia and is characterized by gingivitis, recurrent otitis media, rhinitis, and stomatitis. Hyperimmunoglobulin E syndrome (Job's syndrome) is usually associated with multiple cutaneous abscesses caused by staphylococci, but deep-seated infections and infections due to other organisms such as pseudomonads and *Candida* have also been reported. Wound healing does not appear to be a problem, as it is in CGD. Chemotaxis defects have been reported in patients with congenital ichthyosis and recurrent *T. rubrum* infections.

DEFECTS IN CELL-MEDIATED IMMUNITY (CMI)

Cellular immune dysfunction either may be primary, as in a number of congenital immunodeficiency states, or may occur secondary to other disorders of therapeutic interventions. Defec-

tive CMI may lead to infections caused by bacteria, fungi, viruses, and protozoa. The predominant pathogens are intracellular organisms (those microbes that survive inside of macrophages) and include mycobacteria (both *M. tuberculosis* and atypical mycobacteria), *Legionella, N. asteroides, Salmonella* species, *Cryptococcus neoformans, Histoplasma capsulatum, Coccidioides immitis,* varicella-zoster virus (VZV), herpes simplex virus (HSV), cytomegalovirus (CMV), Epstein-Barr virus (EBV), *Pneumocystis carinii, T. gondii, Cryptosporidium,* and *Strongyloides stercoralis.*

Patients with Malignant Disorders

Hodgkin's disease and the non-Hodgkin's lymphomas are associated with altered CMI not only when the malignancy is active, but in some instances even when the malignancy is in remission.

CMI defects have been postulated to help explain the incidence of atypical mycobacterial infections in patients with hairy cell leukemia and also occur in relatively rare T-cell malignancies such as mycosis fungoides and T-cell CLL. CMI defects exist in children with ALL, as evidenced by their increased susceptibility to infections due to *P. carinii* or disseminated VZV, but it is likely that concurrent therapy plays a major role. Clinically significant impairment of CMI has not been well established for other malignancies.

Patients with Nonmalignant Hematologic Disorders

Impaired CMI is not a prominent feature of nonmalignant hematologic disorders unless associated with therapy or acquisition of HIV-1 infection. Abnormalities in CMI have been best described in patients with hemophilia who have received Factor VIII concentrates even in the absence of apparent HIV-1 infection. Patients with sickle cell anemia have been found to be anergic in association with zinc deficiency and decreased nucleoside phosphorylase activity.

A number of infections may produce impaired CMI either directly (e.g., by infecting key cellular components such as T lymphocytes or macrophages) or by affecting other immunoregulatory mechanisms. The most notable viral infection associated with impaired CMI is HIV-1. Other viral infections that also are associated with CMI defects include CMV, EBV, RSV, hepatitis B, and influenza. Other nonviral infections that have been variably associated with impaired CMI by in vitro testing have included tuberculosis, leprosy, bacterial pneumonia, brucellosis, typhoid fever, coccidioidomycosis, syphilis, and a variety of parasitic diseases.

Noninfectious disorders that have been linked to abnormal CMI include chronic protein-calorie malnutrition, uremia, diabetes mellitus, surgery, anesthesia, sarcoidosis, and cystic fibrosis.

Pharmacologic Agents

Corticosteroids are the pharmacologic agents most often associated with CMI abnormalities, although they may also cause immune suppression owing to effects on other host defense mechanisms. The degree of immunosuppression and the relative risk of infection depend on the dose and duration of corticosteroids as well as the underlying disease. Patients receiving pharmacologic doses of steroids (e.g., brain tumor patients, patients with inflammatory bowel disease, patients with autoimmune disorders) may have impaired CMI and should be considered at risk for mycobacterial, viral, and parasitic infections. Patients who are to be treated with corticosteroids and who have a known history of tuberculosis or a positive PPD skin test should be placed on prophylactic INH to prevent reactivation and potential dissemination of disease.

A number of cytotoxic agents are also associated with impaired CMI, including methotrexate, cyclophosphamide, 6-mercaptopurine, and azathioprine. Cyclosporine is an immunosuppressant used to suppress transplant rejection and is associated with alterations in helper T cells, effector T cells, and NK cells. It has not been established, however, that the use of cyclosporine per se is associated with an increased risk of infection.

Radiotherapy may also result in impaired CMI, especially when used in combination with other immunosuppressive agents or for treatment of patients with underlying diseases associated with intrinsic CMI defects (e.g., as a component of the preparatory regimen for bone marrow transplantation or for treatment of Hodgkin's disease).

Primary Disorders of Cell-mediated Immunity
(see Ch. 244)

Defects in CMI are found as components of mixed primary B- and T-cell abnormalities, including severe combined immunodeficiency disease (SCID), Wiskott-Aldrich syndrome, ataxia-telangiectasia, and certain purine pathway enzyme deficiencies. Infections in patients with these disorders tend to begin early in life and may be caused not only by pathogens associated with CMI abnormalities but also by those seen with humoral defects, such as the encapsulated bacteria.

SCID is associated with a marked decrease in both B- and T-cell numbers and extremely low levels of immunoglobulins. Patients fail to react to skin tests and have a negligible antibody response following immunizations. Failure to thrive and recurrent infections are seen within the first few months of life. Infections are due to S. aureus, S. pneumoniae, H. influenzae, P. carinii, Candida, and herpes group viruses. Affected infants usually die by 2 years of age. A variant of SCID has been described that is associated with chronic skin eruption, hepatosplenomegaly, eosinophilia, and histiocytic infiltration of the lymph nodes (Omenn's disease). P. carinii pneumonia may be a common presenting symptom in this disorder.

In patients with Wiskott-Aldrich syndrome, the major abnormality is an inability to respond to polysaccharide antigens. Infections are caused by polysaccharide-encapsulated bacterial pathogens such as S. pneumoniae and H. influenzae. However, patients may also lose T-cell functions and may have increased susceptibility to pathogens such as HSV and certain fungi and protozoa.

Ataxia-telangiectasia is associated with absent serum and secretory IgA. The thymus is hypoplastic, and thymus-dependent zones in lymph nodes are empty. Infection with encapsulated bacteria predominates, especially recurrent sinopulmonary infections. Many patients have progressive loss of T-cell function over time and may become susceptible to associated pathogens.

Purine pathway enzyme deficiencies (adenosine deaminase deficiency or nucleoside phosphorylase deficiency) may be associated with either combined B- and T-cell defects or isolated B- or T-cell abnormalities. The type of infection depends on the predominant immune defect. Infections may not appear until 6 to 12 months of age.

The primary cellular immunodeficiencies associated with T-cell abnormalities include thymic hypoplasia (DiGeorge's syndrome), combined immunodeficiency with predominant T-cell defect (Nezelof's syndrome), purine nucleoside phosphorylase deficiency, and chronic mucocutaneous candidiasis.

DiGeorge's syndrome develops when the third and part of the fourth pharyngeal pouches fail to develop during embryogenesis, resulting in absence of the thymus and parathyroid glands. Children with DiGeorge's syndrome lack T lymphocytes and have severe depression of CMI, making them susceptible to overwhelming infections due to a variety of organisms, including HSV, VZV, C. albicans, and P. carinii. Nezelof's syndrome can be differentiated from DiGeorge's syndrome by the absence of parathyroid and cardiac involvement.

Cartilage-hair hypoplasia is a form of short-limbed dwarfism associated with a virtual absence of T-cell function. Interestingly, susceptibility to infection is not as pronounced as in other T-cell deficiencies. Overwhelming viral infections due to vaccinia or varicella viruses may occur.

Chronic mucocutaneous candidiasis involves impairment in CMI, and infection is almost always limited to the skin and mucous membranes.

ABNORMALITIES OF HUMORAL DEFENSE MECHANISMS—IMMUNOGLOBULINS AND COMPLEMENT

Immunoglobulins and complement are among the most important components of the humoral immune system, and defects or deficiencies in either may be associated with serious infections. Other proteins that have been classified as part of the humoral defense system include lysozyme, lactoferrin, tuftsin, and fibronectin. Immunoglobulins may be opsonic (enhance phagocytosis) or neutralizing (inhibits replication of viruses) or with complement may lyse microbes or cells. The humoral system functions predominantly against bacterial infections. Patients with either primary or secondary defects or deficiencies in these proteins are at highest risk for developing serious infections due to the encapsulated bacteria and to a lesser extent the enteroviruses and Giardia lamblia.

Patients with Malignant Disorders

The degree of humoral impairment in multiple myeloma appears to be related to the stage of the disease, primarily due to malignant plasma cell induction of a protein that is synthesized by macrophages and that selectively suppresses B-cell function. Myeloma patients are most susceptible to recurrent infections from encapsulated bacteria such as S. pneumoniae or H. influenzae early in the course of the disease. Infections due to enteric gram-negative rods and staphylococci are also encountered, especially in patients with refractory or advanced disease. Sites of recurrent infection are most often the upper respiratory tract, urinary tract, or skin.

Patients with B-cell CLL appear to have an unbalanced immunoglobulin chain synthesis and resultant hypogammaglobulinemia. The incidence of infection correlates with the duration and stage of the disease as well as the serum levels of immunoglobulins (particularly IgG). Encapsulated bacteria predominate, although infections due to staphylococci and enteric gram-negative bacilli also occur. Upper and lower respiratory tract infections are encountered most commonly, although other sites such as urinary tract and skin are frequently involved.

Nonmalignant states (e.g., nephrotic syndrome, burns, protein-losing enteropathy) can be associated with increased immunoglobulin catabolism or loss and may lead to decreased antibody levels and enhanced susceptibility to infection. Clinically significant acquired complement defects are unusual.

Primary Deficiencies

Isolated B-cell immunodeficiency states and their associated risks for infection in children include transient hypogammaglobulinemia of infancy, which is not usually associated with serious infections; sex-linked hypogammaglobulinemia, which is associated with recurrent pyogenic infections and septicemia due to S. pneumoniae, H. influenzae, S. aureus, N. meningitidis, and P. aeruginosa; hypogammaglobulinemia associated with hyperimmunoglobulin M, in which patients have recurrent respiratory, soft tissue, and gastrointestinal infections; selective IgM deficiency, in which patients have severe recurrent infections due to pyogenic bacteria; and selective IgA deficiency, in which certain patients may have increased numbers of upper respiratory tract infections whereas others appear not to be at increased risk. Chronic diarrhea due to G. lamblia is also associated with IgA deficiency. Common variable hypogammaglobulinemia is associated with respiratory tract infections due to S. pneumoniae, H. influenzae, and S. aureus. Diarrhea due to G. lamblia also occurs.

Many patients with B-cell deficiencies, particularly those with congenital hypogammaglobulinemia, appear to be at risk for the development of chronic central nervous system infections due to enteroviruses.

A number of primary defects in complement components have also been described. Although deficiencies of the early classic pathway components (C1, C2, C4) have been reported, associated infection is rare, probably because the alternative pathway remains functional and is able to compensate. Deficiencies of C3 or C5, on the other hand, often lead to severe infections due to encapsulated organisms, enteric gram-negative bacteria, and staphylococci. Absence of the later components (C5b, C6, C7, C8, C9) leads to an increase in infections, primarily due to Neisseria species, both N. gonorrhoeae and N. meningitidis. Although the defects in these later components may be present from birth, infectious episodes do not typically begin until the teenage years. Indeed, any patient with recurrent infections due to Neisseria species should be investigated for the possibility of complement deficiency.

PLATE 9   INFECTIOUS DISEASES

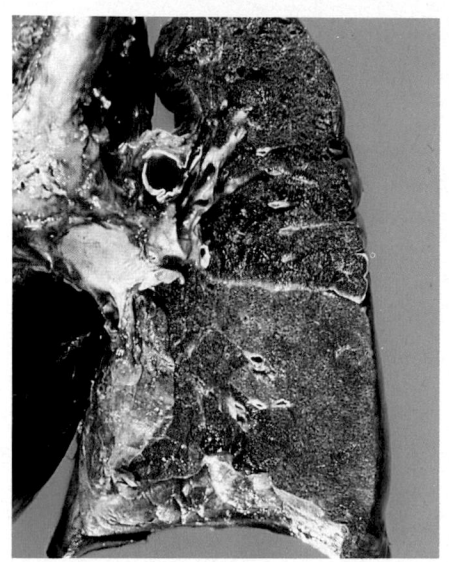

A, Autopsy specimen revealing lobar consolidation (gray and red hepatization) of the left lower lobe due to *Streptococcus pneumoniae.* Note the absence of abscess formation and the presence of dense consolidation extending from the hilum to the pleural surface.

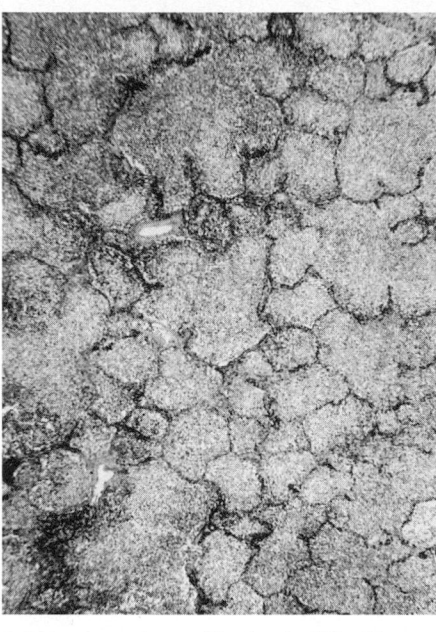

B, Low-powered magnification (×100) of hematoxylin and eosin (H & E) stain of tissue section from left lower lobar pneumonia pictured in A. Note intact alveolar walls and alveoli filled with edema and thick cellular exudate.

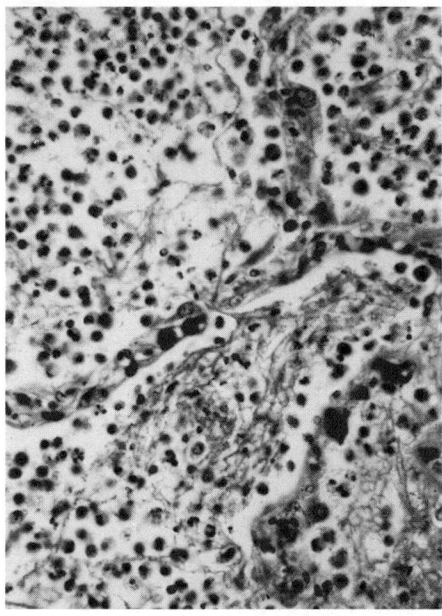

C, Higher magnification (×500) of H & E stain depicted in B. Note heavy infiltrate of polymorphonuclear cells and intact alveolar walls.

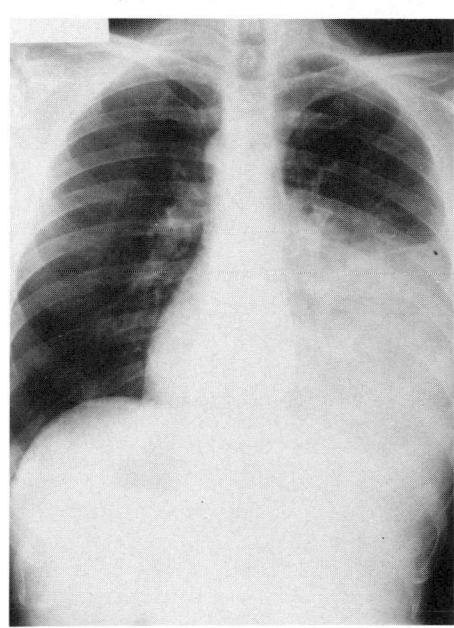

D, Roentgenogram (posteroanterior view) of the chest of a patient with left lower lobar pneumonia due to *S. pneumoniae,* with concomitant pleural effusion. Note obliteration of the left diaphragmatic shadow and the air bronchogram effect seen near the hilum, consistent with air space or alveolar exudative disease.

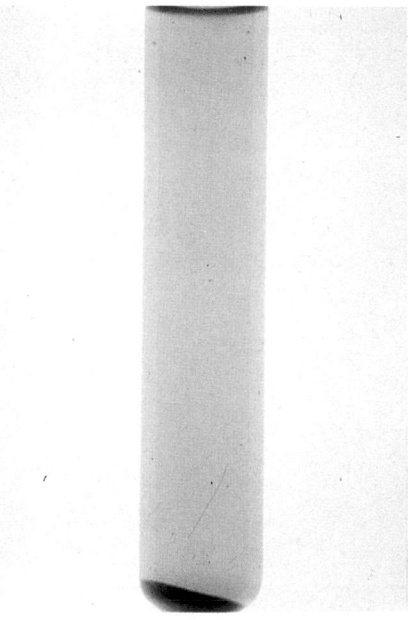

E, Fluid removed from the pleural space in a patient with early pneumococcal pneumonia and pleural effusion. The fluid may be serous, serosanguineous, green, or thick and white.

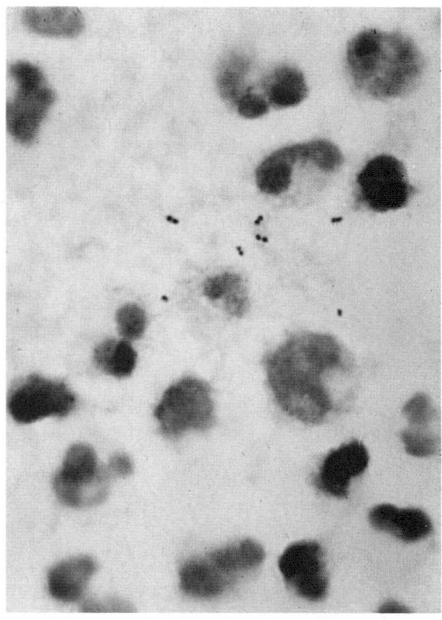

F, Gram's stain of pleural fluid shown in E, revealing the presence of polymorphonuclear cells and typical gram-positive diplococci in pairs, consistent with pneumococci.

G, Erysipeloid. Characteristic indolent, violaceous, nonpurulent lesion on a finger.

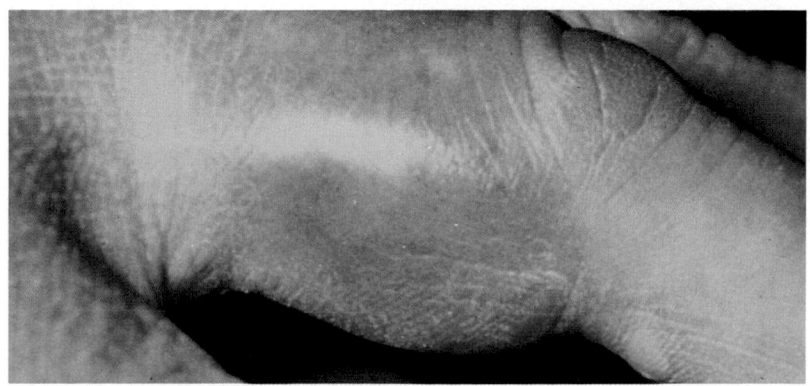

PLATE 10 LYME DISEASE, POLYCHONDRITIS, AND LEISHMANIASIS

A, Erythema chronicum migrans (ECM), the major dermatologic manifestation of Lyme disease. Four days after onset of ECM, this patient has developed secondary annular lesions; some of their borders have merged. (From Steere AC, Bartenhagen NH, Craft JE, et al.: The early clinical manifestations of Lyme disease. Ann Intern Med 99:76–82, 1983; with permission.)

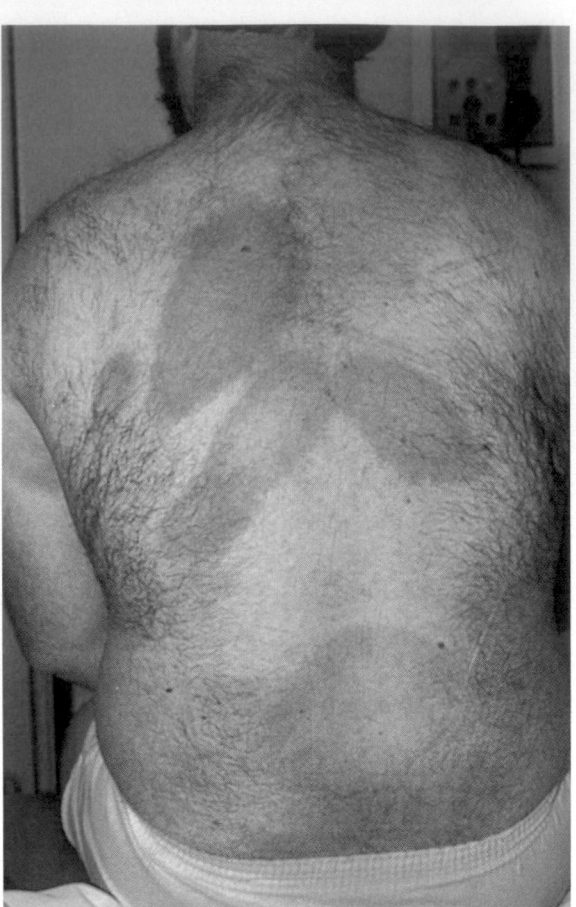

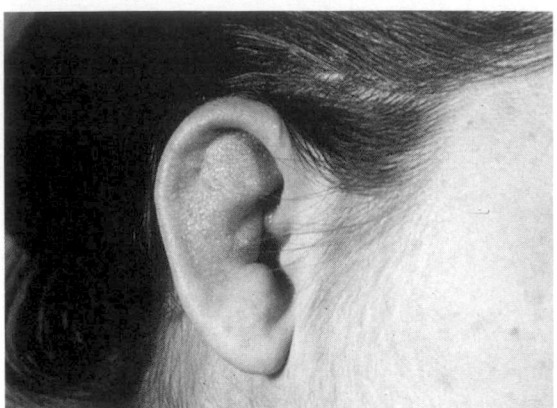

B, Polychondritis. Note nodularity of ear.

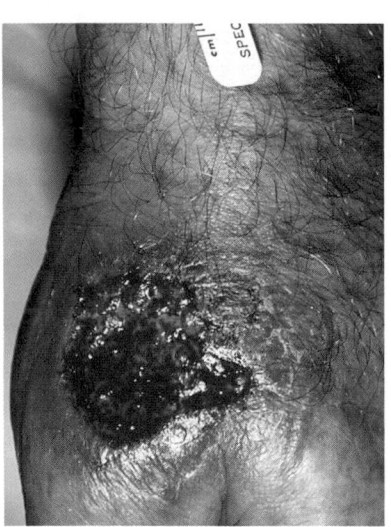

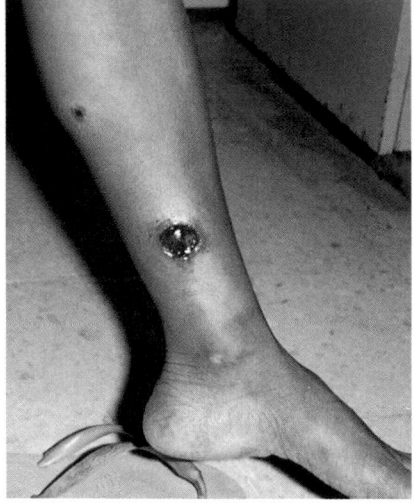

C, Left, Exudative cutaneous leishmanial lesion on the dorsum of the hand (L. braziliensis) acquired in the jungle of southeastern Peru. Right, Cutaneous leishmanial lesion on the lower leg (L. mexicana) of an inhabitant of southern Mexico.

PLATE 11. *See figure on the opposite page*

Protozoan diseases. A to D show various erythrocyte forms of falciparum or vivax malaria (×1500).

A, "Ring forms" of Plasmodium falciparum. Note the delicate rings and an erythrocyte containing two organisms.

B, Trophozoite of Plasmodium vivax. The red cell is enlarged, Schüffner's dots are seen, and the parasite is large and ameboid.

C, Schizont of Plasmodium vivax with at least 18 merozoite nuclei.

D, Gametocyte of Plasmodium falciparum. The crescent or banana shape is characteristic.

E, Trypanosoma rhodesiense in the peripheral blood. It has a nucleus, posterior kinetoplast, undulating membrane, and flagellum (×1500).

F, Spleen smear showing a cell filled with Leishmania donovani. The rod-shaped kinetoplast and large, round nucleus appear as two adjacent red dots.

G, Methenamine silver nitrate stain of clump of Pneumocystis cysts. They appear as black circles against the blue background (×800). It should be noted that Pneumocystis is no longer considered a protozoan.

H, Stool sample observed by light microscopy, showing a motile Entamoeba histolytica moving in a straight line across the field. The ameba contains lucent vacuoles and shows a pseudopod directed to the upper right (×500).

(A, C, D, and F are photographs taken by T. C. Jones from the Cornell Parasitology teaching slides; B is from the collection of H. Zaiman, originally photographed by M. Wittner; E and G were provided by R. B. Roberts; H is a photograph of fresh material provided by T. C. Jones.)

PLATE 11   PROTOZOAN DISEASES

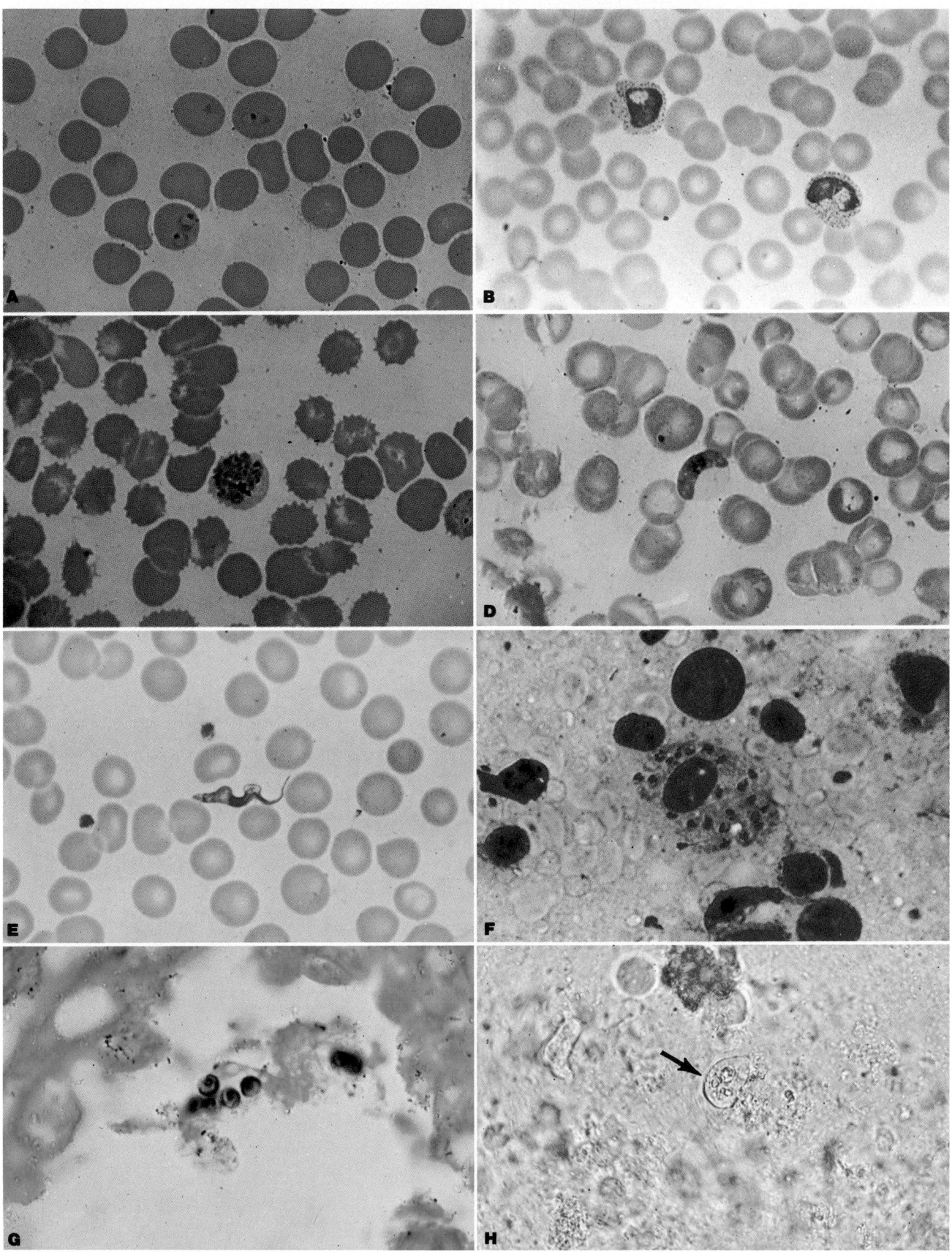

See legend on the opposite page

PLATE 12 HIV AND ASSOCIATED DISORDERS

A to E show dermatologic abnormalities in AIDS.

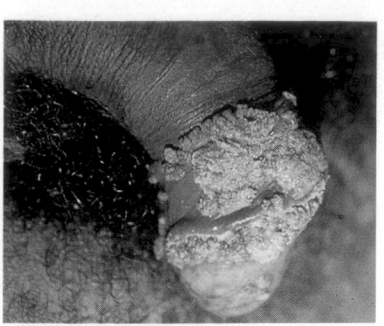

A, Prominent condyloma surrounding the corona and the shaft of the penis.

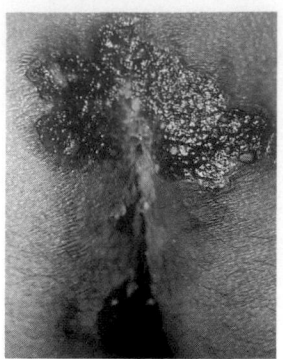

B, Chronic ulcerative herpetic infection is commonly seen in the intergluteal fold.

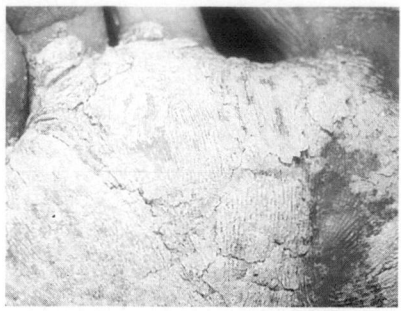

C, Marked hyperkeratosis characterizes keratoderma blennorrhagicum of Reiter's syndrome in HIV-seropositive patients.

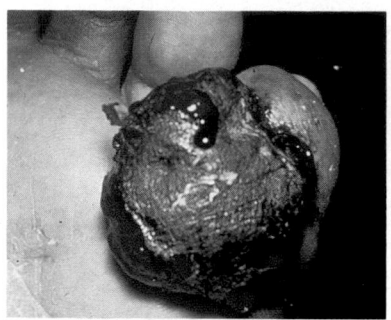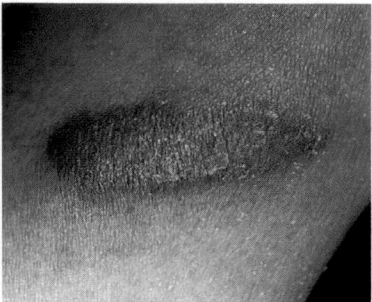

D, *Left,* An exophytic tumor of Kaposi's sarcoma on the sole. *Right,* Lesion demonstrating the linear configuration frequently noted in Kaposi's sarcoma of the skin in patients with AIDS.

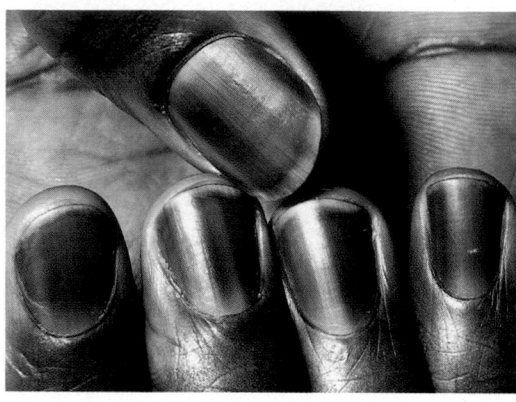

E, Vertical bands in the nail plates developed during treatment with AZT.

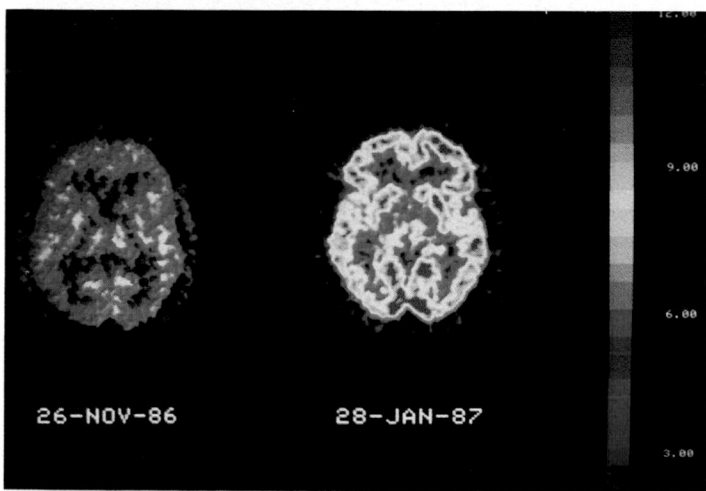

F, Positron emission tomography (PET) scan showing glucose metabolism in the brain of a patient with AIDS dementia before *(left)* and during *(right)* therapy with AZT. This patient had marked improvement in his cognitive function that was associated with a relative normalization of glucose metabolism in the brain. (Reproduced with permission from Brunetti A, Berg G, Di Chiro G, et al.: Reversal of brain metabolic abnormalities following treatment of AIDS dementia complex with 3′ - azido - 2′, 3′ - dideoxythymidine (AZT, zidovudine): A PET - FDG study. J Nucl Med 30:581–590, 1989.)

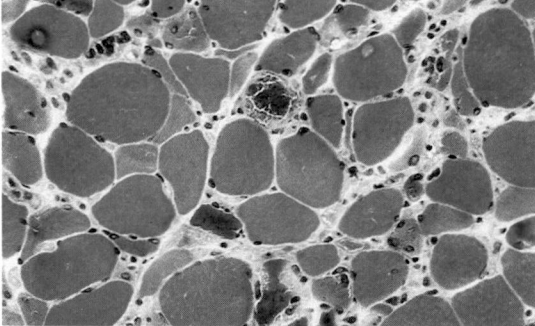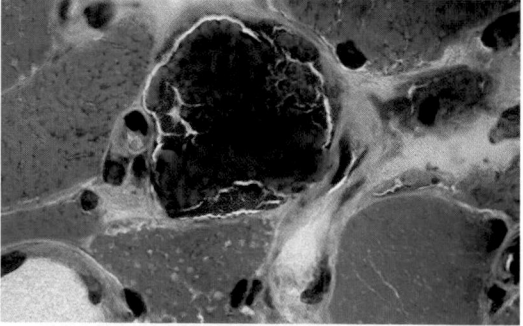

G, Pathologic findings in a patient with AZT-induced myopathy. *Top,* Destructive changes with variation in fiber size and a "ragged-red" fiber. Inflammatory changes can be seen in both AZT-induced myopathy and the myopathy of HIV infection. However, ragged-red fibers are seen only in patients receiving AZT. Transverse section, stained with the modified Gomori trichrome stain (×320). *Bottom,* Detail showing a ragged-red fiber (×900). (Photographs courtesy of Dr. M.C. Dalakos.)

Splenectomy may be performed either as a part of staging or as a therapeutic intervention in a number of disorders, including Hodgkin's disease, agnogenic myeloid metaplasia, paroxysmal nocturnal hemoglobinuria, hereditary spherocytosis, thalassemia, and a variety of autoimmune disorders.

The spleen probably plays an adjunctive role in host defense by removing organisms from the blood that have been ineffectively opsonized by complement. In addition, it participates in the primary immunoglobulin response and is involved in the regulation of the alternative complement pathway, with low levels of immunoglobulins and properdin reported in patients following splenectomy. A decrease in the opsonic peptide tuftsin has also been reported following splenectomy, and alternative pathway defects may be important in patients with sickle cell disease and splenic dysfunction.

The risk of developing serious infection, as well as the types of infections may vary depending on the reason for abnormal splenic function and the presence or absence of other immune abnormalities. Patients who undergo post-traumatic splenectomy appear to be at a lower risk for infection. An increased risk of *Salmonella* infections appears to be unique for the sickle cell population. Most asplenic patients or patients who have undergone splenectomy are at increased risk for serious bacterial infections primarily due to *S. pneumoniae* and *H. influenzae*, as well as *Neisseria* species and the DF2 bacillus. The initial presentation of even overwhelming infection may be deceptively subtle, with fever often being the only sign of infection. Asplenic patients with an underlying hematologic disease who present with fever should be managed initially as potentially septic.

EVALUATION AND MANAGEMENT OF THE FEBRILE GRANULOCYTOPENIC PATIENT: A PARADIGM FOR THE COMPROMISED HOST

A classic tenet of infectious disease is that antibiotic therapy is based on the isolation and identification of a specific organism or on a reliable prediction of a specific organism from a clinically involved site of infection. The overall management of neutropenic patients is based on the use of empiric antibiotics directed against a wider array of potential pathogens. Indeed, it is well accepted that when a neutropenic patient develops a new fever (usually defined as one oral temperature $\geq 38.5°C$, or more than two successive readings of $\geq 38°C$ in a 12-hour period), an empiric broad-spectrum antibacterial regimen should be started expeditiously. The rationale for this approach evolved from the observation that bacteremias in neutropenic patients were rapidly lethal, especially those due to gram-negative organisms, if antibiotic therapy was delayed until an organism was isolated or a site of infection identified. Although the goal of the pre-antibiotic evaluation of a newly febrile neutropenic patient is to identify potential sources, the majority of patients will not have a source of infection identified to explain the fever.

The standard initial evaluation should include a careful physical examination with particular attention to areas that may "hide" an infection, notably the oral cavity and the perianal area. Examination of the perirectal area, including deep palpation, should be performed, and only if there are findings suggestive of a localized inflammatory site (e.g., pain or fluctuance) should a judicious digital examination be performed. At a minimum, two sets of blood samples for culture should be obtained. If the patient has an indwelling intravenous catheter, then at least one set should be drawn through the catheter and another from a peripheral vein. For patients with multilumen intravenous catheters, a culture should be obtained through *each* lumen and the specific lumen clearly identified on the culture bottle. This is important, because catheter infection may be limited to a single lumen. Because of the absence of granulocytes, microscopic examination of the urine may be normal even in the presence of a urinary tract infection. A chest radiograph can serve as a valuable baseline, although some investigators have questioned the use of this procedure in patients without pulmonary symptoms. In addition, accessible sites of potential infection should be aspirated or biopsied, with appropriate material sent for Gram's stain, culture, and histologic examination.

Even with a comprehensive evaluation, an infectious etiology for the fever is found in only 30 to 50 per cent of patients.

Nonetheless, even subtle indications of inflammation must be considered as sites of potential infection in the presence of granulocytopenia. For example, minimal perirectal erythema and tenderness may be harbingers of a perirectal cellulitis. Minimal erythema or serous discharge at the exit site of an indwelling intravenous catheter may herald a tunnel or exit-site infection.

Colonization with microorganisms often precedes development of significant infection. However, routine "surveillance" cultures are not of practical benefit in a neutropenic patient, since colonization of no single body site is consistently predictive and multiple potential pathogens are usually isolated from any single site, making it difficult to predict the organism responsible for infection. Moreover, since empiric broad-spectrum antibiotics are administered under any circumstance, the expense of routine surveillance cannot be justified.

Tests such as nuclear scanning have also been used to define occult sites of infection. Although gallium citrate accumulates in inflammatory lesions because of its avid binding to lactoferrin, this test has not been shown to be useful in granulocytopenic patients. Autologous or allogeneic leukocytes labeled in vitro with indium-111 have been used with some success in the evaluation of febrile granulocytopenic patients.

Because of these diagnostic difficulties, even fevers that are temporally associated with the administration of blood products or with fever-producing antineoplastic agents should be considered potentially infectious in etiology and treated as such. In sum, virtually all new fevers in the neutropenic population warrant careful clinical and microbiologic evaluation, followed by prompt initiation of empiric antibiotic therapy. Conversely, any clinically evident site of potential infection mandates expeditious broad-spectrum therapy, even in the absence of fever.

Since the goal of empiric antibiotic therapy is to protect against the early morbidity and mortality that result from untreated bacterial infections, regimens have been formulated to maximize activity against organisms that are commonly encountered and are particularly virulent. However, empiric regimens cannot realistically be designed to cover every potential bacterial pathogen. Moreover, no regimen is capable of completely eliminating the risk of development of subsequent infections in persistently neutropenic patients.

Management of Indwelling Intravenous Catheters

Although gram-positive bacterial infections (especially staphylococcal) are the most frequent causes of catheter-related infections, other bacterial and nonbacterial species can be encountered, particularly in the neutropenic patient. These include resistant *Corynebacterium*, *Bacillus* species, gram-negative organisms, and fungi. In approaching the patient with a catheter-related infection, it is important to consider the specific type of infection, the location of the infection (i.e., bacteremia versus exit site versus tunnel), the type of access device (e.g., Hickman versus implantable subcutaneous reservoir), and the duration of symptoms.

In general, the vast majority of simple catheter-related bacteremias and exit-site infections can be cleared using appropriate antibiotics and do not necessitate catheter removal. This applies to both neutropenic and non-neutropenic patients. If multilumen devices are used, the antibiotic infusion should be rotated among the ports, since infection may be limited to one lumen (failure to do so can be a cause of persistent infection despite antibiotics). Diagnostic cultures should also be drawn through all ports of any multilumen device. If there is persistent bacteremia after 48 hours of appropriate therapy, the catheter should be removed. Failures of therapy are more common when the infections are due to certain organisms, such as *Bacillus* species or *Candida albicans*, and when these are isolated, the catheter usually should be removed.

Infections extending to involve the tunnel of a Hickman catheter also mandate prompt removal of the device, as antibiotics alone rarely cure this "closed-space" infection, particularly in the granulocytopenic host. Likewise, infections around the reservoir of an implantable subcutaneous device may be difficult to eradicate without catheter removal. Patients with recurrent catheter infections (despite a history of appropriate therapy) are also candidates for prompt catheter removal.

It is unresolved whether a non-neutropenic patient with an indwelling catheter who becomes newly febrile should receive antibiotics empirically. The safest policy is to begin antibiotics (using a third-generation cephalosporin like ceftriaxone or an aminoglycoside plus vancomycin) and continue them pending culture results and clinical response. This approach protects against rapid progression of undetected yet virulent infections (such as *S. aureus*) and may minimize the need for ultimate catheter removal. If by 72 hours the cultures are negative and the patient is stable, antibiotics can be discontinued.

Initial Management of the Neutropenic Patient Who Becomes Febrile

Traditionally, gram-negative bacteria have been the most frequently isolated pathogens in the neutropenic population. Of the gram-negative bacteria, *E. coli, K. pneumoniae,* and *P. aeruginosa* have been the most common. While gram-negative bacteria still predominate at some institutions, there has been a trend in recent years toward more gram-positive infections, and these now comprise the majority of isolates at many centers. In general, the gram-negative infections tend to be more virulent, and early empiric regimens have been formulated to provide protection primarily against these organisms while maintaining a broad spectrum of activity against other potential pathogens. Indeed, adequate coverage of these gram-negative organisms is still an essential property of any empiric regimen.

Although there is no single best regimen or recipe, there are a number of appropriate options. The selection of a specific antibiotic regimen depends on many factors, including institutional sensitivity patterns, individual and institutional experience, and clinical parameters.

The standard approach to the empiric management of the febrile neutropenic patient has been to use combination antibiotic regimens. Until recently, this has been the only way to provide coverage broad enough to encompass the predominant gram-positive and gram-negative organisms. Moreover, some combinations have been considered to provide synergy and to have the potential for decreasing the emergence of resistant isolates. Aminoglycoside–β-lactam combinations were the first empiric regimens with acceptable efficacy in the setting of fever and neutropenia. Such combination regimens are still widely used and represent a standard against which newer regimens are tested. Many variations have been studied and include aminoglycosides combined with either an extended-spectrum penicillin, a cephalosporin, or as a component of a triple-drug regimen. If an aminoglycoside-containing combination regimen is to be employed, the choice of specific antibiotics should be based primarily on the institutional antibiotic sensitivity patterns and secondarily on toxicity and cost differences.

Non–aminoglycoside-containing combination regimens have also been studied. These have consisted of combinations of two β-lactam antibiotics, or so-called double β-lactam regimens, usually consisting of an expanded-spectrum carboxy- or ureido-penicillin plus a third-generation cephalosporin (e.g., piperacillin and ceftazidime).

New or Novel Antibiotics for Neutropenic Patients

The advent of β-lactam antibiotics with broad-spectrum activity which achieve high serum bactericidal levels has made monotherapy another option for the initial empiric therapy of the febrile neutropenic patient (Table 287–3). The third-generation cephalosporins and the carbapenems are the two classes that include potential candidates for empiric single-agent therapy. Ceftazidime has been the most extensively studied of the third-generation cephalosporins as monotherapy because of its superior activity against *P. aeruginosa.*

A large, randomized study evaluating 550 consecutive episodes of fever and neutropenia was conducted at the National Cancer Institute (NCI). In this study, patients with fever and granulocytopenia underwent a standard initial evaluation and then were randomized to receive either a combination of antibiotics (cephalothin, gentamicin, and carbenicillin) or ceftazidime as a single agent. The overall results show that monotherapy compared favorably with a standard combination regimen. Approximately two thirds of the episodes in both groups were successfully treated for the entire duration of their granulocytopenia, without requiring *any* changes in their initial regimen. Another one third of the episodes required some change or modification (such as addition of an antibacterial, antifungal, or antiviral drug) to ensure a successful outcome (see indications for modifications below), and an equally low number in both groups (about 5 per cent) died of infection. None of the deaths was attributable to a specific deficiency in one regimen that was not present in the other.

Two subgroups of patients were identified who required more frequent modifications of the initial regimen in order to achieve a successful outcome: (1) those presenting with a documented source of infection to account for the initial fever, and (2) those having relatively protracted periods of granulocytopenia (> 1 week). The need for modification in these subgroups was identical for those episodes treated with monotherapy and those treated with combination therapy. In this study, these modifications did not represent a failure of either regimen per se but instead were reflective of the limitations of any regimen in treating patients who are at high risk for development of subsequent infections.

Concerns regarding the use of ceftazidime as a single agent for fever and neutropenia include the lack of synergy against documented gram-negative infections, lack of activity against certain gram-positive isolates, poor antianaerobic activity, and the potential for development of resistance.

In addition to the third-generation cephalosporins, other anti-

TABLE 287–3. ACTIVITY OF NEWER ANTIBIOTICS AGAINST BACTERIAL PATHOGENS COMMONLY ENCOUNTERED IN IMPAIRED HOSTS

Antibiotic	Enteric Gram-negative	*P. aeruginosa*	Coagulase-positive Staphylococci	Coagulase-negative Staphylococci	Enterococci	Non-Group D Streptococci	Anaerobes
Ceftazidime	Good	Good	Moderate (poor against methicillin-resistant strains)	Poor against the majority (most are methicillin-resistant)	Poor	Good	Poor
Cefoperazone	Good	Moderate	Moderate (poor against methicillin-resistant strains)	Poor against the majority	Poor	Good	Poor
Other third-generation cephalosporins	Good	Poor	Moderate (poor against methicillin-resistant strains)	Poor against the majority	Poor	Good	Poor to moderate (moxalactam and ceftizoxime have some activity)
Imipenem	Good	Good	Good (poor against methicillin-resistant strains	Poor against the majority	Good	Good	Good
Quinolones	Good	Good	Good (including most methicillin-resistant strains)	Good (limited clinical experience)	Poor to moderate	Poor to moderate	Poor
Aztreonam	Good	Good	Poor	Poor	Poor	Poor	Poor

From Rubin M, Walsh TJ, Pizzo PA: Clinical approaches to the compromised host. *In* Hoffman R, Benz EJ, Shattil SJ, et al. (eds.): Hematology: Basic Principles and Practices. New York, Churchill Livingstone, 1991.

biotics are also being evaluated in neutropenic patients. Imipenem, for example, is a member of the carbapenem class of antibiotics. It is formulated in fixed combination with cilastatin, which inhibits a renal enzyme that can degrade imipenem. Overall, it has the broadest spectrum of activity of any available antibiotic. Of note is its excellent in vitro activity against enterococci as well as many anaerobes.

Early results of two randomized studies appear to corroborate its efficacy in this setting—one comparing it with an aminoglycoside-containing combination and another being performed at the NCI comparing it with monotherapy with ceftazidime. Interestingly, neither of these studies appears to demonstrate superior efficacy for imipenem. Two potential drawbacks to its use include a relatively high incidence of the development of resistant *P. aeruginosa* and its potential to decrease the seizure threshold in patients with central nervous system pathology. In addition, in the ongoing NCI trial, a higher than expected frequency of nausea has been found with imipenem.

Because of the increasing incidence of gram-positive infections in cancer patients during the 1980's and their increased resistance to β-lactam antibiotics, some authorities have recommended that vancomycin be added to empiric regimens. Conversely, it has been argued that since many of these organisms are of relatively low virulence, vancomycin may be safely withheld until the gram-positive isolate has been identified microbiologically.

Although two randomized studies demonstrated a reduction in gram-positive infections in patients receiving a vancomycin regimen, there were no significant differences in outcome or survival when vancomycin was added in a pathogen-directed manner. A retrospective analysis from the NCI also indicated that there was no excess morbidity in delaying the institution of vancomycin by waiting for either a microbiologic or clinical indication for its use (i.e., a positive culture for a resistant gram-positive organism or a clinical infection developing with other antibiotics).

At the present time, it seems reasonable not to routinely include vancomycin in all empiric antibiotic regimens. Its use, however, should be guided by institutional experience and sensitivity patterns. For example, in a center with a high incidence of methicillin-resistant *S. aureus*, routine use of vancomycin is clearly warranted, since this may be a particularly virulent organism if not treated. In addition, fluctuations in patterns of infecting microorganisms may occur over time. For example, penicillin-resistant α-hemolytic streptococci have recently been identified as particularly virulent pathogens in some centers (perhaps related to the use of high-dose cytosine arabinoside). Clearly, the emergence of new pathogens or pathogens with altered sensitivity profiles may force dramatic changes in our use of antibiotics in the future.

The appropriate role for the quinolones in the neutropenic patient has yet to be defined. Because of their relatively poor activity against certain gram-positive organisms, they should not be used for empiric therapy alone. They may, however, be useful for completion of therapy in patients who initially respond to intravenous antibiotics and who have had either a fever of undetermined origin or a susceptible bacterial isolate.

A particularly useful feature of aztreonam is its apparent lack of cross-reactivity with the other β-lactams in patients who have penicillin or β-lactam allergies. In this group of patients empiric therapy might begin with a combination of vancomycin, aztreonam, and an aminoglycoside.

Also recently introduced are combinations of β-lactams with β-lactamase inhibitors (i.e., clavulanic acid and sulbactam). Three preparations are now available, including amoxicillin + clavulanic acid (oral formulation only), ticarcillin + clavulanic acid, and ampicillin + sulbactam. A number of studies have documented the efficacy of ticarcillin + clavulanic acid combined with aminoglycoside for initial empiric therapy of fever in neutropenic patients. The expanded gram-positive coverage may obviate additional anti–gram-positive agents.

APPROACH TO THE PATIENT WITH PROLONGED GRANULOCYTOPENIA

How Long Should Antibiotics Be Continued?

A question of practical importance is how long empiric antibiotics should be continued in persistently neutropenic patients.

Should they always be continued until the granulocyte count recovers, or can they be safely discontinued prior to that time?

The question of duration of therapy can be approached by placing patients in two categories: those whose initial workup (at the time of presentation with fever and neutropenia) did not reveal a source of infection (i.e., a fever of undetermined origin, or FUO) and those whose initial workup revealed an infection to account for the fever (i.e., a positive culture, clinically infected site, or both). The majority of patients (approximately 60 per cent) fall into the FUO category, although this varies with the institution, the therapy, and the patient population (Fig. 287–1).

FUO PATIENTS. There are only limited data that specifically address the issue of duration of empiric therapy in neutropenic patients presenting with an FUO. For patients with an expected short duration of granulocytopenia (e.g., < 1 week), waiting to stop antibiotics until recovery of the counts is practical and effective. However, the real dilemma arises in the population with more prolonged granulocytopenia.

In a study from the NCI, patients with FUO and persistent granulocytopenia were randomized either to discontinue antibiotics on day 7 of therapy or to continue them until the resolution of the neutropenia. Nearly 40 per cent of afebrile patients in whom antibiotics were stopped developed recurrent fever, and 38 per cent of febrile patients whose antibiotics were discontinued developed hypotensive episodes. It was concluded that day 7 was too early to discontinue antibiotics in this group.

A subsequent study randomized persistently neutropenic, afebrile patients to continue or discontinue antibiotics on day 14. Preliminary analysis showed no difference between the two groups: Approximately one third of patients became febrile again regardless of whether they stopped or continued antibiotics. However, those whose fevers recurred following discontinuation of antibiotics responded to a reinstitution of their initial regimen, whereas those remaining on antibiotics required addition of amphotericin B. On this basis, it seems reasonable to discontinue antibiotics and carefully observe FUO patients who are predicted to have a long duration of neutropenia and who have remained afebrile after 14 days of therapy.

PATIENTS PRESENTING WITH DOCUMENTED INFECTIONS. There are even fewer data that address the issue of duration of antibiotics in patients with defined sites of infection. For persistently neutropenic patients who have had clinical and microbiologic resoluton of their infection and who are afebrile at day 14 (for a minimum of 7 days), antibiotics should be discontinued. The ultimate decision of whether to continue or discontinue rests on a number of clinical parameters, such as the degree of or potential for antibiotic toxicity, the predicted duration of neutropenia, the seriousness of the initial infection, and the presence or absence of a continued site of infection or other factors predisposing to subsequent infection. It should be emphasized that any neutropenic patient whose antibiotics are discontinued requires careful, meticulous follow-up in order to quickly detect new fevers or infection.

Modifications of Antibiotic Therapy During the Course of Granulocytopenia

Empiric antibiotics have their greatest impact early in the course of neutropenia. However, it is during a prolonged granulocytopenic episode when the patient is at highest risk for the development of multiple types of secondary infections or superinfections. Many of these dictate specific modifications of the initial regimen (Table 287–4).

Bacterial isolates that are resistant to the initial empiric regimen are invariably encountered when managing neutropenic patients. For example, at most centers, the majority of coagulase-negative staphylococci are resistant to β-lactams, and breakthrough infections might be anticipated. Fortunately, coagulase-negative staphylococci are relatively indolent, and the risk for secondary infection can be balanced accordingly. Thus, for the patient who develops evidence of gram-positive infection while receiving β-lactam or who has evidence of a catheter site infection, vancomycin is an appropriate addition to the initial antibiotic regimen. Similarly, if the coverage of the initial regimen has limited antianaerobic activity, secondary infection with anaerobics might be anticipated.

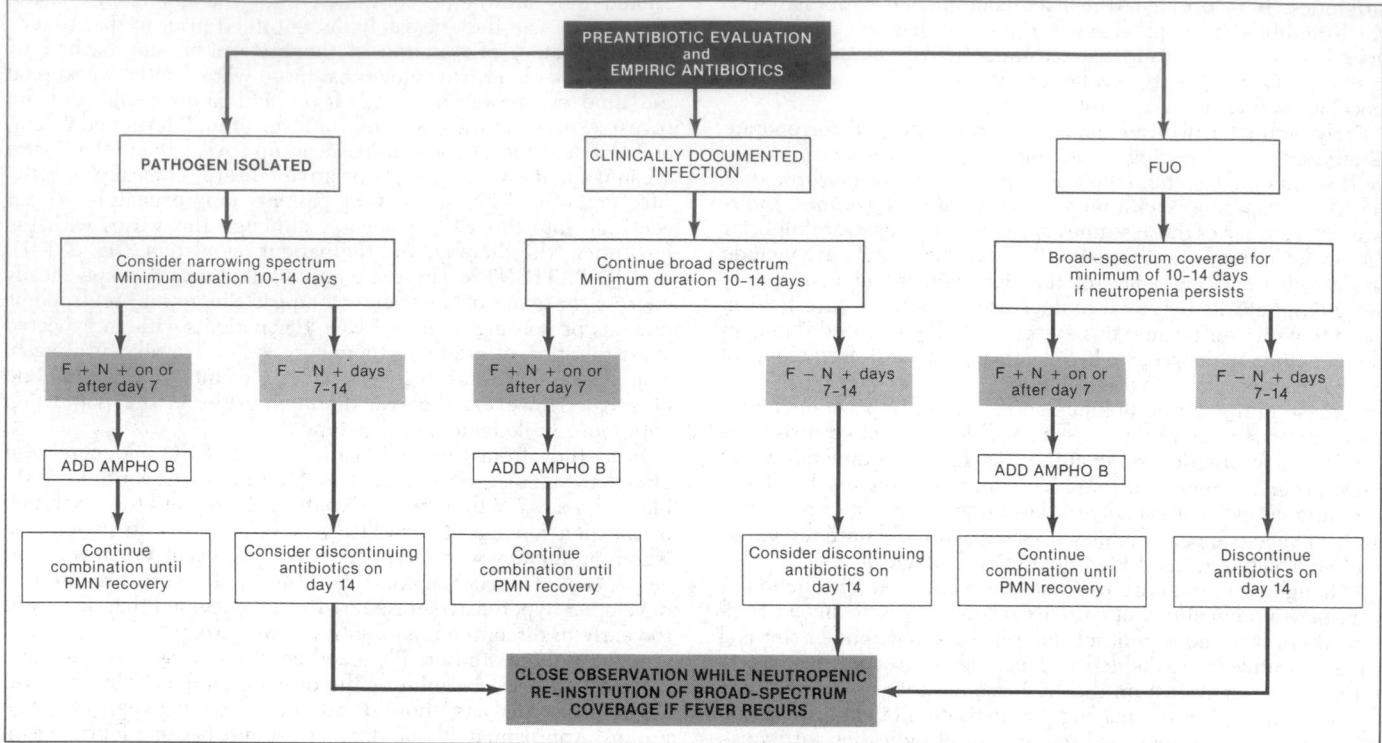

FIGURE 287–1. Management of fever and neutropenia. F + N + = Febrile, neutropenic. F − N + = Afebrile, neutropenic. FUO = No source for fever on preantibiotic evaluation. AMPHO B = Amphotericin B. (From Rubin M, Walsh TJ, Pizzo PA: Clinical approach to the compromised host. *In* Hoffman R, Benz EJ, Shattil SJ, et al. (eds.): Hematology: Basic Principles and Practices. New York, Churchill Livingstone, 1991.)

The appearance of "secondary" resistance is seen more frequently with certain organisms. For example, *Enterobacter* species, *Citrobacter* species, and *Serratia* have inducible β-lactamases, and the appearance of a clinically significant clustering of resistant *Enterobacter* in a neutropenic population has been recently observed. Accordingly, when these organisms are isolated from a patient, careful observation for emergence of resistance is warranted, and for patients receiving monotherapy with a broad-spectrum β-lactam an aminoglycoside should be added. *P. aeruginosa* may develop resistance to imipenem through a relatively novel mechanism involving a change in the porins. Hence, patients receiving single-agent therapy for *P. aeruginosa* infection should also have an aminoglycoside added to their regimens. Secondary development of resistance by gram-positive organisms is somewhat rarer, although it has been described. Of note, recent studies have documented the emergence of vancomycin-resistant coagulase-negative staphylococci and enterococci in patients receiving vancomycin.

The appearance of a new site of infection (e.g., cellulitis or pneumonia) or the progression of a previously documented site of infection is an additional reason for changes or modifications of the antimicrobial regimen. For example, the development of marginal or necrotizing gingivitis is relatively common in patients who have received intensive cytotoxic therapy. Anaerobic organisms contribute to this process, and an antianaerobic agent such as clindamycin or metronidazole should be added to the empiric regimen if gingivitis is diagnosed.

The most common pathogens contributing to perianal cellulitis are the aerobic gram-negative bacilli, enterococci, and bowel anaerobes. Therefore, when it occurs in a patient already receiv-

TABLE 287–4. MODIFICATION OF THERAPY

Clinical Event	Possible Modifications of Therapy
Breakthrough bacteremia	If gram-positive isolate (e.g., *S. epidermidis*), add vancomycin If gram-negative isolate (i.e., presumably resistant), switch to new regimen
Catheter-associated infection	Add vancomycin (as well as gram-negative coverage if not already being given)
Severe oral mucositis or necrotizing gingivitis	Add specific antianaerobic agent (e.g., metronidazole)
Esophagitis	Oral clotrimazole, fluconazole, or IV amphotericin B
Pneumonitis Diffuse or interstitial New infiltrate in a granulocytopenic patient also receiving antibiotics	Trimethoprim-sulfamethoxazole and erythromycin (plus broad-spectrum antibiotics if the patient is granulocytopenic) If granulocyte count is rising, watch and wait If granulocyte count is not recovering, biopsy to establish diagnosis; if biopsy cannot be done, add amphotericin B empirically
Perianal tenderness	If patient is already receiving broad-spectrum antibiotics, add a specific antianaerobic agent If patient is not on antibiotics, begin broad-spectrum therapy with anaerobic coverage
Persistent fever and neutropenia	Continue antibiotics and after 1 week of persistent fever and neutropenia, add systemic antifungal therapy

ing broad-spectrum antibiotics, the addition of an antianaerobic agent as well as a change in the broad-spectrum coverage may be necessary. Similarly, any suspected intra-abdominal site of infection should prompt addition or inclusion of antibiotics active against aerobic gram-negative bacilli, enterococci, and bowel anaerobes.

The development of a new site of infection may also warrant the addition of antimicrobial agents directed at fungi, viruses, or parasites. The appearance of burning retrosternal pain is frequently an indicator of esophagitis, most often caused by cytotoxic therapy, *Candida*, or herpes simplex. The development of pulmonary infiltrates might raise suspicion not only of resistant bacteria, but also of *P. carinii,* fungi, or a viral pneumonia. A new localized infiltrate in a neutropenic patient whose white blood count is rising while receiving broad-spectrum antibiotics with the "new" infiltrate may simply represent an inflammatory reaction at a previous unrecognized site of infection. Close observation without any modification may be appropriate. If, however, the granulocyte count is not rising and the patient has been neutropenic for only a short period of time (≤ 1 week), then a bacterial process is most likely. If the patient has been persistently neutropenic for a more prolonged period, then a fungal pneumonia should also be strongly considered and amphotericin B added while a diagnostic workup is initiated.

Patients who develop hypotension while receiving broad-spectrum antibiotics should be presumed septic with a resistant organism or breakthrough infection. In such patients, changes in the empiric regimen should be made expeditiously and continued for the duration of treatment if an organism is not recovered. So-called culture-negative sepsis may occur when the growth of resistant organisms is suppressed by marginally effective antibiotics or when samples for culture are not drawn during the bacteremic episode.

Empiric Antifungal Therapy

The diagnosis of a disseminated fungal infection is difficult in an immunocompromised patient. Neutropenic patients who remain persistently febrile despite a 4- to 7-day trial of broad-spectrum antibacterial therapy are particularly likely to have a fungal infection. Empiric antifungal therapy might be expected to have a dual effect: the prevention of a fungal overgrowth in patients with prolonged neutropenia and the early treatment of "subclinical" fungal disease.

To date, the only proven agent for empiric therapy has been amphotericin B. Amphotericin B should be begun at 0.5 mg per kilogram per day and administered along with antibiotics until the resolution of neutropenia. A number of new azole and triazole antifungal agents are being evaluated and offer the promise of less toxic alternatives to amphotericin B.

Patients who remain febrile after the resolution of neutropenia should be evaluated for hepatosplenic candidiasis. The diagnosis is suggested by "bull's-eye" lesions on CT scan or ultrasonography of the liver and spleen. MRI scanning of the liver may be even more sensitive. Biopsy and histologic examination are essential. Patients with hepatosplenic candidiasis may require extended courses of antifungal therapy. The average amount of amphotericin B required for resolution of these lesions is approximately 5 grams, often in conjunction with 5-flucytosine (100 mg per kilogram per day).

PREVENTION OF INFECTIONS

Because bacteria account for the majority of infections in compromised patients, prophylactic strategies have focused on these pathogens. The strategies that have been explored include mechanical techniques to prevent acquisition of new pathogens; absorbable or nonabsorbable oral antibiotic regimens to either prevent acquisition or decrease the number of potentially pathogenic colonizing organisms; and methods to improve the host defense matrix, including immunization, and more recently, biologic agents (e.g., the colony-stimulating factors) (Table 287–5).

Perhaps the most important infection prevention strategy of all, however, is hand washing. Although taken for granted, this simple procedure is frequently overlooked to the detriment of the patient.

TABLE 287–5. METHODS FOR PREVENTING INFECTION IN HIGH-RISK PATIENTS

Prevent Acquisition and/or Suppress or Eliminate Microbial Flora	Improve or Modify Host Defenses
Isolation	Immunization
Simple or reverse isolation	Active
Isolation with HEPA air filtration	*Pseudomonas*
	Pneumococcus
Prophylactic antibiotics	VZV
Nonabsorbable antibiotics	Passive
Trimethoprim-sulfamethoxazole erythromycin	J-5 core glycolipid
Selective decontamination	Pooled immunoglobulins
Quinolones	Hyperimmune globulins
Prophylactic antivirals	Monoclonal antibodies
Acyclovir	Cell-component replacement
Amantadine	Leukocyte transfusions
Prophylactic antifungals	Accelerate granulocyte recovery
Nystatin	Lithium
Imidazoles	G-CSF
Triazoles	GM-CSF
Amphotericin B	Immunomodulations
Prophylactic antiparasitics	Interferons
Thiabendazole	Interleukins
Trimethoprim-sulfamethoxazole	
Combination-comprehensive	
Total protective isolation	

Modified from Pizzo PA: Considerations for the prevention of infectious complications in patients with cancer. Rev Infect Dis 11:S1551–1563, 1989.

Neutropenic Patients

MECHANICAL TECHNIQUES. Reverse isolation (i.e., single room with gowns, masks, and gloves) following the onset of neutropenia does not prevent infection. This is because most of the infections arise from the patient's endogenous microbial flora. In addition, having a patient wear a surgical mask outside of his or her room does little to protect against subsequent infection. Although some authorities have recommended that all foods be thoroughly cooked and that fresh fruits and vegetables be avoided to decrease the acquisition of gram-negative bacteria, the value of these measures in preventing infection remains unproven.

The total protective environment (TPE) is a comprehensive regimen designed to reduce the patient's endogenous microbial burden as well as the acquisition of new organisms. The TPE includes a HEPA-filtered laminar airflow room together with an aggressive program of surface decontamination, including the sterilization of all objects that enter the room, and an intensive regimen to disinfect the microbial diet. A number of studies have documented that TPE can reduce infections in profoundly granulocytopenic individuals. However, TPE is expensive, and because of the improvement in treating established infections, it does not offer a current survival advantage to most patients. Thus TPE is not necessary for the routine care of the majority of granulocytopenic patients.

ORAL ANTIBIOTIC REGIMENS. Numerous studies have evaluated both nonabsorbable antibiotics (such as gentamicin, vancomycin, polymyxin, or colistin) and antibiotics that are absorbed from the gastrointestinal tract (e.g., trimethoprim-sulfamethoxazole, erythromycin, or quinolones). The goal of antibiotics has ranged from "total decontamination" of the alimentary tract with oral nonabsorbable antibiotics to "selective decontamination," in which the goal is to eliminate the potentially pathogenic aerobic flora (mostly the enteric gram-negative bacteria) while preserving the majority of anaerobic organisms and thus preserving "colonization resistance." Although the introduction of each new prophylactic regimen has been met with enthusiasm, over time these strategies have failed because of the emergence of resistant organisms.

The fluoroquinolones (mostly norfloxacin and ciprofloxacin) have been used in recent years for prophylaxis in neutropenic patients. These agents are well absorbed and their use may really represent "early treatment" rather than prophylaxis. Although studies evaluating quinolones have demonstrated a reduction in gram-negative infections in the patients who receive them, caution about the widespread use of quinolones for prophylaxis should be underscored. Organisms resistant to the quinolones have already been described, and the indiscriminate use of these agents only accelerates this process. Since the quinolones are useful for the treatment of both immunocompromised and immunocompetent individuals, the use of these antibiotics for prophylaxis should be discouraged.

PATIENTS WITH SICKLE CELL ANEMIA. Since patients with sickle cell anemia are prone to infections with encapsulated organisms (e.g., S. pneumoniae, H. influenzae), especially in young children, the pneumococcal vaccine and prophylactic penicillin have been used to prevent these infections. Unfortunately, the vaccination has not resulted in an effective antibody response. Prophylactic penicillin can, however, significantly reduce the incidence of infection, and it is recommended that penicillin prophylaxis be begun by 4 months of age in children with sickle cell anemia and that it be continued beyond the third birthday.

Prevention of Fungal Infections

Although the increasing incidence of fungal infection makes a preventive strategy desirable, to date no clear evidence of benefit has been demonstrated. It is hoped that newer azole and triazole antifungal agents may improve the ability to control these opportunistic pathogens.

Prevention of Viral Infections

HERPES SIMPLEX. Herpes simplex is a frequent cause of morbidity in compromised patients, particularly in association with bone marrow or renal transplantation or intensive chemotherapy regimens. Several studies have demonstrated that acyclovir administered either orally or intravenously at dosages of 250 mg per square meter every 8 hours can reduce the incidence of herpetic gingivostomatitis. Accordingly, it seems reasonable to administer prophylactic oral or intravenous acyclovir in patients who are HSV seropositive (titers $\geq$1:16) or who have a prior history of infection and are undergoing bone marrow transplantation or intensive therapy for acute leukemia.

VARICELLA-ZOSTER VIRUS. One of the most important ways to prevent VZV transmission is to prevent contact of immunosuppressed individuals with infected individuals. This includes patients with either primary VZV (chicken pox) or secondary VZV (zoster). If a seronegative individual has had contact with an infected individual, passive immunization with ZIG (zoster immune globulin) has been shown to reduce the incidence of pneumonitis and encephalitis. Administration of ZIG (1 vial per 15 kg) must occur within 72 hours after exposure.

A varicella vaccine has been shown to reduce infection in children with leukemia. The live vaccine may be released soon for administration in normal healthy children and if effective should reduce the overall population of infected individuals.

CYTOMEGALOVIRUS. Strategies aimed at prevention of CMV infection have included use of seronegative blood products in seronegative patients, passive immunization, and chemoprophylaxis with acyclovir.

Prevention of Parasitic Infections

The clearest benefit of prophylaxis has been demonstrated in preventing P. carinii pneumonia with trimethoprim-sulfamethoxazole. The decision to administer prophylaxis for P. carinii should be influenced by the patient's underlying disease, the intensity or immunosuppression of the therapy being delivered, and the center where treatment is being administered. Recent studies have demonstrated that trimethoprim-sulfamethoxazole can be effective and safe at a dosage of 75 mg per square meter twice a day given on 3 consecutive days each week. Alternatives include aerosolized pentamidine and dapsone.

Improving Host Defense

Immunization against bacterial and viral pathogens has played an extremely important role in decreasing the incidence and/or severity of many infectious diseases. Unfortunately, active immunization is generally unsuccessful in immunocompromised hosts, since they are unable to mount or to sustain an antibody response to most vaccines.

Passive immunization, on the other hand, involves administration of preformed antibodies to high-risk patients. ZIG, for example, is effective in preventing infection and decreasing the incidence of morbidity and mortality associated with primary chicken pox in susceptible hosts. Another "hyperimmune" preparation that has been investigated in high-risk patients is the so-called J-5 antisera, collected from patients with high titers of antibody directed against the core glycolipid of Enterobacteriaceae. The results of early clinical trials with the J-5 antisera appeared encouraging, although confirmatory studies have not been consistent. Monoclonal antibodies have been developed and suggest that they may reduce morbidity in some patients with gram-negative sepsis. Pooled immunoglobulin preparations do not appear to offer benefit for neutropenic hosts but are of benefit to patients who have either congenital or acquired (e.g., CLL, multiple myeloma) hypogammaglobulinemia.

Perhaps the most exciting new developments will be the therapeutic use of cytokines and lymphokines to enforce the host defense repertoire. Clearly, as new factors become defined, the prospect for restoring function in the compromised host stands as the opportunity for the 1990's.

Graybill JR: Systemic fungal agents—diagnosis and treatment I: Therapeutic agents. Infect Dis Clin North Am 3:805–825, 1988. *Comprehensive review of diagnostic and therapeutic advances in the management of patients with systemic mycoses.*

Hill HR: Infections complicating congenital immunodeficiency syndromes. *In* Rubin RH, Young LS (eds.): Clinical Approach to Infection in the Compromised Host. New York, Plenum Medical Book Company, 1988, pp 407–438. *Practical overview of the serious infectious complications that occur in children with congenital immune deficiency diseases.*

Hirsch MS: Herpes group virus infections in the compromised host. *In* Rubin RH, Young LS (eds.): Clinical Approach to Infections in the Compromised Host. New York, Plenum Medical Book Company, 1988, pp 347–366. *Details the important issues related to the serious infections caused by herpes simplex, varicella-zoster, and cytomegalovirus in immunocompromised hosts.*

Immunization Practices Advisory Committee, CDC. General recommendations on immunization. Guidelines from the Immunization Practices Committee. Ann Intern Med 111:133–142, 1989. *Offers recommendations for immunization practices for adults.*

Leher RJ, Ganz T, Selsted ME, et al.: Neutrophils and host defense. Ann Intern Med 109:127–142, 1988. *Comprehensive review of phagocyte function and its relevance to host defense.*

Mandell GL, Douglas RG, Bennett JE (eds.): Principles and Practice of Infectious Diseases, 3rd ed. New York, Churchill Livingstone, 1990.

Pizzo PA: Considerations for the prevention of infectious complications in patients with cancer. Rev Infect Dis 11:S1551–S1563, 1989. *Provides a critical overview of preventive strategies aimed at suppressing or eliminating the host's microbial burden or at augmenting altered host defenses.*

Pizzo PA, Hathorn JW, et al.: A randomized trial comparing combination antibiotic therapy to monotherapy in cancer patients with fever and neutropenia. N Engl J Med 315:552, 1986. *A large prospective randomized clinical trial that provides a basis for the evaluation of empiric antibiotics for adults and children who become febrile while neutropenic.*

Pizzo PA, Robichaud KJ, Wesley R, et al.: Fever in the pediatric and young adult patient with cancer. A prospective study of 1001 episodes. Medicine 61:153–165, 1982. *Reviews the clinical presentation and outcome of children, adolescents, and young adults with cancer who develop fever.*

Rubin RH, Young LS (eds.): Clinical Approach to Infection in the Compromised Host. New York, Plenum Medical Book Company, 1988.

Rubin M, Walsh, TJ, Pizzo PA: Clinical approaches to infections in the compromised host. *In* Hoffman R, Benz EJ Jr, Shattil SJ, et al. (eds.): Hematology: Basic Principles and Practice. New York, Churchill Livingstone, 1991, pp 1063–1114. *Detailed review of infections in compromised hosts.*

The International Chronic Granulomatous Disease Cooperative Study Group: A controlled trial of interferon gamma to prevent infection in chronic granulomatous disease. N Engl J Med 324:509, 1991. *Demonstrates the clinical benefits of reduced infection frequency when interferon gamma was administered to children with chronic granulomatous disease.*

Walsh T, Pizzo PA: Nosocomial fungal infections: A classification for hospital-acquired fungal infections and mycoses arising from endogenous flora or reactivation. Annu Rev Microbiol 42:517–545, 1988. *Reviews the major fungal pathogens that contribute to infectious complications in cancer patients and provides a system for their classification.*

288 Shock Syndromes Related to Sepsis

John N. Sheagren

Sepsis is defined as the presence of various pus-forming and other pathogenic organisms or their toxins in the blood or tissues. A presumptive diagnosis of sepsis is often made on the basis of historical, physical, and laboratory data even in the absence of proof. The most serious complications are produced when infection spreads from the original focus to the bloodstream. Bacteremia can produce two different types of complications: microbiologic and inflammatory. The microbiologic complications result from the local and systemic proliferation and seeding of the causative organism, which cause direct tissue or organ damage. The inflammatory complications are produced locally and can result in tissue or organ destruction independent of toxic factors produced by the causative organism. Bacteremia triggers intravascular activation of the same inflammatory systems that are protective within tissues but which, during severe sepsis, combine with stress-generated endocrine responses to produce a deleterious sequence of metabolic events. The end stage of these events is systemic vascular collapse, traditionally termed *septic shock*, and/or the constellation of symptoms referred to as the "multiple system organ failure" (MSOF) syndrome. The clinical definition of septic shock is a systolic blood pressure less than 90 mm Hg which has become unresponsive to adequate volume replacement.

Morbidity and mortality associated with septic shock are high: Approximately two thirds of such patients die, and the cause of death is usually progressive failure of one or more vital organs. Prevention of septic shock should be the primary goal. It is possible to recognize clinically the changes that occur in patients in the early stages of septic shock. Intervention at early stages can reduce morbidity and mortality.

INCIDENCE AND EPIDEMIOLOGY. Infections most commonly occur in the hospital setting. Many infected patients become bacteremic. It is estimated that of 100 randomly chosen patients who appear to be infected (septic) in a hospital setting, approximately 90 per cent actually are infected. Of these, about 20 per cent develop some evidence of hemodynamic instability and appear, at least temporarily, "shocky." About half of shocky patients (or about 10 per cent of all septic-appearing patients) go on to frank septic shock and/or manifest serious end-organ malfunction related to the septic episode (MSOF) such as adult respiratory distress syndrome (ARDS), renal failure, or disseminated intravascular coagulation (DIC). Since about 5 per cent of all hospital patients either are admitted with or develop an infection during hospitalization, the number of patients at risk of developing septic shock is large. The clinician must be familiar with the manifestations and differential diagnosis of the septic-appearing patient and have in mind rapid comprehensive diagnostic and therapeutic plans of action.

Shock Related to Gram-Negative as Opposed to Gram-Positive Organisms. Septic shock more commonly follows gram-negative than gram-positive septic episodes, and many textbooks refer to generic septic shock as gram-negative sepsis or endotoxic shock because endotoxin is found only in gram-negative bacterial cell walls. In patients who are bacteremic with gram-negative microbes, the incidence of metabolic complications and shock is high (about 25 per cent). However, about 10 per cent of patients with gram-positive bacteremia, especially those infected with *Staphylococcus aureus*, develop shock. The incidence of suppurative complications (metastatic seeding to bones, joints, viscera, and so on), on the other hand, is much higher with gram-positive microorganisms. Gram-positive bacteria have the capability of adhering to endothelial cells and subendothelial matrix substances (such as fibronectin, laminin, fibrinogen, and endothelial cell proteins) to a much greater degree than do gram-negative organisms, so that seeding to heart valves, to other organs, and especially to foci of trauma and/or pre-existing inflammation is much more common.

PATHOGENESIS. Sepsis can cause shock in many ways, either related to the primary focus of infection or to the systemic effects of bacteremia. These mechanisms of shock are listed in Table 288–1.

The classic *septic shock syndrome* results primarily from the sequence of events triggered by bacteremia during which cell wall bacterial substances (endotoxin in gram-negative organisms, the peptidoglycan/teichoic acid complex in gram-positive organisms, and polysaccharide substances in yeast cell walls) activate the monokine, complement, coagulation, kinin, and ACTH/endorphin systems. Endotoxin (and probably other toxic microbial cell wall substances) is the strongest stimulus known to produce tumor necrosis factor-α (also known as TNF-α and cachectin) (see

TABLE 288–1. MECHANISMS OF SHOCK CAUSED BY SEPSIS

1. Shock related to a localized primary focus of infection
   Hypovolemic shock: severe local infection may
   —cause sufficient local fluid accumulation to produce systemic hypovolemia.
   —produce severe diarrhea with gastrointestinal fluid loss.
   —erode into a local vessel with mycotic aneurysm formation and rupture.
   Cardiogenic shock: extension of a pericardiac infection (usually pneumonia) into the pericardium
   —may cause purulent pericarditis and tamponade.
   Toxigenic shock (the toxic shock syndrome): a toxin is produced locally, causing
   —endothelial cell damage with capillary leakage.
   —cardiodepression.
2. Shock related to bacteremic infections
   Cardiogenic shock: seeding of the organism through the bloodstream may cause
   —valvular malfunction (endocarditis).
   —myocarditis secondary to multiple metastatic myocardial abscesses.
   —purulent pericarditis (metastatic).
   Inflammatory-system–mediated shock: bacterial cell wall substances activate the complement, coagulation, kinin, and ACTH/endorphin systems and thus cause
   —vasodilation (roles of endorphins, kinins, and complement).
   —capillary leakage (primarily due to the intracapillary adherence and aggregation of activated polymorphonuclear leukocytes).
   —disseminated intravascular coagulation.
   —cardiodepression (encephalins, vasopressin, monokines, possibly other substances).

Ch. 286) by macrophages. TNF-α, in high enough concentration, impairs functioning of surrounding cells in multiple ways, and data are now firmly in hand to indicate that TNF-α plays a central role in mediating the toxic effects of endotoxin and other microbial products. All these mediators initiate a series of metabolic events that ultimately may progress to a state of shock.

Severe sepsis produces hemodynamic changes in two phases. Septic patients initially have hemodynamic changes primarily reflecting vasodilation. Systemic vascular resistance is decreased, pulse rate increases to compensate, and cardiac output is dramatically increased. Paradoxically, a state of cardiodepression exists during severe sepsis, and a circulating myocardial depressant factor (MDF) has recently been rediscovered. This MDF turns out probably to be TNF-α. Septic patients develop a fall in cardiac ejection fractions down to 20 to 25 per cent despite the markedly increased cardiac output.

As this hyperdynamic state develops, complement-mediated leukoagglutination combines with other inflammatory mediators (such as bradykinin, histamine, and the endorphins) to cause a severe capillary leak, intravascular volume decreases, blood pressure falls, and cardiac output now further declines. Several additional factors contribute to the decline in cardiac output: Peripheral resistance increases in late septic shock and other cardiodepressants participate such as vasopressin and encephalin. Individual organs may be damaged independently of the hypotensive events; for example, direct pulmonary damage by the activated leukocytes may result in ARDS, or the patient may develop renal malfunction. Presumably these end-organ manifestations are related to localized direct inflammatory damage. It is in this stage that DIC associated with severe hypoperfusion may occur, resulting in extremely high morbidity and mortality.

An important pathophysiologic concept in understanding the damage that occurs during bacteremia or fungemia is that of the syndrome of multiple system organ failure (MSOF). Septicemia is the most important of a number of precipitating causes. Other causes include severe trauma, burns, pancreatitis, and all other causes of shock. Once the syndrome of MSOF is triggered, by whatever cause, the patient becomes febrile and hypermetabolic, exhibits hyperactive hemodynamic measurements, and develops progressive failure of one or more organs. Mortality approaches 90 per cent despite all modern therapeutic measures.

Figure 288–1 outlines the sequence of early events initiated from the localized focus of infection. From these events are derived the various complications of bacteremia, which include metastatic abscess formation and the metabolic complications described earlier. Antibiotics limit metastatic abscess formation (the microbiologic complications of bacteremia). However, the other metabolic events, when initiated and independent of bacterial proliferation, still produce substantial morbidity and mortality. Therefore, therapy in addition to antibiotics is being sought to counter these deleterious metabolic sequelae.

The ACTH/Endorphin System. During systemic stress, increased ACTH release occurs. For each molecule of ACTH produced, a molecule of one of the endorphins or encephalins is also produced. The endorphins provide pain and anxiety relief during severe stress, but high levels of circulating endorphins may contribute to hypotension, changes in vascular permeability, and alterations in mentation.

Coagulation/Kinin System Activation. Bacterial endotoxins and other cell wall materials directly activate the coagulation system both by initiating platelet aggregation and by activating Hageman factor. Subsequently, kinin system activation (see Ch. 256) results in the production of bradykinin, a powerful vasodilator.

Complement System Activation. The complement system is also directly activated by high molecular weight bacterial and fungal polysaccharides, primarily by means of the alternative pathway. A sequence of intravascular events ensues, resulting in histamine release (contributing, to vasodilation), microvascular instability, and activation of circulating polymorphonuclear leukocytes (PMN's). The activated PMN has enhanced bactericidal capabilities but also an enhanced capability of damaging host tissues. The activated PMN possesses increased amounts of lysosomal enzymes and produces a variety of toxic metabolites of molecular oxygen, all of which are both bactericidal and cytocidal. Furthermore, the activated PMN produces both inflammatory prostaglandins and several products of the lipoxygenase system, many of which enhance inflammation by also producing vasodi-

lation, capillary leakage, chemotaxis, and PMN activation. The activated PMN's adhere to each other (the *leukopenic phase* of sepsis during which PMN aggregates form in capillaries) and to endothelial cells to cause severe damage and capillary leakage.

CLINICAL MANIFESTATIONS. The Septic Patient. The clinical situation in which a patient is considered septic (highly likely to be infected) is common. High fever and a chill strongly indicate that bacterial sepsis is occurring. In this setting, the physician must be alert for signs of septic shock. When a clinical diagnosis of septic shock can be made, the mortality rate is high. Therefore, it is important to develop the concept of a "preshock phase of septic shock" predicated on identifying a subgroup of infected patients more likely than others to develop shock. Treatment before shock develops undoubtedly prevents some of the morbidity and mortality associated with sepsis.

Table 288–2 lists several systemic signs and a variety of physical findings likely to be predictive of septic shock. Extremes of body temperature are often associated with shock. Specifically, fever in excess of 40.6° C and hypothermia associated with sepsis should be alerting signs that hypotension may soon follow. Also, in the febrile patient with a distinct change in mentation the mortality rate is higher. In association with such a finding, primary central nervous system infection may be present, and lumbar puncture is often indicated. Febrile patients who have hemodynamic instability (who are orthostatic with a blood pressure decrease of 30 mm Hg or greater) should be considered on the verge of septic shock.

While it is not possible to distinguish between simple dehydration and early septic shock solely on the basis of orthostatic blood pressure changes, hemodynamic monitoring shows an increase in peripheral vascular resistance in the former case and a reduction in the latter. Also, fluid challenge alone rapidly stabilizes the purely hypovolemic patient. Sepsis is associated in the early stages with a state of "warm shock" in which there is an orthostatic decrease in blood pressure but good perfusion in the extremities (they are warm and pink rather than cool and cyanotic). Tachypnea with hypoxemia or metabolic acidosis or both may be predictive of impending ARDS. The development of peripheral edema, often with a suddenly decreased serum albumin concentration, as in toxigenic shock (see Toxic Shock Syndrome in Ch. 300), may be caused by an unrecognized bacteremic event.

Laboratory Data Suggesting Bacteremia or Toxemia. Several laboratory tests are often helpful in the evaluation of a potentially septic patient (Table 288–2). The blood may show hypoxemia and a metabolic acidosis. Serum lactate elevation is highly predictive of deterioration leading to septic shock. Decreasing urine output, often associated with rising blood urea nitrogen and creatinine, may be seen early in sepsis as renal failure occurs. Serum albumin measurements may show decreases in excess of that calculated by catabolism alone. Often such patients show signs of progressive peripheral edema. In early sepsis, the total white count may be low, with most of the decrease in the PMN count, owing to complement-induced leukoaggregation. As white cells aggregate, platelets become caught up in the process. Thrombocytopenia is predictive of high risk of septic shock and ARDS.

In the future, assistance in clinical decision making may be provided by rapid laboratory measurements of the levels of

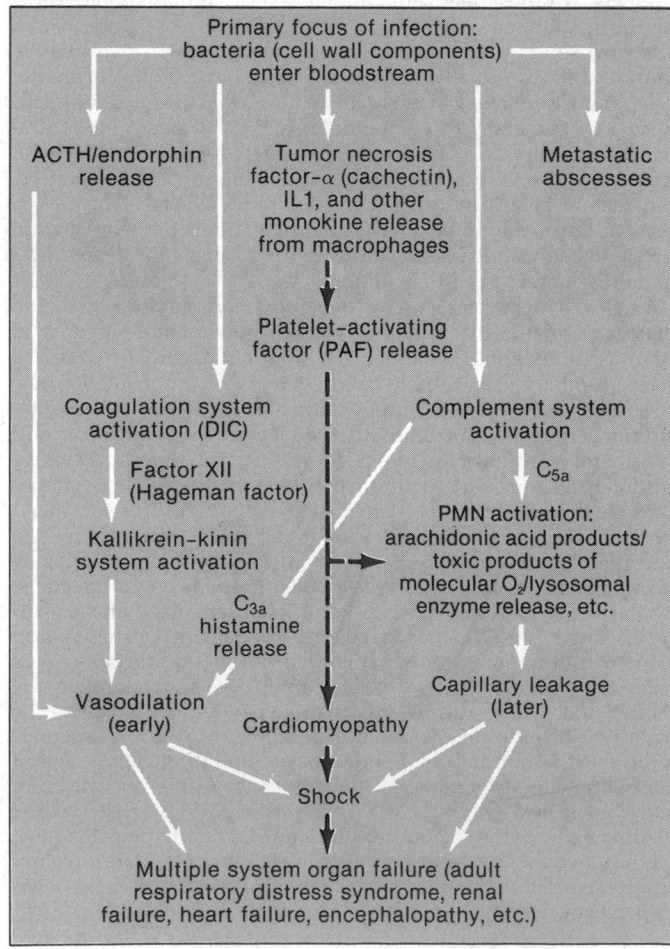

FIGURE 288–1. The complications of severe sepsis.

TABLE 288–2. PHYSICAL SIGNS AND LABORATORY DATA LIKELY TO BE PREDICTIVE OF THE DEVELOPMENT OF SEPTIC SHOCK

1. Extremes of body temperature (fever > 40.6°C or hypothermia)
2. Altered mental status
3. Orthostatic blood pressure decrease (>30 mm Hg) or sustained unexplained hypotension.
4. Decreasing urine output
5. Unexplained edema, usually associated with a falling serum albumin concentration
6. Tachypnea with hypoxemia and/or the development of a metabolic acidosis
7. Elevated serum lactate concentration
8. Development of leukopenia (predominantly neutropenia)
9. Development of thrombocytopenia with or without petechial skin rash
10. Unexplained end-organ failure (e.g., renal, hepatic)

activating bacterial products (e.g., endotoxin) and/or products of the mediator systems shown in Figure 288–1. For example, the rapid identification of an elevated level of TNF-α, a falling total complement level, and elevated levels of C5a, prostaglandins, or endorphins might predict subgroups of septic patients at higher risk of developing shock.

DIAGNOSIS. The presumptive diagnosis of sepsis must be made when the setting and attendant clinical signs are suggestive. In general, patients with fever should be considered septic until proven otherwise. Therapy should always be initiated for high-risk febrile patients in advance of microbiologic confirmation of sepsis.

Evaluation of the Septic Patient. The setting in which the episode is occurring should be evaluated promptly. Crucial to appropriate initial decision making are the background history, which may help to define the type of host defense defect present, and prior cultural data, which might predict the infecting organism. The physical examination should be directed at quickly but thoroughly searching for the septic source as well as signs of end-organ failure that might indicate progression to shock such as altered mental status, progressive edema, hypotension, and so on (Table 288–2). All potentially infected foci should be appropriately sampled, and the material obtained should be Gram-stained and cultured.

Differential Diagnosis of Severe Sepsis. Having done a thorough preliminary evaluation and initiated therapy (see below), one can reassess the clinical situation on subsequent days and stop antibiotic therapy if the episode later turns out not to be infectious. Many nonseptic events can cause high fever with or without hemodynamic instability. For example, a variety of hypersensitivity reactions (often caused by drugs) may mimic sepsis. Vasculitic disease may present with high fever, unstable blood pressure, and altered mentation. Pulmonary emboli occur frequently in the hospital setting, and especially if the patient develops fever, the embolic event initially may be confused with sepsis. Myocardial infarction may result in hemodynamic instability, and in the subset of patients who develop higher than average fever may lead to initial confusion with sepsis.

There are infectious syndromes against which antimicrobials are of no use and in which bacterial sepsis may be suspected. For example, viral syndromes such as those caused by influenza viruses, enteroviruses, adenoviruses, cytomegalovirus, and hepatitis viruses may all produce high fever and be difficult to diagnose. Malaria can be difficult to identify unless the parasite is detected on the peripheral blood smear.

TREATMENT. Possible therapeutic modalities for the septic patient are outlined in Figure 288–2.

Antibacterial Therapy. Broad coverage is required in patients with severe sepsis. It is best to initiate therapy with a combination of antibiotics when the infecting organism is unknown. An aminoglycoside should always be used, and gentamicin remains the aminoglycoside of choice unless other considerations (such as abnormal renal function and known microbial resistance) dictate the use of tobramycin or amikacin. In the granulocytopenic patient, the aminoglycoside should be combined with high doses of piperacillin. In the patient likely to have an anaerobic focus of infection in which *Bacteroides fragilis* is likely to be present, such as an intra-abdominal or gynecologic infection, or decubitus and lower extremity vascular and neuropathic ulcers, clindamycin or cefotetan or cefoxitin is combined with gentamicin. For all other patients, gentamicin plus cefazolin or ceftriaxone is the combination of choice. If β-lactam antibiotic–resistant (methicillin-resistant) staphylococci are possible, then vancomycin must be added to the above combinations. When cultures define the causative microbe(s) or other data point to a specific organism, therapy can be tailored to the most appropriate, most specific, least toxic, and least expensive single antibiotic.

Antishock Therapy. The most important component of the therapy of shock associated with sepsis is volume replacement. Sufficient quantities of an appropriate solute (or, where indicated, a colloid such as albumin or whole blood) should be administered in an attempt to provide adequate volume support. Evidence is accumulating, especially in the surgical literature, that colloid-containing solutions are more efficacious than solute solutions once capillary leakage has developed or after approximately 4 liters of a solute have been administered. Hemodynamic monitoring is mandatory and is preferably carried out in the intensive

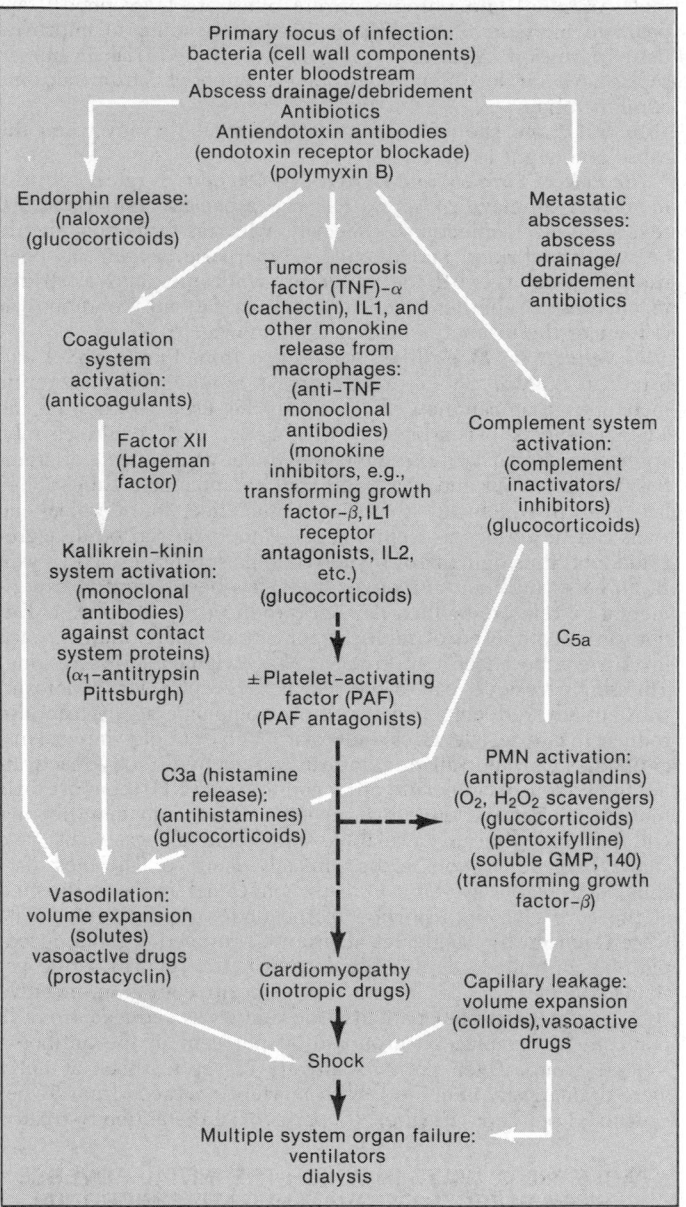

FIGURE 288–2. Therapy for the complications of severe sepsis. Theoretically efficacious but unproven or ineffective therapeutic modalities are in parentheses.

care unit (see Ch. 71). Fluid administration should be just sufficient to bring the pulmonary capillary wedge pressure to the high normal range.

Recently two multicenter studies prospectively compared high doses of methylprednisolone sodium succinate (MPSS) with placebo in a blinded protocol in over 600 severely septic patients. Glucocorticoids were administered within 4 hours of recognition of the septic event. Both studies showed *no* efficacy of MPSS and one study showed *increased* mortality in patients who have mild degrees of renal malfunction (creatinines of 2 mg per deciliter or greater) or who have developed ARDS. Thus, glucocorticoid therapy has no proven role in the treatment of human sepsis.

The use of other anti-inflammatory drugs such as the antiprostaglandins is under active investigation. These agents may selectively suppress inflammatory damage caused by the activated PMN without interfering with the antibacterial capabilities of these important host defense cells.

Some clinicians have tried to use naloxone in severe sepsis on the basis of the contribution of the endorphin system to hemodynamic instability in experimental models of septic shock.

However, in primate models naloxone, like α-agonists (metaraminol [Aramine] and norepinephrine bitartrate [Levophed]), appears to increase blood pressure without leading to improved tissue perfusion. Also, data from small controlled trials in human sepsis have not documented any long-term benefits from naloxone administration.

In DIC, one should not use anticoagulant therapy when the cause is thought to be sepsis.

The Role of Surgery and Hyperbaric Oxygen. Surgical debridement and drainage of septic foci are especially important. All severe localized infections, especially with gas formation, should be widely debrided and drained. Hyperbaric oxygen has been used in patients with the gangrene syndromes and clostridial myonecrosis. Whether or not it stabilizes patients' conditions or influences the ultimate outcome is unknown.

Antiendotoxin Modalities. As derived from Figure 288–1 and listed in Figure 288–2, there are a number of therapeutic modalities that can now theoretically be used to counter the adverse effects of endotoxin. Ultimately, each could also be applied in similar fashion to counter the adverse effects of gram-positive microbial and yeast cell wall components. Table 288–3 lists ways in which the adverse systemic effects of microbial cell walls can be reduced or eliminated. Endotoxin can be disaggregated, and thus detoxified, by polycationic substances. Polymyxin B, an early antibiotic no longer used, has been found in experimental systems to reduce damage produced by endotoxin. Endotoxin is composed of multiple repeating small subunits, each in turn composed of a substituted N-acetylglucosamine residue. The single residue can block the cell receptor for endotoxin, substantially reducing toxicity. Immunobiologic agents can also reduce the toxic effects of endotoxin. For example, monoclonal antibodies can neutralize endotoxin, either by directly inactivating the endotoxin molecule or by countering TNF, the most toxic biologic mediator of endotoxin toxicity. Antiendotoxin antibodies will soon be clinically available, and recent clinical trials have shown two preparations to be clinically effective. The most data thus far available are on a human monoclonal antibody directed at the core glycolipid portion of the endotoxin molecule. Data were reported by Ziegler et al. from a prospective randomized, placebo-controlled, double-blind clinical trial of 543 septic patients, 200 of whom had blood cultures positive for gram-negative bacteria. In those 200 patients, mortality was reduced from 49 per cent in the placebo group to 30 per cent in the antibody-treated group. Even patients already in septic shock at entry were dramatically benefited, with mortality reduced from 57 per cent to 33 per cent. Further, 51 per cent of the antibody-treated

patients survived to be discharged from the hospital, compared with only 29 per cent of the placebo-treated group. Another product, a mouse monoclonal preparation, has also shown efficacy in a randomized, double-blind clinical trial reported in abstract form; mortality in patients with gram-negative sepsis was reduced if the patient was not yet in septic shock. Thus, when released for clinical use (possibly by the time of publication of this text), a dose of one or another of these preparations will be indicated at the point where initial stabilization measures have failed in the course of severely septic patients who are at high risk of being infected with gram-negative microbes.

Finally, as noted above, there may be a therapeutic benefit in neutralizing or in other ways countering the effects of TNF and/or other monokines (especially IL1). A monoclonal antibody preparation that neutralizes TNF can increase survival in animal models of septic shock. There are also a number of biologic antagonists of TNF, such as transforming growth factor-β, IL2, and an IL1 receptor antagonist (see Table 288–3) that could prove useful. Inhibiting any or all of the other mediators generated by the septic event is being explored. For example, the kallikrein-kinin system may play a very important role, and new ways of inhibiting contact system proteins or in other ways impairing bradykinin generation may become clinically feasible (Fig. 288–2).

PROGNOSIS. Most febrile patients lacking other signs of severe sepsis (as described in Table 288–2) will usually do well even when bacteremic. Such patients usually respond quickly to fluid administration, antibacterial therapy, and drainage of the primary focus of infection. However, the presence of shock and/or progressive dysfunction in any organ system dramatically increases morbidity and mortality. Even when the inciting infection is localized, shock (with the exception of the toxic shock syndrome) is associated with a 30 to 50 per cent mortality. Full-blown, bacteremia-associated septic shock has greater than a 50 per cent mortality. A favorable outcome in a patient in frank shock depends on the skill of management in the intensive care unit. Early diagnosis and therapy of severely septic patients decrease morbidity and mortality.

PREVENTION. Prevention of infection, especially in the hospital, is the key to reducing morbidity and mortality associated with septic shock. Strict adherence to the hospital infection control program with avoidance of Foley catheters and meticulous attention to the placement and maintenance of intravascular lines dramatically reduces the incidence of bacteremic infections. The concept of the preshock approach to the therapy of septic shock is useful; in all such patients fluids should be administered and broad antibiotic coverage started early. Controlled studies of anti-inflammatory therapy in severe sepsis are under way, and better guidelines should be forthcoming.

Abraham E, Shoemaker WC, Bland RD, et al.: Sequential cardiorespiratory patterns in septic shock. Crit Care Med 11:799, 1983. *Describes the hemodynamic patterns occurring in patients as they develop septic shock.*

Beutler B: The tumor necrosis factors: Cachectin and lymphotoxin. Hosp Pract 25:45, 1990. *Describes roles of cachectin (TNF-α) and lymphotoxin (TNF-β) in tissue damage during infection.*

Beutler B, Cerami A: Cachectin: More than a tumor necrosis factor. N Engl J Med 316:379, 1987. *Excellent review of the role of cachectin in inflammation, sepsis, and septic shock.*

Bone RC, Fisher CJ, Clemmer TP, et al.: Sepsis syndrome: A valid clinical entity. Crit Care Med 17:389, 1989. *Describes clinical criteria for prospectively identifying a patient population at risk of severe septic complications.*

Cerami A, Beutler B: The role of cachectin/TNF in endotoxic shock and cachexia. Immunol Today 9:28–31, 1989. *Reviews history, structure, mechanism of production and biologic effects of TNF.*

Parillo JE, Parker MM, Natanson C, et al.: Septic shock in humans: Advances in the understanding of pathogenesis, cardiovascular dysfunction and therapy. Ann Intern Med 113:227, 1990. *An excellent review of cardiovascular patterns, pathogenesis, and therapy of septic shock.*

Sibbald WJ, Sprung CL: New Horizons—Perspectives on Sepsis and Septic Shock. Fullerton, CA, Society of Critical Care Medicine, 1986. *A complete review of all basic and clinical aspects of the sepsis and multiple organ system failure syndromes.*

Tracey KJ, Beutler B, Lowry SF, et al.: Shock and tissue injury induced by recombinant human cachectin. Science 234:470, 1986. *Cachectin (tumor necrosis factor) is capable of producing most of the deleterious effects of endotoxin.*

Zeigler EJ, Fisher CJ, Sprung CL, et al.: Treatment of Gram-negative bacteremia and septic shock with HA-1A human monoclonal antibody against endotoxin. N Engl J Med 324:429, 1991. *Conclusively demonstrates that a human monoclonal IgM antibody that binds to the lipid A domain of endotoxin is safe and effective treatment of patients with severe sepsis caused by gram-negative bacteria.*

TABLE 288–3. WAYS IN WHICH THE INITIAL ADVERSE SYSTEM EFFECTS OF GRAM-NEGATIVE MICROBIAL CELL WALLS CAN BE REDUCED OR ELIMINATED

1. **Endotoxin "dissolution":** By administering polymyxin B (a polycationic antibiotic) or other detergents; probably causes disaggregation of the organized complexes or endotoxin, reducing toxicity.

2. **Endotoxin receptor blockade:** Small subunits of disaggregated endotoxin bind to endotoxin receptors on macrophages and, while not causing toxicity themselves, block toxic monokine (TNF-α, IL1, etc.) release.

3. **Antiendotoxin antibodies:** Antibodies can be directed either (1) against the "core endotoxin" moiety, resulting in "detoxification," or (2) against the antigenic polysaccharide side chains ("O-antigens"), resulting in enhanced opsonization and/or antibody-mediated killing of the bacterium.

4. **Monokine neutralization:** Specific monoclonal antibodies directed against TNF-α decrease the systemic effects either of purified endotoxin or of live, whole microbes.

5. **Monokine antagonists:** The effects of TNF-α are inhibited by transforming growth factor-β and IL2. IL1 synergizes with TNF-α, and an inhibitor of IL1 (known as IL1 receptor antagonist) ameliorates the effects of bacteremia. Many other biologic inhibitors of the monokines undoubtedly exist.

6. **Platelet-activating factor (PAF) antagonists:** In some experimental systems, PAF seems to play an important role in the damage produced by monokines. Thus, PAF antagonists may play potential therapeutic roles.

289 Prevention and Control of Hospital-Acquired Infections

William Schaffner

HISTORY. Hospitals are viewed today as institutions where scientific advances are used to provide the most up-to-date diagnostic and therapeutic services for patients. This optimistic view is tempered, however, by the realization that the hospital also can be a dangerous place for patients. The application of technology is not without hazards, and among these hospital-acquired infection has the longest history. When hospitals first were established in Europe during the Middle Ages, they were primarily places where the gravely ill were taken to die. Because facilities were primitive, infections that prompted the admission of some patients were readily spread to others. Hospital typhus and typhoid were commonplace, for example, and hospitals acquired the reputation of pest houses.

These circumstances remained basically unchanged until the mid-nineteenth century, when a Hungarian physician, Ignaz P. Semmelweis, was appointed to direct the obstetric service of the prestigious Allgemeines Krankenhaus (General Hospital) in Vienna. Semmelweis encountered a puzzling situation concerning the hospital's two obstetric wards. They were ostensibly similar and admitted patients on alternate days. Yet the mortality rates on the two wards were strikingly different. Semmelweis performed a seemingly elementary exercise but one that was unique in his time. He tabulated the monthly mortality rates on the two wards and documented that on Ward I the rates regularly were 8 to 10 per cent or even higher, whereas on Ward II they rarely rose above 2 per cent. The cause of this extraordinary mortality was puerperal sepsis (childbed fever), a rapidly fatal septic illness. Semmelweis worked before the formulation of the germ theory of disease, but we now know puerperal sepsis to be caused by the group A β-hemolytic streptococcus. He systematically examined a series of hypotheses attempting to explain the disparate mortality rates, but none proved valid. Among the more far-fetched notions was that the disease was psychosomatic and that intense anxiety was provoked when monks made their rounds, tolling hand-bells in mourning for those recently dead. Semmelweis persuaded the monks not to ring the bells and, of course, the occurrence of puerperal sepsis continued unaffected.

At that point a pathologist cut his finger while performing an autopsy of a woman who had died of puerperal sepsis. He soon developed a fatal illness with a clinical course that was entirely similar to puerperal sepsis. Because the pathologist had been inoculated with trace amounts of material during the autopsy, Semmelweis drew an insightful analogy: Perhaps the obstetric patients also were being inoculated with infectious material. It was then that a seemingly trivial difference between the two obstetric wards became important. The deliveries on the low-mortality ward were performed by midwives; on the high-risk ward they were performed by medical students and physicians. Furthermore, the autopsy room was directly adjacent to the ward and Semmelweis deduced that the unwashed contaminated hands of students and physicians going from autopsies to the delivery room were the vehicles for transmitting infection to patients. Despite protestations from the medical staff, Semmelweis then insisted upon hand washing after autopsies and before the examination of each patient. The mortality rate on Ward I promptly fell to levels even lower than those on the other ward.

Semmelweis is honored as the originator of hospital infection control efforts. His process of systematically gathering data, performing an analysis, and instituting control measures still is followed today. Furthermore, his emphasis on the hands of caregivers as the means for carrying pathogens from patient to patient remains valid. Unfortunately, as in the last century, contemporary physicians still require constant reminders to wash their hands during their patient care duties.

After the acceptance of the germ theory of disease, rapid advances in microbiology, disinfection, and aseptic technique around the turn of the century substantially enhanced the safety of patient care in hospitals. Starting in the 1930's, the introduction of antimicrobials made possible the development of progressively more elaborate surgery. However, predictions that hospital infections soon would become inconsequential have not come true. Rather, the types of hospital infection have changed in response to advancing medical science.

Most recently, the 1950's and 1960's witnessed a global pandemic of hospital infections caused by *Staphylococcus aureus*. Previously very susceptible to penicillin, the new penicillin-resistant epidemic strain (phage type 80/81) became the scourge of hospitals worldwide. It stimulated research into all aspects of hospital-acquired infection and persuaded authorities that every hospital should have a formal infection control program. For reasons that still are not clear, the staphylococcal pandemic waned in the 1970's and gram-negative bacilli, often antibiotic-resistant, became the dominant nosocomial pathogens. In the 1980's there again was a shift; staphylococci returned (now methicillin-resistant), enterococci rose in importance, and *Candida* and other yeast infections caused a larger proportion of nosocomial infections in seriously ill patients. Predictions for the 1990's suggest that antibiotic-resistant organisms of all kinds will assume even greater importance in hospitals. Thus, it seems that there will be no infection-free utopia; each era presents infection control challenges anew as yesterday's saprophyte becomes tomorrow's pathogen.

INTRODUCTION. Infections that are acquired during hospitalization and are neither present nor incubating at the time of hospitalization are defined as *nosocomial** infections. The occurrence of a nosocomial infection does not per se indicate that the hospital or its personnel were at fault or committed an error in caring for the patient. Current preventive measures still cannot prevent many nosocomial infections. Medicolegal liability regarding a nosocomial infection occurs when it can be demonstrated that physicians or hospital personnel have been negligent in not adhering to appropriate standards of care and that an infection resulted from the failure to perform consistent with the standard.

It is estimated that five to eight nosocomial infections occur for every 100 admissions to acute-care hospitals in the United States, resulting in 2 to 4 million such infections annually. Some nosocomial infections are more serious than others, but taken together they are estimated to require over 6 million days of excess hospital stay a year and contribute to the deaths of a substantial number of patients (Table 289-1).

Most studies of nosocomial infections have been performed in the high-technology hospitals of the developed countries. Although less attention has been given to delineating nosocomial infections in developing countries, it is clear that they are an important problem there as well. Hospital outbreaks of measles and shigellosis as well as infections related to a lack of disinfectants and other supplies occur regularly. Because developing countries have only modest resources, it is especially unfortunate that their efforts to provide medical care are so often thwarted by nosocomial infections. The World Health Organization recently has acknowledged that nosocomial infections are a substantial international public health issue.

PREDISPOSING FACTORS. All patients do not have an equal risk of developing a nosocomial infection. The inherent resistance of the patient to infection is probably the most important determinant of risk. The extremes of age, poor nutritional status, the severity of underlying diseases, and breaks in the integrity of the skin and mucous membranes all increase a patient's risk of nosocomial infection.

The second strong influence on risk of nosocomial infection is the array of diagnostic and therapeutic manipulations undertaken for the patient's benefit. Every invasive procedure carries some risk of infection because it violates either a cutaneous or mucosal barrier to microbial invasion. The risk varies with the degree of invasiveness. For example, an intramuscular injection usually has virtually no risk of infection, whereas 15 to 20 per cent of colorectal operations are complicated by wound infections despite meticulous surgical technique, preoperative bowel preparation, and appropriate antibiotic prophylaxis. Thus, physicians should

---

Nosocomial has a derivation from the Greek word for hospital or infirmary.

subject every invasive procedure to an assessment of potential benefits weighed against potential risks. Medical therapy also can make patients extremely susceptible to nosocomial infections. Cancer chemotherapy eliminates virtually all of a patient's circulating neutrophils, and the immunosuppressive regimens used in organ transplantation ablate the normal immune response to invading microorganisms (see Ch. 287). Infection control measures are designed to protect the patient until periods of such exquisite vulnerability have passed and the patient again has normal or nearly normal phagocytic and immune functions. In addition, the antibiotics used to combat infection can be considered a two-edged sword. Although their use does not generally confer an increased risk of complicating infection, when new infections occur in the face of antibiotic therapy, the pathogens often are resistant to the antibiotics being used (so-called suprainfections). Lastly, it follows that the longer a patient remains in the hospital, the more likely it is that a nosocomial infection will occur.

MODES OF TRANSMISSION. Nosocomial pathogens can be found in both the animate and inanimate environment of the hospital. It is not generally appreciated how clean the hospital's inanimate environment has become. The furniture, bedclothes, curtains, and other inanimate surfaces in the hospital only very rarely harbor microorganisms that cause infections in patients. Nevertheless, reservoirs of nosocomial pathogens still can be established in inanimate areas of the hospital occasionally, especially in specialty care areas. For example, if the countertop in the intensive care unit where urine specific gravity determinations are performed remains wet, it may harbor multiresistant gram-negative bacilli. Nurses' hands then become contaminated and the organisms can be carried back to patients in the unit. Although similar infection hazards in the inanimate environment are detected periodically and need to be remedied, we cannot look to enhanced housekeeping of the general hospital environment to reduce nosocomial infection rates further.

Whereas the hospital's general inanimate environment has receded as a source of nosocomial infections, the role of contaminated medical devices has increased substantially; over 100,000 device-related infections are estimated to occur each year. Medical devices are examples of imaginative medical technology that offer new benefits to patients. However, manufacturers often do not consider the potential infection risks of new devices fully and physicians often employ devices in ways that were not initially anticipated. For example, when intravascular pressure transducers first were introduced, their use was associated with outbreaks of bacteremia. Investigations revealed that instruments were being inadequately disinfected because the instruments were very fragile. When appropriate disinfection protocols were developed, this new infection risk associated with technologic innovation was virtually eliminated.

The animate hospital environment consists of the patients and their caregivers. These humans are the sources of most nosocomial pathogens, and the intimacies of patient care often result in their sharing their microbial flora.

A familiar scenario involves *Staphylococcus aureus*, a classic hospital pathogen. Hospital personnel have a higher rate of asymptomatic carriage of *S. aureus* (often over 30 per cent) than does the general population. Staphylococci may be transmitted from hospital workers to patients, where they later can produce, for example, postoperative wound infections. Such "hospital staph" often are more antibiotic-resistant than community-acquired *S. aureus*, providing a distinctive marker that enables their movement to be readily traced. However, hospital personnel are not the only source of resistant microbial flora. Recent

investigations have demonstrated that on admission to the hospital, some patients already may be colonized with small numbers of resistant bacterial strains. After antibiotic treatment, these resistant strains have a survival advantage and multiply to emerge as potential causes of nosocomial infection. Indeed, the endogenous flora is the major source of both the bacterial and viral pathogens that cause nosocomial infections in patients who receive organ transplants and are immunosuppressed for long periods.

Over 100 years have passed since Semmelweis implicated the hands of the students and physicians as the means of spreading pathogens to patients. Nevertheless, such direct contact continues to be the most common way patients are colonized with microorganisms of exogenous origin. At times the microorganisms may be from the caregiver's own flora. Usually, however, the hands of nurses or doctors are contaminated transiently while caring for one patient, and the pathogens then are carried over to the next patient (this process is aptly called "cross-infection" in Britain). Gram-positive skin flora (*S. aureus* and *S. epidermidis*), many gram-negative bacilli (*Enterobacter* and *Serratia*, for example), and even viruses (respiratory syncytial virus, rotavirus) are spread by this means. Over a century ago Semmelweis introduced the most effective way to interrupt transmission by contaminated hands: hand washing. In order to promote hand washing after every patient contact, modern hospitals have located sinks conveniently and have provided disinfectant soap wherever patient examinations and manipulations take place, with special attention to intensive care areas, treatment rooms, and the like. However, persuading medical staff, especially physicians, to routinely wash their hands remains a challenge, especially in the hectic environment of the intensive care unit.

Airborne transmission once was thought to have an important role in the spread of pathogens in the hospital. Today this seems not to be the case, although occasional explosive outbreaks of tuberculosis and chickenpox strongly suggest airborne transmission from a source patient. *Aspergillus* infections have occurred in immunosuppressed patients whose rooms drew air from the vicinity of major construction sites in or adjacent to the hospital. Likewise *Legionella* infections have been produced by the contaminated water spray from an air conditioning cooling tower. Concern about the role of airborne infection in the operating room continues to influence the design and construction of these areas. Most studies indicate that the bacteria causing wound infections originate from the resident flora of either the patients themselves or the operating team. This suggests that transmission likely occurs by direct contact or droplet spread. Nevertheless, because only a few bacteria can incite infection in certain elaborate procedures that implant foreign bodies (such as total joint replacements), such procedures are performed in laminar air flow facilities where the air stream is designed to flow away from the operative field.

ANTIMICROBIAL RESISTANCE. Since the pandemic of the 1950's and 1960's caused by staphylococcal strains newly resistant to penicillin, it has become axiomatic that antibiotic resistance has been a major feature of nosocomial infections. Although antibiotic-resistant bacteria are not inherently more virulent than their susceptible counterparts, they reduce the physician's therapeutic options and often require the use of more expensive antibiotics.

Currently, both gram-positive and gram-negative hospital pathogens have developed patterns of antimicrobial resistance. *S. aureus* infections are resurgent, and many strains now have developed resistance to methicillin and other similar β-lactam antibiotics that have been mainstays of therapy until recently. Many physicians turned to the quinoline antibiotics as alternate therapy, but quinoline-resistant strains were recovered with

TABLE 289–1. IMPACT OF HOSPITAL-ACQUIRED INFECTIONS IN ACUTE CARE HOSPITALS

Anatomic Site	Number of Infections per 100 Admissions	Proportion of All Hospital-Acquired Infections	Estimated Direct Mortality	Estimated Number of Excess Hospital Days per Infection	Proportion of All Excess Hospital Days
Urinary tract	2.5	30–40%	<1%	2	19%
Postoperative wound	1.5	20–25%	1–2%	7	33%
Pulmonary	1	10–20%	5–10%	8	21%
Bloodstream	0.5–1	5–15%	25%	14	16%
Others	1	20–25%	Varies with site	2	12%

extraordinary rapidity in hospitals where these drugs were used widely. *S. epidermidis* has become a notable nosocomial pathogen in some intensive care units; these organisms have a very diverse pattern of antibiotic resistance. Likewise, gram-negative bacilli have developed distinctive resistance profiles in some hospitals; *Enterobacter cloacae, Pseudomonas aeruginosa,* and *Acinetobacter calcoaceticus* particularly have been involved. It has become clear that genes determining antibiotic resistance are often carried on extrachromosomal plasmids that can be transferred among bacterial species. Thus, some medical centers have been subjected to outbreaks of resistant gram-negative bacillary infections that have extended over years. The distinctive antibiotic resistance pattern first was detected in one bacterial species (among *Serratia,* for example) and then over time also was found among other gram-negative nosocomial pathogens (among *Enterobacter* and *Klebsiella* sequentially). Investigations that combine studies of infections in hospital populations with molecular biologic studies of the pathogens have been called "molecular epidemiology."

During the early 1950's bacterial pathogens isolated from infections virtually anywhere in the United States had essentially identical antibiotic susceptibility patterns. Shortly after antimicrobial resistance was recognized, however, it became apparent that different hospitals began to develop antibiotic resistance patterns among their hospital pathogens that were distinctive and different from each other. Thus, one hospital might have a problem with multiresistant *Serratia,* whereas another hospital directly across the street might encounter almost no such isolates. Although never precisely explained, these differences have been attributed to differences in patient populations, severity of illness, length of stay, and, most importantly, patterns and intensity of antibiotic use. Physicians needed to be aware of these differences, so clinical microbiology laboratories maintained surveillance of resistance patterns and reported them periodically to the medical staff. The more sophisticated surveillance systems were able to distinguish resistance patterns between community-acquired and hospital-acquired infections. Just recently it has become clear that such hospital-wide surveillance is insufficient in large, complex medical centers. Rather than a uniform hospital-wide nosocomial flora, there are a number of independent subpatterns that are specific to each special care area. Thus, the burn unit, neonatal intensive care unit (NICU), and surgical intensive care unit each may have a distinctive nosocomial flora, each with its own localized resistance problem. Laboratories have started to adapt their computerized data management systems so that specialty unit–specific surveillance data can be provided to the physicians who practice in each unit.

COMMON NOSOCOMIAL INFECTIONS, BY ANATOMIC SITE (see Table 289–1)

URINARY TRACT INFECTIONS. Urinary tract infections continue to be the most common nosocomial infection, accounting for 30 to 40 per cent of all hospital-acquired infections. They occur so frequently because almost all are linked to prior urinary tract instrumentation, most often with the seemingly innocuous bladder catheter. Even single in-and-out catheterization is associated with 2 to 3 per cent bacteriuria in otherwise healthy persons. The urethral meatus is colonized with bacteria and even after appropriate cleansing, some are inoculated into the bladder during the catheterization process. The healthy bladder almost always rids itself of small numbers of introduced bacteria. If the bladder and urethra are traumatized, however, an infection is more likely to be established. After complicated labor with its associated urethral and bladder trauma, 23 per cent of postpartum women develop a urinary tract infection after only a single catheterization.

Given these risks, the use of indwelling Foley catheters is preferred, and 10 to 20 per cent of hospitalized patients are treated with these devices. Because of their frequent use, Foley catheters are the leading factor predisposing to nosocomial urinary tract infections. The longer the catheter is in place, the more likely it is that an infection will occur; approximately 5 per cent of patients with a catheter develop bacteriuria per day. The infecting strains colonize the urethral meatus. Through movement of the catheter as well as their own motility they gain entrance to the bladder. Contemporary urinary drainage systems are well designed so that ascending infection from the reservoir bag now is quite uncommon.

Most nosocomial urinary tract infections are asymptomatic or mild, clear with little or no therapy after catheter removal, and do not prolong hospital stay very much (an average of 1 to 2 days only). They are important, however, for two reasons. They are occasionally severe, and 1 of every 200 nosocomial urinary tract infections results in bacteremia. In addition, many nosocomial urinary tract infections are caused by antibiotic-resistant bacterial strains. Thus, the infected catheter systems become reservoirs of resistant gram-negative bacilli, especially in intensive care units where they can be spread easily to other very ill patients. The most common organisms producing nosocomial urinary tract infections include *E. coli* (30 per cent), enterococci (16 per cent), *Pseudomonas* (12 per cent), and *Klebsiella* (6 per cent). Pseudomonas and other multiresistant gram-negative bacteria account for a gradually increasing proportion of these infections as the hospitalized population becomes older, is more severely ill, and receives more intensive antibiotic treatment.

The prevention of nosocomial urinary tract infections has received sustained attention and considerable success. Of course, assuring that catheters are used only for patients who genuinely require continuous bladder drainage is the first guiding principle. It follows that catheters should be removed as soon as possible when patients no longer need them. Industry has been very responsive by producing reliable, sturdy, closed drainage systems. In the past, catheters were disconnected from drainage bags to empty the bags, obtain diagnostic urine specimens, and the like. Every such interruption was an opportunity to introduce bacteria into the catheter system. Contemporary designs facilitate maintenance of the system's integrity by allowing the catheter to be aspirated with a needle and syringe.

These systems work so well that catheters need not be changed routinely, nor is catheter irrigation required unless the catheter becomes obstructed. The use of triple-lumen catheters with a closed prophylactic antibiotic irrigation system has been proposed, but these systems offer no great advantage in preventing infection and are difficult to manage by ward nurses. They may be useful in some patients after urologic surgery in order to prevent obstruction by blood clots and proteinaceous debris. There is no need to culture the urine routinely at the time of catheter removal; the practice of cutting off the catheter tip and culturing it has no value.

Regular perineal hygiene and antibiotic-containing creams have not proven to be of value in reducing infection. Likewise, catheters impregnated with a variety of antibacterial materials have offered no substantial advantage. The use of prophylactic systemic antibiotics to "cover" an indwelling catheter has been decried for 30 years, yet some data suggest they may be efficacious for the first 4 days of catheterization. A serious prospective trial has not been undertaken, perhaps because of the fear of selecting antibiotic-resistant strains.

BACTEREMIA. If urinary tract infections are the most frequent nosocomial infections, nosocomial bacteremias are the most serious. Bacteremias may be secondary to recognized infection at some site, or they may be primary and cannot be attributed to an obvious infection in another anatomic location. Identifying the source of a secondary bacteremia permits one to treat it as well as the bacteremia and prevent recurrences.

The occurrence of a primary bacteremia should always prompt a thorough review of all the patient's intravenous infusions as well as other intravascular devices, as they are frequent sources of bloodstream infections. More than 25 per cent of hospitalized patients receive intravenous fluids. Other diagnostic and therapeutic procedures require access to the venous or arterial systems for either brief or prolonged periods. An intravenous pyelogram and cardiac catheterization are examples of abbreviated procedures, whereas intra-arterial pressure monitoring may continue for days. Although all these procedures create an access for bacteria to enter the bloodstream, they are remarkably safe. Nevertheless, the history of intravascular technology is punctuated with many studies of endemic and epidemic bloodstream infections. The procedures that offer an assurance of reasonable safety today were hard won, and any lapse in appropriate care can result in a device-related bacteremia. As more patients have required admission to intensive care units, the rate of nosocomial bacteremia has gradually risen during the 1980's.

Intrinsic contamination of intravenous fluid by the manufacturer is fortunately a rare event. Most episodes of infusion-related sepsis are caused by microorganisms that enter the system during its use (extrinsic contamination). The major locus of contamination is the cannulation site. The longer the catheter is left in place, the more likely it is that infection will occur. The catheter site may be purulent and phlebitis may be evident, but these overt clinical manifestations frequently are not present. Suppurative thrombophlebitis is an unusual event in which a substantial segment of vein becomes a linear abscess, the entire lumen being filled with pus. *S. aureus* and *S. epidermidis* are the most frequently isolated pathogens, but an array of gram-negative bacilli and *Candida* species also regularly are associated with catheter sepsis.

Any indwelling vascular access device can be associated with infection. Hickman-Broviac catheters that are tunneled under the skin of the anterior chest wall before they enter the subclavian vein were developed to provide long-term vascular access (as for cancer chemotherapy) and minimize the risk of infection. They have been largely successful. When infection does occur, it often is possible to treat the infection, leaving the catheter in place. Although such catheters have an enhanced risk for developing another infection, enough time is often gained to complete a course of chemotherapy.

The essentials of prevention begin with meticulous aseptic catheter insertion technique. Because the risk of infection increases with increasing duration of use, strict nursing protocols exist to ensure that all catheters are discontinued on a regular rotation and that new catheters are inserted at different sites. As a reminder, the dressings at the insertion site are dated; peripheral catheters should be left in place no longer than 72 hours unless there is no alternative. If a catheter must remain in place, a note providing the reasons should be written in the chart. Likewise, the infusions themselves also must be changed regularly; infusions should hang no longer than 24 hours. Because most infections originate at the insertion site, in-line filters have not reduced infection rates; they add expense without increasing safety. The catheter insertion site is protected by a single dressing for the duration of the catheter's routine use; daily dressings and antibiotic ointments are no longer considered useful.

NOSOCOMIAL PNEUMONIA. Hospital-acquired lower respiratory tract infections (including pneumonia and bronchitis) account for 10 to 15 per cent of nosocomial infections. Almost 1 per cent of patients admitted to the hospital develop pneumonia. Elderly patients with serious underlying illnesses are at risk, as are all patients receiving mechanical ventilation. These infections usually extend a patient's hospital stay for 7 days or more, produce substantial morbidity, and contribute to the deaths of already seriously ill patients.

In contrast to community-acquired pneumonia in younger patients, nosocomial pneumonia usually is a mixed infection involving more than one organism. Although a hospital's intensive care unit may develop a dominant bacterial respiratory tract pathogen, the list of bacteria associated with nosocomial pneumonia is large. Aerobic gram-negative bacilli are associated with more than half the cases, including *P. aeruginosa, Enterobacter, Klebsiella, E. coli,* and *Acinetobacter*, among others. *Acinetobacter* particularly is associated with ventilated patients in busy intensive care units. Among gram-positive organisms, *S. aureus* is isolated with regularity but may not always have a major pathogenic role. Pneumococci contribute to about 3 per cent of nosocomial pneumonias, usually in elderly patients with predisposing lung disease. Most clinical laboratory routines do not process respiratory tract specimens anaerobically, and even research methods have limitations in ascribing a role for anaerobes in lower respiratory tract infections. Although aerobic pathogens clearly are dominant, most authorities believe that anaerobes are involved in about one third of nosocomial pneumonias. *Legionella pneumophila* can be a vexing problem in some hospitals, where it can be isolated from the water supply. Viral respiratory infections are increasingly recognized as causes of nosocomial pneumonia and as infections predisposing to subsequent bacterial invasion. Respiratory syncytial virus, influenza, and cytomegalovirus are the viruses most commonly identified.

Endotracheal tubes and tracheostomies bypass the upper respiratory tract defense mechanisms and can traumatize mucous membranes. When managed improperly, these devices can provide direct access for the introduction of hospital pathogens on the hands of personnel or by contaminated suction tubing. Ventilator machines often produced contaminated aerosols in past years, but current maintenance protocols have made nosocomial pneumonia due to the machine itself an unusual event.

Aspiration of oropharyngeal secretions is the principal initiating event in nosocomial pneumonia. Patients who have an impaired gag reflex, are sedated, or have altered consciousness are more likely to aspirate. The volume and pH of the aspirate as well as its bacterial population contribute to the likelihood of lung injury. The bacterial population is determined by the organisms colonizing the oropharynx. The flora of the normal pharynx is largely gram-positive. Gram-negative bacillary colonization occurs in older persons with a variety of underlying diseases, after antibiotic therapy, and in patients who are leukopenic.

Gastric alkalinization can permit the multiplication of gram-negative bacteria in the stomach. These bacteria can then become the source of oropharyngeal colonization. Antacids and histamine type-2 (H_2) blockers are often given to patients in ICU's who are being ventilated in order to prevent stress ulcers. Because they raise gastric pH, these drugs promote the growth of bacteria in the stomach and increase the risk of nosocomial pneumonia. Because it does not neutralize gastric acidity, sucralfate is preferred for stress ulcer prophylaxis.

The prevention of nosocomial pneumonia is a daunting challenge. Positioning patients with their heads raised may reduce somewhat the occurrence of aspiration. Scrupulous hand washing inhibits the transmission of nosocomial pathogens. Meticulous maintenance of ventilatory equipment and assiduous pulmonary toilet by nurses reduce risks. The role of selective decontamination of the gastrointestinal tract with combinations of oral and systemic antibiotics currently is being studied.

SURGICAL WOUND INFECTIONS. Postoperative wound infections account for 20 per cent of nosocomial infections. These infections account for a substantial amount of morbidity, increase hospital stay considerably, and are costly. Some postoperative infections extend down from the skin incision to the depths of the surgical field where they can destroy vascular anastomoses or disrupt an implanted prosthetic device. Bacteremia may accompany such infections. The extent of the surgical procedure and its anatomic location, the severity of the patient's underlying illness, and the surgeon's skill are all important determinants of risk. When surgery involves tissues that normally are not subjected to a large microbial population during the procedure ("clean" operations), wound infection rates often are less than 2 per cent. Such operations include inguinal herniorrhaphy and vascular surgery in the neck, for example. When procedures transect mucosal surfaces, such as in a colectomy ("contaminated" operations), up to 20 per cent of patients have a postoperative wound infection. If patients are malnourished, at the extremes of age, or have serious underlying diseases, wound infections are more likely to occur. The longer the duration of the operation, the more likely that a postoperative infection will occur. A surgeon's skill is critical. If tissues are traumatized, the vascular supply is unnecessarily interrupted, devitalized tissue or blood clots are left in the wound, or wound layers are not realigned properly, the risk of wound infection increases.

S. aureus and *S. epidermidis* are the most commonly isolated pathogens from wound infections, reflecting their common residence on human skin. A wide variety of other organisms contribute to these infections, including enterococci, *E. coli, P. aeruginosa*, and *Bacteroides*, largely determined by the organ undergoing surgery. The infecting bacteria most often originate in the patient's own endogenous microbial flora, whether on the skin or on a mucosal surface. A smaller contribution comes from the bacterial flora of the surgeon and other members of the operating team. Even clean wounds are not truly sterile; small numbers of bacteria can be recovered from virtually all wounds at the time of wound closure. Thus, for the most part, the infecting bacteria are in the wound when the patient leaves the operating room, unless there is a drain or packing in the incision. Occasionally bacteremia originating from another infected site implant at the operative site; there have been a few well-described instances in which a wound was infected during postoperative care.

A whole array of techniques are employed to minimize the occurrence of wound infection. The architecture, air handling, and housekeeping in the operating room have made the physical environment very clean. Special laminar flow rooms are used for some procedures, such as implantation of an artificial joint. An elaborate ritual of aseptic practice involves both the patient (shaving the surgical area, baths with disinfectant soap, skin preparation just before surgery, among others) and the surgeon (precise hand scrubbing, operating room gowns and masks, use of sterile gloves, and the like). The importance of the appropriate use of antibiotic prophylaxis cannot be overemphasized. Indeed, some medical historians suggest that the most important consequence of the discovery of antibiotics was that their use permitted the development of the technologically adventurous procedures that characterize contemporary surgery. In recent years it has been amply confirmed that for antibiotics to be effective in preventing wound infection they need to be given only briefly, chosen to be effective against the most commonly expected pathogens at the surgical site, and given in amounts sufficient to provide killing concentrations in the tissues. The brevity of their use (often no longer than 24 hours) results in very little drug toxicity or development of bacterial resistance.

MISCELLANEOUS SITES. In addition to the most commonly occurring infections discussed above, nosocomial infections also occur in numerous other sites and circumstances. The extent of nosocomial infectious diarrhea is only now being recognized. Among children, the most common pathogen is rotavirus; among adults, *Clostridium difficile* colitis is a complication of antibiotic therapy. Epidemics of keratoconjunctivitis due to adenoviruses can be propagated by the contaminated hands of ophthalmologists as well as contaminated tonometers. Meningitis, usually caused by *S. epidermidis*, can follow the placement of shunts in the cerebral ventricles. Meningitis also can occur in immunocompromised organ transplant recipients. In renal transplant patients *Cryptococcus* and *Listeria* are the most frequent pathogens. Transfusions of blood and blood products have resulted in the transmission of hepatitis B virus and human immunodeficiency virus as well as other viruses and bacteria.

INFECTION CONTROL PROGRAMS

Although many efforts were being made to prevent infections in hospitals, most institutions did not have a formal organized program until the 1960's. At that time it became apparent that the previous focus by hospitals on environmental hygiene was insufficient. Strongly influenced by the Centers for Disease Control, the American Hospital Association, and the Joint Commission on Accreditation of Health Care Organizations, every hospital now must have an active infection control program in order to secure accreditation. Central to the program is an Infection Control Committee whose members are broadly representative of hospital administration and the professional disciplines. A physician knowledgeable about infection control is designated the Hospital Epidemiologist. It is recommended that the hospital employ one infection control practitioner (usually a nurse with special infection control training) for every 250 beds. These practitioners organize a wide variety of infection control activities, but all who work in hospitals must realize that the practitioners alone cannot produce the safest milieu for patients. Rather, all who work in hospitals must assume responsibility: Infection control is everyone's business.

A critical element of the program is a system of surveillance for detecting nosocomial infections, analyzing the data, and reporting on distinctive events. Surveillance may involve reviewing microbiology laboratory reports, visiting wards, inspecting surgical wounds, and the like. It now has been well demonstrated that such surveillance provides more pertinent information than routinely culturing features of the environment, a practice that has largely ceased.

The infection control practitioners also orchestrate the institution's control measures, ranging from appropriate isolation systems to responses when an epidemic is detected. Each unit in the hospital contributes its own section of procedures to a hospital-wide infection control manual. Its procedures are reviewed on 1- to 2-year cycles and as needed when new developments occur.

Sophisticated support from the clinical microbiology laboratory is necessary for a successful infection control program. The laboratory provides its routine data for surveillance purposes, may be asked to process extra cultures when an outbreak is under investigation, and may undertake special studies with nosocomial pathogens.

Other hospital service units also provide critical support for the infection control program. Although the role of the inanimate environment has been de-emphasized, the housekeeping department must maintain a high level of cleanliness throughout the institution. They also are responsible for managing and disposing of the hospital's solid waste. Heavily contaminated wastes (such as from the microbiology laboratory) must be incinerated. Solid waste disposal has become a major political issue over the last several years and has become very expensive, so this function has grown in importance.

The central supply operation cleans and either disinfects or sterilizes reusable materials that are employed in the diagnosis and therapy of patients. The laundry collects and launders soiled linen. Linen need be sterilized only for use in operative procedures. The hospital kitchen or outside food service must adhere to strict hygiene standards in preparing the many and varied diets for patients. Fortunately, foodborne outbreaks in hospitals are not common.

The occupational health service has special responsibilities to protect hospital personnel from acquiring an infection from patients while performing their patient-care duties, and, in turn, also to prevent employees from transmitting their own infections to patients. In this regard, several diseases have assumed particular importance.

AIDS (see Part XXI). Although the risk of acquiring HIV infection from occupational exposure is very low, this disease has received great attention from hospital infection control programs over the past several years. AIDS has raised a number of scientific, ethical, social, and legal issues that have had an impact on the ability of the infection control team to devise solutions. Not every issue has as yet been adequately addressed, largely because certain essential data are lacking.

Because HIV is not transmitted through casual contact, routine interactions with patients are not hazardous. Exposures that are associated with a risk of acquiring HIV infection are injuries by "sharps" (needles and scalpels, primarily) contaminated with the body fluid (blood, most commonly) or tissue of an HIV-infected patient. A number of studies have indicated that approximately 1 of every 250 such exposures results in transmission of HIV infection to the health care worker. Transmission is more likely to occur when the exposures are multiple and deep and when a substantial volume of blood is inoculated during the injury. The prospective studies of exposures on skin or mucous membranes have not shown any seroconversions, but there have been anecdotal reports suggesting that such exposures rarely might result in transmission. Much remains to be learned in this regard.

Standard protocols have been developed to manage the hospital worker who sustains an occupational injury involving a patient's blood or other body fluid. These include testing the source patient for HIV infection (if the patient can be identified), counseling the hospital worker, and possibly offering zidovudine prophylaxis. Such injuries often are major anxiety-provoking events, and the cooperation of the occupational health service and the infection control team in the supportive counseling of the hospital worker is extremely important. See Ch. 413 for additional discussion of AIDS prevention and control.

TUBERCULOSIS. Health care workers have always been at greater risk than the general population for acquiring tuberculosis. The patient who is diagnosed with tuberculosis is only a modest hazard. Respiratory isolation techniques and antituberculosis therapy quickly reduce the hazard of nosocomial transmission. Rather, the risk is from the cryptic case, the patient with as yet undiagnosed tuberculosis. After a steady decline for years, tuberculosis is again resurgent because of the recent wave of immigrants from Southeast Asia and Central America and the frequency with which tuberculosis complicates HIV infection.

All hospitals are obliged to have a tuberculosis control program. All personnel receive a tuberculin skin test on employment. Those who are skin test–negative are followed by periodic skin testing, usually at yearly intervals, although high-risk persons may be tested at shorter intervals. Those who convert to a positive skin test are evaluated for active disease and are candidates for isoniazid (INH) preventive therapy. There is no place for annual chest roentgenograms, a now discarded practice.

HEPATITIS B. Like HIV infection, hepatitis B is transmitted in the hospital by exposure to blood and other body fluids that contain the virus. Hospital personnel who are exposed to blood and use needles, scalpels, and other sharp objects are at increased risk of hepatitis B infection. Programs to prevent hepatitis B infection are two-pronged. First, strong attempts must be made to reduce injuries through education, designing safer devices, and providing for the secure disposal of sharps in impervious containers. These precautions help avert not only hepatitis B infections, but all other blood-borne pathogens including retroviruses and other viral hepatitis agents. Secondly, hepatitis B vaccine must be offered to all workers at potential risk. Ideally, all students of the health care professions should be immunized early in their training. In addition, insistent attempts to immunize current health care workers, including physicians and nurses, must continue. After an injury, standard protocols are used by the occupational health service to evaluate the health worker and the source patient and to offer appropriate prophylaxis.

In addition to providing hepatitis B vaccine, hospitals should provide other vaccines for the protection of personnel. Measles, mumps, and rubella have produced outbreaks in hospitals resulting in a great deal of unnecessary illness, turbulence, and expense. In these outbreaks, hospital workers have both acquired these viral infections and transmitted them to patients. It now is recommended that hospital workers born since 1957 receive a second dose of measles vaccine. If this is provided as the combined measles-mumps-rubella (MMR) vaccine, protection is achieved against all three diseases.

Finally, as the United States population ages, as hospitals care for increasingly sicker patients, and as medical technology continues its aggressive advances in organ transplantation and other invasive therapies, the importance of nosocomial infections will likely continue to increase. Infection control programs must be alert to these changes and be prepared to respond to them with equally new and innovative preventive measures.

American Hospital Association: Management of HIV Infection in the Hospital, 3rd ed. Recommendations of the Technical Panel on Infections Within Hospitals. Chicago, American Hospital Association, 1988. *A booklet available from the AHA that discusses aspects of caring for HIV-infected patients in hospitals. Not a clinical text.*

Bennett JV, Brachman PS: Hospital Infections. Boston, Little Brown & Company, 1986. *A comprehensive treatment of hospital infection issues.*

Centers for Disease Control: Guidelines for prevention of transmission of human immunodeficiency virus and hepatitis B virus to health care and public safety workers. MMWR 37(No. S-6):3–37, 1989. *The official recommendations.*

Kaiser AB: Antimicrobial prophylaxis in surgery. N Engl J Med 315:1129–1138, 1986. *A comprehensive review.*

Pugliese G, Lynch P, Jackson MM: Universal Precautions. Policies, Procedures, and Resources. Chicago, American Hospital Publishing Company, 1991. *An excellent resource for practical suggestions.*

Weber DJ, Rutala WA: Nosocomial infections: New issues and strategies for prevention. Infect Dis Clin North Am 3(4):671–929, 1989. *A collection of papers discussing a wide variety of current infection control issues.*

Wenzel RP: Prevention and Control of Nosocomial Infections. Baltimore, Williams & Wilkins, 1987. *A scholarly text on nosocomial infections.*

290 Advice to Travelers

Bruce M. Greene

Overseas travel by U.S. citizens is steadily increasing, including travel to developing countries. Approximately 15 million people from the United States travel overseas each year, including an estimated 7 million to developing countries. It is the latter group, who are exposed to a variety of health hazards as a consequence of overseas travel, that this chapter addresses. Importantly, most of such health problems are entirely or partially preventable.

The precautions that one can recommend to travelers to

developing countries include general preventive health measures, vaccinations, and medications. What is recommended depends greatly on the specific itinerary and living conditions. It is incumbent upon the physician making such recommendations to be cognizant of the most recent epidemiologic information pertinent to the situation.

GENERAL PREVENTIVE HEALTH MEASURES

TRAVELER'S DIARRHEA. Travelers to developing countries frequently experience gastroenteritis. The risk of this problem can be minimized by avoiding indiscriminate consumption of high-risk foods, such as lettuce salads, unpeeled fruits and vegetables, local water and milk, ice cubes made from local water, creamy sauces and other obvious rich foods that serve as a good culture medium, and food prepared and served by sidewalk vendors. Eating food that is prepared in a reputable restaurant, cooked well and served hot, and drinking bottled water, carbonated drinks, or hot tea or coffee reduce the risk of gastroenteritis. Finally, it is important to recall that airline food is usually prepared locally.

Boiling water for 10 minutes at usual elevations (longer at high elevations with low atmospheric pressure) is the most reliable way to purify water. Purification tablets and filtration devices are less effective. Bottled mineral water in which the seal is unbroken is usually safe. For further details of the clinical aspects of this syndrome, see Ch. 319.

MALARIA. Minimizing exposure to mosquito bites is an important precaution for malaria prevention. No prophylactic agent is completely effective, and wearing protective clothing and utilizing appropriate insect repellent (containing DEET) are essential. Mosquito exposure is usually worst in the evening and early morning. In areas with high-intensity exposure to infected mosquitoes, mosquito bed nets and knockdown sprays should be used for sleeping.

Large urban areas usually are malaria transmission–free; however, many urban areas of Africa are exceptions. Travel to a game park even for a day or overnight travel through rural areas is sufficient to create a significant risk of malaria.

Most important, travelers to malaria-endemic areas should be advised that, even though all preventive measures are taken and observed carefully, acquisition of malaria is still a possibility. Therefore, because of the risk of rapidly fatal falciparum malaria, such individuals should be advised to report promptly to an emergency room for unexplained fever that occurs within 6 months of returning. It is imperative to note that the fever associated with falciparum malaria frequently does *not* demonstrate a regular pattern and can even be unremitting.

ACUTE MOUNTAIN SICKNESS. An individual whose travel results in an increase in altitude of greater than approximately 2500 to 3000 meters within a 48- to 72-hour period has a risk of developing acute mountain sickness. This syndrome, associated with headache, nausea, vomiting, diarrhea, and fever, can be extremely debilitating and is preventable. Treatment with acetazolamide, 250 mg three times a day starting 24 hours before travel and continuing for 5 days after arrival, minimizes symptoms. The individual should be warned of the mild diuretic effect of acetazolamide.

ADVICE TO INDIVIDUALS WITH UNDERLYING CARDIOPULMONARY DISEASE. Persons with severe angina pectoris should be advised against air travel. On the other hand, persons with well-compensated, stable ischemic heart disease should be able to travel without undue risk, although it is apparent that access to medical care will be suboptimal during travel.

Individuals with underlying respiratory insufficiency may be able to travel by air, although supplemental oxygen may be required during travel. Guidelines have recently been proposed to assist in making these determinations (see references).

MOTOR VEHICLE ACCIDENTS. One of the most serious threats to visitors to developing countries is motor vehicle accidents. The traveler must exert special vigilance and a high level of individual responsibility in safeguarding against this possibility. In this regard, knowing and having a record of one's blood type may be important.

SPECIAL RISKS. Schistosomiasis can be acquired by even transient exposure to fresh water lakes and ponds. Rabies is quite common in developing countries, and dogs and other vertebrate animals should be avoided. Cysticercosis is a particular threat in some countries, e.g., Mexico, and the usual source is not under-cooked meat, but rather a food handler harboring an adult *T. solium* worm. Similarly, trichinosis is a risk in many countries, and pork may be used as a substitute for other meats in some dishes. In West and West Central Africa, loa loa is a risk and can be prevented with weekly diethylcarbamazine. Finally, individuals who are medication-dependent should pack an extra supply of critical medications and ensure their safe passage by packing strategically.

JET LAG. Individuals traveling to a time zone that is more than 3 hours different from that to which they are accustomed frequently experience extreme fatigue, somnolence, and disordered sleeping patterns. This results in part from lack of adequate sleep in transit and in part from the necessary resetting of the individual's biologic clock. To counter the first problem, short-acting benzodiazepines are helpful and can ensure adequate sleep. Upon arrival in the new time zone, resetting of the biologic clock is facilitated by forcing oneself to live according to the new time schedule. This frequently necessitates increased consumption of coffee or tea and sometimes further use of short-acting hypnotics. There is no clear evidence that more extensive and elaborate programs to avoid jet lag are of value.

PRETRAVEL VACCINATIONS AND OTHER INJECTIONS

It is important to review the individual patient's overall immunization status, including those vaccines addressed below as well as others such as pneumococcal and influenza vaccines that may be indicated for some persons. Prior to administration, full details concerning the injectable reagent, available in the manufacturer's package insert, should be consulted.

IMMUNE SERUM GLOBULIN (GAMMA GLOBULIN). For travel to most developing countries, individuals who have not had hepatitis A infection should receive 0.06 ml per kilogram for a stay of greater than 3 months' duration, to be repeated every 5 months; for travel with a total duration of less than 3 months, a single injection of 0.02 ml per kilogram is adequate. Following deep intramuscular injection, the site usually remains sore for 1 to 3 days. Immune serum globulin has been found to have some efficacy in preventing food-borne non-A, non-B hepatitis.

YELLOW FEVER. This is recommended for travelers to endemic areas in South and Central America and Africa. Although it is a live virus vaccine, yellow fever immunization is not affected by concurrent administration of immune serum globulin preparations in the United States. Occasionally (in 2 to 5 per cent of vaccines), fever, headache, and myalgias develop 6 to 10 days after injection during the phase of virus replication. Because of the time required for virus replication, yellow fever vaccine must be given at least 10 days prior to travel to an endemic area. Administration once every 10 years is required. As with all live virus vaccines, except oral polio vaccine, it is not recommended that yellow fever vaccine be given with known or possible pregnancy. Egg allergy is a contraindication. Further, infants less than 4 months of age and some persons with altered immune status should not receive yellow fever vaccine.

TETANUS. Travelers to developing countries should receive a tetanus booster if they have not been immunized within the previous 5 years. This is because of the risk of hepatitis B and HIV infection associated with needle injection in the event that a tetanus-prone injury is sustained in a developing country. In adults, tetanus-diphtheria (TD) is recommended.

POLIO. Adults who are traveling to developing countries where polio is a risk should receive a polio booster if none has been given since childhood. Those who previously received a primary course of immunization with oral polio vaccine should receive trivalent OPV on one occasion. Those who are uncertain of what they received previously, or who received inactivated polio vaccine, should receive a booster dose of enhanced efficacy inactivated polio vaccine (eIPV). Adults who have no prior history of polio immunization should receive a primary series with eIPV. Refer to the first reference below for further details.

Oral polio vaccine is a live virus and can lead to paralytic polio in nonimmunized adult contacts of those who receive OPV. Further, individuals with immunodeficiency (IgA deficiency, common variable immunodeficiency, acquired immunodeficiency syndrome, and others) *should not* receive OPV.

MEASLES. Because of the recent outbreaks of measles in previously immunized populations, the Immunization Practices Advisory Committee on Measles Prevention has recently changed policy to recommend that every person receive a two-dose vaccination regimen. For adults, it is recommended that, irrespective of any travel plans, every person born after 1956 receive a second dose of measles vaccine. Revised recommendations for children are also available.

For full effect, measles immunization should precede administration of immune serum globulin by at least 2 weeks. As the time interval between measles immunization and administration of immune serum globulin decreases from 4 weeks, measles vaccination efficacy may decrease, and one must consider giving a second dose of measles vaccine 3 months after the last administration of immune serum globulin (or 6 months later if the larger dose of immune serum globulin has been administered). Live measles vaccine, when given as a component of combined measles/rubella or measles/mumps/rubella vaccine should not be given to women known to be pregnant or who are considering becoming pregnant within the subsequent 3 months. Women who are given measles vaccines should not become pregnant for at least 30 days after vaccination. Individuals with severe alterations of immune competence should not be given measles vaccine.

MENINGOCOCCAL MENINGITIS. Outbreaks of meningococcal meningitis occur in epidemic form across sub-Saharan Africa. In addition, recent major outbreaks have occurred in Nepal, northern India, and Saudi Arabia and may occur unpredictably across much of Africa and in Brazil. Meningococcal vaccine is available that protects against the A, C, Y, and W-135 capsular strains. Although the risk to casual visitors to endemic areas is extremely small, it is recommended that meningococcal vaccine be given to individuals who will spend more than simple in-transit time in areas with a risk of major outbreaks.

TYPHOID. Avoiding intake of potentially contaminated food and drink is the most effective means of prevention of typhoid infection. The overall risk to American travelers is less than 1 case in 10,000 trips, but travelers to higher-risk countries such as India have about a fourfold increased incidence. For primary immunization, the newly licensed oral live-attenuated Ty21a vaccine is recommended. One capsule is taken every other day for a total of four doses. Concurrent antibiotic use is contraindicated. For booster immunization, either oral vaccine (as for primary immunization) or heat-phenol–inactivated vaccine, 0.5 cc subcutaneously in adults, can be used. Booster is necessary after 5 years following oral immunization or after 3 years when parenteral immunization has been used. The available typhoid vaccines provide approximately 50 to 90 per cent protection.

CHOLERA. This vaccine, because of its short duration of effect and lack of efficacy (approximately 50 per cent protection), as well as the lack of substantial risk of disease for most U.S. travelers, is no longer recommended. Concomitant administration with yellow fever vaccine may result in a reduced vaccine response to yellow fever virus.

MUMPS. This live vaccine should be given to susceptible persons unless there is a contraindication, such as immune defects and pregnancy or possible pregnancy.

JAPANESE ENCEPHALITIS. This mosquito-borne viral encephalitis occurs in epidemics, primarily in late summer and autumn, in the temperate regions and the northern part of tropical zones in Bangladesh, Burma, China, India, Japan, Kampuchea, Korea, Laos, Nepal, Thailand, Vietnam, and the eastern areas of the USSR. There is a lower risk to visitors to endemic areas, which include the tropical zones of southern India, Indonesia, Malaysia, Philippines, Singapore, Sri Lanka, Taiwan, and southern Thailand. Persons who intend to live for prolonged periods of time in an endemic or epidemic area are at greater risk. Because of fear of litigation, the manufacturer of the vaccine no longer makes it available in the United States, but the American Consulate in many cities in China and in various clinics in other capitals in endemic and epidemic areas can administer the Japanese encephalitis vaccine.

HEPATITIS B. This is indicated for travelers to developing countries who may have blood or other significant body fluid exposure. HIV infection risk must, of course, also be considered.

PLAGUE. This vaccine is rarely indicated and should be reserved primarily for travelers to known endemic areas, particularly Vietnam. Individuals who are at extreme risk of developing plague should be given antibiotic chemoprophylaxis with tetracycline, 500 mg 4 times per day during periods of exposure.

RABIES. Rabies occurs commonly in many developing countries, and travelers should be forewarned about the risk associated with even seemingly totally healthy dogs and other animals. Preexposure vaccination with human diploid cell vaccine (HDCV) is recommended for individuals who will be living or visiting for more than 30 days in countries where rabies is a constant threat. In addition, veterinarians, animal handlers, spelunkers, and some laboratory workers should receive rabies vaccine. Chloroquine phosphate may interfere with developing an antibody response to HDCV, but intramuscular injection can overcome this problem.

RUBELLA. Rubella vaccine is recommended for susceptible, unvaccinated adolescents and adults, particularly females. Even though thought to be safe during pregnancy, this vaccine is not recommended for women known to be pregnant or those who may become pregnant within 3 months of vaccination. In addition, individuals with immunodeficiency should not be given this live vaccine.

SMALLPOX. This vaccine is no longer available and should not be administered, since the last human case in nature occurred in 1977.

TYPHUS. This vaccine is not available in the United States and is only very rarely indicated.

MEDICATIONS

MALARIA PROPHYLAXIS. Because of the explosive spread of chloroquine-resistant strains of *Plasmodium falciparum* and the emergence of resistance to alternative drugs in Asia, East and West Africa, and South America, recommendations regarding chemotherapeutic approaches to prevent malaria are changing rapidly.* In rural Thailand, where chloroquine and dihydrofolate reductase inhibitor resistance is ubiquitous, doxycycline, 100 mg per day orally, has given good results. Mefloquine is the recommended agent for most other areas with drug-resistant *P. falciparum*. Unfortunately, significant central nervous system side effects can be associated with mefloquine. The recommended dosage for prophylaxis is 250 mg per week starting 1 week prior to travel and for 4 weeks after departure from the malarious area. With intensive exposure that may include *P. vivax* and *P. ovale*, chloroquine prophylaxis is recommended, followed by primaquine to eliminate liver stage parasites. See Ch. 424 for further details regarding antimalarial prophylaxis and treatment.

TRAVELERS' DIARRHEA PREVENTION. For short-term (less than 5 days) visitors to developing countries, norfloxacin, 400 mg taken once a day, provides considerable protection. Two tablets of bismuth subsalicylate taken four times per day provide similar results.

Treatment of mild diarrhea consists of restricting intake to fluids (Coca-Cola or hot tea with sugar), soups, and toast. Loperamide is recommended as an effective antiperistaltic agent. Norfloxacin, 400 mg orally twice a day for 5 days, is useful in more severe cases. High fever with diarrhea or bloody diarrhea indicates the need for medical consultation. See Ch. 101 for further details regarding possible etiologies and treatment of diarrheal diseases.

ANTIBIOTICS FOR INFECTED WOUNDS AND OTHER SKIN INFECTIONS. It is recommended that antibiotic ointment (e.g., bacitracin–polymyxin B) and bandages be taken to treat minor cuts and scrapes. For prolonged treks away from civilization, cephalexin tablets may be recommended for pyogenic infections. Because of the frequency of fungal infections in tropical climates, it is advisable for travelers to take antifungal powder and, in the case of females, vaginal antifungal cream or suppositories.

---

*For up-to-date information on malaria prevention from the Centers for Disease Control, U.S. Public Health Service, telephone (404) 639-1610. For other information, telephone (404) 639-3311 (main switchboard).

Centers for Disease Control, Department of Health and Human Services: Health Information for International Travel. Washington, D.C., U.S. Government Printing Office, 1991. *Excellent concise source of current information on health risks in overseas locations, as well as key information on vaccines and drugs. Obtainable from the Superintendent of Documents, U.S. Government Printing Office, Washington, D.C. 20402, telephone (202) 783-3238. Updated yearly.*

Conrad ME, Lemon SM: Prevention of endemic icteric viral hepatitis by administration of immune serum gamma globulin. J Infect Dis 156:84–91, 1987.

Gong H: Advising patients with pulmonary diseases on air travel. Ann Intern Med 111:349–351, 1989.

Hill DR, Pearson RD: Health advice for international travel. Ann Intern Med 108:829–852, 1988. *Authoritative recent review.*

Johnson TS, Rock PB: Current concepts: Acute mountain sickness. N Engl J Med 319:841–845, 1988.

Steffen R, Rickenbach M, Wihelm U, et al.: Health problems after travel to developing countries. J Infect Dis 156:84–91, 1988. *Most detailed study available providing follow-up data on cohorts of travelers to developing countries.*

291 Antimicrobial Therapy

Lowell S. Young

The advent of antimicrobial therapy represented an historic milestone in the cure and control of many infectious diseases. Invariably fatal infections, like bacterial endocarditis, became treatable for the first time. Subsequently, abundant evidence has accumulated that early treatment of localized bacterial infections may obviate further complications. The greatest progress during the modern era of antimicrobial therapy has been in the treatment of acute bacterial infections, although a few chronic diseases such as tuberculosis are usually successfully treated. New developments offer promise in controlling viral diseases and parasitic infections that are a major burden on much of humankind. There have been some modest developments in the antifungal area as well. Nonetheless, the initial enthusiasm that greeted the introduction of new agents with antibacterial activity has been tempered by a more sobering perspective. Antimicrobial agents are not always innocuous to the host, and their widespread usage appears to have fostered increasing drug resistance throughout the world. The growing complexities of antimicrobial therapy appear to be related to the rapid proliferation of agents of several classes, increasing drug resistance, and a greater recognition of interactions between pharmacologic agents.

SOME DEFINITIONS

The terms *antibiotic*, *antimicrobic*, and *chemotherapeutic agent* have often been used interchangeably to designate defined chemical substances that possess activity against specific microorganisms. Indeed, antibiotic was first defined as a substance produced in nature by living microbes that inhibited the growth of other microbial organisms at low concentrations. Viewed in this light, antibiotics seem to be a product of evolution and may confer a selective advantage on the producer in a specific ecosystem. Technically, antibiotics differ from chemotherapeutic agents in that the latter represent the products of chemical synthesis, such as the sulfonamide dyes that were subsequently found to have antibacterial activity. Antibiotics in common use, such as penicillins and aminoglycosides, are derived from natural products but from a functional point of view may be considered interchangeable with chemotherapeutic agents. As the development of new antibacterial agents has proliferated, restrictive technical terms have become outdated. For instance, new penicillins, cephalosporins, and aminoglycosides contain synthetic or semisynthetic modifications of existing structures that confer potent new biologic activity. The term "antimicrobic" has been proposed to describe all substances with antimicrobial activity, whether of natural or synthetic origin, but its acceptance has been variable.

GENERAL PRINCIPLES

The goal of antimicrobial therapy is to kill or inhibit the growth of an infecting pathogen without causing harm to the host. Thus, the basis for such an effect is *selectivity*, whereby the parasite is specifically targeted by virtue of some difference between it and mammalian cells. The first widely used antimicrobial compounds, sulfonamides and penicillins, illustrate this principle very clearly. Sulfonamides are inhibitors of para-aminobenzoic acid, an essential requirement for nucleic acid synthesis in many bacteria but not in humans. Penicillins and related agents that contain a beta-lactam ring act to disrupt the synthesis of peptidoglycan, which gives the bacterial cell wall its shape and strength. Mammalian cells have no cell wall, making penicillin-type drugs the ideal antibacterial agent in terms of selectivity.

Table 291–1 summarizes the mechanism of action of some of the major groups of antibacterial agents. Unfortunately, the selective action of some important compounds on the infecting microbe is not as specific as with penicillin, and important toxic effects on host cells may be encountered. Some drugs like the sulfonamides merely inhibit the growth of organisms and are *bacteriostatic*. When these agents are used, eradication of an infecting agent depends on host defenses such as phagocytic cells and antibodies. Others, like penicillins and the aminoglycosides, inhibit bacteria at relatively low concentration and at higher (but still usually therapeutic) concentrations can kill them; these are *bactericidal* agents. These designations of a bacteriostatic or bactericidal agent may vary, depending on the type of organism: Penicillin G is usually bactericidal for gram-positive cocci but is only static against the enterococcus (*Streptococcus faecalis*), while chloramphenicol is usually bacteriostatic even at very high concentrations but can be bactericidal against *Haemophilus influenzae*. Spectrum refers to range of microorganisms affected by a particular agent, which varies from relatively narrow for low doses of penicillin G to quite broad for large doses of the new cephalosporins. Breadth of spectrum is not necessarily related to mechanism of action.

The interaction between a microbe and therapeutic agent can be complex, and many important variables affect outcome. Intrinsic virulence differs considerably among infecting agents, so that the progression of infection ranges from a very indolent tempo to a fulminating course. Host factors should influence selection of bactericidal versus bacteriostatic agents and the breadth of spectrum of therapy. The site of infection influences dose and duration of treatment. The proliferation of therapeutic choices compels the physician to obtain in-depth knowledge of any agent prescribed. Treatment can be guided by laboratory studies, but therapeutic choices must be based on knowledge of antimicrobial spectrum, mode of action, pharmacology, toxicity, and all major factors that affect drug activity.

IDENTIFICATION OF THE INFECTING AGENT

It is highly desirable to have the infecting agent identified prior to initiation of treatment, but in most circumstances culture confirmation and tests in vitro of antimicrobial susceptibility will not be available for at least a day. Clinical decision making is usually based on a perception of probabilities and on simple tests, the most important of which is the Gram stain. Even the latter

is not necessary in the case of exudative pharyngitis, because the only treatable bacterial causes of the syndrome are hemolytic streptococci and now, rarely, *Corynebacterium diphtheriae*. Other isolates can usually be ignored and therapy with a penicillin initiated. When only a single infecting organism seems likely, therapy with a narrow-spectrum agent is preferable.

In reality, many infectious processes initially begin as mixed infections: The aspiration of secretions into the lung usually results in the deposition of many types of oral microbes that can lead to pneumonia or lung abscess, or the perforation of an abdominal viscus leads to release of millions of aerobic and anaerobic bacteria into the abdominal cavity. What may survive to be cultured in respiratory secretions or from abdominal drainage may well be the hardiest of bacteria, and not necessarily all of those that were associated with initial infectious morbidity. Not all mixed infectious processes require treatment with broad-spectrum agents, but the presence of multiple pathogens might explain clinical failure when a mixed infection is being treated and only one component of that infection is being affected by a particular drug regimen.

Initiation of antibiotic therapy prior to obtaining appropriate cultures is perhaps the leading explanation for the failure to document infecting pathogens. On the other hand, the Gram stain or immunofluorescent staining of secretions can identify the cause of infection after treatment is started. Irrespective of when it is done, the Gram stain can provide valuable semiquantitative information about predominant pathogens and can help the clinician decide whether a subsequent culture result can actually be relied upon. For instance, the validity of a sample of respiratory secretions is greatly enhanced by the detection of phagocytic cells, such as neutrophils or alveolar macrophages. In contrast, the presence of squamous epithelial cells should be the basis for rejecting the validity of expectorated sputum, since they reflect oropharyngeal contamination. With regard to quantitative evaluation of a potentially infected body fluid, isolation of greater than 10^5 organisms per milliliter has been accepted as establishing the validity of a urine culture result. However, microscopic examination of uncentrifuged urine may still yield an approximate idea of the degree of infection (any organism seen corresponds with 10^5 bacteria per milliliter), as well as the nature of the infection that is taking place in the urinary tract. Isolation of organisms in pure culture from blood or normally sterile body fluids (like spinal fluid) is an unambiguous laboratory result that establishes an infectious etiology. Occasionally, some bloodstream infections are polymicrobial. Some blood culture isolates may be rejected as contaminants. The latter are usually skin flora like corynebacteria or coagulase-negative staphylococci. However, repeated isolation of such organisms from blood culture in association with signs of infection calls for careful clinical assessment. Coagulase-negative staphylococci and corynebacteria can be valid pathogens in immunosuppressed subjects and patients with prosthetic devices.

TABLE 291–1. MECHANISM OF ACTION OF ANTIMICROBIAL AGENTS

Agent	Site of Action	Effect	Cidal	Static
Penicillins, cephalosporins	Cell wall	Inhibit crosslinking of peptidoglycan, resulting in spheroplast formation	+	Occasionally
Vancomycin	Cell wall	Block transfer of pentapeptide from cytoplasm to cell membrane	+	Occasionally
Polymyxin B, colistin	Cytoplasmic membrane	Bind phospholipid and disrupt membrane	+	
Aminoglycosides	Ribosome	Bind to 30S ribosomal subunit, thereby inhibiting attachment of messenger RNA; also affect transfer RNA	+	
Tetracyclines	Ribosome	Bind to 30S subunit and inhibit binding of transfer RNA		+
Chloramphenicol	Ribosome	Bind to 50S subunit and inhibit messenger RNA translation	Occasionally	+
Erythromycin, clindamycin	Ribosome	Inhibit messenger RNA translation	Occasionally	+
Rifampin	Nucleic acid synthesis	Impaired RNA formation by inhibiting DNA-dependent RNA polymerase	+	Occasionally
Metronidazole	Nucleic acid synthesis	Damages nucleic acid structure	+	
Quinolones	Nucleic acid synthesis	Inhibit DNA gyrase	+	
Sulfonamides	Nucleic acid synthesis	Competes with para-aminobenzoic acid, thereby blocking formation of thymidine and purines		+

SUSCEPTIBILITY, RESISTANCE, AND ANTIBACTERIAL SPECTRA

Appropriate antimicrobial therapy is based on the results of laboratory tests and validated by the clinical effect of treatment. Test results and treatment are not always consistent: Patients who have excellent or intact host defenses may recover from infection irrespective of whether the antibiotic they receive has an effect on the infecting agent. Nevertheless, in a serious deep-seated or bloodstream infection, laboratory tests do provide an invaluable guide to the selection or adjustment of therapy. Usually a microbe is considered susceptible to an antibacterial agent if it can be inhibited or killed by a concentration of the drug that is realistically achievable at the site of the infection. The levels of drug that must be achieved in the host vary, depending on the site of infection, and could be limited by toxic side effects. A common practice is to set the range of susceptibility at or above realistically achievable blood levels, but there are some notable exceptions. For instance, some agents like nalidixic acid or nitrofurantoin are rapidly excreted in the urine, and only very low blood levels are achieved. Low doses of drugs that are effective for some infections are totally inadequate for deep-seated infections. The best example is the relatively low dose of benzyl penicillin G that is required to cure pneumococcal pneumonia, sometimes less than 100,000 units of penicillin per day, which contrasts with the dose of approximately 20 million units per day that may be necessary to treat pneumococcal endocarditis or meningitis. With aminoglycosides the levels for effective therapy of bloodstream infections have been projected to be in the range of 4 to 6 μg per milliliter of gentamicin or tobramycin, and such concentrations are usually accepted as the upper boundary for susceptibility in vitro. However, it is clear that the peak levels of aminoglycosides like gentamicin and tobramycin are sustained for less than an hour. Nonetheless, that period seems sufficient to achieve rapid killing of many bacterial strains.

Many methods have been introduced to determine the susceptibility of bacteria to antimicrobials in vitro. They have been best standardized for rapidly growing organisms. The most common involve measuring inhibition of growth in a broth medium or around an antibiotic-impregnated disc placed on the surface of agar containing the test strain (disc diffusion test). By varying drug concentrations in a series of test tubes or wells, the broth dilution test yields quantitative data on the drug concentration required to inhibit the organism, the minimum inhibitory concentration, or MIC (usually expressed in micrograms per milliliter). Subcultures of broth media make it possible to determine the concentration of drug that kills the test strain—the minimum bactericidal concentration, or MBC. In the disc diffusion test, only growth inhibition can be determined, but the diameter of the zone of inhibition usually correlates inversely with the MIC. The two methods give generally similar results (with the disc test being perhaps somewhat easier to perform), and for most infections susceptibility results based on inhibitory measurements are satisfactory. In treating endocarditis, meningitis, and septicemias occurring in immunocompromised hosts, MBC data on infecting isolates are desirable. Bactericidal activity appears to be a requisite for cure of enterococcal endocarditis, as penicillin G or ampicillin inhibits but does not kill this group of organisms. The phenomenon of "tolerance" has also been observed: a wide discrepancy, 32-fold or more, between MIC and MBC. Some investigators believe that strains of staphylococci isolated from patients with endocarditis or osteomyelitis that prove to be tolerant to penicillins or vancomycin should be treated with the addition of gentamicin or rifampin, but this policy remains controversial.

Table 291–2 summarizes the susceptibilities of clinically important gram-positive and gram-negative bacteria in vitro and indicates agents of choice and alternative therapies. The darkened squares (resistant or not indicated) may include drug-pathogen combinations for which clinical evidence fails to support an effect in vitro. Susceptibility testing in vitro is needed because no one agent is predictably effective against all categories of bacteria and because of the increasing incidence and changes in patterns of resistance. There are a few exceptions to this dogma, such as the uniform susceptibility of group A streptococci to penicillin. On the other hand, relative resistance (intermediate susceptibility) of pneumococci to penicillin G may be increasing, and it is advisable to test blood and cerebrospinal fluid (CSF) isolates.

Antimicrobial resistance may be absolute, in which case increasing the concentration of the agent has no effect, and relative, in which case it may be overcome by dose augmentation. The basis and mechanisms of resistance have become complex, and the simplest approach is to consider (a) the genetic basis for resistance and (b) the actual mechanisms involved. Chromosomal alterations or mutations were the first basis for resistance recognized. These occurred at a relatively predictable rate. Subsequently, a much more common genetic basis has emerged: Plasmids or extrachromosomal DNA elements include R-factors or genetic elements that encode for synthesis of enzymes that functionally inactivate or modify antibiotics. The rapid spread of resistance in some hospital and community settings has been related to acquisition of plasmids by the process of conjugation among gram-negative bacilli and transduction by phages among gram-positive cocci. The mechanisms of resistance are summarized in Table 291–3. The most familiar are the beta-lactamases that hydrolyze to varying degrees agents possessing the beta-lactam ring (penicillins, cephalosporins, monobactams). A great variety of these have been described, occurring in both cocci and bacilli and having both a constitutive and an inducible nature. The latter poses real problems in laboratory diagnosis, as organisms that are initially thought to be susceptible (like *Enterobacter* species) may harbor inducible enzymes. Beta-lactamases may be of either chromosomal or plasmid origin and are usually responsible for high-level resistance that cannot be overcome by dosage escalation. Inactivation can destroy the usefulness of drugs outside the beta-lactam class. A growing number of R-factor–encoded enzymes have been identified that can modify aminoglycosides by the addition of an adenyl, acetyl, or phosphorylating group to hydroxyl or amino groups on the drug structure. These additions create a sterically altered molecule with ablated or reduced antibacterial activity. Conversely, the design of innovative new antimicrobial agents that prove invulnerable to inactivating enzymes involves further modifications of antibiotic structures that can block the access of inactivating enzymes to target sites. In this sense, the development of new aminoglycosides is analogous to the substitutions that protect the beta-lactam ring from hydrolysis and yield the antistaphylococcal penicillins.

One of the most worrisome mechanisms of resistance involves the ability of bacteria to exclude antimicrobial agents from the cell. Aminoglycosides are actively transported into bacteria, but high-level, multiresistant strains seem to be impermeable to all aminoglycosides. These appear to arise from chromosomal mutation and are selected by aminoglycoside use. The active transport system for aminoglycosides is oxygen dependent. This probably explains the lack of effect of aminoglycosides on anaerobic bacteria, since anaerobic conditions impair the activation of the transport system.

Another type of enzymatic resistance is illustrated by organisms that have acquired a plasmid-encoded "bypass" enzyme that subverts the metabolic block of the sulfonamides.

To have an effect, antibiotics that resist hydrolysis or modification must enter the bacterial cell and reach their target site. Target site alteration explains sudden high-level streptomycin resistance (30S ribosomal subunit) or erythromycin resistance (50S ribosomal subunit). The basis for these changes appears to be chromosomal mutations. A similar basis is postulated for alterations in penicillin-binding proteins, which can result in both low- and high-level resistance.

The indiscriminate use of antimicrobial agents generally favors the emergence of resistance. Antibiotics are not mutagens and do not "create" resistant bacteria. Rather, usage selects for strains that are resistant by virtue of chromosomal mutations or spread of plasmids among the bacterial population. Emergence of resistance during treatment is common with some gram-negative rods such as *Serratia* and *Pseudomonas*. This phenomenon must be distinguished from superinfection, in which a new and usually resistant pathogen becomes a secondary invader. Superinfection may be a consequence of prolonged high-dose therapy and may be avoided by use of narrow-spectrum agents in doses that are not excessive.

Laboratory conditions for testing antibacterial agents may differ strikingly from conditions in vivo. In clinical situations the rates of growth of bacteria may be slow, thus affecting the rapidity with which cell wall–active drugs can work. More important, blood and tissue concentrations fluctuate with frequency and method of dosing, and the concentration of drug at the active site of infection may differ from that in body fluids that are more easily sampled. The distribution of agents even within the same class can vary considerably, as they may be metabolized, inactivated, and eliminated by different pathways. Such factors have a crucial effect on the size of doses, the interval between dosing, and possible drug toxicity. Also, the properties of the infecting agent may affect dosing. After exposure of bacteria to an antibiotic, a certain proportion of the population is killed or inhibited, and there may be a significant lag time before multiplication of bacteria resumes after the drug concentration falls. This time interval for regrowth has been called the "postantibiotic effect." For different organisms and with different antibiotics, there may be varying postantibiotic effects. Thus, intermittent dosing of agents may be quite feasible if there is rapid killing and a long postantibiotic effect. Some of the more recalcitrant organisms like *Pseudomonas* regrow rapidly after exposure to antipseudomonal penicillins, and there is very little postantibiotic effect. This argues for more frequent or even continuous dosing, but for the great majority of clinical situations the latter has proved impractical, and the clinical superiority of continuous dosing has not been established.

Table 291–4 summarizes the recommended doses and some pharmacologic data on most of the commonly used agents. Tissue penetration is linked to serum protein binding. The quantity of drug that diffuses into a site of infection is related to the "peak" or maximum serum concentration of free or unbound drug and the duration that the maximum level is maintained. On the other hand, therapeutic outcome does not always correlate with protein-binding affinity, probably because protein binding is usually easily reversible. Lipid solubility of an antibiotic is another factor affecting tissue penetration and influences the ability of an agent

TABLE 291–2. SUSCEPTIBILITIES OF CERTAIN BACTERIA TO SELECTED ANTIBIOTICS

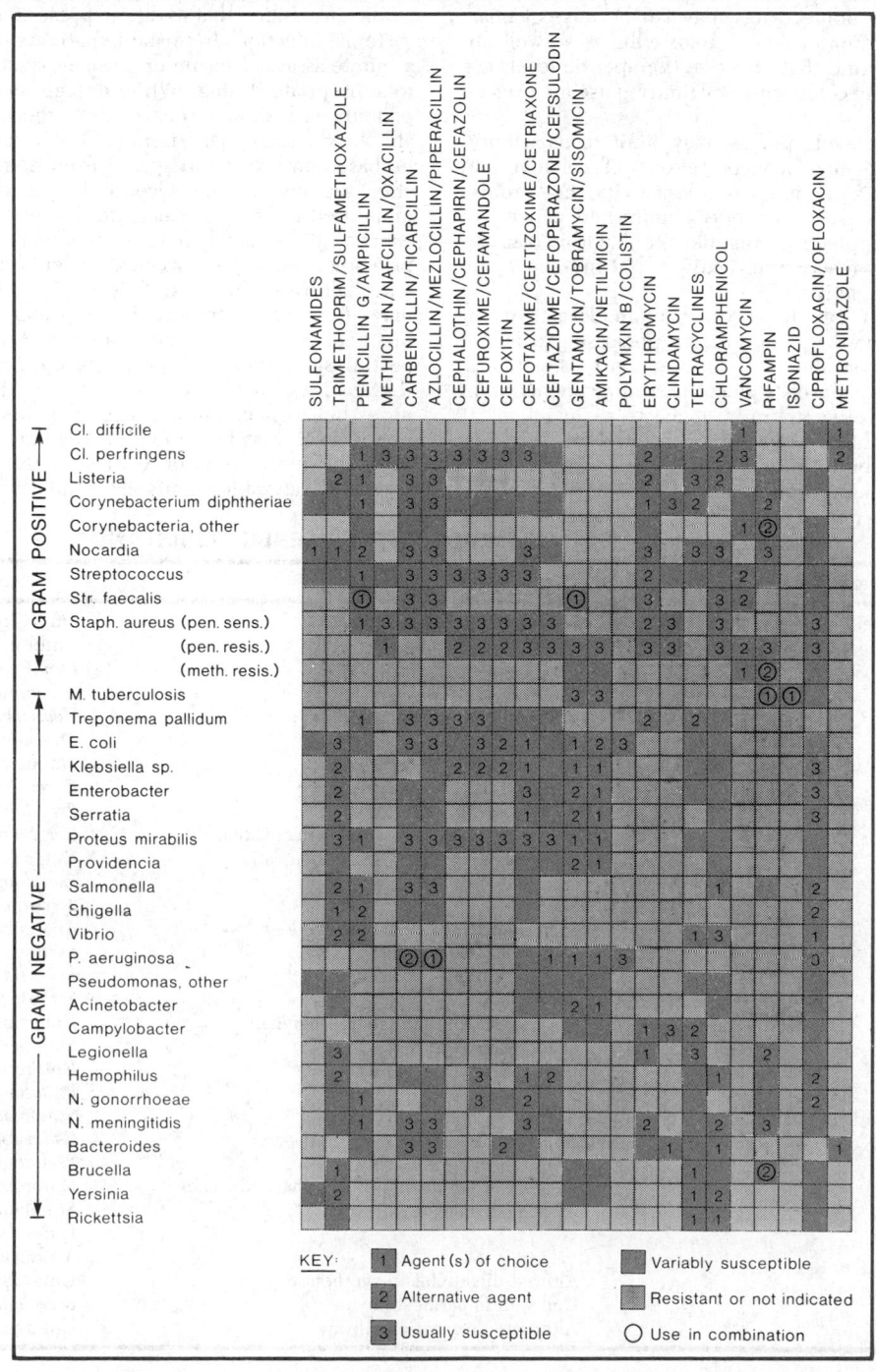

to pass through membranes by nonionic diffusion. Penetration of drug into the spinal fluid is related not only to the drug itself but also to the degree of inflammation in the meninges. Lipid-soluble agents such as chloramphenicol, isoniazid, rifampin, sulfonamides, and metronidazole penetrate spinal fluid well. Aminoglycosides, amphotericin B, and polymyxins do not penetrate well even in the face of inflammation. Penicillins and vancomycin generally penetrate CSF when inflammation is present. Most antibiotics commonly used are excreted primarily through the kidney, but notable exceptions include erythromycin and chloramphenicol. Thus, it may be possible to treat infections of the urinary tract with doses smaller than are required for serious systemic disease, because high urine levels are achieved with most agents. Urine and bile regularly contain higher concentrations of antibiotics than does serum. Penicillins and tetracyclines are concentrated in bile, but aminoglycosides enter bile less well, particularly when liver disease or obstruction is present. Drugs like tetracyclines and clindamycin diffuse readily into bone and have been used successfully in osteomyelitis. Agents that enter prostate tissue well include quinolones, trimethoprim, erythromycin, and doxycycline. Some drugs may fail because of pharmacokinetic properties. For instance, amoxicillin is so well absorbed in the small intestine that effective therapeutic levels are usually not achieved in the colon, thereby limiting use for *Shigella* infections.

Factors besides drug levels per se may limit drug activity. Purulent secretions and high concentrations of calcium and magnesium ions antagonize aminoglycoside activity. Erythromycin and aminoglycosides have markedly diminished activity in acidic environments. Cephalosporins like cephalothin can be metabolized to relatively inactive derivatives, but metabolites of cefotaxime are still quite active.

There is evidence that a high ratio of bactericidal activity in serum (e.g., serum diluted 1:8 or greater possessing a killing effect) against infecting strains is associated with therapeutic success. Such activity may merely reflect the serum concentration required to achieve effective therapy at a site of infection. It should not be assumed that a given dose corrected for weight or body surface area reliability produces the same levels in all patients. With agents like aminoglycosides that are potentially

toxic, therapeutic monitoring is clearly indicated during serious systemic infection. For example, gentamicin peak (postinfusion) levels should exceed 4 μg per milliliter, and trough (or "valley") levels should be less than 2 μg per milliliter. Route of administration is important, since orally administered drugs may be poorly absorbed in serious systemic infections. For patients who are in shock, intramuscular or subcutaneous injections should clearly be avoided, and all medications should be given intravenously.

MODIFICATION OF DRUG DOSES IN RENAL AND HEPATIC FAILURE

Since the majority of antibiotics are excreted via the kidney, dosage adjustment must be considered in moderate to severe renal failure. Many studies have related serum creatinine level or creatinine clearance to degree of dosage modification, and useful nomograms have been derived that may aid in the calculation of dosage. Table 291–4 indicates the agents affected by renal failure and dialysis. Many of these guidelines have been derived by study of patients who are in the "steady state," i.e., patients in renal failure who are on dialysis programs but who may not be infected. Thus, they may not manifest the hemodynamic instability that is often present in patients with serious systemic infection. In unstable patients, there is no substitute for accurate assays of serum or plasma drug concentrations as a guide to appropriate dosing. While dosage modification is indicated in patients with serious renal failure, the initial doses should probably be the same. The timing of the second dose should probably be based on levels anticipated from nomograms, but peak levels after the end of the second dose and third dose should be monitored in order to calculate the next doses. Increased trough concentrations may help to warn of incipient toxicity. As a general principle, many pharmacologic agents are given every three to four half-lives. In renal failure these half-lives are prolonged many-fold. One strategy is to prolong the interval between maintenance doses, which can result in fairly high "peak" or postinfusion levels and rather prolonged (and occasionally subtherapeutic) troughs. Another strategy is to give more frequent doses but to decrease the size of maintenance doses. Subtherapeutic levels may be avoided by the latter tactic, but the approach could be more nephrotoxic (as in the case of aminoglycoside agents). Dialyzable agents are similarly cleared by peritoneal or

TABLE 291–3. MECHANISMS OF ANTIBACTERIAL RESISTANCE

Antimicrobial Agent	Mechanisms	Representative Organisms
Beta-lactams (penicillins, cephalosporins, carbapenems, monobactams)	Destruction by beta-lactamase	*Staphylococcus aureus*
		Enterobacteriaceae
		Pseudomonas aeruginosa
		Haemophilus influenzae
	Alteration of penicillin-binding proteins	*Neisseria gonorrhoeae*
		Streptococcus pneumoniae
		Staphylococcus aureus
	Cell wall impermeability	*Enterobacter* species
		Pseudomonas aeruginosa
Aminoglycosides	Enzymatic modification by *N*-acetylation, *O*-phosphorylation, or *N*-adenylation	*Staphylococcus aureus*
		Enterobacteriaceae
		Pseudomonas aeruginosa
		Streptococcus faecalis
	Membrane transport O$_2$ dependent	Anaerobes
	Cell wall impermeability	*Pseudomonas aeruginosa*
		Serratia species
		Streptococcus faecalis
	Altered 30S ribosome (streptomycin)	Enterobacteriaceae
Chloramphenicol	*O*-acetylation	*Staphylococcus aureus*
	Cell wall impermeability	Enterobacteriaceae
		Pseudomonas aeruginosa
Erythromycin, clindamycin	Alteration of 23S RNA	*Staphylococcus aureus*
Quinolones	Altered DNA gyrase	Enterobacteriaceae
	Cell wall impermeability	*Pseudomonas aeruginosa*
Tetracyclines	Decreased permeation plus enhanced removal	Enterobacteriaceae
Sulfonamides	Altered thymidylate synthetase	*Staphylococcus aureus*
		Enterobacteriaceae
		Neisseria gonorrhoeae
Trimethoprim	Altered dihydrofolate synthetase	Enterobacteriaceae
	Cell wall impermeability	*Pseudomonas aeruginosa*
	Alternate enzymatic pathway	Enterococci

TABLE 291–4. DOSAGE, PHARMACOLOGIC FACTORS, AND ADJUSTMENT IN RENAL AND HEPATIC FAILURE

Class/Agent	Dose — Systemic Infection	Dose — Oral	Protein Binding (%)	Normal Serum Half-Life (hr)	Dose Adjustment — Hepatic Failure	Dose Adjustment — Renal Failure	Serum Levels Affected by Dialysis
Aminoglycosides							
Amikacin	5–7 mg/kg/q8	—	0	2–3	No	Major	Yes
Gentamicin	1.7 mg/kg/q8	—	0	2–3	No	Major	Yes
Netilmicin	1.7 mg/kg/q8	—	0	2–3	No	Major	Yes
Tobramycin	1.7 mg/kg/q8	—	0	2–3	No	Major	Yes
Antifungal Agents							
Amphotericin B	0.7–1 mg/kg/d	—	90	24	No	No	No
Flucytosine	40 mg/kg/q6	Yes	10	3	No	Major	Yes
Ketoconazole	6 mg/kg/d	Yes	98	8	Avoid	No	No
Miconazole	5 mg/kg/q6–8	—	92	2.2	Avoid	No	No
Antituberculous Agents							
Ethambutol	15 mg/kg/d	Yes	10	1.5	No	Major	Yes
Isoniazid	5 mg/kg/d	Yes	10	3	Yes	Minor	Yes
Rifampin	10 mg/kg/d	Yes	70	3	Yes	Minor	No
Cephalosporins							
Cefaclor	7 mg/kg/q6	Yes	20	1	No	Yes	Yes
Cefamandole	30 mg/kg/q6	—	70	1	No	Yes	Yes
Cefazolin	15 mg/kg/q6	—	80	2	No	Major	Yes
Cefotetan	30 mg/kg/q12	—	85	3	No	Major	Yes
Cefoxitin	30 mg/kg/q6	—	70	0.7	No	Yes	Yes
Cephalothin	30 mg/kg/q6	—	70	0.7	Minor	Yes	Yes
Cephalexin	7 mg/kg/q6	Yes	15	1	No	Yes	Yes
Cefoperazone	30 mg/kg/q8–12	—	90	2	Some	Minor	Yes
Cefotaxime	30 mg/kg/q6	—	50	1.2	Some	Minor	Yes
Cefsulodin†	30 mg/kg/q6–8	—	20	1.6	No	Major	Yes
Ceftizoxime	30 mg/kg/q6–8	—	50	1.3	No	Minor	Yes
Ceftriaxone	30 mg/kg/q12–24	—	90	8	No	Yes	Yes
Ceftazidime	30 mg/kg/q8	—	60	2	No	Major	Yes
Moxalactam	30 mg/kg/q8–12	—	50	2	No	Major	Yes
Penicillins							
Amoxicillin	7 mg/kg/q6	Yes	20	1	No	Yes	Yes
Ampicillin	30 mg/kg/q6	Yes	20	1	No	Yes	Yes
Azlocillin	50 mg/kg/q6	—	50	1	Minor	Major	Yes
Carbenicillin	70 mg/kg/q4	—	50	1	Minor	Major	Yes
Cloxacillin	7 mg/kg/q6	Yes	95	0.5	Minor	Minor	Yes
Dicloxacillin	7 mg/kg/q6	Yes	97	0.5	Minor	Minor	No
Methicillin	30 mg/kg/q4–6	—	30	0.5	No	Minor	No
Mezlocillin	50 mg/kg/q6	—	50	1	No	Major	Yes
Nafcillin	30 mg/kg/q4–6	—	90	0.5	Yes	Minor	No
Oxacillin	30 mg/kg/q4–6	—	90	0.5	Yes	Minor	Yes
Penicillin G	0.3–4 million U q4–6	Yes	60	0.5	No	Yes	Yes
Penicillin V	7 mg/kg/q6	Yes	80	1	No	Minor	Yes
Piperacillin	40 mg/kg/q6	—	50	1	Minor	Major	Yes
Ticarcillin	40 mg/kg/q4–6	—	50	1	Minor	Major	Yes
Quinolones							
Ciprofloxacin	10 mg/kg/q12	Yes	30	3	No	Major	Yes
Nalidixic acid	15 mg/kg/q6	Yes	90	1.5	No	Avoid	No
Norfloxacin	6 mg/kg/q12	Yes	15	3	No	Major	No
Tetracyclines							
Chlortetracycline	7 mg/kg/q6	Yes	50	5	Avoid	Avoid	No
Demeclocycline	7 mg/kg/q12	Yes	50	10	Avoid	Avoid	Yes
Doxycycline	1.5 mg/kg/q12–24	Yes	90	15–20	No	No	No
Minocycline	3 mg/kg/q12–24	Yes	90	15	Avoid	Avoid	No
Oxytetracycline	7 mg/kg/q6–12	Yes	35	8	Avoid	Avoid	No
Tetracycline HCL	7 mg/kg/q6	Yes	50	7	Avoid	Avoid	No
Sulfonamides							
Sulfadiazine	15 mg/kg/q6	Yes	50	3	Avoid	Major	Yes
Sulfamethoxazole	12 mg/kg/q8	Yes	50	6	Avoid	Major	Yes
Trimethoprim (used with above)	2.3 mg/kg/q8–12	Yes	60	10	No	Major	Yes
Sulfisoxazole	15 mg/kg/q6	Yes	50	6	Avoid	Major	Yes
Other Agents							
Aztreonam	30 mg/kg/q8	—	60	2.0	No	Major	Yes
Chloramphenicol	7–15 mg/kg/q6	Yes	30	1.5	Some	Minor	Yes
Clindamycin	7 mg/kg/q6	Yes	90	2.5	Some	Minor	No
Colistin	2 mg/kg/q12	—	0	5	No	Avoid	No
Erythromycin	7 mg/kg/q6	Yes	20	1.5	Some	No	No
Imipenem	7.5 mg/kg/q6	—	15	1	No	Avoid	Yes
Metronidazole	15 mg/kg/q6	Yes	20	8	No	No	Yes
Nitrofurantoin	1 mg/kg/q6	Yes	60	0.3	No	Avoid	No
Polymyxin B	1.5 U/kg/q12	—	0	5	No	Avoid	No
Spectinomycin	30 mg/kg	—	0	2	No	Avoid	No
Vancomycin	7 mg/kg/q6	Yes*	10	6	No	No	No

*Not systemically absorbed.
†Not available in the United States.

extracorporeal hemodialysis. Following dialysis, a dose approximately two thirds to three quarters of a maintenance dose should be given, depending upon the degree of removal of the antibiotic by dialysis and the timing of the previous maintenance dose.

Several important antibiotics are metabolized in the liver and are partially excreted in the bile. Agents primarily metabolized by the liver include the sulfonamides, chloramphenicol, and tetracycline. There is usually little reason to alter the dose of penicillin, cephalosporins, and aminoglycosides in patients with liver disease. Even with erythromycin, ethambutol, and clindamycin, there is little evidence that dosage reduction is necessary except in severe hepatic failure. For instance, clindamycin should probably be reduced to half-normal doses after 2 to 3 days of treatment. Chloramphenicol total dosage should be restricted to 1.5 to 2.0 grams per day (adult), and erythromycin should be reduced to perhaps one-half the normal dose after 2 to 3 days of treatment. Drugs to be avoided in hepatic failure include sulfonamides and tetracyclines.

COMBINATION ANTIMICROBIAL THERAPY

Use of combinations of antibacterial agents is exceedingly common. The rationale for their use may be summarized as follows: (1) Prior to the identification of pathogens infecting critically ill subjects, combinations offer a broader, more comprehensive antibacterial spectrum than does a single agent. (2) Use of a drug combination may eradicate an infection that cannot be cured by a single agent, such as the effect of penicillin on enterococci. Addition of an aminoglycoside or a potentiating agent such as rifampin may result in bactericidal activity at a deep-seated focus of infection, as in endocarditis. (3) Combinations are indicated in the treatment of mixed infections, since not all of the pathogens may be susceptible to a single agent. (4) Combinations may decrease the opportunity for emergence of resistance. This has been best documented in tuberculosis. (5) Combinations may interact additively or synergistically against infecting organisms. As a result, there may be an enhancement of antibacterial activity and/or enhanced rate of killing. The latter may lead to more rapid clearing of infection with reduction in duration of therapy. Combinations may permit the use of a lower dosage of one or more components of the regimen, particularly the more toxic component, thereby avoiding undesirable side effects. More rapid killing or greater potency in vivo may be more directly beneficial in patients with impaired host defenses. Some clinical studies suggest an improved clinical response not only when drugs used to treat endocarditis interact synergistically but also in sepsis occurring in immunocompromised patients.

The converse of synergism is antagonism between antimicrobial agents. This is best described for combinations of bactericidal plus bacteriostatic agents. Penicillin-type drugs require cell growth to exert their lethal effect. When penicillins are combined with static drugs like tetracycline, only growth inhibition may result. Clinical studies in humans indicate poorer results in treatment of pneumococcal meningitis with penicillin plus tetracycline than with penicillin alone.

Empiric therapy is presumptive or "blind" therapy given when the clinical severity of a likely infection dictates that treatment be started. It is not necessarily combination therapy, as some single agents can still be quite effective. Intelligent choices in the absence of microbiologic information can be made based on the clinical syndrome and the likely infecting pathogen. Epidemiologic factors as well as host factors enter into the decision. The setting in which the patient develops infection or a prior exposure or travel history can be of considerable value. Pneumonias contracted outside the hospital are usually due to streptococci (and pneumococci) and penicillin-sensitive anaerobes. An "atypical" or diffuse pattern raises the likelihood that community-acquired pneumonia will be better treated with erythromycin than penicillin. Infections that occur in the nosocomial setting or in markedly neutropenic patients should always be initially treated with therapy directed against gram-negative bacilli.

Table 291–5 summarizes recommendations for initial empiric therapy by clinical syndrome.

SPECIFIC ANTIMICROBIAL AGENTS

Table 291–2 summarizes recommended choices of antimicrobial agents for specific infecting agents. The organisms are divided into gram-positive and gram-negative isolates, and antimicrobial agents that are similar are grouped together. Clearly, such a table oversimplifies the appropriate choices for various agents. In some situations, there is no clear-cut agent of first choice, and any member of a class may be appropriate. Differences in pharmacology, cost, and side effects might lead to a selection of one agent in preference to another. There is an increasing divergence in antibacterial spectrum among the newer beta-lactam agents, such as the antipseudomonal penicillins and the third-generation cephalosporins. Among the aminoglycosides, anticipated efficacy may be expressed as follows: While gentamicin and tobramycin remain the most widely prescribed, gram-negative bacilli that are resistant to these agents are more likely to be inhibited by netilmicin and amikacin.

Few oral agents are listed in Table 291–2, but it may be inferred that any of the oral antistaphylococcal agents, such as cloxacillin or dicloxacillin, could be used to treat mild infections due to penicillinase-producing staphylococci. The spectrum of oral cephalosporins such as cephalexin or cephradine mimics that of cephalothin or cefazolin. In the case of group A hemolytic streptococci, it would not be necessary to test for susceptibility of these organisms against penicillin G and related penicillins in vitro, since all would be expected to be susceptible. It would, however, be highly desirable if one were to use a penicillin against the *Klebsiella* species to test that penicillin for susceptibility in vitro; it should probably not be presumed that antibiotics such as piperacillin or mezlocillin will be effective in vitro and in vivo without specific testing. Some agents should always be used in combination to treat serious bloodstream or systemic infections, such as antituberculous therapy (isoniazid plus at least one other agent) or enterococcal sepsis with or without endocarditis (the combination of either a penicillin or a vancomycin with an aminoglycoside). Older agents of the aminoglycoside class, such as streptomycin or kanamycin, are no longer widely used because their activity is more comprehensively covered by newer drugs (gentamicin and amikacin). The exception to this might be in the conventional treatment of disease caused by *Mycobacterium tuberculosis*, for which streptomycin is still indicated.

Sulfonamides and Sulfa-Containing Combinations

Sulfonamides were the first chemotherapeutic agents to be introduced into wide clinical use. They are bacteriostatic and previously were quite active against many gram-positive and gram-negative organisms. They are, however, no longer among the first choices for serious systemic infections, the exception being *Nocardia asteroides* infections. Sulfonamides remain effective therapy for coliform organisms causing community-acquired urinary tract infections, but they are unreliable against hospital-acquired microorganisms. More commonly used to treat a wide variety of more serious bacterial infections is the fixed combination (1:5) of trimethoprim and sulfamethoxazole. Synergism in vitro against many enteric bacteria can be demonstrated with this combination, yet trimethoprim is a highly active agent itself. A major argument in favor of continued use of the fixed combination is that it may reduce the likelihood of the development of resistance to one component in the pair. Trimethoprim-sulfamethoxazole is usually active against enteric bacteria and *H. influenzae* (including most penicillinase-producing strains), and it has been effective against *Pneumocystis carinii*. The diffusion of trimethoprim into prostate fluid makes it a useful agent in prostatic infections. Central nervous system penetration is good. The oral preparation is well absorbed, although a parenteral form is available for patients in whom gastrointestinal absorption may be erratic. Occasional side effects include neutropenia and all of the dermal and systemic hypersensitivity reactions that have been well associated with sulfonamides.

Penicillin G and Related Agents

The primary spectrum of penicillin G (benzyl penicillin) is gram positive, with such organisms as *Streptococcus pyogenes*, *Streptococcus pneumoniae*, and *Streptococcus viridans* remaining exquisitely susceptible. Procaine penicillin is readily administered intramuscularly, and because of slow absorption, dosing of 600,000 units every 12 hours remains effective therapy for pneumococcal pneumonia. Benzathine penicillin is a long-acting (2 to 3 weeks) agent that is slowly released after intramuscular injection and provides therapeutic levels for streptococcal pharyngitis and some forms of syphilis and prophylactic effect against acute rheumatic fever. For oral use in mild respiratory infections, phenoxymethyl penicillin (V) is acid stable and preferable to penicillin G. In large doses penicillin G is still effective against *Neisseria meningitidis*, most *N. gonorrhoeae*, and anaerobic organisms, including *Clostridium* species, but usually not against strains of *Bacteroides fragilis*. Against enterococci, penicillin G or ampicillin should be used in combination with an aminoglycoside such as streptomycin or gentamicin. Ampicillin may be effective in the treatment of *Salmonella* infections, central nervous system infections due to *Haemophilus* strains, and *Listeria monocytogenes* infections. When used in large doses, penicillin G or ampicillin is effective against a few gram-negative organisms, most notably *Proteus mirabilis* (but not other *Proteus* species). Penicillin G and related penicillins should not be used against the great majority of coagulase-producing staphylococci, most of which now produce beta-lactamases.

Antistaphylococcal Penicillins

The antistaphylococcal penicillins are beta-lactamase–stable and relatively narrow in spectrum. Parenteral preparations include methicillin, nafcillin, and oxacillin. There is little choice among this category of agents in terms of antistaphylococcal activity. There may be some differences in side effects, with methicillin possibly associated with more hypersensitivity nephritis and oxacillin with a greater incidence of abnormal serum elevations of hepatic enzymes. When used in appropriate doses, the central nervous system penetration is probably adequate to treat meningitis. The oral antistaphylococcal agents should not be used to treat serious infections, but mild or moderately severe infections may respond to dicloxacillin or cloxacillin. Combination of antistaphylococcal penicillins with an aminoglycoside or rifampin has been recommended for refractory staphylococcal infections or when the isolates demonstrate tolerance. Coagulase-negative staphylococci may produce beta-lactamase like most coagulase-positive *Staphylococcus aureus* organisms. However, serious infections like prosthetic valve endocarditis are better treated with vancomycin plus rifampin or vancomycin plus an aminoglycoside.

Broad-Spectrum Penicillins and Related Compounds

Although ampicillin and amoxicillin are technically classified as broad-spectrum penicillins, the extended spectrum really only includes *Escherichia coli*, *H. influenzae*, *Salmonella*, and *Shigella* species. Even then, amoxicillin should not be used orally for *Shigella* infections because excellent absorption from the upper gastrointestinal tract results in subtherapeutic levels in the lower gut. Other penicillins like carbenicillin, ticarcillin, mezlocillin, azlocillin, or piperacillin are notable for their activity against *Pseudomonas aeruginosa*, most *Proteus* species, and anaerobic pathogens such as *Bacteroides fragilis*. On a weight basis, car-

benicillin and ticarcillin have relatively weak antipseudomonal activity and so must be used in considerably larger doses than most penicillins, in the range of 18 to 30 grams a day for adults (200 to 400 mg per kilogram). The large sodium load given with such doses may aggravate congestive failure and cause electrolyte abnormalities. While these antipseudomonal penicillins are important agents for serious infections, emergence of resistance and variable stability to beta-lactamases has led to the tendency to combine these agents with an aminoglycoside. They are quite active against the coccal organisms that ampicillin usually inhibits, but none of these agents should be used against coagulase-positive staphylococci. The combination of a beta-lactamase inhibitor (clavulanate) with amoxicillin or ticarcillin confers stability on staphylococcal penicillinase and broadens coverage of some gram-negative bacilli. Other potential uses of extended-spectrum penicillins include treatment of infection caused by *Acinetobacter* species, *Listeria*, and a variety of anaerobes. Like the antistaphylococcal penicillins, their half-life is relatively short, but protein binding is low. Thus, frequent dosing at 4- to 6-hour intervals is usually necessary. Newer antipseudomonal penicillins, such as mezlocillin, azlocillin, or piperacillin, are augmented in their antipseudomonal activity, in the case of the last two approximately six- to eight-fold by weight in comparison to carbenicillin when organisms are tested at low inoculum concentrations. On the other hand, the tendency has been to use smaller doses of these more potent penicillins to avoid the side effects associated with large doses of carbenicillin. The result is that no clear-cut clinical differences have been found between these agents when they are used in combination with aminoglycosides. Some of these newer penicillins, such as mezlocillin and piperacillin, have variable activity against *Klebsiella* species and must be tested prior to use.

Newer compounds that possess a beta-lactam nucleus (and thus are related to the penicillins) include (1) imipenem, an agent with very broad activity against gram-positive and gram-negative bacteria; and (2) monobactams, such as aztreonam. The latter compound is devoid of activity against gram-positive bacteria, but like the third-generation cephalosporins, they are potent agents for treatment of gram-negative bacillary infections.

Cephalosporins

Cephalosporins are structurally related to penicillins, yet there are major differences in activity between these agents in vitro and in vivo. The first cephalosporins, such as cephalothin, cephaloridine, and cefazolin, were effective against penicillinase-producing staphylococci as well as pneumococci and streptococci (except enterococci). Additionally, they offered good activity against several important gram-negative pathogens, such as *E. coli*, *Klebsiella*, and *Proteus mirabilis*. Despite activity in vitro, they are not effective against *Salmonella* and *Shigella* and do not

TABLE 291–5. INITIAL EMPIRIC THERAPY FOR SERIOUS INFECTION

Syndrome	Qualifying Factors	Recommended Treatment
Septicemia	Immunocompromised host	
	Neutrophil count >500 µl	Third-generation cephalosporin or
		Cephalosporin (cefalozin) + aminoglycoside (gentamicin, tobramycin)
	Neutrophil count <500 µl	Piperacillin or ceftazidime + aminoglycoside (amikacin, tobramycin)
	Normal host	
	Urinary source	Ampicillin + gentamicin or third-generation cephalosporin
	Biliary source	Ampicillin + gentamicin or imipenem
	Abdominal or pelvic source	Aminoglycoside + clindamycin or cefoxitin, or broad-spectrum penicillin
	No source	Oxacillin + gentamicin or third-generation cephalosporin
	Neonate or child	
	<48 hr old	Ampicillin + either cefotaxime or ceftriaxone
	>48 hr old	Ampicillin + oxacillin + aminoglycoside
Meningitis	<6 yr	Ampicillin + cefotaxime or ceftriaxone
	>6 yr	Ampicillin, penicillin G, or ceftriaxone
Brain abscess		Penicillin G + cefotaxime or ceftriaxone + metronidazole
Pneumonia	Community acquired	Ampicillin or penicillin G ± erythromycin
	Postinfluenzal	Antistaphylococcal penicillin or cephalosporin
	Postaspiration	Ampicillin or clindamycin
	Nosocomial	Azlocillin or piperacillin + aminoglycoside, or third-generation cephalosporin + aminoglycoside

penetrate the blood-brain barrier. The enormous popularity of these agents appears related to a low incidence of side effects, fairly broad coverage against community-acquired respiratory and urinary tract pathogens, and the availability of both oral and parenteral dosing. Nevertheless, these compounds have not been considered the agents of choice for any serious systemic infections. They have been successfully used to treat patients with a history of mild penicillin-type reactions, such as rash, but not urticaria or anaphylaxis. With the development of newer cephalosporins, the principal advantages of these older compounds (often referred to as "the first generation") have been in prophylactic surgical usage and relatively greater activity against penicillinase-producing *Staphylococcus aureus*.

The so-called "second-generation" cephalosporins offer a few improvements over cephalothin and cefazolin. Cefoxitin is a compound with fairly consistent activity against *B. fragilis*. Cefamandole and cefuroxime lack the anaerobic spectrum of cefoxitin but have modestly improved activity against some gram-negative organisms not inhibited by the first generation, such as *H. influenzae* and *Enterobacter* species. Oral agents include cefaclor, which has greater activity against penicillinase-producing *H. influenzae* than does cephalexin.

The newest cephalosporins (often referred to as "third generation") or structurally related compounds such as moxalactam, a 1-oxy-beta-lactam, have markedly enhanced activity against enteric bacteria as well as variable coverage of *P. aeruginosa*. These compounds are stable against the beta-lactamases of *H. influenzae* and *N. gonorrhoeae* and cross the blood-brain barrier in sufficient concentrations to offer effective therapy for gram-negative meningitis (with perhaps the exception of *P. aeruginosa* infection). Among the agents shown to be effective in gram-negative central nervous system infections are cefotaxime, moxalactam, ceftazidime, and ceftriaxone. Several of these agents have a much longer half-life than first-generation cephalosporins, permitting dosing intervals of 8 to 12 hours. In the case of one agent, ceftriaxone, once-a-day dosing has been possible in some infections because of an 8-hour half-life. The antipseudomonal activity of these compounds is variable; nonetheless, newer antipseudomonal cephalosporins like cefsulodin* and ceftazidime represent some of the most potent antipseudomonal agents introduced into clinical practice, and these compounds appear to be significantly safer than aminoglycosides. Table 291–6 summarizes the relative properties of these agents, as well as selected comments. As a general rule, the increased activity against gram-negative pathogens is also coupled with relatively diminished activity against gram-positive cocci. While the gram-positive, particularly antistaphylococcal, coverage of these agents may be satisfactory for initial therapy, serious staphylococcal disease as well as pneumococcal infection is better and certainly more economically

---

*Investigational drug in the United States.

treated with older beta-lactam agents (e.g., oxacillin, penicillin G, respectively). These agents are also not without serious untoward effects, including the triggering of disulfiram reactions, inhibition of platelet adhesiveness, and hypoprothrombinemia. In many patients with community-acquired and mild to moderately severe nosocomial infections, third-generation cephalosporins offer the potential of effective single-agent therapy. The results in immunocompromised hosts suggest that these compounds may still be more efficacious when combined with aminoglycosides.

Chloramphenicol

Chloramphenicol is an oral or parenterally administered drug whose spectrum makes it useful for a wide variety of bacterial and rickettsial infections. The antibacterial spectrum includes gram-positive organisms such as streptococci and staphylococci, but the agent has not been considered to be one of the more potent antistaphylococcal compounds. It is usually bacteriostatic except against *H. influenzae*, against which it is bactericidal. Many enteric organisms are inhibited by chloramphenicol, but *Pseudomonas* strains are usually resistant. Important therapeutic uses include typhoid fever, central nervous system infections, anaerobic infections, intraocular infections, and serious rickettsial infections. Against *B. fragilis*, it remains one of the most useful agents. On the other hand, chloramphenicol can cause severe hematologic toxicity. In the great majority of individuals receiving courses in excess of 1 week of chloramphenicol, there is a dose-dependent inhibition of erythropoiesis. Some patients, estimated at 1 in 50,000, have developed irreversible aplastic anemia following oral or parenteral dosing. While it remains a highly effective agent in selected situations, there are now a number of very reasonable alternatives to chloramphenicol. The unpredictability of the hematologic toxicity should lead physicians to reserve this agent for serious infections in which there are major indications for avoiding alternative drugs.

The Tetracyclines

Tetracyclines inhibit a wide range of gram-positive and gram-negative bacteria as well as *Mycoplasma* species, but they are not agents of choice for any serious bacterial infections. Their activity against gram-positive organisms is static, and the results do not appear to approach those obtained with bactericidal agents. Gram-negative coverage includes *E. coli* and *Klebsiella* species, but there are major gaps in their spectrum, including *Pseudomonas, Serratia* species, and other serious nosocomial pathogens. Tetracycline may be useful in urinary tract infections, rickettsial infections, mycoplasmal infections, and the prophylaxis or treatment of traveler's diarrhea (caused by toxigenic *E. coli*). Older preparations such as chlortetracycline or oxytetracycline have been supplanted by tetracycline HCl, minocycline, or doxycycline. The last-named two preparations have certain pharmacologic advantages, including less frequent dosing, and doxycycline may be used in renal failure.

TABLE 291–6. THIRD-GENERATION CEPHALOSPORINS AND RELATED COMPOUNDS

Agent	Protein Binding (%)	Peak Serum Levels (μg/ml) After 1 gm IV	Half-Life (hr)	Comments
Aztreonam	60	50	2.0	No activity vs. gram-positive organisms
Cefmenoxime*	77	40	1.0	Weak antipseudomonal activity
Cefoperazone	90	125	2.1	Primary excretion is biliary with little dose adjustment in renal failure
Cefotaxime	38	40	1.1	Good CNS penetration but weak antipseudomonal activity
Cefsulodin*	30	65	1.5	Primarily antipseudomonal activity; not much else
Ceftazidime	20	70	1.9	Potent antipseudomonal activity
Ceftizoxime	30	75	1.4	Potent gram-negative activity except for *Pseudomonas*
Ceftriaxone	85	140	8.0	Very long half-life, good CNS penetration, but poor antipseudomonal activity
Imipenem	15	50	0.9	Broad gram-positive and gram-negative activity
Moxalactam	50	60	2.3	Good anaerobe coverage but associated with coagulopathy

*Not available in United States.
CNS = central nervous system.

Erythromycin

This is the most commonly available member of the class of macrolide antibiotics. Traditionally, erythromycin has been regarded as an agent of second choice for streptococcal and staphylococcal infections, to be used in those patients with history of serious penicillin allergy. In this regard, erythromycin remains a useful agent, but its primary appeal in recent years has been its clinical efficacy against several important new causes of infection, such as *Mycoplasma, Legionella, Chlamydia,* and *Campylobacter* species. Against all of these pathogens, erythromycin can be considered the agent of choice. In serious respiratory infections, erythromycin should be administered parenterally, but this use is associated with a high incidence of phlebitis. The compound is one of the safest of all antimicrobials, but mild gastrointestinal disturbances are common. Several oral preparations are available, but none seems clinically superior.

Clindamycin and Lincomycin

Clindamycin and lincomycin mimic some of the spectrum of erythromycin. Their major advantage over erythromycin is greater activity against anaerobes, particularly *B. fragilis.* Nonetheless, the antianaerobic spectrum of these compounds is not complete. In the treatment of intra-abdominal infections, these agents are usually combined with aminoglycosides for gram-negative coverage. A major problem with clindamycin therapy has been antibiotic-associated diarrhea and pseudomembranous colitis. The incidence and severity of this complication vary, and the problem is not always associated with clindamycin. The development of gastrointestinal symptoms on treatment should be a warning to discontinue use of these agents.

Metronidazole

Metronidazole has long been used for the therapy of trichomoniasis, amebiasis, and giardiasis. Subsequently, it has been found to be a highly effective and bactericidal agent against many anaerobic pathogens, including *B. fragilis.* It is available in both oral and parenteral forms and must be considered the therapy of choice for *B. fragilis* infections involving deep-seated foci, such as heart valves and the central nervous system. Many infections involving anaerobes are mixed processes that also involve aerobic organisms. Because it is almost exclusively active against anaerobic pathogens, metronidazole is usually combined with other antimicrobials. The drug must be metabolized to its active form. Its excellent distribution, rapid bactericidal activity, and penetration in "closed spaces" are appealing characteristics, but it also has the potential of inducing disulfiram reactions and potentiating the effects of warfarin (Coumadin). Metronidazole's carcinogenicity in animals and mutagenicity in bacteria have not been demonstrated in humans, but it seems wise to restrict this agent to use in severe infections.

Rifampin

Rifampin is a semisynthetic derivative of rifamycin B and has been used principally for the therapy of tuberculosis. It is one of the most potent and effective antituberculous agents available, with a spectrum that includes both *M. tuberculosis* and atypical organisms. It has been found to be very active against the wide variety of gram-positive and gram-negative organisms, including staphylococci (both coagulase-positive and coagulase-negative types) and *Legionella* species. The compound is one of the few that have been effective in terminating meningococcal carrier state, and it inhibits methicillin-resistant staphylococci. The principal drawback to the use of rifampin is that almost all microorganisms have the ability to develop resistance rapidly. Therefore, even in tuberculosis this drug must be combined with another active agent. It seems useful as an adjunct to other antibacterial agents, such as in combination with antistaphylococcal penicillins to treat "tolerant" strains in endocarditis and meningitis. It inhibits methicillin-resistant staphylococci but is best used with vancomycin. Another potential advantage has been excellent penetration into phagocytic cells. A disadvantage, however, is its potent ability to induce enzymes that decrease the half-life of a number of other pharmacologic agents, including steroids, sulfonylureas, and digitoxin.

Vancomycin

Initially developed during an intense search for agents active against coagulase-producing staphylococci, this agent acquired a reputation for efficacy as well as toxicity to the eighth cranial nerve and to renal function. More modern preparations of vancomycin do not appear to be strongly associated with these side effects. Indeed, the compound has been used effectively to treat serious infections in patients with renal failure because it is not significantly excreted by the kidneys; prolonged bactericidal activity results from widely spaced doses. The spectrum includes not only *Staphylococcus aureus* but also coagulase-negative staphylococci, *Staphylococcus faecalis* (enterococci), and *Corynebacterium* species. Vancomycin has not been considered an agent of primary choice for *Staphylococcus aureus* but is an effective alternative in the penicillin-allergic patient. In prosthetic valve endocarditis caused by coagulase-negative staphylococci, it is often considered the agent of choice in combination with rifampin or gentamicin or both.

Aminoglycosides

Aminoglycosides are rapidly bactericidal against most of the clinically important gram-negative bacilli, including enteric bacteria and *P. aeruginosa.* Most isolates of *Staphylococcus aureus* are also inhibited by aminoglycosides. The initial compounds of this series, like streptomycin, were also shown to be effective against *M. tuberculosis,* and in combination with a penicillin, either streptomycin or gentamicin offers the best available therapy for deep-seated enterococcal infections. Older agents like streptomycin, neomycin, and kanamycin are considerably less useful today because they appear to be relatively more toxic or have been supplanted by agents with greater activity against *P. aeruginosa.* The contemporary aminoglycosides include gentamicin, tobramycin, netilmicin, and amikacin. The last two compounds offer some advantages in that they are stable to inactivation by some of the plasmid-encoded enzymes that acetylate, adenylate, or phosphorylate the older agents. Thus, amikacin or netilmicin may be preferred to treat infections caused by gentamicin- or tobramycin-resistant strains, but susceptibility testing in vitro is necessary because some isolates may be resistant to all agents within this class. Rapid bactericidal effect and good distribution except for the central nervous system make these highly desirable compounds for the treatment of serious systemic gram-negative infections. Unfortunately, aminoglycosides are toxic to renal function, can cause eighth cranial nerve (both cochlear and vestibular function) and renal damage, and occasionally manifest curare-like effects. Pharmacologically, there is a narrow range between the therapeutic levels achievable by dosing every 8 to 12 hours and levels that are associated with toxicity. Aminoglycoside therapy should be closely monitored by frequent blood level determinations in treating serious infections when large doses are used for prolonged courses. These agents are either additive or often synergistic with beta-lactam compounds against pathogens such as *P. aeruginosa, Serratia* species, and other gram-negative rods. For immunocompromised hosts, aminoglycosides remain an important component of therapy, usually as part of a combination with a beta-lactam agent. Aminoglycosides do not adequately penetrate the central nervous system or bone and are not absorbed via the oral route. They are perhaps overused as topical agents, and in that setting the rapid emergence of resistance has been documented. For prophylaxis in colonic surgery, older aminoglycosides like neomycin or kanamycin may suffice in regimens that transiently suppress the growth of aerobic bowel flora.

Spectinomycin also belongs to the aminoglycoside class and is used exclusively for the treatment of gonorrhea when penicillin-type agents have failed. Such antigonococcal activity is shared by other members of the class.

Polymyxin, Colistin (*Polymyxin E*)

Polymyxin B and colistin (polymyxin E) are closely related cationic polypeptide detergents that bind to the lipoproteins of many gram-negative outer cell membranes. They are rapidly bactericidal in vitro, particularly against *P. aeruginosa* and enteric rods except *Proteus* species and *Serratia.* These agents are without effect against gram-positive organisms. Resistance has rarely emerged on therapy. Because of poor clinical results and nephrotoxic potential, the use of these compounds has decreased markedly. Lack of clinical efficacy could be due to properties of poor diffusion and rapid binding to tissues.

Quinolones

The quinolone group of agents includes older compounds like nalidixic acid and newer, more active agents such as ciprofloxacin, norfloxacin, and ofloxacin. Nalidixic acid has few modern uses and may be regarded as a urinary antiseptic for suppression of chronic infection. The newer quinolones have very broad activity against both gram-positive and gram-negative organisms (including *Mycoplasma* and *Legionella*) and can be administered orally. Their use is best defined for urinary tract infection and gastrointestinal infection. Quinolone therapy for serious systemic infections is justified following defervescence achieved with intravenous antibiotics.

Urinary Antiseptics

Mandelamine, nitrofurantoin, and nalidixic acid are agents that are effective only in urinary tract infections and usually as suppressive therapy in chronic infections. Resistance to some of these compounds may emerge rapidly. They may be useful in situations where the goal is suppression rather than a cure because of unremediable anatomic abnormalities. Gastrointestinal side effects have been commonly associated with each of these preparations. Additionally, the optimum antibacterial effect of mandelamine is at urine pH of less than 5.0, so that additional acidification of the urine with acidic substances is required for efficacy.

DURATION OF THERAPY

There are no easy formulas for determining duration of therapy, although a practical guide is treating for 2 to 4 days after defervescence and resolution of signs of infection. The site of infection, host factors, the nature and antimicrobial susceptibility of infecting organisms, the severity of infections, and the response to treatment should be taken into consideration. For bloodstream infections not accompanied by endocarditis or bone involvement, 10 to 14 days is a usual course of treatment. Most respiratory infections are adequately treated in the same interval. Uncom-

plicated meningitis caused by the meningococcus or pneumococcus is probably adequately treated by 7 to 10 days of high-dose parenteral penicillin G. Endocarditis, deep-seated bone infections, and infections involving prostheses require a minimum 4- to 6-week course of treatment but in some cases more. It is important to remember that signs of inflammation, particularly pulmonary infiltration, may persist long after infecting organisms are killed or contained by host defenses, and delayed resolution of lung infiltrates is not uncommon. On the other hand, deep-seated infections like endocarditis and osteomyelitis may have to be treated for periods long after subsidence of signs of infection. Thus, the decision to continue or stop treatment at the end of an appropriate interval must be based on thorough clinical examination and careful reasoning. Patients with impaired host defenses may require longer therapy than those individuals who are basically healthy. A single dose of an effective antimicrobial agent may be adequate to cure lower urinary tract infection involving the bladder, but a much longer duration, on the order of several weeks, is required to ensure therapeutic success in treatment of intrarenal infection.

FAILURE TO RESPOND TO TREATMENT

One of the most important clinical dilemmas is the persistence of fever and other manifestations of infection after a course of costly and potentially toxic therapy has been started. At the same time that every component in antimicrobial therapy is being reassessed, an alternative explanation for fever, pain, and inflammation must also be sought. For instance, tumors or hypersensitivity reactions can incite febrile reactions. Usually, an interval of 2 to 5 days is necessary to judge the efficacy of treatment. At that point, the following are indicated: (1) assessing the accuracy of the diagnosis of infection; (2) determining if the drug selection is appropriate, and particularly if the dose and mode of administration are responsible for the lack of success of therapy; and (3) searching for (a) presence of anatomic abnormalities, (b) foreign body, (c) undrained abscess, (d) infarction of tissue, (e) development of superinfection, (f) emergence of resistance, or (g) presence of a simultaneous infectious process that is not being treated by antibacterial therapy. If these are unrevealing, a noninfectious origin of fever or drug reaction should be considered.

In the severely immunosuppressed host, fever and signs of infection may persist despite appropriate therapy. In these patients clinical failure of drug treatment is more realistically regarded as host failure; if any improvement is possible in this

TABLE 291–7. UNTOWARD EFFECTS OF SOME ANTIMICROBIAL AGENTS

Target	Agent	Mechanism	Manifestation
Endocrine	Ketoconazole	Altered steroid synthesis	Gynecomastia
	Sulfonamides	Block iodine uptake	Goiter
Gastrointestinal	All agents, especially ampicillin, clindamycin	(1) Altered bowel flora	Diarrhea
		(2) Exotoxin of *Clostridium difficile*	Pseudomembranous colitis
	Isoniazid, rifampin, tetracyclines	Hepatocellular necrosis	Hepatitis
	Neomycin	Villous damage	Malabsorption
Hematologic	Chloramphenicol	(1) Protein synthesis inhibition	Reversible anemia, leukopenia
		(2) Idiosyncratic	Aplastic anemia
	Carbenicillin, others	Inhibition of platelet aggregation	Bleeding
	Moxalactam	Impaired prothrombin synthesis	Bleeding
	Penicillins, many others	Impaired leukopoiesis, thrombopoiesis	Neutropenia, thrombocytopenia
	Sulfonamides	Glucose-6-phosphate dehydrogenase (G6PD) deficiency	Hemolytic anemia
Kidney	Aminoglycosides, polymyxins	Tubular damage	Renal failure
	Amphotericin	Tubular damage	Hypokalemia, renal failure
	Carbenicillin	Na-K exchange	Hypokalemia
	Penicillins	Interstitial nephritis	Renal failure
	Sulfonamides	Tubular crystallization	Renal failure
Nervous	Aminoglycosides	(1) Damage to hair cells of Corti	Deafness
		(2) Vestibular damage	Vertigo
		(3) Neuromuscular blockade	Respiratory arrest
	Isoniazid	Pyridoxine antagonism	Neuropathy
	Penicillins, cephalosporins	Cortical irritation	Seizures
	Polymyxins	Neuromuscular blockade	Respiratory arrest
Pulmonary	Nitrofurantoin	Interstitial inflammation	Fibrosis
Skin	Tetracyclines	Bind to dermal structures	Photosensitivity
	Penicillins, sulfonamides, tetracyclines, others	Allergic reactions	Rash, serum sickness, erythema multiforme

difficult situation, it usually correlates with improvement in underlying disease or the immunologic status of the host. If an infection is documented and responds poorly to initially prescribed treatment, then a change to an alternate regimen is indicated. If signs and symptoms progress or new complications appear in spite of seemingly appropriate treatment, a change in therapy is indicated as well as a search for superinfection or an undiagnosed process such as a viral or fungal infection. One of the greatest clinical dilemmas is presented by the patient in whom drug fever or a hypersensitivity reaction is suspected but in whom discontinuing treatment could be dangerous. In such individuals, it is usually prudent to give alternative medication rather than to stop antibacterial therapy completely.

ANTIBIOTIC TOXICITY AND UNTOWARD REACTIONS

A large proportion of drug reactions are related to antimicrobial agents. As many as 10 per cent of patients receiving penicillins and sulfonamides experience some type of toxic or hypersensitivity reaction. These reactions can be fatal, as in the anaphylaxis associated with penicillin or the aplastic anemia due to chloramphenicol. Table 291–7 summarizes some of the major untoward reactions to antibiotics. The majority of toxic reactions are, however, short lived and reversible. Nephrotoxicity secondary to aminoglycosides may be averted by careful therapeutic drug monitoring. A commonly recognized complication of antibiotic therapy is diarrhea and/or pseudomembranous colitis. This is due to bowel overgrowth by *C. difficile*, which elaborates an exotoxin that is responsible for symptoms. Discontinuation of antibiotic therapy will usually lead to resolution of treatment, but some patients require vancomycin or metronidazole.

Besides anaphylaxis, other hypersensitivity reactions include fever, hemolytic anemia, serum sickness, and a wide variety of dermal reactions that include rash and exfoliation. When serious infection is being treated, mild hypersensitivity reactions may be suppressed by a variety of symptomatic medications. Manifestations of hypersensitivity such as rash may fade despite continued treatment, as is common with ampicillin. The decision to continue therapy in the face of such reactions must be based on severity of infection and the lack of reasonable alternatives. Another issue of great clinical importance that is not fully resolved is the potential cross-reactivity between penicillins and cephalosporins. However, the great majority of patients who have only rash following exposure to penicillin, ampicillin, or related penicillins can be safely treated with cephalosporin compounds. The immediate hypersensitivity-type reactions, such as anaphylaxis, wheezing, and urticaria, should be carefully noted. Patients with a history of immediate reactions to penicillin should not be rechallenged with cephalosporins unless they have life-threatening infections and can be observed under close medical supervision.

MAJOR ANTIBIOTIC DRUG INTERACTIONS

An increasing number of interactions have been reported between antimicrobials, or antimicrobials and other pharmacologic agents that seriously ill patients may be receiving. Some of these are summarized in Table 291–8. Some noteworthy examples include the induction of hepatic enzymes by rifampin, which may hasten the metabolism of other antibiotics or drugs. An unexplored area of drug interactions is that which may involve more than two agents. Penicillins like ampicillin or carbenicillin gradually inactivate aminoglycosides like gentamicin in renal failure, when a long half-life for both types of drugs provides opportunity for complexing between the two classes of agents. While this effect is not apparent when patients have normal renal function, the net effect in patients in renal failure is effectively to lower the levels of circulating aminoglycosides and penicillin.

USE OF TOPICAL ANTIBIOTICS

Topical antibiotics or antiseptics have been commonly applied to burns and open wounds, and they are often incorporated into irrigants. A few studies suggest that topical agents can suppress bacteria in burn wounds and reduce sepsis originating from this source. Some topical antiseptics, such as those that contain iodine, are probably too toxic to inflamed tissues, and their local appli-

TABLE 291–8. IMPORTANT ANTIBIOTIC DRUG INTERACTIONS

Antimicrobial Agent	Interacting Drug	Result
Amphotericin B	Curariform drugs	Increased curare-like effect
Aminoglycosides	Neuromuscular blockers (i.e., tubocurarine, pancuronium)	Additive blockade
	Diuretics: ethacrynic acid, furosemide	Increased ototoxicity
	Antibiotics: amphotericin B	Increased nephrotoxicity
	Carbenicillin/ticarcillin (other penicillins)	Inactivation, resulting in reduced activity
Ampicillin/amoxicillin	Allopurinol	Rash
Cephalosporins (cefamandole, cefoperazone, moxalactam)	Alcohol	Disulfiram reaction
Chloramphenicol	Warfarin	Decreased warfarin metabolism and inhibition of vitamin K–producing gut bacteria, thus increasing prothrombin time
	Phenytoin	Decreased phenytoin metabolism levels
	Oral hypoglycemic agents	Increased hypoglycemia
Isoniazid	Warfarin, phenytoin	Increased risk of toxicity by decreased drug metabolism
	Disulfiram	Psychosis
	Rifampin, para-aminosalicylic acid	Additive hepatotoxicity
	Oral contraceptives	Decreased contraceptive effect
Metronidazole	Alcohol	Disulfiram-like reaction (nausea)
	Disulfiram	Psychosis
Nalidixic acid	Warfarin	Increased prothrombin time
Polymyxins	Curariform drugs	Increased curare-like effect
Quinolones	Theophylline	Increased theophylline blood levels
Rifampin	Warfarin, phenytoin	Decreased warfarin, phenytoin effect
	Isoniazid	Additive hepatotoxicity
	Methadone	Withdrawal symptoms
	Oral contraceptives	Decreased contraceptive effect
	Steroids	Decreased steroid effect
Sulfonamides	Procaine	Decreased sulfonamide effect
	Hypoglycemic agents	Hypoglycemia
	Warfarin, phenytoin	Displace drugs from protein-binding sites, causing increased warfarin and phenytoin effects
Tetracyclines	Antacids, oral iron	Decreased tetracycline absorption

cation should be discouraged. Topically applied antibiotics can provide only surface suppression of microbial flora. They also provide ample opportunity for development of resistance, since large numbers of organisms may be present on injured skin. Antibiotics in irrigants may be irritating, may be absorbed in large quantities so as to cause increased toxicity, and may offer little advantage over irrigation per se.

Bennett WM, Aronoff GR, Morrison G, et al.: Drug prescribing in renal failure: Dosing guidelines for adults. Am J Kidney Dis 3:155, 1983. *A highly practical guide to antibiotic dose reduction in renal failure.*

Hooper DC, Wolfson JS: Drug therapy: Fluoroquinolone antimicrobial agents. N Engl J Med 324:384, 1991. *Succinct review of the most important "new" group of antibiotics.*

Krogstad DJ, Moellering RC Jr: Antimicrobial combinations. *In* Lorian V (ed.): Antibiotics in Laboratory Medicine. 2nd ed. Baltimore, The Williams and Wilkins Company, 1986, pp 537–595. *A laboratory-oriented review with practical guidelines for clinicians.*

Lupski JR: Molecular mechanisms for transposition of drug-resistance genes and other movable genetic elements. Rev Infect Dis 9:357, 1987. *An up-to-date summary of a rapidly changing field.*

Neu HC: β-Lactam antibiotics: Structural relationships affecting *in vitro* activity and pharmacologic properties. Rev Infect Dis 8(Suppl 3):237, 1986. *An important and well-written overview of the single most important group of antibiotics.*

Peterson PK, Verhoef J (eds.): The Antimicrobial Agents Annual. Vol 3. Amsterdam, Elsevier, 1988. *One of the most comprehensive reviews of all major categories of antimicrobial agents.*

Siegenthaler WE, Bonetti A, Luthy R: Aminoglycoside antibiotics in infectious diseases. Am J Med 80(Suppl 6B):2, 1986. *Succinct summary of this group of agents, which remain important in modern antimicrobial chemotherapy.*

Young LS: Empirical antimicrobial therapy in the neutropenic host. N Engl J Med 315:580, 1986. *Summarizes, with relevant references, the debate over the merits of combination antimicrobial therapy versus the use of a single agent for empiric treatment of immunocompromised hosts.*

SECTION TWO / BACTERIAL DISEASES

292 Pneumococcal Pneumonia

Richard J. Duma

DEFINITION. Pneumococcal pneumonia is an acute, suppurative infection of the lungs produced by an encapsulated bacterium, *Streptococcus pneumoniae* (pneumococcus). It is the most commonly occurring bacterial pneumonia in the world; in the United States, an estimated 150,000 to 500,000 cases occur annually.

MICROBIOLOGY. Virulent *S. pneumoniae* organisms are encapsulated, gram-positive cocci about 0.8 μm in diameter that occur in chains (streptococci) or pairs (diplococci) (see Color Plate 9*F*). When in pairs, cocci are characteristically described as lancet shaped; i.e., each coccus is pointed at the end like the tip of a lance, and the bases are in juxtaposition. The capsule, which is a polysaccharide and which varies in thickness from strain to strain, is not seen with Gram stain but may be recognized by negative staining (e.g., with India ink or methylene blue). In purulent clinical specimens, some pneumococci stain negatively rather than positively on the Gram stain, as aging, exposure of the cell wall to a variety of destructive host enzymes (e.g., lysozyme), and/or inhibition of cell wall synthesis by antibiotics (e.g., penicillin) result in incomplete or abnormal bacterial cell walls that no longer retain the iodine-fixed crystal violet stain.

Pneumococci are fastidious, facultative bacteria that grow best in the presence of blood or serum and in air supplemented with 10 per cent carbon dioxide. Since they are fermentative and since lactic acid is the usual end-product, concentrations of glucose must be controlled in the culture media and should not exceed 1 per cent. In addition, since they produce hydrogen peroxide (H_2O_2) but not catalase, the addition of a catalase source (e.g., red blood cells) enhances growth. Viability is reduced by drying, a low pH (<6.5), and prolonged incubation.

On blood agar plates after overnight incubation at 37°C, colonies generally appear mucoid, glistening, and dome shaped and are surrounded by an area of greening (α-hemolysis) within the blood agar. With continued incubation, as aged bacteria undergo autolysis, the colony domes of highly encapsulated strains collapse centrally and appear umbilicated. An important biologic feature that distinguishes *S. pneumoniae* from other streptococci is its bile solubility or susceptibility to surface-active agents, such as sodium deoxycholate and ethyl hydrocuprein chloride (optochin). The latter agent (optochin) is incorporated into a standardized 5-μg disc and is utilized worldwide to identify pneumococci rapidly. However, since optochin-resistant pneumococci occur and since some nonpneumococcal, α-hemolytic streptococci are optochin sensitive, for purposes of species determination, the usefulness of this biologic property may be questioned.

Pneumococcal virulence and pneumococcal pneumonia are often studied in the mouse, since this animal is highly sensitive to encapsulated pneumococci (with the exception of type 14). Indeed, the sensitivity of mice to encapsulated pneumococci may be utilized for rapidly and selectively isolating virulent pneumococci from sputum specimens or from clinical materials containing mixtures of other bacteria. If the specimen in question contains pneumococci and is injected into the peritoneal cavity of the mouse, a peritoneal exudate containing pneumococci may be harvested in 24 hours.

Unlike many other streptococci, particularly those belonging to Lancefield group A, and unlike other pyogenic bacteria that may produce pneumonia, *S. pneumoniae* organisms do not possess or produce any clinically important toxins, and particularly none that are tissue destructive. Some strains may elaborate hyaluronidase, and all contain a hemolysin (pneumolysin O) that produces α- or β-hemolysis on blood agar under aerobic or anaerobic conditions, respectively; however, no clinical importance is assigned to any of these substances, and their values are principally for strain identification purposes.

The most important factor defining virulent *S. pneumoniae* is the presence of a high molecular weight, complex polysaccharide capsule, which is a potent inhibitor of neutrophil phagocytosis. At least 84 different immunogenic types of capsules exist, and two different nomenclatures (Danish and American) are used to number them (which is often a source of confusion). Antigenically distinct capsules are easily identified with polyvalent antisera in an agglutination or precipitin test or by the Neufeld quellung reaction, a rapid test based on visualization of refractile swelling of the capsule after application of a polyvalent or monovalent type-specific antiserum to the bacterium in question. Rough or nonencapsulated pneumococci, which are generally avirulent, do not react with antipolysaccharide antisera. Although the identification of pneumococcal capsular antigen in certain body fluids or secretions may suggest active pneumococcal infection (see below), immunologic tests to detect such antigens must be interpreted with caution, since antibodies against some pneumococcal capsular serotypes cross-react with polysaccharides of other streptococci (particularly group B), *Haemophilus influenzae* type B, *Escherichia coli*, *Klebsiella pneumoniae*, *Salmonella* species, and even human ABO blood group isoantigens.

TABLE 292–1. MIC₉₀ OF SOME COMMONLY USED BETA-LACTAM ANTIBIOTICS AGAINST PENICILLIN-RESISTANT PNEUMOCOCCI

Antibiotic	MIC$_{90}$ (μg/ml)* Intermediate Penicillin Resistance	High-Level Penicillin Resistance
Ampicillin	0.5	8
Oxacillin	4.0	31
Methicillin	—	64
Carbenicillin	32.0	64
Ticarcillin	64.0	128
Piperacillin	1.0	8–16
Mezlocillin	1.0–2.0	8–15
Azlocillin	1.0	16
Cephalothin	1.0	8–31
Cefaclor	4.0–16.0	16
Cefonicid	16.0	16
Cefoxitin	4.0–8.0	32–125
Cefamandole	0.5–2.0	8–31
Cefuroxime	0.25–0.44	—
Cefotaxime	0.125–1.0	1–4
Ceftriaxone	0.12–0.5	1
Ceftazidime	3.2–32.0	64
Cefoperazone	1.0–2.0	2–16
Moxalactam	2.0–4.0	128
Imipenem	0.06–1.0	1–2

*MIC$_{90}$ = Minimal inhibitory concentration at which 90 per cent of strains are susceptible.

Adapted with permission from Klugman KP: Pneumococcal resistance to antibiotics. Clin Microbiol Rev 3:171–196, 1990.

The susceptibility of pneumococci to most chemotherapeutic antibacterials is generally excellent. Noteworthy among antipneumococcal drugs are the beta-lactams, especially penicillins, cephalosporins, cefamycins, and carbapenems (but *not* monobactams). In addition, erythromycins, lincosines (e.g., clindamycin), vancomycin, chloramphenicol, and teicoplanins are effective. For penicillin G, the antibiotic against which all other antipneumococcal agents are compared, *susceptibility* is defined as inhibiting the growth of pneumococci at a concentration of less than 0.1 μg per milliliter (referred to as the *minimal inhibitory concentration*, or MIC). Indeed, the MIC of penicillin G worldwide for the vast majority of pneumococcal strains is predictably 0.1 μg per milliliter or less. However, since 1968, when penicillin-resistant strains were first identified in Australia, a significant per cent (in some studies as high as 10 per cent) of isolates may be moderately or intermediately resistant (i.e., the MIC is 0.1 to <2.0 μg per milliliter), and a small per cent may be highly resistant (i.e., the MIC is ≥ 2.0 μg per milliliter). Isolates that are highly resistant to penicillin G are also usually resistant to a wide array of other antibacterials (Table 292–1), although such bacteria are uniformly susceptible to vancomycin and occasionally to third-generation cephalosporins or carbapenems. The resistance of pneumococci to beta-lactams is *not* due to bacterial production of a beta-lactamase and is *not* plasmid mediated, as is so often the case with most other bacteria (especially gram-negative bacilli), but rather it is chromosomally mediated and appears to result from point mutations that dictate the production of target membrane penicillin-binding proteins (PBP's) with an affinity for penicillin G that differs from that of the PBP's of penicillin-susceptible strains.

Pneumococci are relatively resistant to aminoglycosides; in fact, gentamicin is frequently incorporated into primary culture media for selective isolation of pneumococci from sputum, since it suppresses the growth of concurrent or contaminating bacteria. Similarly, quinolones at low or clinically achievable concentrations are generally ineffective in inhibiting the growth of most pneumococci; further, in some studies, more than 50 per cent of pneumococcal isolates are resistant to tetracyclines.

EPIDEMIOLOGY. Pneumococcal pneumonia is a sporadic disease that occurs most often during the coldest months of the year. The vast majority of such pneumonias occur after aspiration of "normal" oropharyngeal secretions that contain encapsulated pneumococci, followed by an inability to clear such bacteria-containing secretions adequately; thus, oropharyngeal carrier rates of pneumococci are important in understanding the dynamics of acquiring pneumococcal pneumonia, its spread, and its frequency of occurrence within a population.

Since most data referable to oropharyngeal carrier rates come from studies performed prior to the development and distribution of a commercially available pneumococcal vaccine, the prevalence of colonization with (or carriage of) certain serotypes and the relative importance of factors that have an impact on carriage must be interpreted with caution. Nevertheless, since most estimates suggest that only 10 per cent of people at increased risk for pneumococcal pneumonia receive pneumococcal vaccine, and since some studies suggest that the presence of pre-existing, type-specific, circulating serum antibody does not prevent oropharyngeal colonization, prevaccine data on carriage rates are probably applicable and useful.

In longitudinal, prevaccine studies of pneumococcal oropharyngeal carriage by people living in temperate zones, serotypes with USA numbers of 23 or less are most frequently encountered, further suggesting that humans are infected by their own endogenous flora, since more than half the cases of pneumococcal pneumonia and bacteremia are caused by these strains. Clustering of one serotype within a family commonly occurs, and the prevalence of carriage does not appear to be affected by sex. Rates of carriage are higher in children, particularly those of a preschool age, than in adults; and among adults, rates are highest in those intimately exposed to preschool children. Oropharyngeal carriage appears to be highest during the coolest months of the year (fall, winter, and early spring), when respiratory infections are common. Although some studies suggest that respiratory infections do not affect pneumococcal carriage rates, others indicate that the spread of carriage within families occurs in association with the appearance of respiratory tract infections due either to the pneumococcus or to certain respiratory viruses, such as the rhinovirus. Although the prevalence of oropharyngeal carriage in the surrounding community or within households affects the risk of individual acquisition, crowding does not appear to be critical or even important, as is the case with infections by group A streptococci. The duration of oropharyngeal carriage of a particular serotype ranges from 2 weeks to years, the mean being 6 to 8 weeks. Reacquisition of the same serotype with no change in risk factors for acquisition commonly occurs. In children, initial acquisition within a family setting is frequently associated with rises in homotypic serum antibody and occasionally with illness, but in adults, both of these phenomena are observed infrequently.

Although epidemics of pneumococcal pneumonia may occur, they are *rare* and generally appear in special populations known to be at high risk for pneumococcal disease, such as domiciliary populations of alcoholics, institutionalized elderly, Navajo Indians, New Guinea highlanders, Alaskan natives, and South African gold miners.

In studies of ambulatory adult populations, a variety of conditions or specific risk factors appear to predispose to the development of pneumococcal pneumonia (Table 292–2): extremes of age, dementia, seizure disorders (aspiration), cigarette smoking, congestive heart failure, cerebrovascular occlusions or severe neurologic impairments (especially those associated with chronic aspiration and paralysis of respiratory muscles or impaired cough reflex), chronic obstructive pulmonary disease, chronic bronchitis, bronchiectasis, malignancies (particularly solid tumors of the lung), institutionalization, immunologic deficiencies (e.g., of immunoglobulins G [IgG] or A [IgA]), recent viral infections (particularly those caused by myxoviruses, such as influenza), and splenic dysfunction (e.g., sickle cell anemia).

IMMUNOLOGY. In nonimmunized, untreated patients, specific anticapsular humoral antibody (immunoglobulin M [IgM] and immunoglobulin G [IgG]) can be detected in the blood 5 to 10 days after infection and correlates with the clearance of pneumococci and eventual recovery. Complement (C3) and type-specific, opsonizing antibody, principally IgG, enhance phagocytosis by polymorphonuclear leukocytes, the major host defense mechanism for eradicating pneumococci. Patients with deficiencies of biologically active IgM, IgG, and, to a lesser degree, IgA (particularly secretory) are more susceptible to developing pneumococcal pneumonia and other pneumococcal infections than are normal persons without such deficiencies. In normal persons,

TABLE 292–2. RISK FACTORS OR UNDERLYING CONDITIONS PREDISPOSING TO THE DEVELOPMENT OF PNEUMOCOCCAL PNEUMONIA OR SERIOUS PNEUMOCOCCAL INFECTIONS

Age (extremes)
Alcoholism
Bone marrow transplantation
Bronchiectasis
Cerebrovascular occlusions or severe neurologic impairment
Chronic bronchitis
Chronic lymphocytic leukemia
Chronic obstructive pulmonary disease (COPD)
Cirrhosis or chronic liver disease
Complement deficiency (particularly C3)
Conditions associated with aspiration (e.g., seizures)
Congestive heart failure
Dementia
Diabetes mellitus
Immunologic deficiencies (acquired, hereditary, or iatrogenic)—humoral (IgG or IgA) or cellular (e.g., acquired immunodeficiency syndrome [AIDS])
Institutionalization
Malignancy (particularly solid tumors of the lung)
Multiple myeloma
Nephrotic syndrome
Neutropenia
Smoking
Splenic dysfunction (e.g., in sickle cell disease) or asplenia
Viral diseases, especially influenza

once specific anticapsular antibodies form, they generally persist for life.

PATHOGENESIS AND PATHOLOGY. Most cases of pneumococcal pneumonia result from the aspiration of oropharyngeal material containing indigenous, virulent pneumococci into terminal bronchioles and alveoli and then the inability to clear such bacteria adequately from these sites. Although microaspiration is a natural, common event that occurs during sleep, pneumonia seldom results, because pulmonary bacterial clearance and/or local host defense mechanisms are adequate and intact and are not defective or suppressed. These important defense mechanisms, which serve as either a barrier against or a clearance for bacteria, are the epiglottic reflex, ciliary escalator and mucous blanket, secretory and humoral immunoglobulins, surfactant, alveolar macrophage and polymorphonuclear leukocyte activity, and lymphatic drainage. When these mechanisms are blunted or overwhelmed by large volumes of aspirated noxious material, by large inocula of pneumococci, by a highly virulent strain, and/or by material containing additional virulent pathogens, pneumonia may result. After aspiration, atelectasis or bronchiole obstruction (which predisposes to or abets infection) may occur, and infection may follow; once infection follows, further atelectasis from inspissated material may result. These events may be modified by the level of type-specific humoral and/or secretory immunity present in the host.

Once virulent pneumococci establish a base in the lung, the first visible evidence of an inflammatory response is localized capillary dilatation and hyperemia, the appearance of serous edema within alveoli, and margination, diapedesis, and chemotaxis of polymorphonuclear cells induced by immunoglobulins and/or activated complement. Fluid-filled alveoli enhance the passage of bacteria through the pores of Kohn and into terminal bronchioles, with spread to contiguous, uninfected alveoli, forming the advancing margins of the disease. If clearance and host immune mechanisms are adequate at this stage, the infection may resolve. However, if not, the disease may spread further until the pleura and interlobar fissures are reached and consolidation with dense infiltrates of polymorphonuclear leukocytes and extravasated red blood cells occurs (see Color Plates 9A to C).

Pneumococcal pneumonia may involve an entire lobe (lobar pneumonia), multiple lobes (multilobar pneumonia), or just segments of a lobe, producing a patchy area (or areas) of pneumonia (pneumonitis). At times, infection spreads concentrically from bronchi (bronchopneumonia), a pattern occasionally seen in infants and in the elderly. In the central and oldest portions of infection, consolidation with massive numbers of polymorphonuclear leukocytes predominates, while peripheral to this are new areas of hemorrhage, infiltrating polymorphonuclear cells, and edema. Early pathologists referred to these areas in the lung as "gray hepatization" and "red hepatization," respectively, because of the gross resemblance of involved lung to liver tissue (see Color Plate 9A). In fully developed, untreated pneumococcal pneumonia, all stages of the cellular inflammatory process may be present.

In 5 to 10 per cent of patients, infection may extend into the pleural space, resulting in an *empyema*, or in 15 to 25 per cent of patients, bacteria may enter the bloodstream (*bacteremia*) via the lymphatics and thoracic duct. Invasion of the bloodstream by pneumococci may lead to serious metastatic or secondary infections at a number of extrapulmonary sites (Table 292–3), the most important and most frequent of which is the subarachnoid space (*meningitis*). Other infections that may occur from bacteremic spread are *septic arthritis, pericarditis, endocarditis* (infection of the heart valves), and, in patients with ascites, *peritonitis* (*spontaneous bacterial peritonitis*, or SBP). In addition, organs of the sinopulmonary system may be concomitantly and acutely infected by pneumococci; involved structures include the air sinuses (*sinusitis*), mastoids (*mastoiditis*), ears (*otitis media*), conjunctivae (pyogenic *conjunctivitis*), epiglottis (*epiglottitis*, particularly in infants), or rarely the soft tissues of the neck or retropharyngeal area (*Ludwig's angina*).

CLINICAL FINDINGS. The presentation of acute bacterial pneumonia due to *S. pneumoniae* may be highly variable, depending on when the patient presents to the physician in the course of the disease, the patient's age, whether or not effective antibiotics were previously administered, the presence or absence of satisfactory host defenses, and the existence of risk factors for dissemination of pneumococci (e.g., asplenia, neutropenia, and agammaglobulinemia). The presentation may be mild or explosive and rapidly lethal. Classically, the onset of acute pneumococcal pneumonia is sudden and is characterized by an abrupt occurrence of cough, chills, high fever (up to 40°C), myalgias, tachypnea, shallow respirations, tachycardia, weakness, and often frank rigors. Initially, the cough may be productive of scant mucopurulent or blood-streaked sputum; later (after 24 to 48 hours), it may be thick, purulent, frankly bloody or rust-colored, and consistent with an alveolar, hemorrhagic, exudative process. If the infecting pneumococcus is highly encapsulated, a gelatinous, blood-tinged sputum may be seen. The presence of pleuritic pain is specific clinical evidence that the pneumonia is probably bacterial and, in the presence of most of the above findings, pneumococcal.

The patient with pneumococcal pneumonia is generally diaphoretic and, in addition, may be dehydrated and hypotensive. Anorexia, nausea, and vomiting are common. If allowed to continue untreated, single-lobe disease may progress to multilobe involvement, and the patient may become dusky, cyanotic, and confused. If bacteremia occurs, chills and rigors may persist, and rarely shock, a disseminated intravascular coagulopathy (DIC), and/or an adult respiratory distress syndrome (ARDS) may supervene and ultimately lead to the patient's death.

A history is frequently elicited of a recent upper respiratory or viral-like illness that has occurred prior to the appearance of

TABLE 292–3. CONCURRENT OR COMPLICATING PNEUMOCOCCAL INFECTIONS OCCURRING IN PNEUMOCOCCAL PNEUMONIA

Otitis media
Sinusitis/mastoiditis
Conjunctivitis (suppurative)
Epiglottitis
Tracheobronchitis
Pleuritis (empyema)
Soft tissue cellulitis (e.g., Ludwig's angina)
Pericarditis*
Endocarditis*
Meningitis*
Arthritis (septic)*
Peritonitis (in presence of ascites)*

*Usually blood borne.

clinical pneumonia, especially during the winter months, when influenza is common. Risk factors for aspiration, such as alcoholism, seizures, or vomiting, or for acquiring pneumococcal pneumonia, may be present (see above).

On physical examination, the acutely ill patient is tachypneic and may be observed to use accessory muscles for respiration (intercostal, abdominal, and sternocleidomastoid) and even to exhibit nasal flaring. If pleuritic pain is severe, reflex splinting of the ipsilateral thorax is observed. Fever and tachycardia are present, and although hypotension may occur, frank shock is unusual, except in the later stages of infection or if DIC occurs.

Auscultation of the chest reveals bronchovesicular or tubular breath sounds and wet rales over the involved lung. As consolidation occurs, vocal and tactile fremitus is increased; however, if a concurrent pleural effusion is present, breath sounds and fremitus may be diminished or absent. A localized, grating pleural friction rub may occasionally be heard.

Examination of the upper respiratory passages may be helpful in suggesting a diagnosis of pneumococcal pneumonia. For example, in children the absence of an exudative pharyngitis and the presence of otitis media might suggest pneumococcal involvement. In older children and adults, the air sinuses and/or mastoids may be acutely infected. (But this infection can also occur in streptococcal, staphylococcal, and *H. influenzae* pneumonia.)

Evidence of extrapulmonary infections may be present, particularly in untreated disease lasting more than 48 hours; for example, signs of meningeal irritation (stiff neck, Kernig's or Brudzinski's signs) with abnormalities in mentation may suggest meningitis; the appearance of pathologic heart murmurs, splenomegaly, and heart failure may be evidence of endocarditis; or the presence of pain, swelling, tenderness, heat, and possibly redness of one or more joints may point toward a septic arthritis of hematogenous origin.

Additional findings unrelated to pneumonia per se, but related, rather, to sepsis and/or toxicity, may be noted: a paralytic ileus with abdominal pain, distention, and loss of bowel sounds; mild jaundice due to a reactive hepatitis or to intrapulmonary hemorrhage associated with the pathology of the disease; frank shock; purpuric lesions resulting from DIC; or symmetric gangrene and purpura of the fingers and/or toes (*purpura fulminans*) associated with bacteremia.

LABORATORY FINDINGS. The peripheral white blood cell (WBC) count is often two to three times the normal value; however, in alcoholics or immunosuppressed patients, it may be normal or low. Of more value is the WBC differential, which consists predominantly of bands and polymorphonuclear leukocytes (left shift). If DIC is suspected, then thrombocytopenia and pleomorphism of red blood cells (schistocytes and helmet cells) are present and may be seen on the peripheral blood smear, prothrombin and partial thromboplastin times are prolonged, and hypofibrinogenemia and circulating fibrin-split products may be detected.

In some patients, the total bilirubin and hepatic cellular enzyme levels may be slightly elevated. Since dehydration and hypovolemia commonly occur (owing to fever, diaphoresis, nausea, and vomiting), the hemoglobin, hematocrit, and serum sodium level may be elevated. When pneumonia is the dominant clinical event, arterial blood gas studies, which reflect pulmonary function and compensatory events, usually reveal hypoxemia (low Po_2), hypocarbia (low Pco_2), and alkalosis (blood pH above 7.4) resulting from hyperventilation and shunting. However, if frank shock intervenes, a metabolic acidosis may result (blood pH less than 7.4); if it is not corrected, death may follow.

Good posteroanterior and lateral chest roentgenograms are important to obtain (see Color Plate 9D), first to confirm the presence and to ascertain the extent and radiographic character of the pneumonia and second to determine if underlying predisposing pulmonary diseases are present, such as bronchiectasis, bronchial obstruction, emphysema, tumor, or tuberculosis. In severely dehydrated or profoundly neutropenic or immunodeficient patients, early inflammatory infiltrates may not be seen radiographically or may be patchy and irregular in appearance; but after hydration or restoration of circulating levels of inflammatory cells, patterns of lobar consolidation may become apparent.

Characteristically, in immunocompetent patients with untreated, frank pneumococcal pneumonia, chest roentgenograms reveal a lobar distribution and an air space (or alveolar exudative) pattern of disease with an air bronchogram effect. However, if prior, partially effective antibiotic usage has occurred, the pattern may be atypical, and a lobar distribution may be the exception rather than the rule. Interlobar fissures may bulge, owing to considerable fluid content within the involved lung associated with large amounts of capsular material. In severe cases, more than one lobe may be involved (multilobar pneumonia). In 30 per cent of cases, a pleural effusion may be present and may be readily detected by a lateral decubitus film. Such effusions may be sterile and represent parapneumonic collections of fluid, or occasionally they may be infected with pneumococci, in which case they are called *empyemas*.

If blunting of the costophrenic angle is noted radiographically, and the finding is believed to represent an effusion, then at least 300 to 500 ml of fluid is probably present, and a thoracentesis is indicated. Unless contraindicated, *every pleural effusion associated with an acute bacterial pneumonia in which the etiology of the pneumonia is unclear should be tapped and the fluid studied for microorganisms* (see Color Plate 9E). Ordinarily, fluid removed from the pleural space is sterile, so that any bacteria seen on a Gram stain or cultured from the fluid represent pathogens until proved otherwise.

Other important laboratory studies *that must be obtained early in the patient's workup* are routine cultures of the blood, a microscopic examination of a Gram stain and a culture *of purulent material from the site of infection* (alveoli, bronchi, or lung), and an examination of any infected material that can be removed from a secondarily infected extrapulmonary focus. In pneumococcal pneumonia, 15 to 25 per cent of blood cultures may be positive for *S. pneumoniae*. However, the results of blood cultures are generally not available for 18 to 24 hours and thus cannot assist the physician in making a presumptive diagnosis or in initially selecting appropriate chemotherapy. Often, in asplenic patients, a high-grade bacteremia occurs, so that examination of the peripheral WBC smear or of the buffy coat for pneumococci may be useful.

Microscopic examination and cultures of expectorated purulent sputum from a patient with acute bacterial pneumonia are essential if a correct presumptive etiologic diagnosis is to be made and an appropriate antibiotic is to be given. Ideally, these tests should be done before therapy is initiated; however, a significant delay in instituting therapy should not be permitted. Attention must also be given to obtaining a diagnostically useful sputum sample; that is, material must be purulent and thus presumed to be from the site of infection. Ideally, saliva or oropharyngeal contamination of the sample should be avoided.

In a patient with the clinical picture of acute bacterial pneumonia, the finding of gram-positive diplococci in expectorated sputum that contains many (≥ 50 bacterial cells per $100\times$ field) polymorphonuclear cells (purulent sputum) and few (<10 squamous cells per $100\times$ field) or no squamous epithelial cells (which indicates little or no oropharyngeal contamination of the specimen) is strong presumptive evidence of pneumococcal pneumonia.

Cultures of expectorated sputum are also important but are not without problems; for example, since *S. pneumoniae* is fastidious, it may fail to grow in culture, but this does not exclude its presence. In addition, pneumococci may be overlooked, since they may be overgrown by other organisms or mixed with similar-appearing, nonpneumococcal, α-hemolytic streptococci, which are normally present in oropharyngeal secretions. On the other hand, since *S. pneumoniae* is often present normally in the oropharynx, its growth from sputum, especially from that which is expectorated, may not be indicative of pneumococcal disease. Perhaps the main value of securing a sputum culture is to confirm or question observations made from the Gram stain and, if pneumococci (and/or other bacteria) are ultimately isolated, to perform antibiotic susceptibility testing.

If the patient is unable to expectorate purulent sputum for microscopic examination and culture, and if other infected materials (e.g., pleural or joint fluid) either are not available or are negative for pneumococci, various procedures for obtaining pus from the infected lung must be considered. Cough can be induced by having the patient inhale an aerosol of warm 3 per cent NaCl;

a plastic catheter can be inserted into the trachea via the nose or throat and suction applied; a direct transtracheal needle and catheter aspiration may be performed (a procedure not without complications); the patient may undergo endoscopy (provided the arterial Po_2 is ≥ 50 mm Hg), and alveolar washings or bronchial brushings may be obtained; or rarely, direct aspiration of the pneumonic infiltrate through the chest wall with a long, "skinny" needle (22 gauge) may be employed (a procedure also not without risks). Open lung biopsies for pneumococcal pneumonia are not indicated, although they may be for certain complications, ill-defined superinfections, or underlying diseases. In any acute bacterial pneumonia, the guiding principles for deciding what procedure, if any, to use for obtaining purulent sputum from the involved lung are as follows: (1) If expectorated sputum is satisfactory (i.e., purulent and relatively free of contaminating oropharyngeal material), further efforts to obtain pus from the deeper recesses of the lung are probably not necessary or indicated; (2) if additional procedures are necessary, one should select first the procedure that is least traumatic and invasive and is risk free and then proceed, if necessary, in a stepwise fashion to the next least invasive, risk-free procedure until satisfactory material is obtained; (3) one should not delay more than several hours before beginning chemotherapy, and if the patient is extremely ill, one must rely on clinical judgment and not delay treatment at all; and (4) one must make every effort to identify the etiologic agent (or agents) responsible for the pneumonia early in the course of the illness, since once this goal is realized, the chances of managing the patient successfully are markedly enhanced.

A variety of other tests may be applied to sputum specimens to identify pneumococci in acute bacterial pneumonia; but in skilled hands, few, if any, are better, less costly, easier to do, and more informative than the Gram stain. All tests done on sputum possess a similar problem in interpretation, namely, determining whether or not bacteria present in the sample are responsible for the pneumonia observed. If blood or pleural fluid cultures are subsequently positive for *S. pneumoniae*, the etiologic agent is confirmed, although the presence of additional pathogenic bacteria within the lung may not be entirely excluded, as, rarely, blood or pleural fluid cultures may yield other bacteria (polymicrobial infection) in addition to pneumococci.

Detection of pneumococcal capsular antigen generally requires the presence of approximately 10^5 bacteria per milliliter, about the same concentration as required to observe an average of one bacterium per $1000\times$ (or an oil immersion field on a standard light microscope) on a Gram stain. Cross-reactions with other antigens of other bacteria are frequent, and with certain serotypes, false-negative results are common. Perhaps the greatest value of capsular antigen detection is to confirm the presence of pneumococci in those patients who have been partially treated and in whom sputum cultures may be negative and a Gram stain may reveal few, if any, intact bacteria.

Colony counts of bacteria from bronchoalveolar lavage (BAL) washings obtained during endoscopy are seldom available early in the course of illness. Specimens must be obtained with a special cuffed endoscope so that oropharyngeal contamination does not occur with insertion of the scope. Generally, counts of colony-forming units (CFU) of bacteria higher than 10^3 to 10^5 per milliliter of fluid removed are considered significant, but this is not invariably so.

DNA hybridization studies may be performed, but as with capsular antigen detection, adequate numbers of bacteria must be present for the test to be positive. Utilization of the polymerase chain reaction (PCR) may amplify pneumococcal DNA and improve the potential for detection; however, such enhanced sensitivity may lead to false-positive tests caused by very small numbers of contaminating pneumococci.

Elastase or elastin fibers in sputum may suggest the presence of a gram-negative bacillary necrotizing pneumonia, particularly that due to *Pseudomonas*, but this test is of little value in the diagnosis of pneumococcal pneumonia (other than the test should be negative), since necrosis of the lung is not produced by pneumococci.

DIFFERENTIAL DIAGNOSIS (see also Ch. 61 and chapters dealing with specific organisms). The clinical picture and many of the routine laboratory and roentgenographic features associated with pneumococcal pneumonia are often indistinguishable from those of other acute bacterial pneumonias. Thus, collecting appropriate microbiologic data is essential if the correct etiologic diagnosis is to be made.

In adults, the second most common community-acquired, acute bacterial pneumonia is that caused by *H. influenzae*. The Gram stain of purulent sputum from such patients often reveals myriads of tiny gram-negative coccobacilli, with the observation of an occasional filamentous form. Such an infection often occurs in a patient with chronic bronchitis or chronic obstructive pulmonary disease and usually is due to nonencapsulated *H. influenzae* (as opposed to highly encapsulated, serotype B strains commonly infecting young children).

Staphylococcus aureus is another bacterium occasionally producing acute pneumonia, but when this kind of pneumonia is community acquired, it usually occurs during or just after an epidemic of viral influenza. In the hospital setting, *S. aureus* may be seen year round, as it is a commonly occurring nosocomial infection. If a highly virulent, toxin-producing strain is responsible, the "toxic shock syndrome" may be observed. On a Gram stain of purulent sputum, clusters of gram-positive cocci and characteristic tetrads of cocci are seen. Late in the clinical course, abscess formation or destruction of the lung occurs.

Group A streptococci (*S. pyogenes*) also produce acute pneumonia, and in such instances, the patient may be more toxic appearing than the extent of involvement of the lung might suggest. Classically, a small, peripherally located, wedge-shaped infiltrate is commonly seen, and a thin, watery, serosanguineous pleural effusion is often present. A roentgenogram of the chest may suggest a pulmonary infarction. An upper respiratory tract infection, particularly an exudative or erythematous pharyngitis or tonsillitis (especially in children), may be present; and an erythematous rash produced by streptococcal erythrogenic toxin (scarlet fever) may be seen. A Gram stain of purulent sputum usually reveals numerous short chains of gram-positive cocci or diplococci. Thus, the Gram stain may not differentiate group A streptococcal from pneumococcal pneumonia.

Moraxella catarrhalis, which in the recent past was referred to as *Neisseria* or *Branhamella catarrhalis*, may produce acute pneumonia, but usually in the elderly and particularly in those with chronic bronchitis or obstructive lung disease. It is a relatively benign infection, compared with those produced by other pyogenic bacteria, and is rarely, if ever, associated with bacteremia. A Gram stain of purulent sputum is again important, and the diagnosis should probably be made only when numerous gram-negative diplococci, in the absence of other potentially pathogenic bacteria, are seen. *N. meningitidis* (meningococci) are morphologically similar to *M. catarrhalis* organisms and must also be included in the differential diagnosis. However, in such instances patients are generally young adults, and the infection is associated with significant toxicity.

Gram-negative bacilli, particularly those belonging to the family *Enterobacteriaceae* (e.g., *E. coli*, *Klebsiella*, *Enterobacter*, *Serratia*, and *Proteus*) must also be considered as causative agents in the differential diagnosis of pneumococcal pneumonia, particularly if the patient is debilitated and is residing in a nursing home or similar institution, and certainly if the patient is hospitalized. Aerobic gram-negative bacilli are often responsible for nosocomial but infrequently for community-acquired pneumonias. This is because gram-negative bacilli rarely colonize the oropharynx of otherwise healthy people in the community, but they are common oropharyngeal residents in debilitated, hospitalized, or institutionalized patients. In addition, the patient in question may exhibit certain risk factors associated with invasion by gram-negative bacilli, such as the receipt of prior antibiotics, corticosteroids, inhalation therapy, or tracheostomy and the existence of profound neutropenia or severe debilitation. The pneumonic process is usually necrotizing, and gas formation may be detected on roentgenograms. A Gram stain of purulent sputum usually reveals many large, bipolar-staining gram-negative rods. Elastin fibrils may also be seen on a KOH preparation of sputum from the site of infection.

Anaerobic bacteria may also produce acute suppurative pneumonia. The anaerobes most frequently involved are *Bacteroides* species (usually *B. melanogenicus*), *Peptostreptococcus*, and *Fusobacterium*. Frequently, anaerobic infections are polymicrobial and may include bacteria other than strict anaerobes (e.g., *S. aureus*). The occurrence of anaerobic infection is usually preceded by gross aspiration and is enhanced if the individual has anaerobic oral infections or solid tumors of the oropharyngeal structures or tracheobronchial tree (tumors that may outstrip their blood supply, necrose, and provide an ideal anaerobic environment). The clinical presentation of anaerobic pleuropneumonic disease may be indolent rather than abrupt, and it may be accompanied by expectorated sputum or empyemas that have fetid and nauseating odors. (However, the absence of such an odor does not exclude the presence of anaerobes.) As with gram-negative bacillary pneumonias, necrosis of the lung with gas formation may be noted.

Mycoplasma pneumoniae, *Chlamydia*, and *Legionella* may also produce acute pneumonias, which are usually best described as atypical. With mycoplasmal pneumonia, patients are ordinarily young, and prolonged communicability, especially within households, may often be documented. The clinical, radiographic, and pathologic features are usually those of an interstitial pneumonia, rather than lobar consolidation and an alveolar exudative process. Serum cold agglutinin levels may be elevated, and the disease is rarely, if ever, fatal. Chlamydial pneumonia, especially that due to *C. psittaci*, is contracted from infected psittacine birds; or in the case of *C. pneumoniae* or TWAR agent (derived from the designation of the first two isolates, TW-183 and AR-39), infection is acquired from other infected humans. *C. pneumoniae* is the most common species producing chlamydial pneumonia in humans, and the clinical picture is usually that of pharyngitis, often with laryngitis, and segmental pneumonia of a single lobe without pleural effusion. Seroepidemiologic studies reveal a higher prevalence of antibodies in males than females and in older adults than children. Legionnaires' disease, which may be produced by a variety of *Legionella* species but principally by *L. pneumophila*, is associated with considerable systemic toxicity (nausea, vomiting, and diarrhea) and may be very difficult to differentiate from pneumococcal pneumonia. However, in the temperate zones, community-acquired legionnaires' disease is usually seasonal, occurring in the warmer months or summer; patients are typically male construction workers and smokers in their fifties whose clinical manifestations include fever, chills, myalgias, headache, dry cough, and nonspecific pulmonary infiltrates. Anti-*Legionella* fluorescein-labeled antibodies, which may be employed to examine sputum for *Legionella*, as well as antigen detection techniques applied to the urine, may be helpful in the early diagnosis of this disease.

Patients with the acquired immunodeficiency syndrome (AIDS) and acute pneumonia present considerable diagnostic problems. Although pneumococcal pneumonia and infections from encapsulated bacteria occur with greater frequency in patients with AIDS than in normal individuals, pneumocystosis and cytomegalovirus pneumonia occur more frequently than pneumococcal pneumonia in these patients and thus must also be excluded.

Finally, not only does pneumonia due to microbes other than the pneumococcus have to be considered in a differential diagnosis, but also a variety of noninfectious conditions may mimic the clinical picture of pneumococcal pneumonia. Pulmonary infarction, with emboli (e.g., in right-sided endocarditis) or without emboli (e.g., in sickle cell anemia), may present a considerable diagnostic challenge, even after differential lung scanning and pulmonary angiography. Chemical pneumonitis, localized or diffuse (Mendelson's syndrome), often caused by aspiration of gastric juice of low pH, may also be difficult to differentiate from pneumococcal or other bacterial pneumonias; however, in the absence of antibiotic therapy, a Gram stain of purulent sputum consistently reveals a paucity of bacteria.

TREATMENT. All patients with suspected pneumococcal pneumonia should be treated as promptly as possible with an effective antimicrobial agent. One should not wait for cultural confirmation of the diagnosis to initiate therapy. Although many patients may recover without antibacterial therapy, effective antimicrobial agents reduce morbidity, mortality, and complications.

At present, *penicillin G* is the therapy of choice, and it is the standard against which all other antipneumococcal agents are compared. Susceptible strains exhibit an MIC of less than 0.1 µg per milliliter, levels that are easily achieved in a variety of tissues with therapeutic dosing of 1.2 to 2.4 million units per day. If complicating pneumococcal bacteremia occurs, only 10 to 15 per cent of untreated patients may be expected to survive; this figure may be increased to 85 to 90 per cent with penicillin G treatment. A variety of other penicillins or related beta-lactam antibiotics are also effective and may be used in special circumstances, as when bacteria other than or in addition to pneumococci are seriously considered in the differential diagnosis or when penicillin-resistant pneumococci are present. Ideally, initial therapy should be parenteral to ensure delivery and adequate serum and tissue levels. If the patient is in shock or has heart failure, the route of delivery should be intravenous. Later in the course of therapy, if the patient's progress is good, the route of administration may be changed to oral. Treatment with any effective agent should be for at least 5 to 7 days.

For patients who are believed to be allergic to penicillin, a variety of other antibacterial agents may be used. Usually, a first-generation cephalosporin is selected, since its molecular configuration is slightly different from that of penicillin G (a six-membered thiazole ring rather than a five-membered one) and since the frequency of serious reactions due to cross-allergenicity appears to be low. However, careful observation of the penicillin-allergic patient during the initial use of a cephalosporin must still be made, since the threat of a serious side effect exists. If the patient has a clear history of a type I (immediate) hypersensitivity reaction, all beta-lactams should be avoided. For such patients, erythromycin is an excellent choice, even though an increasing frequency of resistance (MIC $\geq$ 1.0 µg per millileter) to erythromycin is being observed worldwide. Tetracyclines should be avoided because the frequency of resistant strains is often widespread and high (up to 80 per cent of isolates in some parts of the world). Similarly, quinolones should also not be used because concentrations at which most strains are susceptible are too high to predict a satisfactory outcome.

With the advent of penicillin-resistant pneumococci (see above), different strategies of therapy may have to be devised on the basis of susceptibility or resistance to other agents (Table 292-4). At present, in the United States, such strains are infrequent, sporadic, localized to certain geographic areas, and generally of intermediate resistance (MIC between 0.1 and 2.0 µg per milliliter). Nevertheless, each locale or hospital needs to monitor its own isolates, and therapeutic strategies should be based on these results. If strains are intermediate in resistance, simply increasing the dose of penicillin G to 6 million units per day will suffice (unless the complication of meningitis or endocarditis exists). However, if strains highly resistant to penicillin G (MIC $\geq$ 2.0 µg per milliliter) are repeatedly or frequently isolated, then penicillin G should not be routinely employed as initial therapy. In fact, such highly resistant isolates are generally resistant to most other beta-lactam antibiotics (see Table 292-1), as well as many other antimicrobials, so that agents such as vancomycin, teicoplanin, or rifampin may have to be used (with or without empiric penicillin) until the results of susceptibility data are available. Among currently available beta-lactams, cefotaxime, ceftriaxone, and imipenem appear to be most active against highly resistant pneumococci (see Table 292-1).

If effective antibacterial therapy is employed, the patient's temperature usually falls to or below normal by crisis within 24

TABLE 292-4. CRITERIA FOR RESISTANCE OF S. PNEUMONIAE TO SOME COMMONLY USED ANTIBIOTICS*

Antibacterial Agent	MIC (µg/ml)†
Penicillin G	
Intermediate	$\geq$0.1
High level	$\geq$2.0
Erythromycin	$\geq$1.0
Trimethoprim/sulfamethoxazole	$\geq$1/19
Tetracycline	$\geq$8.0
Rifampin	$\geq$2.0
Chloramphenicol	$\geq$8.0

*Based on criteria established by the National Committee for Clinical Laboratory Standards (NCCLS).

†MIC = Minimal inhibitory concentration.

hours. However, in some instances, perhaps because of the nature of the pathology or complications that occur (e.g., pleural effusion), the patient's temperature may fall by lysis over 2 to 3 days. Resolution and recovery from pneumococcal pneumonia generally result in restoration of normal pulmonary architecture. Occasionally, healing may be via fibrosis, in which instance persistence of pulmonary infiltrates on roentgenograms may be evident for months after clinical recovery.

In addition to effective antibacterial therapy, a variety of supportive measures are generally employed in the initial management of acute pneumococcal pneumonia; these include bed rest, monitoring of vital signs and urine output, insertion of a Swan-Ganz catheter to monitor cardiac output, administration of an occasional analgesic to relieve pleuritic pain to permit more effective breathing and coughing, fluid replacement if the patient is dehydrated, electrolyte correction, oxygen therapy, and relief of an ileus with nasal gastric suctioning. In relieving pleuritic pain or in providing sedation in situations requiring it (e.g., delirium tremens), care should be taken not to use excessively high doses that would depress the respiratory center. Intercostal nerve blocks, which do not interfere with respiratory drive, may be employed. In patients with neuromuscular disorders, particularly those involving defective conduction at the myoneural junction, aminoglycosides should be avoided. If possible, antipyretics should also be avoided, since the use of these agents interferes with the evaluation of fever as a measurement of the patient's progress (or lack of).

COMPLICATIONS. Approximately 5 per cent of patients with pneumococcal pneumonia develop an empyema, although a larger per cent (up to 30 per cent) commonly develop sterile pleural effusions. Most effusions resolve with or after successful antibacterial therapy, although empyemas often require drainage. Empyemas usually consist of thick pus composed of fibrin, serous proteins, large numbers of leukocytes and/or their products, and pneumococci. Initially, such collections may be drained by needle aspiration; however, later, as loculations occur, drainage via chest tubes is usually necessary. Chest roentgenograms with lateral decubitus films are often useful in the early recognition of pleural effusions; however, at a later time and in the course of removal and follow-up, ultrasonography and/or computed tomography (CT) may be necessary. In any acute bacterial pneumonia, pleural fluid that has been removed should be subject to a Gram stain, aerobic and anaerobic cultures, pH determination, cell count and differential, protein and sugar analysis, and a lactate dehydrogenase determination.

If pneumococcal bacteremia occurs, extrapulmonary complications, such as *meningitis, septic arthritis,* and *endocarditis,* must be excluded, since their therapy generally requires higher dosages of penicillin G and, in the case of septic arthritis, may require drainage. A spinal tap with examination of cerebrospinal fluid should be done if meningitis is suspected, and multiple pretreatment blood cultures and echocardiography of the heart valves should be obtained if endocarditis is suspected. Other complications that might occur are *pyogenic pericarditis,* which may produce tamponade and require drainage, and *peritonitis* in those with ascites (e.g., cirrhosis or nephrotic syndrome).

PROGNOSIS. The case fatality rate for untreated pneumococcal pneumonia is about 25 per cent, whereas in those treated promptly with penicillin G, it may be less than 5 per cent. Fatality rates differ considerably among patient groups, depending on such factors as presence or absence of bacteremia, multilobe involvement, neutropenia, asplenism, underlying diseases (particularly of the heart or lung), age of the patient (the prognosis being poor at the extremes), complicating extrapulmonary pneumococcal infections (e.g., meningitis), the occurrence of shock, the serotype of pneumococcus responsible (type 3 being highly virulent), delayed therapy, penicillin susceptibility or resistance, and prior immunization with polyvalent pneumococcal vaccine. However, it is noteworthy that since the advent of penicillin G in the 1940's (but prior to widespread use of the pneumococcal vaccine) the case fatality rate of pneumococcal pneumonia and bacteremia remains essentially unchanged.

PREVENTION. At present, the single most important preventive measure that is readily available is polyvalent pneumococcal vaccine. This vaccine contains 23 antigenic capsular poly-

saccharide types, which in the United States account for up to 90 per cent of bacteremic infections. In immunocompetent populations, it is estimated to be 80 per cent protective, inducing antibodies of the IgG2 subclass, which enhance opsonization, phagocytosis, and killing of pneumococci by polymorphonuclear leukocytes and fixed macrophages. It is virtually free of life-threatening side effects, and obviously it cannot produce a pneumococcal infection in itself, since it contains no viable, intact pneumococci. About 15 to 30 per cent of patients who receive the vaccine may develop fever, localized swelling, and/or pain at the injection site. As with all polysaccharide vaccines, it is poorly immunogenic in infants and may be less immunogenic in the very elderly and in those with a variety of conditions generally associated with poor vaccine responsiveness (e.g., those having uremia, hemodialysis, previously treated Hodgkin's disease, multiple myeloma, AIDS, and splenic dysfunction syndromes, as well as immunosuppressed transplant recipients, to name a few). Nevertheless, the vaccine should probably be given to immunodeficient patients, as mortality may still be reduced in a significant number of vaccine recipients. In normal individuals, if antibodies result from vaccination, they usually persist for more than 5 years and possibly for life. At present, new vaccines in which the capsular antigens are conjugated to proteins are under development and may prove more immunogenic.

The U.S. Public Health Service specifically recommends the currently available pneumococcal vaccine for patients with underlying conditions that are associated with increased susceptibility to pneumococcal infections or increased risk of mortality from such infections, namely, healthy adults 65 years or older and those with chronic cardiac or pulmonary diseases, anatomic or functional asplenia, chronic liver disease, alcoholism, diabetes mellitus, and cerebrospinal fluid leaks. In addition, although antibody responsiveness may be less than desirable, recommendations for receipt of the vaccine also are made for those with chronic renal failure or those on hemodialysis, for those with Hodgkin's disease, chronic lymphocytic leukemia, multiple myeloma, and AIDS; or for those receiving or about to receive chemotherapy for cancer, organ transplantation, or splenectomy.

Antibiotic prophylaxis with penicillin G or similar agents in otherwise healthy patients with viral upper respiratory infections is not routinely indicated, is not cost effective, and may only lead to superinfections with antibiotic-resistant bacteria or to adverse side effects from the antibiotic itself. However, in individuals with seriously compromised pulmonary, cardiac, or immune function, a narrow-spectrum agent, such as penicillin G, may be given in low dosages during a viral syndrome for a limited time to reduce the risk of morbidity and mortality from potentially invasive pneumococci. Such prophylaxis may especially apply to those in households where pneumococcal infections recently occurred.

Finally, it should be appreciated that pneumococcal infections, including pneumonia, are generally not acquired by otherwise normal people from exposure to other patients with pneumococcal pneumonia; thus patients with pneumococcal pneumonia do not require isolation, and prophylaxis for medical staff exposed to such infections is not indicated.

Austrian R: Prevention of pneumococcal infection by immunization with capsular polysaccharides of *Streptococcus pneumoniae:* Current status of polysaccharide vaccines. J Infect Dis 136(Suppl):S38, 1977. *A review of early and more recent studies of successes and difficulties with pneumococcal vaccines by a real authority.*

Austrian R: Life with the Pneumococcus. Notes from the Bedside, Laboratory, and Library. Philadelphia, University of Pennsylvania Press, 1985. *An array of interesting observations, both clinical and laboratory, on pneumococcal infections by an outstanding authority and the father of the modern capsular polysaccharide pneumococcal vaccine.*

Austrian R, Gold J: Pneumococcal bacteremia with especial reference to bacteremic pneumococcal pneumonia. Ann Intern Med 60:759, 1964. *A landmark clinical study that clearly points out the major risk factors involved in pneumococcal pneumonia and bacteremia.*

Burman LA, Norrby R, Trollfors B: Invasive pneumococcal infections: Incidence, predisposing factors, and prognosis. Rev Infect Dis 7:133, 1985. *An analysis of 494 Swedish patients with 508 culturally confirmed pneumococcal infections.*

Coonrod JD: Pneumococcal pneumonia. Semin Respir Infect 4:4, 1989.

Finland M, Barnes MW: Changes in occurrence of capsular serotypes of *Streptococcus pneumoniae* at Boston City Hospital during selected years between 1935 and 1974. J Clin Microbiol 5:154, 1977. *A thorough study of the distribution of pneumococcal serotypes in bacteremia, empyema, and meningitis useful for a complete understanding of vaccine efficacy by world-renowned investigators in the field of pneumococcal disease.*

Heffron R: Pneumonia, with Special Reference to Pneumococcal Lobar Pneumonia. New York, Commonwealth Fund, 1939. *Complete descriptions of the natural history of patients with pneumococcal pneumonia during the preantibiotic era.*

Hook EW III, Horton CA, Schaberg DR: Failure of intensive care unit support to influence mortality from pneumococcal bacteremia. JAMA 249:1055, 1983. *A clinical study that reveals that even intensive care and special units have not influenced the survival rate in pneumococcal pneumonia and bacteremia since the advent of penicillin, thus further emphasizing the need for prevention.*

Jabes D, Nachman S, Tomaz A: Penicillin-binding protein families: Evidence for the clonal nature of penicillin resistance in clinical isolates of pneumococci. J Infect Dis 159:16, 1989. *A study of the molecular abnormalities and mechanisms involved in penicillin-resistant pneumococci by some of the leading investigators in this field.*

Klugman KP: Pneumococcal resistance to antibiotics. Clin Microbiol Rev 3:171, 1990. *A complete, in-depth microbiologic, epidemiologic, and clinical review, evaluation, and update of the problem of penicillin resistance by an authority with considerable experience with such isolates.*

Palmer DL, Jones CC: Diagnosis of pneumococcal pneumonia. Semin Respir Infect 3:131, 1988. *A thorough review of the issues complicating the diagnosis of pneumococcal pneumonia and an update on tests that might be helpful in the future.*

293 Mycoplasmal Infections

Stephen G. Baum

In the late 1930's, a group of pneumonias was delineated that did not resemble typical bacterial lobar pneumonia. Because the cause of the pneumonias was unknown, and because the radiographic appearance and low mortality distinguished these cases from pneumococcal and other bacterial respiratory infections, these were called *primary atypical pneumonias*. In the 1950's, the organism responsible for many cases of so-called atypical pneumonia was isolated by Eaton and was shown to be similar to one causing pleuropneumonia in cattle; hence the names Eaton agent and pleuropneumonia-like organisms (PPLO). In 1962, this agent was reclassified as *Mycoplasma pneumoniae*.

The most significant human infections caused by mycoplasmas are diseases of the respiratory tract, including pharyngitis, tracheobronchitis, and pneumonia. Also, one species of mycoplasmas, *Mycoplasma hominis*, and a closely related organism, *Ureaplasma*, have been etiologically implicated in some diseases of the human urogenital tract and in respiratory disease of the neonate.

The high incidence of mycoplasmal infection is not generally appreciated. Factors responsible for this include lack of familiarity with mycoplasmal syndromes; the absence of specific, rapid tests for diagnosis in the early phases of these diseases; and the relative difficulty of growing the organisms in the diagnostic laboratory.

Accurate etiologic diagnosis of mycoplasmal diseases, however, is of considerable clinical importance. Mycoplasmal infections do not respond to the antimicrobial therapies usually used for respiratory or genital infections, but treatment with erythromycins or tetracyclines leads to amelioration of symptoms, decrease in the likelihood of spread, and eventually, true microbiologic cure.

DESCRIPTION OF THE ORGANISM AND RELATIONSHIP TO PATHOGENESIS. The mycoplasmas, members of the class Mollicutes, represent the smallest free-living forms, i.e., they do not require host cells for replication. For many years the question of whether these organisms were viruses or bacteria was debated. However, it appears that they are neither, and there is no significant DNA similarity between mycoplasmas and any known bacterium or virus.

The average diameter of mycoplasmas (125 to 150 nm) is in the size range of large viruses. They have no cell wall but are bounded by a limiting membrane containing lipid. Absence of a cell wall renders them susceptible to lysis by hypotonic solutions but insensitive to cell wall–active antibiotics, such as the penicillins. Mycoplasmas and *Ureaplasma* can be grown on agar supplemented with serum proteins and sterols. Most *Mycoplasma* species form 200- to 300-μm colonies, which look much like a fried egg. They have a peripheral halo and a thicker central portion lying just below the surface of the agar. *M. pneumoniae* colonies, however, lack the halo and resemble a mulberry. When

M. pneumoniae is grown on agar containing mammalian erythrocytes, it rapidly produces a clear zone of hemolysis similar to β-hemolysis of some bacteria. *M. pneumoniae* also differs from many other mycoplasmas in that it grows more slowly, ferments glucose to produce acid, adsorbs red cells to growing colonies, and reduces the dye tetrazolium under aerobic conditions. All of these characteristics have been exploited to establish a rapid microbiologic diagnosis.

When mycoplasmas contaminate tissue culture systems, as they often do, they are found intracellularly. This fact has led to speculation about the mechanisms of persistence of these organisms in vivo. However, electron microscopic studies using tracheal organ culture systems have demonstrated most of the infecting organisms extracellularly at the base of the cilia of epithelial cells.

Two properties of *M. pneumoniae* seem to correlate extremely well with its pathogenicity in humans. *M. pneumoniae* has a selective affinity for respiratory epithelial cells and produces hydrogen peroxide. The H_2O_2 is thought to be responsible for much of the initial cell disruption in the respiratory tract. H_2O_2 also causes damage to erythrocyte membranes. In the laboratory, this damage results in hemolysis and, in the patient, may alter erythrocyte antigens, thereby stimulating cold agglutinins. These agglutinins appear in the serum of over 50 per cent of patients who develop mycoplasmal pneumonia and are capable of clumping red blood cells in vitro at 4°C. They are different from cold precipitins or cryoglobulins occurring in other diseases. Cold agglutinins are immunoglobulin M (IgM) antibodies directed at the I antigen on the surface of normal erythrocytes. There is increasing evidence that cold agglutinins are antibodies to a glycolipid in the membrane of *M. pneumoniae*, which happens to cross-react with a similar erythrocyte antigen. Cold agglutinins occur rarely in other diseases, including influenza and adenoviral pneumonia.

RESPIRATORY DISEASES CAUSED BY *M. pneumoniae*

DEFINITION. Respiratory infection by *M. pneumoniae* may be asymptomatic or may lead to inflammation of the upper airways (pharyngitis or tracheitis) or lower respiratory tract (bronchitis or pneumonia). In the vast majority of cases, disease is self-limited, but proper antibiotic therapy can shorten the duration of symptoms.

EPIDEMIOLOGY. Each year about one of every thousand people in the United States experiences mycoplasmal pneumonia. The incidence of all other mycoplasmal upper and lower respiratory infections is probably 10 times that of mycoplasmal pneumonia. One quarter to three quarters of all pneumonias occurring in "closed" populations (military recruit camps, boarding schools, and colleges) are caused by *M. pneumoniae*. Patients with hypogammaglobulinemia may have increased susceptibility, and *M. pneumoniae* infection may often exacerbate bronchial asthma.

Mycoplasmal respiratory infection is most common in children and young adults, with a peak incidence in the age range of 5 to 20 years; however, infants and elderly patients are also infected. Distribution is worldwide. Although documented epidemics have occurred primarily in the fall months, this disease does not have the marked seasonal predominance that is found with influenza.

Infection is spread from person to person by respiratory secretions expelled during bouts of coughing. The organism is present in these secretions for several days prior to the onset of symptoms and peaks in titer in the sputum during the first week of clinical illness. *M. pneumoniae* organisms persist in the sputum, albeit in reduced numbers, for weeks after the cessation of appropriate antimicrobial therapy.

In open populations under nonepidemic conditions, the infection seems to be spread most easily among playmates and within the household. The index case is usually a child. The majority of households having an index case will experience secondary infections, and the majority of susceptible family members become infected, with resultant symptomatic disease or asymptomatic seroconversion.

In comparison with viral respiratory disease, the incubation period for mycoplasmal infection is relatively long, averaging 2 to 3 weeks. Therefore, unless two or more people from a household are simultaneously infected from an index case, it is unusual for several family members to be ill at the same time, and the disease may take several months to run its course through a household.

CLINICAL PRESENTATIONS. Mycoplasmal infection of the upper airways is impossible to distinguish clinically from infection by other agents. On the other hand, mycoplasmal pneumonia has several characteristics that may help the physician to diagnose this disease (Fig. 293–1). The onset of mycoplasmal pneumonia is usually insidious, in contrast to the abrupt onset of adenoviral or influenzal pneumonia. Mild fever is usually the first sign of infection. The hallmark of the disease is severe, disabling, paroxysmal cough, which usually becomes prominent 2 or 3 days after the onset of fever and often requires narcotic medication for suppression. Although usually nonproductive, the cough may yield small amounts of whitish sputum. Occasionally, the sputum may contain flecks of blood, but grossly purulent sputum and marked hemoptysis are rare. Production of purulent or bloody sputum is actually more prevalent in tracheobronchitis than in pneumonia.

Headache occurs commonly in conjunction with the cough. During the first week of illness, many patients complain of burning soreness in the chest, though true pleuritic pain is uncommon. Fever rarely exceeds 39.5° C (102 to 103° F), and mild myalgias and malaise occur early in the disease. A history of shaking chills, severe myalgias, or gastrointestinal complaints is unusual.

On physical examination, the pharynx may be slightly injected or inflamed. Much diagnostic emphasis has been placed on the presence of bullous myringitis in patients with mycoplasmal respiratory disease. This finding was noted in fewer than 25 per cent of volunteers experimentally infected with *M. pneumoniae* and is very rare in naturally occurring mycoplasmal infection. Bacteria are much more commonly cultured than are *M. pneumoniae* from patients with bullous myringitis, and the relationship between *M. pneumoniae* infection and bullous myringitis or otitis remains tenuous.

Examination of the chest usually fails to show signs of dense consolidation or fluid accumulation. Auscultation reveals fine rales either unilaterally or bilaterally, which are often not very impressive. Findings from the remainder of the physical examination are usually normal.

The radiographic appearance of the lungs frequently presents a surprise. There is marked patchy infiltration of the lungs consistent with extensive interstitial pneumonia; bilateral involve-

ment is evident in about one quarter of the patients. Infiltration is most prominent at the base of the lungs, although mycoplasmal pneumonia can be seen in any pulmonary segment. There may be slight blunting of the costovertebral angle on the affected side (or sides) in 10 to 20 per cent of patients, but large pleural effusions are rare. If thoracentesis is performed, it yields a serous or serosanguineous transudative fluid.

COMPLICATIONS. Spread of infection within the lung and pleural effusions are the most common pulmonary complications. Involvement of a number of extrapulmonary sites has been attributed to infection with *M. pneumoniae*, usually occurring as complications of pulmonary disease. Occasionally, they have been seen without pneumonia, and mycoplasmal causation has been substantiated on the basis of culture of the organism from involved organs, fourfold or greater rises in mycoplasma-specific antibodies, or demonstration (described later) of less specific cold hemagglutinins.

Three extrapulmonary complications are relatively common (occurring in 2 to 10 per cent of seriously ill patients). These deserve comment because, when present, they help to confirm the diagnosis of mycoplasmal pneumonia.

Erythema Multiforme Major (Stevens-Johnson Syndrome). Some patients with mycoplasmal pneumonia develop blistering lesions involving the mouth, eyes, and skin. Usually, although the lesions look quite severe, they heal with minimal scarring. However, when the cornea is involved, blindness may ensue, and local and systemic steroid therapy is often recommended in these instances. This dermatologic syndrome has many causes, including adverse reaction to drugs. When, however, it occurs in conjunction with interstitial pneumonia in a child or young adult, its presence helps confirm the clinical diagnosis of mycoplasmal pneumonia.

The pathogenesis of this syndrome is unknown. There is one report of isolation of *M. pneumoniae* from skin lesions, but most authorities consider Stevens-Johnson syndrome an allergic reaction. A great variety of other skin rashes in mycoplasmal pneumonia have been described, but these are not diagnostically helpful.

Raynaud's Phenomenon. A second syndrome, occurring in fewer than 5 per cent of mycoplasmal pneumonia patients, is Raynaud's phenomenon. This consists of painful blanching of the distal parts of fingers and toes upon exposure to cold and may occur whether or not the patient has a history of Raynaud's phenomenon unrelated to mycoplasmal infection. The pathogenesis of this complication in *M. pneumoniae* infection is unknown. However, it is tempting to hypothesize that high titers of cold hemagglutinins could play a role by creating minute thrombi in

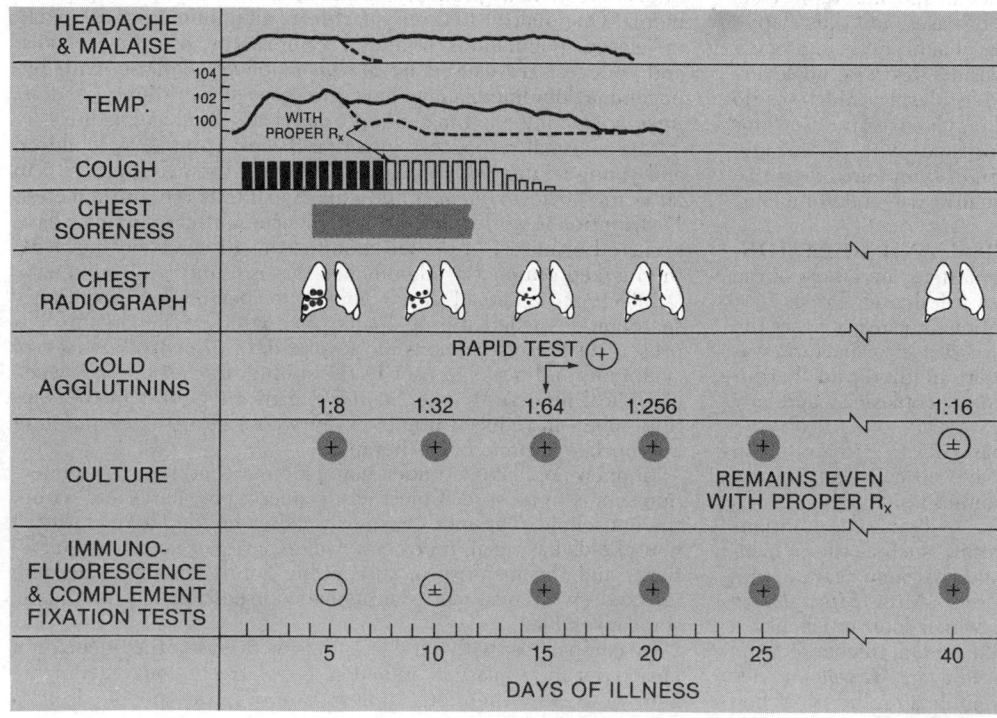

FIGURE 293–1. Major clinical manifestations of mycoplasmal pneumonia.

the microcirculation of the distal extremities when exposed to cold. Patients with sickle cell disease may have particularly severe symptoms when they contract mycoplasmal pneumonia. In the presence of extremely high titers of cold agglutinins (1:20,000), gangrene of the distal parts of fingers and toes in these patients has been reported.

Hemolysis. Patients with cold agglutinin titers of greater than 1:500 may experience rapid and severe hemolysis with decreases of 50 per cent in hematocrit. This complication occurs in fewer than 5 per cent of patients in the second or third week of illness.

LESS COMMON COMPLICATIONS. Among the organ systems reported to be rarely involved in mycoplasmal infection are the cardiovascular, skeletal, and central nervous systems. In a very few cases involving each of these systems, the organism has been cultured directly from the affected organ.

NEUROLOGIC COMPLICATIONS. Aseptic meningitis, meningoencephalitis, cranial nerve neuritis, peripheral neuritis, Guillain-Barré syndrome, transverse myelitis, and psychosis all have been reported as complications of *M. pneumoniae* infection. Most often, etiologic diagnosis is made on the basis of exclusion of other agents and antibody response to *M. pneumoniae*. Spinal fluid cell counts and glucose and protein levels are extremely variable in these cases, ranging from normal to patterns consistent with aseptic meningitis. In some cases, elevated cerebrospinal fluid proteins were found to contain antibodies to *M. pneumoniae*, but these often paralleled serum antibody levels, and it was unclear whether or not cerebrospinal fluid antibody represented diffusion from the serum. There are only two or three reports of isolation of *M. pneumoniae* from cerebrospinal fluid or neural tissue, and the prevailing hypothesis is that mycoplasmal central nervous system disease occurs on the basis of allergic reaction.

Patients with neurologic complications seem to have greater mortality than is commonly associated with mycoplasmal disease. This could either signify a group of patients at increased risk of death from mycoplasmal infection or, alternatively, support the hypothesis that these patients had a second (concurrent) undiagnosed disease with greater inherent mortality.

CARDIOVASCULAR COMPLICATIONS. Pericarditis and myocarditis are the most commonly reported cardiovascular complications of mycoplasmal infection. In general, the major criteria of heart disease have been congestive failure and abnormal electrocardiographic results. Large pericardial effusions have not occurred. There have been a few deaths during the acute phase of the disease, but recovery without sequelae is the rule. In most cases documentation of *M. pneumoniae* infection has been made by noting seroconversion. In one retrospective study based on seroconversion, 8 per cent of patients with *M. pneumoniae* infection had evidence of pericarditis or myocarditis. The average age of these patients was 46 years, considerably greater than the mean for patients with *M. pneumoniae* infection.

MUSCULOSKELETAL COMPLICATIONS. Arthralgias are common in association with mycoplasmal pneumonia, but frank arthritis is rare. When it does occur, arthritis may continue long after the other manifestations of mycoplasmal infection are gone. Large joints seem to be preferentially affected, and the arthritis may be migratory. *Mycoplasma* has not been cultured from joint fluid of immunocompetent patients.

M. pneumoniae and other mycoplasmas have been implicated as the causative agents of a number of other connective tissue diseases, including rheumatoid arthritis, juvenile rheumatoid arthritis, and Reiter's syndrome. Nonhuman mycoplasmas have been shown to cause arthritis in the animals they infect, and *M. pneumoniae* has been cultured on several occasions from the joints of immunocompromised patients. To date, however, there is no evidence that human mycoplasmas cause joint disease, except perhaps as an acute complication of pneumonia.

CLINICAL COURSE. Mycoplasmal respiratory disease is almost invariably self-limited and very rarely results in death. In the absence of treatment, upper respiratory infection usually lasts 1 to 3 weeks, and pneumonia may persist from 4 to 6 weeks. Recovery is gradual, with clinical improvement preceding roentgenographic clearing. Development of any of the severe cardiovascular, dermatologic, hematologic, or neurologic complications described earlier may prolong resolution. Proper treatment, which is often not begun until other antibiotics have failed, would appear to shorten the duration of symptoms by about one half. Results might be even better if treatment were begun earlier.

Relapse occurs in 5 to 10 per cent of patients. In most cases, these patients have received courses of therapy less than 2 weeks in duration.

Two groups of patients commonly appear to develop severe disease. The first group consists of infants who, until recently, were thought not to be particularly susceptible to *M. pneumoniae* infection. Many infants develop severe respiratory distress requiring intubation and supported respiration. Fortunately, despite severe illness the prognosis for these children is excellent. The second group comprises patients with sickle cell disease. In addition to digital gangrene, these patients are prone to develop large multilobar pneumonias and pleural effusions. The possibility of mycoplasmal infection should be considered in a patient with sickle cell crisis and interstitial pneumonia.

PATHOLOGY. Since death is rare in patients with mycoplasmal pneumonia, descriptions of pathologic changes in this disease rest on a very small number of specimens. The tracheobronchial tree and lungs are generally hyperemic. There is evidence of interstitial pneumonia with engorged lungs consistent with the findings on radiographs. Cellular infiltrate, usually minimal, consists mostly of mononuclear elements. Tracheal organ culture systems have been used to demonstrate that infection with *M. pneumoniae* causes a marked decrease of ciliary action, followed by complete loss of cilia and sloughing of epithelial cells.

IMMUNITY. There are varied antibody responses to infection with *M. pneumoniae*. It is unclear what role these immune responses play in the pathogenesis of, and recovery from, infection. Secretory immunoglobulin A (IgA) antibody is thought to be the most protective immunoglobulin in this disease. Individual immunity may be relatively short lived, and there are well-documented instances of recurrent disease within 2 to 10 years following primary infection.

DIAGNOSIS. A clinical diagnosis of mycoplasmal pneumonia should be seriously entertained whenever interstitial pneumonia occurs in a young adult. Examination of the Gram-stained sputum is helpful in that it reveals inflammation but no bacterial organisms. The peripheral leukocyte count may be normal or slightly elevated. There is minimal shift toward immature forms, and mild lymphopenia may exist. The diagnosis is substantiated by finding a cold agglutinin titer greater than 1:32 in the serum.

Hospital bacteriology or serology laboratories titrate cold agglutinins in the patient's serum using Rh-positive, type O erythrocytes to avoid reactions due to major blood group isoantibodies present in the patient's serum. However, a simple, rapid bedside procedure for finding cold agglutinins can be performed using only the patient's blood. One milliliter of freshly drawn blood is placed in a tube containing anticoagulant. The tube used for prothrombin determinations is suitable. The tube is chilled on ice for 2 or 3 minutes and then gently rotated in a horizontal position. Development of small clumps of erythrocytes, similar to those seen when typing blood, which disappear on warming the tube between the hands, indicates the presence of cold agglutinins. The agglutination-dissociation cycle can be repeated many times with the same blood sample. This differentiates the reaction from direct hemagglutination by viruses—a process that generally cannot be recycled. A positive test result correlates with a cold agglutinin titer of 1:64 or greater. When the cold agglutinin titer is extremely high, an easily dissociable clot may form in the tube. Blood from a patient with an unrelated disease should be used as a control. Cold agglutinins are usually found during the second and third weeks of illness and may peak 1 month or more after the onset of symptoms.

Diagnosis of mycoplasmal pneumonia should be further supported by finding rising titers of specific antibodies to the *Mycoplasma* organism. These can be measured by complement fixation, inhibition of metabolism, indirect hemagglutination, or immunofluorescence techniques. In addition, patients with mycoplasmal pneumonia may develop a false-positive test result for syphilis.

Definitive diagnosis of mycoplasmal pneumonia rests, however, on coupling an antibody rise with culturing *M. pneumoniae* from sputum. Although growth on agar may take 2 to 3 weeks, rendering results useless for initiating drug therapy, a more rapid (3 to 4 days) presumptive diagnosis can be based on the use of a diphasic medium available in some diagnostic laboratories.

DIFFERENTIAL DIAGNOSIS. The most common respiratory infections mimicking mycoplasmal pneumonia are influenza and adenoviral and *Legionella* pneumonia. These tend to be more fulminant in onset and are associated with more severe systemic symptoms and greater respiratory insufficiency. Patients with legionnaires' disease are likely to be older men with a history of smoking. Confusion and gastrointestinal disturbance are common in *Legionella* pneumonia. Often one cannot definitively distinguish between these diseases, and a therapeutic trial with erythromycin (which also is used to treat *Legionella pneumophila*) may be warranted. Psittacosis and ornithosis (chlamydial diseases) and Q fever (a rickettsial disease) should also be considered in the diagnosis. In such cases, history of exposure to birds on the one hand and to cattle on the other may prove diagnostically helpful.

THERAPY. Treatment with appropriate antibiotics can terminate symptoms abruptly and usually must be begun on the basis of clinical diagnosis. Penicillins, cephalosporins, and aminoglycosides, such as streptomycin, kanamycin, and gentamicin, have little or no effect against these organisms.

M. pneumoniae is sensitive in vitro and in vivo to erythromycin and to the tetracyclines. These agents appear to be equally effective in diminishing the symptoms of the disease. Because there are fewer adverse effects, especially in children under age 10 years, erythromycin is preferred. The dosage for either drug is 250 to 500 mg four times daily for 2 to 3 weeks. Although erythromycin and the tetracyclines are effective in ending symptoms, *M. pneumoniae* can be isolated from the sputum of patients for several weeks after the onset of therapy. The mechanism of persistence is unknown but does not depend on the emergence of drug-resistant organisms.

PREVENTION. The frequency of mycoplasmal infection makes the development of a vaccine an attractive objective. Inactivated vaccines, while producing rises in serum antibody levels, give little protection.

The possible role of IgA antibodies in combating disease has prompted the trial of intranasally administered vaccines using live temperature-sensitive (ts) mutants of *M. pneumoniae*. The rationale was that these mutants would induce a localized nasopharyngeal immune response but would not replicate in the warmer lower respiratory tree and cause disease. The results of initial trials of these vaccines have been variable.

GENITAL AND NEONATAL INFECTION BY *MYCOPLASMA* AND *UREAPLASMA*

INTRODUCTION. One strain of human mycoplasmas, *M. hominis*, and a closely related organism, *Ureaplasma urealyticum*, frequently colonize the male and female genital tracts. During the past decade, there has been increasing interest in discovering the role these organisms might play in causing disease of the genitourinary system in adults and pulmonary and central nervous system disease in infants.

EPIDEMIOLOGY. *M. hominis* and ureaplasmas can be included in the group of venereally transmitted infectious agents. Infants are colonized during birth, but carriage of the organism is lost during the first year of life. After this, the prevalence of colonization increases with age and sexual experience, as it does for other sexually transmitted organisms. At all ages, females seem to be more readily colonized than males, and colonization is found most frequently in patients from lower socioeconomic groups. *U. urealyticum* carriage may decrease with increasing age over 40 and with hypoestrogenism.

CLINICAL PRESENTATIONS. *M. hominis, U. urealyticum*, or both organisms have been implicated in nongonococcal urethritis (NGU) and inflammatory disease of the prostate, vagina, cervix, upper urinary tract, and female pelvic organs. In addition, colonization by one or both of these organisms has been associated with male and female infertility, habitual abortion, and recurrent production of premature and underweight infants.

INFECTION OF THE LOWER URINARY TRACT. Chlamydia are responsible for a large percentage of cases of NGU. *U. urealyticum* is probably the cause of many of the remaining cases of NGU. Evidence for this stems from the many patients with NGU from whom ureaplasmas are cultured and from these patients' poor clinical response to treatment with sulfa drugs, to which chlamydia are susceptible and to which *Ureaplasma* is not. *M. hominis* probably does not cause urethritis.

INFECTION OF THE UPPER URINARY TRACT. *M. hominis* has been isolated from the kidneys and ureters of patients with clinical pyelonephritis. Antibody to the organism was detected in serum and urine from some of these patients, providing moderately strong evidence that *M. hominis* causes some cases of pyelonephritis. *U. urealyticum* infection may infrequently play a role in urinary calculus formation.

INFECTION OF THE FEMALE GENITAL TRACT. *M. hominis* probably causes a small proportion of the cases of vaginitis and cervicitis. Infection of the uterus and fallopian tubes with this organism has also been documented. *Ureaplasma* rarely, if ever, causes infection in the female pelvis.

MYCOPLASMAS AND REPRODUCTIVE ABNORMALITIES. *U. urealyticum* has been cultured from the sperm of males with fertility disorders. Treatment to eradicate *Ureaplasma* has resulted in increased motility and number of sperm as well as improved morphology. However, recent studies do not indicate a causal role for ureaplasmas in infertility.

Ureaplasma has also been isolated from the internal organs of the products of conception of patients with repeated spontaneous abortions. In addition, in some studies *U. urealyticum* was more often isolated from the genital tracts of women with this syndrome than from control populations. Finally, treatment with tetracycline prior to conception in women with a history of habitual abortion has been reported to increase fetal salvage rate. Unfortunately, few if any of these studies took into account the presence of chlamydia, which might have been responsible for the reproductive disorders.

LOW BIRTH WEIGHT. Prior to the realization that tetracycline is contraindicated in pregnancy, it was shown that tetracycline treatment of mothers who habitually gave birth to underweight fetuses would increase birth weight. In addition, vaginal colonization by ureaplasmas was correlated with decreased birth weight. However, these studies did not take into account the presence or absence of chlamydia. Despite numerous studies, the relationship of genital mycoplasmal colonization to prematurity and abortion remains controversial.

INFECTION OF NEONATES AND INFANTS. *U. urealyticum* has been the most commonly isolated organism from the upper and lower respiratory tract of premature and low birth weight infants with respiratory disease. Infants colonized or infected with this organism at birth, whether or not they manifested respiratory distress at that time, were significantly more likely to develop chronic lung disease than were noncolonized infants. Infection appeared to occur in utero and was also related to neonatal death. The requirement for oxygen therapy in these neonates may have played a role in the pathogenesis of the chronic lung disease. *M. hominis* was the second most commonly isolated organism in preterm infants, but the relationship to disease appears more tenuous.

U. urealyticum and *M. hominis* have also commonly been cultured from the cerebrospinal fluid of premature infants with meningitis, hydrocephalus, and intraventricular hemorrhage.

PUERPERAL INFECTION. *M. hominis* infection and septicemia have been associated with some cases of postpartum fever. This organism has been found in the blood of up to 10 per cent of women with fever after delivery, and antibody response indicating true infection has been noted in many cases.

THERAPY. Mycoplasmas and *Ureaplasma* are all susceptible to the tetracyclines. *U. urealyticum* is sensitive to erythromycin, but *M. hominis* is not. Spectinomycin, an antimicrobial agent used in cases of penicillin-resistant gonococcal disease, appears to be effective against both *M. hominis* and *U. urealyticum*. Since both *U. urealyticum* and *C. trachomatis* are sensitive to tetracycline, it is recommended that patients with NGU be treated with a tetracycline at a dose of 1 to 2 grams daily for 1 to 2 weeks. The patient should abstain from sexual intercourse during this period, and sexual partners should be evaluated for therapy.

In addition, tetracycline therapy prior to conception and erythromycin therapy during pregnancy should be considered for couples with gestational problems who are shown to harbor *U. urealyticum* in the genitourinary tract.

Episodes of postabortal and puerperal fever are usually self-limited and do not require antimicrobial therapy directed at mycoplasmas. Should such therapy be deemed necessary, tetracycline is the drug of choice.

Couch RB: Mycoplasma diseases. *In* Mandell G, Douglas RG, Bennett JE (eds.): Principles and Practice of Infectious Diseases. 3rd ed. New York, Churchill Livingstone, Inc., 1990, pp 1445–1458. *An up-to-date chapter dealing with both clinical and microbiologic aspects.*

Sanchez PJ, Regan JA: *Ureaplasma urealyticum* colonization and chronic lung disease in low birth weight infants. Pediatr Infect Dis J 7:542, 1988. *A prospective study of the relationship of genital mycoplasmas and neonatal lung diseases.*

Taylor-Robinson D, McCormack WM: The genital mycoplasmas. N Engl J Med 302:1003, 1980; 302:1063, 1980. *A comprehensive two-part article on epidemiology, microbiology, clinical presentation, and therapy.*

Waites KB, Rudd PT, Crouse DT, et al: Chronic *Ureaplasma urealyticum* and *Mycoplasma hominis* infections of central nervous system in preterm infants. Lancet 1:17, 1988. *A study showing the high incidence of congenital mycoplasmal central nervous system infection in the newborn.*

294 Pneumonia Caused by Aerobic Gram-Negative Bacilli

Waldemar G. Johanson, Jr.

Over the past 30 years, the group of organisms known collectively as aerobic gram-negative bacilli (GNB) has assumed an increasing importance in clinical respiratory infections. There is no evidence that this phenomenon is due to a change in the virulence of these organisms. Rather, it is due to changes in the human hosts they infect and, to some degree, to changes in the environment induced by antibiotics and other factors, especially in hospitals. Each of the GNB has its place (or places) in nature. Many are regular inhabitants of the human gastrointestinal tract, while others are found in water or other sites in the environment. None is especially virulent for the respiratory tract of healthy mammalian hosts; all are distinctly inferior to the pneumococcus, for example, in that regard. A careful review of the preantibiotic literature reveals that the presence of these organisms in the respiratory tracts of seriously ill patients is not a recent occurrence; rather, the presence of these organisms was disregarded for many years, an approach that was not unjustified, considering the preeminence of the pneumococcus as a cause of fatal pneumonia prior to the availability of highly efficacious antibiotics. The emergence of GNB as respiratory pathogens in recent years is the result of suppression of more aggressive organisms by effective therapy and the long-term survival of people who would have succumbed to other infections or other processes in an earlier era.

PATHOGENESIS. Pneumonias due to GNB are caused by one of three mechanisms: inhalation of contaminated aerosols, hematogenous infection of the lungs from another primary source of infection, or aspiration of oropharyngeal secretions that are colonized by these organisms.

Contamination of respiratory therapy equipment by GNB, usually *Pseudomonas aeruginosa*, was recognized as a major cause of nosocomial pneumonias in the 1960's. With the advent of disposable nebulizers and other control strategies, this problem has been largely eliminated, although sporadic outbreaks remind us that continued vigilance is required. However, as a practical matter, pneumonias due to GNB are rarely caused by inhalation of contaminated aerosols today.

The incidence of pneumonia caused by bacteremic spread to the lungs has probably been overestimated in the literature. *P. aeruginosa* causes a distinctive vasculitis involving pulmonary arteries and veins, and pneumonia in adjacent lung units associated with bacteremia, but this is uncommon with other organisms. It is likely that most instances of bacteremia from a nonpulmonary source, such as the gastrointestinal or urinary tract, associated with pulmonary infiltrates, fever, and hypoxemia, represent noncardiogenic pulmonary edema, or the "adult respiratory distress syndrome," and not actual pneumonia. In fact, pneumonia due to this cause is sufficiently uncommon that the presence of gram-negative bacteremia in association with new pulmonary infiltrates should initiate a vigorous search for a primary site of infection outside the lungs before it is concluded that pneumonia is responsible.

Aspiration of oropharyngeal secretions that contain GNB is the usual event leading to pneumonia caused by these organisms. Colonization of the upper respiratory tract with GNB occurs in 10 per cent or fewer of normal people, but the prevalence of such colonization is markedly increased among patients with acute or chronic diseases. Colonization rates are similar among populations with chronic disease, such as alcoholics and residents of skilled nursing facilities, and previously healthy individuals with acute but severe illnesses or trauma; in both types of patient groups, colonization rates approach 50 per cent. Similarly, colonization of the oropharynx by GNB among healthy persons undergoing elective surgical procedures rises from essentially zero to 35 to 50 per cent within 24 hours following surgery. The organisms responsible for colonization vary from one study to another, but only rarely can this sudden acquisition of GNB be attributed to demonstrable environmental sources. Instead, colonization appears to be caused by a translocation of the patient's fecal flora or the transfer of organisms from one patient to another on the hands of personnel. However, the root cause of this colonization is the great susceptibility of ill patients to the acquisition of GNB from the immediate environment.

Healthy people are resistant to the implantation of GNB in the oropharynx; even gargling a broth culture of GNB fails to produce colonization. This difference between healthy and ill people is related to the ability of GNB to adhere to epithelial cells of the oropharynx. Buccal epithelial cells obtained from healthy subjects adhere few GNB during incubation in vitro, while cells obtained from either acutely or chronically ill patients adhere large numbers. The ability of cells to resist adherence by GNB is directly related to the concentration of fibronectin on the cell surface; loss of cell surface fibronectin, whether removed by proteolytic enzymes experimentally in vitro or by endogenous enzymes in vivo, appears to expose binding sites on the cells to which GNB can adhere and thus achieve colonization.

Once established in the oropharynx, GNB multiply, achieve high concentrations in secretions, and are aspirated in small liquid boluses into the lungs (see Ch. 61). Since lung defenses are often impaired by the same underlying conditions that promote changes in cell resistance to adherence and colonization, the ability of the lungs to handle this bacterial inoculum is insufficient and pneumonia results. The specific lung defense mechanism that might be impaired in a given patient varies with the nature of the underlying illness. For example, patients with chronic airway obstruction have impaired mucociliary transport and alveolar hypoxia that hinders the effectiveness of phagocytic cells. Some data suggest that the bronchial abnormalities in these patients allow persistent colonization of the distal airways by potentially pathogenic bacteria, a factor that affords the bacteria the advantage of access to the distal lung. Patients who are neutropenic are remarkably predisposed to develop pneumonias with GNB, a clinical observation that correlates nicely with the experimental finding that swift recruitment of circulating neutrophils into the lungs is a crucial aspect of host defense against *Pseudomonas* infection. Alcoholism seems to predispose to GNB pneumonias in several ways. Malnutrition promotes colonization of the upper tract by GNB, aspiration is facilitated by episodes of impaired consciousness, and acute alcohol intoxication hinders the ability of phagocytes to migrate to the site of inflammation.

Of the many species of gram-negative aerobic bacilli that colonize human hosts, only *Haemophilus influenzae* can be classified as a true respiratory pathogen, if the ability of the organism to produce infections in previously normal individuals is accepted as a reasonable criterion of pathogenicity. All of the others together, including Enterobacteriaceae (*Escherichia coli, Klebsiella, Enterobacter, Serratia,* and *Proteus*), *Pseudomonas,* and *Acinetobacter,* account for 10 to 20 per cent of community-acquired pneumonias, and these occur almost exclusively in patients with serious underlying disease. The genus *Klebsiella* contains four species, of which only *K. pneumoniae* and *K. oxytoca* cause pneumonia; infections due to *K. pneumoniae* are by far the most common.

Pneumonia caused by *Klebsiella* has been held separate from that caused by other gram-negative bacilli largely for historical reasons. It was the first such organism to be recognized as a pulmonary pathogen, and the pneumonia it caused was distinct from that caused by the pneumococcus, especially in its lack of response to early forms of treatment and its predilection to cause upper lobe pneumonias in alcoholic men. However, the classic features of *Klebsiella* pneumonia as described in the earlier literature, such as "currant jelly" sputum (a mixture of blood and mucus), the bulging fissure associated with upper lobe consolidation, and the syndrome of "chronic cavitary pneumonia," are rarely observed today. While *Klebsiella* remains an important pulmonary pathogen, the illness it causes cannot be clinically differentiated from that caused by other aerobic gram-negative bacilli, and its treatment is similar.

CLINICAL MANIFESTATIONS. Pneumonias caused by GNB may be community acquired or hospital acquired (nosocomial). Virtually all patients with community-acquired pneumonias caused by GNB have serious underlying chronic illnesses, especially chronic obstructive lung disease, alcoholism, or malignancy. Nosocomial pneumonias resulting from GNB occur principally in patients with severe, acute illnesses whether or not they have underlying chronic disease as well. Thus, these infections are most likely to be found in postoperative patients or patients who require intensive care for other reasons. The clinical manifestations of infection are influenced by the nature of the associated processes.

Community-acquired gram-negative bacillary pneumonias share the common features of all bacterial pneumonias—fever, cough productive of purulent sputum, chest pain, and shortness of breath. The illness tends to be abrupt and associated with prominent systemic signs and symptoms, such as mental confusion, vomiting, and hypotension. Physical examination reveals rales in most patients, but the classic findings of dense consolidation are uncommon. Pleural effusion is present in 15 to 20 per cent of patients. Radiographic infiltrates may involve any lobe and are bilateral in about one third of patients. Although cavitation is most likely to occur in pneumonia caused by *Klebsiella*, it also occurs commonly with *Pseudomonas* infections and occasionally with other organisms. Laboratory features include leukocytosis or leukopenia, either of which is characteristically associated with a marked left shift. Leukopenia is a poor prognostic sign.

Nosocomial pneumonia produced by GNB can be an explosive illness similar to the community-acquired form but frequently proceeds with a more indolent but seemingly inexorable course. Often the patient is in respiratory failure, intubated, and receiving mechanical ventilation. GNB are initially found colonizing the oropharynx, and over the subsequent few days appear in tracheal secretions, followed by increasing numbers of neutrophils. Finally, the patient becomes febrile and develops new radiographic infiltrates and worsening hypoxemia. Another common presentation is fever on the second or third postoperative day. Postoperative pneumonias are most common after lateral thoracotomies (especially combined thoracoabdominal procedures) and upper abdominal incisions. When nosocomial GNB pneumonia complicates the course of an already seriously ill patient, it is frequently associated with evidence of impaired function of other organs, commonly the liver, kidneys, hematopoietic system, and central nervous system. Upper gastrointestinal bleeding and impaired coagulation are also common. This phenomenon is referred to as the syndrome of multiple organ failure and is the most common cause of death in patients with protracted serious illness. The occurrence of any of these complications should alert the clinician to the probable presence of bacterial infection. If no apparent site is found elsewhere in the patient, the lungs must be highly suspect even in the absence of strong clinical signs, since such pulmonary infections are often difficult to detect in the setting of serious disease.

DIAGNOSIS. Confirmation that GNB are responsible for pneumonia is a difficult clinical problem created largely by colonization of proximal airways by these organisms. Thus, GNB are often present in the secretions of ill patients whether they have pneumonia or not and whether or not the GNB are the cause of pneumonia. Blood cultures are positive in 20 to 30 per cent of patients with community-acquired infections but in as few as 8 per cent of those with nosocomial pneumonias. Nevertheless, because the information gained from a positive blood culture regarding the causative organism and its antimicrobial susceptibility is so important in patient management, blood cultures should always be obtained when GNB pneumonia is suspected. Similarly, while pleural effusion is usually not present, the yield of positive cultures from such fluid when it is present is about 30 per cent, and a diagnostic thoracentesis should be performed if a sufficient volume of fluid is identified radiographically.

Invasive sampling via the fiberoptic bronchoscope adds significantly to the accuracy of diagnosis, especially among mechanically ventilated patients. The best technique appears to be the "protected specimen brush" (PSB), in which samples are collected from the peripheral lung without contamination by proximal secretions. The PSB sample should be cultured quantitatively. Samples containing more than 10^3 organisms are indicative of pneumonia. This technique may be especially useful in ruling out significant infections. Fewer than one half of mechanically ventilated patients who meet the clinical criteria of pneumonia have positive PSB cultures; those who do not may be safely managed without antimicrobial treatment for pneumonia.

TREATMENT. Recommendations for the antimicrobial treatment of pneumonia due to GNB are changing rapidly as new drugs aimed at this group of organisms are entering clinical practice. It must be remembered that GNB are relatively poor respiratory pathogens and that patients susceptible to infection by them are at even greater risk of pulmonary infection by more virulent organisms, such as the pneumococcus, *Haemophilus*, and *Staphylococcus aureus*. Thus, despite the presence of GNB in sputum, initial treatment of these pneumonias—particularly those acquired outside the hospital or in the absence of concomitant antibiotic therapy—should include coverage of the usual respiratory pathogens. The use of multiple agents is advisable for initial therapy for several reasons: The susceptibility of the infecting organisms is not known, and two agents provide broader coverage; emergence of antibiotic resistance may be retarded by the use of multiple agents; and antibacterial synergism may result from the use of multiple agents. The agents chosen must be given parenterally and in adequate dosage. Metabolic clearance rates of the aminoglycosides in particular vary widely, and standard dosages based on body weight and renal function may result in either excessively high or low plasma concentrations in the individual patient. Improved clinical outcomes in the treatment of pneumonia caused by GNB have been associated with peak plasma levels of 6 μg per milliliter for gentamicin or tobramycin and 28 μg per milliliter for amikacin.

On the basis of the foregoing, a reasonable therapeutic approach to the patient with a community-acquired pneumonia suspected to be of gram-negative bacillary etiology would be to initiate treatment with a beta-lactam agent plus an aminoglycoside, for example, cefuroxime or cephalothin plus gentamicin or tobramycin. This combination provides coverage for the usual respiratory pathogens as well as the most common GNB (*K. pneumoniae* and *E. coli*) in this setting. If the patient has recently received antimicrobial therapy or has been recently hospitalized, a third-generation cephalosporin, such as cefotaxime or ceftazidime, can be substituted for the other beta-lactam agents.

Treatment of nosocomial infection is often made more difficult by previous antimicrobial therapy, and drug susceptibility studies are critically important. However, empiric therapy must usually be initiated before the results of such studies are available. Agents should be chosen on the basis of several factors, including knowledge of local resistance patterns, previous cultures, and prior treatment. For example, resistance of *P. aeruginosa* to gentamicin varies from 5 to 50 per cent in different hospitals, and knowledge of resistance patterns in one's hospital can be very helpful in selecting empiric therapy. Most clinicians choose an aminoglycoside, usually amikacin because of the less frequent resistance to this agent, and a third-generation cephalosporin such as ceftazidime. If *P. aeruginosa* is strongly suspected on the basis of previous cultures or the clinical setting (respiratory failure, neutropenia), an agent with greater antipseudomonas activity, such as piperacillin or ticarcillin, can be substituted for the cephalosporin. Because new beta-lactam agents with good activity against gram-negative bacilli are less active than earlier generation agents against a number of important respiratory pathogens, great care needs to be given to the spectrum of organisms covered until the results of cultures are available.

PROGNOSIS. The mortality of GNB pneumonias remains high—in the range of 30 to 50 per cent. It has been argued that this is the result of the underlying disease usually present in patients who develop these pneumonias. This notion could lead to therapeutic nihilism. Other data clearly indicate that GNB pneumonias increase hospital mortality among patients who have nonlethal disease processes, a finding that would support an aggressive diagnostic and treatment approach. It is probable that both conclusions could be correct, depending on the population of patients studied. There is little doubt that GNB pneumonias represent the terminal event for a number of patients with irreversible and lethal diseases and that such patients form a large fraction of all hospital patients. On the other hand, there is reason to expect recovery rates of 80 per cent or more among patients who develop GNB pneumonias in the context of acute, severe, but nonlethal disease processes, and in these patients aggressive diagnostic maneuvers and intensive therapy are clearly indicated.

COMPLICATIONS. Pneumonias caused by GNB are more likely than other pneumonias to be complicated by one or another adverse event. Important complications include empyema, lung necrosis, superinfections, and multiple organ failure; metastatic seeding of infection to other sites is an uncommon complication.

Empyema occurs in perhaps as many as 30 per cent of patients with GNB pneumonias. Criteria for the diagnosis of empyema, besides the presence of gross pus, include the presence of bacteria on Gram stain, a pleural fluid pH of 7.2 or less, or a pleural fluid white cell count exceeding 30,000 per deciliter. Each of these criteria indicates a condition that is unlikely to respond to antimicrobials alone but that usually requires drainage of the pleural space as well. Thus, the term "complicated effusion" has gained favor over "empyema" to identify pleural fluid collections for which drainage needs to be considered. The occurrence of a complicated effusion generally prevents the recovery of the patient until it is recognized and effectively treated. Signs and symptoms of continuing illness, such as fever, persistent leukocytosis, and the onset of multiple organ failure, in a patient undergoing treatment for a GNB pneumonia should raise suspicion of a complicated effusion. If pleural fluid is identified on upright posteroanterior and lateral chest radiographs, thoracentesis should be performed; useful studies of the fluid obtained include measurements of pH and glucose, white cell count, Gram stain, and cultures for aerobic and anaerobic organisms.

If the fluid qualifies as a complicated effusion, most authorities recommend prompt placement of a thoracostomy tube and drainage. Alternative approaches, principally repeated thoracentesis, are less successful owing to loculation of the pleural space. Surgical drainage of the pleural space, using localized resection of an overlying rib with creation of a larger drainage tract, is reserved for patients who do not respond to tube drainage. Decortication of the pleura may be necessary if the clinical signs of uncontrolled infection are not ameliorated by simple drainage plus antimicrobial therapy. In such patients, radiographic evidence of effusion persists, along with continued fever and leukocytosis. At surgery, the pleural space is found to contain numerous loculated pockets of pus. The timing of intervention with these techniques requires excellent clinical judgment, because the patients are usually seriously ill and poor candidates for surgical treatment of any kind; on the other hand, they will not recover unless the pleural space is adequately drained.

Extensive lung necrosis has been termed "lung gangrene" because of the rapid occurrence of pulmonary cavitation associated with marked systemic toxicity and the appearance of extensive devitalization of lung tissue at necropsy. Occasionally, an entire lung appears to dissolve within a few days, leaving multiple cavities with air-fluid levels. This complication occurs with all of the common GNB, although perhaps more commonly in infections produced by *K. pneumoniae* and *P. aeruginosa*. Lung necrosis may be caused by the extracellular products of these organisms. *P. aeruginosa* makes a number of "virulence factors," including exotoxin A, exoenzyme S, elastase, and a neutral protease. However, *K. pneumoniae* makes none of these, and the propensity of this organism to cause lung necrosis remains unexplained.

Extensive lung necrosis may be followed by massive hemoptysis, continued suppuration because of inadequate drainage of the massively disrupted lung parenchyma, or bronchopleural fistula caused by extension of the necrotizing process through the pleura. The last must be promptly treated with placement of a chest tube because of the attendant pneumothorax. However,

the definitive treatment of extensive lung necrosis is surgical resection of the involved lobe or lobes. As with management of complicated effusion, the timing of such an intervention must be carefully considered in light of the control of the underlying infection, the severity of complicating problems (hemoptysis, air leak, and so on), and the patient's general condition.

Assessment of the patient with multiple organ failure in the context of a serious illness complicated by a GNB pneumonia is always difficult. The major question is usually whether a new complication such as oliguria is due to the underlying disease, to the current treatment, or to the infection. Each of the common manifestations of multiple organ dysfunction—altered liver function, acute renal failure, hematopoietic abnormalities, upper gastrointestinal bleeding, and altered mental state—may be multifactorial in etiology, and the antimicrobial agents used to treat GNB pneumonia may cause most of them. The guiding principles are to treat the infection aggressively and to correct life-threatening complications as they occur.

Superinfections may develop during the treatment of GNB pneumonia, just as GNB pneumonia may occur as a superinfection of a previous pneumonia. Unfortunately, treatment of the patient's pneumonia does not prevent colonization of the oropharynx and tracheobronchial tree by additional GNB or fungi. Thus, the clinician is often faced with evaluating a new set of microorganisms recovered from the patient's secretions. The guiding principle here is to treat patients, not culture results. If the patient is responding well and appears to be improving, the new cultures can be disregarded for the time being. On the other hand, if the new cultural data correspond to a worsening clinical course, the process of evaluation and revision of treatment must be begun again.

Fagon JY, Chastre J, Hance AJ, et al.: Detection of nosocomial lung infection in ventilated patients. Am Rev Respir Dis 138:110, 1988. *A study that documents the usefulness of invasive sampling with the protected specimen brush (PSB) technique in diagnosing or excluding pneumonia.*

Karnad A, Alvarez S, Berk SL: Pneumonia caused by gram-negative bacilli. Am J Med 79(Suppl 1A):61, 1985. *Many well-documented cases are described that indicate clearly the variable clinical presentation of these infections and the generally poor response to treatment.*

Levison ME, Kaye D: Pneumonia caused by gram-negative bacilli: An overview. Rev Infect Dis 7(Suppl 4):S656, 1985. *A thorough review from the standpoint of microbiology and antimicrobial therapy.*

Nolan PE, Bass JB: New drugs for treating lung infection. Chest 94:1076, 1988. *A review of the role of new antimicrobial agents in the treatment of lung infections.*

295 Recurrent Aspiration Pneumonia

Waldemar G. Johanson, Jr.

Categorization of the various syndromes associated with aspiration of liquids into the tracheobronchial tree is not an area distinguished by precise terminology or even consistency in the use of terms. Most of the important syndromes are dealt with elsewhere in this volume: gastric acid aspiration (Ch. 528), anaerobic pneumonias and lung abscess (Ch. 62), lipoid pneumonia (Ch. 66), and hydrocarbon aspiration (Ch. 528). In this chapter, we concentrate on an infrequent but difficult problem: that of recurrent bacterial pneumonias associated with aspiration. Such pneumonias are defined as recurring clinical illnesses characterized by fever, purulent sputum, and new radiographic infiltrates in the lungs in a patient with known or suspected chronic aspiration of oropharyngeal contents.

ETIOLOGY. Most patients afflicted with this problem have serious problems with swallowing for one or another reason. Common predisposing conditions are carcinoma of the esophagus with obstruction, tracheobronchial fistula (usually following treatment for cancer), and neurologic diseases affecting deglutition. Strokes are certainly the most common cause of the latter but amyotrophic lateral sclerosis (including bulbar palsy), multiple sclerosis, and the myopathies may be responsible. Recurrent nocturnal aspiration of gastric contents by patients with esophageal reflux represents the one situation in which the swallowing mechanism may be intact in this syndrome.

Impaired swallowing having neural or myopathic causes is most pronounced when the patient attempts to swallow liquids. By contrast, dysphagia caused by obstruction is always worse with solid foods. Thus, it is not surprising that the patient with myoneural deficits of the pharyngeal musculature repeatedly aspirates oropharyngeal secretions. In patients with esophageal obstruction, secretions accumulate proximal to the obstruction, especially at night, and are aspirated. Gastric contents are normally sterile. However, as the patient with reflux aspirates gastric contents, a certain volume of oropharyngeal secretions is necessarily carried along.

Oropharyngeal secretions are massively contaminated, containing 10^6 to 10^8 aerobic bacteria per milliliter and about 10 times as many anaerobic organisms. Although the majority of organisms composing the normal flora of this region have little invasiveness for the normal host, highly pathogenic organisms, including *Streptococcus pneumoniae*, *Staphylococcus aureus*, and *Haemophilus influenzae*, may be present in the secretions of normal people. Since most of the patients susceptible to recurrent aspiration have serious underlying diseases, their upper respiratory tracts are likely to be colonized by enteric gram-negative bacilli and *Pseudomonas* as well.

Normal individuals aspirate small volumes of oropharyngeal secretions during sleep but do not develop recurrent pneumonias. The difference between normal people and those who do develop recurrent pneumonias is probably the volume of material aspirated and the underlying chronic illnesses of the latter patients; differences in the bacterial flora of secretions may play a role as well.

CLINICAL MANIFESTATIONS. Episodes of recurrent pneumonia associated with aspiration tend not to be acute, fulminant illnesses but rather are characterized by progressive fever, purulent sputum production, shortness of breath, and systemic symptoms (such as loss of appetite and malaise) over a period of days. The frequency of such episodes in an individual prone to recurrent aspiration varies widely. In patients with tracheobronchial fistulas, the episodes are essentially continuous until an effective preventive measure can be implemented or the patient dies. By contrast, patients with esophageal reflux may go years between episodes. The frequency of episodes is usually directly related to the frequency and volume of material aspirated and thus is increased in conditions in which aspiration is a daily event, especially if coupled with a decreased level of awareness, as occurs in some patients following strokes.

Physical findings include those related to the underlying illness and the presence of coarse rhonchi over dependent lung zones. Rales and signs of consolidation may or may not be present. Fever and leukocytosis are regularly present. Radiographs of the chest reveal infiltrates of varying intensity, with a preponderance of change in the dependent zones, i.e., posterior aspects of the lower lobes and posterior segments of the upper lobes. Pleural effusion is uncommon unless anaerobic infection is present.

DIAGNOSIS. Examination of expectorated sputum is helpful in confirming the suspicion of aspiration pneumonia but of little help in defining a specific bacterial etiology. Typically, the sputum of such patients is intensely purulent, with a wide spectrum of bacterial forms present on Gram stain. Culture of this material yields the same flora as in upper respiratory secretions, and the clinical problem consists of trying to discern which of several pathogenic organisms should be treated. Cultures should be obtained, however, since knowledge of the sensitivity of the organisms present may be needed to guide therapy. Blood cultures are rarely positive. The presence of food particles in tracheal secretions is clear evidence of aspiration. In patients receiving enteral feedings, the presence of glucose in secretions may be demonstrable by bedside tests. Since normal secretions contain an undetectable level of glucose, a positive result is highly specific for aspiration. Dietary lipids form large intracellular deposits when ingested by phagocytic cells, and examination of sputum with a lipid stain may confirm the clinical impression of chronic aspiration. The microscopic appearance of the large lipid

deposits is important in differentiating this type of lipid inclusion from the foamy deposit that occurs in macrophages owing to the accumulation of endogenous lipid distal to an obstructing lesion in the airways.

When the diagnosis of recurrent aspiration is in doubt, cineradiographic studies of the patient swallowing a thin, watersoluble contrast material is usually definitive. Thick barium should be avoided, as aspiration of this material compounds the patient's problems and the use of a thick solution is less likely to identify the swallowing difficulty. The procedure may need to be repeated with the patient in the supine position in questionable cases. Follow-up films of the chest reveal the presence of contrast material in the airways.

Patients with infrequent episodes of recurrent pneumonia caused by esophageal reflux and nocturnal aspiration represent a somewhat different problem. The presence of a hiatal hernia or the demonstration of reflux during an upper gastrointestinal contrast study does not necessarily prove that pneumonia was caused by this mechanism, although that would be a reasonable presumption if other aspects of the patient's presentation were compatible with the diagnosis. Probably the best diagnostic test in uncertain circumstances is to monitor the pH in the upper esophagus during sleep. Reflux into the upper esophagus is marked by a sudden fall in pH, an event that is easily captured on a long-term strip chart recorder for review the next morning. Attempts to document aspiration by placing contrast material or radioisotopes in the stomach prior to sleep are of limited value, since such patients do not aspirate every night.

TREATMENT. Initial antibiotic therapy should provide broad coverage. Pending the results of culture and sensitivity studies, therapy with intravenous penicillin and an aminoglycoside is reasonable. Alternatively, a second- or third-generation cephalosporin can be used as long as coverage for gram-positive, gram-negative, and anaerobic organisms is provided. Supportive care, including aggressive tracheobronchial toilet, is required. Nutrition must not be overlooked despite the difficulties encountered in many of these patients. If swallowing is impossible and a small feeding tube cannot be placed in the intestinal tract via the nose or mouth, parenteral nutrition should be provided while a long-term solution to the patient's problem is sought. Failure to address the nutritional deficits of these patients is a common cause of protracted and often lethal complications.

Surgical intervention to prevent esophageal reflux is indicated for the patient in whom recurrent pneumonia can be reasonably attributed to this mechanism. Long-term solutions for the other patients with this syndrome often involve difficult choices. Bypassing the mouth to facilitate feeding can be accomplished with a feeding gastrostomy or enterostomy. The former can be performed noninvasively via fiberoptic gastroscopy, with the feeding tube being passed percutaneously into the stomach. In some patients, cessation of swallowing food diminishes the frequency and severity of aspiration and successfully ameliorates the clinical problem. However, in many it does not because patients must still handle their own secretions. Drug therapy aimed at reducing the volume of secretions in this situation is usually not successful. The only certain preventive measure is tracheostomy with all of the complications attendant to this procedure. Even tracheostomy does not negate the possibility of aspiration around the tube unless the larynx is removed or the vocal cords are sewn together. The latter can be undone at a later date if the patient's condition improves. These procedures should not be contemplated in all patients with the syndrome of recurrent aspiration, since many patients have underlying conditions that will be lethal in a short time. However, if the patient has a reasonable chance of long-term survival in the absence of recurrent episodes of pneumonia, these steps should be considered.

Bartlett JG: The triple threat of aspiration pneumonia. Chest 68:560, 1975. *A useful classification and review of the bacteriology of aspiration pneumonias.*

Lorber B, Swenson RM: Bacteriology of aspiration pneumonia. A prospective study of community and hospitalized cases. Ann Intern Med 81:329, 1974. *Emphasizes the differences in bacteriology among these two groups of patients.*

Shike M, Berner YN, Gerdes H, et al.: Percutaneous endoscopic gastrostomy and jejunostomy for long-term feeding in patients with cancer of the head and neck. Otolaryngol Head Neck Surg 101:549, 1989. *This study documents the safety and benefit of percutaneous endoscopic gastrostomy in patients at risk of aspiration due to cancer.*

Winterbauer R, Durning R Jr, Baron E, et al.: Aspirated nasogastric feeding solution detected by glucose strips. Ann Intern Med 95:67, 1981. *Provides insight into the problem and a simple approach to diagnosis.*

296 Legionellosis

Paul H. Edelstein

DEFINITION. Legionellosis is the term used to describe infections caused by bacteria of the genus *Legionella*. The most important of these diseases is pneumonia, called legionnaires' disease. Either as part of legionnaires' disease or distinct from it, the legionellae may cause infections elsewhere in the body, usually in the form of abscesses. Finally, a type of transient and mild febrile illness, called Pontiac fever, is assumed to be caused by legionellae, though this is unproved.

HISTORY. Legionnaires' disease was first recognized as a distinct entity when it caused epidemic pneumonia among members of the American Legion attending a convention in Philadelphia in 1976; this resulted in 29 deaths and in 182 cases of pneumonia. Despite evidence that people who were not legionnaires became ill during the same epidemic, the disease earned the name "legionnaires' disease." Charles McDade and William Shepard, of the United States Centers for Disease Control, determined that this disease was caused by an ostensibly newly discovered bacterium. The bacterium was named *Legionella pneumophila* to honor the legionnaires who had the disease, as well as to denote the organ that the bacterium infects. It has been subsequently determined that neither the disease nor the bacterium is new. The first documented epidemic of legionnaires' disease occurred in a meat packing plant in Minnesota in 1957, and the first recorded isolation of the bacterium was in 1943. In fact, three different *Legionella* species had been isolated from humans prior to 1976, although they were thought to be rickettsia-like agents. Several unsolved epidemics of pneumonia, including one in Philadelphia in 1974, were recognized to have been due to legionnaires' disease.

BACTERIOLOGY. Twenty-nine *Legionella* species have been recognized to date. About half of these have been isolated from patients with legionnaires' disease, and about half have been isolated only from the environment. The species that most commonly cause disease are *L. pneumophila*, *L. micdadei*, *L. bozemanii*, *L. dumoffii*, and *L. longbeachae*. Fourteen serogroups are recognized for *L. pneumophila*, while several other species contain up to two serogroups. *L. pneumophila* causes up to 90 per cent of cases of legionnaires' disease in nonimmunocompromised individuals, and about 90 per cent of these cases are caused by *L. pneumophila* serogroup 1. *Legionella micdadei* is probably the second most common cause of legionnaires' disease and is a very common cause of legionnaires' disease in immunocompromised patients.

The legionellae are small, gram-negative, obligately aerobic, asaccharolytic, and usually motile bacilli. *Legionella* requires complex growth media, having an absolute nutritional requirement for L-cysteine. Optimal growth occurs on a buffered charcoal yeast extract medium supplemented with iron, L-cysteine, and α-ketoglutarate (BCYEα). These bacteria do not grow on conventional bacteriologic media, such as tryptic soy blood agar, MacConkey's agar, or unsupplemented chocolate agar. Their usual habitat is natural and treated waters, such as lakes, ponds, and tap water. Legionellae are found in highest concentration in warm water, especially in hot water heaters, hot water plumbing fixtures, and cooling towers. They appear to be obligate or facultative parasites of fresh water amoebae, such as *Hartmannella* and *Acanthamoeba*. Humans are very likely accidental hosts of these bacteria.

Virulence factors have been examined for relatively few strains each of *L. pneumophila* and *L. micdadei* and are not well understood. The bacteria produce endotoxins and exotoxins, which may cause tissue damage independently or in concert with the host immune system.

PATHOGENESIS. Legionnaires' disease is acquired by inhalation of aerosolized water containing *Legionella* organisms. It is also possible that some patients acquire disease by pulmonary aspiration of contaminated water. The contaminated aerosols are derived from humidifiers, shower heads, respiratory therapy equipment, industrial cooling water, and cooling towers. Aerosols formed by contaminated water in plumbing systems and in cooling towers are the most common sources of infection. Inhaled organisms are phagocytosed by pulmonary alveolar macrophages, which are unable to kill the bacteria. The bacteria inhibit phagolysosomal fusion and multiply within the phagosome. Eventually, the multiplying bacteria, which produce cytotoxins, kill the macrophage and are released extracellularly. The intracellular infection cycle is reinitiated in another macrophage. Continuing bacterial multiplication and consequent lung damage produce symptoms 2 to 14 days after the initiation of infection. Bacterial uptake and multiplication are curtailed by the action of cytokines (e.g., gamma-interferon), which are produced by macrophages and lymphocytes. Natural killer and lymphokine-activated killer cells probably lyse infected macrophages, aborting the intracellular infection cycle. The role of polymorphonuclear phagocytes is unclear, although they probably have some part in eliminating bacteria, especially after activation by interleukin 2 and tumor necrosis factor. Antibody appears to have little function in host immunity or defense, whereas T lymphocytes play a major role in the immune process. The actual mechanism of pulmonary damage is not well understood and could be due to bacterial toxins, immune reactions to infection, or both. The bacteria may spread to extrapulmonary sites via the lymphatic system and bloodstream; they are likely transported in the blood by infected blood mononuclear cells. The mechanism whereby the pneumonia exerts systemic effects is unknown but could be the result of disseminated bacterial infection, the effect of toxin, or the production of host factors such as tumor necrosis factor.

The pathogenesis of Pontiac fever is still a mystery. On the basis of epidemiologic and microbiologic findings, inhalation of water contaminated with many different types of bacteria, including *Legionella* species, produces the disease. The incubation period of the disease, 12 to 36 hours, is too short to allow for bacterial infection and multiplication. Therefore, it is possible that bacterial or fungal toxins present in the water produce this illness, as has been hypothesized for a closely related disease, humidifier fever. Another possibility is an immune response to one or more of the multiple microorganisms found in the water. Antibody to *Legionella* species found in the contaminated water is present in most disease victims, but it is unclear what this means.

EPIDEMIOLOGY. Legionnaires' disease occurs worldwide but is primarily a disease found in technically advanced countries. Case reports from underdeveloped countries are rare, perhaps because of limited diagnostic facilities and also perhaps because of the infrequent use of air conditioning and complex plumbing systems. Normal children have this disease very rarely. Elderly adults are at increased risk, as are cigarette smokers and those with chronic pulmonary or cardiac disease. Glucocorticosteroid administration, or its endogenous production, is the major risk factor for legionnaires' disease. OKT3 administration may also predispose to this illness, but cyclosporine administration probably does not. Administration of cytotoxic agents does not appear to be a risk factor, nor are hematologic malignancies (except hairy cell leukemia), neutropenia, or acquired immunodeficiency syndrome (AIDS), in the absence of glucocorticoid administration. Patients in the immediate postoperative period appear to be at increased risk of acquiring legionnaires' disease, perhaps because of inhalation of contaminated water aerosols during anesthesia, transient paralysis of local lung defenses, or both. Males get legionnaires' disease about twice as often as females, although this does not hold true for several epidemics of legionnaires' disease. No good evidence exists for person-to-person spread of legionnaires' disease.

Legionnaires' disease may occur in epidemics originating in a single building or area. Outbreaks of the disease have occurred among hotel guests, hospital inpatients and outpatients, office building workers, and factory workers. There appears to be little, if any, increased risk of disease acquisition among people with occupational water exposure.

It is estimated that from 1 to 5 per cent of all pneumonias in adults are due to legionnaires' disease. In some geographic regions, community-acquired legionnaires' disease is more common, with average prevalence rates of 10 to 20 per cent of all pneumonias. When the disease occurs in endemic or epidemic nosocomial form, 1 per cent to as many as 20 per cent of hospitalized patients with pneumonia have this disease.

Pontiac fever has been recognized primarily as an epidemic illness, with attack rates in excess of 90 per cent. It has been noted to occur in office and factory workers and in recreational bathers using spa or Jacuzzi-type baths. The disease very likely has a sporadic form, but the lack of specific diagnostic tests makes diagnosing this form very difficult.

PATHOLOGY. Specific pathologic changes are found only in the lung in the vast majority of fatal cases of legionnaires' disease. Intense inflammation is present in the alveolus, alveolar ducts, respiratory bronchioles, and alveolar septa. The inflammatory process consists of bacteria, polymorphonuclear leukocytes, and macrophages. On occasion, pleuritis, pleural empyema, pericarditis, and cavitary lung disease are found. Very rarely, abscess formation occurs outside the chest cavity; this is characterized by the presence of polymorphonuclear leukocytes.

CLINICAL PRESENTATION. Legionnaires' disease manifests as a febrile systemic illness with pneumonia. Several prospective and retrospective studies of patients with different types of pneumonia have shown that legionnaires' disease has few, if any, characteristic clinical features and that it cannot be distinguished clinically from pneumococcal pneumonia. However, clinical observations during epidemics of legionnaires' disease have often documented characteristic clinical findings. It is probable that the spectrum of clinical presentations is wide, ranging from a "typical" form of legionnaires' disease to one indistinguishable from other causes of pneumonia. This chapter describes the "typical" form of legionnaires' disease, which in reality may be present in the minority of patients. A prodromal illness consisting of malaise, low-grade fever, and anorexia may develop several days before the onset of more severe symptoms. Myalgia, extreme fatigue, and high fever then develop. Gastrointestinal complaints are common, such as generalized or localized abdominal pain, nausea, vomiting, and diarrhea; the diarrhea is generally watery and not dehydrating. Recurrent rigors and prostration may occur. Symptoms referable to the respiratory tract may not develop until later. It is this paucity of respiratory tract symptoms, despite evidence of a systemic febrile illness, that can either be a clue to diagnosis or mislead clinicians. When the patient is pressed for details regarding symptoms, a history of a nonproductive cough, or one productive of nonpurulent, sometimes bloody, secretions, is usually obtained. Production of large amounts of grossly purulent sputum is unusual. Pleuritic chest pain, sometimes in concert with hemoptysis, may be present and may mislead the clinician into considering pulmonary infarction. Mental confusion is reported commonly in some series; obtundation, seizures, and focal neurologic findings may also occur less frequently.

Fever is almost uniformly present in cases of legionnaires' disease, although there are reports of short (days) afebrile periods in some immunosuppressed patients with *L. micdadei* pneumonia. Some patients have pulse-temperature dissociation. Chest examination early in the disease may reveal only scattered rales or evidence of pleural effusion. However, later in the course, most patients have classic findings of consolidating pneumonia. Abdominal examination may reveal generalized or local tenderness and, in rare cases, evidence of peritonitis. Splenomegaly is uncommon. Findings of pericarditis, myocarditis, and focal abscesses are rare. No rash is associated with this disease, except that caused by other factors, such as drug therapy.

The fatality rate of untreated legionnaires' disease is about 10

TABLE 296–1. EXTRAPULMONARY INFECTIONS CAUSED BY LEGIONELLA

Dialysis shunt infection
Sinusitis
Pericarditis
Prosthetic valve endocarditis
Peritonitis
Abscesses
    Skin
    Brain
    Bowel
    Rectum
    Kidney
    Myocardium

to 30 per cent in nonimmunosuppressed patients and up to 80 per cent in immunocompromised ones. Thus, the majority of previously healthy people recover from untreated legionnaires' disease after 7 to 10 days of severe illness; those who do not recover die of progressive respiratory and multisystem failure.

Clinically significant extrapulmonary infection in patients with legionnaires' disease is quite rare (Table 296–1).

Pontiac fever is a nonfatal influenza-like disease, with symptoms of myalgia, fever, headache, and malaise occurring in 60 to 90 per cent of patients. Arthralgia occurs with variable frequency, as do cough, anorexia, and abdominal pain. The illness is generally not severe enough, nor long enough in duration, to cause most patients to seek medical attention. Not much is known about physical findings early in the disease; findings after 3 to 5 days of illness are generally normal except for fever and possibly tachypnea. Pneumonia does not occur. The illness lasts about 3 to 5 days, although some patients may have persistent fatigue or nonfocal neurologic complaints for weeks to months afterward.

CHEST ROENTGENOGRAPHIC FINDINGS. Legionnaires' disease causes alveolar filling infiltrates that usually eventuate in consolidation. Interstitial infiltrates are rare, although they may occur early in the course of disease and then progress to consolidating infiltrates. The infiltrates may be unilateral or bilateral and can spread very quickly to involve the entire lung. Pleural effusion, usually small in volume, occurs commonly and may be the sole abnormal radiographic finding in early disease.

DIAGNOSIS. The results of multiple nonspecific laboratory tests may be abnormal in patients with legionnaires' disease. These abnormal findings include proteinuria, pyuria, hematuria, leukocytosis, leukopenia, and thrombocytopenia. Disseminated intravascular coagulation may be seen in patients with respiratory failure caused by legionnaires' disease. Hyponatremia, hypophosphatemia, hyperbilirubinemia, and elevated serum alanine transaminase (ALT), serum aspartate transaminase (AST), and alkaline phosphatase concentrations may also be found. Elevation of creatine kinase (MM isoenzyme) is common, and some patients develop myoglobinuria and renal failure. The cerebrospinal fluid is usually normal, although rare patients may have 25 to 100 white blood cells per microliter of cerebrospinal fluid.

Legionnaires' disease can be diagnosed using specific laboratory tests (Table 296–2). The most sensitive and specific test is culture of respiratory tract secretions, such as sputum. Sputum culture for *Legionella* should be performed on every patient suspected of having this disease. Serologic testing is more useful to epidemiologists than to clinicians, because of cross-reactions with antibodies to unrelated organisms. No laboratory test currently available is 100 per cent accurate for the diagnosis of legionnaires' disease. Thus empiric therapy must be considered in appropriate clinical settings.

The diagnosis of Pontiac fever is based on demonstration of legionellae in water to which the patient was exposed, significant increases in antibody to the isolated *Legionella* species, and a clinical course compatible with this diagnosis. To be certain about the diagnosis of Pontiac fever, it is almost always necessary to perform extensive studies of unaffected people and their environments. This is because recovery of legionnellae from water and the elevation of antibodies to *Legionella* are relatively common events. Thus, it is nearly impossible to diagnose nonepidemic cases of Pontiac fever specifically.

The differential diagnosis of legionnaires' disease is especially broad, especially in immunosuppressed hosts. Mycoplasmal pneumonia is generally much less severe and causes significant respiratory system complaints. Pneumococcal pneumonia, in contrast to legionnaires' disease, is usually penicillin-responsive. Psittacosis and Q fever can have clinical presentations quite similar to that of legionnaires' disease.

THERAPY. Erythromycin is considered the drug of choice for this disease, on the basis of retrospective studies, which show that the case fatality rate is lowered about fivefold by prompt administration of erythromycin. The drug is given every 6 hours in a dosage of 0.5 to 1.0 gram intravenously until there is clinical improvement, which usually occurs in 2 to 4 days. Therapy can then be changed to oral erythromycin, 0.5 gram every 6 hours for 3 weeks. Possible alternative drugs include doxycycline (100 mg twice daily), sulfamethoxazole-trimethoprim (15 mg per kilogram per day of the trimethoprim component, three times daily), or ciprofloxacin (750 mg twice daily); clinical experience is not

TABLE 296–2. SPECIFIC DIAGNOSTIC TESTS FOR *LEGIONELLA*

Type	Suitable Specimens	Sensitivity (%)*	Specificity (%)	Notes
Culture	Sputum, lung, pleural fluid, blood, abscess contents	—	100	Use of special and selective media required; 3 to 5 days required for growth
Immunofluorescent microscopy	Sputum, lung, pleural fluid, abscess contents	25–75	95–99.9	Species-specific monoclonal antibody available; not helpful for diagnosis of all species; highest specificity for *L. pneumophila;* relatively low specificity for other species; 2 to 3 hours required for testing
DNA probe	Sputum, lung	50–60	99.1–99.9	Genus specific; may have lower sensitivity for detection of some species and for detection of organism in pleural fluid and transtracheal aspirates; 2 to 3 hours required for testing
Urine enzyme-linked immunosorbent assay (ELISA)	Urine	90–95	>99.9	Useful only for detection of *L. pneumophila* serogroup 1, the most common cause of legionnaires' disease; 2 to 3 hours required for testing
Antibody	Serum	60–70	90–99	Requires testing of paired specimens; seroconversion may not occur until 2 to 3 months after infection; most specific for *L. pneumophila* serogroup 1; cross-reactions with antibodies to many other bacteria

*Sensitivity versus culture. Culture is the most sensitive diagnostic technique, but its absolute sensitivity is unknown; reasonable estimates are 80 to 90 per cent.

substantial with any of these alternative drugs and they should not be used unless erythromycin cannot be tolerated, so they remain second choices. Quinolone antimicrobials (ciprofloxacin, pefloxacin) are much more effective than erythromycin in experimental laboratory studies; with further clinical experience, they may become the drugs of choice. Because of its potent in vitro activity and efficacy in experimental models, many clinicians would add rifampin (600 mg twice daily) to erythromycin for the treatment of severe cases of legionnaires' disease. There are no clinical data indicating the superiority of this combination. Penicillins, cephalosporins (first, second, and third generation), and aminoglycosides are ineffective for the therapy of legionnaires' disease. In fact, the failure of pneumonia to respond to these agents should prompt consideration of legionnaires' disease, and perhaps initiation of erythromycin therapy. No effective therapy for Pontiac fever is known.

Most patients with legionnaires' disease respond within 1 to 4 days to specific antimicrobial therapy. The symptoms clearing most rapidly are rigors, mental confusion, myalgia, anorexia, fatigue, and abdominal complaints. Fever may persist for a week after initiation of therapy but starts a downward trend within a few days. Despite this clinical evidence of improvement, other findings may falsely imply disease progression, such as evidence of increased pulmonary consolidation on physical examination and on roentgenography. Weeks to months are required for the resolution of pulmonary infiltrates. Patients with respiratory failure have a relatively poor prognosis and tend to have a much slower response to therapy.

Doebbeling BN, Wenzel RP: The epidemiology of *Legionella pneumophila* infections. Semin Respir Infect 2:206, 1987. *A recent comprehensive review.*

Edelstein PH: The laboratory diagnosis of legionnaires' disease. Semin Respir Infect 2:235, 1987. *Expands on laboratory diagnosis.*

Kirby BD, Snyder KM, Meyer RD, et al.: Legionnaires' disease: Report of sixty-five nosocomially acquired cases and review of the literature. Medicine (Baltimore) 59:188, 1980. *Classic description of the disease.*

Winn WC Jr: Legionnaires' disease: Historical perspective. Clin Microbiol Rev 1:60, 1988. *Good review of most aspects, extensively referenced.*

Streptococcal Diseases

297 Streptococcal Diseases

Richard M. Krause

Streptococci are ubiquitous, gram-positive globular bacteria that grow in chains. They were first described by Billroth in 1874 in purulent exudates from erysipelas lesions and infected wounds. Subsequently they were shown to cause different forms of streptococcal disease, including streptococcal sore throat, scarlet fever, streptococcal skin infections (impetigo or pyoderma), suppurative infections (including abscesses and pneumonia), food poisoning, septicemia, bacterial endocarditis, and urinary tract infections. A single streptococcal species may be responsible for a variety of diseases, and many different kinds of streptococci may be cultured from humans and animals.

The first classification of these organisms was based on their capacity to lyse red blood cells. When streptococci are cultured on blood agar plates, three types of hemolytic reactions are observed. Streptococcal colonies surrounded by a clear zone of hemolysis are termed beta (β), colonies surrounded by green partial hemolysis are termed alpha (α), and the nonhemolytic colonies are termed gamma (γ).

Primarily through the efforts of Lancefield, the β-hemolytic streptococci were further differentiated into a number of serologic categories, designated groups A to H and K to T, on the basis of specific polysaccharide antigens. Most streptococci causing pharyngitis and impetigo belong to group A. Rheumatic fever occurs only after group A pharyngitis. Streptococci belonging to certain other Lancefield groups are now recognized as important causes of infection. α-Hemolytic and gamma streptococci can cause endocarditis and other forms of sepsis with systemic illness.

Group A streptococcal pharyngitis has been intensely studied over the years because it may give rise to the delayed, nonsuppurative sequelae acute rheumatic fever (ARF) and acute glomerulonephritis (AGN). While ARF is less common in the United States today than 30 years ago, it still persists as a common cause of heart disease in the developing world. Pyoderma due to group A streptococci may lead to AGN but not to ARF.

CLASSIFICATION OF STREPTOCOCCI OF CLINICAL IMPORTANCE

The classification of streptococci on the basis of hemolysis patterns on blood agar plates and antigenic composition was a major advance. Nevertheless, it is frequently necessary to employ a combination of features, including growth characteristics and biochemical reactions, to characterize fully these organisms because they are such a heterogeneous group. A classification of streptococci with a clinical orientation for the most important streptococcal infections is presented in Table 297–1. While group A streptococci remain important human pathogens, β-hemolytic non–group A, α-hemolytic, and nonhemolytic streptococci are of increasing importance as the cause of suppurative infections in all regions of the body.

GROUP A INFECTIONS. Group A streptococci are the most common cause of streptococcal pharyngitis. They are recognized by the characteristic group A carbohydrate cell wall antigen, which is identified by serologic reactions to specific rabbit antiserum. In this way they can be distinguished from other β-hemolytic streptococci that are also frequently isolated from the human pharynx, vagina, or skin.

GROUP B INFECTIONS. Group B streptococci are identified serologically by their characteristic cell wall polysaccharide. First recognized as a cause of bovine mastitis, since the 1960's they have emerged as a major cause of neonatal sepsis with or without meningitis. Carriage of group B streptococci in the female genital tract is a major source of these infections.

GROUP D INFECTIONS. Group D streptococci consist of two major categories: enterococci (such as *S. faecalis*) and nonenterococci (such as *S. bovis*). Strains isolated from clinical cultures are usually nonhemolytic or α-hemolytic, but β-hemolytic strains are seen.

Enterococci are present in the normal intestinal flora and are a significant cause of community-acquired and hospital-acquired sepsis and septicemia. Enterococci are a frequent cause of urinary tract infections, particularly in patients with structural abnormalities of the urinary tract. They are also a frequent cause of endocarditis. Enterococci are frequently resistant to many antibiotics, which complicates treatment. For the treatment of enterococcal endocarditis, combined therapy should be employed, including intravenously administered penicillin in high doses plus an aminoglycoside antibiotic. In combination, these drugs have a synergistic killing effect on enterococci.

In contrast to enterococci, nonenterococcal group D streptococci isolated from patients with endocarditis are extremely sensitive to penicillin. Because of these differences in antibiotic sensitivity, it may be necessary to perform additional biochemical tests to differentiate enterococci from nonenterococcal group D organisms. One simple culture procedure employs broth containing 6.5 per cent sodium chloride. Enterococci usually grow under these conditions, whereas other streptococci do not.

OTHER STREPTOCOCCAL INFECTIONS. Not infrequently, the β-hemolytic streptococci cultured from the throat or other sites are identified as groups C or G organisms. Most commonly when they colonize the pharynx, these organisms produce no symptoms or illness. But on occasion pharyngitis occurs, which may be exudative. A rise in the convalescent antistreptolysin O titer indicates that these groups actually can cause an infection of the pharynx and other sites and are not just passively carried. An unexpected event was the occurrence of 10 cases of group C streptococcal sepsis, including meningitis, in New Mexico in the summer of 1983. In addition to groups C and G, case reports indicate that streptococci belonging to most of the other groups can cause sporadic infections, including meningitis, infected heart valves, visceral abscesses, and soft tissue infections following surgical procedures. Furthermore, these less common organisms are now known to cause opportunistic infections in individuals with diminished resistance due to other diseases or treatments.

The predominant aerobic flora of the oral pharynx normally consists of a large variety of streptococci. These are classified as *viridans*, α-hemolytic, or green streptococci. They may play some useful role by maintaining a favorable ecologic balance. However, they can produce disease in abnormal circumstances. They are a common cause of subacute bacterial endocarditis and enter the bloodstream most often from diseased teeth and gums.

Special interest has now centered on a species of these organisms identified as *S. mutans*. These bacteria colonize the oral cavity and have been implicated in the development of dental caries. They produce a mucoid substance that becomes part of the plaque adhering to the tooth enamel. The bacteria remain embedded in the plaque and excrete metabolic products that are a factor in the production of caries. Currently there is evidence that dental caries can be prevented by decreasing sugar in the diet to diminish the growth of these bacteria as well as by practicing proper oral hygiene to remove the plaque containing the *S. mutans* organisms.

Anaerobic streptococci are also a prominent part of the normal flora in the mouth, intestine, and vagina. It is suspected that they maintain an ecologic balance on the surface of these tissues, but the mechanism is unknown. The presence of this normal flora appears to be important, however, because when the ecologic balance is disturbed by the use of antibiotics, pathogens such as *Candida albicans* may cause infections of these sites.

Anaerobic streptococci may cause abscesses in many different regions of the body, including retropharyngeal spaces, paranasal sinuses, dental structures, and the brain. Visceral infections include lung abscesses and empyema fluids, abscesses of the liver and other intra-abdominal viscera, and perirectal and pelvic abscesses. Anaerobic streptococci are especially prone to thrive in dead or devitalized muscle, skin, or subcutaneous tissue. A rapidly progressing necrotizing fasciitis or *progressive synergistic gangrene* is usually produced by these anaerobic streptococci along with *Staphylococcus aureus*. While these anaerobic organisms are frequently sensitive to penicillin, debridement and drainage of abscesses are important aspects of treatment.

GROUP A STREPTOCOCCAL INFECTIONS

BACKGROUND AND PATHOGENESIS. Although streptococci were identified as the cause of scarlet fever and tonsillitis in 1895, it was not until later that a major advance was made in classification, when these organisms were classified serologically into groups by Lancefield and into types by Lancefield and Griffith. With these developments it was possible to identify

TABLE 297–1. CLINICAL CLASSES OF STREPTOCOCCAL INFECTIONS

Lancified Groups	Hemolysis on Blood Agar	Representative Species	Major Clinical Syndromes	Colonization (Carriage)
A	β	*S. pyogenes*	Pharyngitis (scarlet fever), pyoderma, wound infection, sepsis, rheumatic fever, acute glomerulonephritis	Pharynx
B	β	*S. agalactiae*	Perinatal sepsis, newborn meningitis, subacute bacterial endocarditis, urinary tract infection, adult sepsis	Adult urogenital tract, gastrointestinal tract, throat, rectum, pharynx
C and G	β	—	Mild pharyngitis	Pharynx
D	Variable (usually nonhemolytic)	Enterococci (*S. faecalis*)	Subacute bacterial endocarditis, urinary tract infection	Bowel
		Nonenterococci (*S. bovis*)	Subacute bacterial endocarditis	
Nongroupable: viridans streptococci	α (green)	*S. salivarius, S. sanguis, S. mutans*	Subacute bacterial endocarditis, caries	Oropharynx, saliva
Anaerobic (microaerophilic streptococci)	γ (nonhemolytic) or variable	*Peptostreptococcus*	Abscesses, gangrene, necrotizing fasciitis, peritonsillar abscess	Mouth, intestine, vagina

group A streptococci as the most common cause of streptococcal pharyngitis. The ability to measure serologic responses was another important advance. Most widely used has been the antistreptolysin O (ASO) test developed by Todd in 1932. This was a major achievement because a rise in an ASO titer or a markedly elevated titer was found to be indicative of a prior streptococcal infection. These immunologic and bacteriologic developments led to the firm conclusion that ARF and AGN are nonsuppurative sequelae to group A streptococcal infections and that infections by *any* of the other streptococcal groups do not result in such sequelae. The rare exception to this rule is that, on occasion, group C streptococcal infections appear to cause AGN. ARF is observed *only* after group A pharyngitis, but AGN is seen after pharyngitis and pyoderma.

Epidemics of streptococcal disease in the armed forces have been known since the Civil War. The epidemics in World War I, World War II, and the Korean War were studied in detail, and much of the current knowledge concerning the epidemiology of group A streptococcal disease rests on this research. A major advance was the primary prevention of rheumatic fever by penicillin treatment of streptococcal pharyngitis and the use of penicillin prophylaxis to prevent recurrences of ARF. Epidemics of streptococcal sore throat and scarlet fever were once commonly observed among school children, and this resulted in extensive programs for the early detection and treatment of pharyngitis to prevent rheumatic fever. While epidemics of streptococcal pharyngitis are now less common, sporadic outbreaks in schools or other closed populations still occur as minor epidemics. Indeed, during the past several years there has been an unexpected increase in the occurrence of rheumatic fever in school children and military recruits.

Group A streptococci are subdivided into M types on the basis of an antigen known as *M protein*. More than 80 antigenically distinct M types have been identified. This substance plays a very important role in the pathogenesis of group A streptococcal infections. The M protein is a surface component of the streptococcus and is correlated with its ability to resist phagocytosis. Streptococci that have large amounts of M protein are highly resistant to phagocytosis, whereas those with no or a sparse amount of M protein are susceptible to phagocytosis. Following an infection with streptococci of a particular M type, homologous type-specific immunity develops, so that the individual is resistant to infection by organisms of the same M type; this immunity persists for many years. Reinfection with the same M type is rare. Because there are numerous M types of streptococci, repeated streptococcal infections caused by different M types are common, particularly in childhood and early adult life. Penicillin or other antibiotic therapy can suppress the type-specific immune response. For this reason, reinfection with the same M type has been seen since the use of antibiotics.

Because of the importance of M type–specific immunity in resistance to group A streptococcal infections, intensive research has centered on the immunochemistry of the M protein and the immune response to it. The complete chemical structure of several different M proteins is now known, and with the use of recombinant DNA technology, pure type 6 M protein has been produced by *Escherichia coli*. It should now be possible to examine at the molecular level the chemical basis for the anti-phagocytic properties of M protein and to explore the molecular interactions that occur when specific antibody promotes phagocytosis of group A streptococci. While these recent developments on the chemistry of M protein have raised again the possibility of a multivalent streptococcal vaccine for use in regions where streptococcal disease still flourishes, a number of theoretical and practical impediments to the development of such a vaccine have to be overcome.

The T antigen is another streptococcal surface protein that has assisted in the classification of streptococci isolated from clinical material. As with M proteins, there are multiple serotypes of T antigens. While T antigens (unlike M proteins) play no part in virulence, they have become very useful antigenic markers, particularly in the recognition of less virulent strains that have lost their M protein. The T antigen classification also has been useful in identifying strains isolated from patients with pyoderma for which an M protein has not yet been identified.

Group A streptococci grown in vivo and in vitro produce a great variety of antigenic extracellular products, such as the two hemolysins—streptolysin O and streptolysin S—streptokinase, hyaluronidase, nicotinamide adenine dinucleotidase (NADase), and several deoxyribonucleases (DNases). The antibody responses to several of these substances are useful in clinical diagnosis. Streptolysin O is reversibly inhibited by oxygen. Because anaerobic conditions prevail beneath the surface of the blood agar, hemolysis in this region is due to streptolysin O. Streptolysin O is produced by almost all group A strains as well as by many group C and G organisms. Since streptolysin O is a good antigen, titration of ASO antibodies in human sera is the most widely used serologic procedure in clinical practice to detect a prior group A streptococcal infection. In recent years, a test to measure anti-DNase B antibodies has been used in the evaluation of streptococcal pyoderma as well as upper respiratory tract infections. A rise in ASO antibodies is not observed in pyoderma.

The erythrogenic toxins cause the typical erythema of scarlet fever. There are three serologically distinct toxins, each neutralized by its respective antibody. For this reason scarlet fever may occur more than once. Not all strains of streptococci produce an erythrogenic toxin. In the past several years, there have been numerous reports of the occurrence of a toxic shock–like syndrome associated with group A streptococcal infections, but there is still uncertainty if this is due to erythrogenic toxin or some other streptococcal product.

Group A streptococci most commonly infect the tonsils, nasopharynx, and skin. A number of features of streptococcal skin infections set them apart from streptococcal tonsillitis, and for this reason, the clinical features of skin infections are considered separately.

EPIDEMIOLOGY. Streptococcal pharyngitis and tonsillitis are the most common group A streptococcal infections. Their most frequent occurrence is in children between 5 and 15 years of age, but both younger and older persons are still highly susceptible to infection. This is particularly true when special environmental circumstances enhance transmission. For example, mobilization of troops during wartime results in an increased incidence of streptococcal infections in individuals 18 to 25 years of age. The high attack rate in children and military recruits is related to the close contact between susceptible individuals and either infected persons or healthy carriers who carry contagious streptococci in the pharynx. Organisms are transmitted from one person to another on saliva droplets produced by sneezing or coughing.

Untreated patients are the primary source of the spread of streptococcal disease, especially during the period of acute pharyngitis and for the first several weeks of convalescence. Studies of kindergarten and school-age children indicate that an untreated child is often the source of the disease in the classroom as well as in the home. It is therefore important to identify and treat patients as soon as possible to prevent secondary spread of the disease.

Throat cultures of untreated patients obtained during the illness and early convalescence (1 to 3 weeks) usually reveal large numbers of streptococci, and therefore the source of spread. Small numbers of streptococci may be detected in the throat cultures for many weeks or months after an untreated infection. However, individual carriers in whom small numbers of streptococci persist for long periods are an unusual source of secondary spread.

Nasal or throat carriage (or both) of virulent streptococci is also a source of infection of open wounds and skin abrasions as well as of puerperal sepsis. Secondary infection of the lungs may occur, particularly after a respiratory infection such as influenza. Indeed, streptococcal pneumonia may be seen with greater frequency during an influenza epidemic.

A confusing aspect of streptococcal pharyngitis is that a significant number of individuals have "silent" infections that are detected by positive throat cultures *and* a rise in the ASO titer. In early studies it was learned that at least 25 to 30 per cent of all patients who developed ARF had had a preceding silent throat infection. Such silent infections complicate the control of spread of streptococcal disease in a family or community. Epidemiologic studies have shown that patients with subclinical or silent infection are capable of disseminating the streptococci to other individuals, who then may develop overt disease.

Currently there is debate concerning reasons for the declining frequency of severe acute pharyngitis with exudate. Certainly the number of such patients with severe disease is much smaller than it was 30 years ago, while the mild form appears more common. It is unknown whether this change in the clinical picture is due to a decline in the virulence of the streptococci, to host factors, or to the widespread use of antibiotics to treat patients who have been infected with the more virulent forms of streptococci, thus eliminating these organisms from the reservoir of potential pathogens.

A number of epidemiologic factors influence the spread of streptococcal disease. Clearly, socioeconomic factors that promote crowding will result in close contact between individuals and therefore in the spread of streptococci. Climate, season, and geography also can enhance the spread of streptococci because of their influence in bringing people into close contact. It has already been mentioned that military recruits are susceptible because they are clustered in large camps under crowded conditions. Similarly, streptococcal disease is common in civilian populations where poverty and poor housing promote crowding and therefore the spread from one individual to another. It is probable that these factors continue to influence the widespread occurrence of streptococcal disease, and therefore ARF and rheumatic heart disease, in developing countries.

Scarlet fever is now uncommon in the United States. The reasons for this are not clear, because the decline began before the widespread use of antibiotics. Streptococcal strains that produce scarlet fever are the same as those that produce group A infections except that they are lysogenized by a bacteriophage that induces the production of erythrogenic toxin.

Although streptococcal pharyngitis is most common in the winter months, when close contact between individuals is greatest, streptococcal pyoderma occurs in the late summer and early fall. Presumably this is due to exposure of uncovered skin, during the warmer months, to minor trauma and insect bites, which favor skin infections. Although streptococcal pharyngitis and streptococcal pyoderma occur worldwide, geography clearly influences the occurrence of these diseases. Pharyngitis is more common in temperate and cold climates, and pyoderma is more frequent in hot or tropical climates.

The attack rate of ARF after streptococcal infections may vary widely. During the major epidemics of World War II and the Korean War, the attack rate was 3 per cent or more in military recruits with untreated group A streptococcal infections. Since that time, studies of children and other civilian populations, particularly those experiencing the sporadic infections that occur today, have suggested that the attack rate may be as low as 0.3 per cent or less.

The epidemiology and bacteriology of the streptococcal infections that precede ARF differ in important respects from those of the streptococcal infections that precede AGN. In the early years of streptococcal bacteriology, ARF was seen as a complication of epidemic pharyngitis due to nearly all of the different types of group A streptococci. For example, certain M types, such as 1, 3, 5, 6, 14, 18, 19, and 24, have all produced epidemics of pharyngitis in the United States that have resulted in ARF. In contrast, AGN was not a constant complication of these epidemics. The occurrence of AGN has been associated with epidemics of pharyngitis caused by a limited number of M types, such as type 12. Such differences in the bacteriology of ARF and AGN have raised speculation concerning "rheumatogenic" and "nephritogenic" strains of streptococci. However, such designations become blurred on the basis of epidemiologic information. Sporadic outbreaks of AGN caused by types 1, 3, and 6 have been seen, all of which have been associated with ARF. There is no doubt that certain outbreaks of type 12 pharyngitis have resulted in an unusually high incidence of AGN, but type 12 strains in the general population have not consistently resulted in outbreaks of AGN. Therefore, no single M type can be arbitrarily designated "nephritogenic." Clearly the *antecedent* streptococcal infection that results in AGN must be due to an organism that has acquired some special characteristic other than a particular M protein. Despite intensive study, there is no certainty about the nature of this special characteristic. Efforts are under way to identify streptococcal antigens in the immune complexes of patients with AGN that are associated with "nephritogenic" streptococci. It is

tempting to speculate that strains acquire the "nephritogenic" property by some form of gene transfer from those streptococci that already possess the capacity to produce AGN.

As attention was focused on the epidemiology of streptococcal infections and AGN, additional M serotypes that had not been associated with pharyngitis were identified, primarily from skin infections. AGN has been associated with skin infections due to several of these types, such as M types 49, 55, and 57.

Streptococcal Sore Throat

The usual incubation period of streptococcal pharyngitis is between 2 and 4 days. Typically, in both children and adults there is a rather abrupt onset of sore throat. A particular characteristic is pain on swallowing. Hoarseness is rare. Other symptoms include headache, malaise, feverishness, and anorexia. Chilliness is common, but not rigor. Nausea, vomiting, and abdominal pain are common in children. The patient appears mildly to moderately ill, but signs and symptoms depend upon the severity of the illness. Temperature frequently exceeds 38.5°C. In the moderately severe case, examination of the throat reveals diffuse erythema, edema, and lymphoid hyperplasia of the posterior pharynx. The uvula may be edematous. The tonsils are enlarged and reddened. A yellow-gray exudate, when present, may be punctate or confluent. There may be discrete areas of exudate about 1 to 2 mm in diameter on the posterior pharynx. The anterior cervical nodes are usually enlarged and tender. The white blood cell count is usually greater than 12,000 per cubic millimeter. When properly taken, the throat culture usually reveals large numbers of group A β-hemolytic streptococci. Not uncommonly, group A streptococci are the predominant organisms observed on the culture plate. The course of streptococcal pharyngitis is usually self-limited, and the fever and other symptoms abate within 3 to 4 days.

A pharyngitis of the severity just described is typical of the infections seen in earlier years in civilian populations and during military epidemics, but such infections occur less commonly today. Many patients do not have all of the signs and symptoms just described. For example, in mild pharyngitis, there may be no exudate and the throat culture may reveal modest numbers of group A streptococci.

If antimicrobial therapy has not been used, group A streptococci may persist in the pharynx for weeks or months following acute pharyngitis. Some patients who are treated with penicillin will carry the streptococci for several weeks. If the course of antibiotics has been adequate, these patients need not be retreated, since they are unlikely to be a source of spread to other individuals.

The diagnosis of streptococcal pharyngitis in infants and small children presents a special challenge. The disease lacks a well-defined onset. Often rhinorrhea is a dominant manifestation. Fever is low grade. Usually the physical signs in the throat are not helpful in the differential diagnosis. A throat culture is positive when properly taken, as is the culture of the anterior nares. Despite the mildness of the pharyngitis in infants, suppurative complications such as otitis media can occur.

Scarlet Fever

Scarlet fever occurs in those patients with streptococcal pharyngitis in whom the infected organism produces an erythrogenic toxin and who are not immune to the toxin because they have had no prior exposure. The enanthem of scarlet fever includes a tongue that may be bright red with large papillae (raspberry tongue) or coated, with the red papillae protruding (strawberry tongue). These manifestations of the disease are rarely seen in adults. The rash appears shortly after the onset of the sore throat, usually within 2 days, and involves the neck, upper chest, and back and then spreads to the remainder of the trunk and the extremities. The palms and the soles are spared. The rash consists of a diffuse erythema that blanches on pressure, with numerous 1-mm punctate elevations that give a sandpaper texture to the skin. There is a generalized facial flush with a pale area often seen around the mouth, the *circumoral pallor*. The distribution of the rash is variable. The trunk and inner aspects of the arms and thighs are most often affected, but in milder cases the rash is seen only in the axilla or groin. Linear striations of confluent petechiae are known as *Pastia's lines*. A tourniquet applied to the arm for 5 minutes results in large numbers of petechiae distal to the obstruction in nearly all cases (the *Rumpel-Leede sign*). The erythema usually disappears by the sixth to ninth day after the onset of infection. Desquamation of the skin is a characteristic of scarlet fever. It begins with a fine scaling of the face and body and is usually completed during the second week. There then occurs an extensive and characteristic desquamation of the palms and soles. Eosinophilia has been observed, particularly during the period of desquamation.

SUPPURATIVE COMPLICATIONS. The most frequent suppurative complications of streptococcal pharyngitis are perinasal sinusitis, otitis media, and mastoiditis. Suppurative cervical adenitis may occur. Bacteremia was seen more commonly in earlier times prior to the use of antibiotics; this resulted in metastatic lesions in joints, bones, and other sites. Group A streptococcal meningitis is now uncommon.

Recent reports have called attention to unusually severe group A streptococcal infections of skin or wounds, which then extended to soft tissue infection and septicemia, associated with a toxic shock–like syndrome. Cellulitis and fasciitis were common. Most patients developed shock and acute respiratory distress syndrome. The constellation of renal failure, shock, hypocalcemia, and thrombocytopenia is similar to that seen in staphylococcal toxic shock syndrome. In one series, 6 of 20 patients died. The severe complications of these patients are listed in Table 297–2.

An unusual and infrequent complication of streptococcal tonsillitis is *peritonsillar abscess*, or *quinsy*. While it is probable that the streptococcal infection leads to the formation of the abscess, the abscesses themselves do not contain group A streptococci but a variety of oropharyngeal flora, including anaerobic bacteria. This complication should be suspected if there is an abrupt increase in (1) soreness in the throat, (2) swelling in the neck, and (3) fever during or shortly after streptococcal pharyngitis. Inspection of the throat reveals the displacement of the tonsil on the affected side toward the midline. A fluctuant mass may be felt in the affected area with a gloved finger; it should be treated promptly because complications arise when the infection extends farther into the neck and surrounding tissues.

NONSUPPURATIVE COMPLICATIONS. The nonsuppurative complications of streptococcal disease are ARF and AGN. These are discussed in Ch. 298 and 79, respectively.

DIAGNOSIS. Group A streptococcal pharyngitis must be differentiated from pharyngitis due to other bacterial and viral agents. Gonococcal tonsillopharyngitis should be suspected if there is a history of homosexuality or fellatio. *Vincent's angina* usually has an insidious onset without the constitutional symptoms characteristic of a streptococcal sore throat. Signs of this infection, including an exudate, are commonly unilateral, whereas streptococcal pharyngitis is not. *Diphtheria* is now rare, although it should be recognized by the presence of the characteristic diphtheritic membrane as well as the other signs and symptoms of the disease.

TABLE 297–2. COMPLICATIONS OF GROUP A STREPTOCOCCAL SOFT TISSUE INFECTION*

Complication	No. of Patients (%)
Shock	19 (95)
Acute respiratory distress syndrome	11† (55)
Renal impairment	16 (80)
Irreversible	2 (10)
Reversible	14 (70)
Amputation	2 (10)
Desquamation of the skin	4 (20)
Fasciotomy	9‡ (45)
Sepsis	12 (60)
Death	6 (30)

*In a total of 20 patients.
†Diffuse pulmonary edema and hypoxia developed in one patient; both complications were resolved with diuresis and supplemental oxygen.
‡Amputation of a limb was ultimately required in two patients who underwent fasciotomies.
From Stevens DL, Tanner M, Winship J, et al.: Severe group A streptococcal infections associated with a toxic shock–like syndrome and scarlet fever toxin A. N Engl J Med 321:1–7, 1989. Modified by permission of the New England Journal of Medicine.

The major confusion in the differential diagnosis stems from viral respiratory infections, which not only occur more frequently than do streptococcal infections but which also may cause pharyngeal and tonsillar exudate. While many upper respiratory infections have a "common cold–like" quality, the symptoms may overlap considerably with those of streptococcal disease. Adenoviruses can cause an exudative pharyngitis clinically indistinguishable from that due to group A streptococci. A severe exudative pharyngitis with fever and toxicity is seen in infectious mononucleosis. The generalized symptoms and signs associated with infectious mononucleosis, however, should assist in the differential diagnosis. Pharyngitis due to group A coxsackieviruses (herpangina) or to herpes simplex results in the formation of vesicles. When these rupture, they may leave shallow ulcers that can often be differentiated from streptococcal disease by inspection. Because it is frequently not possible to distinguish streptococcal from nonstreptococcal sore throat on clinical grounds, precise diagnosis requires a throat culture.

Before any antimicrobial therapy is administered, swabs should be passed through the mouth under direct vision and a good light and rubbed over the tonsils and posterior pharynx. The swabs should be streaked directly, with a minimum of delay, on a sheep blood agar plate of low dextrose content. After incubation overnight, the number of hemolytic streptococci present should be recorded in a roughly quantitative manner. The organisms are very numerous in most cases if they are the cause of the infection, but in some instances as few as 10 to 20 colonies are observed. The presence of a few colonies does not provide convincing evidence that they are responsible for the illness, because 5 to 10 per cent of the general population (and a higher percentage of children) may be nasopharyngeal carriers of these organisms, so growth of a few colonies is not by itself an indication of infection. Serologic grouping and typing of the isolated organisms are usually not necessary for routine clinical diagnosis. Because the growth of group A streptococci is inhibited in vitro by paper discs containing less than 0.02 unit of bacitracin, some laboratories routinely determine the bacitracin susceptibility of hemolytic streptococci. Hemolytic bacteria resistant to such low concentrations of bacitracin are unlikely to be group A streptococci. On the other hand, approximately 5 per cent of non–group A hemolytic streptococci are also susceptible to this low concentration. New rapid antigen detection systems have been developed to identify group A streptococci directly from the cotton swab, including latex agglutination of throat swab extracts. The specificity of these tests is reasonably good, but when small numbers of streptococci are present, the test is less sensitive than the culture methods. If the test is negative and pharyngitis is suspected on clinical grounds, a throat culture should be done.

If the pharyngitis persists with adequate penicillin therapy, it is unlikely to be due to group A streptococci. However, viral pharyngitis is often of brief duration, and if such patients are treated with penicillin, it may appear that there has been a therapeutic response when in fact the disease has abated spontaneously.

The ASO test is not useful in the diagnosis of streptococcal pharyngitis. An elevation in titer is evidence of a recent infection and is employed in the diagnosis of patients with rheumatic fever and rheumatic heart disease.

TREATMENT. There are four reasons for treating streptococcal pharyngitis: (1) the prevention of suppurative complications; (2) the prevention of the nonsuppurative complications ARF and AGN; (3) the prevention of spread of the disease to family contacts or to persons in small social units, such as school rooms and army barracks, and (4) the relief of symptoms. The recent occurrence of streptococcal pharyngitis followed by rapid onset of a toxic shock–like syndrome that may be fatal is now a compelling reason for early diagnosis and treatment. Prevention of ARF depends upon the eradication of the organism from the pharynx, and this requires treatment for at least 10 days. Because signs and symptoms frequently subside in a few days, there is a tendency to shorten the time antibiotics are given. Brief periods of antibiotic therapy do not eliminate the streptococci from the pharynx. Patients treated briefly have a greater risk of developing ARF than do those who are adequately treated for at least 10 days.

Penicillin is the drug of choice. Group A streptococci are highly susceptible in the action of penicillin. Despite its use for over 40 years, no penicillin-resistant strains have developed. A single intramuscular injection of 1.2 million units of benzathine penicillin G provides a sufficiently prolonged level of penicillin in the blood to eradicate the organism. For children weighing less than 60 pounds, the dose is 600,000 units. If oral therapy is used, 250,000 units of penicillin G or 250 mg of penicillin V, three or four times daily, is the treatment of choice. If penicillin allergy is suspected or known to exist, erythromycin is the drug of choice, 20 mg per pound per day (not to exceed 1 gram per day) for a period of 10 days. Erythromycin resistance is not yet a serious problem in the United States. Many group A streptococci have developed resistance to tetracycline, and it is no longer recommended for treatment of group A infections. Sulfonamides, when used to treat streptococcal pharyngitis, are ineffective in preventing rheumatic fever. They do not suppress the immune response, do not terminate pharyngeal carriage of streptococci, and thus do not reduce the attack rate of subsequent rheumatic fever. They may be used, however, as continuous prophylaxis to prevent new infections in patients who have had an initial attack of rheumatic fever.

Treatment of streptococcal sore throat should be started as soon as a definite diagnosis of streptococcal infection is made. Because of the occurrence of toxic shock–like syndrome with streptococcal infections, if the clinical picture suggests streptococcal pharyngitis, a throat culture should be done and the treatment begun without delay. It has been shown, however, that a short delay while awaiting throat culture results (even for several days) in initiating antimicrobial therapy does not significantly interfere with rheumatic fever prevention. One exception to this statement involves the patient with a history of rheumatic fever. In such a patient, the prevention of rheumatic occurrence is not always possible unless treatment is instituted at the first clinical sign of streptococcal infection. For such a patient, any delay of therapy entails the risk of reactivation of the disease.

If severe suppurative streptococcal infections such as mastoiditis, pneumonia, wound infections, or other forms of sepsis are present, patients should receive 600,000 units of procaine penicillin G twice a day intramuscularly for several days until the illness is under control. Then a shift can be made to benzathine penicillin or oral penicillin. It may be necessary to prolong therapy for several weeks whenever pus or necrosis is present, particularly when adequate debridement is not possible.

STREPTOCOCCAL PNEUMONIA

Streptococcal pneumonia is now uncommon. It can be seen, however, as a complication of influenza, measles, pertussis, or varicella. It is characterized by abrupt onset of fever, chills, myalgia, dyspnea, cough, pleuritic chest pain, and hemoptysis. Patients are severely ill. Radiologically, there is usually bronchopneumonia. Lobar consolidation is less common. One characteristic feature of streptococcal pneumonia is the early and rapid accumulation of a large volume of thin empyema fluid. The pneumonic infection can extend to the mediastinum and pericardium. Bacteremia occurs in 10 to 15 per cent of the cases. Bacteriologic diagnosis depends on recovering group A streptococci from the sputum, empyema fluid, and blood. Because the patient is very ill, treatment should be started promptly. Therapy consists of 4 to 6 million units of parenteral procaine penicillin G given daily; this total daily dose is given in two to four intramuscular injections. There must also be adequate drainage of the empyema fluid. This may require insertion of a chest tube.

STREPTOCOCCAL SKIN INFECTIONS

PYODERMA. Group A streptococci can produce localized purulent skin infections known as pyoderma. While some of the lesions represent secondary infections of wounds or burns, most commonly the infection is primary and is usually referred to as *streptococcal impetigo* or *impetigo contagiosa*. Intensive studies over the past 20 years have revealed a number of important bacteriologic and epidemiologic differences between streptococcal impetigo and streptococcal pharyngitis (Table 297–3). Impetigo occurs in the summer and fall, but pharyngitis is seen in the winter and spring. Children between the ages of 2 and 5 years

TABLE 297–3. COMPARISON OF THE FEATURES OF STREPTOCOCCAL PHARYNGITIS AND PYODERMA*

Features	Pharyngitis	Pyoderma
Clinical illness	Acute	Indolent
Laboratory		
Leukocytosis	Usually present	Often absent
Antistreptolysin O response	Common	Uncommon
Epidemiology		
Seasonal occurrence	Winter and spring	Late summer and early fall
Geographic distribution	More common in temperature or cold climates	Common in hot or tropical climates
Age	School-aged children	Children of preschool age
Transmission	Direct spread from human reservoirs	Unknown; insects may be mechanical vectors
Carrier state	Common in pharynx of many populations	Unusual on skin
Preceding trauma	Not present	May predispose to infection
Complications		
Acute nephritis	Occurs; partially preventable (50%)	Occurs; preventability unknown
Acute rheumatic fever	Occurs; preventable	Does not occur
Treatment		
Local	Not important	Removal of crusts and scrubbing with hexachlorophene soap
Systemic	Single intramuscular injection of benzathine penicillin or oral penicillin for 10 days	May not be necessary; extensive lesions may require intramuscular benzathine penicillin

From Wannamaker LW: N Engl J Med 282:23, 78, 1970. Modified by permission of the New England Journal of Medicine.

are more commonly infected. They are usually from underprivileged families residing in the southern United States or the tropics. Nevertheless, outbreaks can be seen among children of similar circumstances in other areas of the United States, such as those on American Indian reservations.

Epidemiologic studies have not clarified the mode of spread of streptococcal pyoderma, but it is reasonable to assume that personal contact with those infected, and perhaps insect vectors, may be important. Despite the uncertainty about the mode of spread, a number of important epidemiologic and clinical facts have emerged from recent studies. In general, the streptococci that cause pyoderma are the higher numbered M types, whereas pharyngitis is usually due to M types 1 through 40. Children who develop streptococcal impetigo and who carry the higher types on the skin may then develop pharyngeal carriage of these skin strains, which are unlikely to cause pharyngitis. Such pharyngeal carriage must be taken into consideration in the diagnosis of respiratory disease in these children, because carriage of these strains alone is not indicative of streptococcal pharyngitis.

Differences have been seen also in the immune response, depending on the site of the streptococcal infection. While the ASO response is usually brisk following streptococcal pharyngitis, it is weak or absent in patients with impetigo. It has been suggested that inactivation of streptolysin O by the lipids present in the skin accounts for this feeble antibody response. Brisk antibody responses do occur, however, to DNase B in patients with impetigo. M type–specific protective antibodies are almost always produced after streptococcal pharyngitis, but the response to the M type–specific antigens is variable in the case of impetigo. It is not surprising, therefore, that lesions due to the same serotype may persist for months if untreated.

The lesions of streptococcal impetigo occur over the exposed areas of the body. They are more common on the lower extremities, undoubtedly because abrasions of the skin are more common in these areas. The lesions begin as papules but rapidly evolve into vesicles surrounded by erythema. They may be localized but are often multiple. As the papules enlarge, they break down over 5 or 6 days to form a thick crust. The lesions heal slowly, leaving a depigmented area. While there may be some regional lymphadenitis, systemic symptoms are not usually present.

While streptococcal impetigo can be suspected from the history as well as the examination, definite diagnosis requires bacteriologic culture. The crust must be removed to obtain specimens from the base of the lesion after washing the infected area of the skin with sterile water. Soap or other detergents can kill or reduce the number of group A streptococci. Culturing the surface of the lesion itself usually gives a negative result. Culture results may show both group A streptococci and *Staphylococcus aureus*, but it is generally believed that the streptococcus is the primary pathogen. In many instances mild impetigo responds to local treatment. The crusts should be removed and the skin washed with soap and water. Topical antibiotics and other antiseptics have little or no value in treatment or prevention. When the lesions are more extensive, parenteral use of benzathine penicillin G is indicated. The lesions respond well to penicillin therapy. The antibiotic regimen is the same as that used for the treatment of pharyngitis. Even though the *S. aureus* present may produce penicillinase, this does not interfere with penicillin treatment. Prevention of impetigo is achieved with good personal hygiene and liberal use of soap and water.

The importance of streptococcal impetigo beyond the inconvenience and some disfiguration of the skin relates to its association with AGN. Not all strains of group A streptococci that cause impetigo and other forms of pyoderma result in AGN; nevertheless, certain M types, such as 49, 55, and 57, have been associated with sporadic cases as well as large epidemics of pyoderma-associated AGN. These have occurred in many different geographic regions. Although there is evidence to suggest that treatment of streptococcal pharyngitis prevents AGN 50 per cent of the time, there is no conclusive evidence that treatment of an individual case of pyoderma prevents subsequent occurrence of AGN. Nevertheless, treatment of the individual is important, particularly in a setting in which AGN is occurring or has occurred in the past, because this eradicates the streptococcus from the environment. The individual is therefore less of a risk to siblings and other school children.

A more severe ulcerated form of pyoderma is known as *ecthyma*. During the Vietnam conflict, this was seen in combat troops serving in the jungle. The ulcers, located on the ankle or dorsum of the foot, are circular, have a punched-out appearance, and are 0.5 to 3 cm in diameter. They contain purulent material and may be covered with a yellowish-gray crust. They are surrounded by a zone of erythema, and in more severe cases there may be cellulitis and lymphadenitis.

ERYSIPELAS. Erysipelas (St. Anthony's fire) is an acute infection of the skin and subcutaneous tissues caused by group A streptococci. The disease is more common in infants, young children, and elderly people. It is most commonly seen on the face and has a "butterfly" distribution when the bridge of the nose and the cheeks are involved. Eyelids are edematous and often swollen shut. The source of the infection is the patient's nasopharynx. Erysipelas may also develop from streptococcal infections elsewhere on the body, including surgical incisions and wounds. In some cases, the disease has been seen in association with dermatophytosis.

As with streptococcal pharyngitis, the onset is usually abrupt, and similar systemic symptoms are frequently present. The lesion initially begins with an area of mild discomfort at the site of infection. Erythema follows and enlarges rapidly, reaching a maximum in 3 to 6 days. The lesion, pink to deep red in color, has an advancing irregular margin. It is warm to the touch. Vesicles and bullae may appear, which then rupture and become crusted. As the margin advances, the central area begins to clear and the skin returns to a normal appearance, usually with some residual pigmentation.

While recovery is usually seen in a week or 10 days, this varies with the severity of the infection. High fever and bacteremia were often present before antibiotics were available, and mortality was not uncommon, particularly in patients who had bacteremia. Death is rare when the disease is adequately treated with penicillin or another appropriate antibiotic. Early diagnosis and treatment are important in infants and in elderly, debilitated, or immunosuppressed individuals. Death can occur in these cases if treatment is not prompt. Not uncommonly the disease will recur in the same site, particularly if there are areas of lymphatic obstruction.

Large numbers of group A streptococci can usually be cultured from the nasopharynx of patients with early erysipelas. Efforts to culture the streptococci from the edema fluid of the lesion are not always successful. Diagnosis is primarily made on the basis of clinical findings.

PREVENTION AND PROPHYLAXIS OF GROUP A STREPTOCOCCAL DISEASES AND THEIR NONSUPPURATIVE SEQUELAE

Views on the antibiotic treatment of streptococcal pharyngitis to prevent ARF and AGN are undergoing re-evaluation because of the decrease in the severity of streptococcal pharyngitis in recent years and the dramatic decline in the occurrence of ARF. Do the low attack rates of ARF (1 to 2 per 100,000 people per year for the age group 5 to 17 years) justify intensive efforts to detect streptococcal infections by bacteriologic cultures? Do they justify a prolonged course of antibiotic therapy for all patients in whom streptococcal infection is suspected, however mild it may be? There has been some discussion about possible relaxation of the vigorous efforts used in the past to diagnose and treat streptococcal pharyngitis. Any relaxation of efforts to diagnose and treat even mild infections shoud be tempered by consideration of the recent outbreaks of rheumatic fever and severe, even fatal, infection associated with a toxic shock–like syndrome.

From this debate several principles are emerging. While direct proof is lacking, it is probable that the decline in the incidence of ARF and the clinical severity of streptococcal pharyngitis is due at least in part to the widespread use of penicillin to treat this infection during the past 50 years. It is difficult to believe that this decline in disease has occurred as a result of genetic changes in the streptococci. This would have required the simultaneous occurrence of similar genetic events in a large number of different streptococci during this interval, which seems unlikely. Certainly the decline in both diseases has been too precipitous to have been the result of changes in the genetic background of the population that would have enhanced natural immunity. These considerations suggest that the treatment of pharyngitis with penicillin has been a major factor in reducing the incidence of this infection; it follows that penicillin treatment has also influenced the decline in ARF. It seems likely that continuation of treatment in the future will maintain this low incidence. It is known that virulent group A streptococci lurk in the shadows and are the cause of occasional outbreaks of streptococcal pharyngitis and ARF. It is certainly conceivable that such outbreaks would become more common if penicillin treatment were no longer used. Therefore, arguments to discontinue the use of throat cultures for diagnosis and of penicillin to treat streptococcal pharyngitis, even though the disease is generally less virulent today than in previous times, are reminiscent of the arguments to discontinue the use of pertussis or poliomyelitis vaccines now that these diseases are rare. We know that failure to vaccinate will result in the re-emergence of these diseases. It is likely that the failure to treat streptococcal infections will have the same consequences.

Until there is more evidence concerning the benign nature of most streptococcal diseases that are occurring today, it is prudent to maintain vigilance concerning streptococcal infections.

The occurrence of an index case of either ARF or AGN should alert the physician to the possibility that an outbreak of streptococcal disease is occurring in a family or school.

It is apparent from this discussion concerning the infrequency of ARF and the milder nature of most streptococcal disease that there is probably much less risk today of the recurrence of rheumatic fever in patients with prior history of the disease following an untreated streptococcal infection. Continuous antibiotic prophylaxis has been employed in the past to prevent recurrences of rheumatic fever in such patients, and while discussions are under way concerning modification of the recommendations, the three regimens listed below are still recommended at this time, particularly since there has been an unexpected resurgence of rheumatic fever in recent years.

1. Benzathine penicillin G given in a single injection of 1.2 million units every 4 weeks usually provides protection for about 30 days. The disadvantages and discomfort of this regimen should be weighed against the individual patient's susceptibility to

rheumatic occurrences. Those with rheumatic heart disease, those who have had a recent attack of rheumatic fever, and those exposed to an environment in which the incidence of streptococcal infection is frequent deserve the most effective protection. For such patients, benzathine penicillin by monthly injection is recommended.

2. Sulfonamide given daily by mouth in the form of 1.0 gram of sulfadiazine or one of the other sulfapyramidines provides satisfactory prophylaxis, but failures do occur. Toxic reactions may be observed during the first 60 days of continuous treatment. These have been rare, however, with the small doses of sulfadiazine that have been employed extensively.

3. Oral penicillin V is the preferred form because it is relatively resistant to gastric acid. The dose is 125 or 150 mg twice a day. This regimen has not been any more effective, however, than the daily dose of 1.0 gram of sulfadiazine. Indeed, 200,000 units of penicillin twice daily has not proved as yet to be clearly superior to the single dose. It is possible that the oral dose of penicillin may have to be increased to nearly therapeutic proportions to be more effective than sulfonamides, and this would increase further its expense and impracticality.

GROUP B STREPTOCOCCAL INFECTIONS

In the past, group B streptococci were primarily of interest to veterinarians because they were the cause of bovine mastitis. However, in recent years human strains of group B streptococci that appear to be distinct from the bovine strains have received considerable attention because they frequently produce neonatal sepsis. Group B streptococci are subdivided by means of surface polysaccharides into five serotypes: Ia, Ib, Ic, II, and III. Recent evidence suggests that group B streptococci normally colonize the intestine, and it is speculated that there is then secondary spread from the rectum to the vagina. This raises the possibility of sexual transmission of these organisms. Vaginal carriage is asymptomatic in postpubertal women. The incidence of carriage and of neonatal infection varies widely, depending on socioeconomic status and geographic residence.

Infections due to group B streptococci are associated with perinatal events. Maternal infections include chorioamnionitis, septic abortion, and puerperal sepsis. Group B streptococci are now recognized as one of the most frequent causes of neonatal sepsis and meningitis. Extensive clinical and epidemiologic studies have delineated two forms of the disease. "Early-onset disease" primarily involves infection of the lungs. The disease usually occurs within the first 10 days of life, but cases after this period have been reported. The organisms are usually acquired from the maternal genital tract. This infection may be secondary to aspiration of infected amniotic fluid. Septicemia usually is present. Early-onset disease occurs as frequently as 5 in every 1000 live births, although this varies, depending upon the region of the country and the specific hospital reporting. Early-onset disease tends to occur in infants of certain high-risk pregnancies, such as those involving prematurity, prolonged rupture of membranes, and maternal infection. The other form of group B streptococcal neonatal infection has been referred to as "late-onset disease." Affected infants develop meningitis and bacteremia. The infant is usually over 10 days old, but cases have occurred at 4 or 5 days of age. Infection may be due to nosocomial transmission. The disease has a much lower mortality than does early-onset disease. Type III organisms predominate as the cause of early- and late-onset disease.

Because all the evidence suggests that early-onset disease in the newborn infant is acquired by vertical transmission from the mother who has vaginal colonization by group B streptococci, intravenous administration of ampicillin sodium has been used to treat such women during labor in an effort to prevent transmission. While recent reports suggest that the disease in newborns is prevented by selective chemoprophylaxis of the mother, more research remains to be done in this important area.

While group B streptococci frequently may be cultured from the throat, they rarely, if ever, cause pharyngitis. Group B streptococci infection can, however, cause urinary tract infections in both sexes. Infected men are likely to be elderly. Group B streptococci may produce suppurative gangrenous lesions in adults with insulin-dependent diabetes mellitus who have peripheral vascular insufficiency. Any large series of infectious diseases reveals group B streptococci as a cause of endocarditis, pneumonia, empyema, meningitis, peritonitis, and terminal bacteremia in patients with malignancy.

All group B streptococci are susceptible to penicillin. It is the drug of choice for these infections. Thus far, most strains are susceptible to erythromycin. Tetracycline should not be used because the organisms have developed resistance to this antibiotic.

Anthony B: Group B streptococcal infections. In Feigin R, Cherry J (eds.): Textbook of Pediatric Infectious Diseases. 2nd ed. Philadelphia, W.B. Saunders Company, 1987, pp 1322–1336. *A thorough review of the epidemiology, microbiology, and clinical aspects of group B neonatal infections, including medical management.*

Bass JW: Treatment of streptococcal pharyngitis revisited. JAMA 256:740, 1986. *An excellent recent review of current indications for treatment and the choice of therapy.*

Fischetti A: Streptococcal M protein: Molecular design and biologic behavior. Clin Microbiol Rev 21:285, 1989. *A thorough review of the molecular biology of M protein, including the identification of the antigenic epitopes that stimulate type-specific immunity, with a commentary on the biologic and medical implications.*

Kaplan L, Markowitz M: The fall and rise of rheumatic fever in the United States: A commentary. Int J Cardiol 21:3, 1988. *A thoughtful review of the recent "resurgence" of rheumatic fever in the United States, which calls attention to the need for continued vigilance in the diagnosis and treatment of streptococcal pharyngitis.*

Kimura Y, Kotami S, Shiokawa Y: Recent Advances in Streptococci and Streptococcal Diseases. IX Lancefield International Symposium. Bracknell, United Kingdom, Reedbooky, 1985. *Brief reports by international scientists on most aspects of steptococcal bacteriology, immunology, epidemiology, and clinical research on streptococcal disease and pathogenesis.*

McCarty M: Streptococci. In Davis BD, Dulbecco R, Eisen HN, et al. (eds.): Microbiology. 4th ed. New York, Harper & Row, 1990, pp 525–538. *A good brief review of all aspects of streptococcal bacteriology and streptococcal disease.*

Rheumatic Fever Committee, American Heart Association: Prevention of rheumatic fever. Circulation 70:1118A, 1984. *Standard recommendations for the prevention of rheumatic fever, which should be basic knowledge for all physicians.*

Shulman ST (ed.): Management of Pharyngitis in an Era of Declining Rheumatic Fever. Columbus, Ohio, Ross Laboratories, 1984. *A collection of papers that thoroughly reviews the changing patterns of streptococcal diseases and the implications of these changes for treatment.*

Stevens D, Tanner M, Winship J, et al.: Severe group A streptococcal infections associated with a toxic shock–like syndrome and scarlet fever toxin A. N Engl J Med 321:1, 1989. *An excellent recent review of the recent occurrence of this syndrome, which may be lethal and is seen in association with group A streptococcal infections in various sites, accompanied by septicemia and toxic shock.*

Wood HF, Feinstein AR, Taranta A, et al.: Rheumatic fever in children and adolescents. III. Comparative effectiveness of three prophylaxis regimens in preventing streptococcal infections and rheumatic recurrences. Ann Intern Med 60 (S5):31, 1964. *A classic controlled long-term study of the prevention of rheumatic recurrences and the relative effectiveness of the three regimens commonly in use for secondary prophylaxis.*

298 Rheumatic Fever

Alan L. Bisno

DEFINITION. Rheumatic fever is a delayed, nonsuppurative sequel of upper respiratory infection with group A streptococci. The disease is characterized by inflammatory lesions involving primarily the joints, heart, and subcutaneous tissues; its pathogenesis remains obscure. The clinical manifestations include polyarthritis, carditis, subcutaneous nodules, erythema marginatum, and chorea in varying combinations. In its classic form, the disorder is acute, febrile, and largely self-limited. However, damage to heart valves may be chronic and progressive, causing cardiac disability or death many years after the initial episode.

ETIOLOGY. The development of acute rheumatic fever (ARF) requires antecedent infection with a specific organism, the group A *Streptococcus*, at a specific body site, the upper respiratory tract. Cutaneous streptococcal infection, a precursor of poststreptococcal acute glomerulonephritis, has never been shown to cause rheumatic fever.

Strains representing a number of the more than 80 M protein serotypes of group A streptococci are capable of causing ARF.

There is a substantial body of evidence to indicate, however, that group A streptococci vary in their rheumatogenic potential. Analysis of epidemics of ARF caused by a variety of serotypes shows a striking absence of certain highly prevalent types (e.g., type 12) and an overrepresentation of types 5 and 18 and a number of others. Reports from the preantibiotic era document epidemics of streptococcal tonsillitis, even among rheumatic subjects, in which ARF failed to appear. Prospective studies in which poststreptococcal acute glomerulonephritis and ARF occur simultaneously in the same indigent population suggest that the streptococcal strains responsible for each sequel are serotypically distinct.

Streptococci epidemiologically associated with recent ARF outbreaks in the United States belong to the classic "rheumatogenic" serotypes and often exhibit mucoid colonial morphology.

PATHOGENESIS. The mechanism by which group A streptococci elicit the connective tissue inflammatory response that constitutes ARF remains unknown. Various theories have been advanced, including (1) toxic effects of streptococcal products, particularly streptolysins S and O, both of which are capable of initiating tissue injury; (2) inflammation mediated by antigen-antibody complexes, perhaps localized to sites of tissue injury; and (3) "autoimmune" phenomena induced by the similarity of certain streptococcal and human tissue antigens.

Efforts to discriminate among these potential pathogenetic mechanisms have been hampered by the lack of an animal model of rheumatic fever. Most authorities currently favor the theory that ARF is an "autoimmune" disorder, in which tissue damage is mediated by the host's own immunologic responses to the antecedent streptococcal infection. This theory is rendered more credible by the relatively long latent period between the onset of pharyngitis and ARF and by the demonstration of numerous examples of antigenic similarity between somatic constituents of the group A *Streptococcus* and human tissues. The most intensively studied of these antigenic cross-reactions is that between streptococci and human heart. Many patients with ARF (as well as patients with uncomplicated streptococcal infections) have in their sera antistreptococcal antibodies that cross-react with heart tissue in a variety of test systems. Components of the streptococcal cell wall (including group A carbohydrate and M protein) and of the cell membrane contain epitopes that share antigenic determinants with certain constituents of the human heart.

Patients with ARF have, on the average, higher titers of antibodies to streptococcal extracellular and somatic antigens than do patients with uncomplicated streptococcal infections. Data relating to cellular immunity are more limited. ARF patients exhibit an exaggerated cellular reactivity to streptococcal cell membrane antigens, as demonstrated by inhibition in vitro of migration of peripheral blood lymphocytes.

Chronic remittent nodular lesions have been produced in dermal connective tissue following injection into experimental animals of a streptococcal mucopeptide-polysaccharide cell wall complex. Antibodies to the cytoplasm of neurons located in the caudate and subthalamic nuclei of the brain have been identified in sera of patients with Sydenham's chorea, and such antibodies cross-react with group A streptococcal membranes. Streptococcal extracellular products appear to be present in immune complexes circulating in the blood of ARF patients. Taken together, these and other reported immunologic cross-reactions and toxic phenomena could theoretically account for most of the manifestations of ARF. As yet, however, there is no direct evidence that any of them is of pathogenetic significance.

Several observations suggest that development of rheumatic fever may be modulated, at least in part, by the specific genetic constitution of the host. These include (1) the tendency of rheumatic fever to affect more than one member of a given family; (2) the fact that only a small percentage of all individuals experiencing an immunologically significant streptococcal infection develop ARF; (3) the tendency of rheumatic individuals to experience recurrent attacks; (4) the propensity of rheumatic subjects to exhibit exaggerated immunologic responses to streptococcal antigens; and (5) the fact that certain class II histocompatibility antigens are encountered significantly more frequently in ARF patients than in controls. Recently, a unique antigen has been found to be strongly expressed on the B cells of virtually all ARF patients but in fewer than 20 per cent of controls.

EPIDEMIOLOGY. The epidemiology of ARF mirrors that of streptococcal pharyngitis. The peak age of incidence is 5 to 15 years, but both primary and recurrent cases occur in adults. ARF is rare in children less than 4 years of age, a fact that has led some observers to speculate that repetitive streptococcal infections are necessary to "prime" the host for the disease. There is no clear-cut sex predilection, although females are more likely to develop certain manifestations such as Sydenham's chorea and mitral stenosis.

The frequency with which ARF develops following untreated group A streptococcal upper respiratory infection differs with the epidemiologic circumstances. In the years following World War II, careful prospective studies were conducted among personnel in military recruit camps suffering from exudative tonsillitis or pharyngitis caused by M-typable group A streptococci. Under such circumstances, in which cases of streptococcal pharyngitis tend to be clinically severe and to appear in epidemics, approximately 3 per cent of untreated patients developed ARF. Studies of endemically occurring streptococcal infection among open populations of children are complicated by the difficulties of differentiating cases of streptococcal pharyngitis from viral pharyngitis occurring in streptococcal carriers; nevertheless, the ARF attack rate in such circumstances is clearly lower than in the military experience, with an overall attack rate of less than 1 per cent.

Certain features of the antecedent streptococcal infection are associated with an increased risk of ARF. Among these are the magnitude of the antistreptolysin O (ASO) titer rise and the persistence of the infecting organism in the pharynx. Prospective civilian studies indicate that ARF is more likely to occur following clinically severe exudative pharyngitis than following mild, nonexudative illness. On the other hand, one third or more of cases of ARF occur after streptococcal infections that are asymptomatic or so mild as to have been forgotten by the patient.

Patients with a history of ARF are at greatly increased risk of recurrent disease following an immunologically significant streptococcal infection. In long-term prospective studies of rheumatic subjects carried out at Irvington House, a rheumatic fever sanitarium outside New York City, one of every five documented streptococcal infections gave rise to a recurrence of ARF. The risk of recurrence is greater in patients with pre-existing rheumatic heart disease and in those experiencing symptomatic throat infections; the risk declines with advancing age and with increasing interval since the most recent rheumatic attack. Nevertheless, rheumatic patients remain at increased risk well into adult life, perhaps indefinitely.

Rheumatic fever occurs in all parts of the world; there is no known racial predisposition. In temperate climates, ARF peaks in the cooler months of the year, in the winter and early spring or shortly after schools open in the fall. The major environmental factor favoring occurrence appears to be crowding, as in military barracks or similar closed institutions and in large households. Crowding favors interpersonal spread of group A streptococci and perhaps enhances streptococcal virulence by frequent human passage.

ARF remains rampant in developing areas such as the Middle East, the Indian subcontinent, and many nations of Africa and South America. It has been estimated that rheumatic heart disease causes 25 to 40 per cent of all cardiovascular disease in the Third World. In striking contrast, the incidence of ARF and the prevalence of rheumatic heart disease have declined dramatically both in North America and in Western Europe over the past four to five decades. During this time, the disease has become extremely uncommon in the affluent suburbs of many United States cities, while persisting among lower socioeconomic groups, particularly those massed in the densely populated core areas of major urban centers.

The mid-1980's, however, witnessed some startling developments in the epidemiology of ARF in the United States. Outbreaks of the disease were reported in Salt Lake City, Utah; Columbus and Akron, Ohio; Pittsburgh, Pennsylvania; Nashville and Memphis, Tennessee; and a number of other communities. Equally surprising was the fact that, in many of these outbreaks, the victims were predominantly white, middle-class children dwelling in the suburbs. Moreover, ARF epidemics occurred in military training bases in Missouri and California, a phenomenon that had not been observed for two decades. There is as yet no evidence that these events presage a major national resurgence of ARF.

PATHOLOGY. ARF is characterized by exudative and proliferative inflammatory lesions in the connective tissues, especially those of heart, joints, and subcutaneous tissues. The early lesions consist of edema of the ground substance, fragmentation of collagen fibers, cellular infiltration, and fibrinoid degeneration. In the heart, diffuse degeneration and even necrosis of muscle cells may be observed. At a slightly later stage, focal perivascular inflammatory lesions develop. These so-called *Aschoff nodules* (Fig. 298–1), considered virtually pathognomonic of rheumatic fever, consist of a central area of fibrinoid surrounded by lymphocytes, plasma cells, and large basophilic cells, some of them multinucleate. Many of these cells have elongated nuclei with a distinctive chromatin pattern, sometimes called "caterpillar" or "owl-eye" nuclei, depending on their orientation in microscopic cross-section. Cells containing these nuclei are called "Anitschkow myocytes," despite the fact that most authorities believe them to be of mesenchymal origin.

Cardiac findings may include pericarditis, myocarditis, and endocarditis. Foci of coronary arteritis may also be observed. A thickened and roughened area ("MacCallum's patch") is frequently present in the left atrium above the posterior leaflet of the mitral valve. Valvular lesions appear early as small verrucae along the line of closure. Later, as healing occurs, the valves may become thickened and deformed, the chordae shortened, and the commissures fused. These changes result in valvular stenosis or insufficiency. The mitral valve is most commonly involved, followed by the aortic, the tricuspid, and, rarely, the pulmonic.

Pathologically, the *arthritis* of ARF is characterized by a fibrinous exudate and sterile effusion without erosion of the joint surfaces or pannus formation. *Subcutaneous nodules* have many histologic features in common with the Aschoff nodules. These consist of central zones of fibrinoid necrosis surrounded by histiocytes, fibroblasts, occasional lymphocytes, and rare polymorphonuclear cells. Inflammation of the smaller arteries and arterioles may occur throughout the body. Despite pathologic evidence of diffuse vasculitis, aneurysms and thrombosis are not typical features of ARF.

CLINICAL MANIFESTATIONS. Rheumatic fever may involve a number of different organ systems, most notably the heart, joints, skin, and central nervous system. The clinical picture of the disease may thus be quite variable (Table 298–1), depending upon which systems are attacked, whether they are involved singly or in combination, the order in which they are affected, and the severity of the involvement. Five clinical

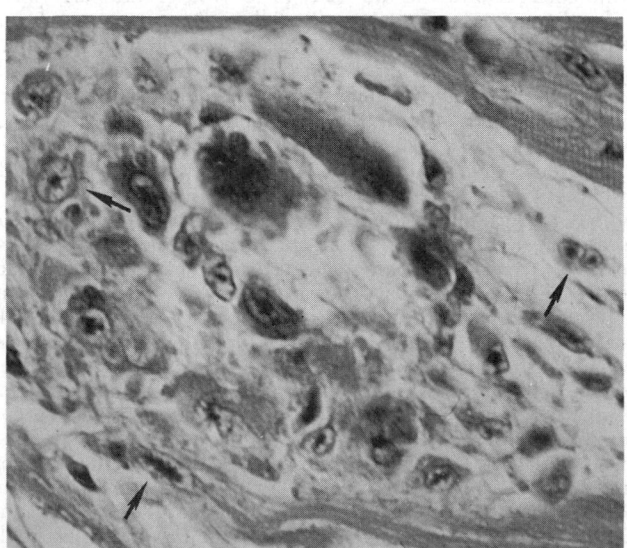

FIGURE 298–1. Myocardial Aschoff nodule demonstrates areas of fibrinoid degeneration and numerous large cells with polymorphous nuclei; several of the nuclei have "owl-eye" or "caterpillar" configurations (*arrows*). × 630. (Courtesy of Robert Peace, M.D.)

TABLE 298–1. THE MANY FACES OF ACUTE RHEUMATIC FEVER: POSSIBLE PRESENTATIONS

High fever, prostration, crippling polyarthritis
Lassitude, tachycardia, new cardiac murmurs
Acute pericarditis
Fulminant heart failure
Sydenham's chorea, without fever or toxicity
Acute abdominal pain, mimicking appendicitis
Varying combinations of the above

features of the disease are so characteristic that they are recognized as "major manifestations" according to the revised Jones criteria (see below) for diagnosis of ARF: carditis, polyarthritis, chorea, subcutaneous nodules, and erythema marginatum. Certain other findings, frequently present but nonspecific, have been designated "minor manifestations." These include arthralgia, fever, history of previous rheumatic fever or evidence of preexisting rheumatic heart disease, and certain laboratory findings (see below).

In cases in which it can be determined, the *latent period* between the antecedent streptococcal infection and the onset of symptoms of ARF ranges between 1 and 5 weeks. The average latent period is 19 days for both primary and recurrent attacks. When acute polyarthritis is the presenting complaint, the onset is often rather abrupt and may be marked by high fever and toxicity. If isolated carditis is the initial manifestation, the onset may be insidious or even subclinical. Between these two extremes, a wide variety of gradations exist in the initial presentation of ARF (Table 298–1). In most attacks, fever and joint involvement are the earliest clinical manifestations, although they may occasionally be preceded by abdominal pain localized to the periumbilical or infraumbilical areas. At times the location and severity of the pain, as well as fleeting signs of peritoneal inflammation, may lead to a misdiagnosis of acute appendicitis. Carditis, if it is to appear, usually does so within the first 3 weeks of the illness. In contrast, chorea tends to occur later in the course of the disease, sometimes after all other manifestations have subsided. Fortunately, chorea and polyarthritis almost never occur simultaneously. Epistaxis may be a feature of ARF, occurring both at the onset and throughout the acute phase of the illness; it may be quite severe.

Overall, arthritis occurs in approximately 75 per cent of first attacks of ARF, carditis in 40 to 50 per cent, chorea in 15 per cent, and subcutaneous nodules and erythema marginatum in fewer than 10 per cent. The incidence of individual manifestations, however, varies with age. Carditis is more frequent in the youngest age groups and is relatively uncommon in first attacks occurring in adults. Chorea occurs primarily in persons between age 5 years and puberty. It is seen more frequently in females and virtually never occurs in adult males. Thus, the majority of ARF attacks occurring in adults are manifested primarily by arthritis.

Arthritis. Joint involvement ranges from arthralgia alone to acute, disabling arthritis characterized by swelling, warmth, erythema, severe limitation of motion, and exquisite tenderness to pressure. The larger joints of the extremities are usually involved—most frequently the knees and ankles, but also the wrists and elbows. The hips and small joints of the hands and feet are affected occasionally. Involvement of shoulders and lumbosacral, cervical, sternoclavicular, and temporomandibular joints occurs in a relatively small percentage of cases. The synovial fluid contains thousands of white blood cells, with a marked preponderance of polymorphonuclear leukocytes; bacterial cultures are sterile.

Characteristically, the articular involvement in ARF assumes a pattern of *migratory polyarthritis*. This does not mean that inflammation in one joint disappears before the next is attacked. Rather, a number of joints are affected in succession, and the periods of involvement overlap. Inflammation in one joint may subside while another is becoming symptomatic, so that the process seems to migrate from joint to joint. In untreated cases, as many as 16 joints may be affected, and about half the patients develop arthritis in more than six joints. When effective antiinflammatory therapy is administered early in the course of the disease, the involvement not infrequently remains monoarticular or pauciarticular.

In most instances, inflammation in any one joint begins to subside spontaneously within a week, and the total duration of involvement is no more than 2 or 3 weeks. The entire bout of polyarthritis rarely lasts more than 4 weeks and resolves completely, leaving no residual joint damage. Some authors have described the rare occurrence of *Jaccoud's arthritis*, so-called chronic post-rheumatic fever arthropathy of the metacarpophalangeal joints, following repetitive bouts of rheumatic polyarthritis. This entity is not a true arthritis but a form of periarticular fibrosis; its relationship to rheumatic fever remains unresolved.

Carditis. Rheumatic fever may involve the endocardium, myocardium, and pericardium (Table 298–2), and thus the disease is capable of inducing a true *pancarditis*. Carditis is the most important manifestation of ARF because it is the only one capable of causing significant permanent organ damage or death. Although the clinical picture may at times be fulminant, it is more frequently mild or even asymptomatic and may escape notice in the absence of more obvious associated findings, such as arthritis or chorea. The diagnosis of carditis requires the presence of one of the following four manifestations: (1) organic cardiac murmurs not previously present, (2) cardiomegaly, (3) pericarditis, or (4) congestive heart failure. In practice, the characteristic murmurs of ARF are almost always present in cases of rheumatic carditis, unless the ability to hear them is obscured (e.g., loud pericardial friction rub, large pericardial effusion, low cardiac output, severe tachycardia). The diagnosis of carditis should be made with caution in the absence of one of the following three murmurs: apical systolic, apical mid-diastolic, and basal diastolic. Such murmurs, if they are destined to develop, do so usually within the first week and almost always within the first 3 weeks of illness. (An exception to this rule may occur in the patient with "pure" chorea; see later discussion.) The *apical systolic murmur* of relative or actual mitral regurgitation encompasses most of systole. It is blowing, relatively high pitched, and heard best at the apex; it radiates to the axilla and at times to the base of the heart or the back. It must be distinguished carefully by quality, location, and radiation from a variety of functional precordial systolic murmurs heard in normal individuals, especially in children. The *apical mid-diastolic* (Carey-Coombs) murmur is a low-pitched sound replacing or immediately following the third heart sound and ending distinctly before the first heart sound. It may be heard in a variety of conditions associated with increased flow across the mitral valve and is thus not pathognomonic of ARF. It may be differentiated from the diastolic rumble of mitral stenosis by the absence of an opening snap, presystolic accentuation, or accentuated first sound at the mitral area. The high-pitched, descrescendo *basal diastolic murmur* of aortic regurgitation is best heard along the upper left sternal border or over the aortic area. It may be brief and faint, best heard after expiration with the patient leaning forward. The prognostic significance, if any, of echocardiographically recorded valvular regurgitation in the absence of audible murmurs remains to be determined.

Other prominent auscultatory findings in patients with active rheumatic carditis include tachycardia, which persists during sleep; protodiastolic, presystolic, or summation gallops; an indistinct or "mushy" quality to the first heart sound (resulting in some cases from first-degree heart block); pericardial friction rub; or muffling of heart tones caused by pericardial effusion. In the early stages of congestive heart failure, rapid distention of the hepatic capsule may lead to right upper quadrant aching and tenderness over the liver. All the usual clinical findings of pericarditis or congestive failure may be observed.

A number of different rhythm disturbances may occur during

the course of ARF. By far the most common is first-degree atrioventricular block. Second- and third-degree heart block, nodal rhythm, and premature contractions may also be observed; atrial fibrillation, on the other hand, is usually a feature of chronic rather than acute rheumatic involvement. Conduction disturbances do not in themselves indicate acute carditis, and their presence or absence is unrelated to the subsequent development of rheumatic heart disease.

In cases of ARF with severe carditis, areas of patchy pneumonitis are sometimes seen. Many observers feel that these pulmonary infiltrates represent a specific *rheumatic pneumonia*. The case is difficult to prove, however, because of the confusion induced by such confounding clinical entities as pulmonary edema, pulmonary embolization, superimposed bacterial pneumonia, and the acute respiratory distress syndrome in these severely ill and toxic patients.

Sydenham's Chorea (Chorea Minor, "St. Vitus' Dance"). This neurologic syndrome occurs after a latent period that is variable but on the average longer than that associated with the other manifestations of ARF. It frequently occurs in "pure" form, either unaccompanied by other major manifestations or, after a latent period of several months, at a time when all other evidence of acute rheumatic activity has subsided. Chorea is characterized by rapid, purposeless, involuntary movements, most noticeable in the extremities and face. The arms and legs flail about in erratic, jerky, incoordinated movements that may sometimes be unilateral (hemichorea). Facial tics, grimaces, grins, and contortions are evident. The speech is usually slurred or jerky. The tongue, when protruded, retracts involuntarily, while asynchronous contractions of lingual muscles produce a "bag of worms" appearance. The involuntary motions disappear during sleep and may be partially suppressed by rest, sedation, or volition.

Patients with chorea display generalized muscle weakness and an inability to maintain a tetanic muscle contraction. Thus, when the patient is asked to squeeze the examiner's fingers, a squeezing and relaxing motion occurs that has been described as "milkmaid's grip." The knee jerk may have a pendular quality. There is no cranial nerve or pyramidal involvement, and sensory modalities are unaffected. The electroencephalogram may display abnormal slow wave activity.

Emotional lability is characteristic of Sydenham's chorea and often may precede other neurologic manifestations, leaving teachers and parents puzzled over apparently inexplicable personality changes.

Subcutaneous Nodules. These are firm, painless subcutaneous lesions that vary in size from a few millimeters to approximately 2 cm. The skin overlying them is freely movable and is not inflamed. The lesions tend to occur in crops over bony surfaces or prominences and over tendons. Sites of predilection include the extensor surfaces of elbows, knees, and wrists; the occiput; and spinous processes of the thoracic and lumbar vertebrae (Fig. 298–2). Nodules are virtually never the sole major manifestation of ARF; they almost always appear in association with carditis, and the cardiac involvement in such cases tends to be clinically severe. Nodules ordinarily do not appear until at least 3 weeks after the onset of an attack, usually lasting 1 to 2 weeks. They may appear in repeated crops in patients with protracted carditis. Similar nodules may be seen in systemic lupus erythematosus and in rheumatoid arthritis. Subcutaneous nodules in the latter disease are larger and more persistent than those in rheumatic fever.

Erythema Marginatum. The rash begins as an erythematous macule or papule, which then extends outward, while the skin in the center returns to normal. Adjacent lesions coalesce, forming circinate or serpiginous patterns. The lesions are neither pruritic nor indurated, and they blanch on pressure. They vary greatly in size and appear mostly upon the trunk and proximal extremities, sparing the face. Erythema marginatum may be raised or flat; the latter was termed *erythema annulare* in the older literature. The lesions are evanescent, migrating from place to place, at times changing before the observer's eyes, and leaving no residual scarring. The erythema may be brought out by the application of heat. Individual lesions may come and go in minutes to hours, but the process may go on intermittently for weeks to

TABLE 298–2. CLINICAL MANIFESTATIONS OF CARDITIS IN ACUTE RHEUMATIC FEVER

Murmurs*
    Apical systolic
    Apical mid-diastolic (Carey-Coombs murmur)
    Basal diastolic
Pericarditis
Cardiomegaly
Congestive heart failure

*At least one of the characteristic murmurs is almost always present in acute rheumatic carditis (see text for details).

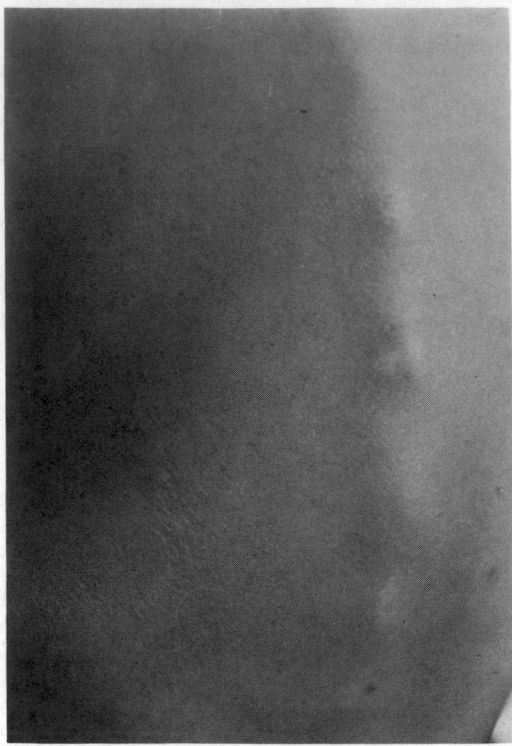

FIGURE 298–2. Subcutaneous nodules over spinous processes on the back of a patient with acute rheumatic carditis. (Courtesy of S. Levine, M.D.)

months uninfluenced by anti-inflammatory therapy; its persistence is not necessarily an adverse prognostic sign. In the great majority of cases, erythema marginatum is accompanied by carditis; it also tends to be associated with subcutaneous nodules.

LABORATORY FINDINGS. No specific laboratory test is diagnostic of ARF. Usually there is a leukocytosis with an increase in the proportion of polymorphonuclear leukocytes. A mild to moderate normocytic normochromic anemia is the rule. In some patients the serum aspartate aminotransferase (AST) level is elevated. Evidence of acute inflammation is prominent, including readily detectable quantities of C-reactive protein in the blood and elevation of the erythrocyte sedimentation rate. An exception is "pure" chorea, which may appear long after indices of inflammation have returned to normal.

The urine may contain protein, white cells, and red cells. Biopsy studies have revealed a variety of renal abnormalities, but the classic proliferative glomerular abnormalities that characterize poststreptococcal acute glomerulonephritis occur quite rarely in ARF. Electrocardiographic and radiographic studies may reveal evidence of rhythm disturbances, pericarditis, or congestive heart failure. Echocardiography may document myocardial and valvular dysfunction and pericardial effusion.

The major laboratory contribution to the workup of ARF is the documentation of recent group A streptococcal infection. Throat culture should always be performed but is positive in only a minority of cases. This is perhaps due to the time lapse of several weeks between the onset of the pharyngeal infection and the throat culture. The serum titer of ASO is elevated in 80 per cent or more of ARF patients. If two streptococcal antibody tests, e.g., ASO plus either anti-DNase B or antihyaluronidase, are performed, an elevated titer of at least one will be found in 90 per cent of ARF patients. A battery of three tests establishes the presence of recent, immunologically significant streptococcal infection in more than 95 per cent of individuals experiencing an acute rheumatic attack. The definition of an "elevated" titer varies, depending upon the test employed, age of the patient, and geographic locale. ASO titers greater than 200 to 250 Todd units per milliliter are generally considered elevated. At times, serial sampling may detect a rising titer of streptococcal antibodies in patients seen early in the course of a rheumatic attack.

COURSE AND PROGNOSIS. The average duration of an untreated attack of ARF is approximately 3 months. The duration tends to be longer, up to 6 months, in patients with severe carditis. Fewer than 5 per cent of patients have continuing rheumatic activity for longer than 6 months. In a few of these the disease is limited to chorea and is otherwise benign. Other patients exhibit evidence of persistent inflammatory activity, including arthritis, carditis, and subcutaneous nodules. "Chronic rheumatic fever" occurs more frequently in patients who have had one or more previous attacks; cardiac involvement in chronic rheumatic fever tends to be frequent and severe.

Death from intractable myocarditis during the acute phase of ARF is now very rare. Once the acute attack has subsided, the only long-term sequel is that of rheumatic heart disease, manifested primarily by insufficiency and/or stenosis of the mitral and aortic valves. The prognosis from a cardiac standpoint is very much dependent upon the clinical findings at the time the patient is first seen. In one large study, for example, 347 patients were examined during an acute rheumatic attack and again 10 years later. Among patients who had been free of carditis during their acute attack, only 6 per cent had residual heart disease on follow-up. Patients with no pre-existing heart disease and with mild carditis during their acute attack (i.e., apical systolic murmur without pericarditis or heart failure) had a relatively good prognosis in that only approximately 30 per cent had heart murmurs 10 years later. About 40 per cent of subjects with apical or basal diastolic murmurs and 70 per cent of subjects with failure and/or pericarditis during their acute attacks had residual rheumatic heart disease. The prognosis was worse in patients with pre-existing heart disease and in those who had experienced recurrent attacks of ARF in the 10-year interval.

The data cited above indicate that patients who do not develop carditis during an acute attack and are protected from ARF recurrences are most unlikely to suffer from rheumatic heart disease. The patient with "pure" chorea represents an exception to this rule. A significant proportion of such patients who have no evidence of carditis when first examined may develop rheumatic valvular disease on prolonged follow-up. Although the explanation for this phenomenon is unknown, it is conceivable that in view of the long latent period associated with chorea, signs of carditis might have been present earlier but subsided by the time the neurologic abnormality became evident.

DIAGNOSIS. Although ARF is readily recognized in the individual who presents with multiple major manifestations or in epidemic circumstances, at other times the disease may be extraordinarily difficult to diagnose with confidence. This is because of the variability of its clinical presentation, the frequency with which only a single major manifestation is detected, and the fact that there is no definitive diagnostic laboratory test. Nevertheless, precise diagnosis is especially important in this disease because of the necessity to advise the patient regarding prolonged antimicrobial prophylaxis (see below).

The diagnostic criteria of T. Duckett Jones, as subsequently modified by a committee of the American Heart Association, attempt to minimize overdiagnosis and underdiagnosis (Table 298–3). Two major manifestations, or one major and two minor manifestations, indicate a high probability of ARF, *provided that there is supporting evidence of recent streptococcal infection.* Although a positive throat culture for group A streptococci technically satisfies this requirement, streptococcal carriage rates of 15 per cent are not uncommon among school-aged children during the fall and winter. Elevated titers of antibodies to streptococcal extracellular products, although not diagnostic of ARF, do indicate a recent, *immunologically significant* streptococcal infection. Conversely, if a battery of streptococcal antibody tests fails to reveal any evidence of recent infection, the diagnosis of ARF must be considered unlikely. This statement does *not* necessarily hold true in patients whose only rheumatic manifestation is Sydenham's chorea. Because of the long latent period associated with chorea, previously elevated antibody titers may have declined to normal.

The modified Jones criteria are, of course, only guidelines. They are most difficult to apply confidently when polyarthritis is the single major manifestation. Under such circumstances, serious consideration must be given to various other entities, including rheumatoid arthritis, Still's disease, viral arthritides (e.g., rubella, hepatitis B), the early prepurpuric phase of Henoch-Schönlein purpura, and septic arthritis, including gonococcal arthritis.

TABLE 298–3. JONES CRITERIA (REVISED) FOR GUIDANCE IN THE DIAGNOSIS OF RHEUMATIC FEVER*

Major Manifestations	Minor Manifestations
Carditis	*Clinical*
Polyarthritis	Previous rheumatic fever or rheumatic
Chorea	heart disease
Erythema marginatum	Arthralgia
Subcutaneous nodules	Fever

Laboratory
Acute phase reactions
Erythrocyte sedimentation rate,
C-reactive protein, leukocytosis
Prolonged PR interval
Plus

Supporting evidence of preceding streptococcal infection (increased ASO or other streptococcal antibodies; positive throat culture for group A *Streptococcus;* recent scarlet fever).

The presence of two major criteria, or of one major and two minor criteria, indicates a high probability of the presence of rheumatic fever if supported by evidence of a preceding streptococcal infection.

*Reprinted from Jones criteria (revised) for guidance in the diagnosis of rheumatic fever. Circulation 69:204A, 1984, by permission of the American Heart Association, Inc.

Serum sickness is frequently a serious consideration, particularly if the patient has received penicillin or other antibiotics for a preceding respiratory infection. Systemic lupus erythematosus, sickle cell hemoglobinopathies, and infective endocarditis may involve the joints and the heart. Other differential diagnostic considerations include congenital heart lesions, viral and idiopathic forms of myocarditis and pericarditis, and functional heart murmurs. Nonfamilial forms of chorea have been described in systemic lupus erythematosus and rarely in association with the use of birth control pills. It remains uncertain how often episodes of chorea occurring during pregnancy ("chorea gravidarum") represent attacks of rheumatic fever. Other disorders that may at times be confused with ARF are gout, sarcoidosis, Hodgkin's disease, and acute leukemia.

Following an episode of acute streptococcal pharyngitis, a small proportion of patients may experience persistent symptoms of malaise, arthralgia, low-grade fever, and lymphadenopathy plus laboratory evidence of mild inflammation. It is difficult to classify such cases, but the affected individuals do not meet the criteria for diagnosis of ARF and, moreover, do not appear to be at risk for the delayed cardiac sequelae of ARF.

TREATMENT. Antibiotics neither modify the course of a rheumatic attack nor influence the subsequent development of carditis. Nevertheless, it is conventional to give a course of antibiotics designed to eradicate any rheumatogenic group A streptococci remaining in the tonsils and pharynx, at least in part to prevent spread of the organism to close contacts. The recommended regimens are those conventionally used for treatment of acute streptococcal pharyngitis (Ch. 297). Benzathine penicillin G is preferred in the non–penicillin-allergic patient. Following completion of this therapy, continuous antistreptococcal prophylaxis should commence (see below).

Treatment with anti-inflammatory agents is effective in suppressing many of the signs and symptoms of ARF. These agents do not "cure" the disease, nor do they prevent the subsequent evolution of rheumatic heart disease. They should be avoided in very mild or equivocal cases because, by suppressing the clinical manifestations, they may obscure the diagnosis. The two drugs most widely used are aspirin and corticosteroids. The former is used in patients with acute polyarthritis, provided that carditis is either absent or mild and there is no evidence of congestive heart failure. Aspirin is very effective in decreasing fever, toxicity, and joint inflammation. It should be given in a dosage of 90 to 100 mg per kilogram per day in children and 6 to 8 grams per day in adults. This is administered in equally divided doses, every 4 hours for the first 24 to 36 hours; thereafter it may be given in four doses during waking hours. A salicylate level of 25 mg per deciliter is usually satisfactory. The incidence of nausea

and vomiting may be minimized by starting somewhat below the optimal dosage level and gradually increasing over a few days. The patient should be observed for evidence of significant gastrointestinal bleeding and for signs and symptoms of salicylism. After 2 weeks, the dosage is reduced to 60 to 70 mg per kilogram per day for an additional 6 weeks. These dosage schedules represent general guidelines only. The precise aspirin dose must be determined by the patient's clinical response, blood salicylate levels, and tolerance of the drug.

Corticosteroids are generally reserved for patients who have severe carditis manifested by congestive heart failure, who are unable to tolerate large doses of salicylates, or whose signs and symptoms are inadequately suppressed by aspirin. As with aspirin, the dosage must be individualized. Prednisone, 40 to 60 mg per day in divided doses, may be used initially; after 2 to 3 weeks it should be withdrawn slowly over an additional 3-week period. In cases of fulminating carditis with profound heart failure, intravenous corticosteroids may be employed. Aspirin should be administered for a month after discontinuation of prednisone. As is the case for other patients receiving corticosteroids, the physician should be alert to problems such as gastrointestinal bleeding, sodium and water retention, and impairment of glucose tolerance. Suppression of the pituitary-adrenal axis or of the host immune system is a potential problem but not ordinarily a major one during this relatively short course of treatment. The role of nonsteroidal anti-inflammatory agents in management of ARF remains to be defined.

Following cessation of anti-inflammatory therapy, clinical or laboratory evidence of ARF may reappear. Such therapeutic "rebounds" occur more frequently after corticosteroid therapy than after treatment with aspirin. They may be minimized by prolonging salicylate therapy for 9 to 12 weeks and, when corticosteroids have been required, by continuing aspirin use for a month after corticosteroids have been discontinued.

Congestive heart failure is managed by the usual measures of bed rest, sodium restriction, diuretics, and, if necessary, oxygen and digitalis. The potential risk of digitalis-induced arrhythmias in the patient with active myocarditis must be borne in mind.

All patients should be kept at bed-chair rest for the first 3 weeks of illness, during which time carditis will usually manifest itself if it is destined to appear. Bathroom privileges may be allowed unless arthritis or chorea makes this infeasible or unless frank heart failure supervenes. Subsequently the level of physical activity should be guided by the patient's clinical status, primarily by the presence and activity of rheumatic carditis. Patients with congestive heart failure should be kept at rest until compensation has been achieved. Patients with Sydenham's chorea require a quiet environment, and sedatives such as phenobarbital may be helpful.

Once the acute attack has subsided completely, the patient's subsequent level of physical activity is dependent upon cardiac status. Patients without residual heart disease may resume full and unrestricted activity. It is important that the patient not be subjected to unwarranted invalidism, either because of his or her own inaccurate perceptions of the nature of the rheumatic process or because of those of parents, teachers, or employers.

PREVENTION. "Primary prevention" of ARF consists of accurate diagnosis and appropriate treatment of streptococcal sore throat (Ch. 297). Although straightforward in theory, primary prevention is often frustratingly difficult to achieve. In many of the densely populated, indigent communities in which the risk of ARF is greatest, children with self-limited illnesses such as sore throats may never come to medical attention, and throat culture services are usually unavailable to aid in diagnosis. Moreover, in one third or more of cases, ARF may arise after a clinically inapparent streptococcal infection.

Perhaps the most effective strategy for avoiding the mortality and chronic cardiac disability associated with ARF is that of "secondary prevention." This strategy focuses upon the group of persons who have already suffered a rheumatic attack and who are inordinately susceptible to a recurrence following an immunologically significant streptococcal upper respiratory infection. Recurrent attacks tend to be mimetic in nature, so that patients who have suffered carditis with their previous attack are likely to have repetitive cardiac involvement and progressive cardiac damage. Because even patients who experienced only arthritis or chorea may develop carditis with recurrent attacks of ARF, *all* patients who have experienced a documented attack of ARF should receive continuous antimicrobial prophylaxis to prevent either symptomatic or asymptomatic streptococcal infections. The specific regimens to be used are indicated in Ch. 297. By far the most effective of these is intramuscular benzathine penicillin G every 4 weeks. Rheumatic recurrences are very unusual in patients faithfully adhering to this regimen.

The total duration of intramuscular or oral rheumatic prophylaxis remains unresolved. Some authorities recommend lifelong prophylaxis. On the other hand, the risk of rheumatic recurrence is known to diminish with increasing age and increasing interval since the most recent rheumatic attack. Patients who escape carditis during their initial attack are less likely to experience rheumatic recurrences and less likely to develop carditis if a recurrence does ensue. These facts suggest that prophylaxis need not be perpetual for all rheumatic subjects. Continuous prophylaxis should be maintained indefinitely for those with clinically significant rheumatic heart disease. Other rheumatic subjects should be protected until reaching adulthood, for at least 5 years after their most recent attack, and if they are in an epidemiologic circumstance that places them at high risk of streptococcal acquisition (e.g., parents of small children, school teachers, military recruits, nurses, pediatricians, or residents of areas with a high incidence of ARF). The decision to remove a rheumatic subject from continuous prophylaxis should be an individualized one, based upon the physician's assessment of the risk and likely consequences of recurrence, and taken with the patient's informed consent. Patients taken off prophylaxis must be instructed to return immediately for medical follow-up whenever symptoms of pharyngitis occur.

Patients with rheumatic valvular heart disease must receive prophylaxis designed to avoid bacterial endocarditis whenever they undergo dental or surgical procedures likely to evoke bacteremia. This is not necessary in the rheumatic subject who is free of residual heart disease. The regimens for prevention of endocarditis (see Ch. 299) are different from those prescribed for prevention of ARF, and the fact that a patient is receiving rheumatic fever prophylaxis does not exempt him or her from endocarditis prophylaxis. This is a frequent point of confusion not only among patients but among physicians and dentists as well.

Bisno AL: The resurgence of acute rheumatic fever in the United States. Annu Rev Med 41:319, 1990. *A review that places in historical perspective the epidemiologic and bacteriologic features of the recent outbreaks of ARF in the United States.*

Committee on Rheumatic Fever, Infective Endocarditis, and Kawasaki Disease, American Heart Association: Prevention of rheumatic fever. Circulation 78:1082, 1988. *Official recommendations of the American Heart Association for primary and secondary prevention of rheumatic fever. Includes specific antimicrobial regimens.*

Stollerman GH: Rheumatic Fever and Streptococcal Infection. New York, Grune & Stratton, 1975. *A comprehensive, extremely readable summary of all aspects of rheumatic fever.*

Endocarditis

299 Infective Endocarditis

David T. Durack

When microbes colonize the endocardium, they cause the disease termed *infective endocarditis*. The organism is usually a common bacterium, the site affected is usually one of the heart valves, and the characteristic lesion is a vegetation. For general use, the term infective endocarditis is more appropriate than *bacterial endocarditis*, because this disease also can be caused by fungi and chlamydia. Serviceable terms in general use include *subacute* and *acute bacterial endocarditis* (SBE and ABE), *native valve endocarditis* (NVE), *prosthetic valve endocarditis* (PVE), and *nonbacterial thrombotic endocarditis* (NBTE).

MICROBIOLOGY. Most of the species of bacteria that can colonize or infect humans have been reported to cause endocarditis. However, a few common gram-positive species account for the great majority of infections. Streptococci and staphylococci dominate the list; together these organisms cause more than 80 per cent of infections on native valves. Table 299–1 shows representative figures for the reported frequency of the main etiologic microbes on native valves, on prosthetic valves, and in drug addicts. Individual and local experience may differ widely.

The Gram-Positive Cocci. The various α-hemolytic (viridans) streptococci together cause more cases of endocarditis than any other bacteria. These relatively avirulent streptococci are found in large numbers in the oropharyngeal and gastrointestinal flora. In order of frequency, the species that cause SBE most often are *Streptococcus sanguis, S. mutans, S. intermedius,* and *S. mitis.* Next in frequency among the streptococci causing endocarditis are the group D streptococci, *S. bovis* and *Enterococcus faecalis. S. bovis* bacteremia and endocarditis are associated with the presence of lower gastrointestinal lesions, including polyps and colonic cancer. Therefore, recovery of this species from blood cultures should be followed up by investigation for colonic tumors, whether or not the patient has any symptoms. *E. faecalis*

(the enterococcus) causes endocarditis in association with infections of the genital and urinary tract in women of childbearing age and of the urinary tract in elderly men with prostatic disease.

S. pneumoniae occasionally causes acute endocarditis. The triad of coexisting pneumococcal pneumonia, meningitis, and endocar-

TABLE 299–1. APPROXIMATE FREQUENCY OF VARIOUS ORGANISMS CAUSING INFECTIVE ENDOCARDITIS ON NATIVE VALVES, IN DRUG ABUSERS, AND ON PROSTHETIC VALVES*

	NVE (%)	Intravenous Drug Abusers (%)	Early PVE (%)	Late PVE (%)
Streptococci	65	15	10	35
Viridans, alpha-hemolytic	35	5	<5	25
S. bovis (group D)	15	<5	<5	<5
E. faecalis (group D)	10	8	<5	<5
Other streptococci	<5	<5	<5	<5
Staphylococci	25	50	50	30
Coagulase-positive	23	50	20	10
Coagulase-negative	<5	<5	30	20
Gram-negative aerobic bacilli	<5	15	15	10
HACEK group	5	<5	<1	<5
Fungi	<5	5	10	5
Miscellaneous bacteria	<5	5	5	5
Diphtheroids, propionibacteria	<1	<5	5	<5
Other anaerobes	<1	<1	<1	<1
Legionella	0	0	0	<1
Rickettsia	<1	<1	<1	<1
Chlamydia	<1	<1	<1	<1
Polymicrobial infection	<1	5	5	5
Culture-negative endocarditis	5	<5	<5	<5

*These are representative figures collated from the literature; wide local variations in frequency are to be expected.

Adapted from Durack DT: Infective and non-infective endocarditis. *In* Hurst JW (ed.): The Heart, 6th ed., pp 1130–1157. Copyright © 1986 by McGraw-Hill, Inc. Used by permission of McGraw-Hill Book Company.

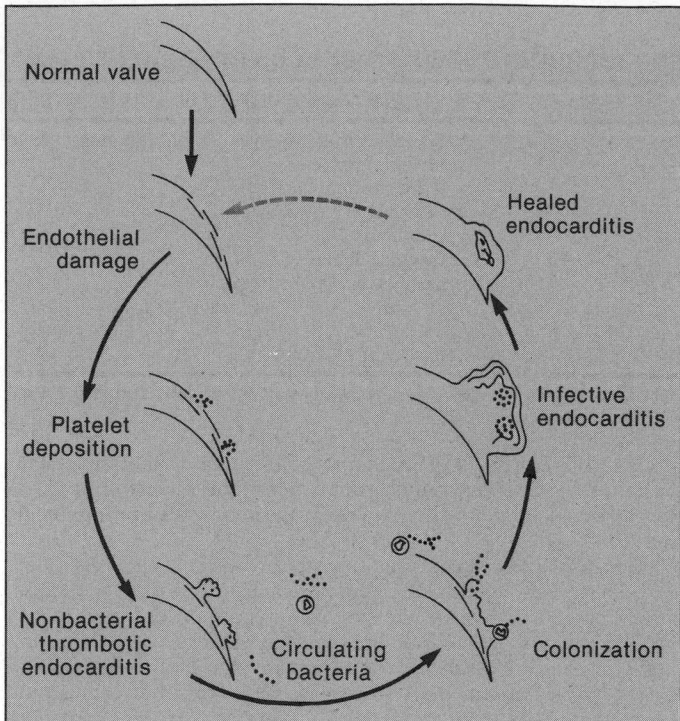

FIGURE 299–1. A diagram to illustrate the main events in pathogenesis of subacute bacterial endocarditis. (Adapted from Durack DT: Infective and non-infective endocarditis. *In* Hurst JW (ed.): The Heart, 5th ed. Copyright © 1982 by McGraw-Hill, Inc. Used by permission of McGraw-Hill Book Company.)

ditis is known as *Austrian's syndrome.* It often occurs in debilitated alcoholics and carries a very poor prognosis.

A few cases of endocarditis are caused by nutritionally dependent streptococci that require media supplemented with L-cysteine or pyridoxine for growth. These fastidious organisms can be difficult to isolate from blood cultures, and the infections they cause are more difficult to cure than infections caused by other streptococci.

Staphylococcus aureus is the leading cause of acute bacterial endocarditis, is the predominant species in narcotic addicts with endocarditis, and is an important cause of PVE (Table 299–1). *Staphylococcus epidermidis* rarely causes NVE, but it is a leading cause of PVE.

Other Etiologic Organisms. Gram-negative and fungal infections are described later. Endocarditis caused by *Haemophilus* species is usually caused by *H. aphrophilus, H. paraphrophilus,* or *H. parainfluenzae,* rarely *H. influenzae. Neisseria gonorrhoeae* causes acute endocarditis; this complication of gonorrhea has become rare since the introduction of penicillin. Cases of endocarditis caused by anaerobic bacteria or by more than one species (polymicrobial infection) also are rare, accounting for less than 1 per cent of cases.

PATHOGENESIS AND PATHOLOGY. Figure 299–1 illustrates the sequence of events in pathogenesis of SBE, which usually develops on previously abnormal heart valves. Forty years ago, the underlying cardiac condition was most often chronic rheumatic valvular heart disease. Today, the leading pre-existing condition for SBE in the United States is congenital heart disease in its

various forms, including mitral valve prolapse. The number of cases engrafted upon rheumatic valvular disease will decline even further in the United States and other developed countries as the prevalence of chronic rheumatic heart disease in the general population continues to fall. Other important predisposing conditions are cardiac surgery (especially if a prosthetic valve has been implanted) and previous episodes of infective endocarditis. ABE can attack previously normal as well as damaged valves and prosthetic valves. Estimates of the frequency of the main underlying heart conditions for patients of various ages with acute or subacute endocarditis are shown in Table 299–2. Table 299–3 ranks the relative risks for endocarditis posed by various cardiac lesions.

The pathogenetic sequence leading to SBE begins with endothelial damage. When subendothelial connective tissue containing collagen fibers is denuded of endothelium, platelets aggregate at the site. These aggregates have been found occasionally on normal valves, but they occur more frequently on the surfaces of valves damaged by congenital or rheumatic disease or by a previous episode of infective endocarditis. These microscopic platelet thrombi may form and resolve harmlessly, but sometimes they are stabilized by deposition of fibrin and grow to form nodular sterile vegetations that are referred to as NBTE. Microscopic examination shows bundles of degenerating platelets held together by strands of fibrin, with few other cells present. This process can be induced in experimental animals by passing a catheter into the heart; NBTE forms at sites where the catheter damages the endothelium. Intracardiac pressure-monitoring catheters produce NBTE in humans in the same way. For unknown reasons, patients with cachexia caused by advanced malignancy or other wasting diseases are prone to form NBTE, which in this setting is usually termed *marantic endocarditis.* The sterile vegetations found in a few patients with systemic lupus erythematosus (Libman-Sacks endocarditis) are another form of NBTE.

The vegetations of NBTE are irregular friable white or tan masses of variable size that are usually found along the lines where valves touch upon closing. They may be so small as to be easily missed on inspection but are frequently rather large. Because there is no inflammatory reaction at the site of attachment, the vegetations of NBTE can often be picked off easily with forceps at necropsy, leaving a normal-looking valve surface. These easily dislodged vegetations embolize frequently, often blocking peripheral arteries and causing infarction in myocardium, spleen, kidney, brain, gut, or extremities.

When NBTE is colonized by circulating bacteria, infective endocarditis results. Two important factors that determine which organisms are most likely to cause endocarditis are (1) the frequency with which they are found in the blood and (2) their ability to adhere to fibrin and platelet thrombi. Viridans streptococci enter the blood from the oral cavity frequently (probably daily) and adhere well to platelets and fibrin. Therefore, it is not surprising that they are the leading cause of SBE (Table 299–1). In contrast, *Escherichia coli* adheres poorly and rarely causes infective endocarditis, even though it is a very frequent cause of bacteremia.

Once lodged upon the surface of NBTE, bacteria multiply rapidly and attain high numbers within the vegetation, after which many enter the stationary or resting phase. The presence of bacteria is a powerful stimulus for further localized thrombosis, which causes vegetations to enlarge by accretion of new layers of fibrin. Because these layers protect bacteria from phagocytes, the

TABLE 299–2. APPROXIMATE FREQUENCY OF THE MAJOR CATEGORIES OF PRE-EXISTING CARDIAC LESIONS IN PATIENTS WITH INFECTIVE ENDOCARDITIS IN THE UNITED STATES

	Children Under 2 Years Old (%)	Children 2 to 15 Years Old (%)	Adults 15 to 50 Years Old (%)	Adults > 50 Years Old (%)	Adults, Intravenous Drug Abusers
No known heart disease	50–70	10–15	10	10	50
Congenital heart disease	30–50	70–80	20–30	10	10
Mitral valve prolapse	Rare	Rare	30	30	10
Rheumatic heart disease	Rare	<10	10	10	<10
Degenerative heart disease	0	0	Rare	10–20	Rare
Prosthetic valve	Rare	<10	10–20	10–20	20
Previous endocarditis	Rare	<5	5	5–10	20

Adapted from Durack DT: Infective and non-infective endocarditis. *In* Hurst JW (ed.): The Heart, 6th ed., pp 1130–1157. Copyright © 1986 by McGraw-Hill, Inc. Used by permission of McGraw-Hill Book Company.

TABLE 299–3. ESTIMATED RELATIVE RISK FOR INFECTIVE ENDOCARDITIS POSED BY VARIOUS CARDIAC LESIONS

Relatively High Risk	Intermediate Risk	Very Low or Negligible Risk
Prosthetic heart valves	Mitral valve prolapse with regurgitation	Mitral valve prolapse without regurgitation
Aortic valve disease	Pure mitral stenosis	Atrial septal defects
Mitral insufficiency	Tricuspid valve disease	Arteriosclerotic plaques
Patent ductus arteriosus	Pulmonary valve disease	Coronary artery disease
Ventricular septal defect	Previous infective endocarditis	Syphilitic aortitis
Coarctation of the aorta	Asymmetric septal hypertrophy	Cardiac pacemakers
Marfan's syndrome	Calcific aortic sclerosis	Surgically corrected cardiac lesions (without prosthetic implants, more than 6 months after operation)
	Hyperalimentation or pressure-monitoring lines that reach the right atrium	
	Nonvalvular intracardiac prosthetic implants	

Adapted from Durack DT: Infective and non-infective endocarditis. *In* Hurst JW (ed.): The Heart, 6th ed., pp 1130–1157. Copyright © 1986 by McGraw-Hill, Inc. Used by permission of McGraw-Hill Book Company.

vegetation provides a sanctuary in which even avirulent bacteria can flourish.

Approximate figures for the frequency with which vegetations are found at various locations in the heart are given in Table 299–4. The frequency with which a cardiac valve is involved by endocarditis is related to the mean blood pressure acting upon it. Accordingly, the aortic and mitral valves are infected far more often than the tricuspid and pulmonary valves. This rule does not hold for acute endocarditis in intravenous drug abusers, in whom tricuspid valve infection is common (Table 299–4).

Endocarditis usually develops at sites where blood flows from a high-pressure source (e.g., the left ventricle) through an orifice (e.g., a ventricular septal defect) into a low-pressure sink (e.g., the right ventricle). Examples of cardiovascular conditions subject to infection that fit these criteria include mitral regurgitation, aortic stenosis, ventricular septal defect, patent ductus arteriosus, and coarctation of the aorta. Vegetations are usually located on the "downstream" side of these anatomic abnormalities, where pressure effects and turbulence favor deposition of bacteria from the swift stream of blood. Vegetations also may develop at sites where a turbulent regurgitant jet of blood strikes the wall of a cardiac chamber, causing endothelial roughening and reactive endocardial fibrosis. These are called *jet lesions*.

The vegetations of infective endocarditis are variable in appearance. Some are small warty nodules, whereas others have the cauliflower-like polypoid appearance that gave rise to the descriptive term *vegetation*. Some are less than 1 sq mm in size, whereas others are so large as to block valve orifices and cause functional stenosis. They may be white, red, tan, or gray. Vegetations on the tricuspid valve are often larger than those on left-sided valves. Microscopic examination shows colonies of bacteria or masses of fungal hyphae embedded in fibrin and platelets. Infected vegetations usually contain surprisingly few leukocytes. Inflammatory cells may accumulate at the base of the vegetation, where it attaches to the valve. This distorts the valve, superimposing new damage on any pre-existing pathology. If this reaction is severe, the valve may perforate, or an abscess may develop in adjacent tissues. Abscess formation is common in ABE and PVE but not in SBE.

Antibodies to many of the commensal organisms that cause SBE are present in low titer before infection occurs, increase in titer during the course of SBE, and decrease after successful treatment. These antibodies do not arrest the progress of SBE and do not provide immunity to future endocardial infection.

The healing process begins even in untreated endocarditis but reaches completion only if antibiotic treatment kills the bacteria. Host cells move in to organize the vegetation; macrophages ingest bacterial and cellular debris; and fibroblasts lay down new collagen. The vegetations gradually shrink over a period of weeks or months and become endothelialized. Recognizable but nonviable bacteria can sometimes be found in sections of valves resected at operation or necropsy, months after infection has been eradicated. The healed valve is often scarred, thickened by fibrosis, and calcified. It may be perforated, and the supporting structures may be damaged. Residual hemodynamic dysfunction, mild or severe, is therefore likely. This condition may worsen over time, even though the bacteria had been eradicated long before by antibiotic treatment. The scarred valve remains susceptible to reinfection for life.

CLINICAL FEATURES. All the clinical and laboratory manifestations of infective endocarditis reflect the effects of an intravascular infection and the patient's physiologic and immunologic reaction to it.

History. The onset of subacute endocarditis is usually insidious, with nonspecific complaints, general malaise, anorexia, weakness, and fatigue. This nonspecific syndrome is often described as a "a flu-like illness." Low-grade intermittent fevers with chills and night sweats are usual. Headaches, myalgias, arthralgias, and back pain are common. A history of heart murmur, congenital heart disease, rheumatic fever, or cardiac surgery may help identify the underlying lesion. The patient may conceal intravenous drug abuse, which should be kept in mind during both interview and examination as a likely mode of infection.

Symptoms of heart failure must be carefully sought because their presence is of great prognostic significance. Embolization and infarction can cause sudden onset of neurologic syndromes, such as hemiparesis, or abdominal pain due to infarction of spleen, kidney, or gut. Embolization of a coronary artery can cause silent or symptomatic myocardial infarction. Perforation of a valve or rupture of chordae tendineae can cause sudden onset of severe heart failure.

Physical Examination. Patients with subacute endocarditis may have nonspecific symptoms of subacute systemic infection including pallor, asthenia, and sweating. A variety of interesting peripheral signs may be found on further examination, including petechiae, splinter hemorrhages, Roth's spots, Osler's nodes, Janeway lesions, and clubbing of the fingers. Some of the characteristics of these signs are summarized in Table 299–5.

Examination of the spleen often shows moderate enlargement, usually without notable tenderness unless there is a splenic abscess or recent embolic infarction.

On examination of the cardiovascular system, the peripheral pulse is often rapid because of fever, heart failure, or both. A collapsing pulse may be present, indicating aortic incompetence

TABLE 299–4. FREQUENCY WITH WHICH ANATOMIC SITES ARE INVOLVED IN SUBACUTE ENDOCARDITIS, ACUTE ENDOCARDITIS, AND ENDOCARDITIS IN INTRAVENOUS DRUG ABUSERS

	SBE (%)	ABE (%)	Endocarditis in Intravenous Drug Abusers (%)
Left-sided valves	85	65	40
Aortic	15–26	18–25	25–30
Mitral	38–45	30–35	15–20
Aortic *and* mitral	23–30	15–20	15–20
Right-sided valves	5	20	50
Tricuspid	1–5	15	45–50
Pulmonary	1	Rare	2
Tricuspid *and* pulmonary	Rare	Rare	3
Left- *and* right-sided sites	Rare	5–10	5–10
Other sites (patent ductus, VSD, coarctation, jet lesions)	10	5	5

Adapted from Durack DT: Infective and non-infective endocarditis. *In* Hurst JW (ed.): The Heart, 6th ed., pp 1130–1157. Copyright © 1986 by McGraw-Hill, Inc. Used by permission of McGraw-Hill Book Company.

associated with pre-existing aortic valve disease, or new aortic insufficiency associated with endocarditis. Individual peripheral arteries may be occluded by emboli, or they may be the site of a mycotic aneurysm.

One or more cardiac murmurs are present in virtually all patients with endocarditis. Murmurs may be caused by pre-existing heart disease, by endocarditis itself, or by both. Up to 15 per cent of patients do not have a heart murmur when first examined, but nearly all develop a murmur before the disease has run its course. New murmurs and changing murmurs are more likely to occur in acute endocarditis than in subacute disease. Development of a new murmur of aortic insufficiency during a febrile illness of unknown origin strongly suggests the diagnosis of infective endocarditis.

COMPLICATIONS. Heart failure is by far the most important complication of infective endocarditis; it exerts more influence on prognosis and treatment than any other. In one representative series, some degree of heart failure was present in 75 per cent of patients with aortic valve disease and endocarditis, in 50 per cent with mitral valve involvement, and in 19 per cent with tricuspid disease.

Arterial embolization is diagnosed in about one third of patients with subacute endocarditis and in up to two thirds of patients with acute endocarditis. Many small or large arterial emboli go undetected. Any artery may be affected. In order of frequency, arteries supplying the brain, lung, myocardium, spleen, and extremities are involved.

Neurologic manifestations of endocarditis are common and clinically important. These include toxic confusional states, stroke, meningoencephalitis, cranial or peripheral nerve lesions, and psychiatric symptoms. About 10 per cent of patients with endocarditis have complaints involving the central nervous system at presentation, and 30 to 50 per cent have nervous system involvement at some point during the course of the disease. Cerebral infarction is usually caused by embolism, while cerebral hemorrhage, which is less common than infarction, may be associated with emboli or rupture of a mycotic aneurysm. Heparin therapy increases the risk that an intracranial hemorrhage will occur during the course of infective endocarditis.

Cerebritis secondary to impaction of infected emboli or hematogenous spread of bacteria is quite common, especially in acute bacterial endocarditis caused by *S. aureus.* Cerebritis may progress to form a frank cerebral abscess, which is found in 1 to 5 per cent of cases of acute endocarditis. However, brain abscesses rarely complicate subacute endocarditis.

In up to 15 per cent of patients, examination of the cerebrospinal fluid may show reactive changes consisting of the presence of polymorphonuclear leukocytes and moderately elevated protein concentration. Such reactions are particularly common in acute staphylococcal endocarditis. In most cases cerebrospinal glucose concentrations do not decrease, cultures are negative, and true bacterial meningitis does not develop, except in a few patients with acute pneumococcal or staphylococcal endocarditis.

Mycotic aneurysm is an unusual but important complication that is diagnosed in 3 to 5 per cent of patients. The true incidence is probably higher, but a number pass undetected, especially small aneurysms in the brain. Mycotic aneurysms are caused by an inflammatory reaction in the arterial wall associated with septic microemboli to vasa vasorum or with impaction of an infected embolus in the arterial lumen. The site most often involved is the proximal aorta, including the sinuses of Valsalva, followed by arteries to the viscera, extremities, and brain. Living organisms are seldom found in the wall of these aneurysms, even when the underlying endocardial infection is still active. Presumably, the damage that weakened the arterial wall was caused by an inflammatory reaction to infected emboli. If an aneurysm enlarges to a certain critical size (probably about 1 cm in diameter), it is likely to continue to enlarge and eventually rupture as a result of the physical forces exerted by the arterial pressure, despite eradication of the infecting organisms by antimicrobial therapy.

Many patients with subacute endocarditis show abnormalities in the urinary sediment. In some cases this is due to glomerulonephritis, a relatively common complication that occasionally causes significant renal failure. Glomerulonephritis is caused by deposition of immune complexes on the glomerular basement membrane. Other inflammatory manifestations of subacute infective endocarditis that may be mediated by immune complexes include arthritis, tenosynovitis, and possibly pericarditis, Osler's nodes, and Roth's spots. In a few patients with long-term SBE, glomerulonephritis is severe enough to necessitate dialysis. Renal function usually recovers steadily within a few weeks after the start of effective treatment.

TABLE 299–5. CHARACTERISTICS OF SOME PERIPHERAL SIGNS OF INFECTIVE ENDOCARDITIS

	Petechiae	Splinter Hemorrhages	Roth's Spots	Osler's Nodes	Janeway's Lesions	Clubbing
Appearance	Tiny red hemorrhagic spots	"Splinters" under nails; red when fresh, then brown or black	Small bright red patches with white centers	Pea-sized red or purplish nodules	Red macules	Curvature of the nails in two planes, with swelling of the terminal phalanges
Distribution	Anywhere, especially above clavicles, in mouth and in conjunctivae	Distal third of nails	Retinae	Fingers and toes; occasionally hands and feet	Palms and soles; occasionally on flanks, forearms, ankles, feet, ears	Fingers and/or toes
Incidence	Common, in both SBE and ABE	Common, in both SBE and ABE	Infrequent; usually in SBE	Infrequent; usually in SBE	Infrequent; usually in ABE	Rare; in SBE only
Pathology	Increased capillary permeability; microemboli	Blood in avascular squamous epithelium under nail; due to microemboli or increased capillary fragility	Inflammation and hemorrhage	Intracutaneous local vasculitis; bacteria rarely found; occasional abscess formation; probably embolic in origin	Origin uncertain; possibly embolic or allergic in origin	Soft tissue proliferation, occasionally periosteal new bone formation
Pain	None	None	None	Mild to moderately severe	None	Usually none; sometimes painful
Duration	Days	Weeks	Days	Days	Several hours to days	Weeks to months
Diagnostic significance	Nonspecific; also found in septicemia, after cardiac surgery, and in many other disorders	Nonspecific; found in up to 10% of normal people and up to 40% of patients with mitral stenosis	Strongly suggestive of endocarditis but not diagnostic	Almost pathognomonic for endocarditis	Unusual in bacteremia without endocarditis	Nonspecific; found in many cardiopulmonary disorders; can be congenital

Adapted from Durack DT: Infective and non-infective endocarditis. *In* Hurst JW (ed.): The Heart, 5th ed., pp 1250–1277. Copyright © 1982 by McGraw-Hill, Inc. Used by permission of McGraw-Hill Book Company.

SPECIAL FORMS OF INFECTIVE ENDOCARDITIS

ACUTE BACTERIAL ENDOCARDITIS. Several important features distinguish acute from subacute bacterial endocarditis. The clinical course is usually measured in days rather than in weeks or months. The associated systemic illness is more severe, and early mortality is higher than in subacute endocarditis. The diagnosis is usually made within 7 days from onset of symptoms.

Acute endocardial infection is usually caused by primary pathogens capable of producing invasive infection at other sites. *S. aureus* is the most common cause of acute endocarditis. This species alone accounts for 50 to 70 per cent of cases. The patient is more likely to suffer rapid destruction of the valve, including perforation, so the likelihood that valve replacement will be required is greater. Patients with acute bacterial endocarditis are also more likely to have one or more focal infections outside the heart—in brain, bone, lungs, or other sites. Such foci could be either primary infections (that is, the portal of entry for the organism causing endocarditis) or secondary hematogenous infections. In contrast, the organisms that cause subacute bacterial endocarditis rarely cause localized hematogenous infection elsewhere in the body.

Abscesses in the fibrous cardiac skeleton or myocardium are much more likely to form in acute than in subacute endocarditis. If such abscesses are adjacent to the fibers of the conduction system, they may cause conduction defects. Abscesses may be responsible for antibiotic treatment failure.

Because acute bacterial endocarditis is caused by invasive organisms and progresses rapidly, treatment should not be delayed until blood culture results are available. It is important to clear the bloodstream of circulating organisms as soon as possible, both to reduce the risk of death from septicemia and to lessen the chances that metastatic infection will develop elsewhere. When acute endocarditis is strongly suspected, empiric antibiotic therapy should be started immediately after three blood samples have been drawn for culture.

ENDOCARDITIS IN DRUG ADDICTS. Endocarditis is the most important of the many bacterial infections experienced by intravenous drug abusers. Salient features that distinguish endocarditis in this subgroup from the disease in general include a younger age of onset, a higher proportion of acute cases, a correspondingly higher proportion of cases involving normal cardiac valves, and a high frequency of tricuspid valve infection. The etiologic organisms can gain entry into the bloodstream in various ways: directly, by injection of contaminated drugs; or indirectly, from the patient's skin flora, from cellulitis caused by subcutaneous injection of drugs, or from suppurative thrombophlebitis or drug-related infections in other sites such as the lungs. *S. aureus* is the leading etiologic organism. Addicts also have an increased incidence of endocardial infection with gram-negative bacilli, especially *Pseudomonas* species, and fungi.

Drug addicts with acute endocarditis usually experience a brief, severe illness, with heavily positive blood cultures. Because the etiologic organisms are often primary pathogens, hematogenous infections at other sites in the body are common. A frequent finding on admission is multiple patches of pneumonitis visible on chest radiography. These are caused by septic pulmonary emboli arising from vegetations on the tricuspid or occasionally the pulmonary valve. Although acute disease is typical, subacute endocarditis also is common in addicts, especially in those who have had previous episodes of endocarditis.

The prognosis for young drug addicts with right-sided *S. aureus* infection is good, with mortality rates being less than 5 per cent. Factors that worsen the prognosis include left-sided involvement, particularly aortic, and infection with gram-negative bacilli or fungi. Recurrent episodes of endocarditis are common in addicts who continue to use drugs after their first episode of endocarditis, especially if a prosthetic valve has been inserted.

PROSTHETIC VALVE INFECTION. Prosthetic valve endocarditis should be regarded as a special category, because it differs in many ways from other forms of endocarditis. By arbitrary definition, early PVE occurs within 60 days of valve placement and late PVE more than 60 days postoperatively. Early PVE occurs at a rate of about 0.5 per cent, although this figure varies between hospitals. Late PVE is estimated to occur at an overall rate of about 1 per cent per year. The rate for infection of aortic valve prostheses is three to five times higher than for mitral prostheses.

The progress of PVE may be either acute or subacute, but this cannot be predicted reliably from the infecting organism. For example, even *S. epidermidis*, a "nonpathogen" that causes indolent chronic disease on native valves, can cause an acute syndrome in early PVE.

The spectrum of organisms causing PVE is quite distinct. *S. epidermidis*, which rarely infects native valves, is a leading cause of both early and late prosthetic valve infection. Gram-negative bacilli and fungi infect prosthetic valves notably more often than they do native valves, especially in early onset cases. The later the onset of PVE after operation, the more nearly the spectrum of etiologic organisms resembles that of native valve endocarditis.

In addition to forming vegetations, infection may spread around the circumference of the sewing ring of the prosthesis, often causing partial dehiscence and paravalvular leaks. Abscess formation in fibrous tissue or myocardium adjacent to the sewing ring is common. Despite these adverse factors, when a prosthetic valve is replaced because of infection, early reinfection with the same organism is uncommon.

In general, PVE is harder to cure than most other forms of endocarditis (Table 299–6). This is due partly to the increased frequency of antibiotic-resistant organisms in PVE, partly to the fact that a foreign body is present at the site of infection, and partly to the high frequency of perivalvular abscesses. Not surprisingly, the risk of relapse after antibiotic therapy is much higher for PVE than for native valve infection. Valve replacement is often necessary to achieve cure. Antibiotic treatment usually must be continued for a minimum of 4 to 6 weeks, sometimes for many months. In some cases in which repeated valve replacement is contraindicated, cure cannot be achieved but suppressive antibiotic therapy is continued indefinitely.

GRAM-NEGATIVE BACTERIAL ENDOCARDITIS. This term usually refers to infection with enteric or environmental gram-negative aerobic bacilli such as *Klebsiella*, *Pseudomonas*, *Serratia*, *Enterobacter*, and *E. coli*. (*Haemophilus* species are not considered in this group.) Gram-negative endocarditis is a rare disease except in two settings: early prosthetic valve infection and intravenous drug addiction. In these two groups, gram-negative bacilli can account for up to 15 per cent of cases.

TABLE 299–6. ESTIMATED BACTERIOLOGIC CURE RATES FOR ETIOLOGIC ORGANISMS TREATED WITH ANTIMICROBIAL THERAPY ALONE OR ANTIMICROBIALS PLUS SURGERY*

Native Valve Endocarditis	Antimicrobial Therapy Alone	Antimicrobial Therapy Plus Surgery
Viridans streptococci, group A streptococci, *S. bovis*, pneumococci, gonococci	98	98
E. faecalis	90	>90
S. aureus (in young drug addicts)	90	>90
S. aureus (in elderly patients with chronic underlying diseases)	50	70
Gram-negative aerobic bacilli†	40	65
Fungi	<5	50

Prosthetic Valve Endocarditis	Early PVE (No Surgery)	Late PVE	Early PVE (With Surgery)	Late PVE
Viridans streptococci, group A streptococci, *S. bovis*, pneumococci, gonococci	‡	80	‡	90
E. faecalis	‡	60	‡	75
S. aureus	25	40	50	60
S. epidermidis	20	40	60	70
Gram-negative aerobic bacilli†	<10	20	40	50
Fungi	<1	<1	30	40

*Morbidity and mortality will be significantly greater than these figures for *bacteriologic* cure indicate.

†Excluding *Haemophilus* species, which carry a better prognosis.

‡Insufficient data to estimate rate.

Adapted from Durack DT: Infective and non-infective endocarditis. *In* Hurst JW (ed.): The Heart, 5th ed., pp 1250–1277. Copyright © 1982 by McGraw-Hill, Inc. Used by permission of McGraw-Hill Book Company.

Gram-negative endocarditis often progresses acutely. Patients may develop septic shock. The mortality rate is higher than for gram-positive infections, approaching that of fungal endocarditis. Antibiotic treatment alone is often unsuccessful, so valve replacement is frequently necessary. Treatment with combinations of two or more antibiotics for 6 weeks or more is often necessary. Relapse after antibiotic treatment is much more common than for gram-positive infection.

HACEK ENDOCARDITIS. The acronym HACEK refers to a group of unusual organisms that share some characteristics and, taken together, cause a significant number of cases of infective endocarditis. They are *Haemophilus* species (but usually not *H. influenzae*), *Actinobacillus actinomycetemcomitans*, *Cardiobacterium hominis*, *Eikenella corrodens*, and *Kingella* species. These are fastidious gram-negative bacteria that have a tendency to cause subacute endocarditis with large vegetations. They are more likely to be sensitive to β-lactam antibiotics, especially ampicillin and ceftriaxone, than other aerobic gram-negative bacilli. Endocarditis caused by these organisms has a fairly good prognosis and often can be cured without valve replacement, even in some cases of prosthetic valve infection.

FUNGAL ENDOCARDITIS. Like gram-negative endocarditis, fungal infection of the endocardium is rare except in two groups of patients: those with prosthetic valves and intravenous drug addicts. Although a wide variety of fungal species have been recovered from patients with endocarditis over the years, only two predominate: *Candida* and *Aspergillus* species. *C. albicans* endocarditis occurs in patients with central intravascular lines, especially hyperalimentation lines that are allowed to reach the level of the tricuspid valve. Therefore, these infections often involve the right side. *C. parapsilosis* and *C. tropicalis* are more likely to occur in drug addicts and can infect valves on either side of the heart. Fungal vegetations tend to be bulky and often cause infarctions as a result of embolization of peripheral arteries. Because blood cultures are commonly negative in fungal endocarditis (see earlier discussion), surgical removal of a large embolus from an artery to one of the limbs may be diagnostic as well as therapeutic. Histologic examination may show hyphae of the infecting fungus in tissue sections.

Few drugs are available for treatment of fungal endocarditis. Amphotericin B is generally used, but the chance of achieving cure with drug therapy alone is extremely low. Cure rates can be increased by surgical removal of vegetations and valve replacement, but mortality remains relatively high compared with that for other forms of endocarditis (Table 299–6).

ENDOCARDITIS IN INFANTS AND CHILDREN. Infective endocarditis is an unusual occurrence in infants. When it does occur, it is most often only one component of systemic bacterial infection caused by an invasive organism such as *S. aureus*. The endocardial infection is likely to follow an acute course, being discovered unexpectedly at necropsy in an infant who has died with bacterial infection. Often a normal cardiac valve is involved, as in other forms of acute endocarditis. The remaining cases are associated with congenital cardiac defects. Because the diagnosis is often delayed or missed, endocarditis in infants has a higher mortality than in other age groups.

In children more than 1 year old, infective endocarditis is not rare. Most affected children have subacute disease involving congenital cardiac defects. The spectrum of etiologic organisms and the approach to diagnosis and treatment are similar to those in adults with infective endocarditis. However, the age and physical size of children must be carefully considered when choosing the best time for cardiac surgery, especially when prostheses must be implanted.

ENDOCARDITIS IN OBSTETRIC AND GYNECOLOGIC PRACTICE. Pregnancy itself poses little increased risk for infective endocarditis. Septic abortion or pelvic infection related to intrauterine contraceptive devices can lead to endocarditis in susceptible patients. Occasionally, infective endocarditis develops during delivery or in the puerperium. If the mother has pre-existing valvular disease, bacteremias associated with perinatal infective complications such as amnionitis, endometritis, parametritis, septic thrombophlebitis, or urinary tract infection can seed the endocardium. The leading etiologic organisms in this setting are *E. faecalis*, *S. agalactiae* (group B), *S. aureus*, and only occasionally *Bacteroides* or gram-negative enteric bacilli.

NOSOCOMIAL ENDOCARDITIS. Intensive medical care can predispose to endocarditis in many ways. Endothelial damage can be caused by intracardiac surgery, pressure-monitoring catheters, ventriculoatrial shunts, and hyperalimentation lines if they reach into the right atrium. Portals of entry for microorganisms are provided by wounds, burns, biopsy sites, intravenous and arterial catheters and pacemakers, hemodialysis access sites, urinary catheters, and intratracheal airways. Nosocomial bacteremias are common in seriously ill patients. Therefore, it is not surprising that hospital-acquired infective endocarditis has become increasingly common in the past two decades, as intensive care units have proliferated. Perhaps the highest risk is found in severely burned patients, who may sustain repeated episodes of bacteremia while pressure-monitoring catheters are kept in the right side of the heart for long periods. In contrast, diagnostic right heart catheterization over brief periods in patients in a coronary care unit, who seldom develop bacteremia, presents a very low risk for infective endocarditis.

The microbes likely to cause nosocomial endocarditis are staphylococci, *Candida* species, and gram-negative bacilli. The prognosis is worse than for most other forms of infective endocarditis. This is because the patients have serious pre-existing diseases that may obscure the symptoms and signs, thus delaying diagnosis. Also, nosocomially acquired organisms are more likely to be resistant to antibiotics.

CULTURE-NEGATIVE ENDOCARDITIS. This term refers to the situation in which the endocardium is infected, but blood cultures remain persistently negative. Possible causes include antibiotic therapy, and infection by slow-growing or fastidious microorganisms that are missed because of suboptimal blood culture technique. Culture-negative endocarditis is an uncommon disease. Therefore, when blood cultures from a patient not receiving antibiotics remain *persistently* negative in the absence of antibiotic therapy, that patient probably does not have endocarditis. Fungal endocarditis is an exception. Blood cultures are positive in only about half of patients with *Candida* endocarditis and in less than one fifth of those with *Aspergillus* infection. When culture-negative disease does occur, it is much more likely to follow a subacute than an acute course.

If the clinical findings strongly support the diagnosis of culture-negative endocarditis, a therapeutic trial of antibiotic therapy may be given. This usually consists of a penicillin plus an aminoglycoside for subacute infection, a combination that covers viridans streptococci, enterococci, HACEK organisms (see above), and diphtheroids. If the disease is acute, treatment for *S. aureus* must be included. To be of any diagnostic value, a proper therapeutic trial must be continued for at least 2 weeks, unless new diagnostic information changes the clinical situation.

INFECTIVE ENDARTERITIS. An infection located within an artery can mimic infective endocarditis. Possible sites of vegetations include patent ductus arteriosus, coarctation of the aorta, arteriovenous fistulas, and prosthetic vascular grafts. In the past, about one quarter of all patients with an uncorrected patent ductus arteriosus eventually developed bacterial endarteritis. Because many of the underlying lesions are surgically correctable, infective endarteritis is now uncommon in developed countries, with the exception of infections in arteriovenous shunts constructed for the purpose of hemodialysis. When bacterial endarteritis occurs in an aneurysm, the etiologic organisms are usually found within a multilayered thrombus in the lumen of the aneurysm rather than in vegetations.

RECURRENT ENDOCARDITIS. The term *recurrent endocarditis* includes both *relapses* and *reinfections*. Recurrent endocarditis has been reported in 2 to 30 per cent of cases. This wide variation is partly explained by variable duration of follow-up. Intravenous drug abusers are at higher risk than any other group for recurrent endocarditis. A few patients with more than four separate episodes of infective endocarditis have been reported.

The likelihood of relapse after treatment of different forms of infective endocarditis can be predicted from published experience (Table 299–6). Because occasional relapses occur even after optimal treatment, careful follow-up for several months after treatment is mandatory. Most relapses occur within a few days or weeks of ending treatment, but occasional late relapses occur as a result of a few organisms surviving in a metabolically inactive state deep within vegetations.

Reinfection means that a new episode of endocarditis has developed after cure of a previous episode. Reinfections have become more common in recent years, as more patients are followed for longer periods after a first episode. Usually a different species or strain of etiologic organism is involved, but if the second organism is a common viridans streptococcus that appears identical to the first, one cannot be certain, without special tests, whether an episode of recurrent endocarditis represents reinfection or relapse.

DIFFERENTIAL DIAGNOSIS. The differential diagnosis of endocarditis is very wide because its manifestations are numerous and often nonspecific. SBE must be considered in the evaluation of every patient with fever of unknown origin. It can be confused with rheumatic fever, osteomyelitis, tuberculosis, meningitis, intra-abdominal infections, salmonellosis, brucellosis, glomerulonephritis, myocardial infarction, stroke, endocardial thrombi, atrial myxoma, connective tissue diseases, vasculitis, occult malignancy (especially lymphomas), congestive heart failure, pericarditis, and even psychoneurosis. ABE shares many manifestations with septicemias caused by *S. aureus, Neisseria,* pneumococci, and gram-negative bacilli in patients who do not have endocarditis. ABE may mimic pneumonia, meningitis, brain abscess, stroke, malaria, acute pericarditis, vasculitis, and disseminated intravascular coagulation.

INVESTIGATIONS. *Routine Tests.* Results of urinalysis are abnormal in about 50 per cent of cases, showing microscopic hematuria or slight proteinuria or both. Gross hematuria suggests that renal infarction may have occurred. Red cell casts and heavy proteinuria indicate that immune complex glomerulonephritis may be present.

The automated blood count shows only nonspecific abnormalities. Anemia is usual in SBE and fairly common in ABE. Anemia is most often of the hypoproliferative type, with a normochromic normocytic smear. ABE may cause acute hemolysis.

A moderate leukocytosis with some immature forms apparent on smear is often found in SBE, but in many cases the leukocyte count is normal. Patients with ABE often show neutrophilia with band forms, vacuoles, Döhle bodies, and toxic granulation. In a few cases, careful examination of a Gram-stained smear of the buffy coat reveals organisms within neutrophils.

The erythrocyte sedimentation rate is usually elevated, except in a few acute cases of brief duration.

Blood Culture. This is the single most important investigation in diagnosis of endocarditis. Blood cultures should be drawn from all patients with fever and heart murmur unless their illness is clearly due to another diagnosed disease or the fever resolves quickly without recurrence. Blood cultures should also be taken if a patient with a heart lesion susceptible to endocarditis has other symptoms or signs consistent with infection.

The bacteremia of infective endocarditis is usually continuous, with between 1 and 100 organisms per milliliter of blood in subacute cases. Therefore, it is seldom necessary to draw a large number of blood cultures. The causative organism can be recovered from culture samples taken on the first day of admission in over 90 per cent of patients with culture-positive endocarditis. No more than three separate venous blood cultures should be drawn on the first day. If these show no growth by the second day, two or three further culture samples may be drawn. If the patient has received prior antibiotic therapy, further blood samples may be taken over the following week in a search for recrudescence of bacteremia after antibiotic effect has passed. Otherwise, repeated blood cultures are likely to be uninformative and wasteful.

After careful skin cleansing, 10 to 20 ml of blood should be drawn for each culture. Skin preparation is especially important because common skin flora (*S. epidermidis* and diphtheroids) can cause endocarditis, and their isolation from blood cultures can cause diagnostic confusion. Pour plates can help to distinguish contaminants from true positive cultures. The culture medium should be adequately supplemented to allow growth of fastidious, nutritionally variant bacteria. When endocarditis is suspected, cultures should be incubated for at least 3 weeks and stains made at intervals even if no growth is apparent on inspection.

Subacute endocarditis stimulates the humoral immune system to produce both nonspecific and specific antibodies. A positive test for rheumatoid factor is found in 40 to 50 per cent of subacute cases, but rarely in ABE. This can provide a useful diagnostic clue in culture-negative cases. A polyclonal increase in gamma globulins is characteristic. Occasional false-positive serologic test results for syphilis occur. Hemolytic complement levels may be moderately elevated, normal, or low. The lowest levels are found in patients with immune complex glomerulonephritis. Circulating immune complexes are present in more than 80 per cent of patients with either ABE or SBE. All these immunologic findings revert to normal after eradication of the organisms.

Electrocardiography. Electrocardiography may reveal evidence of myocardial infarction due to embolization of a vegetation to a coronary artery. When a disturbance of conduction develops during the course of endocarditis, extension of infection into the myocardium may have occurred. This could be focal myocarditis or an abscess located close to the conduction system.

Echocardiography. Modern echocardiographic imaging is essential for optimal management of infective endocarditis. Serial two-dimensional studies with color flow Doppler can detect most vegetations and provide valuable additional data on underlying heart conditions and cardiac function. Introduction of transesophageal imaging has greatly improved sensitivity for detection of small vegetations, prosthetic valve infections, and abscesses. Echocardiography, valuable though it is, does have some limitations in this application. Because the sensitivity for small vegetations is not perfect, a negative echocardiogram cannot rule out endocarditis, especially when a prosthetic valve is present. Occasional false-positive readings for vegetations occur, particularly in cases with myxomatous changes affecting a valve. Finally, the echocardiographic appearance of vegetations during and after therapy is not a reliable criterion for success or failure of antibiotic therapy.

Radiography. The chest radiograph is most useful as a means of providing evidence of congestive heart failure. Multiple small patchy infiltrates in the lungs of an intravenous drug abuser with fever strongly suggest the diagnosis of septic emboli arising from right-sided infective endocarditis. Valvular calcification may identify a valve affected by chronic rheumatic or congenital disease. A mycotic aneurysm could cause widening of the aorta.

Abnormal motion of a prosthetic valve can be detected by fluoroscopy, indicating presence of a vegetation or partial dehiscence of the valve from the aortic root. This information can indicate that valve replacement is needed during management of PVE.

Computerized axial tomography can be very useful to define the cause of focal neurologic lesions in patients with endocarditis. Such lesions could be caused by various complications, including cerebritis, infarction, hemorrhage from a mycotic aneurysm, or brain abscess. Angiography is occasionally necessary to demonstrate mycotic aneurysms in the brain or elsewhere.

Cardiac catheterization and cineangiography are not necessary for most patients who respond well to antimicrobial therapy without developing cardiac failure. When treatment seems to be failing and/or operation is considered, cardiac catheterization can provide vital information. In one study of 35 patients who underwent cardiac catheterization during active endocarditis, the precatheterization assessment was significantly modified for 23, the diagnosis of site of valve involvement was altered for 14, and six valve ring abscesses were revealed. Surgery was postponed or cancelled for six patients when catheterization indicated only mild hemodynamic abnormalities. There were no serious complications. This study suggests that catheterization for selected patients with endocarditis provides such important information that it should not be avoided for fear of dislodging emboli.

TREATMENT. _General Measures._ The patient should be informed of the diagnosis and treatment plan and comforted. Heart failure, if present, should be managed with bed rest, salt restriction, and drug treatment as necessary. High temperatures and headaches can be treated symptomatically.

Antibiotic Therapy. For optimal antibiotic therapy, certain microbiologic information on the infecting organism is necessary. For most bacteria, both the minimal inhibitory concentration (MIC) and minimal bactericidal concentration (MBC) of the antibiotics likely to be used should be determined. This forms the basis for choice of curative therapy.

The serum bactericidal titer (SBT or Schlichter test) is frequently used and is sometimes useful in the management of endocarditis. The infecting organism is exposed in vitro to the patient's serum, which is drawn while antibiotic therapy is being administered, to determine the maximum dilution of serum that will inhibit and kill the organism. The SBT provides assurance that the antibiotic(s) present in the patient's serum is actually capable of killing the infecting organism. Clinical experience indicates that the SBT should be 1:8 or higher at intervals during each day of treatment. For gram-positive organisms the serum usually can kill the organism without difficulty, and SBT's are often very high (1:128 to 1:1024). In such cases, SBT's need not be measured repeatedly. SBT's for gram-negative bacilli are usually rather low (1:2 to 1:16). The SBT is most likely to be clinically helpful when the physician is treating an unusual organism, using unusual antibiotics, using an unusual regimen (such as oral treatment), or encountering treatment failure. If treatment with unusual combinations of antibiotics is needed, further laboratory tests should be performed to find out whether they are synergistic, indifferent, or antagonistic in combination.

Bactericidal antibiotics should be used for treatment of endocarditis whenever possible. Some patients have been cured with bacteriostatic drugs, but results of treatment with these agents are usually poor, presumably because host defense mechanisms are inadequate in the vegetations. With respect to treatment, the vegetations of infective endocarditis provide a contrast to bacterial pneumonia, in which phagocytes are plentiful and bacteriostatic antibiotics are usually effective. Curative antibiotic therapy for endocarditis must eradicate organisms completely, without the help of phagocytes to eliminate microbes that are relatively resistant to antibiotics because they are in the resting phase.

Clinical experience with treatment of the common forms of bacterial endocarditis caused by gram-positive cocci is so extensive that specific therapeutic regimens can be recommended with confidence. Standard regimens for streptococcal and staphylococcal endocarditis are listed in Table 299–7. Regimens for treatment of endocarditis caused by less common organisms are not listed. For these, treatment must be chosen on the basis of more limited published experience, together with the results of tests performed upon the infecting organism in the microbiology laboratory. One of the β-lactam antibiotics should be included in the regimen whenever possible.

Empiric Therapy. When the causative organism is unknown, the choice of empiric therapy depends upon whether the patient has acute or subacute disease. For ABE, broad-spectrum therapy that will cover *S. aureus* as well as many species of streptococci and gram-negative bacilli is required. For SBE, a regimen that will treat most streptococci including *E. faecalis* is appropriate. To meet these requirements, the following regimens are suggested:

1. For ABE, a combination of nafcillin, 2 grams intravenously every 4 hours, plus ampicillin, 2 grams intravenously every 4 hours, plus gentamicin, 1.0 mg per kilogram intravenously every 8 hours.

2. For SBE, a combination of ampicillin, 2 grams intravenously every 4 hours, plus gentamicin, 1.0 mg per kilogram intravenously every 8 hours.

These regimens should be adjusted if and when the causative organism is identified.

Duration of Therapy. Because infective endocarditis carries significant mortality even when well managed, it is important that treatment be continued long enough to ensure that relapse will not occur. On the other hand, patients with the most easily treated forms of endocarditis should not be subjected to unnecessarily long and expensive treatment in hospital. Extensive experience with treatment of the streptococci provides sufficient grounds for firm recommendations on duration of therapy for these organisms (Table 299–7).

In contrast, the natural history of *S. aureus* endocarditis is more variable. Some patients recover swiftly without complications, whereas others remain febrile for several weeks, sometimes owing to manifestations of disseminated staphylococcal disease such as osteomyelitis. While 4 weeks of therapy is adequate for most cases, this must not be regarded as a rigid rule because some patients require treatment for 6 to 8 weeks or longer to achieve cure. In general, the less extensive the published experience with a particular infective agent, the more one should lean toward prolonging treatment in order to provide a reasonable margin of safety. Guidelines on duration of treatment for other organisms are not listed because the duration required varies greatly according to individual circumstances.

Anticoagulants. Although the infected vegetation is essentially a thrombotic lesion, there is no evidence that anticoagulants provide any useful therapeutic effect in endocarditis. In fact, simultaneous treatment with antibiotics plus heparin carries a higher risk of serious or fatal intracerebral hemorrhage from mycotic aneurysm or infarction than treatment with penicillin alone. However, Coumadin can be given to most patients with endocarditis without excessive risk.

It is therefore best to avoid use of heparin entirely in endocarditis and to discontinue or avoid anticoagulation therapy if possible. However, Coumadin may be given if there is a clear-cut indication, taking care not to allow the prothrombin time to rise above 1.5 times normal values. An antibiotic treatment regimen that does not require intramuscular injections should be used if the patient is receiving anticoagulant therapy.

Surgical Treatment. Modern operative treatment constitutes the greatest advance in management of endocarditis since the advent of antibiotics. Surgical consultation should be obtained early, so that prompt operative intervention is available if needed.

Aortic or mitral valvular incompetence with consequent acute left ventricular failure can occur without warning, even in the most favorable forms of endocarditis. These patients need valve replacement in order to reverse cardiac failure resulting from new or worsening valvular dysfunction. Replacement of an infected prosthesis is often necessary for cure because prosthetic valve infection is more difficult to eradicate with antibiotics than is native valve infection. Repeated major emboli constitute a relative indication for valve replacement. Occasionally, a patient remains septic despite antibiotic therapy. Operation may then be required for infection control rather than for the hemodynamic consequences of infection. Operation to close a patent ductus arteriosus or septal defect, to excise a coarctation of the aorta, or to relieve asymmetric septal hypertrophy may be required as part of treatment of endocarditis engrafted upon these lesions.

Good surgical management for endocarditis depends on correct timing for valve replacement. If operation is undertaken too soon, unnecessary operative mortality and early and late morbidity of valve replacement may result. Some patients respond quickly to medical therapy, so that operation can be postponed indefinitely. If time is available for treatment of septicemia, renal failure, pneumonia, myocarditis, conduction defects, or other complications before valve replacement, ventricular function will improve and operative risk will be correspondingly lower. Given for a few days, antibiotic therapy should eradicate or at least greatly reduce the population of organisms on the valve, thus increasing the chance that an artificial valve can be inserted without itself becoming infected. However, if surgery is delayed too long patients may die suddenly, or their hemodynamic status may deteriorate so that operation is no longer feasible. This is a tragic error, because some of these patients could have been saved by earlier operation.

Frequent re-examination of the patient, together with echocardiography and/or cardiac catheterization to extend the clinical findings, is indicated in every case in which operation may be needed. The natural history of the type of endocarditis being treated should be taken into account. Penicillin-sensitive streptococcal endocarditis can almost always be bacteriologically cured (see Table 299–6), and the prognosis is good if cardiac failure does not occur. Thus, operation should usually be considered only for patients with cardiac failure who do not respond to medical treatment. Similarly, narcotic addicts with acute staphylococcal endocarditis have a relatively good prognosis, so operation should be reserved for those who develop serious heart failure. At the other end of the spectrum, the likelihood that fungal prosthetic valve endocarditis can be eradicated with antifungal drugs alone is negligible, even in the absence of heart failure (see Table 299–6). Such patients usually should undergo valve replacement early, without waiting to test the remote possibility that antifungal treatment could eradicate the infection. Aortic valve involvement, staphylococcal infection in patients other than drug addicts, gram-negative infection, prosthetic valve infection, and extension of infection into the myocardium should be regarded as other relative indications favoring early valve replacement.

For selected cases, excision of vegetations with valve repair is a desirable option that can avoid the morbidity associated with a prosthetic valve.

PROGNOSIS. Infective endocarditis is unusual among infectious diseases in that it is always fatal if untreated. Most of the rare cases of apparent recovery reported in the preantibiotic era probably did not have infective endocarditis, which can be diagnosed with absolute certainty only at operation or necropsy. The median interval between onset of symptoms and death in patients with untreated subacute endocarditis was about 6 months, with wide individual variation. Almost all patients with acute infective endocarditis died in less than 4 weeks.

Favorable prognostic factors include infection with penicillin-sensitive streptococci, a youthful patient, absence of serious pre-existing diseases, and early diagnosis and treatment. The rate of recovery for many young drug addicts with *S. aureus* infection of the tricuspid valve is excellent—greater than 95 per cent.

Heart failure is by far the most important adverse prognostic factor. Other adverse factors include aortic valve involvement, renal failure, culture-negative disease, gram-negative or fungal infection, prosthetic valve infection, and presence of an abscess in the valve ring or myocardium.

Today, bacteriologic cure can be achieved in most patients with bacterial endocarditis (see Table 299–6). This is not true for infection with resistant gram-negative bacilli and fungi, but fortunately these are uncommon. Despite the ability to eradicate most organisms, both early and long-term mortality and morbidity of infective endocarditis remain significant because of damage already done before treatment. Follow-up of patients cured of infective endocarditis shows a 5-year survival of only 60 to 70 per cent.

PREVENTION. Because endocarditis is a serious disease, antibiotics are usually given to susceptible patients during medical and dental procedures known to cause bacteremia, in an attempt to prevent this infection. Unfortunately, there is no proof that this practice is effective. Meaningful cost-benefit ratios cannot be calculated, and any recommendations are therefore necessarily empiric.

One approach is to consider two factors in each situation: (1) the relative risk for endocarditis posed by the patient's heart condition and (2) the relative risk for endocarditis posed by the procedure. If both risks are judged to be significant, prophylactic antibiotics should be given. If one or both of these risk factors are judged to be negligible, prophylaxis should be omitted. The first of these two questions can be approached by using a ranking like that shown in Table 299–3. The second can be approached

TABLE 299–7. TREATMENT REGIMENS

Organism	Antibiotic Regimen	Duration (Weeks)	Comments
Alpha-hemolytic (viridans) streptococci, *S. bovis*	1. Penicillin G, 10–20 million U/day IV in six equal doses, plus gentamicin, 1 mg/kg IV or IM q 8 h	2	For patients <65 years old without renal failure, eighth-nerve defects, or serious complications
	2. Penicillin G, 10–20 million U/day IV in six equal doses, plus gentamicin, 1 mg/kg IV or IM q 8 h (for first 2 weeks only), *or*	4	For patients with complicated disease, e.g., CNS involvement, shock, moderately penicillin-resistant organism, failed previous treatment
	3. Penicillin G, 10–20 million U/day IV in six equal doses, *or*	4	For patients >65 years old or with renal failure or eighth-nerve defect
	4. Ceftriaxone, 2 grams IV or IM once daily, *or*	4	For patients allergic to penicillin
	5. Vancomycin, 15 mg per kilogram (not to exceed 1 gram) q 12 h IV	4	For patients allergic to penicillin
Group A streptococci, *S. pneumoniae*	1. Penicillin G, 2 million U q 6 h IV, *or*	2–4	These organisms are usually highly sensitive to penicillin; 2–3 weeks will be adequate for most cases
	2. Cefazolin, 2 grams q 8 h IV	2–4	
E. faecalis, other penicillin-resistant streptococci	1. Ampicillin, 2 grams q 4 h IV, *plus* gentamicin, 1 mg per kilogram q 8 h IV, *or*	4–6	Four weeks will be adequate for most cases; serum levels must be checked and dose adjusted accordingly
	2. Vancomycin, 15 mg per kilogram (not to exceed 1 gram) q 12 h IV, *plus* gentamicin, 1 mg/kg IV or IM q 8 h	4–6	Four weeks will be adequate for most cases; the dose of streptomycin may have to be reduced as treatment progresses, to avoid toxicity
S. aureus	1. Nafcillin, 2 grams q 4 h IV, *or*	4 or longer	Standard regimen
	2. Nafcillin as above *plus* gentamicin, 1.0 mg per kilogram q 8 h IV for the first 3–5 days, *or*	4 or longer	For patients with severe disseminated staphylococcal disease, gentamicin synergy may be advantageous during early stages of treatment
	3. Cephalothin, 2 grams q 4 h IV, *or*	4 or longer	For patients allergic to penicillin
	4. Vancomycin, 15 mg per kilogram (not to exceed 1 gram) q 12 h IV	4 or longer	For patients allergic to penicillin and cephalosporin; for resistant organisms
HACEK group	1. Ampicillin, 2 grams q 4 h IV, *plus* gentamicin, 1 mg/kg q 8 h IV or IM, *or*	4	Standard regimen
	2. Ceftriaxone, 2 grams IV or IM once daily	4	For patients allergic to penicillin, or for outpatient therapy

TABLE 299–8. AUTHOR'S RECOMMENDATIONS FOR PROPHYLAXIS OF ENDOCARDITIS*

	Indications	Drug and Dosage
Standard regimen	For dental procedures and oral or upper respiratory tract surgery	Amoxicillin, 3 grams orally 1 hour before, then 1.5 grams 6 hours later†
Special regimens	Parenteral regimen for high-risk patients; also for gastrointestinal or genitourinary tract procedures	Ampicillin, 2 grams IM or IV, *plus* gentamicin, 1.5 mg per kilogram IM or IV, 0.5 hour before†, then 1.5 grams amoxicillin orally 6 hours later
	Parenteral regimen for penicillin-allergic patients	Vancomycin, 1 gram IV *slowly* over 1 hour, starting 1 hour before; *add* gentamicin, 1.5 mg per kilogram IM or IV, if gastrointestinal or genitourinary tract is involved†
	Oral regimen for penicillin-allergic patients (oral and respiratory tract procedures)	Erythromycin, 1 gram orally 2 hours before, then 0.5 gram 6 hours later,† *or* clindamycin, 300 mg orally 1 hour before, then 150 mg 6 hours later
	Oral regimen for minor gastrointestinal or genitourinary tract procedures	Amoxicillin, 3 grams orally 1 hour before, then 1.5 grams 6 hours later†
	Parenteral regimen for cardiac surgery including prosthetic valve placement	Cefazolin, 2 grams IV on induction of anesthesia, repeated 8 and 16 hours later,‡ *or* Vancomycin, 1 gram IV *slowly* over 1 hour, starting on induction of anesthesia, then 0.5 gram IV 8 and 16 hours later‡

*These are empiric suggestions. No regimen has been proven effective, and prevention failures may occur with any regimen. These recommendations are not intended to cover all clinical situations; practitioners should use their own judgment on safety and cost-benefit issues in each individual case. Several additional doses may be given if the period of risk for bacteremia is prolonged, but prophylaxis should not be extended for days.

†Pediatric dosages: ampicillin, 50 mg per kilogram; erythromycin, 20 mg per kilogram for first dose, then 10 mg per kilogram; gentamicin, 2 mg per kilogram; vancomycin, 20 mg per kilogram; penicillin V, cefazolin, and amoxicillin for children weighing more than 60 pounds, use same dose as for adults; for children weighing less than 60 pounds, use half the adult dose.

‡Gentamicin, 1.5 mg per kilogram IV, may be given with each dose only if postoperative gram-negative infections have occurred with significant frequency.

Adapted from Durack DT: Nine controversies in the management of endocarditis. *In* Petersdorf RG, et al. (eds.): Update V. Harrison's Principles of Internal Medicine, pp 35–46. Copyright © 1984 by McGraw-Hill, Inc. Used by permission of McGraw-Hill Book Company.

by knowing something of the frequency of bacteremia after the procedure in question and the number of cases of endocarditis attributed to it. For example, if a patient with aortic stenosis were to have dental extraction or urologic surgery, attempted prevention with antibiotics would be appropriate. If the same patient were to undergo gastroscopy, antibiotics would not be indicated because that procedure poses very little risk for endocarditis.

Prophylaxis for endocarditis is not required to cover the most common gastrointestinal diagnostic procedures such as endoscopy or radiocontrast studies, nor for normal delivery, therapeutic abortion, dilation and curettage, insertion or removal of intrauterine contraceptive devices in the absence of local infection, cardiac catheterization, insertion of pacemakers, endotracheal intubation, or bronchoscopy. However, some physicians choose to cover even these low-risk procedures in patients with prosthetic valves because they are at higher risk for endocarditis.

The indication for prophylactic antibiotics in patients with mitral valve prolapse remains controversial. MVP increases an individual's risk for endocarditis by five to eight times and underlies a significant proportion of cases of subacute bacterial endocarditis. However, mitral valve prolapse is very common in the general population, while endocarditis is relatively uncommon, so prolapse should be regarded as a low-risk lesion for endocarditis. Many authorities currently recommend prophylaxis for patients with prolapse, especially those with mitral regurgitation, but an estimate of benefits in relation to costs has indicated that parenteral prophylaxis for prolapse is probably not cost-effective. In the author's opinion, it is reasonable to give oral antibiotic prophylaxis to MVP patients undergoing procedures that cause significant bacteremia because the costs and risks of oral penicillin therapy for an individual are very low, and a serious disease may occasionally be prevented. However, use of antibiotics in this setting should be considered optional rather than mandatory. Parenteral prophylaxis for MVP patients probably should be avoided to reduce the risk of anaphylaxis.

Specific recommendations for prophylaxis of endocarditis are listed in Table 299–8.

Bisno AL: Treatment of Infective Endocarditis. New York, Grune & Stratton, 1982. *This book deals with many aspects of endocarditis besides treatment. It provides a good source for references.*

Bisno AL, Dismukes WE, Durack DT, et al.: Antimicrobial treatment of infective endocarditis due to viridans streptococci, enterococci, and staphylococci. JAMA 261:1471–1477, 1989. *A resource paper from the American Heart Association Committee appointed to review and recommend therapy for the common forms of endocarditis caused by gram-positive cocci. This is a detailed publication with seven large tables that list definitive recommendations for most situations involving infective endocarditis caused by gram-positive cocci.*

Durack DT: Infective and non-infective endocarditis. *In* Hurst JW (ed.): The Heart, 7th ed. New York, McGraw-Hill Book Company, 1990, pp 1230–1225. *A general review of infective and noninfective endocarditis in a leading cardiology textbook (204 references).*

Durack DT: Prophylaxis of endocarditis. *In* Mandell GL, Douglas RG, Bennett JE (eds.): Principles and Practice of Infectious Diseases, 3rd ed. New York, John Wiley & Sons, 1990, pp 716–721. *This chapter analyzes the problems of endocarditis prophylaxis in detail and reviews current recommendations (74 references).*

Karchmer AW, Dismukes WE, Buckley MJ, et al.: Late prosthetic valve endocarditis: Clinical features influencing therapy. Am J Med 64:199, 1978. *This paper reports on patients with late prosthetic valve endocarditis, comparing survival according to etiologic organisms and medical as opposed to surgical treatment. Various features that carry a poor prognosis are identified, and relative indications for surgery are discussed.*

Rahimtoola SH: Infective Endocarditis. New York, Grune & Stratton, 1978. *A heavily referenced book, with good material on pathogenesis, pathology, and endocarditis in addicts and fungal endocarditis.*

Reisberg BE: Infective endocarditis in the narcotic addict. Prog Cardiovasc Dis 22:193, 1979. *A useful review of infective endocarditis in narcotic addicts. The importance of tricuspid valve infection and the effect of different infecting organisms and the sites involved on prognosis are analyzed.*

Reller LB: The serum bactericidal test. Rev Infect Dis 8:803, 1986. *A concise analysis of the strengths and weaknesses of the SBT as a means to monitor therapy.*

Weinstein L: Infective endocarditis. *In* Braunwald E (ed.): Heart Disease. A Textbook of Cardiovascular Medicine. Philadelphia, W. B. Saunders Company, 1988. *A long, detailed chapter in a major cardiology textbook (approximately 400 references).*

Staphylococcal Infections

300 Staphylococcal Infections

John N. Sheagren

Staphylococci are ubiquitous in nature. All humans are colonized by "nonpathogenic" staphylococci. In addition the "pathogenic" coagulase-producing *Staphylococcus aureus* is present transiently in a high percentage of people and is chronically carried by about 15 per cent of the normal population.

S. aureus itself is one of the most important bacterial pathogens of man. It can be aggressively invasive, spreading rapidly through soft tissues, directly invading bones and other support structures, and ultimately, under conducive circumstances, seeding the bloodstream to produce septic shock and disseminated intravascular coagulation. Conversely, *S. aureus* can lie dormant deep within tissues for years without causing disease. The balance between host and parasite that results in infection with a given strain of staphylococci is not known and continues to be the subject of active research.

Staphylococci rank only behind *Escherichia coli* in overall incidence of infections in the hospital setting. In the community, staphylococci, particularly *S. aureus*, are the leading cause of acute, serious, and progressive skin, soft tissue, and post-traumatic infections. A thorough understanding of the pathogenetic mechanisms and clinical manifestations of staphylococcal infections is crucial to the care of septic patients in every medical environment.

BACTERIOLOGY. Staphylococci are members of the family Micrococcaceae, of which there are two genera of major clinical importance, the micrococci and the staphylococci. These two genera are both catalase positive, but only staphylococci can anaerobically ferment glucose to produce acid. The staphylococci in turn have three clinically important species: *S. aureus*, *S. epidermidis*, and *S. saprophyticus*. *S. aureus* alone has the capacity to produce coagulase. Most laboratories label all coagulase-negative organisms as "*S. epidermidis*," which results in the failure to differentiate at least one clinically important subspecies, *S. saprophyticus*. *S. saprophyticus* ferments mannitol and can also be identified by resistance to novobiocin. *S. saprophyticus* is a frequent cause of urinary tract infections, almost always in young women; these organisms are sensitive to all generally prescribed urinary tract antibiotics.

The word *aureus* comes from the Latin word meaning gold and refers to the fact that most *S. aureus* colonies develop a bright golden-yellow color on blood agar media. However, *S. aureus* speciation is now assigned to all strains producing coagulase, whether or not they are golden in color. In addition, almost all strains of *S. aureus* ferment mannitol and contain deoxyribonuclease (DNAase). Staphylococci grow well both anaerobically and aerobically: thus, both aerobic and anaerobic bottles in a blood culture set from a truly bacteremic patient are usually positive.

The name *staphylococcus* comes from the Greek word "staphyle" (literally, "a bunch of grapes") for these organisms grow in "grape-like" clusters in liquid or semisolid media or within tissues when causing infection. However, in material obtained from abscesses, the organisms can sometimes be confusing in morphology, being quite variable in size, shape, and tendency toward clustering. Occasionally the organisms may grow in pairs or even chains, and confusion with streptococci is possible. Nonetheless, to the trained eye the size and general characteristics of the organism usually permit an accurate diagnosis of a pure staphylococcal lesion when the stained smear is carefully examined.

No reproducible serologic typing schemes are available to classify staphylococci. However, bacteriophage typing has been extremely useful in identifying strain characteristics of *S. aureus* and in providing epidemiologic data. Recently, bacteriophage typing has begun to be applied to *S. epidermidis*, and over 50 per cent of recovered strains can now be typed by this system. Recent techniques of plasmid profile analysis have been very useful in studying the epidemiology of hospital-associated *S. aureus* and *S. epidermidis* infections. Plasmid (the extrachromosomal DNA in staphylococci) analysis using electrophoretic techniques provides distinctive patterns for individual strains of staphylococci.

EPIDEMIOLOGY. Staphylococci may colonize almost all animal species, and *S. epidermidis* is universally present on the human skin. The carrier state of *S. aureus* is clinically important. Humans carry *S. aureus* predominantly in the nasopharynx, although some individuals can be heavily colonized in the axillae, groin, and perineal region. The heavily colonized individual may become a source of recurrrent infections both to himself and to surrounding contacts. Most humans probably carry a few *S. aureus* organisms among the normal flora of every body site but at such a low level that routine cultures rarely reveal the organism. About 15 per cent of normal, non–hospital-associated persons more or less chronically carry a heavy growth of *S. aureus* in their noses.

The definition of the carrier state is a simple one: from swab culture of the anterior nares of a carrier, multiple colonies of *S. aureus* are visually identified on a blood agar culture plate. Clearly this definition is imprecise, because the more intensely one focuses attention on the organism the higher will be the percentage of normal individuals found to carry it. Nonetheless, colony counts of the nasopharyngeal flora consistently indicate a small group of persons who harbor relatively large numbers of the organism.

The factors that result in high growth rates and numbers of *S. aureus* in the nares of certain individuals and not in others are unknown. There is no evidence that the immune response to the organism (for example, secretory immunoglobulins or other inhibitory substances) plays a major role in the acquisition and loss of the organism from the nose and throat, as is the case for the meningococcus. Data indicate that the teichoic acid moiety in the cell wall of *S. aureus* mediates the adherence of the organism to nasal mucosal cells, a phenomenon of major import in mucous membrane colonization. Also, it is highly probable that the carrier state is influenced by the ability of other members of the normal bacterial flora of the nose, throat, and skin to suppress growth of a given strain of *Staphylococcus*. Most probably, other staphylococci or micrococci (or both) will turn out to be instrumental in controlling the growth of a newly introduced staphylococcal strain. In fact, clinical use of this concept has already been attempted via the process termed *bacterial interference*. Bacterial interference is the concept that a nonpathogenic strain of *Staphylococcus*, once established, seems to reduce the likelihood of acquisition of another, more pathogenic strain (see later section).

There is an interesting association between the nasal carriage of *S. aureus* and any condition associated with small breaks in the skin and mucous membranes. It has been known for a long time that patients with a variety of dermatoses, especially atopic dermatitis, are very likely to be heavily colonized with *S. aureus*. In fact, patients with eczematous skin diseases may be heavily colonized in the lesions but have few organisms on the intervening normal skin. Possibly related to these observations is the fact that patients who regularly use needles have an increased rate of carriage of *S. aureus*. Drug addicts, diabetics injecting insulin, patients on hemodialysis, and even patients receiving brief courses of allergy shots all have an increased rate of nasal carriage of *S. aureus*. Recently, AIDS patients have been identified as frequent carriers of *S. aureus* (probably because of the frequency of chronic dermatologic conditions), and serious *S. aureus* infections are being increasingly recognized in AIDS patients. Another group of patients recently described as having a high risk of

S. aureus bacterium are those treated with interleukin 2 (IL2, an immunotherapeutic agent now available for melanoma, renal cell carcinoma, lymphoma, and some other solid tumor therapy). About 20 per cent of IL2-treated patients develop bacteremia, the vast majority of which (approx. 70 per cent) are caused by *S. aureus*. Probably, dermal IL2 toxicity leads to increased colonization followed by invasion and dissemination. In addition, IL2 produces an acute defect in polymorphonuclear leukocyte (PMN) chemotaxis which undoubtedly contributes to its propensity to cause bacterial infections, especially with *S. aureus*.

The carrier state, especially of *S. aureus*, is clinically important, because the organism carried in the nose and throat is often identical to that in the bloodstream of drug-abusing patients with endocarditis. Similarly, studies done years ago demonstrated that patients who entered hospitals for surgical procedures and who were carriers of *S. aureus* had increased rates of wound infections with the carried organism. The same phenomenon has recently been shown for hemodialysis patients, 60 to 80 per cent of whom are colonized in the nose with *S. aureus*. The colonizing organism often causes recurrent infections. Prophylaxis of the nasal carrier state in hemodialysis patients with rifampin significantly reduces the subsequent incidence of infections (see later section on Treatment of Chronic Carriers).

Thus, the sequence of events leading to infection with *S. aureus* seems to be the following: Persons who for whatever reason begin to carry the organism in the nose are at risk of seeding the organism to other bodily sites and to breaks in the skin (for example, wounds or points of insertion of intravascular catheters). From such colonized peripheral sites, the organism may invade and cause destructive and rapidly progressive local and systemic septic complications.

Carriage of staphylococci within the gastrointestinal tract has not been extensively studied. However, normally a few staphylococci can usually be isolated. *S. epidermidis* is not uncommonly isolated from the stool but probably represents contamination from the perianal skin. Staphylococci, especially *S. aureus*, may grow to very high titers in the gastrointestinal tract in the presence of antibiotic therapy and cause gastrointestinal symptoms; the presumption is that antibiotics suppress the more sensitive normal floral components that are responsible for inhibiting the growth of *S. aureus*. This rationale is similar to that for the emergence of *C. difficile* in the syndrome of antibiotic-associated colitis (see Ch. 308).

Newborn infants rapidly experience an increasing rate of colonization following birth. It is not uncommon within nurseries to note infant colonization rates of 25 to 30 per cent. Most infants remain asymptomatic; on occasion, however, outbreaks of disease within nurseries may occur, sometimes traceable to a common carrier. Adult patients become increasingly colonized with *S. aureus* the longer they remain in the hospital. Once a hospitalized individual becomes a carrier (especially individuals with open, actively infected lesions), the nasally carried organisms may spread to other anatomic sites, to clothing and other items within the room, and to individuals with whom the patient has contact. The most effective technique for stopping transmission of staphylococci from person to person, especially in a hospital setting, is to wash one's hands meticulously immediately before and after examining each patient. This process is particularly important when examining a patient with a gross, obviously staphylococcal lesion or with a chronic exudative dermatosis. Such patients should always be appropriately isolated while they are hospitalized.

PATHOGENESIS. Whether or not an infection develops with any microorganism depends on the balance between the aggressiveness of the organism and the level of defense provided by the host. Thus, organisms that are highly virulent may regularly infect normal hosts and, conversely, nonpathogenic (saprophytic) organisms usually cause infection only in the face of a significant impairment of host defense. The following paragraphs first describe those microbial characteristics that lead to the presence or absence of virulence and then the primary mechanisms by which the host attempts containment.

Microbial Virulence. The factor that makes certain strains of staphylococci virulent and others nonpathogenic is unknown. Several extracellular enzymes are produced by *S. aureus*, many probably participating in the pathogenic capabilities of the organism. For example, as in the case of streptococci, hyaluronidase probably assists the organism in its rapid spread through tissues. A variety of other enzymes may also degrade other tissue elements, may lyse inflammation-associated coagulation (coagulase), and may be directly toxic to either white cells (leukocidins) or platelets. Studies in experimental models have shown a high correlation between coagulase production and organism virulence.

The ability of *S. aureus* to adhere to damaged endothelial surfaces explains why the organism has a high likelihood of seeding to traumatized or inflamed tissues. Adherence is mediated by receptors on the surface of *S. aureus* for laminin and fibronectin (components of the subendothelial matrix), fibrin and fibrinogen (coagulation factors), and endothelial cell surface protein components.

Numerous toxins are produced by *S. aureus*. Some have endotoxic capabilities when injected into tissues (for example, the α and β toxins). *S. aureus* frequently produces an enterotoxin, and at present six enterotoxins (A through F) have been described. Enterotoxin F is identical to pyrogenic exotoxin C, the toxin found to be involved in the toxic shock syndrome and now called "toxic shock syndrome toxin-1" (abbreviated TSST-1). Another well-described toxin is the exfoliative toxin responsible for the staphylococcal scalded skin syndrome.

The capsular and cell wall components of *S. aureus* clearly participate in the pathogenesis of certain clinical syndromes produced by the organism. Many *S. aureus* strains have a polysaccharide capsule covering the complex rigid cell wall matrix that consists of peptidoglycan and teichoic acid (ribitol in *S. aureus* and predominantly glycerol in *S. epidermidis*), and recent data suggest that the encapsulated strains of staphylococci are major causes of bacteremic episodes. In most strains of *S. aureus*, a unique substance, *protein A*, is also part of the cell wall. Protein A is an immunologically active substance having high affinity for the Fc fragment of immunoglobulins, particularly subgroups of IgG. Thus, protein A binds to and aggregates IgG molecules and, interestingly, fixes complement in the process. Protein A has emerged as an extremely useful immunochemical substance for extraction and quantitation of IgG molecules from biologic specimens. Whether protein A plays a role in any of the clinical syndromes produced by *S. aureus* is unknown.

The presence of a capsule varies greatly from strain to strain and may explain some of the biologic differences between organisms as they invade tissues or the bloodstream. The capsule inhibits phagocytosis by interfering with the interaction between the underlying teichoic acid–peptidoglycan complex and complement, which is activated primarily via the alternative pathway. Thus, encapsulated strains are protected in tissues from the complement-mediated attack by PMN leukocytes. Along with the enzymes described above, the capsule undoubtedly increases the ability of *S. aureus* to protect itself as it spreads through tissues and therefore is an important virulence factor for tissue infections. Paradoxically, while unencapsulated organisms are more likely to be contained in tissues, should the bloodstream be reached (for example in a narcotics addict directly injecting carried organisms into the blood stream), the syndrome of septic shock and disseminated intravascular coagulation (DIC) may result. The syndrome of septic shock follows massive intravascular activation of monokines (especially tumor necrosis factor-α [TNF-α] and the complement, coagulation, and kinin systems (Ch. 243 and 285). In such a situation, unencapsulated strains of *S. aureus* produce septic shock exactly like gram-negative bacteria wherein the cell wall lipopolysaccharide (endotoxin) activates the responsible inflammatory systems.

Host Defense Aspects. The primary mechanism by which the host defends against staphylococci, especially *S. aureus*, is via the nonspecific defense system. The specific antibody and T cell–mediated host defenses appear to participate very little, if at all, in defense against *S. aureus*. Thus, antibodies are of theoretical value against encapsulated strains of *S. aureus*, and at present, attempts to induce anticapsular antibodies as therapeutic modalities are being revived. Previous attempts to develop vaccines against the organism, however, have not yielded documented clinical benefits.

The nonspecific host defense system consists of the barrier systems (skin and mucous membranes) plus the complement-mediated PMN leukocyte assault on invading organisms. Patients with defects in intracellular killing of bacteria by the PMN (for example, as in the chronic granulomatous disease of childhood or the Chédiak-Higashi syndrome) are particularly prone to develop serious infections with *S. aureus*. AIDS patients probably also have a subtle bactericidal defect in their PMN's as well as frank neutropenia in the end stage of the disease.

Certain pathologic states with highly elevated levels of IgE predispose the patient to recurrent, chronic infections with *S. aureus*. *Job's syndrome* is a condition wherein an elevated IgE level associated with eczematous skin changes somehow predisposes the patient to recurrent soft tissue infections. No one knows how or why staphylococcal infections are enhanced by highly elevated levels of IgE. The theory is that mast cell activation in the neighborhood of a focus of *S. aureus* infection somehow impairs normal PMN-mediated defense mechanisms. Some recent studies have shown that antihistamines may at least partially correct the defect demonstrated in these patients. Interestingly some AIDS patients have increased IgE production associated with a chronic, diffuse dermatitis, a combination of events strongly predisposing to infection with *S. aureus*.

The presence of a foreign body has a dramatic effect on the development of staphylococcal infections. For example, infections with *S. epidermidis* strains are particularly common in patients harboring foreign bodies such as prosthetic heart valves, cerebrospinal fluid shunts, and artificial joints. As for *S. aureus*, the inoculum required experimentally to produce a skin infection in a healthy individual is very large (10^6 to 10^7 organisms); however, the presence of even a small foreign body such as a suture reduces the dose required to produce an infection to less than 100 organisms. Thus, foreign bodies must provide a nidus of chronic inflammation in which leukocyte accumulation and function are impaired.

CLINICAL MANIFESTATIONS

This section reviews two broad categories of human diseases produced by staphylococci: first, diseases related to the production of toxins by staphylococci (exclusively *S. aureus*) and, second, diseases related to direct organism invasion.

TOXIN-PRODUCED DISEASES. Clinically, the most important toxins produced by *S. aureus* are the enterotoxins and exfoliative toxin. The distinction between the different types of toxins is becoming less clear: For example, the toxin involved in the toxic shock syndrome (pyrogenic exotoxin C) has recently been shown to be identical to enterotoxin F; furthermore, that toxin clearly has exfoliative properties.

Staphylococcal Gastroenteritis. Most cases of gastroenteritis caused by *S. aureus* follow the ingestion of foods containing a preformed toxin. The toxin itself is not produced within the gastrointestinal tract. A number of extracellular toxins are produced in large amounts when the culture media contain high amounts of carbohydrate (as in sugary and starchy foods contaminated by *S. aureus*) and when such a mixture is incubated at appropriate conditions of temperature and acidity. Toxin ingestion results in increased intestinal peristalsis, profuse nausea, vomiting, diarrhea, and in some cases fever. The organism and its preformed toxin can usually be identified in point source outbreaks from the epidemiologically implicated foodstuff. Toxin-mediated staphylococcal gastroenteritis is usually self-limited, lasting anywhere from 12 to 24 hours; however, supportive therapy (fluid and electrolyte maintenance) may on occasion be required. Antibiotics are not useful.

The Toxic Shock Syndrome (TSS). TSS is almost certainly caused by the production of one or more toxins at the site of a localized, often relatively asymptomatic or unnoticed infection with any strain of *S. aureus* capable of toxin production. The most common site of infection is still the vagina, usually in association with tampon usage. About 25 per cent of TSS cases reported to the CDC in 1989 were not associated with infection of the female genital tract; most of those were associated with infected foreign bodies (such as sutures) in surgical wounds, or other sites, often relatively asymptomatic, of *S. aureus* colonization and/or infection. As stated earlier, the toxin responsible for TSS is now named TSST-1, although recent data also implicate staphylococcal

enterotoxin-A (SEA) in some cases of TSS. TSST-1 production by strains of *S. aureus* isolated from cases of TSS has been shown to be related to lysogeny, the presence of a temperate bacteriophage. Presumably, the clinical manifestations of the syndrome are produced when the toxin is absorbed either through mucous membranes or from a subcutaneous tissue site of colonization or infection. TSST-1 production by toxigenic strains of *S. aureus* is markedly enhanced in Mg^{++}-depleted media; further, superabsorbent tampon materials chelate Mg^{++} and/or in other ways result in ideal conditions for toxin production, explaining the relationship between superabsorbent tampon introduction and the TSS. The toxin probably produces its systemic effects both by directly damaging cell membranes in peripheral tissues and by stimulating production of monokine mediators, especially TNF-α. Interestingly, TNF-α production by mononuclear cells is triggered because TSST and SEA bind specifically to MHC class II molecules.

The clinical syndrome that results is dramatic. The patient, almost always unaware of the focus of toxin production, experiences the abrupt onset of high fever, myalgias, and profuse nausea, vomiting, and watery diarrhea. Within the first several days, a sunburn-like rash appears, and the conjunctivae become injected. On biopsy of the skin lesions, the epidermis exhibits cleavage in the basilar layers, differentiating it from the staphylococcal scalded skin syndrome (discussed later) and from viral and drug eruptions. The patient often becomes progressively more ill and is frequently in frank shock when presenting for care. A diffuse capillary leak syndrome rapidly develops, and the serum albumin concentration often plummets to less than 2 grams per 100 ml. Hypotension and frank shock are common and are often associated with the adult respiratory distress syndrome (ARDS), acute renal failure, and abnormalities in literally every organ system evaluated. For example, almost all patients exhibit an altered state of mentation, hepatocellular malfunction, elevated levels of muscle enzymes, thrombocytopenia, and a low serum calcium concentration (far out of proportion to the hypoalbuminemia). Highly elevated levels of calcitonin are present for which no explanation currently exists.

Therapy is both supportive and specific. Identification of site of infection, drainage thereof (most frequently consisting of removal of contaminated tampons), and antibiotic therapy with β-lactamase–resistant antistaphylococcal agents are all indicated. Antibiotics do not change the course of the initial illness but seem to prevent relapse, at least in tampon-associated cases. Patients with TSS are rarely bacteremic, and therefore this type of shock syndrome is different from bacteremic, inflammatory system-mediated shock (see Ch. 286), wherein complement, coagulation, and kinin system activation seem to be primary events.

The prognosis in TSS is favorable despite the fact that most patients are critically ill for a period of time in the hospital. In the early 1980's, between 5 and 10 per cent of patients studied died; in 1989, no deaths were reported to the CDC among women with menstrual TSS. Since recurrences, generally milder, are relatively common following tampon-associated TSS (up to 10 per cent over the subsequent three menstrual cycles), women who have recovered from TSS should avoid tampon use for at least 6 months following the illness.

The Staphylococcal Scalded Skin Syndrome (SSSS). SSSS is another toxin-mediated disease produced by certain strains of *S. aureus*, usually of phage group II. These organisms produce an exfoliative toxin that when injected experimentally into infant mice produces dramatic skin desquamation and mimics in every way the clinical syndrome seen in human infants. The human disease is produced by a toxin originating in a distant focus of infection. The exfoliative toxin is absorbed and disseminated systemically and causes cleavage of the middle layers of the epidermis, bulla formation, and ultimately slippage of the superficial layer of the epithelium on gentle pressure (a positive *Nikolsky's sign*). The skin is often tender and very erythematous, producing a sunburn-like rash during the initial phase. Infants are most commonly involved, and outbreaks of this syndrome have occurred in nurseries after introduction of a toxin-producing strain. Often mild or asymptomatic omphalitis is the source. In older children, the portal of infection can be any minor skin abrasion, furuncle, or some other infected local site. The conjunctival sac may be the source as a result of mild conjunctivitis, and this source often goes undetected. The syndrome has occasionally been reported in adults. The rash proceeds rapidly to desquamation, but healing is rapid and is related to how promptly the peripheral site has been treated. Mortality of SSSS is very low.

Differentiation of SSSS from viral exanthems and drug allergies is very important. The most important disease with which SSSS can be confused is *toxic epidermal necrolysis (TEN)*, an often fatal variant of erythema multiforme usually caused by a drug allergy (see Ch. 525). The two illnesses can be differentiated on skin biopsy, and therapy is very different for each: Local care and antibiotics suffice to cure SSSS, whereas high-dose systemic glucocorticoids are indicated in TEN, with mortality still remaining high.

DISEASES RELATED TO DIRECT INVASION AND SYSTEMIC SPREAD OF STAPHYLOCOCCI. In the following subsections, the classic clinical manifestations of invasive staphylococcal infection, bacteremia, and endocarditis are described.

Dermal Infections. Most minor skin infections in man are caused by either *S. aureus* or group A β-hemolytic streptococci. There is no way clinically to differentiate between diseases produced by the penicillin-sensitive streptococci and *S. aureus*; obviously, this is an important point, for all skin infections in which antibiotic therapy seems indicated therefore require the use of a β-lactamase–resistant antibiotic. Direct invasion through minor breaks in skin and mucous membranes is the hallmark of disease produced by *S. aureus*. A wide variety of dermal and soft tissue infections may result, including cellulitis, local abscess formation (furuncles and carbuncles), lymphangiitis, and lymphadenitis. Direct extension can occur to deep support structures such as bones and joints and result in primary osteomyelitis and septic arthritis. Even dermal staphylococcal infections that appear minor are important to recognize because they may become a source of bacteremia. When a patient with a localized *S. aureus* skin infection manifests fever and chills, bacteremia must be assumed to be present, and prompt diagnosis and therapy should be initiated.

Diagnosis of dermal infections is usually relatively easy. The aspirate of a large, well-developed abscess (furuncle or carbuncle) almost always reveals typical, creamy, yellow pus; and on Gram's stain the clustered cocci are mixed with inflammatory debris. One should perform Gram's stains of materials from every dermal infection because occasionally gram-negative organisms may cause a clinical picture similar to that of gram-positive infections, especially in immunocompromised hosts, and obviously the initial therapeutic approach will be very different.

Therapy must always be initiated with a β-lactamase–resistant antibiotic if antimicrobial therapy is indicated at all. In fact, the backbone of therapy of dermal staphylococcal infections continues to be debridement and drainage. Only large lesions associated with signs of surrounding cutaneous spread or systemic clinical symptoms need be treated with antibiotics. It is usually wise, however, before incising a large staphylococcal abscess (even when localized) to treat the patient with an oral dose of a penicillinase-resistant antibiotic (e.g., 250 mg of dicloxacillin). Such a dose should be administered 30 minutes to 1 hour before incision and drainage are carried out.

The prognosis for most localized infections is excellent, but infections due to *S. aureus* often recur. Population surveys have found that each year most persons develop one to several isolated local lesions, most probably caused by *S. aureus*. However, not infrequently an individual may suffer from recurrent crops of extremely debilitating local skin lesions. In this situation the patient is usually found to be carrying the causative organism in the anterior nares, axilla, groin, or perirectal region. Most such individuals are nasal carriers, and an attempt to eradicate nasal carriage is worth making (see later section on Treatment of Chronic Carriers).

Bone and Joint Infections. Through a variety of mechanisms *S. aureus* commonly involves bone (osteomyelitis, see Ch. 304) and joints (see Ch. 260 on septic arthritis). Direct inoculation by *S. aureus* can occur in trauma or penetrating wounds. Bone and joint infections can also result from bacteremia. In children and young adults it is assumed that bacteremia originates from a minor dermal source (such as folliculitis) or from heavily colonized mucous membranes. Seeding of *S. aureus* from the blood tends to occur to areas previously traumatized or harboring foreign

bodies. In young children, the organism tends to seed into the diaphyseal plates of the long bone, areas of greatest vascularity. The affected area (usually on the ankle, knee, or shin) becomes acutely warm and swollen and may appear at first to be a primary cellulitis. Fever and shaking chills are common. Blood cultures are usually positive. In adults, the syndrome of hematogenous osteomyelitis is usually less acute, often involving the lumbar vertebrae. The individual begins to develop low-grade fever, night sweats, and back pain that gradually becomes localized to an area of point tenderness. In such cases, *S. aureus* may be grown from the blood, but more commonly the organism is isolated from an aspirate of the bone or intervertebral space obtained by an orthopedic surgical consultant.

Staphylococcal septic arthritis usually involves a joint afflicted by pre-existing chronic arthritis (such as rheumatoid arthritis or osteoarthritis). Again, an episode of bacteremia causes seeding to a previously inflamed joint. The only indication in some patients is the development of increasing symptoms in one joint, usually accompanied by fever. Joint aspiration reveals a purulent effusion; Gram's stains may be negative, but the organism can usually be cultured. *S. epidermidis* increasingly is being described as a cause of chronic osteomyelitis, especially in debilitated patients such as those on hemodialysis or with underlying neoplastic diseases.

The diagnosis of staphylococcal bone and joint infections depends on recovering the organism from an aspirate of the involved site; every effort should be made, with the assistance of an orthopedic surgeon, to aspirate or biopsy the involved area *before* antibiotics are started. Newer techniques permit core biopsies to be obtained from deep tissues and may in the future permit more frequent definitive bacteriologic diagnosis of low-grade, chronic bone and joint infections. The diagnosis becomes especially difficult if patients have been treated with antibiotics before appropriate culture material has been obtained. In such cases a rising or significantly elevated teichoic acid antibody titer may assist in diagnosing deep infections due to *S. aureus* (see later section on The Teichoic Acid Antibody Assay).

Treatment of osteomyelitis in adults must be prolonged. While it is becoming customary to treat children with a brief course of parenteral antibiotics, adults on oral antibiotics tend to relapse if a prolonged parenteral course of antibiotics is not administered. Four weeks of parenteral therapy is the minimum acceptable course, and most clinicians prefer to treat for 6 to 8 weeks. Much of such a course of prolonged parenteral therapy can be administered at home. An oral antistaphylococcal agent (for example, dicloxacillin 2 grams daily) should be continued for several weeks following completion of the parenteral course. Gradual reduction of the dose of oral antibiotic over a 3- to 6-month period may leave the patient symptom-free for an extended period of time. Some clinicians treat isolated septic arthritis for only 2 weeks; however, it is extremely difficult to differentiate septic arthritis *without* bone involvement from that with osteomyelitis. Therefore, a 4-week course of therapy with appropriate parenteral antibiotics is recommended. Staphylococcal osteomyelitis tends to relapse even after years of quiescence, and one can never be sure of complete eradication of the disease. Once a relapse has occurred, chronic recurrence will be the rule. In such situations carefully planned surgical debridement and drainage under the cover of a prolonged parenteral and oral course of antibiotics may result in extended quiescence or even apparent cure. The availability of microsurgical techniques to apply muscle grafts over areas of chronic osteomyelitis now permits healing to occur even in some extraordinarily recalcitrant cases. Some of the newer β-lactam antibiotics have favorable pharmacokinetics, permitting once-daily parenteral therapy to be administered long term to outpatients. The most widely used such antibiotic is ceftriaxone.

Staphylococcal Pneumonia and Empyema. Although most cases of *S. aureus* pneumonia follow acute viral infections of the lower respiratory tract (especially influenza), the disease occasionally occurs de novo in elderly and debilitated individuals. *S. aureus* pneumonia is most often acquired in the hospital. Primary staphylococcal pneumonia is most common in children and usually evolves radiologically from patchy pulmonary infiltrates into harder nodules and then pneumatoceles. Rapid development of pleural effusions and empyema often accompanied by pneumothorax may occur. Staphylococcal bronchitis and recurrent pneumonias are also seen in children and young adults with cystic fibrosis, and a young adult suffering from recurrent bronchitis from which *S. aureus* and/or *Pseudomonas aeruginosa* (usually with mucoid colonial morphology) are isolated should have a sweat test evaluation.

Adult patients with influenza have an increased incidence of *S. aureus* pneumonia. The patient is usually recovering from typical symptoms of influenza when the rapid onset of fever, chills, and chest pain supervenes. Gram's stain of the sputum in such cases reveals large clumps of gram-positive cocci. Therapy must be intense with appropriate antibiotics. Nonetheless, such patients often do poorly and frequently develop secondary infections with gram-negative organisms, chronic respiratory failure, and progressive debility. Mortality rates remain high. Even in young people, morbidity is substantial, related to serious, rapidly progressive pulmonary disease often with empyema as well as the sequelae of the accompanying bacteremia.

In particular, pleural effusions accompanying *S. aureus* pneumonia require early drainage to prevent empyema formation. If thorough drainage cannot be accomplished by needle aspiration, a chest tube must be inserted. Every effort should be made to avoid the debilitating, prolonged sequelae that result from an extensive, multiloculated *S. aureus* infection of the pleural space.

Staphylococcal Meningitis, Cerebritis, and Brain Abscess. Meningitis due to *S. aureus* most commonly develops as a complication of a central nervous system diagnostic or neurosurgical procedure. Occasionally, however, meningitis may develop during an episode of bacteremia from a peripheral site. Many patients with staphylococcal bacteremia, with or without endocarditis, develop transient but sometimes focal central nervous system symptoms. On lumbar puncture, such patients commonly have a PMN pleocytosis with elevated protein but a normal to low normal glucose concentration and a *negative* Gram's stain. These individuals probably have begun to develop multiple perimeningeal foci or areas of cerebritis (or both) and not yet frank meningitis. Almost certainly, if left untreated such patients would develop frank brain abscesses or fulminant staphylococcal meningitis. On occasion, such a patient may also exhibit purpura, disseminated intravascular coagulation, and shock in which the differentiation from *meningococcal meningitis* (see Ch. 302) is difficult. Treatment of such patients is particularly difficult, for the initial inclination is to use penicillin, an inappropriate antibiotic choice. Thus, for any patient whose Gram's stain of the spinal fluid does not reveal identifiable organisms (such as meningococci or pneumococci), a β-lactamase–resistant antibiotic must be included in the initial antibiotic coverage.

Brain abscesses in general are usually caused by anaerobes, but not infrequently *S. aureus* is found to accompany them. Therefore, antistaphylococcal drugs should be included with antianaerobic antibiotics in the initial coverage of such individuals. For example, nafcillin plus metronidazole is an excellent combination for the patient who has a brain abscess with the source and causative organisms not yet defined. Surgical drainage is required only if the abscess is large and encapsulated.

Therapy of staphylococcal meningitis and cerebritis is usually that of the underlying syndrome (for example, endocarditis). However, even in the rare patient with an uncomplicated case of pure meningitis, therapy should be prolonged, at least 4 weeks parenterally, in contrast to the customary 10 to 14 days of therapy for patients with uncomplicated meningitis caused by *S. pneumoniae* or *N. meningitides*.

Staphylococcus epidermidis may cause meningeal signs and symptoms, almost always in a patient with a central nervous system shunt in place. In such instances, the infection has originated in the shunt, and the organism has proliferated and seeded back into the spinal fluid. In many such cases, the individual known to have a shunt in place simply has fever with few if any central nervous system signs. Only an aspirate of the shunt itself reveals the organism. Therapy may result in suppression of symptoms, but removal of the infected shunt is almost always required before cure can be accomplished.

Staphylococcal Urinary Tract Infections. Here the species spectrum changes, and coagulase-negative staphylococci become the more common infecting organisms. *S. epidermidis* may occasionally cause urinary tract infections, especially in elderly hospital-ized men with obstructive urinary tract pathology or indwelling Foley catheters.

Staphylococcus saprophyticus accounts for between 5 and 10 per cent of urinary tract infections in otherwise healthy young women. Presumably the organism colonizes the genitalia and for reasons not yet ascertained may ascend the urethra to involve the bladder and cause symptomatic cystitis. *S. saprophyticus* is easily treated, being sensitive to essentially all commonly used antibiotics, including penicillin, ampicillin, sulfonamides, and cephalosporins.

S. aureus may involve the urinary tract by either of two mechanisms: First, the organism may seed to the renal cortex during an episode of staphylococcal bacteremia; second, usually in patients with lower urinary tract pathology or indwelling Foley catheters, the organism may ascend to cause a primary lower urinary tract infection. Approximately 10 per cent of patients with staphylococcal bacteremia eventually excrete the organism in the urine; other studies have found that about 25 per cent of patients with a defined urinary tract infection caused by *S. aureus* had had a preceding bacteremic episode. Thus, small cortical abscesses must occur frequently during bacteremia and ultimately rupture in some patients into the tubules and the urine. Most such patients respond promptly to therapy for the underlying disease, and renal carbuncles are now rare.

Conversely, about 5 per cent of patients with a primary staphylococcal urinary tract infection may develop secondary bacteremia. In some patients, the renal infection may seed to the perinephric and retroperitoneal structures, with resultant chronic infection and fibrosis. Frank perinephric abscess is a complication associated with high morbidity and mortality. This condition occurs most frequently in patients with chronic underlying renal diseases who are also often diabetic. Aggressive drainage along with prolonged antibiotic therapy is required for cure.

Staphylococcal Endocarditis. This condition follows staphylococcal bacteremia during which a nidus of infection becomes established on one or more heart valves. Endocarditis consists of two clinical syndromes (see Ch. 299): The first is "subacute" bacterial endocarditis, and the second is "acute" bacterial endocarditis.

Subacute Bacterial Endocarditis. The patient presents with a history of days to weeks of low-grade fever with or without chills, myalgias, night sweats, and weight loss. The word *subacute* refers to the clinical manifestations: The clinical course is one of a chronic, febrile illness. The patient almost always has a history of pre-existing organic valvular heart disease, and the species of *Staphylococcus* involved is usually *S. epidermidis*. *S. epidermidis* accounts for approximately 5 per cent of all cases of subacute endocarditis, the vast majority being caused by streptococcal species. *S. epidermidis* is the most common cause, however, of endocarditis occurring in association with prosthetic heart valves (see Ch. 299). The organism, being a contaminant from the patient's or surgeon's skin flora, is inoculated at the time of the surgical valve replacement. Most such infections occur within the initial 2 months after surgery. In such instances, the outlook for therapy with antibiotics alone is poor, and reoperation with removal of the infected valve or valve ring is often required. More than half of such patients die.

Acute Bacterial Endocarditis. The word *acute* refers to the clinical presentation of the patient who experiences the rapid onset of fever, chills, and myalgias, often with back pain or some gastrointestinal symptoms. The fever is often quite high (103 to 105° F), and the individual at first has the feeling of developing a very bad case of the flu. In the majority of cases, the individual has not had a history of pre-existing valvular heart disease, although it is assumed that many of these individuals have had asymptomatic organic valvular lesions (such as a fenestrated or bicuspid aortic valve, mitral valve prolapse, and so forth). Frequently, therapy for such individuals, who previously had been well, is delayed because the patient and the physician do not realize the gravity of the situation.

S. aureus is almost always the cause of the syndrome of acute endocarditis, and recent data suggest that this syndrome is *increasing* in frequency. At the time of presentation, the patient may not have an obvious heart murmur or show evidence of embolic phenomenon. Thus, the differentiation between primary staphylococcal bacteremia, which may remain uncomplicated, and acute staphylococcal bacterial endocarditis is clinically difficult. The physician must closely follow every patient whose blood samples grow *S. aureus* and must examine carefully each day for the presence of a new murmur, the signs of embolic phenomena, or the observable development of vegetation(s) by echocardiography. Valve destruction, especially of the aortic valve, may progress quite rapidly, and surgery may be necessary even within the first few days of presentation.

S. aureus endocarditis in the drug addict is almost always on one of the right-sided heart valves, usually the tricuspid valve. Therefore, pleuritic chest pain and pulmonary infiltrates are common occurrences due to embolization. In drug-abusing patients who have surreptitiously taken antibiotics, the syndrome may be of a much lower grade and may mimic that of subacute bacterial endocarditis.

The treatment of bacterial endocarditis must be prolonged (see Ch. 299). Four weeks of parenteral therapy is the minimum for staphylococcal endocarditis, although some authors have reported that 2 weeks may suffice for the drug addict, usually a young, otherwise healthy individual with right-sided endocarditis. All staphylococcal infections should be treated with a "cidal" antibiotic, and serum bactericidal levels must be monitored to guide effective therapy. For infections caused by β-lactam antibiotic–resistant staphylococci, whether *aureus* or *epidermidis* species, a cephalosporin is not adequate therapy (see later discussion of treatment), although data may indicate sensitivity to the cephalosporins in vitro. As noted earlier, patients with prosthetic valve endocarditis often require surgery to eradicate the infection. Even those patients with prosthetic valve infections who respond to antibiotics alone probably should be treated with a prolonged course of an appropriate oral antistaphylococcal drug following the 6-week course of parenteral therapy in the hospital.

The prognosis for patients with staphylococcal endocarditis is guarded. Patients with prosthetic valve endocarditis have about a 50 per cent mortality rate. Patients with acute bacterial endocarditis caused by *S. aureus* on native valves do well if they are young and otherwise healthy and especially if the vegetations are on the right-sided valves. The older the patient with left-sided valvular involvement, the higher the mortality (approaching 60 to 80 per cent). Pre-existing symptomatic heart disease is a particularly ominous prognostic sign. The patients who have the subacute syndrome due to *S. epidermidis* not on prosthetic valves, in which the organism is susceptible to the usual antibiotics, usually do quite well: Survival rates are comparable to those of patients with streptococcal endocarditis (in the range of 90 per cent).

Staphylococcal Bacteremia. Sustained true bacteremia due to *S. epidermidis* is uncommon: Although blood cultures frequently yield the organism, 80 to 90 per cent of the time it is a contaminant. True, sustained *S. epidermidis* bacteremia is usually caused by infection of an intravascular line or a prosthetic valve. The most common species causing true bacteremia, especially in the hospital, is *S. aureus*.

There are two varieties of *S. aureus* bacteremia: primary and secondary. Primary bacteremia exists when a patient presenting with fever and chills grows *S. aureus* out of multiple blood cultures but does *not* have an identifiable primary focus of infection. The patient usually has unrecognized endocarditis and should be treated accordingly. Secondary bacteremia is that associated with an obvious, peripheral focus of infection, for example, an intravascular line. Many such patients have a benign clinical course after line removal and a brief course of antibiotic treatment. The problem is to select from the overall group of such patients those who have not developed metastatic septic complications. Patients without metastatic sequelae usually do well with a short (14-day) course of therapy. The typical patient who develops *S. aureus* bacteremia has usually been hospitalized for some other medical problem and has had a neglected peripheral or central venous or arterial access line in place. The patient suddenly develops fever and chills with or without signs of local infection at the site of the line. Other common sources are hemodialysis access shunts, postsurgical or traumatic wounds, and decubitus ulcers. The diagnosis of staphylococcal bacteremia is made when *S. aureus* grows from several blood cultures obtained before an empiric course of antibiotics is begun. Some patients already have an obvious metastatic complication of the bacteremic episode when first examined.

TABLE 300–1. CRITERIA FOR ANTIBIOTIC THERAPY FOLLOWING *STAPHYLOCOCCUS AUREUS* BACTEREMIA

1. Host defenses are normal.
2. The patient has no seedable sites (pre-existing valvular heart lesions, implanted prostheses, chronic arthritis).
3. The primary focus of infection is obvious and easily managed.
4. There is a prompt, complete response to the initial course of antimicrobial therapy.
5. The *S. aureus* recovered is fully sensitive to the antibiotics initially chosen.
6. No clinical evidence of a metastatic, suppurative complication is found during 10–14 days of careful follow-up examinations.

The complications of an episode of *S. aureus* bacteremia are of two varieties: The first type is *nonsuppurative*, i.e., patients who exhibit the septic shock syndrome, some also developing disseminated intravascular coagulation; the second type is *suppurative*, involving the metastatic spread of the organism via the bloodstream to heart valves or other organs. The development of endocarditis in this setting is distinctly uncommon; most suppurative spread occurs to bones, joints, and kidneys, occasionally to other deep viscera, and rarely to the meninges. Following the episode of bacteremia, the patient is placed first on broad, empiric and later on specific antistaphylococcal antibiotic therapy. Throughout this period, the patient must be examined carefully each day for metastatic suppurative sites. Laboratory evaluation may also be helpful, yielding pyuria and the organism from the urine, abnormalities of liver function, and other data. Vegetations may become demonstrable by echocardiography. Radionuclide scans may reveal infectious foci within bones, joints, or soft tissues.

Those patients who develop a clinically evident metastatic focus are treated as dictated by the type of complication that has evolved. Approximately 20 per cent of previously healthy persons who acquire *S. aureus* bacteremia develop some type of complication. Administration of an oral antistaphylococcal drug (dicloxacillin) should be continued for several weeks if there is any doubt about the possibility of residual metastatic abscesses.

If the criteria listed in Table 300–1 are present, such patients usually do well with a short course (14 days) of antibiotic therapy following an episode of *S. aureus* bacteremia.

Septic Shock Syndromes Due to Staphylococci. Staphylococci can produce shock by five mechanisms (Table 300–2). Massive local infection due to staphylococci is uncommon, and such infections usually involve several organisms, usually anaerobes coinfecting with *S. aureus*. *S. epidermidis* may be a part of the flora in these infections but is probably not pathogenic. Specifically, patients with one of the gangrene syndromes (for example, necrotizing fasciitis or synergistic gangrene) may develop shock not caused by bacteremia but by fluid accumulation in the infected area. Such individuals require massive fluid and albumin replacement, extensive local debridement, and broad antibiotic coverage, including effective antianaerobic drugs.

Diarrhea, nausea, and vomiting may be so severe in some patients with staphylococcal food poisoning that shock may develop from hypovolemia secondary to gastrointestinal fluid loss. Hospitalization with fluid replacement may be required.

TABLE 300–2. MECHANISMS OF SHOCK CAUSED BY STAPHYLOCOCCI

1. The local infection can generate a massive inflammatory reaction resulting in sufficient "third spacing" (i.e., fluid accumulation into the area of infection) to lead to hypovolemic shock.
2. Enterotoxin-producing *S. aureus* occasionally causes diarrhea severe enough to cause hypovolemia and shock.
3. Cardiogenic shock can be produced by staphylococci by causing either valve malfunction (usually aortic), multiple myocardial abscesses, or purulent pericarditis.
4. Endotoxic-like shock can be produced via inflammatory mediator activation (see Ch. 288).
5. Toxigenic shock—the toxic shock syndrome—can produce shock, probably both by activating inflammatory mediators and by direct capillary endothelial and end-organ damage.

Cardiogenic shock is self-explanatory (see Ch. 41).

During acute sepsis *S. aureus* may produce shock that mimics that produced by endotoxin during gram-negative organism septicemia (see Ch. 288). Briefly, the primary event in endotoxic shock is the following: On entering the bloodstream, endotoxin activates a sequence of endocrine and inflammatory events leading first to vasodilation and subsequently to a monokine (especially TNF-α)-, complement-, and PMN-mediated capillary leak syndrome resulting in full-blown septic shock. The coagulation and kinin systems also become activated, and such patients may suffer frank DIC. The presence or absence of a capsule seems to be a major factor determining whether or not a particular strain of *S. aureus* in the bloodstream will cause an endotoxic shock–like syndrome. Encapsulated organisms are virulent in tissues and are *more* likely to reach the bloodstream in the course of a peripheral infection. However, once there they are *less* likely to produce the septic shock syndrome. Unencapsulated strains activate inflammatory mediators readily in tissues and therefore are *more* likely to be contained and are least likely to reach the bloodstream and to cause bacteremia. Yet, these are the organisms that can cause shock when directly inoculated into the bloodstream, as by a parenteral drug user or when having colonized an intravascular line.

For a discussion of the toxigenic shock caused by *S. aureus*, refer to the earlier section on the toxic shock syndrome.

Miscellaneous Staphylococcal Infections. This section focuses on several relatively unusual infections that require special diagnostic and therapeutic considerations.

Staphylococcal Pyomyositis. This malady is primarily a tropical disease of malnourished persons, rare enough to be reportable in the United States. The patient develops pain, warmth, and swelling over a muscle region, usually of the lower extremities and buttocks. The overlying skin may appear quite normal or may look like a mild cellulitis; however, when drainage is attempted, the surgeon discovers that the infection extends into muscle, often with extensive destruction.

S. Aureus Epidural Abscess. This infection is often related to the presence of vertebral osteomyelitis wherein periosseus inflammation extends into the epidural space. The inflammation causes localized tenderness over the spine at point of infection followed by weakness and progressive neurologic signs of paraplegia. Effective therapy depends on early diagnosis and *prompt* surgical intervention and drainage.

DIAGNOSIS. Knowledgeable interpretation of the Gram's stain of an adequately obtained specimen usually suggests the presence of staphylococci. Culture of such a specimen almost always yields the responsible staphylococcus, and confirmation is provided by positive blood cultures. Some judgment is required in deciding whether *S. epidermidis* in blood cultures is a contaminant or a true infection. The presence of the organism in *more than two* consecutive blood cultures and associated with proper clinical circumstances (the presence of an indwelling intravascular catheter or a prosthetic device) strongly suggests true bacteremia. The vast majority (80 to 90 per cent) of *S. epidermidis* isolated from blood culture bottles are single organisms, usually in only one of the two bottles in a set, and are contaminants. While *S. aureus* may on occasion contaminate blood cultures, the clinician must consider the isolation of *S. aureus* from the blood under any condition to be significant until proven otherwise. In most cases multiple blood cultures are positive, and there is no question about the diagnosis of the true bacteremic state. If there is any doubt as to the origin of *S. aureus* either in blood, urine, or other fluid specimens, appropriate therapy should be continued.

The Teichoic Acid Antibody (TA-AB) Assay. This assay measures the presence (and titer) or absence of antibodies to staphylococcal cell wall teichoic acids. It is of no use in diagnosing infections with *S. epidermidis* because it only identifies antibodies to the ribitol teichoic acid moiety in the wall of *S. aureus*. Approximately 90 per cent of patients with *S. aureus* endocarditis develop a significant titer of teichoic acid antibodies. The test is fairly sensitive but only moderately specific for other types of serious, deep-seated *S. aureus* infections. The major role of the TA-AB assay is not primarily to diagnose *S. aureus* infections, most of which are diagnosed on clinical grounds, but to assist the clinician

in deciding how long to treat bacteremic patients. Patients with *S. aureus* bacteremia who develop disseminated or metastatic abscesses usually develop an increase in the titer of TA-AB acid antibodies as opposed to those with benign, self-limited bacteremias. The predictive value of a negative assay in someone who has experienced an episode of *S. aureus* bacteremia is high; therefore, the test may be useful in *ruling out* metastatic infections in such patients. In general, however, clinical parameters suffice in such clinical decision-making, and the TA-AB assay rarely provides additional, helpful information.

TREATMENT. Effective therapy of staphylococcal infections depends on early, effective debridement and drainage of the primary focus of infection along with the selection of antibiotics to which the organisms are susceptible. At present, more than 90 per cent of all organisms, whether nosocomial or community-acquired, are resistant to penicillin. Therefore, no patient suspected of having an infection with *S. aureus* should be started on any penicillinase-susceptible penicillin. Most staphylococci are still susceptible to nafcillin and oxacillin; methicillin is an antiquated drug, more toxic than either of the aforementioned parenteral alternatives. Usual doses of nafcillin and oxacillin are in the range of 6 to 12 grams daily, and patients with endocarditis should receive between 9 and 12 grams daily. In the penicillin-allergic individual, the cephalosporins can be used in the absence of a history of an anaphylactic type of penicillin hypersensitivity; however, the most effective alternative continues to be vancomycin. Vancomycin is used in a dose of 2 to 4 grams per day parenterally and has been considered equal to the penicillins and cephalosporins in terms of therapeutic efficacy. Recently, however, some studies have shown relatively poorer clinical responses to vancomycin than to the β-lactam antibiotics, and a switch to nafcillin or oxacillin in patients not infected by a β-lactam–resistant strain of staphylococcus is probably indicated.

β-Lactam Antibiotic–Resistant Staphylococci (BLARS). These organisms are usually referred to as "methicillin-resistant staphylococci." However, methicillin is simply the drug used to determine resistance of these organisms and many methicillin-resistant organisms remain sensitive to the cephalosporins in vitro. However, the clinical responses to the cephalosporins of cephalosporin-sensitive but methicillin-resistant organisms have not been good. Thus, when any species of staphylococcus has been identified as being methicillin-resistant (or, therefore, nafcillin- or oxacillin-resistant) it should be considered resistant to *all* β-lactam antibiotics regardless of contrary data in vitro. The drug of choice in the treatment of BLARS continues to be vancomycin. Alternative drugs include rifampin and trimethoprim-sulfamethoxazole (TMS). Some BLARS remain sensitive to the aminoglycosides, and aminoglycosides may provide a synergistic effect with whatever other antibiotic is used. Newer antibiotics that will be effective against BLARS are teichoplanin* and the quinolones, although recent data indicate increasing quinolone resistance. A new β-lactam–like antibiotic, imipenem (a carbapenem), should probably not be used against BLARS, despite sensitivity in vitro. These recommendations hold true both for *S. aureus* and *S. epidermidis*. Fusidic acid, an antibiotic which inhibits ribosomal GTPase (elongation factor), has been used for many years in England and Canada. It should be thought of when one encounters a serious, resistant *S. aureus* infection in a patient who is intolerant of the glycopeptide antibiotics or who requires an oral agent to treat such infections.

Treatment of Chronic Carriers. Certain individuals may suffer recurrent staphylococcal infections of the skin (furunculosis), and eradication of the nasal carrier state may be required to terminate the series of infections. Nasal carriage termination may be difficult by local, topical measures. Traditionally, individuals so afflicted have been advised to observe meticulous personal hygienic measures such as frequent bathing or showering, using pHisoHex or other bactericidal soap preparations, and the application of an antibacterial ointment such as bacitracin to the anterior nares. While such a treatment program clears a portion of chronic carriers, many relapse and continue to develop recurrent crops of boils. One drug very helpful in this situation is rifampin, known to be excreted in bactericidal concentrations in external (nasal) secretions. Rifampin should always be used with another

---

*Investigational drug.

oral antistaphylococcal drug that, even though present in low concentrations, will delay the emergence of rifampin resistance. Thus, a 5-day course of rifampin* (600 mg twice daily) plus, for example, dicloxacillin (125 mg four times a day) or in the penicillin-allergic patient cephalexin or TMS is very effective in eliminating nasal carriage of S. aureus and the associated dermal infections. A percentage of individuals reacquire the organism and the course of therapy may have to be repeated; the physician should be sure to ascertain that the carried organism is still sensitive to rifampin. As discussed earlier, 5 days of rifampin treatment administered every 3 months to colonized hemodialysis patients significantly reduced the incidence of subsequent infections with S. aureus. Another agent recently introduced for topical use is mupirocin (Bactroban). Application of mupirocin ointment to the anterior nares 3 times a day for 5 days rapidly eliminates nasal carriage; however, 10 per cent relapse occurs in 3 weeks and 40 per cent by 14 weeks. Some mupirocin resistance may be developing. Other antibiotics that may help clear nasal carriage include the oral quinolones and clindamycin.

Bacterial Interference. Bacterial interference is the process of recolonizing an individual with an organism in order to displace a more pathogenic microbe. Initially, investigators found that patients heavily colonized with an aggressive strain of S. aureus that was associated with recurrent infections (boils, omphalitis, or conjunctivitis) could be helped by being recolonized with a nonpathogenic strain (designated strain 502A) of the organism. Reports in the 1960's and 1970's attested to the efficacy of bacterial interference. However, from time to time, there were reports of a serious infection caused by the 502A strain of S. aureus. The use of bacterial interference to treat recurrent infections due to a carried strain of S. aureus therefore has declined. The potential usefulness of this process should be kept in mind as one considers therapeutic approaches to patients with recurrent furunculosis recalcitrant to repeated courses of therapy.

PREVENTION. Prevention of nosocomial staphylococcal infections depends on breaking the chain of transmission between a carrier and a susceptible noncarrier. Transmission from person to person is effectively interrupted by thorough handwashing before and after examination of each patient. Certain other

hospital infection control recommendations and procedures apply in particular to staphylococcal infections. For example, hospitals are required to have specific recommendations about the placement and maintenance of intravascular catheters; such instructions should be followed *meticulously*. Staphylococci are among the leading causes of infection of indwelling intravascular catheters, and proper catheter maintenance substantially reduces the incidence of nosocomial infections with these organisms.

While in theory vaccines containing capsular polysaccharides might enhance host defenses against the encapsulated strains of staphylococci, vaccines developed in the past were not shown to be of major clinical benefit. It is probable that some acquired immunity does develop against staphylococci, since the incidence of S. aureus infections decreases with increasing age. Also, recent data have shown that anticapsular antibodies facilitate opsonization of encapsulated strains. New monoclonal antibody technology will revitalize attempts to develop passive and possibly active immunization of patients at high risk of S. aureus bacteremia.

Bergdoll MS, Chesney PJ: Toxic Shock Syndrome. Boca Raton, Fla., CRC Press, in press. *New volume addressing all aspects of the toxic shock syndrome.*

Brumfitt W, Hamilton-Miller J: Methicillin-resistant *Staphylococcus aureus*. N Engl J Med 320:1188–1196, 1989. *Up-to-date review of all aspects of infections with β-lactam antibiotic–resistant staphylococci.*

Chambers HF, Korzeniowski OM, Sande MA: *Staphylococcus aureus* endocarditis. Clinical manifestations in addicts and nonaddicts. Medicine 62:170–177, 1983. *Data from a prospective, multicenter study describe and contrast the clinical presentation of the syndromes in addicts and nonaddicts.*

Esperson F, Frimodt-Møller N: *Staphylococcus aureus* endocarditis: A review of 119 cases. Arch Intern Med 146:1118–1121, 1986. *Excellent review of the syndrome of acute bacterial endocarditis with emphasis on community-acquired cases.*

Haley RW: Methicillin-resistant *Staphylococcus aureus:* Do we just have to live with it? Ann Intern Med 114:162–164, 1991. *Succinct review of the problem of nosocomial MRSA infections.*

Musher DM, McKenzie SO: Infections due to *Staphylococcus aureus*. Medicine 56:383–409, 1977. *A nice review of most clinical aspects of* S. aureus *infections; still relevant today.*

Sheagren JN: *Staphylococcus aureus*—the persistent pathogen. N Engl J Med 310:1368–1372, 1437–1442, 1984. *A complete review of all aspects of infections with* S. aureus.

Yu VL, Goetz A, Wagener M, et al.: *Staphylococcus aureus* nasal carriage and infection in patients on hemodialysis. Efficacy of antibiotic prophylaxis. N Engl J Med 315:91–96, 1986. *The rate of infection in hemodialysis patients can be decreased by treating the nasal carrier state.*

---

*This use of rifampin is not listed in the manufacturer's directive.

Bacterial Meningitis

Morton N. Swartz

301 Bacterial Meningitis

Meningitis is an inflammation of the arachnoid, the pia mater, and the intervening cerebrospinal fluid. The inflammatory process extends throughout the subarachnoid space about the brain and spinal cord and regularly involves the ventricles. Pyogenic meningitis, considered in this chapter, is usually an acute infection with bacteria that evoke a polymorphonuclear response in the cerebrospinal fluid (CSF). One of its major forms, that caused by meningococci, is considered in Ch. 302; less acute forms of bacterial meningitis, characterized by a mononuclear cell response in the CSF, are discussed in Ch. 332 and 456.

ETIOLOGY AND INCIDENCE. Approximately 20,000 to 25,000 cases of bacterial meningitis occur annually in the United States. If all cases are included regardless of the age of patients, data from the Centers for Disease Control indicate that *Haemophilus influenzae* type b is the most frequent bacterial cause (48 per cent), followed by *Neisseria meningitidis* (19 per cent) and *Streptococcus pneumoniae* (13 per cent). About 70 per cent of all cases occur in children under 5 years of age. The relative frequencies with which the different bacterial species cause meningitis are age related (Table 301–1). In the newborn, gram-

negative bacilli (most frequently *Escherichia coli*, but also other enteric bacilli and *Pseudomonas*) and group B streptococci are the principal causes. In the past 25 years the group B *Streptococcus* has increased in importance in neonatal meningitis; in some hospitals it is the single most frequent etiology, surpassing *E. coli*. Beyond the first month of life and extending through childhood, *H. influenzae* and *N. meningitidis* are the most fre-

TABLE 301–1. BACTERIAL CAUSES OF MENINGITIS

	Neonates (≤1 month) (%)	Children (1 month–15 years) (%)	Adults (>15 years) (%)
S. pneumoniae	0–5	10–20	20–40
N. meningitidis	0–1	25–40	10–20
H. influenzae	0–3	40–60	2–4
Streptococci	20–40*	2–4	5–10
Staphylococci	5	1–2	5–15
Listeria	2–10	1–2	5–10
Gram-negative bacilli	50–60†	1–2	10–20

*Almost all isolates from neonatal meningitis are group B streptococci.

†Of all cases of neonatal meningitis, *E. coli* accounts for about 40 per cent and *Klebsiella-Enterobacter* for about 8 per cent.

quent causes of bacterial meningitis. In adults *S. pneumoniae*, *N. meningitidis*, and gram-negative bacilli are responsible for most cases. Meningococcal meningitis is the only type that occurs in outbreaks; its relative frequency among the meningitides depends on whether statistics have been gathered in a hyperendemic area or during an epidemic period. In about 10 per cent of patients with pyogenic meningitis the bacterial cause cannot be defined. Simultaneous mixed meningitis is rare, occurring in the setting of neurosurgical procedures, penetrating head injury, erosion of the skull or vertebrae by adjacent neoplasm, or intraventricular rupture of a cerebral abscess; the isolation of anaerobes should strongly suggest the latter two of these.

Important changes have occurred in the frequencies of several types of bacterial meningitis over the past 25 years. Gram-negative bacillary meningitis has doubled in frequency in adults, probably reflecting more frequent and extensive neurosurgical procedures as well as other nosocomial factors. *Listeria monocytogenes* has increased eight- to tenfold as a cause of bacterial meningitis in urban general hospitals, reflecting the enlarging immunosuppressed population at particular risk. *Listeria* infections appear to be food borne (dairy products, uncooked vegetables) and involve particularly organ transplant recipients, other patients receiving corticosteroids and cytotoxic drugs, patients with liver disease, pregnant women, and neonates. Meningitis due to *Staphylococcus epidermidis*, essentially unheard of 30 years ago, now represents about 3 per cent of cases in large urban hospitals. It occurs as a complication of neurosurgical procedures and may present a particular therapeutic problem due to methicillin resistance of many of the *S. epidermidis* strains.

CLINICAL SETTINGS. The clinical setting in which meningitis develops may provide a clue to the specific bacterial cause. Meningococcal disease, including meningitis, may occur sporadically and in cyclic outbreaks. In the past, military recruits were particularly susceptible, but now meningococcal vaccine (polysaccharides of groups A, C, Y and W135) is employed for protection. Large urban outbreaks can occur.

Certain predisposing factors are frequently associated with the development of *pneumococcal meningitis. Acute otitis media* (±*mastoiditis*) occurs in about 30 per cent of patients. *Pneumonia* is present in about 15 per cent of patients with pneumococcal meningitis, a much higher frequency than in meningitis caused by *H. influenzae* or *N. meningitidis. Acute pneumococcal sinusitis* is occasionally the initial focus from which infection spreads to the meninges. A significant head injury (recent or remote) has occurred in about 10 per cent of patients with pneumococcal meningitis. CSF rhinorrhea (usually caused by a defect or fracture in the cribriform plate) is present in about 5 per cent of patients with pneumococcal meningitis. Meningitis occurring in young children with sickle cell anemia is most likely to be caused by *S. pneumoniae*. A variety of defects in host defenses (primary or acquired immunoglobulin deficiencies, the asplenic state) may predispose to severe pneumococcal disease, particularly bacteremia and meningitis. Alcoholism is an underlying problem in 10 to 25 per cent of adults with pneumococcal meningitis in urban hospitals.

S. aureus meningitis is seen most commonly as a complication of a neurosurgical procedure, following penetrating skull trauma, or occasionally secondary to staphylococcal bacteremia and endocarditis. Meningitis caused by *gram-negative bacilli* takes one of three forms: neonatal meningitis, meningitis following trauma or neurosurgery, or spontaneous meningitis in adults (e.g., bacteremic *Klebsiella* meningitis in a patient with diabetes mellitus). The most common causes of gram-negative bacillary meningitis in the adult are *E. coli* (about 30 per cent) and *Klebsiella-Enterobacter* (about 40 per cent). The most frequent causes of bacterial meningitis in patients with neoplastic disease are gram-negative bacilli (particularly *Pseudomonas aeruginosa* and *E. coli*), *Listeria monocytogenes, S. pneumoniae*, and *S. aureus*. Meningitis caused by *group A streptococci* is uncommon but occasionally occurs following acute otitis media.

The age-related incidence (children under 5 years) of *H. influenzae* type b meningitis is so striking that the occurrence of this disease in an adult should raise the question of the presence of an underlying anatomic or immunologic defect, circumventing the usual barrier interposed by serum bactericidal mechanisms.

Neonatal Meningitis. The incidence of meningitis is higher in the first month of life than in any other single month. The principal cause, *E. coli* strains containing the K1 capsular antigen, is usually acquired by the neonates from their mothers who carry the organism in their stool. In the newborn the group B *Streptococcus* can produce either an "early onset" (occurring within 8 days of delivery and characterized by a fulminant illness with septicemia, severe respiratory distress, and sometimes meningitis) or a "late onset" (occurring 10 days to 2 months after delivery and presenting a more insidious, slowly progressive illness which usually includes meningitis) infection.

The clinical signs in neonatal meningitis suggest sepsis but not necessarily central nervous system involvement: fever (in only 60 per cent), jaundice, diarrhea, lethargy, poor feeding or vomiting, respiratory distress (including apnea), seizures, irritability, bulging fontanel (in only 30 per cent), and nuchal rigidity (15 per cent). Frequently, only by examination of the CSF can the presence of meningitis be ruled in or out.

PATHOLOGY. The purulent exudate is distributed widely in the subarachnoid space, most abundant in the basal cisterns and about the cerebellum initially, but also extending into the sulci over the cerebrum. There is no direct invasion of cerebral tissue by the infecting organism or the inflammatory exudate, but the subjacent brain becomes congested and edematous. The effectiveness of the pial barrier accounts for the fact that cerebral abscess does not complicate bacterial meningitis. Indeed, when these two processes coexist, the sequence usually has been that of an initial abscess subsequently leaking its contents into the ventricular system, producing meningitis. There are two possible exceptions to the aforementioned generalization: (1) neonatal meningitis due to *Citrobacter*, in which the organisms appear to invade the brain after producing a necrotizing vasculitis of small penetrating blood vessels; (2) *Listeria* rhombencephalitis, a very rare process in which brain stem infection can occur simultaneously with *Listeria* meningitis (or alone). Structures adjacent to the meninges may show a variety of pathologic changes secondary to bacterial meningitis. *Cortical thrombophlebitis* results from venous stasis and adjacent meningeal inflammation. Infarction of cerebral tissue may follow. *Involvement of cortical and pial arteries* with peripheral aneurysm formation and vascular occlusion occurs occasionally in bacterial meningitis. Rarely, narrowing of the supraclinoid portion of the internal carotid artery at the base of the brain occurs as a result of arteritis and arterial spasm. In fulminating cases (particularly meningococcal meningitis), *cerebral edema* may be marked even though the CSF pleocytosis is only moderate. Rarely such patients develop temporal lobe and cerebellar herniation, resulting in compression of the midbrain and medulla. *Damage to cranial nerves* occurs in areas where dense exudate accumulates; the third and sixth cranial nerves are also vulnerable to damage by increased intracranial pressure. *Ventriculitis* probably occurs in most cases of bacterial meningitis; rarely this progresses to the accumulation of pus, *ventricular empyema. Hydrocephalus* can develop during meningitis from obstruction to CSF flow within the ventricular system (obstructive hydrocephalus) or extraventricularly (communicating hydrocephalus). *Subdural effusions* are sterile transudates that develop over the cerebral cortex in about 15 per cent of infants with bacterial meningitis. Rarely such effusions become infected, producing a subdural empyema. In the past the diagnosis has been made almost exclusively in infants, in whom abnormal transillumination or increasing head size can be detected. Now, sterile or infected (showing peripheral contrast enhancement) subdural collections can be demonstrated readily by CT scan as low-density areas about the cerebrum.

PATHOGENESIS. Bacteria may reach the meninges by several routes: (1) systemic bacteremia, (2) direct ingress from the upper respiratory tract or skin through an anatomic defect (e.g., skull fracture, eroding sequestrum, meningocele), (3) passage intracranially via venules in the nasopharynx, or (4) spread from a contiguous focus of infection (infection of the paranasal sinuses, leakage of a brain abscess). Bacteremic spread to the meninges is probably the most frequent path of infection. However, not all bacteremic organisms have the same likelihood of causing meningitis. Most bacterial species causing meningitis (*H. influenzae* b, *N. meningitidis, S. pneumoniae, E. coli* K1, group B *Streptococcus*) have definable capsules which are antiphagocytic. Whether the capsular polysaccharide confers some special meningeal tropism, possibly through surface receptors, is not known. The primary focus initiating the bacteremia is usually in the upper respiratory tract or lung (pneumonia) but may be in the heart (endocarditis) or the gastrointestinal or urinary tracts. Experiments in infant primates infected with *H. influenzae* suggest that the initial site of inflammation in the central nervous system may be the choroid plexus. Once established in any part of the meninges, infection quickly extends throughout the subarachnoid space. Bacterial replication proceeds relatively unhindered, since CSF levels of complement are low early in meningeal inflammation, resulting in minimal opsonic and bactericidal activity (or none), and since surface phagocytosis of unopsonized organisms is meager in such a fluid environment. A secondary bacteremia may follow meningeal infection and itself contribute to continuing further inoculation of the cerebrospinal fluid.

Acute meningeal inflammation can be induced in animal models by intracisternal inoculation of pneumococcal cell wall components or of *H. influenzae* type b lipopolysaccharide, probably through the release of inflammatory cytokines such as interleukin 1, tumor necrosis factor (TNF), or prostaglandins. Increased CSF levels of TNF have been found in bacterial, but not viral, meningitis.

CLINICAL MANIFESTATIONS. *History.* An acute onset of fever, generalized headache, vomiting, and stiff neck are common to many types of meningitis. The majority of patients with pyogenic meningitis of the three common causes have had an antecedent or accompanying upper respiratory tract infection, acute otitis (or mastoiditis), or pneumonia. Myalgias (particularly in meningococcal disease), backache, and generalized weakness are common symptoms. The illness usually progresses rapidly with development of confusion, obtundation, and loss of consciousness. Occasionally the onset may be less acute, with meningeal signs present for several days to a week.

General Physical Findings. Evidences of meningeal irritation (drowsiness and decreased mentation, stiff neck, Kernig's and Brudzinski's signs) are usually present. In certain patients the findings of meningitis may be easily overlooked; infants, obtunded patients, or elderly patients with congestive failure or pneumonia may develop meningitis without prominent meningeal signs. Their lethargy should be investigated carefully and meningeal signs should be sought; if any doubt exists, examination of the CSF is indicated.

The presence of a petechial, purpuric, or ecchymotic rash in a patient with meningeal findings almost always indicates meningococcal infection and requires prompt treatment because of the rapidity with which this infection can progress (see Ch. 302). Rarely, extensive petechial and purpuric lesions occur in meningitis caused by *S. pneumoniae* or *H. influenzae*. Very rarely skin lesions almost indistinguishable from those of meningococcal bacteremia occur in patients with acute *S. aureus* endocarditis who also have meningeal signs and a CSF pleocytosis (secondary either to staphylococcal meningitis or to embolic cerebral infarction). Usually one or two of the lesions in such a patient are those of purulent purpura; aspiration of material reveals staphylococci on Gram's stain. In the summer months viral aseptic meningitis may produce meningeal signs, macular and petechial skin lesions, and a CSF pleocytosis of several hundred cells, sometimes with neutrophils predominating initially.

Neurologic Findings and Complications. Cranial nerve abnormalities, involving principally the third, fourth, sixth, or seventh nerves, occur in 10 to 20 per cent of patients with bacterial meningitis. These usually disappear shortly after recovery. Persistent sensorineural hearing loss occurs in 10 per cent of children with bacterial meningitis. In another 16 per cent a transient conductive hearing loss develops. The most likely sites of involvement in persistent sensorineural deafness appear to be the inner ear (infection or toxic products possibly spreading from the subarachnoid space along the cochlear aqueduct) and the acoustic nerve. In children permanent hearing impairment is more common following meningitis due to *S. pneumoniae* than to *H. influenzae* or *N. meningitidis.*

Seizures (focal or generalized) occur in 20 to 30 per cent of patients and may result from readily reversible causes (high fever in infants; penicillin neurotoxicity when large doses are administered intravenously in the presence of renal failure) or from focal cerebral injury. Seizures can occur during the first few days or can appear with associated focal neurologic deficits caused by

cortical vein phlebitis 7 to 10 days after the onset of the meningitis. In adults with seizures accompanying meningitis, *S. pneumoniae* is more commonly the cause, but alcoholism is a confounding factor.

Brain swelling and increased CSF pressure are associated with seizures, third nerve dysfunction, abnormal reflexes, coma, hypertension, and bradycardia. Two anatomic features of brain capillaries account for the functioning of the blood-brain barrier in controlling the concentration of substances in brain interstitium. They are the presence of tight junctions fusing brain capillary endothelial cells together and the paucity of pinocytotic vacuoles in the same cells. With bacterial meningitis, separation of intercellular junctions occurs, and pinocytotic vacuoles increase, probably accounting for the development of complicating cerebral edema. In approximately one quarter of fatal cases of community-acquired meningitis in adults, cerebral edema accompanied by temporal lobe herniation is observed at autopsy.

Papilledema is rare in bacterial meningitis even with high CSF pressures. Its presence should indicate the possibility of some other associated or independent suppurative intracranial process (subdural empyema, brain abscess). Marked central hyperpnea sometimes occurs in patients with severe bacterial meningitis; CSF acidosis (principally caused by increased lactic acid levels) provides much of the respiratory stimulus.

Focal cerebral signs (principally hemiparesis, dysphasia, visual field defects, and gaze preference) occur in about 25 per cent of adults with community-acquired bacterial meningitis. They may develop during early meningitis secondary to occlusive vascular processes or some days later. Also, cerebral blood flow velocity may be decreased in the presence of increased intracranial pressure and lead to temporary or lasting neurologic dysfunction. It is important to distinguish lateralizing findings resulting from postictal changes (Todd's paralysis), which usually persist for no more than several hours.

Prompt treatment of bacterial meningitis usually results in rapid recovery of neurologic function. Persistent or late-onset obtundation and coma without focal findings suggest development of brain swelling, subdural effusion (in the infant), hydrocephalus, loculated ventriculitis, cortical thrombophlebitis, or sagittal sinus thrombosis. The last three are commonly associated with fever and continuing CSF pleocytosis.

Residual neurologic damage remains in 10 to 20 per cent of patients who recover from bacterial meningitis. Developmental delay and speech defects are each observed in about 5 per cent of children. In infants surviving neonatal meningitis, significant sequelae are much more frequent (30 to 50 per cent).

LABORATORY DIAGNOSIS. *Cerebrospinal Fluid Examination.* Initial CSF pressure is usually moderately elevated (200 to 300 mm H_2O). Striking elevations (over 450 mm) occur in occasional patients with acute brain swelling complicating meningitis in the absence of an associated mass lesion.

Gram-Stained Smear. By the time of hospitalization, most patients with pyogenic meningitis have large numbers (at least 10^5 per milliliter) of bacteria in the cerebrospinal fluid. Careful examination of the Gram-stained smear of the spun sediment of CSF reveals the etiologic agent in 70 to 80 per cent of cases. In most instances when gram-positive diplococci (or short chaining cocci) are observed on stained CSF smear they are pneumococci. In certain clinical settings it is important to distinguish this organism from the relatively penicillin-resistant *Enterococcus,* which would require the addition of an aminoglycoside to penicillin in treatment. This can be done by identifying pneumococcal polysaccharide in the CSF by latex particle agglutination (or by employing the quellung reaction). Culture of the cerebrospinal fluid reveals the etiologic agent in 80 to 90 per cent of patients with bacterial meningitis.

Special Immunologic and Serologic Procedures. In patients in whom the etiologic agent is not identified on Gram-stained smear of the CSF, rapid diagnosis may often be made by detection of specific bacterial antigens by latex agglutination (LA) or countercurrent immunoelectrophoresis (CIE). These techniques have been employed most extensively in the rapid diagnosis of meningitis caused by *H. influenzae* type b, but have also been used in the diagnosis of meningococcal (groups A,B,C, and Y) and pneumococcal meningitis, and meningitis due to group B streptococci. Antigen detection by LA is more sensitive and provides results more rapidly than CIE. Since *E. coli* K1 and *N. meningitidis* serogroup B share a common antigenic determinant, immunologic cross-reactivity may cause a false-positive reaction with the group B meningococcal reagent. Since the bacterial cause can be found on Gram-stained smear in most cases of bacterial meningitis, the role of latex agglutination appears to be as an adjunct in rapid diagnosis when no organisms are observed or in providing a specific rather than a morphologic (Gram's stain) diagnosis.

The limulus gelation assay for endotoxin is positive in the CSF of patients with meningitis caused by gram-negative but not by gram-positive bacteria.

Cell Count. The cell count in untreated meningitis usually ranges between 100 and 10,000 per cubic millimeter, with polymorphonuclear leukocytes predominating initially (80 per cent or more) and lymphocytes appearing subsequently. Extremely high cell counts (>50,000 per cubic millimeter) may occur rarely in primary bacterial meningitis but should also raise the possibility of intraventricular rupture of a cerebral abscess. Cell counts as low as 10 to 20 may be observed early in bacterial meningitis (particularly that caused by *N. meningitidis* and *H. influenzae*). Occasionally, in granulocytopenic patients or in the elderly with overwhelming pneumococcal meningitis, the CSF may contain very few leukocytes and yet may appear grossly turbid because of the presence of myriads of organisms. Meningitis caused by several bacterial species (*M. tuberculosis*, *B. burgdorferi*, *T. pallidum*) characteristically produces a lymphocytic pleocytosis. *Listeria monocytogenes* meningitis in infants may produce a primarily lymphocytic response in the CSF; in the adult there is usually a polymorphonuclear response, but rarely lymphocytes predominate.

Glucose. The CSF glucose is reduced to values of 40 mg per deciliter or below (or less than 50 per cent of the simultaneous blood level) in 50 per cent of patients with bacterial meningitis; this finding can be very valuable in distinguishing bacterial meningitis from most viral meningitides or parameningeal infections. A normal CSF glucose does not exclude the diagnosis of bacterial meningitis. The simultaneous blood glucose level should be determined, because patients with diabetes mellitus (or who are receiving intravenous glucose infusions) have an elevated level of glucose in the CSF, and its significance can be appreciated only on comparison with the simultaneous blood level. However, it may take 90 to 120 minutes for equilibration to occur after major shifts in the level of glucose in the circulation. The hypoglycorrhachia characteristic of pyogenic meningitis appears to be due to interference with normal carrier-facilitated diffusion of glucose.

Protein. The level of protein in the CSF is usually elevated above 100 mg per deciliter, and the higher values are more commonly observed in pneumococcal meningitis. Extreme elevations, 1000 mg per deciliter or more, indicate subarachnoid block secondary to the meningitis.

Other Abnormalities in the CSF. Elevated levels of lactic acid occur in pyogenic meningitis. Although lactic dehydrogenase levels are higher in patients with bacterial meningitis than in those with viral infections of the central nervous system, these alterations are not of help in determining the specific etiologic agent involved. C-reactive protein is increased in about 95 per cent of patients with bacterial meningitis and is not increased in most patients with viral meningitis. However, it does not seem to provide more information than the CSF cell count, is not helpful in diagnosing bacterial meningitis in newborns, and does not provide clues to the bacterial species involved.

Other Laboratory Tests. Blood and Respiratory Tract Cultures. Bacteremia is demonstrable in about 80 per cent of patients with *H. influenzae* meningitis, 50 per cent of those with pneumococcal meningitis, and 30 to 40 per cent of those with meningococcal meningitis. Cultures of the upper respiratory tract are not helpful in establishing an etiologic diagnosis. Determination of serum creatinine and electrolytes is important in view of the gravity of the illness, the occurrence of specific abnormalities secondary to the meningitis (syndrome of inappropriate secretion of antidiuretic hormone), and problems in therapy in the presence of renal dysfunction (seizures and hyperkalemia with high-dose

penicillin therapy). In patients with extensive petechial and purpuric skin lesions, evaluation for coagulopathy is indicated.

Radiologic Studies. In view of the frequency with which pyogenic meningitis is associated with primary foci of infection in the chest, nasal sinuses, or mastoid, roentgenograms of these areas should be taken at the appropriate time after institution of antimicrobial therapy. Computerized tomography (CT) scans are not indicated in most patients with bacterial meningitis. If a mass lesion (cerebral abscess, subdural empyema) is suspected by history, clinical setting, or physical findings (papilledema, focal cerebral signs), then CT scans should be performed. *Bacterial meningitis is a medical emergency requiring immediate diagnosis and rapid institution of antimicrobial therapy.* Delay in performing a diagnostic lumbar puncture in order to obtain a CT scan should be avoided except on the basis of findings indicative of a parameningeal collection or other intracranial mass lesion. Changes may be observed on CT scan during meningitis itself: cerebral edema, enlargement of the subarachnoid spaces; contrast enhancement of the leptomeninges and the ependyma; or patchy areas of diminished density caused by associated cerebritis and necrosis. Patients with meningitis rarely have significant CT abnormalities in the absence of focal neurologic findings. In the patient with meningitis whose clinical status deteriorates or fails to improve, the CT scan may be helpful in demonstrating suspected complications: sterile subdural collections or empyema; ventricular enlargement secondary to communicating or obstructive hydrocephalus; prominent persisting basilar meningitis; extensive areas of cerebral infarction resulting from occlusion of major cerebral arteries or veins; or marked ventricular wall enhancement, suggesting ventriculitis or ventricular empyema.

DIAGNOSIS. Diagnosis of bacterial meningitis is not difficult in a febrile patient with meningeal symptoms and signs developing in the setting of a predisposing illness. The diagnosis may be less obvious in the elderly, obtunded patient with pneumonia or the confused alcoholic patient in impending delirium tremens. Examination of the CSF should be carried out promptly whenever there is any question of meningitis.

Headache, fever, vomiting, stiff neck, and CSF pleocytosis are features of meningeal inflammation and are common to many types of meningitis (e.g., bacterial, fungal, viral) and also to some parameningeal processes. The CSF findings are most helpful in distinguishing among these processes (see Ch. 471). In the patient with meningitis whose CSF does not reveal the etiologic agent on examination of Gram-stained smear, particularly when the CSF glucose is normal and the polymorphonuclear pleocytosis is atypical, certain treatable processes which can mimic bacterial meningitis should be considered in differential diagnosis: (1) *Parameningeal infections.* The presence of infections (chronic ear or nasal accessory sinus infections, lung abscess) predisposing to brain abscess, epidural (cerebral or spinal) abscess, subdural empyema, or pyogenic venous sinus phlebitis should be sought. Neurologic findings may appear in the course of primary bacterial meningitis, but their presence should alert the physician to the need for close scrutiny for the presence of a space-occupying infectious process in the central nervous system. Neurologic symptoms or findings antedating the onset of meningeal symptoms should suggest the possibility of a parameningeal infection. The isolation of an anaerobic organism should suggest the possibility of intraventricular leakage of a cerebral abscess. (2) *Bacterial endocarditis.* Bacterial meningitis may occur during bacterial endocarditis caused by pyogenic organisms such as *S. aureus* and enterococci. In subacute bacterial endocarditis sterile embolic infarctions of the brain may occur and produce meningeal signs and a CSF pleocytosis containing several hundred cells, including polymorphonuclear leukocytes. A history of dental manipulation, fever, and anorexia antedating the meningitis should be sought; careful examination for heart murmurs and peripheral stigmata of endocarditis is indicated. (3) "*Chemical*" *meningitis.* The clinical and CSF findings (polymorphonuclear pleocytosis and even reduced glucose level) of bacterial meningitis may be produced by chemically induced inflammation. Acute meningitis following a diagnostic lumbar puncture or spinal anesthesia may be due to bacterial or chemical contamination of equipment or anesthetic agent. Endogenous chemical meningitis resulting from leakage into the subarachnoid space of material from an epidermoid tumor or a craniopharyngioma can produce a polymorphonuclear pleocytosis and hypoglycorrhachia. Birefringent material may be seen on polarizing microscopy of the CSF sediment.

Rarely, a patient develops meningitis characterized by subacute onset and persistent neutrophilic CSF pleocytosis lasting weeks or months without ready bacteriologic diagnosis. The etiologic agent in such cases of *chronic neutrophilic meningitis* has usually been either a fungus (*Aspergillus, Candida, Blastomyces*, etc.) or a bacterium such as *Nocardia* or *Actinomyces* species.

NON-NEUROLOGIC COMPLICATIONS. Shock. When shock occurs in pyogenic meningitis it is usually a manifestation of an accompanying intense bacteremia, as in fulminant meningococcemia, rather than of the meningitis itself. Management is guided by the principles of septic shock therapy with appropriate modifications for myocardial failure (see Ch. 302).

Coagulation Disorders. Coagulopathies are frequently associated with the intense bacteremias (usually meningococcal, occasionally pneumococcal) and hypotension which can accompany meningitis. The changes may be mild such as thrombocytopenia (with or without prolongation of prothrombin and partial thromboplastin times) or more marked with clinical evidences of disseminated intravascular coagulation (see Ch. 302).

Septic Complications. **Endocarditis.** Previously, 5 to 10 per cent of patients with pneumococcal meningitis, particularly those with bacteremia and pneumonia as well, developed acute endocarditis, most commonly on the aortic valve. The incidence is currently much lower, as a result of earlier treatment of the initiating infection. In such patients, febrile relapse and a new murmur may appear shortly after completion of antimicrobial therapy for meningitis.

Pyogenic Arthritis. Septic arthritis may result from the bacteremia associated with meningitis caused by *S. pneumoniae, N. meningitidis*, or *H. influenzae*.

Prolonged Fever. With appropriate antimicrobial treatment of meningitis of the three most common bacterial causes, patients become afebrile within 2 to 5 days. Sometimes fever persists beyond this or recurs after an afebrile period. In the patient with persisting headache, obtundation, and cerebral findings, inadequate drug therapy or neurologic sequelae (cortical venous thrombophlebitis, ventriculitis, subdural collections) are important considerations. Re-evaluation of the CSF, particularly Gram-stained smear and culture, is essential under these circumstances. Drug fever may be responsible in the patient who continues to show clinical improvement in all other respects. Metastatic infection (septic arthritis, purulent pericarditis, thoracic empyema, endocarditis) may be the cause of continuing or recurrent fever.

A syndrome consisting of fever, arthritis, and pericarditis 3 to 6 days after initiation of effective antimicrobial therapy of meningococcal meningitis occurs in about 10 per cent of patients (see Ch. 302).

RECURRENT MENINGITIS. Repeated episodes of bacterial meningitis generally indicate a host defect, either in local anatomy or in antibacterial and immunologic defenses (e.g., recurrent *N. meningitidis* infections in patients with congenital or acquired deficiencies of complement, particularly late-acting components). Eleven per cent of patients with pneumococcal meningitis have had more than one episode, whereas 0.5 per cent of patients with meningitis caused by other organisms have had recurrent attacks. *S. pneumoniae* is the cause of one third of episodes of community-acquired recurrent meningitis; various streptococci, *H. influenzae*, and *N. meningitidis* are the causes of another one third of episodes. In contrast, in nosocomial recurrent meningitis, gram-negative bacilli and *S. aureus* are the causes of about 60 per cent of episodes. A history of head trauma is much more frequent in patients with recurrent meningitis. Organisms may directly enter the subarachnoid space, through a defect in the cribriform plate (the most common site), in association with the empty sella syndrome, via a basilar skull fracture, through an erosive sequestrum of the mastoid, through congenital dermal defects along the craniospinal axis (usually evident before adult life), or as a consequence of penetrating cranial trauma or neurosurgical procedures. The anatomic defect may produce a frank CSF leak (rhinorrhea or, less commonly, otorrhea) or may entrap a vascular cuff of meninges which might subsequently serve as a direct route for organisms to reach the meninges. CSF rhinorrhea may be intermittent, and meningitis may occur months or years after head injury.

Any patient with bacterial meningitis, particularly if meningitis is recurrent, should be evaluated carefully for any congenital or post-traumatic defects. The presence of CSF rhinorrhea should be sought at admission and subsequently (rhinorrhea may clear during active meningitis only to recur when inflammation has resolved). Clinical clues suggesting the presence of a CSF fistula through the cribriform plate, pericranial air sinuses, or temporal bone include (1) salty taste in the throat, (2) positionally dependent rhinorrhea (rhinorrhea only in the lateral recumbent or prone position suggests an otic or sphenoid origin), (3) anosmia (cribriform plate leak), and (4) hearing loss or full feeling in the ear, often with a finding of fluid or bubbles behind the tympanic membrane (leakage into the middle ear). Demonstration of glucose in nasal secretions with glucose oxidase "sticks" (Dextrostix) suggests the presence of CSF. Quantitative determination of glucose and chloride content of nasal secretions can definitively establish the presence of CSF rhinorrhea.

Recurrent pneumococcal meningitis may occur without apparent predisposing circumstances, and cryptic CSF leaks should be sought actively in such patients by polytomography of the frontal and mastoid regions and by radioisotope techniques. (Radioiodine-labeled albumin is introduced intrathecally, and pledgets of cotton placed in the nares are subsequently examined for the radionuclide. Radioisotopic cisternography has been used successfully recently.) Intrathecal introduction of fluorescein as a visual tracer (under ultraviolet light) can be employed similarly in detecting active leaks. Surgical closure of CSF fistulas should be carried out to prevent further episodes of meningitis. Newer extracranial approaches via the ethmoid sinuses for repair of cribriform plate or sphenoid sinus dural defects are successful and avoid the higher morbidity associated with craniotomy.

In most patients with CSF otorrhea and rhinorrhea following an acute head injury, the leak ceases in 1 or 2 weeks. *Persistent rhinorrhea for more than 4 to 6 weeks is an indication for surgical repair.* Prolonged administration of penicillin does not prevent pneumococcal meningitis and may encourage infection with more drug-resistant species.

Rarely, recurrent meningitis of nonbacterial etiology may mimic bacterial meningitis. *Mollaret's meningitis* consists of repeated febrile episodes of mild meningeal symptomatology, usually without neurologic abnormalities. Initially, large "endothelial" cells may be seen in the CSF along with polymorphonuclear leukocytes, which subsequently are replaced by lymphocytes. *Behçet's syndrome*, characterized by relapsing oral and genital ulcers and ocular lesions (hypopyon), may exhibit a variety of neurologic abnormalities, including recurrent meningitis.

PROGNOSIS. The introduction of antimicrobial agents has converted bacterial meningitis from a disease that was almost always fatal to one in which the majority of patients survive without significant neurologic residua. The mortality rate for community-acquired bacterial meningitis varies with the etiologic agent and the clinical circumstances. With current antimicrobial therapy the mortality rate for *H. influenzae* meningitis is below 5 per cent and that for meningococcal meningitis is about 10 per cent. The highest mortality is with pneumococcal meningitis, in which the rate is about 25 per cent. The mortality rate for gram-negative bacillary meningitis in adults has been 20 to 30 per cent, but it appears to be decreasing in the past 5 to 10 years. The mortality rate for recurrent community-acquired meningitis in adults (about 5 per cent) is strikingly lower than the 20 per cent rate for nonrecurrent episodes. Poor prognostic factors include advanced age, presence of other foci of infection, underlying diseases (leukemia, alcoholism), coma, and delay in instituting appropriate therapy.

TREATMENT. Antimicrobial Agents. Antimicrobial therapy should be begun promptly in this life-threatening emergency. Treatment should be aimed at the most likely causes based on clinical clues (age of the patient, presence of a purpuric rash, a recent neurosurgical procedure, CSF rhinorrhea). If the infecting organism is observed on examination of the Gram-stained smear of the CSF sediment, specific therapy is initiated. If the etiologic agent is not seen on smear (or not detected by latex agglutination), treatment for bacterial meningitis of unknown etiology should be carried out (see below).

With the exception of chloramphenicol, the commonly employed antimicrobial agents do not readily penetrate the normal blood-brain barrier; but the passage of penicillin and other antimicrobials is enhanced in the presence of meningeal inflammation. Antimicrobial drugs should be administered intravenously throughout the treatment period; reduction in dosage as the patient improves should be avoided, because normalization of the blood-brain barrier during recovery reduces the CSF levels of drug that are achievable. Bactericidal drugs (penicillin, ampicillin, third-generation cephalosporins) are preferred whenever possible in the treatment of meningitis caused by susceptible bacteria. In animal models of bacterial meningitis CSF levels of antibiotics at least 10 to 20 times the minimal bactericidal concentration appear to be needed for optimal therapy. Several antimicrobial drugs (first- or second-generation cephalosporins, clindamycin) do not provide effective levels in the cerebrospinal fluid and should not be used.

Meningitis of Specific Bacterial Cause. The treatment of choice for pneumococcal meningitis in the adult is penicillin (24 million units daily in divided doses every 2 to 3 hours) or ampicillin (12 grams daily in divided doses every 2 to 3 hours). In the patient with a major penicillin allergy, chloramphenicol (4 to 6 grams intravenously daily in the adult) is a reasonable alternative. However, several points of caution should be made: (1) resistance to chloramphenicol has been reported from Spain in 45 per cent of pneumococcal strains, (2) the response to chloramphenicol of granulocytopenic patients may be suboptimal, and (3) recently, isolates of S. pneumoniae that are relatively resistant (minimum inhibitory concentration [MIC] of 0.1 to 1.0 μg per milliliter) or highly resistant (South African strains with MIC of 2 to 8 μg per milliliter) to penicillin have been identified. In the United States, relative pneumococcal resistance to penicillin, not due to β-lactamase production but rather to alterations in penicillin-binding proteins, occurs in 0 to 2 per cent of clinical isolates (in a few geographic areas the figures are as high as 6 to 8 per cent). (In one area of Spain 50 per cent of pneumococcal isolates have been reported to be penicillin resistant.) In addition to cases of meningitis due to highly penicillin-resistant S. pneumoniae that occurred during the outbreak in South Africa in the late 1970's, seven cases of meningitis due to moderately penicillin-resistant strains (including two that were multiply resistant) have been described in the United States and abroad. Thus, antimicrobial susceptibilities should be determined for all pneumococcal isolates from cerebrospinal fluid, blood, or sterile body fluids. If the isolate is, or is suspected to be, relatively penicillin resistant, a third-generation cephalosporin (e.g., cefotaxime or ceftriaxone) or chloramphenicol (provided the strain is not multiply resistant) is a reasonable alternative to penicillin G. If the isolate should prove to be highly penicillin resistant, vancomycin is the antimicrobial of choice.

The treatment of meningococcal meningitis is the same as for pneumococcal meningitis (see Ch. 302).

At present 30 per cent of isolates of H. influenzae b in the United States are ampicillin resistant. Thus, cefotaxime (200 mg per kilogram intravenously daily in divided doses every 4 to 6 hours for children; 12 grams daily in adults) or ceftriaxone (loading dose of 75 mg per kilogram intravenously followed by 50 mg per kilogram intravenously every 12 hours in children; not to exceed a total of 4 grams daily) is appropriate therapy for H. influenzae b meningitis. The combination of chloramphenicol (100 mg per kilogram intravenously daily for a child; 4 grams intravenously daily for an adult) and ampicillin (300 to 400 mg per kilogram intravenously per day for a child; 12 grams intravenously per day for an adult) is an acceptable alternative. If the isolate proves susceptible to ampicillin, the chloramphenicol may be discontinued. Although in Spain over 50 per cent of isolates are chloramphenicol resistant, less than 1 per cent have been resistant in the United States. Cefuroxime, a second-generation cephalosporin, has been used extensively the past half-dozen years, but the third-generation cephalosporins are preferable because of reports indicating slower sterilization of CSF and a higher incidence of sensorineural hearing loss with cefuroxime.

Adult meningitis caused by methicillin-sensitive S. aureus should be treated with a penicillinase-resistant penicillin (nafcillin, 10 to 12 grams intravenously per day). Rifampin (600 mg orally or intravenously daily), because adequate CSF levels can be achieved and because of its capacity to penetrate leukocytes and kill intracellular organisms, may be added as a second antimicrobial in difficult cases. In the penicillin-allergic patient, vancomycin (2.0 grams intravenously in divided doses every 6 hours) is the alternative of choice. Since penetration of vancomycin into the CSF is limited, adjunctive intrathecal therapy (5 to 20 mg of vancomycin in 10 ml of 5 per cent dextrose–0.85 per cent NaCl slowly in the adult)* has been used when CSF cultures have remained positive after 48 hours of intravenous therapy alone. For adult meningitis due to methicillin-resistant S. aureus, intravenous vancomycin (with adjunctive intrathecal vancomycin as needed) is the treatment of choice. In refractory cases the addition of another drug for systemic therapy (rifampin or gentamicin) may be warranted.

Treatment of enterococcal meningitis in the adult involves the use of intravenous penicillin (24 million units daily) or ampicillin (12 grams daily), supplemented with parenterally administered gentamicin (3 to 5 mg per kilogram daily in divided doses every 8 hours). In the patient who fails to respond promptly to parenteral therapy, adjunctive intrathecal therapy with gentamicin (3 to 5 mg per day) should be considered.

Cefotaxime (12 grams daily intravenously in divided doses every 4 hours in adults) or ceftriaxone is now being used extensively in the treatment of meningitis known to be due to susceptible gram-negative bacilli (E. coli, Klebsiella, Proteus, etc.). It should not be used in the treatment of meningitis due to less susceptible species such as Pseudomonas aeruginosa and Acinetobacter. Initial treatment (on the basis only of findings on Gram-stained smear of CSF) of adults with gram-negative bacillary meningitis involves the combination of cefotaxime (or ceftazidime) with an aminoglycoside (e.g., gentamicin, 5 mg per kilogram daily intravenously in divided doses every 8 hours). Adjunctive intrathecal therapy with gentamicin (3 to 5 mg administered at intervals of 24 hours for the first few days) may be indicated as well if there is no response to initial systemic therapy. Following identification of the specific pathogen and determination of its drug susceptibilities, alterations in antimicrobial therapy may be indicated. If the organism is Pseudomonas aeruginosa, a third-generation cephalosporin with antipseudomonal activity, ceftazidime (2 grams intravenously every 6 or 8 hours in an adult), is combined with parenteral (and intrathecal, if needed) aminoglycoside in treatment. If necessary, alternative therapy would be a combination of an antipseudomonal penicillin (e.g., piperacillin or azlocillin, 3 to 4 grams intravenously every 4 to 6 hours in an adult) with an aminoglycoside.

Bacterial Meningitis of Unknown Etiology. Initial treatment of meningitis when the etiologic agent cannot be identified on Gram-stained smear of cerebrospinal fluid is based on available clinical clues. *In the neonate,* a wide range of gram-positive (group B streptococci, Listeria) and gram-negative organisms (E. coli, Klebsiella, H. influenzae) may be the cause, indicating the intravenous use of combined therapy with drugs such as ampicillin with gentamicin (or amikacin), or ampicillin with cefotaxime (or ceftriaxone), until results of cultures become available. *In children,* therapy is directed at the three most frequent pathogens: H. influenzae, S. pneumoniae, and N. meningitidis. The appearance of ampicillin resistance among strains of H. influenzae almost two decades ago necessitated the shift from single-drug therapy (ampicillin) to a two-drug approach (ampicillin-chloramphenicol) in the treatment of meningitis of unknown cause in this age group, pending results of culture. Now, ceftriaxone (same dosage as for H. influenzae meningitis) or cefotaxime is most commonly employed in many pediatric centers. *In adults,* therapy with ampicillin or penicillin is directed at the most common community-acquired pathogens (S. pneumoniae and N. meningitidis; L. monocytogenes in older adults and in the previously mentioned high-risk groups). In the highly penicillin-allergic individual, trimethoprim-sulfamethoxazole is a suitable alternative in the treatment of Listeria meningitis. Because H. influenzae type b infections appear to be increasing in adults, and because of the increased incidence of gram-negative bacillary and staphylococcal meningitis in certain clinical settings, broader initial therapy may be indicated if clinical features suggest unusual organisms.

Duration of Therapy. The frequency of cerebrospinal fluid examinations depends on the clinical course, but a repeat exam-

---

*Intrathecal use is not mentioned in the manufacturer's package insert approved by the U.S. Food and Drug Administration. Therefore its use in these circumstances must be considered investigational.

ination should be done in 24 to 48 hours if there has not been satisfactory improvement. Routine "end-of-treatment" CSF examination is unnecessary in most patients with the common types of community-acquired bacterial meningitis. Meningococci are rapidly eliminated from the circulation and CSF with appropriate antimicrobial therapy, which should be continued for 5 to 7 days after the patient becomes afebrile. If the patient has responded well, a follow-up lumbar puncture is not necessary. *H. influenzae* meningitis should be treated for 10 days (at least for 7 days after the patient becomes afebrile). Follow-up CSF examination may be omitted in those patients who have responded with rapid clinical resolution of the meningitis. In pneumococcal meningitis antimicrobial treatment should be continued for 10 to 14 days and follow-up examination of the CSF should be done. More prolonged therapy is indicated with concomitant parameningeal infection. Treatment of gram-negative bacillary meningitis with parenteral antimicrobials is prolonged, usually for a minimum of 3 weeks (particularly in patients with a recent neurosurgical procedure) in order to prevent relapse. Repeated examinations of the CSF are necessary both during and at the conclusion of treatment to determine whether bacteriologic cure has been achieved.

Other Aspects of Treatment. Occasional patients with acute bacterial meningitis develop marked brain swelling (CSF pressure exceeding 450 mm H_2O), which may lead to temporal lobe or cerebellar herniation following lumbar puncture. To reduce this increased pressure, an intravenous infusion of 20 per cent mannitol solution (0.25 to 0.5 gram per kilogram) is administered over 20 to 30 minutes. Continued control of increased intracranial pressure, if needed thereafter, may be effected with mannitol, dexamethasone (10 mg intravenously, followed by 4 mg every 6 hours), or both. Brain swelling is about the only current indication for the use of corticosteroids in the treatment of pyogenic meningitis in adults; they should be employed only when the appropriate antimicrobial drugs are administered. Fluid restriction (1200 to 1500 ml daily in adults) is advisable during the first 24 to 48 hours to minimize brain swelling.

In a recent placebo-controlled trial of adjunctive dexamethasone therapy in community-acquired childhood bacterial meningitis, those treated with the corticosteroid became afebrile earlier and were less likely to have complicating bilateral sensorineural hearing loss. However, complicating gastrointestinal bleeding occurred in several patients, dictating caution if this approach is considered in the treatment of severe childhood meningitis. In mild cases of bacterial meningitis use of dexamethasone to reduce the incidence of sensorineural hearing loss should await results of confirmatory studies. There is no evidence in adults, as yet, of a similar reduction in the incidence of sensorineural hearing loss with adjunctive corticosteroids.

Patients with acute bacterial meningitis should receive constant nursing attention to ensure prompt recognition of seizures and to prevent aspiration. If seizures occur, they should be treated acutely with diazepam (Valium) administered slowly intravenously in a dose of 5 to 10 mg in the adult. Maintenance anticonvulsant therapy can be continued thereafter with intravenous phenytoin (Dilantin) until the medication can be administered orally. Sedation should be avoided because of the danger of respiratory depression and aspiration.

Surgical treatment of an accompanying pyogenic focus such as mastoiditis should be carried out when complete recovery from the meningitis has occurred, but under continuing antibiotic administration. Rarely, the mastoid infection (e.g., Bezold abscess) is so hyperacute that early drainage may be required after 48 hours or so of antibiotic therapy when the acute meningeal process has subsided somewhat.

Berk SL, McCabe WR: Meningitis caused by gram-negative bacilli. Ann Intern Med 93:253, 1980. *Good descriptions of gram-negative bacillary meningitis occurring spontaneously and after surgery.*

Del Rio M, Skelton S, Chrane D, et al.: Ceftriaxone versus ampicillin and chloramphenicol for treatment of bacterial meningitis in children. Lancet 1:1241, 1983. *A clinical and bacteriologic study of meningitis in 78 children showing the equivalence of ceftriaxone treatment to that of the heretofore conventional regimen.*

Dodge PR, Davis H, Feigin RD, et al.: Prospective evaluation of hearing impairment as a sequela of acute bacterial meningitis. N Engl J Med 311:869, 1984. *An excellent detailed prospective study of deafness as a complication of childhood meningitis. A model study of this sort.*

Durack DT, Spanos A: End-of-treatment spinal tap in bacterial meningitis. Is it worthwhile? JAMA 248:75, 1982. *Places in perspective the role of end-of-treatment CSF examination.*

Geiseler PJ, Nelson KE, Levin S, et al.: Community-acquired purulent meningitis: A review of 1316 cases during the antibiotic era, 1954–1976. Rev Infect Dis 2:725, 1980. *Extensive experience at one of the last contagious disease hospitals in the United States is recounted. Effects of prior antibiotic therapy on culture results are particularly well studied.*

Hyslop NE Jr, Montgomery WW: Diagnosis and management of meningitis associated with cerebrospinal leaks. *In* Remington JS, Swartz MN (eds.): Current Clinical Topics in Infectious Diseases, 3. New York, McGraw-Hill Book Company, 1982, pp 254–285. *Most complete review of the bacteriology, anatomy, diagnostic approach, and surgical repair of CSF leaks associated with meningitis.*

Lebel MH, Freij BJ, Syrogiannopoulos GA, et al.: Dexamethasone therapy for bacterial meningitis. Results of two double-blind, placebo-controlled trials. N Engl J Med 319:964, 1988. *Results from a controlled trial involving 200 infants and children with bacterial meningitis indicate that dexamethasone as adjunctive therapy with antibiotics (ceftriaxone or cefuroxime) reduced the incidence of moderate or severe bilateral sensorineural hearing loss.*

New PFJ, Davis KR: The role of CT scanning in diagnosis of infections of the central nervous system. *In* Remington JS, Swartz MN (eds.): Current Clinical Topics in Infectious Diseases, 1. New York, McGraw-Hill Book Company, 1980, pp 1–33. *Comprehensive review of the changes on CT scan in a wide variety of CNS infections. Large number of illustrative scans with good descriptions.*

Saez-Llorens X, Ramilo O, Mustafa MM, et al.: Molecular pathophysiology of bacterial meningitis: Current concepts and therapeutic implications. J Pediatr 116:671, 1990. *A thorough review of the bacterial components implicated in initiating toxic effects in the central nervous system, the cytokines involved in enhancing the inflammatory response in the subarachnoid space, and potential therapeutic interventions.*

Sande MA, Smith AL, Root RL (eds.): Bacterial Meningitis. New York, Churchill–Livingstone, 1985. *A collection of articles reviewing current issues and recent progress in understanding bacterial meningitis. Provides valuable insights in pathogenesis and pathophysiology.*

Schaad UB, Suter S, Gianella-Borradori A, et al.: A comparison of ceftriaxone and cefuroxime for the treatment of bacterial meningitis in children. N Engl J Med 322:141, 1990. *This study of 106 infants and children with bacterial meningitis indicates that in a direct comparison ceftriaxone produces more rapid sterilization of CSF and is less frequently complicated by sensorineural hearing loss than is cefuroxime.*

Swartz MN, Dodge PR: Bacterial meningitis—a review of selected aspects. N Engl J Med 272:725, 779, 842, 898, 954, 1003, 1965. *Detailed account of experience at the Massachusetts General Hospital. Particularly good on clinical aspects, neurologic complications, and differential diagnosis.*

Tunkel AR, Wispelwey B, Scheld WM: Bacterial meningitis: Recent advances in pathophysiology and treatment. Ann Intern Med 112:610, 1990. *An up-to-date and comprehensive review of the pathogenesis, pathophysiology, and treatment of bacterial meningitis. Practical therapeutic guidelines are presented.*

302 Meningococcal Disease

DEFINITION. Meningococcal infections are caused by *Neisseria meningitidis*. The best known syndromes are *meningococcal meningitis* ("epidemic cerebrospinal meningitis") and *fulminant meningococcemia*. Infections also occur in the upper and lower respiratory tracts, joints, pericardium, eyes, and genitourinary tract.

ETIOLOGY. *N. meningitidis* is a gram-negative coccus that appears on smears of infected fluids as biscuit-shaped diplococci, located either extracellularly or within polymorphonuclear leukocytes. Colonies are best isolated on blood, "chocolate," or enriched Mueller-Hinton agar in an atmosphere of 3 to 10 per cent CO_2. Modified Thayer-Martin selective medium is useful in detection of meningococcal carriers or in initial isolation of *N. meningitidis* from areas with an extensive indigenous flora. The organism is susceptible to drying or chilling, and specimens should be inoculated and incubated promptly. Sodium polyethylolesulfonate, frequently included in commercial blood culture media as an anticoagulant and to neutralize inhibitory factors in human blood, may inhibit isolation of occasional strains of *Neisseria* species.

Since other *Neisseria* species and related organisms (*Moraxella catarrhalis*), as well as morphologically similar gram-negative coccobacilli (e.g., other *Moraxella* species, *Acinetobacter*, *Kingella*), may be isolated from clinical specimens, biochemical and immunologic methods are needed for identification. *Neisseria* species are oxidase positive. Whereas *N. gonorrhoeae* ferments only glucose (but not maltose or lactose) to acid, *N. meningitidis* ferments both glucose and maltose (but not lactose). *N. lactamica*, a species sometimes present in throat cultures, may be mistaken for the meningococcus, since it too ferments both glucose and maltose; however, it also utilizes lactose. Occasional maltose-negative strains of *N. meningitidis* have been noted; fluorescent antibody or coagglutination tests or electrophoretic analysis of hexokinase isoenzymes may be helpful in distinguishing such strains from *N. gonorrhoeae*, particularly when isolated from atypical locations.

N. meningitidis are classified by serogroup and further defined by serotype. There are 13 serogroups, including groups A, B, C, D, X, Y, Z, 29E, and W135; they differ in the structures of their capsular polysaccharides and can be identified by agglutination reactions with specific antisera. Most meningococcal disease is due to strains belonging to groups A, B, C, and Y. Twenty to 50 per cent of isolates from carriers are nongroupable (unencapsulated). Subcapsular protein antigens located in the outer bacterial membrane have been used to identify 20 serotypes among the various serogroups, providing a classification useful in epidemiologic studies. Serotype 2 (2a, 2b) strains are responsible for most cases of meningococcal disease due to group B (50 per cent) and group C (80 per cent) organisms (and also are associated with groups Y and W135), but they are rarely isolated from carriers not in direct contact with clinical cases. In contrast, other serotypes are commonly isolated, but primarily from carriers. More detailed differentiation between strains can be carried out by including lipopolysaccharide typing in addition. Group A meningococcal strains show no variation in their outer membrane proteins and are unrelated serologically to the serotypes of other groups.

Strains of *N. meningitidis* produce extracellular proteases that cleave the IgA1 heavy chain in the hinge region. Although the role of this protease in infection is unknown, its elaboration also by the other principal causes of bacterial meningitis (*H. influenzae*, *S. pneumoniae*) and the importance of IgA in mucosal immunity at the pharyngeal portal for these organisms suggest a possible role in pathogenicity.

Fresh isolates of *N. meningitidis* from the pharynx of carriers and from patients with meningococcal disease contain pili, which appear to have an important role in attachment to nonciliated columnar human nasopharyngeal cells.

Meningococci contain endotoxins, and these lipopolysaccharides may play a role in the purpura and other clinical features of meningococcemia.

INCIDENCE. *N. meningitidis* is second only to *H. influenzae* as a cause of bacterial meningitis in this country. In the period 1984 to 1990, 2400 to 2700 cases of meningococcal infection were reported annually in the United States.

EPIDEMIOLOGY. The natural reservoir of *N. meningitidis* is the human nasopharynx, and transmission occurs principally through airborne droplets or close contact. Infection may occur as the *asymptomatic carrier state* (the most common form), *endemic disease* (sporadic cases occurring at a relatively stable rate), *hyperendemic disease* (cyclic waves of increased incidence), or *epidemic disease* (major outbreaks involving large portions of the population or focal outbreaks involving particularly lower socioeconomic groups).

Carrier State. Nasopharyngeal carrier rates may fluctuate widely. The rate varies with age: 0.5 to 1.0 per cent in children 3 to 48 months of age, 5 per cent in those 14 to 17 years of age, and 20 to 40 per cent in young adults. In the nonepidemic setting carriage usually lasts weeks to months. The carrier rate in close family contacts of a case of meningococcal disease is increased and may reach 40 per cent. In crowded populations (e.g., military training camps) the carrier rate has ranged between 20 and 60 per cent and has reached 90 per cent during epidemics. Although it has often been stated that meningococcal outbreaks occur when the rate of nasopharyngeal carriage exceeds 20 per cent in a military camp, there is in reality no clear relation between the overall carriage rate in a community and the occurrence of meningococcal disease. The strain (serotype)-specific acquisition rate appears to be a more reliable indicator of an outbreak than the group-specific carriage rate.

Spread of disease appears to be mediated by carriers rather than by direct case-to-case transmission. An adult family member generally is the one who brings *N. meningitidis* into a household, where it spreads to others and often colonizes younger children and infants last. As yet unknown host and environmental factors are of decisive importance in determining whether the organism will be confined to the nasopharynx or dissemination will take place.

Meningococcal Disease. The annual attack rate for meningococcal disease in the United States in recent years has been about 1.2 cases per 100,000 population. The highest incidence is in the first year of life (17.1 per 100,000), declining in the 1- to 4-year age group (5.2 per 100,000), and ultimately reaching the level of 0.3 per 100,000 in adults. During epidemics of meningococcal disease, overall annual attack rates of 5 to 24 cases per 100,000 are observed (as high as 370 per 100,000 in Sao Paulo, Brazil, in 1974), and the age incidence tends to shift to older children and young adults. The peak incidence is in the winter and early spring.

During a nonepidemic period the risk of meningococcal illness for household contacts of an initial case is about 3 per 1000 (500- to 1000-fold higher than the overall endemic rate for meningococcal disease) and stems from the higher carriage rate in this setting. The secondary attack rate appears to be age related, with most cases occurring in younger children.

Major meningococcal epidemics, caused primarily by group A strains, tend to recur at 20- to 30-year intervals (e.g., as occurred during World Wars I and II). More circumscribed outbreaks have taken place in interepidemic periods, as in Detroit in 1929, when about 750 cases occurred. Aside from several minor urban outbreaks, particularly among alcoholics, group A strains have only rarely been implicated in meningococcal disease in North America during the past decade. However, serious epidemics caused by group A meningococci have occurred in Finland in 1973, in Brazil in 1974, and in northern Nigeria in 1977. The outbreak in Nigeria is but one of many that have occurred about once every 10 years in the "meningitis belt" in sub-Saharan Africa. In the 1948–49 epidemic, about 93,000 cases were reported, with over 14,000 deaths. Although group A meningococci had been susceptible to sulfonamides in the past, resistant strains first appeared in the epidemics in Africa in the late 1960's and subsequently in Brazil and Finland.

Although group A meningococci have been involved in the most extensive epidemics of meningococcal disease, groups B and C have been responsible for focal outbreaks and for *endemic disease* both in this country and abroad. In the United States in 1963 and 1964, outbreaks caused by group B meningococci (noteworthy for their frequent resistance to sulfonamides) occurred in military camps. By 1967 serogroup B was responsible for the majority of infections occurring in military and civilian populations. By the early 1970's serogroup C strains were those most frequently isolated, only to be supplanted by group B in the mid 1970's. Currently, serogroup B accounts for 50 to 55 per cent of cases; serogroup C, for 20 to 25 per cent; serogroup W135, for 15 per cent; serogroup Y, for 10 per cent; and serogroup A, for 1 to 2 per cent.

Just as serogrouping of meningococcal strains has been invaluable in the study of major epidemics and in the development and use of polysaccharide vaccines, serotyping can be helpful in evaluating changes in ambient strains. Between epidemics sporadic cases are caused by heterogeneous strains belonging to many serogroups and a variety of serotypes. In military recruit populations, the serogroup carried is not a valid indicator of epidemic potential. At intervals of 5 to 10 years a single serotype (e.g., serotype 2, present in most disease-related strains of groups B and C and in some strains of groups Y and W135 during this past decade) becomes pre-eminent, producing *hyperendemic disease*, sometimes accompanied by scattered small outbreaks.

Meningococci can be further subdivided by clonal analysis based on the electrophoretic mobilities of a series of cytoplasmic isoenzymes and outer membrane proteins. In an analysis of over 400 serogroup A strains of diverse epidemiologic origins isolated from around the world from 1915 to 1983 (including 23 outbreaks or epidemics since 1960), seven clones have been identified as responsible for sets of epidemics. At least two of these sets represent mutually exclusive pandemics, involving numerous epidemics between 1967–75 and 1973–83, respectively. Case strains showed little clonal diversity during individual epidemics, indicating that such a typing scheme can be useful in defining the etiology of outbreaks.

Similarly, several serogroup B epidemics have involved changes in serotypes from 2a to 2b. This change did not result from antigenic drift or genetic recombination among strains, but rather represented clonal replacement, since these serotypes are linked to distinctive groups of clones.

Nosocomial transmission of infection occasionally occurs. Meningococcal meningitis has developed in several physicians who gave mouth-to-mouth resuscitation to infected patients. Group Y meningococci particularly have been implicated in meningococcal pneumonia, and such patients, if not isolated, may be responsible for nosocomial spread of infection.

Immunity. The age-specific incidence of meningococcal disease is inversely proportional to the prevalence of antimeningococcal bactericidal antibodies (against serogroups A, B, C). At birth, over 50 per cent of infants have bactericidal antibody as a result of transplacental transfer. Group B organisms present a special problem that accounts for the occurrence of group B meningococcal disease in neonates. Because the capsular polysaccharide of group B meningococci is a polymer of α 2–8–linked sialic acid and is immunologically identical to oligosaccharides of several human glycoproteins (including brain gangliosides), immunologic tolerance for this molecule exists in humans. IgM antibody can be induced but without the usual switch to IgG. As a result, maternal antibody to group B capsular antigen is entirely IgM and cannot be passed transplacentally. All infants are born lacking antibody to group B (but not to other common serogroup) capsular antigens. Because the capsular polysaccharide of E. coli K1 is the same, infants are born also lacking antibody to this organism, the major cause of neonatal sepsis and meningitis.

From 6 to 24 months of age, the prevalence of antibodies is lowest, and thereafter it increases to early adulthood, when over 70 per cent of individuals have bactericidal activity. The protective role of bactericidal antibodies against N. meningitidis was demonstrated during an outbreak of group C meningitis among army recruits in 1968. Eleven per cent of recruits lacked serum antibody against the outbreak-associated strain, and one quarter of these susceptibles acquired this strain during their training period. Of the susceptibles exposed, 38 per cent developed systemic meningococcal disease; in contrast, only 1 per cent of the entire trainee group developed disease.

IgA antibody to meningococcal polysaccharide may have a paradoxic effect. When a large part of an individual's antibodies to a meningococcal serogroup is of this class, serum complement-mediated immune lysis by IgM is blocked, enhancing susceptibility to meningococcal disease. This was demonstrated in several outbreaks. Sera drawn from susceptibles at the time of acute meningococcal infection lacked bactericidal activity for the infecting strain; removal of IgA restored this activity which was in the IgM class. This odd phenomenon is observed for a short time following the induction of IgA by asymptomatic carriage of N. meningitidis or an immunologically related organism.

Following meningococcal meningitis serum bactericidal antibody develops, and the patient is immune to clinical reinfection with the same serogroup. However, this is not the usual means of acquiring immunity. Nasopharyngeal carriage of N. meningitidis is an effective immunizing process, producing rises in bactericidal antibody within 5 to 12 days of acquisition of the organism. About 90 per cent of carriers of group B, C, or Y meningococci develop increased serum bactericidal titers, primarily to the colonizing strain but also to heterologous strains. Similarly, nasopharyngeal carriage of nongroupable meningococci, strains rarely causing human disease, can induce antibodies against various groupable pathogenic isolates.

The group-specific capsular polysaccharides of group A and group C meningococci are good immunogens and have been used in successful vaccines. The capsular polysaccharide of group B meningococci is a very poor immunogen because of its immunologic identity with oligosaccharides of several human glycoproteins, and this likely contributes to the failure to develop an effective group B vaccine.

In young children, colonization with N. lactamica may induce cross-reactive antibodies to N. meningitidis and thus contribute to natural immunity. N. lactamica is relatively avirulent and has only rarely been involved in systemic infections. During the first 8 years of life the age-related prevalence of meningococcal carriage is between 0.5 and 2 per cent, whereas that of N. lactamica is considerably higher (4 to 20 per cent).

In addition to antibody, complement is an important component of serum bactericidal activity. Isolated congenital deficiency of one of the late complement components (C5–C8) is rare and has been associated with recurrent or, occasionally, chronic (chronic meningococcemia) infections with N. meningitidis. Repeated episodes of meningococcal meningitis have occurred in patients with late complement component deficiencies in the absence of enhanced susceptibility to organisms other than N. meningitidis. Measurement of total hemolytic complement is helpful for screening purposes in a patient with recurrent systemic Neisseria infections. The course of infection, whether meningitis or meningococcemia, is not unusual, and the response to antimicrobial treatment is satisfactory. Complement deficiency may be an important risk factor, as well, for the occurrence of first episodes of endemic meningococcal disease. Although the latter occur in persons with deficiencies of early-acting components (C2–C4), which are often due to complement-depleting underlying diseases (systemic lupus, multiple myeloma, C3 nephritic factor, hepatic failure), their frequencies are similar to those of infections caused by other encapsulated bacteria. In contrast, essentially the only clinical features of deficiency of late components are meningococcal infections. Fulminant meningococcal disease has also occurred in several members of a family with properdin deficiency. Preliminary evidence suggests that immunization with meningococcal vaccine can correct the bactericidal defect in sera of affected male members with familial properdin deficiency.

PATHOGENESIS AND PATHOLOGY. The factors that determine whether initial exposure to N. meningitidis will result in benign nasopharyngeal carriage or serious invasive infection are unclear. Binding by pili to microvilli of nonciliated columnar mucosal cells of the nasopharynx may allow surface multiplication and colonization by N. meningitidis. Transport across these specialized mucosal cells appears to occur within phagocytic vacuoles and provides a potential mechanism for invasive meningococcal disease. About one third of patients with invasive infection have had antecedent symptoms referable to the upper respiratory tract. Whether these prodromal symptoms are produced by N. meningitidis or a predisposing viral respiratory infection is difficult to determine, particularly since many cases of meningococcal disease occur in winter when viral respiratory infections are frequent. A simultaneous outbreak of meningococcal disease and influenza A2 infection has occurred in a closed institutional setting. The predisposing role of influenza for meningococcal lower respiratory infections may be clearer (e.g., numerous cases of meningococcal pneumonia complicating influenza during the 1918–19 pandemic).

The incubation period from initiation of nasopharyngeal infection to bloodstream dissemination is probably under 10 days. The incubation period may be quite short, judging by the fact that the interval between primary and secondary cases in the same household is often only 1 to 4 days. Also, among prospectively studied military recruits cultured within 7 days preceding hospitalization for meningococcal disease, only about 20 per cent were carriers of the implicated strain. Once the organism has entered the circulation, the predominant (over 90 per cent) clinical expression is meningitis or meningococcemia.

The pathologic findings in acute meningococcemia are observed when shock and disseminated intravascular coagulation have occurred. The skin lesions show evidence of fibrin thrombi and vasculitis in small blood vessels. N. meningitidis can be seen in endothelial cells and in neutrophils surrounding damaged vessels. The prominent purpura has been attributed to the enhanced capacity to elicit the dermal Shwartzman reaction of its endotoxin compared to endotoxin from enteric gram-negative bacilli. Hemorrhagic adrenal infarction is often observed in patients with fulminant meningococcemia (Waterhouse-Friderichsen syndrome). Shock in this disease is a consequence of bacteremia and not of adrenal failure, since (1) fulminant meningococcemia can occur without adrenal hemorrhage, (2) serum cortisol levels are normal or elevated, and (3) patients who have recovered have not developed Addison's disease. It has been suggested that the shock, purpura, and widespread microvascular thrombi are consequences of an endotoxin-initiated generalized Shwartzman-like reaction or endotoxin-activated disseminated intravascular coagulation. Increased levels of circulating endotoxin are associated with the development of severe septic shock and death in systemic meningococcal disease. Serum levels of tumor necrosis factor, a cytokine induced in macrophages by endotoxin, correlate with the severity of meningococcemia. Depressed levels of complement components are found in some patients with acute meningococcemia and may reflect complement activation by circulating endotoxin. Interstitial myocarditis is observed in about 70 per cent of cases of fatal meningococcal disease.

CLINICAL MANIFESTATIONS. Overt illness develops when the initial, often minimally symptomatic nasopharyngeal infection has progressed to bloodstream invasion. The subsequent clinical picture may be mild, or sudden in onset and fulminant, and may reflect principally the bacteremia or features referable to metastatic localization of infection. The most common clinical syndromes are acute meningococcemia, acute purulent meningitis, and a combination of the two (meningococcemia-meningitis).

Meningitis. Most cases occur in children between 3 months of age and adolescence. Isolated meningitis is less common than meningococcemia-meningitis. The clinical picture may be dominated by manifestations of either meningococcemia or meningitis. In the latter instance the findings are similar to those of meningitis caused by any of the common pyogens (see Ch. 301). Predisposing acute otitis media or pneumonia is unusual in contrast to *H. influenzae* or pneumococcal meningitis. The onset of meningeal symptomatology (1) may be rapid (less than 24 hours) without premonitory symptomatology, (2) may follow an upper respiratory infection of 1 or 2 weeks' duration, or (3) may evolve gradually over several days of upper respiratory or nonlocalizing symptoms. Rarely, the clinical course with fever and meningismus may be indolent and persist unchanged for a week or longer, suggesting the diagnosis of "aseptic" meningitis. In the last-named instance CSF examination during this period may reveal minimal or no increase in cell count and no organisms on Gram-stained smear, but *N. meningitidis* may be isolated, indicating early meningeal involvement. A "clear" CSF in this setting should *not* preclude careful culture. The rapid onset of delirium is seen occasionally in bacterial meningitis (more frequently meningococcal), but it also may occur with a temporal lobe abscess or encephalitis. The neurologic features and complications of meningococcal meningitis are generally the same as for other bacterial meningitides.

The course of meningococcal meningitis may differ from that of other pyogenic meningitides in the occasional occurrence during convalescence of a nonseptic arthritis-pericarditis syndrome.

Meningococcemia. About 20 per cent of patients with meningococcal disease have meningococcemia without meningitis. The clinical expression of meningococcemia varies from an acute process (mild systemic illness or rapidly lethal course) to a chronic, indolent, relapsing disease that may go on for months.

Mild Acute Meningococcemia. This is the most common form of meningococcemia, characterized by the rapid development of malaise, fever, chills, myalgias, and arthralgias, often following a minor upper respiratory infection. In a few patients diarrhea has been an early symptom. The subsequent course may follow one of several paths: (1) Symptoms may abate in 2 or 3 days, and the diagnosis is made in retrospect when *N. meningitidis* is isolated from a blood culture. (2) Initial symptomatology is followed over 24 to 48 hours by recurrent chills and the appearance of erythematous macular lesions, particularly on the extremities, often accompanied by petechiae. In more severe infections, purpura and ecchymotic areas with gunmetal gray necrotic centers appear. Tachycardia and tachypnea are prominent. Mild hypotension may be present, and shock is a feature if fulminant meningococcemia ensues. In some patients headache may appear and confusion and stiff neck develop; the syndrome then becomes one of combined *meningococcemia-meningitis*. A meningoencephalopathic picture has been described in up to 15 per cent of patients. This probably represents a heterogeneous group (some with meningitis and others with fulminant meningococcemia and central nervous system changes secondary to shock), in whom confusion, delirium, or coma is striking. (3) Occasionally, initial malaise, fever, and arthralgias (accompanied by a few macular and petechial skin lesions) may persist for about a week, during which one or more joint effusions may develop. Blood cultures reveal *N. meningitidis*, and all manifestations promptly subside on treatment with penicillin.

Fulminant Meningococcemia. This is the most dramatic form of infection, with an abrupt onset and extraordinarily rapid progression (occasionally less than 10 hours from onset to fatal termination). It occurs in about 10 per cent of patients with meningococcal disease. Violent chills, high fever, dizziness, headache, and profound weakness develop over a few hours. Petechiae appear initially on the extremities; they rapidly increase in number and coalesce as new ones appear in the conjunctivae and buccal mucosa. Hypotension with peripheral vasoconstriction quickly appears. Purpura soon develops (Fig. 302-1). At this point the patient may still be febrile or may have become hypothermic. As shock supervenes, restlessness, mental obtundation, and coma may follow in rapid succession. Disseminated intravascular coagulation (DIC) is commonly present, with enlarging hemorrhagic areas in the skin and sometimes mucosal and gastrointestinal bleeding. Cardiac (myocarditis) and respiratory ("shock lung") failure may be terminal events. *The relentless course, once shock develops, makes mandatory early diagnosis*

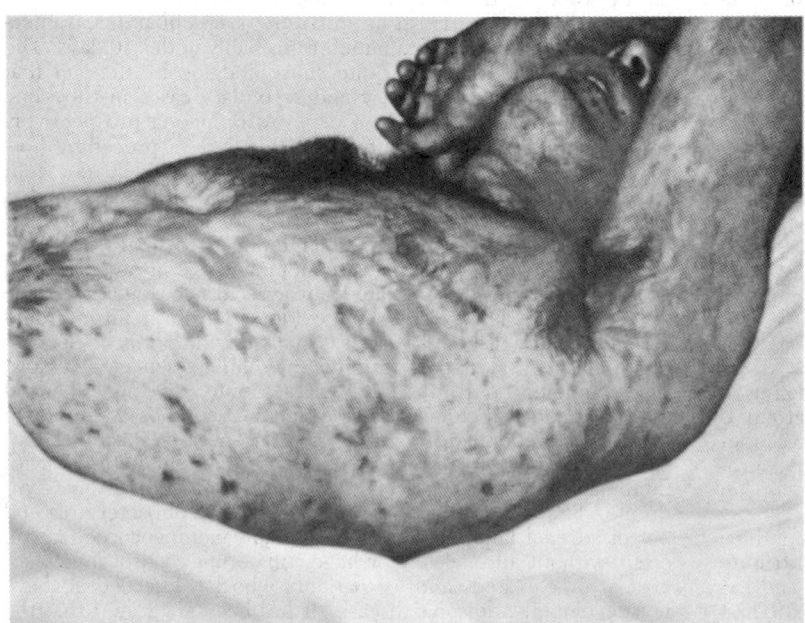

FIGURE 302-1. Skin lesions in fulminating meningococcemia. (Courtesy of Dr. Worth B. Daniels.)

and immediate institution of antibiotic treatment even while parts of the initial examination are being performed.

Chronic Meningococcemia. This uncommon form of meningococcemia is characterized by intermittent febrile episodes lasting 1 to 6 days, or, rarely, by sustained fevers for several weeks. It begins with chills, migratory arthralgias (or occasionally mild arthritis), and headache, but minimal toxicity. A transient polymorphous (erythematous macules and papules, rare petechiae, and purpuric nodules) nonpruritic rash appears with each febrile episode. The total number of skin lesions is small, and Gram's stain and culture only rarely reveal the etiologic agent. Biopsy reveals a leukocytoclastic angiitis, which may be mistaken for a collagen disease or allergic vasculitis. Splenomegaly is observed in 20 per cent of patients. Blood cultures are not positive during apyrexial periods and may not yield the organism until the second or third febrile episode.

Untreated, about 20 per cent of patients ultimately develop meningitis. Rarer complications include endocarditis and epididymitis.

Where the organism resides between episodes is unclear. Throat cultures frequently have not revealed meningococci. The occurrence of chronic meningococcemia in several patients with congenital late complement component deficiencies suggests a possible factor in pathogenesis.

Upper Respiratory Tract Infection. How frequently nasopharyngeal infection is symptomatic is unclear. Nasopharyngeal symptoms preceding some systemic meningococcal infections may be due to this organism or to ambient viral respiratory infections.

Pneumonia. Meningococcal pneumonia is much more often of bronchogenic than of hematogenous origin. Other than during the 1918 influenza pandemic, it has been reported only rarely until this past decade. Primary meningococcal pneumonia is most often due to group Y; 15 years ago among recruits pneumonia caused by group Y was the most common form of meningococcal disease. Primary meningococcal pneumonia may be segmental, lobar, or bronchopneumonic in pattern. It sometimes follows antecedent influenza or adenoviral infection. Clinical features are similar to those of community-acquired pneumonias. The onset may be gradual or abrupt. Lower lobes are usually involved. Bacteremia occurs in about 15 per cent of cases. In some patients purulent sputum is produced, containing numerous gram-negative diplococci; in others sputum is scanty, and diagnosis is made on a transtracheal aspirate or by blood culture. Response to treatment with penicillin is prompt.

Meningococcal pneumonia occasionally develops in the course of clinical meningococcemia or meningitis, but the clinical picture is dominated by the extrapulmonary aspects.

To be distinguished from meningococcal pneumonia are pulmonary infections due to *Moraxella catarrhalis* (gram-negative biscuit-shaped diplococci) or rarely to other usually noninvasive *Neisseria* species (e.g., *N. sicca*). Such infections usually take the form of acute exacerbations of chronic bronchitis or of pneumonia, occurring particularly in immunodeficient individuals, patients with chronic pulmonary disease, or as a nosocomial infection. *M. catarrhalis* can also be the cause of acute sinusitis, bacteremia, and, rarely, meningitis. In children this organism, after *S. pneumoniae* and *H. influenzae*, is the third most common cause of acute otitis media. β-Lactamase production occurs in 75 per cent of strains isolated currently from children. Alternatives to ampicillin or penicillin for therapy, based on in vitro susceptibilities, include trimethoprim-sulfamethoxazole, amoxicillin-clavulanic acid, chloramphenicol, tetracycline, and cefuroxime.

Arthritis. Arthritis complicates 2 to 16 per cent of acute meningococcal illness and may take several forms: (1) *Isolated, acute suppurative meningococcal arthritis* is a rare type occurring in the absence of meningitis or clinical meningococcemia. The joint fluid has the characteristics of septic arthritis. (2) *Early onset (first 2 to 3 days) arthritis* during meningococcal meningitis or meningococcemia is the most common form. It is a polyarthritis with acutely inflamed joints; effusions are small or absent. It responds promptly to penicillin. (3) *Late onset (fourth to tenth day, when meningitis is subsiding) arthritis* is commonly a subacute mono- or oligoarthritis accompanied by joint effusions. It is associated with recrudescence of fever, pleuropericarditis, and, occasionally, new papulobullous skin lesions. Synovial and pericardial fluids are characteristically serosanguineous (but sometimes purulent) and sterile. Immunopathologic study of synovial lesions implicates immune complex formation in their genesis. Treatment involves joint aspiration and the use of anti-inflammatory agents.

Pericarditis. Pericarditis complicates 2 to 20 per cent of meningococcal disease. It may take several forms: (1) *Early onset pericarditis*, appearing in the first several days of clinical meningococcemia or meningitis, may be purulent and may be due to invasion by *N. meningitidis*. (2) *Late onset pericarditis*, developing 4 to 10 days after onset of meningitis, may cause large sterile, serosanguineous effusions. The favorable response to anti-inflammatory agents and adrenal corticosteroids supports the proposed role of hypersensitivity in pathogenesis. (3) *Isolated purulent pericarditis*, occurring in the absence of meningitis or clinical meningococcemia, is the least common form of meningococcal pericarditis and usually presents with a purulent effusion and tamponade requiring surgical intervention.

Other Meningococcal Infections. Ocular involvement (panophthalmitis, conjunctivitis) occurs in less than 1 per cent of patients with meningococcal disease. Primary conjunctivitis, an acute purulent process, is even less common. Since dissemination develops in 10 per cent of children with primary meningococcal conjunctivitis, systemic therapy with penicillin should be employed along with topical antimicrobials.

Genital tract and anal infections with *N. meningitidis* occasionally occur, the latter in homosexual males. In the female symptomatic or asymptomatic infections of the cervix and vagina may be associated with salpingitis or subsequent clinical meningococcemia. Urethral infection is less common than anal infection but is usually symptomatic. Treatment, as for gonococcal infection, is warranted to eliminate symptomatic disease and to prevent the rare instance of disseminated infection.

COURSE AND COMPLICATIONS. Acute meningococcemia may run a varied course, from that of mild disease to that of fulminant illness with death in a day or less. Certain features (particularly if present simultaneously) indicate a poor prognosis: (1) petechiae for less than 12 hours prior to hospitalization (rapid development of crops of new petechiae and purpura from one hour to the next is ominous); (2) shock; (3) fever above 40° C; (4) absence of meningitis; (5) leukopenia; (6) thrombocytopenia or evidence of DIC; and (7) extremes of age.

Extensive purpura, acral cyanosis, hemorrhagic bullae, and peripheral gangrene are features of fulminant meningococcemia, usually occurring in the presence of shock and DIC. DIC may be evident on hospitalization or may develop precipitously in some patients who are stable initially. In acute DIC platelets, fibrinogen, prothrombin, and Factors V, VII, and VIII are reduced. Abnormalities in three screening tests (prothrombin time prolongation, platelet count reduction, hypofibrinogenemia) aid in detection of DIC, which occurs to some extent in about one quarter of patients with meningococcemia. The partial thromboplastin time may also be prolonged. Confirmation is provided by demonstration of circulating fibrin degradation products in concentrations greater than 40 μg per milliliter. These coagulation defects can result in upper gastrointestinal bleeding, hematuria, and bleeding from the respiratory tract. Despite all therapeutic interventions, some patients show progressive deterioration with marked tachycardia, hyperventilation, refractory shock, metabolic acidosis, deepening coma, and "shock lung." Myocardial involvement may be manifest as either transient electrocardiographic changes or left ventricular failure.

In those who recover, resolution of the hemorrhagic or gangrenous lesions is slow and may require skin grafting. Areas of the hands and feet may remain edematous, cold, and cyanotic and may show demarcation after some weeks.

DIAGNOSIS. Laboratory Findings. Bacteriologic diagnosis is established by the finding of organisms on stained smears from an infected area (in an appropriate clinical setting), by isolation of *N. meningitidis* from blood or infected body fluids, or by demonstration by latex agglutination of group A, B, C, or Y polysaccharide antigen in blood or CSF. Blood cultures reveal *N. meningitidis* in about one third of patients with meningococcal meningitis and in 50 to 75 per cent with clinical meningococcemia or meningococcemia-meningitis. In rare patients with fulminant meningococcemia, diplococci can be seen on Gram-stained smears of blood or buffy coat. Demonstration of organisms on scrapings from skin lesions in acute meningococcemia has been variable: 70 per cent in one study, but much lower in more recent experience.

Since *N. gonorrhoeae* can be isolated from the pharynx and *N. meningitidis* can occasionally be found in the anogenital area, since both species may invade the bloodstream, and since gonococci and *N. lactamica* have on rare occasions been implicated in meningitis, accurate bacteriologic identification is important. However, 0.5 to 5 per cent of meningococci are maltose negative and may thus resemble gonococci and cause confusion.

Meningococcal polysaccharide antigen is demonstrated in the CSF of about 70 per cent of patients with meningococcal meningitis. Antigen is detected in the blood of 10 to 25 per cent of patients with meningococcemia, and its presence is associated with a poorer prognosis and higher incidence of late onset arthritis.

The CSF findings in meningococcal meningitis are those of pyogenic meningitis.

Differential Diagnosis. The differential diagnosis of meningococcal meningitis in the absence of clinical meningococcemia is that of acute meningitis with a purulent CSF formula. With the meningococcemia-meningitis syndrome it should be remembered that very rare instances of meningitis caused by *H. influenzae* and *S. pneumoniae* may be accompanied by petechial skin lesions. Occasional patients with enteroviral meningitis may have a brisk CSF pleocytosis (up to several thousand cells, with as many as 50 to 80 per cent neutrophils and a maculopetechial rash). Rarely, acute bacterial endocarditis caused by *Staphylococcus aureus* can produce a clinical picture almost indistinguishable from that of meningococcemia-meningitis, with a polymorphonuclear CSF pleocytosis and petechial and purpuric skin lesions. In *S. aureus* endocarditis there are a few skin lesions of purulent purpura which show the etiologic agent on Gram-stained smear. Occasionally measles or other viral exanthems may resemble early meningococcemia. Rocky Mountain spotted fever may mimic meningococcemia, but the absence of meningitis in the former, epidemiologic considerations, and demonstration of the etiologic agent aid in distinguishing between these processes.

Chronic meningococcemia, because of its protean manifestations, may be mistaken for Henoch-Schönlein purpura, acute vasculitis, gonococcemia, rheumatic fever, and subacute bacterial endocarditis.

TREATMENT. Antibiotic Management. As soon as the diagnosis is made, the patient should be put on respiratory isolation to minimize nosocomial spread of infection. Whereas practically all meningococci isolated prior to 1963 were susceptible to sulfadiazine (formerly the treatment of choice), since that time isolates resistant to sulfonamides have become common. Sulfonamide resistance in this country peaked in 1970, when 67 per cent of strains were resistant, and has since decreased (1980) to 12 per cent (8 per cent of group B, 30 per cent of group C, 4 per cent of group W135; all group Y strains susceptible). Should resistance to sulfonamides decline to less than 10 per cent, sulfonamides may again become appropriate drugs for prophylaxis.

Antimicrobial therapy should be initiated *immediately* in patients with suspected meningococcal meningitis or clinical meningococcemia because of the rapidity with which the illness may progress. Intravenous penicillin G is the drug of choice (24 million units daily in the adult in divided doses every 2 to 3 hours) for meningococcal meningitis. Alternatively, intravenous ampicillin can be employed in the adult (12 grams daily in divided doses every 2 to 3 hours). In patients allergic to penicillin, intravenous chloramphenicol (4 to 6 grams daily in the adult) is the recommended alternative, with appropriate monitoring of the hematopoietic system. Third-generation cephalosporins such as cefotaxime and ceftriaxone are active in vitro against *N. meningitidis* and have been used successfully in treatment of meningococcal meningitis. They may now provide an alternative when the use of chloramphenicol is considered. The duration of treatment of meningococcal meningitis and the management of complications are considered in Ch. 301.

Until the mid 1980's clinical isolates were uniformly susceptible to penicillin and ampicillin. However, in the past 5 years penicillin-resistant *N. meningitidis* (Groups B and C) have been isolated from blood and CSF of patients in Spain (up to 5 per cent of isolates), England, Ireland, and South Africa. Almost all of these isolates have been relatively penicillin resistant (non–β-lactamase–producing) strains, with minimum inhibitory concentrations of 0.25 to 0.7 µg per milliliter due at least in part to altered forms of penicillin-binding protein 2. Three isolates (β-lactamase–producing) have been highly penicillin resistant, and at least one of these contained a β-lactamase plasmid. Although high doses of penicillin have been effective in treatment of meningococcemia due to relatively resistant strains, this treatment might not be effective for meningitis due to similar strains or for invasive infections due to β-lactamase–producing strains. Alternative antimicrobial agents in such situations include cefotaxime and chloramphenicol.

Intravenous penicillin G is the treatment for acute clinical meningococcemia without meningitis. Although 8 to 10 million units daily is usually adequate to sterilize the blood and most areas of metastatic infection, it may not provide therapeutic CSF levels in the patient with incipient meningitis. For this reason, initial therapy with "meningitis" doses is often employed. Treatment is continued until the patient has been afebrile for 5 days. Penicillin (5 to 8 million units daily intravenously in the adult) is effective treatment for chronic meningococcemia.

Other Aspects of Treatment. Treatment of severe meningococcemia requires supportive measures to deal with shock and other complications (DIC, congestive failure, metabolic acidosis, "shock lung"). These include cardiovascular monitoring in an intensive care setting, initial volume expansion, use of vasoactive agents, attention to fluid balances, maintenance of adequate oxygenation, and possible use of digoxin. A central venous pressure (CVP) catheter is placed (a flow-directed pulmonary catheter for evaluation of left atrial and ventricular filling pressures may be necessary if cardiac decompensation develops). Volume expansion (dextrose-saline infused rapidly) is necessary initially to assure that intravascular volume is optimal. If there is no sudden or progressive rise in CVP, then volume expansion (utilizing both crystalloid and colloid) is continued until shock is corrected or fluid overload (increased CVP, rales) develops. Urine output should be monitored and maintained at 40 to 50 ml per hour.

If rapid improvement does not follow volume expansion or if the CVP exceeds appropriate limits, a catecholamine should be added to enhance cardiac output and raise arterial pressure to the range of 90 to 100 mm Hg. Dopamine has been widely used because of its ability to increase renal blood flow (at dosage below 6 µg per kilogram per minute) while increasing cardiac contractility. It is administered by continuous intravenous (initial rate of 2 to 5 µg per kilogram per minute) infusion at a rate sufficient to maintain an adequate arterial pressure and urine volume.

Controlled multicenter clinical trials have not shown a beneficial effect of adrenal corticosteroids in high dosage (30 mg per kilogram of methylprednisolone or 6 mg per kilogram of dexamethasone) as adjunctive therapy in sepsis or septic shock. One or two pharmacologic doses (3 mg per kilogram of dexamethasone or 30 mg per kilogram of methylprednisolone intravenously) have been used in patients not responding to the aforementioned initial measures. Smaller maintenance doses do not appear beneficial, and continued administration predisposes to superinfection. If adrenal insufficiency is suspected, replacement doses of corticosteroids are indicated.

Adequate oxygenation is essential in a patient with shock, particularly if meningitis is also a feature (in which hypoxia can aggravate cerebral edema). Oxygen administration, and intubation with ventilatory assistance if needed, should be an integral part of therapy aiming at restoring the arterial Po_2 to appropriate levels (80 to 120 mm Hg). Acidosis should be corrected by intravenous administration of sodium bicarbonate (45 mEq) as needed. Digoxin is not of value in meningococcemic shock but may have a role if fluid overload complicates volume expansion or secondary myocarditis. Generally, diuretics such as furosemide have been of more value in this acute situation.

The initial enthusiasm for heparin treatment of DIC in meningococcemia and septic shock has waned, since evidence of efficacy in reducing mortality has been conflicting despite improvement in coagulation factors. Heparin treatment on the basis of laboratory abnormalities alone is inadvisable. Reversal of hypotension is often associated with improvement in laboratory evidences of

DIC and a halt in further clinical progression of the coagulopathy. Only if bleeding into deep tissues or thrombotic manifestations occur in the presence of DIC might heparinization be considered. After initiation of heparin therapy coagulation factor deficiencies can be repaired by administration of fresh frozen plasma. Once heparin is started, prothrombin time and partial thromboplastin time determinations are no longer helpful in following laboratory evidences of DIC; levels of fibrin degradation products, fibrinogen, and platelets are of greatest assistance.

PREVENTION. *Chemoprophylaxis.* Close contacts (e.g., same household or daycare center, medical personnel exposed by intimate contact prior to institution of proper isolation precautions) of a patient with meningococcal disease are at increased risk of developing systemic disease and should receive chemoprophylaxis. Since secondary (or coprimary) cases usually occur within 4 days of the initial case, prophylactic treatment should begin as soon as the initial case is identified. Rifampin has been shown to be 80 to 90 per cent effective in eliminating meningococci from the nasopharynx of asymptomatic carriers, and minocycline has been almost as effective. Because of reports of vestibular side effects with minocycline, rifampin is the recommended drug for chemoprophylaxis. It is administered for 2 days: to adults at a dosage of 600 mg orally every 12 hours; to children (1 month of age or older) at a dosage of 10 mg per kilogram every 12 hours; and to children under 1 month of age, at a dosage of 5 mg per kilogram every 12 hours. Since even the high doses of penicillin used to treat meningococcal meningitis or meningococcemia may not eradicate nasopharyngeal carriage, rifampin should be administered also to the index patient prior to discharge from hospital. Rifampin-resistant strains appear readily and would be selected if use of the drug for prophylaxis were widespread. Preliminary evidence indicates that ciprofloxacin also is effective in eradicating pharyngeal carriage of *N. meningitidis*.

Meningococcal Vaccine. A quadrivalent (groups A, C, Y, W135) vaccine is now commercially available. A previous serogroup A vaccine showed efficacy of 85 to 95 per cent and was helpful in controlling epidemics; similar clinical efficacy has been demonstrated for a serogroup C vaccine in military recruits and in an epidemic. The polysaccharide vaccines are immunogenic in adults but do not induce a good antibody response in children under 2 years of age. A vaccine against serogroup B, the major cause of meningococcal disease in the United States, is not available.

The principal indication for use of meningococcal vaccines is the presence of outbreaks of meningococcal disease caused by *N. meningitidis* belonging to serogroup A or C (or more recently Y and W135).

The routine immunization of individuals against meningococcal disease is not recommended because of the low risk of disease in the absence of outbreaks. However, immunization would be advisable for high-risk groups such as those with complement deficiencies or with anatomic or functional asplenia. Also, vaccination should be considered for travelers to countries in which there is epidemic meningococcal disease. Since about 50 per cent of secondary cases among close contacts occur more than 5 days following the primary case, consideration should be given to the use of immunization as an adjunct to chemoprophylaxis to extend protection if the latter has been unsuccessful.

PROGNOSIS. The mortality from meningococcal meningitis before any treatment was available was about 75 per cent, and residual neurologic damage in the survivors was extensive. The advent of the sulfonamides brought a dramatic reduction in mortality to 5 to 15 per cent. Despite the emergence of sulfonamide-resistant *N. meningitidis*, mortality has been kept at the same low level through the use of high doses of penicillin G or ampicillin. The case-fatality ratio for patients with meningococcemia without accompanying meningitis is higher (25 per cent) than for meningococcal meningitis and reflects the fulminant course in some patients. The case-fatality ratio is highest in children under 2 years of age and in adults over 50.

Band JD, Chamberland ME, Platt T, et al.: Trends in meningococcal disease in the United States, 1975–1980. J Infect Dis 148:754, 1983. *Review of incidence of meningococcal disease in the United States, with emphasis on the role of various serogroups and the prevalence of sulfonamide resistance.*

Benoit FL: Chronic meningococcemia. Case report and review of the literature. Am J Med 35:103, 1963. *The best review of the clinical features of this fascinating entity.*

DeVoe IW: The meningococcus and mechanisms of pathogenicity. Microbiol Rev

46:162, 1982. *Comprehensive review of the biologic properties of* N. meningitidis *and of the epidemiologic and immunologic aspects of meningococcal disease.*

Duerden BI (ed.): Meningococcal infection. J Med Microbiol 26:161, 1988. *A series of papers reviewing newer aspects of the epidemiology, pathogenesis, and immunology of meningococcal infections based on the recent European experience.*

Feldman HA: Meningococcal infections. Adv Intern Med 18:117, 1972. *The best overview of the major aspects of meningococcal disease, including epidemiology, clinical aspects, treatment, and prevention. Authoritative; very well referenced.*

Goldschneider I, Gotschlich EC, Artenstein MS: Human immunity to the meningococcus. I. The role of humoral antibodies. J Exp Med 129:1307, 1969. *A most important paper, relating susceptibility to meningococcal infection to the lack of serum bactericidal activity against N. meningitidis. A lucid presentation of the basic facts necessary to understand the epidemiology of meningococcal disease.*

Goldschneider I, Gotschlich EC, Artenstein MS: Human immunity to the meningococcus. II. Development of natural immunity. J Exp Med 129:1327, 1969. *A second landmark paper by these authors on immunity to meningococcal infection. The role of the carrier state as an immunizing process is clearly demonstrated.*

Griffiss JM, Brandt BL: Nonepidemic (endemic) meningococcal disease: Pathogenetic factors and clinical features. In Remington JS, Swartz MN (eds.): Current Clinical Topics in Infectious Disease, 7. New York, McGraw-Hill Book Company, 1986, pp 27–50. *Provides important insights into the endemic and hyperendemic forms of meningococcal disease in the United States. The role of host-parasite interactions is emphasized.*

Koppes GM, Ellenbogen C, Gebhart RJ: Group Y meningococcal disease in United States Air Force recruits. Am J Med 62:661, 1977. *A very good description of the spectrum of disease produced by group Y meningococci. The importance of pneumonia in a recruit population is emphasized.*

Olyhoek T, Crowe BA, Achtman M: Clonal population structure of *Neisseria meningitidis* serogroup A isolated from epidemics and pandemics between 1915 and 1983. Rev Infect Dis 9:665, 1987. *An extensive and thorough study of serogroup A isolates from around the world over a period of about 70 years, indicating that most epidemics have been associated with a single or predominant clone. Seven predominant clones have been identified as causing groups of epidemics worldwide since 1915.*

Peltola H: Meningococcal disease: Still with us. Rev Infect Dis 5:71, 1983. *Authoritative evaluation of the status of meningococcal disease around the world.*

303 Infections Caused by *Haemophilus* Species

DEFINITION. *Haemophilus* infections involve primarily the upper respiratory tract and the bronchopulmonary system. Invasive infections (bacteremia, meningitis, pericarditis, septic arthritis, cellulitis) may sometimes ensue; they occur predominantly in young children and are almost aways due to one species, *H. influenzae* type b. Endocarditis is occasionally caused by *Haemophilus* species other than *H. influenzae* b. One *Haemophilus* species (*H. ducreyi*) is the cause of chancroid (see Ch. 339).

GENERAL MICROBIOLOGIC FEATURES. The various *Haemophilus* species (Table 303–1) are similar in morphology (small, pleomorphic, gram-negative bacilli) and growth requirements (facultatively aerobic, media supplemented with blood). *H. influenzae* requires for aerobic growth both the X factor (hematin) and the V factor (NAD, NADP, or nicotinamide nucleoside) present in erythrocytes. Since some strains of *H. influenzae* grow best in 5 to 10 per cent carbon dioxide and other *Haemophilus* species have a CO_2 dependence, clinical specimens

TABLE 303–1. DIFFERENTIAL PROPERTIES OF *HAEMOPHILUS* SPECIES

| Species | Growth Factor Requirement | | | Hemolysis |
	X	V	CO_2 Dependence	
H. influenzae	+	+	−	−
H. parainfluenzae	−	+	−	−
H. aphrophilus	−, +	−	+	−
H. paraphrophilus	−	+	+	−
H. hemolyticus	+	+	−	+
H. ducreyi	+	−	−	−

should be incubated in a CO_2 incubator. Media for isolation of *Haemophilus* species include chocolate agar, agar containing horse (*not* sheep) blood, or enrichment agar (Levinthal).

H. hemolyticus rarely is isolated from sites outside the upper respiratory tract and is of dubious pathogenicity.

INFECTIONS DUE TO *HAEMOPHILUS INFLUENZAE.*

Etiology. *H. influenzae* strains are either encapsulated (typable) or unencapsulated (nontypable). The former consist of six distinguishable types, designated a to f. Type b capsular polysaccharide contains both ribose and ribitol phosphate (PRP). In children 95 per cent of *H. influenzae* strains causing meningitis and bacteremia belong to type b, and the remaining strains are mainly nontypable. However, encapsulated strains make up only a small percentage of all clinical isolates of *H. influenzae*. Nontypable strains are more likely to be implicated in localized or surface infections such as otitis media in children and lower respiratory tract infections (exacerbations of chronic bronchitis and pneumonia) in adults. *H. influenzae* bacteremia is uncommon in adults, but when it occurs only about 30 per cent of isolates are type b strains and the remainder are mostly nontypable. Encapsulated strains can be identified by a variety of methods employing antisera to their capsular antigens (immunofluorescence; production of immunoprecipitin halos ringing colonies on agar plates containing antiserum; demonstration by counterimmunoelectrophoresis or latex particle agglutination of capsular antigen in culture supernatants). The outer membrane of *H. influenzae* strains contains a lipopolysaccharide with the properties of endotoxin. A classification of *H. influenzae* b into 21 subtypes based on differences in outer membrane proteins has been developed and is of use in epidemiologic studies.

H. aegyptius (Koch-Weeks bacillus) is a cause of sporadic or epidemic summer conjunctivitis. It has the same growth factor requirements as *H. influenzae*, and, since it shares over 70 per cent nucleotide sequence homology with *H. influenzae*, it is now designated *H. influenzae* biogroup *aegyptius*. It is nonencapsulated. Strains of this biogroup have been responsible for an invasive bacteremic illness, Brazilian purpuric fever (BPF), which resembles meningococcemia and occurs in Brazil, often following conjunctivitis. Strains of biogroup *aegyptius* from BPF appear to be more virulent in animal models than strains of this biogroup isolated from patients with only conjunctivitis.

Genetic relationships (clonality) between strains of *H. influenzae* differing both geographically and temporally in isolation can be identified by electrophoretic studies of cytoplasmic enzymes and outer membrane proteins. Examination by such multilocus enzyme electrophoresis of numerous isolates from around the world suggests certain conclusions: (1) most invasive disease caused by *H. influenzae* type b is caused by a limited number (about nine) of clones; (2) some geographic variation in clonal composition of serotype b *H. influenzae* populations exists on a continental or regional basis; (3) nontypable strains belong to distinctive clone clusters (much more diverse as a group than clones of type b) rather than represent variants that have simply lost the capacity to elaborate polysaccharide capsule; (4) no clear associations of clone groups with clinical manifestations have been defined with the possible exceptions of certain clones of nontypable *H. influenzae* involved in meningitis and bacteremia in neonates and in urogenital disease in women.

Smears of clinical specimens usually show pleomorphic gram-negative coccobacilli. Occasionally, in underdecolorized Gram-stained smears of spinal fluid, bipolar concentration of stain may incorrectly suggest gram-positive diplococci.

Incidence and Prevalence. Nontypable *H. influenzae* are commonly carried in the nasopharynx of asymptomatic individuals. Rates of carriage for encapsulated strains (usually type b) are much lower (less than 5 per cent of children and less than 1 per cent of adults). However, the carriage rate of household contacts, at the time of hospitalization of a child with invasive *H. influenzae* b, is much higher, 20 to 25 per cent (50 per cent in children under 5 years). Nasopharyngeal carriage of *H. influenzae* b may develop in some persons in the presence of circulating antibody to PRP, and successful antibiotic treatment of *H. influenzae* meningitis may not eliminate it from the upper respiratory tract. The carrier state may persist for weeks to months.

H. influenzae b is the principal (estimated 8000 to 11,000 cases annually) cause of bacterial meningitis in the United States. It is estimated to cause an additional 6000 cases per year of other invasive diseases such as bacteremia, epiglottitis, pneumonia, and cellulitis. By 5 years of age, one in every 200 children has had a systemic infection from *H. influenzae* b. In the past decade many clinicians have had the impression that systemic disease caused by *H. influenzae* b has become more frequent in adults. Systemic infection with *H. influenzae* probably should be considered in the adult in the proper setting more frequently than was formerly the case. *H. influenzae* type f is probably the second most frequent encapsulated *H. influenzae* pathogen in adults.

Epidemiology. Infections in the first 2 months of life are rare, probably because of transplacental transfer of maternal antibody. Most cases (about 80 per cent) of meningitis and invasive infections caused by *H. influenzae* in the United States occur in children under 2 years of age. The mean age of children with epiglottitis is 3 to 5 years. Host factors appearing to contribute to increased susceptibility include immune globulin deficiencies, sickle cell disease, CSF fistulas, splenectomized states, and chronic pulmonary infections. Alcoholism appears to be a risk factor in adults. In certain racial groups (Eskimos, American Indians, blacks) children are at higher risk of invasive *H. influenzae* infection; socioeconomic factors undoubtedly play a role.

Unlike *Neisseria meningitidis*, *H. influenzae* b does not cause epidemics in the community, but it is responsible for an increased incidence of secondary cases among susceptibles in families or possibly in daycare centers exposed to an index case. The risk of serious *H. influenzae* illness among exposed household contacts of a child with *H. influenzae* meningitis is age dependent: 4 per cent among children under 2 years of age, 2 per cent among children 2 to 3 years of age, and 0.1 per cent among children 4 to 5 years of age. The risk of infection in household contacts represents a 600-fold increase over the age-adjusted risk in the population at large.

Pathogenesis and Immunity. Most nasopharyngeal infections with *H. influenzae* are unrecognized and occur by age 5 years. Type b strains may occasionally invade locally, producing epiglottitis, pneumonia, or buccal cellulitis, or may be disseminated directly from the nasopharynx via the bloodstream, producing meningitis. Intense ($>10^3$ organisms per milliliter of blood) sustained bacteremia resulting from intravascular bacterial replication (rather than growth at a focal site of initial infection) appears to be a prerequisite for the development of meningitis. Pathogenicity of type b strains owes principally to the antiphagocytic activity of its PRP capsule. Nonencapsulated strains rarely produce bacteremic infection but can produce disease involving the upper (otitis media, sinusitis) and lower (pneumonia, exacerbations of chronic bronchitis) respiratory tracts.

In Finland, studies of anti-PRP antibodies by radioimmunoassay indicate an inverse correlation between age-related antibody levels and incidence of bacteremic *H. influenzae* disease (confirming Fothergill and Wright); 90 per cent of children (3 to 12 months of age) had antibody levels below 150 ng per milliliter, whereas all adults had higher levels. In the presence of complement, IgG class antibodies to PRP are not only bactericidal (bacteriolytic) but are also opsonic. Such antibodies are protective in vivo. Antibodies to outer membrane proteins also play a role in immunity, but they appear to be protective primarily against strains of the same subtype.

The antibody response to *H. influenzae* b meningitis is age related (infants responding poorly and older children and adults developing high titers) and related to PRP load and clearance rate. Antigenemia may persist for as long as several weeks in younger children; an antibody response may be delayed until antigenemia has cleared. Anti-PRP antibody responses are observed within about 3 months in about 80 per cent of children with meningitis.

Failure of specific anti-PRP antibody response occurs in individuals with agammaglobulinemia and with IgG_2 subclass deficiency. In addition, during the first 1 or 2 years of life polysaccharide antigens such as PRP vaccine are not efficient immunogens. The rare recurrence of *H. influenzae* b meningitis in the first 24 months of life may reflect failure even of invasive infection to elicit a protective antibody response.

It has been suggested that the age-related acquisition of anti-PRP antibodies is too rapid and extensive to be accounted for by the low incidence of *H. influenzae* b carriage or disease, and that cross-reacting *E. coli* strains in the intestine may serve as the primary immunogen.

Clinical Manifestations. In one survey of children with serious *H. influenzae* infections, meningitis was the most common manifestation (about 50 per cent), followed by pneumonia (15 per cent), bacteremia without definable portal (10 per cent), cellulitis (10 per cent), epiglottitis (10 per cent), and pericarditis (4 per cent).

Among adults with *H. influenzae* bacteremia, pneumonia is the most common cause. Other sources of *H. influenzae* bacteremia in adults include obstetric infections (nontypable strains), meningitis, occult bacteremias, cellulitis, acute sinusitis, and epiglottitis. Metastatic *H. influenzae* infections in the adult include septic arthritis and purulent pericarditis.

Meningitis (See Ch. 301). *H. influenzae* type b is the preeminent cause of bacterial meningitis in childhood, most cases occurring between age 4 months and 2 years. The clinical features are not distinctive except as they relate to pyogenic meningitis occurring at that age. The manifestations may be nonspecific (fever, irritability, listlessness, poor feeding, vomiting) initially, especially in the younger child, and there may be only minimal nuchal rigidity. If the fontanel is still open, it may not be tense, particularly if the infant is dehydrated. Subdural effusions occur more frequently (20 to 30 per cent) with *H. influenzae* meningitis, but this is related to age and ease of detection by transillumination.

Anemia is more frequent in children with *H. influenzae* b meningitis and invasive infections than in those with comparable meningococcal or pneumococcal illnesses. It appears, in patients with prolonged antigenemia coinciding with production of antibody to PRP, to be a consequence of splenic removal of PRP-coated erythrocytes to which antibody and complement have been bound, or of intravascular hemolysis.

In adults *H. influenzae* b causes only about 4 per cent of cases of bacterial meningitis, and a CSF leak is a predisposing factor in about half of such cases.

Epiglottitis. This pediatric otolaryngologic emergency begins abruptly with a severe sore throat, fever, and dysphagia; progression is swift, usually requiring hospitalization (and intubation) within 12 hours of onset. In the adult the onset of epiglottitis may be more prolonged and respiratory difficulty less pronounced initially despite severe pharyngitis and dysphagia; occasionally, the clinical picture may be mistaken for that of asthma. Airway obstruction in the child develops early with a sensation of choking, inspiratory (but not expiratory) distress, drooling, and anxiety. Speech is muffled, but the barking cough observed in croup is uncommon. The patient sits leaning forward with arms, back, and neck hyperextended to provide maximal airway. Pneumonia occurs in 15 to 25 per cent of patients, but simultaneous meningitis is uncommon. *Intraoral examination of the child (particularly in the supine position) may precipitate a cardiorespiratory arrest and should be performed only with the means of establishing an airway immediately at hand.* The pharynx is reddened; the epiglottis is bright red and markedly swollen. Lateral radiographs of the neck can demonstrate swelling of the epiglottis, but are of less value in acute cases (the procedure may delay establishment of an adequate airway) than in subacute ones.

Viral croup may resemble epiglottitis but occurs in younger children (3 to 36 months), has a more gradual onset, and frequently is preceded by an upper respiratory infection; the airway obstruction is subglottic.

Pneumonia. Most cases occur in children, are caused by type b, and are accompanied by bacteremia. Lobar consolidation occurs more commonly than bronchopneumonia, and pleural effusions (or empyema) are present in 75 per cent of cases. Lung abscess is rare. Meningitis occurs in about 15 per cent of patients.

In the adult, *H. influenzae* pneumonia occurs more frequently in the setting of chronic lung disease, alcoholism, immunologic deficiency, or following viral respiratory tract infection, but it may develop in previously healthy individuals. The majority of sputum isolates are nontypable, as are most blood isolates from the approximately 20 per cent of patients in whom bacteremia occurs. The radiologic pattern is usually that of bronchopneumonia. Small sterile parapneumonic effusions are common. The diagnosis can be suspected on the basis of findings on Gram-stained smears of sputum, but confirmation requires isolation of the organism from blood, pleural fluid, or lower respiratory tract.

Bronchitis. *H. influenzae* (nontypable) has been associated with purulent sputum and clinical exacerbations (dyspnea, wheezing, low-grade fever) of chronic bronchitis. Gram-stained smears of sputum show numerous neutrophils and small pleomorphic gram-negative bacilli. A direct etiologic role may be difficult to establish because of the frequent (20 to 80 per cent) carriage of these organisms in the upper respiratory tract of normal adults.

Bacterial Tracheitis. This acute upper airway infection particularly of children is characterized by fever, stridor, subglottic edema without epiglottal involvement, and abundant purulent tracheal secretions. Inspissation of the latter may lead to pseudomembrane formation requiring removal. This bacterial infection, often due to *H. influenzae* but even more often due to *Staphylococcus aureus*, is usually secondary to a primary parainfluenza virus respiratory infection.

Cellulitis. *H. influenzae* b causes cellulitis in children below 2 years of age, but may also cause cellulitis on rare occasions in older adults. The cheek, periorbital area, head, and neck are the most common sites. An associated ipsilateral otitis media or upper respiratory infection is a frequent precursor. It begins with fever, local pain, and increasing toxicity. The lesion develops within a few hours and progresses rapidly; it is poorly demarcated, tender, and edematous. Although usually described as having a distinctive bluish purple color, the lesion is commonly erythematous like other types of cellulitis. Bacteremia occurs in 80 per cent of cases. Diagnosis is made on the basis of the appearance and location of the lesion, the patient's age, Gram-stained smears and culture of an aspirate, and blood cultures.

Bacteremia Without Obvious Portal. *H. influenzae* b is responsible for about 20 per cent of cryptogenic bacteremias occurring in febrile children with mild nonspecific illnesses. Such patients are at considerable risk for subsequent serious localized infection (meningitis, pneumonia, epiglottitis). Unsuspected *H. influenzae* bacteremia also occurs in patients with neoplastic disease undergoing chemotherapy. Fulminant *H. influenzae* bacteremia with fatal shock and disseminated intravascular coagulation can develop in splenectomized patients.

Skeletal Infections. Septic arthritis accounts for 1 to 8 per cent of cases of invasive *H. influenzae* b infection in children. It is the cause of pyogenic arthritis in about one half of cases in children under 2 years of age. Weight-bearing joints are most often involved. Most commonly pyarthrosis is secondary to bacteremic spread from an upper respiratory tract infection, but joint involvement may result from direct spread of adjacent osteomyelitis in the first year of life.

A "reactive" arthritis has recently been described in children in association with *H. influenzae* b meningitis. Whereas the articular manifestations of pyogenic arthritis are usually present within the first day of admission with meningitis, the joint findings in the "reactive" form usually appear about a week following institution of appropriate antimicrobial therapy. Gram's stains and cultures of repeated synovial fluid aspirates are negative. Whether this process is comparable to the reactive arthritis of meningococcal meningitis, in which immune complexes are present in blood and synovial fluid, is not known. Joint effusions with a neutrophilic pleocytosis occurring in this setting should be considered to be those of pyogenic arthritis until results of repeated bacteriologic studies are available.

H. influenzae is a rare cause of osteomyelitis in children, usually occurring in the first year of life.

Pericarditis. *H. influenzae* b is the cause of 10 to 15 per cent of cases of purulent pericarditis in children. It is a rare cause of pericarditis in adults. Over one half of the children have an associated pneumonia. The hemodynamic manifestations of cardiac tamponade are commonly present. Treatment involves pericardiocentesis for diagnosis followed by surgical drainage (closed catheter drainage or anterior pericardectomy), along with antimicrobial therapy. With treatment 85 to 95 per cent of patients recover.

Otitis Media and Sinusitis. *H. influenzae* is second in frequency to *Streptococcus pneumoniae* as the cause of acute otitis media in children. In most instances the *H. influenzae* strains are not typable, but type b strains can be isolated in 10 per cent of cases. Serous middle ear fluid in children with chronic low-grade otitis media with effusion may be colonized by *H. influenzae*, which may contribute to its persistence. *H. influenzae* also appears to be a significant cause of otitis media in older children and adults. The manifestations of acute otitis media caused by *H. influenzae* are indistinguishable from those caused by other pyogens: otalgia, fever, hyperemia of the tympanic membrane, and middle ear fluid. Tinnitus, vertigo, and nystagmus may develop.

Acute sinusitis is more common in adults than in children. In about 25 per cent of cases *H. influenzae* (nontypable) is the cause. Facial pain, frontal headache, purulent nasal discharge or nasal obstruction, anosmia, and nasal speech are common features. Sinus tenderness and opacity on transillumination are helpful findings.

Conjunctivitis. *H. influenzae* biogroup *aegyptius* mucopurulent conjunctivitis occurs principally in children, particularly in the summer. The findings of acute catarrhal conjunctivitis are present, but petechial hemorrhages on the tarsal and epibulbar conjunctivae are suggestive of *H. influenzae* or a pneumococcal cause. Diagnosis is made on the basis of Gram-stained smears of conjunctival scrapings and culture of the outer eye.

H. influenzae biogroup *aegyptius* conjunctivitis is often self-limited, clearing in 7 to 14 days. Treatment consists of moist soaks to keep the eyelids clean and topical antimicrobials (e.g., 10 to 30 per cent sulfacetamide eyedrops).

Brazilian Purpuric Fever (BPF). This recently recognized, frequently fatal infection of young children in Brazil usually follows recovery from purulent conjunctivitis that began 1 or 2 weeks earlier. Clinical features include acute onset with fever and toxicity, abdominal pain and vomiting, rapidly followed by the appearance of petechiae, purpura, hypotension, and shock. *H. influenzae* biogroup *aegyptius*, previously identified only with cases of purulent conjunctivitis worldwide, is responsible for this bacteremic illness resembling meningococcemia. The fulminant clinical picture associated with BPF is consistent with the lack of close genetic relatedness of BPF strains with other isolates of the same biogroup and with the greater pathogenicity of BPF strains of biogroup *aegyptius* in infant rats compared with control conjunctival isolates of the same biogroup.

Other Infections. *H. influenzae* is a very rare cause of endocarditis and brain abscess. *H. influenzae* may occasionally be the cause of nonexudative pharyngitis (with prominent pain and dysphagia), but its presence in the pharynx often merely represents colonization. Rare cases of genital tract infections (salpingitis, endometritis, puerperal sepsis) and urinary infections have occurred.

Diagnosis. Certain serious infections (purulent meningitis, epiglottitis, facial and orbital cellulitis) in young children should suggest the possibility of *H. influenzae* b as the cause. In meningitis the presence of gram-negative pleomorphic coccobacillary forms in smears of CSF is highly suggestive of *H. influenzae*, but other organisms (*Pasteurella multocida, Acinetobacter*) which only rarely cause meningitis may have a similar appearance. Rapid and sensitive methods of antigen (PRP) detection such as latex particle agglutination (LPA), coagglutination (CoA), countercurrent immunoelectrophoresis (CIE), and enzyme-linked immunosorbent assay (ELISA) have detected *H. influenzae* b antigen in initial CSF specimens of 60 to 90 per cent of cases of *H. influenzae* meningitis; they are particularly helpful in early diagnosis and in the diagnosis of patients whose cultures may be negative because of prior antibiotic therapy. LPA is positive in 90 to 95 per cent of culture-confirmed cases of *H. influenzae* b meningitis and has the advantages over CIE and ELISA of being easier to perform and more rapid. Antigenemia can be demonstrated in 60 to 100 per cent of patients with *H. influenzae* b meningitis but much less frequently in children with epiglottitis and cellulitis. False-positive reactions may occur owing to cross-reactive antigens in other bacteria such as *E. coli*, but these are infrequent.

Bacteremia is commonly demonstrable in patients with invasive infections (at least 80 per cent of children with meningitis, epiglottitis, or cellulitis) caused by *H. influenzae* b. *H. influenzae* is generally isolated on cultures of the epiglottis, joint fluid, and empyema fluid when it is the cause of infection in those areas.

Treatment. Currently, about 30 per cent of strains of *H. influenzae* b isolated in this country from systemic infections are ampicillin resistant. Resistance to chloramphenicol is found in less than 1 per cent of strains. Regional variations in resistance patterns exist. In a pediatric hospital in Barcelona, Spain, 60 per cent of meningeal isolates are ampicillin resistant; 66 per cent are resistant to chloramphenicol; and 57 per cent are resistant to both drugs. Most ampicillin-resistant *H. influenzae* strains are resistant by virtue of plasmid-encoded β-lactamase production. Detection of β-lactamase production is commonly employed to determine ampicillin resistance. Recently rare isolates of ampicillin-resistant *H. influenzae* that are resistant because of alterations in penicillin-binding proteins rather than β-lactamase production have been detected. Since routine testing for β-lactamase would indicate incorrectly such strains to be ampicillin susceptible, special disc or agar-dilution testing would be required if this were suspected. About 15 per cent of strains (usually nontypable) associated with childhood otitis media are ampicillin resistant, as are 8 to 20 per cent of strains (mostly nontypable) isolated from adults with invasive infections or chronic bronchitis.

Because of the prevalence of ampicillin resistance, ampicillin should not be used as single-drug therapy of systemic illnesses caused by *H. influenzae* b unless it has been established that the organism is ampicillin susceptible (a non–β-lactamase producer). Several forms of initial therapy are currently being employed (see Ch. 301). These include a third-generation cephalosporin such as ceftriaxone or cefotaxime; chloramphenicol (alone, or in combination with ampicillin until testing for ampicillin resistance has been performed); and, for nonmeningeal infections, cefuroxime (a second-generation cephalosporin resistant to many β-lactamases). Ceftriaxone or cefotaxime would be the drug of choice, particularly in areas where resistance to both chloramphenicol and ampicillin exists or when such resistance is suspected on the basis of clinical response to other therapy.

Amoxicillin (20 to 40 mg per kilogram per day in three divided doses) or ampicillin (50 to 100 mg per kilogram per day in four divided doses), because each is active against *S. pneumoniae* and most strains of *H. influenzae*, is still the drug of choice for initial treatment of otitis media in children. Alternatives include amoxicillin-clavulanate, trimethoprim (TMP)-sulfamethoxazole (SMX) (8 mg per kilogram of TMP and 40 mg per kilogram of SMX per 24 hours, given in two divided doses every 12 hours), the combination of penicillin (or erythromycin) with a sulfonamide, cefaclor or cefuroxime-axetil. Treatment should be continued for 10 to 14 days. Initial treatment of *H. influenzae* pneumonia in the adult should be with ampicillin or amoxicillin, since these infections are infrequently caused by ampicillin-resistant strains, and there is sufficient time to shift therapy (cefuroxime, amoxicillin-clavulanate, chloramphenicol) if the response is unsatisfactory. Based on the bacteriology (*S. pneumoniae* and *H. influenzae* are frequently identified) of acute sinusitis, ampicillin is a reasonable initial antibiotic choice. (In the patient with rapidly progressive frontal sinusitis, *S. aureus* must be considered as a cause as well, and a penicillinase-resistant penicillin should be included in the initial therapeutic program.)

Prevention. A vaccine (*Haemophilus* b polysaccharide vaccine) against invasive infection with *H. influenzae* b was licensed in 1985 for use in the United States in children who are 24 months or older. This vaccine was demonstrated in Finland to have 90 per cent efficacy among children 18 to 71 months of age. It was not possible statistically to demonstrate efficacy in children immunized at 18 to 23 months of age. The vaccine was ineffective in children under 18 months of age. Subsequent case-control studies in the United States of children of 24 months and older indicate that this vaccine is somewhat less effective in this country than would have been anticipated from results of the Finnish trial, suggesting possible regional differences in vaccine efficacy. Consideration may be given to immunization of children in high-risk groups (sickle cell disease, asplenic states, malignancies associated with immunosuppression) at 18 months of age even though efficacy has not been established in this age group. If this is done, a booster dose within 18 months may be necessary.

Since the majority of cases of *H. influenzae* meningitis occur in the first 18 to 24 months of life, when the current polysaccharide vaccine is not efficacious, other vaccines have been developed. Since there appears to be an age-specific defect in the response of infants to polysaccharide antigen (thymus-independent), attempts have been made to overcome this limitation by linking the PRP antigen to a protein (e.g., diphtheria toxoid), thus invoking T cell participation and establishing immunologic memory. A large-scale Finnish field trial of *H. influenzae* type b polysaccharide–diphtheria toxoid conjugate vaccine in infancy (administered at 3, 4, 6, and 14 months of age) indicated that the vaccine afforded 83 per cent protection. A recent comparable study of the same vaccine in Alaskan native infants showed only very limited protective efficacy, suggesting again unexplained possible regional variation in vaccine efficacy. This conjugate vaccine is currently approved for immunization of children as young as 15 to 18 months of age. Other *H. influenzae* polysaccharide–protein conjugate vaccines, employing as the protein moiety either *N. meningitidis* outer membrane protein or a nontoxic antigenically identical mutant diphtheria toxin, are being developed for immunization of younger infants.

The rate of secondary cases among young children who are close household contacts of a patient with invasive *H. influenzae* b infection indicates the need for an effective prophylactic antibiotic program. Since rifampin has efficacy in eliminating nasopharyngeal carriage of *H. influenzae* b, the following management of household contacts has been recommended: (1) if another child less than 4 years of age resides in the household of an index case, all household members (including adults) should receive rifampin (20 mg per kilogram orally once daily for 4 days, with a maximal daily dose of 600 mg); (2) rifampin in the same dosage should also be administered to the index patient prior to discharge from the hospital, since nasopharyngeal carriage may reappear after discontinuation of antimicrobial therapy for systemic infection; (3) rifampin prophylaxis is probably not indicated if over 2 weeks have elapsed since illness began in the index patient or if the youngest child in the household is 4 years of age or older.

Whether the risk of subsequent invasive *H. influenzae* infection is increased in contacts of patients in daycare facilities is controversial; the risk may vary from region to region. If 2 or more cases occur in a daycare center within 60 days, rifampin prophylaxis should be given to all contacts in the facility, including adults. Whether to do likewise if only one case has occurred is controversial. However, if any of the exposed classroom contacts is under 2 years of age, institution of chemoprophylaxis seems warranted.

INFECTIONS CAUSED BY OTHER *HAEMOPHILUS* SPECIES. *Haemophilus parainfluenzae.* This *Haemophilus* species is part of the normal flora of the nasopharynx and is found in dental plaque. It is very uncommonly responsible for human disease. It has been a rare cause of meningitis, epiglottitis, otitis media, puerperal bacteremia, brain abscess, and pneumonia in adults. Ampicillin is the drug of choice, except when ampicillin resistance is present (6 per cent of isolates), in which case a third-generation cephalosporin or chloramphenicol is an alternative. The most common association of *H. parainfluenzae* with disease has been with infective endocarditis. It may take as long as 14 to 18 days to grow out of blood cultures. The only distinctive clinical feature (also observed with *H. aphrophilus* endocarditis) appears to be the frequent occurrence of embolic occlusion of large arteries. For endocarditis in the adult, treatment with ampicillin (12 grams daily intravenously) alone or in combination with gentamicin (4 mg per kilogram per day in divided doses every 8 hours intravenously) for 4 to 6 weeks has been employed successfully.

Haemophilus aphrophilus. This organism is part of the normal gingival flora and is a rare cause of disease, generally acting as an "opportunist." The infections it produces, often following oropharyngeal foci of infection or trauma, include abscesses (particularly brain abscess), bacteremia, and endocarditis. Most strains are susceptible to penicillin, ampicillin, third-generation cephalosporins, chloramphenicol, and gentamicin. Successful treatment of endocarditis has involved the use of ampicillin or penicillin, alone or in combination with streptomycin, for 4 to 6 weeks.

Haemophilus ducreyi. See Ch. 339.

Haemophilus influenzae

Campos J, Garcia-Tornel S, Gairi JM, Fabregues I: Multiply resistant *Haemophilus influenzae* type b causing meningitis: Comparative clinical and laboratory study. J Pediatr 108:897, 1986. *Summarizes the extent of a major endemic problem in Spain of resistance to ampicillin and chloramphenicol in* H. influenzae *strains. Alternative therapeutic approaches are suggested.*

Cherry JD: Acute epiglottitis, laryngitis, and croup. *In* Remington JS, Swartz MN (eds.): Current Clinical Topics in Infectious Disease, 2. New York, McGraw-Hill Book Company, 1981, pp 1–30. *Provides a particularly vivid clinical picture of acute* H. influenzae *epiglottitis. Valuable points on differential diagnosis and treatment are emphasized. A very well organized and thoroughly referenced presentation.*

Dajani AS, Asmar BI, Thirumoorthi MC: Systemic *Haemophilus influenzae* disease. J Pediatr 94:355, 1979. *This is a thorough review of an extensive pediatric experience with systemic* H. influenzae b *infections. It provides helpful data on the relative frequencies of the various clinical syndromes and an extensive bibliography.*

Eskola J, Peltola H, Takola AK, et al.: Efficacy of *Haemophilus influenzae* type b polysaccharide–diphtheria toxoid conjugate vaccine in infancy. N Engl J Med 317:717, 1987. *This article describes a 5-month follow-up of a very large trial in Finland of the type b capsular polysaccharide–diphtheria toxoid vaccine, which protected children from 7 to 14 months of age against invasive* H. influenzae *infection.*

Fothergill LD, Wright J: Influenzal meningitis: Relation of age incidence to bactericidal power of blood against causal organism. J Immunol 24:273, 1933. *This is the original and "classic" study demonstrating an inverse relationship between the presence of serum bactericidal antibody and the incidence of* H. influenzae *meningitis at various ages.*

Granoff DM, Ward JI: Current status of prophylaxis for *Hemophilus influenzae* infections. *In* Remington JS, Swartz MN (eds.): Current Clinical Topics in Infectious Disease, 5. New York, McGraw-Hill Book Company, 1984. *Provides excellent background regarding secondary spread of* H. influenzae *infections and concrete recommendations for chemoprophylaxis of close family and daycare center contacts.*

Mayo-Smith MF, Hirsch PJ, Wodzinski SF, et al.: Acute epiglottitis in adults. An eight year experience in the state of Rhode Island. N Engl J Med 314:1133, 1986. *A clinical and bacteriologic review of 56 cases of acute epiglottitis (supraglottitis) in adults, indicating that* H. influenzae *is an important cause in this age group (28 per cent of published cases in which blood cultures were obtained). Practical management issues are considered.*

Murphy TF, Apicella MA: Nontypable *Haemophilus influenzae:* A review of clinical aspects, surface antigens, and the human immune response to infection. Rev Infect Dis 9:1, 1987. *A detailed review of the antigenic nature and biologic properties of nonencapsulated* H. influenzae. *The role of such strains in clinical infections in adults and children is very thoroughly covered.*

Musser JM, Kroll JS, Granoff DM, et al.: Global genetic structure and molecular epidemiology of encapsulated *Haemophilus influenzae*. Rev Infect Dis 12:75, 1990. *This represents an enormous study by multilocus electrophoresis of over 2200 isolates of encapsulated* H. influenzae *from around the world. It provides insights into the clonal population structure of this species and indicates patterns of intercontinental and regional geographic distribution.*

Peltola H, Kayhty H, Virtanen M, et al.: Prevention of *Hemophilus influenzae* type B bacteremic infections with the capsular polysaccharide vaccine. N Engl J Med 310:1561, 1984. *This article describes a long-term follow-up of a very well conducted, large scale trial of the type b capsular polysaccharide vaccine, which protected against bacteremic* H. influenzae b *disease in children older than 24 months of age.*

Shurin SB, Anderson P, Zollinger J, et al.: Pathophysiology of hemolysis in infections with *Hemophilus influenzae* type b. J Clin Invest 77:1340, 1986. *In a careful laboratory study the authors demonstrate that the anemia observed in invasive* H. influenzae b *infections is hemolytic in origin and may be due to coating of PRP on erythrocytes and their subsequent immune destruction.*

Spagnuolo PJ, Ellner JJ, Lerner PL, et al.: *Haemophilus influenzae* meningitis: The spectrum of disease in adults. Medicine 61:74, 1982. *These 15 cases represent the largest series of cases of* H. influenzae *meningitis reported in the past 20 years. Particular emphasis is on predisposing factors in this unusual form of meningitis in adults.*

Wallace RJ Jr, Musher DM, Septimus EJ, et al.: *Haemophilus influenzae* infections in adults: Characterization of strains by serotypes, biotypes, and β-lactamase production. J Infect Dis 144:101, 1981. *This is a detailed review of 103 cases of* H. influenzae *bacteremia or meningitis. Noteworthy is the frequency of nontypable strains among blood isolates in adults and the infrequency of ampicillin resistance in the same group.*

Haemophilus parainfluenzae and Haemophilus aphrophilus

Bieger RC, Brewer NS, Washington JA II: *Haemophilus aphrophilus:* A microbiologic and clinical review and report of 42 cases. Medicine 57:345, 1978. *A comprehensive review of the bacteriologic features, ecologic niche, and clinical impact of this uncommon cause of human disease.*

Oill PA, Chow AW, Guze LB: Adult bacteremic *Haemophilus parainfluenzae* infections: Seven reports of cases and a review of the literature. Arch Intern Med 139:985, 1979. *The type of infection (exclusive of endocarditis) caused by* H. parainfluenzae *and the antibiotic susceptibilities of this organism are summarized concisely.*

Osteomyelitis

304 Osteomyelitis

Francis A. Waldvogel

DEFINITION. Osteomyelitis is an infection by microorganisms that invade and destroy bone. Osteomyelitis is a well-known, albeit rare, consequence of bacteremia. In most situations nowadays, open fractures, wounds, and orthopedic procedures allow the microorganism to gain access to bone from a contaminated or infected contiguous structure. Peripheral bones can also be invaded by contiguity in cases of severe vascular insufficiency. In the latter case, metabolic and neurologic factors often play an important contributory role.

ETIOLOGY. Most cases of osteomyelitis are of bacterial origin. Of all pathogenic organisms, *Staphylococcus aureus* is still the most common offending agent, whatever the mechanism of the infection. However, *S. epidermidis* has emerged in recent years as a frequent offender as well, for instance, in hematogenous spread to a vertebral body from an infected intravenous line. *S. epidermidis* is also responsible for many bone infections secondary to implantation of prosthetic material, such as total hip prosthesis, where it can account for up to 30 per cent of the cases.

Other etiologic agents include gram-negative enteric organisms, which are often responsible for hematogenous vertebral osteomyelitis, certain *Salmonella* species that cause hematogenous disease in patients with sickle cell anemia, and often *Pseudomonas aeruginosa*, which can involve the spine in heroin addicts. Anaerobic organisms, most often in mixed cultures, have been isolated from infected bone in the vicinity of an anaerobic reservoir (mandible, sinuses, sacrum), after human or animal bites, or from infected extremities in diabetic patients. *Mycobacterium tuberculosis* should always be considered a diagnostic possibility in osteomyelitis of the spine, especially in patients presenting with limited periosteal reactions, and in nonhealing bone infections. Various fungi can cause osteomyelitis under exceptional conditions, such as hematogenous spread from a chronically infected intravenous device or in connection with prosthetic material. Finally, exceptional cases of viral osteomyelitis have been described after chickenpox.

All causes of osteomyelitis have not yet been discovered. Thus, multifocal hematogenous osteomyelitis is a syndrome occurring in children and young adults characterized by multiple, lytic inflammatory bone lesions in patients with various skin conditions such as pustulosis palmoplantaris and acne fulminans. Bacterial cultures of biopsy specimens are negative, and the disease usually evolves toward cure without specific antibacterial therapy.

INCIDENCE, PREVALENCE, AND EPIDEMIOLOGY. Hematogenous osteomyelitis has a biphasic incidence, occurring mainly in children, in whom it shows a predilection for the metaphysis of long bones, and in adults beyond the age of 50 years, in whom it most often involves the spine. Any factor favoring bacteremia (urinary tract infection, prostatitis, various skin infections, prolonged intravenous therapy, or repeated injections) can occasionally lead to hematogenous osteomyelitis of the spine. Osteomyelitis secondary to a contiguous focus varies in frequency acccording to the primary trauma, the invasive procedure performed, the type of material inserted, the underlying disease, and the degree of contamination of the wound. For instance, in well-planned aseptic interventions such as total hip replacement, the risk of infection is usually around 0.4 per cent; insertions of total knee prostheses, on the other hand, are associated with a higher risk of infection, particularly in patients with rheumatoid arthritis; at the other end of the spectrum, the prevalence of postoperative osteomyelitis can reach 15 per cent after comminuted fracture.

PATHOGENESIS AND PATHOLOGY. The development of

experimental models and the collection of better morphologic data have shed some new light on the mechanisms leading to bone destruction in osteomyelitis. The porous structure of bone, its canaliculi filled with capillaries and/or osteoblast cytoplasmic extensions, and the space between these organic structures and the mineral constituents, account for a nonnegligible fluid volume in bone, in the range of 5 per cent. In hematogenous osteomyelitis, microorganisms settle probably first in this fluid phase, where they stimulate an active inflammatory reaction. Whether microorganisms have to adhere on the hydroxyapatite surface or on collagen to escape host defense mechanisms, as suggested by other infection models, is currently suggested by some experimental data. Since microorganisms per se are unable to destroy bone tissue, one has to postulate that the inflammatory reaction, the metabolic alterations, and the vascular changes triggered by the bacterial invasion play predominant roles in the development of an osteomyelitic focus, i.e., in bone destruction and regeneration. From a morphologic point of view, the following major alterations can be identified: (1) bone necrosis, with death of the cellular constituents and disappearance of bone mass. Sometimes devitalized bone persists as a dead fragment called a sequestrum; (2) a heavy inflammatory reaction, in which granulocytes predominate initially but are replaced over time by a mononuclear infiltrate; (3) new bone apposition, originating from periosteal activation. In some cases, this bone apposition can be exuberant and lead to bridging of two adjacent bone structures, as in vertebral osteomyelitis. In other cases, bone apposition is very modest, and radiographic examination may show only an intraosseous, punched-out radiolucent lesion, as in subacute hematogenous osteomyelitis (Brodie's abscess) (Fig. 304–1).

CLINICAL MANIFESTATIONS. Acute hematogenous osteomyelitis involving long bones usually does not pose any major diagnostic problems: It starts as an acute episode with chills and fever, the young patient usually complaining of severe pain in the affected bone, most often the tibia or femur, more rarely the humerus. Clinical examination of the affected limb is usually unremarkable, except for pain on palpation of the affected area, usually the metaphysis. Characteristically, the adjacent joint is freely mobile and painless. If the infection is caused by an organism less virulent than *S. aureus*, however, the onset can be protracted, the pain less severe, and the fever moderate.

In hematogenous osteomyelitis of the spine, the clinical pres-

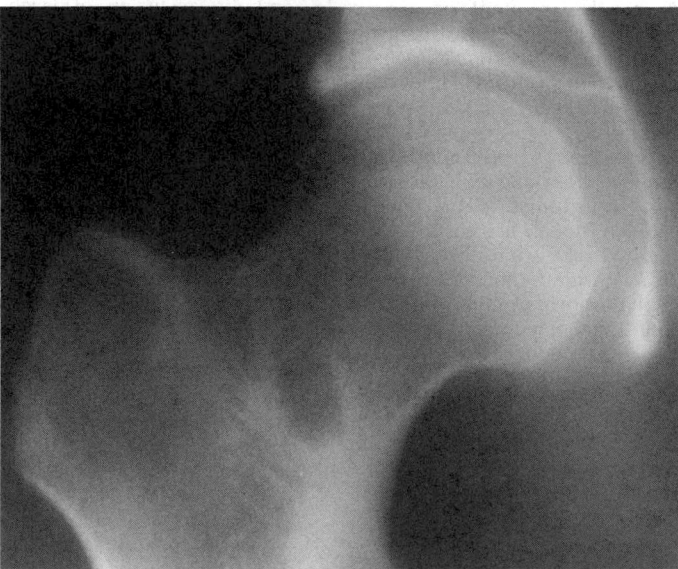

FIGURE 304–1. Subacute osteomyelitis (Brodie's abscess), hematogenous, in the right femur of a 31-year-old male.

entation is often characterized by progressive, ill-defined pain with low fever, following, for instance, an episode of urinary tract infection, bacteremia, or skin infection. The dull pain is usually located in the lower dorsal or lumbar segments of the spine ("febrile lumbago"). Any vertebral body can occasionally become involved by the disease, even the cervical spine ("febrile torticollis"). On physical examination, the mildly febrile patient usually has vertebral and paravertebral tenderness, but the overlying skin is normal. At this stage, there is no radicular pain and no sign of pyramidal tract involvement. Either of the two latter findings suggests a spinal epidural abscess, a dreaded complication of vertebral osteomyelitis calling for immediate neuroradiologic evaluation, surgical decompression, and appropriate antibiotic therapy (see Spinal Epidural Abscess in Ch. 471).

Under exceptional circumstances, a patient with hematogenous osteomyelitis—usually of long bones—will present only with pain in the affected area, without fever. Radiographs show a punched-out lesion, without expansion beyond cortical bone. Without biopsy, it is difficult to differentiate such a lesion (Brodie's abscess) from benign or even malignant tumors.

Osteomyelitis secondary to a contiguous focus of infection after open trauma or secondary to orthopedic reconstructive surgery is a diagnostic challenge, since pain, low-grade fever, local signs of low-grade inflammation, and radiographic findings are compatible with both postoperative repair and infection. Recurrence of mild fever 1 week after surgery or trauma, increasing pain on weight bearing after total joint prosthetic replacement (Fig. 304–2), poor healing of the incision, and drainage of increased amounts of serosanguineous fluid should alert the physician to the possibility of ongoing infection.

DIAGNOSIS AND DIFFERENTIAL DIAGNOSIS. In hematogenous osteomyelitis, blood cultures are positive in about 25 to 30 per cent of cases, yielding most frequently S. aureus. Positive cultures for S. epidermidis should not be discarded as

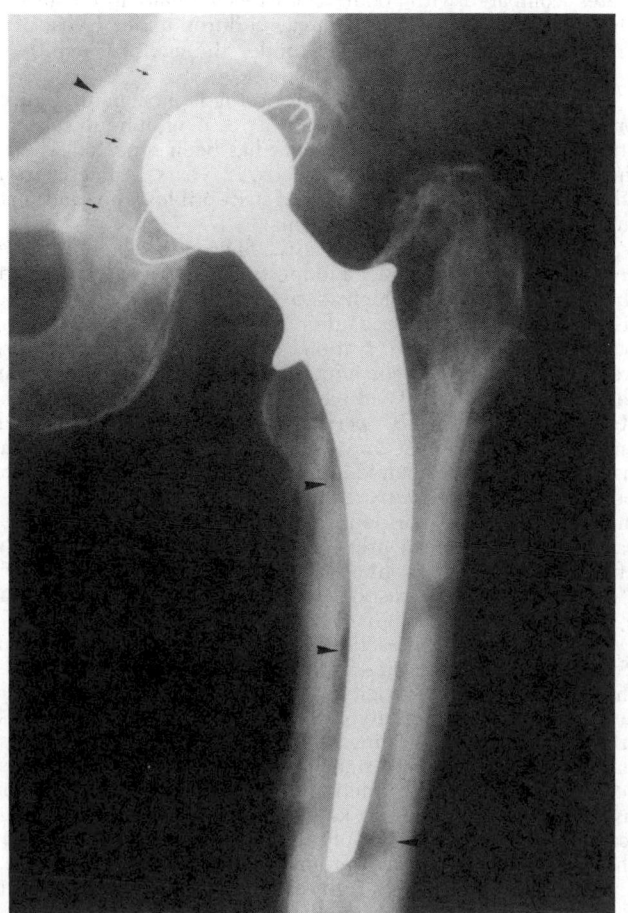

FIGURE 304–2. Osteomyelitis secondary to a contiguous focus of infection (arrows): infection after placement of a total hip prosthesis in a 63-year-old patient.

contaminants, but the organism should be further characterized as to sensitivity patterns, biotype, even plasmid contents, since this organism—often nosocomial—has become a common pathogen in bone infection. If the blood cultures remain negative, a direct aspiration and/or bone biopsy should be done for full microbiologic diagnosis. This is particularly true for vertebral osteomyelitis, which can be due to a great variety of microorganisms.

In osteomyelitis secondary to a focus of infection, the clinician is often tempted to perform a local superficial aspiration or to culture the fistulous tract for microbiologic diagnosis. Such cultures often yield multiple organisms, and it is often difficult to differentiate the pathogenic organisms from contaminants. Deep bone aspiration and/or biopsy is of greater value under these circumstances, and usually yields the offending organism in pure culture. For all cases of osteomyelitis, other laboratory tests are noncontributory: Erythrocyte sedimentation rate is usually increased; the white blood cell count is normal or high; and blood chemistry values are normal.

Radiologic changes are delayed, appearing several weeks after the onset of the disease. In hematogenous osteomyelitis of long bones, periosteal elevation and subsequent bone destruction are the first changes to be observed. In vertebral osteomyelitis, progressive piecemeal destruction of two adjacent vertebral plateaus, narrowing of the intervertebral space, and progressive anterior periosteal bridging are the hallmarks of the disease, bone sclerosis being a late event. All of these changes occur over several weeks. In tuberculous osteomyelitis of the spine, the changes just mentioned are delayed and occur over several months, periosteal reaction usually being absent.

In most cases of hematogenous osteomyelitis, ^{99m}Tc-pyrophosphate uptake, although nonspecific, can be of great diagnostic help by identifying the suspected areas of infection for appropriate tomograms at a stage when conventional radiographic results are still normal. In osteomyelitis secondary to a contiguous focus of infection, radiologic techniques and bone scanning are less helpful, since they cannot distinguish between normal bone reaction and infection. When detailed radiologic information is mandatory, such as in identifying an abscess in acute osteomyelitis, demonstrating sequestra in chronic osteomyelitis, or searching for a possible paraspinal abscess in vertebral body infection, CT scanning can offer additional diagnostic help. However, besides identifying such complications, this procedure has not been helpful in decreasing the delay in early diagnosis of osteomyelitis. In vertebral osteomyelitis, magnetic resonance imaging studies (MRI) have been particularly helpful in identifying infection and assessing its extension within and beyond osseous structures.

Acute hematogenous osteomyelitis of long bones must be differentiated clinically from septic arthritis, bursitis, and cellulitis. These more superficial infections are accompanied by local skin changes, and radiographic results remain normal. Osteomyelitis of the spine is a diagnostic challenge and has to be differentiated from bone tumors such as myeloma and metastases, which usually do not involve two adjacent vertebral plateaus. In case of doubt, bone biopsy is usually indicated.

TREATMENT. The therapeutic approach to osteomyelitis is both surgical and medical. For instance, although acute hematogenous osteomyelitis is usually treated medically, an orthopedic surgeon should be ready to intervene in case of abscess or sequestrum formation, pathologic fracture, etc. Conversely, osteomyelitis after total hip replacement will need surgical intervention for debridement, and possibly prosthetic replacement, under coverage of antibiotic therapy.

Appropriate medical treatment of osteomyelitis presupposes isolation of the offending organism and a complete assessment of its antibiotic sensitivities. In case of S. aureus sensitive to oxacillin, nafcillin should be used at a dosage of 1.5 grams to 2 grams every 4 hours parenterally. In case of an S. aureus or S. epidermidis resistant to oxacillin, vancomycin at a dosage of 1 gram given every 12 hours as a slow infusion is the treatment of choice. Dose adjustment is required for patients with renal dysfunction. For all other organisms, a similar rule can be applied: Those parenteral antibiotics usually effective for the treatment of septicemia due to a particular organism are also appropriate for osteomyelitis, provided that they are administered over a 4- to

6-week period. Thus, osteomyelitis of the spine caused by a gram-negative organism will be cured by a 4- to 6-week course of ampicillin, a first- or second-generation cephalosporin, an aminoglycoside, or a fluoroquinolone, depending on the sensitivity pattern. Bed rest is usually recommended until all signs of inflammation have abated, pain has subsided, and radiographs show signs of improvement. This is particularly true for osteomyelitis of the spine. Surgery is generally unnecessary in hematogenous infection, except for drainage of intramedullary abscesses, removal of sequestra, and decompression if neurologic signs supervene in vertebral osteomyelitis. In osteomyelitis secondary to a contiguous focus of infection, however, careful evaluation of the situation by a skilled orthopedic surgeon is mandatory. In case of infected fractures or prostheses, stable union is a prerequisite for bacteriologic cure. Union should be achieved first despite sepsis, and infection is controlled subsequently by antibiotic therapy after removal of the foreign material. In case of nonunion of a fracture or loosening of the prosthesis, the foreign material should be removed and, if possible, replaced by an external fixation device. Infected prostheses should also be removed and the infected focus cleaned out, with reinsertion of new material in a one-step or two-step procedure.

PREVENTION. At present, there is no preventive treatment available for hematogenous osteomyelitis, since the occurrence of the disease after bacteremia is unpredictable. Infection rates after insertion of hip prostheses have been shown to be markedly decreased by short-term coverage (1 to 2 days) with parenteral antistaphylococcal antibiotics. Such coverage should also be considered in high-risk operations, such as reduction of comminuted fractures, open fractures, and insertion of joint prostheses in high-risk patients.

Kido D, Bryan D, Halpern M: Hematogenous osteomyelitis in drug addicts. Ther Nucl Med 118:356, 1973. *A concise study of 32 cases, most of them due to Pseudomonas species. Discusses their clinical and radiologic manifestations.*

Larde D, Mathieu D, Frija J, et al.: Vertebral osteomyelitis: Disk hypodensity on CT. AJR 139:963, 1982. *Thirty-six cases of vertebral osteomyelitis, investigated by CT scan for early diagnosis of complications.*

Norden CW (ed.): Osteomyelitis. Infect Dis Clin North Am 4:361, 1990. *A comprehensive, up-to-date monograph that focuses on epidemiologic, clinical, diagnostic, and therapeutic aspects of osteomyelitis (12 chapters).*

Waldvogel FA: Use of quinolones for the treatment of osteomyelitis and septic arthritis. Rev Infect Dis 11 (Suppl 5):S1259–1263, 1989.

Waldvogel FA, Medoff G, Swartz MN: Osteomyelitis: A review of clinical features, therapeutic considerations and unusual aspects I. II. III. N Engl J Med 282:198, 260, 316, 1970. *A retrospective review of 247 cases of osteomyelitis, their clinical and radiologic presentations, and their treatment.*

Waldvogel FA, Vasey H: Osteomyelitis: The past decade. N Engl J Med 303:360, 1980. *A review update of newer approaches in diagnosis and treatment of osteomyelitis, with emphasis on a combined surgical and medical approach.*

Wing VW, Jeffrey RB, Federle MP, et al.: Chronic osteomyelitis examined by CT. Radiology 154:171, 1985. *The additional information obtained by CT scanning in case of sequestra is well illustrated in 14 out of 25 patients with chronic osteomyelitis.*

Whooping Cough

305 Whooping Cough (Pertussis)

Richard B. Johnston, Jr.

DEFINITION. Whooping cough (synonym, pertussis) is a noninvasive, highly communicable bacterial respiratory illness. It occurs at all ages but is most common and most severe in infants and young children. The etiologic agent of the syndrome is usually *Bordetella pertussis*. The descriptive name derives from a distressing, prolonged inspiratory effort that follows paroxysmal coughing. Whooping cough is estimated to cause 600,000 to 1 million deaths yearly in infants from areas where pertussis immunization is not practiced.

ETIOLOGY. When first isolated, *Bordetella pertussis* is a small, nonmotile, weakly staining, gram-negative coccobacillus, 0.5 to 1.0 μm in length. Capsules can be demonstrated by special procedures, and bipolar metachromatic granules are present. The complex medium containing blood originally employed by Bordet and Gengou is still used (in modified form) for cultivation. *Primary isolates do not grow on conventional laboratory media.*

An estimated 5 to 10 per cent of clinical whooping cough is caused by *B. parapertussis*. The animal pathogen *B. bronchiseptica* is responsible for a minor percentage of cases. These organisms can be differentiated from *B. pertussis* by growth requirements, enzyme production, and presence of species-specific antigens. It has been suggested that adenoviruses, alone or in concert with *B. pertussis*, and *Chlamydia trachomatis* may play an etiologic role in some cases of whooping cough.

EPIDEMIOLOGY. In nonimmune households the attack rate is 80 to 90 per cent. Transmission is by droplet infection. Carriers of *B. pertussis* are found infrequently, but persons previously immunized have been shown during outbreaks of disease to excrete the organism in the absence of clinical symptoms or in the presence of mild or atypical illness.

The mortality rate from whooping cough has fallen since the beginning of the twentieth century owing to improved supportive therapy. The incidence of whooping cough, however, did not change until after the 1940's, when immunization of young children became standard practice. In the 1940's, approximately 200,000 cases of pertussis were reported annually in the United States, compared with about 4000 cases annually in recent years. Over 70 per cent of deaths occur in children under 1 year of age. The case fatality rate in infants under the age of 6 months is 1 per cent.

Neither immunization against pertussis nor natural disease provides lifelong protection. In the case of immunization, an attack rate greater than 50 per cent has been reported when the interval after immunization exceeds 12 years. Adolescents and adults represent a large reservoir of susceptibles who can transmit the disease to unimmunized infants.

PATHOGENESIS. *B. pertussis* adheres to ciliated epithelial cells of the respiratory tract and multiplies there without invading the tissues. Yet this colonization leads to profound changes in tissues which persist long after the responsible bacteria have been cleared. Such observations suggest that a toxin or toxins from the bacteria play an important part in the pathogenesis of the syndrome. A variety of biologic activities have been demonstrated by injecting *B. pertussis* products into experimental animals. An endotoxin and a heat-labile toxin that can cause tissue necrosis have been identified among these bacterial factors, but the exotoxin *pertussis toxin* (PT) is the best candidate at the moment for a major virulence factor. Immunization with chemically detoxified PT can prevent severe whooping cough with an efficacy similar to that achieved with the standard cellular vaccine. PT is believed to be responsible for the characteristic lymphocytosis of whooping cough.

PT is a protein composed of five noncovalently linked subunits (S1–S5). The subunits S2–S5 form a nontoxic unit that binds to the cell membrane; toxicity is mediated by the enzymatically active subunit, S1. Activity of S1 inhibits a subclass of guanosine triphosphate (GTP)–binding proteins (G proteins) that are essential for transmembrane signaling and, thus, certain types of receptor-mediated cell functions. Genetic engineering has been used to replace one or two key amino acids within the enzymatically active S1 subunit, resulting in a stable nontoxic form of PT that can be used as a safe immunogen.

Adherence of *B. pertussis* to respiratory epithelium is required for the pathogenesis of whooping cough. Adherence appears to involve a bacterial outer membrane protein with a molecular weight of 69 kilodaltons, termed 69kD outer membrane protein (OMP), P69, or pertactin. An antigenically similar protein exists on *B. parapertussis* and *B. bronchiseptica*. Injection of this protein into mice or humans elicits agglutinating antibody to *B. pertussis* and protects the mice against lethal *B. pertussis* respiratory challenge. Synthesis of 69kD OMP is controlled by a regulatory gene at the *vir* (virulence) locus, which modulates synthesis of PT and additional factors that may contribute to pathogenesis, including filamentous hemagglutinin.

PATHOLOGY. Lesions caused by *B. pertussis* are found principally in the bronchi and bronchioles, but changes are also seen in the nasopharynx, larynx, and trachea. Masses of bacteria and mucopurulent exudate are intertwined with the cilia of the columnar epithelium. There is necrosis of the midzonal and basilar epithelium with infiltration of polymorphonuclear leukocytes and macrophages. The most frequent findings in the lung are bronchopneumonia, interstitial pneumonitis, and numerous small areas of atelectasis. The brain can show edema and scattered petechiae at autopsy.

CLINICAL MANIFESTATIONS. The incubation period lasts 7 to 14 days (rarely over 2 weeks). It is customary to divide the clinical course into three stages.

Catarrhal Stage. Whooping cough begins with symptoms indistinguishable from those of a mild viral upper respiratory infection. Sneezing is frequent, conjunctivae are injected, and a nocturnal cough appears. The temperature may be slightly elevated. Infectivity is greatest at this stage.

Paroxysmal Stage. Seven to 14 days after onset, the cough becomes more frequent, then paroxysmal. In a typical paroxysm there is a series of 15 to 20 short coughs of increasing intensity, and then a deep inspiration, making the "whoop." A tenacious mucous plug is usually expelled, and vomiting frequently follows. Paroxysms may occur as often as every half hour and are accompanied by signs of increased venous pressure, including deeply engorged conjunctivae, periorbital edema, petechial hemorrhages, particularly about the forehead, and epistaxis. During the attack the infant may be cyanotic until the crowing whoop occurs. Between paroxysms the child usually feels well, although justifiably apprehensive. This phase lasts 2 to 4 weeks.

Physical examination of the chest is often unremarkable except for scattered rhonchi. The chest roentgenogram sometimes reveals hilar and mediastinal nodal enlargement. The presence of fever should immediately suggest the development of a secondary infectious process.

Convalescent Stage. The paroxysms gradually become less frequent and less intense; vomiting ceases, and slow recovery ensues. Convalescence requires 4 to 12 weeks. For many months even a mild, unrelated respiratory infection can induce a return of paroxysmal cough and whoop.

In infants less than 6 months old the paroxysms and the whoop are often absent; choking spells and apneic episodes may be the major manifestations. Second attacks of whooping cough as well as disease occurring in previously immunized individuals often present simply as an upper respiratory illness or bronchitis.

Complications. Recurrent vomiting can lead to metabolic alkalosis or malnutrition. Central nervous system changes can result from cerebral anoxia or hemorrhages consequent to the elevated venous pressure. Rarely, cortical degeneration occurs, but the exact pathogenesis of the encephalopathy is unknown. A serous meningitis with lymphocytosis of the cerebrospinal fluid has been described. Pneumothorax and interstitial emphysema are infrequently seen. Secondary bacterial otitis media occurs frequently. The major cause of death in whooping cough is pneumonia, either primary or caused by other bacteria or viruses.

DIAGNOSIS. There is little difficulty in making the clinical diagnosis of whooping cough in a patient who, after a period of coryzal symptoms, develops paroxysmal coughing with a terminal inspiratory whoop. Lymphocytosis often occurs toward the end of the catarrhal stage or early in the spasmodic phase. Characteristically the leukocyte count ranges from 15,000 to 30,000 per microliter or higher, and 80 per cent of the cells are small lymphocytes. Polymorphonuclear leukocytosis suggests a secondary bacterial complication.

Microbiologic identification of the organisms may be required to make the diagnosis in abortive or mild cases or in young infants. During the early stages *B. pertussis* can be isolated from approximately 90 per cent of patients. By the third or fourth week the organism can be recovered in only 50 per cent of cases, and in the convalescent stage it is unusual to obtain a positive culture.

Specimens for culture are best obtained by pernasal swab rather than by the cough plate method. A sterile cotton swab wrapped about a flexible copper wire is passed through the nares, and mucus is obtained from the posterior pharynx. *B. pertussis* is readily killed by desiccation, so the specimen should be quickly plated onto fresh medium, to which penicillin has been added to prevent overgrowth of adventitious organisms.

A fluorescent antibody staining procedure can be applied directly to clinical specimens or organisms grown in culture. It greatly accelerates the identification of cultured organisms after isolation but is less reliable with nasopharyngeal swabs or other clinical material.

Serologic procedures are of little help in the diagnosis of whooping cough because a rise in titer of most antibodies does not occur until at least the third week of illness. Tests are not well standardized, and few laboratories perform them.

TREATMENT. *Supportive Therapy.* Young infants, particularly those under 6 months of age, should be hospitalized. Supportive measures combined with careful nursing care are of paramount importance. Specific attention must be devoted to the maintenance of proper water and electrolyte balance, adequate nutrition, and sufficient oxygenation. Constant alertness for the presence of secondary infectious complications such as pneumonia is required. Mild cases require only supportive treatment.

Antimicrobials. Specific therapy of severe whooping cough has been disappointing despite the in vitro susceptibility of *B. pertussis* to various antimicrobial agents. Antimicrobials given in the catarrhal stage may ameliorate the disease. In the established paroxysmal stage the organisms can be readily eliminated by antimicrobials, but the course of the illness is unaltered. Antibiotics may be justified in order to render the patient noninfectious. Erythromycin is the drug of choice. The daily dose is 50 mg per kilogram of body weight given in four divided doses. The organism is eliminated after a few days of therapy, but because bacteriologic relapse may occur, treatment should be continued for 14 to 21 days. Trimethoprim-sulfamethoxazole (8 mg per kilogram and 40 mg per kilogram per day in two doses) is a possible alternative for patients who do not tolerate erythromycin.

PREVENTION. Unfortunately, the diagnosis is usually not made until the end of the catarrhal stage, and by then spread of the disease has already occurred. Exposed susceptibles should receive erythromycin prophylaxis, and close (household, daycare, classroom) contacts under 7 years of age who have been previously immunized should receive a booster dose of vaccine in addition to erythromycin. Booster doses of vaccine have been used to protect adults, such as hospital staff, but side effects tend to be frequent, and erythromycin chemoprophylaxis may be preferable.

Active Immunization. Women of childbearing age generally do not have significant levels of protective antibody in their sera, and most newborns have received no passive protection. Consequently, active immunization is begun as early as is practicable. At present, it is recommended that the infant receive three injections of pertussis vaccine (inactive *B. pertussis* organisms) at 8-week intervals commencing at age 2 months. The pertussis suspension is mixed with alum-precipitated diphtheria and tetanus toxoids (DTP). A fourth injection is given 6 to 12 months after the third dose (15 to 18 months of age), and a booster is given before entering kindergarten. Administration of pertussis vaccine to those over 6 years of age is not generally recommended because of an apparent increased incidence of untoward reactions and the diminished risk of the illness itself in the older child. However, low doses have been administered to adults without incident.

As previously noted, immunization does not confer lifelong protection. Approximately 80 per cent of those vaccinated within 4 years of exposure are protected, whereas 80 to 90 per cent of a matched unimmunized group with similar exposure contract pertussis. The prophylactic efficacy of pertussis vaccine was clearly demonstrated when epidemics occurred in the United Kingdom in 1977–79 and 1982 following a 3- to 5-year period during which vaccine acceptance had declined to very low levels. More than 170,000 cases of whooping cough were reported, including 42 deaths, principally among children under 5 years of age. Similar outbreaks have followed diminished vaccine utilization in Japan and Sweden.

Reactions at the injection site as well as fever and hyperirritability occur commonly after injection of pertussis vaccine. The incidence of postinjection encephalopathy is uncertain, and it is not clear whether the vaccine can cause permanent neurologic damage. A recent British study suggests a risk of 1 in 140,000 immunizations for previously normal infants, with residual neurologic damage in 1 in 330,000 immunizations. This estimated risk of neurologic complications from pertussis immunization is far less than the hazards of whooping cough in the young child. Nevertheless, in infants with a personal history of convulsions or other neurologic disorders, pertussis immunization should be deferred until the condition has stabilized. Acellular vaccines containing various combinations of pertussis toxin, 69kD OMP, filamentous hemagglutinin, or other *B. pertussis* products are being studied. Acellular vaccines cause far fewer reactions than does the whole bacterial cell vaccine. If tests currently under way of their immunogenicity and prophylactic efficacy are convincing in field use, acellular vaccines should replace the killed whole-cell vaccine.

Geller RJ: The pertussis syndrome: A persistent problem. Pediatr Infect Dis J 3:182, 1984. *A succinct state-of-the-art presentation of diagnosis, clinical picture, and management.*

Griffin MR, Ray WA, Mortimer EA, et al.: Risk of seizures and encephalopathy after immunization with the diphtheria-tetanus-pertussis vaccine. JAMA 263:1641, 1990. *A careful (and unrevealing) search for neurologic sequelae associated with DTP immunization. Accompanying editorial, p. 1679.*

Manclark CR (ed.): Proceedings of the Sixth International Symposium on Pertussis. Department of Health and Human Services, United States Public Health Service, Bethesda, Md. DHHS Publication No. (FDA) 90-1164, 1990. *Comprises a review of recent research on virulence factors, surface proteins, host-parasite interactions, genetic regulation of virulence factors, epidemiology, diagnosis, and clinical aspects.*

Pittman M: The concept of pertussis as a toxin-mediated disease. Pediatr Infect Dis J 3:467, 1984. *A thorough review of pathogenesis, immunity, and immunization.*

Wardlaw AC, Parton R (eds.): Pathogenesis and Immunity in Pertussis. New York, John Wiley and Sons, 1988. *A superb source of current information on clinical and microbiologic aspects of whooping cough and on pertussis vaccines.*

Diphtheria

306 Diphtheria

Erik L. Hewlett

Diphtheria is an acute, toxin-mediated infectious disease caused by toxigenic *Corynebacterium diphtheriae*. Classically, the infection usually localizes to the pharynx, larynx, and nostrils, with skin infection representing an increasing proportion of cases in developed nations. Severe systemic disease and mortality occur most frequently in patients with pharyngeal infection and are largely attributable to an exotoxin released by the bacteria at the site of localized infection. The disease, but not necessarily the local infection, is preventable by immunization with diphtheria toxoid.

ETIOLOGY. *C. diphtheriae* is a pleomorphic, non–spore-forming, non–acid-fast, nonmotile gram-positive rod that on smears is often seen in palisades or configurations resembling Chinese characters. Its club-end appearance is the origin of the name *Corynebacterium*, from the Greek "korynee," meaning club. The heterogeneous morphology of corynebacteria makes diagnosis on the basis of stained smear unreliable. *C. diphtheriae* grows well on tellurite agar or Loeffler's serum slants under aerobic conditions and is distinguished from related corynebacteria by fermentation of glucose and maltose but not sucrose. Although the organisms are killed by mild heating (56°C for 10 minutes), they are strikingly resistant to damage from drying and can be cultured from floor dust for 5 weeks or longer.

The species is divided into three stable biotypes, named *gravis*, *intermedius*, and *mitis*, to indicate their relative virulence in epidemics during the early twentieth century. Although biotypes are still used to characterize strains, there is not a direct correlation between biotype and severity of disease. In fact, the *intermedius* biotype is most frequently toxigenic (98.9 per cent), followed by *gravis* (84.0 per cent) and *mitis* (34.1 per cent). Recently, DNA hybridization, using an insertion sequence probe, has enabled identification and epidemiologic tracking of strains in a population.

The major virulence determinant is an exotoxin that is produced by organisms infected by a lysogenic β-phage. The toxin structural gene is carried in the genome of the phage, and toxin is produced by lysogenized *C. diphtheriae* only after depletion of the iron in the medium. Toxigenicity of an isolate can be determined in vitro by ELISA or by the Elek test, in which the clinical isolate is streaked at right angles to an antitoxin-impregnated strip of filter paper on a plate. If the strain is toxigenic, a precipitin line of toxin-antitoxin complex forms during culture. Toxigenicity testing in vivo involves intraperitoneal injection of a suspension of organisms into naive and antitoxin-treated guinea pigs. Death of the test animal, but not the antitoxin recipient, in 1 to 4 days indicates toxin production.

EPIDEMIOLOGY. Diphtheria is a highly contagious infection that is spread most easily under socioeconomic conditions in which there is poor personal hygiene, crowding, and limited access to medical care. The primary route of transmission has been by aerosol or other transfer of respiratory secretions from an infected individual. As illustrated by several outbreaks among adults in the United States, however, spread from cutaneous lesions of subjects with little or no systemic disease by direct contact or by fomites (such as unclean blankets) is of increasing importance epidemiologically. The skin infections of these carriers may occur in many different forms, such as purulent punched-out ulcers, impetiginous lesions, and wound infections. As a result, it is often difficult to make the diagnosis of diphtheria without classic symptoms in their contacts. Furthermore, the diagnosis may be missed because of the presence of a mixed infection with staphylococci or streptococci. Such localized infections with limited toxin absorption are postulated to be the source of acquired immunity among nonimmunized children in the tropics. Although infections of animals, especially cattle, can be the source of human disease, this is an uncommon mechanism of transmission and there are no known reservoirs in nature. Molecular epidemiologic studies indicate that among toxigenic strains, some may be more virulent than others, and severe disease results from transmission of more virulent strains in a population.

Immunization status influences susceptibility to infection and severity of disease in the individual patient. When disease does occur in immunized or partially immunized patients, mortality (1.3 per cent) is 10-fold lower than in nonimmunized individuals (13.4 per cent). Herd immunity has a major impact on patterns of transmission and carriage of *C. diphtheriae*. Although it was expected by some that immunization with diphtheria toxoid would increase the rate of carriage of *C. diphtheriae* in a population, the opposite is true. The selective advantage of toxigenicity is lost, and fewer toxigenic strains are found in an immunized population. Serologic surveys indicate a high proportion of susceptible adults in many populations. Although clinical diphtheria is at its lowest level ever, with no cases reported in the United States in 1986, the potential exists for disease in the setting of unrecognized exposure.

PATHOGENESIS. Following arrival of *C. diphtheriae* at the site of infection, organisms proliferate and elaborate toxin. As with other bacterial diseases that are mediated in large part by exotoxins, the rapidity of onset, severity of disease, and ultimate outcome are determined by the rate of production, absorption, and dissemination of the toxin. The determinants of these variables include the site of infection, the virulence of the strain (quantity of toxin produced and availability of ancillary factors to facilitate toxin absorption), and the status of host immunity. For example, individuals with *C. diphtheriae* infection of the skin, middle ear, or anterior nares—sites from which toxin absorption is less than across the pharyngeal mucosa—may have little or no systemic disease. Prior immunity, by virtue of immunization or prior infection, may prevent systemic manifestations of disease without affecting the localized carriage of the organism.

Diphtheria toxin, among the best studied of all bacterial toxins, is synthesized as an inactive single polypeptide of 61,000 molecular weight. It is activated by proteolytic cleavage and reduction of the interchain disulfide bonds, yielding two subunits (A or active subunit and B or binding subunit). Upon reaching the host cell, the B subunit attaches to a specific glycoprotein receptor, a step that is required for internalization by receptor-mediated endocytosis. Within mammalian cells, the A subunit catalyzes the transfer of the adenosine diphosphate ribose (ADPR) portion of nicotinamide adenine dinucleotide (NAD) to a specific target amino acid (modified histidine named diphthamide because of this reaction) on a single protein, elongation factor 2, which is required for protein synthesis. The consequence to the cell is interruption of protein synthesis, disruption of cell processes requiring new proteins, and, ultimately, cell death. The consequences to the infected host depend upon the types of cells intoxicated and the extent of intoxication.

CLINICAL MANIFESTATIONS. The manifestations of infection with *C. diphtheriae* can range from a single, localized lesion without systemic signs or symptoms to a rapidly progressive, fatal illness. In general, the severity of the disease is correlated with the magnitude and site of the local lesion, and, in fact, the different clinical presentations have been classified on the basis of the primary site of infection.

Symptoms begin after an incubation period of less than 1 week. Patients with cutaneous, anterior nasal, or middle ear infection with *C. diphtheriae* are generally well, with little or no local pain and often only purulent drainage from the involved site. Occasionally, a thin membrane with associated crusting can be seen. Because of the infrequent occurrence of systemic toxicity, these lesions can become chronic, providing a source for transmission to contacts. This presentation is now the predominant one in developed countries.

Tonsillar or faucial diphtheria, although not frequently life-threatening, can be associated with severe complications. At the time of presentation, patients are moderately ill, with complaints of low-grade fever, fatigue, headache, and sore throat. The typical adherent, grayish green membrane may be localized to one tonsil or may extend across the midline and anteriorly. Such patients have the potential for abrupt deterioration and warrant close observation.

Pharyngeal diphtheria, especially associated with laryngeal and bronchial extension, represents an extreme in the spectrum of clinical presentations. The patient is gravely ill with weak pulse, restlessness, and confusion, but at the same time may be afebrile. The diphtheritic membrane may be extensive, covering the posterior pharynx and extending upward into the nasopharynx, forward onto the hard palate, and downward through the larynx. The thick, partially necrotic membrane is difficult to remove and is the source of the classic, but not diagnostic, foul odor associated with this disease. Development of anterior cervical warmth and edema resulting in the "bull neck" appearance is not uncommon in extensive pharyngeal disease. Patients in whom the membrane extends to the larynx and beyond experience airway obstruction with stridor and cyanosis.

Clinical diphtheria may be associated with dysfunction of a variety of tissues, especially heart and nerve, and these complications are the major cause of morbidity and mortality. Myocarditis, for example, occurs in 50 per cent of patients with moderately severe disease, apparently as a result of direct toxin action on myocardial cells and perhaps subsequent inflammation and fibrosis. The onset may be slow, with manifestations after the local pharyngeal lesion is improving. There are concurrent abnormalities of the cardiac conducting system, as indicated by electrocardiographic (ECG) abnormalities such as ST-T wave changes, arrhythmias, and heart block. The rapid onset of ECG changes, circulatory collapse, and congestive heart failure indicates a high level of systemic intoxication and a very poor prognosis.

Functionally significant intoxication of neural tissue occurs in 10 to 20 per cent of patients and is manifested by cranial nerve palsies, peripheral neuropathies, and frank paralysis. Patients may experience difficulty swallowing, with regurgitation and aspiration of liquids, extremity weakness, and even respiratory failure. These deficits may be first recognized 4 or more weeks after onset of the illness, but, if the patient survives, are generally slowly reversible.

DIAGNOSIS. Although bacteriologic identification is a critical feature of diphtheria diagnosis, therapy for this life-threatening illness must not await culture confirmation. Gram-stained or fluorescent antibody–stained material can be used to increase the index of suspicion but is not adequate for definitive diagnosis. Swabs from nose and pharynx or other sites should be cultured on Loeffler's slants and the more selective tellurite agar as well as blood agar. All clinical isolates of *C. diphtheriae* should be tested for toxigenicity by ELISA or Elek test. Since coinfection with staphylococci and streptococci can occur, the presence of these organisms does not rule out diphtheria.

In milder cases, the diphtheritic membrane may not be striking and other physical findings are not distinguishing. Although the sore throat is generally less than with a streptococcal infection, the differential diagnosis should include streptococcal pharyngitis, oral candidiasis, infectious mononucleosis, and Vincent's angina.

TREATMENT AND PREVENTION. The goals of therapy in a patient with presumed or documented diphtheria are neutralization of free toxin, elimination of further toxin production, control of the local infection, support during the course of the systemic intoxication phase, and prevention of transmission. The mainstays of treatment, therefore, are (1) equine diphtheria antitoxin (human diphtheria immune globulin is not available in the United States), (2) antibiotics, (3) supportive intervention directed at complications such as respiratory compromise, congestive heart failure, cardiac arrhythmias, neuropathies, renal failure, and bleeding diatheses, and (4) strict isolation.

Presumptive diagnosis of diphtheria is adequate justification for use of diphtheria antitoxin, since the severe life-threatening complications are the result of toxin action at distal sites and immediate neutralization of circulating toxin is essential. The dose of antitoxin is based upon the site and extent of local infection and the severity and duration of symptoms at the time of presentation. Patients with cutaneous infection generally do not experience toxicity, but a low dose of antitoxin (20,000 units) is sometimes given. A dose of 20,000 to 40,000 units of antitoxin is recommended for patients with limited pharyngeal disease of 2 days' or less duration. Patients with more extensive nasopharyngeal involvement, especially of greater than 3 days' duration and associated with bull neck and other complications, require 80,000 to 100,000 units of antitoxin. The antitoxin is most effective when given intravenously, but because it is of equine origin, patients must be tested for hypersensitivity before administration and desensitized as necessary.

Antibiotics are required for prevention of further toxin production, control of local infection, and reduction of transmission, as untreated convalescent carriage can persist for weeks. Treatment with penicillin or erythromycin should be followed by repeat culture to document elimination of the organism because resistance to erythromycin has been observed. Since the consequences of toxin action within target cells cannot be reversed pharmacologically, patients with life-threatening complications need intensive monitoring and specific supportive therapy as indicated. For example, myocarditis with arrhythmias and congestive heart failure may necessitate salt restriction, digitalis, antiarrhythmics, and even temporary pacing during the height of illness. As with other toxin-mediated diseases, there may not be a sufficient immune response to provide future protection, and convalescent individuals should receive diphtheria toxoid immunization.

All contacts should be cultured. Those immunized 5 or more years previously should receive a booster, and those never immunized should be treated prophylactically with antibiotics. All asymptomatic carriers should be treated with antibiotics to eliminate the organism and immunized with either a primary series or booster as indicated.

The only effective measure for prevention of clinical diphtheria is immunization with diphtheria toxoid. The primary series is three doses given in conjunction with tetanus toxoid and pertussis vaccine during the first 6 months of life. Boosters are given at 15 months and 4 to 6 years of age. In order to maintain immunity during adolescence and adulthood, boosters are needed at 10-year intervals using a preparation containing a reduced amount of the diphtheria toxoid, owing to adverse reactions related to some prior immunity. The reduced dose for adults is available alone or in combination with tetanus toxoid (Td).

Although not commonly determined at the present time except as an epidemiologic research tool, susceptibility of an individual to clinical diphtheria can be assessed by quantitation in vitro of toxin-neutralizing antibody in the serum or by the Schick test, which involves injection of a low dose of native diphtheria toxin intradermally and observation for evidence of local toxin damage (redness, edema at 48 to 96 hours). A positive reaction indicates lack of neutralizing antibody and susceptibility to disease.

Björkholm B, Böttiger M, Christenson B, et al.: Antitoxin antibody levels and the outcome of illness during an outbreak of diphtheria among alcoholics. Scand J Infect Dis 18:235, 1986. *Illustration of the reduced level of immunity in adult population and significance of "protective" antibody levels.*

Dixon JMS, Noble WC, Smith GR: Diphtheria; other corynebacterial and coryneform infections. *In* Smith GR, Easmon CSF (eds.): Topley and Wilson's Principles of Bacteriology, Virology and Immunity. 8th ed. Vol. 3. London, Edward Arnold, 1990, pp 55–79. *Useful compilation of microbiologic and epidemiologic data.*

Harnisch JP, Tronca E, Nolan CM, et al.: Diphtheria among alcoholic urban adults. A decade of experience in Seattle. Ann Intern Med 111:71, 1989. *Extensive summary of diphtheria in the United States in the last 20 years.*

Hewlett EL: Selective primary health care: Strategies for control of disease in the developing world. XVIII. Pertussis and diphtheria. Rev Infect Dis 7:426, 1985. *Review of approaches to control of diphtheria, compared and contrasted with pertussis.*

Pappenheimer AM: Diphtheria: Studies on the biology of an infectious disease. The Harvey Lectures, Series 76. New York, Academic Press, 1982, pp 45–73. *Detailed description of the cellular and molecular biology of toxin structure and function.*

Rappuoli R, Perugini M, Falson E: Molecular epidemiology of the 1984–1986 outbreak of diphtheria in Sweden. N Engl J Med 318:12–14, 1988. *Demonstration of the utility of a molecular probe and the concept of alternative virulence factors it raises.*

Clostridial Diseases

John G. Bartlett

307 Clostridial Myonecrosis and Other Clostridial Diseases

Clostridia are gram-positive, spore-forming anaerobic bacteria that are widely distributed in soil and in the normal intestinal microflora of humans and animals. Sporulation permits survival in adverse conditions so that these organisms can be isolated with ease from almost any environmental source. Concentrations vary considerably, but any fertile loam is expected to contain at least 10^3 clostridia per gram. Clostridia have been found in the intestinal tract of almost all animals examined. Most humans harbor 10^9 to 10^{10} clostridia per gram of stool; these organisms are less commonly found in the normal flora of the skin, oral cavity, and female genital tract. *Clostridium perfringens*, the most frequent clinical isolate, is found in virtually all soil samples and, along with *C. ramosum*, is the most frequent clostridial species found in the intestinal flora of humans. Nevertheless, there are over 60 recognized species, and about 30 species have been found in human infections. Most clinical laboratories do not perform the extensive biochemical testing necessary to speciate clostridial isolates, and even when this is done, many organisms do not fit current taxonomic schema.

Clostridia cause diverse disease processes including bacteremia, localized infections at various anatomic sites, and the histotoxic clostridial syndromes. The latter refer to diseases caused by toxins elaborated under appropriate cultural conditions by specific clostridial species (Table 307–1). The most commonly encountered histotoxic species is *C. perfringens*, which is divided into five types designated A to E on the basis of the production of the four major lethal toxins designated alpha, beta, epsilon, and iota. All *C. perfringens*, and many other species of clostridia (Table 307–1), produce alpha toxin, a phospholipase that splits lecithin to phosphoryl choline and a diglyceride. Intravenous administration of alpha toxin in experimental animals causes massive hemolysis, platelet destruction, and widespread capillary damage. Other clostridial toxins cause diseases of the intestine (enteric toxins) or of the nervous system (neurotoxins). The toxins of *C. botulinum* and *C. tetanus* are lethal to mice in doses of 1 ng. By extrapolation, the lethal dose in the bloodstream of humans is approximately 10^{-9} mg per kilogram body weight, making these toxins the most potent microbial poisons known. The toxins of *C. difficile* and the alpha toxin of *C. perfringens* are about 100 to 1000 times less potent in mouse lethality testing.

Smith LDS: The Pathogenic Anaerobic Bacteria, 2nd ed. Springfield, IL, Charles C Thomas, 1975, pp 109–324. *The author, a noted authority in the field, provides a scholarly review of clostridia, including a description of the species, their natural habitat, their toxins, and their role in disease.*

CLOSTRIDIAL MYONECROSIS

DEFINITION. Clostridial myonecrosis, or gas gangrene, is a life-threatening infection involving muscle caused by toxins produced by clostridia, usually *C. perfringens*.

ETIOLOGY. Clostridial myonecrosis usually follows wounding from trauma or surgery, contamination with histotoxic clostridia, and toxin elaboration. It is estimated that 30 to 80 per cent of serious, traumatic, open wounds are contaminated by clostridia, although gas gangrene remains a relatively rare infection. This experience emphasizes the decisive role of local conditions that promote toxin production primarily by decreasing the oxidation-reduction potential. Contributing factors to tissue hypoxia include vascular insufficiency, the presence of foreign bodies, tissue necrosis, and concurrent infection involving other microbes.

The most frequent pathogen, *C. perfringens*, is found in approximately 80 per cent of cases with positive cultures. Other clostridial species implicated include *C. novyi*, *C. septicum*, *C. histolyticum*, *C. bifermentans*, and *C. fallax*. In many instances, there are several clostridial species isolated from the infected site. Species causing gas gangrene produce over 20 exotoxins,

TABLE 307–1. HISTOTOXIC CLOSTRIDIAL SYNDROMES

Disease	Agent	Toxin
Enteric diseases		
Food poisoning	*C. perfringens*, type A	Enterotoxin
Antibiotic-induced diarrhea or colitis	*C. difficile*	Toxins A and B
Enteritis necroticans	*C. perfringens*, type C	Beta toxin
Neurologic syndromes		
Botulism	*C. botulinum*	Botulinal toxins A, B, E, F, and G
Tetanus	*C. tetanus*	Tetanospasmin
Myonecrosis (gas gangrene)	*C. perfringens*, *C. novyi*, *C. septicum*, *C. histolyticum*, *C. bifermentans*, *C. fallax*	Multiple toxins, especially alpha toxin

including seven that are lethal to experimental animals. In appropriate environmental conditions, vegetative forms of the histotoxic clostridia replicate and elaborate toxins that diffuse into adjacent soft tisssue to promote local spread as well as extensive systemic effects.

CLINICAL MANIFESTATIONS. Gas gangrene is a devastating infection characterized by prominent findings at the site of injury and profound systemic toxicity. Most cases occur in association with wounding from trauma or surgery. The usual clinical settings are (1) traumatic injury or penetrating wound; (2) surgery, especially intestinal or biliary tract operations; (3) uterine gas gangrene, which most frequently follows delivery or septic abortions; (4) soft tissue lesions associated with vascular insufficiency; (5) intestinal gas gangrene, which is most commonly found in compromised hosts, especially patients with leukemia or colonic carcinoma; and (6) "spontaneous gas gangrene," a rare form of the disease in which there is no readily identifiable predisposing condition. During peacetime in the United States approximately 50 per cent of cases follow severe traumatic injury and 40 per cent follow surgery. The most frequent traumatic injuries are car accidents, crush injuries, industrial accidents, and gunshot wounds. The most frequent antecedent surgical procedures are colon resection and biliary tract surgery. About two thirds of cases involve extremities, and one third involve the abdominal wall.

The usual incubation period from the time of wounding to the onset of symptoms is 1 to 4 days, with a range of 8 hours to several weeks. The first symptom is usually sudden and severe pain at the site of injury. Observations at this time typically show tense edema and tenderness. Gas may be noted in the soft tissues by palpation, radiography, computed tomography, or ultrasound studies. The skin is initially pale and then progresses to a magenta or bronze discoloration, and there is often cutaneous necrosis with hemorrhagic bullae. As the lesion evolves, there may be a thin, serosanguineous discharge with characteristic sweet odor. The systemic findings that accompany the evolving changes at

the wound are profound. These include diaphoresis, low-grade fever, and tachycardia. Common complications include hemolytic anemia, hypotension, and renal failure. The patient is typically anxious throughout the disease but remains alert despite profound systemic toxicity.

DIAGNOSIS. The diagnosis of clostridial myonecrosis is based on a constellation of clinical findings and supporting microbiologic data. Roentgenographic studies often show gas bubbles in the soft tissue, computed tomography shows gas and myonecrosis, and Gram's stains of discharge typically show large, gram-positive or gram-variable bacilli with blunt ends and a paucity of polymorphonuclear leukocytes. Approximately 15 per cent of patients have clostridial bacteremia. Nevertheless, the findings of Gram's stain and the detection of gas in the soft tissue cannot be considered specific, and most patients with clostridial bacteremia do not have myonecrosis. The definitive diagnostic procedure is surgical incision to expose muscle that may appear pale and edematous, beefy-red, or, in the most advanced stages, black and friable. The muscle is nonviable, it fails to contract with stimulation, and the cut surface does not bleed.

The differential diagnosis includes a number of soft tissue infections that may also involve clostridia, or occur in association with severe systemic toxicity, tissue necrosis, a fulminant course, or gas formation. Important findings in the differential diagnosis are summarized in Table 307-2. This classification includes two anatomic patterns: infections involving the enveloping fascia and infections within the fascial compartment. The latter category includes infections associated with myonecrosis which are classified by microbiologic pattern as streptococcal myonecrosis, synergistic necrotizing cellulitis due to mixtures of aerobic and anaerobic bacteria, and gas gangrene. None of these infections is common, but all require aggressive treatment including early surgical intervention. Clinical clues suggesting these devastating conditions include severe systemic toxicity, severe pain that is

TABLE 307–2. DEEP AND SERIOUS SOFT TISSUE INFECTIONS

	Gas-Forming Cellulitis	Synergistic Necrotizing Cellulitis	Gas Gangrene	"Streptococcal" Myonecrosis	Necrotizing Fasciitis	Infected Vascular Gangrene	Streptococcal Gangrene
Predisposing conditions	Traumatic	Diabetes, prior local lesion, perirectal lesion	Traumatic or surgical wound	Trauma, surgery	Diabetes, trauma, surgery, perineal infection	Arterial insufficiency	Traumatic or surgical wound
Incubation period	>3 days	3–14 days	1–4 days	3–4 days	1–4 days	>5 days	6 hours–2 days
Etiologic organism(s)	Clostridia, others	Mixed aerobic-anaerobic flora	Clostridia, esp. *C. perfringens*	Anaerobic streptococci	Mixed aerobic-anaerobic flora	Mixed aerobic-anaerobic flora	*S. pyogenes*
Systemic toxicity	Minimal	Moderate to severe	Severe	Minimal until late in course	Moderate to severe	Minimal	Severe
Course	Gradual	Acute	Acute	Subacute	Acute or subacute	Subacute	Acute
Wound findings							
Local pain	Minimal	Moderate to severe	Severe	Late only	Minimal to moderate	Variable	Severe
Skin appearance	Swollen, minimal discoloration	Erythematous or gangrenous	Tense and blanched, yellow-bronze, necrosis with hemorrhagic bullae	Erythema or yellow-bronze	Blanched, erythema, necrosis with hemorrhagic bullae	Erythema or necrosis	Erythema, necrosis
Gas	Abundant	Variable	Usually present	Variable	Variable	Variable	No
Muscle involvement	No	Variable	Myonecrosis	Myonecrosis	No	Myonecrosis limited to area of vascular insufficiency	No
Discharge	Thin, dark, sweetish or foul odor	Dark pus or "dishwater," putrid	Serosanguineous, sweet or foul odor	Seropurulent	Seropurulent or "dishwater," putrid	Minimal	None or serosanguineous, no odor
Gram stain	PMN's, gram-positive bacilli	PMN's, mixed flora	Sparse PMN's, gram-positive bacilli	PMN's, gram-positive cocci	PMN's, mixed flora	PMN's, mixed flora	PMN's, gram-positive cocci in chains
Surgical therapy	Debridement	Wide filleting incisions	Extensive excision, amputation	Excision of necrotic muscle	Wide filleting incisions	Amputation	Debridement of necrotic tissue

spontaneous (tenderness suggests a more superficial infection such as cellulitis), bullae, gas in the soft tissue, and rapid extension. Computed tomography or magnetic resonance imaging often demonstrates the tissue plane of involvement, and deep aspirates and blood cultures may reveal microbiologic patterns. However, surgery provides a definitive diagnosis.

TREATMENT. The most important facet of treatment is extensive surgical debridement with wide excision of involved muscle, amputation when an extremity is involved, or hysterectomy with uterine gas gangrene. The preferred antibiotic is aqueous penicillin G given intravenously in doses of 10 to 40 million units daily for adults. Alternative antimicrobial agents include intravenous metronidazole (2 grams per day), chloramphenicol (2 grams per day), or clindamycin (1800 mg per day). Cephalosporins are generally less active against clostridia. The therapeutic value of hyperbaric oxygen is controversial. Advocates claim that this clearly demarcates the necrotic tissue to simplify surgery and improve survival rates. Nevertheless, controlled studies to document efficacy are not available, and there may be major problems in transferring critically ill patients to centers with this type of facility. Surgery should not be delayed. Supportive measures include fluid and electrolyte replacement, control of acidosis, transfusions for severe anemia, and appropriate measures for renal failure.

PROGNOSIS. Clostridial myonecrosis is a devastating infection that often requires mutilating surgery and prolonged hospital courses. The overall mortality rate in 116 reports summarizing over 1200 cases is 25 per cent. However, many reported cases actually represent other types of soft tissue infections involving clostridial species, and the mortality rate for true gas gangrene is probably far higher.

PREVENTION. The inoculum of *C. perfringens* required to produce gas gangrene is reduced by 10^6 organisms in experimental animals if the organism is delivered into devitalized muscle containing dirt instead of normal tissue. As noted earlier, contamination of wounds by clostridia either from soil sources or from the endogenous fecal flora is common with both traumatic injuries and surgical incisions. The incidence of clostridial myonecrosis following battlefield injury was 10 per cent in World War I, 1 per cent in World War II, and 0.01 per cent (22 cases in 139,000 battle injuries) in the Vietnam War. These figures reflect improvements in the management of battlefield injuries with major emphasis on prompt and thorough debridement. There should also be care in preserving the vascular supply, particularly with the use of tourniquets and casts. Judicious decisions regarding closure of traumatic wounds and the prophylactic use of antibiotics are also important. There is no effective means of active immunization.

Baxter CR: Surgical management of soft tissue infections. Surg Clin North Am 52:1483, 1972. *Soft tissue infections are reviewed using three categories: infections requiring incision and drainage, infections requiring excision of tissue, and infections not requiring extensive surgery.*

Dellinger EP: Severe necrotizing soft tissue infections. JAMA 246:1717–1721, 1981. *The author reviews management principles for severe soft tissue infections and emphasizes the differential diagnosis based on clinical presentation, Gram's stain, and operative inspection.*

Heimbach RD: Gas gangrene: Review and update. HBO Review 1:41, 1980. *The author reviews gas gangrene and presents an endorsement for hyperbaric oxygen treatment which may be overly enthusiastic.*

Stevens DL, Maier KA, Laine BM, et al.: Comparison of clindamycin, rifampin, tetracycline, metronidazole, and penicillin for efficacy in prevention of experimental gas gangrene due to *Clostridium perfringens.* J Infect Dis 155:220, 1987. *A provocative report showing multiple antimicrobial agents to be superior to penicillin in an animal model of gas gangrene.*

Weinstein L, Barza M: Gas gangrene. N Engl J Med 289:1129, 1972. *A review of clinical features and management recommendations for gas gangrene.*

OTHER CLOSTRIDIAL DISEASES

SEPTICEMIA. Clostridia account for up to 3 per cent of all positive blood cultures in most clinical microbiologic laboratories. The most frequent species is *C. perfringens,* which accounts for 50 to 60 per cent. Most patients have other conditions and the significance of the clostridia is enigmatic. Less frequently there is an associated mixed infection, such as an intra-abdominal abscess, that represents the presumed portal of entry. Gas gangrene is rare and this diagnosis should be based on compatible clinical features. Special notation must be made for bacteremia with *C. septicum.* Many of these patients have leukemia in relapse, neutropenia, or colonic carcinoma. The usual portal of entry is the distal ileum or cecum ("neutropenic enterocolitis"), most patients are acutely ill, the mortality rate is high, and aggressive resectional surgery combined with intravenous penicillin is indicated. *Clostridium tertium* may cause a similar syndrome, but the mortality rate is low and most patients respond to antibiotics without surgery.

MISCELLANEOUS INFECTIONS. Clostridia are frequently isolated from infections involving the host's normal flora. This situation especially applies to cases in which the infecting flora originates in the colon, such as in intra-abdominal sepsis, wound infections after intestinal surgery, and wounds such as ischemic ulcers, diabetic ulcers, or decubitus ulcers located on the lower trunk or lower extremities. These organisms are especially common in infections associated with gas formation such as emphysematous cholecystitis, emphysematous cystitis, and crepitant cellulitis. Clostridia are also found in 5 to 10 per cent of anaerobic pulmonary infections and with similar frequency in nonvenereal infections of the female genital tract. Such infections usually involve a mixture of aerobic and anaerobic bacteria so that the role of clostridia is uncertain. Penicillin G is generally considered the preferred antibiotic for clostridial infections, although increasing resistance is noted with some species other than *C. perfringens.* Alternative agents include imipenem, metronidazole, chloramphenicol, or a β-lactam–β-lactamase inhibitor.

CLOSTRIDIA ENTEROTOXEMIAS. Clostridia cause three different types of enteric disease, each of which is ascribed to a unique toxin (Table 307–1). *C. difficile,* the major cause of antibiotic-associated colitis, is discussed in Ch. 308.

C. perfringens is commonly responsible for foodborne outbreaks of a self-limited enteric disease. More recent studies show that this organism may also cause diarrhea in other settings such as sporadic diarrhea, antibiotic-associated diarrhea, and diarrhea in chronic care facilities. The mechanism is an enterotoxin produced by some type A strains during sporulation. Requirements for the foodborne form are (1) ingestion of at least 10^8 viable vegetative cells; (2) enterotoxigenic potential of the ingested strain; and (3) sporulation with toxin production in the alkaline medium of the small bowel. The usual symptoms are diarrhea and abdominal cramps ascribed to fluid secretion, morphologic damage to the intestinal mucosa, and altered motility in the small bowel. Less frequent symptoms are nausea, vomiting, and fever. The usual vehicle in outbreaks is meat or food made with meat, such as stews, meat pies, gravies, or casseroles. The attack rate among exposed persons is usually 30 to 60 per cent, and the incubation period ranges from 7 to 15 hours. The diagnosis is suspected in any outbreak of gastrointestinal disease associated with typical symptoms and incubation period among persons sharing a common and likely food source. Confirmation requires the recovery of *C. perfringens* in concentrations of at least 10^5 per gram of epidemiologically implicated food, recovery of at least 10^6 spores per gram of stool obtained within 48 hours after onset of symptoms from victims, or, preferably, detection of enterotoxin in stool. Nearly all patients have spontaneous resolution of symptoms within 6 to 24 hours and do not require any specific form of therapy.

Enteritis necroticans is a serious gastrointestinal disease caused by the beta toxin of *C. perfringens,* type C. This disease, once called "darmbrand," occurred in epidemic form in malnourished individuals from Norway and Germany at the end of World War II. More recently, the same condition, known locally as "pigbel," has been found to be endemic in the highlands of New Guinea. Sporadic cases have been reported in Africa, Southeast Asia, China, and western countries. In New Guinea, most victims are children who have participated in pig feasts. The toxin is susceptible to proteolytic enzymes including trypsin. However, toxin inactivation in the small bowel fails because of enzyme deficiency ascribed to protein malnutrition, excessive consumption of sweet potatoes, which contain trypsin inhibitors, or colonization with *Ascaris lumbricoides,* which secretes trypsin inhibitors. The predilection for children presumably reflects antigenic naiveté. Pathologically, enteritis necroticans is a segmental disease of the small bowel which is characterized by mucosal infarction, edema, hemorrhage, and infiltration with polymorphonuclear cells. In advanced stages the bowel is thinned, friable, and subject to perforation. Medical therapy consists of intestinal decompression, penicillin or chloramphenicol, and intravenous fluid support. About half of the patients require resectional surgery, and the overall mortality rate is 15 to 40 per cent. Prevention is achieved with a beta-toxoid vaccine that is currently recommended for children in the endemic area.

Editorial: *Clostridium septicum* and neutropenic enterocolitis. Lancet 2:608, 1987. *The authors review "typhlitis" with C. septicum bacteremia.*

Gorbach SL, Thadepalli H: Isolation of *Clostridia* in human infections: Evaluation of 114 cases. J Infect Dis 131:S81–S85, 1975. *The authors review their experience with 152 strains of clostridia recovered from 144 patients at Cook County Hospital. Sixty-five patients had soft tissue infections or intra-abdominal sepsis, and 84 per cent of these had polymicrobial infections. Clostridia bacteremia in 49 patients usually occurred with no apparent relation to the clinical setting.*

Larson HE, Borriello SP: Infectious diarrhea due to *Clostridium perfringens*. J Infect Dis 157:390, 1988. *The authors review diarrhea due to enterotoxin-producing strains of C. perfringens, calling attention to some unique clinical features such as a prolonged clinical course and the potential utility of stool analysis for enterotoxin.*

Lawrence G, Walker PD: Pathogenesis of enteritis necroticans in Papua New Guinea. Lancet 1:125–126, 1976. *The authors, noted authorities in the field, provide a postulate for the pathophysiology of pigbel.*

Ramsay AM: The significance of *Clostridium welchii* in the cervical swab and blood stream in postpartum and postabortum sepsis. J Obstet Gynecol Br Commonwealth 56:247–258, 1949. *The author refers to C. perfringens (welchii) as a "harmless saprophyte" in a discussion of 28 women with bacteremia, since most had minimal clinical disturbance despite the fact that the majority were studied before antibiotics were available.*

Shaudera WX, Tacket CO, Blake PA: Food poisoning due to *Clostridium perfringens* in the US. J Infect Dis 147:167–170, 1983. *The authors review the Centers for Disease Control's experience with C. perfringens food poisoning.*

Van Damme–Jongsten M, Rodhouse J, Gilbert RJ, et al.: Synthetic DNA probes for detection of enterotoxigenic *Clostridium perfringens* strains isolated from outbreaks of food poisoning. J Clin Microbiol 28:131, 1990. *The DNA probes described proved useful in identifying enterotoxin-producing strains of C. perfringens.*

308 Pseudomembranous Colitis

DESCRIPTION. Pseudomembranous colitis is a severe gastrointestinal disease characterized by exudative plaques on the colonic mucosa.

ETIOLOGY. Pseudomembranous colitis is usually found in association with other conditions, although occasional cases occur in healthy persons with no identifiable risk factors. The great majority of cases represent a complication of antimicrobial use, and the etiologic agent in nearly all cases of antibiotic-associated pseudomembranous colitis is *Clostridium difficile*. The pathophysiologic mechanism is elaboration of toxins during replication of vegetative forms of *C. difficile*, a process that is presumably promoted by suppression of the competitive flora.

INCIDENCE. The incidence of antibiotic-associated pseudomembranous colitis depends on the frequency with which endoscopy is performed to establish the diagnosis, antimicrobial use patterns, and epidemiologic patterns. Nearly all antimicrobials with an antibacterial spectrum of activity have been implicated. The most frequent are ampicillin, clindamycin, and cephalosporins. Less frequent are penicillins other than ampicillin, erythromycin, and sulfamethoxazole-trimethoprim. Drugs rarely implicated include tetracyclines, chloramphenicol, sulfonamides, quinolones, and parenterally administered aminoglycosides. *C. difficile*–induced diarrhea or colitis may occur sporadically or in clusters within institutions. Epidemiologic studies indicate that *C. difficile* may be found in the colonic flora of about 3 per cent of healthy adults, is widely distributed in the environment, and is especially common in areas subject to fecal contamination from patients who have *C. difficile*–induced diarrheal complications. This last observation provides an explanation for focal outbreaks of the disease in hospitals and nursing homes where there is clustering of vulnerable patients, mainly the elderly and antibiotic recipients.

MECHANISM. *C. difficile*–induced colitis is a toxin-mediated enteric disease in which there is no microbial invasion of the intestinal mucosa. Toxin A appears to be responsible for the clinical features of the intestinal disease; toxin B is strongly cytopathic and accounts for positive results in the tissue culture assay. Most strains of *C. difficile* produce both toxins, although there is substantial strain variation in the quantities of toxins produced.

CLINICAL MANIFESTATIONS. Virtually all patients are at risk for antibiotic-associated pseudomembranous colitis, although there appears to be an increased risk with increasing age. The most common symptom is diarrhea consisting of watery or semiliquid stools without visible blood. Stool examination may show fecal leukocytes, but this is inconsistent and nonspecific. Many patients also have fever, which is usually moderate but may reach 40° C. Other common findings are abdominal cramps, lower quadrant tenderness, leukocytosis, and hypoalbuminemia. Systemic symptoms and abdominal findings are not invariably present, and some patients simply have annoying diarrhea. Complications in severe cases include dehydration, hypoalbuminemia with anasarca, electrolyte disturbances, toxic megacolon, and colonic perforation. Symptoms may begin at any time during the course of antimicrobial treatment or up to 6 weeks after antimicrobials have been discontinued. The differential diagnosis includes acute and chronic diarrhea caused by enteric pathogens other than *C. difficile*, an adverse reaction to drugs other than antibiotics, intra-abdominal sepsis, and idiopathic inflammatory bowel disease.

DIAGNOSIS. The preferred method to establish the anatomic diagnosis is colonoscopy to demonstrate typical punctate, raised, yellowish-white plaques with "skip areas" of a normal mucosa or a mucosa showing erythema or edema. The plaques are usually 2 to 10 mm wide but may enlarge and coalesce over extensive segments of the colon in the late stages. Microscopic examination of colonic biopsies shows epithelial necrosis, goblet cells distended with mucus, and infiltration of the lamina propria with polymorphonuclear cells and eosinophilic exudate. The pseudomembrane is attached to the surface epithelium and is composed of fibrin, mucin, and polymorphonuclear cells.

The preferred diagnostic test to implicate *C. difficile* is a tissue culture assay of stool to demonstrate a cytopathic toxin that is neutralized by antitoxin to *C. difficile* or *C. sordellii*. Antitoxin neutralization with antisera to *C. sordellii* reflects antigenic cross-reactivity. Toxin titers may also be performed using serial dilutions of stool specimens, although there is little correlation between the toxin titer and the severity of the disease. Alternative methods to detect *C. difficile* toxins, including the latex agglutination assay, are considered less reliable. Stool cultures for *C. difficile* often show high rates of false-positive results due to carrier rates of 10 to 30 per cent among hospitalized patients and persons receiving antibiotics without diarrheal complications. However, cultures of stool or rectal swabs are appropriate for evaluating epidemics of *C. difficile*–associated enteric disease.

Anatomic changes in the colonic mucosa noted in patients with the diarrheal complications of antibiotic use include an entirely normal colonic mucosa; erythema or edema; colitis with friability, ulceration, or hemorrhage; and pseudomembranous colitis. The toxin of *C. difficile* has been implicated in the entire spectrum of anatomic changes, but the frequency of this toxin correlates to a large extent with the severity of the disease process. Tissue culture assays for *C. difficile* toxin are positive in over 90 per cent of patients with pseudomembranous colitis and in approximately 20 per cent of those with antibiotic-associated diarrhea and an entirely normal colonic mucosa. Thus, the tissue culture assay defines the etiologic agent and does not establish the anatomic diagnosis. There is no identifiable pathogen in most patients with antibiotic-associated diarrhea or colitis in whom the assay for *C. difficile* toxin is negative, except for occasional cases that may involve *S. aureus*, Salmonella, or *C. perfringens*.

TREATMENT. Most important is discontinuation of the implicated antibiotic. This often results in resolution of symptoms with no necessity for further diagnostic tests or therapy. Patients with severe or persistent symptoms should have stool examination to detect *C. difficile* cytotoxin. Patients with severe fluid, albumin, or electrolyte depletion often require intravenous replacement and may require hyperalimentation. The role of corticosteroids and attempts to manipulate the flora, as with oral lactobacilli or fecal enemas, is not established. Antiperistaltic drugs are contraindicated.

Specific therapy is available for diarrhea caused by *C. difficile*, using cholestyramine to bind the toxin or antibiotics to inhibit the pathogen. The preferred agent for seriously ill patients is orally administered vancomycin, 125 to 500 mg four times daily for 7 to 14 days. Vancomycin is active against virtually all strains of *C. difficile*, the levels in the colon with oral administration are extremely high, and systemic toxicity is nil owing to poor absorption. The major problems with vancomycin are high cost, noxious taste, and relapses in 15 to 35 per cent of patients when vancomycin is discontinued. Relapses are characterized by the recurrence of typical symptoms, positive tissue culture assays for *C. difficile* cytotoxin, and stool cultures that yield vancomycin-sensitive strains of *C. difficile*. The frequency of relapses is not influenced by the dose of vancomycin, the duration of treatment, or the selection of vancomycin versus metronidazole.

Alternative and less expensive treatments are anion exchange resins that bind *C. difficile* toxins, such as cholestyramine (4 gm packet orally three times daily for 5 to 10 days) and metronidazole (500 mg orally 3 or 4 times daily for 7 to 14 days). These drugs should be reserved for less seriously ill patients. Patients with relapses may be treated with metronidazole or vancomycin for 10 to 14 days, followed by cholestyramine (above doses) or low dose vancomycin (125 mg on alternate days) for 3 weeks.

PROGNOSIS. *C. difficile* causes a disease spectrum ranging from asymptomatic carriers of the toxin to patients with life-threatening pseudomembranous colitis. The most common clinical expression is "simple diarrhea" that resolves when the implicated antibiotic is discontinued. Even patients with PMC usually recover without specific forms of therapy. However, symptoms may be prolonged and debilitating, with persistent diarrhea for several weeks or months. Reports that focus on more seriously ill patients indicate mortality rates of 10 to 30 per cent. With early institution of vancomycin therapy there is a prompt symptomatic response, and virtually all patients recover. The incidence of relapse following vancomycin or metronidazole treatment is 15 to 35 per cent, and some patients suffer multiple relapses following each course of treatment.

PREVENTION. The most important preventive measure is judicious use of antimicrobial agents. Patients with *C. difficile*–induced diarrhea or colitis should be isolated and placed on enteric precautions to limit spread to susceptible hosts within institutions. Additional maneuvers sometimes suggested in facilities where this complication is endemic or epidemic include sequestering *C. difficile* carriers, restriction of afflicted patients to rooms with private bathrooms, antibiotic control programs, and treatment of carriers with oral vancomycin.

Bartlett JG, Gorbach SL: Pseudomembranous colitis. Adv Intern Med 22:455, 1977. *Review of the topic with extensive reference list for publications prior to evidence implicating* C. difficile.

Bartlett JG: Treatment of *Clostridium difficile* colitis. Gastroenterology 89:1192, 1985. *Editorial review of treatment strategies.*

Bartlett JG: Clostridium difficile: Clinical considerations. Rev Infect Dis 12(Suppl 2):S243, 1990. *Review of the topic including clinical features, diagnostic tests, and therapy.*

Fekety R, Kim K-H, Brown D, et al.: Epidemiology of antibiotic-associated colitis. Am J Med 70:906, 1981. *A survey of the epidemiology of* C. difficile.

McFarland LV, Mulligan ME, Kwok RYY, Stamm WE. Nosocomial acquisition of *Clostridium difficile* infection. N Engl J Med 320:210, 1989. *The authors document the frequency of* C. difficile *as a nosocomial pathogen, although most of the colonized patients remained asymptomatic.*

Price AB, Davis DR: Pseudomembranous colitis. J Clin Pathol 30:1, 1977. *A review of histopathologic changes.*

309 Botulism

DEFINITION. Botulism is a severe neuroparalytic disease caused by botulinal toxin produced by clostridial species, usually *C. botulinum*. There are four recognized disease categories: (1) foodborne botulism, (2) infant botulism, (3) wound botulism, and (4) unclassified cases.

ETIOLOGY. *C. botulinum* is a gram-positive, spore-forming obligate anaerobe that is widely distributed in nature and frequently found in soil, marine environments, and agricultural products. Adults regularly ingest *C. botulinum* spores from fresh agricultural products without deleterious consequences, and this organism is not recognized as a component of the normal fecal flora. Each strain produces one of eight antigenically distinct toxins of approximately 150,000 daltons, designated A through H. Human disease is caused by types A, B, E, and rarely by F and G. *C. barati* and *C. butyricum* have been implicated in infant botulism with production of type F and E toxins, respectively. Botulinal toxins are hematogenously disseminated to peripheral cholinergic synapses where they bind irreversibly and block acetylcholine release. The result is hypotonia with a descending symmetric flaccid paralysis. Botulinal toxin is the most potent poison of man; it has an estimated lethal dose in the bloodstream of 10^{-9} mg per kilogram. Type A botulinum toxin is now available for injection as treatment for ocular muscle disorders, such as strabismus and blepharospasm, and dystonias, such as torticollis and hemifacial spasm.

FOOD POISONING. Foodborne botulism results from the ingestion of preformed toxin in inadequately prepared food, although *C. botulinum* in the intestine may be responsible or may serve as a continuing source of toxin. There are an average of 15 "outbreaks" annually in the United States, most of which involve a single case. The most frequently implicated vehicle in the United States is home-canned foods, which usually have a putrefactive odor. Meat and meat products are more commonly responsible in Europe, and preserved fish is most frequent in Japan, Scandinavia, and Russia. Type A and B organisms predominate in the United States, type A west of the Mississippi River and type B in eastern states. Type E organisms are usually, but not exclusively, associated with an aquatic source in northern latitudes, where they are found in coastal waters, lakes, and intestines of fish that inhabit these areas.

CLINICAL MANIFESTATIONS. The incubation period is usually 18 to 36 hours but may be as short as 2 hours or as long as 8 days. Persons with the shortest incubation period usually have the most severe disease. The bulbar musculature is affected first, with resultant diplopia, difficulty in focusing to a near point, dysphonia, dysarthria, and dysphagia. Involvement of the cholinergic autonomic nervous system may cause decreased salivation with a dry mouth and sore throat, ileus, or urinary retention. Common gastrointestinal symptoms include nausea, vomiting, and abdominal pain. Neurologic examination shows lateral rectus muscle weakness (cranial nerve VI), ptosis, dilated pupils with sluggish reaction, decreased gag reflex, or medial rectus paresis. This is followed by descending involvement of the motor neurons to peripheral muscles, including the muscles of respiration. Some patients have only mild illness, whereas others have severe paralysis that may require intensive supportive care for weeks. Mentation remains clear, there is no fever, and neurologic dysfunction is bilateral but not necessarily symmetric. The principal causes of death are respiratory or bulbar paralysis and infectious complications during the period of supportive care.

DIAGNOSIS. The usual laboratory test in suspected cases is analysis of serum, stool, gastric contents, and/or food for botulinum toxin and analysis of stool and/or food for *C. botulinum*. The classic toxin test is a mouse assay in which specimens are injected intraperitoneally to demonstrate a lethal toxin that is neutralized by type-specific antitoxin. Alternative antigen assays, such as the enzyme-linked immunoassay, have been developed, but are not widely available. Among patients with clinical evidence of botulism, the toxin is detected in sera from one third, the toxin is found in the stool from one third, and the organism is recovered in stool from 60 per cent.

Botulism should be suspected in patients with acute flaccid paralysis, especially when there is bilateral sixth cranial nerve dysfunction, associated gastrointestinal symptoms, prior ingestion of possibly contaminated food, and typical symptoms in other persons who shared this food. The differential diagnosis includes myasthenia gravis, Guillain-Barré syndrome, tick paralysis, cerebrovascular accident involving branches of the basilar artery, trichinosis, the Eaton-Lambert syndrome, hypocalcemia, hypermagnesemia, organophosphate poisoning, atropine poisoning, paralytic poisoning caused by shellfish or puffer fish, and psychiatric syndromes. Electromyography using repetitive stimulation at 40 Hz or greater is useful in differentiating botulism from other neurologic syndromes. This shows a diminished amplitude of muscle action potentials with a single supramaximal stimulus and facilitation of action potentials using paired or repetitive stimuli. These findings do not appear until the patient develops peripheral muscle weakness and are most likely to be positive in an affected limb.

TREATMENT. Sudden respiratory arrest is the most important serious complication, so that patients must be carefully observed with monitoring of vital capacity and liberal use of ventilatory support. Elimination of the toxin from the gastrointestinal tract may be facilitated using gastric lavage, cathartics, and enemas early in the course. Antitoxin is usually given irrespective of the duration of illness, since the toxin may persist in the blood for extended periods. Treatment is initiated using two vials of the trivalent antitoxin, each containing 7500 IU type A, 5500 IU type B, and 8500 IU type E antitoxin; one vial is given intravenously, one is given intramuscularly, and the two-vial treatment is then repeated at 2 to 4 hours. The antitoxin is horse serum and is associated with a 20 per cent incidence of hypersensitivity reactions, the most serious being anaphylaxis in 3 to 5 per cent. Efficacy of the antitoxin is most clearly established with type B and type E botulism. Other therapeutic considerations include guanidine hydrochloride (15 to 50 mg per kilogram daily) to enhance acetylcholine release, but efficacy has not been established. Some advocate penicillin to help eradicate *C. botulinum* from the intestine, since this represents a potential source of additional toxin.

PROGNOSIS. The case fatality rate for foodborne botulism was formerly 60 to 70 per cent. Improved methods of management, especially support of respiratory function, have reduced the fatality rate to less than 10 per cent. Patients who survive generally have complete recovery.

PREVENTION. Foodborne botulism is caused by germination of spores in food with toxin produced by vegetative forms, although the toxin may also be produced in vivo by simultaneous ingestion of spores. The disease may be prevented by destruction of spores in the original food source, inhibition of germination, or destruction of preformed toxin. Specific measures are as follows:

1. Destruction of spores with heat or irradiation. Spores of types A and B may survive boiling for several hours, especially at high altitudes (such as in Colorado) where the boiling point may be substantially lower. These spores may be destroyed if kept at 120°C for 30 minutes using pressure cookers. Spores of type E are most heat-labile and are killed with heating at 80°C for 30 minutes.

2. Germination may be inhibited by a reduction in pH, refrigeration, freezing, drying, or addition of salt, sugar, or other inhibitory substances such as sodium nitrite.

3. Inactivation of preformed toxin is accomplished by terminal heating for 20 minutes at 80°C or 10 minutes at 90°C.

INFANT BOTULISM. Infant botulism results from production of botulinal neurotoxin in vivo following colonization of the gastrointestinal tract in children ages 1 to 9 months. This is the most common form of botulism in the United States, where 30 to 80 cases are documented annually. Spores of *C. botulinum* (but not the toxin) have been found in about 10 per cent of honey supplies, which presumably account for one third of cases. The disease spectrum varies considerably, ranging from "failure to thrive" or mild changes in bowel habits to the sudden infant death syndrome or "crib death." The most commonly recognized form of the disease is the "floppy baby syndrome." Initial symptoms are lethargy, diminished suck, constipation, weakness, feeble cry, and diminished spontaneous activity with loss of head control. This is followed by extensive flaccid paralysis. The diagnosis is established with the recovery of *C. botulinum* or its toxin in stool. The toxin has rarely been detected in the serum. Fecal carriage of the organism and the toxin may persist for weeks to months following clinical improvement and hospital discharge. The major therapeutic need is supportive care with special attention to nutrition and maintenance of respiratory function. The role of antitoxin, guanidine, and antibiotics in this form of botulism has not been established, and generally their use is not advised. The mortality rate for hospitalized patients given supportive care is only 2 per cent.

WOUND BOTULISM. This is a rare form of botulism in which a traumatic wound is infected by *C. botulinum* with toxin production in vivo. Types A and B have been implicated, reflecting their presence in soil. Clinical features are identical to those of foodborne botulism except that the incubation period from the time of injury is 4 to 14 days and there is a paucity of gastrointestinal symptoms. The diagnosis is established by recovering *C. botulinum* from the wound or by detection of the toxin in serum. Management includes wound debridement and other treatments described for foodborne botulism except for bowel cleansing.

UNCLASSIFIED BOTULISM. This category includes persons over the age of 12 months who have typical symptoms and signs of botulism with no identifiable vehicle. It is possible that some cases result from production of toxin in vivo by organisms colonizing the intestine in a fashion comparable to the mechanism described for infant botulism.

SPECIAL NOTE. Physicians who suspect foodborne botulism or wish to receive botulinal antitoxin should contact the state health department (daytime and 24-hour numbers listed in JAMA 256:1105, 1986) or contact the CDC 24-hour number (404-329-2888).

Arnon SS: Infant botulism: Anticipating the second decade. J Infect Dis 154:201, 1986. *An authoritative review of infant botulism based on the 10-year experience following its original report in 1976.*

Botulinum toxin for ocular muscle disorders. The Medical Letter 32:100, 1990. Medical Letter *consultants review the uses of botulinum toxin (Oculinum) for ocular muscle disorders and other dystonias, a growing role of this potent toxin.*

Chia JK, Clark JB, Ryan CA, et al.: Botulism in an adult associated with food-borne intestinal infection with *Clostridium botulinum*. N Engl J Med 315:239, 1986. *This is a case report of an adult with the infant form of botulism and an accompanying editorial that places this observation in perspective.*

Dowell VR Jr, McCroskey LM, Hathaway CL, et al.: Coproexamination for botulinal toxin and *Clostridium botulinum*. JAMA 238:1829, 1977. *Reviews methods to establish the diagnosis in foodborne botulism.*

Merson MH, Hughes JM, Dowell VR, et al.: Current trends in botulism in the United States. JAMA 229:1305, 1974. *Summary of the CDC experience with foodborne botulism.*

Tacket CO, Shandera WX, Mann JM, et al.: Equine antitoxin use and other factors that predict outcome in type A foodborne botulism. Am J Med 76:794, 1984. *A review supporting the previously controversial role of antitoxin in type A botulism in adults.*

310 Tetanus

DEFINITION. Tetanus is a neurologic syndrome caused by a neurotoxin elaborated at the site of injury by *Clostridium tetani*.

ETIOLOGY. *C. tetani* is an anaerobic, gram-positive, slender, motile bacillus. The sporulated form has a characteristic drumstick or tennis racket shape with a terminal spore. The vegetative form produces tetanospasmin, a protein neurotoxin with a molecular weight of approximately 150,000. Tetanospasmin ranks with botulism toxin as the most potent known microbial toxin; 1 mg is capable of killing 50 to 70 million mice. The vegetative forms of *C. tetani* are highly susceptible to heat, disinfectants, and other adverse environmental conditions, but the spores are highly resistant and can survive in soil for months to years. Killing of spores requires boiling for at least 4 hours or autoclaving for 12 minutes at 121°C.

EPIDEMIOLOGY. *C. tetani* can be found in 20 to 65 per cent of soil samples, the highest yields being in cultivated land and the lowest yields, in virgin soil. The organism can also be found in stool from a variety of animals, house dust, operating rooms, and contaminated heroin. Approximately 10 per cent of humans harbor *C. tetani* in the colon.

Tetanus is most common in warm climates and in highly cultivated rural areas. The greatest problem is in economically deprived countries, owing to poor immunization standards and unhygienic practices. An example is the practice of dressing the umbilical stump with animal dung or "dusting powder," a local dried clay sold for cosmetic purposes, after childbirth by unimmunized mothers. It is estimated that the annual toll from neonatal tetanus in developing countries is 1 million. In the United States, there are 40 to 60 reported cases annually, and almost all occur in unimmunized or inadequately immunized persons. Of these cases 60 to 80 per cent are associated with acute wounds, 15 to 20 per cent represent complications of chronic wounds, 3 to 10 per cent are complications of parenteral drug abuse, and 5 to 10 per cent have no clearly identified source. Over 70 per cent of these patients are 50 years of age or older, and less than 4 per cent are under 20 years; there is only about one case of neonatal tetanus per year. This predilection for the disease in the elderly appears to reflect waning immunity associated with aging.

PATHOGENESIS. Clinical tetanus requires a source of the organism, local tissue conditions that promote toxin production, and immunologic naiveté. The usual portals of entry are traumatic wounds, surgical wounds, subcutaneous injection sites, burns, skin ulcers, infected umbilical cords, and otitis media with tympanic membrane perforation. The spores are ubiquitous in the environment, and most cases reflect contamination from exogenous sources, although endogenous infection is conceivable in occasional cases that follow intestinal surgery. Important factors at the site of injury are necrotic tissue, suppuration, and the presence of a foreign body. These are responsible for a reduction in the local oxidation-reduction potential (eH), thus promoting reversion of spores to the vegetative forms that produce tetanospasmin. Tetanospasmin is taken up by the peripheral nerve terminals and carried intra-axonally within membrane-bound vesicles to spinal neurons at a transport rate of approximately 250 mm per day. Upon reaching the perikarya of the motor neurons the toxin passes to the presynaptic terminals where it blocks release of neurotransmitters, including glycine, which is the neurotransmitter used by group 1A inhibitory afferent motor neurons. Loss of the inhibitory influence results in unrestrained firing with sustained muscular contraction. The result with spinal cord neurons is rigidity. In severe cases there is also involvement of the sympathetic chain causing autonomic dysfunction.

CLINICAL FEATURES. Forms of tetanus include generalized, localized, cephalic, and neonatal.

Generalized tetanus is the most common. The extent of the associated trauma varies from a rather trivial injury that may be forgotten by the patient to a severe, contaminated crush injury. The usual incubation period is 7 to 21 days, depending largely on the distance of the site of injury from the central nervous system. The "onset period" refers to the time from the first clinical symptoms of tetanus to the first generalized spasm. An incubation period of less than 9 days and an onset period of less than 48 hours appear to be associated with more severe symptomatology. Trismus is the presenting complaint in 75 per cent of cases, so the patient is often initially seen by a dentist or oral surgeon. Other early features include irritability, restlessness, diaphoresis, and dysphagia with hydrophobia and drooling. Sustained trismus may result in a characterisic sardonic smile, or "risus sardonicus," and persistent spasm of the back musculature may cause opisthotonos. These early manifestations reflect involvement of the bulbar muscles and paraspinous muscles, possibly because they are innervated by the shortest axons. Waves of opisthotonos are highly characteristic of the disease. With progression, the extremities become involved in episodes characterized by painful flexion and adduction of the arms, clenched fists, and extension of the legs. Noise or tactile stimuli may precipitate spasms and generalized convulsions, although they occur spontaneously as well. Involvement of the autonomic nervous system may result in severe arrhythmias, oscillation in the blood pressure, profound diaphoresis, hyperthermia, rhabdomyolysis, laryngeal spasm, and urinary retention. In most cases the patient remains lucid. Complications include fractures from sustained contractions and convulsions, pulmonary emboli, bacterial infections, and dehydration.

Localized tetanus refers to involvement of the extremity with a contaminated wound and shows considerable variation in severity. In the more severe cases there are intense, painful spasms that usually progress to generalized tetanus. Cases that remain localized tend to be less severe. This is a relatively unusual form of tetanus, and the prognosis for survival is excellent.

Cephalic tetanus generally follows a head injury or occurs with *C. tetani* infection of the middle ear. The clinical symptoms consist of isolated or combined dysfunction of the cranial motor nerves, most frequently the seventh cranial nerve. This may remain localized or progress to generalized tetanus. Again, this is a relatively unusual form of tetanus, but the incubation period is only 1 or 2 days, and the prognosis for survival is extremely poor.

Tetanus neonatorum refers to generalized tetanus resulting from *C. tetani* infection in neonates. This occurs primarily in underdeveloped countries where various contaminated materials are used to sever or dress the umbilical cord in newborn infants of unimmunized mothers. The usual incubation period following birth is 3 to 10 days, and it is sometimes referred to as "the disease of the seventh day," reflecting the average incubation period. The child typically shows irritability, facial grimacing, and severe spasms with touch. The mortality rate exceeds 70 per cent.

DIAGNOSIS. The diagnosis of tetanus is usually made on the basis of clinical observations. The putative agent, *C. tetani*, is infrequently recovered with cultures of the wound. A confirmed history of immunization or a serum antitoxin level of 0.01 units per deciliter or higher makes tetanus very unlikely. Spinal fluid analysis is entirely normal, and the electroencephalogram generally shows a sleep pattern. The differential diagnosis depends on the dominant clinical features and includes oculogyric crisis secondary to phenothiazine toxicity, meningitis, dental abscess, seizure disorder, subarachnoid hemorrhage, hypocalcemic or alkalotic tetany, alcohol withdrawal, and strychnine poisoning. Strychnine poisoning produces very similar symptoms but differs from tetanus in that patients usually recover rapidly following supportive care.

TREATMENT. *Surgery.* Debridement of any associated wound. (This may pose a problem in "skin poppers," who often have multiple possibly infected sites.)

Antibiotics. Penicillin G should be given parenterally in doses of 1 to 10 million units daily for 10 days; tetracycline, erythromycin, and chloramphenicol are alternative agents for penicillin-allergic patients.

Antitoxin. Human tetanus immunoglobulin (TIG) should be given as soon as possible to neutralize toxin that has not entered neurons. The dose is arbitrary, ranging from 500 to 6000 units, and the route of administration may be intramuscular or as split doses intramuscularly and by infiltration into the wound. Some authorities advocate intrathecal administration of 250 units of TIG. Equine tetanus immune globulin (10,000 to 100,000 units intravenously or intramuscularly) is equally effective, but the rate of reactions is high owing to the equine source. Epinephrine 1:1000 should be readily available for severe reactions. This preparation is far less expensive and is consequently used most extensively in underdeveloped countries.

Active Immunization. Natural infection does not result in detectable levels of circulating antibody, so a full course of immunization with tetanus toxoid in three doses should be given.

Muscle Spasms. Chlorpromazine (50 to 150 mg every 4 to 8 hours in adults), meprobamate (400 mg every 3 to 4 hours in adults*), or diazepam (2 to 20 mg intravenously every 2 to 8 hours) are given to control spasms and convulsions, and short-acting barbiturates are useful for sedation. Overuse of these agents may lead to hypoventilation. When muscle spasms are severe or interfere with ventilation, therapeutic paralysis should be introduced using pancuronium bromide or metocurine combined with mechanical ventilation.

Supportive Care. Trismus, dysphagia, laryngeal spasm, respiratory muscle spasm, and sedatives all contribute to the high frequency of pulmonary complications. Maintenance of a patent airway is imperative, often with intubation followed by a tracheostomy. The patient may then be maintained with mechanical ventilation in conjunction with diazepam in intravenous doses titrated to relieve rigidity without excessive sedation.

Patients with dysphagia should be fed via a nasogastric tube. Fluid balance needs to be followed assiduously, since large losses may occur and may be difficult to measure owing to profuse sweating. Autonomic nervous system involvement may result in tachycardia and hypertension with high cardiac output and cardiac arrhythmias. Alpha- and beta-adrenergic blocking agents were used formerly, but beta blockade was sometimes complicated by cardiac arrest. Other considerations with autonomic instability include morphine, epidural blockade, or magnesium sulfate in-

---

*May exceed manufacturer's recommended dosage.

TABLE 310–1. GUIDELINES FOR TETANUS PROPHYLAXIS IN WOUND MANAGEMENT

History of Adsorbed Tetanus Toxoid	Clean and Minor Wounds		Other Wounds*	
Number of Doses	Td†	TIG‡	Td†	TIG‡
Unknown or less than three	Yes§	No	Yes§	Yes
Three or more	Yes if over 10 years since last dose	No	Yes if over 5 years since last dose	No

*Included but not limited to wounds contaminated with dirt, feces, soil, saliva, puncture wounds; avulsions; and wounds resulting from missiles, crushing, burns, and frostbite.

†Td: Tetanus and diphtheria toxoids adsorbed. Children under 7 should receive DPT (diphtheria and tetanus toxoids and pertussis vaccine adsorbed). Too frequent booster doses of tetanus toxoid have been associated with hypersensitivity reactions.

‡TIG: Tetanus immune globulin in a dose of 250 to 500 units intramuscularly. The usual dose is 250 units. The usual prophylactic dose of equine tetanus immune globulin is 1500 to 5000 units intramuscularly. When tetanus toxoid is given concurrently there should be separate syringes and injection sites.

§Unimmunized or incompletely immunized persons (1 or 2 doses of toxoid) should receive complete immunization with Td at time 0, 4–8 weeks later, and 6–12 months later.

fusions. Additional concerns are pulmonary emboli requiring anticoagulation, gastrointestinal bleeding that may be prevented with sucralfate, rhabdomyolysis with myoglobinuria and renal failure that may require dialysis, superimposed infections requiring judicious use of antibiotics, hyperthermia requiring a cooling blanket, and hypotension requiring pressor agents.

PROGNOSIS. The overall mortality rate for generalized tetanus is 25 to 50 per cent even in modern medical facilities with extensive resources. Important prognostic features are the form of tetanus, as described above, the incubation period, the onset period, patient's age, and severity of symptoms. Patients with mild disease have only trismus with or without minor and brief muscle spasms. Moderate disease is characterized by trismus, dysphagia, rigidity, and intermittent muscle spasms. With severe tetanus there are generalized convulsions. Patients with moderate or severe generalized tetanus generally require 3 to 6 weeks for recovery. They may require intensive care during most of this time, but if they survive their recovery is usually complete. The highest mortality rates are at the extremes of age. The most frequent cause of death is pneumonia, but many patients have no obvious findings at autopsy, suggesting that death was directly due to the neurotoxin.

PREVENTION. Nearly all cases of tetanus occur in unimmunized or inadequately immunized individuals. The Immunization Practices Advisory Committee recommends active immunization of infants and children with DPT (diphtheria and tetanus toxoids and pertussis adsorbed) at 2 months, 4 months, 6 months, 15 months, and 4 to 6 years. Tetanus toxoid is a highly effective antigen and protective levels of serum antitoxin in persons who complete the primary series persist for at least 10 years. Td (tetanus and diphtheria toxoids adsorbed for adult use) is re-

commended every 10 years at mid-decade ages (15 years, 25 years, 35 years, etc.). This is commonly neglected as disclosed by serosurveys showing that 40 per cent of persons over 60 years in the United States lack protective levels of tetanus antitoxin. The recommended primary immunization series for unimmunized persons over 7 years is Td at time 0, 4 to 8 weeks, 6 to 12 months after the second dose, and then every 10 years. Nearly all states now require DPT immunization for school enrollment. About 95 per cent of tetanus cases in the United States occur in persons who have not received the primary series of tetanus toxoid. Immunized childbearing women confer protection on their infants through transplacental maternal antibody.

Prevention of tetanus after injury requires appropriate wound management, assurance of adequate immunity, and consideration of antibiotic prophylaxis. The aim of surgery is to eliminate necrotic tissue, purulent collections, and foreign bodies that promote the environmental conditions necessary for spore germination. Guidelines for immunoprophylaxis based on immunization status and wound characteristics are summarized in Table 310–1. Passive immunization is recommended only for "tetanus prone" wounds, preferably with TIG prepared from plasma of adults hyperimmunized with tetanus toxoid. The alternative is tetanus antitoxin equine prepared from hyperimmunized horses. The horse serum is associated with a high reaction rate including pain at the injection site, serum sickness, and anaphylactic shock. Equine antitoxin also generates immune complexes that are rapidly excreted so that larger doses are required to produce sustained blood levels. The definition of *tetanus-prone* depends on the interval between injury and treatment, the degree of contamination, the extent of devitalized tissue or foreign bodies within the site of injury, and the depth of the injury. Antimicrobial agents such as penicillin, erythromycin, or metronidazole may be given to inhibit replication of the vegetative forms of *C. tetani*, but immunization and wound cleansing are considered more important, so the use of antibiotics is generally dictated by other considerations.

Armitage P, Clifford R: Prognosis in tetanus: Use of data from therapeutic trials. J Infect Dis 138:1–8, 1978. *Data for 1385 patients with tetanus in India are reviewed to propose a prognostic classification.*

Bizzini B: Tetanus toxin. Microbiol Rev 43:224, 1979. *An extensive discussion of tetanus toxin.*

Centers for Disease Control: Tetanus—United States 1987 and 1988. MMWR 39:37–41, 1990. *A review of the clinical experience with tetanus in the United States and the revised guidelines for tetanus prophylaxis.*

Dowell VR Jr: Botulism and tetanus: Selected epidemiologic and microbiologic aspects. Rev Infect Dis 6(Suppl 1):202, 1984. *A review of the reported experience in the United States for these neurologic syndromes.*

Faust RA, Vickers OR, Cohn L Jr: Tetanus: 2,449 cases in 68 years at Charity Hospital. J Trauma 16:704–712, 1976. *The authors review a large clinical experience with tetanus in a United States hospital.*

Griffin JW: Local tetanus. Johns Hopkins Med J 149:84–88, 1981. *A good review of local tetanus and the pathophysiology of tetanospasmin.*

Olsen KM, Hiller FC: Management of tetanus. Clin Pharm 6:570, 1987. *A review of management guidelines with emphasis on the important role of benzodiazepines.*

Schofield F: Selective primary health care: Strategies for control of disease in the developing world XXII. Tetanus: A preventable problem. Rev Infect Dis 8:144, 1986. *The author reviews the tetanus problem in the developing world.*

Anaerobic Bacteria

311 Diseases Caused by Non–Spore-forming Anaerobic Bacteria

Sherwood L. Gorbach

DEFINITIONS. Anaerobic bacteria are the major constituents of the microflora that colonizes the gastrointestinal tract, upper

respiratory tract, skin, and vagina. Under normal circumstances these organisms exist in a *commensal* (literal meaning "dining at the same table") relationship with their host. Anaerobic bacteria require reduced oxygen tension for growth; the more fastidious strains cannot survive exposure to atmospheric oxygen for more than 5 minutes. As a general rule, anaerobes associated with infectious processes are relatively aerotolerant. Teleologically, aerotolerance provides anaerobic bacteria with a survival advantage in mammalian tissues, since the extremely oxygen-sensitive forms perish almost immediately upon escape from their natural ecologic niche, whereas aerotolerant forms can establish a septic focus.

Regardless of the organ site, anaerobic infections have three characteristics in common. First, such infections are truly endogenous, since the pathogens originate from the normal flora of the host. Second, certain pathogenic conditions predispose to anaerobic infections by initiating spread of the normal flora beyond the confines of mucosal barriers. These inciting events also produce a low *oxidation-reduction potential* (Eh) in the tissues, thereby favoring the growth of anaerobic organisms. Compromised vascular supply, trauma, tissue destruction, and antecedent infections caused by aerobic bacteria or viruses that result in necrosis are among the situations that precede anaerobic infection. Third, the infecting flora is highly complex. Abdominal infections, for example, harbor an average of five different bacterial species, usually three anaerobes and two aerobic or facultative strains.

ANAEROBIC GRAM-NEGATIVE BACILLI. *Bacteroides.* *B. fragilis* is the pre-eminent anaerobic pathogen in humans. This distinction is based on its virulence, its ubiquity in various organ sites, and its resistance to many conventional antimicrobial drugs. The organism frequently produces abscesses and causes tissue destruction. The *B. fragilis* group has been divided into five distinct species, based on biochemical differences and DNA homology: *B. fragilis, B. distasonis, B. vulgatus, B. ovatus,* and *B. thetaiotaomicron.* Although these organisms are recognized pathogens, they all lack one of the prime virulence factors of other gram-negative organisms, endotoxin. *Bacteroides* strains do possess a surface *lipopolysaccharide* (LPS), but this substance differs in chemical composition from LPS of other gram-negative organisms. In addition, *B. fragilis* LPS lacks the biologic activities of classic endotoxin, such as production of septic shock and vascular collapse in experimental animals. On the other hand, *B. fragilis* contains on its outer cell membrane a specific, large molecular weight capsule composed of polysaccharide. In a purified form the capsular material is highly antigenic, and it can produce abscesses when it is injected into experimental animals.

B. fragilis causes infections in the abdominal cavity that are associated with contamination by the intestinal flora. These organisms also are found in female pelvic infections and in mixed infections of skin and soft tissue such as decubitus ulcer, diabetic foot ulcer, and gangrene of the perineum.

B. bivius and *B. disieus* are frequent isolates in female pelvic infections. These organisms often are resistant to conventional penicillins and cephalosporins.

The *Bacteroides oralis/B. melaninogenicus* group and the asaccharolytic *Bacteroides* are found in the normal flora but may be associated with various infections. The major distinguishing feature of the asaccharolytic *Bacteroides* is the production of a brown-black pigment, formed in the colony after 5 to 7 days of growth on blood agar. Many strains require blood and vitamin K or its analogues for growth. Infections caused by these organisms are most commonly found in the respiratory tract, head and neck region, and female pelvic area.

Fusobacterium. The major species found in clinical specimens are *F. nucleatum* and *F. necrophorum.* In Gram-stained preparations, these organisms take up stain poorly and appear as slender spear-shaped bacilli with parallel sides and tapered ends. The LPS of *F. nucleatum* causes septic shock and vascular collapse when injected intravenously into rabbits, in contrast with the material found in *B. fragilis,* which is biologically inactive in this model. *Fusobacterium* species are regular constituents of the normal flora of the oral cavity, gastrointestinal tract, and female genital tract. Among the infectious processes, these organisms are major causes of pleuropulmonary infections and various abscesses of the head and neck region. They are also responsible for bacteremia. The most common sites of origin are the female genital tract, orofacial region, and lower respiratory tract.

ANAEROBIC GRAM-POSITIVE COCCI. This diverse group of organisms ranks second in importance to *Bacteroides* in frequency of isolation from infected sites. The major genera are *Peptostreptococcus,* which includes strains formerly classified as *Peptococcus.* Anaerobic streptococci, a disease group of aerotolerant and anaerobic organisms, are distinguished by producing mainly lactic acid. (There are also gram-negative cocci known as *Veillonella,* that are only rarely involved as pathogens.)

Anaerobic gram-positive cocci are important components of the normal flora of humans. Within the oral cavity these organisms represent a significant percentage of the anaerobic isolates in saliva and dental plaque. They are also among the leading components of the fecal flora and the vaginal flora. As pathogenic organisms these anaerobic cocci are found in virtually all sites where anaerobes have been identified. Approximately 50 per cent of such isolates in a clinical bacteriology laboratory are from surgical wounds, mostly associated with abdominal operations and hysterectomies. The gram-positive cocci are also found in skin and soft tissue infections and in blood cultures. About one third of anaerobic pleuropulmonary infections are associated with these gram-positive cocci. In the female genital tract they are probably the most important cause of salpingitis and are frequently isolated in cases of pelvic abscess.

GRAM-POSITIVE NON–SPORE-FORMING BACILLI. The two leading isolates are *Propionibacterium acnes* and various species of *Eubacterium.* *P. acnes* is the most frequent anaerobe found on normal skin. This organism is commonly recovered from blood cultures, most often as a contaminant, or from wound infections as part of a mixed flora. Although these organisms have little intrinsic pathogenicity, they are important causes of infection in patients with artificial heart valves, vascular grafts, orthopedic prostheses, or ventricular shunts. *Eubacterium* is isolated from wound infections, particularly in association with *Bacteroides.* Insofar as can be determined, *Eubacterium* plays no pathogenic role in the infective process. A newly described genus, *Mobiluncus,* consists of gram-variable or gram-negative curved rods that are implicated in vaginal infections.

PATHOGENESIS OF ANAEROBIC INFECTIONS. *Unitarian Compared with Synergistic Infections.* Our theoretical models of infections are based on concepts of microbial monoetiology. Pasteur established that certain microorganisms are responsible for a specific disease state. His theory was formalized by Robert Koch in his famous postulates. Finally, Erhlich created the concept of a single drug, the "magic bullet," designed for a specific infection. Thus, the principle states: one microbe, one disease, one drug. This concept applies to classic infections such as typhoid fever, diphtheria, and cholera. However, the classic design does not fit most infections associated with anaerobic bacteria, since these processes harbor multiple strains of organisms with varying oxygen sensitivities and undefined pathogenic potentials. Anaerobic infections follow the model of bacterial synergy, in which several bacteria behave in a cooperative fashion to produce infection. In experimental model systems of mixed infection, various microbial components contribute virulence factors or growth substances that permit other more pathogenic forms to invade the tissues. Most clinical anaerobic infections are mixed, containing several species of bacteria. Because it is not clear which are the primary pathogens and which are the symbionts and commensals, it is often necessary to treat all of the potential pathogens.

Virulence Factors. The microenvironment of an anaerobic abscess has features that ensure its own survival. An abscess has an Eh of -250 mv, with an extremely low concentration of oxygen. Anaerobiosis is a hostile condition for host-defense mechanisms. Within this oxygen-free zone, neutrophils are unable to kill bacteria by their oxidative metabolic pathway. Low oxygen tension also inhibits the activity of aminoglycoside antibiotics, since they require an oxidative transport system to cross the bacterial cell envelope. The abscess itself contains a large concentration of microorganisms, approximately 10^8 to 10^9 per milliliter. A high inoculum and a relatively low growth rate are adverse conditions for the activity of β-lactam antibiotics. Thus, host defenses and antibiotic interventions are hindered in an anaerobic abscess.

Individual anaerobic microorganisms possess virulence factors that promote their survival in the host's tissues. *B. fragilis* elaborates a polysaccharide capsule that provides protection against phagocytosis by neutrophils. Membrane-associated enzymes are found in many virulent anaerobes, including β-lactamases and superoxide dismutase (SOD). The β-lactamases destroy antibiotics such as penicillin and cephalosporin. SOD, an enzyme present in virtually all pathogenic anaerobes studied thus far, seems to protect the organism in its initial exposure to oxygenated tissues.

Immunologic factors are affected by anaerobic bacteria. Several species of anaerobes are more resistant to phagocytosis than coliforms and other facultative organisms. Anaerobic bacteria can also interfere with phagocytosis of aerobes when both organisms are present in a mixed infection. Infection with *B. fragilis* induces T cells of CD4$^+$8$^+$ phenotype, leading to abscess formation. Thus, abscess is related to cellular, rather than humoral immune mechanisms.

Role of Facultative Organisms. Facultative or aerobic organisms are frequent partners in anaerobic infections. In some settings these organisms seem to initiate the infective process, perhaps by promoting early tissue necrosis or by consuming oxygen in the tissues. In abdominal infections coliforms and *Bacteroides* are often isolated together.

An animal model of intra-abdominal infection has delineated the role of these pathogens in the septic process. Following intestinal perforation, the initial phase consists of peritonitis, bacteremia, and septic shock. This phase is caused, at least in the animal model, by coliforms such as *E. coli* and *Proteus*. The later abscess formation is associated with anaerobes, particularly *Bacteroides*. Antimicrobial drugs active only against coliforms suppress the initial septicemic and shock phase but have no effect on abscess formation. Similarly, antianaerobic drugs do not protect against coliform bacteremia, but they do suppress formation of abscess. The clinical picture is complex, with overlapping of the septic shock stage and the abscess stage. However, the therapeutic implications are clear: Both components of abdominal sepsis should receive appropriate antimicrobial attention.

ANAEROBIC BACTERIA IN VARIOUS INFECTIONS. Aerobic and facultative microorganisms have been traditionally considered the major pathogens in infectious diseases. Recent improvements in laboratory techniques have facilitated the identification of anaerobic bacteria, and it has become clear that these oxygen-sensitive organisms share responsibility for a significant number of infections seen in clinical practice (Table 311–1).

Intra-abdominal Infections. Infections within the peritoneal cavity usually are related to contamination by the intestinal flora. The microflora of the upper intestine, from the stomach to the upper ileum, consists of sparse numbers of facultative gram-positive organisms derived from the oropharynx. Relatively few coliforms and obligate anaerobes are encountered. The lower bowel, on the other hand, harbors a luxuriant flora in which anaerobes outnumber facultative organisms such as coliforms by a factor of 1000 to 1. Hence, injuries to the upper intestinal tract, such as perforated ulcer or trauma, result in a small inoculum of microorganisms and a low risk of infection. But colonic perforations release a large inoculum of bacteria, causing a high rate of infection.

TABLE 311–1. PRINCIPAL TYPES OF ANAEROBIC INFECTIONS

Location	Type of Infection
Head and neck	Brain abscess
	Gingivitis
	Chronic sinusitis
	Chronic otitis media
	Odontogenic and oropharyngeal-space infections
Respiratory tract	Aspiration pneumonia
	Necrotizing pneumonia
	Lung abscess
	Empyema (adults)
Gastrointestinal tract	Peritonitis
	Intra-abdominal abscess
	Liver abscess
Female genital tract	Tubo-ovarian abscess
	Salpingitis (30–50% of cases)
	Septic abortion and endometritis
	Bartholin's gland abscess
	Bacterial vaginosis
Skin and soft tissue	Crepitant cellulitis
	Necrotizing fasciitis
	Myonecrosis (gas gangrene)
	Decubitus ulcer
	Diabetic foot ulcer
	Bite wounds

From Styrt B, Gorbach SL: Recent developments in the understanding of the pathogenesis and treatment of anaerobic infections. N Engl J Med 321:240–246, 1989. Reprinted by permission of the New England Journal of Medicine.

Peritonitis and intra-abdominal abscess are associated with anaerobic bacteria in 95 per cent of cases. The most frequent finding is a mixture of aerobes and anaerobes. (Infection by a single facultative organism such as *E. coli* is uncommon and usually is seen in *primary peritonitis* associated with cirrhosis of the liver.) In a large series of intra-abdominal infections, an average of five different organisms were isolated from each patient, including three types of anaerobes and two aerobes. Of the anaerobes, *Bacteroides*, *Clostridium*, anaerobic cocci, and *Fusobacterium* are the major pathogens. The specific site of infection does not determine the flora, since the same pathogens are found in peritonitis, appendicitis, subphrenic abscess, and diverticular abscess.

Anaerobic Pleuropulmonary Infections. Anaerobic infections of the lower respiratory tract produce four clinical conditions: *aspiration pneumonia, lung abscess, necrotizing pneumonia,* and *empyema.* The pathogenesis of these conditions is aspiration of oropharyngeal contents, a situation associated with compromised state of consciousness, obstruction of the esophagus, and neurologic deficits. The oral flora is permitted admission to normally sterile regions of the lower respiratory tract. Approximately 90 per cent of patients with aspiration pneumonia have anaerobes as the major infecting flora. The situation applies to patients who have aspirated outside the hospital or shortly after admission, since they harbor normal oral flora. When the aspiration event occurs after hospitalization or after treatment with antibiotics, at which time the oral flora becomes colonized by gram-negative facultative organisms, the aspirated flora assumes a different character consisting of coliforms and *Pseudomonas.* Lung abscess is associated with anaerobic bacteria in over 90 per cent of cases. The aerobes that occasionally cause a solitary lung abscess include *Klebsiella* and *S. aureus*. Necrotizing pneumonia is actually an earlier stage of lung abscess in which a specific segment or lobe of the lung is extensively damaged with multiple small abscesses. In the more advanced stage these abscesses coalesce to form a single large cavity, leaving in its wake a large area of destroyed lung. Necrotizing pneumonia is a more aggressive condition than lung abscess, with higher mortality. Anaerobes are responsible for the vast majority of cases. Empyema is an infection usually associated with underlying pneumonitis or lung abscess. Nearly 75 per cent of the cases of empyema are associated with anaerobes, most frequently in patients with chronic infection. The remaining cases are caused by the classic aerobic pathogens such as staphylococci, group A streptococci, and pneumococci; these organisms produce an acute onset and a more virulent course. Formerly, most cases of empyema were caused by these aerobic gram-positive organisms, but the situation has been reversed with the advent of antimicrobial agents.

Anaerobic pleuropulmonary infections involve multiple bacterial species including *B. melaninogenicus, F. nucleatum,* and anaerobic gram-positive cocci. *B. fragilis* is found in 15 per cent of cases. The fact that these organisms are found in the same relative concentrations in the various clinical cases suggests that the inoculum of oral contents is similar in each setting.

Obstetric and Gynecologic Infections. The source of infections of the female upper genital tract is the vaginal flora, which has aerobic and anaerobic bacteria as normal constituents. The clinical conditions in which anaerobes are frequently encountered include tubo-ovarian abscess, pelvic abscess, septic abortion, endomyometritis, and postoperative wound infection (following hysterectomy). Polymicrobic bacteremia is a frequent occurrence in patients with severe pelvic infections. The major anaerobic pathogens are *Bacteroides, Peptostreptococcus, Fusobacterium,* and *Clostridium.* Pelvic inflammatory disease, also known as salpingitis, is a milder condition that is caused by an array of organisms, including gonococci, *Chlamydia,* and anaerobes, particularly *Peptostreptococcus.*

Head and Neck Infections. Because the anaerobic bacteria in the normal flora of the upper airways have limited invasive properties, they require an antecedent event that permits their movement into deeper structures. Dental manipulation, trauma, prior bacterial or viral infections, and operative interventions can provide the initiating circumstance. Necrotizing infections of the gingiva and endodontal infections are usually associated with oral strains of *Bacteroides* and *Fusobacterium.* Spirochetes have been found at the advancing border of inflammation in histologic sections of acute ulcerative gingivitis, noma, and lung abscess. Since these organisms cannot be grown in subculture, their role in pathogenesis cannot be assessed. In patients with *sinusitis*, anaerobes are recovered from 50 per cent of patients with chronic processes. However, acute or subacute sinusitis, lasting 3 months or less, is rarely associated with anaerobes. *Otitis media* may be either acute or chronic. As in sinusitis, anaerobes may be present in the chronic forms but are rarely present in the more acute cases. *Space infections*, occurring in the potential spaces formed by fascial planes of the head and neck, are usually associated with three types of organisms: either *S. aureus*, *Streptococcus pyogenes*, or anaerobic bacteria. The first two organisms occur in space infections related to overlying skin processes such as boils or impetigo. Anaerobes are associated with space infections that arise from diseases of the mucous membrane, dental manipulations, or in those cases that occur spontaneously. *Ludwig's angina* is an example of a space infection associated with anaerobes.

Of the central nervous system infections, *brain abscess* is the one most frequently associated with anaerobic bacteria. These organisms are isolated from 85 per cent of suppurative brain abscesses unrelated to trauma or operative procedures. Grampositive cocci, followed in frequency by *Fusobacterium* and *Bacteroides*, are the most common strains, often in association with facultative streptococci and coliforms. *Subdural empyema* may also be caused by anaerobes, particularly when it occurs in association with a parameningeal focus in an ear or nasal sinus. Classic pyogenic meningitis, however, is rarely caused by anaerobes.

Skin, Bone, and Soft Tissue Infections. The predisposing factors in anaerobic skin and soft tissue infections are trauma, ischemia, and surgery. The organisms often derive from the fecal or oral flora, particularly in wounds associated with intestinal surgery, decubitus ulcer, and human bites. The clinical presentations are *crepitant cellulitis*, *synergistic gangrene* or *cellulitis*, and *necrotizing fasciitis*. Anaerobes are also regularly encountered in *diabetic foot ulcers*; 75 per cent of such lesions are associated with *Bacteroides*, anaerobic cocci, and *Clostridium*, usually in mixed culture. Anaerobic *osteomyelitis* is associated with trauma or prior surgery, although some cases arise from hematogenous spread.

CLUES TO PRESUMPTIVE DIAGNOSIS OF ANAEROBIC INFECTION. Clinicians should suspect the diagnosis of an anaerobic infection before the bacteriologic results are available on the basis of the following features: (1) Any infection that is contiguous or in proximity to a mucosal surface normally harboring an anaerobic flora—the gastrointestinal tract, female genital tract, and oropharynx. (2) A foul-smelling discharge; this odor is pathognomonic evidence of anaerobic infection. The absence of odor, however, is not helpful, because 50 per cent of anaerobic infections lack the characteristic odor. (3) The presence of severe tissue necrosis, abscess formation, fasciitis, or gangrene. (4) Gas in the tissue, which is highly suggestive, although not absolutely diagnostic. (5) A mixed infection, indicated by a Gram's stain of exudate showing a polymorphic array of organisms. Certain anaerobes have a characteristic appearance under the microscope, especially *Clostridium*, *Fusobacterium*, *Actinomyces*, and certain strains of *Bacteroides*. (6) The failure to recover organisms by conventional aerobic culture in the presence of clinical infection. (7) Failure to respond to antibiotics that have poor anaerobic activity, such as aminoglycosides and certain penicillins and cephalosporins.

TREATMENT STRATEGIES FOR ANAEROBIC INFECTIONS. Successful therapy for anaerobic infections involves rational antibiotic selection in conjunction with judicious surgical resection and drainage. The operative approach may be ultimately decisive, but it should be emphasized that surgical intervention alone may be inadequate. Anaerobic infection can continue to simmer with intermittent sepsis and insidious extension of the process unless appropriate antimicrobial agents are employed. Selection of initial antibiotic therapy should be based on knowledge of the pathogens likely to be present in a specific clinical setting. Because many anaerobic infections tend to be mixed with coliforms and other facultative organisms, it is advisable to use antimicrobial drugs active against both components. With regard

to the anaerobic components, important differences are seen in infections above and below the diaphragm. Anaerobic infections above the diaphragm, including those in the central nervous system, head and neck region, and pleuropulmonary area, tend to involve organisms sensitive to penicillin. This observation is not invariably true, since certain organisms, especially *Bacteroides*, can elaborate β-lactamases, which inactivate penicillins and cephalosporins. Anaerobic infections below the diaphragm, such as those in the abdominal cavity and female genital tract, commonly involve the *B. fragilis* group as a major pathogen. Because these organisms are commonly resistant to several antimicrobial agents, infections in these sites require special consideration for choice of antimicrobial drugs.

TREATMENT. The range of choice among antimicrobial drugs is somewhat limited with regard to anaerobic bacteria in general and even more so with members of the *B. fragilis* group. A United States survey of antibiotic susceptibility among strains of *B. fragilis* from eight medical centers was conducted from 1981 to 1986. Among the β-lactam antibiotics, imipenem and ticarcillin–clavulanic acid were the most active, followed by piperacillin, cefoxitin, and moxalactam. Since high blood levels can be achieved with these drugs, they can be used to treat clinical infections caused by this organism. Disappointing results were seen with penicillin, carbenicillin, ticarcillin, cephalothin, cefamandole, cefotetan, and certain third-generation cephalosporins such as cefotaxime and cefoperazone. The drugs in this grouping are not considered good choices for infections associated with *B. fragilis*. Clostridia, fusobacteria, and gram-positive cocci are usually sensitive to several drugs, including penicillins, cephalosporins, clindamycin, and metronidazole.

The explanation for variations in activity of the β-lactam drugs against anaerobes is the presence in certain strains of constitutive β-lactamases. This enzyme is found in most strains of *Bacteroides* and in occasional strains of *Fusobacterium* isolated from clinical sources. The increased activity of cefoxitin, imipenem, and ticarcillin–clavulanate against *Bacteroides* is based on their resistance to hydrolysis by β-lactamase elaborated by anaerobic organisms.

Metronidazole, a bactericidal drug, has excellent activity against *Bacteroides*, *Fusobacterium*, *Clostridium*, and most strains of anaerobic cocci. Resistance to metronidazole among *Bacteroides* is extremely rare. Since the drug has a spectrum limited almost exclusively to anaerobes, another agent such as an aminoglycoside or a cephalosporin should be included for facultative organisms. In clinical trials metronidazole has produced excellent results in intra-abdominal infections, female pelvic infections, brain abscess, and anaerobic osteomyelitis. Many failures, however, have been noted in anaerobic pleuropulmonary infections, probably related to the relatively poor activity against microaerophilic organisms that may accompany this infectious process.

Clindamycin is highly active against most anaerobic isolates with resistance rates among *Bacteroides* running at about 5 per cent. Some resistant isolates of *Clostridium* and *Fusobacterium* have been encountered, but they have been relatively uncommon in clinical practice. The drug is also active against streptococci, both aerobic and anaerobic, and most strains of *S. aureus*. Because it has very little activity against coliforms and other facultative gram-negative organisms, a second drug is used in mixed anaerobic infections. Clindamycin has produced excellent results in intra-abdominal infections, female pelvic infections, and skin and soft tissue infections. Some authorities consider it the drug of choice for anaerobic pleuropulmonary infections, preferring it to penicillin because of apparent failures associated with penicillin treatment. Erythromycin is less active than clindamycin, although resistance patterns commonly overlap. The problem with erythromycin is the difficulty in administering it parenterally. By the oral route only low serum levels of erythromycin are obtained, often below the amount needed to inhibit many anaerobic bacteria.

Tetracyclines were once touted as drugs of choice for anaerobic infections, but their performance against *Bacteroides* and many gram-negative cocci has considerably altered this view. Widespread tetracycline resistance has been noted. As a result, this class of compounds is not recommended for treatment of anaerobic infections. Chloramphenicol shows excellent activity in vitro against *Bacteroides* and most other anaerobic pathogens. It also has activity against coliforms, staphylococci, and streptococci.

Whereas some clinical trials have shown good results with chloramphenicol, others have encountered therapeutic failures. In addition, animal models of anaerobic infection have shown poor results with chloramphenicol treatment.

Aminoglycoside and quinolone antimicrobial drugs, as well as aztreonam and ceftazidime, are inactive against most anaerobic bacteria. These drugs are included in antimicrobial regimens for therapy of mixed infections, although their role is clearly to suppress the facultative gram-negative components.

PROGNOSIS. Prognosis of anaerobic infections is related to the site of infection, the type of pathogen, the underlying condition of the patient, and the choice of antimicrobial therapy. In general, anaerobic pleuropulmonary infections have a good outcome, especially when adequate drainage can be achieved. Penicillin G has been successful in treating these infections in the past, curing up to 95 per cent of patients with aspiration pneumonia or lung abscess, for example. Some failures have been noted with penicillin, and in such instances clindamycin has been used to advantage. Metronidazole treatment has been associated with failures in lung abscess.

Severe intra-abdominal infections have a failure rate of 10 to 20 per cent even with optimal surgery and antimicrobial therapy. Higher failure rates in controlled clinical trials have been associated with treatment regimens using antimicrobial agents with poor activity against *B. fragilis* such as cephalothin, doxycycline, cefamandole, and cefoperazone. Infections of the female genital tract generally have a good prognosis, since most patients tend to be rather healthy prior to the onset of the septic process. Good results have been reported with cefoxitin, clindamycin,

and metronidazole, usually in association with another antibiotic. In one clinical trial penicillin combined with gentamicin produced a poor result in endomyometritis when compared with the alternative regimen of clindamycin and gentamicin.

In general, clinical trials with new antimicrobial agents have corroborated the findings in animal models and susceptibility testing in vitro. Because of the vast array of anaerobic organisms and their varying patterns of susceptibility, it is best to base empiric therapy on known sensitivity patterns and performance of the specific drugs in controlled clinical trials.

Bartlett JG, Louie TJ, Gorbach SL, et al.: Therapeutic efficacy of 29 antimicrobial regimens in experimental intra-abdominal sepsis. Rev Infect Dis 3:535, 1981. *An experimental model of intra-abdominal infections that explains the pathophysiologic events and the rationale for antimicrobial treatments.*

Cuchural GJ, Tally FP, Jacobus NV, et al.: Comparative activities of newer β-lactam agents against members of the *Bacteroides fragilis* group. Antimicrob Agents Chemother 34:479, 1990. *Seven medical centers in the United States collaborated on this survey of antibiotic efficacy against the pre-eminent anaerobic pathogens.*

Finegold SM, George WL (eds.): Anaerobic Infections in Humans. New York, Academic Press, 1989. *A collection of authoritative articles by the "Who's Who" in anaerobic bacteriology.*

Kasper DL, Onderdonk AB (eds.): International Symposium on Anaerobic Bacteria and Bacterial Infections. Rev Infect Dis 12:S2, 1990. *Complete clinical, laboratory, and therapeutic aspects, presented by foremost experts in the field.*

Styrt B, Gorbach SL: Recent developments in the understanding of the pathogenesis and treatment of anaerobic infections. N Engl J Med 321:240–246, 298–302, 1989. *An update of advances, with an extensive bibliography.*

Enteric Infections

312 Introduction

Bruce M. Greene

Included in this section are bacteria that are pathogenic in humans as a consequence of their intraintestinal localization and multiplication, and biologic properties that lead to disease through toxin production and its physiologic effects, direct damage to intestinal epithelial cells, or invasion across the mucosa into lymphoid tissues with subsequent multiplication and dissemination. Although the major global impact of most of these pathogens is in developing countries, in the aggregate they represent a major and poorly controlled threat to human health in many developed countries, including the United States. Furthermore, diarrhea in travelers to developing countries, most commonly due to strains of *Escherichia coli*, is a major health problem, affecting one third to one half of those who spend significant time abroad.

The clinical manifestations associated with this group of pathogens are quite diverse. Typhoid fever is dominated by systemic manifestations in the majority of cases, particularly early in the infection, and in only approximately one third of cases is diarrhea a significant manifestation. Intestinal perforation and hemorrhage are frequent. Conversely, at the other end of the spectrum, cholera is manifest almost exclusively as a secretory diarrhea, with systemic manifestations reflecting fluid loss. Shigellosis shows a combination of febrile and toxic manifestations as well as fluid loss reflecting damage to colonic epithelium. Nontyphoidal salmonellae may cause classic enteric fever as well as severe diarrheal syndromes. Strains of diarrheogenic *E. coli* vary considerably in their mode of pathogenesis and consequently in the associated clinical manifestations. Campylobacter enteritis is a febrile illness associated with diarrhea that is frequently bloody.

Differential diagnostic features of this group of infections are indicated in Table 312–1. Importantly, in addition to these agents it may be difficult to exclude amebic dysentery from consideration, as well as rotavirus enteritis, giardiasis, yersinia infection, and food poisoning due to other bacterial pathogens such as *Bacillus cereus*, clostridia, *Vibrio parahemolyticus*, and *Staphylococcus aureus*. Therefore, specific epidemiologic features in an individual case may be crucial in establishing the correct diagnosis and in instituting proper therapy. Furthermore, the presence of

TABLE 312–1. DIAGNOSTIC FEATURES OF COMMON ENTERIC INFECTIONS

Causative Agent(s)	Typical Clinical Manifestations	Signs and Laboratory Manifestations	Epidemiologic Features
Salmonella typhi	Fever, intestinal perforation, or hemorrhage	Rose spots, relative leukopenia	Travel to or residence in endemic areas
Vibrio cholera	Severe watery diarrhea; dehydration	Fecal leukocytes absent	Residence in endemic areas
Shigella species	Fever, cramps, explosive diarrhea	Abundant fecal leukocytes	Travel to developing countries; residence in a custodial institution
Nontyphoidal salmonellae	a. Fever, diarrhea b. Typhoidal fever	a. Fecal leukocytes (moderate) b. Relative leukopenia	Consumption of undercooked poultry, eggs, processed meats; nursing homes
Diarrheogenic *E. coli*	a. Fever, diarrhea b. Hemorrhagic diarrhea	Fecal leukocytes prominent in enteroinvasive forms	Travel to developing countries; consumption of inadequately cooked processed food
Campylobacter jejuni	Fever, diarrhea	Fecal leukocytes present	Consumption of undercooked poultry, unpasteurized milk, contaminated water

immunodeficiency, especially AIDS, necessitates consideration of multiple additional pathogens and reordering of the likelihood of causative agents (see Ch. 416 for clinical manifestations of AIDS).

313 Typhoid Fever

Thomas Butler

DEFINITION. Typhoid fever is a bacterial disease caused by *Salmonella typhi*. It is characterized by prolonged fever, abdominal pain, diarrhea, delirium, rose spots, and splenomegaly and complicated sometimes by intestinal bleeding and perforation. Enteric fever is synonymous with typhoid fever, which is occasionally caused also by *S. enteritidis* bioserotype paratyphi A or B.

ETIOLOGY. The typhoid bacillus is a motile gram-negative rod in the family Enterobacteriaceae. It possesses a flagellar (H) antigen, a cell wall (O) lipopolysaccharide antigen, and a polysaccharide virulence (Vi) antigen located in the cell capsule. The polysaccharide side chain of the O antigen confers serologic specificity to the organism and is essential in virulence because salmonellae other than *S. typhi* and *S. enteritidis* bioserotype paratyphi A or B do not produce enteric fever in humans. These antigens play critical roles in permitting the organisms to invade lymphoid tissue from the gut lumen and to multiply within macrophages.

INCIDENCE AND PREVALENCE. Typhoid fever has been almost eliminated from developed countries because of sewage and water treatment facilities but remains a common disease in developing countries. In 1980, the number of cases occurring yearly was estimated as about 7 million in Asia, over 4 million in Africa, and 0.5 million in Latin America. About 500 cases are diagnosed each year in the United States, and over half of these are in recently arrived travelers who contracted their infections abroad.

EPIDEMIOLOGY. Adults and children of all ages and both sexes appear equally susceptible to infection. In developing countries, most cases occur in school-age children and young adults. Although acquired immunity provides some protection, reinfections have been documented. Typhoid fever occurs during all seasons.

Transmission is by the fecal-oral route through contaminated water or food. The main human sources of infection in the community are asymptomatic fecal carriers and cases during either disease or convalescence. Females and older males are prone to become chronic fecal carriers because underlying cholecystitis enables them to harbor chronic infection in the gallbladder. *S. typhi* is resistant to drying and cooling, thus allowing bacteria to survive prolonged periods in dried sewage, water, food, and ice.

Vi-phage typing of *S. typhi* is a useful epidemiologic tool to trace cases of typhoid fever to a carrier or food source. Single-source outbreaks of typhoid fever are rare. In endemic situations, multiple phage types are present, and several phage types may be responsible for an epidemic.

PATHOGENESIS AND PATHOLOGY. After ingestion of *S. typhi*, the part of the inoculum that survives the acidity of the stomach enters the small intestine, where bacteria penetrate the mucosa and enter mononuclear phagocytes of ileal Peyer's patches and mesenteric lymph nodes. Inocula of at least 10^5 bacteria are necessary to initiate disease, and inocula of 10^7 and more cause disease regularly. The incubation period ranges from 8 to 28 days, depending on inoculum size and immune status of the host. Bacteria proliferate in mononuclear phagocytes and spread by way of the blood to the spleen, liver, and bone marrow, where further proliferation in macrophages occurs. The earliest symptoms of fever and chills (Table 313-1) are associated with bacteremia. Inflammatory reactions occur in the spleen, liver, bone marrow, Peyer's patches mainly in the terminal ileum, and skin, consisting of mononuclear cell infiltration, hyperplasia, and focal necrosis. Focal collections of mononuclear leukocytes are called "typhoid nodules." Fever and other constitutional symptoms are probably caused by the release of interleukin 1 (endogenous pyrogen) from infected mononuclear phagocytes. Endotoxemia does not occur in typhoid fever. Intestinal manifestations are caused by hyperplasia of Peyer's patches with ulcerations of overlying mucosa, resulting in pain, diarrhea, bleeding, or perforation.

CLINICAL MANIFESTATIONS. In the first days of illness the nonspecific symptoms of fever, chills, and headache are mild and in the typical case build up in intensity during the first week, resulting in prostration. The evolution of disease syndromes occurs stepwise over 1 to 3 weeks (Table 313-1) but may be variable in the time of appearance. The early symptoms of fever, abdominal pain, and prostration tend to persist throughout the illness, which in untreated cases lasts a month or longer. Abdominal pain occurs in more than half of patients and is frequently diffuse or located in the right lower quadrant over the terminal ileum. Diarrhea occurs in about a third of patients and consists of either watery stools or semisolid stools described as "pea soup." Melena occurs less commonly. Rose spots occur in more than half of light-skinned individuals but are often not visible in dark-skinned patients. The rash is seen most commonly on the shoulders, thorax, and abdomen and rarely affects the extremities. The lesions are erythematous macules or papules about 1 to 5 mm in diameter which typically blanch with pressure but may become hemorrhagic. They fade quickly after a few days of treatment. Many patients display abnormal behavior or altered mental status that may be out of proportion to the severity of the systemic illness. Among the common presentations are "toxic" staring, delirium, aphonia, and coma. Seizures are common in children. Patients are rarely jaundiced.

In about 5 per cent of patients, intestinal bleeding or intestinal perforation occurs, usually after the second week of illness. Bleeding occurs from ileal ulcers and may present as melena or bright red blood in stools. Brisk bleeding develops rarely but is an occasional cause of death. Intestinal perforation presents as the sudden onset of more severe abdominal pain, distention, and tenderness. Bowel sounds are diminished and the abdominal radiograph usually reveals free air. Perforation most often occurs unexpectedly after a few days of treatment when a patient has started to improve. Other complications of typhoid fever include pneumonia, which develops as a superinfection due to other bacteria, myocarditis, acute cholecystitis, and acute meningitis.

Relapses occur in about 10 to 20 per cent of patients treated with chloramphenicol. Patients with relapses experience the reappearance of typical symptoms about 7 to 14 days after the

TABLE 313-1. EVOLUTION OF TYPICAL SYMPTOMS AND SIGNS OF TYPHOID FEVER

Disease Period	Symptoms	Signs	Pathology
First week	Fever, chills gradually increasing and persisting; headache	Abdominal tenderness	Bacteremia
Second week	Rash, abdominal pain, diarrhea or constipation, delirium, prostration	Rose spots, splenomegaly, hepatomegaly	Mononuclear cell vasculitis of skin, hyperplasia of ileal Peyer's patches, typhoid nodules in spleen and liver
Third week	Complications of intestinal bleeding and perforation, shock	Melena, ileus, rigid abdomen, coma	Ulcerations over Peyer's patches, perforation with peritonitis
Fourth week and later	Resolution of symptoms, relapse, weight loss	Reappearance of acute disease, cachexia	Cholecystitis, chronic fecal carriage of bacteria

end of treatment. Relapses tend to be less severe than the initial episode.

DIAGNOSIS. The preferred method of diagnosis is isolation of *S. typhi* from a blood culture, which is positive in most patients during the first 2 weeks of illness. Urine and stool cultures are positive less frequently but should be taken to increase the diagnostic yield. The bone marrow culture is the most sensitive test, positive in nearly 90 per cent of cases, and can be used when a bacteriologic diagnosis is crucially needed or in patients who have been pretreated with antibiotics. The duodenal string test to culture bile has also been used with success in typhoid fever.

The Widal test for agglutinating antibodies against the somatic (O) and flagellar (H) antigens of *S. typhi* is widely used for serodiagnosis. An O agglutinin titer of $\geq 1:80$ or a fourfold rise supports a diagnosis of typhoid fever, whereas the H agglutinins are more often nonspecifically elevated by immunization or previous infections with other bacteria. Serodiagnosis is of limited value because false-positive results are often obtained in endemic areas and false-negative results occur in some cases of bacteriologically proven typhoid fever.

Other laboratory findings are anemia of variable severity and a white blood cell count that is normal or decreased with an increased percentage of band forms. Platelets are often diminished, and signs of disseminated intravascular coagulation are present. Liver function tests frequently show elevated aminotransferases and bilirubin concentrations. Renal failure is an infrequent complication. In patients with diarrhea, the stool shows fecal leukocytes.

The differential diagnosis depends on infections that are endemic in the area where an individual contracted the infection. For returned travelers from developing countries, the common possibilities are malaria, hepatitis, typhus, amebic liver abscess, shigellosis, nontyphoid salmonellosis, and leptospirosis. In the United States one must consider septicemias originating from the urinary tract, GI tract, or gallbladder as well as influenza, infectious mononucleosis, meningococcemia, miliary tuberculosis, and bacterial endocarditis.

TREATMENT. Chloramphenicol has remained the drug of choice since its introduction in 1948 because no other drug has been demonstrated to cause more rapid or consistent improvement of disease. Resistance to chloramphenicol mediated by plasmid R factors has been reported only occasionally in patients who acquired infections in Mexico, India, and Thailand. Chloramphenicol is given orally in a dose of 50 to 60 mg per kilogram of body weight per day in four equal portions every 6 hours. After defervescence and clinical improvement the dosage can be reduced to 30 mg per kilogram per day to complete a 14-day course. In patients unable to take oral medication the same dosage should be given intravenously until the patient can take capsules.

Alternative drugs should be considered when *S. typhi* resistant to chloramphenicol is isolated or strongly suspected. Several are nearly equal to chloramphenicol in efficacy. Trimethoprim-sulfamethoxazole is effective in a standard adult dose of 160 mg trimethoprim and 800 mg sulfamethoxazole given orally or intravenously twice a day for 14 days. Other drugs that are effective include ampicillin (intravenously), amoxicillin, cefoperazone, and ceftriaxone.

Patients who are dehydrated, anorectic, or suffering from diarrhea should receive intravenous saline with attention to electrolyte and acid-base disturbances. Patients with brisk intestinal bleeding require blood transfusion. Patients with suspected perforation should have an abdominal radiograph to look for free air and peritoneal fluid. Laparotomy should be undertaken as early as possible to suture the perforation, and gentamicin should be added to broaden coverage for polymicrobial peritonitis.

In some high-risk patients with delirium, coma, or shock, high-dose dexamethasone in addition to antibiotics reduces mortality. The dose should be 3 mg per kilogram initially, followed by 1 mg per kilogram every 6 hours for 48 hours. One must be cautious with this therapy because signs and symptoms of perforation are masked by steroids. Antipyretic drugs such as aspirin should be administered with caution because they occasionally cause marked reductions in blood pressure.

Patients with relapses of typhoid fever should be treated the same as patients with a first attack. Chronic fecal carriers (asymptomatic excretion for a year or longer) should be given high doses of ampicillin or amoxicillin, 100 mg per kilogram per day, plus probenecid 30 mg per kilogram per day for 4 to 6 weeks. Trimethoprim-sulfamethoxazole is also effective. Patients with gallstones or cholecystitis may require cholecystectomy for eradication of the carrier state. Chloramphenicol neither prevents nor effectively treats the chronic carrier state.

PROGNOSIS. Typhoid fever carried a case fatality rate of about 12 per cent in the preantibiotic era which was reduced to about 4 per cent after chloramphenicol became available. Case fatality rates over 10 per cent continue to be reported in developing countries despite availability of antibiotics, whereas developed countries show case fatality rates less than 1 per cent. After treatment with chloramphenicol or other effective drug, most patients become afebrile in 4 to 7 days. In the preantibiotic era about 10 per cent of recovered patients had relapses, and chloramphenicol treatment has not reduced this rate. Intestinal bleeding or perforation occurs in about 5 per cent of patients and may not be prevented by antibiotic treatment. Thus, bleeding or perforation is occasionally detected after patients have defervesced during treatment. About 1 to 3 per cent of patients become chronic fecal carriers after recovery.

PREVENTION. Travelers to developing countries should avoid consuming untreated water, drinks served with ice, peeled fruits, and other food that is not served hot. American international travelers face an overall risk of developing typhoid fever of less than 1 case in 10,000 trips, but travelers to high-risk countries like India and Pakistan have a probability of about 4 in 10,000 trips of getting typhoid fever. Travelers wishing immune protection should receive either live oral vaccine Ty21a (Berna Products [1-800-533-5899]) given as one capsule every other day for a total of four capsules or typhoid vaccine, U.S.P., administered as two subcutaneous injections of 0.5 ml each at intervals of 4 weeks, with booster doses given every 3 years if needed. These vaccines give only partial protection, and thus vaccinated persons should still exercise dietary precautions. The traditional method of controlling typhoid is to follow stool cultures of convalescent cases and report positive cultures to the Health Department. The Health Department investigates nonimported typhoid cases to identify possible food sources or contact with a chronic carrier.

Butler T, Islam A, Kabir I, et al.: Patterns of morbidity and mortality in typhoid fever dependent on age and gender: Review of 552 hospitalized patients with diarrhea. Rev Infect Dis 13:85, 1991. *Severe and fatal disease in Bangladesh was more common in young children and adults and was correlated with high incidences of seizures, delirium or coma, intestinal perforation, and pneumonia.*

Hornick RB: Selective primary health care: Strategies for control of disease in the developing world. XX. Typhoid fever. Rev Infect Dis 7:536, 1985. *A useful review of pathogenesis, epidemiology, and prevention of this infection.*

Islam A, Butler T, Nath SK, et al.: Randomized treatment of patients with typhoid fever by using ceftriaxone or chloramphenicol. J Infect Dis 158:742, 1988. *Study of treatment in Bangladesh showed that chloramphenicol remains the treatment of choice because of low cost and rapid defervescence, but newer cephalosporins are good alternatives.*

Klotz SA, Jorgensen JH, Buckwold FJ, et al.: Typhoid fever: An epidemic with remarkably few clinical signs and symptoms. Arch Intern Med 144:533, 1984. *In 34 patients in Texas who were infected after eating Mexican food at a restaurant, illness was characterized by fever without localizing signs and symptoms; there were no deaths or complications.*

Levine MM, Ferreccio C, Black RE, et al.: Large-scale field trial of Ty21a live oral typhoid vaccine in enteric-coated capsule formulation. Lancet 1:1049, 1987. *In Chilean school children, three capsules given every other day conferred 67 per cent protection during 3 years; oral vaccination is preferred to parenteral vaccine because of absence of toxic reactions.*

314 Salmonella Infections Other Than Typhoid Fever

Donald Kaye

DEFINITION. *Salmonella,* a genus of the family Enterobacteriaceae, can cause an asymptomatic intestinal carrier state or clinical disease in both humans and animals. In humans the most common clinical manifestation is enterocolitis with diarrhea as the major symptom. Some patients develop bacteremia without gastrointestinal manifestations. Localization from bacteremia may result in osteomyelitis, a mycotic aneurysm, or other localized infection. *S. typhi*, a pathogen of humans only, causes enteric fever. Enteric fever produced by *S. typhi* is called typhoid fever, whereas enteric fever caused by other salmonellae is named paratyphoid fever.

An asymptomatic intestinal carrier state of variable duration may follow inapparent or symptomatic infection. Most carriers are transient carriers. A chronic carrier state, defined as lasting more than 1 year, is usually permanent and is most often related to persistent infection in the gallbladder. With the exception of *S. typhi*, in which a human carrier is always implicated, most salmonella infections are acquired from food products derived from infected animals (e.g., eggs, poultry, meat, milk).

ETIOLOGY. Salmonellae are motile, gram-negative, non–spore-forming members of the family Enterobacteriaceae. They are differentiated from other Enterobacteriaceae by biochemical tests. They ferment glucose, maltose, and mannitol but not lactose or sucrose. Almost all salmonellae produce acid and gas with fermentation and are ornithine- and trehalose-positive. Exceptions to the rules which are helpful in identification are the following: *S. typhi* does not produce gas and is ornithine-negative; *S. choleraesuis* is trehalose-negative; and *S. gallinarum-pullorum* is nonmotile. As another confounding exception, lactose-fermenting strains of salmonellae have been isolated.

Salmonellae can be differentiated into over 2000 serotypes by their somatic (O) antigens, which are composed of lipopolysaccharides and are part of the cell wall, and flagellar (H) antigens. Proper nomenclature has divided the salmonellae into three species: *S. typhi*, *S. choleraesuis*, and *S. enteritidis*. The first two consist of only one serotype each, whereas the third contains all the rest of the serotypes. These latter serotypes are recognized as *S. enteritidis* serotype _____(e.g., *S. enteritidis* serotype typhimurium). However, in a less confusing and cumbersome system, each serotype is commonly referred to as a separate species and is so indicated in this chapter. In this system, using common O antigens, salmonellae have been divided into five major groups, A through E. Some of the important serotypes and their groups are *S. typhi* (group D), *S. choleraesuis* (Group C₁), *S. typhimurium* (group B), and *S. enteritidis* (group D).

S. typhimurium is the most common cause of human disease and represents about 25 per cent of *Salmonella* isolates in the United States reported to the Centers for Disease Control (CDC). Other common isolates are *S. enteritidis*, *S. heidelberg*, *S. newport*, *S. hadar*, *S. infantis*, *S. agona*, *S. montevideo*, *S. thompson*, and *S. braenderup*. In 1987, these 10 serotypes accounted for 73 per cent of the human isolates reported to the CDC. Recently, *S. enteritidis* outbreaks related to eggs have been increasing.

EPIDEMIOLOGY. *S. typhi*, *S. paratyphi* A, *S. schottmuelleri* (*S. paratyphi* B), *S. hirschfeldii* (*S. paratyphi* C), and *S. sendai* are either solely or almost always pathogens in man only, and human-to-human transmission is important.

The remaining serotypes of salmonellae are widely spread in the animal kingdom, and salmonellae have been isolated from virtually all species, including birds, poultry, mammals, reptiles, amphibians, and insects. Salmonella infection in man usually occurs from ingestion of contaminated animal food products, most often eggs, poultry, and meat. Eggs usually become contaminated from feces on the surface of the egg, with small cracks allowing entry into the egg. However, infection of the ovary allows primary incorporation of salmonellae into the egg. Meat and poultry become widely contaminated at the slaughterhouse with salmonellae spread from carcass to carcass, usually on the surface. *S. choleraesuis* is associated with pig products and *S. dublin* with cattle and consumption of unpasteurized milk from cattle. Salmonellae may survive cooking at relatively low temperatures in the center of eggs or turkeys, or food may be contaminated after cooking from kitchen utensils or from the hands of food preparers who handle raw food.

Salmonella infections have been acquired following contamination of food or water with feces of pet turtles, chicks, birds, dogs, cats, and many other species. These pets become infected from their food.

Salmonella infection can also be acquired by eating food or less commonly drinking water contaminated by a human carrier who has not washed his hands adequately. Infection has been spread by the fecal-oral route in children, by contaminated enema and fiberoptic instruments, and by diagnostic and therapeutic preparations made from animal or insect products (e.g., pancreatic extract, carmine dye).

Outbreaks of salmonellosis occur in institutionalized patients, who are probably more prone to develop salmonella infections for three reasons. First, there are more underlying diseases which decrease host defense mechanisms against salmonellae such as disorders of gastric acidity and intestinal motility; second, use of antimicrobial agents reduces the normal, protective intestinal flora; and third, institutional food prepared in bulk is more likely to be contaminated than individually prepared meals. Outbreaks in nurseries and in the elderly in nursing homes have the highest mortality rates (i.e., over 5 per cent).

Most cases of salmonella infection occurring in the United States are sporadic rather than related to outbreaks. However, when an infection occurs in a family, other members of the household also tend to have positive stool cultures. About 40,000 cases of salmonella infection have been reported to the CDC in recent years, a marked increase over the past 30 years. However, this undoubtedly represents only a fraction of actual cases. It has been estimated that over 1 million cases actually occur each year. A disproportionate number of infections occur in July through October, probably related to the warm weather. Salmonella infections are most common in infants and children under 5 years of age.

Salmonellae have become increasingly resistant to antibiotics, with many strains now resistant to ampicillin. Resistance to ampicillin and other antibiotics is usually by means of bacterial acquisition of resistance transfer factors. It is believed that much of the resistance has been related to widespread use of antimicrobial agents in farm animals.

PATHOGENESIS. Following ingestion of organisms, the determinants of whether or not infection results, as well as the severity of infection, are the dose and virulence of the *Salmonella* strain and the status of host defense mechanisms. Large inocula such as 10^7 bacteria are usually required to produce clinical infection in the normal host. Smaller inocula are more likely to result in no infection or to produce a transient intestinal carrier state. Gastric acid serves as a host defense mechanism by killing many of the ingested organisms, and intestinal motility is also probably a host defense mechanism. In the absence or decrease of gastric acidity (as in the elderly, following gastrectomy, vagotomy or gastroenterostomy, with H₂-receptor antagonists, and with antacids) and with decreased intestinal motility (as with antimotility drugs), much smaller inocula can produce infection and the infection tends to be more severe.

Administration of antimicrobial agents prior to ingestion of salmonellae can markedly reduce the size of inoculum needed to produce infection, presumably by reducing the protective bowel flora.

While any *Salmonella* serotype can produce any of the salmonella syndromes (transient asymptomatic carrier state, enterocolitis, bacteremia, enteric fever, and chronic carrier state), each serotype tends to produce certain syndromes much more often than others. For example, *S. anatum* usually causes asymptomatic intestinal infection, whereas *S. typhimurium* usually causes enterocolitis. *S. choleraesuis* is more likely to produce bacteremia (often with metastatic infection) than asymptomatic infection or enterocolitis, and some serotypes such as *S. typhi* are most likely to cause enteric fever as well as the chronic carrier state. Fortunately, most *Salmonella* serotypes are of relatively low pathogenicity for man, and therefore, although food products are commonly contaminated, large outbreaks occur only when more virulent serotypes are involved.

In order to produce infection (even asymptomatic intestinal infection), enteric pathogens (including salmonellae) must first adhere to intestinal mucosal epithelial cells. Pili on the surface of salmonellae adhere to specific receptor sites on the epithelial cells. Following adherence, invasion of the mucosal cell may result, or multiplication may occur without invasion, resulting in asymptomatic infection. When the organisms reach the lamina propria, polymorphonuclear leukocytes serve as a defense mechanism to prevent invasion of lymphatics. Certain serotypes seem more able than others to invade lymphatics and subsequently produce bacteremia. For example, *S. dublin*, which has been isolated from unpasteurized milk, commonly produces bacteremia following intestinal infection. Both the small intestine and colon are involved in the inflammatory process. The diarrhea in salmonella enterocolitis results from the inflammation. In addition, watery stools may occur, apparently the result of secretion of water and electrolytes by small intestinal epithelial cells in response to an enterotoxin secreted by some of the *Salmonella* strains or in response to tissue mediators of inflammation.

Patients with diseases that impair host defense mechanisms seem to have an increased frequency of severe salmonella infection. For many years, a striking association has been recognized between diseases producing hemolysis and salmonella bacteremia. Specifically, salmonella bacteremia is common in patients with sickle cell disorders, malaria, and bartonellosis. In fact, because of the frequency of salmonella bacteremia in sickle cell diseases and the underlying bone disease in these patients to which salmonellae localize, these organisms are the most common cause of osteomyelitis in patients with sickle cell disorders. Prolonged salmonella bacteremia occurs in patients with hepatosplenic schistosomiasis, probably related to localization on and in the intravascular schistosomes. Patients with lymphoma and leukemia also are more prone to develop salmonella bacteremia. Recently, prolonged and recurrent refractory salmonella bacteremia has been observed in patients with AIDS.

CLINICAL SYNDROMES. *Asymptomatic Intestinal Carrier State.* The asymptomatic intestinal carrier state may result from inapparent infection, which is the most common form of salmonella infection, or may follow clinical disease (convalescent carrier). The carrier state is usually self-limited to several weeks to months, with the incidence of positive stool cultures rapidly decreasing. By 1 year far less than 1 per cent still have positive stools. The major exception is with *S. typhi*: About 3 per cent of those infected excrete the organism for life. A patient who has had *Salmonella* in his or her stool for 1 year (chronic carrier) is likely to become a lifelong carrier. Patients with *Schistosoma haematobium* infections are predisposed to become chronic urinary carriers of *Salmonella*.

Enterocolitis. After an incubation period, which is usually 12 to 48 hours, the illness starts suddenly with crampy abdominal pain and diarrhea. A chill is common. Although occasional patients have nausea and vomit once or twice, vomiting is not persistent. The diarrhea may be watery and of large volume or small volume. The stools may contain mucus and occasionally blood. Polymorphonuclear leukocytes are present in the stool. Diarrhea may be mild or may be severe with up to 20 to 30 stools a day. Fever is present in most patients and may reach 40°C (104°F) or higher. The abdomen is tender to palpation. Transient bacteremia may occur and is most likely in infants, the elderly, and patients with impaired host defense mechanisms.

Symptoms usually improve over a period of days, with fever lasting no more than 2 to 3 days and diarrhea no more than 5 to 7 days. However, these symptoms may occasionally persist for up to 14 days.

Enteric Fever. Paratyphoid fever is an enteric fever syndrome identical to typhoid fever but produced by a serotype other than *S. typhi* (most often *S. paratyphi* A, *S. schottmuelleri*, or *S. hirschfeldii*). On occasion, it may immediately follow classic enterocolitis caused by the same organism. The syndrome, characterized by prolonged sustained fever, relative bradycardia, splenomegaly, rose spots, and leukopenia, is described in Ch. 313. Enteric fever produced by serotypes of *Salmonella* other than *S. typhi* is usually milder than typhoid fever, and the chronic carrier state follows less commonly than after typhoid fever.

Bacteremia. Patients with the syndrome of salmonella bacteremia usually complain of fever and chills for a period of days to weeks. Gastrointestinal symptoms are unusual, but in some patients the syndrome of salmonella bacteremia follows classic enterocolitis. Other symptoms are nonspecific such as malaise, anorexia, and weight loss. Metastatic infection of bones, joints, mycotic aneurysm (particularly of the abdominal aorta), meninges (mainly in infants), pericardium, pleural space, lungs, heart valves, cysts, uterine myomas, malignancies, and other sites is common, and symptoms may be related to the site of metastatic infection. Stool cultures are usually negative for *Salmonella*, but blood cultures are positive.

Although any *Salmonella* serotype can produce the syndrome of bacteremia, *S. choleraesuis* is most likely to cause this syndrome; over 50 per cent of *S. choleraesuis* infections are bacteremic. *S. choleraesuis* infection also has the highest mortality rate of infection caused by any *Salmonella*.

Salmonella bacteremia occurs with increased frequency in infants and the elderly and in patients with diseases associated with hemolysis (such as sickle cell diseases, malaria, and bartonellosis), with lymphoma, and with leukemia. Localization to bone is common in patients with sickle cell diseases.

Prolonged salmonella bacteremia lasting for months occurs in patients with hepatosplenic schistosomiasis. Patients with AIDS develop recurrent, relapsing salmonella bacteremia that is difficult to cure with antibiotics.

DIAGNOSIS. The diagnosis of salmonella infection is made by isolation of the organism from the stool in enterocolitis, from the blood in bacteremia, from blood and stool in enteric fever, and from the local site in localized infection. Serologic studies are of little clinical value in salmonella infections other than typhoid fever, but they may be of use in epidemiologic studies. The white blood cell count is usually normal in enterocolitis, normal or low in enteric fever, and normal in bacteremia. A stained smear of the stool usually demonstrates polymorphonuclear leukocytes in patients with salmonella enterocolitis.

The differential diagnosis of salmonella enterocolitis includes all causes of acute diarrhea, including invasive bacteria such as *Campylobacter jejuni*, *Shigella* species, invasive *E. coli*, *Yersinia enterocolitica*, and *Vibrio parahaemolyticus*; toxigenic bacteria such as *Vibrio cholerae*, enterotoxigenic *E. coli*, *S. aureus*, *B. cereus*, *C. perfringens*, and *C. difficile*; viruses; and protozoa such as *E. histolytica*, *G. lamblia*, and *Cryptosporidium* species. Invasive bacterial causes of diarrhea and *C. difficile* infection are also associated with polymorphonuclear leukocytes in the stool, whereas bacterial toxigenic causes (other than *C. difficile*), viruses, and protozoa generally are not. The bacterial toxigenic causes of diarrhea other than *C. difficile* do not produce fever.

Stool culture is definitive for the diagnosis of salmonella enterocolitis, but by the time the results of the stool culture are available, most patients are recovering.

The differential diagnosis of salmonella bacteremia includes all acute infectious and noninfectious causes of fever, including bacteremia caused by other organisms.

The differential diagnosis of enteric fever is the same as discussed in Ch. 313.

TREATMENT. *Enterocolitis.* The primary approach to treatment of salmonella enterocolitis is fluid and electrolyte replacement. Oral fruit juices and carbonated sodas are useful for those who can take fluids orally. Intravenous fluids are necessary in those who are unable to take oral fluids or who are severely dehydrated, most often the very young and the elderly.

Drugs with antiperistaltic effects such as loperamide or diphenoxylate with atropine can relieve cramps but should be used sparingly, as they can prolong the diarrhea.

Salmonella enterocolitis is self-limited, and the large majority of cases do not require antimicrobial therapy. However, infants, the elderly, and those with sickle cell disease, lymphoma, leukemia, or other serious underlying diseases who are severely ill and may have bacteremia may benefit from antimicrobial therapy. Amoxicillin, 1 gram every 6 hours orally, or trimethoprim-sulfamethoxazole, one double-strength tablet every 12 hours orally in adults, can be used in those who are able to take oral drugs. Ampicillin, 1 to 2 grams IV every 6 hours, and trimethoprim-sulfamethoxazole, 10 mg per kilogram per day IV of the trimethoprim component, have been used in those who are more severely ill. Antibiotic susceptibility studies should be performed on the isolates, as many strains are now resistant to ampicillin. Therapy is continued for 5 days.

There has been a reluctance to treat salmonella enterocolitis, as antibiotic therapy has been reported to have no effect on the clinical course and furthermore to prolong the period of time that salmonellae are excreted in the stool. In addition, most patients are improving by the time that salmonellae or other bacterial pathogens are isolated from the stool. Perhaps most important, effective, single-drug therapy active against *Salmonella*, *Shigella*, *Campylobacter*, and other bacterial causes of diarrhea has been lacking until recently, and early empiric antimicrobial therapy for diarrhea suspected to be of bacterial origin has therefore been problematic.

In the past few years, the availability of norfloxacin and ciprofloxacin has changed some of these factors. These agents are active against virtually all bacterial pathogens that cause diarrhea except for *C. difficile* and can be used empirically in the early therapy of severe diarrhea of presumed bacterial etiology. Furthermore, several preliminary studies indicate that these agents decrease the duration of the clinical course of salmonella enterocolitis but may increase the duration of fecal excretion. These observations of efficacy must be confirmed and extended before routine use of these agents can be advocated for suspected salmonella enterocolitis.

Bacteremia and Enteric Fever. The major therapeutic agents are chloramphenicol, 50 mg per kilogram per day in four equally divided doses orally or IV, or ampicillin, 2 grams IV every 6 hours. With resistant organisms or when these agents cannot be used for other reasons, trimethoprim-sulfamethoxazole IV may be substituted at a dose of 10 mg per kilogram per day of the trimethoprim component. Ampicillin is preferred when localized infection (especially intravascular) is present. After response, oral amoxicillin or oral trimethoprim-sulfamethoxazole can be given in the doses described under enterocolitis. In patients infected with salmonellae resistant to these agents, third-generation cephalosporins such as cefotaxime, ceftizoxime, ceftriaxone, and ceftazidime may be useful. First- and second-generation cephalosporins such as cephalothin and cefamandole do not seem to be acceptably effective. With further experience, ciprofloxacin may also prove to be a very useful agent. Therapy is continued for 2 weeks for enteric fever and bacteremia without localization of organisms and for much longer periods of time with localization to bone, aneurysms, heart valves, and various other sites. Surgical drainage or removal of foreign bodies is often necessary for cure of localized infection.

Cure of the schistosomiasis in patients with salmonella bacteremia may cure the bacteremia. Patients with AIDS tend to relapse repeatedly after treatment courses for salmonella bacteremia. Long-term suppressive therapy has been recommended by some.

Carriers. Chronic carriers (i.e., over 1 year) of salmonellae other than *S. typhi* are rare. Stools of convalescent carriers spontaneously become negative over a period of weeks to months, and no therapy should be given. The rare chronic carrier of non–*S. typhi* serotypes (usually infected with *S. paratyphi* A, *S. schottmuelleri*, or *S. hirschfeldii*) may be treated with 4 to 6 grams of ampicillin plus 2 grams of probenecid orally each day in four divided doses for 6 weeks. Strains resistant to ampicillin may respond to ciprofloxacin. Patients who relapse usually have gallbladder disease (most often calculi) and will not be cured with antimicrobial therapy. Cholecystectomy plus antimicrobial therapy may cure these patients, but it is doubtful that the carrier state per se is a sufficient indication for cholecystectomy.

PROGNOSIS. Mortality in salmonella enterocolitis is rare; infants and the elderly are at greatest risk, with death occurring from dehydration and electrolyte imbalance. Mortality from salmonella bacteremia or enteric fever is not uncommon and is most likely to occur in the very young and the very old. *S. choleraesuis* bacteremia has the highest mortality rate of any *Salmonella* serotype, as high as 20 to 30 per cent.

PREVENTION. Salmonella infection is best prevented by proper management of the water supply and sewage disposal, cooking and refrigeration of foods made from animal products, pasteurization of milk and milk products, and handwashing before preparing foods and after handling animals and uncooked animal products. Despite these precautions, because of the widespread presence of salmonellae in the animal kingdom, it is unlikely that the frequency of salmonella infections will be significantly diminished.

There is no vaccine for any salmonellae other than *S. typhi*.

Asperilla MO, Smego RA Jr, Scott LK: Quinolone antibiotics in the treatment of salmonella infections. Rev Infect Dis 12:873–889, 1990. *A review of the effectiveness of the newer quinolones in salmonella infections.*
Centers for Disease Control Salmonella Surveillance. Annual Survey 1987. U.S. Public Health Service, 1988, pp 1–90. *A compilation of the serotypes of* Salmonella *isolated from human and nonhuman sources in the United States.*
Fischl MA, Dickinson GM, Sinave C, et al: Salmonella bacteremia as manifestation of acquired immunodeficiency syndrome. Arch Intern Med 146:113–115, 1986. *A paper illustrating the refractoriness of salmonella bacteremia in patients with AIDS.*
Neill MA, Opal SM, Heelan J, et al.: Failure of ciprofloxacin to eradicate convalescent fecal excretion after acute salmonellosis: Experience during an outbreak in health care workers. Ann Intern Med 114:195–199, 1991. *A study demonstrating a high relapse rate of fecal excretion of salmonella with a prolonged carriage state after ciprofloxacin treatment of convalescent carriers.*
Soe GB, Overturf GD: Treatment of typhoid fever and other systemic salmonelloses with cefotaxime, ceftriaxone, cefoperazone and other new cephalosporins. Rev Infect Dis 9:719–736, 1987. *A review of use of third-generation cephalosporins in systemic salmonella infections.*

315 Shigellosis

Thomas Butler

DEFINITION. Shigellosis is an acute bacterial infection caused by the genus *Shigella* resulting in colitis affecting predominantly the rectosigmoid colon. Bacillary dysentery is synonymous with shigellosis. The disease is characterized by diarrhea, dysentery, fever, abdominal pain, and tenesmus. Shigellosis is usually limited to a few days. Early treatment with antimicrobial drugs results in more rapid recovery.

ETIOLOGY. Shigellae are nonmotile gram-negative bacilli belonging to the family Enterobacteriaceae. Four species of shigellae are recognized on the basis of antigenic and biochemical properties: *S. dysenteriae* (group A), *S. flexneri* (group B), *S. boydii* (group C), and *S. sonnei* (group D). Among these species there are over 40 serotypes, each of which is designated by the species name followed by a specific Arabic number. *S. dysenteriae* 1 is called the Shiga bacillus and causes epidemics with higher mortality than other serotypes. With the exception of *S. flexneri* 6, they do not ferment lactose.

Serotypes are determined by the O polysaccharide side chain of the lipopolysaccharide (endotoxin) in the cell wall. Endotoxin is detectable in the blood of severely ill patients and may be responsible for the complication of the hemolytic-uremic syndrome. To be virulent, shigellae must be able to invade epithelial cells, as tested in the laboratory by keratoconjunctivitis in the guinea pig (Sereney test) or HeLa cell invasion. Bacterial invasion of cells is genetically governed by three chromosomal regions and a 140 Mdal plasmid. Shiga toxin is produced by *S. dysenteriae* 1 and in lesser amounts by other serotypes. It inhibits protein synthesis and has enterotoxic activity in animal models, but its role in human disease is uncertain.

INCIDENCE AND PREVALENCE. In the United States in 1988, there were over 30,000 reported cases of shigellosis. The predominant species in the 1980's was *S. sonnei* (64 per cent), followed by *S. flexneri* (31 per cent), *S. boydii* (3 per cent), and *S. dysenteriae* (2 per cent). Most cases were in young children, and a large proportion occurred in population groups living in homes for the mentally ill or in nursing homes. A large outbreak occurred in 1987 in Tennessee affecting more than 1000 persons camping under unsanitary conditions at a mass gathering.

Worldwide most cases of shigellosis occur in children of developing countries, where *S. flexneri* is the predominant species. During the past 20 years, major epidemics due to *S. dysenteriae* 1 have occurred in Central America, Central Africa, India, and Bangladesh.

EPIDEMIOLOGY. Shigellosis is transmitted by the fecal-oral route. Crowded living conditions, low standards of personal hygiene, poor water supply, and inadequate sewage facilities all contribute to an increased risk of infection. Transmission most often occurs by close person-to-person contact through contaminated hands. During clinical illness and for up to 6 weeks after recovery, organisms are excreted in the feces. Although the organisms are sensitive to desiccation, they may survive several months in food or water, which are occasional vehicles of transmission.

Children between 1 and 4 years of age have the greatest risk of developing shigellosis. Inhabitants of custodial institutions, such as homes for retarded children, are at highest risk. Intrafamilial spread follows often when the initial case has occurred in a pre-school child. In young adults the incidence is higher in women than men, which probably reflects closer contact of women with children. The male homosexual population in the United States is at increased risk for shigellosis, which is one of the causes of the "gay bowel syndrome."

Humans and higher primates are the only known natural reservoirs of shigellosis. Transmission shows variable seasonal patterns in different regions. In the United States, the peak incidence is in late summer and early autumn.

PATHOGENESIS AND PATHOLOGY. Since the microorganisms are relatively resistant to acid, shigellae pass the gastric barrier more readily than other enteric pathogens. In volunteer studies, as few as 200 ingested bacilli regularly initiate disease in 25 per cent of healthy adults. This contrasts strikingly with the much larger numbers of typhoid or cholera bacilli required to produce disease in normal individuals. During the incubation period, usually 12 to 72 hours, the organisms traverse the small bowel, penetrate colonic epithelial cells, and multiply intracellularly. An acute inflammatory response ensues in the colonic mucosa attended by prodromal symptoms (Table 315–1). Epithelial cells containing bacteria are lysed, resulting in superficial ulcerations and shedding of shigella organisms into stools. The mucosa is friable and covered with a layer of polymorphonuclear leukocytes. Advancing inflammation causes the formation of crypt abscesses. Initially the inflammation is confined to the rectosigmoid colon but after about 4 days of illness may advance to involve the proximal colon also. In severe cases, there may be pancolitis with extension of inflammation into the terminal ileum; a pseudomembranous type of colitis may develop. Diarrhea results because of impaired absorption of water and electrolytes by the inflamed colon.

Although the colonic inflammation is superficial, bacteremia occurs occasionally, especially in S. *dysenteriae* 1 infections. Susceptibility of organisms to serum complement–mediated bacteriolysis may explain the infrequency of bacteremia and disseminated infection. Colonic perforation is a rare complication during toxic megacolon. Children with severe colitis due to S. *dysenteriae* 1 are prone to develop the hemolytic-uremic syndrome. In this complication fibrin thrombi are deposited in the renal glomeruli, causing cortical necrosis and fragmentation of red cells.

CLINICAL MANIFESTATIONS. Most patients with shigellosis begin their illness with a nonspecific prodrome (Table 315–1). The height of the temperature varies, and children may have febrile convulsions. The initial intestinal symptoms soon follow as cramps, loose stools, and watery diarrhea, which usually precede the onset of dysentery by 1 or more days. The average fecal output is about 600 grams a day for adults. The dysentery consists typically of flecks and small clots of bright red blood and mucus in stools that are small in volume. Frequency of passage is often as high as 20 to 40 times a day, with excruciating rectal pain and tenesmus during defecation. Some patients develop rectal prolapse during severe straining. The amount of blood in stools varies widely but usually is small because of the superficial colonic ulcerations. Abdominal tenderness is often most marked in the left lower quadrant over the sigmoid colon but may also be generalized. The fever is likely to abate after a few days of dysentery, making afebrile bloody diarrhea an occasional clinical presentation. After 1 to 2 weeks of untreated disease, spontaneous improvement occurs in most patients. Some patients with mild disease develop only the prodrome or experience only watery diarrhea without dysentery.

Complications include dehydration, which can be a cause of death, especially in children and the elderly. Shigella septicemia occurs mainly in malnourished children with S. *dysenteriae* 1 infections. The leukemoid reaction and hemolytic-uremic syndrome may develop in children late in the course after antimicrobial treatment when the dysentery has started to improve. Neurologic manifestations can be striking and include delirium, seizures, and nuchal rigidity.

The important postdysenteric syndromes are arthritis and Reiter's triad of arthritis, urethritis, and conjunctivitis (see Ch. 259). These are nonsuppurative phenomena that occur in the absence of viable *Shigella* organisms about 1 to 3 weeks after resolution of dysentery.

DIAGNOSIS. Shigellosis should be considered in any patient with acute onset of fever and diarrhea. Examination of the stool is essential. Blood and pus are grossly apparent in severe bacillary dysentery; even in milder forms of the disease, microscopic examination of the stool often reveals numerous leukocytes and erythrocytes. The fecal leukocyte examination should be performed with a portion of liquid stool, preferably containing mucus. A drop of stool is placed on a microscopic slide, mixed thoroughly with two drops of methylene blue, and overlaid with a coverslip. The presence of abundant polymorphonuclear leukocytes helps in distinguishing shigellosis from diarrheal syndromes caused by viruses and enterotoxigenic bacteria. The fecal leukocyte examination is not helpful in distinguishing shigellosis from diarrheal illnesses caused by other invasive enteric pathogens (nontyphoidal *Salmonella*, *Campylobacter*, and *Yersinia*). Amebic dysentery is excluded by the absence of trophozoites on a microscopic examination of fresh stool under a cover slip. The peripheral white cell count is of little diagnostic value, since it may range from less than 3,000 to more than 30,000. Sigmoidoscopic examination reveals diffuse erythema with a mucopurulent layer and friable areas of mucosa with shallow ulcers 3 to 7 mm in diameter.

Definitive diagnosis depends upon isolating shigellae by selective media. A rectal swab, a swab of a colonic ulcer obtained by sigmoidoscopic examination, or a freshly passed stool specimen should be inoculated immediately on culture plates or into carrying media. Since isolation rates of shigellae from freshly passed stools of patients with shigellosis may be as low as 67 per cent, culturing for 3 successive days is recommended. Stool cultures are generally positive within 24 hours after onset of symptoms and may remain positive for several weeks in the absence of antimicrobial therapy. Appropriate culture media include blood, desoxycholate, and Salmonella-Shigella (S-S) agars. Selected colonies should be diagnosed by agglutination with polyvalent *Shigella* antisera. S-S agar is inhibitory for S. *dysenteriae* 1.

Definitive bacteriologic diagnosis becomes of critical importance in distinguishing the more severe and prolonged cases of shigellosis from ulcerative colitis, with which it may be confused both clinically and on sigmoidoscopic examination. Patients with

TABLE 315–1. EVOLUTION OF CLINICAL SYNDROMES IN SHIGELLOSIS

Stage	Time of Appearance After Onset of Illness	Symptoms and Signs	Pathology
Prodrome	Earliest	Fever, chills, myalgias, anorexia, nausea, vomiting	None or early colitis
Nonspecific diarrhea	0–3 days	Abdominal cramps, loose stools, watery diarrhea	Rectosigmoid colitis with superficial ulceration, fecal leukocytes
Dysentery	1–8 days	Frequent passage of blood and mucus, tenesmus, rectal prolapse, abdominal tenderness	Colitis extending sometimes to proximal colon, crypt abscesses, inflammation in lamina propria
Complications	3–10 days	Dehydration, seizures, septicemia, leukemoid reaction, hemolytic-uremic syndrome, ileus, peritonitis	Severe colitis, terminal ileitis, endotoxemia, intravascular coagulation, toxic megacolon, colonic perforation
Postdysenteric syndromes	1–3 weeks	Arthritis, Reiter's syndrome	Reactive inflammation in HLA-B27 haplotype

shigellosis have been subjected to colectomy because of a mistaken diagnosis of ulcerative colitis; a positive culture should prevent such a misadventure.

TREATMENT. The effectiveness of antimicrobial agents in treating shigellosis has been well established. Appropriate antimicrobial therapy instituted early may decrease the duration of symptoms by 50 per cent and decrease the duration of excretion of shigellae (an important epidemiologic factor) by a far greater percentage. Because of the increasing frequency of plasmid-mediated antimicrobial resistance to *Shigella* infections, drug susceptibility testing is important. Trimethoprim-sulfamethoxazole administered in standard doses twice daily for 5 days is now the treatment of choice for *Shigella* strains of unknown antibiotic sensitivity in both adults and children. Alternative drugs include ampicillin, tetracycline, nalidixic acid, norfloxacin, and ciprofloxacin.

Fluid losses in shigellosis are qualitatively similar to those in other infectious diarrheal diseases, and the patient should be treated with appropriate intravenous or oral electrolyte repletion fluids in quantities adequate to correct clinical signs of saline depletion. The requirement for fluids is generally small, but fluid repletion is lifesaving in exceptional cases.

Agents that decrease intestinal motility should not be used. Such preparations as diphenoxylate and paregoric may exacerbate symptoms, presumably by retarding intestinal clearance of the microorganisms. There is no convincing evidence that pectin- or bismuth-containing preparations are helpful.

PROGNOSIS. The mortality rate in untreated shigellosis is dependent upon the infectious strain and ranges from 10 to 30 per cent in certain outbreaks caused by *S. dysenteriae* 1 to less than 1 per cent in most *S. sonnei* infections. Even with infection caused by *S. dysenteriae* 1, mortality rates should approach zero if appropriate fluid replacement and antimicrobial therapy are initiated early.

About 2 per cent of patients may develop arthritis or Reiter's syndrome weeks or months after recovery from shigellosis.

PREVENTION. Individuals excreting shigellae should be excluded from all phases of food handling until negative cultures have been obtained from three successive stool specimens collected after completion of antimicrobial therapy. In institutional outbreaks, strict and early isolation of infected individuals is mandatory. Targeted antimicrobial chemoprophylaxis has been disappointing. The most important control measure is scrupulous handwashing by all individuals involved in handling of food. Reporting of shigellosis cases to health authorities should be mandatory.

For the traveler to countries with major *Shigella* problems, no chemoprophylactic agent is an adequate substitute for good personal hygiene and the avoidance of contaminated food and water. A variety of vaccines has been developed and tested, but no vaccine is now commercially available.

Bennish ML, Harris JR, Wojtyniak BJ, et al.: Death in shigellosis: Incidence and risk factors in hospitalized patients. J Infect Dis 161:500, 1990. *Among more than 9000 infected inpatients, 9 per cent died, with death more likely in infants, the malnourished, and patients with low serum protein concentrations and thrombocytopenia.*

Butler T, Islam MR, Azad MAK, et al.: Risk factors for development of hemolytic uremic syndrome during shigellosis. J Pediatr 110:894, 1987. *In children with S. dysenteriae 1 infection, hemolytic-uremic syndrome developed after antibiotic therapy, which was usually inappropriate for the susceptibilities of the isolated bacterial strains.*

Butler T, Speelman P, Kabir I, et al.: Colonic dysfunction during shigellosis. J Infect Dis 154:817, 1986. *Studies perfusing the human colon showed diminished colonic water absorption, increased potassium secretion, and normal ileocecal flow rates.*

Haltalin KC, Kusmiesz HT, Hinton LV, et al.: Treatment of acute diarrhea in outpatients. Am J Dis Child 124:554, 1972. *An unequivocal demonstration of the value of appropriate antimicrobial therapy in the management of shigellosis.*

Levine MM: Bacillary dysentery. Mechanisms and treatment. Med Clin North Am 66:623, 1982. *A good review of microbiologic and clinical aspects of shigellosis.*

Wharton M, Spiegel RA, Horan JM, et al.: A large outbreak of antibiotic-resistant shigellosis at a mass gathering. J Infect Dis 162:1324, 1990. *Poor sanitation at a campsite in Tennessee led to an attack rate of more than 50 per cent in several thousand attendees; the Shigellosis was caused by multiresistant S. sonnei.*

316 *Campylobacter* Enteritis

Richard L. Guerrant

Enteric infection with a member of the genus *Campylobacter* usually results in an inflammatory, occasionally bloody diarrhea or dysentery syndrome. In industrialized, temperate areas, *Campylobacter jejuni* is often the most commonly recognized cause of inflammatory enteritis. The diarrhea may also be watery, especially in developing, tropical areas. An enterocolitis or proctocolitis syndrome similar to that seen with *C. jejuni* is also increasingly appreciated in homosexual males with several "*Campylobacter*-like organisms." The other major *Campylobacter* species that infects humans is *C. fetus*, a relatively uncommon cause of bacteremia and occasional intravascular infection in immunocompromised hosts. Finally, *Helicobacter pylori* (previously called *Campylobacter pylori*) has been increasingly associated with histologic gastritis and peptic ulcer disease.

ETIOLOGY. *Campylobacter* (meaning curved rod) is a curved or spiral, motile, non–spore-forming, gram-negative rod measuring 1.5 by 3.5 μ which is distinguished from Enterobacteriaceae by its inability to ferment or oxidize carbohydrates. It was formerly called a vibrio, but is now recognized as a separate genus, on the basis of its distinctive DNA content. It is both oxidase- and catalase-positive and is a microaerophilic organism that requires reduced oxygen (5 to 10 per cent) and increased carbon dioxide (3 to 10 per cent). The organism does not grow at either aerobic or strictly anaerobic conditions. Perhaps reflecting its avian reservoir, *C. jejuni* also requires an increased temperature to 42°C for optimal growth. *C. jejuni* is distinguished from *C. fetus* by its higher growth temperatures, cephalothin resistance, and nalidixic acid sensitivity. As shown in Table 316–1, the additional *Campylobacter* species that infect humans include *C. laridis*, a thermophilic organism commonly found in healthy sea gulls which has been reported in children with mild recurrent diarrhea and in an elderly patient with sepsis and terminal multiple myeloma. The weak or non–catalase-producing *C. upsaliensis* may cause diarrhea or bacteremia and *C. hyointestinalis*, like *C. fetus*, causes occasional bacteremia in compromised hosts. These organisms are also inhibited by cephalothin that is in some selective culture media. Up to three distinct species of "*Campylobacter*-like organisms" (including proposed species names *C. fennelliae* and *C. cinaedi*) are associated with proctocolitis in homosexual males and occasionally with bacteremia or diarrhea in women and children. Like *C. fetus*, these *Campylobacter*-like organisms do not grow at 42°C or in the presence of cephalosporin antibiotics and may require several days to a week or more to

TABLE 316–1. HUMAN *CAMPYLOBACTER* INFECTIONS

Species	Growth Temperature	Reservoir	Clinical Manifestations
C. jejuni/coli	37–42°C	Poultry, mammals	Common cause of dysentery/diarrhea
C. fetus (sub sp. fetus, old sub sp. intestinalis)	25–37°C	Cattle, sheep	Uncommon, bacteremia; intravascular infections in debilitated hosts
C. laridis	30–42°C	Sea gulls	Uncommon, childhood diarrhea, one case of sepsis
C. upsaliensis	37–42°C	Dogs	Occasional diarrhea
C. hyointestinalis	37°C	Swine	Occasional bacteremia in compromised hosts
"Campylobacter-like organisms": (including C. cinaedi, C. fennelliae)	37°C	?	Proctocolitis, rarely sepsis, in homosexual males
Helicobacter pylori (formerly C. pylori)	37°C	?	Histologic gastritis, peptic ulcer disease

grow in culture. *C. jejuni* is further subdivided into over 90 serotypes on the basis of heat-stable O antigens or over 50 serotypes on the basis of heat-labile capsular and flagellar antigens, markers that are helpful in tracing the epidemiology of this common enteric pathogen.

EPIDEMIOLOGY. Although the frequency of other *Campylobacter* infections is either low or unclear, *C. jejuni* infections are extremely common throughout the world. In many studies, the frequency of *Campylobacter* enteritis exceeds that of *Salmonella* or *Shigella* infections, and it has been estimated that as many as 2 million *Campylobacter* enteritis cases occur annually in the United States. The reservoirs of *C. jejuni/coli* include a wide range of mammalian species. Thirty to 100 per cent of chickens, turkeys, and water fowl may be infected asymptomatically in their intestinal tracts, and commercially prepared poultry in supermarkets can often be shown to be culture positive. In addition, swine, cattle, sheep, horses, and even household pets and rodents may carry *Campylobacter jejuni*, *C. coli*, or *C. fetus*. Enteric symptoms may be found, particularly in puppies, kittens, calves, or lambs, which may have diarrhea when infected. Furthermore, the organisms survive days to weeks in fresh or salt water and in milk and are killed most effectively by pasteurization, chlorination, drying, or freezing.

The transmission of *Campylobacter* infections is likely via the fecal-oral route. Fecal-oral spread may occur by contact among animals, homosexual males, and those in day care centers. However, secondary transmission is relatively infrequent and the infectious dose appears to vary from 500 to over 1 million organisms. The majority of infections, however, are probably acquired via ingestion of contaminated food, water, or milk vehicles. Many cases and outbreaks are associated with ingestion of inadequately cooked poultry, unpasteurized milk, inadequately treated water, and even cake icing, salads, beef, and clams.

The majority of those infected in well-described outbreaks are symptomatic. Asymptomatic infection appears to be relatively infrequent in temperate climates and in adults. An exception is among young children in certain tropical developing areas such as Bangladesh, where as many as 39 per cent of children under the age of 2 years may be infected asymptomatically (Table 316–2). These frequent asymptomatic infections in tropical areas raise important questions about possible strain differences in virulence, host susceptibility, and protective immunity against disease that might be acquired very early in developing areas.

Throughout the world, *Campylobacter* infections appear to predominate during the warmer or wet season. As with diarrheal illnesses in general, the highest age-specific attack rate is in young children. However, the greatest proportion of positive fecal cultures occurs in older children and young adults. There is little if any sexual predominance of recognized *C. jejuni* infections.

PATHOGENESIS AND PATHOLOGY. *C. jejuni* and *C. coli* are reasonably susceptible to gastric acidity. However, the reported variation in infectious dose suggests considerable host or strain variability. After an incubation period of 1 to 7 (median 4) days, symptoms of the enteric infection begin. *C. jejuni* organisms are attracted toward mucus and fucose in bile, and the flagellae may be important in both chemotaxis and adherence to epithelial cells or mucus. Adherence may also involve lipopolysaccharide or other outer membrane components. Several laboratories around the world have documented the production by *C. jejuni* of a cholera-like, heat-labile enterotoxin that binds to ganglioside and is neutralized by anticholera toxin antiserum. However, the genetic code and role of this toxin in disease remain elusive to date. Studies from Mexico have shown that antitoxic immunity

develops after infection, often with watery diarrhea, suggesting that this toxin is significant in those infections.

However, more characteristic in temperate areas is a diffuse, often bloody exudative enteritis involving the ileum and colon. These pathologic changes may include nonspecific crypt abscesses that on colonoscopy and histopathology may mimic the changes seen with inflammatory bowel disease. Such invasive pathology is also seen in rabbit, chick, mouse, dog, and monkey models of infection. Although *C. jejuni* is negative in the Sereny test for guinea pig conjunctivitis, some have reported the production of cytotoxins by certain strains of *C. jejuni* that may be involved in the pathogenesis of the invasive colitis. The relative infrequency of bloodstream invasion by *C. jejuni*, compared with *C. fetus*, likely relates to the relative serum sensitivity of most *C. jejuni* strains and to the rapid development of bactericidal antibody with infection in normal individuals. Volunteer studies suggest that effective immunity develops to rechallenge with the homologous strain, and animal studies suggest that protective immunity may be transferred in immune milk to suckling offspring. Additional evidence of effective immunity comes with the decreasing illness:infection ratio among children in endemic areas as well as among regular consumers of raw milk.

Once patients are infected, they shed 10^7 to 10^9 organisms per gram of stool for a median duration of 2 to 3 weeks, if not treated with effective antibiotics. Although some may continue to excrete the organism for 2 to 3 months, chronic asymptomatic intestinal carriage is rare.

CLINICAL MANIFESTATIONS. As noted in Table 316–1, the major recognized disease with human *Campylobacter* infections is the characteristic diarrheal illness seen with *C. jejuni* or *C. coli* infections. Although asymptomatic infections and watery, noninflammatory diarrhea are seen with *C. jejuni* infections in tropical, developing areas as shown in Table 316–2, *C. jejuni* is characteristically associated with an inflammatory, febrile enteritis in industrialized countries throughout the world. After an incubation period of 1 to 7 days, a brief prodrome of fever, headache, and myalgias lasting for 12 to 24 hours is promptly followed in a case of *C. jejuni* enteritis in a child or young adult with the symptoms of acute enteritis. These characteristically include crampy abdominal pain, fever to 39 or 40°C, and diarrhea with up to 10 or more loose, often bloody bowel movements per day. Occasionally the crampy abdominal pain may predominate as an appendicitis-like syndrome, with mesenteric adenitis or terminal ileitis being the predominant pathology. On physical examination the abdomen is diffusely tender and may mimic appendicitis. Although the acute febrile enteritis is usually self-limited to 5 to 7 days, 10 to 20 per cent of cases may last longer than 1 week and 5 to 20 per cent of untreated cases may relapse with a similar illness.

Complications, particularly if antimotility agents are used, include toxic megacolon, pseudomembranous colitis, and colonic hemorrhage. In addition hemolytic-uremic syndrome, postinfectious polyneuritis, or Guillain-Barré syndrome may follow *C. jejuni* enteritis. As with many inflammatory colitis syndromes, reactive arthritis and full-blown Reiter's syndrome may follow weeks after *Campylobacter* enteritis. Bacteremia may occur relatively rarely (< 1 per cent of cases), particularly in the very young or the elderly, in whom meningitis, endocarditis, cholecystitis, urinary tract infections, and pancreatitis have been described. In patients with hypogammaglobulinemia or HIV infection, *C. jejuni* infections may be prolonged or severe despite appropriate antimicrobial therapy.

In striking contrast to *C. jejuni*, the slow-growing *C. fetus* is primarily an uncommon cause of bacteremia, often in immunocompromised hosts. Although *C. fetus* would be missed on most routine stool cultures for *C. jejuni*, studies with filtration methods suggest that it is a relatively infrequent cause of diarrhea. Instead, *C. fetus* tends to cause intravascular, meningeal, or localized infections such as arthritis, cellulitis, abscesses, cholecystitis, and urinary, placental, or pleural infections, often in elderly or debilitated hosts. As it does in animals, *C. fetus* may cause stillbirth or septic abortions more often than generally recognized in humans. *C. fetus* infections are often recognized only by astute clinical microbiology technicians who methodically examine or subculture specimens of blood or other body fluids after 1 week

**TABLE 316–2. CLINICAL PRESENTATIONS OF
CAMPYLOBACTER JEJUNI INFECTION**

	Industrialized Countries	Developing Countries
Per cent of all diarrhea with *C. jejuni*	5–13	2–35
Per cent of *C. jejuni* diarrhea with:		
Fecal PMN	78–93	22–46
Blood in stool	60–65	5–17
Asymptomatic infection rates (%)	<2	0–39*

*Depending on age—39% if less than 2 years old.

in the laboratory. The clinical course of *C. fetus* bacteremia is often related to its recognition and appropriate treatment as well as to the underlying disease.

DIAGNOSIS. The diagnosis of *Campylobacter* infections is related to a careful history for exposure or characteristic clinical syndromes, direct stool examination, and selective culture methods. *C. jejuni* enteritis should be suspected in anyone presenting with a febrile enteritis, especially if there is a history of recent ingestion of inadequately cooked poultry, unpasteurized milk, or untreated water. As suggested in Figure 316–1, such a history should prompt the obtaining of a fecal specimen in a cup if at all possible and direct microscopic examination using methylene blue or Gram's stain for leukocytes as well as gross and/or occult blood. In many industrialized areas, the presence of blood or fecal leukocytes with fever strongly suggests the presence of a cultivable enteric pathogen such as *C. jejuni*, *Salmonella*, or *Shigella*, with *C. jejuni* being most common. Additional imme-

diate clues to *C. jejuni* infection may be seen on darkfield or phase microscopy for characteristic darting motility or on a carbol-fuchsin Gram's stain of stool for characteristic curved rods or sea gull morphology. However, darkfield and Gram's stains, while reasonably specific with trained observers, are each only 50 to 66 per cent sensitive. Patients with febrile enteritis, particularly with blood and leukocytes in the stool, should be cultured for *C. jejuni*.

Additional differential diagnostic possibilities for febrile inflammatory enteritis include *Salmonella* and *Shigella* infections, for which one should seek a history of an outbreak or contact exposure (such as in day care centers or among homosexual males, respectively). If the patient has recently taken antibiotics, *C. difficile* colitis or *Salmonella* enteritis should be considered. Recent ingestion of raw seafood should prompt investigation for *Vibrio* infection that may present with either inflammatory or noninflammatory diarrhea. A history of sick pet exposure, persisting abdominal pain, or unexplained inflammatory diarrhea should also prompt consideration of *Yersinia enterocolitica* infections, and

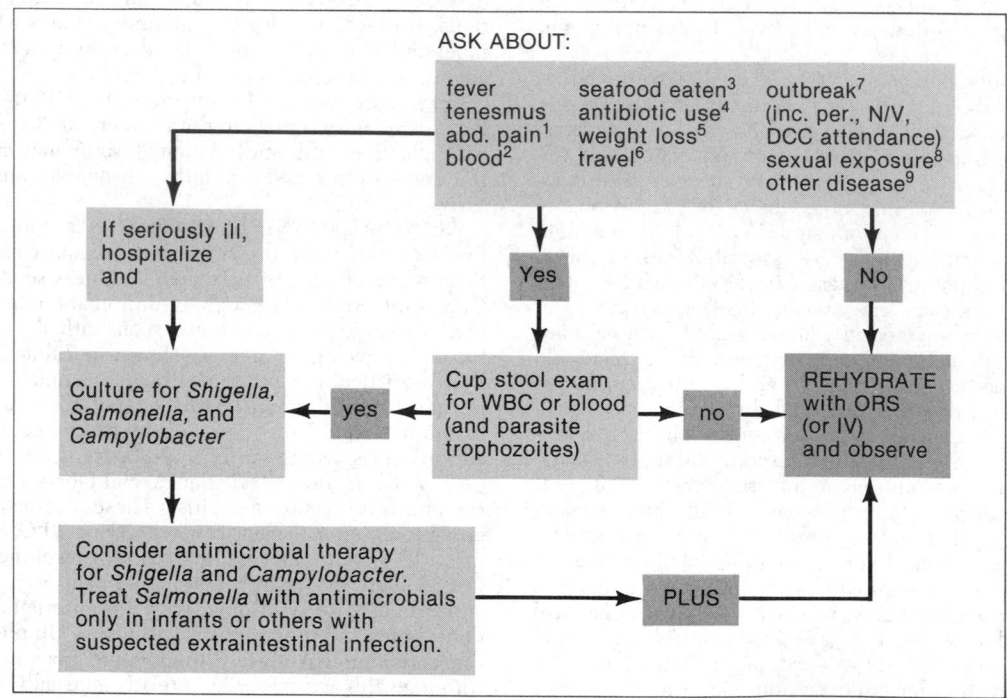

FIGURE 316–1. Approach to the diagnosis and management of acute infectious diarrhea.

1. If unexpected abdominal pain and fever persist or suggest an appendicitis-like syndrome, culture for *Yersinia enterocolitica*.

2. Bloody diarrhea, especially if without fecal leukocytes, suggests enterohemorrhagic (Shiga toxin–producing) *E. coli* 0157 or amebiasis (where leukocytes are destroyed by the parasite).

3. Ingestion of inadequately cooked seafood should prompt consideration of *Vibrio* infections or Norwalk-like viruses.

4. Associated antibiotics should be stopped if possible and cytotoxigenic *C. difficile* considered.

5. Persistence (> 10 days) with weight loss should prompt consideration of giardiasis or cryptosporidiosis.

6. Travel to tropical areas increases the chance of enterotoxigenic *E. coli* as well as viral (ex. Norwalk-like or rotaviral), parasitic (ex. *Giardia; Entamoeba, Strongyloides, Cryptosporidium*), and, if fecal leukocytes are present, invasive bacterial pathogens as noted in the algorithm.

7. Outbreaks should prompt consideration of *S. aureus, B. cereus, Anisakis* (incubation period < 6 hours), *C. perfringens*, ETEC, *Vibrio, Salmonella, Campylobacter, Shigella* or EIEC infection. If unexplained, consider saving *E. coli* for LT, ST, invasiveness, adherence testing, and serotyping, and save stool for rotavirus and stool + paired sera for Norwalk-like virus testing.

8. Sigmoidoscopy in symptomatic homosexual males should distinguish proctitis in the distal 15 cm only (caused by herpesvirus, gonococcal, chlamydial, or syphilitic infection) from colitis [*Campylobacter, Shigella, C. difficile*, or chlamydial (LGV serotypes) infections] or noninflammatory diarrhea (due to giardiasis).

9. Immunocompromised hosts should have a wide range of viral (ex. CMV, HSV, coxsackie, rotavirus), bacterial (ex. *Salmonella, Mycobacterium avium-intracellulare, Listeria*), fungal (ex. *Candida*), and parasitic (ex. *Cryptosporidium, Strongyloides, Entamoeba*, and *Giardia*) agents considered.

(Adapted from Guerrant RL, Shields DS, Thorson SM, et al.: Evaluation and diagnosis of acute infectious diarrhea. Am J Med 78:91–98, 1985.)

travel exposure to tropical areas or residence in an institution where careful hygiene is difficult should prompt an examination of stool and possibly rectal biopsy specimens for *E. histolytica* (which often destroys fecal leukocytes). Another frequent diagnosis that is considered, especially if *Campylobacter* enteritis has relapsed once or twice, is inflammatory bowel disease. However, it is imperative that anyone who is being considered for that diagnosis have treatable causes such as *Campylobacter* enteritis or amebiasis excluded by appropriate cultures or stains, as treatment with steroids may worsen *Campylobacter* or amebic enteritis with potentially devastating consequences. Additional noninfectious causes of bloody diarrhea with abdominal pain include intussusception and vascular insufficiency.

The diagnosis of *H. pylori* infections is best made by documenting the organism by culture and histology of gastric biopsies. Additional clues may be provided by urease tests of biopsies, breath tests for urease degradation of ingested urea, or serologic tests for anti–*H. pylori* antibody.

THERAPY. The most important treatment for *Campylobacter* enteritis, as with all diarrheal illnesses, is adequate rehydration and maintenance fluid therapy, which can often be accomplished with oral glucose-electrolyte solutions. The effectiveness of specific antimicrobial therapy remains debated. Although most *C. jejuni* strains are sensitive to erythromycin as well as to tetracyclines, chloramphenicol, clindamycin, quinolones, and aminoglycosides, they are characteristically resistant to penicillin, ampicillin, cephalosporins, and sulfamethoxazole-trimethroprim. Indications for antibiotic treatment remain controversial. Several studies have failed to show a significant reduction in the duration of illness with erythromycin treatment despite its prompt eradication of the organism from the stool. Some reserve antimicrobial treatment for those with particularly severe symptoms of high fever, bloody or severe diarrhea, young children in day care centers, or prolonged or relapsing illnesses. Antimotility agents should be avoided in *Campylobacter* enteritis, as with any inflammatory diarrhea.

It should be remembered that erythromycin orally may not be adequate for systemic *C. jejuni* or *C. fetus* endovascular infections, which probably warrant 2 to 4 weeks of parenteral bactericidal antimicrobial therapy.

H. pylori infections, although difficult to eradicate with a single agent, may be eradicated by combinations of agents such as bismuth compounds plus metronidazole, provided that the organism is susceptible.

PROGNOSIS. The prognosis of *C. jejuni* enteritis is generally quite good, and the disease is usually self-limited with or without specific therapy.

PREVENTION. As most *Campylobacter* infections arise from fecal contamination, often from animal reservoirs, many if not most *Campylobacter* infections are potentially preventable by education. The most common recognized vehicles of spread are inadequately cooked food, unpasteurized milk, and inadequately treated water. Consequently, thorough cooking of meats, careful handwashing after food preparation, pasteurization of milk, and adequate chlorination of drinking water should greatly reduce the frequency of *Campylobacter* infections. Parents should be warned that sick pet kittens or puppies may harbor potential human pathogens such as *C. jejuni* and keep them away from small children and practice careful hygienic measures in their care.

Blaser MJ: *Helicobacter pylori* and the pathogenesis of gastroduodenal inflammation. J Infect Dis 161:626–633, 1990. *Excellent overview of the rapidly emerging work on this important, newly recognized pathogen.*

Blaser MJ, Wells JG, Feldman RA, et al.: *Campylobacter* enteritis in the United States. Ann Intern Med 98:360–365, 1983. *Critical analysis of the presentation of* C. jejuni *and other enteritides in the United States.*

Butzler JP, Skirrow MB: *Campylobacter* enteritis. Clin Gastroenterol 8:737–765, 1979. *Good review of cultivation methods, epidemiology, clinical presentation, and models of* C. jejuni *infections.*

Guerrant RL, Lahita RG, Winn WC, et al.: Campylobacteriosis in man: Pathogenic mechanisms and review of 91 bloodstream infections. Am J Med 65:584–592, 1978. *Review of both* C. fetus *and* C. jejuni *infections and their presentations as bacteremic illnesses.*

Guerrant RL, Shields DS, Thorson SM, et al.: Evaluation and diagnosis of acute infectious diarrhea. Am J Med 78:91–98, 1985. *Review of a more cost-effective approach to selecting patients for stool culture who are likely to have an identifiable bacterial pathogen, such as* C. jejuni.

Perlman DM, Ampel NM, Schiffman RB, et al.: Persistent *Campylobacter-jejuni* infections in patients infected with the human immunodeficiency virus: Association with abnormal serological response to *C. jejuni* and emergence of erythromycin resistance during therapy. Ann Intern Med 108:540–546, 1988. *Report of persistent, severe* C. jejuni *enteritis and occasional bacteremia in patients with HIV infection who fail to mount a serum antibody response.*

Quinn TC, Corey L, Chaffee RG, et al.: The etiology of anorectal infections in homosexual men. Am J Med 71:395–406, 1981. *Review of the clinical manifestations and diagnostic approach to the wide range of enteric infections commonly seen in promiscuous homosexual males.*

Ruiz Palacios GM, Torres J, Torres NI, et al.: Cholera-like enterotoxin produced by *Campylobacter jejuni*. Lancet 2:250–252, 1982. *Original report of evidence for production of a cholera-like enterotoxin by* C. jejuni *in a developing area.*

Walker RI, Caldwell MB, Lee EC, et al.: Pathophysiology of *Campylobacter* enteritis. Microbiol Rev 50:81–94, 1986. *Excellent recent review of the virulence traits, pathogenic mechanisms, and animal models of* C. jejuni *infections.*

317 Cholera

William B. Greenough, III

DEFINITION. Cholera is an acute watery diarrheal disease caused by *Vibrio cholerae*, serogroup 1, which occurs both sporadically and as large outbreaks. Fluid loss may be extreme, exceeding 1 liter per hour. In such cases loss of solute-rich body fluids in stools rapidly depletes circulating plasma volume, producing vascular collapse and death in hours. Without treatment, mortality approaches 60 per cent of those affected; however, mild cases and carriers also occur and participate in the spread of disease.

ETIOLOGY. *V. cholerae* are short, slightly curved, rapidly motile, uniflagellate gram-negative bacteria that grow aerobically at 37°C on relatively simple media. They are currently classified as Enterobacteriaceae and are members of a very large group of surface water organisms distributed in all parts of the world, especially favoring brackish or salt-fresh water interfaces. There are many O serogroups of *V. cholerae*, but only serogroup 1 causes epidemic human disease. It occurs as two major serotypes, Ogawa and Inaba, with a less common Hikojima variant occasionally observed. There are also two main biotypes, "classic" and "eltor." The eltor biotype is recognized by its resistance to polymyxin B and by characteristic vibriophage susceptibility. These markers are of use epidemiologically. *V. cholerae* produces a potent exotoxin (choleragen) that binds to intestinal epithelium, producing a chloride ion–driven secretion and malabsorption of sodium ion and water. Other vibrios can produce exotoxins but do not have other biologic characteristics that lead to spreading epidemic disease.

EPIDEMIOLOGY. Cholera is thought to be a disease of antiquity, with clear written descriptions dating before 500 BC. The present global spread (seventh pandemic) has been due to an eltor biotype first recognized in 1911 at the El Tor quarantine station in the Persian Gulf. Epidemics due to this organism first appeared in the Celebes in the 1930's, spreading westward through Southeast Asia and reaching the Mediterranean and Africa in the 1970's. In 1991, for the first time in a century, a large epidemic struck the Western Hemisphere, involving more than 20,000 people in Peru and Ecuador in less than 6 weeks. However, in the Ganges delta, epidemics of classic *V. cholera* were replaced by eltor late in the 1960's. There have been small but regular outbreaks of cholera in the United States in the Mississippi delta regions since 1973. The eltor strains isolated have not been the same as the global epidemic strain. If special methods are applied, *V. cholerae* serogroup 1 can be isolated from many waters and may be associated in an altered state with phytoplankton. The main puzzle of where the interepidemic reservoir of *V. cholerae* is in nature has yet to be solved.

Mode of Spread. During epidemics cholera is mainly waterborne. Large numbers of vibrios enter many water sources from the voluminous liquid stools that soak clothing and linens and contaminate the environment. The setting for epidemics is often extreme poverty with lack of safe water supplies. However, an outbreak in Portugal affected the most careful travelers who used only bottled water, which unfortunately had been supplied from a spring contaminated with *V. cholerae*. Occasionally, contaminated foods spread disease. Most often raw or undercooked shellfish or fresh vegetables washed with contaminated water are responsible. There is a high risk of secondary spread in families or institutions in which water and food are shared. Contamination of household food and water sources is the rule. It is easy to understand how this occurs when an adult patient may produce 30 to 50 liters of stool in 2 to 3 days and is usually too weak to use a commode or toilet. Mild cases and rare convalescent carriers probably spread the disease between communities. True long-term carriers are rare enough to be reportable.

Susceptibility to Cholera. In areas where cholera occurs each year, children under 5 years are the main victims. Older children and adults in such endemic areas have acquired a lasting and strongly protective local intestinal immunity. Breast-fed infants in such circumstances do not get cholera and are solidly protected by antibodies from their mother's milk. When cholera attacks a population that has not experienced it for many years, as was true in recent spread to the Philippines and Africa, all ages are attacked equally, but morbidity and mortality are greatest among the very young and very old. Individuals with low gastric acid production, who are on acid-suppressing medications, or who have had gastrectomies are especially vulnerable, since *V. cholerae* is quite sensitive to acid. Cholera tends to attack persons of blood group O with greater severity, whereas individuals with AB blood group have less severe disease. People with a safe, piped water supply and effective disinfected waste disposal are at least risk regardless of host susceptibility.

PATHOGENESIS. After ingesting *V. cholerae*, vomiting and diarrhea may begin as early as 12 hours or not appear for more than a week. Illness occurs when viable organisms reach the duodenum and jejunum where favorable conditions, such as alkaline pH, nutrients, and bile salts, exist for growth. Multiplication occurs rapidly, with a doubling time of 20 to 30 minutes. Actively motile vibrios penetrate mucous layers and attach to the brush border of the intestinal epithelium where they secrete a potent exotoxin. This toxin is a protein of 84,000 daltons consisting of five B subunits that bind irreversibly to a specific chemical receptor on the cell surfaces (GM1-ganglioside). The toxic moiety or A subunit is linked to the B aggregate and gains entry once binding has occurred. It catalyzes an ADP ribosylation reaction that results in increased adenylate cyclase activity and consequent raised cyclic AMP levels in the enterocytes or any other affected cells. The most visible result in the small intestine is the profuse watery diarrhea resulting from abolition at the villous tips of the normal absorption of sodium ion and with it anions and water, and stimulation of crypt cells to secrete chloride, drawing with them cations and water from the bloodstream into the gut lumen. The resulting solute-rich stream originating in the duodenum and jejunum is profuse, eliciting vomiting as it progresses cephalad and diarrhea as it flushes through the colon. The fluid lost in cholera is a slightly fishy-smelling nonfecal whitish mucous-flecked liquid ("rice water stool"). There is no cellular damage and no inflammation or loss of plasma proteins or formed elements of the blood. There is also increased secretion of hepatic and pancreatic fluids, prostaglandin, and other intestinal hormones. All signs and symptoms of cholera derive from the fluid losses, which approach in composition an ultrafiltrate of plasma enriched in potassium and bicarbonate (Table 317–1). There is no evidence

for systemic effects by cholera toxin itself, since *V. cholerae* does not invade the body. It exerts all of its effects topically by adhering to the intestinal lining and producing toxin that is bound at cell surfaces.

CLINICAL MANIFESTATIONS. In its most dramatic presentation cholera can reduce a perfectly healthy robust adult to shock and death in 4 to 6 hours. More usually death ensues in 18 or more hours. In rare instances "cholera sicca" shock and death occur before diarrhea appears, the voluminous secretions pooling in distended loops of bowel and not escaping as either diarrhea or vomiting. Despite the capacity of cholera to cause severe illness, many of the infected patients have only a mild diarrhea indistinguishable from that of ordinary gastroenteritis. In epidemics about half of those infected have either no symptoms or very mild illness.

Without fluid replacement cholera patients demonstrate signs of severe volume depletion—sunken eyes, poor skin turgor, hoarse voice, extreme thirst, faint heart sounds, weak or absent peripheral pulses, and severe muscle cramps. Patients are oriented but appear apathetic except for thirst. If patients survive and have not received adequate hydration, fever secondary to sepsis and pneumonia is common and pulmonary edema can ensue with even modest fluid replacement.

In children, unconsciousness and/or convulsions may signal hypoglycemia. In both children and adults, adequate early volume replacement with a correctly formulated oral hydration solution can prevent all signs and symptoms except diarrhea. Initial laboratory values from depleted cholera patients (Table 317–1) reflect the loss of isotonic fluid without larger molecules such as albumen. This results in increased concentrations of plasma proteins and blood cells. Loss of bicarbonate leads to acidosis with a low arterial pH and bicarbonate. Potassium depletion is not reflected by low plasma values until acidosis has been corrected.

DIAGNOSIS. Cholera should be ruled out in any patient with acute watery diarrhea. Travel or residence in a cholera-endemic area should raise the index of suspicion. In clusters of acute watery diarrhea, particularly where sanitation is poor, it is especially important to recognize cholera early to permit advance actions to prevent deaths of large numbers of people.

Treatment does not depend on an etiologic diagnosis. Fluid replacement should be started without delay as soon as diarrhea begins. After initiating treatment, stool should be examined directly for red and white blood cells. Except in mixed infections with invasive organisms, which do occur in cholera outbreaks, fecal red and white cells are not a feature of cholera. If phase or darkfield microscopy is available, the characteristic darting motility of vibrios can be recognized in fresh wet preparations. To be certain that these motile bacteria are *V. cholerae*, serogroup 1 antisera can be applied to wet preparations, immobilizing the organisms in a rapid and specific diagnostic test. For greater sensitivity of this test, a stool sample or rectal swab can be incubated in an enrichment medium for vibrios, such as alkaline peptone water, for 12 to 18 hours. Stool culture is best done on a selective medium, since colonies of *V. cholerae* may be overgrown or are easily missed on standard enteric media. A simple method uses thiosulfate-citrate-bile salt-sucrose (TCBS) agar, which is very stable and selective for vibrios. Opaque flat yellow colonies form on TCBS agar in 18 hours at 37°C. Confirmation of serogroup and serotype can be done by direct slide agglutination with specific antisera. Biotyping requires more elaborate procedures, but resistance to polymyxin B is a quick way to recognize the eltor biotype.

Although the first line of immune defense is local at the intestinal epithelium, circulating antibodies occur to the specific O antigens. Testing for these is of use only as an epidemiologic tool to judge prevalence of disease in a specific population.

TREATMENT. Early and complete replacement of fluid losses averts death and all complications. It does not decrease diarrhea, however, unless an advanced oral hydration solution based on food polymers is used. In all except the most severe cases, oral rehydration therapy is sufficient to treat cholera, especially if started as soon as diarrhea begins. All varieties of watery diarrhea lose fluid of similar composition, depending principally on the rate of loss. Oral hydration therapy is the treatment of choice in all situations except when a patient has been permitted to become depleted and is in vascular collapse or is comatose. It is as

TABLE 317–1. TYPICAL CHEMICAL VALUES IN STOOL AND PLASMA FROM PATIENTS WITH SEVERE CHOLERA

| | | Plasma | |
	Stool	Untreated	Treated†
Sodium*	138 (105)	141	142
Chloride*	102 (90)	107	106
Potassium*	18 (25)	4.5	3.6
Bicarbonate*	45 (30)	9	21
Arterial pH	—	7.21	7.43
Plasma specific gravity	—	1.040	1.026

*Milliequivalents per liter. Stool values in parentheses are for children less than 10 years old.

†Four hours after water and electrolyte replacement.

TABLE 317–2. CHOLERA AND ACUTE DIARRHEA TREATMENT SOLUTIONS (ORAL AND INTRAVENOUS)

	Substrate (g/L)	Na+	K+ (millimoles/L)	*Base	Cl⁻	Osmolarity
Oral						
WHO/UNICEF	20 (glucose)	90	20	30	80	330
Pedialyte	25 (glucose)	45	20	30	35	300
Rice solution	80 (rice)	90	20	30	80	240
Ricelyte	30 (rice digest)	50	25	30	45	200
Intravenous						
Dhaka solution	0	134	13	48 (bicarbonate)	99	294
Ringer's†	0	130	4	28 (lactate)	109	271

*Citrate is generally used but bicarbonate is equally effective, and lactate or acetate are used in intravenous solutions.
†Also contains calcium, 3.0 mEq per liter.

appropriate to use oral rehydration therapy in hospitals as at home or in the field, as it entails fewer risks, is much less costly, does not require trained medical personnel for administration, and is equally effective. The discovery that absorption of sodium by cotransport pathways of intestinal mucosa is spared during cholera and other diarrheal diseases opened the way for a safe, inexpensive, and effective oral replacement solution. Glucose, amino acids, and small peptides, when absorbed by separate cotransport pathways of the intestine, carry with them sodium ions. Water and anions follow down the osmotic and electochemical gradients from the gut lumen to the bloodstream. Originally oral rehydration solutions were based only on glucose, and these were and remain very effective but do not diminish diarrheal fluid losses. Recent use of complex carbohydrates and proteins in foods, such as rice and other starchy foods, as the source for cotransporting substances has resulted in oral rehydration solutions that not only replace losses but also markedly reduce diarrhea. The composition of available oral rehydration solutions is listed in Table 317–2, together with some standard intravenous solutions.

Intravenous fluid replacement should be reserved for neglected patients who have not received oral replacement and are in shock or close to it. In a cholera epidemic it is essential that all individuals at risk be thoroughly familiar with oral rehydration therapy and use it early to minimize deaths and the need of intravenous fluids. Thirst and urination are adequate guides to oral replacement therapy even in small children. This eliminates the need for accurate intake and output measurements and weighings, which even in excellent hospitals are difficult and are out of the question under epidemic conditions. Intravenous replacement for patients who are depleted and in shock should be given rapidly through a large-bore needle to ensure infusion rates of 50 to 100 ml per minute until a strong radial pulse has been achieved. Remaining fluid deficits may then be replaced less rapidly over 2 hours. The fluid deficit in a severely depleted patient is about 10 per cent of body weight (for a 50-kg patient— 5 liters). As soon as patients are strong enough to drink, oral rehydration therapy should begin, preferably with a rice- or other cereal-based solution of the proper solute composition. If this is done adequately, no further intravenous fluids are needed. In semicomatose patients who are unable to cooperate, nasogastric intubation permits adequate enteral replacement. For both intravenous and oral solutions the composition is of critical concern and should be within a range to properly replace losses of solutes and water (Table 317–2). It should be noted that many drinks ordinarily given to diarrhea patients are not adequate, although they may be allowed as a complement to intravenous or oral rehydration therapy. Vomiting is not a contraindication for use of oral rehydration therapy.

If a commercial preparation of oral rehydration salts is not available, a home solution can be prepared. The safest and most effective of these is a thick but drinkable suspension prepared from rice or other suitable ground starchy foods. If precooked products are available, these are very convenient but not essential. To a quart of water with cereal thickly suspended, a half level teaspoon (two three-finger pinches of salt) are added and the mixture cooked only long enough to soften the ground cereal powder. The mixture should be used within 6 hours and may be taken warm or cold. In cholera it may be necessary to drink a great deal of fluid every hour for the first day. The patient must be offered a small cup every few minutes to minimize overloading the stomach and consequent vomiting. This is labor intensive but does not require medical skills. Especially in epidemics, family members are essential and effective participants in the treatment program.

In treating either children or adults, fluid therapy should be guided by thirst, observations on the circulation, urine output, and presence of edema or rales at the lung bases. Feeding is important and should be initiated immediately. Breast feeding is especially useful in affected infants, although few breast-fed babies contract cholera except in nonendemic areas where maternal milk lacks protective antibodies. Feeding should be with appetizing complex carbohydrates and proteins culturally adapted to the taste of the patient.

Adjunctive antibiotic therapy shortens diarrhea. This varies with the epidemic strain, but tetracycline and doxycycline have been effective when resistance is not present.

PREVENTION. Safe water supplies and appropriate disposal of human waste prevent spread of cholera but may not be achievable. *V. cholerae* is a fragile organism and cannot withstand drying, mild oxidation, or acid conditions. Thus a wide variety of disinfectants are effective for soiled articles. Bleaching powder is frequently used. Handwashing with soap before food handling is important.

There are no effective vaccines currently available, but several oral vaccines are in experimental use and have proven effective. Antibiotic prophylaxis has not been useful and encourages the emergence of resistant strains.

Barua D, Greenough WB III: Cholera. New York, Plenum Scientific Publishing Co., 1991. *A broad review of all aspects of cholera.*

Carpenter CCJ, Mitra PP, Sack RB: Clinical studies in Asiatic cholera. Parts I–VI. Bull Johns Hopkins Hosp 118:165, 1966. *This is an excellent series of reports concerning the pathophysiology of cholera, rational fluid replacement, and the value of antibiotic therapy.*

Hirschhorn N: The treatment of acute diarrhea in children. An historical and physiologic perspective. Am J Clin Nutr 33:637, 1980. *A thorough review of the special concerns that surround treatment of acute diarrhea, including cholera, in children. The review serves to "bridge" the traditional pediatric literature and the recent literature on cholera and related diarrheal diseases.*

Johnston JM, Martin DL, Perdue J, et al.: Cholera on a Gulf Coast oil rig. N Engl J Med 309:523, 1983. *Describes outbreaks of cholera along the coast of the Gulf of Mexico.*

Layseca CV: Cholera—Peru 1991. MMWR 40:108–110, 1991.

Rabbani GH, Greenough WB III: Cholera. *In* Lebenthal E, Duffey H (eds.): Textbook of Secretory Diarrhea. New York, Raven Press Ltd., 1990. *An up-to-date review of current knowledge about cholera.*

318 Enteric *Escherichia coli* Infections

Richard L. Guerrant

Escherichia coli is the predominant aerobic, coliform species in the normal colon. However, *E. coli* can also be an enteric pathogen and cause intestinal disease, usually diarrhea. Diarrhea caused by *E. coli* may be watery, inflammatory, or bloody, depending on which genetic codes for virulence traits the organism happens to possess. Consequently, diarrheogenic *E. coli* must be defined more specifically according to its virulence traits. Specific virulence traits determine the type of disease the organism causes, such as enterotoxigenic, enteroinvasive, enterohemorrhagic, enteropathogenic, or enteroadherent *E. coli* diarrhea. Each of these categories is being further resolved by the type of enterotoxin (such as the cholera-like, heat-labile toxin, LT, or the heat-stable toxin, ST) or adherence (such as close, focal, epithelial cell effacing, or diffuse) it causes. Taken separately, organisms such as enterotoxigenic *E. coli* constitute major bacterial causes of diarrhea morbidity and mortality on a global scale, particularly among children in tropical, developing areas and in travelers. Taken together, the varied types of *E. coli* diarrhea not only constitute the major category of bacterial enteric pathogens, but illustrate the wide array of ways that enteric pathogens can cause disease.

As noted in Table 318–1, at least three different types of *E. coli* enterotoxins may cause intestinal secretion (ETEC), others are enteroinvasive (EIEC), still others cause food-borne hemorrhagic colitis (EHEC) and produce large amounts of Shiga-like toxin (EHEC), while the classically recognized enteropathogenic *E. coli* (EPEC) serotypes are neither enterotoxigenic nor invasive but may focally attach and efface the epithelium. Further information is emerging on additional types of enteroadherent *E. coli* (EAEC) that exhibit autoaggregating (EAggEC) or diffuse adherence (DAEC) traits and may be associated with prolonged diarrhea among children in tropical developing areas.

ETIOLOGY. *Escherichia coli* is a small, catalase-positive, oxidase-negative, gram-negative bacillus in the family Enterobacteriaceae. It characteristically reduces nitrates, ferments glucose and usually lactose, and is either motile (with peritrichate flagella) or nonmotile. It gives a positive methyl red reaction and negative reactions with Voges-Proskauer, urease, phenylalanine deaminase, and citrate agents. *E. coli* constitutes the predominant facultative gram-negative bacillus in the intestinal tract of humans and other mammals. As with other gram-negative organisms, the lipopolysaccharide cell wall contains lipid A and 2-keto-3-deoxy-octanate (KDO), a core glycolipid that has been used in vaccine development to provide cross-protection against systemic infections with other gram-negative organisms. Smooth (S) forms of *E. coli* have O specific carbohydrate chains attached to this core glycolipid to provide 169 O serogroups as well as at least 60 heat-labile protein flagellar (H) antigens by which strains are currently serotyped. Historically some 80 variably heat-labile capsular (K) antigens have also been described (L, B, and A), not to mention the more recently appreciated numerous adherence, enterotoxin, cytotoxin, and invasiveness factors that may be gained or lost by a particular serotype, as they are characteristically encoded on transmissible genetic elements such as plasmids or bacteriophages. Consequently, this common inhabitant of the normal human intestinal tract becomes a pathogen when it houses one or more specific traits that contribute to its colonization and virulence in the intestinal tract. Other traits such as O and H serogroup appear also to be important for certain enteropathogenic and enteroinvasive organisms. For reasons that remain obscure, only a few O serogroups tend to predominate in the normal human colon (O groups 1, 2, 4, 6, 7, 8, 18, 25, 45, 75, and 81), while others noted in Table 318–1 tend (albeit not absolutely) to be associated with specific virulence traits and thus different types of pathogenesis in the intestine. The O antigens of invasive *E. coli* often cross-react with various *Shigella* species, suggesting further that, in addition to the 140 Mdal plasmid, serotype also has a role in pathogenesis.

EPIDEMIOLOGY. Enteric *E. coli* infections are essentially acquired by the fecal-oral route, reflecting primarily a human reservoir for most recognized types of *E. coli* enteropathogens. Enterotoxigenic *E. coli* is also an important veterinary pathogen, especially in calves and piglets. However, the attachment traits of animal strains are different from those that infect humans and likely substantially influence their epidemiology.

The infectious doses of enterotoxigenic *E. coli* and enteroinvasive *E. coli* have been determined in volunteers to be 10^6 to 10^8, numbers that usually require multiplication in contaminated food or water vehicles for their transmission. Heavy contamination with enterotoxigenic *E. coli* has been documented in foods prepared in homes, restaurants, and at street vendors as well as in drinking water in many tropical areas, and contaminated water and foods likely represent the major sources of their acquisition, primarily in the warm or wet season. In the United States, major outbreaks of water- or food-borne *E. coli* diarrhea of different

TABLE 318–1. DIFFERENT TYPES OF ENTERIC *E. COLI* INFECTIONS

Type	Mechanism	Predominant O Serogroups	Genetic Code	Detection	Clinical Syndromes
Enterotoxigenic E. coli (ETEC):					
1. Cholera-like, heat-labile toxin (LT)	Activates intestinal adenylate cyclase & adhesin fimbriae	6, 8, 11, 15, 20, 25, 27, 63, 80, 85, 139	Plasmid	ELISA, RIA, PIH, CHO, Y1 cells, 18 h loops, gene probe	Watery diarrhea, Travelers' diarrhea
2. Heat-stable toxin (STa: STh or STp)	Activates intestinal guanylate cyclase & adhesin fimbriae	12, 78, 115, 148, 149, 153, 159, 166, 167	Plasmid (transposon)	ELISA, RIA, suckling mice, 6 h loops, gene probes	Watery diarrhea, Travelers' diarrhea
3. Heat-stable toxin (STb)	?; Not cAMP or cGMP		Plasmid	Piglet loops, gene probe	?
Enteroinvasive E. coli (EIEC):					
4. Enteroinvasive E. coli (EIEC)	Invasive	11, 28ac, 29, 124, 136, 144, 147, 152, 164, 167	Plasmid (140 Mdal, pWR110)	Sereny test, gene probe, (lys⁻, NM, oft. lactose⁻)	Inflammatory dysentery
Enterohemorrhagic E. coli (EHEC):					
5. Enterohemorrhagic E. coli (EHEC)	Shiga-like toxin(s) & adhesin fimbriae	26, 39, 113, 121, 128, 139, 145, 157, occ 55, 111	Phage(s) & adhesin plasmid(s)	Serotype, HeLa, Vero cells, sorbitol	Bloody noninflammatory diarrhea; hemolytic-uremic syndrome
Enteropathogenic E. coli (EPEC):					
6. Focal attaching and effacing EPEC	Attach, then efface the mucosa	55, 111, 119, 125, 126, 127, 128, 142, 158	Plasmid (50 Mdal, pMAR2)	Serotype, focal HEp2 adhesion, gene probes for EAF or eae	Infantile diarrhea
7. Other EPEC	?	44, 86, 114	?	Serotype	?
Enteroadherent E. coli (EAEC):					
8. Enteroadherent-aggregating E. coli (EAggEC)	Colonize; ? toxin(s)		? Plasmid	HEp2 cell adherence; AA or DA probes	? Prolonged diarrhea
9. Diffusely adherent E. coli (DAEC)			? Plasmid		

types have been documented in the last 10 to 15 years. A large water-borne outbreak of diarrhea at a popular national park was found to be caused by enterotoxigenic *E. coli* (ETEC), and a widespread outbreak of enteroinvasive *E. coli* (EIEC) enteritis was traced to consumption of French Camembert cheese. More recently, bloody, noninflammatory diarrhea was noted in two states in association with enterohemorrhagic *E. coli* (EHEC) (O157) in specialty hamburgers in a fast-food chain. Occasional nosocomial outbreaks of enterotoxigenic *E. coli* and enteropathogenic *E. coli* serotypes (EPEC) have also occurred in hospitalized infants in the United States and other industrialized countries.

As with most diarrheal illnesses, the highest age-specific attack rates of enterotoxigenic *E. coli* infections are in young children, especially at the time of weaning, when enterotoxigenic *E. coli* account for 15 to 50 per cent of illnesses. Like immunologically inexperienced young children, the traveler visiting tropical areas has a 30 to 50 per cent chance of acquiring travelers' diarrhea over a 2- to 3-week stay unless untreated water or ice and uncooked foods such as salads are strictly avoided. The most commonly recognized pathogen associated with travelers' diarrhea around the world is enterotoxigenic *E. coli* that produces either the STa, LT, or both enterotoxins (see Ch. 319).

Of potential immunologic significance is the continued occurrence of symptomatic infections with *E. coli* which produce the less immunogenic STa in adult residents of tropical or other areas endemic for enterotoxigenic *E. coli* infections. In contrast, adult residents in endemic areas often carry LT-producing *E. coli* asymptomatically, suggesting that they may be protected from symptoms, if not from colonization.

Limited data on invasive *E. coli* suggest that the infectious doses are relatively high. As with enterotoxigenic *E. coli* infections, such large numbers have been readily spread in food with high attack rates. Enteropathogenic *E. coli* have been recognized primarily in urban areas, especially among hospitalized infants in their first year of life, with apparent cross-infection in hospital nurseries. While sporadic cases still occur, nosocomial outbreaks of EPEC diarrhea during summer months appear to have become less common and less severe in industrialized countries in the last decade or two.

PATHOGENESIS AND PATHOLOGY. The pathogenesis of enteric *E. coli* infections begins with the ingestion of the organism in contaminated food or water, which then faces the normal gastric acid barrier. Both enterotoxigenic *E. coli* and enteroinvasive *E. coli* appear to be sensitive to gastric acid; neutralization by gastric acid reduces the infectious dose by 100- to 1000-fold. This is followed by an incubation period of 2 to 7 days, during which colonization of the involved part of the intestinal tract and enterotoxin production or invasion takes place. Best characterized is the colonization by enterotoxigenic *E. coli* in the upper small bowel which involves one of at least three major colonization factor antigen groups (which are fimbriate or fibrillar protein structures on the surface of the organism). The colonization fimbriae bind the organism to cell surface receptors in the upper small bowel where the enterotoxin is delivered to reduce normal absorption and cause net electrolyte and water secretion. The heat-labile toxin (LT) with a molecular weight of about 86,000 has a binding and active subunit that, like choleratoxin, binds to a monosialoganglioside (Gml) receptor. Also like choleratoxin, the active subunit ADP-ribosylates the regulatory subunit of adenylate cyclase to activate adenylate cyclase. The consequently increased chloride secretion and reduced sodium absorption combine to cause net isotonic electrolyte loss that must be replaced to prevent severe dehydration and hypotension and its potential consequences. Other strains produce the heat-stable toxin (STa), a much smaller molecule of 18-19 amino acids (molecular weight less than 2000) which activates intestinal particulate guanylate cyclase. Like cyclic AMP, the cyclic GMP thus formed also causes net secretion. A third type of *E. coli* enterotoxin (STb) causes secretion in porcine intestine without activating adenylate or guanylate cyclase; STb has no known role in human disease. Both the colonization traits and enterotoxin production are encoded on transmissible plasmids. Besides the complications of dehydration, the only significant pathologic change is depletion of mucus from intestinal goblet cells.

Other *E. coli*, often of certain serogroups noted in Table 318-1, have the capacity, analogous to *Shigella*, to invade and multiply in epithelial cells, cause conjunctivitis in guinea pigs (Sereny

test), and cause inflammatory colitis and dysenteric or bloody diarrhea. As seen with shigellosis, there is a striking inflammatory response with sheets of polymorphonuclear leukocytes in the stool. The colon shows patchy, acute inflammation in the mucosa and submucosa with focal denuding of the surface epithelium but usually without deeper invasion or systemic spread. While epithelial cell invasiveness in both enteroinvasive *E. coli* and *Shigella* appears to be encoded on a large 120-140 Mdal plasmid, several chromosomal determinants, including the O antigen, are critical for full invasive virulence.

Classically recognized enteropathogenic *E. coli* serotypes often fail to produce known enterotoxins or to be invasive. Nevertheless, they are well established causes of infantile diarrhea. Recent studies document at least two separate mechanisms by which different EPEC serotypes may cause diarrhea. The first, demonstrable with the majority of classically recognized EPEC serotypes such as O55 and O111, is a plasmid-encoded adherence to epithelial cells. This close adherence is associated with dissolution of the glycocalyx, disruption and effacement of the microvilli, villus atrophy, mucosal thinning, inflammation in the lamina propria, and variable crypt cell hyperplasia. These morphologic changes are associated with a reduction in the mucosal brush border enzymes and may contribute to the impaired absorptive function and diarrhea.

Other *E. coli*, notably of serogroups O26, 39, and 157, have been associated with food-borne outbreaks of bloody, noninflammatory diarrhea and with the hemolytic-uremic syndrome. These organisms produce large amounts of Shiga-like toxin that may be responsible for the characteristic colonic mucosal inflammation, edema, and hemorrhage. Sigmoidoscopy usually reveals only moderately hyperemic mucosa, and barium enema may reveal a thumb-print pattern of submucosal edema in the ascending and transverse colon. Some patients have superficial ulceration with mild neutrophil infiltration in the edematous submucosa.

Still other EPEC serotypes have historically been associated with diarrhea and have caused diarrhea in volunteers without recognized attachment, enteroadherence, enterotoxin, or enteroinvasiveness traits to date, suggesting that still other mechanisms remain to be unraveled for *E. coli* strains that cause diarrhea. The roles of a recently recognized LT-like toxin (which activates adenylate cyclase but is immunologically distinct from LT), of STb (a unique large heat-stable toxin that causes secretion without altering cyclic AMP or cyclic GMP in porcine intestine), or of colonization alone offer three additional potential types of enteric *E. coli* infections for which roles in human disease remain unclear at present.

CLINICAL MANIFESTATIONS. The most common clinical manifestation of enteric *E. coli* infections is the watery diarrhea that characterizes enterotoxigenic *E. coli* infections, particularly in young children and travelers to tropical or developing areas. This may range from mild to severe, cholera-like diarrhea that may be life-threatening, especially in small children and elderly patients who are particularly prone to suffer the most severe consequences of dehydration, undernutrition, and electrolyte imbalance (especially hypokalemia and acidosis).

The incubation period (2 to 7 days) varies with the size of the inoculum. Characteristic symptoms include malaise, abdominal cramping, anorexia, and watery diarrhea, occasionally associated with nausea, vomiting, or low-grade fever. The illness is usually self-limited to 1 to 5 days and rarely extends beyond 10 days or 2 weeks. Infections with *E. coli* which produce both ST and LT or ST alone may be more severe than those with only LT-producing *E. coli*. The persistence of impaired mucosal absorptive capacity for 1 to 3 weeks may further compound the cycle of malnutrition that complicates diarrheal illnesses in children in developing, tropical areas.

Infection with enteroinvasive *E. coli* is characterized by inflammatory colitis, often with abdominal pain, high fever, tenesmus, and bloody or dysenteric diarrhea essentially like that seen with *Shigella*, to which this organism is closely related. The incubation period is usually 1 to 3 days with the duration usually self-limited to 7 to 10 days.

Outbreaks of enteropathogenic *E. coli* infections in newborn nurseries have ranged from mild transient diarrhea to severe and rapidly fatal diarrheal illnesses, especially in premature or otherwise compromised infants. The more severe illnesses appear to have been more common in industrialized countries prior to 1950. However, more recent outbreaks and sporadic cases are well documented.

Recently recognized outbreaks of hemorrhagic colitis associated with the Shiga-like toxin producing E. coli (EHEC) O157:H7 and O26:H11 have been characterized by grossly bloody diarrhea with remarkably little fever or inflammatory exudate in the stool. Although the diarrheal illnesses have been self-limited, a significant number of children have subsequently developed a hemolytic-uremic syndrome. In addition, outbreaks of hemorrhagic colitis due to EHEC in nursing homes may be quite severe and more common than previously appreciated. The incubation period in two outbreaks has been 3 to 4 days (range 1 to 7 days), and the illness is characteristically self-limited to 5 to 12 days (mean 7.8).

DIAGNOSIS. A definitive etiologic diagnosis of E. coli diarrhea requires the documentation of a specific virulence trait such as enterotoxin, invasiveness, enteroadherence, or serotype, which usually requires specialized immunologic, tissue culture, animal bioassay, or gene probes that are available only in research and reference laboratories. Such tests are rarely cost effective or clinically indicated, except in outbreak or research situations. Fortunately, a likely diagnosis can often be suspected by the clinical and epidemiologic setting. For example, self-limited, noninflammatory diarrhea in tropical, developing areas is most likely due to enterotoxigenic E. coli, rotaviruses (young children), or Norwalk-like viruses (older children and adults). Noninflammatory diarrhea in winter months in temperate areas in older children or younger adults is more likely to be due to Norwalk-like viruses. Specific tests for the respective virulence traits of different types of E. coli are noted in Table 318–1. One should also consider Vibrio infections in areas endemic for cholera or in any coastal area where inadequately cooked seafood may be eaten. If noninflammatory diarrhea persists, especially with weight loss, one should also consider Giardia lamblia or Cryptosporidium infection. In outbreaks of food poisoning, S. aureus, Clostridium perfringens, and Bacillus cereus should be considered.

Inflammatory colitis with high fever, tenesmus, and leukocytes, mucus, and blood in the stool may well be due to enteroinvasive E. coli but should prompt a stool culture for more common invasive pathogens such as Campylobacter jejuni, Shigella, and Salmonella or even Clostridium difficile, Yersinia enterocolitica, or non-cholera Vibrio (see Ch. 316). On the other hand, bloody diarrhea without high fever or fecal leukocytes should prompt consideration of the Shiga-like toxin producing enterohemorrhagic E. coli (EHEC) such as strain O157:H7. This organism is often suspected as a sorbitol-negative E. coli, which may require further study for serotype or Shiga-like toxin production.

THERAPY. As with all diarrheal illnesses, the primary treatment is replacement and maintenance of water and electrolytes. Losses of water and electrolytes may be particularly severe and even life-threatening with enterotoxigenic E. coli and can usually be replaced with a simple oral rehydration solution that employs the intact, sodium-coupled glucose, and/or amino acid absorption to replace fluid losses, as described in Ch. 317. This oral rehydration solution should be given ad libitum with free water and, in breast-fed infants, continued breast feeding and early refeeding to compensate for the nutritional losses.

Because most E. coli diarrhea is self-limited, the role of antimicrobial agents is debated and remains of secondary importance to rehydration. In areas where the enterotoxigenic E. coli remains sensitive, early initiation of sulfamethoxazole-trimethoprim, tetracycline, or new quinolone derivatives may reduce a 3- to 5-day illness to a 1- to 2-day illness if started with the first loose stool in travelers to endemic, tropical areas (see Ch. 319). The use of antimotility agents should be tempered by the potential added risk of worsening or prolonging inflammatory diarrheas and by their lack of effectiveness in reducing fluid loss even though abdominal cramping and overt diarrhea may be temporarily reduced. Because of the potential severity of the disease in infants, some pediatricians use neomycin, 100 mg per kilogram per day P.O., divided into three daily doses for 5 days, for documented enteropathogenic E. coli infections in neonates.

Bismuth subsalicylate may reduce symptoms in travelers' diarrhea but should be used with caution to avoid toxic doses of salicylate. A number of pharmacologic agents have been shown to enhance absorption or reduce secretion with experimental diarrhea but remain inadequately studied or too toxic for recommended use to date.

PROGNOSIS. The overall prognosis in E. coli diarrheas of the various types noted, if fully and adequately treated, is generally excellent. However, the impact of E. coli and other common diarrheas on mortality and morbidity (particularly with repeated infections compounding malnutrition in developing young children) remains one of the major health problems on a global scale; this problem may actually be worsening in some transitional areas.

PREVENTION. The prevention of E. coli enteric infections is ultimately related to basic economic development and adequate sanitary facilities and wide availability of sufficient quality and quantity of water. In the interim, especially in areas where adequate water supplies and sanitary facilities are not available, such measures as breast feeding for at least 6 to 12 months and hygienic measures like handwashing should reduce the likelihood of acquiring E. coli enteric infections. Travelers to developing or tropical areas should avoid drinking untreated or unboiled water or ice and eating uncooked fruits or vegetables that may have been "freshened" with highly contaminated water. Although a number of antimicrobial agents have been documented to be effective over short periods of time when taken prophylactically, their effectiveness is sharply limited by the rapidly emerging resistance to antimicrobial drugs as well as by the potential side effects of their indiscriminate, widespread use. For example, tetracycline resistance among enterotoxigenic E. coli is common, and combined sulfamethoxazole-trimethoprim resistance is rapidly emerging around the world. Finally, currently developing toxoid or colonization factor vaccines hold considerable promise for the prevention of enterotoxigenic E. coli diarrhea.

Bhan MK, Raj P, Levine MM, et al.: Enteroaggregative Escherichia coli associated with persistent diarrhea in a cohort of rural children in India. J Infect Dis 159:1060–1064, 1989. *A first report of a clinical role for new types of enteroadherent* E. coli.

Black RE, Merson MH, Hug I, et al.: Incidence and severity of rotavirus and Escherichia coli diarrhoea in rural Bangladesh. Implications for vaccine development. Lancet 1:141–143, 1981. *Concise report of community-based studies of enterotoxigenic* E. coli *and rotaviral diarrhea in a rural area of Bangladesh.*

Carter AO, Borczyk AA, Carlson AK, et al.: A severe outbreak of E. coli O157:H7 associated hemorrhagic colitis in a nursing home. N Engl J Med 317:1496–1500, 1987. *A common source outbreak with secondary, probable person-to-person spread, of this serious cause of bloody diarrhea and hemolytic-uremic syndrome in the institutionalized elderly.*

DuPont HL, Formal SB, Hornick RB, et al.: Pathogenesis of Escherichia coli diarrhea. N Engl J Med 285:1–9, 1971. *Classic early clinical, pathologic, and pathogenetic studies of enterotoxigenic and enteroinvasive* E. coli *diarrhea in human volunteers.*

Guerrant RL, Kirchhoff LV, Shields DS, et al.: Prospective study of diarrheal illnesses in northeastern Brazil: Patterns of disease, nutritional impact, etiologies and risk factors. J Infect Dis 148:986–997, 1983. *A detailed study of endemic diarrhea in a tropical area, including seasonality, risk after weaning, and nutritional impact, as well as relationship of enterotoxigenic* E. coli *to other pathogens.*

Guerrant, RL, Hughes JM, Lima NL, Crane JK: Diarrhea in developed and developing countries: Magnitude, special settings and etiologies. Rev Infect Dis 12:S41–S50, 1990. *Overview of community-based and hospital-based studies of diarrhea that reviews the relative importance of* E. coli *among other pathogens in developing and developed countries.*

Levine MM, Edelman R: Enteropathogenic Escherichia coli of classic serotypes associated with infant diarrhea: Epidemiology and pathogenesis. Epidemiol Rev 6:31–51, 1984. *A thorough historical review of classic enteropathogenic* E. coli *diarrhea as well as an update on recent volunteer studies and pathogenesis.*

Levine MM: Escherichia coli that cause diarrhea: Enterotoxigenic, Enteropathogenic, Enterohemorrhagic, and Enteroadherent. J Infect Dis 155:377–389, 1989. *A good overview of major pathogenic mechanisms of* E. coli *diarrhea.*

Microbial Toxins and Diarrheal Diseases. CIBA Foundation Symposium No. 112, 1985. *Thorough review of the mechanisms of enterotoxin action, relating the pharmacology of* E. coli *toxins (LT, STa, STb, Shiga) to those of other enteric pathogens like* V. cholerae, Shigella, and C. difficile.

NIH Consensus Development Conference on Traveler's Diarrhea. JAMA 253:2700–2704, 1985. *A balanced critical appraisal of the epidemiology, etiologies, presentation, and treatment of concise travelers' diarrhea.*

Sansonetti PJ, Hale TL, Oaks EV: Genetics of virulence in enteroinvasive Escherichia coli. Microbiology, 1985, pp 67–82. *One of a series of three brief reviews that offer a considerable amount of new information on the pathogenesis of the major types of* E. coli *enteric infection including ETEC, EIEC, EPEC, and EHEC.*

319 The Diarrhea of Travelers

R. Bradley Sack

Travelers from the developed world who visit the developing world are highly susceptible to an acute diarrheal illness known as "travelers' diarrhea" or by more colorful names that fit the locale in which the travelers find themselves incapacitated. Although at one time this condition was blamed on a change in diet, minerals in the water, and travel fatigue, it is now known to be an acute infection, caused by enteric pathogens that are endemic throughout the areas of the world where sanitation is less than optimal. In those areas the diarrhea produced by these pathogens is primarily a childhood disease that decreases markedly in incidence after the first few years of life, because of the development of protective immunity. Travelers are, in a sense, immunologically naive "children" who are suddenly placed in an endemic area of infection and therefore are highly susceptible to the disease. The predictable, high attack rates of diarrhea in travelers make this syndrome one that can be conveniently and intensively studied by investigators attempting to prevent and treat it. Perhaps other than a common source outbreak of diarrheal disease, the attack rates among travelers are the highest known in any identifiable population. Among travelers from the United States to the developing world, attack rates vary from about 25 to 75 per cent during the first 3 weeks of stay, with rates decreasing markedly as immunity develops.

By way of contrast, travelers from developing countries who visit other developing countries usually have a considerably lower attack rate, based on their prior exposure to these organisms. However, they are still susceptible to "new" agents that they may not have encountered previously. Visitors from the developing countries who visit the developed world, on the other hand, have a very low attack rate of diarrhea, as would be expected.

ETIOLOGY. Multiple studies have now been done on the etiology of this syndrome throughout the world, and it is clear that enterotoxigenic *Escherichia coli* (Ch. 318) is the predominant organism. Other bacteria, viruses, and protozoa are also involved, but with lesser frequency (Table 319–1). In different geographic areas, the rank order of these pathogens varies, but *E. coli* heads the list; because of this observation, studies of treatment and prophylaxis have been possible by focusing on this single group of organisms. However, a considerable percentage of episodes is undiagnosed etiologically, in spite of the best available laboratory techniques; evidence from studies employing antimicrobials suggests that a large number of these are also bacterial in origin. Contrary to "popular" notions about travelers' diarrhea, relatively few cases are caused by protozoa, particularly *Entamoeba histolytica*.

PATHOGENESIS AND CLINICAL PICTURE. The clinical syndrome of travelers' diarrhea is typically that of a secretory watery diarrhea caused by the enterotoxins of *E. coli* (see Ch. 318). The entire process is analogous to the pathogenesis of cholera (Ch. 317). The watery diarrhea usually lasts 3 to 4 days, and when most severe, may result in watery stools as frequent as 15 to 20 times per day, with significant water and electrolyte loss, leading to clinical signs of dehydration. Although deaths due to this illness are extremely rare, definitive replacement of fluid

TABLE 319–1. ETIOLOGIC AGENTS OF TRAVELERS' DIARRHEA

Agent	Percentage
Enterotoxigenic *E. coli*	30–70
Shigella	5–10
Salmonella	<5
Campylobacter	<5
Enteroadherent *E. coli*	5–10
Rotavirus	<5
Giardia lamblia	<5
Entamoeba histolytica	<3
Cryptosporidium	<5
Unknown agents	30–40

and electrolytes lost in the stool may be necessary, and hospitalization may be required. The vast majority of illnesses are much milder, however, consisting of only three to five diarrheal stools per day, and are of importance primarily because of limitation of activities.

Those episodes due to *Shigella* organisms are usually typical of a dysentery-like illness, with abdominal pain, fever, and blood and inflammatory cells in the stool.

Nearly all episodes are self-limited, but a few (less than 1 per cent) may become persistent and require evaluation following return home.

Although the clinical syndrome in children traveling to the developing world has been less well studied, there are a number of reports of severe, persistent diarrhea and marked nutritional wasting following visits to high-risk areas.

TRANSMISSION. The transmission of the enteric pathogens occurs almost exclusively through fecally contaminated food and water. Of highest risk to the traveler are foods that are not cooked or peeled and are consumed raw. Foods obtained from road-side vendors or foods kept unrefrigerated for long periods of time are also in the highest risk category.

PREVENTION. Since the mode of transmission is known, prudent attention to the ingestion of uncontaminated food and water should entirely prevent the disease. This has been shown in the military and on board cruise ships, where all food is hygienically prepared and packaged. For the usual traveler, however, food must be obtained from local sources, and contamination cannot be entirely prevented. Even the "best" hotels in the developing world may have unsanitary kitchens, and "first class" travelers are therefore not exempt.

A number of studies have been carried out in an attempt to prevent the disease with drugs, and many agents have been shown to be highly protective. The most protective are antimicrobials directed against the most common etiologic agents, the enterotoxigenic *E. coli*. Either doxycycline (100 mg), trimethoprim-sulfamethoxazole (160 + 800 mg), norfloxacin (400 mg), or ciprofloxacin (500 mg), taken once daily for a period of up to 3 weeks, has provided a high degree of protection against travelers' diarrhea, in the neighborhood of 75 to 90 per cent. Because the antibacterial spectrum of norfloxacin and ciprofloxacin includes *Campylobacter jejuni*, these drugs may theoretically provide a broader spectrum of coverage against the known etiologic agents of travelers' diarrhea. A nonantimicrobial drug, bismuth subsalicylate taken four times a day, has also given a significant degree of protection (approximately 60 per cent). Other antimicrobial drugs have also been used successfully (erythromycin, mecillinam, trimethoprim alone) but have not been tested as extensively. Drugs that have been tested and found to be of little or no benefit include neomycin, streptotriad, hydroxyquinolines, and *Lactobacillus* preparations.

The main questions relating to the use of prophylactic medications are not the efficacy, but rather the side effects; this issue will be further discussed later.

THERAPY. Therapy is based on recognition of clinical disease and a general knowledge of the causative organisms, since identity of specific etiologic agents will usually not be known (Table 319–1). The therapy of travelers' diarrhea falls under three general categories: (1) replacement of fluid and electrolytes lost to prevent and treat the resulting dehydration, (2) symptomatic therapy directed at relieving the frequency of stooling or the attendant abdominal cramps, and (3) specific antimicrobial therapy directed at the causative agent, in order to decrease the severity and shorten the duration of the illness.

Replacement therapy is done best with the oral glucose-electrolyte solutions developed for therapy of all dehydrating diarrheas, regardless of etiologic agent or age of the patient. These are now available commercially in packets, which can be carried by the traveler and used as required by mixing the contents with the appropriate volumes of potable water.

Symptomatic therapy may be useful for travelers with a typical secretory diarrhea who need to participate in certain vital events, such as long bus rides or important business or social occasions. The drugs used (loperamide, diphenoxylate) primarily interfere with intestinal motility and therefore can decrease the rate of stooling in persons with mild disease. However, because of this action, there is the possibility of actually intensifying the clinical illness due to invasive bacteria, since they are more slowly cleared from the bowel.

Preparations of bismuth subsalicylate have also been shown to give mild symptomatic relief, although the mechanism of action is unknown. Kaolin/pectin preparations are of no significant effect in treatment.

Specific antimicrobial therapy has been shown to be highly effective for this illness. The same drugs used for prophylaxis—trimethoprim-sulfamethoxazole (160–180 mg), norfloxacin (400 mg), ciprofloxacin (500 mg), and doxycycline (100 mg) in twice-daily doses—are also effective in shortening the duration of the disease to 24 to 36 hours. A 3-day course of therapy is sufficient.

THE STRATEGY OF MANAGING THE PROBLEM OF TRAVELERS' DIARRHEA. The questions relating to the prevention and treatment of travelers' diarrhea were reviewed at an NIH Consensus Conference, which should be consulted for further details. The most difficult issue is who, if anyone, should receive prophylactic antimicrobials. Since antimicrobials are widely available as over-the-counter medications throughout the developing world, the small addition to the antimicrobial pool by tourists is thought to be inconsequential to the larger issue of antibiotic pressure on a worldwide basis. Of more importance is the issue of adverse reactions to the drugs being taken for prophylaxis. Although none of the published controlled studies demonstrated any significant side effects, all were done using primarily young healthy adults. Since these drugs have significant side effects, although at low frequency, they are not recom-

mended for routine prophylaxis. For the short-term individual traveler, however, who is advised of the possible side effects and who wishes to avail him/herself of the protection, these drugs can be considered for use.

Since the same drugs can be taken as treatment, the preferred strategy in most cases would be to have the traveler carry along sufficient medication, so that he or she can administer appropriate treatment when indicated. Oral rehydration therapy should be given simultaneously for the prevention of dehydration. For milder episodes of diarrhea, drugs like bismuth subsalicylate or antimotility drugs can be taken for symptomatic relief.

The problem of travelers' diarrhea will continue until the general sanitation of the developing world approaches that of the industrialized countries or until effective vaccines against the major diarrheal pathogens are available. Neither of these occurrences is expected soon, and therefore this common syndrome will need to be addressed for some time; this can now be done rationally and effectively based on our knowledge of etiologies and modes of transmission.

Consensus Conference: Travelers' Diarrhea. JAMA 253:2700, 1985. *A summary of the NIH conference in which all aspects of the problem were reviewed; a complete publication of the conference is given in Rev Infect Dis 8:(Suppl 2), 1986.*

DuPont HL, Reves RR, Galindo E, et al.: Treatment of travelers' diarrhea with trimethoprim/sulfamethoxazole and with trimethoprim alone. N Engl J Med 307:841, 1982. *A controlled therapeutic study showing marked efficacy of these drugs.*

Sack RB: Treatment and prevention of travelers' diarrhea. *In* Holmgren J, Lindberg A, Mollby R (eds.): Development of Vaccines against Diarrhea, 11th Nobel Conf., Stockholm 1985, pp 289–301. Lund, Sweden, Studentlitteratur, 1986. *A comprehensive review of all controlled studies of prophylaxis and treatment.*

Other Bacterial Infections

320 Extraintestinal Infections Caused by Enteric Bacteria

Elizabeth J. Ziegler

Bacteria constitute over half the dry weight of stool. *Bacteroides* species far outnumber other genera, at 10^{12} organisms per gram. Other anaerobes such as *Fusobacterium, Clostridium,* and peptostreptococci also are abundant. Among the facultative bacteria, members of the family Enterobacteriaceae predominate, at about 10^9 organisms per gram. Pseudomonads, enterococci, other nonhemolytic streptococci, and yeasts are present as well.

These bacteria that normally inhabit the human gastrointestinal tract perform important functions beneficial to the host. *Bacteroides fragilis, Clostridium,* and enterococci deconjugate bile acids for participation in fat metabolism. Some intestinal bacteria synthesize menaquinone, or vitamin K, a cofactor for blood coagulation. Normal gut flora discourage colonization of the bowel with primary pathogens and overgrowth of bacteria usually present in small numbers. Colonization resistance is not understood completely, but it must involve bacteriocins, regulation of local oxidation-reduction potential, and balance of nutrients as well as unknown factors. Breakdown of colonization resistance is illustrated by the increase in susceptibility of antibiotic-treated animals to *Salmonella* and by the emergence of fecal *Pseudomonas aeruginosa* and *Candida* in patients receiving antimicrobial agents.

PATHOGENESIS OF INFECTIONS

Enteric bacteria are not primary pathogens but cause disease when they escape from their usual gastrointestinal habitat. Direct penetration of the bowel wall by surgical, traumatic, or spontaneous rupture spills fecal contents into the peritoneal cavity and

into open wounds. Gut bacteria on the perineal skin gain access to the urinary tract and proliferate there, especially when the flushing action of urine flow is disrupted by mechanical obstruction or neurologic dysfunction. When the biliary tract is obstructed by gallstones or tumor, the upper small bowel, which normally is sterile, becomes colonized with facultative bacteria (*Escherichia coli, Klebsiella,* enterococci) or, less often, with *Bacteroides* and *Clostridium,* which then infect the gallbladder and bile ducts. Intestinal flora can be introduced into the respiratory tract from contaminated skin or the environment; they proliferate there under the influence of antibiotics and in the presence of underlying pulmonary disease and tracheal instrumentation. Penetrating foreign bodies, such as intravenous catheters and intraventricular cerebral pressure monitors, become colonized by gut flora on the skin and in respiratory secretions and then induce infection in adjacent tissues. In burns, destruction of the skin barrier, the rich culture medium of oozing tissue fluid, and a shift of surface flora by application of local and systemic antibacterial agents result in local necrotizing infection of the burn wound with gut flora and frequent secondary gram-negative bacteremia.

In the absence of mechanical and surface abnormalities such as those outlined above, systemic resistance to enteric bacteria is very strong. The mainstay of this resistance is the polymorphonuclear neutrophil, destruction or malfunction of which leads almost inevitably to bloodstream invasion by bowel bacteria. Serum complement must be protective against invasion of some organisms, since very few of the gram-negative bacilli isolated from blood are sensitive to complement-mediated bacteriolysis, whereas many enteric rods in feces are susceptible. Newborn infants, whose neutrophils and complement activity have not fully matured, are at high risk of disseminated infections with facultative enteric rods. Microbial factors are important, too. Although anaerobes predominate over facultative bacteria and aerobes in the gut, these anaerobes rarely cause bacteremia or metastatic infection even in neutropenia. The presence of certain bacterial polysaccharide capsules (e.g., *E. coli* K1) or production of large amounts of capsule (e.g., by *Klebsiella pneumoniae* in hyperglycemic or glycosuric diabetics) predisposes to systemic invasion by these organisms.

Infections with enteric bacteria have increased dramatically during the past four decades. The reasons should be apparent from the discussion above. Advances in surgical and intensive care, trauma and burn management, blood transfusion, antimicrobial and cancer chemotherapy, transplantation, and immunosuppression all create opportunities for these infections. The average lifespan has lengthened, so that those receiving medical attention carry the added risks of advanced age. The majority of extraintestinal infections with enteric bacteria now arise in the hospital, and they exact a high toll in mortality and increased hospital costs. Furthermore, they jeopardize the success of the advanced treatments we have worked so hard to develop. For these reasons, physicians should understand the pathogenesis of each infection so that they can effect a cure and prevent recurrence if possible.

SPECIFIC LOCAL INFECTIONS WITH ENTERIC BACTERIA

The diagnosis and management of each of the following gram-negative infections are discussed in depth in the appropriate section elsewhere in the textbook. A few points are emphasized here.

PERITONITIS (see Ch. 110). It can be difficult to recover bacteria from patients with spontaneous bacterial peritonitis; large volumes of fluid should be submitted for culture. Patients undergoing chronic peritoneal dialysis frequently develop peritonitis. If the same organism is isolated from repeated episodes and especially if it is an enteric rod or *Pseudomonas*, infection of the subcutaneous catheter tunnel should be suspected. A radio-labeled white blood cell scan can be helpful in detecting such infections so that the infected catheter can be removed.

PYELONEPHRITIS (see Ch. 84). Urinary tract infections localized to the bladder or kidneys can have important implications for therapy. Symptoms may be misleading, selective ureteral catheterization carries considerable risk, and examination of urine for antibody-coated bacteria is not practical in routine laboratories. A simple culture technique can differentiate between upper and lower urinary tract infections in difficult cases in which parenteral antibiotics would be required for kidney infection. In brief, the test (Fairley, 1967) employs a newly placed three-way bladder catheter through which a combination antibiotic and enzyme mixture (fibrinolysin and DNase) is instilled to sterilize the bladder. Neomycin is employed for most organisms; polymyxin can be used for *Pseudomonas* and amphotericin for yeast. Bladder instillation is followed by a large-volume sterile water wash. Then the catheter is clamped, and three 10-minute specimens are collected. Increasing bacterial counts after the wash point to pyelonephritis. If infection is limited to the bladder, the Fairley procedure can cure it. The test is unreliable in patients with low urinary output, and it should not be performed in patients with neutropenia.

PROSTATITIS (see Ch. 223). Most antibiotics available for treatment of infections with enteric bacilli do not penetrate the prostate well. For this reason, chronic prostatitis rarely is cured. However, the role of chronic prostatitis as a nidus of recurrent acute urinary tract infection in males can be curbed by low levels of suppressive antibiotics in bladder urine, achieved by a single tablet of an oral antibiotic given daily.

MENINGITIS (see Ch. 301). Enteric rods, especially *E. coli* and *Klebsiella*, are a frequent cause of neonatal meningitis. In adults, meningitis with enteric bacilli is exceedingly rare except in cases of head trauma or neurosurgery. Bacteria may be infrequent and difficult to see on stained smears of spinal or ventricular fluid. Treatment with a third-generation cephalosporin that penetrates the blood-brain barrier at high dose may be sufficient, but infections with organisms resistant to such drugs may require chloramphenicol or a combination of intravenous and intrathecal aminoglycosides. Infected foreign bodies must be removed.

PNEUMONIA (see Ch. 61, 294, 295). Seeing gram-negative rods in respiratory secretions or growing them from the secretions does not necessarily imply infection. Susceptible patients often have severe chronic lung disease with abnormal chest radio-graphs. Many are on respirators with inflammation around endotracheal tubes and have abnormal gram-negative nasopharyngeal flora. Evidence of increasing infiltrates, fever, increasing leukocytosis, and/or worsening respiratory function should be sought before the diagnosis of gram-negative pneumonia is made in such cases.

INFECTIONS OF INTRAVENOUS CATHETERS. Patients who are critically ill may have limited numbers of sites for placement of intravenous catheters. If catheter infection is suspected, it may be impractical or impossible to remove all the lines. Comparison of quantitative blood cultures drawn through each catheter and from one peripheral vein can identify the infected site and preserve the uninfected catheters in place.

INFECTIONS IN NEUTROPENIA (see Ch. 287). The most common bowel infection in neutropenia is perirectal abscess. Inflammation may be modest, but patients complain of severe pain. Examination can cause bacteremia. Surgical drainage may not be required unless neutropenia resolves and fluctuance develops. A less common but much more serious condition is typhlitis, an infection of the cecum associated with gas in the bowel wall, peritonitis, perforation, and bacteremia. This condition can be fatal within hours. Surgical resection has been helpful in a few cases, but surgical mortality is very high. Aggressive antibiotic therapy should be directed against *E. coli* and *P. aeruginosa*, the most common etiologic agents.

Necrotic skin lesions can accompany gram-negative bacteremia in neutropenic patients. These lesions are called ecthyma gangrenosum, and they are seen most frequently in *Pseudomonas* bacteremia. Cases have been reported with other gram-negative rods and with *Candida* and *Aspergillus* septicemia as well. The lesions can be scraped to search for the organism on smear. If nothing is seen, a punch biopsy for culture and histologic section can be done safely even in severe thrombocytopenia. In fungemia, the histologic section may be the only premortem diagnostic specimen obtained.

GRAM-NEGATIVE BACTEREMIA AND ENDOTOXIC SHOCK

Gram-negative bacteria gain access to the bloodstream from foci of tissue infection or, when host resistance is depressed, from sites of heavy colonization and minor trauma. Although bacteremia creates the opportunity for metastatic infections, a more immediate and serious consequence of gram-negative bacteremia is septic shock. The incidence of gram-negative bacteremia has risen steadily during the past three decades. It is estimated that at least 200,000 episodes occur in the United States each year, of which 20 to 60 per cent are fatal. Mortality varies with the severity and nature of underlying disease, the source of bacteremia, and the incidence of serious sequelae of sepsis, such as the adult respiratory distress syndrome (ARDS) and disseminated intravascular coagulation (DIC). Death is caused by either irreversible hypotension or damage to vital organs such as lung or kidney, which cannot be salvaged despite recovery from circulatory collapse.

Rates of shock vary in different series from less than 20 per cent to more than 50 per cent. In comparable groups, shock is somewhat more frequent in gram-negative bacteremia than in gram-positive bacteremia or fungemia. However, gram-negative bacteremia is distinguished from the other septicemias by the fact that very small numbers of circulating bacteria are associated with hypotension. It is generally agreed that the principal trigger of gram-negative shock is endotoxin, a major structural component of the gram-negative bacterial cell wall, for the abnormalities seen in endotoxic shock can be duplicated with intravenous infusions of pure endotoxin in experimental animals. Endotoxin is a lipopolysaccharide (LPS) consisting of a long chain of strain-specific repeating sugar subunits at one end, some connecting core sugars in the middle, and lipid A, a fatty acid– and phosphate-substituted diglucosamine, at the other end, embedded in the cell wall. Lipid A, the biologically active portion of the molecule, is highly conserved with little variation among gram-negative bacteria. An exception is *Bacteroides fragilis*, which makes an unusual lipid A; its LPS is virtually nontoxic and pure *B. fragilis* bacteremia is infrequently associated with shock.

Endotoxin has been detected in the plasma of patients with gram-negative bacteremia who are sick enough to exhibit signs of peripheral hypoperfusion. There is evidence that antibiotics, especially those directed at the cell wall, release substantial amounts of LPS from bacteria while killing them; this may explain the transient worsening of hypotension occasionally seen after the first dose of antibiotics.

The human is one of the species most sensitive to endotoxin. Subnanogram quantities of LPS stimulate beneficial host responses, such as lymphocyte activation and fever (interleukin 1). However, nanogram quantities given intravenously can elicit a panoply of toxic reactions, including complement activation, production of procoagulant factors with DIC, neutrophil aggregation, lung capillary damage, and perturbation of circulatory control with splanchnic pooling of blood, hypotension, and metabolic acidosis. Many mediators are involved in these toxic reactions; recent work suggests that tumor necrosis factor, a small protein produced by endotoxin-stimulated macrophages, may be responsible for many of the phenomena leading to death from endotoxin (see Ch. 285, 286). High levels of interleukin 6, another cytokine, have been correlated with a fatal outcome in septic shock. It has not yet been determined whether interleukin 6 mediates some of the toxic reactions or whether it is an "alarm hormone" that merely reflects the severity of cell injury in sepsis.

CLINICAL MANIFESTATIONS (see also Ch. 288). Since focal infections usually precede bloodstream invasion, patients are likely to have had fever and leukocytosis for several days before the sudden deterioration that marks the onset of gram-negative bacteremia. The temperature may suddenly increase or it may fall to subnormal levels, especially in elderly patients or those who are debilitated. Rarely, fever is obliterated by chronically administered high-dose steroids. There may be frank shaking chills. Patients may exhibit new anxiety, agitation, or confusion. The first clue to sepsis in an already critically ill patient may be an increase in cardiac output or an inability to absorb enteral nutrition. For some reason, patients with burns often develop unexplained ileus as one of the few signs of bacteremia on a background of fever, leukocytosis, and vascular instability associated with the burn itself. Even though blood pressure still may be normal, orthostatic pulse and blood pressure changes may be seen. Resting tachycardia and/or increased respiratory rate is helpful (unless the patient has a pacemaker, is on drugs that affect heart rate, or is on a respirator at controlled rate). In patients under less strict surveillance, the first symptom of hypotension may be a significant decrease in urine output. When the blood pressure is obtained, it is important to consult the medical record for the patient's normal reading. Formerly hypertensive patients will suffer poor perfusion at levels of blood pressure that are normal for most individuals. In general, the traditional distinction between "warm" and "cold" shock has not been helpful in separating gram-positive from gram-negative shock, and no reliance should be placed on it. When measured, cardiac output generally is high and systemic resistance is low in cases of endotoxic shock uncomplicated by other diseases. In late stages of untreated or irreversible shock, patients exhibit intense vasoconstriction, then cyanosis. Symptoms of shock-induced organ failure—bleeding, ARDS, azotemia, and infarcts of brain, heart, and bowel—will appear and may dominate the picture.

DIAGNOSIS. The term "sepsis" has come to denote a syndrome in which there is a systemic response to infection in the form of fever or hypothermia, tachycardia, tachypnea, and either hypotension (in 50 per cent of cases) or evidence of hypoperfusion of one or more organ systems. Analysis of clinical series suggests that 30 to 50 per cent of patients with the sepsis syndrome have gram-negative bacteremia documented by blood culture. Many of those without gram-negative bacteremia have gram-negative focal infections. Most patients with measurable endotoxin in the blood have gram-negative bacteremia, but a few do not. Figure 320–1 is a schematic representation of these relationships. Other considerations in the differential diagnosis of sepsis include infection of the bloodstream by gram-positive bacteria and fungi, staphylococcal toxic shock syndrome, clostridial shock, pulmonary embolus, acute allergic reactions, myocardial infarction, and a long list of less common conditions.

For therapeutic purposes, the diagnosis of gram-negative bac-

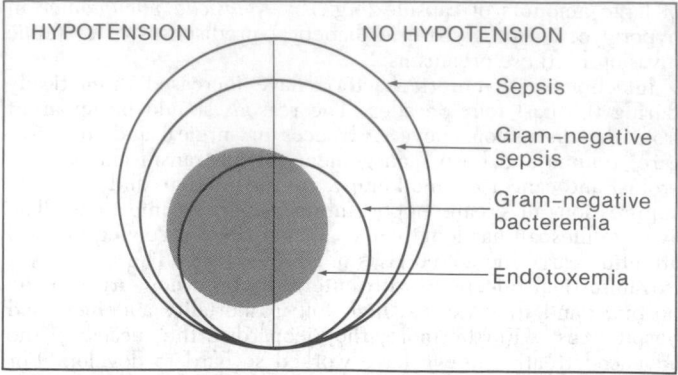

FIGURE 320–1. Schematic representation of etiologies of the sepsis syndrome. (Courtesy of Craig R. Smith.)

teremia cannot await the results of blood cultures but must be made on clinical grounds alone. The clinical setting is very helpful. A diagnosis of gram-negative bacteremia should be considered when sudden deterioration occurs in patients with focal infections usually caused by gram-negative bacteria (e.g., pyelonephritis, cholecystitis), in patients with significant focal infections from which gram-negative bacteria already have been isolated, and in patients with compromise in host defenses (e.g., neutropenia, burn injury), rendering them susceptible to their own bacterial flora. Neutropenic patients rarely have physical signs to localize the source of their bacteremia, but careful conversation often reveals a history of minor trauma, slight pain, or diarrhea.

Gram-negative bacteremia and endotoxin infusion both cause transient neutropenia followed by neutrophilic leukocytosis. Large "toxic" vacuoles are seen. The first leukocyte count often is obtained after the leukopenic phase, but patients recovering from chemotherapy may have limited leukocyte reserves and thus exhibit only an apparent reversal of marrow recovery. Isolated thrombocytopenia or full-blown disseminated intravascular coagulopathy is not diagnostic of gram-negative bacteremia but, if present, is good supporting evidence. Arterial blood gas determinations may reveal unexplained hypoxemia without overt pulmonary disease, followed by metabolic acidosis.

TREATMENT. Three elements are essential in the management of gram-negative bacteremia: physiologic support, antibiotics, and identification of the source so that it can be eradicated. These are listed in the order in which they should be addressed, but all three should be considered urgently, generally within 1 hour. If the patient is in shock or impending shock, physiologic monitoring in an intensive care unit should be applied if available. Good intravenous access should be obtained and a bladder catheter placed for hourly measurement of urine flow.

The aim of physiologic support is to restore adequate tissue perfusion. This is judged most easily by urine flow and mental status; perfusion of vital organs may be adequate when systolic blood pressure remains low and there is marked peripheral vasoconstriction. The principles of management of septic shock are the same as those used for other kinds of shock. If urine flow is less than 0.5 ml per kilogram per hour, fluids should be infused at the maximum rate tolerated by the patient. The composition, infusion rate, and total amount of fluid must be tailored to individual cardiovascular capacity. If urine flow is not restored with the pulmonary artery wedge pressure at the upper limits of normal or if the wedge pressure cannot be raised by fluids, a sympathomimetic amine, such as dopamine or dobutamine, should be administered without delay. If excessive quantities of fluid are used, severe pulmonary edema may develop just as the patient is recovering from septic shock. Dopamine is diluted to a concentration of 0.8 to 1.6 mg per milliliter and is given intravenously at an initial rate of 1 to 5 μg per kilogram per minute. At the lowest dose, dopamine acts only on dopaminergic receptors to cause vasodilation in renal, mesenteric, and other peripheral vascular beds. In patients with severe hypotension, the infusion may be started at 5 μg per kilogram per minute and gradually increased by 5 to 10 μg per kilogram per minute up to 20 to 50 μg per kilogram per minute as needed. At higher doses, dopamine acts on β-adrenergic and then α-adrenergic receptors to raise blood pressure. Dobutamine may be preferable in patients with congestive heart failure because it does not increase the pulmonary artery wedge pressure; however, in contrast to dopamine, it does not produce renal vasodilation. Therefore, dopamine is preferable in profound, prolonged shock. If shock is not responsive to dopamine, isoproterenol and then norepinephrine should be tried. If pressors are used for many days, patients may require very slow weaning; continued hypotension does not necessarily imply continuing infection.

The correct choice of antibiotics is crucial to successful treatment of gram-negative bacteremia. When inappropriate drugs are used or the doses are too low, outcome is poor. It is never wise to give a single antibiotic to a patient at the onset of a bacteremic episode, even if the diagnosis and etiology seem certain. Many other infections can mimic gram-negative bacteremia, as discussed. Sometimes more than one bacterial species is involved. In neutropenia, the outcome of *Pseudomonas* bacteremia is much better if more than one effective antibiotic is used. The choice of empiric antibiotics should be made on the basis of the site of the focal infection (or infections) present, the known antimicrobial sensitivities of previous isolates from the patient and of agents of recent nosocomial infections in the hospital, and the patient's underlying diseases. At the present time the best regimen seems to be a combination of an aminoglycoside with a third-generation cephalosporin. An antistaphylococcal drug should be added if *S. aureus* infection is likely. If bowel perforation or infarction has occurred, *Bacteroides fragilis* must be covered. If *Clostridium perfringens* is suspected to be part of a mixed infection, concomitant high-dose penicillin should be used. (*C. perfringens* decolorizes easily in the Gram stain and may be distinguishable from gram-negative rods only by its boxlike rectangular shape.) A common mistake in the use of aminoglycosides is to tailor the initial regimen to the first renal function tests. If azotemia is acute and attributable to poor perfusion, initial low doses will give inadequate levels as soon as hypotension is reversed. Renal toxicity from these drugs rarely occurs early; it is far more important to treat infection effectively in the first 24 hours than to avoid aminoglycoside toxicity.

Gram-negative bacteremia cannot be cured without eradication of the source of bacteremia. In cases of infection associated with ureteral or biliary obstruction, bacteremia and shock may persist in the face of adequate antibiotics until the obstruction is relieved. All likely sites of infection should be cultured, if possible, before antibiotics are given. However, antibiotic treatment should not be delayed for this reason. Wound cultures often remain positive after blood and urine have been sterilized. The physician should not be content until he or she has found a satisfactory explanation for bacteremia. New fever or clinical deterioration can signal a new infection in a susceptible patient, the emergence of resistant bacteria, spread of the original focal infection, inadequate antibiotic levels, or a drug reaction. Such an episode requires complete re-evaluation with physical examination and repeat cultures.

Several modes of adjunctive treatment for endotoxic shock are being evaluated at the present time. High-dose corticosteroids were used empirically for many years because of beneficial effects seen in experimental animal models of septic shock, but two recent large clinical trials have demonstrated no benefit and a possible deleterious effect on resolution of secondary infections. Nonsteroidal anti-inflammatory drugs also are being studied in endotoxic shock. Because endotoxin seems to play a central role in the evolution of gram-negative shock, several groups have raised antibodies to LPS determinants common to most gram-negative bacteria and have found these anti-endotoxin antisera effective in preventing LPS toxicity and bacteremic death in experimental gram-negative infections. A controlled clinical trial of human anti-LPS antiserum to treat established bacteremia showed a lower bacteremic death rate in patients given antiserum than in those given preimmunization control serum; the protective effect extended to patients in profound endotoxic shock. In an extension of this work, two double-blind, placebo-controlled trials of monoclonal antibodies to lipid A in patients with gram-negative sepsis have recently been completed. In one study, a therapeutic effect of a murine monoclonal antibody has been reported in some patients with gram-negative sepsis. In the other study, treatment with a human monoclonal antibody resulted in a 39 per cent decrease in mortality among patients with gram-

negative bacteremia, compared with placebo treatment, and the antibody was effective in patients who were in septic shock. Adjunctive immunotherapy with antiendotoxin monoclonal antibody may soon become part of the standard regimen for treating patients in sepsis who have gram-negative bacteremia.

Bone RC, Fisher CJ Jr, Clemmer TP, et al.: Sepsis syndrome: A valid clinical entity. Crit Care Med 17:389, 1989. *A description of the clinical presentation of patients in sepsis, many of whom have gram-negative bacteremia.*

Fairley KF, Bond AG, Brown RB, et al.: Simple test to determine the site of urinary tract infection. Lancet 1:427, 1967. *A brief description of the details of the Fairley test.*

Hack CE, DeGroote ER, Felt-Bersma RJF, et al.: Increased plasma levels of interleukin 6 in sepsis. Blood 74:1704, 1989. *A good analysis of cytokine dynamics in sepsis.*

Kreger BE, Craven DE, Carling PC, et al.: Gram-negative bacteremia. III. Reassessment of etiology, epidemiology and ecology in 612 patients. Am J Med 68:332, 1980. *A recent classic clinical description of gram-negative bacteremia in an academic hospital setting, with emphasis on the pathogenesis and the influence of the underlying condition on outcome.*

Tracey KJ, Beutler B, Lowry SF, et al.: Shock and tissue injury induced by recombinant human cachetin. Science 234:470, 1986. *An excellent review of tumor necrosis factor and experimental evidence of its role in the shock of gram-negative bacteremia.*

Van Deventer SJH, Buller HR, ten Cate JW, et al.: Endotoxemia: An early predictor of septicemia in febrile patients. Lancet 1:606, 1988. *Use of the Limulus lysate test to show endotoxin in the circulation of septic patients, most of whom had gram-negative bacteremia.*

Ziegler EJ, Fisher CJ Jr, Sprung CL, et al.: Treatment of gram-negative bacteremia and septic shock with HA-1A human monoclonal antibody against endotoxin. N Engl J Med 324:429, 1991. *Description of the randomized, double-blind, placebo-controlled trial of human monoclonal IgM anti–lipid A antibody in gram-negative bacteremia, with a review of previous work.*

321 *Yersinia* Infections

Thomas Butler

PLAGUE

DEFINITION. Plague is a bacterial infection of animals and humans caused by *Yersinia pestis*. The most common clinical form is *acute regional lymphadenitis*, called *bubonic plague*. Less common forms include *septicemic, pneumonic, cutaneous,* and *meningeal plague*. Mortality is high in untreated cases, but antibiotic treatment administered early in the course of the disease markedly reduces fatalities.

HISTORY. *Y. pestis* has caused devastating pandemics with high mortality rates throughout history. The fourth great pandemic in the world is currently under way. The first three are believed to have occurred in the following times: the first originated in Egypt in 542 A.D. and spread to Turkey and Europe. The second started in the 14th century in Asia Minor and Africa; after spreading to Europe the black death killed about a fourth of the continent's people. The third occurred in Europe during the 15th to 18th centuries. The present fourth pandemic began around 1860 in the Chinese province of Yunnan. It spread to the southern coast of China, reaching Hong Kong in 1894. Subsequently plague was carried by ship to India, other countries of Asia, Brazil, and California. An estimated 10 million deaths were caused by this disease in India during this century. The plague bacillus was discovered by Alexandre Yersin in 1894 in Hong Kong and was called *Pasteurella pestis* until 1970. Transmission by flea bites was suggested by Ogata in 1897.

ETIOLOGY. The causative agent, *Y. pestis*, belongs to the family of bacteria Enterobacteriaceae. It is virulent by virtue of plasmid-mediated V and W antigens, which confer calcium dependency and are believed to enable the plague bacillus to proliferate inside mammalian mononuclear phagocytic cells. In the capsular envelope there is an antiphagocytic protein called Fraction 1 antigen. In the cell walls there is a potent lipopolysaccharide endotoxin, which produces fever, disseminated intravascular coagulation, and complement activation. In addition, *Y. pestis* elaborates *murine toxin*, which produces β-adrenergic blockade, but the role of this exotoxin in human disease is unclear.

DISTRIBUTION AND EPIDEMIOLOGY. During 1980 to

1986, 4522 cases of human plague were reported to the World Health Organization. Countries reporting the most cases were Vietnam, Brazil, Peru, Tanzania, Burma, Madagascar, and United States. In the United States, plague is limited almost entirely to the Southwestern states of New Mexico, Arizona, Colorado, Nevada, and California.

Plague is a zoonotic infection that is transmitted among animal reservoirs by flea bites or by ingestion of contaminated animal tissues. Throughout the world domestic and urban rats are the most important reservoirs. In sylvatic foci of plague, however, as occur in the United States, reservoirs are the ground squirrel, rock squirrel, and prairie dog. Humans are an accidental host in the natural cycle of plague, when rodent fleas bite people, and appear to play no role in the maintenance of plague in nature. Only rarely, during epidemics of pneumonic plague, is the infection passed directly from person to person. Occasionally, the infection develops in humans by the direct handling of contaminated animal tissues, as when hunters skin dead rabbits.

The incidence of plague in humans for any particular locality is a function of both the frequency of infection in local rodent populations and the intimacy with which the people live with the infected rodents and their fleas. In the United States, the season for plague is April to September, when people are out of doors. Off-season cases often involve hunters who handle their prey.

PATHOGENESIS AND CLINICAL FEATURES. The most common clinical form is bubonic plague, which presents a distinctive clinical picture (Table 321–1). During an incubation period of 2 to 8 days following a bite by an infected flea, bacteria proliferate in the regional lymph nodes. Patients are typically affected by the sudden onset of fever, chills, weakness, and headache. Usually at the same time, or after a few hours or the next day, patients notice the *bubo*, which is signaled by intense pain in one anatomic region of lymph nodes, usually the groin, axilla, or neck. A swelling evolves that is so tender that the patient typically avoids any motion that would provoke tenderness of the affected nodes. The bubo contains acute inflammatory cells, a high density of bacteria, and hemorrhagic necrosis.

The buboes of patients with plague are oval swellings varying from about 1 to 10 cm in length and elevating the overlying skin, which may appear stretched or erythematous. They appear either as a smooth, uniform, egg-shaped mass or as an irregular cluster of several nodes. There is warmth of the overlying skin and an underlying, firm, tender, nonfluctuant mass. Usually around the lymph nodes there is considerable edema, which can be gelatinous or pitting in nature. Occasionally, edema extends into the skin region drained by the affected lymph nodes. Although infections other than plague can produce acute lymphadenitis, plague is unique for the suddenness of onset of the fever and the bubo, the rapid development of intense inflammation in the bubo, and the fulminant clinical course that can produce death as quickly as 2 to 4 days after the onset of symptoms. The bubo of plague is also distinctive for the usual absence of a detectable skin lesion and likewise for the absence of an ascending lymphangitis nearby.

In uncomplicated *bubonic plague*, the patients are typically prostrate and lethargic and often exhibit restlessness or agitation. Occasionally, they are delirious with high fever, and seizures are common in children. Temperature is usually in the range of 38.5 to 40.0°C, and the pulse rate is increased. Blood pressure is characteristically low, in the range of 100/60 mm Hg. Pressure determinations may be unobtainable if shock ensues. The liver and spleen are often palpable and tender. Abdominal pain, vomiting, and diarrhea are common.

The majority of patients with bubonic plague do not have skin

TABLE 321–1. PLAGUE SYNDROMES

Syndrome	Features
Bubonic	Fever, painful lymphadenopathy (bubo)
Septicemic	Fever, hypotension without bubo
Pneumonic	Cough, hemoptysis with or without bubo
Cutaneous	Pustule, eschar, carbuncle, or ecthyma gangrenosum usually with bubo
Meningitis	Fever, nuchal rigidity usually with bubo

lesions. About a fourth of patients in Vietnam, however, did show pustules, vesicles, eschars, or papules near the bubo or in the anatomic region of skin that is lymphatically drained by the affected lymph nodes. These presumably represent sites of flea bite inoculations. When these lesions are opened, they usually contain white cells and plague bacilli. These skin lesions rarely progress to extensive cellulitis or abscesses. Ulceration may lead, however, to a larger plague carbuncle. Another kind of skin lesion in plague is purpura, which may become necrotic, resulting in gangrene of distal extremities that is the probable basis of the term "black death." These purpuric lesions result from vasculitis and thrombosis.

A distinctive feature of plague is the propensity for massive growth of bacteria in the blood. In the early acute stages of bubonic plague, all patients probably have intermittent bacteremia. Single blood cultures obtained at the time of hospital admission from Vietnamese patients were positive in 27 per cent of cases. A hallmark of moribund patients with plague is high-density bacteremia, so that a blood smear revealing characteristic bacilli has been used as a prognostic indicator in this disease. Occasionally in the pathogenesis of plague infection, bacteria are inoculated and proliferate in the body, producing bacteremia without a bubo. This syndrome has been termed *septicemic plague*.

One of the feared complications of bubonic plague is secondary pneumonia. The infection reaches the lungs by hematogenous spread from the bubo. In addition to the high mortality, plague pneumonia is highly contagious by airborne transmission. It is characterized by fever and lymphadenopathy with cough, chest pain, and often hemoptysis. Radiographically, there is patchy bronchopneumonia or confluent consolidation. The sputum is usually purulent and contains plague bacilli. *Primary inhalation pneumonia* is rare now but is a potential threat to the individual exposed to a patient with plague who has a cough.

Plague meningitis is a rarer complication and typically occurs more than a week after inadequately treated bubonic plague. Less commonly, plague meningitis appears as a primary infection without antecedent lymphadenitis. Bacteria are frequently demonstrable with a Gram stain of spinal fluid sediment.

LABORATORY FEATURES. The white blood cell count is typically elevated in the range of 10,000 to 20,000 cells per cubic millimeter, with a predominance of immature and mature neutrophils. Blood platelet counts may be normal or low in the early stages of bubonic plague. Although a generalized bleeding tendency from profound thrombocytopenia is rare, disseminated intravascular coagulation (DIC) is common. Fibrinogen-fibrin degradation products in the serum that are indicative of DIC were detected in elevated titers in most patients tested in Vietnam.

DIAGNOSIS. Plague should be suspected in febrile patients who have been in known endemic areas. A bacteriologic diagnosis is readily made in most patients by smear and culture of a bubo aspirate. The aspirate is obtained by inserting a 20-gauge needle on a 10-ml syringe containing 1 ml of sterile saline solution into the bubo and aspirating several times until the saline solution has become blood tinged. It may be necessary to inject some of the saline solution and to reaspirate it immediately. Drops of the aspirate should be placed on microscope slides. The Gram stain reveals polymorphonuclear leukocytes and gram-negative coccobacilli and bacilli. Smears of blood, sputum, or spinal fluid can be handled similarly.

The aspirate, blood, and other appropriate fluids should be inoculated onto blood and MacConkey's agar plates and into infusion broth. For definitive identification, cultures can be mailed in double containers to the Centers for Disease Control, Plague Branch, P.O. Box 2087, Fort Collins, Colorado 80422 (telephone no.: 303–221–6450). At this same laboratory, a serologic test, the passive hemagglutination test utilizing Fraction 1 of *Y. pestis*, can be performed on acute and convalescent phase serum. For patients with negative cultures, a fourfold or greater increase in titer or a single titer of greater than or equal to 1:16 is presumptive evidence for plague infection.

The differential diagnosis of bubonic plague includes tularemia, streptococcal and staphylococcal lymphadenitis, secondary syphilis, and lymphogranuloma venereum. For pneumonia, the physician should also consider common forms of bacterial and viral pneumonia. For meningitis and septicemia, the common bacterial causes need to be assessed by age groups.

TREATMENT AND PROGNOSIS. Untreated plague has an estimated mortality of greater than 50 per cent. Therefore, the early institution of effective antibiotic therapy is mandatory. In 1948, streptomycin was identified as the drug of choice for the treatment of plague by reducing mortality to less than 5 per cent. No other drug has been demonstrated to be more efficacious or less toxic. Streptomycin should be administered intramuscularly in two divided doses daily, totaling 30 mg per kilogram of body weight per day for 10 days. Most patients improve rapidly and become afebrile in about 3 days. If the serum creatinine concentration rises significantly, the dose of streptomycin should be reduced. In mild renal failure, the recommended dose is about 20 mg per kilogram per day and in advanced renal failure, 8 mg per kilogram every 3 days.

For patients allergic to streptomycin or for whom an oral drug is strongly preferred, tetracycline is a satisfactory alternative. It is administered orally in a dose of 2 to 4 grams per day in four divided doses for 10 days. For patients with meningitis who require a drug that penetrates the cerebrospinal fluid effectively and for patients with profound hypotension in whom an intramuscular injection may not be well absorbed, chloramphenicol should be administered intravenously with a loading dose of 25 mg per kilogram of body weight followed by 60 mg per kilogram per day in four divided doses. After clinical improvement, oral chloramphenicol administration should be continued to complete a total course of 10 days; the dosage may be reduced to 30 mg per kilogram per day to reduce the magnitude of bone marrow suppression. The three antibiotics streptomycin, tetracycline, and chloramphenicol given alone are clinically very effective, and relapses are exceedingly rare. Therefore, there is no rationale for using multiple antibiotics to treat plague.

Because patients are febrile and often have nausea or vomiting, hypotension, and dehydration, intravenous 0.9 per cent saline solution should be given to most patients for the first few days of the illness or until improvement occurs. Patients in shock require additional quantities of fluid, with hemodynamic monitoring.

The buboes usually recede without need of local therapy. Occasionally, however, they may enlarge or become fluctuant during the first week of treatment and require incision and drainage. The aspirated fluid should be cultured for evidence of superinfection, but this material is usually sterile.

PREVENTION. All patients with suspected plague should be reported to the local health department. Those with cough or other signs of pneumonia must be placed in strict respiratory isolation for at least 48 hours after the start of antibiotic therapy or until the sputum culture is negative. The bubo aspirate and blood must be handled with gloves. Standard bacteriologic techniques that safeguard against skin contact with and aerosolization of infected fluids and cultures should be adequate to protect laboratory personnel.

Persons living in endemic areas should protect themselves against rodents and fleas. Measures include living in ratproof houses, reducing opportunities for rodent harborage near homes, wearing shoes and garments to cover the legs, and application of insecticide dusts to houses and household pets. A formalin-killed vaccine, plague vaccine U.S.P. (Cutter Laboratories, Berkeley, California 94710) is available for travelers to epidemic areas, for individuals who must live and work in close contact with wild rodents, and for laboratory workers who must handle live *Y. pestis* cultures. A primary series of two injections is recommended, with a 1- to 3-month interval between them. Booster injections are given every 6 months for as long as exposure continues.

Butler T: Plague and other *Yersinia* infections. New York, Plenum Publishing, 1983. *This monograph gives full clinical description and contemporary literature citations.*

Hull HF, Montes JM, Mann JM: Septicemic plague in New Mexico. J Infect Dis 155:113, 1987. *One fourth of 71 recent cases of plague in New Mexico were septicemic without a bubo. To prevent the observed 33 per cent mortality rate, earlier empiric antibiotic treatment is advised.*

Welty TK, Grabman J, Kompare E, et al.: Nineteen cases of plague in Arizona. West J Med 142:641, 1985. *This paper describes clinical features of recent cases in Arizona.*

OTHER *YERSINIA* INFECTIONS

DEFINITION. The nonplague yersinioses are caused by *Yersinia enterocolitica* and *Y. pseudotuberculosis*. These gram-neg-ative rod bacteria produce fever, diarrhea, and abdominal pain that can mimic acute appendicitis. The common pathologic lesions in yersiniosis are acute enteritis and mesenteric lymphadenitis. Extraintestinal disease may result from septicemia or may appear as arthritis and erythema nodosum.

ETIOLOGY. Of the 34 different O serotypes of *Y. enterocolitica* that have been identified, the ones most commonly associated with human disease are types 3, 8, and 9. All virulent strains possess a plasmid that encodes the V and W antigens, which confer calcium dependency on the bacteria. Like other gram-negative bacteria, the yersiniae contain a lipopolysaccharide endotoxin in the cell wall that may be responsible, in part, for the fever and inflammation.

EPIDEMIOLOGY. The yersinioses are distributed worldwide. Large numbers of confirmed cases have been reported in Europe, Canada, the United States, and Japan. In the United States, infection with *Y. enterocolitica* appears to be rare when compared with infection with *Salmonella* and *Shigella* species. Both adults and children are susceptible to infection. Males acquire the infection more commonly than do females. The natural reservoirs of *Y. enterocolitica* are farm animals, especially pigs and goats, and other domestic animals, including dogs and cats. The natural reservoirs of *Y. pseudotuberculosis* include birds and other diverse domestic and farm animals. These animals harbor the bacteria in their intestines and excrete them in feces. Humans become infected by ingesting food or water contaminated by animal feces or directly by the ingestion of certain fomites. Person-to-person transmission seems to be rare. Blood transfusion has transmitted infections. Well-defined outbreaks of *Y. enterocolitica* infection have occurred in children in Georgia whose caregivers handled raw pork intestines, in a New York school at which chocolate milk was the source of infection, in members of a Brownie scout troop in Pennsylvania who ate infected bean sprouts, and in persons who drank milk from a dairy in Tennessee. There are no clear seasonal patterns of infection.

PATHOGENESIS OF CLINICAL SYNDROMES. An inoculum with as many as 10^9 organisms may be required to produce infection. During the incubation period, estimated at 4 to 10 days, bacteria proliferate in the small bowel; invade the mucosa, especially that of the ileum; and elicit an acute inflammatory response. Ulcerations may occur, and polymorphonuclear leukocytes appear in the stool. Some bacteria migrate via the lymphatics to the mesenteric lymph nodes, where inflammation occurs. The initial symptoms include fever and either diarrhea or abdominal pain. In these instances, the corresponding pathologic finding is terminal ileitis or mesenteric lymphadenitis or both. The colon is less frequently affected, but aphthoid ulcers and hemorrhagic colitis have been described in yersiniosis. The tissues are affected by acute inflammation, thrombosis of blood vessels, hemorrhage, and necrosis. The diarrhea results from the mucosal invasion by bacteria or the action of an enterotoxin. Diarrhea varies from semisolid or watery to grossly bloody. In some patients the abdominal pain is severe and located in the right lower quadrant and may be mistaken for appendicitis; the appendix is usually normal. A few days later, some patients may develop extraintestinal complications of arthralgias, arthritis, and erythema nodosum. Synovial fluid contains bacterial antigen, and an immunologic reaction has been postulated to explain the pathogenesis of these complications. Arthritis, including sacroileitis, is more likely to occur in individuals of haplotype HLA-B27, and erythema nodosum occurs more commonly in women. Septicemia is a rare complication that occurs in the setting of prior liver disease, malignancies, immunosuppressive therapy, or after blood transfusion. Rarer clinical forms of yersiniosis include pneumonia, pharyngitis, and meningitis. Antibodies appear in the blood against the O and other antigens of *Y. enterocolitica*, and nearly all infections are self-limited. However, fatalities have occurred from extensive ulceration and necrosis of the intestine and septicemia.

DIAGNOSIS. The diagnosis requires the isolation of yersiniae from stool, blood, or surgical specimens. The number of bacteria in stool may be small, and a cold-enrichment technique has been used. A rectal swab or piece of stool is placed into 0.067M phosphate-buffered saline solution at a pH of 7.6 and incubated at 4°C for 4 weeks. Most other stool bacteria die, whereas *Y.*

enterocolitica grows. At weekly intervals, subcultures should be made on MacConkey's agar. A presumptive diagnosis can be made from serologic test results by showing a rise in agglutinin titer in paired serum specimens. The existence of cross-reacting antigens in the genera *Brucella*, *Vibrio*, and *Salmonella* indicates that false-positive serologic results sometimes occur.

TREATMENT AND PROGNOSIS. Yersiniosis is usually self-limited and so rarely diagnosed that it is impossible to assess the possible benefits of antibiotic treatment. Most isolates of *Y. enterocolitica* are susceptible to streptomycin, gentamicin, tetracycline, chloramphenicol, and sulfamethoxazole-trimethoprim and resistant to the penicillins and cephalosporin antibiotics. *Y. pseudotuberculosis* isolates usually have been susceptible to penicillin. It is important to suspect the diagnosis in patients with severe abdominal pain to avoid unnecessary surgery for appendicitis. The recognition that early fever accompanies yersiniosis may be helpful, as is epidemiologic information pertaining to outbreaks in the community.

PREVENTION AND CONTROL. The presumed origin of *Y. enterocolitica* infection in farm and domestic animals suggests that transmission may be similar to that of *Salmonella*. Meat and dairy products and other farm produce should periodically be examined for *Y. enterocolitica* content. During outbreaks, public health authorities should identify sources of infection in food (especially milk and pork), water, or persons.

Cover TL, Aber RC: *Yersinia enterocolitica*. N Engl J Med 321:16, 1989. *This comprehensive review covers epidemiology, clinical features, diagnosis, and treatment and has 201 references.*

Lee LA, Taylor J, Carter GP, et al.: *Yersinia enterocolitica* 0:3: An emerging cause of pediatric gastroenteritis. J Infect Dis 163:660, 1991. *Outbreaks of diarrhea are being recognized, and some involve black children whose caregivers are exposed to raw pork intestines during holiday seasons.*

Tertti R, Vuento R, Mikkola P, et al.: Clinical manifestations of *Yersinia pseudotuberculosis* infection in children. Eur J Clin Microbiol Infect Dis 8:587, 1989. *In an outbreak affecting 34 Finnish school children, fever and abdominal pain led to unnecessary laparotomies in 3 cases.*

322 Tularemia

Richard B. Hornick

DEFINITION. Tularemia is a rare infectious disease caused by a small gram-negative pleomorphic rod, *Francisella tularensis*. This organism is acquired from an animal reservoir, frequently cottontail rabbits, by direct contact with diseased animal tissues, the bite of an infected tick or deer fly, ingestion of contaminated food or water, and inhalation of aerosolized bacteria. Clinical manifestations usually include a cutaneous ulcer with enlargement of regional lymph nodes. Rarely, a pneumonitis results from inhalation of *F. tularensis* or secondary spread from the skin ulcer and lymph nodes. Confirmation of the diagnosis by cultural technique is not advocated because of the high contagion risk to personnel handling this organism. The therapeutic response to effective antibiotic therapy is rapid.

The typhoidal form of tularemia was first described in Japan in 1818. A clear description of the organism occurred in 1906 when McCoy uncovered a "plaguelike" disease among ground squirrels in Tulare County, California. In Japan, tularemia may be referred to as Ohara's disease or Yato-byo (wild hare disease).

ETIOLOGY, SPECIFIC LABORATORY DIAGNOSIS, AND EPIDEMIOLOGY. *F. tularensis* is a small gram-negative pleomorphic rod-shaped bacterium. Organisms are not seen in smears of infected tissue unless special staining techniques are used. Fluorescent antibody conjugate staining and modified Dieterle staining are the best methods for demonstrating them. All tularemia strains are serologically identical, but there are biochemical and virulence differences for mammals that have allowed differentiation of two strains. These are called Jellison A and B; the former, found only in North America, is lethal for domestic rabbits (*Oryctolagus*) and causes severe disease in humans. The unique biochemical capabilities of this strain—e.g., it ferments

glycerol and contains citrulline ureidase—do not explain its increased virulence. Strain B lacks these biochemical features, is not lethal for cottontails, causes milder disease in humans, usually is isolated from rodents or from water, and is distributed over Europe, Asia, and North America. Reasons for the differences in virulence are unknown.

Culture Methods. The direct isolation of *F. tularensis* from blood (rarely), pus from ulcers or buboes, sputum, or pharyngeal or gastric aspirations in a patient with pneumonitis can be achieved by two methods. This is a class 4 organism requiring an effective hood or an adequate isolation laboratory to prevent human disease or epizootics. The two methods for isolation are intraperitoneal inoculation of guinea pigs and direct plating of a specimen onto glucose cysteine blood agar, cystine heart agar, or eugon agar. As few as one to five viable organisms will cause the death of guinea pigs in 5 to 10 days. Appropriate facilities are needed to prevent spread of the disease to other animals. The media employed to isolate the organism usually contain drugs to suppress other flora and allow the tularemia colonies to be visible. Useful additions are 0.1 mg of cycloheximide and 20 units of penicillin per milliliter of media. The colonies are small on these media; they appear in 48 to 72 hours of incubation at 37°C.

Serologic Diagnosis. The measurement of serum agglutinating antibodies is a useful and safer method of diagnosing tularemia. Titers begin to rise in about 7 to 10 days and peak in 3 to 4 weeks. Paired serum specimens obtained 2 weeks apart and demonstrating a fourfold or greater rise are diagnostic of tularemia. However, a single specimen with a titer of 1:160 or greater in a patient thought to have tularemia on clinical grounds is diagnostic. Antibiotic therapy does not appear to dampen the antibody response. Titers remain elevated for 6 to 8 months and then decline in the subsequent 1 to 1.5 years to low or undetectable levels. There is a cross-reaction with brucella antigen during the early phase of the antibody response. The brucella titer falls off faster than and is never so high as the tularemia titer.

Skin Testing. A skin test antigen has proved to be reliable for diagnostic and epidemiologic purposes. A positive test result, similar in appearance to a tuberculin test response, is present during the first week of illness, frequently before the agglutinins are detectable, and remains positive for years. There is no known cross-reacting skin test antigen. The antigen is derived from *F. tularensis* by ether extraction; however, it is not commonly available. It can be obtained from the Centers for Disease Control, Atlanta. In 10 per cent of patients, the skin test antigen may boost pre-existing agglutinating antibody titers. Skin test reactivity can be shown to be associated with sensitized lymphocytes.

Epidemiology. Tularemia is a sporadic disease; humans acquire it when bitten by an infected tick or deer fly or when handling an infected animal. In the process of dressing a rabbit or skinning a muskrat, the hands may become contaminated with infected blood, subcutaneous abscesses, or liver and spleen that contain millions of organisms. The act of eviscerating the animal can create an aerosol that can be inhaled. The ingestion of contaminated water or food is the least likely method of acquiring tularemia. Many carnivores such as dogs, cats, bull snakes, and others may feed on diseased rabbits. This results in contamination of the teeth and saliva. These animals are relatively resistant to tularemia. Contact with the teeth of a pet dog or cat has resulted in ulceroglandular tularemia. Studies in volunteers have quantified the susceptibility of humans to infection and disease and the virulence of *F. tularensis* for humans. As few as 50 type A organisms injected subcutaneously cause ulceroglandular disease. Pneumonic tularemia can be induced by a similar inoculum size if the aerosolized and inhaled particles are small (less than 5 μm). Type B organisms require an inoculum about 1000 times larger to induce ulceroglandular or respiratory disease in humans.

The incidence of tularemia is low, 150 to 300 cases a year having been reported in each of the past 20 years. The peak incidence was in 1939, when almost 2300 cases were reported. Laws passed at that time prohibited the sale of wild rabbits, especially cottontails, and this legislation plus increased public awareness of the danger of handling sick or dying wild animals has contributed to the decline. Most cases occur in the Midwest, but the disease is not restricted to any one geographic location in the United States. Cottontail rabbits in urban and suburban areas throughout the country provide the reservoir from which tularemia can occur. Epizootics among these or other animals can cause epidemics in humans. Tularemia has been reported only north of the 30th parallel. The cottontail rabbit is not found in Europe; various rodents such as voles, muskrats, and hares carry *F. tularensis* (Jellison B type) in that part of the world. Diseased jackrabbits, found west of the Mississippi River, may be an important source of contamination of ticks and deer flies.

In the summer months, most cases of tularemia are caused by tick or deer fly bites. Ulceroglandular disease begins with an ulcer at the site of the bite, e.g., groin, axilla, or scalp. In the fall, during hunting season, sporadic cases, usually ulceroglandular, occur among hunters and trappers. In the Scandinavian countries, epidemics have occurred in the winter months when farmers handling stored hay contaminated by diseased voles inhaled *F. tularensis* and developed pneumonic tularemia.

MECHANISMS OF INFECTION AND PATHOLOGY. The most common form of tularemia results from the penetration of *F. tularensis* into the skin. This penetration may be through hair follicles or minute areas of trauma. The development of the subsequent disease takes 2 to 6 days, depending upon the number of bacteria and their virulence. The organisms multiply in the dermis and induce a marked inflammatory process consisting primarily of mononuclear cells with a perivascular distribution. This process produces an erythematous tender papule. The inflamed area continues to swell until the induced ischemia causes the skin to ulcerate. The base of the ulcer becomes black and depressed. The edges are sharply demarcated. At the time of penetration, some organisms may be phagocytized and transported in the lymph to regional nodes. There is no clinically apparent lymphangitis. The nodes enlarge and become painful when caseation occurs. Histologic sections reveal geographic necrosis and disruption of the capsule. Fluctuation of the node is a late and rare event. It may then rupture. The necrotic, purulent, painful lymph node is termed a bubo. Healing of a bubo takes months even with appropriate antibiotic treatment. Aspiration of an unruptured node may lead to an indolent draining sinus tract. *F. tularensis* may remain in the necrotic tissue and purulent drainage for many weeks. The ulcer heals slowly and usually leaves a depigmented, rounded area in the skin.

Oculoglandular tularemia may occur when the conjunctival sac is infected from an ulcer or contaminated finger. Small yellowish granulomatous lesions develop on the palpebral conjunctivae, accompanied by enlargement of the preauricular lymph nodes. In untreated patients the cornea may perforate.

Inhaled small particle aerosols (<5 μm in diameter) containing *F. tularensis* (usually type A) are ultimately deposited in the terminal bronchioles and alveoli, although infection of the trachea and large bronchi also occurs. A peribronchial inflammation develops, with infiltration by neutrophils and mononuclear cells. This produces necrosis of alveolar walls and results in localized pneumonitis. In humans, small areas of pneumonitis represent the most common findings on chest roentgenograms. Often these are ill defined and difficult to interpret. Lobar consolidation or lung abscesses represent extensive spread and necrosis. These are infrequent in humans. Mediastinal and peritracheal lymph nodes enlarge and may be apparent on chest x-ray films. They may be partially responsible, along with the bronchitis, for the substernal burning that is common in patients with tularemic pneumonia. The incubation period for this form of tularemia varies inversely with the size and virulence of the inhaled inoculum. Following an inoculum of 10 to 50 organisms, disease appears in about 4 to 7 days in volunteers.

Typhoidal tularemia follows systemic spread of *F. tularensis* from the oropharynx and probably the gastrointestinal tract when a huge inoculum is swallowed. Enlargement of cervical lymph nodes, and presumably nodes in the mesentery, occurs. This latter process causes abdominal pain and is associated with an ileus. This is the most unusual form of tularemia in this country.

CLINICAL MANIFESTATIONS. Disease initiated by a tick bite is manifested by an ulcer at the site or adjacent to it. The tick defecates after feeding, and the infected feces may be scratched into the epidermis. Usually the lesion is in the inguinal, axillary, or scalp skin. If contact with tularemia organisms results from the handling of an infected animal, an ulcerative lesion evolves in the skin of the hands, frequently around a fingernail. This lesion may be so trivial that it is ignored by the patient.

The ulcer is depressed into the dermis, has sharply demarcated edges, and gradually develops a black base. In the initial stage of development the lesion produces a thick, yellowish exudate. Regional lymph nodes enlarge and are tender to palpation. Fever and chills are common. The temperature curve is usually remittent or continuous in character. Without antibiotic therapy, most patients remain febrile for several weeks, the ulcer heals slowly over weeks to months, and the enlarged lymph nodes persist for months. Untreated patients may occasionally develop a secondary necrotizing pneumonia as a consequence of bacteremia. These patients may be acutely ill.

Primary tularemia pneumonia presents with the sudden development of substernal burning and a nonproductive paroxysmal cough associated with fever and chills. Headache, myalgia, photophobia, malaise, and prostration are common findings. The temperature elevates quickly to 39.4 to 40°C and remains at that level (continuous fever curve) until antibiotic treatment is given. Sixty to 70 per cent of patients survive without specific therapy, and in these a slow defervescence occurs over several months. Radiographs of the lungs may reveal ill-defined, scattered oval areas of infiltration, with enlarged peritracheal lymph nodes. Pleural effusions, lobar consolidation, and lung abscess are other manifestations of this form of tularemia. Cervical lymph nodes are palpable and tender.

DIAGNOSIS AND DIFFERENTIAL DIAGNOSIS. The diagnosis of ulceroglandular tularemia is made on the basis of the clinical manifestations and serologic studies. Paired serum specimens collected over a 2- to 3-week period are required to demonstrate a fourfold rise in titer. A baseline agglutinin titer of 1:160 in a patient with a history of an indolent ulcer for 2 or more weeks is diagnostic of tularemia. Culture of an ulcer and blood should be performed only if the hospital laboratory has appropriate protective isolation hoods. Patients with sporotrichosis or *Mycobacterium marinum* infections may have ulcers suggestive of tularemia but are usually afebrile. Enlarged lymph nodes extending centripetally as a beaded chain are a characteristic finding in sporotrichosis. Lesions of the fingers infected with staphylococci or β streptococci usually produce more pus and may be associated with lymphangitis. *Bacillus anthracis* can produce an ulcer (anthrax) with black-based, sharply demarcated edges similar to that initiated by *F. tularensis*. A careful history and serologic data help in the differential diagnosis. In patients in whom any form of tularemia is suspected, the use of the skin test antigen is helpful. The test result is usually positive prior to the development of agglutinating antibodies.

Tularemia pneumonia must be differentiated from the more common bacterial, viral, and mycoplasmal pneumonias. The history and the presence of ulceroglandular disease are helpful. Skin testing and serologic studies are diagnostic. The chest radiographs may yield suggestive findings consisting of ill-defined, small, oval, multiple infiltrates but is not diagnostic.

Patients infected with *F. tularensis* usually have a normal leukocyte count with an elevation of the sedimentation rate. The white count is elevated when a bubo or a lung abscess is present.

COMPLICATIONS. Pericarditis and meningitis are rare events that usually occur in patients who have been misdiagnosed and have received inappropriate treatment. Pericarditis results from direct extension of the infection from the purulent, necrotic mediastinal lymph nodes or the involved lung. Constrictive pericarditis has been reported. Meningitis develops rarely, represents a seeding of the meninges during bacteremia, and is characterized by a lymphocytic pleocytosis in the cerebrospinal fluid.

TREATMENT. Patients with all forms of tularemia respond to the following antibiotics: streptomycin, gentamicin, tetracycline, and chloramphenicol. The aminoglycoside antibiotics are recommended, since they produce a prompt cure of patients with the most severe form of tularemia. Patients with pneumonitis are afebrile within 24 to 48 hours and do not relapse. Ulcers and tender lymph nodes heal in 7 to 10 days. Gentamicin, 5 mg per kilogram per day in divided doses, is given for 10 days. Streptomycin was the principal drug for treating tularemia before gentamicin; 1 gram is given every 12 hours for 10 days. Treatment with tetracycline or chloramphenicol may produce an equally rapid response, but relapses occur in 15 to 20 per cent of the patients. These drugs are not recommended unless gentamicin and streptomycin are contraindicated. Doses of 3 to 4 grams of tetracycline or 3 grams of chloramphenicol daily for 10 days can be employed. Naturally acquired resistance to any of these antibiotics has not been found.

Patients with ulceroglandular tularemia respond well to these antibiotics. Fluctuant lymph nodes should not be aspirated until the patient has finished the course of the antibiotic treatment. Isolation of patients with any form of tularemia is not required; there is no evidence of person-to-person spread.

PROGNOSIS. The mortality for untreated ulceroglandular disease is about 5 per cent. Patients infected with type B strains and untreated probably have a mortality less than 1 per cent. Many of these patients probably go undiagnosed, as the disease is mild and self-limiting. Treatment with antibiotics prevents death and promotes healing in a week to 10 days.

The mortality for pneumonic tularemia in the preantibiotic period was 30 to 40 per cent. Treatment with streptomycin or tetracycline has lowered this figure to less than 1 per cent. Healing occurs without residual lung damage or deficits in pulmonary function.

PREVENTION. Patients who recover from tularemia have a high degree of resistance to reinfection. If *F. tularensis* is reintroduced into the skin, a positive skin test reaction ensues without ulceration. Resistance to pulmonary disease may be associated with sensitized lymphocytes and alveolar macrophages.

A live attenuated strain of *F. tularensis* has been prepared as a vaccine. This can be administered by the acupuncture route, and it produces excellent immunity. The vaccine can be obtained from the Commander, U.S. Army Medical Research Institute of Infectious Diseases, Frederick, Maryland 21701. Its use is limited to persons considered at high risk, such as selected laboratory workers, forest rangers, game wardens, and perhaps others known to be exposed during an outbreak. The vaccine exerts its effect through the stimulation of cellular immune mechanisms. Circulating agglutinins are not associated with resistance to disease.

Buchanan TM, Brooks GF, Brachman PS: The tularemia skin test; 325 skin tests in 210 persons: Serologic correlation and review of the literature. Ann Intern Med 74:336, 1971. *This study is an extension of the study reported by Young et al. (see below). It clearly presents proof of the efficacy of the skin test as a diagnostic test for tularemia. In addition, it shows the amount of antigen stimulation needed to cause a conversion to a positive reactor.*

Evans ME, Gregory DW, Schaffner W, et al.: Tularemia: A 30-year experience with 88 cases. Medicine 64:251, 1985. *An excellent summary of the clinical presentations of F. tularensis disease.*

Penn RL, Kinasewitz GT: Factors associated with a poor outcome in tularemia. Arch Intern Med 147:265, 1987. *A retrospective study of the factors leading to poor outcomes. One significant factor was delay in diagnosis and treatment.*

Young LS, Bicknell DS, Archer BG, et al.: Tularemia epidemic: Vermont, 1968. Forty-seven cases linked to contact with muskrats. N Engl J Med 280:1253, 1969. *This represents one of the largest outbreaks occurring in the United States in the past 20 years. It is one of the best described epidemiologic studies of infection caused by the Jellison type B organism.*

323 Anthrax

Jonas A. Shulman

DEFINITION. Anthrax is a zoonotic disease caused by *Bacillus anthracis*, a large gram-positive, spore-forming bacillus that is transmitted to humans by contact with infected animals or contaminated animal products. Other names for anthrax include woolsorter's disease, Siberian ulcer, malignant pustule, charbon, malignant edema, and ragsorter's disease. In 1877, Koch described *B. anthracis* as one of the first microbes identified as a cause of a specific disease, thereby making anthrax the prototype for Koch's postulates and the first disease to satisfy them. Anthrax has all but disappeared from North America, Western Europe, and Australia since being nearly eradicated in livestock following extensive veterinary programs, including vaccination. The disease is still prevalent in many developing countries, however, especially Asia, Africa, and Central America, where livestock are only

marginally subjected to veterinary control and where environmental conditions are favorable for an animal-to-soil-to-animal cycle.

Anthrax occurs primarily in herbivorous animals, especially cattle, goats, and sheep, but many other animals, including pigs, buffalo, and elephants, have also been infected with the disease. Cattle are particularly susceptible to the systemic form of anthrax and clinically progress to death in 24 to 48 hours. The large numbers of organisms found in infected cattle may contaminate not only the animal but also its products and environs, thereby allowing infection to occur in animals more resistant to anthrax, such as humans.

The primary forms of anthrax in humans are cutaneous, inhalation, gastrointestinal, and oropharyngeal. Septicemia and meningitis may occur from any of these primary foci. By far, the most common form of the disease in the United States is the cutaneous lesion, which accounts for more than 95 per cent of clinical cases. Inhalation anthrax has occurred only rarely in the United States in the past 25 years, and gastrointestinal anthrax has never been reported in this country.

ETIOLOGY. *Bacillus anthracis* is a large gram-positive, nonmotile, spore-forming bacillus (1 to 1.3 × 3 to 8 μm). Although spores of *B. anthracis* do not form in living tissue, they are induced by aerobic conditions in the external environment and may persist for years in the soil, in animal products, or in an appropriate industrial setting. The organism grows well aerobically on ordinary laboratory media at 35° to 37°C. The colonies produced are especially sticky (positive tenacity test, positive string of pearls test) and have a tendency to stand up in stalagmite fashion when lifted with a bacteriologic loop. The colonies are nonhemolytic, rough, and flat, with many comma-shaped outgrowths on blood agar. Microscopic examination of organisms growing on artificial media shows long, parallel chains of organisms frequently described as having a rather characteristic "boxcar" appearance. Spores are oval and occur either centrally or paracentrally but cause no swelling of the bacillus. Material from fresh lesions reveals single or short chains of two or three bacilli, which may appear encapsulated, the ends of which are slightly rounded.

Anthrax organisms can be differentiated from the saprophytic *Bacillus* species by fluorescent antibody staining, lysis with a specific γ bacteriophage, and virulence for mice, guinea pigs, and rabbits. Parenteral inoculation into these species results in death in 1 to 3 days.

INCIDENCE AND PREVALENCE. *Bacillus anthracis* is a soil organism that has a worldwide distribution. Animal anthrax is endemic in some areas of Asia, Africa, and Latin America, especially in the less socioeconomically developed regions that have inadequate animal vaccination programs and poor animal husbandry. These countries are more likely to have a number of human cases as well. Certain areas within the United States and other parts of the world may provide a particularly favorable environment for large numbers of resistant spores to survive in the soil for many years. In fact, a number of epizootics related to focal regions of heavily contaminated soil have occurred.

Since no reliable reporting of anthrax exists, and in many instances the diagnosis may never be made, the actual worldwide incidence of anthrax is not known. Estimates in the past have ranged between 20,000 and 100,000 human cases per year, but these figures have more recently been estimated at 2000 to 20,000 cases per annum. In the United States, approximately one case of human anthrax per year was reported between 1970 and 1985, but only two cases have been documented since 1984. Reports of human anthrax have been especially frequent in areas of the world such as Turkey, Pakistan, Iran, Haiti, and several Asian and African countries. There are probably many parts of the world with significant endemic problems but from which data are not available.

The potential for large outbreaks in animals and humans continues to exist, especially when economic or political upheaval is present. One of the largest epidemics of anthrax was reported in Zimbabwe between 1978 and 1980, when nearly 10,000 human cases of cutaneous anthrax and a few cases of gastrointestinal anthrax occurred, resulting in approximately 100 deaths. This outbreak was related to an extensive epizootic infection in cattle. Another major outbreak of anthrax occurred in Siberia in 1979. It was initially thought by some to be related to inhalation, but more recently the route of infection has been identified as the ingestion and handling of infected "black market" meat. The source of anthrax in the cattle in this epidemic appeared to be a single 29-ton lot of bone meal used as animal feed that likely was made from the bones of animals that had died of anthrax the previous year.

Very rare cases of inhalation anthrax have developed in workers exposed to aerosolized anthrax spores generated during the processing of contaminated materials such as woolens, hides, or bone meal, and even more rarely in people who have simply been in the vicinity of a wool-processing mill or tannery but who were not directly involved in the processing of the product. Cases have even been reported in home weavers, such as those using contaminated goat yarn, or in individuals working with contaminated bone meal fertilizer.

In the United States, the average annual occurrence has diminished. From 1977 to 1988, the number of cases was only 0.8, as opposed to 127 cases reported to occur annually between 1916 and 1925. The case fatality rate of the 221 U.S. cases of cutaneous anthrax from 1955 to 1986 was approximately 5.0 per cent (11 of 221), whereas the case fatality rate was 82 per cent in the patients with inhalation anthrax (9 of 11). The overall mortality rate in these 232 American cases of anthrax was 8.6 per cent.

EPIDEMIOLOGY. Cases of anthrax are classified generally as either agricultural or industrial. Most of the agricultural cases of human anthrax result from direct contact with contaminated discharges from infected animals. Occasional human cases have been transmitted by bites of flies that have fed on the carcasses of animals that have died of anthrax. Industrial cases usually result from contact with anthrax spores contaminating animal products, such as goat hair, wool, hides, and skin, and animal bones, especially those imported from areas of high endemicity. Transmission usually occurs during the processing of these animal products, either by direct contact with the contaminated raw material or by indirect contact with a contaminated environment; rarely, transmission may occur via airborne particles produced during the manufacturing process. Because the *B. anthracis* spores can survive for long periods, a wide variety of unusual products have been associated with human infection, such as imported bongo drums made with goat skins, shaving brushes, various leather or woolen blankets, and ivory piano keys. Laboratory-acquired infections have been reported; however, human-to-human transmission of anthrax is not thought to occur.

Most cases of anthrax in the United States are sporadic, but occasional epidemics have been reported. In 1957, the largest and most serious of these occurred in New Hampshire, where nine employees of a textile mill acquired anthrax while processing a batch of contaminated goat hair imported from Asia. This outbreak included four cutaneous cases and five inhalation cases, with four fatalities reported in the latter group.

PATHOGENESIS. The virulence of *B. anthracis* is determined by both a plasmid-mediated group of exotoxins and another plasmid-mediated antiphagocytic polydiglutamic acid capsule. Three toxic proteins (exotoxins) have been identified and cloned, including a protective antigen (PA), an edema factor (EF), and a lethal factor (LF). A combination of two of these proteins (PA and EF) has been demonstrated to decrease polymorphonuclear neutrophil function, suggesting that in this way host susceptibility to infection with *B. anthracis* may be increased.

In cutaneous anthrax, the organism is introduced either through a wound or by means of infected animal fibers that disrupt the skin. The organism is not known to penetrate intact skin. Once in the subcutaneous tissue, the anthrax spore is thought to germinate, multiply, and produce both its exotoxin and the antiphagocytic capsular material. The toxins are capable of provoking a marked edematous response and tissue necrosis with a paucity of neutrophil invasion. Phagocytosis of the organisms by local macrophages occurs, and these bacilli are then spread to regional lymph nodes, where further production of toxins produces a hemorrhagic, necrotic, and edematous lymphadenitis. Bacilli may enter the circulation, at times producing meningitis, pneumonia, and systemic toxicity.

Inhalation anthrax is fortunately a very uncommon clinical presentation of anthrax, as it is associated with close to 100 per cent mortality. In the United States, inhalation anthrax is now essentially obsolete, with only two cases reported during the past 20 years; however, this is still a cause of significant disease in many parts of the world. Inhalation anthrax, commonly known as "woolsorter's disease," occurs not as a result of direct contact with infected animals but rather by inhalation of an aerosol of spores in particle sizes less than 5 μm. These aerosols have usually occurred during the processing of contaminated material. In humans, spores are inhaled, reach the alveoli, and may then eventually be phagocytized by macrophages and carried by these cells to the mediastinal lymph nodes. Germination, growth, and toxin formation at this site can produce a severe, massive hemorrhagic lymphadenitis and mediastinitis. *B. anthracis* may also directly affect the pulmonary capillary endothelium, causing thrombosis and respiratory failure. Pleural effusion is common. Anthrax is not thought to cause a primary pneumonia, but secondary bacterial pneumonia may complicate inhalation anthrax. *Bacillus anthracis* may also enter the bloodstream from this site, with the evolution of an intense bacteremia. The number of organisms per milliliter of blood may be so great that the organism may be seen on smears of the peripheral blood. In some instances, a hemorrhagic meningitis ensues. Respiratory failure, shock, and pulmonary edema are frequent causes of death.

Ingestion of markedly contaminated, poorly cooked meat may result in either the oropharyngeal or the gastrointestinal form of infection. When oropharyngeal anthrax occurs, there is localized swelling of the pharynx, sometimes causing tracheal obstruction, and marked cervical adenopathy with overlying brawny edema. Similarly, the organism may reach the small and large intestines and cause a gastrointestinal syndrome. In this case, the spores that are deposited in the submucosa of the intestinal tract may germinate, multiply, and produce toxin, again resulting in marked edema, hemorrhage, and necrosis. Regional mesenteric lymphadenopathy is common, and findings associated with the syndrome include fever, vomiting, abdominal pain and distention, massive bloody diarrhea, mesenteric adenitis, hemorrhagic ascites, and septicemia. Gastrointestinal anthrax is a very severe form of the disease, has a high mortality rate (25 to 75 per cent), and is rarely diagnosed during life except in the setting of an epidemic.

It is important to note that although antimicrobial agents may rapidly eradicate the organism, the persistence of the toxin that has been produced may result in continued development of the disease process until the toxin is metabolized. Thus, although the mortality rate may be diminished by appropriate antibiotic therapy, especially in the cutaneous form of the disease, the clinical process may continue to progress even after the institution of antimicrobial therapy. Antitoxins have been tried by some in the past, but such antitoxins are not currently available.

CLINICAL MANIFESTATIONS. Cutaneous anthrax is the most common form of the disease in humans, accounting for more than 95 per cent of cases. After an incubation period of 1 to 5 days, the infection generally begins with a small, somewhat pruritic papule at the site of an abrasion, which over the next several days develops into a vesicle containing serosanguineous fluid teeming with organisms. The lesion generally occurs on the upper extremities, especially the arms and hands, or on the face, neck, or other areas that are likely to be exposed to the contaminated animal product or infected soil. As the lesion progresses, ulceration occurs, with formation of a necrotic ulcer base that is frequently surrounded by smaller vesicles. The characteristic black eschar evolves over several weeks to a size of several centimeters, gradually separating and leaving a scar. This black eschar accounts for the name "anthrax," which comes from the Greek word for coal. The edema is frequently nonpitting, gelatinous, and brawny and is very striking. It may be quite extensive, spreading over a wide area in severe cases. With involvement near the eye, periorbital swelling may be especially intense. The edema may be so dramatic that hypotension occurs in part owing to the loss of intravascular volume as fluid enters the subcutaneous tissues. This edema, in combination with the vesicle progressing to the necrotic black eschar, forms the lesion that is highly characteristic of anthrax. Despite the dramatic appearance of the lesion, it is frequently painless.

In association with the localized cutaneous lesion, most patients present with minimal constitutional findings, such as fever, malaise, myalgias, and headaches. In those with extensive edema, the systemic symptoms may be more severe. Localized lymphadenopathy may occur at times and may be complicated by bacteremia and even meningitis. Death is rare if appropriate antimicrobial therapy is instituted; in untreated cases of cutaneous anthrax, however, the mortality rate remains about 25 per cent.

Bacterial adenitis due to staphylococci and streptococci, tularemia, plague, orf, cat scratch disease, localized herpes, and ecthyma gangrenosum are diagnostic considerations, and lesions seen in these diseases may be confused with those of anthrax. The diagnosis of cutaneous anthrax will rarely be missed if the disease is considered in any patient who has had exposure to an appropriate animal or animal product and who develops a painless ulcer surrounded by small vesicles, along with marked edema and eschar formation. Gram stains of the vesicular fluid and lesion usually readily demonstrate the characteristic gram-positive bacilli, as the organisms are present in large numbers in these lesions and are readily isolated by culture. Informing the bacteriology laboratory of the possibility of the diagnosis of anthrax is important to prevent the organism from being discarded as merely a probable contaminant of *Bacillus* species, which is frequently not fully characterized. At times, secondary bacterial infection may occur in these ulcers. Rarely, more than one lesion may be present, resulting from co-primary infections.

Inhalation anthrax is very rare, usually fatal, and extremely difficult to diagnose. The incubation period in this syndrome is generally 1 to 6 days, and the illness is generally biphasic. Initially, a brief, nonspecific "influenza-like" illness occurs, manifested by high fever, fatigue, myalgias, malaise, a nonproductive cough, and at times some chest discomfort. Few physical findings are noted at this time; however, within several days after a short period of clinical improvement, the patient becomes much more ill. This second phase is manifested by severe dyspnea, cyanosis, hypoxia, hemoptysis, stridor, chest pain, and diaphoresis. Physical examination may reveal some crepitant rales and evidence of pleural effusions. Some subcutaneous brawny edema of the chest wall and neck may be noted. The chest radiograph in these patients shows a rather distinctive clinical finding, namely, a widened mediastinum. Bacteremia, shock, and meningitis are frequently present, and death generally follows within 1 to 2 days of the onset of the respiratory distress. The mortality rate is 80 to 100 per cent, even with appropriate therapy.

Inhalation anthrax should be considered in patients with an appropriate exposure to an animal product, such as in a weaver using imported goat hair or a textile mill worker. The most important clue is the presence of an appropriate epidemiologic history in a patient developing severe respiratory distress and a rapidly enlarging mediastinum.

Gastrointestinal anthrax is an extremely rare disease and has an incubation period of 2 to 5 days, although there are some cases in which a more prolonged incubation period has been postulated. The diagnosis is rarely suspected before death except in areas where anthrax is highly endemic and in which multiple human cases are occurring. The symptoms include severe abdominal pain, hematemesis, melena, rapid onset of ascites, and at times marked diarrhea. Paracentesis may reveal hemorrhagic ascites, and sometimes these cases may simulate acute surgical abdomens. The disease usually progresses to bacteremia, toxemia, shock, and eventually death in many patients. No cases of intestinal anthrax have been reported in the United States.

Oropharyngeal anthrax presents as severe sore throat with neck swelling, adenopathy, dysphagia, and at times tracheal compression and dyspnea. Cervical and submandibular lymphadenopathy is common. Again, bacteremia and its complications may ensue.

The meningitis caused by anthrax is a complication of any of the forms of anthrax and almost never is found without a primary focus of infection. It is frequently hemorrhagic and most often fatal.

DIAGNOSIS. The clinician who elicits a careful epidemiologic history and who has a high index of suspicion of anthrax will not have problems establishing the diagnosis in cutaneous anthrax and will even be alert to the rarer and more difficult to recognize cases of inhalation, gastrointestinal, or oropharyngeal anthrax.

Inhalation anthrax is rarely suspected before death and only if an epidemiologic history of aerosol exposure is obtained or if an epidemic is recognized. The major finding in the clinical evaluation, other than epidemiologic history, is the presence of a widened mediastinum or at times hemorrhagic pleural effusions or an associated hemorrhagic meningitis. Ordinarily, Gram stains of sputum and cultures do not demonstrate *B. anthracis*. These patients frequently do develop bacteremia, however, and in these cases the organism can be readily isolated and sometimes seen on stains of the peripheral blood.

A number of serologic tests are available to diagnose anthrax retrospectively, but many of these very ill patients die so quickly that the initial serologic studies may not be especially helpful to the clinician. In some cases, however, serology has been a helpful diagnostic tool, especially when prior antibiotics have eradicated the bacteria before cultures or smears were obtained. Current serologic tests considered to be of value include an enzyme-linked immunosorbent assay (ELISA), which detects antibodies to the capsular antigen, and an electrophoretic immunotransblot test, which detects antibodies to the PA exotoxin. Both of these serologic tests are quite sensitive and specific enough to be useful, but the test for antibody to the PA exotoxin may be more specific.

TREATMENT. Penicillin G is the drug of choice for treatment of anthrax. Only a few isolates of *B. anthracis* have been identified as resistant to penicillin G. In cutaneous anthrax, cultures of the infected blisters have become negative for the organism within 5 hours of receiving 2 million units of penicillin G. As previously mentioned, however, the presence of the toxin may persist, and the cutaneous lesion frequently goes through its various phases of evolution, even though the organism has been eradicated and the mortality rate reduced.

For cutaneous anthrax, intravenous penicillin G is given, 2 million units every 6 hours for several days, followed by a 7- to 10-day course of oral penicillin G. In patients presenting with severe, overwhelming edema, corticosteroids have been thought by some to be helpful, although no controlled studies of its use have been performed. Severe neck swelling may require intubation or tracheostomy. In patients who are allergic to penicillin, effective alternatives include streptomycin, erythromycin, tetracycline, and chloramphenicol. No local surgery should be performed on these patients, since no pus requiring drainage is usually present and since excision of the lesion has been reported to increase the severity of symptoms and the spread of the organism. The lesion should be covered with a sterile dressing. There have been no definite cases of spread of anthrax from human to human.

In inhalation, gastrointestinal, or oropharyngeal anthrax or in anthrax meningitis, high dosages of intravenous penicillin G, in the range of 24 million units per day, are recommended, along with excellent supportive care for the problems of hypotension and respiratory distress. Some authors encourage the addition of parenteral streptomycin in a dosage of 1 to 2 grams per day to the penicillin G therapy in these cases. When the patient is hospitalized, good infection control practices are required. Soiled dressings must be incinerated or autoclaved.

PROGNOSIS. Inhalation anthrax is considered to be fatal in 80 to 100 per cent of cases, and gastrointestinal anthrax has a case fatality rate of 25 to 75 per cent. The case fatality rate for cutaneous anthrax is about 20 to 25 per cent without treatment but generally is less than 1 per cent with appropriate treatment.

PREVENTION. Control of anthrax in animals is essential to control of the disease in humans. All cases of animal anthrax, as well as human anthrax, should be reported to the state health department or the appropriate veterinary agency. Live avirulent animal vaccines are effective and may help control anthrax in endemic areas. Animals dying of anthrax should be cremated or buried, and care must be taken at autopsy to avoid additional contamination of the environment by infected blood and tissues. Prevention of human anthrax can be partially accomplished through proper disposal of the infected animals. In addition, formaldehyde has been used successfully to decontaminate raw wool and hair. A cell-free filtrate vaccine has been shown to protect humans from anthrax and is available from the Michigan State Department of Health. This vaccine should be offered to workers likely to be exposed to contaminated animal products in high-risk industries. Newer vaccines are being evaluated, such as a protective antigen (PA) toxoid vaccine and a protective antigen (PA)–producing live vaccine. In the Soviet Union, in addition to the chemical vaccine, a live anthrax spore vaccine has been widely used for prophylaxis against anthrax in both humans and animals. Good personal hygiene, as well as the use of protective clothing and respirators when contaminated aerosols are likely to be encountered, may also prove to be helpful preventive measures. Gastrointestinal anthrax can be prevented by proper cooking of meat and by avoiding ingestion of potentially contaminated meat.

Care must be taken in the laboratory when working with *B. anthracis*, since cases of anthrax have been acquired in this setting.

Brachman PS: Anthrax. *In* Evans A, Feldman H (eds.): Bacterial Infections of Humans: Epidemiology and Control. New York, Ms. Hilary Evans Publishing Company, 1982, pp 63–74. *Comprehensive summary of all aspects of anthrax, with emphasis on the epidemiology.*

Brachman PS: Inhalation anthrax. Ann NY Acad Sci 353:83, 1980. *A review of all aspects of inhalation anthrax.*

Gold H: Anthrax. Arch Intern Med 96:387, 1955. *Excellent clinical summary.*

Harrison LH, Ezzell JW, Abshire TG, et al.: Evaluation of serologic tests for diagnosis of anthrax after an outbreak of cutaneous anthrax in Paraguay. J Infect Dis 160:706, 1989. *Newer serologic methods for diagnosis and detection of immunity.*

Ivins BE, Welkos SL: Recent advances in the development of an improved human anthrax vaccine. Eur J Epidemiol 4:12, 1988. *New approach to vaccines for anthrax.*

Knudson GB: Treatment of anthrax in man: History and current concepts. Milit Med 151:71, 1986. *Reviews the history of anthrax with emphasis on treatment.*

Little SF, Knudson GB: Comparative efficacy of *Bacillus anthracis* live spore vaccine against anthrax in guinea pigs. Infect Immun 52:509, 1986. *Compares two different anthrax vaccines and discusses ELISA testing.*

Plotkin SA, Brachman PS, Utell M, et al.: An epidemic of inhalation anthrax, the first in the twentieth century. I. Clinical features. Am J Med 29:992, 1960. *Summarizes the clinical features of an epidemic of inhalation anthrax in the United States.*

324 Diseases Caused by Pseudomonads

Stephen C. Schimpff

PSEUDOMONADS

Pseudomonads are gram-negative aerobic bacilli that prefer moist environments and are relatively noninvasive, yet can cause serious and often fatal infection when the host defense mechanism is damaged or deficient. Each species is different in its pathogenic properties, each causes somewhat different types of infection, and each invades as a result of different host defense defects, but with each pseudomonad, the environmental source is usually water, moist soil, or a contaminated medical device, infusion, or injection.

Pseudomonads are divided into five major groups based upon RNA/DNA homology (Table 324–1). For purposes of discussion,

TABLE 324–1. CLASSIFICATION OF PSEUDOMONADS THAT HAVE BEEN ISOLATED FROM CLINICAL SPECIMENS

Group/Subgroup	Genus and Species
RNA group I	
Fluorescent group	P. aeruginosa
	P. fluorescens
	P. putida
Nonfluorescent group	P. stutzeri
	P. alcaligenes
	P. pseudoalcaligenes
RNA group II	P. mallei
	P. pseudomallei
	P. cepacia
	P. pickettii
RNA group III	P. acidovorans
	P. testosteroni
RNA group IV	P. diminuta
	P. vesicularis
RNA group V	Xanthomonas maltophilia

this chapter considers *Pseudomonas mallei* (the cause of melioidosis), *Pseudomonas pseudomallei* (the cause of glanders), *Pseudomonas aeruginosa* (which principally causes bacteremia, endocarditis, pneumonia, keratitis, and urinary tract infections), and *Pseudomonas cepacia* and *Pseudomonas (Xanthomonas) maltophilia* (which cause bacteremia, pseudobacteremia, endocarditis, and urinary tract infections).

Pseudomonas pseudomallei. This organism causes melioidosis, which is often characterized as a glanders-like infectious disease. It was first described in Rangoon among debilitated morphine addicts. The term "melioidosis" means "a similarity to distemper of asses." Despite the clinical resemblance to glanders, it has a totally different epidemiology. Melioidosis occurs in animals and humans in endemic areas of southeast Asia and northern Australia and has now been recognized to occur in epidemic-like form in specific areas, given the combination of the environment (an appropriate rainy season with water-covered rice paddies) and a susceptible host (abraded skin in barefoot farmers who have a high prevalence of diabetes mellitis and renal calculi).

P. pseudomallei is a gram-negative, motile, aerobic bacillus that is small and may grow in filamentous chains. Staining with methylene blue or Wright's stain shows a bipolar "safety pin" pattern. *P. pseudomallei* has a characteristic wrinkling appearance of the colonies on agar if held long enough. The organism, like most pseudomonads, can be isolated from soil and water and particularly streams, rice paddies, and ponds of the endemic areas and on plants, including commonly consumed vegetables. Most human infection probably occurs through skin abrasions. However, laboratory animals have been found to become infected by the respiratory route, so inhalation may be a possible human route of acquisition, which would explain the occurrence of primary pneumonia.

At the conclusion of American involvement in the Vietnam War, 343 cases were reported, with 36 deaths among the American military; however, serologic surveys suggest that either mild or inapparent infection may be fairly common, with positive serologies found in 1 to 2 per cent of healthy, nonwounded U.S. Army troops returning to the United States. This would suggest that as many as 225,000 Americans may have had subclinical infection with *P. pseudomallei*. The importance of this observation is that recrudescence of disease has been observed many years after primary infection.

In addition to inapparent infection or asymptomatic pulmonary infection, the frequently observed forms of melioidosis are an acute, localized, suppurative soft tissue infection, an acute pulmonary infection, and an acute septicemic presentation. The localized infections are probably related to skin abrasion, with the development of a nodule with secondary lymphangitis and regional lymphadenitis. It is likely that this is the form of infection that progresses to the acute septicemic phase. An apparent primary pulmonary infection ranges from bronchitis to necrotizing pneumonia. For the patient with pneumonia, there is usually high fever and signs and symptoms of consolidation, ordinarily in an upper lobe. It is an acute pyogenic process, frequently leading to early cavitation and giving a pulmonary appearance consistent with tuberculosis. Progression to bacteremia is rare.

Patients with the acute septic form characteristically present with a short history of fever and no clinical evidence of focal infection. Most are profoundly ill, with signs of sepsis, such as tachypnea or Kussmaul's breathing, and occasional evidence of septic shock. Clinical and radiologic evidence frequently demonstrates progression to diffuse bilateral and patchy pulmonary infiltrate, which progresses to abscess and cavity formation if the patient survives. Subcutaneous abscesses are relatively uncommon but can occur at multiple sites, as can visceral abscesses, such as in the liver or spleen.

The diagnosis should be considered in any patient living in an endemic area who has a febrile illness and especially one who is occupationally at risk and, perhaps, who is at further risk of sepsis because of diabetes or renal disease. The diagnosis should be highly suspected in such an individual who presents with a rapidly progressive, extensive pulmonary process if there are subcutaneous lesions or in one whose condition progresses to a cavitary form indistinguishable from tuberculosis. A Gram stain of pulmonary or abscess exudate shows small gram-negative bacilli, and methylene blue staining shows the bipolar "safety pin" characteristic. The organism grows on standard media and is usually detected in blood cultures within 48 hours.

In northeast Thailand, a report from a hospital that serves a population of nearly 2 million rural rice farming families determined that about 20 per cent of all community-acquired bacteremias were caused by *P. pseudomallei* and that during the rainy season, when the paddy fields are under water (from June to September), *P. pseudomallei* was the single most common organism isolated from blood culture, representing nearly one half of all documented cases of community-acquired bacteremia in the month of August (Fig. 324–1). An interesting observation was the higher than expected frequency of both diabetes mellitus and renal calculi in patients with sepsis who are from this region, where both diabetes and calculi are common.

Treatment of pulmonary or suspected septic forms should probably begin with a combination of agents. The standard recommended treatment has been a combination of chloramphenicol, doxycycline, and trimethoprim-sulfamethoxazole. These agents, however, are bacteriostatic rather than bactericidal and do not represent a regimen one would wish to use for suspected community-acquired bacteremia. Although clinical data remain limited, the third-generation cephalosporin ceftazidime is now likely the drug of choice, with carbapenem, imipenem, piperacillin, or amoxicillin–clavulanic acid as reasonable alternatives. The addition of an aminoglycoside during empiric therapy might be appropriate until culture results are known. Treatment apparently needs to be prolonged, including intravenous therapy (ceftazidime, imipenem, or piperacillin) for 2 to 4 weeks, followed by oral therapy (perhaps amoxicillin–clavulanic acid) for 6 months or longer to prevent recrudescence.

The prognosis for patients with localized disease should be excellent with appropriate therapy. However, those with the septicemic form are often gravely ill at the time of admission, and the mortality rate reported in 1989 was 68 per cent. Some groups of patients with the highest mortality were those who were hypothermic, azotemic, or unable to produce a leukocytosis. It should be pointed out that in the reported survey only 27 per cent of the patients with septicemic melioidosis were given an antibiotic active against *P. pseudomallei* as part of the initial empiric regimen. Thus, it remains unclear what the survival rate would be in patients treated promptly with an appropriate agent, especially ceftazidime, imipenem, or amoxicillin–clavulanic acid.

Evidence also exists that melioidosis may be more frequent

among immunocompromised individuals. In a report from Bangkok, Thailand, 49 cases of melioidosis seen over a 12-year period occurred exclusively among patients with diabetes mellitus, collagen vascular disorders, leukemia, lymphoma, or aplastic anemia. Twenty-nine of the 49 had the disseminated, or septic, form of the infection. Some associated infections included tuberculosis, candidiasis, aspergillosis, cytomegalovirus infection, and Epstein-Barr virus infection, all being infections associated with depressed cellular immunity. Among these patients, the mortality in those with localized melioidosis was low, whereas it was high in those with disseminated disease. An interesting finding among a subgroup of these patients demonstrated that the four patients with localized melioidosis who were evaluated had normal numbers of lymphocytes, including T-helper and T-suppressor lymphocytes, whereas the seven evaluated patients with disseminated melioidosis had a marked reduction in total lymphocytes and one third of the lower limit of normal for T-helper lymphocytes. This finding suggests that dissemination of *P. pseudomallei* is at least in part a function of an effective cellular arm of the immune system.

Pseudomonas mallei. *P. mallei* can cause an infection in horses, mules, and donkeys that occasionally has been transmitted to humans. The name "glanders" comes from the prominent pulmonary involvement, although the infection can, instead, be characterized by subcutaneous ulcerative lesions or lymphatic thickening with nodules (known as farcy).

Glanders was never a common human infection, and with the decline in the use of horses for day-to-day activities and with improved sanitation, glanders has become a very rare disease. Apparently, there have been no naturally acquired infections in the United States since 1938, although the occasional case occurs in other countries.

Like melioidosis, glanders tends to occur as an acute localized suppurative infection, an acute pulmonary infection, an acute septicemic infection, or a chronic suppurative infection. An abraded area of skin may lead to a local nodule with acute lymphangitis. Inoculation into an abraded mucous membrane can lead to extensive ulcerating granulomatous lesions. These forms of infection seem to have an incubation period of 1 to 5 days; in contrast, after inhalation, a primary pneumonia tends to develop 10 to 14 days later. Symptoms are relatively nonspecific and include fever, occasional rigors, malaise, fatigue, and headache. Examination findings depend upon the form of infection. Leukocytosis is common. Chest radiographs of the acute pulmonary form usually show densities consistent with early lung abscess; however, lobar or bronchopneumonia-type infiltrates are common. Chronic suppurative disease involves multiple subcutaneous and intramuscular abscesses, especially on the extremities, with lymphatic involvement and, in many, a nasal discharge with or without ulceration.

The organism is usually difficult to find in exudates, but, when seen with a Gram stain or methylene blue, appears similar to *P. pseudomallei*. The organism is reasonably easy to cultivate.

The treatment of glanders is uncertain because of the rarity of the disease and therefore the inability to carry out clinical trials. A reasonable recommendation is to initiate therapy with regimens found effective for melioidosis, recognizing that the acute septicemic form has been uniformly fatal in the past and suggesting that the full dosage of intravenous combinations of agents be given initially.

Pseudomonas aeruginosa. The name "aeruginosa" comes from the flourescent blue-green pigment pyocyanin, produced by many, but not all, strains. Other pigments produced by *P. aeruginosa* include pyoverdin (green) and, occasionally, pyorubin (deep red) and pyomelanin (black). Like other pseudomonads, *P. aeruginosa* grows well in multiple moist settings with limited nutrients. Found in soil, in water, and on plants, it can also be a normal commensal in animals and humans. Colonization in humans usually takes place in moist areas, such as perineum, auditory canal, axillae, and the lower alimentary canal. It is commonly found in sink traps, ice machines, and kitchen settings in the hospital; it can become a particular problem when it contaminates medications or medical devices with a moist environment, such as ventilators, endoscopes, pressure monitors, and the like. It can withstand many disinfectants and is resistant to a broad variety of antimicrobial agents. In the nonhospital setting, infections have been related to growth in swimming pools, contact lens solutions, and hot tubs.

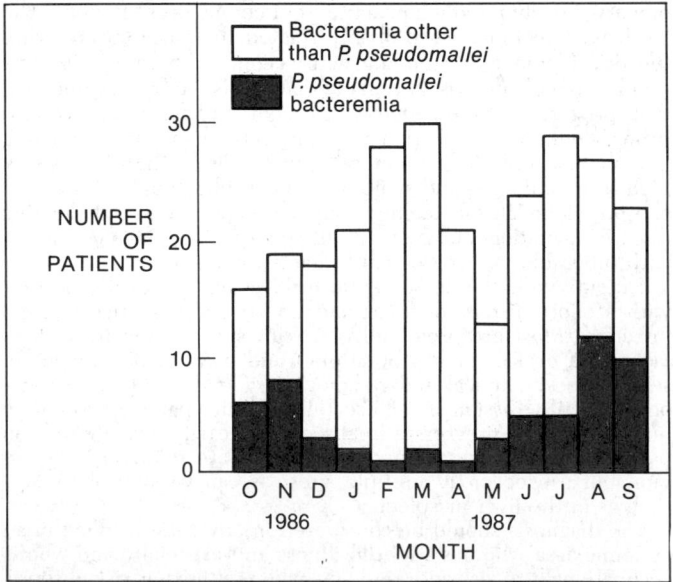

FIGURE 324–1. Number of persons with community-acquired bacteremia caused by *P. pseudomallei* and other organisms, in northeast Thailand from October 1986 to September 1987. (From Chaowagul W, White NJ, Dance DAB, et al.: Melioidosis: A major cause of community-acquired septicemia in northeastern Thailand. J Infect Dis 159:890–899, 1989; by permission of the University of Chicago Press, 1989.)

Infection with *P. aeruginosa* has become, to a large degree, a by-product of medical advances in technology. In the 20 years prior to 1960 at the Johns Hopkins Hospital, only 91 cases of *P. aeruginosa* bacteremia occurred. Today, *P. aeruginosa* is the fourth most common cause of primary nosocomial gram-negative bacteremia and is the fourth most frequently isolated nosocomial pathogen, causing about 10 per cent of all hospital-acquired infections, 13 per cent of all nosocomial pneumonias, 12 per cent of urinary tract infections, and 7 per cent of surgical wound infections.

The most common infections caused by *P. aeruginosa* include nosocomial bacteremia; nosocomial pneumonia; nosocomial urinary tract infection; surgical wound infection; endocarditis related to intravenous drug abuse or placement of artificial heart valves; respiratory infection associated with cystic fibrosis; external otitis, including "malignant" external otitis (see Ch. 471); corneal keratitis; and uncommon occurrences of spinal osteomyelitis in heroin addicts (see Ch. 304) and rare cases of meningitis or brain abscess. A common origin of bacteremia in the granulocytopenic patient is infection along the alimentary canal, especially perianal cellulitis, colonic lesions, and, occasionally, pharyngitis or esophagitis. Finally, extensive burns are commonly colonized by *P. aeruginosa*, with progression to sepsis and death.

P. aeruginosa almost never causes infection in the absence of (1) damage to a normal host defense mechanism (e.g., cancer chemotherapy–induced mucosal damage to the alimentary canal or extensive third-degree burns); (2) deficiency or alteration in a defense mechanism (e.g., the progressive respiratory tract changes of cystic fibrosis); or (3) bypass of a normal defense mechanism (e.g., respiratory assist device directly inoculating organisms into the bronchial tree while concurrently limiting or damaging the mucociliary mechanism, or insertion of an indwelling urinary catheter, circumventing the normal bladder clearance mechanism). Thus, infections with *P. aeruginosa* are most commonly seen in patients with a urinary catheter; those neutropenic from disease, chemotherapy, or both; those with cystic fibrosis; those with extensive thermal injuries; those in the intensive care unit who are subjected to any number of invasive procedures; those with head trauma, allowing entry either directly or via a pressure monitoring device; those with artificial heart valves or damaged endocardium from contaminants in illicit drugs; and those who have had extensive surgery, particularly when there is consequent need for open drainage.

Pollack has pointed out three distinct stages of *Pseudomonas* infection: stage I—bacterial attachment and colonization; stage II—local invasion; and stage III—bloodstream dissemination and systemic disease. Stage I is a prerequisite to stage II, which, in turn, is a prerequisite to stage III, although obviously not all colonized individuals have local invasion and not all those with local invasion progress to dissemination or systemic disease. The three stages relate to the fact that this organism is both invasive and toxigenic. Colonization in a normal person is relatively uncommon at most sites, although over time, a fair proportion of the population will have transient colonization of the colon. However, hospitalized patients have a much higher frequency of colonization, related, in part, to changes in host defenses, as discussed above, and, in part, to the frequency of hospital reservoirs of this organism. In addition, broad-spectrum antimicrobial therapy suppresses other normal microbial flora, especially along the alimentary canal. This suppression reduces the body's normal mechanism of colonization resistance, so that an organism such as *P. aeruginosa* or other species resistant to the antibiotics used can more readily colonize multiple locations in high concentration. Additional specific factors further predispose to colonization by *P. aeruginosa*. These include the presence of pili for attachment, flagella for motility, and exoproducts, especially proteinases. Also involved is the secretory protease-induced loss of fibronectin from epithelial cells during serious illness (among patients hospitalized or not), which, in turn, allows the pili or fimbriae to adhere to the oral, pharyngeal, and respiratory epithelium. Thus, the illness determinants of protease production are major modulators of the oral flora. This colonization, in turn, can be accentuated by local damage caused by an endotracheal tube, by viral infection (such as influenza), by thermal injury, or by cancer chemotherapy and is exacerbated by antibiotics. *P. aeruginosa*, in some settings, can help protect itself from defense mechanisms by the production of a glycocalyx, a carbohydrate produced by many bacteria, which, by surrounding the cell and anchoring it to epithelial cells or invasive devices, such as an intravascular or urinary catheter, protects the bacterium from antibody, complement, and polymorphonuclear leukocytes or macrophages.

After colonization, *P. aeruginosa* can invade in the appropriate setting through the effect of extracellular enzymes (toxins). These include elastase, alkaline protease, and perhaps also cytotoxin and hemolysins. Elastase and protease have been demonstrated to cause necrotizing lesions in the skin, lung, and cornea, along with small vessel necrotizing lesions, which cause the characteristic skin finding known as ecthyma gangrenosum. It is this combination of local necrosis and blood vessel destruction that is the essence of the initial invasive characteristic of *P. aeruginosa*.

The third stage of *Pseudomonas* infection, dissemination and systemic disease, is due, in the first case, to these same extracellular enzymes and, in the second case, to *Pseudomonas* liposaccharide (endotoxin) and exotoxin A. As with other septicemias caused by gram-negative bacilli, endotoxin is thought to be a critical factor in the activation of the clotting, fibrinolytic, kinin, and complement systems, along with the production of prostaglandins and leukotrienes, the release of β-endorphins, and the release of cytokines, including tumor necrosis factor. By some interaction of many or all of these factors come fever, shock, disseminated intravascular coagulation (which is relatively uncommon with *Pseudomonas* bacteremia), and the adult respiratory distress syndrome. The other factor, exotoxin A, is similar to diphtheria toxin in that it inhibits protein synthesis. It causes local necrosis and encourages bacterial dissemination to the systemic circulation and, in itself, has been shown to produce shock in animal models.

Pseudomonas bacteremia occurs most commonly in cancer patients who are receiving intensive chemotherapy that produces granulocytopenia in patients with extensive third-degree burns, and, occasionally, in patients with immunoglobulin or hypocomplementemia states. It is also a common cause of bacteremia in the patient with urinary catheterization. It is the fourth most frequent cause of primary hospital-acquired gram-negative bacteremia. Sepsis in burn patients arises from the thermally damaged skin. Bacteremia in neutropenic patients arises principally from the lower intestinal tract and occasionally from primary pneumonia. Surveillance cultures have documented that granulocytopenic patients frequently become colonized, and nearly all colonized patients will develop bacteremia if profound (<100 per microliter) granulocytopenia persists for more than a few days. Ecthyma gangrenosum, usually a sign of fairly advanced systemic infection, is not pathognomonic but is most frequently associated with *P. aeruginosa* bacteremia. These skin lesions at first are small and indurated, and then they rapidly enlarge, become necrotic, and may ulcerate. Bacteria, on histologic section, are seen to be invading small arteries and veins, with remarkably minimal evidence of inflammation. A histologically similar lesion can be found in the lungs as a secondary consequence of bacteremia. The mortality of *Pseudomonas* sepsis is high, with the underlying status of the patient's host defenses and the promptness of institution of empiric antibiotic therapy being the two critical factors affecting survival. The presence of septic shock, the evidence of septic metastases, or both, at the initiation of antibiotic administration are usually considered adverse prognostic signs but, in reality, represent another measure of late institution of therapy.

The standard approach to suspected gram-negative sepsis, including that caused by *P. aeruginosa*, is a combination employing an antipseudomonal β-lactam (penicillin or cephalosporin) with an aminoglycoside. Two newer drugs, imipenem or the antipseudomonal quinolones—again, in combination with an aminoglycoside—are also effective. Although in some cases, such as in the febrile, neutropenic patient, monotherapy has been recommended with agents such as ceftazidime or imipenem, a two-drug regimen is advised for initial empiric therapy. A number of studies suggest that survival is improved when two antibiotics to which the organism is susceptible are administered immediately and that survival is further improved if the two agents prove to be synergistic in activity. For the future, we must look also to immunologic approaches to bacteremia prevention and treatment, such as monoclonal antibodies to lipopolysaccharide.

Respiratory tract infections (see also Ch. 294) can take the form of a primary pneumonia, a secondary pneumonia due to bacteremia, or a chronic infection with intermittent exacerbations. Primary pneumonia occurs almost exclusively in hospitalized patients whose oropharynx or tracheobronchial tree is colonized by *P. aeruginosa* as a result of intubation. Frequently, *Pseudomonas* pneumonia occurs in the setting of additional pulmonary damage, such as blunt trauma, substantial atelectasis, or hemothorax. Atelectasis appears to be a key contributing pathogenic factor. Early, aggressive physiotherapy for the chest sometimes clears what appears to be a pneumonia but, in fact, is atelectasis that has resulted in fever, purulent sputum production, and a positive chest radiograph. However, once actual pneumonia has begun, the prognosis is poor, and early empiric therapy is critical.

The pneumonia that follows bacteremia is usually fulminant, with multiple areas of hemorrhage around small and medium-sized pulmonary arteries and lesions caused by necrosis of the small muscular arteries and veins in a fashion similar to ecthyma gangrenosum. Survival is limited even with prompt, aggressive therapy.

Chronic *Pseudomonas* respiratory infections are largely limited to patients with cystic fibrosis (see also Ch. 64), with the frequency of this infection increasing with age, so that, ultimately, almost all patients will have significant *Pseudomonas* pulmonary infection. The age differential is probably related to the progressive development of airway obstruction, which seems to be a critical factor in the development of *Pseudomonas* infection. This chronic infection is associated with chronic cough, nutritional losses, and progressive loss of pulmonary function. The standard treatment has been an antipseudomonal penicillin plus an aminoglycoside. The development of resistance is common, so therapy must therefore be based on susceptibility patterns. Ceftazidime, imipenem, or a quinolone may also be considered. Acute exacerbations may be reduced or even prevented with intermittent therapy a number of times each year, irrespective of whether the infection is currently quiescent.

OTHER PSEUDOMONADS

Pseudomonas cepacia. This species of *Pseudomonas* can grow as well in distilled water as it can in trypticase soy broth; it is resistant to many of the commonly used hospital disinfectants; it can use penicillin as a carbon source; and it is resistant to many of the commonly used antimicrobials. Its virulence properties are not understood.

Community-acquired infections are, without doubt, rare. However, certain hosts are at substantially increased risk. Endocarditis has occurred among intravenous drug abusers; skin infections related to extensive burns have occurred; a necrotizing, occasionally recurrent pneumonia has occurred among patients with the phagocytic dysfunction of chronic granulomatous disease; and an emerging problem for cystic fibrosis patients has been a relentless, often fulminating pneumonia caused by *P. cepacia*.

Nosocomial infections and pseudoinfections are considered

together because of a common origin and because it is sometimes difficult to distinguish between the two. The source of *P. cepacia* in the hospital setting is usually a moist or water-based reservoir, which, given the technologic advances of medicine in recent decades, suggests that *P. cepacia* has the potential to become a not infrequent cause of infection and pseudoinfection in the high-technology or intensive care setting. *P. cepacia* has been found to cause pneumonitis, endocarditis, wound infections, and urinary tract infections, along with primary bacteremia. The origins of iatrogenic bacteremia can be conveniently divided into those related to contaminated solutions, injectables, and medical devices. Among the contaminated solutions that have been implicated in bacteremia or pseudobacteremia have been disinfectant solutions, heparinized flushing solutions, distilled water, topical anesthetics, and intravenous infusates, including human serum albumin and cryoprecipitate. Contaminated injectables have included saline, methylprednisolone, and fentanyl. The implicated devices all have the common property of including a moist environment where the organism can multiply; pressure monitoring devices, respiratory assist devices, peritoneal dialysis machines, reusable hemodialysis coils, and blood gas analyzers have been documented as point sources.

Figure 324–2 shows an epidemic of *P. cepacia* bacteremia among patients at the Clinical Center of the National Institutes of Health. The figure indicates that *P. cepacia*–positive blood cultures were uncommon in the years preceding this outbreak and that the majority during the epidemic occurred within the medical intensive care unit. A blood gas analyzer in an adjoining laboratory was found to be contaminated, and this served as the point source for this series of bacteremias. Although some were apparently pseudobacteremias, (i.e., the blood culture became positive owing to contamination by skin or other sources), others were true bacteremias with significant morbidity. Indeed, among those highly compromised patients, many with cancer and significant immune suppression, the mortality resulting from the *P. cepacia* infection itself was 38 per cent.

P. cepacia is resistant to many of the commonly used broad-spectrum antibiotics but does usually tend to be susceptible to trimethoprim-sulfamethoxazole.

Pseudomonas maltophilia (Xanthomonas maltophilia). *X. maltophilia* is atypical of the other pseudomonads in that the oxidase test is negative or equivocal. It is probably a fairly common commensal and a part of the transient flora, especially of hospitalized patients. In the hospital environment, it is not infrequently found in moist or wet settings. The organism is resistant to most of the first- and second-generation cephalosporins, semisynthetic penicillins, and aminoglycosides, although it has variable susceptibility to the antipseudomonal penicillins. It is generally susceptible to many of the third-generation cephalosporins, trimethoprim-sulfamethoxazole, and rifampin. Synergy has been noted with trimethoprim-sulfamethoxazole plus carbenicillin and with the triple regimen of trimethoprim-sulfamethoxazole plus carbenicillin and rifampin.

X. maltophilia is an uncommon cause of a wide spectrum of diseases that, in general, are less severe than infections caused

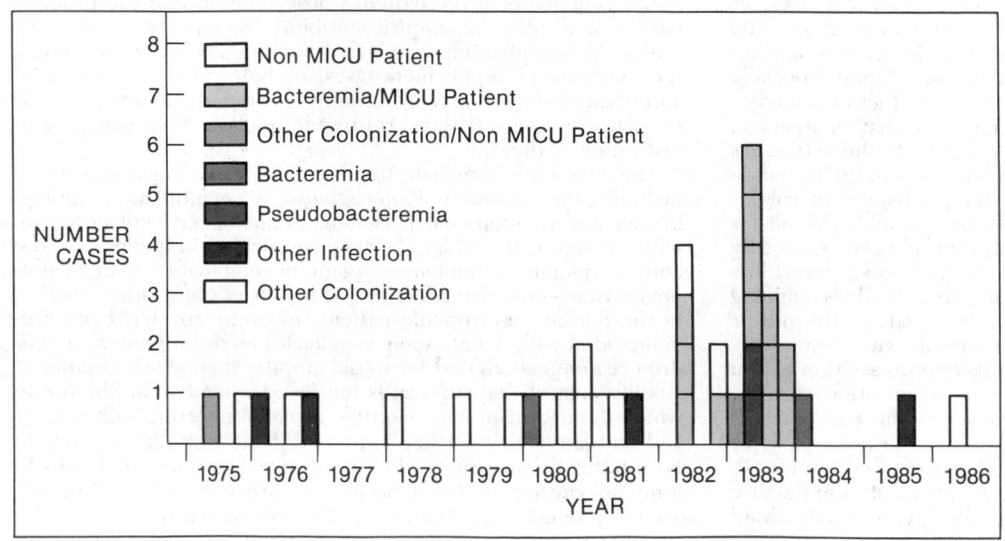

FIGURE 324–2. An epidemic of *Pseudomonas cepacia* bacteremia among patients at the Clinical Center of the National Institutes of Health. MICU = medical intensive care unit. (Reprinted with permission from Henderson DK, Baptiste R, Parillo J, et al.: Indolent epidemic of *Pseudomonas cepacia* bacteremia and pseudobacteremia in an intensive care unit traced to a contaminated blood gas analyzer. Am J Med 84:75–81, 1988.)

by other gram-negative bacilli in similar locations. Currently, *X. maltophilia* infections are relatively responsive to antimicrobial therapy. The most common types of infection are pneumonia, endocarditis, urinary tract infection, and iatrogenic bacteremia or pseudobacteremia. Cholangitis and meningitis have been reported but are quite unusual, and wounds, although a common site for *X. maltophilia* isolation, are rarely infected by this organism. Pneumonias tend to occur in debilitated patients with prior antibiotic therapy in a nosocomial setting, but they are very uncommon, and the organism should be questioned as causative in the absence of a pure culture via bronchoscopy, thoracentesis, or blood. Endocarditis in the community occurs among intravenous drug abusers and in the hospital as a complication of open heart surgery, usually among those with abnormal valves.

X. maltophilia bacteriuria is found somewhat often in patients with indwelling long-term catheters; however, only rarely has the organism been shown to cause clinical infection. When infection has occurred, it has usually been in association with significant instrumentation, genitourinary surgery, or both. The morbidity has tended to be low, and therapy, especially with trimethoprim-sulfamethoxazole, has frequently been effective.

Iatrogenic bacteremia and pseudobacteremia caused by this organism have been reported often. In one epidemic of 25 patients with positive blood cultures, it was determined that these cases were pseudobacteremias due to contaminated blood collection tubes. In another setting, eight children were found to have bacteremia after open heart surgery, apparently as a result of contamination of the monitoring transducers in the intensive care unit. *X. maltophilia* has been found to contaminate the deionized water used for diluting disinfectants, and the organism can even survive in the diluted disinfectant. It is important to emphasize that not all of these bacteremias have been "pseudobacteremias"; for example, two fatal cases of endocarditis have been noted as a result of bacteremia caused by a contaminated device or solution.

Bodey GP, Jadeja L, Elting L: *Pseudomonas* bacteremia: Retrospective analysis of 410 episodes. Arch Intern Med 145:1621, 1985. *A review of* P. aeruginosa *bacteremia.*

Curtin JA, Petersdorf RG, Bennett IL: Pseudomonas bacteremia: Review of ninety-one cases. Ann Intern Med 54:1077, 1961. *A classic paper describing* P. aeruginosa *bacteremia.*

Dance DAB, Wuthiekanun V, Chaowagul W, et al.: The antimicrobial susceptibility of *Pseudomonas pseudomallei*. Emergence of resistance *in vitro* and during treatment. J Antimicrob Chemother 24:295, 1989. *New data on the antimicrobial susceptibility of* P. pseudomallei *to the newer antibiotics, with reference to clinical trials.*

Henderson DK, Baptiste R, Parillo J, et al.: Indolent epidemic of *Pseudomonas cepacia* bacteremia and pseudobacteremia in an intensive care unit traced to a contaminated blood gas analyzer. Am J Med 84:75, 1988. *A nice review of bacteremia and pseudobacteremia due to* P. cepacia.

Marshall WF, Keating MR, Anhalt JP, Steckelberg JM: *Xanthomonas maltophilia*: An emerging nosocomial pathogen. Mayo Clin Proc 64:1097, 1989. *A thorough review of infection due to* Pseudomonas (Xanthomonas) maltophilia.

Palleroni NJ: Family Pseudomonadaceae. *In* Kreig NR, Holt JG (eds.): Bergey's Manual of Systematic Bacteriology. Vol. 1. Baltimore, The Williams and Wilkins Company, 1984, pp 141–219. *Basic reference manual for taxonomy of bacteria.*

Pollack M: *Pseudomonas aeruginosa*. *In* Mandell GL, Douglas RG Jr, Bennett JE (eds.): Principles and Practice of Infectious Diseases. 3rd ed. New York, Churchill Livingstone, 1990, pp 1673–1691. *A very thorough discussion of the microbiology, epidemiology, pathogenic factors, and clinical syndromes of* P. aeruginosa.

Sanford JP: Pseudomonas species (including melioidosis and glanders). *In* Mandell GL, Douglas RG Jr, Bennett JE (eds.): Principles and Practice of Infectious Diseases. 3rd ed. New York, Churchill Livingstone, 1990, pp 1692–1696. *Broad discussion of melioidosis and glanders by an expert in infections of importance to the U.S. military.*

325 Listeriosis

Alan M. Stamm

DEFINITION. Listeriosis is an infectious disease caused by the bacterium *Listeria monocytogenes*. The majority of afflicted patients are immunocompromised and present with meningoencephalitis.

ETIOLOGY. *Listeria monocytogenes* is a gram-positive bacillus but may stain unevenly and/or appear coccoid. It is facultatively anaerobic, non–spore forming, and β-hemolytic on blood agar. It grows optimally at 35 to 37°C, grows less well at temperatures as low as 4°C, and exhibits tumbling motility at 20 to 25°C.

Although at least 16 serotypes of *L. monocytogenes* are identified, each of the types 1/2a, 1/2b, and 4b accounts for about 30 per cent of human disease in the United States. These serotypes are uniformly distributed throughout this country. Six other species of *Listeria* exist, but they are rarely pathogenic for humans.

EPIDEMIOLOGY. *Listeria monocytogenes* is distributed widely in nature throughout the world. It is recovered from water, soil, decaying vegetation, silage, sewage, insects, crustaceans, fish, birds, and wild and domestic mammals. Sporadic as well as epizootic disease, manifest as meningitis, encephalitis, or spontaneous abortion, occurs in sheep, cattle, and goats. Asymptomatic human intestinal carriage is present in 1 to 5 per cent of normal adults and in 20 to 25 per cent of case contacts.

Neonates and the elderly have the highest attack rates of listeriosis. The sexes are equally represented. The incidence of disease is not significantly different across the United States or from one continent to another. Consistent seasonal patterns are noted, with disease occurring most commonly in domestic animals in late winter to early spring and in humans in late summer to early fall. However, the correlation between the number and location of animal cases and human cases is poor in any one region, and direct animal-to-human transmission of disease is rarely documented.

Epidemiologic investigations of outbreaks of listeriosis have demonstrated their frequent foodborne etiology. Manure from infected sheep was used to fertilize cabbage plants in the Maritime Provinces of Canada; 41 cases of human disease in 1980–1981 were linked to the ingestion of cole slaw prepared from these cabbages. Milk from cows was pasteurized but nonetheless implicated in 49 cases of listeriosis in Massachusetts in 1983; whether the microorganism survived pasteurization or contaminated the product afterward remains controversial. The largest epidemic occurred in southern California in 1985; 142 cases were associated with the consumption of soft, Mexican-style cheese made with unpasteurized milk. Similarly, an outbreak of 122 cases in Switzerland during 1983–1987 was attributed to a soft cheese. During periods of increased disease activity, the organism causing an epidemic is differentiated from those causing sporadic disease by serotyping, phage typing, or electrophoretic enzyme typing. All four of these outbreaks were due to *L. monocytogenes* serotype 4b.

Further evidence for foodborne acquisition of *L. monocytogenes* is provided by recent microbiologic investigations. The microorganism has been identified as a fairly common contaminant of raw and pasteurized milk; ice cream; raw beef, pork, and lamb; ready-to-eat meat products, including salami, sausages, and hot dogs; retail poultry; cooked shrimp and crab; raw vegetables such as cabbage, cucumbers, potatoes, and radishes; and packaged salads. Studies to date have not shown contamination of eggs or fruits. Although commercial food production methods may effectively kill the microorganism, products may become contaminated during subsequent processing and packaging before leaving the production facility.

PATHOGENESIS. The majority of adults with listeriosis have impaired cell-mediated immunity caused by cytotoxic chemotherapy for malignancy, immunosuppressive therapy for organ transplantation, or pregnancy. Both helper and suppressor T cells are centrally involved, whereas immunoglobulin and complement play lesser roles as opsonins. The gastrointestinal tract is the usual portal of entry. Bacteria are taken up from the lumen by endocytosis of epithelial cells covering intestinal villi. The inoculum required to cause disease may depend on the immunologic health and gastric acidity of the host as well as the virulence characteristics of the microorganism.

Dissemination occurs via simple bacteremia and/or circulation of infected monocytes. *Listeria monocytogenes* is a facultative intracellular parasite capable of multiplying within the nonimmune monocyte-macrophage. Listeriolysin O, a hemolysin structurally similar to streptolysin O, may be an important virulence factor in this process. Phagocytosis of the bacterium stimulates its production; it binds to cholesterol in cell membranes, leading to their disruption. This feature may allow the microorganism to escape from phagolysosomes but to persist and multiply within macrophages, ultimately leading to their destruction.

Factors external to the human host and the bacterium may also be important. Investigation of an outbreak of 36 cases of listeriosis in Philadelphia in 1986–1987 identified no predominant serotype. It is hypothesized that an epidemic co-infection may have triggered disease through an effect on the mucosal barrier or on intestinal motility in those previously merely colonized by *L. monocytogenes*.

Transmission from the pregnant woman to the fetus may occur either transplacentally or at the time of vaginal delivery. Listeriolysin O may increase uterine contractility and contribute to fetal loss.

CLINICAL MANIFESTATIONS. The incubation period between acquisition of infection and onset of disease varies from days to weeks. The clinical presentation of listeriosis is as meningitis in 50 to 60 per cent of cases; bacteremia without evident localized disease in 25 to 30 per cent; parenchymal disease of the central nervous system (CNS), with or without meningitis, in 10 per cent; and endocarditis in 5 per cent. Infrequent manifestations due to hematogenous dissemination include anterior uveitis, endophthalmitis, cervical lymphadenitis, pneumonia, empyema, pericarditis, peritonitis, hepatitis, liver abscess, cholecystitis, mycotic aneurysm, osteomyelitis, and arthritis.

Listeria monocytogenes is the etiologic agent in about 1 per cent of cases of acute bacterial meningitis. However, among patients with cancer, it is responsible for more than one fifth of episodes. Conversely, among patients with *Listeria* meningitis, 25 per cent have a malignancy; 25 per cent are transplant recipients; 20 per cent have another underlying disorder, such as diabetes mellitus or cirrhosis, or are receiving glucocorticosteroids; and 30 per cent have no predisposing condition. Two thirds of patients experience a fairly sudden onset of symptoms, but one third note an insidious progression over several days. No features distinguish *Listeria* meningitis. High fever is almost always reported. Headache, meningismus, and a decreased level of consciousness are present in more than one half of patients. Focal neurologic deficits and seizures are found in about one fourth. Most patients have 100 to 10,000 white blood cells per cubic millimeter of cerebrospinal fluid (CSF), with two thirds of them being polymorphonuclear cells. The CSF glucose level is less than 50 mg per deciliter in one half of cases, and the protein level is usually 50 to 300 mg per deciliter. The Gram stain of CSF is interpreted as revealing gram-positive bacilli in only 25 per cent of cases. Cultures of blood are positive in 60 to 75 per cent. The differential diagnosis includes disease due to *Streptococcus pneumoniae*, a gram-negative bacillus, or *Cryptococcus neoformans*.

Parenchymal disease of the CNS is associated with clinical and CSF findings of meningitis in only 50 per cent of cases. Anatomically, the spectrum of disease includes diffuse and localized cerebritis, brain stem meningoencephalitis (rhombencephalitis), and macroscopic abscess formation in the brain or spine. All patients are febrile; other common symptoms and signs are decreased consciousness in two thirds of patients, headache and hemiparesis in one half, and seizures and cranial nerve palsies in one third. *Listeria* rhombencephalitis merits special mention. Eight of the first 11 reported victims have been previously healthy. The illness has a biphasic course: A 3- to 10-day prodrome of fever, headache, and vomiting is terminated by the abrupt onset of palsies of cranial nerves V, VI, VII, IX, and/or X. In patients without concurrent meningitis, the analysis of CSF is usually normal or reveals only a mild pleocytosis and increased protein; Gram stain and culture are rarely positive. Blood cultures are positive in most patients with parenchymal CNS disease. The differential diagnosis includes tuberculosis, toxoplasmosis, nocardiosis, mycoses, and stroke.

Bacteremia without evident localized disease (primary bacteremia) occurs in patients with hematologic malignancies (33 per cent of cases), organ transplant recipients (25 per cent), pregnant women (13 per cent), and individuals suffering from alcoholism or cirrhosis (11 per cent). *Listeria* bacteremia has no distinguishing features. Up to one fourth have premonitory gastrointestinal symptoms: nausea, vomiting, abdominal pain, and/or diarrhea. Less frequently, upper respiratory symptoms may precede the onset of fever, chills, hypotension, tachycardia, and malaise.

Endocarditis occurs not in immunocompromised hosts but usually in those with underlying valvular heart disease. The aortic valve is involved in two thirds of cases and the mitral valve in one third, and prosthetic valve disease is well described. The onset of illness is subacute, with a median duration of symptoms prior to hospitalization of 5 weeks. Fever is cited in 75 per cent of reported cases, a new or changing murmur in 40 per cent, splenomegaly in 35 per cent, and hepatomegaly, CNS emboli, and pulmonary emboli each in 25 per cent.

One third of all cases of listeriosis are associated with pregnancy. Most commonly, in the third trimester, the mother develops a "flulike" illness with fever, sore throat, myalgias, crampy abdominal pain, and diarrhea. After 3 to 7 days, premature labor or abortion ensues. Transplacental transmission of disease becomes clinically evident in the newborn within hours of delivery; this severe septicemic illness is known as granulomatosis infantisepticum. Babies may also acquire infection in the birth canal or nosocomially in the nursery; at a mean of 14 days of life, disease presents as anorexia, fever, or meningismus. *Listeria monocytogenes* is the third most common cause of neonatal sepsis and meningitis after *Escherichia coli* and group B streptococci.

The complete spectrum of listeriosis is seen among patients with acquired immunodeficiency syndrome (AIDS), but the cumulative prevalence is much less than 1 per cent. Chemoprophylaxis of pneumocystosis with trimethoprim-sulfamethoxazole may prevent listeriosis.

TREATMENT. Ampicillin is the antimicrobial agent of choice for listeriosis. Although no comparative trials have been conducted, it has an established record of efficacy and can be administered safely even during pregnancy and infancy. The standard dosage in patients with meningitis is 200 mg per kilogram per day in six divided doses given intravenously. The duration of therapy necessary to effect a cure consistently is 3 weeks. Seriously ill and immunocompromised patients are treated with ampicillin plus gentamicin; the latter drug is administered intravenously in doses sufficient to yield peak serum concentrations of 5 to 8 μg per milliliter and predictable CSF concentrations of 1 to 2 μg per milliliter. The majority of the data from in vitro studies and animal model trials suggest that these two drugs act synergistically against *L. monocytogenes*.

Trimethoprim-sulfamethoxazole has emerged as the preferred therapy for patients allergic to penicillins. The combination is bactericidal at achievable serum and CSF concentrations. Ten case reports have appeared in the literature, including those of immunocompromised patients with CNS disease, and all 10 were cured. Experience to date suggests an initial dosage of 160 mg of trimethoprim plus 800 mg of sulfamethoxazole given intravenously every 12 hours in adults with normal renal function. Erythromycin and tetracycline are alternative therapies.

The inordinate number of treatment failures and relapses among patients treated with cephalosporins or chloramphenicol indicates that these agents are not to be used. Newer β-lactams, including imipenem, are not as active as ampicillin against *L. monocytogenes*. The quinolones do not appear to be sufficiently active at achievable concentrations to be useful clinically. There has been no significant change in the antimicrobial susceptibility profile of *L. monocytogenes* over the past two decades.

DIAGNOSIS. The microbiologic diagnosis of listeriosis is established by culture of blood, CSF, or tissue. In cases of granulomatosis infantisepticum, meconium, amniotic fluid, and lochia are cultured. Initial growth in the laboratory may be slow and may require several days. Unwary technicians may misinterpret these gram-positive bacilli as diphtheroids and label them contaminants.

PROGNOSIS. The overall mortality rate of *Listeria* meningitis is 30 per cent, being higher in patients with cancer, hypoglycorrhachia, or bacteremia and lower in previously healthy individuals. Parenchymal CNS disease and endocarditis are fatal in 50 per cent of cases.

PREVENTION. Individuals at increased risk should avoid raw milk, wash raw vegetables carefully, and cook meats thoroughly. In the hospital, patients with listeriosis should be isolated from immunocompromised hosts.

Carvajal A, Frederiksen W: Fatal endocarditis due to *Listeria monocytogenes.* Rev Infect Dis 10:616, 1988. *A detailed survey of 44 cases.*

Gellin BG, Broome CV: Listeriosis. JAMA 261:1313, 1989. *An excellent analysis focusing on pathogenesis and epidemiology.*

Nieman RE, Lorber B: Listeriosis in adults: A changing pattern. Report of eight cases and review of the literature, 1968–1978. Rev Infect Dis 2:207, 1980. *A comprehensive review of the clinical aspects of disease in 186 patients.*

Schlech WF III: Virulence characteristics of *Listeria monocytogenes.* Food Technol 42:176, 1988. *A concise discussion relating virulence factors to epidemiology.*

Schwartz B, Hexter D, Broome CV, et al.: Investigation of an outbreak of listeriosis: New hypotheses for the etiology of epidemic *Listeria monocytogenes* infections. J Infect Dis 159:680, 1989. *Description of an outbreak that may have been precipitated by a co-infecting organism.*

Stamm AM, Dismukes WE, Simmons BP, et al.: Listeriosis in renal transplant recipients: Report of an outbreak and review of 102 cases. Rev Infect Dis 4:665, 1982. *An extensive review of disease in an immunocompromised population.*

WHO Working Group: Foodborne listeriosis. Bull WHO 66:421, 1988. *An in-depth analysis of this problem.*

326 Erysipeloid
W. Edmund Farrar

DEFINITION. Erysipeloid is a localized skin infection that is almost always limited to the fingers and hands and is caused by *Erysipelothrix rhusiopathiae.* The term "erysipeloid" was coined by Rosenbach to distinguish the lesion from that of human erysipelas. Usually, only a single lesion is present, but diffuse skin involvement and endocarditis occur rarely.

ETIOLOGY. *E. rhusiopathiae* is a straight or slightly curved, thin, non–spore-forming gram-positive rod that grows readily on most ordinary laboratory media. It is nonmotile, catalase negative, nonhemolytic, or α-hemolytic on blood agar and able to form hydrogen sulfide on triple sugar iron (TSI) slants; these properties help to distinguish it from corynebacteria (diphtheroids) and *Listeria monocytogenes.*

EPIDEMIOLOGY. Human infection with *E. rhusiopathiae* almost always results from exposure to infected animals. Infection occurs worldwide in many species of wild and domestic animals, including, especially, swine, sheep, rodents, and birds. Disease in swine, sheep, turkeys, and ducks is of substantial economic importance. Although the organism appears not to cause disease in fish, it can grow and persist for long periods in the mucoid exterior slime of these animals. It can survive for months in soil after initial contamination and may remain viable in foods after salting, pickling, and smoking, but it is killed within 15 minutes by moist heat at 55°C. Most human cases are related to occupational exposure; individuals at greatest risk include butchers, fishermen, fish handlers, abattoir workers, veterinarians, and homemakers.

CLINICAL MANIFESTATIONS. Most human cases probably occur via scratches or puncture wounds of the skin. Within a few days after inoculation, itching, pain, and a characteristic violaceous erythema appear (see Color Plate 9*G*). The lesion may spread slowly to involve other fingers but rarely progresses beyond the wrist. Systemic effects are uncommon. Low-grade fever and arthralgias or arthritis occur in approximately one tenth of cases, and lymphangitis and lymphadenopathy occur in about a third. The absence of suppuration, along with the violaceous color, lack of pitting edema, and disproportionate pain, helps to distinguish erysipeloid from staphylococcal or streptococcal infection. Erysipeloid is a self-limited disease, and the lesions usually resolve within 3 or 4 weeks without therapy.

Approximately 50 cases of systemic infection with *E. rhusiopathiae* have been reported; 90 per cent of the patients had endocarditis. All but one involved native valves. Compared with endocarditis due to other microorganisms, infection with *E. rhusiopathiae* is more likely to occur in males (probably reflecting occupational exposure), is more likely to involve the aortic valve, and results in a higher mortality rate (38 per cent). In nearly 60 per cent of patients, endocarditis due to *E. rhusiopathiae* develops on previously normal heart valves. The clinical picture with respect to fever, peripheral skin stigmata of endocarditis, emboli, splenomegaly, hematuria, and mycotic aneurysm is similar to

that produced by other bacterial organisms. Antecedent or concurrent skin infection has been noted in only about a third of cases of endocarditis.

TREATMENT. Most strains of *E. rhusiopathiae* are highly susceptible to penicillins, cephalosporins, erythromycin, and clindamycin; most strains are resistant to sulfonamides, trimethoprim-sulfamethoxazole, aminoglycosides, and vancomycin. Although skin lesions usually heal spontaneously within 4 weeks, healing is hastened by antibiotic therapy. Oral penicillin V is probably the best choice for therapy.

Endocarditis or septicemia due to *E. rhusiopathiae* should be treated with large dosages of penicillin G (12 to 20 million units per day), given by the intravenous route, for 4 to 6 weeks. Cephalosporins may be used in patients who are allergic to penicillins. The resistance of *E. rhusiopathiae* to vancomycin is noteworthy because this agent is often used in empiric therapy for prosthetic valve endocarditis and in the treatment of native valve endocarditis caused by gram-positive organisms in individuals who are allergic to penicillins.

Barnett KJ, Estes SA, Wirman JA, et al.: Erysipeloid. J Am Acad Dermatol 9:116, 1983. *A good review of the clinical features and appearance of the lesions on electron microscopy and enunciation of the hypothesis that L-forms may play a role in the pathogenesis of the infection.*

Gorby GL, Peacock JE: *Erysipelothrix rhusiopathiae* endocarditis: Microbiologic, epidemiologic and clinical features of an occupational disease. Rev Infect Dis 10:317, 1988. *An up-to-date review that compares this infection with endocarditis due to other bacteria.*

Klauder JV: Erysipeloid as an occupational disease. JAMA 111:1345, 1938. *An account of the epidemiology of the infection in 100 patients, together with a vivid, illustrated clinical description.*

Reboli AC, Farrar WE: *Erysipelothrix rhusiopathiae*: An occupational pathogen. Clin Microbiol Rev 4:354, 1989. *A concise review of epidemiology, clinical features, and bacteriology.*

327 Actinomycosis
Ward E. Bullock

DEFINITION. Actinomycosis is a chronic bacterial infection that induces both a suppurative and a granulomatous inflammatory response. It spreads contiguously through anatomic barriers and frequently forms external sinuses, from which may extrude "sulfur granules" that are characteristic but not pathognomonic. The most common clinical forms are cervicofacial, thoracic, abdominal, and, in females, genital.

ETIOLOGY. Members of the genus *Actinomyces* are prokaryotes with cell walls that contain both muramic acid and diaminopimelic acid. Unlike the cell walls of fungi, the cell walls of these organisms do not contain sterols and are insensitive to polyene antibiotics. *Actinomyces israelii* is the species most often recovered from human cases of actinomycosis. However, *A. naeslundii, A. odontolyticus, A. viscosus, A. meyeri,* and a related genus, *Arachnia propionica,* cause identical clinical infections and bear close resemblance in primary culture. *Actinomyces bovis* produces "lumpy jaw" in cattle but is not a human pathogen. These gram-positive bacteria are filamentous (0.5 to 1.0 μm in diameter) with branching and are non–acid fast, with a tendency to break up into coccobacilli. They require anaerobic to microaerophilic conditions for growth, which is quite slow; usually, 3 to 10 or more days are required before these organisms can be macroscopically detected in culture.

EPIDEMIOLOGY. Actinomycosis is observed throughout the world, and its prevalence is unrelated to climate, occupation, race, or age. The disease has been reported more commonly in men than in women (3:1). However, since the recognition of pelvic actinomycosis in association with the use of intrauterine contraceptive devices (IUCD's), the male prevalence ratio may be decreasing. The number of cases of actinomycosis reported annually to the Centers for Disease Control is fewer than 100. These infections are not easily recognized by clinicians, and the organisms are fastidious; therefore, it is likely that the true incidence is substantially greater. Although many animal species are susceptible to actinomycosis, infection is neither transmissible from animal to human nor transmissible from person to person. *Actinomyces* species are part of the indigenous microbiota colonizing the teeth and oral cavity. They may also be found in the tonsillar crypts of asymptomatic individuals, in the fecal flora, and within the female reproductive tract.

PATHOGENESIS AND PATHOLOGY. The *Actinomyces* maintain their niche within the microbial community of the mouth by adherence to oral surfaces, especially to dental plaque, a thin film of salivary proteins and glycoproteins that coats the enamel surface. Adherence is achieved by complex protein-protein stereochemical interactions and by lectin-carbohydrate interactions, the latter of which also mediate cellular coaggregation of oral *Actinomyces* with *Streptococcus milleri*, *Streptococcus sanguis*, and other mouth flora. This propensity for coaggregation may explain, in part, why actinomycotic infections often are polymicrobic, with "associate" mouth flora frequently isolated from cervicofacial, thoracic, and central nervous system abscesses. The associate flora may play a synergistic role in infection by maintaining the low oxygen tension necessary for growth of the *Actinomyces*. To cause disease, these organisms must be introduced into tissue through a break in the mucous membrane resulting from dental infections and manipulations or from aspiration of infected dental debris. They may enter the abdominal cavity by perforation of the lower gastrointestinal tract or by ascending infection of the genital tract in women.

Actinomycotic infection evokes a combination of suppurative and granulomatous inflammatory responses that are accompanied by intense fibrosis. Plasma cells and multinucleated giant cells often are observed within lesions, as may be large macrophages with foamy cytoplasm around purulent centers. The infection spreads through fascial planes and ultimately may produce draining sinus tracts, especially in infections of the pelvis and abdomen. Sulfur granules within lesions and sinus drainage are a typical feature, though not always present. These granules are gritty aggregates of organisms measuring 1 to 2 mm in diameter; the centers have a basophilic staining property, with eosinophilic rays terminating in pear-shaped "clubs" on the surface. They contain calcium phosphate, probably as a result of phosphatase activity of both the host and the organisms.

CLINICAL MANIFESTATIONS. Cervicofacial actinomycosis comprises 50 to 60 per cent of reported cases. Infection is usually observed in a setting of poor oral hygiene with tooth decay, periodontal disease, or gingivitis, in which mucosal integrity is disrupted by dental manipulations or other injury. The infection generally evolves as a chronic or subacute soft tissue swelling or mass involving the submandibular or paramandibular region. The swelling may have a ligneous consistency that is caused by tissue fibrosis. More rapidly developing lesions often simulate pyogenic infections. Trismus may be present, and advanced lesions may discharge odorless pus containing "sulfur granules" through one or more sinuses. Fever, pain, and leukocytosis may be present. The infection can extend to the tongue, salivary glands, pharynx, and larynx. Bone (most commonly the mandible) may be invaded from the adjacent soft tissue. Cervical spine or cranial bone infection may lead to subdural empyema and invasion of the central nervous system. The differential diagnosis includes tuberculosis (scrofula), fungal infections, nocardiosis, suppurative infections by other organisms, and neoplasms.

Thoracic actinomycosis comprises 15 to 30 per cent of the disease spectrum and usually results from aspiration of infective material from the oropharynx. Less commonly, thoracic infection may be introduced by esophageal perforation, by extension into the mediastinum from the neck, or by spread from an abdominal site; hematogenous spread to the lung is rare. Pulmonary actinomycosis commonly spreads from an early pneumonic focus across lung fissures to involve the pleura and the chest wall, with eventual fistula formation and drainage containing sulfur granules (Fig. 327–1). Granules rarely are present in the sputum. The incidence of this complication, as well as the destruction of thoracic vertebrae and adjacent ribs, has declined in the antibiotic era.

The complaints of patients with thoracic actinomycosis are nonspecific. The most common of these are a productive cough,

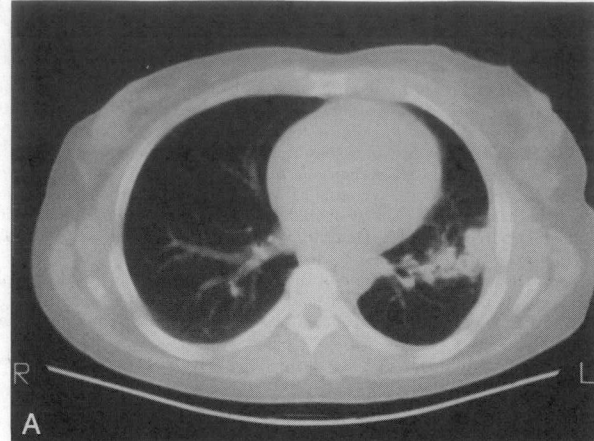
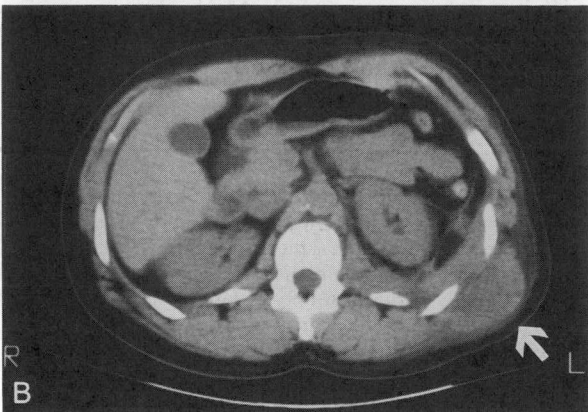

FIGURE 327–1. Thoracic computed tomographic (CT) scan of a 43-year-old woman with pulmonary actinomycosis. There is consolidation within the left lung and pleural thickening adjacent to the parenchymal disease (*A*). Abscess extended into the left breast and inferiorly to the costophrenic sulcus, to the retroperitoneum, and into the lateral abdominal wall (*arrow*) (*B*).

dyspnea, weight loss, fever, and chest pain. Anemia, mild leukocytosis, and an elevated sedimentation rate are relatively common. There often is a history of underlying lung disease, and patients rarely present in an early stage of infection. The pulmonary lesions may resemble tuberculosis, especially when cavity formation occurs, and blastomycosis, which may destroy ribs posteriorly but rarely form sinuses. Nocardiosis, bronchogenic carcinoma, and lymphoma can also mimic thoracic actinomycosis.

ABDOMINAL-PELVIC ACTINOMYCOSIS. Actinomycosis of the abdomen and pelvis is a chronic, localized inflammatory process that often is preceded weeks or months by surgery for acute appendicitis with perforation or for perforated colonic diverticulitis, or by emergency surgery upon the lower intestinal tract after trauma. Occasionally, abdominal actinomycosis may manifest without identifiable predisposing factors. The ileocecal region is involved most frequently, with the formation of a mass lesion. The infection extends slowly to contiguous organs, especially the liver, and may involve retroperitoneal tissues, the spine, or the abdominal wall. Persistent draining sinuses may form, and those involving the perianal region can simulate Crohn's disease or tuberculosis. The extensive fibrosis of actinomycotic lesions, presenting to the examiner as a mass, often suggests tumor. Constitutional symptoms and signs are nonspecific; the most common are fever, weight loss, nausea, vomiting, and pain.

An association has been recognized between long-term use of IUCD's and actinomycosis of the genital tract. Manifestations of infection may range from a chronic vaginal discharge to pelvic inflammatory disease with tubo-ovarian abscesses or pseudomalignant masses. No association exists between actinomycotic infection and the type of IUCD employed. Accurate data on the prevalence and incidence of infection among IUCD users are sparse, since cytologic criteria and fluorescent antibody staining techniques are the principal means of detecting *Actinomyces* in vaginal smears and other genital tract specimens. Anaerobic cultures of the female genital tract generally are unsuccessful.

Currently, it is generally agreed that *Actinomyces* species may be part of the indigenous genital tract flora of females and that demonstration of their presence by morphologic criteria and fluorescent antibody stains does not predict disease. However, colonization of the endometrium appears to require the presence of an IUCD. Although many cases of genital-pelvic actinomycosis associated with IUCD use have been reported, the actual incidence of disease appears to be low relative to the millions of those who use IUCD's.

Central nervous system (CNS) and disseminated actinomycosis are very uncommon. Most infections of the CNS manifest as encapsulated brain abscesses that are indistinguishable from those caused by other organisms. Most actinomycotic infections of the CNS are thought to be seeded hematogenously from a distant primary site; however, direct extension of cervicofacial disease is well recognized. Sinus formation is not a characteristic of CNS disease. The rare meningitis caused by *Actinomyces* is chronic and basilar in location, and the pleocytosis usually is lymphocytic. Thus, it may be misdiagnosed as tuberculous meningitis.

Unlike *Nocardia* species, *Actinomyces* usually are not opportunistic in the immunocompromised host. To date, few systemic actinomycotic infections have been reported among patients with the acquired immunodeficiency syndrome (AIDS).

DIAGNOSIS. Critical to the diagnosis of actinomycosis is a high index of suspicion that is communicated to the microbiology diagnostic laboratory, along with material from draining sinuses, from deep needle aspiration, or from biopsy specimens. Anaerobic culture is required, and no selective media are available to restrict overgrowth of the slow-growing *Actinomyces* by associated microflora. The presence in pus or tissue specimens of non–acid-fast, gram-positive organisms with filamentous branching is very suggestive of the diagnosis. The characteristic morphology of "sulfur granules" and the presence of gram-positive organisms within are helpful. However, the granules must be distinguished from similar structures that are sometimes produced in infections and that are caused by *Nocardia, Monosporium, Cephalosporium, Staphylococcus* (botryomycosis), and others. *Actinomyces* and *Arachnia* generally can be differentiated from other gram-positive anaerobes by means of growth rate (slow), by catalase production (negative, except *A. viscosus*), and by gas-liquid chromatographic detection of acetic, lactic, and succinic acids produced in peptone-yeast-glucose broth. Direct fluorescent antibody conjugates can be employed to detect *Actinomyces* in clinical material or culture but are not readily available to clinical microbiology laboratories. There are no reliable serologic tests or skin tests.

TREATMENT. Penicillin G is the drug of choice for treatment of infection caused by any of the *Actinomyces*. It is given in high dosage over a prolonged period, since the infection has a tendency to recur, presumably because antibiotic penetration to areas of fibrosis and necrosis and into "sulfur granules" may be poor. Most deep-seated infections can be expected to respond to intravenous penicillin G, 10 to 20 million units per day given for 2 to 6 weeks, followed by an oral phenoxypenicillin in a dosage of 2 to 4 grams per day. A few additional weeks of oral penicillin therapy may suffice for uncomplicated cervicofacial disease; complicated cases and extensive pulmonary or abdominal disease may require treatment for 12 to 18 months. To date, little evidence exists of acquired resistance to penicillin G by *Actinomyces* during prolonged therapy. Radical excision of large sinus tracts should be considered in some cases. Alternative first-line antibiotics for treatment of infection caused by *Actinomyces* include tetracycline, erythromycin, and clindamycin. First-generation cephalosporins and imipenem also are highly effective. Antifungal drugs are not active against these organisms. In vitro antibiotic sensitivity testing of *Actinomyces* is difficult, and the results may not be predictive of antibiotic activity in vivo.

The need to employ combination antibiotic therapy to attack microorganisms that are isolated in association with *Actinomyces* has not been established. The generally good results obtained with penicillin G alone over nearly three decades indicate that monotherapy is effective in most cases. In complicated infections of the lower abdomen, where anaerobic gram-negative organisms, among others, may be the "associates," combination antibiotic therapy is appropriate.

The presence of organisms presumed to be *Actinomyces* on a Papanicolaou smear, obtained from an asymptomatic female with or without an IUCD in place, is not an indication for therapy. When patients experience well-defined IUCD-related symptoms and Papanicolaou smears demonstrate *Actinomyces* by specific fluorescent-labeled antibody, the device should be removed. Antibiotic administration for a 2-week period may be indicated. More serious infections require prolonged therapy as recommended above.

PROGNOSIS. The advent of antibiotics has greatly improved the prognosis for all forms of actinomycosis. At present, cure rates are high, and neither deformity nor death is common.

Bennhoff DF: Actinomycosis: Diagnostic and therapeutic considerations and a review of 32 cases. Laryngoscope 94:1198, 1984. *A helpful general review.*

Bernardi RS: Abdominal actinomycosis. Surg Gynecol Obstet 149:257, 1979. *A thorough review of all aspects of actinomycosis, with emphasis on the abdominal form.*

Cisar JO, Sandberg AL, Clark WB: Actinomycosis of the central nervous system. Rev Infect Dis 9:855, 1987. *A good review of 70 cases of CNS actinomycosis.*

Flynn MW, Felson B: The roentgen manifestations of thoracic actinomycosis. AJR 110:707, 1970. *An outstanding guide to roentgenographic diagnosis of pulmonary actinomycosis.*

Nayar M, Chandra M, Chitraratha K, et al.: Incidence of actinomycetes infection in women using intrauterine contraceptive devices. Acta Cytol 29:111, 1985. *Ten of 350 women using intrauterine contraceptive devices (IUD's) had Actinomyces-like organisms in Papanicolaou-stained smears; 8 of the 10 were symptomatic. Seven of the 10 patients had been using an IUD for more than 2 years.*

Richtsmeier WJ, Johns ME: Actinomycosis of the head and neck. CRC Crit Rev Clin Lab Sci 11:175, 1979. *An excellent review, with an emphasis on infection of the head and neck.*

Smego RA Jr: Molecular aspects of adherence of Actinomyces viscosus and Actinomyces naeslundii to oral surfaces. J Dent Res 68:1558, 1989. *A brief summary for those wishing to know more about adherence mechanisms.*

328 Nocardiosis

Ward E. Bullock

DEFINITION. Nocardiosis is a subacute or chronic bacterial infection that evokes a suppurative response. The most common sites of primary infection are, first, the lung and then the skin, from which bacteria may disseminate hematogenously to the central nervous system and other tissues. The infection often pursues a more acute and aggressive course in immunosuppressed patients.

ETIOLOGY. *Nocardia* species are gram-positive, aerobic actinomycetes, many of which are weakly acid fast in tissue or on initial isolation. They reproduce by filamentous branching, with fragmentation into bacillary and coccoid forms. *Nocardia* species are distributed widely in nature and commonly are found in soil, grasses, and rotting vegetation. Of the three species that cause most infections in humans, *N. asteroides* is by far the predominant pathogen. *N. caviae, N. farcinica,* and *N. brasiliensis* also produce pulmonary and disseminated infections, but much less frequently. *N. brasiliensis* is the most common cause of actinomycetoma in Latin and South America.

INCIDENCE AND PREVALENCE. A 1976 survey estimated the incidence of nocardiosis in the United States to be 500 to 1000 new cases per year. At present, the incidence undoubtedly is higher as a consequence of an expanding population of individuals who are immunosuppressed iatrogenically or by underlying diseases. Nocardiosis has been reported worldwide in all ages and races, and is two to three times more common in men than in women. No occupation-related risks have been found. Thus, possible hormonal effects on bacterial growth or virulence have been postulated.

EPIDEMIOLOGY. The majority of infections caused by *N. asteroides* are encountered in patients with impairment of cell-mediated immunity (CMI). However, the organism clearly is capable of infecting apparently normal persons. Nocardiosis presumably is acquired by inhalation of airborne bacteria, since the primary site of infection is the lung in the majority of cases. Other mammals can be infected. However, no well-established evidence exists for animal-to-person transmission or for person-to-person transmission. Occasional clusters of nocardial infection have been reported among immunosuppressed hospital patients, suggesting possible nosocomial acquisition. *Nocardia asteroides* has been recovered from the sputum, skin, and other body regions of patients who do not have apparent disease. Nevertheless, repeated isolation of *Nocardia* species from any immunocompromised person should be considered evidence of infection rather than colonization, and treatment should be initiated. Nocardiosis can manifest as a primary cutaneous infection (especially *N. brasiliensis*) after inoculation through local injury and may disseminate to other organs.

PATHOGENESIS AND PATHOLOGY. The typical nocardial lesion within the lung and other tissues is one of liquefactive necrosis with abscess formation. Polymorphonuclear leukocytes predominate in association with varying proportions of macrophages and lymphocytes. Granuloma formation is infrequent, and in contrast with actinomycotic lesions, fibrosis is rare. Confluent daughter abscesses are common. Sulfur granules are not present in visceral lesions, as they are in actinomycosis. However, they may be seen in nocardial lesions of the skin.

That CMI plays a major role in host defense against nocardiosis is suggested by the fact that immunocompromised patients are prone to this infection. The importance of antigen-specific T lymphocyte immune function is illustrated by the increased susceptibility of athymic nude mice to *Nocardia* infection and by the capacity of T lymphocytes from rabbits immunized with *N. asteroides* to augment phagocytosis and growth inhibition of these organisms by macrophages. Neutrophils exhibit poor nocardicidal activity in vitro but may inhibit growth of organisms during an early phase of infection prior to maturation of cellular immune responses.

Among the mechanisms that may be employed by *N. asteroides* to counter host defenses are inhibition of lysosome-phagosome fusion that enables phagocytic cells to kill ingested bacteria, production of superoxide dismutase and catalase, and the capacity to block the acidification of parasitized phagosomes.

Nocardia species are not visible in tissue specimens stained by hematoxylin and eosin or by the periodic acid–Schiff procedure. They can be visualized by a tissue Gram stain or after slight overstaining by the Gomori methenamine silver method, which demonstrates the filamentous structure of the organisms. Many *Nocardia* are weakly acid fast and can be seen on a modified Ziehl-Neelsen stain.

CLINICAL MANIFESTATIONS. Pulmonary infection is the most frequent manifestation of nocardiosis (about 75 per cent of the reported cases). The clinical manifestations are nonspecific and include fever, cough, weight loss, and dyspnea. The range of pulmonary involvement extends from transient or inapparent infection to confluent bronchopneumonia with complete consolidation. Radiographic examination of the chest may reveal one or more of the following: fluffy infiltrates, multiple abscess formation with cavitation in 10 to 20 per cent of cases, bulging fissures, masses, nodules, and empyema. Hilar involvement and calcification are infrequent. *Nocardia* can disseminate to other organs from pulmonary lesions, especially in patients who are immunosuppressed following organ transplantation. Patients who have received extensive x-irradiation and chemotherapy for malignancies and those who are treated with steroids in high dosage also are prone to metastatic infection, and evidence thereof should be sought aggressively.

In 20 to 40 per cent of patients with pulmonary nocardiosis, dissemination to the central nervous system occurs, and therefore, computed tomography (CT) scanning of the head should be considered. Loculated brain abscesses, either singular or multiple, are common and are often accompanied by headache and focal neurologic findings; meningitis is infrequent. Other common sites of dissemination include the skin and subcutaneous tissues, kidneys, eyes, liver, and lymph nodes. In cases of apparently localized nocardial lesions of skin, it is important to distinguish between the possibilities of primary inoculation and hematogenous dissemination to the skin from another site.

DIAGNOSIS. The clinical and radiographic findings in pulmonary nocardiosis are nonspecific. Consequently, it may be confused with a variety of other bacterial infections of the lung, including actinomycosis and tuberculosis, as well as fungal infections and malignancies. Alertness to the possibility of nocardiosis can expedite the diagnostic workup, especially in immunosuppressed patients, in whom the disease may coexist with other opportunistic infections. Cultures and stains should be done on specimens of sputum, pleural fluid, and bronchial lavage fluid, as well as on percutaneous lung aspirates or open lung biopsy specimens. Needle biopsy of cerebral mass lesions should be considered strongly in patients with the acquired immunodeficiency syndrome (AIDS) who have pulmonary nocardiosis because of the multiplicity of infections and tumors that can manifest in a similar manner.

Skin lesions should be aspirated if fluctuant, or biopsied, and specimens should be submitted for culture and the smear preparations or histologic sections examined for organisms. Nocardiosis can often be diagnosed with a high degree of confidence by direct examination of sputum or purulent material. The presence of gram-positive, filamentous branching rods that stain unevenly with crystal violet to give a beaded appearance is highly suggestive of either *Actinomyces* or *Nocardia*. If the organisms are acid fast on a modified Ziehl-Neelsen stain, the probability of *Nocardia* is high. However, lack of acid-fast staining does not exclude *Nocardia*.

Nocardia species are not fastidious and grow aerobically, though slowly, on routinely used media. Characteristic heaped, waxy colonies, often colored tan, orange, or even purple, may be seen after 2 to 7 days of culture. Longer times may be required. Thus, the microbiology laboratory should be advised of possible nocardiosis to ensure that plates are held for 10 to 14 days and that steps are taken to limit overgrowth by microbial contaminants, particularly in sputum samples. The use of defined carbon-free medium to which paraffin is added may enhance the chances of isolating *N. asteroides* from sputum because it can utilize paraffin as a sole source of carbon, in contrast to most other organisms. Several simple tests can assist in the presumptive differentiation of *Nocardia* from other aerobic actinomycetes and from rapidly growing *Mycobacteria*, as, for example, the decomposition of casein, xanthine, tyrosine, and 1 per cent ethylene glycol. However, most clinical laboratories should rely on reference facilities for definitive taxonomic designations.

TREATMENT. The sulfonamides are equally efficacious and are first-line agents for treatment, as is the combination of trimethoprim-sulfamethoxazole (TMP-SMX). Typically, sulfadiazine should be given in a dosage of 6 to 10 grams per day, with adjustment as needed to achieve peak serum levels of 12 to 15 mg per deciliter. These antimicrobials penetrate the central nervous system and other body compartments well. A high percentage of *Nocardia* isolates are sensitive to sulfonamides and to TMP-SMX by in vitro testing. However, the techniques of in vitro sensitivity testing with *Nocardia* have not been standardized, in part because of technical difficulties created by slow growth in culture and problems in obtaining a homogeneous suspension of cells for standardization of the inoculum. Thus, the results of in vitro tests frequently are poor predictors of in vivo efficacy and should be interpreted with caution.

Not all patients respond to sulfonamide or TMP-SMX therapy. Acquisition of resistance to the sulfonamides during therapy has been documented, and metastatic lesions can appear during the course of apparently successful treatment. Hypersensitivity reactions or hemopoietic toxicity induced by these drugs may force discontinuation of treatment, especially in patients with AIDS. The alternative antibiotics that have proved to be most efficacious, both in vitro and clinically, are minocycline, amikacin, and imipenem. Ceftriaxone, cefuroxime, and cefotaxime display in vitro activity against many strains of *Nocardia*. However, it remains to be determined if the last-named three antibiotics will prove valuable for treatment of nocardiosis. Although some in vitro studies indicate that certain combinations of antibiotics may exert synergistic activity against *Nocardia*, no good clinical evidence exists that combination antibiotic regimens are superior to single-agent therapy.

Treatment should be prolonged, since relapse of nocardiosis is common. In patients with intact host defenses, treatment should be continued for 6 weeks after clinical recovery. In those who have AIDS or who are otherwise immunocompromised, treatment should be continued for a year or more. As a rule, it is necessary to perform surgical drainage of brain abscesses, empyema, and subcutaneous abscesses. Patients with cerebral nocardiosis or other deep abscesses should be monitored by serial CT scans. If patients are receiving immunosuppressive drugs, the dosage should be reduced if at all possible.

PROGNOSIS. The prognosis for clinical cure of nocardiosis is influenced by the location of the infection, by pre-existing impairment of cellular immunity from underlying disease or drug therapy, and by the aggressiveness of the patient's management. Mortality rates range from near 0 per cent in patients with isolated skin lesions to more than 40 per cent in cases of central nervous system involvement. The overall mortality rate in patients with pulmonary disease is in the range of 15 to 30 per cent, even in those who are immunocompromised.

Barnicoat MJ, Wierzbicki AS, Norman PM: Cerebral nocardiosis in immunosuppressed patients: Five cases. Q J Med 268:689, 1989. *Presentation of five cases with a good bibliography on the topic.*

Feigin DS: Nocardiosis of the lung: Chest radiographic findings in 21 cases. Radiology 159:9, 1986. *A good descriptive study.*

McNeil MM, Brown JM, Jarvis WR, et al.: Comparison of species distribution and antimicrobial susceptibility of aerobic actinomycetes from clinical specimens. Rev Infect Dis 12:778, 1990.

Palmer DL, Harvey RL, Wheeler JK: Diagnostic and therapeutic considerations in *Nocardia asteroides* infection. Medicine 53:391, 1974. *A comprehensive literature review of 243 cases of nocardiosis (including 13 patients in the authors' own experience).*

Smego RA Jr, Moeller MB, Gallis HA: Trimethoprim-sulfamethoxazole therapy for *Nocardia* infections. Arch Intern Med 143:711, 1983. *This article provides an extensive literature review and discusses TMP-SMX in depth.*

Wallace RJ Jr, Steele LC, Sumter G, et al.: Antimicrobial susceptibility patterns of *Nocardia asteroides.* Antimicrob Agents Chemother 32:1776, 1988. *An examination of antibiotic sensitivity patterns among 78 clinical isolates of N. asteroides by a group experienced in the complexities of in vitro sensitivity testing with these organisms.*

Wilson JP, Turner HR, Kirchner KA, et al.: Nocardial infections in renal transplant recipients. Medicine 68:38, 1989. *A current and well-written review of nocardiosis, with emphasis upon disease manifestations in renal transplant patients.*

329 Brucellosis

Robert A. Salata

DEFINITION. Bacteria of the genus *Brucella* cause disease with protean manifestations. Transmission of infection to humans from animals occurs as a consequence of occupational exposure or ingestion of contaminated milk products. Despite the attempt to institute effective control measures, brucellosis remains a significant health and economic burden in many countries.

ETIOLOGY. Brucellae are slow-growing, small, aerobic, nonmotile, nonencapsulated, non–spore-forming, gram-negative coccobacilli. *B. abortus, B. suis, B. melitensis,* and *B. canis* are known to infect humans and are typed on the basis of biochemical, metabolic, and immunologic criteria. There are differences in virulence among these four species. *B. abortus,* with a reservoir in cattle, usually is associated with mild sporadic disease; suppurative or disabling complications are rare. *B. suis* infection, resulting from swine contact, is often associated with destructive, suppurative lesions and may have a prolonged course. *B. melitensis,* with a reservoir in sheep and goats, may cause severe, acute disease and disabling complications. *B. canis,* spread to humans from infected dogs, causes disease with an insidious onset, frequent relapse, and a chronic course that is indistinguishable from infection related to *B. abortus.*

EPIDEMIOLOGY. Over 500,000 cases of brucellosis are reported yearly to the World Health Organization. *B. melitensis* infection, distributed primarily in the Mediterranean region, Latin America, and Asia, accounts for the majority of cases. *B. abortus* infection occurs worldwide but has been effectively eradicated in several European countries, Japan, and Israel. *B. suis* occurs mainly in the midwestern United States, South America, and Southeast Asia, whereas *B. canis* infection is most common in North and South America, Japan, and Central Europe.

In association with effective control programs in animals, human brucellosis has decreased dramatically in the United States, from over 6000 cases in 1947 to fewer than 200 cases

since 1980 (Fig. 329–1). States reporting the greatest number of cases include Texas, California, Virginia, and Florida. In North America, brucellosis occurs mainly in spring and summer and is most common in adult males, usually related to occupational exposure.

Brucella infection in the United States most frequently occurs in high-risk groups, including slaughterhouse workers, farmers and dairymen, veterinarians, travelers to endemic areas, and laboratory workers handling the organisms. Over one half of reported cases occur in the meat-processing industry, particularly in the kill areas, where infection is spread through abraded or lacerated skin and the conjunctiva, possibly by aerosolization, and rarely by ingestion of infected tissue. Many cases of *B. abortus* infection in veterinarians have accidentally occurred from the strain 19 vaccine used to immunize cattle. In American travelers or immigrants, Mexico has been the most frequent source of *B. melitensis* infection, transmitted through the ingestion of goat's milk cheese. *Brucella* infections associated with unpasteurized milk and accidental strain vaccine injections may account for an increasing proportion of cases reported in the United States.

Brucellosis in children accounts for only 3 to 10 per cent of all reported cases, is most common in endemic areas, and is often a mild, self-limited process. There is no convincing evidence to associate *Brucella* infection with abortion in humans.

PATHOGENESIS AND IMMUNITY. After penetrating the epithelial cells of human skin, conjunctiva, pharynx, or lung, *Brucella* organisms initially induce an exuberant polymorphonuclear neutrophil response in the submucosa. Following ingestion of organisms by neutrophils and tissue macrophages, spread to regional lymph nodes occurs. If host defenses within the lymph nodes are overwhelmed, bacteremia follows. The usual incubation period between infection and bacteremia is 1½ to 3 weeks. Bacteremia is accompanied by phagocytosis of free *Brucella* organisms by neutrophils and localization of bacteria primarily to the spleen, liver, and bone marrow, with the formation of granulomas.

If the inoculum is large and the patient is untreated, large granulomas may form, suppurate, and serve as a source of persistent bacteremia with the potential for multiorgan spread.

Both virulent and attenuated strains of *Brucella* are readily phagocytized by neutrophils after opsonization with normal human serum. Whole bacteria and extracts of *Brucella* species may inhibit neutrophil oxidative burst activity and degranulation. Intracellular killing of ingested bacteria has been demonstrated

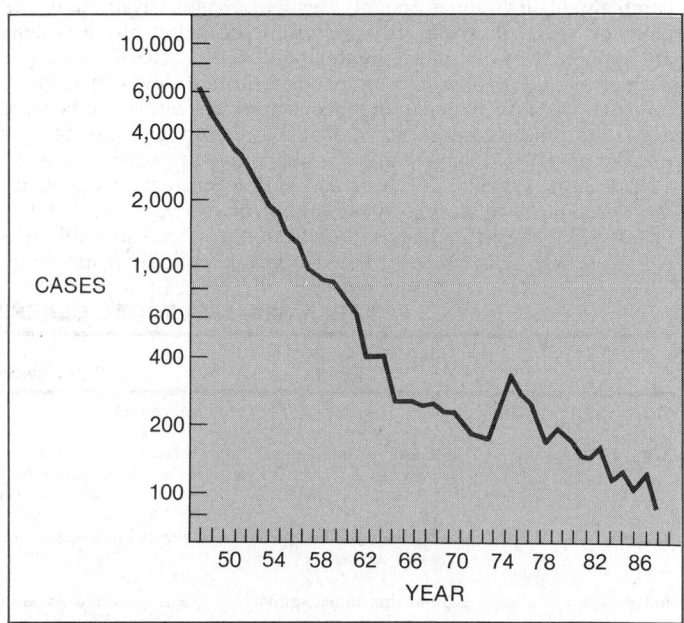

FIGURE 329–1. Incidence of human brucellosis, United States, 1947 to 1988. Following the implementation of eradication programs in cattle, the incidence of human brucellosis in the United States has steadily declined from 6321 cases in 1947 to fewer than 100 cases in 1988.

with *B. abortus* but not *B. melitensis*; this may explain differences in pathogenicity between these species.

Humoral factors may be important in the host defense against *Brucella*. Even in the absence of specific agglutinating antibody, normal human serum is bactericidal for *Brucella* organisms; *B. abortus* is more susceptible to serum lysis than is *B. melitensis*. The intracellular location of the organism may provide a means for the bacteria to escape the lethal effects of serum. Specific serum agglutinating antibody has opsonic activity but does not correlate with the development of protective immunity.

A role for mononuclear phagocytes and cell-mediated immunity in brucellosis has been demonstrated. Protection against *Brucella* infection in animals is associated with preceding infection with *Listeria monocytogenes* or *Mycobacterium tuberculosis*, both of which stimulate cell-mediated immune mechanisms. Skin testing with *Brucella* proteins elicits a typical delayed hypersensitivity response in infected individuals. Macrophages, activated with lymphokines, kill *Brucella* in vitro. In some cases of chronic brucellosis, depressed proliferative responses to classic T cell mitogens or to *Brucella* antigen occur. An increased incidence of *Brucella* infection has been seen in patients with Hodgkin's disease and other lymphomas.

CLINICAL MANIFESTATIONS. Clinically, human brucellosis may be conveniently divided into subclinical illness, acute/subacute disease, localized disease and complications, relapsing infection, and chronic disease (Table 329–1).

Subclinical Illness. Detected only by serologic testing, asymptomatic or clinically unrecognized human brucellosis often occurs in high-risk groups, including slaughterhouse workers, farmers, and veterinarians. Greater than 50 per cent of abattoir workers and up to 33 per cent of veterinarians have high anti-*Brucella* antibody titers but no history of recognized clinical infection. Children in endemic areas frequently have subclinical illness. Subclinical cases outnumber clinically evident cases of brucellosis by 12 to 1.

Acute and Subacute Disease. After an incubation period of several weeks or months, acute brucellosis may occur as a mild, transient illness (with *B. abortus* or *B. canis*) or as an explosive, toxic illness with the potential for multiple complications (with *B. melitensis*). Approximately 50 per cent of patients have an abrupt onset over days, while the remainder have an insidious onset over weeks. Symptoms in brucellosis are protean and nonspecific. Over 90 per cent of patients experience malaise, chills, sweats, fatigue, and weakness. More than 50 per cent of patients have myalgias, anorexia, and weight loss. Fewer patients complain of arthralgias, cough, testicular pain, dysuria, ocular pain, or visual blurring. Likewise, few localizing physical signs are apparent. Fever, often greater than 39.4°C (103°F), occurs in 95 per cent. An undulating or intermittent fever pattern is unusual. Because *Brucella* organisms are intracellular pathogens, a relative pulse-temperature deficit may occur. Splenomegaly is present in 10 to 15 per cent, lymphadenopathy occurs in up to 14 per cent (axillary, cervical, and supraclavicular locations are most frequent, related to hand-wound or oropharyngeal routes of infection); hepatomegaly is less frequent. Acute/subacute disease is usually associated with a significant serologic response by the standard tube agglutination assay. Other laboratory findings in acute or subacute disease may include mild anemia, lymphopenia or neutropenia (especially with bacteremia), lymphocytosis, thrombocytopenia, or (rarely) pancytopenia. The majority of infected individuals recover completely without sequelae if the diagnosis is appropriately made and prompt therapy is initiated.

Localized Disease and Complications. *Brucella* organisms may localize in almost any organ, most commonly in bone, central nervous system, heart, lung, spleen, testes, liver, gallbladder, kidney, prostate, and skin. Localized disease may occur simultaneously at multiple sites. Localized complications most often appear in association with a more chronic course of illness, although complications may occur with acute disease due to *B. melitensis* or *B. suis*. In the United States, localized disease is most frequently related to *B. suis*.

Relapsing Infection. Up to 10 per cent of patients with brucellosis relapse after antimicrobial therapy. This probably results from the intracellular location of the organisms, which protects the bacteria from certain antibiotics and host defense mechanisms. Relapses occur most frequently within months after initial infection but may occur as long as 2 years after apparently successful treatment. Relapsing infection is difficult to distinguish from reinfection in high-risk groups with continued exposure. Nearly all relapsed cases respond to a repeated course of antimicrobial agents.

Chronic Disease. Disease with a duration greater than 1 year has been called chronic brucellosis. A majority of patients classified as having chronic brucellosis really have persistent disease caused by inadequate treatment of the initial episode, or they have focal disease in bone, liver, or spleen. About 20 per cent of patients diagnosed as having chronic brucellosis complain of persistent fatigue, malaise, and depression. These symptoms frequently are not associated with clinical, microbiologic, or serologic evidence of active infection.

DIAGNOSIS. Many more common illnesses mimic the clinical presentation of brucellosis. The most conclusive means of establishing the diagnosis of brucellosis is by positive cultures from normally sterile body fluids or tissues. Special media are necessary because of the unusual metabolic requirements and slow growth of *Brucella*. The culture of *Brucella* organisms is potentially hazardous to laboratory personnel; a laboratory should not undertake isolation and identification of *Brucella* unless Biosafety Level 3 facilities are available. Therefore, most cases of brucellosis are diagnosed by serologic testing.

In acute brucellosis, positive blood cultures are obtained in 10 to 30 per cent of cases (as high as 85 per cent with *B. melitensis*). Blood culture positivity decreases with increasing duration of illness. With *B. melitensis* infection, bone marrow cultures are of higher yield than are blood cultures. Blood cultures processed in radiometric detection systems may yield positive cultures in less than 10 days. With localized brucellosis (e.g., lymph nodes, spleen, liver, or skeletal system), cultures of purulent material or tissues usually yield *Brucella* organisms. Culture of cerebrospinal fluid is positive in 45 per cent of patients with meningitis. Antibody against *Brucella* may be demonstrated in cerebrospinal fluid by enzyme-linked immunosorbent assay (ELISA).

Most patients mount significant serologic responses to *Brucella* infections. The most frequently utilized test is the standard tube

TABLE 329–1. CLINICAL CLASSIFICATION OF HUMAN BRUCELLOSIS

	Duration of Symptoms Before Diagnosis	Major Symptoms and Signs	Diagnosis	Comments
Subclinical	—	Asymptomatic	Positive (low titer) serology, negative cultures	Occurs in abattoir workers, farmers, and veterinarians
Acute and subacute	Up to 2–3 mo and 3 mo to 1 yr	Malaise, chills, sweats, fatigue, headache, anorexia, arthralgias, fever, splenomegaly, lymphadenopathy, hepatomegaly	Positive serology, positive blood or bone marrow cultures	Presentation can be mild, self-limited (*B. abortus*), or fulminant with severe complications (*B. melitensis*)
Localized	Occurs with acute or chronic untreated disease	Related to involved organs	Positive serology, positive cultures in specific tissues	Bone/joint, genitourinary, hepatosplenic involvement most common
Relapsing	2–3 mo after initial episode	Same as acute illness but may have higher fever, more fatigue, weakness, chills, and sweats	Positive serology, positive cultures	May be extremely difficult to distinguish relapse from reinfection
Chronic	Greater than 1 yr	Nonspecific presentation but neuropsychiatric symptoms and low-grade fever most common	Low titer or negative serology, cultures negative	Most controversial classification; localized disease may be associated

agglutination (STA) test, measuring antibody to *B. abortus* antigen. A fourfold or greater rise in titer to 1:160 or higher is considered significant. A presumptive case is one in which the agglutination titer is positive ($\geq$1:160) in single or serial specimens, with symptoms consistent with brucellosis. By 3 weeks of illness, over 97 per cent of patients demonstrate serologic evidence of infection. Several problems exist, however, with the STA test. This test equally detects antibodies to *B. abortus, B. suis,* and *B. melitensis,* but not to *B. canis.* Serologic confirmation of *B. canis* infection requires *B. canis* or *B. ovis* antigen. Despite adequate antibiotic treatment, significant STA titers can persist for up to 2 years in 5 to 7 per cent of cases. As the STA titer may remain elevated, it is not useful in differentiating relapsing infection from other febrile illnesses in patients with past *Brucella* infections. Individuals with subclinical infection may demonstrate significant STA titers. In chronic localized brucellosis, STA titers may appear absent or low owing to a prozone phenomenon. This prozone effect appears to be related to the presence of immunoglobulin G (IgG) or immunoglobulin A (IgA) blocking antibodies; it can be eliminated if dilutions are carried out to at least 1:1280. False-positive STA titers due to immunologic cross-reactivity have been associated with *Brucella* skin testing, cholera vaccination, or infections due to *Vibrio cholerae, Francisella tularensis,* or *Yersinia enterocolitica.*

Immunoglobulin M (IgM) is the major agglutinating antibody formed in the first few weeks following infection with *Brucella* organisms. Thereafter, IgG levels also rise. The STA test measures both IgM and IgG. With prompt and adequate therapy, IgG antibody levels usually become undetectable after 6 to 12 months. If therapy is given, those patients who develop persistent *Brucella* infection usually maintain elevated IgG agglutinins. The addition of 2-mercaptoethanol (2-ME) to the STA test results in the detection of only IgG antibodies. In the absence of rising STA titers, a single elevated 2-ME *Brucella* agglutination titer ($\geq$1:160) suggests either current or recent infection. Since a substantial number of patients maintain elevated IgM antibodies for years after treatment, the 2-ME agglutination test helps to identify those patients who have been cured, as IgG titers usually disappear within 6 months of adequate treatment. Certain newer antibody tests, including an ELISA and radioimmunoassay (RIA), are more sensitive than the STA; these methods have not been widely employed, and agglutination tests remain the standard for serologic diagnosis.

TREATMENT. Antibiotic treatment of *Brucella* infections is complicated by a number of complex issues, including the requirement for antibiotics that penetrate intracellularly, for prolonged therapy to prevent relapse, and for bactericidal antibiotics in treating central nervous system infection and endocarditis, as well as the lack of controlled, randomized, double-blind studies comparing different antimicrobial regimens. Debate is still considerable regarding which antibiotic regimens are clearly superior.

Patients treated with single agents such as tetracycline, streptomycin, chloramphenicol, rifampin, or trimethoprim-sulfamethoxazole have a 10 to 40 per cent chance of failure or relapse. Therefore, most authorities consider that combination antibiotic therapy for brucellosis is indicated. In acute brucellosis, without evidence of endocarditis or central nervous system involvement, the antibiotic regimen of tetracycline (2 grams per day) for 6 weeks plus streptomycin (1 gram per day) for 3 weeks has been used widely and has a low rate of relapse. Intramuscular administration of streptomycin makes this therapy difficult in some circumstances. Currently, doxycycline (200 mg per day) plus rifampin (600 to 900 mg per day) for 6 weeks is considered the antibiotic regimen of choice by the World Health Organization. Acute brucellosis in children can be treated with trimethoprim-sulfamethoxazole.

In central nervous system brucellosis, the combination of a third-generation cephalosporin with rifampin should be considered. In localized brucellosis, surgical drainage of abscesses should be pursued in conjunction with antimicrobial therapy for 6 or more weeks. *Brucella* endocarditis, which accounts for the highest mortality rates among *Brucella* infections, requires bactericidal drugs; early valve replacement is often necessary because of aortic valve destruction and/or major arterial emboli.

PROGNOSIS. Brucellosis appropriately treated within the first month of symptom onset is curable. Acute brucellosis often produces severe weakness and fatigue, and patients are frequently unable to work for up to 2 months. Immunity to reinfection follows initial *Brucella* infection in the majority of individuals. With early antimicrobial therapy, cases of chronic brucellosis or localized disease and complications are rare. Of patients who die of brucellosis, 84 per cent have endocarditis involving a previously abnormal aortic valve, often associated with severe congestive heart failure.

PREVENTION. The control of human brucellosis relates directly to prevention programs in domestic animals and avoidance of unpasteurized milk and milk products. With control in animals and the resultant marked decrease in human cases, the need for a vaccination program in humans has been less pressing. In other countries, the experience with human vaccination has shown a narrow range between efficacy and toxicity. In slaughterhouses, important means of prevention include careful wound dressing, protective glasses and clothing, prohibition of raw meat ingestion, and the use of previously infected (immune) individuals in high-risk areas. Eradication of human cases requires elimination of disease in animals and a greater awareness by the physician of the epidemiology, nuances of clinical presentation, and available diagnostic and treatment strategies in *Brucella* infections.

Ariza J, Gudiol F, Valverde J, et al.: Brucella spondylitis: A detailed analysis based on current findings. Rev Infect Dis 7:656, 1985. *The epidemiologic, clinical, diagnostic, and therapeutic features of spondylitis due to* B. melitensis *are detailed in 20 patients included in a 10-year prospective study from Barcelona, Spain.*

Arnow PM, Smaron M, Ormiste V: Brucellosis in a group of travelers to Spain. JAMA 251:505, 1984. *Describes the risk of brucellosis in travelers to endemic areas and the value of epidemiologic investigation to detect unrecognized cases.*

Bouza E, Garcia de la Torre M, Parris F, et al.: Brucella meningitis. Rev Infect Dis 9:810, 1987. *An excellent review about the variable clinical manifestations and approaches to the diagnosis and treatment of meningitis due to* Brucella.

Buchanan TM, Faber LC, Feldman RA: Brucellosis in the United States, 1960–1972: An abattoir-associated disease. I. Clinical features and therapy. Buchanan TM, Sulzer CR, Frix MK, et al.: II. Diagnostic aspects. Buchanan TM, Hendricks SL, Patton CM, et al.: III. Epidemiology and evidence for acquired immunity. Medicine 53:403, 415, 427, 1974. *A very complete description of all aspects of brucellosis derived from a study of 160 patients in a large Iowa slaughterhouse.*

Fernandez-Guerrero ML, Martinell J, Agaudo JM, et al.: Prosthetic valve endocarditis. Arch Intern Med 147:1141, 1987. *Highlights the expanding spectrum of brucellosis to include prosthetic valve infections and issues regarding management.*

Gazapo E, Gonzalez Lahoz J, Subiza JL, et al.: Changes in IgM and IgG antibody concentrations in brucellosis over time: Importance for diagnosis and follow-up. J Infect Dis 159:219, 1989. *Patterns of antibody responses correlating with successful treatment, chronic disease, or drug relapses and failures were followed prospectively and proved clinically useful.*

Gotuzzo E, Carrillo C, Guerra J, et al.: An evaluation of diagnostic methods for brucellosis—the value of bone marrow culture. J Infect Dis 153:122, 1986. *The high yield of bone marrow culture in patients with* B. melitensis *infection is emphasized.*

Hall WH: Modern chemotherapy for brucellosis in humans. Rev Infect Dis 12:1060, 1990. *A comprehensive analysis of the world's literature related to therapy of brucellosis that stresses that prolonged combined chemotherapy in conjunction with surgery, where indicated, is the key to successful treatment.*

Jacobs F, Abramowicz D, Vereerstraeten P, et al.: Brucella endocarditis: The role for combined medical and surgical treatment. Rev Infect Dis 12:740, 1990. *A review of 39 cases of cured* Brucella endocarditis.

330 Cat Scratch Disease

Andrew M. Margileth

DEFINITION. Cat scratch disease is characterized by tender regional chronic lymphadenopathy that is frequently preceded by a primary skin lesion related to cat contact or scratches. The disease is usually benign, and the adenopathy resolves spontaneously in 3 weeks to several months. In about 3 per cent of patients, severe systemic disease (pulmonary hilar adenopathy, hepatosplenomegaly with granuloma, neuroretinitis, encephalopathy, angiomatoid papules) has occurred.

ETIOLOGY. Since 1983, studies by Wear et al. have continued to identify a pleomorphic gram-negative rod-shaped bacterium in tissue from patients with clinical and histopathologic criteria of cat scratch disease. These specimens include about 900 lymph nodes, 10 primary inoculation skin lesions, and over 12 from patients with ocular granulomas. Recently, a gram-negative pleomorphic bacillus was cultured from over 20 patients with subacute cat scratch disease. Further identification of this organism is pending.

EPIDEMIOLOGY. Since the initial description by Debré (1950), over 3000 patients with cat scratch disease have been reported. Cat scratch disease may occur in preschool children and in adults, but over 60 per cent of cases present between ages 5 and 21 years. An estimated 2000 unreported cases occur annually in the United States. The disease is worldwide, occurring in all races, with a predominance in males (55 per cent). In temperate zones, most cases have occurred during fall and winter. Seasonal variation is minimal in warmer climates. There is a familial clustering in 5 per cent of cases.

TRANSMISSION AND COMMUNICABILITY. The mode of transmission is presumably by direct contact, since the bubo usually follows a scratch, bite, or lick from a young cat. Cat contact occurs in 94 per cent of patients. The disease has also developed after a dog bite or scratch and rarely after a scratch from a thorn, wood splinter, or fish bone or after insect bites. Person-to-person transmission has not been reported. Attempts to isolate an infectious agent from cat saliva or claws have been unsuccessful. The healthy cat—often a kitten—apparently acts as a mechanical vector for the infective agent, for skin tests with cat scratch antigen on the implicated cats have been nonreactive. Studies in family outbreaks have shown that the family cat usually transmits the causative agent no longer than 2 to 3 weeks.

PATHOGENESIS AND PATHOLOGY. No serologic test is available to measure antibodies to the causative agent. Fortunately, the cat scratch skin test is reliable and has a high degree of specificity; the reaction is a delayed hypersensitivity type. A positive reaction is usually detected at the time the clinical diagnosis is suspected; however, conversion may be delayed up to 4 weeks thereafter. Cutaneous reactivity lasts up to 10 years. Recurrent lymphadenopathy has been reported recently in three adults.

Histopathologic findings of biopsied lymph nodes may show a broad spectrum of reactions: arteriolar proliferation and widening of arteriolar walls, reticulum cell hyperplasia, multiple microabscesses, frank abscess formation, and round or stellate granulomas. Other than the vascular changes, similar histopathologic findings may be found in tularemia, brucellosis, tuberculosis, lymphogranuloma venereum, and the solid granulomas in sarcoidosis. One presentation, reticulum cell hyperplasia and granulomas, is suggestive of Hodgkin's disease. Cat scratch bacilli were best demonstrated by the Warthin-Starry silver impregnation stain in nodes removed during the first 3 to 4 weeks of the illness. In early lesions these bacteria were abundant in clumps or filaments and were most readily found in vessel walls, collagen fibers, and microabscesses. The bacilli ranged in size from 0.2 to 0.3 μm in diameter and 0.5 to 1.5 μm in length.

CLINICAL MANIFESTATIONS. The patient usually is not ill in spite of impressive lymphadenopathy; however, malaise, fever, fatigue, headache, and anorexia may be present. Three to 10 days elapse from the time of the scratch or contact until a primary skin papule or pustule forms. One or more erythematous papules may be observed. Unilateral conjunctival granuloma or conjunctivitis occurred in 6 per cent of the author's 1237 patients. An inoculation site (a scratch or a primary lesion, or both) may be detected in 64 to 96 per cent of patients, depending on the thoroughness of the examination and the duration of the bubo. Most primary lesions persist for 1 to 3 weeks, rarely for months, and heal without scar formation. Regional lymphadenopathy usually develops about 2 weeks after the scratch (range, 5 to 50 days). Lymphangitis has not been observed. Tender nodes, present in 80 per cent of patients for the first 1 or 2 weeks, are commonly found in the head, neck, or axilla. Epitrochlear, inguinal, femoral, or occipital areas are involved less frequently. Multiple site involvement occurred in one third of the author's cases. Node size varies from 1 to 8 cm. Enlargement persists for 2 to 4 months, rarely for 6 to 24 months. Suppuration occurs in

about 10 per cent of patients seen in office practice and in about 25 per cent of those admitted to hospitals.

About one half of patients have no clinical signs other than lymphadenopathy. About one third have fever (38.3 to 41.2°C) lasting for 5 to 9 (range, 1 to 60) days; 30 per cent have malaise or an influenza-like syndrome lasting about 4 (range, 1 to 21) days. Less common manifestations include splenomegaly (11 per cent), the oculoglandular syndrome of Parinaud (6 per cent), central nervous system involvement (2 per cent), and severe chronic systemic disease (2 per cent) (see Tables 330–1 and 330–2). Rarely, thrombocytopenic purpura, hepatosplenomegaly, breast tumor, and osteomyelitis have been reported.

Central or peripheral nervous system involvement may develop in all age groups. Encephalopathy, meningitis, neuroretinitis, radiculitis, polyneuritis, or myelitis with paraplegia has been observed in over 110 patients. Onset of neurologic symptoms is sudden, usually with fever, and occurs within 1 to 6 weeks of the

TABLE 330–1. CLINICAL FEATURES IN 1237 PATIENTS WITH CAT SCRATCH ADENOPATHY AND A POSITIVE SKIN TEST (APRIL 1975 TO JANUARY 1990)

Category	Percentage of Patients
Animal contact	
Cat	94
Dog	5
None	1
Animal scratch	
Cat	75
Dog	2
None	23
Primary lesion	
Skin papule or pustule	54
Eye granuloma	6
Mucous membrane	4
Symptoms and signs	
None except adenopathy	48
Fever (38.3–41.2°C)	32
Malaise/fatigue	30
Headache	14
Anorexia/emesis/weight loss	15
Splenomegaly	11
Sore throat	8
Exanthem	5
Parotid swelling	1.3

TABLE 330–2. CAT SCRATCH LYMPHADENOPATHY IN 1237 PATIENTS: CLINICAL CHARACTERISTICS OF INVOLVED NODES AND DURATION OF ADENOPATHY (APRIL 1875 TO JANUARY 1990)

Adenopathy (N = 1237)	Per Cent	Size (cm) (N = 1237)	Per Cent
Single node	42.5	1.0 to <3.0	41.4
Multiple nodes	24	3.0 to <5.0	39
Multiple sites	33	≥5.0	19.6
Tender nodes	79		
Suppuration	16		

Location (N = 1636*)	Per Cent	Duration of Node (N = 818)	Per Cent
Head: total (N = 286†)	17.5	Prior to diagnosis‡	
Submandibular	12	1 to <4 weeks	45
Preauricular	5	1 to <2 months	31
Neck: total (N = 634)	39	2 to <4 months	15
Posterior	14	4 to <6 months	3
Anterior	21	6 to <12 months	3
Supraclavicular	3	Regression (months, <1.0 cm)§ (N = 1235)	
Extremities: total (N = 712)	43.5	1 to <2	15
Axillary	25	2 to <6	63
Epitrochlear/brachial	7.3	6 to <12	14
Inguinal	7	12 to <24	5
Femoral	4.3	≥24	0.8

*Mediastinal = 3, breast = 2, pancreas = 1, mesenteric = 1: N = 7 (0.5%).
†Occipital = 16 (1%).
‡Duration ≥12 months = 22 (3%).
§2 to 4 weeks = 27 (2.2%).

onset of adenopathy. There may be cerebrospinal fluid pleocytosis, elevated protein levels, or both. Electroencephalograms are abnormal in most patients. Severe manifestations last for 1 to 2 weeks, with complete recovery in 1 to 12 months.

Cat scratch disease in individuals with acquired immunodeficiency syndrome (AIDS) is less well recognized and is often confused with other clinical manifestations related to AIDS. Although cat scratch disease in children with AIDS has not been reported, the syndrome in adults has unusual manifestations and responds to antibiotic therapy. Recently, the first case of culture-proven cat scratch disease in an AIDS patient was reported. The patient with AIDS often presents with numerous lesions ranging from pink to deep reddish-purple papules to sessile nodules or pedunculated nodules on any part of the body. The skin lesions occur most frequently on the head, trunk, or extremities but may also occur on the conjunctival, oral, or nasal mucosa. The nodules are firm, indurated, and usually nontender and range in size from 1 mm to 6 cm in diameter. Clinically, the lesions are indistinguishable from Kaposi's sarcoma, histiocytoid hemangioma, epithelioid hemangioma, or pyogenic granuloma. Radiographs of lesions over bone may show increased bone loss and periostosis and a marked increase in soft tissue mass.

DIAGNOSIS. Regional lymphadenopathy developing 2 weeks after cat contact, and especially if a primary inoculation papule or pustule followed a scratch, suggests cat scratch disease. Three of the four following manifestations would confirm the diagnosis in a typical case, whereas all four would be necessary in an atypical case: (1) a history of animal (usually cat) contact, with the presence of a scratch or a primary dermal, eye, or mucous membrane lesion; (2) negative laboratory studies (serology, cultures of aspirated pus or lymph node, PPD-T, and PPD-Battey) for other causes of lymphadenopathy; (3) a positive skin test result to one or two cat scratch antigens; (4) node biopsy revealing typical histopathology, especially if pleomorphic rod-shaped bacilli can be demonstrated with the Warthin-Starry silver stain.

If a negative skin test result is found to one or two different cat scratch antigens applied simultaneously and again 4 weeks later, and if results of other studies are negative, a biopsy must be considered to rule out a benign tumor or lymphoma. The presence of tenderness favors cat scratch or a pyogenic or mycobacterial adenopathy rather than a neoplasm. Ultrasonography has been very useful in deciding whether or not to aspirate nontender or nonfluctuant cervical masses. It may also aid needle placement for cyst or abscess aspiration.

Skin Tests. A skin test using cat scratch antigen is positive in 98 per cent of patients who are clinically suspected of having cat scratch disease. A negative result often occurs if the duration of illness is less than 3 or 4 weeks, and 1 to 2 per cent of patients with typical cat scratch disease have negative test results with one or two different antigens. The positive reaction consists of a wheal or papule with 5 mm or more of induration, with or without erythema, occurring 48 to 72 hours after intradermal inoculation of 0.1 ml of antigen. Induration may persist for 5 to 6 days or longer. A positive test result may be obtained for years (10 to 28) after the initial episode.

Positive reactions have been reported in veterinarians (12 to 29 per cent), healthy persons (5 per cent), and family contacts (18 per cent); the overall incidence is 5 per cent. Thus the limit of confidence for a positive reaction in a person suspected of having cat scratch disease is about 95 per cent. If the reaction is negative at 4-week intervals, the disease can be excluded with reasonable certainty, especially if two different antigens are used. Repeated skin testing with cat scratch antigen in the same patients has not produced positive reactions.

Since cat scratch antigen is not available commercially, aspirated pus from affected nodes should be saved to prepare test antigen. Cat scratch antigen for medical diagnosis is usually available from the author upon written request.

Laboratory Data. Laboratory tests are not diagnostic. Eosinophilia has been reported. At the onset there may be a mild leukocytosis. The erythrocyte sedimentation rate is usually elevated during the first few weeks of adenopathy.

DIFFERENTIAL DIAGNOSIS. Cat scratch disease should be considered in all patients with persistent lymphadenopathy (over 3 weeks), because it is the most common cause of chronic regional lymphadenitis in children or adolescents. The presence of an inoculation (dermal or ocular) lesion strongly suggests cat scratch disease. Other less common causes are sporotrichosis, primary syphilis, lymphogranuloma venereum, typical or atypical tuberculosis, other bacterial adenitis, tularemia, brucellosis, histoplasmosis, coccidioidomycosis, sarcoidosis, toxoplasmosis, infectious mononucleosis, and benign or malignant tumors. In atypical forms of cat scratch disease, one may observe benign parotid lymphosialadenopathy, Parinaud's oculoglandular disease, encephalitis, pneumonia, thrombocytopenic purpura with or without anemia, erythema nodosum, angiomatoid papules, and osteomyelitis, as well as fluctuant lymphadenopathy simulating cystic hygroma or a thyroglossal duct cyst. If cat scratch skin test reactions, appropriate cultures, and serologic and PPD-T and PPD-Battey skin tests are negative, a node biopsy will usually determine the cause.

TREATMENT. The best therapy is reassurance that the adenopathy is benign and in most cases will subside spontaneously within 2 or 3 months. Management consists of appropriate follow-up examination, analgesics for pain, and aspiration if suppuration occurs. Commonly used antimicrobials are usually ineffective. Gentamicin or trimethoprim-sulfamethoxazole (TMP-SMX) may be effective. Gentamicin sulfate is given intramuscularly, 5 mg per kilogram per 24 hours in divided doses. TMP-SMX is given orally, 6 to 12 mg of TMP and 30 to 60 mg of SMX per kilogram twice daily for 7 days. In the child whose node suppurates, needle aspiration on an ambulatory basis is preferred to incision and drainage. After washing with povidone-iodine (Betadine) cleanser, a needle (18 or 20 gauge) is inserted through normal unanesthetized skin at the base of the mass to avoid a chronic sinus tract in the event that a tuberculous lesion is present. Aspiration provides material for skin test antigen, relieves painful adenopathy, and usually allows the patient to become symptom free within 24 to 48 hours. If fluid recurs, reaspiration may be necessary. Application of moist soaks to the primary lesion may facilitate drainage and shorten the duration of lymphadenopathy. The efficacy of steroid therapy is questionable, and it is not recommended. Excisional biopsy of the node may be necessary in selected patients because of persistent pain or for diagnostic purposes.

Paradoxically, patients with human immunodeficiency virus (HIV) infection and associated skin, bone, liver, or spleen lesions, lymphadenopathy, and associated systemic illness due to cat scratch disease have responded promptly to common antibiotics (erythromycin, doxycycline, antimycobacterial drugs). In vitro studies have shown the English-Wear bacillus to have microbial susceptibility to aminoglycosides, cefoxitin sodium, cefotaxime sodium, netilmicin sulfate, and mezlocillin sodium.

PROGNOSIS. The prognosis is excellent; lymphadenopathy usually regresses spontaneously in 2 to 4 months. One attack appears to confer lifelong immunity. Three adults had a recurrence of cat scratch disease. Complications and sequelae are almost nonexistent. Rarely, patients have been observed to have chronic adenopathy for 2 to 3 years.

PREVENTION. Because of the number of household pets (50 million cats in the United States), cat scratch disease is difficult to prevent. Disposal of the suspect cat is not recommended, because the cat involved is invariably well. Four to 9 per cent of family members scratched by the same cat may develop cat scratch disease. The patient with the disease does not require isolation or quarantine. Active or passive protection is not available.

Bogue CW, Wise JD, Gray GF, et al.: Antibiotic therapy for cat-scratch disease? JAMA 262:813, 1989. *Three patients with cat scratch disease were treated successfully with intramuscular gentamicin sulfate. Two patients had extensive hepatic involvement, and one had marked inguinal lymphadenitis.*

Carithers HA, Margileth AM: Cat scratch disease: Acute encephalopathy and other neurologic manifestations. AJDC 145:98, 1991. *Sixty-one patients developed encephalopathy within one-half to 6 weeks of the onset of cat scratch disease. The average age of the patients was 10.6 years (1 to 66 years). Convulsions occurred in 46 per cent and combative behavior in 40 per cent. Lethargy with or without coma was accompanied by variable neurologic signs. The "English-Wear" bacillus was demonstrated in 10 of 14 biopsy specimens. All 61 patients recovered within ½ to 12 months.*

Collipp PJ: Cat scratch disease therapy. AJDC 143:1261, 1989. *Eleven patients with proven CSD responded to oral TMP-SMX therapy within 1 week.*

English CK, Wear DJ, Margileth AM, et al.: Cat scratch disease: Isolation and culture of the bacterial agent. JAMA 259:1347, 1988. *A gram-negative bacterium or its cell wall defective variants were isolated from lymph nodes of 10 patients with cat scratch disease. Vegetative bacteria produced lesions in the skin of an armadillo identical to early lesions in human skin. These vegetative bacteria were recovered from the lesions in the armadillo.*

Kemper CA, Lombard CM, Deresinski SC, et al.: Visceral bacillary epithelioid angiomatosis. Am J Med 89:216, 1990. *Two adults, one HIV infected and one not HIV infected, are reported. The HIV-infected patient had bacillary epithelioid angiomatosis of liver and bone marrow, causing hepatic failure. The cardiac transplant recipient had fever of unknown origin with hepatic and splenic bacillary epithelioid angiomatosis, with positive Warthin-Starry cat scratch–like stain.*

Koehler JE, LeBoit PE, Egbert BM, et al.: Cutaneous vascular lesions and disseminated cat-scratch disease in patients with the acquired immunodeficiency syndrome (AIDS) and AIDS-related complex. Ann Intern Med 109:449, 1988. *Four patients with AIDS developed angiomatous nodules involving skin and bone, two of whom were scratched by a cat. Numerous bacteria were noted in these nodules by the Warthin-Starry stain and electron microscopy. Rapid resolution of skin and osseous lesions occurred after treatment with erythromycin, doxycycline, or antimycobacterial antibiotics.*

Relman DA, Loutit JS, Schmidt TM, et al.: The agent of bacillary angiomatosis. N Engl J Med 323:1573, 1990. *Tissue from three unrelated patients with bacillary angiomatosis yielded a unique 16S gene sequence. These 16S sequences belong to a previously uncharacterized microorganism, most closely related to Rochalimgea quintana, a rickettsia-like organism.*

Schlossberg D, Morad Y, Krouse TB, et al.: Culture-proved disseminated cat-scratch disease in acquired immunodeficiency syndrome. Arch Intern Med 149:1437, 1989. *An HIV-positive adult with cat scratch disease developed papillitis and retinitis that responded to TMP-SMX and dexamethasone. Subsequently, epithelioid hemangioma, liver abscesses, pleural effusion, and gingival Kaposi's sarcoma developed. Cultures of lymph node, pleural fluid, and liver yielded gram-negative bacilli believed to be the causative agent of cat scratch disease.*

331 Bartonellosis

C. Glenn Cobbs

DEFINITION. Bartonellosis (Carrión's disease) is an insect-borne bacterial disorder characterized by two well-defined clinical stages. It has a striking geographic restriction, occurring only on the western coast of South America at altitude. The first stage, Oroya fever, was recognized in the nineteenth century when it caused an outbreak of febrile hemolytic anemia among railway workers in Peru. Even before that time, the cutaneous stage, verruga peruana, had been described. The common bacterial etiology of the two forms of the disease was established in 1885 by Daniel Carrión, a Peruvian medical student, when he died of acute hemolytic anemia 39 days after inoculation with material from a verruga lesion.

ETIOLOGY. In 1909, Barton described the causative microorganism, *Bartonella bacilliformis*, a small, motile, pleomorphic bacillus that can be grown on various enriched media.

EPIDEMIOLOGY. Bartonellosis is generally restricted to the habitat of its main vector, the sandfly, *Phlebotomus verrucarum*. Other *Phlebotomus* species have rarely been associated with transmission. The sandfly breeds and transmits the infection in river valleys of the Andes Mountains at an altitude between 2500 and 9000 feet. Humans provide the only known reservoir of the microorganism. Convalescent individuals may have low-grade bacteremia for months to years after infection, and *B. bacilliformis* may be recovered from 5 to 10 per cent of apparently healthy persons in an endemic area. These carriers present the greatest epidemiologic threat.

Similar hemotropic bacterial species have occasionally been described in other geographic locales, but these microorganisms are distinguishable from *B. bacilliformis*.

PATHOLOGY. After inoculation by the vector, the bacteria replicate in the human host and invade erythrocytes and endothelial cells. Red cell parasitization results in increased fragility of red cells and increased phagocytosis by the reticuloendothelial system. In severe cases, as many as 90 per cent of the circulating erythrocytes may be parasitized. The hemolytic anemia that ensues results in fever, anemia, and weakness. Peripheral blood smears reveal a normochromic macrocytosis, striking polychromasia, Howell-Jolly bodies, Cabot rings, and nucleated erythrocytes. The Coombs test and other assays for red cell agglutinins and hemolysins are usually negative. Cells of the reticuloendothelial system may demonstrate intracellular organisms, presumably as a result of erythrophagocytosis, and reactive hyperplasia of lymphatic tissue is common.

Most untreated patients who survive the acute hemolytic anemia go on to develop the chronic cutaneous lesions of verruga peruana. These hemangiomatous nodules consist of proliferating small vessels infiltrated by lymphocytes and macrophages. Verrugas may also occur in the viscera, bone, and central nervous system.

CLINICAL MANIFESTATIONS. Within 2 to 6 weeks after the sandfly bite, the nonimmune host develops Oroya fever, characterized by the insidious onset of myalgias and low-grade fever, followed by high fever, headache, and painful muscles and joints. Tender lymphadenopathy is common, but splenomegaly should suggest some other disorder. Erythrocyte counts decrease rapidly within a few days and many fall as low as 1 million per cubic millimeter. The combination of anemia and jaundice results in a lemon color in light-skinned individuals. In some patients, the disease is characterized by a febrile crisis, followed by rapid resolution of symptoms and signs, increased erythropoiesis, and gradual reduction in fever. Recurrence of fever after initial improvement suggests secondary infection. *Salmonella* disease is an especially important complication of bartonellosis, as it is in other disorders associated with hemolysis, such as sickle cell anemia.

After resolution of the febrile hemolytic anemia, immunity develops, and relapses or reinfections are distinctly unusual. After a latent period, which ranges in untreated patients from weeks to months, many patients manifest the second stage of bartonellosis, verruga peruana. This disorder is characterized by hemangiomatous nodules that are reddish-purple, are 1 to 2 cm in diameter, and typically evolve over 1 to 2 months in crops on exposed skin but also on mucous membranes and internal organs. The lesions are usually nontender and morphologically may vary, appearing as ulcers or secondarily infected pustules. In some instances, these may be mistaken for Kaposi's sarcoma or other malignant disorders of skin. The verrugas may persist for months to years in untreated patients.

DIAGNOSIS. The diagnosis is made by examining the peripheral blood film. There bacilli may be seen within red cells, either singly or in pairs or clusters. With a Giemsa stain, the bacilli appear as 0.3- to 1.5-μm red or reddish-purple rods with some pleomorphism. The microorganism may be cultured from blood if appropriate media are utilized. Identification of the microorganisms in the verrucal lesion is possible but more difficult.

TREATMENT AND PROGNOSIS. The mortality in untreated Oroya fever approaches 50 per cent and is a result of both acute hemolytic anemia and secondary infectious disorders, such as *Salmonella* disease, as noted above. Malaria, amebiasis, and tuberculosis also appear to be more common in these patients. Penicillin, chloramphenicol, and possibly tetracycline or streptomycin all seem to be clinically effective. Chloramphenicol, at a dose of 2 to 4 grams daily for 7 or more days, is the therapy of choice because of the frequent association of *Salmonella* infection. In patients so treated, fever generally disappears within 2 to 3 days, although blood smears may remain positive for some time longer.

PREVENTION. Insecticides, particularly those with dichlorodiphenyl trichloroethane (DDT), are of use in eradicating the vector.

Schultz MG: A history of bartonellosis (Carrión's disease). Am J Trop Med Hyg 17:503, 1980. *A fascinating summary of the initial historical accounts, medical descriptions, and investigations into the etiology and epidemiology of the disease.*

Diseases Due to Mycobacteria

332 Tuberculosis

Emanuel Wolinsky

DEFINITION. Tuberculosis is a chronic infectious disease caused by mycobacteria of the "tuberculosis complex," mainly *Mycobacterium tuberculosis.*

INCIDENCE. During the Industrial Revolution of the eighteenth and ninteenth centuries, the disease was known as the *white plague.* It was the leading cause of death in young people all over the world. Today, despite great progress in its treatment and control, it remains an important medical problem in many developing countries. There are still 4 to 10 million new cases and about 1 million deaths each year from tuberculosis. In the United States tuberculosis mortality decreased from a rate of 202 per 100,000 in 1900 to less than 1 in 1982. The new case rate has also declined from about 60 per 100,000 in 1950 to 9 in 1985. During the last few years, however, there has been little decline, and even an upsurge in 1986, in the number of new cases reported, thought to be primarily related to the association of tuberculosis with the acquired immunodeficiency syndrome (AIDS).

The rate of infection as determined by skin test surveys remains high in many developing countries. In the United States the rate has become increasingly difficult to estimate because of the abandonment of large-scale testing in cities. Information obtained in 1977 from selected urban areas of the country indicated that the rate of infection varied from less than 3 per cent in young children to 14 to 40 per cent in adults over the age of 65. Tuberculosis is becoming more and more a disease of middle-aged and older nonwhite men in residual urban pockets of disease associated with poverty and overcrowding.

ETIOLOGY. The microorganism that causes tuberculosis belongs to the genus *Mycobacterium,* which is classified in the family Mycobacteriaceae of the order Actinomycetales. Taxonomists do not agree on the further classification of the genus, but a useful concept is that of the tuberculosis complex to include *M. tuberculosis, M. bovis,* and probably *M. africanum.* Some taxonomists would subdivide *M. bovis* into European, Afro-Asian, and African variants. A few suggest that there should be just one species, *M. tuberculosis,* with subclassifications of bovine type, African type, and so forth.

M. tuberculosis is an obligate intracellular parasite that shares with other mycobacteria a characteristic staining quality. The popular abbreviation *AFB* for *acid-fast bacilli* is based on this quality. Acid-fastness is the result of retention of carbol fuchsin (or certain fluorochrome dyes) after washing with acid, alcohol, or both. It is not unique to mycobacteria, since *Nocardia* and certain *Corynebacterium* strains may also be acid fast. Mycobacterial cell walls are rich in lipids, existing mainly as complexes with peptides and polysaccharides. Certain stains can form a stable complex with one of these lipid compounds, mycolic acid, provided that the latter is contained within an intact cell wall structure.

In addition to the members of the tuberculosis complex, the genus *Mycobacterium* may be divided into about 30 species. Again, there is disagreement among the taxonomists on the definition of some of these species (see Ch. 333).

PATHOLOGY AND PATHOGENESIS. Tuberculosis is derived from the word *tubercle,* meaning a small lump or nodule. Histopathologically, the tubercle is a more or less discrete focus of granulomatous inflammation consisting of lymphocytes, epithelioid cells, macrophages, and giant cells. The granulomas seen in tuberculosis are characterized by a form of tissue necrosis known as *caseation,* so called because the caseum has the consistency of soft cheese. Prior to the time of necrosis the lesion may heal completely by resolution, but once necrosis and caseation have occurred it heals by fibrosis, encapsulation, calcification, and scar formation. Breakdown of the pulmonary lesion occurs when the caseum softens and liquefies and is expelled through the bronchial system. This process results in the formation of a cavity in the lung. Spread of disease may occur by local extension, by an intrabronchial route, or through the lymphohematogenous pathway. Early in the primary infection the organisms are transported to the draining lymph nodes and may be widely disseminated throughout the body. In the apical posterior areas of the upper lobes the seeded organisms may remain dormant in inactive lesions for many years only to reactivate during a period of lowered host immunity. The processes of healing and breakdown may occur sequentially and repeatedly so that various stages of the inflammatory reaction are seen in different areas.

The primary lesion in a nonsensitized individual consists of an area of nonspecific pneumonitis in a middle or lower lung zone at the site of deposition of the inhaled droplet nuclei carrying tubercle bacilli. The initial inflammatory response is the same as that seen in any bacterial pneumonia and consists mainly of fibrin, edema, and polymorphonuclear leukocytes. The extent of this primary exudative response varies with the number and virulence of the bacilli inhaled, the native resistance of the host, and the effectiveness of the immune response. The change to a granulomatous type of reaction occurs coincidentally with the development of delayed hypersensitivity after 2 or 3 weeks. The mechanisms of cellular immunity may allow the host to wall off the lesion and to halt the lymphohematogenous spread. It is the softening and liquefaction of the caseous focus that leads to further trouble and the provision of a favorable environment for the rapid multiplication of the mycobacteria. In the encapsulated lesion that does not soften, the bacilli slowly lose their viability.

Stages in the natural history of untreated pulmonary tuberculosis, especially as it occurs in childhood, may be described as follows:

1. During the primary phase and throughout the development of the lesions there are usually no symptoms. Even in the so-called manifest primary stage, symptoms may be mild or absent despite parenchymal lesions and enlarged hilar or mediastinal lymph nodes. Pleurisy with effusion may occur. Life-threatening complications at this stage are meningitis and miliary disease.

2. The primary disease usually heals, leaving evidence of its presence in the form of a calcified pulmonary scar along with calcifications in the draining lymph nodes, which together are known as a *Ghon's complex.*

3. The third stage is one of latency, during which the bacilli remain dormant but still viable within inactive lesions. This situation may exist for the remainder of the patient's life.

4. Reactivation may occur in a relatively small proportion of infected individuals. This is the mechanism by which tuberculosis in the adult usually develops, either in the lung or in an extrapulmonary site.

5. Exogenous reinfection occasionally may be documented by the demonstration of bacilli with a different phage type or drug sensitivity pattern from those of the primary infection.

EPIDEMIOLOGY. Infection is usually transmitted from person to person by the inhalation of infective droplet nuclei that result from the aerosolization of respiratory secretions. The source of the infected material usually is an adult with cavitary pulmonary tuberculosis. The most important determinants of infectivity are the concentration of organisms in the sputum and the closeness and duration of contact with the index case. Other factors of importance are the cough frequency and the personal habits of the index case, the efficiency with which aerosols are produced by such activities as singing, loud talking, and laughing, and the air circulation and ventilation in the area of contact. A situation favorable to acquisition of infection would be an overcrowded and poorly ventilated house in which there were several young children and an adult with highly positive sputum.

Ingestion is no longer a common pathway for infection, although in the days of unpasteurized milk and widespread tuberculosis in cattle this was a common route of infection for *M. bovis*, especially for the production of tuberculosis of the tonsils and subsequent involvement of the submandibular lymph nodes. Another route of infection that still may be observed, however, is primary inoculation through the skin. Laboratory workers may inoculate themselves with actively growing cultures via needle puncture or broken glass, and pathologists may sustain a penetrating injury while doing a postmortem examination.

Many localized outbreaks or miniepidemics have been reported in the past and continue to be observed today (Lincoln, 1967; Stead, 1979). The pattern of airborne transmission in a closed environment is well described in these accounts of infections aboard ships, in day care centers, nursing homes, prisons, industrial school dormitories, and school buses, and among members of a choir.

Tuberculosis Control. Tuberculosis is perpetuated by the repeated cycle of new infections that result from the inhalation of infected droplet nuclei coughed into the air by adults with cavitary pulmonary disease. This cycle may be attacked at several points. Case-finding efforts are needed to recognize individuals with active disease so that they may be placed under treatment to terminate the infectivity. Large-scale roentgenographic surveys have been abandoned in favor of contact investigation, recognition of symptomatic cases at entry points to the medical care system, and surveillance of high-risk groups such as hospital personnel, prisoners, and nursing home patients.

Protection from the complications of primary disease may be afforded by vaccination with bacille Calmette-Guérin (BCG). This was a strain of *M. bovis* attenuated by many passages on artificial media. There are now many different strains, each unique, maintained in laboratories across the world. Vaccination has been utilized mainly in areas that have a high rate of tuberculosis infection. Although vaccination may protect the individual, it does not reduce the overall rate of infection in the community, since it does not prevent the transmission of infection. Its effectiveness depends on an enhancement of the immune response, which enables the host to eliminate most of the bacilli before tissue destruction and dissemination occur. The efficacy of BCG is controversial. It has not been used extensively in the United States because it interferes with the subsequent use of the tuberculin test in recognizing tuberculosis infection and because the major source of morbidity is people already infected. Nevertheless, a case could be made for BCG in certain special circumstances such as to protect the infant whose noncompliant mother has active disease and to prevent infection in close contacts of an index case with drug-resistant bacilli.

Chemoprophylaxis may prevent infection in close contacts with negative skin tests, prevent disease in those already infected, and prevent subsequent recurrences in individuals with inactive pulmonary disease. The recommended drug for prophylaxis is isoniazid, once daily, in a dosage of 300 mg for adults and 10 mg per kilogram (not to exceed 300 mg) for children. When taken for 1 year, such treatment results in a reduction of at least 70 per cent in the appearance of primary disease in household contacts. Protection is about 90 per cent in those who actually take the drug as prescribed, and it continues for many years. There is some evidence that isoniazid for only 9 months is almost equally effective, and even shorter two-drug courses are being investigated. The two principal drawbacks to this method of control are isoniazid-related hepatitis and the failure of about 30 per cent of patients to take the prescribed medication.

The risk of developing active disease in recent tuberculin converters of any age is about 3 to 5 per cent in the first year after infection. From 5 to 15 per cent may progress to active disease within 5 years. The risk is greater in infants. Chemoprophylaxis is recommended for close contacts of patients with recently diagnosed active disease; for persons with recent infection documented by skin test conversion within the past 2 years; for individuals with positive skin test results, radiographic findings consistent with inactive tuberculous disease, and neither positive bacteriologic findings nor a history of adequate chemotherapy;

and for individuals with positive skin test results who have additional risk factors (such as malignancy or severe diabetes) or who are undergoing prolonged immunosuppressive or corticosteroid therapy. Although chemoprophylaxis is one of the important methods of tuberculosis control in this country, it has not been accepted in many other parts of the world. Isoniazid does not prevent disease resulting from infection with isoniazid-resistant bacilli. Rifampin alone, or combined with pyrazinamide for a few months, has been suggested as an alternative.

IMMUNOLOGY. Tuberculosis is the classic example of disease caused by an intracellular parasite. Protection is afforded by the mechanisms of cell-mediated immunity rather than by those associated with antibodies. Immunity may be natural or acquired, but in either case it is the macrophage that assumes the major burden of protection. Polymorphonuclear leukocytes have the ability to phagocytize but not to destroy mycobacteria. Although the results of some experiments are contradictory, most researchers have been able to demonstrate that macrophages from an immunized animal kill the bacilli more efficiently and at a more rapid rate than do control cells. Macrophages may be activated by immunologically specific mechanisms as well as by nonspecific stimulation. Specific stimulation occurs when sensitized T lymphocytes contact mycobacterial antigens that have been properly processed by macrophages. The lymphocytes then release a number of active chemical substances known as *lymphokines*, one variety of which activates macrophages.

Native immunity certainly has played a role in the global aspects of tuberculosis. Good examples exist in the animal kingdom; the rat and the cat are quite resistant to infection with *M. tuberculosis*, in contrast to the guinea pig and the monkey, which are highly susceptible. Lurie was able to breed two races of rabbits, one susceptible and one resistant to infection. Although it is difficult to separate the factors of social and economic conditions from those of race, the Eskimo peoples and blacks are considered by some researchers to be more susceptible. The forces of natural selection probably contributed to the decline of tuberculosis prior to the introduction of chemotherapy, although improved socioeconomic conditions played an important role. Acquired immunity may occur as a result of natural infection or by vaccination. Recovery from tuberculosis confers protection against reinfection with a new inoculum, even though the original bacilli may remain latent for many years and be capable of producing recrudescent disease. Whether acquired by natural infection or vaccination, the protection is only relative and may be overwhelmed by a sufficiently large infecting dose.

The relationship between delayed hypersensitivity and immunity is still controversial. The two functions appear at about the same time after infection and are intimately related thereafter. Nevertheless, it has been shown in experimental animals that immunity may remain despite abolition of a positive skin test result by desensitization and that immunity may be induced by ribosome preparations that do not induce a positive skin reaction.

The balance between the reactions of delayed hypersensitivity and those of the humoral antibody response is very important in determining the clinical presentation and prognosis in leprosy. A similar but less dramatic situation exists in tuberculosis. A more favorable prognosis may be expected for patients who have strong reactivity in their cell-mediated immune functions than for those who are hypoergic and have abundant antibody production. Patients with nonreactive tuberculosis tend to have disseminated disease with almost unopposed multiplication of the organisms in reticuloendothelial cells and a lack of granulomatous response. The question of whether the anergic state is the cause or the result of severe tuberculosis is moot. Recovery of the compromised cell-mediated immune functions, including delayed hypersensitivity, usually accompanies clinical improvement. A patient's location in the immune spectrum usually is dynamic and changeable rather than fixed.

The Tuberculin Skin Test. The biologically active material in the liquid medium after growth of *M. tuberculosis* was named *tuberculin* by Robert Koch. This crude material was later called *Old Tuberculin (OT)*. A purified protein derivative of tuberculin *(PPD)* was made by Siebert in 1924 by precipitation with saturated ammonium sulfate. The World Health Organization adopted a large batch, designated *PPD-S*, as the international standard tuberculin. Five tuberculin units *(TU)* was defined as the biologic activity contained in a specified weight of PPD-S. Solutions with much greater stability were achieved by the addition of a wetting agent. All preparations of PPD commercially available in this country must be bioequivalent to 5 TU of PPD-S as demonstrated by comparative testing in humans.

The intracutaneous, or Mantoux, test is performed by injecting 5 TU contained in 0.1 ml of solution intracutaneously with needle and syringe. This is known as the intermediate-strength test. It corresponds to 0.1 µg of the standard preparation. A more dilute solution containing 1 TU is available to test those who may be expected to have a very strong reaction, especially children. This preparation is known as first-strength PPD and is essentially a fivefold dilution of the 5 TU material. Second-strength PPD contains what is calculated to be 250 TU.

In the sensitized individual a reaction of redness, swelling, and induration begins at about 6 hours, reaches a maximum intensity at 36 to 60 hours, and then fades over the next several days. A positive result usually is defined as 10 mm or more of induration at 48 hours. This arbitrary definition is based on results of large-scale testing that showed that a reaction of 10 mm best separated those with from those without tuberculosis. The reading of the test is a subjective evaluation, with wide observer variation. It is only by averaging multiple readings made blindly by at least two expert readers that an accuracy within 3 mm may be approached.

It is unwise to have an arbitrary definition of a positive reaction in the diagnostic evaluation of a sick patient. Many factors may diminish the response in a nonspecific manner. They include virus infections or live virus vaccination; immunosuppression by disease, drugs, or steroids; malnutrition; overwhelming infection of any kind; and old age. It is best to measure the induration as accurately as possible and, in addition, to describe the intensity of both the erythema and the induration. Well-defined erythema that persists for 72 hours is usually indicative of a positive reaction. In case of doubt, it is often useful to repeat the test using 250 TU. If there is no reaction to the second-strength material, the odds against the diagnosis of nondisseminated tuberculosis are overwhelming. It is helpful to determine the reaction to other antigens utilizing the so-called *anergy panel*. The most useful are mumps, *Candida*, trichophytin, tetanus toxoid, and a streptococcal antigen such as streptokinase. Failure to react to the panel indicates a generalized state of cutaneous anergy, which may be expected to include tuberculin. Several multiple puncture devices are available for performing a tuberculin test. They should all be regarded as screening tests, and any doubtful or positive reactions should be tested with the Mantoux technique.

Intradermal administration of tuberculin in the recommended dosage does not induce an immunologic response even after repeated injections. However, a second injection from 2 weeks to 12 months after an original negative reaction may produce a booster response from recall of waning delayed hypersensitivity. To avoid the assumption that the positive reaction represents a new infection, it has been suggested that negative reactors be retested up to a week later in surveillance programs such as those for hospital personnel. Infection with any mycobacterium and probably with organisms of related genera, such as *Nocardia* and *Corynebacterium*, may give cross-reactions with the tuberculin test materials available today. Tuberculin reactivity is a quantitative function that may vary in intensity from time to time in a given person.

Factors Modifying the Course of Tuberculosis.

Before chemotherapy, tuberculosis patients were considered to be at risk for recrudescent disease for the rest of their lives. Mitchell was able to follow over 2000 patients for 15 to 25 years after their moderately or far advanced disease had become inactive. He found a relapse rate of 28 per cent. Even with modern drug therapy relapse occasionally may occur, depending mainly on whether or not the patient was cooperative in taking medication. A study of 20,000 cases reported to the Centers for Disease Control in 1980 revealed that 7 to 8 per cent represented recurrent disease.

Many conditions are known to increase the risk for the recurrence of tuberculosis. Among these are emotional stress, malnutrition, drug addiction, alcoholism, immunosuppression by diseases that interfere with cell-mediated immunity, and the use of drugs such as corticosteroids. Gastric resection is a risk factor, presumably in relation to malnutrition. A risk over 10 times that of suitable controls has been documented for patients with chronic renal failure on maintenance dialysis or for those with renal transplants. Influenza, pneumonia, and cancer of the lung may cause local reactivation of dormant lesions. Another local factor is pneumoconiosis, especially silicosis and coal worker's pneumoconiosis.

CLINICAL DESCRIPTION. *Pulmonary Tuberculosis.* Tuberculosis may involve any organ system, but the lung is the usual site of the primary lesion and the principal organ involved. In roughly one half of patients with extrapulmonary disease, however, the original pulmonary lesions may not be discernible clinically or radiographically.

Primary Tuberculosis. Primary tuberculosis refers to disease in a person not previously infected with a virulent mycobacterium of the tuberculosis complex. Primary tuberculosis formerly was seen almost exclusively in children and was known as the childhood type. At present it is not uncommon in adults of all ages. Most primary infections are subclinical and not detectable by ordinary radiographic procedures. They may be recognized, however, by a documented tuberculin skin test conversion. When accompanied by symptoms or radiographic evidence, or both, the disease is called manifest or overt primary tuberculosis. Enlarged hilar lymph nodes are almost always seen. Complications of the primary infection include pleurisy with effusion, miliary disease, meningitis, bone and joint disease, and progressive primary infection. In progressive primary disease the lesions enlarge, caseate, liquefy, and cavitate. Primary disease in adults is especially prone to progression and cavity formation.

The morbidity and mortality associated with primary infection are related to age. Although usually benign in older children and adults, it is life threatening when it occurs in infants. In a New York City study before the development of chemotherapy, tuberculosis in children less than 6 months of age had a mortality rate of 50 per cent. Congenital tuberculosis, often fatal, may be acquired from a mother with active disease by the hematogenous route or by the aspiration or ingestion of contaminated amniotic fluid. A unique finding in primary tuberculosis of young children is the development of consolidated and collapsed segmental lesions resulting from a combination of bronchial compression from enlarged hilar lymph nodes and extrusion of caseous contents into the bronchial lumen. This situation usually is clinically benign despite the alarmingly unhealthy appearance of the chest roentgenogram. The spectrum of primary tuberculosis in adults was documented by Stead and colleagues in 1968. In almost half of 37 adults the disease progressed without interruption into chronic pulmonary tuberculosis.

Reactivation Tuberculosis. This term refers to the pattern of disease in adults. It usually results from the reactivation of dormant foci in the posterior portions of the upper lobes that had been seeded by the bloodstream during the early primary infection. Occasionally adult disease is the result of a new inoculum of tubercle bacilli in a person already sensitized by a previous infection (*exogenous reinfection*). Adult disease is characterized by chronicity, caseation, sloughing of liquefied caseous material, cavity formation, and the simultaneous occurrence of healing and progression in different areas of the lung. Lymph node involvement is usually minimal or absent, at least in those nodes that directly drain the pulmonary foci. Phage typing of strains recovered from different areas of the body and correlation between antimicrobial susceptibility patterns and the history of drug intake have been used to document both recrudescence of an old infection and exogenous reinfection.

The onset of disease may be *insidious, catarrhal, hemoptoic,* or *acute.* With insidious onset there is gradual development of fatigue, anorexia, weight loss, and other vague complaints. Later, a low-grade intermittent fever may develop that is commonly associated with excessive sweating at night. The temperature elevation tends to occur in the late afternoon. The catarrhal onset is characterized by an increasingly productive cough and occasional blood streaking of the sputum. Fever and night sweats may also be noted. In the hemoptoic variety, the presenting symptom is hemoptysis either with or without other symptoms already mentioned. Occasionally, the onset is acute and influenza-like with high fever, chills, myalgia, and productive cough. Pleuritic pain may be the presenting complaint, often without pleural fluid but sometimes ushering in the appearance of an effusion. Many cases of adult-type pulmonary tuberculosis in the past were discovered by routine chest films in asymptomatic persons. Some individuals might recall minor symptoms, such as slight pleurisy, night sweats, or tiredness, but others would deny all warning signs despite the presence of advanced disease. Before the advent of chemotherapy it was not unusual for the patient to have hoarseness or perirectal abscess—both conditions being secondary to the long-term presence of highly positive sputum.

Diagnosis. A careful history and physical examination often suggest the diagnosis of pulmonary tuberculosis before any laboratory test is ordered. The most characteristic physical findings of adult-type disease are rales heard posteriorly near the apex of one or both lungs. The chest radiographs then confirm the presence of disease in the posterior portion of the upper lobes. Visualization of one or more cavities strengthens the diagnosis. In primary tuberculosis the initial pneumonic area may be anywhere in the lung, especially in the middle or lower lobes, with enlargement of the draining lymph nodes at the lung root. These characteristic patterns are not always seen, however. In a report from a large teaching hospital, the diagnosis of tuberculosis was not suggested by the radiologist in 26 per cent of 100 consecutive cases. A wide variety of unusual patterns may be encountered, from mass lesions resembling malignancy to widespread interstitial disease of a nonspecific nature. Diabetics are more likely than nondiabetics to have lower lobe disease, which may also be noted as a bronchogenic spread from apical cavities. Nonapical, noncavitary, and thoracic lymph node disease is common in AIDS patients with tuberculosis.

Confirmation of the diagnosis should be sought by bacteriologic examination of the sputum. It may be necessary to obtain specimens by the inhalation of nebulized distilled water or saline solution or by gastric lavage. In addition to properly stained smears and cultures for acid-fast bacilli, it is useful to search for elastic fibers by unstained potassium hydroxide wet mounts. The presence of these fibers indicates destruction of lung tissue and should be accompanied by smears positive for AFB. Occasionally, it may be necessary to resort to bronchoscopy and even to lung biopsy to establish the diagnosis.

The tuberculin skin test is very useful in diagnosis, despite the fact that 5 to 20 per cent of those with newly diagnosed cases may have a negative response to the initial test. Transient depression of cell-mediated immune reactions either may be specific for tuberculin or may take the form of a generalized anergy to all skin test antigens. For immediate diagnostic purposes in such cases, it is useful to apply a second-strength PPD containing 250 TU, which will give a false-negative reaction in no more than 2 or 3 per cent of patients without disseminated disease or severe debility.

Recent innovations in laboratory tests include automated radiometric culture methods that allow for more rapid results and simultaneous differentiation of *M. tuberculosis* from other mycobacteria; immunoassays and polymerase chain reaction for specific antigens in sputum and body fluids; DNA probes specific for organisms of the tuberculosis complex applied to growing cultures (available now) and to sputum (investigational); and serodiagnosis by enzyme-linked immunosorbent assay to detect antibodies against specific *M. tuberculosis* antigens.

Differential Diagnosis. Many subacute and chronic pulmonary conditions, both infectious and noninfectious, may be confused with tuberculosis. Some pulmonary mycoses, especially histoplasmosis, may present with a similar clinical and radiologic picture. Pyogenic lung abscess as well as pneumonia with a delayed resolution may be confused with tuberculosis. A pyogenic lung abscess is likely to have more fluid within it, hence a higher air-fluid level, and more dense consolidation around it. When repeated examinations of the sputum are negative for AFB, one should increase efforts at establishing another diagnosis. Tuberculomas may be confused with similar lesions arising from several different fungal infections and with pulmonary neoplasms. Sarcoidosis and tuberculosis may have similar manifestations. One third of cases of fever of unknown origin are due to infection, and extrapulmonary tuberculosis is still prominent among these cases.

TREATMENT. *Historical Perspective.* For many decades the physician relied upon nonspecific measures to treat tuberculosis.

These measures included fresh air, good food, bed rest, and graded exercise, among others. The idea of the cottage sanatorium was started in this country in 1884 to accommodate these feeble attempts at treatment. Measures designated to collapse cavities and to put diseased portions of the lungs "at rest" included artificial pneumothorax, pneumoperitoneum, phrenic nerve crush, and various forms of thoracoplasty. Resectional surgery became popular after the introduction of effective drug therapy.

The era of chemotherapy began in 1945 with Waksman's discovery of streptomycin. In 1949 it was shown that treatment with the combination of streptomycin and para-aminosalicylic acid (PAS) delayed the emergence of streptomycin-resistant tubercle bacilli. With the introduction of isoniazid in 1952 it became possible to treat the disease with two drugs given by mouth. A course of 18 to 24 months was recommended by studies of relapse rates and the bacteriology of lesions removed at lung resection as related to duration of treatment. Ethambutol, marketed in 1961, replaced PAS because of its relative lack of annoying side effects. These drugs rendered all previous modes of therapy obsolete, and most sanatoriums in this country were closed by 1960. A study done in India in 1960 demonstrated that home treatment was not risky for the patient or his or her family. It was documented in 1973 that supervised intermittent treatment twice a week was just as beneficial as daily treatment, especially for the ambulatory continuation phase after a period of daily drug therapy. Such intermittent treatment is especially suited for uncooperative patients. The introduction of rifampin in 1966 provided not only another very powerful antituberculosis agent, but also the opportunity to shorten the duration of therapy by at least one half. Published reports on short-course chemotherapy began to appear in 1972. With proper combinations and rhythm of administration it is now possible to achieve excellent results with 6 months of treatment, provided that all doses are consumed as prescribed.

The Antituberculosis Drugs. *Isoniazid (INH)* is the most important drug in original treatment regimens. It is easily synthesized, highly stable, inexpensive, and well tolerated. The drug is well absorbed when given by mouth and also may be administered parenterally. It is widely distributed throughout the body, including the central nervous system, and it reaches bacilli within cells. The drug exerts a bactericidal effect on actively multiplying bacilli. Adverse reactions may occur in approximately 5 per cent of cases with a dose of 5 mg per kilogram per day, usually given as 300 mg once daily for adults. A common toxicity is peripheral neuropathy, based on interference with the metabolism of pyridoxine. It is directly related to the dose and blood level and is more likely to be seen in genetically constituted slow acetylators and in malnourished individuals. Neuropathy can be prevented by the administration of 25 mg of pyridoxine daily and is not likely to occur when ordinary doses of INH are used in nonalcoholic, nondiabetic, well-nourished, and relatively young patients. The most important adverse reaction is hepatitis of the hepatocellular variety. Although approximately 10 per cent of healthy individuals may have asymptomatic elevations of aminotransferases within the first 2 months of treatment, the enzyme levels usually return to normal despite the continued administration of the drug. The risk of hepatitis is related to age, being less than 1 per cent in those under 35 and increasing with age to 2.3 per cent at age 60. Hepatitis usually occurs within the first few months of treatment but occasionally appears in later stages. Heavy alcohol intake is associated with a greater risk of hepatitis. Several fatalities from INH hepatitis have been reported, mainly in patients whose reaction occurred late and in those who continued to take the drug despite progressive symptoms.

Some rare untoward effects include encephalopathy, loss of memory, optic atrophy, convulsions, hemolytic anemia, and purpura. The usual hypersensitivity reactions such as drug fever and skin rash occasionally may be seen. Isoniazid is one of several drugs that can produce a lupus-like syndrome. Although INH is excreted promptly and mainly by the kidneys, the half-life is prolonged only slightly in patients with renal failure.

Rifampin (RMP) is comparable to INH in its bactericidal effect on metabolically active bacilli. It is an antibiotic of the rifamycin family and is much more expensive than INH. Well absorbed when taken orally in a fasting state, the drug is widely distributed and penetrates well into cells and into the central nervous system when the meninges are inflamed. It differs from most of the antituberculosis drugs in that it has good activity against a variety of gram-positive and gram-negative bacteria. Its activity depends upon inhibition of DNA-dependent RNA polymerase activity. Rifampin is well tolerated by most patients in a dosage of 10 mg per kilogram per day, usually given to adults as 600 mg once daily by mouth. An intravenous preparation recently has become available. Hepatitis is the most important adverse effect, occurring in about 1 per cent of patients. There are conflicting reports on the risk of hepatitis when INH and RMP are given together. Most studies now indicate no excessive risk. An exception occurs in the treatment of children, for whom a dosage of greater than 10 mg per kilogram per day of INH given with RMP is associated with a high risk of hepatitis.

Allergic reactions occasionally occur, especially in those individuals who take the drug irregularly or in those who are given intermittent treatment twice weekly in a dosage greater than 600 mg. These reactions include chills and fever and more rarely acute renal failure, thrombocytopenia, and massive hemolysis. Rifampin may induce enzymes in the liver that increase metabolic degradation of several other drugs, such as oral contraceptive agents and anticoagulants. The drug is excreted mainly by the liver and biliary tract and therefore must be given with caution to patients with liver failure.

Ethambutol (EMB) is a synthetic chemical compound that is well absorbed when given by mouth and is excreted mainly in the urine. Thus, the drug should be given with great care to patients with poor renal function, for whom dosage must be reduced and blood levels followed carefully. Aside from its principal toxicity, optic neuritis, there are very few adverse effects. Optic nerve toxicity is directly related to dosage and blood levels. At the recommended dosage of 15 mg per kilogram per day, optic neuritis is very rare, but some physicians administer 25 mg per kilogram per day for the first 2 or 3 months, at which dosage approximately 3 per cent of patients may have impaired visual acuity. When the higher dose is used, periodic examinations for visual acuity are indicated. The toxicity usually is reversible if administration of the drug is discontinued promptly.

Pyrazinamide (PZA) is an important drug because of its excellent tissue-sterilizing ability when used in combination with other bactericidal drugs. It is well absorbed from the gastrointestinal tract, is widely distributed throughout the body water, and penetrates well into the central nervous system. The drug is active against only one species of *Mycobacterium, M. tuberculosis*, and then only at the low pH of 5.0 to 5.5. It is especially useful to kill tubercle bacilli within macrophages, into whose acidic environment it penetrates well. It is excreted mainly by way of the kidneys. Allergic reactions are rare, but joint pains and occasionally gout may occur as the result of a hyperuricemic effect. Hepatitis may occur in about 1 per cent of patients receiving the recommended daily dose of 20 to 30 mg per kilogram, usually 1.5 grams for small and 2.0 grams for large adults, given by mouth once daily.

Streptomycin (SM) is an aminoglycoside antibiotic that has been chemically defined and synthesized. It is not absorbed when given by mouth. The principal method of elimination is through the kidneys, so that dosage adjustment is necessary when renal function is reduced. It is distributed largely in the extracellular fluid and does not enter appreciably into the central nervous system or into macrophages. The dosage is 10 to 15 mg per kilogram per day, given intramuscularly, usually as 0.75 to 1.0 gram once daily in adults with normal renal function. As with other aminoglycosides, damage to the renal tubules is common, as manifested by cylindruria, but renal function is not compromised unless blood levels of the drug are excessive. The major toxicity is exerted against the eighth nerve, of which the vestibular division is more likely to be affected, although deafness may also be produced. The seriousness of these reactions makes periodic testing of renal and eighth nerve function advisable, especially in the elderly. Measurements of blood levels should be obtained whenever renal function is in question. Allergic reactions are fairly common, as are paresthesias of the lips and extremities immediately after injection. The drug is bactericidal against tubercle bacilli. The maximum effect is exerted at a pH of 7.7.

Kanamycin and *capreomycin* are used as substitutes for SM when the organisms are resistant to that drug or on the rare occasions when the patient cannot tolerate SM. Dosages, methods of administration, and adverse reactions are similar to those of SM. More care is needed with kanamycin, since it is slightly more ototoxic and nephrotoxic than SM, especially on the cochlear division of the eighth nerve.

Ethionamide and *cycloserine* are not used for initial therapy but are reserved for retreatment cases and for special situations of drug intolerance and bacillary resistance. Both drugs are given by mouth in dosages of 10 to 15 mg per kilogram per day. The administration of ethionamide is accompanied by rather severe gastrointestinal upset and occasionally by hepatitis, and allergic reactions are common. Allergic reactions with cycloserine are rare, but aberrations of mental function and seizures are quite common. Other drugs under investigation include the quinolones ciprofloxacin and ofloxacin, rifabutin, and several long-acting rifamycins (rifapentine is one that has a name).

Drug Regimens. Until the landmark short-course chemotherapy studies of the British Medical Research Council and its cooperative investigators, the conventional drug regimens for initial treatment consisted mainly of INH and EMB for 1.5 to 2 years, supplemented by RMP or SM for the first month or two in patients with far-advanced disease. An intermittent schedule of supervised twice-weekly drug administration often was used after the initial 2 or 3 months of daily treatment for noncompliant patients. The main problems were those related to compliance with and cost of the long-term administration of two or more drugs. The conventional regimen has been all but abandoned in favor of short-course treatment.

Short-Course Treatment. The first report of successful short-course treatment was published in 1968 and involved experience in East Africa. From the results of many other trials conducted since then, it appears that the minimum requirements include therapy with INH and RMP for at least 9 months. The addition of a third drug—EMB, SM, or PZA—for the first 1 to 3 months of intensive treatment guards against the eventuality of infection with INH- or RMP-resistant bacilli. To shorten the course to 6 months, a third drug is necessary. That drug should be PZA for the initial 2 months. Treatment may then be continued with daily INH plus RMP for the remaining 4 months. When the patient is in a high-risk group for infection with INH-resistant or RMP-resistant organisms, use of a four-drug regimen has been suggested for the first 2 months (INH/RMP/PZA/SM), followed by administration of two or three drugs, depending on drug susceptibility, for 4 months. Even shorter regimens consisting of INH/RMP/PZA/SM daily for 4 months may be advisable for problem patients for whom ambulatory treatment of any kind is unsuitable, with expected success rates of 70 to 80 per cent.

Short-course treatment has the obvious advantages of smaller amounts of drugs used and less time needed at the ambulatory health facility for supervision of treatment. Another benefit is more rapid sputum conversion. In addition, if relapse occurs following short-course treatment, it is usually caused by drug-susceptible organisms. The main disadvantage of intensive three- and four-drug regimens, drug toxicity, has proved to be less troublesome than was predicted. Many experts believe that the 6-month INH/RMP regimen supplemented with PZA for the first 2 months should be the standard initial treatment for tuberculosis. Directly observed, twice-weekly therapy for the last 4 months should be utilized for poorly cooperative individuals.

The remarkable success of short-course treatment has been attributed to special characteristics of certain drugs, e.g., the ability of INH, RMP, and PZA to penetrate macrophages and to kill rapidly growing bacilli; the effectiveness of PZA in the acid environment of the phagolysosome; and the more rapid bactericidal activity of RMP during periods of intermittent growth of otherwise dormant bacilli.

Results of Treatment. The success of treatment may be judged by clinical assessment, decreased bacillary count of the sputum, and clearing of the lungs as shown on radiographs. The temperature usually returns to normal within a week or two, but in some patients who are highly febrile, defervescence may not occur for many weeks. The speed of radiographic improvement depends upon the nature and extent of pulmonary disease and the age of the patient. Chronic, cavitary, and fibrotic lesions do not clear rapidly. The sputum should be examined at frequent intervals during the first few months of treatment, since a decreasing number of acid-fast bacilli is the surest indication of successful treatment. The best of regimens in patients with far-advanced disease takes 4 to 6 weeks to convert sputum cultures to negative in 50 per cent of cases; to convert 75 per cent of cases usually requires about 10 weeks. The rate of conversion depends on the same factors that determine the rate of radiographic clearing. Failure of the sputum to convert to negative or a rise in the bacillary count after an initial decrease represents a treatment failure. Such failures are usually the result of poor compliance on the part of the patient but occasionally are related to bacillary drug resistance or an inappropriate drug regimen. The aim of chemotherapy is an initial success rate of 100 per cent without relapses. When relapse occurs, it is usually within a year of the completion of therapy. Rarely, relapses may occur with decreasing frequency up to 5 to 10 years after completion of therapy. This is so infrequent after adequate drug therapy that it is no longer necessary for the local health department to carry out periodic follow-up examinations.

Corticosteroids. Corticosteroids may be a useful adjunct to chemotherapy for selected patients. They usually produce a dramatic reversal of overwhelming sepsis and prompt defervescence in those patients who remain febrile, anorectic, and debilitated despite apparently adequate drug treatment. Absorption of the fluid may be hastened in tuberculous pleurisy and pericarditis, although there is no evidence that late complications in the pleural and pericardial spaces are prevented. Steroids should be given for as short a time as possible, preferably for no longer than 3 or 4 weeks. A more controversial issue is whether or not to use INH prophylaxis to cover the administration of steroids in the patient with a history of tuberculosis or with a positive tuberculin skin test result. This situation is most likely to occur in patients receiving steroids to prevent rejection of transplanted organs, to help control lymphoma or leukemia, or to control severe asthma. One year of INH preventive therapy is recommended when steroids are used on a long-term basis.

Reversal of Infectiousness. Some experts believe that it takes only about 2 weeks of effective chemotherapy to render patients noninfectious to others, even when large numbers of viable acid-fast bacilli are still present in the sputum. The evidence for this is inconclusive, and it is more reasonable to consider a patient with smear-positive sputum to represent a gradually diminishing risk until the smears are negative.

Drug Resistance. The phenomenon of clinical bacillary resistance was recognized soon after SM was tried as single drug therapy. The emergence of drug-resistant strains was at least delayed, if not prevented, by the use of two or more drugs in combination. Resistant populations emerge by a selective process in which resistant cells are favored which have arisen by spontaneous random mutation at the rate of about 1×10^{-8} to 1×10^{-10} per bacterium per generation.

Modern drug regimens are designed to prevent the emergence of drug resistance unless the patient is noncompliant or infection occurs with strains already resistant to one or more drugs—a situation known as *primary drug resistance*. The rate of primary drug resistance in a community influences the choice of drug regimens for initial treatment. In this country the overall rate is 7 per cent and varies in different locations from 3 to 15 per cent, depending mainly on the relative numbers of Asian and Hispanic individuals in the population. Age is another important factor; the highest rate is seen in young children. The highest single drug rate is for INH, with SM second. In a 1980 study from the Centers for Disease Control, 41 per cent of unsuccessfully treated patients harbored strains resistant to at least one drug. In the face of known or suspected drug-resistant bacilli, it is preferable to use at least three drugs until susceptibility test results are available.

Retreatment. The choice of proper therapy for initial treatment failures and disease that relapses after apparently successful treatment requires special expertise. Accurate drug susceptibility testing is a prerequisite for devising the best drug regimen, but while awaiting test results the following guidelines may be followed: A single new drug should not be added to a regimen that has failed, since rapid emergence of resistance to the new drug may occur. Instead, the new regimen should contain at least two drugs that the patient has never received previously.

In selecting the proper drugs, all available information should be gathered from the patient, the patient's family and former physicians, and health departments. It may be necessary to use combinations of four or more drugs, some of which have high rates of adverse reactions. After two or three relapses, especially when the infecting strain is resistant to INH, RMP, and SM, the chances of success are slim. The best approach to retreatment of patients with multiply resistant strains is to prevent this unfortunate turn of events by proper supervision of the initial course of drug therapy.

Patients with Impaired Renal and Hepatic Function. Isoniazid is excreted mainly in the urine, and it has been reported that the drug will accumulate in patients with markedly impaired renal function. However, the drug is dialyzable, and others have reported that the half-life is prolonged only slightly in patients with renal failure. It is probably not necessary to reduce the dosage, but pyridoxine supplementation should be given and patients should be monitored for hepatitis and peripheral neuropathy. It may also be advisable to assay INH serum concentrations from time to time. Rifampin is metabolized in the liver and excreted mainly in the bile. When hepatic function is impaired, the drug may accumulate to toxic levels. It is only slightly, if at all, dialyzable. Both EMB and SM are cleared by dialysis and are excreted mainly through the urine. The dosage of SM must be reduced in proportion to the renal function; serum levels should be checked frequently, and the patient should be monitored for signs of eighth nerve toxicity. In a similar fashion, the dosage of EMB must be reduced, serum levels checked, and the visual acuity monitored. Since about 20 per cent of EMB is metabolized in the liver, it would be wise to check serum levels when there is hepatic failure. There is insufficient information upon which to base recommendations for use of PZA, ethionamide, and cycloserine in patients with impaired renal or hepatic function. Since PZA and cycloserine are excreted mainly by the kidneys, the dosage should be reduced and blood levels monitored when these drugs are used in patients with poor kidney function. It is not known how ethionamide is metabolized; only a very small amount may be found unchanged in the urine. Drug levels should be monitored to avoid accumulation.

Treatment of Pregnant Women. Ethionamide and SM should be avoided, the first because of teratogenic potential and the second because eighth nerve damage has been reported in the offspring. Cycloserine and PZA should also be avoided because of a lack of information on possible adverse effects. Although rifampin crosses the placental barrier readily and inhibits ribonucleic acid (RNA) polymerase, there is no evidence of its association with fetal damage. Recommended treatment for pregnant women with active tuberculosis is INH/RMP for 9 months, supplemented with EMB if necessary.

Treatment of Children. There are conflicting recommendations for drug regimens and dosages of individual drugs for treatment of children with tuberculosis. The most suitable combination is INH 10 mg per kilogram daily (maximum of 300 mg daily) and RMP 15 mg per kilogram daily (maximum of 600 mg daily). A third drug should be added if there is risk of infection with drug-resistant organisms. The third drug, given for the first 2 or 3 months of therapy, may be SM, EMB,* or PZA. All three drugs have drawbacks: SM has a high rate of adverse effects and must be given by injection; young children cannot be monitored for the major toxicity of EMB, optic neuritis; and experience with PZA is limited. Directly observed, twice-weekly therapy should be considered for a poorly cooperative family. Nine months has been suggested for duration of treatment, perhaps reduced to 6 months when PZA is used as a third drug.

Surgical and Collapse Procedures. The need for collapse procedures such as pneumothorax, pneumoperitoneum, and phrenic nerve crush and for excisional surgery with or without thoracoplasty has been virtually eliminated by the success of chemotherapy. The surgeon may still be called upon to correct late complications of previous attempts at treatment such as bronchopleural fistula, persistent empyema, and hemoptysis from bronchiectasis or aspergilloma.

EXTRAPULMONARY DISEASE. In contrast to the declining incidence of pulmonary tuberculosis, there has been little change

---

*Not recommended for use in children under 13 years of age.

in the number of extrapulmonary cases reported in the United States since 1964, about 4000 per year. This may be partially explained by the higher rate of infection in the immunocompromised states associated with old age, renal failure (including dialysis and transplant patients), cirrhosis, malnutrition, hematologic malignancies, and AIDS. In England, extrapulmonary disease is reported mainly in recent immigrants from the Asian subcontinent.

Thoracic Cavity and Chest Wall. Tuberculosis of the pleura is almost always associated with disease of the lung, arising by contiguous spread or rupture of a subpleural tubercle. It usually begins as a localized fibrinous inflammation, which produces pleuritic chest pain. Pleurisy with effusion is often associated with primary infection. When this occurs in young adults who are untreated, approximately 75 per cent may be expected to develop overt pulmonary tuberculosis within 5 years. The onset may be either abrupt or insidious, with cough and fever accompanying the chest pain. Pain and friction rub often disappear as pleural fluid accumulates. Most primary tuberculous pleural effusions resorb spontaneously, sometimes within a week or two, but the diagnosis can be made on the basis of a positive tuberculin skin test result, the exudative characteristics of the fluid, and the preponderance of lymphocytes. Tubercle bacilli are usually very scarce in the fluid so that stained smears may be negative and cultures only weakly positive. Imprints and cultures made from pleural tissue removed by closed needle biopsy are more likely than the fluid to be positive. Histologic examination also may be helpful. Pleural effusions in young adults who have positive tuberculin skin test results are best treated as tuberculosis unless some other cause can be identified. The fluid should be aspirated for diagnosis and perhaps once or twice more if it accumulates rapidly. Chest tube drainage should be avoided. Corticosteroids should not be used routinely but may be given in selected cases to hasten symptomatic improvement and absorption of the fluid. Pleural effusion may also occur in disseminated tuberculosis with multiple organ and serous membrane involvement. Tuberculous empyema may be secondary to involvement of the vertebral column or result from a bronchopleural fistula.

Endobronchial tuberculosis commonly accompanies pulmonary disease but now rarely results in identifiable symptoms and signs. In primary tuberculosis of children it is the pressure of enlarged lymph nodes together with ulceration and rupture through the bronchial wall that produces endobronchial disease. Endobronchial disease in adults usually starts as inflammatory lesions from repeated implantations of tubercle bacilli originating in lung parenchyma. These lesions may progress to ulceration and narrowing of the bronchi and eventually to cicatricial stenosis. Secondary changes include atelectasis and obstructive pneumonitis, tension cavity from involvement of the distal small bronchi or bronchioles, and accumulation of fluid within cavities. The symptoms of endobronchial disease are spasmodic coughing and a localized wheeze. Bronchial ulceration or erosion of a caseating lymph node may cause positive sputum in the absence of recognizable pulmonary disease. Bronchoscopy usually serves to identify the lesions.

Although tuberculosis of the endocardium and myocardium has been described, the most common involvement of the heart is *pericarditis*. Rupture into the pericardium of nearby caseous lymph nodes is the common route of infection, although lymphohematogenous dissemination may occur. The serofibrinous pericardial effusion usually is associated with substernal pain, fever, pericardial friction rub, and left-sided pleural effusion. Cardiac tamponade occasionally develops in the acute stage. A search for tuberculosis elsewhere and a tuberculin skin test should be performed. A thorough examination of the pericardial fluid obtained by needle aspiration or surgical drainage also may be helpful. Obtaining a pericardial biopsy sample in the operating room may be justified in obscure cases because of the importance of early drug treatment. The differential diagnosis includes benign or viral pericarditis, pyogenic infection, other granulomatous inflammations, connective tissue disease, and malignant effusion. The diagnosis is made more difficult by the facts that the skin test reaction is negative in a sizable minority; the fluid rarely contains enough organisms to be positive by smear and often not even by culture; the characteristics of the fluid are nonspecific; and about half of the individuals have no other obvious sites of tuberculosis. The administration of corticosteroids may be bene-

ficial, but antituberculosis drugs should be used in addition even when tuberculosis is only suspected.

The most important sequela is constrictive pericarditis, which usually occurs 2 to 4 years after the acute disease. At this stage the heart is small and relatively immobile and there is a paradoxical pulse and obstruction of venous return to the heart, with congestion of the liver, peripheral edema, and later ascites. Calcification of the pericardium may be seen on x-ray films. Treatment consists of removal of the pericardium, although it is preferable to perform the operation at an earlier stage.

The chest wall may be the site of one or more subcutaneous abscesses as a result of hematogenous dissemination or sometimes as the peripheral manifestation of an empyema necessitatis as it burrows through the chest wall. Chest wall abscesses may also result from drainage of underlying caseous lymph nodes along the intercostal lymphatics.

Extrathoracic. Lymphatic. Tuberculous lymphadenitis is the most common manifestation of extrathoracic disease throughout the world, and the most frequently involved nodes are cervical. The disease in this location was known as *scrofula*, or the *King's Evil*. The latter name was used because the condition was supposedly amenable to cure by the royal touch. Although it was once thought that infection with *M. bovis* was responsible for most cases of scrofula, a recent study from England emphasized that *M. tuberculosis* accounted for more cases than did the bovine organism, although the latter is relatively more common in lymphatic tuberculosis than in other forms of the disease. Infection of the tonsils through the ingestion of contaminated milk was the usual route of infection for the tonsillar node high in the neck, near the angle of the jaw. At present, scrofula in young children is mainly due to infection with mycobacteria other than *M. tuberculosis* and *M. bovis* (see Ch. 333). Supraclavicular node involvement usually arises by lymphatic spread from mediastinal disease. Affected nodes elsewhere in the neck, as well as those in the axilla and inguinal area, the other common sites of involvement, may be the result of drainage from a primary site or from hematogenous spread. Both intra- and extrathoracic node involvement is common in tuberculosis of AIDS patients.

The infected nodes are usually detectable by sight and palpation. Although the nodes usually are not painful, they may be tender during the phase of rapid enlargement early in the infection. Later they become matted together and eventually soften, slough, and drain. Draining sinuses may persist for many months, sometimes for years, with intermittent healing and breakdown. The diagnosis may be made by bacteriologic study of the pus from draining sinuses or by biopsy together with bacteriologic studies. The presence of calcific densities in the neck and axilla as seen in the chest radiograph may provide evidence of healed tuberculous adenitis.

Lymphatic tuberculosis tends to heal but often not completely, so that relapse is common even many years after the primary infection. Treatment with antituberculosis drugs is usually successful, although the tendency to late relapse may still be seen. Good results have been reported with short-course regimens. Excision of large caseous nodes in accessible sites sometimes is advisable.

Genitourinary. The second most common site of infection is the genitourinary tract. Disease is usually centered in the kidney, which becomes seeded either during the primary infection or later. These foci may remain dormant for many years. When reactivation occurs, one or more renal abscesses are produced, followed by spread to the remainder of the urinary tract. Extensive scarring of the ureters eventually occurs. This scarring produces obstructive hydronephrosis, which together with renal caseation may destroy the kidney completely. Specific symptoms may be lacking until the hydronephrotic kidney becomes secondarily infected or until the development of tuberculous cystitis manifested by frequency and dysuria. Long before the onset of symptoms, the examination of the urine may show hematuria, pyuria, and albuminuria, along with cultures negative for pyogens. The diagnosis is made by radiographic examination of the urinary tract, cystoscopy, and demonstration of tubercle bacilli by cultures of first morning voided urines. It was found that approximately 10 per cent of a general tuberculosis patient population had positive urine cultures, and in 7 per cent of these patients the urinary tract disease was completely unanticipated. Renal tuberculosis responds well to drug treatment. According to recent recommendations, conventional long-term regimens may be replaced by 6- to 9-month courses of INH, RMP, and a third drug (either EMB or PZA). The role of surgery remains controversial. Some urologists would remove destroyed kidneys and repair strictures of the ureter, while others claim that surgery is almost never indicated.

Genital tuberculosis in the male may involve the prostate, seminal vesicles, and epididymis. The acute inflammation is later replaced by induration and hard nodules, sometimes followed by obstruction, calcification, and chronic draining sinuses of the scrotum. The diagnosis is made by finding tubercle bacilli in the urine, sinus drainage, or biopsied tissues. In the female, tuberculous salpingitis is the common manifestation, followed by disease of the uterus and ovaries. Sterility almost always results, and peritonitis may occur secondarily. The symptoms are those of chronic pelvic inflammatory disease. Diagnosis should be based on examination of tissue from the endometrium and from lesions visible through the laparoscope and cultures of the menstrual fluid or vaginal discharge. As with renal tuberculosis, drug therapy usually is successful, but excisional surgery may be indicated for residual lesions or persistently draining sinuses.

Skeletal Tuberculosis. The presence of a gibbus or hunchback deformity of the thoracic spine (Pott's disease) has served as a marker of tuberculosis since prehistoric times. *Tuberculous spondylitis* is still the most common manifestation of bone and joint infection. At present, it is mainly a disease of adults that arises by reactivation of dormant foci. The common areas of involvement are thoracic and lumbar; the cervical spine may be involved in 2 to 3 per cent of cases. The destructive process usually begins in the intervertebral discs, where it first produces narrowing of the disc space, then destruction of the two adjacent vertebral bodies through the bony end-plates. Sometimes, however, the anterior portion of the vertebral body is destroyed first. Inflammation often extends into the soft tissues surrounding the spine, either in the form of a spreading, phlegmonous reaction or as a cold abscess that may be paravertebral, in and around the psoas muscle, or retropharyngeal, depending upon the site of disease. The symptoms are usually dominated by back pain, sometimes followed by the neurologic manifestations of compression of the spinal cord and nerve roots. There may be fever. Active tuberculosis of the lungs may be absent, although some evidence of past disease usually is seen.

Radiographic examination of the spine shows destructive lesions in the commonly involved sites. The paraspinal involvement appears as widening of the mediastinum or an oval-shaped density behind the heart. It may be manifested as a psoas abscess, a retropharyngeal abscess, or a mass in the groin or in the supraclavicular area. A similar radiographic appearance may occur in pyogenic infection of the spine. A needle biopsy sample usually is necessary to establish the proper diagnosis. Occasionally open biopsy of the vertebral body may be necessary. Imaging of the spine by magnetic resonance and computed tomography is valuable in the differential diagnosis and to delineate the extent of disease.

The disease has a natural tendency to heal by spontaneous fusion of the vertebral bodies. Treatment consists of antituberculosis chemotherapy according to the modern regimens described under Treatment. Preliminary results with short-course treatment are encouraging, but they cannot be recommended for routine use until further experience has accumulated. Prolonged bed rest, immobilization of the spine, and spinal fusion usually are not necessary, although some indications still exist for surgical procedures: evidence of cord compression and other major neurologic deficits, instability of the spine, and involvement of the upper and midthoracic spine.

Tuberculous arthritis occurs mainly in hips and knees but also may involve many other joints, including elbows, shoulders, and the joints of the hands and feet. The patient usually has chronic monoarticular arthritis. Diagnosis is made by synovial biopsy and bacteriologic study of tissues and pus. The process usually responds to antituberculosis chemotherapy without the necessity for operative procedures, but occasionally excision of extensively destroyed synovium and temporary immobilization may be beneficial.

Tuberculous tenosynovitis is usually secondary to involvement of adjacent bone. At least two distinctive processes may result from involvement of the hand: carpal tunnel syndrome, and compound palmar ganglion, a distinctive bilobed swelling on either side of the volar carpal ligament. Chemotherapy often needs to be supplemented by debridement and evacuation of fibrinous material.

Abdominal Tuberculosis. *Intestinal tuberculosis* secondary to chronic pulmonary disease once was so common that patients were routinely screened by radiography of the small bowel upon admission to the sanatorium. This situation continued long after the ingestion of *M. bovis* was brought under control by the pasteurization of milk. Lately, the emphasis has been on primary intestinal disease in the absence of recognizable pulmonary lesions. The route of infection in these cases remains unknown. Tuberculosis may involve all parts of the alimentary canal from top to bottom, but by far the most common location is in the ileocecal area. The predominant tissue reaction may be either ulcerative or hyperplastic, with accompanying bleeding, perforation, fistula formation, obstruction, or combinations of two or more of these processes. The early symptoms are nonspecific, consisting mainly of anorexia, loss of weight, abdominal pain, and alternating periods of diarrhea and constipation. The clinical picture is not unlike that of Crohn's disease, especially since a fibrogranulomatous tissue reaction is characteristic of both. Tuberculosis of the colon also may occur and needs to be distinguished from carcinoma, diverticulitis, and inflammatory bowel disease of nonspecific nature. Perirectal abscess and fistula formation may result from lower colon lesions. The disease usually responds well to antituberculosis chemotherapy, but surgical correction may be necessary for the complications described earlier. The diagnosis often is made unexpectedly at surgery or autopsy.

Tuberculous peritonitis may result from bloodborne infection or by extension of disease from the intestine, mesenteric lymph nodes, or fallopian tubes. The classic form is that of a chronic adhesive peritonitis that produces a doughy, tender abdomen, abdominal masses, low-grade fever, anorexia, and weight loss. A much more common manifestation is painless ascites. When this occurs in adults with alcoholic cirrhosis and ascites, it makes for a difficult differential diagnosis. Tuberculosis should be suspected when the combination of fever, ascites, and a positive tuberculin skin test reaction is found. Examination of the fluid is helpful. A high total protein concentration with a moderate number of leukocytes, mostly lymphocytes, is suggestive of tuberculosis. A more definitive diagnosis may be obtained by laparoscopy or laparotomy. Usually the entire peritoneal surface is studded with tubercles that are easily differentiated from carcinomatosis histologically. The fluid is rarely positive for AFB by stained smear and even by culture is positive in somewhat less than 50 per cent of cases. Response to antituberculosis chemotherapy is good.

Isolated tuberculosis of the liver or spleen occasionally has been described. These organs are usually involved in disseminated or miliary tuberculosis, but occasionally a liver biopsy done in an attempt to explain enlargement of the liver, jaundice, or abnormal liver function studies leads to a diagnosis of tuberculosis when there is apparently no disease elsewhere.

Central Nervous System. In the past, *tuberculous meningitis* was one of the most dreaded complications of primary tuberculosis in young children, appearing in about one in a thousand cases and almost always resulting in fatality. It usually occurred 2 to 6 months after the primary infection in infants and was commonly associated with miliary tuberculosis. In this country it is now more likely to be seen in adults than in children. Invasion of the meninges occurs by direct extension from subjacent caseous foci in the cerebral cortex, cerebellum, choroid plexus, middle ear, or spine. Brain infarcts secondary to tuberculous arteritis sometimes occur. The syndrome of inappropriate secretion of antidiuretic hormone may accompany the meningitis.

The inflammatory reaction is concentrated around the base of the brain, where the thick exudate may eventually obstruct the basal foramina to produce hydrocephalus. Examination of the spinal fluid reveals a characteristic pattern of high protein, low sugar, and a moderate number (up to a few hundred) of leukocytes, most of which are lymphocytes. However, early in the course of the disease neutrophils may predominate; rarely the shift to a lymphocytic exudate does not occur; the sugar level may be normal or only slightly decreased; and the number of leukocytes may reach several thousand. Occasionally the protein content is high enough that a thin web or pellicle appears in undisturbed refrigerated fluid. Acid-fast bacilli may be seen in this web, although they are not visible in the sedimented fluid. Stained smears of the fluid are usually positive in no more than 25 per cent of samples, but there are a few colonies of tubercle bacilli in cultures in about 75 per cent of cases. The larger the sample of spinal fluid submitted, the greater the chance of finding the organism. The tuberculin skin test should be positive in approximately 75 per cent of cases, provided that those nonreactive to 5 TU are retested with 250 TU. A careful search reveals evidence of tuberculosis elsewhere in the majority of cases, although the disease in the lungs may appear to be inactive.

The onset is usually insidious, extending over a period of many weeks. Occasionally, however, there is a much more acute onset that resembles pyogenic or aseptic meningitis. The most common symptoms are headache, fever, lethargy, and confusion. Later, focal neurologic signs appear in the form of ocular palsies, other cranial nerve palsies, and increasing stupor progressing to coma. Stiffness of the neck is common. The outcome of therapy depends mainly on the stage of disease at the time treatment is instituted. Treatment should start immediately when tuberculous meningitis is suspected, without waiting for confirmation of diagnosis. A triple-drug regimen including INH and RMP is recommended. Ethionamide and PZA achieve therapeutic concentrations in spinal fluid even in the absence of an inflammatory reaction. Ethambutol penetrates reasonably well through inflamed meninges. It should be remembered that SM does not appear in therapeutic concentrations and that infections with INH-resistant organisms occur more often in children than in adults. Treatment should be continued for at least 1 year, although administration of the third drug may be discontinued after 2 or 3 months once it has been determined that drug resistance is not a problem. The use of corticosteroids is controversial, but should be considered in the presence of coma or spinal fluid block. Intrathecal treatment is usually not necessary.

Tuberculomas of the brain may be seen at any age. Cases involving children still predominate in the developing countries, while in the United States they occur mainly in adults. The clinical presentation is that of a brain tumor with signs and symptoms of increased intracranial pressure, focal seizures, and focal neurologic defects. Indications of infection, such as fever, often are absent. Lesions may be single or multiple and must be differentiated from tumor and abscess. The spinal fluid may show slight lymphocytosis and elevated protein concentration, but often it is normal. The correct diagnosis may be suggested by radiographic or magnetic resonance scanning techniques, a positive tuberculin skin test reaction, and the presence of tuberculosis elsewhere, but the definitive procedures are needle aspiration through a burr hole and craniotomy for open biopsy. Drug treatment similar to that used for tuberculous meningitis should be used.

Miscellaneous. Almost every organ and tissue of the body can be involved in tuberculosis. In the upper respiratory tract and oral cavity, the larynx and the middle ear are most prone to infection. *Tuberculous laryngitis* used to be a rather common complication that was considered to be secondary to longstanding highly positive sputum associated with chronic cavitary disease. It was extremely painful and resulted in such difficulty in swallowing that severe inanition resulted. Response to drug treatment, even to administration of SM alone, was rapid and dramatic. The new face of tuberculous laryngitis is that of a primary laryngeal lesion that must be distinguished from carcinoma. Tuberculous middle ear disease, formerly common, is now rare. It was usually associated with advanced pulmonary or disseminated disease. Involvement of the eye is in the form of chronic uveitis, such as chorioretinitis, iridocyclitis, or iritis. Phlyctenular conjunctivitis produces small, yellowish vesicles. Direct inoculation into the eye may produce conjunctivitis or keratitis. The specific origin of eye disease is difficult to prove. Cutaneous tuberculosis has all but disappeared, except for lesions associated with direct inoculation in laboratory workers and pathologists. Other manifestations include lesions like lupus vulgaris, in which tubercle bacilli may be located, and the tuberculids that are considered to be hypersensitivity reactions, in which the organisms usually are not found. The larger blood vessels may harbor infections in their walls. Tuberculosis is a rare cause of aortic aneurysm. At one time tuberculosis of the adrenal gland was a common cause of adrenal insufficiency. Occasional cases of tuberculosis of the thyroid, breast, and soft tissues elsewhere than in the chest wall are still being reported.

DISSEMINATED AND MILIARY TUBERCULOSIS. These terms are used synonymously, although miliary tuberculosis is but one form of disseminated tuberculosis in which the widely dispersed small tubercles resemble millet seeds. During life these lesions usually are first recognized in the chest roentgenogram as very small nodules of uniform size that are evenly distributed throughout both lungs. The acute form was predominantly an early complication of untreated primary tuberculosis, occurring mainly in young children and often associated with meningitis. During the past three decades the predominant age group has changed to the elderly, and the disease has become more subacute in its progression.

The diagnosis often is missed because it is difficult to distinguish the tuberculosis symptoms from those of the many underlying conditions that could be responsible for the weight loss, increasing fatigue, and low-grade fever. Skin test anergy and frequent absence of chronic pulmonary tuberculosis may compound the difficulty. This sort of subacute disseminated tuberculosis has been called *cryptic* or *nonreactive tuberculosis*. In a series of autopsied cases analyzed by Slavin and colleagues in 1980, only 15 per cent of patients admitted during the antibiotic era had the correct diagnosis made ante mortem. A composite of such a case would be an elderly anergic patient without previously recognized tuberculosis who presented to the hospital with malignancy, renal failure, a renal transplant, or chronic alcoholism. Constitutional symptoms would be nonspecific, mainly fever, loss of weight, and increasing fatigue. Examinations would reveal no obvious tuberculosis in lungs or other organs, no hepatosplenomegaly, and no enlarged peripheral lymph nodes. There would be moderate anemia, a slight elevation of alkaline phosphatase, and a negative initial bacteriologic workup. The correct diagnosis depends upon a high index of suspicion and the demonstration of characteristic microscopic lesions and mycobacteria by biopsy. The most productive tissue is the liver, usually sampled by needle biopsy, with bone marrow next in line. Blood cultures should be obtained, since they are sometimes positive at this stage of disease. At a later stage choroidal tubercles may be seen and radiographs of the lungs may show the typical miliary pattern.

Miliary tuberculosis almost always results from the discharge of infected caseous material into the bloodstream, usually from a well-hidden lymph node in the mediastinum or the abdomen. When multiple bacteremic episodes occur, the process may be protracted. The patient may have serositis manifested by pleural effusion, pericardial effusion, or ascites. Hematologic abnormalities may be so prominent that a primary blood disease is suspected. The most common abnormality is a leukemoid reaction, although leukopenia, thrombocytopenia, and hemolytic anemia may occur. More commonly the primary disease is hematologic, complicated by a secondary tuberculosis dissemination, especially when large doses of corticosteroids have been given.

Treatment should consist of an intensive antituberculosis drug regimen using at least three drugs. After a few months, when a good response has occurred and after the drug susceptibility pattern of the infecting strain is known, the third drug can be discontinued. The total duration of therapy has not been established, but it probably should be at least 1 year.

TUBERCULOSIS AND AIDS. The pandemic of AIDS has had a major impact on the worldwide tuberculosis problem. The incidence of tuberculosis in AIDS patients has been reported to be 5 to 21 per cent in New York, Newark, and Florida, and 3.8 per cent nationwide. Those at highest risk are intravenous drug users. In addition, analysis of patients with active tuberculosis revealed an HIV seropositivity rate of 40 per cent in Zaire and 30 per cent in Florida. The association of the two infections accounts for the failure of the tuberculosis case rate curve to move downward since 1984.

Tuberculosis usually occurs early in the course of AIDS and may even be the sentinel infection. Diagnosis is difficult because the characteristic pulmonary symptoms, signs, and radiographic appearance often are absent. Disease tends to be extrapulmonary, disseminated, and lymphatic. Pulmonary lesions, when present, often are noncavitary and nonapical. Skin test reactions are not dependable. Diagnosis may depend upon biopsies of lymph node, liver, and bone marrow, blood cultures, and bronchoscopy. Modern chemotherapy regimens usually are successful but probably should be continued for a year. All patients with risk factors for HIV infection or with ARC should be skin tested and, if positive, given a course of the best preventive chemotherapy available. See also Part XXI.

NEW DIAGNOSTIC TESTS. Several innovative techniques have been proposed for the rapid diagnosis of tuberculosis. The most promising are (1) specific antigen detection by enzyme-linked immunosorbent assay (ELISA) or antibody-sensitized latex particles, (2) detection of DNA sequences by probes and polymerase chain reaction, and (3) demonstration of tuberculostearic acid by chromatography and mass spectrometry, which is especially useful for body fluids such as cerebrospinal fluid (CSF).

Abernathy RS: Tuberculosis in children and its management. Sem Respir Infect 4:232, 1989. *The latest thorough review of this subject.*

Anonymous: Tuberculosis in chronic renal failure. Lancet 1:909, 1980. *A short leading article documenting an incidence 10 times as high as in a control population.*

Ben-Dov I, Mason GR: Drug resistant tuberculosis in a southern California hospital; trends from 1969 to 1984. Am Rev Respir Dis 135:1307, 1987. *Resistance to at least one drug was found in 35 per cent of 281 hospitalized patients. Resistance was primary in 23 per cent, acquired in 59 per cent.*

Centers for Disease Control: Primary resistance to antituberculosis drugs—United States. MMWR 32:521, 1983. *The final report of a 7-year study in which 20 selected laboratories throughout the country submitted over 12,000 cultures to the CDC laboratory to be tested for drug susceptibility in a uniform manner.*

Chapman M, Murray RO, Stoker DJ: Tuberculosis of the bones and joints. Semin Roentgenol 14:266, 1979. *This is a thorough clinical review, replete with excellent pictures, from the Royal National Orthopaedic Hospital in London.*

Daniel TM, Debanne SM: The serodiagnosis of tuberculosis and other mycobacterial diseases by enzyme-linked immunosorbent assay. Am Rev Respir Dis 135:1137, 1987. *This state-of-the-art review takes us from the early work of Arloing in 1898 through many decades of failures up to the present, when we can look forward to having soon a useful clinical diagnostic test.*

Dannenberg AM Jr: Macrophages in inflammation and infection. N Engl J Med 293:489, 1975. *This study utilizing skin lesions in rabbits demonstrates the dynamic nature of mycobacterial lesions. Macrophages enter the arena as novices, become activated locally by interaction with immune lymphocytes, ingest bacilli, die, and are replaced by fresh cells recruited from the circulation.*

DeWit D, Steyn L, Shoemaker S, et al: Direct detection of *Mycobacterium tuberculosis* in clinical specimens by DNA amplification. J Clin Microbiol 28:2437, 1990. *Specific DNA was detected in specimens of CSF, pleural and pericardial fluid, and tissue. The test was "at least as sensitive as conventional culture techniques."*

Edwards D, Kirkpatrick CH: The immunology of mycobacterial disease. Am Rev Respir Dis 134:1062, 1986. *A relatively brief state-of-the-art review that brings this subject up to date.*

Elias J, DeConing JP, Vorster SA, et al.: The rapid and sensitive diagnosis of tuberculous meningitis by the detection of tuberculostearic acid in cerebrospinal fluid using gas chromatography–mass spectrometry with selective ion monitoring. Clin Biochem 22:463, 1989. *In this study from South Africa, the authors document a satisfactory 5-hour test using 35 samples of spinal fluid.*

Fertel D, Pitchenik AE: Tuberculosis in acquired immune deficiency syndrome. Semin Respir Infec 4:198, 1989. *An excellent review of tuberculosis in AIDS from a well-informed Miami team.*

Fine PEM: BCG vaccination against tuberculosis and leprosy. Br Med Bull 44:691, 1988. *The author reviews the history and the public health impact of BCG vaccines. He concludes that they have had a substantial impact.*

Fox W: The chemotherapy of tuberculosis: A review. Chest 76S:785, 1979. *An excellent review of antituberculosis drug treatment up to 1979.*

Jacobs RF, Abernathy RS: Management of tuberculosis in pregnancy and the newborn. Clin Perinatol 15:305, 1988. *A valuable review for coverage of clinical management as well as drug therapy.*

Kallo JR, Pulliam L: The BACTEC radiometric system for detection and rapid identification of mycobacteria. Lab Med 20:692, 1989. *The automated system compared favorably with culture controls in over 1,000 specimens, confirming several previously reported large-scale studies.*

Lichtenstein IH, MacGregor RR: Mycobacterial infections in renal transplant recipients: Report of 5 cases and review of the literature. Rev Infect Dis 5:216, 1983. *Among the cases were two that probably represented reactivation tuberculosis in the transplanted kidney. A survey of 26 transplantation centers revealed a tuberculosis rate of 480 cases per 100,000.*

Lifeso RM, Weaver P, Harder EH: Tuberculous spondylitis in adults. J Bone Joint Surg 67A:1405, 1985. *Experience with 107 cases from Saudi Arabia allows the authors to reach valid conclusions regarding the role of surgery. They report good results with chemotherapy and selected anterior decompression and fusion.*

Lincoln EM: Epidemics of tuberculosis. Arch Environ Health 14:473, 1967. *A review of 109 epidemics in 12 countries, the majority of them occurring in schools.*

Mackay AD, Cole RB: The problems of tuberculosis in the elderly. QJ Med 53:497, 1984. *The case rate of tuberculosis is increasing among the elderly, and physicians should understand the special problems of diagnosis and management so well presented in this report.*

O'Brien RJ: Present chemotherapy of tuberculosis. Semin Respir Infect 4:216, 1989. *An excellent presentation from the Division of Tuberculosis Control, CDC.*

Omari B, Robertson JM, Nelson RJ, Chiu LC: Pott's disease, a resurgent challenge to the thoracic surgeon. Chest 95:145, 1989. *Recounts good results with combined medical and surgical treatment of 19 patients from Los Angeles.*

Rieder HL, Snider DE Jr, Cauthen GM: Extrapulmonary tuberculosis in the United States. Am Rev Respir Dis 141:347, 1990. *The latest statistics on all varieties of extrapulmonary disease from the Division of Tuberculosis Control, CDC.*

Sahn SA, Lakshminarayan S: Tuberculosis after corticosteroid therapy. Br J Dis Chest 70:195, 1976. *This review emphasizes the usefulness of preventive therapy with isoniazid in patients already infected with M. tuberculosis.*

Schofield PF: Abdominal tuberculosis (leading article). Gut 26:1275, 1985. *The author gives a good discussion of all aspects of abdominal disease as it is seen today.*

Slavin RE, Walsh TJ, Pollack AD: Late generalized tuberculosis: A clinical pathologic analysis and comparison of 100 cases in the preantibiotic and antibiotic eras. Medicine 59:352, 1980. *This study, from the Department of Pathology at Johns Hopkins University, consists of an analysis of 200 autopsied cases. It contains a wealth of useful information on one form of disseminated tuberculosis.*

Stead WW: Control of tuberculosis in institutions. Chest 76 (suppl):797, 1979. *Reviews recent outbreaks in nursing homes, prisons, schools, and hospitals and suggests common-sense methods of control.*

Stead WW, Kerby GR, Schlueter DP, et al.: The clinical spectrum of primary tuberculosis in adults. Ann Intern Med 68:333, 1968. *Primary pulmonary disease was documented in 37 adults, of whom 9 had only minor symptoms, 11 developed pleural effusion, and 16 showed progression to adult-type chronic pulmonary disease.*

Stead WW, Senner JW, Reddick WT, Lofgren JP: Racial differences in susceptibility to infection by Mycobacterium tuberculosis. N Engl J Med 322:422, 1990. *The authors provide convincing epidemiologic evidence that blacks are more readily infected than whites, at least in the nursing home setting. Once infected, the progression to clinical disease was not different.*

333 Other Mycobacterioses

Emanuel Wolinsky

Organisms of the tuberculosis complex are not the only mycobacteria associated with human disease. The most popular label at present for these other mycobacteria is "nontuberculous." They have become more prominent in the total picture of mycobacterial disease because of the declining incidence of tuberculosis and a greater awareness and recognition of the other mycobacterioses. Indeed, there is evidence that the frequency of nontuberculous pulmonary disease may be increasing in certain areas of the country. In addition, disseminated mycobacterial infection is now recognized much more frequently as an opportunistic infection in immunosuppressed individuals, especially in those with the acquired immunodeficiency syndrome (AIDS). Infection with other mycobacteria has been blamed, perhaps unfairly, for the apparent failure of bacille Calmette-Guérin (BCG) vaccination to protect adults in South India from subsequent tuberculosis. Leprosy, also a mycobacterial disease, is discussed in Ch. 334.

Although the existence of nontuberculous mycobacteria was recognized in the late 1800's, they were first identified as causes of human disease in the mid 1950's.

MYCOBACTERIA. **_Mycobacterium avium-intracellulare (MAI)._** Mycobacteria of this species or complex constitute the most important agents of nontuberculous mycobacteriosis throughout the world. The organism known as the avian tubercle bacillus was described in 1890, although tuberculosis of chickens had been recognized for 22 years before that time. Supposedly quite resistant to infection with *M. avium*, people with documented *M. avium* disease were the subjects of occasional literature reports. Recognition of the expanded role of these mycobacteria in pulmonary and disseminated disease occurred in the 1950's, when the organism was misnamed *Nocardia intracellularis* and given the common name of Battey bacillus. The official name of *Mycobacterium intracellulare* was assigned in the 1960's. The realization that *M. intracellulare* could not be distinguished from *M. avium* in most laboratories dictated another change to the term MAI or *M. avium complex*. In this complex one can recognize 28 types by seroagglutination, of which types 1 to 3 represent the classic *M. avium* strains. By using DNA probes, one can differentiate *M. avium* (serotypes 1–6, 8–11, 21) from *M. intracellulare* (types 7, 12–20). Strains of MAI grow slowly; usually are nonpigmented or slightly yellow, becoming more highly pigmented with age but independently of light; are resistant to most antituberculosis drugs; and often produce colony variants of two or three types, including smooth translucent, smooth domed, and rough opaque. Of the three variants, the translucent colonies are usually most drug resistant and most virulent for experimental animals. Strains of MAI may be associated with all varieties of mycobacterial disease, especially pulmonary disease, childhood lymphadenitis, and disseminated infection in patients who have AIDS. AIDS-associated strains tend to be deeply pigmented and, in the United States, are mainly serotypes 1, 4, and 8.

Mycobacterium scrofulaceum. This is a scotochromogenic mycobacterium similar in many ways to MAI. The pigmentation varies from light yellow to dark orange. In some publications these organisms are lumped together with MAI, and the combination is called the *MAIS complex.* The name derives from the fact that the organism was recognized as the cause of scrofula in young children. Rarely, *M. scrofulaceum* may be associated with pulmonary disease in adults. Most of the disease-associated strains belong to one of three seroagglutination types, but it is not uncommon to see a strain of *M. scrofulaceum* agglutinate in one of the MAI serotypes.

Mycobacterium kansasii. The "yellow bacillus" was described in 1953 in Kansas City and was later given the official name of *M. kansasii.* It is responsible for a large number of pulmonary mycobacteriosis cases in some areas of the world. The organisms may be recognized in the initial sputum smears as large cross-barred acid-fast bacilli. Positive cultures may be identified by their distinctive photochromogenicity. The yellow color is light dependent, developing within hours after the colonies have been exposed to light. Most strains are fully susceptible to rifampin and only slightly resistant to isoniazid, ethambutol, and streptomycin. *M. kansasii* is not found in nature except occasionally in samples of water.

Mycobacterium fortuitum-chelonae. Strains of this group grow rapidly, even on ordinary laboratory media. They are sometimes spoken of as the *M. fortuitum complex,* but it is better to retain at least two separate species because they can be distinguished from each other readily in the laboratory, and *M. chelonae* tends to be much more drug resistant than *M. fortuitum.* Both species are pathogenic for mice and resistant to the usual antituberculosis drugs. Long known for their ability to produce injection site abscesses and severe infections of traumatic wounds, strains of this group recently have become prominent as the cause of sternal osteomyelitis after cardiac surgery, of wound infection after implantation of silicone breast prostheses, of disseminated and localized infection in dialysis patients, of prosthetic valve endocarditis, and of disseminated infections with skin lesions in the immunosuppressed host.

Mycobacterium marinum. This organism is distinctive by virtue of its photochromogenicity and an optimal growth temperature of 30 to 33° C. It was named and recognized as a pathogen of fish in 1926. It is a common contaminant in fresh and salt water, accounting for the frequent occurrence of skin infection in individuals who work or play in a marine environment, including those with home aquariums. Deep infections of the hand may also occur. Almost all strains are resistant to isoniazid but susceptible to rifampin and ethambutol. The organisms are also susceptible to tetracycline and sulfonamides.

Other Slow-Growing Species. *Mycobacterium xenopi* has an optimal growth temperature of 43° C and has been found as a contaminant in hot water generators and storage tanks. From these sites several outbreaks have occurred of respiratory tract colonization and pulmonary disease in the hospital environment. Other species that may cause disease are *M. simiae, M. szulgai,* and *M. malmoense.* Two species that may be associated with superficial soft tissue disease but not with pulmonary disease are *M. ulcerans* and *M. hemophilum.*

Species of Low Pathogenic Potential. A few cases have been reported in which strains of the *M. terrae* complex (including *M. triviale)* were the cause of pulmonary disease, arthritis, or tenosynovitis. Strains of this complex may be found in the soil. An organism long associated with water and considered to be saprophytic is *M. gordonae.* Documented infections with this organism now range from bursitis to widely disseminated disease. Cases of pulmonary disease and synovitis also have been ascribed to *M. flavescens,* an organism with an intermediate growth rate that was previously considered to be nonpathogenic for humans.

EPIDEMIOLOGY. In contrast to tuberculosis, the other mycobacterioses are not transmitted from person to person but are acquired from the environment by mechanisms that are not well understood. For *M. xenopi* and *M. kansasii* the evidence points to the inhalation of aerosols of infected water. Strains of MAI may be found in domestic animals, soil, dust, and water. There is evidence that infected droplet nuclei may be produced along coastlines. Still largely unexplained is the geographic variability in the incidence of other mycobacterioses and the relative proportion of these infections attributable to each of the two most important agents of disease, MAI and *M. kansasii.* In this country the highest rates of *M. kansasii* disease have been reported from New Orleans, Dallas, Houston, Kansas City, and Chicago, while Milwaukee and the states of Georgia and Florida have reported a predominance of MAI disease. From one institution in St. Louis, 27 per cent of newly diagnosed cases of mycobacterial pulmonary disease were associated with an equal proportion of MAI and *M. kansasii.* Australia, Israel, and Japan have reported an overwhelming predominance of MAI infections over those caused by *M. kansasii.* In the Scandinavian countries, southeast England, and the Canadian province of Ontario, *M. xenopi* is an important pathogen. These figures refer to pulmonary disease; they do not reflect the distribution of disseminated infections. A recent increase in MAI and a concomitant decrease in *M. kansasii* pulmonary disease have been reported from Virginia and have been noted elsewhere, as well.

PATHOGENESIS. The localization of disease in the lungs suggests that the inhalation of infectious aerosols represents the primary route of infection. In many cases infection occurs by inoculation as a result of surgery, puncture wounds, lacerations, and foreign bodies. The question of whether the disease in adults usually represents primary infection or recrudescence of dormant foci cannot be answered at this time. The alimentary tract may be the route of infection in AIDS, since the intestinal tract is so often involved.

CLINICAL DESCRIPTION. *Pulmonary Disease.* The classic description is that of chronic cavitary disease resembling tuberculosis that occurs in a middle-aged rural man who has one or more of the following predisposing conditions: pneumoconiosis, healed tuberculosis, chronic bronchitis and emphysema, bullous disease, bronchiectasis, and malignant disease. However, there are many exceptions: The disease may be seen in all age groups except rarely in children, in either sex, and in some individuals without any apparent predisposing factor. It sometimes appears as an acute condition in which there is an infected bulla or cyst or in a case resembling pneumonia. Solitary pulmonary nodules also have been described.

The diagnosis may be suspected from the clinical appearance and the x-ray film, but it is the laboratory that must supply the correct identification of the mycobacterial agent. Skin tests are not helpful owing to a lack of adequately standardized antigens and the poor specificity of the currently available reagents. Pulmonary changes are characterized by one or more thin-walled cavities with little or no pleural disease or spread to the basal segments of the lungs. The sputum usually contains many acid-fast bacilli visible on smear and yields a heavy growth of the infecting agent. It may be possible to recognize the large banded forms of *M. kansasii* in the direct smear. A single positive culture result in which there are only a few colonies usually represents environmental contamination. Repeatedly positive specimens may be indicative of transient or long-term colonization of the respiratory tract when they are not associated with new or enlarging cavities and a compatible clinical picture.

Treatment for *M. kansasii* disease usually is highly successful, provided that rifampin is included in the regimen. It is recommended that isoniazid, rifampin, and ethambutol be given for 1 year after the sputum becomes negative for the organism. Results of preliminary trials of short-course treatment have not been encouraging.

Therapy for MAI disease, on the other hand, has proved to be difficult. Most strains are resistant to the available antituberculosis drugs as well as the other anti-infectives, and the drug regimens recommended up to now have been chosen empirically. The necessity for treatment must first be established by an observation period to determine the stability of disease and the rate of progression if it is advancing. During this period the sputum should be examined at frequent intervals, and the patient should receive a comprehensive course of bronchial hygiene, including cessation of smoking, bronchodilator therapy, chest physiotherapy, and antibiotics if there are purulent secretions. These maneuvers have served to eliminate the organism from the sputum of some patients with chronic pulmonary disease. It may be necessary to initiate therapy immediately in certain cases of severe acute disease with a new cavitary lesion and no other apparent cause. Drug treatment may be considered at three levels. Level 1 is a triple-drug regimen consisting of isoniazid, rifampin, and ethambutol for a duration of at least 2 years provided there is some response within the first few months. This level would be suitable for a patient who had chronic stable disease with consistently positive sputum test results and in whom the mycobacterial infection was adding to the burden of pulmonary disease. Level 2 treatment consists of the same three drugs plus daily streptomycin administration for at least 2 years. Administration of streptomycin may be reduced to two or three times a week after an initial response has been demonstrated. This treatment level would be suitable for a patient who had slowly progressive disease, who had a poor response to level 1 treatment, or who had a relapse after discontinuation of level 1 drug therapy. Drug treatment at level 3 may be empiric combinations of five or six drugs or, more reasonably, a regimen based on drug susceptibility studies: drugs used for level 2 with the addition of ethionamide, cycloserine, ciprofloxacin, or clofazimine (available); and rifabutin and other rifamycin derivatives or new macrolides (investigational).

The response to drug treatment depends to a large extent on the underlying chronic lung disease and on the rate of progression of the mycobacterial infection. For those patients who have rapidly progressive infection in lungs that are already severely damaged, the prognosis is poor even with level 3 treatment. Some of these individuals have defects in cellular immune functions, especially those associated with T cells. Resectional surgery should be considered after a few months of treatment for those patients who have adequate pulmonary function and sufficiently localized mycobacterial disease. Treatment is not necessary for solitary pulmonary nodules that result from MAI infection, usually recognized after resection.

Disease caused by *M. xenopi* and *M. szulgai* usually is amenable to drug therapy. The exact combinations of drugs to be used depend on the drug susceptibility patterns in vitro. Suggested for *M. xenopi* disease is a regimen consisting of isoniazid, rifampin, and streptomycin and for *M. szulgai*, rifampin, ethambutol, and either ethionamide or streptomycin.

Infections associated with *M. scrofulaceum*, *M. simiae*, and *M. fortuitum-chelonae* are more difficult to control because of natural drug resistance. Strains of *M. simiae* usually are resistant to all of the antituberculosis drugs except cycloserine and ethionamide. Limited information on susceptibility of *M. scrofulaceum* suggests that ethionamide, rifampin, and ethambutol are most likely to be active in vitro. The same considerations as those described for MAI infection are applicable to these resistant infections. Although pulmonary infections with *M. fortuitum-chelonae* are quite rare, there is some information about the response to drug treatment from cases of extrapulmonary disease. Before sensitivity test results are available, full doses of amikacin should be given intramuscularly, together with one or more of the following drugs: doxycycline, erythromycin, ciprofloxacin, cefoxitin, and a sulfonamide.

Lymphadenitis. Mycobacterial lymphadenitis is almost exclusively a disease of children of preschool age. Data from British Columbia published in 1974 indicated that the case rate for this new kind of scrofula was 0.37 per 100,000 persons per year, about 10 times higher than for that caused by *M. tuberculosis*. Involved nodes may be found in the femoral, inguinal, epitrochlear, and axillary areas, although the most common location is

around the angle of the jaw. The route of infection to the groin area is a penetrating injury or splinter entry into an extremity. The cervical nodes probably become infected by mucous membrane penetration in the mouth or pharynx. Examination shows a child who has had a painless localized swelling for several weeks and who is otherwise healthy. An unknown proportion of cases goes on to suppuration and breakdown. Draining sinuses, whether spontaneous or following incision and drainage, may persist for many months. *M. scrofulaceum* was the most common cause of this infection, with MAI the second. However, there has been a recent reversal of this ratio so that strains of MAI now are the most common isolates from these infected nodes. Rare cases caused by several other species have been reported.

Correct diagnosis depends on the physician's familiarity with the disease, a positive tuberculin skin test result (sometimes requiring the use of second-strength purified protein derivative), the absence of a history of contact with tuberculosis, absence of thoracic disease, and the location as well as the appearance of the involved nodes. Other conditions that need to be differentiated are tuberculosis, pyogenic lymphadenitis, cat scratch disease, congenital cyst, and lymphoma. The treatment of choice is excision of the involved nodes. In about 10 per cent of cases there is a recurrence of the infection in another group of nodes near the original site, occasionally on the other side. Rarely there may be a third episode. Recurrences should be treated in the same manner as the original infection. There is no convincing evidence that drug treatment is beneficial. It should be remembered that as a result of this infection a child may have a positive tuberculin skin test reaction for many years.

Skin and Soft Tissue Infections. **Cutaneous Granuloma.** Localized groups of papules have been called swimming pool granuloma or fish tank granuloma, depending on the source of infection. In another form of the disease there is a local abscess at the inoculation site, usually on the hand, followed by a series of secondary nodules that progress centrally along the lymphatics in a manner not unlike that seen in sporotrichosis. A few deep hand infections have also been described; such cases should be referred to a hand surgeon. The infection is not uncommon as an occupational or recreational illness in people who work or play in a marine environment. With few exceptions, the etiologic agent is *M. marinum*. Most superficial infections are self-limited. When treatment is deemed necessary, the physician may use a combination of rifampin and ethambutol, rifampin alone, one of the tetracyclines, or trimethoprim-sulfamethoxazole. All of these regimens have been reported to be successful.

Local Abscess. Many cases of local abscess following subcutaneous or intramuscular injection have been reported, some in outbreaks. The trouble usually is traced to a contaminated multiple injection vial, and the etiologic agent usually is *M. fortuitum-chelonae*. Incision and drainage usually will suffice to control the infection.

Local Trauma. Most of these infections caused by *M. fortuitum-chelonae* occur as a result of penetrating or lacerating wounds contaminated with soil. Expert surgical handling is necessary, along with appropriate drug therapy as outlined under Pulmonary Disease.

Disseminated Nodules. Multiple nodules and abscesses may be associated with widely disseminated mycobacterial disease, almost always in an immunocompromised host. The species most often isolated is *M. fortuitum-chelonae*. In addition, such nodules have been described in renal transplant patients as a result of infection with *M. hemophilum*.

Buruli Ulcer. This deeply penetrating ulcer caused by *M. ulcerans* is confined mainly to Africa, Papua New Guinea, Malaysia, and Australia. The treatment is difficult and controversial.

Skeletal Infections. The synovia, tendon sheaths, and bursae are involved more often than other parts of the skeletal system in nontuberculous mycobacterial infections. A wide variety of species may be associated, including environmental strains with little pathogenicity for humans, such as *M. terrae*, *M. gordonae*, and *M. flavescens*. Leading the list of etiologic agents is *M. kansasii*, with *M. fortuitum-chelonae* and MAI following in that order. Many of these infections follow trauma in which the wound is contaminated with soil or water. Others have occurred after injections of corticosteroids into arthritic joints; in these cases it is difficult to determine which condition was primary. The most common site is the hand, where the infection produces an indolent but persistent tenosynovitis, including the carpal tunnel syndrome. Osteomyelitis may occur in the form of multifocal lesions from hematogenous dissemination, often as a slowly progressive rather than a fulminant infection. The principal etiologic agent in these cases is MAI.

Treatment for skeletal infection usually demands close cooperation between a skilled surgeon and a physician specializing in infectious disease. Drug therapy depends on the etiologic agent (refer to earlier discussion).

Postsurgical Infections. Infections following surgery mainly are caused by *M. fortuitum-chelonae.* They include prosthetic valve endocarditis, sternal wound infection and osteomyelitis after open heart surgery, wound infection after augmentation mammoplasty, and infections associated with hemodialysis and peritoneal dialysis.

Disseminated Disease. Patients who develop disseminated disease usually are severely immunocompromised from the standpoint of cellular immune functions. The arrival of AIDS has been associated with a dramatic increase in disseminated mycobacterial infections, since up to 50 per cent of such patients coming to autopsy in several cities have been found to have disseminated MAI infections. Prior to 1980 there were relatively few cases of disseminated mycobacterial disease reported throughout the world. They usually involved patients who had underlying hematologic malignancies or who were under treatment with corticosteroids, or both. Both children and adults were affected, and the most common etiologic agents were *M. kansasii* and MAI. The case fatality rate was very high, even with the most intensive multiple-drug treatment. Diagnosis is most commonly made by biopsy and culture of liver, bone marrow, or lymph nodes. Cultures of the blood are often positive. Skin lesions or subcutaneous nodules or abscesses should be biopsied and examined for acid-fast bacilli. Strains of *M. fortuitum-chelonae* often are associated with these superficial lesions. The tissues may show a nonspecific necrotizing reaction in which macrophages are loaded with acid-fast bacilli, rather than a granulomatous reaction. In AIDS patients, disseminated infection usually occurs in the late stages of the disease, and the diagnosis may be made quickly by finding AFB in the stool or in the buffy coat.

Treatment for disseminated disease is based on the same principles as those outlined for pulmonary disease. Infections caused by drug-sensitive organisms such as *M. kansasii* can usually be brought under at least temporary control provided that the human host is able to provide an adequate immune response. For infections related to MAI a multiple-drug regimen is usually chosen as outlined earlier, with the realization that, for the AIDS patient, the response usually is poor and the side effects may be severe.

Chester AC, Winn WC Jr: Unusual and newly recognized patterns of nontuberculous mycobacterial infection with emphasis on the immunocompromised host. Pathol Ann 21:251, 1986. *This is an extensive review, well referenced, and presented from the standpoint of the pathologist.*

Davidson PT: The diagnosis and management of disease caused by *M. avium* complex, *M. kansasii,* and other mycobacteria. Clin Chest Med 10:431, 1989. *An excellent contribution from an established leader in the clinical mycobacterial arena.*

Grange JM, Yates MD: Infections caused by opportunist mycobacteria: A review. J R Soc Med 79:226, 1986. *A succinct, informative account of mycobacteriosis as seen in England.*

Grange JM, Yates MD, Boughton E: The avian tubercle bacillus and its relatives. J Appl Bacteriol 68:411, 1990. *The important historical, ecological, and microbiological facts are presented admirably.*

Horsburgh CR Jr, Mason UG III, Farhi DC, et al.: Disseminated infection with *Mycobacterium avium-intracellulare:* A report of 13 cases and a review of the literature. Medicine 64:36, 1985. *A thorough analysis of 13 cases from the National Jewish Hospital and 24 cases from the literature, with emphasis on response to treatment. Patients with AIDS were excluded.*

Lichtenstein IH, MacGregor RR: Mycobacterial infections in renal transplant recipients: Report of five cases and review of the literature. Rev Infect Dis 5:216, 1983. *Renal transplant recipients have a high risk of disseminated mycobacteriosis, and 34 per cent of reported cases have been attributed to nontuberculous species.*

Marchevsky AM, Damsker B, Green S, et al.: The clinicopathological spectrum of nontuberculous mycobacterial osteoarticular infections. J Bone Joint Surg 67A:925, 1985. *A report of eight cases, attributed to five different species, with a good literature review. Infection of bone, synovium, and tendon sheaths may be seen.*

Margileth AM, Chandra R, Altman RP: Chronic lymphadenopathy due to mycobacterial infection: Clinical features, diagnosis, histopathology, and management. Am J Dis Child 138:917, 1984. *From Washington and New York comes this informative report of 153 cases, of which 86 per cent were due to*

nontuberculous mycobacteria. Unfortunately, no speciation of the positive cultures is presented.

Moran JF, Alexander LG, Staub EW, et al.: Long-term results of pulmonary resection for atypical mycobacterial disease. Ann Thorac Surg 35:597, 1983. *This report documents the good results of resectional surgery in 37 patients seen by the surgical group at Duke University from 1967 to 1981. All disease was attributed to* M. avium-intracellulare.

O'Brien RJ: The epidemiology of nontuberculous mycobacterial disease. Clin Chest Med 10:407, 1989. *This is a unique review dealing with such features as ecology of the organisms, mechanisms of transmission, and prevalence of disease (roughly 2 per 100,000 in the United States).*

Roth RI, Owen RL, Keren DF, et al.: Intestinal infection with *Mycobacterium avium* in AIDS: Histological and clinical comparison with Whipple's disease. Dig Dis Sci 30:497,1985. *A good account of the fascinating similarity of some MAI intestinal infections to Whipple's disease.*

Wallace RJ Jr: The clinical presentation, diagnosis, and therapy of cutaneous and pulmonary infections due to the rapidly growing mycobacteria, *M. fortuitum* and *M. chelonae.* Clin Chest Med 10:419, 1989. *Dr. Wallace has been at the forefront of clinical research in diseases associated with rapidly growing mycobacteria. This review is excellent.*

Wallace RJ Jr, O'Brien R, Glassroth J, et al.: Diagnosis and treatment of disease caused by nontuberculous mycobacteria. Am Rev Respir Dis 142:940, 1990. *This is an authoritative review and an official statement of the American Thoracic Society.*

Wolinsky E: Nontuberculous mycobacteria and associated diseases. Am Rev Respir Dis 119:107, 1979. *A state-of-the-art review of the entire subject.*

Woodring JH, Vandiviere HM, Melvin IG, Dillon ML: Roentgenographic features of pulmonary disease caused by atypical mycobacteria. South Med J 80:1488, 1987. *A retrospective study of 40 cases, with good radiographic pictures.*

Woods GL, Washington JA: Mycobacteria other than *Mycobacterium tuberculosis:* Review of microbiologic and clinical aspects. Rev Infect Dis 9:275, 1987. *From the Cleveland Clinic comes this helpful review of the epidemiologic, pathologic, and clinical features of each species.*

Young LS, Inderlied CB, Berlin OG, Gottlieb MS: Mycobacterial infections in AIDS patients, with an emphasis on the *Mycobacterium avium* complex. Rev Infect Dis 8:1024, 1986. *A good exposition of the subject from Los Angeles, which includes a section on the authors' laboratory studies of potentially useful combination drug regimens.*

334 Leprosy—Hansen's Disease

Zanvil A. Cohn and Gilla Kaplan

DEFINITION. Leprosy is a bacterial disease of great chronicity and low infectivity which occurs worldwide. The primary host is the human, in whom the causative agent *Mycobacterium leprae* accumulates largely in the skin and peripheral nerves, leading to a variety of cutaneous lesions and loss of nerve conduction. Serious disfigurement and loss of digits and extremities may result and represent the stigmata of this biblical disease. The clinical manifestations are largely governed by the ability of the host to mount a cell-mediated immune (CMI) response to the organism and its antigens. Patients unable to generate an immune attack develop widely distributed skin lesions of the *lepromatous* state and allow unrestricted growth of bacilli. In contrast, a moderate to vigorous immune response leads to the local cutaneous lesions of the *tuberculoid* form. In addition to these polar states there are intermediate forms that demonstrate gradations in reactivity. Modulation of the disease toward more polar forms can occur and may lead to tissue damage via humoral (immune complex) and cellular (CMI) mechanisms. Therapy with multiple drugs leads to a prompt reduction in viable organisms and transmissibility but must be maintained for long periods for the disappearance of skin lesions and a reduction in bacterial load.

TRANSMISSION. Little detailed information is available about how the bacillus is transmitted from one individual to another. This deficit in our understanding is related to the long incubation period (>3 years) and the absence of adequate techniques to identify the organism in the environment. Other than in humans the disease has been discovered in feral armadillos studied in Louisiana and Texas. These animals contain large numbers of acid-fast bacilli in parenchymatous organs which by DNA hybridization and restriction fragment length polymorphism analysis techniques are identical to bacilli obtained from humans. The sooty mangabey, a new world monkey, can become infected naturally in the wild or when injected with human bacilli. In both armadillos and monkeys it takes 18 to 24 months for the injected bacilli to reach high numbers. These infections are quite unlike the spectrum of human disease.

The localized lesions of tuberculoid leprosy and the generalized distribution of lepromatous disease are in keeping with suggested pathways for the introduction of bacilli. Direct inoculation via such means as trauma and puncture wounds might lead to an initial focus with environmental bacilli. Some suggest that the initial route may be through the respiratory or gastrointestinal tract. Biting insects have been considered, but no clear evidence exists regarding them as an intermediate vector. It seems reasonable, however, that at some point during the infection in lepromatous leprosy patients, hematogenous spread occurs with wide seeding of the body.

It is likely that the number of environmental bacilli is correlated with transmission. The incidence of the disease within a household containing an infected tuberculoid or lepromatous index patient may be four to eight times that of the general population. In particular, lepromatous patients with lesions in the nasal mucosa discharge large numbers of organisms. Bacilli recovered from dry nasal discharges retain some viability for up to 7 to 10 days, with somewhat greater viability under conditions of higher humidity. Transmission of the disease from an untreated, infected mother to an infant is not uncommon and should always be considered. In general, clinical wisdom indicates that disease transmission takes place only after years of exposure. Little likelihood of transmission is present in a ward or hospital setting and patients are now cared for on an ambulatory basis with a minimum of precautions.

SUSCEPTIBILITY. Leprosy occurs worldwide and in individuals of all ages. It appears more frequently in young adults, but this may be related to a parental index case and the long period of incubation. The incidence of the disease is greater in males than in females. However, it is unlikely that this represents differences in gender but possibly reflects the greater likelihood that males seek and obtain medical attention in the Third World.

A large number of studies suggest, but do not prove, that the overall susceptibility to leprosy is not controlled by immune response genes and their expressed major histocompatibility class II antigens. Early analysis of the disease incidence and susceptibility in identical twins has not been conclusive. More recent studies suggest that the type of leprosy rather than overall disease susceptibility may be controlled by HLA determinants. No clearcut conclusions on the genetic basis of susceptibility can therefore be accepted at this time. In this context, environmental factors such as nutrition and coincident microbial and parasitic infections must be considered as alternatives.

The physiologic immunodeficiency of the newborn may lead to an early colonization with the bacillus. The AIDS pandemic has been associated with a rise in the incidence of other mycobacterial diseases, and this association may become more apparent in leprosy in the future.

EPIDEMIOLOGY. The worldwide number of leprosy cases has been estimated to be between 12 and 15 million. In many countries valid statistics are not available, and the incidence in outlying, rural areas is poorly documented. The highest prevalence rates are in Asia and Africa, followed by Central and South America and Oceania. The highest rates do not usually exceed 55 per 1000 but may be as high as 200 per 1000 in selected villages. Many accept the fact that with effective chemotherapy the worldwide incidence is dropping and will continue to do so with advanced diagnostic and public health methods.

The majority of leprosy cases are found in tropical areas. Socioeconomic condition, availability of health care, and body exposure to the environment may all contribute. The disease also occurs in the colder climates of Tibet, Nepal, Korea, and Siberia. In the previous centuries the disease occurred more commonly in Scandinavia and those countries bordering the North Sea. Small numbers (300 to 500 per year) of cases currently occur in the United States. The majority of these are in immigrant groups from Asia and South America, although occasional cases are seen in the southern states and those bordering Mexico.

The nature of the disease varies considerably with geographic distribution. African and Asian countries have a predominance of tuberculoid leprosy, and 20 per cent or fewer of the cases are of the lepromatous type. In contrast, larger numbers of lepromatous cases are reported in Brazil and Venezuela. Early infection and/or sensitization with cross-reacting antigens of other mycobacteria has been considered as an explanation for the variation in type of leprosy with which an individual presents.

ETIOLOGIC AGENT. *Mycobacterium leprae* is the causative agent of human leprosy, and no evidence of strain variation has been noted by DNA–DNA hybridization or restriction fragment length polymorphism. The organism is acid-alcohol fast when stained by the Ziehl-Neelsen method. *M. leprae* is an obligate intracellular parasite and has never been cultivated extracellularly in laboratory media. It is a resident of the phagolysosomes of macrophages, Schwann cells, and endothelial cells. *M. leprae* is classified as a mycobacterium and contains mycolic acid, arabinogalactan, and phenolic glycolipid. The latter molecule is the only *M. leprae*–specific component. Most other carbohydrates, peptidoglycans, and proteins share antigenic determinants with other mycobacterial species, making serologic diagnosis especially difficult.

The absence of a culture system for *M. leprae* has complicated any investigations of the physiology and pathogenicity of the organism. Many advances in this field have resulted from the ability of the armadillo to support the growth of the mycobacteria. Eighteen to 24 months after inoculation, large numbers of bacilli (10^9 per gram) can be purified from liver and spleen and serve as a source for antigenic and chemical analysis. *M. leprae* is one of the few pathogenic mycobacteria which lacks the enzyme catalase and is susceptible to killing by oxygen metabolites such as hydrogen peroxide. Many of the metabolic activities of *M. leprae* appear to be low compared with other mycobacteria, and de novo purine biosynthesis appears to be missing. *M. leprae* replicates very slowly within host cells and has a doubling time of approximately 13 days. It prefers ambient temperatures below 37°C and grows selectively in cooler portions of the body such as skin, testes, and nasal mucosa.

Within the vacuolar apparatus, the bacillus is surrounded by a loose matrix of secreted phenolic glycolipid which also serves as a scavenger of oxygen intermediates. Specific *M. leprae* proteins have been identified by direct chemical analysis and through recombinant DNA technology. Other polypeptides are cross-reactive with those of *M. tuberculosis* and other mycobacteria.

The determination of bacillary viability and resistance to chemotherapeutic agents depends upon its slow growth in the foot pads of mice—a bioassay taking about 12 months. Accelerated growth occurs in the athymic nude mouse but still requires 6 or more months. These properties impose severe restrictions on rapid diagnosis. Application of the polymerase chain reaction, in which selected DNA sequences are amplified a millionfold, may lead to the specific identification of as few as 10 bacilli within a few days.

IMMUNOLOGIC CONSIDERATION. A major immunologic defect occurs in patients with lepromatous leprosy. This is expressed as a selective unresponsiveness of T cells to *M. leprae* and is evident in skin test anergy and the in vitro lymphocyte transformation test to *M. leprae* antigens (Table 334–1). Patients

TABLE 334–1. IMMUNOLOGIC FEATURES OF LEPROSY PATIENTS

	Tuberculoid	Borderline Tuberculoid	Mid Borderline	Borderline Lepromatous	Lepromatous
Acid-fast bacilli in skin lesion	−	−/+	+	+ + +	+ + +
Lepromin (Mitsuda) reaction	+ + +	+ +	−	−	−
Lymphocyte transformation test	15%	5.7%	2%	0.4%	0.3%
Anti–*M. leprae* antibodies	−/+	−/+ +	+ +	+ + +	+ + +
CD4+/CD8+ T-cell ratio in skin	1.35	1.11	NT	0.48	0.20

with the tuberculoid form of the disease respond normally, and in neither form of the disease are there abnormalities in humoral immunity. The association between cell-mediated, T cell–directed immunity and the number of *M. leprae* in the tissues is shown in Figure 334–1. These two parameters are inversely related. In the absence of *M. leprae*–specific T-cell reactivity, lymphokine formation is depressed or absent and tissue macrophages fail to be activated into an antimicrobial state. Normally, macrophage activation occurs largely through the local release of interferon-γ (IFN-γ), a lymphokine that enhances the production of toxic oxygen intermediates in these cells. Bacilli taken up by "resting" and "aged" macrophages of the skin are able to multiply intracellularly, leading in the case of lepromatous disease to multibacillary vacuoles. In tuberculoid forms, the bacilli are largely destroyed and only small numbers survive to perpetuate the cell-mediated immune reactions.

Lepromatous patients, although unresponsive to *M. leprae* antigen, develop adequate reactions to other antigens to which they have been sensitized. These include skin test antigens such as PPD, mumps, *Candida*, trichophytin, and tetanus toxoid. The highly selective anergy of leprosy may be related to the loss of T cells with surface recognition receptors rather than suppressor cell phenomena.

CLINICAL DIAGNOSIS. Patients with leprosy are first seen and followed by dermatologists because the cutaneous lesions are often the presenting complaint. The range in immunity to *M. leprae* is reflected clinically by a wide variation of skin lesions and peripheral nerve involvement. In this section we review the characteristics of the major polar forms.

Polar Tuberculoid Leprosy (TT). This form presents as one to three plaques or macules defined by a sharp, raised border. In dark-skinned patients they are often hypopigmented centrally with a more erythematous border. The central area is scaly, lacks hair, and is anesthetic. Nerves may be palpably enlarged in and adjacent to the plaque, and these are commonly found leading to the area of the ear, elbow, and knee. Almost any area of the skin may be affected except for the warmer regions of the scalp, axilla, and perineum.

Borderline Tuberculoid Leprosy (BT). As the body burden of antigen increases, in association with a partial reduction in immunity, the number, distribution, and nature of the cutaneous lesions increase in complexity and the sequelae of peripheral nerve damage increase in severity. The skin exhibits a polymorphic array of macular, erythematous, hypopigmented lesions involving the trunk, extremities, and face. These vary in number and distribution in a seemingly random fashion. Larger nerve trunks are involved with a granulomatous reaction, leading to foot drop, flexion contractions of the digits, and corneal abrasions.

The anesthesia of hands and feet and the resulting damage from burns, trauma, and secondary infection leads to loss of digits, plantar ulcerations, and blindness. These widely dispersed lesions suggest hematogenous spread and a cell-mediated reaction that is not capable of fully controlling bacillary growth.

Lepromatous Leprosy (LL). Here there is little or no CMI, and tremendous numbers of organisms are dispersed throughout the body. Again the lesions are pleomorphic but often are less "angry" or erythematous than in borderline disease. Macules, papules, and nodules may cover wide areas of the trunk and extremities, and lesion distribution is often symmetric. Almost any area of affected or "normal" looking skin contains bacilli. Often there are no obvious lesions but the skin looks shiny and "full," as the dermis is expanded with macrophages containing bacilli. This is particularly prominent on the ears, eyebrows, and face, giving rise to an appearance called leonine facies. Eyebrow loss is frequent; a saddle nose deformity may result from cartilage destruction; gynecomastia from reduced testosterone levels secondary to testicular damage may be present; and blindness and iridocyclitis, laryngeal stenosis, loss of incisor teeth, and loss of digits may occur. These results of long-term untreated lepromatous leprosy are the stigmata that ostracized the leper from his community and necessitated custodial care. This is almost never the case today, and patients undergoing chemotherapy remain members of their households. Nerve damage in lepromatous leprosy is more slowly progressive but is eventually severe and diffuse and leads to a sensory polyneuropathy. Rigid, swollen nerves are palpable in many locations.

REACTIONAL STATES. *Erythema Nodosum Leprosum (ENL).* The release of *M. leprae* antigen, often following the initiation of therapy in multibacillary patients with or without the formation of immune complexes, results in an acute reactional state that may lead to death. Suddenly, painful, erythematous nodules and papules arise diffusely and may eventually lead to necrosis and suppuration. These symptoms, accompanied by fever and malaise, can continue for months, are extremely debilitating, and are often accompanied by acute inflammation of the eyes, testes, nerves, lymph nodes, and joints. Some patients develop glomerulonephritis with the deposition of complement and immune complexes in the glomeruli. This serious complication requires prompt diagnosis and therapy.

Reversal Reactions. This reactional state may also occur after chemotherapy but differs from ENL in that tissues are infiltrated with newly recruited T lymphocytes. The acceleration of the local cell-mediated reaction, observed mostly in borderline patients of the tuberculoid as well as the lepromatous type, is accompanied by widespread erythema and induration of pre-existing lesions as well as systemic symptoms, e.g., pyrexia. The onset of this state is slower, takes weeks to months, and may persist for many months if not properly treated. Rapid progression of pre-existing peripheral nerve damage may take place. These irreversible changes in nerve conduction should be considered a medical emergency and treated accordingly.

LABORATORY DIAGNOSIS. In addition to clinical manifestations the primary method for the diagnosis of leprosy is the identification of acid-fast bacilli in the skin. The slit smear technique is used throughout the world. Skin is incised with a scalpel, squeezing the area to maintain a bloodless field. The edges of the slit are scraped with the edge of the scalpel, smeared on a slide, fixed, and stained by the Ziehl-Neelsen method. A microscopic logarithmic score (1+ to 6+), (5+ equals 100 to 1000 acid-fast bacilli per high-power field), is used to quantitate the bacterial load. Usually six sites on the ear lobes, eyebrows, elbow, knee, and a lesion are prepared. This simple method when skillfully applied is as sensitive as any diagnostic procedure.

A more definitive estimate of bacillary numbers in the skin comes from biopsy material. Biopsies are fixed, sectioned, and stained for acid-fast organisms as well as the background host cells. A logarithmic score is made by counting the number of bacilli in high-power fields. This ranges from 1+ to 6+ and is a useful index in following the response of patients to therapy in terms of bacillary numbers and histopathologic classification. (Bacterial Index: 0—no bacilli in 100 microscopic fields ($\times 100$); 1+ = 1 to 10 bacilli in 100 fields; 2+ = 1 to 10 bacilli in 10 fields; 3+ = 1 to 10 bacilli per field; 4+ = 10 to 100 bacilli per

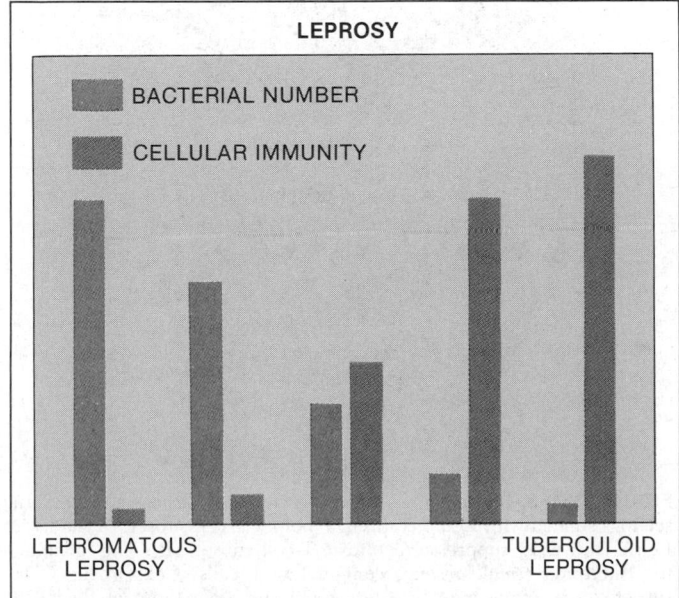

LEPROSY

BACTERIAL NUMBER

CELLULAR IMMUNITY

LEPROMATOUS LEPROSY

TUBERCULOID LEPROSY

FIGURE 334–1. Cellular immunity and bacterial numbers across the clinical spectrum of leprosy.

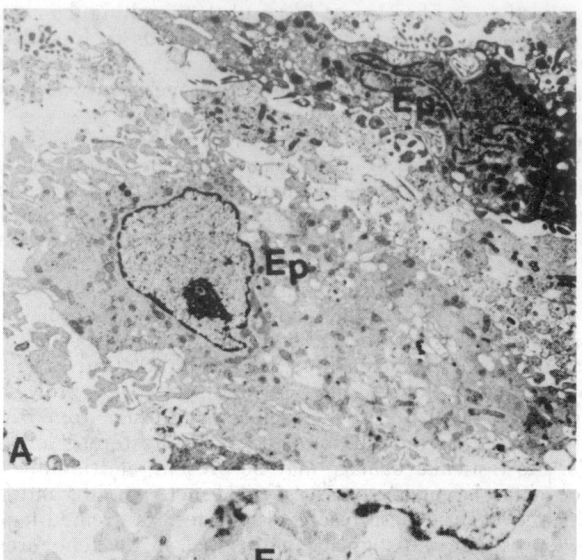

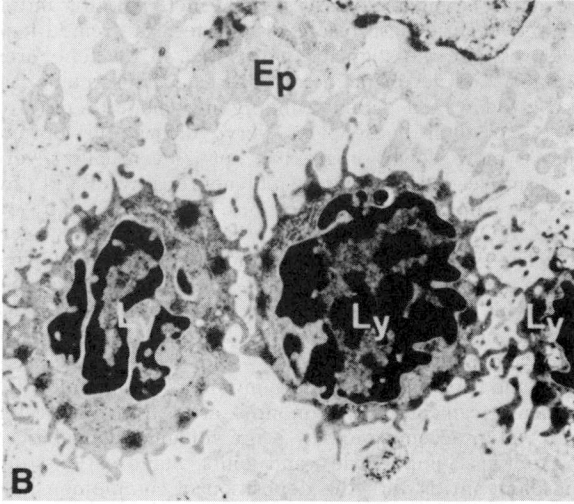

FIGURE 334–2. Transmission electron photomicrographs of cutaneous granulomas from a patient with tuberculoid leprosy. *A,* The granuloma contains large epithelioid cells (Ep) with multiple cytoplasmic organelles (× 4500). *B,* Three T lymphocytes (Ly) and an epithelioid cell are observed (× 9000).

field; 5+ = 100 to 1000 bacilli per field; and 6+ = many 1000s per field.)

A skin test may be employed which distinguishes the immunologically reactive (tuberculoid) and nonreactive (lepromatous) poles of the disease. A crude antigen consisting of heat-killed bacilli from lepromatous skin nodules is injected and induces local induration and the formation of granulomas in 3 to 4 weeks in most tuberculoid patients. Patients with lepromatous leprosy fail to react to the antigen and may remain unresponsive long after effective chemotherapy.

Serologic tests are useful in assaying the level of anti–*M. leprae* antibodies in multibacillary lepromatous but not in the paucibacillary tuberculoid forms. However, the many cross-reactive antigenic epitopes shared with other mycobacteria complicate interpretation and differential diagnosis. ELISA tests, which recognize antibodies against the carbohydrate moieties of the phenolic glycolipids, the only molecule that is *M. leprae*–specific, are positive in patients with lepromatous but not tuberculoid disease and decline after the initiation of chemotherapy. Patients with lepromatous leprosy have a polyclonal hypergammaglobulinemia, acute phase reactants such as C-reactive protein, and immune complexes in the circulation. Ten per cent give false-positive tests for syphilis and 30 per cent have cryoglobulinemia.

HISTOPATHOLOGY AND IMMUNOPATHOLOGY. Microscopic analysis of tissue plays a primary role in diagnosing and classifying the various clinical forms of leprosy and employs the standardized classification described by Ridley and Jopling. Five groups have been defined spanning the spectrum from polar tuberculoid (TT) to polar lepromatous (LL) and include borderline

(BB) as well as borderline tuberculoid (BT) and borderline lepromatous (BL). Our discussion focuses on the polar forms, and the details pertaining to the intermediate manifestations can be found in more specialized texts.

Lesions of the Skin. **Tuberculoid Leprosy.** Microscopic examination of H & E–stained sections of biopsies obtained from a TT macular plaque reveals heavy infiltration of the dermis by mononuclear leukocytes organized in well-developed granulomas. These contain large numbers of lymphocytes scattered between and surrounding other components of the granulomatous response, including macrophage-derived epithelioid cells and Langhans-type multinucleated giant cells (Fig. 334–2). Occasional plasma cells but no granulocytes are found. Langhans cells are found within the dermal infiltrate in significant numbers. Staining with monoclonal antibodies shows that the majority of lymphocytes are T cells and that the CD4+ "helper type" phenotype predominates over CD8+ "suppressor/cytotoxic" cells.

The epidermis overlying the dermal infiltrate is thickened (two- to threefold), and individual keratinocytes are enlarged. The keratinocytes display large amounts of MHC class II determinants on their surface. This is a response to the local production of IFN-γ in the dermis and is accompanied by the expression of other IFN-γ–induced molecules by keratinocytes and other cell types.

Acid-fast staining of sections reveals an occasional bacillus or bacillary remnants within macrophages. Borderline tuberculoid (BT) lesions are similar except that acid-fast bacilli are more readily seen.

Lepromatous Leprosy. In contrast to TT lesions, the lepromatous lesion contains only small numbers of lymphocytes, predominantly of the CD8+ phenotype, scattered through a background of loosely organized dermal macrophages and collagen (Fig. 334–3). The macrophages often have a pale, foamy cytoplasm and may contain large clumps of *M. leprae* called globi (Fig. 334–4). By electron microscopy these organisms are seen to reside within large cytoplasmic vacuoles, embedded in a lucent matrix that contains a phenolic glycolipid. Remnants of the osmiophilic bacilli are always present along with structurally intact organisms (Fig. 334–4*B* and *C*). A gram of skin may contain 10⁹ bacilli. The small proportion of lymphocytes is predominantly

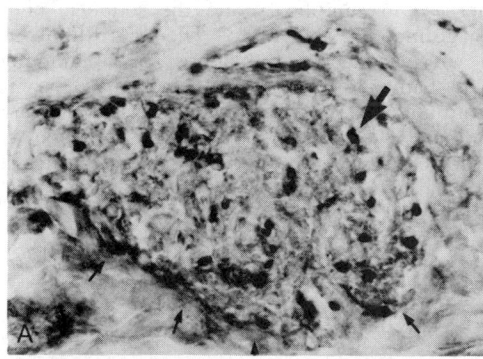

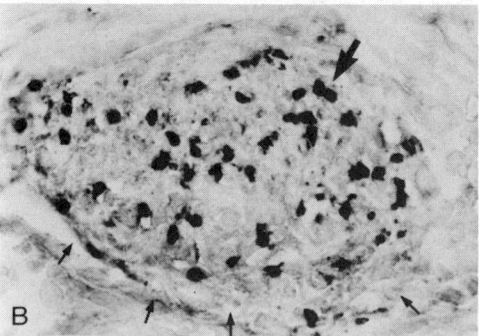

FIGURE 334–3. Lepromatous leprosy—cutaneous lesion. Frozen serial sections stained with Leu 3 (anti CD4–helper T-cell subset) *(A)* and with Leu 2 (anti CD8–suppressor/cytotoxic T-cell subset) *(B).* The inflammatory infiltrates *(small arrows)* contain few T cells. Cells of the CD4+ subset *(large arrow* in *A)* are less numerous than those of the CD8+ subset *(large arrows* in *B).* Immunoperoxidase, counterstained with hematoxylin (× 200).

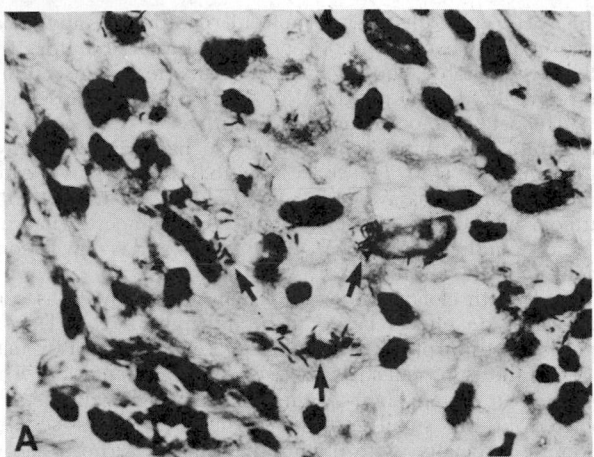

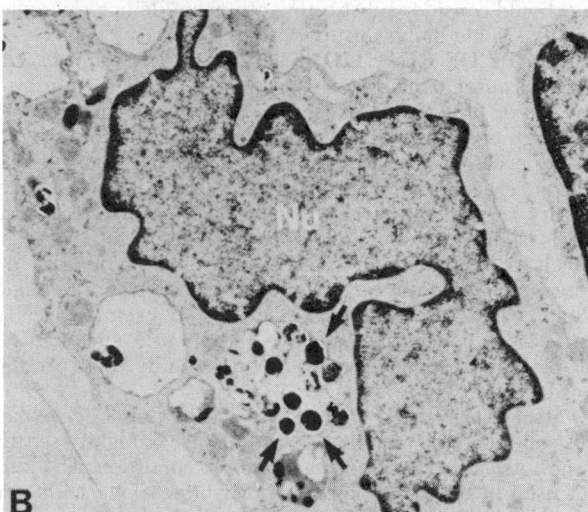

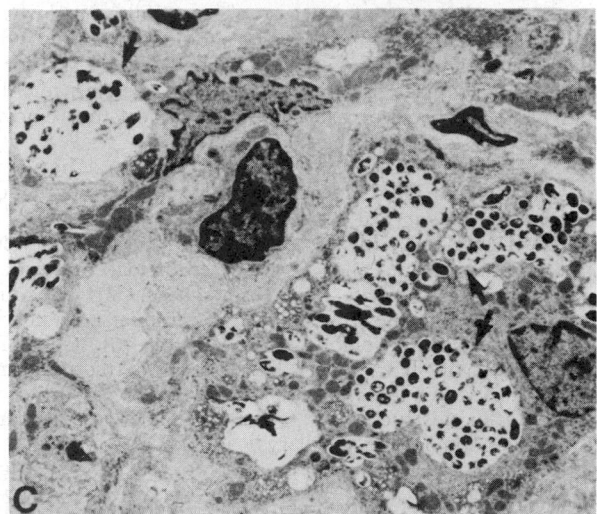

FIGURE 334–4. Lepromatous leprosy—cutaneous lesions. Acid-fast staining of histologic section (A) and transmission electron photomicrographs (B and C) of M. leprae–parasitized foamy macrophages (arrows). The phagocytes have large nuclei and many light and electron lucent vacuoles containing darkly staining bacteria (A, × 500; B, × 9000; C, × 3000).

of the CD8⁺ subset, and very small numbers of CD4⁺ helper cells are present. Langhans cells are rarely seen in the dermis; the overlying epidermis is thin and atrophic and fails to show surface MHC class II antigens usually associated with local IFN-γ production.

The loose infiltrates of LL and its bacilli are present in almost every area of the skin examined and individual infected macrophages may be observed surrounded by collagen bundles.

Lesions of Peripheral Nerve. Tuberculoid Leprosy. The pau-

cibacillary granulomatous response is associated with significant destruction of peripheral nerve fascicles and late in the disease may lead to caseous necrosis of nerve trunks. Large numbers of T cells and mononuclear phagocytes breach the perineurium and lead to destruction of Schwann cells and axons alike. By the time the skin lesion is apparent, nerve damage and sensory loss have occurred. The mechanism of the nerve damage in TT is unclear but is related to the granulomatous response.

Lepromatous Leprosy. Many bacilli are observed within Schwann cells and macrophages surrounding and within the perineural sheath in a reaction involving the majority of subcutaneously placed nerve trunks (Fig. 334–5). Nerve damage is relatively slow as compared to TT but more extensive and insidious. Few if any lymphocytes are part of the lesion. Eventually more enlargement and displacement by connective tissue result. Schwann cells are particularly capable of taking up M. leprae and serve as permissive hosts for their replication (Fig. 334–5).

Other Organs. Granulomatous lesions can be seen in the lymph nodes, liver, spleen, bone marrow, endocrine organs, and eye. These contain bacilli but are not considered to be an important source of infection. Patients with untreated multibacillary disease can have a constant bacteremia of 10⁵ AFB per milliliter, all of which are present within monocytes. The total body burden of M. leprae can reach 10¹².

Lesions of Reactional States. **Erythema Nodosum Leprosum (ENL).** Patients with BL and LL disease maintain high levels of circulating anti–M. leprae antibodies as well as high antigen levels in tissue depots. Following effective chemotherapy a prompt and extensive kill of bacilli takes place, and large amounts of soluble antigens are liberated extracellularly. More than 50 per cent of such patients develop ENL and present with painful erythematous skin nodules, fever, iridocyclitis, neuritis, glomerulonephritis, and other systemic manifestations. Examination of the skin nodules shows extensive infiltration of neutrophils, mononuclear cells, and tissue necrosis. Immune complexes are evident and there is a panvasculitis of dermal arteries and veins. These are all hallmarks of an extensive acute inflammatory response resulting in tissue damage.

Reversal Reactions. Patients with BT, BB, or BL leprosy, who are partially responsive to M. leprae antigens, occasionally undergo an upgrading reaction after several months of therapy. This differs from ENL in the migration of a predominantly T-cell infiltrate into pre-existing inflammatory sites. Many of the T cells are of the helper phenotype and are secreting lymphokines into

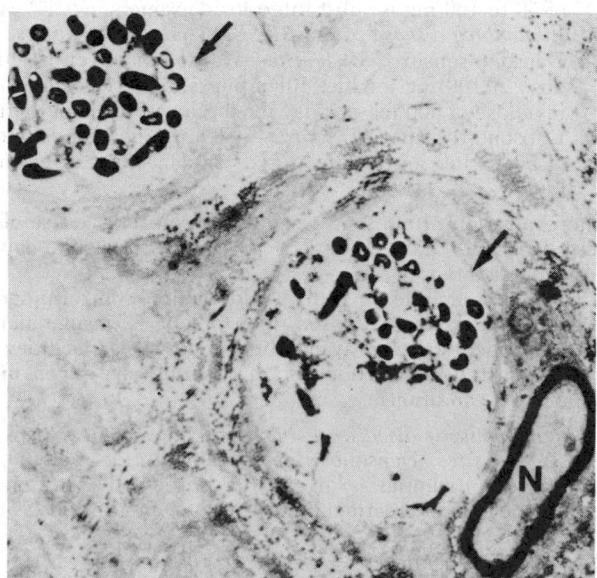

FIGURE 334–5. Transmission electron micrograph of an infiltrated peripheral nerve of a cutaneous lesion from a lepromatous leprosy patient. The myelinated neuron (N) and two M. leprae–infected Schwann cells (arrows) are observed (× 9000).

their environment. T-cell migration into skin lesions is associated with mononuclear phagocyte differentiation into organized granuloma and is often associated with the rapid progression of peripheral nerve damage. This enhancement of CMI leads to limited bacillary destruction. Such reactions may continue for weeks or months and are associated with severe morbidity leading to serious sequelae.

PATHOGENESIS. Recovery from infections with obligate intracellular parasites such as *M. leprae* requires the host to mount an effective CMI response. For this purpose, antigen-presenting dendritic cells must recognize and cluster with appropriate T cells, leading to T-cell stimulation, differentiation, and replication. T cells then follow two distinct pathways. In the first, helper cells synthesize and secrete a variety of hormone-like lymphokines which seem to enhance the microbicidal activity of monocytes and macrophages as well as stimulate other cells in the environment, e.g., keratinocytes, endothelial cells, and fibroblasts. A second pathway leads to the development of T cells which are of the CD4$^+$ phenotype and are antigen specific and MHC class II restricted. Along with NK (natural killer) and LAK (lymphokine-activated killer) cells, they serve as potent specific and nonspecific cytotoxic effector cells.

In lepromatous leprosy and in the absence of local lymphokine production, bacilli multiply in macrophages that have neither the capacity to kill the organism nor to be activated by lymphokines. To modify this fertile intracellular culture environment, the host must destroy the heavily parasitized macrophage, liberating its contents into the extracellular milieu. Here newly emigrated monocytes ingest, kill, and degrade *M. leprae* with the help of a lymphokine stimulus. This is the situation which applies in the tuberculoid form of the disease and is lacking in the lepromatous state. The immunomodulation necessary to mobilize host defense in lepromatous disease is discussed in a later section.

RECOMMENDED TREATMENT SCHEDULES. The most commonly used drug in the therapy of leprosy is 4,4'-diamino-diphenylsulfone (dapsone, DDS). Because of the widespread emergence of dapsone-resistant strains of *M. leprae*, all patients now receive multidrug therapy. The components and schedules vary depending upon the presence of dapsone-sensitive strains and the part of the world in which the patient resides. In the United States the following regimens are employed:

1. *Paucibacillary disease of the TT and BT categories.*
   a. Dapsone-sensitive *M. leprae*—Dapsone is given in a daily dose of 100 mg for 4 to 7 years and rifampin at a daily dose of 600 mg for 6 months.
   b. Dapsone-resistant *M. leprae*—Clofazimine at a daily dose of 50 to 100 mg is substituted for dapsone.
2. *Multibacillary disease of the BB, BL, and LL categories.*
   a. Dapsone-sensitive *M. leprae*—Dapsone is given in a daily dose of 100 mg for life. Rifampin is given in combination in a dose of 600 mg per day for the first 3 years of therapy.
   b. Dapsone-resistant *M. leprae*—Clofazimine at a daily dose of 50 to 100 mg is substituted for dapsone and given for life.

The evaluation of dapsone sensitivity requires the use of the mouse foot pad assay and is a procedure available only in specialized facilities.

A modified schedule for third world country control programs was issued in 1982 and is based upon practical consideration by the WHO, including the availability of slit smear facilities and financial constraints. Portions of the therapy are given under unsupervised conditions.

1. *Paucibacillary disease—a bacillary index of less than 2+ at all six skin sites.* Dapsone is given daily at a dose of 100 mg, unsupervised. Rifampin is given at a dose of 600 mg once a month, supervised. Treatment is given for 6 months and is then discontinued.
2. *Multibacillary disease—a bacillary index of more than 2+ at any one of six skin sites.* Dapsone is given daily at 100 mg with clofazimine 50 mg daily, unsupervised. Rifampin 600 mg and clofazimine 300 mg are given once monthly, supervised. This therapy is continued for 2 years or preferably until slit smears are negative.

The WHO schedule for intermittent rifampin therapy is based in part upon its expense and upon clinical and laboratory trials. It should be noted, however, that many leprologists employ rifampin at 450 to 600 mg daily for 2 to 3 years. Relapses under the WHO schedule occur not infrequently.

Rifampin is the most rapidly effective bactericidal agent and kills the majority of *M. leprae* within 2 to 3 weeks. This is evident by mouse foot pad assays and occurs only after 2 to 6 months of treatment with dapsone or clofazimine. Resistance to rifampin is well known in the therapy of *M. tuberculosis* and is now becoming evident with *M. leprae*.

Therapy with clofazimine, a phenazine derivative, has certain unpleasant side effects based upon its lipophilicity. The compound is a red-purple dye taken up and concentrated by macrophages of the skin, causing increased skin pigmentation. This is distressing to certain light-skinned patients. Clofazimine is also deposited in the small intestine, where it causes segmental thickening associated with crampy pain and diarrhea. The physician should consider substituting ethionamide or prothionamide at 250 to 375 mg daily, unsupervised.

THERAPY OF REACTIONS. *Erythema Nodosum Leprosum.* The acute onset of ENL may be mild enough to require only salicylates or other cyclo-oxygenase inhibitors. With severe episodes, high doses of corticosteroids (prednisone 60 to 80 mg per day) are necessitated and should be tapered off as soon as feasible. However, exacerbations occur frequently and repeated dosing is necessary. A particularly useful drug in severe ENL is thalidomide. It is given initially at 200 mg twice a day and then tapered to levels of 50 to 100 mg per day. Thalidomide is a potent teratogen and should be assiduously avoided if pregnancy is possible. Clofazimine has also been found useful in ENL but requires 4 to 6 weeks to achieve therapeutic effects. ENL in some patients responds poorly to thalidomide, and prednisone and/or clofazimine is employed.

Reversal Reactions. The chronicity and potential nerve damage of this cell-mediated reaction require the use of high-dose steroids and careful evaluation of peripheral nerve condition. Thalidomide is not used in this condition but clofazimine along with steroids allows the more rapid withdrawal of prednisone.

Other Complications. A variety of surgical procedures are available at specialized leprosy hospitals to help correct foot drop, hand deformities, madarosis, and lagophthalmos. Plastic surgical procedures can replace nasal septa and aid in the closure of large plantar ulcerations. On occasion patients request the removal of glandular tissue for gynecomastia.

The presence of a cold abscess of a peripheral nerve with sudden increase in pain and functional loss requires immediate decompression by surgical drainage.

IMMUNOMODULATION. The availability of recombinant lymphokines that can enhance the microbicidal properties of macrophages and stimulate the expression of CMI may find a place in the care of leprosy patients. Preliminary studies with the T-cell mitogen interleukin 2 (IL2) have already been carried out in patients with lepromatous leprosy. The intradermal injection of IL2 leads to a local cell-mediated reaction associated with induration, the destruction of parasitized macrophages, and a marked reduction in the bacillary load. Trials with more prolonged administration have demonstrated that a systemic response can be achieved.

PROGNOSIS. Tuberculoid leprosy is usually self-limited and responds well to chemotherapy. Nerve damage is, however, irreversible. In lepromatous disease, prolonged courses of multiple drugs arrest the progression of the illness when compliance is good. It is the ability of the public health infrastructure to monitor compliance that is central to effective therapy. Recurrences due to poor maintenance therapy are not infrequent.

PREVENTION AND PROPHYLAXIS. Education of the general public plays an important role in sensitizing individuals to the nature of leprosy lesions and the ability to cure the illness with medication. Once a case has been identified in a household, careful physical examination of all contacts with the biopsy of suspicious lesions should be carried out. The threat of contagion is much higher in children under 16 years of age. In this adolescent category the prophylactic use of dapsone should be considered.

A number of vaccine trials are currently underway, many sponsored by the World Health Organization. These are employing BCG vaccine with and without heat-killed *M. leprae* or other mycobacteria in highly endemic areas of Africa, Asia, and India. There is suggestive evidence that BCG alone may reduce the incidence of disease.

Guinto RS, Abalos RM, Cellona RV, Fajardo TT: An Atlas of Leprosy. Sasakawa Memorial Health Foundation, 1983. *Excellent pictorial presentation of diagnostic signs.*

Hansen GA: Causes of leprosy. Norsk Laegevidensk 4:76–79, 1874. *The classic work on leprosy.*

Hastings EC: Leprosy. New York, Churchill Livingstone, 1985.

Hastings RC, Franzblau SG: Chemotherapy of leprosy. Annu Rev Pharmacol Toxicol 28:231–245, 1988. *Current update of therapy and complications thereof.*

Job CK: Nerve damage in leprosy. XIII Leprosy Congress State of the Art Lectures. Int J Leprosy 57:532–539, 1989. *Good discussion of mechanisms of nerve damage.*

Kaplan G, Britton WJ, Hancock GE, et al.: The systemic influence of recombinant interleukin 2 on the manifestations of lepromatous leprosy. J Exp Med, in press. *Systemic modulation of CMI with IL-2.*

Kaplan G, Kiessling R, Teklemariam S, et al.: The reconstitution of cell-mediated immunity in the cutaneous lesions of lepromatous leprosy by recombinant interleukin 2. J Exp Med 169:893–907, 1989. *Discussion of our current understanding of the immunopathology of leprosy.*

Sexually Transmitted Diseases

P. Frederick Sparling

335 Introduction and Common Syndromes

Sexually transmitted diseases (STD's) are a diverse group of infections, caused by biologically dissimilar microbial agents, which are grouped together because of certain common clinical and epidemiologic features. In recent years there has been a remarkable accumulation of information about venereal infections. Advent of the acquired immunodeficiency syndrome (AIDS) has heightened public awareness of the importance of STD's and the dangers of unsafe sexual practices. New knowledge has accumulated rapidly about old diseases; for instance, it is now clear that cervical carcinoma is a complication of certain human papillomavirus (genital wart virus) infections. Some relatively less severe infections, such as chlamydial ones, are known to be alarmingly prevalent in young persons. This chapter discusses certain common features of some of these infections, as well as the differential diagnosis and management of several of the common syndromes of genital infections.

DEFINITIONS. Those infectious agents that are frequently transmitted by sexual contact, and for which sexual transmission is epidemiologically important, are considered sexually transmitted diseases. In some cases, such as gonorrhea and genital herpes simplex virus infection, sexual transmission is the only important mode of transmission, at least between adults. In others, such as the hepatitis viruses, giardiasis, shigellosis, and amebiasis, there are also important nonsexual means of acquiring infection. Table 335–1 lists the important infectious agents that are commonly transmitted sexually, as well as their known or probable disease syndromes. "Sexual" includes the full range of heterosexual or homosexual behavior, including genital, oral-genital, oral-anal, and genital-anal contact.

EPIDEMIOLOGIC CONSIDERATIONS. Sexually transmitted infections are prevalent in many segments of society, but, for obvious reasons, are most prevalent in the groups with the most promiscuous sexual activity. It is not sexual activity per se but the number and type of different sexual partners that determine the risk of acquiring STD. The highest rates of gonorrhea are found in the young (15 to 30) and unmarried and in groups of low educational and socioeconomic status. Rates of gonococcal infection may be 50-fold higher in young, single inner-city persons than in married middle- to upper-middle-class persons. Decisions regarding the cost-effectiveness of screening for STD should be governed by these considerations; screening is most effective in high-risk groups.

Multiple infections are frequent in patients with sexually transmitted infection. In venereal disease clinics, about 20 per cent of men with gonorrhea also have urethral chlamydial infection, and 30 to 50 per cent of women with gonorrhea also have cervical chlamydial infection. In women with vaginitis, one study showed that 16 per cent of cases were caused by mixed infection with various combinations of *Candida, Trichomonas,* and *Gardnerella vaginalis.* However, there is no convincing evidence that one sexually transmitted infection directly increases the risk of acquiring others. Rather, the frequent coexistence of multiple sexually acquired infections probably reflects the frequency of these organisms and the multiplicity of sexual partners among patients who were the subjects of these studies.

Control of sexually transmitted infections is complicated by the frequent lack of significant symptoms. The majority of gonococcal and chlamydial infections in women probably are associated with few symptoms. From 10 to 50 per cent of urethral gonococcal infections in men are oligo- or asymptomatic. Urethral chlamydial infections of men are more common than gonococcal infections and frequently are asymptomatic. The importance of the asymptomatic male is underscored by the repeated observation that women with gonococcal pelvic inflammatory disease have male partners whose infection is asymptomatic. Thus, one of the crucial issues in management is proper diagnosis and treatment of the asymptomatically infected partner.

STD IN HOMOSEXUAL MALES. Homosexual males are recognized as a group at particularly high risk of acquiring sexually transmitted disease, including human immunodeficiency virus (HIV) infection. HIV is but one of many STD-related problems in homosexual males, however. Syphilis remains a serious problem in homosexual males, although it also is a problem in drug-abusing heterosexuals. Some homosexual males are exceptionally promiscuous and are at high risk of acquiring not only syphilis but also gonococcal urethritis, proctitis, and pharyngitis; herpes genitalis and proctitis; hepatitis A and B; and a variety of enteric infections that are rarely transmitted in heterosexual sex, including giardiasis, amebiasis, and shigellosis. These enteric infections are probably transmitted by oral-anal or anal-penile-oral contact. In recent years, however, the incidence of some STD's, such as gonorrhea, has declined in homosexual males owing to adoption of changed and safer sex practices (fewer partners, condoms) resulting from the fear of acquiring AIDS. Homosexual women apparently do not have increased rates of STD.

INCIDENCE OF STD's. The true incidence of the STD's is not known in the United States because of serious problems of under-reporting. Gonorrhea is the most common of the reported infectious diseases in the United States, with over 1,000,000 reported infections annually. Although genital chlamydial infections generally are not reported, their prevalence certainly exceeds that of gonorrhea. Herpes simplex virus (HSV) and human papillomavirus (HPV) infections also are more prevalent than gonorrhea. The relative incidence of STD is quite variable in different areas of the world. For instance, chancroid is currently uncommon in the United States but is about as common as gonorrhea in certain areas of the Far East.

COMMON SYNDROMES. Urethritis in Males. Urethritis in males is a very common syndrome. It is ordinarily classified as either gonococcal or nongonococcal urethritis (NGU), depending on whether the presence of gonococci can be demonstrated by

TABLE 335–1. SEXUALLY TRANSMITTED AGENTS AND THEIR SYNDROMES*

Microorganism	Syndromes
Bacteria	
Neisseria gonorrhoeae	Urethritis, cervicitis, bartholinitis, proctitis, pharyngitis, salpingitis, epididymitis, conjunctivitis, perihepatitis, arthritis, dermatitis, endocarditis, meningitis, amniotic infection syndrome
Mobiluncus species and *Gardnerella vaginalis*	"Nonspecific" vaginosis
Treponema pallidum	Syphilis (multiple clinical syndromes)
Haemophilus ducreyi	Chancroid
Calymmatobacterium granulomatis	Granuloma inguinale
Shigella species	Enteritis in homosexual men
Campylobacter species	Enteritis in homosexual men
Group B *Streptococcus*	Neonatal sepsis and meningitis
Chlamydiae	
Chlamydia trachomatis	Nongonococcal urethritis, purulent hypertrophic cervicitis, epididymitis, salpingitis, conjunctivitis, trachoma, pneumonia, perihepatitis, lymphogranuloma venereum, Reiter's syndrome
Mycoplasmas	
Ureaplasma urealyticum	Nongonococcal urethritis, ? premature rupture of membranes and abortion
Mycoplasma hominis	Postpartum fever, pelvic inflammatory disease
Viruses	
Herpes simplex virus (HSV)	Genital herpes, proctitis, meningitis, disseminated infection in neonates
Hepatitis A virus	Hepatitis in homosexual men
Hepatitis B virus	Hepatitis, ? periarteritis nodosa, hepatoma; especially prevalent in homosexual men
Cytomegalovirus	Congenital infection (birth defects, infant mortality, mental deficiency, hearing loss); mononucleosis syndrome
Human papillomavirus (HPV)	Condyloma acuminatum; cervical carcinoma
Molluscum contagiosum virus	Molluscum contagiosum
Human immunodeficiency virus (HIV)	Acquired immunodeficiency syndrome and related illnesses
Protozoa	
Trichomonas vaginalis	Trichomonal vaginitis, occasional urethritis
Entamoeba histolytica	Enteritis in homosexual men
Giardia lamblia	Enteritis in homosexual men
Fungi	
Candida albicans	Vaginitis, balanitis
Ectoparasites	
Phthirus pubis	Pubic lice infestation
Sarcoptes scabei	Scabies

*The relative importance of sexual transmission in the epidemiology of several of these agents remains to be defined; these include Group B streptococci, hepatitis A virus, cytomegalovirus, *Candida albicans*, and others.

Gram's stain or culture. In venereal disease clinics, the prevalence of gonococcal and nongonococcal urethritis is similar, but NGU is considerably more common in private practice and in college infirmaries. Several recent studies of asymptomatic sexually active young persons found a prevalence of up to 15 per cent of genital chlamydial infection.

A large number of studies have established *Chlamydia trachomatis* as a cause of approximately 40 per cent of cases of NGU. Case-control studies have provided suggestive evidence that *Ureaplasma urealyticum* (formerly "T-strain" mycoplasma) is a

significant factor in chlamydia-negative NGU. In addition, urethral inoculation of volunteers with pure cultures of *U. urealyticum* produced rather typical NGU. In practice, however, it is difficult to define the importance of *Ureaplasma* infection in patients with urethritis, because up to 70 per cent of asymptomatic sexually active persons are colonized by these organisms. A very small proportion of cases of NGU in men is due to *Trichomonas vaginalis* or herpes simplex virus infection.

Diagnosis of urethritis requires demonstration of an inflammatory urethral exudate. A discharge may not be evident if the patient has recently voided, and patients preferably should be examined several hours after their last urination. The discharge may be present only in the morning, prior to urination. Demonstration of discharge often requires urethral "milking" and may require insertion of a small calcium alginate or similar swab into the anterior urethra, with examination of a direct Gram-stained smear of the swab for leukocytes. Presence of an average of at least five polymorphonuclear leukocytes per high power (100×) field suggests the diagnosis of urethritis.

The patient should be questioned for past history of urethritis and for symptoms suggestive of systemic diseases such as Reiter's syndrome or disseminated gonococcal infection. Examination should be made for signs of conjunctivitis, arthritis, dermatitis, and epididymitis. Prostatitis is rarely present unless there are symptoms of perineal, suprapubic, or rectal discomfort, and rectal examination is not routinely indicated. Rectal examination and urine culture are indicated in men with dysuria but without signs of anterior urethral discharge.

Laboratory studies are ordinarily limited to a Gram's stain of urethral exudate. Demonstration of typical gram-negative diplococci, many of which are inside neutrophils, establishes the diagnosis of gonococcal urethritis. At least 90 per cent of men with symptomatic culture-proven urethral gonorrhea have a positive Gram's stain. In occasional patients, especially those with equivocal Gram's stain, it may be necessary to culture the anterior urethra or freshly voided urine sediment for gonococci. This is particularly important in asymptomatic male contacts of patients with disseminated gonococcal infection or gonococcal salpingitis, since Gram's stain of urethral contents is positive in only about 60 per cent of men with asymptomatic urethral gonorrhea.

Diagnosis of NGU usually is made by exclusion of gonorrhea. Monoclonal antibodies are available for diagnosis of chlamydiae in secretions; results indicate a sensitivity of over 90 per cent compared with culture, with nearly 100 per cent specificity. This test requires use of a fluorescence microscope, and cost considerations preclude widespread use. Other immunoassays are available, with comparable efficacy. A DNA hybridization test recently was introduced. Culture for *Chlamydia* is now more widely available than in the past and is the best (but expensive) test. There is no serologic test that is clinically useful. Tests for *Ureaplasma* are not readily available and rarely are indicated. Examination of a saline suspension of urethral exudate occasionally may reveal motile trichomonads in patients with recurrent urethritis who fail to respond to appropriate therapy. A serologic test for syphilis should be obtained, but the diagnostic yield is low.

Management is outlined in Figure 335–1 and is discussed further in Ch. 336. Sexual partners of men with gonococcal or nongonococcal urethritis should be treated both to prevent reinfection of the patient and to prevent development of complications in the partners.

The syndrome of *postgonococcal urethritis* (persistence or crudescence of urethritis after administration of therapy that has eradicated gonococcal infection) is usually due to concomitant urethral chlamydial infection that was not eradicated by the original treatment. This syndrome is more common after therapy with a β-lactam antibiotic than after a regimen of tetracycline, undoubtedly because of the greater efficacy of tetracycline for treating chlamydial infections. Accordingly, there is considerable merit to use of oral tetracycline to follow up ceftriaxone therapy for genital gonorrhea.

Genital Ulcer Syndrome. Genital skin lesions may be either ulcerative or nonulcerative. In patients seen in a venereal disease clinic, the most common sexually transmitted nonulcerative genital lesions are due to scabies, genital warts, molluscum contagiosum, or *Candida* species, but differential diagnosis includes a long list of dermatologic conditions.

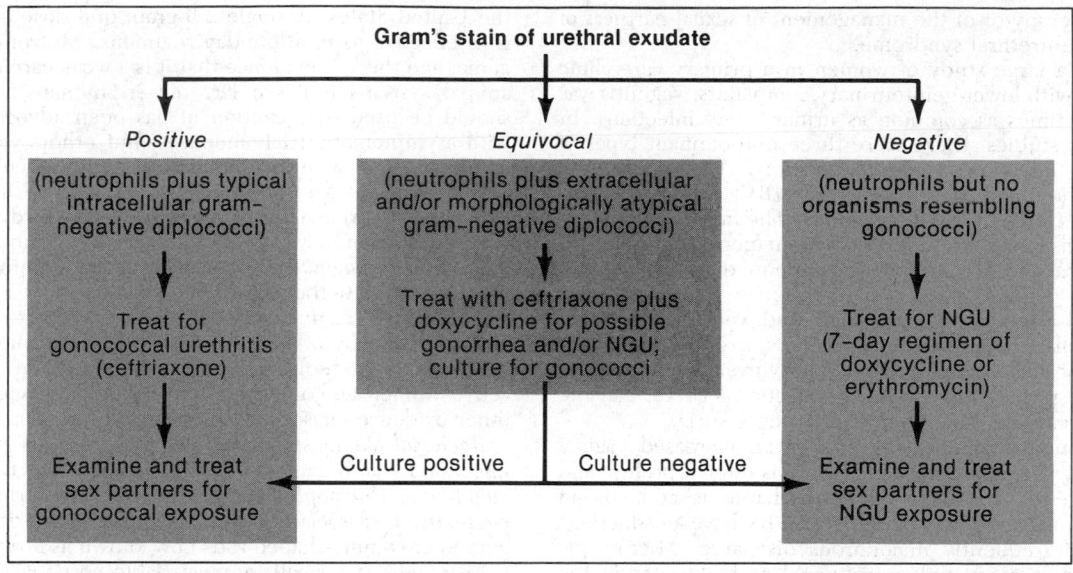

FIGURE 335–1. Management of male patients with urethritis.

The most common cause of ulcerative genital lesions in patients in the United States is herpes simplex virus, but differential diagnosis includes syphilis, chancroid, lymphogranuloma venereum (LGV), granuloma inguinale (GI), and trauma. Chancroid is becoming more common in certain cities in the United States; LGV and GI are rare. The most important distinction is between syphilis, genital herpes, and chancroid. Sometimes, the appearance is virtually diagnostic: Grouped, painful, superficial vesicles are nearly diagnostic of herpes, whereas a single, clean-based, nonpainful ulcer with indurated margins suggests primary syphilis. In recent studies, only about 60 per cent of penile syphilitic chancres had this classic appearance. Painful ulcers suggest herpes or chancroid. Genital herpes may present as a single ulcer, particularly in patients with recurrent herpes, and syphilis may present with multiple ulcers. Secondarily infected lesions of primary syphilis may be painful.

It is a useful rule to obtain a serologic test for syphilis on all patients with genital ulcers, and, if the initial serology is negative and if the diagnosis remains uncertain, to obtain a second serology about 2 weeks later. A darkfield examination for syphilis should also be done, and it should be repeated twice on successive days if syphilis is seriously suspected and the initial examination is negative.

Infection by herpes simplex virus may be efficiently diagnosed by viral culture or by immunofluorescent methods, but these are frequently unavailable in practice. Papanicolaou's smear is suggestive of herpes in about two thirds of culture-positive cases. Giemsa's or Wright's stain of cells scraped from the base of a vesicle may reveal multinucleate giant cells (Tzanck's test), but this test is particularly insensitive in herpetic lesions that have become ulcerated. Serologic tests for herpesvirus are not helpful in management but may indicate persons with latent infection. Referral of patients to centers with capability of viral culture may be indicated in diagnostically difficult patients.

In addition to herpesvirus infection, chancroid should be suspected in patients with painful genital ulcers. Chancroid is occurring in epidemics in certain United States cities, particularly among crack house clients. Attempts should be made to isolate the causative agent, *Haemophilus ducreyi;* selective culture media are an improvement over previously available methods. No serologic tests are available.

Therapy clearly depends on the correct diagnosis. Topical antibiotics are never indicated. Initial genital herpes (first infection) is best treated with topical or oral administration of acyclovir or intravenous administration for severe infections. Therapy of chancroid is with co-trimoxazole, erythromycin, or ceftriaxone. Occasional empiric trials of oral co-trimoxazole or erythromycin are warranted in patients with persistent genital ulcers not readily attributable to herpesvirus or syphilis, but repeated attempts to isolate *H. ducreyi* should be made in such instances. It is not possible to arrive at an unequivocal diagnosis of the cause of genital ulcers in all patients.

Lower Genital Tract Infections in Women. Infections of the female genitourinary tract produce a variety of syndromes, often with overlapping symptoms (dysuria, vaginal discharge, vulvar irritation). These infections are very common, relatively poorly understood by most physicians, sometimes difficult to treat, and often frustrating for both doctor and patient. However, the various syndromes usually can be distinguished on relatively simple clinical and laboratory grounds, and a precise microbial etiology often can be established.

It is most helpful first to determine the primary anatomic site of infection: urethra or bladder, endocervix, or vagina. This can sometimes be accomplished by history; women with urinary tract infection (UTI) usually experience "internal" dysuria, whereas women with dysuria associated with vaginitis usually experience "external" dysuria owing to passage of urine over inflamed labia. Cervicitis is diagnosed by physical examination; there are mucopurulent secretions emanating from the endocervical canal, and there is often a hypertrophic, mucoid, reddened "cobblestone" appearance to the cervical mucosa. Patients with cervicitis may also have urethritis or vaginitis. Vaginitis is associated with increased vaginal discharge of several types, as discussed below, and frequently there are associated signs and symptoms of vaginal, vulvar, and perineal irritation (dyspareunia, external dysuria, itching, pain). In patients with lower genitourinary infection, it is important to determine whether there is involvement of the upper genitourinary tract (pyelonephritis, salpingitis).

The Urethral Syndrome. Bacterial cystitis with or without pyelonephritis is usually diagnosed in women with dysuria, urinary frequency, and pyuria if they have colony counts of at least 10^5 bacteria per milliliter of urine. If similar symptoms are present but routine cultures grow less than 10^4 bacteria per milliliter of voided urine, the "urethral syndrome" is likely.

In a study of sexually active young women who presented to walk-in clinics with dysuria and urinary frequency, and who did not have vaginitis or active herpes simplex infection, 43 per cent had the urethral syndrome (urethritis). Among women with urethritis, 25 per cent had positive urethral cultures for *Chlamydia trachomatis*. Isolation of chlamydiae from the urethra was uncommon in women without urethritis. In other studies, gonococci also were shown to cause this syndrome. Thus, women as well as men may present with urethritis caused by gonococci and chlamydiae.

Management of patients with the urethral syndrome has not been carefully evaluated. Patients with symptoms of urinary tract infection who do not have bacteriuria should have urethral and cervical cultures for *Neisseria gonorrhoeae*. If these cultures are also negative, a therapeutic trial may be made with a tetracycline or a sulfonamide for approximately 7 days. There are no controlled trials of such therapy or of the management of sexual partners of women with the urethral syndrome.

Vaginitis. In a large study of women in a primary care clinic who presented with lower genitourinary complaints, vaginitis was more than five times as common as urinary tract infections. In this and similar studies, there were three predominant types of vaginitis: yeast infection (*Candida albicans*), trichomonas (*T. vaginalis*) infection, and bacterial vaginosis (BV) caused by organisms other than *Candida* and *T. vaginalis*. The incidence of these types of vaginitis varies in different patient populations, but in general *Candida* and BV are more common than *T. vaginalis* vaginitis.

Symptoms of vaginitis include increased volume of vaginal discharge, which is often abnormally yellow or green in appearance and may be malodorous. Vaginal and vulvar itching may be troublesome, especially in *Candida* infection. There may be vaginal tenderness and pain, dyspareunia, or dysuria.

The most common sign of vaginitis is an increased vaginal discharge. In *T. vaginalis* infections, there is often a profuse and frothy discharge. A curdlike, white discharge is common in *Candida* infections, and many patients with BV have an adherent, often gray, and frequently malodorous discharge. Microscopic examination shows many polymorphonuclear leukocytes in the discharge in all but BV. Speculum examination may show signs of endocervicitis as well, with purulent discharge issuing from the cervical os. In occasional patients, no objective signs of vaginal inflammation are found despite the presence of troublesome symptoms. See Table 335–2.

Candida Vaginitis. Most vaginal yeast infections are due to *C. albicans*. Diagnosis is usually made by visualizing yeasts or pseudohyphae by microscopic examination of vaginal secretions suspended in normal saline or 10 per cent KOH. Microscopic examination is less sensitive than culture. However, many asymptomatic women have positive vaginal cultures for *C. albicans*, and therefore some authorities advocate using microscopy in preference to culture. The discharge in *Candida* vaginitis is not malodorous and has a pH of less than 4.5 when a drop is applied to pH paper with a range of 4.0 to 5.5.

Therapy of *Candida* vaginitis is with one of the imidazole compounds (e.g., clotrimazole, miconazole, butaconazole, or teraconazole) once each night for 3 to 7 days intravaginally. There is no convincing evidence that attempts to eradicate yeast from the gastrointestinal tract have a significant effect on rates of cure or relapse of *Candida* vaginitis. There is no evidence to warrant therapy of sexual partners. Attempts should be made to correct ancillary conditions that increase susceptibility to vaginal candidiasis: antibiotic therapy, diabetes, or oral anovulatory steroids. Relapse is a significant problem in some patients. No therapy is indicated for asymptomatic vaginal carriers of *C. albicans*.

T. vaginalis Vaginitis. Diagnosis is made ordinarily by visualizing motile trichomonads in a normal saline suspension of vaginal secretions. The organisms are easily seen at high-dry (100×) magnification, and may usually be seen under low-power magnification. The saline suspension should be examined promptly. Culture is more sensitive, but about 80 to 90 per cent of culture-positive cases are detected by microscopy. Addition of a drop of 10 per cent KOH to vaginal secretions usually results in liberation of a detectable fishlike odor, attributed to release of volatile amines. The pH of vaginal secretions is usually greater than 5.0. In these latter two respects, *T. vaginalis* vaginitis is similar to BV.

Therapy of trichomoniasis is with one of the nitroimidazoles,

either metronidazole or newer compounds such as tinidazole. The latter is extensively used in Europe but is not approved in the United States. A single 2.0-gram oral dose of metronidazole is as effective as multiple-day regimens. Metronidazole is mutagenic, and there is evidence that it is a weak carcinogen in certain animal systems (but, so far, not in humans). Accordingly, it should be used with caution; it has been advocated for women with asymptomatic trichomoniasis, but others would reserve its use for women with symptomatic infections because of possible adverse effects. Metronidazole should not be used in the first trimester of pregnancy. Since over one third of male sexual partners of women with trichomoniasis are asymptomatic urethral carriers of *T. vaginalis*, the male partners should also be treated with a single 2.0-gram dose of metronidazole.

Although *T. vaginalis* can be transmitted sexually, it probably is transmitted by other means as well. This conclusion is based on prevalence studies that show one peak in young, sexually active women and a second peak in older women who have no other evidence for sexually transmitted infection.

Bacterial Vaginosis (BV). This syndrome is probably due to infection by an organism formerly called either *Corynebacterium vaginale* or *Haemophilus vaginalis*, but now termed *Gardnerella vaginalis*, in association with anaerobic bacteria, including the curved or comma-shaped rods now known as *Mobiluncus* species. *G. vaginalis* is a small, gram-variable coccobacillus that can be grown quite successfully on partially selective enriched media. Among women with abnormal vaginal discharge who do not have yeast infection or trichomoniasis, over 90 per cent grow *G. vaginalis*, whereas fewer than 10 per cent of matched controls grow the same organism. There usually are increased numbers of anaerobic vaginal bacteria as well, and decreased numbers of the normal vaginal lactobacilli. Development of full symptoms may require both *G. vaginalis* and vaginal anaerobes, although the precise pathophysiology of this syndrome is still under investigation.

Diagnosis of bacterial vaginosis is by exclusion of trichomoniasis, candidiasis, and purulent cervicitis. Abnormal cells termed "clue cells" are often seen in a wet mount of vaginal secretions in normal saline; these are stippled, granular-appearing vaginal epithelial cells that contain large numbers of adherent *G. vaginalis*. Few polymorphonuclear leukocytes are present. Addition of a drop of 10 per cent KOH usually results in production of an unpleasant fishy odor. The pH of the vaginal secretions is nearly always greater than 5.0.

Optimal therapy is being investigated. Metronidazole has only borderline activity in vitro against *G. vaginalis*, but in a dose of 500 mg by mouth twice daily for 7 days it was effective in eradicating both *G. vaginalis* and the symptoms of vaginitis from 80 of 81 patients in one trial; similar results have been obtained in other trials. This suggests that the principal cause of this syndrome is an anaerobe, since metronidazole is principally effective against anaerobes. Clindamycin (300 mg orally twice daily for 7 days) also is effective. Over 90 per cent of male partners are urethral carriers of *G. vaginalis* and therefore probably should be treated with the same regimen as the patient, although data to support this are lacking at present.

Mixed Vaginitis. In 2 to 16 per cent of patients, vaginitis may be due to polymicrobial infection with two or three organisms. Such mixed infection may account for some instances of treatment failure. Particular care should be given to identification of all causative organisms in patients who have recurrent or relapsing vaginitis.

Cervicitis. Two organisms are recognized as probable causes of mucopurulent endocervicitis: *N. gonorrhoeae* and *C. trachomatis*. Women who are sexual partners of men with chlamydia-positive NGU have a much higher rate of isolation of chlamydiae from the cervix than do women who are partners of men with chlamydia-negative NGU, and they also have significantly higher rates of mucopurulent cervicitis. Herpes simplex virus can also cause cervicitis, especially in primary infection. However, the clinical appearance in herpetic cervicitis is different, with cervical vesicles and ulcers rather than mucopurulent cervicitis.

True cervicitis should not be confused with cervical ectopy, which is merely the appearance of endocervical columnar epithelium on the exposed, visible exocervix. This results in a red-appearing cervix and may result in increased production of a mucoid vaginal discharge but does not require therapy.

TABLE 335–2. DIFFERENTIAL DIAGNOSIS OF VAGINITIS

Characteristics of Vaginal Discharge	Organism Causing Vaginitis		
	C. albicans	*T. vaginalis*	BV
pH	4.5	>5.0	>5.0
White curd	Usually	No	No
Odor with KOH	No	Yes	Yes
Clue cells	No	No	Usually
Motile trichomonads	No	Usually	No
Yeast cells	Yes	No	No

Diagnosis of mucopurulent endocervicitis requires visualization of purulent discharge from the cervical os. There often is a roughened "cobblestone" appearance to the cervix. Gram's stain is about 60 per cent sensitive and over 90 per cent specific for gonorrhea if typical intracellular gonocoddi are seen, but cultures for *N. gonorrhoeae* should be taken. Tissue culture for isolation of *C. trachomatis* may be employed if available. Cytology is not sufficiently sensitive to warrant widespread use. New immunoassays for *C. trachomatis* allow rapid, sensitive, specific diagnosis from patient secretions and undoubtedly should be more widely employed to document etiology and to initiate proper treatment for cervicitis due to chlamydiae.

Antibiotic therapy appears to result in clinical improvement in mucopurulent cervicitis. Patients with negative cultures for the gonococcus probably should be treated with doxycycline (100 mg twice daily for 7 days) or erythromycin in a dose of 500 mg four times daily for at least 7 days; their sexual partners probably should be treated similarly. One should recognize that only modest data support these recommendations. No other form of cervicitis has been shown to respond to antimicrobial therapy.

Upper Genital Tract Disease in Women: Salpingitis. Full coverage of this important topic is precluded by space considerations. This is a very important clinical problem, resulting in considerable morbidity in the estimated 250,000 to 500,000 women who are affected yearly in the United States.

Etiology. The gonococcus may account for as many as 50 per cent of cases in the United States, particularly among women with relatively severe and first-episode salpingitis. About 15 to 20 per cent of women with gonococcal cervicitis probably subsequently develop salpingitis. Strong evidence now implicates genital chlamydial infections as another significant cause of salpingitis; in Sweden, more cases of salpingitis are due to *C. trachomatis* than to *N. gonorrhoeae*. Salpingitis due to genital chlamydial infections may be mild, and patients may not seek medical care. Nevertheless, complications may follow, particularly tubal scarring and infertility. There is less convincing evidence that *Mycoplasma hominis* may occasionally cause a similar syndrome. Many cases of salpingitis are caused by mixed infection with microaerophilic streptococci and enteric bacilli, often including *Bacteroides* species. These polymicrobial infections appear to be more common in recurrent attacks of salpingitis.

Diagnosis. Clinical diagnosis of salpingitis is inexact. Perhaps only 20 per cent of patients have the classic syndrome of lower abdominal pain and tenderness, cervical tenderness, fever, leukocytosis, and elevated sedimentation rate. The most common findings are lower abdominal tenderness, which is usually bilateral, and adnexal and cervical tenderness. Patients with gonococcal salpingitis are more likely to present with fever, and more commonly have onset near the menses, whereas patients with nongonococcal salpingitis more commonly present with adnexal masses. Laparoscopy is commonly used to diagnose salpingitis in certain countries but is invasive and requires general anesthesia. In the United States, laparoscopy is usually used only in selected patients whose differential diagnosis includes ectopic pregnancy, appendicitis, ruptured abscess, or other potential emergencies.

Complications. Complications are primarily infertility and ectopic pregnancies. Rates of involuntary infertility are about 15 per cent after one attack of salpingitis and about 75 per cent after three or more attacks. Total hysterectomy may eventually be necessitated by symptoms of chronic salpingitis.

Therapy. Recommendations from the Centers for Disease Control suggest initial therapy of outpatients with cefoxitin 2.0 grams intramuscularly along with probenecid 1.0 gram orally, followed by doxycycline 100 mg orally twice daily for 10 to 14 days. There are no controlled data on efficacy of various regimens used for hospitalized patients. Current recommendations call for doxycycline 100 mg twice daily plus cefoxitin 2.0 grams intravenously four times daily; or clindamycin 900 mg intravenously three times daily plus gentamicin 1.5 mg per kilogram three times daily. After discharge, doxycycline should be given in a dose of 100 mg twice daily to complete 10 to 14 days of therapy. Patients should usually be hospitalized if they are very ill, are pregnant, have significant adnexal masses, or have failed previous therapy, or if the differential diagnosis includes surgical emergencies such as appendicitis or ectopic pregnancy.

Prevention. Sexual partners of women with gonococcal salpin-gitis must be identified, examined, and treated to prevent subsequent reinfection of the patient. About one half of the infected male partners of women with gonococcal salpingitis are asymptomatic. Treatment of women with tetracycline (as compared with penicillin) to eradicate chlamydiae from the cervix reduces the incidence of post-therapy salpingitis (Rees, 1980), which suggests that increased emphasis on treatment of chlamydiae in the male and female genital tract might reduce the incidence of salpingitis.

Bowie WR, Wang S-P, Alexander ER, et al.: Etiology of nongonococcal urethritis: Evidence for *Chlamydia trachomatis* and *Ureaplasma urealyticum.* J Clin Invest 59:735, 1977. *An excellent epidemiologic and clinical study of the etiology and therapy of nongonococcal urethritis in males.*

Brunham RC, Paavonen J, Stevens CE, et al.: Mucopurulent cervicitis—the ignored counterpart in women of urethritis in men. N Engl J Med 311:1, 1984. *Genital chlamydial infection causes mucopurulent cervicitis, and proper diagnosis leads to effective treatment.*

Holmes KK, Mårdh P-A, Sparling PF, et al. (eds.): Sexually Transmitted Diseases, 2nd ed. New York, McGraw-Hill, 1990. *The definitive textbook on STD's, heavily referenced.*

Mårdh P-A, Møller BR, Paavonen J: Chlamydial infection of the female genital tract with emphasis on pelvic inflammatory disease. A review of Scandinavian studies. Sex Transm Dis 8(Suppl):140, 1981. *Review of the role of chlamydiae in pelvic inflammatory disease.*

Nettleman MD, Jones RB, Roberts SD, et al.: Cost-effectiveness of culturing for *Chlamydia trachomatis*: A study in a clinic for sexually transmitted diseases. Ann Intern Med 105:189, 1986. *Cultures were most cost effective in low-risk women. In high-risk groups, empiric therapy is suggested.*

Pheifer TA, Forsyth PS, Durfee MA, et al.: Nonspecific vaginitis: Role of *Haemophilus vaginalis* and treatment with metronidazole. N Engl J Med 298:1429, 1978. *A clinical and therapeutic study of nonspecific vaginitis, showing that both G. vaginalis and vaginal anaerobes are probably important in causation of the syndrome and also that metronidazole is effective therapy.*

Rees E: The treatment of pelvic inflammatory disease. Am J Obstet Gynecol 138:1042, 1980. *Treatment of women with chlamydial infection of the cervix with tetracycline compared with penicillin reduced the incidence of subsequent salpingitis.*

Stamm WE, Harrison HR, Alexander ER, et al.: Diagnosis of *Chlamydia trachomatis* infections by direct immunofluorescence staining of genital secretions: A multicenter trial. Ann Intern Med 101:638, 1984. *Immunofluorescence was reasonably sensitive (89 to 92 per cent) and specific (96 to 99 per cent) in the diagnosis of genital chlamydial infection in symptomatic men and women, compared with culture. Other reports show less sensitivity in asymptomatic screening.*

Stamm WE, Koutsky LA, Benedetti JK, et al.: *Chlamydia trachomatis* urethral infections in men: Prevalence, risk factors, and clinical manifestations. Ann Intern Med 100:47, 1984. *Asymptomatic male urethral carriers of chlamydiae are very common.*

Stamm WE, Wagner KF, Amsel R, et al.: Causes of the acute urethral syndrome in women. N Engl J Med 303:409, 1980. *Females may also develop a form of nongonococcal urethritis resulting from infection with Chlamydia trachomatis.*

Tait IA, Rees E, Hobson D, et al.: Chlamydial infection of the cervix in contacts of men with nongonococcal urethritis. Br J Vener Dis 56:37, 1980. *Chlamydia trachomatis is shown to cause mucopurulent cervicitis, and appropriate antibiotic therapy results in clinical improvement.*

Taylor-Robinson D, Csonka GW, Prentice MJ: Human intraurethral inoculation of ureaplasmas. Q J Med 46:309, 1977. *Inoculation of the investigator's urethra with ureaplasmas resulted in nonspecific urethritis.*

336 Gonococcal Infections

INTRODUCTION. *Neisseria gonorrhoeae* is a common sexually transmitted organism that causes anterior urethritis in males and endocervicitis and urethritis in females. Other types of primary infection include pharyngitis, proctitis, conjunctivitis, and vulvovaginitis; the last-named disorder occurs principally in prepubescent females. Complications may occur by direct extension of infection, including epididymitis, prostatitis, Bartholin gland abscess, salpingitis, and perihepatitis. Bacteremia may occur, with production of characteristic cutaneous lesions, arthritis, and tenosynovitis; rare complications include endocarditis and meningitis. Conjunctival infection formerly was a common cause of blindness in neonates.

Gonorrhea is the most common reportable infectious disease in the United States, with about 1 million reported cases annually. The true incidence is probably at least 2 million cases annually.

EPIDEMIOLOGY. The only natural hosts for *N. gonorrhoeae* are humans. The organism normally resides on the columnar epithelium of mucosal surfaces and is usually transmitted by intimate sexual contact.

The prevalence of gonorrhea varies greatly in different groups. As many as 5 per cent of persons in high-risk populations may be infected at any time. Surveys of private practices in the United States in the 1970's showed that about 2 per cent of sexually active young women had positive endocervical cultures for the gonococcus. Highest prevalence was found in young (15 to 30) single persons of low socioeconomic and educational status, probably because these factors correlate positively with sexual promiscuity.

The risk of acquiring infection depends on the type of contact with an infected person. About 60 to 80 per cent of females in contact with a male with urethral gonorrhea develop gonococcal cervicitis. By contrast, it is estimated that only 20 to 30 per cent of males having sex with an infected female develop gonorrhea. This difference may be due to exposure of females to a larger inoculum of gonococci. A person having oral sex with a male with gonococcal urethritis has considerable risk of acquiring pharyngeal gonorrhea. Transmission of infection by oral contact with the genitals of an infected female is rare. Infection is apparently efficiently spread by penile-rectal contact.

Gonococci die rapidly upon drying, and transmission by fomites is rare. Epidemics were reported in prepubertal females living in close proximity in orphanages, but such episodes are now very uncommon.

Control of gonorrhea is difficult because of the frequency of asymptomatic infection. Perhaps 50 per cent of infections in females are asymptomatic or only minimally symptomatic, and at least 10 per cent of infected males are asymptomatic.

In past years there was considerable emphasis on case finding by endocervical culture of young, sexually active females. The merit of this strategy depends on the prevalence of infection in the community and the lifestyle of the patient. A more cost-effective method for finding infected patients is to culture patients about 6 weeks after treatment for gonorrhea; as many as 15 to 20 per cent of such persons are culture positive, usually because of reinfection.

THE ORGANISM. *N. gonorrhoeae* is a gram-negative, aerobic diplococcus. Many strains require 3 to 10 per cent CO_2 for optimal growth. They are highly autolytic and die rapidly when outside their normal human environment. They are sensitive to fatty acids and grow best on media with added starch to inhibit fatty acids present in agar. Several partially selective media are available; most employ antibiotics such as trimethoprim, vancomycin, colistin, and nystatin to inhibit growth of other microorganisms. Replacement of vancomycin with lincomycin seems to improve the rate of isolation of gonococci.

Presumptive identification in vitro is made by colonial morphology, Gram's stain, and a positive oxidase test. Differentiation from the closely related meningococcus and the various nonpathogenic *Neisseria* is ordinarily by patterns of utilization of various simple carbohydrates; gonococci use glucose but not maltose or sucrose.

Gonococci are highly variable and occur in a number of different colonial forms. Small colonial types are piliated and more virulent in humans than the larger, nonpiliated variants. Variation is also found in certain outer membrane proteins. Gonococci undergo rapid variation in the antigenic type of pilus expressed, which probably contributes to prolonged infections without treatment and to the ability of persons to acquire repeat infections after treatment. The importance of surface components of the gonococcus in the pathogenesis of infection is under intense investigation.

Gonococci can be serotyped on the basis of antigenic differences in pili, outer membrane proteins, and other antigens. They also can be reliably biotyped by definition of their nutritional requirements on defined agar media ("auxotypes"). These tests are not routinely available at present.

PATHOGENESIS. The minimal infective dose of gonococci for establishment of urethritis in male volunteers is between 100 and 1000 colony-forming units. Surface pili undoubtedly help to attach the bacteria to the mucosal surface, and they also help prevent ingestion and killing by polymorphonuclear leukocytes. Typical urethral infections result in a moderately severe inflammatory response, which is probably due to release of toxic lipopolysaccharide from gonococci and to production of chemotactic factors that attract neutrophilic leukocytes. Certain strains are likely to cause asymptomatic urethral infection for reasons not completely understood. These strains are usually penicillin sensitive, resistant to the bactericidal effects of normal human serum, and particularly likely to cause bacteremia and septic arthritis.

In the preantibiotic era, symptoms usually persisted for 2 to 3 months before host defenses finally succeeded in eradicating the infection. Host defenses include serum opsonic and bactericidal antibodies, as well as local (mucosal) antibodies of the IgG and IgA classes. All gonococci produce an enzyme, IgA protease, which cleaves the major class of secretory IgA, perhaps contributing to persistence of local gonococcal infections.

Serum bactericidal antibodies are undoubtedly important in prevention of bacteremic infection. The best evidence for this has been provided by patients who suffer from homozygous deficiency of one of the complement components C6, C7, C8, or C9. This results in deficiency of serum bactericidal activity but no alteration of serum opsonic activity. Such individuals are particularly prone to recurrent bacteremic gonococcal infection or to recurrent meningococcal meningitis or meningococcemia.

CLINICAL PATTERNS OF DISEASE. *Gonorrhea in Males.* Gonococcal urethritis in males ("the clap" or "the strain") is characterized by a yellowish, purulent urethral discharge and dysuria. The usual incubation period is 2 to 6 days. The discharge of gonorrhea is slightly more copious and purulent than in nongonococcal urethritis (NGU). Symptoms are probably produced by 90 per cent of infections, although asymptomatic infections do occur and may persist for many months. Males with asymptomatic infection do not seek treatment, whereas those with symptomatic infection are usually promptly treated and cured. This is the probable explanation for prevalence studies that show that up to 50 per cent of infected males are asymptomatic. Asymptomatic infection in males and females is of great epidemiologic importance, since such carriers may continue to spread infection to new sexual partners for months if they are not properly diagnosed and treated.

Complications of gonococcal urethritis in males are now rare. Urethral stricture was formerly a common complication but was probably due in part to the use of caustic treatment regimens. Epididymitis and prostatitis, relatively common complications in the past, are seen only occasionally today. The principal complication is disseminated gonococcal infection, which is estimated to affect about 1 per cent of men with gonorrhea. This entity is discussed below.

The differential diagnosis of gonococcal urethritis is discussed in Ch. 335.

Gonococcal infections of the pharynx and rectum are common problems in homosexual males. Most patients with pharyngeal infection are asymptomatic, but occasional patients have exudative pharyngitis with cervical adenopathy. Gonococcal infection of the rectum causes a wide spectrum of symptoms, ranging from asymptomatic carriers to severe proctitis with tenesmus and bloody, mucopurulent discharge. Although approximately 40 per cent of females with cervical gonorrhea also have positive rectal cultures, symptoms of proctitis in females are unusual. This has suggested that the trauma of rectal intercourse may contribute to the proctitis observed in males. Sigmoidoscopy may be indicated to exclude ulcerative colitis, Crohn's colitis, rectal lacerations, or other infections such as shigellosis, amebiasis, or syphilis, all of which are common in male homosexuals.

Gonococcal epididymitis is usually unilateral. Both *Chlamydia trachomatis* and the gonococcus are significant causes of epididymitis in men under 35 years, whereas coliform bacteria are the usual cause in older males. The differential diagnosis includes trauma, tumor, and torsion of the testicle, the last of which is suggested by sudden onset and elevation of the testicle. If there is question of testicular torsion, consultation with a urologist is necessary. In epididymitis there is often a urethral exudate, which should be cultured for gonococci and other bacteria. Treatment of gonococcal epididymitis includes scrotal elevation and 7 to 10 days of appropriate antibiotics, as indicated in Table 336–1.

Gonorrhea in Females. In prevalence studies, approximately one half of women infected with the gonococcus are asymptomatic or have so few symptoms that they do not seek medical care. The most commonly involved site is the endocervix (80 to 90 per cent), followed by the urethra (80 per cent), rectum (40 per cent), and pharynx (10 to 20 per cent). Most pharyngeal, urethral, and rectal infections cause few or no symptoms. Cervical infection may result in vaginal discharge or abnormal menstrual bleeding. Neither of these symptoms is specific for gonococcal infection. Gonococcal urethritis may mimic cystitis caused by enteric bacilli, although standard urine cultures are negative because gonococci do not grow on culture media ordinarily used to diagnose urinary tract infection. Culture methods are discussed below under Laboratory Diagnosis. The differential diagnosis of cervicitis, vaginitis, and the urethral syndrome is discussed in Ch. 335.

The most important complication of gonorrhea is salpingitis. The less precise term "pelvic inflammatory disease" (PID) is often used synonymously. Although many other organisms can cause a similar syndrome, the gonococcus accounts for about half of the estimated 500,000 annual cases of PID in the United States. About 15 per cent of women with gonococcal cervicitis develop PID, often in close proximity to a menstrual period. Symptoms usually include abdominal pain, and often there is fever. Physical examination usually discloses cervical motion tenderness and bilateral adnexal tenderness; in a small proportion of cases the disease may be unilateral, causing confusion with appendicitis or ectopic pregnancy. There may be signs of generalized peritonitis. Laboratory studies often show an elevation of the white blood cell count and sedimentation rate. The diagnosis of PID is inexact, as shown by laparoscopic examination; many patients with PID are missed if undue reliance is placed on presence of fever or elevation of white blood cell count or sedimentation rate.

Although PID is uncommon in pregnancy, it may be particularly severe, and pregnant patients with PID should probably be hospitalized. The incidence of gonococcal PID is increased about threefold in women using an intrauterine device (IUD) for contraception.

A single attack of gonococcal PID seems to increase twofold the risk of developing another bout of PID with subsequent gonococcal cervicitis. About half of the male sexual partners of women with gonococcal PID are infected, and half of these infections are asymptomatic. Failure to diagnose and treat properly the male partners exposes the patient to the risk of further attacks of PID. After the patient has been effectively treated, it often is wise to refer her and her sexual partners to a public health clinic for follow-up.

The major complication of gonococcal PID is tubal scarring and infertility. The incidence of involuntary infertility is estimated as 15 per cent after one attack of PID and about 50 per cent after three attacks. The incidence of ectopic pregnancy is increased from seven- to tenfold in women with previous salpingitis, with resultant increased fetal and maternal mortality. Treatment is indicated in Table 336–1.

Gonococci may spread upward to the liver, causing perihepatitis (Fitz-Hugh-Curtis syndrome). Gonococcal perihepatitis causes tenderness and pain in the region of the liver, mimicking acute cholecystitis. However, it resolves promptly with appropriate antibiotic therapy. Peritoneoscopy may be indicated rarely for diagnostic purposes; "violin-string" adhesions between the liver capsule and the peritoneum are seen.

Gonorrhea in Children. Infants born to a mother with cervicovaginal gonorrhea may develop a gonococcal conjunctivitis, although routine use of prophylactic 1 per cent silver nitrate eye drops (or, in some hospitals, topical erythromycin or tetracycline) has markedly reduced the incidence of this problem. Neonates may also acquire pharyngeal, respiratory, or rectal infection and may develop gonococcal sepsis. Older children up to 1 year of age usually acquire conjunctival or vaginal infection by accidental contamination from an adult, whereas from 1 year to puberty most childhood gonorrhea is the result of purposeful sexual abuse by an adult.

Gonococcal Bacteremia. Approximately 1 per cent of adults with gonorrhea develop the syndrome of gonococcal bacteremia, dermatitis, and arthritis, or disseminated gonococcal infection (DGI). In most series, the majority of patients with DGI are women. The regional incidence of DGI probably varies because of geographic differences in prevalence of the usually antibiotic-sensitive, serum-bactericidal-resistant strains of *N. gonorrhoeae* that cause this syndrome. The severity of the syndrome is variable, from a slowly evolving mild illness with little or no fever, mild arthralgias, and few skin lesions to a fulminant illness with high fever and prostration. Most episodes of DGI are relatively mild in comparison with meningococcemia.

Many patients with DGI have no local symptoms of gonococcal infection. Initial manifestations are usually migratory asymmetric polyarthralgias and skin lesions that are often accompanied by fever. Many patients have tenosynovitis, typically involving the flexor tendon sheaths of the wrist or the Achilles tendon (colloquially known as "lover's heels"). Skin lesions are few in number (fewer than 30 usually), are acral in distribution (fingers, toes, extremities), and may be painful before they are visible. The individual lesions may be papules, pustules, or bullae on an erythematous base; less commonly seen are petechiae or necrotic lesions. The rash is not pathognomonic but is sufficiently typical that it should strongly suggest DGI when seen in young patients with polyarthralgia. Blood cultures are often positive at this stage, and circulating immune complexes may be present. Gram's stain of the skin lesions is positive in only about 5 per cent of patients, but gonococcal antigens can be detected in these lesions in about two thirds of patients by use of immunofluorescent-labeled antigonococcal antibody.

The early stage of gonococcemia may subside spontaneously or may merge indistinctly after about 1 week into a second stage of septic arthritis. Skin lesions have usually disappeared by this time, and blood cultures are nearly always negative. Septic

TABLE 336–1. ANTIBIOTIC REGIMENS RECOMMENDED FOR GONOCOCCAL INFECTION

Diagnosis	Treatment
Uncomplicated genital, rectal, or pharyngeal infection of men and women	Ceftriaxone, 250 mg IM once, plus doxycycline, 100 mg orally twice daily for 7 days *or* Spectinomycin, 2.0 grams IM once, plus doxycycline, 100 mg orally twice daily for 7 days
Treatment failure (patients should be recultured and isolates tested for production of β-lactamase)	Spectinomycin, 2.0 grams IM *or* Ceftriaxone, 250 mg IM
Gonorrhea in pregnancy	Ceftriaxone, 250 mg IM once, plus erythromycin base, 500 mg orally four times daily for 7 days *or* Spectinomycin, 2.0 grams IM plus erythromycin (as in ceftriaxone regimen)
Salpingitis—outpatient	Cefoxitin, 2.0 grams IM, plus doxycycline, 100 mg orally twice daily for 10–14 days (see text)
Salpingitis—inpatient	Doxycycline, 100 mg IV twice daily, plus cefoxitin, 2.0 grams IV four times daily until improved, followed by doxycycline, 100 mg PO twice daily to complete 14 days of therapy; alternative regimens include clindamycin plus an aminoglycoside (see text)
Disseminated gonococcal infection	Ceftriaxone, 1 gram IM every 24 hours *or* Spectinomycin, 2 grams IM every 12 hours (see text)

arthritis may occur without preceding skin lesions or polyarthralgia. One large joint (elbow, wrist, hip, knee, ankle) is usually involved, although some series report involvement of two joints in a significant minority of patients. On infrequent occasions symmetric involvement of the fingers may mimic acute rheumatoid arthritis. Physical examination typically discloses a swollen, warm joint with evident intra-articular fluid. Aspiration of the joint often reveals a marked neutrophilic leukocytosis (50,000 to 100,000 leukocytes per cubic millimeter), although early in the development of the septic joint the synovial leukocyte count may be much lower. Cultures of joint fluid are often positive if the leukocyte count is 80,000 or greater but are often negative when leukocyte counts are 20,000 or less.

Other complications of gonococcal bacteremia include mild hepatitis, myocarditis, the Fitz-Hugh-Curtis syndrome, meningitis, and endocarditis. In the preantibiotic era gonococcal infection accounted for up to 10 per cent of all endocarditis, but it is now rare. Gonococcal endocarditis is often a rapidly progressive infection with severe valvular damage; it should be suspected in patients with a new murmur, severe prostrating illness, severe myocarditis, or evidence of renal failure, or in the presence of stigmata of peripheral embolization.

The differential diagnosis of the gonococcal bacteremia arthritis syndrome includes Reiter's syndrome, rheumatic fever, rheumatoid arthritis, systemic lupus erythematosus, other infectious or postinfectious arthritis, subacute bacterial endocarditis, meningococcemia, and viral hepatitis. In young males, Reiter's syndrome is the principal consideration. Conjunctivitis is rarely seen in gonococcemia but is common in Reiter's syndrome. In the absence of typical skin lesions, DGI may not be suspected until culture results are known.

Diagnosis of DGI is secure when gonococci are recovered from the blood, skin lesions, or synovial fluid. The diagnosis of DGI is probably correct in patients in whom the only positive cultures are from local mucosal surfaces but in whom there are both typical skin lesions and a prompt response to antigonococcal therapy.

LABORATORY DIAGNOSIS. Gram's stain of urethral exudate in symptomatic males has a sensitivity of 90 to 98 per cent and a specificity of 95 to 98 per cent. Accordingly, urethral cultures are not ordinarily indicated in untreated symptomatic males. Since the sensitivity of the Gram stain is only about 60 per cent in asymptomatic male urethral infection, cultures of the anterior urethra or fresh urine sediment are recommended when epidemiologic evidence suggests possible asymptomatic urethral infection. Gram's stain of the endocervix is about 50 to 60 per cent sensitive and about 82 to 97 per cent specific in women with positive cervical cultures for N. gonorrhoeae. Care must be taken to avoid mistaking normal endocervical flora and neutrophils for gonorrhea; only smears showing several neutrophils with multiple, typical intracellular gram-negative diplococci should be read as presumptively positive for gonorrhea. All women should be cultured for N. gonorrhoeae, even if the Gram's stain appears positive.

Cultures should be plated immediately if possible onto chocolate agar or chocolate agar containing selective antibiotics (e.g., modified Thayer-Martin medium, MTM). Holding media such as Amies' or Stuart's transport media may be used if necessary, but viability of gonococci drops after 12 to 24 hours in such media. In infected women, a single endocervical culture on MTM is about 80 to 90 per cent sensitive, as judged by yields obtained with multiple cultures from multiple sites. About 3 to 5 per cent of women have their only positive culture at the pharyngeal, urethral, or rectal site. The yield from these sites is too low to warrant routine pharyngeal, urethral, or rectal cultures. Urethral cultures are indicated in women with the urethral syndrome. Both cervical and rectal cultures should be obtained as part of the test of cure in women after treatment, since inclusion of the rectal culture increases the diagnostic yield of treatment failures by as much as 50 per cent. Pharyngeal cultures should be obtained from patients with symptomatic pharyngitis or from persons exposed by fellatio to infected males. Patients with possible disseminated gonococcal infection should have culture samples taken from all possible mucosal sites (pharynx, urethra, cervix, rectum), as well as blood and synovial fluid.

Cultures of the cervix should be taken under direct visualization during speculum examination, using a cotton-tipped swab. Lubricant jellies may be deleterious to gonococci and should be avoided. Cultures of tampons can be used if speculum examination is not possible. Cultures of the anterior urethra of males should be taken with calcium alginate swabs or a sterile wire loop.

Positive cultures from the pharynx or rectum should be carefully evaluated by the microbiology laboratory to avoid confusion between gonococci and meningococci. Meningococci are more common than gonococci in throat cultures. Male homosexuals apparently transmit meningococci sexually, and positive rectal cultures for meningococci are relatively common in this group.

A variety of inexpensive office kits are available for culturing gonococci. These offer the advantages of media with long shelf life. They are approximately equal to standard cultures when their use is limited to urethral or cervical samples; the currently available systems should not be used for pharyngeal or rectal cultures.

A variety of serologic tests for gonorrhea have been developed in the past, and more are being tested currently. No test available in 1991 is sufficiently sensitive and specific to merit use for screening purposes. Patients with complications of gonorrhea usually have detectable serum antibodies against crude or purified gonococcal antigens, but none of the tests is routinely available at present.

TREATMENT. Gonococci frequently have chromosomal mutations that result in relative resistance to penicillin, tetracycline, and other antibiotics. The resistance in these strains is relatively low and usually can be overcome by appropriate doses of penicillin. Recently, strains with slightly higher levels of chromosomally mediated resistance (CMRNG strains) have become prevalent in certain areas of the United States and are more common in parts of Asia. These strains do not respond to penicillin but do respond to spectinomycin or ceftriaxone. As many as 5 to 10 per cent of all gonococci in the United States now are CMRNG.

Gonococci that carry a β-lactamase (penicillinase) plasmid recently emerged in the Far East and elsewhere in 1975 and have spread to much of the world. Penicillinase-producing gonococci (PPNG) account for about 30 per cent of all gonorrhea in certain cities in the Africa and the Far East but are less common in the United States. The prevalence of PPNG is about 1 to 5 per cent in the United States and seems to be rising. There are two closely related gonococcal penicillinase plasmids of either 3.2 or 4.4 × 10⁶ daltons; each encodes a typical enteric-type TEM β-lactamase. The gonococcal plasmids are similar to penicillinase plasmids found in Haemophilus species. PPNG are resistant to clinically attainable doses of penicillins but are sensitive to spectinomycin and to certain cephalosporins (cefuroxime, cefoxitin, ceftriaxone). PPNG are known to cause DGI and salpingitis.

Quite recently, a new problem has arisen: plasmid-encoded tetracycline resistance, Tcʳ. These strains do not respond to tetracycline but do respond to spectinomycin or ceftriaxone and may respond to penicillin. Prevalance of Tcʳ gonococci is increasing and approximates 5 to 15 per cent in various cities in the United States.

The antibiotic regimens recommended for gonorrhea in the United States are summarized in Table 336–1. Ceftriaxone now has replaced penicillin and ampicillin, because of the prevalence of CMRNG and Pcʳ strains. Tetracyclines no longer are acceptable therapy for gonorrhea because of the prevalence of Tcʳ strains. Because gonococcal infections commonly are associated with genital chlamydial infection, most authorities now recommend a 7-day course of a tetracycline (usually doxycycline) for all patients with gonorrhea as follow-up to initial ceftriaxone therapy.

Each of the recommended regimens is highly effective for genital gonorrhea. If patients fail to respond to therapy, they should be cultured so that their isolates can be tested for production of penicillinase, and spectinomycin should be used for retreatment. However, most apparent failures are really reinfections. Some studies show that 15 per cent of patients are reinfected within 6 weeks of successful therapy. On this basis, many authorities recommend that patients should be recultured 6 weeks after treatment.

In the absence of an effective vaccine, control of this disease depends on proper diagnosis and treatment of patients' sexual contacts. If patients are given simple instructions, many bring their contacts to the physician for examination. There are sound epidemiologic reasons for treating contacts immediately. Local health departments are not utilized sufficiently for help in examination and treatment of contacts.

Treatment of salpingitis (PID) has not been studied adequately (see Table 336–1). Most authorities recommend removal of intrauterine devices in women with PID. It is crucial to examine and treat all sexual partners of women with gonococcal PID.

Therapy of gonococcal arthritis is ordinarily highly successful with each of the recommended regimens (Table 336–1). Failure to improve in 3 days suggests that the patient does not have DGI. Septic joints should be aspirated, both to make the initial diagnosis and to remove inflammatory exudate. Open drainage is rarely indicated, except in infection of the hip in childhood. Repeat closed aspiration may be necessary if joint fluid rapidly reaccumulates, but most patients require only one or a few joint aspirations. Antibiotics should not be injected into the joint space. Most patients with DGI should be hospitalized initially, but outpatient therapy may be used occasionally in carefully selected, compliant patients with a definite diagnosis and only mild infection. Antibiotics indicated in this situation include cefuroxime, 500 mg orally twice daily, or ciprofloxacin, 500 mg orally twice daily. Therapy should be continued for 7 days.

Gonococcal conjunctivitis should be treated by immediate saline irrigation and intravenous ceftriaxone.

PREVENTION. Although vaccines are currently under intense study, an effective gonococcal vaccine is still only a hope. Condoms prevent most infection, but those who need them most often do not use them. Certain contraceptive foams have antigonococcal activity but are of unproven efficacy clinically.

Barlow D, Phillips I: Gonorrhoea in women: Diagnostic, clinical, and laboratory aspects. Lancet 1:761, 1978. *A concise description of the clinical and laboratory findings in a large group of women.*

Collier AC, Judson FN, Murphy VL, et al.: Comparative study of ceftriaxone and spectinomycin in the treatment of uncomplicated gonorrhea in women. Am J Med 77:68, 1984. *Ceftriaxone was effective in a single dose of 125 mg intramuscularly without probenecid for oropharyngeal and genital infections. Spectinomycin resulted in a 50 per cent failure rate in oropharyngeal infection, in agreement with earlier reports.*

Dans PE, Judson F: The establishment of a venereal disease clinic. II. An appraisal of current diagnostic methods in uncomplicated urogenital and rectal gonorrhea. J Am Vener Dis Assoc 1:107, 1975. *A critical examination of the utility of various diagnostic methods, including multiple cultures and Gram's stains.*

Eisenstein BI, Sox T, Biswas G, et al.: Conjugal transfer of the gonococcal penicillinase plasmid. Science 195:998, 1977. *Gonococci contain a conjugal plasmid that enables them to transfer sexually their penicillinase plasmid with efficiency.*

Faruki H, Kohmescher RN, McKinney WP, et al.: A community-based outbreak of infection with penicillin-resistant *Neisseria gonorrhoeae* not producing penicillinase (chromosomally mediated resistance). N Engl J Med 313:607, 1985. *Drug resistance among gonococci is an increasing problem everywhere.*

Handsfield HH, Lipman TO, Harnisch JP, et al.: Asymptomatic gonorrhea in men: Diagnosis, natural course, prevalence and significance. N Engl J Med 290:117, 1974. *Asymptomatic infection of the male urethra by gonococci is carefully described and is shown to be much more common than previously recognized.*

Handsfield HH, Murphy VL: Comparative study of ceftriaxone and spectinomycin for treatment of uncomplicated gonorrhoea in men. Lancet 2:67, 1983. *Among newer antibiotics, ceftriaxone appears most promising for single-dose therapy of penicillin-resistant gonorrhea.*

Handsfield HH, Wiesner PJ, Holmes KK: Treatment of the gonococcal arthritis-dermatitis syndrome. Ann Intern Med 84:661, 1976. *This is probably the best evaluation of the efficacy of various regimens for therapy of disseminated gonococcal infection.*

Hook EW, Holmes KK: Gonococcal infections. Ann Intern Med 102:229, 1985. *An excellent, clinically relevant review.*

Lebedeff DA, Hochman EB: Rectal gonorrhea in men: Diagnosis and treatment. Ann Intern Med 92:463, 1980. *This paper briefly reviews the clinical findings, diagnostic methods, and efficacy of various methods of treatment for gonococcal proctitis in men.*

Luciano AA, Grubin L: Gonorrhea screening: Comparison of three techniques. JAMA 243:680, 1980. *Culture of the first-voided urine in asymptomatic males is shown to be a highly reliable method for diagnosis.*

337 Lymphogranuloma Venereum

Lymphogranuloma venereum (LGV) is an acute to chronic sexually transmitted disease caused by strains of *Chlamydia trachomatis*. LGV typically produces transient genital lesions followed by significant regional lymphadenopathy, which may progress to late fibrosis and tissue destruction in untreated cases.

ETIOLOGY. The organisms causing LGV are closely related to the *C. trachomatis* strains that cause trachoma (serotypes A–C) or nongonococcal urethritis (serotypes D–K). By use of a microimmunofluorescent procedure the LGV strains have been grouped into three serotypes (L1, L2, and L3), of which L2 is apparently the most common. On one occasion the related organism *Chlamydia psittaci* caused a similar syndrome. All chlamydiae contain a common group antigen, but an LGV-specific protein antigen has been partially characterized. As is the case with all chlamydiae, the LGV strains can be isolated only in tissue culture or in yolk sac culture.

EPIDEMIOLOGY. LGV is more common in tropical and subtropical climates but does occur in relatively low incidence throughout the Western world. The true incidence is unknown. Screening of patients in venereal disease clinics with the LGV complement fixation test has sometimes shown 10 per cent with positive serologies; however, this may merely reflect cross-reactions between antibodies directed against the *Chlamydia trachomatis* serotypes D–K (the causes of nongonococcal urethritis and related syndromes) and the LGV serotypes L1, L2, and L3.

The disease is almost always transmitted by sexual contact. The site of primary infection is usually around the genitals but may be anal or oral, depending on the mode of sexual practice.

PATHOGENESIS AND PATHOLOGY. The incubation period is uncertain but has been estimated to be anywhere from a few days to several weeks. In approximately one fourth of patients a small, evanescent primary lesion develops at the site of inoculation, but in the other three fourths of patients no primary lesion is clinically evident. Occasional patients may have symptoms of nonspecific urethritis, presumably owing to intraurethral infection. Approximately 2 to 6 weeks after sexual contact most patients develop significant regional lymphadenopathy. Primary infection of the anterior vulva or penis results in inguinal adenopathy, whereas primary infection of the vagina or posterior vulva or rectum results in primary perirectal or pelvic adenopathy. Most patients seen in venereal disease clinics are males with inguinal adenopathy. In about one third of patients the adenopathy is bilateral. Involvement of lymphatic tissue may result in significant lymphedema and, if untreated, may lead to elephantiasis of the external genitalia. Chronic infection of the perirectal tissues may lead to rectal strictures. The histologic appearance of involved tissues is nonspecific with acute and chronic inflammation.

CLINICAL MANIFESTATIONS. The transient primary lesion usually appears as an infiltrated papule or small erosion. It may mimic herpes but is frequently unnoticed or not present. In its earlier stages the adenopathy syndrome is manifested by discrete, tender, movable nodes. After several days the nodes become matted, with an ovoid, firm, lobulated swelling with adherent, erythematous overlying skin. In about 10 to 20 per cent of patients, nodes are involved above and below the inguinal ligament, and fibrosis may result in the so-called "groove sign" (linear depressions parallel to the inguinal ligament). The nodes may undergo necrosis, and, if not aspirated, spontaneous fistula tracts may develop. Lymphatic obstruction may result in vulvar edema or polypoid masses around the anal orifice. In early stages anal masses may resemble hemorrhoids. There may be fever, chills, and headache, associated with other nonspecific systemic symptoms such as nausea and weight loss. Infrequently, there is generalized rash, polyarthralgia, splenomegaly, generalized lymphadenopathy, or meningismus. Cutaneous manifestations may include erythema nodosum, erythema multiforme, urticaria, or a scarlatiniform eruption.

Late complications are usually limited to strictures or scarring of the rectum. This complication is more common in women but is now fortunately rare. There is often no preceding adenopathy syndrome. The strictures may be bandlike or may involve extensive areas of the lower large bowel.

DIAGNOSIS. LGV must be considered in patients with enlarged inguinal lymph nodes, draining inguinal fistulas, and rectal strictures. Differential diagnosis includes reactive nodes secondary to distal sites of pyogenic infection on the extremities (which may be small and not noticed unless careful examination is performed), chancroid, granuloma inguinale, syphilis, and a variety of other diseases associated with adenopathy or adenitis. Diagnosis is made by one of two methods: either by direct demonstration of LGV organisms in lesion material or by appropriate serologic tests. Material may be obtained for culture from affected lymph nodes by inserting a needle into the area of fluctuance, being careful to insert the needle through normal skin. The aspirated pus is characteristically extremely viscous. Organisms may sometimes be directly demonstrated in this material by immunofluorescence, although this test is not routinely available. Culture may be performed in yolk sacs or in tissue cell culture. A complement fixation test, using group-specific antigen, is widely available for serologic diagnosis. In the presence of a compatible clinical syndrome, a titer greater than or equal to 1:16 is strongly suggestive of LGV. Serial samples frequently show a fourfold or greater rise in titer in the acute stage of the disease. Most patients with LGV develop peak titers of at least 1:64. Other serologic tests are under development, including indirect immunofluorescence and counterimmunoelectrophoresis; each of these tests uses antigens specific for LGV, but neither is widely available at present. A direct immunofluorescence test employing monoclonal antibodies against *C. trachomatis* serotypes L1, L2, and L3 offers promise for rapid specific diagnosis, but it is not yet widely available.

Other laboratory tests are of little help. Many patients have a modest elevation in total leukocyte count with predominance of lymphocytes. There may be a reversal of the albumin globulin ratio, and some patients have elevated cryoglobulins or rheumatoid factor.

TREATMENT. Both tetracycline and sulfonamide drugs are effective. Usual therapy for adults is tetracycline, 500 mg four times daily for at least 3 weeks. When tetracycline is contraindicated, as in pregnancy, sulfisoxazole may be given in a dose of 500 mg four times daily for at least 3 weeks. Tense nodes should be aspirated through normal skin to prevent formation of fistulous tracts. Patients with early stages of the disease respond well to therapy, but those with late complications, including chronic lymphatic obstruction and rectal stricture, respond poorly or not at all to antibiotic therapy. Surgery may be needed to correct rectal stricture. After an initial course of treatment, patients should be seen at least every 3 months for 1 year, and the titer of the LGV complement fixation test should be followed. Retreatment should be given if there is a fourfold increase in serologic titer or if there is clinical evidence of relapse. Sexual contacts should be treated similarly.

PREVENTION. There are no specific data regarding modes of prevention. Presumably, use of condoms would help to prevent transmission. An effective vaccine is not available.

Klotz SA, Drutz DJ, Tam MR, et al.: Hemorrhagic proctitis due to lymphogranuloma venereum serogroup L2: Diagnosis by fluorescent monoclonal antibody. N Engl J Med 308:1563, 1983. *LGV may cause hemorrhagic proctitis that mimics ulcerative colitis in homosexual males; monoclonal antibodies provide rapid diagnosis.*
Schachter J: Lymphogranuloma venereum and other nonocular *Chlamydia trachomatis* infections. *In* Hobson D, Holmes KK (eds.): Nongonococcal Urethritis and Related Infections. Washington, D.C., American Society for Microbiology, 1977, pp 91–97. *An excellent short review of the biology of the organism and the clinical manifestations of the disease.*
Sowmini CN, Gopalan KN, Chandrasekhara RG: Minocycline in the treatment of lymphogranuloma venereum. J Am Vener Dis Assoc 2:19, 1976. *Tetracyclines were effective in infected military personnel in Vietnam.*

338 Granuloma Inguinale (Donovanosis)

Granuloma inguinale, also known as donovanosis, is a slowly progressive ulcerative disease involving principally the skin and subcutaneous tissues of the genital, inguinal, and anal regions. It is primarily transmitted sexually, but probably can be transmitted by nonsexual contact as well. Multiple sexual contacts with an infected partner seem necessary for transmission of infection.

The disease is uncommon in the United States, with less than 100 recorded cases annually. It is quite common, however, in certain other areas of the world, especially Papua New Guinea.

ETIOLOGY. The causative organism is *Calymmatobacterium granulomatis*, a gram-negative bacterium which is immunologically related to certain *Klebsiella* strains. Current evidence suggests that *C. granulomatis* is not a member of the *Klebsiella-Enterobacter-Serratia* family; its exact taxonomic status is uncertain. The organism can be grown in yolk sacs, but only with great difficulty on artificial medium. It is apparently a facultative intracellular parasite, since in infected lesions it is found primarily in histiocytes or other mononuclear cells.

CLINICAL MANIFESTATIONS. The initial lesion usually appears as a subcutaneous nodule that erodes through the surface and develops into a beefy, elevated granulomatous lesion. This usually is painless and unassociated with systemic symptoms. Secondary bacterial infection may cause a necrotic painful ulcerative lesion that may be rapidly destructive. A cicatricial form may also occur with a depigmented elevated area of keloid-like scar containing scattered islands of granulomatous tissue. Lesions in the genital area are commonly associated with pseudobuboes in the inguinal region; these swellings are usually not due to involvement of the inguinal lymph nodes but rather to granulomatous involvement of the subcutaneous tissues. Metastatic infection of bones or other viscera is occasionally seen. Clinical experience suggests that secondary carcinomas may be a complication of granuloma inguinale.

DIFFERENTIAL DIAGNOSIS. The differential diagnosis includes tumor, lymphogranuloma venereum, chancroid, syphilis, and other ulcerative granulomatous diseases. Chancroid is usually differentiated by its irregular undermined borders, which are not seen in the usual cases of granuloma inguinale. Darkfield examination and serologic tests should help to distinguish syphilis. Biopsies may be necessary to distinguish granuloma inguinale from certain tumors.

DIAGNOSIS. Diagnosis is made by demonstrating intracellular "Donovan bodies" in histiocytes or other mononuclear cells from lesion scrapings or biopsies. Wright's stain and Giemsa's stain of fresh impression smears or unfixed biopsies usually demonstrate the bacilli relatively easily, although multiple biopsies may be necessary in chronic cases. Culture is not practical at present. A serologic test has been devised but is not clinically available. Histologic examination of biopsies shows mononuclear cells with some infiltration by polymorphonuclear leukocytes but no giant cells.

TREATMENT. Treatment consists of tetracycline or sulfisoxazole in a dose of 0.5 gram four times daily for at least 3 weeks. Other regimens that have proved effective include ampicillin, chloramphenicol, gentamicin, or co-trimoxazole. Limited experience suggests that lincomycin may be used successfully. Patients should be followed for at least several weeks after discontinuation of treatment because of the possibility of relapse. Although the risk of communicability appears to be low, sexual contacts should also be examined; at present, treatment of contacts is not indicated in the absence of clinically evident disease.

PREVENTION. No effective prevention is known.

Breschi LC, Goldman G, Shapiro SR: Granuloma inguinale in Vietnam: Successful therapy with ampicillin and lincomycin. J Am Vener Dis Assoc 1:118, 1975. *Ampicillin was frequently effective in patients previously unresponsive to tetracycline.*
Garg BR, Lal S, Sivamani S: Efficacy of co-trimoxazole in donovanosis. A preliminary report. Br J Vener Dis 54:348, 1978. *Trimethoprim and sulfamethoxazole were effective.*
Kuberski T: Granuloma inguinale (donovanosis). Sex Trans Dis 7:29, 1980. *An excellent short review.*
Maddocks I, Anders EM, Dennis E: Donovanosis in Papua New Guinea. Br J Vener Dis 52:190, 1976. *A description of the epidemiology and clinical manifestations in an endemic area of granuloma inguinale.*
Rosen T, Tschen JA, Ramsdell W, et al.: Granuloma inguinale. J Am Acad Dermatol 11:433, 1984. *An American epidemic of this relatively rare disease is described.*

339 Chancroid

Chancroid is a sexually transmitted infection caused by the gram-negative bacillus *Haemophilus ducreyi*.

EPIDEMIOLOGY. On a worldwide basis chancroid is considerably more common than syphilis, and in parts of Africa and in Southeast Asia is nearly as great a problem as gonorrhea. In the United States it is an uncommon disease, but the incidence is rising. Epidemics have been documented in several cities in North America in recent years. The majority of reported cases occur in males. An outbreak in Greenland was exceptional in that about 40 per cent of cases were noted in women. It is quite likely that there has been significant underdiagnosis in women in the past.

CLINICAL MANIFESTATIONS. The usual incubation period is 2 to 5 days but may be up to 14 days. In the Greenland outbreak the incubation period averaged nearly 2 weeks in women. The initial clinical manifestation is an inflammatory macule that then becomes a vesicle-pustule and finally a sharply circumscribed, somewhat ragged, and undermined painful ulcer. The base is moist and may be covered with a grayish necrotic exudate. Removal of the exudate reveals purulent granulation tissue. There is usually surrounding cutaneous erythema. Lesions typically are single but may be multiple, possibly owing to autoinoculation of nearby tissues. There are rarely systemic symptoms. Inguinal adenopathy is noted in one half of patients, approximately two thirds of whom have unilateral adenopathy. Lesions are usually noted on the shaft or glans of the penis or around the anal orifice in males. In females lesions may occur on the cervix, vagina, vulva, or perianal area. Lesions may occasionally occur primarily on or spread to the abdomen, thigh, breast, fingers, or lips. Intraoral lesions are uncommon.

There are reports of a transient genital ulcer, followed by significant inguinal adenopathy. This may be difficult to distinguish from lymphogranuloma venereum. Other uncommon clinical variants include the *phagedenic type* of ulcer with secondary suprainfection and rapid tissue destruction; *giant chancroid*, which is characterized by a very large single ulcer; *serpiginous ulcer*, which is characterized by rapidly spreading, indolent, shallow ulcers on the groin or the thigh; and a *follicular* type with multiple small ulcers in a perifollicular distribution.

DIFFERENTIAL DIAGNOSIS. The differential diagnosis includes syphilis, herpes genitalis, lymphogranuloma venereum, traumatic ulcers, and granuloma inguinale. Of these the most commonly confused are syphilis and herpes genitalis. Multiple infections are relatively common. Outpatients with suspected chancroid should have a serologic test for syphilis and preferably a darkfield examination as well.

DIAGNOSIS. The diagnosis of chancroid is made on the basis of the clinical appearance of the lesions plus either morphologic demonstration of typical organisms in the lesions or recovery of *H. ducreyi* by culture. Culture is the preferred method. Positive cultures can be obtained in over 80 per cent of cases. Best culture results seem to be obtained with a chocolate agar medium containing 3 µg per milliliter of vancomycin. Necrotic debris should be removed from the ulcer with physiologic saline. The base and edges of the ulcer should be swabbed with a cotton-tipped swab and inoculated directly onto the culture plate if possible; swabs may be put into Amies transport medium if culture plates are not immediately available. Smears obtained from the undermined edges should be gently rolled onto a slide. *H. ducreyi* is a small gram-negative bacillus with rounded ends, which typically forms chains or parallel aggregates in lesions. Typical organisms are seen in 50 to 80 per cent of cases. Organisms may also be obtained by aspiration of inguinal nodes. Nodes should be aspirated by placing the needle through normal skin to avoid formation of fistulous tracts. Nodes should not be incised. There is no serologic test for chancroid.

TREATMENT. The drug of choice is probably erythromycin, in a dose of 500 mg orally four times daily for 7 to 10 days. A single intramuscular dose of ceftriaxone (250 mg) is curative. Combinations of trimethoprim and sulfamethoxazole (co-trimoxazole) usually are effective. Ciprofloxacin, 500 mg orally twice daily for 3 days, is highly effective. Ampicillin should not be used, since some strains of *H. ducreyi* produce a typical TEM-type β-lactamase and are quite ampicillin resistant. Interestingly, the plasmids containing the gene for production of β-lactamase are very closely related to the penicillinase plasmids found recently in *H. influenzae* and *Neisseria gonorrhoeae*. Tetracycline resistance is common. All regular sexual partners should be examined and epidemiologically treated with a similar regimen.

PREVENTION. No vaccine is available. Use of a condom is presumably helpful. There are no data regarding efficacy of antibiotic prophylaxis.

Blackmore CA, Limpakarnjanarat K, Rigau-Perez JG, et al.: An outbreak of chancroid in Orange County, California: Descriptive epidemiology and disease-control measures. J Infect Dis 151:840, 1985. *A very large continental United States outbreak is described. Sulfa and tetracycline resistance was common, but erythromycin and co-trimoxazole were effective.*

Hammond GW, Slutchuk M, Scatliff J, et al.: Epidemiologic, clinical, laboratory, and therapeutic features of an urban outbreak of chancroid in North America. Rev Infect Dis 2:867, 1980. *An excellent summary of a recent epidemic in Winnipeg.*

Lykke-Olesen L, Larsen L, Pedersen TG, et al.: Epidemic of chancroid in Greenland 1977–78. Lancet 1:654, 1979. *A remarkable epidemic, affecting 3 per cent of the adult population. Tropical climates are not necessary for disease transmission or expression.*

Plummer FA, D'Costa LJ, Nsanze H, et al.: Antimicrobial therapy of chancroid: Effectiveness of erythromycin. J Infect Dis 148:726, 1983. *Documents the efficacy of erythromycin.*

Taylor DN, Pitarangsi C, Echeverria P, et al.: Comparative study of ceftriaxone and trimethoprim-sulfamethoxazole for the treatment of chancroid in Thailand. J Infect Dis 152:1002, 1985. *Ceftriaxone appears to be effective for this infection as well, in a single intramuscularly administered dose of 250 mg.*

340 Syphilis

DEFINITION. Syphilis is a subacute to chronic infectious disease caused by the bacterium *Treponema pallidum*. It is usually acquired by sexual contact with another infected individual. Syphilis is remarkable among infectious diseases in its large variety of clinical presentations. It progresses, if untreated, through primary, secondary, and tertiary stages. The early stages (primary and secondary) are infectious. Spontaneous healing of early lesions occurs, followed by a long latent period. In about 30 per cent of untreated patients, late disease of the heart, central nervous system, or other organs ultimately develops. At one time this disease was termed "the great imitator." Although the disease is less common now than previously, it remains a great challenge to the clinician because of its protean manifestations and is of great interest to biologists as well because of the long and tenuous balance between the host and the invading spirochete.

ETIOLOGY. The etiology of syphilis was discovered in 1905 by Schaudinn and Hoffman when they visualized spirochetal organisms in early infectious lesions. The causative agent of syphilis, *Treponema pallidum*, is closely related to other pathogenic spirochetes, including those causing yaws (*Treponema pertenue*) and pinta (*Treponema carateum*).

T. pallidum is a thin, helical cell approximately 0.15 µ wide and 6 to 50 µ long. Ordinarily there are approximately 6 to 14 spirals. The organism is tapered on either end. It is too thin to be seen by ordinary Gram's stain but can be visualized in wet mounts by darkfield microscopy (see below) or by silver stains or fluorescent antibody methods.

The organism bears considerable structural resemblance to gram-negative bacteria. A superficial hyaluronic acid slime layer is formed around the organism and may contribute to virulence. Beneath the slime layer is the outer membrane, or outer envelope, which is structurally similar to the outer membrane of gram-negative bacteria. Between the outer membrane and the peptidoglycan cell wall are six axial fibrils. The axial fibrils are attached three at each end and overlap in the center of the organism. They are structurally and biochemically similar to flagella and may be in part responsible for the motility of the organism.

It is possible to culture *T. pallidum* in vitro, but yields are very low; culture is of limited use in research but of no use in clinical practice. *T. pallidum* can be maintained by serial passage in rabbits without loss of virulence. Only a few strains have been isolated in rabbits and carefully studied, and little evidence is available regarding the genetic diversity of the organism. All studied isolates have been susceptible to penicillin and are similar antigenically. Immunity to the homologous strain develops after prolonged infection in rabbits. The only known natural hosts for *T. pallidum* are humans and certain monkeys and higher apes.

PATHOGENESIS AND HOST RESPONSE. *T. pallidum* may penetrate through normal mucosal membranes and also through minor abrasions of epithelial surfaces. In experimental rabbit syphilis, spirochetes can be found in the lymphatic system within 30 minutes of inoculation and are found in blood shortly thereafter. There have been occasional instances in humans of transfusion syphilis resulting from use of blood from a donor who was in the incubation stage of the disease. Therefore it seems clear that syphilis is a systemic disease from the onset in humans as well. However, the first lesions appear at the site of primary inoculation, presumably because of the large numbers of treponemes implanted at this site. In laboratory animals, there is an inverse relationship between numbers of treponemes inoculated and time required for development of the primary cutaneous lesion. The minimal number of treponemes required to establish infection is not known but may be as low as one treponeme. Multiplication of organisms is very slow, with a division time in rabbits of approximately 33 hours. Similarly slow growth of treponemes in humans probably accounts in part for the protracted nature of the illness and for the relatively long incubation period.

T. pallidum is not known to produce any toxins. Although the outer membrane structurally resembles those of gram-negative bacteria, there is no biologically active endotoxin in *T. pallidum*. Treponemes are capable of specific attachment to host cells, but it is not known whether attachment results in damage to host cells. Most treponemes are found in intercellular spaces, but occasional treponemes can be seen within phagocytic cells. However, there is no evidence for intracellular survival of treponemes.

The primary pathologic lesion of syphilis is a focal endarteritis. There is an increase in adventitial cells, endothelial proliferation, and presence of an inflammatory cuff around affected vessels. Lymphocytes, plasma cells, and monocytes predominate in the inflammatory lesion, and in some cases polymorphonuclear cells are seen as well. The vessel lumen is frequently obliterated. With healing there is considerable fibrosis. Treponemes may be seen in most early lesions of syphilis and in some of the late lesions such as the meningoencephalitis of general paresis.

Granulomatous reaction is also frequent in secondary syphilis and in late syphilis. The granuloma is histologically nonspecific, and cases of syphilis have been incorrectly diagnosed as sarcoidosis or other granulomatous diseases. Human inoculation studies suggest that the pathogenesis of the gumma, which is a granulomatous lesion, involves hypersensitivity to small numbers of virulent treponemes introduced into a previously sensitized host.

Intracutaneous inoculation of patients with syphilis in various stages with partially purified antigens of *T. pallidum* showed that delayed cellular hypersensitivity developed only in late secondary syphilis but was uniformly present in latent syphilis. There may be temporary hyporesponsiveness of lymphocytes from patients with primary and secondary syphilis to treponemal antigens. It is possible but not proved that the unusual waxing and waning of lesions in early syphilis depend on the balance between development of effective cellular immunity and suppression of thymus-derived lymphocyte function.

The host also responds to infection with production of numerous antibodies, and in some instances circulating immune complexes may be formed. The nephrotic syndrome has been recognized occasionally in secondary syphilis, and renal biopsies from such cases have shown membranous glomerulonephritis characterized by focal subepithelial basement membrane deposits. The deposits contain both IgG and C3, and treponemal antibody.

Rarely patients may develop paroxysmal cold hemoglobinuria. This is due to production of an IgG antibody that binds to the red cell at 4°C and, upon rewarming of the blood in the presence of complement, results in hemolysis. Thus patients may develop massive hemolysis and hemoglobinuria after cold exposure. This was formerly usually due to congenital syphilis but is now almost always due to other infections. Treatment with penicillin usually stops the attacks.

Antibodies useful in diagnosis are discussed under Serologic Tests, below.

EPIDEMIOLOGY. Syphilis, with the exception of congenital syphilis, is acquired almost exclusively by intimate contact with the infectious lesions of primary or secondary syphilis (chancre, mucous patches, condylomata lata). This is usually through sexual intercourse, including anogenital and orogenital intercourse. Health workers have sometimes been infected during unsuspecting examination of patients with infectious lesions. Infection by contact with fomites is extremely uncommon.

Syphilis is most common in large cities and in young, sexually active individuals. The highest rate in both men and women occurs at ages 20 to 24, followed by ages 25 to 29 and 15 to 19 years. Among predominantly rural areas in the United States the disease is most prevalent in the southeast.

Syphilis spares no class, race, or group but is more prevalent in the United States among the poorly educated and economically deprived than among more prosperous groups. Increased numbers of different sexual partners and perhaps indiscriminate choice of partner increase the risk of acquiring sexually transmitted disease. Patients with primary and secondary syphilis name on the average nearly three different sexual contacts within the previous 90 days. A cornerstone of syphilis control is epidemiologic investigation of sexual contacts of patients with primary or secondary lesions, and of patients with early latent disease. Recent evidence suggests that syphilis is strongly correlated with drug use and anonymous sex, and epidemiologic investigations are less efficacious in this situation.

In recent years male homosexuals have accounted for an increasing proportion of the total cases of infectious syphilis. The ratio of male:female cases of primary and secondary syphilis in the United States rose from 1.6:1.0 in 1965 to 2.5:1.0 in 1975 and about 3:1 in the mid 1980's. Currently, more than half of all white males with infectious syphilis name at least one male sexual partner during the recent past. In contrast, only 2 per cent of primary and secondary syphilis in females occurs in women who name a female sexual contact. Similar trends have been noted in other countries. Unfortunately, syphilis increased dramatically in 1989–1990 in many parts of the United States, particularly among nonwhite heterosexuals, many of whom probably exchanged sex for drugs. In many cities, incidence of infectious syphilis increased 50 to 100 per cent in 1990, which is worrisome both because syphilis is a serious disease and because it is a cofactor for acquisition of HIV.

The annual incidence of syphilis has generally declined worldwide for approximately 100 years with the exception of periods of extensive war. With the introduction of penicillin there was a rapid decline in primary and secondary syphilis after World War II, to annual rates of approximately 4 cases per 100,000 in 1957. This resulted in declining federal expenditure for syphilis control, however, and there was a subsequent resurgence in infectious primary and secondary syphilis in the United States, reaching peaks of over 12 cases per 100,000 several times in the period 1965–1983. Since many cases of syphilis are not reported, the true incidence is much higher, perhaps 75,000 to 100,000 annually.

Reported deaths from syphilis declined from 2434 in 1965 to 200 in 1976. Infant deaths from syphilis fell by 98 to 99 per cent by 1980, but rose sharply in 1988–1990. Patients with clinically manifest late syphilis, particularly those with gummas, are becoming less common, perhaps as a result of the effectiveness of penicillin therapy for early syphilis. However, surveys indicate that there still are significant numbers of patients with untreated cardiovascular and neurologic syphilis, especially among older age groups. There is suggestive evidence that neurosyphilis may be presenting with atypical clinical manifestations and therefore may not be easily recognized. There is considerable clinical evidence that early syphilis is more severe and more difficult to treat in patients with HIV infection.

NATURAL COURSE OF UNTREATED SYPHILIS. The incubation period from time of exposure to development of the primary lesion at the place of initial inoculation of treponemes averages approximately 21 days but ranges from 10 to 90 days. A painless papule develops and gradually breaks down to form a clean-based ulcer with raised, indurated margins. This persists for 2 to 6 weeks and then heals spontaneously. Several weeks later the patient characteristically develops a secondary stage characterized by low-grade fever, headache, malaise, generalized lymphadenopathy, and a mucocutaneous rash. There may be involvement of visceral organs. The secondary eruption may occur while the primary chancre is still healing or several months after the disappearance of the chancre. The secondary lesions heal spontaneously within 2 to 6 weeks, and the infection then enters latency. Some patients may later develop relapsing lesions similar to those of the secondary stage; rarely the relapse takes the form of recurrence of the primary chancre. About one third of untreated patients eventually develop late destructive tertiary lesions involving one or more of the eyes, central nervous system, heart, or other organs, including skin. These may occur at any time from a few years to as late as 25 years following infection.

The incidence of late complications of untreated syphilis is currently unknown but seems less than noted previously. Cases of gumma are at present so rare as to be reportable.

CLINICAL MANIFESTATIONS. *Primary Syphilis.* The typical lesion of primary syphilis is the chancre, a painless, clean-based, indurated ulcer. The chancre starts as a papule, but then superficial erosion occurs, resulting in the typical ulcer. The borders of the ulcer are raised, firm, and indurated. Occasionally, secondary infections change the appearance, resulting in a painful lesion. Most chancres are single, but multiple ulcers are sometimes seen, particularly when skin folds are opposed ("kissing chancres"). The untreated chancre heals in several weeks, leaving a faint scar. The chancre is usually associated with regional adenopathy, which may be either unilateral or bilateral. The regional nodes are movable, discrete, and rubbery. If the chancre occurs in the cervix or in the rectum, the affected regional iliac nodes are not palpable. See Figure 340–1.

It was formerly taught that 90 per cent of chancres occurred in the genital region. Currently, a much higher proportion of nongenital chancres is observed, particularly among male homosexuals, in whom chancres in or near the rectum are common. Rectal chancres may have an atypical appearance, mimicking rectal fissures or other more benign lesions, and are frequently overlooked. Conversely, they have also been mistaken for malignant disease. In general it is reasonable to assume that any ulcer occurring in the genital area or, in male homosexuals, around the rectum is syphilitic until proved otherwise. Chancres may also be seen in the pharynx, on the tongue, around the lips, on the fingers, on the nipples, or in diverse other areas. The morphology depends in part on the area of the body in which they occur and also on the host immune response. Chancres in previously infected individuals may be small and may remain papular. Chancres of the finger may appear more erosive and may be quite painful.

The *differential diagnosis* of a genital ulcer should include genital herpes. Herpetic ulcers can usually be distinguished because they are multiple, superficial, and, if seen early, vesicular. They are often painful. Herpetic ulcers, unlike syphilitic ulcers, may yield positive findings on Tzanck's test—multinucleated giant cells in the base of the ulcer. The ulcers of chancroid are usually painful, often multiple, and frequently exudative and nonindurated. Lymphogranuloma venereum may produce a small papular lesion associated wtih a regional adenopathy. Other conditions that must be distinguished include granuloma inguinale, drug eruptions, carcinoma, superficial fungal infections, traumatic lesions, and lichen planus. Final distinction in most cases is made on the basis of darkfield examination, which is positive only in syphilis.

Secondary Syphilis. Approximately 4 to 8 weeks following the appearance of the primary chancre, patients typically develop lesions of secondary syphilis. They may complain of *malaise, fever, headache, sore throat,* and other systemic symptoms. Most patients have generalized lymphadenopathy, including the epitrochlear nodes. Approximately 30 per cent of patients have evidence of the healing chancre, although many patients, including male homosexuals and women, give no history of a primary lesion.

At least 80 per cent of patients with secondary syphilis have cutaneous lesions or lesions of the mucocutaneous junctions at some point in their illness. The diagnosis is usually first suspected on the basis of the cutaneous eruption. The rash is often minimally symptomatic, however, and many patients with late syphilis do not recall either primary or secondary lesions. The rashes are quite varied in their appearance but have certain characterisitc features. The lesions are usually widespread and are symmetric in distribution. They often are pink, coppery, or dusky red, particularly the earliest macular lesions. They usually are nonpruritic, although occasional exceptions have been noted, and are almost never vesicular or bullous in adults. They are indurated except for the very earliest macular lesions and frequently have a superficial scale (papulosquamous lesions). They tend to be polymorphic and rounded, and on healing they may leave residual pigmentation or depigmentation. The lesions may be quite faint and difficult to visualize, particularly on dark-skinned individuals.

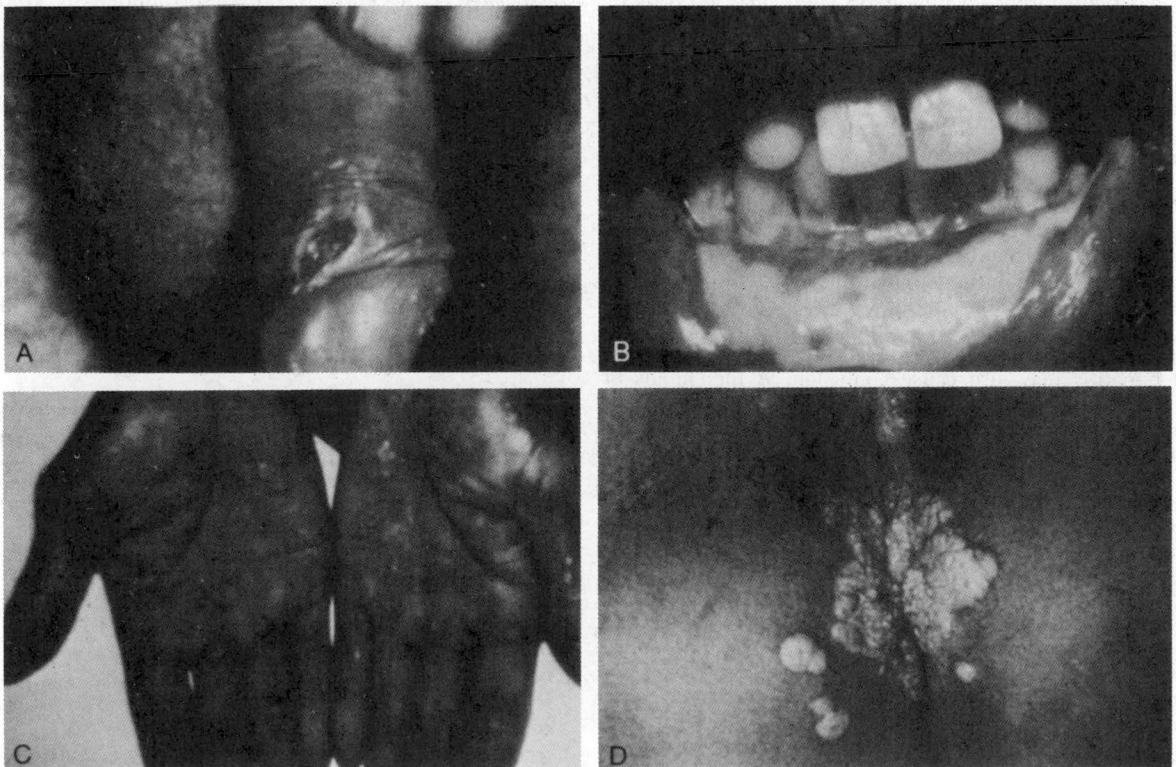

FIGURE 340–1. *A,* Primary syphilis, chancre. *B,* Secondary syphilis, mucous patch. *C,* Secondary syphilis, papulosquamous rash. *D,* Secondary syphilis, condylomata lata.

The earliest pink macular lesions are frequently seen on the margins of the ribs or the sides of the trunk with later spread to the rest of the body. The face is often spared except around the mouth. Subsequently a papular rash appears, which is usually generalized but is *quite marked on the palms and soles.* These rashes frequently are associated with a superficial scale and may be hyperpigmented. When the rash occurs on the face, it may be pustular, resembling acne vulgaris. On occasion the scale may be so great as to resemble psoriasis. Deep nodular lesions may cause confusion. Ulceration may occur, producing lesions resembling ecthyma. In malnourished or debilitated patients extensive destructive ulcerative lesions with a heaped-up crust may occur, the so-called rupial lesion. Lesions around the hair follicles may result in patchy alopecia of the beard or of the scalp.

Ringed or annular lesions may occur, especially around the face, particularly on black individuals. Lesions at the angle of the mouth or the corner of the nose may have a central linear erosion (the so-called "split papule").

In warm, moist areas such as the perineum, large, pale, flat-topped papules may coalesce to form condylomata lata. These may also be seen in the axilla and rarely in a generalized form. They are extremely infectious. They are not to be confused with the common venereal warts (condylomata acuminata), which are small, often multiple, and more sharply raised than condylomata lata.

Other lesions of the mucous membranes are common. The palate and pharynx may be inflamed. Approximately 30 per cent of patients develop the so-called mucous patch. This is a slightly raised oval area covered by a grayish-white membrane, which when raised reveals a pink base that does not bleed. These may be seen on the genitalia, in the mouth, or on the tongue and, like condylomata lata, are highly infectious.

Other manifestations of secondary syphilis include hepatitis, which has been reported in up to 10 per cent of patients in some series. Jaundice is rare, but an elevated alkaline phosphatase is common. Liver biopsy reveals small areas of focal necrosis and mononuclear infiltrate or periportal vasculitis. Spirochetes can often be visualized with silver stains. Periostitis with widespread lytic lesions of bone has been reported occasionally; use of bone scans appears to be a sensitive test for early syphilitic osteitis. An immune complex type of nephropathy with transient nephrotic syndrome has been rarely documented. There may be iritis or an anterior uveitis. From 10 to 30 per cent of patients have pleocytosis in the cerebrospinal fluid, but symptomatic meningitis is seen in less than 1 per cent of patients. Symptomatic gastritis may be present.

Differential diagnosis of secondary syphilis includes a large number of diseases. The cutaneous eruptions may be mimicked by pityriasis rosea, which can be differentiated by the occurrence of lesions along lines of skin cleavage and frequently by the presence of a herald patch. Drug eruptions, acute febrile exanthems, psoriasis, lichen planus, scabies, and other diseases must also be considered in some cases. The mucous patch may superficially resemble oral candidiasis (thrush). Infectious mononucleosis may appear very similar to secondary syphilis, with sore throat, generalized adenopathy, hepatitis, and a generalized rash. Infectious hepatitis may also cause confusion. A high index of suspicion is required to make the diagnosis of syphilis in some cases. Unfortunately even classic cases with widespread, hyperpigmented, papulosquamous lesions involving the palms and the soles are not infrequently misdiagnosed in the current era. Fortunately, if the serologic tests for syphilis are obtained, they are positive in 99 per cent of patients. The condylomata lata and mucous patches contain large numbers of treponemes on darkfield examination. Aspiration of lymph nodes may occasionally reveal motile *T. pallidum.*

Relapsing Syphilis. Condylomata lata are likely to recur. The skin manifestations tend to be unilateral, the eruptions more dense, marked, with fewer lesions, and sometimes solitary. They are also more infiltrated and of somewhat longer standing and have some characteristics that resemble the skin lesions in late syphilis. This reflects the increasing immunity with the duration of the early disease. Neurorecurrences, as well as ophthalmic and other relapsing manifestations, may occur. If the patient has been inadequately treated, relapses may be delayed.

Latent Syphilis. By definition latent syphilis is that stage in which there are no clinical signs of syphilis and the cerebrospinal fluid is normal. Latency begins with the passing of the first attack of secondary syphilis and may last for a lifetime thereafter. It is usually detected by positive specific treponemal antibody tests for syphilis. The test must be shown to be reactive on more than one occasion to rule out technical errors. Diseases known to cause occasional false-positive treponemal reactions for syphilis, such as systemic lupus erythematosus, must be excluded. In addition, congenital syphilis must be excluded before the diagnosis of latent syphilis can be made. Patients may or may not have a history of earlier primary or secondary syphilis, although such history is obviously helpful in making a firm diagnosis of latent syphilis.

Latency has been divided into two stages: *early* and *late latency.* Evidence suggests that most relapses occur in the first year, and epidemiologic evidence shows that the most infectious spread of syphilis occurs during the first year of infection. *Therefore early latency in the United States is defined as the first year after infection.* Late latent syphilis is ordinarily not infectious except for the case of the pregnant woman, who may transmit infection to her fetus after many years.

Late Syphilis. Late, or tertiary, syphilis is the destructive stage of the disease and can be crippling. Late syphilitic complications are still important medical problems, but newly recognized cases of late syphilis have been declining steadily in the United States since World War II. Although the incidence of late syphilis is unknown, the prevalence of various types of late syphilis has been approximated (Table 340–1).

Late syphilis is usually very slowly progressive, although certain neurologic syndromes may have sudden onset owing to endarteritis and thrombosis in the central nervous system. Late syphilis is noninfectious. Any organ of the body may be involved, but three main types of disease may be distinguished: late benign (gummatous), cardiovascular, and neurosyphilis.

Late Benign Syphilis. Late benign syphilis, or gumma, was the most common complication of late syphilis in the Oslo Study of untreated patients (1891–1951). In the penicillin era gummas are rare. They typically develop from 1 to 10 years after the initial infection and may involve any part of the body. Although they may be very destructive, they respond rapidly to treatment and therefore are relatively benign. Histologically the gumma is a granuloma. The histologic findings are nonspecific and may be associated with central necrosis surrounded by epithelioid and fibroblastic cells and occasionally giant cells. There is sometimes vasculitis. *T. pallidum* is ordinarily not demonstrable by silver stains but can sometimes be recovered by inoculation of rabbits.

Gummas may be solitary or multiple. They are usually asymmetric and are often grouped. They may start as a superficial nodule or as a deeper lesion that breaks down to form punched-out ulcers. They are ordinarily indolent and slowly progressive with curving or polycyclic borders. They are indurated on palpation. There often is central healing with an atrophic scar surrounded by hyperpigmented borders. Cutaneous gummas may resemble other chronic granulomatous ulcerative lesions caused by tuberculosis, sarcoidosis, leprosy, and other deep fungal infections. Precise histologic diagnosis may not be possible. However, the syphilitic gumma is the only such lesion to heal

TABLE 340–1. NEWLY DIAGNOSED TERTIARY SYPHILIS IN 105 PATIENTS IN DENMARK, 1961–1970

Type of Tertiary Syphilis	Number Observed*
Neurosyphilis	72
Asymptomatic	45
Tabes dorsalis	11
General paresis	13
Meningovascular	1
Optic atrophy	2
Cardiovascular syphilis	44
Aortic insufficiency	16
Aortic aneurysm	13
Uncomplicated aortitis†	15
Late benign syphilis (gumma)	4

*Some patients had more than one form of late syphilis.
†Autopsy diagnoses only.

dramatically with penicillin therapy. Another form of gumma is papulosquamous and may mimic psoriasis.

Gummas may also involve deep visceral organs, of which the most common are the respiratory tract, the gastrointestinal tract, and bones. In earlier centuries gummas of the nose and palate commonly resulted in septal perforations and disfiguring facial lesions. Gummas may also involve the larynx or the pulmonary parenchyma. Gumma of the stomach may masquerade as carcinoma of the stomach or lymphoma. Gummas of the liver were once the most common form of visceral syphilis, presenting often with hepatosplenomegaly and anemia, occasionally with fever and jaundice. Skeletal gummas typically produce lesions in the long bones, skull, and clavicle. A characteristic symptom is nocturnal pain. Radiologic abnormalities, when present, include periostitis and either lytic or sclerotic destructive osteitis.

Cardiovascular Syphilis. The primary cardiovascular complications of syphilis are aortic insufficiency and aortic aneurysm, usually of the ascending aorta. Less commonly other large arteries may be involved, and rarely involvement of the coronary ostia results in coronary insufficiency. These complications in all cases are due to obliterative endarteritis of the vasa vasorum with resultant damage to the intima and media of the great vessels. This results in dilatation of the ascending aorta and eventually in stretching of the ring of the aortic valve, producing aortic insufficiency. The valve cusps remain normal. Death may eventually result from congestive heart failure. There has been some success with placing prosthetic heart valves in patients with syphilitic aortic insufficiency. Aneurysms occasionally present as a pulsating mass bulging through the anterior chest wall. Syphilitic aortitis may involve the descending aorta, but this is almost always proximal to the renal arteries, unlike atherosclerotic aneurysms, which typically involve the descending aorta below the renal arteries.

The disease usually begins within 5 to 10 years after initial infection but may not become clinically manifest until 20 to 30 years after infection. Cardiovascular syphilis is thought to be more common in men than in women and possibly in blacks than in whites. Cardiovascular syphilis does not occur after congenital infection—a phenomenon that remains unexplained.

Asymptomatic aortitis is best diagnosed by visualizing linear calcifications in the wall of the ascending aorta by radiography. The signs of syphilitic aortic insufficiency are the same as for aortic insufficiency of other causes. In aortic insufficiency resulting from dilatation of the aortic ring, the decrescendo murmur is often loudest along the *right* sternal margin. Syphilitic aneurysms may be fusiform but are more typically saccular and do not lead to aortic dissection. Approximately 10 to 25 per cent of patients with cardiovascular syphilis have coexistent neurosyphilis, and it is therefore mandatory to do a lumbar puncture in all patients with cardiovascular syphilis.

At present, syphilis is a relatively more common cause of aortic insufficiency among the elderly than among younger patients; this is due to the progressively decreasing incidence of new cases of late cardiovascular syphilis.

Neurosyphilis. Neurosyphilis may be divided into four groups: asymptomatic, meningovascular, tabes dorsalis, and general paresis. These are more fully described in Ch. 472. Division is not absolute, and there may be considerable overlap between syndromes. Current cases of neurosyphilis are more likely than heretofore to be variants of the classic syndromes, possibly as a result of use of antimicrobials for other diseases.

Asymptomatic Neurosyphilis. Asymptomatic neurosyphilis is diagnosed when there is a positive VDRL* in the cerebrospinal fluid (CSF) in the absence of signs and symptoms of neurologic disease. False-positive VDRL test results are very rare in CSF in the absence of a traumatic tap. The CSF usually shows an increased total protein and a lymphocytic pleocytosis. If the CSF is normal 2 or more years after the initial infection, the patient is not likely to develop a positive CSF later. Although up to 30 per cent of patients with untreated secondary syphilis have an abnormal CSF, penicillin therapy apparently prevents progression to late symptomatic neurosyphilis. Because of this, routine lumbar punctures for examination of CSF are not indicated in early syphilis unless the patient is known to have HIV infection.

---

*See Serologic Tests, below. Also refer to Table 340–2.

Unfortunately, it has become common practice to avoid lumbar punctures in later stages of syphilis as well. Instead, patients are treated with doses of penicillin thought to be effective for neurosyphilis, if present. As a result, there are few data on the present frequency and course of asymptomatic neurosyphilis.

Some laboratories perform an FTA-ABS* test on spinal fluid. Interest in tests such as this has been prompted by good evidence that patients with untreated neurosyphilis may have a negative CSF-VDRL. There are published reports of positive FTA-ABS test results in the CSF of patients with otherwise normal spinal fluid, in whom there were clinical signs and symptoms compatible with neurosyphilis. However, the CSF FTA-ABS test has not been standardized, and there is some evidence that positive CSF test results are caused by passive transfer of serum antibody into spinal fluid. At present no diagnosis of asymptomatic (or symptomatic) neurosyphilis should be based solely on the CSF FTA-ABS* test.

Meningovascular Syphilis. An acute to subacute aseptic meningitis may occur at any time after the primary stage but usually within the first year of infection. It frequently involves the base of the brain and may result in unilateral or bilateral cranial nerve palsies. In about 10 per cent of cases, the onset of meningitis coincides with the rash of secondary syphilis. The spinal fluid shows a lymphocytic pleocytosis with increased protein and usually normal glucose concentration. The CSF-VDRL is nearly always positive. Rarely CSF glucose concentration is decreased. This syndrome can mimic tuberculous or fungal meningitis or nonpurulent meningitis of various causes.

In other patients, the meningeal involvement may be less prominent, but there is sufficient endarteritis and perivascular inflammation to result in cerebrovascular thrombosis and infarction. This usually occurs 5 to 10 years after the initial infection and is more common in males. There often is an associated aseptic meningitis as well. Most cerebrovascular accidents are not due to syphilitic arteritis even in patients with a positive serologic test for syphilis. However, syphilis should be considered as the cause in young patients with a history of syphilis and without other causes for cerebrovascular accidents.

Tabes Dorsalis. Tabes dorsalis is a slowly progressive degenerative disease involving the posterior columns and posterior roots of the spinal cord, resulting in progressive loss of peripheral reflexes, impairment of vibration and position sense, and progressive ataxia. There may be chronic destructive changes in the large joints of the affected limbs in far-advanced cases (Charcot's joints). Incontinence of the bladder and impotence are common. Sudden and severe painful crises of uncertain cause are a characteristic part of the syndrome. These may involve the larynx, vagina, rectum, or other organs. Not infrequently severe, sharp abdominal pains lead to exploratory surgery. Lightning pains in the extremities may require opiates for relief. These may be triggered by exposure to cold or other stresses or may arise with no obvious precipitating cause.

Optic atrophy is seen in 20 per cent of cases. The pupils are abnormal in 90 per cent of cases, with bilaterally small pupils that fail to constrict further in response to light but that do constrict normally to accommodation (Argyll Robertson pupils).

The cause of tabes dorsalis is unclear. Spirochetes cannot be demonstrated in the posterior column or dorsal root.

Onset of the disease is usually delayed, often 20 to 30 years after initial onset of infection. It is thought to be more common in whites and in males. Typical cases of patients presenting with lightning pains, ataxia, Argyll Robertson pupils, absent deep tendon reflexes, and loss of posterior column function are easy to diagnose. Atypical cases may be more troublesome, particularly because the VDRL test result in the serum is normal in as many as 30 to 40 per cent of patients, and 10 to 20 per cent of patients (even before the advent of penicillin) have normal CSF-VDRL results as well. The FTA-ABS test in serum is nearly always positive.

Treatment is unsatisfactory. Penicillin does not reverse the symptoms, although it does usually result in clearing of the abnormal spinal fluid. Carbamazepine in doses of 400 to 800 mg per day has been reported to be effective in treatment of the lightning pains.

Tabes dorsalis is now thought to be uncommon, although a

survey of newly diagnosed late syphilis in Denmark in the decade 1961 to 1970 showed that in approximately 10 per cent of all persons with late syphilis and 40 per cent of all with clinical neurosyphilis there was evidence of tabes dorsalis.

General Paresis. This form of neurosyphilis is a chronic meningoencephalitis resulting in gradually progressive loss of cortical function. It typically occurs 10 to 20 years after the initial infection. Pathologically there is a perivascular and meningeal chronic inflammatory reaction with thickening of the meninges, a granular ependymitis, degeneration of the cortical parenchyma, and abundant spirochetes in the tissues.

The most devastating effect of general paresis is on the mind. With effective penicillin therapy this disease has become much less common; in the United States, first admissions to mental hospitals because of syphilitic psychosis declined from 7694 in 1940 to 154 in 1968, the last year for which definite figures are available.

In its early stages general paresis results in nonspecific symptoms such as irritability, fatigability, headaches, forgetfulness, and personality changes. Later there is impaired memory, defective judgment, lack of insight, confusion, and often depression or marked elation. The patients may be delusional, and seizures are sometimes seen. There may also be loss of other cortical functions, including paralysis or aphasia.

Physical signs are primarily those of the altered mental status. Cranial nerve palsies are uncommon. Optic atrophy is rare. The complete Argyll Robertson pupil is also uncommon, but irregular or otherwise abnormal pupils are not infrequent. Peripheral reflexes are often somewhat increased.

The CSF is nearly always abnormal with lymphocytic pleocytosis and increased total protein. The VDRL is usually reactive in both spinal fluid and serum. The disease responds well to penicillin therapy if administered early, although as many as a third of treated patients may develop progressive neurologic decline in later years. Fever therapy induced with malaria was formerly an effective adjunct to treatment with arsenicals but has now been abandoned.

Even though classic general paresis is now infrequent, it remains reasonable to suspect syphilis as the cause of undiagnosed neurologic illness. Since the VDRL may be negative in patients with late neurologic syphilis, the FTA-ABS test on serum must be performed before syphilis can be excluded.

Congenital Syphilis. Congenital syphilis results from transplacental hematogenous spread of syphilis from the mother to the fetus. The incidence of congenital syphilis among newborns or infants under 1 year of age in the United States rose from 180 cases in 1957 to 422 cases in 1972 but declined to about 100 cases annually thereafter. Unfortunately, the recent rise in heterosexually acquired syphilis has been accompanied by a rise in congenital syphilis as well. Each case of congenital syphilis represents a tragedy that could have been prevented by better case reporting and by proper prenatal care. A VDRL should be obtained in all expectant mothers at the beginning and near the end of pregnancy.

Spirochetes can be found in abortuses of as little as 9 to 10 weeks' gestation. The risk of fetal infection is greatest in the early stages of untreated maternal syphilis and declines slowly thereafter, but the mother may infect her fetus during at least the first 5 years of her infection. Adequate treatment of the mother prior to the sixteenth week usually prevents manifest clinical illness in the neonate. Later treatment may not prevent late sequelae of the disease in the child. Untreated maternal infection may result in stillbirth, neonatal death, prematurity, or syndromes of early or late congenital syphilis among surviving infants.

Manifestations of early congenital syphilis are often seen in the perinatal period but may not develop until the infant has been discharged from the hospital. The disease resembles secondary syphilis of the adult except that the rash may be vesicular or bullous, which is extremely rare in adults. There often is rhinitis, hepatosplenomegaly, hemolytic anemia, jaundice, and pseudoparalysis (immobility of one or more extremities) resulting from painful osteochondritis. There may be thrombocytopenia and leukocytosis. The early stages of congenital syphilis must be differentiated from rubella, cytomegalovirus infection, toxoplasmosis, bacterial sepsis, and other diseases.

Late congenital syphilis is defined as congenital syphilis of more than 2 years' duration. The disease may remain latent with no manifest late damage. Cardiovascular alterations have not been observed in congenital syphilis. Neurologic manifestations are common, and there may be eighth cranial nerve deafness and interstitial keratitis. The latter occurs in over 10 per cent of patients but may not be manifest until the tenth year of life or later. Periostitis may result in prominent frontal bones, depression of the bridge of the nose ("saddle nose"), poor development of the maxilla, and anterior bowing of the tibias ("saber shins"). There may be late-onset arthritis of the knees (Clutton's joints). The permanent dentition may show characteristic abnormalities known as Hutchinson's teeth; the upper central incisors are widely spaced, centrally notched, and tapered in the manner of a screwdriver. The molars may show multiple poorly developed cusps (mulberry molars). Some of the late manifestations such as interstitial keratitis and Clutton's joints may be due to hypersensitivity responses and are benefited by corticosteroids in some cases.

DIAGNOSIS. *Darkfield Examination.* The most definitive means of making a diagnosis is finding spirochetes of typical morphology and motility in lesions of early acquired or congenital syphilis. The darkfield examination is almost always positive in primary syphilis and in the moist mucosal lesions of secondary and congenital syphilis. It may occasionally be positive in aspirates of lymph nodes in secondary syphilis. Problems arise, however, because of false-negative results in primary syphilis owing to application by the patient of soaps or other toxic compounds to the lesions. A single negative result is therefore insufficient to exclude syphilis. Patients with suspicious lesions but with an initially negative darkfield examination should be instructed to avoid washing the lesion and to return daily for two successive examinations. Confusion may also arise because of the presence of spirochetes that are morphologically indistinguishable from *T. pallidum* in the mouth, particularly around the gingival margins. For lesions in these areas, therefore, diagnosis often depends upon clinical appearance, history, and serologic testing.

To perform the darkfield examination, the surface of the suspected ulcerative lesion should be cleaned with saline solution and gauze without production of bleeding. The presence of red cells in the specimen makes it difficult to visualize small numbers of *T. pallidum*. Squeezing of the lesion (with gloves on) may help produce serous fluid, which is picked up on a glass slide, covered with a coverslip, and examined with the darkfield microscope. Living *T. pallidum* organisms demonstrate gradual motion to and fro, rotational movement around the long axis, and rather sudden 90-degree bending near the center of the organism. Since most physicians do not have the proper equipment and are not familiar with the techniques of darkfield microscopy, the state public health authorities can be called for assistance.

T. pallidum may also be demonstrated in biopsies or pathologic specimens by fluorescent antibody stains or by silver stains.

Serologic Tests. Two basic types of humoral antibody are stimulated by infection with *T. pallidum:* nonspecific antibody directed against diphosphatidylglycerol (cardiolipin), which is a normal component of many tissues; and specific treponemal antibodies. Nonspecific antibodies against cardiolipin were formerly designated "reagin," a term that should be discarded to avoid confusion with another "reagin," IgE. The kinds of tests used in syphilis are summarized in Table 340–2.

Nonspecific Tests. Anticardiolipin antibodies were first discovered by Wassermann in 1907, using extracts of congenitally syphilitic livers as the antigen for a complement fixation test. Subsequently it was shown that normal livers contained the same antigen as do many other tissues; the antigen for this class of test is now extracted from beef heart. As yet there is no convincing explanation for why patients infected with *T. pallidum* develop increasing titers of antibody against a normal tissue component.

The Wassermann test has now been replaced by related tests. The standard test in use today for detection of anticardiolipin antibody is the Venereal Disease Research Laboratories (VDRL) test, which is an easily quantified slide flocculation test. Many similar tests, including the rapid plasma reagin (RPR) test and the unheated serum reagin (USR) test, are frequently used for screening for syphilis.

The VDRL and related tests are simple, well standardized, cheap, and the screening tests of choice. The VDRL is the test

TABLE 340–2. SEROLOGIC TESTS FOR SYPHILIS

Type	Use
Nonspecific (anticardiolipin) antibodies:	
VDRL (slide flocculation)	Screening, quantitation, following response to treatment
RPR (circle-card) (agglutination)	Screening
Specific treponemal antibodies:	
FTA-ABS (immunofluorescence with absorbed serum)	Confirmatory, diagnostic, not for routine screening
MHA-TP (microhemagglutination)	Similar to FTA-ABS but can be quantified and automated

VDRL = Venereal Disease Research Laboratories test.
RPR = Rapid plasma reagin test.
FTA-ABS = Fluorescent treponemal antibody absorption test.
MHA-TP = Microhemagglutination assay for *T. pallidum*.

of choice for following the response of patients to treatment. Since the VDRL detects antibody against a normal tissue component, it may be falsely positive in a significant number of patients. The relative proportion of patients with a false-positive VDRL depends on the prevalence of syphilis in the community; the lower the prevalence of syphilis, the higher the proportion of positive VDRL tests that are due to nonsyphilitic causes.

The VDRL test begins to turn positive 1 to 2 weeks after the onset of the chancre. In large series of patients with primary syphilis, approximately two thirds have had a positive VDRL test result. Obviously, then, a negative VDRL test does not exclude primary syphilis, particularly if the lesion is less than 2 weeks old. The VDRL is positive in 99 per cent of patients with secondary syphilis, the only exceptions being patients with such high titers of antibody that they are in antibody excess; dilution of the serum will then paradoxically result in conversion of a negative test to positive. There is some evidence that AIDS delays or diminishes the serologic response in early (primary and secondary) syphilis. VDRL reactivity tends to diminish in later stages of the disease, and only about 70 per cent of patients with cardiovascular or neurosyphilis have a positive VDRL test result.

The *quantitative titer* of the VDRL test is somewhat useful in diagnosis and quite useful in following therapeutic response. The titer is reported as the highest dilution that gives a positive response. Most patients with secondary syphilis have titers of at least 1:16. Most patients with false-positive VDRL tests have titers of less than 1:8. No single titer is in itself diagnostic. Significant rises (fourfold or greater) in paired sera, however, are strongly indicative of acute syphilis.

Treponemal Tests. There are many varieties of specific treponemal antibody tests. The most widely used is the fluorescent treponemal antibody absorption (FTA-ABS) test. Patient serum is absorbed with extracts of nonpathogenic cultivable treponemes to remove cross-reacting group treponemal antibody. Agglutination of red cells to which *T. pallidum* antigens have been fixed is the basis of the microhemagglutination assay for *T. pallidum* (MHA-TP).

The precise nature of the antigens involved in these tests is not known. Characterization of the antigens of *T. pallidum* has been greatly hindered by inability to grow the organism in cell-free culture. Recent success in cloning *T. pallidum* antigens into *Escherichia coli* may circumvent this problem. Antibodies reactive in the various tests are found in all major immunoglobulin classes (IgG, IgM, IgA). A modification of the FTA-ABS test has been developed using fluorescein-labeled anti–human IgM (IgM FTA-ABS). The IgM FTA-ABS test is of some use in the diagnosis of early congenital syphilis but is of no use in distinguishing acute disease from old infections in adults.

The FTA-ABS test is best used as a confirmatory test. It is somewhat more difficult to perform than the VDRL test and cannot be easily quantified. It is sensitive and has a high degree of specificity, being positive in only approximately 1 per cent of normal individuals. It is positive in 85 per cent of patients with primary syphilis, 99 per cent with secondary syphilis, and at least 95 per cent with late syphilis. It may therefore be the only test positive in patients with cardiovascular or neurologic syphilis. In late syphilis the FTA-ABS test usually remains positive for life despite adequate therapy. It (as well as the MHA-TP) is positive in other treponemal diseases, such as pinta, yaws, and bejel.

The FTA-ABS test is reported in terms of relative brilliance of fluorescence, from borderline to 4+. Borderline reactivity has the same meaning as nonreactive for clinical purposes. Most laboratories report 1+ positive tests as reactive, but some studies have shown that such tests may be difficult to reproduce. Occasional laboratories therefore only report as positive tests with 2+ or greater reactivity. In patients lacking historical or clinical evidence of syphilis but with a reactive FTA-ABS test, one should repeat the FTA-ABS test. Use of another treponemal test such as the MHA-TP may be helpful in problem cases.

The MHA-TP test is less sensitive than either the VDRL or the FTA-ABS test in primary syphilis. Its sensitivity and specificity otherwise are nearly identical to those of the FTA-ABS test, being positive in nearly all patients with secondary syphilis and in 95 per cent or more of patients with late syphilis. The reactivity of serologic tests for syphilis in various stages of disease is shown in Table 340–3.

False-Positive Serologic Test Results for Syphilis. The VDRL or RPR test may be positive in a variety of diseases other than syphilis. A false-positive result is defined as a reproducible positive test in a patient with no clinical or historical evidence of syphilis and whose serum FTA-ABS or MHA-TP test is negative. *"Acute" (less than 6 months) false-positive VDRL test* results occur with low frequency in atypical pneumonia, malaria, and other bacterial or viral infections and may occur after smallpox or other vaccinations as well. *Chronic false-positive VDRL tests* (lasting longer than 6 months) are relatively common in autoimmune disorders such as systemic lupus erythematosus (SLE), in narcotic addicts, in leprosy, and in aged persons. From 8 to 20 per cent of patients with SLE have been reported as having a false-positive VDRL test, and the false-positive result may develop many years prior to the onset of other manifestations of the disease. A chronic false-positive VDRL test in females age 20 or younger carries a significant risk of future development of SLE, thyroiditis, or other autoimmune disorders, and such patients should be followed carefully for a considerable period of time. As many as one third of patients with narcotic addiction have a false-positive VDRL test. Over 1 per cent of patients aged 70 and 10 per cent of patients over age 80 have a low-titer false-positive VDRL test. Most false-positive VDRL tests have a titer of 1:8 or less, although occasional patients with lymphoma and other diseases have been described with very high-titer false-positive VDRL tests.

A positive FTA-ABS result is usually indicative of recent or past syphilis. However, there is an increased incidence of false-positive FTA-ABS results in SLE and in other chronic diseases associated with hyperglobulinemia, including rheumatoid arthritis, biliary cirrhosis, and others. False-positive results are of two kinds in SLE: The most common is one with a beaded pattern of fluorescence, which has been shown to be due to anti-DNA antibodies; there also may be homogeneous fluorescence of the treponeme indistinguishable from a true positive result in syphilis. Patients with SLE who have a false-positive FTA-ABS result almost always have a negative VDRL result (and conversely, patients with SLE with a positive VDRL usually have a negative FTA-ABS).

Occasionally one encounters reproducible positive FTA-ABS results in patients with no clinical or historical evidence of syphilis and in whom there is no evidence of diseases associated with false-positive FTA-ABS results. It may be wise to obtain CSF for examination of total protein, cells, and VDRL reactivity in order to rule out neurosyphilis. If in doubt and if the patient is not allergic to penicillin, it is often wisest to treat such patients for possible syphilis.

IgM FTA-ABS Test for Congenital Syphilis. Mothers with a positive VDRL or FTA-ABS deliver infants with a positive VDRL

TABLE 340–3. FREQUENCY OF POSITIVE SEROLOGIC TESTS IN UNTREATED SYPHILIS

Stage	VDRL (%)	FTA-ABS (%)	MHA-TP (%)
Primary	70	85	50–60
Secondary	99	100	100
Latent or late	70	98	98

and FTA-ABS because of passive transfer of the IgG antibodies reactive in these tests. Since many infants with congenital syphilis are clinically normal at birth but develop serious symptomatic disease some weeks later, it is important to determine whether a newborn with a positive VDRL or FTA-ABS test has passively transferred maternal antibody or is actively infected. Since maternal IgM antibodies are not passively transferred to the fetus, an IgM FTA-ABS test has been developed to detect syphilis in the newborn. Unfortunately there is approximately a 35 per cent incidence of false-negative IgM FTA-ABS test results in delayed-onset congenital syphilis. There also is a false-positive rate of approximately 10 per cent. For these reasons the IgM FTA-ABS test is of limited use in the diagnosis of neonatal syphilis.

If the mother has been adequately treated for syphilis during pregnancy and the infant is clinically normal at birth, one may elect to follow the infant carefully by serial examination and VDRL titers. If the positive VDRL in the infant is due to passively transferred maternal antibody, the titer of reactivity falls markedly in the first 2 months of life. A rising titer indicates active disease and the need for treatment. Many physicians are unwilling to risk failure of proper follow-up of VDRL-positive but clinically normal neonates and instead administer effective therapy immediately. The risk of penicillin allergy in neonates is very low.

TREATMENT. *T. pallidum* is highly susceptible to penicillin, being inhibited by less than 0.01 μg of penicillin G. Since treponemes divide slowly, and since penicillin acts only on dividing cells, it is necessary to maintain serum levels of penicillin for many days. Studies in animals and in humans show that more therapy is required as the length of infection increases. Current recommendations for treatment of syphilis are summarized in Table 340–4.

Early (Less Than 1 Year) Infectious Syphilis. Early syphilis may be treated with a single injection of 2.4 million units of *benzathine penicillin G*, which provides low but effective serum levels for over 2 weeks. Extensive studies in the 1940's and 1950's with regimens that provided similar serum levels and duration of therapy showed that approximately 95 per cent of patients were cured by such treatment. Many of the remaining 5 per cent who had clinical or serologic evidence of relapse may actually have been reinfected. It is not necessary to examine the CSF at this stage because penicillin prevents development of later neurosyphilis. Motile treponemes disappear from primary lesions in 24 hours.

A single injection of 2.4 million units of *aqueous procaine penicillin*, which provides relatively high serum levels for a brief period, is ineffective in established early syphilis but is curative if the disease is still in the incubating stage. The ceftriaxone regimen currently useful for gonorrhea probably is curative for incubating syphilis, but data are few, and careful follow-up is indicated if there is reason to suspect exposure to syphilis in a patient treated for gonorrhea with ceftriaxone. The incidence of incubating syphilis in gonorrhea patients is 2 per cent or more in several series.

For patients allergic to penicillin, tetracycline hydrochloride may be given in a total dose of 30 grams over 15 days, or doxycyline 100 mg twice daily for 14 days. Particularly careful follow-up is necessary in patients treated with drugs other than penicillin, because patients may not be fully compliant with these prolonged courses of oral therapy and these regimens have been less fully evaluated clinically. Ceftriaxone, 2 gram IM daily for 10 days, may be effective but has not been well studied. Chloramphenicol is of equivocal efficacy and for this reason, as well as because of the risk of toxicity, should not be used. Spectinomycin has essentially no effect on syphilis. Erythromycin is of questionable efficacy.

Syphilis of More Than 1 Year's Duration. Larger doses of penicillin are needed for *neurosyphilis* (see Ch. 472) than for syphilis of less than 1 year's duration. In general, patients with general paresis respond better to treatment than do patients with tabes dorsalis, although patients with paresis should be expected to show residual effects of the infection. This is particularly true in advanced cases. Meningovascular syphilis usually responds well, except for residual damage to cranial nerves or cortical function resulting from ischemic infarcts. Published studies show that a total of 6.0 to 9.0 million units of penicillin G results in a

TABLE 340–4. PENICILLIN TREATMENT PRACTICE IN SYPHILIS AS RECOMMENDED BY UNITED STATES PUBLIC HEALTH SERVICE

Indications for Syphilis Therapy†	Dosage and Administration*	
	Benzathine Penicillin G	***Aqueous Benzyl Penicillin G or Procaine Penicillin G***
Primary, secondary, and early latent syphilis (<1 year); epidemiologic treatment	Total of 2.4 million units; single IM dose of two injections of 1.2 million units in one session	Total of 4.8 million units IM in doses of 600,000 units daily for 8 consecutive days
Late latent (>1 year) or when CSF was not examined in "latency"; asymptomatic neurosyphilis (HIV negative), cardiovascular syphilis, late benign (cutaneous, osseous, visceral gumma)	Total of 7.2 million units IM in doses of 2.4 million units at 7-day intervals, over 21 days	Total of 9 million units IM in doses of 600,000 units daily over 15 days
Symptomatic neurosyphilis or asymptomatic neurosyphilis in an HIV-positive patient	2 to 4 million units of aqueous (crystalline) penicillin G intravenously every 4 hours for at least 10 days	2 to 4 million units procaine penicillin IM daily and probenecid, 500 mg orally 4 times daily for 10–14 days
Congenital Infants	CSF normal: Total of 50,000 units per kilogram IM in a single or divided dose at one session	CSF abnormal: Total of 50,000 units per kilogram IM per day for 10 consecutive days‡
Older children	CSF normal: Same as for early congenital syphilis, up to 2.4 million units	CSF abnormal: 200,000–300,000 units/kg/day IV aqueous crystalline penicillin for 10–14 days

*Individual doses can be divided for injection in each buttock to minimize discomfort.

†In *pregnancy*, treatment is dependent on the stage of syphilis.

‡For aqueous penicillin, give in two divided IV doses per day; for procaine penicillin, give as one daily dose IM.

satisfactory clinical response in approximately 90 per cent of patients with neurosyphilis, in the absence of HIV infection.

Currently used benzathine penicillin regimens have received relatively little study in neurosyphilis. Benzathine penicillin G in a total dose of 7.2 million units given as 2.4 million units weekly for 3 successive weeks is effective in most patients. However, there are reports of patients who have failed standard penicillin therapy for neurosyphilis but who responded to intensive intravenous therapy that provided high serum levels of penicillin. Benzathine penicillin does not provide measurable levels of penicillin in the spinal fluid or aqueous humor of the eye. There are anecdotal reports of increased treatment failures in patients with concomitant HIV infection. *Therefore in cases of symptomatic central nervous system syphilis, which is a serious disease, or in asymptomatic neurosyphilis in HIV-positive patients there is considerable rationale to treatment with intravenous penicillin G (20 million units per day for at least 10 days in hospital).* Therapy of neurosyphilis not infrequently results in increased CSF pleocytosis for 7 to 10 days after starting treatment and may transiently convert a normal CSF to abnormal.

Limited evidence suggests that treating *latent syphilis* with 7.2 million units total dose of benzathine penicillin is curative even if the patient has asymptomatic neurosyphilis. However, because of the possible lack of the efficacy of benzathine penicillin in some patients with central nervous system syphilis, it is desirable to examine CSF in all patients with latent syphilis to exclude asymptomatic neurosyphilis. This is particularly important in

HIV-positive patients. Alternatively, one may reasonably elect to perform a lumbar puncture at the conclusion of the follow-up period (2 years); if the CSF is normal, the patient can be reassured that neurosyphilis will not develop.

There is no evidence that therapy with antimicrobial drugs is clinically beneficial to patients with *cardiovascular syphilis*. Nevertheless, treatment of cardiovascular syphilis is recommended in order to prevent further progression of disease and because approximately 15 per cent of patients with cardiovascular syphilis have associated neurosyphilis.

There is no evidence regarding the efficacy of other antimicrobials in the treatment of later syphilis. Therefore if patients are allergic to penicillin, it is mandatory that the CSF be examined before therapy is undertaken. Either tetracycline or doxycycline taken for 4 weeks is probably effective.

Syphilis in Pregnancy. All pregnant women should be examined with a VDRL or RPR test during pregnancy; if they are at high risk for syphilis, a second test should be obtained before delivery. Because of the risk to the fetus, evaluation and treatment of the VDRL-positive patient should be done as rapidly as possible, particularly for patients first seen in the later stages of pregnancy. If a confirmatory FTA-ABS is positive and the patient has not been treated, penicillin should be administered in doses appropriate for early or late syphilis as outlined above. Penicillin-allergic patients should not be treated with tetracycline or erythromycin because of toxicity (tetracycline) or lack of efficacy (erythromycin). Penicillin desensitization may be considered but also carries risks. For patients who are VDRL positive but FTA-ABS negative and who have no clinical signs of syphilis, treatment may be withheld. In such patients a quantitative VDRL test and another FTA-ABS test should be repeated in 4 weeks. If the VDRL titer has risen by fourfold or more, or if clinical signs of syphilis have developed, the patient should be treated. If after repeat examination the diagnosis remains equivocal, the patient should be treated to prevent possible disease in the neonate. After treatment a quantitative VDRL titer should be followed monthly; if it rises fourfold, the patient should be treated a second time.

Congenital Syphilis. Proper treatment of the mother usually prevents active congenital syphilis in the neonate. However, infected infants may be clinically normal at birth, and the infant may be seronegative if the mother's infection was acquired late in pregnancy. The infant should be treated at birth if the mother has received no or inadequate treatment, or has been treated with drugs other than penicillin, or if the infant cannot be carefully followed up for several months after birth. The CSF should be examined before treatment of the infant. If the CSF is normal, treatment may be with a single injection of 50,000 units per kilogram of benzathine penicillin G. If the CSF is abnormal, treatment should be with aqueous penicillin G, 50,000 units per kilogram intramuscularly or intravenously daily, given in two divided doses, for a minimum of 10 days. Alternatively, a single daily intramuscular injection of procaine penicillin G, 50,000 units per kilogram, may be given for 10 days. These recommendations are based upon the failure of benzathine penicillin to provide adequate treponemicidal levels in spinal fluid and on evidence that aqueous or procaine penicillin does provide adequate CSF levels of penicillin. Many experts believe that all syphilis in infected infants should be treated with either procaine or aqueous penicillin to ensure adequate CSF levels. Tetracycline should not be used to treat children of less than 8 years of age. Antimicrobial agents other than penicillin are not recommended for treatment of congenital syphilis.

Follow-up Examinations. All patients with early syphilis or congenital syphilis should return for quantitative VDRL titers and clinical examination 3, 6, and 12 months after treatment. Patients with late latent syphilis should be examined also at 24 months after therapy; if CSF was not examined prior to therapy, a lumbar puncture should be done prior to discharge to rule out inadequately treated asymptomatic neurosyphilis.

The quantitative VDRL titer should return to normal within 12 months after therapy of primary syphilis or 24 months after therapy of secondary syphilis. In a small percentage of patients with early syphilis, the VDRL remains reactive in low titer for long periods of time. Chronic low-titer VDRL reactivity after therapy is much more common in late syphilis and should not be viewed with alarm. The FTA-ABS test usually remains positive

for years, despite adequate therapy. The influence of therapy on serologic tests is shown in Table 340–5. A fourfold or greater rise of VDRL titer after therapy is sufficient evidence for retreatment. Patients with treated early syphilis are fully susceptible to reinfection, and many clinical and serologic relapses after therapy are probably reinfections. As such they represent failures of proper epidemiologic case finding and of preventive therapy of the patient's sexual contacts.

Patients with neurosyphilis should be followed with serologic tests for at least 3 years and with repeat examination of CSF at 6-month intervals. The CSF pleocytosis is the first abnormality to disappear, but cell counts may not be normal for 1 to 2 years. The elevated CSF protein level falls more slowly, followed by the positive CSF-VDRL test, which may take years to become negative. It is not known whether use of high-dose intravenous penicillin therapy accelerates the return of CSF to normal. Rising CSF cell counts, protein, and VDRL titer obtained at follow-up are an indication for retreatment.

Epidemiologic Investigation and Treatment. All patients with syphilis should be reported to public health authorities. In the absence of an effective vaccine, control of syphilis depends on finding and treating persons with infectious lesions of primary and secondary syphilis before they can further transmit the disease and on finding and treating persons with incubating syphilis before they develop infectious lesions. All patients with early syphilis (less than 1 year) should be carefully interviewed by qualified persons to determine the nature of their recent sex contacts. Approximately 16 per cent of the named recent contacts of patients with early syphilis are found to have active untreated syphilis on examination, and a similar proportion of individuals named as suspects or associates also have active syphilis.

Most authorities, particularly in the United States, recommend treatment of sexual contacts of patients with early syphilis even if the contacts are clinically and serologically normal on examination. This is justifiable, because 30 per cent of clinically normal individuals named as contacts of persons with infectious lesions of syphilis within the previous 30 days go on to develop syphilis if untreated. In general, preventive treatment is given to all sexual contacts of the past 90 days, although nearly all cases of syphilis in contacts develop within 60 days of exposure.

Jarisch-Herxheimer Reactions. Up to 60 per cent of patients with early syphilis, and a significant proportion of patients with later stages of syphilis, experience a transient febrile reaction after therapy for syphilis. This usually occurs in the first few hours after therapy, peaks at 6 to 8 hours, and disappears within 12 to 24 hours of therapy. Temperature elevation is usually low grade, and there is often associated myalgia, headache, and malaise. The skin lesions of secondary syphilis are often exacerbated during the Herxheimer reaction, and cutaneous lesions that were not visible may become visible. It is usually of no clinical significance and may be treated with salicylates in most cases. In patients with syphilis of the coronary ostia or of the optic nerve, there is a theoretic risk that local inflammation coincident with the Herxheimer reaction could precipitate serious damage. This is the subject of much discussion in the old literature, but there is little current evidence that "local Herxheimer rections" constitute a significant risk to the patient. Corticosteroids have been used to prevent adverse effects of the Herxheimer reaction, but there is no evidence that they are

TABLE 340–5. EFFECT OF RECOMMENDED TREATMENT SCHEDULES ON SEROLOGIC TESTS FOR SYPHILIS

Stage of Disease When Treated	Time to Follow-up (years)	Frequency of Positive Serologic Tests (%)	
		VDRL†	FTA-ABS
Primary (seropositive)*	2	0–3‡	>80
Secondary	2	0–24	>80
Late latent or tertiary	5–13	56–70	98

*Patients with primary syphilis and a positive VDRL test.

†Positive VDRL tests after treatment are almost always *low titer* unless reinfection or relapse has occurred.

‡The range of results reflects inclusion of data from several series, using different patient selection and treatment regimens.

clinically beneficial (other than reducing fever) or necessary. Institution of treatment with small doses of penicillin does not prevent the Herxheimer reaction.

The pathogenesis of the Herxheimer reaction is unclear. It may be due to liberation of antigens from the spirochetes. There is evidence of activation of the complement cascade, including transient consumption of C3, C4, C6, and C7, and of transient decrease in treponemal antibodies coincident with the Herxheimer reaction. There is also evidence for endotoxemia, obtained by positive limulus amebocyte gelatin tests, at the time of the Herxheimer reaction, although *T. pallidum* does not contain biologically active endotoxin. These seemingly contradictory observations could be explained if the reaction resulted in release of endogenous endotoxin from the gut.

Persistence of Treponemes After Treatment. Studies in humans and in rabbits have shown that spiral forms may be visualized by silver stains in lymph nodes after effective treatment. Living virulent treponemes have occasionally been recovered by rabbit inoculation from lymph nodes, CSF, or ocular fluids after effective treatment has been given. These documented cases of treponemal persistence are very rare, however. At present there is little reason to worry about persistence of virulent treponemes after therapy with penicillin, with the possible exception of central nervous system syphilis, which needs further evaluation. There is no evidence for selection of penicillin-resistant mutants of *T. pallidum* to date.

PROSPECTS FOR PREVENTION. Solid immunity develops in rabbits following prolonged infection with virulent *T. pallidum.* It has not yet been possible to transfer immunity passively in laboratory animals by either immune serum or immune lymphocytes alone, suggesting that both cellular and humoral systems are necessary for immunity. Rabbits have been effectively immunized with multiple injections of treponemes that have been rendered avirulent by irradiation or by exposure to cold. However, a very large number of injections and a large mass of treponemes are necessary to effect immunity in the laboratory animal. For this reason and since *T. pallidum* cannot yet be grown in a virulent state in cell-free medium, there is no immediate prospect for a vaccine. However, significant immunity does develop in humans after prolonged infection. For the present, control depends entirely on clinical awareness on the part of physicians, adequate reporting to public health authorities, and vigorous application of epidemiologic investigation and preventive treatment of sexual contacts.

Drusin LM, Singer C, Valenti AJ, et al.: Infectious syphilis mimicking neoplastic disease. Arch Intern Med 137:156, 1977. *A fascinating and frightening account of diagnostic problems caused by oral, rectal, or lymphatic syphilis, nearly leading to cancer surgery.*

Feher J, Somogyi T, Timmer M, et al.: Early syphilitic hepatitis. Lancet 2:896, 1975. *A description of the frequency and histology of early syphilitic hepatitis.*

Fischer A, Kristensen JK, Husfelt V: Tertiary syphilis in Denmark 1961–1970. A description of 105 cases not previously diagnosed or specifically treated. Acta Dermatovener 56:485, 1975. *One of few studies of the prevalence of newly diagnosed late syphilis in the antibiotic era.*

Gamble CN, Reardan JB: Immunopathogenesis of syphilitic glomerulonephritis: Elution of antitreponemal antibody from glomerular immune-complex deposits. N Engl J Med 292:449, 1975. *Clear evidence for an immune-complex etiology of syphilitic nephrosis.*

Gjestland T: The Oslo study of untreated syphilis: An epidemiologic investigation of the natural course of the syphilitic infection based upon a re-study of the Boeck-Bruusgaard material. Acta Derm Venereol 35:Suppl 34, 1955. *A medical classic, in which the long-term course of untreated syphilis is evaluated.*

Holmes KK, Märdh P-A, Sparling PF, et al.: Sexually Transmitted Diseases, 2nd ed. New York, McGraw-Hill Book Company, 1990. *The definitive text on sexually transmitted diseases.*

Lee TJ, Sparling PF: Syphilis. An algorithm. JAMA 242:1187, 1979. *An algorithm for management of patients who present with a positive VDRL or similar test.*

Lugar A, Schmidt B, Spendlingwimmer I, et al.: Recent observations on the serology of syphilis. Br J Vener Dis 56:12, 1980. *A current evaluation of the merits of serologic tests for syphilis.*

Magnuson HJ, Thomas EW, Olansky S, et al.: Inoculation syphilis in human volunteers. Medicine 35:33, 1956. *A classic paper, in which prison volunteers were inoculated with virulent T. pallidum. Immunity to inoculation syphilis was observed only in individuals who had congenital or late syphilis.*

Raskind MA, Eisdorfer C: Screening for syphilis in an aged psychiatrically impaired population. West J Med 125:361, 1976. *Syphilitic disease of the central nervous system may be more prevalent than hospital surveys suggest.*

Tramont EC: Persistence of *Treponema pallidum* following penicillin G therapy: Report of two cases. JAMA 236:2206. *At least one of the cases of neurosyphilis probably was a true penicillin treatment failure.*

Wilner E, Brody JA: Prognosis of general paresis after treatment. Lancet 2:1370, 1968. *Neurosyphilis frequently shows clinical progression despite what is probably adequate therapy.*

Spirochetal Diseases Other Than Syphilis

341 Nonsyphilitic Treponematoses*

Thomas Butler

DEFINITION. The nonsyphilitic treponematoses are the skin diseases called *yaws, bejel,* and *pinta.* They occur predominantly in tropical regions and are transmitted by skin contact with infected persons. Disfiguring ulcerations of the skin may be produced, and invasion of bone and other tissues has been described. Treatment with benzathine penicillin G is effective, and the World Health Organization has carried out extensive treatment campaigns in endemic areas.

ETIOLOGY. Yaws is caused by *Treponema pertenue;* pinta is caused by *T. carateum;* and bejel is caused by a treponeme that is indistinguishable from other species. Like *T. pallidum,* these treponemes are spirochetal bacteria with helical structures and measure about 0.2 μ in diameter and 10 μ in length. They are visible by darkfield microscopy but cannot be cultivated in vitro.

DISTRIBUTION AND EPIDEMIOLOGY. Yaws is prevalent in rural areas of tropical Africa, the Americas, Southeast Asia, and Oceania. The highest incidence is in children between ages 2 and 5 years. Bejel occurs in Africa, in Eastern Mediterranean countries, on the Arabian peninsula, in Central Asia, and in Australia. It is most prevalent in arid regions. Pinta occurs in rural areas of tropical Central and South America. Pinta affects mostly older children and adolescents. Humans are the only known carriers of the nonsyphilitic treponematoses. The portal of entry is the skin, which must be broken, as by a scratch or insect bite, before the spirochete can enter. Transmission is believed to occur by contacting the skin directly or indirectly by contaminated hands or fomites and is facilitated by conditions of poor personal hygiene and crowding.

CLINICAL FEATURES. *Yaws* produces a skin papule at the site of inoculation after an incubation period of 3 to 4 weeks. The most common sites are the legs and buttocks. The papule enlarges, ulcerates, and develops a serous crust from which treponemes can be recovered. Regional lymphadenitis may accompany the papule, which will heal spontaneously within 6 months. A generalized secondary rash will occur before or after healing of the initial lesion, and these rashes are also papular and often covered with brown crusts. Relapsing crops of lesions can occur. Papillomas may result, and the plantar surfaces of the feet are involved with hyperkeratotic lesions. Periostitis of long bones leads to tender bones, and fever may be present. Relapsing lesions may occur over several years, resulting in chronic ulcerations and destructive gummatous lesions affecting the skin and bones.

Bejel produces patches on the mucous membranes of the oral cavity and pharynx and can cause split papules at the mucocutaneous junction of the oral angles. Anal, genital, and other

---

*The author acknowledges the contribution of Dr. Thorstein Guthe on this subject in the 16th edition of the *Cecil Textbook of Medicine,* pages 1584–1589, and refers the interested reader to this more complete treatment of the subject, which includes photographs of skin lesions.

intertriginous skin areas can be affected by lesions that resemble secondary syphilis. Regional lymphadenitis is common, and generalized rashes are rare. Healing of these early lesions is followed by latency manifested by seropositivity or by late lesions that resemble tertiary syphilis. These include nodular ulcers of skin, deformities of bones, and gummatous lesions that can perforate the palate.

Pinta starts similarly as a cutaneous papule with regional lymphadenitis that is followed by a generalized maculopapular eruption. One to 3 years after healing of the initial lesion, large hyperpigmented macules that are brown or blue develop and subsequently lose their pigment and become white. The time required for lesions to pass through these stages varies, so that the same patient may have coexisting areas of increased pigment and loss of pigment.

DIAGNOSIS. By darkfield microscopy, the causative spirochetes from early skin lesions can be observed directly. Spirochetes have been demonstrated also in lymph node aspirates. Serologic tests for syphilis detect cross-reacting antibodies in these diseases. The VDRL test, the serologic test for syphilis, and the fluorescent treponemal antibody absorption test all give positive results if serum is taken at least 2 weeks after the appearance of initial lesions.

TREATMENT AND PROGNOSIS. Long-acting benzathine penicillin G given as 1.2 million units intramuscularly is the preferred treatment for patients with early lesions. For patients with late manifestations, this therapy should be repeated twice at approximately 7-day intervals. The early lesions heal rapidly, and most seropositive patients convert to seronegative status. Late destructive lesions take longer to show improvement.

PREVENTION. The prevalence of these diseases has been reduced in several areas of the world by mass treatment campaigns using penicillin. The World Health Organization has treated about 53 million cases of yaws and 350,000 cases of pinta in the field with good results. These campaigns, however, are not adequate to eradicate the disease. It has been suggested that reduction in transmission requires improvements in the sanitation and economic standards of people living in endemic areas.

Guthe T: Clinical serological and epidemiological features of framboesia tropica (yaws) and its control in rural communities. Acta Dermatovener 49:343, 1969.
Hackett CJ, Lowenthal LJA: Differential Diagnosis of Yaws. WHO Monograph Series No. 45. Geneva, WHO, 1960.
Kantor I, Wilentz JM, Berger BB: Yaws. Arch Dermatol 103:546, 1971.
Vorst FA: Clinical diagnosis and changing manifestations of treponemal infection. Rev Infect Dis 7(Suppl 2):S327, 1985. *This paper shows that yaws in populations after mass treatment with penicillin assumes attenuated forms characterized by shorter duration of papillomas and lower antibody titers.*

342 Relapsing Fever

Thomas Butler

DEFINITION. Relapsing fever is an acute febrile illness caused by blood spirochetes belonging to *Borrelia* species. The two major kinds of relapsing fever are *louse-borne relapsing fever*, for which the human is the reservoir and the body louse is the vector, and *tick-borne relapsing fever*, for which rodents and other animals are the predominant reservoirs and ticks are the vectors. The clinical course consists of one or more phases of fever and spirochetemia, which last for several days and are separated by afebrile intervals of several days without spirochetemia. The relapsing fevers are effectively treated with antibiotics, but after treatment patients often experience a Jarisch-Herxheimer–like reaction.

ETIOLOGY. Relapsing fevers are caused by spirochetes of *Borrelia* species, which belong to the order of bacteria Spirochaetales. *Borrelia* species differ from the other two genera of pathogenic spirochetes, *Leptospira* and *Treponema*, by structure, biochemical characteristics, and antigenic determinants. *Borrelia* spirochetes are spiral organisms that measure 5 to 40 μ in length and about 0.5 μ in diameter. They are too thin to be seen reliably by light microscopy of wet preparations, but they are visible by darkfield or phase contrast microscopy and display corkscrew-like motility. They are stainable with aniline dyes, such as Wright's or Giemsa's stains, and can be visualized well in tissue by the application of silver stains. Between the cell wall and the cytoplasmic membrane there are 15 to 20 flagella, which are anchored to the ends of the spirochete and wrap around its body until they meet at the middle region. *Borrelia* spirochetes are microaerophilic and fermentative in their growth characteristics. They require long-chain fatty acids for growth and are cultivable in Kelly's medium.

The species names of the tick-borne *Borrelia* are derived from the species names of *Ornithodorus* tick vectors that carry them. The more common ones in North America are *B. turicatae*, *B. hermsii*, and *B. parkeri* and in Africa *B. duttonii*. Louse-borne disease is caused solely by *B. recurrentis*. *Borrelia* spirochetes produce fever when injected into rabbits but do not possess endotoxin.

The relapsing feature of *Borrelia* infection has been attributed to antigenic variation in the infecting population of spirochetes. In experimental infections of rats with *B. hermsii*, three separate serotypes emerged sequentially during relapses, and specific antibody appeared in response to each of the antigenic variants.

DISTRIBUTION AND EPIDEMIOLOGY. The two types of relapsing fever, louse-borne and tick-borne, differ so much in their epidemiology that they must be considered separately. *Epidemic relapsing fever* refers to the louse-borne kind and *endemic* or *sporadic relapsing fever* to the tick-borne variety. For louse-borne relapsing fever, the cycle of infection is from person to person via the louse. Body lice acquire the infection by feeding on a spirochetemic person, and they remain infected for their entire lifespan, which is 10 to 61 days under laboratory conditions. Spirochetes do not reach the salivary glands or ovaries of the lice. Therefore, infection is not transmitted to humans by bites of lice. Infection is believed to be transmitted to humans by the crushing of lice on the skin, which allows liberated spirochetes to penetrate through a bite site or through intact skin.

The persons at greatest risk for acquiring louse-borne relapsing fever are those living under crowded, unhygienic conditions that favor infestation with body lice. Migrant workers and soldiers in war are particularly prone to develop this infection. Males are at much greater risk than females. A strain-specific, short-lived acquired immunity develops following infection. This immunity helps to explain why migrant workers coming into an endemic area are more susceptible to infection than are the permanent inhabitants. In some endemic areas, such as Addis Ababa, Ethiopia, there is an increased incidence during the cool winter season when people wear heavier clothing that becomes louse infested.

The vectors for tick-borne relapsing fever are argasid soft ticks of the genus *Ornithodorus*. The major reservoirs of tick-borne relapsing fever are wild rodents, including squirrels, deer mice, rats, chipmunks, and rabbits. The infection is passed between the reservoir animals by tick bites, and humans are accidental hosts when they come into contact with infected animal ticks.

Ticks acquire the infection by biting and sucking blood from a spirochetemic animal. Transmission of the infection to animals or to humans follows injection of infected saliva through the bite site or intact skin. Ticks are more durable vectors than body lice, being able to survive as long as 15 years between blood meals and to harbor viable spirochetes for years. In addition, female ticks can pass *Borrelia* spirochetes transovarially to their offspring, thus permitting ticks to be infective without having previously bitten an infected host.

Persons at greatest risk of infection are those who come in contact with infected ticks from wild rodents. The largest outbreak of tick-borne relapsing fever occurred in 62 campers and employees in the National Park at the Northern Rim of the Grand Canyon, Arizona, in 1973. They had all slept in log cabins that were inhabited by wild rodents. Another outbreak in Washington State affected 42 boy scouts who also camped in a log cabin.

CLINICAL SYNDROMES AND PATHOGENESIS. Following an incubation period of 4 to 18 days after exposure to ticks or lice, illness begins abruptly with shaking chills, fever, headache, and fatigue. Most patients have these symptoms almost continuously throughout the day, whereas some patients report intermittent symptoms several times a day. Patients complain frequently of myalgias, arthralgia, anorexia, dry cough, and abdominal pains. These symptoms are usually mild on the first day of illness and increase in intensity over a few days, until they result in prostration and a visit to a physician. The nonspecific nature of the symptoms leads the patient or the physician to believe the illness is flulike.

The temperature is elevated in the range of 38.5° to 40°C, and the pulse rate is increased. The blood pressure is lowered to about 105/70 mm Hg. Patients appear lethargic or may be delirious. Common physical signs are conjunctival injection, petechial skin rash that is more apparent on the trunk than on the extremities, and palpable liver and spleen. Jaundice is occasionally present. Generalized muscle weakness is common. Some patients have nuchal rigidity.

The white blood cell count is usually normal, with increased band forms and decreased eosinophils. The platelet counts are often less than 50,000 per cubic millimeter, and there may be prolongation of prothrombin and partial thromboplastin times. Liver function test results are frequently abnormal, with elevations in concentrations of serum alanine aminotransferase and bilirubin that are evenly divided between the conjugated and unconjugated fractions. Renal function studies often show mild abnormalities of the serum urea nitrogen and creatinine values, and patients may have proteinuria and microscopic hematuria.

DIAGNOSIS. The diagnosis of relapsing fever depends on the demonstration of spirochetemia. In most patients, this is readily accomplished by obtaining peripheral blood by either fingerstick or venipuncture methods and preparing a thin film on a microscope slide. *Borrelia* spirochetes are stained blue by aniline dyes. Thus a routine blood smear stained with Wright's or Giemsa's stain is adequate. Blood smears, thin or thick, prepared for examination for malaria parasites, are also satisfactory. Spirochetes lie in the plasma spaces between blood cells or may overlie the blood cells. Febrile patients with relapsing fever typically have large numbers of spirochetes in the blood, approximately 10^6 to 10^8 per milliliter, or several per high-power field. Patients who are afebrile in the interval between relapses have smears negative for *Borrelia* and should be re-examined when the fever reappears. Spirochetemia also may be detected by darkfield or phase contrast microscopy. A drop of fresh blood is diluted with another drop of 0.9 per cent NaCl and overlaid with a coverslip. Spirochetes are readily identified by their characteristic rotational motility.

TREATMENT AND PROGNOSIS. The relapsing fevers are effectively treated with tetracycline and erythromycin. Tetracycline is the treatment of choice except in children less than 7 years old and in pregnant women, in whom tetracycline may stain developing fetal teeth. Recent studies in Ethiopia indicate that a single oral dose of tetracycline, 500 mg, is as effective in clearing spirochetemia and preventing relapse as a longer course of treatment. Erythromycin, 500 mg given orally as a single dose, is equally effective and is a satisfactory alternative to tetracycline. For patients unable to take oral medication, intravenous injections of 250 mg of tetracycline or erythromycin are curative. For children weighing less than 30 kg, the dosage of tetracycline or erythromycin should be reduced to approximately 10 mg per kilogram. Penicillin G has been used to treat relapsing fever, but its use has been associated with slow clearance of spirochetes and relapses following treatment.

In most patients with louse-borne relapsing fever and in some with tick-borne relapsing fever, a distressing Jarisch-Herxheimer–like reaction occurs within 4 hours after antibiotic treatment. During the reaction, the patient is extremely uncomfortable, feeling very cold with severe headache and myalgia. The blood leukocyte and platelet counts sharply decrease, and spirochetes disappear from the plasma. The patient may require intravenous infusions of 0.9 per cent NaCl to maintain adequate blood pressure. Over several hours, the temperature declines and the patient's condition improves. Attempts to ameliorate the severity of the reaction by giving antipyretic or anti-inflammatory drugs have not been entirely successful. The best approach is to anticipate the reaction and to provide intensive nursing care and intravenous fluid support during the first day of treatment.

The prognosis is favorable for complete recovery in 95 per cent or more of treated cases of relapsing fever. Bad prognostic signs are the presence of jaundice, high spirochete counts in the blood,

and hypotension. The prognosis of untreated disease is grave in the case of louse-borne relapsing fever, for which mortality rates of 40 per cent have been reported during recent epidemics. Causes of death include liver failure, cerebral hemorrhage, and cardiac arrhythmia due to myocarditis. Untreated patients experience relapses. In louse-borne relapsing fever, the first attack lasts about 6 days and is followed by an afebrile period of about 9 days. There usually is one relapse, which lasts only about 2 days. In tick-borne relapsing fever, the first attack lasts about 3 days and is followed by an interval of about 7 days, after which an average of three relapses occur, each lasting about 2 days. Relapses are usually milder in intensity than the first attacks.

PREVENTION. Available approaches for the control of relapsing fevers include the detection and treatment of human cases, vector control, rodent control, and public health education. Delousing of clothing and bodies with insecticides such as DDT (chlorophenothane) can be employed, as can the application of insect repellents. In known epidemic situations, prophylactic antibiotics are a temporary measure to contain spread of infection to persons at high risk. For tick-borne relapsing fever, campers and hikers going into endemic areas should be advised to avoid cabins that are inhabited by rodents and ticks and to apply topical tick repellents to the skin.

Barbour AG, Hayes SF: Biology of *Borrelia* species. Microbiol Rev 50:381, 1986. *Review of recent knowledge about this genus of spirochetes and similarity of relapsing fever and Lyme disease.*

Butler T: Relapsing fever: New lessons about antibiotic action. Ann Intern Med 102:397, 1985. *Reviews clinical research in Ethiopia relating to mechanisms of Jarisch-Herxheimer reaction.*

Horton JM, Blaser MJ: The spectrum of relapsing fever in the Rocky Mountains. Arch Intern Med 145:871, 1985. *This report of 23 recent cases indicated an increased incidence of the disease in Colorado. Severe Jarisch-Herxheimer reactions occurred in four patients.*

343 Lyme Disease

Stephen E. Malawista

Lyme disease is a tick-borne inflammatory disorder caused by a newly recognized spirochete, *Borrelia burgdorferi*. Its clinical hallmark is an early expanding skin lesion, *erythema chronicum migrans* (ECM), which may be followed weeks to months later by neurologic, cardiac, or joint abnormalities. Symptoms may refer to any one of these four systems alone or in combination. All stages of Lyme disease may respond to antibiotics, but treatment of early disease is the most successful. Although cases of the illness are concentrated in certain endemic areas, foci of Lyme disease are widely distributed within the United States and Europe.

"Lyme arthritis" was recognized in November 1975 because of unusual geographic clustering of children with inflammatory arthropathy in the region of Lyme, Connecticut. It soon became clear that this was a multisystem disorder (Lyme *disease*) occurring at any age, in both sexes, and often preceded by a characteristic expanding skin lesion, *erythema chronicum migrans* (ECM). In Europe ECM had been associated with the bite of the sheep tick, *Ixodes ricinus*, and with tick-borne meningopolyneuritis. In the Lyme region, a closely related deer tick, *Ixodes dammini*, was implicated as the principal disease vector on epidemiologic grounds. In 1982, Burgdorfer and associates isolated a spirochete, now called *Borrelia burgdorferi*, from *Ixodes dammini* and linked it serologically to patients with Lyme disease. It was soon recovered from patient specimens.

DISTRIBUTION AND EPIDEMIOLOGY. Lyme disease is widespread. In the United States there are three distinct foci: the Northeast from Massachusetts to Maryland, the Midwest in Wisconsin and Minnesota, and the West in California, southern Oregon, and western Nevada. However, the illness has been reported in 43 states, as well as throughout Europe and Asia. The earliest known cases in the United States occurred on Cape Cod in 1962 and in Lyme, Connecticut, in 1965; annual cases now number in the thousands. Disease can occur at any age and in either sex. Onset of illness is generally between May 1 and November 30, with the peak in June and July.

The primary vectors of Lyme disease are tiny ixodid ticks. Major foci of disease correspond to the distribution of *I. dammini* (Northeast, Midwest), *I. pacificus* (West), *I. ricinus* (Europe, western USSR), and *I. persulcatus* (Asian USSR, China, Japan), but other vectors, including the Lone Star tick, *Amblyomma americanum*, are likely in some areas. In one United States study, 31 per cent of 314 patients recalled a tick bite at the skin site where ECM developed days to weeks later. The six ticks that were saved were invariably nymphal *I. dammini*, whose peak questing period is May through July; the nymphal stage is primarily responsible for transmission of disease. Preferred hosts for *I. dammini* nymphs are white-footed mice and, for adults, white-tailed deer, in whose fur they mate.

The rising incidence of Lyme disease in recent years in the United States may be explained by multiple factors including an increase in the numbers of ixodid ticks, the outward migration of residential areas into previously rural woodlands (habitats favored by ixodid ticks and their hosts), an exploding deer population, and increased recognition.

In areas endemic for Lyme disease, the prevalence of *B. burgdorferi* in nymphal *I. dammini* ranges from about 20 per cent to over 60 per cent (cf. *I. pacificus*, 1 to 3 per cent). The organism has been isolated, or specific antibody found, in blood and tissues of a wide variety of large and small animals, including domestic dogs and birds. Indiscriminate feeding on a variety of animals by immature *I. dammini* may favor the spread of infection.

PATHOGENESIS. Recovery of *B. burgdorferi* is straightforward from the tick but difficult from patients, in part because of a relative paucity of organisms in specimens of tissue and fluids from the latter. Nevertheless, rare positive cultures are reported at all stages of the illness—from blood (early), *erythema chronicum migrans*, secondary annular lesions, meningitic cerebrospinal fluid, heart, joint fluid, and even a late skin lesion, *acrodermatitis chronica atrophicans*, that had been present for 10 years. Spirochetes have been identified by silver stain or by immunofluorescence in some histologic sections of ECM and rarely of secondary annular lesions, synovium, brain, eye, heart, striated muscle, liver, spleen, kidney, and bone marrow.

From these data, combined with clinical (see below) and epidemiologic features of Lyme disease, the following pathogenetic sequence is likely. *B. burgdorferi* is transmitted to the skin of the host via the tick vector. After an incubation period of 3 to 32 days, the organism migrates outward in the skin (ECM), spreads in lymph (regional adenopathy), or disseminates in blood to organs (e.g., central nervous system, joints, heart, and presumably liver and spleen) or other skin sites (secondary annular lesions; see below). Maternal-fetal transmission is distinctly uncommon. Although organisms are hard to find in later stages of Lyme disease, it is likely that persistent live spirochetes are driving the illness throughout its course. Evidence for this interpretation includes the responsiveness of many patients to antibiotics, the rare sightings of spirochetes in affected tissues, and an expansion of the antibody response to additional spirochetal antigens over time.

Lyme disease is associated with characteristic immune abnormalities. At disease onset (ECM), almost all patients have evidence of circulating immune complexes. At that time, the findings of elevated serum immunoglobulin M (IgM) levels and cryoglobulins containing IgM predict subsequent nervous system, heart, or joint involvement—i.e., early humoral findings have prognostic significance. Serial determinations of serum IgM are often the single most helpful laboratory indicator of disease activity. These abnormalities tend to persist during neurologic or cardiac involvement. Later in the illness, when arthritis is present, serum IgM levels are more often normal. By then, immune complexes are usually lacking in serum but are present uniformly in joint fluid, where their titers correlate positively with the local concentration of polymorphonuclear leukocytes. Mononuclear cells from peripheral blood increase their antigen-specific proliferative response as the disease progresses, but the greatest reactivity to antigen is seen in cells from inflamed joints. Adjacent to that joint fluid, one sees on biopsy a proliferative synovium often replete with lymphocytes and plasma cells that are presumably capable of producing immunoglobulin locally. Thus, an initially disseminated, immune-mediated inflammatory disorder becomes in some patients localized and propagated in joints.

In addition to factors related to the pathogenicity of specific isolates of *B. burgdorferi*, immunogenetic make-up may play a role in whether an infected individual is able to rid himself of spirochetes. Patients with chronic arthritis have been reported to have an increased frequency of the B-cell alloantigen HLA DR4 or DR2, and individuals with another late manifestation, *acrodermatitis chronica atrophicans*, have an increased frequency of DR2.

CLINICAL CHARACTERISTICS. Lyme disease is conveniently divided into three clinical stages, but the stages may overlap, most patients do not exhibit all of them, and, in fact, seroconversion can occur in asymptomatic individuals. The illness usually begins with ECM and associated symptoms (stage 1), sometimes followed weeks to months later by neurologic or cardiac abnormalities (stage 2) and weeks to years later by arthritis (stage 3). Chronic neurologic and skin involvement may also occur years after onset.

Early Manifestations. *Erythema chronicum migrans*, the unique clinical marker for Lyme disease, begins as a red macule or papule at the site where the tick vector, usually long gone, had engorged. As the area of redness expands to 15 cm or so (range, 3 to 68 cm), there is usually partial central clearing. The outer borders are red, generally flat, and without scaling. The centers are occasionally red and indurated, even vesicular or necrotic. Variations may occur—multiple rings, for example. The thigh, groin, and axilla are particularly common sites. The lesion is warm to touch, but not often sore, and is easily missed if out of sight. Routine histologic findings are nonspecific: a heavy dermal infiltrate of mononuclear cells, without epidermal change except at the site of the tick bite.

Within days of onset of ECM, one half of United States patients develop multiple annular secondary lesions (see Color Plate 10A; Table 343–1). They resemble ECM itself but are generally smaller, migrate less, and lack indurated centers; they are not associated with the sites of previous tick bites. Individual lesions may come and go, and their borders sometimes merge. Other occasional skin lesions are noted in Table 343–1. In addition, benign lymphocytoma cutis has been reported in Europe. *Erythema chronicum migrans* and secondary lesions fade in 3 to 4 weeks (range, 1 day to 14 months). They may recur.

Skin involvement is often accompanied by flulike symptoms—malaise and fatigue, headache, fever and chills, myalgia, and arthralgia (Table 343–2). Some patients have evidence of meningeal irritation or mild encephalopathy—for example, episodic attacks of excruciating headache and neck pain, stiffness, or pressure—but typically lasting only for hours at this stage of the illness, and without spinal fluid pleocytosis or objective neurologic deficit. Except for fatigue and lethargy, which are often constant, the early signs and symptoms are typically intermittent and

TABLE 343–1. EARLY SIGNS OF LYME DISEASE

Signs	No. of Patients	
	N = 314	(%)
Erythema chronicum migrans	314	(100)*
Multiple annular lesions	150	(48)
Lymphadenopathy		
Regional	128	(41)
Generalized	63	(20)
Pain on neck flexion	52	(17)
Malar rash	41	(13)
Erythematous throat	38	(12)
Conjunctivitis	35	(11)
Right upper quadrant tenderness	24	(8)
Splenomegaly	18	(6)
Hepatomegaly	16	(5)
Muscle tenderness	12	(4)
Periorbital edema	10	(3)
Evanescent skin lesions	8	(3)
Abdominal tenderness	6	(2)
Testicular swelling	2	(1)

*Erythema chronicum migrans was required for inclusion in this study.

From Steere AC, Bartenhagen NH, Craft JE, et al.: The early clinical manifestations of Lyme disease. Ann Intern Med 99:76, 1983.

TABLE 343–2. EARLY SYMPTOMS OF LYME DISEASE

Symptoms	No. of Patients	
	N = 314	(%)
Malaise, fatigue, and lethargy	251	(80)
Headache	200	(64)
Fever and chills	185	(59)
Stiff neck	151	(48)
Arthralgias	150	(48)
Myalgias	135	(43)
Backache	81	(26)
Anorexia	73	(23)
Sore throat	53	(17)
Nausea	53	(17)
Dysesthesia	35	(11)
Vomiting	32	(10)
Abdominal pain	24	(8)
Photophobia	19	(6)
Hand stiffness	16	(5)
Dizziness	15	(5)
Cough	15	(5)
Chest pain	12	(4)
Ear pain	12	(4)
Diarrhea	6	(2)

From Steere AC, Bartenhagen NH, Craft JE, et al.: The early clinical manifestations of Lyme disease. Ann Intern Med 99:76, 1983.

changing. For example, a patient may have meningitic attacks for several days, a few days of improvement, and then the onset of migratory musculoskeletal pain. This last may involve joints (generally without swelling), tendons, bursa, muscle, and bone. The pain tends to affect only one or two sites at a time and to last a few hours to several days in a given location. The various associated symptoms may occur several days before ECM (or without it) and last for months (especially fatigue and lethargy) after the skin lesions have disappeared.

Later Manifestations. Neurologic Involvement. Within several weeks to months of the onset of illness, about 15 per cent of patients develop frank neurologic abnormalities, including meningitis, encephalitis, chorea, cranial neuritis (including bilateral facial palsy), motor and sensory radiculoneuritis, or mononeuritis multiplex, in various combinations. The usual pattern is fluctuating meningoencephalitis with superimposed cranial nerve (particularly facial) palsy and peripheral radiculoneuropathy, but Bell's palsy may occur *alone*. By now, patients with meningitic symptoms have a lymphocytic pleocytosis (about 100 cells per cubic millimeter) in cerebrospinal fluid and sometimes diffuse slowing on electroencephalogram. However, the neck is rarely stiff except on extreme flexion; Kernig's and Brudzinski's signs are absent. Neurologic abnormalities typically last for months but usually resolve completely (late neurologic complications are noted below).

Cardiac Involvement. Also within weeks to months of onset, about 8 per cent of patients develop cardiac involvement. The most common abnormality is fluctuating degrees of atrioventricular block (first-degree, Wenckebach, or complete heart block). Some patients have evidence of more diffuse cardiac involvement, including electrocardiographic changes compatible with acute myopericarditis, radionuclide evidence of mild left ventricular dysfunction, or, rarely, cardiomegaly, None has had heart murmurs. Cardiac involvement is usually brief (3 days to 6 weeks), but it may recur.

Arthritis. From weeks to as long as 2 years after the onset of illness, about 60 per cent of patients develop frank arthritis, usually characterized by intermittent attacks of asymmetric joint swelling and pain primarily in large joints, especially the knee, one or two joints at a time. Affected knees are commonly more swollen than painful, often hot, and rarely red; Baker's cysts may form and rupture early. However, both large and small joints may be affected, and a few patients have had symmetric polyarthritis. Attacks of arthritis, which generally last from weeks to months, typically recur for several years, decreasing in frequency with time. Fatigue is common with active joint involvement, but fever or other systemic symptoms at this stage are unusual. Joint fluid white cell counts vary from 500 to 110,000 cells per cubic

millimeter, with an average of about 25,000 cells per cubic millimeter, mostly polymorphonuclear leukocytes. Total protein ranges from 3 to 8 grams per deciliter. The C3 and C4 levels are generally greater than one-third, and glucose levels usually greater than two-thirds, that of serum. Rheumatoid factor and antinuclear antibody are absent.

In about 10 per cent of patients with arthritis, involvement in large joints may become chronic, with pannus formation and erosion of cartilage and bone. Synovial biopsy findings may mimic those of rheumatoid arthritis: surface deposits of fibrin, villous hypertrophy, vascular proliferation, and a heavy infiltration of mononuclear cells. In addition, there may be an obliterative endarteritis and (rarely) demonstrable spirochetes. In vitro, *B. burgdorferi* stimulates mononuclear cells to produce interleukin 1, and concentrations of this cytokine have been elevated in synovial fluid. In one patient with chronic Lyme arthritis, synovium grown in tissue culture produced large amounts of collagenase and prostaglandin E_2. Thus, in Lyme disease the joint fluid cell counts, the immune reactants (except for rheumatoid factor), the synovial histology, the amounts of synovial enzymes released, and the resulting destruction of cartilage and bone may be similar to those in rheumatoid arthritis.

Other late findings (years) associated with this infection include a chronic skin lesion—*acrodermatitis chronica atrophicans*—well known in Europe but still rare in the United States. One sees violaceous infiltrated plaques or nodules, especially on extensor surfaces, that eventually become atrophic. Uncommon late chronic neurologic disease includes transverse myelitis, diffuse sensory axonal neuropathy, and demyelinating lesions of the central nervous system. Mild memory impairment, subtle mood changes, and chronic fatigue states may also occur.

LABORATORY TEST RESULTS. The diagnosis of Lyme disease is based on the recognition of clinical features of the illness in a patient with a history of possible exposure to the causative organism. Culture of *B. burgdorferi* from patients is definitive but has rarely been successful except from skin biopsy specimens. Recently, the organism was isolated from blood in a significant minority of patients with systemic manifestations of early disease (it grows very slowly). Special tissue staining techniques generally have a low yield and are not readily available. Determination of specific antibody titers is currently the most helpful adjunctive test for Lyme disease. In serum, specific IgM antibody titers against *B. burgdorferi* usually reach a peak between the third and sixth weeks after the onset of disease; specific immunoglobulin G (IgG) antibody titers rise more slowly and are generally highest months later when arthritis is present (Fig. 343–1). Individuals with Lyme disease of more than 6 weeks' duration can be expected to have elevated levels of specific antibodies. However, the tests employed are not yet standardized, and results from different commercial laboratories may vary, especially for boderline elevations. The vast majority of individuals with established Lyme arthritis have elevated specific IgG titers. This finding makes antibody titers against *B. burgdorferi* particularly useful in differentiating Lyme disease from other rheumatic syndromes, especially when ECM is missed, forgotten, or absent. This antibody cross-reacts with other spirochetes, including *Treponema pallidum*, but patients with Lyme disease do not have positive VDRL test results.

Other tests under development seek to identify spirochetal material in host fluids or tissues. They include a test for spirochetal protein in urine and use of the polymerase chain reaction to detect spirochetal DNA in host material; neither has been perfected for clinical use as of this writing.

The most common nonspecific laboratory abnormalities, particularly early in the illness, are a high erythrocyte sedimentation rate, an elevated serum IgM level, or an increased serum glutamic-oxaloacetic transaminase (SGOT) level. The enzyme levels generally return to normal within several weeks. Patients may be mildly anemic early in the illness and occasionally have elevated white cell counts with shifts to the left in the differential count. A few patients have had microscopic hematuria, sometimes with mild proteinuria (dipstick); values for creatinine and blood urea nitrogen have been normal. Throughout the illness, serum C3 and C4 levels are generally normal or elevated. Rheumatoid factor and antinuclear antibodies are usually absent.

DIFFERENTIAL DIAGNOSIS. *Erythema chronicum migrans* is the unique herald lesion of Lyme disease (see Color Plate

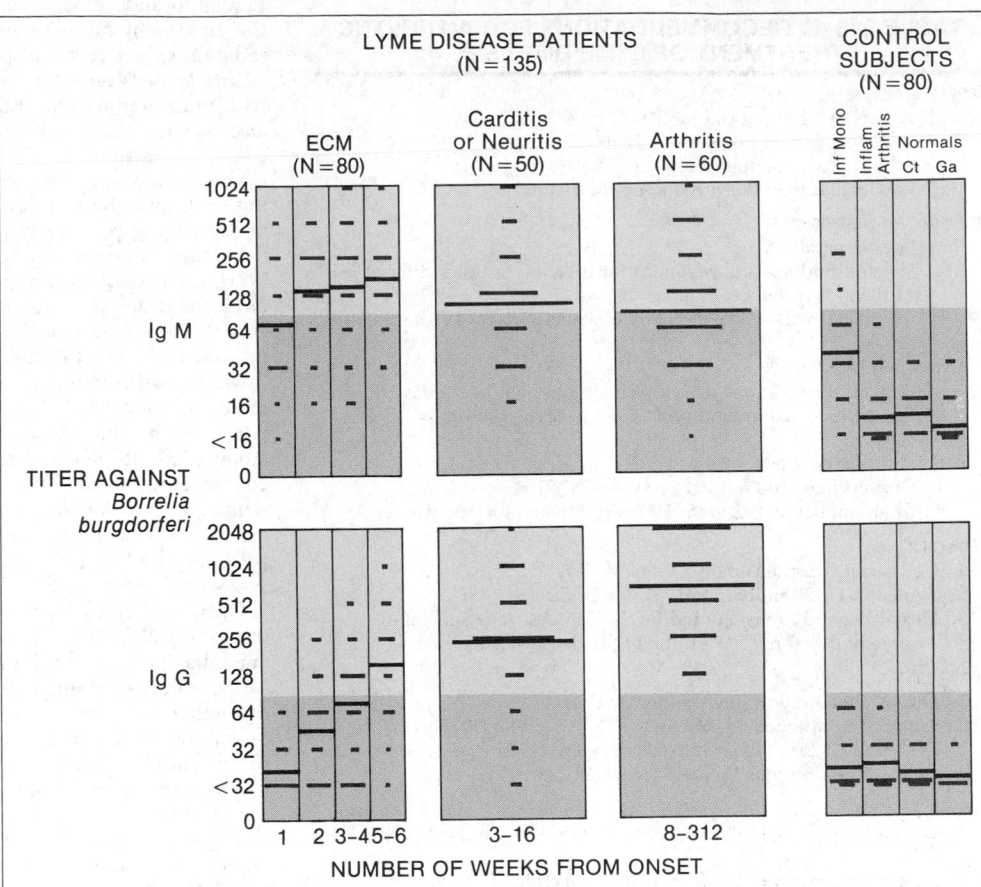

FIGURE 343–1. Antibody titers against *Borrelia burgdorferi* are shown in serum samples from 135 patients with different clinical manifestations of Lyme disease, and from 80 control subjects with infectious mononucleosis, inflammatory arthritis, or no disease (titers determined by indirect immunofluorescence). The black bar shows the geometric mean titer for each group; the pink shaded areas indicate the range of values generally observed in control subjects. Note that all patients with Lyme arthritis have elevated IgG antibody titers. (Adapted from Steere AC, Grodzicki RL, Kornblatt AN, et al: The spirochetal etiology of Lyme disease. N Engl J Med 308:733–740, 1983. Reprinted by permission of the New England Journal of Medicine.)

10A). When present in its classic form, there is little else that might be confused with it. However, some patients are not aware of having had ECM, and in others, its appearance is not always characteristic. Secondary lesions might suggest *erythema multiforme*, but blistering, mucosal lesions, and involvement of the palms and soles are not features of Lyme disease. Malar rash may suggest systemic lupus erythematosus; an urticarial rash, hepatitis B infection or serum sickness. Evanescent blotches and circles may resemble *erythema marginatum*, but those of Lyme disease do not expand.

Early flulike symptoms may be misleading, especially when *erythema chronicum migrans* is absent or missed or is not the first manifestation. Severe headache and stiff neck may suggest aseptic meningitis; abdominal symptoms, hepatitis; and generalized tender lymphadenopathy and splenomegaly, infectious mononucleosis. As in the last infection, profound fatigue in Lyme disease may be a major and persistent complaint.

In later stages, Lyme disease may mimic other immune-mediated disorders. Like rheumatic fever, Lyme disease may be associated with sore throat followed by migratory polyarthritis and carditis, but without evidence of valvular involvement or of a preceding streptococcal infection. Migratory pain in tendons and joints may also suggest disseminated gonococcal disease. An isolated facial weakness may mimic Bell's palsy of other causes. Late neurologic involvement may suggest multiple sclerosis (transverse myelitis), Guillain-Barré syndrome (symmetric peripheral neuropathy), primary psychosis, or brain tumor. In adults with Lyme arthritis, the large knee effusions can resemble those in Reiter's syndrome, and the occasional symmetric polyarthritis, that of rheumatoid arthritis. In children, the attacks of arthritis, although generally shorter, may be identical to those seen in the oligoarticular form of juvenile rheumatoid arthritis, but without iridocyclitis.

TREATMENT. The major goal of therapy in Lyme disease is to eradicate the causative organism. Like other spirochetal diseases, Lyme disease is most responsive to antibiotics early in its course. Treatment regimens have evolved over time based on both controlled clinical data and on clinical experience. Because

of the difficulty in proving that bacteria have been eradicated and the common persistence of some symptoms long after treatment, the endpoint of antibiotic therapy is not always clear. The treatment regimens presented here represent guidelines that will no doubt be refined in time (Table 343–3).

Early Lyme Disease. If patients are treated early with oral antibiotics, *erythema chronicum migrans* typically resolves promptly, and major later sequelae (myocarditis, meningoencephalitis, or recurrent arthritis) usually do not occur. Prompt treatment is therefore important, even though such patients may be susceptible to reinfection. For adults, antibiotic choices in order of preference include oral doxycycline, 100 mg twice a day; amoxicillin, 500 mg three times a day; and erythromycin, 250 mg four times a day, each for 10 to 21 days depending on the rapidity of clinical response. Failures are more common with erythromycin than the other two agents. In children younger than 9 years, amoxicillin, 30 mg per kilogram per day (not less than 1 gram or more than 2 grams per day), is given in divided doses for the same period or, in cases of penicillin allergy, erythromycin, 30 mg per kilogram per day, in divided doses for 10 to 21 days.

About 10 per cent of patients with early Lyme disease experience a Jarisch-Herxheimer–like reaction (higher fever, redder rash, or greater pain) during the first 24 hours of antibiotic therapy. Whichever drug is given, 30 to 50 per cent of patients have brief (hours to days) recurrent episodes of headache, musculoskeletal pain, and fatigue which may continue for extended periods. The etiology of these symptoms is unclear at present; they may result from undegraded spirochetal antigen(s) rather than persistence of live spirochetes. It is clear, however, that the risk of delayed resolution is greatest in individuals with disseminated manifestations of disease (multiple skin lesions, headache, fever, lymphadenopathy, or Bell's palsy) prior to the institution of antibiotics.

Later Lyme Disease. For Lyme meningitis, with or without other neurologic manifestations (cranial neuropathy or radiculoneuropathy), intravenous ceftriaxone, 2 grams daily in a single dose, or intravenous penicillin G, 20 million units a day in six divided doses, each for 10 to 21 days, is effective therapy.

TABLE 343–3. RECOMMENDATIONS FOR ANTIBIOTIC TREATMENT OF LYME DISEASE*

Early Lyme disease†
1. Doxycycline, 100 mg bid for 10–21 days
2. Amoxicillin, 500 mg tid for 10–21 days
3. Erythromycin, 250 mg qid for 10–21 days
(less effective than doxycycline or amoxicillin)

Neurologic manifestations
Facial nerve paralysis
1. Isolated finding: oral regimens for early disease, used for at least 21 days, may suffice.
2. Associated with other neurologic manifestations: IV therapy (see below)
Lyme meningitis‡
1. Ceftriaxone, 2 grams daily by single dose for 14–21 days
2. Penicillin G, 20 million units daily in divided dose for 10–21 days
Possible alternatives
1. Doxycycline, 100 mg PO or IV for 14–21 days
2. Chloramphenicol, 1 gram IV every 6 hours for 10–21 days

Lyme carditis
1. Ceftriaxone, 2 grams daily IV for 14 days
2. Penicillin G, 20 million units IV for 14 days
3. Doxycycline, 100 mg PO bid for 14–21 days, may suffice§
4. Amoxicillin, 500 mg PO tid for 14–21 days, may suffice§

Lyme arthritis
1. Doxycycline, 100 mg PO bid for 30 days
2. Amoxicillin/probenecid, 500 mg each PO qid for 30 days
3. Penicillin G, 20 million units IV daily for 14–21 days
4. Ceftriaxone, 2 grams IV daily for 14–21 days

Pregnancy
1. Localized early Lyme disease: amoxicillin, 500 mg tid for 10–21 days
2. Late or disseminated Lyme disease: penicillin G, 20 million units daily for 14–21 days
3. Asymptomatic seropositivity: no treatment necessary

*These are guidelines, to be modified by new findings and to be applied always with close attention to the clinical context of individual patients.

†Shorter courses are reserved for disease that is limited to a single skin lesion only.

‡Regimens for radiculoneuropathy, peripheral neuropathy, and encephalitis are the same as those for meningitis.

§Oral regimens have been reserved for mild cardiac involvement (first-degree heart block, normal ventricular function), but there is no substantiation that more severe degrees of heart involvement require more aggressive antibiotic therapy.

Reprinted with permission from Rahn DW, Malawista SE: Lyme disease: Recommendations for diagnosis and treatment. Ann Intern Med 114:472, 1991.

Headache and stiff neck usually begin to subside by the second day of therapy and disappear by 7 to 10 days; motor deficits and radicular pain frequently require 7 to 8 weeks for complete recovery but do not require longer antibiotic courses. Possible alternative oral regimens are listed in Table 343–3. For Bell's palsy alone, oral regimens may suffice, but these patients may be at higher risk of later sequelae than are individuals with early disease without neurologic dissemination.

Despite the generally benign course of Lyme carditis in most patients, intravenous antibiotics are commonly employed for all but the mildest forms of cardiac involvement (first-degree atrioventricular block of less than 0.4 second; Table 343–3). This practice is warranted by the knowledge that *B. burgdorferi* can invade myocardium directly and by the frequency of other manifestations of dissemination in these patients. Prednisone, 40 to 60 mg a day in divided doses, has, in the past, seemed to hasten resolution of high-grade heart block, but one should hesitate to institute glucocorticoids during antibiotic administration, as they may impede eradication of infecting organisms. If second- or third-degree heart block is present, patients should be admitted to hospital for cardiac monitoring; temporary pacing is occasionally required for complete heart block.

In clinical practice, ceftriaxone (2 grams daily for 14 to 21 days) has largely replaced penicillin for the therapy of disseminated Lyme disease. Arguments in favor of this practice are a once-daily administration schedule which is amenable to outpatient intravenous antibiotic programs, and improved penetration of the cerebrospinal fluid in comparison with that noted with penicillin. Penicillin and cefotaxime have been found equally effective for the treatment of acute neurologic Lyme disease (meningitis or radiculitis) in a group of patients studied in Germany.

Late Lyme Disease. Lyme arthritis has been successfully treated with both oral and parenteral antibiotics, but failures occur with any regimen chosen. Unless central nervous system involvement coexists, first-line treatment with a month-long course of doxycycline, 100 mg twice a day, or amoxicillin plus probenecid, 500 mg each four times a day, is recommended. Roughly two thirds of patients appear to respond to these oral regimens, but the frequency of definitive cures will await long-term follow-up. During treatment, the affected joint should be kept at rest and effusions drained by needle aspiration as for any infected joint. In a double-blind placebo-controlled trial, 7 of 20 patients given intramuscular benzathine penicillin, 2.4 million units weekly for 3 weeks, were cured (mean follow-up 33 months), versus none of 20 control patients. This regimen provides low serum levels of penicillin for about 6 weeks. High-dose intravenous penicillin G (above), which yields much higher serum levels over its 10-day course, cured 11 of 20 patients, including two in whom benzathine penicillin had failed. In one comparative trial, ceftriaxone (2 grams daily for 14 days) outperformed intravenous penicillin. In patients who fail one or more courses of antibiotics, arthroscopic synovectomy can result in a long-term response and perhaps cure.

Optimal therapy for the later neurologic complications of Lyme disease is also not yet clear. The frequency of subtle chronic encephalopathy and peripheral neuropathy is debated at present. These entities, when suspected, should be carefully documented through neurologic, neuropsychological, and electrophysiologic testing before aggressive or prolonged antibiotic therapy is instituted. Although some current thinking favors longer periods of the highest tolerated oral doses of amoxicillin (with probenecid), doxycycline, or even intravenous antibiotics in difficult cases, there is no controlled experience with courses of antibiotics longer than 1 month for any manifestation of Lyme disease. The infiltrative lesions of acrodermatitis chronica atrophicans are usually cured by 3 weeks of oral phenoxymethyl penicillin, 2 to 3 grams daily in divided doses.

Pregnancy. Because the spirochetes that cause relapsing fever and syphilis can cross the placenta, there has been concern regarding this possibility in Lyme disease. Maternal-fetal transmission of *B. burgdorferi* resulting in either neonatal death or stillbirth has been reported in rare instances in which symptomatic early Lyme disease occurred early in pregnancy and was either untreated or inadequately treated. In follow-up studies conducted by the Centers for Disease Control, maternal Lyme disease was not directly implicated as a cause of fetal malformations. There have been no cases of fetal infection occurring when currently recommended antibiotic regimens for Lyme disease have been used during pregnancy. A lower threshold for initiating therapy for suspected Lyme disease in pregnancy is understandable, but women acquiring the illness during pregnancy should be reassured that the vast majority of infants born to women in these circumstances have been entirely well.

Tick Bites. A final treatment issue regards the advisability of administering antibiotics prophylactically to individuals sustaining ixodid tick bites in endemic areas. The single study completed to date has not supported this common practice. Because nymphal ixodid ticks must, in general, feed for a day or more before transmitting spirochetes (at least in mice), ticks removed prior to this time are unlikely to have transmitted *B. burgdorferi* even if infected. Tick bite sites should be observed for development of ECM and patients cautioned regarding the common associated symptoms of early Lyme disease.

Malawista SE, Steere AC, Hardin JA: Lyme disease: A unique human model for an infectious etiology of rheumatic disease. Yale J Biol Med 57:473, 1984. *The larger significance of Lyme disease, a disorder that is infectious in origin but inflammatory or "rheumatic" in expression.*

Rahn DW, Malawista SE: Lyme disease: Recommendations for diagnosis and treatment. Ann Intern Med 114:472, 1991. *Critical review of the literature supplemented by 15 years of clinical experience with this illness.*

Steere AC, Green J, Schoen RT, et al.: Successful parenteral penicillin therapy of established Lyme arthritis. N Engl J Med 312:869, 1985. *Cure by antibiotics of a rheumatoid "look-alike."*

Steere AC, Grodzicki RL, Kornblatt AN, et al.: The spirochetal etiology of Lyme disease. N Engl J Med 308:733, 1983. Borrelia *recovered from blood, ECM, and cerebrospinal fluid of patients.*

Steere AC, Malawista SE, Syndman DR, et al.: Lyme arthritis: An epidemic of oligoarticular arthritis in childen and adults in three Connecticut communities. Arthritis Rheum 20:7, 1977. *The first description of a new nosologic entity, recognized because it clusters geographically; rheumatoid arthritis does not.*

Steere AC, Pachner AR, Malawista SE: Neurologic abnormalities of Lyme disease: Successful treatment with high-dose intravenous penicillin. Ann Intern Med 99:767, 1983. *Meningitis, formerly treated with high-dose prednisone tapered over months, responds to penicillin in days.*

344 Leptospirosis

J. Bruce McClain

The term *leptospirosis* designates an infection with any serovar of *Leptospira interrogans*, regardless of the syndrome. Old names such as canicola fever, Fort Bragg fever, Weil's disease, or peapicker's disease are potentially confusing and should be avoided.

ETIOLOGY. *Leptospira* consists of three species: *interrogans*, which is pathogenic, and *biflexa* and *parva*, which are saprophytic. Serotyping and serogrouping have established over 170 serovars in the species *L. interrogans*. The proper designation of a serovar is *L. interrogans* serovar Pomona, not *L. pomona*. The latter usage, although widespread, represents serovars as species and is incorrect. The organism is a tightly coiled spirochete with one axial filament. It is gram-negative but with a diameter of 0.15 μm it is difficult to see on light microscopy and so is usually visualized by phase contrast or darkfield techniques. It is easily cultured on Fletcher's medium and is an obligate aerobe.

EPIDEMIOLOGY. Leptospirosis is a ubiquitous enzootic disease. Reservoirs of infection include rodents, skunks, foxes, domestic livestock, dogs, and frogs. Many animals exhibit a prolonged urinary shedding of the organism without clinical illness. When humans contact infected tissues, fluids, or contaminated waters they contract the illness. Transmission may occur through cuts, mucous membranes, and possibly unabraded skin. In earlier series, illness was reported associated with occupational exposure such as among sanitation, dairy, slaughterhouse, and fishing workers. The epidemiology has changed over the last 15 years owing to the advent of multiuse land development, with farmlands draining into recreational bodies of water. More recent reports indicate that at least one half of cases result from nonvocational exposure. There has been a corresponding decrease in the age of persons infected, although males still comprise 80 per cent of cases. In the United States between 50 and 150 cases are reported annually.

The national attack rate is 0.05 per 100,000, although rates as high as 1 per 100,000 occur in Hawaii. The disease is probably substantially under-reported. Leptospirosis peaks annually in the summer months and displays a 4- to 5-year periodicity in attack rate over the last 25 years.

PATHOLOGY AND PATHOGENESIS. Gross anatomic findings in patients dying from leptospirosis are (1) widespread hemorrhage in skin, mucosa, serosa, heart, lungs, spleen, liver, and kidneys; (2) hepatomegaly without prominent splenomegaly; (3) bile staining and enlargement of the heart and kidneys. Histologic examination of the liver in autopsy material shows nonspecific inflammatory changes, bile stasis, and disruption of the limiting plate. Biopsy material under light and electron microscopic examination shows similar features with less destruction of architecture.

Kidneys in autopsy series show a spectrum of changes that reflect an initial tubular injury that is acellular. As the disease progresses and antibodies appear, inflammatory changes occur that represent an overt interstitial nephritis with disruption of the tubular architecture. Biopsy series show similar changes to a lesser degree. The glomeruli have foot process fusion and mesangial hypertrophy but are otherwise spared. Leptospiras are seen in most of the renal material. Hemorrhagic manifestations are associated with areas of capillary wall damage and necrosis with perivascular round cell infiltration. Striated muscle is frequently involved with degeneration of individual fibrils and loss of architecture associated with inflammation. This pattern is considered specific for leptospirosis. The myocardium is affected with similar changes. In one fourth of autopsy cases myocarditis is listed as serious enough to be a contributing cause of death.

The mechanism by which *Leptospira* organisms cause damage to tissues is obscure. Toxic factors have been identified in culture supernatants, but organisms that do not produce some of these factors may cause serious disease. Early in the illness the evidence favors direct toxicity to certain tissues, while late in the illness damage secondary to inflammation is more pronounced.

CLINICAL FEATURES. Most natural infections appear 7 to 14 days after the exposure, although the incubation period ranges from 2 to 20 days. The length of the incubation period has no prognostic significance. Clinical findings vary among reported series, but a general description includes fever and headache, 95 per cent; myalgia and conjunctival suffusion, 80 per cent (in nonmilitary series suffusion is reported less often); gastrointestinal symptoms (nausea, vomiting, or abdominal pain), 60 per cent; cough or pharyngitis, 40 per cent; lymphadenopathy, 25 per cent; hepatomegaly, 15 per cent; rash, 10 per cent; and jaundice and gastrointestinal hemorrhage, 5 per cent each. Less commonly reported symptoms are splenomegaly, uveitis, and diarrhea. About one half of patients exhibit a "brutal beginning," with an abrupt onset of symptoms over a 1- to 2-hour period. The clinical picture that should bring leptospirosis to mind is a febrile patient with severe muscle aches and pain who is nauseated or vomiting. The presence of conjunctival suffusion may be helpful in detecting the illness in military populations. It is not conjunctivitis as seen in allergic or viral conjunctivitis but rather a *pericorneal reddening or hyperemia*. The fever is high, usually above 38°C and frequently up to 40°C, and is accompanied by chills. Headache is severe and is characterized as retro-orbital or occipital. The presence of headache, high fever, and neck stiffness or pain due to profound myalgia suggests meningitis and may necessitate a lumbar puncture. Spinal fluid is usually acellular in the first 5 to 7 days of illness, although leptospiras may be seen. With the onset of antibody in the serum, an aseptic meningitis may occur in up to 90 per cent of patients, but only one half have meningeal symptoms. Other neurologic manifestations such as changes in the level of consciousness, encephalitis, and cranial nerve palsies have been reported less often. The muscle pains and tenderness are truly remarkable. The severity of myalgia may even prevent the patient from standing. The presence of nausea, vomiting, and anorexia with abdominal tenderness caused by muscle involvement can mimic pancreatitis. Acute dilatation of the gallbladder and cholecystitis can occur in leptospirosis and make the clinical evaluation of an ill patient very difficult, especially since there is already laboratory evidence of inflammation.

The illness usually lasts 4 to 9 days. During that period all clinical findings resolve simultaneously, and both doctor and patient are surprised at how quickly the recovery has taken place and at how well the patient feels. In about 15 per cent of patients the illness persists beyond the ninth day. It rarely may last 6 to 7 weeks.

Leptospirosis is generally a monophasic illness. In a minority of patients after an initial illness there is a period of apparent recovery, after which symptoms worsen. This second phase is termed the immune phase. It lasts 2 to 4 days in most patients. It differs from initial illness in being more variable. Fever is not so high, myalgia and gastrointestinal symptoms are not so severe, but meningitis and abnormal spinal fluid and iridocyclitis are more common. The immune phase is so named because of its correlation with the onset of antibodies to leptospirosis in the blood, the disappearance of leptospiremia, and the increased positivity of urine cultures for the germ.

The term *Weil's syndrome* is applied to one pole of a continuum of illness. It is not a specific subgroup of leptospirosis; it is simply severe leptospirosis. Any of the several manifestations of Weil's syndrome may occur alone. The clinical findings of intense jaundice, mental status changes, hemorrhage, purpura or petechiae, and renal insufficiency occurring in a previously normal patient are so memorable that this syndrome stimulated the search for leptospiras. The first manifestation of severe illness is usually jaundice that develops between the fifth and ninth days. The intensity of jaundice has no prognostic significance. Renal insufficiency may develop concomitantly with jaundice. Oliguria is a grave prognostic sign. Hemorrhagic manifestations may develop: Purpura and petechiae may appear on the oral, vaginal, or conjunctival mucosa. A biphasic pattern may be seen, although the stages tend to merge into a single severe illness. Convalescence is rapid in most patients but has taken up to 10 weeks. Several reports in the Far Eastern literature describe a distinctive presentation of severe leptospirosis seen in China and Korea, where the dominant syndrome is an influenzal illness. These pneumonias may be frankly hemorrhagic.

Childhood Disease. A recent report of nine pediatric cases reiterated the close contact of children to a common reservoir such as dogs. The pediatric syndrome shares many features of adult disease but is more intense, with several atypical features such as shock, hydrops of the gallbladder, skin desquamation, and chest radiographic abnormality.

LABORATORY FEATURES. Leukocyte counts are usually below 15,000 per cubic millimeter but may be as high as 50,000 per cubic millimeter. There is almost always neutrophilia. Hematocrit is normal in anicteric illness, but in prolonged illness anemia is common. The causes of anemia are many, with blood loss, microangiopathy, and leptospiral hemolysin all implicated in clinical cases. Thrombocytopenia is seen in severe cases. Coagulation studies occasionally demonstrate a vitamin K–reversible prolongation of prothrombin time. However, this is not responsible for the hemorrhagic diathesis of severe leptospirosis. The sedimentation rate is elevated in one half of the cases.

Liver function tests reveal a mean serum glutamic-oxaloacetic transaminase/serum glutamic-pyruvate transaminase (SGOT/SGPT) elevation of 5 times normal, with occasional patients having elevations up to 20 times normal. The direct bilirubin concentration may rise as a manifestation of severe disease and may reach 64 mg per deciliter, but in most icteric cases it is below 20 mg per deciliter. The pattern is one of intrahepatic cholestasis.

Early in the illness 80 per cent of patients have abnormal urine findings, the most common of which are microscopic hematuria, pyuria, and 2+ proteinuria. Gross hematuria rarely has been reported. One fourth of patients demonstrate elevations of the blood urea nitrogen between 20 and 100 mg per deciliter. The most common electrolyte abnormality is hyperkalemia, primarily in patients with renal failure.

The chest radiograph appears abnormal in one fourth to two thirds of patients, including anicteric cases. The most common abnormality is patchy bronchopneumonia. A small pleural effusion is seen in 10 per cent of patients. Recent reports from the Far East indicate a distinctive pulmonary presentation with radiographic abnormalities in 64 per cent of cases.

Electrocardiographic abnormalities occur in 10 to 40 per cent of patients, with bradycardia and low voltage accounting for one half of abnormalities. The remainder consist of nonspecific ST-T wave changes.

Cerebrospinal fluid may be abnormal in up to 90 per cent of patients. In 70 per cent of specimens the total cell count is below 500 per cubic millimeter, with frequent presence of neutrophils. Protein ranges from 50 to 110 mg per deciliter in 80 per cent of cases. The glucose concentration is usually normal. IgM antibodies may be detected in blood by day four or five of illness in most patients.

DIAGNOSIS. A diagnosis of leptospirosis must be suspected in any patient with fever, myalgia, headache, and nausea or vomiting. The presence of conjunctival suffusion is an early and helpful sign. The most common misdiagnosis of a patient with leptospirosis is aseptic meningitis followed by viral hepatitis, viral syndrome, fever of unknown origin, bronchitis, influenza, nephritis, and rickettsiosis. The following differential points aid the clinician: (1) The myalgias of leptospirosis are not a prominent feature of viral hepatitis; (2) creatine kinase is frequently elevated in leptospirosis, and this seldom occurs in viral hepatitis; (3) liver enzyme values in viral hepatitis may average 10 to 15 times higher than normal, but the average is 5 times higher in leptospirosis; (4) conjunctival suffusion is very helpful in separating leptospirosis from other processes; (5) in the first 3 days of leptospirosis, although spirochetes are present in the cerebrospinal fluid, the cytology is usually normal; early in the course of aseptic meningitis the cytology is usually abnormal.

The diagnosis may be confirmed by culture (on Fletcher's semisolid medium) of the blood in the first week of illness or of the urine thereafter. Cultures are usually positive in 2 weeks but may take up to 8 weeks to become positive. Since leptospiras may be excreted in the urine for prolonged periods, the diagnosis may be established by urine culture in untreated patients even after clinical illness is over. Direct examination of the urine and blood is not sufficient to establish the diagnosis. Some artifacts may be mistaken for leptospiras as well as nonpathogenic spirochetes. When cultures are performed three or four times, organisms are recovered with regularity. The diagnosis may be established serologically by two methods. The macroagglutination method is a screening test that uses pooled antigens from all of the serogroups of leptospirosis. Diagnosis is made by a fourfold rise in titer. This test is broadly available but does not detect infecting serovars that are not included in the pooled test antigens. Microagglutination requires a live pathogenic leptospiral culture and therefore is performed mainly in reference laboratories. Techniques for detecting genus-specific antibody or antigen using hemolytic assays and counterimmunoelectrophoresis have been published and are available as research tools. The most promising test for early diagnosis is a genus-specific antibody detection system.

PROGNOSIS. In most untreated cases this is a nonfatal, self-limited illness. The reported mortality of leptospirosis varies greatly among series. In military populations is around 0.1 per cent. In civilian series it ranges from 5 to 10 per cent. In both military and civilian series mortality is related to age and the presence of jaundice. Thirty per cent of patients over age 60 die. Jaundiced patients have a 15 per cent mortality. The differences in mortality may have to do with the underlying health of the host and the bias toward reporting more serious cases. In the military series, involving large groups of well men, high attack rates have been documented and physicians are sensitive to the diagnosis. If the patient lives, sequelae are uncommon even in severe cases. When sequelae occur, they consist of focal cerebral or peripheral nerve deficits or ocular problems caused by persistent uveitis. Several patients have been reported with persistent renal abnormalities.

THERAPY AND PREVENTION. Antibiotics are effective in the therapy of leptospirosis, although patients have died despite therapy. Tetracycline and doxycycline (in controlled trials) are both effective in shortening the course of anicteric leptospirosis when they are given in the first 2 to 4 days of illness. Penicillin G, even given late in the course of severe leptospirosis in a blinded controlled trial, has been shown to be effective in shortening illness. Both doxycycline and penicillin prevent leptospiruria in infected patients. Chloramphenicol is not effective therapy. Although in vitro activities within the achievable levels have been demonstrated for penicillin, cephalosporins, erythromycin, gentamicin, and quinolones, they have not been studied in a controlled trial. Vancomycin and daptomycin lack activity. Ceftriaxone is effective in animal studies. The balance of therapy in leptospirosis consists of careful attention to the details of care in patients with renal, hepatic, hematologic, and central nervous system complications.

Doxycycline, 100 mg once a week, prevents leptospirosis in high-risk groups for 3 weeks. Efficacy in longer periods of exposure has not been studied. There are no licensed human vaccines, although effective animal vaccinations are available.

Feigin RD, Anderson DC: Human leptospirosis. CRC Crit Rev Clin Lab Sci 5:413, 1975. *The most comprehensive review of leptospirosis, including history, microbiology, pathogenesis, clinical findings, and therapy.*

Im J, Yeon KM, Han MC, et al.: Leptospirosis of the lung: Radiographic findings in 58 patients. AJR 152:955, 1989. *A description of radiographic findings seen in the Far Eastern pulmonary presentation of leptospirosis.*

McClain JBL, Ballou WR, Harrison SH, et al.: Doxycycline therapy of leptospirosis. Ann Intern Med 100:696, 1984. *A placebo-controlled trial of oral doxycycline in the therapy of anicteric leptospirosis.*

Takafuji ET, Kirkpatrick JW, Miller RN, et al.: An efficacy trial of doxycycline chemoprophylaxis against leptospirosis. N Engl J Med 310:497, 1984. *A placebo-controlled trial of oral doxycycline demonstrated efficacy in preventing illness in American soldiers.*

Watt G, Padre LP, Tuazon ML, et al.: Placebo-controlled trial of intravenous penicillin for severe and late leptospirosis. Lancet 1:433, 1988. *A placebo-controlled blinded trial demonstrating the effectiveness of penicillin G in patients who were ill for over 5 days with renal and hepatic impairment.*

Watt G, Padre LP, Tuazon M, et al.: Limulus lysate positivity and Herxheimer-like reactions in leptospirosis: A placebo controlled study. J Infect Dis 162:564, 1990. *A description of these reactions in treated patients.*

Diseases Caused by Chlamydiae

Walter E. Stamm

345 Introduction

Because of their obligate intracellular growth cycle, chlamydiae were originally considered large viruses and were variously called *Bedsonia* or *TRIC* (for *trachoma-inclusion conjunctivitis*) agents. These terms have been discarded, and chlamydiae now constitute a separate order (Chlamydiales), family (Chlamydiaceae), and genus (*Chlamydia*). All members of the genus are obligate intracellular pathogens, but they more closely resemble bacteria than viruses in that they possess both deoxyribonucleic acid (DNA) and ribonucleic acid (RNA), divide by binary fission, have bacterial ribosomes and a cell wall not unlike that of Enterobacteriaceae, and can be inhibited by antibiotics. Compared with other bacteria, they have a small genome of 6 to 8 × 10⁵ base pairs. They also lack adenosine triphosphate (ATP)–generating enzymes and hence depend entirely upon host cell metabolism for energy production.

The genus *Chlamydia* originally contained two species, *C. psittaci* and *C. trachomatis*. The former is a ubiquitous cause of infection in birds and lower mammals, with humans being occasional accidental hosts, while *C. trachomatis* infects humans and has no apparent natural animal hosts. Characteristically, *C. psittaci* produces long-lived, persistent infections of birds and mammals. Transmission to humans occurs via exposure to infected animal tissues or secretions. Persistent infections caused by *C. trachomatis* in humans may also be common but have been less well documented. In most of the developed world, *C. trachomatis* is transmitted sexually and from mother to infant at the time of birth. Trachoma, still endemic in arid parts of the developing world but rare in industrialized countries, spreads within families via close nonsexual contact. Recently, Grayston and colleagues described a fastidious new strain of chlamydia that was originally called the TWAR agent. Subsequent genetic studies have identified this organism as a new chlamydial species, *Chlamydia pneumoniae*. *C. pneumoniae* appears to be a common cause of both upper respiratory tract infections and pneumonia worldwide and often occurs episodically in community-wide epidemics. No animal reservoirs have been identified, and the mode of transmission is presumed to be from person to person via respiratory droplets and secretions.

All three chlamydia species possess a genus-specific, heat-stable lipopolysaccharide antigen that serves as the basis for the widely available complement fixation serologic test. Species- and immunotype-specific antigens have also been described, and the latter serve as the basis for subdividing *C. trachomatis* into 15 immunotypes using the microimmunofluorescence test of Wang and Grayston. Specific immunotypes tend to cause particular clinical syndromes. Types A, B, Ba, and C produce endemic trachoma (see Ch. 346). Types D, E, F, G, H, I, J, and K cause oculogenital infections in adults (see Ch. 335) and ocular, respiratory, and genital infections in infants. Types L1, L2, and L3 produce lymphogranuloma venereum (LGV) (see Ch. 337) and proctocolitis, primarily in homosexual men (see Ch. 103). LGV strains of *C. trachomatis* possess properties that distinguish them from non-LGV strains biologically, including more efficient cell entry and cell-to-cell infectivity in tissue culture, as well as increased mouse lethality upon intracerebral injection. Only one serovar of the new species, *C. pneumoniae*, has been identified to date.

Chlamydiae replicate by means of a unique life cycle unlike that of other bacteria. The 300-nm elementary body (the infective and extracellular form of chlamydia) initiates infection by attachment to receptors in the susceptible host cell's outer membrane. Subsequently, the elementary body enters the host cell by endocytosis. Within the resulting phagosome, the elementary body reorganizes within 6 hours into the larger 800- to 1000-nm and more metabolically active reticulate body. These reticulate bodies undergo repeated binary division until a large inclusion occupying much of the cell's cytoplasm and containing many reticulate bodies is formed. Reticulate bodies possess many ribosomes and synthesize deoxyribonucleic acid (DNA), ribonucleic acid (RNA), proteins, and other molecules but cannot generate ATP. After 24 hours, some of the reticulate bodies condense to form compact elementary bodies in the mature inclusion, and the latter are released into the extracellular environment to begin the cycle anew by infecting adjacent cells.

C. trachomatis preferentially infects columnar epithelial cells. In most patients, *C. trachomatis* infections remain superficial, involving mucosal surfaces of the eye, nasopharynx, cervix, urethra, and rectum (Table 345–1). Many of these infections produce few or no symptoms and tend to be subacute in nature and mild in terms of the signs they produce. Ascending infections of the endometrium, fallopian tube, liver capsule, epididymis, or lung produce more severe symptoms and signs and can be regarded as more extensive or invasive infections. Infection of the upper genital tract in women is of particular importance, often leading to tubal scarring with resultant complications of infertility and ectopic pregnancy. LGV strains of *C. trachomatis* infect lymphoid cells and macrophages as well as epithelial cells and cause the most invasive disease, manifested either by proctocolitis or by painful inguinal adenopathy and fever. *C. trachomatis* occasionally causes nongenital systemic infection, including culture-negative endocarditis, peritonitis, and pneumonia in adults. Both *C. pneumoniae* and *C. psittaci* preferentially infect respiratory epithelial cells, but the latter has a broader host range that includes macrophages (see Ch. 348). *C. psittaci* also causes culture-negative endocarditis.

Since many chlamydial infections produce either no symptoms or nonspecific symptoms and signs, laboratory confirmation of infection should be sought. Available techniques include direct microscopic examination of tissue scrapings or secretions for typical inclusions or for elementary bodies; isolation of the

TABLE 345–1. CLINICAL SPECTRUM OF C. TRACHOMATIS INFECTIONS*

Males	Females	Infants
Uncomplicated Infections		
Urethritis (NGU, PGU)	Cervicitis	Conjunctivitis
	Urethritis	Pharyngitis
Proctitis	Proctitis	Asymptomatic rectal
Conjunctivitis	Conjunctivitis	and vaginal carriage
Pharyngitis	Pharyngitis	
	Bartholinitis	
Invasive Infections		
Proctocolitis	Endometritis	Pneumonia
Lymphogranuloma venereum	Salpingitis	? Otitis media
	Perihepatitis	
Epididymitis	Postpartum endometritis	
? Prostatitis		
Complications	Infertility	? Chronic pulmonary impairment
Reiter's syndrome	Ectopic pregnancy	
Rectal strictures	Chronic salpingitis	
? Urethral strictures	Complications of pregnancy (? prematurity, stillbirth)	
? Sterility		

*Excludes trachoma.
NGU = nongonococcal urethritis; PGU = postgonococcal urethritis.

organism in cell culture; and assessment of antichlamydial antibody in serum or secretions. Adoption of cell culture techniques for isolation of *C. trachomatis* from patients' secretions or biopsies (replacing the more cumbersome embryonated yolk sac method) has been a major factor contributing to recognition of the wide spectrum of infections caused by *C. trachomatis*. Inclusions formed in cell culture monolayers can be visualized using iodine, Giemsa's, or immunofluorescent staining procedures. Despite widespread use in research laboratories, cell culture procedures for isolation of *C. trachomatis* have not been generally available to clinicians because of their expense and technical difficulty. Lack of an available confirmatory diagnostic test and the inability to screen high-risk populations for infection have been major factors contributing to the increasing incidence of genital and neonatal *C. trachomatis* infections in this country. Newer immunodiagnostic procedures that detect chlamydial antigen in patients' secretions have recently been developed and can be used for diagnostic confirmation and for screening where cultures are not available. These tests utilize monoclonal or polyclonal antichlamydial antibodies to demonstrate the presence of chlamydial antigens in infected secretions by either enzyme-linked immunosorbent assay (ELISA) or immunofluorescence techniques, and have approximate sensitivities of 80 to 90 per cent and specificities of 97 to 99 per cent compared with culture in high-risk populations. Nucleic acid hybridization tests using chlamydia-specific DNA and RNA probes have also been developed and have similar sensitivity and specificity. Neither cultures, specific antigen detection, nor nucleic acid probes are routinely available for the diagnosis of *C. pneumoniae* and *C. psittaci* infections; hence, these infections must be diagnosed serologically.

Chlamydial infection stimulates both a humoral and a cellular immune response, but neither appears to be completely protective against subsequent infection with either homologous or heterologous strains. Both local and systemic antibody can be demonstrated after acute infection, and immunoglobulin G (IgG) antibody neutralizes infective elementary bodies. Some have advocated that the immune response actually participates in the disease process by producing continued inflammation. Serodiagnosis of chlamydial infections has limited applicability except in specific circumstances. The complement fixation test, available in most health department laboratories, should be used for confirmation of suspected psittacosis or LGV. A titer of 1:64 or greater in a patient with a clinical syndrome compatible with LGV can be regarded as diagnostic. In patients with pneumonia, however, the complement fixation test does not distinguish between *C. psittaci* and *C. pneumoniae* infection (see Ch. 348). The microimmunofluorescence test is useful in the diagnosis of infant pneumonia, pelvic inflammatory disease, or Fitz-Hugh-Curtis syndrome as well as suspected LGV or *C. pneumoniae* infection but is available only in research laboratories. Uncomplicated genital infections evoke only low titer-antibody responses, and acute infections cannot be easily distinguished from pre-existing antibody in many patients.

C. trachomatis infections can be treated with a variety of antimicrobial agents. Those with greatest activity in cell culture assays and in clinical studies include the tetracyclines (tetracyline HCl, doxycycline, and minocycline), erythromycin, sulfonamides, sulfamethoxazole-trimethoprim, and rifampin. Ofloxacin, a new fluoroquinolone antibiotic, has in vitro activity against chlamydia and has been effective in clinical trials of uncomplicated infection. The β-lactam antibiotics produce abnormal inclusions in cell culture and inhibit replication but have been largely ineffective in clinical treatment trials. The aminoglycosides, vancomycin, and spectinomycin have no activity against chlamydiae. In general, chlamydial infections require 7 to 21 days of antibiotic treatment; single-day regimens have been largely ineffective. Treatment failure usually indicates noncompliance, reinfection, or inadequate duration of drug therapy. Clinically significant resistance to tetracycline or erythromycin has not been described.

Bowie WR, Caldwell HD, Jones RP, et al. (eds.): Chlamydial Infections. Cambridge, Cambridge University Press, 1990, pp 1–601. *Excellent source of most recent knowledge on all aspects of chlamydial infection, including 13 comprehensive review articles.*

Grayston JT: *Chlamydia pneumoniae*, Strain TWAR. Chest 95:664–669, 1989. *Excellent overview of knowledge regarding this new pathogen.*

Stamm WE: Diagnosis of *Chlamydia trachomatis* genitourinary infections. Ann Intern Med 108:710–717, 1988. *Review of clinical criteria and new diagnostic tests for common chlamydial infections.*

346 Trachoma

Chlamydia trachomatis causes two epidemiologically distinct patterns of ocular infection. In trachoma-endemic parts of the world, *C. trachomatis* immunotypes A, B, Ba, and C cause trachoma, a chronic eye disease that may lead to severe visual impairment or blindness. In nonendemic areas, immunotypes D through K produce a milder, self-limited conjunctivitis in infants born to mothers with cervical infection or in adults who acquire ocular infection after secondary spread from genital sites.

Since antiquity, trachomatous infection has been recognized in the Mediterranean basin and in the Orient, and it remains prevalent in Africa and Asia. Although the incidence has been decreasing over the last 30 years, millions have eye infections with chlamydiae, with millions blinded as a result. Trachoma flourishes in hot, dry areas that have a shortage of available water and poor hygienic customs. Initial infection usually occurs in early childhood, and in certain parts of the world virtually the entire population is infected with chlamydiae before reaching adulthood. Specific chlamydia antigens may stimulate a local immune response resulting in a hypersensitivity reaction. Repeated exposure to chlamydiae and the high prevalence of bacterial superinfection with *Haemophilus* spp., pneumococci, staphylococci, and Enterobacteriaceae in these populations contribute to the severity of the resulting eye disease. In the United States, trachoma is occasionally seen on Indian reservations in the Southwest, in Mexican-Americans, and in immigrants from endemic areas, but such cases rarely result in major visual impairment.

Persons with active trachoma shed chlamydiae in desquamated conjunctival cells, in conjunctival exudate, and in tears, which then may be transmitted by fingers, fomites, and perhaps flies. In endemic areas, transmission by these routes occurs through close personal contact, especially within family units and in groups of young children. Patients with early active infection shed more infective chlamydiae than those with chronic infection. However, even patients with long-term eye disease unaccompanied by signs of current activity may shed chlamydiae and thus serve as a source of infection.

Typically, trachoma in children begins insidiously at about age 2 as a follicular conjunctivitis, most noticeable in the conjunctiva of the upper lid and the tarsal plate. Histologically, inclusion bodies appear within the conjunctival epithelial cells, polymorphonuclear leukocytes infiltrate the epithelium, and subepithelial lymphoid follicles develop. Reinfection is common during this period. Next the cornea becomes involved, with epithelial keratitis and subepithelial corneal infiltration resulting in opacities. Blood vessels from the limbus, accompanied by fibroblasts, invade the cornea to form a pannus. Progression of the inflammatory response leads to necrosis and scarring of the conjunctiva and gradual corneal vascularization from the upper limbus downward. Eventually a dense fibrovascular pannus extends over part or all of the cornea to grossly impair vision. Linear or stellate scars appear on the conjunctiva. Progressive scarring of the subepithelial tissues leads to deformation of the tarsal plate and results in entropion, trichiasis, and further corneal damage. Destruction of the conjunctival goblet cells and lacrimal ducts and gland produces xerosis. The latter changes often follow secondary bacterial infection, which may also produce corneal ulceration and accelerate loss of vision. Typically there are no systemic symptoms or signs of infection. Active infection with chlamydia is common between the ages of 2 and 5, but then resolves. The disease process may evolve over about 10 years in hyperendemic areas, but is milder and more slowly progressive in most cases, evolving over 20 to 40 years.

The traditional diagnostic criteria for trachoma include lymphoid follicles on the upper tarsal plate, limbal follicles, typical conjunctival scars, and vascular pannus. Early in the disease the last two can be detected only by slit-lamp examination. The presence of any two of these features confirms the diagnosis. Laboratory confirmation of trachoma is based on (1) identification of typical inclusions in epithelial cells from a conjunctival swab or scraping (usually done by Giemsa's or immunofluorescence staining); (2) cultivation of chlamydiae from a conjunctival specimen in cell culture; (3) microimmunofluorescent antibody in high titer in tears; or (4) demonstration of chlamydia using noncultural tests such as antigen detection or nucleic acid hybridization. Approximately 20 to 60 per cent of children with early inflammatory trachoma have Giemsa-positive scrapings; higher yields result from cultures of chlamydiae.

In the differential diagnosis of ocular chlamydial infection, epidemic keratoconjunctivitis (usually caused by adenovirus type 8 or type 19), herpetic keratoconjunctivitis, Newcastle disease virus conjunctivitis, acute hemorrhagic conjunctivitis caused by enterovirus type 70 or coxsackievirus, reactions to allergens and irritating chemicals, and other bacterial causes of conjunctivitis must be considered. Some of these entities may coexist with chlamydial infections, and repeated ophthalmologic examinations and extensive laboratory evaluation may be required to establish a correct diagnosis.

Adult inclusion conjunctivitis caused by *C. trachomatis* usually presents as an acute follicular conjunctivitis with preauricular lymphadenopathy. Untreated, it regresses slowly, but keratitis with marginal infiltrates, subepithelial opacities, and corneal neovascularization may develop in the conjunctiva. Unlike trachoma, adult inclusion conjunctivitis rarely impairs vision permanently.

Control of chronic trachoma in endemic areas has been attempted using tetracycline or erythromycin ointment in the eyes of all affected children in the community for 21 to 60 days. Oral administration of erythromycin has been used as an alternative. Antibiotic therapy usually suppresses clinical activity and chlamydial as well as bacterial growth but may not eradicate chlamydiae permanently. However, in endemic areas, repeated courses of drug treatment are beneficial because they reduce severity of eye disease and thus avoid progression toward blindness. Even one dose per month of doxycycline, 300 mg (2.5 to 4 mg per kilogram), can provide clinical benefit by converting severe to mild eye disease. Drug therapy has no influence on scars or pannus. Surgical correction is required for serious entropion or trichiasis. Topical corticosteroids and caustic substances have no place in therapy. For acute adult inclusion conjunctivitis, tetracycline HCl, 2.0 grams given orally daily in divided doses, or erythromycin, 2.0 grams given orally daily in divided doses for 1 to 2 weeks, successfully treats genital tract as well as ocular involvement. Sulfisoxazole, 4 grams daily, may also be effective. Sexual partners must be treated simultaneously in order to avoid reinfection.

The potential measures to prevent trachoma include efforts to increase the supply of water; practices to maintain cleanliness, such as frequent handwashing and avoidance of use of common towels; and measures to reduce flies. The disease has disappeared in many areas coincident with improved hygienic conditions. It is important to detect mild early infection in young children in endemic areas and to apply effective drug treatment repeatedly to prevent the blinding progression of the disease. Detection and treatment of adults who already have visual impairment probably can reduce the source of infection for children. Entire family groups or communities should be treated simultaneously. Efforts to prevent trachoma with a vaccine have been unsuccessful.

Dawson CR: Eye disease with chlamydial infection. *In* Oriel D, Ridgway G, Schachter J, et al. (eds.): Chlamydial Infections. Cambridge, Cambridge University Press, 1986, pp 135–144. *Excellent overview of all aspects of trachoma.*

Schachter J, Dawson CR: Epidemiology of trachoma predicts more blindness in the future. Scand J Infect Dis Suppl 69:55–62, 1990. *Reviews trends in the epidemiology and control of trachoma.*

347 Neonatal Chlamydial Infections

Between 5 and 22 per cent of pregnant women have *Chlamydia trachomatis* infection of the cervix, with neonatal infection occurring when the infant passes through the infected birth canal. Ascending intrauterine infection of the fetus has not been demonstrated. After birth, 30 to 50 per cent of infants born to infected mothers have cultural evidence of infection, 25 per cent manifest clinically apparent conjunctivitis, and 10 to 15 per cent acquire nasopharyngeal infection, which in some cases progresses to chlamydial neonatal pneumonitis. Otitis media and symptomatic nasopharyngitis may be caused by *C. trachomatis* in some infants. Untreated neonatal infections may become chronic and persist over many months.

Neonatal *C. trachomatis* inclusion conjunctivitis typically begins 5 to 14 days after birth. In infants given ocular prophylaxis, however, onset may be delayed for weeks or months. The infection must be differentiated from gonococcal ophthalmia (which has a shorter incubation period of 1 to 3 days) and from other common causes of neonatal conjunctivitis (*Streptococcus pneumoniae, Haemophilus influenzae, Staphylococcus aureus,* and group D streptococci). Typical manifestations include lid and conjunctival swelling, mucopurulent ocular discharge, conjunctival hyperemia, and membrane formation. Untreated, the disease persists 3 to 12 months but usually heals without sequelae. Rarely, conjunctival scarring and corneal neovascularization occur. Neonates with inclusion conjunctivitis frequently have concomitant chlamydial infection of the nasopharynx, rectum, urethra, and vagina, usually without associated clinical manifestations at these sites.

The diagnosis can be rapidly established by demonstration of chlamydial inclusions or elementary bodies in conjunctival scrapings stained by Giemsa's stain or immunofluorescence. Alternatively, demonstration of chlamydial antigen in ocular secretions by ELISA or cultures for *C. trachomatis* can be used if available.

The relative effectiveness of topical ocular prophylaxis for chlamydial eye infection using silver nitrate, erythromycin ointment, or tetracycline ointment has become increasingly unclear. Early studies suggested that topical erythromycin was most effective and silver nitrate least effective, but more recent studies have found little difference among these three regimens. Many health departments currently recommend the use of topical erythromycin. However, topical erythromycin prophylaxis does not cure concomitant nasopharyngeal or rectal infection. Thus, a better preventive approach would be screening and treatment of pregnant women for *C. trachomatis* infection before term. This approach essentially eliminates *C. trachomatis* infections in neonates and should be the strategy of choice in high-risk women.

Since many infants with inclusion conjunctivitis have concomitant nasopharyngeal, rectal, and vaginal *C. trachomatis* infection, systemic rather than topical therapy should be used. In addition, relapses often follow topical therapy. Erythromycin, 40 to 50 mg per kilogram per day in four divided doses for 14 to 21 days, cures more than 80 per cent of cases. Both parents should be examined for *C. trachomatis* infection and should be treated with tetracycline or erythromycin (for nursing mothers) if cultures or immunodiagnostic tests are not available.

Approximately 10 per cent of infants born to infected mothers develop a distinctive subacute chlamydial pneumonia between the first and fourth months of life. Typically, tachypnea, a staccato cough, inspiratory rales, elevated serum globulin concentrations, and eosinophilia are seen, but fever is absent. Hyperinflated lungs with scattered interstitial infiltrates are evident on chest radiographic examination. The disease lasts for weeks to months but is mild in most infants and resolves without specific therapy. However, marked hypoxemia and apnea have been reported in some cases. Lung biopsies have demonstrated chlamydial inclusions, alveoli with inflammatory exudate, and a lymphocytic interstitial infiltration of the bronchial submucosa. In some cases, *C. trachomatis* has been recovered from lung tissue. Diagnosis in most instances can be suspected on clinical grounds and confirmed by the demonstration of chlamydial inclusions or elementary bodies on Giemsa- or immunofluorescent-stained smears of the conjunctivae or nasopharynx. *C. trachomatis* should be sought by cell culture of eye scrapings, nasopharyngeal swabs, or rectal swabs if they are available. Rising high-titer immunoglobulin M (IgM) microimmunofluorescent antibody to *C. trachomatis* can be demonstrated in the majority of infants with pneumonia. Erythromycin, 50 mg per kilogram per day in four divided doses for 14 to 21 days, has been recommended for treatment of pneumonia in infants, although there are no control trials demonstrating the benefits of this regimen. Chronic respiratory impairment and persistent pulmonary symptoms may develop in some patients.

Hammerschlag MR, Cummings C, Roblin PM, et al.: Efficacy of neonatal ocular prophylaxis for the prevention of chlamydial and gonococcal conjunctivitis. N Engl J Med 320:769–772, 1989.

Harrison HR: Chlamydial infection in neonates and children. *In* Oriel D, Ridgway G, Schachter J, et al. (eds.): Chlamydial Infections. Cambridge, Cambridge University Press, 1986, pp 283–292. *Excellent review.*

Laga M, Plummer FA, Piot P, et al.: Prophylaxis of gonococcal and chlamydial ophthalmia neonatorum: A comparison of silver nitrate and tetracycline. N Engl J Med 318:653–657, 1988. *Good discussion of the issues of ocular prophylaxis.*

348 Infections Due to *Chlamydia psittaci* and *Chlamydia pneumoniae**

PSITTACOSIS

Psittacosis (ornithosis), an infection of birds caused by *Chlamydia psittaci*, can produce asymptomatic infection, a transient influenza-like illness, or serious pneumonic disease when transmitted to humans.

Parrots and parakeets are common carriers and until recently were the major source of human infection. With better control of psittacine disease in aviaries, other birds now cause more human infections, including turkeys, pigeons, ducks, and other fowl. Persons working with birds are at greatest risk, notably pet shop employees, pigeon handlers, and poultry workers. There is no risk associated with eating poultry products.

The agent is present in the blood, tissue, feathers, and discharges of infected birds. Although avian disease can be fatal, infected birds frequently show only minimal evidence of illness. Birds having active infections are most likely to transmit the disease, but asymptomatic carriers are common, and birds can transmit the agent for months.

Psittacosis is generally acquired by the respiratory route through inhalation of infected dried bird excreta or by handling of infected birds. Cases have been reported after only brief exposure to birds, and 20 per cent of patients can recall no history of exposure to birds. Person-to-person transmission of psittacosis is rare.

PATHOLOGY. In birds, the principal sites of disease are the liver, spleen, and pericardium. In humans, the lung is most commonly involved. *C. psittaci* gains access to the human body via the respiratory route, rapidly enters the blood, and reaches the reticuloendothelial cells of the liver and spleen. After replication in these sites, invasion of the lung occurs via hematogenous spread. Lobar pneumonitis results from inflammation and progressive edema of the alveoli, often accompanied by small hemorrhages. Thick, gelatinous plugs of mucus may fill major and minor bronchi and account for the severe cyanosis and progressive anoxia seen in fatal cases. Foci of necrosis may occur in more severely affected parts of the lung and are sometimes associated with capillary thrombi. The process is generally most severe in

dependent bronchopulmonary segments. Monocytes and macrophages containing cytoplasmic inclusion bodies, which represent the agent (LCL bodies), are characteristic. Hyperplasia and monocytic infiltration of pulmonary and hilar lymph nodes and splenic enlargement with occasional areas of focal necrosis occur. Rarely the liver shows intralobular focal necrosis and swollen Kupffer's cells containing psittacosis elementary bodies. Pathologic changes in the myocardium, heart valves, pericardium, meninges, brain, adrenal glands, pancreas, and kidneys have been reported.

CLINICAL MANIFESTATIONS. Wide variations can occur in the clinical picture. The incubation period ranges from 7 to 15 days but may be longer. Asymptomatic or mild influenza-like infections probably are the rule. Moderate or severe infections, although less frequent, are more commonly diagnosed. The onset of illness may be insidious, but it often starts with chills and a fever that rises slowly to 39 to 40.5°C during the first week of illness. The pulse may be slow relative to the level of the fever. Headache is severe. Malaise, anorexia, nausea, vomiting, severe myalgias, particularly in the neck and back, and arthralgias are common. Cough is generally prominent but may be delayed until late in the first week. Small amounts of mucoid sputum with occasional blood streaking are the rule. Changes in mentation are often seen. Delirium or stupor may occur in severe cases toward the end of the first week and usually are associated with severe pulmonary involvement, cyanosis, and anoxia. Other neurologic manifestations are uncommon. A macular rash (Horder's spots) resembling that seen in typhoid has occasionally been described. Jaundice and progressive renal failure have been reported in severe cases. Severe dyspnea, tachypnea, tachycardia, cyanosis, jaundice, delirium, and stupor are all poor prognostic signs.

The physical findings of pneumonia are usually sparse. Chest roentgenograms often reveal infiltrates not detected at the bedside. Examination may reveal only fever, painful muscle groups, an elevated respiratory rate, and a relative bradycardia. Fine, crepitant rales may be heard in localized areas over the lungs, but true consolidation is less common. Pleurisy with effusion occurs but is unusual. Mild hepatomegaly is frequent. A palpable spleen has been noted in a substantial number of patients. Splenomegaly in a patient with undiagnosed acute pneumonitis should raise the consideration of psittacosis. An erythematous pharynx may be noted. In rare instances there may be signs of pericarditis or myocarditis. In prolonged, severe illness, thrombophlebitis and pulmonary infarction have been reported as late complications.

Patients with mild cases may recover in 7 days. More severe infections may last 12 to 21 days without specific treatment. Defervescence is generally slow, and a prolonged convalescence is common. Relapses have been reported even after appropriate treatment. Reinfections have been described. Occasional cases of endocarditis caused by *C. psittaci* in patients with sterile blood cultures have been described.

LABORATORY FINDINGS. The leukocyte count is usually normal or slightly elevated. The erythrocyte sedimentation rate is generally elevated. Chest roentgenograms show soft, patchy infiltrates radiating outward from the hilum, which tend to be more prominent in dependent lobes or segments. Occasionally diffuse miliary, nodular, or frank lobar distribution of infiltrates is seen.

A specific diagnosis can be made only by isolation of the agent or by serologic studies. The agent is present in the blood and sputum during the first 2 to 3 weeks, but owing to the high risk of laboratory-acquired infection, isolation is hazardous and should not be attempted except in special laboratories. Diagnosis is generally made by a fourfold rise in complement-fixing antibodies. A significant change in antibody titers is generally present by the twelfth to fourteenth day of disease; the titers are usually maximal by 30 days, then slowly wane. Treatment can delay or suppress antibody response. A serum complement-fixation titer of 1:32 during the acute illness is presumptive evidence of psittacosis. However, the complement fixation test is also positive in infections with LGV strains of *C. trachomatis* and with *C. pneumoniae* infections (see below). False-positive complement-fixation tests have been reparted with Q fever, brucellosis, and legionnaires' disease.

DIFFERENTIAL DIAGNOSIS. Establishing a specific diag-

---

*Portions of this chapter are based upon "Psittacosis (Ornithosis, Parrot Fever)" by William Schaffner, in the 17th edition of the *Cecil Textbook of Medicine*.

nosis of psittacosis is of importance because of its potential severity, its response to antimicrobials, and the public health significance of psittacosis. All cases should be reported to the local health department. The syndrome of idiopathic pneumonia accompanied by protracted high fever, usually severe headache, and relative bradycardia should suggest psittacosis. Often a history of contact with birds is the only clue to diagnosis and may be elicited only by repeated questioning of the patient and family. When pneumonic symptoms are prominent, psittacosis must be differentiated from legionnaires' disease, viral pneumonias, mycoplasmal pneumonia, influenza, Q fever, tularemia, tuberculosis, fungal infection, and other bacterial pneumonias. If pneumonic symptoms are not prominent, psittacosis can be confused with other systemic febrile illnesses such as typhoid fever, brucellosis, infectious mononucleosis, infectious hepatitis, miliary tuberculosis, or the viral meningoencephalitides.

TREATMENT. The tetracyclines are the drugs of choice, and early diagnosis and initiation of treatment may be lifesaving. After institution of therapy with 2 to 3 grams daily, both fever and symptoms are generally controlled within 48 to 72 hours, although the response may be indolent. Although the disease apparently responds to penicillin in doses above 2 million units daily and to erythromycin, tetracycline remains the drug of choice. Treatment should be continued for at least 10 days after defervescence to prevent relapse. With treatment, mortality rates as low as 1 to 5 per cent can be achieved.

CHLAMYDIA PNEUMONIAE (Strain TWAR)

A new species of chlamydia, *Chlamydia pneumoniae*, has recently been established. Current evidence indicates that *C. pneumoniae* (formerly called the TWAR organism) is a frequent cause of upper and lower respiratory tract infection in both children and adults. Seroprevalence studies show that about 40 per cent of most adult populations tested worldwide have evidence of prior infection with this agent. Infections are uncommon in children under the age of 5 but are frequent in children between the ages of 8 and 15 and in young adults. *C. pneumoniae* has been identified as a cause of epidemics of respiratory infection in closed populations such as military recruits. The organism may be transmitted in communities in a cyclic fashion. Thus, in some years many infections occur, whereas in other years very few are noted. Studies to date have failed to identify an animal reservoir for *C. pneumoniae*. It is believed to be an exclusively human pathogen that is transmitted from person to person via respiratory secretions in much the same way as many viral respiratory infections and *M. pneumoniae*. Transmission has been demonstrated within households, schools, and military barracks.

Chlamydia pneumoniae is an obligate intracellular pathogen with 10 per cent or less DNA relatedness to *C. psittaci* or *C. trachomatis*. Like other chlamydiae, it produces cytoplasmic inclusions in infected cells. *C. pneumoniae* has unique pear-shaped elementary bodies and forms dense oval inclusions that do not contain glycogen. Only a single serovar of *C. pneumoniae* has been recognized to date. The organism can be cultured in HeLa 229 and McCoy cells but has been difficult to isolate from patients with suspected infection. More recently, HL cells have been identified as a more sensitive cell line for isolation of *C. pneumoniae*.

Clinically, *C. pneumoniae* produces a spectrum of respiratory infections that differ somewhat in manifestations by age. In children, teenagers, and young adults, the most common manifestations are bronchitis, sinusitis, and mild pneumonia. Occasionally, pharyngitis is seen. It is thought that many infections are asymptomatic or produce mild nonfebrile upper respiratory tract infections. *C. pneumoniae* infection, however, may frequently be prolonged, lasting for several weeks. Clinically, the pneumonia produced by *C. pneumoniae* generally resembles that seen with mycoplasma infection. Chest radiographs most commonly show small, single, subsegmental infiltrates, and more extensive consolidation is rarely seen. In adults, pneumonia may be more severe and bronchitis and sinusitis more prolonged. With most infections due to *C. pneumoniae*, the white blood cell count is normal.

Specific diagnosis of infection due to *C. pneumoniae* is difficult. Although the organism can be cultivated in HL cells and other cell lines, it is not easily grown and most laboratories are not equipped to undertake cultures. Similarly, specific serologic testing is not widely available. The complement fixation test for chlamydiae can be utilized and is available to most clinicians. A fourfold titer rise or a single titer of 1:64 or greater suggests the diagnosis. However, antibodies to *C. psittaci* or *C. trachomatis* infection are also measured by this test, and hence it is not specific for *C. pneumoniae*. The microimmunofluorescence test for *C. pneumoniae* provides a specific means of diagnosis but is not widely available. Using this test, a fourfold titer rise, an IgM of 1:16 or greater, or a single IgG titer of 1:512 or greater supports the diagnosis. More sensitive and easily performed methods for diagnosis of *C. pneumoniae* infection are clearly needed.

In vitro, tetracyclines and erythromycin are the most effective drugs against *C. pneumoniae*. Sulfonamides are not effective. Although no controlled trials have been conducted, it is currently recommended that therapy with tetracycline or erythromycin, 2 grams per day, be provided for 10 to 14 days.

Grayston JT: *Chlamydia pneumoniae*, strain TWAR. Chest 95:664–669, 1989.

Grayston JT, Wang SP, Kuo CC, Campbell LA: Current knowledge of *Chlamydia pneumoniae* strain TWAR, an important cause of pneumonia and other acute respiratory diseases. Eur J Clin Microbiol Infect Dis 8:191–202, 1989. *Reviews current knowledge of* C. pneumoniae.

Jariwalla AG, Davies BH, White J: Infective endocarditis complicating psittacosis: Response to rifampicin. Br Med J 1:155, 1980. *Endocarditis caused by psittacosis is reviewed concisely.*

Macfarlane JT, Macrae AD: Psittacosis. Br Med Bull 39:163, 1983. *A well-written review.*

Schaffner W, Drutz DJ, Duncan GW, et al.: The clinical spectrum of endemic psittacosis. Arch Intern Med 119:433, 1967. *Good descriptions of clinical presentations.*

Rickettsial Diseases

Richard B. Hornick

349 Introduction

The rickettsiae are small obligate intracellular, gram-negative pathogens. They do not have a symbiotic relationship with human host cells and therefore cause metabolic derangements that result in cell death. Infections with the typhus and spotted fever groups of rickettsiae involve endothelial cells. This host-pathogen interaction results in a perivasculitis. Q fever induces granulomas in the liver plus interstitial pneumonia. Ehrlichiosis is a new human disease caused by a rickettsial organism that has long been associated with disease in dogs. *Ehrlichia canis* appears to be transmitted by ticks, can be demonstrated rarely inside leukocytes, and induces antibodies. Fortunately, these small, gram-negative organisms are susceptible to tetracycline and chloramphenicol antibiotics so that patients recover quickly once the drugs are administered.

Each of the rickettsiae is transmitted to humans by ticks, mites, lice, fleas, or aerosols originating from animal products (placentas, Q fever) or from feces of the aforementioned insects. In the United States, there are relatively few cases of rickettsial infections. Rocky Mountain spotted fever is the most prevalent, 600

TABLE 349–1. SUMMARY OF SOME EPIDEMIOLOGIC FEATURES OF SELECTED RICKETTSIAL DISEASES OF HUMANS

| Disease | Organism | Natural Cycle | | Usual Mode of Transmission to Humans | Common Occupational or Environmental Association | Geographic Distribution |
		Arthropod Vector	Reservoir/ Mammalian Host			
Typhus group						
Murine typhus	*Rickettsia mooseri* (*R. typhi*)	Flea	Rodents	Infected flea feces into broken skin or aerosol to mucous membranes	Rat-infected premises (shops, warehouses, grain elevators)	Scattered foci, worldwide
Epidemic typhus	*R. prowazekii*	Body louse	Humans*	Infected crushed louse of feces into broken skin or aerosol to mucous membranes	Lousy human population with louse transfer	Worldwide
Brill-Zinsser disease	*R. prowazekii*	Recrudescence months to years after primary attack of louse-borne typhus			Unknown; ?stress	Worldwide
Spotted fever group (selected examples)						
Rocky Mountain spotted fever	*R. rickettsii*	Ixodid ticks	Ticks/small mammals	Tick bite, mechanical transfer to mucous membranes, ?airborne	Tick-infested terrain, houses, dogs	Western hemisphere
Ehrlichiosis	*Ehrlichia canis*	Ticks	?Dogs	Tick bite	Tick-infested areas	At least 12 states in US, primarily southern states
Boutonneuse fever	*R. conorii*	Ixodid ticks	Ticks/rodents, dogs	Tick bite	Tick-infested terrain, houses, dogs	Mediterranean littoral, Africa, ?Indian subcontinent
Rickettsialpox	*R. akari*	Mouse mite	Mite/mice	Mouse mite bite	Unique mouse- and mite-infested premises (incinerators)	United States, U.S.S.R., Korea, ?Central Africa
Scrub typhus Tsutsugamushi disease	*R. tsutsugamushi* (multiple serotypes)	Chigger	Chigger/?rodents	Chigger bite	Chigger-infested terrain; secondary scrub, grass airfields, golf courses	Asia, Australia, New Guinea, Pacific Islands
Q fever	*Coxiella burnetii*	?Ticks	Ticks/mammals	Inhalation of dried airborne infective material; ?tick bite	Domestic animals or products, dairies, lambing pens, slaughterhouses	Worldwide
Trench fever	*Rochalimaea quintana*	Body louse	Humans	Infected crushed louse or feces into broken skin; ?aerosol to mucous membranes	Lousy human population with louse transfer	Africa, Mexico, ?South America, ?Eastern Europe

*Recent isolations of putative *R. prowazekii* from flying squirrels in the eastern United States have not been evaluated as reservoirs for human infection. Previous claims of involvement of domestic animals are now largely discounted.

to 700 cases having been reported annually from 1985 to 1989. Fewer cases of Q fever and murine typhus are identified each year. Certain other rickettsial infections are major public health problems in developing countries but are not found in the United States, e.g., scrub typhus. The potential for tourists to return to the United States with an emerging rickettsial infection is increasing. Because of the rarity of rickettsial infections in the United States, diagnosis may be delayed. Delays in diagnosing these illnesses can adversely affect the potential for recovery.

In this introductory chapter, three tables are included that summarize, first, the epidemiologic features of rickettsial infections; second, the host cells involved in the pathogenesis of the clinical manifestations of the disease; and third, those clinical features that will assist in differentiating the various forms of rickettsial infections. The following chapters provide additional details on the major rickettsial infections that are found in this country or that represent potential threats to persons traveling abroad.

TABLE 349–2. RICKETTSIA TARGET CELL RELATIONSHIPS, PATHOLOGIC LESIONS, AND CLINICAL MANIFESTATIONS OF HUMAN RICKETTSIOSES*

Disease	Target Cell	Host-Cell Association	Basic Lesion	Clinical Manifestations
Typhus-like fevers				
Typhus group	Endothelial	Free intracytoplasmic	Vasculitis	Acute self-limited fever
Scrub typhus	Endothelial	Free intracytoplasmic	Vasculitis	Acute self-limited fever
Spotted fever group	Endothelial, smooth muscle	Free intracytoplasmic and intranuclear	Vasculitis	Acute self-limited fever
Ehrlichiosis	Leukocytes	Intracytoplasmic inclusion body	Leukopenia, thrombocytopenia, liver cell damage	Acute self-limited fever
Q fever	Reticuloendothelial	Intracytoplasmic vacuole	Granulomas	Acute self-limited fever, "atypical pneumonia," subacute hepatitis, subacute endocarditis
Trench fever	Unknown	Pericellular (in louse and cell culture)	Unknown	Recurring febrile episodes

*Adapted from Stickland (ed.): Hunter's Tropical Medicine. Philadelphia, W. B. Saunders Company, 1984.

TABLE 349–3. SOME CLINICAL FEATURES OF SELECTED RICKETTSIAL DISEASES

Disease	Usual Incubation Period (Days)	Eschar	Rash Onset, Day of Disease	Rash Distribution	Rash Type	Usual Duration of Disease* (Days)	Usual Severity†	Fever After Chemotherapy (Hours)
Typhus group Murine typhus	12 (8–16)	None	5–7	Trunk → extremities	Macular, maculopapular	12 (8–16)	Moderate	48–72
Epidemic typhus	12 (10–14)	None	5–7	Trunk → extremities	Macular, maculopapular, petechial	14 (10–18)	Severe	48–72
Brill-Zinsser disease	—	None		Trunk → extremities	Macular	7–11	Relatively mild	48–72
Spotted fever group Rocky Mountain spotted fever	7 (3–12)	None	3–5	Extremities → trunk, face	Macular, maculopapular, petechial	16 (10–20)	Severe	72
Ehrlichiosis	7–21	None	Rare?	Unknown	Petechial	7 (3–19)	Mild	72
Boutonneuse fever	5–7	Often present	3–4	Trunk, extremities, face, palms, soles	Macular, maculopapular, petechial	10 (7–14) 7	Moderate	—
Rickettsialpox	?9–17	Often present	1–3	Trunk → face, extremities	Papulovesicular	7 (3–11)	Relatively mild	—
Scrub typhus (tsutsugamushi disease)	1–12 (9–18)	Often present	4–6	Trunk → extremities	Macular, maculopapular	14 (10–20)	Mild to severe	24–36
Q fever	10–19	None		None		(2–21)	Relatively‡ mild	48 (occasionally slow)

*Untreated disease.
†Severity can vary greatly.
‡Occasionally subacute infections occur (e.g., hepatitis, endocarditis).

350 The Typhus Group

This group of conditions includes three established clinical and epidemiologic entities: epidemic louse-borne typhus fever, the oldest disease known to be caused by rickettsiae; Brill-Zinsser disease, a classic example of reactivation of a latent infection; and flea-borne murine typhus. The first two conditions are induced by *Rickettsia prowazekii*, a pathogen transferred from person to person by the bite of body lice. Persons who have recovered from epidemic typhus have persistent rickettsiae in various host cells, presumably in the reticuloendothelial cells; stresses that cause a defect in the suppressive lymphocytes will, years later, permit these rickettsiae to be reactivated, resulting in a mild typhus-like illness, called Brill-Zinsser disease. In 1975, *R. prowazekii* was isolated from flying squirrels in the southeastern

United States. A number of persons acquired typhus fever from squirrels living in their attics and probably harboring infected fleas or lice or both.

Flea-borne murine typhus, caused by *R. typhi*, is a mild form of typhus fever occurring in this country and elsewhere. It is transmitted by fleas from rodents (Fig. 350–1). *R. canada* is a tick-borne (mouse-rabbit reservoirs), rickettsial organism, formerly classified with the typhus group. It is distinct from the typhus, as well as the spotted fever group. Whether it is a significant human pathogen requires more study. It has been implicated by serologic means as the cause of acute febrile cerebrovasculitis in one patient.

EPIDEMIC LOUSE-BORNE TYPHUS

INTRODUCTION. Synonyms include classic, historic, and European typhus; jail, war, camp, and ship fever; *Flichfieber* (German); *typhus exanthematique* (French); and *tifus exantematico* and *tabardillo* (Spanish). Many of these names indicate the

FIGURE 350–1. Flea-borne (endemic, murine) typhus fever: cases, by year in the United States from 1955 to 1988. For 1988, 54 cases of murine typhus were reported from 10 states. Thirty of the cases were reported from Texas, 10 from California, and 7 from Hawaii.

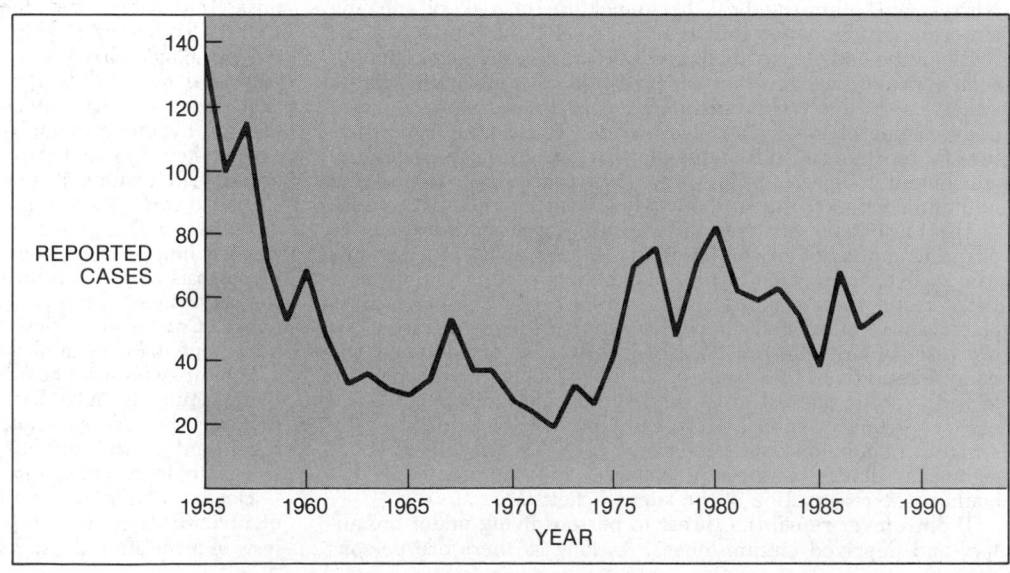

location of the outbreaks—military and concentration camps, crowded ships with poor and starved immigrants, outbreaks in persons living in occupied countries during wartime, and so forth. Each implies crowded, unsanitary living conditions where bathing and laundry facilities are inadequate. These conditions allow for the breeding and propagation of body lice. The impact of typhus fever on military campaigns and immigration patterns is a fascinating and provocative story. The reader is referred to Woodward for an introduction to the effects of this disease on history.

DEFINITION. Classic typhus fever is manifested by the sudden onset of headache, fever, rash, and an altered mental state. (Typhus is derived from the Greek word meaning cloudy or misty. Applied to typhus, it describes the obtunded, lethargic state of mind.) *R. prowazekii* is transmitted by human body lice (*Pediculus humanus humanus*).

ETIOLOGY. *R. prowazekii* is a small obligate intracellular, gram-negative bacillus. In cells it stains red when exposed to Gimenez's stain. Viable rickettsiae stimulate the endothelial cell to act like a phagocyte to engulf the rickettsiae in a phagosome and internalize it. If rickettsiae do not break out of the phagosome promptly, they begin to disintegrate, perhaps owing to enzymatic activities. The rickettsiae have an enzyme, phospholipase A, that enables them to lyse the phagosome wall and to multiply freely in the cytoplasm. *R. prowazekii* escape from the cell by destroying it. The necrotic cell stimulates an inflammatory response that leads to the vasculitis and subsequent clotting abnormalities.

TRANSMISSION AND EPIDEMIOLOGY. The unique feature of infection with *R. prowazekii* is that no animal reservoir has been implicated, at least until its isolation from the flying squirrel (*Glaucomys volans*). It is still uncertain how significant the flying squirrel will be in amplifying the incidence of this disease. Very few, if any, cases of classic typhus occur each year in this country (Centers for Disease Control does not have an active surveillance for it). Fifteen cases were reported in 1980 and 1981, all in persons having contact with flying squirrels.

Classic typhus is a disease of humans. An individual with rickettsemia can infect body lice. The lice acquire the organisms in their blood meal. These ectoparasites may then find another person to whom they transmit the rickettsiae via infected feces. Body lice do not survive the ingestion of rickettsiae. The organisms multiply in the gut of the louse, destroy the epithelial cells, and the louse dies (usually in 1 to 3 weeks). However, during the period of infection, the louse passes feces heavily laden with rickettsiae. Either the human host scratches the site of the bite and thereby self-inoculates the rickettsiae, or the feces and rickettsiae can contaminate minute apertures in the epidermis, allowing the organisms to find cells in which to multiply. Dried, contaminated feces can also become airborne, e.g., by shaking out one's clothes loaded with lice and feces and thereby creating an infectious aerosol. When inhaled, the rickettsiae can penetrate the mucosal cells and enter endothelial cells. Laboratory accidents frequently generate aerosols that induce infection in technicians. Nurses and other medical personnel are at risk of inhaling airborne particles when they remove the clothing from a patient.

When the body louse obtains a blood meal containing antibody-coated rickettsiae, the louse may modify the infectivity of the rickettsiae-antibody combination by partially digesting the antibody coating of the organism in its gut. This digestion destroys the Fc portion of the antibody that would have permitted attachment to macrophages. The rickettsia is then free of the inhibiting action of the antibody when it infects the next person.

The louse does not transmit *R. prowazekii* transovarially to offspring and is not an amplifier for further propagation. Patients who recover from classic typhus have the opportunity to develop Brill-Zinsser disease and at that time have rickettsemia and are able again to infect body lice. However, this happens rarely, for few cases of Brill-Zinsser disease have been detected among the many hundreds of thousands of soldiers who acquired typhus in World War II; one estimate suggested a rate of 10 per 100,000 cases of primary typhus. More cases may be recognized as the geriatric population continues to increase. This group will have significant illness, surgical procedures, and chemotherapy that could cause reactivation of the latent rickettsiae.

Typhus fever remains a threat to persons living under unsanitary and deprived circumstances. As long as there are persons who are latent reservoirs for *R. prowazekii*, an epidemic can erupt. One country with persistent typhus is Ethiopia. There, prolonged drought, poverty, and malnutrition contribute to the perpetuation of the disease.

PATHOLOGY. The rickettsiae invade only endothelial cells, as described in Ch. 351. This leads to vasculitis, with differing pathologic changes in various organs. There is no eschar in this disease. The rash appears to have its origin in the leakage of blood and fluid from the damaged capillaries. The damage to the endothelial cells results in cell death, and at these sites platelet-fibrin thrombi form, platelet-active substances are released, and vasoconstriction and occlusion of small vessels occur. These changes can lead to infarcts in various organs, edema of tissue, leakage of inflammatory cells around small blood vessels ("typhus nodules" of the brain, for instance), stimulation of clotting mechanisms, and the development of shock. Almost all organs are involved in patients with untreated disease. The inflammatory exudate consists of mononuclear cells, plasma cells, histiocytes, and polymorphonuclear leukocytes. Gangrene of skin and limbs occurs in the presence of extensive thrombotic activity.

CLINICAL MANIFESTATIONS AND COURSE. The incubation period is about 7 days on the average but can range from 6 to 15 days. The onset is abrupt with intense headache, chills, fever, and myalgia. There is back or leg pain—presumably due to the muscle damage secondary to the vasculitis. Bites of lice may cause pruritus, and persons infested with lice may have numerous scratches in the skin. Sometimes the skin has a yellow-gold hue because of frequent louse bites. The headache is described as the "worst ever," and the pain is unremitting unless treated with narcotic analgesics. The temperature rises quickly during the first 2 days and persists for about 2 weeks, maintaining a continuous fever pattern if not altered by antibiotics or antipyretic medications. During the first week, there is a bradycardia relative to the temperature elevations of 39° to 41°C. Conjunctivae are injected, and photophobia is present. Deafness, tinnitus, and sometimes vertigo are prominent features. The patient appears to be in a toxic state, with a flushed face, obtundation, and profound weakness. There may be a cough, but no rales are apparent on auscultation of the lungs. The pharyngeal mucous lining is dry and inflamed.

The rash, characteristic of the typhus group, appears on the fourth to seventh day of disease. The lesions appear first on the trunk and axillary folds (areas of skin stress) and spread to the extremities but spare the palms and soles of the feet. The lesions are reddish-pink macules that fade on pressure. With treatment or in mild cases, the rash disappears within several days. In untreated patients, it can spread and coalesce, leading to gangrene of portions of the skin, especially over regions of bony prominences. In 5 to 10 per cent of patients, the rash may not be present.

These and other manifestations of the disease occur because of the initial unchecked multiplication and spread of the rickettsiae, involving ever-enlarging segments of the endothelial surface. The resulting damage to the organs evolves because of the compromised circulation and the associated acute inflammatory responses. Whether rickettsial toxin or endotoxin contributes to the pathologic changes is still a debated point. Whatever processes are involved, certain organs are regularly involved: the skin, heart, kidneys, and skeletal muscle. In patients with severe disease, hypotension and renal failure portend a fatal outcome.

The altered mental status that occurs as the disease progresses (in untreated patients) is striking. The patient may progress from stupor to coma. The stupor may be interrupted by brief periods of delirium. The patient may have to be restrained in order to protect him or her from trauma. At this stage, lymphocytic pleocytosis of the cerebrospinal fluid may be present. Despite the seriousness of the patient's condition, complete recovery can ensue. Cranial nerve lesions are common. There are also temporary mental aberrations.

Patients who have acquired typhus fever in this country from flying squirrels have had signs and symptoms of the classic disease. The rash was noted in 8 of 15, and it was evanescent. Significant central nervous system involvement was reported in five patients; two had coma and three had confusion or delirium.

Death in untreated patients occurs between the ninth and eighteenth days. Recovery from the disease begins with a rapid lysis of fever after about 2 weeks of disease. With the disappearance of fever, mental function returns quickly. Recovery of a sense of well-being is protracted owing to the need to counter the stresses of prolonged negative nitrogen balance, inanition, and loss of muscle mass.

Brill-Zinsser disease is manifested in a manner similar to classic typhus. All signs and symptoms are milder, presumably because the host has well-developed immune mechanisms that can regain control in a short time. Serologic studies in these patients demonstrate immunoglobulin G (IgG) rather than immunoglobulin M (IgM) antibodies. Occasionally, patients with unrecognized Brill-Zinsser disease die. An underlying disease or procedure may permit activation of the latent rickettsiae, and this combination can culminate in death. Reactivation has been noted following surgical procedures and the use of immunosuppressive drugs. In experimental animals that have recovered from the primary disease, isolation of rickettsiae at a future date is facilitated by the administration of steroids.

PROGNOSIS. The fatality rate in untreated groups of patients with classic typhus is 10 to 60 per cent. Children usually have a mild illness with minimal risk of death. Patients over 60 years of age have the highest mortality rate. Recovery is the rule with appropriate antibiotic treatment.

TREATMENT. *R. prowazekii* responds well to tetracycline and chloramphenicol antibiotics. Doxycycline, 200 mg as a single oral dose, is the treatment of choice. Tetracycline, 25 mg per kilogram daily in four doses, or chloramphenicol, 50 mg per kilogram daily in four doses, is an effective alternative. Therapy should be continued for 2 to 3 days after the fever has defervesced. Most patients are afebrile within 48 to 72 hours and improve quickly from the debilitating headache or mental aberrations or both. Relapses occur in persons who are treated early, on day 1 or 2 of illness. Such patients do not develop the required immune mechanisms to contain the proliferation of the residual rickettsiae. Furthermore, both antibiotics are rickettsiostatic and do not eradicate all of these intracellular parasites even with the introduction of specific immune mechanisms. Recovery from disease without the assistance of antibiotic therapy also allows rickettsiae to remain in cells, later to be activated and cause Brill-Zinsser disease. In the severely ill patient, fluid therapy and proper nutrition are mandatory. Fortunately, antibiotic therapy has simplified the need for supportive care.

PREVENTION AND CONTROL. To prevent and control the spread of classic typhus, the body lice (and feces) associated with patients and their clothes must be destroyed. The clothing should be carefully placed in plastic bags and sealed and carefully removed only in the area where they are to be treated. Clothes that can sustain boiling are boiled, and the rest should be subjected to steam and dry heat. It is also possible to kill the lice (also the eggs present in seams and elsewhere—these eggs will hatch in a week) with insecticides. Formerly, 10 per cent DDT (chlorophenothane) was used, but lice are now generally resistant to it. Resistance has also become a problem with 1 per cent lindane dust. Malathion (1 per cent) and 2 per cent temefos (Abate) are effective in most areas. These dusts are applied to the fully clothed individual. This approach controls the acute outbreaks of disease when applied to all persons in the community. Long-time use of insecticides is not effective because of the development of resistance, because long-term compliance is difficult, and because the insecticides may have a deleterious effect on the ecology of the region. Control requires improvement of sanitary conditions and standards of living as well as health education.

Health personnel who encounter patients with classic typhus are at risk for acquiring the disease from lice picked up from the patient or his or her clothes. There is no risk of direct human-to-human transfer of the rickettsiae other than by aerosolized, dried, contaminated feces. Once the patient has been deloused, no isolation barriers are required.

No vaccine is currently available for preventing classic typhus. Travelers to endemic areas are rarely at risk unless, for example, they work in camps for displaced persons or carry out relief work that brings them in contact with persons with lice. Decontaminating the clothing overnight with insecticides or wearing insect repellent–treated clothes provides some protection. Prophylactic doxycycline has been effective when given weekly to prevent scrub typhus and would be expected to be effective in preventing *R. prowazekii* infections. This drug should

be used only for short periods, 2 to 4 weeks. It is important under these circumstances to monitor the temperature for 2 weeks at least, as the drug may have masked the initial infection and delayed the onset of symptoms. Retreatment with doxycycline at the onset of the fever is curative.

MURINE TYPHUS

DEFINITION. Murine typhus, a milder form of classic typhus, is caused by *Rickettsia typhi* and is transmitted from rodents to humans by means of the rat flea (*Xenopsylla cheopis*). It is the only disease of the typhus group that occurs regularly in the United States, albeit in small numbers.

ETIOLOGY. *R. typhi* is a small, gram-negative, obligate, intracellular pathogen. Like *R. prowazekii*, it can penetrate into endothelial cells by induced phagocytosis. Its disease potential resides in its ability to multiply in these cells, destroy them, and initiate a vasculitis. *R. typhi* is catalogued with the typhus group because it shares common antigens with *R. prowazekii* and *R. canada*. In addition, there is cross-immunity between *R. prowazekii* and *R. typhi* induced by infections. Despite these similarities, it is clear from deoxyribonucleic acid (DNA) homology studies that the two are not closely related.

TRANSMISSION AND EPIDEMIOLOGY. *R. typhi* causes disease worldwide. Wherever there are large rodent populations, there is the potential for outbreaks. The rat and other small animals serve as reservoirs of this disease. *Rattus rattus* and *Rattus norvegicus* are two species of rats that can sustain the *R. typhi*, serve as a source of rickettsiae for the rat flea, and have no obvious illness from carrying this human pathogen. The rat flea disseminates the infection not through its bite but by placing contaminated feces on the skin. These may be rubbed or scratched into the skin; they can be carried to the conjunctival sac or mucous membranes on the fingers, where the rickettsiae can invade; or they can be aerosolized after drying and cause infection if inhaled. In the flea, the rickettsiae multiply in the enterocytes in the gut, do not kill the flea, and continue to be shed in the feces for the life of the flea. The rickettsiae are not transmitted by fleas to their offspring.

The numbers of cases reported to the Centers for Disease Control (CDC) from 1955 to 1988 are shown in Figure 350–1. Fifty-four cases were reported in 1988, most from Texas and California. These numbers probably represent an under-reporting of the true incidence. There was a dramatic drop in the number of reported cases after the mid 1940's. In 1944 there were over 5400 cases. By 1954 there were 163. This decline was due to intensive efforts at rodent control. Most of the cases occur in the warmer months, when rat fleas are plentiful.

PATHOLOGY. Descriptions of the pathologic lesions in this disease are few because of the rarity of fatal cases. Since the rickettsiae are known to invade endothelial cells, the pathologic consequences should mimic those seen in other rickettsial infections. The reasons for the differences in virulence of these rickettsiae and the varying severity of illnesses produced are unknown.

CLINICAL MANIFESTATIONS AND COURSE. Headache, fever, and myalgia are the principal symptoms and signs associated with illness produced by *R. typhi*. These appear after an incubation period of about 1 to 2 weeks. A faint macular-papular pink-colored rash appears in about 80 per cent of patients after 4 to 5 days of illness. It may be difficult to see in poor light. When present, it may be visible for 4 to 8 days before it gradually fades.

Rarely are there any significant complications of this infection, but as it is an infection of the endothelial cells, there is a vasculitis that can cause widespread organ derangement. The patients, especially if older, are debilitated by the infection when not treated. They may remain febrile, with a temperature of 39 to 40°C for 2 weeks. This metabolic stress necessitates prolonged convalescence. Antibiotic therapy brings about a prompt recovery.

DIAGNOSIS. This disease has no distinguishing characteristics during the early days of symptoms. The rash appearing on the fourth or fifth day of illness should alert the physician to the possibility of a rickettsial infection. The history of a possible exposure to areas where rats are known to exist, e.g., grain elevators, port facilities, and farm buildings, provides useful information. Flea bites, if seen early, are discrete and may have a central hemorrhagic punctum. The location and grouping of flea bites are important diagnostic features. They occur in covered parts of the body, in irregular groups of several to a dozen or more. They may be in the region of the belt, shoulders, and hips or on the legs.

Differentiating this disease from Rocky Mountain spotted fever (RMSF) may be difficult. The rash of RMSF usually begins on the wrists and palms and on the soles of the feet and then extends to the skin of the thorax and abdomen. In murine typhus the lesions are on the skin of the chest and abdomen and rarely on the extremities. The history of a tick bite or exposure provides evidence for a clinical diagnosis of RMSF.

Serologic studies confirm the rickettsial infection. Weil-Felix OX-19 reaction is positive in most patients who have not received antibiotic treatment. This test, however, does not distinguish murine typhus from the spotted fever group of infections. The indirect immunofluorescent test can be used to identify *R. typhi* infections. However, because of the common antigens shared with *R. prowazekii*, the serum requires cross-absorption with special antigens from these two rickettsia strains. Isolation of the organism is possible but should be done only in special laboratories where containment facilities are available.

PROGNOSIS. The mortality rate is less than 5 per cent in untreated patients. Appropriate antibiotic treatment results in prompt cure, and the mortality rate is reduced almost to zero. One death was reported between 1977 and 1986.

TREATMENT. Tetracycline and chloramphenicol are effective drugs for treating this rickettsial infection. A 5- to 7-day course of either is effective. The usual dosage of 25 mg per kilogram of tetracycline per day in four doses or chloramphenicol, 50 mg per kilogram per day in four doses, effects a prompt cure. The organisms are sensitive to these antibiotics. No resistant strains have been identified. Relapses do occur when antibiotics are administered early in the course of the illness. Retreatment with the antibiotic of choice provides prompt response.

PREVENTION AND CONTROL. There is no vaccine to prevent this disease. Control of rats has been shown to be very effective. When rat control programs are instituted, appropriate insecticides should be simultaneously used to prevent the fleas from seeking humans for feeding as the rat population is decreased.

Bozeman FM, Maisello SA, Williams MG, et al.: Epidemic typhus rickettsia isolated from flying squirrels. Nature 225:545, 1975.
Duma RJ, Sonenshine DE, Bozeman FM, et al.: Epidemic typhus in the United States associated with flying squirrels. JAMA 245:2318, 1981. *These two papers provide a good background on the discovery of the flying squirrel as a reservoir of* R. prowazekii *and the disease associated with exposure to these animals and their ectoparasites.*
Gaon JA, Murray ES: The natural history of recrudescent typhus (Brill-Zinsser disease) in Bosnia. Bull WHO 35:133, 1966. *Classic paper describing the studies conducted to prove that Brill-Zinsser disease is truly a recrudescence of classic typhus fever.*
Linneman CC, Pretzman CI, Peterson ED: Acute febrile cerebrovasculitis. A non–spotted fever group rickettsial disease. Arch Intern Med 149:1689, 1989. *An intriguing case report and discussion of the probable role of* R. canada *in causing this clinical entity.*
Walker TS: Rickettsial interactions with human endothelial cells in vitro: Adherence and entry. Infect Immun 44:205, 1984.
Wohlbach SB, Todd JI, Palfrey FW: The Etiology and Pathology of Typhus. Cambridge, Mass., Harvard Press, 1922. *This book provides the reader with an excellent description of the natural course of classic typhus fever.*
Woodward TE: A historical account of the rickettsial diseases with a discussion of unsolved problems. J Infect Dis 127:5, 1973.

351 Rocky Mountain Spotted Fever

SYNONYMS. Rocky Mountain spotted fever (RMSF) is also known as typhus fever, tick-borne, by the Centers for Disease Control (CDC), *fiebre manchada* (Mexico), *fiebre petequial* (Colombia), and *febre maculosa* or Sao Paulo typhus (Brazil).

DEFINITION. Rocky Mountain spotted fever is a sometimes fatal systemic infection manifested by fever, severe headache, rash, and other organ disease caused by the vasculitis induced by *Rickettsia rickettsii.* The organism is usually transmitted to humans from animal reservoirs by a tick bite.

ETIOLOGY. *R. rickettsii* organisms are small, gram-negative, coccobacillary bacteria that can grow only inside eukaryotic host cells. They cannot be isolated on cell-free culture media. In human infections the rickettsiae invade and multiply within endothelial cells of arteries and veins. Different strains of *R. rickettsii* vary in virulence in human as well as animal hosts. Mortality rates appear to be higher in Montana than on the Eastern seaboard. Attempts to correlate virulence with structural components in the polysaccharide portion of the cell wall have been unsuccessful. However, two surface proteins, with molecular weights of 120,000 and 155,000, have been identified as possible virulence factors (protective antigens), and the latter has been produced from cloned genes in *Escherichia coli.* The antigenic material protects mice from lethal infection and will be studied as a potential vaccine.

DISTRIBUTION AND INCIDENCE. This disease was named for the geographic site of its original discovery; the causative agent was named for the discoverer, Howard T. Ricketts. By the 1940's the disease had become more common on the East Coast than in the West. The incidence rose sharply beginning in 1971 and peaked at 1.91/100,000 population in 1980 in the eight South Atlantic states. Subsequently, it has fallen to a value similar to that of 1970. A total of 603 cases of RMSF were reported in 1989 in the United States (Fig. 351–1).

Serologic surveys in children and adults in North Carolina, the state with the highest number of reported cases, demonstrate that subclinical infections occur. Almost 20 per cent of the children had OX-19 agglutination titers in the diagnostic range, and a smaller number had positive indirect fluorescent antibody titers, a more specific test. None of these children was previously diagnosed as having had Rocky Mountain spotted fever.

TRANSMISSION AND EPIDEMIOLOGY. Ninety-five per cent of reported cases occur between April 1 and September 30, with two thirds in May, June, and July. Children and young adults account for about 40 per cent of cases. Ninety per cent of patients give a history of a tick bite or attachment or of having been in a tick-infested area 14 days prior to onset of illness. Infected ticks are found in urban as well as rural areas. A park in New York City was the source of ticks that transmitted *R. rickettsia* to four children, one of whom died.

Rocky Mountain spotted fever occurs in humans when an infected tick bites and injects *R. rickettsii* into the skin. Probably fewer than 10 organisms injected intradermally are sufficient to induce disease.

Several species of ticks are commonly involved in transmission of disease: *Dermacentor andersoni,* the wood tick, in the Rocky Mountain states; *Dermacentor variabilis,* the dog tick, in the East and Oklahoma; *Amblyomma americanum* in Texas and Oklahoma; and *Rhipicephalus sanguineus* in Texas and Mexico. These ticks feed on small mammals such as ground squirrels and rabbits as well as on larger animals such as bear and deer. Dogs serve as a reservoir to infect ticks and then other animals or humans. Figure 351–2 shows the distribution of cases of Rocky Mountain spotted fever by state in the United States in 1989.

Laboratory-acquired infections have occurred in persons exposed to droplets from accidental generation of aerosols from solutions of the organism. However, even in circumstances conducive to airborne transmission, person-to-person transmission does not occur. Rocky Mountain spotted fever can also be acquired by the transfusion of contaminated blood.

PATHOLOGY. The basis of the pathologic changes in this disease, as in other rickettsial infections, is the inflammatory response stimulated by the irreparable damage of the endothelial cells. In patients dying within 3 to 5 days of onset of disease, significant coagulation abnormalities are present. Causes may include damage to the endothelial cells with release of Factor VIII; and stimulation of the release of platelet factors by damage to the endothelium or by activation of the kallikrein-kinin system by the Hageman factor. Microinfarcts result from occlusions of small vessels, and edema and hemorrhages occur secondary to increased permeability of the vasculature. Such lesions can be found in the heart, kidneys, adrenals, lungs, brain, skin, spleen, and subcutaneous tissues.

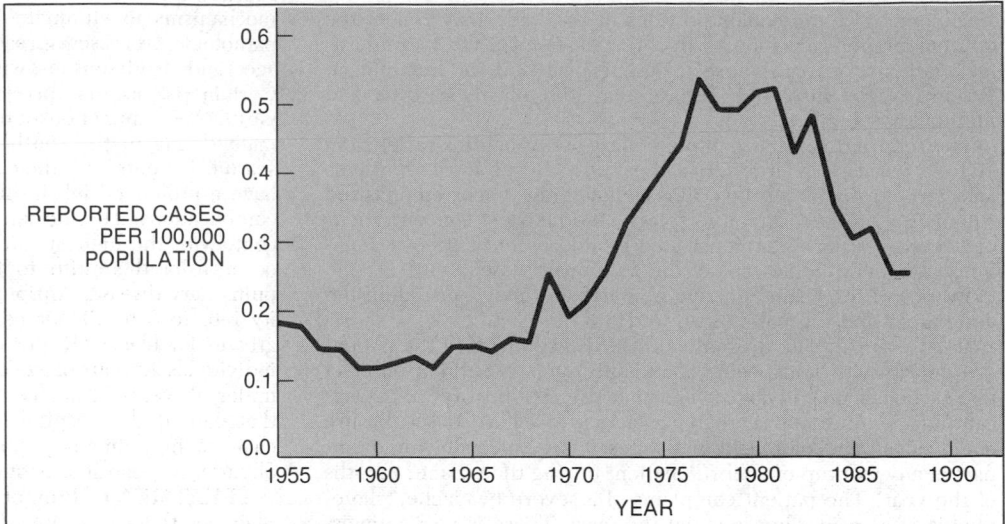

FIGURE 351–1. Rates of reported Rocky Mountain spotted fever cases, by year, in the South Atlantic states and all other states, from 1955 to 1988.

The rash is thought to result from the vasculitis and the associated permeability changes. Petechial lesions are caused by microhemorrhages secondary to the vasculitis and thrombocytopenia.

Patients with glucose-6-phosphate dehydrogenase (G6PD) deficiency appear to be prone to severe infections caused by *R. rickettsii* and other rickettsial agents. These patients have severe hemolytic reactions and significant thrombotic lesions in the glomeruli, resulting in oliguria.

CLINICAL MANIFESTATIONS. The incubation period of naturally acquired disease has a range of 2 to 14 days with an average of 7 days. The onset of disease in the typical case is sudden, with a severe headache, often retrobulbar in location, chills, fever, myalgia, malaise, nausea and vomiting, conjunctival injection, and photophobia. Tenderness may be present in large muscle groups. The duration of fever in untreated cases is about 2 weeks, but recovery from the debilitating effects of the disease requires several additional weeks.

Rash appears in 80 to 90 per cent of patients—usually on the third or fourth day of fever, rarely after 5 or more days. It consists of pink macules, 2 to 5 mm, often noted first about the wrists and ankles. Lesions then spread to arms, chest, face, feet, and abdomen. Rarely does the rash involve the mucous membranes. Initially, these lesions blanch with pressure, but after 2 to 3 days they become fixed and turn dark red or purple and then slowly disappear during convalescence. The latter lesions represent microhemorrhages. Lesions on the palms and soles of the feet, in conjunction with the rash elsewhere, and petechial lesions in the skin folds of the axillae and around the ankles, constitute the classic distribution of the rash. Biopsy of the rash reveals perivascular round cell infiltration. Staining of the specimens of skin with fluorescent tagged antibodies to *R. rickettsii* reveals the intracellular organisms.

In patients with unrecognized and inappropriately treated disease, the rash coalesces as the spread of the infectious process involves additional and larger vessels. This can result in large ischemic and gangrenous lesions. Especially susceptible is the skin of the tip of the nose, ear lobes, digits, and scrotum.

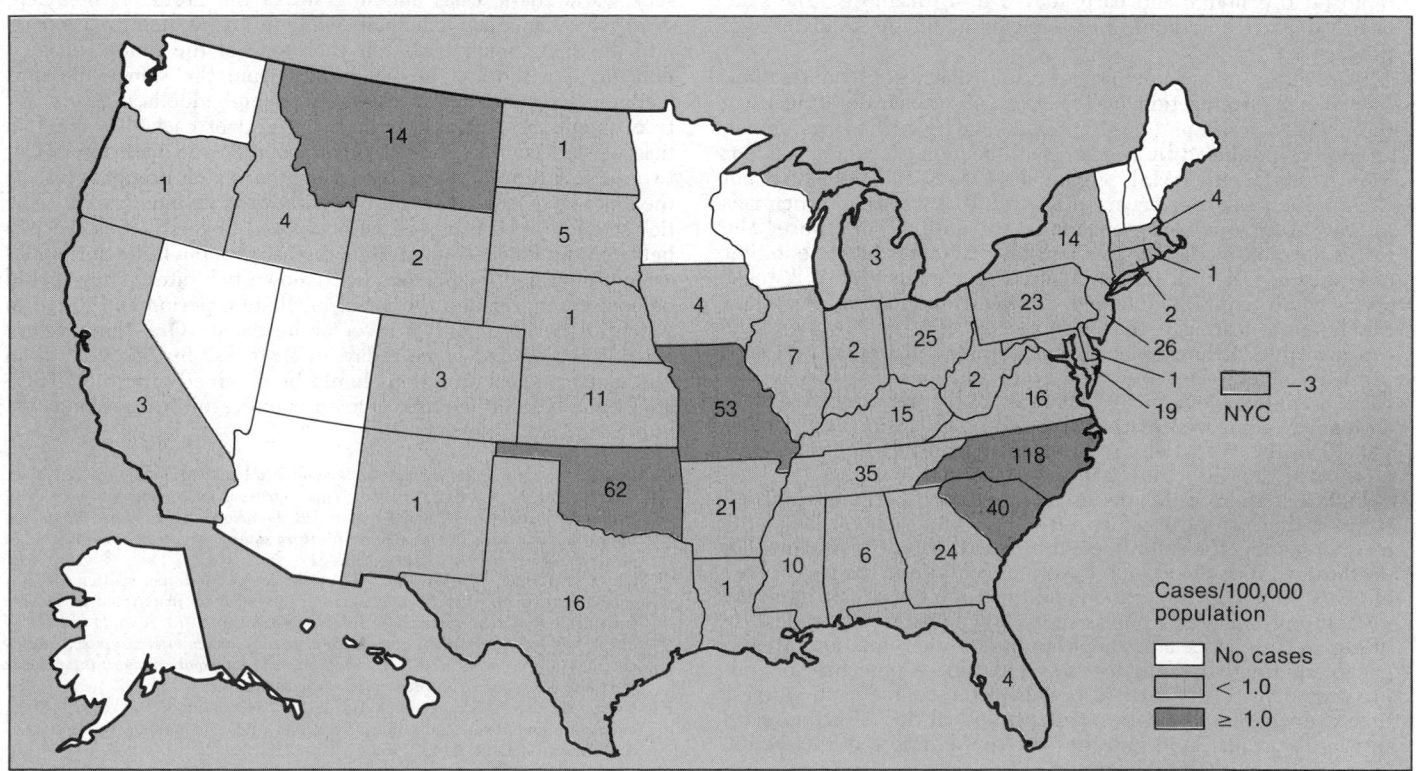

FIGURE 351–2. Rocky Mountain spotted fever: Cases, by state, in the United States in 1989.

Involvement of the cooler portions of the body may reflect the optimal temperature for growth of *R. rickettsii* (32°C). Thrombosis of larger arteries can cause gangrene of a limb or hemiplegia. Patients with untreated disease may die of myocarditis and pulmonary edema.

The reported incidence of pulmonary abnormalities varies from 10 to 40 per cent in large series of patients. Respiratory symptoms and signs as part of this illness have not been emphasized sufficiently. In fact, after the spleen, the heaviest concentrations of rickettsiae can be demonstrated by fluorescent antibody staining in the endothelial cells of the pulmonary vasculature.

Edema of the brain and ring hemorrhages may cause delirium and stupor and ultimately lead to death.

DIAGNOSIS. The diagnosis of RMSF is difficult in the patient presenting with nonspecific complaints such as sudden onset of fever, headache, myalgia, and malaise. A history of travel, camping, or outdoor recreational activities where tick exposure could occur and of recent tick bites is an especially important part of any workup of a febrile patient during the warmer months of the year. The patient complains of a severe headache, photophobia, and pain when moving the eyes. There is no meningismus. Lumbar puncture usually reveals normal cerebrospinal fluid (CSF). Patients with stupor or coma may demonstrate elevated CSF protein and a few mononuclear cells. The presence of a faint, pink-colored rash on wrists and ankles should raise a suspicion of RMSF. Helpful in making the diagnosis is the knowledge that the rash appeared after the fever.

A search for an attached tick should concentrate on the scalp and groin. Hard body ticks such as *D. andersoni* tend to remain attached for long periods. The finding of an engorged tick should provide the needed information for a clinical diagnosis. There usually is no ulceration or scar from the tick bite.

Most patients have thrombocytopenia but not significant clotting abnormalities. In severe cases, disseminated intravascular coagulopathy (DIC) occurs with hypofibrinogenemia and prolonged prothrombin and partial thromboplastin times. Other laboratory studies are not helpful in making a diagnosis. The white blood cell count is usually normal.

Confirmation of RMSF is achieved by immunofluorescence staining of tissue specimens and by serologic analyses. The detection by immunofluorescence of rickettsiae in tissues, such as skin or rash biopsies, is the one test that can provide the most rapid (4 to 6 hours) and early (day 3 to 4) diagnosis. The state health department should be contacted about the availability of this test.

Serologic tests do not provide rapid diagnostic confirmation. The Weil-Felix reaction utilizes the polysaccharide antigens of three *Proteus* strains (OX-19, OX-2, and OX-K) to agglutinate antibodies produced by a rickettsial infection. Serum specimens from patients with RMSF agglutinate OX-19 and OX-2, but not OX-K. The peak titer occurs at about 2 to 3 weeks and then falls rapidly. Antibiotic treatment blunts the antibody response. The test is inexpensive, and with a fourfold or greater increase in titer of OX-19 or OX-2, or both, in paired specimens (drawn 2 weeks apart) confirmation is obtained. Indirect immunofluorescent antibody (IFA) testing is the most specific and sensitive serologic test available. It has replaced the complement fixation test and, in many laboratories, the Weil-Felix reaction. The IFA is now used in epidemiologic surveys because of the persistence of these antibodies compared with the short-lived antibodies demonstrated in the Weil-Felix reaction. A diagnostic rise (fourfold or greater) in titer also takes 2 to 3 weeks.

Differentiation of this disease from other infections is difficult without the history of a tick bite or the information about the fever preceding the rash. In children measles and atypical measles (in those who received killed vaccine) can mimic the early phase of RMSF illness. The location and type of lesions making up the rash, the presence of Koplik's spots, and a history of measles-like illness in close associates should permit a differentiation. Meningococcemia with meningitis usually produces petechiae or purpura, or both, in the patient earlier in the course of the disease than expected in all but rare patients with RMSF. Furthermore, the cerebrospinal fluid indicates the septic nature of the meningitis caused by the meningococci.

PROGNOSIS. Patients with RMSF have a serious infectious disease that involves endothelial cells throughout the host. Prompt antibiotic therapy is necessary to assist cellular immune mechanisms to eliminate the pathogen. In some patients, the pathologic processes spread rapidly and cause irreversible damage, and death ensues within 3 to 5 days (fulminant disease). Certain risk factors correlate with severe diseases: presence of G6PD/A−, time of onset of specific antibiotic therapy, and black males living in the southeastern United States during the tick season. Patients with the classic form of RMSF who are untreated have a prolonged febrile illness lasting 2 to 3 weeks with many complications. The mortality rate in such patients is 20 to 30 per cent, with the highest rate occurring in the elderly. Death may occur from the ninth to the fifteenth day, often from severe pulmonary disease. Antibiotic treatment has lowered the mortality rate to 3 to 10 per cent. The 1985 case fatality rates were greater for blacks (16 per cent) than whites (3 per cent) and for individuals 40 years of age or older (9 per cent) than for individuals under 40 years (2 per cent). This is a serious disease requiring that patients be hospitalized and carefully monitored to detect changes in pulmonary findings and evidence of hypotension, oliguria, myocarditis, or increasing intracranial pressure.

TREATMENT. Prompt initiation of tetracycline or chloramphenicol therapy is mandatory to ensure optimal chances for recovery. Tetracycline (25 to 50 mg per kilogram per day), doxycycline (100 mg every 12 hours in adults), and chloramphenicol (50 mg per kilogram per day) are the drugs of choice. Usually the fever abates in 2 to 3 days, and concurrently a sense of well-being is restored. Antibiotic treatment can be discontinued 2 to 3 days thereafter. No instances of strains resistant to the tetracyclines or chloramphenicol have been reported. The newer third-generation cephalosporins or the aminoglycoside antibiotics have not been evaluated in RMSF. Evaluation of four aminoquinolone antibiotics in various infected tissue culture cell lines have revealed antibacterial activity equal to that of tetracyclines. Clinical evaluations are not available. Relapses after tetracycline or chloramphenicol treatment are uncommon.

PREVENTION AND CONTROL. Immunity to reinfection after recovery from RMSF appears to be complete. No naturally acquired second cases have been reported. There is no effective vaccine.

The best method for preventing disease is to avoid contact with ticks. Ticks are brushed off leaves or blades of grass onto clothes or skin as one comes in contact with such vegetation. Ticks usually remain stationary until the host is quiet. They then seek warm, dark areas and migrate to the groin or the scalp, where they can grasp hair shafts while inserting their mouth parts into the skin. Small barbs on each side of the mouth make it difficult to withdraw the whole tick from the skin while it is feeding; the mouth parts may remain embedded. A search for ticks should be accomplished at the end of each day spent in tick-infested country. They should be removed with forceps or tweezers. A drop of acetone or a lighted match brought close to the tick may ensure that the tick withdraws its mouth parts. The tick should not be removed with exposed fingers. A tick crushed between the fingers may induce disease. Prophylactic antibiotics are not indicated for persons with known tick bites. They should be advised concerning the usual incubation period and urged to watch for development of fever or headache. Oral temperature should be recorded twice a day for 2 weeks. In the event of an elevation, medical attention should be obtained promptly. Therapy begun before the onset of fever could result in a prolongation of the incubation period.

Donohue JF: Lower respiratory tract involvement in Rocky Mountain spotted fever. Arch Intern Med 140:223, 1980. *This retrospective review of pulmonary findings in patients with RMSF points out the delays that occurred in making the correct diagnosis because the respiratory symptoms were not considered to be a part of the clinical picture of RMSF.*

DuPont HL, Hornick RB, Dawkins AT, et al.: Rocky Mountain spotted fever: A comparative study of the active immunity induced by inactivated and viable pathogenic *Rickettsia rickettsii*. J Infect Dis 128:340, 1973. *A study of induced disease in volunteers that demonstrated the minimal effectiveness of killed vaccines in preventing RMSF. In addition, new information about the number of rickettsiae required to cause diseases was obtained.*

Kaplowitz LG, Lange JV, Fischer JJ, et al.: Correlation of rickettsial titers, circulating endotoxin, and clinical features in Rocky Mountain spotted fever. Arch Intern Med 143:1149, 1983.

Marx RS, McCall CE, Abramson JS, et al.: Rocky Mountain spotted fever: Serological evidence of previous subclinical infection in children. Am J Dis

Child 136:16, 1982. Wilfert CM, MacCormack JN, Kleeman K, et al.: The prevalence of antibodies to *Rickettsia rickettsii* in an area endemic for Rocky Mountain spotted fever. J Infect Dis 151:823, 1985. *Two good studies attempting to assess the specificity and sensitivity of various serologic tests in measuring antibodies as an indicator of subclinical infections.*

Rao AK, Schapira M, Clements ML, et al.: A prospective study of platelets and plasma proteolytic systems during the early stages of Rocky Mountain spotted fever. N Engl J Med 318:1021, 1988. *An excellent presentation of the events that lead to the pathologic changes in patients with RMSF.*

Silverman D: *Rickettsia rickettsii*—induced cellular injury of human vascular endothelium in vitro. Infect Immun 44:545, 1984. *Electron microscopic study of cellular derangements caused by* R. rickettsii.

352 Other Tick-Borne Rickettsioses

DEFINITIONS. *Mediterranean spotted fever,* also known as North African tick typhus, Kenya tick-bite fever, Indian tick typhus, and boutonneuse fever, is caused by *Rickettsia conorii.* A second disease, called North Asian tick-borne rickettsiosis, is induced by *Rickettsia siberica.* A third tick-borne rickettsial infection, called Queensland tick typhus, is caused by *Rickettsia australis.* The disease produced by these agents consists of headache, fever, rash, myalgia, and malaise. The rickettsiae induce disease by invading endothelial cells and producing a vasculitis. The outcome of disease is usually favorable. The illnesses are mild compared with Rocky Mountain spotted fever (RMSF). One other difference is the usual presence of a depressed, black ulcer—the site of the tick bite. This is the *tache noire,* or eschar, and has been likened to a cigarette burn.

ETIOLOGY, DISTRIBUTION, AND EPIDEMIOLOGY. Mediterranean spotted fever (MSF) occurs in countries bordering the Mediterranean Sea, but also in the Middle East, India, and Pakistan. Several species of ticks are involved. The brown dog tick, *Rhipicephalus sanguineus,* is the main vector, but ticks common to wild animals transmit *R. conorii* in African countries. Italian epidemiologists have demonstrated a dramatic increase in the incidence of this disease in Italy, Spain, and Israel. The assumption is that the suburbanization of cities and towns resulted in increased opportunities for humans to contact ticks.

The distribution of *R. siberica* extends from European Russia through Siberia to the Soviet Far East and south into the Indo-Pakistan subcontinent. Several species of hard, or ixodid, body ticks appear to be the vectors: *Haemaphysalis concinna, Dermacentor sylvarum,* and *Dermacentor nuttallii.* Transovarian transmission occurs in these three naturally infected ticks.

Queensland tick typhus is one of several rickettsial infections found in Australia. The *R. australis* is carried by the tick *Ixodes holocyclus,* and marsupial animals are among known animal reservoirs.

PATHOLOGY. These three rickettsiae are very similar to *R. rickettsii.* There is greater than 90 per cent homology by DNA hybridization between the latter strain and *R. conorii.* All share group-specific antigens but have species-specific antigens as well that allow for their identification. These strains invade endothelial cells and cause cell death, resulting in a vasculitis (see Ch. 351). Each of these three strains produces an eschar (*tache noire*) at the site of the tick bite.

SYMPTOMS, LABORATORY FINDINGS, AND DIAGNOSIS. The onset of disease caused by each of these three rickettsiae is sudden and characterized by fever, headache, malaise, myalgia, and conjunctival injection. These symptoms and signs appear about 5 to 7 days after the tick bite. The eschar is the distinguishing sign that confirms the diagnosis. It should be looked for in the scalp, axillae, and groin area, regions of the body favored by ticks. Because of the necrotic nature of the eschar, lymph nodes draining the region of the eschar are enlarged. The lesion has been appropriately likened to a cigarette burn, about 2 to 5 mm in diameter with a black center and a raised, erythematous rim. The lesion is only mildly tender.

As with RMSF, a rash appears on the fourth to fifth day. The faint pink macular-papular lesions represent small hemorrhages into the skin. The rash is generalized, including the palms and soles of the feet. The duration of the disease is about 2 weeks. Mortality is unusual.

The Weil-Felix reaction demonstrates agglutinating antibodies to OX-19 antigen in most patients; these appear in the second to third week of disease. The microimmunofluorescence test for detection of antibodies to *R. conorii* is the serologic test of choice, if available.

A skin biopsy stained with immunofluorescent antibody stain is the most rapid and earliest diagnostic procedure. This approach is indicated only when the diagnosis of spotted fever is suspected and a *tache noire* eschar is not present.

TREATMENT. Tetracycline and chloramphenicol are the drugs of choice. Defervescence occurs within 2 days. Therapy (see Ch. 351) should be continued for at least 2 days after the patient becomes afebrile.

PROPHYLAXIS. Prevention of human disease requires avoidance of tick bites. Travelers into wild game country of Africa should check their clothes and skin carefully for ticks. Tourists traveling to southern European countries should search for ticks if they go on hiking tours through suburban and rural areas during the spring and summer months.

Recovery from these rickettsial infections imparts solid immunity. In experimental animals *R. conorii* is relatively avirulent compared with most strains of *R. rickettsii.* However, animals recovered from infections with the former strain are protected against challenge with virulent *R. rickettsii.* This protection is mediated by T lymphocytes that recognize antigens on other species of rickettsial agents of the spotted fever group.

HUMAN EHRLICHIOSIS (SPOTLESS ROCKY MOUNTAIN SPOTTED FEVER). The first recognized case occurred in 1986. The organism *Ehrlichia canis* is catalogued in the family Rickettsiaceae. As the species name indicates, it causes disease in canines and is known to be transmitted by ticks (*R. sanguineus*—brown dog tick). The reservoir of *E. canis* is unknown. Much of what is known of this disease has been acquired through retrospective serologic studies and prospective studies of hospital admissions who present with signs and symptoms suggestive of the disease, as well as comparisons of human illness with induced and acquired disease in dogs.

Serologic surveys of febrile hospitalized patients have demonstrated an equal or greater incidence than RMSF. Oklahoma and Georgia surveys in 1987 and 1988 revealed an estimated incidence of 3.3 and 5.3 cases, respectively, per 100,000 persons per year. The Centers for Disease Control reported an informal, laboratory-based survey from 1989 in which 38 cases were detected. Only 4 cases were from Oklahoma and 2 from Georgia. Each state had many more cases of RMSF (see Fig. 351–1). The other 32 cases were from Missouri (14), Virginia (10), Washington (2), Arkansas (1), Illinois (1), Louisiana (1), and Texas (1). Serologic surveys have revealed low titers (1:40 or less) of antibodies in 96 per cent of normal persons. The significance of these low titers is uncertain but may suggest that the infection is more common than RMSF and that many infections must be asymptomatic. As with RMSF, peak incidence is in spring and early summer months.

E. canis has not yet been isolated from patients who have been diagnosed by serologic tests and/or visualization of the organism in leukocytes. Although this does not satisfy Koch's postulates, the serologic evidence is compelling, and the electron microscopic pictures of the organisms in white blood cells are morphologically compatible with *E. canis.* The demonstration of the organisms in inclusion bodies in leukocytes (most likely in lymphocytes, but also in monocytes and neutrophils) is rare. These bodies are round or ovoid, purple to dark blue (Leishman stain), and 2 to 5 μm in diameter. One to four bodies have been seen per infected cell. The electron microscope reveals these bodies to contain a few to as many as 40 microorganisms. Their size of 0.2 to 0.8 μm is consistent with that of rickettsiae and of *E. canis.*

Infected humans (and dogs) present with fever, thrombocytopenia, leukopenia (lymphopenia), and anemia. Bone marrow biopsies reveal hypocellularity and occasional noncaseating granulomas. Evidence of liver cell damage appears subsequently; in dogs this is thought to be due to enlargement of cells of the reticuloendothelial system with compression of adjacent parenchyma. Many patients are asymptomatic and are diagnosed only by serologic surveys. A few hospitalized patients have had significant disease; the manifestations may have been due to hemorrhage into various part of the body, perhaps a vasculitis (seen in dogs) or secondary infections. Fever is usually short-lived (3 to 7 days), but one untreated patient was febrile for 19 days. Rash is unusual, but petechial lesions are likely with thrombocytopenia. Myalgia, headache, asthenia, nausea, or vomiting are common complaints. Physical findings are minimal; the presence of fever, petechial rash, and history of tick bite plus leukopenia is very suggestive of RMSF and of ehrlichiosis. The absence of a rash, but with the other characteristics, should suggest *E. canis* infections. Therapy is the same—tetracycline or chloramphenicol. This treatment for patients thought to have RMSF, but with minimal or no rash and subsequently no serologic response, probably cured many patients with ehrlichiosis. Diagnosis is made by demonstrating a fourfold rise in antibody titer. Single titers of 1:160 or greater have been interpreted as indicative of recent infection. An indirect fluorescent antibody (IFA) test using *E. canis* grown in primary canine monocyte blood cultures has been the discriminating serologic standard.

De Micco C, Raoult D, Toga M: Diagnosis of Mediterraneam spotted fever by using an immunofluorescence technique. J Infect Dis 153:137, 1986.

Raoult D, De Micco C, Gallais H, et al.: Laboratory diagnosis of Mediterranean spotted fever by immunofluorescent demonstration of *Rickettsia conorii* in cutaneous lesions. J Infect Dis 150:145, 1984. *These investigators studied two groups of patients to demonstrate the usefulness of the technique and then to establish the sensitivity and specificity of the procedure.*

Fishbein D, Kemp A, Dawson JE, et al.: Human ehrlichiosis: Prospective active surveillance in febrile hospitalized patients. J Infect Dis 160:803–810, 1989.

Harkess JR, Ewing SA, Crutcher JM, et al.: Human ehrlichiosis in Oklahoma. J Infect Dis 159:576–579, 1989. *These two papers provide important epidemiologic evidence about the incidence of E. canis infections in Georgia and Oklahoma. They also compare the incidence to that of RMSF in those states.*

Harris RL, Kaplan SL, Bradshaw MW, et al.: Boutonneuse fever in American travelers. J Infect Dis 153:126, 1986. *Excellent color print of eschar. Provides warning to American physicians to be alert to the tick-borne rickettsial disease that tourists can acquire overseas.*

Maeda K, Markowitz N, Hawley RC, et al.: Human infection with *Ehrlichia canis*, a leukocytic rickettsia. N Engl J Med 316:851–856, 1987. *The first reported case of ehrlichiosis. This patient had intracytoplasmic inclusion bodies in leukocytes that led eventually to the correct diagnosis.*

Mansueto S, Tringali G, Walker DH: Widespread simultaneous increase in the incidence of spotted fever group rickettsiosis. J Infect Dis 154:539, 1986.

Vicente V, Alegre A, Ruiz R, et al.: Kinin-prekallikrein system in Mediterranean spotted fever. J Infect Dis 154:541, 1986. *These authors carefully studied the kinin system and found that unlike in RMSF, it was not activated in MSF; additional laboratory evidence confirmed the lesser virulence of R. conorii.*

353 Rickettsialpox

DEFINITION. Rickettsialpox is a rare mite-borne infectious disease caused by *Rickettsia akari*. This mild, self-limited illness consists of headache, fever, an eschar at the site of the mite bite, and a papulovesicular rash.

ETIOLOGY. *R. akari* is classified with the spotted fever group of rickettsia. It is a small, gram-negative, coccobacillus-shaped, obligate intracellular organism.

DISTRIBUTION AND INCIDENCE. Rickettsialpox was first described in 1946. In the subsequent few years, more than 500 cases were diagnosed, primarily in New York City. Since the early 1950's, only one outbreak has occurred, again in New York City. The disease is virtually unknown throughout the rest of the United States.

TRANSMISSION AND EPIDEMIOLOGY. The original description of this disease included the isolation of *R. akari* from persons with the disease, from mites (*Allodermanyssus sanguineus*) that feed on rodents, and from house mice (*Mus musculus*). Engorged mites were occasionally found on the mice; attachment was usually around the rump. The mites remain in the nest, where access to mice is readily available. Intrusion into this animal-ectoparasite cycle by humans can result in an infected mite's biting and inducing disease. The ecologic range of *A. sanguineus* covers most of the United States, and mice are ubiquitous animals. Thus the elements for potential epidemics exist. Isolated cases may develop from unusual exposure to mice, as in persons working in land fills or in homeless persons sleeping in abandoned buildings.

Rickettsialpox is fairly common in some urban areas of the Ukraine, where rats appear to be the animal reservoir. In Korea small field mice are infected.

PATHOLOGY. The known pathologic changes are limited to the skin, since this is a nonfatal infection. Histologic examination of the eschar (site of mite bite) reveals intense inflammation with necrosis. Other findings are similar to those in Rocky Mountain spotted fever: thrombosis and necrosis of capillaries, edema, and a monocytic perivascular infiltrate. The characteristic rash in this disease is papulovesicular. The lesions contain fluid that may yield *R. akari* on culture.

CLINICAL MANIFESTATIONS AND COURSE. The bite of the mite is not painful and goes unnoticed. This site undergoes a localized inflammatory reaction over the next week to 10 days. During this time the edema and cellular components of the reaction create a slowly enlarging, firm, erythematous papule, which may reach 1 to 1.5 cm in diameter. The involved skin separates gradually, creating a vesicle that finally breaks down to form an ulcer. The base of the ulcer is usually black and is surrounded by a rim of erythematous skin. This progression occurs over a 3- to 7-day period, at the end of which there is the sudden onset of fever, chills, sweats, headache, backache, and malaise. The lymph nodes draining the area of the eschar enlarge but are nontender. These symptoms and signs may be present for a week if no specific antibiotic treatment is administered.

As with other members of the spotted fever group, a rash appears after 2 to 3 days of illness. Initially the lesions are maculopapular, few in number, and distributed mostly on the trunk and abdomen, rarely involving the palms or soles. The lesions evolve quickly and uniformly into vesicular lesions; the vesicle appears to sit on top of an erythematous papule. These lesions persist for about a week; the fluid in the vesicle is slowly absorbed, and a scab forms, which leaves a brownish discoloration in the skin after it falls off. This gradually clears without leaving a scar. There is no significant internal organ involvement.

DIAGNOSIS. The diagnosis is made by clinical observation; the unique lesions of the rash, the presence of the eschar, and a history that suggests contact with rodents in the past 2 weeks provide sufficient evidence to make the diagnosis. Serologic studies confirm the diagnosis; complement-fixing antibody titers have been the standard, but indirect immunofluorescent antibodies are more specific, when available. Confusion exists regarding whether the Weil-Felix reaction can be used to diagnose rickettsialpox. In about 10 per cent of patients in small series, significant titer rises to OX-19 and OX-2 have been observed. The test lacks sensitivity for confirming the diagnosis. The organism can be isolated from the vesicular fluid or from clotted blood specimens. These materials must be injected into animals or embryonated eggs. Laboratory tests are of no diagnostic help, although leukopenia is common.

The rash may be confused with the lesions of chickenpox, but no eschar is present in chickenpox. In addition, the lesions of chickenpox are usually in various stages of maturity, whereas the character of those in rickettsialpox is more uniform. Finally, the vesicle of rickettsialpox appears to sit on a papule, whereas those of chickenpox lack such a base.

PROGNOSIS. Rickettsialpox is a benign illness, and recovery occurs without therapy.

TREATMENT. Treatment with tetracycline or doxycycline shortens the febrile period and hastens recovery. Antibiotic treatment need only be administered for 3 to 4 days to ensure a cure. No relapse will occur.

PREVENTION AND CONTROL. Rickettsialpox is a zoonosis involving a common house pest, the mouse. Control of this reservoir through elimination of mouse harborages and the application of residual acaricides to walls adjacent to mice-infested areas should control mite populations. There is no available vaccine.

Brettman LR, Lewin S, Holzman RS: Rickettsialpox: Report of an outbreak and a contemporary review. Medicine 60:363, 1981. *Good summary of clinical features of recent outbreak.*

Dolgopol VB: Histologic changes in rickettsialpox. Am J Pathol 24:119, 1948.

Greenberg M, Pelliteri O, Klein IF, et al.: Rickettsialpox—a newly recognized rickettsial disease. II. Clinical observations. JAMA 133:901, 1947. *Original clinical description of a newly recognized spotted fever group infection.*

Huebner RJ, Stamps P, Armstrong C: Rickettsialpox—a newly recognized rickettsial disease. I. Isolation of the etiological agent. Public Health Rep 61:1605, 1946. *Excellent description of the discovery of rickettsialpox.*

Lackman DH: A review of information on rickettsialpox in the United States. Clin Pediatr 2:296, 1963. *A resource for information on rickettsialpox in the United States.*

354 Scrub Typhus

DEFINITION. Scrub typhus is an acute febrile illness caused by *Rickettsia tsutsugamushi* (from the Japanese: *tsutsuga,* "dangerous"; *mushi,* "bug"). This rickettsia is inoculated into humans during the bite by a chigger. The site of the bite develops into an eschar.

ETIOLOGY. *R. tsutsugamushi (R. orientalis)* is a small, gramnegative, obligate intracellular organism. Unlike other rickettsial infections, infection with *R. tsutsugamushi* does not induce solid protection against additional bouts of scrub typhus. This results from the variable antigenic compositions of the strains.

This is the only rickettsia whose polysaccharides bear an antigenic relationship to *Proteus* OX-K. This *Proteus* strain is used in serologic tests to confirm scrub typhus.

DISTRIBUTION. This disease occurs almost exclusively in the large triangular region extending from the northern islands of Japan southwest to Australia and southeast to the South Pacific Islands. This region contains the larval form of mites that are both vector and reservoir of rickettsiae.

TRANSMISSION AND EPIDEMIOLOGY. *R. tsutsugamushi* is transmitted to humans by the bite of the larva of trombiculid mites (chiggers). Chiggers are the only stage in the life cycle of these mites (*Leptotrombidium deliensis* and others) that can feed on humans. Chiggers are almost microscopic, often brilliantly colored (red bugs). The chiggers feed on rats and other small rodents. The word "scrub" was applied because of the type of vegetation—transitional between forests and clearings—that maintains the chigger-mammal relationship. But other regions (semiarid, sandy beaches, and so on) also support rodents and mites. Humans encounter scrub typhus when they enter such areas to build roads, to clear fields or forests, or on military expeditions. Circumscribed regions are highly endemic, a reflection of the lack of mobility of the chiggers and their rodent hosts. Mites transmit the rickettsiae to their offspring via the ova. In this fashion they can serve as vector and reservoir of the etiologic agent.

This disease has been called river or flood fever because of the increased incidence during the rainy seasons. Chiggers and mites proliferate in warm, wet environments.

PATHOLOGY. *R. tsutsugamushi* invades endothelial cells to produce a vasculitis (see Ch. 351). The serious pathologic manifestations in untreated patients are predominantly myocarditis, meningoencephalitis, and pneumonitis. Coagulopathy develops but is less severe than in Rocky Mountain spotted fever or typhus.

The site of the chigger bite develops into a papular lesion that ulcerates to form an eschar. This is associated with regional and later generalized lymphadenopathy.

CLINICAL MANIFESTATIONS AND COURSE. The incubation period for development of the primary papular lesion ranges from 6 to 18 days. This lesion can occur anywhere on the body. It enlarges, undergoes central necrosis, and crusts to form the eschar. As the eschar matures, the patient has the sudden onset of headache, fever, chills, and malaise. Over the next several days, these symptoms increase in severity with further elevation of the temperature. The patient, if untreated, may become stuporous as meningoencephalitis develops. Signs of cardiac dysfunction, including minor electrocardiographic abnormalities such as first-degree heart block and inverted T waves, can appear. The rash of scrub typhus appears at the end of the first week of disease. This is a faint, pink maculopapular rash appearing first on the trunk and spreading to the extremities.

Physical findings late in the first week of illness include generalized lymphadenopathy and palpable spleen and occasionally liver. Pulmonary findings are often absent despite radiographic evidence of interstitial pneumonia. In those patients with myocarditis, there may be a gallop rhythm, poor-quality heart sounds, and systolic murmurs.

Various cranial nerve deficits have been noted in untreated patients. Deafness, dysarthria, and dysphagia may occur but are usually transient, although deafness can last for several months.

All of 87 (nonimmune) soldiers in Vietnam who developed scrub typhus had fever and headache, 46 per cent had an eschar, and 35 per cent had a rash. Eighty-five per cent had generalized lymph node enlargement. It is not surprising that many were misdiagnosed as having infectious mononucleosis.

Laboratory studies reveal leukopenia early in the disease with subsequent increase of white blood cell counts to normal levels. Coagulopathies can be demonstrated, but only rare patients develop the disseminated intravascular clotting syndrome. Liver enzyme values may be elevated, indicating hepatocellular damage. Proteinuria is common.

Patients with untreated disease remain febrile for about 2 weeks and have a long convalescence of 4 to 6 weeks thereafter.

DIAGNOSIS. The variable presentations in this disease make the clinical diagnosis difficult. The eschar and rash should suggest a rickettsial infection, but these may be found in fewer than one half of patients. Furthermore, the eschar and rash may suggest other rickettsial infections, such as tick-borne typhus. A knowledge of the endemic foci of scrub typhus and determination of whether the patient has traveled or worked in such areas constitute important epidemiologic information. A therapeutic trial of tetracycline or chloramphenicol is indicated in patients in whom the diagnosis of scrub typhus is suspected. Defervescence should occur within 24 hours.

The specific serologic test is the detection of significant increases (greater than fourfold) of indirect immunofluorescent antibodies in paired serum specimens obtained 2 weeks apart. The *Proteus* OX-K antigen test is readily available and inexpensive, so that it is frequently employed in endemic areas. About 50 per cent of patients have diagnostic titers. In Malaya, the sensitivity and specificity of both tests were found to be about the same, but their usefulness was enhanced when they were used concurrently.

R. tsutsugamushi can be isolated from a patient's blood by inoculating it, intraperitoneally, into white mice. The rickettsiae can be demonstrated in the tissues of the mice.

PROGNOSIS. Without treatment, the mortality rate ranges from 0 to 30 per cent depending upon virulence and resistance factors; with treatment, survival is the expected outcome. Second or third attacks of scrub typhus, caused by different serotypes, usually result in a mild illness, usually with no eschar or rash.

Persistence of *R. tsutsugamushi* in lymph node tissues has been demonstrated 1 year after recovery. This finding raises the possibility of reactivation of disease during immunosuppression.

TREATMENT. Tetracycline, doxycycline, and chloramphenicol are all effective. The drug should be continued for at least 2 days after the patient has become afebrile.

PREVENTION AND CONTROL. Vaccines were developed and tested during and after World War II. Some were effective against homologous strains. However, no single antigen has been identified that induces protection against all of the antigenically diverse strains of *R. tsutsugamushi*. In military populations in endemic areas, weekly doses of doxycycline protect against scrub typhus.

Avoidance of chigger attachment can be accomplished by insect repellents applied to the skin and by wearing protective clothing impregnated with benzyl benzoate. Diethyltoluamide preparations such as OFF and DEET are also effective if sprayed on clothing and exposed skin but are removed rapidly by water. Application of this chemical to socks is especially important in preventing chigger bites.

Berman SJ, Kunidin WD: Scrub typhus in South Vietnam: A study of 87 cases. Ann Intern Med 79:26, 1973. *A good analysis of the clinical features of scrub typhus appearing in United States troops. Helpful in assessing potential for disease in tourists returning from endemic areas.*

Brown GW, Saunders JP, Singh S: Single dose doxycycline therapy for scrub typhus. Trans R Soc Trop Med Hyg 72:412, 1978. *Clinical investigation on the feasibility of a single dose of drug to treat scrub typhus.*

Traub R, Wisseman CL Jr: The ecology of chigger-borne rickettsiosis (scrub typhus) (review article). J Med Entomol 11:237, 1974. *Excellent summary by two experts who have clarified much of what is now known about the ecology of this disease.*

355 Trench Fever

DEFINITION. Trench fever is caused by a louse-borne rickettsial organism *Rochalimaea quintana*. Patients have a self-limited but relapsing illness characterized by headache, fever, and severe pain in bones, joints, and muscles. Because of these latter complaints, the disease has been called shin-bone fever. Other synonyms include Volhymia fever and 5-day or quintan fever.

ETIOLOGY AND EPIDEMIOLOGY. *R. quintana* is distinct from other rickettsia because it can be grown extracellularly and can be cultivated on cell-free blood agar. It is transmitted to humans by the body louse *Pediculus humanus humanus*. The organism lives in the digestive tract of lice, a permanent carrier state, and is excreted in the feces. It is the deposition of the feces on scratched or abraded skin that allows the organisms to penetrate into the human host. Once in the bloodstream, *R. quintana* may persist for months to years. This rickettsemia serves as a source of infection for other lice and may be associated with relapses of disease, or the host may remain asymptomatic despite it. Late relapses may be precipitated by stresses to the immune system such as other infections, malignancies, or vaccine administration.

Trench fever is rarely diagnosed in the United States. Epidemics occurred during World Wars I and II in Europe. Cases have been reported from Mexico and Bolivia and in Africa and Asia. Diagnosis of the disease is usually made during epidemics.

PATHOLOGY AND CLINICAL MANIFESTATIONS. Little is known of the pathologic changes associated with this disease. The rash that occurs has been biopsied and these specimens revealed perivascular infiltrates consisting of lymphocytes, but no endothelial damage has been seen. It is not known where the organism resides in the human host.

The clinical manifestations are variable and nonspecific. The incubation period ranges from 14 to 35 days (average 22 days). Most patients have the sudden onset of fever with chills, headache, retro-orbital pain, especially on moving the eyes, and pain in joints, bones, and muscles. Bone pain is often severe in the shin, thighs, and back. The temperature may rise to 39.5° to 40°C and persists for several days to a week. There may be an evanescent erythematous macular rash; the lesions blanch with pressure. Only a few lesions are present on the chest, back, and abdomen, and they disappear within 24 hours.

On physical examination, the spleen and liver may be enlarged and the conjunctivae are injected. Laboratory findings are of no diagnostic help; white blood cell count is variable, and proteinuria and polyuria are common.

Relapses of disease occur in 50 per cent of patients. These are associated with a short, variable, febrile course. Multiple relapses are not unusual.

DIAGNOSIS. Isolated cases in immigrants or travelers are difficult to diagnose. The finding of body lice in clothing or on the patient should alert the physician to the diagnosis. Blood cultivated on agar containing 10 per cent fresh defibrinated horse blood yields *R. quintana*. Serologic tests are available in some state laboratories or at the Centers for Disease Control. The disease can be confused with influenza, relapsing fever, louse-borne typhus, malaria, dengue, leptospirosis, and typhoid fever.

TREATMENT AND PROGNOSIS. No therapeutic regimen has been proven in clinical trials. Tetracycline and chloramphenical are antibacterial in in vitro testing. Tetracycline therapy appears to control the acute phase of the disease. Relapses,

however, do occur despite this treatment. Mortality, even without antibiotic treatment, is very rare. Eventual recovery does occur in most patients; the remainder continue to have recurrences for months or years.

PREVENTION. Control of body lice is the key. Obviously, preventing the acquisition of lice through bathing and clean clothing would be effective, but not practical in times of war. Dusting of clothing, especially the seams, with DDT 10 per cent, Allethrin, or Abate 2 per cent, may be done. The lice that may be present on the patient should be removed with Kwell Shampoo and/or lotion or cream.

Hurst A: Trench fever. Br Med J 2:318, 1942. *A good resource document outlining the variety of clinical manifestations of trench fever.*

Vinson JW: *In vitro* cultivation of the rickettsial agent of trench fever. Bull WHO 35:155, 1966.

356 Q Fever

DEFINITION. Q fever is a systemic infection caused by the inhalation of small numbers of *Coxiella burnetii*. Domestic animals and pets are the usual sources of infection for humans. This highly infectious rickettsial agent induces mild febrile illness, occasionally associated with pneumonitis, but in a few patients causes chronic hepatitis and life-threatening endocarditis.

ETIOLOGY. *C. burnetii* is unique among the rickettsiae in the following ways: It is not transmitted to humans by arthropod vectors; rather, it is readily disseminated by aerosols. No rash ensues despite the similarity of the infection of endothelial cells (vasculitis) as occurs with *Rickettsia rickettsii*. The organism resides uniquely inside the phagolysosome in the cytoplasm of the infected cell. *C. burnetii* does not have cross-reacting antigens with *Proteus vulgaris*, and, therefore, antibodies developed during infection do not agglutinate in the Weil-Felix test. These rickettsiae are resistant to destruction by environmental stresses, e.g., sunlight, humidity.

Isolation of *C. burnetii* from pulmonary secretions, liver biopsies, and surgical cardiac valve specimens is possible but not recommended unless appropriate laboratory facilities are available. This is a highly infectious agent that can readily cause laboratory-acquired infections. These materials are injected into eggs and/or guinea pigs. In the latter, the production of agglutinating antibodies confirms the presence of the organism. *C. burnetii* can exist in two phases. Phase I organisms are usually associated with chronic, severe clinical illnesses, such as endocarditis. Phase II organisms evolve (through the loss of mono- and polysaccharide chains of the lipopolysaccharide surface antigens) following multiple transfers in eggs. Phase II is equivalent to the rough and Phase I to the smooth form of gram-negative bacteria. Antibodies to Phase II organisms are predominant in the majority of patients with Q fever. However, patients with endocarditis have higher titers of antibodies to Phase I organisms, specifically IgA and IgG; the latter two types of antibodies are diagnostic for this entity.

Three different types of plasmids have been found in *C. burnetii*. These may account for the variations in virulence of strains but do not account for the phase variation, since plasmids are found in organisms in either phase. Persons with mild infections have isolates that contain different plasmids from those isolated from patients with endocarditis. These plasmids control the production of proteins that may be involved in the infectious process. Another virulence factor appears to be the lipopolysaccharide antigens. These antigens are variable, but are strain-specific and thus are unique for those strains associated with chronic disease, such as endocarditis. Similarly, other specific antigens are on strains that cause mild disease.

EPIDEMIOLOGY. Human disease is acquired by inhalation of aerosols containing *C. burnetii*. The organisms are disseminated from domestic and pet animals (cats). The placentas from these animals contain huge concentrations of rickettsiae. During delivery of the placenta, aerosols are generated which may be wind borne to contaminate soil, clothing, and the wool or fur of other animals or may be transmitted hundreds of yards to susceptible persons. Trucks carrying sheep appear to disseminate organisms to persons passed on the streets. Sheep regularly transported to research laboratories through hallways in a medical center caused an epidemic that persisted for 6 months. Organisms are also found in the mammary glands and milk of sheep and cows, amniotic fluid, and feces. The ability of *C. burnetii* to form sporelike structures that resist environmental destruction allows these organisms to cause disease long after the initial contamination occurs and at sites distant from the original source.

The animals are infected by ticks. There are ticks that transmit the organisms among wild animals, such as the kangaroo in Australia. Spread to domestic animals occurs when the two populations of animals intermingle. Ticks have not been implicated in the transmission from animals to humans. Q fever is a mild and inapparent infection in animals. It may be responsible for placental deficiencies that lead to stillbirth of kittens and lambs.

Various volunteer studies, designed to evaluate vaccine effectiveness, have demonstrated that very few organisms, probably less than 10, are sufficient to induce disease. For this reason, as well as the ability to survive in most environments, *C. burnetii* is a hazardous organism with which to work. In one laboratory 21 of 50 cases diagnosed over a 15-year period occurred in persons working in laboratories (or offices) not directly involved in Q fever research. Presumably, these persons were infected by widely disseminated aerosols from laboratory accidents or from contaminated clothing of workers socializing outside their laboratory. Despite the infectious nature of the organism and its presence in sputum, human-to-human transmission does not occur and respiratory isolation for infected patients is not needed.

In the United States and Canada, *C. burnetii* (and antibodies) have been found in milk from numerous herds of cattle. Despite this evidence, documented cases of Q fever occurring after the ingestion of unpasteurized milk from such cows have not been identified. The ingestion of 10^5 organisms by mouth by volunteers failed to induce disease. If disease occurs, it could originate from aerosols created in the act of pouring the milk into a glass.

The incubation period varies indirectly with inoculum size. Large doses result in disease at about 7 days. Most persons develop symptoms at 13 to 18 days.

PATHOLOGY. Knowledge of the pathologic changes is greatest for the more severe form of this disease. For example, microscopic examinations of liver biopsies and autopsy material from patients dying of chronic hepatitis and from heart valves infected with *C. burnetii* are available. Patients with pneumonitis usually have a mild illness so tissue specimens are scarce. Animal studies have provided complementary pathohistologic data.

Hepatitis. Granulomas with fatty necrosis are typical microscopic findings. These granulomas are doughnut-shaped. While they are common in Q fever, they also are seen in patients with tuberculosis. Fatty metamorphosis is also seen. Patients with mild forms of Q fever may have elevated liver enzyme values indicative of minimal liver cell damage.

Subacute and Chronic Endocarditis. This is a life-threatening disease because of the difficulty in eradicating the infection. These patients may have large vegetations on the aortic valve and less likely on the mitral valve. They have negative blood cultures and frequently have a history of a febrile illness with or without pneumonitis months previously. The vegetations have a histologic picture similar to that in other forms of endocarditis, an avascular collection of fibrin and platelets. These patients also have enlarged livers and spleens, plus signs of vasculitis associated with endocarditis, e.g., splinter hemorrhages, Roth spots, and petechiae.

Pneumonitis. In the few autopsies performed, consolidation similar to that of other bacterial pneumonias was the gross finding. The microscopic examination revealed an exudate loaded with histocytes and no polymorphonuclear leukocytes. This inflammatory response is compatible with a nonbacterial process. The histologic features have been described as those of a "severe intra-alveolar, focally necrotizing, hemorrhagic pneumonia with associated necrotizing bronchitis and bronchiolitis."

The portal of entry of *C. burnetii* is the respiratory tract; small particles less than 3 to 5 μ in diameter can reach the terminal bronchioles. The pneumonia does not appear until the third or fourth day of fever. In a mouse model, the rickettsia enter pneumatocytes, histiocytes, and fibroblasts. The self-limiting nature of this infection is probably related to the destruction of the organisms in the macrophages. However, *C. burnetii* can persist for 2 months inside those cells. Some of the macrophages can be damaged by *C. burnetii*, leading to an inflammatory response. Cellular immune mechanisms attack these damaged cells. Numerous factors are involved in the pathogenesis of pneumonia—the number and virulence of the rickettsiae, particle size, and the functional status of the macrophages and parenchymal cells of the lung.

CLINICAL MANIFESTATIONS. The onset of Q fever is very abrupt; the manifestations are not specific. The patient develops a high fever that is associated with headache, chills, myalgia, and malaise. This flulike syndrome differs from influenza disease because of the height of the temperature, frequently 39.4° to 40°C. The fever also persists for 10 to 14 days. No rash occurs. Retro-orbital pain, common in other rickettsial infections, is reported in 10 to 15 per cent of patients.

Patients may have a dry, nonproductive cough indicative of the bronchiolitis and the minimal pneumonitis produced by the invading *C. burnetii*. Physical findings of consolidated lung are lacking early in the course of the pneumonia. There may be decreased breath sounds, but rales are unlikely until resolution of the lesion(s) begins. The chest films reveal patchy infiltrates that frequently are multiple round, segmental opacities. These are discrete lesions. Larger areas of the lung may show consolidation, and linear atelectatic lesions occur in about half the patients with pneumonia. Resolution of the lesions is slow. The incidence of pneumonitis varies from 4 to 97 per cent in series of cases reported from the United States (28 per cent), Australia (4 to 75 per cent), and Switzerland (97 per cent). The reasons for these variations are unknown.

Most patients (85 per cent) with Q fever have hepatic involvement as measured by abnormal liver cell enzymes. Hepatomegaly is noted in about 65 per cent of patients, but few patients (10 per cent) have liver tenderness. Jaundice is unlikely (about 5 per cent of cases) unless chronic hepatitis ensues, a very rare manifestation. Liver biopsies have demonstrated, by direct immunofluorescent studies, rickettsia residing in hepatic cells. Q fever may account for a few cases of acute hepatitis. Patients with a strong exposure history should be evaluated for infection by *C. burnetii*.

The clinical manifestations of Q fever endocarditis are characteristic of those associated with the syndrome of endocarditis, e.g., splenomegaly, splinter hemorrhages, and heart murmurs. In the United States, endocarditis caused by *C. burnetii* is an extremely rare condition. Evidence of endocarditis in a patient occurs years after the acute infection. This fact, plus the lack of positive blood cultures, leads to a delay in diagnosis. The diagnosis is made by serologic means, demonstrating a high titer or a rising titer of Phase I antibodies, especially IgA and IgG classes. The level of Phase I antibodies is higher than that of Phase II, a reversal of what is seen in the common forms of Q fever. Presumably, the polysaccharide nature of the Phase I antigens is the reason they are poor immunogens, but their chronic presence leads finally to high antibody production.

DIAGNOSIS. The key to making a diagnosis of Q fever in a patient with a debilitating febrile illness is obtaining a history of contact with sheep, cattle, goats, or cats or the skins or wool from these animals. This history should be compelling enough to initiate antibiotic treatment and to obtain acute and convalescent serum for serologic studies. These latter studies are the practical and definitive diagnostic aids. Phase II antibodies (complement fixing [CF] or indirect fluorescent antibody [IFA]) are present in two thirds of patients at the end of 2 weeks of illness and in 90 per cent at 1 month. Phase I antibodies, if present, are found in titers lower than Phase II antibodies. IFA is more sensitive than CF in detecting early antibody formation (IgM) and also in demonstrating persistence of antibody at 1 year or longer. The presence of Phase I antibodies in excess of Phase II, and specifically Phase I IgA, is diagnostic of Q fever endocarditis.

The nonspecific clinical manifestations of early symptoms and signs of Q fever, e.g., headache, fever, myalgia, suggest numerous infectious diseases. Influenza infections are seasonal, the temperature is less than that of Q fever, and liver function tests are normal. The white blood cell count is not helpful, as it is normal in both infections. Other diseases such as typhoid fever and brucellosis can be diagnosed by bacterial cultures. Viral hepatitis can be mistaken for Q fever. Appropriate serologic studies and liver biopsy provide diagnostic evidence. In those patients with pneumonitis, the differential diagnosis includes viral or mycoplasmal etiologies, tularemia, psittacosis, and *Legionella pneumophila*. Serologic and culture results identify these organisms.

TREATMENT AND PROGNOSIS. *C. burnetii* is known to be susceptible to a number of antibiotics. Sensitivity studies have been conducted in eggs, guinea pigs, and recently in acute and chronically infected tissue culture cells. Tetracycline and doxycycline or chloramphenicol have been effective in vitro as well as in clinical studies. Early institution of tetracycline (within 3 days of onset) reduces the febrile course by half. Tetracycline, 500 mg four times a day, or doxycycline, 100 mg twice a day, should be continued for at least 1 week after the patient becomes afebrile (usually 2 to 3 days). The prognosis with such therapy is excellent, with no mortality expected. Those patients who receive no antibiotics also do well, with a recovery rate of over 99 per cent. If a febrile relapse occurs, retreatment with the same antibiotic is effective.

The recommended treatment of patients with Q fever endocarditis is not settled. Long-term therapy (1 year or more) with combinations of antibiotics has been effective in small numbers of patients. Tetracycline plus trimethoprim-sulfamethoxazole and rifampin plus doxycycline are two such combinations. Evidence from tissue culture studies indicates that the quinoline antibiotics in combination with rifampin may offer a therapeutic advance. Surgical resection of infected valves is usually required because the large vegetations cause hemodynamic deficiencies in cardiac function.

PREVENTION. There is no commercially available vaccine for Q fever. Experimental vaccines using either Phase I or Phase II organisms have been effective in preventing disease in volunteers and in several field trials. For those persons at high risk, such as researchers working with sheep, veterinarians, or exposed laboratory workers, vaccine can be obtained under an investigational new drug (IND) application.

Focusing on controlling disease in the workplace is more effective than attempting to control the disease in animals. Three recommended measures include knowledge of the serologic status of the employees, not permitting pregnant women or persons with valvar heart disease to be in the high-risk jobs, and confining the research on sheep to a building dedicated solely to that purpose. Vaccination of employees should also be attempted.

Derrick EH: "Q" fever, a new fever entity: Clinical features, diagnosis and investigation. Med J Aust 2:281, 1937. *The original description of Q fever.*

Khavin T, Tabibzadeh S: Histologic, immunofluorescence, and electron microscopic study of infectious process in mouse lung after intranasal challenge with *Coxiella burnetii*. Infect Immun 56:1792, 1988.

Meikeljohn G, Reimer EG, Graves PS, et al: Cryptic epidemic of Q fever in a medical school. J Infect Dis 144:107, 1981. *A good epidemiologic study of Q fever originating in a research laboratory.*

Millar JK: The chest film findings in "Q" fever—a series of 35 cases. Clin Radiol 29:371, 1978.

Sawyer LA, Fishbein DB, McDade JE: Q Fever: Current concepts. Rev Infect Dis 9:935, 1987. *An excellent review of recent investigations concerning Q fever.*

Urso FP: The pathologic findings in rickettsial pneumonia. Am J Clin Pathol 64:335, 1975.

Yeaman MR, Roman MJ, Baca OG: Antibiotic susceptibilities of two *Coxiella burnetii* isolates implicated in distinct clinical syndromes. Antimicrob Agents Chemother 33:2053, 1989. *A new method to evaluate sensitivities of Q fever isolates to antibiotics.*

Zoonoses

357 Zoonoses

J. Bruce McClain

Many infectious diseases are zoonoses with which we come into contact by way of occupation, avocation, or bad luck. Since the manifestations of disease change with each species, a mild infection for one species can be lethal for another. Many zoonoses are treated fully elsewhere in this book. This chapter is an attempt to inform practitioners of diseases contracted from animals which may deserve mention although not extensive description and are treated more fully and properly in subspecialty textbooks.

There are still three main venues where zoonotic illness is contracted: agriculture, laboratory work, and pets. Laboratory-acquired disease depends on the agents in the laboratory as well as agents proper to the species. A review summarizing the experience from several large research institutions dealing in biomedical research indicated that the most common occupational illnesses are, in decreasing order, brucellosis, Q fever, typhoid, infectious hepatitis, tularemia, tuberculosis, dermatomycoses, Venezuelan equine encephalitis, typhus, and psittacosis. Common pet-acquired illnesses are toxoplasmosis, toxocariasis, dermatomycoses, psittacosis, salmonellosis, cat scratch disease, campylobacteriosis, and lymphocytic choriomeningitis. Common agricultural illnesses are brucellosis, hydatid disease, leptospirosis, Q fever, yersinosis, cryptosporidiosis, campylobacteriosis, and anthrax. Brief descriptions of zoonoses not covered elsewhere in this text are found in Table 357–1.

Donham KJ: Zoonotic diseases of occupational significance in agriculture: A review. Int J Zoon 12:163, 1985. *An extensive description of 40 of the most important zoonoses.*

Miller CD, Songer JR, Sullivan JF: A twenty-five year review of laboratory-acquired human infection at the National Animal Disease Center. Am Ind Hyg Assoc J 48:271, 1987. *A summary of all major reports from large research institutions on occupational zoonoses.*

Stehr-Green JK, Schantz PM: The impact of zoonotic diseases transmitted by pets on human health and the economy. Vet Clin North Am: Small Anim Pract 17:1, 1987. *A description of the number of cases and fatality of pet-transmitted disease.*

TABLE 357–1. CHARACTERISTICS OF SELECTED ZOONOSES

Microorganism	Common Name(s)	Epidemiology	Syndrome	Mode of Transmission	Reservoir	Diagnosis	Treatment	Prevention
Corynebacterium ovis	Pseudotuberculosis	12 cases in agricultural workers of sheep and goats	Lymphadenitis	Mechanical inoculation from infected animals	Sheep and goats, 10–80% of herds	BI blood agar 10% CO_2	Penicillin, erythromycin, resistant to TMX	B
Pasteurella multocida	—	14,000 cases/year in pet owners and laboratory workers	Cellulitis, respiratory infection, bacteremia, similar to *H. influenzae*	Animal bites, contact with oral secretion	Dogs, cats, other domestic and wild mammals	BI	Oral AMP, TCN, IM/IV PEN G, CEF	B
Rhodococcus equi	*Corynebacterium equi*	19 cases in immunosuppressed patients	F, Mal, C, L, lung abscess	Aerosol	Cattle, pigs, sheep, cats	BI	CHL, VAN, GEN	None
Streptobacillus moniliformis	Rat-bite fever, Haverhill fever	1–2 cases/year; 12% mortality untreated	HA, N&V, My, R, arthritis 70%, endocarditis	Rat bite, trauma, food contamination	Rats, mice, weasels, dogs, pigs	Isolation on special medium, SC	PEN G, AMP, TCN, CHL × 10 days	B
Spirillum minus	Rate-bite fever, sodoku	<1 case/year; 7% mortality untreated	Local eschar, F, HA, N&V, R	Subcutaneous inoculation of infected secretion	Rodents and other mammals	Animal passage, darkfield of peripheral blood	PEN × 25 days	B
Herpesvirus simiae	Virus W	Laboratory workers, 24 cases reported, 18/24 fatal	Encephalitis, preceded by local itching or numbness	Skin defect in contact with infected saliva or animal tissues. Human-to-human transmission has occurred.	*Macaca mulatta*; lethal epizootics have occurred in bonnet macaques, pata, and colobus monkeys	SC, VI	Hyperimmune globulin not useful. ACY used in 2 human cases; ACY effective in animal model	?ACY, B
Parapoxvirus infections	Orf, milker's nodule, bovine papular stomatitis[a]	Agricultural workers	Granulomatous ulcerative lesions with regional adenopathy	Contact with infected secretions or trauma from virus-contaminated objects	Goats, cows	Histopathology, VI, electron microscopy	None	B
Paramyxovirus	Newcastle disease	Poultry workers	Follicular conjunctivitis, F, C, Mal	Direct contact with infected birds or environmental aerosols	Poultry and other birds	SC, VI	None	B, mask
Orthopox virus	Monkeypox (mouse pox, cow pox, buffalo pox[b])	Agricultural, laboratory workers, pets	L, F, R, skin pox, fever, HA, Mal, like smallpox	Direct contact	Multiple species	SC to specific virus, VI	None	B
Rhabdovirus	Vesicular stomatitis virus	Agricultural and veterinary workers	F, My, N&V, Mal, oral vesicles	Direct contact with infected animal	Horses, cattle, wild and domestic swine, plus others	SC, VI from blood	None	B
Animal herpes virus	Pseudorabies, mad itch	7 cases with animal contact	Dysphagia, altered taste and smell, cutaneous dysesthesia, paresthesia, pruritus, cranial nerve palsy	Skin and mucous membrane contact	Pigs, cats, livestock	SC, VI	None; cases resolved	B
Arenavirus	Lymphocytic choriomeningitis virus	Outbreaks from pets and labs	Aseptic meningitis	Aerosols and direct contact	Mice, hamsters	SC, VI	None	Extermination

[a]There are subtle differences between isolates from the above three diseases, but the lesions and virions are morphologically indistinguishable and serology is not useful, so the name depends on the epidemiologic setting.

[b]These are distinct viruses and the syndromes differ, but the histopathology of the lesions is similar.

Abbreviations

ACY	= acyclovir	CEF	= cephalosporin	N&V	= nausea and vomiting
AMP	= ampicillin	CHL	= chloramphenicol	PEN	= penicillin
B	= barrier techniques taken to mean physical separation and or quarantine for affected animals	F	= fever	R	= rash
		GEN	= gentamicin	SC	= seroconversion
		HA	= headache	TCN	= tetracycline
		L	= lymphadenopathy	TMX	= sulfa/trimethoprim
BI	= bacterial isolation	Mal	= malaise	VAN	= vancomycin
C	= cough	My	= myalgia	VI	= virus isolation

SECTION THREE / VIRAL DISEASES

358 Introduction to Viral Diseases

R. Gordon Douglas, Jr.

Viruses are among the simplest and smallest of all forms of life. They are obligate intracellular parasites that require host cell structural and metabolic components for replication. They infect bacteria as well as plants and animals. More than 400 distinct viruses infect humans. They produce diseases ranging from subclinical infections and mild, self-limited, localized infections to common systemic infections and overwhelming, highly lethal infections such as meningoencephalitis or hemorrhagic fever with shock.

CHARACTERISTICS OF VIRUSES

Essentially, virus particles, or virions, consist of nucleic acid enclosed in a protein coat. They lack metabolic activity and do not possess ribosomes or most enzymes necessary for replication. In addition, some possess a lipid envelope. Both the lipid and the protein coats protect the nucleic acid from enzymatic degradation. The nucleic acid may be either deoxyribonucleic acid (DNA) or ribonucleic acid (RNA). It may code for only a few or, in some cases, several hundred proteins. The protein coat, or capsid, consists of repeating, identical subunits called capsomeres. The capsid and nucleic acid together are called the nucleocapsid. The smallest (parvoviruses) are only 18 nm in diameter, whereas some poxviruses may be as large as 450 nm in diameter.

There are two major types of structure of virus particles. In the first type, capsomeres are arranged as a regular polyhedron with 20 triangular faces and 12 corners. Such a virus exhibits icosahedral symmetry. Many nonenveloped viruses are of this type. Other viruses exhibit helical symmetry in which a helix is formed of ribonucleoprotein and nucleic acid. Helical viruses are always enveloped, whereas icosahedral viruses may be enveloped

or nonenveloped. The envelope is derived from host cell membranes and modified by insertion of one or more spike-like glycoproteins. These and other proteins on the surface of enveloped or nonenveloped viruses are important for two reasons: They provide specific interaction with receptors on host cells, and they serve as the major antigens of the virus.

Figure 358–1 demonstrates schematically the marked variety in size, shape, and structure of human viruses. In addition, there is great diversity in the structure of the viral genome: Either RNA or DNA may be single stranded or double stranded. The genome may be linear or circular and may exist as single or multiple segments.

Viruses are classified by the International Committee on Taxonomy of Viruses according to the scheme presented in Table 358–1. The following order of virion characteristics is used: nucleic acid type, presence or absence of envelope, genome replication strategy, positive- or negative-sense genome, and genome segmentation.

As a result of the variety of structures of viruses and the complexities of genomes, mechanisms of replication are diverse and dependent upon the structure of the virus and its genome. Following a random collision between a virus particle and a cell surface, attachment occurs by binding of a surface protein of a virus to a host cell virus receptor. Penetration of the plasma membrane of the cell occurs by endocytosis, a process similar to receptor-mediated endocytosis of nonviral ligands, or by nonendocytic pathways such as direct translocation across the plasma membrane. Following acidification of the endosome, fusion of the viral membrane with that of the vesicle occurs, releasing the nucleocapsid. After uncoating of the viral nucleic acid, macromolecular synthesis of nucleic acid and protein occurs. The strategy for genome replication is dependent on the type of nucleic acid. Assembly of virus components then occurs, with release of mature viruses by budding, in the case of enveloped viruses, or by lysis of the cell, in the case of some nonenveloped viruses. Such released virions are infectious for other cells.

Viruses cause cell injury by a number of mechanisms: directly by lysis resulting from viral replication, by lysis induced by

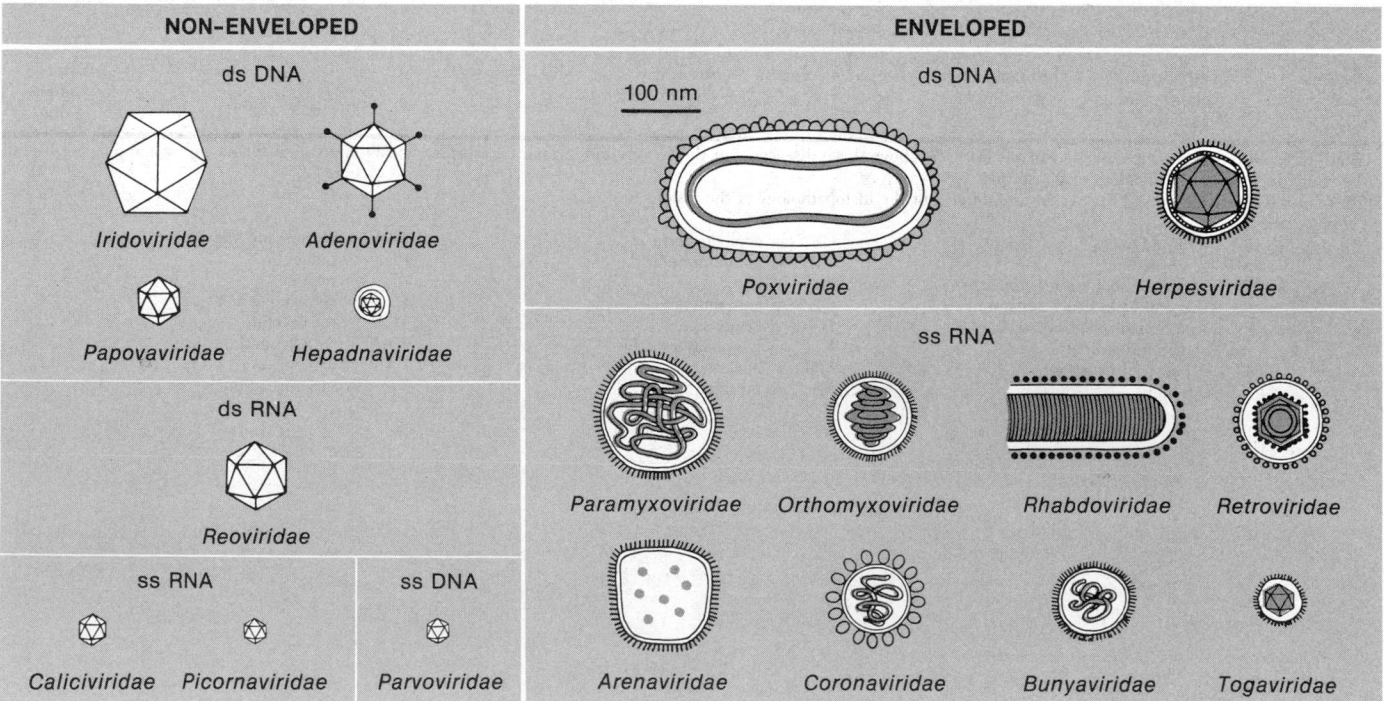

FIGURE 358–1. Structure and relative size of human virus families. (Modified from Matthews REF: Intervirology 12:158, 1979.)

TABLE 358–1. CLASSIFICATION OF HUMAN VIRUSES

Dividing Characteristics	Virus Families	Important Human Viruses
DNA Viruses		
dsDNA, enveloped	Poxviridae	Variola (smallpox) virus
		Vaccinia virus
	Herpesviridae	Herpes simplex virus types 1 and 2
		Varicella-zoster virus
		Human cytomegalovirus
		EB virus
		Human herpesvirus type 6
dsDNA, nonenveloped	Adenoviridae	Human adenovirus
	Papovaviridae	Papillomavirus
	Hepadnaviridae	Hepatitis B virus
ssDNA, nonenveloped	Parvoviridae	Parvovirus B19
RNA Viruses		
dsRNA, nonenveloped	Reoviridae	Colorado tick fever virus
		Human rotaviruses
ssRNA, enveloped		
No DNA step in replication		
Positive-sense genome	Togaviridae	Alphavirus: Eastern equine encephalitis, Western equine encephalitis
		Rubivirus: Rubella virus
	Flaviviridae	Yellow fever virus
		Dengue viruses
		St. Louis encephalitis
	Coronaviridae	Human coronaviruses
Negative-sense genome		
Nonsegmented genome	Paramyxoviridae	Parainfluenza virus
		Measles virus
		Respiratory syncytial virus
	Rhabdoviridae	Rabies virus
	Filoviridae	Marburg and Ebola viruses
Segmented genome	Orthomyxoviridae	Influenza A and B virus
	Bunyaviridae	California encephalitis virus
	Arenaviridae	LCM virus
		Lassa virus
DNA step in replication	Retroviridae	HTLV I, II
		HIV I, II
ssRNA, nonenveloped	Picornaviridae	Polioviruses, coxsackieviruses, echoviruses, rhinoviruses
	Caliciviridae	Norwalk virus

EB = Epstein-Barr; LCM = lymphocytic choriomeningitis; ss = single stranded; ds = double stranded.

From Murphy FA: Virus taxonomy. *In* Fields BN: Virology. New York, Raven Press, 1985. With permission.

antiviral antibody and complement, or by cell-mediated immune mechanisms recognizing infected host cells. As virus infection spreads and sufficient numbers of cells are injured, disease results. A role for viral toxins has never been established, and such enzymes that are virus coded have a role in viral replication, but not directly in cellular injury, and they do not affect host tissues at distant sites. However, release of products of inflammation from sites of cell injury and circulating interferon and other lymphokines may contribute to the signs and symptoms of viral infection.

In addition to lytic effects on cells, viral infection may transform cells so that they proliferate continuously, and in vertebrates, mammals, and humans, may produce tumors, sometimes as a result of the occurrence of viral oncogenes in such viruses.

HOST DEFENSE MECHANISMS

In addition to nonspecific barriers such as skin, respiratory epithelium, gastric acidity, and so on, three main host defense mechanisms against viral infections have been described: (1) production of specific antiviral antibody; (2) development of specific cell-mediated immunity involving cytotoxic T cells and nonspecific effector cells such as natural killer (NK) cells; and (3) proliferation of macrophages that restrict virus replication and dissemination and can also destroy infected cells.

Antiviral antibodies develop in response to viral infection and to immunization with attenuated or inactivated virus or viral components. In the serum, antibodies of all classes and subclasses of immunoglobulins are found; in addition, secretory antibodies consisting predominantly of immunoglobulin A (IgA) molecules develop on mucosal surfaces in response to infection of their surfaces. They are of critical importance in diseases in which the primary site of inoculation is a mucosal surface.

The immune system may interact with extracellular (free) virus or cell-associated virus. Specific antibody inactivates (neutralizes) extracellular virus, and this activity may be enhanced by complement. Thus, it can prevent initial infection or restrict cell-to-cell spread of virus through extracellular fluids. It cannot, however, penetrate into cells and neutralize intracellular virus. Thus, virus may escape the effects of antibody by direct cell-to-cell transfer. Virus-infected cells possess viral antigens on their surface and may be lysed by specific antibody and complement, by specific cytotoxic T cells, or by nonspecific cells such as NK cells or macrophages. Virus released in the process may be neutralized by antiviral antibody.

Cytotoxic T cells (Tc), which are HLA class I antigen restricted, also develop in response to infection or immunization (Ch. 242). They are important in limiting the growth of certain viruses in the infected host. This has been most clearly shown for influenza infections in mice, and Tc are undoubtedly important in a number of viral infections in humans.

Natural killer cells are another important host defense mechanism against viral infections. During early stages of viral infection, the numbers of natural killer cells and their activity are greatly augmented by virus-induced interferon. Mice deficient in NK cells are more sensitive to cytomegalovirus infection, and NK activity has been demonstrated in a number of human infections.

Virus-induced interferons (α and β) have important roles in protection against virus infection through their ability to prevent viral replication in many cells throughout the body and by means of their regulatory function in the immune system. In experimental infections in animals in which interferon activity is neutralized by specific antibody, potentiation of viral infection occurs. In humans, in a number of infections, development of endogenous

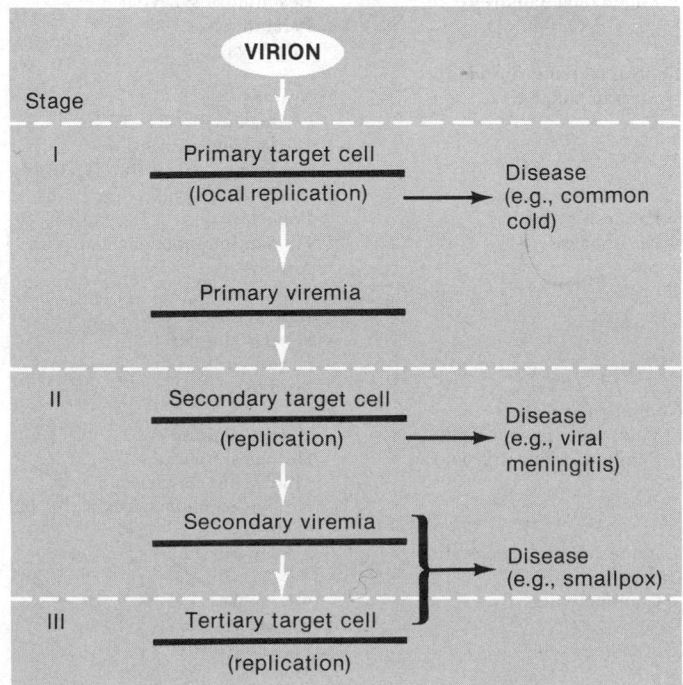

FIGURE 358–2. Stages of viral pathogenesis. Initial invasion may involve only primary target cells or may lead to secondary or tertiary target cell invasion, which results in the characteristic disease. (Courtesy of ED Kilbourne.)

interferon in serum or secretions correlates with recovery: decreasing virus titers and amelioration of symptoms. Since administration of interferon to humans produces a number of side effects, such as fever, leukopenia, and myalgias, interferon may also account, in part, for some of the systemic signs and symptoms that accompany viral infections.

Interferon-γ is induced as a result of immune stimulation. It also has antiviral effects and is a major immune regulatory protein that induces Tc, activates macrophages and NK cells, and regulates antibody production by B cells.

MECHANISMS OF PATHOGENESIS

Infection is initiated, often when one or a very few virus particles are deposited in the respiratory tract, gastrointestinal tract, or genitourinary tract or are injected percutaneously or pass transplacentally. As shown in Figure 358–2, human viral infections may be classified according to mechanisms of pathogenesis. Many infections are limited to cells at the portal of entry, and dissemination does not occur. Conjunctivitis due to adenovirus type 8 and common colds due to rhinoviruses and to other respiratory viruses are excellent examples of this type of pathogenesis.

Other virus infections spread hematogenously to distal sites. Infection at the primary site may or may not result in symptoms, but viral replication in the distal site usually results in the characteristic illness associated with such a virus infection. Enteroviruses such as coxsackievirus and echovirus infect the gastrointestinal tract as their primary site, and this infection is usually clinically silent but produces a primary viremia, following which encephalitis, meningitis, or other central nervous system disease may occur as these tissues are infected.

In other infections, viral replication in the secondary site produces a viremia that results in replication in still other sites. Such was the case with smallpox and may be the case with measles. Rash may be a manifestation of either primary or secondary viremia.

Many virus infections have clinical characteristics that permit diagnosis: measles, mumps, chicken pox, and poliomyelitis. However, many others do not, and many syndromes have multiple etiologies, as is shown in Table 358–2. In fact, as many as 200 serologically distinct viruses may cause the common cold and related disorders. In the case of some syndromes—for example, atypical pneumonia—the etiology may be shared with other infectious organisms: *Mycoplasma pneumoniae, Chlamydia pneumoniae,* and *Legionella pneumophila.* Others, however, are exclusively viral in etiology.

TABLE 358–2. VIRUSES COMMONLY ASSOCIATED WITH DIFFERENT SYNDROMES

Disease Category	Common Associated Virus	Disease Category	Common Associated Virus
Respiratory Tract		*Immune System*	
Upper respiratory infection (including common cold and pharyngitis)	Rhinoviruses	Acquired immunodeficiency syndrome	Human immunodeficiency virus I
	Coronaviruses	*Gastrointestinal Tract*	
	Parainfluenza 1–3	Gastroenteritis	Rotavirus
	Influenza A, B		Norwalk-like agents
	Herpes simplex		Adenovirus
	Adenoviruses		
	Echoviruses	Hepatitis	Hepatitis A
	Coxsackieviruses		Hepatitis B
	Epstein-Barr virus		Hepatitis C
	Respiratory syncytial		Delta virus
Croup	Parainfluenza 1–3		Hepatitis E
	Influenza A, B		Epstein-Barr virus
	Respiratory syncytial		Cytomegalovirus
Bronchiolitis	Respiratory syncytial	*Skin*	
	Parainfluenza 1–3	Maculopapular rash	Measles
Pneumonia (adults)	Influenza A		Rubella
Pneumonia (children)	Respiratory syncytial		Parvovirus B19
	Parainfluenza 1–3		Echoviruses
	Influenza A		Coxsackievirus A16
Central Nervous System			Enterovirus 71
Aseptic meningitis	Mumps	Hemorrhagic rash	Herpesvirus G
	Coxsackievirus B1–5		Alphavirus
	Coxsackievirus A9		Bunyavirus
	Echovirus 4, 6, 9, 11, 14, 18, 30, 31		Flaviviruses
		Localized lesions	Herpes simplex
Paralysis	Polio 1–3		Human papillomavirus 1, 2, 4, 41
Encephalitis	Human immunodeficiency virus I		Molluscum contagiosum
	Alphaviruses	*Neonatal*	
	Flaviviruses	Teratogenic effects	Rubella
	Bunyaviruses		Cytomegalovirus
	Herpes simplex 1	Disseminated disease	Coxsackievirus B1–5
	Enterovirus 71		Echoviruses
	Mumps		Hepatitis B
Genitourinary Tract			Parvovirus B19
Vulvovaginitis, cervicitis	Herpes simplex 2		Cytomegalovirus
Penile and vulvar lesions	Herpes simplex 2		Herpes simplex
	Molluscum contagiosum	Lower respiratory disease	Respiratory syncytial
	Human papillomavirus 6, 10, 11, 40–45, 51		Influenza
		Enteritis	Rotavirus
Acute hemorrhagic cystitis	Adenovirus 11	*Other*	
Ocular		Arthritis	Rubella
Conjunctivitis	Adenovirus 3, 4, 7, 8, 19		Parvovirus B19
	Herpes simplex		Hepatitis B
	Varicella-zoster	Myositis	Togaviruses
	Measles		Influenza B
Acute hemorrhagic conjunctivitis	Enterovirus 70	Carditis	Coxsackievirus B
	Coxsackievirus A 24	Parotitis, pancreatitis, and orchitis	Mumps

Modified from Menegus MA, Douglas RG Jr: Viruses, rickettsia, chlamydiae, and mycoplasmas. *In* Mandell GL, Douglas RG, Jr, Bennett JE: Principles and Practice of Infectious Diseases, 3rd ed. New York, Churchill Livingstone, 1990.

Recent advances in antiviral chemotherapy have produced a number of specific antivirals that are available and effective for prophylaxis or treatment, or both, of certain viral diseases. Drugs such as trifluridine, amantadine, ribavirin, acyclovir, vidarabine, zidovudine, and ganciclovir are available in the United States. For many other viral infections, however, no specific therapy exists. Proper use of antivirals requires specific viral diagnosis. Fortunately, in the case of herpes zoster, the diagnosis can usually be made clinically, and in influenza, the diagnosis can often be made on clinical and epidemiologic grounds; however, for many infections, viral diagnosis is required. Viral diagnostic laboratories are more common than in the past, and rapid techniques are gaining acceptance.

Vaccines are available for a number of viral infections, and many have greatly affected morbidity and mortality due to specific infections. Antibodies induced by vaccination may block initiation of infection in a primary site, as in the case in influenza. Others, such as inactivated poliomyelitis vaccine, are designed to prevent primary viremia after initial infection has occurred. Live attenuated viruses induce cell-mediated as well as humoral immune response.

Fields BN (ed.): Virology, 2nd ed. New York, Raven Press, 1990. *Excellent recent definitive textbook of basic virology.*

Mandell GL, Douglas RG Jr, Bennett JE (eds.): Principles and Practice of Infectious Diseases, 3rd ed. New York, John Wiley & Sons, 1990. *Excellent reference work about clinical aspects of viral infections; both syndromes and specific viruses are discussed, as well as vaccines, antivirals, and diagnostic virology.*

359 Antiviral Therapy

Mark Middlebrooks and Richard J. Whitley

Compared with the progress made in the treatment of bacterial infections over the past four decades, advances in the chemotherapy of viral diseases have come much more slowly. In the United States, only a few antiviral agents of proven clinical value are available and for a limited number of indications. The problems associated with the development of antiviral agents can be summarized as follows: (1) viruses are obligate intracellular parasites that utilize biochemical pathways of the infected host cell, so that it is difficult to achieve clinically useful antiviral activity without also adversely affecting host cell metabolism; (2) early diagnosis of viral infection is crucial for effective antiviral therapy, yet by the time symptoms appear several cycles of viral multiplication may have occurred and replication has begun to wane; (3) precise diagnosis is difficult for many viral infections because of the lack of specificity of symptoms; and (4) since many of the disease syndromes caused by viruses are common, relatively benign, and self-limiting, the therapeutic index (ratio of efficacy to toxicity) must be extremely high for therapy to be acceptable.

As with all infectious diseases, the effectiveness of therapy is related to host defenses. Not only is the incidence of reactivation of certain viral diseases high in the immunocompromised host, but these infections are often much more severe. These patients require high doses of antiviral agents for long periods of time and have a high morbidity and mortality with currently approved antiviral therapy.

ANTIVIRALS FOR HERPESVIRUS INFECTIONS

Vidarabine

MECHANISM OF ACTION. Also known as vira-A or adenine arabinoside (9-β-D arabinofuranosyl adenine), vidarabine is a purine nucleoside analogue that is phosphorylated intracellularly to its active triphosphate derivative. This compound competitively inhibits DNA-dependent DNA polymerases of some DNA viruses approximately 40 times more than those of host cells. In addition, it is incorporated into DNA, thus inhibiting elongation. Although viral DNA synthesis is blocked at lower doses of drug than is host cell DNA synthesis, large doses of vidarabine are cytotoxic to dividing host cells.

LICENSED USES. Vidarabine is licensed currently for intravenous treatment of herpes simplex encephalitis (HSE), neonatal herpes simplex virus (HSV) infections, and varicella-zoster virus (VZV) infections in immunocompromised patients. In addition, vidarabine 3 per cent ophthalmic ointment is approved for the treatment of HSV keratoconjunctivitis and recurrent epithelial keratitis.

TOXICITY AND ADVERSE CLINICAL EFFECTS. When therapeutic doses are given intravenously, vidarabine causes few adverse effects in most patients. The most common side effects (10 to 15 per cent incidence) are gastrointestinal disturbances (e.g., anorexia, nausea, vomiting, diarrhea), which are usually mild. Central nervous system disturbances occasionally include tremors, dizziness, confusion, hallucinations, ataxia, and psychoses. An elevated aspartate aminotransferase level and blood urea nitrogen may also be seen. Doses of 20 mg per kilogram per day may cause more pronounced central nervous system effects as well as leukopenia and thrombocytopenia. Vidarabine is a relatively insoluble drug that requires continuous administration in large volumes of fluid given over 12 hours. This relative difficulty in administration as compared with acyclovir, as well as acyclovir's more favorable safety profile, has resulted in the latter becoming the drug of choice for virtually all HSV and VZV infections.

Vidarabine should be recognized historically as the first drug licensed for systemic use in the treatment of a viral infection. Although it is efficacious for a number of herpesvirus infections, for the most part it has been replaced by acyclovir.

Acyclovir

MECHANISM OF ACTION. Acyclovir, 9-((2-hydroxyethoxy)methyl) guanine, is an acyclic analogue of guanosine. Virus-specified thymidine kinase phosphorylates acyclovir to its monophosphate derivative, an event that does not occur in uninfected cells to a significant extent. Acyclovir is then further phosphorylated by cellular enzymes to its triphosphate derivative. Acyclovir triphosphate binds viral DNA polymerase, acting as a DNA chain terminator. Because acyclovir is taken up selectively by virus-infected cells, the concentration of acyclovir triphosphate is 40 to 100 times higher in infected than in uninfected cells. Furthermore, viral DNA polymerase exhibits a 10- to 30-fold greater affinity for acyclovir triphosphate than do cellular DNA polymerases. The higher concentration in infected cells plus the affinity for viral polymerases results in the very low toxicity of acyclovir for normal host cells. Although Epstein-Barr virus (EBV) and cytomegalovirus (CMV) do not have virus-specific thymidine kinases, acyclovir does have minimal activity against these viruses.

LICENSED USES. Acyclovir is available in ointment, capsule, and intravenous formulations. In the topical form, acyclovir is licensed for the management of primary herpes genitalis in both immunocompetent and immunocompromised hosts as well as in limited, non–life-threatening mucocutaneous HSV infections in immunocompromised hosts. It is less active topically than when delivered by other routes.

Oral acyclovir is indicated in the management of most cases of primary or initial genital herpes in all patient populations and as suppressive therapy in normal hosts with frequently recurrent genital herpes (six or more recurrences a year). Oral acyclovir is also used as prophylaxis and treatment in immunocompromised patients with a history of HSV infections, e.g., herpes labialis or genital herpes. High-dose oral acyclovir (i.e., 800 mg five times per day) has recently been approved for use in immunocompetent patients with localized herpes zoster. However, there has been no conclusive demonstration of a decrease in the incidence of postherpetic neuralgia after treatment with acyclovir.

Intravenous acyclovir is indicated in severe initial herpes genitalis of immunocompetent patients and in the treatment of some initial and recurrent mucocutaneous infections in immunocompromised patients, as well as in the treatment of HSE (licensure pending). Recently, intravenous acyclovir was approved for treatment of VZV infections in immunocompromised hosts. Oral high-dose administration for the treatment of VZV infections in immunocompromised patients is currently under investigation.

TABLE 359–1. DOSAGE ADJUSTMENT FOR INTRAVENOUS ACYCLOVIR IN PATIENTS WITH IMPAIRED RENAL FUNCTION

Creatinine Clearance (ml/min/1.73 M²)	Percentage of Standard Dose	Dosing Interval (Hours)
>50	100	8
25–50	100	12
10–25	100	24
0–10*	50	24

*Administered after hemodialysis.

TOXICITY. Acyclovir has an excellent safety profile and is well tolerated. The major adverse effect of acyclovir is alteration of renal function. High-dose bolus injection of acyclovir can cause crystallization in renal tubules and subsequent acute tubular necrosis, or simply a reversible elevation of serum creatinine. Dehydration, pre-existing renal insufficiency, and higher doses of acyclovir are risk factors for renal toxicity. Dosage alterations are required with renal impairment (Table 359–1). In addition, there have been a few brief reports suggesting CNS toxicity after intravenous administration of acyclovir. Oral acyclovir has not been associated with renal toxicity, even when given in high doses (800 mg five times a day).

Because acyclovir is a nucleoside analogue that can be incorporated into both viral and host-cell DNA, it has been studied extensively for its potential as a carcinogen, teratogen, and mutagen. There is no significant evidence that acyclovir is a carcinogen in humans, and animal studies indicate that acyclovir is not a significant teratogen in clinically used doses. Acyclovir is not a significant mutagen in vitro but seems to be able to induce chromosomal events in a manner similar to that of caffeine. Because of the many possible indications for acyclovir during pregnancy, as well as the likelihood of frequent first-trimester exposures to drug before pregnancy is established, it is extremely important to define the risk of acyclovir in pregnancy. An "Acyclovir in Pregnancy Registry" has been established to gather data on all reported prenatal exposures to oral acyclovir. Although no significant risk to the mother or fetus has been documented, the total number of monitored pregnancies remains too small to detect any risk that is not overwhelming. The safety of acyclovir in pregnancy, therefore, has not been unequivocally established. Since acyclovir crosses the placenta and can concentrate in amniotic fluid, there is valid concern about the potential for renal toxicity in the fetus.

RESISTANCE TO ACYCLOVIR. Resistance to acyclovir develops through mutations in one of two HSV genes, namely those specifying viral thymidine kinase (TK) or DNA polymerase. Clinical isolates resistant to acyclovir are almost uniformly deficient in TK. Until recently such resistance has been rare; all such mutants had reduced neurovirulence and did not readily establish latency. However, acyclovir-resistant HSV mutants are being reported more frequently in the immunocompromised patient population. These mutants are deficient in viral TK and sensitive to vidarabine and foscarnet, drugs that do not require viral TK for activation. Importantly, a small number of isolates are fully neurovirulent and able to establish latency in a murine model, a finding somewhat unusual for TK-deficient viruses. With the growing population of immunocompromised patients (due to both HIV infection and therapeutic immunosuppression) who suffer from frequent and severe herpesvirus infections, it is expected that acyclovir resistance will become more prevalent.

Ganciclovir

MECHANISM OF ACTION. Ganciclovir, also known as DHPG, is an acyclic nucleoside analogue of acyclovir that has increased in vitro activity against all herpesviruses as compared with acyclovir, including an 8 to 20 times greater antiviral activity against CMV. Like acyclovir, the activity of ganciclovir in HSV-infected cells depends upon phosphorylation by virus-specific TK. Also like acyclovir, ganciclovir monophosphate is further converted to its di- and triphosphate derivatives by cellular kinases. In cells infected by HSV-1 or HSV-2, the triphosphate (DHPG-TP) competitively inhibits the incorporation of guano-sine-TP into viral DNA and terminates chain synthesis. The mode of action of ganciclovir against CMV and EBV (which do not produce virus-specific TK) is not entirely known, but it has been suggested that these viruses may induce a cellular TK or other kinase that efficiently promotes the obligatory initial phosphorylation of ganciclovir to its monophosphate.

LICENSED USES. Ganciclovir has been licensed by the United States Food and Drug Administration for the treatment of CMV retinitis and life-threatening CMV diseases in AIDS and other immunocompromised patients.

TOXICITY. The most important side effects of ganciclovir are the development of neutropenia and thrombocytopenia. Neutropenia occurs in approximately 35 per cent of patients and is usually (but not always) reversible with dose adjustment or discontinuation. Thrombocytopenia occurs in about 20 per cent of patients. Numerous other side effects possibly related to ganciclovir, such as nausea, vomiting, dizziness, and headache, are usually not of clinical significance. Agents with significant myelotoxicity, such as antimetabolites or alkylating agents, cannot be used concomitantly with ganciclovir. Zidovudine (azidothymidine, or AZT) may be used cautiously in low doses in patients receiving ganciclovir, but hematologic parameters must be monitored closely.

Ganciclovir also has significant gonadal toxicity in animal screening systems, most notably as a potent inhibitor of spermatogenesis. As an agent affecting DNA synthesis, ganciclovir has carcinogenic potential.

CLINICAL USE. Ganciclovir has been the most widely tested drug for the treatment of CMV infections. There is support for clinical benefit in immunocompromised patients with CMV retinitis and gastrointestinal infection. Benefit is suggested but has been less dramatic for CMV pneumonia in AIDS patients and organ transplant recipients. There are many issues requiring further study to determine the optimal use of ganciclovir, including the indications, dose, duration of maintenance therapy, prophylactic use, usefulness of other modalities in combination (e.g., immunoglobulin therapy), and use in treatment of other life-threatening herpesvirus infections.

Idoxuridine and Trifluorothymidine

Idoxuridine and trifluorothymidine are analogues of thymidine. When administered systemically, these nucleosides are phosphorylated by both viral and cellular TK to active triphosphorylate derivatives that inhibit both viral and cellular DNA synthesis. The result is antiviral activity but also sufficient host cytotoxicity to prevent the systemic use of these drugs. Toxicity of these compounds is not significant, however, when applied topically to the eye in the treatment of HSV keratitis. Both idoxuridine and trifluorothymidine, as well as vidarabine, ophthalmic ointments are effective and licensed for such treatment. Acyclovir as an ophthalmic preparation also appears to be effective but is not yet licensed. Trifluorothymidine appears to be the most efficacious of these compounds. Although these agents are not of proven value in the treatment of stromal keratitis and uveitis, trifluorothymidine is more likely to penetrate the cornea. Some forms of stromal keratitis and uveitis are thought to be caused by immune mechanisms and thus would not respond to antiviral drugs. The ophthalmic preparations of idoxuridine, vidarabine, and trifluorothymidine may cause local irritation, photophobia, edema of the eyelids and cornea, punctual occlusion, and superficial punctate keratopathy.

ANTIVIRALS FOR RESPIRATORY VIRAL INFECTIONS

It is difficult to overestimate the impact of respiratory viral illnesses on human health. Almost 90 per cent of the population experiences one of these illnesses each year, resulting in a staggering number of days lost from work and school, as well as significant potential for serious morbidity and even death. Nonetheless, since these conditions in most patient populations are self-limited and rarely fatal, the requirements for new drugs are stringent: an extreme degree of safety, moderate to high effectiveness, ease of administration, and low cost. Accordingly, only two such antivirals are approved for use in the United States, each with fairly limited indications. Because of the number of developmental programs identifying new antivirals for treatment of respiratory viruses, it seems likely that an expanded armamentarium will be forthcoming.

Amantadine and Rimantadine

MECHANISM OF ACTION. Amantadine has a narrow spectrum of activity, and at concentrations achievable in humans it is useful only against influenza A infections. Although amantadine was the first antiviral to be approved in the United States, its mechanism of action is not yet completely understood. Influenza A viruses differ in their susceptibility to amantadine, and the drug may have different actions depending upon the concentration and virus strain. Early studies indicated that amantadine acted by preventing the penetration of the virus and/or by uncoating it. In more recent studies, low concentrations of the drug were shown to inhibit virus assembly by interacting with hemagglutinin; high concentrations appear to inhibit an early stage of the infection involving fusion between the virus envelope and the membrane of secondary lysosomes.

LICENSED USES. As an antiviral agent, amantadine is licensed for both the chemoprophylaxis and the treatment of influenza A infections. Amantadine can be used for any unimmunized member of the general population who wishes to avoid influenza A, but prophylaxis with amantadine is especially recommended for control of presumed influenza outbreaks in institutions housing high-risk persons. High-risk individuals include adults and children with chronic disorders of the cardiovascular or pulmonary systems requiring regular follow-up or hospitalization during the preceding year, as well as residents of nursing homes and other chronic-care facilities. In these instances, amantadine should be administered to all residents of the institution, whether or not they received influenza vaccination the previous fall. To reduce spread of virus and to minimize disruption of patient care, it is also recommended that amantadine prophylaxis be offered to unvaccinated staff who care for high-risk patients. Amantadine prophylaxis is also recommended in the following situations:

1. As an adjunct to late immunization of high-risk individuals. Amantadine does not interfere with antibody response to the vaccine.
2. For persons who have not been immunized and who care for high-risk persons in home settings, both to reduce spread of virus and to allow persons to maintain care for high-risk persons in the home setting.
3. For immunodeficient persons, who may be expected to have a poor antibody response to vaccine.
4. For persons for whom influenza vaccine is contraindicated, e.g., for persons hypersensitive to egg protein.

Amantadine is also indicated in the treatment of uncomplicated respiratory illness caused by influenza A. Studies have shown a beneficial effect on the signs and symptoms of acute influenza, as well as a significant reduction in quantity of virus in respiratory secretions. Because of the short duration of disease, amantadine must be administered within 48 hours of symptom onset to show benefit. The effect of amantadine on the prevention of complications in high-risk groups is under evaluation.

Rimantadine is a structural analogue of amantadine, with the same spectrum of activity, mechanism of action, and clinical indications. Rimantadine is used extensively in the Soviet Union and has been widely tested in the United States. It is anticipated that this drug will be licensed soon in the United States. Rimantadine is somewhat more effective than amantadine against influenza type A viruses at equal concentrations. Absorption of rimantadine is delayed when compared with amantadine, and, furthermore, equivalent doses of rimantadine produce lower plasma levels than does amantadine. The lower plasma levels may explain the lower incidence of side effects at similar doses. Rimantadine has similar CNS side effects even though, unlike amantadine, this drug does not affect CNS catecholamine release and is not effective in the treatment of Parkinson's disease. The efficacy of rimantadine in both the prophylaxis and treatment of influenza A infections is similar to that of amantadine. There has been a recent report of rimantadine-resistant strains of influenza isolated from patients treated for acute influenza A.

TOXICITY. Amantadine is reported to cause side effects in 5 to 10 per cent of healthy young adults taking the standard adult

TABLE 359–2. DOSAGE ADJUSTMENT FOR ORAL AMANTADINE IN PATIENTS WITH IMPAIRED RENAL FUNCTION

Creatinine Clearance (ml/min/1.73 M²)	Suggested Oral Maintenance Regimen After 200 mg (100 mg bid) on the First Day
≥ 80	100 mg bid
60–80	100 mg bid alternating with 100 mg daily
40–60	100 mg daily
30–40	200 mg (100 mg bid) twice weekly
20–30	100 mg 3 times each week
10–20	200 mg (100 mg bid) alternating with 100 mg every 7 days
<10	100 mg every 7 days

dose of 200 mg per day. These side effects are usually mild, cease soon after amantadine is discontinued, and often disappear even with continued use of the drug. Central nervous system side effects are most common and include difficulty in thinking, confusion, lightheadedness, hallucinations, anxiety, and insomnia. Activities requiring mental alertness (e.g., driving) should be avoided until it is reasonable to assume that these symptoms will not occur. More severe adverse effects, e.g., mental depression and psychosis, are usually associated with doses exceeding 200 mg daily. About 5 per cent of patients complain of nausea, vomiting, or anorexia. Older individuals are more likely to experience side effects. Rimantadine appears to be somewhat better tolerated.

Patients with renal disease should receive doses based on their creatinine clearance (Table 359–2). Doses for older people and children are usually lower as well. Persons with an active seizure disorder may be at increased risk for seizures when amantadine is given at standard doses.

Ribavirin

MECHANISM OF ACTION. Ribavirin is a nucleoside analogue whose mechanisms of action are poorly understood and probably not the same for all viruses; however, its ability to alter nucleotide pools and the packaging of mRNA appears to be important. This process is not totally virus specific, but there is a certain selectivity in that infected cells produce more mRNA than noninfected cells. The capacity of viral mRNA to support protein synthesis is markedly reduced by ribavirin. High concentrations also inhibit cellular protein synthesis.

LICENSED USES. The development of a mechanism to deliver ribavirin via a small-particle aerosol greatly enhanced the potential usefulness of this drug for respiratory viral infections. At this time ribavirin is licensed for the treatment, by aerosol administration, of carefully selected hospitalized infants and young children with severe lower respiratory tract infections caused by respiratory syncytial virus (RSV). The vast majority of infants and children with RSV infection have disease that is mild and self-limited and do not require ribavirin.

TOXICITY AND CLINICAL PROBLEMS. No adverse effect has been clearly attributable to aerosol therapy with ribavirin, although reports of adverse effects during or following therapy of infants with RSV have included bronchospasm, pulmonary function test changes, pneumothorax in ventilated patients, apnea, cardiac arrest, hypotension, and concomitant digitalis toxicity. Precipitation of drug within the ventilatory apparatus of patients on mechanical ventilation can be a serious problem. When proper precautions are taken, such as frequent changes in ventilator tubing, safe delivery of ribavirin to ventilated patients can be accomplished. Reticulocytosis, rash, and conjunctivitis have been associated with the use of ribavirin aerosol. Although there are no pertinent human data, ribavirin has been found to be teratogenic and mutagenic in nearly all species in which it has been tested. This drug is, therefore, contraindicated in women who are or may become pregnant. Some concern has been expressed about the risk to persons in the room with infants being treated with ribavirin aerosol, particularly females of childbearing age. Although this risk seems to be minimal with limited exposure, awareness and caution are warranted.

FUTURE ANTIVIRALS

Advances in molecular virology continue to define those sites of viral replication which may be vulnerable to attack without harm to the host cell. Further characterization of the viral DNA polymerase, required for replication but not utilized by the host cell, is a major research focus. In addition, classes of compounds, many of them nucleoside analogues, are being systematically evaluated in order to identify more efficacious and less toxic antivirals. A description of some of the most promising drugs follows.

Several compounds have activity against the herpesviruses, including foscarnet sodium (trisodium phosphonoformate, PFA), 1-β-D-arabinofuranosyl-E-5-(2-bromovinyl) arabinosyluracil (BV-araU), fluoroidoarabinosyl cytosine (FIAC), and (S)-1-((3-hydroxy-2-phosphonylmethoxy)propyl) adenine (HPMPA).

Foscarnet, a pyrophosphate analogue of phosphonoacetic acid (PAA), has potent in vitro and in vivo activity against herpesviruses. Unacceptable toxicity was demonstrated with PAA (deposition in bone), but foscarnet has been less toxic. These drugs inhibit the DNA polymerase of all human herpesviruses by blocking the pyrophosphate binding site and preventing chain elongation. Unlike acyclovir, which requires activation by a virus-specific thymidine kinase, foscarnet acts directly on the virus DNA polymerase. Thymidine kinase–deficient, acyclovir-resistant herpesviruses remain sensitive to foscarnet. Foscarnet has recently attracted attention as an inhibitor of HIV replication and is undergoing evaluation in patients with AIDS. It is in clinical trials as a treatment for CMV infection. The lack of marrow toxicity of foscarnet offers an advantage over ganciclovir. Renal toxicity, however, has been demonstrated.

Bromovinyl arabinosyl uracil, BV-araU, is a potent inhibitor of HSV-1 and EBV. More importantly, it is exquisitely active against VZV, being over 1000 times more potent than acyclovir. Like acyclovir, the mechanism of action of BV-araU is based upon the phosphorylation of the parent compound by herpesvirus TK, which restricts its action to virus-infected cells. BV-araU appears to have a favorable toxicity profile and will soon begin clinical trials in the United States.

Fluoroiodoarabinosyl cytosine (FIAC) and fluoroiodoarabinosyl uracil (FIAU), its principal metabolite, are both potent selective inhibitors of herpesviruses. Like acyclovir and BV-araU, their activity depends on phosphorylation by herpesvirus TK. The parent compound is converted rapidly to the triphosphate in infected cells, selectively utilized by virus DNA polymerase, and incorporated into viral DNA, resulting in the formation of very short DNA chains. In vitro, FIAC has greater activity than acyclovir against HSV-1; it is also active against HSV-2, VZV, and CMV. Because of its oral bioavailability, FIAC is thought to have potential usefulness in the treatment of CMV retinitis in patients with AIDS.

HPMPA is a potent, broad-spectrum antiviral agent that is one of a new class of nucleotide analogues structurally characterized as phosphonylmethyl ethers of acyclic nucleoside derivatives. The associated guanine and cytosine analogues are designated HPMPG and HPMPC. HPMPA has in vitro activity against HSV-1, HSV-2, CMV, VZV, EBV, adenovirus, and a retrovirus. The mechanism of action of HPMPA is thought to be similar to that of acyclovir, i.e., the triphosphate analogue inhibiting viral DNA polymerase. The difference, however, is that HPMPA is a monophosphate equivalent and does not require phosphorylation by a virus-specific TK, allowing HPMPA to have an expanded spectrum of activity. Of all these compounds, HPMPC is emerging with the most clinical potential. Although its in vitro potency is only moderate, HPMPC exhibits impressive potency in vivo.

INTERFERONS

HISTORY AND INTRODUCTION. Interferons (IFN) are glycoprotein cytokines (intracellular messengers) with a complex array of immunomodulating, antineoplastic, and antiviral properties. The name *interferon* was derived from landmark experiments by Isaacs and Lindemann in 1957, demonstrating the existence of a biologic substance that "interfered" with viral replication in infected cells. Interferons are currently classified as α, β, or γ, with natural sources of these classes, in general, being leukocytes, fibroblasts, and lymphocytes, respectively. Each type of IFN can now be produced via recombinant DNA technology. The complexity of the response to IFN, including the variability of dose response, duration of therapy, and combination with other treatments, creates enormous challenges to determine appropriate clinical scenarios in which IFN might be a worthwhile therapeutic agent.

MECHANISM OF ACTION. Binding of IFN to the intact cell membrane is the first step in establishing an antiviral effect. Interferon binds to specific cell surface receptors; IFN-γ appears to have a different receptor from either IFN-α or -β, which may explain the purported synergistic antiviral and antitumor effects sometimes observed when IFN-γ is given with either of the other two IFN species.

A prevalent view of IFN action is that, following binding, there is synthesis of new cellular RNA's and proteins, which mediate the antiviral effect. The antiviral state is not fully expressed until these primed cells are infected with virus. In addition to their antiviral effect, IFN's have a number of other biologic activities, including inhibition of cell proliferation and enhancement of the cytotoxic activities of lymphocytes, the expression of cell surface antigens, and the phagocytic and tumoricidal activities of macrophages. These properties may play an important role in the in vivo antiviral and antitumor effects of the IFN's.

LICENSED USES. Although promising for a number of viral infections and HIV-associated conditions, the only licensed use of IFN as an antiviral is its intralesional administration in the treatment of condyloma acuminatum, or genital warts, which are caused by human papillomaviruses. Only IFN-α is licensed.

TOXICITY AND CLINICAL PROBLEMS. Side effects are frequent with IFN administration and are usually dose-limiting. Influenza-like symptoms, i.e., fever, chills, headache, and malaise, commonly occur, but these symptoms usually become less severe with repeated treatments. At doses used in the treatment of condyloma acuminatum, these side effects rarely cause termination of treatment and may be reduced in severity by pretreatment with acetaminophen. For local treatment (intralesional injection) pain at the injection site does not differ significantly from that in placebo-treated patients and is short-lived. Leukopenia is the most common hematologic abnormality, occurring in up to 26 per cent of patients treated for condyloma. Leukopenia is usually modest, not clinically relevant, and reversible upon discontinuation of therapy. Increased alanine aminotransferase levels may also occur, as well as nausea, vomiting, and diarrhea.

At higher doses of IFN, neurotoxicity is encountered, as manifested by personality changes, confusion, loss of attention, disorientation, and paranoid ideation. Early studies with IFN-γ show similar side effects as treatment with IFN-α and -β but with the additional side effects of dose-limiting hypotension and a marked increase in triglyceride levels.

CLINICAL TRIALS. Interferon has potential use against virtually all viral infections. Its ultimate utility depends on a number of factors, including the acceptability of side effects, cost, and the availability of other antivirals. Of the many viral infections in which IFN has been tested, treatment of condyloma acuminatum, chronic hepatitis B, chronic hepatitis C, and recurrent respiratory papillomatosis and prophylaxis of rhinovirus and coronavirus upper respiratory infection have been promising.

Condyloma Acuminatum. Several large controlled trials have demonstrated the clinical benefit of IFN-α therapy of condyloma acuminatum. These studies have demonstrated clearance rates of treated lesions from 36 to 62 per cent. Up to one third of lesions treated with IFN recur. Much research remains to be done to examine the effects of different routes of administration, prolonged therapy, repeated courses of treatment, and combined treatment with other therapeutic modalities (i.e., cryotherapy, podophyllin, and laser ablation).

Respiratory Papillomatosis. Recurrent respiratory papillomatosis is a disease in which squamous papillomata relentlessly recur within the larynx and trachea of both children and young adults. Standard management consists of careful microendoscopic excision, usually with a CO_2 laser. In recent years, there have been numerous case reports and uncontrolled studies supporting benefit from IFN as an adjunct to surgical treatment. Results of placebo-controlled trials have suggested benefit.

Hepatitis. The inhibitory effect of human leukocyte IFN-α on hepatitis B virus (HBV) replication was first reported more than

TABLE 359–3. INDICATIONS FOR THE USE OF AVAILABLE ANTIVIRAL AGENTS

Indication	Antiviral Agent	Route	Dose	Comments
Respiratory syncytial virus infection (infants)	Ribavirin	Aerosol	Diluted in sterile water to a concentration of 20 mg/ml, then delivered via aerosol for 12–18 hrs/day for 3–7 days	Only for infants at high risk
Life- or sight-threatening CMV infections in immunocompromised hosts	Ganciclovir	IV	5.0 mg/kg q12h × 14 days	Maintenance therapy of 5.0 mg/kg/day recommended for AIDS patients. Leukopenia is a frequent complication; in bone marrow transplant patients with CMV pneumonia, CMV immune globulin may be a useful adjunct
Condyloma acuminatum	Interferon-α	Intralesional	1.0 million units injected into the base of each lesion, up to 3 times per week for 3 weeks	Flu-type symptoms may occur with administrations
Influenza A infection	Amantadine	Oral	Adults: 100–200 mg/day for 5–7 days Children ≤ 9 years: 4.4–8.8 mg/kg/day for 5–7 days not to exceed 150 mg/day	Normal person >65 years of age should receive 100 mg/day
Prophylaxis against influenza A virus infection	Amantadine	Oral	Adults: 100–200 mg/day Children ≤ 9 years: 4.4–8.8 mg/kg/day (not to exceed 150 mg/day)	Continued for the duration of the epidemic or for 2 weeks in conjunction with influenza vaccination (until vaccine-induced immunity develops); normal persons >65 years of age should receive 100 mg/day
Herpes simplex virus (HSV) encephalitis	Acyclovir	IV	10 mg/kg (1 hour infusion) every 8 hours for 10–14 days	Morbidity and mortality are significantly lower in patients treated with acyclovir than with vidarabine
Neonatal herpes	Vidarabine or Acyclovir	IV IV	30 mg/kg/day (continuous infusion over 12 hours) for 10 days 10 mg/kg (1 hour infusion) every 8 hours for 10 days	Efficacy of vidarabine is established; vidarabine and acyclovir show equal efficacy
Mucocutaneous HSV in immunocompromised hosts	Acyclovir or Acyclovir or Acyclovir	IV Oral Topical	250 mg/M² or 6.2 mg/kg (1 hour infusion) every 8 hours for 7 days 400 mg 5 times/day for 10 days 5% ointment; 4–6 applications/day for 7 days or until healed	Choice of topical, oral, or intravenous preparation depends upon clinical severity and setting; topical acyclovir is appropriate only when it can be applied to all lesions; it does not affect untreated lesions or systemic symptoms Least desirable
Prophylaxis against mucocutaneous HSV during intense immunosuppression	Acyclovir or Acyclovir	Oral IV	200 mg 3–4 times/day 250 mg/M² every 8 hours or 5 mg/kg every 12 hours (1 hour infusion)	Oral therapy most convenient; lesions recur when therapy stops Lesions recur when therapy stops
Treatment of initial genital HSV infections	Acyclovir or Acyclovir	Oral IV	200 mg 5 times/day for 10 days 5 mg/kg (1 hour infusion) every 8 hours for 5–7 days	Drug of choice in most clinical settings; treatment has no effect on subsequent recurrence rates For patients requiring hospitalization or with neurologic or other visceral complications
Recurrent genital herpes	Acyclovir	Oral	200 mg 5 times/day for 5 days	No effect on subsequent recurrence rates; efficacy greater if used early in attack
Prophylaxis against frequently recurring genital herpes	Acyclovir	Oral	200 mg 3–5 times/day	Occasional "breaking through" attacks and/or asymptomatic virus shedding during treatment; re-evaluation every 6 months recommended
Treatment of HSV keratitis	Trifluorothymidine or Vidarabine or Idoxuridine	Topical Topical Topical	One drop of 0.1% ophthalmic solution every 2 hours while awake (up to 9 drops/day) One-half-inch ribbon of 3% ophthalmic ointment 5 times/day One-half-inch ribbon of 0.5% ophthalmic ointment 5 times/day	3% acyclovir ointment (ophthalmic) is equal or superior to idoxuridine, vidarabine, and trifluridine for treatment of HSV keratitis but is not available in the United States
Localized herpes zoster in immunocompetent hosts	Acyclovir	Oral	800 mg 5 times/day for 7–10 days	Shortens time to lesion healing, but not shown to decrease the incidence of postherpetic neuralgia
Chickenpox in immunocompromised hosts	Acyclovir or Vidarabine	IV IV	500 mg/M² (1 hour infusion) every 8 hours for 7 days 10 mg/kg/day (continuous infusion over 12 hours) for 5 days	In the absence of comparative data, acyclovir is preferred because of its ease of administration and lower toxicity.
Treatment of severe localized or disseminated herpes zoster in immunocompromised hosts	Acyclovir or Vidarabine	IV IV	500 mg/M² or 12.4 mg/kg (1 hour infusion) every 8 hours for 5–7 days 10 mg/kg/day (continuous infusion over 12 hours) for 5–7 days	Comparative trials in severe localized and disseminated herpes zoster are under way; pending results, acyclovir is preferred because of its ease of administration and lower toxicity

10 years ago. Treatment with IFN-α in chronic hepatitis B subsequently has been investigated in several large, randomized, controlled trials. The earlier studies were encouraging, but the response rate was low at approximately 30 per cent.

In an attempt to enhance the efficacy of antiviral therapy, combinations of IFN with other agents have also been studied. Vidarabine and acyclovir have been used in such studies with little success. It has been observed, however, that the use of a short course of corticosteroids before treatment with IFN-α results in "immunologic rebound" after prednisone withdrawal. This phenomenon, which seems to be directed at virus-infected hepatocytes, is characterized by an acute hepatitis-like elevation of serum aminotransferases and a transient decline in levels of HBV DNA polymerase and HBV DNA. The results of a large multicenter trial comparing patients randomly assigned to receive one of two doses of IFN-α versus prednisone followed by IFN-α, or no treatment, were recently published. The authors found that a 4-month treatment regimen of subcutaneous IFN-α in a dose of 5 million units daily resulted in a complete response (loss of serum HBeAg and HBV DNA) in nearly 40 per cent of patients, and that reactivation of infection within 6 months after treatment was no greater than 2 per cent. The beneficial effect of pretreatment with a tapering dose of prednisone was limited to patients with low baseline levels of alanine aminotransferase (less than 100 units per liter). The best predictor of response in this study was the HBV DNA level before treatment, with approximately half of the patients having levels less than 100 pg per milliliter experiencing a complete response. Long-term follow-up studies are required to determine the duration of antiviral effect and the impact on survival.

The efficacy of IFN for treatment of chronic hepatitis C (non-A, non-B hepatitis) has also recently been investigated. Both acyclovir and corticosteroids have been ineffective, but preliminary reports suggest benefit with the use of IFN. The first large, randomized, placebo-controlled study of IFN-α therapy in patients with chronic hepatitis C showed that the serum alanine aminotransferase levels declined to normal in 38 per cent of patients treated with 3 million units of IFN-α for 6 months, compared with 4 per cent of untreated patients. However, only 52 per cent of the patients who initially responded to treatment remained in remission during 6 months of follow-up.

Respiratory Infections. The upper respiratory infection known as the "common cold" has a multitude of possible viral causes (see Ch. 360). It has been demonstrated that nasal spray or drops of IFN-α provide prophylaxis against the common cold caused by rhinovirus or coronavirus infection. Although clinical benefit was demonstrated in these studies, administration of IFN-α for 2 to 3 weeks led to hemorrhage of nasal mucosa.

IMMUNOGLOBULIN THERAPY

Efficacy has been established for prophylactic immunoglobulin administration for several viral infections, but the use of immunoglobulin alone for therapy of established disease has not been proven unequivocally beneficial for any viral infection. Benefit has been shown for the administration of intravenous immunoglobulin or CMV hyperimmune globulin when combined with ganciclovir in the treatment of CMV pneumonia in bone marrow transplant recipients. Survival was increased to 52 to 79 per cent, which is significantly better than that of historical controls treated with either agent alone. Currently active areas of research include the efficacy of CMV hyperimmune globulin for prevention and treatment of disease in bone marrow, kidney, and heart transplant patients, and that of CMV monoclonal antibody in the treatment of established CMV disease in AIDS patients.

CONCLUSION

Although relatively few antiviral drugs are licensed for use at this time, there is significant interest in the development of antiviral compounds. Table 359–3 summarizes the use of currently available antivirals for indications other than therapy of HIV infections. Systematic approaches have revealed a number of promising new drugs and biologic agents that are in various stages of evaluation. A better understanding of the molecular biology of virus replication and pathogenesis should elucidate agents with enhanced virus-specific activity.

Buhles WC, Mastre BJ, Tinker AJ, et al.: Ganciclovir treatment of life- or sight-threatening cytomegalovirus infection: Experience in 314 immunocompromised patients. Rev Infect Dis 10:495–503, 1988. *Describes the clinical efficacy of ganciclovir when used to treat infections of the retina, gastrointestinal tract, and lungs.*

Couch R: Respiratory diseases. *In* Galasso G, Whitley R, Merigan T (eds.): Antiviral Agents and Viral Diseases of Man, 3rd ed. New York, Raven Press, 1990, pp 327–372. *This chapter contains a summary of the published work regarding the efficacy and toxicity of amantadine, rimantadine, and ribavirin for influenza and respiratory syncytial virus infections.*

Davis GL, Balart LA, Schiff ER, et al.: Treatment of chronic hepatitis C with recombinant interferon alfa. N Engl J Med. 321:1501–1506, 1989. *The first large, randomized, placebo-controlled trial of interferon therapy of chronic hepatitis C.*

Dorsky DI, Crumpacker CS: Drugs five years later: Acyclovir. Ann Intern Med 107:859–874, 1987. *A detailed analysis of the chemistry, antiviral activity, and clinical efficacy of acyclovir.*

Hayden FG, Belshe RB, Clover RD, et al.: Emergence and apparent transmission of rimantadine-resistant influenza A virus in families. N Engl J Med 321:1696–1702, 1989. *Postexposure prophylaxis with rimantadine in families was not as effective as pre-exposure prophylaxis during community outbreaks.*

Hirsch MS, Kaplan JC: Antiviral Agents. *In* Fields BN, Knipe DM, Chanock E (eds.): Virology, 2nd ed. New York, Raven Press, 1990, pp 441–468. *A comprehensive text which includes a detailed analysis of antiviral therapy.*

Matthews T, Boehme R: Antiviral activity and mechanism of action of ganciclovir. Rev Infect Dis 10:490–494, 1988. *A concise description of the antiviral activity and mechanism of action of ganciclovir.*

Perrillo RP, Schiff ER, Davis GL, et al.: A randomized, controlled trial of interferon alfa-2b alone and after prednisone withdrawal for the treatment of chronic hepatitis B. N Engl J Med 323:295–301, 1990. *A multicenter study of combination therapy for chronic hepatitis B.*

Reichman RC, Oakes D, Bonnez W, et al.: Treatment of condyloma acuminatum with three different interferons administered intralesionally. Ann Intern Med 108:675–679, 1988. *Intralesional injections of three different interferon preparations were found to be efficacious in the treatment of condyloma acuminatum.*

Reines ED, Gross PA: Antiviral agents. Med Clin North Am 72:691–721, 1988. *An excellent review of the principles and applications of antiviral chemotherapy.*

Viral Infections of the Respiratory Tract

360 The Common Cold

Albert Z. Kapikian

DEFINITION. Although the term "common cold" does not denote a precisely defined disease, it has an almost universally comprehended meaning of an acute, self-limited, common illness of all age groups, in which the major clinical manifestations involve the upper respiratory tract, with nasal discharge (coryza) or nasal obstruction as the predominant symptom.

ETIOLOGY. Although it was known since 1914 that bacteria-free filtrates of nasal secretions from patients with a common cold could induce a similar illness in volunteers inoculated intranasally, the discovery of etiologic agents from common colds eluded scientists for many years. Despite the isolation of numerous viruses that were associated etiologically with acute respiratory illnesses, such as influenza virus in 1933, and the adeno-, parainfluenza, and respiratory syncytial viruses in the 1950's, it was clear that the major etiologic agent or agents of the common cold had not yet been discovered. However, beginning gradually in the 1950's and escalating rapidly in the 1960's, about 100 distinct common cold viruses were discovered and shown to be the major causative agents of the common cold. These heretofore fastidious agents were named rhinoviruses (rhin- is Greek for nose), because they caused predominantly nasal symptoms. Shortly thereafter, another group of fastidious viruses, the coronaviruses, were discovered and shown to be the second most important etiologic agents of the common cold and related diseases.

Rhinoviruses have emerged as the major known etiologic agents of adult upper respiratory illnesses such as common colds. They have been isolated from approximately 15 to 40 per cent of adults with these illnesses (Table 360–1). The isolation rate is lower in children with upper respiratory tract illnesses, as only about 5 per cent are rhinovirus positive. Rhinoviruses are classified as a genus in the picornavirus family and possess certain common characteristics, including small size (approximately 27 nm), ribonucleic acid (RNA) core, ether resistance, and complete or almost complete inactivation at pH 3. The last property is a major characteristic distinguishing rhinoviruses from another genus of the picornaviruses, the enteroviruses (poliovirus, coxsackievirus, and echovirus), which are stable at pH 3. There are now 100 officially designated rhinovirus serotypes and a single subtype, and it appears that this number includes most circulating strains.

The second most important etiologic agents of common colds are the coronaviruses, which are associated with 10 to 20 per cent of common colds in adults. Their importance as etiologic agents of common colds in infants and young children has not been determined. The human coronaviruses possess certain common characteristics, including (1) a unique electron microscopic appearance characterized by pleomorphic 100- to 150-nm enveloped particles possessing relatively widely spaced club- or pear-shaped surface projections (reminiscent of the solar corona, from which the name coronavirus is derived); (2) an RNA genome; and (3) ether and acid lability. There are at least three distinct human coronavirus serotypes, designated B814, 229E, and OC43. As a result of difficulties in propagating these fastidious agents, fewer than 50 isolates have been recovered since their discovery; most epidemiologic studies have thus relied on serologic studies with the 229E and OC43 viruses, for which suitable antigens could be prepared. As shown in Table 360–1, many other viruses, such as influenza, parainfluenza, respiratory syncytial, adeno-, echo-, and coxsackieviruses, can also cause common cold–like symptoms. These other agents are described in other sections of this text. A determination of the etiology of a common cold cannot be made clinically, since the agents causing the syndrome are so numerous. In addition, about one third to one half of common colds have yet to be associated with an etiologic agent.

INCIDENCE AND PREVALENCE. The common cold is probably the most frequently occurring illness in humans worldwide. The National Center for Health Statistics estimated that in the United States in 1988 the population experienced more than 68 million common colds for an incidence of 28.5 per 100 persons per year. Common colds represented 16.3 per cent of all acute conditions and were estimated to cause over 175 million days of restricted activity. The incidence of common colds was estimated to be 70.8 per 100 infants and young children under 5 years of age.

TABLE 360–1. PERCENTAGE OF COMMON COLDS ASSOCIATED WITH SPECIFIC ETIOLOGIC AGENTS IN ADULTS*

Rhinoviruses (100 serotypes)	15–40%
Coronaviruses (at least 3 serotypes)	10–20%
Influenza viruses A, B, C Parainfluenza viruses (4 serotypes) Respiratory syncytial virus (1 serotype) Adenoviruses (various serotypes)	5–10%
Coxsackieviruses (various serotypes) Echoviruses (various serotypes)	1–2%
Group A β-hemolytic streptococci	2–10%
No specific agent known but presumed to be viral	30–50%

*Each of these agents can also cause common colds in the pediatric age group, but their relative roles are not clearly defined. Viruses associated with specific syndromes such as rubeola, rubella, and varicella have also been associated with common cold–like symptoms in the pediatric age group.

In the Cleveland Family Study, which spanned a period of about 10 years and included close surveillance of over 25,000 illnesses, common respiratory diseases accounted for 60 per cent of all illnesses. The overall incidence of common respiratory diseases (which included illnesses diagnosed as the common cold, rhinitis, laryngitis, bronchitis, and other undifferentiated acute respiratory illnesses) was 5.6 per person per year. Children under 1 year of age experienced about seven respiratory illnesses per year; the highest incidence occurred in the 1-year age group (8.3 cases per year) and the incidence remained rather high through age 5 (7.4 cases per year). A progressive decrease was observed beginning at age 6. As expected, adults had relatively fewer common respiratory illnesses than children (adults averaged over four per year). The average incidence was slightly greater in boys than in girls, whereas in adults, mothers experienced higher rates than fathers. In addition, the incidence of common respiratory diseases was greater in young children attending school than in those of the same age who were not in school; also, preschool siblings of school children had more respiratory illnesses than preschool siblings without brothers or sisters attending school. The incidence of common respiratory diseases increased progressively as family size increased from three to seven members. Such illnesses were introduced into the home most frequently by school children under 6 years of age, followed in order of decreasing frequency by preschool children, school children 6 years of age and over, mothers, and fathers. Analysis of secondary attack rates in families revealed that on the average 25 per cent of all exposures in the home were followed by illness; 1- and 2-year-olds experienced the highest secondary attack rates (about twice the average).

In a more recent survey of acute respiratory illnesses over a 6-year period in Tecumseh, Michigan, the mean incidence of respiratory illnesses per person per year was 3. The highest incidence was in the 1-year age group (6.1) and the next highest in the 1- to 2-year age group (5.7). A viral or potentially pathogenic bacterial agent was isolated from about 25 per cent of the specimens collected, with rhinoviruses accounting for 38.5 per cent of the total number of isolates, a figure representing more than twice the number of isolates of the next most frequently detected group, the parainfluenza viruses.

Studies of the prevalence of neutralizing antibodies in serum against various rhinovirus serotypes have revealed a gradual acquisition of antibody beginning early in childhood and reaching a maximum of at least 50 per cent in the fifth decade. The prevalence of serum antibody to specific serotypes was not consistent. Although all individuals studied had neutralizing antibodies to each of the 55 serotypes tested, the prevalence of antibody to each serotype varied from about 10 to 80 per cent. Limited surveys of the prevalence of neutralizing antibody to rhinoviruses in various developed and developing countries, including several tropical areas, indicated a generally worldwide presence of rhinovirus antibody.

The prevalence of coronavirus serum antibody has been difficult to determine, because only two serotypes, 229E and OC43, can be cultivated with consistency in cell cultures and, in addition, results have been variable in different locations with these two viruses. For example, in one study in the United States, 29 per cent of children and 69 per cent of adults had serum complement-fixing (CF) antibody to OC43 virus. Such antibody to 229E virus was present very infrequently in children, whereas about one third of adults were antibody positive. However, in the United Kingdom, about 25 per cent of children and 41 per cent of adults had neutralizing antibody to 229E virus. In United States marine recruits, over 80 per cent had serum hemagglutination inhibition antibody to OC43 virus and 12 per cent had CF antibody to 229E virus. By recently developed enzyme- or radio-immunoassays, the prevalence of serum antibody to 229E and OC43 or related coronaviruses was over 80 per cent in adults in different geographic areas. A true evaluation of the prevalence of antibody to the coronavirus group must await the development of serologic assays for other members of this fastidious group of agents.

EPIDEMIOLOGY. In the temperate climates common colds occur most frequently in the colder months of the year. For example, in the Cleveland Family Study a consistent pattern of a low summer and high winter incidence of common respiratory diseases was documented. In September, a rise in respiratory illnesses to about six cases per person-year from a summer low of three cases per person-year was observed. After a slight dip in October an average rate of about seven cases per person-year was observed for each month from November through March.

Rhinoviruses are spread from person to person by aerosol, direct contact, or indirect contact involving environmental objects (fomites) via virus-contaminated respiratory secretions. In early volunteer studies, rhinoviruses induced common colds when administered in nasal drops or by swabbing the nasal mucosa or conjunctiva but not by swabbing the throat. More recent volunteer studies have yielded conflicting views on the most efficient mode of transmission of rhinovirus-induced common colds. One view highlights a mode of transmission that involves self-inoculation of the nasal mucosa or conjunctiva with a rhinovirus-contaminated finger. Virus was recovered in 15 of 16 trials from fingers that were rubbed on plastic surfaces contaminated with rhinovirus 1 to 3 hours previously. In addition, rhinovirus dried on volunteers' fingers could be transferred to uncontaminated fingers of other volunteers following skin contact, in three of five trials. The efficiency of transmission of infection from experimentally infected volunteers to susceptible volunteers by hand-to-hand contact followed by self-inoculation was compared with that of transmission by large- and small-particle aerosols. It was striking that 11 of 15 hand-to-hand exposures initiated infection, whereas only 1 of 12 large-particle exposures (donor and contact in social setting) and none of 10 small-particle exposures (donor and contact separated by double mesh barrier) induced such infection. In contrast, another view stresses the major role of aerosol transmission since following exposure to rhinovirus-infected "donors," 10 of 18 restrained volunteers (i.e., they could not touch their faces) and a similar number (12 of 18) of unrestrained volunteers developed common colds. However, none of 12 unrestrained individuals exposed to presumably rhinovirus-contaminated fomites (playing cards, etc.) developed illness. Thus, under the conditions of these separate volunteer studies, aerosol, direct contact, and indirect contact with fomites were capable of inducing common colds. However, the relative importance of each mode of transmission is still a matter of controversy.

In another study, rhinovirus communicability was evaluated in childless married couples who lacked serum neutralizing antibody to the challenge viruses. The overall transmission of a rhinovirus-related cold between partners was 38 per cent, which is similar to the secondary attack rate in the Cleveland Family Study or to those in epidemiologic studies of naturally occurring rhinovirus infections. Transmission rarely occurred unless (1) at least 1000 $TCID_{50}$ (50 per cent tissue culture infective doses) of virus were present in the donor's nasal washing, (2) the donor's hands and anterior nares were rhinovirus positive, (3) the donor had at least moderate symptoms, and (4) the partners spent many hours together (at least 122 hours during a 7-day period). Virus in saliva was not strongly associated with transmission.

The effect of exposure to cold temperatures on the course of common colds was evaluated in volunteers who were challenged with rhinovirus by small-particle aerosol or intranasal instillation. Exposure to the cold environment did not have a significant effect on host resistance to rhinovirus infection and illness. Exposure to cold temperature did not induce a common cold in uninoculated volunteers. This finding is consistent with results of early studies on the epidemiology of common colds on the island of Spitzbergen. These studies demonstrated that very few colds occurred during the bitter Arctic winter, but sharp outbreaks began shortly after the first ship arrived at the end of May. Thus, cold weather by itself did not induce common colds; the ingredient needed to initiate the outbreak was exposure to infected individuals. In early volunteer studies using common cold virus–like agents for challenge, fatigue and sleep deprivation caused an insignificant increase in the frequency with which colds occurred; however, in females, susceptibility was related to the menstrual cycle, with attempts to induce colds during menstruation being relatively unsuccessful.

The incubation period of rhinovirus-related common colds is quite short, ranging from 1 to 5 days with a mean of 2 days. Virus shedding generally begins with the onset of symptoms and continues for 1 week or even longer. Although there are 100 distinct rhinovirus serotypes, no one serotype has assumed special importance because numerous serotypes usually circulate at the same time. Rhinoviruses can be detected during most months of the year but reach peak prevalence during the fall and spring seasons. They are least prevalent during the cold winter months of December, January, and February, when common colds still occur frequently. However, coronavirus infections have been found to be prevalent during the late fall, winter, and early spring, when rhinovirus infections occur less frequently. Thus, coronaviruses can be considered to be the major known etiologic agents of the common cold in the winter.

A cyclic pattern in infection rates of coronaviruses 229E and OC43 has been described. With the 229E virus, infections appear to occur in the same years in various locations, including Chicago, Maryland, Virginia, and Michigan; a 2-year cycle of activity has been suggested. For OC43 virus, a 2- to 4-year cycle was found that did not coincide in all locations. The 229E virus was shed in nasal washings of volunteers for 1 to at least 4 days after challenge; the peak frequency of virus excretion generally coincided with the peak of clinical symptoms. Virus shedding was also detected in certain volunteers who did not develop colds after challenge. Reinfections have also been observed frequently with coronaviruses under natural conditions; however, volunteers inoculated with the same coronavirus strain 8 to 12 months after initial challenge failed to develop illness on rechallenge.

It appears that serum antibody to a specific rhinovirus serotype correlates with protection against natural or experimental challenge with that serotype. However, serum antibody may not in itself be responsible for protection but may be a reflection of the level of specific nasal secretory antibodies. In one volunteer study in which the protective effects of neutralizing antibody in serum and in nasal secretions were compared, it was found that only nasal secretory antibody was associated with resistance to rhinovirus infection and illness.

PATHOLOGY. The pathologic mechanisms whereby a common cold is induced by a virus are not known. However, the pathology of viral rhinitis in general has been described. In the initial acute period of viral rhinitis the nasal mucosa is thickened and edematous and, depending on the degree of hyperemia, is pale gray to red in color and covered by a thin, watery mucoid discharge. The nasal cavities are narrowed by the enlargement of the turbinates. Histologically, there is extreme edema of the mucosal tissue, which is also infiltrated sparsely with neutrophils, lymphocytes, plasma cells, and eosinophils. Secretory hyperactivity of the mucus-secreting submucosal glands is also observed. The edematous nasal mucosa can cause obstruction of the orifices of the accessory air sinuses and lead to sinusitis. Extension of bacterial superinfections can result in serious sequelae, including osteomyelitis, cavernous sinus thrombophlebitis, epidural or subdural abscess, meningitis, or brain abscess. However, such complications are exceedingly rare.

Information on the pathologic findings in acute rhinovirus infections is extremely limited. Biopsies of nasal epithelium obtained from volunteers with experimentally induced rhinovirus colds failed to demonstrate consistent histologic changes. However, sloughed ciliated epithelial cells are found in nasal secretions.

CLINICAL MANIFESTATIONS. The major clinical manifestation of common colds occurring under natural or experimental conditions is coryza or nasal congestion. The most common complaints in naturally occurring rhinovirus-positive respiratory illnesses in 139 civilian adults were rhinorrhea and sneezing, which were recorded in one half to two thirds of the cases. The next most frequent complaint was sore throat, which occurred in nearly one half, whereas hoarseness and cough were less common, being present in one quarter to one half of the cases. Temperature elevation was unusual. An oral temperature of 99.6°F (37.6°C) or greater at the time of study was documented in less than 1 per cent of the cases. Nonrespiratory complaints were not common except for headache, which occurred in approximately one quarter of the cases. The mean duration of symptoms was about 9 days with a median of 7.4 days and a mode of 4 days.

The clinical manifestations of coronavirus 229E–like infections under natural conditions in adults are quite similar. Of nine patients who shed this agent, all had coryza, eight had nasal congestion, seven had sneezing, and five had sore throat at the time of study. Less common manifestations were headache (in four), cough (in three), muscular or general aches (in three), and chills and fever (in two). Coryza or nasal congestion was the chief complaint in eight of the nine patients.

Administration of rhinoviruses or coronaviruses to volunteers has provided an opportunity to define the clinical manifestations associated with these agents under carefully controlled conditions (Table 360–2). The mean incubation period of colds induced by coronaviruses was significantly longer (about 1 day), the duration of the illness somewhat shorter, and the mean maximum number of paper tissues used per day (for nasal discharge) greater than in rhinovirus-induced illnesses. In later studies, each of six other coronavirus strains was also administered by the nasal route to volunteers: cumulatively, 35 of 49 volunteers developed common cold–like illnesses. Thus, the ability to induce common colds in adults under experimental conditions is now as firmly established for the coronaviruses as for the rhinoviruses.

Rhinoviruses also cause common colds in children. The role of rhinoviruses as etiologic agents of bronchitis, bronchiolitis, bronchopneumonia, pneumonia, and croup in the pediatric age group is unclear. However, it appears certain that rhinoviruses are not important causes of these syndromes, even though nasal inhalation of a rhinovirus by small-particle aerosol induces a tracheobronchitis in volunteers. Rhinoviral respiratory illness has also been implicated as an important precipitant of asthmatic attacks in children with a history of asthma. Rhinoviruses have been recovered from certain hospitalized pediatric patients with lower respiratory tract disease; most of these patients had significant underlying disease involving the immune or cardiopulmonary system. In addition, rhinoviruses were recovered from patients with cyanosis and apnea in an intensive care nursery. Coronaviruses can also cause common cold–like illnesses in children. In one study, coronavirus 229E was recovered from two infants with pneumonia, and serologic evidence of coronavirus infection was demonstrated in 8.2 per cent of pediatric patients hospitalized with lower respiratory tract disease. However, in other studies such an association was not found. Coronavirus infection has been associated with exacerbations of wheezing in young children with asthma. Coronavirus OC43 and rhinovirus infections also were observed in several military trainees with pneumonia with pleural reaction and with atypical pneumonia, respectively. The etiologic significance of such associations is not known. Rhinovirus and coronavirus infections have been associated with exacerbations of chronic bronchitis in adults. A transient decrease in pulmonary function has also been observed in volunteers infected with rhinovirus. Rhinovirus has also been recovered from the lung of an adult patient with a fatal pulmonary infection and other underlying disease involving the immune system. Other complications of common colds include sinusitis, otitis media, and extension of infection into the central nervous or vascular system, as noted in the pathology section. Rhinovirus has been recovered from sinus and middle ear fluids. The role of bacteria acting in concert with the virus infection in certain of these complications must be kept in mind in establishing therapeutic regimens.

DIAGNOSIS. Since most respiratory viruses can induce common colds, an etiologic diagnosis cannot be made on clinical grounds. Specific viral diagnosis of the common cold is essentially a research procedure that requires tissue or organ cultures for virus isolation or antigens for certain serologic studies. Serologic evidence of rhinovirus infection is demonstrated by an antibody rise to a specific serotype by neutralization assay in tissue culture. Complement fixation (229E, OC43), hemagglutination-inhibition (OC43), enzyme-linked immunosorbent assay (229E), or radioimmunoassay (OC43) can be performed in order to detect serologic evidence of infection with certain coronaviruses. However, antigens for such tests are not generally available. Molecular biologic techniques are being introduced for the diagnosis of rhinovirus or coronavirus infection. The most important test for a patient with a common cold–like illness is a throat culture for group A β-hemolytic streptococci because symptoms of illnesses associated with the common cold viruses and the streptococcus may overlap. Appropriate antibiotic therapy is available for treatment of this bacterial infection.

TREATMENT AND PREVENTION. There is no specific treatment for patients with the common cold. Only symptomatic treatment measures should be employed. At this time, it appears that acetylsalicylic acid (aspirin) should not be used in children with colds because of the epidemiologic association of this drug with Reye's syndrome (see Ch. 480) when the drug is administered during a viral illness, usually influenza or varicella, both of which can cause symptoms resembling those of the common cold (Table 360–1).

Antibiotics have no value in the therapy of the uncomplicated common cold. Clinical trials evaluating the efficacy of antihistamines for treatment of common colds have yielded inconsistent, inconclusive results. Thus, it appears from currently available evidence that the routine use of antihistamines for treatment of the common cold is not indicated. Previous tonsillectomy did not significantly affect the number of common respiratory illnesses or the induction of experimental colds in volunteers in the Cleveland Family Study. Available evidence indicates that vitamin C does not reduce the number of episodes of respiratory illness but does decrease somewhat the total number of days of disability. The routine use of large doses of vitamin C for preventive treatment of common colds does not appear to be warranted from evidence available at this time. The efficacy of steam (heated, humidified air) inhalation for the treatment of common colds has yielded variable results and needs further evaluation.

Currently 100 serotypes of rhinovirus are known to exist, and no one serotype or group of serotypes appears to be consistently more important than others. Experimental rhinovirus vaccines against single serotypes have been made and shown to be effective in preventing or modifying illnesses induced by the serotype present in the vaccine. Although some heterotypic antibody responses have been observed with experimental decavalent rhinovirus vaccines, the production of a rhinovirus vaccine appears to be impractical because of the multiplicity of serotypes. Until the number of serotypes of coronaviruses can be elucidated and the role of antibody in preventing or modifying illnesses can be established, consideration of a coronavirus vaccine is premature.

Since the three-dimensional structure and the cellular recep-

TABLE 360–2. COMPARISON OF THE CLINICAL FEATURES OF COMMON COLDS PRODUCED BY INTRANASAL ADMINISTRATION OF CORONAVIRUSES OR RHINOVIRUSES

	Coronaviruses		Rhinoviruses	
	229E	B814	Type 2 (HGP or PK)	DC
Number of volunteers inoculated	26	75	213	251
Number getting common colds	13 (50%)	34 (45%)	78 (37%)	77 (31%)
Incubation period (days)				
Mean	3.3	3.2	2.1	2.1
Range	2–4	2–5	1–5	1–4
Duration (days)				
Mean	7	6	9	10
Range	3–18	2–17	3–19	2–26
Maximum number of tissues used daily				
Mean	23	21	14	18
Range	8–105	8–120	3–38	3–60
Malaise	46%	47%	28%	25%
Headache	85%	53%	56%	56%
Chill	31%	18%	28%	15%
Pyrexia	23%*	21%	14%	18%
Mucopurulent nasal discharge	0	62%	83%	80%
Sore throat	54%	79%	87%	73%
Cough	31%	44%	68%	56%
Number of volunteers with common colds of indicated severity				
Mild	10 (77%)	24 (71%)	63 (80%)	36 (47%)
Moderate	2 (15%)	7 (20%)	12 (15%)	28 (36%)
Severe	1 (8%)	3 (9%)	4 (5%)	13 (17%)

*Between 99.2°F (37.3°C) and 100.4°F (38°C) (oral). After Bradburne, Bynoe, Tyrrell: Br Med J 3:767, 1967.

tors of rhinovirus have been determined recently, it may be possible to design effective and practical antiviral compounds based on these findings. In addition, there has been renewed interest in the use of interferon to prevent common colds, since interferon can now be produced by recombinant deoxyribonucleic acid (DNA) techniques. Interferon applied topically by nasal spray was effective in reducing the number of symptomatic illnesses when given prophylactically to volunteers challenged with rhinovirus or following natural exposure to a rhinovirus cold in a family setting. Nasal irritation from interferon was minimized by short-term application. However, in a recent study, another interferon preparation was not effective for prophylaxis of naturally occurring common colds when administered as a nasal spray. Interferon nasal sprays are not effective as treatment for common colds caused by rhinovirus after symptoms have begun. Prophylactic interferon nasal spray has also been shown to shorten the duration and reduce the severity of coronavirus (229E)–induced cold symptoms. The use of interferon for prophylaxis of common colds does not appear practical for general usage but may be beneficial under special circumstances.

One method available for preventing rhinovirus-induced colds may be the application of rigid personal hygienic measures when a family member has a common cold. This would entail handwashing and avoidance of finger-eye and finger-nose contact.

Recently, the use of virucidal paper handkerchiefs has been shown to interrupt the transmission of rhinovirus-induced colds. This intervention awaits further evaluation in various settings.

Committee on Infectious Diseases of the American Academy of Pediatrics (Fulginiti VA, Brunell PA, Cherry JD, Ector WL, Gershon AA, Gotoff SP, Hughes WT, Mortimer EA Jr, Peter G): Special Report: Aspirin and Reye syndrome. Pediatrics 69:810, 1982. *After weighing the available evidence, this Committee has made a strong recommendation against the use of aspirin under usual circumstances in children with varicella or influenza (both of which can cause common cold–like symptoms).*

Couch RB: Rhinoviruses. In Fields BN, et al. (eds.): Virology, 2nd ed. New York, Raven Press, 1990, pp 607–629. *An up-to-date review of the rhinoviruses (196 references).*

Dick EC, Jennings LC, Mink KA, et al.: Aerosol transmission of rhinovirus colds. J Infect Dis 156:442–448, 1987. *Presents evidence of the importance of aerosol transmission of rhinovirus-induced common colds in a volunteer setting.*

Fox JP, Cooney MK, Hall EC, et al.: Rhinoviruses in Seattle families, 1975–1979. Am J Epidemiol 122:830, 1985. *A comprehensive epidemiologic study of rhinovirus infections in families in Seattle, Washington.*

Gaffey MJ, Kaiser DL, Hayden FG: Ineffectiveness of oral terfenadine in natural colds: Evidence against histamine as a mediator of common cold symptoms. Pediatr Infect Dis J 7:215–220, 1988. *A study demonstrating the lack of effect of an antihistamine on the treatment of naturally occurring common colds. Describes the inconsistent results in the evaluation of antihistamines in the treatment of common colds.*

Greve JM, Davis G, Meyer AM, et al: The major human rhinovirus receptor is ICAM-1. Cell 56:839–847, 1989. *Describes continued progress in the elucidation of cellular receptors of rhinoviruses, which may lead to the development of antiviral compounds.*

Hendley JO, Gwaltney JM Jr: Mechanism of transmission of rhinovirus infections. Epidemiol Rev 10:242–258, 1988. *Reviews the various modes of transmission of rhinovirus common colds (60 references).*

Kim S, Smith TJ, Chapman MS, et al.: Crystal structure of human rotavirus serotype 1A (HRV1A). J Mol Biol 210:91–111, 1989. *A basic paper describing further advances in determining the structure of rhinoviruses and the application of this information to the development of antiviral compounds.*

Lowenstein SR, Parrino TA: Management of the common cold. Adv Intern Med 32:207–233, 1987. *A balanced, careful description of the management of common colds (121 references).*

Macknin ML, Mathew S, Medendorp SV: Effect of inhaling heated vapor on symptoms of the common cold. JAMA 264:989–991, 1990. *A recent study describing the ineffectiveness of steam (heated, humidified air) inhalation on common cold symptoms. Includes a review and references which demonstrate the variable results with this therapy.*

McIntosh K: Coronaviruses. In Fields BN, et al. (eds.): Virology, 2nd ed. New York, Raven Press, 1990, pp 857–864. *An up-to-date review of the coronaviruses (74 references).*

Remington PL, Rowley D, McGee H, et al.: Decreasing trends in Reye syndrome and aspirin use in Michigan, 1979 to 1984. Pediatrics 77:93, 1986. *The decreasing use of aspirin in children with colds or influenza and the decrease in Reye syndrome in Tecumseh, Michigan, is evaluated.*

Sperber SJ, Hayden FG: Chemotherapy of rhinovirus colds. Antimicrob Agents Chemother 32:409–419, 1988. *A review of various approaches—experimental and available—for treating the rhinovirus common cold (119 references).*

Sperber SJ, Levine PA, Sorrentino JV, et al.: Ineffectiveness of recombinant interferon-β serine nasal drops for prophylaxis of natural colds. J Infect Dis 160:700–705, 1989. *Demonstrates the variability of results of efficacy of interferon in prophylaxis of common colds.*

Tyrrell DAJ: Common colds. Intervirology 25:177–189, 1986. *A review of common colds from a historical perspective by a pioneer in this field.*

361 Viral Pharyngitis, Laryngitis, Croup, and Bronchitis

Maurice A. Mufson

DEFINITION. Viral infections that localize to the upper and middle respiratory passages produce an acute inflammatory response and, depending upon the anatomic site involved, evoke the clinical manifestations of pharyngitis, laryngitis, croup (laryngotracheobronchitis), and bronchitis. These infections do not ordinarily involve the pulmonary alveoli. Pharyngitis, laryngitis, and bronchitis can occur in persons of any age. Croup occurs exclusively in children and mainly during the second year of life. These illnesses usually begin abruptly with predominant upper respiratory tract signs and symptoms and limited systemic findings, and the uncomplicated illness abates after 5 to 10 days. Croup can be a life-threatening illness; the most common complications include respiratory failure and pneumonia.

ETIOLOGY. The major viral pathogens of the respiratory tract that can cause pharyngitis, laryngitis, croup, and bronchitis include members of the myxoviruses (influenza, parainfluenza, and respiratory syncytial viruses), adenoviruses, coronaviruses, picornaviruses (rhinoviruses and enteroviruses), and herpesviruses (Table 361–1). However, they differ in their propensity to cause these illnesses (Table 361–2). An etiologic diagnosis requires either isolation of virus or visualization of viral antigen in respiratory secretions by immunofluorescence, detection of antigen by enzyme immunoassay, or demonstration of a rise in antibody during convalescence.

Pharyngitis also can occur as part of systemic viral illnesses associated with *Epstein-Barr virus* (see Ch. 373) or *cytomegalovirus* (see Ch. 372) infection, and laryngitis and bronchitis occur in *measles* virus infection (see Ch. 367). When coryza represents the main feature of an upper respiratory infection, the term *common cold* (see Ch. 360) prevails. When the infecting virus is an influenza virus, the designation *influenza* describes an acute respiratory tract infection with fever and prostration (see Ch. 364).

INCIDENCE AND PREVALENCE. Most children and adults experience three to five viral infections of the upper respiratory tract each year. Croup is a serious illness of infants and children; the incidence of croup peaks in the second year of life, as high as 47 cases per 1000 children per year, and by age 4 to 5 it declines to under 15 cases per 1000 children per year (Denny, 1983).

EPIDEMIOLOGY. Viral pharyngitis, laryngitis, croup, and bronchitis occur during all months of the year, with peaks of occurrence paralleling epidemics of individual viruses. Respiratory syncytial virus, influenza A and B viruses, and parainfluenza virus type 1 occur in epidemics, mainly in the late fall, winter, and spring (see Table 361–3). The other viral pathogens occur endemically or sporadically. Virus infections of the respiratory tract spread by direct person-to-person contact, by infectious aerosols, or by fomites.

CLINICAL MANIFESTATIONS. *Viral Pharyngitis.* Acute viral pharyngitis is characterized by a scratchy and sore throat, but pain upon swallowing is not a prominent or constant feature. Dysphagia occurs infrequently in viral pharyngitis. Cough is not a feature of acute viral pharyngitis. Fever and malaise accompany influenza and adenovirus infections, but these findings are infrequent with the other respiratory viral pathogens. Pharyngeal erythema and edema and enlarged and tender lymph nodes may

TABLE 361—1. VIRUSES THAT CAUSE PHARYNGITIS, LARYNGITIS, CROUP, AND BRONCHITIS

Virus	Serotype
Influenza	Types A, B
Parainfluenza	Types 1, 2, 3
Respiratory syncytial	Subgroups A, B1, B2
Adenovirus	Types 1, 2, 3, 4, 5, 6, 7 (also others)
Coronavirus	Types 229E, OC43 (also others)
Rhinovirus	Most or all of more than 100 serotypes
Enterovirus	At least some of more than 75 serotypes
Herpes simplex	Type 1

TABLE 361–2. RELATIVE IMPORTANCE OF VIRUSES CAUSING PHARYNGITIS, LARYNGITIS, CROUP, AND BRONCHITIS

Virus	Occurrence in Indicated Illness*			
	Pharyngitis	*Laryngitis*	*Croup*	*Bronchitis*
Influenza A	+ + + +	+ + + +	+	+ + +
B	+ +	+ +		+ +
Parainfluenza 1	+ +	+ +	+ + + +	+ +
2	+	+	+ + +	+
3	+ +	+ +	+ + + +	+ +
Respiratory syncytial	+		+	+ + +
Adenovirus	+ + + +	+ +		+ +
Coronavirus	+	+		+ + +
Rhinovirus	+ + + +	+		+
Enterovirus	+			
Herpes simplex	+ +			+

*Graded from minimal (+) to major (+ + + +) importance; blank means unlikely occurrence.

be the only physical findings. Adenovirus pharyngitis may be associated with conjunctivitis. Exudative tonsillitis occurs in adenovirus infections, infectious mononucleosis associated with Epstein-Barr virus infection, herpetic pharyngitis (with or without vesicles or small ulcers), as well as streptococcal pharyngitis. Exudative tonsillitis alone does not distinguish these infections. Bronchospasm occurs as a feature of herpes tracheobronchitis in elderly persons.

Viral Laryngitis. In acute viral laryngitis, hoarseness predominates, associated with difficulty in talking, pain on clearing respiratory secretions, and often fever, depending upon the infecting virus. Cough and pharyngitis may be present. The larynx is erythematous and edematous, and the regional lymph nodes are slightly enlarged and tender. Wheezes may be audible upon auscultation.

Viral Croup. The clinical picture of croup characteristically includes inspiratory stridor, hoarseness, and a brassy cough. This distinctive triad of symptoms reflects the acute and intense edema and mucoid exudative secretions of the larynx and associated obstruction of the subglottic portion of the upper airway. These symptoms develop acutely, accompanied by fever, cough, tachypnea, and wheezing. Retractions of the chest wall occur. Hemoptysis does not occur. Rhonchi, rales, or wheezes, alone or in combination, may be audible upon auscultation of the lungs. Radiographic examination of the neck can demonstrate subglottic narrowing, and a chest roentgenogram may show hyperinflation of the lungs. In the uncomplicated case, the findings resolve in several days, but some children develop respiratory failure and pneumonia. Children who perviously experienced multiple episodes of croup manifest hyperreactive airways several years later.

Viral Bronchitis. In acute viral bronchitis, cough, with or without sputum production, and fever are the main features. The sputum is slightly mucoid or watery and white. Other common symptoms include hoarseness, nonpleuritic substernal chest pain, and malaise. Rhonchi or rales may be heard upon auscultation of the chest. The chest roentgenogram may show increased intensity of the vascular pattern, but pulmonary infiltrates do not occur. Acute bronchitis associated with influenza or coronavirus infection occurs often as an exacerbation of chronic bronchitis.

TREATMENT AND PROGNOSIS. Viral pharyngitis, laryngitis, and bronchitis are self-limited illnesses, and not severe, except for herpes tracheobronchitis infections. The symptoms of these illnesses should be treated with analgesics, fluids, and rest.

Persistent cough can be treated with suppressant preparations. Antibiotics are not indicated, except when secondary bacterial infection occurs; it is likely to develop mainly with influenza virus infections. In pharyngitis, pharyngeal pain or dysphagia should be treated with analgesics and fluids.

The less serious cases of croup can be managed by having the child rest in bed at home. Vaporizers that produce a mist of moist air may be beneficial. Children with severe croup require hospitalization, supportive treatment, and constant monitoring for the development of respiratory distress. If hypoxemia develops, oxygen therapy is essential; hypoxemia requiring oxygen can develop even before cyanosis becomes evident. Subglottic edema may be reduced by the administration of racemic epinephrine. Administration of corticosteroids in the treatment of croup may have limited benefit. Antiviral drug therapy is available for influenza A, respiratory syncytial, and herpes simplex viruses (Table 361–4). Ribavirin lessens the severity of serious respiratory syncytial virus infection in the infant and child. Herpes tracheobronchitis can be successfully treated with acyclovir. Influenza virus vaccine must be administered to persons in the high-risk group (unless contraindicated) to diminish the chance of infection (see Ch. 16).

Avila MM, Carballal G, Rovaletti H, et al.: Viral etiology in acute lower respiratory tract infections in children in a closed community. Am Rev Respir Dis 140:634, 1989. *One fifth of 94 children with bronchitis had virus infections; respiratory syncytial virus and adenoviruses were the most common.*

Houvinen P, Lahtonen R, Ziegler T, et al.: Pharyngitis in adults: The presence of coexistence of viruses and bacterial organisms. Ann Intern Med 110:612, 1989. *About one fourth of 106 adults with pharyngitis had virus infections; respiratory syncytial and influenza A viruses were most common.*

Mufson MA, Örvell C, Rafnar B, et al.: Two distinct subtypes of human respiratory syncytial virus. J Gen Virol 66:2111, 1985. *New description of two subtypes (or subgroups) of respiratory syncytial virus recognized by their pattern of reaction with monoclonal antibodies generated against the major proteins of the virus.*

Sherry MK, Klainer AS, Wolff M, et al.: Herpetic tracheobronchitis. Ann Intern Med 109:229, 1988. *Successful treatment of adults with severe herpes infection of trachea and bronchi with intravenous acyclovir.*

Thom DH, Grayston JT, Wang SP, et al.: *Chlamydia pneumoniae* strain TWAR, *Mycoplasma pneumoniae*, and viral infections in acute respiratory disease in a university student health clinic population. Am J Epidemiol 132:248, 1990. *One tenth of college students with either bronchitis or pharyngitis had virus infections; influenza A and B viruses predominated.*

TABLE 361–3. EPIDEMIOLOGY OF VIRUSES THAT CAUSE PHARYNGITIS, LARYNGITIS, CROUP, AND BRONCHITIS

Epidemic	Endemic	Sporadic
Parainfluenza 1*	Parainfluenza 3	Parainfluenza 2
Influenza A†	Adenovirus	Herpes simplex
Influenza B	Coronavirus	
Respiratory syncytial‡	Rhinovirus	
	Enterovirus	

*Alternate years, usually.
†Epidemic and pandemic.
‡Annual epidemics.

TABLE 361–4. ANTIVIRAL DRUG THERAPY OF VIRUSES THAT CAUSE PHARYNGITIS, LARYNGITIS, CROUP, AND BRONCHITIS

Virus	Drug	Dose (Duration)	Route
Influenza A	Amantadine*	200 mg daily (10 days)	Oral
	Rimantidine*	200–300 mg daily (10 days)	Oral
Respiratory syncytial	Ribavirin	20 mg/ml solution (12–18 hours)	Aerosol
Herpes simplex†	Acyclovir	8 mg/kg q8hr (7–10 days)	IV

*More commonly used for prophylaxis at same daily dose over longer periods of time until the virus leaves the community.
†Herpes simplex tracheobronchitis treated with IV acyclovir.

362 Respiratory Syncytial Virus

Robert M. Chanock

DEFINITION. Respiratory syncytial virus (RSV) is the most important cause of viral lower respiratory tract disease in infants and children. This ubiquitous virus causes an extensive epidemic every year during fall, winter, or early spring. During these epidemics there is a dramatic increase in admission to hospitals of infants and young children with severe lower respiratory tract disease. Older children and adults commonly undergo reinfection, but disease is usually milder than that experienced during infancy and early childhood.

ETIOLOGY. RSV, an enveloped virus that belongs to the family Paramyxoviridae, genus *Pneumovirus*, resembles the parainfluenza viruses of the genus *Paramyxovirus* but differs from them in morphology of its nucleocapsid, in failure to agglutinate erythrocytes (hemagglutination), and in absence of a neuraminidase enzyme. The RSV negative ($-$) strand RNA genome, approximately 15,000 bases in length, is transcribed as a series of 10 separate messenger ribonucleic acids (mRNAs), each of which is translated into a separate viral protein. One of these proteins, nucleocapsid protein, coats the viral RNA to form a helical nucleocapsid. This structure is enclosed within a bilayer lipid membrane that is studded with two different viral glycoproteins. One of these, the fusion protein, lyses the host cell membrane, permitting entry of virus into the cell. This protein is also responsible for fusion of infected cells to neighboring cells, a process that results in syncytium formation, a prominent feature of the virus during its growth in tissue culture.

Although antigenic variation among strains has been noted, it does not appear to have major epidemiologic significance. A related RSV is a common cause of respiratory disease in calves, but this virus does not appear to infect humans.

EPIDEMIOLOGY. Whenever appropriate studies have been performed, RSV has been found to be the major pediatric respiratory tract viral pathogen. The highest incidence of severe lower respiratory tract disease is observed in infants between 1 and 6 months of age, with a peak incidence at 2 months. Serious lower respiratory tract disease occurs more commonly in males than in females and in nonblack than in black infants. Approximately 50 per cent of infants who live through a single RSV epidemic become infected. In certain settings, such as day care centers, the attack rate approaches 100 per cent during an outbreak.

Reinfection occurs with high frequency during childhood. Adults are also reinfected frequently, particularly when there is exposure to a large amount of virus. For example, in families into which virus is introduced, spread of RSV among older siblings and parents occurs with high frequency (40 per cent). In individuals of all ages, reinfection is usually symptomatic, and adults exposed to a large amount of virus may develop an influenza-like disease.

Most individuals infected with RSV have upper respiratory illness. However, a surprisingly large proportion of infants (25 to 40 per cent) also develop lower respiratory tract disease. Hospitalization of infants for RSV disease varies with environmental and socioeconomic conditions. Overall, 1 in 120 to 1 in 200 infants requires hospital care for RSV pneumonia or bronchiolitis during the first year of life. RSV is responsible for approximately 50 to 75 per cent of bronchiolitis and for 20 to 25 per cent of pneumonias that necessitate admission of infants and young children to hospital.

In developed countries, severe RSV lower respiratory tract disease is rarely fatal (0.5 to 2.5 per cent). Fatal RSV disease occurs most often in infants with other underlying illnesses, particularly congenital heart disease (37 per cent), bronchopulmonary dysplasia, serious renal disease, and diseases such as cancer that are treated with immunosuppressive drugs. In a British study of 46 infants and children who died with lower respiratory tract disease, 13 were infected with RSV. In addition, a number of babies dying of sudden infant death syndrome are infected with RSV.

RSV has a clear seasonality in temperate zones of the world. In urban centers, epidemics occur yearly in the late fall, winter, or spring but not during the summer. In the northern hemisphere, the virus is rarely isolated during August or September. Each RSV epidemic lasts approximately 5 months, with 40 per cent of infections occurring during the peak month in the temporal center of the outbreak. In the northern hemisphere, most outbreaks peak in February or March, but the peak may occur as early as December or as late as June. RSV is spread by infected respiratory secretions in the form of large droplets or through fomite contamination.

During epidemic intervals, RSV is one of the most common causes of hospital-acquired infection on pediatric wards. The risk of infection increases as the hospital stay is extended beyond 1 week. The mortality in such hospital-acquired infections is considerably higher than in community-acquired infections because the patients involved are frequently at high risk from other diseases, malnourishment, or immunosuppressive drugs.

Since reinfection with RSV is common and often associated with disease, it is clear that immunity is neither permanent nor complete. However, multiple reinfections induce temporary immunity to infection and a more long-term resistance to severe RSV lower respiratory tract disease. Studies in adult volunteers indicate that immunity to induced upper respiratory tract infection correlates better with the level of nasal neutralizing immunoglobulin A (IgA) antibodies than with serum antibodies. On the other hand, there is some epidemiologic evidence that the high levels of maternally derived RSV antibodies possessed by many small infants provide protection from serious lower respiratory tract disease. However, lower levels of such antibodies present in the serum of older infants are not protective.

CLINICAL MANIFESTATIONS. During infancy, RSV infection usually causes upper respiratory symptoms. In 25 to 40 per cent of infections the respiratory tract below the larynx is also involved. Lower respiratory tract signs are preceded by a prodromal phase of rhinorrhea that is sometimes accompanied by a decrease in appetite. Low-grade fever is common. Cough is often accompanied by wheezing, and if disease is mild, symptoms may not progress beyond this stage. Examination usually reveals moderate tachypnea, diffuse rhonchi, fine rales and wheezes, as well as profuse rhinorrhea and intermittent fever. Otitis media is also common. The chest radiograph usually appears normal. In most instances, uneventful recovery occurs after 7 to 12 days.

In more severe cases, coughing and wheezing progress and the child becomes dyspneic and refuses feedings. Hyperexpansion of the chest is evident, and there may be intercostal and subcostal retractions. Severe tachypnea is common even in the absence of visible cyanosis, and in advanced disease, as the child tires and hypoxia becomes more extreme, listlessness and apnea occur. The chest may appear normal on radiographic examination, but often there is a combination of air trapping (hyperexpansion) and peribronchial thickening or interstitial pneumonia. Segmental or lobar consolidation is also occasionally seen, usually involving the right upper lobe. Pleural effusion is rare. In infants with underlying cardiac or respiratory disease, the progression of symptoms may be rapid. In these instances, respiratory failure requiring intubation and ventilation may appear on the second or third day of illness.

Almost all infants who require hospitalization are hypoxemic on admission and remain so for a prolonged period—up to several weeks—although recovery has ensued. The hypoxemia reflects an abnormally low ventilation-perfusion ratio. Hypercarbia may also be present.

In infants who were born prematurely, and sometimes in normal infants under 6 weeks of age, apneic spells may develop during RSV infection. These often occur in the absence of significant respiratory signs and may be the predominant symptom bringing the infant to medical attention. Such apneic spells, while often recurrent during acute infection, are usually self-limited and rarely cause neurologic or systemic damage. However, exceptions to this pattern occur, and such episodes are an indication for hospitalization and careful medical supervision. Apnea at the peak of severe illness is a poor prognostic sign.

In the newborn infant, most RSV infections produce only upper respiratory symptoms. Bronchiolitis is rare, and severe infection is more often characterized by lethargy, irritability, and fever or unstable body temperature than by specific respiratory signs.

Children who have apparently recovered completely from RSV bronchiolitis or pneumonia may still retain both measurable and symptomatic respiratory abnormalities for many years. A study of 23 children examined 10 years after an episode of bronchiolitis found that although all were symptom free (a criterion for admission to the study), 20 had some measurable physiologic abnormality of lung function or arterial blood gases.

Acute RSV infections are common in adults, particularly in medical personnel or in those caring for small children. These reinfections are occasionally asymptomatic but usually are associated with rhinorrhea, pharyngitis, cough, constitutional symptoms of headache and fatigue, and fever. Disease usually lasts about 5 days but may be more prolonged, particularly in hospital staff. Alterations in pulmonary function, such as elevated total respiratory resistance and increased airway reactivity, often last for 8 weeks. There is some evidence that RSV infection in the elderly is a cause of febrile bronchitis and severe or even fatal pneumonia.

DIAGNOSIS. Presumptive diagnosis of RSV infection can often be made on the basis of the clinical syndrome in relation to the time of year and other epidemiologic features. Definitive diagnosis depends upon the laboratory. In older children and adults, an increase in serum RSV antibody concentration, either complement fixing (CF) or neutralizing, is a fairly sensitive index of reinfection with RSV. Serologic tests in infants are less sensitive, particularly in patients under 4 months of age. In young infants, only 2 to 15 per cent of RSV infections are detectable by CF and 2 to 20 per cent by neutralization assay. Antibody measurement by solid-phase immunoassay (enzyme-linked immunosorbent assay, or ELISA) recently has been shown to be a more sensitive indicator of infection in small infants than CF or neutralization. At all ages, however, isolation of virus or detection of antigen in respiratory secretions is the procedure of choice. Specimens are best obtained by aspiration or gentle washing out of nasopharyngeal secretions. These may be examined by inoculation of tissue culture, immunofluorescence, or ELISA. Infectivity of RSV in secretions is labile; hence samples should be placed on wet ice while being transported to a tissue culture laboratory.

TREATMENT AND PREVENTION. Treatment of RSV infections of the lower respiratory tract consists primarily of supportive care: mechanical removal of secretions, proper positioning of the infant, administration of humidified oxygen, and in severe cases respiratory assistance. When wheezing is an important symptom, some patients, particularly those over a year of age, benefit from the use of theophylline or adrenergic drugs.

Ribavirin (1β D-ribofuranosyl-1,2,4-triazole-3-carboxamide), delivered by small-particle aerosol to high-risk infants, is now licensed for treatment of severe RSV disease in young infants. The drug has a beneficial effect on illness and diminishes virus shedding. Recently, intravenous inoculation of 2 grams per kilogram of human IgG containing a high titer of RSV neutralizing antibodies was shown to decrease virus shedding and improve oxygenation. In the case of both ribavirin and human IgG it remains to be shown that treatment decreases duration of hospitalization.

Because immunity to RSV is neither permanent nor complete, the goal of immunoprophylaxis is prevention of severe lower respiratory tract disease. It should be possible to achieve this through the cumulative effect of repeated vaccination. Efforts to develop an effective vaccine have been frustrated by the ineffectiveness of formalin-inactivated virus and by the genetic instability of satisfactorily attenuated temperature-sensitive mutants that initially showed promise as live virus vaccine strains. Perhaps recent success in preparing purified RSV surface glycoproteins and in constructing vaccinia virus or adenovirus recombinants that express RSV surface glycoproteins may open the way to effective immunoprophylaxis for this virus because each of these experimental vaccines induces significant resistance to RSV infection in experimental animals.

Groothuis JR, Woodin KA, Katz R, et al.: Early ribavirin treatment of respiratory syncytial viral infection in high-risk children. J Pediatr 117:792, 1990. *Early administration of ribavirin by small-particle aerosol to high-risk infants and children with RSV lower respiratory tract disease had a beneficial effect on severity of clinical illness and oxygenation but did not reduce duration of hospitalization.*

Hall CBH, Geiman JM, Biggar R, et al.: Respiratory syncytial virus infections within families. N Engl J Med 294:414, 1976. *Longitudinal surveillance of RSV infections in families. During an epidemic, infection occurred in 44 per cent of families; within these families the infection rate was 62 per cent in infants and 43 per cent in adults, the latter rate representing reinfection.*

Hemming VG, Rodriguez W, Kim HW, et al.: Intravenous immunoglobulin treatment of respiratory syncytial virus infections in infants and young children. Antimicrob Agents Chemother 31:1882–1886, 1987. *Intravenous inoculation of 2 grams per kilogram of human IgG with a high titer of RSV neutralizing antibodies effected a significant reduction in virus shedding and an improvement in oxygenation.*

Henderson FW, Collier AM, Clyde WA Jr, et al.: Respiratory-syncytial-virus infections, reinfections and immunity. N Engl J Med 300:530, 1979. *Longitudinal surveillance of children in a day care center demonstrated high frequency of reinfection; also, after several reinfections partial immunity developed to RSV.*

McIntosh K, Chanock RM: Respiratory syncytial virus. In Fields B, Knipe D (eds.): Virology. New York, Raven Press, 1990, pp 1045–1072. *A summary of biologic properties of RSV as well as its epidemiology and the pathogenesis of the disease.*

Olmsted RA, Elango N, Prince GA, et al.: Expression of the F glycoprotein of respiratory syncytial virus by a recombinant vaccinia virus: Comparison of the individual contributions of the F and G glycoproteins to host immunity. Proc Natl Acad Sci USA 83:7462, 1986. *Immunization of cotton rats with a vaccinia virus—RSV surface glycoprotein gene recombinant induces resistance to RSV infection in the lungs.*

363 Parainfluenza Viral Diseases

Robert M. Chanock

DEFINITION. Infection with parainfluenza viruses occurs early in life and is an important cause of *pediatric respiratory tract disease*. The spectrum of illness varies from mild upper respiratory disease to severe croup, pneumonia, or bronchiolitis. Reinfection is common in later life and is associated with mild respiratory tract disease.

ETIOLOGY. The parainfluenza viruses are enveloped viruses that belong to the family Paramyxoviridae, genus *Paramyxovirus*. The single-stranded ribonucleic acid (RNA) viral genome has negative polarity (antimessenger sense) and is approximately 15,000 bases in length. Its genetic information is expressed as a series of messenger RNA's (mRNA's) transcribed from the viral genome that codes for eight or nine viral-specific proteins. One of these proteins, nucleocapsid protein, coats the viral RNA to form a helical nucleocapsid. This structure is enclosed within a lipid bilayer envelope that is studded with the two viral glycoprotein surface antigens, the hemagglutinin-neuraminidase, and the fusion protein. Parainfluenza viruses share many properties with the influenza viruses, but they differ from these agents in their wider RNA nucleocapsid (18 nm as compared with 9 nm) and in the distribution of hemagglutination and neuraminidase functions on their surface glycoproteins. Both parainfluenza hemagglutinin and neuraminidase are located on the same surface glycoprotein, whereas these functions reside on separate surface glycoproteins of the influenza viruses. The parainfluenza viruses have common antigens that are not shared by the influenza viruses. Mumps virus shares the foregoing properties, as well as related antigens, with the parainfluenza viruses.

There are four antigenically distinct serotypes of human parainfluenza virus. Related parainfluenza viruses cause respiratory disease in mice (Sendai virus, a subtype of type 1), dogs (SV5, a subtype of type 2), calves (bovine shipping fever virus, a subtype of type 3), and birds (seven distinct serotypes not closely related to human parainfluenza viruses). Animal and avian parainfluenza viruses are distinct antigenically from human parainfluenza viruses and do not appear to infect humans.

EPIDEMIOLOGY. The four parainfluenza virus types have wide geographic distribution. The first three types have been identified in most areas where appropriate tissue culture and hemadsorption techniques have been applied to the study of childhood respiratory tract diseases. So far, type 4 viruses (subtypes 4A and 4B), which are more difficult to recover in tissue culture, have been isolated in fewer areas, but serologic studies suggest that they are also relatively ubiquitous.

The parainfluenza viruses are exceeded only by *respiratory syncytial virus (RSV)* as an important cause of lower respiratory tract disease in young children. These viruses, particularly type 3, commonly reinfect older children and adults to produce upper respiratory tract disease. Illness usually occurs less often and is less severe during reinfection than during primary infection.

There is considerable diversity in both epidemiologic and clinical manifestations of infections caused by the parainfluenza viruses. Parainfluenza virus type 1 is the principal cause of croup (laryngotracheobronchitis) in children, and parainfluenza virus type 3 is second only to RSV as a cause of pneumonia and bronchiolitis in infants less than 6 months of age. Parainfluenza virus type 2 resembles type 1 virus in clinical manifestations but causes serious illness less frequently. Infections with parainfluenza virus type 4 are detected infrequently, and associated illnesses are usually mild.

The parainfluenza viruses are most important as respiratory tract pathogens during infancy and childhood, when they (types 1 through 3) cause a spectrum of effects ranging from inapparent infection to life-threatening lower respiratory tract disease. Studies in different parts of the world indicate that types 1, 2, and 3 are associated with approximately 40 to 70 per cent of severe croup. In addition to croup, these three viruses are also responsible for a smaller but appreciable percentage of other acute respiratory tract diseases of infancy and early childhood. Eighty per cent of individuals undergoing primary infection with type 3 virus develop a febrile illness, and in one third there is involvement of the lower respiratory tract. Approximately one half of initial type 1 virus infections and two thirds of initial type 2 virus infections produce a febrile illness. Severe croup, although the most dramatic and serious manifestation of initial parainfluenza virus infection, is noted in only 2 to 3 per cent of primary type 1 or type 2 virus infections.

Primary parainfluenza virus infection generally occurs early in life. Type 3 virus often causes illness during the first months of life while infants still possess circulating neutralizing antibodies derived from their mothers. In contrast, in young infants, maternally derived antibodies appear to prevent both infection and severe disease caused by type 1 and type 2 viruses. After age 4 months, there is an increase in the incidence of croup and other lower respiratory tract diseases caused by type 1 and type 2 viruses. This high incidence continues until approximately 6 years of age, after which there is a much lower incidence. It is unusual for type 1 or type 2 virus to cause lower respiratory tract illness during adolescence or adult life, although this does occur on occasion.

At present, type 1 and type 2 virus epidemics are synchronous, occurring during the autumn of odd-numbered years. For many years, type 3 virus exhibited an endemic pattern, with infection occurring during all seasons of the year. Within this endemic pattern, small outbreaks occurred, but there was no predictable periodicity. Within the past 10 years, there has been a shift toward yearly spring epidemics of type 3 virus infection. Nosocomial infection of infants and young children with the parainfluenza viruses, particularly type 3 virus, is common and often leads to serious lower respiratory tract disease.

Transmission of parainfluenza viruses is by direct person-to-person contact or large droplet spread. The high rate of infection early in life, coupled with the high frequency of reinfection, suggests that these viruses spread readily from person to person. Reinfected individuals appear to be infectious, and a relatively small inoculum is able to initiate infection. Type 3 virus appears to be the most transmissible of the parainfluenza viruses.

In experimental infection of adult volunteers, the interval between administration of type 1, 2, or 3 virus and onset of upper respiratory tract symptoms ranged from 3 to 6 days. The incubation period in pediatric infections has not been defined; however, the interval between exposure to type 3 virus and the subsequent initial shedding of this virus is 2 to 4 days. Resistance to type 1 or type 2 parainfluenza virus infection and associated upper respiratory disease appears to be a function of local respiratory tract, secretory, immunoglobulin A (IgA)–neutralizing antibodies. Infants may also be partially protected from infection and lower respiratory tract disease by serum antibodies. This protective relationship is suggested by the relative sparing of young infants from type 1 and type 2 virus infection and associated disease at a time when they possess serum antibodies passively acquired from their mother. Also, the risk of infection with type 3 virus during the first 4 months of life is inversely related to the level of neutralizing antibodies present in cord serum at birth. However, the protective effect of passive immunity is less than that observed for type 1 and type 2 viruses, since a significant number of infants with moderately high levels of maternally derived serum antibody become infected with type 3 virus and develop severe illness.

CLINICAL MANIFESTATIONS. In children, the most common type of illness consists of rhinitis, pharyngitis, and bronchitis, usually with fever. The most common initial symptoms are cough, hoarseness, and fever. The cough may be croupy, but respiratory distress is not present. Approximately three fourths of such ill children have a temperature above 37.8°C; fever usually lasts 2 to 3 days. Coarse breath sounds, rhonchi, erythema of the pharyngeal mucous membranes, and rhinitis are characteristic physical findings. Cervical adenopathy is uncommon.

When croup develops, the initial symptoms of rhinitis, pharyngitis, fever, and cough progress. After several days, the cough worsens and becomes brassy, seal-like, or barking, and stridor ensues. At this stage, most children recover uneventfully after 24 to 48 hours, but in some air hunger develops, with cyanosis, sternal and intercostal retractions, and progressive airway obstruction. The lateral radiograph of the neck (which should be obtained only under carefully controlled medical supervision, if at all) shows glottic and subglottic narrowing (the "steeple sign") and differentiates this disease from epiglottitis.

When bronchiolitis or pneumonia develops, fever persists and the cough progresses and becomes somewhat productive. It is accompanied by wheezing, tachypnea, and retractions and in severe cases by cyanosis. The x-ray film shows interstitial or perihilar infiltrates and air trapping. In some patients a combined bronchopneumonia-croup syndrome occurs.

DIAGNOSIS. Presumptive diagnosis of parainfluenza virus infection can be made on the basis of age, history, clinical findings, and relation to known or characteristic prevalence of virus in the community. Definitive diagnosis, however, requires recovery of the virus from appropriate specimens taken from the respiratory tract or identification of viral antigens in respiratory tract secretions by immunofluorescence or another form of immunoassay. Serodiagnosis by hemagglutination inhibition, complement fixation, or neutralization can establish that infection with a member of the parainfluenza virus group has occurred, but frequent heterotypic responses make type-specific diagnosis by serology extremely difficult.

TREATMENT. Symptomatic treatment of croup usually includes humidification of air by ultrasonic nebulizer and periodic inhalation of racemic epinephrine. Antibiotics are usually contraindicated. The use of corticosteroids is controversial, but many physicians prescribe high doses of dexamethasone if croup is severe. Specific antiviral treatment or effective vaccines for prevention of parainfluenza virus disease are not available.

Chanock RM, McIntosh K: Parainfluenza viruses. *In* Fields B (ed.): Virology. New York, Raven Press, 1990, pp 963–988. *Summary of natural history of parainfluenza virus infection and pathogenesis of disease.*

Chanock RM, Parrott RH, Johnson KM, et al.: Myxoviruses: Parainfluenza. Am Rev Respir Dis 88:152, 1963. *A discussion of the importance of parainfluenza viruses in pediatric respiratory tract disease and the first description of pattern of spread and reinfection.*

Denny FW, Murphy TF, Clyde WA, Jr, et al.: Croup: An 11-year study in a pediatric practice. Pediatrics 71:871, 1983. *Eleven-year evaluation of the role of parainfluenza viruses in croup. These viruses accounted for 74 per cent of all virus isolates from croup patients.*

Fox JP, Hall CE: Infections with other respiratory pathogens: Influenza, mumps, and respiratory syncytial viruses; *Mycoplasma pneumoniae*. *In* Fox JP (ed.): Viruses in Families. Littleton, MA, John Wright/PSG Inc, 1980, pp 335–381. *Longitudinal surveillance of families for parainfluenza virus infection and illness. Infection rate was 44 per 100 person-years for all ages, while attack rate for illness associated with parainfluenza virus infection was 76 per cent for babies under age 2 years and 25 per cent for adults.*

Glenzen WP, Denny FW: Epidemiology of acute lower respiratory disease in children. N Engl J Med 288:498, 1973. *Excellent summary of contribution of parainfluenza viruses to pediatric respiratory disease.*

364 Influenza

R. Gordon Douglas, Jr.

DEFINITION. Influenza is an acute, usually self-limited febrile illness that occurs in outbreaks of varying severity almost every winter. The causative virus is transmitted by the respiratory route; however, systemic symptoms are out of proportion to those in the respiratory tract. Infection with influenza virus can produce several other clinical syndromes common with infection with respiratory viruses, such as common colds, pharyngitis, croup, tracheobronchitis, bronchiolitis, or pneumonia. Conversely, infections with other respiratory viruses, such as respiratory syncytial virus, rhinovirus, or adenovirus, may produce sporadic cases indistinguishable from those of typical influenza. In addition to enormous morbidity and loss of time from school and work, influenza epidemics are associated with substantial mortality caused in large part by pulmonary complications

Since the year 1510, 31 pandemics of respiratory disease similar to modern influenza have been described, 5 of which have occurred in the twentieth century (1900, 1918, 1957, 1968, and 1977). Of these, the pandemic of 1918 was the most severe, accounting for at least 21 million deaths. Over 500,000 deaths have occurred in the United States from epidemic influenza in the past 20 years.

ETIOLOGY. Influenza viruses belong to the family Orthomyxoviridae. Influenza A virus constitutes one genus and influenza B virus another. The virion is a medium-sized (80 to 100 nm in diameter) enveloped spherical or elongated particle covered with surface projections that are glycoproteins possessing either hemagglutinin (H) or neuraminidase (N) activity (Fig. 364–1). The envelope is composed of a lipid bilayer, on the inner surface of which is the matrix (M) protein. Within the envelope are eight segmented pieces of nucleocapsid, formed by a single species of protein, the nucleoprotein (NP), and single-stranded ribonucleic acid (RNA). Three polymerase (P) proteins and three nonstructural (NS_1, NS_2, and M2) proteins of unknown function are found within the envelope. The H is responsible for binding of the virus to the cell. Antibody to this protein neutralizes viral infectivity and thus is the major determinant of immunity. The viral N is instrumental in release of virus from cells. Antineuraminidase antibody is not neutralizing but limits viral replication and therefore the severity of infection. The M protein plays a role in stability of the membrane and in organization of the virion

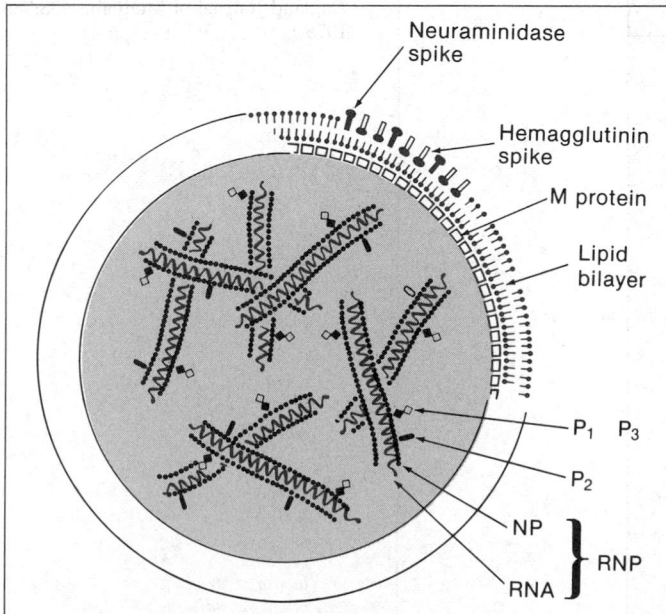

FIGURE 364–1. Schematic model for influenza virus virions. (Modified from Ginsberg HS: Orthomyxoviruses. *In* Davis BD, Dulbecco R, Eisen HN, Ginsburg HS [eds.]: Microbiology, 3rd ed. Hagerstown, MD, Harper & Row, Publishers, 1980, p 1119.)

during assembly. The three polymerases are important in viral replication. The internal M, NP, and P proteins are antigenically indistinguishable in all influenza A viruses but vary from those found in influenza B and C viruses. Thus, type-specific (A, B, or C) distinction of influenza viruses depends on serologic reactions mediated by these internal antigens. However, the surface proteins (H and N) do vary, not only among influenza virus types but also among subtypes of influenza A.

The viral *genome* comprises eight segments of RNA, each of which codes for one or two viral proteins. Reassortment of gene segments occurs frequently during coinfection of cells with two influenza A viruses. Influenza B and C viruses have been studied much less but appear to be structurally similar to influenza A virus. Antigenic variation is much less frequent with influenza B, and it may not occur with influenza C.

EPIDEMIOLOGY. *Antigenic Variation.* One of the unique and most remarkable features of influenza virus is the frequency with which changes in antigenicity occur. Such changes help explain why influenza continues to be a major epidemic disease in humans. As noted previously, antigenic variation involves only the H and N proteins among the proteins of influenza virus. The H is the more important, since it is more frequently involved in antigenic variation than the N protein and since antibody to this protein neutralizes infection. Antigenic variation is referred to as *antigenic drift* or *antigenic shift*, depending on whether the variation is small or great.

Antigenic Drift. Antigenic drift refers to relatively minor changes that occur frequently (every year or every few years) within an influenza A subtype. Each subtype is named by its hemagglutinin and neuraminidase. To date, three hemagglutinins (H1, H2, and H3) and two neuraminidases (N1 and N2) have been recognized in humans. The former designations, HO and HSW, are now classified as variants of H1. Each strain within the subtype is identified by site and year of isolation. Thus, influenza A/Bangkok/79/H3N2 indicates an influenza virus of type A and subtype H3N2 that was isolated in 1979 in Bangkok. The original H3N2 variant, A/Aichi/68/H3N2, was isolated in Aichi, Japan, in 1968. All isolates worldwide for the next 3 years were serologically identical. Subsequent antigenic drifts resulted in recovery of variants possessing minor differences: A/England/72/H3N2, A/Port Chalmers/73/H3N2, A/Scotland/74/H3N2, A/Georgia/74/H3N2, A/Victoria/75/H3N2, A/Texas/77/H3N2, A/Bangkok/79/H3N2, A/Philippines/2/82/H3N2, A/Mississippi/1/85/H3N2, A/Shanghai/11/87/H3N2, and so on. Antigenic drift results from point mutations that usually affect the RNA segment coding for the hemagglutinin, resulting in an alteration in protein structure that involves one or a few amino acids. Four antigenic sites have been described and complete nucleotide sequencing of hemagglutinins of several H3 strains has been determined, in support of this hypothesis. There is immunologic selection in which a new virus is favored over the old for person-to-person transmission because of the less frequent presence of antibody in the population to the new virus.

Antigenic Shift. Major antigenic shifts result from genetic reassortment when two influenza viruses simultaneously infect a single cell. Such an event results in a hemagglutinin or neuraminidase, or both, that is completely new in comparison with the previously circulating strain. Because of the high level of immunity to the old strain and lack of immunity to the new strain within the human population, the new strain, provided that it possesses intrinsic viral properties such as virulence and transmissibility, can readily cause a major outbreak of influenza.

Epidemic Influenza. An epidemic is an outbreak of influenza confined to one location such as a city, town, or country. In a given community, epidemics of influenza A virus infection have a characteristic pattern. A graphic description of an epidemic due to an A/Victoria/75/H3N2–like virus, which occurred in 1976 in Houston, Texas, is shown in Figure 364–2. Such localized epidemics begin rather abruptly, reach a sharp peak in 2 to 3 weeks, and last 5 to 6 weeks. Reports of increased numbers of children with febrile respiratory illness are often the first indication of influenza in a community. This is soon followed by the occurrence of influenza-like illnesses among adults. The next event is increased hospital admissions of patients with pneumonia, exacerbation of chronic obstructive pulmonary disease, croup, and congestive heart failure. There are increases in school and industrial absenteeism and in the number of deaths caused by pneumonia and influenza. Although the latter finding is a highly specific indicator of influenza, it invariably lags behind the others. Viral isolation studies show a peak that parallels that of acute febrile respiratory illness. Year-round studies indicate that almost all isolates are obtained during the epidemic period. It is rare to recover influenza virus during other periods of the year, although occasionally there is serologic evidence of infection during other months.

Epidemics occur almost exclusively during the winter months—October through April in the northern hemisphere and May through September in the southern hemisphere. When observed in large countries such as the United States or Australia, regional differences in the time of occurrence of influenza outbreaks are apparent. It is not uncommon to have major outbreaks occurring in some communities or regions while others are experiencing no activity whatsoever. Often those so spared experience similar outbreaks at a later time, particularly if the prevalent virus demonstrates significant antigenic variation compared with previously prevalent viruses. During epidemics, the average overall attack rates are estimated to be 10 to 20 per cent;

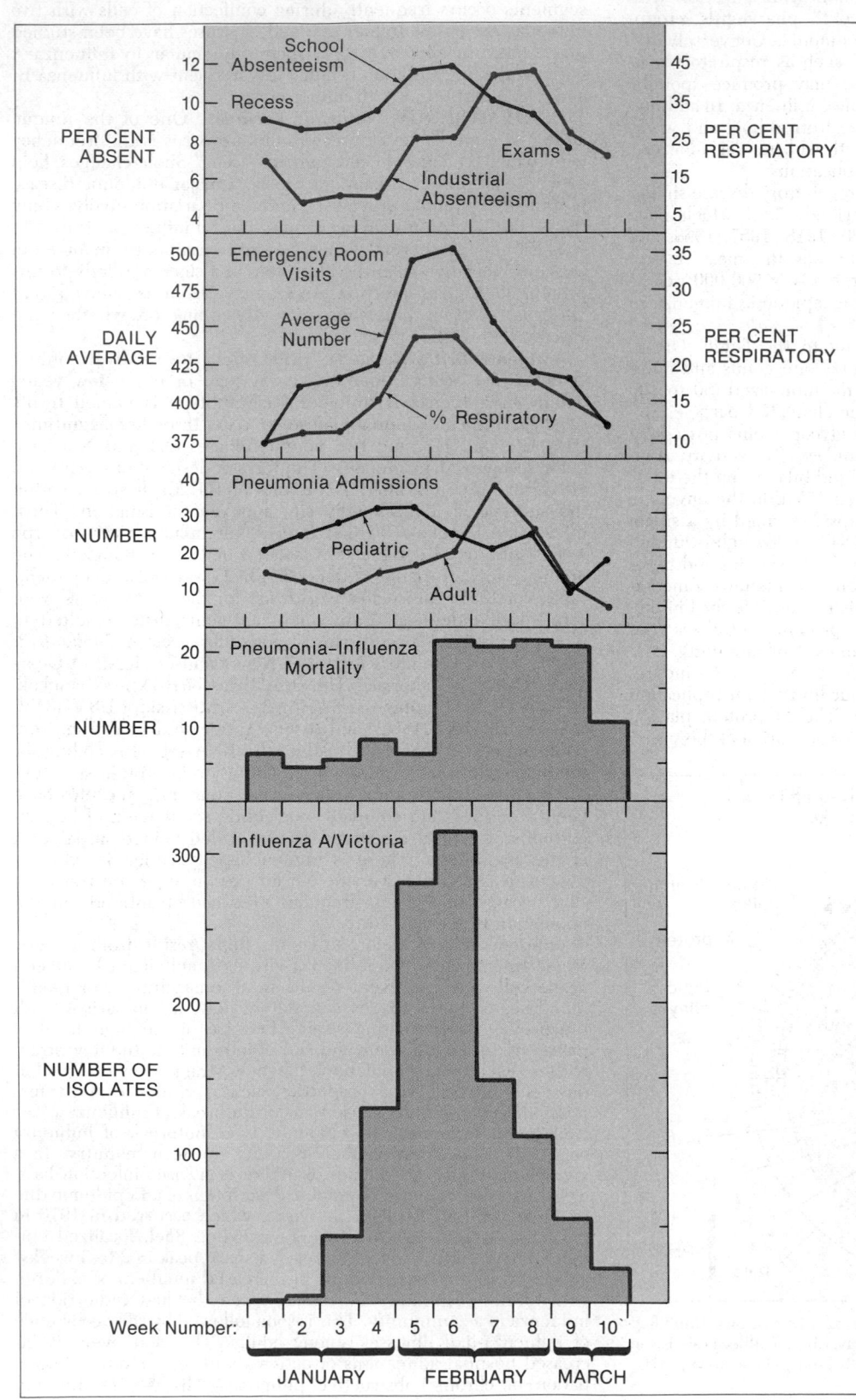

FIGURE 364–2. Correlation of the nonvirologic indexes of epidemiologic influenza with the number of isolates of influenza A/Victoria virus according to week, Houston, 1976 (industrial absenteeism is indicated by percentage with respiratory complaints). (Modified, by permission, from the New England Journal of Medicine 298:589, 1978.)

however, in selected populations of age groups, attack rates of 40 to 50 per cent are not uncommon. For many years it had been thought that during an epidemic of influenza a single strain of influenza virus prevailed and that other respiratory viruses were diminished or disappeared. However, we now know that two different strains within a single subtype, for example, A/Victoria/3/75/H3N2 and A/Texas/1/77/H3N2, or two different influenza virus subtypes, H1N1 and H3N2, may cocirculate. Furthermore, outbreaks of influenza A and B or simultaneous outbreaks of influenza A and respiratory syncytial virus infection have been demonstrated. Studies indicate that strains circulating at the end of one season's epidemic are most likely to be responsible for the next season's outbreak (the so-called *herald wave phenomenon*).

Pandemic Influenza. Pandemics of influenza result from the emergence of a new virus to which the overall population contains no immunity, so that epidemics of influenza progress to involve all parts of the world. The association of different subtypes of influenza A virus with pandemic influenza for the past 80 years is shown in Table 364–1. The pandemics of 1957, 1968, and 1977 all began in mainland China and then spread east and west, but primarily to the USSR and Western Europe before reaching the American continent. The interval between pandemics is variable and unpredictable, and this fact, in part, led to the national immunization program against swine influenza, when a small outbreak of A/H1N1 infection was detected at Fort Dix, New Jersey. This virus, A/New Jersey/76/H1N1, was very similar to the virus responsible for the 1988 outbreak. The most severe pandemics have resulted when there were major antigenic alterations in both of the major surface antigens. A striking exception to this occurred when A/USSR/77/H1N1 did not cause a severe pandemic in 1977 to 1978, despite major shifts in both surface glycoproteins. This discrepancy may reflect that much of the world's population in 1977 had been alive during the previous H1N1 era and thus possessed partial protective immunity. Furthermore, it appears that transmissibility from person to person and intrinsic virulence are virus-coded functions that vary much as does antigenicity. Intrinsic virulence with H1N1 viruses appears to be milder than with H3N2 viruses.

Proposed Mechanism of Epidemic Behavior. When a new virus with appropriate characteristics of virulence and transmissibility is introduced into a population lacking appropriate antibody, pandemic influenza results. After one or more waves of pandemic influenza, the level of immunity in the population increases. Such a chain of events provides a setting for emergence of a variant showing antigenic drift, since the level of immunity to it is less than that to the original strain. Repeated epidemics caused by strains showing antigenic drift within the subtype occur in subsequent years. After 10 to 40 years of circulation of variants within this given subtype, the population's immunity to all variants within the subtype is very high, and the conditions for the spread of a new virus are favorable. Such a virus originates by genetic reassortment. It possesses an H or N, or both, that is markedly different from the prior subtype. When such a virus circulates, the next pandemic occurs. Antigenic variation does not provide the entire explanation. Virus factors also contribute to virulence and transmissibility. Furthermore, other than the association of influenza outbreaks with colder seasons, the factors that allow an epidemic to develop or those responsible for the tapering off of an epidemic after 5 or 6 weeks, when only a

TABLE 364–1. ANTIGENIC SUBTYPES OF INFLUENZA A VIRUS ASSOCIATED WITH PANDEMIC INFLUENZA

Year	Interval (Years)	Designation	Extent of Antigenic Change in Indicated Surface Protein*	Severity of Pandemic
1870	—	H2N?	?	Moderate
1889	19	H3N8	H + + +N?	Severe
1918	29	H1N1†	H + + +N + + +	Severe
1957	39	H2N2	H + + +N + + +	Severe
1968	11	H3N2	H + + +N −	Moderate
1977	9	H1N1	H + + +N + + +	Mild

* + = Minor change; + + = moderate change; + + + = major change; − = no change.

†Former designation was Hsw1N1 (35).

portion of susceptible persons is infected, are unknown. Finally, where the virus resides between epidemics is not understood.

Mortality. Pneumonia and influenza deaths fluctuate annually in predictable fashion, with peaks in the winter and troughs in the summer. When pneumonia and influenza deaths exceed the predicted number, this is due to influenza A or occasionally to influenza B virus activity. Although mortality is greatest during pandemics, substantial mortality occurs with epidemics, and the cumulative mortality from epidemics may exceed that of pandemics. Excess deaths due to influenza in the United States average 30,000 per epidemic (Fig. 364–3).

PATHOGENESIS and PATHOLOGY. Influenza virus infection is acquired by transfer of virus-containing respiratory secretions from an infected to a susceptible person. Small-particle aerosols (less than 10 μ mass medium diameter) may be most significant in such person-to-person transmission. Once the virus has been deposited in the respiratory tract epithelium, unless it is prevented by specific secretory antibody, nonspecific mucoproteins, or mechanical actions of the mucociliary blanket, it attaches to and penetrates columnar epithelial cells by pinocytosis. Viral replication lasts 4 to 6 hours, and virus release continues for several hours before cell death ensues. Infection of adjacent and nearby cells follows, so that within a few replication cycles large numbers of cells in the respiratory tract are infected. The duration of the incubation period until onset of illness and virus shedding, which occur in close proximity, varies from 18 to 72 hours, depending in part on the inoculum size. Quantitation of virus in respiratory tract specimens reveals a characteristic pattern that correlates with severity of illness, suggesting that a major mechanism in the production of illness is cell death resulting from viral replication. Serum or secretory antibody or cell-mediated immune mechanisms are not detectable at this time, indicating that immunologic mechanisms are probably not involved in production of illness, with the exception of circulating interferon, which may contribute to systemic symptoms and fever. Viremia is rare.

Interferon is frequently detected in respiratory tract and serum specimens. Shedding of virus precedes by 1 to 2 days the appearance of interferon, which is correlated with improvements of signs and symptoms and decrease of virus titer, suggesting that interferon is active in the recovery process.

Neutralizing, hemagglutination-inhibiting (HAI), antineuraminidase, complement-fixing, enzyme-linked immunosorbent assay (ELISA), and immunofluorescent antibodies begin to develop in the sera of persons with primary influenza virus infection during the second week after exposure to antigen and reach a peak by 4 weeks. Secretory antibodies develop in the respiratory tract after influenza infection and consist predominantly of immunoglobulin A (IgA) antibodies that reach peak titers in 14 days. Protection against infection is afforded by serum HAI titers of 1:40 or greater, serum-neutralizing titers of 1:8 or greater, or nasal-neutralizing antibody titers of 1:4 or greater.

Nasal and bronchial biopsy specimens from persons with uncomplicated influenza reveal desquamation of the ciliated columnar epithelium. Individual cells show shrinkage, pyknotic nuclei, and loss of cilia. In addition, the lungs in fatal influenza show extensive hemorrhage, hyaline membrane formation, and paucity of polymorphonuclear cell infiltration. Patients with secondary bacterial pneumonia have the changes characteristic of bacterial pneumonia in addition to the tracheobronchial findings of influenza in the tracheobronchial tree.

CLINICAL FINDINGS. Many patients can pinpoint the hour of onset. Initially, systemic symptoms predominate and include feverishness, chilliness or frank shaking chills, headache, myalgias, malaise, and anorexia. In more severe cases, prostration is observed. Usually myalgias or headaches are the most troublesome symptoms, and their severity is related to the level of the fever. Arthralgias are commonly observed. Ocular symptoms, although less commonly present, are helpful diagnostically and include photophobia, tearing, burning, and pain on moving the eyes. Respiratory symptoms, particularly dry cough and nasal discharge, are usually also present at the onset but are overshadowed by the systemic symptoms. Nasal obstruction, hoarseness, and dry sore throat may also be present.

Fever is the most important physical finding. The temperature usually rises rapidly to a peak of 38 to 40°C and occasionally to 41°C within 12 hours of onset, concurrently with the development of systemic symptoms. Fever is usually continuous but may be intermittent, especially if antipyretics are administered. On the second and third days of illness, the temperature elevation is usually less than on the first day. As fever subsides, the systemic symptoms diminish. Typically, the duration of fever is 3 days, but it may last from 1 to 5 or more days. In a few cases, a second fluctuation in fever occurs on the third or fourth day, resulting in a biphasic fever curve. Early in the course of illness, the patient appears toxic, the face is flushed, and the skin is hot and moist. The eyes are watery and reddened. Clear nasal discharge is common, but nasal obstruction is uncommon. The mucous membranes of the nose and throat are hyperemic, but exudate is not observed. Small, tender cervical lymph nodes are often present, and transient, scattered rhonchi or localized areas of rales are found in less than 20 per cent of cases.

As systemic signs and symptoms diminish, respiratory complaints and findings become more apparent. Cough is the most frequent and troublesome of these symptoms and may be accompanied by substernal discomfort or burning. Nasal obstruction, discharge, pharyngeal pain, and injection are also common. Such symptoms and signs usually persist 3 to 4 days after fever subsides; however, cough, lassitude, and malaise may persist for 1, 2, or more weeks before full recovery.

This pattern of illness just described occurs with any type or subtype of influenza A or B virus. Attack rates are higher in children than in adults, although the incidence of pulmonary complications is lower in children. Maximum temperatures are higher in children, cervical adenopathy may be more frequent, and croup occurs only among children.

PULMONARY COMPLICATIONS. Three kinds of pulmonary complications are well recognized: *primary influenza viral pneumonia, secondary bacterial pneumonia,* and *mixed viral and bacterial pneumonia.* In addition, during an outbreak of influenza, less distinct and milder pulmonic syndromes often occur that may represent viral tracheobronchitis, localized viral pneumonia, or possibly mixed viral and bacterial infection.

Primary Influenza Viral Pneumonia. This syndrome first became well documented in the pandemic of 1957 to 1958. However, it is clear that many of the deaths in the 1918 to 1919 outbreak were due to this syndrome in healthy young adults. Primary influenza viral pneumonia has occurred predominantly among persons with cardiovascular disease, especially rheumatic heart disease with mitral stenosis. Although this syndrome occurs in healthy young adults in every large outbreak, other chronic disorders and pregnancy have been implicated as risk factors in some epidemics. Following a typical onset of influenza, there is rapid progression to fever, cough, dyspnea, and cyanosis. Physical examination and chest roentgenograms reveal bilateral findings consistent with the adult respiratory distress syndrome. Blood gas studies show marked hypoxia. Gram's stain of the sputum fails to reveal significant bacteria, and bacterial culture yields sparse growth of normal flora. Viral cultures of sputum or tracheal aspirates yield high titers of influenza virus. Such patients do not respond to antibiotics, and mortality is high.

Secondary Bacterial Pneumonia. Bacterial superinfection is often clinically distinguishable from primary viral pneumonia. The patients are most often elderly or have chronic pulmonary, cardiac, metabolic, or other diseases. Following a typical influenza illness, a period of improvement lasting from 1 to 4 days may occur. Recrudescence of fever is associated with symptoms and signs of bacterial pneumonia, such as cough, sputum production, and a localized area of consolidation apparent on physical and chest roentgenogram examination. Gram's stain and sputum culture reveal predominance of a bacterial pathogen, most often *Streptococcus pneumoniae, Staphylococcus aureus,* or *Haemophilus influenzae.* Such patients usually respond to specific antibiotic therapy.

Mixed Viral and Bacterial Pneumonia. During an outbreak of influenza, many cases are observed that do not clearly fit into either of the categories just described. The disease is not relentlessly progressive, and yet the fever pattern may be persistent and not biphasic. These patients may have a milder form of primary viral, secondary bacterial, or mixed viral and bacterial infection. Many respond to antibiotics. Milder forms of primary viral pneumonia involving only one lobe or segment have been described that do not invariably lead to death. Such cases are more likely to be confused with a pneumonia due to *Mycoplasma pneumoniae* than to that produced by bacterial infection. Pneumonia may occur in children, but it is less common than in adults. In addition, bronchiolitis and croup may be caused by influenza A or B virus infection.

Exacerbation of Chronic Obstructive Pulmonary Disease. In

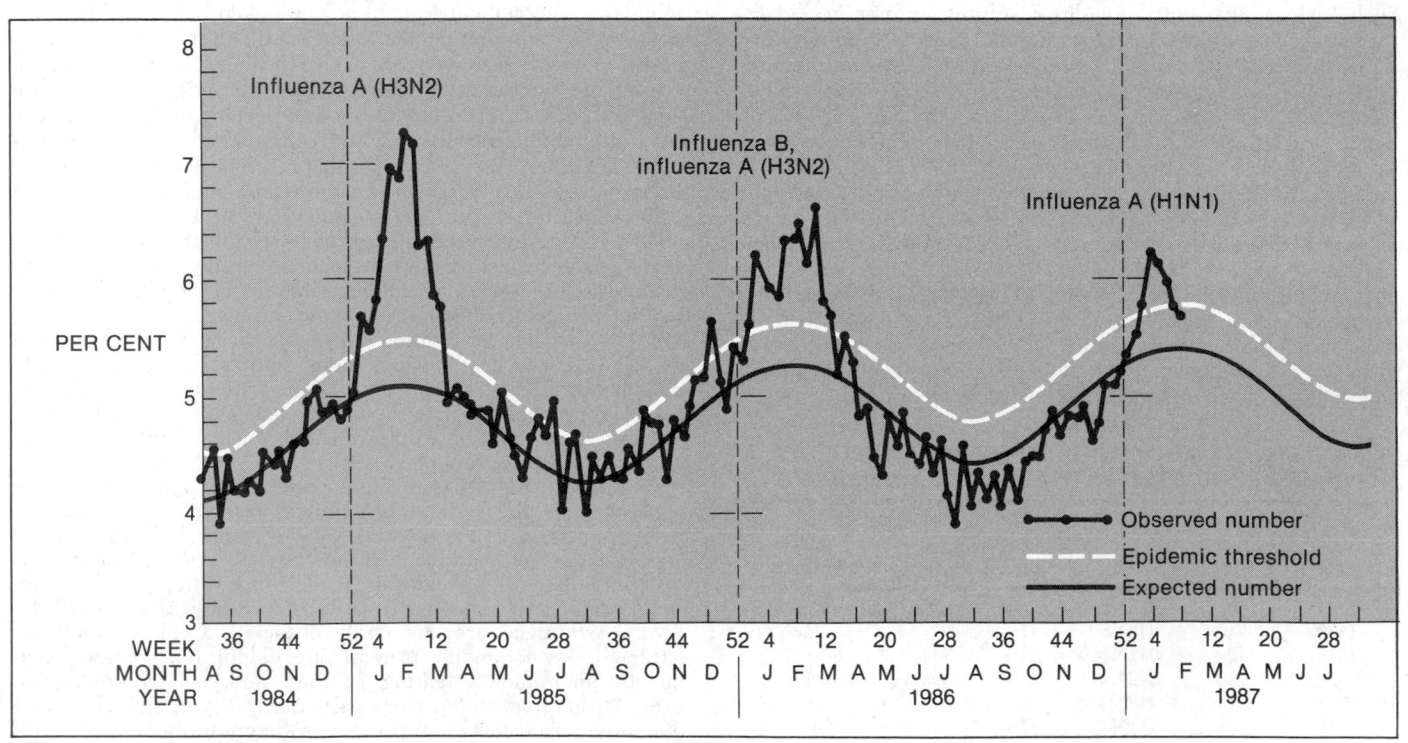

FIGURE 364–3. Pneumonia and influenza deaths as a percentage of total deaths in 121 cities from August 1984 through February 1987. (From Centers for Disease Control: Update: Influenza activity—United States. MMWR 36:116, 1987.)

adults with chronic obstructive pulmonary disease, influenza A or B virus infection may lead not only to pneumonia but also to acute exacerbation of chronic bronchitis, a syndrome that is associated with other respiratory viruses and bacteria as well.

NONPULMONIC COMPLICATIONS. *Reye's Syndrome.* Reye's syndrome is a frequently recognized hepatic and central nervous system complication of influenza A and B infection. Reye's syndrome is discussed in Ch. 480.

Other Complications. Myositis and myoglobinuria with tender leg muscles and elevated serum creatine kinase (CK) levels have been reported, mostly occurring in children. Myocarditis, pericarditis, and myocardial infarction rarely have been associated with influenza A and B virus infection. Gullain-Barré syndrome has been reported to occur after influenza A, but no definite causal relationship has been established. Transverse myelitis and encephalitis have also been reported rarely. Toxic shock syndrome due to infection of the respiratory tract with toxin-bearing S. *aureus* has been reported.

DIAGNOSIS. In an individual case, influenza often cannot be distinguished from infection with a number of other viruses and bacteria that produce headache, muscle aches, fever, and cough. On occasion, other respiratory viruses can produce an influenza-like illness, as can streptococcal pharyngitis. In the summer months, enteroviruses produce a clinically indistinguishable picture, and the acute manifestations of many other infections, such as dengue, may mimic influenza. On the other hand, in the context of an epidemic, influenza may be readily distinguished from other acute infections. When local, state, or national health authorities report an epidemic of influenza A or B virus infection in a given community, and a patient is seen with the acute onset of fever, headache, muscle aches, and cough, it is highly likely that these symptoms are caused by an influenza virus infection.

Definitive diagnosis depends on detection of infectious virus or viral antigen in secretions from patients or the detection of a serum antibody response. Influenza virus is readily isolated from throat or nasal specimens, sputum, or tracheal secretion specimens in the first 2 or 3 days of illness. Usually infectivity is detected within 48 to 72 hours in cell cultures. Viral antigen may be detected more rapidly in such specimens by use of immunofluorescence or ELISA. Serologic methods are less useful clinically because they require a convalescent serum obtained 10 to 14 days after the onset of infection. However, they are of great use in epidemiologic studies and to document the occurrence of an outbreak. A fourfold increase in antibody titer, comparing an acute with a convalescent phase, is diagnostic. The complement fixation antibody test is most useful for diagnosis because it is not dependent on strain or subtype variation, as is hemagglutination inhibition.

TREATMENT. Amantadine shortens the duration of fever and of systemic and respiratory symptoms by about 50 per cent. The dose is 100 to 200 mg per day orally for 3 to 5 days. Rimantadine, although not yet licensed, has a similar effect and reduces the likelihood of the mild, transient central nervous system side effects that occur with amantadine. Other symptomatic measures include antipyretics and cough suppressants. Many authorities consider that aspirin should not be used, especially for persons under 16 years of age, because of its association with the occurrence of Reye's syndrome. There is no evidence that amantadine or rimantadine is effective in treatment of pulmonary complications of influenza.

Currently, primary influenza viral pneumonia in its severe stages is best managed in an intensive care unit with supportive measures such as respiratory therapy, supplemental oxygen, and fluids. Secondary bacterial pneumonia should be treated with appropriate antibiotics. When studies of the sputum do not clearly indicate which bacterium may be infecting the patient, coverage should include antibiotics that are effective against S. *aureus*, S. *pneumoniae*, and H. *influenzae*.

PREVENTION. The mainstay of prevention is the use of inactivated influenza virus vaccines. These vaccines provide about 80 per cent protective efficacy. The antigenic composition is reviewed annually so that the vaccine contains the most recently circulating strains. Usually the vaccine is a trivalent product containing one or more subtypes of influenza A and influenza B virus. The recent vaccines have been purified by density gradient centrifugation or chromatography and have very low reaction rates. One to two per cent of persons vaccinated have fever and systemic symptoms peaking at 8 to 12 hours after vaccination, and up to 25 per cent may have mild local reactions at the site of vaccination. "Split" virus (subvirion) vaccines contain antigens with disrupted virus and may be less reactigenic than "whole" virus vaccines. The highest priority for vaccination should be given to persons with cardiac or pulmonary conditions requiring ongoing medical care and to residents of nursing homes and other chronic care facilities. Physicians, nurses, and other personnel including home health-care providers who have extensive contact with high-risk patients constitute the next priority for vaccination. Finally, persons over age 65 and persons with other chronic disease of any age should be vaccinated. Vaccine may also be given to well persons under age 65 who wish to reduce the likelihood of acquiring influenza. Vaccine should be administered each year in the fall prior to the influenza season.

Amantadine and rimantadine are also effective in preventing influenza A and should be used to supplement vaccine programs. Persons who are not vaccinated in the fall should be placed on amantadine when an outbreak occurs or throughout the influenza season for the highest risk group. If vaccine is available, persons may be vaccinated simultaneously, and amantadine therapy should be stopped after 14 days. Alternatively, if vaccine is not available, amantadine administration may be continued for the duration of the outbreak, the dose being 100 to 200 mg per day orally. In the family setting, prophylaxis may fail owing to emergence of resistant viruses. Amantadine, administered to patients and staff alike, is very helpful in managing nosocomial outbreaks.

Arden NH, Patriarca PA, Fasano MB, et al.: The roles of vaccination and amantadine prophylaxis in controlling an outbreak of influenza A (H3N2) in a nursing home. Arch Intern Med 148:865–868, 1988. *Useful data to manage a common problem.*

Barker WH, Mullooly JP: Pneumonia and influenza deaths during epidemics: Implications for prevention. Arch Intern Med 142:85–89, 1982. *Best study of the devastating effects of an influenza epidemic.*

Centers for Disease Control: Prevention and Control of Influenza. Part I. Vaccines. MMWR 38:297–298, 303–311, 1989. *Details of extensive revisions of recommendations for use of influenza vaccine as well as a summary of recent epidemiology.*

Dolin R, Reichman RC, Madore HP, et al.: A controlled trial of amantadine and rimantadine in the prophylaxis of influenza A infection. N Engl J Med 307:580, 1982. *Definitive study comparing prophylactic efficacy of amantadine and rimantadine.*

Douglas RG Jr.: Prophylaxis and treatment of influenza. N Engl J Med 322:443–450, 1990. *Recent review of vaccines and antivirals for influenza.*

Hayden FG, Belshe RB, Clover RD, et al.: Emergence and apparent transmission of rimantidine resistant influenza A virus in families. N Engl J Med 321:1696–1702, 1989. *A problem possibly limiting usefulness of antiviral prophylaxis.*

Kendel AP, Patriarca PA (eds.): Options for the Control of Influenza. New York, Alan R. Liss, 1986. *Excellent recent review of rationale for vaccine and amantadine use. In addition, an up-to-date summary of epidemiology.*

Younkin SW, Betts RF, Roth FK, et al.: Reduction in fever and symptoms in young adults with aspirin or amantadine. Antimicrob Agents Chemother 23:577, 1983. *Study comparing therapeutic effects of amantadine and aspirin.*

365 Adenovirus Diseases

Stephen G. Baum

The most clinically significant diseases caused by adenoviruses are infections of the respiratory system and the eye. Recently, adenoviruses have been shown to play a significant role in causing diarrheal disease in children and respiratory infections in immunocompromised patients. Adenoviruses are the object of intensive research efforts because they possess several fascinating and important biologic capabilities, including oncogenesis and latency. Today they are perhaps the best characterized human virus group.

ETIOLOGIC AGENT. Adenoviruses are double-stranded DNA viruses that average 70 nm in diameter and have a unique outer structure, which permits their morphologic identification by electron microscopic examination. The virus is icosahedral with 20 equilateral triangular faces and 12 vertices. The faces are made up of hexon subunits, and the vertices each contain a penton subunit. From each vertex, an antenna-like structure, the fiber, projects with a knob at the end. Each class of these surface subunits differs antigenically from the others. The hexon contains group-specific and type-specific antigens. Forty-seven serotypes of human adenovirus have been identified (types 1 to 47). Many of the serotypes have been associated with specific syndromes, but over half the adenovirus types have not been shown to cause disease. The 47 serotypes have been divided into six groups by DNA homology and four groups according to ability to agglutinate different erythrocytes. The latter grouping correlates well with the ability of different serotypes to cause specific syndromes and to induce tumors in animals.

In acute infections, adenoviruses cause cell death and lysis with release of new progeny virions. The mechanisms of latency and animal oncogenesis are not completely understood, although many of the functions of adenovirus have been accurately mapped on the deoxyribonucleic acid (DNA) genome. Adenoviruses can form a family of hybrid viruses with an unrelated DNA virus, SV40. Portions of the DNA of adenovirus and SV40 are covalently linked within an adenovirus outer coat. The hybrid virus has unique biologic and oncogenic capabilities in vitro and in animals in vivo. Neither adenovirus alone nor the hybrid viruses have been shown to cause cancer in humans.

A small defective DNA parvovirus has been isolated from some adenovirus preparations and from some patients with adenovirus infection. This *adeno-associated virus (AAV)* requires adenovirus for its replication. It is not known to cause disease by itself and does not appear to contribute to adenovirus pathogenesis. A related parvovirus (B19) has recently been implicated as the cause of erythema infectiosum (fifth disease), aplastic crisis in patients with hemoglobinopathies, and arthropathy in adults.

EPIDEMIOLOGY. Most people experience an adenovirus infection during the first decade of life. The initial infecting serotype and the syndrome it causes are a function of the age of the patient and the route of infection. Studies of large populations show that adenoviruses cause 3 to 5 per cent of all clinically apparent infections in children. Adenoviruses are the most common viral isolates in this age group, and at least half of these isolations are associated with subclinical infections. Respiratory infection is transmitted by person-to-person contact or through contaminated swimming water.

Conjunctival infection may be transmitted directly, through water, or by fomites such as towels or ophthalmologic equipment and solutions. Pneumonia and urinary tract infection in immunocompromised patients may be acquired exogenously or may represent reactivation of latent infection. There are many adenoviruses that infect other animals and birds, but these play no known role in human disease.

CLINICAL PRESENTATIONS OCCURRING MOSTLY IN CHILDREN. Respiratory Infection. Infants most commonly manifest adenovirus infections as coryzal symptoms, but occasionally adenovirus type 7 causes fulminant bronchiolitis and pneumonia in this age group. Recently, Reye's syndrome has been reported as a complication of severe adenovirus infection in infants. In older children, pharyngitis and tracheobronchitis are most prevalent. Adenoviruses are the most common viral isolate from children with the whooping cough syndrome. It is not known whether this virus contributes to the pathogenesis of *Bordetella pertussis* infection or whether adenovirus alone can cause the syndrome.

Pharyngoconjunctival Fever. This syndrome occurs in small epidemics in summer camps where it is probably spread in swimming water. Adenovirus type 3 has been the most common isolate. The onset of symptoms is acute and includes pharyngitis, rhinitis, conjunctivitis, cervical adenitis, and elevation in temperature to about 38°C. The bulbar and palpebral conjunctivae have a granular appearance. The symptoms last 3 to 5 days. Permanent sequelae are rare, and there is no specific therapy.

Intestinal Disease. Immunoelectron microscopy has revealed viruses in the stool in many cases of infantile diarrhea. The most common viruses visualized are rotaviruses and adenoviruses. These adenoviruses appear to be defective in their replication and require special cells for isolation in tissue culture. Serotypes 40 and 41 have been found most often in this situation. Intussusception in children has also been linked to adenovirus types 1,

2, 3, and 5, although a causal role is unproven. Many of the children with this syndrome have intercurrent adenoviral respiratory infection.

Hemorrhagic Cystitis. Adenovirus types 11 and 21 have been associated with hemorrhagic cystitis in as many as 20 to 50 per cent of American and Japanese children with this syndrome. Boys are affected more often than girls, in contrast to the situation with bacterial cystitis. Gross and microscopic hematuria may persist for 1 to 2 weeks.

CLINICAL PRESENTATIONS OCCURRING MOSTLY IN ADULTS. Respiratory Infection. The first isolation of adenoviruses directly from sick patients occurred during an epidemic of acute respiratory disease in military recruits. This population seems extremely susceptible to infection with types 4 and 7, as it is to infection with *Mycoplasma pneumoniae* and the meningococci. In general, the manifestations are those of atypical pneumonia, of which up to 40 per cent of cases are caused by adenovirus. Fever to 39°C, cough, pharyngitis, rhinorrhea, and pulmonary rales are the most common signs and symptoms. Radiographic examination of the chest shows patchy interstitial infiltrates that are unilateral in most cases. Small pleural effusions can occur.

In nonepidemic situations, it is impossible to make a definitive clinical diagnosis of adenoviral pneumonia. Some factors useful in comparing adenoviral with mycoplasmal pneumonia are lower incidence of cold agglutinins, shorter incubation period, and better correlation of radiographic and physical findings in the chest in adenovirus infection. Influenza and parainfluenza viruses produce similar syndromes. Adenoviral pneumonia usually lasts about 1 week. There is no specific therapy, and bacterial superinfection and death are rare.

Adenoviruses have been isolated from the lungs and urine of immunocompromised patients including renal transplant recipients and patients with acquired immunodeficiency syndrome (AIDS). Several of the higher serotypes were first isolated from such patients. In these instances, adenovirus operates as an opportunistic agent.

Neurologic Disease. Central nervous system infection, most often appearing as meningoencephalitis, has been attributed to adenovirus. It sometimes occurs in minor epidemic form and is frequently associated with recent respiratory infection. The clinical presentation is that of encephalitis or aseptic meningitis. There are no pathognomonic findings.

Epidemic Keratoconjunctivitis. The initial epidemic of adenoviral keratoconjunctivitis involved shipyard workers who sustained minor eye trauma from paint and rust fragments. Adenovirus type 8 was isolated in this and many other epidemics. Serotypes 19 and 37 have caused keratoconjunctivitis that was spread by fomites such as roller towels. Contaminated ophthalmic solutions have also transmitted infection. The incubation period is from 3 to 24 days. The onset is insidious, and both eyes often are affected. Eye irritation and exudation may last 1 to 4 weeks. Preauricular adenopathy often occurs early. Corneal involvement is a late complication and may persist for a month or more with blurring of vision. Residual blindness is unusual. There is no specific antiviral therapy as there is for herpes keratitis. Secondary spread to household contacts occurs in about 10 per cent of cases, varying with the duration of the index case.

DIAGNOSIS. Diagnosis is usually made on clinical grounds alone. In the case of diarrheal illness, immunoelectronmicroscopy and DNA hybridization assays have proved useful, but these are not at present generally available. Antibody and nucleic acid probes have also been developed for diagnosis of adenovirus keratoconjunctivitis. Virus culture is, of course, the definitive assay.

TREATMENT AND PREVENTION. There is no effective antiviral chemotherapy for human adenoviral infections. Live, enteric-coated oral adenovirus vaccines of types 4 and 7 have been effective in immunizing military populations. In epidemic situations, mass immunization with the live virus vaccine promptly interrupts the epidemic. The vaccine is not recommended or available for civilians because of the low incidence and sporadic occurrence of infection with adenovirus types 4 and 7.

Baum SG: Adenovirus. *In* Mandell A, Douglas RA, Bennet JE (eds.): Principles and Practice of Infectious Diseases. 3rd ed. New York, Churchill Livingstone

Inc., 1990, pp 1185–1191. *An expanded version of the material in this chapter, containing correlative tables, fully referenced.*

Horwitz MS: Adenoviridae and their replication. *In* Fields BN, Knipe DM (eds.): Virology, 2nd ed. New York, Raven Press, 1989, pp 1679–1721. *An encyclopedic chapter on the molecular biology of the adenoviruses.*

366 Viral Gastroenteritis

Albert Z. Kapikian

DEFINITION

Viral gastroenteritis (acute infectious nonbacterial gastroenteritis, epidemic diarrhea, winter vomiting disease, sporadic infantile gastroenteritis) is a common acute infectious disease of all age groups, characterized by vomiting or watery diarrhea, or both, that may be accompanied by fever, nausea, anorexia, and malaise. It ranges from a mild, self-limited illness of short duration to life-threatening dehydration, especially in infants and young children.

The importance of this disease in a developed country was highlighted in the Cleveland Family Study, in which infectious gastroenteritis, presumably nonbacterial, was the second most common disease experience, accounting for 16 per cent of some 25,000 illnesses in a period of almost 10 years. In developing countries the impact of diarrheal illnesses is staggering: In Asia, Africa, and Latin America, 3 to 5 billion cases of diarrhea and 5 to 10 million diarrhea-associated deaths occur annually, with the major impact in infants and young children. In addition, diarrheal illness was ranked first among infectious diseases in incidence and mortality in these developing areas.

In spite of major discoveries in bacteriology and parasitology in the past century, the etiology of most acute diarrheal illnesses remained elusive for many years. In the 1940's and 1950's, oral administration of bacteria-free stool filtrates from patients with acute diarrhea induced illness in volunteers, but the suspected viral etiologic agent could not be identified. In 1972, Kapikian and colleagues, employing immune electron microscopy (IEM), discovered virus-like particles in a stool suspension derived from a gastroenteritis outbreak in Norwalk, Ohio. In 1973, Bishop and associates, employing electron microscopy (EM), discovered rotavirus particles in duodenal biopsies from infants and young children hospitalized with acute gastroenteritis.

ETIOLOGY

NORWALK VIRUS GROUP. The Norwalk virus is the prototype strain of a group of fastidious, nonenveloped particles usually named after the geographic location of the gastroenteritis outbreak from which they are recovered. They share these common characteristics: (1) a diameter of approximately 27 nm; (2) indistinct morphology; (3) presence in feces; (4) noncultivable in vitro; (5) unknown nucleic acid content; and (6) a characteristic buoyant density of 1.36 to 1.41 grams per cubic centimeter in cesium chloride. The group includes at least four serotypes —Norwalk, Hawaii, Ditchling, and Snow Mountain agents—and several other strains (Montgomery County, "W," cockle, Taunton, and Parramatta) that share an antigenic relationship with one of the known serotypes or have not been characterized. Classification of these fastidious viruses into a virus family has not been feasible. However, the protein composition of Norwalk and Snow Mountain viruses resembles that of the caliciviruses, since they each possess a single primary virion-associated protein with an approximate molecular weight of 60,000. The Norwalk virus was recently cloned and found to contain a positive sense single-stranded ribonucleic acid (RNA) genome.

ROTAVIRUS. Rotaviruses are classified as a genus in the family Reoviridae and are etiologic agents of diarrhea in humans and in numerous animal and a few avian species. They are 70 nm in diameter, with a genome consisting of 11 segments of double-stranded RNA, and possess a distinctive double-layered capsid. The name rotavirus (rota = wheel) was adopted because the sharply defined circular outline of the outer capsid was reminiscent of the rim of a wheel placed on short spokes radiating from a wide hub (the inner capsid). The virions (see Fig. 366–1)

have a density of 1.36 grams per cubic centimeter in cesium chloride and are antigenically distinct from the three reovirus serotypes. Rotaviruses possess three important antigenic specificities—group, subgroup, and serotype—which are mediated by different proteins: group specificity prominently by VP6 and subgroup by VP6 alone (encoded by RNA segment 6). Serotype specificity has been defined by VP7, a glycoprotein that is one of the two major neutralization antigens located on the outer capsid (encoded by RNA segment 7, 8, or 9). The other outer capsid protein VP4 (formerly designated VP3), which is encoded by RNA segment 4 and which protrudes from the smooth outer surface as a spike of about 12 nm in length, also induces neutralizing antibodies. VP4 is the hemagglutinin in certain strains. Antibodies to both VP4 and VP7 are associated with protection against rotavirus illness. There are seven human rotavirus serotypes as defined by VP7, of which those numbered 1 to 4 are of epidemiologic importance. Several human and animal rotavirus strains share VP7 serotype specificity. Most animal and human rotaviruses share the common group antigen and are thus classified as group A rotaviruses, and these are further divided into subgroups. The human rotaviruses have only recently been grown efficiently in cell culture. Several human and animal rotavirus strains have been discovered that do not share the common group antigen and are classified as non–group A rotaviruses (groups B to G). They were formerly designated "pararotaviruses." In this chapter, when the term rotavirus is used, it is meant to describe only those rotaviruses belonging to group A, unless specified otherwise.

OTHER AGENTS. Other viral agents have been associated with gastroenteritis and include enteric adenoviruses belonging to types 40 and 41 (70 to 80 nm in diameter); caliciviruses (30 to 40 nm); astroviruses (28 to 30 nm); small, round viruses other than the Norwalk virus group (20 to 30 nm); putative coronavirus–like particles (100 to 150 nm); the Otofuke, Sapporo, and Osaka agents (33 to 40 nm); the "minireoviruses" (30 nm); the pleomorphic, fringed, Breda or Berne virus-like particles (toroviruses) (100 to 140 nm); 35 nm "picobirnavirus"; and a pestivirus antigen. The role of these viruses as etiologic agents of severe infantile diarrhea appears to be minor, with the exception of the enteric adenoviruses, which are associated with approximately 5 to 10 per cent of the diarrheal illnesses of infants and young children requiring hospitalization. In addition, the role of these other agents in epidemic viral gastroenteritis appears to be minor. Additional studies are needed to assess the role of these other agents in gastroenteritis. It should be noted that about one third to one half of gastroenteritis episodes have yet to be associated with an etiologic agent.

EPIDEMIOLOGY

NORWALK VIRUS GROUP. The Norwalk group of viruses comprises major etiologic agents of acute nonbacterial gastroenteritis, which typically occurs as a sharp outbreak affecting adults, school-age children, and family contacts. The location or source of contamination responsible for these outbreaks includes various settings such as schools, camps and recreational areas, nursing homes, swimming facilities, cruise ships, and restaurants. For example, the Norwalk virus was derived from an outbreak in an elementary school in Norwalk, Ohio, in which 50 per cent of the students and teachers developed gastroenteritis within a 2-day period. Norwalk virus has been linked with 42 per cent of 74 nonbacterial gastroenteritis outbreaks investigated from 1976 to 1980 and approximately 10 per cent of all acute gastroenteritis outbreaks. In the United States, antibody to the Norwalk virus is usually acquired gradually in childhood and somewhat more rapidly in the adult years, so that by age 50 at least 50 per cent of individuals have serum antibody. In developing countries, infants and young children acquire Norwalk antibody at an earlier age, and the virus is associated with mild gastroenteritis in this age group.

Norwalk virus is most likely transmitted via the fecal-oral route; however, it has also been detected in vomitus. Although sporadic cases attributed to person-to-person transmission may occur, the explosive nature of outbreaks associated with the Norwalk virus group often suggests a common source of infection, such as water or food. Common-source outbreaks have been attributed to contamination of community and noncommunity public water systems, stored water on cruise ships, or recreational swimming water and to ingestion of tainted oysters, cockles, lettuce, or cake frosting. Secondary person-to-person transmission to contacts is relatively common. The incubation period ranges from 10 to 51 hours, with a mean of 24 hours, and symptoms usually last 24 to 60 hours. Norwalk virus outbreaks occur throughout the year without a peak season.

Norwalk virus infections have been detected in individuals with travelers' diarrhea. However, this agent is not considered to be an important cause of this disease.

ROTAVIRUS. Rotaviruses are the major known etiologic agents of severe diarrhea in infants and young children in most areas of the world and are usually associated with sporadic infantile gastroenteritis, which differs from epidemic viral gastroenteritis associated with the Norwalk virus group in the following characteristics: (1) it usually does not occur in sharp outbreaks; (2) it is associated with a severe diarrheal illness in infants and young children; (3) it does not usually cause illness in adults; and (4) the attack rate among family contacts of index cases is low, although subclinical infections occur frequently in contacts.

The most compelling evidence for the importance of rotaviruses in severe infantile gastroenteritis has emerged from numerous cross-sectional studies in developed and developing countries. In developed countries, including the United States, rotaviruses are associated with approximately 35 to 52 per cent of acute diarrheal illness requiring hospitalization of infants and young children. The contribution of other enteric pathogens is consistently relatively minor. A similar pattern is also usually observed in developing countries, where rotaviruses are the most frequently detected pathogens in children less than 2 years of age who have severe gastroenteritis; however, bacterial agents also play an important role in such areas. It is estimated that in developing countries 873,000 infants and young children under 5 years of age die from rotavirus diarrhea each year. It should be noted that during longitudinal studies in a community setting where all diarrheal episodes are monitored, the incidence of rotavirus diarrhea is lower than that of diarrhea caused by other pathogens, but dehydration is more often associated with rotavirus disease than with illness caused by other agents.

In temperate climates, rotavirus gastroenteritis has a characteristic seasonal occurrence during the cooler months of the year with peak prevalence in the winter months. In tropical countries it occurs throughout the year, with less pronounced peaks. Rotavirus diarrhea occurs most frequently in children between 6 months and 24 months of age. Infants less than 6 months of age have the next highest frequency, although in certain studies the highest frequency is observed in this age group. The low frequency of clinical illness in neonates who undergo rotavirus infection is an unusual paradox that has not been explained.

Rotavirus gastroenteritis occurs infrequently in adults, but subclinical infections are common.

Rotaviruses are likely transmitted by the fecal-oral route, although respiratory transmission remains a possibility, since there is such a rapid acquisition of serum antibody during the first 2 years of life regardless of hygienic conditions. Nosocomial rotavirus infections occur frequently. The incubation period of rotavirus illness is approximately 2 to 4 days. There are seven recognized human rotavirus serotypes of which those numbered 1 to 4 appear to be of clinical importance. Group B rotavirus is responsible for widespread outbreaks of gastroenteritis in adults in China, and a relatively small number of group C rotaviruses have been recovered from individuals with gastroenteritis in various countries. With the exception of the group B rotaviruses in China, the role of the non–group A rotaviruses in other regions of the world appears to be relatively minor at this time.

Rotavirus infections have been observed in individuals with travelers' diarrhea. However, rotaviruses are not considered to be an important cause of this illness.

PATHOLOGY AND PATHOGENESIS

NORWALK VIRUS GROUP. Histopathologic lesions following Norwalk or Hawaii virus infections are characterized by a reversible involvement of the upper jejunum. The jejunal mucosa remains intact with marked broadening and blunting of the villi and shortening of the microvilli, along with mononuclear cell infiltration and cytoplasmic vacuolization. Functional alterations may include a transient malabsorption of fat, D-xylose, and lactose and a significant decrease in levels of small intestinal brush border enzymes (alkaline phosphatase and trehalase). Adenylate cyclase activity in the jejunum is not elevated. Delay in gastric emptying may be responsible for the nausea and vomiting associated with these agents.

The nature of immunity to Norwalk virus is perplexing, because a high percentage (~50 per cent) of adults are susceptible to both natural and experimental illness. In addition, although immunity has been observed in approximately 50 per cent of adults, it appears to correlate inversely with the level of serum or local jejunal antibody.

ROTAVIRUS. The major histopathologic lesions are characterized by reversible involvement of the proximal small intestine. The mucosa remains intact, with shortening of the villi, mononuclear cell infiltration in the lamina propria, distended cisternae of the endoplasmic reticulum, mitochondrial swelling, and sparse, irregular microvilli. Functional alterations may include impaired D-xylose absorption and depressed levels of disaccharidases (maltase, sucrase, and lactase).

The mechanism of immunity to human rotaviruses is not completely clear. Although serum antibodies correlate with resistance to illness, the role of local intestinal immunity has not been elucidated. Animal studies indicate that antibody in the small intestine is the major determinant of resistance to illness. A high rate of subclinical infection in neonates is well documented and may be related to passively acquired maternal antibody, host

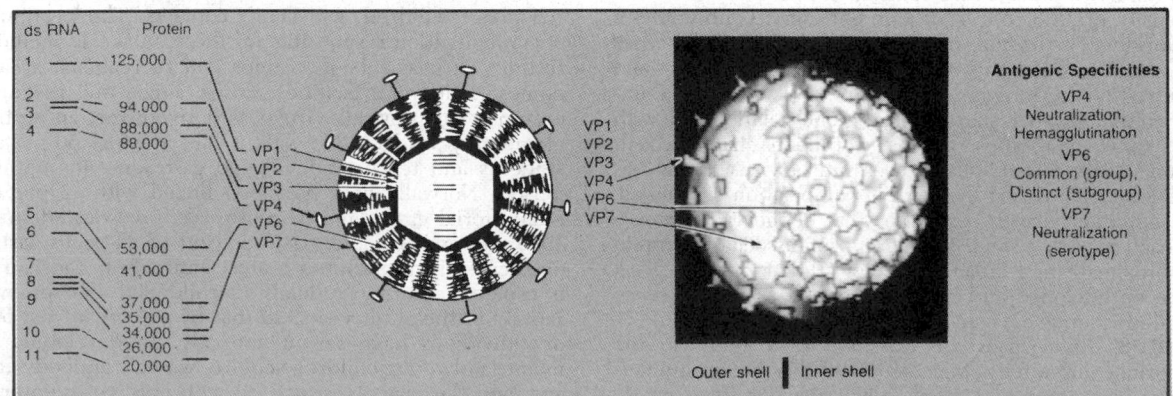

FIGURE 366–1. *Left,* Schematic representation of the rotavirus double-shelled particle. *Right,* Surface representations of the three-dimensional structures of a double-shelled particle (on the left half) and a particle (on the right half) in which most, if not all, of the outer shell and a small portion of the inner shell mass have been removed. (From Kapikian AZ, Chanock RM: Rotaviruses. *In* Fields BN, et al. (eds.): Virology, 2nd ed. New York, Raven Press, 1990; with permission. Figure on right from Prasad BV, Wang GJ, Clerx JP, et al.: Three-dimensional structure of rotavirus. J Mol Biol 199:269–275, 1988; with permission.)

factors, or naturally attenuated rotaviruses that are able to persist in newborn nurseries.

CLINICAL MANIFESTATIONS

NORWALK VIRUS GROUP. Clinical characteristics of illness induced by the Norwalk group of viruses include nausea, vomiting, diarrhea, anorexia, or abdominal discomfort, or any combination. Accompanying clinical manifestations may also include myalgias, low-grade fever, headache, and chills. In children, vomiting occurs more often than diarrhea, whereas in adults the opposite is observed. The onset of illness may be abrupt, marked by vomiting, diarrhea, or both. The illness is usually mild and lasts about 24 to 60 hours. However, severe gastroenteritis has been observed in middle-aged patients and has contributed to the death of elderly, debilitated individuals. The stools are characteristically loose and watery; blood, mucus, and leukocytes are not typically present. A transient decrease in the T, B, and null cell lymphocyte subpopulations has been observed.

ROTAVIRUS. Rotavirus infection can produce a variety of responses in infants and young children, ranging from subclinical infection and mild diarrhea to a severe and occasionally fatal dehydrating illness. Clinical characteristics include vomiting, diarrhea, abdominal discomfort, or fever, or any combination. Fever and vomiting often develop before the diarrhea. Accompanying clinical manifestations may include dehydration, irritability, and pharyngeal or tympanic membrane erythema. In hospitalized patients, the mean duration of confinement is 4 days, with a range of 2 to 14 days. The stools are characteristically loose and watery and only infrequently contain blood or leukocytes.

Although rotaviruses can cause severe or fatal dehydrating illnesses in developing countries, deaths have also been documented in developed countries. In a study in Canada, rotavirus gastroenteritis was implicated in the deaths of 21 children 4 to 30 months of age (mean 11 months) over a period of about 5 years. Twenty children were dead or moribund upon arrival at hospital, and one child was infected nosocomially. With the exception of the latter patient and one other, each child was considered healthy prior to the rotaviral illness. Death occurred within 1 to 3 days of onset of symptoms. Dehydration and electrolyte imbalance leading to cardiac arrest were believed to be the major cause of death in 16 patients; aspiration of vomitus was the cause of death in 3 patients; and seizures were a contributing factor in the remaining 2 patients.

Rotavirus can also induce chronic symptomatic diarrhea with prolonged fecal shedding of the virus and antigenemia in patients with primary immunodeficiency diseases. Infections with rotaviruses or other viral and bacterial enteric pathogens may be especially severe in individuals who are immunosuppressed for bone marrow transplantation. In one study, 8 of 78 such patients (average age of entire group, 20.5 years) shed rotavirus in stools and 5 of the 8 died. In addition, a non–group A rotavirus was associated with severe gastroenteritis in an 8-year-old bone marrow transplant patient. Rotavirus infections have also been persistent and severe in children with severe combined immunodeficiency. Rotavirus infections have also been associated with necrotizing enterocolitis and hemorrhagic gastroenteritis in neonates.

Outbreaks of rotavirus gastroenteritis have occurred in elderly individuals in nursing homes with several fatalities.

DIAGNOSIS

NORWALK VIRUS GROUP. Since a specific diagnosis of infection with this group cannot be made by clinical observation, the diagnosis must be made in the laboratory and relies on the detection of virus in the stool or a serologic response to a viral-specific antigen. These tests include IEM (for the entire group), radioimmunoassay (Norwalk and Snow Mountain agents), and enzyme-linked immunosorbent assay (ELISA) (Norwalk, Snow Mountain, and Hawaii viruses). These are still research procedures, because reagents are not generally available. Virus shedding is maximal at or shortly after onset of illness and minimal at 72 hours following onset. The characteristic absence of fecal leukocytes in Norwalk infection may be helpful for differentiation from *Shigella* or *Salmonella* enteritis.

Although a specific clinical diagnosis of infection with Norwalk

virus cannot be made in the individual patient, a tentative diagnosis of infection can be made during an outbreak if certain criteria are met: (1) bacterial or parasitic pathogens are not detected; (2) vomiting is present in at least 50 per cent of cases; (3) incubation period is 24 to 48 hours; and (4) mean or median duration of illness is 12 to 60 hours.

ROTAVIRUS. The clinical manifestations of rotavirus gastroenteritis are not distinctive enough to enable diagnosis. Thus, diagnosis requires either detection of the virus or demonstration of a significant serologic response to rotavirus in paired acute and convalescent sera. The epidemiologic pattern relating to the age of the patient, the temporal occurrence of illness, and the signs and symptoms of illness, however, may suggest the diagnosis. In addition, the usual absence of fecal leukocytes in rotavirus diarrhea may help in early differentiation from *Shigella* or *Salmonella* enteritis.

Stools obtained from the first to fourth day of illness are optimal for rotavirus detection, but virus shedding may continue up to 21 days. Virus is characteristically present in stools during the early phase of diarrhea, but diarrhea may continue for 2 to 3 days after the cessation of virus shedding.

Over 25 assays have been developed for the detection of rotavirus in stools. The most rapid method is still direct EM because in negatively stained preparations these agents have a distinctive morphologic appearance and are present in large amounts. The non–group A rotaviruses, which do not share the common group antigen, can also be detected by EM. However, an electron microscope may not be readily available, and its use may be impractical when evaluating a large number of specimens. Thus, other rapid and highly effective methods for virus detection have been developed, including ELISA, counterimmunoelectroosmophoresis (CIEOP), radioimmunoassay (RIA), reverse passive hemagglutination assay (RPHA), latex agglutination (LA), RNA electrophoresis, dot hybridization, and recently by utilizing the polymerase chain reaction. Commercial kits are now available for the ELISA, LA, RPHA, and RNA electrophoresis assays. A popular method is the confirmatory ELISA because it is simple to perform, is sensitive, does not require specialized equipment, and has a negative serum antibody control for detecting nonspecific reactions. An ELISA using monoclonal anti-VP7 antibody is also available. The non–group A rotaviruses cannot be detected by these assays, because they lack the common group antigen; however, an ELISA for group B rotaviruses has recently been developed. Diagnosis of group A rotavirus infection by growth in cell cultures is not practical.

There are many methods for measuring a serologic response to rotavirus infection, including IEM, complement fixation (CF), immunofluorescence, immune adherence hemagglutination assay, ELISA, neutralization, hemagglutination-inhibition (HI), and inhibition of RPHA. Complement fixation is an efficient assay for detecting a serologic response to rotavirus in patients 6 to 24 months of age but is not as effective in adults or infants below 6 months of age.

Detection of rotavirus or demonstration of a serologic response does not necessarily establish an etiologic association with the patient's illness, especially in newborns and adults, who frequently undergo subclinical infection.

TREATMENT

NORWALK VIRUS GROUP. Since the Norwalk group of viruses characteristically causes a mild, self-limited gastroenteritis, replacement of fluid and electrolyte loss with orally administered isotonic fluids is usually sufficient. However, if severe vomiting or diarrhea occurs, parenteral fluid replacement may be necessary. Oral administration of bismuth subsalicylate significantly reduces the severity of abdominal cramps, with a decrease in the median duration of gastrointestinal symptoms from 20 hours to 14 hours. However, the number, weight, and water content of stools and the level of virus excretion are not affected significantly.

ROTAVIRUS. Because rotavirus gastroenteritis may lead to severe dehydration in infants and young children, the early replacement of fluids and electrolytes is essential. Intravenous fluids have been used effectively in the treatment of dehydration.

However, in many parts of the world where such treatment is not feasible, efforts have been made to evaluate the effectiveness of an oral rehydration salts (ORS) solution. In a double-blind study comparing ORS with intravenous fluids in children with rotavirus gastroenteritis, ORS solution containing either glucose (20 grams per liter) or sucrose (40 grams per liter) plus electrolytes was found to be as effective as intravenous therapy for rehydration. Glucose electrolyte solutions are recommended for optimal results. The recommended World Health Organization (WHO) ORS solution is made by adding the following to 1 liter of water: sodium chloride, 3.5 grams; trisodium citrate, dihydrate, 2.9 grams; potassium chloride, 1.5 grams; and glucose, anhydrous, 20 grams. Sodium bicarbonate, 2.5 grams, may be substituted for the trisodium citrate, dihydrate. The efficacy of oral glucose-electrolyte solutions that contained either 90 mmol of sodium per liter (as in the WHO formula above) or 50 mmol of sodium per liter, plus additional electrolytes, was examined in well-nourished ambulatory or hospitalized children with mild or moderate dehydrating diarrheal illnesses of varied etiology (including rotavirus but excluding cholera), and each was found to be safe and effective. After the initial calculated fluid deficit is corrected by the ORS, water or fluids without added electrolytes, such as breast milk or some other form of low-solute feeding, should be given orally in addition to the ORS solution, to replace both continued diarrheal fluid and electrolyte losses and to provide normal daily fluid requirements. If oral rehydration fails to correct the fluid and electrolyte loss or if the patient is severely dehydrated or in shock, intravenous therapy must be given.

In a recent study, rice-based ORS solution was found to be effective in the rehydration of infants and young children hospitalized with mild to moderate dehydration caused by diarrhea associated with various pathogens, including rotavirus. Although either a glucose-based or a rice-based ORS solution was effective in rehydration, the latter was associated with decreased stool output and greater absorption and retention of fluid and electrolytes when compared with the glucose-based solution.

In a limited study, chronic rotavirus illness in immunodeficient children has been treated effectively by oral feeding of pooled human milk that contained rotavirus antibody. However, oral administration of preparations containing rotavirus antibody is not effective for treatment of normal children during episodes of rotavirus gastroenteritis.

PREVENTION

NORWALK VIRUS GROUP. There are no specific methods for the prevention of illness by the Norwalk virus group. However, because of the extremely infectious nature of these agents, careful handwashing and proper disposal of contaminated material should minimize transmission. In addition, hygienic preparation of food and measures to decrease contamination of drinking water or swimming facilities should limit the frequency of Norwalk virus outbreaks. Active immunization against this group of viruses is not yet feasible.

ROTAVIRUS. Epidemiologic studies indicate the global need for a rotavirus vaccine to prevent rotavirus diarrhea in the first 2 years of life, when illness is most severe. Current efforts are focused on developing a live, attenuated oral vaccine that is effective against all serotypes. A promising initial strategy involved the "Jennerian" approach, in which a related rotavirus from a nonhuman host (a bovine or rhesus rotavirus strain) was used as the immunizing agent. Efficacy trials of several such candidate rotavirus vaccines gave variable results and it soon became clear that these vaccines did not induce satisfactory heterotypic immunity in infants not primed by previous rotavirus infection. The rhesus rotavirus vaccine (a VP7 serotype 3 strain) induced protection against rotavirus diarrhea in the 1- to 4-month age group in a study in which VP7 serotype 3 was predominant, but it failed in other studies to protect unprimed infants against illnesses caused by other than serotype 3 rotaviruses. Thus, the "Jennerian" approach has been modified with the goal being a quadrivalent vaccine composed of rhesus rotavirus (serotype 3) and three reassortant rotaviruses each containing 10 rhesus rotavirus genes and a single human rotavirus gene that encodes VP7 serotype 1, 2, or 4 specificity. Efficacy trials of this vaccine are underway.

Finally, a non-Jennerian approach to rotavirus vaccination is also being evaluated. It involves the use of a neonatal rotavirus strain, M37, that appears to be naturally attenuated. The feasibility of this approach is based on the observation in an Australian study that neonates who developed a subclinical rotavirus infection in the first 14 days of life were protected against severe rotavirus diarrhea during a 3-year follow-up.

Breast milk is generally considered to confer some degree of protection against clinically significant rotavirus diarrhea during infancy. The prophylactic oral administration of human serum globulin containing rotavirus antibody to low birth weight neonates provides significant protection against rotavirus diarrhea. In addition, passive oral immunization of infants and young children with bovine colostrum that contained antibodies to human rotavirus was effective in preventing rotavirus illness when compared with a control group.

Chiba S, Yokohama T, Nakata S, et al.: Protective effect of naturally acquired homotypic and heterotypic rotavirus antibodies. Lancet 2:417, 1986. *An important study that examines the relationship of serotype-specific and heterotypic rotavirus neutralizing antibodies to immunity against rotavirus gastroenteritis.*

Ciba Foundation Symposium 128: Novel Diarrhea Viruses. Chichester, John Wiley and Sons, 1987. *An entire volume by various contributors, with special emphasis on non-group A rotaviruses, enteric adenoviruses, caliciviruses, astroviruses, Berne and Breda or Breda-like viruses, the Norwalk virus and rotavirus vaccines.*

Estes MK, Cohen J: Rotavirus gene structure and function. Microbial Rev 53:410-449, 1989. *A review of the molecular biology of rotaviruses with application to an understanding of the natural history of rotavirus infection. Has extensive bibliography of 358 references.*

Green KY, Taniguchi K, Mackow ER, Kapikian AZ: Homotypic and heterotypic epitope specific antibody responses in adult and infant rotavirus vaccines. J Infect Dis 161:667–679, 1990. *An analysis of serologic responses to various rotavirus vaccines by an epitope blocking assay and by neutralization. Demonstrates the influence of prior rotavirus infection on the response to vaccination and the role this might have on vaccination strategy.*

Jiang X, Graham DY, Wang K, Estes MK: Norwalk virus genome cloning and characterization. Science 250:1580–1583, 1990. *A study describing the cloning of the fastidious Norwalk virus.*

Kapikian AZ, Chanock RM: Norwalk group of viruses. In Fields BN, et al. (eds.): Virology, 2nd ed. New York, Raven Press, 1990, pp 671–693. *A detailed current review of the Norwalk group of viruses from a virologic, epidemiologic, and clinical point of view. Has extensive bibliography with 219 references.*

Kapikian AZ, Chanock RM: Rotaviruses. In Fields BN, et al. (eds.): Virology, 2nd ed. New York, Raven Press, 1990, pp 1353–1404. *A detailed current review of rotaviruses from a virologic, epidemiologic, and clinical point of view. Has extensive bibliography with 780 references.*

Kapikian AZ, Flores J, Midthun K, et al.: Strategies for the development of a rotavirus vaccine against infantile diarrhea with an update on clinical trials of rotavirus vaccines. Adv Evp Biol Med 257:67–89, 1989. *A perspective on various approaches to rotavirus vaccination with a description of several field trials.*

Kaplan JE, Gary WG, Barron RC, et al.: Epidemiology of Norwalk gastroenteritis and the role of Norwalk virus in outbreaks of acute nonbacterial gastroenteritis. Ann Intern Med 96:756, 1982. *A review of outbreaks of viral gastroenteritis associated with the Norwalk virus from 1976 to 1980.*

Matsui SM, Kim JP, Greenberg HB, et al.: The isolation and characterization of a Norwalk virus specific cDNA. J Clin Invest 87:1456–1461, 1991. *A study describing the cloning of the fastidious Norwalk virus.*

Matsui SM, Machow ER, Greenberg HB: Molecular determinant of rotavirus neutralization and protection. Adv Virus Res 36:181–214, 1989. *A review of the rotavirus proteins involved in neutralization and protection (116 references).*

Perez-Schael I, Garcia D, Gonzalez M, et al.: Prospective study of diarrheal diseases in Venezuelan children to evaluate the efficacy of rhesus rotavirus vaccine. J Med Virol 30:219–229, 1990. *A detailed description of a field trial with a rotavirus vaccine candidate.*

Pizarro D, Posada G, Sandi L, Moran JB: Rice-based oral electrolytic solutions for the management of infantile diarrhea. N Engl J Med 324:517–521, 1991. *A study evaluating the efficacy of two rice-based rehydration solutions and a conventional glucose-based solution.*

Prasad BUV, Burns JW, Marietta E, et al.: Localization of VP4 neutralization sites in rotavirus by three-dimensional structure of a rotavirus and Fab fragments. Nature 343:476–479, 1990. *Demonstrates the three-dimensional structure of a rotavirus and Fab fragments of a rotavirus-neutralizing monoclonal antibody directed at VP4. Identifies the spikes as VP4.*

Rodriguez WJ, Kim HW, Arrobio JO, et al.: Clinical features of acute gastroenteritis associated with human reovirus-like agent in infants and young children. J Pediatr 91:188, 1977. *A comprehensive description of the clinical features of rotavirus gastroenteritis from a clinical, epidemiologic, and laboratory point of view.*

Santosham M, Burns B, Nadkarni V, et al.: Oral rehydration therapy for acute diarrhea in ambulatory children in the United States: A double-blind comparison of four different solutions. Pediatrics 76:159, 1985. *A evaluation of various oral rehydration solutions in infants and young children with diarrhea and mild dehydration. Of special interest to the clinician.*

Santosham M, Daum RS, Dillman L, et al.: Oral rehydration therapy of infantile diarrhea. A controlled study of well-nourished children hospitalized in the United States and Panama. N Engl J Med 306:1070, 1982. *An evaluation of oral glucose-electrolyte rehydration solutions containing different sodium con-*

centrations in children hospitalized with diarrhea. *An important study for the clinician.*

Tyrrell DAJ, Kapikian AZ (eds.): Virus Infections of the Gastrointestinal Tract. New York, Marcel Dekker, Inc., 1982. *An entire volume on viral infections of the gastrointestinal tract by numerous contributors. Includes relevant data on viral agents associated with gastroenteritis with extensive references.*

367 Measles *(Morbilli, Rubeola)*

Philip A. Brunell

DEFINITION. Measles is an acute, highly contagious disease characterized by fever, coryza, cough, conjunctivitis, and both an enanthem and an exanthem.

ETIOLOGY. The virus is an enveloped, negative-stranded RNA paramyxovirus (genus *Morbillivirus*) measuring 120 to 250 mm in diameter, similar to other members of the Paramyxovirus family but lacking neuraminidase. Its single antigenic serotype has been remarkably stable throughout the world for many years with no variation noted. The virus contains six major polypeptides, which are responsible for a number of structural and functional properties, including hemagglutination (of primate erythrocytes), hemolysis, cell fusion, and others. Isolation of virus from clinical specimens is most successful with primary kidney cell cultures of human or simian origin. Selected laboratory strains grow well in other continuous cell lines of mammalian origin.

EPIDEMIOLOGY. With the introduction of routine immunization against measles in the United States in 1963, the incidence of measles fell by about 99 per cent. Smaller outbreaks have occurred at increasing intervals in 1971, 1976, and 1986. A somewhat larger outbreak started in 1989. Prior to the advent of measles vaccine, almost every child got measles, most before school entry. The frequency increased every other year. This pattern still is seen in developing countries where measles in the very young is common. It is estimated that there are from 1 to 2 million deaths annually worldwide. Many developed countries have a less stringent policy toward measles immunization than does the United States.

During the 1989 epidemic in the United States, the highest attack rate was in preschool children, which was more than twice that of 15- to 19-year-olds, the group with the second highest incidence. Most of the former were immunized, whereas the majority of the older group had received measles vaccine. There were more than 400 cases in those born prior to 1957. About 30 per cent of the deaths occurred in the latter group; most occurred in those who were immunocompetent. Almost all of the remaining deaths occurred in those under 5 years of age, most of whom were unimmunized and otherwise normal.

Communicability. Measles is one of the most highly contagious infections. Almost all unprotected household contacts are infected. Demonstration of virus in nasopharyngeal secretions during the prodromal, pre-eruptive phase and in the first days of rash is in accord with epidemiologic evidence of contagiousness. Close physical proximity or direct person-to-person respiratory droplet contact is the usual requisite for infection, although airborne transmission has been documented.

Immunity. An unmodified attack of measles is followed by lifelong immunity. Passively transferred maternal antibody protects the young infant during the early months of life.

PATHOLOGY AND PHYSIOLOGIC RESPONSES. Pathologic changes in fatal measles usually represent the compound effect of viral and secondary bacterial infection. Pneumonia is almost invariably present; it is most frequently interstitial. More representative are changes of the uncomplicated viral diseases within the tonsillar, nasopharyngeal, and appendiceal tissue removed during the prodrome. These changes consist of round cell infiltration and the presence of multinucleated giant cells. Giant cells also are observed in tissue cultures infected with measles virus. The skin and mucous membranes contain perivascular round cell infiltrates with congestion and edema. Koplik's spots are inflammatory lesions of the submucous glands with similar microscopic features.

Simultaneous with the onset of rash, measles-specific antibodies are detectable in serum. Leukopenia is observed on the first day of rash mainly owing to a decrease in lymphocytes; subsequently, granulocytopenia ensues as well. Measles virus replicates in lymphoid tissues (spleen, thymus, lymph nodes), can multiply in vitro in peripheral blood T and B lymphocytes and monocytes, and can be isolated from blood leukocytes during the course of the disease. The virus is propagable in a suspension of leukocytes in vitro.

Immunosuppressive Effects of Measles. It has long been known that cell-mediated immunity is impaired during measles. There is transient suppression of the tuberculin reaction (observed also with measles vaccines); improvement in eczema and allergic asthma and the induction of remissions in nephrosis have been described. Infection of activated lymphocytes may explain the depression of cell-mediated immunity during the acute disease. In severe disease, the magnitude of depression of the total lymphocytes has been positively correlated with a lessened chance of recovery.

CLINICAL MANIFESTATIONS. After an incubation period that averages 11 days, measles becomes clinically manifest with symptoms of fever, malaise, myalgia, and headache. Within hours *ocular symptoms* of photophobia and conjunctival injection occur. The palpebral and, to a lesser extent, the bulbar conjunctivae are involved. There is usually no exudate. Sneezing, coughing, and nasal discharge occur almost simultaneously. Less commonly, hoarseness and aphonia may reflect laryngeal involvement. In this prodromal stage of 1 to 4 days' duration, tiny white spots on the buccal mucosa may herald the appearance of skin rash. The white lesions described by Koplik characteristically occur lateral to the molar teeth and typically are mounted on a bluish-red areola of injected mucosa, superimposed on a diffuse red background. They generally appear a day or so prior to rash and disappear within 2 days after its appearance. They constitute a pathognomonic diagnostic sign. The enanthem may involve other mucous membranes such as the palpebral conjunctiva and vaginal lining.

The *rash* of measles follows the prodromal symptoms by 2 to 4 days, occasionally as late as 7 days. It first appears behind the ears or on the face and neck as a blotchy erythema, spreads downward to cover the trunk, and finally is manifest on the extremities. The hands and feet may escape involvement. Initially, the eruption consists of discrete red macules that blanch with pressure. Subsequently, these lesions become papular, tend to coalesce, and may develop a red, nonblanching component. In adults the rash generally is more extensive, with a greater tendency to become confluent and slightly raised and redder than in children. This is particularly true on the face. The rash fades in the order of its appearance; its disappearance about 5 days after onset may be attended by a fine, powdery desquamation that spares the hands and feet. In adults malaise may continue for 1 to 2 weeks.

The *fever* of measles may persist for about 6 days and frequently reaches 40 or 41°C. Throughout the febrile period, productive cough and auscultatory evidence of bronchitis may be evident. These manifestations may persist after defervescence, and cough is often the last symptom to disappear. Bronchopulmonary symptomatology is an integral part of the primary viral infection; roentgenographic evidence of pulmonary involvement is frequently seen in the uncomplicated disease in the absence of leukocytosis and obvious bacterial infection. Generalized lymphadenopathy accompanies the acute febrile illness and may persist for several weeks thereafter. Nausea and, less commonly, emesis appear to be more common in adults. Diarrhea may also be present.

COMPLICATIONS. The persistence or recurrence of fever and development of leukocytosis are presumptive evidence of the common bacterial sequela of otitis media or pneumonia. Pneumococcus and Group A streptococcus are the most common secondary invaders.

Serious complications directly related to the measles virus are rare. Laryngitis of sufficient severity to embarrass respiration has been observed and may warrant tracheostomy. Keratoconjunctivitis is part of the acute phase but rarely progresses to actual corneal ulceration. Electrocardiographic abnormalities may be found in as many as 30 per cent of children, but clinical evidence of cardiac disease is absent. Abdominal pain or diarrhea may be related to invasion of lymphoid tissue of the appendix or Peyer's patches. These symptoms may lead to unnecessary surgery before the appearance of the typical rash.

Encephalomyelitis. A rare (0.1 per cent) but serious consequence of measles is a demyelinating encephalomyelitis that may appear from 1 to 14 days after the onset of infection. This complication is associated with recurrence of fever and headache, vomiting, and stiff neck. Stupor and convulsions usually follow. Localizing neurologic symptoms may be present. Death ensues in about 10 per cent of patients; more than half of survivors suffer permanent residuals of varying severity. Abnormal electroencephalograms were recorded in about half of children with measles without clinical signs of encephalitis. In some of the children the abnormal encephalographic findings were persistent. Infection of brain cells results in an incomplete viral replicative cycle with production of defective virions lacking the matrix (M) measles virus protein. Studies of patients with acute measles encephalomyelitis and those with late-onset subacute sclerosing panencephalitis show high titers in serum and cerebrospinal fluid of antibodies to all the measles virus proteins except M.

Other late sequelae of measles are thrombocytopenic purpura and exacerbation or activation of pre-existing pulmonary tuberculosis. The late complication of subacute sclerosing panencephalitis is discussed in Ch. 478.4.

Giant-Cell Pneumonia. In patients who are immunocompromised, e.g., those with AIDS, measles virus may induce an interstitial pneumonia characterized by giant cells and intracellular inclusion bodies. The disease is usually fatal.

Measles Modified by Antibody Administration. Attenuation of the natural disease by antibody prophylaxis may result in an illness of lessened severity comparable to the milder infection as seen in infants with illness modified by maternally acquired antibody. Fever alone may be observed, but some degree of exanthem is usually apparent. Koplik's spots may not appear. In general, the course is truncated and relatively uncomplicated. Lasting immunity is uncertain. Later routine immunization of these individuals is probably indicated.

Atypical Measles. From 1963 to 1967, two types of measles vaccine, one live attenuated, the other inactivated or "killed," were available in the United States. The live attenuated vaccine has been the sole product licensed and used in this country since 1967. A severe illness was reported in killed vaccine recipients after exposure to natural measles. These patients had high fever, pneumonia with pleural effusion, obtundation, and an unusual rash. The exanthem was hemorrhagic and was most marked on the extremities. In some instances vesicular, macular, or maculopapular phases have been observed. The rash is sometimes accompanied by edema of hands and feet. Concomitantly these patients' sera revealed extraordinarily high titers of measles-specific antibodies.

Subsequent investigations showed that patients who had received inactivated measles vaccines failed to develop antibodies to the fusion (F) protein of the virus. Lack of antibodies to the cell fusion factor is believed to have permitted these patients to support measles infection. Thus, the atypical measles syndrome

is believed to be due to an anamnestic antibody response in the face of an abundance of measles antigens.

In addition to the rash and pulmonary findings, these patients may have elevated liver enzymes, disseminated intravascular coagulation, and marked myalgia. Nodular pulmonary changes have persisted in some patients. Some cases of pneumonia are reported to have occurred in the absence of rash. Initial diagnoses on presentation have included Rocky Mountain spotted fever and meningococcemia because of the similarities of rash and toxicity. Since inactivated vaccines were available only from 1963 through 1967, the past recipients are now young adults. This atypical measles syndrome is of increasing importance to the internist. Atypical measles has been reported in some patients who received live vaccine alone or after killed vaccine. Recipients of killed vaccine who later received live vaccine may have severe local and systemic reactions to reimmunization.

DIAGNOSIS. The diagnosis should be suspected during an epidemic or following history of exposure. Prior to the appearance of rash, the diagnosis may be difficult unless Koplik's spots are present. Finding in a darkened room an uncomfortable patient who has conjunctivitis, coryza, and cough should make one suspect measles. The rash in adults may be more violaceous, confluent, slightly raised, and more extensive than in children. A history of having received measles vaccine does not preclude the diagnosis, as most individuals with measles of school age have had the vaccine.

Differential diagnosis (Table 367–1) includes consideration of rubella, scarlet fever, infectious mononucleosis, secondary syphilis, drug eruptions, toxic shock syndrome, and Kawasaki's disease. Of value in excluding these possibilities are the milder course, postauricular nodes, and pinker rash of rubella; the sore throat, eventual desquamation, strawberry tongue, and leukocytosis of scarlet fever; and serologic tests for infectious mononucleosis. Fever, enanthem, and catarrh are uncommon with the cutaneous manifestations of drug hypersensitivity. Erythema infectiosum is usually an afebrile illness with rash on the cheeks, arms, and legs. There is no prodrome or accompanying respiratory tract involvement. Kawasaki's disease is rare in adults.

Specific Diagnosis. Virus isolation is technically difficult. Increase in specific antibody may be detected as early as the first or second day of rash. Generally, acute and convalescent sera are required. Demonstration of measles IgM is available in some laboratories.

Presumptive diagnosis may be made if giant cells are detected in stained smears of nasal exudate in the pre-eruptive period.

PROGNOSIS. Uncomplicated measles is rarely fatal, and complete recovery is the rule. Fatalities are almost always the result of pneumonia, occurring in adults or in children below the age of 2 years. Congestive cardiac failure is a common cause of death in patients over 50 years old. The prognosis is particularly poor in patients with AIDS or other immunocompromised patients (see Ch. 410).

Antimicrobial drugs effective against the usual secondary invaders have reduced the case fatality rate of measles sharply. They have proved effective in therapy of bacterial complications, but not in prophylaxis.

Encephalitis occurs as frequently in mild as in severe measles (i.e., about one in 1000 cases); subacute sclerosing panencephalitis

TABLE 367–1. A GUIDE TO THE DIFFERENTIAL DIAGNOSIS OF MEASLES

	Conjunctivitis	Rhinitis	Sore Throat	Enanthem	Leukocytosis	Specific Laboratory Tests Available
Measles	+ +	+ +	0	+	0	+
Rubella	±	±	±	±	0	+
Exanthem subitum	±	±	0	0	0	0
Enterovirus infection	0	±	±	0	0	+
Adenovirus infection	+	+	+	0	0	+
Scarlet fever	±	±	+ +	0	+	+
Infectious mononucleosis	0	0	+ +	±	±	+
Drug rash	0	0	0	0	0	0

  0 Not usually present; no test available.
  ± Variable in occurrence.
  + Present; test available (virus or bacterial culture, serology).
  + + Present and severe.

occurs about 7 years after measles and has essentially disappeared with widespread vaccine use.

TREATMENT. There is no specific antiviral therapy for measles with demonstrated efficacy.

Symptomatic Therapy. In the absence of complications, bed rest is the essence of treatment in this self-limited disease. Codeine sulfate may be useful in the amelioration of headache and myalgia and is effective in the management of cough. Analgesics and antipyretics many be useful. Fluids should be encouraged. Bright light is not an ocular hazard, but photophobia may require darkening of the patient's room.

Antimicrobial Prophylaxis. The course of uncomplicated measles is not influenced by antimicrobial drugs, and their use during the acute illness has resulted in no decrease of secondary bacterial complications (otitis, sinusitis, pneumonia). Instead, the same rates of complications (about 10 to 15 per cent) have been observed, but with organisms resistant to the antibiotics used during the viral illness. If careful observation of the patient is possible, rational therapy is based on the prompt recognition and etiologic definition of complications, followed by initiation of the appropriate antimicrobial drug in proper dosage.

PREVENTION. Vaccination. A highly effective vaccine available for the prevention of measles is derived from the Edmonston strain of virus isolated originally in the laboratory of Dr. John Enders. This live virus vaccine produces immunity by infection. A second dose now is recommended routinely. In children over 1 year of age, seroconversion after vaccination in recent years is about 98 to 99 per cent. Measles vaccine usually is given as a single preparation as measles, mumps, and rubella (MMR) vaccine. Failure of measles immunization was much more common prior to 1980. The reasons for this are unclear. It may be due to poor recall or faulty documentation of immunization, age of immunization, use of immune globulin with the vaccine, receipt of killed rather than live vaccine, or the type of live vaccine.

Vaccine recommendations vary depending upon the measles experience in the community. The first dose is usually given at 15 months of age as MMR. In hyperendemic areas it is given at 12 months of age. During epidemics it may be given as monovalent measles vaccine to infants as young as 6 months of age. In the latter case, it should be repeated in combination with mumps and rubella (MMR) after the first birthday. The second routine dose of MMR is given between 5 and 12 years of age. All entering college students and beginning health care workers born after 1956 should show evidence of measles immunity, e.g., positive serologic test, physician-documented measles, or receipt of two doses of measles vaccine or preferably MMR. The immune status of those contemplating foreign travel should be reviewed. A large number of military personnel have been reimmunized without significant side effects.

Contraindications to live virus vaccine include pregnancy, immunodeficiency, leukemia, and other systemic malignant diseases, active tuberculosis, and administration of resistance-depressing drugs such as corticosteroids and antimetabolites.

Annunziato D, Kaplan MH, Hall WW, et al.: Atypical measles syndrome: Pathologic and serologic findings. Pediatrics 70:203, 1982. *Excellent clinical description and explanation of a syndrome now seen in young adults.*

Centers for Disease Control: Measles prevention: Recommendations of the Immunization Practices Advisory Committee (ACIP). MMWR 38:1–18, 1989. *Everything you want to know about the use of measles vaccine.*

Gilad M.: Measles in adults: A prospective study of 291 consecutive cases. Br Med J 295:1313, 1987. *A brief summary of findings in a large number of adults.*

Gremillioin DH, Crawford GE: Measles pneumonia in young adults. Am J Med 71:539–542, 1981. *A large series of cases of measles pneumonia in young adults and other features of measles in this group.*

Gustafson TL, Brunell PA, Lievens AW, et al.: Measles outbreak in a "fully-immunized" secondary school population. N Engl J Med 316:771–774, 1987. *School outbreaks are described in a presumably well-immunized population.*

Katz SL, Krugman S, Quinn TC (eds.): International symposium on measles immunization. Rev Infect Dis 5:389, 1983. *An all-inclusive presentation of measles and its prevention throughout the world.*

Panum PL: Observations Made During the Epidemic of Measles on the Faroe Islands. Delta Omega Society, 1940. *A classic clinical epidemiologic description of measles introduced into an isolated population with disease among all susceptibles born since the previous epidemic 65 years earlier.*

368 Rubella *(German Measles)*

Philip A. Brunell

DEFINITION. Rubella is an acute, usually benign infectious disease characterized by a 3-day rash, generalized lymphadenopathy, and minimal or no prodromal symptoms. Since 1941 it has been known to cause congenital malformations when infection occurs during the early months of pregnancy.

ETIOLOGY. Rubella is a small, spherical, enveloped virus containing single-stranded RNA of positive polarity. The structural proteins consist of membrane glycoproteins and a nucleo-capsid protein. The virus is classified as a togavirus, genus rubivirus. It multiplies in a variety of primary cell culture systems and in some continuous cell lines in most systems without detectable cytopathic effects. Hemagglutination of avian erythrocytes provides a convenient method for virus assay, and by inhibition of this hemagglutination the presence and titer of antibody are readily measured.

EPIDEMIOLOGY. Prior to the availability of rubella vaccines, the disease was worldwide in distribution, produced major epidemics at 6- to 9-year intervals, and was recognized mainly in school-age children; it also produced outbreaks in settings such as military recruit bases and college campuses where large numbers of susceptible young adults gathered in relatively crowded conditions. Since licensure in 1969 in the United States there has been strikingly altered epidemiology. There has been no major epidemic since 1964–1965. In other nations, where rubella vaccine has not been widely utilized, the epidemiology has remained unchanged. Because the disease may be quite nonspecific clinically, with nearly one third of adults undergoing infection without rash, epidemiologic reporting tends to underestimate its prevalence. Since 1966, congenital rubella has been a reportable disease. It is probable that rubella is spread by the respiratory route and by close and sustained personal contact. The incubation period in experimentally infected individuals was found to be 12 to 19 days, with most cases occurring 14 to 15 days following exposure. Although virus was isolated as early as 7 days prior to and as late as 21 days following onset of rash, infectivity probably is greatest throughout the period of prodromal symptoms and for as long as 7 days after the appearance of rash. Infants with congenitally acquired infection may excrete virus in respiratory secretions and in urine for months after birth and are contagious during this time. In hospital environments, especially in nurseries, the congenital rubella baby has been a source of nosocomial infection of personnel involved in his care.

Immunity is lifelong in duration after initial infection. Authenticated second attacks are exceedingly rare and require serologic documentation because of the nonspecific nature of the clinical syndrome. Subclinical reinfection demonstrated by increase in IgG serum antibody has been documented. Such reinfections are not associated with viremia and thus pose little threat to pregnant women. IgM response has been used to distinguish primary infection from reinfection. Immunity that follows artificial immunization with live virus vaccine is apparently of equal duration even though the antibody titers induced may be somewhat lower.

PATHOLOGY. Death from postnatal rubella is usually due to encephalitis. Thus, most autopsies describe only the brain findings. Since 1962 it has been possible to investigate the pathogenesis and to correlate clinical findings with virologic events. After initial invasion of the upper respiratory tract, virus spreads to local lymphoid tissue, where it multiplies and initiates a viremia of approximately 7 days' duration. Respiratory tract shedding of virus and the viremia rise to peak levels until the onset of rash, at which time the latter becomes undetectable, whereas respiratory secretions contain diminishing quantities of virus over the succeeding 5 to 15 days. Specific serum antibodies can be demonstrated with the onset of rash, and circulating immune complexes are detectable soon thereafter.

Congenital Rubella. Necropsies of fetal and neonatal victims of intrauterine infection have shown a variety of embryonal defects related to developmental arrest involving all three germ layers.

The virus establishes chronic persistent infection of many tissues, with resultant intrauterine growth retardation. Delayed and disordered organogenesis produces embryopathic structural defects of the eye, brain, heart, and large arteries; continued viral infection during the fetal and postnatal period causes organ and tissue damage, e.g., hepatitis, nephritis, myocarditis, pneumonia, osteitis, meningitis, cochlear degeneration, and pancreatitis.

CLINICAL MANIFESTATIONS. *Postnatally Acquired Rubella.* Twelve to 19 days after exposure, the onset of rubella is manifested by the appearance of a rash with mild accompanying constitutional symptoms of malaise and occasionally sore throat. Enlargement of the postauricular and suboccipital nodes generally appears about a week prior to rash. Moderate fever, coryza, and faint conjunctivitis may accompany or precede the rash. Generalized peripheral lymphadenopathy and, more rarely, splenomegaly may occur.

The exanthem of rubella is usually apparent within 24 hours of the first symptoms as a faint macular erythema that first involves the face and neck. Characterized by its brevity and evanescence, it spreads rapidly to the trunk and extremities, sometimes leaving one site even as it appears at the next. The pink macules that constitute the rash blanch with pressure and rarely stain the skin. Rubella virus has been isolated from the skin lesions as well as from uninvolved sites. The truncal rash may coalesce, but the lesions on the extremities remain discrete. The eruption usually vanishes by the third day. Rubella may occur without rash. In the absence of an epidemic and of serologic or virologic confirmation, the clinical diagnosis of rubella is not reliable.

COMPLICATIONS. Recovery is almost always prompt and uneventful. In contrast to measles, secondary bacterial infections are not encountered in rubella. Transient polyarthralgia and polyarthritis are more common among adolescents and adults with rubella, particularly females. They appear 3 or more days after onset of rash and may last 5 to 10 days. The knees and joints of the hands and wrist are most often involved. Surveys during urban epidemics have revealed rates of 5 to 15 per cent in males and 10 to 35 per cent in females.

Thrombocytopenia, when sought by serial platelet counts, is common but rarely of clinical consequence. A meningoencephalitis of short duration may occur 1 to 6 days after the appearance of rash. Its incidence is estimated at 1 in 5000 cases, and it is fatal in approximately 20 per cent of those afflicted. Rubella encephalopathy is not associated with demyelinization, in contrast to other postviral encephalitides. Survivors may have electroencephalographic abnormalities, but intellectual function seems to be preserved. A progressive panencephalitis following congenital or postnatal rubella has been described. Its onset generally is during the second decade.

Congenital Rubella. Congenital transplacental infection of the fetus occurs as a consequence of maternal infection, usually in the first 4 months of pregnancy. Virus is demonstrable in placental and fetal tissues obtained by therapeutic abortion at that time. If pregnancy is not interrupted, fetal infection persists, and upon delivery of the infant, virus is recoverable from the throat, urine, conjunctivae, bone marrow, and cerebrospinal fluid of the living infant and from most organs at autopsy. From 20 to 80 per cent of infants born to mothers infected in the first trimester of pregnancy have stigmata of infection readily recognizable in the first year of life. These include cardiac lesions and eye defects, e.g., cataracts, glaucoma, retinitis, microphthalmia. Many infants in whom virus is detectable do not have evidence of disease at birth or may simply have intrauterine growth retardation. In others, more severe disease occurs. Most prominent of these manifestations is thrombocytopenic purpura, which disappears soon after birth. Hepatosplenomegaly with active hepatitis may persist for months. Other involvement includes interstitial pneumonia, meningoencephalitis, hearing loss of varying extent, and lesions of the long bones. Recently, a progressive panencephalitis simulating subacute sclerosing panencephalitis has been observed in the second decade following congenital infection. The long-term sequelae for infants with congenital rubella include psychomotor retardation, hearing loss, retinopathy, and diabetes.

A striking finding has been the persistence of virus in the pharynx, urine, and cerebrospinal fluid for as long as 1 year after birth in 7 per cent of infants. Infective virus was found in a congenital cataract after 3 years and in the urine of a victim of congenital rubella 29 years after her birth. This evidence of continuing viral synthesis occurs coincidentally with circulating antibody. The character of the antibody changes during the first months from maternal IgG to IgM, indicating a primary response of the infant to the persisting viral antigen. Studies of older infants and children with stigmata of congenital rubella show them to be free of demonstrable virus and to possess the IgG immunoglobulins that characteristically persist after other viral infections.

DIAGNOSIS. Rubella may be diagnosed clinically with assurance only during an epidemic. Distinction from measles may be made on the basis of fainter, nonstaining rash, the milder course, and the minimal or absent respiratory complaints. Sore throat is a more prominent complaint in scarlet fever; the course of infectious mononucleosis is often more protracted, and splenomegaly is more frequent than in rubella. Specific diagnosis of rubella is made by isolation of the virus in any of several cell culture systems or by demonstration of a rise in hemagglutination-inhibiting (HI), ELISA, or complement-fixing antibody during infection.

PROGNOSIS. Complete recovery from postnatally acquired rubella is almost invariable. The rare deaths attributable to rubella follow the infrequent complication of meningoencephalitis. Infection in pregnancy constitutes a grave hazard to the fetus but not to the mother.

TREATMENT. There is no specific antiviral therapy. Few patients suffer discomfort severe enough to warrant symptomatic medication. Headache and myalgia or arthritis may be controlled by analgesics.

PREVENTION. *Passive Immunization.* Administration of gamma globulin to the pregnant woman may only mask her symptoms of infection and not protect the fetus from viral invasions. Thus, its use may only obscure the picture and confound decision about the need to terminate the pregnancy if this is an option.

Active Immunization. Rubella may be prevented in children and adults by the parenteral administration of attenuated live virus vaccines produced in cell cultures. Seroconversion rates after immunization are at least 98 per cent with the current RA 27/3 vaccine. Joint symptoms are less common than with the older HPV 7-DE strain, occurring in about 2.5 per cent of adults. Arthritis occurs 13 to 19 days following immunization and lasts 2 to 11 days. The fingers are most often affected, with the wrists and knees less commonly involved. Arthralgias generally begin 10 to 25 days following vaccination and last 1 to 9 days. Joint symptoms are less common in men than in women. In children, vaccination is attended by little or no reaction.

It was initially recommended in the United States that immunization be carried out principally in childhood. There now is a more aggressive attempt to immunize those remaining susceptible women and adolescent girls. Current policy recommends vaccination of all such persons who have no history of previous rubella immunizations. Postpartum immunization of those found to be seronegative during pregnancy is encouraged. Although there occasionally has been transmission of vaccine virus to the newborn by breast milk, this has proven to be of little consequence. Only nonpregnant individuals should be immunized, and contraception, when appropriate, should be carried out for at least 3 months after vaccination. The inadvertent administration of vaccine to pregnant women has occasionally resulted in attenuated vaccine virus infection of the fetus. In more than 500 such cases studied, no infant has been observed with congenital malformations as a result. The frequency of fetal infection with the RA 27/3 vaccine currently used is less than with the previous rubella vaccine. The use of vaccine in the United States prevented a large epidemic of rubella expected in the early 1970's and has reduced the reported annual occurrence from more than 50,000 cases annually, with epidemic peaks of 200,000 to 500,000, to an all-time low in 1988 of 221 cases.

Burke JP, Hinman AR, Krugman S (eds.): International symposium on prevention of congenital rubella infection. Rev Infect Dis 7(Suppl):1, 1985. *Fifteen years of vaccine use summarized by investigators from the developed nations.*

Centers for Disease Control: Rubella and congenital rubella syndrome—United States. MMWR 38:173, 1989. *A summary report of progress in rubella "eradication" in the United States.*

Gregg NM: Congenital cataract following German measles in the mother. Trans Ophthal Soc Aust 3:35, 1941. *The original "classic" report associating rubella in pregnancy with congenital malformations.*

Proceedings of the International Conference on Rubella Immunization. Am J Dis Child 118, July 1969. *A compendium on rubella and congenital rubella.*

Sherman FE, Michaels RH, Kenny FM: Acute encephalopathy (encephalitis) complicating rubella. JAMA 192:675, 1965. *A clinical, pathologic, and epidemiologic study of rubella encephalitis.*

Townsend JJ, Stroop WG, Baringer JR, et al.: Neuropathology of progressive rubella panencephalitis after childhood rubella. Neurology 32:185, 1982. *A review of the clinical and neuropathologic findings.*

Weibel RE, Vilarejos VM, Klein EB, et al.: Clinical and laboratory studies of live attenuated RA 27/3 and HPV 77-DE rubella virus vaccines (40931). Proc Soc Exper Biol Med 165:44, 1980. *A description of the clinical and serologic response to rubella vaccine.*

369 Foot-and-Mouth Disease

John W. Gnann, Jr.

Foot-and-mouth disease virus (FMDV) is an extremely important pathogen of cloven-hoofed animals (e.g., cattle, swine, sheep, and goats) and a rare cause of disease in humans. Foot-and-mouth disease (FMD) should not be confused with hand-foot-and-mouth disease caused by coxsackieviruses. FMD is endemic in parts of Europe, Asia, Africa, and South America but is not currently present in North America or Australia. Strict regulations are in place to prevent importation of FMDV or FMDV-infected animals into the United States.

Because of the huge economic impact of FMD on the livestock industry, FMDV has been intensively studied and consequently is one of the best-characterized animal viruses. The three-dimensional ultrastructure of FMDV has been determined by x-ray diffraction studies. A highly immunogenic synthetic peptide based on a FMDV coat protein (VP1) sequence may prove to be the basis for an enhanced FMD vaccine. FMD is currently controlled among livestock herds either by test-and-slaughter procedures or by use of an inactivated virus vaccine.

FMDV is a member of the family Picornaviridae and the genus *Aphthovirus*. FMDV is a nonenveloped icosahedral virus with a diameter of about 25 to 30 nm. The genome consists of one linear molecule of positive-sense single-stranded RNA. Seven major serotypes have been identified; most well-documented human infections have been caused by type O.

FMD is extremely contagious and spreads rapidly among susceptible animals. Infected animals develop papular and vesicular eruptions of the mouth and other mucous membranes and of the skin around the hooves. FMDV can be isolated from the skin lesions, saliva, urine, and milk of infected animals. Although not usually fatal, infection renders the animal economically worthless.

Humans are not very susceptible to infection by FMDV, as evidenced by the rarity of infection among veterinarians, abattoir workers, and laboratory personnel who study the virus. Older literature contains many case reports of human infection with FMDV, but these were not confirmed serologically or virologically. However, there have been several cases of human FMD which have been documented by viral isolation. FMDV can apparently be transmitted to humans by direct skin contact with infected animal materials, by ingestion of virus (e.g., in contaminated milk), or possibly by inhalation. Following an incubation period of 3 to 8 days, human infection is characterized by fever, malaise, increased salivation, and vesicles in the mouth, on the perioral area, and sometimes on the hands and feet. The vesicles ulcerate, then slowly heal over a period of 10 days to 2 weeks. Virtually all infected individuals recover without sequelae. Human-to-human transmission of FMDV has not been documented. The diagnosis can be established either by isolation of the virus from vesicle fluid or by serologic testing. No specific therapy is available.

Armstrong R, David J, Hedger RS: Foot-and-mouth disease in man. Br Med J 4:529, 1967. *Report of a culture-proven case of human FMD.*

Bittle JL, Houghten RA, Alexander H, et al.: Protection against foot-and-mouth disease by immunization with a chemically synthesized peptide predicted from

the viral nucleotide sequence. Nature 298:30, 1982. *Immunization of animals with synthetic VP1 peptides induces serotype-specific virus-neutralizing antibody.*

370 Mumps

John W. Gnann, Jr.

Mumps is an acute systemic viral infection that is usually self-limited, occurs most commonly in school-age children, and is clinically characterized by nonsuppurative parotitis.

VIROLOGY. Mumps virus is classified as a member of the family Paramyxoviridae in the genus *Paramyxovirus*. Mumps virions are pleomorphic, roughly spherical, enveloped particles with an average diameter of 200 nm. Glycoprotein spikes project from the surface of the envelope, which encloses a helical nucleocapsid composed of RNA and nucleoproteins. The mumps virus genome is contained in a linear molecule of nonsegmented, single-stranded, negative-sense RNA. The virus is composed of five major proteins: Nucleocapsid protein (NP) is the major structural protein; polymerase protein (P) appears to have RNA-dependent RNA-polymerase activity; matrix (M) protein is important in the assembly of virions; and two surface glycoproteins mediate hemagglutinin-neuraminidase (HN) and fusion (F) activity. An additional large (L) nucleocapsid-associated protein has been observed by some investigators. There is only one serologic strain of mumps virus.

Humans are the only known natural hosts for mumps virus, although infection can be experimentally induced in a wide variety of mammalian species. In vitro, mumps virus can be cultured in many mammalian cell lines, including monkey kidney, BSC-1, Vero, and HeLa cells, as well as in embryonated hens' eggs.

EPIDEMIOLOGY. In unvaccinated urban populations, mumps is a disease of school-age children. Mumps infrequently occurs in infants less than 1 year of age, presumably because of transplacentally acquired antibody. The largest number of mumps cases occurs in children between 4 and 7 years of age. By age 15, 92 per cent of children have mumps antibodies. Prior to the release of the live attenuated mumps vaccine in the United States in 1967, mumps was an endemic disease with a seasonal peak of activity between January and May. Mumps epidemics occurred at 2- to 5-year intervals. The largest number of cases reported in the United States was in 1941, when the incidence of mumps was 250 cases per 100,000 population. In 1968, when the live attenuated vaccine was first entering clinical usage, the incidence of mumps was 76 cases per 100,000 population. In 1985, a total of only 2982 cases of mumps was reported, an incidence of 1.1 per 100,000 population, representing a 98 per cent decline from the number of cases reported in 1967.

Between 1985 and 1987, the incidence of mumps in the United States increased fivefold to 5.2 cases per 100,000 population. More than one third of the cases reported between 1985 and 1987 occurred in adolescents and young adults, reflecting the slow acceptance of universal mumps vaccination during the 1970's when this cohort of children grew up. This is an important trend, since mumps generally causes a more severe disease in adults than in children. The increased incidence of mumps in susceptible young adults was most prominent in those states without comprehensive school immunization laws.

PATHOGENESIS. Mumps can be experimentally transmitted by inoculation of virus onto the nasal or buccal mucosa, suggesting that most natural infections result from droplet spread of upper respiratory secretions from infected individuals. The average incubation period for mumps is 18 days. During this interval, primary viral replication is thought to take place in epithelial cells of the upper respiratory tract, followed by spread of virus to regional lymph nodes and subsequent viremia and systemic dissemination. Virus can be isolated from saliva for 5 to 6 days before and up to 5 days after the onset of clinical symptoms, meaning that an infected individual is potentially able to transmit mumps for a period of about 10 days.

Mumps is highly contagious, although some studies have suggested that it is less contagious than varicella or measles. This clinical observation may be skewed by the fact that up to 30 per cent of all mumps infections are subclinical and asymptomatic. Over 90 per cent of adults who give negative histories for mumps are seropositive when tested for mumps antibody, indicating prior subclinical infection.

CLINICAL MANIFESTATIONS. *Parotitis.* Mumps is a systemic infection, and the virus has been demonstrated to replicate in epithelial cells of multiple visceral organs. Mumps usually begins with a short prodromal phase characterized by low-grade fever, malaise, headache, and anorexia. Young children may initially complain of ear pain. The patient then develops the typical salivary gland enlargement and tenderness. The parotid glands are most commonly involved, although other salivary glands may occasionally be enlarged. Parotitis may initially be unilateral, with swelling of the contralateral parotid gland occurring 2 to 3 days later; bilateral parotitis eventually develops in most patients with symptomatic salivary gland involvement. Painful parotid gland enlargement progresses over about 3 days, lifting the ear lobe outward and obscuring the angle of the mandible. The orifice of Stensen's duct is often edematous. Parotid gland swelling and tenderness peak on about the third day of the illness, followed by defervescence and resolution of parotid pain and swelling within about 7 days. Long-term sequelae of parotitis are uncommon.

Meningitis. Symptomatic meningitis occurs in 15 per cent of cases and is the second most common manifestation of mumps. Studies with animal models indicate that mumps virus is clearly neurotropic and replicates well in the ependymal cells of the choroid plexus. Studies have shown that half of patients with mumps parotitis without signs or symptoms of meningitis have cerebrospinal fluid (CSF) pleocytosis. Mumps virus can be recovered from CSF.

Symptoms of meningeal irritation (headache, neck stiffness, vomiting, and lethargy) usually develop 4 to 5 days after the onset of parotitis, although the meningitis may occasionally precede the parotitis. Indeed, 40 to 50 per cent of all cases of documented mumps meningitis occur in patients who never develop clinical parotitis. Symptomatic central nervous system involvement with mumps is 2 to 3 times more common in males than in females. Examination of the CSF usually reveals a normal opening pressure and a mononuclear cell pleocytosis with an average cell count of 250 per cubic millimeter, although cell counts as high as 1000 to 2000 per cubic millimeter are not uncommon. A polymorphonuclear leukocyte predominance may be seen in some patients early during the course of mumps meningitis. The CSF protein is usually normal or mildly elevated (<100 mg per 100 ml). Hypoglycorrhachia, which is not usually seen in viral meningitis, may be present in 10 to 30 per cent of patients with meningitis due to mumps virus. Although the symptoms of mumps meningitis usually resolve within a week, the CSF abnormalities may persist for up to 5 weeks. The meningitis is usually benign, and significant neurologic complications are rare.

Encephalitis. The spectrum of mumps-induced central nervous system disease ranges from mild "aseptic" meningitis (which is common) to severe encephalitis (which is relatively rare). The pathogenesis of mumps encephalitis is not precisely understood. Some cases of encephalitis develop concurrently with the parotitis and are thought to result from direct extension of viral infection from the choroid plexus ependyma into parenchymal neurons. Other cases of mumps encephalitis occur 1 to 2 weeks after the onset of parotitis and may represent an autoimmune parainfectious encephalitis. Clinical findings in mumps encephalitis include obtundation (and less commonly delirium), generalized seizures, and high fever. Other neurologic findings, including focal seizures, aphasia, paresis, and involuntary movements, have been reported. Recovery from mumps encephalitis is usually complete, although complications such as aqueductal stenosis with hydrocephalus, seizure disorders, and psychomotor retardation have been noted. The overall mortality from mumps encephalitis is 0.5 to 2.3 per cent.

Orchitis. Epididymo-orchitis is rare in boys with mumps but occurs in 25 to 30 per cent of postpubertal men with mumps infection. Orchitis results from replication of mumps virus in seminiferous tubules with resulting lymphocytic infiltration and edema. Orchitis is most often unilateral, but bilateral involvement occurs in 17 to 38 per cent of cases. Orchitis typically develops within 1 week after the onset of parotitis, although orchitis (like mumps meningitis) can develop prior to or even in the absence of parotitis. Mumps orchitis is characterized by marked testicular swelling and severe pain, accompanied by fever, nausea, and headache. The pain and swelling resolve within 5 to 7 days, although residual testicular tenderness can persist for weeks. Testicular atrophy may follow orchitis in about 35 to 50 per cent of cases, but sterility is an uncommon complication even among patients with bilateral orchitis.

Other Manifestations. Mumps can cause inflammation of other glandular tissues, including pancreas and thyroid. Oophoritis and mastitis have been reported in postpubertal women with mumps. Renal function abnormalities are common in mumps, and virus can be readily isolated from urine, but significant renal damage is rare. Other infrequent manifestations of mumps include sensorineural deafness (either transient or permanent), arthritis, myocarditis, and thrombocytopenia.

Mumps During Pregnancy. Maternal mumps infection during the first trimester of pregnancy results in an increased frequency of spontaneous abortions. However, no clear association between congenital malformations and maternal mumps has been demonstrated.

IMMUNE RESPONSE. Transient IgM antibody responses are detected early in the course of mumps infection, followed by the appearance of IgG antibody and cytotoxic T lymphocytes (CTL). The relative contributions of humoral and cell-mediated immunity to viral clearance have not been precisely determined. Life-long immunity follows natural infection. Patients who report more than one episode of mumps probably had parotitis due to infection with a different virus.

A variety of serologic tests have been designed to determine susceptibility to mumps. The neutralizing antibody (NA) assay has been considered the "gold standard" test but is technically demanding. The hemagglutination inhibition (HAI) assay is simple to perform but less specific owing to cross-reactivity with other paramyxoviruses. Detection of complement fixing (CF) antibodies against V antigen (hemagglutinin-neuraminidase) has previously been the routine method for determining immune status but is being replaced by a sensitive and specific enzyme-linked immunosorbent assay (ELISA). The mumps skin test is not a reliable indicator of immune status.

DIAGNOSIS. The diagnosis of mumps is most often made on clinical grounds in a patient who presents with parotitis, particularly if the individual is known to be susceptible and has been exposed to mumps during the preceding 2 to 3 weeks. However, an atypical clinical presentation (e.g., meningitis or orchitis without parotitis) may require laboratory confirmation. Culturing for mumps virus is definitive but frequently not available. Testing of paired acute and convalescent sera should demonstrate a diagnostic fourfold rise in mumps antibody titer. Alternatively, demonstration of mumps IgM antibody provides good evidence of recent infection. In the past, a CF test for detecting antibodies against S (nucleocapsid) and V antigens has been the most commonly used diagnostic test, but ELISA is now becoming the standard assay.

Parotitis can be caused by other viruses such as influenza A, parainfluenza virus, coxsackievirus, lymphocytic choriomeningitis virus, and bacteria such as *Staphylococcus aureus*. Parotid gland enlargement can also be associated with Sjögren's syndrome, sarcoidosis, thiazide ingestion, iodine sensitivity, tumor, or salivary duct obstruction. A careful examination should distinguish parotitis from lymphadenopathy.

THERAPY. Management of the patient with mumps consists of conservative measures to provide symptomatic relief and to ensure adequate hydration and nutrition. Therapy of orchitis includes bed rest, scrotal support, analgesics, and ice packs. Patients with significant central nervous system involvement require hospitalization for observation and supportive care. There is currently no established role for antiviral drugs, steroids, or passive immunotherapy.

PREVENTION. Children with mumps are usually isolated for about 1 week after the appearance of parotitis, although this practice is of dubious benefit to classmates, since the virus is known to be excreted for several days prior to the onset of clinical symptoms. The cornerstone of mumps prevention is active immunization using the live attenuated mumps vaccine. This vaccine is administered in the United States to infants during the second year of life and produces protective antibody levels in more than 97 per cent of recipients. The vaccine is given subcutaneously in combination with the live measles and rubella vaccines and has virtually no side effects. Booster immunizations are not required.

Administration of the live mumps vaccine is relatively contraindicated in pregnant women, in persons with a history of anaphylactic reaction to eggs or neomycin (the vaccine is produced in chick-embryo cell culture), in persons who have received immunoglobulin therapy within the preceding 3 months (which might interfere with the immune response to the vaccine), or in persons with severe systemic immunosuppression. Mumps immunization is recommended for asymptomatic HIV-infected children.

Questions regarding prevention often arise when an individual with no history of mumps (typically an adult male) is exposed to a patient with active mumps. The immune status of the exposed individual can be determined by serologic testing, although this may involve some delay. Mumps vaccine can be safely administered to an individual of unknown immune status, although vaccine given to a susceptible individual after exposure to mumps may not provide protection. Mumps immune globulin is not of proven value and is no longer commercially available. The vast majority of adults born in the United States before 1957 have been naturally infected and are therefore immune.

ACIP: Mumps prevention. MMWR 38:388, 1989. *Current vaccination recommendations from the Immunization Practices Advisory Committee.*

Shehab ZM, Brunnell PA, Cobb E: Epidemiologic standardization of a test for susceptibility to mumps. J Infect Dis 149:810, 1984. *Development of an ELISA for detection of mumps antibody.*

371 Herpes Simplex Virus Infections

Mark Middlebrooks and Richard J. Whitley

Herpes simplex virus (HSV), a member of the family Herpesviridae, has been implicated in human infections since descriptions of cutaneous spreading lesions in ancient Greek times. Scholars of Greek civilization define the word *herpes* to mean "to creep or crawl," in reference to the spreading nature of the observed skin lesions. More recent scholars have further described the spectrum of illnesses caused by HSV and have made significant discoveries in the molecular biology of HSV infection. A major advance was the detection of differences between herpes simplex virus types. Although suggested by clinical and laboratory observation for many years, it was not until 1968 that well-defined antigenic and biologic differences were demonstrated between herpes simplex virus type 1 (HSV-1) and herpes simplex virus type 2 (HSV-2). Nahmias and Dowdle demonstrated that HSV-1 was more frequently associated with nongenital infection and HSV-2 with genital disease. Further study has revealed that, of all the herpesviruses, HSV-1 and HSV-2 are the most closely related, with approximately 60 per cent genomic homology. These two viruses can be distinguished most reliably by DNA restriction enzyme analyses; however, differences in antigen expression and biologic properties also serve as methods for differentiation.

STRUCTURE. Membership in the family Herpesviridae is based on the structure of the virion (Fig. 371–1). Herpes simplex virus contains double-stranded DNA at the central core, has a molecular weight of approximately 100 million, and encodes at least 70 polypeptides. The DNA core is surrounded by a capsid that consists of 162 capsomers, arranged in icosapentahedral symmetry. The capsid is approximately 100 to 110 nanometers in diameter. Tightly adherent to the capsid is the tegument, which appears to consist of amorphous material. Loosely surrounding the capsid and tegument is a lipid bilayer envelope derived from host cell membranes. The envelope consists of polyamines, lipids, and glycoproteins. These glycoproteins confer distinctive properties to the virus and provide unique antigens to which the host is capable of responding. Notably, glycoprotein G (gG) provides antigenic specificity to HSV and therefore results in an antibody response that allows for the distinction between HSV-1 (gG-1) and HSV-2 (gG-2).

A fascinating feature of HSV DNA is its genomic sequence arrangement. The genome consists of two components, L (long) and S (short), each of which contains unique sequences that can invert upon themselves, leading to four isomers. The ability to exist as one of four isomers is a unique property of HSV. Viral DNA extracted from virions of infected cells consists of four equimolar populations, differing only with respect to the relative orientation of the two unique components. The biologic relevance of this phenomenon is unknown.

REPLICATION. Replication of HSV is a multistep process (Fig. 371–2). Following the onset of infection, DNA is uncoated and transported to the nucleus of the host cell. This is followed

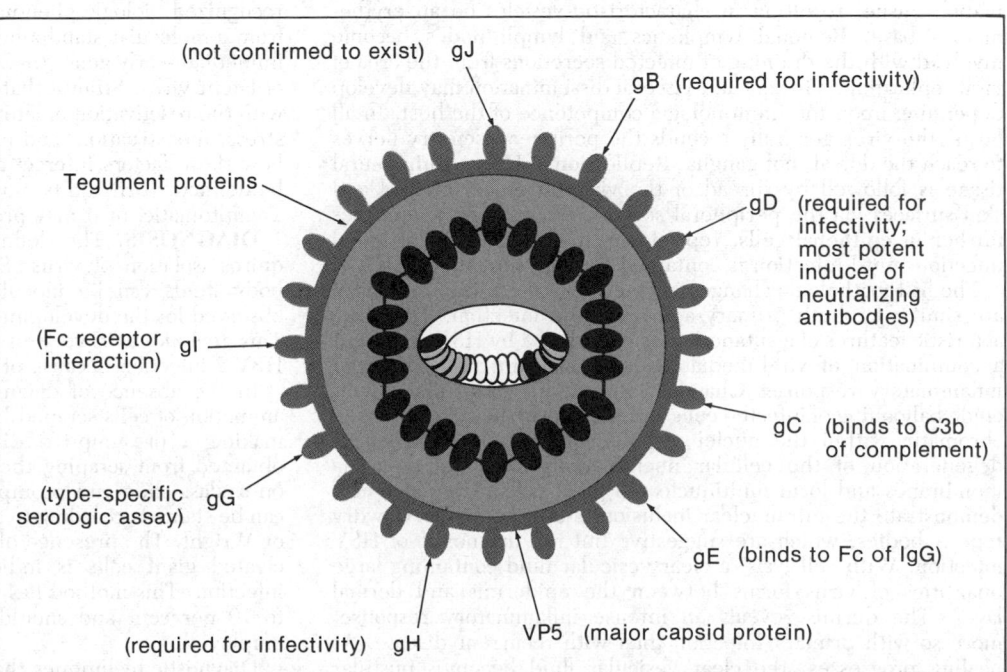

FIGURE 371–1. Schematic diagram of the HSV virion.

(not confirmed to exist) gJ

gB (required for infectivity)

Tegument proteins

gD (required for infectivity; most potent inducer of neutralizing antibodies)

(Fc receptor interaction) gI

(type–specific serologic assay) gG

gC (binds to C3b of complement)

gE (binds to Fc of IgG)

(required for infectivity) gH

VP5 (major capsid protein)

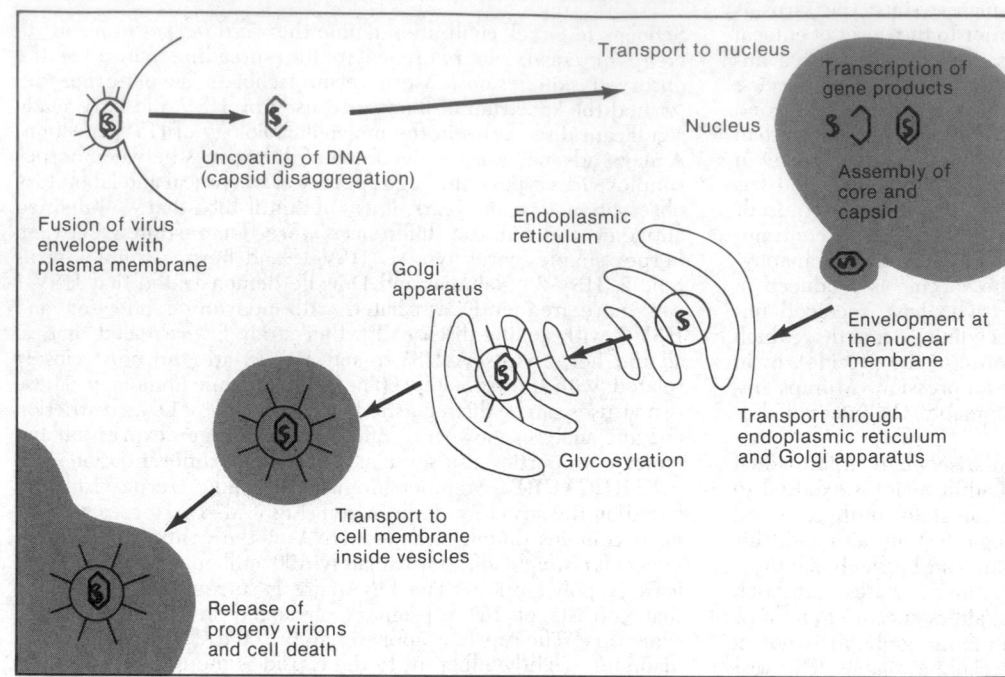

FIGURE 371–2. Schematic diagram of HSV replication.

Labels in figure:
Transport to nucleus
Transcription of gene products
Nucleus
Uncoating of DNA (capsid disaggregation)
Assembly of core and capsid
Fusion of virus envelope with plasma membrane
Endoplasmic reticulum
Golgi apparatus
Envelopment at the nuclear membrane
Transport through endoplasmic reticulum and Golgi apparatus
Glycosylation
Transport to cell membrane inside vesicles
Release of progeny virions and cell death

by transcription of immediate-early genes, which encode for the regulatory proteins. Expression of immediate-early gene products is followed by the expression of proteins encoded by early and then late genes. These proteins include enzymes necessary for viral replication and structural proteins.

Assembly of the viral core and capsid takes place within the nucleus. This is followed by envelopment at the nuclear membrane and transport out of the nucleus through the endoplasmic reticulum and the Golgi apparatus. Glycosylation of the viral membrane occurs in the Golgi apparatus. Mature virions are transported to the outer membrane of the host cell inside vesicles. Release of progeny virus is accompanied by cell death. Replication for all herpesviruses is considered inefficient, with a high ratio of noninfectious to infectious viral particles.

PATHOGENESIS AND LATENCY. A critical factor for transmission of HSV, regardless of virus type, is intimate contact between a person who is shedding virus and a susceptible host. With inoculation onto the skin or mucous membrane, HSV replicates in epithelial cells; the incubation period is 4 to 6 days (Fig. 371–3). As replication continues, cell lysis and local inflammation ensue, resulting in characteristic vesicles on an erythematous base. Regional lymphatics and lymph nodes become involved with the draining of infected secretions from the area of viral replication. Viremia and visceral dissemination may develop depending upon the immunologic competence of the host. In all hosts, the virus generally ascends the peripheral sensory nerves to reach the dorsal root ganglia. Replication of HSV within neural tissue is followed by spread of the virus to other mucosal and skin surfaces via the peripheral sensory nerves. Virus replicates further in epithelial cells, reproducing the lesions of the initial infection, until infection is contained through host immunity.

The histopathologic changes induced by the replication of HSV are similar for both primary and recurrent infection. The characteristic features of a cutaneous lesion induced by HSV represent a combination of viral-mediated cellular death and associated inflammatory response. Changes induced by viral infection include ballooning of infected cells and the appearance of condensed chromatin within the nuclei of cells, followed by subsequent degeneration of the cellular nuclei. Cells lose intact plasma membranes and form multinucleated giant cells. They also may demonstrate the intranuclear inclusion bodies known as Cowdry type A bodies, which are suggestive but not diagnostic of HSV infection. With cell lysis, a clear vesicular fluid containing large quantities of virus forms between the epidermis and dermal layer. The dermis reveals an intense inflammatory response, more so with primary infection than with recurrent disease. As healing progresses, the clear vesicular fluid becomes pustular

with the recruitment of inflammatory cells. The pustule then forms a scab, with scarring being uncommon.

The vascular changes in the area of infection include perivascular cuffing and hemorrhagic necrosis. These changes are particularly prominent when organs other than skin are involved, as is the case with herpes simplex encephalitis or disseminated neonatal HSV infection. Local lymphatics can show evidence of infection with intrusion of inflammatory cells due to the draining of infected secretions from the area of viral replication. As host defenses are mounted, an influx of mononuclear cells can be detected in infected tissue.

A unique characteristic of the herpesviruses is their ability to establish latent infection, persist in an apparently inactive state for varying amounts of time, and then be reactivated (Fig. 371–4). The latent viral genome may be either extrachromosomal or integrated into host-cell DNA.

Latency is established when HSV reaches the dorsal root ganglia after retrograde transmission via sensory nerve pathways. Latent virus may be reactivated and enter a replicative cycle at any point in time. The reactivation of latent virus is a well-recognized biologic phenomenon but not one that is understood from a molecular standpoint. An antisense message to one of the immediate-early genes (α-O) may be involved in the maintenance of latent virus. Stimuli that have been observed to be associated with the reactivation of latent herpes simplex virus have included stress, menstruation, and exposure to ultraviolet light. Precisely how these factors interact at the level of the ganglia remains to be defined. It should be noted that reactivation may be clinically asymptomatic, or it may produce life-threatening disease.

DIAGNOSIS. The definitive diagnosis of HSV infection requires isolation of virus. Swabs of clinical specimens or other body fluids can be inoculated into susceptible cell lines and observed for the development of characteristic cytopathic effects. This technique is very useful for the diagnosis of HSV-1 and HSV-2 infection because of the short replicative cycles.

In the absence of diagnostic virology facilities, cytologic examination of cells scraped from a clinical lesion may be useful in making a presumptive diagnosis of HSV infection. Material obtained from scraping the base of a lesion should be smeared on a glass slide and promptly fixed in cold enthanol. The slide can be stained according to the methods of Papanicolaou, Giemsa, or Wright. The presence of intranuclear inclusions and multinucleated giant cells is indicative, but not diagnostic, of HSV infection. This method has a sensitivity of only approximately 60 to 70 per cent and should not be the sole diagnostic method employed.

Diagnostic techniques that are still being evaluated for clinical

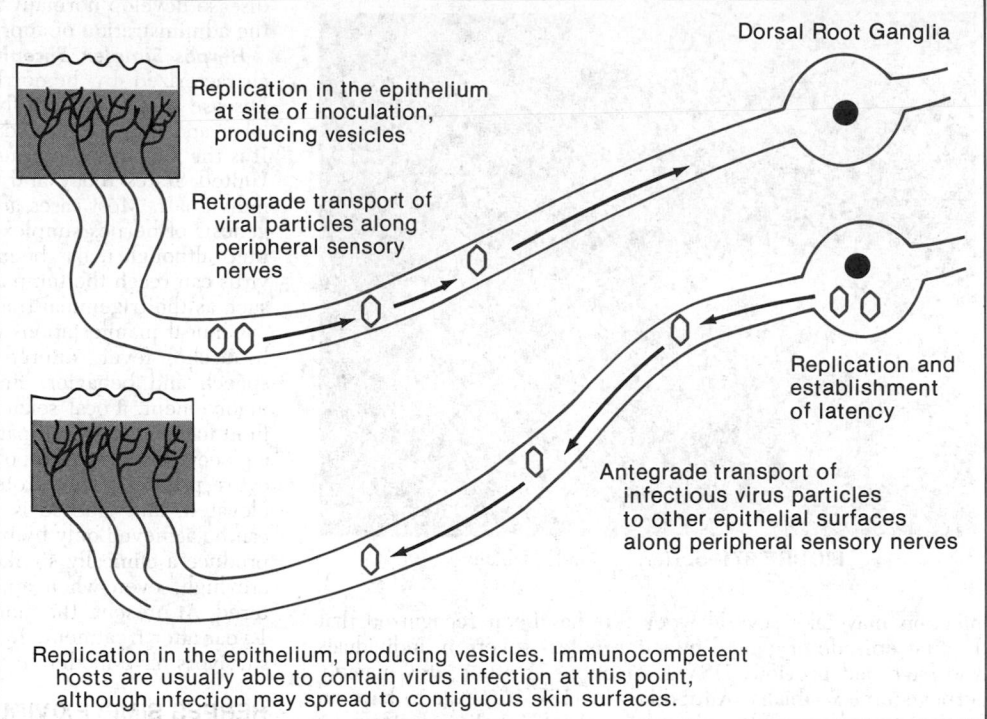

FIGURE 371–3. Schematic diagram of primary HSV infection.

Dorsal Root Ganglia

Replication in the epithelium at site of inoculation, producing vesicles

Retrograde transport of viral particles along peripheral sensory nerves

Replication and establishment of latency

Antegrade transport of infectious virus particles to other epithelial surfaces along peripheral sensory nerves

Replication in the epithelium, producing vesicles. Immunocompetent hosts are usually able to contain virus infection at this point, although infection may spread to contiguous skin surfaces.

utility include in situ and dot-blot hybridization, as well as DNA amplification by polymerase chain reaction. The potential for DNA amplification is significant, owing to its ability to detect small amounts of specific genomic material. However, its applicability to diagnostic assays is not well defined at the present time. A concern of many investigators is the specificity of these reactions owing to the possible amplification of contaminant DNA, which leads to false-positive results.

In addition to new tests for virus gene products and viral DNA, improved serologic assays are also becoming available. However, these tests are useful only for making a diagnosis in retrospect.

CLINICAL MANIFESTATIONS. *Mucocutaneous Infections.* **Gingivostomatitis.** Gingivostomatitis, which is usually caused by HSV-1, occurs most frequently in children less than 5 years of age. This illness is characterized by fever, sore throat, pharyngeal edema, and erythema, followed by the development of vesicular

or ulcerative lesions on the oral and pharyngeal mucosa. Recurrent HSV-1 infections of the oropharynx are most frequently manifest as herpes simplex labialis (cold sores) and usually appear on the vermillion border of the lip (Fig. 371–5). Intraoral lesions as a manifestation of recurrent disease are uncommon.

Genital Herpes. Genital herpes is most frequently caused by HSV-2. Primary infection in women usually involves the vulva, vagina, and cervix. In men, initial infection is most often associated with lesions on the glans penis, prepuce, or penile shaft. In individuals of either sex, primary disease is associated with fever, malaise, anorexia, and bilateral inguinal adenopathy. Women frequently have dysuria and urinary retention due to urethral involvement. As many as 10 per cent of individuals develop an aseptic meningitis with primary infection. Sacral radiculomyelitis may occur in both men and women, resulting in neuralgias, urinary retention, or obstipation. The complete healing of primary

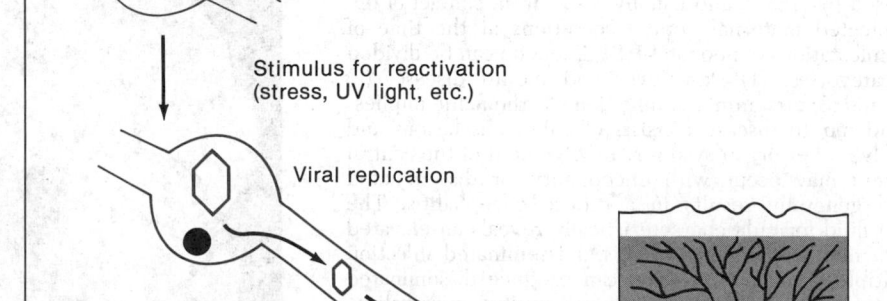

FIGURE 371–4. Schematic diagram of HSV latency and reactivation.

Dorsal Root Ganglia

Latent viral genome (may be integrated or extrachromosomal)

Stimulus for reactivation (stress, UV light, etc.)

Viral replication

Transport along peripheral sensory nerves

Replication in the epithelium with the production of vesicles

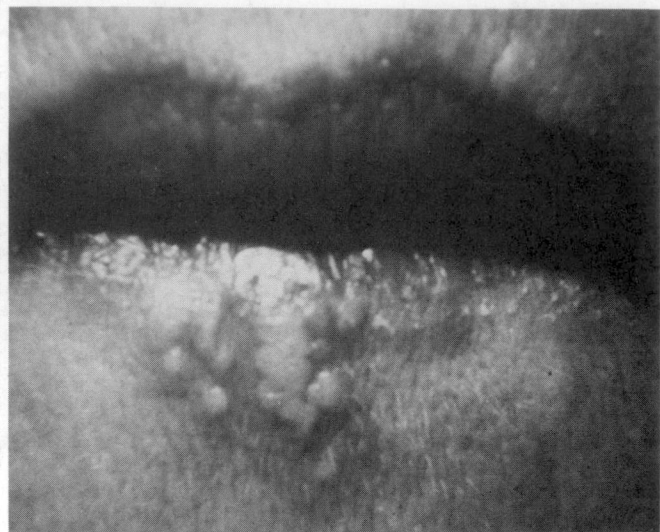

FIGURE 371–5. Herpes simplex labialis.

infection may take several weeks. It has been recognized that the first episode of genital infection is less severe in individuals who have had previous HSV-1 infections at other sites, namely herpes simplex labialis. Antibodies to HSV-1 appear to have an ameliorative effect on the expression of HSV-2 clinical disease.

Recurrent genital infections in either men or women can be particularly distressing. The frequency of recurrence varies significantly from one individual to another. It has been estimated that one third of individuals with genital herpes have virtually no recurrences, one third have approximately three recurrences per year, and another third have more than three per year. Seroepidemiologic studies have found that between 25 and 65 per cent of individuals in the United States in 1978 had antibodies to HSV-2 and that seroprevalence is correlated with the number of sexual partners.

Herpetic Keratitis. Herpes simplex keratitis is usually caused by HSV-1 and is accompanied by conjunctivitis in many cases. It is considered the most common infectious cause of blindness in the United States. The characteristic lesions of herpes simplex keratoconjunctivitis are dendritic ulcers best detected by fluorescein staining. Deep stromal involvement has also been reported and may result in visual impairment.

Other Cutaneous Manifestations. Herpes simplex virus infections can manifest at any skin site. Common among health care workers are lesions on abraded skin of the fingers, known as herpetic whitlows. Similarly, wrestlers, because of physical contact, may develop disseminated cutaneous lesions known as herpes gladiatorum.

Neonatal Herpes Simplex Virus Infection. Neonatal HSV infection is estimated to occur in approximately one in 3500 deliveries in the United States each year. Approximately 70 per cent of cases are caused by HSV-2 and usually result from contact of the fetus with infected maternal genital secretions at the time of delivery. Manifestations of neonatal HSV infection can be divided into three categories: (1) skin, eye, and mouth disease, (2) encephalitis, and (3) disseminated infection. As the name implies, skin, eye, and mouth disease consists of cutaneous lesions and does not involve other organ systems. Involvement of the central nervous system may occur with encephalitis or disseminated infection and generally results in a diffuse encephalitis. The cerebrospinal fluid formula characteristically reveals an elevated protein and a mononuclear pleocytosis. Disseminated infection involves multiple organ systems and can produce disseminated intravascular coagulation, hemorrhagic pneumonitis, encephalitis, and cutaneous lesions. Diagnosis can be particularly difficult in the absence of skin lesions, which occur in as many as 36 per cent of cases. The mortality rate for each disease classification varies from zero for skin, eye, and mouth disease to 15 per cent for encephalitis and 60 per cent for neonates with disseminated infection, even with appropriate antiviral treatment. In addition

to the high mortality associated with these infections, morbidity is significant in that children with encephalitis or disseminated disease develop normally in only 40 per cent of cases, even with the administration of appropriate antiviral therapy.

Herpes Simplex Encephalitis. Herpes simplex encephalitis is characterized by hemorrhagic necrosis of the temporal lobe. Disease begins unilaterally, spreads to the contralateral temporal lobe, and is characterized by hemorrhagic necrosis (Fig. 371–6). It is the most common cause of focal, sporadic encephalitis in the United States today and occurs in approximately 1 in 150,000 individuals. Most cases are caused by HSV-1. The actual pathogenesis of herpes simplex encephalitis requires further clarification, although it has been speculated that primary or recurrent virus can reach the temporal lobe by ascending neural pathways, such as the trigeminal tracts or the olfactory nerves.

Clinical manifestations of herpes simplex encephalitis include headache, fever, altered consciousness, and abnormalities of speech and behavior, findings characteristic of temporal lobe involvement. Focal seizures may also occur. The cerebrospinal fluid formula for these patients is variable but usually consists of a pleocytosis with both polymorphonuclear leukocytes and monocytes present. The protein concentration is characteristically elevated, and glucose is usually normal. A definitive diagnosis can be achieved only by brain biopsy, since other pathogens may produce a clinically similar illness. The mortality and morbidity are high, even when appropriate antiviral therapy is administered. At present, the mortality rate is approximately 30 per cent 1 year after treatment. In addition, approximately 50 per cent of survivors have moderate or severe neurologic impairment.

HERPES SIMPLEX VIRUS INFECTIONS IN THE IMMUNOCOMPROMISED HOST

Herpes simplex virus infections in the immunocompromised host are usually due to reactivation of latent infection and are clinically more severe, may be progressive, and require a longer time to heal. Manifestations of HSV infections in this patient population include pneumonitis, esophagitis, hepatitis, colitis, and disseminated cutaneous disease. Individuals suffering from human immunodeficiency virus infection may have extensive perineal or orofacial ulcerations. Herpes simplex virus infections are also noted to be of increased severity in individuals with extensive burns.

EPIDEMIOLOGY. Herpes simplex viruses are distributed worldwide and have been reported in both developed and underdeveloped countries. Animal vectors for human HSV infections have not been described, and there is no seasonal variation in the incidence of HSV infections. The virus is transmitted from infected to susceptible individuals during close personal contact, and virus must come in contact with mucosal surfaces or abraded skin for infection to be initiated. Since approximately one third of the world's population has recurrent HSV infections, and

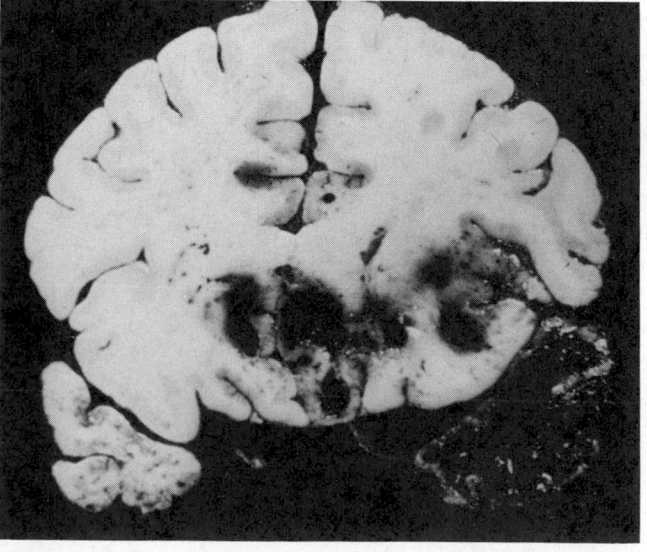

FIGURE 371–6. Hemorrhagic necrosis in herpes simplex encephalitis.

because infection is rarely fatal, a large reservoir of HSV exists in the community.

Although HSV-1 and HSV-2 are usually transmitted by different routes and involve different areas of the body, there is a great deal of overlap between the epidemiology and clinical manifestations of infections caused by these viruses. The mouth and lips are clearly the most common sites of HSV-1 infection. Primary HSV-1 infection in the young child is usually asymptomatic but may be manifest as gingivostomatitis. Primary infection in young adults has been associated with pharyngitis and sometimes a mononucleosis-like syndrome. Seroprevalence studies have demonstrated that acquisition of HSV-1 infection is related to socioeconomic factors. Antibodies, which indicate past infection, are found early in life among individuals of lower socioeconomic groups. This presumably is a consequence of crowded living conditions that provide a greater opportunity for direct contact with infected individuals. As many as 75 to 90 per cent of individuals from lower socioeconomic populations develop antibodies by the end of the first decade of life. In contrast, only 30 to 40 per cent of persons in middle and upper socioeconomic groups are seropositive by the middle of the second decade of life.

Because infections with HSV-2 are usually acquired through sexual contact, antibodies to this virus are rarely found until the onset of sexual activity. There is a progressive increase in infection rates with HSV-2 in all populations beginning in adolescence. As with HSV-1 infections, the rate of acquisition of HSV-2 infection appears related to socioeconomic factors. The number of sexual contacts is also an important risk factor for the acquisition of HSV-2. Importantly, genital herpes infection has recently been found to be a risk factor for another sexually transmitted virus, the human immunodeficiency virus (HIV).

Localized, recurrent HSV-2 infection is the most common form of HSV infection during gestation. Transmission of infection to the fetus is most frequently related to the shedding of virus at the time of delivery. Since HSV infection of the fetus is usually the consequence of contact with infected maternal genital secretions at the time of delivery, the determination of viral excretion at this time is of utmost importance. The incidence of cervical shedding in pregnant women with asymptomatic HSV infection is approximately 1 per cent. Interestingly, most infants who develop neonatal disease are born to women who are completely asymptomatic for genital HSV infections at the time of delivery and who have neither a past history of genital herpes nor a sexual partner reporting a genital vesicular rash. These women account for 60 to 80 per cent of all women whose children develop neonatal HSV infection.

PREVENTION. At present, there are no licensed vaccines directed against HSV. However, experimental vaccines for HSV-1 and HSV-2 entered phase 1 and phase 2 trials in mid-1990. Acyclovir is currently being given to recipients of solid organ and bone marrow transplants in the immediate post-transplant period in an effort to prevent reactivation of latent disease.

TREATMENT. Infections caused by HSV-1 and HSV-2 are amenable to therapy with antiviral drugs (see Ch. 359). Both vidarabine and acyclovir have proved useful for the management of specific infections caused by these viruses. At present, acyclovir is the treatment of choice for mucocutaneous HSV infections in the immunocompromised host, herpes simplex encephalitis, and neonatal herpes simplex virus infections. Intravenous administration is preferred for therapy of life-threatening disease. Intravenous acyclovir is also recommended for treatment of clinically severe initial genital herpes in the immunocompetent host. This includes patients with complications such as urinary retention or aseptic meningitis, and they should receive 5 mg per kilogram every 8 hours for 5 to 7 days. Caution must be exercised when acyclovir is used intravenously, because it may crystallize in the renal tubules when given too rapidly or to dehydrated patients.

Immunocompromised individuals with mucocutaneous HSV infections that are not life-threatening may be given oral acyclovir. Oral acyclovir is also useful in the treatment of initial genital herpes. Recurrent episodes, however, are not as responsive to acyclovir. For individuals who experience severe or frequent recurrences of genital herpes, a "suppressive" regimen of acyclovir in doses of 600 to 800 mg per day may be useful. The efficacy of acyclovir for the treatment of primary or recurrent oropharyngeal HSV in the immunocompetent host has not been well established.

Corey L, Spear P: Infections with herpes simplex viruses. N Engl J Med 314:686–691, 749–757, 1986. *This two-article series is a concise review of herpes simplex virus infections.*

Goldsmith SM, Whitley RJ: Herpes simplex encephalitis. *In* Lambert HP (ed.): Infections of the Central Nervous System. Philadelphia, B. C. Decker, 1991, pp 283–299. *This chapter describes the clinical presentations, diagnostic evaluation, and treatment of herpes simplex virus encephalitis.*

Nahmias AJ, Lee FK, Bechman-Nahmias S: Sero-epidemiological and sociological patterns of herpes simplex virus infection in the world. Scand J Inf Dis 69:19–36, 1990. *A comprehensive analysis of herpes simplex virus seroepidemiology, utilizing new techniques for HSV-2–specific antibody.*

Roizman B: Herpesviridae: A brief introduction. *In* Fields BN, Knipe DM, Chanock E, et al. (eds.): Virology, 2nd ed. New York, Raven Press, 1990, p 1787. *This chapter provides an overview of the herpes family of viruses.*

Straus SE: Clinical and biological differences between recurrent herpes simplex virus and varicella-zoster virus infections. JAMA 262:3455–3458, 1989. *A concise article that emphasizes the distinctions between recurrent herpes simplex virus infections and recurrent varicella-zoster virus infections.*

Whitley RJ: Herpes simplex viruses. *In* Fields BN, Knipe DM, Chanock E, et al. (eds.): Virology, 2nd ed. New York, Raven Press, 1990. *A comprehensive text that includes a detailed analysis of the molecular biology and clinical manifestations of herpes simplex virus.*

372 Cytomegalovirus Infection

David J. Lang

DEFINITION. Infections caused by cytomegalovirus (CMV) may be asymptomatic or may cause disseminated and even fatal multisystem disease, depending upon the mode and timing of virus acquisition and the immunocompetence of the host. CMV infections occur commonly, although with variable severity, in the fetus, the neonate, and immunocompromised individuals.

ETIOLOGY. CMV is a species-specific member of the herpesvirus group. Like other herpesviruses, CMV has the capacity to replicate persistently in the face of normal host immunity and to establish latent infections subject to reactivation. Replication of the virus in vitro yields characteristic focal cytopathology and is largely limited to cell cultures of species-specific fibroblasts. In vivo, however, CMV replicates in epithelial as well as fibroblastic elements. Subtypes of CMV can be distinguished, although the variants do not seem to be associated with a unique clinical presentation.

EPIDEMIOLOGY. CMV is worldwide in distribution, and infection shows no seasonal preference. Persistence, latency, and reactivation of CMV make it difficult to interpret the etiologic significance of the recovery of the virus.

The age of acquisition of CMV is variable. In less developed parts of the world, CMV infection is acquired universally in infancy, probably at or shortly after parturition. Where interpersonal contact is reduced and sanitation is more advanced, acquisition of CMV infection is delayed and occurs gradually through infancy, childhood, and adulthood. Transmission of CMV is associated with close interpersonal (including sexual) contact or with direct introduction of cells or body fluids. CMV has been recovered from virtually all organs and tissues and can be found in urine, saliva, blood, semen, milk, secretions of the uterine cervix, and stool. CMV is opportunistic; it reactivates in, is transmitted to, and spreads from hosts whose defenses are compromised. Since these patients are often found in hospital settings, this virus poses a theoretic risk for nosocomial spread. However, no substantial evidence has been found for patient-to-patient or patient-to-staff transmission.

Transmission of CMV occurs with blood (estimated 5 per cent of whole-blood units) and with a proportion of organ transplants. Horizontal interpersonal transmission of CMV occurs, but not in epidemics. Young children, infected as neonates from blood or as toddlers by contact in day care centers, can serve as a source of family infection. Thus in a reversal of the usual pattern, the child attending day care may prove a risk factor for the pregnant, previously seronegative mother. Day care workers experience the acquisition of CMV infections more frequently than do matched controls. Young women working in a day care setting should be appropriately counseled about the risks of CMV infection and means to reduce that risk.

Prenatal CMV infection is the most common known congenital infection of humans. It occurs in about 1 per cent of infants born in the United States (0.5 to 8 per cent depending upon the population studied). Most of these infections reflect prenatal transmission of CMV reactivated during pregnancy in otherwise healthy immune women. As many as 30 per cent of pregnant women may shed CMV at some time and from some site during pregnancy.

PATHOGENESIS AND PATHOLOGY. CMV replicates slowly in vitro. Infected cells swell and develop characteristic intranuclear and paranuclear inclusions. CMV infections in vitro are accompanied by some changes associated with morphologic transformation. It has been possible to transform cells permanently by infecting with irradiated virus and in this way interfering selectively with the full cycle of virus replication and cytopathology. These CMV-transformed cells have malignant potential in certain animals. Whether CMV plays a role in the pathogenesis of malignancy in humans is unresolved.

CMV can and frequently does reactivate in immune hosts. When immune function is immature or compromised, reactivated virus can spread, causing significant injury and functional impairment. The pathogenesis of transplacental spread in the presence of intact maternal immunity remains unclear.

That CMV is carried in circulating cells of healthy individuals appears certain on the basis of epidemiologic observations. Nevertheless, it has been difficult to recover this virus from the circulating cells of healthy individuals. The use of CMV antibody–negative blood units has been recommended for transfusion in high-risk groups such as selected newborns (especially premature infants) and patients with compromised cell-mediated immunity (including those on chemotherapy and allograft recipients). There is evidence that certain blood filters can substantially reduce the risk of CMV transmission with transfusions.

CLINICAL MANIFESTATIONS. Postnatal CMV Infection in Normal Hosts. In healthy individuals CMV infection is usually asymptomatic or unrecognized. Occasionally primary CMV infection is accompanied by a self-limited, mononucleosis-like syndrome characterized by fever, splenomegaly, mild hepatocellular dysfunction, lymphoid hyperplasia (including the presence of atypical lymphocytes), occasional thrombocytopenia, hemolysis, and inconsistent skin rash. Pharyngitis may occur. The fever may range from 39°C to over 40°C and in some instances is accompanied by night sweats and chills. Between febrile episodes the patient, although tired, does not feel very ill.

Some cases of mild to moderate hepatitis have been associated with CMV infection, and infrequently a normal host experiences an interstitial pneumonitis caused by this virus. There have been reports associating prior CMV infection with the Guillain-Barré syndrome. CMV infections have also been associated with isolated thrombocytopenia, hemolytic anemia, and ulcerative gastrointestinal disease.

Postnatal CMV Infection in Abnormal Hosts. Individuals undergoing open heart surgery requiring perfusion and others receiving multiple units of blood may experience a mononucleosis-like illness about 3 to 6 weeks later. The illness can be mistaken for bacterial sepsis or endocarditis, a particularly important distinction in recipients of cardiac prostheses.

CMV infections have been a major problem for allograft recipients. Latent virus may be reactivated in connection with the response to the allograft (either host-versus-graft or graft-versus-host). Immunosuppression limits the ability of the host to restrict virus spread. CMV infections may enhance graft rejection, although the mechanism mediating this process remains uncertain. CMV infections have been prominently associated with bone marrow transplantation (BMT), and CMV interstitial pneumonitis has been an important cause of mortality following BMT. Viremia has been shown to be predictive of clinical disease in BMT recipients. CMV infections occur frequently among recipients of all forms of allograft, and infection can be associated with interstitial pneumonitis, hepatitis, encephalitis, retinitis, and diffuse cytomegalic inclusion disease. Both newly acquired (from transplant, blood cell components, or both) and endogenous (reactivated in host) CMV infections occur. The progress and effect of these infections may be mediated by direct cytopathology or by immunopathologic mechanisms.

CMV infections are very common among male homosexuals and have been found prominently in the acquired immunodeficiency syndrome (AIDS), which occurs in response to infection with human immunodeficiency virus (HIV). Evidence indicates that reciprocal interactions may exist between CMV and HIV infections such that CMV may transactivate HIV and HIV infections may be associated with reactivation of CMV. Overall, CMV infections associated with AIDS are likely to be opportunistic, although since CMV infections are often associated with some depression of the helper-suppressor T-cell ratio, as well as suppression of natural killer (NK) cell activity and depression of T-cell proliferation, the precise distinction between cause and effect, opportunism and pathogenesis, remains to be elucidated. Much of the morbidity and some mortality associated with AIDS has been ascribed to CMV infections of the liver, brain (associated with glial nodules), gastrointestinal tract (ulcerative lesions), lungs (diffuse interstitial pneumonitis often coexisting with *Pneumocystis carinii* infection), and eyes (retinitis).

It has been proposed that CMV may play a role in atherogenesis, and supportive epidemiologic data have been presented. CMV infections can be shown to infect and injure endothelial cells of arterial walls, and it has been hypothesized that this may be followed by local cellular proliferation, injury, and cholesterol deposition.

Prenatal and Perinatal CMV Infection. Prenatal CMV infections were first appreciated through retrospective pathologic studies, and it was initially concluded that these infections were rare and always fatal. The severe, disseminated infection was termed *cytomegalic inclusion disease* (CID). Subsequently, cytologic and virologic techniques identified CMV infection in living infants, and it became apparent that infants congenitally infected with CMV could survive. In some cases these infected infants exhibited intracerebral calcifications, hepatosplenomegaly, chorioretinitis, thrombocytopenia with purpura, macular rash, hemolytic anemia, and a variety of structural and functional organ impairments.

Prospective studies determined that congenital infections with CMV were not rare. Overall, about 1 per cent of babies were found to be prenatally infected with CMV. Women who are immune prior to conception may give birth to CMV-infected infants. The birth to a woman of more than one CMV-infected infant with identical viral strains has been documented. Most prenatal CMV infections are acquired from latent maternal virus reactivated during gestation, and most CMV-infected infants appear normal at birth. Nonetheless, as many as 10 to 20 per cent of these apparently healthy babies ultimately display learning disabilities, hearing impairment, or evidence of cognitive dysfunction. In contrast, primary maternal infection during pregnancy, a much less common event, is associated in some cases with devastating CID.

Perinatal acquisition of CMV infection (from infected cervix, breast milk, or saliva) is usually asymptomatic. However, an infant born to a CMV-seronegative woman may develop significant postnatal pneumonia or hepatitis if infected with CMV via transfusion. This is a particularly important risk among markedly premature infants who may acquire no maternal immunoglobulins.

DIAGNOSIS. The laboratory isolation of CMV is accomplished in tissue culture and requires the prompt transportation of refrigerated specimens to a prepared virus laboratory. Weeks can be required for recovery and identification of virus. However, although the evolution of cytopathology may be slow, some viral antigens appear rapidly (hours) in inoculated cells. Furthermore, CMV replication in cell culture can be enhanced by centrifugation of specimens on monolayers in shell vials. The use of monoclonal antibodies to early CMV antigens, coupled with labeled antiglobulin preparations applied to inoculated centrifuged shell vials, can provide rapid and specific virus detection. The recovery of cloned subgenomic fragments of CMV DNA has permitted detection of CMV directly and specifically by hybridization procedures. Currently the polymerase chain reaction (PCR) is being explored as a means for rapid and specific CMV isolation and identification.

Regardless of the technique used, occasional prolonged shedding of virus and the intermittent reactivation of latent CMV can confuse the interpretation of virus recovery. The isolation of

CMV at certain times (from urine taken during the first days of life) or from unusual sites (blood, spinal fluid, or tissues specifically involved in the disease process) makes the etiologic association of virus and clinical condition more likely. Demonstration of simultaneous seroconversion or significant (fourfold or greater) serologic change further strengthens the association. CMV serology may be assessed by complement fixation, immunofluorescence, and enzyme-linked immunosorbent assay (ELISA) procedures. The detection of CMV-specific IgM serology is useful to identify recent infections.

DIFFERENTIAL DIAGNOSIS. Postnatally acquired CMV infections in normal hosts may be difficult to distinguish from those caused by Epstein-Barr virus (EBV). However, EBV mononucleosis is often associated with a positive heterophil-agglutination reaction, whereas CMV mononucleosis is always heterophil-negative. CMV mononucleosis tends to occur in older individuals and is associated with more prominent fever and night sweats and less adenopathy than EBV mononucleosis. Hepatitis associated with CMV infection is generally milder than that associated with hepatitis A, B, or C or other hepatitis viruses. The ultimate distinction between these conditions depends upon the results of virus-specific tests.

CMV interstitial pneumonitis, similar to that caused by *Pneumocystis carinii*, cannot be identified on clinical grounds alone but requires the use of virologic studies applied to clinical samples, especially those from lung biopsies, needle aspirations, bronchoscopy, and bronchoalveolar lavage. Accurate and rapid identification of CMV infections may be made in these specimens by application of histologic and cytologic techniques as well as by procedures employing monoclonal antibodies, immunofluorescence, DNA hybridization, and PCR.

Congenital infections caused by toxoplasmosis, rubella, syphilis, and herpes simplex virus (HSV) may be difficult to distinguish from those caused by CMV. All may be associated with intrauterine growth retardation, hepatic and splenic enlargement, purpura, thrombocytopenia, and hemolysis. Congenital toxoplasmosis can be associated as well with chorioretinitis and intracerebral calcifications.

Congenital rubella is associated with glaucoma, microphthalmia, cataracts, and cardiac malformations more frequently than is congenital CMV infection. The retinitis of congenital rubella, unlike that of CMV, is often marked by punctate retinal pigmentation.

HSV can be transmitted transplacentally, although usually neonatal HSV infection reflects perinatal acquisition. HSV infections are often associated with vesicular skin lesions, although systemic visceral and central nervous system infection may occur without rash.

In all of these instances the distinctions are made ultimately by laboratory studies. Specific IgM determinations are available for CMV, toxoplasmosis, rubella, and HSV. The presence of a positive test for specific IgM to only one of these agents is usually diagnostic. The recovery of the specific agent in the case of CMV, rubella, or HSV is also a rigorous means of identification. Differentiation of all of these conditions is important, since specific treatment is available for HSV and toxoplasmosis, and specific anti-CMV therapy is becoming available and is already applicable in some clinical settings. The distinction between congenital syphilis and bacterial sepsis, other potentially confusing entities in the neonate, is also important to facilitate specific therapy.

PROGNOSIS. Among individuals with acquired CMV infections, the prognosis depends upon the immune status of the host. In otherwise healthy persons, acquired CMV infections are self-limited and generally not associated with late complications. Among immunocompromised individuals, including patients with AIDS, those with disseminated neoplasms, and transplant recipients, the outlook may vary from those who recover, maintain (allograft) function, and are without sequelae, to those who die with progressive interstitial pneumonitis. Disseminated CMV may also predispose to significant life-threatening bacterial infections.

The outlook for normal development is variable in infants who are infected prenatally with CMV. Even among those with apparently symptomless congenital CMV infections, by school age as many as 20 per cent may manifest significant sensorineural dysfunction.

TREATMENT. Until recently, a variety of nucleoside analogues, other antiviral drugs, transfer factor, antiserum, and steroids have been administered in an effort to treat CMV infections without any conclusive success. The most that was achieved was the transient depression of virus titer without alteration of the clinical condition or ultimate course of the virus infection. The intensive use of interferon in renal transplant recipients has reduced the shedding of virus and apparently improved the associated clinical conditions. Withdrawal of immunosuppression has been used as a means to control CMV infections in allograft recipients. Recent preliminary studies have shown improvement in some immunodeficient patients with severe CMV infections when treated with 9-(1,3 dihydroxy-2-propoxymethyl) guanine (DHPG). Those who received DHPG for retinitis or gastrointestinal disease fared better than did patients with CMV pneumonitis. Foscarnet, a pyrophosphate analogue, is an investigational antiviral agent that inhibits CMV DNA polymerase and is being explored as a therapeutic alternative to DHPG in CMV retinitis. Concomitant treatment with DHPG and azidothymidine (AZT) is also under study in CMV-infected AIDS patients.

PREVENTION. CMV infections have been prevented in seronegative at-risk patients (newborns, allograft recipients) by the use of CMV-seronegative blood products and allografts. The administration to BMT patients of acyclovir (given to prevent HSV and varicella-zoster virus infections) has been shown to reduce the risk of CMV-associated disease and to improve survival. The use of CMV-specific intravenous immunoglobulin with and without DHPG has been associated in some studies with the reduction of CMV-associated symptoms in BMT recipients. Attenuated CMV vaccine strains have been produced in England, the United States, and France. These candidate vaccine strains have been administered to volunteers, including health care workers, and to some individuals prior to allograft. The vaccines are immunogenic and have not been associated with detectable virus shedding or reactivation. Inoculated individuals who later received transplants and were immunosuppressed did nevertheless experience CMV reinfection and associated virus shedding but seemed to have fewer sequelae of the infections.

Since evidence indicates that immunity does ameliorate, if not prevent, prenatal and postnatal CMV infections, and since some questions and concerns are associated with the production and use of attenuated CMV strains, attention is also being directed to the development of subunit and peptide immunogens.

Emanuel D: Treatment of cytomegalovirus disease. Semin Hematol 27(2)(Suppl 1):22–27; discussion 28–29, 1990. *Review of the treatment of CMV infections especially as they impact bone marrow transplantation.*

Ho M: Cytomegalovirus: Biology and Infection. New York, Plenum Publishing Corporation, 1982. *Treatise covering all aspects of CMV infection in humans. Small but thorough section pertinent to murine CMV. Very comprehensive bibliography.*

Jacobson MA, Mills J: Serious cytomegalovirus disease in the acquired immunodeficiency syndrome (AIDS). Clinical findings, diagnosis, and treatment. Ann Intern Med 108(4):585–594, 1988. *Experience with CMV-associated disease in patients with AIDS. Attention is given to therapeutic modalities, current and anticipated.*

Melnick JL, Adam E, DeBakey ME: Possible role of cytomegalovirus in atherogenesis. JAMA 263:2204–2207, 1990. *Hypothesis and review of evidence for the role of CMV in atherogenesis.*

Meyers JD, Reed EC, Shepp DH, et al: Acyclovir for prevention of cytomegalovirus infection and disease after allogeneic marrow transplantation. N Engl J Med 318:70–75, 1988. *Demonstration that prophylaxis with intravenous acyclovir significantly reduces the risk of CMV infection and disease and improves survival.*

Meyers JD: Management of cytomegalovirus infection. Am J Med 85(2A):102–106, 1988. *Management of CMV infections among immunocompromised patients from a center with extensive experience.*

Meyers JD, Ljungman P, Fisher LD: Cytomegalovirus excretion as a predictor of cytomegalovirus disease after marrow transplantation: Importance of cytomegalovirus viremia. J Infect Dis 162:373–380, 1990. *This study demonstrates that viremia in bone marrow transplant recipients is predictive of clinical disease.*

Pass RF: Daycare centers and transmission of cytomegalovirus: New insight into an old problem. Semin Pediatr Infect Dis 1:245–251, 1990. *A current review with complete discussion of background, mechanisms, means for control, and a complete reference list.*

Rubin RH (ed.): Cytomegalovirus infections: Epidemiology, diagnosis, and treatment strategies. Rev Infect Dis 12(Suppl 7):S691–S860, 1990. *An up-to-date series of reviews.*

373 Infectious Mononucleosis (Epstein-Barr Virus Infection)

Elliott D. Kieff

DEFINITION. Infectious mononucleosis is a clinical syndrome characterized by malaise, fever, pharyngitis, pharyngeal lymphatic hyperplasia, lymphadenopathy, atypical lymphocytosis, and heterophil antibody. The syndrome occurs most commonly in adolescents and young adults.

ETIOLOGY. Primary Epstein-Barr virus (EBV) infection is the cause of almost all typical infectious mononucleosis syndromes. EBV is a herpesvirus. In vitro, it infects only human B lymphocytes. Virus infection results in B lymphocyte proliferation and immunoglobulin secretion. EBV usually remains latent in the infected B lymphocyte.

EPIDEMIOLOGY. The usual mode of EBV infection is oropharyngeal inoculation. Virus in saliva from infected persons is infectious in nonimmune persons. Infection in infancy commonly results from eating food premasticated by an infected mother, whereas infection in adolescents or adults is usually from salivary transfer during kissing. Virus survival in expectorated saliva is probably brief, since infection does not spread to susceptible roommates. Spread among young children sharing toys has not been studied.

Following salivary inoculation, the virus replicates in oropharyngeal epithelial cells, including salivary gland epithelium. Although the amount of virus in saliva is highest in the months following primary infection, virus replication in the oropharynx persists indefinitely. EBV has also been found in cervical secretions, suggesting hematogenous dissemination to other epithelial surfaces. In the course of primary oropharyngeal infection, EBV infects tonsillar and peripheral blood B lymphocytes. Virus persists indefinitely in a small fraction of the peripheral blood B lymphocytes. Transfusion of whole blood, bone marrow, blood fractions, or tissue containing viable B lymphocytes to susceptible (nonimmune) persons may result in symptomatic primary infection. Following bone marrow transplantation, the donor's virus may predominate in the recipient, indicating that a bone marrow or blood cell is a site of persistent or latent infection. Previously infected normal persons are immune to the development of infectious mononucleosis. In less industrialized societies or among lower socioeconomic groups in industrialized societies, most children experience primary infection in the first decade of life. Among middle and higher socioeconomic groups, primary infection usually occurs as a consequence of adolescent or postadolescent kissing. More than 90 per cent of adults in all human populations have serologic evidence of EBV infections and are carriers. Although EBV infection is limited to humans, each Old World primate species is endemically infected with a related virus characteristic of that species. New World primates are free of EBV-related viruses and can be experimentally infected. Experimental infection of some species with a sufficient EBV inoculum results in acutely fatal lymphoproliferation.

CLINICAL MANIFESTATIONS. The syndrome of infectious mononucleosis was a distinctive clinical entity for at least 40 years before the discovery of its etiologic agent. After a 2- to 5-week incubation period, most infected nonimmune adolescents and young adults develop malaise, fever, pharyngitis, and lymphadenopathy lasting from one to several weeks. Temperatures may reach 40°C. Tonsillar or cervical lymph nodes may be quite enlarged, painful, and tender. Laboratory findings include a relative or absolute lymphocytosis and a high titer of heterophil antibody to horse or ox red blood cells. A substantial fraction of the peripheral lymphocytes is an atypical large cell with unusually abundant cytoplasm, large pale nucleus, and variable nuclear shape. Other common manifestations include splenomegaly (50 per cent), mild hepatitis or hepatomegaly (20 per cent), headache (20 per cent), vomiting (20 per cent), jaundice (5 per cent), palatal petechiae, skin rash (4 per cent), and albuminuria (10 per cent). Less frequent (0.5 to 1 per cent) manifestations include cough,

pneumonitis, neck stiffness, aseptic meningitis, cerebritis, cerebellar dysfunction, mono- or polyneuritis, transverse myelitis, Guillain-Barré syndrome, uveitis, subcapsular splenic hemorrhage or rupture, myocarditis, pericarditis, cardiac conduction abnormalities, diarrhea, hemolytic anemia with anti-I antibody, thrombocytopenia, agranulocytosis, pancytopenia, or a hemophagocytic syndrome. Malaise or weakness may recur over several months. Rashes are significantly more common in patients with primary EBV infection receiving penicillin or ampicillin treatment than in untreated patients or patients with other diseases who are treated with penicillin. Persistence of illness beyond several months is unusual. Almost all normal people completely recover from acute infectious mononucleosis. Persistent hematalogic, neurologic, or cardiac abnormalities are rare.

Outside of the adolescent and young adult populations, primary EBV infection frequently does not result in the full infectious mononucleosis syndrome. In younger children, fever and pharyngitis from primary EBV infection may be clinically indistinguishable from upper respiratory tract infections caused by other viruses, mycoplasma, or streptococci. At any age cerebritis, neuritis, pneumonitis, hepatitis, carditis, or autoimmune hemolytic anemia or thrombocytopenia may be the predominant clinical manifestation. Atypical lymphocytosis or heterophil antibody may be less prominent or absent.

Severe, progressive, and sometimes fatal primary EBV infections occur in children with X-linked lymphoproliferative disease (Duncan's syndrome). Non–X-linked, sporadic cases also occur. Although these children have no obvious pre-existing immune deficiency, primary EBV infection leads to massive lymphoproliferation, fever, anemia, hepatitis, or fulminant hepatic necrosis. The proliferating B lymphocytes are EBV-infected cells that express EBV latent infection associated proteins. The early proliferation is polyclonal. Fulminant hepatic failure is a frequent cause of death. Recovery may be accompanied by persistent anemia, hypogammaglobulinemia, or pancytopenia. Some patients present with agammaglobulinemia, anemia, or pancytopenia. Oligoclonal or uniclonal EBV-infected B lymphomas may occur during primary infection or after recovery. Similar illnesses occur in other immunosuppressed patients with primary EBV infection. The administration of high-dose cyclosporine as part of immunosuppressive regimens for organ or bone marrow transplantation has also been associated with severe EBV infection. Moreover, children with human immunodeficiency virus (HIV) infection are also at risk for severe EBV infection and lymphoproliferative disease (see Ch. 419). Lymphocytic interstitial pneumonitis may be prominent in such patients. In AIDS patients, replicating EBV has also been found in hairy leukoplakia of the tongue, a proliferative epithelial lesion.

Rare cases of chronic progressive primary EBV infection in young adults have been well documented. These patients have severe acute mononucleosis which persists, with clinical manifestations that include lymphadenopathy or visceral organ involvement and abnormally high antibody titers to EBV replicative cycle antigens. Some patients have lacked antibody to EBV nuclear antigens. Most patients eventually recover without specific treatment. In one patient, acycloguanosine treatment produced a clinical remission. Persistent active EBV infection was initially proposed to be the cause of a more common chronic mononucleosis or chronic fatigue syndrome. This syndrome is characterized by recurrent episodes of malaise and weakness, sometimes accompanied by myalgias, arthralgias, pharyngitis, lymphadenitis, or mild fever. Careful documentation of the lack of significant objective clinical or laboratory abnormalities distinguishes most patients with this poorly defined syndrome from those with known infectious, autoimmune, oncologic, metabolic, or neurologic diseases. EBV-specific antibody titers in most patients with the chronic fatigue syndrome do not differ significantly from those of normal infected adults (see below). Thus, there is little to support the initial hypothesis that EBV is a frequent cause of this syndrome.

Longstanding EBV infection is associated with B lymphomas in immunosuppressed patients, with Burkitt-type lymphoma in African children, and with anaplastic nasopharyngeal carcinoma. A substantial fraction of B lymphomas occurring in immunocompromised patients have EBV DNA in the tumor cells. In B lymphomas in which the virus is latent in all of the tumor cells, the virus probably provided an initial stimulus for cell proliferation. Malignant conversion in these late postinfection lymphomas requires at least one additional factor, since these cells also have a chromosome translocation that enhances c-*myc* oncogene expression. In a prospective study of African children, a correlation was noted between the EBV antibody response in the years between infection and tumor onset and the Burkitt tumor incidence, suggesting that the extent of EBV replication is an important parameter in tumor induction. In retrospective and prospective clinical studies, high levels of IgA antibody to EBV antigens have been closely associated with anaplastic nasopharyngeal carcinoma. EBV has also been uniformly found in each of the tumor cells of anaplastic nasopharyngeal carcinomas. The uniclonality of the virus genomes in these tumor cells indicates that the tumors arise in a single virus-infected cell. The virus is, therefore, likely to be necessary for this oncogenic conversion. Chinese and some native North American populations have a high incidence of nasopharyngeal carcinoma. Other factors in the pathogenesis of nasopharyngeal carcinoma have not been defined.

PATHOLOGY AND PATHOGENESIS. EBV first infects pharyngeal epithelial cells and then spreads to subepithelial circulating B lymphocytes. Infection may be confined to epithelial and B lymphocyte tissues, since only these cells have EBV receptors. The EBV receptor is also the receptor for the C3d fragment of complement. Tonsils and regional and systemic lymph nodes enlarge because of follicular hyperplasia, due in part to virus-infected B lymphocytes, and, because of infiltration of sinuses and paracortex with reactive, atypical T lymphocytes. Loss of normal architecture and the presence of Reed-Sternberg–like cells may make EBV infection difficult to distinguish from Hodgkin's disease. Similar changes occur in the spleen. In patients with significant hepatitis, hepatic lobules or portal areas may be infiltrated with mononuclear cells. The bone marrow is usually unaffected. Early in the illness, up to 1 or 2 per cent of the circulating leukocytes may be EBV-infected B lymphocytes. The predominant atypical lymphocyte in the peripheral blood, however, is a reactive T cell. EBV-infected B lymphocytes can be detected by their expression of EBV nuclear proteins (EBNA's) or by their ability to proliferate continuously in vitro or in SCID mice, a property that normal B lymphocytes lack. EBV infection of B lymphocytes stimulates both B-cell proliferation and Ig secretion, particularly IgM.

Lymphoproliferation following EBV infection of normal B lymphocytes in vitro is associated with the expression of six EBNA proteins, two membrane proteins (LMP's), and two small RNA's. The same repertoire of genes appears to be expressed in EBV-associated lymphoproliferative diseases. In vivo, primary infection results in transient hypergammaglobulinemia. The hypergammaglobulinemia results from direct and indirect effects of virus infection on B lymphocytes. The induction of antibodies that react with a heterologous erythrocyte glycoprotein antigen is the basis for the heterophil test. The pre-existence of B lymphocytes with heterophil antibody specificity remains an enigma, perhaps explainable by cross-reactivity of some of these antibodies with bacterial polysaccharides. The acute, non–B lymphocyte response to EBV infection is multifunctional. Some T lymphocytes suppress both B lymphocyte proliferation and Ig secretion. Other peripheral blood T lymphocytes and natural killer cells from patients with infectious mononucleosis are cytotoxic to autologous EBV-infected B cells. The cytotoxic T lymphocytes are largely CD8+ and recognize EBNA or LMP epitopes in the context of class I histocompatibility molecules. Other T lymphocytes may augment the T and B lymphocyte immune responses. Two EBV types are endemic in humans. These two types differ in their EBNA proteins and in their ability to transform B lymphocytes in vitro. Some cytotoxic T lymphocyte clones are specific for EBNA proteins. Some of these EBNA-specific cytotoxic T lymphocytes recognize only the EBNA protein of one virus type.

After recovery from acute infectious mononucleosis, the proportion of circulating B lymphocytes infected with EBV is one in 10^5 to 10^6. Latently infected B lymphocytes or B-lymphocyte precursors are likely to be the site of virus persistence, since long-term suppression of virus replication with antiviral chemotherapy does not decrease the number of circulating EBV-infected B lymphocytes; and following bone marrow transplantation, the donor's rather than the recipient's virus may persist. T lymphocytes also circulate which can suppress or kill HLA-related EBV-

infected cells that express EBNA's or LMP's. EBV-infected B lymphocytes and reactive T cells circulate in the peripheral blood indefinitely after primary infection. Cyclosporine indirectly inhibits the EBV-specific T lymphocyte immune response, thereby enabling EBV-infected B lymphocytes to overgrow in transplantation recipients receiving high doses of cyclosporine and other immunosuppressive drugs. In this patient group EBV-associated lymphoproliferative diseases have been a significant, albeit unusual, problem.

DIAGNOSIS. In normal adolescents, the diagnosis of acute infectious mononucleosis can usually be made on clinical grounds and confirmed by the laboratory findings of atypical lymphocytosis and heterophil antibody to ox or horse erythrocytes. Bacterial throat culture should be done in patients with significant pharyngitis to exclude concomitant β-hemolytic streptococcal infection. The rapid heterophil tests are more than 95 per cent sensitive and more than 95 per cent specific in an adolescent or young adult population. Titers are substantially diminished by 3 months after primary infection and not detectable by 6 months. In patients with equivocal or absent heterophil antibodies, EBV-specific serologic testing should be done. The differential diagnosis may include streptococcal (pharyngeal) or gonococcal infection, cytomegalovirus, hepatitis virus A or B, HIV, HHV6, adenovirus, or toxoplasma infection, leukemia, and lymphoma. Most heterophil-negative infectious mononucleosis with pharyngitis is also caused by EBV. In the absence of pharyngitis, however, cytomegalovirus, toxoplasmosis, hepatitis virus, or HIV infections are likely causes of heterophil-negative or low-titer heterophil-positive infectious mononucleosis. In some patient populations, acute HIV infection is a significant cause of typical or atypical infectious mononucleosis syndromes. HIV antigen or nucleotide sequence–specific detection may be necessary to diagnose HIV infection early in the illness. Later, seroconversion may establish the diagnosis.

Specific serologic testing for EBV infection involves determining antibody titers to latently infected (anti-EBNA), early replication cycle (anti-EA), or late replication cycle (anti-VCA) viral proteins. This is usually done by indirect immunofluorescence microscopy or by enzyme-linked immunoassay. With acute primary infection, EA and IgM VCA titers are high and IgG VCA and EBNA titers are low. Patients recovering from primary infection have lower EA or IgM VCA titers, higher IgG VCA titer, and low EBNA titer. After several months, EA and IgM VCA titers are low or negative, whereas IgG VCA and EBNA titers are high. The high IgG VCA and EBNA titers frequently persist for many years. Those rare patients with chronically progressive EBV infection tend to have abnormally high titers of antibodies to some or many EBV antigens. On the other hand, serologic diagnosis may be misleading in immunosuppressed patients, including children with X-linked immunodeficiency. These infected children may have high or low antibody titers. EBV serologies are helpful in following patients with anaplastic nasopharyngeal carcinoma or in screening for early detection of this malignancy in high-risk populations. Patients at risk for primary anaplastic nasopharyngeal carcinoma or for recurrences have high IgG or IgA EA antibody titers.

TREATMENT. No treatment is necessary for most EBV infections. Rest during the period of acute symptoms and slow return to normal activity are commonly advised, although the therapeutic efficacy of this regimen has not been firmly established. Patients with splenomegaly should restrict their involvement in sports to avoid traumatic rupture. Acetaminophen or aspirin may be used to reduce temperature and pharyngeal pain. Very brief courses of glucocorticoid treatment (e.g., 60 mg prednisone per day for 4 days followed by rapidly decreasing doses) have been effective in shrinking obstructing tonsils, probably by ameliorating an overactive T-cell response. Autoimmune hemolytic anemia, granulocytopenia, and thrombocytopenia usually respond to longer courses of glucocorticoid therapy. The use of glucocorticoids for other manifestations of EBV infection is less certain to be beneficial. Glucocorticoids have no antiviral activity and are contraindicated in most herpesvirus infections. A few patients with severe hemorrhagic thrombocytopenia refractory to glucocorticoids have responded to intravenous immunoglobulin. Early plasmapheresis is indicated in patients with Guillain-Barré syndrome. Acycloguanosine and its derivatives have activity against EBV in vitro but are not approved for use against EBV. These drugs should not be used in normal patients with EBV infections but can be considered for AIDS patients with oral hairy leukoplakia or for patients with well-documented chronically progressive EBV infection. Acycloguanosine has not affected the outcome of EBV-associated lymphoproliferative syndromes in immunosuppressed patients. No effect on EBV DNA in latently infected cells has been seen. Partial restoration of immune function by lowering immune suppression has been beneficial. In one patient with X-linked lymphoproliferative disease, recombinant interferon-γ produced a rapid clinical remission.

Duncombe AS, Amos RJ, Metcalfe P, Pearson TC: Intravenous immunoglobulin therapy in thrombocytopenic infectious mononucleosis. Clin Lab Haematol 11(1):11–15, 1989. *Effect of Ig in two cases of refractory hemorrhagic thrombocytopenia.*

Ernber I, Andersson J: Acyclovir efficiently inhibits oropharyngeal excretion of Epstein-Barr virus in patients with acute infectious mononucleosis. J Gen Virol 67:2267–2272, 1986. *Effect of acycloguanosine on EBV infection.*

Kieff E, Liebowitz D: Epstein-Barr virus and its replication. *In* Fields B, Knipe D (eds.): Virology, 2nd ed. New York, Raven Press, 1990, pp 1889–1920. *Review of the biochemistry of Epstein-Barr virus and its effect on lymphocytes.*

Miller G: Epstein-Barr virus: Biology, pathogenesis and medical aspects. *In* Fields B, Knipe D (eds.): Virology, 2nd ed. New York, Raven Press, 1990, pp 1921–1958. *Review of EBV-associated diseases.*

Schooley RT, Carey RW, Miller G, et al.: Chronic Epstein-Barr virus infection associated with fever and interstitial pneumonitis. Clinical and serologic features and response to antiviral chemotherapy. Ann Intern Med 104:636–643, 1986. *Illustrative case of chronic EBV.*

374 Varicella

Philip A. Brunell

DEFINITION. Varicella, or chickenpox, is an acute communicable disease characterized by a generalized vesicular rash. Because it is highly contagious, most individuals contract it in childhood. Herpes zoster, due to reactivation of varicella-zoster virus (VZV), is a dermatomal cutaneous eruption (see Ch. 476.3).

ETIOLOGY. Varicella is caused by VZV, a member of the α-herpesvirinae subfamily. This enveloped herpesvirus contains at least five glycoproteins, some of which bear some homology to those of other members of the human herpesvirus group. The double-stranded DNA has a molecular weight of approximately 80 million. There is some diversity in the restriction enzyme patterns among wild isolates; there is only a single serotype. Although the human is the only known natural host, a closely related virus has been identified in a simian species.

EPIDEMIOLOGY. Varicella is a highly contagious disease. After continuing household exposure, as would occur in a family, almost all susceptibles are infected. The subclinical attack rate is believed to be no more than 4 per cent. The results of nonhousehold exposure are less certain. Although chickenpox is believed to be contagious prior to the onset of rash, this has been difficult to prove. Virus has not been isolated from respiratory secretions prior to onset of rash and is difficult to isolate following rash. Chickenpox is contagious for as long as 5 days after the appearance of the first lesion. Patients are customarily isolated for 5 days. The incubation period is usually about 14 days. Ninety-nine per cent of the cases occur 10 to 20 days following exposure. The disease is known to be spread by direct contact. Airborne spread also has been demonstrated, most notably in hospitals.

Nosocomial spread of varicella has been well documented. This has occurred room to room by airborne spread as well as by patient-to-patient or staff-to-patient contact. Adults with herpes zoster who are hospitalized are less likely to cause secondary cases of chickenpox among adult contacts than among children. The reason is that hospitalized children are more likely to be susceptible to chickenpox than hospitalized adults. Strict isolation is recommended for hospitalized patients with varicella and for children or immunocompromised adults with herpes zoster.

Adults with localized herpes zoster require less stringent isolation procedures.

Most cases of chickenpox occur in childhood. Most children contract chickenpox either in day care situations or shortly after they enter school. Fewer than 2 per cent of the cases occur following the second decade. Approximately 2.5 per cent of entering professional students were found to be seronegative. Approximately 10 per cent of hospital workers with a negative history are seronegative. Almost all individuals with a positive history are seropositive. A single attack of chickenpox usually confers lifetime immunity.

There appears to be more efficient transmission of disease in temperate than in tropical climates. The reason for this is uncertain but may be due to temperature rather than urbanization. Varicella occurs most commonly during the late winter and spring months, the peak being about in March. Sporadic cases occur into the early summer and start in late fall.

Varicella is more common than other childhood diseases during the early months of life. In this situation the disease is generally mild. Maternal antibody transferred across the placenta may not be as effective in protecting infants against this disease as are antibodies against other viruses. However, nursery outbreaks have been rare. Children who develop varicella during the early months of life, or are exposed in utero, have a greater risk of developing herpes zoster in childhood.

PATHOGENESIS. VZV produces a disseminated rash, which indicates that bloodstream distribution must have occurred. Virus has been isolated from white blood cells just prior to and during the first 1 or 2 days following the appearance of rash. After clinical recovery, the virus infection continues in the absence of clinical symptoms in a latent phase. During this time, virus deoxyribonucleic acid (DNA) or messenger ribonucleic acid (RNA) can be demonstrated in non-neuronal cells in dorsal root ganglia. The segmental distribution of herpes zoster (see Ch. 476.3), which usually occurs decades after the initial VZV infection, is consistent with a dorsal root ganglion site for the latent virus. In uncomplicated chickenpox, rises in serum transaminase levels have been demonstrated. This suggests that there is visceral involvement in the normal course of this disease.

The vesicular lesions of varicella contain a predominance of polymorphonuclear leukocytes even during the early phase of vesicle formation. Multinuclear giant cells are occasionally found in the base of the lesions, often containing eosinophilic intranuclear inclusions. Large amounts of virus can be demonstrated in vesicular fluid by electron microscopy.

Postmortem descriptions of patients with varicella have usually involved immunocompromised subjects. In these cases inflammatory changes are usually found in multiple organs, including the lung, liver, spleen, and skin, together with anoxic changes in the brain. Similar involvement is found in the newborn. Focal areas of necrosis and intranuclear eosinophilic inclusions in mononuclear cells are common. Changes in otherwise normal individuals usually include myocardial and pulmonary lesions. On microscopic examination, the brain has demonstrated edema with some lymphocyte cuffing around the cerebral vessels.

CLINICAL MANIFESTATIONS. Varicella is characterized by a generalized eruption that is centripetal in distribution; erythematous macules, papules, vesicles, and scabbed lesions may be present at the same time. The vesicles are superficial, with varying amounts of erythema at their bases. Adults tend to have considerably more erythema than children. During the early phase of the eruption, lesions are found on the face, scalp, and trunk. By running the fingers through the hair, one often detects lesions that were not visible. Later, new lesions appear on the extremities. By this time, the earlier lesions have dried and crusted. Excoriations are common, attesting to the pruritic nature of the lesions. Mucous membranes of the conjunctiva, oropharynx, and vagina are more frequently involved in adults than in children. New lesions continue to appear over a 3- or 4-day period, after which the rate of their appearance decelerates markedly.

There is a striking variation in the extent of systemic symptoms associated with varicella. Most children have a mild illness with few systemic complaints and an average maximal temperature of about 38.3°C. It is more common for adults to have considerable malaise, muscle ache, arthralgia, and headache. These may precede the first skin lesions by 24 to 48 hours.

In the immunocompromised subject, the disease often is very severe. Approximately 30 per cent of children with leukemia or lymphoma who get varicella develop "progressive varicella." Vesicles continue to erupt into the second week of illness, accompanied by high fever. Lesions tend to be deep seated rather than superficial. Toward the end of the first week and the beginning of the second week, the lesions are more common on the extremities than on the trunk. Indeed, the distribution and lesions may resemble those with smallpox. Visceral involvement occurs in about 30 per cent of these patients. The lung, liver, pancreas, and brain may be involved. Death occurs in about 9 per cent of immunocompromised patients who develop varicella. The death usually is due to pulmonary involvement.

Varicella in pregnant women is believed to be more serious than in nongravid females; fatalities have been reported. The rate of fetal wastage is not increased. Seven to 9 per cent of infants born to mothers who have had varicella early in pregnancy, however, have been found at birth to have "varicella embryopathy." These infants are born with cerebral damage and a variety of ocular findings and characteristically have a scarred, atrophic limb. They are generally small for gestational age and may have other abnormalities as well. When mothers develop chickenpox within a few days of delivery, "varicella of the newborn" may occur. If the onset of varicella is between 5 and 10 days after birth, it is associated with a higher risk of serious disease and even death.

Bacterial infections of the skin are the most common complication of chickenpox in childhood. The rate of complications is much higher in adults than in children. Although fewer than 2 per cent of the reported cases occur after the second decade, almost a quarter of the deaths occur in this group. A disproportionate rate of hospitalization also is found in adults. The major complications of varicella in adults are encephalitis and pneumonia.

Approximately 1 in 400 adults with chickenpox are hospitalized for pneumonia. In a prospective study, however, it was found that only 6 per cent of young adults with chickenpox had respiratory symptoms, whereas 16 per cent had roentgenographic evidence of pulmonary involvement.

Infection produces a diffuse interstitial type of pneumonia with hypoxia resulting from poor diffusion of gases. Diffuse calcification of the lung parenchyma may be found years after recovery.

Encephalitis in childhood is most commonly manifested by a cerebellitis, which usually occurs at the end of the first week or during the second week following onset of rash. This complication is almost always self-limited. In contrast, an acute form of encephalitis usually occurring soon after the onset of rash often has a fulminating course; it is characterized by severe brain swelling. It has been estimated that as many as 20 per cent of cases of Reye's syndrome may be preceded by chickenpox. A variety of other neurologic complications, including optic neuritis, transverse myelitis, and Guillain-Barré syndrome, may be associated with chickenpox. Hemorrhagic complications of chickenpox include thrombocytopenic purpura and purpura fulminans. Nephritis, myocarditis, and arthritis also have been described.

DIAGNOSIS. There is usually little difficulty in recognizing typical forms of chickenpox, particularly if there has been a history of exposure. The disease is seen more commonly by pediatricians than internists. The latter may not consider the diagnosis or may be less familiar with its clinical characteristics. The diagnosis may be more difficult in immunocompromised hosts, as they may have features of progressive varicella with visceral involvement. Modified cases of chickenpox may occur following passive or active immunization. These cases may require laboratory confirmation. The most common sources of confusion are insect bites; generalized herpes in the immunocompromised host; rickettsialpox; or "hand, foot, and mouth disease" caused by an enterovirus. The differentiation of disseminated herpes zoster from chickenpox may be difficult. The former usually has dermatomal involvement initially. Generalization usually does not occur until 3 to 5 days after onset of the zosteriform rash. In severely immunocompromised patients, e.g., bone marrow recipients, generalization may occur earlier and the clinical differentiation may be difficult.

The Tzanck smear is a frequently used laboratory aid for diagnosis. Multinucleated giant cells identify the lesions as being caused by one of the herpesviruses, but this is not specific for varicella. A properly stained smear also contains eosinophilic intranuclear inclusions. Virus can usually be isolated during the first 3 or 4 days after the onset of lesions. The virus is quite labile; it must be stored at $-70°C$ if cultures cannot be inoculated immediately. Our preference is to collect vesicular fluid in unheparinized capillary tubes and put the specimen directly into human embryonic lung fibroblasts at the bedside. A high isolation rate is found during the first 3 days of rash. Specimens from throat, urine, or stool are of little value for isolation of virus. PCR has been used to identify virus in vesicular fluid and respiratory secretions.

Serologic confirmation of diagnosis can be made using a variety of techniques. The enzyme-linked immunosorbent assay (ELISA) and complement fixation are the most generally available. The laboratory director should be consulted regarding appropriate time of collection of specimens as well as interpretation of data. Because complement-fixing antibody generally does not persist, a single high titer often is confirmatory evidence of recent infection.

Determining the immune status of contacts can be done with the ELISA or fluorescent antibody against membrane antigen (FAMA). The ELISA is a much simpler and technically less demanding test. Because complement-fixing antibody is lost rapidly after infection, it cannot be used for determining susceptibility. Fluorescence antibody tests using fixed cells sometimes yield false-positive results. A number of laboratories have developed tests for VZV immunoglobulin M (IgM). It was hoped that these might differentiate varicella from herpes zoster in cases in which this was unclear. Unfortunately, these tests have not been very useful, as VZV IgM is present in the sera of many patients with acute herpes zoster.

TREATMENT. Major therapeutic objectives are the prevention of superinfection and relief of pruritus. The latter can be accomplished frequently by application of calamine lotion. Occasionally this does not suffice, and a systemic antipruritic agent such as trimeprazine may be necessary. It is advisable to trim and file nails to reduce the damage from scratching. Bacterial superinfection can best be prevented by encouraging daily bathing with soap or hexachlorophene. Following this with a colloidal starch bath may also be useful in relief of pruritus.

Relief of systemic symptoms may require additional medication such as acetaminophen. Salicylates are contraindicated, as there is an association between their use and development of Reye's syndrome in children. Special care should be taken to be certain that over-the-counter medications containing salicylates are avoided.

Some patients, particularly those who are immunocompromised, may require antiviral therapy. Acyclovir has been shown to be effective in immunocompromised children with varicella. A dose of 500 mg per square meter repeated every 8 hours has been used. VZV is generally less sensitive to acyclovir than herpes simplex. For this reason, larger doses are probably required. Doses of 10 to 20 mg per kilogram have been shown to shorten the course of varicella by about 1 day if used early. The rate of complications was not affected. Patients who are sick enough to require antiviral therapy probably should be treated with parenteral rather than oral medication. In comparative studies, acyclovir appears to be somewhat safer and probably more effective than vidarabine.

Patients on high doses of steroids or other immunosuppressive drugs who have been exposed to chickenpox are at high risk of developing progressive varicella. Steroids appear to be most deleterious when given during the incubation period. They have been used without any obvious deleterious effects in the treatment of pneumonia after the eruption has occurred.

PREVENTION. Immune serum globulin does not prevent varicella. Massive doses are required to produce measurable modification. If prevention or modification is indicated, varicella zoster immune globulin (VZIG) should be given. Candidates are those who (1) are susceptible, (2) are at high risk of developing complicated varicella, and (3) have had an adequate exposure to the disease. Any individuals fulfilling the first two criteria who have had a household exposure should receive prophylaxis. It is often difficult to judge the degree of intimacy in other types of exposure. Reference to guidelines published by the Academy of Pediatrics or Centers for Disease Control (CDC) may be helpful.

Patients considered at high risk are (1) those who are immunocompromised by virtue of either disease or immunosuppressive therapy, (2) infants born to mothers who have had varicella less than 5 days prior to or 2 days following delivery, (3) premature infants of mothers with no history of varicella, (4) bone marrow transplantation recipients regardless of susceptibility, and (5) certain adults.

A history of varicella is usually reliable in both adults and children. Children who have a negative history are usually susceptible. Serologic testing of adults who have a negative history is useful if it does not delay administration of VZIG. VZIG should be given as soon as possible following exposure and should not be delayed more than 96 hours.

Nosocomial infection following herpes zoster or varicella has been well documented. These outbreaks may result in significant morbidity and cause disruption of hospital routine. These situations are best managed by serologic screening of personnel and by permitting only those who are seropositive to care for patients with varicella or herpes zoster. Patients who are hospitalized with varicella should be isolated for 7 days. Susceptible persons who are exposed to active cases should be isolated from the tenth to the twenty-first day after the last exposure if they cannot be discharged. Whenever possible, patients with chickenpox should be isolated in a room with negative pressure in order to prevent dissemination of infectious virus to other patients. Airborne spread in hospitals has been documented.

An attenuated live vaccine has been licensed for use abroad and is being considered for licensure in the United States. Susceptible adults who receive the vaccine have some local reactions and occasionally develop a varicelliform rash. Protection against infection is less complete than in children. In normal children, the vaccine is virtually benign and appears to offer very good protection. Initial data suggest that herpes zoster would be no more frequent and perhaps less common following immunization than following natural infection. Live varicella vaccine also has been used to protect children with acute lymphocytic leukemia. Protection is less complete than in normal children. Some of these vaccinated children develop a varicelliform illness from the vaccine.

Advisory Committee on Immunization Practice: Varicella-zoster immune globulin for the prevention of chickenpox. MMWR 33:84, 95, 1984. *Guidelines for passive immunization against chickenpox.*

Brunell PA: Fetal and neonatal varicella-zoster infections. Semin Perinatol 7:47, 1983. *A critical review of fetal, neonatal, and maternal varicella.*

Brunell PA: Varicella vaccine—where are we? Pediatrics 78:721, 1986. *A symposium on the epidemiology, cost burden, and complications of varicella and on varicella vaccine.*

Shehab ZM, Brunell PA: Varicella-zoster virus. *In* Rose NR, Friedman H, Fahey JL (eds.): Manual of Clinical Laboratory Immunity, 3rd ed. Washington, DC, American Society for Microbiology, 1986, pp 502–503. *A review of serologic tests for varicella-zoster antibody.*

Takahashi M: Chickenpox virus. Adv Virus Res 28:285, 1983. *A comprehensive review of both basic science and information on the vaccine.*

Varicella-zoster infections. Report of the Committee on Infectious Diseases, 21st ed. Evanston, IL, American Academy of Pediatrics, 1988, pp 456–462. *A useful guide to management of patients exposed to varicella, including control of nosocomial infection.*

Weller TH: Varicella and herpes zoster. N Engl J Med 309:1362, 1983. *A review of immunology, immunization, and therapy.*

375 Variola and Vaccinia

Donald A. Henderson

The Thirty-third World Health Assembly "declares solemnly that the world and all its peoples have won freedom from smallpox . . . an unprecedented achievement in the history of public health. . . ." (Resolution 33.3, May 8, 1980, Geneva, Switzerland).

This announcement was made some 30 months after the last known endemic case, in Somalia, on October 26, 1977. In 1978, two additional cases of smallpox occurred in Birmingham, England, as a result of a laboratory infection, but except for these cases no others have been found.

To confirm that eradication had been achieved, each country where smallpox had been endemic since 1967 and those at risk of importations conducted a search for cases for at least 2 years after the last known case. At the end of this period, World Health Organization (WHO)–appointed International Commissions reviewed the records of work and conducted extensive field visits to confirm the results. Between 1973 and 1979, 21 different commissions visited and certified eradication in 49 countries.

Finally, a Global Commission for the Certification of Smallpox Eradication reviewed the findings and made special field visits. After satisfying itself that eradication had been achieved, the commission reported its findings to the World Health Assembly. The assembly members concurred and recommended that "smallpox vaccination be discontinued in every country except for investigators at special risk," and advised that "an international certificate of vaccination against smallpox should no longer be required of any traveller."

Thus concluded the first successful global program to eradicate a disease—one that had proved to be one of the most devastating known to man.

HISTORY. Because of the need for variola virus to spread continually from person to person to survive, historians speculate that it emerged after the first agricultural settlements, about 10,000 B.C. A distinctive smallpox rash has been identified on the mummy of Pharaoh Ramses V (1160 B.C.). In ancient times, only a few populated areas, probably in India, could have sustained its transmission. In the early Christian era descriptions suggestive of smallpox appear in historical accounts of western Asia, and by the eighth century it had established itself in Europe. Central and southern Africa were probably infected sometime later. In 1520, Spanish conquistadors brought the disease to the Americas.

Case-fatality rates of 20 per cent and greater were characteristic, and where population densities permitted the disease to become endemic virtually all persons eventually contracted smallpox. At the end of the eighteenth century, it was killing an estimated 400,000 Europeans each year and was responsible for one third of all cases of blindness.

VACCINATION. Edward Jenner discovered in 1796 that smallpox could be prevented by "vaccination" with material from a cowpox lesion. Before his discovery, the only defense against smallpox was deliberately to inoculate (variolate) scabs or pustular material from smallpox patients into the skin of susceptible persons. The resulting infection was usually less severe than infection acquired naturally by inhalation. Although case-fatality rates among those with induced infection were sometimes as low as 1 per cent, they readily transmitted infection to others.

Within 3 years after Jenner first published his findings, more than 100,000 had been vaccinated in England. By 1803, the new vaccine had been transported to the Americas, Asia, and Africa. During the nineteenth century, vaccination was increasingly widely practiced in temperate-climate countries, but the difficulties of sustaining the virus through arm-to-arm inoculation resulted in an uncertain supply. The discovery, late in the nineteenth century, that vaccinia virus could be propagated on the flank of a calf was an important advance. However, such vaccine remained viable for only a few days at ambient temperature. Finally, in the 1950's a commercially feasible technique was developed for producing a dried, heat-resistant vaccine.

In the industrialized countries, smallpox incidence declined steadily, and Europe and North America succeeded in interrupting smallpox transmission after World War II. In these areas, the impetus for vaccination had diminished early in the century when a less virulent strain, variola minor, with a case-fatality rate of about 1 per cent, replaced variola major. In most of Africa, however, 5 to 15 per cent died of smallpox, and in Asia the virulent variola major prevailed. Neither in Africa nor in Asia was vaccination widely practiced.

ERADICATION OF SMALLPOX. Smallpox was a problem to all countries. Even those without disease feared importations and conducted vaccination programs. Although the global control of smallpox was in everyone's best interests, progress was slow. Finally, in 1959, the World Health Assembly decided that a global eradication program should be undertaken. During the succeeding 7 years, a number of countries undertook campaigns, but few succeeded in interrupting smallpox transmission.

In 1966, the assembly decided that one further effort should be made. A 10-year goal was proposed. The program commenced on January 1, 1967 (Fenner and colleagues). In 1967, smallpox was endemic in 31 countries, and 13 additional countries reported importations. Although 131,768 cases were officially reported, the true number was about 10 to 15 million. Four geographic reservoirs of smallpox were identified: (1) Africa south of the Sahara; (2) a group of Southeast Asian countries, extending from Bangladesh through India, Nepal, Pakistan, and Afghanistan; (3) Indonesia; and (4) Brazil. The estimated population of these countries was more than 1 billion persons.

WHO's strategy called for each country to undertake a program of vaccination with the objective of reaching at least 80 per cent of the population during a 2- to 3-year period. During this time, a reliable reporting system was to be developed to identify foci of smallpox that would be eliminated by isolation of patients and vaccination of contacts. Extensive vaccination was believed necessary to increase population immunity and so reduce the number of cases to permit disease surveillance and containment activities to be effective.

Experience soon showed that the surveillance-containment strategy was more effective than had been thought, and this proved to be a key to success. In part, this was due to the unique characteristics of smallpox. An infected patient was able to transmit infection only from the time of first appearance of rash until the last scabs had separated. There were no chronic carriers or individuals with latent, transmissible infection and no animal reservoir. The rash was sufficiently characteristic to be diagnosed with a high degree of accuracy. The presence or absence of smallpox in an area could thus be reliably determined without laboratory studies. Moreover, approximately two thirds of recovered patients had characteristic residual facial scars. Thus, it was possible to determine both the present status of smallpox and its past history in an area.

To persist, smallpox virus had to be transmitted from patient to susceptible contact. By isolation of the patient and by vaccination of contacts, a barrier to transmission was created. In small villages and in scattered populations, chains of transmission often terminated without intervention. Because smallpox did not spread rapidly, and then only to those in close contact, secondary cases usually were found among neighbors and relatives. A patient rarely infected more than two to three others. Because of these factors, early detection of outbreaks and their containment proved effective in stopping transmission.

Smallpox vaccine that conferred excellent and durable immunity was an important factor in the program's success. Studies revealed vaccine efficacy ratios of more than 90 per cent after 20 years. Because the lyophilized vaccine retained its potency after incubation at 37°C for at least 1 month, the logistics of vaccine storage and distribution were comparatively simple. Vaccination was greatly facilitated by the inexpensive, newly developed bifurcated needle. Vaccine was held between the tines by capillarity. Fifteen rapid punctures were made with the needle held perpendicular to the skin. The technique was learned quickly and produced a high proportion of successful vaccinations.

PROGRESS IN THE PROGRAM. By 1969, eradication programs were in progress in all of the infected and immediately adjacent countries except for Ethiopia, whose program began in 1971. By 1970, the number of endemic countries had decreased from 31 to 18. Brazil registered its last case in 1971 and Indonesia and Afghanistan in 1972. By 1973, all of Africa had become smallpox free except for Ethiopia and Botswana. In Asia, there remained only four smallpox-endemic countries: India, Pakistan, Nepal, and Bangladesh. However, the population of these four was over 700 million, and the techniques of surveillance and containment that had been applied in other areas proved to be less successful.

A new strategy in India began in the autumn of 1973 (Basu and colleagues). Far more rapid case detection and more effective containment of outbreaks were required. Accordingly, for 1 week each month more than 100,000 health workers were mobilized to search house by house to detect cases. Hundreds of special teams contained the outbreaks that were found. Between searches, the teams asked questions at markets and in schools to uncover rumors of cases. By the summer of 1974, new cases began to decline, and a cash reward was offered to anyone who reported a case. In May 1975 the last case was detected in India, and on October 16, 1975, the last case in Asia.

The only remaining endemic country was Ethiopia. With the end of smallpox in Asia, resources were shifted to Ethiopia. In August 1976, the last case was isolated. Unfortunately, Somalian guerrilla forces had meanwhile introduced the disease into neighboring Somalia, and yet another year was to elapse before finally, on October 26, 1977, the last case occurred.

POSSIBLE SOURCES FOR A RETURN OF SMALLPOX. As of 1990, variola virus was known to exist in only two laboratories, where it was kept under high-security conditions.

Extensive studies had been conducted since 1967 to discover a possible animal or other natural reservoir of the virus. None was found. However, some 400 cases of a newly recognized disease that is clinically indistinguishable from smallpox but caused by the related monkeypox virus occurred in seven central and west African countries between 1970 and 1990. Genome maps of this and other animal poxviruses reveal many differences between them and variola, suggesting that mutation to variola would be highly unlikely.

The recurrence of smallpox resulting from a deliberate release of variola virus cannot be ruled out. However, the potential damage of such an act should not be exaggerated. Smallpox does not spread rapidly, and an outbreak caused in this manner should be able to be contained within 3 to 4 weeks.

As insurance against unforeseen events, WHO has established vaccine storage reserves of some 200 million doses of vaccine. Additional stocks are being retained by a number of governments.

Barring improbable circumstances, a human case of smallpox will never again be seen. However, the problem of mistaken diagnosis is a real one. For this reason, WHO medical officers with expertise in diagnosis remain on call to investigate rumors, and an expertise in laboratory diagnosis is maintained by WHO Diagnostic Reference Laboratories (Centers for Disease Control, Atlanta, and the Institute for Virus Preparations, Moscow).

VARIOLA (Smallpox)

ETIOLOGY. Variola virus is one of a group of orthopoxviruses that includes vaccinia, monkeypox, rabbitpox, cowpox, camelpox, buffalopox, and ectromelia. The poxviruses are the largest viruses so recognized. The virions are brick-shaped structures with a diameter of about 200 mμ. The genome consists of a single molecule of a double-stranded DNA.

INCIDENCE AND PREVALENCE. The disease was declared to be eradicated on May 8, 1980.

PATHOLOGY AND PATHOGENESIS. The site of entry of the smallpox virus was probably the respiratory tract. In the 12-day incubation period the virus multiplied in the regional lymphoid tissues. Viremia occurred at the onset of fever and continued during the first 2 or 3 days of the pre-eruptive phase. During this time, the virus localized in mucous membranes, skin, and internal tissues. Virus multiplication in the epithelial cells of the skin and mucous membranes caused pustulation. Antibodies appeared as early as the fourth day of disease.

CLINICAL MANIFESTATIONS. The incubation period of smallpox was about 12 days with a range of 7 to 17 days. The illness began with severe malaise, prostration, head- and backache, and high fever lasting 2 to 5 days (Rao). Following the initial febrile period, a macular rash developed, which quickly became papular, and within 2 days the papules developed into vesicles and then pustules. On the eighth or ninth day of rash, crusting began. The scabs separated over the succeeding 2 to 3 weeks, leaving pigment-free skin. Subsequently, scarring or pitting developed. The eruption was characteristically more severe on the face and the distal parts of the arms and legs, and less severe over the trunk and abdomen. Lesions were often found on the palms of the hands and the soles of the feet.

VARIOLA MINOR AND INTERMEDIATE FORMS. In the early twentieth century, a milder clinical form of smallpox (variola minor, or alastrim) became prevalent in the Americas, Europe, and parts of southern and eastern Africa. Case-fatality rates were 1 per cent or less. Variola major and minor were distinct although at times coexisting. Each of the two types gave rise to illnesses with a wide spectrum of severity. There was cross-protection between each of these forms and vaccinia.

DIFFERENTIAL DIAGNOSIS. Most cases of smallpox could

readily be identified by the typical deep-seated rash, the centrifugal distribution of lesions, and the fact that in any area on the body all lesions were at the same stage of development. The infrequent severe hemorrhagic cases were frequently mistakenly diagnosed as meningococcemia, acute leukemia, or drug toxicity. Mild cases with few lesions were confused with varicella. Most problematic were severe cases of chickenpox in adults. Of help in diagnosis, however, was the fact that in any outbreak 80 per cent or more of the cases were clinically typical.

LABORATORY TESTS. Diagnosis of a poxvirus infection can be rapidly established by electron microscopic identification of virus particles in vesicular or pustular fluid or scabs. Differentiation among poxviruses requires that the virus be isolated on chick chorioallantoic membrane and its properties characterized by specific biologic tests. WHO Reference Laboratories are prepared to undertake necessary diagnostic studies. For patients who have recovered, neutralizing antibody in serum specimens serves to identify which poxvirus was responsible for the illness.

TREATMENT. No specific treatment is available.

IDENTIFICATION OF A SUSPECT CASE OF SMALLPOX. Because smallpox has been eradicated, the occurrence of a single case has profound international implications. Should a suspect case be identified, *immediate notification of local, state, and national health officials is essential.* Most suspected cases in recent years have been cases of varicella in adults. Should a case prove to be smallpox, the source of virus must be assumed to be inadvertent or deliberate release from a laboratory. A suspect patient should be placed under strict isolation. Additional measures will be dictated by epidemiologic circumstances.

VACCINIA (Vaccination)

No countries now require international certificates of vaccination, and none conducts civilian vaccination programs. Several countries, including the United States, continue to vaccinate military personnel. Vaccination is recommended only for investigators who are working with poxviruses in the laboratory.

THE VACCINE. Vaccinia virus is grown in tissue culture or on the scarified flank of a calf. After purification and the addition of stabilizing agents, the suspension is freeze dried. Inoculated intradermally, vaccinia virus induces a mild infection and confers protection against all orthopoxviruses known to infect man—monkeypox, variola, and cowpox.

VACCINE PROTECTION. Following successful vaccination, protection against variola is virtually complete for 5 years, but effectiveness wanes over time. In poxvirus laboratories, vaccination at least every 3 years has been customary.

RISKS OF VACCINATION. Those who are candidates for vaccination are adults, a diminishing proportion of whom have received primary vaccinations as children. Although the risk of complications following revaccination is very low, primary vaccination of adults has been thought to be associated with a higher incidence of serious complications. However, a special study of vaccination complications among military recruits failed to document any cases of the most important, postvaccinal encephalitis, among an estimated 2 million primary vaccinees.

FIRST VACCINATION (PRIMARY TAKE). Three days after vaccination a papule appears at the vaccination site; the papule changes to a vesicle and by the seventh day is a fully developed pustule. It is whitish, umbilicated, and multilocular and contains clear lymph. An erythematous areola expands to reach a maximal diameter about 9 days after vaccination. A crust forms and falls off about 3 weeks after vaccination, leaving a scar.

REVACCINATION. When persons are vaccinated a second time, a gradation of cutaneous responses is observed. Individuals who have not been vaccinated for several decades may develop what appears to be a primary take. In persons with an intermediate level of immunity, development of the lesion is more rapid, and the maximal diameter of erythema is reached in 3 to 7 days. In the highly immune person, virus multiplication may not occur. In such persons, a hypersensitivity response to vaccinial protein may occur. A papule and sometimes a vesicle with erythema may develop, reaching its peak in 48 hours.

To distinguish the hypersensitivity type of reaction, which may be caused by heat-inactivated vaccine, from one in which virus multiplication has taken place, the site of inoculation is examined between the sixth and eighth days. If there is evidence of induration or congestion, virus multiplication may be assumed.

CONTRAINDICATIONS. Four groups of persons are at special risk of complications: (1) persons with eczema or other forms of chronic dermatitis; (2) pregnant women; (3) patients with leukemia, lymphoma, other reticuloendothelial malignancies and the acquired immunodeficiency syndrome (AIDS); and (4) those receiving immunosuppressive drugs, especially glucocorticosteroids. Vaccinees in close contact with persons with eczema may infect them, sometimes with serious consequences. If vaccination is required for persons at special risk, vaccinia immune globulin (0.3 ml per kilogram intramuscularly) should be administered simultaneously.

COMPLICATIONS. *Postvaccinal Encephalitis.* Encephalitis following vaccination is a rare event and occurs between the eighth and fifteenth days. Paralysis, when it occurs, is generally spastic in type. Residual paralysis and other central nervous system symptoms may persist. There is no treatment. Studies conducted in the United States in 1963 and 1968 (Neff and colleagues, Lane and associates) revealed 28 cases, 9 fatal, among 11.3 million primary vaccinees. No cases occurred among 16.3 million revaccinees.

Progressive Vaccinia (Vaccinia Gangrenosa). Progressive vaccinia is an exceedingly rare but often fatal complication among vaccinated persons who have deficient immune responses. The initial vaccinial lesion fails to heal and progresses to involve adjacent skin with necrosis of tissue. Dissemination may result in metastatic vaccinial lesions in other parts of the skin, bones, or viscera. Treatment with vaccinia immune globulin is beneficial.

Eczema Vaccinatum. Eczema vaccinatum is sometimes a serious complication, which may occur in vaccinated persons with active or healed eczema, or in subjects in contact with recent vaccinees. The disease tends to localize at sites where eczematous lesions are or have been present. Vaccinia immune globulin is of help in therapy.

Generalized Vaccinia. Generalized vaccinia represents a secondary eruption resulting from bloodborne dissemination of vaccinia virus. Almost all cases occur after primary vaccination. The lesions become evident between 6 and 9 days after vaccination. The number of lesions may range from a few to a generalized involvement of the skin. It is a self-limited illness, and complete recovery occurs without specific therapy.

Fetal Vaccinia. Fetal vaccinia results from a bloodborne dissemination of vaccinia virus in the pregnant woman given primary vaccination. It may occur during any trimester of pregnancy and frequently results in death of the fetus.

Miscellaneous Complications. A great variety of rashes have been reported to be caused by vaccination. Most common are erythema multiforme and variously distributed urticarial, maculopapular, blotchy erythematous eruptions.

Basu RN, Jerek Z, Ward NA: The Eradication of Smallpox from India. New Delhi, India, World Health Organization, 1979. *A well-written, detailed, profusely illustrated book describing the epidemiologic and operational aspects of the program in India.*

Fenner F, Henderson DA, Jerek Z, et al.: Smallpox and its Eradication. Geneva, Switzerland, World Health Organization, 1988. *This 1400-page, extensively illustrated and referenced book is the definitive text, providing an historical account of smallpox control and eradication as well as a summary of current knowledge regarding the epidemiology, virology, and pathogenesis of the disease.*

Hopkins DR: Princes and Peasants: Smallpox in History. Chicago, University of Chicago Press, 1983. *The only comprehensive history of smallpox prepared in this century, this interesting and readable book complements the book by Fenner and associates.*

Lane JM, Ruben FL, Neff JM, et al.: Complications of smallpox vaccination, 1968. N Engl J Med 281:138, 1969. *With the paper by Neff and co-workers, one of the few detailed studies of the frequency of complications following smallpox vaccination.*

Neff J, Lane JM, Pert JH, et al.: Complications of smallpox vaccination. N Engl J Med 276:1, 1967. *With the paper by Lane and associates, one of the few detailed studies of the frequency of complications following smallpox vaccination.*

Rao AR: Smallpox. Bombay, India, Kothari Book Depot, 1972. *Written by a clinician who treated more than 3000 cases, this book is an excellent reference on the clinical aspects of variola major.*

376 Retroviruses That Cause Human Disease*

William A. Blattner

The decade of the 1980's ushered in a new age of medical virology with the discovery and characterization of human oncornaviruses and lenti-retroviruses. These discoveries began with the search for human cancer viruses in the early decades of this century and were propelled by the studies of cancer-causing retroviruses in mammals from the 1950's to 1970's. During the 1960's and 1970's molecular retrovirology established the replication cycle and the nature and function of viral genes and proteins, along with basic technology to assay reverse transcriptase and grow key target cells using newly discovered growth factors such as interleukin 2 (IL2). Within a few years of the first detection of a human retrovirus, HTLV-I in 1978, systems for their study in vitro were developed; their modes of transmission and geographic prevalence were determined; their genomes were analyzed and some novel genes were found; the mechanism of their effects on cells was partly unraveled; and, most importantly, some were causally linked to fatal human diseases, including diverse malignancies and the pandemic of acquired immunodeficiency syndrome (AIDS). In this chapter, some of the general properties of this remarkable virus class are considered.

DEFINITION, GENERAL FEATURES, AND CLASSIFICATION. Retroviruses are ribonucleic acid (RNA) viruses consisting of an outer envelope and an inner core that contains two molecules of a single-stranded RNA. The genome is relatively small (8.0 to 9.5 Kb) and simple (three to eight genes). Envelope and core structural proteins of the virus are produced from spliced viral RNA coded message and as the virus assembles at the cell membrane, the envelope incorporates the cell's lipid

---

*This chapter is based in part on a chapter written by Dr. Robert C. Gallo and his colleague Dr. Howard Z. Streicher in the 18th edition of the *Cecil Textbook of Medicine*. They have given permission to update portions of that chapter and have assisted, in conjunction with Drs. Dani Bolognasi and Thomas Palker of Duke University, in the preparation of this chapter.

bilayer during the budding process, producing an infectious virion of about 100 nm. The life cycle of a human retrovirus is schematically portrayed in Figure 376–1.

The hallmark of a retrovirus is the replication of viral RNA through a deoxyribonucleic acid (DNA) intermediate called a provirus. The initial step in virus infection is attachment of the virus envelope glycoproteins to a cell surface receptor. For HIV-1 the receptor is the CD4 molecule, but other components including major histocompatibility molecules may also play a role in this high-affinity binding step. In addition to T lymphocytes, monocyte/macrophages that express CD4 may also be infected. The other human retroviruses, HTLV-I and -II, which preferentially infect and transform CD4+ cells, use another as yet unknown receptor. Following uptake and uncoating, viral RNA is transcribed by reverse transcriptase into double-stranded DNA. This unique mechanism is catalyzed by viral *reverse transcriptase*, an RNA-dependent DNA polymerase that is complexed to the RNA in the core of the virus particle. This double-stranded viral DNA is integrated by the virally encoded integrase into the host cell nucleus, resulting in cell infection that may be lifelong. Essential to integration are the viral long terminal repeat (LTR) elements. Depending on the specific retrovirus, the LTR's are sequences of 300 to 900 nucleotides that flank both ends of the viral genome. They form the sites of covalent attachment of the provirus to cellular DNA and are the site of important viral regulatory elements. The virus may remain "hidden" (unexpressed, nonreplicative) in cells for very long periods, and this may contribute to the long interval (sometimes many years to decades) between the time of infection and disease. Factors that control viral replication (viral regulatory genes, cell stimulation, and possibly coinfections) may also be cofactors in disease progression. When the DNA provirus is expressed (transcribed by a cellular RNA polymerase), viral genomic and messenger RNA and subsequently viral proteins are made by the cell. These assemble at the cell membrane to be packaged and released, thereby completing the replication cycle.

Retroviruses are found in many different vertebrates. Their principal target cells in most animals are those of the hematopoietic, immune, and central nervous systems. Consequently, they induce a wide range of diseases, including malignancies, which chiefly consist of leukemias and lymphomas. Yet retrovirus

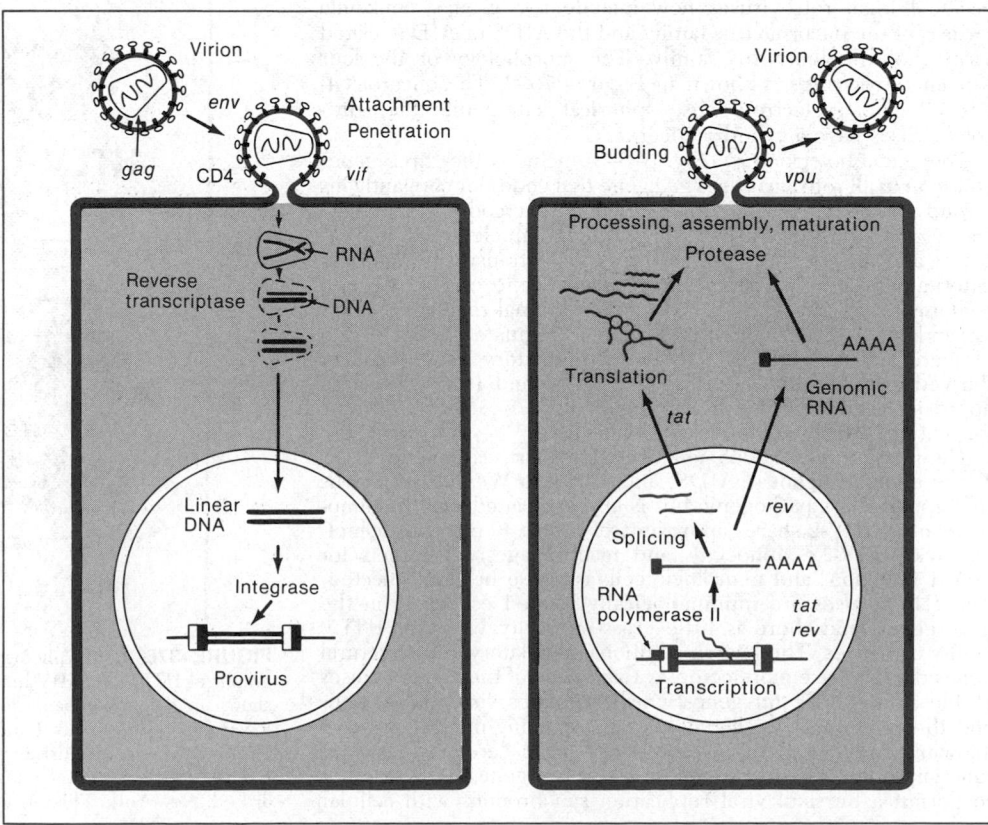

FIGURE 376–1. Life cycle of HIV. *Left,* Attachment of the virus involves binding to the CD4 receptor of the cell. The virus uncoats in an endosome transcribed to double-stranded viral DNA. Linear viral DNA is transported to the nucleus and integrated into host genome by virally encoded integrator. The proviral DNA can remain latent in the cell or serve as a template for production of new virions *(right)*. Under the influence of viral regulatory proteins *tat* and *rev*, viral message is expressed either as structural proteins involving translation or as genomic RNA. New virions are produced with the viral protease modulating processing, assembly, and maturation. Particles bud through the cell membrane and incorporate into the cell lipid bilayer in which are embedded the viral transmembrane and external proteins. (Reprinted with permission from Gallo RC: Mechanism of disease induction by HIV. J AIDS 3:380–389, 1990.)

infection can produce quite the opposite effect. Sometimes they interfere with cell growth, leading to aplasias of various cell types (e.g., aplastic anemia of feline leukemia virus). Some infections are cytopathic, killing the infected cells (AIDS), and some may alter cell function. The kind of disease induced by a retrovirus depends in part upon its major target cell, (which is determined by viral envelope binding to cell receptor) and sometimes upon interaction of proviral LTR regulatory elements with cellular genes (e.g., *cis* activation of a cellular oncogene).

Retroviruses are named and classified according to their species, their mode of transmission (endogenous, exogenous), the type of disease produced (e.g., leukemia viruses, sarcoma viruses), their morphology and mode of maturation (types C,D,B, foamy, and lenti), the organization of their genome, and the genetic relatedness of one to another. Many of these terms and descriptions are no longer useful and are not considered here. For example, the ubiquitous endogenous retroviruses, sometimes known as spuma or foamy virus of the chimpanzee, are transmitted in the germ line as genetic elements and have no known role in the origin of disease except in a few highly inbred strains of laboratory mice. By contrast, exogenous viruses are transmitted by infection of a somatic cell like any other virus and frequently cause disease.

There are three general groups of retroviruses. The first are those with the three genes necessary for virus replication (*gag* gene for core proteins, *pol* gene for reverse transcriptase, and *env* gene for envelope). The majority of known animal retroviruses are of the first type. The mechanisms by which they induce disease often involve extensive replication of the virus and random integration of transcribed DNA into target-cell DNA with occasional chance integration in a region in which the viral LTR may promote altered expression of one or more nearby cellular genes important to cell growth or differentiation. This process is sometimes called *cis*-activation and may result in leukemia. The second group are those carrying a cellular *onc* gene that codes for a protein that transforms each infected cell; viruses belonging to this second type are rare and usually defective and have never been found in humans. The third group contains the three requisite genes for viral replication plus one or more additional genes (e.g., *tax* of HTLV-I) that regulate virus expression and also may directly or indirectly alter cell function. This third type includes all of the known human retroviruses.

The human retroviruses now include two groups, leukemia viruses of the oncornavirus family and the AIDS or AIDS-related viruses of the lentivirus family. The morphology of the four human retroviruses is shown in Figure 376–2. The oncoronaviruses have an electron-dense spherical core while the lentiretroviruses have a cylindrical core.

Their genetic structure (Fig. 376–3) includes the three genes common to all retroviruses: a *gag* gene that codes for core antigens (group-associated antigens); a *pol* gene that codes for reverse transcriptase (polymerase), integrase (endonuclease), and protease; and an *env* gene which codes for a transmembrane and external envelope glycoprotein. The *env* gene of HTLV-I also contains a "pX" region that codes for additional regulatory genes *tax* and *rex*, which function in concert to regulate the expression of mature virions. These additional regulatory genes are not derived from cellular genes. The HTLV-I and II viruses share approximately 60 per cent homology (Fig. 376–3) and are tropic for mature, usually CD4+ T lymphocytes.

The human immunodeficiency family of viruses includes HIV-1, the etiologic agent of AIDS, and HIV-2, a West African virus that appears less pathogenic but is also associated with immunodeficiency. HIV-2 shares approximately 30 to 40 per cent homology with HIV-1. Monocytes and macrophages are targets for HIV-1 infection, and neurologic cells can also become infected. The HIV viruses are immunologically related especially in the *gag* region, and there is little cross-reactivity with the HTLV family of viruses. The known additional regulatory and structural genes of HIV-1 are more complex than those of the HTLV viruses (Table 376–1). The *tat* gene, which regulates virus production, and the *rev* gene, which regulates the splicing of viral message allowing larger structural proteins to form, are analogous in function to the *tax* and *rex* genes. These two genes work together to permit a burst of viral replication synchronous with cellular

replication. They are essential for viral expression and may provide targets for future therapy. The function of other expressed small viral genes has been deduced primarily from deletion mutations and are essential in some cases for mature virion expression.

EPIDEMIOLOGY AND MODES OF TRANSMISSION OF HUMAN RETROVIRUSES. *Origin of Human Retroviruses.* The origin of human retroviruses is unclear. Retroviruses related to HTLV-I/II and HIV-1/2 have been isolated from several primate species, especially from Africa, suggesting the possibility of enzootic transmission to man. An African origin of HTLV-I is also supported by the fact that HTLV-I clusters among persons of African descent in the Caribbean but not in other populations. However, clusters of HTLV-I in southern Japan and northeastern Iran as well as elsewhere make the origin of this class of virus more difficult to discern. Although HTLV-I often appears in endemic clusters in a population, the pattern for HIV-1 is that of an epidemic contagion that is spreading worldwide. HIV-1 may be derived from a older virus, since its replicated mechanisms of cell infection and pathogenic function are highly evolved and adapted to complex human T-cell structures such as the CD4 molecule. Yet surveys of many populations have identified no evidence for widespread HIV-1 infection prior to the mid-1970's, when the epidemic of positivity first became evident in high-risk U.S. populations. There are only sporadic examples of putative infection in some rare individuals as early as the 1960's in Africa, a single putative positive in the United States with a possible history of male homosexual contact in the late 1960's, and a polymerase chain reaction–proven case of a British seaman from 1959.

Features of HTLV. The epidemiology of retroviruses has been largely defined through the use of antibody testing. Since virus-positive antibody-negative individuals could be missed by antibody tests, the true prevalence of virus may be underestimated. However, small-scale surveys employing polymerase chain reaction have not detected large numbers of virus-positive, antibody-

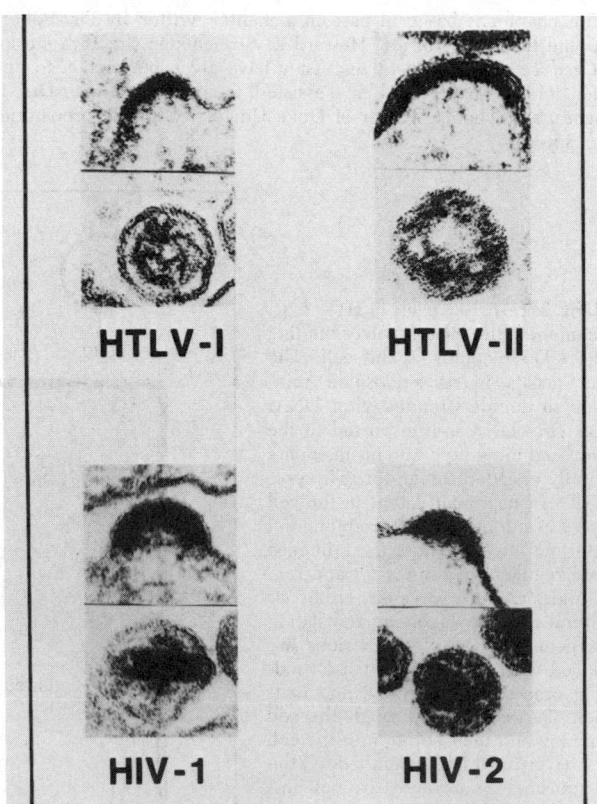

FIGURE 376–2. Morphology of human retroviruses. Electron micrographs of HTLV and HIV human retroviruses. The budding particles are shown in the upper panel for each virus and the mature virion in the lower panel. The HTLV-I and -II viruses have a spherical core and HIV-1 and -2 have a cylindrical core. (From Blattner WA: Retroviruses. *In* Evans A (ed.): Viral Infections of Humans, Epidemiology and Control, 3rd ed. New York, Plenum Publishing, 1989, pp 545–592.)

FIGURE 376–3. Genomic structure of human retroviruses. LTR = Long terminal repeat, which is organized into three regions: U5, R, and U3, which house the polyadenylation site; and the *rev*—responsive element—and the transactivating response (TAR) element, which are involved in controlling virus expression. *gag* = Gene for core protein. *pol* = Gene for reverse transcriptase, integrase, and protease. *env* = Envelope gene. *tax/tat* = Transactivating genes of HTLV and HIV. *rex/rev* = Viral regulatory genes involved in promoting genomic RNA production. *vif, vpr, vpu, vpx,* and *nef* = Additional regulatory genes whose functions are summarized in Table 376–1. (Reprinted by permission from *Nature,* Vol. 333, p. 504. Copyright © 1988 Macmillan Magazines Limited.)

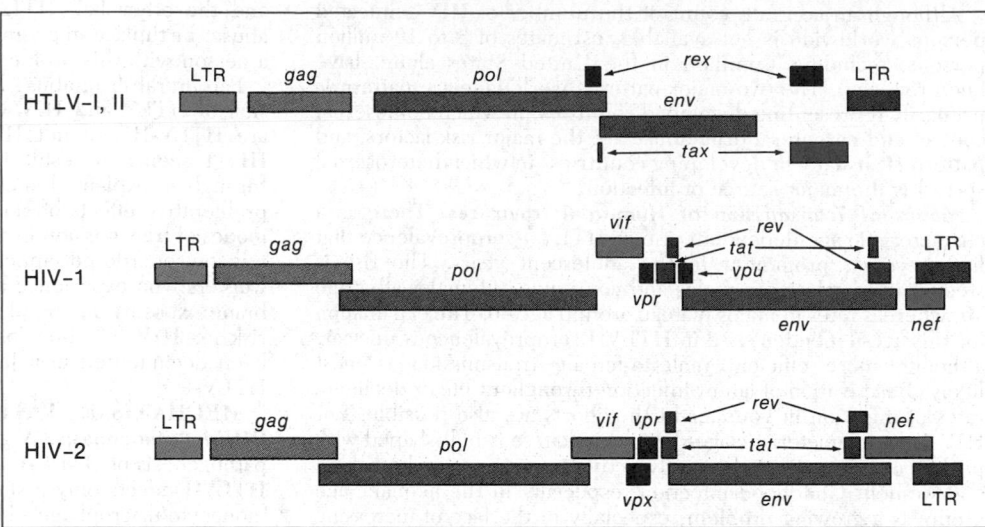

negative individuals, although some instances have been reported. Epidemiologic studies of HTLV-I are complicated by the inability of current serologic assays to distinguish HTLV-I from the closely related HTLV-II virus.

The distribution of antibody positivity in populations varies by region and risk group. Geographic clustering of HTLV-I is exemplified by endemic foci of HTLV-I in southern Japan (Kyushu, Shikoku, and the islands of the Ryukyu chain, including Okinawa) but not in Honshu and other areas of Japan. Extensive surveys of China, Korea, Taiwan, and Vietnam are also largely negative; high rates are reported from Papau New Guinea, but serologic and epidemiologic data raise the possibility that this reactivity is associated with a new variant of HTLV I. A major focus of HTLV-I infection occurs in the Caribbean region. In Trinidad and Tobago, seropositivity is restricted almost exclusively to persons of African descent, even though individuals of Indo-Asian ethnic background have shared a common environment for over 100 years. In Jamaica highest rates of positivity are observed in the lowland, high-rainfall areas. In Colombia, HTLV-I clusters along the Pacific Coast in an area with an unusually high rate of the associated neurologic syndrome. Other areas of South America with documented foci of HTLV-I include Brazil, Venezuela, Surinam, and Guyana. In Panama, a cluster of HTLV-II was recently reported in an isolated Indian population, representing the first known endemic focus for this orphan virus.

Recent surveys of the African continent (Nigeria, Zaire, Kenya, Tanzania) document that rates of HTLV-I seropositivity are similar to those in the Caribbean region, with documented examples of a microgeographic clustering in Zaire. Recently a focus of HTLV-I was found among Iranian Jews from northeastern Iran residing in Israel and New York.

Migrant populations often acquire infection early in life and carry their virus infection to nonendemic areas where disease may appear years later. Migrant populations from Okinawa to Hawaii and from the Caribbean to the United States and the United Kingdom are risk groups for HTLV positivity, as are Americans who experience exposure through sexual contact or transfusion in viral endemic areas.

Appearance and Nature of AIDS (see Ch. 412). Acquired immunodeficiency syndrome was recognized as a new disease among United States homosexual males in 1981. The disease was associated with a loss of T4 cells, progressive immunodeficiency manifesting with opportunistic infections, frequent development of certain tumors (particularly the peculiar multifocal proliferation known as Kaposi's sarcoma), and frequent impairment of the central nervous system. It was soon learned that the causal agent could also be transmitted by blood, plasma, and Factor VIII concentrate, and additional risk groups were identified (hemophiliacs, recipients of blood, and intravenous drug abusers and their sexual partners). The same disease was reported in central Africa and in Haiti, largely affecting sexually active heterosexual populations. By 1983 there were many theories on the cause of AIDS. One of these, the hypothesis that AIDS was caused by a new human T4 lymphotropic retrovirus, was proposed in 1982 and turned out to be correct. This idea was based on information derived from experiences with HTLV-I (and II) and from the feline leukemia virus. The latter virus causes a T-cell leukemia of cats, but a minor variant (of the envelope gene) causes an AIDS-like disease in cats. With the use of the same basic technology that had been employed for the isolation of HTLV-I, a new retrovirus termed LAV was identified in a patient with lymphadenopathy in 1983. In early 1984, numerous isolates of a new human retrovirus (termed HTLV-III) were described, and the virus was characterized, produced in permanent cell lines, used for development of a successful test to screen blood prior to transfusion, and unambiguously shown to be the cause of AIDS. In addition, reagents specific for this virus were developed and the virus was shown to be the same as the isolate obtained in 1983. The virus could now properly be called the AIDS virus or the human immunodeficiency virus (HIV-1).

TABLE 376–1. ROLE OF THE HIV ACCESSORY GENES FOR VIRUS REPLICATION

	Immunogenicity	Size	Cellular Localization	Function	Replication Competence of (−) Mutants
Viral infectivity factor (*vif*)	+	p23	Cytoplasm/inner membrane	Infectivity	±
Transactivating protein gene (*tat*)	+	p14	Nucleus/nucleolus	Transcriptional and post-transcriptional activation	−
Regulation of expression of virion gene (*rev*)	+	p19	Nucleus/nucleolus	Expression of structural proteins; modulation of transcription	−
Negative regulator factor gene (*nef*)	+ +	p27	Cytoplasm	Negative regulator	+ +
Viral protein R gene (*vpr*)	+	p18	Nucleus	Rapid viral growth (?)	+ +
Viral protein U gene (*vpu*) (HIV-1)	+	p15	Cytoplasm/membrane	Assembly and release (?)	+
Viral protein R gene (*vpx*)	+	p15	Cytoplasm	?	+ +

Although an accurate count of the number of HIV-1 infected persons worldwide is not available, estimates of 5 to 10 million persons, including 1 million in the United States alone, have been reported. The two major patterns worldwide are pattern I, primarily representing developed countries, in which homosexual contact and parenteral drug abuse are the major risk factors, and pattern II, usually in developing countries, in which heterosexual spread is the major source of infection.

Modes of Transmission of Human Retroviruses. There is a characteristic age-dependent rise in HTLV-I seroprevalence that first becomes prominent in the adolescent years. The rise is steeper in females than males and continues in females after age 40, whereas rates in males plateau around age 40. The explanation for this age-dependent rise in HTLV-I seroprevalence is unclear, although more efficient male-to-female transmission is most likely. Reactivation of latent infection throughout life or declining rates of infection in younger birth cohorts are also possible. For HIV-1 the characteristic age-dependent curve is bell-shaped with peak occurrence in the sexually active age group for both men and women. Childhood infection, especially in the neonatal age group, is a growing problem, especially in the face of increasing heterosexual spread. Summarized in Table 376–2 are the routes, cofactors, and viral characteristics associated with transmission of human retroviruses. The basic modes of transmission of HTLV-I are quite analogous to those of HIV-1.

Sexual transmission of HTLV-I from male to female and female to male as well as from male to male has been documented. HIV-1, which can be transmitted cell free (whereas HTLV-I is cell-associated) appears to be at least an order of magnitude more infectious than HTLV-I. Another cofactor for sexual transmission of HTLV and HIV is the coincidence of other sexually transmitted diseases, particularly ulcerative genital lesions such as occur in syphilis. Higher HIV-1 virus load, as measured by free p24 virus antigen and by quantitative PCR, is associated with heightened efficiency of transmission. For HTLV-I, elevated antibody titer, which also may correlate with virus load, is linked to heightened transmission.

The second major route of transmission is from mother to child. For HTLV-I, breast feeding, as documented from Japanese studies, is more efficient than perinatal transmission. For example, whereas 20 per cent of breast-fed infants seroconvert to HTLV-I, only 1 to 2 per cent of bottle-fed infants of HTLV-I–positive mothers become infected. In this regard HTLV-I differs from HIV-1 because perinatal transmission of HIV-1 appears to be associated with up to 30 per cent of neonatal (transplacental and/or perinatal) infections. The rate of breast milk–associated HIV-1 transmission is unknown because most HIV-1–positive mothers in the United States are discouraged from breast feeding.

A third major route of transmission is parenteral, via either transfusion or intravenous drug abuse. In the case of transfusion transmission, cellular components are associated with transmission of HTLV-I, whereas HIV-1 can be transmitted by cells, plasma, or plasma products. Approximately one half of recipients of HTLV-positive blood seroconvert, while for HIV-1 the percentage is over 95 per cent. Whereas AIDS results from HIV-1 transfusion transmission in a large percentage of cases, the only documented illness linked to HTLV-I transfusion transmission is the HTLV-associated demyelinating neurologic syndrome de-

TABLE 376–2. MODES OF HUMAN RETROVIRUS TRANSMISSION

Route
  Sexual: Male-to-female, female-to-male, and male-to-male
  Parenteral: Transfusion or IV drug abuse
  Mother-to-child transplacental, perinatal, and breast feeding
Cofactors
  Sexual
    Large number of sexual partners
    Traumatic sexual practice
    Coincident sexually transmitted diseases
  Needle sharing
Infectivity
  Virus replication
  Immune status—activated T-cell targets

scribed below. Among blood donors in the United States who are confirmed HTLV positive (approximately half are HTLV-I and the other half HTLV-II), the major risk factors are drug abuse, birthplace in a viral endemic area, and sexual contact with a person with this profile.

Parenteral drug abuse has also been associated with transmission of HTLV and HIV virus. The majority of HTLV positives are HTLV-II and not HTLV-I. Coinfection with HTLV-I and HIV-1 seems to result in a more rapid progression to AIDS through unexplained mechanisms possibly related to the cell-proliferative effects of HTLV-I on HIV-I infected T cells. Other modes of transmission involving "casual contact," mosquito transmission, etc. do not appear to occur. Health care and laboratory workers who experience a needle stick or skin or mucous membrane exposure in the absence of protective barriers are at low risk for HIV infection; only a single case of such infection has been documented in a Japanese health care worker exposed to HTLV-I.

MECHANISM, PATHOGENESIS, AND PATHOLOGY. **HTLV-I Pathogenesis.** A great deal has been learned about the pathogenesis of HTLV-I–associated leukemia. Early in infection, HTLV-I infects only a small number of T cells and perhaps the monocyte/macrophage. The DNA provirus randomly integrates into the DNA of infected cells. Whereas HTLV-I may exist as a latent virus, the genes of the virus promote cell proliferation by direct and indirect mechanisms including various lymphokine pathways. For example when lymphocytes from HTLV-I–infected normal persons are placed in tissue culture, they undergo spontaneous (in the absence of exogenous antigens or mitogens) lymphocyte proliferation. At some point, a clone of transformed, but not malignant, cells emerges, probably from a polyclonally transformed population. Such polyclonal, oligoclonal, and monoclonal expansions have been noted to appear and sometimes disappear spontaneously. After a long latent period (years to several decades), a monoclonal malignancy may develop, presumably involving additional oncogenic mutations. The reasons why only a small percentage of infected individuals develop malignancy (1 to 3 per cent lifetime risk), the disease takes so long to develop, and T4 cells are selectively involved (although T8 cells can also be infected) remain unknown. When malignancy develops, the HTLV-I provirus is found integrated in the DNA of the leukemic cells in a clonal fashion. The tumor contains one copy (or occasionally two copies) of the provirus integrated in the same chromosomal location in each cell. This means that the tumor was derived from a single transformed cell and that the virus infection occurred before transformation and clonal expansion, rather than later as a passenger virus. Tumors from different patients, however, have the provirus in different locations. This means that the mechanism cannot be a *cis*-activation of a nearby cellular gene by the LTR of the virus, as occurs with some animal leukemia viruses. It is postulated that transformation may involve at some stage the viral up-regulatory *tat* protein encoded by the px gene of HTLV-I. The *tat* protein induces expression of cellular genes critical for T-cell proliferation, including IL2 and its receptor (IL2R). The cells apparently both produce and respond to these growth factors (autocrine or autostimulation). This is probably the first step in leukemogenesis, and it leads to polyclonal T-cell proliferation. For the development of malignancy, one or more additional genetic changes are probably required because these cells become independent of IL2 requirements for growth. The continued expression of these growth factor receptors is likely to be a major abnormality in this leukemia. The nature and cause of the additional genetic changes are unknown, but these changes do not appear to require unique environmental factors, since the incidence of ATL is similar, for example, in the Caribbean region and Japan.

The pathogenesis of the HTLV-associated demyelinating neurologic syndrome, tropical spastic paraparesis/HTLV-associated myelopathy (TSP/HAM), is uncertain but appears to occur with a much shorter latency (sometimes acutely following transfusion-associated infection) than does ATL. Some researchers postulate a direct mechanism involving infection of nervous system cells, whereas others suggest an indirect mechanism involving immune- and autoimmune-mediated responses due to HTLV-I infection of regulatory T-cell populations.

Pathogenesis and Mechanisms of HIV-1. HIV-1 may be transmitted either as free extracellular virus or by virus-infected cells.

When transmitted by an infected cell, this "donor" cell may contact a target cell, the viral genes may then become activated, and virus is transmitted directly to the recipient cell. This route could avoid immune detection or exposure of the virus to antibodies. This mechanism may explain documented cases of virus-positive antibody-negative individuals as detected by virus culture and PCR. The duration of this latency is controversial and may vary from weeks to months. However, in general several weeks to months after exposure, a humoral immune response usually develops. High titers of antibodies are often made against every viral protein. This includes antibodies to the envelope of the virus, but the critical neutralizing antibodies (against one or more epitopes of the envelope) made after infection do not appear to prevent disease, presumably because the titers are too low or the response is too late, or both. Furthermore, it is now well documented that certain epitopes of the viral external envelope are hypervariable so that a series of quasispecies of viruses emerge which are resistant to immune inactivation. Cellular immunity (T-cell cytotoxicity against infected cells) has been well documented and appears to involve, among other sites, the same hypervariable neutralizing epitope that is shared by antibodies. The major target cells of HIV are the T4 cell and the monocyte/macrophage. Cells of the reticuloendothelial system, such as the Langerhans cells of the skin and follicular dendritic cells of the lymph node germinal centers and neuroglial cells of the brain, may also be infected. It appears that most target cells have CD4 on the cell surface. The mechanism by which HIV brings about destruction of the immune system is complex. In contrast to the immunostimulating effects of HTLV, HIV is immunoablative through both direct and probably indirect mechanisms.

For example, when the CD4 cell containing integrated HIV-1 DNA is immunostimulated, the HIV-1 provirus is activated, virus particles are formed, the CD4 + cell dies, and the virus spreads to reinitiate the process, which in time leads to a progressive depletion of the T4 cells. Other indirect mechanisms involving subversion of T-cell regulatory pathways, autoimmune phenomena, and immune paralysis have also been invoked to explain the discrepancy between the relatively small number of infected cells and the severity of the immune defect associated with HIV-1 infection. Infected macrophages may bring the virus to the brain, or free virus may cross the blood-brain barrier and infect microglial and possibly other non-neuronal cells. These cells may release factors that cause the major pathologic changes in the brain.

For HIV, the incubation period between infection and disease is estimated to range from 2 to 15 years or more, with a median of 8 to 10 years. In contrast to HTLV, which has a relatively low attack rate (3 to 5 per cent lifetime risk), HIV is projected to cause serious morbidity in over 60 to 80 per cent or more of infected persons. Prospective cohort studies document that 90 per cent of infected people progress from their presenting stage to a more advanced disease stage within 1.5 to 3 years. The major cofactor influencing progression is age. Newborns tend to progress more rapidly than adults, and older children and adolescents progress more slowly than adults or infants. The adolescent–young adult group tends to progress more slowly to immune depletion (e.g., CD4 count less than 200) than do adults, and once impaired they tend to take much longer to manifest clinical disease. A role for other cofactors has been postulated, including the occurrence of other viral infections, variation in HIV strain, difference in dose of inoculum, and nutritional status. Interestingly HTLV-I, perhaps owing to its shared regulatory structure or its immunostimulating effects, appears to accelerate progression to AIDS in HIV/HTLV-coinfected individuals. Some herpesviruses, including cytomegalovirus and human virus type 6 (HHV-6), may also accelerate progression, but the findings are controversial. Ultimately the fact that progression to AIDS shows a similar curve (controlling for age) in all risk groups suggests that most cofactor effects are less important than HIV-1 infection itself.

CLINICAL MANIFESTATIONS AND DIAGNOSIS. The list of HTLV-I–associated diseases has grown since adult T-cell leukemia/lymphoma (ATL) was first etiologically linked to HTLV-I (Table 376–3). The most common malignancy caused by HTLV-I is adult T-cell leukemia/lymphoma (ATL). The worldwide prevalence of these HTLV-I–associated leukemias is unknown; the incidence in any population depends on the prevalence of viral infection. In endemic areas such as southern Japan and the

TABLE 376–3. HTLV-ASSOCIATED DISEASE

Diagnosis	Nature of Syndrome	Strength of Association
Adult T-cell leukemia/lymphoma	Aggressive lymphoproliferative malignancy of mature T lymphocytes	Strong
B-cell chronic lymphocytic leukemia	Tumor-associated immunoglobin reacts to HTLV antigen	2 cases reported
Tropical spastic paraparesis (TSP)/HTLV-associated myelopathy (HAM)	Chronic progressive demyelinating syndrome of long motor tracks of spinal cord	Strong
Polymyositis	Degenerative inflammatory syndrome of skeletal muscles	Probable
Infective dermatitis	Chronic generalized eczema of skin; potential for preleukemia and immunodeficiency	Probable
Immune deficiency	Anecdotal reports of AIDS-like illness in HTLV-I positives; subclinical (e.g., decreased PPD response) or clinical (e.g., poor response to therapy for symptomatic strongyloidiasis)	Possible
Miscellaneous clinical conditions	Case reports or case series of polyarthropathy, interstitial pneumonitis, small cell lung cancer with monoclonal HTLV-I integration, and invasive cervical cancer in Japan	Uncertain

Caribbean islands, the annual incidence of virus-associated leukemia is approximately 3 per 100,000 per year and may account for one half of adult lymphoid malignancies in HTLV-I–endemic areas. The chance of an infected individual's developing malignancy over a lifetime is 1 to 5 per cent, with early-life exposure associated with the greatest risk for subsequent disease.

As further experience with ATL has been gained in viral endemic areas, the breadth of clinical variants has become more evident. The acute form of ATL as first described in Japan is characterized by an aggressive mature T-cell lymphoma whose clinical course is often associated with high white count, hypercalcemia, and cutaneous involvement. Other cases resemble T-cell chronic lymphocytic leukemia and are termed chronic ATL. Smoldering ATL may clinically resemble mycosis fungoides/Sezary syndrome with cutaneous involvement presenting as erythema or as infiltrative plaques or tumors. Sometimes a long prodrome of symptoms is noted before transformation to an acute, rapidly fatal form of disease occurs. Sometimes ATL presents as a T-cell non-Hodgkin's lymphoma with no clinical features of ATL except monoclonal integration of HTLV-I in proviral DNA in the tumor cells. Most patients with acute ATL die within 6 months of diagnosis. The cause of death is usually an explosive growth of tumor cells, hypercalcemia, and various opportunistic infections including *Pneumocystis carinii* pneumonia and other infections observed in AIDS patients. The age group ranges from adolescence to a peak in middle-aged adults. The diagnosis should be considered in adults with mature T-cell lymphoma and hypercalcemia and/or cutaneous involvement, particularly if the individual is from a known risk group or known endemic region. The diagnosis is established by testing serum for HTLV-I antibodies and finding leukemic T cells with the provirus in the blood or in biopsy specimens.

Other HTLV-I–Associated Diseases. An association between HTLV-I and some cases of B-cell chronic lymphotropic leukemia is now recognized. In this case, the role of the virus appears to be indirect. No viral sequences are found in the tumor, but the immunoglobulins of the tumor cell react to HTLV-I–specific antigens. It may be that chronic stimulation of B-cell proliferation by viral antigens, coupled with virus-induced impairment of T4-cell function, leads to an increase in the probability of malignant transformation in B cells.

HTLV-I has been linked to a neurologic syndrome called TSP/HAM. This disease is characterized by the usually chronic, slowly progressive development of spastic paraparesis resulting from the demyelination of the long motor neurons of the spinal cord. Symptoms often begin with a stiff gait progressing (usually slowly) to increasing spasticity and weakness, with incontinence and impotence developing later during the course of the illness. Sometimes ataxia develops. On nuclear magnetic resonance scan isolated lesions of the central nervous system are detected in some cases. The syndrome differs from classic multiple sclerosis because of the generally slow, progressive course and absence of waxing and waning of symptomatology. However, some cases are acutely progressive and such cases are sometimes associated with the transfusion of HTLV-I–positive blood. The incidence of disease is thought to be approximately twice that of ATL, and an indirect mechanism of pathogenesis, possibly immune-mediated, has been postulated, although direct viral infection of nervous system tissue has not been ruled out. The diagnosis is suspected in unexplained central nervous system disease with loss of pyramidal tract functions and is confirmed by testing sera for HTLV-I antibodies. There is no known treatment. Recently HTLV-I has also been linked to some cases of polymyositis of skeletal muscle in viral endemic areas. There are no features of these cases which distinguish this syndrome from polymyositis seen in HTLV-I–nonendemic areas. Possible links of HTLV-I to immunosuppression come from clinical and laboratory observations. Cases from Japan of patients with AIDS-like illnesses associated with HTLV-I (in the absence of underlying malignancy) have been reported. The association of HTLV-I with parasitic infestations (e.g., strongyloides) refractory to treatment have also been interpreted to suggest that HTLV-I may have immunosuppressive effects. Decreased skin test response to recall antigens has also been reported among HTLV-infected, especially older, individuals. The infective dermatitis syndrome in Jamaica may represent the first childhood HTLV-I syndrome, and immunosuppression and preleukemia are possible features. Other clinical syndromes mentioned as possible HTLV-associated diseases include large joint polyarthropathy and interstitial pneumonitis. A case of small cell lung cancer with monoclonal HTLV integration is of interest as well as the finding in Japan that invasive cervical cancer may also be HTLV-I–associated.

HTLV-II and Leukemia. This virus has been found in several cases of T-cell hairy cell leukemia and frequently among parenteral drug abusers. Recently a focus of HTLV-II was reported in an isolated tribe of Central American Indians in Panama. While molecular biologic studies of the leukemia cells from the HTLV-II–positive leukemia cases strongly suggest that HTLV-II is causally involved, surveys of hairy cell leukemia including some with T-cell phenotype have failed to document an association. HTLV-II, like HLTV-I, induces spontaneous lymphocyte proliferation in vitro but at a lower level than HTLV-I. HTLV-II remains a true orphan virus without clear disease association. The recognition of a naturally occurring endemic focus of HTLV-II in Panama and the development of new techniques for distinguishing HTLV-I from HTLV-II should make it feasible in coming years to characterize the epidemiology and clinical outcomes of infection.

CLINICAL MANIFESTATIONS OF HIV INFECTIONS. The spectrum of clinical outcomes, particularly opportunistic infection linked to HIV infection, is quite broad as detailed in Part XXI. While contributing to a relatively smaller percentage of AIDS-associated morbidity and mortality, certain malignancies such as Kaposi's sarcoma, B-cell lymphomas, and some carcinomas are more common in HIV-infected persons in association with varying levels of immune impairment. These malignancies are not directly due to HIV as a transforming virus, since viral genes are not present in the DNA of the cells of any of these tumors. Kaposi's sarcoma associated with HIV is composed of endothelial cells, fibroblasts, and other infiltrating cells, and recently indirect HIV-mediated growth factors have been defined which contribute to pathogenesis. Since Kaposi's sarcoma is very common in HIV-1–infected homosexuals but much less so in other HIV-infected individuals, another still unknown etiologic factor may be involved. The B-cell lymphomas are of several types, including some with rearranged c-*myc* genes in association

with Epstein-Barr virus analogous to the pattern reported in Burkitt's lymphoma. Recently, a new virus called human herpesvirus type 6 (HHV6) was isolated from some cases, but its pathogenic role is unclear. The study of HIV-associated lymphomas provides a unique opportunity to gain fundamental etiologic insights, especially since the number of lymphoma cases may be increasing in association with prolonged survival in HIV-infected persons on antiretroviral therapy.

TREATMENT AND PREVENTION. HTLV-I. There is no proven effective therapy for ATL; however, some cases do respond, occasionally with prolonged remission, to multidrug regimens for advanced-stage aggressive lymphoma. Exciting experimental approaches that employ monoclonal antibodies to the IL2 receptor which can be linked with cell toxins, selectively targeted to the leukemic cells, are one example. Other approaches involving antiretroviral therapy and various lymphokines are under consideration. Treatment of the complicating hypercalcemia often responds to standard methods but may be refractory, and opportunistic infections are frequent. Prevention is achieved by avoiding infection: testing blood prior to transfusion, care in sexual practices, and avoidance of mother-infant transmission by discouraging breast feeding.

Vaccines containing recombinant HTLV-I envelope produced in *Escherichia coli* and vaccinia virus–based expression vectors have been used successfully to prevent HTLV-I infection in monkeys and rabbits. Various sites that represent important biologic and immunologic epitopes of HTLV-I envelope have been mapped. The envelope gene of HTLV-I encodes a 63- to 67-kilodalton (kd) glycoprotein precursor that is proteolytically processed to give rise to a mature gp46 external envelope glycoprotein and a 21-kd transmembrane protein designated as p21E. Using rabbit antisera to the N- and C-terminal portions of HTLV-I gp63 envelope precursor, Japanese investigations have neutralized both American and Japanese HTLV-I isolates in vitro. Results indicate the presence of at least two neutralizing sites on HTLV-I envelope, one associated with the external gp46 envelope glycoprotein and a second associated with the p21E transmembrane glycoprotein. A vaccine consisting of an envelope subunit of HTLV generated protective immunity in cynomolgus monkeys against primary infection by HTLV-I. Of interest is that this study employed HTLV-I–infected cells as the challenge vehicle, which is a step closer to natural transmission than free virus itself. Protection correlated with the presence of neutralizing antibodies, indicating that humoral immunity can be an effective barrier against infection. More intensive studies are currently being carried out in a rabbit model of HTLV-I infection. This approach enables the optimization of candidate HTLV vaccines in terms of immunogenicity and efficacy. Since human or animal antisera to Japanese and American HTLV-I envelope cross-neutralize, it is likely that the envelope antigens of HTLV-I represent a single serotype worldwide. Thus, unlike the isolate-specific neutralizing epitopes of HIV, a synthetic vaccine against one HTLV-I isolate should protect against other HTLV-I isolates.

HIV. As detailed in Ch. 411, an understanding of the fundamental biology of HIV has also led to therapeutic breakthroughs. Nucleotide analogues, which can be used as antimetabolites against the error-prone virus reverse transcriptase, have already resulted in substantial benefit to patients with AIDS and ARC and with depressed T cells. Examples of this class of drugs with proven efficacy include azidothymidine (AZT) and dideoxyinosine (DDI). Combinations of these and other drugs may also show the type of benefit first noted in combination chemotherapy for cancer. Other promising approaches, such as hybrid moleculars that block CD4 binding of the virus, are the subject of ongoing therapeutic research. The major preventive strategies for HIV, in the absence of an effective vaccine, are to promote public health programs that decrease the likelihood of transmission. This includes educational campaigns which emphasize that HIV is a sexually transmitted agent. For parenteral drug abusers, elimination of needle sharing or, better yet, elimination of needle use through drug abuse treatment, as well as safe sex has also been promoted. A successful prevention strategy has been the implementation of screening of the blood supply for HIV, which has virtually eliminated this source of infection for hemophiliacs and blood recipients. HIV-1–positive women, whose children have a risk of infection from perinatal transmission of approximately 30 per cent, are encouraged not to breast feed their babies if they do conceive.

The goal of vaccine development is to generate an immune response that will be broadly reactive against all variants of the AIDS virus. A variety of approaches, including whole virus and subunit vaccines based on viral envelope proteins and *gag* antigen, are being tried (see Ch. 413). Type-specific neutralizing antibodies can be induced in many species, including primates, using native envelope glycoprotein, but no broadly reactive immunity has yet been achieved in animal studies. There are some early indications that some vaccine approaches are working in primate models. However, results are not yet reproducible, and the variation in virus strains, particularly at critical neutralizing sites, presents formidable barriers that need to be overcome.

SUMMARY

The story of human retrovirology is in its infancy, but it is already one of the most fascinating and important chapters in contemporary medicine. These viruses seem destined to open many doors to our knowledge of disease causation and provide conceptual advances in our understanding of disease pathogenesis. The human retroviruses—or viruses with similar properties of long latency, minimal replication, lymphotropism, and neurotropism—may be at the heart of some of our important unexplained autoimmune, immunodeficiency, and neurologic diseases. Some may be involved in other human malignancies.

Blattner WA (ed.): Human Retrovirology: HTLV. New York, Raven Press, 1990. *Comprehensive update of human T-cell leukemia virus, including chapters on virology, immunology, epidemiology, clinical features, and management.*

Bolognasi D: Immunobiology of the HIV envelope and its relativity to vaccine strategies. Mol Biol Med 7:1–15, 1990. *An updated review of HIV vaccine prospects and pitfalls.*

Ensoli B, Salahuddin SZ, Gallo RC: AIDS-associated Kaposi's sarcoma: A molecular model for its pathogenesis. Cancer Cells 1:93–96, 1989. *In this paper are reviewed new concepts of growth factor–mediated Kaposi's sarcoma carcinogenesis.*

Gallo RC, Montagnier L: AIDS in 1988. Sci Am 259:41–48, 1988. *The entire October, 1988 issue of Scientific American provides a readable and well-illustrated review of AIDS and HIV-related issues.*

Gallo RC, Wong-Staal F (eds.): Retrovirus Biology and Human Disease. New York, Marcel Dekker, Inc., 1990. *This scholarly book includes comprehensive reviews of the biology and molecular biology of human retroviruses.*

Goedert JJ, Kessler CM, Aledort LM, et al.: A prospective study of human immunodeficiency virus type 1 infection and the development of AIDS in subjects with hemophilia. N Engl J Med 321:1141–1148, 1989. *The natural history of HIV infection, particularly the role of age in progression to AIDS, is analyzed in this paper.*

Mitsuya H, Yarchoan R, Broder S: Molecular targets for AIDS therapy. Science 249:1533–1544, 1990. *A comprehensive review of current and future approaches to anti-HIV therapy which evaluates the basic molecular biology of the virus and the potential targets for therapeutic benefit.*

377 Enteroviral Diseases

Michael N. Oxman

Enteroviruses, so named because they generally infect the alimentary tract and are shed in the feces, cause a wide variety of diseases in humans and lower animals. They comprise one of the four major genera of the *Picornavirus* (*pico*, small; *rna*, ribonucleic acid) *Family*. The other picornavirus genera, distinguished from each other primarily by difference in sensitivity to acid and in buoyant density in cesium chloride, are *rhinoviruses*, which inhabit the upper respiratory tract and include the principal recognized etiologic agents of the common cold (see Ch. 360); *cardioviruses*, recovered chiefly from rodents and only very rarely implicated in human disease; and *aphthoviruses*, named for the vesicular lesions that they produce in cloven-footed animals. Only the enterovirus and rhinovirus genera contain important human pathogens.

Enteroviruses are differentiated from rhinoviruses primarily by their resistance to acid; they are fully infectious at pH 3 or even lower. Consequently, enteroviruses that have undergone limited replication in the oropharynx survive passage through the stomach and implant in the lower intestinal tract, where they undergo more extensive multiplication. In contrast, rhinoviruses are acid labile; they begin to lose infectivity at pH 6 and are completely inactivated at pH 3. They are further distinguished from enteroviruses by their lower optimal temperature of replication (33°C versus 37°C for enteroviruses) and higher buoyant density in cesium chloride. Since rhinoviruses inhabit the nasopharynx, they have no obvious need for acid stability, and their preferential replication at lower than body temperature probably reflects their adaptation to the cooler nasal passages.

Species of enteroviruses are distinguished immunologically by the ability of specific antisera to neutralize only the homotypic virus. There are now 68 recognized human enterovirus species (*serotypes* or *immunotypes*), as well as numerous enteroviruses of lower animals. Humans appear to be the only natural host for the human enteroviruses, and, in general, the enteroviruses of lower animals are not natural pathogens for humans.

Historically, human enteroviruses have been subclassified into *polioviruses*, group A and group B *coxsackieviruses*, and *echoviruses* on the basis of antigenic relationships, differences in host range, and type of disease produced (Table 377–1). By 1969, 67 species (serotypes) of human enteroviruses had been identified and classified according to these criteria, although reclassification and redundancy have reduced this number to 63. The distinguishing characteristics of these enterovirus subgroups are outlined below.

Polioviruses. The first human enteroviruses to be recognized, polioviruses produce characteristic lesions when inoculated into the central nervous system of primates. Clinical isolates replicate only in primates and in primate cell cultures (see Ch. 475). There are three poliovirus serotypes.

Coxsackieviruses. In contrast to polioviruses, coxsackieviruses produce paralysis and death when inoculated into suckling mice. This property was responsible for their detection and differentiation from polioviruses when they were first recovered in 1948 from the feces of two children in the village of Coxsackie, New York, who were suffering from a poliomyelitis-like paralytic illness. With the isolation of additional serotypes, it was recognized that when inoculated into suckling mice, some coxsackieviruses, designated *group A coxsackieviruses*, produced generalized myositis of skeletal muscles that resulted in flaccid

TABLE 377–1. CLASSIFICATION OF HUMAN ENTEROVIRUSES[a]

Enterovirus Group	Number of Serotypes	Numerical Designation	Growth in Primate Cell Culture	Pathogenicity for Suckling Mice	Pathogenicity for Monkeys
Poliovirus	3	1–3	+	−	+
Coxsackievirus, group A	23	A1–22, A24[b]	+/−[c]	+	−[d]
Coxsackievirus, group B	6	B1–6	+	+	−
Echovirus	31	1–9, 11–27, 29–34[e]	+	−	−
Enterovirus	5	68–72[f]	+[g]	Variable[h]	Variable[i]

[a]Many enterovirus strains have been isolated that do not conform to these criteria.

[b]Coxsackievirus A23 has been reclassified as echovirus 9.

[c]Except for a few serotypes (e.g., A7, A9, A16), primary isolates of group A coxsackieviruses grow poorly or not at all in cell culture; virus isolation requires inoculation of suckling mice.

[d]Coxsackievirus A7 is neurovirulent in monkeys.

[e]Echovirus 10 has been reclassified as reovirus type 1. Echovirus 28 has been reclassified as rhinovirus 1A.

[f]Hepatitis A virus has been classified as human enterovirus 72.

[g]Enterovirus 72 (hepatitis A virus) replicates in monkey kidney cell cultures without producing cytopathic effects.

[h]Enteroviruses 70 and 71 are pathogenic for suckling mice.

[i]Enteroviruses 70 and 71 are neurovirulent in monkeys.

paralysis, whereas others, designated *group B coxsackieviruses*, produced only focal myositis but caused an encephalitis that resulted in spastic paralysis and a generalized infection that involved the myocardium, brown fat, pancreas, and other organs. Moreover, group B coxsackieviruses could be readily propagated in primate cell cultures, whereas group A coxsackieviruses grew poorly or not at all. Twenty-three group A and six group B coxsackievirus serotypes have been identified.

Echoviruses. The use of the cell culture techniques developed by Enders and his associates led to the recovery from the feces of healthy children of additional enteroviruses that produced cytopathic effects in primate cell cultures but failed to produce disease in suckling mice or in the central nervous system of primates. There agents, initially considered "orphan" viruses because they were unrelated to any disease, were called *echoviruses* (*e*nteric *c*ytopathic *h*uman *o*rphan). Echoviruses have now been associated with a variety of diseases, and 31 serotypes have been identified. Most echoviruses are readily propagated in primate cell cultures.

The detailed comparison of enterovirus genomes supports the validity of this classification scheme. Different serotypes within the same human enterovirus subgroup, e.g., group B coxsackieviruses, generally have 30 to 50 per cent of their nucleotide sequences in common, whereas serotypes from different subgroups generally share fewer than 20 per cent of their nucleotide sequences. About 5 per cent of the nucleotide sequences are conserved among all human enteroviruses.

Over the years, however, an increasing number of enterovirus isolates were identified that could not be subclassified unambiguously by these criteria (e.g., viruses serologically related to known echoviruses but with a host range characteristic of coxsackieviruses). Consequently, it was agreed in 1970 that newly recognized human enteroviruses would be simply designated "enterovirus" and numbered sequentially, beginning with enterovirus 68. To avoid confusion with the older literature, the original classification (poliovirus, group A and group B coxsackievirus, and echovirus) has been retained for the first 63 serotypes. Since adoption of this simplified taxonomic scheme, five new human enteroviruses, enteroviruses 68 to 72, have been recognized.

Enteroviruses 68 to 72. Enterovirus 68 was initially isolated from the throat of an infant with bronchiolitis and pneumonia. Few isolates have since been reported, and the agent is little studied. Enterovirus 69 was recovered from the feces of an asymptomatic child, and this serotype has not yet been associated with disease. Enterovirus 70 is the principal cause of acute hemorrhagic conjunctivitis, a disease that was first recognized in 1969 and has subsequently affected tens of millions of persons throughout the world. Enterovirus 70 has an unusually broad host range; it causes meningoencephalitis in humans and experimentally infected monkeys and infects both primate and nonprimate cell cultures. Genome analysis and serologic surveys raise the possibility that it may be a zoonotic enterovirus that has recently extended its host range to include humans. Enterovirus 70 is discussed in Ch. 381. Enterovirus 71, first recognized as the cause of an outbreak of aseptic meningitis and encephalitis in California between 1969 and 1972, is neurovirulent in monkeys and produces a myositis in suckling mice typical of that produced by group A coxsackieviruses. Enterovirus 71 has been recovered throughout the world in association with a variety of clinical manifestations and many fatal infections. These have included respiratory infections, aseptic meningitis, hand-foot-and-mouth disease, maculopapular exanthems, encephalitis, and poliomyelitis-like paralytic disease. Hepatitis A virus has been classified as enterovirus 72 on the basis of its physical, biochemical, and biologic characteristics. However, differences between the nucleotide sequence of its genome and the genomes of other enteroviruses suggest that it may belong in a separate genus. Hepatitis A virus (enterovirus 72) is discussed in Ch. 117.

The enteroviruses have many features in common, and thus they are discussed as a group before considering the special features of individual members. Since polioviruses are the subject of Ch. 475, this discussion is limited to the nonpolio viruses.

CHARACTERISTICS OF NONPOLIO ENTEROVIRUSES

PHYSICAL AND BIOCHEMICAL CHARACTERISTICS.

The enteroviruses share with all picornaviruses certain important physical and biochemical characteristics: They are small, spherical, nonenveloped viruses approximately 30 nm in diameter. Their genome consists of a linear, single-stranded, unsegmented molecule of RNA with a molecular weight of about 2.6×10^6 daltons (approximately 7500 nucleotides) which has the same polarity as messenger RNA; i.e., it is plus (+) stranded and is thus infectious and can also be translated in vitro. The viral genome is tightly packed within an icosahedral protein shell or *capsid* composed of 60 identical subunits or *protomers,* each of which has a molecular mass of 90,000 to 100,000 daltons and is itself composed of four nonidentical virus-encoded polypeptides (VP1, VP2, VP3, and VP4). VP1, VP2, and VP3 are exposed on the virion surface, whereas VP4 lies buried in association with the RNA core. Like all picornaviruses, enteroviruses exhibit a unique pattern of replication in which the viral genome is translated into a single giant *polyprotein*, which is then cleaved by endogenous viral proteinases into the individual viral structural and nonstructural proteins.

Enteroviruses are stable over a wide range of pH (pH 3 to 10) and retain infectivity for days at room temperature, weeks at refrigerator temperature, and indefinitely when frozen at $-20°C$ or lower. They are readily inactivated at temperatures above 50°C, but this inactivation is inhibited by molar magnesium chloride, which greatly enhances the stability of enteroviruses at all environmental temperatures. Thus, magnesium chloride is widely employed as a stabilizer for oral poliovirus vaccines.

Enteroviruses are resistant to proteolytic enzymes and to inactivation by organic solvents (e.g., ether, alcohol, chloroform), disinfectants (e.g., Lysol, quaternary ammonium compounds), deoxycholate, and various detergents that destroy lipid-containing enveloped viruses such as herpesviruses, orthomyxoviruses, and paramyxoviruses. Enteroviruses are inactivated by formaldehyde, chlorination, and ultraviolet light but are protected from inactivation by dissolved organic matter, the formation of virus aggregates, and adsorption to particulate matter. Consequently, enteroviruses survive secondary sewage treatment and chlorination as generally practiced and are abundant in urban sewage and treated waste water. The agricultural use of treated sewage and recycled waste water may thus contaminate food and water supplies. Since sewage treatment that destroys fecal coliform bacteria does not eliminate enteroviruses, the use of fecal coliform counts to assess the sanitary quality of water is inadequate with respect to its potential for transmission of enteroviral diseases. Enteroviruses are often detectable in samples of recreational water judged acceptable on the basis of fecal coliform counts. Although person-to-person (fecal-oral) spread is the dominant mode of transmission, and waterborne outbreaks of enterovirus infection have rarely been documented, the hazard associated with the discharge of virus-laden sewage into coastal waters is demonstrated by the occurrence of shellfish-associated outbreaks of hepatitis A (caused by enterovirus 72). Clams, mussels, and oysters are filter-feeders that concentrate virus and function as passive virus carriers. Most of the enteroviruses in sewage are associated with suspended solids, and virus adsorbed to sediment remains infectious for long periods in the marine environment. The reintroduction of specific enteroviruses into coastal populations when marine sediments are disturbed by storms or dredging might explain the sudden occurrence of epidemics and the reappearance of certain enterovirus serotypes after years of absence from the human population.

EPIDEMIOLOGY. Human enteroviruses are worldwide in distribution, and humans are their only known reservoir. The prevalence of enterovirus infection varies markedly with season and climate and with the age and socioeconomic status of the population studied. In tropical and semitropical regions, enterovirus infections are frequent throughout the year. In temperate climates, the incidence of infection is markedly increased in the summer and early fall; 80 to 90 per cent of enterovirus isolates are recovered during the period from June through October, with peak recovery in August. Even within the United States, climatic and socioeconomic factors can be seen to affect the prevalence of enterovirus infections. Enterovirus isolation rates from young children are two- to threefold higher in southern than in northern cities and three- to sixfold higher in lower than in middle and upper socioeconomic districts. In developed countries, usually only one to three enterovirus serotypes are highly prevalent in a given community each year, with different serotypes prevalent in different years, and isolation rates in young children rarely exceed 10 per cent. In developing countries with poor sanitation, a greater number of enterovirus serotypes circulate simultaneously, and isolation rates in children regularly exceed 75 per cent, with many fecal specimens yielding three or more enterovirus serotypes.

Some enteroviruses appear to be endemic, being isolated at low frequency in the same locality each year, whereas others produce local or regional epidemics and then disappear, only to return again years later. Occasionally, an enterovirus spreads worldwide, infecting tens of millions of persons and producing pandemic disease. This pattern was observed with echovirus 9 in the late 1950's and with enterovirus 70, which caused a pandemic of acute hemorrhagic conjunctivitis beginning in 1969 (see Ch. 381).

Enteroviruses exhibit a high rate of mutation during replication in the human gastrointestinal tract, and this can lead to the appearance of antigenic variants, as well as virus strains with altered tissue tropism, host range, and virulence. Such mutations are readily detected within days after the administration of attenuated poliovirus vaccines to normal children. They have also been observed in a number of nonpolio enteroviruses. Recently isolated strains of several coxsackieviruses, echoviruses, and enterovirus 70 have been found to differ in many epitopes from the corresponding *prototype* strains isolated more than a decade earlier, a pattern of "antigenic drift" not unlike that seen with influenza viruses. In addition, recombination between the genomes of different enterovirus serotypes is a frequent occurrence in multiply infected individuals, e.g., in young children in developing countries, and in recipients of trivalent oral poliovirus vaccines. Antigenic changes and alterations in cell tropism produced by mutation and recombination may help to account for the ability of individual enterovirus serotypes to persist in nature and to cause a variety of clinical syndromes.

Transmission of human enteroviruses is chiefly by the fecal-oral route directly from person to person or via fomites; spread by respiratory secretions plays a lesser role. After infection by most serotypes, virus can be recovered from the oropharynx and intestine of both symptomatic and asymptomatic individuals, but virus is shed in greater amounts and for a longer period (a month or more) in the feces.

Young children have the highest rates of infection, and enteroviruses are most efficiently disseminated by infected children less than 2 years of age. Spread is from child to child and then within family groups, and it is facilitated by crowding and poor hygiene. Introduction of virus into the household by one family member results in a high rate of infection among others lacking type-specific neutralizing antibodies; family surveillance studies have demonstrated secondary attack rates of approximately 90 per cent for polioviruses, 75 per cent for coxsackieviruses, and 50 per cent for echoviruses. Middle-class parents with children in day care centers are at particular risk. Reared in circumstances that minimized their childhood exposure, they are likely to be susceptible to infection by many of the enteroviruses brought home from day care centers by their asymptomatically infected toddlers. This is well illustrated by day care center–based outbreaks of hepatitis A (see Ch. 117).

Although the epidemiology of most enteroviruses is similar, patterns of infection with some serotypes are distinctive. Enterovirus 70 and coxsackievirus A24, etiologic agents of acute hemorrhagic conjunctivitis (see Ch. 381), are transmitted by direct inoculation of the conjunctivae by fingers and fomites contaminated with infected tears. Replication of these viruses in the alimentary tract, if it occurs at all, is limited. Coxsackievirus A21 is also shed primarily from the upper respiratory tract, where it produces a rhinovirus-like illness.

The incubation period for illnesses caused by enteroviruses may vary from less than 1 day to more than 4 weeks, but it is generally 2 to 10 days. It is shortest when symptoms are the direct result of virus replication at the portal of entry (e.g., acute hemorrhagic conjunctivitis caused by enterovirus 70) and longest when they reflect tissue injury that involves immunopathology in target organs infected following viremia (e.g., hepatitis A and some forms of coxsackievirus myocarditis).

PATHOGENESIS. The pathogenesis of enterovirus infections is best understood for polioviruses, which have been extensively studied in experimentally infected primates and in humans infected with attenuated vaccine strains. The pathogenesis of most nonpolio enterovirus infections appears to be similar, except for the principal target organs affected.

Following ingestion of fecally contaminated material by individuals lacking type-specific neutralizing antibodies, virus implants and replicates in susceptible tissues of the pharynx and distal small intestine. These probably include mucosal epithelial cells and lymphoid tissues in the lamina propria, tonsils, and Peyer's patches. Within a day or two virus spreads to regional lymph nodes, and on about the third day small quantities escape into the blood stream (the "minor viremia") and are disseminated throughout the reticuloendothelial system (liver, spleen, bone marrow, lymph nodes) and to other receptor-bearing target tissues. None of the replicative events up to this point produce symptoms and, in most cases, infection is contained by host defense mechanisms without further progression, resulting in asymptomatic infection. In a minority of infected persons, replication continues in reticuloendothelial tissues, producing, by about the fifth day, a heavy sustained viremia (the "major viremia") that coincides with the "minor illness" of poliovirus infection (see Ch. 475) and with the "nonspecific febrile illness" caused by other human enteroviruses. The major viremia also disseminates large amounts of virus to target organs, such as the spinal cord, brain, meninges, heart, and skin, where further virus replication results in inflammatory lesions and cell necrosis. In most such patients, host defense mechanisms quickly terminate the major viremia and halt virus replication in target organs; only rarely is virus replication in target organs extensive enough to be clinically manifest. Although other host defense mechanisms (e.g., macrophages, interferon production) are doubtless involved, neutralizing antibodies play a major role in terminating viremia and limiting enterovirus multiplication in target tissues. Serotype-specific neutralizing antibodies may be detected in the serum within 4 or 5 days of the infection, and they generally persist for life. Evidence for the critical role of antibodies in terminating infection is provided by the occurrence of chronic persistent enterovirus infections in agammaglobulinemic children. Host defenses do not, however, terminate virus replication in the intestine, and fecal shedding continues for weeks after both symptomatic and asymptomatic enterovirus infections. Reinfection (i.e., virus excretion by a person with pre-existing homotypic antibodies) is relatively uncommon. When it occurs, infection is confined to the alimentary tract and is not associated with illness, and the duration of virus shedding is markedly reduced.

The clinical syndrome(s) caused by a given enterovirus reflects the particular target organs and tissues that it infects, i.e., its *cell tropism*. All of the determinants of cell tropism have not been elucidated, but a major factor is the presence on the cell surface of specific *receptor* molecules to which the virus attaches. Different groups of enteroviruses utilize different receptors, most or all of which are encoded by genes on human chromosome 19. Distinct receptors have already been identified for the polioviruses, a subset of group A coxsackieviruses, group B coxsackieviruses, and echoviruses, as well as for two subsets of human rhinoviruses.

The presence and density of various receptor molecules on the surface of cells are profoundly influenced by such factors as species, cell type, physiologic state, degree of differentiation, innervation, and exposure to extracellular signals such as hormones, lymphokines, and growth factors. Thus, for example, the susceptibility of primates and the resistance of mice to poliovirus infection are correlated with the presence of poliovirus receptors only on primate cells; and the ability of group A coxsackieviruses to produce myositis only in suckling mice is correlated with the presence of specific receptors on differentiating myoblasts, but not on the fully differentiated myocytes of older animals.

Several of the enterovirus receptors that have been characterized are members of the immunoglobulin superfamily; for example, intracellular adhesion molecule-1 (ICAM-1), which binds to an integrin (LFA-1) on lymphocytes and promotes their adherence to a variety of nonlymphoid cells, serves as the receptor for several of the group A coxsackieviruses as well as for the majority of human rhinoviruses. These receptor molecules appear to extend from the cell surface and mediate virus attachment by binding to a specific site located on the floor of canyon-like depressions on the surface of the virus capsid. Because these canyons are too narrow to admit antibody molecules, neutralizing antibodies are not directed at the receptor attachment site itself but at epitopes on or near the canyon rim. Antibody molecules bound to these epitopes prevent virus attachment indirectly by preventing the receptor molecule from reaching its attachment site within the canyon. Since these "neutralizing" epitopes are unique in each enterovirus serotype, neutralizing antibodies are serotype-specific (e.g., antibody to coxsackievirus B2 does not neutralize coxsackievirus B5) despite the fact that a number of enterovirus serotypes (e.g., all group B coxsackieviruses) share the same cellular receptor. In contrast to virus-specific neutralizing antibodies, monoclonal antibody to a cellular receptor can prevent infection by all of the enterovirus serotypes that utilize it. Similarly, soluble preparations of receptor molecules can neutralize the infectivity of all enterovirus serotypes that utilize that particular receptor. These observations suggest new approaches to the prevention and treatment of enteroviral diseases.

CLINICAL MANIFESTATIONS. The majority of nonpolio enterovirus infections (50 to 80 per cent) are asymptomatic. Most symptomatic infections consist of "undifferentiated febrile illnesses" ("summer grippe"), often accompanied by upper respiratory symptoms. These are generally mild and last only a few days. This syndrome is totally nonspecific; it can be caused by virtually any enterovirus serotype, as well as by members of several other virus families (e.g., adenoviruses, paramyxoviruses, orthomyxoviruses). The so-called characteristic enterovirus syndromes, such as aseptic meningitis, hand-foot-and-mouth disease, and pleurodynia, are in fact unusual manifestations of enterovirus infection. They represent the "very small tip of a very large iceberg."

Some clinical syndromes are highly associated with certain enterovirus serotypes or subgroups (e.g., hand-foot-and-mouth disease with coxsackievirus A16, myopericarditis with group B

TABLE 377–2. CLINICAL MANIFESTATIONS OF NONPOLIO ENTEROVIRUS INFECTIONS[a]

Clinical Syndrome	Group A Coxsackieviruses[b]	Group B Coxsackieviruses	Echoviruses	Enteroviruses
Asymptomatic infection	All serotypes	All serotypes	All serotypes	All serotypes
Undifferentiated febrile illness ("summer grippe") with or without respiratory symptoms	All serotypes	All serotypes	All serotypes	68, 70, 71
Aseptic meningitis	1, 2, 3, 4, 5, 6, 7, 8, 9, 10, 11, 14, 16, 17, 18, 22, 24	1, 2, 3, 4, 5, 6	1, 2, 3, 4, 5, 6, 7, 8, 9, 10, 11, 12, 14, 16, 17, 18, 19, 20, 21, 22, 23, 25, 30, 31, 33	70, 71
Encephalitis	2, 4, 5, 6, 7, 9, 10, 16	1, 2, 3, 4, 5	2, 3, 4, 6, 7, 9, 11, 14, 17, 18, 19, 22, 25, 30, 33	70, 71
Paralytic disease (poliomyelitis-like)	4, 5, 6, 7, 9, 10, 11, 14, 16, 21	1, 2, 3, 4, 5, 6	1, 2, 4, 6, 7, 9, 11, 14, 16, 17, 18, 19, 30	70, 71
Myopericarditis	1, 2, 4, 5, 7, 8, 9, 14, 16	1, 2, 3, 4, 5, 6	1, 2, 3, 4, 6, 7, 8, 9, 11, 14, 16, 17, 19, 22, 25, 30	
Pleurodynia	1, 2, 4, 6, 9, 10, 16	1, 2, 3, 4, 5, 6	1, 2, 3, 6, 7, 8, 9, 11, 12, 14, 16, 19, 23, 24, 25, 30	
Herpangina	1, 2, 3, 4, 5, 6, 7, 8, 9, 10, 16, 22	1, 2, 3, 4, 5	6, 9, 11, 16, 17, 22, 25	
Hand-foot-and-mouth disease	4, 5, 7, 9, 10, 16	2, 5		71
Exanthems	2, 4, 5, 6, 7, 9, 10, 16	1, 2, 3, 4, 5	2, 4, 5, 6, 9, 11, 16, 18, 25	71
Common cold	2, 10, 21, 24	1, 2, 3, 4, 5	2, 4, 9, 11, 20, 25	
Lower respiratory tract infections (broncheolitis, pneumonia)	7, 9, 16	1, 2, 3, 4, 5	4, 8, 9, 11, 12, 14, 19, 20, 21, 25, 30	68, 71
Acute hemorrhagic conjunctivitis[c]	24			70
Generalized disease of the newborn	3, 9, 16	1, 2, 3, 4, 5	3, 4, 6, 7, 9, 11, 12, 14, 17, 18, 19, 20, 21, 22, 30	

[a]A great many enterovirus serotypes have been implicated in most of these syndromes, at least in sporadic cases. The serotypes listed are those that have been clearly and/or frequently implicated. Serotypes with the strongest association are underlined.

[b]Because isolation of many of the group A coxsackieviruses requires suckling mouse inoculation, they are likely to be underreported as causes of illness.

[c]Conjunctivitis without hemorrhage is frequently seen in association with other manifestations in patients infected with many group A and group B coxsackieviruses and echoviruses, especially coxsackieviruses A9, A16, and B1 to 5; and echoviruses 2, 7, 9, 11, 16, and 30.

coxsackieviruses), but these associations are not specific. The same syndrome may be caused by a number of enterovirus serotypes. Conversely, a single enterovirus serotype may cause several different syndromes, even within the same outbreak (Table 377-2). The more important syndromes are discussed below.

Aseptic meningitis is the most common significant illness caused by nonpolio enteroviruses, and these viruses are responsible for more than 80 per cent of the cases of aseptic meningitis in which an etiologic agent is identified. Almost every enterovirus serotype has been implicated, but those most frequently associated include coxsackieviruses A2, A4, A7, A9, A10, and B1 to 5; echoviruses 3, 4, 6, 9, 11, 14, 16 to 19, 25, 30, and 33; and enteroviruses 70 and 71, all of which have been responsible for outbreaks as well as sporadic cases. Attack rates are generally highest in children, but cases also occur in adults, especially during larger outbreaks. Initial symptoms, which are typical of *undifferentiated febrile illness* (e.g., fever, headache, malaise, myalgias, and sore throat) are followed, usually within a day, by signs and symptoms of meningitis, including a more severe headache that is often retrobulbar, photophobia, meningismus, stiffness of the neck and back, and nausea and vomiting, especially in children. The illness is sometimes biphasic like poliomyelitis. In some cases, especially those caused by echoviruses and enterovirus 71, meningitis may be accompanied by a rash which, if petechial, may raise the specter of meningococcemia. The cerebrospinal fluid is clear and under slightly increased pressure. The total cell count, which can vary from less than 10 per cubic millimeter to more than 3000 per cubic millimeter, averages 50 to 500 per cubic millimeter. Initially, neutrophils may predominate (although they rarely exceed 90 per cent), but they are quickly replaced by mononuclear cells. The glucose concentration is usually normal, and the protein concentration is normal or slightly elevated (<100 mg per deciliter). Fever and signs of meningeal inflammation subside in 3 to 7 days, although cerebrospinal fluid pleocytosis may persist for an additional week or more. The great majority of children and adults recover fully without sequelae. However, enteroviral meningitis during the first year of life may, in up to 10 per cent of affected infants, result in permanent neurologic damage as evidenced by reduced head circumference, spasticity, and impaired intellectual function.

Paralytic disease may occur in the course of many nonpolio enterovirus infections, but it is generally less severe than that caused by polioviruses. Muscle weakness is far more common than frank paralysis and recovery is nearly always complete, although occasional patients suffer cranial nerve palsies or severe, sometimes fatal, bulbar involvement. Frequently implicated serotypes include coxsackieviruses A7, A9, and B2 to 5; echoviruses 2, 4, 6, 9, 11, and 30; and enteroviruses 70 and 71. In contrast to paralytic poliomyelitis, which in the prevaccine era occurred in epidemics, cases of paralysis associated with nonpolio enteroviruses are generally sporadic. However, several nonpolio enteroviruses produce paralytic disease with sufficient frequency to cause local outbreaks and epidemics. A variant of coxsackievirus A7 has caused outbreaks, as well as numerous sporadic cases of paralytic disease. In fact, it was once thought to be a fourth serotype of poliovirus. Paralytic disease resembling poliomyelitis, with a significant incidence of residual paralysis and muscle atrophy, has been observed in patients with acute hemorrhagic conjunctivitis caused by enterovirus 70 (see Ch. 381). Enterovirus 71 has caused outbreaks and epidemics of cutaneous and central nervous system disease in temperate regions around the world since its initial isolation in California in 1969. These have included epidemics of poliomyelitis-like paralytic disease with residual flaccid paralysis and of encephalitis, with significant mortality.

Encephalitis is a well-recognized but uncommon manifestation of enterovirus infection. Thus, despite their prevalence, enteroviruses account for only 10 to 20 per cent of the cases of encephalitis of proven viral etiology in the United States. The most frequently implicated serotypes include coxsackieviruses A9, B2, and B5; echoviruses 4, 6, 9, 11, and 30; and enterovirus 71. In most cases, encephalitis complicates the course of aseptic meningitis; parenchymal involvement is indicated by the onset of confusion, coma, abnormalities of motor function, hemiparesis, vasomotor instability, cranial nerve palsies, cerebellar ataxia, and focal or generalized seizures, singly or in various combinations. Cerebral involvement is usually generalized, but focal encepha-

litis does occur and may occasionally be clinically indistinguishable from herpes simplex encephalitis. Recovery is usually complete, although neurologic sequelae and deaths occur, especially in young infants and during enterovirus 71 epidemics.

Other neurologic complications, including Guillain-Barré syndrome, transverse myelitis, and Reye syndrome, have been reported in patients with enterovirus infections. However, no clear epidemiologic or etiologic linkage to enteroviruses has been established and, given the high prevalence of enterovirus infections, the associations may be only coincidental.

Enterovirus infections tend to be more severe in the newborn infant than in older children and adults. Asymptomatic infections and undifferentiated febrile illnesses are still common, but many infections, especially those caused by group B coxsackieviruses and echovirus 11, result in a fulminant, frequently fatal, generalized disease. This *generalized disease of the newborn* is often clinically indistinguishable from bacterial sepsis or neonatal herpes simplex virus infection. Manifestations include myocarditis, meningoencephalitis, hepatitis, pancreatitis, adrenal involvement, and disseminated intravascular coagulation with hemorrhage and circulatory collapse. Virus is frequently acquired transplacentally when the mother is infected just prior to birth, but it may also be acquired by contact during delivery or nosocomially in the newborn nursery. Once an enterovirus is introduced into a newborn nursery, usually by a transplacentally infected infant, it is often spread to other infants on the hands of nursery personnel.

Enteroviruses, primarily echoviruses, have been responsible for a syndrome of chronic meningoencephalitis in patients with inherited or acquired defects in B-lymphocyte function, most often children with X-linked agammaglobulinemia. The majority of these patients have a dermatomyositis-like syndrome and many also have chronic hepatitis. Surprisingly, despite the presence in their cerebrospinal fluid of abundant virus, a lymphocytic pleocytosis and an elevated protein concentration, these patients generally exhibit few if any clinical signs of meningitis. The pathogenesis of this often fatal disease remains to be elucidated.

Several important syndromes caused by nonpolio enteroviruses are discussed in subsequent chapters and thus are not considered here. These include epidemic pleurodynia (Ch. 378), myopericarditis (Ch. 379), a variety of exanthems and enanthems (Ch. 380), and acute hemorrhagic conjunctivitis (Ch. 381).

A number of enteroviruses have been associated with mild upper respiratory tract illness in children and adults, especially coxsackieviruses A21, A24, and B1 to 5; and echoviruses 2, 4, 9, 11, 20, and 25. Enteroviruses have also been associated with lower respiratory tract illnesses in infants and children, although rarely in adults. These include tracheitis, bronchitis, croup, bronchiolitis, and pneumonia. Frequently implicated serotypes include coxsackieviruses A9, A16, and B1 to 5; echoviruses 4, 8, 9, 11, 12, 14, 19 to 21, 25, and 30; and enterovirus 68. In addition, respiratory tract symptoms frequently accompany the undifferentiated febrile illnesses ("summer grippe") caused by most enteroviruses. The respiratory illnesses caused by enteroviruses are clinically indistinguishable from similar illnesses caused by viruses more commonly considered to be respiratory tract pathogens, such as rhinoviruses, influenza viruses, parainfluenza viruses, respiratory syncytial virus, and adenoviruses. However, infections with these viruses occur most frequently during the winter, whereas enterovirus infections occur primarily in the summer and early fall.

DIAGNOSIS. The enteroviral etiology of a disease may be suspected on clinical and epidemiologic grounds, but the multiplicity of agents capable of causing most clinical syndromes makes it impossible to establish a specific etiologic diagnosis on the basis of such information alone. Virus isolation and/or serologic evidence is required. Most enteroviruses can be isolated from the pharyngeal secretions and feces of infected patients. However, the high prevalence of asymptomatic enterovirus infections and the prolonged period (up to 3 months) of virus shedding following both symptomatic and asymptomatic infections make it difficult to assess the etiologic significance of an enterovirus isolated concurrently with an episode of disease; it may merely reflect an etiologically unrelated antecedent or intercurrent infection. The development of serotype-specific antibodies, demonstrated by assay of acute and convalescent sera, indicates that the enterovirus infection occurred concurrently with the episode of disease, but even this does not prove that the enterovirus was causal. The following criteria are generally used to establish the etiologic association of an enterovirus with a given disease: (1) There is a much higher rate of isolation of the virus from patients with the disease than from healthy controls matched for age, socioeconomic status, area of residence, and time; (2) antibodies against the virus develop during the course of the disease; (3) virologic and serologic evidence of concurrent infection by other agents known to cause a similar clinical syndrome is negative; (4) the virus is isolated from pathologically involved tissues or body fluids that are not normally sites from which asymptomatic virus shedding occurs (e.g., from cerebrospinal fluid in patients with aseptic meningitis; from the myocardium in patients with myopericarditis). Only the isolation of virus from pathologically involved tissues constitutes proof of causation. An alternative to the isolation of virus from pathologically involved sites is the identification in these sites of viral proteins or viral RNA. It is now possible to detect enteroviral RNA in tissues directly by nucleic acid hybridization or following amplification by the polymerase chain reaction (PCR) using probes and primers from regions of the genome that are common to all human enteroviruses.

In the individual patient, the diagnosis of enterovirus infection is most readily established by virus isolation. Rising titers of serotype-specific neutralizing antibodies in paired acute and convalescent sera are confirmatory, but serologic diagnosis cannot generally substitute for virus isolation. This is because group-reactive antigens are lacking, and it is impractical to perform serotype-specific tests (e.g., neutralization tests) for each of the 68 recognized human enteroviruses. Of necessity, serologic assays are generally limited to neutralization tests against the patient's virus isolate (if one has been obtained), against one or two serotypes then prevalent in the community, or against a very limited number of enterovirus serotypes suspected on the basis of the nature of the clinical illness, e.g., the three poliovirus serotypes in a patient with paralytic disease, coxsackievirus A24 and enterovirus 70 in a patient with acute hemorrhagic conjunctivitis, or coxsackieviruses B1 to 6 in a patient with myopericarditis. Because of the importance of demonstrating seroconversion, or at least a marked rise in antibody titer, it is imperative that specimens of acute serum be obtained as early in the course of disease as possible; convalescent serum is obtained 2 to 4 weeks later. Serotype-specific IgM assays, already developed for enteroviruses 70 and 72 (hepatitis A virus), and the use of new techniques for the detection of enterovirus RNA, can be expected to improve the speed and accuracy of enteroviral diagnosis.

TREATMENT AND PREVENTION. Specific antiviral chemotherapy and chemoprophylaxis are not yet available for enterovirus infections. Treatment is symptomatic and, in severe disease, supportive. Corticosteroids, which have a deleterious effect on coxsackievirus-infected mice, should not be administered during acute enterovirus infections. Strenuous exercise and intramuscular injections, both of which appear capable of precipitating paralysis of the involved muscles during poliovirus and enterovirus 70 infections, should probably also be avoided during the acute, presumably viremic, phase of symptomatic enterovirus infections. Administration of immune serum globulin, which contains high titers of neutralizing antibodies to many enteroviruses, appears to have been useful in some agammaglobulinemic patients with chronic enteroviral meningoencephalitis. Immune serum globulin may also have a role in the treatment of enteroviral infections in other patients with severely compromised B-lymphocyte function. Infants with generalized neonatal enterovirus infections are unlikely to have received antibodies to the causative virus from their mothers. Consequently, it seems reasonable to administer immune serum globulin to such infants in an attempt to terminate their viremia and limit virus replication in infected tissues.

Live attenuated and inactivated poliovirus vaccines have been remarkably successful in preventing paralytic poliomyelitis (see Ch. 16), and live, inactivated, and synthetic vaccines produced by recombinant DNA technology are being developed for hepatitis A (caused by enterovirus 72). However, the large number of nonpolio enterovirus serotypes and the benign nature of most

nonpolio enterovirus infections have precluded the development of vaccines for these agents. Pre-exposure administration of immune serum globulin reduces the risk of paralytic poliomyelitis. Since immune serum globulin also contains neutralizing antibodies to many nonpolio enteroviruses, it would probably prevent many nonpolio enteroviral diseases as well. This approach has proven effective for pre- and postexposure prophylaxis of hepatitis A and probably reduces the frequency of severe enteroviral infections in agammaglobulinemic patients receiving replacement therapy. However, the benign nature of most enterovirus infections, the fact that exposures are rarely recognized (most result from contact with an asymptomatically infected person), and the relatively short half-life of exogenous immune serum globulin make this approach to prevention impractical in most situations. Nursery outbreaks of severe enteroviral disease provide an exception; the administration of immune serum globulin to all infants in the nursery offers protection to those infants without transplacentally acquired neutralizing antibody who have not yet been infected.

In general, control of enterovirus infections is best effected by hygienic measures, such as handwashing, and improvements in sanitation. Isolation of patients with enteroviral illnesses is generally not helpful because of the simultaneous existence of a large reservoir of unidentified asymptomatically infected patients who are excreting virus.

Cherry JD: Enteroviruses: Polioviruses (poliomyelitis), coxsackieviruses, echoviruses, and enteroviruses. In Feigin RD, Cherry JD (eds.): Textbook of Pediatric Infectious Diseases. Philadelphia, W.B. Saunders, 1987, pp 729–790. *A thorough review of enteroviral diseases with an emphasis on infections of children and newborn infants and a comprehensive bibliography.*
McKinney RE, Katz SL, Wilfert CM: Chronic enteroviral meningoencephalitis in agammaglobulinemic patients. Rev Infect Dis 9:334–356, 1987. *An excellent review of this interesting syndrome with thoughtful discussion of pathogenesis and management.*
Melnick JL: Enteroviruses. In Fields BN, et al. (eds.): Virology, 2nd ed. New York, Raven Press, 1990, pp 549–605. *An authoritative review with an extensive bibliography and an emphasis on epidemiology.*
Modlin JF: Coxsackieviruses, echoviruses, and newer enteroviruses. In Mandel GL, Douglas RG Jr, Bennett JE (eds.): Principles and Practice of Infectious Diseases. New York, Churchill Livingstone, 1990, pp 1367–1383. *An extensive review of the epidemiology and clinical manifestations of nonpolio enterovirus infections, with an excellent bibliography.*
Rotbart HA: Nucleic acid detection systems for enteroviruses. Clin Microbiol Rev 4:156–168, 1991. *A practical and authoritative review of the newest and most promising approaches to the diagnosis of enteroviral diseases.*
Rueckert RR: Picornaviridae and their replication. In Fields BN, et al. (eds.): Virology, 2nd ed. New York, Raven Press, 1990, pp 507–548. *A detailed summary of our current knowledge of picornavirus structure, replication, and virus-cell interactions.*

378 Epidemic Pleurodynia (Bornholm Disease)

Michael N. Oxman

DEFINITION. Epidemic pleurodynia is an acute febrile viral illness characterized by the sudden onset of intense paroxysmal lower thoracic or abdominal pain. Synonyms include Bornholm disease, devil's grip, epidemic myalgia, epidemic benign dry pleurisy, and Sylvest's disease. The name *pleurodynia* (*pleura*, side; *odyne*, pain) reflects the characteristic intercostal location of the pain and does not connote disease of the pleura. Pleurodynia is usually an epidemic disease, but sporadic cases do occur.

ETIOLOGY. The enteroviral etiology of epidemic pleurodynia was established in 1949. Group B coxsackieviruses, especially B3 and B5, are the principal cause. Other viruses associated with epidemic disease include echoviruses 1 and 6. Sporadic cases have also been associated with these viruses, as well as with many other enteroviruses, including coxsackieviruses A1, A2, A4, A6, A9, A10, and A16 and echoviruses 2, 3, 7 to 9, 11, 12, 14, 16, 19, 23, 24, 25, and 30.

EPIDEMIOLOGY. Epidemics of pleurodynia have been recognized in Scandinavian countries for more than two centuries, but the disease was little known elsewhere until 1933, when a

Danish physician, Ejnar Sylvest, published a classic monograph describing an epidemic on Bornholm, a Danish island in the Baltic Sea. Since then, epidemics and sporadic cases have been recognized in many parts of the world. As with other enteroviral infections, the majority of illnesses occur in summer and early fall. However, in contrast to the annual outbreaks of enteroviral aseptic meningitis, epidemics of pleurodynia are much less frequent, generally occurring at intervals of 10 to 20 years.

Transmission is primarily from person to person, and multiple family members may be attacked almost simultaneously or in rapid succession at intervals of 2 to 5 days. In epidemics, disease is observed in children and adults of both sexes. The peak age of incidence is somewhat older than with other enterovirus syndromes, but the majority of cases occur in persons under 30 years of age. The incubation period is generally 2 to 5 days.

PATHOGENESIS. Pleurodynia is a disease of skeletal muscle, not of the pleura or peritoneum. As in most enteroviral diseases, infection is initiated in the alimentary tract. Skeletal muscle is probably most often infected during the primary ("minor") viremia, although it may be infected later, during the "major" viremia in the minority of patients in whom pleurodynia is preceded by a prodromal illness. Host immune responses terminate viremia and halt virus replication in the tissues, but they also contribute to the severity of local inflammation. Muscle tenderness and occasionally swelling can be detected at the site of pain, and characteristic paroxysms of pain can often be elicited by pressure on the affected muscles. In contrast, pleural friction rubs have been infrequently noted, and peritonitis has generally not been observed in patients who have come to laparotomy. Histopathologic data in humans is lacking because of the benign nature of the disease, but studies in murine models of coxsackievirus infection suggest that the myositis results from a combination of direct virus-induced cytolysis and immunopathology mediated by sensitized T lymphocytes.

CLINICAL MANIFESTATIONS. Pleurodynia is characterized by the abrupt onset of fever and sharp, paroxysmal pain over the lower ribs or upper abdomen. In about 25 per cent of patients, this is preceded by a 1- or 2-day prodrome of headache, malaise, anorexia, sore throat, and diffuse myalgia. The pain varies in intensity but is often severe. It is accentuated, sometimes elicited, by deep breathing, coughing, and movement. The pain of pleurodynia has been described as "catching" (a "stitch" in the side), "stabbing," "knife-like," "lancinating," "crushing," or "vice-like." In adults, the pain is primarily in muscles of the thorax, especially the intercostals. In children, abdominal muscles are more often involved. Occasionally, it may involve muscles in the neck or limbs. The pain is often unilateral and is generally experienced in only one or two locations.

During paroxysms of severe pain, the patient lies still in bed, sweating profusely and appearing acutely ill and apprehensive. Respiration, limited by pain, is shallow, rapid, and grunting, suggesting pneumonia or pleural inflammation. Fever of 38 to 40°C is present at the onset of pain, reaches its peak during the episode, and resolves between paroxysms. Multiple paroxysms of pain occur, each lasting from a few minutes to several hours. The initial paroxysm is usually the most severe, and patients frequently appear relatively well between paroxysms.

The acute illness generally lasts for 2 to 6 days, with a range of 12 hours to 3 weeks. The disease is often biphasic; the initial pain and fever resolve and the patient is asymptomatic for a day or more, and then the pain and fever recur, frequently at the same site. Rarely, patients have several recurrences over a period of several weeks or have a late recurrence after being symptom-free for a month or more.

LABORATORY DIAGNOSIS. A specific diagnosis can be established by isolating virus (usually a group B coxsackievirus) from the throat or feces during the acute illness and demonstrating the concurrent development of serotype-specific neutralizing antibodies by testing acute and convalescent sera. Virus is most readily isolated from samples taken early in the illness. The level of creatine phosphokinase in the serum may be elevated, reflecting injury to striated muscle. Other laboratory values are usually normal, although there may be a mild leukopenia in some patients.

DIFFERENTIAL DIAGNOSIS. The most useful distinguishing feature of pleurodynia is the intermittent paroxysmal character of the pain. Epidemiologic information, such as the occurrence of similar illnesses in family members or in the community, may also suggest the diagnosis. Nevertheless, depending upon the location of the pain, pleurodynia may be confused with any of a number of more serious diseases. When the pain is thoracic, these include pneumonia, pulmonary infarction, rib fracture, costochondritis, and myocardial infarction. The absence of physical and roentgenographic evidence of fracture, costochondritis, or pulmonary parenchymal disease; lack of sputum production; absence of leukocytosis; and normal electrocardiogram help to exclude these diagnoses. When the pain is abdominal, it can be difficult to differentiate pleurodynia from serious causes of acute abdominal pain, such as peritonitis, cholecystitis, appendicitis, perforated peptic ulcer, and acute intestinal obstruction. Thus, during epidemics of pleurodynia, it is common to have as many children with the disease admitted to surgical wards as to medical wards, and in one epidemic 9 of 49 of these children underwent laparotomy with negative findings before the nature of their disease was recognized. The absence of signs of peritonitis and the normal white blood cell count are helpful in excluding these diagnoses, as are normal ultrasound and roentgenographic studies. Pleurodynia may also be confused with the pain of pre-eruptive herpes zoster, herniated intervertebral disc, and renal colic. However, the pain of pre-eruptive herpes zoster is usually more constant, and the localization of pain and tenderness to the affected muscle, normal roentgenographic and neurologic examinations (except, perhaps, for a local area of hyperesthesia over the affected muscle), and the absence of hematuria help to exclude the other two diagnoses.

TREATMENT AND PREVENTION. Treatment of pleurodynia is symptomatic. Episodes of pain can usually be controlled with salicylates or other mild analgesics, but opiate analgesics are recommended for severe pain once serious intra-abdominal processes have been excluded. Application of heat to affected muscles may also be useful. Despite the tendency of the disease to relapse, patients with epidemic pleurodynia eventually recover completely. Occasionally, convalescence may be prolonged, with malaise or asthenia persisting for several months. Complications, which reflect dissemination of virus to other tissues, are relatively uncommon. When they do occur, they generally become apparent within several days after the onset of the disease. Aseptic meningitis is observed in approximately 5 per cent of cases and orchitis in a similar proportion of postpubertal males. Pericarditis and myocarditis are rare complications of epidemic pleurodynia.

Bain HW, McLean DM, Walker SJ: Epidemic pleurodynia (Bornholm disease) due to coxsackie B5 virus. The interrelationship of pleurodynia, benign pericarditis and aseptic meningitis. Pediatrics 27:889–903, 1961. *A good discussion of epidemic pleurodynia and its complications.*

Fin JJ Jr, Weller TH, Morgan HR: Epidemic pleurodynia: Clinical and etiologic studies based on one hundred and fourteen cases. Arch Intern Med 83:305, 1949. *An excellent clinical review of epidemic pleurodynia.*

Huebner RJ, Risser JA, Bell JA, et al.: Epidemic pleurodynia in Texas: A study of 22 cases. N Engl J Med 248:267–274, 1953. *Demonstration of the viral etiology of a local epidemic of pleurodynia.*

Pickles NW: Sylvest's disease (Bornholm disease). N Engl J Med 250:1033, 1954. *A vivid account of the clinical presentation of epidemic pleurodynia.*

Sylvest E: Epidemic Myalgia: Bornholm Disease. Transl. by H. Andersen. London, Oxford University Press, 1934, pp 1–155. *The classic monograph and still the best clinical description of the disease.*

Warin JF, Davies JBM, Sanders FK, et al.: Oxford epidemic of Bornholm disease, 1951. Br Med J 1:1345–1351, 1953. *An excellent description of an epidemic of pleurodynia, including its complications.*

Weller TH, Enders JF, Buckingham M, et al.: The etiology of epidemic pleurodynia: A study of two viruses isolated from a tropical outbreak. J Immunol 65:337–346, 1950. *The original study establishing the viral etiology of epidemic pleurodynia.*

379 Myocarditis and Pericarditis Caused by Enteroviruses

Michael N. Oxman

Myocarditis and pericarditis have long been known to occur in association with epidemic viral diseases, including measles, mumps, rubella, varicella, influenza, poliomyelitis, and pleurodynia. As many of these diseases have been controlled by the use of vaccines, enteroviruses have emerged as the major recognized infectious cause of myocarditis and pericarditis in North America and Western Europe. The pathogenesis, clinical manifestations, and outcome of enteroviral infections of the heart vary markedly depending upon properties of the virus and characteristics of the host, especially age. Neonatal infections frequently result in severe myocarditis, widespread involvement of other organs, and high mortality, whereas in older children and adults, pericarditis often predominates, and the disease is generally benign and self-limited. In fact, it appears that the clinical manifestations are generally so subtle that cardiac involvement during enteroviral infections is often unrecognized. However, there is increasing evidence that idiopathic dilated cardiomyopathy may, in many cases, be a late sequela of both recognized and unrecognized enteroviral myocarditis.

ETIOLOGY. The evidence linking specific enteroviruses with myocarditis or pericarditis varies markedly. Proof of causation requires the isolation of virus from, or the demonstration of viral proteins or nucleic acids in, the myocardium, pericardium, or pericardial fluid. Except in neonatal myopericarditis, virus is rarely isolated from cardiac tissue or pericardial fluid, and detection of viral proteins has been difficult, primarily because lack of specificity has led to false-positive results. However, the increasing use of endomyocardial biopsy and the application of new techniques for the detection and amplification of enteroviral nucleic acid should significantly improve our ability to establish the etiology in cases of myocarditis and pericarditis. In most instances, the association of a particular enterovirus with myocarditis or pericarditis is based upon the isolation of virus from noncardiac sources (e.g., feces) and/or serologic evidence of recent or concurrent enterovirus infection. Because of the high prevalence of enteroviral infections and the prolonged period of fecal virus shedding, these associations may often be coincidental rather than causal. On the other hand, because routine serologic testing is available for group B but not for group A coxsackieviruses or echoviruses, and because many group A coxsackieviruses are not readily isolated by routine cell culture techniques, the true contribution of group A coxsackieviruses and echoviruses is probably underestimated.

Coxsackieviruses B1 to 6, A4, and A16, and echoviruses 9, 11, and 22 have been proven to cause myopericarditis in children and adults. Coxsackieviruses A1, A2, A5, A7 to A9, and A14, and echoviruses 1 to 4, 6 to 8, 14, 16, 17, 19, 25, and 30 have also been implicated. The group B coxsackieviruses are the most common etiologic agents of myocarditis and pericarditis. They appear to account for approximately 50 per cent of sporadic cases of acute myocarditis and for virtually all cases that have occurred in epidemics. Group B coxsackieviruses also appear to account for 30 per cent or more of sporadic cases of acute nonbacterial pericarditis.

The newborn is particularly susceptible to severe, frequently fatal, enteroviral infections (*generalized disease of the newborn*), and myocarditis is invariably a major component. These overwhelming systemic enterovirus infections occur in nursery epidemics and as sporadic cases. They are most frequently caused by coxsackieviruses B2 to 5 and echovirus 11, but other echoviruses have also been implicated, including echoviruses 4, 6, 7, 9, 12, 14, 17 to 22, and 31. Coxsackieviruses A3, A9, and A16 have occasionally been associated with sporadic cases.

EPIDEMIOLOGY. Enteroviral myocarditis and pericarditis occur most frequently in the summer and early fall. Idiopathic myopericarditis also peaks during this period of maximum enterovirus prevalence, an observation that is consistent with the notion that most cases of idiopathic myopericarditis are caused by enteroviruses. The incidence of myocarditis and pericarditis has been observed to increase during periods of group B coxsackievirus prevalence, and epidemics of myopericarditis were observed during coxsackievirus B5 epidemics in a number of countries in 1965. However, except in the newborn, epidemic myopericarditis is unusual; most reported cases of enteroviral myopericarditis beyond the neonatal period have been sporadic.

The incidence of myopericarditis during enteroviral infections depends upon the virus and characteristics of the host, especially age. Myopericarditis has been the predominant manifestation of infection in only about 3 per cent of group B coxsackievirus infections reported to the World Health Organization. However, 5 to 10 per cent of infected adults and children over 9 years of age who sought medical care during coxsackievirus B5 epidemics were found to have evidence of acute myopericarditis. The incidence of myocarditis and disseminated disease during group B coxsackievirus infection is very high during the neonatal period. It drops to a minimum (e.g., 1 per cent or less of symptomatic coxsackievirus B5 infections) in children 1 to 9 years of age and then increases again in older children and adults. Thus, despite the higher frequency of enterovirus infections in younger children, enteroviral myopericarditis is primarily a disease of adolescents and young adults. At least two thirds of the cases occur in males, but the risk of cardiac involvement also appears to be increased during pregnancy and immediately following delivery. An unknown but probably significant proportion of enteroviral myopericarditis appears to be asymptomatic or unrecognized. Postmortem examinations have revealed evidence of previously unsuspected myopericarditis in 2 to 10 per cent of unselected cases, with a higher incidence in young persons who have died suddenly. However, questions have been raised about the pathologic criteria employed, and thus the significance of these observations is unclear. The application of new techniques for detection and amplification of enteroviral nucleic acid may help clarify the situation.

Transmission of enteroviruses associated with myocarditis and pericarditis is the same as that of enteroviruses in general (see Ch. 377). In children and adults, it is primarily fecal-oral. The majority of neonatal enteroviral infections are acquired perinatally from an infected mother. Virus is frequently acquired transplacentally when the mother is infected shortly before birth, but it may also be acquired by contact during or after delivery. During nursery epidemics, virus is transmitted nosocomially on the hands of nursery personnel.

PATHOGENESIS. Enteroviruses reach the heart during the viremia that follows infection and replication in the alimentary tract. When enteroviral infections involve the heart they almost always cause an inflammatory response in both the myocardium (*myocarditis*) and the pericardium (*pericarditis*). Although one or the other usually predominates, the term *myopericarditis* best describes the pathologic process. The hallmark of enteroviral myopericarditis is injury to myocytes with an adjacent inflammatory infiltrate. The pathologic changes may be acute or chronic, and they vary in extent depending upon the severity of the disease and the point in its course at which tissue is obtained. Early in infection there are often hypereosinophilic myocytes, widespread edema, and only a few inflammatory cells, many of which are polymorphonuclear leukocytes. Later there is loss of striation, nuclear degeneration, and fragmentation of myocytes. The degenerating and partially necrotic myocytes are surrounded by lymphocytes, plasma cells, and macrophages. The acute process may resolve completely or progress. Healing and progression are reflected by the development of interstitial fibrosis and loss of myocytes. Enteroviral pericarditis is almost always accompanied by focal subepicardial myocarditis, which has these same pathologic characteristics.

The inflammatory process may affect myocytes, vascular elements, the conducting system, autonomic nerves, and/or the interstitium. One or more of at least four mechanisms appear to be involved: (1) cytolytic enteroviral infection; (2) cytotoxicity caused by infection-induced immune responses; (3) indirect nonspecific damage to myocytes caused by adjacent interstitial inflammation; and (4) indirect damage to myocytes caused by infection and inflammation of small blood vessels. Cardiac myocytes, which bear receptors that are shared by all six group B coxsackievirus serotypes, are infected and lysed by these viruses. Interestingly, this same receptor is utilized by several adenoviruses, which have also been implicated in some cases of myocarditis. It appears that other cell types are also infected, e.g., vascular endothelial cells.

Mouse models of myocarditis induced by coxsackievirus B3 have revealed several possible pathogenic mechanisms. Susceptibility to coxsackievirus B3–induced myocarditis is age dependent and genetically determined. Mechanisms of injury vary in different mouse strains. In susceptible animals, acute myocarditis results from direct infection and cytolysis of myocytes. In surviving animals, neutralizing antibody, perhaps in conjunction with interferon, macrophages, and natural killer (NK) cells, appears to terminate virus replication within 7 to 9 days after infection. Exercise and corticosteroids markedly enhance mortality during the early stages of infection, and nonsteroidal anti-inflammatory agents may also have deleterious effects. Mice surviving the acute replicative phase of infection may recover completely or go on to develop severe myocarditis in the absence of recoverable virus. This second phase of virus-induced myocardial destruction depends upon the presence of cytolytic T lymphocytes, which appear as virus replication ceases. Some of these cytolytic T lymphocytes recognize and lyse both infected and uninfected myocytes, and their presence correlates with myocardial damage. The severity of myocardial damage caused by this immune mechanism is greatest in male and pregnant female mice and is reduced in castrated males. In some strains of mice less prone to myocarditis, suppressor T lymphocytes appear to inhibit this cytolytic T-lymphocyte response. Variants of coxsackievirus B3 that do not elicit cytotoxic T lymphocytes directed at both infected and uninfected myocytes fail to cause myocarditis, even though they are indistinguishable from myocarditic strains in their ability to replicate in the myocardium and stimulate the production of interferon and neutralizing antibodies. Mice infected with coxsackievirus B3 also develop antibodies that react with cardiac tissue but do not cross-react with the virus, and these antibodies may contribute to myocyte destruction in some mouse strains. Certain strains of mice infected with coxsackievirus B3 go on to develop chronic dilated cardiomyopathy, primarily as a result of ongoing immunopathology that occurs in the absence of detectable virus. Enterovirus-associated myopericarditis in humans appears to involve a comparable spectrum of pathogenic mechanisms and outcomes.

In neonatal enteroviral myopericarditis, the relatively short incubation period, the widely disseminated infection, and the presence of high titers of virus in the heart and other organs indicate that the primary pathogenic mechanism is direct cytolytic virus infection of the tissues involved. In myopericarditis in older children and adults, the longer incubation period, the presence of virus specific antibodies and T lymphocytes at clinical presentation, the low frequency of virus isolation from the heart and pericardial fluid, and the later occurrence of relapses suggest that immunopathologic mechanisms are involved. Idiopathic dilated cardiomyopathy may represent the end stage of an immunologically mediated chronic progressive enteroviral myocarditis. This notion is supported by observations in the mouse model of coxsackievirus B3 myocarditis, by the development of chronic cardiomyopathy in approximately 10 per cent of patients followed long term after group B coxsackievirus myocarditis, by the demonstration of progressive fibrosis in such patients by serial endomyocardial biopsies, and by the failure to isolate enterovirus from these biopsy specimens. The association of idiopathic dilated cardiomyopathy with group B coxsackievirus myocarditis has been further strengthened by the recent demonstration of group B coxsackievirus RNA in some myocardial biopsies obtained from patients with the disease. These observations need to be confirmed and extended.

CLINICAL MANIFESTATIONS. Although the term *myopericarditis* best describes the pathologic process observed in enteroviral infections of the heart, *myocarditis* or *pericarditis* usually predominates, and the two syndromes are sufficiently distinct in clinical presentation and pathophysiology to warrant separate consideration. They are discussed in detail in Ch. 50 and 51.

Neonatal Myocarditis. Most severe neonatal enterovirus infections begin during the first week of life; the infant's mother has frequently been infected shortly before delivery and has transmitted the virus transplacentally or by contact during or soon after delivery. However, the disease can be present at birth or, when acquired later, may present at any time during the first 3 months of life following a 2- to 8-day incubation period. The disease usually begins with the abrupt onset of fever, listlessness, and anorexia. This is often followed within a day or two by respiratory distress, rapid tachycardia, cardiomegaly, systolic murmur, and electrocardiographic evidence of myocarditis, which may rapidly progress to circulatory collapse and congestive heart failure manifested by cyanosis, hepatomegaly, pulmonary hemorrhage, and edema. Symptomatic meningoencephalitis usually accompanies myocarditis in fatal cases, and there is virus dissem-

ination to other organs, including the liver, lungs, pancreas, and adrenal glands. The disease is biphasic in about one third of patients; the initial symptoms are followed by 1 to 7 days of relative well-being, after which the signs and symptoms of myocarditis develop. The syndrome of neonatal myocarditis is simply a common manifestation of generalized enteroviral disease of the newborn, which is usually caused by group B coxsackieviruses, but it is also seen with echovirus 11 infection and is occasionally associated with other enteroviruses. The mortality in recognized infections appears to be nearly 50 per cent. Death usually occurs within a week of onset, but it can occur within hours in fulminant cases. In survivors, improvement is rapid following defervescence. A second syndrome, characterized by increasing jaundice, hypotension, profuse hemorrhage, and hepatic necrosis, with mortality exceeding 80 per cent, has been described in newborns with disseminated echovirus infections (usually echovirus 11). Severe myocarditis is present at postmortem examination, together with involvement of many other organs. These life-threatening neonatal enterovirus infections are more common in males and in premature infants.

Myocarditis and Pericarditis in Older Children and Adults. In contrast to the neonate, enteroviral infections of the heart in older children and adults often present clinically as pericarditis rather than myocarditis, although the myocardium is almost always involved to some degree. Approximately 60 per cent of older children and adults with symptomatic group B coxsackievirus–associated heart disease present with a clinical diagnosis of pericarditis; approximately 40 per cent present with a clinical diagnosis of myocarditis. More than two thirds of the patients are male. The clinical features of myocarditis and pericarditis are discussed in Ch. 50 and 51.

In 60 to 70 per cent of patients, a mild influenza-like illness with fever, malaise, myalgia, arthragias, and often upper respiratory tract symptoms precedes the manifestations of heart disease by 7 to 10 days. Presenting signs and symptoms may be those of pericarditis, progressive heart failure, or coronary artery occlusion. Some patients present with a nonspecific febrile illness and no signs or symptoms of heart disease; they are diagnosed only when typical electrocardiographic abnormalities are detected. The most common symptoms are chest pain, dyspnea, malaise, fever, and tachycardia, each of which occurs in the majority of patients. Chest pain is present in most patients who present with pericarditis. It is typically retrosternal and radiates to the left trapezius ridge, shoulder, and neck. It is usually exacerbated by breathing, swallowing, and lying supine, and relieved by sitting up and leaning forward. The classic physical finding is the three-component pericardial friction rub that reflects cardiac motion during atrial systole, ventricular systole, and rapid diastolic ventricular filling. The three-component rub is heard in 50 per cent of patients presenting with acute enteroviral pericarditis, and one or more component can be heard in more than 90 per cent. The rub is often intermittent, position-dependent, and brought out by maximum inspiration or expiration, and it may disappear as pericardial effusion accumulates. Patients presenting with acute myocarditis may also have chest pain. This is often dull and oppressive, but it may also resemble the pain of angina or have the character of pericardial pain when there is coexistent pericarditis. Many patients with enteroviral myocarditis present only with signs and symptoms of heart failure or with arrhythmias. Supraventricular tachycardia and ventricular extrasystoles are common, and varying degrees of heart block signal involvement of the conducting system and are responsible for the occurrence of sudden death in patients with enteroviral myopericarditis. Cardiomegaly is present in about 50 per cent of patients with enteroviral myopericarditis, reflecting either pericardial effusion or cardiac dilatation. Pleural effusions, generally left-sided, are present in about one third of patients. Other clinical manifestations of systemic enteroviral infection sometimes accompany myopericarditis, including aseptic meningitis, rash, pleurodynia, and orchitis. Death may occur as a consequence of arrhythmia or congestive heart failure, but this is uncommon in acute enteroviral myopericarditis.

LABORATORY DIAGNOSIS. The enteroviral etiology of myopericarditis is established by isolating virus from, or detecting viral proteins or nucleic acid in, the myocardium, pericardium, or pericardial fluid. Isolation of virus from the throat or feces, together with serologic evidence of recent or concurrent infection with the same enterovirus serotype, provides circumstantial evidence associating enterovirus infection with the cardiac disease.

Diagnosis of neonatal enteroviral infection is most rapidly accomplished by isolating virus, which is present in high titer and widely disseminated. Virus is readily recovered from the throat, feces, and urine. It can also be recovered from the blood, cerebrospinal fluid, ascitic fluid, and multiple tissues obtained by biopsy or at postmortem examination. Characteristic cytopathic effects can often be seen in cell culture within 2 or 3 days of inoculation. Serologic diagnosis is readily accomplished in surviving infants if a viral isolate has been obtained or if a particular enterovirus serotype is suspected.

In older children and adults, etiologic diagnosis of enteroviral myopericarditis is difficult. Virus is rarely isolated from the heart or pericardial fluid, and patients present late in the course of enterovirus infection when virus shedding has ceased and high stable levels of antiviral antibody are already present. The increasing use of endomyocardial biopsy combined with the application of new methods for the detection and amplification of enteroviral nucleic acid, as well as the increasing use of serotype-specific IgM antibody assays, should improve significantly our ability to establish the etiology of viral myopericarditis.

Electrocardiographic (ECG) abnormalities are present in virtually every patient with enteroviral myopericarditis. In pericarditis there is a characteristic progression of abnormalities. Initially, ST-segment elevation is observed in multiple leads without change in QRS morphology, reflecting diffuse subepicardial inflammation. There may also be depression of the PR segment. After a few days, the ST segment returns to baseline and there is T-wave flattening or inversion, which may persist for months. Large pericardial effusions may be associated with reduced QRS voltage and electrical alternans. The presence of nonspecific ST-segment and T-wave abnormalities is frequently used as the basis for the diagnosis of myocarditis. However, these same changes are often seen, in the absence of myocarditis, with fever, hypoxia, tachycardia, and electrolyte disturbances. Thus acceptance of ECG abnormalities alone as sufficient evidence of myocarditis may result in overdiagnosis. In severe myocarditis, Q waves, tachyarrhythmias, ventricular extrasystoles, and conduction disturbances are seen. Serum levels of myocardial enzymes are usually elevated in patients with severe myocarditis. Echocardiography is extremely useful for detecting and quantitating impaired ventricular function, identifying and quantitating pericardial effusion, and demonstrating early hemodynamic compromise.

The widespread use of endomyocardial biopsy was expected to compensate for the difficulty in clinically diagnosing myocarditis, but the introduction of this technique may have created as many problems as it has solved. In addition to the problem of sampling error, the question of whether small foci of lymphocytic infiltration, which have been observed on postmortem examination in 4 to 10 per cent of healthy young accident victims, are a manifestation of viral myocarditis or a normal finding is crucial but as yet unanswered. On the one hand, scattered small collections of inflammatory cells with focal necrosis of myocytes may occur in response to stress or the administration of vasopressors, and their presence in patients with heart failure may not be indicative of viral myocarditis. On the other hand, a single small focus of myocarditis in the conducting system may be responsible for a fatal arrhythmia in someone with little or no evidence of myocarditis elsewhere in the myocardium.

DIFFERENTIAL DIAGNOSIS. Neonatal myocarditis is sometimes mistaken for congenital heart disease, but fever, electrocardiographic evidence of myocarditis, and the involvement of other organ systems help to differentiate the two. Neonatal myocarditis and the generalized enteroviral infection that usually accompanies it are often indistinguishable from bacterial sepsis. Antimicrobial chemotherapy should be initiated and continued until bacterial sepsis is ruled out by appropriate cultures. Neonatal myocarditis is also difficult to distinguish from neonatal herpes simplex virus infection with visceral dissemination if cutaneous lesions are absent. In this situation, therapy with acyclovir should be initiated until herpes simplex virus

infection can be ruled out by virus isolation and antigen detection assays.

PROGNOSIS. With aggressive supportive therapy, the mortality of neonatal myocarditis appears to be less than 50 per cent. Long-term follow-up of survivors is lacking, but the frequent involvement of other organ systems, including the central nervous system, suggests that sequelae are likely to occur.

The majority of children and adults with enteroviral myopericarditis recover without obvious sequelae. Acute mortality is low (0 to 5 per cent), and deaths occur as a result of arrhythmias or congestive heart failure in patients with myocarditis; cardiac tamponade is rare in enteroviral pericarditis.

Approximately 20 per cent of patients experience one or more episodes of recurrent myopericarditis within 1 year of their initial illness, and persistent electrocardiographic abnormalities are observed in 10 to 20 per cent of patients. Cardiomegaly persists in 5 to 10 per cent of patients, and long-term follow-up suggests that 10 per cent or more may develop chronic cardiomyopathy. Constrictive pericarditis rarely occurs following enteroviral pericarditis.

TREATMENT AND PREVENTION. Specific antiviral chemotherapy is not yet available for enterovirus infections. Infants with neonatal myocarditis are unlikely to have received antibodies to the causative virus from their mothers. Thus it seems reasonable to administer human immune serum globulin, which contains high titers of neutralizing antibodies to a number of enterovirus serotypes, in an attempt to terminate viremia and limit further virus replication in infected tissues.

Treatment of enteroviral myopericarditis in older children and adults is primarily supportive. It should include control of pain with analgesics; careful monitoring for arrhythmias, heart failure, and hemodynamic compromise; and prompt treatment of these complications if they arise. Bed rest is an important component of therapy because of clear evidence in mice with coxsackievirus B3 myocarditis that exercise markedly increases the extent of myocardial necrosis and mortality during the acute phase of the disease. Adequate oxygenation should be assured and fluid overload avoided and promptly treated if it develops. In severe cases cardiac-assist devices may be lifesaving.

Corticosteroids should not be administered to patients with suspected enteroviral myocarditis or pericarditis. Their use during the acute phase of viral myocarditis has been associated with rapid clinical deterioration, and their deleterious effects have been clearly demonstrated during the acute phase of coxsackievirus B3 myocarditis in mice.

In uncontrolled trials, some patients with myocarditis who have been treated with immunosuppressive agents have shown improvement, but others have not, and early immunosuppressive therapy has increased myocardial damage in murine coxsackievirus myocarditis. Thus, because of the potential for harm, the use of immunosuppressive therapy for enteroviral myopericarditis should await the results of controlled trials now in progress.

Older children and adults with enteroviral myopericarditis do not require isolation. In neonatal myocarditis, the infected infant should be isolated and careful attention given to routine nursery infection control procedures, especially handwashing before and after handling each infant, in order to prevent nosocomial transmission. In nursery outbreaks, human immune serum globulin should be administered to all infants in an attempt to prevent disease.

Billingham M: Acute myocarditis: A diagnostic dilemma. Br Heart J 58:6–8, 1987. *A clear and concise discussion of the problems inherent in the use of endomyocardial biopsies for the diagnosis of myocarditis.*

Kaplan MH, Klein SW, McPhee J, Harper RG: Group B coxsackievirus infections in infants younger than three months of age: A serious childhood illness. Rev Infect Dis 5:1019–1032, 1983. *A thorough account of the clinical presentation, course, and outcome of neonatal myocarditis caused by group B coxsackieviruses.*

Koontz CH, Ray CG: The role of coxsackie group B virus infections in sporadic myopericarditis. Am Heart J 82:750–758, 1971. *A clinical and serologic study of 63 consecutive patients with suspected myopericarditis*

Savoia MC, Oxman MN: Myocarditis, pericarditis and mediastinitis. In Mandel GL, Douglas RG Jr, Bennett JE (eds.): Principles and Practice of Infectious Diseases. New York, Churchill Livingstone, 1990, pp 721–732. *A well-referenced review of the etiology, pathogenesis, clinical manifestations, and diagnosis of myocarditis and pericarditis.*

Woodruff JF: Viral myocarditis: A review. Am J Pathol 101:427–478, 1980. *A comprehensive review of all aspects of viral myocarditis.*

380 Mucocutaneous Syndromes Caused by Enteroviruses

Michael N. Oxman

Enteroviruses are the leading cause of exanthematous disease in the United States and most other developed countries. Almost all enteroviruses can cause maculopapular eruptions, and most serotypes are occasionally responsible for petechial or papulovesicular exanthems and enanthems as well. Moreover, a given enterovirus may cause more than one pattern of mucocutaneous disease, even within a single infected household. Consequently, except for hand-foot-and-mouth disease, which is usually caused by coxsackievirus A16 or enterovirus 71, there are no clinical or epidemiologic characteristics of any given enteroviral rash that point to a specific enterovirus as its cause.

EPIDEMIOLOGY. The epidemiology of enteroviral exanthems and enanthems is the epidemiology of enteroviral infections in general (see Ch. 377). The vast majority occur during the summer and early fall. The incidence of enanthems and exanthems in infected persons varies among different enteroviruses and even among different strains of the same enterovirus. For example, enanthems and exanthems are often seen in more than 50 per cent of infected children during outbreaks of infection caused by echovirus 9 or coxsackievirus A16 but are rare during outbreaks caused by echovirus 6 or coxsackievirus A7. Host factors, especially age, are also important; infants and young children are more likely to develop mucocutaneous lesions, whereas other manifestations of enterovirus infection, such as aseptic meningitis, are more likely to develop in older children and adults. Thus, during outbreaks of echovirus 9 infection, rash is often seen in the majority of infected children under 5 years of age but in less than 5 per cent of infected adults, and it is not uncommon when evaluating an adult with aseptic meningitis and no rash to find that a child in the same household is convalescing from an illness characterized by a maculopapular rash. Enteroviral exanthems and enanthems occur in outbreaks and as sporadic cases. Asymptomatic infections are common and are often the source of virus for symptomatic infections. Attack rates are highest in young children, who frequently introduce the virus into households where several members may become infected simultaneously or sequentially, with an incubation period of 3 to 10 days.

PATHOGENESIS. Enteroviral lesions in the oropharyngeal mucosa and skin are manifestations of a systemic virus infection. They result from the secondary infection of endothelial cells of small vessels in the underlying lamina propria and dermis, which occurs during the viremia that regularly follows enteroviral infection and replication in the alimentary tract. Their pathogenesis thus resembles that of the mucocutaneous lesions of measles, rubella, and varicella and contrasts with the pathogenesis of the lesions of acute herpetic gingivostomatitis, human papillomavirus infections (warts), and acute hemorrhagic conjunctivitis, which are the direct result of exogenous virus infection and replication in epithelial cells at the portal of entry. The nature of the enteroviral lesions reflects the nature and extent of local inflammatory changes in and around these small vessels. Vascular dilatation alone produces an erythematous macular eruption. Vascular dilatation plus edema and cellular infiltration results in erythematous papules. Endothelial damage with extravasation of red blood cells produces a petechial eruption. Infection and necrosis of cells in the surrounding dermis or overlying epidermis, together with the influx of fluid and inflammatory cells, produces vesicular lesions. When a vesicle forms in the mucosa of the oropharynx, the overlying layer of epithelial cells is rapidly macerated, producing a shallow ulcer that is usually surrounded by a zone of erythema. Although cytolytic virus replication is the predominant factor in the pathogenesis of enteroviral enanthems and exanthems, damage may be accentuated, at least in some cases, by host immune responses to enterovirus antigens in the infected tissues.

The obligatory occurrence of alimentary tract replication and viremia prior to the development of mucocutaneous lesions explains the 3- to 10-day incubation period and the frequent occurrence of prodromal signs and symptoms. Moreover, the simultaneous dissemination of virus to a number of target organs explains the concurrent appearance of other manifestations of enterovirus infection, such as aseptic meningitis and pericarditis.

CLINICAL MANIFESTATIONS. Enanthems. The oropharyngeal mucosa is involved to some degree during most symptomatic enteroviral infections. This is usually manifest by mild pharyngitis and mucosal erythema, but it may also result in a variety of enanthems. These may consist of macules, papules, vesicles, petechiae, or ulcers, and they may occur alone or in association with exanthems and other manifestations of systemic enteroviral infection. They are often transient and frequently unrecognized, but they occasionally lead to diagnostic confusion, for example, when they resemble Koplik's spots and accompany a morbilliform exanthem in a child infected by echovirus 9. Two enanthems are sufficiently unique to warrant separate description:

Herpangina (*herpes*, vesicular eruption; *angina*, inflammation of the throat) is a syndrome characterized by the sudden onset of fever, sore throat, pain on swallowing, and a vesicular enanthem of the posterior pharynx. It is seen primarily in children between 3 and 10 years of age. The disease begins abruptly, after a 3- to 10-day incubation period, with fever ranging from 38 to 41°C, sore throat, and pain on swallowing. Fever tends to be higher in younger children, who may suffer febrile convulsions; older children and adults frequently complain of headache and myalgia. On examination, there is pharyngeal erythema but little or no tonsillar exudate. The characteristic lesions are discrete 1- to 2-mm vesicles and ulcers surrounded by 1- to 5-mm zones of erythema. Lesions are few in number, averaging four or five per patient, with a range of 1 or 2 to 20. They occur most frequently on the anterior tonsillar pillars, the posterior edge of the soft palate and the uvula, and less frequently on the tonsils, the posterior pharyngeal wall, and the posterior buccal mucosa. They begin as small papules, progress to vesicles, and ulcerate within 24 hours. The shallow ulcers, which are moderately painful, may enlarge over the next day or two to a diameter of 3 to 4 mm. Symptoms generally disappear in 3 or 4 days, but the ulcers may persist for up to a week. Most cases are mild and resolve without complications, but herpangina is occasionally associated with exanthems, aseptic meningitis, or other serious manifestations of enterovirus infection. Outbreaks of herpangina are common during the summer, and sporadic cases are also observed. Group A coxsackieviruses (A1 to 6, A8, A10, and A22) account for the majority of outbreaks, but outbreaks have also been caused by other enteroviruses, including coxsackievirus B1 and echoviruses 16 and 25. In addition, these viruses, as well as coxsackieviruses A7, A9, A16, and B2 to 5, and echoviruses 6, 9, 11, 17, and 22, have been isolated from sporadic cases. A variant of herpangina has been described in children infected with coxsackievirus A10. The lesions have the same distribution as in typical cases of herpangina, but instead of evolving into vesicles and ulcers they remain papular and are infiltrated with lymphocytes to form 2- to 3-mm gray-white nodules surrounded by narrow zones of erythema. The disease, which has been called *acute lymphonodular pharyngitis*, is otherwise indistinguishable from herpangina.

Hand-foot-and-mouth disease (vesicular stomatitis with exanthem) is a mild enteroviral disease characterized by a vesicular eruption in the mouth and over the extremities. It occurs most frequently in children less than 5 years of age. After an incubation period of 3 to 6 days, the disease begins with mild fever ranging from 38 to 39°C, anorexia, malaise, and often a sore mouth. Within a day or two, vesicular lesions appear in the oral cavity, most frequently on the anterior buccal mucosa and the tongue but also on the labial mucosa, gingivae, and hard palate. The oral lesions begin as erythematous macules and quickly evolve into 2- to 4-mm vesicles surrounded by zones of erythema. Some vesicles ulcerate, forming 4- to 6-mm shallow painful ulcers surrounded by erythema; others coalesce to form bullae; and still others are absorbed without ulcerating. In the majority of preschool children, but in only about 10 per cent of infected adults, the oral lesions are accompanied by vesicular skin lesions, most often on the dorsal or lateral surfaces of the hands and feet and on the fingers and toes, but not infrequently on the palms and soles. Less often, lesions occur on the buttocks or more proximally on the extremities, and rarely on the genitalia. They are generally 3 to 7 mm in diameter and surrounded by a narrow zone of erythema. They range in number from two or three to 30 or more and consist of subepidermal vesicles containing a mixed inflammatory infiltrate of lymphocytes, monocytes, and neutrophils and accompanied by acantholysis and cellular degeneration in the overlying epidermis. The cutaneous lesions are generally not pruritic or painful, and they resolve without ulcerating, crusting, or scarring within about a week. Hand-foot-and-mouth disease is caused most frequently by coxsackievirus A16, less frequently by enterovirus 71 and coxsackieviruses A5, A9, and A10, and occasionally by coxsackieviruses A4, A7, B2, and B5. Outbreaks and sporadic cases occur primarily in the summer and early fall. Attack rates are highest in young children, and during epidemics more than half of the children in affected households may develop disease. Hand-foot-and-mouth disease itself is benign, but it may occasionally be associated with one of the more severe manifestations of systemic enterovirus infection, such as aseptic meningitis, encephalitis, or myocarditis. This has been especially true during epidemics of enterovirus 71 infection, in which a number of patients with hand-foot-and-mouth disease also developed serious central nervous system disease.

Exanthems. Enterovirus exanthems themselves are benign, but they are clinically important for at least three reasons: (1) They constitute direct evidence of enterovirus dissemination and thus provide a clue to the presence and the etiology of coexistent disease referable to other potentially infected target organs, such as the heart and the central nervous system; (2) they represent the "tip of an iceberg" of enterovirus infection in the community; and (3) they are often confused with other infectious exanthems, some of which have more serious consequences, require specific control measures, or are amenable to specific anti-infective therapy. Since enteroviral rashes are not sufficiently distinctive to permit an etiologic diagnosis to be made on clinical grounds, identification of the responsible agent requires laboratory diagnosis. However, the problem of confusing enteroviral rashes with other infectious exanthems can be approached by comparing the enterovirus rashes to the nonenterovirus rashes that they resemble.

The most common cutaneous manifestation of enterovirus infection is an erythematous maculopapular rash that appears together with fever and other manifestations of systemic infection. This is also a common manifestation of infection by a variety of other organisms, but it is more often caused by enteroviruses than by any other infectious agent. Only certain enteroviruses (e.g., echovirus 9) cause this syndrome with high frequency, but almost all can produce it, at least occasionally. The rash begins on the face and quickly spreads to the neck, trunk, and extremities. It consists of 1- to 3-mm erythematous macules and papules that may be discrete (*rubelliform*, resembling rubella) or confluent (*morbilliform*, resembling measles). It usually lasts for 2 to 5 days and does not itch or desquamate. Enteroviral exanthems are generally not accompanied by significant posterior cervical, suboccipital, or postauricular lymphadenopathy, but there are many exceptions. For example, posterior cervical and suboccipital lymphadenopathy similar to that seen in rubella has been observed in many children with exanthems caused by coxsackievirus A9.

When the enteroviral rash consists of discrete erythematous macules and papules (i.e., when it is rubelliform), it is most likely to be confused with rubella. When the lesions are confluent (i.e., when the rash is morbilliform), it is more likely to be confused with measles. Confusion with measles is accentuated when the rash is accompanied by an enanthem that resembles Koplik's spots, something that has often been seen in children infected with echovirus 9 and is occasionally seen in children infected with a number of other enteroviruses.

Enteroviral rashes are sometimes petechial and occasionally purpuric. Although this pattern is seen most frequently in echovirus 9 and coxsackievirus A9 infections, it is observed occasionally with many other enterovirus serotypes. When an enteroviral infection is accompanied by a petechial or purpuric rash, it is easily confused with meningococcemia, and when it is also associated with aseptic meningitis, as it often is in echovirus 9 and coxsackievirus A9 infections, it is clinically indistinguishable

from meningococcal meningitis. In this situation it is usually prudent to initiate antimicrobial chemotherapy pending the results of laboratory investigations.

Vesicular exanthems are most often seen as a component of hand-foot-and-mouth disease (see above), but several enteroviruses, including echovirus 11 and coxsackievirus A9, cause vesicular exanthems without an associated enanthem. The lesions resemble those caused by varicella-zoster and herpes simplex viruses. In contrast to varicella, however, vesicular rashes caused by enteroviruses are usually peripheral in distribution and consist of relatively few lesions that heal without crusting. When they are not associated with hand-foot-and-mouth disease, vesicular lesions caused by enteroviruses are often confused with insect bites or poison ivy. Echovirus 11 and several coxsackievirus serotypes have been associated with skin lesions resembling papular urticaria, lesions that usually result from insect bites.

Enteroviral rashes are generally accompanied by fever; they develop at or within a day or two of its onset. In some cases, however, the rash does not develop until the fever subsides, a pattern resembling that of *roseola infantum* (exanthem subitum), a benign sporadic disease of infants 6 to 24 months of age now known to be caused by human herpesvirus 6. These roseola-like enterovirus infections are typified by the "Boston exanthem," caused by echovirus 16 and first described during an epidemic in Boston in 1951. It is characterized by fever (to 38 to 39°C) lasting 2 to 4 days, followed by defervescence and then by the appearance of a salmon-pink maculopapular rash on the face and upper chest. The rash resolves in 1 to 5 days without sequelae. Frequently, multiple cases occur sequentially in households; the illness is mild in children and more severe in adults, who often develop high fever and aseptic meningitis without rash. In addition to echovirus 16, a number of other enterovirus serotypes have occasionally been associated with roseola-like illnesses.

DIFFERENTIAL DIAGNOSIS. Herpangina is most often confused with bacterial pharyngitis or tonsillitis or with pharyngitis caused by other viruses. Other considerations include hand-foot-and-mouth disease, herpes simplex virus infections, and herpes zoster involving the palate. In bacterial pharyngitis and tonsillitis there is usually a more extensive tonsillar exudate, more prominent cervical lymphadenopathy, and more signs of systemic illness. Bacterial pharyngitis and pharyngitis caused by most viruses other than enteroviruses are not ordinarily associated with vesicular lesions. However, in individual cases, bacterial pharyngitis may be difficult to distinguish from enteroviral pharyngitis on clinical grounds, and the two may even coexist. Thus, throat cultures and assays for group A β-hemolytic streptococcal antigens are often warranted. Herpangina is a disease of the posterior oropharynx, whereas hand-foot-and-mouth disease and primary herpes simplex gingivostomatitis involve the anterior oropharynx. The former is also generally accompanied by cutaneous lesions, and herpetic gingivostomatitis is characterized by more extensive and painful lesions, prominent gingivitis, cervical lymphadenopathy, and more severe systemic signs and symptoms. Recurrent herpes simplex (herpes labialis) generally involves the vermilion border of the lip or the adjacent skin rather than the palate, and it is often preceded by tingling or burning neuralgia. There is also usually a history of recurrent episodes. Palatal herpes zoster may sometimes mimic herpangina, but it generally occurs in older individuals, is preceded and accompanied by pain and sensory abnormalities, and is unilateral. Vesicular lesions caused by herpes simplex and varicella-zoster viruses contain multinucleated giant cells, which are not present in enteroviral lesions.

The vesicular lesions of hand-foot-and-mouth disease resemble those caused by herpes simplex and varicella-zoster viruses. Patients with primary herpetic gingivostomatitis are usually more toxic and have cervical lymphadenopathy and more prominent gingivitis. Their cutaneous lesions are usually perioral but may occasionally involve a finger that has been in the mouth. Lesions of herpes labialis usually involve the vermilion border of the lip or the adjacent skin, are rarely accompanied by lesions on the hands or feet, often have a neuralgic prodome, and frequently have a history of recurrent episodes. The cutaneous lesions of varicella are generally more extensive and are centrally distributed, sparing the palms and soles. Oral lesions are far less prominent in varicella, and its prevalence in winter and spring further distinguishes it from hand-foot-and-mouth disease.

Aphthous stomatitis is distinguished from hand-foot-and-mouth disease by the absence of fever and other signs of systemic illness, the absence of cutaneous lesions, and often a history of recurrence.

Maculopapular exanthems caused by enteroviruses are distinguished from measles and rubella by their summertime occurrence, the usual absence of posterior cervical, suboccipital, and postauricular lymphadenopathy, and their relatively short incubation period. The absence of significant coryza and conjunctivitis further distinguishes the typical enteroviral exanthems from measles. In addition, the probability of measles and rubella is markedly reduced in persons with a well-documented history of adequate immunization.

When enteroviral rashes are maculopapular they may be confused with drug reactions; when they are petechial they may be confused with bacterial or rickettsial rashes. In addition to obvious differences in epidemiologic and exposure histories, the maculopapular and petechial (but not vesicular) rashes caused by enteroviruses are distinguished by their tendency to spare the palms and soles, which are usually involved in drug reactions and bacterial and rickettsial rashes.

When enteroviral rashes are petechial, it is impossible to rule out meningococcemia on clinical grounds alone. Laboratory investigation is required, even during proven outbreaks of enteroviral disease, because concurrent enteroviral and meningococcal infections can occur.

Vesicular rashes caused by enteroviruses can be confused with varicella, herpes simplex virus infections, insect bites, and poison ivy. They can be distinguished from varicella by their occurrence during the summer and early fall, their relatively short incubation period, their peripheral distribution, and their tendency to heal without crusting. The various forms of herpes simplex virus infection have unique characteristics that distinguish them from enteroviral infections. Cutaneous dissemination occurs occasionally in patients with primary genital herpes or acute herpetic gingivostomatitis, but the clinical picture is dominated by genital or oral signs and symptoms. Primary cutaneous herpes simplex infections are uncommon, and the lesions are localized at the site of inoculation. Recurrent cutaneous herpes simplex (e.g., herpetic whitlow) is generally localized within a single dermatome and accompanied by neuralgia but not by fever or other signs of systemic infection. The vesicles of recurrent herpes simplex are grouped, whereas those of enteroviral exanthems are scattered, and there is often a history of previous episodes at the same site. The presence of fever and other signs of systemic infection distinguishes enteroviral exanthems from insect bites and poison ivy, whether the enteroviral rash is vesicular or urticarial.

Roseola-like enteroviral infections can be distinguished from roseola infantum by their occurrence in outbreaks and epidemics during the summer and early fall and by the involvement of older children and adults.

LABORATORY DIAGNOSIS. As with other enterovirus infections, the etiology of mucocutaneous syndromes caused by enteroviruses is established by virus isolation and demonstration of the concurrent development of serotype-specific neutralizing antibodies (see Ch. 377). Virus can be isolated from the throat, feces, blood, and vesicular lesions early in the disease, and it can also be isolated from the cerebrospinal fluid of many patients with aseptic meningitis. Vesicular lesions can be differentiated from those caused by herpes simplex and varicella-zoster viruses by the absence of multinucleated giant cells on Tzanck smears, as well as by immunofluorescent or immunoperoxidase staining for viral antigens. It is often essential to exclude other potential pathogens, such as *Neisseria meningitides* and the group A β-hemolytic streptococcus, by using appropriate cultures and antigen detection tests.

TREATMENT AND PREVENTION. Enteroviral enanthems and exanthems are benign, self-limited illnesses that require only symptomatic therapy for headache and sore throat. More serious manifestations of disseminated infection, such as aseptic meningitis or encephalitis, may require supportive treatment. When illness mimics meningococcemia or meningococcal meningitis, antimicrobial chemotherapy should be initiated until bacterial infection is ruled out by appropriate cultures and antigen detection assays.

Control of enterovirus infections is best accomplished by hygienic measures such as handwashing and improved sanitation.

Isolation of patients with enteroviral enanthems or exanthems is generally not helpful because of the simultaneous existence of a large reservoir of asymptomatically infected persons who are excreting virus. The generally benign nature of these infections and the large number of enterovirus serotypes that cause them preclude the development of vaccines.

Adler JL, Mostow SR, Mellin H, et al.: Epidemiologic investigation of hand-foot-and-mouth disease. Infection caused by coxsackievirus A16 in Baltimore, June through September, 1968. Am J Dis Child 120:309–313, 1970. *A detailed investigation of an outbreak of hand-foot-and-mouth disease caused by coxsackievirus A16.*

Cherry JD: Skin infections: Cutaneous manifestations of systemic infections. *In* Feigen RD, Cherry JD (eds.): Textbook of Pediatric Infectious Diseases. Philadelphia, W. B. Saunders, 1987, pp 786–817. *An excellent review of the etiology and differential diagnosis of the mucocutaneous manifestations of systemic infections.*

Cherry JD, Jahn CL: Herpangina: The etiologic spectrum. Pediatrics 36:632–634, 1965. *A review of herpangina and its various enteroviral causes.*

Hall CB, Cherry JD, Hatch MH, et al.: The return of Boston exanthem: Echovirus 16 infections in 1974. Am J Dis Child 131:323–326, 1977. *An excellent description of the roseola infantum–like disease produced by echovirus 16.*

Huebner RJ, Cole RM, Beeman EA, et al.: Herpangina. Etiologic studies of a specific infectious disease. JAMA 145:628–633, 1951. *The initial association of herpangina with group A coxsackievirus infections.*

Neva FA, Feemster RF, Gorbach IJ: Clinical and epidemiological features of an unusual epidemic exanthem. JAMA 155:544–548, 1954. *The original description of the Boston exanthem.*

Robinson CR, Doane FW, Rhodes AJ: Report of an outbreak of febrile illness with pharyngeal lesions and exanthem, Toronto, summer 1957-isolation of a group A Coxsackie virus. Can Med Assoc J 79:615–621, 1958. *An early description of hand-foot-and-mouth disease and its association with coxsackievirus A16.*

Sabin AB, Krumbiegel ER, Wigand R: ECHO type 9 virus disease. Virologically controlled clinical and epidemiologic observations during a 1957 epidemic in Milwaukee with notes on concurrent similar diseases associated with coxsackie and other ECHO viruses. Prog Pediatr 96:197–219, 1958. *A detailed review of the spectrum of disease associated with echovirus 9 infections and a comparison with diseases caused by other enteroviruses.*

381 Acute Hemorrhagic Conjunctivitis

Michael N. Oxman

DEFINITION. Acute hemorrhagic conjunctivitis (AHC) is an acute, highly contagious, self-limited disease of the eye characterized by the sudden onset of pain, photophobia, conjunctivitis, swelling of the eyelids, and prominent subconjunctival hemorrhages. Since its first appearance in 1969, AHC has occurred in explosive epidemics throughout the world. The disease was initially nicknamed "Apollo 11 disease" because its appearance in Ghana coincided with the Apollo 11 moon landing.

ETIOLOGY. Enterovirus 70, a new enterovirus isolated from patients during the initial pandemic of AHC that began in Ghana in 1969, has been responsible for tens of millions of cases that have occurred in widespread epidemics during the past 20 years. A variant of coxsackievirus A24, which first appeared at about the same time as enterovirus 70, has been responsible for hundreds of thousands of cases of the disease that have occurred in a number of more circumscribed epidemics during the same period. Both viruses have been involved concurrently in some epidemics. To date, coxsackievirus A24 has been responsible for fewer cases of epidemic conjunctivitis than enterovirus 70, and it does not cause subconjunctival hemorrhages in as high a proportion of patients. Nucleic acid hybridization and serologic studies have shown that the two viruses are genetically and antigenically unrelated.

EPIDEMIOLOGY. Although mild conjunctivitis may occur as a minor manifestation of infection by many enteroviruses, especially in children, its occurrence as the major clinical manifestation of enterovirus infection was not observed until 1969, when explosive epidemics of AHC occurred in Ghana and almost simultaneously in Indonesia. The responsible agent proved to be a new enterovirus, designated enterovirus 70. Over the next 2 years the disease assumed pandemic proportions, with large epidemics occurring in many areas of Africa, Southeast Asia, the Far East, India, and Japan and involving tens of millions of people. A number of smaller outbreaks also occurred in Europe. Scattered epidemics of AHC continued to occur in these same areas during the remainder of the decade, and the recurrence of epidemics in the same geographic areas suggests that immunity to AHC may be short-lived. In 1981 a new pandemic began, with epidemics again occurring in Africa and Asia, but this time it extended to Australia and the South Pacific, and to the Americas, including the United States, where its arrival was marked by an explosive outbreak of AHC in Miami, Florida. Some outbreaks in Europe and the United States have been initiated by infected travelers and then spread nosocomially within eye clinics.

Another enterovirus, subsequently identified as a variant of coxsackievirus A24, was responsible for a large epidemic of AHC in Singapore in 1970. This virus has subsequently been responsible for a number of epidemics in many of the same regions invaded by enterovirus 70, including Africa, Southeast Asia, India, the Far East, and the Americas. Both viruses have been involved together in several epidemics.

AHC is a highly contagious disease. In contrast to most enteroviral infections, it is transmitted by direct inoculation of the conjunctivae with virus-contaminated fingers or fomites (i.e., transmission is eye-finger or fomite-eye). Enterovirus 70 and the coxsackievirus A24 variant are both naturally occurring, temperature-sensitive viruses that replicate optimally at 33 to 35°C, the temperature of the conjunctivae. There appears to be little or no virus replication in the alimentary tract. Virus is abundant in the conjunctivae and in the ocular exudate, from which it can be readily isolated early in infection. Virus is less readily isolated from pharyngeal secretions and only very rarely recovered from feces. In contrast to most other enteroviruses, there does not appear to be a prolonged period of virus excretion following acute infection. Transmission is favored by crowding and unhygienic living conditions and also by warm, humid coastal climates. During epidemics all age groups are affected; attack rates of clinical illness are highest in young adults, but infection rates are highest in children under 10 years of age, many of whom experience mild or inapparent infections. Infection rates are also substantially higher among the poor than in middle and upper socioeconomic groups. School-age children are most likely to introduce infection into households, where secondary attack rates often exceed 50 per cent. During the 1969–1971 pandemic, postepidemic serologic surveys revealed enterovirus 70 neutralizing antibody prevalence rates to be nearly 50 per cent in affected populations in Ghana, Indonesia, and other developing countries, but only about 5 per cent in affected populations in Japan and other developed countries. These results were consistent with the more limited spread of AHC observed when the disease was introduced into developed countries, and they also confirmed the widespread occurrence of subclinical infections.

Enterovirus 70 is a most unusual enterovirus. In addition to being a naturally occurring temperature-sensitive virus that causes disease at its portal of entry and is not transmitted by the fecal-oral route, it has an exceptionally broad host range. It replicates in a wide variety of nonprimate as well as primate cells and causes paralytic disease in monkeys. Moreover, neutralizing antibodies to enterovirus 70 have been detected in a number of animal species, including cattle, sheep, goats, swine, chickens, dogs, and wild monkeys. Oligonucleotide mapping of a series of epidemic strains suggests that they all evolved from a hypothetical ancestor strain that was not in existence before 1967. Serologic studies have reinforced the notion that enterovirus 70 has only recently emerged as a human pathogen; neutralizing antibodies to enterovirus 70 have generally not been found in human sera collected prior to 1969, even sera from elderly persons. Detailed analysis of the enterovirus 70 genome, which has recently been cloned and sequenced, shows that except for its 5' noncoding region, which is very similar to that of poliovirus type 3, the enterovirus 70 genome is more closely related to the genomes of bovine enteroviruses and swine vesicular disease virus than to the genomes of other human enteroviruses. Finally, neutralizing antibodies to enterovirus 70 have been detected in animal sera from Japan and West Africa collected prior to 1969, indicating that enterovirus 70 or a very similar virus was circulating in animals before the first appearance of AHC in humans. Taken together, these observations suggest that enterovirus 70 may represent a zoonotic picornavirus that extended its host range to humans, perhaps as a consequence of recombination with poliovirus type 3.

PATHOGENESIS. In contrast to other enteroviral infections (see Ch. 377), AHC is transmitted by direct inoculation of the conjunctivae with virus on contaminated fingers or fomites (e.g., ophthalmologic instruments, shared towels). Disease results from local virus replication at the portal of entry; prior replication in the alimentary tract and viremia are not required to disseminate virus to ocular tissues. This explains the unusually short incubation period, which is generally 24 hours or less (range, 12 to 72 hours). There is, in fact, little evidence of alimentary tract infection or fecal virus shedding in AHC, and constitutional symptoms are observed in only a small minority of cases. This behavior is consistent with the preferential growth of enterovirus 70 (and coxsackievirus A24) at 33 to 35°C, which would be expected to limit its capacity to replicate and spread systemically. Conjunctival infection terminates spontaneously within 4 to 7 days of onset.

The major complication of AHC is a poliomyelitis-like flaccid paralysis, which occurs rarely in patients with AHC caused by enterovirus 70, but apparently not at all in patients with AHC caused by coxsackievirus A24. The pathogenesis of this AHC-associated paralytic disease is not clear. While enterovirus 70 has not been isolated from the cerebrospinal fluid, all of the affected patients have aseptic meningitis and evidence of local production of antibodies to enterovirus 70 within their central nervous system, findings not observed in patients with uncomplicated AHC. This suggests that AHC-associated paralytic disease probably reflects enterovirus 70 infection and destruction of motor neurons. The relatively high frequency of bulbar involvement (see below) further suggests that the route of infection of the central nervous system may be axonal rather than viremic.

CLINICAL MANIFESTATIONS. AHC begins with the sudden onset of eye pain and foreign body sensation, lacrimation, photophobia, blurred vision, and bulbar conjunctivitis. Signs and symptoms rapidly increase in severity with the development of palpebral conjunctivitis, conjunctival edema, swelling of the eyelids, subconjunctival hemorrhages in the bulbar conjunctivae, and a serous or seromucoid ocular discharge containing large numbers of polymorphonuclear leukocytes. The subconjunctival hemorrhages, which are the hallmark of the disease, range from discrete petechiae to confluent hemorrhages that occupy virtually the entire bulbar conjunctiva. They are present, usually within 24 hours of onset, in 70 to 90 per cent of patients with AHC caused by enterovirus 70, but are much less frequent in AHC caused by coxsackievirus A24. AHC often begins unilaterally, but it rapidly spreads to the other eye. Signs and symptoms peak within 24 to 36 hours of onset, by which time most patients have also developed hypertrophy of palpebral follicles and papillae, preauricular lymphadenopathy, and punctate epithelial keratitis with tiny corneal erosions that are often seen only by slit lamp examination after fluorescein staining. Clinical improvement usually begins by the second or third day, and recovery is generally complete without sequelae within 7 to 10 days. Constitutional symptoms, including headache, low-grade fever, and malaise, occur in a minority of patients.

A poliomyelitis-like motor paralysis occurs as a rare complication of AHC caused by enterovirus 70, but not in AHC caused by coxsackievirus A24. It occurs predominantly in adult males. The neurologic disease generally does not begin until 2 to 5 weeks after AHC (range, 5 to 60 days or more), and thus its relationship to the conjunctivitis is often overlooked by physicians, as well as by patients themselves. Radicular pain and paresthesia, usually accompanied by headache, fever, and malaise, are followed in 1 to 3 days by acute asymmetric areflexic paresis or paralysis of one or more limbs. Proximal muscles are usually affected more than distal muscles and lower limbs more than upper limbs. Bulbar involvement, as evidenced by paralysis of one or more cranial nerves, is observed in one third or more of affected patients. The cerebrospinal fluid is characterized by a mononuclear pleocytosis and elevated protein concentration. Permanent paralysis and muscular atrophy occur in approximately 25 per cent of affected patients. More than 200 cases have been reported to date, and the long interval between AHC and paralysis almost certainly accentuates underreporting. Nevertheless, in view of the many tens of millions of cases of AHC that have occurred since 1969, the incidence of this neurologic complication is probably less than 1 in 10,000 cases of AHC.

DIFFERENTIAL DIAGNOSIS. During major epidemics, AHC is unlikely to be confused with other eye infections. However, small outbreaks and sporadic cases may be mistaken for adenovirus infections, either acute follicular conjunctivitis or the more severe epidemic keratoconjunctivitis (EKC). This is especially likely when subconjunctival hemorrhages are not a prominant feature, as is often the case when AHC is caused by coxsackievirus A24. In addition, some outbreaks involve more than one agent (e.g., enterovirus 70 and adenovirus 11). Acute follicular conjunctivitis may occur as a separate entity or as one component of pharyngoconjunctival fever (PCF), in which case fever, malaise, pharyngitis, and cervical lymphadenopathy are prominent features. The adenovirus infections are more gradual in onset; in AHC, conjunctivitis generally reaches its peak within a day of onset and resolves in less than a week, whereas in adenovirus infections conjunctivitis slowly increases in intensity over several days and lasts for 2 weeks or more. Preauricular lymphadenopathy and conjunctival follicular hypertrophy are usually more prominent in adenovirus infections than in AHC, and in EKC epithelial keratitis is much more extensive than it is in AHC and is associated with subepithelial corneal opacities that persist for weeks to months after the epithelial lesions have resolved. Subconjunctival hemorrhages and eyelid ecchymosis may develop in EKC, producing an appearance suggesting previous eye trauma, but these manifestations do not appear until at least 4 or 5 days after onset, by which time AHC is always well on its way to resolution. EKC, which is often transmitted nosocomially during ophthalmic procedures such as tonometry or slit-lamp examination, is frequently unilateral, whereas AHC is almost always bilateral. Adenovirus is readily cultured from conjunctival scrapings or swabs in both EKC and acute follicular conjunctivitis.

Conjunctivitis caused by herpes simplex virus is most often associated with primary infection. Herpetic vesicles and ulcers often appear on the eyelids, and acute herpetic gingivostomatitis is typically present before the onset of the eye infection. Extensive subconjunctival hemorrhages are not a characteristic feature of herpes simplex virus infections of the eye. Recurrent ocular herpes usually produces characteristic dendritic corneal ulcers and little or no conjunctivitis. Tzanck smears of corneal scrapings reveal multinucleated giant cells, which are not observed in AHC, and herpes simplex virus is readily cultured from conjunctival swabs.

Bacterial and chlamydial infections are quite different from AHC in their epidemiology, presentation, and clinical course. A variety of noninfectious conditions can produce the signs and symptoms of conjunctivitis. These include chemical and radiation exposure (e.g., ultraviolet light from sunlamps or welders arcs), overwearing of contact lenses, and foreign bodies. Although none of these produces the extensive subconjunctival hemorrhages typically seen in AHC, their symptoms are sufficiently like the initial symptoms of AHC to cause confusion. The presence of a foreign body should be ruled out by careful examination, including eversion of the upper lid and fluorescein staining to highlight areas of epithelial disruption.

LABORATORY DIAGNOSIS. Enterovirus 70 and coxsackievirus A24 can be isolated from conjunctival swabs and scrapings in a high proportion of patients with AHC if these specimens are obtained during the first 2 or 3 days of illness. In contrast to other enteroviral infections, virus is only occasionally isolated from the throat and almost never from the feces. The diagnosis is supported by the development of serotype-specific neutralizing antibodies, demonstrated by assay of acute and convalescent sera.

In AHC-associated paralytic disease, virus cannot be isolated from the cerebrospinal fluid or from the eye, throat, or feces. Serum antibodies to enterovirus 70 have generally already reached their maximum level before the onset of neurologic symptoms. The enterovirus 70 etiology of the paralytic disease can be supported by demonstrating serotype-specific antibodies in the cerebrospinal fluid at levels indicative of local central nervous system production and by documenting the absence of serologic evidence of poliovirus infection.

Appropriate cultures, conjunctival smears, and serologic assays can be used to exclude other infectious agents.

TREATMENT AND PREVENTION. AHC almost always resolves spontaneously without sequelae, and treatment is symptomatic. Topical application of antihistamine/decongestant eye drops and cold compresses may be used to reduce discomfort. Antimicrobial agents are not indicated unless there is bacterial superinfection (which should be documented by Gram's stain and culture). Corticosteroids, a component of many topical ophthalmic preparations, are contraindicated.

Transmission of AHC can be prevented by careful handwashing, avoidance of contaminated washcloths and towels, and sterilization of all ophthalmologic instruments. These practices should be routine in eye clinics.

Specific antiviral chemotherapeutic agents are not currently available, nor are vaccines for either enterovirus 70 or coxsackievirus A24.

Christopher S, Theogaraj S, Godbole S, et al.: An epidemic of acute hemorrhagic conjunctivitis due to coxsackievirus A24. J Infect Dis 146:16–19, 1982. *Clinical description and virologic studies of AHC caused by coxsackievirus A24*

Hierholzer JC, Hilliard KA, Esposito JJ: Serosurvey for "acute hemorrhagic conjunctivitis" virus (enterovirus 70) antibodies in the southeastern United States, with review of the literature and some epidemiologic implications. Am J Epidemiol 102:533–544, 1975. *A detailed review of the seroepidemiology and spread of enterovirus 70 infection*

Kono R: Apollo 11 disease or acute hemorrhagic conjunctivitis: A pandemic of a new enterovirus infection of the eyes. Am J Epidemiol 101:383–390, 1975. *An excellent description of the first pandemic of AHC.*

Kono R, Miyamura K, Tajiri E, et al.: Virologic and serologic studies of neurological complications of acute hemorrhagic conjunctivitis in Thailand. J Infect Dis 135:706–713, 1977. *Description of the poliomyelitis–like paralytic disease associated with AHC caused by enterovirus 70.*

Patriarca PA, Onorato I, Sklar VEF, et al.: Acute hemorrhagic conjunctivitis. Investigation of a large-scale community outbreak in Dade County, Florida. JAMA 249:1283–1289, 1983. *Excellent description of an epidemic of AHC in Miami, Florida.*

Ryan MD, Jenkins O, Hughes PJ, et al.: The complete nucleotide sequence of enterovirus type 70: Relationships with other members of the Picornaviridae. J Gen Virol 71:2291–2299, 1990. *A detailed comparison of the genome of enterovirus 70 to the genomes of other human and animal enteroviruses, with evidence for its unique nature and origin.*

Wadia NH, Katrak SM, Misra VP, et al.: Polio-like motor paralysis associated with acute hemorrhagic conjunctivitis in an outbreak in 1981 in Bombay, India: Clinical and serologic studies. J Infect Dis 147:660–668, 1983. *Description of the poliomyelitis-like paralytic disease associated with AHC and evidence linking it to enterovirus 70.*

Arthropod-Borne Viral Diseases

382 Introduction

Robert E. Shope

Arthropod-borne viruses (arboviruses) are transmitted biologically by an arthropod to a vertebrate host, either a human or a lower animal. The viruses replicate during an extrinsic incubation period in the arthropod, which may be a mosquito, tick, phlebotomine sandfly, or culicoid midge. The viruses are then transmitted by bite to the vertebrate, which becomes viremic and is in turn capable of infecting another biting arthropod. Some arboviruses also are transmitted vertically through the egg of the arthropod and may be maintained this way between seasons.

There are nearly 500 arthropod-borne viruses and at least 100 of these infect humans. These viruses contain RNA and all except the Reoviridae have lipid-containing envelopes. They are classified by biologic, physical, and chemical properties. Most fit into five families—Togaviridae, Flaviviridae, Bunyaviridae, Rhabdoviridae, and Reoviridae. Within each family are one or more genera, the genus usually corresponding to an antigenic group. These groups are important, because the clinician must rely heavily on the laboratory for a serologic diagnosis or identification of an isolate.

Table 382–1 lists some of the arboviruses that cause disease in humans. The viruses described in this section were selected as a few of the more important of approximately 100 that are known to infect people.

Most infections are inapparent. The remainder are associated with one or more of four major syndromes: (1) undifferentiated fever, (2) fever with rash and/or arthritis, (3) encephalitis, and (4) hemorrhagic fever (see Ch. 390).

The diseases described in this section are nearly all zoonoses (i.e., diseases caused by viruses transmitted from animals to man). The diseases are more prevalent in the tropics and subtropics and are usually focal because of ecologic restrictions on their transmission (Table 382–1). Diagnosis depends on a careful

TABLE 382–1. SOME PROPERTIES OF RNA VIRUSES CAUSING FEVER, ARTHRITIS, ENCEPHALITIS, OR HEMORRHAGIC FEVER

Family (*Genus*) Virus	Human Disease	Distribution	Vector
Togaviridae (*Alphavirus*)			
Mayaro	Fever, arthritis, rash	South America	Mosquito
Ross River	Arthritis, rash, sometimes fever	Australia, S. Pacific	Mosquito
Chikungunya	Fever, arthritis, hemorrhagic fever	Africa, Asia, Philippines	Mosquito
Eastern encephalitis	Fever, encephalitis	Americas	Mosquito
Western encephalitis	Fever, encephalitis	Americas	Mosquito
Venezuelan encephalitis	Fever, sometimes encephalitis	Americas	Mosquito
Flaviviridae (*Flavivirus*)			
Dengue (4 types)	Fever, rash, hemorrhagic fever	Worldwide (tropics)	Mosquito
Yellow fever	Fever, hemorrhagic fever	Tropical Americas, Africa	Mosquito
St. Louis encephalitis	Encephalitis, hepatitis (rare)	Americas	Mosquito
Japanese encephalitis	Encephalitis	Asia, Pacific	Mosquito
West Nile	Fever, rash, hepatitis, encephalitis	Asia, Europe, Africa	Mosquito
Kyasanur Forest	Hemorrhagic fever, meningoencephalitis	India	Tick
Omsk hemorrhagic fever	Hemorrhagic fever	U.S.S.R.	Tick
Tick-borne encephalitis	Encephalitis	Europe, Asia	Tick
Bunyaviridae (*Bunyavirus*)			
LaCrosse encephalitis	Encephalitis	North America	Mosquito
Oropouche	Fever	Brazil, Panama	Midge
Bunyaviridae (*Phlebovirus*)			
Sandfly fever viruses	Fever	Asia, Africa, tropical Americas	Sand fly, mosquito
Rift Valley fever	Fever, hemorrhagic fever, encephalitis, retinitis	Africa	Mosquito
Bunyaviridae (*Nairovirus*)			
Crimean-Congo hemorrhagic fever	Hemorrhagic fever	Asia, Europe, Africa	Tick
Bunyaviridae (*Hantavirus*)			
Hantaan	Hemorrhagic fever, renal syndrome	Asia	Rodent-borne
Puumala	Hemorrhagic fever, renal syndrome	Europe	Rodent-borne
Arenaviridae (*Arenavirus*)			
Junin	Hemorrhagic fever	Argentina	Rodent-borne
Machupo	Hemorrhagic fever	Bolivia	Rodent-borne
Lassa	Hemorrhagic fever	West Africa	Rodent-borne
Reoviridae (*Orbivirus*)			
Colorado tick fever	Fever	Western U.S.A.	Tick
Filoviridae (*Filovirus*)			
Marburg	Hemorrhagic fever	Africa	Unknown
Ebola	Hemorrhagic fever	Africa	Unknown

history encompassing exposure to vertebrate animals and arthropod vectors, age, season, and travel, including geographic site of exposure. The physician must have a high index of suspicion. Fevers may often be diagnosed erroneously as malaria; indeed, in malaria-endemic regions the patient frequently has malaria concomitantly with an arboviral infection.

Laboratory confirmation of infection is essential. Classically the virus was isolated from acute phase serum or whole blood in laboratory animals such as the mouse or in tissue culture. The neutralization, complement fixation, and hemagglutination-inhibition tests of acute and 3-week convalescent sera also led to the correct diagnosis. Now the fluorescent antibody and enzyme-linked immunosorbent assays (ELISA) are supplanting the classic techniques. Antigen detection and IgM capture ELISA permit diagnosis on the initial visit to the physician in many cases, and at least within a week of onset of the illness in most cases.

Control can be achieved by interrupting the cycle, including vaccination of reservoir animals, vector control, and education on methods to avoid the vector. Vaccines are available or under development for some of the agents such as Rift Valley fever, Venezuelan encephalitis, yellow fever, Japanese encephalitis, and dengue.

Beaty BJ, Calisher CH, Shope RE: Arboviruses. *In* Schmidt NJ, Emmons RW (eds.): Diagnostic Procedures for Viral, Rickettsial and Chlamydial Infections, 6th ed. Washington, D.C., American Public Health Association, 1989, pp 797–855. *Detailed description of diagnostic technology with clearly defined explanation of indications and limitations of procedures.*

Karabatsos N (ed.): International Catalogue of Arboviruses Including Certain Other Viruses of Vertebrates, 3rd ed. San Antonio, TX, American Society of Tropical Medicine and Hygiene, 1985. *Encyclopedic listing of 504 arboviruses and rodent-borne viruses with detailed description of epidemiologic, serologic, biochemical, and physical properties.*

383 Dengue

Jay P. Sanford

DEFINITION. Dengue is an acute arbovirus infection that presents chiefly with fever, malaise, lymphadenopathy, and rash. The first epidemic of a disease resembling dengue, which occurred in Philadelphia in 1780, was described by Benjamin Rush. Epidemics which now occur worldwide over large areas of the tropics and subtropics, including the Pacific basin, Southeast Asia, and Africa, were also common in North America in the nineteenth and early twentieth centuries, although many of these outbreaks more likely were Chikungunya virus disease. Outbreaks recurred in the Caribbean, including Puerto Rico and the U.S. Virgin Islands, in 1969. Indigenous infections were recognized in the continental United States for the first time in 35 years in 1980. Transmission by the mosquito *Aedes aegypti* was initially described by Bancroft (1906). *A. aegypti* has reappeared along the U.S. Gulf Coast; hence, the threat of reappearance of dengue in the United States again is real.

ETIOLOGY. Dengue viruses, members of the family Flaviviridae, are single-stranded, nonsegmented RNA viruses. There are four distinct serogroups of dengue viruses, types 1 through 4, each of which has now been documented in the western hemisphere.

EPIDEMIOLOGY. The cycle of dengue virus transmission involves primarily humans and mosquitoes. *A. aegypti* is the most important vector, but other species of *Aedes* are involved in Asia and the Pacific. *A. aegypti* is peridomestic, biting humans readily or even preferentially. Feeding is frequently interrupted, with the female taking multiple blood meals and thus enabling multiple infections by a single mosquito. Breeding occurs in small collections of water such as backyard litter, especially tires. Surveys in Texas have revealed containers with water in which *A. aegypti* were breeding in up to 25 per cent of premises. Zoonotic cycles of dengue virus transmission involving monkeys and forest *Aedes* species occur in Malaysia and West Africa. The mechanism for maintenance of the virus between epidemics has not been defined, but vertical transmission in *Aedes* has been experimentally documented. Nonimmune individuals are uniformly susceptible, and susceptibility is not influenced by age, sex, or race. During outbreaks attack rates in nonimmune individuals may be high; in Puerto Rico and the U.S. Virgin Islands, the overall rate of clinical disease was 20 per cent, with infection rates as determined by serologic surveys as high as 79 per cent. Immunity against homotypic reinfection is complete and probably lifelong, but cross-protection between different serotypes lasts less than 3 months.

PATHOLOGY. Dengue viruses multiply in the midgut epithelium and salivary glands of mosquitoes without producing pathologic changes. Mosquitoes remain infectious for life. The virus replicates in the female mosquito genital tract and may enter the ovum, enabling vertical transmission. In humans, in whom the classic disease is self-limited, biopsy of skin lesions shows swelling of endothelial cells and perivascular mononuclear cell infiltrates.

CLINICAL FEATURES. Dengue virus infection is often inapparent. When disease occurs, three overlapping clinical forms are recognized: classic dengue, a mild atypical form; dengue hemorrhagic fever (DHF), a severe form; and the dengue shock syndrome (DSS). Classic dengue (breakbone fever) occurs primarily in nonimmune individuals who are often nonindigenous children and adults. Disease begins abruptly after a 2- to 7-day incubation. Initial symptoms include a severe splitting headache, retro-orbital pain, backache especially in the lumbar area, leg pain, and arthralgia. At least three fourths of patients complain of pain on moving their eyes. True rigors are common during the illness but usually do not herald the onset. Other common symptoms include insomnia, nausea, anorexia with taste aberrations, cutaneous hyperesthesia, and generalized weakness. Mild rhinopharyngitis occurs in one fourth of patients. Findings on examination include a relative bradycardia, scleral injection (30 to 90 per cent), tenderness on pressure on the ocular globes, and pharyngeal injection. A transient macular rash may occur on the first or second day. Within 2 to 3 days after onset, the temperature may decrease to nearly normal and other symptoms subside. The remission typically lasts 2 days. Fever then recurs, giving the "saddle-back" or biphasic course. During the second phase, symptoms may return, although they are generally less severe. On the third to fifth day (with the second phase) a more definite maculopapular rash usually appears on the trunk and then spreads to the arms and legs while sparing the palms and soles. The rash is often characterized by 2- to 5-mm "islands of white in a sea of red." The rash is accompanied in some cases by complaints of burning in the palms of the hands and soles of the feet. On resolution, the rash may desquamate. Concurrently, generalized nontender lymphadenopathy, typically including posterior cervical, epitrochlear, and inguinal chains, develops. The biphasic febrile course is considered characteristic but often is not encountered. The entire illness lasts 5 to 7 days and terminates abruptly. Complaints of fatigue and depression for an additional several weeks are common.

In addition to the classic syndrome, an atypical mild illness characterized by fever, anorexia, headache, myalgia, and evanescent rashes occurs. The atypical syndrome is usually not associated with lymphadenopathy.

At the onset in both classic and mild dengue, leukocyte counts may be normal or low; however, by the third to fifth day leukocyte counts are decreased (less than 5000 per cubic millimeter with granulocytopenia). Thrombocytopenia (less than 100,000 per cubic millimeter) also may be a feature. Urinalysis may show moderate albuminuria.

DIAGNOSIS. A history of travel to dengue-endemic areas and occurrence of other cases in a community are important reminders to include dengue in the differential diagnosis. Specific diagnosis depends upon virus isolation or serologic tests. Viremia can be detected for the initial 3 to 5 days with dengue types 1, 2, and 3 by inoculation of mosquito tissue cell cultures. Viral titers in patients with dengue 4 are considerably lower than in patients with types 1, 2, and 3, making viral isolation less common. Of serologic tests, plaque-reduction neutralization is most specific. IgM antibodies indicate recent dengue infection but do not provide a type-specific diagnosis and cross-react with other flavivirus antibodies, including those following immunization with yellow fever vaccine.

TREATMENT. Treatment is entirely symptomatic—bed rest, antipyretics, and analgesics.

PROGNOSIS. In the absence of dengue hemorrhagic fever or the dengue shock syndrome, mortality is nil.

PREVENTION. Live attenuated vaccines against types 1, 2, and 4 are in various stages of development, but all are still investigational. Prevention of epidemics relies principally on reduction or eradication of *A. aegypti* by breeding site elimination and use of larvacides. Ultra low volume aerial spraying of organophosphate insecticides (malathion) to reduce the population of adult female mosquitoes has been used successfully for emergency control of epidemics.

Carey DE: Chikungunya and dengue: A case of mistaken identity. J Hist Med 26:243–262, 1971. *An in-depth review emphasizing clinical features. Not only interesting but provides useful clinical information.*

Ehrenkranz NJ, Ventura AK, Cuadrado RR, et al.: Pandemic dengue in Caribbean countries and the Southern United States—past, present and potential problems. N Engl J Med 285:1460–1469, 1971. *Summarizes the recent Caribbean pandemic and potential for reintroduction into the United States.*

Halstead SB: Pathogenesis of dengue: Challenges to molecular biology. Science 239:476–481, 1988. *The pathobiology of DHF and DSS versus that of classic dengue has remained unproved. Dr. Halstead reviews alternative hypotheses.*

Sabin AB: Research on dengue during World War II. Am J Trop Med Hyg 1:30–50, 1952. *This old paper still provides the best available summary of clinical features.*

384 West Nile Fever

Jay P. Sanford

DEFINITION. West Nile fever, like dengue, is a mosquito-transmitted, acute, self-limited illness that presents chiefly with fever, malaise, lymphadenopathy, and rash.

ETIOLOGY. West Nile fever virus is a member of the flaviviruses—single-stranded, nonsegmented RNA viruses. Viral strains from Africa, Europe, the USSR, and the Middle East are antigenically distinct from strains isolated in India and the Far East.

EPIDEMIOLOGY. The cycle of West Nile fever virus transmission involves mosquitoes and wild birds, with mammals, including man, as incidental end-stage hosts. The mosquito vector species vary between areas: *Culex univittatus*, *C. pipiens*, and *C. molestus* in the Middle East and Africa, *Mansonia metallicus* in Uganda, and *C. tritaeniorhynchus* in Asia. In many areas, human infections are extremely common, with over 60 per cent of young adults having antibodies. This indicates that in endemic areas there is a high prevalence of inapparent or undifferentiated febrile illness in children. There is no sex predominance.

CLINICAL FEATURES. Following an incubation period of 1 to 6 days, the onset is usually abrupt without prodromal symptoms. The temperature rises quickly to 38.3 to 40°C, with rigors in one third of patients. Symptoms include drowsiness, severe frontal headache, ocular pain, myalgia, and pain in the abdomen and back. A small number of patients have dryness of the throat, anorexia, and nausea. Cough is uncommon. Examination shows facial flushing, conjunctival injection, and coating of the tongue. The prominent finding is generalized lymphadenopathy. Nodes are of moderate size and nontender and usually include the occipital, axillary, and inguinal chains. The spleen and liver are occasionally slightly enlarged. The temperature curve may be biphasic. In one half of patients a pale roseolar maculopapular rash, predominantly truncal and on the upper arms, appears from the second to fifth day. The rash may be evanescent (several hours) or persist until defervescence. It clears without desquamation. Rarely vesicular lesions may occur. The illness is self-limited and lasts 3 to 5 days in 80 per cent of patients. Generally the illness in children is milder than in adults.

Infection may also result in aseptic meningitis or meningoencephalitis, especially in the elderly. Spinal fluid examinations may reveal a lymphocytic pleocytosis with some increase in protein concentration. Other rare complications include myocarditis, pancreatitis, and hepatitis. Convalescence is often prolonged, lasting several weeks with prominent symptoms of fatigue. Lymph node enlargement requires several months to regress. Laboratory findings include leukopenia (less than 4000 per cubic millimeter in one third of patients).

DIAGNOSIS. Clinically West Nile fever resembles dengue. West Nile virus can be isolated from blood of three fourths of patients on the first day, with viremia persisting but decreasing over 5 days. Serologic diagnosis is possible using a number of tests; however, cross-reactions with other flaviviruses complicate interpretation.

TREATMENT AND PROGNOSIS. Treatment is symptomatic. Ribavirin has activity against West Nile fever virus, but since the disease is self-limited and almost never fatal its use does not seem indicated.

PREVENTION. There is no vaccine.

Flatau E, Kohn D, Daher O, et al.: West Nile fever encephalitis. Isr J Med Sci 17:1057–1059, 1981. *A brief but adequate description of encephalitis in older patients.*

Marberg K, Goldblum N, Sterk VV, et al.: The natural history of West Nile fever. 1. Clinical observations during an epidemic in Israel. Am J Hyg 64:259–269, 1956. *A good description of the clinical illness.*

Southam CM, Moore AE: Induced virus infections in man by the Egypt isolates of West Nile virus. Am J Trop Med Hyg 3:19–50, 1954. *A detailed paper that includes clinical and laboratory features of West Nile fever.*

385 Phlebotomus Fever

Jay P. Sanford

DEFINITION. Phlebotomus (sandfly, pappataci, or 3-day fever) is an acute, relatively mild, self-limited infection transmitted by *Phlebotomus* flies. It is characterized by fever, malaise, headache, and myalgia and caused by at least five immunologically distinct phleboviruses (Naples, Sicilian, Punto Toro, Chagres, and Candiru).

ETIOLOGY. The sandfly fever group of viruses, within the *Phlebovirus* genus, are enveloped, single-stranded, trisegmented RNA viruses.

EPIDEMIOLOGY. Phlebotomus fever viruses are transmitted by phlebotomine flies. In the Mediterranean, Middle East, and northwest India, *Phlebotomus papatasii*, which breeds in dry sandy areas and feeds in early evening, is the principal vector. In Central America, *Lutzomyia*, a forest-dwelling species, is the principal vector. In interepidemic intervals sandfly fever viruses are presumably maintained in a vector-host wildlife cycle, but this has not been defined. During epidemics man may act as the major host. Transovarial transmission probably serves as an alternative mechanism for virus perpetuation. Sandflies are small (2 to 3 mm), which enables them to penetrate screens and mosquito netting. There is no pain or itching after the bite; hence only about 1 per cent of patients remember being bitten. Epidemics occurred among allied troops in Italy in 1942–1944.

CLINICAL FEATURES. The best descriptions of clinical illness come from the study of experimentally infected human volunteers (Sabin). After an incubation period of 2 to 6 days, symptoms develop abruptly in over 90 per cent. Temperatures rise to 37.8 to 40.1°C. Headache is nearly always present and often is accompanied by pain on ocular movement and retro-orbital pain. Myalgia is common and may be localized, for example to the abdomen; if to the chest it resembles pleurodynia. Other symptoms include vomiting, photophobia, alteration or loss of taste, and arthralgia. Conjunctival injection is seen in one third of patients. With severe illness, mild papilledema has been seen. Small vesicles occur on the palate. Macular or urticarial rashes may occur. The spleen is rarely palpable and lymphadenopathy is absent. The pulse is proportional to the temperature on the first day; subsequently there is a relative bradycardia. Fever persists for 2 to 4 days in most patients, with gradual defervescence. Weakness and feelings of depression are common during convalescence. Second attacks occur 2 to 12 weeks after the first in 15 per cent of cases. Aseptic meningitis may occur. In one series, 12 per cent of patients had lumbar punctures; findings included pleocytosis (average cell counts of 90 per cubic millimeter with either mononuclear or neutrophilic leukocytes).

Laboratory findings include leukopenia (less than 5000 per cubic millimeter) in 90 per cent of patients. The leukopenia may not occur until the third day. Early there is lymphopenia with an increase in band neutrophils. Subsequently a relative lymphocytosis (40 to 65 per cent) occurs. Urinalyses are usually normal.

DIAGNOSIS. Diagnosis is made on clinical and epidemiologic findings. Sandfly fever viruses replicate and produce plaques in Vero cell cultures. Serologic tests are not available.

TREATMENT AND PROGNOSIS. Treatment is symptomatic. No fatalities have been reported.

PREVENTION. During World War II phlebotomus fever was controlled in the Mediterranean theater by the use of DDT, to which sandflies are sensitive.

Sabin AB, Philip CB, Paul JR: Phlebotomus (pappataci or sandfly) fever: A disease of military importance. JAMA 125:603–606, 693–699, 1944.

Oldfield EC, Wallace MR, Hyams KC, et al.: Endemic infectious diseases of the Middle East. Rev Infect Dis 13(Suppl 3):S199–S217, 1991. *The most recent review, which includes investigational use of oral ribavirin in experimentally infected volunteers.*

386 Rift Valley Fever

Jay P. Sanford

Rift Valley fever (RVF) is an acute disease principally of livestock—sheep, goats, cattle, and camels—caused by the Rift Valley fever virus, an RNA virus that is transmitted by mosquitoes. It belongs to the genus *Phlebovirus*, which contains more than 30 viruses. The other medically important phleboviruses are the sandfly fever (phlebotomus fever) group of viruses. RVF was originally recognized as a cause of epizootic hepatitis in sheep in 1912. In cattle and sheep, most pregnant ewes and cows abort, and mortality in newborn lambs is over 90 per cent. It was first described in humans in 1930 during an extensive epizootic of hepatitis in sheep in Kenya. During an epizootic in South Africa in 1950–1951, an estimated 20,000 humans were infected. Fatal human disease, four cases of hemorrhagic disease and hepatitis, was first reported during an epizootic in South Africa in 1975. In 1977–1978 Rift Valley fever virus appeared for the first time in Egypt with a major outbreak involving cattle, sheep, goats, and buffalo. Two hundred thousand cases of human disease were estimated, with 598 deaths reported in 1977. RVF appears to have disappeared from Egypt after 1981.

ETIOLOGY. Rift Valley fever virus is an enveloped, single-stranded, trisegmented RNA virus. The virus multiplies readily in most common cell cultures, is cytopathic, and forms plaques.

EPIDEMIOLOGY. Rift Valley fever virus can be transmitted by a number of mosquito species; in Egypt *Culex pipiens*, in South Africa *C. theileri*, and in East Africa *Aedes* species are the major vectors. Epizootics in large domestic animals have been associated with particularly wet rainy seasons and high mosquito density. A wildlife-mosquito cycle during interepizootic periods has been postulated but not confirmed. Transovarial vertical transmission is an alternative. During an epizootic, disease occurs first in animals and then in humans. Direct transmission to man by contact with blood or tissues of infected animals may be more important than mosquito transmission. Laboratory-acquired infections presumably due to aerosols are common. In addition to eastern and southern Africa, Rift Valley fever virus has been isolated in West Africa. Zinga virus, a cause of sporadic human disease in central Africa, has been shown to be a strain of Rift Valley fever virus.

CLINICAL FEATURES. The incubation period is usually 3 to 6 days. It is an influenza-like illness with an abrupt onset, malaise, occasionally rigors, headache, myalgia, and backache. The temperature rises rapidly to 38.3 to 40°C. Later complaints include anorexia, loss of taste, photophobia, and epigastric pain. On examination findings may include flushing of the face and conjunctival injection. The course of fever is often saddle-back, with the initial elevation lasting 2 to 3 days, followed by remission and then a second febrile period. The total duration of fever is usually about 1 week. Convalescence is usually rapid. Prior to

the outbreak in Egypt, RVF was considered to be a benign illness with almost no fatalities. In Egypt, approximately 1 per cent of patients developed severe complications—meningoencephalitis, retinopathy, or hepatic or hemorrhagic manifestations. Encephalitis with intense headache, confusion, and stupor appeared as the acute infection subsided. The cerebrospinal fluid showed a lymphocytic pleocytosis with normal CSF glucose values. Some survivors had severe residuals. Ocular complications were characterized by visual loss occurring 2 to 7 days after the onset. Findings on ophthalmoscopic examination included macular edema, cotton-wool exudates on the macula, hemorrhages, retinitis, and vascular occlusion. One half of such patients had some permanent loss of visual acuity. Hepatic and hemorrhagic manifestations also occurred during the acute illness. Deaths from massive hepatic necrosis occurred 7 to 10 days after onset. Hemorrhagic manifestations include epistaxis, hematemesis, melena, and intracranial hemorrhage. The fatality ratio in severely ill patients exceeded 50 per cent. Laboratory features include initial normal to increased total leukocyte counts followed by leukopenia with granulocytopenia but an increase in band forms. Thrombocytopenia and clotting defects occur.

DIAGNOSIS. The diagnosis is confirmed by isolating virus from blood by inoculation of mice. Three fourths of patients are viremic (up to 10^8 mouse intraperitoneal lethal doses per milliliter of blood) at onset of illness. Neutralizing antibodies appear as early as 4 days.

TREATMENT. Treatment has been symptomatic. In patients with hemorrhagic manifestations, transfusion of platelets and fresh frozen plasma may be beneficial. In experimentally infected animals, ribavirin has been partially protective. Given the experience including minimal toxicity with intravenous ribavirin in patients with Lassa fever and Korean hemorrhagic fever (Hantaan), one might consider administration of ribavirin in similar dosage (2.0-gram loading dose IV, then 1.0 gram IV every 6 hours for 4 days, then 0.5 gram IV every 8 hours for 6 days) to patients with severe disease.

PREVENTION. Because the virus can be spread by contact with blood and tissues, and humans show high levels of viremia, blood and needle precautions are essential. An inactivated Rift Valley fever vaccine, although not yet licensed for man, has been produced and is protective in animals.

Kark JD, Aynor Y, Peters CJ: A Rift Valley fever vaccine trial. I. Side effects and serologic response over a six-month follow-up. Am J Epidemiol 116:808–820, 1982.

Kende M, Alving CR, Rill WL, et al.: Enhanced efficacy of liposome-encapsulated ribavirin against Rift Valley fever virus infection in mice. Antimicrob Agents Chemother 27:903–907, 1985.

Laughlin LW, Meegan JM, Strausbaugh LH, et al.: Epidemic Rift Valley fever in Egypt: Observations of the spectrum of human illness. Trans Roy Soc Trop Med Hyg 73:630–633, 1979. *If you are going to read one paper on RVF, this one provides the best overall recent experience.*

Siam AL, Meegan JM, Gharbawi KF: Rift Valley fever ocular manifestations: Observations during 1977 epidemic in Egypt. Br J Ophthalmol 64:366–374, 1980.

387 Alphaviruses Associated with Polyarthritis

Jay P. Sanford

DEFINITION. The alphaviruses (previously designated group A arboviruses) are a genus within the Togaviridae family. They are single-stranded RNA viruses with common antigenic determinants. At least nine alphaviruses, including six which cause acute arthropathy, have been associated with epidemics. The cycle for all is mosquito-vertebrate-mosquito. Those alphaviruses associated with systemic febrile illness (Venezuelan equine encephalitis) and primarily encephalitis (eastern equine encephalitis and western equine encephalitis) are discussed in Ch. 389.

This section reviews the epidemiology and clinical features of the alphaviruses associated with acute arthropathy.

CHIKUNGUNYA VIRUS

DEFINITION. The name chikungunya is a local tribal word, "that which bends up," which was used to describe an epidemic of acute arthropathy in Tanzania in 1952–1953.

EPIDEMIOLOGY. Today Chikungunya (CK) virus is of major importance in Africa and Asia. It was probably responsible for disease in the southern United States in the early nineteenth century. In Africa CK virus is transmitted by *Aedes* mosquitoes. In the forests of tropical Africa the mosquitoes belong to the subgenera *Stegomyia* and *Diceromyia*. The vertebrate hosts are nonhuman primates—monkeys or baboons. Transmission occurs primarily in the rainy season. Human involvement is largely secondary. In villages and urban areas, *Aedes aegypti* also serves as a vector. In these circumstances humans may serve as the vertebrate host. In sub-Saharan Africa, except in the dry areas and below 18° latitude, antibody prevalence surveys range from 20 to greater than 90 per cent. In Asia, transmission is primarily human to human by *A. aegypti*. CK virus is present in India, Southeast Asia, and the Philippines. Seroprevalence rates in Bangkok of 31 per cent were observed. The potential for CK virus transmission outside of the current distribution, i.e., Central and South America as well as the southern United States, exists.

CLINICAL FEATURES. The incubation period is usually 2 to 3 days but may be as long as 12 days. The onset is usually abrupt, with temperatures rising to 38.3 to 40°C, often accompanied by rigors and incapacitating arthralgia. The arthralgias are polyarticular and migratory, involving predominantly the small joints of the hands, wrists, ankles, and toes. Pain is increased with motion and worse in the morning. Joint swelling is common, but effusions are uncommon. The arthralgia is associated with generalized myalgia. Other symptoms include headache, photophobia, sore throat, anorexia, and vomiting, but these do not dominate the clinical picture. Cutaneous manifestations are typical. At onset there is flushing of the face and neck. Other signs include conjunctival injection and lymphadenopathy. A maculopapular rash usually involving the trunk and limbs typically occurs on the second to fifth day. The rash lasts 1 to 5 days and may just fade or may desquamate. On the second or third day, the fever may remit for 1 to 2 days, then recur, giving a biphasic "saddle-back" course. However, the biphasic course is not as striking as that seen with dengue. Laboratory findings include occasional leukopenia with relative lymphocytosis, although most leukocyte counts are normal. Mild thrombocytopenia may occur. The joint symptoms may persist for long periods, only one third of individuals being asymptomatic within a few weeks. About 5 per cent of patients have persistent joint pain, stiffness, and recurrent effusions. Persistence may be more common in HLA B27 positive patients. In African children disease is milder, with arthralgia less prominent. In Asia CK virus is responsible for a hemorrhagic fever syndrome closely resembling dengue hemorrhagic fever or the dengue shock syndrome. About 8 per cent of patients with the hemorrhagic fever syndrome had CK virus. Other features may include encephalitis and myocarditis.

DIAGNOSIS. CK virus disease should be suspected clinically given the appropriate epidemiologic history and the triad of fever, acute arthralgia/arthritis, and rash. Viremia is present in most patients during the first 48 hours. Hemagglutination inhibition (HI) antibodies appear by day 5 to 7.

TREATMENT. Treatment is symptomatic.

PREVENTION. A promising live attenuated vaccine is under clinical investigation.

Deller JJ Jr, Russell PK: Chikungunya disease. Am J Trop Med Hyg 17:1007–1111, 1968.

Fourie ED, Morrison JGL: Rheumatoid arthritis syndrome after chikungunya fever. S Afr Med J 56:130–132, 1979.

Halstead SB, Udomsakdi S, Singharaj P, et al.: Dengue and chikungunya virus infection in man and virologic observations on disease in non-indigenous white persons. Am J Trop Med Hyg 18:984–996, 1969.

Robinson MC: An epidemic of virus disease in Southern Province Tanganyika Territory in 1952–53. I. Clinical features. Trans R Soc Trop Med Hyg 49:28–32, 1955.

O'NYONG-NYONG VIRUS

DEFINITION. O'nyong-nyong (ON) virus first appeared in February 1959 as an epidemic of polyarthritis in Uganda. The name *o'nyong-nyong* means "weakening of the joints." The epidemic spread to involve at least 2 million people, with clinical attack rates of 9 to 78 per cent in different villages. The epidemic ceased in the mid-1960's, although the virus was again isolated from mosquitoes in Kenya in 1978.

EPIDEMIOLOGY. The vectors of ON virus are mosquitoes, *Anopheles funnestus* and *A. anogambiae*. The nonhuman vertebrate reservoir, if there is one, is unknown.

CLINICAL FEATURES. The clinical features are similar to those of chikungunya virus disease. The incubation period may be somewhat longer, at least 8 days. Fever is less prominent, exceeding 38.3°C in only one third of patients. Rash occurred in 60 to 70 per cent. In contrast to CK virus disease, generalized lymphadenopathy was a common feature. There appears to be less residual arthropathy with ON than CK disease.

DIAGNOSIS. Diagnosis is based on virus isolation. Patients seroconvert by hemagglutination inhibition assays, but cross-reactions with CK virus make interpretation difficult.

Shore H: O'nyong-nyong fever: An epidemic virus disease in East Africa. III. Some clinical and epidemiological observations in the northern province of Uganda. Trans R Soc Trop Med Hyg 55:361–373, 1961.

MAYARO VIRUS

DEFINITION. Mayaro (MY) virus has been associated with epidemics of acute polyarthritis in Brazil and Bolivia.

EPIDEMIOLOGY. MY virus has been recognized in the forested areas of Central and South America with annual infection rates of 10 to 60 per cent. There is usually a 2:1 male predominance. The vectors for MY virus are *Haemagogus* mosquitoes. The virus causes high-level viremia in marmosets and other primates. Whether or not marmosets are the major vertebrate host has not been confirmed.

CLINICAL FEATURES. The incubation period is about 1 week. Ages of patients have ranged from 2 to 62 years with both sexes involved. Illness begins abruptly with fever, chills, severe frontal headache, myalgia, and dizziness. Arthralgia occurs uniformly and is very prominent and occasionally incapacitating and in some patients precedes the fever. Small joints, wrists, fingers, ankles, and toes predominate. Temperatures usually exceed 40°C. Other initial symptoms (less than one third of patients) include nausea, vomiting, and diarrhea. Initial clinical features include occasional conjunctival suffusion, inguinal lymphadenopathy (one half of patients), and joint swelling (one quarter of patients). About the fifth day maculopapular rash develops over the chest, back, arms, and legs. Rash appeared in 90 per cent of children and one half of adults and lasted about 3 days. The clinical course is usually 3 to 5 days except for the arthralgia, which may persist for several months. Laboratory findings include leukopenia (as low as 2500 per cubic millimeter). Urinalyses revealed albuminuria (2+) in one fourth of patients. Some patients showed increases in SGOT levels. In Brazil no relapses were observed and no deaths have been recognized. In Bolivia, several fatalities have been reported.

DIAGNOSIS. Diagnosis is confirmed by virus isolation, preferably in Vero cells. MY-specific IgM responses have been observed.

Pinheiro FP, Freitas RB, Travassos da Rosa JF, et al.: An outbreak of Mayaro virus disease in Belterra, Brazil. I. Clinical and virological findings. Am J Trop Med Hyg 30:674–681, 1981.

ROSS RIVER VIRUS

DEFINITION. Epidemics of fever, polyarthritis, and rash were noted in rural Australia in 1928.

ETIOLOGY. Ross River (RR) virus is a typical alphavirus.

EPIDEMIOLOGY. Outbreaks occur almost entirely between December and June. RR virus infection was limited to Australia, New Guinea, and the Solomon Islands until 1979, when a major outbreak occurred in Fiji and then spread to the Samoan, Cook, and some Melanesian Islands. The natural vector-reservoir relationships have not been well established. *Culex annulirostris* is probably the major vector, although other species of mosquitoes may be involved. Several mammalian species, especially the New Holland mouse and wallabys, are important hosts in Australia. In the Pacific outbreak *Aedes vigilax* may also have been an important vector. In the Pacific, man-mosquito-man transmission was likely. In the Fiji outbreak, infection rates were equal at all ages and in both sexes, but clinical disease rates were 4 per cent in patients under 20 years of age and 42 per cent in those over 20 years of age. The clinical attack rate of males to females was 1:1.7.

CLINICAL FEATURES. In Australia, the incubation is estimated to be 7 to 9 days, while in the Pacific the incubation period was shorter. The illness at onset is characterized by headache, myalgia, nausea and vomiting, and occasionally tenderness of the palms of the hands and soles of the feet. Initially fever may be absent or minimal (highest 38°C). In about one half of patients arthritis involving mainly the small joints, wrists, and ankles occurs. Knee involvement also is common. The joint swelling and paresthesias may precede a rash by 1 to 15 days. In the other half of patients the rash precedes the arthralgia. The rash, which is usually maculopapular, appears on the cheeks and forehead, occasionally spreads to the trunk, or may be restricted to extremities. The rash may be pruritic. Vesicles occur rarely. Tender lymphadenopathy occurs in one fifth of patients. Most patients are unable to work. Recovery is slow, only one half being able to return to work by 1 month and 10 per cent still having joint symptoms at 3 months. Laboratory findings are not striking; leukocyte counts are normal or minimally decreased. The erythrocyte sedimentation rate is increased acutely but normalizes over several weeks even with continued joint symptoms. Antinuclear antibodies and rheumatoid factor tests are negative. Synovial fluid changes are not striking—cell counts of 1,000 to 60,000, predominantly mononuclear, normal viscosity. Urinalyses are normal, although recently RR virus has been associated with segmental sclerosing glomerulonephritis.

DIAGNOSIS. The diagnosis is usually based on clinical features. In Australia patients seldom have viremia on presentation, while in the Pacific outbreak viremia was readily detected. Hemagglutination inhibition antibodies appear early.

TREATMENT. Treatment is symptomatic.

Aaskov JG, Mataika JU, Lawrence GW, et al.: An epidemic of Ross River virus infection in Fiji, 1979. Am J Trop Med Hyg 30:1053–1059, 1981.

Clarke JA, Marshall ID, Gard G: Annually recurrent epidemic polyarthritis and Ross River virus activity in the coastal area of New South Wales. I. Occurrence of the disease. Am J Trop Med Hyg 22:543–550, 1973.

Davies DJ, Moran JE, Niall JF, et al.: Segmental necrotising glomerulonephritis with antineutrophil antibody: Possible arbovirus etiology. Br Med J 285:606, 1982.

Fraser JRE: Epidemic polyarthritis and Ross River virus disease. Clin Rheum Dis 12:369–388, 1986. *If one is reading only one paper on RR virus, this is the most inclusive.*

SINDBIS VIRUS (Okelbo Disease, Pogosta Disease, Karelian Fever)

DEFINITION. Sindbis virus, a prototype alphavirus, was isolated from *Culex* mosquitoes collected in the Egyptian village of Sindbis in 1952. Initially it was thought only rarely to produce clinical disease. It has now been recognized elsewhere in Africa, in Europe, and in Australia. In the U.S.S.R. it is known as Karelian fever, in Sweden as Okelbo disease, and in Finland as Pogosta disease.

EPIDEMIOLOGY. The vector-host relationships have been best defined in Africa and the Middle East. *Culex univittatus* is the principal vector. The major hosts are birds. Human infection is common where birds and *Culex* mosquitoes are in close proximity. Human antibody rates are commonly 20 to 30 per cent in the Nile Valley of Egypt. Since Sindbis and West Nile fever virus share the same transmission cycles, Sindbis transmission often parallels West Nile fever virus. In northern Europe symptomatic disease is recognized between 60° and 65° north latitude. The virus has been isolated from *Culiseta, Aedes,* and *Culex* mosquitoes. In Europe it occurs in late summer in adults with forest occupations. The host has not been defined.

CLINICAL FEATURES. The incubation period has not been defined. Disease more closely resembles Ross River virus disease than chikungunya or o'nyong-nyong disease. Clinically fever is low grade and accompanied by malaise, myalgia, rash, and arthralgia. Joint involvement is multiple, involving wrists, ankles, knees, and elbows. Periarticular involvement and tendinitis are common. The rash begins on the trunk as scattered macules and spreads to the extremities, palms, and soles. The rash may precede or follow the joint symptoms by 1 to 2 days. Unlike that caused by other alphaviruses, the rash frequently becomes vesic-

ular, especially on the feet and hands. The rash fades within a week. In Europe, persistence of joint complaints is a common feature. In Sweden more than 20 per cent had joint symptoms longer than 1 month after onset.

DIAGNOSIS. Antibodies can be detected by hemagglutination inhibition tests within 7 to 10 days of onset.

TREATMENT. Treatment is symptomatic.

Espmark A, Niklasson B: Okelbo disease in Sweden: Epidemiological, clinical and virological data from the 1982 outbreak. Am J Trop Med Hyg 33:1203–1211, 1984.

Lvov DK, Skvortsova TM, Berezina LK, et al.: Isolation of Karelian fever agent from *Aedes communis* mosquitoes. Lancet 2:399–400, 1984.

Malherbe H, Strickland-Cholmley M: Sindbis virus infection in man. S Afr Med J 37:547–552, 1963.

IGBO-ORA VIRUS

DEFINITION. Igbo-ora virus is a closely related alphavirus isolated from a child in Nigeria. The virus was also isolated from a Peace Corps volunteer with a clinical illness resembling chikungunya disease.

Moore DL, Causey OR, Carey DS, et al.: Arthropod-borne viral infections of man in Nigeria, 1964–1970. Ann Trop Med Parasitol 69:49–64, 1975.

388 Colorado Tick Fever

Theodore C. Eickhoff

DEFINITION. Colorado tick fever (CTF) is an acute, benign, tick-transmitted viral infection that occurs throughout the Rocky Mountain area and is characterized by headache, myalgia, a biphasic febrile course lasting about 1 week, and leukopenia.

ETIOLOGY. CTF virus is an RNA virus in the orbivirus genus of the reoviruses; it is unrelated to other major arbovirus groups. The virus is transmitted to humans by the bite of the hard-shelled wood tick, *Dermacentor andersoni.* Human cases appear to be limited to the combined geographic distribution of the tick vector and the major mammalian rodent reservoirs, ground squirrels and chipmunks. Some antigenic variation of CTF virus has been documented.

EPIDEMIOLOGY. The disease occurs during the spring and summer months, when tick exposure in the mountains is common. Disease activity appears to follow springtime in the mountains, for cases occur at lower altitudes during April and May, and at higher altitudes during June and July, presumably reflecting the slower emergence of ticks at higher altitudes. Most patients give a history of having found attached ticks, but others are not aware of the tick attachment and bite, even though they may have seen ticks on their body or clothing. Cases may occasionally be encountered in other areas of the country as a result of travel outside the endemic area during the incubation period or accidental transportation of infected adult ticks in clothing or bedding.

CTF virus has been recovered from as many as 14 per cent of *Dermacentor andersoni* collected in endemic areas. The virus overwinters in hibernating nymphal and adult ticks and in infected hibernating rodent hosts. Infected nymphal ticks feed on ground squirrels and chipmunks in the spring, and since the resulting viremia in the rodent reservoirs lasts for weeks or months, the virus is amplified in a cycle involving larval and nymphal ticks and the chipmunk and ground squirrel hosts. Humans are accidental hosts, resulting from the bite of an adult tick.

INCIDENCE AND PREVALENCE. The disease has been reported from most states in the Rocky Mountain area and from western Canadian provinces. Several hundred cases are diagnosed annually in the endemic area, but it is likely that this represents only a fraction of the total. Mild or wholly subclinical infections probably do occur, but their frequency has not been systematically evaluated.

The virus has been isolated from other species of ticks and

from numerous species of small mammals, suggesting that the disease may occur over a wider geographic area than is currently appreciated.

PATHOGENESIS. There is no unusual local reaction at the site of the tick bite inoculation, and the site of initial localization of the virus is unknown. The virus replicates in hematopoietic stem cells. Symptoms begin 3 to 6 days after tick exposure. Viremia can be demonstrated at the time of onset of fever, not only persisting during the febrile illness itself, but remarkably persisting in red blood cells long after the virus has disappeared from serum and neutralizing antibody has appeared. The virus can be demonstrated within erythrocytes by fluorescent antibody staining for up to 120 days and has been grown from washed erythrocytes 100 days after the original infection. Transfusion-transmitted CTF has been documented.

Few pathologic data in humans are available, since fatal cases are rare. In experimental animals, the heart, lungs, spleen, bone marrow, and lymph nodes are important sites of viral replication. Occasional patients have clinical evidence of central nervous system or meningeal involvement, and CTF virus has been recovered from cerebrospinal fluid.

CLINICAL MANIFESTATIONS. The disease begins abruptly, with chilly sensations, fever of 38 to 40°C, myalgias most prominent in the back and legs, headache, retro-orbital pain, and photophobia. Malaise and nausea may occur, but vomiting is uncommon. Physical findings during the first 2 to 3 days of illness are nonspecific. The patient may be flushed, with conjunctival and pharyngeal erythema. Lymphadenopathy is not prominent, although mild splenomegaly is sometimes present. Rashes have been reported in up to 12 per cent of patients, commonly macular or maculopapular and distributed over the entire body, sometimes petechial and involving primarily the extremities. Tachycardia is in proportion to the temperature elevation.

In approximately one half of cases, a distinctly biphasic illness occurs, the so-called "saddleback" fever. Symptoms abate after 2 to 3 days, temperature becomes normal or nearly so, and the patient feels relatively well for 1 or 2 days, following which there is an abrupt return of fever, headache, and back pain, often more intense than in the first phase. The second phase lasts 2 to 4 days and then subsides, leaving the patient with weakness and lassitude that disappear during the succeeding week or two. Convalescence may be prolonged in patients over 30 years of age to 3 weeks or more. Some patients do not exhibit the typical biphasic course and experience only one bout of fever or have a typical illness but with a third phase of fever or have a single prolonged febrile illness lasting 5 to 8 days.

Central nervous system involvement has occurred in some patients, usually children. The presenting findings have been those of aseptic meningitis with nuchal rigidity and mononuclear pleocytosis or of encephalitis with a depressed sensorium or stupor. Hemorrhagic manifestations have been described in a few children with encephalitis.

Laboratory findings very early in the illness are generally not helpful, but leukopenia is usually present by the third day of illness and becomes even more pronounced during the second phase, reaching levels as low as 1000 per cubic millimeter. The most striking decrease is in the granulocyte series, with a relative lymphocytosis, and there is frequently an accompanying thrombocytopenia. Atypical, vacuolated lymphocytes are frequently observed. Bone marrow examination reveals a maturation arrest in the granulocyte series. The white blood count returns to normal during convalescence.

DIAGNOSIS. The diagnosis should be suspected in any person with a history of tick exposure in the endemic area 3 to 7 days prior to the onset of a febrile illness. Findings during the first phase, however, cannot be differentiated from many other acute febrile illnesses. A brief symptom-free interval followed by a second febrile illness should strongly suggest CTF. Profound leukopenia is usually present by that time and lends support to the diagnosis.

The diagnosis is confirmed by isolation of the virus from red blood cells, via inoculation of suckling mice, or in tissue culture. More rapid diagnosis is possible by direct immunofluorescent staining of virus in the patient's erythrocytes. A diagnostic rise in antibody titers can be detected by indirect immunofluorescence or by neutralization test; an enzyme-linked immunoassay is available also.

The differential diagnosis can be troublesome, inasmuch as Rocky Mountain spotted fever is transmitted in the tick fever endemic area by the same vector, *Dermacentor andersoni*. Paradoxically, Rocky Mountain spotted fever has become an unusual disease in the state of Colorado and is outnumbered by CTF in Colorado by at least 20-fold. Nevertheless, differential diagnosis may be impossible early in the course of disease, before the characteristic rash of Rocky Mountain spotted fever appears. A relatively symptom-free interval after 2 or 3 days would be most unusual in Rocky Mountain spotted fever and strongly favors the diagnosis of CTF.

TREATMENT. Therapy is entirely supportive, there being no specific therapy. Salicylates or acetaminophen may be necessary to minimize headache and myalgias but are neither required nor advisable in most patients.

PROGNOSIS. The disease is almost invariably benign, and the prognosis is excellent. Severe illness, complicated by central nervous system involvement, is seen infrequently and only in children.

PREVENTION. Both inactivated and live attenuated vaccines have been studied, but the modest number of cases and the benign nature of the disease suggest little need for active immunization.

The most effective means of preventing the disease is the use of protective clothing or repellents by people outdoors in endemic areas during the spring and summer months, together with frequent body inspection and prompt removal of ticks. Transfusion-associated disease can be prevented by exclusion of convalescent donors for a minimum of 6 months.

Anderson RD, Entringer MA, Robinson WA: Virus-induced leukopenia: Colorado tick fever as a human model. J Infect Dis 151:449, 1985. *An interesting exploration of the pathogenesis of the profound leukopenia observed in CTF.*

Emmons RW: Ecology of Colorado tick fever. Annu Rev Microbiol 42:49–64, 1988. *A comprehensive recent review.*

Goodpasture HC, Poland JD, Francy DB, et al.: Colorado tick fever: Clinical, epidemiologic and laboratory aspects of 228 cases in Colorado in 1973–1974. Ann Intern Med 88:303, 1978. *The most recent descriptive clinical study.*

Oshiro LS, Dondero DV, Emmons RW, et al.: The development of Colorado tick fever virus within cells of the haematopoietic system. J Gen Virol 39:73, 1978. *Recommended for those interested in the unusual host-parasite relationship in CTF.*

389 Arthropod-Borne Viral Encephalitides

R. Gordon Douglas, Jr.

Arboviral encephalitis is a significant health problem in Europe, the Soviet Union, parts of Asia, and Central and South America but not Africa. The disease is of particular concern in the Americas, not only because of its multiple etiologic agents and widespread occurrence, but also because of its concurrent affliction of domestic animals and humans and its potential for epidemic spread.

Only a few of the more than 500 arboviruses belonging to the Togaviridae, Bunyaviridae, and Reoviridae families are responsible for epidemic or endemic encephalitis (Table 389–1). These viruses, which circulate in the blood of vertebrate hosts, are transmitted between wild or domestic animals by mosquitoes or ticks. Once replication of the virus has taken place in the salivary glands of the arthropod vector (a week or more after ingestion of infectious blood), transmission by bite can occur. Humans are not essential hosts. Only a small fraction of persons experience severe central nervous system manifestations, and human infection is most often subclinical (Table 389–2). The ratio of inapparent to clinically overt infections is a distinctive, age-dependent quality of each disease. The neurologic disease usually begins after a variable period of nonspecific systemic symptoms and may take the form of aseptic meningitis, meningoencephalitis, or encephalitis. These syndromes are not distinguishable on clinical grounds alone from similar syndromes caused by other infectious agents.

PATHOLOGY AND PATHOGENESIS. Two pathologic processes are common to the arboviral encephalitides: (1) neuronal and glial damage mediated by intracellular viral infection, and (2) migration of immunologically active cells into the perivascular space and brain parenchyma. Endothelial cell swelling and proliferation, destruction of myelin sheaths in deep white matter areas, and vasculitis are present in some arboviral encephalitides.

After a bite by an infected arthropod, viral replication occurs in local tissues and in regional lymph nodes. Viremia, which seeds extraneural tissues, occurs and persists depending on the extent of replication in extraneural sites, the rate of viral clearance by the reticuloendothelial system, and the appearance of humoral antibodies. Sites of extraneural infection vary from virus to virus. Many alpha- and flaviviruses involve striated muscle and vascular endothelium, whereas Venezuelan encephalitis virus is associated with myeloid and lymphoid tissue invasion. During this viremia, the neural parenchyma may be invaded, but the mode of penetration of virus across the blood-brain barrier is not completely understood. Possible mechanisms include passive movement of virus across vascular membranes and virus replication in cerebral capillary endothelial cells. Factors that increase vascular permeability promote neuroinvasion. In experimental animals infected

TABLE 389–1. ARTHROPOD-BORNE VIRUSES THAT CAUSE ACUTE CENTRAL NERVOUS SYSTEM INFECTION AND ENCEPHALITIS

Virus by Group	Mode of Transmission	Geographic Distribution	Disease in Domestic Livestock
Viruses principally associated with the encephalitis syndrome; epidemic and endemic			
Togaviridae, alphavirus			
Eastern equine encephalitis	Mosquito	Eastern North America, Caribbean, South America	Equines, penned pheasants
Western equine encephalitis	Mosquito	Western North America, South America	Equines
Venezuelan equine encephalitis	Mosquito, possibly other modes (see text)	Florida, Central and South America	Equines
Flaviviridae, flavivirus			
St. Louis encephalitis	Mosquito	North America, Caribbean, Central and South America	None
Japanese encephalitis	Mosquito	East and Southeast Asia, India	Equines, swine
Rocio encephalitis	Mosquito	Brazil	None
Murray Valley encephalitis	Mosquito	Australia	(Equines)*
Tick-borne encephalitides: Russian spring-summer and Central European encephalitis	Tick, ingestion of milk	Europe, U.S.S.R.	None
Louping ill	Tick	British Isles	Sheep, equines, cows
Powassan	Tick	North America	None
Bunyaviridae, California subgroup			
California encephalitis, LaCrosse, Jamestown Canyon, snowshoe hare	Mosquito	North America, China, U.S.S.R.	None
Viruses principally associated with other syndromes, but occasionally causing encephalitis; epidemic and endemic			
Togaviridae, alphavirus			
Sindbis (febrile illness with rash)	Mosquito	Africa, Europe	None
Semliki Forest (febrile illness)	Mosquito	Africa, Southeast Asia	(Equines)*
Flaviviridae, flavivirus			
West Nile (febrile illness with rash)	Mosquito	Africa, Middle East	(Equines)*
Kyasanur Forest disease†	Tick	India	None
Omsk hemorrhagic fever†	Tick	Central Asia	None
Bunyaviridae, phlebovirus			
Rift Valley fever (febrile illness, hemorrhagic fever, retinitis)	Mosquito, direct contact	Africa	Sheep, cows, goats
Crimean hemorrhagic fever†—Congo	Tick	Eastern Europe, U.S.S.R., Africa	None
Reoviridae, orbivirus			
Colorado tick fever (febrile illness)	Tick	Western North America	None
Rare and sporadic infections associated with encephalitis			
Flaviviridae, flavivirus			
Ilheus‡	Mosquito	South America	None
Negishi	Tick	Japan, China	None
Langat†	Tick	Asia	None
Orthomyxovirus			
Thogoto	Tick	Africa	None

*Disease rare or suspected but not well documented.
†Tick-borne hemorrhagic fevers.
‡Encephalitis recorded in laboratory infections or experimental infections of cancer patients only; significance in naturally acquired infections unknown.

with some flaviviruses, virus enters the central nervous system by way of the olfactory neuroepithelium.

The immature brain is more susceptible to damage by Western equine, Venezuelan equine, and California encephalitis viruses (Table 389–2). St. Louis encephalitis principally affects the elderly, whereas Japanese encephalitis and eastern equine encephalitis have a bimodal incidence, striking both children and elderly persons. In endemic areas, immunity accumulated with increasing age may reduce the incidence of disease in older persons for some viruses; however, the reasons for increased severity of illness with other viruses are unknown.

DIFFERENTIAL DIAGNOSIS. The most important consideration in diagnosis is to differentiate arthropod-borne viral encephalitis from acute central nervous system infection due to treatable organisms. The early prodromata resemble those of influenza, dengue, or other influenza-like illness. Bacterial meningitis (especially early or partially treated), infective bacterial endocarditis, brain abscess, subdural empyema, and cerebral thrombophlebitis may mimic viral encephalitis, and cerebrospinal fluid changes are sometimes similar. Other infections that occasionally cause meningoencephalitis resembling arthropod-borne viral encephalitis include tuberculosis, cryptococcosis, histoplasmosis, coccidioidomycosis, Rocky Mountain spotted fever, leptospirosis, falciparum malaria, trichinosis, *Naegleria* meningitis, typhoid fever, Lyme disease, and *Mycoplasma* pneumonia.

Acute meningoencephalitis may result from infections with other viruses, including herpesviruses, human immunodeficiency virus, mumps virus, enteroviruses, lymphocytic choriomeningitis virus, rabies, influenza, and the exanthematous viral infections of childhood. Exposure history, presence of an outbreak of similar disease in the community, and summer-fall occurrence are principal clues to an arboviral etiology. Enteroviruses also cause summer-fall outbreaks, but the predominant syndrome is aseptic meningitis, and the occurrence of rash or pleurodynia is a helpful clue. Herpes simplex encephalitis presents an important diagnostic challenge, since chemotherapy is available. The presence of localizing neurologic signs, localizing findings on computed tomography or magnetic resonance imaging scans, or brain biopsy may help distinguish herpes simplex encephalitis from that due to arthropod-borne viral encephalitides.

Noninfectious diseases of the central nervous system such as *cerebrovascular accident* may be confused with viral encephalitis. For example, St. Louis encephalitis, a disease of the elderly, has been misdiagnosed as a stroke. Subarachnoid hemorrhage produces meningismus, fever, headache, and neurologic signs that mimic an infectious etiology. *Metabolic encephalopathies* may present features suggesting infectious encephalitis. *Neoplastic* or *granulomatous diseases* involving the central nervous system and a variety of diseases of uncertain etiology (cat scratch disease, Behçet disease, Reye syndrome, acute multiple sclerosis, and systemic lupus erythematosus) must be considered in the differential diagnosis as well.

WESTERN EQUINE ENCEPHALITIS (WEE)

ETIOLOGIC AGENT. WEE virus is a member of the alphavirus genus of the Togaviridae family.

EPIDEMIOLOGY. *Incidence and Prevalence.* Since 1955, the number of cases of WEE reported annually in the United States has varied from 0 to 200. Most affected in recent years has been the area from the Mississippi River west to the Rocky Mountains. Mixed outbreaks of WEE and St. Louis encephalitis are common. Epidemics occur in early or midsummer and may follow heavy snow melt or flooding, conditions favorable for breeding of mosquitoes. Cases of encephalitis in equines often precede the appearance of human disease. The disease principally affects residents of rural communities, and the incidence is higher in males than in females. WEE is most severe in infants and young children. The case-fatality rate is between 3 and 5 per cent. The ratio of inapparent to apparent infection is also age-dependent, ranging from about 1:1 in infants under 1 year, to 58:1 in children 1 to 4 years old, to over 1000:1 in persons over 14 years of age.

WEE virus also occurs in South America. Equine epizootics in Argentina have been associated with human cases.

Transmission. WEE virus circulates between wild birds and *Culex tarsalis* mosquitoes. *C. tarsalis* is responsible for infection of humans and equines, which develop low or undetectable viremias and do not perpetuate the chain of transmission. In temperate areas, transmission ceases during the winter months.

CLINICAL FEATURES AND PATHOLOGY. The disease usually begins with an influenza-like illness consisting of fever, headache, malaise, and myalgias lasting 1 to 4 days. Somnolence, lethargy, photophobia, vomiting, and neck stiffness may follow; neurologic involvement may rapidly progress to stupor, coma, and convulsions. Paresis, cranial nerve deficits, tremors, and abnormal reflexes may be present. In fatal cases, patients die 1 to 2 days after development of coma. Survivors generally experience a sudden and rapid recovery. However, about one third of surviving infants suffer retardation, cerebellar damage, choreoathetosis, and spastic paralysis. Children with protracted illnesses who develop convulsions during the acute stage are more likely to suffer long-term neurologic impairment. Adults may have a prolonged convalescent syndrome, but objective residua are rare. Congenital infections are documented and result in severe and progressive neurologic deterioration.

Leukocytosis and shift to the left are common. The cerebrospinal fluid contains less than 500 white cells (at first polymorphonuclear, then mononuclear) per cubic millimeter and elevated protein concentration (usually 90 to 110 mg per deciliter).

Pathologic examination of the brains of infants reveals massive neuroparenchymal destruction; children dying months or years after the acute insult often have large cystic lesions in many areas of the brain. In older children and adults, acute WEE is characterized by focal necrosis and perivascular cuffing, predominantly in the basal ganglia and thalamic nuclei but also in deep cerebral white matter.

DIAGNOSIS. Viral isolation from blood or cerebrospinal fluid is almost never successful. Diagnosis is achieved by demonstration of a rise in hemagglutination inhibition (HI), fluorescent, complement-fixing (CF), enzyme-linked immunosorbent assay (ELISA), or neutralizing antibody titers in appropriately timed (10 to 14 days apart) paired sera. Demonstration of immunoglobulin M (IgM) antibodies in serum or cerebrospinal fluid by ELISA provides a presumptive diagnosis.

TABLE 389–2. DIFFERING FEATURES OF ARTHROPOD-BORNE ENCEPHALITIDES IMPORTANT IN THE UNITED STATES

	Western Equine Encephalitis	Eastern Equine Encephalitis	Venezuelan Equine Encephalitis	St. Louis Encephalitis	California Encephalitis
Incidence	0–200/year, mostly infants and children	15/year	Rare in U.S.; mostly children	0–2000/year, mostly adults	50–100/year, mostly children
Time of year	Early or midsummer	Late summer, early fall	Summer	Mid- to late summer	July–September
Case-fatality	3–5% in children	50–70%, highest in children <15 years and adults >55 years	35% in children <10% in older persons	9% overall; 0% <20 years, 30% >65 years	<1%
Residual damage	33% in infants	30–50%, especially in children	Frequent in children	Frequent in elderly	Probably rare
Cerebrospinal fluid	<500 cells	500–2,000 cells PMNs*	<500 cells	<500 cells	<500 cells

*Polymorphonuclear leukocytes.

TREATMENT. As with most types of arboviral encephalitis, there is no specific therapy for WEE. Supportive care is essential and may reduce mortality. Control of high fever, convulsions, fluid and electrolyte imbalances, and airways is critical. Prevention and treatment of secondary bacterial infections, good pulmonary toilet, and care of urinary catheters also are essential. If clinical signs suggest cerebral edema or if the cerebrospinal fluid pressure is very high (>400 mm H_2O), measures to reduce brain swelling are indicated.

PREVENTION AND CONTROL. An experimental formalin-inactivated vaccine grown in chick embryo cell cultures has been used for protection of laboratory workers but is not indicated for others. In threatened or ongoing epidemics, residents should be advised to use protective clothing, insect repellents, and window screens and to restrict outdoor activity in the early morning, late afternoon, and evening (times of greatest mosquito activity). Public health measures include spray applications of insecticides aimed at the adult *C. tarsalis* vector.

EASTERN EQUINE ENCEPHALITIS (EEE)

ETIOLOGIC AGENT. EEE virus is a member of the Togaviridae family, alphavirus genus.

EPIDEMIOLOGY. *Incidence and Prevalence.* The disease in humans is relatively rare, with fewer than 15 cases occurring each year in the Gulf Coast and Atlantic states, usually associated with a predominantly equine epizootic involving 100 to 300 animals. Outbreaks usually occur during the late summer and early fall. The occurrence of equine cases or outbreaks of fatal encephalitis in penned exotic birds (pheasants, chukar partridges) precedes the appearance of human cases by several weeks or more. Epizootics of EEE have been reported in the Caribbean (Hispaniola) and South America.

Despite the small size of EEE epidemics, the severity is high. The case-fatality rate is 50 to 70 per cent. Incidence and mortality are highest in children under 15 and in persons over 55 years, with no sex predilection.

Transmission. In temperate areas, EEE virus circulates between wild birds and *Culiseta melanura* mosquitoes in freshwater swamp habitat. Equine epizootics and associated human cases result from extension of the transmission cycle to involve *Aedes* and *Coquillettidia* mosquitoes, which feed on horses and humans.

CLINICAL FEATURES AND PATHOLOGY. The disease is more acute and rapidly progressive than the other arboviral encephalitides. Onset is abrupt, with high fever, vomiting, and somnolence. Stupor, coma, myoclonus, and generalized convulsions appear within 24 to 48 hours. Autonomic disturbances (sialorrhea) may be prominent, and respiratory difficulty and cyanosis are frequent. In children, facial, periorbital, or generalized edema may be present. Death usually occurs during the first week; in surviving patients, recovery begins during the second week and may progress rapidly. Good functional recovery is associated with a long prodromal course and absence of coma. Residual damage, found in 30 to 50 per cent of the patients, is often severe, especially in children, and is characterized by retardation, spastic paralysis, and atrophy of brain substance.

A striking peripheral leukocytosis and shift to the left are frequent findings in patients with EEE. Examination of the cerebrospinal fluid reveals 500 to 2000 white cells (predominantly polymorphonuclear) per cubic millimeter. As the total cell count falls, polymorphonuclear cells persist as a significant fraction. Red blood cells may be present, the protein is elevated, and glucose is normal.

In contrast to St. Louis encephalitis and WEE, the brain is grossly edematous and congested, and the inflammatory response is predominantly polymorphonuclear. The areas most affected are basal ganglia, thalamus, hippocampus, and frontal and occipital cortex. Focal vasculitis, endothelial cell swelling, intravenous and arteriolar thrombus formation, demyelination, necrosis, neuronolysis, and neuronophagia are prominent.

SPECIFIC DIAGNOSIS. Isolation of virus from blood and spinal fluid is rarely successful. Serologic diagnosis by demonstration of a rise in antibody titer using appropriately timed paired sera is the most practical and available test. Because of the rapid course of the clinical disease, sera should be obtained at 2- to 3-day intervals during the acute phase of illness.

TREATMENT. Treatment is supportive (see previous discussion of WEE).

PREVENTION AND CONTROL. An experimental formalin-inactivated chick embryo cell culture vaccine is used to protect laboratory and field workers. Reduction of mosquito populations by appropriate use of insecticides may be effective in threatened or established outbreaks.

VENEZUELAN EQUINE ENCEPHALITIS (VEE)

ETIOLOGY. The causative agent of VEE is a member of the Togaviridae family, alphavirus genus. Six antigenic subtypes (I to VI) and multiple antigenic variants of subtypes I and III are recognized by serologic tests. Subtypes IAB and IC are responsible for epidemics involving humans and equines. In Florida, subtype II is enzootic and produces sporadic human disease.

EPIDEMIOLOGY. *Incidence and Prevalence.* Prior to 1973, large equine epizootics occurred at 5- to 10-year intervals in Venezuela, Columbia, Ecuador, and Peru, involving many thousands of animals and incurring mortality rates as high as 40 per cent. Associated human morbidity also was great (up to 32,000 clinical cases). No outbreaks of equine or human disease have been recognized in over 12 years.

The predominant syndrome is a self-limited influenza-like illness; only about 4 per cent of infected persons, principally children under 15 years, develop encephalitis. Subclinical infections are rare. The case-fatality rate in children up to 5 years old with encephalitis is approximately 35 per cent, but in older persons it is less than 10 per cent. Laboratory infections are common in unvaccinated persons working with the virus or infected animals.

Transmission. A large variety of mosquito vectors, including species of the genera *Aedes*, *Psorophora*, and *Mansonia*, transmit subtypes IAB and IC during epizootic epidemics. Equines are the principal viremic hosts. Virus may be present in pharyngeal excretions of human patients; contact or aerosol person-to-person spread, although possible, is not epidemiologically important.

The other members of the VEE viral complex, including subtype II in Florida, have enzootic transmission cycles involving *Culex* (*Melanoconion*) species mosquitoes and small forest rodents and marsupials. Equines are not involved in transmission. Human disease is sporadic and relatively uncommon.

CLINICAL FEATURES AND PATHOLOGY. After an incubation period of 2 to 5 days, there is sudden onset of fever, chills, malaise, and headache, followed by myalgias, nausea, vomiting, and occasionally diarrhea. Physical examination reveals fever, tachycardia, conjunctival injection, and, in some cases, nonexudative pharyngitis. The acute illness generally subsides in 4 to 6 days, and convalescent symptoms may last up to 3 weeks. A biphasic course has sometimes been noted; acute symptoms reappear after a brief remission, within a week after the initial onset.

Some patients exhibit evidence of mild central nervous system involvement (photophobia, somnolence, confusion) during the typical influenza-like illness. When it occurs, severe encephalitis is characterized by meningeal signs, convulsions, tremor, stupor, coma, spastic paralysis, abnormal reflexes, cranial nerve palsies, and central respiratory failure. Residual neurologic damage occurs in severe cases. Infections of pregnant women acquired during the first and second trimesters may result in fetal encephalitis and death.

The peripheral leukocyte count is often low, with decrease in both lymphocytes and neutrophils, or normal, with a relative lymphopenia. In patients with central nervous system signs, the cerebrospinal fluid contains up to 500 cells, predominantly lymphocytes, per cubic millimeter. The serum lactic dehydrogenase and glutamic-oxaloacetic transaminase levels may be elevated.

Pathologic changes in the central nervous system include edema, congestion, meningeal and perivascular inflammation, intracerebral hemorrhages, neuronal degeneration, and vasculitis. In addition, hepatocellular degeneration and necrosis, widespread lymphoid depletion and follicular necrosis, and interstitial pneumonitis are frequent findings. In the congenitally infected fetus, there are massive and widespread necrosis of brain tissue, hemorrhages, and resorption of brain material, resulting in hydranencephaly.

DIAGNOSIS. In contrast to the other arthropod-borne encephalitides, VEE virus can be isolated from the blood or from throat swabs or washings during the first 3 or 4 days of illness. Serodiagnosis is usually more practical and is achieved by testing appropriately timed paired sera by HI, CF, ELISA, neutralization, or IgM immunoassay.

TREATMENT. No specific therapy is available, and treatment of encephalitis cases is supportive (see WEE discussion).

PREVENTION AND CONTROL. An experimental live attenuated vaccine made from subtype IAB is used for adult laboratory personnel. It provides solid immunity to subtype IAB and its closest relative (IC) but incomplete protection against infection with other heterologous VEE viruses. Epidemics and epizootics can be prevented by effective vaccination of equines. Spraying insecticides to reduce adult (infective) mosquito populations is the only means of immediate control in the face of an ongoing epidemic. Individual protection against mosquitoes also is advised (see WEE discussion).

ST. LOUIS ENCEPHALITIS (SLE)

ETIOLOGY. St. Louis encephalitis virus, a member of the family Flaviviridae, shares close antigenic relationships with Japanese encephalitis, Murray Valley encephalitis, and West Nile viruses and is related to yellow fever and dengue viruses. Strains associated with *Culex pipiens*–borne epidemics in the eastern United States are distinct from endemic strains transmitted by *C. tarsalis* in the western states.

EPIDEMIOLOGY. Incidence and Prevalence. The virus is present in all parts of the western hemisphere, but epidemics occur only in North America and some Caribbean islands. During epidemic years, the virus has been responsible for up to 80 per cent of all reported cases of encephalitis of known etiology in the United States. In recent years, epidemics of up to 2000 cases have taken place, mainly in urban-suburban localities of the Ohio-Mississippi River basin, in eastern and central Texas, and in Florida. Small outbreaks also have occurred in the western United States. Epidemics usually occur between July and September but may arise later in the year in warm areas such as Florida. Prior exposure and immunity to dengue may provide a degree of cross-protection against clinical SLE.

The overall case-fatality rate is approximately 9 per cent. Mortality is negligible in persons under 20 years but rises steeply after age 55 to approximately 30 per cent in patients over 65 years of age. The ratio of inapparent to apparent infection is 800:1 in children up to 9 years, 400:1 in persons 10 to 49 years, and 85:1 in persons over 60 years.

Transmission. In most of the eastern United States, SLE virus circulates between wild birds and *C. pipiens* mosquitoes, which breed in polluted water. In Florida and in parts of the Caribbean, *C. nigripalpus* is the principal vector. The cycle in the western United States also involves wild birds, but the vector is *C. tarsalis*, the vector of WEE. Because of the similar ecology of SLE and WEE viruses in the west, mixed outbreaks occur, mostly in rural, agricultural areas.

Above-average summer temperatures and conditions such as deficient rainfall, which create stagnant pools suitable for *C. pipiens* breeding, are associated with epidemics in the eastern United States. SLE in the western states is favored by warm spring temperatures, heavy snow melt, and flooding (see WEE).

CLINICAL FEATURES AND PATHOLOGY. Three clinical syndromes are recognized: febrile headache, aseptic meningitis, and encephalitis. After an incubation period of 4 to 21 days, a variable period of nonspecific symptoms occurs, including fever (38 to 41°C), headache, malaise, drowsiness, myalgias, and sore throat. This may be followed by the acute or subacute onset of meningeal or encephalitic signs or both. Nausea, vomiting, and photophobia are common. Neurologic abnormalities occur in up to 25 per cent of patients. Extrapyramidal abnormalities (tremor of tongue, face, and limbs) and an altered state of consciousness are the most significant findings. Others include altered sensorium, meningismus, cranial nerve deficits (particularly of cranial nerve VII), abnormal reflexes, tremors, myoclonic twitching, nystagmus, and ataxia. Motor abnormalities are infrequent and sensory changes extremely uncommon. Convulsions occur in 10 per cent of patients and are a poor prognostic sign, as is a

persistent high temperature of 40 to 41°C. Signs of markedly increased intracranial pressure are very unusual. Guillain-Barré syndrome has occasionally been associated with SLE, both as an acute presentation and during the convalescent period. Approximately half of the patients with fatal outcome succumb during the first week and 80 per cent within 2 weeks after onset.

In uncomplicated cases of SLE, there is a moderate peripheral neutrophilic leukocytosis and shift to the left. Cerebrospinal fluid pressure is elevated, protein mildly elevated, and sugar normal. Pleocytosis up to 500 cells per cubic millimeter is present. Polymorphonuclear cells predominate early, the change to lymphocytes occurring within several days. Serum creatinine phosphokinase, glutamic-oxaloacetic transaminase, and serum aldolase are frequently elevated. The electroencephalogram typically shows amorphous δ-wave activity and diffuse generalized slowing most prominently in the frontal and temporal regions, but brain scans are normal. Inappropriate secretion of antidiuretic hormone is present in one third of patients.

Genitourinary tract symptoms (urgency, frequency, incontinence, and retention), microscopic hematuria, pyuria, and proteinuria, and elevated blood urea nitrogen are frequent. SLE viral antigen in cells of the urinary sediment has been detected by fluorescent techniques and virus-like particles in urine by immunoelectronmicroscopy.

A convalescent syndrome, characterized by weakness, fatigue, nervousness, tremulousness, sleeplessness, irritability, depression, difficulty in concentrating, and headaches, occurs in 30 to 50 per cent of older persons and clears in 80 per cent of these within 3 years.

Pathologic changes in fatal cases are limited to microscopic findings. Leptomeningitis is characterized by lymphocytic inflammation. Parenchymal changes consist of lymphocytic perivascular cuffing, cellular nodule formation, and neuronal degeneration. Changes are most pronounced in substantia nigra, thalamus and hypothalamus, cerebellar cortex, cerebral cortex, and basal ganglia.

DIAGNOSIS. SLE virus is rarely isolated from blood or spinal fluid obtained during the acute phase of illness. Serologic diagnosis is achieved by demonstration of changing antibody titers; the HI, fluorescent, ELISA, and neutralizing tests demonstrate antibody within the first week after onset, and titers rise during the ensuing 2 weeks. CF antibodies appear 10 to 20 days after onset. Rapid, early diagnosis is possible by detection of IgM antibodies by ELISA in serum and cerebrospinal fluid. Serologic cross-reactions may occur in persons with prior exposures to dengue and other related flaviviruses.

TREATMENT. Treatment is supportive (see WEE).

PREVENTION AND CONTROL. No vaccine is available for SLE. Surveillance of viral activity in vectors and avian hosts is used to define the risk of human infection and initiate vector control efforts. In an established outbreak, avoidance of mosquito bites and spraying to reduce infected adult mosquitoes are the only effective means of control (see WEE discussion).

CALIFORNIA ENCEPHALITIS

ETIOLOGY. At least four members of the California serogroup of the Bunyaviridae family (*Bunyavirus* genus)—LaCrosse, California encephalitis, Jamestown Canyon, and snowshoe hare virus—cause encephalitis. California encephalitis virus occurs in the western United States (California, New Mexico, Utah, Texas) and has been implicated in only three human cases. In contrast, LaCrosse virus, distributed more widely in the eastern half of the United States and southern Canada, is a major human pathogen. Recently, Jamestown Canyon and snowshoe hare viruses have been implicated in sporadic human encephalitis cases in the northern central United States and Canada. California serogroup viruses have been implicated in human disease in the People's Republic of China and the U.S.S.R.

EPIDEMIOLOGY. Incidence and Prevalence. California encephalitis occurs as an endemic rather than an epidemic disease, with individual or small clusters of cases scattered across the affected areas. An average of 80 cases are reported each year, generally occurring between July and September with peak incidence in August. The virus primarily affects persons less than 15 years of age living in rural and suburban areas characterized by deciduous hardwood forests. It is most prevalent in the northern central states, where it is responsible for as many as 20 per cent of cases of acute central nervous system infection in children. Focal "hot spots" (communities, even backyards) of recurrent summertime viral activity are recognized. The case-fatality rate is less than 1 per cent. The ratio of inapparent to apparent infection has been estimated variably at between 26:1 and 157:1.

Transmission. The vector of LaCrosse virus is *Aedes triseriatus*, which breeds both in forest tree-holes and in peridomestic artificial containers. The vector also serves as a reservoir of LaCrosse virus. Wild rodents (squirrels, chipmunks) contribute to a cycle of transmission as viremic hosts. Humans acquire the disease through the bite of an infected mosquito.

Aedes communis, A. stimulans, A. triseriatus, and possibly anopheline mosquitoes are involved in transmission of Jamestown Canyon virus, and deer are the principal vertebrate hosts.

CLINICAL FEATURES. The clinical spectrum of California virus infection includes nonspecific febrile illness, aseptic meningitis, and meningoencephalitis. The disease begins with fever, headache, sore throat, and gastrointestinal symptoms, with appearance of the neurologic disorder within 1 to 3 days. In mild cases, central nervous system signs appear on the third day after onset and subside within 7 to 8 days. In the more severe form, neurologic signs appear within 24 to 48 hours of onset, usually in the form of generalized seizures and altered consciousness, and are more prolonged. Papilledema or abnormal optic disc margins have been noted. Encephalitis may be quite severe in the acute stage, but the disease is almost always self-limited and death is extremely uncommon. The question of permanent sequelae is unsettled. Many researchers believe LaCrosse virus infection is responsible for residual psychologic problems, emotional lability, hyperkinesis, infantilism, compulsive behavior, and auditory and visual perceptual problems. There are case reports of hemiparesis and persistent seizure disorders.

The peripheral white cell count is elevated, with a predominance of polymorphonuclear cells and a shift to the left. The cerebrospinal fluid contains up to 500 lymphocytes per cubic millimeter, normal or mildly elevated protein, and normal glucose concentrations. The electroencephalogram reveals generalized slowing in the δ and θ range, indicating diffuse cortical dysfunction. Focal δ-wave activity related to cortical destruction or focal seizures is also a common finding.

Histopathologic features in the central nervous system are qualitatively similar to those of other viral encephalitides; however, absence of inflammatory lesions in cerebellum, medulla, and spinal cord has been postulated to be a distinguishing feature of LaCrosse infection.

DIAGNOSIS. The virus cannot be recovered from blood or spinal fluid obtained during the acute phase. Diagnosis is best achieved by tests for antibody in paired acute and convalescent sera using counterimmunoelectrophoresis, HI, CF, fluorescent, ELISA, and neutralization tests. The most practical, sensitive, and reliable methods are the HI test using the LaCrosse viral antigen and IgM antibody-capture ELISA.

TREATMENT. Treatment is supportive (see WEE).

PREVENTION AND CONTROL. There is no vaccine for California encephalitis. Vector-control methods are of uncertain usefulness in this disease. In defined "hot spots" of recurrent viral activity, efforts to eliminate breeding sites for *A. triseriatus* should be made. Parents should protect children by limiting exposure and using mosquito repellents (see WEE).

JAPANESE ENCEPHALITIS (JE)

ETIOLOGY AND EPIDEMIOLOGY. Incidence and Prevalence. Japanese encephalitis virus is a member of the Flaviviridae family. It causes epizootics of clinical encephalitis in equines. The disease occurs throughout Asia, including Japan, the Korean peninsula, Taiwan, People's Republic of China, Okinawa, Vietnam, the Philippines, Burma, Malaysia, Bangladesh, east and south India, Sri Lanka, Thailand, and Indonesia. Over 30,000 cases occur annually. JE is a summertime disease in temperate areas but occurs sporadically year-round in the tropics. Epidemics have been most frequent at the northern fringe of the tropical zone. JE is predominantly a rural disease, and the incidence in males is often higher than in females. In hyperendemic areas, over 70 per cent of adult populations surveyed have antibodies,

and children under 15 years old principally are affected by the disease. In areas without a high prevalence of background immunity (e.g., northern India), however, all age groups are affected. In Japan, where school children have been protected by vaccination campaigns targeted at this age group, occurrence of encephalitis in the elderly has become prominent. The ratio of inapparent to apparent infection is over 500:1 in children and decreases with age; in Korea, the ratio among American servicemen was estimated at 25:1. The case-fatality rate probably is about 25 per cent, but rates of 50 per cent or more have been reported, which may reflect underrecognition of nonfatal cases.

Transmission. The natural cycle involves *Culex* mosquito vectors and wild birds and swine. Humans and equines are incidental hosts.

CLINICAL FEATURES AND PATHOLOGY. Manifestations of JE include febrile headache, aseptic meningitis, and meningoencephalitis. Onset is abrupt, with fever, headache, and gastrointestinal symptoms. Meningeal irritation develops within 24 hours and is followed on the second or third day by the appearance of irritability, impaired consciousness, convulsions (especially in children), muscular rigidity, masklike facies, ataxia, coarse tremor, involuntary movements, cranial nerve deficits, paresis, hyperactive deep tendon reflexes, and pathologic reflexes. Weight loss and dehydration are often striking findings. In mild cases, fever subsides after the first week and neurologic signs resolve by the end of the second week after onset. In severe cases, hyperpyrexia, progressive neurologic dysfunction, and coma result in death, usually between the seventh and tenth days. About 25 per cent of patients undergo a prolonged recovery, often leaving permanent sequelae. Cardiorespiratory complications are frequent during the acute stage in these patients. A poor prognosis is associated with protracted high fever, frequent or prolonged seizures, high protein content in the cerebrospinal fluid, Babinski signs, and early appearance of respiratory depression. Fetal death and abortion due to transplacental JE infection have been reported.

The occurrence of sequelae correlates with severity of the acute stage of illness. Young children are most susceptible, and sequelae such as mental impairment, emotional lability, choreoathetosis, tremor, parkinsonism, autonomic disturbances, motor paralysis, and pathopsychologic syndromes (including schizophrenia) have been reported in up to 75 per cent of patients.

A moderate peripheral leukocytosis and neutrophilia occur early in the disease. Cerebrospinal fluid pleocytosis, protein elevation, and normal glucose are usual findings.

Neuropathologic changes and distribution of lesions are similar to those described for St. Louis encephalitis (see earlier discussion of SLE).

DIAGNOSIS. Isolation of JE virus from blood is uncommon; virus may be recovered from cerebrospinal fluid of about one third of patients who progress to a fatal outcome, but rarely from patients who live. HI and neutralizing antibodies appear during the first and CF antibodies during the second week after onset. Cross-reactions with other flaviviruses make serodiagnosis difficult. Specific IgM antibodies in serum or cerebrospinal fluid are detectable by immunoassays in over three fourths of patients at the time of hospital admission.

TREATMENT. Treatment is supportive (see WEE). Uncontrolled trials of intrathecal interferon suggest a beneficial effect but require confirmation.

PREVENTION AND CONTROL. Inactivated, partially purified mouse brain vaccines produced in Japan are safe and effective in preschool- and school-age children. Although not yet licensed for use in the United States, a vaccine produced in Japan is available on a limited scale to United States citizens traveling to high-risk areas. Information should be sought from state health departments or the Centers for Disease Control. Since three doses of the inactivated vaccine are used, and approximately 1 month is required to confer protection, vaccination is not a practical measure in the face of an ongoing epidemic. Live attenuated vaccines are under study in China. Reduction of vector mosquito populations by application of insecticides may help to abort outbreaks (see WEE). Immunization of swine is an ancillary control strategy.

MURRAY VALLEY ENCEPHALITIS AND ROCIO ENCEPHALITIS

Murray Valley encephalitis and Rocio encephalitis are similar to Japanese encephalitis in pathogenesis and clinical features and are caused by closely related flaviviruses. Murray Valley encephalitis has occurred in small epidemics in the Murray and Darling River valleys of Victoria and New South Wales, Australia. The virus is endemic in northern Australia and New Guinea, where it is maintained in a bird-mosquito cycle. Rocio encephalitis has caused epidemics of 1000 cases in São Paulo State, Brazil.

TICK-BORNE ENCEPHALITIS (TBE)

ETIOLOGIC AGENTS. A complex of six antigenically related tick-borne flaviviruses cause encephalitis: Powassan, tick-borne encephalitis, louping ill, Kyasanur Forest disease (KFD), Omsk hemorrhagic fever (OHF), and Langat viruses. The predominant syndrome in KFD and OHF is hemorrhagic fever (see Ch. 393), but meningoencephalitis may be a component of the disease spectrum. Two subtypes of TBE virus (Central European encephalitis and Russian spring-summer encephalitis) are distinguished by special serologic tests, are ecologically distinct, and differ in virulence for humans. Powassan and louping ill viruses are rare causes of encephalitis in North America and the British Isles, respectively. These viruses are serologically easily distinguished from mosquito-borne flaviviruses but induce cross-reactions within the complex.

Tick-borne Encephalitis (TBE). TBE occurs in Europe (including European Russia), southern Scandinavia, and the far eastern U.S.S.R. during summer months, corresponding to peak tick vector populations. Several hundred to 2000 cases are reported annually, with morbidity rates of up to 20 per 100,000 inhabitants. Inapparent infections are common. Adults over 20 years are mainly affected, and persons frequenting wooded areas that are heavily tick infested are at highest risk. In Europe, the disease is relatively mild (case-fatality rate 1 to 2 per cent), but in the Far East, it is severe (20 to 25 per cent).

In Europe, the vector of TBE is *Ixodes ricinus*, and in the Far East, *I. persulcatus*. The tick vector also serves as a reservoir of the virus. Larval ticks parasitize small rodents, which serve as amplifying viremic hosts during the spring and summer. Large vertebrates (goats, sheep, cattle) are hosts for nymphal and adult ticks. Outbreaks have occurred in families or groups of individuals ingesting unpasteurized milk or cheese from goats or sheep.

TBE in Europe typically (but not invariably) has a diphasic course, beginning 7 to 14 days after exposure with an influenza-like illness lasting 1 week, followed by a period of clinical remission for several days, and then abrupt onset of aseptic meningitis or meningoencephalitis. The latter is usually benign, although severe paralytic illness, myelitis, myeloradiculitis, and bulbar forms may occur. Convalescence is often prolonged, and residual paralysis may follow in severe cases. In the Far East, TBE begins suddenly with fever, headache, and gastrointestinal symptoms, followed rapidly by appearance of depressed sensorium, coma, convulsions, and paralysis. Bulbar paralysis and cervical myelitis are frequent findings. In fatal cases, death occurs in the first week after onset. Survivors have a high incidence of residual paralyses, especially lower motor neuron paralysis of upper extremities or shoulder girdle. Aseptic meningitis and milder forms of encephalitis also occur. Chronic forms of TBE have been described, with active clinical and pathologic abnormalities a year or more after onset.

In TBE, virus isolation from blood is also possible during the early phase of illness. Serologic diagnosis is achieved by the HI, CF, N, or ELISA techniques.

Treatment is supportive (see WEE).

In eastern Europe and the U.S.S.R., TBE vaccines are used in high-risk groups (forestry and agricultural workers, military personnel). In Austria, immunization of the general population has resulted in a marked decline in incidence. Avoidance of tick exposure by use of protective clothing and repellents may be recommended in areas of high TBE activity.

Louping ill Encephalitis. Louping ill causes encephalitis in sheep (rarely in cattle, horses, and swine) in Scotland and in northern England and Ireland. Sporadic human cases have been recognized. Louping ill virus is maintained in nature by *I. ricinus* ticks and a variety of hosts, including small mammals, ground-dwelling birds (grouse), and probably sheep. The clinical features of louping ill resemble the European form of TBE.

Powassan Virus Encephalitis. Powassan virus encephalitis has been documented in a total of 15 cases in the northeastern United States and eastern Canada, with a case-fatality rate of 50 per cent. The virus is not associated with animal disease. The transmission cycle of Powassan virus involves *I. cookei*, *I. marxi* (and possibly other tick species), and mammals, particularly rodents and carnivores. Powassan encephalitis is characterized by fever and nonspecific symptoms, followed by encephalitic signs, which are frequently severe. Residual paralysis may occur. Peripheral blood and cerebrospinal fluid changes are similar to those described in other forms of flaviviral encephalitis.

Calisher CH, Thompson WH (eds.): California Serogroup Viruses. New York, Alan R. Liss, Inc., 1983. *Symposium covering all aspects of this virus group.*

Day JF, Curtis GA, Edman JD: Rainfall-directed oviposition behavior of *Culex nigripalpus* (Diptera: Culicindae) and its influence on St. Louis encephalitis virus transmission in Indian River County, Florida. J Med Entomol 27(1):43–50, 1990. *Correlation between rainfall patterns and transmission of SLE virus by infected mosquitoes in the field.*

Hardy JL, Winkelstein W Jr, Milby MM (eds.): Symposium: The epidemiology of mosquito-borne virus encephalitis in the United States, 1943–1987. Am J Trop Med Hyg 37:1S–100S, 1987. *A thorough discussion of mosquito-borne viral encephalitis.*

Hoke CH, Nisalak A, Sangawhipa N, et al.: Protection against Japanese encephalitis by inactivated vaccines. N Engl J Med 319(10):608–614, 1988. *Report of protective efficacy of Japanese encephalitis vaccines. This study and the accompanying editorial (see Monath) raise the question of the advisability of widespread vaccination in Asia as well as vaccination of travelers to Asia.*

Holmgren EB, Forsgren M: Epidemiology of tick-borne encephalitis in Sweden 1956–1989: A study of 1116 cases. Scand J Infect Dis 22(3):287–295, 1990. *A recent description of epidemiologic and clinical factors of tick-borne encephalitis.*

Matthews CG, Chun RWM, Grabow JD, et al.: Psychological sequelae in children following California arbovirus encephalitis. Neurology 18:1023, 1968. *Useful to the physician facing questions from patients about sequelae in children recovering from this infection.*

Monath TP: Japanese encephalitis—a plague of the Orient (editorial). N Engl J Med 319(10):641–643, 1988. *See comment under Hoke.*

Monath TP (ed.): The Arboviruses: Epidemiology and Ecology. Boca Raton, CRC Press, 1988. *An up-to-date source of critical information.*

Monath TP (ed.): Saint Louis Encephalitis. Washington, D.C., American Public Health Association, 1980. *Encyclopedic coverage of all aspects of St. Louis encephalitis, including clinical features and differential and definitive laboratory diagnosis. Contains references to all previously published studies.*

Przelomski MM, O'Rourke E, Grady GF, et al.: Eastern equine encephalitis in Massachusetts. Neurology 38:736–739, 1988. *Review of 16 cases of EEE in Massachusetts showing increased frequency in older persons.*

Rosato RR, Mancasaet FF, Jahrling PB: Enzyme-linked immunosorbent assay detection of immunoglobulins G and M to Venezuelan equine encephalomyelitis virus in vaccinated and naturally infected humans. J Clin Microbiol 26(3):421–425, 1988. *Use of ELISA to detect antibody to VEE induced by injection or vaccination.*

Schlesinger S, Schlesinger MJ (eds.): The Togaviridae and Flaviviridae. New York, Plenum Publishing, 1986. *An authoritative source of epidemiologic and virologic information.*

Viral Hemorrhagic Fevers

Robert E. Shope

390 Introduction

The viral hemorrhagic fevers encompass syndromes that vary from febrile hemorrhagic disease with capillary fragility to acute severe shock leading rapidly to death. The causative agents include arthropod-borne and rodent-borne viruses. The rodent-borne viruses do not require an arthropod vector but are transmitted directly to vertebrates by aerosol spread or contact with infected excreta or body secretions of the rodent. The reservoir and natural mode of transmission for the African hemorrhagic fever viruses, Marburg and Ebola, are not known.

There are at least 15 viruses that cause human hemorrhagic fevers (see Table 382–1). They are in the families Flaviviridae, Bunyaviridae, Arenaviridae, and Filoviridae. All contain RNA, and all are zoonoses.

The hemorrhagic fevers form a special group of diseases characterized by viral replication in lymphoid cells, followed by fever and myalgia and leading to hemorrhagic manifestations and hypovolemic shock. The basic physiologic defect in most is capillary leakage. In some, such as yellow fever, hepatocellular damage is prominent. In others, such as hemorrhagic fever with renal syndrome, renal lesions are striking. The mortality rates may be high, and the pathogenesis is poorly understood. Disseminated intravascular coagulopathy (DIC) is a feature in some cases, but probably not all. Antigen-antibody complexes may lead to release of mediators of shock in some cases, and direct effects of viral replication on capillary permeability in some have not been ruled out. It is important to understand the pathogenetic mechanism in order to manage the patient, but our knowledge is sparse at present.

Control can be achieved by interrupting the cycle, including peridomestic rodent control (Bolivian hemorrhagic fever), and, in those that are arboviruses, by vaccination of reservoir animals (Rift Valley fever), vector control, and education on methods to avoid the vector (dengue). Vaccines are available or under development for some of the agents such as Rift Valley fever, yellow fever, dengue, and Junin viruses. For others such as Lassa virus, we now have an antiviral drug, and for still another (Junin) pre-exposure and postexposure protection is afforded by human immune plasma.

391 Yellow Fever

DEFINITION. Yellow fever is an acute viral disease caused by infection with yellow fever virus. The disease is exemplary of the viral hemorrhagic fevers described in the following sections (Table 391–1). The infection is often subclinical but may lead to disease whose severity varies from mild and self-limited to a fulminant fatal outcome. Classic yellow fever is characterized by sudden onset, moderately high fever, nausea, bradycardia, prostration, vomiting of altered blood, jaundice, oliguria, and albuminuria. Natural cycles of the infection occur periodically in mosquitoes and primates of tropical South America as far north as Panama and in tropical west, central, and east Africa.

ETIOLOGY. Yellow fever virus is in the genus *Flavivirus* of the family Flaviviridae. Members of the family are single-stranded, negative-sense RNA viruses, spherical and approximately 40 nm in diameter. Particles form in the cytoplasm in close association with endoplasmic reticulum. They contain a lipid envelope and replicate in both arthropod and vertebrate cells. Other members of the Flaviviridae, including dengue, West Nile, and St. Louis encephalitis, cross-react with yellow fever virus in serologic tests and may confound the diagnosis. Minor antigenic differences exist between strains of yellow fever virus from Africa and South America, and among strains from different regions of Africa; however, the 17D yellow fever vaccine protects against all strains. The virus can be isolated in mosquitoes, arthropod and vertebrate tissue cultures, baby mice, and several monkey species. Rhesus monkeys regularly succumb following experimental inoculation and mimic severe human disease.

EPIDEMIOLOGY. Two epidemiologic types of yellow fever are distinguished: the urban and the sylvan (jungle) forms. Urban yellow fever is transmitted by *Aedes aegypti* mosquitoes from person to person, whereas sylvan yellow fever is maintained in a forest cycle of monkeys and forest-canopy mosquitoes; humans are infected when they enter the forest. The two types do not differ clinically.

A. aegypti is a peridomestic mosquito that breeds in abandoned tires, jars, cans, water storage containers, roof catchments, and drains in and around houses. Urban yellow fever was a major killer until the early 1900's, when mosquito control in Havana, Rio de Janeiro, Guayaquil, and the other large urban centers eliminated the disease. The last recorded urban case in the Americas was in Trinidad in 1954. *A. aegypti* continues to be prevalent in African cities, and *A. aegypti*–transmitted outbreaks still occur there. Major epidemics were recorded in Ethiopia, 1960–1962; Nigeria, 1969; Senegal, 1965 and 1979; Gambia, 1978; and Ghana and Burkina Faso, 1983. In 1986, an epidemic involving at least 3000 persons occurred in Nigeria, in Benue and Cross River States, and extended into Oyo and Niger States in 1987. An estimated 39,000 cases, with 8400 deaths, were recorded.

Yellow fever virus in Africa is transmitted by *A. aegypti* not only in the cities but also in semirural areas. In addition, some African epidemics are maintained by other *Aedes* species, such as *simpsoni* and the tree hole–breeding *africanus*, *leuteocephalus*, and *furcifer-taylori*, which transmit the virus in savannah and the transition forest-savannah zones of west Africa.

Sylvan yellow fever was recognized initially in Brazil in 1932. After urban yellow fever had been controlled in the Americas, sporadic cases continued to occur in persons exposed to mosquitoes in the jungles of South America and Africa. This sylvan form is maintained in tropical America by *Haemagogus* mosquitoes and forest primates, and sometimes by other sylvan animals. Evidence favors the hypothesis that the virus moves through the forest, cycling in one place until the monkeys are immune, then dying out and moving to areas where there are susceptible monkeys. People entering the forest are at risk. Sylvan yellow fever extends periodically outside the enzootic zone into forests such as those in Panama and Central America. The virus can be maintained over dry periods by transovarial transmission in mosquitoes, although it remains to be shown whether maintenance in mosquito eggs is more than a temporary mechanism.

The sylvan cycle in Africa is more complicated than in the Americas; in tropical Africa the virus cycles between *A. africanus* and monkeys. Another African mosquito, *A. simpsoni*, which feeds on both humans and monkeys, serves in some areas as a link between primates in the deep forest and people in the African villages.

A. aegypti was once carried on sailing ships between tropical ports and into temperate-zone cities. Modern ocean-going ships no longer harbor mosquito breeding sites, but the mosquito continues to travel by small boats, airplanes, cars, and especially in the form of dried eggs transported by used tires. Cities such as Rio de Janeiro, which were once freed of the mosquito, are now reinfested. Dengue fever reappeared there in 1986. To control the mosquito again in this area will be difficult because of insecticide resistance and the high price of labor and materials. Jungle yellow fever continues to cycle, reappearing in the same locale every 5 to 40 years. The scene is thus set again for emergence of the virus from the jungle to reinitiate the urban cycle in the Americas.

A. aegypti is easily identified. It has white thoracic scales in the shape of a lyre and black legs with white bands. Mosquitoes that have fed on a viremic vertebrate become infective after an extrinsic incubation period of 9 to 30 days, the shorter periods correlating with higher ambient temperatures. This extrinsic incubation period in the mosquito accounts for the delay from the first human infection in an urban outbreak to subsequent clusters of infection.

Yellow fever is not found in Asia, although large areas harbor A. aegypti that are capable of transmitting the virus, should it be introduced. India and other Asian nations require vaccination of travelers from yellow fever–endemic regions.

All age groups and races are susceptible. However, sylvan yellow fever is found almost always in young males because they are the individuals who venture into the forest. Immunity following vaccination or infection is long-lasting. During an epidemic, the population at risk, therefore, may be limited to age groups not covered by prior immunization or those born since a prior outbreak. There is also some evidence that persons may be protected by antibody to heterologous flaviviruses.

During the 24-year period from 1965 to 1988, there were 3324 cases of yellow fever reported in the Americas, and 7701 in Africa. The numbers of cases are greatly underestimated, probably by a factor of at least 10. Case-fatality rates are usually about 20 per cent but are higher in some epidemics. Ratios of apparent to inapparent infection, estimated at 1:10, may vary greatly.

PATHOLOGY AND PATHOGENESIS. The lesions of yellow fever involve primarily the liver, heart, kidneys, and lymphoid tissues. Grossly, the skin is icteric, and there may be multiple hemorrhages or petechiae of the skin, mucous membranes, and multiple organs. The liver is normal in size, icteric, and fatty. The heart is soft and flabby, and the kidneys are swollen and a pink-gray color. Small peritoneal and pleural effusions are sometimes observed.

Histology is often characteristic in patients who die before the ninth day of illness, but the lesions are not always pathognomonic. The most striking lesion is the eosinophilic degeneration and coagulation of hepatocytes (Councilman's bodies). Hepatocyte destruction is most marked in the midzone of the lobule, with relative sparing of the central vein and portal areas. Intranuclear eosinophilic granular inclusions or enlarged nucleoli (Torre's bodies) are also described. Both microvacuolar- and multivacuolar fatty changes are prominent, especially after the first week of illness. Inflammation is uncommon, and the reticulum framework is unaffected, probably accounting for the absence of postnecrotic fibrosis in convalescence and the regeneration of hepatocytes in recovered cases. The kidneys show cloudy swelling of tubular epithelium leading to acute tubular necrosis. The glomeruli are not obviously affected, but special stains indicate Schiff-positive

alterations in the basal membranes, and proteinaceous material accumulates in the capsular spaces and lumina of the proximal tubules. The myocardium is characterized by granular or fatty infiltration of muscle fibers and of the atrioventricular (AV) conduction system and cloudy swelling and degeneration of myocytes without inflammation. Large monocytes replace lymphocytic cells in the splenic follicles and lymph nodes. Encephalitis is rare, although petechial hemorrhage in the brain stem and cerebral edema are observed.

Knowledge of the pathogenesis of yellow fever is sparse. Yellow fever cases occur in remote areas, and pathophysiologic studies of yellow fever patients are usually done with only rudimentary laboratory facilities. The virus replicates in the hepatocytes and myocytes, and it is presumed that lesions in these target cells are a direct effect of the virus. Jaundice and prolonged prothrombin time can be explained by hepatocellular damage; bradycardia and arrhythmias, by myocyte and AV node perturbation. The etiology of renal tubular necrosis is not clear, but it may be secondary to hepatic changes. Some, but not all, fatal cases are associated with thrombocytopenia; increased prothrombin, partial thromboplastin, and thrombin times; diminished factor VIII and fibrinogen; and the presence of fibrin split products. The bleeding in these cases may be secondary to disseminated intravascular coagulopathy, but this is not generally accepted by all investigators. Hypoglycemia, metabolic acidosis, and hyperkalemia characterize the terminal stage and are probably the result of multiple organ system failure.

CLINICAL MANIFESTATIONS. Severe yellow fever is a fulminant febrile illness with 50 per cent or greater mortality. There is a great deal of variation, however; most cases are mild with a better prognosis, and only about 10 to 20 per cent are in the severe category. The intrinsic incubation period is 3 to 6 days, exceptionally as long as 10 days.

The clinical syndrome is classified as very mild, mild, moderately severe, or malignant. Patients with very mild cases have fever and headache, and the patient recovers in 48 hours or less. Those with mild cases have sudden fever and headache with nausea, sometimes bleeding of the gums or epistaxis, bradycardia, or albuminuria. The patient recovers in 2 or 3 days. Those with moderately severe cases have more marked manifestations of bleeding, definite bradycardia in relation to the fever, nausea and vomiting, jaundice, and striking albuminuria. The illness may be aborted after 3 to 4 days or may develop serious hemorrhagic manifestations, such as black vomit, melena, and metrorrhagia. Moderately severe yellow fever may last 1 week or even longer.

Classic yellow fever is characterized as malignant and is divided into three periods. The period of infection involves sudden onset of fever and headache, with initial rapid pulse, but by day 2, the pulse slows in spite of continued fever (Faget's sign). Headache, back, and muscle pain may be severe, blood oozes from the gums, and other signs of bleeding become prominent. The face is flushed, the tongue is reddened (strawberry tongue), and the conjunctivae are injected; the patient is irritable, unable to sleep, and frequently constipated. The temperature is often 40°C or higher. On the third day of illness, there is nausea, vomiting of coffee-ground material, and notable albuminuria. The bleeding

TABLE 391–1. CLINICAL PARAMETERS OF VIRAL HEMORRHAGIC FEVERS

| Disease | Viral Agent | Incubation Period (Days) | Clinical Syndromes | | | | Case-Fatality Rate (%) |
			Hemorrhage	Hepatitis	Encephalitis	Nephropathy	
Yellow fever	Yellow fever	3–6	major	major	absent	moderate	2–20
Dengue hemorrhagic fever	Dengue 1–4	5–8	moderate	moderate	absent	absent	2–5
Rift Valley fever	Rift Valley fever	3–6	major	major	moderate	absent	30–50
Crimean-Congo hemorrhagic fever	Crimean-Congo hemorrhagic fever	2–9	major	major	minor	absent	30–50
Kyasanur Forest disease	Kyasanur Forest disease	3–8	minor	minor	moderate	absent	5–10
Omsk hemorrhagic fever	Omsk hemorrhagic fever	3–8	minor	minor	moderate	absent	0.4–2.5
Hemorrhagic fever with renal syndrome	Hantaan	2–42	moderate	rare	minor	major	2–5
Argentine hemorrhagic fever	Junin	10–14	minor	rare	moderate	minor	1–15
Bolivian hemorrhagic fever	Machupo	7–14	moderate	rare	moderate	minor	15–30
Lassa fever	Lassa	3–16	minor	major	minor	minor	10–25
African hemorrhagic fever	Marburg	3–9	major	major	minor	absent	20–30
	Ebola	3–18	major	major	minor	absent	60–90

is usually gastric, not lower intestinal. In the period of remission, often on day 4, the patient feels better, the fever drops, and headache and nausea subside. Remission lasts a few hours to 2 days. It is followed by the period of intoxication in which the classic signs of fever, epigastric tenderness with vomiting of altered blood, nosebleeds, and albuminuria leading to oliguria or anuria occur. Dehydration may predispose to suppurative parotitis; the lungs are usually normal; but bacterial pneumonia may complicate the disease. Intoxication lasts from 3 days up to 2 weeks and may be accompanied by heart failure with drop in blood pressure, hiccough, coma, and death. Sometimes the patient is lucid until the end.

The clinical syndrome may be predominantly one of hepatic, renal, or cardiac failure. Meningoencephalitis has also been recorded. Death usually occurs between the seventh and the tenth day of illness. Patients who survive generally recover completely, although the convalescence may be prolonged, and late death from cardiac failure or arrhythmias is a rare complication.

CLINICAL LABORATORY FINDINGS. Early in the course there may be leukopenia with relative neutropenia (but sometimes with normal or elevated leukocyte count), decreased prothrombin time, and elevation of the serum bilirubin level. After the third day of illness, full-blown yellow fever is associated with abnormalities referable to the liver, kidneys, and heart. The total and conjugated bilirubin concentration values are elevated and rise together. The mean bilirubin value is 9 to 10 mg per deciliter but averages 15 to 20 mg per deciliter in severe cases and may be much higher. There are increased prothrombin and partial thromboplastin times and decreased platelets, blood glucose, and clotting factors II, V, VII, IX, and X. Alkaline phosphatase levels are normal. Aminotransferase levels are of prognostic value; serum aspartate aminotransferase and alanine aminotransferase levels are consistently elevated in jaundiced patients.

Albuminuria usually appears on the fourth day, reaching levels of 3 to 5 mg per liter (in severe cases much higher). Blood urea averages 109 mg per deciliter, and creatinine averages 5.9 mg per deciliter in fatal cases; the averages are 59 and 2.6 mg per deciliter, respectively, in nonfatal yellow fever. The urine may contain bile and casts. Electrocardiogram abnormalities are sometimes present, including abnormal ST-T waves and prolonged PR and QT intervals. The cerebrospinal fluid is under increased pressure and may contain increased protein with normal cell counts.

DIAGNOSIS. Diagnosis can be made by histopathologic examination of the liver, by isolation of yellow fever virus from blood during life and from liver and other tissues post mortem, by demonstration of specific nucleic acid, or by serologic tests. Yellow fever should be suspected in any febrile patient from endemic zones of Africa and the Americas and in areas of high *A. aegypti* prevalence where yellow fever may be introduced. Diagnosis post mortem by examination of liver taken by a viscerotome was successfully used in South America routinely for many years. Liver biopsy should not be attempted because of the danger of uncontrolled bleeding.

Yellow fever virus can be isolated from serum and blood during the first 4 days of fever by inoculation intracerebrally into baby mice or onto mammalian or mosquito cell cultures. Mice are observed for death; the virus causes cytopathic effect in Vero cells and is detected by immunofluorescence tests in mosquito cells 3 to 6 days after inoculation. The most rapid method of diagnosis is detection of antigen in acute phase blood by the antigen-capture enzyme-linked immunosorbent assay (ELISA). The test can be completed in a few hours, although detection of antigen by ELISA is less sensitive than virus isolation.

Serologic diagnosis is made by demonstrating immunoglobulin M (IgM) by the antibody-capture ELISA. Since IgM is relatively specific and is detectable for only a short time after infection, this technique is reliable using a single convalescent serum specimen. Alternatively, tests of sera collected during the acute and convalescent phases are diagnostic if they show a fourfold or greater rise (or fall) of yellow fever antibody. The neutralization test is highly specific, but the complement fixation, hemagglutination-inhibition, and ELISA methods are usually used because they are quicker and lend themselves to field laboratory use. The laboratory must also rule out cross-reacting antibody by related viruses such as dengue. A radiolabeled RNA probe detected yellow fever RNA in fixed human liver stored for more than 20 years.

DIFFERENTIAL DIAGNOSIS. The mild form of yellow fever is not clinically distinguishable from other tropical fevers. Severe yellow fever simulates viral hepatitis, including delta hepatitis; other hemorrhagic fevers; leptospirosis; rickettsial fevers; malignant malaria; and drug- and toxin-related conditions.

PROGNOSIS. Two to 20 per cent of patients with clinically evident yellow fever die, although as many as 50 per cent of severely ill patients succumb. It is not clear whether these patients would survive if they received the most modern supportive treatment, because most cases are treated in primitive clinics in Africa and South America. Patients who enter the period of intoxication have a guarded prognosis, especially if they develop anuria, high levels of albuminuria and bilirubinemia, a prothrombin time prolonged beyond 25 per cent of normal, a rapid, weak pulse, uncontrolled bleeding, persistent hiccough, delirium, hypotension, or coma.

TREATMENT. The treatment consists of complete bed rest, fluid and blood replacement, and supportive care, including monitoring of vital signs. Analgesics and antiemetics may be useful, but aspirin is contraindicated because it may exacerbate bleeding. Patients are placed under bed nets to prevent possible mosquito transmission to other patients and to hospital personnel. Malaria and bacterial complications should be treated if diagnosed. Electrolyte imbalance should be corrected. Dialysis has not been used in cases of renal tubular damage but on theoretical grounds may benefit patients in renal failure. If disseminated intravascular coagulopathy is evident by laboratory tests, heparin may be used cautiously, although there is insufficient experience to date to predict its efficacy. Interferon and other antiviral substances have not been tried in patients with yellow fever.

PREVENTION AND CONTROL. Yellow fever can be prevented by inoculation of 17D attenuated vaccine. This vaccine is safe and in over 90 per cent of vaccinees induces antibody that persists at least 10 years, and usually for life. The vaccine is produced in eggs and should not be given to persons with egg allergies. Travelers should be vaccinated at least 10 days before arrival in yellow fever–endemic areas. Since the presence of yellow fever often goes undetected and unreported in tropical Africa and South America, the vaccine should be given to travelers whether or not there is known active transmission. Human immunodeficiency virus (HIV) infection is not a contraindication to vaccination. Unless the risk of exposure to yellow fever is great, vaccine is not recommended during pregnancy; however, it is not known to have caused fetal damage. In an epidemic, mosquito control measures and use of bed nets and repellents are recommended until vaccine can be obtained.

392 Hemorrhagic Fever Caused by Dengue Viruses

DEFINITION. Dengue hemorrhagic fever (DHF) is an acute febrile illness characterized by decreased platelet counts and hemoconcentration in patients infected with any one of the four serotypes of dengue virus. The disease affects children mainly and, sometimes, adults. Capillary permeability and coagulation defects lead to hemorrhagic manifestations and, in the more severe cases, to hypovolemic shock (dengue shock syndrome), with death in 40 to 50 per cent of untreated shock syndrome patients. The disease has been endoepidemic in Southeast Asia since 1953 and is increasing in prevalence. It was restricted to Asia and the Pacific until 1981, when epidemic DHF appeared in Cuba; it reappeared in Venezuela in 1990.

ETIOLOGY. DHF is caused by infection with dengue viruses, but it is not yet established why one patient develops hemorrhagic fever and another develops classic dengue fever. Initially, it was hypothesized that strains of dengue virus that caused DHF were more virulent than others; another current theory holds that infection is enhanced and the disease is more severe when the host has been sensitized by a prior dengue infection of different serotype.

EPIDEMIOLOGY. The epidemiology of DHF is that described for dengue fever with some added features. Epidemics of DHF are limited to Southeast Asia, the Pacific Islands, and, since 1981, the Caribbean and northern South America. It is estimated that fewer than 5 per cent of individuals with dengue develop DHF. The attack rate in Thailand is highest in children, with a minor peak in infants, when maternal antibody is waning, and a major peak at 4 to 12 years of age, when second dengue infections are most common; adults as well as children develop DHF in some outbreaks, such as that in Cuba in 1981. Well-nourished children in Southeast Asia appeared to be at higher risk than the undernourished, and blacks in the Cuban epidemic had milder illness than whites; well-controlled studies are needed to substantiate these observations.

PATHOLOGY. Post mortem there are focal hemorrhages, vascular congestion, and edema in multiple organs. The spleen and lymphoid tissues show marked lymphocytolysis and phagocytosis of lymphocytes, primarily in the T cell–dependent zones. There is also proliferation of lymphoblasts and young plasma cells. Monocytic and lymphocytic nonnecrotizing perivascular infiltration is found in skin lesions, resembling an antibody-dependent Arthus reaction.

PATHOGENESIS. Dengue virus infects the macrophages, lymphocytes, and endothelial cells. On rare occasions, DHF occurs in primary dengue, indicating that direct infection of these cells with the virus can lead to the syndrome; however, the vast majority of cases are secondary infections. In these cases there is a rapid anamnestic antibody response, with formation of antigen-antibody complexes. Experimentally, formation of complexes enhances infectivity of the virus for monocytes through attachment of complexes at the Fc receptor site and entry of virus into the cell. Between 0.05 and 0.1 per cent of monocytes in the peripheral blood can be visualized carrying dengue antigen. The replication of dengue virus in the monocyte is postulated to be the effector pathway leading to vascular permeability. Monocyte infection is presumably responsible for the observed complement activation and consumption via the classic and perhaps the alternate pathway. This process may result in formation of C3a and C5a, which are anaphylatoxins, or some other as yet unknown mediator of vascular permeability may be activated. Another effector pathway leads to coagulation defects, including thrombocytopenia and abnormal clotting. The entire process is rapid. It may evolve in a few hours to shock and death or, if managed effectively, to complete recovery. Although the pathogenesis is not understood, the pathophysiologic events are known and can be treated rationally.

CLINICAL MANIFESTATIONS. DHF usually starts with sudden onset of high fever and the signs and symptoms of dengue fever, which include facial flush, anorexia, headache, nausea, and pains in the muscles and joints. Hepatic tenderness, epigastric or generalized abdominal pain, and sore throat are frequent. The liver is usually palpable, and the spleen is characteristically prominent on radiographs. The temperature continues high for 2 days to a week. A positive tourniquet test result, easy bruising, and fine petechiae on the face, soft palate, and extremities indicate a hemorrhagic disorder. Sometimes gum bleeding and epistaxis are noted. The majority of cases are moderately severe or mild, and the patients recover after lysis of fever. The lysis may be associated with sweating, coolness of extremities, and transient lowering of blood pressure.

More severe cases are associated with shock. The fall in blood pressure occurs suddenly on the third to the seventh day of illness and is accompanied by cool, blotchy skin, circumoral cyanosis, and tachycardia. The patient becomes restless and may complain of acute abdominal pain. The pulse pressure drops to 20 mm Hg or less, and in severe cases the blood pressure and pulse may not be detectable. Uncorrected shock may lead to metabolic acidosis and severe bleeding from the gastrointestinal tract and other sites. Death or recovery usually occurs in 12 to 24 hours. Surviving patients do not usually have sequelae. The white blood cell count is normal or slightly elevated, with lymphocytosis and atypical lymphocytes commonly seen. There is hemoconcentration and elevated serum aspartate aminotransferase and blood urea nitrogen levels.

DIAGNOSIS. The laboratory diagnosis is that of dengue fever, which is usually made retrospectively. DHF with shock syndrome is a medical emergency, and therefore early clinical diagnosis is essential. DHF presents with (1) acute onset of fever, which is high, continuous, and lasts 2 days or more; (2) positive tourniquet test result, with spontaneous petechiae or ecchymoses; bleeding from gums or nose; hematemesis or melena; (3) hepatomegaly, observed in more than 90 per cent of Asian patients; (4) hypotension with cold, clammy skin, restlessness, and pulse pressure less than 20 mm Hg; (5) thrombocytopenia; (6) hematocrit increased 20 per cent over the convalescent value; and (7) radiographic evidence of pleural effusion. Fever, hemorrhagic phenomena, thrombocytopenia, and hemoconcentration are the hallmarks of DHF, and, with hypotension or narrow pulse pressure, of dengue shock syndrome (DSS). Hepatoencephalopathy sometimes develops as a late manifestation. Bacterial endotoxic shock and meningococcemia can mimic DHF/DSS.

TREATMENT. There is no specific treatment. The object of therapy is to maintain hydration, to combat acidosis, and to correct coagulation abnormalities. Salicylates may contribute to bleeding and acidosis and are contraindicated. Paracetamol may be used. Steroids should not be used. Hematocrit should be determined frequently, at least daily, to measure the degree of plasma loss and the need for intravenous fluid. Fluid should be started at 20 ml per kilogram of body weight. One third to one half of fluid should be physiologic saline and the remainder, 5 per cent glucose in water. If acidosis is present, one quarter of fluid should be 0.167 mol per liter of sodium bicarbonate. In shock cases, one should use Ringer's lactate, 5 per cent glucose in physiologic saline, 5 per cent glucose in one-half physiologic saline, 5 per cent glucose in one-half Ringer's lactate, or 5 per cent glucose in one-third physiologic saline (depending on degree of dehydration and age). One should monitor for signs of cardiac failure during rapid fluid administration.

In case of shock, one should administer fluid rapidly and under pressure if necessary. One should give plasma or another volume expander if shock persists and should follow the vital signs and hematocrit. The hematocrit should decline with fluid therapy, which is continued until the hematocrit is under 40 per cent, urine output is adequate, and the appetite returns. If electrolytes and blood gases indicate acidosis, sodium bicarbonate should be administered. Heparin for intravascular coagulopathy (prolonged prothrombin and partial thromboplastin times) is usually not needed but may be used cautiously in refractory cases. Chloral hydrate for sedation, oxygen for shock, and blood should be administered as needed.

PROGNOSIS. Case fatality from DHF is 2 to 10 per cent; deaths occur in shock cases. Most patients survive when treated early by experienced health care workers. Recovery is rapid and without sequelae.

PREVENTION. Prevention is as described for dengue fever.

393 Tick-Borne Flavivirus Diseases: Kyasanur Forest Disease and Omsk Hemorrhagic Fever

DEFINITION. Kyasanur Forest disease (KFD) of India and Omsk hemorrhagic fever (OHF) of western Siberia are tick-transmitted flavivirus fevers characterized by hemorrhage or encephalitis. Some patients manifest both syndromes.

ETIOLOGY. KFD and OHF viruses belong to the tick-borne complex of flaviviruses, which also encompasses the closely related viruses of central European tick-borne encephalitis, Russian spring-summer encephalitis, and Powassan encephalitis of North America and Asia.

EPIDEMIOLOGY. KFD was originally limited to the forests of Shimoga District of Karnataka State, India, but since its discovery in 1957 it has spread in an unpredictable fashion to three other neighboring forested districts. The largest and most recent outbreak occurred during 1982–83 in a new focus in Nidle Forest. Many tick species are involved in transmission, especially nymphal *Haemaphysalis spinigera*. Small terrestrial mammals as well as birds and bats are infected in nature. When the forest is felled for plantations, the ecology is upset. Cattle brought in to graze at the forest fringe are not infected but serve as hosts that greatly increase the numbers of ticks. Infected ticks feed on black-faced langur monkeys and South Indian bonnet macaques, which become viremic, serve as amplifiers of infection, and often die. At the same time, epidemics occur in persons involved in forest occupations. People are infected incidentally and do not form part of the transmission cycle.

OHF occurs in the forest-steppe areas of the lake region of western Siberia. Epidemics of as many as 600 cases were recorded in the 1940's, but in recent years the disease has virtually disappeared. Numbers of cases peak in May and again in August and September. The virus is transmitted by *Dermacentor pictus* ticks and is maintained in small-mammal populations. Muskrats, which were introduced for hunting in the 1920's, are susceptible and apparently transmit OHF virus to other muskrats and to hunters by direct contact. Lake water contaminated by dead muskrats is said to be responsible for water-borne disease. Both KFD and OHF are transmitted transovarially and trans-stadially in ticks.

CLINICAL MANIFESTATIONS AND PATHOLOGY. The incubation period is 3 to 8 days. Onset is sudden, with fever up to 40°C, headache, papulovesicular lesions of the soft palate, myalgia, and prostration lasting 1 to 2 weeks. In more severe cases, there may be nasal, enteric, uterine, or pulmonary hemorrhage. Leukopenia, thrombocytopenia, and albuminuria are found. Some patients have a diphasic course, with a more severe illness and meningoencephalitis after a 1- or 2-week afebrile period. The second phase is characterized by fever, severe headache, meningismus, mental disturbances, and tremors. Hemorrhagic manifestations or pneumonia may also be prominent in the second phase. The case fatality rate of KFD is 5 to 10 per cent; that of OHF is 0.4 to 2.5 per cent. There are no sequelae. Infections in laboratory workers are common but are usually mild. Histopathology is minor in comparison to the gravity of the clinical disease. Findings include extravasation of red blood cells, edema, and thrombi in the small vessels.

DIAGNOSIS AND TREATMENT. Diagnosis is by isolation of virus from the blood during the first 10 days of illness and by demonstration of antibody rise or presence of specific immunoglobulin M (IgM) during convalescence. There is no specific treatment, but fluid and electrolyte balance should be maintained and blood transfused if needed. Analgesics other than aspirin may be indicated.

PREVENTION. Tick repellents, protective clothing, and spraying of forest tracts with acaricides are the only measures available for prevention.

---

394 Crimean-Congo Hemorrhagic Fever

DEFINITION. Crimean-Congo hemorrhagic fever (CCHF) is an acute febrile hemorrhagic tick-borne disease of Asia, Europe, and Africa. Mortality is high and hospital-based outbreaks are common.

ETIOLOGY. The disease is caused by CCHF virus of the *Nairovirus* genus, family Bunyaviridae. The virus kills baby mice and replicates in CER cells and several other cell culture systems.

EPIDEMIOLOGY. CCHF virus is transmitted in nature principally by hard ticks of the genus *Hyalomma*, but also by ticks in the genera *Rhipicephalus*, *Boophilus*, and *Amblyomma*. Virus is maintained by transovarial and trans-stadial passage in the tick and is amplified by hares and possibly hedgehogs, sheep, and cattle. Giraffe, rhinoceros, eland, buffalo, kudu, zebra, and dogs in southern Africa have antibody to CCHF virus.

The virus or its antibody is found in the distribution of *Hyalomma* ticks. Foci occur in the Soviet Union, the Balkan nations, Iraq, Iran, Pakistan, Afghanistan, western China, the Middle East, and most of sub-Saharan Africa, including South Africa. Outbreaks occur among military personnel, campers, and persons tending sheep and cattle. Medical workers are at high risk because of frequent spread in hospitals from infected human blood and tissues.

CLINICAL MANIFESTATIONS. The incubation period is usually between 2 and 9 days. Onset is sudden, with severe headache, fever, chills, myalgia, especially in the back and legs, sore throat, abdominal pain, nausea, vomiting, diarrhea, photophobia, and conjunctival injection. The fever is constant but may be remitting. The patient is often confused or aggressive with a marked mood change. Leukopenia and thrombocytopenia are usually observed. On days 3 to 6, hemorrhagic manifestations and a petechial rash on the trunk, limbs, and oral cavity appear. Epistaxis, hematemesis, melena, and uterine bleeding may be severe and require transfusion. The liver is sometimes enlarged and tender. In severe cases, hepatorenal failure or multiple organ system failure leads to death, usually on days 6 to 14 of illness. Death may also result from blood loss, cerebral hemorrhage, dehydration after diarrhea, or pulmonary edema. Patients recover gradually starting on day 10 when the rash fades. Asthenia may last for a month or more. Recovery is usually complete, although neuritis may persist for months. Liver function tests are abnormal, especially the aspartate aminotransferase, and serum bilirubin levels are often elevated late in the illness. Abnormal prothrombin, activated partial thromboplastin, and thrombin times, as well as increased fibrin degradation products, are indicative of disseminated intravascular coagulation (DIC).

DIAGNOSIS. Virus is easily isolated during the first 8 days of illness. Antibodies are detectable by the immunofluorescence and enzyme-linked immunosorbent assays in surviving patients. Specific immunoglobulin M (IgM) and immunoglobulin G (IgG) are present by days seven to nine of illness.

TREATMENT AND PROGNOSIS. Patients suspected of having CCHF should be housed in an isolation facility with needle and blood precautions. Health care personnel should use respirators and protective clothing. Treatment is supportive, including monitoring and correction of fluid and electrolyte imbalance and treatment of DIC. The vital signs and hematocrit should be tested frequently, and blood should be replaced by transfusion. Case-fatality rates range from 30 to 50 per cent.

PREVENTION. Protection from tick bites and care in handling blood and tissues of sick sheep and cattle are the only preventive measures available in the case of exposure in natural foci.

---

395 Hemorrhagic Diseases Caused by Arenaviruses *(Argentine and Bolivian Hemorrhagic Fevers and Lassa Fever)*

DEFINITION. Argentine and Bolivian hemorrhagic fevers and Lassa fever are acute febrile diseases characterized by hemorrhagic diatheses, marked myalgia, and, in severe cases, shock. Case-fatality rates are between 5 and 30 per cent.

ETIOLOGY. The diseases are caused by the viruses Junin (Argentina), Machupo (Bolivia), and Lassa (West Africa) of the family Arenaviridae.

EPIDEMIOLOGY. The reservoirs are rodents that excrete virus in urine and possibly other body fluids. The rodents involved are Junin virus, *Calomys musculinus*, *Calomys laucha*, and *Akodon arenicola*; Machupo virus, *Calomys callosus*; and Lassa virus, *Mastomys natalensis*. People are believed to be infected by inhaling or eating contaminated excreta or by passage of virus through abraded skin or mucous membranes. In Argentina, exposure to Junin virus is primarily in workers harvesting corn in Cordoba and Buenos Aires provinces in the north. In Bolivia, domestic and peridomestic exposure to Machupo virus occurs in Beni province. Lassa virus is endemic in west and central Africa, especially in Liberia, Sierra Leone, and parts of Nigeria, where it is transmitted in and around homes that have an abundance of domestic rats.

Argentine hemorrhagic fever epidemics involving hundreds to thousands of farm workers are recorded annually. Bolivian hemorrhagic fever epidemics were common in the 1960's, but after institution of rodent control measures, the disease has not been reported since 1974. Lassa fever was recognized first in 1969 in a nosocomial outbreak in Nigeria. Several other nosocomial outbreaks were subsequently diagnosed, but studies in Sierra Leone established the basic endemic nature of the disease. In the eastern province, 8 to 52 per cent of the population have antibody, and the annual seroconversion rate in susceptible subjects ranges between 5 and 22 per cent. It is estimated that 5 to 14 per cent of the fevers are Lassa virus infections and that Lassa fever accounts for 10 to 16 per cent of the adult hospital admissions.

PATHOGENESIS AND PATHOLOGY. The diseases are characterized by multiple organ impairment, yet specific lesions are absent. The prominent findings are focal diapedesis and capillary hemorrhage, but inflammation is minimal. Focal areas of liver necrosis in Lassa fever are not sufficient to account for the profound shock and death. It is postulated that the virus infects cells of the reticuloendothelial system, including the B and T cells. It causes temporary inhibition of immune cell function leading to prolonged and high-titered viremia. It is not known whether subsequent capillary damage and parenchymal edema are direct or indirect effects of the virus.

CLINICAL MANIFESTATIONS. The three diseases have many similarities. The incubation period of Lassa fever is 3 to 16 days; of Argentine hemorrhagic fever, 10 to 14 days; and of Bolivian hemorrhagic fever, 7 to 14 days. Onset is insidious, initially with fever, chills, malaise, asthenia, headache, retroocular pain, anorexia, nausea, vomiting, and muscle pain, (especially at the costovertebral angle in the South American forms and the legs in Lassa fever). Fever is nonremitting between 39° and 40.5°C. Sore throat is not prominent in the Argentine and Bolivian diseases, but purulent pharyngitis and aphthous ulcers are common in Lassa fever.

Signs include conjunctivitis, facial edema, enanthem with pharyngeal vesicles, exanthem of the face, neck, and upper thorax, tenderness of thighs, laterocervical and other polyadenopathy, and petechiae, especially in the axillae. There is no jaundice or hepatosplenomegaly. Leukopenia, thrombocytopenia, and albuminuria with casts are characteristic.

Late in the first week of illness, the signs and symptoms become more pronounced. Signs of dehydration, decreased blood pressure, and relative bradycardia are prominent. Hemorrhage from the gums, nose, stomach, intestines, uterus, and urinary tract indicates a severe hemorrhagic diathesis. Bleeding was observed commonly in the South American forms, but in only 17 per cent of Lassa fever cases. Blood loss is not massive enough to account for the shock. The acute phase usually lasts 7 to 15 days. Death is the result of uremia or hypovolemic shock, usually in the second week of illness. Recovery is heralded by lysis of fever; there is usually a prolonged convalescence marked by periods of sweating, flush, and postural hypotension, but patients suffer no permanent nonneurologic sequelae.

Neurologic signs are prominent in Bolivian hemorrhagic fever; nearly 50 per cent of patients have an intention tremor of the tongue and hands at about the fifth day of illness, and 25 per cent of these progress to more serious encephalopathy with delirium and convulsions. The cerebrospinal fluid is normal in these patients. A similar syndrome is occasionally seen in Lassa fever, and about 5 per cent of patients develop unilateral or bilateral eighth cranial nerve damage, which may be permanent. Other transient complications are loss of hair and Beau's lines of the nails.

Most patients have leukopenia with depression of both lymphocytes and neutrophils; however, some Lassa fever patients have markedly elevated white counts. Thrombocytopenia is present during the first week of illness.

DIAGNOSIS. The diagnosis can be made definitively only with laboratory tests. Fever, muscle pain, and diminished white cell count in the endemic areas should alert the physician to the diagnosis. Virus can be isolated in Vero cells from blood, cerebrospinal fluid, and throat washings during life and from most tissues at necropsy. Virus is recoverable even in the presence of antibody. Isolation of virus from Bolivian hemorrhagic fever cases is more difficult than from the Argentine or West African form. Virus isolation should be attempted only in laboratories with high biosecurity containment equipment because of the risk of infection of laboratory workers. Serologic diagnosis is made by the immunofluorescence test. Immunoglobulin G is present in 53 per cent of Lassa fever patients on admission to hospital and immunoglobulin M (IgM), in 67 per cent. The IgM test is useful for early and rapid diagnosis.

TREATMENT. Supportive therapy, including attention to electrolyte and fluid balance, is essential. Hematocrit and urine protein measurements aid in detection of hypovolemic shock. Plasma expanders are effective if used early but may precipitate pulmonary edema late in the clinical course.

Specific Junin virus–immune human plasma given during the first 8 days of Argentine hemorrhagic fever reduced the case-fatality rate from 16 to 1 per cent. A neurologic illness was observed about 3 weeks after the acute attack in some patients receiving this therapy. Most of these persons recovered completely.

Ribavirin given to Lassa fever patients early in the illness significantly reduced mortality. The drug was administered intravenously, 60 mg per kilogram per day for the first 4 days, and then orally, 30 mg per kilogram per day for 6 days more. Immune plasma was not effective in Lassa fever patients in controlled trials.

PROGNOSIS. In Lassa fever, bleeding manifestations, high levels of circulating virus in the blood, and elevated aspartate aminotransferase levels in serum are predictive of death. There are no such predictors for the South American arenavirus hemorrhagic fevers. Shock or abnormal neurologic findings indicate a poor prognosis.

PREVENTION AND CONTROL. Environmental sanitation, including rodent-proofing of homes, and proper storage of grains and other foods to diminish rodent populations are the only community control measures now available. An experimental vaccine for Junin virus has proved efficacious in Argentina. Barrier nursing with use of gloves and gowns should be instituted in suspected cases of arenaviral hemorrhagic fevers. Blood and other tissues are infective and should be decontaminated.

396 African Hemorrhagic Fever (Marburg-Ebola Disease)

DEFINITION. African hemorrhagic fever is an acute, often fatal, hemorrhagic disease. Fever, rash, hemorrhage, hepatic and pancreatic inflammation, and prostration are hallmarks of the illness.

ETIOLOGY. The disease is caused by Marburg and Ebola viruses of the family Filoviridae. The two viruses are distinct antigenically but of very similar morphology.

EPIDEMIOLOGY. Marburg disease was described in 1967 in Germany and Yugoslavia, where workers in vaccine manufacturing facilities sickened and died after they were exposed to infected tissues of African green monkeys from Uganda. Where the monkeys became infected is not known, although Marburg virus is indigenous to Africa. (Additional isolated cases in South Africa and Kenya are recorded.) Ebola virus epidemics in Sudan and Zaire in 1976 were traced to contact with infected patients and, in Zaire, to spread by needle. The disease recurred in Sudan in

1979, and there was an isolated case in Kenya in 1980. The source of the outbreaks is unknown, and the natural history remains a mystery. A third filovirus, most closely related to Ebola virus, was isolated in 1989 from sick cynomolgus monkeys recently imported to the United States from the Philippines. Animal handlers in the United States seroconverted to the virus without associated illness.

PATHOLOGY. African hemorrhagic fever is a systemic disease with multiple organ involvement, most prominently the lymphatic system, testes, ovaries, and liver. Liver cell necrosis with eosinophilic inclusions, unlike that in yellow fever, is random and focal. Fibrin deposits are found in the renal glomeruli, consistent with disseminated intravascular coagulopathy. There is edema and diffuse inflammation in the brain.

CLINICAL MANIFESTATIONS. The incubation period is 3 to 9 days for Marburg virus infection and 3 to 18 days for Ebola. Onset is abrupt, with severe headache, backache, muscle pains, and sometimes abdominal pain. At this stage, the disease is not readily differentiated from malaria, typhoid fever, and other bacterial, rickettsial, or viral illnesses. On about the third day, nausea, vomiting, and profuse watery diarrhea with mucus and blood commence. Diarrhea may continue for several days. A maculopapular rash appears on the trunk and spreads to the rest of the body. On day 4 or 5, the patient's status becomes critical, with high, unremitting fever and an altered mental state, including confusion, aggression, or lethargy. There is spontaneous bleeding from injection sites, hematemesis, melena, hemoptysis, and, in pregnant patients, abortion, often with massive blood loss. Renal failure may be a terminal event. Death occurs from day 8 to 17, often on day 8 or 9. Recovery is marked by fatigue, anorexia, weight loss, hair loss, and, sometimes, psychological problems.

The pathophysiology is characterized by leukopenia, thrombocytopenia, increased prothrombin time, and other abnormalities in the liver function tests, increased serum amylase, proteinuria, and electrocardiographic changes indicative of myocardial disease. Disseminated intravascular coagulopathy has been documented in some cases.

DIAGNOSIS. Virus is isolated from acute phase blood, liver, and other organs by inoculation into guinea pigs or cell culture. The immunofluorescence assay becomes positive during the second week of illness.

TREATMENT AND PROGNOSIS. There is no specific treatment. Supportive therapy consists of maintenance of fluid and electrolyte balance and administration of blood, platelets, or fresh frozen plasma to control bleeding. Peritoneal dialysis for renal failure and heparin for disseminated intravascular coagulopathy have been recommended, but their value in African hemorrhagic fever is not established. The presence of bleeding indicates a poor prognosis. The case-fatality rate under relatively sophisticated hospital conditions in Marburg, Germany, was 22 per cent in 1967, and under Third World rural conditions in Zaire during 1976, it was 90 per cent.

PREVENTION. Control activities are not carried out because the natural reservoir is unknown. Nosocomial spread can be minimized by barrier nursing and handling of blood and tissues in isolator laboratory units with proper decontamination.

397 Hemorrhagic Fever with Renal Syndrome

DEFINITION. Hemorrhagic fever with renal syndrome (HFRS) is a disease of Europe and Asia characterized by fevers, capillary dilatation, leakage of blood leading to hemorrhagic manifestations, and, in severe cases, shock and renal tubular disease.

ETIOLOGY. HFRS is caused by any one of several closely related viruses of the genus *Hantavirus*, family Bunyaviridae. The prototype is Hantaan virus, originally isolated from *Apodemus agrarius* field mice in the endemic region of Korea.

EPIDEMIOLOGY. The virus is transmitted from rodents. *Apodemus agrarius* in Korea and other parts of Asia, *Clethrionomys glareolus* in Finland and west of the Ural Mountains, and *Rattus rattus* and *R. norvegicus* in cities of Japan, Korea, and Belgium serve as reservoirs. The rodent excretes virus in urine, saliva, and feces for weeks, and sometimes for months, after infection. Transmission is presumably by respiratory spread or direct contact with fomites contaminated by rodent excretions. Persons at risk include soldiers in field operations, campers, farmers, woodsmen, and, especially in the winter, family groups in houses harboring field rodents that seek shelter from the cold. Outbreaks have also occurred in laboratories housing field rodents or housing laboratory rats that carry the virus as an inapparent infection. Nosocomial infections are not reported. Viruses of the genus *Hantavirus* have been isolated from rodents in the Americas, but HFRS is absent.

PATHOLOGY. Patients who die of shock in the early stages demonstrate retroperitoneal gelatinous edema. There are macroscopic hemorrhages in the pituitary and right auricle. The renal medulla is congested and hyperemic, and patients who die later in the course of the disease have marked renal tubular necrosis. Petechial hemorrhages found in the skin and in multiple organs indicate widespread capillary fragility.

CLINICAL MANIFESTATIONS AND PATHOLOGIC PHYSIOLOGY. The incubation period ranges from 2 to 42 days but is usually about 2 weeks. Eighty per cent of cases are mild (demonstrating only fever, facial flush, backache, and muscle aches) or moderate (fever plus proteinuria, and petechial hemorrhages). The remaining 20 per cent are severe. They progress through five characteristic phases: febrile, hypotensive, oliguric, diuretic, and convalescent. The febrile phase lasts about 5 days, during which fever, facial flush, conjunctival injection, and backache precede the appearance of petechial hemorrhages and albuminuria. In the hypotensive phase, the temperature returns to baseline, and the patient manifests nausea, vomiting, abdominal pain, and about 3 days of capillary leakage with a rising hematocrit, heavy proteinuria, leukocytosis, thrombocytopenia, and decreased renal clearance. This is followed for about 4 days by the oliguric phase, when extravascular fluid is resorbed, leading to relative hypervolemia, hypertension, metabolic acidosis, and sometimes pulmonary edema and/or acute renal failure. The diuretic phase is accompanied by return of renal clearance to normal, but with marked electrolyte and fluid imbalance, which may lead to death if not adequately managed. The convalescent phase may last 1 to 3 months, with slowly recovering renal function. The clinical diagnosis may be reliable during an outbreak with classic severe cases but not with mild infections; serologic confirmation is obtained by the immunofluorescence and neutralization tests, which become positive at the end of the first week of illness. Antibody titers peak at 2 weeks and last for many years.

TREATMENT AND PROGNOSIS. Management includes careful monitoring of electrolytes and fluid intake and output with correction, especially during the oliguric and diuretic phases. Plasma expanders can be used for shock, and hemodialysis in cases of renal failure with hyperkalemia. Ribavirin improves survival if given within 5 days of onset. The case fatality in Korea is about 5 per cent with hospital management; the disease in northern Europe is milder with a more favorable prognosis.

PREVENTION. Rodent control should be practiced where feasible, especially in urban settings.

Halstead SB: In vivo enhancement of dengue virus infection in rhesus monkeys by passively transferred antibody. J Infect Dis 140:527, 1979. *The definitive experimental evidence conferring credibility to the secondary infection hypothesis of dengue hemorrhagic fever.*

Hoogstraal H: The epidemiology of tick-borne Crimean-Congo hemorrhagic fever in Asia, Europe, and Africa. J Med Entomol 15:307, 1979. *Extensive description and bibliography of natural history of CCHF.*

Maiztegui JI, Fernandez NJ, deDamilano AJ: Efficacy of immune plasma in treatment of Argentine hemorrhagic fever and association between treatment and a late neurological syndrome. Lancet 2:1216, 1979. *Definitive study showing that immune plasma is efficacious for treatment of Argentine hemorrhagic fever.*

Monath TP: Lassa fever—new issues raised by field studies in West Africa. J Infect Dis 155:433, 1987. *An up-to-date perspective on Lassa fever surveillance, treatment, and research.*

Monath TP: Yellow fever: A medically neglected disease. Report on a seminar. Rev Infect Dis 90:165, 1987. *Excellent summary of state-of-the-art yellow fever case management and diagnosis.*

Pattyn SR (ed.): Ebola Virus Haemorrhagic Fever. New York, Elsevier/North-Holland, 1978. *Descriptions of the outbreaks of African hemorrhagic fever in 1976 in Zaire and Sudan.*

Reviews of Infectious Diseases, Vol. II, Suppl 4, May-June 1989, pp 5669–5896. *A comprehensive compilation of reviews of the viral hemorrhagic fevers, including DHF, Crimean-Congo hemorrhagic fever, arenaviral hemorrhagic fevers, African hemorrhagic fevers, and HFRS.*

Strode GK (ed.): Yellow Fever. New York, McGraw-Hill Book Company, 1951. *Classic description of history, epidemiology, and clinical details of yellow fever cases.*

Swanepoel R, Shepherd AJ, Leman PA, et al.: Epidemiologic and clinical features of Crimean Congo hemorrhagic fever in Southern Africa. Am J Trop Med Hyg 36:120, 1987. *Current clinical description and review of recent CCHF literature.*

Symposium on epidemic hemorrhagic fever. Am J Med 16:617, 1954. *Detailed information on the pathophysiology of HFRS.*

WHO Expert Committee Report: Viral Haemorrhagic Fevers. WHO Tech Rep Ser No 721, 1985. *Excellent review of hemorrhagic fevers by an international group of experts with detailed guide to management of patients, investigation of outbreaks, and vector control.*

WHO Scientific Group Report: Arthropod-borne and rodent-borne viral diseases. WHO Tech Rep Ser No. 719, 1985. *Authoritative discussion of epidemiologic principles, laboratory safety, vector control, and epidemic preparedness.*

WHO Technical Advisory Group Report: Dengue haemorrhagic fever: Diagnosis, treatment and control. Geneva, World Health Organization, 1986. *A most comprehensive manual for the physician faced with management of DHF patients.*

SECTION FOUR / THE MYCOSES

398 Introduction

William E. Dismukes

Fungi are classified as eukaryotic microorganisms, in contrast to bacteria, which are considered prokaryotic. Eukaryotes, such as fungi, possess a discrete nuclear membrane and a nucleus that contains several chromosomes, whereas prokaryotes have no nucleus or nuclear membrane and possess only a single chromosome. Fungi also differ from bacteria in the ability of the former to reproduce sexually or asexually. Most fungi reproduce by asexual spore formation. When sexual mating of two closely related species, e.g., *Cryptococcus neoformans*, serotypes A and D, takes place, the "perfect state" (*Filobasidiella neoformans* var. *neoformans*) is produced. Fungi for which a perfect state has not been identified are referred to as Fungi Imperfecti (e.g., *Candida albicans* and *Coccidioides immitis*). The cell walls of fungi are rigid, usually containing chitin and polysaccharides, another feature that distinguishes fungi from bacteria. In addition, the inner cytoplasmic membrane of fungi contains sterols, which are the site of action of the polyene antifungal agents amphotericin B and nystatin.

The terms "fungal diseases" and "mycoses" are used interchangeably. Fungal infections that involve only the skin and its appendages are referred to as cutaneous or superficial mycoses (e.g., ringworm of the scalp or groin and tinea versicolor). By contrast, fungal infections that are acquired primarily by inhalation and spread via lymphohematogenous dissemination to involve one or more organs, such as the lungs, skin, liver, spleen, and central nervous system, are referred to as systemic mycoses (e.g., blastomycosis, coccidioidomycosis, cryptococcosis, and histoplasmosis). Candidiasis is a mycosis that may cause superficial disease (e.g., intertrigo, oral thrush, and vaginitis) or systemic disease (e.g., candidemia and hepatosplenic candidiasis).

Fungi causing systemic disease may also be classified by the morphologic or structural form of the organism. For example, *Aspergillus* species and zygomycetes (*Mucor* and *Rhizopus* species) are molds that grow as a hyphal structural form both in the laboratory (and nature) and in humans. By contrast, other fungi are dimorphic, i.e., they have the ability to transform morphologically into either a mold or a yeast form, depending on the environmental conditions. *Blastomyces dermatitidis*, *C. immitis*, *Histoplasma capsulatum*, *Paracoccidioides brasiliensis*, and *Sporothrix schenckii* exist as hyphal or filamentous forms in nature, but as yeasts (*B. dermatitidis*, *H. capsulatum*, *S. sporothrix*) or endosporulating spherules (*C. immitis* and *P. brasiliensis*) in humans. *Cryptococcus neoformans* is a true yeast, growing as the same spherical form in both nature and humans.

The route (or routes) of transmission and the geographic distribution of the major systemic mycoses are shown in Table 398–1. Detailed discussions of these epidemiologic features of each mycosis are provided in the individual chapters that follow. As a rule, mycoses are not transmissible from human to human. The natural habitat of several fungal pathogens is limited to specific geographic areas. Consequently, persons living in these areas are at highest risk of acquiring infection. The diseases caused by such organisms are referred to as endemic mycoses. As shown in Table 398–1, the endemic systemic mycoses are blastomycosis, coccidioidomycosis, histoplasmosis, and paracoccidioidomycosis. These diseases, which are acquired by inhalation of spores, typically are associated with asymptomatic or mild pulmonary infection that heals spontaneously. Progressive pulmonary infection or spread to extrapulmonary sites occurs less frequently.

TABLE 398–1. EPIDEMIOLOGIC FEATURES OF COMMON SYSTEMIC MYCOSES

Disease	Geographic Distribution	Route of Transmission
Candidiasis	Worldwide (part of normal flora of skin, oropharynx, gastrointestinal tract, vagina)	Endogenous Contact (less commonly)
Cryptococcosis	Worldwide (avian habitats)	Respiratory
Aspergillosis	Worldwide (ubiquitous in nature)	Respiratory Cutaneous (rarely)
Zygomycosis (Mucormycosis)	Worldwide (ubiquitous in nature)	Respiratory Cutaneous (rarely)
Blastomycosis	South and North Central United States Mexico, Central and South America, Africa (occasionally)	Respiratory Cutaneous (rarely)
Coccidioidomycosis	Southwestern United States, Mexico, Central and South America	Respiratory
Histoplasmosis	Worldwide (along river basins, especially Mississippi, Tennessee, Ohio, and St. Lawrence—bird and bat habitats)	Respiratory
Paracoccidioidomycosis	Mexico, Central and South America	Respiratory
Sporotrichosis	Worldwide (soil and vegetation)	Cutaneous Respiratory (rarely)

TABLE 398–2. ALTERED HOST DEFENSE AND OPPORTUNISTIC FUNGAL DISEASE

Alteration in Host Defense	Opportunistic Fungal Disease
Interruption of mechanical barriers or indwelling foreign bodies	Candidiasis
Granulocyte dysfunction (quantitative or qualitative)	Aspergillosis Candidiasis Zycomycosis
Depressed cell-mediated immunity	Candidiasis (mucosal) Coccidioidomycosis Cryptococcosis Histoplasmosis

Some fungal organisms are considered opportunistic pathogens and are especially prone to cause disease in the setting of altered host defense (Table 398–2). Common predisposing conditions or factors include interruptions in anatomic barriers (burns and endotracheal tubes) or indwelling foreign bodies (arterial or central venous catheters, urinary catheters, and prosthetic heart valves or joints); granulocyte dysfunction secondary to hematologic malignancies (leukemia) or cytotoxic chemotherapy; and depressed cell-mediated immunity associated with organ transplantation, acquired immunodeficiency syndrome (AIDS), or immunosuppressive therapy, such as corticosteroids and azathioprine. Other conditions that may predispose to systemic mycoses include diabetic ketoacidosis (rhinocerebral mucormycosis) and intravenous drug abuse (*Candida* endocarditis and basal ganglia mucormycosis).

Culture for fungus and histopathologic studies using special stains of infected body fluids (sputum, blood, urine, and cerebrospinal fluid [CSF]) and tissues (skin, lung, liver, bone marrow, and lymph nodes) are the mainstays of diagnosis of the mycoses. If fungal disease is suspected, the microbiology laboratory should be alerted to use appropriate culture media. Skin testing with fungal antigens has no place in the diagnosis of individual infections, although skin tests are useful as indicators of prior infection in epidemiologic studies of prevalence. Although most serologic tests for mycoses have limited value in diagnosis because of either low sensitivity and specificity or poor standardization of assay reagents and methods, there are two exceptions. A positive latex agglutination test for cryptococcal antigen in CSF or blood

TABLE 398–3. THERAPY FOR THE COMMON SYSTEMIC MYCOSES

Disease	First Choice	Alternative(s)
Aspergillosis	Amphotericin B ± rifampin or flucytosine	Itraconazole*
Zygomycosis (Mucormycosis)	Amphotericin B	None
Candidiasis		
Candidemia, invasive, disseminated	Amphotericin B ± flucytosine	? Ketoconazole ? Fluconazole
Urinary tract	Fluconazole	Amphotericin B Flucytosine
Cryptoccocosis	Amphotericin B ± flucytosine	Fluconazole Itraconazole*
Coccidioidomycosis	Amphotericin B or ketoconazole	Fluconazole Itraconazole* Miconazole
Blastomycosis	Amphotericin B or ketoconazole	Itraconazole* ? Fluconazole
Histoplasmosis	Amphotericin B or ketoconazole	Itraconazole* ? Fluconazole
Paracoccidioidomycosis	Amphotericin B or ketoconazole	A sulfonamide Miconazole Itraconazole*
Sporotrichosis		
Cutaneous	Potassium iodide	Itraconazole* ? Fluconazole
Extracutaneous	Amphotericin B	Itraconazole*

*Investigational.
Adapted with permission from The Medical Letter 32:58–60, 1990.

is a highly reliable indicator of cryptococcal disease; similarly, a positive titer for complement-fixing antibody in serum or CSF is a reliable marker of coccidioidal disease. Widely available serologic tests that are both sensitive and specific would be very useful in the diagnosis of invasive aspergillosis and candidiasis.

Table 398–3 provides an overview of the currently recommended treatment regimens for the common systemic mycoses. Although amphotericin B remains the "gold standard" of therapy for most fungal diseases, much progress in antifungal therapy has been made over the past two decades, especially with regard to antifungal azoles. Miconazole, the first of this class of drugs and a parenteral formulation, is associated with considerable toxicity, which has limited its usefulness. The approval in 1981 of ketoconazole represented a major breakthrough. Ketoconazole is an oral formulation with broad-spectrum activity and less toxicity than either miconazole or amphotericin B. Fluconazole, approved in 1990, possesses several advantages over ketoconazole, including availability as either an oral or a parenteral preparation, significant urinary excretion of active drug, good to excellent penetration into CSF (60 to 80 per cent of serum concentrations), and minimal toxicity, with no documented suppression of endogenous steroid synthesis. Promising investigational azole compounds include itraconazole and saperconazole.

The only other antifungal drug currently approved for the treatment of systemic mycoses is flucytosine, an oral preparation, which is often used in combination with amphotericin B to provide a synergistic effect against *C. neoformans* and *Candida* species and sometimes used alone as therapy for chromomycosis. Unfortunately, flucytosine is potentially toxic to the bone marrow and liver; in addition, its use, especially as a single agent, may be associated with rapid emergence of resistant organisms. Research efforts are currently ongoing to standardize and commercially prepare new formulations of amphotericin B, either encapsulated in liposomes or complexed with lipids. Preliminary evidence indicates that these investigational lipid preparations will offer several advantages over currently available amphotericin B (Fungizone), including less toxicity, increased tropism for reticuloendothelial organs, and possibly increased dosing of active drug.

Gallis HA, Drew RH, Pickard WW: Amphotericin B: 30 years of clinical experience. Rev Infect Dis 12:308, 1990. *A practical up-to-date review of the pharmacology, clinical uses, and adverse effects of amphotericin B, the most important systemic antifungal agent (190 references).*
Rippon JW: Medical Mycology. 3rd ed. Philadelphia, W.B. Saunders Company, 1988. *A comprehensive text that considers most fungal pathogens and their diseases, including the superficial mycoses.*

399 Histoplasmosis

William E. Dismukes

DEFINITION. Histoplasmosis, the most common endemic systemic mycosis in the United States, is associated with a variety of clinical syndromes, the most frequent of which is an asymptomatic or self-limited influenza-like respiratory infection. Less frequently, histoplasmosis manifests as chronic cavitary pulmonary disease, progressive disseminated disease involving multiple organs, or immune-mediated disease of the mediastinum or eye.

ETIOLOGY. *Histoplasma capsulatum* is the imperfect state of a dimorphic fungus that grows as a mycelial form at temperatures below 35°C in the laboratory and in soil, its natural habitat, and as a yeast form at 37°C and in infected hosts. The perfect state is *Emmonsiella capsulata*. The mycelial form bears two types of infectious spores, macroconidia and microconidia, both of which are readily airborne, but the smaller microconidia (2 to 6 μm versus 8 to 14 μm) more easily reach alveoli or small bronchioles upon inhalation. The oval yeast cells (2 to 3 × 3 to 4 μm) reproduce by single narrow-based buds, are unencapsulated, and are usually found within macrophages in viable tissue. A variant strain, *H. capsulatum* var. *duboisii*, which is found solely in

Central Africa, is characterized by a larger yeast form (7 to 15 μm).

EPIDEMIOLOGY. Results of skin test surveys using histoplasmin antigen indicate that histoplasmosis is worldwide in distribution, with greatest prevalence in tropical and temperate zones. The disease is endemic in the South Central and North Central United States, especially along the Mississippi, Tennessee, Missouri, Ohio, and St. Lawrence River basins. A high prevalence has also been noted in selected areas of the eastern United States. In these endemic areas, over 80 per cent of persons are infected by 20 years of age. *Histoplasma capsulatum* can be readily recovered from soil, especially that enriched by bird and bat guano. Because of high body temperatures, birds are not infected, whereas bats are. Soil contaminated by chicken, pigeon, blackbird, or starling droppings and areas frequented by bats, such as caves, hollow trees, old buildings, and attics, are frequently identified sources of outbreaks. The disturbance of soil or sites by wind, bulldozing, demolition, or other construction-related activities may greatly increase the number of airborne spores and result in exposure of both nearby and distantly located persons. Although *H. capsulatum* is more prevalent in bird- or bat-related microenvironments, aerosolized microconidia are commonly present as "air pollutants" in endemic areas and may account for the majority of sporadic infections.

Pulmonary infection does not convey protective immunity; consequently, reinfection may occur. However, reactivation of quiescent or dormant disease appears to be more likely than reinfection as an explanation for second-episode disease or disease that develops after a person has left an endemic area. Person-to-person transmission of histoplasmosis is not known to occur. Although age, sex, and race do not significantly affect susceptibility to infection, middle-aged white men with pre-existing chronic obstructive pulmonary disease appear to be at highest risk of developing chronic pulmonary histoplasmosis. Over recent years, *H. capsulatum* has emerged as an opportunistic fungal pathogen, especially in hosts with altered cellular immunity secondary to organ transplantation, corticosteroid or cytotoxic drugs, or infection with human immunodeficiency virus (HIV). In some endemic areas, disseminated histoplasmosis is the most common acquired immunodeficiency syndrome (AIDS)–defining opportunistic infection.

PATHOGENESIS AND PATHOLOGY. Aerosolized microconidia of *H. capsulatum*, after inhalation into the lungs, undergo transformation into yeast forms at body temperature and are promptly phagocytized by macrophages. In nonimmune persons, macrophages are initially unable to kill the yeasts, which multiply intracellularly. These infected macrophages migrate to the mediastinal lymph nodes and to other organs of the mononuclear phagocyte system (reticuloendothelial system), such as the spleen. Recent evidence indicates that L3T4$^+$ cells are a critical determinant of an effective host response to *H. capsulatum*. In normal hosts, once antigen-specific cellular immunity becomes established, infection is usually contained by a sequence of events including a vasculitic response, granuloma formation with caseation necrosis, enlargement of regional lymph nodes followed by fibrosis, and, ultimately, calcification. By contrast, in persons with impaired cell-mediated immunity, the mononuclear phagocyte system is unable to contain the infection, and viable *H. capsulatum* organisms disseminate widely to macrophage-rich tissues, including liver, spleen, visceral lymph nodes, and bone marrow. In these individuals, because the normal reaction of host tissue to parasitized macrophages is either minimal or absent, infection goes unchecked, and progressive disseminated disease ensues. The pathogenesis of mediastinal fibrosis and ocular histoplasmosis, two uncommon but clinically significant complications of infection with *H. capsulatum*, is presumed to be immune mediated, at least in part. Mediastinal fibrosis appears to develop in hypersensitive persons with a large antigen load in caseous mediastinal nodes. Exuberant fibrous encapsulation of nodes and adjacent tissues may lead to bronchial or vascular occlusion or erosion.

In histopathologic specimens stained with periodic acid–Schiff (PAS), Giemsa, or Gomori methenamine silver (GMS), the characteristic ovoid yeast forms of *H. capsulatum*, surrounded by a clear space resembling a capsule but actually due to fixation artifact, are generally found in macrophages. Organisms are more difficult to visualize in tissue stained with hematoxylin-eosin. The likelihood of identifying organisms in tissue sections is directly related to the effectiveness of cellular immunity in a given host. In immune individuals with an intact host defense, fungi are rare, granuloma formation is well developed, and extent of disease is limited. By contrast, in compromised hosts with impaired cellular immunity, macrophages, including those in peripheral blood, are filled with intracellular yeasts; granulomas are poorly developed or absent; and disease is extensive.

CLINICAL MANIFESTATIONS. Pulmonary disease in histoplasmosis is conveniently classified into acute and chronic forms. Acute disease, which results from primary infection, most often resolves spontaneously but may be associated with early and late complications.

Acute Pulmonary Infection. The vast majority of primary infections with *H. capsulatum* are either asymptomatic or associated with a flulike illness, manifested by fever, chills, headache, nonproductive cough, pleuritic or substernal chest pain, malaise, and myalgias. The incubation period and severity of illness are directly related to the inoculum of inhaled spores and the prior immune status of the individual. In nonimmune persons with a heavy exposure, respiratory symptoms tend to be more severe and progressive and include severe dyspnea. Radiologic findings also vary, depending on the inoculum size and the pre-exposure immunity of the host. A normal chest x-ray film is most common, but abnormalities range from one or two patchy infiltrates, with or without mediastinal and hilar adenopathy, to diffuse miliary opacities, which frequently heal in a pattern of "buckshot" calcifications. Pleural effusion and cavitation are uncommon. Extrapulmonary symptoms and signs, including arthralgias, erythema nodosum, and erythema multiforme, may be present, especially in young women. Early and late complications of acute or primary pulmonary infection may result from vigorous host reactions causing enlarged mediastinal or hilar nodes and exuberant encapsulating fibrosis, which in turn lead to compression or erosion of adjacent mediastinal structures. These rare complications include acute pericarditis; tracheal, bronchial, or esophageal obstruction; esophageal diverticuli; bronchoesophageal fistula; broncholithiasis (secondary to erosion of a calcification into a bronchus); mediastinal granuloma; mediastinal fibrosis or fibrosing mediastinitis; and enlarging histoplasmoma (usually located in the peripheral lung parenchyma and recognized by concentric laminations of calcium). Mediastinal granuloma, which tends to develop more often in the right paratracheal area, is more circumscribed, smaller in size, and associated with fewer sequelae than is mediastinal fibrosis. Both entities are recognized causes of superior vena cava syndrome.

Chronic Pulmonary Infection. Chronic pulmonary histoplasmosis often occurs in men with underlying chronic obstructive pulmonary disease and resembles pulmonary tuberculosis in symptomatology and radiographic manifestations, although the course of this type of histoplasmosis tends to be milder and more indolent than that of tuberculosis. The pathogenesis and course of chronic pulmonary histoplasmosis are highly complex; pathologic studies indicate two basic lesions. An interstitial pneumonitis featuring mononuclear infiltration, periarteriolar inflammation, areas of infarct-like necrosis, and few organisms is characteristic of the early lesion. The inflammatory process often surrounds apical emphysematous blebs and bullae. In contrast, the chronic lesion is manifested by organization of diseased tissue, with prominence of giant cells and progressive cavitation. Cavities are surrounded by an area of vascular granulation tissue, and their inner linings are often necrotic. Organisms are typically found in the necrotic lining or in surface exudate. In the thicker walled cavities, infection is persistent, with continuing necrosis, leading to progressive cavity enlargement (marching cavity) at the expense of the surrounding lung parenchyma. In general, the symptoms and roentgenographic findings reflect the two types or stages of disease, namely, pneumonitis and progressive cavitation. Although symptoms overlap, they tend to be more abrupt in onset, with more severe constitutional symptoms, such as fever, night sweats, and malaise, in the pneumonitis stage; hemoptysis and progressive dyspnea are more typical of the cavitation stage. In 80 per cent of cases, the pneumonitis stage tends to resolve spontaneously over 2 to 3 months, with a small fibrotic residuum, whereas the cavitation stage, especially that associated with thick-walled cavities, tends to be relentlessly progressive, leading to destruction and diminution of lung parenchyma, fibrosis, and, eventually, respiratory insufficiency.

Disseminated Histoplasmosis. This less common form of histoplasmosis develops primarily in persons with defective host immunity, including infants with immature immune systems; compromised hosts, such as corticosteroid-treated organ recipients and HIV-infected persons; and individuals with either no measurable defect or a highly selective defect, such as the failure of host lymphocytes to undergo in vitro blast transformation upon exposure to *H. capsulatum* antigen. The severity of the symptoms and signs of disseminated disease and the attendant histopathologic findings in a given patient mirror the level of immunocompetence of the individual. For example, in patients with the mildest and most chronic forms of disseminated disease, well-developed tuberculoid granulomas, typical of the response in normal hosts, can be found in reticuloendothelial tissues. In contrast, in patients with overwhelming multiorgan histoplasmosis superimposed on a severely immunocompromising condition, such as AIDS, the host response is suboptimal, with the pathologic findings consisting of large numbers of diffusely scattered macrophages filled with yeast forms and minimal or no granuloma formation.

Fever, chills, and other nonspecific constitutional symptoms, including malaise and weight loss, predominate. On initial presentation, many patients satisfy criteria for fever of unknown origin. Enlargement of the liver and spleen is common; less frequently, peripheral lymphadenopathy is present. Mucous membrane ulceration, especially of the oropharynx, occurs in about 25 to 75 per cent of patients with subacute disease and should alert the physician to the possibility of histoplasmosis. Laboratory clues may include anemia, leukopenia and thrombocytopenia as evidence of impaired bone marrow function or replacement of the marrow, elevated alkaline phosphatase levels, elevated erythrocyte sedimentation rate, and electrolyte abnormalities suggestive of adrenal insufficiency. In some patients, adrenal hypofunction may not be clinically manifest until years later. Chest x-ray films may be normal or show findings suggestive of earlier primary infection or an interstitial pneumonitis consistent with hematogenous spread of infection. Unusual syndromes, including cardiac involvement with culture-negative endocarditis associated with large emboli, gastrointestinal involvement with bleeding secondary to mucosal ulceration, or central nervous system involvement with chronic lymphocytic meningitis, occasionally dominate the clinical course. Cutaneous lesions, manifested by diffusely scattered papulonodules on an erythematous base, and central nervous system disease are more likely in HIV-positive persons. In some AIDS patients, disseminated histoplasmosis represents reactivation of dormant foci, as evidenced by the development of symptoms and signs during a period of residence in a nonendemic area, years after having lived in an endemic region.

Ocular Histoplasmosis. Vision loss associated with the triad of punched-out choroidal lesions or "spots," macular neovascular membranes, and peripapillary atrophy or scarring, in the absence of inflammatory changes in the vitreous or anterior chamber, has been labeled presumed ocular histoplasmosis syndrome (POHS). Although no direct relationship to active ongoing infection with *H. capsulatum* has been established, POHS is believed to represent a localized hypersensitivity response to *Histoplasma* antigen. In almost all instances, the syndrome occurs in young adults with no evidence of pulmonary or disseminated histoplasmosis. Antifungal therapy, either systemic or intraocular, is not indicated. Laser photocoagulation appears to be the most beneficial therapeutic modality to prevent or reduce vision impairment.

DIAGNOSIS. The diagnostic approach varies in part with the clinical syndrome under consideration. Histoplasmosis in many ways resembles tuberculosis and is as clinically diverse in its myriad manifestations. Special features or presentations that should raise suspicion of histoplasmosis include atypical pneumonia syndrome that occurs in a resident of an endemic area, right paratracheal adenopathy, superior vena cava syndrome secondary to adenopathy or a mediastinal mass, an oral ulcer resembling carcinoma, chronic progressive upper lobe cavitation associated with negative sputum smears and cultures for tuberculosis, adrenal insufficiency, "buckshot" calcifications in the lungs or spleen, and persistent unexplained fever in an HIV-infected person. In most instances, diagnosis should be based on demonstration of *H. capsulatum* by culture or by histopathologic study of involved organs. The histoplasmin skin test, while important in epidemiologic studies, is not recommended for diagnostic purposes, owing to the high positivity rate among persons residing in endemic areas. In addition, the skin test may falsely elevate titers of serum antibodies.

Among the three serologic tests to detect serum antibody to *H. capsulatum*, complement fixation is the most widely used. Although a titer of 1:32 or more or a fourfold rise in titer provides presumptive evidence of active infection, a negative or lower titer does not exclude histoplasmosis. Similarly, titers do not parallel disease activity, correlate with response to therapy, or predict outcome. Testing of serum by immunodiffusion to detect precipitin bands to M and H antigens appears to be a more specific but less sensitive serologic method than complement fixation. The presence of both bands, while infrequent, is highly specific, provided the patient has not been previously skin tested with histoplasmin. A positive M band alone is more frequent than a positive H band and is moderately specific. The M band may persist for several years, while the H band usually clears within 6 months; thus, a positive H band signifies active infection. Radioimmunoassay is the most sensitive of the three methods for detection of antibody but is also the least specific. All three methods are associated with frequent false-positive reactions to *Histoplasma* antigens among patients with tuberculosis and other fungal diseases, especially blastomycosis and coccidioidomycosis. Because these cross-reactions are most commonly observed by testing with radioimmunoassay, this methodology for detecting antibody cannot be recommended over complement fixation and immunodiffusion. On the other hand, use of radioimmunoassay to detect *H. capsulatum* polysaccharide antigen in body fluids such as serum and urine appears to provide a relatively sensitive and specific marker of disseminated histoplasmosis. Antigen levels fall with treatment; consequently, this test is useful for both diagnosis and evaluation of response to therapy. At present, the availability of the antigen test is limited because of technical difficulties.

The diagnosis of primary pulmonary histoplasmosis should be suspected on the basis of clinical, radiographic, and epidemiologic clues, e.g., an acute febrile respiratory illness accompanied by scattered patchy infiltrates and hilar adenopathy in an individual with high risk of exposure to *Histoplasma* spores. An elevated complement fixation titer and/or precipitin bands in serum provide presumptive evidence. Whereas sputum cultures are rarely positive (only 10 to 20 per cent) in primary pulmonary disease, the likelihood of positive sputum cultures is significantly higher in chronic pulmonary histoplasmosis. Among patients with chronic disease, about 60 per cent with marching thick-walled cavities have positive cultures, and a significant percentage of these also have positive smears of stained sputum. Although serologic tests for antibody are only moderately helpful (positive results in only 50 per cent of cases), an elevated complement fixation titer in a patient with characteristic radiographic findings provides strong supportive evidence. Definitive diagnosis of chronic pulmonary histoplasmosis must be based on a positive sputum culture or smear or on histopathologic studies and special stains of lung tissue obtained by bronchoscopy.

The diagnosis of disseminated histoplasmosis depends on either demonstration of intracellular yeast forms by histopathologic study or a positive culture of blood, bone marrow, lymph node, skin or mucous membrane, liver, lung, or other involved site. A Wright-stained smear of peripheral blood is positive in more than 50 per cent of acute or subacute cases. If possible, serum and urine should be examined for *H. capsulatum* antigen by radioimmunoassay. The cerebrospinal fluid of patients with chronic unexplained culture-negative lymphocytic meningitis should be tested by complement fixation for antibodies to *H. capsulatum*.

TREATMENT. For most patients with primary pulmonary histoplasmosis, no antifungal therapy is necessary. For those with severe or progressive primary infection, short-course intravenous amphotericin B (a total dose of around 1000 mg) or oral ketoconazole, 400 mg daily for 3 to 6 months, is recommended, although neither therapeutic regimen has been prospectively evaluated in this setting. The treatment of chronic pulmonary histoplasmosis is less standardized, in large part owing to the relative difficulty in clinically and radiologically distinguishing the pneumonitic and cavitary stages of disease. While the early pneumonitic form of chronic pulmonary disease has been reported to resolve spontaneously in 80 per cent of cases, rest and inactivity clearly promote healing. Traditionally, antifungal therapy has been advocated only for patients with progressive or marching cavitary disease, manifested by persistent or enlarging thick-walled cavities larger than 2 mm. Both amphotericin B (total dose, 2.0 to 2.5 grams) and ketoconazole (400 mg daily for at least 6 months) are effective therapy. There may be merit in liberalizing criteria for treatment in patients with chronic pulmonary disease. Rather than reserving therapy only for patients with advanced cavitary disease, some authorities suggest that oral ketoconazole or a newer, better tolerated oral triazole may be indicated for all patients with chronic pulmonary disease, regardless of the stage.

In contrast to the somewhat controversial guidelines regarding therapy for pulmonary histoplasmosis, there is no question that all patients with disseminated histoplasmosis should be treated. For patients with severe, life-threatening disease, immunocompromised hosts, such as organ transplant recipients or corticosteroid-treated patients, and the rare patients with central nervous system or cardiac histoplasmosis, amphotericin B (total dose, 2.0 to 2.5 grams) is the drug of choice. Ketoconazole, 400 mg daily for 6 to 12 months, is an effective alternative in immunocompetent patients with mild to moderate subacute disease. Experience over the past decade with histoplasmosis in AIDS patients indicates that a more aggressive approach to treatment is necessary to prevent relapse. Intensive "induction" therapy with intravenous amphotericin B (total dose, 1.0 to 2.0 grams) is used to gain control of disease and reduce the organism load and is followed by lifelong maintenance or suppressive therapy with either weekly amphotericin B (1 mg per kilogram) or an oral antifungal azole, given daily. Among the azole drugs, itraconazole, an investigational triazole, appears to be the most promising therapy for AIDS patients. Ketoconazole is an inadequate primary or maintenance therapy in patients with AIDS. The approach of initiating therapy with intravenous amphotericin B and completing it with an oral agent may prove applicable to selected other patients with either chronic pulmonary or disseminated histoplasmosis.

The management of mediastinal fibrosis presumed secondary to *H. capsulatum* infection is largely unsatisfactory, as evidenced by progressive morbidity in many patients and a mortality rate of at least 30 per cent. Antifungal chemotherapy is generally not recommended. In selected cases, surgical extirpation may be beneficial in alleviating entrapment or obstructive syndromes.

PROGNOSIS. Although primary pulmonary histoplasmosis may be associated with acute or chronic intrathoracic complications, this form of disease is usually self-limited. In contrast, chronic cavitary pulmonary histoplasmosis is usually progressive, resulting in respiratory insufficiency and death. Disseminated histoplasmosis is variable in its severity and course, depending on the immune status of the host. Although a single course of therapy may be curative in some patients, long-term maintenance therapy to prevent relapse is required in others, especially HIV-positive individuals.

Dismukes WE, Cloud G, Bowles C, et al., National Institute of Allergy and Infectious Diseases Mycoses Study Group: Treatment of blastomycosis and histoplasmosis with ketoconazole: Results of a prospective randomized clinical trial. Ann Intern Med 103:861, 1985. *This study showed that ketoconazole is effective therapy for immunocompetent patients with non–life-threatening, nonmeningeal forms of histoplasmosis.*

Goodwin RA, Owens FT, Snell JD, et al.: Chronic pulmonary histoplasmosis. Medicine (Baltimore) 55:413, 1976. *This monograph, which describes the clinical, radiographic, and pathologic findings in 228 cases, remains the definitive commentary on this complex form of histoplasmosis.*

Loyd JE, Tillman BF, Atkinson JB, et al.: Mediastinal fibrosis complicating histoplasmosis. Medicine (Baltimore) 67:295, 1988. *An excellent review, with emphasis on clinical and radiographic manifestations plus management of this immune-mediated syndrome.*

McKinsey DS, Gupta MR, Riddler SA, et al.: Long-term amphotericin B therapy for disseminated histoplasmosis in patients with the acquired immunodeficiency syndrome (AIDS). Ann Intern Med 111:655, 1989. *A report of the results of amphotericin B treatment in 22 patients, indicating efficacy of long-term maintenance therapy in the prevention of relapse.*

Wheat LJ: Diagnosis and management of histoplasmosis. Eur J Clin Microbiol Infect Dis 8:480, 1989. *A comprehensive, up-to-date review that includes an excellent perspective on the currently available serologic tests used to detect either antibody or antigen; includes 78 references.*

Wheat LJ, Connolly-Stringfield PA, Baker RL, et al.: Disseminated histoplasmosis in the acquired immunodeficiency syndrome: Clinical findings, diagnosis, treatment, and review of the literature. Medicine (Baltimore) 69:361, 1990. *A thorough, thoughtful, and current review that is especially valuable to physicians caring for AIDS patients at risk for histoplasmosis.*

400 Coccidioidomycosis

John N. Galgiani

DEFINITION. Coccidioidomycosis is a systemic infection due to *Coccidioides immitis*, a fungus that is endemic to certain desert regions of the Western Hemisphere.

ETIOLOGY. *C. immitis* is dimorphic, both forms of which grow asexually. Outside humans or other mammalian hosts, mycelia with true septations mature to produce arthroconidia, single-cell structures approximately 2 to 5 μm in length. After infection, an arthroconidium sheds its outer wall and enlarges as spherules, sometimes to as much as 75 μm in diameter, and undergo septation internally to produce scores of endospores. When spherules rupture, packets of endospores are released, and these produce more spherules in infected tissue or revert to mycelia if removed from the body.

EPIDEMIOLOGY. *C. immitis* can be recovered from the soil of the low deserts of Arizona; the Central Valley of California; parts of other states, including New Mexico and Texas; and parts of Central and South America. Endemic regions follow the climatologic Sonoran life zone, which is characterized by modest rainfall, mild winters, and low humidity. In such regions, *C. immitis* grows in a soil layer a few centimeters below the surface, and disruption of the dirt by windstorms or construction equipment increases the release of fungal particles into the air. The risk of sporadic exposure is seasonally more likely in dry periods. Primary infection outside the endemic regions has rarely occurred from exposure to contaminated soil carried on bales of cotton or other fomites. Person-to-person transmission of coccidioidomycosis has not been reported, and isolation precautions for patients are unnecessary.

INCIDENCE AND PREVALENCE. Dermal hypersensitivity to coccidioidal antigens is an indicator of prior infection. The frequency of skin test conversion is approximately 3 per cent per year within strongly endemic areas. This represents a lower estimate than that of 40 years ago, and the change is presumed to be the result of urbanization and the concurrent reduction of exposure to dust. However, in situations where exposure is unusually intense, such as at archeology sites or during military maneuvers within endemic regions, infections can develop in the majority of persons exposed for only a matter of days. The prevalence of reactive coccidioidal skin tests ranges as high as 60 per cent in certain populations, depending upon factors such as age, occupational exposure, and years of residence within the endemic area.

PATHOGENESIS AND PATHOLOGY. Virtually all coccidioidal infections are the result of inhalation of arthroconidia into the lung, and only rarely does direct cutaneous inoculation of the skin occur. Within the small airways, proliferation engenders both acute inflammation, including eosinophils, associated with spherule rupture, and granulomatous inflammation, associated with mature, nonproliferating spherules. Tissue damage results from the consequences of inflammation rather than the elaboration of specific fungal toxins. Focal pneumonia is often associated with ipsilateral hilar adenopathy, and less frequently, infection produces enlargement of peritracheal, supraclavicular, and cervical nodes. Lesions occurring elsewhere are the result of hematogenous dissemination from a pulmonary source and usually develop within months of the initial infection. Although extrapulmonary lesions occur in well below 1 per cent of all those infected, subclinical spread of the fungus beyond the chest may not be rare, since as many as 8 per cent of persons with self-limited infection are left with chorioretinal scars. In most persons, immunity develops within weeks after infection, arresting fungal proliferation and allowing inflammation to resolve. Despite apparent control of the infection, immunity may not sterilize lesions, and *C. immitis* may persist for long periods in a dormant state. The precise mechanisms responsible for these events are not understood but require competent T lymphocytes. Reactivation of dormant infection or second infections are infrequent, except in patients whose cell-mediated immunity becomes deficient.

CLINICAL MANIFESTATIONS. Two of every three infections are subclinical and are detectable by finding dermal hypersensitivity to coccidioidal antigens. Those who become ill usually experience a self-limited pulmonary syndrome. However, a minority of patients develop complications or progressive forms of infection that display a broad variety of manifestations and pose difficult problems for the clinician.

Primary Pulmonary Infections. Five to 21 days after exposure, symptoms develop; these may include fever, weight loss, fatigue, a dry cough, or pleuritic chest pain, and they are difficult to differentiate from those caused by other respiratory pathogens. Arthralgias without associated joint effusions are also frequent. Skin manifestations may also occur as a short-lived nonpruritic maculopapular rash, erythema multiforme, or erythema nodosum. The arthritic and dermatologic manifestations are thought to be mediated by circulating immune complexes or other immunologic phenomena and are referred to as "desert rheumatism." Roentgenographs of the chest may show no abnormalities or may demonstrate pulmonary infiltrates, either segmental or lobar. Hilar adenopathy is often a distinctive finding. Peripneumonic pleural effusions may occur and usually resolve without intervention, even though *C. immitis* is usually recoverable from the pleura. Eosinophilia is frequently a prominent finding in differential leukocyte counts of peripheral blood, and the erythrocyte sedimentation rate is usually elevated. Symptoms may persist for several weeks before improvement is clearly under way, and the illness, especially lassitude, may persist for months.

The primary pulmonary process produces a variety of sequelae. The most frequent is the development of a pulmonary nodule (Fig. 400–1*A* and *B*), typically measuring 1 to 4 cm and lying

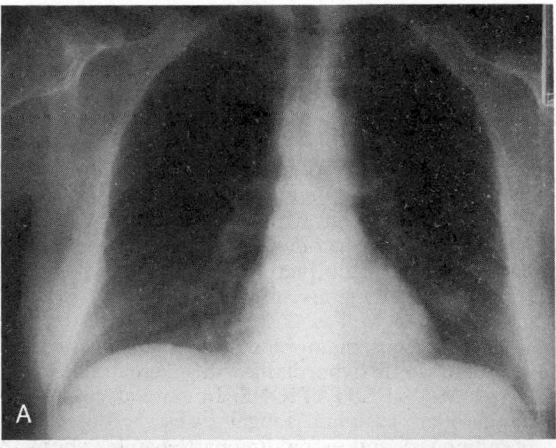

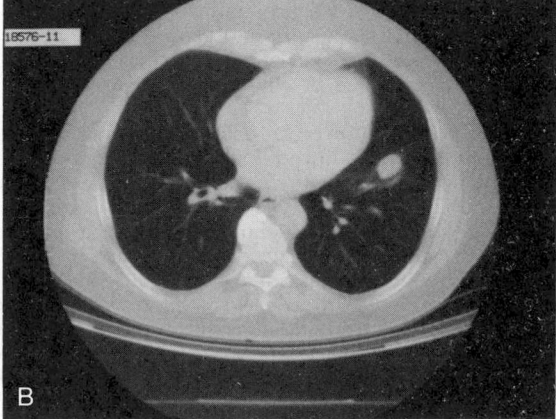

FIGURE 400–1. *A,* Benign nodule due to coccidioidomycosis. *B,* Computed tomographic (CT) image of the nodule shown in *A.*

within 5 cm of the hilus. Despite their harmless nature, coccidioidal nodules may engender concern because of their similarity to a malignant mass. For this reason, management usually requires percutaneous needle aspiration or resection. Another consequence of pulmonary coccidioidomycosis is cavitation of the infiltrate, which occurs in approximately 5 per cent of pneumonias. Cavities are usually single, thin walled, in an upper lobe, and close to the pleura; they may cause pain, produce hemoptysis, or develop associated infiltrates. Infrequently, a cavity ruptures, forming a pyopneumothorax. This usually is the first symptom of coccidioidal infection and commonly occurs in otherwise healthy young males. An air-fluid level, detectable by roentgenography in the pleural space, often helps differentiate this problem from a spontaneous pneumothorax. Surgical resection of the cavity with closure of the bronchopleural fistula is the preferred treatment for this complication. The least common pulmonary complication is persistent fibrocavitary infection that progresses from one lobe to another, involving both lungs.

Extrapulmonary Dissemination. Coccidioidomycosis usually results in dissemination beyond the lungs in immunosuppressed patients, such as organ recipients or those with acquired immunodeficiency syndrome (AIDS) or lymphoma. However, some patients have no underlying disease and do not manifest heightened susceptibility to other infections. The most common locations for disseminated lesions are skin (cutaneous papules or subcutaneous nodules); joints (especially the knee); bones, including vertebrae; and the basilar meninges. Such infections may produce one or many lesions and frequently are subacute or chronic in their presentation. When infections are more fulminant, they are usually in broadly immunosuppressed patients and produce fungemia detectable with blood cultures and diffuse reticulonodular embolic pulmonary infiltrates. Although the kidneys and the urinary bladder are rarely involved, *C. immitis* may be recovered from concentrated specimens of urine, because of either transient fungemia or focal dissemination to the prostate. In contrast to histoplasmosis, the gastrointestinal tract is rarely involved in coccidioidomycosis.

DIAGNOSIS. The diagnosis is firmly established by recovering *C. immitis* from clinical specimens. Growth of the fungus is supported by most routinely available microbiology media and may be evident by the first week of incubation. Spherules can be seen as large structures with doubly refractile walls and internal organization in KOH preparations or cytologic stains of respiratory secretions and also on hematoxylin-eosin, silver, or periodic acid–Schiff stains of histologic preparations. The Gram stain does not detect spherules. Except in the case of coccidioidal meningitis, in which positive cerebrospinal fluid (CSF) cultures are usually negative, isolation of the fungus is nearly always possible in patients with infections sufficiently severe to warrant therapy. In contrast, recovery of *C. immitis* may be difficult in patients who have only scant respiratory secretions associated with the initial pneumonia.

The presumptive diagnosis of coccidioidal infection is often based on detecting specific antibodies in serum. Within the first weeks of initial infection and occasionally with recurrent infections, a precipitin-type antibody is detected, usually by immunodiffusion techniques. Later in the course of infection, complement fixing (CF)–type antibodies are often detected. When reported quantitatively, CF antibodies generally are found to be highest in the most extensive infections and decrease in concentration in patients whose infections are controlled. An important means of diagnosing coccidioidal meningitis is by detection of CF antibodies in the CSF, along with other abnormalities, such as leukocytosis, elevated protein concentration, or low glucose concentration.

TREATMENT. Treatment has been limited to those with more serious forms of coccidioidal infection, since the primary pneumonia is usually self-limited, and until recently, amphotericin B was the only antifungal drug available. Amphotericin B has been used successfully in cumulative doses of 1.0 to 3.0 grams for treating all types of coccidioidomycosis. However, it has not been uniformly effective and frequently has produced treatment-limiting morbidity and toxicity. Treatment of coccidioidal meningitis has necessitated intrathecal administration, which imposes additional toxicity and risks. Binding amphotericin

B in liposomes or lipid complexes has been explored as a means of improving the therapeutic to toxic profile. However, to date, such efforts have been hindered by difficulties in producing stable, uniform material for clinical trials and hence remain investigative.

During the past 15 years, azole antifungals have been extensively studied as alternative therapy for coccidioidomycosis. Miconazole was found to be effective, but its use has necessitated multiple daily parenteral administrations, and frequent relapses were found upon cessation of therapy. Ketoconazole has also been found to be effective and is administered orally. However, absorption is variable; gastrointestinal intolerance is frequent; dose-dependent hormonal suppression and gynecomastia occur in some patients, especially at dosages above 400 mg per day; and as with miconazole, relapses after stopping therapy remain a significant limitation. Currently, triazoles such as itraconazole and fluconazole are under investigation and show promise. Although these agents appear nearly identical in terms of their mechanism of action, they differ significantly in their metabolism and disposition. Fluconazole achieves CSF concentrations approximately 80 per cent of that in serum during chronic therapy, and this finding has prompted hopes that triazole antifungals may be useful therapy for coccidioidal meningitis. It is not known if the use of ketoconazole or any other oral agent shortens the course of the primary coccidioidal pneumonia or changes the likelihood of later complications.

PROGNOSIS. After resolution of the initial untreated infection, most patients maintain lifelong immunity, and second infections are very infrequent. Similarly, late recurrence is unlikely in the absence of intercurrent profound immunosuppression. The disease in those who are unable to resolve the initial infection frequently follows a protracted course. Although infection is more debilitating than fatal, fulminant respiratory failure can occur, and if untreated, coccidioidal meningitis is nearly always fatal within 2 years.

Ampel NM, Wieden MA, Galgiani JN: Coccidioidomycosis: Clinical update. Rev Infect Dis 11:897, 1989. *Major review of recent literature of coccidioidomycosis. A previous comprehensive review was Drutz DJ, Catanzaro A: Coccidioidomycosis. State of the art. Am Rev Respir Dis 117:559, 727, 1978.*

Fish DG, Ampel NM, Galgiani JN, et al.: Coccidioidomycosis during human immunodeficiency virus (HIV) infection: A retrospective review of 77 patients. Medicine (Baltimore) 69:384, 1990. *In Arizona, coccidioidomycosis is the third most common opportunistic infection in patients with AIDS. Manifestations are usually severe in patients with CD4 counts less than 0.250 × 10⁶ cells per liter.*

Graybill JR, Stevens DA, Galgiani JN, et al.: Itraconazole treatment of coccidioidomycosis. Am J Med 89:282, 1990. *Itraconazole is the first of several triazole antifungals likely to prove effective for the treatment of coccidioidomycosis.*

Labadie EK, Hamilton RH: Survival improvement in coccidioidal meningitis by high-dose intrathecal amphotericin B. Arch Intern Med 146:2013, 1986. *Cure of coccidioidal meningitis with intrathecally administered amphotericin B appears to be more likely if higher doses are given. This report antedates more recent experience using suppressive therapy with oral triazole antifungal agents such as fluconazole.*

Pappagianis D, Zimmer BL: Serology of coccidioidomycosis. Clin Microb Rev 3:247, 1990. *Authoritative review of serologic testing in relation to the clinical manifestations of coccidioidomycosis.*

401 Blastomycosis

William E. Dismukes

DEFINITION. Blastomycosis (North American blastomycosis, Gilchrist's disease) is an endemic systemic mycosis that occurs primarily in noncompromised hosts. As with the other important endemic mycoses, such as coccidioidomycosis and histoplasmosis, infection follows inhalation of the aerosolized spore form of the fungus. Clinical disease most commonly involves the lungs, skin, skeletal system, and male genitourinary tract.

ETIOLOGY. *Blastomyces dermatitidis*, the imperfect or asexual stage of *Ajellomyces dermatitidis*, is a dimorphic fungus, growing as a mycelial form in the environment and in the laboratory at room temperature and as a yeast form in mammalian tissue and in the laboratory at 37°C. The yeast cells, which are identical in vitro and in vivo in tissue and fluid specimens, vary from 8 to 15 μm in diameter, have a thick, highly refractile cell wall, and reproduce by single broad-based buds. In the laboratory, growth of *B. dermatitidis* is somewhat slow; mold colonies may not appear for 1 to 3 weeks.

EPIDEMIOLOGY. Because no sensitive and specific skin test exists, the epidemiology of blastomycosis is less well understood than that of coccidioidomycosis and histoplasmosis. The incidence of clinical disease as a manifestation of blastomycosis appears to be lower than the incidence of clinical disease associated with the two other endemic mycoses. The prevalence of subclinical blastomycosis is largely unknown. Isolated cases of blastomycosis have been reported worldwide, including Africa and Central and South America; however, the disease is concentrated or endemic in the South and North Central United States, especially in areas bordering the Mississippi and Ohio River basins, and the Great Lakes. In these endemic areas, small point-source outbreaks of blastomycosis have been associated with recreational or occupational activities occurring in wooded areas along waterways. Current evidence indicates that *B. dermatitidis* exists in warm, moist soil enriched by organic debris, including decaying vegetation or wood. It is not surprising, therefore, that persons with occupational or avocational exposure to soil and the outdoors appear to be at highest risk of acquiring infection. Data from point-source outbreaks indicate that the median incubation period from exposure to infection is about 43 days. Animals, especially dogs and horses, are also susceptible to infection, which may progress to clinical disease. Among humans, clinical illness is most common among middle-aged men. *Blastomyces dermatitidis*, in contrast to the other dimorphic fungi, rarely is an opportunistic pathogen in immunosuppressed hosts, e.g., human immunodeficiency virus (HIV)–infected individuals. This observation and other limited data suggest that reactivation blastomycosis is uncommon.

PATHOGENESIS AND PATHOLOGY. Humans and animals, for the most part, acquire infection by inhalation of aerosolized conidia that convert to the yeast form in the lungs at body temperature. Percutaneous inoculation of *B. dermatitidis* has been documented rarely, as a result of either a laboratory accident or a dog bite. The clinical manifestations of disease at body sites other than lung (and rarely skin) result from the hematogenous spread of organisms.

Cell-mediated immunity appears to be the most important arm of host defense against *B. dermatitidis*. Recent in vivo and in vitro studies indicate that macrophages, stimulated by lymphokines, are more effective in inhibiting or killing the organism than are granulocytes. A growth-inhibiting or protective role of humoral immunity in blastomycosis has not been established. The typical histopathologic picture of pulmonary blastomycosis and other nonmucocutaneous sites of disease consists of noncaseating granulomas as well as clusters of neutrophils. By contrast, cutaneous and mucous membrane lesions are characterized by pseudoepitheliomatous hyperplasia with microabscesses.

CLINICAL MANIFESTATIONS. In general, blastomycosis is a chronic indolent systemic fungal disease associated with a variety of pulmonary and extrapulmonary manifestations. Among the latter, cutaneous disease predominates, occurring in about 40 to 80 per cent of cases. Multiple organ involvement occurs in approximately 50 to 60 per cent of cases. Extrapulmonary disease may occur in the absence of clinical or radiologic evidence of lung disease.

Pulmonary. Although precise data are not available, most primary infections are believed to be either asymptomatic or unrecognized as being due to *B. dermatitidis* on the basis of nonspecific flulike symptoms. In patients with proven acute pulmonary blastomycosis, the radiologic findings usually consist of infiltrative or nodular air space opacities, most often in the lower lobes. Pulmonary blastomycosis usually manifests as a chronic pneumonia syndrome, characterized by productive cough, pleuritic chest pain, hemoptysis, weight loss, and low-grade fever. Although there are no distinguishing radiologic characteristics, one or more fibronodular infiltrates or mass lesions with or without cavitation are common, often mimicking the findings in other granulomatous diseases or bronchogenic carcinoma. Although hilar adenopathy and pleural effusions occur, they are uncommon. Rarely, patients with fulminant hematogenous dissemination may develop a miliary pattern on the chest radiograph and clinical evidence of acute respiratory distress syndrome.

Skin. The cutaneous lesions, which often prompt the patient with blastomycosis to seek medical evaluation initially, are of two general types, verrucous and ulcerative; both types tend to occur more commonly on exposed parts. The verrucous lesions, which begin as papulopustules, are more characteristic; these progress slowly over weeks to months to become crusted, heaped-up, and warty in appearance, often with a reddish-black or violaceous hue, an area of central healing and scarring, and a well-circumscribed outer border. Microabscesses, manifested by black dots on the surface, are typically located at the periphery of verrucous lesions; removal of the crusted eschar often reveals purulent material in which the yeast form of the organism can be demonstrated by wet preparation. Ulcerative lesions overlying a bed of friable red granulation tissue are less common. Occasionally, mucosal ulcerations may be found in the mouth, nose, or larynx, mimicking the mucocutaneous lesions of histoplasmosis. Lymphadenopathy in the region corresponding to the skin lesion or lesions is distinctly uncommon in patients whose cutaneous disease is secondary to hematogenous spread of organisms from a primary pulmonary focus.

Other. After lung and skin disease, bone and joint involvement is next most common and is seen in 10 to 50 per cent of cases. Osteolytic lesions, with or without sclerotic margins, are typically located in long bones and vertebrae. Often, patients with bone disease present as a result of overlying chronic draining sinuses or contiguous soft tissue lesions rather than bone pain. Septic arthritis, which is much less common than osteomyelitis, is frequently secondary to contiguous extension. Up to one third of men with blastomycosis have genitourinary tract disease, manifested most commonly by prostatic enlargement with obstructive symptoms and less frequently by epididymitis. Central nervous system disease in the form of either granulomatous meningitis or a mass lesion (intracerebral blastomycoma) occurs in fewer than 5 per cent of cases. Clinically apparent blastomycotic involvement of other organs, e.g., gastrointestinal tract, liver, spleen, adrenals, and kidneys, is unusual, except in patients with fulminant disseminated disease.

DIAGNOSIS. As is true for all systemic mycotic diseases, the definitive diagnosis of blastomycosis requires a positive fungal culture from clinical specimens. A presumptive diagnosis may be based on the finding of characteristic yeast forms in a wet preparation of sputum, pus, or other body fluid or in a histopathologic section of tissue, e.g., skin, lung, bone, or prostate. *Blastomyces dermatitidis* in wet preparations of fluid specimens mixed with 10 per cent KOH appears as a broad-based single budding yeast and in fixed-tissue specimens stained with hematoxylineosin or periodic acid–Schiff (PAS) reagents as single or budding yeast cells with a doubly refractile cell wall. Because a presumptive clinical diagnosis based on "characteristic" skin lesions or radiologic findings is associated with an unacceptably high error rate, obtaining fluids or tissue from involved sites for culture and histopathologic study is mandatory in the evaluation of all patients with suspected blastomycosis. Moreover, documented cutaneous and/or pulmonary disease should signal the possibility of bone or genitourinary disease and lead to appropriate diagnostic studies, such as bone scan and prostate examination and massage. As a diagnostic test, the blastomycin skin test lacks sensitivity and specificity and should not be used. Similarly, the complement fixation assay for serum antibody is highly cross-reactive and of no diagnostic value. Recent studies suggest that immunodiffusion or enzyme immunoassay tests for the A antigen of *B. dermatitidis* have potential as serologic markers of disease.

TREATMENT. At present, two drugs, amphotericin B and ketoconazole, are approved for the treatment of blastomycosis. Although intravenous amphotericin B has been traditionally considered the drug of choice for all forms of disease, studies and experience gained over the past decade indicate that oral ketoconazole is highly effective, especially in patients with chronic indolent disease and noninvolvement of the central nervous system. Oral ketoconazole should be initiated at a dosage of 400 mg per day, advanced by 200-mg increments at monthly intervals, up to a maximum of 800 mg per day in patients with progressive disease, and continued for a minimum of 6 months. Amphotericin B, a total dose of 1.5 to 2.5 grams, should be reserved for patients with overwhelming life-threatening or central nervous system disease, those rare patients who are immunocompromised, and those in whom ketoconazole has failed. In selected situations, some investigators advocate an induction course of amphotericin B (total dose of approximately 500 mg) for a rapid fungicidal effect to gain control of disease, followed by maintenance or "consolidation" therapy with ketoconazole for 3 to 6 months. Newer oral antifungal azoles, such as itraconazole and fluconazole, show promise and appear to be less toxic than ketoconazole. Although controversy exists about whether or not to treat patients with acute pulmonary blastomycosis who are identified as part of point-source outbreaks, available data suggest that most such patients do not require therapy. However, careful long-term follow-up of untreated patients is important to monitor for evidence of disease activity.

PROGNOSIS. In contrast to the past, now most patients with blastomycosis are identified and treated before the development of overwhelming or fatal disease. Both amphotericin B and ketoconazole are associated with cure rates of 80 per cent or better and relapse rates of less than 10 per cent. Relapse in a few ketoconazole-treated patients has been manifested by either central nervous system or genitourinary disease, not surprising in view of the poor penetration of ketoconazole into cerebrospinal fluid and the low level of active drug in urine.

Bradsher RW: Blastomycosis. Infect Dis Clin North Am 2:877, 1988. *A comprehensive, up-to-date review, with a nice perspective on treatment and 116 references.*

Dismukes WE, Cloud G, Bowles C, et al., National Institute of Allergy and Infectious Disease Mycoses Study Group: Treatment of blastomycosis and histoplasmosis with ketoconazole: Results of a prospective randomized clinical trial. Ann Intern Med 103:861, 1985. *Results of this study of 80 patients with blastomycosis indicate that ketoconazole is effective therapy for immunocompetent patients with non–life-threatening, nonmeningeal disease.*

Klein BS, Vergeront JM, Davis JP: Epidemiologic aspects of blastomycosis, the enigmatic systemic mycosis. Semin Respir Infect 1:29, 1986. *A valuable review that focuses on seven point-source epidemics and the ecologic niche of the organism.*

Sarosi GA, Davies SF, Phillips JR: Self-limited blastomycosis: A report of 30 cases. Semin Respir Infect 1:40, 1986. *This study provides evidence that acute pulmonary blastomycosis in most patients resolves spontaneously without therapy and with no sequelae.*

402 Paracoccidioidomycosis

William E. Dismukes

DEFINITION. Paracoccidioidomycosis is a chronic granulomatous disease typically involving the lungs, skin, mucous membranes, and lymph nodes and limited to an endemic area extending from Mexico south to Argentina.

ETIOLOGY. The causative agent, *Paracoccidioides brasiliensis*, is a dimorphic fungus that grows as a mycelial form in nature and as an oval or round yeast form in tissues or at 37°C. Identification of characteristic multiple budding or "pilot wheel," thick-walled yeast cells, 10 to 40 μm in diameter, in tissue provides presumptive evidence of disease. Because the organism grows slowly on primary isolation, fungal cultures should be held for at least 4 weeks before discarding.

EPIDEMIOLOGY. Most cases occur in persons living in or with a history of prior exposure to southern Mexico, Central America, or South America; in these areas, paracoccidioidomycosis is the most common systemic mycosis. Owing to the long period of latency, overt disease may develop in persons many years after they have left the endemic region. Infection is acquired via inhalation of spores. Neither human-to-human transmission nor common-source outbreaks have been documented. The majority of cases occur in adult males, especially those who labor in the outdoors. The preponderance of cases in men may also be related to the observation that estrogens inhibit the mycelium-to-yeast transformation of the organism. Although cases have been reported in compromised hosts, in general, paracoccidioidomycosis is not considered an opportunistic fungal disease.

PATHOGENESIS AND PATHOLOGY. After inhalation of

spores, infection may remain confined to the lungs or may spread by lymphohematogenous dissemination to multiple organs. The host pathologic response caused by *P. brasiliensis* is similar to that caused by tissue invasion with *Blastomyces dermatitidis* and *Coccidioides immitis*, i.e., both granulomas and suppuration may develop. The type of tissue pathology and the spectrum of clinical disease are in large part dictated by the integrity of the cell-mediated defenses of the host.

CLINICAL MANIFESTATIONS. Pulmonary paracoccidioidomycosis may be asymptomatic or result in symptomatic acute or chronic disease. Whereas the acute form of pulmonary paracoccidioidomycosis is usually nonspecific and indistinguishable from other influenza-like illnesses, the clinical and radiographic features of the chronic form often resemble those of chronic pulmonary coccidioidomycosis. Any or all lobes may be infected, but the upper lobes tend to be less frequently involved. In addition, cavities, if present, are usually small (so-called microcavities). Extrapulmonary disease, especially in persons less than 30 years old, may be acute in onset, is often manifested by lymphadenopathy and hepatosplenomegaly, and carries a poor prognosis. More typically, extrapulmonary disease in older adults is an indolent illness, manifested by oropharyngeal and laryngeal mucous membrane ulcers; verrucous, ulcerative, or nodular skin lesions, often on the face or mucocutaneous borders; and enlarged or necrotic, draining lymph nodes, especially in the cervical region. Other sites of less frequent involvement are the gastrointestinal tract, adrenal glands, testes, epididymis, and skeletal system. Central nervous system and eye disease secondary to *P. brasiliensis* are rare. A few cases of paracoccidioidomycosis have been observed in human immunodeficiency virus (HIV)–infected persons.

DIAGNOSIS. Demonstration of the characteristic "pilot wheel," multiple-budding *P. brasiliensis* yeast cells by wet mounts or KOH preparations of sputum, pus, or other body fluids or by special fungal stains of biopsy or cell-block specimens provides presumptive evidence of paracoccidioidomycosis. A positive culture of body fluid or tissue specimens is diagnostic. Two different serologic tests (agar gel immunodiffusion and complement fixation) are available through the Centers for Disease Control in Atlanta. Precipitin bands appear early in the course of active infection and may persist for years, even after successful therapy. Complement-fixing antibodies appear later and are more useful in evaluating response to treatment. Both tests have high specificity. Alternative serologic tests, including enzyme-linked immunosorbent assay (ELISA) and counterimmunoelectrophoresis (CIE) as well as newer ones for detection of a 43-kD glycoprotein antigen and for antibodies to this antigen, are under investigation. Skin tests have no role in diagnosis.

TREATMENT. In the past, oral sulfonamides were the mainstay of therapy; however, these have two major drawbacks, namely, a high rate of relapse even after prolonged suppression therapy and a high frequency of adverse reactions, especially skin rashes. Intravenous amphotericin B is effective therapy and is usually employed for more severe forms of paracoccidioidomycosis, such as pulmonary or disseminated multiorgan disease, and for more refractory cases. Follow-up chronic suppression therapy with sulfonamides is recommended. Oral antifungal azole drugs represent a significant advance in the treatment of this disease. Ketoconazole, an imidazole, is highly effective in both in vivo animal models and humans. Cure is usually achieved with dosages of 200 to 400 mg per day, given for at least 1 year. Recent trials indicate that itraconazole, a triazole, given in a dosage of 50 to 100 mg daily for 6 to 12 months, is as effective as ketoconazole and better tolerated. Because of the tropism of *P. brasiliensis* for the adrenal glands and the possibility of adrenal insufficiency during active disease or even after discontinuation of therapy, periodic tests of adrenal function are recommended.

PROGNOSIS. Untreated disseminated paracoccidioidomycosis is generally fatal. In general, the more common indolent forms of adult disease, usually associated with reactivation, are amenable to prolonged therapy, given over months to years.

Franco M: Host-parasite relationships in paracoccidioidomycosis. J Med Vet Mycol 25:5, 1987. *A thorough discussion of virulence factors, mechanisms of host defense, and granuloma morphogenesis, with 71 references.*

Naranjo MS, Trujillo M, Munera MI, et al.: Treatment of paracoccidioidomycosis with itraconazole. J Med Vet Mycol 28:67, 1990. *Forty-five of 47 patients had the chronic form of disease. Itraconazole, 100 mg per day, given for a mean duration of 6 months, was highly effective, as measured by radiographic and cultural responses, falling serologic titers, and improvement in clinical severity scores.*

Negroni R, Palmieri O, Koren F, et al.: Oral treatment of paracoccidioidomycosis and histoplasmosis with itraconazole in humans. Rev Infect Dis 9 (Suppl 1):S47, 1987. *Another study demonstrating the efficacy of itraconazole in 25 patients with paracoccidioidomycosis.*

Restreppo A, Robledo M, Giraldo R, et al.: The gamut of paracoccidioidomycosis. Am J Med 61:33, 1976. *An older review with emphasis on pulmonary and extrapulmonary manifestations.*

Sugar AM: Paracoccidioidomycosis. Infect Dis Clin North Am 2:913, 1988. *A recent comprehensive review.*

403 Cryptococcosis

William E. Dismukes

DEFINITION. Cryptococcosis is a systemic mycosis that most often involves the lungs and central nervous system and, less frequently, the skin, skeletal system, and prostate gland. *Cryptococcus neoformans*, the causative organism, is the most common etiologic agent of fungal meningitis, and since the onset of the acquired immunodeficiency syndrome (AIDS) epidemic in the early 1980's, it has been increasingly recognized as an opportunistic fungal pathogen.

ETIOLOGY. *Cryptococcus neoformans* is a yeastlike round or oval fungus, 4 to 6 μm in diameter, which is surrounded by a polysaccharide capsule and reproduces by budding. There are four different serotypes—A, B, C and D—based on the antigenic specificity of the capsule; biochemical differences also exist in serotypes. Nomenclature of the perfect or sexual states is based on mating properties. For example, serotypes A and D, which include the majority of clinical isolates, can be mated to produce the perfect state (*Filobasidiella neoformans* var. *neoformans*). In the laboratory on solid media, *C. neoformans* grows at 37°C as smooth yellow or tan colonies, usually within a week after inoculation. By contrast, nonpathogenic *Cryptococcus* species do not grow at 37°C. Other characteristics used to distinguish *C. neoformans* from nonpathogenic species include no pseudomycelial growth on cornmeal or rice-Tween agar, glucose assimilation but not fermentation, use of creatinine as a nitrogen source, and production of melanin and urease.

EPIDEMIOLOGY. Cryptococcosis is worldwide in distribution. Serotypes A and D are found in soil and other environmental areas, especially those contaminated by pigeon droppings; pigeons themselves are not infected. Less is known about the ecologic niche of serotypes B and C. Although humans and animals acquire infection after inhalation of aerosolized spores, clusters of cases or mini-outbreaks of cyptococcosis rarely occur, as they do in aerosol-transmitted mycoses such as blastomycosis and histoplasmosis. Animal-to-human and human-to-human transmission of cryptococcosis has not been documented, with one exception; active cryptococcosis in a corneal transplant donor is believed to have resulted in cryptococcal endophthalmitis in the recipient. There is no obvious age, sex, or occupational predilection. Conditions or factors that predispose to cryptococcosis include corticosteroid therapy, lymphoreticular malignancies (especially Hodgkin's disease), sarcoidosis (even in the absence of corticosteroid therapy), human immunodeficiency virus (HIV) infection, and perhaps diabetes mellitus (data are conflicting). The association of cryptococcosis and organ transplantation probably relates in large part to immunosuppression with corticosteroids. Cyclosporine, at least in a murine model, inhibits growth of *C. neoformans*. Among HIV-positive individuals, the incidence of cryptococcosis varies from 5 to 10 per cent, and *C. neoformans* ranks in frequency behind only *Pneumocystis carinii*, cytomegalovirus, and mycobacteria as an opportunistic systemic pathogen in this high-risk population group. Although cryptococcosis frequently occurs in immunosuppressed hosts, approximately one third of patients with the disease have no apparent underlying condition or predisposing factor.

PATHOGENESIS AND PATHOLOGY. After inhalation of aerosolized spores, most infections begin with an asymptomatic pulmonary focus. Subsequently, hematogenous spread to extrapulmonary organs occurs. Initially, neutrophils and, later, monocytes clear cryptococci from inflammatory sites. Phagocytosis by neutrophils and macrophages is mediated in part by complement, interferon, and other T cell–derived lymphokines. Cryptococcal polysaccharide capsule is a major virulence factor and may be immunosuppressive, induce T-suppressor cells, suppress both specific and nonspecific antibody response, inhibit phagocytosis, and impair migration of leukocytes. Paradoxically, cryptococcal polysaccharide has also been shown to activate the alternative complement pathway. In general, immunity depends on functioning, sensitized T cells and an intact cell-mediated arm of host defense. Consequently, patients with defective or altered T cell immunity, such as those with HIV infection, are highly susceptible to infection with *C. neoformans* and progressive disease. The preferential involvement of *C. neoformans* for the central nervous system is explained partially by the absence of complement and soluble anticryptococcal factors (present in normal serum) in normal cerebrospinal fluid (CSF), as well as a decreased to absent inflammatory response to cryptococci in brain tissue. As a result, well-formed granulomas are generally absent in histopathologic sections of infected tissue. The characteristic lesion in cryptococcal meningoencephalitis consists of cystic clusters of fungi; the basal ganglia and the cortical gray matter are the sites of heaviest involvement. In other organs such as the lung, the inflammatory response varies in intensity from minimal to heavy and consists of an array of cells, including organism-containing macrophages, giant cells, plasma cells, and lymphocytes. No necrosis is present, and tissue is usually displaced by multiplying organisms. Yeastlike cryptococci with characteristic narrow-based buds stain poorly with hematoxylin-eosin but are easily visualized with Gomori methenamine silver (GMS) or periodic acid–Schiff (PAS) stains. Mucicarmine stain further aids in identification by giving a rose color to the polysaccharide capsule.

CLINICAL MANIFESTATIONS

Pulmonary Cryptococcosis. The pattern of pulmonary cryptococcal infection is highly variable, ranging from the extremes of saprophytic airway colonization without clinical or radiographic evidence of disease to full-blown acute respiratory distress syndrome in compromised hosts, such as AIDS patients. More typically, radiographic findings include either patchy pneumonitis or solitary or multiple small nodules in asymptomatic persons or those with mild to moderate symptoms, e.g., fever, malaise, cough, scant sputum, pleuritic pain, or rarely hemoptysis. Although tumor-like masses mimicking carcinoma are not uncommon, cavitation and pleural effusions are less likely. The course of pulmonary cryptococcosis is also variable. In patients with normal host defenses, spontaneous regression of both clinical and radiographic manifestations is the rule, although chronic stable infection is known to occur. In contrast, pulmonary cryptococcosis in immunocompromised patients is more likely to progress and therefore requires antifungal therapy. Pulmonary disease may occur in the absence of extrapulmonary cryptococcosis, and, conversely, extrapulmonary disease, such as meningitis, may develop in the absence of apparent lung involvement.

Central Nervous System Cryptococcosis. Meningitis, usually subacute or chronic in nature, is the most common manifestation of central nervous system (CNS) cryptococcosis. Complications include hydrocephalus, encephalitis, involvement of the optic pathways, brain stem vasculitis, and mass lesions (cryptococcomas) of the brain parenchyma or spinal cord. The clinical presentation and course of cryptococcal meningitis vary greatly, related in part to the underlying condition and immune status of the host. In "normal" hosts, the onset is usually insidious, whereas in compromised hosts, such as HIV-infected or corticosteroid-treated patients, the onset tends to be more acute and the course more rapidly progressive. The most common symptoms are headache and alteration in mental status, e.g., confusion, lethargy, obtundation or coma, and personality change. Nausea and vomiting are frequent; fever and stiff neck are less common. Ocular symptoms, such as blurred vision, photophobia, vision loss, and diplopia, secondary to perineuritic adhesive arachnoiditis, papilledema, optic nerve neuritis, chorioretinitis, or retino-

vitreal abscess, are present in 30 to 50 per cent of patients. Other findings include hearing deficits, seizures, ataxia, aphasia, and choreoathetoid movements. Dementia is important to recognize as a potential sequela, since it may be curable. Because cryptococcomas reportedly accompany cryptococcal meningitis in as many as 20 per cent of cases, an imaging study (computed tomography [CT] or magnetic resonance imaging [MRI]) should be considered in the evaluation of all patients. Rarely, CNS cryptococcomas can be seen in the absence of meningeal disease. The mortality rate varies from 20 to 30 per cent; most deaths occur in the first 6 weeks of illness in patients with fulminant deterioration.

Miscellaneous. After the lungs and CNS, the next most commonly involved organs in patients with disseminated cryptococcosis are the skin and skeletal system. Cutaneous manifestations occur in 10 to 15 per cent of cases and usually take the form of papules, pustules, nodules, ulcers, or draining sinuses. Typically, cellulitis with prominent erythema and induration is seen in corticosteroid-treated transplant recipients, and umbilicated papules resembling molluscum contagiosum are observed in AIDS patients. Oral mucosal chancres have been reported rarely. Osteomyelitis is more common than septic arthritis. Less commonly involved sites of cryptococcal disease include pericardium, myocardium, muscle, liver, peritoneum, adrenal glands, kidneys, and prostate gland. Infections of these organs are being increasingly identified in AIDS patients. For example, the prostate has been reported to be a nidus of residual infection in this population group.

DIAGNOSIS. As with other systemic mycoses, the definitive diagnosis of cryptococcosis depends on demonstration of the characteristic yeastlike organism with its surrounding capsule in tissue or fluid obtained from involved sites, together with cultural confirmation. In addition, in patients with suspected cryptococcosis, the latex agglutination test for detection of cryptococcal polysaccharide antigen in serum and CSF is an extremely important adjunct to diagnosis, unlike the situation for most other fungal diseases, in which serologic tests lack specificity and sensitivity. Cryptococcal antigen is found in CSF in more than 90 per cent and in serum in about 75 per cent of patients with meningitis, especially if serial specimens are examined over time. Titers are particularly high in patients with AIDS. In patients with extraneural cryptococcal disease, antigen is detected in only 25 to 50 per cent of cases. Proper controls are necessary to eliminate rheumatoid factor, which may give rise to a false-positive result. Serum of patients with disseminated infection caused by *Trichosporon beigelii* may also test positive for cryptococcal antigen. False-negative tests for cryptococcal antigen may be due to low numbers of cryptococcal organisms invading tissue or in CSF, unencapsulated or poorly encapsulated strains, or a prozone phenomenon. Tests for cryptococcal antibody are not useful for diagnosis.

Pulmonary cryptococcosis is difficult to diagnose in most cases without obtaining lung tissue via bronchoscopy or open lung biopsy. Wet preparations of sputum are only occasionally helpful, and sputum cultures are positive for *C. neoformans* in only 20 per cent of cases. In patients with pleural effusions, test of the fluid for cryptococcal antigen may be positive, thereby obviating a more invasive procedure. In every patient with established pulmonary cryptococcosis, a lumbar puncture should be performed, whether or not CNS disease is apparent. Blood cultures and tissue for culture and histopathologic study of any other suspected sites of involvement, e.g., skin or bone, should also be obtained.

The diagnosis of cryptococcal meningitis is easier to establish than the diagnosis of cryptococcal pulmonary disease. Once the diagnosis of meningitis is considered, a lumbar puncture should be performed. Most patients, except for those with AIDS, have significant CSF abnormalities, including elevated opening pressure, depressed glucose levels (hypoglycorrhachia) in half the cases, elevated protein levels, and a low-grade lymphocytic pleocytosis. The India ink preparation of centrifuged CSF to detect budding yeast cells and surrounding capsule is positive in 50 to 75 per cent of cases; because the incidence of false-positive smears is high, confirmation of findings by culture is imperative. Culturing of centrifuged sediment of large volumes (5 to 10 ml) of CSF obtained by repeated lumbar punctures is associated with a positive culture rate of 90 to 95 per cent. In AIDS patients, the CSF formula is often normal or only minimally abnormal, owing to a diminished or absent inflammatory response. Yet in most cases, cultures are positive, cryptococcal antigen titers are high, and India ink preparations reveal organisms. The chest roentgenogram may or may not be abnormal. Blood should be cultured and tested for antigen in all patients. In addition, CT or MRI of the head is indicated in most patients, especially those with coma, suspected hydrocephalus, focal neurologic findings, seizures, or clinical deterioration after initial improvement. Cisternal puncture for CSF analysis, culture, and cryptococcal antigen testing may be rewarding in patients with chronic lymphocytic meningitis in whom an etiology has not been established over a period of weeks to months, despite serial testing of lumbar CSF.

TREATMENT. Approaches to therapy for cryptococcosis vary according to the site (or sites) of involvement and the underlying host status. Whereas all patients with CNS cryptococcosis or other forms of extrapulmonary disease require treatment, the majority of cases of pulmonary cryptococcosis alone, especially in the "normal" host, resolve without antifungal therapy. Every patient with pulmonary disease deserves thorough evaluation for the possibility of disseminated infection. In addition, malignancy such as bronchogenic carcinoma or metastases must be excluded. In the absence of extrapulmonary cryptococcal disease in the normal host, therapy may be safely withheld, provided careful follow-up evaluation can be done. By contrast, other patients with pulmonary cryptococcosis, including immunocompromised patients, those with accompanying extrapulmonary disease, and those with progressive disease, require antifungal therapy. Although specific guidelines are poorly defined, amphotericin B (total dose, 1.0 to 1.5 grams) is generally recommended. Fluconazole, recently approved by the Food and Drug Administration for treatment of cryptococcal meningitis (see below), appears to be more effective against C. neoformans than does ketoconazole, the other orally available antifungal azole. Fluconazole (200 to 400 mg per day for 3 to 6 months) is a promising alternative to amphotericin B, especially in patients with mild to moderate forms of pulmonary disease; however, data about its efficacy in this form of cryptococcosis are limited. Controversy also exists over the management of patients who have undergone thoracotomy with resection of a nodule or mass lesion that is subsequently proved to be caused by C. neoformans. In the past, if evidence of extrapulmonary infection was lacking, no antifungal therapy was advocated. Now, with the availability of a well-tolerated and potentially effective oral agent such as fluconazole, this approach deserves reconsideration; a 2- to 6-month course of fluconazole may be merited.

In terms of chemotherapy, cryptococcal meningitis has been more extensively studied than any other systemic fungal disease. Data indicate that (1) all patients require treatment; (2) a combination of amphotericin B and flucytosine for 4 to 6 weeks is the regimen of choice; and (3) combination therapy is more effective than therapy with amphotericin alone. Although recommendations are based on studies using a 0.3 mg per kilogram per day dosage of amphotericin B and a 150 mg per kilogram per day dosage of flucytosine, dosing regimens should be individualized, balancing the risk of toxicities associated with higher doses versus the potential benefits of enhanced efficacy. For example, some authorities recommend higher dose amphotericin B (0.5 to 0.7 mg per kilogram per day) and lower dose flucytosine (100 mg per kilogram per day). Regardless of regimen, both renal function and serum flucytosine levels should be closely monitored, and flucytosine doses should be regulated to maintain serum concentrations in the range of 50 to 100 µg per milliliter. Potential toxic effects of flucytosine include bone marrow suppression, hepatitis, diarrhea, and rash. Intrathecal therapy with amphotericin B is usually reserved for patients who relapse or whose disease is refractory to prolonged courses of high-dose intravenous amphotericin B.

Because cryptococcal meningitis in AIDS patients may be highly refractory and associated with a relapse rate of 50 to 60 per cent if therapy is stopped, more aggressive primary or initial therapy, as well as long-term maintenance therapy, is required.

For primary therapy, higher dose amphotericin B (0.5 to 1.0 mg per kilogram per day), preferably with flucytosine (approximately 100 mg per kilogram per day), should be administered until there is clinical and mycologic response. Some AIDS patients may not tolerate flucytosine because of a high incidence of drug-induced cytopenias, often superimposed upon pre-existing bone marrow suppression secondary to zidovudine, cytotoxic chemotherapy, and opportunistic infectious diseases. In addition, flucytosine should not be used unless serum levels can be monitored. Recent studies indicate that fluconazole (200 to 400 mg per day) may be an effective alternative to amphotericin B as primary therapy. Although limited clinical data also suggest a potential role for itraconazole, another triazole, fluconazole, is favored in cryptococcal meningitis because of its pharmacologic properties, including water solubility, minimal protein binding, and good to excellent penetration into CSF (60 to 80 per cent of serum concentration). In addition, an intravenous formulation of fluconazole is available. A major disadvantage of fluconazole is less rapid sterilization of CSF when compared with amphotericin B. As a result, amphotericin B should be preferentially used as primary therapy in more seriously ill patients, such as those who are obtunded or comatose or those who have widespread disseminated cryptococcosis.

Ventricular shunting of CSF should be performed in obtunded or comatose patients with hydrocephalus demonstrated by imaging studies. Since not all patients with abnormal mental status, blindness, hearing loss, or other neurologic complications have documented hydrocephalus, serial lumbar punctures or temporary ventricular drainage with monitoring of intracranial pressure plus observation of clinical response is often indicated in this setting.

Once primary therapy has sterilized the CSF, i.e., converted the fungal culture from positive to negative, some form of maintenance therapy should be initiated. Recent evaluation of maintenance therapy in AIDS patients with cryptococcal meningitis indicates that fluconazole (200 mg daily) is more effective in preventing relapse than is amphotericin (1 mg per kilogram per week) and is much better tolerated, resulting in better patient compliance. Regardless of which drug is used, chronic suppressive therapy must be continued for life.

PROGNOSIS. The outcome of cryptococcosis is significantly worse in AIDS patients than in the non-AIDS population. The mortality rate of treated cryptococcal meningitis approaches 30 per cent and is even higher among AIDS patients. Among non-AIDS patients treated with amphotericin B, the relapse rate is 20 per cent. Because the relapse rate of cryptococcal disease in persons with AIDS is 50 per cent or more, all such individuals must receive lifetime maintenance therapy. Prognostic factors, in addition to HIV infection, that adversely affect outcome include corticosteroid therapy or lymphoreticular cancer; absence of headache as a presenting symptom; pretreatment altered mental status, as evidenced by obtundation, stupor, or coma; a pretreatment CSF white cell count that is 20 per cubic millimeter or less; pretreatment cryptococcal serum antigen titer that is 1:32 or higher and end-of-therapy CSF and serum antigen titers that are 1:8 or higher; and positive India ink preparation at end of therapy. Some, but not all, studies indicate that high pretreatment CSF antigen titers also predict a poor outcome. Abnormalities of CSF, such as hypoglycorrhachia and elevated protein levels, may persist for months after therapy has been discontinued and do not appear to correlate with relapse.

PREVENTION. Because an environmental source of infection cannot be determined in the vast majority of patients who develop cryptococcal disease, attempts at elimination of C. neoformans from soil or other habitats are not feasible or practical. With the availability of effective, safe, orally administered antifungal agents, future consideration may be given to their use as prophylactic agents in groups at high risk of developing cryptococcosis, such as HIV-positive persons.

Bozette SA, Larsen RA, Chin J, et al.: A placebo-controlled trial of maintenance therapy with fluconazole after treatment of cryptococcal meningitis in the acquired immunodeficiency syndrome. N Engl J Med 324:580, 1991.
Chuck SL, Sande MA: Infections with Cryptococcus neoformans in the acquired immunodeficiency syndrome. N Engl J Med 321:794, 1989. A retrospective review of 106 cases of cryptococcosis in AIDS patients, with emphasis on management.
Dismukes WE, Cloud G, Gallis HA: Treatment of cryptococcal meningitis with

combination amphotericin B and flucytosine for four as compared to six weeks. N Engl J Med 317:334, 1987. *The largest prospective clinical trial (194 patients) reported to date that deals with therapy for a systemic fungal disease. Focuses primarily on non-AIDS patients.* Stamm AS, Diasio RB, Dismukes WE, et al.: Toxicity of amphotericin B plus flucytosine in 194 patients with cryptococcal meningitis. Am J Med 83:236, 1987. *The companion paper, which addresses toxicity of the two mainstay drugs, amphotericin B and flucytosine.*

Miller GP: The immunology of cryptococcal disease. Semin Respir Infect 1:45, 1986. *A concise overview of the complex interaction between* C. neoformans *and host.*

Perfect JR: Cryptococcosis. Infect Dis Clin North Am 3:77, 1989. *A comprehensive, up-to-date review with 244 references.*

404 Sporotrichosis

William E. Dismukes

DEFINITION. Sporotrichosis is a chronic mycotic disease that typically involves skin, subcutaneous tissue, and regional lymphatics as a result of cutaneous inoculation of *Sporothrix schenckii*. Extracutaneous disease secondary to either lymphohematogenous dissemination or inhalation of organisms is rare.

ETIOLOGY. *Sporothrix schenckii* is a dimorphic fungus that grows in nature and in the laboratory on Sabouraud's agar as a white mold, which, with time, becomes brownish black. In tissue and at 37°C, the organism exists as yeastlike cells, which appear as round, spherical, or cigar-shaped budding forms, 2 to 6 μm in size.

EPIDEMIOLOGY. Sporotrichosis is worldwide in distribution. *Sporothrix schenckii* appears to be ubiquitous in soil and in both living and decaying vegetation. Although the organism does not appear to infect plants, it may infect animals, especially cats and dogs, as well as humans, especially those who frequently handle or come in contact with mulch, sphagnum moss, hay, timber, and thorny bushes. Consequently, sporotrichosis is considered an occupational disease of certain groups, including farmers, nursery or forestry workers, gardeners, florists, landscapers, and carpenters. Transmission almost always results from the percutaneous introduction of organisms. In the majority of patients with extracutaneous disease, the route of acquisition is unclear. Rarely, pulmonary sporotrichosis may result from inhalation of aerosolized conidia. Although person-to-person transmission is not known to occur, transmission from animals, especially cats, to humans has been documented. The number of cases of cutaneous disease in males and females is similar; gender and age appear to play less of a role than does environmental exposure. By contrast, extracutaneous sporotrichosis is more common in males. *Sporothrix schenckii* is not considered an opportunistic fungal pathogen, although sporotrichosis in compromised hosts is being increasingly recognized. For example, cases have been observed in human immunodeficiency virus (HIV)–infected persons.

PATHOGENESIS AND PATHOLOGY. Cutaneous inoculation may follow either inapparent or obvious penetrating trauma. In the majority of patients, clinical disease does not extend beyond the site of inoculation or the draining lymphatics. Localized disease may persist for years, and cell-mediated immunity appears to be responsible for preventing or limiting the spread to extracutaneous sites. Conversely, multiorgan disease involving skin and distant sites, such as lungs, bones, and joints, is more common in immunosuppressed hosts.

The basic histopathologic pattern in cutaneous sporotrichosis is a combination of suppuration and granulomas, often accompanied by pseudoepitheliomatous hyperplasia. This pattern is not diagnostic, as it may also be seen in malignancy as well as other fungal diseases, such as blastomycosis, coccidioidomycosis, and chromomycosis. Since the yeastlike cells, typical of *S. schenckii*, are uncommonly identified in tissue sections, cultural confirmation is usually necessary for diagnosis. The finding of large asteroid bodies (radiate eosinophilic material surrounding fungal yeast cells) provides presumptive evidence of sporotrichosis.

CLINICAL MANIFESTATIONS. Sporotrichosis is manifested by two distinctive clinical forms of cutaneous and extracutaneous disease, which differ in management and prognosis.

Cutaneous. This form of sporotrichosis can be further divided into two types: plaque (or fixed) and lymphocutaneous. Plaque sporotrichosis, which is less common, consists of a single ulcerative or nodular lesion at the site of primary inoculation, usually on an exposed extremity or the face. The lesion begins as a small, painless, red papule, which gradually enlarges and finally ulcerates (sporotrichotic chancre). A violaceous hue and intermittent serosanguineous drainage are characteristic. Lymphocutaneous sporotrichosis, which is the more typical type and is found in about 75 per cent of cases, represents an extension of the primary lesion. Subcutaneous nontender nodular lesions appear proximally along thickened lymphatics over days to weeks and occasionally ulcerate. Lymph nodes are rarely enlarged. Similarly, constitutional symptoms, such as fever and chills, are usually absent. This type of sporotrichosis, which usually remains confined to the primary site and its regional lymphatics, may wax and wane over years if untreated. Lymphohematogenous spread to distant organs is uncommon.

Extracutaneous. The pathogenesis of the majority of cases of extracutaneous sporotrichosis is uncertain, since most cases are not accompanied by clinically apparent cutaneous disease. The skeletal system is the most commonly involved extracutaneous organ. Although indolent monarticular arthritis of the knees, ankles, wrists, and elbows is most frequent, osteomyelitis (especially of the tibia), tenosynovitis, and carpal tunnel syndrome have been reported. Multiarticular arthritis is more likely in compromised hosts with widespread hematogenous spread to multiple organs. Pulmonary sporotrichosis is far less common than osteoarticular disease. Fewer than 100 cases of pulmonary disease have been reported. This form of insidious infection occurs primarily in older male alcoholics and mimics reactivation tuberculosis. Thin-walled cavitary lesions in a single upper lobe are characteristic; bilateral fibrocavitary disease may be seen occasionally. Extrapulmonary spread of disease is uncommon. Ocular sporotrichosis results from traumatic inoculation of the conjunctiva or cornea; endophthalmitis is unusual. Chronic lymphocytic meningitis may be a complication of sporotrichosis, even in the absence of obvious extraneural disease. Testing of cerebrospinal fluid (CSF) for antibody to *S. schenckii* should be performed in any patient with chronic meningitis of unknown etiology.

DIAGNOSIS. As a rule, the diagnosis of sporotrichosis must be based on cultural demonstration of the organism in tissue or fluid obtained from involved sites, e.g., skin, subcutaneous nodule, joint, or lung. Histopathologic findings are usually nonspecific, and the characteristic yeastlike cells are often not identified by special stains such as Gomori methenamine silver (GMS) or periodic acid–Schiff (PAS). Direct immunofluorescence, if available, may be helpful. Although testing of serum of CSF by latex agglutination or enzyme immunoassay for antibody to *S. schenckii* may be useful, especially in patients suspected of having extracutaneous disease, positive low-level antibody titers may be observed in normal persons. No skin test is commercially available.

TREATMENT. Conventional therapy for cutaneous sporotrichosis is saturated solution of potassium iodide, which is begun at a dosage of 5 drops three times a day and increased in a dropwise fashion (3 to 5 drops per day) up to a maximum of 120 drops per day or until the development of iodine toxicity (manifested by rash, lacrimation, parotid swelling, or nonspecific gastrointestinal symptoms). Iodide therapy should be continued for at least 1 month after clinical resolution of the disease. Itraconazole, an investigational oral triazole, in a dosage of 100 to 200 mg per day, is more effective than ketoconazole, an imidazole; is better tolerated than potassium iodide; and offers promise as the drug of choice for cutaneous sporotrichosis. Amphotericin B should be given to patients with cutaneous disease in whom iodide or azole therapy fails and to all patients with extracutaneous disease (total dose, 2.0 to 3.0 grams). Cure rates may be improved in selected patients with bone and joint disease or single-cavity pulmonary disease by surgical resection of synovial tissue, bone, or lung, as an adjunct to amphotericin B. Intra-articular amphotericin B may also be useful. The role of itraconazole in the treatment of extracutaneous disease has not been established.

PROGNOSIS. Although untreated cutaneous sporotrichosis may remit and relapse for years, and rarely disseminate, the likelihood of cure with iodide or itraconazole therapy is high. In contrast, extracutaneous disease is more refractory, even to therapy including amphotericin B and surgery; significant morbidity and mortality are frequent sequelae.

Dunstan RW, Langham RF, Reimann KA, et al.: Feline sporotrichosis: A report of five cases with transmission to humans. J Am Acad Dermatol 15:37, 1986. *Seven humans exposed to five cats developed disease, illustrating the potential importance of animal-to-human transmission.*

Pluss JL, Opal SM: Pulmonary sporotrichosis: Review of treatment and outcome. Medicine (Baltimore) 65:143, 1986. *A comprehensive review of 58 cases, with emphasis on management.*

Restreppo A, Robledo J, Gomez I, et al.: Itraconazole therapy in lymphangitic and cutaneous sporotrichosis. Arch Dermatol 122:413, 1986. *Total resolution without relapse was achieved in 82 per cent of patients treated for 3 to 5 months with 100 mg per day.*

Scott EN, Kaufman L, Brown A, et al.: Serologic studies in the diagnosis and management of meningitis due to Sporothrix schenckii. N Engl J Med 317:935, 1987. *A description of seven cases, all of whom had antibody to S. schenckii in CSF and serum.*

Winn RE: Sporotrichosis. Infect Dis Clin North Am 2:899, 1988. *An up-to-date literature review, emphasizing the varied clinical manifestations of sporotrichosis. Includes 74 references.*

405 Candidiasis

William E. Dismukes

DEFINITION. *Candida* species can cause a variety of clinical syndromes that are generically termed candidiasis and are usually categorized by site of involvement. Broadly speaking, the two most common syndromes are mucocutaneous candidiasis (e.g., stomatitis or thrush, esophagitis, and vaginitis) and invasive or deep organ candidiasis (e.g., fungemia, endocarditis, and endophthalmitis). In most patients, candidiasis is an opportunistic disease.

ETIOLOGY. Among more than 150 recognized species of *Candida*, *C. albicans* is the most commonly identified pathogen in humans. Other clinically important species include *C. tropicalis*, *C. parapsilosis*, *C. krusei*, *C. pseudotropicalis*, and *C. guilliermondi*. *Candida* organisms share two morphologic features: small, spherical yeast forms (4 to 6 μm), which reproduce by budding; and pseudohyphae (pseudomycelia), which are chains of elongated yeasts separated by constrictions. In body fluids or tissue, both budding cells and fragments of pseudohyphae may be visualized. Identification and speciation in the microbiology laboratory are based on both morphologic characteristics and results of metabolic tests. The ability of *C. albicans* to produce germ tubes in serum allows presumptive identification. The yeast form of *Torulopsis glabrata* resembles the yeast forms of other *Candida* species; because it does not produce a pseudomycelial form, *T. glabrata* is generally not considered a member of the genus *Candida*.

EPIDEMIOLOGY. Candidiasis occurs worldwide. *Candida albicans* is part of the normal human flora of the mouth, gastrointestinal tract, and vagina; normally lives in balance with other microorganisms in the body; and, in most individuals, exists as a saprophytic colonizer or commensal. When various drugs or conditions, such as broad-spectrum antibiotics, corticosteroids, diabetes mellitus, or human immunodeficiency virus (HIV) infection, upset this balance, *C. albicans*, arising from an endogenous source, may assume the role of pathogen and cause either mucocutaneous or deep disease. *Candida albicans* may also be recovered from soil, hospital environments, food, and other substrates. In contrast to *C. albicans*, the other *Candida* species that are pathogenic for humans may colonize skin but usually not the gastrointestinal tract or vagina of normal individuals. These species more often reside in the environment and on inanimate objects and thus reach the body from exogenous sources; consequently, they are generally regarded as opportunistic fungal pathogens. Unlike other fungi, *Candida* species may be transmitted from person to person, e.g., between sexual partners, by hands of medical personnel, and during birth from colonized vagina to neonatal oropharynx.

Candidiasis, both mucocutaneous and deep forms, has emerged as the most common opportunistic fungal disease over recent decades, owing to the progressively increasing use of antibiotics (both prophylactic and therapeutic); immunosuppressive and cytotoxic drugs; indwelling foreign bodies, including prosthetic heart valves, prosthetic joints, and intravascular monitoring devices; venous, arterial, urinary, and peritoneal catheters; and organ transplantation. In addition, the ongoing acquired immunodeficiency syndrome (AIDS) epidemic has been highly contributory.

PATHOGENESIS AND PATHOLOGY. Several components of the host defense system are important in protecting against infection with *Candida* species. An intact integumentary barrier, including skin and mucous membranes, prevents invasion of normally colonizing organisms, which possess adherence properties as yet not fully understood. *Candida albicans* and *C. tropicalis* appear to be more adherent than other species, accounting in part for the frequency of these organisms as pathogens. Disruption or loss of normal barriers as a consequence of percutaneous catheters, endotracheal tubes, severe burns, or abdominal surgery is a common predisposing factor, especially to deep invasive or disseminated disease. Polymorphonuclear leukocytes and monocytes are the major cellular defenses against *Candida* species; intracellular killing is largely dependent upon the myeloperoxidase, hydrogen peroxide, and superoxide anion systems. While the role of tissue macrophages is unclear, lymphocytes and cell-mediated immunity appear to play a role. Abnormalities of host defense include T cell dysfunction, which predisposes to mucocutaneous disease (oropharyngeal or esophageal candidiasis in HIV-infected persons as well as chronic mucocutaneous candidiasis), and granulocytopenia secondary to underlying disease or therapy, which predisposes to deep disease (candidemia or invasive candidiasis). In cutaneous candidiasis, histopathologic evidence of chronic dermatitis with yeasts confined to the stratum corneum is characteristic. By contrast, microabscesses interspersed in normal tissue are the characteristic pathologic finding in visceral candidiasis. Neutrophils appear initially, followed by histiocytes and giant cells and, in some cases, a readily apparent granulomatous response. In severely immunocompromised patients, the inflammatory response may be minimal or absent. Both yeasts and pseudohyphae can usually be visualized by special stains, such as periodic acid–Schiff (PAS) or Gomori methenamine silver (GMS).

CLINICAL MANIFESTATIONS

Mucocutaneous Infections. Thrush or oropharyngeal candidiasis is manifested by creamy white curdlike exudative patches on the tongue, buccal mucosa, palate, or other oral mucosal surfaces. These patches are actually pseudomembranes, which, upon removal, may leave a raw, bleeding, painful surface. Poorly fitting dentures may be a predisposing factor. Cheilosis, an inflammatory reaction at the corners of the mouth, and atrophic changes, either acute or chronic, are less common presentations of oropharyngeal disease. Esophagitis, which may occur as an extension of thrush or may occur in the absence of thrush in up to one third of patients, is manifested typically by odynophagia, dysphagia, or substernal chest pain and uncommonly by bleeding. Thrush or esophagitis, occurring in the absence of any known predisposing condition, should raise the suspicion of HIV infection. Gastrointestinal candidiasis involving the mucosa of the stomach and small and large bowel is most common in patients with cancer and is an important source of disseminated infection.

Intertrigo, a cutaneous *Candida* infection involving warm, moist surfaces, such as the axillae, gluteal and inframammary folds, and groin, may be variable in appearance but is usually manifested as well-marginated, erythematous, exudative patches surrounded by satellite vesicles or pustules. Paronychia, a painful, tense, reddened swelling at the base of the nail or along the sides, is commonly caused by *Candida* species, especially in diabetics and persons whose hands are chronically immersed in water. Although *Candida* species may cause onychomycosis, this chronic deforming infection of the nails is most frequently due to one of the genera of superficial dermatophytes, such as *Trichophyton* or *Epidermophyton*. Vulvovaginitis, probably the most common *Candida* mucocutaneous infection in women, especially in association with pregnancy, antibiotic therapy, and diabetes, is characterized by thick, creamy vaginal discharge, erythematous labia, and intense pruritus. Balanitis in males, often acquired through sexual intercourse, is manifested by superficial vesicles and exudative patches, usually on the glans penis. *Candida* cystitis, which at cystoscopy resembles oral thrush, is most often a complication of an indwelling bladder catheter. Chronic mucocutaneous candidiasis, a rare condition manifested by a heterogeneous group of persistent, often disfiguring *Candida* infections involving skin, mucous membranes, hair, and nails, occurs primarily in persons with altered T cell function or an endocrinopathy such as hypoparathyroidism or hypoadrenalism.

Deep Organ Candidiasis. Numerous diagnostic categories or labels for serious or deep *Candida* infection exist, including candidemia, disseminated candidiasis, systemic candidiasis, invasive candidiasis, visceral candidiasis, and terms indicating involvement of specific organs, such as hepatosplenic candidiasis and ocular candidiasis. Here, discussion focuses on two major categories: candidemia, which may or may not be associated with visceral organ involvement; and disseminated candidiasis, which implies systemic multiorgan disease and encompasses other subgroups, such as visceral, invasive, and hepatosplenic disease.

Candidemia. Candidemia, which is usually defined as more than one positive blood culture for *Candida* species, may occur in the presence or absence of clinical manifestations, e.g., fever or skin lesions. The incidence of candidemia has risen dramatically over recent years in association with the increased number of compromised hosts (e.g., those with AIDS, cancer, or burns, those in the postsurgical intensive care unit, and organ transplant recipients) managed by aggressive interventions, including empiric antibiotics, cytotoxic chemotherapy, hemodialysis, intravenous and intra-arterial catheters, other intravascular devices, and parenteral alimentation. In many hospitals, *Candida* has become one of the three to five most common microorganisms isolated from blood cultures. Previously, "transient candidemia" was used to imply short duration (<24 hours) of fungemia and indicate either clearing of the candidemia upon removal of an infected intravascular catheter or a benign condition that did not require antifungal therapy. Recent data argue against this concept and suggest that catheter removal alone is insufficient, even in the noncompromised patient, to prevent metastatic hematogenous dissemination to visceral organs. Accordingly, most investigators now believe that all patients with candidemia, regardless of duration or circumstances, deserve some form of antifungal treatment. Controversy at present centers on which drug, at what dose, and for how long (see Treatment below).

Candida albicans is the most common species identified in blood. Studies from multiple medical centers indicate that *C. tropicalis* is the most likely species in the leukemic population, while *C. parapsilosis* fungemia occurs most frequently in patients with solid tumor or nononcologic diseases, especially in association with cannula-related sepsis and hyperalimentation. *Torulopsis glabrata* resembles *C. parapsilosis* in its predilection for patients with solid tumors or nononcologic disorders.

Cannulas of various types are the most important portals of entry, accounting for more than one half of the episodes of candidemia. In almost all cases, removal of cannulas, either peripheral or central, is necessary for eradication of candidemia. Other common sources of infection are the gastrointestinal tract, especially in granulocytopenic patients, and surgical wounds. The urinary and respiratory tracts, while frequently colonized by *Candida* species, are less common sources of bloodstream infection. The mortality rate of candidemia caused by all species is high, ranging from 40 to 80 per cent; *T. glabrata* is associated with the highest mortality. The mortality rate in cannula-associated candidemia is lower than in candidemia related to other sources.

The frequency with which candidemia results in localized single-organ disease (e.g., ocular candidiasis) or widespread disseminated multiorgan disease is unknown. Premortem diagnosis of invasive or disseminated candidiasis must be based on histopathologic demonstration of *Candida* organisms invading tissue. Since blood cultures are negative in at least 50 per cent of patients with disseminated candidiasis and there are no other reliable markers, such as serologic tests, systemic *Candida* disease

may not be suspected and appropriate invasive diagnostic procedures may not be performed. Autopsy series indicate that disseminated disease involving kidneys, liver, spleen, brain, myocardium, and eyes is most likely in patients with some rapidly fatal underlying disease, such as leukemia complicated by neutropenia, and is least likely in patients with candidemia in the setting of nononcologic disease, especially cannula-related sepsis. In addition, patients whose candidemia is treated are less likely to develop disseminated disease.

Cutaneous Lesions of Disseminated Candidiasis. Papulopustules or macronodules on an erythematous base, usually widely distributed over the trunk and extremities, are the hallmark lesions associated with persistent candidemia. Hemorrhagic bullae have also been reported.

Ocular Candidiasis. This form of localized candidiasis may result from either hematogenous spread or direct inoculation, e.g., after cataract extraction or implantation of an intraocular lens. Any eye structure may be infected; endophthalmitis is the most fulminant manifestation and may result in blindness. Single or multiple fluffy white cotton ball–like chorioretinal lesions, often extending into the vitreous, are characteristic. These lesions can be easily recognized on fundoscopic examination and should be serially looked for in all patients with known candidemia.

Renal Candidiasis. Infection of the kidneys may be secondary to ascending extension from the bladder (*Candida* cystitis), resulting in papillary necrosis, caliceal invasion, or formation of a fungus ball in the ureter or renal pelvis. More commonly, renal candidiasis is secondary to hematogenous spread, in patients with either documented or undocumented candidemia, resulting in pyelonephritis with diffuse cortical and medullary abscesses. The triad of candidemia, candiduria, and *Candida* organisms within casts in urinary sediment provides presumptive evidence of upper urinary tract involvement.

Hepatosplenic Candidiasis. This visceral form of deep infection occurs most commonly in patients with hematologic malignancies, especially leukemia, who are in remission after prolonged chemotherapy-induced neutropenia. Gastrointestinal candidiasis complicated by portal fungemia is the source in most patients; documented candidemia or evidence of disease in other organs is usually absent. Persistent unexplained fever, right upper quadrant tenderness and pain, elevated alkaline phosphatase levels and multiple, scattered "bull's eye" lesions in the liver and spleen, demonstrated by abdominal ultrasonographic examination or computed tomography (CT), are features. Diagnosis is established by characteristic histopathology on liver biopsy.

Pulmonary Candidiasis. Whereas colonization by yeasts of the tracheobronchial tree is common in seriously ill, debilitated intensive care unit patients on ventilators, bona fide pneumonia caused by *Candida* species is rare. Diagnosis should be based on histopathologic evidence of yeast invasion.

Cardiac Candidiasis. Disseminated candidiasis is complicated frequently by *Candida* myocarditis (more than 50 per cent of cases) and occasionally by *Candida* pericarditis. *Candida* is the most common cause of fungal endocarditis and should be suspected in the setting of indwelling cardiac prostheses, intravenous drug abuse, and prolonged use of central intravenous catheters for chemotherapy, hyperalimentation, or hemodynamic monitoring. Because fungal valvular vegetations are large and friable, major embolic events involving the central nervous system, coronary arteries, and large peripheral arteries are common.

Central Nervous System Candidiasis. Meningitis and intracerebral microabscesses as well as macroabscesses frequently complicate disseminated candidiasis. Cerebrospinal fluid pleocytosis, most often lymphocytic, hypoglycorrhachia, and elevated protein levels are typical; yeast organisms can be identified by wet preparation, Gram stain, or culture, in fewer than one half of cases. *Candida* meningitis may be a complication of ventricular shunt infection.

Musculoskeletal Candidiasis. Manifestations include myositis (abscess) in neutropenic patients and costochondritis, arthritis, and osteomyelitis (special predilection for vertebrae and intervertebral discs) in intravenous drug users. All of these complications may develop in any patient with disseminated candidiasis, whatever the setting or source.

DIAGNOSIS. Mucocutaneous lesions are diagnosed on the

basis of clinical appearance and by examination of potassium hydroxide wet mounts or Gram-stained smears of lesion material obtained by scraping or swabbing. Masses of spherical budding yeast forms and pseudohyphae are characteristic. Patients suspected of having *Candida* esophagitis should undergo not only endoscopy and brushing but also biopsy in an attempt to demonstrate, histopathologically, mucosal invasion of *Candida* organisms. Esophagitis caused by either herpes simplex virus or cytomegalovirus may mimic the symptoms and appearance of *Candida* esophagitis; infection in a single patient caused by more than one microorganism is not unusual. Fungal blood cultures in patients with suspected candidemia or disseminated candidiasis should be performed using the highly sensitive lysis centrifugation method; this technique also allows more rapid detection of growth. Multiple serial cultures should be obtained. A patient with a single positive blood culture for *Candida* species poses a difficult clinical dilemma. Such a patient should be carefully evaluated for evidence of disseminated disease; foreign bodies, especially intravascular catheters, should be removed and additional blood cultures obtained. Two or more positive blood cultures should be assumed to represent clinically significant disease, which warrants antifungal therapy. The finding of heavy growth of *Candida* species in cultures of sputum, tracheal aspirate, wounds, or urine may increase the likelihood of bloodstream invasion but does not prove that dissemination has occurred. Since blood cultures may be negative in as many as 50 per cent of patients with disseminated candidiasis, diagnosis must often depend on the results of histopathologic study and fungal cultures of tissue obtained by biopsy. Diagnostic procedures that should be considered include CT of the head, thorax, and abdomen; echocardiography; thoracentesis; arthrocentesis; lumbar puncture; and biopsy of skin, liver, kidney, myocardium, bone, muscle, or lung. Although quantitative or semiquantitative cultures of selected tissue specimens have been advocated as useful predictors of disseminated disease, no correlative data support this concept. Skin testing with *Candida* antigen may be useful in assessing for anergy but has no role in diagnosing candidiasis. Although much effort has been devoted to the development of reliable, simple, sensitive, and specific serologic assays for detection of serum antibodies to *Candida* or circulating *Candida* antigen, controversy persists about the value of these serodiagnostic procedures. Because false-positive and false-negative results are common, the decision to initiate treatment cannot be based on results of serologic tests alone.

TREATMENT. In most patients with mucocutaneous infections, any one of several topical preparations, including nystatin, clotrimazole, miconazole, econazole, butoconazole, and ketoconazole, provides effective therapy. Nystatin suspension and clotrimazole troches appear to be equal in efficacy as therapy for oral thrush, but clotrimazole is better tolerated. Although the clinical manifestations of *Candida* vulvovaginitis are usually eliminated by local topical therapy with nystatin, clotrimazole, butoconazole, or miconazole administered for 3 to 7 days, the disease tends to recur frequently in some patients. Newer approaches to the management of acute vulvovaginitis utilize single-dose therapy, e.g., clotrimazole, 500-mg vaginal pessary; miconazole, 1200-mg ovule; or fluconazole, 150-mg oral tablet. In refractory cases, prolonged therapy with a topical agent or an orally absorbed azole, such as ketoconazole or fluconazole, provided that pregnancy has been excluded, may be beneficial. Oral ketoconazole, 200 to 400 mg daily, is the treatment of choice for chronic mucocutaneous candidiasis and must be continued indefinitely to avoid relapse. HIV-infected patients with mucocutaneous forms of candidiasis respond less rapidly than other patient groups and often with incomplete clearance of exudative patches. Nystatin suspension appears to be less effective than either clotrimazole troches or an oral drug, e.g., ketoconazole or fluconazole, in AIDS patients with oropharyngeal or esophageal candidiasis. Fluconazole appears to be more effective than ketoconazole. In refractory cases with severe disease, low-dose intravenous amphotericin B can be employed.

Therapy for serious *Candida* disease, such as candidemia or disseminated candidiasis, remains highly controversial. Although most authorities consider amphotericin B to be the mainstay of treatment, there have been no large prospective clinical trials to delineate optimal daily dose, total dose, or duration of amphotericin B therapy. Consequently, present guidelines are largely empiric. In most patients with catheter-related candidemia, the catheter, if still present, should be removed. In patients with suppurative peripheral thrombophlebitis, surgical segmental venous resection may be necessary. Because of the high risk of metastatic complications of candidemia, such as endophthalmitis, osteomyelitis, arthritis, and endocarditis, there is increasing evidence to support the approach that all patients with candidemia, even nonneutropenic hosts, should have a course of antifungal chemotherapy. Both low-dose amphotericin B regimens, 0.3 to 0.4 mg per kilogram per day or a 200- to 400-mg total dose, and high-dose regimens, 0.5 to 0.8 mg per kilogram per day or a 500- to 800-mg total dose, have been advocated. Until clearer guidelines are forthcoming from ongoing prospective studies, the decision regarding which regimen to employ must be based on the host defense status of the patient, underlying conditions, predisposing factors, and results of serial blood cultures and physical examinations to search for complications of candidemia.

Patients with documented disseminated disease, manifested either as localized deep disease (hepatosplenic candidiasis, central nervous system candidiasis, renal candidiasis, or *Candida* endocarditis) or as multiorgan disease, should be treated with amphotericin B (total dose, 2.0 to 3.0 grams) plus flucytosine (100 to 150 mg per kilogram per day). Because flucytosine may be associated with significant toxicity, including bone marrow suppression, hepatitis, diarrhea, and rash, serum flucytosine levels should be regularly monitored and the dosage adjusted to maintain levels in the range of 50 to 100 μg per milliliter. Valve replacement is a necessary adjunct to chemotherapy in patients with *Candida* endocarditis.

Current data do not justify the treatment of candidemia or disseminated candidiasis with newer oral antifungal azoles such as fluconazole. Prospective studies are ongoing to address this issue. Similarly, the role of immunomodulators, e.g., human granulocyte colony-stimulating factor, in the therapy of serious *Candida* disease has not yet been defined.

Candida cystitis, in contrast to renal candidiasis, can be cured by removal of the bladder catheter in the majority of cases. Therapeutic options available for the management of candiduria that is persistent after catheter removal or in diabetic patients include oral flucytosine, 75 to 100 mg per kilogram per day for 7 to 10 days, or oral fluconazole, 100 to 200 mg per day for 7 to 10 days. Although both of these antifungal agents are excreted by the kidneys, fluconazole is preferred because it is less toxic. Eradication of candiduria in patients whose condition justifies a persistent indwelling catheter can be attempted with amphotericin B (50 μg per milliliter) or miconazole (50 μg per milliliter) bladder rinses.

Therapy for *Candida* peritonitis, which most often is a complication of peritoneal dialysis, is less straightforward. Ideally, the peritoneal catheter should be discontinued, and either intravenous amphotericin B or oral fluconazole should be administered until clinical symptoms and signs resolve and cultures become negative. For patients in whom the catheter must be maintained, instillation of amphotericin B, 2 to 4 μg per milliliter in the dialysate fluid, has been successfully employed.

The management of ocular candidiasis requires close cooperation with an ophthalmologist experienced in eye infections. Although reports indicate that hematogenously acquired *Candida* eye disease not involving the vitreous may heal spontaneously, for most cases, systemic amphotericin B, with or without flucytosine, plus vitrectomy to remove vitreous abscesses is required. Findings at vitrectomy may also be used to confirm the diagnosis. Oral ketoconazole is reportedly effective, especially in endophthalmitis secondary to intravenous heroin use, but ketoconazole cannot be recommended over amphotericin B.

PREVENTION. Given the increasing incidence of nosocomial candidemia, with its high mortality rate, excess length of hospital stay, and potential for multiorgan complications, focus on awareness of the problem and development of measures aimed at prevention assume increasing importance. In selected clinical situations as discussed above, suspicion of candidemia or deep organ candidiasis should be high, and appropriate diagnostic studies pursued. Once the diagnosis is established, intensive antifungal therapy must be given. In addition, factors that predispose to *Candida* disease should be controlled or avoided, whenever possible. For example, the frequency and duration of use of intravascular catheters and monitoring devices should be reduced, and central catheters should be changed at least weekly. Special care should be paid to long-term access devices for chemotherapy, such as Hickman or Broviac catheters. Similarly, the frequency, breadth, and duration of courses of antibiotics should be reduced. Prophylactic regimens of oral nystatin, clotrimazole, ketoconazole, or fluconazole are widely employed in granulocytopenic patients to prevent *Candida* infection. Two problems, however, are associated with their use. First, their efficacy has not been unequivocally established. Second, azole-containing regimens may be associated with development of resistance of *Candida* species to amphotericin B.

Crislip MA, Edwards JE Jr: Candidiasis. Infect Dis Clin North Am 3:103, 1989. *A comprehensive, up-to-date review, with a nice perspective on clinical syndromes and treatment and 182 references.*

Jones JM: Laboratory diagnosis of invasive candidiasis. Clin Microbiol Rev 3:32, 1990. *A thorough, thoughtful perspective on the role of the microbiology laboratory, with a good analysis of the current status of serologic tests for candidiasis. Includes 131 references.*

Komshian SV, Uwaydah AK, Sobel JD, et al.: Fungemia caused by *Candida* species and *Torulopsis glabrata* in the hospitalized patient: Frequency, characteristics, and evaluation of factors influencing outcome. Rev Infect Dis 11:379, 1989. *Detailed univariate and multivariate analyses of the risk factors for development of candidemia and predictors of outcome among 135 cases occurring between 1983 and 1986. The findings lead the authors to argue against the concept of cannula-related candidemia as a benign disease.*

Thaler M, Behram P, Shawker T, et al.: Hepatic candidiasis in cancer patients: The evolving picture of the syndrome. Ann Intern Med 108:88, 1988. *A review of 68 cases with emphasis on diagnosis and therapy.*

Wey SB, Mori M, Pfaller MA, et al.: Hospital-acquired candidemia: The attributable mortality and excess length of stay. Arch Intern Med 148:2642, 1988. Wey SB, Mori M, Pfaller MA, et al.: Risk factors for hospital-acquired candidemia: A matched case-control study. Arch Intern Med 149:2349, 1989. *Two comparison papers that further our understanding of this increasingly recognized nosocomial infection.*

406 Aspergillosis

David A. Stevens

DEFINITION. Aspergillosis refers to infection with any of the species of the genus *Aspergillus*. These are in mold form in the environment, on artificial media, and when invading tissues.

ETIOLOGY AND EPIDEMIOLOGY. Aspergilli are ubiquitous in the environment and have been isolated with ease from fertile soil and air, and even swimming pools and saunas. They are associated with decaying matter and may grow well in any self-heating organic composting process; these processes attain temperatures of 40 to 50°C. The ease with which they are isolated from sewage sludge composting, from silos, and from the cooling canals of nuclear power plants has been an environmental and industrial concern. They are easily isolated from the human habitat, e.g., in houses, particularly from basements, crawl spaces, bedding, and house dust; and in surveys they have been found in, for example, 94 per cent of pasta samples and 92 per cent of marijuana samples. This pervasiveness should not make it surprising that they are found in 16 per cent of normal expectorated sputa. They are important pathogens of insects (of economic importance to beekeepers) and of birds, both domesticated and wild, in which the air sacs and lungs are targets. They are also important because of the production of toxins, particularly aflatoxin, one of the most potent carcinogens known, which are products of their growth and which contaminate the food chain, posing a risk to animals and humans. Their threat to hospitalized patients has been revealed in outbreaks of infection, particularly pulmonary infection in compromised hosts, associated with renovation and new construction. The suspected vector has been unfiltered air, as from inlets contaminated with bird excreta and fireproofing materials.

The most common species infecting humans are *A. fumigatus*, *A. flavus*, *A. niger*, and *A. terreus*. Some are speciated by the clinical laboratory only with difficulty, and they may be reported to the clinician only as "*Aspergillus* species." In tissues they may be seen as septate hyphae, dichotomously branched (resembling the divergence of fingers from one another), and they may produce their characteristic conidia in tissues or artificial media, which is one means of their differentiation. If the septation can be seen, they can be differentiated from the zygomycetes; they may be confused with *Pseudallescheria boydii*, however, unless the characteristic terminal spores of the latter are seen.

Aspergillosis generally results from airborne conidia and is not contagious.

SYNDROMES. The main forms of clinical aspergillosis are shown in Table 406–1.

The *invasive* form of the disease is generally a problem of immunocompromised hosts (Ch. 287), and more aggressive immunosuppression and anticancer therapy are the most important factors contributing to the rise of *Aspergillus* infections. Series have reported an incidence as high as 41 per cent in those with acute leukemia at autopsy, and in 89 per cent of these cases it played a significant role in the death of the patient. In 97 per cent, pulmonary involvement was present, and in 25 per cent, the infection was disseminated widely to various organs. Similarly, in a group of heart transplant patients, the incidence of infection was 28 per cent. This is also a problem in diabetics and patients with the neutrophil defect of chronic granulomatous disease. Diagnosis is difficult because aspergilli are frequently contaminants in sputum and even in other cultures when handled in the laboratory. In patients with leukemia, there is particularly an association with relapses of the malignancy, and usually three or four of the following factors are present: leukopenia, steroid therapy, cytotoxic chemotherapy, and broad-spectrum antibacterials. In addition, hypogammaglobulinemia is common. The classic picture is that of fever and pulmonary infiltrates or nodules, especially progressing to a cavity (usually when granulocytopenia is reversed), or wedge-shaped densities resembling infarcts. The pulmonary pathology in all these entities is that of hemorrhagic infarction and pneumonia. Pulmonary emboli are common because of the organism's tendency to invade blood vessel walls. These processes often combine to produce a "target lesion" pathologically, consisting of a necrotic center surrounded by a ring of hemorrhage. The sputum culture is positive in only 8 to 34 per cent of cases, and obtaining tissue is necessary to make the diagnosis. Prospective culturing of the nose of granulocytopenic patients has been of some value, because a positive nasal culture (and particularly the presence of nasal *Aspergillus* lesions) has led to the early diagnosis of concurrent pulmonary disease. However, negative nasal cultures are common in pulmonary aspergillosis.

Targets of *disseminated disease* include the central nervous system, where abscesses are characteristic. The cerebrospinal fluid (CSF) glucose level is normal, and cultures of the CSF are negative. Mycelia invading blood vessels may produce a microangiopathic hemolytic anemia. Dissemination can result in Budd-Chiari syndrome, myocardial infarction, gastrointestinal disease, or skin lesions. Esophageal ulcers may produce gastrointestinal bleeding. Abscesses are common in the kidney, liver, and myocardium.

Seventy-two per cent of *endocarditis* cases have occurred after cardiac surgery, and 69 per cent of these were associated with prostheses. Intravenous drug addicts are also susceptible. Eighty-three per cent of affected individuals have major arterial emboli, and neurologic presentations are common. Only 8 per cent have positive blood cultures, and this positivity is usually delayed 14 to 20 days, contributing to the poor record of diagnosis ante mortem (23 per cent), which is usually made on histologic examination of an embolus. Overall survival is about 5 per cent, or 22 per cent of those diagnosed ante mortem, and these individuals have had valve replacement. The disease should be suspected in any post–cardiac surgery patient who presents with endocarditis or emboli and negative blood cultures.

TABLE 406–1. ASPERGILLOSIS SYNDROMES

Invasive disease	Allergic bronchopulmonary disease
Aspergilloma (mycetoma)	Pleural disease
Superficial bronchial disease	Local disease
Extrinsic allergic alveolitis	Endocarditis
Mixed disease	

The typical picture of a *mycetoma* (aspergilloma) is a fungus ball (matted hyphae and debris) in a cavity in an upper lobe (Fig. 406–1). The mycetoma has been reported as a complication in as many as 11 per cent of old tuberculous cavities. The patients present with cough (87 per cent), hemoptysis (81 per cent), dyspnea (61 per cent), weight loss (61 per cent), fatigue (61 per cent), chest pain (31 per cent), or fever (25 per cent). The sputum culture is positive in most. Total immunoglobulin G (IgG) and immunoglobulin A (IgA) levels are elevated. Invasion of the parenchyma is rare.

Pleural disease is associated with tuberculosis and bronchopleural fistulas. It may occur after surgery or spontaneously.

Allergic bronchopulmonary aspergillosis is usually seen superimposed on a background of chronic asthma (see Ch. 57) or cystic fibrosis. It is characterized by episodic airway obstruction, fever, eosinophilia, mucous plugs, positive sputum cultures, and the presence of grossly visible brown flecks in the sputum (hyphae), transient infiltrates and parallel "tram-line" or ring markings on chest radiographs, proximal bronchiectasis, upper lobe contraction, and elevated levels of total IgA and immunoglobulin E (IgE) (especially when the patient is symptomatic). It is more common in agricultural areas and in the winter, presumably representing an association with stored agricultural products (especially moldy hay) and spore production. The eosinophilia is present in blood, sputum, and the lung on biopsy. The mucous plugs contain mycelia, and the plugs may be the cause of the infiltrates, with collapse and inflammation occurring peripherally, or inflammatory edema may be responsible. The parallel or ring markings are caused by thickened ectatic bronchi, and the upper lobe changes are a result of progressive apical fibrosis. The infiltrates may be nonsegmental and transient, with a clinical presentation of "eosinophilic pneumonia" and asthma, with eosinophils in blood and sputum; alternatively, they may be segmental, associated with the blocking of bronchi by plugs, and asthma and eosinophilia may be absent. A biphasic skin test response may assist in the diagnosis. A scratch test with *Aspergillus* antigens produces an immediate type I wheal and flare reaction, mediated by IgE and blocked by antihistamines, but not by corticosteroids. An intracutaneous test with the antigens produces a later (6 to 8 hours) Arthus-type reaction, mediated by IgG antibody and complement and blocked by steroids. Similarly, bronchial challenge with the antigens can produce a biphasic response. Immediate, short-lived wheezing may result, reproducing the asthmatic symptoms and associated with increased airways resistance; this can be blocked by isoproterenol, antihistamines, and cromolyn, but not by steroids. There may be a later (2 to 6 hours) reaction, of two types. One is increased airways resistance, as described. The other is a restrictive defect occurring peripherally, which may be associated with influenza-like symptoms, fever, leukocytosis, and infiltrates. These reactions are associated with IgG precipitins and are believed to account for some transient infiltrates.

Extrinsic allergic alveolitis is an unusual form of *Aspergillus* lung disease and has been most associated with A. *clavatus* in malt workers. The patients develop dyspnea and fever 4 hours after exposure, and the clinical picture resembles that of the better known bird-fancier's lung or farmer's lung (due to other allergens). Diffuse micronodular infiltrates may be present at the time of symptoms. The patients have IgG precipitins and cell-mediated immune reactions against *Aspergillus* antigens, and granulomas are present on biopsy. Eosinophilia is not a feature. The scratch test is negative, although an intradermal test produces a reaction in 4 hours, with immunoglobulins and complement present on biopsy. Bronchial challenge produces a reaction in 4 hours, with systemic symptoms and a restrictive defect but without airways resistance. The entity can progress to irreversible fibrosis. The same pathophysiology may be involved in episodes following massive inhalation of spores, usually in farm environments. Symptoms are present within 24 hours, and granulomas are found on biopsy.

Superficial bronchial disease, with features similar to those of acute or chronic bronchitis due to bacterial pathogens, may occur. Brown-flecked sputum and positive sputum cultures are associated. The allergic bronchopulmonary, alveolitis, and superficial forms rarely progress to invasive disease. *Chronic necrotizing pulmonary aspergillosis* is a poorly defined entity that usually occurs in patients with underlying lung disease, often with features of invasive disease and mycetoma.

Examples of *locally invasive disease* abound and are usually severe. These include invasion of burn wounds, keratitis or external otitis (particularly in the tropics), sinusitis (particularly in immunosuppressed and/or granulocytopenic hosts), and osteomyelitis or endophthalmitis (after fungemia, trauma, or surgery). Cutaneous ulcers have been associated with the use of adhesive tape. Bloodborne disease in addicts can produce foci of dissemination that are similar to those associated with the invasive pulmonary form of the disease. A noninvasive form of sinus disease with a predominantly allergic component and eosinophilia, responsive to drainage and corticosteroids, has also been described.

DIAGNOSIS. Some of the modalities of diagnosis have been mentioned in connection with specific syndromes. Common to several of the syndromes mentioned is the use of serodiagnosis. Antibody assays have been reported most commonly using radioimmunoassay, complement fixation, and immunodiffusion, but techniques such as immunofluorescence, counterimmunoelectrophoresis, passive hemagglutination, and enzyme-linked immunosorbent assay (ELISA) also show promise. A variety of methods for preparing antigen have been used. Data from the more commonly reported techniques suggest a high degree of sensitivity in allergic disease or aspergillomas, but generally a low sensitivity in invasive disease. As the frequency of false-positive reactions, even in the presence of other mycoses, is low (although a majority of marijuana smokers in one study had precipitins, a positive test in invasive disease may be useful. IgE antibody specific to *Aspergillus* antigens is another serodiagnostic adjunct in allergic disease. Detection of antigenemia, most commonly studied by radioimmunoassay, and detection of antigen in bronchoalveolar lavage fluid are also promising in the diagnosis of invasive disease. The problem at present with all serodiagnostic modalities is the lack of a generally available, standardized technique. The physician should know the background data for the laboratory to which the specimens may be sent, i.e., the sensitivity and specificity of the assay in the various syndromes. Serial antibody testing in groups of patients predisposed to aspergillomas (i.e., those with lung cavities), to endocarditis (cardiac surgery patients), or to invasive disease may increase the utility of otherwise problematic serodiagnostic methods.

In invasive disease, an aggressive, invasive approach, as well as making a tissue diagnosis early in the illness, appears to be a key to survival. In the appropriate clinical setting, a positive bronchial lavage or other endobronchial culture, or a repeated isolation of the same species in culture, correlates with invasive disease and may have to be the stimulus for therapy if invasive procedures cannot be done. Negative cultures (other than tissue) do not rule out invasive disease.

THERAPY. In invasive disease, prompt, aggressive chemotherapy has produced superior survival statistics at some institutions, although recovery from neutropenia is a necessary accompaniment of recovery in almost every success. The role of granulocyte transfusions is unclear. In endocarditis, in addition to prompt, aggressive chemotherapy, valve replacement appears necessary. Locally invasive disease in other sites also requires

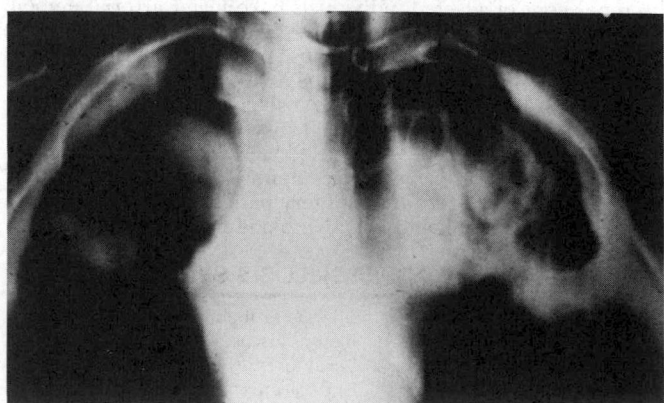

FIGURE 406–1. Tomogram of pulmonary aspergillosis mycetomas.

systemic or local chemotherapy, particularly intravitreal therapy or nephrostomy irrigation in renal disease. Surgical excision has an important role in the invasion of bone, burn wounds, epidural abscesses, vitreal disease, sinus disease of noncompromised hosts, and removal of catheters for peritonitis and of silk sutures in bronchial stump (postpneumonectomy) aspergillosis. It may have a function in invasive pulmonary disease for which chemotherapy has failed.

In cases involving mycetoma, there is evidence that patients with fever, cough, weight loss, malaise, and hemoptysis have an element of allergy, which can be demonstrated by bronchial challenge or the presence of cytophilic IgG and IgE. These patients symptomatically improve if given steroids. Intravenous amphotericin B therapy of patients with mycetoma produces results no better than those with routine pulmonary toilet. Intracavitary amphotericin, instilled through a catheter, is a heroic form of therapy that has been attempted in some patients. The role of surgery in this entity is controversial. Seven to 10 per cent of mycetomas undergo spontaneous lysis. The overall operative mortality aggregated from several series is 7 per cent but may be as high as 14 per cent in some large series. The frequency of various operative complications is 22 per cent, aggregated from several series, with a range of 7 to 60 per cent. Furthermore, new aspergillomas have later developed after surgical successes. On the other hand, in various series, 18 to 26 per cent of patients with adequate follow-up treated without surgery died of disease complications, usually hemoptysis, whereas 50 per cent have shown significant improvement symptomatically and radiographically. If any consensus exists, it is that surgical resection has a role in recurrent, significant hemoptysis. An alternative therapy, particularly for the nonsurgical patient, is selective bronchial arterial embolization to the bleeding vessel.

In pleural disease, local instillation of nystatin, amphotericin, or miconazole has resulted in successes. In allergic disease, measures that have *not* worked include hyposensitization, avoidance of sites in the environment, and aerosolized corticosteroids. Cromolyn is inadequate in most patients. Aerosolized antifungals have produced remissions but do not prevent recurrences. Treatment of the clinical disease is more complicated than the effects of drug blockade demonstrable in challenge tests. The continuous use of systemic corticosteroids can prevent the infiltrates and some accompanying symptoms. Intermittent use of steroids, or raising the dose in patients on chronic therapy, can produce rapid resolution of marked symptomatic episodes. The long-term beneficial effects of steroids are less clear; they are not so useful in arresting dyspnea or wheezing in the long term, and they do not prevent the development of the accompanying bronchiectasis. The proper approach to extrinsic alveolitis is avoidance of the stimulus.

For those entities in which systemic chemotherapy is indicated, almost all clinical experience has been with amphotericin B. Its track record is generally poor in invasive or disseminated disease in compromised hosts (especially so in those with cerebral or hepatic disease or in bone marrow transplant patients). In the compromised host, it should be used aggressively, with prompt progression to a full therapeutic dose, which should be about 1 mg per kilogram per day, if tolerated. Prophylactic therapy may have a role in patients who have survived invasive disease and will become neutropenic again. Rifampin almost always, and flucytosine sometimes, potentiates the activity of amphotericin in vitro against aspergilli. Moreover, animal models have shown an enhanced effect of combinations of these drugs over that with amphotericin alone. Clinical data to support combination therapy are limited, but given the poor record of amphotericin alone in invasive disease, combination therapy appears a logical avenue to explore, particularly if synergy can be demonstrated. A few cures have been reported in invasive disease with flucytosine (which may have a role in cerebral or renal disease) or miconazole alone. Of the new azole drugs, itraconazole is clearly the most promising and as sole therapy has produced responses in invasive disease. Other azoles, lipid-complexed amphotericin B, and other classes of drugs have demonstrated anti-*Aspergillus* activity in vitro, in models, and in a few patients and may represent future avenues of exploration. Comparative clinical trials are needed to assess all alternative forms of systemic therapy.

Denning DW, Stevens DA: The treatment of invasive aspergillosis. Rev Infect Dis 12:1147, 1990. *Reviews and tabulates data from more than 2000 published cases in 497 articles to give a current picture of therapeutic results.*

Gerson SL, Talbot GH, Hurwitz S, et al.: Discriminant scorecard for diagnosis of invasive pulmonary aspergillosis in patients with acute leukemia. Am J Med 79:57, 1985. *The Pennsylvania group published several studies defining the presentation of disease in the granulocytopenic patient. This paper ties many of their observations together in a useful form, presenting an approach to diagnosis when invasive procedures are not possible.*

Patterson R, Greenberger PA, Halwig JM, et al.: Allergic bronchopulmonary aspergillosis: Natural history and classification of early disease by serologic and roentgenographic studies. Arch Intern Med 146:916, 1986. *A recent review of diagnosis and treatment.*

Young RC, Bennett JE, Vogel CL, et al.: Aspergillosis: The spectrum of the disease in 98 patients. Medicine (Baltimore) 49:147, 1970. Meyer RD, Young LS, Armstrong D, et al.: Aspergillosis complicating neoplastic disease. Am J Med 54:6, 1973. *These classic reviews focus on the invasive form of the disease.*

407 Zygomycosis (Mucormycosis)

Sandy F. S. Chun and David A. Stevens

DEFINITION. Zygomycosis is generally an acute and rapidly developing fungal infection caused by fungi of the class Zygomycetes. In healthy hosts, these organisms seldom cause infection. However, in debilitated or immunosuppressed hosts, they produce a fulminant opportunistic infection resulting in marked tissue destruction. Several predisposing conditions have been identified. The infection is most commonly associated with the acidotic patient, especially those in diabetic ketoacidosis. Prolonged treatment with antibiotics, corticosteroids, and cytotoxic drugs and, most recently, the use of deferoxamine in the dialysis patient have also been associated, as have severe malnutrition, hematologic malignancies, and extensive burns.

THE PATHOGENS. The pathogenic zygomycetes are largely in the order Mucorales, which is related to the older (and more familiar) term for this infection, mucormycosis. Phycomycosis is another older term in the literature describing the same infections. The zygomycetes are morphologically distinct. Their hyphae are nonseptated, broad, and variable in size and shape. Furthermore, the branching of the hyphae is usually irregular and at right angles. Species of the genera *Rhizopus* and *Mucor* are the common pathogens of this group. Other genera, including *Absidia, Cunninghamella, Rhizomucor, Mortierella, Saksenaea, Syncephalastrum, Entomophthera,* and *Apophysomyces,* have also been reported to cause disease. These fungi cannot be differentiated histopathologically. Further speciation requires culturing of the pathogen and characterization of the isolates by their morphologic and physiologic features.

EPIDEMIOLOGY. The zygomycetes are ubiquitous saprophytic fungi and are abundant in nature. They have been recovered from bread, fruits, vegetables, soil, and manure. These fungi have been isolated from the nose, stool, and sputum of healthy individuals. Despite their widespread distribution, they cause disease infrequently. Fortunately, even in the severely immunocompromised hosts, zygomycosis remains a rare opportunistic infection. The disease is not contagious.

PATHOGENESIS AND PATHOLOGY. Currently, there is no unifying concept of the pathogenesis of zygomycosis. In diseases of the airways (sinus, lung), the infection is presumed to originate from inhaled spores, although the lung may also be involved secondary to bloodstream invasion. Diabetic patients appear to be more frequently colonized. While normal human serum can inhibit their growth, serum obtained from patients with diabetic ketoacidosis is not inhibitory and may even promote fungal growth. Undefined defects of macrophages and neutrophils contribute to the loss of immunity against this infection in the susceptible host. Corticosteroids weaken normal inhibitors of spore germination in tissue. Unlike most pathogenic fungi, these can grow in the absence of oxygen.

Invasion, thrombosis, and necrosis are the characteristic findings in this disease. Once the fungal spores have germinated at the site of infection, the hyphal elements are very aggressive and tend to invade blood vessels, nerves, lymphatics, and tissues. The infarction leads to further tissue hypoxia and acidosis, resulting in a vicious cycle enhancing rapid growth and infection. The paucity of a granulomatous reaction is quite characteristic. The fungal hyphae sometimes have little or no inflammation around them. In contrast to most fungi, these organisms are readily seen in hematoxylin and eosin–stained tissue. The Gomori methenamine silver stain is usually adequate, but some special fungus stains, such as periodic acid–Schiff, do not demonstrate the organism well.

CLINICAL MANIFESTATIONS. Zygomycosis can be manifested as at least six distinct clinical entities, dependent upon the types of predisposing factors of the patient and the portal of entry of the organism (Table 407–1).

Rhinocerebral zygomycosis is the most frequent form of presentation, accounting for more than 75 per cent of the cases in the literature. It commonly affects the poorly controlled diabetic patient who is also in ketoacidosis. It has also been reported in patients with hematologic malignancies who have been neutropenic for an extended period and who have received broad-spectrum antibacterial drugs or immunosuppressive therapy, in other acidotic patients, and in those with azotemia. This is one of the most rapidly fatal fungal diseases if left undiagnosed. Hyphae invade the paranasal sinuses and palate from the oronasal cavity. From the sinuses, especially the ethmoid sinus, the infection spreads to involve the retro-orbital region or the central nervous system. Epistaxis, severe unilateral headache, alteration in mental status, and eye symptoms such as lacrimation, irritation, or periorbital anesthesia are common symptoms. Examination of the nose may reveal the classic black necrotic turbinates (too often mistaken for dried blood) or even nasal septum perforation. However, at the early stage of infection, the nasal mucosa may appear only inflamed and friable. Facial cellulitis and palatal necrosis may be seen. The early eye findings include mild proptosis, periorbital edema, decreased visual acuity, or lid swelling. In more advanced orbital involvement, exophthalmos, complete ophthalmoplegia, conjunctival hemorrhage, blindness, fixed and dilated pupil, and corneal anesthesia may be found. These conditions result from fungal invasion of the roof of the orbit, affecting the nerves (third, fourth, and sixth cranial nerves and the ophthalmic branch of the fifth cranial nerve), muscles, and orbital vessels, a condition also known as the orbital apex syndrome. The infection can spread through the superior orbital fissure or the cribriform plate to involve the brain. Cavernous sinus thrombosis is a frequent complication usually resulting from hematogenous spread from the ophthalmic veins.

This hematogenous spread leads to additional cranial nerve involvement outside the orbital apex, specifically the trigeminal nerve ganglion and the root of the facial nerve, leading to ipsilateral paresthesia of the face or peripheral facial palsy. Internal carotid artery thrombosis, from retrograde spread from the ophthalmic artery or invasion from the cavernous sinus, is another late complication, leading to cerebral infarction. The middle ear may be involved via the blood, cerebrospinal fluid, or eustachian tube.

The radiographic manifestations are nonspecific. Plain roentgenograms of the sinuses and orbits may reveal nodular thickening of the mucosa of multiple sinuses, usually without air-fluid levels, or spotty destruction of the bone through the walls of the sinuses or into the orbit. Computed tomography is useful in better defining the bone destruction and soft tissue involvement, which could be important in guiding subsequent surgical intervention. The cerebrospinal fluid findings are usually nonspecific and often normal even in the presence of central nervous system involvement. The common findings are pleocytosis, with about 50 per cent polymorphonuclear cells and slight protein elevation; hypoglycorrhachia is rare. Smear and culture of cerebrospinal fluid are usually negative for fungus even in cases with documented meningeal involvement. Several infectious diseases can present

a similar picture. Black necrotic lesions may also be seen with invasive aspergillosis and with infections by *Pseudomonas aeruginosa* or *Pseudallescheria boydii*. The only definitive method of differentiating between these possibilities is by examination of tissue. Cavernous sinus thrombosis due to *Staphylococcus aureus*, as well as rhinoscleroma, aggressive orbital tumor, midline granuloma, and other fungal infections, can mimic the disease as well.

Pulmonary zygomycosis occurs most frequently in patients with hematologic malignancies being treated with antibacterial drugs or immunosuppressive therapy. The presentation is usually acute, and the patients are often profoundly ill, with variable complaints of cough, fever, and sputum production. There is no specific lobar predilection. Pulmonary vascular thrombosis and infarction are universal findings. No pathognomonic clinical or radiographic findings exist. Sputum culture is usually negative. In fact, antemortem diagnosis is seldom made because of the acuteness of the illness, the lack of consideration of the diagnosis, and the need for tissue to establish the diagnosis.

Invasive pulmonary candidiasis, aspergillosis, or nocardiosis, other bacterial infections, such as *Pseudomonas* infection, malignant invasion, hemorrhage, or pulmonary embolism and infarction may mimic the presentation of pulmonary mucormycosis.

Cutaneous zygomycosis is rare and is primarily a nosocomial infection in burn victims. Local infection has also resulted from the use of contaminated elastic bandages. The involved area is erythematous and painful, with varying degrees of central necrosis. This form of infection can also occur as a result of dissemination from another site of involvement. Skin and subcutaneous infection in diabetics can occur.

Gastrointestinal zygomycosis is the rarest form of infection. It is seen primarily in patients suffering from intrinsic abnormalities of the gastrointestinal tract or severe malnutrition. The infection is thought to arise from fungi entering the body with food. Any part of the gastrointestinal tract is susceptible to infection, with the stomach, terminal ileum and colon being the most common sites. Wall invasion, ischemic infarction, and ulceration are characteristic. The diagnosis is frequently made at autopsy.

Disseminated zygomycosis is defined as infection occurring in two or more noncontiguous organ systems. The distant sites are infected by bloodstream invasion from a local site. Although any organ can be affected, the lungs and central nervous system are the two common sites. The outcome of this infection is almost invariably fatal.

Isolated central nervous system zygomycosis results from hematogenous spread and is seen primarily in intravenous drug addicts.

DIAGNOSIS. The diagnosis of any form of zygomycosis is dependent on direct and histologic examinations of scrapings and biopsies of necrotic material. Fixed tissue can be stained with hematoxylin and eosin, and fungal hyphae can be seen with this routine histologic stain. However, a more rapid but preliminary diagnosis can sometimes be made by demonstrating hyphal elements after potassium hydroxide digestion of fresh tissue scraping. The alkali digests some of the tissue debris, but not the fungus, and makes the identification of the fungi easier. Swabs of discharge or abnormal tissue are not adequate and can give erroneous information. Fungal cultures are occasionally positive, but a negative culture result does not exclude the diagnosis nor make it less likely. The media used for culturing these fungi should not contain cycloheximide. At present, no skin tests or serologic methods are adequate for diagnosing zygomycosis. Blood cultures are not helpful.

THERAPY. The hallmarks of successful outcome in this aggressive infection rely on early diagnosis by invasive procedures, immediate correction of the underlying predisposing condition, aggressive surgical debridement, and early rapid systemic amphotericin therapy. Amphotericin B is the only drug with proven clinical efficacy, and a high therapeutic dosage (such as 1.0 to 1.5 mg per kilogram per day, if tolerated) should be achieved as soon as possible. This may be reduced to alternate-day dosing once the patient is stabilized. Typically, a cumulative dose of 2 to 5 grams may be needed to achieve cure. Although local irrigation of infected sites with amphotericin is an unproven adjunct, given the difficulties in perfusion of infected areas because of the tendency to thrombosis, this measure seems logical. Similarly, potentiation of amphotericin with other drugs (such as rifampin, flucytosine) is of unproven benefit, but given the poor results

TABLE 407–1. CLINICAL MANIFESTATIONS OF ZYGOMYCOSIS

Rhinocerebral	Gastrointestinal
Pulmonary	Widely disseminated
Cutaneous	Central nervous system

with conventional therapy, this should be considered if susceptibility testing can be done in vitro with the patient's isolate to show synergy and exclude antagonism. The newer orally administered azole derivates have no proven activity against these fungi. Improvement of survival may necessitate repeated major surgical debridement of necrotic tissue, resulting in significant disfiguring. If the patient survives, major reconstructive surgery may be needed.

PROGNOSIS. Since its first description by Paltauf in Germany in 1885, zygomycosis remains a disease with guarded prognosis. It is difficult to ascertain accurately the effectiveness of any therapeutic approach because the disease is relatively rare and there is a general bias toward reporting cases only if therapy is effective. With the introduction of amphotericin B in 1961, it is generally accepted that the survival rate significantly improved. Rhinocerebral zygomycosis is the most common form of infection and is thought to have an overall mortality rate of about 50 per cent. Patients who develop hemiplegia, facial necrosis, or nasal deformity have a higher mortality. Pulmonary or disseminated zygomycosis frequently escapes antemortem diagnosis, and only a handful of patients have been reported to recover from these infections.

At this time, the most aggressive approach we can take toward this lethal disease is rapid diagnosis and immediate institution of surgical debridement plus systemic and local chemotherapy.

Bigby TD, Serota ML, Tierney LM, et al.: Clinical spectrum of pulmonary mucormycosis. Chest 89:435, 1986. *This review emphasizes the pulmonary form and includes discussion of the microbiology, pathology, predisposing factors, clinical presentation, diagnosis, and treatment.*

Ferry AP, Abedi S: Diagnosis and management of rhino-orbitocerebral mucormycosis. Ophthalmology 90:1096, 1983. *This article reports the personal experience of the senior author with 16 patients. All the patients had one or more predisposing factors, with diabetes mellitus being the most common.*

Ingram CN, Sennesh J, Cooper JN, et al.: Disseminated zygomycosis: Report of four cases and review. Rev Infect Dis 11:741, 1989. *A presentation of four cases of disseminated disease and a comprehensive review of 181 cases reported in the English language literature. Hematologic malignancy is the major predisposing factor for dissemination. More than 90 per cent of disseminated infections were diagnosed at autopsy.*

408 Mycetoma

Michael S. Saag

DEFINITION. Mycetoma is a chronic, localized, subcutaneous infection characterized by draining sinus tracts that frequently discharge purulent material containing granules. The disease most often affects the lower extremities, with the majority of cases involving the foot. Originally described in the mid-1800's, the disease was initially referred to as "Madura foot," named after the region in India where it was first identified. Although still referred to as maduromycosis, the preferred name and the term used most often to describe the disorder is mycetoma.

ETIOLOGY. More than 20 species of fungi and bacteria have been implicated as etiologic agents of mycetoma. Approximately 40 per cent of cases are due to true fungi (eumycetoma), and 60 per cent are caused by aerobic actinomycetes (actinomycetoma). The organisms are distributed throughout the world, and the predominant organisms responsible for disease are subject to regional variation. Etiologic agents of eumycetoma and actinomycetoma may be presumptively identified based on the characteristic pigment of their granules. A listing of the predominant causative organisms is given in Table 408–1.

EPIDEMIOLOGY. Mycetomas have been reported from all over the world but are endemic in tropical regions of Africa, India, Central and South America, and the Far East. The geographic distribution of the disease is more related to rainfall than any other climatic factor. Most of the etiologic agents have been cultured from the soil in endemic areas, and occasionally organisms have been identified on plant thorns, which may be responsible for intradermal inoculation. *Pseudallescheria boydii* is the most common cause of mycetoma in the United States and is readily isolated from the soil in the United States and Canada.

TABLE 408–1. CAUSATIVE ORGANISMS OF MYCETOMA AND THE CHARACTERISTIC PIGMENT OF THEIR ASSOCIATED GRANULES

Eumycetoma	Actinomycetoma
White to yellow grains	
Pseudallescheria boydii	Nocardia brasiliensis
Acremonium species	Nocardia asteroides
Trichophyton species	Nocardia cavae (tiny grains)
Microsporum species	Actinomadura madurae (large
Fusarium species	grains)
Aspergillus nidulans	
Yellow to brown grains	
Neotestudina (Zophia) rosatii	Streptomyces somaliensis
Black grains	
Madurella mycetomatis	Streptomyces paraguayensis
Madurella grisea	
Exophiala jeanselmei	
Leptosphaeria senegalensis	
Leptosphaeria thompkinsii	
Red to pink grains	
	Actinomadura pelletieri

Nocardia brasiliensis and *Actinomadura madurae* are the most frequently isolated organisms in Central America, South America, and the Caribbean.

The majority of cases occur in males, many of whom are field laborers or herdsmen who encounter repeated trauma to their feet while in wet or swampy soil. Although the disease afflicts people of all ages, most cases are reported in young adults. Person-to-person transmission is not believed to occur, and the disease is unrelated to animal contact.

PATHOGENESIS AND PATHOLOGY. In contrast to systemic mycoses, which are usually established via the respiratory route, mycetomas are initiated through direct inoculation of the organism into the skin or mucosal surface, frequently as a consequence of trauma. Although the foot is the most common site of infection, direct inoculation of organisms into the hand, back, neck, and back of the head can occur in individuals who carry loads contaminated with soil.

The precise mechanism of pathogenesis remains unknown. Once inoculated, the organism induces a subacute to chronic suppurative inflammatory response that is primarily neutrophilic in nature but that may be associated with a granulomatous reaction. Over time, localized necrosis, fibrosis, abscess formation, and, frequently, bone and joint disease ensue. Deep sinuses with fistulas commonly develop and present as draining sinus tracts on the skin surface. The purulent drainage from those tracts often contains grains or granules, which consist of the causative organism embedded in a host-derived, proteinaceous matrix. The size, character, and color of the granules suggest the underlying etiologic agent (Table 408–1).

The inflammatory process usually extends along fascial planes and may result in substantial regional destruction of deep tissues and bone. Distal spread of disease via the lymphatics or the bloodstream may occur but is distinctly uncommon.

CLINICAL MANIFESTATIONS. Most cases of mycetoma present late in the course of a longstanding, chronic inflammatory disease. The initial lesion appears as a small, painless nodule several weeks to months after primary inoculation. The patient generally cannot recall a precipitating event or specific traumatic incident. The lesions slowly extend into deep tissues, and the resultant lymphatic obstruction, fibrosis, and tissue thickening give the foot a shortened, raised appearance. Skin nodules may break down, yielding granulomatous tissue with serosanguineous to purulent discharge. Later in the course of disease, sinus tracts begin to appear through which the characteristic fungal granules are expelled onto the skin surface. The sinus tracts spontaneously heal, only to be replaced by new tracts at nearby sites. Eumycetomas tend to be more circumscribed, remain localized, and progress more slowly than actinomycetomas, which have less well defined margins, merge with surrounding tissue, and progress more rapidly. The lesions tend to remain painless until deep bone involvement occurs, although many patients may complain of a deep itching sensation during active disease progression. Systemic involvement is rare, and patients feel remarkably well even in the presence of advanced localized disease.

DIAGNOSIS. The definitive diagnosis of mycetoma depends on culture of the causative organism from tissue specimens. The disease is suspected in the appropriate clinical setting, especially when grains are identified in the purulent discharge. Examination of the grains can establish a differential diagnosis of eumycetoma or actinomycetoma based on the presence of characteristic broad (fungal) or narrow (actinomycete) filaments. The characteristics of the granules, when combined with geographic and epidemiologic information, can yield a presumptive identification of the specific organism. However, cultural data are required for confirmation. Serologic tests are not routinely available.

TREATMENT. The response to therapy is dependent on the underlying etiologic agent. Eumycetomas are unresponsive to antimicrobial therapy, although partial responses to amphotericin B, miconazole, ketoconazole, and thiabendazole have been reported. Fortunately, eumycetomas tend to be well circumscribed, yielding ready access to surgical approaches. If the lesion is not removed in its entirety and residual disease is present, relapse is inevitable.

Actinomycetomas are more responsive to antimicrobial therapy. Regimens consisting of high-dose penicillin (10 to 12 million units per day), sulfadiazine (3 to 10 grams per day), or minocycline (150 mg twice daily) have been reported to have some effect. The most successful regimens consist of trimethoprim-sulfamethoxazole (160 mg of trimethoprim and 800 mg of sulfamethoxazole given twice daily), combined with either streptomycin (1 to 3 grams per day for 3 weeks) or rifampin (600 mg per day for 3 to 4 months); or dapsone (100 mg twice daily) combined with streptomycin (1 gram per day for 1 month, given intramuscularly). The dapsone regimen is often preferred owing to its low cost. The duration of therapy with either the trimethoprim-sulfamethoxazole or the dapsone regimen is usually 9 months, depending on response.

PROGNOSIS. If the disease is diagnosed early, the prognosis for mycetoma is good. Unfortunately, many cases are not identified until late in the course of disease, when response to therapy is limited, and amputation may be required. When disease is located on the back, neck, trunk, or abdomen, very little therapeutic intervention can be offered. The prognosis for survival is quite good; however, the quality of life may be dramatically lessened.

Magana M: Mycetoma. Int J Dermatol 23:221, 1984. *A thorough review of clinical aspects of mycetoma and therapeutic approaches.*

Mahgoub ES: Medical management of mycetoma. Bull WHO 54:303, 1976. *Summarizes general principles of diagnosis and management.*

Smego RA Jr, Gallis HA: The clinical spectrum of *Nocardia brasiliensis* infection in the United States. Rev Infect Dis 6:164, 1984. *An important review of the pathogenesis, diagnosis, and therapy of the most common cause of mycetoma worldwide.*

Tight RR, Bartlett MS: Actinomycetoma in the United States. Rev Infect Dis 3:1139, 1981. *A comprehensive review that focuses on diagnosis, antibiotic susceptibility, and protracted therapy in disease management.*

409 Dematiaceous Fungal Infections

Michael S. Saag

DEFINITION. The term "dematiaceous" is applied to fungi that produce an intrinsic characteristic pigment. Diseases caused by dematiaceous fungi are divided into two groups: chromomycosis (chromoblastomycosis) and phaeohyphomycosis.

ETIOLOGY. Chromomycosis is caused by several species of related fungi, most notably *Fonsecaea, Phialophora, Cladosporium,* and *Acrotheca* species. These agents are brown-pigmented saprophytes commonly found in soil and wood. The clinical appearance, which is virtually identical for all of the causative agents, consists of thick-walled, dark brown bodies ("sclerotic cells" or "copper pennies"), which may be single or clustered. Sclerotic cells represent an intermediate form between yeasts and hyphae and multiply by horizontal and vertical separation, not by budding.

Phaeohyphomycosis may be caused by several organisms, frequently referred to as "black" fungi. They differ from the agents of chromomycosis in their clinical appearance and the absence of sclerotic cells. The black fungi usually exist in tissues as yeastlike cells (solitary or in small chains), as septated hyphae (branched or unbranched), or as a combination of yeast and hyphae. The hyphal forms are frequently confused with *Aspergillus* species but may be distinguished by using the Fontana-Masson staining procedure (a melanin-specific stain) or via in vitro culture. The most common agents of phaeohyphomycosis identified in humans include *Curvularia* species, *Bipolaris* species, *Exserohilum* species, *Alternaria* species, *Mycocentrospora* species, *Pyrenochaeta* species, *Trichomaris* species, *Wangiella* species, *Xylohypha* species, and *Exophiala* species.

EPIDEMIOLOGY AND PATHOGENESIS. The organisms causing chromomycosis and phaeohyphomycosis are worldwide in distribution. Chromomycosis occurs predominantly in young males and is usually inoculated into the skin via thorns, splinters, and other penetrating wounds. The disease is more prevalent in rural populations, especially among those with suboptimal nutritional status and personal hygiene. Chromomycosis appears to be endemic in certain areas, such as Madagascar and Costa Rica.

Phaeohyphomycosis is becoming an important disease among immunocompromised hosts. Despite the ubiquity of black fungi in the environment, disease due to these organisms had, in the past, been sporadic. More recently, however, clusters of cases have been reported from major medical centers as opportunistic infections in transplant recipients, especially bone marrow transplant patients.

CLINICAL MANIFESTATIONS. Chromomycosis initially manifests as a wart-like papule that slowly enlarges into a verruciform plaque. The lesions may progress to ulceration with or without an exudate. Over time, the lesions become dry and crusted with a raised border, which may be serpiginous. Large plaques frequently develop central scarring. Occasionally, the lesions become pedunculated and acquire a cauliflower-like appearance. Systemic spread to distal sites is distinctly uncommon, although spread through autoinoculation or via lymphatic drainage may occur. Rarely, widespread disseminated disease to the pancreas, liver, bowel, lymph nodes, meninges, and brain is noted.

Phaeohyphomycosis may occur as a wide spectrum of clinical disease. Superficial phaeohyphomycosis is the most benign and is found in the stratum corneum or around the hair shaft. Tinea nigra and black piedra are examples of this disorder. More invasive skin disease involving nonliving layers of keratinized epithelium include the dermatomycoses and onychomycoses. Mycotic keratitis may result in extensive corneal damage and subsequent blindness. Subcutaneous disease usually results from direct inoculation of fungi through intact skin. Cystic lesions with well-defined walls and central abscess formation, occasionally surrounding a foreign body such as a splinter, are characteristic.

Invasive phaeohyphomycosis is a potentially life-threatening disease that occurs predominantly in immunocompromised hosts. Localized invasive disease frequently occurs in the paranasal sinuses, lower respiratory tract, and bone. Disease due to *Cladosporium, Curvularia, Bipolaris, Xylohypha,* and *Exserohilum* species is especially prone to invade the central nervous system.

DIAGNOSIS. The diagnosis of chromomycosis and phaeohyphomycosis is made by histopathologic examination of tissue biopsy specimens or KOH (10 per cent) preparations. The brown sclerotic cells of chromomycosis are readily identified, and special stains are not usually required. Phaeohyphomycosis is best diagnosed using the Fontana-Masson technique, which distinguishes organisms producing phaeohyphomycoses from *Aspergillus* species. Cultures are required to identify the specific genera causing chromomycosis and phaeohyphomycosis. All cultures should be held for at least 8 weeks, since some of the organisms grow slowly. No serologic or skin tests are available.

TREATMENT. Surgical excision, when feasible, is the most effective mode of therapy for subcutaneous or deeply invasive disease. Unfortunately, unless lesions are diagnosed and treated early, the rate of relapse is high. Systemic antifungal therapy with amphotericin B is often used; however, the results are generally disappointing. Flucytosine (5-FC; 150 mg per kilogram per day) has been used on an investigational basis in patients with chromomycosis, with some success (16 of 23 patients cured); however, resistance developed in several treated patients. The response to therapy of phaeohyphomycosis is highly dependent on the causative organism. Many black fungi are resistant to 5-FC, and amphotericin B therapy yields variable results. Newer triazole antifungal agents show some promise as effective agents.

Adam RD, Paquin ML, Petersen EA, et al.: Phaeohyphomycosis caused by the fungal genera *Bipolaris* and *Exserohilum*. Medicine 65:203, 1986. *These fungi have been previously misclassified as* Helminthosporium *or* Drechslera *species, but the latter fungi appear not to produce human disease. This paper serves as an excellent review.*

Anaissie EJ, Bodey GP, Rinaldi MG: Emerging fungal pathogens. Eur J Microbiol Infect Dis 8:323, 1989. *An up-to-date overview of phaeohyphomycoses prevention in immunocompromised patients.*

Bennett JE, Bonner H, Jennings AE, et al.: Chronic meningitis caused by *Cladosporium trichoides*. Am J Clin Pathol 59:398, 1973. *Comprehensive review of cerebral infection with dematiaceous fungi.*

McGinnis MR: Chromoblastomycosis and phaeohyphomycosis: New concepts, diagnosis and mycology. J Am Acad Dermatol 8:1, 1983. *Clear-cut exposition of clinical and mycologic criteria for these diagnoses. A very important review.*

PART XXI

HIV AND ASSOCIATED DISORDERS

Introduction

Michael S. Saag

In June 1981 the sentinel cases of the acquired immune deficiency syndrome (AIDS) were reported. Throughout the remainder of that year, additional cases were identified in the major metropolitan centers of the United States. By 1982, the syndrome was beginning to be identified with certain "high-risk" groups, including homosexual men, heroin users, hemophiliacs, and Haitians (the four H's). As details from carefully performed epidemiologic studies became available, it was clear that the epidemic was most likely due to an infectious agent that was transmissible through intimate sexual contact or blood contact. In 1983, the human immunodeficiency virus (HIV-1; previously referred to as LAV, HTLV-III, and ARV) was identified, and by 1985 a blood test was established that could identify HIV-infected individuals prior to the development of AIDS. As a result, the term *AIDS* became important primarily as a useful epidemiologic description, but most clinicians began to think of the disorder as HIV disease, a spectrum of illness that ranges from asymptomatic seropositivity to full-blown AIDS.

The latest epidemiologic evidence strongly indicates continuing spread of the disease into rural areas of the United States and continued spread of infection through all types of sexual contact, both homosexual and heterosexual. As the number of cases continues to grow, it is inevitable that every primary care physician will encounter an HIV-infected patient in his or her practice. The approach to diagnosis and treatment in HIV-infected patients is no different than for uninfected patients: a careful history and physical examination, appropriate use of laboratory tests, development of a differential diagnosis, and initial approach to therapy are all still required. Although some of the opportunistic pathogens that are so common in HIV infection may be unfamiliar to the practicing primary care physician, information regarding current approaches to diagnosis and therapy of these pathogens is contained within this part. Still, the care of HIV-infected patients does present some unique challenges. The vast array of journal articles related to the care of AIDS patients can overwhelm a busy clinician in practice. Office staff and perhaps physicians themselves may be apprehensive in providing care for HIV-infected patients owing to fear of becoming infected. Most notably, however, providing care for HIV-infected patients is complicated by social problems that are unique to that group. Many patients encounter discrimination in the workplace, at schools, in housing, and in obtaining access to care. There are many psychological hurdles patients must overcome to truly focus on *living* with their infection in a positive way.

In the latter part of the 1980's, information regarding the natural history of the disease, approaches to the common manifestations of HIV-related disorders, and clinical experience in caring for HIV-infected patients began to grow in proportion to the exponential growth of the epidemic itself. New therapeutic modalities, earlier interventions of therapy, and application of preventive therapy led to a substantial increase in overall survival and improved quality of life for HIV-infected patients. The dramatic accumulation of knowledge, however, created problems for clinicians who were providing care. Publications, books, audio and video cassettes, and monographs regarding AIDS have

flooded into physicians' offices at unprecedented rates. It is difficult, if not impossible, for even the "AIDS specialist" to keep up with state-of-the-art therapies for HIV infection. Owing to the rapid rate of development of new knowledge, sources of information regarding care of AIDS patients become rapidly outdated, sometimes even before the pages hit the press. In short, it is difficult to find a single best source for updated HIV information.

The goal of this part is to provide state-of-the-art information regarding the care of HIV-infected patients—"a single best source" of information on HIV infection for the practicing clinician. The chapters provide information on the basic biology of the virus, the epidemiology of its transmission and spread, approaches to antiretroviral therapy, common clinical manifestations of HIV-related disorders, approaches to therapy by organ systems, and approaches to prevention and counseling. HIV disease is indeed a spectrum of illness that challenges the physician to develop both breadth and depth of knowledge in science and medicine as well as psychosocial and political issues—a dynamic blend of the science and art of medicine.

410 Immunology Related to AIDS

Bruce D. Walker

Since the first cases of the acquired immune deficiency syndrome (AIDS) were reported in 1981, infection with the human immunodeficiency virus 1 (HIV-1) has become a global medical crisis. An estimated 5 to 10 million persons worldwide have become infected with HIV-1 and related retroviruses through sexual, parenteral, or perinatal exposure. The vast majority of infected individuals, if not all, can be expected eventually to develop symptomatic disease, characterized by progressive and ultimately profound immunosuppression. The clinical consequences of infection are due to the ability of this virus to disarm the host immune system, a process that occurs by virtue of the fact that the primary target for the virus is the helper-inducer subset of lymphocytes. This lymphocyte subset, defined by its surface expression of the CD4 molecule, acts as the pivotal orchestrator of myriad immune functions (see Ch. 242). HIV infection can therefore be considered a disease of the immune system, characterized by the progressive loss of CD4+ lymphocytes, with ultimately fatal consequences for the infected host.

Despite this immunosuppression induced by HIV, a number of specific immunologic defenses against the virus are generated in infected individuals and may contribute to the long asymptomatic phase following infection by keeping the virus at least partially contained. The potential significance of such responses is also underscored by the recent demonstration in animal AIDS models that a state of vaccine-induced protective immunity can be achieved against retroviruses related to HIV. An understanding of the immunology related to HIV provides insight not only into the clinical sequelae of infection but also into the prospects for development of an effective vaccine against HIV.

THE VIRUS LIFE CYCLE (see also Ch. 376, 411, and 421)

The basic molecular structure of HIV is similar to that of other retroviruses, with three major genes termed *gag* (group-specific antigen), *pol* (polymerase), and *env* (envelope), in addition to a number of regulatory genes (*nef, rev, tat*) and others (*vif, vpu, vpr*) with as yet undetermined function. The ability of HIV to infect cells is mediated through the viral envelope protein. The envelope gene encodes a precursor protein gp160, which is subsequently proteolytically cleaved to two smaller proteins, gp41 and gp120, which associate at the infected cell surface. Gp41 is a transmembrane protein that serves as a membrane anchor for gp120, the mature exterior envelope glycoprotein. The first step in virus infectivity is the binding of gp120 to the CD4 (also called T4) cell surface protein, which is the specific cellular receptor for the virus. The CD4 protein is found predominantly on the helper-inducer subset of lymphocytes but also to a lesser degree on monocytes/macrophages and some other nucleated cells (Fig. 410–1). Following binding to CD4, the viral membrane fuses with the host cell membrane and the virus is uncoated and enters the cell cytoplasm. The viral enzyme reverse transcriptase then transcribes the viral RNA into DNA. This double-stranded DNA can remain unintegrated in the cellular cytoplasm or can become integrated into the host chromosomal DNA, in which case it is termed proviral DNA. Through processes of transcription and translation, new viral RNA and proteins are produced, which are subsequently assembled into new virions. As the newly synthesized envelope precursor gp160 is glycosylated and cleaved, mature envelope glycoprotein knobs (gp41/gp120) are embedded in the cellular membrane. As mature capsid proteins containing viral RNA bud at the cell surface, the envelope coating is completed and mature infectious virions are released.

The majority of cell-associated virus in blood is contained within CD4+ lymphocytes. Despite a numerical decline in the absolute number of these cells with disease progression, the actual proportion of cells infected with HIV increases. In patients with AIDS, as many as 1 per 100 CD4+ lymphocytes have been demonstrated to harbor the provirus. Viral replication occurs continuously in HIV-infected persons, and there appears to be no truly latent phase when replication ceases altogether. A number of factors may, however, act to increase viral production in vitro by infected cells. Among these are other viruses (cytomegalovirus [CMV], Epstein-Barr virus [EBV], HTLV-I, and human herpesvirus VI [HHV-6]), mitogens, and lymphokines (GM-CSF, TNF-α, and interleukin 6), suggesting that these may serve as cofactors in disease induction.

HIV-INDUCED IMMUNOSUPPRESSION

The hallmark of HIV infection is progressive depletion of the CD4 helper-inducer subset of lymphocytes. Owing to the central role of these cells in immunologic functioning, the clinical disease manifestations of immunosuppression and susceptibility to opportunistic infections and neoplasms are not surprising. The immunologic deficits associated with HIV infection are wide-spread and involve numerous interdependent effector arms of the immune system, involving both cellular and humoral elements.

DIRECT IMMUNOSUPPRESSIVE PROPERTIES OF VIRAL PRODUCTS. Protein products of a number of retroviruses have been shown to have direct immunosuppressive properties independent of viral infection. A synthetic peptide corresponding to a highly conserved region in the HIV-1 gp41 transmembrane protein has been demonstrated to inhibit lymphocyte proliferative responses to mitogenic or antigenic stimuli in vitro. This region is analogous to a highly conserved immunosuppressive protein of HTLV-I, and similar inhibitory transmembrane proteins have been identified in other animal retroviral infections such as feline leukemia virus (FeLV). Whether such a phenomenon contributes to the global immunosuppression seen in HIV-infected individuals has not been determined, but the possibility that HIV proteins may be immunosuppressive has raised concerns about inclusion of such sequences in potential HIV vaccine candidates.

T-LYMPHOCYTE ABNORMALITIES. Lymphocyte abnormalities associated with HIV infection can be classified as both quantitative and qualitative. Qualitative deficiencies become apparent soon after infection and before CD4 depletion is evident and are largely related to intrinsic functional defects in the helper-inducer subset of lymphocytes. Studies using purified subpopulations of lymphocytes from AIDS patients have demonstrated a selective defect in soluble antigen (e.g., tetanus toxoid) recognition, although these cells are still able to undergo a normal degree of blast transformation and lymphokine production after exposure to mitogen (e.g., phytohemagglutinin). In other words, the weapon is loaded, but only mitogens and not antigens cause the trigger to be pulled. These studies also indicate that the central defect is the lack of helper cell function rather than an overabundance of suppressor cell activity. Other lymphocyte abnormalities observed with HIV infection include decreased lymphokine production, decreased expression of interleukin 2 (IL2) receptors, decreased alloreactivity, and decreased ability to provide help to B cells. The functional T-lymphocyte abnormalities also likely contribute to the loss of delayed-type hypersensitivity reactions, which become more prevalent as disease progresses.

The quantitative abnormality of T lymphocytes is the result of a progressive depletion of the CD4+ helper T-lymphocyte population, which begins soon after primary infection (Table 410–1). This downhill trend continues until the normal levels of 800 to 1200 CD4 cells per cubic millimeter drop below 50 and sometimes below 10 cells per cubic millimeter in the later stages of disease. CD4 cell depletion cannot be attributed solely to direct cytotoxic effects of virus infection, as only a minority of

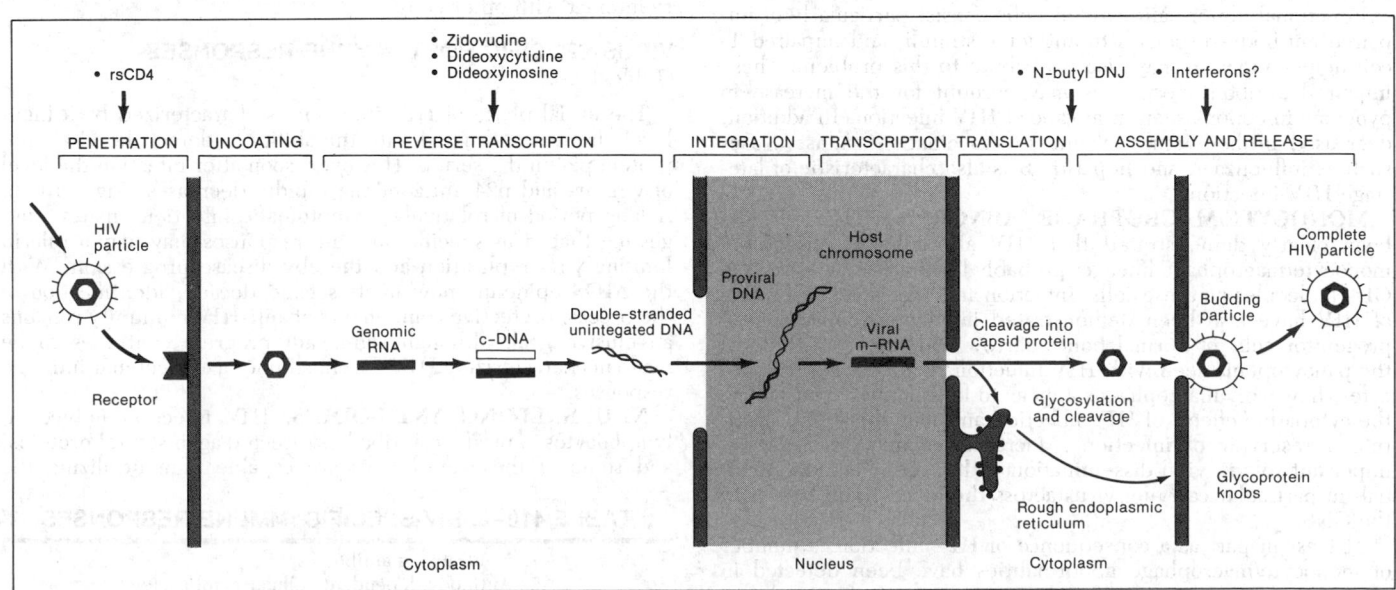

FIGURE 410–1. The life cycle of HIV. The target sites for antiretroviral agents are listed. (Reprinted from Johnson VA, Hirsch MS: *In* Volberding P, Jacobson M (eds.): AIDS Clinical Review 1990. New York, Marcel Dekker, 1990, p 238. By courtesy of Marcel Dekker, Inc.)

TABLE 410–1. POTENTIAL CAUSES OF CD4 CELL DEPLETION

1. Direct toxic consequences of infection
2. Syncytia formation
3. Innocent bystander destruction of cells with adsorbed gp120
4. HIV infection of stem cells
5. Autoimmune destruction

helper cells are actually infected, even in later stages of illness. Other factors potentially contributing to CD4 depletion include (a) syncytia formation, in which a single infected cell fuses via its surface gp120 with the CD4 molecule on uninfected cells, forming multinucleated giant cells, (b) "innocent bystander" destruction of uninfected CD4 cells that have bound free gp120 to the CD4 molecule, rendering them susceptible to immune attack, (c) HIV infection of stem cells, resulting in decreased helper cell production, and (d) autoimmune mechanisms, whereby cross-reactive antibodies or cellular immune responses to the virus result in killing of uninfected CD4 cells. Whatever the mechanisms of the CD4 cell depletion, the resultant consequence to immune function is so profound that total CD4 number is currently the best measure of disease progression. The risk of certain opportunistic infections increases significantly when the total CD4 cell number is less than 200 per cubic millimeter, which is why routine prophylaxis against *Pneumocystis carinii* pneumonia is instituted at this stage. At levels below 100 per cubic millimeter the risk for other complications, such as disseminated *Mycobacterium avium* or CMV infection, increases dramatically.

B-LYMPHOCYTE ABNORMALITIES. As with T-lymphocyte abnormalities in HIV infection, the B-lymphocyte abnormalities are both quantitative and qualitative. Most characteristic, particularly in the early stages of infection, is an intense polyclonal activation of B cells, evidenced clinically by elevated levels of immunoglobulins G and A, the presence of circulating immune complexes, and an increased number of peripheral blood B lymphocytes that secrete immunoglobulin spontaneously. These B-cell abnormalities are unlikely to be a direct consequence of HIV infection of B cells. Whereas B cells can express low levels of CD4 and have been infected in vitro, there are no conclusive data indicating that these cells became infected in vivo. Rather, the virus itself or viral proteins appear to interact directly with and stimulate uninfected cells. Other potential contributors to this polyclonal activation include concurrent viral infections. For example, CMV and EBV infections occur with greatly increased frequency in HIV-infected individuals and can lead to B-cell hyperactivity.

Functional abnormalities of B cells consist particularly of impaired antibody responses to antigenic stimuli, and impaired T-cell helper function may also contribute to this problem. These impaired antibody responses may account for the increase in pyogenic infections seen in advanced HIV infection. In addition, decreased antibody responsiveness to vaccination against viruses such as influenza A and hepatitis B is also characteristic of late-stage HIV infection.

MONOCYTE/MACROPHAGE ABNORMALITIES. It has been clearly demonstrated that HIV also infects cells of the monocyte/macrophage lineage, probably by attachment to surface CD4 molecules on these cells. Infection and high-level replication of HIV have also been demonstrated in monocyte/macrophage progenitor cells of normal bone marrow and may contribute to the pancytopenia seen with HIV infection. Unlike CD4 lymphocytes, however, macrophages appear to be relatively resistant to the cytopathic effects of HIV infection and may therefore constitute a reservoir of infection. Macrophages may also play an important role in viral dissemination within the infected individual, in particular carrying virus across the blood-brain barrier to the CNS.

At least in part as a consequence of HIV infection, a number of monocyte/macrophage abnormalities have been detected in HIV-seropositive persons. The ability of monocytes/macrophages to act as antigen-presenting cells is impaired, particularly in later stages of illness. Some defects in these cells in AIDS patients may be a consequence of chronic in vivo activation, such as

increased IL2 receptor expression, IL1 secretion, and increased chemotactic ligand receptor expression. The reasons for this chronic activation are likely multifactorial and may relate to exposure to viral proteins or lymphokines or to direct effects of HIV infection. These abnormalities may have immunopathogenic consequences, since defects in the ability to present antigens could ultimately impair the ability to sustain an immune response against HIV or other pathogens.

In the brain, cells of the macrophage lineage appear to be the major cell type infected with HIV and directly or indirectly may contribute to the CNS dysfunction observed in this disease. In the lung, infected alveolar macrophages may stimulate HIV-specific immune responses, the by-products of which have been postulated to contribute to the observed alveolitis. Deficient T4 helper cell function may also indirectly contribute to the observed defects in monocytes/macrophages, since a minority of monocytes/macrophages appear to be actually productively infected in vivo.

NATURAL KILLER CELL ABNORMALITIES. Natural killer (NK) cells are thought to be an important component of immunosurveillance against virus-infected cells, allogeneic cells, and tumor cells. NK cells are typically large granular lymphocytes that recognize foreign antigens on cells, resulting in activation of lytic machinery. NK cells are phenotypically and numerically normal in AIDS patients, but they are functionally defective. This may relate in part to an observed defect in the trigger mechanism necessary to deliver the lethal blow to a target cell. In addition, defective lymphokine production in HIV-infected persons may also contribute to NK cell dysfunction. However, addition of IL2 to these cells in vitro only partially restores NK function.

AUTOIMMUNE ABNORMALITIES. Autoimmune phenomena are also part of the immunologic derangement in HIV infection and may also contribute to the disease manifestations seen clinically. When sensitive assays are used, circulating immune complexes can be detected in the majority of HIV-infected individuals. These may help to explain the occurrence of HIV-related arthralgias, myalgias, renal disease, and vasculitis. Anti-HIV antibody complexes attached to platelets of persons with HIV-related thrombocytopenia may be the cause of this defect, although specific antiplatelet membrane antibodies have also been proposed as the cause of this thrombocytopenia.

Autoimmune mechanisms may also directly contribute to the immune suppression seen in AIDS. Sequence similarities exist between the HIV envelope transmembrane protein and HLA Class II proteins, and antibodies that cross-react with these two proteins have been detected in HIV-infected persons. Such autoantibodies could impair functioning of cells bearing Class II antigens, either by directly eliminating these cells through antibody-dependent cellular cytotoxicity or by inhibiting their ability to interact with other cells.

VIRUS-SPECIFIC HOST IMMUNE RESPONSES
(Table 410–2)

The initial phase of HIV infection is characterized by a high-level viremia, associated with the ability to detect the viral core protein p24 in the serum. However, soon after infection the level of viremia and p24 antigenemia rapidly decreases (Fig. 410–2). A long period of relatively asymptomatic infection ensues, suggesting that virus-specific immune responses may play a role in limiting viral replication and thereby disease progression. With the AIDS epidemic now in its second decade, identification of the precise protective components of anti-HIV immunity remains an elusive goal, although significant progress continues to be made in characterizing HIV-specific humoral and cellular immune responses.

NEUTRALIZING ANTIBODIES. HIV infection induces B lymphocytes to produce antibodies directed against viral proteins, and some of these antibodies are capable of neutralizing the

TABLE 410–2. HIV-SPECIFIC IMMUNE RESPONSES

1. Neutralizing antibodies
2. Antibody-dependent cellular cytotoxicity
3. Natural killer cells
4. Cytotoxic T cells
5. Cellular proliferative responses

virus. Antibody responses are typically observed 1 to 3 months following infection, although longer periods before the development of antibody responses have been documented in rare instances. Neutralizing antibodies directly neutralize free virus at a stage before the virus has entered the cell and become uncoated. In a number of viral infections, neutralizing antibody induced by immunization correlates with protection from subsequent viral infection. HIV-1 infection results in the production of HIV-specific antibodies directed at a number of viral proteins, and some of these antibodies demonstrate neutralizing activity. The primary target of neutralizing antibodies is the envelope glycoprotein, in particular a loop structure within a relatively hypervariable region of the gp120 glycoprotein termed the principal neutralizing domain.

Neutralizing antibodies have been demonstrated to be present at all stages of HIV infection, and although titers are generally lower in later stages of illness, attempts to correlate neutralizing antibody titers with disease progression have yielded conflicting results. In one study, chimpanzees given high-titered neutralizing antibody intravenously were not protected from subsequent challenge with HIV-1, although a possible explanation for this lack of protection is that the high virus inoculum used to challenge these animals may have overwhelmed the amount of neutralizing antibody present. In addition, titers of antibodies directed at the principal neutralizing domain were low in the immunoglobulin preparation used in this experiment.

The ability of HIV-specific neutralizing antibodies to confer protection may be impaired in part by the high degree of antigenic variation exhibited by HIV. This antigenic variation is particularly pronounced in the envelope region of the virus, and virus variants may emerge within an infected individual which are neutralization resistant. This antigenic variation also has significant implications for vaccine design, since neutralizing antibodies generated in response to a single immunizing strain of virus are likely to neutralize only very closely related viruses, a phenomenon known as type specificity.

Antibodies also constitute the first line of defense at mucosal surfaces, in the form of secretory IgA. Such secretory antibodies have been found in blood, saliva, and other body fluids of persons infected with HIV, but their potential role as a protective immune response in HIV infection remains undetermined.

In sharp contrast to proposed protective attributes, HIV-specific antibodies have also been shown to promote HIV infection under certain experimental conditions. Antibody binds to virions, and this complex appears to be taken up by some cells by binding of antibody through the cellular Fc receptor. This in vitro evidence for antibody-dependent enhancement is orders of magnitude less than what is observed, for example, in dengue virus infection, and the clinical significance of this phenomenon is not known.

ANTIBODY-DEPENDENT CELLULAR CYTOTOXICITY (ADCC). Another mechanism whereby the immune system can act to limit the spread of infection is ADCC, which involves both cellular and humoral components. ADCC is a process in which virus-specific antibodies bind directly to viral proteins expressed on the surface of infected cells, thereby sensitizing these cells for

lysis by cells that bind to the exposed Fc portion of the antibody. The cells mediating this response are typically NK cells, which express the CD16 Fc receptor for IgG. Antibodies capable of mediating ADCC have been identified in the majority of HIV-infected individuals; these are present soon after seroconversion and are maintained throughout the disease course. The major ADCC target antigens are the envelope glycoproteins gp120 and gp41; *gag* proteins may also be involved. It has been postulated that ADCC may limit cell-to-cell spread of virus by providing an early cytotoxic host defense. ADCC may correlate with better clinical stage in children born to infected mothers, and ADCC titers have been shown to be higher in early stages of infection in some studies. However, the contribution of this immune response to protection from disease remains unclear.

NATURAL KILLER CELLS. In vitro evidence suggests that NK-type cells are not only important in ADCC, but also may bind free HIV-specific antibodies through their Fc receptors, arming them for attack against HIV-infected cells.

CYTOTOXIC T LYMPHOCYTES (CTL). Cytotoxic T lymphocytes have been demonstrated to be one of the protective host defenses generated in response to a number of viral infections. CTL's are able to kill virus-infected cells by recognizing viral protein fragments on the infected cell surface, where these proteins form a binary complex with a surface human leukocyte antigen (HLA) molecule (see Ch. 250). CTL recognition of this complex leads to lysis and elimination of the infected cell.

Although the hallmark of HIV infection is the development of profound immunosuppression, extremely vigorous HIV-specific CTL responses have been detected in the peripheral blood of infected individuals. These responses are directed not only against the major viral structural proteins, but also against the reverse transcriptase protein and regulatory proteins such as *vif* and *nef*. These responses appear to be mediated predominantly by CD8+ lymphocytes, which recognize processed HIV proteins on the surface of infected cells in conjunction with HLA Class I (A, B, C) molecules. In addition to this so-called HLA-restricted CTL population, other cells capable of recognizing HIV envelope protein on infected cells in an HLA-unrestricted fashion also appear to exist. These cells may be T cells or cells of the NK phenotype. Some studies have also suggested the existence of HIV-specific, CD4+ CTL restricted by HLA Class II molecules.

Although a protective role for CTL has been demonstrated in numerous experimental models of viral infection, the question remains unresolved as to the possible protective role of CTL in HIV infection. There is at least indirect evidence to suggest that the CTL response might indeed retard disease progression. For example, CD8+ lymphocytes from HIV-infected individuals are able to inhibit HIV replication in autologous CD4 lymphocytes in vitro. Similar inhibitory CD8 cells have also been identified in the simian immunodeficiency virus (SIV)–infected macaque monkeys, and since cell contact is necessary for this inhibition to occur, it suggests that the cell mediating this response may be a classic CTL. Other indirect evidence that CTL may be important in retarding disease progression stems from studies quantifying

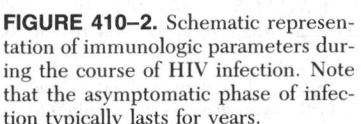

FIGURE 410–2. Schematic representation of immunologic parameters during the course of HIV infection. Note that the asymptomatic phase of infection typically lasts for years.

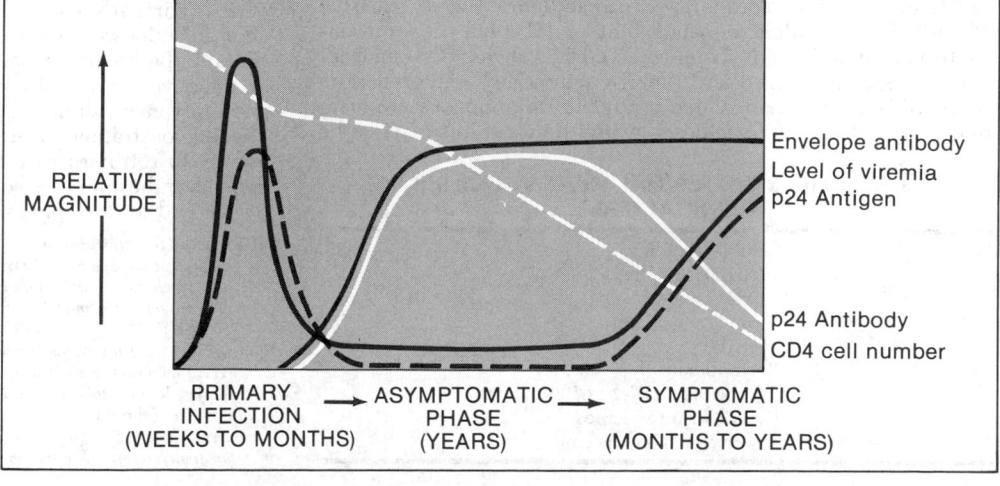

HIV-specific CTL in infected persons. As clinical disease progresses, CTL numbers decline, which could help to explain the increase in viremia observed in later stages of illness.

Conversely, HIV-specific CTL's have also been postulated by others to be deleterious to the host. These cells have been recovered from the lungs of subjects with lymphocytic alveolitis, suggesting that they may be inducing the alveolitis by attacking HIV-infected alveolar macrophages. In addition, CTL's have been detected in the CSF of HIV-infected individuals with neurologic disorders, prompting the hypothesis that CTL-mediated inflammatory reactions may contribute to the observed neurologic dysfunction. CTL's could also contribute to the progressive decline in CD4 cells by eliminating those cells that become HIV infected.

CELLULAR PROLIFERATIVE RESPONSES. T-cell immunity to viral pathogens consists not only of cytotoxic T lymphocytes, but also helper T-cell proliferation and cytokine production in specific response to viral antigens. This CD4+ proliferative response is generally triggered by recognition of viral antigen in association with Class II (HLA-D) molecules on the surface of antigen-presenting cells or B cells to be helped. Although HIV-specific proliferative responses are characteristically depressed in HIV-infected individuals, a number of epitopes eliciting these responses have been identified, particularly in the envelope glycoprotein gp120. Unfortunately, as with other HIV-specific immune responses, the precise contribution as a protective mechanism remains unclear.

PROSPECTS FOR VACCINE DEVELOPMENT
(Table 410–3)

Ultimate global control of the HIV epidemic likely will require a vaccine capable of eliciting protective immunity. Although efforts to define the components of protective immunity in infected persons have been unsuccessful thus far, recent data from animal models of retrovirus infection indicate that a state of protective immunity may be an attainable goal. When immunized with formalin-inactivated whole SIV, eight of nine rhesus monkeys were protected from infection when subsequently challenged with live SIV. The one animal that became infected developed a clinically attenuated form of disease, indicating a protective effect of the vaccine even when it is unable to prevent infection.

Despite these promising results in the SIV model of HIV infection, a number of potential obstacles exist to the development of an effective AIDS vaccine (Table 410–4). Foremost among these is the diversity of the viral genome. Most of this diversity occurs in the envelope gene, with as much as 20 per cent divergence in nucleotide sequence among field isolates. Even within a single individual, multiple divergent strains of virus have been identified, reflecting an extremely high intrinsic mutation rate for the virus. The implications of such diversity for vaccine development are profound, since the virus acts as a moving target for any immune response that is generated. Another obstacle to be overcome is the type specificity of immune responses generated to candidate vaccines, since immune responses generated by an immunogen representing a single field isolate are unlikely to cross-react with all field isolates. The issue of antibody-dependent enhancement of HIV infection remains controversial and needs to be resolved so that high-risk individuals are not immunized and thereby potentially rendered more susceptible to infection. Once candidate immunogens are identified, animal testing for efficacy would be ideal but may not be

TABLE 410–3. POTENTIAL HIV-1 VACCINES IN CLINICAL TRIALS

Soluble proteins
  gp160
  p24
  p17
  gp120
Recombinant live vaccines
  Vaccinia–HIV-1 gp160
Pseudovirion vaccines
Inactivated HIV vaccine

TABLE 410–4. POTENTIAL OBSTACLES TO HIV VACCINE DEVELOPMENT

Diversity of the viral genome
Type specificity of immune responses
Potential generation of enhancing antibodies
Lack of animal models of HIV infection and
  AIDS
Field trials to demonstrate efficacy
Indemnification of vaccinees from discrimination

possible for a number of reasons. Unfortunately there is no good animal model of HIV infection. Although chimpanzees become infected with HIV, they do not develop disease. Rhesus macaques develop an immunodeficiency disease similar to AIDS when infected with SIV but cannot be infected with HIV, are expensive to maintain, and are in limited supply. The potential utility of immunodeficient mice reconstituted with human fetal tissues, providing them with a "human" immune system, remains to be demonstrated. Perhaps the biggest obstacle will be demonstration of efficacy, which will require large field trials in populations demonstrating a high enough incidence of new infection that statistically significant data can be generated in a reasonable period of time. Demonstration of efficacy in one population may not translate to other populations. For example, protection of persons infected by sexual exposure will not necessarily imply that such a vaccine would protect intravenous drug abusers as well, who may be exposed to a higher initial inoculum of virus. As with HIV-infected persons, the potential for discrimination against vaccinees due to a positive serology will have to be addressed.

Although these obstacles exist, a number of preliminary clinical trials are already under way with a variety of vaccine candidates. These include soluble *gag* or envelope proteins, recombinant vaccina virus containing the HIV-1 envelope gene, pseudovirion vaccines that resemble whole HIV particles but are modified to exclude the viral genome or render it harmless, and whole killed virus vaccines. The latter approach is currently being investigated as an immunotherapy in HIV-infected persons. Combinations of some of these approaches are also under investigation. In subjects immunized with vaccinia–HIV-1 gp160, dramatic increases in HIV-1 envelope antibodies were observed when vaccines were boosted with recombinant gp160 protein. Other approaches in various stages of preclinical development include the use of recombinant BCG-HIV vectors and the use of attenuated salmonella-HIV recombinants.

SUMMARY

Since the identification of HIV as the cause of AIDS, it has been firmly established that the virus is able to induce disease because of its ability to disarm the host immune response. Despite this profound degree of immunosuppression, both humoral and cellular immune responses have been shown to be triggered by this infection, and these defenses may contribute to the prolonged asymptomatic period characteristic of this infection by keeping the virus at least partially contained. The precise components of protective immunity against HIV infection are yet to be determined, and an effective immunogen is yet to be identified. Given what is currently known about host responses to this and other viral infections, most would agree that vaccines designed to generate both cellular and humoral responses are most likely to be effective. Immunotherapies designed to bolster HIV-specific immunity may ultimately help those persons already infected. The demonstration in animal models that vaccine-induced immunity to retroviruses related to AIDS can be protective offers hope that the immune response can ultimately be harnessed to put an end to this epidemic.

Fauci AS: The human immunodeficiency virus: Infectivity and mechanisms of pathogenesis. Science 239:617–622, 1989. *An excellent review of viral infectivity, mechanisms of immunosuppression, cellular tropism, pathogenesis of neuropsychiatric manifestations of disease, and the interaction of cytokines with HIV.*

Fauci AS, et al.: Immunopathogenic mechanisms in human immunodeficiency virus (HIV) infection. Ann Intern Med 114:617, 1991.

Javerherian K, Langlois AL, McDanal C, et al.: Mapping the principal neutralizing domain of the HIV-1 envelope protein. Proc Natl Acad Sci USA 86:6768–6772, 1989. *Deletion of the principal neutralizing determinant of the HIV envelope protein renders the envelope unable to elicit neutralizing antibodies.*

Koff WC, Schultz AM: AIDS vaccines 1990: A brief update. AIDS 4(Suppl 1):S179–S184, 1990. *A review of vaccine trials in progress or planned.*

Levy JA: Changing concepts in HIV infection: Challenges for the 1990's. AIDS 4:1051–1058, 1990. *A review of recent advances in understanding of the immunopathogenesis of HIV infection and AIDS.*

Murphy-Corb M, Wyand MS, Kodama T, et al.: A formalin-inactivated whole SIV vaccine confers protection in macaques. Science 246:1293–1297, 1989. *Evidence of vaccine protection against a retrovirus related to HIV.*

Schnittman SM, Psallidopoulous MC, Lane HC, et al.: The reservoir for HIV-1 in human peripheral blood is a T cell that maintains expression of CD4. Science 245:305–308, 1989. *The major cell infected with HIV is the CD4-expressing helper T lymphocyte, and evidence indicates that these cells are present in higher numbers in later stages of illness.*

Shioda T, Levy JA, Cheng-Mayer C: Macrophage and T cell line tropism of HIV-1 are determined by specific regions of the envelope gp 120 gene. Nature 345:167–169, 1991.

Walker BD, Plata F: Cytotoxic T lymphocytes against HIV-1. AIDS 4:177–184, 1990. *A review of cell-mediated immune function in HIV infection, with discussion of the potential protective versus pathogenic role of such cells.*

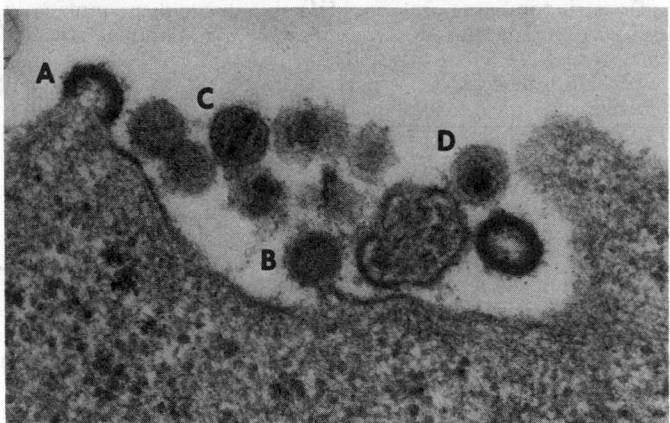

FIGURE 411–1. Transmission electron micrograph of HIV-1. Virions are shown at all stages of morphogenesis: early (A) and late (B) budding forms and cell-free mature virions (C and D) with condensed central cores. The diameter of virions is approximately 110 nm.

411 Biology of Human Immunodeficiency Viruses

George M. Shaw

DISCOVERY OF HUMAN IMMUNODEFICIENCY VIRUSES

The identification of HIV-1 as the causative agent of AIDS just 3 years after the initial description of the clinical syndrome represents a remarkable scientific achievement that had its roots in earlier discoveries of animal and human retroviruses. In the early 1900's, Ellerman, Bang, and Rous first showed that cell-free filtrates from tissues of leukemic chickens could induce leukemias and sarcomas in normal animals. Forty years later, Gross isolated the first mammalian retrovirus (murine leukemia virus) from inbred mice, and Jarrett observed that household cats were infected by a retrovirus, feline leukemia virus, that caused both leukemia and an AIDS-like immunosuppressive disease. However, it was not until 1970 when Temin and Baltimore independently reported the discovery of the retroviral enzyme reverse transcriptase that the unique replicative life cycle of these viruses was elucidated (RNA→DNA→RNA) and the molecular tools were made available to search for human retroviruses.

The first human retrovirus, human T-cell leukemia virus type I (HTLV-I), was discovered by Gallo in 1979 and has since been shown to be the causative agent of adult T-cell leukemia and a myelopathy termed tropical spastic paraparesis. In 1982, Gallo and co-workers reported the discovery of a second human retrovirus, HTLV-II, which is genetically related to HTLV-I but whose clinical significance is currently unknown. This conceptual framework of a family of phylogenetically related human retroviruses and the experimental approaches developed for their isolation in T-lymphocyte cultures were instrumental in the subsequent discovery of HIV-1 as the causative agent of AIDS.

Early suggestions that AIDS might be caused by an infectious agent were supported by epidemiologic evidences: (1) The AIDS epidemic was new in 1981; (2) the disease first appeared in a limited geographic region and subsequently spread to other areas; (3) the disease occurred in socially, economically, and geographically disparate groups that shared a propensity for communicable diseases; (4) clusters of disease were identified in individuals linked by common sexual contacts and by receipt of blood products; (5) children of affected individuals developed AIDS despite having no other risk factors for infection; (6) filtered Factor VIII coagulant transfused to hemophiliacs resulted in disease transmission. That AIDS might be caused by a retrovirus was suggested by the selective loss of CD4+ helper T lymphocytes in patients with the disease, implicating an agent with T-lymphocyte cell tropism reminiscent of infection with HTLV-I and HTLV-II. AIDS originated in Africa, where other human and simian retroviruses were known to be endemic. And a retrovirus in cats, feline leukemia virus, was known to cause an AIDS-like illness as well as leukemia. Based on this circumstantial evidence, investigative teams led by Montagnier at the Pasteur

Institute in Paris and by Gallo at the National Institutes of Health undertook studies to isolate and identify retroviruses from patients with AIDS and pre-AIDS conditions. In 1983-84, the two groups reported the isolation and serologic detection of a novel retrovirus, at that time designated HTLV-III or LAV but now denoted HIV-1, in patients with AIDS and pre-AIDS conditions. As expected for an etiologic agent, HIV-1 was shown to be uniformly present in subjects with AIDS and to reproduce the hallmark of disease, destruction of T lymphocytes, in tissue culture.

GENERAL BIOLOGIC PROPERTIES OF HIV-1

Soon after its discovery, HIV-1 was shown to be biologically, structurally, and genetically distinct from HTLV-I and HTLV-II. Unlike the leukemia viruses, which lead to immortalization of lymphocytes in vitro and in vivo, HIV-1 exhibits pronounced cytopathic properties for lymphocytes, causing syncytia formation and cell death. Morphologically, HIV-1 differs from HTLV-I and other type C oncogenic retroviruses and more closely resembles the lentivirus subfamily of retroviruses, which exhibit a characteristic dense, cylindrical core surrounded by a lipid envelope (Fig. 411–1).

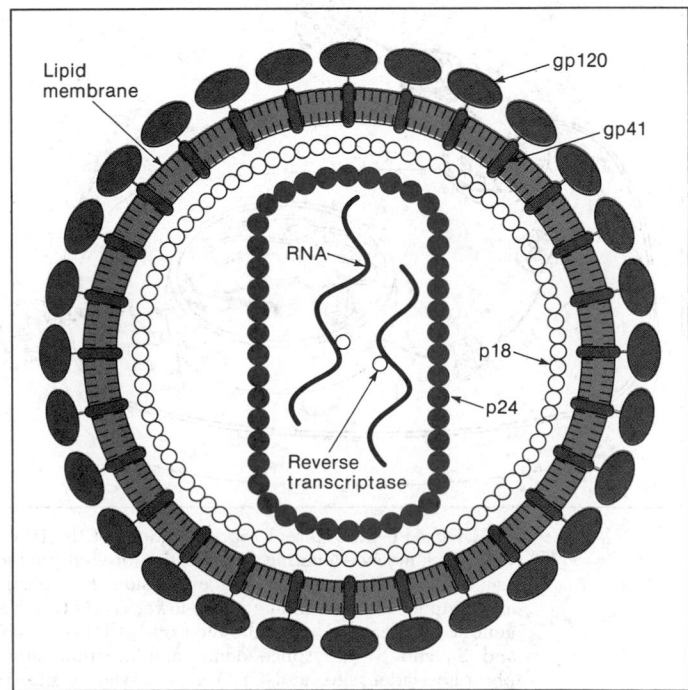

FIGURE 411–2. Structure of HIV-1. (Adapted from R.C. Gallo. Copyright © 1987 by Scientific American, Inc. All rights reserved.)

The structural organization of HIV-1 is shown diagrammatically in Figure 411–2. Like all retroviruses, HIV-1 is a single-stranded plus-sense RNA virus. The RNA-dependent DNA polymerase, or reverse transcriptase, is packaged within the virion core and is responsible for replication of the single-stranded RNA genome through a double-stranded DNA intermediate, which in turn serves as the precursor molecule for proviral integration within the host cell genome. The major structural core proteins of HIV-1 are the p24 capsid protein and the p18 matrix protein, as shown. Surrounding the viral core protein structures is a bilayered lipid envelope that is derived from the outer limiting membrane of the host cell as the virus buds from the cell surface during replication. Studding this outer viral membrane are the envelope glycoproteins, gp120 and gp41, which are encoded by viral-specific genes and are responsible for cell attachment and entry.

The life cycle of HIV-1 is shown diagrammatically in Figure 411–3. Features of this life cycle distinguish retroviruses from all other viruses. The cell-free virion first attaches to the target cell through a specific interaction between the viral envelope and the host cell membrane. The specificity of this interaction between virus and cell has been shown to be due to a high-affinity specific interaction between the viral gp120 envelope glycoprotein and the target cell–associated CD4 molecule. Following virus adsorption, fusion of the viral and cellular membranes occurs, resulting in internalization of the nucleoprotein viral complex. Reverse transcription catalyzed by the viral reverse transcriptase generates a linear double-stranded DNA copy of the viral RNA within the nucleoprotein complex, and this migrates to the nucleus where covalent integration of viral DNA into the host chromosomes leads to formation of the provirus. Subsequent expression of viral DNA is controlled by a combination of viral and host cellular proteins that interact with viral DNA and RNA regulatory elements. Transcribed viral mRNA is translated into viral proteins, and new virions are assembled at the cell surface where genomic-length viral RNA, reverse transcriptase, structural and regulatory proteins, and envelope glycoproteins are assembled. Because the HIV-1 provirus is covalently integrated within the host cell chromosome, it represents a stable component of the host genome and is replicated and transmitted to daughter cells in synchrony with cellular DNA. Relevant to subsequent discussions of viral pathogenesis, the integrated provirus is thus permanently incorporated into the host cell genome and may remain transcriptionally latent or may exhibit high levels of gene expression with explosive production of progeny virus.

MOLECULAR STRUCTURE AND FUNCTION OF HIV-1

The genomic organization of HIV-1 is shown diagrammatically in Figure 411–4. The HIV-1 genome, like other retroviral genomes, is diploid, consisting of two identical viral RNA molecules assembled in a hydrogen-bonded 70S complex. These genomic subunits are plus strands of viral RNA in that they have the same

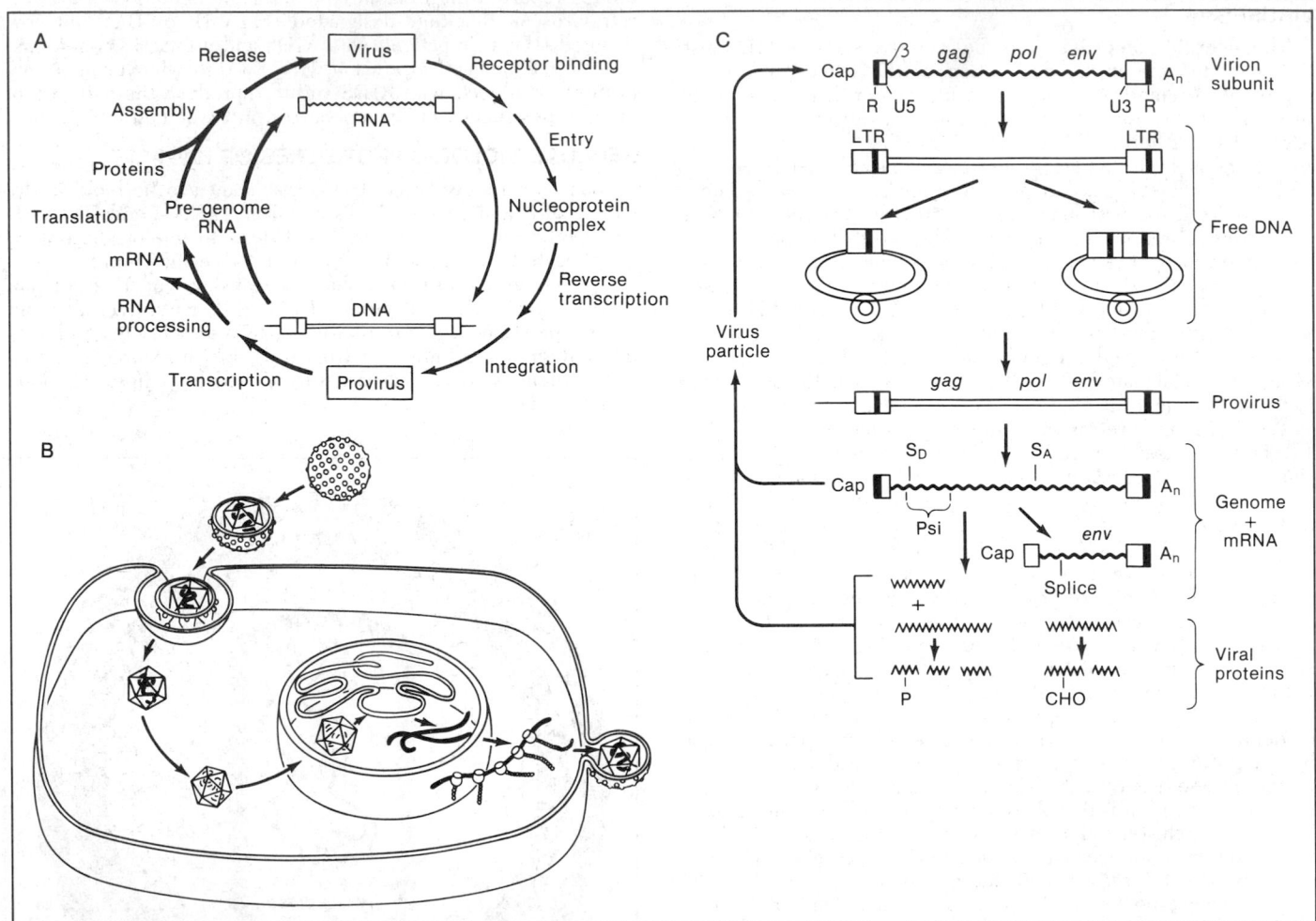

FIGURE 411–3. Different representations of the HIV-1 life cycle. *A,* An outline of the virus life cycle is shown, with thick arrows denoting amplification of viral products that may occur in the latter half of the replication cycle as a result of stimulation of virus expression. *B,* A pictorial overview of the virus life cycle outlined in *A,* beginning at the upper left and ending at the lower right. *C,* A detailed illustration of the major transformations of retroviral genetic information during the life cycle of HIV-1. Cap denotes the 5′ methyl-G-nucleotide, A$_n$ the poly (A) tract, and S$_D$ and S$_A$ the splice donor and acceptor sites. Psi denotes the viral packaging signal sequence, P a phosphorylation site, and CHO a glycosylation site. (See text for discussion.) (Reprinted with permission from Varmus H, Brown P: Retroviruses. *In* Berg DE, Howe MM [eds.]: Mobile DNA. Washington, D.C., American Society for Microbiology, 1989, pp 53–108.)

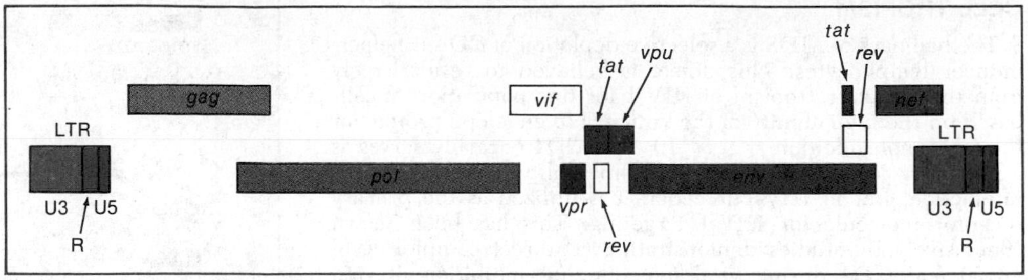

FIGURE 411–4. Genomic organization of HIV-1.

chemical polarity as the mRNA from which viral products are translated. Like eukaryotic mRNA's, the genomic viral RNA contains a 5' methylated-G nucleotide, a poly(A) tract of 100 to 200 nucleotides at its 3' end, and a number of methylated(A) residues. Host cell–derived tRNA incorporated within the virion is base paired over a stretch of 18 nucleotides to the primer binding site of the genomic viral RNA near its 5' terminus and serves to prime the synthesis of minus-strand DNA during the initial stages of viral replication following infection.

The HIV-1 genome is bounded by long terminal repeat (LTR) elements and contains genes encoding structural and enzymatic proteins (gag, pol, and env) found in all other replication-competent retroviruses. In addition to these, however, HIV-1 contains genes (tat, rev, vif, vpu, and nef) encoding other viral functions unique to this family of viruses that are responsible for their biologic behavior.

The LTR sequences of HIV-1 direct and regulate expression of the viral genome (Fig. 411–5). Deletion mutant studies of the LTR have identified at least five regions important for gene expression, including the TATA box and promotor where RNA polymerase binds and transcription is initiated (+1); a negative regulatory element (NRE) located between nucleotides −340 and −185, deletion of which increases the level of gene expression directed by the viral LTR; enhancer elements (NFκB and Sp1) located between nucleotides −137 and −17; and a trans-acting responsive region (TAR) located between nucleotides +1 and +80 which represents the putative binding region for regulatory factors responsible for tat-mediated transcriptional activation.

The gag gene encodes a precursor protein of 53 kDa (pr 53) which is cleaved into four smaller products with the linear order NH₂-p18-p24-p7-p9-COOH. These proteins constitute the core protein structure of the virus and also subserve nucleic acid and lipid membrane binding functions. The gag proteins of HIV-1, like those of other retroviruses, are synthesized as a polyprotein precursor that is subsequently cleaved during the viral maturation process. This facilitates the assembly of the different components of the virus core structure into a three-dimensional configuration that, when cleaved by a specific virus-derived protease, acquires the specialized functions characteristic of the mature virion. The polymerase gene products are translated from the same genomic RNA message as the gag proteins but in a different, overlapping reading frame as a result of ribosomal frame shifting. The pol gene encodes three proteins that are cleaved from a larger precursor polypeptide. These genes include NH₂–protease(p13)–reverse transcriptase (p66/p51)–integrase(p31)–COOH. The HIV-1 protease plays a critical role in virus biology, acting specifically to cleave gag and pol precursor polypeptides into functionally active proteins. The reverse transcriptase of HIV-1 is a magne-

sium-requiring RNA-dependent DNA polymerase responsible for replicating the RNA viral genome. The integrase protein is required for proviral integration into the host cell genome. The envelope gene (env) encodes a glycosylated polypeptide precursor (gp160) that is processed to form the exterior envelope glycoprotein (gp120) and the transmembrane glycoprotein (gp41), which anchors the envelope complex to the virus surface. It is the viral envelope that is responsible for CD4 binding, fusion, and virus entry.

Within the HIV-1 genome, there are additional genes that serve important viral functions and which distinguish HIV-1 and its related viruses from other retroviruses. These include the vif, vpr, and vpu genes located between pol and env; the nef gene located 3' to the env and extending into the U3 region of the viral LTR; and the tat and rev genes, both of which exist as bipartite coding exons in the central and 3' end of the virus. The tat gene encodes a 14-kDa protein that is essential for HIV-1 replication, upregulating HIV-1 expression at both transcriptional and post-transcriptional levels. The target sequence for tat-mediated upregulation of HIV-1 expression is the TAR region of the LTR, which apparently interacts with cellular factors induced by tat, since the tat protein itself has not been shown to bind TAR directly. The rev gene is also absolutely required for HIV-1 replication, facilitating transport of unspliced viral mRNA species from the nucleus to cytoplasm. In the absence of rev, gag and env mRNA transcripts are multiply-spliced such that gag and env proteins are not made. Recent studies have also shown that rev may possess an additional function of downregulating viral mRNA transcription when it is expressed at high levels. The vif gene encodes a protein product of 23 kDa, which, although not part of the virion itself, is required for the production of virions that are fully infectious. The vpr gene encodes a protein of 15 kDa which exhibits transactivating properties on viral and heterologous promoter sequences. The vpu gene encodes a 16-kDa protein that is involved in virus assembly and release. The nef gene encodes a 27-kDa protein that interacts with the NRE region of the LTR to downregulate viral transcription in vitro but whose function in vivo is uncertain. Interestingly, the nef protein shares structural homology with the ATP-binding site of protein kinases, is phosphorylated by protein kinase C, displays GTPase, autophosphorylation, and GTP binding activities, and has been reported to downregulate CD4 expression.

In summary, HIV-1 encodes the usual structural and enzymatic proteins typical of other replication-competent retroviruses, including gag, pol, and env, but in addition it encodes a group of at least six additional regulatory proteins (vif, vpr, vpu, tat, rev, and nef) whose activities are critically important in regulating the life cycle and pathogenesis of the virus.

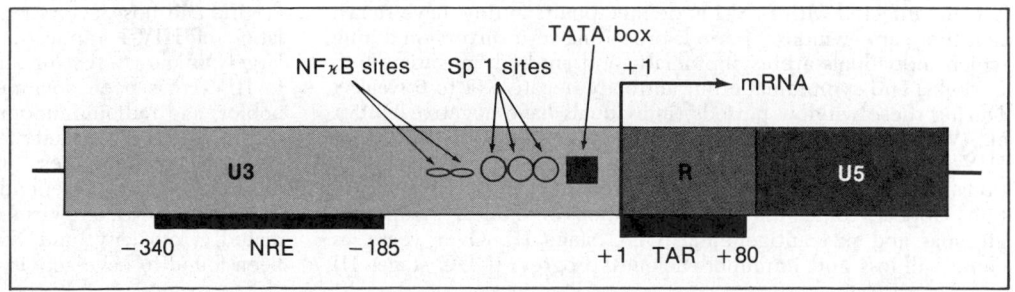

FIGURE 411–5. Regulatory regions in the long terminal repeat (LTR) of HIV-1.

CELL TROPISM

The hallmark of AIDS is a selective depletion of CD4+ helper-inducer lymphocytes. This defect is believed to result largely from the selective tropism of HIV-1 for this population of cells based on the high affinity of the viral gp120 envelope protein for the CD4 molecule (km = 4×10^{-9}M). CD4 normally serves as a ligand for MHC II (major histocompatibility complex type II) interaction, but in HIV-1 infection it is utilized as the primary receptor molecule for HIV-1 targeting. This has been shown conclusively by studies demonstrating (1) direct complexing of gp120 and CD4 during viral infection; (2) inhibition of viral attachment and infection by anti-CD4 monoclonal antibodies that prevent gp120 binding; (3) the ability of recombinant CD4 to confer susceptibility to HIV-1 infection to transfected human cells that normally do not express CD4 (e.g., HeLa cells).

A variety of cell types other than helper-inducer lymphocytes are known to express CD4 on their surface and are capable of replicating HIV-1. These include blood monocytes, tissue macrophages, follicular dendritic cells in lymph nodes, Langerhans cells in skin, and microglial and multinucleated giant cells in the central nervous system. These cells generally express smaller amounts of CD4 on their cell surface but nonetheless have been shown to represent important reservoirs for HIV-1 in vivo. Infection of such cells, in fact, may play an important role in the pathogenesis of AIDS by sequestration of the virus as described for other lentiviruses such as visna. Other cell types, including neurons, glial cells, B lymphocytes, colorectal epithelial cells, and myeloid precursors, which may or may not express small amounts of CD4 or CD4-related mRNA, have occasionally been shown to support HIV-1 replication, but the pathophysiologic significance of such findings in regard to viral pathogenesis in vivo is uncertain. However, such studies have raised the possibility of the existence of cellular receptor molecules for HIV-1 in addition to CD4.

VIRAL PATHOGENESIS

Retroviral diseases are typically characterized by restricted viral gene expression, latency, and lifelong persistence of virus in the face of substantial host immune responses. These features are characteristic of natural infections with visna virus in sheep, equine infectious anemia virus in horses, caprine arthritis-encephalitis virus in goats, and HTLV-I and HTLV-II infection in humans. From cohort studies of individuals infected with HIV-1 at known points in time, it is estimated that between 26 and 36 per cent of infected individuals develop AIDS within 7 years of infection and that an additional 40 per cent develop lesser signs of immune dysfunction. This protracted clinical course suggests that expression of the HIV-1 genome in vivo is downregulated as compared to in vitro infection by lymphocytes by HIV-1, which is characterized by explosive lytic viral infection.

Figure 411–6 depicts the natural history of HIV-1 infection of humans in relationship to clinical symptoms, immune function, and viral replication. Initial infection with HIV-1 frequently causes an acute viral syndrome (CDC stage I) with protean manifestations most frequently characterized by fever, lymphadenopathy, pharyngitis, and rash. Other symptoms and signs that may occur with acute HIV-1 infection include myalgias and arthralgias, leukopenia, thrombocytopenia, nausea, diarrhea, headache, and encephalopathy. During this primary phase of infection, symptoms are accompanied by high-level HIV-1 plasma viremia, with peak virus titers reaching 10^3 to 10^4 infectious units per milliliter. Viremia is also accompanied by high levels of circulating HIV-1 p24 antigen. Studies of individuals who have become infected with HIV-1 at defined points in time have shown that there are "window" periods preceding seroconversion during which individuals are asymptomatic and antibody negative (0 to 2 weeks) and symptomatic but antibody negative (2 to 6 weeks). During these window periods, individuals have negative ELISA and Western blot antibody tests (screening and confirmatory) for HIV-1, yet they are virally infected and their tissues are infectious. Subsequently, antibodies to viral core and envelope proteins appear coincident with resolution of clinical symptoms, viremia, and p24 antigenemia (CDC stage II). Over years, as clinical illness and immunodeficiency progress (CDC stages III

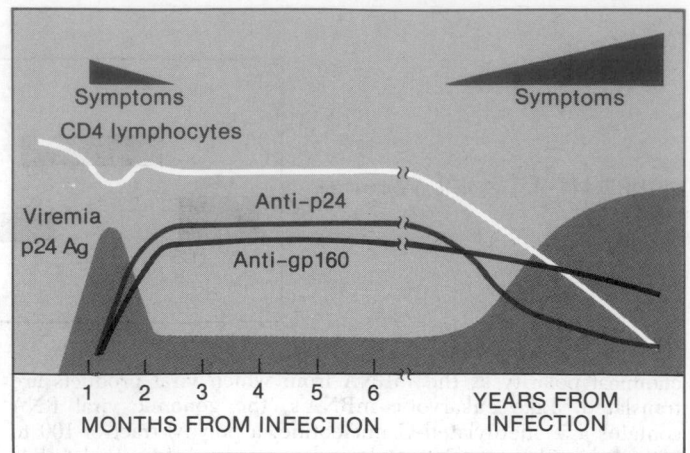

FIGURE 411–6. Natural history model for HIV-1 infection. Viremia denotes cell-free infectious virus in plasma, p24 Ag denotes circulating viral p24 antigen in plasma, and anti-p24 and anti-gp 160 correspond to antibodies to viral core and envelope proteins.

and IV), plasma viremia, p24 antigenemia, and intracellular virus burden increase.

The protracted clinical course of HIV-1 infection raises clinically relevant questions regarding viral pathogenesis: What are the molecular mechanisms responsible for CD4+ cell loss in vivo? What are the viral and host mechanisms underlying the chronicity of HIV-1 infection? The precise biologic mechanisms responsible for the cytopathic effects of HIV-1 in vivo are not known. Molecularly cloned HIV-1 proviral DNA, transfected into human cells, has been shown in cell culture experiments to contain all necessary information to generate infectious and cytopathic virus. Thus, there is no question that HIV-1 alone has the potential for direct cytopathic activity against CD4+ lymphocytes in vitro and in vivo. Expression of only the HIV-1 envelope on lymphocytes is sufficient for inducing fusion of cells with normal uninfected CD4+ bystander cells, suggesting that syncytium formation mediated by gp120–CD4 interaction may also contribute to cell loss in vivo. However, the relatively low proportion of virally infected cells in vivo at any one time has suggested that other mechanisms of CD4 cell loss may also be operative. Cell-free HIV-1 gp120 envelope protein has been shown to adsorb to CD4+ cells and serve as an effective antigen for mediating antibody-dependent cell-mediated cytotoxicity, and when processed by antigen-presenting cells, to constitute a target for direct T-cell cytotoxicity. The possibility has also been raised that since both HIV-1 gp120 and the cellular MHC class II molecule bind to the same ligand, CD4, the two molecules could share certain antigenic determinants. If so, then antibodies directed to gp120 could cross-react with MHC class II molecules, resulting in autoimmunity. Such autoantibodies reactive both with the HIV-1 gp120 and gp41 glycoproteins and with MHC II have been described. The relative importance of these processes to CD4 cell loss in vivo remains to be determined. Viral pathogenesis within the central nervous system of infected individuals, wherein the predominant cell types infected with HIV-1 are cells of the monocyte/macrophage lineage, is likely to involve additional mechanisms. Possibilities include the elaboration of cytotoxic factors from infected cells, interference with neurotropic factors, direct viral infection of neurons or oligodendrocytes, and stimulation of other viral infections. Although a great deal has been learned about the molecular structure and biology of HIV-1, the actual mechanisms of disease pathogenesis are still unclear.

Viral and host factors responsible for the apparent downregulation of HIV-1 replication following initial infection are also largely unknown. A strong humoral and cellular immune response to HIV-1 has been documented on the basis of ELISA, immunoblot, and radioimmunoprecipitation assays of patient sera and cell-mediated cytotoxicity to target cells displaying viral antigens. Neutralizing antibodies, antibody-dependent cell-mediated cytotoxicity, antibody-dependent complement-mediated cytotoxicity, MHC-restricted virus-specific cytotoxic T-lymphocyte–mediated cytotoxicity, and NK cell–mediated cytotoxicity have all been found to have activity against HIV-1 in vitro and may play an important role in the initial downmodulation of viral replication. However, the relative efficacy of the various immune effector arms and the changes that occur with time which eventually allow uncontrolled viral replication are unknown. Another factor believed to influence viral replication of HIV-1 in vivo, aside from the immune response, is the level of cell activation and the interaction of the normal immune cytokine network with viral transcriptional elements in infected cells. The importance of cell activation in the expression and propagation of HIV-1 has been demonstrated by treatment of lymphocytes and lymphoid cell lines with mitogens, antigens, and anti-CD3 monoclonal antibodies. Activation of HIV expression by mitogens is believed to follow a pattern similar to that of eukaryotic gene regulation with cellular transcription factors interacting with specific regions of gene promotors and enhancers, resulting in increased mRNA synthesis. Activation of T lymphocytes involves the induction of cellular factors that bind to specific enhancer elements, termed NFκB, present in both interleukin 2 and interleukin 2 receptor genes as well as in the LTR region of HIV-1 (see Fig. 411–5). Thus, mitogen and antigen activation of T cells resulting in the induction of NFκB binding proteins also stimulates HIV-1 enhancer elements to initiate transcription of viral mRNA. The induction of HIV-1 expression by T-cell activating mitogens and antigens also raises the possibility that specific cytokines may be directly involved in the activation of HIV-1. TNF-α and TNF-β (tumor necrosis factor) along with IL6 and GM-CSF have been shown to induce HIV-1 expression. TNF-α, in particular, is suspected to play an instrumental role in HIV-1 activation in vivo, since it is produced by monocytes/macrophages in response to naturally occurring infections and has been shown to act in both an autocrine and a paracrine fashion to activate macrophages and to further stimulate mitogen- and antigen-induced proliferation of T cells. Elevated levels of TNF-α are produced by monocytes from HIV-1–infected individuals, and such patients have elevated levels of TNF-α in their blood. Infection by other viruses such as herpes simplex virus, cytomegalovirus, Epstein-Barr virus, and HTLV-I and HTLV-II frequently coincides with HIV-1 infection and, by stimulating TNF-α and other cytokines, may enhance HIV-1 replication. In addition, coinfection of cells by HIV-1 and these other viruses may increase HIV-1 replication directly by heterologous enhancement of viral transcription.

One of the most striking properties of HIV-1 is the extent of genetic variability evident in independent isolates of the virus. The variability of the HIV-1 genome is characteristic of retroviruses in general, since reverse transcription of viral RNA into proviral DNA and transcription of proviral DNA into genomic viral RNA are not subject to cellular proofreading mechanisms, and the rate of nucleotide misincorporation by the viral reverse transcriptase is of the order of 10^{-4} per nucleotide per replication cycle. Since the HIV-1 genome is 10^4 nucleotides in length, this high rate of nucleotide misincorporation means that virtually no two viruses are identical and that HIV-1 isolates must, by definition, be described in terms of a "quasispecies" composed of populations of highly related but distinct viral genomes. Direct nucleotide sequence analysis of uncultured, virally infected human tissues using polymerase chain reaction amplification has confirmed these findings. Different genomic regions of HIV-1 typically vary among independent isolates by 5 to 20 per cent in amino acid sequence, with gene products that correspond to structural or enzymatic proteins being more highly conserved than others such as envelope. During natural infection, different viral genomes evolve in parallel and result in the emergence of multiple distinct genotypic forms. Such variation of HIV-1 is comparable to that found for another lentivirus, equine infectious anemia virus, for which it is clear that such genotypic changes are responsible for biologically important alterations in viral antigenicity, allowing the virus to elude host immune defenses. For HIV-1, the full significance of HIV-1 variation has not yet been determined. However, virus strains have been isolated from patients before and after treatment with zidovudine, demonstrating the emergence of drug-resistant variants. Thus, it is believed that genotypic variability of HIV-1 may serve as an important source of antigenic and biologic variation relevant to immunologic control and to vaccine and antiviral drug development.

HUMAN IMMUNODEFICIENCY VIRUS TYPE II

Following the discovery of HIV-1 as the cause of epidemic AIDS in the United States, Europe, and central Africa, patients in West Africa with AIDS-like symptoms were identified whose sera reacted more strongly with an immunodeficiency virus (SIV_{MAC}) isolated from captive rhesus macaques in United States primate centers than with HIV-1. The identification of patients with serologic reactivity for SIV_{MAC} raised the possibility that certain African human and simian populations could be infected with immunodeficiency viruses distinct from HIV-1. An extensive survey of African primate species for such viruses led to the identification of distinct SIV species present in African green monkeys (SIV_{AGM}), mandrills (SIV_{MND}), sooty mangabeys (SIV_{SM}), and chimpanzees (SIV_{CPZ}) (Fig. 411–7). West African patients with AIDS-like symptoms and healthy individuals at risk for AIDS were identified who were infected with a virus closely related to SIV_{SM}. This virus was isolated, molecularly cloned and characterized, and shown to represent a second major class of human immunodeficiency viruses termed HIV-2. Although originally limited geographically to West Africa, HIV-2 has now been

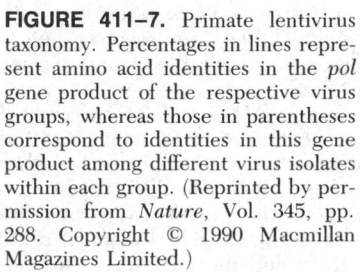
FIGURE 411–7. Primate lentivirus taxonomy. Percentages in lines represent amino acid identities in the *pol* gene product of the respective virus groups, whereas those in parentheses correspond to identities in this gene product among different virus isolates within each group. (Reprinted by permission from *Nature*, Vol. 345, pp. 288. Copyright © 1990 Macmillan Magazines Limited.)

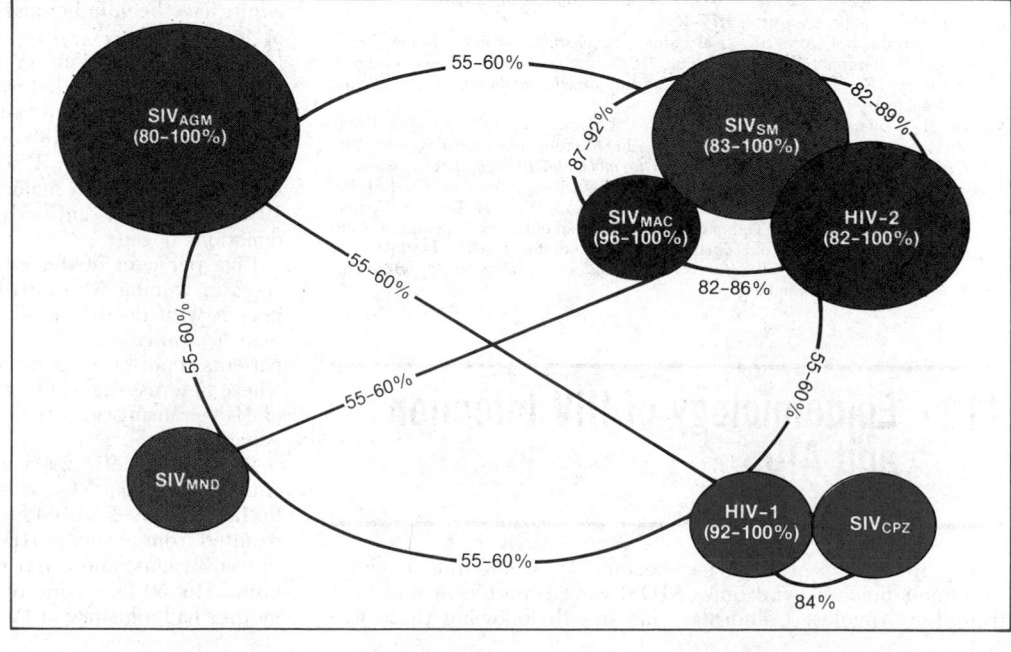

identified infrequently in AIDS patients in Europe, the United States, and South America. HIV-2 is approximately 40 to 50 per cent similar to HIV-1 in overall nucleotide sequence homology. There are two major differences in the genomic organization of HIV-1 and HIV-2. The *vpu* gene of HIV-1 is not present in HIV-2, and HIV-2 contains an additional gene, *vpx*, in its central region that is not present in HIV-1. Although the function of *vpx* is not entirely clear, HIV-2 strains deficient in *vpx* replicate less well in primary lymphocyte cultures. Antigenically, HIV-2 and HIV-1 are distinct, with greatest cross-reactivity in structural proteins and least in envelope proteins. Like HIV-1, HIV-2 selectively infects CD4+ cells. Of clinical relevance, although HIV-2 can cause profound immunodeficiency and an AIDS syndrome indistinguishable from that caused by HIV-1, there is evidence to suggest that HIV-2 may in general be less virulent than HIV-1 and cause disease over a more prolonged period of time. Also, because of the antigenic differences between HIV-1 and HIV-2, currently licensed serologic tests for identification of HIV-1 detect only about half of individuals infected with HIV-2. It is anticipated that in the future diagnostic tests will be developed and licensed that will detect both HIV-1 and HIV-2 infections and distinguish them from each other.

The identification of SIV's in African primates that are genetically closely related to HIV-1 (SIV_{CPZ}) and HIV-2 (SIV_{SM}) (Fig. 411–7) suggests the possibility of a simian origin for these viruses followed by cross-species transmission. At the present time, genetic sequence information of virus strains from wild-caught African monkey species is insufficient to prove conclusively the pattern or timing of cross-species transmission of these viruses. However, such issues are fundamentally important to the elucidation of the origin of the current AIDS epidemic, the molecular basis for the pathogenicity of HIV's and SIV's in natural and unnatural host species, and an explanation for the relatively recent appearance of AIDS as an epidemic.

Barre-Sinoussi F, Chermann JC, Rey F, et al.: Isolation of a T-lymphotropic retrovirus from a patient at risk for acquired immune deficiency syndrome (AIDS). Science 220:868, 1983. *First description of HIV-1.*

Clark SJ, Saag MS, Decker WD, et al.: High titers of cytopathic virus in plasma of patients with symptomatic primary HIV-1 infection. N Engl J Med 324:954, 1991. *First study describing virologic determinants of HIV-1 natural history and the clinical findings associated with acute HIV-1 infection.*

Fauci AS: The human immunodeficiency virus: Infectivity and mechanisms of pathogenesis. Science 239:617, 1988. *Excellent review of immunopathogenic mechanisms of HIV-1 infection.*

Gallo RC, Salahuddin SZ, Popovic M, et al.: Frequent detection and isolation of cytopathic retroviruses (HTLV-III) from patients with AIDS and at risk for AIDS. Science 224:500, 1984. *Initial report conclusively identifying HIV-1 as the etiologic agent responsible for AIDS.*

Greene WC: The molecular biology of human immunodeficiency virus type 1 infection. N Engl J Med 324:308, 1991. *Excellent review of HIV-1 molecular biology and pathogenesis.*

Popovic M, Sarngadharan MG, Read E, et al.: Detection, isolation, and continuous production of cytopathic retroviruses (HTLV-III) from patients with AIDS and pre-AIDS. Science 224:497, 1984. *First description of the large-scale production and biologic analysis of HIV-1.*

Shaw GM, Hahn BH, Arya SK, et al.: Molecular characterization of human T-cell leukemia (lymphotropic) virus type III in the acquired immunodeficiency syndrome. Science 226:1165, 1984. *First description of the molecular cloning and analysis of the HIV-1 provirus.*

Varmus H, Brown P: Retroviruses. *In* Berg DE, Howe MM (eds.): Mobile DNA. Washington, D.C., American Society for Microbiology, 1989, pp 53–108. *Detailed and comprehensive review of the molecular biology of retroviruses.*

Weiss R, Teich N, Varmus H, Coffin J (eds.): RNA Tumor Viruses. Cold Spring Harbor, NY, Cold Spring Harbor Laboratory, 1982. Weiss R, Teich N, Varmus H, Coffin J (eds.): RNA Tumor Viruses 2/Supplements and Appendixes. Cold Spring Harbor, NY, Cold Spring Harbor Laboratory, 1985. *Textbooks on current knowledge of all retroviruses, including the three major groups of onco-, lenti- and spumaviruses.*

412 Epidemiology of HIV Infection and AIDS

James W. Curran

The first cases of what has become known as the acquired immunodeficiency syndrome (AIDS) were reported in mid-1981 from Los Angeles, California. One month following these five reports of *Pneumocystis carinii* pneumonia (PCP) in young homosexual men, 26 cases of Kaposi's sarcoma (KS) in homosexual men in New York and California and additional cases of PCP and other opportunistic infections were reported. Reports of cases in the United States continued to rise, and soon the occurrence of PCP, KS, or other serious opportunistic infections in a person with unexplained immune dysfunction became known as AIDS. In retrospect, sporadic cases may have occurred in the United States, Europe, or Africa as much as three decades earlier, but the worldwide epidemic was not apparent until much later. Extensive retrospective surveillance in the United States revealed several cases diagnosed in 1978 or 1979 with a clear increase in 1980–1981. For all practical purposes, AIDS was a new disease in the United States and throughout the world.

The initial occurrence of AIDS in homosexual men and intravenous drug users suggested by 1982 that a transmissible agent was the likely cause. In the absence of proof, other hypotheses abounded. The transmissible agent hypothesis gained credence by early 1983 with the documented occurrence of AIDS in persons with hemophilia and in recipients of blood transfusions. Within a year, the retrovirus, now termed human immunodeficiency virus (HIV), was isolated and shown to be the cause of AIDS.

HIV INFECTION AND AIDS IN THE UNITED STATES

Since 1981, more than 300,000 cases of AIDS have been reported from 156 countries. Slightly over half of these were reported from the United States, reflecting the relatively high incidence of the syndrome here and a well-established national active surveillance system. All 50 states require reporting of AIDS to state health departments, and subsequently without names to the Centers for Disease Control (CDC). The surveillance case definition for AIDS was initially developed before the etiology of AIDS was known but was revised following the development of diagnostic tests for HIV infection. The current definition provides a consistent method to accurately monitor trends of serious HIV-associated morbidity and mortality (Table 412–1). Patients infected with HIV exhibit a spectrum of manifestations ranging from no symptoms to AIDS. Systems have been developed to classify these manifestations in children and adults (Table 412–2). In states that require reporting of all HIV infections, use of a standardized classification system is encouraged.

INCIDENCE AND TRENDS OF AIDS IN THE UNITED STATES

By March 1991, 167,803 cases of AIDS in adults and children had been reported to the CDC; 106,361 (62 per cent) were reported to have died, including over 80 per cent of those diagnosed before 1987. Nearly sixty per cent of reported cases in adults have been in homosexual or bisexual men without a history of intravenous (IV) drug use, and 7 per cent have been in homosexual or bisexual IV drug users. More than 63 per cent of the reported cases in heterosexual men and women had a history of IV drug use, including slightly over half of the cases in women. One per cent of adults with AIDS had hemophilia or other coagulation disorders; 2 per cent of cases were associated with transfusions, the vast majority of which had been received before 1985, when HIV antibody screening of all blood and plasma donations began.

Five per cent of the total cases of AIDS and 34 per cent of cases in women were attributed to heterosexual contact with a person with documented HIV infection or in one of the other main transmission categories. Also included in this category are patients reported with no other risk who were born in countries where heterosexual contact has been shown to be the major route of HIV transmission (such as Haiti and most countries in sub-Saharan Africa).

By March 1991, 2903 cases of AIDS had been reported in children less than 13 years of age, with over 51 per cent reported to have died. Eighty-four per cent of pediatric AIDS cases resulted from perinatal HIV infection, 9 per cent were attributed to transfusions, and 5 per cent occurred in children with hemophilia. In 50 per cent of the perinatally acquired cases, the mother had a history of IV drug use, and in an additional 21 per

TABLE 412–1. SURVEILLANCE DEFINITION FOR AIDS, CENTERS FOR DISEASE CONTROL (REVISED SEPTEMBER 1987)*

A. Indicator diseases diagnosed definitively in the absence of other causes of immunodeficiency and laboratory tests for HIV
   Candidiasis of the esophagus, trachea, bronchi, or lungs
   Cryptococcus, extrapulmonary
   Cryptosporidiosis with diarrhea >1 month
   Cytomegalovirus disease exclusive of liver, spleen, or lymph nodes in patients >1 month of age
   Herpes simplex virus infection causing a mucocutaneous ulcer >1 month or bronchitis, pneumonitis, or esophagitis in patients >1 month of age
   Kaposi's sarcoma in patients <60 years of age
   Lymphoma of the brain (primary) in patients <60 years of age
   Lymphoid interstitial pneumonia and/or pulmonary lymphoid hyperplasia in patients <13 years of age
   Mycobacterium avium complex or *M. kansasii* disease, disseminated *Pneumocystis carinii* pneumonia
   Progressive multifocal leukoencephalopathy
   Toxoplasmosis of the brain in patients >1 month of age

B. Indicator diseases diagnosed definitively regardless of other causes of immunodeficiency and laboratory evidence of HIV present
   All indicator diseases listed in Section A
   Specified bacterial infections, recurrent or multiple, in patients <13 years of age that are caused by *Haemophilus*, *Streptococcus*, or other pyogenic bacteria
   Coccidioidomycosis, disseminated
   HIV encephalopathy
   Histoplasmosis, disseminated
   Isosporiasis with diarrhea >1 month
   Kaposi's sarcoma at any age
   Primary lymphoma of the brain at any age
   Non-Hodgkin's lymphoma of B cell or unknown immunologic phenotype, including small noncleaved lymphoma or immunoblastic sarcoma
   Mycobacterial disease exclusive of *M. tuberculosis*, disseminated
   M. tuberculosis, extrapulmonary
   Salmonella septicemia, recurrent
   HIV wasting syndrome

C. Indicator diseases diagnosed presumptively with laboratory evidence of HIV infection
   Candidiasis, esophageal
   Cytomegalovirus retinitis with loss of vision
   Kaposi's sarcoma
   Lymphoid interstitial pneumonia and/or pulmonary lymphoid hyperplasia in patients <13 years of age
   Mycobacterial disease, disseminated
   Pneumocystis carinii pneumonia
   Toxoplasmosis, brain, in patients >1 month of age

D. Indicator diseases diagnosed definitively in the absence of other causes of immunodeficiency and negative laboratory test results for HIV
   Pneumocystis carinii pneumonia
   Other indicator diseases listed in Section A and T helper-inducer (CD4) lymphocyte count <400 cubic millimeter

*From MMWR 36(Suppl 1):1–15, 1987.

cent, the mother was reported to be the sexual partner of an IV drug user.

AIDS has disproportionately affected black and Hispanic minority populations in the United States. Twenty-seven per cent of adult and 52 per cent of pediatric cases were blacks and 15 per cent of adult and 26 per cent of pediatric cases were Hispanic. In contrast, blacks and Hispanics are estimated to account for 11.6 per cent and 6.5 per cent of the United States population, respectively. This disproportionate AIDS rate for black and Hispanic Americans to a large extent reflects the much higher rates of reported AIDS cases in black and Hispanic IV drug users, their heterosexual partners, and infants (Table 412–3). The relatively higher rates of AIDS in blacks were greatest in the northeast and southeast regions of the country and in Hispanics among Puerto Rican Americans from the same regions. This reflects the high prevalence of HIV infection in IV drug–using populations in these areas.

Three quarters of cases of AIDS are reported among young adults in the 25- to 44-year-old age group, leading to substantial decreases in life expectancy. In 1988, AIDS accounted for 11 per

TABLE 412–2. CLASSIFICATION SYSTEM FOR HUMAN IMMUNODEFICIENCY VIRUS INFECTIONS IN ADULTS AND ADOLESCENTS (CENTERS FOR DISEASE CONTROL, 1986)*

Group I.	Acute infection
Group II.	Asymptomatic infection
Group III.	Persistent generalized lymphadenopathy
Group IV.	Other diseases
Subgroup A.	Constitutional disease including HIV wasting syndrome in the CDC surveillance definition for AIDS
Subgroup B.	Neurologic disease including HIV encephalopathy in the CDC surveillance definition for AIDS
Subgroup C.	Secondary infectious diseases
Category C-1.	Specified secondary infectious diseases in the CDC surveillance definition for AIDS
Category C-2.	Other specified secondary infectious diseases
Subgroup D.	Secondary cancers in the CDC surveillance definition for AIDS
Subgroup E.	Other conditions

*From MMWR 35:334–339, 1986.

cent of deaths in men and 3 per cent of deaths in women in these age groups. In 1987, HIV infection and AIDS ranked seventh among contributors to premature mortality nationally, behind unintentional injuries, cancer, heart disease, suicide/homicide, congenital anomalies, and premature birth.

TRENDS IN AIDS AND PROJECTIONS FOR THE FUTURE

Reported cases of AIDS continued to increase in the United States throughout the 1980's. Cases diagnosed and reported in 1989 exceeded those in the previous year by 14 per cent. Although reported cases increased in all groups, proportional increases were greater for blacks and Hispanics than whites and substantially greater for women than men. Cases associated with heterosexual contact and pediatric cases resulting from perinatal transmission had the largest increases in the late 1980's.

Long-term trends in AIDS cases are depicted in Figure 412–1. Beginning in mid-1987, trends in reported AIDS cases in the United States shifted, primarily reflecting a slowdown in the increase in reported cases in homosexual/bisexual men (Fig. 412–1A). This slowing of the upward trend in AIDS cases that occurred in 1987, particularly in homosexual/bisexual men, is thought to be due to a combination of factors, including (1) a decline in the incidence of new HIV infections in homosexual/bisexual men in the early 1980's, leading to a subsequent decline in AIDS incidence; (2) use of antiretroviral and other therapies by mid-1987, leading to a lengthening of the incubation period from

TABLE 412–3. ANNUAL INCIDENCE (PER MILLION POPULATION) OF AIDS AND RELATIVE RISK BY RACIAL AND ETHNIC GROUPS, AGE, AND TRANSMISSION CATEGORY, 1989*

Category	White	Black	Hispanic	Other
Adult/adolescent men	243.9 (1.0)	788.1 (3.2)†	586.8 (2.4)†	121.8 (0.5)†
Adult/adolescent women	12.5 (1.0)	163.8 (13.1)†	80.1 (6.4)	14.1 (1.1)
Adult/adolescent total‡	124.4 (1.0)	454.8 (3.7)	331.4 (2.7)	66.3 (0.5)†
Homosexual men	177.9 (1.0)	289.0 (1.6)†	256.6 (1.4)†	64.7 (0.4)†
Bisexual men	30.2 (1.0)	106.5 (3.5)†	71.9 (2.4)†	23.0 (0.8)†
Heterosexual IV drug abusers	11.4 (1.0)	181.7 (15.9)†	117.0 (10.2)†	8.0 (0.7)†
Hemophilia	1.6 (1.0)	0.8 (0.5)†	1.3 (0.9)	0.9 (0.6)
Transfusion	3.6 (1.0)	5.5 (1.5)†	4.6 (1.3)†	2.2 (0.6)
Pediatric, total‡	3.5 (1.0)	47.9 (13.6)†	27.4 (7.8)†	4.2 (1.2)
Mother, IV drugs	1.3 (1.0)	19.9 (15.4)†	11.2 (8.7)†	0.5 (0.4)
Mother's partner, IV drugs	0.5 (1.0)	7.3 (14.9)†	7.0 (14.3)†	0.5 (1.0)
Transfusion-associated	0.7 (1.0)	1.1 (1.6)	1.1 (1.6)	0.5 (0.7)
Hemophilia	0.5 (1.0)	0.7 (1.4)	0.6 (1.2)	1.1 (2.2)

*Relative risk, shown in parentheses, is the ratio of the incidence in each race or ethnic group to the incidence in whites.
†Relative risk significantly different from 1.0 (P < 0.05).
‡For all men, homosexual men, and bisexual men, the denominator consisted of all men ≥13 years; for all women, the denominator was all women ≥13 years. For pediatric categories, the denominator consisted of all children <13 years.

infection to AIDS; and (3) possible decreases in the completeness or timeliness of reporting. Cases in adult transmission recipients and persons with hemophilia had likely reached their peak by 1989, reflecting the dramatic decline in new HIV infections from blood transfusions after 1985 (Fig. 412–1B). By 1989, a dramatic decline had been noted in pediatric cases of AIDS associated with blood transfusions. In contrast, cases associated with IV drug use (Fig. 412–1A), heterosexual transmission (Fig. 412–1C), and perinatal transmission (Fig. 412–1D) continued to increase.

Cases of AIDS are projected to continue to increase through 1993 in each of the principal transmission categories (Fig. 412–2). Including adjustments for underreporting, it was estimated that 390,000 to 480,000 persons will be diagnosed with AIDS by the end of 1993, including 61,000 to 98,000 cases in that year alone (Table 412–4). A minimum of 250,000 deaths are projected to have resulted from AIDS in the United States by 1993, just 12 years after the syndrome was first reported.

PREVALENCE AND INCIDENCE OF HIV INFECTION IN THE UNITED STATES

Trends in reported AIDS cases do not provide a complete picture of the prevalence of the public health problem HIV infection poses for a population group, community, or nation, since HIV infection per se precedes the clinical diagnosis of AIDS by many years. In some groups, reported AIDS continues to increase after HIV infection has declined. For example, despite very dramatic declines in HIV incidence associated with blood and plasma transfusions after 1985, when antibody screening of blood donations was instituted in the United States, reported cases of AIDS associated with transfusions and in persons with hemophilia continued to increase until 1989. Conversely, reported AIDS case rates may grossly underestimate the future impact of HIV infection, especially in communities or populations more recently affected by the epidemic. Most notable are the emerging epidemics of HIV infection in Thailand, India, and other areas of Asia where few cases of AIDS have reached the clinical horizon. For this reason, AIDS surveillance must be accompanied by carefully conducted HIV serosurveys to accurately monitor the public health problem.

The U.S. Public Health Service estimated that approximately 1 million persons were infected with HIV in the United States by the end of 1989, up from approximately 750,000 in 1986. These estimates were based both on available HIV seroprevalence data and on statistical models utilizing AIDS surveillance data and information on the natural history of infection.

National data on HIV prevalence are directly measured from HIV testing of first-time blood donors, military recruit applicants, job corps applicants, and surveys of antibody status of newborn infants. The prevalence of HIV infection in both military recruit applicants and blood donors grossly underestimates true HIV prevalence rates, since homosexual men, IV drug users, and persons with hemophilia are discouraged from applying for military service and actively deferred from donating blood.

Extensive analyses of HIV prevalence rates in military recruit applicants have been published. The crude HIV seroprevalence rates were similar to reported AIDS rates for 1989, with a remarkable similarity in geographic distribution (Fig. 412–3). After age adjustment, HIV prevalence rates in applicants are higher than AIDS rates but still greatly underrepresent the magnitude of the HIV problem. HIV prevalence rates were two to three times higher in male than female applicants and three to ten times higher in black and Hispanic than in white applicants. In limited studies of risk factors in military recruit applicants and blood donors, more than 85 per cent of those interviewed had recognized risk factors for HIV.

The highest HIV prevalence rates detected have been among homosexual or bisexual men, IV drug users, and persons with hemophilia. Prevalence rates in these groups ranged widely in studies—homosexual/bisexual men (10 to 70 per cent), IV drug users (0 to 70 per cent), and persons with hemophilia (15 to 90 per cent). Since most surveys in homosexual men and IV drug users were conducted among persons seeking medical care for sexually transmitted diseases (STD's) or treatment for drug abuse, the data may not be completely representative of these popula-

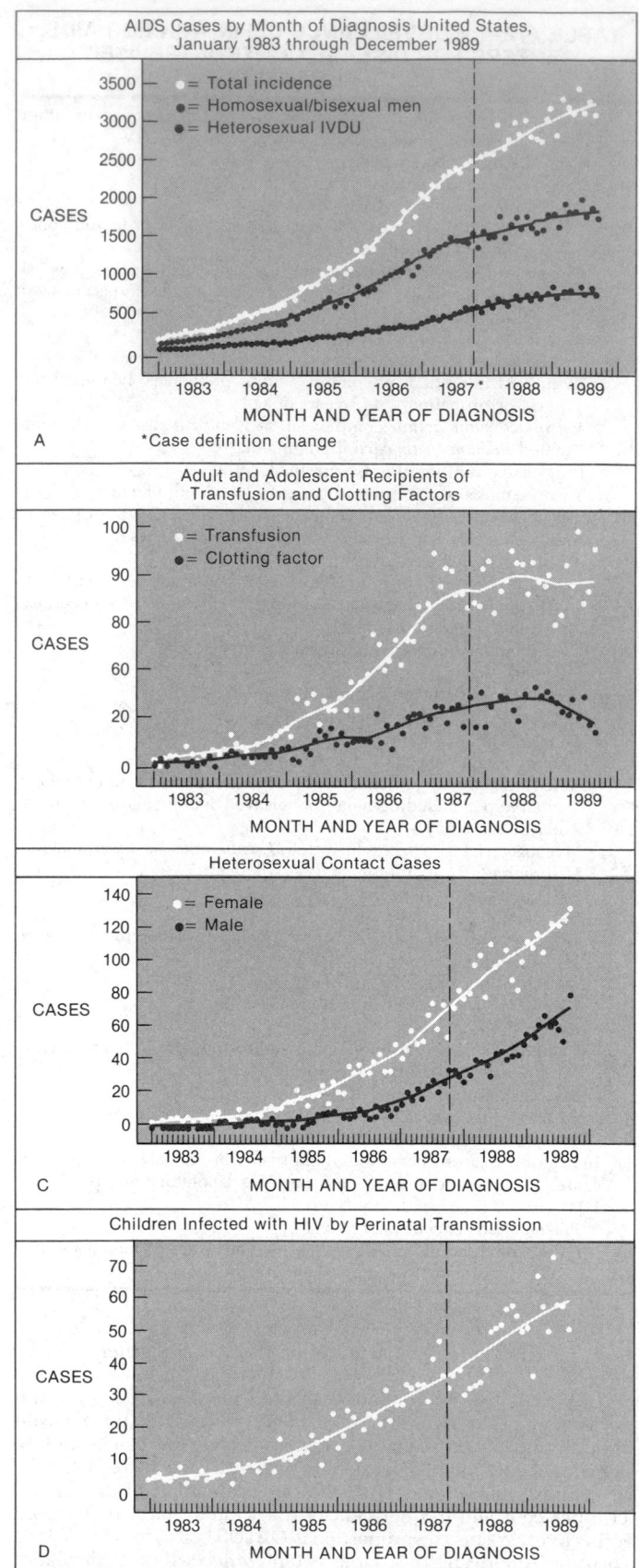

FIGURE 412–1. AIDS cases by month of diagnosis, United States, January 1983 through December 1989. Figures have been adjusted for reporting delays, by mode of transmission. Points represent monthly incidence; lines represent smoothed incidence. The vertical lines depict the date of change in the AIDS case definition. *A*, All cases, homosexual/bisexual men, and heterosexual intravenous drug users (IVDU). *B*, Adult and adolescent recipients of transfusions and clotting factors. *C*, Men and women infected with HIV through heterosexual contact (excludes persons born in countries where heterosexual transmission predominates). *D*, Children infected with HIV by perinatal transmission.

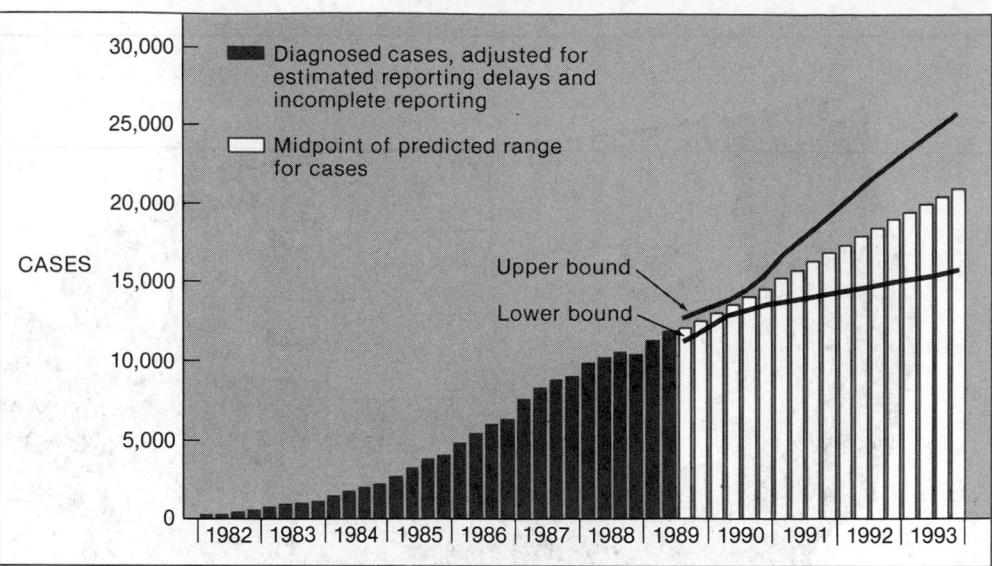

FIGURE 412–2. Cases of AIDS in the United States with projections through 1993. The projections, made for a U.S. Public Health Service meeting in late October 1989, are based on cases diagnosed through June 1989 and reported through September 1989. Projections were made as a range; for comparison with reported cases (*shaded bars*), the midpoint of the range is also shown (*open bars*). The range shown is the range of predictions obtained from two analyses using extrapolation and five analyses using back-calculation. Reported cases have been adjusted for estimated delays in reporting. Reported cases and projections include an adjustment for incomplete reporting of diagnosed cases, based on an assumption that 85 per cent of diagnosed cases are eventually reported.

tions. HIV prevalence rates in persons with hemophilia A and B were directly related to the amount of clotting factor received prior to 1985 and were, hence, highest in those with severe hemophilia. HIV seroprevalence rates among female prostitutes varied widely from 0 to over 50 per cent, with the differences largely attributed to the extent of IV drug use in the population surveyed and the HIV prevalence among IV drug users in the community at that time. HIV prevalence rates in male prostitutes parallel rates in homosexual and bisexual men seen in STD clinics in the same communities.

HIV seroprevalence rates in childbearing women have been measured by blinded testing of blood samples collected on filter paper from newborns to measure maternal antibody. Seroprevalence rates varied widely among states, from less than one per thousand to greater than 1 to 3 per cent in northeastern urban areas. The survey results in New York State (HIV prevalence of 0.67 per cent statewide and greater than 1.4 per cent in New York City in childbearing women in 1989) resulted in a state policy that encourages HIV counseling of all women of childbearing age and offers counseling and HIV testing to women contemplating pregnancy or already pregnant.

Because incident HIV infections seldom cause persons to seek medical care, direct measurement of HIV incidence is very difficult in most populations. Using a combination of approaches, the U.S. Public Health Service estimated that between 40,000 and 80,000 new HIV infections occurred in adults and adolescents in 1989 and 1500 to 2000 HIV-infected infants were born that same year. HIV incidence estimates must be refined to measure

TABLE 412–4. PROJECTED NUMBERS OF AIDS CASES, DEATHS ATTRIBUTABLE TO AIDS, AND LIVING PERSONS WITH AIDS, UNITED STATES, 1989–1993*

Year	AIDS Cases		Deaths
	New Cases†	*Alive‡*	
1989	44,000–50,000	92,000–98,000	31,000–34,000
1990	52,000–57,000	101,000–122,000	37,000–42,000
1991	56,000–71,000	127,000–153,000	43,000–52,000
1992	58,000–85,000	139,000–188,000	49,000–64,000
1993	61,000–98,000	151,000–225,000	53,000–76,000
Through 1993§	390,000–480,000		285,000–340,000

*Projections are adjusted for unreported diagnoses of AIDS by adding 18 per cent to projections obtained from reported cases (corresponding to 85 per cent of all diagnosed cases being reported: 1/0.85 = 1.18) and rounded to the nearest 1000.
†Number of cases diagnosed during the year.
‡Persons with AIDS alive during the year.
§Rounded to the nearest 5000. Includes an estimated 120,000 AIDS cases diagnosed through 1988, 48,000 persons alive with AIDS at the end of 1988, and 72,000 deaths in diagnosed patients through 1988.
Adapted from MMWR 39:110–112; 117–119, 1990. CDC: Estimates of HIV prevalence and projected AIDS cases: Summary of a workshop.

the growth of the epidemic as well as the effectiveness of prevention efforts.

MODES OF TRANSMISSION OF HIV

HIV is transmitted primarily through sexual contact, parenteral exposure to blood or blood products, and perinatally from infected mothers to their infants.

Sexual Transmission

The predominant mode of HIV transmission throughout the world is sexual contact. The risk of acquiring HIV infection during a single sexual contact depends upon several factors. Most important, of course, is the likelihood that the contact is with an HIV-infected partner. Since the prevalence of HIV varies widely among populations within countries as well as among countries, the rates of sexual transmission also vary. Other factors affecting the efficiency of sexual transmission include the type of sexual practice, the infectivity of the source partner, coexisting genital infections, particularly those causing genital ulceration, and possibly others. HIV transmission has been attributed to vaginal, anal, and, less frequently, oral intercourse.

In epidemiologic studies among homosexual men, the risk of HIV acquisition increases with the number of sexual partners and the frequency of receptive anal intercourse, and practices associated with rectal trauma such as receptive "fisting" and anal douching. No sexual activity potentially involving the exchange of semen or blood, however, should be considered without risk. The relative efficiency of HIV transmission through various sexual practices was difficult to estimate precisely, since most HIV-infected homosexual men in epidemiologic studies had engaged in multiple practices. Although the frequency of female-to-female transmission would seem to be quite low, such HIV infections associated with traumatic sexual practices have been reported.

Most heterosexual transmission of HIV occurs during vaginal intercourse, although some studies suggest that receptive anal intercourse increases the risk of HIV transmission from an infected man to a woman. Some infected persons may be more efficient transmitters than others, perhaps owing to differences in viral strains or other factors. Transmission efficiency is probably inversely related to the immunologic status of the infected partner. In studies conducted among spouses and other steady sexual partners of HIV-infected persons with hemophilia, male-to-female sexual transmission of HIV increased as the index partner's T-helper lymphocyte numbers declined. These findings are not surprising, since the quantity of HIV in blood (and probably semen) increases as the disease progresses and the immune system weakens. Several studies have documented that infections such as *Haemophilus ducreyi*, *Treponema pallidum*, herpes simplex virus, and other pathogens causing genital or anal ulcers facilitate acquisition or transmission of HIV through sexual

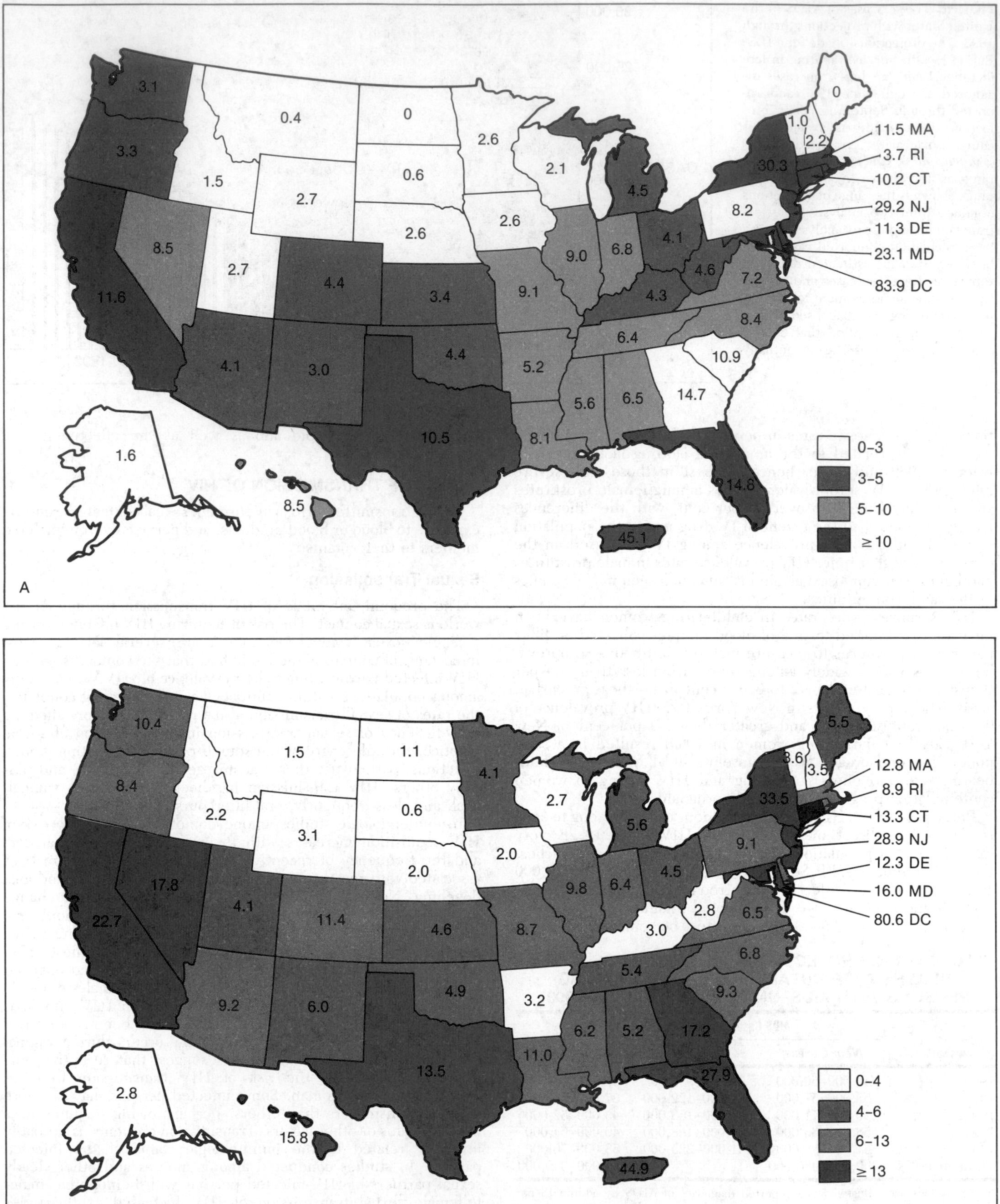

FIGURE 412–3. *A*, HIV seroprevalence in U.S. military recruit applicants, by state, 1989. *B*, Reported annual incidence of AIDS, by state, 1989. Rates shown are per 100,000 population (AIDS) or per 100,000 population tested (HIV); recruit applicants data are sex-adjusted.

contact, most likely by disrupting the genital or anal skin and mucous membranes. Undoubtedly, the higher rates of untreated genital ulcer disease contribute to the high rates of sexual transmission of HIV observed in some areas of the developing world. Not yet confirmed are preliminary observations associating increased risks of HIV acquisition for women with cervical infections with *Neisseria gonorrhoeae* or *Chlamydia trachomatis* and with cervical ectopy. To the extent that coexisting sexually transmitted infections increase the rate of HIV transmission, populations throughout the world with higher rates of these infections will be at higher risk of HIV infection. Conversely, prevention and treatment of other sexually transmitted infections should have a beneficial effect on preventing HIV transmission.

Transmission Through Parenteral Exposure to Blood or Blood Products

HIV is transmitted to IV drug users by parenteral exposure to contaminated injection equipment, including needles. Risk factors for infection include frequency of needle sharing, duration of IV drug use, use of drugs in "shooting galleries," and living in a community with a high prevalence of HIV infection in IV drug users. HIV has been transmitted by whole blood, plasma, cellular components, and clotting factors but not by other products produced in the United States from blood. No HIV transmission has been linked to receipt of immune serum globulin, hepatitis B immune globulin, Rh_o (O) immune globulin, or hepatitis B vaccine. The latter products have been produced by fractionation and other processes that remove and inactivate HIV. On the other hand, receipt of whole blood, packed cells, or plasma from an HIV-infected donor has been shown to transmit HIV virtually 100 per cent of the time. It has been estimated that over 12,000 living persons in the United States were infected with HIV through blood transfusions and that several thousand additional persons with hemophilia were infected from clotting factor concentrates between 1978 and 1985. In the United States and most industrialized countries, screening of all donated blood and plasma for HIV donor deferral procedures and heat treatment of clotting factor concentrates have minimized the risk of HIV transmission through transfusions. The exceptions occur largely in donors very recently infected who have yet to develop detectable antibody. The rate of HIV transmission from HIV-seronegative donors is estimated to range from 1 in 40,000 to 1 in 250,000 units transfused. Since HIV transmission has been reported in recipients of organs, tissue, and semen from HIV-infected donors, the U.S. Public Health Service recommends that potential donors be screened for HIV antibody and that organs, tissue, and semen not be used for transplantation or insemination.

Health Care and Laboratory Workers

Exposure to HIV-infected blood poses a definite occupational risk of HIV infection for health care, laboratory, and theoretically other workers. Large prospective collaborative studies have found the risk of seroconversion following needle stick or other parenteral exposures to the blood of HIV-infected persons to be approximately 0.3 per cent. In addition, there are a few well-documented and published reports of infections in health care workers following mucous membrane or extensive skin exposures. Such transmission can occur, but since transmission has not been observed following mucous membrane or skin exposures to HIV-infected blood in thousands of exposures in prospective studies, the risk is much lower than that following parenteral exposures. Finally, three cases of transmission of HIV from a single dentist to patients during an invasive procedure have been published. The epidemiologic and laboratory investigations, which involved comparison of the viral DNA sequences from the patients and the dentist, indicated that transmission during the invasive dental procedure was the most likely source of the patients' infections.

The risk of transmission of HIV, hepatitis B and C viruses, and other bloodborne pathogens to and from health care workers and patients can be minimized by close adherence to recommendations, which include universal precautions when caring for all patients.

Perinatal Transmission

HIV is transmitted from an infected woman to her fetus or newborn during pregnancy or delivery or through breast feeding.

Detection of HIV in fetal tissues and the isolation of HIV in cord blood provide suggestive evidence that most transmission occurs in utero, but definitive evidence is lacking. There are several reports of mothers who were infected through postpartum transfusions and subsequently transmitted HIV to their infants through breast feeding. For that reason, the U.S. Public Health Service strongly recommends that HIV-positive mothers avoid breast feeding in the United States where nutritionally adequate and safe substitutes are available. In prospective studies, perinatal transmission rates have varied from 15 to 40 per cent. In one study, the risk of perinatal transmission increased with the progression of HIV clinical illness and immunosuppression in the mothers. Obtaining precise estimates of perinatal transmission rates has been hampered by the lack of a reliable test to diagnose HIV infection in the newborn infant. The polymerase chain reaction (PCR) and specific serologic techniques are being applied in attempts to predict perinatal outcome during pregnancy as well as to rapidly diagnose HIV infection in the newborn.

Other Modes of Transmission

Throughout the world, the above routes of transmission have accounted for the overwhelming majority of HIV infections, but there has been considerable concern about other theoretical modes of transmission, especially through "casual" contact with HIV-infected persons, exposure to saliva or aerosols, or insect vectors. More than 700 nonsexual household contacts of adults or children with HIV infection have been evaluated in prospective studies. In thousands of person-years of close contact, including sharing bathroom and kitchen facilities, and frequent personal interactions including kissing and hugging, no transmission other than sexual or perinatal occurred. HIV has been isolated from saliva but less frequently than in blood. There have been no documented transmissions of HIV from exposure to saliva alone, either through kissing or through occupational exposures in dental, medical, or laboratory settings. Although a single case report of HIV transmission between siblings suggested a bite as the possible route of transmission, the precise mode of transmission in this case was unclear, since seroconversion was not documented and the bite did not break the skin or result in bleeding. Other small studies have failed to document HIV transmission following bites. Available evidence suggests that the risk of HIV transmission through normal exposures to saliva is extremely low, if it occurs at all. However, since saliva can contain other pathogenic organisms, appropriate precautions for health care and dental workers remain important, including universal precautions if gross contamination with blood is present. Aerosols have never been reported to transmit bloodborne pathogens such as HIV or hepatitis B in the health care or other settings. Extensive laboratory and epidemiologic studies of hepatitis B have failed to detect HBsAg in respirable particles in air samples in dental operatories or dialysis units during procedures on infected patients when aerosols were generated. Since the concentration of HBsAg in body fluids is much higher than that of HIV, it is unlikely that HIV would be detected. Extensive laboratory studies have failed to demonstrate replication of HIV in insects who were fed high concentrations of HIV or injected with HIV-contaminated blood. Epidemiologic studies in the United States, Haiti, and central Africa show no evidence of insect-borne HIV transmission.

The possibility of previously unrecognized modes of HIV transmission cannot be entirely excluded, but they are likely to be rare, if found.

NATURAL HISTORY OF HIV INFECTION

The time period between HIV infection and the development of severe immunosuppression and AIDS is long and variable. In a cohort study of homosexual men conducted at the San Francisco City Clinic, approximately 50 per cent of men were diagnosed with AIDS after 10 years of follow-up. An additional 30 per cent of infected homosexual men had less severe signs or symptoms and only 20 per cent were asymptomatic after 10 years. In contrast to studies in homosexual men, 49 per cent of patients infected with HIV through blood transfusions and followed in a national collaborative study developed AIDS after only 7 years

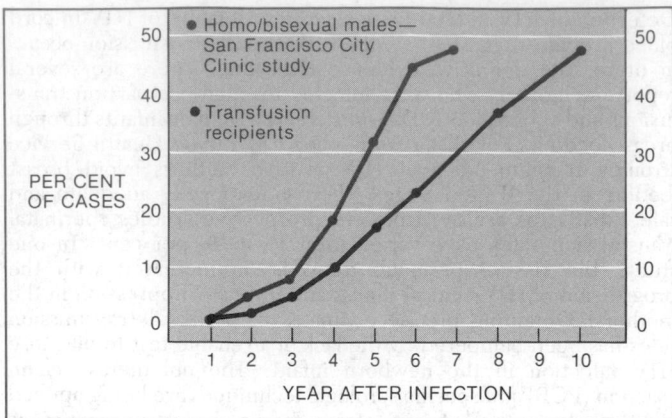

FIGURE 412–4. Estimate of the risk for development of AIDS, by year, after HIV infection in infected adult transfusion recipients and homosexual/bisexual men.

(Fig. 412–4). The authors of the latter study also found that transfusion recipients developed clinical illness more quickly if they had received transfusions from HIV-infected donors who themselves developed AIDS shortly after the donation. They hypothesized that these recipients received a larger inoculum of HIV and that the size of the inoculum affects disease progression, or, alternatively, that they had been inoculated with a more pathogenic strain of HIV. The more rapid rates of progression to AIDS in transfusion recipients may reflect the inoculum size, the older age, the immunologic status of the infected recipient, or all of these factors. Progression rates to AIDS are similar for persons with hemophilia over age 21 years to those observed in homosexual men. In contrast, children and adolescents with hemophilia and HIV infection progressed at a slower rate. Prospective studies of HIV infection in intravenous drug users and persons living in central Africa suggest progression rates at least as rapid as those in homosexual men, but the data are insufficient to make accurate comparisons.

Infants infected with HIV perinatally progress faster than adults. Whereas relatively few infected adults develop AIDS during the first 3 years after infection, the highest incidence of perinatally acquired AIDS occurs during the first year of life, with the median period of progression to AIDS thought to be 3 to 5 years. This difference is thought to reflect the immaturity of the fetal or neonatal immune system at the time of HIV infection. The incidence of AIDS in the first year of life is higher among children born to infected mothers than among children transfused as neonates, perhaps providing indirect evidence for in utero transmission, although other nutritional and socioeconomic factors may play a role.

Several clinical and/or laboratory findings have been shown to predict more rapid progression to AIDS among adults with HIV infection. Persons with oral or severe vaginal candidiasis, hairy leukoplakia, or severe disseminated herpes zoster developed AIDS more rapidly than infected persons without these findings. The single best laboratory predictor of disease progression is the T4 lymphocyte count. Persons with low T4 lymphocytes (e.g., T4 < 200 cells/cubic millimeter) progress much more rapidly to AIDS than those with normal (e.g., > 500 cells/cubic millimeter) counts, while persons with intermediate T4 counts progress at an intermediate rate. Other laboratory markers directly associated with disease progression include persistent HIV antigen in the blood, reductions in antibody to p24 (core protein), and elevated serum β_2-microglobulin, plus others. Other than age, and perhaps route of transmission, there are very few data to support specific cofactors relating to disease progression. Factors studied include coinfection with other organisms, behavioral factors, and genetic factors.

Population-based epidemiologic studies of HIV-infected homosexual men or active duty military personnel with HIV infection showed that the majority of infected adults already showed evidence of immunosuppression secondary to HIV infection. By 1989, approximately 58 to 64 per cent of persons with HIV infection had T4 lymphocyte counts below 500 per cubic millimeter.

In the future, the progression rates to AIDS as well as survival rates for those already diagnosed with AIDS will likely be favorably affected by antiviral therapy and the prophylactic treatment of opportunistic infections in those groups with access to these interventions.

AIDS AND HIV INFECTION OUTSIDE THE UNITED STATES

Within 3 years after recognition of the syndrome in the United States, cases of AIDS were reported from every continent. By July 1990, over 270,000 cases had been reported from 157 countries to the World Health Organization (WHO) (Table 412–5). AIDS case reports from North America, Europe, and Oceania fulfill the CDC/WHO surveillance definition of AIDS (see Table 412–1). The less sensitive and specific WHO clinical definition is often used in developing countries where facilities or resources are less adequate to consistently diagnose opportunistic infections, cancers, or HIV infection. AIDS case reporting from developing countries is often delayed and much less complete than in industrialized countries. Extensive HIV serosurveys in Africa and South and Central America provide evidence that AIDS case reports greatly underestimate the magnitude of the HIV problem in many countries in these regions. Serosurveys in drug users and prostitutes have recently revealed extensive epidemics of HIV infection in Thailand and India, foretelling major public health problems related to AIDS in the future in these regions of Asia.

Modes of transmission of HIV are similar throughout the world, but the relative frequency varies considerably between countries and regions. In North America, Europe, Australia, New Zealand, and some areas of South America, the majority of HIV infections have occurred in homosexual men and IV drug users; heterosexual and perinatal transmission has resulted mostly from transmission from IV drug users and their partners. In most countries in Africa and some in the Caribbean and South America, most HIV infections have occurred through heterosexual transmission. HIV seroprevalence rates are highest in urban prostitutes and sexually active young adults. High rates of infection in young women translate into a substantial perinatal transmission. In some areas of Africa, pediatric HIV infection has significantly increased already high infant mortality rates. In many developing countries, transfusion of HIV-infected blood remains a substantial problem owing to inadequate blood banking and serologic testing capacity. Reuse of nonsterile needles and syringes and other medical practices have caused major HIV outbreaks in the Soviet Union and Romania. Such transmission accounts for an undetermined but probably small proportion of HIV infection in developing countries. In Asian countries such as Thailand and India, emergence of HIV infection as a major public health problem began in IV drug users and prostitutes, respectively. In yet other countries, primarily in Eastern Europe, the Middle East, Asia, and the Pacific region, HIV has not yet been recognized as an important public health problem. The future course of HIV in these countries may depend upon their ability to anticipate and respond to the problem; it can be approximately predicted by the extent and pattern of sexually transmitted and transfusion-associated infections and the extent of IV drug use which currently exists in each country.

A second human immunodeficiency virus, HIV type 2 (HIV-2), was first described in asymptomatic West Africans with AIDS

TABLE 412–5. ACQUIRED IMMUNODEFICIENCY SYNDROME (AIDS) REPORTED TO THE WORLD HEALTH ORGANIZATION THROUGH JULY 1990

Continent	Number of Countries or Territories Reporting		Total Number of Cases Reported
	Zero Cases	One or More Cases	
Africa	2	51	66,978
Americas	0	44	167,014
Asia	12	25	665
Europe	1	29	36,635
Oceania	8	8	2,133
TOTALS	23	157	273,425

in 1986. HIV-2 infection remains most prevalent in West Africa, although well-documented cases have been reported from Western Europe, Canada, Brazil, the United States, and central Africa. HIV-1 and HIV-2 are closely related; tests for antibody for one virus often cross-react with the other. For example, licensed enzyme immunoassays for detecting HIV-1 detect HIV-2 antibody in 60 to 90 per cent of infected patients. As of 1990, HIV-2 infection remained rare in the United States, with nearly all cases detected in persons from West Africa.

SUMMARY

HIV infection and AIDS are already major causes of morbidity and mortality throughout the world. Owing to the large number of persons already infected and continuing high transmission rates, worldwide mortality will continue to increase for the foreseeable future. In both developed and developing countries, long-term commitments are needed to prevent further sexual contact, IV drug use, and perinatal transmission.

AIDS and human immunodeficiency virus infection in the United States: 1988 Update. MMWR 38(S-4):1–38, 1989. HIV infection in the United States: A review of current knowledge. MMWR 36(S-6):1–48, 1987. Gwinn M, Pappaionou M, George JR, et al.: Prevalence of antibody to the human immunodeficiency virus in women delivering infants in the United States. JAMA, in press. The sentinel HIV seroprevalence surveys—special section. Pub Health Rep 105:113–172, 1990. *These articles summarize recent methods and data on HIV seroprevalence throughout the United States.*

Castro KG, Berkelman RL, Jaffe HW, et al.: Revised classification system for human immunodeficiency virus infection in adolescents and adults. MMWR, in press. Redfield RR, Wright DC, Tramont EA: The Walter Reed staging classification for HTLV-III/LAV infection. N Engl J Med 314:131–132, 1986. *These are the most widely used classification systems in the United States. The systems are subject to revision.*

Estimates of HIV prevalence and projected AIDS cases: Summary of a workshop. MMWR 39:110–119, 1990. Karon JM, Devine OJ, Morgan WM: Predicting AIDS incidence by extrapolating from recent trends. *In* Castillo-Chavez C (ed.): Mathematical and Statistical Approaches to AIDS Epidemiology. Lecture Notes in Biomathematics 83:58–88, 1989. Gail MH, Rosenberg PS, Goedert JJ: Therapy may explain recent deficits in AIDS. J AIDS 3:296–306, 1990. Update: AIDS—United States, 1989. MMWR 39:81–86, 1990. *These papers detail recent trends and future projections of AIDS in the United States.*

Goedert JJ, Eyster EE, Biggar RJ, et al.: Heterosexual transmission of HIV: Association with severe depletion of T-helper lymphocytes in men with hemophilia. AIDS Res Hum Retroviruses 3:355–361, 1988. Holmberg SD, Horsburgh CR, Ward JW, et al.: Biologic factors in the sexual transmission of human immunodeficiency virus. J Infect Dis 160:116–125, 1989. *These papers summarize available information on factors related to the heterosexual transmission of HIV.*

Lifson AR, Rutherford GW, Jaffe HW: The natural history of HIV infection. J Infect Dis 158:1360–1367, 1988. Eyster ME, Gail MH, Ballard JO, et al.: Natural history of HIV infection in hemophiliacs: Effects of T-cell subsets, platelet counts, and age. Ann Intern Med 107:106, 1987. Ward JW, Bush TJ, Perkins HA, et al.: The natural history of transfusion-associated infection with HIV. N Engl J Med 321:947–952, 1989. *These manuscripts summarize data and factors associated with progression to AIDS in HIV-infected persons.*

Update: Universal precautions for prevention of transmission of HIV, hepatitis B virus, and other bloodborne pathogens in health care setting. MMWR 37:337–388, 1988. Public Health Service statement on management of occupational exposure to HIV including considerations regarding zidovudine postexposure use. MMWR 39(RR-1):1–14, 1990. Possible transmission of HIV to a patient during an invasive dental procedure. MMWR 39:489–493, 1990. Update: Transmission of HIV infection during an invasive dental procedure—Florida. MMWR 40:21–33, 1991. *These documents summarize data on transmission of HIV in the health care setting and list recommended precautions.*

413 Prevention of HIV Infection

Michael S. Saag

Prevention of HIV infection requires a thorough understanding of the modes of viral transmission, the populations at risk, and the established guidelines to avoid high-risk exposures. HIV has been identified in virtually every body fluid and tissue, including blood, semen, vaginal secretions, saliva, tears, breast milk, cerebrospinal fluid, amniotic fluid, urine, and fluid obtained from bronchoalveolar lavage. In most instances, the virus resides in lymphocytes present within body fluids; therefore, any fluid that contains lymphocytes could be implicated theoretically in the spread of the virus. Nonetheless, no cases of HIV transmission

have been documented through any body fluids except blood and fluids grossly contaminated with blood, semen, vaginal secretions, and, rarely, breast milk. HIV has been transmitted through transplanted organs, including kidney, liver, heart, pancreas, and bone.

MODES OF HIV TRANSMISSION AND PREVENTION

SEXUAL TRANSMISSION. HIV infection is a sexually transmitted disease (STD). Like other STD's, HIV spreads bidirectionally and appears to be transmitted from male to female and female to male with approximately equal efficiency. Although the majority of sexually transmitted cases reported in the United States occur via male homosexual activity, heterosexual transmission is one of the fastest growing modes of transmission reported in the United States and is the primary mode of disease acquisition in many African countries, where male-to-female prevalence ratios are approximately 1.1:1.

Certain cofactors are associated with an increased risk of acquiring HIV infection. Among homosexual men, receptive anal intercourse and contact with a large number of different sexual partners are the most important risk factors. Activities that may lead to damage of the rectal mucosa, such as rectal douching, manual penetration of the rectum ("fisting"), and concomitant ulcerative STD's, increase the likelihood of disease acquisition. Insertive rectal intercourse, fellatio, and ingestion of semen are associated with HIV transmission to a lesser degree. The likelihood of heterosexual acquired disease increases with a higher number of sexual partners, contact with intravenous drug users (IVDU's), prostitution, sexual practices that damage vaginal or rectal mucosa, and a previous history of other STD's. Female-to-female transmission has been reported via orogenital contact.

Prevention. Abstinence is the only absolute way of preventing sexual acquisition of HIV infection. Persons who have been engaged in a mutually monogamous relationship since the mid-1970's are at extremely low risk of acquiring disease; however, the assurance that both partners have remained "faithful" is sometimes difficult to confirm. For the majority of sexually active individuals it should be assumed that their partner is seropositive until demonstrated otherwise. Verbal claims of seronegativity should be viewed with skepticism. When a couple, heterosexual or homosexual, is establishing a long-term relationship, it may be recommended that they undergo serologic testing to determine their HIV status. However, the decision to be tested should be of mutual consent and viewed in the context that exposures outside the relationship may lead to seropositivity in the future.

In situations in which a decision to engage in sexual activity has been made and the HIV status of the partner is unknown or in doubt, safe sexual practices ("safe sex") should be implemented (Table 413–1). Mutual masturbation is considered "safe," assuming it is nontraumatic and not followed by ingestion of body fluids such as semen or vaginal secretions. Transmission of HIV has never been documented to occur through saliva; however, no group of patients has ever been studied who engage in deep "French" kissing as their sole means of sexual activity. Since HIV exists in saliva, albeit in very low titers, deep French kissing cannot be considered absolutely safe even though the likelihood of HIV transmission is extremely low. Condom use is the most

TABLE 413–1. SAFE AND UNSAFE SEXUAL PRACTICES IN ORDER OF "SURENESS" OF SAFETY

Safe
 Abstinence
 Monogamous relationship with confirmed seronegative partner
 Manual sex (mutual masturbation)
 Kissing
 Intercourse with latex condom (used in combination with nonoxynol-9)

Unsafe
 Intercourse with "natural skin" condom
 Intercourse with latex condom lubricated with petroleum-based lubricants
 Unprotected orogenital sex
 Unprotected vaginal intercourse
 Unprotected anal intercourse

effective means of preventing HIV infection among individuals who engage in vaginal or anal intercourse. To be effective, however, the condom should be made of latex and must be used properly. Natural skin condoms have been shown to leak in laboratory studies, whereas latex condoms maintain their integrity and are more durable. Nonoxynol-9, a spermicide with some antiviral activity, enhances the protective effects of condoms and should be used in conjunction with condoms either as a spermicidal jelly or impregnated into the latex condom itself. Petroleum-based lubricants enhance the likelihood of latex condom rupture and should be avoided. If needed, water-based lubricants such as K-Y Jelly should be used.

Both partners should be knowledgeable about the correct use of condoms. Discussions regarding condom use should occur before the need arises, and ideally, condom placement should be practiced in advance. A new condom should be used for each act of intercourse and each condom should be used only one time. Even under the best of circumstances, a 5 to 15 per cent failure rate has been noted among couples using condoms as their sole means of contraception, and HIV transmission has been reported in discordant couples using condoms. Condom ineffectiveness is most often due to improper placement, falling off during intercourse, and rupture. Therefore, while condom use during intercourse is considered "safer" sex, it is not absolutely safe.

HIV TRANSMISSION IN INTRAVENOUS DRUG USERS. The primary mode of HIV transmission in IVDU's is sharing of contaminated needles and syringes. Sharing of injection paraphernalia ("works") is commonplace among IVDU's and is reinforced by the cultural, economic, and legal environment in the IVDU community. Users often purchase and inject drugs in so-called shooting galleries, underground locations where addicts feel insulated from police surveillance. "Works" are rented or shared among several individuals and, in certain instances, sharing equipment represents an important social bond between users. The risk of HIV transmission is highest among IVDU's who share needles and use drugs that are injected more often, such as cocaine. HIV is frequently transmitted from IVDU's to their sexual partners through both heterosexual and homosexual activity, and ultimately, the virus may be transmitted to their children via perinatal exposure. Many cases of heterosexual transmission, including transmission from prostitutes, are associated with intravenous drug use.

Prevention. The primary mode of preventing HIV transmission in IVDU's is to prevent the use of intravenous drugs in the first place. Education programs that are culturally sensitive and geared to young audiences have the best chance of preventing drug use. Access to treatment centers is the best approach for those individuals already using IV drugs. Unfortunately, there is a critical shortage of such centers throughout the United States, and those that do exist are frequently understaffed, underfunded, and overworked. For those IVDU's who do not wish to seek treatment or who are unable to gain access to treatment, the most effective way to prevent HIV infection is to avoid sharing needles and works. Where works are in short supply, needles and syringes should be cleaned after each use, preferably with readily accessible virucidal cleansers such as chlorine bleach (diluted 1:100). Some communities have adopted programs that provide free needles and syringes for IVDU's. Voluntary HIV testing and outreach programs that rigorously maintain confidentiality can be effective in reducing transmission to sexual partners of IVDU's. In order to be effective, antibody testing should be combined with intensive pretest and post-test counseling.

The efficacy of many community programs is limited, however, by cultural barriers, including lack of trust, fear of prosecution, misconceptions regarding the prevalence of HIV infection within the local drug-using population, and the use of ineffective language in delivering anti-HIV messages by program staff. When combined with the relative paucity of IV drug treatment resources, HIV education among IVDU's which ultimately results in behavioral changes represents the most challenging HIV prevention goal.

TRANSMISSION OF HIV THROUGH BLOOD PRODUCTS. HIV has been transmitted via transfusion of single-donor blood and blood products, including whole blood, fresh frozen plasma, packed red blood cells, cryoprecipitate, clotting factors, and platelets. Prior to May, 1985, when the Red Cross began testing the blood supply for evidence of HIV antibodies, an estimated 10,000 to 12,000 individuals received blood products from HIV-infected donors. Most recipients develop infection after transfusion with HIV-tainted blood products, and recent data suggest that the time to development of advanced disease is shorter among transfusion recipients than among those who acquired their disease via sexual contact.

Since 1985, the rate of HIV transmission through transfusion has dropped precipitously. The current estimated rate of transmission is 1 in 40,000 to 1 in 200,000 units of blood, depending on the prevalence of HIV infection in the community where the blood was collected. Pooled plasma components often require 2000 to 30,000 donors per lot and represent a higher potential risk of transmission than single-donor blood products if the pooled product is not treated to eliminate infectious virus.

Prevention. Aggressive efforts by the American Red Cross have greatly reduced the risk of HIV transmission via transfusion in the United States. Voluntary self-deferral of donors at risk for HIV acquisition in the community was initiated in 1983. The effectiveness of self-deferral is limited, however, by social pressures. Some high-risk individuals view blood donation as a means of being tested for HIV and provide erroneous screening information in order to receive free, confidential evaluation of their HIV status. Other at-risk individuals may be coerced to participate in blood donation drives at work. Potentially infected donors may feel uncomfortable excusing themselves from donation and provide false information on screening in order to avoid possible disclosure of a high-risk lifestyle to their co-workers. Self-deferral programs are most effective when free, voluntary testing centers are readily available elsewhere in the community and when blood drives encourage potential donors to come to donation centers by themselves and not in groups.

The institution of HIV antibody testing of donated blood and blood products in 1985 has had the most dramatic effect on lowering the incidence of transfusion-related transmission. When used in combination with voluntary self-deferral, the blood supply has become relatively free of HIV. The use of heat inactivation processes for cryoprecipitate and clotting factor concentrates has virtually eliminated transmission of HIV through use of these products. Other products, such as immune globulin preparations and hepatitis B vaccines, are produced via methods that inactivate HIV and have never been associated with transmission of HIV.

TRANSMISSION OF HIV TO HEALTH CARE WORKERS. Transmission of HIV in the health care delivery setting has been the subject of intense investigation throughout the course of the epidemic. Retrospective analysis of over 53,000 AIDS cases with known employment histories revealed that 5.3 per cent of the reported cases occurred in individuals who worked in a health care or laboratory setting; by comparison, health care workers made up 5.7 per cent of the work force during the same time period. Other epidemiologic studies provide additional evidence of the low likelihood of HIV transmission in the health care setting. The percentage of health care workers with AIDS who have "no identified risk" for HIV infection has remained low (<10 per cent) and has not increased over time, despite the dramatic increase in the number of AIDS cases and concomitant exposure of health care workers to patients with HIV disease. More importantly, detailed studies examining the risk of specific exposures, such as needle stick injuries and mucous membrane exposures, have demonstrated very low risk of disease acquisition in the workplace. Over 1300 health care workers have been examined prospectively in carefully designed surveillance studies at 10 high-incidence medical centers. The overall risk of seroconversion after a percutaneous needle stick from a known HIV-positive source is 0.30 per cent per exposure (95 per cent confidence interval 0.13 to 0.70 per cent). Although mucous membrane exposures to HIV-positive blood have resulted in seroconversion in at least three health care workers, prospective studies of over 900 splash exposures have failed to identify any seroconverters, implying that the risk of infection is even less after mucous membrane exposure than through percutaneous needle stick. To date, no transmission has occurred after exposure to body fluids other than blood or fluids heavily contaminated with blood. When combined with studies of household contacts demonstrating no transmission of HIV to family members living with an infected patient through usual activities of daily living, available evidence strongly argues against "casual contact" as a mode of HIV transmission. Therefore, while the potential for HIV transmission to health care providers clearly exists, the risk of infection is inherently low and can be further minimized by following routine precautions to prevent transmission.

Prevention. In August 1987, the Centers for Disease Control (CDC) published guidelines designed to minimize health care worker exposure to blood and body fluids which may be infected with blood-borne pathogens, such as HIV. These so-called universal precautions are based on the premise that any patient may be infected with blood-borne infectious agents and it may be difficult, if not impossible, to differentiate those with infection from their uninfected counterparts. Thus, all specimens containing blood or blood-tinged fluids obtained from *any* patient should be considered hazardous and handled as such (Table 413–2).

Handwashing is the cornerstone of universal precautions, as it is with all infection control practices. Gloves should be worn when spillage of blood or body fluids is likely. Gloves should *never* be washed and should be changed after soiling or after gross contamination, with handwashing immediately after the gloves are removed. Gowns, protective eyewear, and masks are usually not needed except in circumstances in which splattering or splashing of blood-containing fluids is likely to occur. Masks should always be worn in situations in which eyewear is required. Reusable equipment should be cleansed of visible organic material, placed in an impervious bag, and returned to central supply for decontamination. Although heat is the single best decontamination method, chemical agents that possess mycobactericidal activity are effective against both hepatitis B and HIV and are acceptable alternatives when heat inactivation is impractical. Blood spills should be cleaned with appropriate caution. After placement of gloves and other appropriate barrier precautions, excess blood should be removed with absorbent materials (e.g., paper towels), the area then cleaned with soap and water, and the area disinfected with a 1:10 solution of sodium hypochlorite (household bleach) and water. Health care workers with denuded skin, open lesions, or active dermatitis should avoid direct patient contact and should not process contaminated equipment or materials. Private rooms are generally not required for patients known to be HIV infected unless a concomitant opportunistic disease is present which requires respiratory, enteric, or contact isolation. Food service should be provided as usual on reusable dishware.

Since *all* blood and body fluids should be handled as potentially hazardous and *all* patients presumed to be infected, it makes little sense to identify infected patients or their specimens with

TABLE 413–2. SUMMARY OF UNIVERSAL PRECAUTIONS

Specimens, including blood, blood products, and body fluids, obtained from *all* patients should be considered hazardous and potentially infected with transmissible agents.

Handwashing should be performed before and after patient contact; after removing gloves; and immediately if hands are grossly contaminated with blood.

Gloves should be worn when hands are *likely* to come in contact with blood or body fluids.

Gowns, protective eyewear, and masks should be worn when splashing, splattering, or aerosolization of blood or body fluids is *likely* to occur.

Sharp objects ("sharps") should be handled with great care and disposed of in impervious receptacles.

Needles should never be manipulated, bent, broken, or recapped.

Blood spills should be handled via initial absorption of spill with disposable towels, cleaning area with soap and water, followed by disinfecting area with 1:10 solution of household bleach.

Contaminated reusable equipment should be decontaminated using heat sterilization, or when heat is impractical, using a mycobactericidal cleanser.

Pocket masks or mechanical ventilation devices should be available in areas where cardiopulmonary resuscitation procedures are likely.

Health care workers with open lesions or weeping dermatitis should avoid direct patient contact and should not handle contaminated equipment.

Private rooms are not required for routine care; select circumstances, however, such as the presence of concomitant transmissible opportunistic diseases, may warrant respiratory, enteric, or contact isolation.

"blood and body fluid" labels. The use of such labels on *known* infected patients implies that unlabeled specimens or specimens from patients of unknown status are less hazardous and may be handled with less care. Indeed, studies have shown that over half of the specimens containing antibodies to either HbsAg or HIV went to the laboratory unlabeled. The handling of sharp instruments ("sharps") represents the greatest risk of HIV transmission to health care workers. Although sharp injuries cannot be entirely eliminated, the number of exposures can be reduced substantially by adhering to guidelines put forth in universal precautions. Before a sharp instrument is used, thought should be given regarding where the instrument will be disposed after use. Impervious containers should be readily available in all patient care areas and identified by the health care worker *prior to* "sharp" utilization. The containers should be checked frequently and should not be allowed to overfill. Used needles should never be manipulated, bent, broken, or recapped. Recapping of needles is the single most common activity that results in needle stick injuries.

Despite their logical basis and relative ease of implementation, universal precautions have not been accepted by many medical centers and health care providers. Recent studies have shown that over 50 per cent of health care workers engage in inadequate infection control practices, even in high-impact AIDS centers, and up to 40 per cent of the needle stick exposures were judged to be preventable. Although lack of adequate education may partly explain these findings, implementation of infection control practices has been generally poor historically. Between 200 and 400 health care workers die each year as a result of hepatitis B infection acquired on the job. The use of universal precautions helps minimize the transmission of many transmissible diseases in addition to HIV.

Even in the best of circumstances, accidental mucous membrane and percutaneous exposures to blood from HIV-infected patients do occur. Each institution and health care facility should adopt procedures for management of these exposures based on guidelines published by the CDC. The essential elements of management following needle stick or mucous membrane exposure include definition of the type of exposure, appropriate evaluation of the donor (patient) and recipient (health care worker) at the time of exposure, and follow-up of the health care worker for at least 1 year after exposure.

Proposed definitions of the types of exposure are summarized in Table 413–3. Health care workers with any kind of parenteral exposure should be counseled and evaluated for possible acquisition of HIV and receive routine prophylaxis against hepatitis B. The source patient (donor) should be evaluated for HIV infection; if the donor's HIV status is unknown, the donor should be informed abut the incident and encouraged to allow voluntary, confidential screening of his blood for HIV and hepatitis B antibody. If the patient refuses or cannot give consent, he should be considered to be infected. In cases where exposure to HIV is documented or presumed to have occurred, the health care worker should be evaluated serologically for the presence of HIV as soon as possible after the exposure (baseline) and again at 6 weeks, 12 weeks, 24 weeks, and 1 year after the exposure to determine whether HIV transmission has occurred. The health care worker should report any acute illnesses that occur during the follow-up period, especially during the first 6 to 12 weeks after exposure. Exposed workers should follow the recommended guidelines for preventing HIV transmission, including use of safe sexual practices, refraining from blood, semen, and organ donation, and avoidance of breast feeding. If the source patient is seronegative for HIV and has no clinical manifestations of HIV disease, no further follow-up of the exposed health care worker is necessary, although some workers prefer follow-up for their own peace of mind. Serologic testing should be made available to all health care workers who are concerned about potential on-the-job exposure.

The use of zidovudine (AZT) prophylaxis following parenteral exposure to HIV remains controversial. Many clinicians favor use of prophylactic AZT after massive or definite exposures based on the proven antiviral effect of AZT, the relatively infrequent and apparently reversible nature of serious adverse drug effects, and the demonstration in some animal models of retroviral infection

TABLE 413–3. DEFINITIONS OF EXPOSURES TO BLOOD AND BODY FLUIDS FROM HIV-INFECTED PATIENTS*

Massive parenteral exposure
  Transfusion of blood
  High-inoculum injection of blood (>1 ml) or laboratory materials
    containing high viral titers
Definite parenteral exposure
  Deep intramuscular injury with a needle contaminated with blood or
    a body fluid
  Small volume injection of blood or body fluid (<1 ml)
  Laceration caused by instrument contaminated with blood or body fluids
  Laceration inoculated with blood, body fluids, or virus samples
    (research materials)
Possible parenteral exposure
  Subcutaneous or superficial injury with an instrument or needle
    contaminated with blood or body fluids
  Injury with a contaminated instrument or needle which does not
    cause visible bleeding
  Previous wound or skin lesion contaminated with blood or body fluids
  Mucous membrane exposure to blood or body fluids
Doubtful parenteral exposure
  Subcutaneous injury by instrument or needle contaminated with
    noninfectious fluids†
  Contamination of a wound, previous skin lesion, or mucous
    membrane with noninfectious fluids
  Intact skin visibly contaminated with blood

*Modified from Gerberding JC, Conte JE: Counseling and Testing Service, Center for Municipal Occupational Safety and Health, San Francisco General Hospital, University of California San Francisco, and the California Consortium for Health Care Workers. In Geberding JL: AIDS and Health Care Workers. Chicago, American Medical Association, 1989, pp 35–46; with permission.

†Body fluids considered to be potentially infectious include blood, blood products, cerebrospinal fluid, amniotic fluid, menstrual discharge, inflammatory exudates, pleural fluid, peritoneal fluid, pericardial fluid, and any fluid visibly contaminated with blood. All other fluids are considered noninfectious.

that AZT, when given early after inoculation, modifies the course of disease. Others believe that AZT should not be administered based on the absence of postexposure prophylaxis data, the lack of information regarding toxicity in uninfected individuals, and the unknown long-term carcinogenic potential of AZT use. Unfortunately, it is unlikely that any clinical trials will be able to resolve the issue owing to the large number of participants required (based on low rates of seroconversion) and the difficulty of enrolling exposed health care workers into placebo-controlled studies. Although zidovudine prophylaxis cannot be considered an established standard of practice at this time, the option of zidovudine prophylaxis should be offered to all health care workers with massive or definite exposures and discussed with those encountering possible parenteral exposures. Health care workers with doubtful parenteral or nonparenteral exposures generally should not take zidovudine prophylaxis. Those workers with massive or definite exposures who elect to take zidovudine prophylaxis should sign an informed consent that outlines the risks and benefits of AZT prophylaxis prior to initiation of therapy. The optimal timing and dosage of AZT prophylaxis are unknown; however, animal studies suggest that higher doses given as soon as possible after exposure have the best chance of being effective. Therefore, most centers that offer zidovudine prophylaxis to their employees have established mechanisms whereby the health care worker can be evaluated and the drug administered within 2 to 4 hours after the exposure. Dosing regimens vary from center to center but usually consist of 100 mg to 200 mg of AZT every 4 hours, with or without a 4 A.M. dose, for 4 to 6 weeks.

VACCINE DEVELOPMENT

Education is the only means of HIV prevention currently available. Over the past few years significant efforts have been directed toward the development of an effective vaccine against HIV. Although substantial progress has been achieved, several obstacles still remain. Despite enormous advances in understanding the immunopathogenesis of HIV infection, the precise mechanism of protective immunity remains unknown. Without such knowledge, it is difficult to develop vaccines that are assured of targeting the appropriate arm of the immune system that confers long-term protective immunity. Another obstacle is that no animal

models currently exist to test the effectiveness of candidate vaccines. Therefore, even if an effective vaccine were available it would take years of human testing to demonstrate its effectiveness. Moreover, once a candidate vaccine is in human trials, the relatively low rate of HIV transmission, and in some cases, the difficulty in determining whether HIV infection has actually occurred will complicate the evaluation process. Nonetheless, several candidate vaccines have been developed and are now entering Phase I trials. Recombinant gp160 vaccines expressed in a baculovirus vector and a vaccinia virus vector have been developed. A whole killed HIV vaccine is being evaluated in HIV-infected patients.

In view of the enormous progress made in vaccine development over the last few years, the establishment of an effective vaccine is a viable possibility; unfortunately, it will take several more years before efficacy can be established. Until such time, education remains the primary mode of HIV prevention. Never before has so much been known about an epidemic during the time it was occurring. The challenge is to disseminate the knowledge to populations at risk in language they can understand and, ultimately, to modify activities so that the risk of transmission is minimized.

Brickner PW, Torres RA, Barnes M, et al.: Recommendations for control and prevention of human immunodeficiency virus infection in intravenous drug users. Ann Intern Med 110:883–887, 1989. *Thoughtful discussion of unique problems associated with prevention of HIV transmission in IVDU's.*

Centers for Disease Control: Recommendations for prevention of HIV transmission in health care settings. MMWR 36(2S), 1987. *Original description of universal precautions. Critical reading for all health care workers.*

Centers for Disease Control: Public health service statement on management of occupational exposure to human immunodeficiency virus, including considerations regarding zidovudine post-exposure use. MMWR 39 (RR-1), 1990. *State-of-the-art review of issues regarding use of prophylactic zidovudine after needle stick exposure to HIV.*

Fauci AS, Gallo RC, Koenig S, et al.: Development and evaluation of a vaccine for human immunodeficiency virus infection. Ann Intern Med 110:373–385, 1989. *Overview of HIV vaccine development: progress, obstacles, and future directions.*

Henderson DK, Fahey BJ, Willy M, et al.: Risk for occupational transmission of human immunodeficiency virus type-I associated with clinical exposures. Ann Intern Med 113:740–746, 1990. *Prospective study of health care workers at risk for HIV infection. Establishes risk of transmission to be 0.3 per cent per needle stick exposure.*

Sacks HS, Rose DN: Zidovudine prophylaxis for needle stick exposure to human immunodeficiency virus: A decision analysis. J Gen Intern Med 5:132–137, 1990. *A helpful discussion of how to approach risk analysis of zidovudine use after needle sticks.*

Wofsy CB: Prevention of HIV transmission. *In* Sande MA, Volberding PA (eds.): The Medical Management of AIDS. Philadelphia, W.B. Saunders, 1988, pp 29–43. *A practical review of HIV prevention in different risk groups with specific recommendations for counseling those at risk.*

414 Neurologic Complications of HIV-1 Infection

Richard W. Price

The neurologic complications of HIV-1 infection are both common and varied. Indeed, only rarely do the central and peripheral nervous systems of HIV-infected patients remain unaffected through the course of their disease. Because each of the individual neurologic disorders is discussed in more detail elsewhere in this volume, the major purpose of this chapter is to provide an overview and a general guide to differential diagnosis. It is important to emphasize that differential diagnosis in these patients is far from an "academic exercise," since many of these conditions can be reversed, stabilized, or even cured with specific therapy.

Although the major susceptibility to neurologic complications occurs in the late phase of HIV-1 infection, at the time when immunosuppression leads to a marked increase in vulnerability to a host of conditions, patients may also manifest certain neurologic afflictions early in infection. Because the neurologic complications of early and late HIV-1 infection differ, they are considered separately. Indeed, because of these stage-related differences in susceptibility, when approaching diagnosis in HIV-infected patients it is important to characterize their "background" systemic HIV-1 infection, either clinically with respect to the presence or absence of previous opportunistic infections indicating compromised immunity or by assessment of surrogate markers, particularly the blood CD4+ lymphocyte count.

EARLY HIV-1 INFECTION

Although less common than in the late stages of HIV-1 infection, the nervous system may also be afflicted earlier, indeed as early as the stage of primary infection and seroconversion. Thus, individual reports have described examples of focal or diffuse encephalopathy, ataxia, myelopathy, and meningitis presenting either within the context of the mononucleosis-like HIV-1 seroconversion reaction or with minimal associated systemic symptoms. These conditions appear to evolve acutely or subacutely, to pursue a monophasic course, and to be followed by good, although not always complete, recovery. Peripheral nervous system disorders, including mononeuropathy involving cranial or segmental nerves, brachial plexopathy, and polyneuropathy, have also been reported during this phase. At times these peripheral and central nervous system (CNS) disorders occur together.

Subsequently, during the "asymptomatic seropositive" phase of infection, several neurologic conditions have been reported. Among these is the Guillain-Barré syndrome and its more protracted counterpart, chronic idiopathic demyelinating polyneuropathy (CIDP), both of which are clinically indistinguishable from demyelinating polyneuropathies affecting non–HIV-1–infected individuals, except for higher cerebrospinal fluid (CSF) cell counts and perhaps a poorer prognosis. Response to treatment with corticosteroids and plasma exchange has been noted, supporting presumption of an autoimmune pathogenesis. Because of the potential hazards of corticosteroids, plasma exchange is the preferred therapy.

An additional important aspect of HIV-1 infection, with both diagnostic and pathogenetic implications, is the early development of CSF abnormalities, which presumably relate to early *asymptomatic HIV-1 infection of the CNS* soon after initial systemic infection. Several prospective studies have reported that the majority of asymptomatic HIV-1–infected individuals exhibit mild CSF changes, including elevations in the cell count and protein and immunoglobulin levels as well as evidence of local "intra–blood-brain barrier" synthesis of anti–HIV-1 antibody. Additionally, in a substantial number of asymptomatic patients HIV-1 can be isolated from the CSF using culture techniques. These findings have not been shown to have an adverse prognostic significance for the subject; indeed, it is clear that patients with such abnormalities can continue to function without symptoms or signs of neurologic impairment. These "background" abnormalities may confound CSF analysis.

LATE HIV-1 INFECTION

The evolving, and eventually severe, impairment of immune defenses caused by HIV-1 renders the nervous system highly vulnerable to a broad spectrum of disorders. The following overview emphasizes general principles of pathogenesis and approach to diagnosis.

Pathophysiology

A number of pathophysiologic processes may lead to neurologic dysfunction in the late phase of HIV-1 infection (Table 414-1). These include conditions that distinguish the AIDS patient from other groups, such as *opportunistic infections, opportunistic neoplasms,* and several conditions that appear to relate to more *direct effects of HIV-1* itself. AIDS patients are also susceptible to the neurologic conditions that affect other acute and chronically ill populations, including metabolic brain disease resulting from systemic organ dysfunction, stroke related to nonbacterial thrombotic endocarditis or coagulopathies, toxic effects of medications, and primary psychiatric disturbances. Here we focus on the first group of disorders, those that particularly distinguish AIDS patients.

OPPORTUNISTIC NERVOUS SYSTEM INFECTIONS. As with other organ systems, the spectrum of opportunistic infections of the nervous system results from the intrinsic vulnerabilities of the tissue (fertile soil) and the pattern of immunosuppression, in

TABLE 414–1. PATHOPHYSIOLOGIC CLASSIFICATION OF THE NEUROLOGIC COMPLICATIONS OF LATE HIV-1 INFECTION

Underlying Process	Examples
Opportunistic infections	Cerebral toxoplasmosis
	Cryptococcal meningitis
	Progressive multifocal leukoencephalopathy
	Cytomegalovirus encephalitis, polyradiculitis
Opportunistic neoplasms	Primary central nervous system lymphoma
	Metastatic lymphoma
Conditions possibly related to HIV-1 itself	AIDS dementia complex
	Aseptic meningitis
	Predominantly sensory polyneuropathy
Metabolic and vascular complications of systemic disease	Hypoxic, sepsis-related encephalopathies
	Stroke (nonbacterial thrombotic endocarditis, coagulopathies)
Toxic reactions	Dideoxyinosine, dideoxycytidine neuropathies
	Zidovudine myopathy
Functional (psychiatric) disorders	Anxiety disorders
	Psychotic depression

this case impaired T-cell/macrophage defenses. The patient's long-term history of exposure to particular organisms is also important because most of the opportunistic infections result from reactivation of latent infections rather than from new encounters with pathogens. An important implication of the pre-eminence of reactivated infection relates to serologic testing. Serology is most useful for assessing prior exposure to an organism and hence susceptibility to clinically important reactivation, but not for defining active infection. For example, patients with cerebral toxoplasmosis virtually always exhibit antecedent positive *Toxoplasma gondii* blood serology, and therefore a negative serum IgG antibody titer mitigates against this diagnosis; on the other hand, these serum antibody titers most often do not rise before or during the course of disease and therefore a fourfold increase cannot be relied upon to establish disease activity. Moreover, as long as immunosuppression persists and therapy remains incapable of eliminating latent infection, suppressive antibiotic therapy must be maintained for the remainder of the patient's life.

The reason for the intrinsic vulnerability of the nervous system to certain infections (e.g., *T. gondii*) and not others (e.g., *Pneumocystis carinii*) in many cases remains uncertain. However, in some instances susceptibility relates to the capacity of local cells to support intracellular replication. Thus, the virus causing progressive multifocal leukoencephalopathy (PML), JC virus, causes a productive and lytic infection of oligodendrocytes and hence leads to spreading infection and demyelination as the processes of these myelin-producing cells disappear. In the case of HIV-1, productive infection appears to involve monocyte-derived macrophages and perhaps local microglial cells.

The circumscribed nature of the immunologic defect in AIDS determines the range of opportunistic infections, which therefore differs somewhat from that of other immunosuppressed states. For example, AIDS patients are particularly susceptible to cerebral toxoplasmosis but, unlike patients with certain organ transplants, are very unlikely to develop cerebral *Candida* or *Aspergillus* infections. For this reason, AIDS patients present a unique set of disease probabilities.

OPPORTUNISTIC NEOPLASMS. The major consideration in this category is primary brain lymphoma. These B-cell lymphomas arise in the CNS, usually are multicentric (at least microscopically), and only rarely metastasize systemically. Characteristically, they develop late in HIV-1 infection when blood CD4+ lymphocytes are low, i.e., in the same setting as major opportunistic infections. Radiation therapy usually results in tumor regression, but overall prognosis is poor, principally because of the development of other complications; the role of chemotherapy is uncertain, but aggressive treatment is often not possible because of reduced bone marrow reserves. Systemic lymphoma can also spread to the CNS, although usually to the leptomeninges rather than brain parenchyma. Although Kaposi's sarcoma has been reported to metastasize to brain, this is exceedingly rare.

EFFECTS OF HIV-1 ON THE NERVOUS SYSTEM. Several disorders have been suggested to relate in a more direct or fundamental way to HIV-1 infection. These include the AIDS dementia complex, aseptic meningitis, and perhaps predominantly sensory neuropathy. While there is still considerable uncertainty regarding their etiology and pathogenesis, the seeming uniqueness of these conditions in HIV-1–infected compared with other immunosuppressed patients, as well as more direct evidence of virus infection in some patients with the AIDS dementia complex, lends support to this contention.

Diagnosis: Neuroanatomic Approach

As with other neurologic disease, diagnosis in AIDS patients begins with localization of symptoms and signs and hence involves neuroanatomic classification (Table 414–2).

MENINGITIS AND HEADACHE. Several disorders may involve the leptomeninges in patients with advanced HIV-1 disease. The most important of these is infection by *Cryptococcus neoformans* (see Ch. 403). This condition usually presents sub-

---

TABLE 414–2. NEUROANATOMIC CLASSIFICATION OF THE LATE COMPLICATIONS OF HIV-1 INFECTION

Meningitis and headache
  Cryptococcal meningitis
  Aseptic meningitis (HIV-1)
  Idiopathic, "HIV-1–related" headache
  Tuberculous meningitis (*Mycobacterium tuberculosis*)
  Syphilitic meningitis
  Lymphomatous meningitis (metastatic)
Diffuse brain diseases
  With preservation of consciousness
    AIDS dementia complex
  With concomitant depression of arousal
    Metabolic encephalopathies (alone or as an exacerbating influence)
    Toxoplasmosis ("encephalitic" form)
    Cytomegalovirus encephalitis
    Herpes encephalitis
Focal brain diseases
  Subacute
    Cerebral toxoplasmosis
    Primary CNS lymphoma
    Progressive multifocal leukoencephalopathy
    Tuberculous brain abscess (*M. tuberculosis*)
    Cryptococcoma
    Varicella-zoster virus encephalitis
    Herpes encephalitis
  Acute
    Vascular disorders
Myelopathies
  Subacute/chronic, progressive
    Vacuolar myelopathy
    HTLV-I–associated myelopathy
  Acute/subacute
    Transverse myelitis
      Varicella-zoster virus (herpes zoster)
      Spinal epidural or intradural lymphoma
    With polyradiculopathy
      Cytomegalovirus
Peripheral neuropathies
  Predominantly sensory polyneuropathy
  Toxic neuropathies (dideoxycytidine, dideoxyinosine)
  Autonomic neuropathy
  Cytomegalovirus polyradiculopathy
  Mononeuritis multiplex
  Herpes zoster
  Mononeuropathies associated with aseptic meningitis
  Mononeuropathies secondary to lymphomatous meningitis
Myopathies
  Polymyositis
  Noninflammatory myopathy
  Zidovudine myopathy

---

acutely with headache, nausea, vomiting, and confusion, just as in non-AIDS patients. However, importantly, in some patients initial symptoms can be remarkably benign, with only mild headache or fever. Likewise, the CSF findings may be bland, with few or no cells and little or no perturbation in either glucose or protein levels. For this reason the clinician should have a low threshold for lumbar puncture and should routinely examine CSF for *Cryptococcus* (India ink stain, cryptococcal antigen determination, culture). Initial treatment is usually gratifying, although sterilizing the CSF is difficult and continued chronic therapy is required.

The syndrome of aseptic meningitis, presumably relating to direct HIV-1 infection of the leptomeninges, may complicate advanced HIV-1 infection but most often develops in the period of transition from AIDS-related complex (ARC) to AIDS. Both acute and chronic forms are accompanied by headache and meningeal symptoms, whereas signs of meningeal irritation are more characteristic of the acute group. Cranial nerve palsies affecting the seventh and, less often, the fifth and eighth nerves may complicate the course. The CSF shows a modest mononuclear pleocytosis, usually with normal glucose and mildly elevated protein. The presumption that this condition is due to direct HIV-1 infection of the meninges derives from the fact that the virus can be readily isolated from the CSF and no other cause has been identified. The syndrome itself is characteristically benign but may imply a poor prognosis in relation to impending progression to AIDS. The efficacy of antiretroviral or other therapies in this disorder has not been studied.

Other, less common meningeal disorders (including meningeal lymphoma, tuberculous meningitis, meningovascular syphilis) resemble their counterparts in the non-AIDS patient. A number of other conditions may present with symptoms resembling meningitis; for example, parenchymal brain diseases such as toxoplasmosis and primary CNS lymphoma may initially manifest with headache as an important symptom. More common, however, is the development of headache of uncertain cause. Although not well studied, headache is a common symptom in late HIV-1 infection and at times can be a severe, debilitating problem. While acute headache in some patients may relate to the onset of systemic infection such as *P. carinii* pneumonia, in others the explanation is elusive.

PREDOMINANTLY FOCAL BRAIN DISORDERS. In approaching diagnosis of parenchymal brain disease, it is useful to separate the conditions that cause predominantly focal symptoms and signs from those producing more generalized brain dysfunction. Patients in the former group present with hemiparesis, aphasia, apraxia, hemisensory abnormalities, visual field loss, and the like, as a result of focal macroscopic lesions in cortical or subcortical brain regions. The most important of these are cerebral toxoplasmosis, which complicates the course of AIDS in 7 to 15 per cent of patients, primary cerebral lymphoma developing in up to 5 per cent, and PML, which occurs in perhaps 3 per cent. Less common are a miscellany of other infections and cerebrovascular disorders.

Although the three major focal disorders all characteristically have a subacute onset and may be clinically indistinguishable, they tend to have somewhat different temporal profiles (Table 414–3). Thus, cerebral toxoplasmosis typically progresses most rapidly (over a few days) and progressive multifocal leukoencephalopathy (PML) evolves most slowly (over a few weeks), with primary CNS lymphoma somewhere in between. Each may cause similar neurologic deficits, but there are often differences in the associated findings. Thus, toxoplasmosis commonly presents with a combination of focal deficit and generalized encephalopathy with confusion or clouding of consciousness; fever and headache may also be present. This contrasts with PML, at least at onset, in which focal neurologic deficits are unaccompanied by either diffuse brain dysfunction or evidence of a systemic toxic state. CNS lymphoma, when accompanied by significant mass effect or when deep in the frontal or periventricular region, may cause more global mental dysfunction, but, again, these patients are usually afebrile without constitutional symptoms or signs.

Once the focal nature of patient's symptoms and signs is recognized, use of neuroimaging techniques, including computed tomography (CT) and more recently magnetic resonance imaging (MRI), is critical both to confirm the presence of macroscopic focal disease and to determine the nature of the abnormalities

TABLE 414–3. COMPARATIVE CLINICAL AND RADIOLOGIC FEATURES OF CEREBRAL TOXOPLASMOSIS, PRIMARY CNS LYMPHOMA, AND PROGRESSIVE MULTIFOCAL LEUKOENCEPHALOPATHY

	Clinical Onset			Neuroradiologic Features		
	Temporal Profile	*Level of Alertness*	*Fever*	*Number of Lesions*	*Type of Lesions*	*Location of Lesions*
Cerebral toxoplasmosis	Days	Reduced	Common	Multiple	Spherical, ring-enhancing	Basal ganglia, cortex
Primary CNS lymphoma	Days to weeks	Variable	Absent	One or few	Irregular, weakly enhancing	Periventricular
Progressive multifocal leuko-encephalopathy	Weeks	Preserved	Absent	Multiple	Nonenhancing	White matter

(Table 414–3). Multiple lesions involving the cortex or deep brain nuclei (thalamus, basal ganglia) surrounded by edema strongly favor cerebral toxoplasmosis. In most cases *Toxoplasma* abscesses exhibit ringlike contrast enhancement on CT scan. Double-dose contrast CT studies, or preferably MRI, may help in more clearly defining these lesions and detecting additional characteristic spherical lesions. Cerebral lymphoma may produce a similar CT appearance, although the lesions of lymphoma are usually less numerous (one or two definable lesions), commonly exhibit more diffuse or less clear-cut contrast enhancement, and are more often located in the white matter adjacent to the ventricles. PML characteristically involves the white matter, most often adjacent to the cortex, and is without mass effect or contrast enhancement on CT.

After neuroimaging, the next step in diagnosis of focal mass lesions often involves a trial of anti-*Toxoplasma* therapy. Pyrimethamine and sulfa therapy characteristically results in clinical improvement within a few days and distinct reduction of lesions on neuroimaging by 1 or 2 weeks. This rapid and consistent improvement allows treatment response to serve as a basis for diagnosis and thereby obviates the need for brain biopsy in virtually all patients with toxoplasmosis. Biopsy is then reserved for cases with atypical clinical or laboratory features (including atypical neuroimaging appearance or negative *Toxoplasma* blood serology) along with those who fail to improve with treatment. It is important in the context of such therapeutic trial that, if possible, corticosteroids be avoided. Since the signs and symptoms, and even the CT or MRI abnormalities, of cerebral lymphoma may improve with corticosteroids, such treatment can confuse interpretation of the anti-*Toxoplasma* therapeutic trial. However, if cerebral edema threatens brain herniation, judicious short-term corticosteroids may be instituted along with appropriate specific therapy and subsequently tapered rapidly once the patient improves.

PREDOMINANTLY NONFOCAL BRAIN DISORDERS. The disorders presenting with more general or diffuse brain dysfunction and without focal features can be further divided into those in which consciousness remains fully preserved and those accompanied by a concomitant decrease in alertness. Most important among the former is the *AIDS dementia complex,* a clinical syndrome characterized by cognitive, motor, and, at times, behavioral dysfunction. A number of terms have been used to encompass this clinical syndrome, including the recent designation by the World Health Organization (WHO) as the HIV-1–associated cognitive/motor complex, with three subtypes: HIV-1–associated dementia, HIV-1–associated myelopathy, and HIV-1–associated minor cognitive/motor disorder.

Both the incidence and severity of the AIDS dementia complex increase with advancing immunosuppression. The clinical syndrome is somewhat variable, and its pathologic substrate is heterogeneous. At least in part, it appears to relate to effects of HIV-1 infection on the CNS rather than involving secondary opportunistic infection. Its early, mild form is usually characterized by impaired concentration and attention along with reduced mental agility, resulting in complaints of forgetfulness and slowness in performing complex mental tasks. In those who progress to more severe involvement, cognitive dysfunction worsens and involves other domains, and motor dysfunction becomes clinically manifest with gait unsteadiness and difficulty with rapid, fine movements of the hands. Personality change with apathy, lack of

initiative, or, at times, hyperactivity and agitation may be part of the syndrome. In its most severe form, global dementia, paraplegia, and virtual mutism may evolve with resultant incapacity. Although it is in part a diagnosis of exclusion, the symptoms and signs of the AIDS dementia complex are sufficiently distinct to allow bedside diagnosis in most patients on the basis of their stereotypy. Neuroimaging using CT or MRI characteristically reveals cerebral atrophy, and MRI may additionally demonstrate increased signal in white matter or basal ganglia. Several studies now suggest that zidovudine can partially reverse the symptoms and signs of the AIDS dementia complex. Whether newer antiretroviral drugs will demonstrate a similar therapeutic effect remains to be evaluated.

In the AIDS dementia complex there is relative preservation of alertness in relation to cognitive loss. This contrasts with most metabolic encephalopathies developing as sequelae of the systemic diseases suffered by AIDS patients; for example, hypoxia and sepsis are characteristically accompanied by a degree of lethargy and confusion which parallels the decline in cognition. Likewise, CNS-active drugs often cloud mentation and alertness together. While such metabolic and toxic disorders may present alone, they also commonly have an exacerbating or unmasking influence on the AIDS dementia complex, resulting in a mixture of the two conditions. HIV-1–infected patients may also be more sensitive to neuroleptics and thereby manifest parkinsonian or other movement disorders as side effects at seemingly low doses.

Brain infections may also produce diffuse brain dysfunction. Although CNS toxoplasmosis characteristically causes focal neurologic symptoms and signs, in some patients generalized encephalopathy predominates. Similarly, CNS lymphoma may infiltrate deep structures and impair cognition and motor function without prominent focal symptoms or signs. The clinical importance of CNS cytomegalovirus (CMV) infection in this regard remains imprecisely defined. Scattered CMV infection of the brain is common at autopsy, but the clinical correlate of this finding is not clear, and likely it is often silent or mild. On the other hand, in a small number of patients CMV encephalitis may be severe with subacute clouding of consciousness and, at times, seizures. Herpes simplex virus types 1 and 2 may also cause subacute nonfocal encephalitis.

MYELOPATHIES. The most common spinal cord affliction in AIDS patients is the pathologically defined vacuolar myelopathy, which has been included within the broader clinical designation of the AIDS dementia complex because it is usually accompanied by evidence of concomitant brain dysfunction. The disorder is generally of subacute or slow onset and progression with painless gait disturbance characterized by ataxia and spasticity. Bladder and bowel difficulty usually follow deterioration of gait, and sensory symptoms and signs are less prominent than gait dysfunction unless there is concomitant neuropathy. Patients do not manifest a distinct sensory or motor "level" as in transverse myelopathies but rather distal loss of large-fiber modalities accompanied by increased deep tendon reflexes (again, in the absence of neuropathy) and Babinski signs. The efficacy of zidovudine or other antiretrovirals in this subgroup of AIDS dementia complex patients is uncertain.

An additional, emerging cause of clinically similar myelopathy in HIV-1–infected patients relates to coinfection with a second retrovirus, human T-lymphotropic virus I (HTLV-I). Double infection results from the convergent epidemiologies of these infections related to intravenous drug abuse. Although pathologically distinct, clinical differentiation of vacuolar myelopathy and HTLV-I–associated myelopathy (HAM) may be very difficult. Diagnosis begins with suspicion based on risk and is supported by serologic documentation of HTLV-I infection, but the relative clinical contributions of the two viruses is problematic antemortem. In AIDS patients with myelopathy, laboratory diagnostic studies are principally directed at ruling out spinal cord disease other than vacuolar myelopathy. Neither myelography nor spinal MRI has allowed clear imaging of vacuolar myelopathy or HAM. However, these procedures are often needed to document focal intraspinal processes, including epidural masses.

PERIPHERAL NEUROPATHIES. The most common neuropathy in the late stages of HIV-1 infection is a distal, predominantly sensory, axonal neuropathy. Characteristically, sensory symptoms exceed both sensory and motor dysfunction. Although its prevalence has not been well defined, likely a mild form of this type of neuropathy is very common. In some patients these sensory symptoms become severe, and painful paresthesias and "burning feet" are disabling. Although suspected to relate to direct HIV-1 infection of nerve or dorsal root ganglia, this has not been directly confirmed, and the pathogenesis of this neuropathy is uncertain. Anecdotal experience suggests that it does not generally respond to zidovudine, and treatment therefore relies on symptom management with tricyclics and analgesics. Autonomic neuropathy has also been reported in AIDS patients, with presentation ranging from postural hypotension to cardiovascular collapse in the setting of surgery.

Likely to be of increasing importance in the next several years are the toxic neuropathies caused by some of the newer antiretroviral nucleoside drugs, including dideoxyinosine and dideoxycytidine. These drugs cause dose-dependent axonal neuropathies with clinical features very similar to the AIDS-related sensory polyneuropathy discussed above, often heralded by distal extremity pain.

CMV causes an uncommon but therapeutically important infection of nerve roots. This polyradiculopathy is usually of subacute but fulminant onset, with pain and sacral sensory loss followed by ascending progression to flaccid paralysis. The CSF reveals a characteristic pleocytosis with polymorphonuclear cell predominance. Early diagnosis and prompt institution of ganciclovir treatment can lead to arrest and clinical improvement.

Less common than these polyneuropathies is mononeuritis multiplex, with onset most commonly in the setting of ARC rather than far-advanced AIDS. Favorable response to plasma exchange has been reported.

MYOPATHIES. Several types of myopathy may complicate HIV-1 infection. Although classification and characterization of these conditions remain imprecise, both inflammatory and noninflammatory myopathies have been described, ranging in severity from asymptomatic creatine kinase elevation to severe proximal weakness. Improvement of patients with inflammatory, polymyositis-like illness has been reported following steroid therapy.

Zidovudine can also cause proximal weakness and loss of muscle mass. This toxic myopathy appears to develop only after prolonged use of the antiretroviral and perhaps relates to the drug's effect on mitochondria; muscle biopsy may reveal excessive or abnormal mitochondria. Drug discontinuation usually results in clinical improvement.

Baumbartner JE, Rachlin JR, Beckstead JH, et al.: Primary central nervous system lymphomas: Natural history and response to radiation therapy in 55 patients with acquired immunodeficiency syndrome. J Neurosurg 73:206–211, 1990. *Describes an extensive experience with primary CNS lymphoma in AIDS.*

Berger JR, Kaszovitz B, Post JD, et al.: Progressive multifocal leukoencephalopathy associated with human immunodeficiency virus infection. Ann Intern Med 107:78, 1987. *A review of experience with PML in AIDS.*

Dalakas MC, Illa I, Pezeshkpour GH, et al.: Mitochondrial myopathy caused by long-term zidovudine therapy. N Engl J Med 322:1098–1105, 1990. *Describes zidovudine myopathy and considers other myopathies in AIDS patients.*

Hollander H, Stringari S: Human immunodeficiency virus–associated meningitis: Clinical course and correlations. Am J Med 83:813, 1987. *Describes the aseptic meningitis complicating HIV-1 infection.*

Miller RG, Storey JR, Greco CM: Ganciclovir in the treatment of progressive AIDS-related polyradiculopathy. Neurology 40:569–574, 1990. *Reports experience in CMV-related polyradiculopathy and also discusses other neuropathies in HIV-1–infected patients; full bibliography.*

Navia BA, Cho ES, Petito CK, et al.: Cerebral toxoplasmosis complicating the acquired immune deficiency syndrome: Clinical and neuropathological findings in 27 patients. Ann Neurol 19:224, 1986. *Describes clinical features of cerebral toxoplasmosis in AIDS.*

Navia BA, Jordon BD, Price RW: The AIDS dementia complex. I. Clinical features. Ann Neurol 19517, 1986. *Report characterizing the clinical features of the AIDS dementia complex.*

Petito CK, Navia BA, Cho ES, et al.: Vacuolar myelopathy pathologically resembling subacute combined degeneration in patients with acquired immunodeficiency syndrome (AIDS). N Engl J Med 312:874, 1985. *Describes clinical and pathologic findings associated with vacuolar myelopathy.*

Price RW, Brew B: Management of the neurologic complications of HIV-1 infection and AIDS. *In* Sande MA, Volberding PA (eds.): The Medical Management of AIDS. Philadelphia, W.B. Saunders Company, 1990, pp 161–181. *An expanded general review with full bibliography.*

Zuger A, Louie E, Holzman RS, et al.: Cryptococcal disease in patients with the acquired immunodeficiency syndrome: Diagnostic features and outcome of treatment. Ann Intern Med 104:234–240, 1986. *Describes the clinical features of cryptococcal meningitis in AIDS.*

415 Pulmonary Manifestations of AIDS: Special Emphasis on Pneumocystosis

Fred R. Sattler

Protozoan, viral, fungal, and bacterial infections and tumors such as Kaposi's sarcoma cause most of the deaths in patients with AIDS. All of these complications may involve the lung and often require initial treatment in the hospital. Chest tightness, breathlessness, hacking cough, pleuritic pain, high fevers, drenching sweats, drug-induced rashes, and secondary bacterial infections result in considerable discomfort and anxiety for patients, their partners, and their families. Pneumothoraces, which may occur spontaneously or after bronchoscopy, often prolong hospitalization and contribute further morbidity.

Patients with AIDS are hospitalized two or three times per year for management of these complications. The cost for each hospitalization ranges from $10,000 to $20,000; in many large urban-metropolitan areas where AIDS is highly endemic, medical personnel and hospital services are being consumed and rapidly depleted. Prompt diagnosis and early treatment of these complications facilitates early discharge from the hospital by hastening clinical response and reducing the risks and severity of toxic drug effects. Of equal import, as prophylactic therapies for various infections are established to be effective for HIV-positive patients, the incidence of these pulmonary complications will be reduced. It is imperative, therefore, that medical providers implement a global strategy of prevention and early therapy of these life-threatening complications if the human suffering and progressive depletion of health care resources caused by AIDS are to be alleviated.

PATHOGENESIS AND RISK FOR INFECTION

The risk for HIV-positive persons developing opportunistic pulmonary complications is related to deficiencies in their T-helper (CD4 surface phenotype) lymphocytes, since these cells control or regulate virtually all components of immunity (see Ch. 242 and 410). Thus, host defenses become progressively compromised as the CD4 cells are destroyed during the course of HIV infection. Figure 415–1 shows that the CD4 lymphocyte count is generally below 100 cells per cubic millimeter (or less than 10 per cent of the total T lymphocytes, latter data not shown) for pneumonia due to *Pneumocystis carinii*, Kaposi's sarcoma, *Mycobacterium avium* complex, cytomegalovirus, and *Cryptococcus neoformans*. By contrast, nonspecific interstitial pneumonitis occurs at various levels of CD4 immunity, and pulmonary infection due to *Mycobacterium tuberculosis* most often occurs in HIV-positive persons when their CD4 count is in the range of 200 to 400 cells per cubic millimeter. Thus, the absolute or relative concentration of CD4 lymphocytes is related to the pathogenesis of many of the pulmonary complications and is

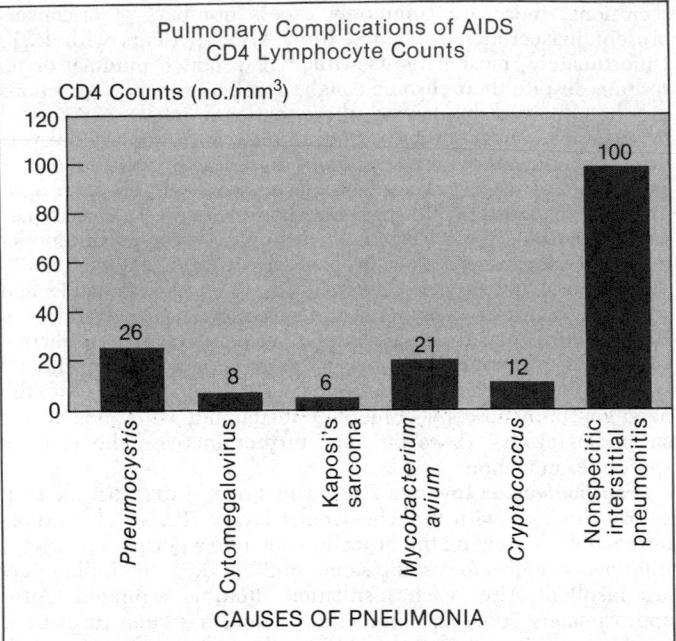

Figure 415–1. Median number of CD4 lymphocytes for various opportunistic pulmonary complications occurring in patients with AIDS. (Adapted from Masur H, Ognibene FP, Yarchoan R, et al.: CD4 counts as predictors of opportunistic pneumonias in human immunodeficiency virus (HIV) infection. Ann Intern Med 111:223–231, 1989.)

useful in assessing the relative risk of the various pulmonary disorders in HIV-positive patients.

Pneumocystis carinii Pneumonia (PCP)

Pneumonia due to *P. carinii* is the most common pulmonary complication in patients infected with HIV. Since the beginning of the epidemic in the United States, PCP has occurred in 50 to 60 per cent of patients as the initial opportunistic complication resulting in the Centers for Disease Control case definition of AIDS. Ultimately 70 to 80 per cent of AIDS patients experience one or more episodes of PCP, and without prophylaxis approximately 60,000 AIDS-related cases will occur in the year 1991 alone. Moreover, 10 to 50 per cent of episodes are fatal, depending on the severity of illness at presentation. In fact, PCP accounts for nearly half of the deaths due to opportunistic complications in patients with AIDS. Thus, considerable emphasis is given here to the diagnosis, treatment, and prevention of this devastating infection.

ETIOLOGY. *P. carinii* was long believed to be a protozoan organism because of its morphologic features and response to drugs used to treat other protozoan infections. However, the genetic composition of the ribosomal RNA of this organism suggests that it is similar to a fungus and phylogenetically may belong to the Ascomycetes yeasts. The immediate importance of this observation is unclear, since PCP does not respond to available antifungal drugs. Better understanding of the molecular composition of *P. carinii* will, however, ultimately provide valuable insights into pathogenic mechanisms and development of better therapies for infections caused by this organism.

CLINICAL SYNDROME. The onset of PCP in AIDS patients is usually insidious. The cardinal manifestation is chronic cough, which often has been present for weeks and sometimes months. The cough is usually nonproductive but occasionally is associated with mucoid sputum. Retrosternal chest tightness, which is intensified with inspiration and coughing, is a second nearly global symptom. Fever occurs in 80 to 90 per cent of patients but may have been present for a shorter duration than the cough and chest tightness. Dyspnea on exertion and breathlessness at rest occur late in the infection when oxygenation is moderately to severely impaired.

Abnormalities on physical examination are usually limited and nonspecific. Elevated temperature and respiratory rate may be present. With mild episodes there may be no tachypnea, but patients with severe episodes are often in respiratory distress and

are using their accessory chest wall muscles. The lungs are frequently clear to auscultation, as rales are detected in only 30 to 40 per cent of cases and are usually a late finding in severe episodes. Indeed, absence of adventitial breath sounds should not be used to exclude the possibility of PCP in persons who are at risk for AIDS.

Physical findings outside the lung are even less specific, but their presence or absence may assist the clinical assessment. For example, in patients with a forme fruste presentation who have not been treated with topical or oral antifungal drugs, a thick coating of thrush on the dorsal aspect of the tongue is a nearly universal finding. Seborrheic dermatitis involving the face between the brows, forehead, and upper cheeks is also common with PCP and unusual with other pulmonary complications of AIDS. By contrast, generalized adenopathy with lymph nodes greater than 1 cm in diameter is rare, since patients with PCP usually have severe immune deficiency and their lymph nodes are hypoplastic. Thus, the presence of large lymph nodes should suggest the occurrence of other opportunistic complications, although concurrent infection with *P. carinii* may occur.

EXTRAPULMONARY PNEUMOCYSTOSIS. *P. carinii* infection outside the lung may occur without prior or concurrent PCP, although most cases have occurred during prophylaxis with aerosolized pentamidine and the lung is frequently involved. It is unlikely that pentamidine is directly related to the pathogenesis of extrapulmonary pneumocystosis. Rather, it is probably an epiphenomenon associated with the lack of protection provided by aerosolized pentamidine for sites of infection outside the lung. Clinical presentations have included external auditory polyps, mastoiditis, choroiditis, digital necrosis secondary to vasculitis, obstruction of the small intestine, ascites with gross nodules in the stomach and duodenum, hepatitis, splenitis, hilar or mediastinal lymphadenopathy, and involvement of the bone marrow. Disseminated infection may also occur in virtually every organ including brain, heart, kidneys, and adrenal glands. Histologic examination of affected organs shows a striking resemblance to the pathology usually found in the lung. There are typical foci of eosinophilic frothy exudates which upon special staining reveal the presence of *P. carinii* cysts. Unlike the lung, these lesions are often calcified and there may be vasculitis with invasion of vessel walls by *P. carinii* organisms.

Signs and symptoms of extrapulmonary pneumocystosis are nonspecific, and the diagnosis usually requires histologic confirmation. *P. carinii* choroiditis is, however, associated with unique features. Lesions consist of slightly elevated, yellow-white plaques, generally limited to the choroid without evidence of intraocular inflammation. Identification of these typical lesions may provide the first clue to the diagnosis of *P. carinii* infection and mandates that therapy include systemic drugs active against *P. carinii*.

LABORATORY ABNORMALITIES. Most patients with PCP are anemic because of the advanced stage of their HIV infection, other concurrent diseases, or treatment with myelosuppressive drugs such as zidovudine. For similar reasons the white blood cell count (WBC) is usually depressed or in the low normal range. An elevated WBC or marked increase in the percentage of band forms should suggest a bacterial pneumonia or other pyogenic process. The serum albumin is often depressed by 0.5 to 1.0 gram per deciliter below normal and is probably a reflection of the poor overall nutritional status of these patients. Serum lactate dehydrogenase (LDH) is a sensitive but not specific marker of PCP and is elevated in more than 90 per cent of patients with PCP, whereas LDH values are usually only minimally elevated or normal in individuals with other pulmonary complications of AIDS.

The absolute or relative number of CD4 lymphocytes is the single most useful test in evaluating patients at risk for PCP. As shown in Figure 415–1 and confirmed by several other studies, more than 90 per cent of individuals when first diagnosed with PCP have less than 200 CD4 lymphocytes per cubic millimeter. However, in one large natural history investigation of ambulatory subjects at risk for AIDS, 26 per cent of individuals had CD4 counts above 200 (all but one had counts between 201 and 350) within 6 months prior to the diagnosis of PCP. The diagnosis is very unlikely in an individual with a normal or nearly normal (generally > 500) number of CD4 cells.

PULMONARY FUNCTION TESTS. Hypoxemia with PaO_2 less than 80 torr occurs in more than 80 per cent and an alveolar-arterial oxygen difference $[(A-a)DO_2]$ of greater than 15 torr occurs in more than 90 per cent of patients with PCP. In patients with PCP in whom these tests are normal or nearly normal, oxygen desaturation can be documented with pulse oximetry during exercise and the $(A-a)DO_2$ generally widens. The carbon monoxide diffusing capacity (DL_{CO}) is less than 80 per cent of predicted in nearly all patients with PCP, since the transmembrane diffusion of carbon monoxide is impaired (alveolar capillary block) by the intra-alveolar exudate associated with this infection. The test is not specific, since it may be abnormal in other pulmonary disorders and in patients who use intravenous drugs. However, in patients with respiratory symptoms whose arterial blood gases and chest radiographs are not helpful, a normal DL_{CO} makes PCP unlikely at that time. The test is also helpful in AIDS patients with asthma, since results should be normal in subjects whose hypoxemia is due to bronchospasm.

RADIOGRAPHIC ABNORMALITIES. Typically in PCP, infiltrates on chest radiographs are interstitial and begin in the perihilar areas and spread to the lower and upper lung fields, although the apices are usually spared. As the disease progresses, an alveolar pattern with air bronchograms may be superimposed on the interstitial process, although alveolar patterns may be the initial presentation in up to 10 per cent of cases. In 10 to 30 per cent of cases the radiographic presentation is atypical, with asymmetric or predominantly upper lobe infiltration, lobar or segmental consolidation, cystic lesions (with a honeycombed appearance), overt cavitation, and rarely solitary parenchymal nodules or postobstructive infiltration secondary to endobronchial nodules of *P. carinii*. Pleural effusions and hilar adenopathy have only rarely been documented to be due to *P. carinii*, although both have reportedly disappeared during therapy for PCP, whereas Kaposi's sarcoma frequently involves the pleural space and hilar nodes may be enlarged with mycobacterial infection and cryptococcosis.

Lung cavitation is not uncommon in AIDS patients with PCP. Lesions are generally thin walled without air-fluid levels and may be solitary or more generalized, resulting in regional areas of honeycombed lung. These lesions may occur in nonsmokers, at initial presentation of the first episode of PCP, prior to bronchoscopy, prior to aerosol therapy, and prior to intubation. Thus, in most cases cavitation is not due to underlying lung disease, specific diagnostic or therapeutic interventions, or barotrauma. It may be due to activated pulmonary macrophages and release of elastase as a consequence of chronic infection with *P. carinii* per se. Regardless of the mechanism, cavitation and cystic lesions, which occurred in just over 10 per cent of patients in one large series, may be complicated by spontaneous pneumothoraces and bronchopleural fistulas that are refractory to closure. Moreover, cavitation is unusual in HIV-positive patients with pulmonary tuberculosis. Thus, radiographic appearance of cavitation or cystic disease should not be a deterrent to pursuing a diagnosis of PCP.

Ten to 20 per cent of patients with documented PCP have had normal chest radiographs at presentation. These patients generally have early, mild episodes and respond well to appropriate and prompt therapy. Thus, every effort should be made to diagnose PCP early when there is minimal or no infiltration present on the chest radiograph.

Gallium-67 accumulates in areas of lung inflammation, but pulmonary uptake is not specific for PCP. Specificity is reportedly improved if scans are designated positive only when gallium uptake in the lungs equals or exceeds that in the liver. However, patients with mild PCP may have minimal or no lung uptake, and other pulmonary complications may produce positive scans. In addition, the test is expensive and images are not produced until 48 to 72 hours after patients have been injected with gallium. However, gallium imaging is useful for patients with chronic lung disease who have worsening respiratory symptoms, since blood gases and radiographs are often not useful in these patients, and for detecting relapses when other tests are not diagnostic.

DIAGNOSIS. *Sputum Induction.* Unlike PCP in other immunocompromised patients in whom organisms are often difficult to find in lung tissue and are rarely present in tracheobronchial secretions, there are commonly excess numbers of organisms present in secretions obtained from AIDS patients with PCP. Unfortunately, most patients with PCP produce minimal or no sputum despite their chronic cough. Tracheobronchial secretions can be obtained by having these patients inhale aerosols of hypertonic saline generated by ultrasonic nebulization. However, even concentrates of such specimens are difficult to examine after adequate staining because of background debris. Thus, to optimize the diagnostic yield, patients should cleanse their oropharynx by brushing their teeth and gargling prior to sputum induction, and specimens should be treated with mucolytic agents to dissolve oral debris prior to staining. When this is done and slides are reviewed by experts, the procedure has a sensitivity of 50 to 80 per cent but only a 39 to 63 per cent negative predictive value. The procedure is laborious for respiratory therapists and laboratory technicians, but positive specimens usually obviate the need for bronchoscopy. Fluorescent staining with monoclonal antibodies against *P. carinii* may further increase the yield of sputum examination.

Bronchoalveolar Lavage. The cornerstone of diagnosis of PCP is bronchoscopy with bronchoalveolar lavage (BAL). This procedure involves wedging the bronchoscope into a peripheral airway. Aliquots of nonbacteriostatic saline of 20 to 30 cubic millimeters are instilled. After each instillation, fluid is aspirated. After approximately 50 cubic millimeters of fluid has been recovered, the specimen is centrifuged and the pellet is stained for *P. carinii*. In 86 to 97 per cent of cases *P. carinii* organisms are detected by this procedure.

Transbronchial Biopsy. When transbronchial biopsies are obtained and specimens are without crush artifact and contain at least 25 alveoli, this procedure results in a diagnostic yield similar to that achieved with BAL. If both BAL and transbronchial biopsies are obtained, the diagnostic sensitivity is additive and approaches 100 per cent. However, pneumothoraces or bleeding may occur in up to 10 per cent of subjects undergoing transbronchial biopsy. Thus, many pulmonologists prefer to perform only BAL with the initial bronchoscopy. If the first procedure fails to provide a diagnosis, BAL is repeated and transbronchial biopsies are obtained. If specimens from both procedures are adequate and fail to show *P. carinii* organisms with standard histologic and cytologic stains, the diagnosis is confidently excluded.

Open Lung Biopsy. Open lung biopsy is rarely needed in AIDS patients to diagnose PCP because of the high yield of sputum induction and bronchoscopy. It is usually reserved for patients in whom bronchoscopy has been nondiagnostic because of technical problems with the procedure or transbronchial biopsies are contraindicated because of bleeding disorders or concurrent management with mechanical ventilation. Open lung biopsy is safer than bronchoscopy for patients with abnormal coagulation, since hemostasis is more reliably achieved intraoperatively than at bronchoscopy.

TREATMENT. *Initial Therapy.* The key to successful treatment of PCP is early therapy, since mild episodes are more likely to respond favorably. In particular, patients with minimal infiltration on their chest radiographs, minimal elevation of serum LDH, and normal or nearly normal $(A-a)DO_2$ generally have greater than 90 per cent chance of responding to treatment. By contrast, patients with extensive infiltration, LDH in excess of 500, and $(A-a)DO_2$ greater than 35 torr have a risk for death during treatment that is greater than 40 per cent. If the $(A-a)DO_2$ exceeds 55 to 60 torr, the risk for a fatal outcome is in the range of 60 to 80 per cent.

Since sputum induction and bronchoscopies are generally not done at night or on weekends or holidays and results of cytologic stains are often not available for 24 hours or more after specimens have been collected, most patients with typical clinical features of PCP should be treated empirically, especially if there is moderate to severe impairment in gas exchange as measured by the PaO_2 or $(A-a)DO_2$. This does not impair the ability to make a histologic or cytologic diagnosis, as large numbers of *P. carinii* cysts and trophozoites remain in lung tissues and pulmonary secretions for weeks to months after the onset of therapy. There are several reasons why every effort should be made to confirm the diagnosis even if the patient appears to be responding promptly to treatment. Bacterial bronchopneumonia may respond to the antibiotic properties of the sulfonamide and sulfone drugs used to treat PCP, and nonspecific interstitial pneumonitis may

TABLE 415–1. TREATMENTS FOR *PNEUMOCYSTIS CARINII* PNEUMONIA

	Dosages*
Standard drug therapies	
Trimethoprim-sulfamethoxazole (IV or oral)	5 mg/kg q6h or q8h of trimethoprim
Pentamidine (IV or IM)	4 mg/kg/day
Trimethoprim-dapsone (both oral)	5 mg/kg q8h of TMP 100 mg/day of dapsone
Adjunctive corticosteroids (prednisone)†	60–80 mg/day for 5–7 days with tapering doses over 2–3 weeks
Experimental therapies	
Aerosolized pentamidine	600 mg/day via Respirgard II jet nebulizer
Trimetrexate-leucovorin (IV or IV/oral)	45 mg/M²/day of trimetrexate 20 mg/M²/q6h of leucovorin
Eflornithine (DFMO) (IV and oral)	100 mg/kg/q6h intravenously 75 mg/kg/q6h orally
Primaquine-clindamycin (oral-parenteral/oral)	15–30 mg/day primaquine base 0.6–0.9 gram IV or 450–600 mg orally of clindamycin q6–8h

*Dosages are once daily unless designated otherwise.
†To be administered concurrently with specific anti-*Pneumocystis* therapy for patients who present with (A-a)DO₂ > 35 mm Hg or PaO₂ < 70 mm Hg.

improve spontaneously. Both situations give the false impression that the patient has responded to anti-*Pneumocystis* therapy. Moreover, bacterial pneumonia can often be treated with a brief course of oral antibiotic therapy, and nonspecific interstitial pneumonitis should not be treated with antimicrobial agents.

Mycobacteriosis, cytomegalovirus pneumonia, and Kaposi's sarcoma may also closely resemble PCP. However, each of these pulmonary complications requires a different therapy. In addition, by the time patients fail to respond to empiric therapy for PCP, they may be too ill for bronchoscopy or open lung biopsy, thus denying them the opportunity to receive specific therapy.

For psychological reasons it is important for patients and their loved ones to know for certain whether they have AIDS. Results of empiric therapy may provide presumptive evidence for the diagnosis, although the uncertainties may be emotionally devastating for individuals who have not met the rigorous U.S. Public Health Service case definition for AIDS. Moreover, access to many community services and financial benefits requires a definitive diagnosis of AIDS, which can usually be established by documenting the presence of a pulmonary opportunistic complication (other than tuberculosis).

Finally, standard therapies for PCP are associated with a high rate of adverse and often serious drug reactions, which may prolong hospitalization. It is difficult to justify these toxic reactions and additional hospitalization for patients who do not have PCP. Thus, there are compelling reasons to establish a definitive diagnosis whenever possible.

Initial therapy should be given parenterally for patients with severe impairment in oxygen exchange as arbitrarily defined by an (A-a)DO₂ of greater than 30 torr. In non-AIDS patients with PCP, trimethoprim (TMP) and sulfamethoxazole (SMX), which have nearly complete bioavailability when administered orally, were erratically absorbed from the gut in subjects with severe hypoxemia. Patients who failed treatment often had serum TMP concentrations less than 5 μg per millileter. The problem is further complicated by the fact that AIDS patients may have nonspecific malabsorption in the absence of overt diarrhea. The principle of beginning initial treatment with parenteral drugs for moderate to severe episodes should also apply to other anti-*Pneumocystis* therapies. Table 415–1 shows the drugs and dosages generally prescribed to treat PCP.

Trimethoprim-sulfamethoxazole. The antifolate combination of TMP-SMX was the first therapy licensed by the U.S. Food and Drug Administration for the therapy of PCP. In the largest prospective controlled study involving AIDS patients with moderate to severe PCP, subjects were prospectively randomized to receive a full 3-week course of either TMP-SMX or pentamidine without being crossed over to the opposite therapy for apparent treatment failure or adverse drug reactions. This allowed the relative efficacy and inherent toxicities of these two therapies to be fully assessed. In this investigation, 86 per cent of individuals

treated with TMP-SMX survived, compared to 61 per cent treated with pentamidine; this difference was statistically significant. An average of 2.4 adverse reactions were ascribed to study therapy in 89 per cent of individuals treated with TMP-SMX. Severe hematologic toxicities were prevented through pharmacokinetic monitoring. By reducing the initial dose of 15 to 20 mg per kilogram per day of the TMP component to maintain serum TMP concentrations in the 5 to 8 μg per milliliter range, dosage-terminating neutropenia or thrombocytopenia did not occur. With this approach the final average dosage was 12 mg per kilogram per day, yet efficacy was not compromised. In addition, therapy was continued despite hypersensitivity reactions of drug-induced fever or morbilliform rash. This was accomplished by concurrent therapy with acetaminophen for fever and antihistamines for rashes. In each case fever ultimately subsided and rashes coalesced and faded, although this occasionally took several weeks. There were no severe complications such as Stevens-Johnson syndrome or exfoliative dermatitis, and other adverse effects associated with TMP-SMX were tolerable. The spectrum and frequency of these toxic drug reactions are shown in Table 415–2. The approach of dosage reduction based on pharmacokinetic monitoring and continuing treatment despite manageable hypersensitivity reactions allowed patients to be switched to oral TMP-SMX once their respiratory status was improved and to complete therapy on an outpatient basis.

Pentamidine. Parenteral pentamidine is the other licensed therapy for PCP. In the aforementioned study involving individuals with moderate to severe PCP, survival was inferior with pentamidine compared to TMP-SMX. However, the dosage of pentamidine was reduced when nephrotoxicity occurred such that the final average dosage was approximately 3 mg per kilogram per day. It is possible that dosage reduction compromised outcome. In one study involving individuals with less severe PCP, 3 mg per kilogram per day resulted in a good outcome. However, until rigorous controlled studies are done to compare this lower dosage with the standard dosage, the initial dosage of pentamidine should be 4 mg per kilogram per day, especially for more severe episodes.

Toxic reactions are also frequent with parenteral pentamidine (Table 415–2). In the study mentioned earlier, an average of 2.9 adverse drug effects occurred in 97 per cent of the individuals treated with pentamidine. Nephrotoxicity (64 per cent), hypotension (27 per cent), and hypoglycemia (21 per cent) were the most frequent serious adverse effects. Impaired renal function, which

TABLE 415–2. TOXIC SIDE EFFECTS ASSOCIATED WITH TREATMENTS FOR *PNEUMOCYSTIS CARINII* PNEUMONIA*

Adverse Effect†	Trimethoprim-Sulfamethoxazole (%)	Pentamidine (parenteral) (%)
Fever (>37.7°C)	78	82
Leukopenia (<4 × 10⁹/L)	72	47
Rash—generalized	44	15
Anemia (↓ >3 g/dl)	39	24
Nausea/vomiting	25	24
Elevated ALT (↑ >5X)	22	15
Azotemia‡	14	64
Thrombocytopenia (<100 × 10⁹/L)	3	18
Hypotension (sys. <80 mm Hg)	0	27
Hypoglycemia (<70 mg/dl)	0	21
Hypocalcemia (<7 mg/dl)	0	3
Total percentage of subjects with adverse reactions	89	97
Average number of reactions per subject (range)	2.4 (0–5)	2.9 (0–7)

*Adapted from Sattler FR, Cowan R, Nielsen DM, Ruskin J: Trimethoprim-sulfamethoxazole compared with pentamidine for treatment of *Pneumocystis carinii* pneumonia in the acquired immunodeficiency syndrome: A prospective noncrossover study. Ann Intern Med 109:280–287, 1988. Thirty-six patients were treated with TMP-SMX and 33 with pentamidine.
†Adverse effects occurring during treatment (e.g., fever = increase in temperature >37.7°C after patient had been afebrile more than 24 hours).
‡Azotemia = increase in serum creatinine greater than 0.5 mg/dl if less than 2.0 at baseline or increase by greater than 1.5 if baseline value was greater than 2.0 mg/dl.

does not usually occur until the second week of therapy and may occasionally progress to renal failure, generally resolves after therapy is discontinued. Hypotension usually occurs in association with intravenous infusions and lasts up to several hours, although modestly low blood pressures may persist for several months after the last dose. The acute drop in blood pressure is corrected by placing the patient in the supine position and providing hydration therapy.

Hypoglycemia, which occurs in 10 to 30 per cent of AIDS patients treated with pentamidine, is a consequence of sudden increases in serum insulin concentrations due to lysis of pancreatic β cells. This is potentially the most serious complication of therapy for *P. carinii* pneumonia. The risk of hypoglycemia is directly related to the cumulative dose of drug administered, since the drug is bound avidly to tissues and is released intact slowly over weeks to months. Therefore, the risk increases with the duration of therapy and the number of courses of treatment. Symptoms are frequently absent until serum glucose concentrations decline to less than 20 mg per deciliter. Moreover, this toxic effect may occur precipitously up to 2 weeks after the last dose has been administered. When any degree of hypoglycemia is detected in patients receiving pentamidine, treatment with the drug should be discontinued and the patient should be monitored closely for several weeks with capillary glucose measurements taken several times daily. These patients must also be instructed to ingest extra glucose whenever symptoms of hypoglycemia occur or glucose measurements are low. Occasionally, patients must remain in the hospital to receive concentrated infusions of glucose for up to several weeks to keep their serum glucose concentrations above 40 mg per deciliter. Depletion of pancreatic insulin may also result in the ultimate need for treatment with oral hypoglycemic agents. Ketoacidosis and hyperosmolar coma have also occurred in some patients after treatment with pentamidine.

When the drug is administered intramuscularly, painful sterile abscesses occur frequently and often limit the usefulness of this mode of therapy for outpatient treatment. Other toxic effects occur less frequently and have included myositis and myoglobinuria, gross hematuria, fatal pancreatitis, ventricular tachycardia, and torsades de pointes.

EXPERIMENTAL THERAPIES. Severe Episodes. For severe episodes of PCP (defined as [A-a]DO$_2$ greater than 30 torr) which are associated with high case fatality rates, more potent therapies are needed. Trimetrexate, eflornithine, and adjunctive therapy with corticosteroids are undergoing evaluation for such episodes. Trimetrexate (an antifolate, anticancer drug similar to methotrexate) binds the dihydrofolate reductase of *P. carinii* approximately 1500 times more avidly than TMP and because of its high lipid solubility is concentrated in protozoan cells. In an open study, 69 per cent of patients treated initially with 30 mg per square meter of intravenous trimetrexate once daily and 80 mg per square meter per day of leucovorin had a favorable response. In a dosage range investigation, 45 mg per square meter per day of trimetrexate and 80 mg per square meter per day of leucovorin proved to be the best regimen for initial therapy, resulting in a 92 per cent survival rate for episodes of various severity. In addition, all patients were able to receive a full 21-dose course of treatment; hypersensitivity reactions and hematologic toxicity were tolerable. Multicenter studies are underway to prospectively compare trimetrexate with TMP-SMX.

Eflornithine (also known as DFMO) is an irreversible decarboxylase inhibitor with efficacy against murine PCP. When this drug was administered to 345 patients who had failed or were intolerant to standard therapies, 66 per cent of nonventilated patients survived. However, only 10 per cent of respirator-dependent patients survived. The most serious toxicities have been thrombocytopenia, which may occur in up to 50 per cent of recipients, and a clinically relevant hearing loss in approximately 10 per cent. Eflornithine has not been adequately tested as initial therapy for PCP and should not be used for that purpose.

Use of corticosteroids as adjunctive therapy appears to benefit patients when instituted early in the course of therapy. In one unblinded study involving 326 patients who were treated with standard therapies, subjects were randomized within 36 hours of beginning therapy for PCP to receive 40 mg of prednisone twice daily for 5 days with tapering doses over the next 2 to 3 weeks or no treatment with corticosteroids. Patients treated with prednisone were significantly less likely to develop oxygenation failure or require intubation, and their chance for survival was increased from 80 per cent to 90 per cent after 31 days and 12 weeks. In a smaller study of similar design that was conducted in Canada, acute clinical respiratory failure defined by a decrease in oxygen saturation of more than 10 per cent occurred significantly less often in patients who received 60 mg of prednisone each day for 7 days followed by tapering doses over the next 14 days than in individuals who did not receive steroid therapy. In both studies there was no difference in the rate of secondary opportunistic complications, nosocomial infections, or adverse drug effects in the treatment groups.

By contrast, there is currently no evidence that corticosteroids are beneficial for "salvage" therapy. A double-blind comparison of adjunctive therapy with 60 mg of intravenous methylprednisolone every 6 hours versus placebo initiated anytime in the course of therapy (generally more than 3 days after beginning specific anti-*Pneumocystis* treatment) when the PaO$_2$ declined to less than 50 torr resulted in a different outcome. The trial was discontinued after 41 patients had been enrolled. There was no difference in survival between the two groups, but more secondary opportunistic infections occurred in patients receiving methylprednisolone. However, the power to determine clinically relevant differences in survival was severely limited by the small sample size.

Mild Episodes. For mild episodes (defined by an [A-a]DO$_2$ less than 30 torr), new treatments should be relatively nontoxic and suited for home therapy, since these patients have at least a 90 per cent response rate to standard therapy with TMP-SMX or pentamidine. Aerosolized pentamidine is one such therapy. Drug is delivered directly to the alveolar airspaces, which are the primary sites of infection, and very little drug is absorbed systemically. Thus, systemic toxicities occur infrequently. In a multicenter investigation, 364 patients were randomized to receive either 600 mg of aerosolized pentamidine once daily via the Respirgard II jet nebulizer or TMP-SMX at 15 mg per kilogram per day (TMP). There was no difference in survival between the two groups after 21 days of treatment, but there were more deaths in the group receiving TMP-SMX by day 35. In addition, drug-related toxicities occurred significantly more often in patients treated with TMP-SMX. By contrast, PaO$_2$ improved significantly faster in patients treated with TMP-SMX. Aerosolized pentamidine alone is not well suited for patients who develop appreciable tachypnea, since alveolar deposition is related to minute ventilation and decreases significantly in individuals with rapid shallow breathing. Moreover, deposition is likely to be impaired in areas of densely consolidated lung. In fact, in two smaller studies, parenteral pentamidine was more effective than aerosol therapy in more severe episodes. In light of these data, aerosolized pentamidine should be prescribed as primary therapy only for patients who are not severely tachypneic and have mild PCP.

Dapsone (a sulfone drug used to treat leprosy and dermatitis herpetiformis) has potent activity against murine PCP. In uncontrolled studies, dapsone alone at 100 mg per day was not as effective as historical use of TMP-SMX, and 200 mg per day has been associated with a high rate of severe methemoglobinemia and respiratory distress. Thus, dapsone should not be used alone to treat PCP. However, at a dosage of 100 mg per day dapsone has been highly effective and well tolerated when combined with 20 mg per kilogram per day of TMP. In one comparative trial, this combination was as effective as TMP-SMX, which caused severe neutropenia and liver test abnormalities significantly more often. In addition, concentrations of dapsone were 40 per cent higher and TMP levels were 48 per cent higher when the drugs were used in combination than when patients were treated with either agent alone. This suggests that there is a bidirectional interference with clearance of both agents and that lower dosages may be effective and may reduce the risk for toxic reactions with the combination. Studies are under way to determine whether this combination is as effective as TMP-SMX and associated with less toxicity.

Clindamycin plus the antimalarial compound primaquine is another promising combination. In tissue cultures and the rat model of PCP, neither agent is effective alone but the combination has excellent activity. In the first clinical investigation of this combination, 23 of 25 patients treated with 600 mg of clindamycin intravenously every 6 hours and 15 mg of primaquine once daily were cured. However, 17 of the subjects had been treated with conventional therapies and the contribution of these other therapies to the ultimate outcome could not be ascertained. In a study of 22 patients with (A-a)DO$_2$ less than 30 torr, 900 mg of clindamycin intravenously every 8 hours and 30 mg of primaquine base orally once daily improved 20 patients by day 7 of treatment. These patients received no other anti-*Pneumocystis* therapies. Generalized rash was the most common toxicity and occurred in 15 cases but required cessation of therapy in only 3 patients. Whether this toxicity will limit the usefulness of this promising treatment is unknown.

OUTCOME AND PROGNOSIS. Several clinical parameters have been associated with an increased risk for a fatal outcome. These include at presentation an elevated serum LDH generally in excess of 500 IU per deciliter, a baseline (A-a)DO$_2$ greater than 35 torr on room air, and BAL neutrophils in excess of 10 per cent at presentation. Lack of clinical improvement and progressive increase in serum LDH during therapy have also been associated with ultimate fatality. During therapy it is often difficult to know when a given patient is failing a specific treatment and is destined for a fatal outcome. Persistence of fever is a poor indicator of treatment failure, since fever may be due to other opportunistic infections, nosocomial bacterial complications, HIV infection per se, drug allergy even in the absence of rash or eosinophilia, and catheter-associated phlebitis as well as PCP. Lack of improvement on chest radiographs is common, and persistence or progression of infiltrates frequently occurs even in patients who ultimately are cured. Repeat bronchoscopy in a patient failing to improve often is not helpful unless a second infection is detected, since *P. carinii* organisms may be present for weeks to months even after successful therapy. Patients are often switched from their initial therapy on a purely empiric basis. It may be that alveolar damage, as with the adult respiratory distress syndrome, which has a similar histologic pattern, is the most important determinant of outcome, and failure to improve promptly is not the result of antibiotic failure per se. Indeed, patients with more severe episodes often continue to deteriorate for 7 to 10 days before they stabilize and begin to show improvement, whether the initial therapy is continued or changed. The fact that nearly 90 per cent survived in one study of moderate to severe episodes despite continuation of TMP-SMX in the face of apparent early failure in many patients supports this contention. Switching therapy may serve only to expose patients to additional drug toxicities. Admittedly, except for patients who rapidly develop respiratory failure, it is often difficult to know when to change therapy.

For patients who survive their episodes, approximately 5 per cent per month, or 60 per cent after 1 year, have a recurrent bout of PCP despite therapy with zidovudine. Thus, effective prophylaxis is needed for such patients.

PROPHYLAXIS. The most desirable approach to therapy is to prevent PCP. Two controlled studies have suggested that the attack rate can be reduced by 5- to 10-fold in HIV-infected patients who are at highest risk, namely those individuals with less than 200 CD4 lymphocytes and those who have already experienced an episode of PCP.

The most compelling study involved 408 high-risk subjects at 14 community treatment centers in San Francisco who were randomly assigned to one of three dosage regimens of aerosolized pentamidine given by the Respirgard II jet nebulizer. A subset of these subjects had already experienced an episode of PCP. Three hundred milligrams once monthly was significantly more protective than the other two dosages in patients with prior episodes. Of equal import, toxicity was limited to transient dysgeusia and cough which generally lasted no more than 1 to 2 hours after treatment. More prolonged coughing and even bronchospasm may occur occasionally, but these toxicities are generally limited to smokers and patients with asthma and are usually prevented by pretreatment with an aerosol bronchodilator. Although very little pentamidine is absorbed into the systemic circulation during aerosol therapy, pancreatitis and hypoglycemia have occurred. Contact dermatitis on the face, conjunctiva, and upper torso may also occur. However, these other toxicities are exceedingly uncommon with aerosol pentamidine. The disadvan-

tages of aerosolized pentamidine include the cost of the drug, need for supervised therapy and a compressed air source for the jet nebulizers, lack of systemic prophylaxis against extrapulmonary *P. carinii* infection, and incomplete protection provided for patients who have already experienced PCP (20 per cent of patients treated with 300 mg once monthly in the San Francisco study relapsed within 12 months).

The need for supervised therapy and compressed air is obviated with the use of portable ultrasonic nebulizers. In a double-blind, placebo-controlled study conducted in Canada using the Fisons ultrasonic nebulizer, a dosage of 60 mg twice monthly was superior to placebo. Whether use of different, more efficient nebulizers or different dosage regimens will improve the efficacy of aerosolized pentamidine for secondary prophylaxis remains to be determined.

By contrast, TMP-SMX is inexpensive, is well suited for self-administration at home, and has been established to provide complete protection against PCP in pediatric cancer patients. The combination has been studied less well for prophylaxis in AIDS. In one study involving patients with Kaposi's sarcoma who were receiving chemotherapy, there were no episodes of PCP in subjects receiving one double-strength tablet twice daily, compared with 16 episodes in 30 subjects who received no prophylaxis. Of concern, gastric intolerance or rash occurred in 50 per cent of subjects treated with TMP-SMX, but these "toxicities" also occurred to a lesser extent in patients who were not given preventive therapy. Unfortunately, the protective efficacy and tolerability of TMP-SMX, especially in combination with zidovudine, which like the antifolate drugs is also myelosuppressive, is currently under examination in controlled studies of other HIV-infected populations. Whether treatment with 5 or 10 mg of oral folinic acid each day can prevent the neutropenia commonly associated with TMP-SMX is unknown.

Other antifolate drugs, dapsone and pyrimethamine-sulfadoxine (Fansidar, used for malaria prophylaxis), have also appeared highly protective in uncontrolled studies involving patients at high risk for PCP. The most serious potential toxicities associated with dapsone are hemolytic anemia and methemoglobinemia, although the exact frequency of these adverse effects in patients infected with HIV is unknown. In contrast to dapsone and TMP-SMX, hematologic toxicities have been relatively infrequent with pyrimethamine-sulfadoxine. However, fatalities have resulted from Stevens-Johnson syndrome during prophylaxis for malaria (although this has occurred in only one patient infected with HIV), which has dampened enthusiasm for prophylaxis with this combination.

The relative efficacy of aerosolized pentamidine and the antifolate drugs for prophylaxis of PCP will be determined in two large multicenter studies sponsored by the National Institutes of Health. The results of these trials should be available in 1991 or 1992. Until then physicians should follow guidelines outlined by the U.S. Public Health Service which currently endorse either aerosolized pentamidine or oral TMP-SMX for patients at high risk for PCP. The selection of either therapy depends in part on the patient's tolerance of these agents, health insurance and patient resources, and individual preferences of physicians and patients.

For patients with 200 to 500 CD4 lymphocytes per cubic millimeter, specific prophylaxis for PCP does not appear necessary if patients are taking 500 to 600 mg of zidovudine daily. Two large placebo-controlled trials established that zidovudine significantly reduced the risk for asymptomatic patients or those with early ARC who had 200 to 500 CD4 cells per cubic millimeter from progressing to advanced ARC or AIDS. Protection against PCP was excellent, thereby obviating the need for specific prophylaxis until CD4 counts decline to less than 200 per cubic millimeter or the percentage of CD4 cells decreases to less than 20 per cent.

KAPOSI'S SARCOMA

Kaposi's sarcoma (see Ch. 163) is the second most common opportunistic complication resulting in a case definition of AIDS in persons infected with HIV and occurs in 20 to 25 per cent of patients with AIDS. The lung is clinically involved in approximately 20 per cent of these patients, commonly when there are extensive cutaneous lesions, although pulmonary involvement has been documented in up to 50 per cent of cases at autopsy. Pulmonary Kaposi's sarcoma occasionally occurs when there is no mucocutaneous involvement.

CLINICAL SYNDROME. The majority of patients with pulmonary Kaposi's sarcoma have nonproductive cough, dyspnea, and fever, although any of these findings have been absent in up to 40 per cent of cases. Large endobronchial lesions may cause localized wheezing, and laryngeal involvement may result in stridor. Owing to the propensity of these lesions to bleed, some patients may present with hemoptysis. Moderate to severe hypoxemia, widened $(A-a)DO_2$, and impaired DL_{CO} (less than 80 per cent of normal) are associated with Kaposi's sarcoma in most patients, although lung volumes are usually normal.

RADIOGRAPHIC ABNORMALITIES. Interstitial infiltrates are the most common abnormalities detectable on chest radiographs and are present in approximately 80 per cent of patients with Kaposi's sarcoma. Pulmonary nodules with or without interstitial infiltrates are present in 20 to 60 per cent, pleural effusions in 20 to 90 per cent, and hilar or paratracheal adenopathy in 50 to 90 per cent of cases. Gallium imaging of the lung has little utility. However, nodules, effusions, and adenopathy not present on plain radiographs may be demonstrable by computed tomography.

DIAGNOSIS. In patients with pleural effusions due to Kaposi's sarcoma, thoracentesis usually produces an exudative fluid but rarely yields a diagnosis, since there is not a particular cell type associated with the tumor. Diagnosis requires the presence of a characteristic histologic architecture. However, pleural biopsies are rarely positive, perhaps owing to the patchy involvement of the pleural surfaces as detected at autopsy.

Bronchoscopy is the single most useful test in confirming the suspicion of pulmonary Kaposi's sarcoma. In most cases one or more typical violaceous or cherry red, plaquelike lesions are distributed throughout the tracheobronchial tree. Despite their raised appearance these lesions are generally submucosal, and, thus, superficial bronchial biopsies frequently are not diagnostic. Transbronchial biopsy of parenchymal disease is also unfruitful, with yields as low as 10 per cent, probably owing to the fact that lung infiltration is patchy with lesions generally less than 1 cm in diameter. In addition, endobronchial lesions may bleed profusely if biopsied. Thus, if typical endobronchial lesions are seen during bronchoscopy and there is histologic confirmation of Kaposi's sarcoma elsewhere, this is sufficient evidence of pulmonary involvement and biopsy is not indicated. In cases in which there are no endobronchial lesions, open lung biopsy may be necessary to establish the diagnosis.

TREATMENT. Most patients with pulmonary Kaposi's sarcoma survive only several months after the diagnosis is established, whereas patients who present with limited cutaneous disease generally have higher CD4 counts and often survive for several years until serious complications of AIDS occur. In one investigation, chemotherapy with bleomycin and vincristine with or without doxorubicin increased survival from 6 to 10 months in responders versus nonresponders. Survival was shortened in patients with pleural effusions and CD4 counts less than 100 per cubic millimeter. Total lung irradiation improved symptoms and pulmonary function tests in one series. Thus, palliative therapy is available for some patients with pulmonary Kaposi's sarcoma and supports a reasonably aggressive approach to establish the diagnosis.

MYCOBACTERIUM AVIUM COMPLEX

EPIDEMIOLOGY. *Mycobacterium avium* complex (*M. avium–M. intracellulare*) (see Ch. 333) appears to be the most frequent cause of systemic bacterial infection in patients with AIDS. This organism is ubiquitous in soil and water. The portal of entry probably involves either the gastrointestinal tract (macrophages laden with acid-fast bacilli are frequently identified in the lamina propria of the small bowel) or the respiratory tract (since the organism was isolated from respiratory secretions in 17 of 23 patients in one study).

Infection is generally widespread at the time of clinical diag-

nosis. Although disseminated disease is AIDS defining or results in the initial case definition of AIDS in only 4 per cent of patients with AIDS, this infection is ultimately documented ante mortem in 18 to 29 per cent and is detected in 53 to 79 per cent of AIDS patients at autopsy. Moreover, the organism was recovered from the lung in 11 (34 per cent) of 32 patients with systemic infection documented at autopsy.

CLINICAL SYNDROME. *M. avium* complex generally causes disease late in the course of AIDS when patients are severely immunocompromised. Thus, patients are often coinfected with other opportunistic pathogens, making it difficult to ascertain whether various symptoms, clinical signs, or radiographic abnormalities are specifically related to *M. avium* complex. However, a systemic illness with fever, sweats, and weight loss and a gastrointestinal disorder with diarrhea and abdominal pain appear to be the most commonly associated clinical syndromes. However, cough was reported to have been present in 36 (70 per cent) of 51 patients and dyspnea in 27 (57 per cent) of 47 patients in one retrospective study.

RADIOGRAPHIC ABNORMALITIES. Chest radiographs may show interstitial, alveolar, or nodular infiltrates. Hilar or mediastinal adenopathy may occur together with or isolated from parenchymal abnormalities. Cavitation and pleural effusions are rare. It is difficult to know precisely how frequently these abnormalities are due specifically to *M. avium* complex because of other concurrent opportunistic complications.

DIAGNOSIS. Recovery of *M. avium* complex from standard automated blood cultures is the sine qua non of disseminated infection, with isolation rates of 90 to 100 per cent. Similarly, the organism is readily recovered from sputum. In one study 23 (92 per cent) of 25 patients with evidence of pulmonary disease had positive sputum cultures, although smears for acid-fast bacilli were positive in only 4 (16 per cent) of the patients. It is possible that some patients with negative blood but positive sputum cultures have infection limited to the lung. However, a positive culture from respiratory secretions may only indicate colonization if there is no clinical or radiographic evidence of disease. It is unknown whether such patients are more likely to develop a pneumonic illness or disseminated disease than those not colonized.

TREATMENT. Treatment of patients with positive blood cultures has provided conflicting results. Initial studies showed that treatment had minimal effect on the clinical illness or numbers of organisms in the blood of these patients. More recently, uncontrolled studies of four- and five-drug regimens indicate that treatment may be beneficial in terminating fever and sweats and decreasing the number of organisms in blood by several logarithms. Whether such therapies will increase survival in AIDS patients infected with *M. avium* complex must be determined in controlled studies.

For patients with pulmonary infiltrates and *M. avium* complex identified in respiratory secretions or specimens of lung in the absence of other identifiable opportunistic pathogens, consideration may be given for treatment. In vitro and in the immunodeficient beige mouse, ethambutol, ansamycin, clofazamine, quinolones (ciprofloxacin and sparfloxacin), macrolides (clarithromycin and azithromycin), and amikacin have activity against the majority of isolates at concentrations achievable in humans. Isoniazid and pyrazinamide have little to no activity as single agents or in combination, although rifampin (structurally similar to ansamycin) does improve the inhibitory effect of other drugs. Based on such laboratory data and several pilot studies showing efficacy, two regimens that are being tested clinically include ethambutol (15 mg per kilogram per day), rifampin (600 mg per day), clofazimine (100 or 200 mg per day), and ciprofloxacin (500 mg twice daily) with or without amikacin (10 mg per kilogram per day 5 days per week for 20 doses). Before the physician prescribes one of these or a similar regimen, patients should be advised that such therapy is unproven, may increase their risk for drug toxicity, but could improve their quality of life.

OTHER ATYPICAL MYCOBACTERIA

M. kansasii, *M. haemophilum*, *M. scrofulaceum*, *M. fortuitum*, *M. flavescens*, *M. xenopi*, and *M. gordonae* have caused disseminated disease in AIDS patients. Clinical manifestations are similar to those associated with *M. avium* complex, with involvement of the lung, liver, and bone marrow being especially common. Effective treatment regimens have not been established for these infections. However, the Centers for Disease Control and American Thoracic Society have recommended that disease caused by *M. kansasii* should be treated with isoniazid, rifampin, and ethambutol for a minimum of 18 months, or 15 months after culture conversion.

MYCOBACTERIUM TUBERCULOSIS (see Ch. 332)

EPIDEMIOLOGY. During the latter half of the 1980's, the annual incidence of tuberculosis increased compared to declining rates in the first half of the decade. The excess cases were focused largely in geographic areas where AIDS is highly endemic. Overall, nearly 4 per cent of AIDS patients have had tuberculosis, which represents an attack rate that is several hundred–fold greater than the average annual incidence in HIV-negative persons during the same period. The risk of tuberculosis has been greatest in AIDS patients who are black, Hispanic, Haitian, or intravenous drug users. The proportion of AIDS patients with tuberculosis composed of racial or ethnic minorities has ranged from 35 to 100 per cent in various areas of the United States; 7 to 69 per cent have been intravenous drug users.

PATHOGENESIS. Since latent tuberculous infection is contained by an intact cell-mediated immune system, it is not surprising that tuberculosis is common in AIDS patients. The fact that 14 per cent of HIV-positive intravenous drug users who were PPD positive developed tuberculosis over 2 years compared to no cases in HIV-positive persons with negative skin tests suggests that this opportunistic complication most often occurs as a reactivation process, although person-to-person spread also occurs.

Unlike *M. avium* complex, *M. tuberculosis* generally causes disease when cell-mediated immunity is normal or only modestly depressed. The median CD4 lymphocyte count was 354 cells per cubic millimeter in one study and the mean count in another investigation was 170 cells per cubic millimeter. In fact, tuberculosis occurred before the first nonmycobacterial AIDS-defining event in 48 (87 per cent) of 55 patients with AIDS and concurrently with an AIDS-defining event in the other 7 (13 per cent) patients in one study. This implies that *M. tuberculosis* is more virulent than *P. carinii* or *M. avium* complex, which generally do not cause disease in HIV-positive patients until CD4 counts are severely depressed.

CLINICAL SYNDROME. Pulmonary tuberculosis is the most common manifestation of tuberculous disease in HIV-positive patients. When tuberculosis precedes the diagnosis of AIDS, disease is usually confined to the lung, whereas, when tuberculosis is diagnosed after the onset of AIDS, the majority of patients also have extrapulmonary tuberculosis, most commonly involving the bone marrow or lymph nodes, or have disease confined to sites outside the lung. Fever, night sweats, wasting, cough, and dyspnea occur in the majority of patients but may be due to infection with HIV per se or other opportunistic infections. Lymphadenopathy, especially in patients with severe immune deficiency (namely, CD4 lymphocyte counts less than 200 per cubic millimeter), is likely to be due to tuberculosis or another opportunistic complication, since lymph nodes are generally hypoplastic at this stage of HIV infection. Other physical findings are rarely helpful.

RADIOGRAPHIC ABNORMALITIES. Although pulmonary tuberculosis in HIV-positive persons is usually a reactivation process, the radiographic abnormalities are more characteristic of primary infection and include hilar or mediastinal adenopathy with or without focal consolidation, which is frequently in the mid to lower lung fields. Upper lobe infiltrates, cavitation, and pleural effusions, which are typical of reactivation disease in HIV-negative persons, generally occur in less than 10 to 15 per cent of cases. In patients with more advanced immune deficiency, when extrapulmonary and disseminated infection are common, the chest radiograph may show a miliary pattern or diffuse interstitial infiltrates indistinguishable from PCP.

DIAGNOSIS. Although most patients with AIDS are anergic, 40 to 80 per cent of HIV-positive patients with tuberculosis have greater than 5 mm cutaneous induration in response to 5 tuberculin units. The "relatively" high rate of cutaneous reactivity likely reflects the fact that HIV-positive patients with tuberculosis

are often only modestly immunocompromised. Examination of respiratory secretions shows acid-fast bacilli in 50 to 80 per cent of patients with pulmonary tuberculosis. With disseminated disease, aspirates from 90 per cent of lymph nodes have shown acid-fast bacilli, and cultures of blood and diarrheal stools have each grown *M. tuberculosis* in approximately 40 per cent of patients.

TREATMENT. The U.S. Public Health Service and the American Thoracic Society recommend that HIV-positive patients with tuberculosis be treated with 10 to 15 mg per kilogram per day of isoniazid, 10 to 15 mg per kilogram per day of rifampin, and for the first 2 months of therapy, pyrazinamide (25 mg per kilogram per day) and/or ethambutal (25 mg per kilogram per day). Therapy with isoniazid should be continued for at least 9 months and at least 6 months after the last positive culture. Patients with extrapulmonary disease should be treated for at least 12 to 18 months.

Since *M. tuberculosis* and *M. avium* complex are indistinguishable morphologically, patients with body fluids containing acid-fast bacilli should be treated presumptively for tuberculosis. Some experts prescribe a regimen of isoniazid and rifampin along with several agents known to be active against *M. avium* complex and then modify the regimen when identification of the mycobacteria and drug susceptibilities have been established.

PREVENTION. In HIV-negative persons with latent infection due to *M. tuberculosis*, the risk of developing tuberculosis is approximately 10 per cent over the remainder of their lifetime and greatest in the first year after infection. The risk is likely to be greater in HIV-positive persons. Thus, the Centers for Disease Control and the American Thoracic Society have recommended that all HIV-positive patients be screened with the Mantoux skin test. Persons who have not been serotested for HIV but who are in risk groups for AIDS, especially intravenous drug users, should also be tested for tuberculous infection. Those with greater than 5 mm of cutaneous induration should have a chest radiograph and sputum induction for acid-fast bacilli and mycobacterial cultures. If there is no evidence of active disease, patients with positive skin tests should receive preventive therapy with 300 mg of isoniazid daily for 6 to 12 months.

PERSON-TO-PERSON TRANSMISSION. The potential for person-to-person transmission is great among AIDS patients. Since individuals receiving inhaled pentamidine frequently cough vigorously during and after treatment, patients with unsuspected tuberculosis are at risk of spreading this infection to other patients and medical personnel, especially in poorly ventilated areas. Thus, patients should be screened by skin testing (if not done previously) and chest radiographs prior to receiving aerosolized pentamidine.

FUNGAL INFECTIONS (see Ch. 398)

Generally fungi cause primary infection in the lung relatively infrequently in AIDS patients, unlike *P. carinii* or *M. tuberculosis*. However, they do cause pulmonary disease as part of disseminated fungal infection in these patients.

Histoplasma capsulatum

EPIDEMIOLOGY AND PATHOGENESIS. Progressive disseminated histoplasmosis occurs as a complication of impaired cell-mediated immunity in HIV-positive persons. As with tuberculosis, this infection occurs early in the course of HIV disease. In fact, disseminated histoplasmosis was the first manifestation of AIDS in 50 to 61 per cent of two groups totalling 125 patients. This suggests that *H. capsulatum*, like *M. tuberculosis*, is more virulent than other opportunistic pathogens, which generally cause infection only when CD4 immunity is more compromised.

Most cases are believed to result from reactivation of prior infection. Many cases have occurred outside the major endemic areas of the Mississippi and Ohio River valleys. However, these patients frequently have a history of travel or residence in other endemic areas such as Puerto Rico, the Dominican Republic, or South America. By contrast, histoplasmosis occurred with high frequency in AIDS patients during an outbreak in the midwestern United States, indicating that disseminated disease may also occur as a consequence of primary infection.

CLINICAL SYNDROME. Patients with disseminated histoplasmosis have usually been ill for 4 to 8 weeks with fever and weight loss. In one series involving 125 patients, respiratory symptoms were limited to cough in 28 per cent and dyspnea in 16 per cent, although both occurred in 60 per cent of the 72 patients with abnormal chest radiographs. Other patients present acutely with septic shock and disseminated intravascular coagulopathy. Important physical findings have included splenomegaly in 32 per cent, hepatomegaly in 26 per cent, and skin lesions in 7 per cent. Anemia, leukopenia, or thrombocytopenia has occurred in 30 per cent. The average PaO_2 is in the range of 84 torr, despite extensive involvement of the lung.

RADIOGRAPHIC ABNORMALITIES. Of the 72 patients described with reports of chest radiographs, 56 per cent have had either diffuse interstitial or diffuse small nodular infiltrates. Of note, 23 (31 per cent) of patients with these radiographic abnormalities had no respiratory symptoms. In addition, unlike disseminated histoplasmosis in HIV-negative persons, there are rarely pulmonary or splenic calcifications.

DIAGNOSIS. *H. capsulatum* has been recovered from the bone marrow in 54 to 70 per cent, blood in 37 to 55 per cent, lung or pulmonary secretions in 36 to 69 per cent, and other organs or body fluids less often. Isolation from blood is increased when lysis centrifugation is used to release *H. capsulatum* from circulating mononuclear cells. It is noteworthy that the organism is infrequently detected microscopically in smears of bronchoalveolar lavage fluid. Since *H. capsulatum* often takes 2 to 3 weeks to be identified in culture, transbronchial biopsy is also advocated by some investigators when histoplasmosis is suspected, since the yeast can be identified in up to 69 per cent of lung tissue sections. The polysaccharide antigen of *H. capsulatum* was detected in the urine of 98 per cent and serum of 75 per cent of 40 patients with histoplasmosis in one study. If the test becomes commercially available, it should facilitate diagnosis.

TREATMENT. Amphotericin B is the treatment of choice for disseminated histoplasmosis. Treatment with a cumulative dose of 2 grams or more results in a significantly greater survival than lower doses. Although ketoconazole alone has been ineffective, another oral triazole, itraconazole, has shown promise in a small number of patients. Studies are needed to determine if the new, inherently less toxic oral azoles are as effective as amphotericin B.

Relapse is common after completion of treatment with amphotericin B, suggesting that chronic suppressive therapy may be necessary. Weekly infusions of 50 to 100 mg of amphotericin B prevented relapse in 13 of 14 patients treated in this manner for a median of 9.5 months in one study. The role of newer oral agents for suppressive therapy is currently under study.

Cryptococcus neoformans

Cryptococcosis occurs in approximately 10 per cent of AIDS patients. Lung involvement has been documented in 4 to 39 per cent of these patients. More than 90 per cent of patients with pulmonary cryptococcosis also have meningitis or disseminated infection. Less than 10 per cent have primary lung infection. The most common symptoms are fever, headache, weight loss, cough, and dyspnea occurring in 42 to 66 per cent. These symptoms may have been present for a few days to a few months. Lymphadenopathy, which is unusual in AIDS patients, was present in 7 of 12 patients in one series and 3 also had splenomegaly without other cause. Patients are usually not severely tachypneic, as their average PaO_2 on room air is in the 70 torr range. Their chest radiographs show either diffuse or focal interstitial infiltrates in more than 90 per cent, with or without hilar or mediastinal adenopathy. Focal areas of consolidation, lung abscess, pleural effusion, and isolated adenopathy may also be detected on radiographs.

Diagnosis is usually not difficult. Cryptococcal antigen has been detected in serum, often in high titers, in virtually all patients with pulmonary cryptococcosis, and BAL specimens have been positive in each case. Moreover, the organism can be recovered from blood cultures in more than 90 per cent of cases. As with histoplasmosis, amphotericin B is the treatment of choice; 5-fluorocytosine may be added for patients who also have meningeal involvement. In a large multicenter comparison of ampho-

tericin B versus fluconazole, an oral triazole, for treatment of cryptococcal meningitis in AIDS patients, fluconazole resulted in a high failure rate during the first 2 weeks, although late failure rates were similar in the two groups. However, in a different study fluconazole prevented relapse in 14 of 15 patients following therapy with amphotericin B, which is comparable to weekly infusions of amphotericin B for suppressive therapy.

Coccidioides immitis

Coccidioidomycosis does not appear to occur as commonly as histoplasmosis or cryptococcosis in patients with AIDS, but it may involve the lung as part of disseminated infection in these patients. The clinical syndrome is, therefore, similar to that associated with histoplasmosis or cryptococcosis. However, cough and dyspnea have been reported in the majority of patients. Radiographs usually reveal diffuse nodular or interstitial infiltrates. Occasionally, isolated nodular lesions, cavities, or pulmonary adenopathy may be the only radiographic abnormalities detected. Complement or tube precipitin antibodies are detectable in most cases, and the fungus can usually be recovered from bronchoscopy specimens.

Other Fungi

Aspergillus, *Candida*, and other fungi are relatively infrequent causes of pulmonary complications in AIDS patients. Care must be taken not to ascribe pulmonary disease to *Aspergillus* or *Candida* when these fungi are cultured from bronchoscopy specimens, since *Aspergillus* is an ubiquitous environmental saprophyte and specimens may be contaminated with *Candida* from the oropharynx. A diagnosis of invasive fungal infection should not be made unless these fungi are demonstrated histologically within pulmonary tissues.

PYOGENIC BACTERIA

PATHOGENESIS AND EPIDEMIOLOGY. Pyogenic bacteria are responsible for 2 to 10 per cent of pulmonary complications in AIDS patients. HIV-associated defects in T cell–mediated immunity result in impaired activation and chemotaxis of macrophages and neutrophils. In addition, B cell–mediated antibody production necessary for opsonization and killing of certain bacteria is impaired in patients with AIDS. It is not surprising, therefore, that patients with AIDS have an increased incidence of pneumonias caused by encapsulated bacteria, in particular *Streptococcus pneumoniae* and *Haemophilus influenzae*. In fact, the attack rate of pneumococcal pneumonia is approximately sixfold greater and the incidence of pneumococcal bacteremia is increased nearly 100-fold in HIV-positive persons. The risk may be even greater in intravenous drug users, as 10 per cent of 144 HIV-seropositive patients had bacterial pneumonias, compared to only 2 per cent of 289 seronegative patients who also used intravenous drugs. Hospital-acquired pneumonias due to staphylococci and gram-negative bacilli are common in patients infected with HIV, but it is uncertain whether these nosocomial infections are more frequent than in HIV-negative patients.

CLINICAL SYNDROME. Fever and cough are nearly universal symptoms in HIV-positive patients with pyogenic pneumonia. Purulent sputum occurs in the majority and distinguishes these patients from those with other causes of pneumonia, albeit opportunistic complications such as PCP can occur together with pyogenic infection of the upper or lower respiratory tract. Unlike other pulmonary infections in AIDS patients, more than half of patients with bacterial pneumonia have lung signs of consolidation.

Most patients have white blood cell (WBC) counts of 6,000 to 12,000 per cubic millimeter with predominantly band forms. By contrast, in most other pulmonary complications of AIDS (other than tuberculosis) the WBC count is usually less than 5000 without a left shift. The serum LDH is minimally elevated in up to one third of patients, and oxygenation is modestly impaired, with room air PaO_2 averaging 60 to 80 torr.

RADIOGRAPHIC ABNORMALITIES. Focal infiltrates with lobar or segmental consolidation occur in 60 to 80 per cent. Infiltrates may be bilateral and there may be pleural effusions, but the frequency of these latter complications has not been established in HIV-positive patients. By contrast, diffuse infiltrates typical of other opportunistic processes are relatively common if the pneumonia is caused by *H. influenzae.*

DIAGNOSIS. The presence of polymorphonuclear neutrophils in sputum is useful in distinguishing bacterial pneumonia from other pulmonary complications. A predominance of either gram-positive or gram-negative bacteria in the presence of PMN's is helpful in selecting initial therapy. The yield of sputum cultures for bacterial pathogens has not been established in AIDS and ARC patients, but 50 to 80 per cent of patients reported to have pneumococcal pneumonia and 5 to 25 per cent with *H. influenzae* pneumonia have had positive blood cultures.

Other bacteria frequently isolated from sputum and occasionally blood of HIV patients with community-acquired infections include *S. pyogenes,* other streptococcal species, *Moraxella catarrhalis,* nonencapsulated *Haemophilus* species, and in intravenous drug users, *Staphylococcus aureus* (see Ch. 302). In hospitalized patients infected with HIV, the most common organisms associated with nosocomial pneumonias have been staphylococci and gram-negative bacteria, as with other patient populations.

TREATMENT. Initial treatment should be directed by the Gram's stain and whether the pneumonia was acquired in the community or the hospital. Ambulatory patients who are stable may be treated with oral antibiotics, since mortality with the most potentially lethal community-acquired bacterial pneumonia, bacteremic pneumococcal pneumonia, has been less than 10 per cent. With appropriate therapy most patients become afebrile with improvement in respiratory symptoms within 5 to 7 days. Patients with severe tachypnea and hypoxemia or evidence of sepsis should be hospitalized for intravenous therapy.

PREVENTION. Bacterial pneumonia may recur in HIV-infected patients, as with other populations who have defective humoral immunity. Thus, the Advisory Committee on Immunization Practices has recommended that all HIV-positive patients receive pneumococcal vaccine, although type-specific protective antibodies are infrequently produced in patients with less than 400 CD4 lymphocytes per cubic millimeter.

ATYPICAL BACTERIAL INFECTIONS

Legionella, Chlamydia, and other atypical bacteria have been associated with pneumonic illnesses in patients with AIDS, although these infections have been infrequent in this population (see Ch. 296 and 345).

CYTOMEGALOVIRUS AND OTHER VIRUSES

Cytomegalovirus, herpes simplex virus, varicella-zoster virus, and respiratory syncytial virus have all been documented to cause pneumonia in patients with AIDS (see Ch. 362, 371, 372, and 374). Although each of these viruses appears to cause opportunistic pulmonary disease only infrequently in HIV-infected patients, their identification as sole pulmonary pathogens is important, since effective therapies are available for these viruses. Influenza and other respiratory viruses such as the adenoviruses may also cause community-acquired pneumonia in AIDS patients, but whether these infections occur more frequently or are more severe in this population than in immunocompetent persons is unknown. HIV per se (and possibly Epstein-Barr virus) has been associated with lymphoid interstitial pneumonitis in children but probably has a limited role in the direct pathogenesis of pulmonary complications in adults.

Cytomegalovirus Pneumonia

Distinguishing actual disease caused by cytomegalovirus from clinically insignificant infection is often difficult in HIV-positive patients. The virus is nearly universal in AIDS patients. Cytomegalovirus viremia was documented in 56 per cent of these patients in one study. Moreover, the virus is commonly cultured from pulmonary secretions (especially bronchoalveolar lavage fluid) and lung tissue in the absence of histologic evidence of cytomegalovirus pneumonia and is often recovered in the presence of other pathogens such as *P. carinii.* Presumably many specimens are contaminated by virus shed in salivary secretions.

Even cytopathologic evidence of infection does not establish with certainty that cytomegalovirus is causally related to pulmonary illness in AIDS patients. In one multicenter study the virus was identified by culture or presence of characteristic cytologic abnormalities in 74 (17 per cent) of 441 bronchoscopy specimens.

Yet, cytomegalovirus was the sole pathogen identified in only 4 per cent of specimens. Similarly, cytomegalovirus infection has been detected at postmortem examination in 50 to 90 per cent of AIDS patients, and there was evidence of lung involvement in 58 per cent of 81 patients with cytomegalovirus infection in one autopsy series. However, another opportunistic infection or neoplasm was found in every patient and in no case was cytomegalovirus infection ascertained to be the direct cause of death. Thus, it is often difficult to know what role cytomegalovirus has in causing pulmonary disease in AIDS patients. Moreover, results of studies differ as to whether cytomegalovirus infection in the lung increases the morbidity or mortality of concurrent opportunistic complications such as PCP.

Strict criteria should, therefore, be defined to establish the diagnosis of cytomegalovirus pneumonia before instituting treatment for this infection with potentially toxic drugs. In particular, patients with hypoxemia (or widened $[A-a]DO_2$) and interstitial pulmonary infiltrates should have cytologic (namely, presence of typical intranuclear and intracytoplasmic inclusion bodies) or histochemical evidence of cytomegalovirus infection and histologic documentation of interstitial pneumonitis in the absence of other opportunistic pulmonary pathogens. All of these elements should be present, since some patients with typical cytomegalovirus inclusion bodies in lung tissue improve during specific treatment for other opportunistic pulmonary complications. With this strict definition, very few patients actually have disease caused by cytomegalovirus alone.

It is clear that antiviral therapy is effective for cytomegalovirus-related disease in other organs of AIDS patients, which also provides indirect evidence of the pathogenic potential of this virus in these patients. In fact, induction therapy with ganciclovir or foscarnet results in improvement of 70 to 90 per cent of patients with cytomegalovirus retinitis or colitis. For lung infection 30 (64 per cent) of 47 patients were reported to respond to treatment with ganciclovir. To what degree these patients would meet a rigorous case definition for cytomegalovirus pneumonia is uncertain. Until controlled studies are conducted to establish the effectiveness of specific antiviral therapy for this pulmonary complication of AIDS, most experts advise treating patients with ganciclovir or foscarnet when there is unequivocal cytomegalovirus pneumonia.

Other Viruses

The epidemiology, pathogenesis, clinical syndrome, severity and mortality, and response to therapy of other viral pulmonary infections have not been well defined in HIV-positive persons. Varicella-zoster, herpes simplex, influenza, respiratory syncytial, and adenoviruses have all been associated with nonproductive cough, dyspnea, hypoxemia, and diffuse interstitial radiographic infiltrates (occasionally mimicking *P. carinii* pneumonia) in other patient populations, including severely immunocompromised persons without HIV infection. By inference, these pathogens are likely to cause similar illnesses in patients with AIDS.

Pulmonary infection with varicella-zoster should be suspected in HIV-positive patients who present with lower respiratory symptoms and either primary varicella or disseminated zoster infection. Unlike findings in PCP, the radiographic infiltrate may be more reticulonodular. Herpes simplex infection must be considered in a patient with a *Pneumocystis*-like illness and hemoptysis, especially if tracheobronchial ulcerations are found at bronchoscopy. Community-acquired infections such as influenza, respiratory syncytial virus, and adenovirus are often associated with "flu"-like illnesses occurring in the winter months. Infection with these viruses should be sought, since specific therapy is available for all except adenovirus and the pulmonary complications caused by these viruses are likely to be more severe in AIDS patients, again emphasizing the need for early intervention. With influenza it is unlikely that amantadine will have much benefit if instituted more than several days after the onset. Thus, preventive therapy through vaccination is the most desirable approach, despite the fact that immunodeficient patients infected with HIV have defective antibody response to various immunogens.

INTERSTITIAL PNEUMONITIS

At least two forms of noninfectious interstitial pneumonitis occur in patients with AIDS and may mimic PCP and other opportunistic infections that cause diffuse infiltrates in these patients.

Nonspecific Interstitial Pneumonitis

In one study 32 per cent of 152 episodes of pneumonitis were associated with this entity. Typically, patients have nonproductive cough, dyspnea, fever, and mild to moderate widening of the (A-a)DO_2. The chest radiographs most commonly show interstitial infiltrates that are usually diffuse but may be focal. Infiltrates may also be reticulonodular or even alveolar. Approximately 50 per cent have no abnormalities on their chest radiographs. Lung biopsies generally reveal mild alveolar damage with interstitial edema, mononuclear cell infiltration, and type II alveolar cell proliferation. The clinical course is characterized by ultimate stabilization or resolution without specific therapy. The etiology is not clear, as opportunistic pathogens are not detectable in most cases and there is no evidence of local HIV infection by in situ hybridization, although approximately half of the cases have been associated with concurrent pulmonary Kaposi's sarcoma and other cases have occurred in patients who have used intravenous drugs or received experimental therapies, suggesting a role for antigenic stimulation.

Lymphoid Interstitial Pneumonitis

Lymphoid interstitial pneumonitis occurs in 10 to 40 per cent of children with AIDS and is case-defining in persons under 13 years of age but occurs in only 1 to 2 per cent of adult patients with AIDS and pulmonary complications. The clinical syndrome and radiographic abnormalities are indistinguishable from those associated with nonspecific interstitial pneumonitis. However, the histopathology of the lymphoid form differs and includes extensive infiltration of the alveolar septae with nonmalignant lymphocytes and plasma cells. In addition, HIV RNA has been detected in the lung of one patient and EBV DNA was present in the pulmonary tissue of 8 of 10 children with lymphoid interstitial pneumonitis, suggesting a possible etiologic role for these two viruses.

SUMMARY

Many of the opportunistic pulmonary complications described in this chapter cannot be distinguished on clinical grounds alone. Most cases require bronchoscopy for a definitive or expeditious diagnosis so that specific treatments can be administered and unnecessary toxic therapies avoided.

Conte JE Jr, Chernoff D, Feigal DW, et al.: Intravenous or inhaled pentamidine for treating *Pneumocystis carinii* pneumonia in AIDS. A randomized trial. Ann Intern Med 113:203, 1990. *One of two controlled studies suggesting that aerosolized pentamidine may be inferior for primary therapy of PCP compared with parenteral therapy.*

DeLorenzo LJ, Huang CT, Maguire GP: Roentgenographic patterns of *Pneumocystis carinii* pneumonia in 104 patients with AIDS. Chest 91:323, 1987. *Comprehensive description of the radiographic manifestations of PCP.*

Gill PS, Akil BA, Colletti P, et al.: Pulmonary Kaposi's sarcoma: Clinical findings and results of therapy. Am J Med 87:57, 1989. *Best overview of the clinical presentation, treatment, and survival of patients with pulmonary Kaposi's sarcoma.*

Hopewell PC: *Pneumocystis carinii* pneumonia: Diagnosis. J Infect Dis 157:1115, 1988. *Concise review of issues relating to the diagnosis of PCP.*

Johnson PC, Hamill RJ, Sarosi GA: Clinical review: Progressive disseminated histoplasmosis in the AIDS patient. Semin Respir Infect 4:139, 1989. *Most complete overview of histoplasmosis in AIDS patients.*

Masur H, Lane HC, Kovacs JA, et al.: Pneumocystis pneumonia: From bench to clinic. Ann Intern Med 111:813, 1989. *Discusses the immunologic, epidemiologic, taxonomic, diagnostic, and therapeutic aspects of PCP.*

Masur H, Meier P, McCutchan A, et al.: Consensus statement on the use of corticosteroids as adjunctive therapy for pneumocystis pneumonia in the acquired immunodeficiency syndrome. N Engl J Med 323:1500, 1990. *Reviews five controlled studies of adjunctive corticosteroid therapy for Pneumocystis pneumonia and summarizes the United States Public Health Service recommendations for this therapy.*

Medina I, Mills J, Leoung G, et al.: Oral therapy for *Pneumocystis carinii* pneumonia in the acquired immunodeficiency syndrome. A controlled trial of trimethoprim-sulfamethoxazole versus trimethoprim-dapsone. N Engl J Med 323:776, 1990. *Describes the relative efficacy and safety of two all-oral therapies for treatment of Pneumocystis pneumonia in AIDS patients.*

Modilevsky T, Sattler FR, Barnes PF: Mycobacterial disease in patients with human immunodeficiency virus infection. Arch Intern Med 149:2201, 1989. *Compares the clinical, laboratory, and radiographic features of tuberculosis and M. avium infection in patients with HIV.*

Murray JF, Felton CP, Garay SM, et al.: Pulmonary complications of the acquired immunodeficiency syndrome: Report of a National Heart, Lung, and Blood Institute workshop. N Engl J Med 310:1682, 1984. *Excellent description of types and frequency of pulmonary disorders in 441 patients with AIDS and the yield of diagnostic tests.*

Phair J, Munoz A, Detels R, et al.: The risk of *Pneumocystis carinii* pneumonia among men infected with human immunodeficiency virus type I. N Engl J Med 322:161, 1990. *Describes the relationship of CD4 counts over time and the occurrence of fever and oral thrush to the risk of PCP.*

Pitchenik AE, Fertel D, Bloch AB: *Mycobacterial* disease: Epidemiology, diagnosis, treatment, and prevention. Clin Chest Med 9:425, 1988. *Best overview of the epidemiology and treatment of tuberculosis and M. avium infections in patients with HIV.*

Sattler FR, Allegra CJ, Verdegem TD, et al.: Trimetrexate-leucovorin dosage evaluation study for treatment of *Pneumocystis carinii* pneumonia. J Infect Dis 161:91, 1990. *Establishes the dosage of trimetrexate and leucovorin resulting in the least dosage-modifying toxicity and excellent efficacy for PCP.*

Sattler FR, Cowan R, Nielsen DM, Ruskin J: Trimethoprim-sulfamethoxazole compared with pentamidine for treatment of *Pneumocystis carinii* pneumonia in the acquired immunodeficiency syndrome: A prospective noncrossover study. Ann Intern Med 109:280, 1988. *Only study comparing efficacy and toxicities of TMP-SMX to pentamidine when patients are not crossed over for failure or drug toxicity.*

Suffredini AF, Ognibene FP, Lack EE, et al.: Nonspecific interstitial pneumonitis: A common cause of pulmonary disease in the acquired immunodeficiency syndrome. Ann Intern Med 107:7, 1987. *Describes incidence, clinical features, and histologic findings of nonspecific interstitial pneumonitis in AIDS patients with pneumonia.*

United States Public Health Service: Guidelines for prophylaxis against *Pneumocystis carinii* pneumonia for persons infected with human immunodeficiency virus. MMWR 38 (S-5):1, 1989. *Summarizes risk factors and effective therapies for prevention of PCP in HIV-positive patients.*

Wallace JM: Pulmonary infection in human immunodeficiency disease: Viral pulmonary infections. Sem Respir Infect 4(2):147, 1989. *Excellent overview of viral lung infections in AIDS.*

416 Gastrointestinal Manifestations of AIDS

John G. Bartlett

The gastrointestinal tract is an especially common site for clinical expression of HIV infection and represents an important factor in morbidity, including malnutrition. Large-scale studies indicate that most patients with AIDS have oral candidiasis, many have severe periodontal infections, up to one third have perirectal lesions due to herpes simplex, 30 to 60 per cent complain of chronic or intermittent diarrhea, and the average weight loss following an AIDS-defining diagnosis is 12 to 15 kg. Most of these complications represent opportunistic infections that occur only with advanced stages of immunosuppression when the T4 lymphocyte count is less than 300 per cubic millimeter.

ORAL LESIONS. Oral candidiasis ("thrush") is encountered at some time in 80 to 90 per cent of all patients with advanced stages of HIV infection. The usual finding is white patches that show yeast forms and pseudohyphae on KOH preparation. The diagnosis is usually made by visual appearance. Thrush is the most common form of AIDS-related complex (ARC), and when found in an otherwise asymptomatic person with HIV infection heralds the probability of an AIDS-defining diagnosis within 2 to 3 years. The lesions usually respond to nystatin, clotrimazole troches, ketoconazole, or fluconazole, but relapse rates are high so that continuous therapy is often necessary. Oral hairy leukoplakia (OHL) is a newly recognized condition found almost exclusively in persons with HIV infection. The cause is unknown, but in situ hybridization implicates Epstein-Barr virus. Typical lesions are patches of white fibrillar projections that are usually located on the tongue and often confused with thrush. OHL is usually asymptomatic, but occasional patients complain of pain or voice changes and respond to treatment with acyclovir. Herpes simplex virus often causes painful oral lesions that have the typical appearance of vesicles on an erythematous base and break down to form ulcers. Herpetic lesions tend to be more severe and prolonged in patients with HIV infection. The usual treatment is acyclovir given orally or parenterally. The major source of confusion is aphthous ulcers of unknown etiology that seem to respond best to topical or systemic administration of corticosteroids. Patients with Kaposi's sarcoma often have involvement of the oral cavity, most frequently with typical erythematous purplish raised lesions on the palate, although any site in the oral cavity may be involved. Most are asymptomatic; symptomatic lesions generally respond to radiation or laser treatments. Periodontal disease is relatively common with either gingivitis or periodontitis. Treatment consists of topical chlorhexidine (Peridex) or systemically administered metronidazole.

ESOPHAGITIS. Dysphagia or odynophagia generally indicates an esophageal lesion. The most common cause is candidiasis, and most patients also have thrush. Alternative causes include herpes simplex, cytomegalovirus, or aphthous ulcers. The diagnosis is optimally made with endoscopy showing grayish white plaques, and smears or biopsy to demonstrate the etiologic agent. A presumptive diagnosis of *Candida* esophagitis is made in patients with thrush combined with dysphagia. Preferred drugs for *C. albicans* esophagitis are ketoconazole or fluconazole by mouth, or a brief course of amphotericin B by vein. Herpes simplex may be treated with acyclovir, cytomegalovirus often responds to ganciclovir, and aphthous ulcers are optimally treated with systemic corticosteroids.

GASTRIC LESIONS. Patients with AIDS often have gastric achlorhydria; less common gastric lesions are Kaposi's sarcoma and opportunistic infections.

SMALL BOWEL AND COLON LESIONS. Acute and/or chronic diarrhea is a frequent complication, usually in the relatively late stages of HIV infection. In many instances, diarrhea is accompanied by severe weight loss, a combination referred to as "diarrhea-wasting syndrome" that is now included as an AIDS-defining diagnosis according to WHO and CDC definitions. The frequency of chronic diarrhea is usually reported at 30 to 60 per cent for patients with AIDS, many have intermittent symptoms, and the small bowel is the most common site of pathologic changes. The most common opportunistic pathogens responsible for chronic diarrhea are *Cryptosporidium*, Microsporida, *Mycobacterium avium*, and cytomegalovirus (CMV).

Cryptosporidia tend to cause intermittent diarrhea that persists for months and may be responsible for severe fluid losses, dehydration, and electrolyte abnormalities. Small bowel biopsies show villous atrophy, crypt hyperplasia, and intraepithelial lymphocytes with typical schizonts that appear adherent to the brush border. Functional tests show D-xylose malabsorption and stools show no fecal leukocytes. The usual diagnostic test is a stool examination for oocysts that appear like yeast but are easily detected using modified acid-fast stains. Complications include papillary stenosis and obstruction of the common bile duct. No therapy has proven effective.

Microsporidia are a group of extremely small unicellular parasites, with the most frequent species in AIDS patients being *Enterocytozoon bieneusi*. The organism cannot be easily detected in stool, so small intestinal biopsy with electron microscopy is often required. Histopathologic changes are similar to those noted with cryptosporidiosis except for the unique morphologic features and location of the organism within the cytoplasm of the enterocyte. No treatment has established merit.

M. avium may cause pathologic changes in the small bowel which appear identical to those of Whipple's disease, with foamy macrophages distended by vesicles containing periodic acid–Schiff (PAS)–positive material in the lamina propria. However, unlike Whipple's disease, the putative agents in the macrophage are acid fast and do not cross-react with antibacterial typing sera. *M. avium* is resistant to most antimicrobial agents, and the utility of aggressive treatment using multiple drugs in combination is controversial.

CMV commonly causes disseminated infection in the late stages of HIV infection at any level of the gastrointestinal tract including the mouth, esophagus, stomach, small bowel, colon, and perirectal region. The most common is a diffuse colitis with superficial ulcerations. Symptoms ascribed to this infection include diarrhea, abdominal pain, or bloody stools. Less common are a solitary ulcer, toxic megacolon, or intestinal perforation. The diagnosis is generally established by demonstrating typical viral inclusions in intestinal biopsies, but the role of this organism as a cause of symptomatic disease is often controversial even when seen. A large number of inclusion bodies per square millimeter of tissue and the presence of high-grade inflammation or typical CMV

vasculitis are possible important correlates in interpretation. Ganciclovir is sometimes effective, although many patients do not respond.

Another enteric pathogen that is found with increased frequency among patients with advanced stages of HIV infection is *Isospora belli*, a protozoan parasite that may cause symptoms similar to those described for cryptosporidiosis. The diagnosis is established by recognition of large acid-fast oocysts (20 to 30 × 10 to 20 μm) in stool. This organism responds well to treatment with trimethoprim-sulfamethoxazole, although the relapse rate is high, so that long-term maintenance treatment is often necessary. With regard to other protozoa, *Entamoeba histolytica* and *Giardia lamblia* are occasionally encountered in this population and both represent treatable pathogens. *Blastocystis hominis* is found in stools of 10 to 15 per cent of healthy heterosexual persons and 35 to 50 per cent of asymptomatic homosexual men; its role as an enteric pathogen is unclear. Nonpathogenic ameba (*E. hartmani, E. coli, E. nana*, and *Iodamoeba butchii*) play no established role in diarrhea in persons with or without HIV infection.

Among bacterial pathogens, *Salmonella*, especially *S. typhimurium*, is found at least 20-fold more frequently in patients with AIDS than in the general population. Unusual features include the lack of an identifiable source of infection in most, a high rate of bacteremia (enteric fever), and the propensity of the infection to recur when treatment is discontinued. The favored drugs include ampicillin or amoxicillin, trimethoprim-sulfamethoxazole, third-generation cephalosporins, and quinolones. Antibiotic-associated diarrhea or colitis is also relatively common in patients with HIV infection owing to their high rate of antibiotic consumption. Additional bacterial agents to consider in this patient population include *Shigella*, *Campylobacter jejuni*, and other *Campylobacter* species including *C. fetus*, *C. laridis*, *C. cinaedi*, and *C. fennelliae*.

Tumors of the gastrointestinal tract associated with HIV infection include Kaposi's sarcoma, non-Hodgkin's lymphoma, cloacogenic carcinoma of the rectum, and squamous cell carcinoma of the rectum and anus. The most common of these is Kaposi's sarcoma, which has been found in gut tissue at autopsy in 40 to 50 per cent of persons with typical cutaneous lesions. Endoscopy typically shows raised red nodules, but histologic confirmation is difficult owing to the depth of pathologic changes. The great majority are asymptomatic; less common presentations include diarrhea, subacute intestinal obstruction, protein-losing enteropathy, and rectal ulcer. The lymphomas associated with HIV infection are usually high-grade B-cell lymphomas that are extranodal in origin. The gastrointestinal tract is affected in up to 20 per cent, and there may be involvement of any site from the oral cavity to the rectum.

AIDS ENTEROPATHY. Endoscopy in patients with advanced AIDS often shows morphologic changes in the small bowel in the absence of evidence for a superimposed opportunistic infection. Characteristic features are villous blunting, a reduced villus:crypt ratio, and an inappropriately low number of mitotic figures. In the absence of an enteric pathogen the findings are sometimes referred to as "AIDS enteropathy." Studies of gastrointestinal function in the presence of AIDS enteropathy usually show malabsorption with abnormal D-xylose and ^{14}C-glycerol-tripalmitin absorption tests. The cause of these changes is not known, but the major considerations include direct invasion by HIV, an opportunistic infection that has not been detected, or a consequence of immune suppression.

MANAGEMENT GUIDELINES FOR PATIENTS WITH DIARRHEA. Recommended tests should be tailored to the specific clinical findings and likely etiologic agents. For most patients with HIV infection and diarrhea that is severe or prolonged, the initial evaluation should include cultures for bacterial pathogens (*Salmonella, Shigella* and *Campylobacter jejuni*), direct examination for ova and parasites, and a *Clostridium difficile* toxin assay. Previous studies indicate that a likely etiologic agent will be detected in 30 to 50 per cent of patients, the most common in chronic diarrhea being *Cryptosporidium*. Those with persistent and unexplained diarrhea or disabling abdominal pain may undergo additional testing, including radiography with contrast, abdominal computerized tomography, and/or endoscopy. Extensive use of upper or lower endoscopy in this setting is controversial, since the conditions most often found cannot be readily treated, giving a poor cost-benefit ratio. These conditions include AIDS enteropathy and infections with cytomegalovirus, *M. avium*, and Microsporida. The treatment of diarrhea in the patient with advanced infection should include appropriate antimicrobial agents directed against identified pathogens (Table 416–1). Nonspecific agents such as imodium or loperamide, indomethacin, somatostatin, or bismuth salts are sometimes useful. Nutritional consequences of chronic diarrhea need to be addressed as described below.

NUTRITIONAL SUPPORT. The average patient with AIDS loses 15 to 20 per cent of his or her baseline weight during the course of the infection. Protein-calorie malnutrition is a common and important sequela to late disease that may accelerate progressive immunosuppression. Contributing factors to malnutrition include a hypermetabolic state associated with chronic infection (especially with fever), oral lesions causing pain, esophageal lesions resulting in dysphagia, reduced taste sensation, depression, HIV-associated subcortical dementia, gastrointestinal side effects of medications, and enteropathy. Therapeutic approaches are optimally based on the cause. Patients with chronic diarrhea should receive small, frequent meals that are low in fiber, residue, lactose, fat, and caffeine. These patients often require additional nutritional support. Enteral feedings are preferred using the oral route, transnasal feeding tubes, or percutaneous endoscopic jejunostomy. Supplementary enteral nutritional feedings may include polymeric formulas or, for patients with severe enteropathy, elemental formulas.

"GAY BOWEL SYNDROME." This term is used in reference to the enteric and perirectal infections that are commonly encountered in homosexual men. Relevant in the context of HIV infection is the fact that the homosexual lifestyle is a risk category for both. However, the pathogens observed with gastrointestinal lesions in immunocompetent homosexual men and immunosuppressed patients with HIV infection are very different (Table 416–2). The former includes a number of sexually transmitted diseases combined with several conventional enteric pathogens. By contrast, the listing for patients with HIV infection is largely restricted to opportunistic infections and opportunistic tumors, reflecting immunosuppression. The single pathogen encountered in both lists is herpes simplex virus, although this infection is distinctive in the two groups; herpes simplex virus infections in patients with AIDS are usually more extensive, more severe, and more prolonged.

HEPATOBILIARY DISEASE. The prevalence of markers for hepatitis B (HBsAg, anti-HBs, or anti-HBc) is 35 to 80 per cent in AIDS patients, reflecting their prevalence among homosexual

TABLE 416–1. TREATMENT OF ENTERIC PATHOGENS IN AIDS

Pathogen	Treatment
Candida albicans	
Thrush	Nystatin, clotrimazole, or ketoconazole
Esophagitis	Ketoconazole, fluconazole, or amphotericin B
Herpes simplex	Acyclovir
Cytomegalovirus	
Esophagitis	Ganciclovir
Enteritis/colitis	Ganciclovir (?)
Oral hairy leukoplakia	Acyclovir (symptomatic only)
Mycobacterium avium	Clofazimine, ethambutol, rifampin, ciprofloxacin ± amikacin (?)
Salmonella species	Ampicillin/amoxicillin, quinolone, trimethoprim-sulfamethoxazole, or third-generation cephalosporin
Clostridium difficile	Metronidazole or vancomycin
Campylobacter species	Erythromycin or quinolone
Entamoeba histolytica	Metronidazole + diloxanide
Giardia lamblia	Quinacrine or metronidazole
Isospora	Trimethoprim-sulfamethoxazole
Cryptosporidium	None

TABLE 416–2. GASTROINTESTINAL LESIONS IN HOMOSEXUAL MEN AND PATIENTS WITH HIV INFECTION

Site	Immunocompetent Homosexual Men	Immune Deficiency with HIV Infection
Oral cavity	*Neisseria gonorrhoeae*	*Candida albicans*
	Herpes simplex	Oral hairy leukoplakia
		Herpes simplex
		Aphthous ulcers
		Necrotizing gingivitis
		Kaposi's sarcoma
Esophagitis		*Candida albicans*
		Cytomegalovirus
		Herpes simplex
		Aphthous ulcers
Small bowel	*Giardia*	*Cryptosporidium*
		Isospora
		Microsporida
		Mycobacterium avium
		Cytomegalovirus
		Salmonella typhimurium
		"AIDS enteropathy"
		Lymphoma, B cell
Colon	*Chlamydia trachomatis* LGV serovars	Cytomegalovirus
	Campylobacter species	
	Shigella	
	Entamoeba histolytica	
Anus, rectum	*Neisseria gonorrhoeae*	Herpes simplex
	Treponema pallidum	Cytomegalovirus
	Condyloma acuminatum	
	Herpes simplex	

men, intravenous drug abusers, and hemophiliacs. Hepatitis surface antigen (HBsAg) is found in 5 to 10 per cent. Nevertheless, chronic active hepatitis and cirrhosis are relatively unusual, possibly reflecting the role of cell-mediated immunity in hepatitis B–associated hepatocellular damage. Other viral causes of hepatitis include herpes simplex virus and CMV. Granulomatous hepatitis is most often due to *M. avium;* less common are histoplasmosis and cryptococcosis. Hepatotoxic drugs commonly taken by HIV-infected patients include sulfonamides, ketoconazole, isoniazid, and rifampin. Cholestasis due to papillary stenosis and sclerosing cholangitis are most often due to *Cryptosporidium* or cytomegalovirus.

ABDOMINAL SURGERY. The most common clinical syndromes in persons with HIV infection that require abdominal surgery are peritonitis associated with perforation due to CMV infection; lymphoma of the gut (most frequently with involvement of the terminal ileum with obstruction or bleeding); Kaposi's sarcoma; and *M. avium* infection involving retroperitoneal lymph nodes or spleen. Patients with cholangiopathy due to CMV or cryptosporidiosis often respond to endoscopic retrograde cholangiopancreatography. The experience to date indicates that patients with HIV infection tolerate surgical procedures well and do not have an unusually high incidence of postoperative complications.

Greenson JK, Belitsos PC, Yardley JH, et al.: AIDS enteropathy: Occult infections and duodenal mucosal alterations in chronic diarrhea. Ann Intern Med 114:366, 1991. *The authors review histopathologic changes in AIDS patients with chronic diarrhea.*

Johanson JF, Sonnenberg A: Efficient management of diarrhea in the acquired immunodeficiency syndrome (AIDS). Ann Intern Med 112:942–948, 1990. *Review of efficacy and cost-effectiveness of various strategies for evaluating diarrhea in AIDS patients suggests that endoscopy and other costly tests are infrequently warranted.*

Kotler DP, Clayton F, Scholes JV, Orenstein JM: Small intestinal injury and parasitic diseases in AIDS. Ann Intern Med 113:444–449, 1990. *The authors review histopathologic findings including electron microscopy in AIDS patients with cryptosporidiosis and microsporidiosis.*

Laughon BE, Druckman DA, Vernon A, et al.: Prevalence of enteric pathogens in homosexual men with and without acquired immunodeficiency syndrome. Gastroenterology 94:984–993, 1988. *This is an exhaustive study of stool to detect bacterial, viral, fungal, and parasitic pathogens in homosexual men without AIDS, with AIDS, and with proctitis or diarrhea.*

Soave R, Johnson WD Jr: *Cryptosporidium* and *Isospora belli* infections. J Infect Dis 157:225–229, 1988. *The authors review Cryptosporidium and Isospora with particular attention to their causing infections in AIDS patients.*

417 Cutaneous Signs of AIDS

Neal S. Penneys

Cutaneous signs and symptoms associated with AIDS are primarily those found with more advanced disease. However, initial infection by human immunodeficiency virus (HIV) may produce a transient macular roseola-like eruption. Infectious processes and neoplastic disease are most commonly seen as the infection progresses. Occasionally, patients have symptoms such as pruritus without visible skin lesions.

Cutaneous infections are a common feature of AIDS. Common superficial infectious processes may be extensive and may have altered appearances because of the immunosuppression associated with HIV infection. Disseminated scabetic infestations may resemble Norwegian scabies. Cutaneous dermatophyte infections have a range of clinical appearances and need not be annular or have an associated scale. These infections may not be clinically recognizable (tinea incognito) or may occur in unusual areas such as the face. Superficial fungal infections may coexist with other pathogens such as herpesvirus or cytomegalovirus (CMV) to produce unusual complex cutaneous infections. These lesions are analogous to oral hairy leukoplakia in that there is more than one infectious agent present in the lesion.

Cutaneous viral infections may also have bizarre presentations. Molluscum contagiosum occurs commonly and is persistent. Lesions may become quite large. A variety of papillomavirus-induced lesions occurs. Persistent common warts occur. Plantar warts may be quite large, painful, and difficult to treat. Anal/genital warts may be a marker of HIV infection. Huge condylomata have been described (see Color Plate 12A). Verrucae may be widespread and have the clinical and histologic morphology of epidermodysplasia verruciformis. Molluscum contagiosum and papillomavirus lesions frequently occur in cosmetically sensitive areas. Locally destructive treatment methods such as curettage and cryotherapy are effective, but lesions almost always recur or new lesions develop.

Herpesvirus infections produce the most significant cutaneous findings in HIV-seropositive patients (see Color Plate 12B). Coinfection by herpesvirus may activate HIV and alter its expression in an infected cell. The development of herpes zoster may be a reliable sign of progression of HIV infection in an otherwise asymptomatic person. With the diminution of the immune response, herpetic infections may become chronic and fail to heal. Chronic herpetic lesions may not exhibit the characteristic morphology of acute lesions in immunocompetent individuals. Both herpes simplex and herpes zoster viruses may produce disseminated skin lesions in HIV-infected individuals. The diagnosis of herpetic infections can be made by morphology of the clinical lesion, Tzanck preparation, skin biopsy, and/or viral culture. For localized persistent herpetic infection, topical acyclovir has some benefit. For symptomatic or severe herpetic infections, systemic acyclovir therapy is helpful. Lastly, viral processes that normally do not affect the skin can occur in the skin of patients with AIDS. Examples include CMV and disseminated vaccinia infections involving the skin.

Unusual primary and disseminated infections occur in the skin. Mucosal and cutaneous lesions of histoplasmosis and cryptococcosis can be signs of disseminated infection in AIDS patients. Mycobacterial infections produced by *M. tuberculosis, M. avium-intracellulare, M. haemophilum,* and others affect the skin in patients with AIDS. Unusual or unique infections such as disseminated amebiasis, sporotrichosis, *Strongyloides* infection, alternariosis, and superficial phaeohyphomycosis have also occurred. Reiter's syndrome is found with increased frequency in patients with AIDS. These patients have all of the characteristics normally associated with Reiter's syndrome, including keratoderma blennorrhagicum (see Color Plate 12C). The treatment approach to Reiter's syndrome in these patients must be cautious. Patients have developed Kaposi's sarcoma and fulminant AIDS after receiving methotrexate as therapy for Reiter's syndrome. It is safe to predict that unusual presentations of disseminated infectious diseases will continue to be described in the skin of AIDS patients.

Mucous membranes are commonly affected by infectious processes in patients with HIV infection. Oral candidiasis may be present and is one harbinger of the progression of HIV infection. White plaques of yeast can be confluent on the palate. Papillomavirus and herpesvirus can produce lesions in the oral cavity. Oral hairy leukoplakia, a mixed infectious process, produces a characteristic "hairy" appearance to the sides of the tongue. This infection contains several pathogens, including Epstein-Barr virus, herpesvirus, and others. Lastly, disseminated infectious disease can affect the mucous membranes.

Neoplastic processes have been associated with AIDS. The most common is Kaposi's sarcoma, and the skin is the most common location for initial recognition of this neoplasm (see Color Plate 12D). In patients with AIDS, however, lesions may be solitary or disseminated, variable in color from light tan to deep purple; variable in appearance from macules to tumor nodules; arranged in a follicular, zosteriform, or linear pattern; and are generally atypical when compared to the lesions of Kaposi's sarcoma occurring in non-AIDS individuals. Kaposi's sarcoma found in AIDS patients frequently affects the mucosae. The risk of development of Kaposi's sarcoma in patients with AIDS does not appear to be uniformly distributed, being highest in homosexual men and lowest in blacks. Other malignant tumors have an increased incidence in these patients, including squamous cell carcinoma and a variety of lymphomas, and these may have cutaneous involvement.

A number of poorly classified eruptions occur in AIDS patients. The best known is seborrheic dermatitis, which occurs in the usual locations but can be persistent and difficult to treat. Patients with AIDS may also have persistent pruritic eruptions that resemble papular urticaria, annular eruptions that resemble granuloma annulare, folliculitis, yellow nail syndrome, vasculitis, alopecia areata, vitiligo, prophyria cutanea tarda, eosinophilic pustular folliculitis, and hypertrichosis of the eyelashes. Certain well-characterized dermatoses such as psoriasis and atopic dermatitis appear to be worsened by the presence of HIV infection. Lastly, many AIDS patients receive a panoply of therapeutic agents that in turn produce a spectrum of cutaneous reactions ranging from macular eruptions to toxic epidermal necrolysis. The etiologic agents that produce certain reactions, such as discolored nails from azidothymidine and interferon (see Color Plate 12E) therapy and palmoplantar thickening from glucan administration, are readily identifiable.

Greenspan J, Greenspan D, Lennette E, et al.: Replication of Epstein-Barr virus within the epithelial cells of oral "hairy" leucoplakia, an AIDS-associated lesion. N Engl J Med 313:1564–1571, 1985.

Klein RS, Harris CA, Butkus-Small C, et al.: Oral candidiasis in high-risk patients as the initial manifestation of the acquired immunodeficiency syndrome. N Engl J Med 311:354–358, 1984.

Lindskov R, Lindhardt BO, Weissmann K, et al.: Acute HTLV-III infection with roseolalike rash. Lancet 1:447, 1986.

Melbye M, Grossman RJ, Goedert JJ, et al.: Risk of AIDS after herpes zoster. Lancet 1:728–730, 1987.

Penneys NS: Skin Manifestations of AIDS. London, Martin Dunitz, 1990.

Redfield RR, Wright C, James WD, et al.: Disseminated vaccinia in a military recruit with human immunodeficiency virus (HIV) disease. N Engl J Med 316:673–676, 1987.

418 Ophthalmologic Manifestations of AIDS

Mark A. Jacobson

Infectious or noninfectious ocular disorders, some of which may lead to severe visual impairment, have been reported in 40 to 90 per cent of patients with AIDS referred for formal ophthalmoscopy. The true incidence of ophthalmic complications of AIDS is difficult to assess because of selection bias in most reported series. For example, in a population of 200 AIDS patients referred to ophthalmologists at Johns Hopkins University, 28 per cent had cytomegalovirus retinitis diagnosed. Smaller referral series have reported even higher percentages. However, the prevalence of this disease in 1986 was only 5.7 per cent in a population-based study of 760 patients with AIDS at San Francisco General Hospital.

The differential diagnosis of HIV-associated ocular disease is best considered by its anatomic location.

DISEASES OF THE CHOROID, RETINA, AND VITREOUS

RETINAL MICROVASCULAR DISEASE (Table 418–1). The most common ophthalmologic complication observed in patients with HIV infection is retinal microvascular disease, which usually manifests as asymptomatic cotton-wool spots or small retinal hemorrhages. Cotton-wool spots have been reported in at least half of patients with AIDS and in up to 40 per cent of patients with ARC. Histopathologically, these lesions represent areas of retinal ischemia. Both immune complex deposition and direct HIV retinal infection have been implicated in the pathogenesis of cotton-wool lesions. On funduscopic examination, they typically appear as white spots with feathered edges on the surface of the retina. A common location is near major posterior retinal vessels, and these lesions can have small associated retinal hemorrhages. It may be difficult to differentiate between cotton-wool spots and early lesions of cytomegalovirus retinitis, which can have a very similar appearance. Sometimes the distinction can be made only by serial ophthalmoscopic examination. Cotton-wool spots remain stationary or resolve, whereas the lesion of cytomegalovirus retinitis increases in size over time. Since cotton-wool spots virtually never cause symptomatic loss of vision and often spontaneously resolve, no treatment is indicated.

Small retinal hemorrhages and other microvascular abnormalities have been reported in up to 40 per cent of patients with AIDS. These lesions also are asymptomatic, except in the rare case where perifoveal involvement may result in visual blurring.

CYTOMEGALOVIRUS (CMV) RETINITIS. CMV retinitis is the most common sight-threatening ocular opportunistic infection in patients with AIDS. It usually occurs in patients with advanced AIDS; and among patients with CMV retinitis at San Francisco General Hospital, it was the index AIDS diagnosis in only 9 per cent. The typical appearance is a white, cottage cheese–like retinal exudate often associated with hemorrhage and frequently located adjacent to major retinal vessels. In tissue sections, full-thickness retinal necrosis and swollen retinal cells containing intranuclear and intracytoplasmic inclusions are observed.

Patients with CMV retinitis typically present with complaints of painless visual impairment—either blurred vision, decreased visual acuity, or visual field defects—almost always affecting one eye more than the other. Several studies of untreated CMV retinitis have demonstrated a natural history of progressive retinal destruction caused by new retinal lesions or increasing size of previous lesions, which is usually evident within 1 month of initial diagnosis.

CMV retinitis is diagnosed primarily by its typical clinical appearance. The differential diagnosis includes cotton-wool spots, retinal hemorrhages, choroidal granulomas, acute retinal necrosis syndrome, and toxoplasmic and syphilitic retinitis. Because dif-

ferentiating between these entities may be difficult and the therapy of CMV retinitis is expensive, time-consuming, and toxic, the diagnosis of CMV retinitis must be confirmed by an experienced ophthalmologist. In a majority of patients with advanced AIDS, cytomegalovirus can be isolated from urine or blood; hence, viral cultures are of value only in monitoring the efficacy of specific anti-CMV therapy.

The current standard therapy for CMV retinitis is ganciclovir, a nucleoside analogue prodrug that is preferentially phosphorylated within CMV-infected cells to an active drug, ganciclovir triphosphate, which inhibits CMV replication. Although intravenous ganciclovir therapy is effective in halting retinitis progression in 80 to 90 per cent of cases, most AIDS patients progress within 1 month after discontinuing therapy. Hence, therapy must be given indefinitely to minimize further visual impairment. Recently, ganciclovir-resistant strains of CMV have emerged and have been associated with therapeutic failure. Foscarnet, a pyrophosphate analogue that does not require phosphorylation for activity, may be effective in controlling retinitis in such cases and in patients who cannot tolerate ganciclovir therapy because of drug toxicity (Table 418–2).

Since atrophy occurs in areas of active CMV retinitis, patients are susceptible to rhegmatogenous retinal detachment (resulting from a scar in a thinned portion of the retina). This complication often occurs during the healing stage, even in patients whose active retinitis has been controlled with antiviral therapy.

TOXOPLASMIC CHORIORETINITIS. Toxoplasmic chorioretinitis is rare compared with cytomegalovirus retinitis but may complicate up to 20 per cent of cases of AIDS-associated toxoplasmic encephalitis. Unlike toxoplasmic retinitis in immunocompetent individuals, which typically results from reactivation of congenitally acquired cysts latent in the retina, AIDS-associated toxoplasmic chorioretinitis does not appear to originate in preexisting retinochoroidal scars but from dissemination of organisms from nonocular sites of disease. Necrotizing retinal lesions are often bilateral and multifocal, and (as in cytomegalovirus retinitis) may result in rhegmatogenous retinal detachment. Vitreous inflammation and anterior uveitis are more common and associated hemorrhage less common than in cytomegalovirus retinitis. Since nearly all cases of toxoplasmic chorioretinitis are associated with toxoplasmic encephalitis, a computed tomographic or magnetic resonance scan of the brain should be done whenever this diagnosis is considered. Specific antiparasitic therapy (pyramethamine and sulfadiazine, or pyramethamine and clindamycin, in the same doses used to treat toxoplasmic encephalitis) is usually effective in preventing further retinal necrosis, but chronic maintenance therapy must be continued indefinitely to prevent relapse.

ACUTE RETINAL NECROSIS SYNDROME. Widespread, often bilateral, necrotizing retinitis caused by herpes simplex or varicella-zoster virus is now a well-characterized, although rare, AIDS-associated condition. Unlike cytomegalovirus retinitis, this disease is often associated with ocular pain and concomitant keratitis or iritis. Many individuals have had recent or concurrent trigeminal zoster or orolabial herpes simplex infection, and evidence of concurrent viral meningoencephalitis may be present. On funduscopic examination, widespread, pale or gray, peripheral retinal lesions are noted. Although intravenous acyclovir is effec-

TABLE 418–1. DIAGNOSTIC FEATURES OF IMPORTANT CAUSES OF HIV-ASSOCIATED RETINITIS*

Feature	Cytomegalovirus	Acute Retinal Necrosis (VZV, HSV)	Toxoplasmosis	Syphilis
Ocular symptoms	Floaters, visual field defect, or decreased visual acuity. Painless.	Floaters, visual field defect, or decreased visual acuity. Pain common.	Floaters, visual field defect, or decreased acuity. ± Photophobia.	Floaters, visual field defect, or decreased acuity. ± Photophobia.
Associated clinical findings	AIDS	Orolabial herpes, trigeminal herpes zoster	AIDS, encephalitis	Rash, hearing loss
Typical retinal lesion	Cottage-cheese exudate with hemorrhage	Confluent, gray or pale retina	White or yellow exudate	Variable
Typical retinal location	Adjacent to major vessel	Peripheral	Multifocal	Focal or posterior retina
Risk of retinal detachment	+ + +	+ + + +	+ +	+
Serology, culture	Not helpful	Viral culture of skin lesion	*Toxoplasma gondii* IgG titer	VDRL, FTA-ABS

*Modified from Culbertson WW: Infection of the retina in AIDS. Int Ophthalmol Clin 29:108–118, 1989.

TABLE 418–2. GANCICLOVIR THERAPY FOR CYTOMEGALOVIRUS (CMV) RETINITIS

TABLE 418–2. GANCICLOVIR THERAPY FOR CYTOMEGALOVIRUS (CMV) RETINITIS

I. Standard ganciclovir dosing regimen for CMV retinitis
  A. Induction therapy: 5 mg/kg IV q12h × 14 days
  B. Chronic maintenance therapy: 5–6 mg/kg every day or 5 days per week
II. Common adverse effect of ganciclovir
  A. Granulocytopenia (absolute neutrophil count < 500 cells/μl occurs in 16% of patients)
  B. Thrombocytopenia (platelet count < 20,000 cells/μL occurs in 5% of patients)
  C. Azoospermia
III. Clinical considerations for initiating ganciclovir therapy
  A. Proximity of retinal lesions to critical anatomic areas (fovea, optic nerve head)
  B. Patient's baseline absolute neutrophil count and marrow reserve
  C. Necessity for concurrent therapy with other myelosuppressive drugs
  D. Practicality of caring for a chronic indwelling venous catheter

tive in preventing further retinal necrosis, subsequent retinal detachment is a frequent, sight-threatening complication.

OTHER CAUSES OF CHORIORETINITIS AND VITRITIS. Cases of syphilitic retinitis have been reported in individuals with AIDS, ARC, and asymptomatic HIV infection. There is no characteristic ophthalmologic appearance, but nearly all reported cases have had markedly positive serologic tests for active syphilis and dermatologic or central nervous system manifestations of secondary syphilis. Generally, response to intravenous penicillin therapy has been good. Disseminated pneumocystosis and *Mycobacterium avium* complex infections with choroidal infiltrates have been described, but these lesions generally have not been sight-threatening. Recently, several cases of indolently progressive retinitis have been attributed to endogenous bacterial infection on the basis of retinal histopathology and response to broad-spectrum antibiotics. Also, vitritis (i.e., endophthalmitis) due to disseminated candidiasis may occur in parenteral drug users who are HIV infected or AIDS patients with indwelling central venous catheters.

OPTIC NEUROPATHY

Opportunistic infectious diseases affecting the optic nerve of patients with ARC or AIDS may result in visual impairment or blindness. The most common cause of optic neuropathy is CMV infection. When CMV retinitis involves the optic disc, swelling of the optic nerve head (papillitis) leads to decreased visual acuity. This may occur in the presence or absence of other areas of retinitis and alternatively may affect the intraorbital optic nerve (optic neuritis) or retrobulbar nerve (retrobulbar neuritis). The acute retinal necrosis syndrome caused by herpes simplex or varicella-zoster virus infection may cause papillitis, and syphilis may cause papillitis, optic neuritis, or retrobulbar neuritis in patients at any stage of HIV disease. The most serious ocular complication of cryptococcal meningitis is an arachnoiditis compressing the retrobulbar optic nerve and occasionally causing blindness. The cause of optic neuropathy can usually be established by seeking the other characteristic features of the specific infection. However, specific antimicrobial therapy for the cause of optic neuropathy often fails to improve vision once significant visual loss has occurred.

ANTERIOR UVEITIS

Severe anterior uveitis is uncommon in patients with HIV disease, but when such cases occur, syphilis or varicella-zoster virus infection is the most common cause. Mild, asymptomatic anterior uveitis commonly is observed in patients with CMV retinitis, but inflammation severe enough to cause symptoms is extremely rare. Occasional cases of toxoplasmic anterior uveitis have also been reported.

KERATITIS

Inflammatory disease of the cornea (keratitis) is most frequently caused by varicella-zoster or herpes simplex virus, and the clinical features usually make diagnosis relatively simple. Patients with advanced HIV disease who develop this complication may require intravenous acyclovir therapy in addition to topical trifluridine.

DISEASES OF THE CONJUNCTIVA AND ADNEXA

Kaposi's sarcoma has a predilection to involve ocular structures. Twenty of 100 patients with Kaposi's sarcoma examined at UCLA had ophthalmic lesions, 16 involving the eyelid and 7 the conjunctiva. In four of these patients, the ophthalmic lesion was the first and only clinically identified manifestation of Kaposi's sarcoma. Conjunctival Kaposi's lesions appear as bright red subepithelial nodules, and small lesions may be mistaken for subconjunctival hemorrhages. Periorbital edema may be caused by lymphangitic Kaposi's sarcoma, even in the absence of apparent ocular or cutaneous lesions. Most ocular lesions respond to local irradiation.

Nonspecific, nonpurulent conjunctivitis that often is self-limited has been reported in up to 10 per cent of AIDS patients. Topical steroid and sulfa therapy may be beneficial for this condition. Other rare causes of conjunctivitis include syphilis and molluscum contagiosum infection. Orbital Kaposi's sarcoma or Burkitt's lymphoma may present with ptosis and diplopia.

Bloom JN, Palestine AG: The diagnosis of cytomegalovirus retinitis. Ann Intern Med 109:963–969, 1988. *Reviews the clinical presentation and natural history of CMV retinitis.*

Jabs DA, Green WR, Fox R, et al.: Ocular manifestations of acquired immune deficiency syndrome. Ophthalmology 96:1092–1099, 1989. *A series of 200 AIDS patients evaluated for ophthalmologic disease.*

Jacobson MA: Ganciclovir therapy for opportunistic cytomegalovirus disease in AIDS. *In* Volberding PA, Jacobson MA (eds.): AIDS Clinical Review 1990. New York, Marcel Dekker, 1990, pp 149–163. *Reviews clinical pharmacology and rational therapeutic use of ganciclovir.*

Krieger AE, Holland GN: Ocular involvement in AIDS. Eye 2:496–505, 1988. *A practical clinical review that organizes ophthalmic complications of AIDS by pathogenic mechanisms (microvascular disease, opportunistic infections, neoplasms, and neuro-ophthalmic abnormalities).*

Winward KE, Hamed LM, Glaser JS: The spectrum of optic nerve disease in human immunodeficiency virus infection. Am J Ophthalmol 107:373–380, 1989. *A series of four patients with HIV-associated optic neuropathies (syphilitic, CMV, varicella-zoster virus, and cryptococcal).*

419 Hematology/Oncology in AIDS

Jerome E. Groopman and David T. Scadden

HEMATOLOGIC ASPECTS OF HIV INFECTION

Hematologic abnormalities are frequent in HIV infection, and their pathogenesis is a subject of intense study. Cytopenias are often the limiting factors in delivery of anti-infective and antineoplastic therapy for patients with AIDS and ARC. Several newly available recombinant hematopoietic growth factors have been employed to ameliorate anemia and neutropenia and are likely to be important components of therapeutic regimens for such patients.

CYTOPENIA. HIV infection is associated most prominently with a decline in the number of CD4 lymphocytes over time. However, other cytopenias are also frequent, with anemia reported in 60 per cent, thrombocytopenia in 40 per cent, and neutropenia in 50 per cent of patients with AIDS. These cytopenias occur in conjunction with progressive deterioration of immune function and are less common in the earlier stages of HIV infection. Thrombocytopenia is the exception to this generalization and may constitute a manifestation of HIV infection during the asymptomatic phases. Multiple etiologies are frequently operative in causing the cytopenia in advanced HIV infection. Direct and indirect effects of HIV, opportunistic infections, neoplasms, and toxic antiretroviral, antimicrobial, or antitumor chemotherapy are the major factors to be considered. The differential diagnosis of cytopenia in HIV infection should primarily consider these etiologies. Evaluation of patients with low blood counts should focus on infectious processes and attendant myelotoxic effects of therapy. In addition to the usual laboratory approaches to diagnosis of cytopenia based on impaired production, excess consumption, and/or sequestration, blood and marrow cultures and stains for fungi and mycobacteria, and buffy coat cultures for cytomegalovirus (CMV) should be performed. *Mycobacterium avium-intracellulare* (MAI), *Mycobacterium tuberculosis*, *Cryptococcus neoformans*, and *Histoplasma capsulatum* may be found within the marrow and lead to hematologic abnormalities. CMV does not generally cause specific histopathologic changes of the bone marrow but may suppress hematopoiesis and is best cultured from the circulating buffy coat. Neoplastic involvement of the marrow by B-cell lymphoma is frequent in AIDS patients with this malignancy, whereas Kaposi's sarcoma has only rarely been found in the bone marrow.

Bone marrow aspirate and biopsy in HIV-infected patients with low blood counts is recommended, particularly in cases of fever of otherwise unknown cause and in staging of patients with non-Hodgkin's lymphoma.

Morphologic abnormalities of myeloid and erythroid lineages are often present in the bone marrow of patients with AIDS and ARC in the absence of infection or neoplasm. These changes are nonspecific and include hypercellularity, dysplasia with frequent megaloblastosis, lymphoid aggregates, and increased eosinophils, plasma cells, and reticulin. The pathogenetic mechanisms for these morphologic abnormalities and the associated impaired hematopoiesis are not well defined. Laboratory studies of hematopoiesis in HIV infection have yielded variable and differing results. Bone marrow cell progenitor number has been quantitated using in vitro colony growth assays. Normal or decreased numbers of progenitors have been reported in such assays using marrow cells from HIV-infected patients. Although differences in experimental methods may account for these contradictory findings, a significant decrease in progenitor cell number due to HIV does not appear to occur. Similarly, the susceptibility to direct HIV infection of bone marrow progenitors bearing the CD34 surface antigen was reported, but subsequent studies indicated that such infection occurs rarely if at all.

The stage of myeloid maturation during which cells may be infected with HIV is not yet rigorously defined. Similarly, the issue as to HIV infection of bone marrow progenitors with resultant direct impairment of blood cell development is unresolved.

The dysregulation of expression of trophic and/or suppressive factors important in control of hematopoiesis has been postulated to occur in HIV infection. T cells and macrophages are important cellular components of the bone marrow which produce such regulatory factors (cytokines) and are major in vivo targets of HIV (see Ch. 242). In vitro, another source of hematopoietic growth regulatory cytokines, the bone marrow fibroblast, may also be infected with HIV. Again, there are conflicting studies on alteration of cytokine production by these cells due to HIV infection. Growth-suppressive factors that impair hematopoiesis have been reported, including an inhibitor within the immunoglobulin fraction of AIDS patients' serum in one study and an 84-kDa glycoprotein derived from AIDS patients' mononuclear cells in another study. T-cell depletion of AIDS patients' bone marrow prior to in vitro culture has been reported to increase colony growth, suggesting that T cells may elaborate inhibitory factors. Further investigation is needed to delineate the pathogenesis of impaired hematopoiesis due to HIV given the lack of consensus from these initial studies.

THROMBOCYTOPENIA (see Ch. 154). Thrombocytopenia may be a presenting laboratory finding in an otherwise asymptomatic HIV-infected person. Consideration should be given to HIV infection in the differential diagnosis of thrombocytopenia, and the medical history should include questions regarding risk factors for this retrovirus. Clinically asymptomatic but thrombocytopenic HIV-infected patients have a similar rate of progression to ARC and AIDS as asymptomatic HIV-seropositive persons without thrombocytopenia. Thrombocytopenia is not a criterion for more advanced HIV disease according to the staging system developed by the Centers for Disease Control. Multiple etiologies need to be considered in evaluating thrombocytopenia in HIV infection. Immune-mediated destruction and ineffective hematopoiesis may both be operative. In addition, cases of AIDS with apparent hemolytic-uremic syndrome or thrombotic thrombocytopenic purpura have been described but are rare. Isolated thrombocytopenia is most often clinically similar to classic autoimmune thrombocytopenic purpura. Bone marrow examination reveals an increased number of megakaryocytes, and there are elevated levels of bound immunoglobulin on the platelet surface. Both platelet-bound immune complexes and a specific antibody against a 25-kDa platelet-associated antigen have been described. The immune complexes may contain anti-HIV antibodies and antibodies directed against them. Several platelet-associated autoantibodies appear to be anti-idiotypic antibodies. The detection of such immune complexes or antiplatelet antibodies does not correlate with low platelet numbers in HIV-infected patients. One possible explanation for normal platelet numbers despite coating of platelets with immune complexes or autoantibodies is dysfunction of the reticuloendothelial system in HIV infection. Impaired Fc receptor–mediated clearance of coated platelets could allow sufficient compensatory production in some patients to sustain a normal platelet count.

The thrombocytopenia in HIV-infected patients has similar sequelae to classic immune thrombocytopenia, yet special attention to the issue of thrombocytopenia should be given in HIV-infected hemophiliacs. The pathogenesis of thrombocytopenia in HIV-infected hemophiliacs appears similar to that in other groups of HIV-infected patients, and the diagnostic study of bone marrow aspiration and biopsy should be performed following administration of factor component, as for other invasive procedures. Complications from thrombocytopenia may be more severe in the setting of hemophilia, so that therapy may need to be initiated at a higher platelet count than in HIV-infected patients without other coagulation defects.

An important observation has been the improvement in platelet count due to treatment with zidovudine (AZT) in HIV-infected patients with significant thrombocytopenia, regardless of risk group. Nearly half of such patients may respond to antiretroviral therapy and increase their platelet counts (mean of threefold increase) within 12 weeks of initiating treatment. If there is no response to zidovudine, then several treatment modalities may be considered, including splenectomy, corticosteroids, danazol, intravenous gamma globulin, anti-RhD preparations, or vincristine. Many of these have been successful in classic immune thrombocytopenia, particularly corticosteroids. There is a theoretical risk of steroid use in an HIV-infected individual, including exacerbation of fungal infection, Kaposi's sarcoma, and activity of HIV itself. Nonetheless, most patients have tolerated corticosteroids for short treatment intervals in studies reported to date. Their long-term use in HIV-associated thrombocytopenia is problematic and cannot be recommended.

ANEMIA. Anemia increases in incidence in HIV-infected patients as their degree of immune dysfunction worsens. The anemia is usually characterized as normochromic and normocytic, and iron studies are either normal or indicative of chronic disease. Occasionally the vitamin B_{12} level is decreased. The anemia rarely is due to vitamin B_{12} deficiency; rather, transcobalamin transport may be altered and therapy with the vitamin does not lead to improved erythropoiesis. Should a low vitamin B_{12} level be found, then a true deficiency needs to be ruled out by a Schilling test and other studies (see Ch. 128).

The Coombs' test (antiglobulin) may be positive in the majority of patients with AIDS or ARC and in about a third of asymptomatic HIV-infected individuals. Although anti-i or other specific antibodies may occur, nonspecific binding of antiphospholipid antibodies or immune complexes to erythrocytes is more common. True hemolysis is unusual in HIV-infected patients as a cause of anemia.

Impaired erythropoiesis accounts for anemia in most HIV-infected individuals. Serum erythropoietin levels are often disproportionately low for the degree of anemia in the patient without renal abnormalities and is of unclear etiology. Parvovirus infection has been reported in HIV-infected patients and may result in red cell aplasia. Gamma globulin therapy has been reported to reverse this unusual cause of severe anemia.

The impairment in erythropoiesis due to HIV infection per se may be due to release of inhibitors and/or impaired production of trophic cytokines, as discussed above. Drug-induced anemia is frequent in HIV-infected patients. Zidovudine is associated with both dose-related and idiosyncratic suppression of erythropoiesis. In the AZT Collaborative Working Group Study, anemia occurred in one third of AIDS patients following 6 weeks of treatment. This occurred at relatively high doses of zidovudine, and patients with severe immunosuppression were least tolerant of the drug. In other studies of zidovudine at doses of 300 to 600 mg per day, the decline in hemoglobin levels was less severe and the need for transfusion less frequent. The reductions in the recommended dosing of zidovudine have reduced the frequency and severity of anemia, but the toxicity profile for prolonged (longer than 2 years) usage at lower doses is not yet defined.

Macrocytic changes occur in the erythrocytes with zidovudine therapy. The mechanism of impaired erythropoiesis due to the drug appears to be impairment of DNA synthesis in developing progenitors. Recombinant erythropoietin therapy may decrease the transfusion requirement and increase the hemoglobin in anemic AIDS patients on zidovudine therapy. The response to recombinant erythropoietin treatment is most clearly seen in patients with pretreatment serum erythropoietin levels below 500 mμ per ml. Some anemic AIDS patients receiving zidovudine have developed red cell aplasia that does not improve with recombinant erythropoietin therapy.

NEUTROPENIA. Neutropenia occurs in the HIV-infected patient in concert with decreases in other cell counts with progressive deterioration of the immune system. As with the other cytopenias, neutropenia may be caused by impaired production and/or increased destruction of leukocytes. Antibody bound to granulocyte membrane structures has been observed in nearly one third of HIV-infected individuals. The presence of neutrophil-associated antibodies has not predicted the development of neutropenia. Impaired hematopoiesis is presumed to be the major etiology of neutropenia due to HIV. In addition to neutropenia, neutrophil destruction has been reported in AIDS and ARC. The extent to which neutrophil defects, particularly in microbial killing, contribute to host immune impairment is unknown, but infections associated with other clinical states of neutrophil dysfunction are unusual in AIDS patients, suggesting that dysfunction is rarely of clinical significance.

Neutropenia is most commonly caused by myelosuppressive therapy in AIDS patients. Zidovudine treatment is at times limited by neutropenia. Other important therapies including trimethoprim-sulfamethoxazole for *Pneumocystis carinii* pneumonia, pyrimethamine-sulfadiazine for CNS toxoplasmosis, ganciclovir (DHPG) for CMV retinitis, and acyclovir for disseminated herpes simplex or herpes zoster may be myelotoxic and result in neutropenia.

HEMATOPOIETIC GROWTH FACTORS. Suppression of leukocyte, as well as erythrocyte, production is a major issue in treatment of both HIV infection and its complicating infectious or neoplastic diseases. This problem may become less limiting as new antiretroviral therapies are developed and hematopoietic growth factors are employed to override myelotoxicity. Several studies have been conducted on the activity and safety of hematopoietic growth factors used to increase blood cell number in cytopenic HIV-infected individuals. The results of these studies have been quite encouraging with respect to the erythroid growth factor, erythropoietin, and the myeloid growth factors, granulocyte colony stimulating factor (G-CSF) and granulocyte macrophage colony stimulating factor (GM-CSF). It is clear that in most patients with anemia due to HIV infection and/or concomitant zidovudine therapy, with baseline serum erythropoietin concentrations that are inappropriately low compared with the degree of anemia, recombinant erythropoietin increases the hemoglobin and reduces the transfusion requirement. In many patients, this allows for treatment with zidovudine that would otherwise be difficult to sustain. The use of the myeloid growth factors, G-CSF or GM-CSF, to ameliorate leukopenia due to HIV infection and/or therapy with zidovudine, interferon-α, or ganciclovir has also been relatively successful. The myelotoxicity of these agents can be overcome using relatively low doses of G-CSF or GM-CSF. It is clear that with the myeloid growth factors as well as with erythropoietin, there is no sustained increase in blood cell production, so that therapy with the growth factor must be continued so long as the myelotoxic agent is administered.

The side effects of growth factor therapy seen in patients with AIDS or ARC have been similar to those in other patients treated with these recombinant proteins. The major issue in the safety profile of the myeloid growth factors relates to their potential effects on replication of HIV. The preponderance of data indicate the stimulation of HIV replication in vitro by GM-CSF but not G-CSF. This is most clearly seen when isolates of HIV that are tropic for monocytes are studied. One clinical report has provided data suggesting increased serum HIV antigen levels during GM-CSF therapy. On the other hand, there is also laboratory evidence that the antiretroviral effects of zidovudine in monocytes can be significantly augmented by the presence of GM-CSF. It appears that the growth factor increases the uptake and phosphorylation of zidovudine, resulting in higher intracellular concentrations of active drug. It is believed that GM-CSF should be considered for therapy only in combination with zidovudine based on these in vitro studies. G-CSF and erythropoietin do not appear to alter HIV expression and have been successfully combined with zidovudine, as stated above. Further clinical trials are required to demonstrate that addition of the erythroid or myeloid growth factor not only will allow for concomitant therapy with myelotoxic agents but will significantly alter the natural history of patients with AIDS or ARC.

Karpatkin S, Nardi M, Lennette ET, et al.: Anti-human immunodeficiency virus type 1 antibody complexes on platelets of seropositive thrombocytopenic homosexuals and narcotic addicts. Proc Natl Acad Sci USA 85:9763, 1988. *Detailed study of immune complexes in HIV-associated thrombocytopenia.*

Koyanagi Y, O'Brian WA, Zhao JQ, et al.: Cytokines alter production of HIV-1 from primary mononuclear phagocytes. Science 241:1673, 1988. *Important laboratory study of cytokine effects on HIV in monocytes.*

Ratner L: Human immunodeficiency virus–associated autoimmune thrombocytopenic purpura: A review. Am J Med 86:194, 1989. *Excellent review of mechanisms and management.*

Richman DD, Fischi MA, Grieco MH, et al.: (AZT Collaborative Working Group): The toxicity of azidothymidine (AZT) in the treatment of patients with AIDS and AIDS-related complex: A double-blind, placebo-controlled trial. N Engl J Med 317:192, 1987. *A major study detailing the hematologic side effects of zidovudine therapy.*

Scadden DT, Zon LI, Groopman JE: Pathophysiology and management of HIV-associated hematologic disorders. Blood 74:1455, 1989. *A comprehensive review with emphasis on pathophysiology; extensive bibliography.*

Stricker RB, Abrams DI, Corash L, Shuman MA: Target platelet antigen in homosexual men with immune thrombocytopenia. N Engl J Med 313:1375, 1985. *Report of antiplatelet antibody in HIV infection.*

Volberding PA, Lagakos ST, Koch MA, et al.: Zidovudine in asymptomatic human immunodeficiency virus infection: A controlled trial in persons with fewer than 500 CD4-positive cells per cubic millimeter. N Engl J Med 322:941, 1990. *An important trial of zidovudine demonstrating improved hematologic tolerance at lower but effective doses.*

Walker RE, Parker RI, Kovacs JA, et al.: Anemia and erythropoiesis in patients with the acquired immunodeficiency syndrome (AIDS) and Kaposi's sarcoma, treated with zidovudine. Ann Intern Med 108:372, 1988. *Detailed clinical and pathologic study focusing on anemia.*

ONCOLOGIC MANIFESTATIONS OF AIDS

Neoplasms, particularly Kaposi's sarcoma and B-cell lymphoma, are frequent in HIV-infected persons. Their development demonstrates the relationship of immune function to suppression of certain oncogenic events and provides a model to study the pathogenesis of these tumors. Clinical management of AIDS-associated neoplasia is complex, since therapy should optimally address HIV and concurrent opportunistic infections as well as the tumors.

KAPOSI'S SARCOMA (see Ch. 109, 154, 417, and 525). Kaposi's sarcoma is the most frequent neoplastic manifestation of HIV infection. Indeed, it forms one of the Centers for Disease Control criteria that define an HIV-infected individual as having AIDS. Kaposi's sarcoma has been recognized in a number of other clinical and epidemiologic settings. The "classic" form of the neoplasm was described over a century ago in predominantly elderly men of Mediterranean and Jewish extraction. It generally involves lower extremities and is an indolent neoplasm. This form of Kaposi's sarcoma was also recognized in association with other malignancies, particularly lymphoma. This latter observation led to the hypothesis that immune surveillance was important in restricting the development of Kaposi's sarcoma. Another form of Kaposi's sarcoma was recognized in certain geographic locations of Central Africa and has been termed the "endemic" form of the neoplasm. This occurrence in Africa was not related to infection with HIV. Again, the neoplasm was more frequently seen in men than in women but was generally more aggressive and involved lymph nodes and viscera.

Patients receiving immunosuppressive therapy, particularly for renal and hepatic transplants, were recognized to have a markedly increased incidence of Kaposi's sarcoma. This further supported the hypothesis that immunocompetence is important with respect to pathogenesis of this neoplasm. Of particular note has been well-documented resolution of Kaposi's sarcoma upon discontinuation of immunosuppressive therapy in these patients. Other disorders of the immune system, including systemic lupus erythematosus and pemphigus vulgaris, have also been associated with Kaposi's sarcoma.

Epidemiologic studies in classic Kaposi's sarcoma, endemic African Kaposi's sarcoma, and among transplant patients all suggest that there are likely to be genetic and environmental factors involved in tumorigenesis in addition to the level of immune competence per se. The clearest genetic association has been with the HLA DR-5 phenotype in classic Kaposi's sarcoma.

The incidence of Kaposi's sarcoma has been estimated to be 20,000 times greater among HIV-infected individuals than in the general population. Although the neoplasm was originally diagnosed in 40 per cent of AIDS patients when first reported in 1981, the incidence may be declining and is believed to constitute 15 per cent of all AIDS patients in the United States diagnosed in 1989. It is not believed that this reduced incidence of the neoplasm is simply due to incorrect diagnosis or altered reporting patterns. AIDS-associated Kaposi's sarcoma is more frequently seen among homosexual or bisexual men with HIV than in other risk groups with the virus. This suggests that HIV infection itself is not sufficient to account for the increased incidence of the disease, but there may be other factors important in the pathogenesis of the neoplasm. Early in the AIDS epidemic, it was suggested that cytomegalovirus infection or the use of volatile nitrites could potentiate the development of Kaposi's sarcoma. However, careful studies have not verified the importance of such candidate cofactors in the development of the neoplasm. A current hypothesis is that other cofactors of an infectious nature may be transmitted in tandem with HIV during intercourse and possibly during use of intravenous drugs. Molecular studies have failed to demonstrate HIV or cytomegalovirus genome in Kaposi's sarcoma lesions. A model of a neoplasm that distantly resembles Kaposi's sarcoma has been established in transgenic mice using the *tat* gene of HIV, but the significance of this to clinical Kaposi's sarcoma in AIDS is still unclear. It has been speculated that certain cytokines, such as interleukin 6, may be elaborated by the Kaposi's sarcoma cells and lead to autocrine proliferation. The recent reports of the development of Kaposi's sarcoma in homosexual men who are not infected with HIV has provided further support to the hypothesis of an independent sexually transmitted infectious agent as an important cofactor in this neoplasm.

Histopathologically, these lesions are a mixture of different cell types. Endothelial cells are quite prominent within the Kaposi's sarcoma lesions, and there is usually a prominent spindle cell proliferation surrounded by extravasated erythrocytes and macrophages. The cell of origin of the neoplasm is still debated, but permanent cell lines derived from the lesions suggest that the spindle cell is the primary neoplastic cell and is of mesenchymal origin. Others have suggested that the primary neoplastic cell is an endothelial cell originating from lymphatic endothelium.

Kaposi's sarcoma usually presents as a cutaneous nonblanching red macule. As lesions increase in size, they often have surrounding ecchymoses and become more of a violet hue than red. At times, the lesions may become nodular, pedunculated, or even necrotic. In advanced disease, the lesions may become confluent with large plaques developing, particularly on the legs. There is no orderly pattern of tumor progression, and presentation may be with lesions at multiple sites. There is no effect on the subsequent appearance of lesions if the primary lesion is excised. The rate of growth of the primary lesions, as well as the appearance of new lesions, can be quite variable from patient to patient. The control of the growth of lesions and of the distribution of lesions is not understood. The lesions may occur on any cutaneous site. Lymphatic involvement is not unusual, and Kaposi's sarcoma may present as lymphadenopathy. Visceral involvement, particularly of trachea, lungs, and gastrointestinal tract, may occur. Clinical symptoms associated with pulmonary involvement include dyspnea and fever and with gastrointestinal involvement, nonspecific abdominal complaints and low-grade blood loss. The most striking morbidity associated with Kaposi's

sarcoma is that of lymph node involvement and consequent lymphedema involving the lower extremities, groin, and head and neck.

The diagnosis of Kaposi's sarcoma is relatively straightforward in HIV-infected individuals presenting with an erythematous or violaceous cutaneous or mucosal lesion. On the other hand, the lesions may initially appear unimpressive and often are misdiagnosed as an insect bite, bruise, or inflammatory reaction. Biopsy is indicated to confirm the clinical diagnosis. Histopathology is generally diagnostic, although there are no specific stains that differentiate the neoplastic spindle cell in Kaposi's sarcoma from that of other proliferative lesions. Following diagnosis, an assessment should be made of the rate of growth and distribution of the lesions. The presence of visceral disease does not necessarily correlate with poor response of lesions to therapy, so that an extensive evaluation for gastrointestinal or lymphadenopathic Kaposi's sarcoma is not indicated unless there are specific symptoms referable to such involvement. It should be pointed out that AIDS patients in general do not die of Kaposi's sarcoma, except for pulmonary Kaposi's sarcoma, but usually succumb to infectious complications of immunosuppression. Thus, staging systems of the neoplasm have emphasized immunologic status and systemic symptoms in addition to the extent of the neoplasm. Recently, a classification system has been adopted by the AIDS Cooperative Trial Group (ACTG) and appears particularly useful in evaluation of such patients. This system proposes a tumor (T), immunologic status (I), and systemic symptoms (S) staging (Table 419–1).

The clinician should pursue therapy of Kaposi's sarcoma in patients with symptomatic visceral disease or rapidly evolving lesions associated with edema. Such patients usually require chemotherapy. The most active chemotherapeutic drugs appear to be doxorubicin, etoposide, vinblastine, bleomycin, and vincristine. Combinations of these agents, particularly doxorubicin, bleomycin, and vincristine, have been associated with a response rate of 50 per cent or greater. The combination of bleomycin and vincristine has been recommended for patients with borderline marrow function, since the drugs are minimally myelotoxic and may be given in conjunction with zidovudine. Response to chemotherapy usually occurs within the first few weeks of treatment. Unfortunately, the lesions regrow when the chemotherapy is stopped so that treatment needs to be chronic.

Patients with Kaposi's sarcoma who do not have rapidly progressive disease and therefore do not require immediate intervention may be treated with several other approaches. These include observation, single-agent interferon-α, local radiation, intralesional chemotherapy, or combinations of these. Zidovudine alone is not effective as an antineoplastic therapy for Kaposi's sarcoma. Selection of the optimal therapeutic approach involves

TABLE 419–1. KAPOSI'S SARCOMA (KS): RECOMMENDED STAGING CLASSIFICATION

	Good Risk (0) (All of the Following)	Poor Risk (1) (Any of the Following)
Tumor (T)	Confined to skin and/or lymph nodes and/or minimal oral disease*	Tumor-associated edema or ulceration Extensive oral KS Gastrointestinal KS KS in other non-nodal viscera
Immune system (I)	CD4 cells ≥ 200/μl	CD4 cells < 200/μl
Systemic illness (S)	No history of OI† or thrush No "B" symptoms‡ Performance status ≥ 70 (Karnofsky)	History of OI and/or thrush "B" symptoms present Performance status < 70 Other HIV-related illness (e.g., neurologic disease, lymphoma)

*Minimal oral disease is non-nodular KS confined to the palate.
†OI = Opportunistic infection.
‡"B" symptoms are unexplained fever, night sweats, >10% involuntary weight loss, or diarrhea persisting more than 2 weeks.
Modified from Krown SE, Metroka C, Wernz J: Kaposi's sarcoma in the acquired immune deficiency syndrome: A proposal for uniform evaluation, response, and staging criteria. J Clin Oncol 7:1201–1207, 1989.

determining the clinical status of the patient, particularly utilizing the ACTG staging classification, as well as lifestyle issues. Patients who are categorized as "good risk" by the TIS staging system are also excellent candidates for response to interferon-α. Interferon-α has been shown to have not only antineoplastic but also anti-HIV effects. Therapy of Kaposi's sarcoma with single-agent interferon-α requires relatively high doses of the agent (18 to 36 million units daily). Recently, it has been recognized that similar benefit may be obtained utilizing lower doses of interferon-α in combination with zidovudine, although hematologic toxicity may be dose limiting. Such hematologic side effects may be overcome by use of myeloid and erythroid growth factors. Interferon-α is associated with flulike side effects, and many patients were not able to tolerate prolonged therapy. It is unclear whether the antiviral as well as the antitumor properties of interferon-α make it a superior agent in the therapy of AIDS-associated Kaposi's sarcoma compared with chemotherapy alone or zidovudine in combination with chemotherapy (Table 419–2).

"Poor risk" patients by TIS staging should be given antiretroviral therapy, since their major life-threatening complication of AIDS is related to immune suppression and opportunistic infection. Local treatment of disfiguring Kaposi's sarcoma lesions may be achieved using radiation therapy (either photon or electron beam) or chemotherapy in these patients. Radiotherapy should be used in low-dose fractions, since the skin of many AIDS patients is unusually sensitive. Radiotherapy is often avoided for oral Kaposi's sarcoma lesions, since severe mucositis may result.

NON-HODGKIN'S LYMPHOMA. B-cell lymphoma frequently occurs in immunosuppressed individuals. Genetic disorders of the immune system such as Wiskott-Aldrich syndrome, as well as immunosuppressive therapy used in organ transplantation, are associated with malignant transformation of B cells and an oligoclonal or monoclonal lymphoma. Non-Hodgkin's B-cell lymphoma is emerging as a frequent manifestation of HIV infection as individuals with the retrovirus live longer as a result of AZT and anti-infective prophylaxis. The initial relative risk of lymphoma in HIV-infected individuals compared with matched uninfected controls was 850 times; it is likely that this is an underestimate of the current risk. Thus, we expect to see an increasing incidence of B-cell lymphoma in this population.

Etiologic factors operative in the development of lymphoma in AIDS are likely to be multiple (see Ch. 147). The Epstein-Barr virus has been suggested as an important agent that induces B-cell proliferation, leading initially to polyclonal expansion of the B-cell population (see Ch. 373). This expanded population may provide targets for genetic abnormalities that lead to malignant transformation and emergence of several dominant clones. The oligoclonal populations of malignant B cells seen in some HIV-infected individuals with lymphoma support such a model. Ultimately, a single malignant clone may emerge, leading to a monoclonal neoplasm. The chromosomal abnormalities frequently seen in B-cell lymphoma involve chromosome 8 and chromosomes 14 and 22, with translocation of loci encoding the immunoglobulin genes. There is often overexpression of the c-myc oncogene. Genomic evidence of Epstein-Barr virus is found in about one third to one half of B-cell lymphomas in AIDS patients. Cytogenetic abnormalities are found in the majority of such individuals. There is likely to be a number of interacting factors that are important in the pathogenesis of lymphoma in individuals with HIV infection.

Clinically, B-cell lymphoma in AIDS patients tends to be of high-grade histologic pattern and follows an aggressive clinical course. Small, noncleaved or immunoblastic histologies are most frequent and account for nearly three fourths of all lymphomas in this setting. The remaining are usually a diffuse, large-cell type of more intermediate grade. The lower-grade lymphomas reported among HIV-infected individuals may represent background rather than neoplasm directly associated with immunosuppression. Rarely, B-cell acute lymphoblastic leukemia has been reported.

The majority of patients have extranodular disease involving the gastrointestinal tract, central nervous system, liver, soft tissues, and bone marrow. In one large series, nearly two thirds of all patients diagnosed with B-cell lymphoma in AIDS had nonnodular involvement. Lymphoma strictly confined to lymph nodes is uncommon. Gastrointestinal lymphoma may occur anywhere from the esophagus to the anus. Primary central nervous system lymphoma is usually immunoblastic in histologic type (see Ch. 414). Such patients generally present with solitary mass lesions in the parenchyma of the brain, whereas central nervous system involvement in conjunction with systemic lymphoma is more often meningeal in location. All AIDS patients diagnosed with systemic non-Hodgkin's lymphoma should undergo careful assessment of the central nervous system.

The majority of AIDS patients with B-cell lymphoma are classified as having stage III (involving both sides of the diaphragm without visceral involvement) or stage IV (visceral involvement). Systemic "B" symptoms are frequent, but fever should not be immediately ascribed to lymphoma in AIDS patients and secondary infectious etiologies need to be ruled out. Staging of patients should follow the approach used in other settings of non-Hodgkin's lymphoma, with particular attention to the gastrointestinal tract, bone marrow, and central nervous system. It is not clear in the setting of AIDS that prognosis of lymphoma is better among stage III than among stage IV patients.

The major differential diagnosis to be considered with primary central nervous system lymphoma is *Toxoplasma gondii* infection or progressive multifocal leukoencephalopathy (PML) (see Ch. 414). PML can usually be distinguished from central nervous system lymphoma by its lack of enhancement with gadolinium on MRI. Central nervous system lesions due to lymphoma may be isodense or hypodense and contrast-enhancing on CT scan, and enhance on MRI, thereby resembling toxoplasmosis. Nonetheless, toxoplasmosis usually presents with multiple lesions throughout the neuraxis, whereas primary CNS lymphoma tends to be a single lesion located in a paraventricular site. Accessible lesions should be biopsied to distinguish between lymphoma and toxoplasmosis; lesions that are difficult to approach surgically may be empirically treated with antitoxoplasmal therapy for a limited period of time, generally 1 to 2 weeks. If no response is seen, then lymphoma becomes more likely.

The treatment of AIDS-related B-cell lymphoma is controversial owing to the poor prognosis of the neoplasm and the limited tolerance of aggressive chemotherapy in this patient population. Both opportunistic infection and bone marrow suppression often limit the delivery of adequate dosage of chemotherapy on schedule. Patients with prior AIDS-defining illness, particularly a history of opportunistic infection, have a poor prognosis compared with patients who present with lymphoma as their initial mani-

TABLE 419–2. TREATMENT OF KAPOSI'S SARCOMA

Interferon-α		
Single agent	Alpha-2a (Roche)	18–36 mU SC daily for 8 weeks, then three times weekly
	Alpha-2b (Schering)	30 mU SC three times weekly
Combined therapy	Zidovudine	Zidovudine 100 mg PO every 4 hours while awake, interferon-α 5–10 mU SC three times weekly
Chemotherapy		
Single agent	Doxorubicin	20–40 mg/m² IV every 3 weeks
	VP-16	100 mg/m² IV every 3 weeks
	Vinblastine	4–8 mg IV weekly
Combined therapy	Vincristine/vinblastine	2 mg IV vincristine every 2 weeks 4–8 mg IV vinblastine on alternate weeks
	Doxorubicin/bleomycin/ vincristine	Doxorubicin 10–20 mg/m² IV every 3 weeks Bleomycin 15 mg/m² IV every 3 weeks Vincristine 2 mg IV every 3 weeks
	Bleomycin/vincristine	Bleomycin 15 mg/m² IV every 2–3 weeks Vincristine 2 mg IV every 2–3 weeks

festation of AIDS. Similarly, more severely immunocompromised patients with low CD4 cell numbers have a poor outcome and are less tolerant of chemotherapy than are those patients with more intact immune function.

Among "good prognosis" patients with relatively intact immune function and/or those presenting with lymphoma as their AIDS manifestation, aggressive therapy with combination regimens is indicated. For those patients who do not have central nervous system involvement at the time of presentation, it is not clear that prophylactic therapy to the central nervous system offers any long-term benefit. The response rate in these good-prognosis patients is similar to that of non-Hodgkin's lymphoma patients of stage IIIB or IVB without HIV (see Ch. 421), but the long-term survival rate is still poor. Nonetheless, some patients have survived 12 months or longer disease free following complete remission.

Patients with poor prognosis based on severe immune suppression and/or complicating opportunistic infections pose a particularly complex treatment dilemma. Some patients have opted for palliative therapy with corticosteroids, since intensive chemotherapy may lead to further immune compromise and infection. Yet lymphoma is generally rapidly growing and fatal in patients who are not aggressively treated. Thus, the clinician needs to pursue therapy in such patients only with an informed discussion of the risks and benefits of treatment, honestly emphasizing the poor prognosis with or without chemotherapy.

Addition of zidovudine to chemotherapeutic regimens has been difficult owing to myelosuppression. Nonetheless, this approach has appeal in that it provides one way to potentially limit HIV spread and stabilize immune function. As less myelotoxic anti-retroviral drugs are developed, or as results of current experimental programs incorporating erythroid or myeloid growth factors into lymphoma therapy are available, this particular approach is likely to become feasible.

The outlook is generally poor for patients with lymphoma, and the majority die within 6 months. No chemotherapeutic regimen has been identified as superior to others for AIDS patients with this neoplasm. The survival is even poorer for those with primary central nervous system lymphoma, on the order of 2 to 4 months. Therapy for central nervous system lymphoma may lead to complete response but does not necessarily alter survival outcome.

OTHER MALIGNANCIES. There is currently active clinical surveillance to determine whether neoplasms other than Kaposi's sarcoma and B-cell lymphoma may ultimately arise at an increased incidence in immunocompromised patients with HIV infection. The incidence of Hodgkin's disease is not clearly increased among HIV-infected individuals. Nonetheless, there may be important differences in the course of Hodgkin's lymphoma in such patients, including a higher incidence of advanced disease, mixed cellularity histology, and extranodular disease. Furthermore, HIV-infected individuals with Hodgkin's disease appear to tolerate chemotherapy less well and have a higher incidence of tumor relapse than do those without HIV infection. This is likely due to their impaired hematopoiesis and the potential for opportunistic infections in such patients. In general, patients have a survival of less than 12 months when presenting with HIV infection and Hodgkin's disease. Further work is needed to better understand the altered pattern of Hodgkin's disease in the setting of HIV infection.

Therapy of Hodgkin's disease among HIV-infected patients is similar to that of uninfected individuals (see Ch. 148). The major difference is to incorporate prophylaxis against opportunistic infections, particularly *Pneumocystis carinii* pneumonia, and to be particularly alert to infectious complications during therapy.

There has been speculation that anal cancer and cervical cancer, neoplasms associated with papillomavirus infection, may increase in incidence in HIV-infected patients. This is due to the high prevalence of papillomavirus infection in groups at risk for HIV (see Ch. 335). A careful cervical examination including colposcopy is indicated in HIV-infected women to detect early malignant change. Ongoing surveillance programs of HIV-infected individuals using Pap smears on cells from the transitional zone of the anus and cervix should provide important data as to the increased incidence, if any, of this cancer in this population.

Although anecdotal reports abound of other malignancies in HIV-infected individuals, it is unclear whether these occur above that of the background prevalence in the general population. Nonetheless, consideration should be given to the significance of the HIV infection in clinical management. These patients have a propensity to develop opportunistic infections upon initiation of chemotherapy or radiotherapy and, in general, have fared poorly because of these infectious complications.

Ensoli B, Nakamura S, Salahuddin SZ, et al.: AIDS-Kaposi's sarcoma–derived cells express cytokines with autocrine and paracrine growth effects. Science 243:223, 1989. *Characterization of Kaposi's sarcoma cells; interesting basic science study.*

Gill PS, Levine AM, Krailo M, et al.: AIDS-related malignant lymphoma: Results of prospective treatment trials. J Clin Oncol 5:1322, 1987. *Detailed analysis of therapeutic trials in AIDS lymphoma.*

Groopman JE, Scadden DT: Interferon therapy for Kaposi's sarcoma associated with the acquired immunodeficiency syndrome (AIDS). Ann Intern Med 110:335, 1989. *Balanced discussion of treatment options in Kaposi's sarcoma.*

Krown SE, Metroka C, Wernz J: Kaposi's sarcoma in the acquired immune deficiency syndrome: A proposal for uniform evaluation, response, and staging criteria. J Clin Oncol 7:1201, 1989. *Kaposi's sarcoma staging system presented and explained.*

Levine AM: Lymphoma in acquired immunodeficiency syndrome. Semin Oncol 17:104, 1990. *Review of lymphoma in AIDS; excellent bibliography.*

Ziegler JL, Beckstead JA, Volberding PA, et al.: Non-Hodgkin's lymphoma in 90 homosexual men: Relationship to generalized lymphadenopathy and acquired immunodeficiency syndrome (AIDS). N Engl J Med 311:565, 1984. *Large clinical study describing lymphoma in AIDS.*

420 Renal, Cardiac, Endocrine, and Rheumatologic Manifestations of HIV Infection

Michael S. Saag

Infection with the human immunodeficiency virus type 1 (HIV) is a multisystem disease that affects every organ system. Manifestations of pulmonary, gastrointestinal, neurologic, hematologic, and oncologic disease are well described in the literature, owing in large part to their high prevalence and often dramatic modes of presentation. In contrast, HIV-related renal, cardiac, endocrine, and rheumatologic diseases are more insidious in presentation. As overall survival of HIV-infected individuals continues to improve and therapeutic regimens become more sophisticated, clinicians will undoubtedly encounter disorders of the latter organ systems with increasing frequency.

RENAL DISEASE

Renal disease associated with HIV infection may present as fluid-electrolyte and acid-base abnormalities, acute renal failure, coincidental renal disorders, or a glomerulopathy directly related to underlying HIV infection, the so-called HIV-associated nephropathy (HIVAN). Originally observed in patients with AIDS and referred to as AIDS-associated nephropathy, recent studies have described the characteristic renal changes of HIVAN in both asymptomatic HIV-infected individuals and those with AIDS-related complex (ARC), thereby broadening the definition to include all HIV-infected patients.

FLUID, ELECTROLYTE, AND ACID-BASE DISORDERS. Fluid-electrolyte disorders are common in patients with advanced HIV infection. Hyponatremia is noted in up to 40 per cent of hospitalized AIDS patients and occurs in the setting of both hypovolemia and euvolemia. Hypovolemia, most often due to gastrointestinal fluid losses, is the most common cause of hyponatremia among this group of patients. The syndrome of inappropriate antidiuretic hormone release (SIADH) is responsible for the majority of cases of euvolemic hyponatremia and is most often due to underlying *Pneumocystis carinii* infection, malignancy, or central nervous system disease. The presence of hyponatremia is associated with increased morbidity and mortality, especially in conjunction with certain opportunistic infections, such as cryptococcosis.

Adrenal insufficiency is a less frequent cause of hyponatremia. Although abnormalities of the adrenal glands are frequently reported at autopsy, overt adrenal insufficiency occurs in less than 5 per cent of patients. The typical findings of hyponatremia, hyperkalemia, non–anion gap metabolic acidosis, hypovolemia, renal salt wasting, and mild renal insufficiency are usually present in some combination.

Drugs are an important cause of fluid and electrolyte disorders in HIV-infected patients and can mimic the abnormalities associated with adrenal dysfunction. Hyperkalemia and non–anion gap metabolic acidosis have been noted in patients receiving parenteral pentamidine. Amphotericin B is associated with hypokalemia, hypomagnesemia, renal tubular acidosis, and renal insufficiency. Chemotherapeutic agents used to treat AIDS-associated malignancies may lead to fluid and electrolyte disturbances through direct nephrotoxicity or gastrointestinal losses associated with prolonged vomiting or diarrhea.

ACUTE RENAL FAILURE. As with most chronic illnesses, acute renal dysfunction may develop as a complication in the management of HIV-infected patients. Prerenal azotemia often results from hypovolemia secondary to poor fluid intake, increased gastrointestinal losses, or both. Acute tubular necrosis can be ischemic in origin, usually secondary to hypotension or sepsis, or due to nephrotoxic agents. Acute interstitial nephritis is another complication associated with drugs used to treat HIV-related diseases. A listing of agents with nephrotoxic potential commonly used in HIV-infected patients is presented in Table 420–1.

Opportunistic infections, invasion of renal parenchyma with lymphoma or Kaposi's sarcoma, and amyloidosis, which occurs as a complication of subcutaneous narcotic abuse, all may result in interstitial nephritis. Other renal lesions, such as hepatitis B–induced membranous glomerulonephritis, acute glomerulonephritis secondary to bacterial infection, direct infection of the renal parenchyma with cytomegalovirus, fungi, or mycobacteria, and the hemolytic-uremic syndrome, have all been associated with renal dysfunction in HIV-infected individuals. The diagnosis and management of acute renal failure are no different in HIV-infected patients than in their uninfected counterparts.

HIV-ASSOCIATED NEPHROPATHY. *Definition.* HIV-associated nephropathy (HIVAN) was first established as a unique clinical entity in 1984. Because it was originally called AIDS-associated nephropathy (AAN), many investigators questioned whether AAN was indeed a unique manifestation of AIDS or simply represented heroin-associated nephropathy (HAN) occurring in intravenous drug users who also happened to be infected with HIV. Although the lesions and clinical manifestations of HAN are similar to those of AAN, further studies have established clear distinctions between the two entities. Of note, AAN occurs in individuals, including children, who have never used intravenous drugs. More recently, the manifestations of AAN have been reported in a significant number of HIV-infected patients who are otherwise asymptomatic. Therefore, HIV-associated nephropathy (HIVAN) has replaced AIDS-associated nephropathy (AAN) as the most appropriate name for this entity.

Epidemiology. The first cases of HIVAN were described in major urban centers, such as New York and Miami, which also had a large proportion of intravenous drug users among their HIV patient population. In contrast, centers whose HIV population consisted primarily of homosexual and bisexual men, such

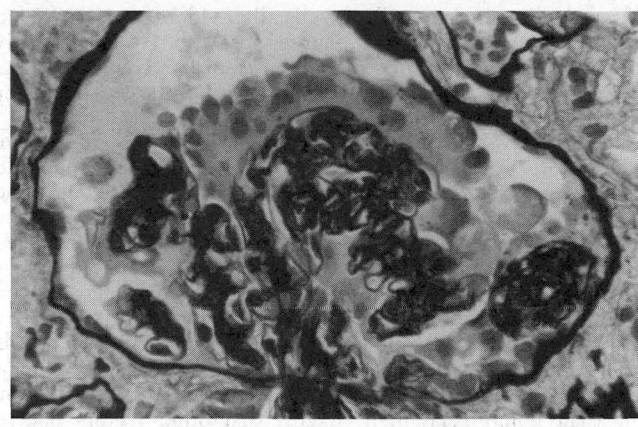

FIGURE 420–1. Glomerulus from a patient with HIV-associated nephropathy demonstrating global collapse of the glomerular capillaries, increased mesangial sclerosis, and a proliferative "cap" of visceral epithelial cells. (Silver methenamine; magnification × 400. Courtesy of Dr. William L. Clapp.)

as San Francisco and the National Institutes of Health, were not observing the renal changes of HIVAN in their patients, thereby implying that HIVAN was a manifestation of HAN. More recent epidemiologic data indicate that 60 per cent of patients with HIVAN are IV drug users, with the remaining cases occurring in homosexual and bisexual men, immigrants from Haiti, women who have acquired HIV from heterosexual contacts, and children born to infected mothers, many of whom did not use intravenous drugs.

Over 90 per cent of patients with HIVAN are black. No explanation regarding the high prevalence of cases among blacks has been established, although many investigators have speculated that cofactors such as superimposed infection(s) or specific immune response genes may be responsible.

Pathology and Pathogenesis. Focal and segmental glomerulosclerosis (FSGS) is the characteristic renal lesion identified in patients with HIVAN, occurring in 80 to 90 per cent of patients. On gross inspection, the kidneys are usually enlarged and the cortical surface is smooth, even in advanced uremia. Microscopic examination of early lesions reveals diffuse mesangial hyperplasia with minimal glomerular sclerosis over time. A variable number of glomeruli develop segmental sclerosis characterized by hyperplastic visceral epithelial cells with coarse cytoplasmic vacuoles, collapsed capillary walls or capillaries obliterated by protein deposits (hyalinosis), and foam cells (lipid-filled monocytes) in the lumina (Fig. 420–1). Bowman spaces are usually dilated and tubular damage is universal. Microcystic dilation of tubules is a unique feature of HIVAN not reported in the FSGS of HAN (Fig. 420–2). Interstitial changes consisting of mild edema with

TABLE 420–1. DRUGS WITH NEPHROTOXIC POTENTIAL COMMONLY USED IN THE TREATMENT OF HIV-RELATED DISEASE

Acyclovir	Nonsteroidal anti-inflammatory
Aminoglycosides	agents
Amphotericin B	Penicillins
Aspirin	Pentamidine
Cephalosporins	Phenytoin
Cimetidine	Rifampin
Cis-platinum	Spiramycin
Dapsone	Sulfonamides
Ethambutol	Tetracyclines
Foscarnet*	Thiazides
Ganciclovir	Trimethoprim

*Investigational

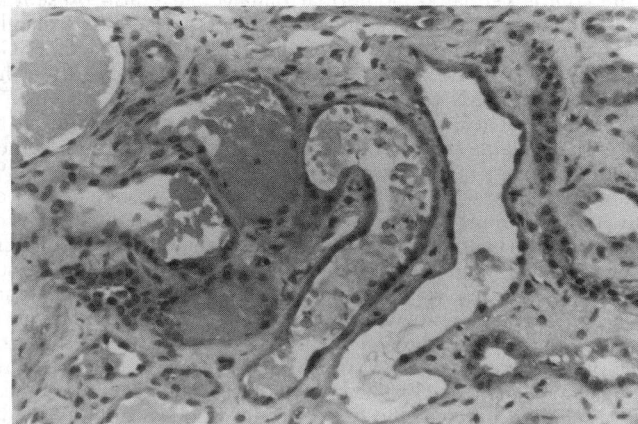

FIGURE 420–2. Dilated degenerated tubules demonstrating flattened epithelium and loss of nuclei and containing proteinaceous casts from a patient with HIV-associated nephropathy. (Hematoxylin-eosin; magnification × 200. Courtesy of Dr. William L. Clapp.)

scattered mononuclear cells are usually evident in HIVAN kidneys but not nearly to the degree noted in HAN. Similarly, although interstitial fibrosis may be present in advanced HIVAN disease, it is not nearly as prominent as the marked interstitial fibrosis noted in HAN disease.

The etiology of HIVAN remains unknown; however, many investigators suspect that an infectious agent is responsible. Ultrastructural studies have demonstrated tuboloreticular structures in vascular endothelium as well as in circulating and tissue lymphocytes. Other findings, such as a large number of nuclear bodies existing as budding forms in renal and lymphoid tissues, have been interpreted by some investigators to suggest a viral etiology. In situ hybridization studies have demonstrated proviral HIV DNA in renal tubular and glomerular epithelial cells, implicating HIV as the causative agent. However, the predominance of HIVAN in blacks and the relative paucity of cases among Caucasian homosexual men suggest that other factors not yet identified must play a role in the pathogenesis of HIVAN.

Clinical Manifestations. HIVAN is characterized by the development of proteinuria, nephrotic syndrome, and rapidly progressive irreversible azotemia. The proteinuria is typically heavy and presents as an early manifestation. The time to the development of end-stage renal disease (ESRD) from the initial diagnosis of proteinuria is 4 to 16 weeks in patients with HIVAN, compared to 20 to 40 months among patients with HAN. Another clinical distinction between HIVAN and HAN is the relative absence of significant hypertension among patients with HIVAN. Accelerated hypertension is a hallmark of HAN. Peripheral edema and anasarca are conspicuously absent in a large number of HIVAN patients with high-grade proteinuria and hypoalbuminemia.

Nephropathy has been documented in patients months to years before the onset of clinical symptoms of ARC or AIDS. In some studies up to 50 per cent of the patients with HIVAN were either asymptomatic or in early stages of ARC. HIVAN is being reported with increasing frequency among HIV-infected children and appears to be independent of the risk factors for HIV infection in their mothers. It is anticipated that the incidence of HIVAN will continue to grow and should be considered as a diagnostic possibility in any HIV-infected patient who presents with unexplained proteinuria regardless of the stage of disease.

Diagnosis. Quantitative measurement of the amount of protein excreted in the urine along with estimation of the creatinine clearance via a 24-hour urine collection should be performed early in the course of evaluation. Other reversible causes of renal insufficiency such as bacterial infection, crystalluria, and obstructive uropathy should be ruled out using urine culture, urinalysis, and ultrasonography. The kidneys are enlarged early in HIVAN and remain enlarged throughout the course of disease. The decision to perform renal biopsy should be made on a case-by-case basis depending on the clinical presentation, the likelihood of other diagnoses, and the therapeutic options available. Since a variety of other renal lesions, such as membranous nephropathy related to hepatitis B, membranoproliferative disease, and immune complex–related glomerular damage, may also present as nephrotic syndrome in HIV-infected patients, renal biopsy should be encouraged. The presence of the typical features of FSGS with tubular involvement as described above establishes the diagnosis of HIVAN when renal tissue is obtained.

Treatment. The lesions of HIVAN respond poorly if at all to currently available treatment regimens. Corticosteroids and other immunosuppressive agents usually have no effect on FSGS. Therefore the treatment of HIVAN is largely supportive in nature. Nutritional support along with appropriate dosage adjustments of nephrotoxic drugs is critical in daily management. Hemodialysis is of marginal benefit in prolonging survival of patients with advanced HIV disease once they have reached end-stage renal disease. Among patients with AIDS, hemodialysis provides short-term prolongation of life for 3 to 11 months. Patients who are asymptomatic or have ARC survive longer, with some patients living over 2 years on chronic hemodialysis. The use of peritoneal dialysis should be considered in patients who are suitable candidates. Chronic ambulatory peritoneal dialysis (CAPD) may offer several advantages over hemodialysis, including avoidance of leukopenia caused by the hemodialysis membranes, fewer problems with anemia, and theoretical advantages of less stimulation

of HIV-infected T lymphocytes via membrane-induced cytokine release. A potential disadvantage of CAPD is the higher incidence of peritonitis. Renal transplantation is not considered a viable option in HIV-infected patients owing to the intensive immunosuppressive regimens required to prevent rejection. In some patients with advanced HIV infection or AIDS who develop HIVAN it may be appropriate to withhold dialysis support based on the generally poor prognosis. As always, such decisions should be individualized, taking into account the wishes of the patient, the family, and significant others.

CARDIAC DISEASE

A wide variety of cardiac abnormalities have been reported in HIV-infected patients, including ventricular dysfunction, myocarditis, pericarditis, endocarditis, and arrhythmias. Most often, cardiac involvement is clinically silent and is noted as an incidental finding at autopsy. When clinical symptoms are present, however, disease manifestations can be debilitating, and, in many cases, life threatening. Unlike HIV-associated renal disease, no specific cardiac syndrome or disease state has been described.

Epidemiology. Cardiac abnormalities have been observed in 25 to 75 per cent of HIV-infected patients studied at autopsy. Myocardial disease is noted most frequently, occurring in over 90 per cent of subjects with cardiac findings. Pericardial disease, often with adjacent myocardial involvement, is observed in over 20 per cent of cases with cardiac abnormalities. Endocarditis is evident histologically in 3 to 5 per cent of cases reported in autopsy series. No characteristic epidemiologic factor, such as age, sex, race, or means of acquiring HIV infection, has been identified which predisposes patients to develop cardiac disease. Although cardiac abnormalities are observed more frequently in AIDS patients, up to 30 per cent of patients with ARC are noted to have abnormal findings on echocardiograms and electrocardiograms.

Pathology and Pathogenesis. HIV-related heart disease may result from metastatic extension of a concomitant opportunistic infection or malignancy but most often is seen as lymphocytic infiltration of the myocardium or as an unspecified myocarditis. The mechanism responsible for the myocarditis remains unknown, although many investigators believe that HIV itself may be directly responsible. Preliminary reports have demonstrated immunologic evidence of HIV antigens (p17, p24, and gp120) in cardiac tissue, molecular evidence of HIV in heart tissue using Southern blot techniques, and virologic evidence of myocardial involvement through culturing HIV-1 from an endocardial biopsy obtained from an AIDS patient with end-stage cardiomyopathy. None of these studies clearly establishes HIV-1 as an etiologic agent of cardiomyopathy, however, since the virus is known to exist in the lymphocytes that invade the myocardium. Other viruses, such as cytomegalovirus, may be responsible for the development of myocarditis, although the typical "owl's eye" inclusion bodies are rarely seen in patients with HIV-associated cardiomyopathy. Additional mechanisms, such as postviral myocarditis or catecholamine-induced myocarditis, have been postulated, but little evidence exists to support their role.

A broad range of opportunistic infections and malignant diseases has been described in cardiac tissue examined at autopsy. Among the infectious disorders, fungal and viral pathogens are identified most often, followed by bacterial and protozoal infections (Table 420–2). Although the invading pathogen is frequently diagnosed at another primary site ante mortem, cardiac involvement is rarely (<2 per cent) identified prior to autopsy. This is due in large part to the clinically silent nature of cardiac disease in HIV infection and a low index of suspicion by clinicians. Kaposi's sarcoma and metastatic lymphoma are the most common neoplastic diseases reported which invade the heart. Primary cardiac lymphoma has been reported rarely.

Pericardial disease is almost invariably associated with adjacent myocardial involvement. Pericarditis is usually nonspecific in origin, but when an etiologic process is identified, Kaposi's sarcoma or a pathogen such as *Mycobacterium tuberculosis* or *Cryptococcus neoformans* is responsible most often. Drugs used to treat HIV-associated disorders, such as doxorubicin for Kaposi's sarcoma, may cause myocardial damage. Other toxins, vitamin deficiencies, or metabolic abnormalities (e.g., hypothyroidism) may also result in myocardial dysfunction or pericardial disease.

TABLE 420–2. INFECTIOUS CAUSES OF CARDIAC DISEASE IN HIV-INFECTED PATIENTS

Bacteria
Bacteria (endocarditis)
Mycobacterium tuberculosis
Mycobacterium avium-intracellulare
Nocardia asteroides
Actinomyces
Fungi
Cryptococcus neoformans
Histoplasma capsulatum
Coccidioides immitis
Candida species
Aspergillus species
Viruses
Cytomegalovirus
Herpes simplex virus
Human immunodeficiency virus
Protozoa
Toxoplasma gondii
Pneumocystis carinii

Endocardial disease has been described in up to 3 per cent of cases studied at autopsy and usually presents as either nonbacterial thrombotic (marantic) endocarditis or healed bacterial endocarditis. The precise etiology of marantic endocarditis is unknown, but it has been reported in other long-term wasting illnesses and malignant diseases. Vegetations are usually located on the mitral valve, although lesions on the tricuspid valve have been noted in up to 29 per cent of AIDS patients with this disorder. Significant embolization to the spleen and brain was noted in over 50 per cent of patients with marantic endocarditis studied at autopsy. Bacterial endocarditis is reported rarely in AIDS patients. Healed lesions from previous bouts of bacterial endocarditis have been reported in autopsy series but are of little clinical significance.

Clinical Findings. Most cardiac disease in HIV-infected patients is clinically silent. When symptoms are present they usually consist of the ordinary findings noted in non–HIV-infected patients with myocarditis or pericarditis, such as fever, dyspnea, chest pain, fatigue, cough, and orthopnea. Hepatomegaly and jugular venous distention are the most common signs noted on physical examination, followed by rales, systolic murmurs, and the presence of an S3 gallop. Signs of advanced pericardial disease with impending tamponade are among the most common clinical manifestations observed in patients who present with clinical symptoms of cardiac disease.

Diagnosis. The demonstration of cardiomegaly on a chest roentgenogram is an important marker of underlying cardiac disease in HIV-infected patients. Right ventricular enlargement is usually the result of pulmonary artery hypertension, which in AIDS patients is often due to severe or recurrent opportunistic pneumonia. Left ventricular or biventricular enlargement is a characteristic finding of congestive cardiomyopathy due to any cause. Echocardiography is a more sensitive and specific noninvasive test that is used to assess the degree of ventricular dysfunction and to characterize the extent of pericardial effusion, if present. Several series have demonstrated echocardiographic abnormalities in up to 50 per cent of HIV-infected patients who had no cardiac symptoms at the time of study. Ventricular enlargement, pericardial effusion, and ventricular hypokinesis were the abnormalities noted most frequently. In view of the overall silent nature of cardiac disease, the high likelihood that infiltrative processes will be evident and diagnosed at another site, and the often limited therapeutic options available for treating cardiac disease in HIV-infected patients, routine echocardiography should be discouraged in patients without cardiac symptoms. The experience with endomyocardial biopsies in HIV-infected patients is quite limited; however, in those individuals who show signs of cardiac disease and have not had a specific diagnosis established, endomyocardial biopsy is a viable option that may lead to a definitive diagnosis.

Treatment. Supportive treatment consisting of diuretic therapy, preload and afterload reduction when appropriate, and correction of cardiac arrhythmias is the obvious initial approach to the treatment of myocardial disease. Pericardial disease requires careful volume management with avoidance of aggressive diuresis or preload reduction. In the case of pericardial tamponade, surgical intervention is warranted. When the underlying etiology of the cardiac disease is known, appropriate targeted therapy directed at the specific infectious agent or malignancy is indicated.

ENDOCRINE DISORDERS

Endocrine dysfunction has not been a prominent clinical manifestation of HIV infection. Nonetheless, all glands of the endocrine system may be infiltrated with opportunistic infections or malignancies or may be affected by drugs used to treat HIV-related disorders. The subtle presentations of endocrine diseases create difficult diagnostic challenges.

ADRENAL GLAND DYSFUNCTION. The adrenal gland is the endocrine gland most commonly affected in patients with AIDS examined at autopsy, although clinical evidence of adrenal insufficiency is observed in less than 8 per cent of AIDS patients. Widespread lipid depletion and varying degrees of adrenal necrosis are the most prevalent pathologic findings in postmortem examinations. Adrenal invasion by cytomegalovirus is noted in up to 50 per cent of patients with adrenal pathology. *Mycobacterium avium* complex, Kaposi's sarcoma, *C. neoformans*, and *Histoplasma capsulatum* involve the adrenal glands in 5 to 12 per cent of cases. Drug therapy with agents such as ketoconazole or rifampin may also result in adrenal dysfunction. Fatigue, anorexia, nausea, vomiting, orthostatic hypotension, and hyponatremia are symptoms frequently noted in many HIV-infected patients; however, only a few patients with these symptoms are actually adrenal insufficient when evaluated using standard laboratory criteria.

Basal 8 A.M. plasma cortisol levels are usually higher in patients with advanced HIV disease than in ARC patients and uninfected healthy controls. However, other ACTH-dependent steroids, such as desoxycorticosterone (DOC), compound B, and 18-hydroxy-DOC, are not elevated and show a blunted response to ACTH stimulation, implying subnormal adrenal reserves. Patients who fail to achieve plasma cortisol levels greater than 20 μg per deciliter 60 minutes after corticotropin (ACTH) stimulation should be considered to have, or be at high risk of developing, adrenal insufficiency. Plasma corticotropin levels are frequently normal or subnormal even when plasma cortisol levels are depressed, suggesting that adrenal insufficiency in some HIV-infected patients is due to a primary pituitary or central nervous system disorder. Treatment of adrenal insufficiency in HIV-infected patients is no different than in other individuals with abnormal adrenal function.

HYPOGONADISM. The most common abnormality of endocrine function noted clinically is hypogonadism. Decreased libido occurs in over one half of male patients with AIDS, and impotence, usually associated with low serum testosterone levels, is reported in up to 30 per cent of AIDS patients. Serum gonadotropin levels may be below normal or inappropriately within normal limits in hypogonadal men with AIDS. When pituitary responsiveness to gonadotropin-releasing hormone is assessed in these hypogonadotropic males, normal release of luteinizing hormone (LH) and follicle-stimulating hormone (FSH) has been observed, suggesting a hypothalamic basis for the central hypogonadotropism. Other studies have demonstrated appropriately elevated levels of LH and FSH in hypogonadal men, implying primary testicular dysfunction. Studies of gonadal function in women are limited, although menstrual irregularities are common in women with advanced HIV disease.

THYROID DISEASE. Thyroid function remains remarkably normal throughout the course of HIV disease. Low levels of thyroxine (T_4), triiodothyronine (T_3), and free-thyroxine index (FTI) in the setting of low concentrations of thyrotropin (TSH), the so-called euthyroid sick syndrome, are remarkably uncommon among ambulatory HIV-infected patients. Decreased levels of T_3 resin uptake and elevated levels of T_4-binding globulin are frequently noted in ambulatory patients with advanced disease; however, concentrations of T_3 and T_4 are most often within normal limits. Invasive disease due to cytomegalovirus, *P. carinii*, *C. neoformans*, Kaposi's sarcoma, and lymphoma has been described in the thyroid. Remarkably, even patients with infiltrating opportunistic diseases of the thyroid gland usually remain euthyroid throughout the course of their disease. Nonetheless, despite the relative infrequency of clinical disease, hypothyroidism represents a potentially reversible cause of fatigue, malaise, altered mental status, and "failure to thrive" in HIV-infected individuals and should be routinely evaluated.

Less common causes of hypothyroidism in HIV-infected patients include adverse effects of medications. Ketoconazole has been associated with primary hypothyroidism on rare occasions. In addition, drugs that are strong inducers of hepatic microsomal enzymes, such as rifampin, may lead to increased clearance of T_4.

METABOLIC ABNORMALITIES. Hyponatremia is the most common electrolyte disturbance noted in HIV-infected individuals (see discussion in renal section). Disorders of carbohydrate metabolism have been reported in association with direct pancreatic invasion by opportunistic processes and with drug therapy. Pancreatic lesions caused by cytomegalovirus, toxoplasmosis, Kaposi's sarcoma, and lymphoma are noted in up to 35 per cent of cases at autopsy. Yet the development of type I diabetes mellitus has been reported in only a few instances. Hypoglycemia is the most common alteration in glucose metabolism. Direct toxic effects of drugs may induce premature release of insulin by β cells, resulting in hypoglycemic episodes that may be severe and prolonged. Pentamidine isothionate is the most common cause of hypoglycemia, occurring in 4 to 33 per cent of treated patients. Renal insufficiency is a predisposing factor in the development of pentamidine-induced hypoglycemia. Although most hypoglycemic episodes result from parenteral administration of pentamidine, several cases have been reported in patients receiving aerosolized drug.

Disorders of calcium metabolism are relatively uncommon but do occur. Hypercalcemia is associated with HIV-related leukemia and lymphoma. Hypocalcemia usually is the result of drug therapy with agents, such as amphotericin B and aminoglycosides, which induce magnesium wasting. Cytomegalovirus has been observed in parathyroid tissue; however, CMV-induced hypoparathyroidism is extremely rare.

RHEUMATOLOGIC DISEASE

Rheumatologic manifestations of HIV disease are being recognized with increased frequency. Musculoskeletal complaints are reported in 33 to 75 per cent of HIV-infected patients and may present as a wide variety of rheumatologic disorders (Table 420–3). The severity of disease ranges from intermittent arthralgias to debilitating arthritis and vasculitis. An array of autoimmune antibodies, including antinuclear, antiplatelet, antilymphocyte, antigranulocyte, and antiphospholipid (anticardiolipin and lupus anticoagulant) antibodies, are associated with HIV infection along with circulating immune complexes, rheumatoid factor, and cryoglobulins. Despite the presence of these antibodies in some patients, the precise mechanisms by which the rheumatologic abnormalities develop have not been elucidated and most likely are different for each particular disorder.

ARTHRALGIAS. Arthralgia is a common manifestation of acute HIV seroconversion, in addition to fever, myalgia, headache, sore throat, abdominal cramps, and lymphadenopathy. Generalized arthralgias are reported in up to one third of HIV-infected patients with minimally symptomatic disease. Some patients develop arthralgias and myalgias upon initiation of zidovudine therapy; however, these symptoms are usually self-limited and abate within 4 to 6 weeks after starting treatment. The "painful articular syndrome" is characterized by severe articular pain of 2 to 24 hours' duration. Although uncommon, this disorder is quite incapacitating and usually unresponsive to oral nonsteroidal anti-inflammatory agents or narcotic analgesics. The etiology of this disorder remains unknown. With the exception of the painful articular syndrome, most of the arthralgias associated with HIV disease are treated with nonsteroidal agents.

MYOPATHIES. Polymyositis-like illnesses, characterized by myalgias, proximal muscle weakness, and wasting, have been reported in several HIV-infected patients and have been the initial HIV-defining presentation in a few. The findings of creatinine phosphokinase (CPK) elevation (greater than five times

TABLE 420–3. RHEUMATOLOGIC DISEASES ASSOCIATED WITH HIV INFECTION

Autoimmune phenomena
Anticardiolipin antibodies
Antigranulocyte antibodies
Antilymphocyte antibodies
Antinuclear antibodies
Antiplatelet antibodies
Circulating immune complexes
Cryoglobulins
Rheumatoid factor
Dermatologic disorders
Dermatomyositis
Malar flush
Psoriasis
Joint disease
Arthralgias
Arthritis
Enthesopathies
HIV-associated arthritis
"Painful articular syndrome"
Psoriatic arthritis
Reactive arthropathy
Reiter's disease
Septic arthritis
Systemic lupus erythematosus (lupus-like syndrome)
Myopathies
Infectious (septic) myositis
Myalgias
    Idiopathic
    Zidovudine-associated
Necrotizing, noninflammatory myopathy
Nemaline rod polymyositis
Polymyositis
Sjögren's syndrome
Sicca complex
Vasculitis
Central nervous system angiitis
Eosinophilic vasculitis
Leukocytoclastic vasculitis
Polyarteritis nodosa

normal) and abnormal electromyography are indistinguishable from those of idiopathic polymyositis. Muscle biopsies reveal necrosis, fibrosis, and inflammation, but usually to a lesser extent than is noted in non–HIV-infected individuals. The presence of nemaline rods, often noted in muscle biopsies of older adults with myositis, suggests the likelihood of underlying HIV infection when noted in biopsy specimens obtained from younger adults, especially in the absence of inflammation.

Although virus-like particles have been demonstrated on rare occasions in synovial tissue and HIV p24 antigen has been noted in the cytoplasm of degenerating muscle cells, no specific viral etiology has been determined. All attempts to culture HIV-1 from muscle tissue of patients with myositis have been unsuccessful.

Patients receiving long-term zidovudine therapy may develop myositis characterized by muscle weakness, elevated CPK levels, myalgias, and evidence of myopathy with a paucity of inflammatory cells on biopsy. Zidovudine-associated myositis usually responds to drug discontinuation and may recur on rechallenge. No definitive therapy exists for HIV-associated polymyositis, although corticosteroid therapy has been successful in reversing symptoms in some patients. If corticosteroid therapy is contemplated, the potential risks of superimposing immunosuppressive therapy on an immunocompromised host must be considered.

REITER'S SYNDROME. Reiter's syndrome is noted in up to 10 per cent of HIV-infected patients who develop arthritis, and an additional 10 to 20 per cent of patients are classified as having "reactive arthritis" because they lack the nonarticular features of Reiter's. Severe, persistent oligoarticular arthritis associated with urethritis, conjunctivitis, painless oral ulcerations, keratoderma blennorrhagicum, or circinate balanitis is the hallmark of Reiter's disease in both HIV-infected and noninfected individuals. Clinical manifestations of Reiter's syndrome may precede or occur at the time of the initial diagnosis of HIV infection but most often follow the onset of immunodeficiency. HLA-B27 positivity is noted in

65 to 75 per cent of HIV-infected patients with Reiter's syndrome. However, studies of African HIV patients with Reiter's disease or reactive arthritis revealed no increased incidence of HLA-B27, suggesting involvement of other gene markers in this group (see Ch. 259). *Shigella, Campylobacter, Ureaplasma*, and other bacterial species associated with the development of reactive arthropathies are rarely described in HIV patients with Reiter's syndrome. However, underlying concomitant sexually transmitted disease(s) may prove to be an important etiologic factor.

Treatment options for HIV patients with Reiter's disease are quite limited. Responses to nonsteroidal anti-inflammatory agents are minimal, and more potent immunosuppressive agents, such as methotrexate and azathioprine, frequently lead to the development of opportunistic diseases and Kaposi's sarcoma shortly after initiation of therapy.

SJÖGREN'S SYNDROME. Xerophthalmia and xerostomia, the characteristic symptoms of Sjögren's syndrome (SS), have been reported with increasing frequency in AIDS patients. Features that closely resemble idiopathic SS, including sicca symptoms, a positive Schirmer test, abnormal salivary gland emptying, and abnormal salivary gland biopsies, have been reported in HIV-infected patients. As a result, it has been suggested that AIDS be an exclusionary disease for the diagnosis of idiopathic SS. The predominance of male patients, the absence of anti-Ro/SS-A and anti-La/SS-B antibodies, the absence of a well-defined connective tissue disease, the presence of HLA-DR52 and DR5 alleles instead of the characteristic A1, B8, DR3, DR2, and DQ1/DQ2 antigens, and a predominance of CD8+ lymphocytes instead of CD4+ cells infiltrating salivary tissue are the characteristic features of AIDS-associated SS, which differs from classic idiopathic SS. Treatment is primarily symptomatic.

SEPTIC ARTHRITIS. Joint space infection is remarkably uncommon in HIV-infected patients. Sporadic case reports have been published of septic arthritis due to fungal pathogens, such as *C. neoformans, H. capsulatum*, and *S. schenkii*, mycobacteria, and routine pyogenic organisms. The approach to diagnosis and treatment of septic arthritis is no different for HIV-infected patients than non–HIV-infected individuals.

HIV-ASSOCIATED ARTHROPATHY. A relatively uncommon arthritis has been described in patients with moderately advanced HIV disease who demonstrate no other signs of any recognizable rheumatologic disease. The so-called HIV-associated arthropathy (HIVAA) presents as a mono- or pauciarticular arthritis. The arthritis is usually severe, affects primarily the knees and ankles, and lasts from 1 week to 6 months. No extra-articular manifestations have been noted. The synovial fluid is noninflammatory in nature, although a mild synovitis consisting of a chronic mononuclear cell infiltrate is noted on biopsy. Rheumatoid factor, antinuclear antibodies, anti-DNA antibodies, and antibodies against RNP, Sm, Ro/SS-A, and La/SS-B are negative. No predominant HLA pattern has been described. Nonsteroidal anti-inflammatory agents are of some benefit, but some patients require intra-articular steroid injections.

VASCULITIS. Several varieties of vasculitis have been reported in association with HIV infection. Necrotizing vasculitis of the polyarteritis nodosa type is reported most commonly and presents as a peripheral sensory or sensorimotor neuropathy. The vasculitis involves the medium-sized vessels of the nerves, skin, and muscle. None of the reported patients with HIV-related PAN were hepatitis B surface antigen positive. Primary angiitis of the central nervous system has been noted in two patients, one of whom had persistent varicella-zoster virus infection. Lymphomatoid granulomatosis has also been reported in HIV-infected patients.

It is unclear whether HIV-associated vasculitis is the result of direct HIV invasion of the vessels, an immunologic reaction to an underlying viral infection, or a response to an opportunistic viral pathogen that invades vascular tissue. As with other serious rheumatologic manifestations of HIV disease, treatment options are limited by the underlying immunodeficiency of the host.

Acierno LJ: Cardiac complications in acquired immunodeficiency syndrome (AIDS): A review. J Am Coll Cardiol 13:1144–1154, 1989. *An in-depth review of potential pathogenic mechanisms responsible for HIV-associated cardiac disease.*

Aron DC: Endocrine complications of the acquired immunodeficiency syndrome. Arch Intern Med 149:330–333, 1989. *An overview of common endocrine disorders in HIV-infected patients.*

Calabrese LH: The rheumatic manifestations of infection with the human immunodeficiency virus. Semin Arthritis Rheum 18:225–239, 1989. *Comprehensive review of rheumatologic disease in HIV-infected patients with special emphasis on autoantibodies and disease pathogenesis.*

Dobs AS, Dempsey MA, Ladenson PW, et al.: Endocrine disorders in men infected with human immunodeficiency virus. Am J Med 84:611–616, 1988. *A review of AIDS-related endocrine abnormalities with special emphasis on hypogonadism and pituitary function.*

Glassock RJ, Cohen AH, Danovitch G, et al.: Human immunodeficiency virus (HIV) infection and the kidney. Ann Intern Med 112:35–49, 1990. *A comprehensive overview of renal disorders associated with HIV infection.*

Kaye BR: Rheumatologic manifestations of infection with human immunodeficiency virus (HIV). Ann Intern Med 111:158–167, 1989. *Clinically relevant review of rheumatologic diseases in AIDS patients.*

Nyamathi A: AIDS-related heart disease: A review of the literature. J Cardiovasc Nurs 3(4):65–76, 1989. *A thorough review of the cardiac manifestations of HIV infection.*

Sreepada Rao TK, Friedman EA: AIDS (HIV)-associated nephropathy; does it exist? Am J Nephrol 9:441–453, 1989. *A nice discussion comparing HIVAN to HAN; it establishes a strong argument for HIVAN as a distinct entity.*

421 Treatment of AIDS and Related Disorders

Robert Yarchoan and Samuel Broder

The last several years have seen a dramatic change in the approach to the treatment of AIDS and related disorders. In 1984, therapy was either entirely supportive or directed at a bewildering array of infectious and oncologic complications. Since that time, the identification of human immunodeficiency virus (HIV) as the causative agent of AIDS and the elucidation of the life cycle of this virus has enabled the development of specific antiretroviral therapy. Such therapy is now recognized as central to the treatment of these diseases. In addition, there is now an intense effort to evaluate new agents and combinations of agents, and the majority of AIDS patients at least consider experimental treatment at some time in the course of their illness. In this chapter, we review the current recommendations for AIDS therapy. In addition, we discuss certain experimental approaches that are now under active clinical development. In AIDS as perhaps in no other disease, the line between approved and experimental therapy is difficult to draw.

The immunodeficiency in AIDS results, either directly or indirectly, from the progressive destruction of the immune system by HIV. In addition, HIV infection affects other organ systems (such as the central nervous system). T lymphocytes bearing CD4 antigen on their surface (CD4 cells or T4 cells), monocytes, macrophages, and monocyte-derived cells such as microglial cells are now recognized as the principal cellular targets for HIV. Although other cells are also susceptible to infection, the clinical significance of this phenomenon is unclear. In infected individuals, the development and progression of disease require at least some level of ongoing infection of new cells by HIV. Thus, one could reason that interference with HIV replication in vivo could halt or even reverse the progression of disease to AIDS. Indeed, the successful development of antiretroviral therapy has shown this to be the case.

AZIDOTHYMIDINE (ZIDOVUDINE) AND OTHER DIDEOXYNUCLEOSIDES

The first antiretroviral drug to be developed and approved for the therapy of HIV infection was 3'-azido—2',3'-dideoxythymidine, also called azidothymidine, zidovudine, or AZT (Fig. 421–1). This drug was initially synthesized by Jerome Horwitz as an anticancer drug in 1964. At the National Cancer Institute in 1985 it was found to inhibit HIV replication in human T cells in vitro and was later found to have anti-HIV activity in monocytes and macrophages. AZT is a member of a family of compounds called dideoxynucleosides, in which the 3'-hydroxy (-OH) group is replaced by another group that does not form phosphodiester linkages. In the case of AZT, the 3'-hydroxy group of thymidine

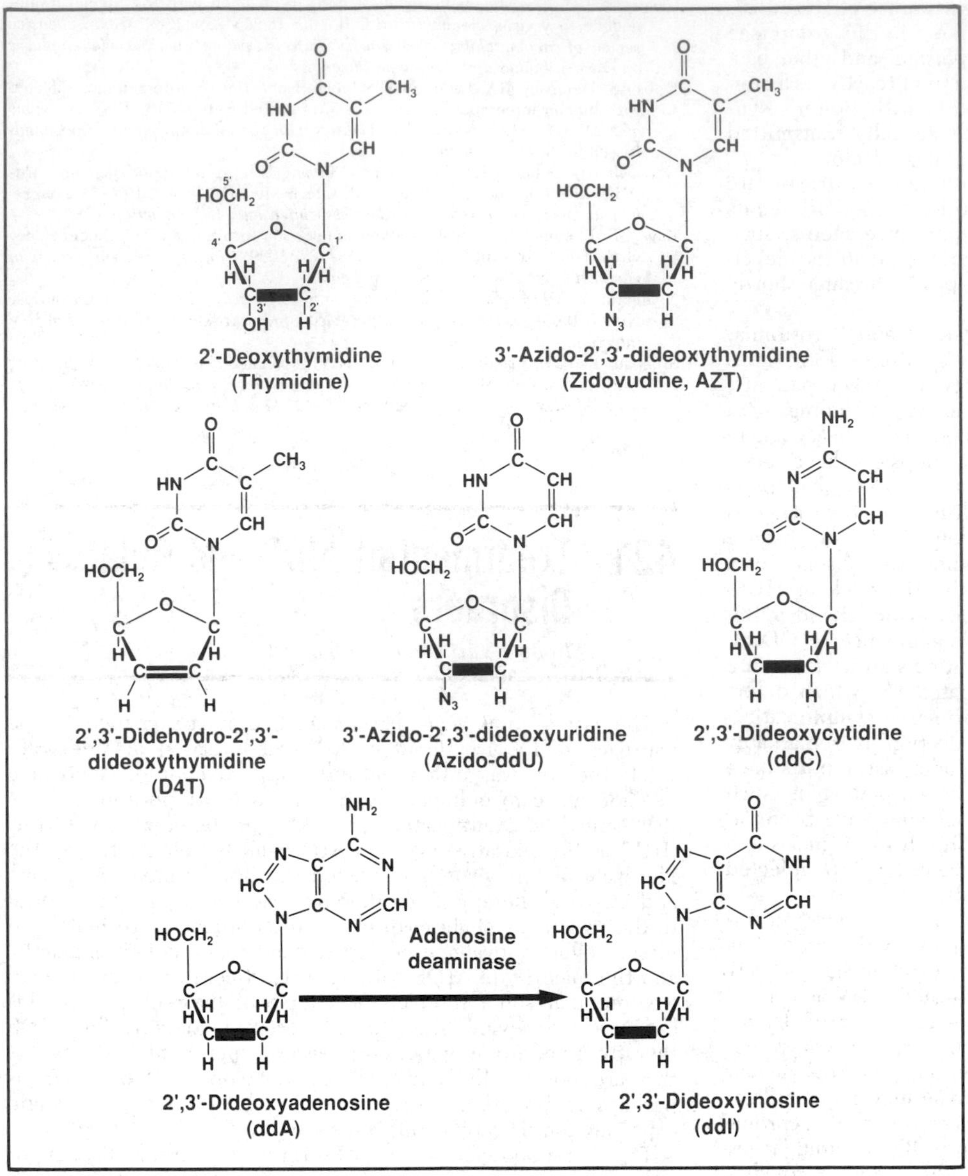

FIGURE 421–1. *Top,* Structures of thymidine (*left*) and AZT (*right*). The 3'hydroxy (-OH) group of thymidine is replaced by an azido (-N$_3$) group to form AZT. *Middle,* Three other dideoxypyrimidines undergoing clinical testing as anti-AIDS drugs. *Bottom,* Two dideoxypurines undergoing clinical testing as anti-AIDS drugs. Dideoxyadenosine (ddA) is rapidly converted to dideoxyinosine (ddI) by the ubiquitous enzyme adenosine deaminase, and these can be considered alternate forms of the same drug for many purposes. (Modified from Yarchoan R, Mitsuya H, Myers CE, Broder S: Clinical pharmacology of 3'-azido-2',3'-dideoxythymidine (zidovudine) and related dideoxynucleosides. N Engl J Med 321:726–738, 1989. Reprinted by permission of the New England Journal of Medicine.)

is replaced by an azido (-N$_3$) group. A number of members of this family have been found to be potent inhibitors of HIV replication in vitro, and several, including AZT, have been shown to have clinical activity in patients with HIV infection.

Upon entering human cells, AZT and other dideoxynucleosides are activated (phosphorylated) to form a 5'-triphosphate moiety. This activation process, called anabolic phosphorylation, utilizes a series of enzymes (kinases) which usually serve to phosphorylate deoxynucleosides (Fig. 421–2). There are substantial differences in the rates at which human cells phosphorylate these compounds and in their enzymatic pathways, and these differences may be important in their antiretroviral activity and differing toxicity profiles. AZT, for example, is much more potent than 2',3'-dideoxythymidine (ddT) in human cells because of differences in the rate of phosphorylation. Also, the rates of phosphorylation vary markedly between species, and one cannot draw conclusions about the activity of dideoxynucleosides in human cells on the basis of animal models.

As triphosphates, dideoxynucleosides act as inhibitors at the level of HIV DNA polymerase (reverse transcriptase). This unique viral enzyme catalyzes the conversion of HIV genetic information from RNA to DNA and subsequently catalyzes the formation of a second viral DNA strand, i.e., a copy complementary to the first. The activity of reverse transcriptase is essential for HIV replication to occur. As 5-triphosphates, dideoxynucleosides are believed to inhibit reverse transcriptase in two ways. First, they

can act as DNA chain terminators: Once added to the end of a growing chain of viral DNA, the chain is elongated by exactly one residue and no further nucleotides can be added because of the 3'-modification. Also, as triphosphates they act as competitive inhibitors for the binding of the physiologic nucleoside-5'-triphosphates to relevant sites within reverse transcriptase. Reverse transcriptase, but not mammalian DNA polymerase α, preferentially utilizes dideoxynucleoside-5'-triphosphates in place of the respective physiologic 5'-triphosphates, and this is most likely the basis for their selective antiretroviral activity. However, human mitochondrial DNA polymerase (γ) is relatively sensitive to inhibition by certain of these drugs, and this may be a basis for certain toxicities. As with virtually any explanation for the mechanism of action for a new drug, the physician should always bear in mind that new knowledge could modify or supplant any working theory.

Clinical Activity of AZT (Zidovudine)

Phase I and II clinical trials of AZT conducted during the years 1985 and 1986 convincingly showed that the drug could be administered to patients and was effective at reducing morbidity and mortality in patients with severe HIV infection (Fig. 421–3). Patients with AIDS or severe ARC had an increase in the number of T4 cells, improved immunologic function, and a decrease in the viral load (as assessed by HIV p24 antigenemia) upon receiving AZT. In addition, patients had increased appetite, gained

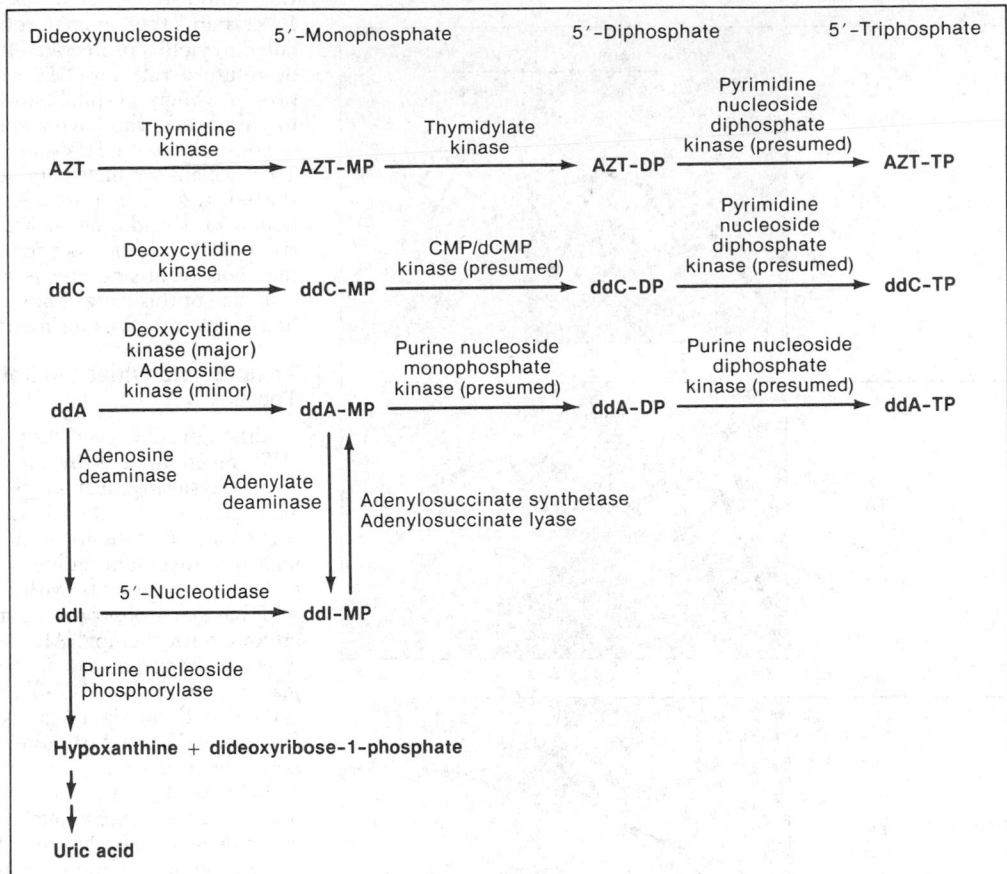

FIGURE 421–2. Activation pathways for AZT, ddC, ddA, and ddI to the active triphosphate moieties in human cells. MP = 5'-monophosphate; DP = 5'-diphosphate; TP = 5'-triphosphate.

weight, and often reported feeling better at least temporarily. In a multicenter randomized trial in which AZT was compared with placebo, patients who had severe ARC or who had had *Pneumocystis carinii* pneumonia (PCP) were found to have a markedly reduced mortality and incidence of opportunistic infections upon receiving AZT as compared with patients on the placebo arm. Some (but not all) of this reduced mortality could be attributed to the T4 increases induced by AZT. Based on these studies, AZT was initially approved for patients with severe HIV infection at a recommended dosage of 200 mg every 4 hours (1200 mg per day) around the clock. Since that time, it has been found that a maintenance regimen of 100 mg every 4 hours (600 mg per day), initiated after a month's therapy with 200 mg every 4 hours, is as effective as the initially recommended regimen and is associated with less toxicity. This is the currently recommended dosage schedule. Many physicians are now suggesting that their patients omit waking up to take their nighttime dose; however, while this 500-mg daily regimen has been found to be effective in asymptomatic patients with fewer than 500 T4 cells per cubic millimeter (see below), it has not formally been proven in patients with AIDS. Studies are now underway to examine the effectiveness of even lower dosages of AZT, and physicians should be keenly alert for possible future modifications of the recommended dosage of this drug.

The pharmacokinetic profile of AZT is one of the factors that guides its usage. AZT is well absorbed by mouth; the average oral bioavailability is 63 per cent. The circulating half-life is approximately 1.1 hours. It is because of this relatively short half-life that a dosing schedule of every 4 hours was initially recommended. However, other dosing regimens are now being examined. Fifteen to 20 per cent of an administered dose of AZT is excreted unchanged in the urine, while approximately 75 per cent undergoes glucuronidation to an inactive form in the liver. AZT glucuronidation can be inhibited by certain other drugs, such as probenecid, which share this pathway, and these drugs can prolong the half-life of AZT. However, certain other drugs that undergo hepatic glucuronidation (e.g., acetaminophen) have no such effect. Studies are underway to evaluate the interactions of other drugs with AZT. Finally, AZT penetrates effectively into the cerebrospinal fluid.

Two large randomized studies recently conducted by the AIDS Clinical Trials Group of the National Institutes of Allergy and Infectious Diseases showed that AZT could reduce the short-term progression to AIDS or severe ARC in patients with 200 to 500 T4 cells per cubic millimeter. One of these trials involved asymptomatic patients, and the other involved patients with minimal symptoms. As a result of these studies, AZT (100 mg every 4 hours) is now recommended for HIV-infected patients with less than 500 T4 cells per cubic millimeter. Physicians should be aware, however, that patients in those studies were followed only for 3 months to 2 years and that no improvement in overall survival was formally proven. As noted above, a formal survival benefit had been shown in advanced AIDS or ARC. Long-term AZT therapy may be associated with cumulative toxicity and the development of viral resistance, and it is not proven at this point whether early intervention with AZT improves long-term survival. We will return to these points below.

AZT was made widely available in the United States in the fall of 1986 for patients who had had PCP, and it was approved as a prescription drug in the spring of 1987. There are epidemiologic data that the widespread use of AZT since that time has played a role in substantially lengthening the survival of patients with AIDS. In New York State, the 18-month survival of homosexual men with AIDS increased from 34.8 per cent in patients diagnosed in 1985 to 62.9 per cent in patients diagnosed in 1987. It is likely that other advances in the diagnosis, prevention, and treatment of complications of AIDS (particularly chemoprophylaxis for PCP) have contributed to this effect. However, where this specific factor has been looked at, the effect of AZT on survival has been observed over and above any contribution from *Pneumocystis* prophylaxis. Also, although AZT has only recently been approved specifically for patients with 200 to 500 T4 cells per cubic millimeter, it has been widely used in such patients during the past several years by physicians practicing in the community. There is now epidemiologic evidence that by delaying the development of fulminant AIDS in HIV-infected individ-

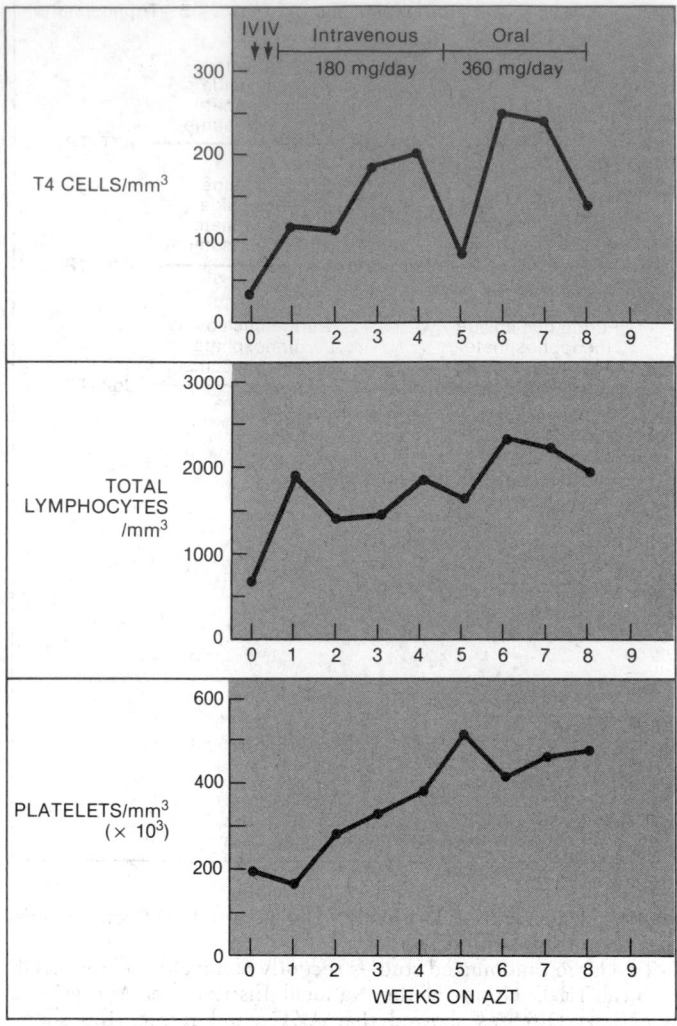

FIGURE 421–3. Course of the first patient ever to receive AZT. This patient, who had recently recovered from *Pneumocystis carinii* pneumonia, was treated on the National Cancer Institute service of the National Institutes of Health Clinical Center with 180 mg per day of AZT intravenously for 4 weeks, followed by 360 mg per day orally for 4 weeks.

uals, this early use of AZT may have led to an unexpected decline in the incidence of new AIDS cases (Fig. 421–4).

As mentioned above, AZT can penetrate into the cerebrospinal fluid. Several studies have shown that AZT can reverse HIV-induced cognitive dysfunction or even frank dementia. Patients have been observed to have improvement on psychometric testing, and, in several cases studied by positron emission tomography, there has been a normalization of the pattern of glucose metabolism in the brain (see Color Plate 12F). The reversal of HIV dementia has been particularly striking in HIV-infected children. In this population, neurologic dysfunction is a particularly prominent feature of HIV infection. It is possible that the ability of AZT to reverse HIV-induced dementia results in part from its ability to protect monocyte-derived cells in the brain (such as microglial cells) from HIV infection. However, much more needs to be learned about the pathogenesis of HIV dementia and the mechanism of AZT's effect on this disorder.

An unresolved question at present is whether AZT given at the time of exposure can protect against HIV infection. In several animal retroviral systems, a short course of AZT given at the time of inoculation was found to prevent infection from occurring. More recently, this issue has been examined by McCune and colleagues in mice with genetically determined severe combined immunodeficiency disease reconstituted with a human immune system (SCID-hu mouse). When a 2-week course of AZT was administered to such mice within 2 hours of an intravenous inoculum of HIV, no evidence of viral infection was detected. In

certain instances, protection was conferred even when the drug was administered as late as 36 hours after the viral inoculation. In certain other animal retroviral systems, however, AZT has failed to yield a protective effect, and there are no data to confirm or refute a role for AZT as a prophylactic drug in humans at present. Many hospitals now offer a 4- to 6-week course of AZT to employees who have a substantial exposure to HIV, such as a needle stick with HIV-infected blood or a laboratory accident. The available animal data suggest that if used, AZT should be started as soon as possible after the exposure, ideally within 2 hours. In considering such therapy, physicians should weigh the risk of HIV infection occurring (about 1 in 200 for a needle stick), the short-term side effects of AZT, and the unknown long-term sequelae of this drug. They should also be aware that this should be considered an experimental use of AZT.

Toxicity and Other Limitations of AZT (Zidovudine) Therapy

Although AZT has clearly been shown to benefit patients with HIV infection, it is by no means a perfect drug. As with any drug, physicians must weigh the risks versus benefits of therapy. The long-term use of AZT is associated with a number of toxicities, particularly in patients with advanced AIDS. Also, the immunologic improvement induced by AZT may be only temporary, especially in patients with AIDS, and a reduced sensitivity to AZT has been observed in strains of HIV isolated from patients on long-term therapy. Also, AZT does not cure AIDS.

The most frequent toxicity associated with AZT therapy is bone marrow suppression (Table 421–1). The earliest sign is often anemia with marked macrocytic changes; a mean corpuscular volume of 110 to 120 cubic microns is not uncommon. AZT is now a leading cause of macrocytosis in several medical centers. Some patients have been observed to develop hypocellular or (rarely) aplastic bone marrows while receiving AZT. This can occur even in the absence of macrocytosis. Later in the course of AZT therapy, patients may become neutropenic or thrombocytopenic. In some patients, the platelet count remains stable or paradoxically increases for some time, perhaps reflecting an effect against underlying HIV-induced thrombocytopenia. AZT-induced bone marrow suppression is most common in patients with advanced AIDS, low T4 counts, pretherapy anemia, and pretherapy neutropenia. It is less problematic with the recently recommended dosage of 600 mg per day; however, even with this dosing schedule, it can occur in 30 per cent or so of patients with advanced disease during the first year of therapy. It is unclear at the present time whether it is preferable to continue the same dose of AZT once patients become anemic and to provide transfusion therapy or to reduce the dose of AZT. It is possible that monitoring of HIV p24 antigenemia will be found to be useful in guiding individual therapy in such situations. HIV-infected patients often have vitamin deficiencies, particularly of vitamin B_{12}, and megaloblastic anemia from folic acid or vitamin B_{12} deficiency bears a certain similarity to AZT toxicity. It may thus be prudent to measure serum levels of folic acid and vitamin B_{12} and give replacement therapy if they are low; however, this intervention has not been shown to prevent or reverse AZT toxicity. It has been shown that administration of genetically engineered erythropoietin (epoetin alfa) can partially ameliorate AZT-induced anemia, particularly in patients who do not have markedly elevated erythropoietin levels. For such patients (with erythropoietin levels of <500 mU per millimeter) epoetin alfa should be considered at starting doses of 100 U per kilogram administered intravenously or subcutaneously three times per week. Other hematopoietic cytokines are now being investigated for AZT-induced marrow suppression.

Myalgias are also common in patients receiving AZT. In addition, after long-term therapy (e.g., a year or more), a subset of patients may develop frank myopathy with muscle wasting and sometimes (but not always) elevations of creatine kinase. In rare cases, this side effect can lead to a catastrophic failure of systemic muscles. AZT-induced myositis can usually be distinguished from myositis caused by HIV by the presence of "ragged red" fibers on biopsy, indicative of abnormal mitochondria (see Color Plate 12G). Paracrystalline inclusions in the mitochondria can be seen on electron microscopy. It is believed that this toxicity results from the inhibitory effect of AZT-5'-triphosphate on mammalian

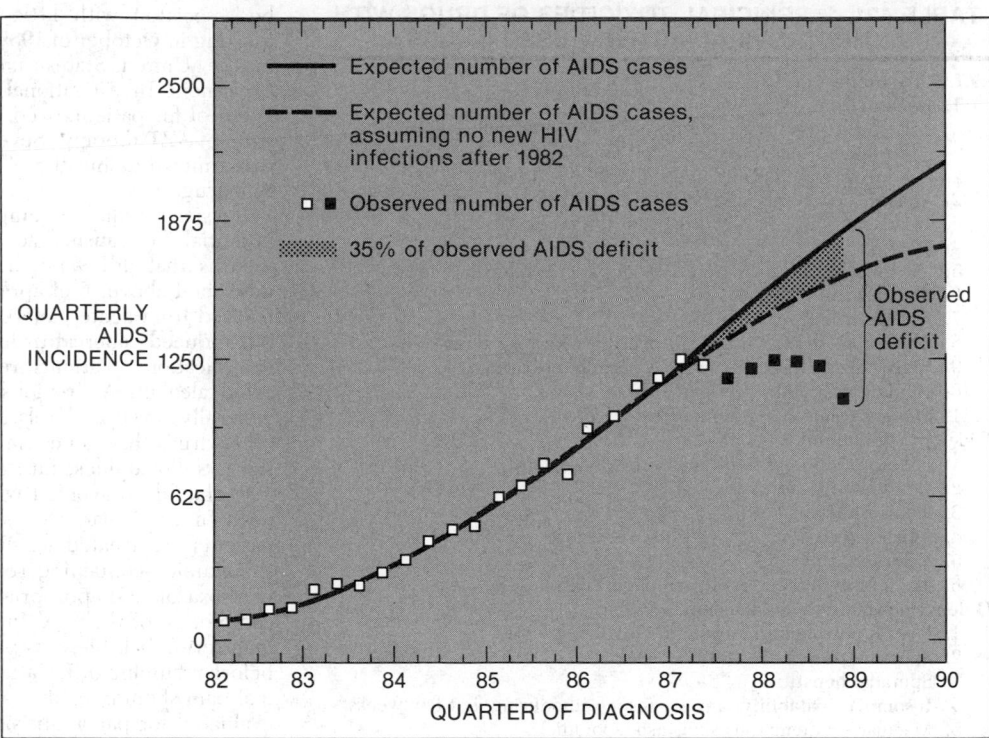

FIGURE 421-4. Decrease in the observed number of cases of AIDS in homosexual men in San Francisco, Los Angeles, and New York since the middle of 1987. The solid line depicts the number of AIDS cases expected. The dashed line depicts the number of AIDS cases that would be expected if one makes the extreme assumption that, as a result of safe sex practices and other public health measures, no patients became infected with HIV after 1982. It was about this time that sexual practices began to change in response to the awareness that AIDS was a sexually transmitted disease. As can be seen, the deficit in AIDS cases since the middle of 1987 is largely attributed to changes in the therapy of HIV-infected individuals before they develop AIDS, including the administration of AZT. Only 35 per cent of the AIDS deficit could be explained by an absence of new infections with HIV after 1982. AZT became a prescription drug in March, 1987. (Reproduced with permission from Gail MH, et al: J AIDS 3:296–306, 1990.)

γ DNA polymerase, an enzyme found in the mitochondrial matrix. Some patients with this toxicity respond to a nonsteroidal anti-inflammatory drug, with or without a reduction in the dose of AZT. In other cases, it may be necessary to discontinue the AZT. Certain patients who do not respond to the above interventions have been reported to respond to therapy with prednisone (40 to 60 mg daily). However, this potentially dangerous immunosuppressive drug should be used only as a last resort in severe cases.

Patients receiving AZT frequently complain of malaise, fatigue, nausea, or headaches. These often become less severe after several weeks on the drug. However, in a subset of patients, these symptoms are intolerable. Some patients, particularly blacks, develop bluish fingernail coloration as a result of AZT therapy (see Color Plate 12E). Finally, clinicians should be aware that AZT has been found in animal studies to be mutagenic and to cause an increased incidence of vaginal tumors in rodents administered life-long high-dose drug. At the present time, the implications of such findings to the treatment of HIV infection are still unclear; however, they do suggest that AZT should not be casually administered to patients without specific indications or outside of an approved clinical trial. AZT should be used in pregnant HIV patients with great caution and preferably only in the context of a clinical trial.

Improved survival from antiretroviral therapy may permit AIDS patients to live long enough to develop certain HIV-related complications. In particular, an unexpectedly high incidence of non-Hodgkin's lymphoma, in some instances approaching 10 per cent of patients per year, has been observed in AIDS patients who have been followed for several years on AZT-containing regimens. These are almost certainly not caused by AZT, but instead appear to represent the development of opportunistic tumors in immunosuppressed patients. The situation is analogous to that of certain genetic immunodeficiency diseases in which the cumulative incidence of tumors was observed to increase when survival is enhanced by improved anti-infective therapy.

Even in patients who tolerate AZT, there are limitations to its long-term use. Although a majority of patients have increases in the number of T4 cells during the first several weeks of therapy, the increases are often transient, particularly in patients with advanced AIDS. In the original Phase II trial of AZT, there was no final difference in the number of T4 cells between the AZT-treated group and the placebo-treated group after 6 months of

therapy. It is conceivable that lower-dose regimens (perhaps by reducing cumulative toxicity in lymphocytes) could yield better performance in this regard.

Some patients who initially have a decrease in their p24 antigenemia upon starting AZT may have late increases while continuing on therapy. Isolates of HIV from patients who have received AZT for over 1 year frequently have reduced sensitivity to AZT. There is suggestive evidence that this may occur as a result of a defined set of mutations in the reverse transcriptase. Interestingly, strains of HIV which have become resistant to AZT have been found to preserve their sensitivity to most other dideoxynucleosides. The clinical significance of these changes in in vitro sensitivity is not clear at this time.

Clinicians frequently ask whether AZT should be continued in patients on long-term therapy who had initial T4 rises but subsequent falls to or below baseline on long-term treatment. There are at present no controlled trials to address this issue. However, one could argue that as long as the drug is reasonably tolerated, suppression of HIV replication to some degree is probably beneficial and AZT therapy should be continued. Such patients will of course be likely beneficiaries of any new effective anti-HIV therapies that may become available.

Other Dideoxynucleosides

As noted above, AZT is one member of the family of compounds called dideoxynucleosides (see Fig. 421-1). More than a score of other dideoxynucleosides have been found to be active against HIV in the laboratory. Of these, 2′,3′-dideoxycytidine (ddC), 2′,3′-dideoxyadenosine (ddA), 2′,3′-dideoxyinosine (ddI), 2′,3′-didehydro-2′,3′-dideoxythymidine (D4T), and 3′-azido-2′,3′-dideoxyuridine (azido-ddU) have entered clinical testing, and trials of others are planned. Several halogenated congeners of these drugs are quite interesting. As noted above, these compounds are believed to inhibit HIV by the same general mechanism as AZT. However, because of differences in their intracellular or extracellular metabolism and effects on normal nucleotides, various dideoxynucleosides may have fundamentally different activity and toxicity profiles. Each must be considered a different drug.

ddC, the first of these other dideoxynucleosides to be tested in vivo, was found to reduce the viral load and improve virologic parameters in patients with AIDS or ARC. The drug has excellent bioavailability. Patients receiving ddC generally did not develop bone marrow suppression. However, a reversible painful periph-

TABLE 421–1. PRINCIPAL TOXICITIES OF DRUGS WITH ANTIRETROVIRAL ACTIVITY USED IN AIDS

AZT (Zidovudine)
1. Bone marrow suppression
   Red cells usually affected more than white cells or platelets
   Prominent increase in red cell mean corpuscular volume
   Marrow may become hypocellular
2. Malaise, fever, fatigue (especially during first few weeks)
3. Headaches (especially during first few weeks)
4. Myalgias
5. Myositis (in approximately 10% of patients after long-term use)
6. Seizures (can be fatal)
7. Nausea, vomiting
8. Confusion, tremulousness (especially with high doses)
9. Bluish pigmentation of nails (especially in blacks)
10. Hepatic transaminase elevations
11. Stevens-Johnson syndrome (very rare)

Dideoxycytidine (ddC)
1. Painful peripheral neuropathy (involving feet)
2. Aphthous stomatitis
3. Skin rash (transient)
4. Fevers, malaise
5. Diarrhea
6. Thrombocytopenia, neutropenia (at high doses)

Dideoxyinosine (ddI, didanosine)
1. Painful peripheral neuropathy (involving feet)
2. Sporadic pancreatitis (can be fatal)
3. Sporadic hepatitis
4. Insomnia, irritability, anxiety (especially during first few weeks)
5. Macular erythematous skin rash (sporadic)
6. Increases in uric acid (from ddI metabolism)
7. Hyperamylasemia, hypertriglyceridemia
8. Diarrhea, hypokalemia (from citrate/phosphate/sucrose vehicle)
9. Neutropenia, thrombocytopenia (rare, relationship to drug unclear)
10. Seizures (relationship to drug unclear)
11. Dry mouth
12. Confusion (especially when administered with triazolam)

Interferon-α
1. Flulike symptoms very common (fatigue, fever, chills, myalgias)
2. Headaches (common)
3. Nausea, vomiting, anorexia, weight loss (common)
4. Diarrhea (common)
5. Bone marrow suppression
6. Hepatitis, hepatic transaminase and alkaline phosphatase elevations
7. Rash, dry skin, pruritus
8. Congestive cardiopathy (sporadic)
9. Decreased mental status, depression, visual disturbances
10. Hypotension
11. Inflammation at injection sites

eral neuropathy was found to be the dose-limiting toxicity. Additional studies have shown that the development of this neuropathy can be delayed or prevented by administration of a carefully selected regimen of low-dose ddC or through intermittent dosing. Some patients receiving ddC also developed aphthous stomatitis or skin rashes; these generally subsided even with continued ddC administration. ddC is now being studied further, both as a single agent and in combination with AZT. In addition, it is being made available, under the mechanism of an open label protocol, to certain patients with advanced disease who have failed or cannot tolerate AZT.

Another dideoxynucleoside, ddI, was also found in initial clinical testing to be well absorbed by the oral route when given with appropriate buffers (oral bioavailability 40 per cent) and to have antiviral activity in patients with AIDS or ARC. In addition, patients not heavily pretreated with AZT had increases in T4 cells upon receiving ddI. At high doses, ddI was found to cause painful peripheral neuropathy. The drug can also cause acute pancreatitis. ddI can be catabolized to hypoxanthine and subsequently to uric acid, and asymptomatic hyperuricemia has been observed in some patients receiving very high doses of ddI. Other adverse reactions were generally not severe enough to warrant discontinuation of therapy (Table 421–1). In contrast to AZT, bone marrow toxicity was not prominent, even in patients

receiving high doses. Also, intermediate doses of ddI (e.g., 500 to 750 mg per day) were found to have anti-HIV activity but to be associated with little long-term toxicity in most patients. Starting in October of 1989, ddI was made available to physicians in the United States under the regulatory mechanisms of a Treatment Investigational New Drug Program or Open Label Protocol for patients who cannot tolerate AZT or were failing in spite of AZT therapy. Several large studies of ddI were begun at that time to define the efficacy and long-term toxicity profile of this drug.

Physicians who contemplate using ddI should be aware of its potential for causing acute pancreatitis. During the initial 6 months that ddI was made available under the two programs described above, 6 of approximately 7000 patients receiving ddI expired from acute pancreatitis. It can be difficult to distinguish ddI-induced pancreatitis from that caused by HIV infection or its complications. Patients receiving ddI should be counseled to avoid alcohol. A previous history of pancreatic disease should generally serve as a relative contraindication for ddI use. Also, other drugs that can cause pancreatitis, such as systemic pentamidine, sulfonamides, furosemide, and thiazide diuretics (see Ch. 106) should be avoided whenever possible in patients receiving ddI. In particular, ddI should be temporarily stopped when patients are treated for PCP with intravenous pentamidine or sulfonamide-containing regimens (including trimethoprim-sulfamethoxazole). If appropriate, ddI can then be restarted after the completion of therapy. In the case of pentamidine, which has a long serum half-life, it is probably prudent to wait at least 1 week before resuming ddI. Patients receiving ddI who develop abdominal pain should be advised to stop the drug immediately and be evaluated for pancreatitis. Physicians should probably avoid administering cimetidine or ranitidine along with ddI, as those drugs have the potential of increasing the absorption of ddI and can cause pancreatitis in their own right. Although ddI has a serum half-life of only 40 minutes, it remains a long time in lymphocytes after being metabolized to a triphosphate. For these reasons, it is currently being administered every 12 hours. The recommended oral doses of ddI for adults are now 334 to 750 mg per day, depending on the patient's weight. However, it is likely that the recommendations for ddI therapy will be modified as we learn more about this drug.

OTHER ANTI-HIV THERAPIES

The development of anti-HIV therapy is currently an area of intense laboratory and clinical research activity, and developments are occurring at a rapid rate. There are now many ongoing clinical trials of anti-AIDS drugs, and physicians who treat AIDS patients may be called upon to counsel their patients about the advisability of entering a particular experimental protocol. A basic knowledge of the strategies being considered to inhibit HIV replication at various steps in its life cycle may therefore be of use (Table 421–2).

As described in Ch. 411, the first step in the infection of a cell by HIV is its binding to a cellular receptor. The principal receptor for HIV binding is the first domain of CD4 glycoprotein. CD4 is an important molecule found on helper T cells and certain other cells. There is some experimental evidence that under certain circumstances, CD4-independent entry mechanisms may exist, although the clinical significance of this finding is unknown. Several groups have shown that genetically engineered soluble recombinant CD4 (containing the extracellular domains) can prevent the binding and infection of cells by laboratory strains of HIV in vitro. These preparations were generally safe to administer to patients. However, recombinant soluble CD4 was found to have a short serum half-life, and it has proved difficult to maintain levels associated with anti-HIV activity in vivo. More recently, hybrid proteins combining the pertinent domain(s) of CD4 with the constant portion of immunoglobulin heavy chain have been created. Such molecules, which are often referred to as immunoadhesins, likewise had anti-HIV activity in the laboratory. In addition, they were found to have substantially longer serum half-lives than unmodified soluble CD4. Initial clinical trials, however, have not shown clear evidence of anti-HIV activity in vivo. It has been found that fresh isolates of HIV are relatively resistant to these agents, and this may in part explain their lack of clinical activity. As another approach, CD4 has been linked

TABLE 421–2. SELECTED DRUGS (EXPERIMENTAL AND APPROVED) FOR THE THERAPY OF AIDS

Site of Effect	Name	Status (Spring 1991)	Comments
Viral binding	Soluble CD4	Experimental	Genetically engineered HIV receptor
	CD4-IgG chimera (immunoadhesin)	Experimental	Longer half-life than CD4
	CD4-toxin hybrids	Preclinical	May selectively kill HIV-producing cells
	Dextran sulfate	Experimental	Poor oral absorption; prototype for polyanionic polysaccharides with anti-HIV activity
	Anti-HIV antibodies	Experimental	May block HIV fusion and entry
Reverse transcriptase	AZT (zidovudine)	Approved	Optimal use still under study
	ddA and ddI	Treatment IND	Available for patients who cannot tolerate or have failed AZT therapy; can cause pancreatitis or peripheral neuropathy at high doses
	ddC	Open label protocol	Peripheral neuropathy is dose-limiting toxicity
	D4T	Experimental	Can cause peripheral neuropathy
	Azido-ddU	Experimental	Cross-reactive resistance with AZT
	Phosphonoformate (Foscarnet)	Experimental	Also has activity against cytomegalovirus
	TIBO derivatives	Experimental	Benzodiazepine derivatives
Replicative efficiency	Tat inhibitors	Experimental	Inhibitors of Tat, a virally encoded protein required for efficient replication
Protein modification	Protease inhibitors	Experimental	An intense effort is now under way to identify selective inhibitors of HIV protease
	Castanospermine and other trimming glucosidase inhibitors	Experimental	Affects sugar moiety of HIV envelope, reducing its ability to infect new cells
Viral budding	Interferon-α	Approved for Kaposi's sarcoma	Antitumor activity against Kaposi's sarcoma; may also have anti-HIV activity

with certain toxins (such as ricin or *Pseudomonas* endotoxin) with the idea of selectively killing cells that are producing HIV. Other approaches being considered to inhibit HIV binding or fusion include polyanionic polysaccharides (such as dextran sulfate or pentosan) or anti-HIV antibodies. In regard to the latter, however, it should be remembered that patients can progress to AIDS in spite of having neutralizing antibodies against HIV.

As discussed above, much of the effort in developing anti-AIDS drugs has focused on reverse transcription. All of the dideoxynucleosides (as triphosphates) are thought to act at this step. In addition, phosphonoformate (Foscarnet), a drug originally developed for the treatment of cytomegalovirus, inhibits HIV replication at the level of reverse transcription. Finally, several benzodiazepine derivatives (TIBO derivatives) have been found to have potent anti-HIV activity and are believed to act at this step.

There is now a substantial research effort directed at inhibiting certain late steps in HIV replication. The proteins of HIV are first produced as large polyproteins and later undergo a variety of modifications to form active proteins or glycoproteins. One of these steps is cleavage by an HIV protease. In the absence of effective protease activity, infectious virions cannot be produced. The structure of this enzyme has recently been determined by x-ray crystallography, and several selective inhibitors have been identified. Clinical trials of these agents are now under way.

HIV replication is regulated by certain genetic elements (long terminal repeats) on either end of the viral genome and by several small proteins encoded by the viral genome. Efficient viral replication requires the proper function of these regulatory elements, and as such they may also be targets for therapy. An inhibitor of the transactivating protein (Tat) has been identified and is expected to enter clinical trials in the near future. Another approach to this step has been the construction of "antisense" segments of modified DNA (e.g., phosphorothioate oligodeoxynucleotides). These are strands of DNA, modified to prevent degradation by cellular nucleases, with sequences complementary to those of HIV RNA. They are believed in part to prevent the movement of ribosomes along the RNA and thus prevent viral proteins from being formed. Phosphorothioate oligodeoxynucleosides can also inhibit HIV replication in a sequence-nonspecific manner.

The last step in the replication of HIV is viral budding. There is evidence that interferon-α can prevent HIV replication in vitro, in part by acting on this final step. Interferons may have other sites of activity as well. Interferon-α has been found to have antitumor activity against Kaposi's sarcoma, particularly in patients with over 100 T4 cells per cubic millimeter who have

disease limited to the skin, and it has recently been approved for HIV-associated Kaposi's sarcoma. It has been found to have synergistic anti-HIV activity with AZT in vitro, and this combination is now being explored in patients with HIV infection.

A final word should be said about strategies to boost the immune system of individuals with HIV infection. The progression of HIV infection to fulminant AIDS represents an interplay between the infective potential of the virus and the ability of the immune system to interfere with this process. In most if not all patients, the virus eventually prevails in the absence of specific therapy and fulminant AIDS develops. Even so, the immune response against HIV certainly slows down this process, and a boosting of the immune system (or of the specific response to HIV) might prove to be advantageous to HIV-infected patients. However, there are also some theoretical considerations to suggest that T-cell activation could trigger viral replication and thereby harm the patient. A variety of experimental approaches to this have been explored, including administration of cytokines (such as interleukin 2) and immunostimulatory drugs. Trials of some of these approaches are still ongoing, but none has so far been definitively shown to offer clinical benefit. Recently, progress has been made in understanding the specific aspects of the immune response which control HIV infection and in eliciting such responses, and it is possible that such an approach will be found to be beneficial in combination with antiretroviral therapy.

Combinations of drugs may potentially offer several advantages over a given single agent. Indeed, it is likely that as individual drugs are developed, combination regimens will become the mainstay of therapy for HIV infection. The use of several agents may help delay the development of HIV resistance. Also, certain combinations, particularly those that act at different steps in the viral replicative cycle, may have synergistic anti-HIV activity. Moreover, combinations of drugs with different toxicity profiles, for example AZT and ddC, may permit a sustained anti-HIV effect with reduced toxicity from either drug. The various agents could be administered either sequentially (e.g., alternating weekly) or simultaneously, and clinical studies will be needed to sort out the relative merits of these approaches. For example, an alternating regimen of AZT and ddC may provide rest periods from each drug, while there is some evidence that they may be synergistic if used simultaneously. Certain drugs may be useful in suppressing certain opportunistic infections and thus have a secondary effect on HIV infection. For example, acyclovir can suppress herpesviruses and might thus indirectly reduce HIV infection (a nuclear regulatory protein of herpesviruses can activate HIV replication). The combination of AZT and acyclovir is usually tolerated and is now used by a number of physicians, particularly for patients who are troubled by recurrent herpes infection. However, it remains to be seen whether this regimen offers any advantages over AZT as a single drug. Combination therapy of AIDS will be an important area for clinical investigation in the near future. However, physicians should be cautioned against ad hoc experimentation in this area, as unexpected drug interactions may occur.

CLINICAL TRIALS OF AIDS DRUGS

Since AIDS-related therapeutics is a rapidly evolving field, it may be worthwhile to provide a brief summary of some principles for developing new drugs and biologics. The clinical evaluation of new drugs generally involves three phases of clinical trials. The first, called Phase I, typically involves toxicity testing. Groups of three to six patients are each administered increasing doses of the drug until a toxic dose is reached; the dose immediately below that level is considered the "maximal tolerated dose." Phase II studies conventionally involve determinations of activity in small groups of patients using doses selected from the Phase I experience. Phase III studies involve definitive testing of efficacy in large groups of patients and generally involve comparison with placebo or with accepted treatment. Such trials also provide useful information on the long-term toxicity profile of the drug in large numbers of patients.

Because of the urgent need to develop effective drugs for AIDS, this process has been compressed somewhat. Phase I studies of new AIDS drugs are now often examined for evidence of a possible anti-HIV effect (activity) in addition to toxicity data. Changes in the number of T4 lymphocytes or other measures of immune function are monitored. HIV p24 antigenemia or related measures of viremia have been useful in detecting effects of HIV replication. Other tests, such as quantitative polymerase chain reaction analyses for HIV genome or plasma culture of HIV, are now being studied for their ability to detect an anti-HIV effect. Laboratory tests per se, however, as "surrogate markers" for a clinical effect, have generally not yet been accepted by regulatory agencies for demonstrating the efficacy of AIDS drugs. Clinical endpoints, such as an effect on survival, disease progression, or the development of opportunistic infections, have so far been required. However, this issue is now being actively studied. There are recent data, for example, to indicate that patients receiving AZT-based therapy in a research setting rarely die until their T4 count falls below 50 cells per cubic millimeter.

Along with the extraction of activity data from Phase I trials, there is a trend toward combining Phase II and Phase III trials for anti-AIDS drugs so that potentially the agents can be approved after two rounds of testing. In the case of AZT, for example, Phase I testing provided strong evidence that the drug had anti-HIV activity. A 282-patient randomized placebo-controlled trial subsequently showed clear evidence that patients taking AZT had a survival advantage over those taking placebo, and the drug was approved at that point. There are a number of risks to patients and society at large from such an accelerated drug development, and clinical researchers are at present trying to grapple with the best balance between speed, safety, and accuracy in developing AIDS drugs, as well as the imperative to provide compassionate therapy for dying patients.

Before the development of AZT, there was no effective anti-retroviral therapy for AIDS, and the Phase II AZT trial was designed to show a difference between patients taking AZT and those taking placebo with respect to survival and the development of opportunistic infections. Trials of new therapies may now be designed to show that the therapy is superior to AZT (or other standard therapy) or alternately may be designed to show that the new treatment is equivalent to the standard treatment but may possess fewer side effects or offer other benefits. In efficacy studies, it is important that each patient be followed for a sufficiently long period of time for potential differences to appear. For example, there are data to suggest that AZT requires 6 weeks or so to bring about immunologic improvements, and only after this period can a difference in the development of opportunistic infections be observed.

In determining the optimal sample size for such efficacy studies, it is important to consider two potential types of error

which may occur. The first, called a type I error, happens when investigators conclude that two treatments have different effects when in fact the effects are equivalent. In general, studies are designed and carried out so that the probability of a type I error (called α) is 5 per cent or less. This is usually denoted as $P < 0.05$. The second type of error, called type II, occurs when an investigator concludes that two treatments have the same effect when in fact they are different. The probability that this will occur (called β), depends on the specified difference in outcome required in order for the results to be considered different and on the number of subjects entered into the study. A trial may be designed, for example, to permit a 20 per cent type II error in detecting a 10 per cent survival difference at 1 year. This means there is one chance in five of not observing a difference, even though there is a "real difference" between the drugs under study. In such a case the "power" of the study to detect this 10 per cent difference in 1-year survival is $1 - \beta$, or 80 per cent. Studies with a power of less than 80 per cent run the serious risk of missing real differences between treatments. Careful study design, including appropriate numbers of patients, can ensure an adequate power in a clinical trial.

Once one has estimated the likelihood of events occurring in the control population in a given period of time, chosen the differences in event rates required to conclude that the treatments are different, and chosen rates of type I and type II errors which one will accept, it is possible to estimate the sample size required. It is important to remember, however, that even in large studies, there is always some possibility of an incorrect conclusion being reached, and clinicians should be aware of these limitations. Such considerations are particularly important in the testing of AIDS drugs, in which there has been an attempt to compress the development process.

GENERAL RECOMMENDATIONS

At the present time, AZT is the only specific antiretroviral therapy formally approved for HIV infection. It is recommended for patients with HIV infection with less than 500 T4 cells per cubic millimeter. For adults with symptomatic HIV infection, including AIDS, the recommended dose is 200 mg every 4 hours for 1 month and then 100 mg every 4 hours. For patients with asymptomatic HIV infection and less than 500 T4 cells per cubic millimeter, a dose of 100 mg administered every 4 hours while awake (500 mg per day) is recommended. There is clear-cut evidence that AZT can increase survival when administered to symptomatic HIV-infected patients with less than 200 T4 cells per cubic millimeter. There is also evidence that short-term progression to AIDS or severe ARC can be decreased by administration of AZT to patients with 200 to 500 T4 cells per cubic millimeter. For patients who develop toxicity on AZT, dose reductions may be necessary. Epoetin alfa can be considered for those patients who develop anemia and have circulating erythropoietin levels of less than 500 mU per milliliter.

In addition to AZT, interferon-α (which may have anti-HIV activity) is approved for its anti-Kaposi's activity, and ddC and ddI are now available under restricted conditions for patients who cannot tolerate or who have failed AZT. AIDS patients may develop many complications that require therapy in their own right, and physicians should be vigilant to monitor unexpected drug interactions.

Yearly vaccinations with killed influenza virus are advisable; however, vaccinations with attenuated viruses should generally be avoided in this population. Because of the high incidence of cervical carcinoma in sexually active HIV-infected women, yearly pelvic examinations and Pap tests are advised in this population. Chemoprophylaxis for PCP, generally with aerosolized pentamidine or trimethoprim-sulfamethoxazole, is now recommended for patients with less than 200 T4 cells per cubic millimeter. Finally, some physicians have found megestrol acetate to be useful in stimulating the appetite of patients with progressive wasting. Perhaps most importantly, physicians should be attuned to diagnose and treat the myriad complications that can develop in this immunosuppressed population (see Ch. 422 as well as other relevant chapters for specific complications).

Through the combination of antiretroviral therapy and improvements in the prevention, diagnosis, and treatment of the complications of HIV infection, much progress has been made in the last several years. Given the agents now in laboratory and clinical development, physicians will likely have an expanding armamentarium of anti-AIDS drugs in the near future. The pace of research in this area is rapid, and physicians treating patients with AIDS should remain alert to ongoing developments that may dramatically alter accepted medical practice with very little advance notice.

Review Articles

Hirsch MS, Kaplan JC: Treatment of human immunodeficiency virus infections. Antimicrob Agents Chemother 31:839–843, 1987. *Overview of approaches to AIDS therapies.*

Mitsuya H, Yarchoan R, Broder S: Molecular targets for AIDS therapy. Science 249:1533–1544, 1990. *Detailed review article discussing the variety of approaches that can be taken to inhibit HIV infection.*

Yarchoan R, Mitsuya H, Myers CE, Broder S: Clinical pharmacology of 3′-azido-2′,3′-dideoxythymidine (zidovudine) and related dideoxynucleosides. N Engl J Med 321:726–738, 1989. *Review article stressing the metabolism and clinical pharmacology of dideoxynucleosides. Extensive bibliography.*

In Vitro Studies of Dideoxynucleosides

Furman PA, Fyfe JA, St. Clair M, et al.: Phosphorylation of 3′-azido-3′-deoxythymidine and selective interaction of the 5′-triphosphate with human immunodeficiency virus reverse transcriptase. Proc Natl Acad Sci USA 83:8333–8337, 1986. *Describes the anabolic phosphorylation of AZT and its effects on cellular kinases.*

Hartshorn KL, Vogt MW, Chou T-C, et al.: Synergistic inhibition of human immunodeficiency virus in vitro by azidothymidine and recombinant alpha A interferon. Antimicrob Agents Chemother 31:168–172, 1987. *Discussion of synergy in anti-HIV therapy.*

Mitsuya H, Broder S: Inhibition of the in vitro infectivity and cytopathic effect of human T-lymphotropic virus type III/lymphadenopathy virus-associated virus (HTLV-III/LAV) by 2′,3′-dideoxynucleosides. Proc Natl Acad Sci USA 83:1911–1915, 1986. *Description of potent anti-HIV activity of a variety of dideoxynucleosides.*

Mitsuya H, Weinhold KJ, Furman PA, et al.: 3′-Azido-3′-deoxythymidine (BW A509U): An antiviral agent that inhibits the infectivity and cytopathic effect of human T-lymphotropic virus type III/lymphadenopathy-associated virus in vitro. Proc Natl Acad Sci USA 82:7096–7100, 1985. *Description of in vitro anti-HIV activity of AZT.*

Clinical Studies of AZT (Zidovudine)

Dalakos MC, Illa I, Pezeshkpour GH, et al.: Mitochondrial myopathy caused by long-term zidovudine therapy. N Engl J Med 322:1098–1105, 1990. *Description of the clinical and pathologic features of AZT-induced myopathy.*

Dournon E, Matheron S, Rozenbaum W, et al.: Effects of zidovudine in 365 consecutive patients with AIDS or AIDS-related complex. Lancet 2:1297–1302, 1988. *Discussion of the activity and toxicity profile of AZT therapy in a general AIDS population.*

Fischl MA, Richman DD, Grieco MH, et al.: The efficacy of azidothymidine (AZT) in the treatment of patients with AIDS and AIDS-related complex: A double-blind, placebo-controlled trial. N Engl J Med 317:185–191, 1987. *Efficacy data from the Phase II trial of AZT that demonstrated an effect on the survival of patients with AIDS.*

Fischl M, Parker C, Pettinelli C, et al.: A randomized controlled trial of a reduced daily dose of zidovudine in patients with acquired immunodeficiency syndrome. N Engl J Med 323:1009–1014, 1990. *Article providing the basis for the current dose recommendation of AZT in AIDS.*

Fischl M, Richman DD, Hansen N, et al.: The safety and efficacy of zidovudine (AZT) in the treatment of subjects with mildly symptomatic human immunodeficiency virus type I (HIV) infection. A double-blind, placebo controlled trial. Ann Intern Med 112:727–737, 1990. *Data that AZT reduces the short-term progression to AIDS in mildly symptomatic patients with 200 to 500 T4 cells per cubic millimeter.*

Larder BA, Darby G, Richman DD: HIV with reduced sensitivity to zidovudine (AZT) isolated during prolonged therapy. Science 243:1731–1734, 1989. *Presents evidence that HIV isolated from patients on long-term AZT therapy often has reduced sensitivity to AZT.*

Pizzo PA, Eddy J, Falloon J, et al.: Effect of continuous intravenous infusion zidovudine (AZT) in children with symptomatic HIV infection. N Engl J Med 319:889–896, 1988. *Effect of AZT on HIV infection and in particular HIV-induced neurologic dysfunction in children with HIV infection.*

Richman DD, Fischl MA, Grieco MH, et al.: The toxicity of azidothymidine (AZT) in the treatment of patients with AIDS and AIDS-related complex: A double-blind, placebo-controlled trial. N Engl J Med 317:192–197, 1987. *Data on AZT toxicity from the Phase II trial.*

Volberding PA, Lagakos SW, Koch MA, et al.: Zidovudine in asymptomatic human immunodeficiency virus infection. A controlled trial in persons with fewer than 500 CD4-positive cells per cubic millimeter. N Engl J Med 322:941–949, 1990. *Describes the efficacy of AZT in preventing progression to AIDS when administered to asymptomatic HIV-infected patients.*

Yarchoan R, Berg G, Brouwers P, et al.: Response of human-immunodeficiency-virus–associated neurological disease to 3′-azido-3′-deoxythymidine. Lancet 1:132–135, 1987. *Describes the activity of AZT on AIDS dementia and its ability to reverse HIV-induced abnormalities of cerebral glucose metabolism.*

Yarchoan R, Klecker RW, Weinhold KJ, et al.: Administration of 3′-azido-3′-deoxythymidine, an inhibitor of HTLV-III/LAV replication, to patients with

AIDS or AIDS-related complex. Lancet 1:575–580, 1986. *First description of the clinical activity of AZT.*

Clinical Studies of Other Dideoxynucleosides

Butler KM, Husson RN, Balis FM, et al.: Dideoxyinosine (ddI) in symptomatic HIV-infected children: A phase I–II study. N Engl J Med 324:137–144, 1991. *Data showing effect of ddI on HIV infection and in particular on HIV-induced neurologic dysfunction in children.*

Cooley TP, Kunches LM, Saunders CA, et al.: Once-daily administration of 2′,3′-dideoxyinosine (ddI) in patients with the acquired immunodeficiency syndrome or AIDS-related complex. N Engl J Med 322:1340–1345, 1990. *Study showing the short-term activity and toxicity of ddI given once daily.*

Lambert JS, Seidlin M, Reichman RC, et al.: 2′,3′-Dideoxyinosine (ddI) in patients with the acquired immunodeficiency syndrome or the AIDS-related complex. A Phase I trial. N Engl J Med 322:1333–1340, 1990. *A study showing the short-term activity and toxicity profile of ddI given twice daily.*

Merigan TC, Skowron G, Bozzette SA, et al.: Circulating p24 antigen levels and responses to dideoxycytidine in human immunodeficiency virus (HIV) infections. Ann Intern Med 110:189–194, 1989. *More detailed profile of the effect of ddC on HIV p24 antigenemia in patients with severe HIV infection.*

Yarchoan R, Pluda JM, Thomas RV, et al.: Long-term toxicity/activity profile of 2′,3′-dideoxyinosine in AIDS or AIDS-related complex. Lancet 2:526–529, 1990. *Data showing the long-term toxicity profile of ddI and its ability to induce sustained T4 elevations.*

Yarchoan R, Perno CF, Thomas RV, et al.: Phase I studies of 2′,3′-dideoxycytidine in severe human immunodeficiency virus infection as a single agent and alternating with zidovudine (AZT). Lancet 1:76–81, 1988. *Data from Phase I trial of ddC.*

Other Agents

Capon DJ, Chamow SM, Mordenti J, et al.: Designing CD4 immunoadhesions for AIDS therapy. Nature 337:525–531, 1989. *Discussion of rCD4-IgG immunoadhesions and the general approach of engineered CD4 as a therapy for AIDS.*

Lane HC, Kovacs JA, Feinberg J, et al.: Anti-retroviral effects of interferon-alpha in AIDS-associated Kaposi's sarcoma. Lancet 2:1218–1222, 1988. *Article showing evidence of an anti-HIV effect of interferon in certain patients with Kaposi's sarcoma.*

Meek TD, Lambert DM, Dreyer GB, et al.: Inhibition of HIV-1 protease in infected T-lymphocytes by synthetic peptide analogues. Nature 343:90–92, 1990. *Discussion of the approach of inhibiting HIV protease.*

Effects of Therapy on the Epidemiology of HIV Infection

Gail MH, Rosenberg P, Goedert J: Therapy may explain recent deficits in AIDS incidence. J AIDS 3:296–306, 1990. *Describes a decline in the incidence of AIDS in homosexual men since 1987 and provides evidence that this is an effect of improvements in therapy, particularly the introduction of AZT.*

Lemp GF, Payne SF, Neal D, et al.: Survival trends for patients with AIDS. JAMA 263:402–406, 1990. *Shows improvement in survival in patients with AIDS since 1986 and a correlation of this effect with AZT therapy.*

Clinical Trial Methodology

Freiman JA, Chalmers TC, Smith H Jr, Kuebler RR: The importance of beta, the type II error and sample size in the design and interpretation of the randomized clinical trial. Survey of 71 "negative" trials. N Engl J Med 299:690–694, 1978. *Good discussion of type I and type II errors and the power of the statistical test of significance in clinical trials.*

422 Chronic Management and Counseling for Persons with HIV Infection

John A. Bartlett

HISTORICAL PERSPECTIVE

The clinical syndrome of Kaposi's sarcoma and *Pneumocystis carinii* pneumonia (PCP) occurring in previously healthy young homosexual men was originally described in 1981. For the next 3 years efforts focused upon the epidemiology of this immunodeficiency state and identification of the responsible infectious agent. The clinical care for these patients was extremely limited and consisted of the delayed treatment of complications with little ability to provide early intervention, preventive treatment, or treatment aimed at the underlying retroviral infection. The past 10 years have witnessed an unprecedented growth of knowledge about AIDS and its causative agent, human immunodeficiency virus (HIV). Early treatment aimed at HIV or the complications of the immunodeficiency state can now delay the onset of full-blown AIDS. For persons with severe AIDS-related complex (ARC) or AIDS, zidovudine can prolong survival, with the preservation of meaningful and productive time. For example, the median survival for a patient with PCP prior to the advent of zidovudine or PCP prophylaxis was 10.5 months; the same patient now has an almost 90 per cent chance of survival at 1 year. AIDS has truly become an illness to be "managed" medically on a chronic basis.

INTRODUCTION

Providing health care to persons with HIV infection represents a tremendous challenge to the involved medical personnel. This challenge is very broad and contains facets involving significant medical, psychological, and social issues. The optimal care for persons with HIV infection must include a comprehensive approach to all of these issues, and therein lies the essential principle for their successful clinical management.

Between 1 and 1.5 million Americans are infected with HIV, and to date only 10 per cent of those infected have been diagnosed with AIDS. As HIV infection progresses within this population and as new HIV infections occur, the burden of their health care needs will increase tremendously. It is doubtful that any health care provider will not have the opportunity to care for HIV-infected persons in the coming 10 years.

NATURAL HISTORY

Understanding the natural history of HIV infection is essential prior to beginning a discussion of medical management. HIV infection is a chronic viral illness characterized by progressive immunologic impairment. The immunologic damage can be directly measured through the determination of lymphocyte subsets, specifically in the absolute number and percentage of CD4 (or T-helper) lymphocytes. The CD4 lymphocyte is the primary target of HIV infection, and declines in the number and percentage of CD4 lymphocytes correlate most closely with clinical progression of HIV infection. It must be emphasized that HIV infection is a chronic illness with a median delay of approximately 10 years between acute infection and progression to AIDS (Fig. 422–1). Full-blown AIDS is a clinical syndrome defined by the occurrence of complicating opportunistic infections and neoplasms and severe HIV-related symptoms. It is simply a clinical manifestation of the underlying immunologic deficit and repre-

sents the end-stage of many years of progressive immunologic damage. Once an individual has been diagnosed with AIDS, there is an anticipated series of complications which can occur. Grossly these can be categorized into relatively early and late complications (Fig. 422–2). Although significant advances have occurred in the treatment of AIDS and its complications, it remains a fatal illness.

MEDICAL MANAGEMENT

Based upon the understanding of the natural history of HIV infection, the medical management of HIV infection focuses upon two major goals: delay in the progression of HIV infection to AIDS and improvement in the quantity and quality of life for persons who have progressed to AIDS. Four aspects of medical management are discussed: the initial evaluation, assessing the need for antiretroviral therapy, assessing the need for preventive therapy, and evaluating the febrile patient with HIV infection.

Initial Evaluation

Each person with HIV infection should undergo an initial comprehensive evaluation of his or her HIV infection to serve as a foundation for subsequent decisions (Table 422–1). Obviously this evaluation begins with a careful history. Specific points to be addressed include the duration of HIV infection, previous evaluations, HIV-related symptoms, HIV-related complications, history of sexually transmitted diseases, previous tuberculin testing or tuberculosis exposure, previous residential and travel history, and medication allergies. Because HIV infection and its complications involve all organ systems, a thorough physical examination is essential. The areas of greatest concern include the skin, eyes, oropharynx, lymphatics, genital and perirectal areas, and neurologic system.

The initial laboratory examination should include a complete blood count with differential, electrolytes, liver and kidney chemistries, lymphocyte subset analysis, and VDRL. Persons with a past history of a negative PPD more than 1 year previously should have a 5TU PPD placed. Persons with a current or past positive PPD should receive 1 year of isoniazid owing to their high risk of tuberculosis reactivation. Persons with HIV infection are at an increased risk for pneumococcal disease and complications of influenza. Currently both vaccinations are recommended, although the serologic response of this population has not been well documented. Based upon this initial evaluation of HIV infection, careful staging can be performed and the relevant therapeutic issues addressed.

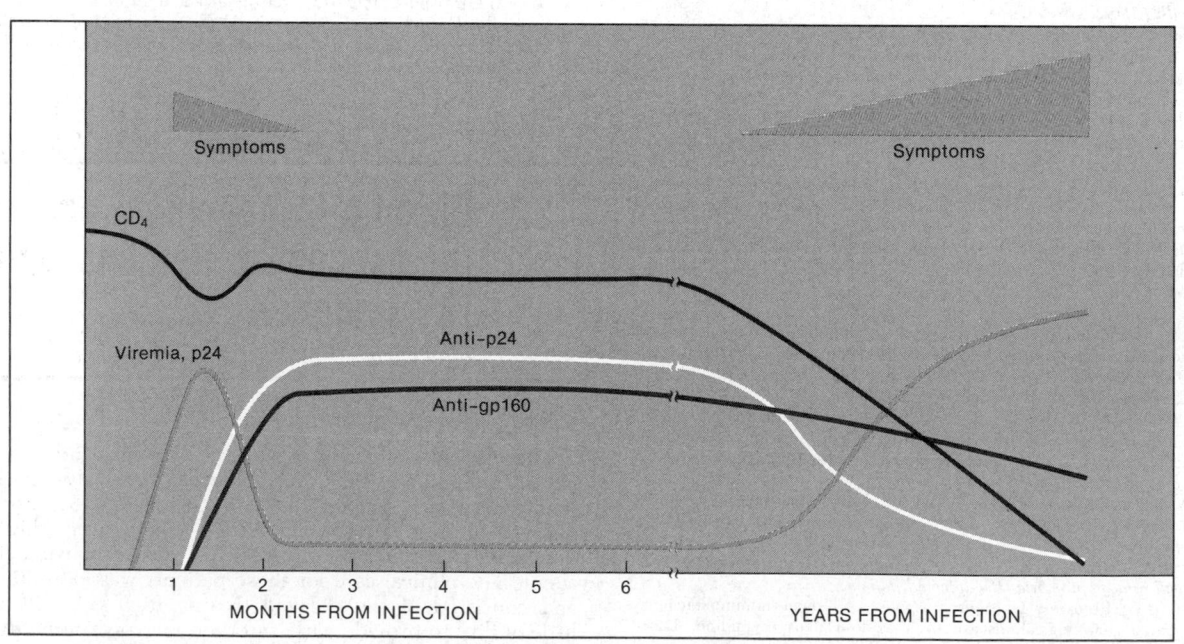

FIGURE 422–1. Model of the time course of HIV-1 infection. (Modified from Clark SJ, et al.: High titer of cytopathic virus in plasma of patients with symptomatic primary HIV-1 infection. N Engl J Med 324:954–960, 1991. By permission of the New England Journal of Medicine.)

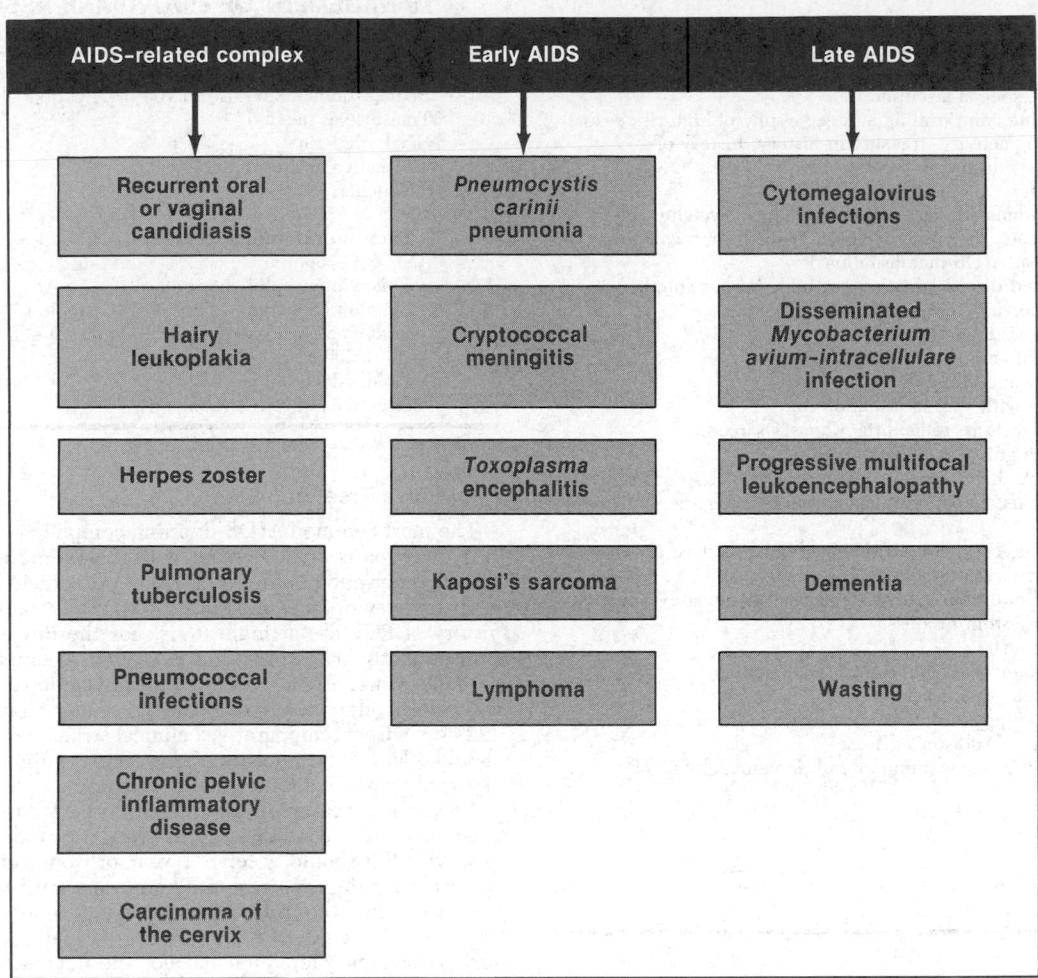

AIDS-related complex	Early AIDS	Late AIDS
Recurrent oral or vaginal candidiasis	*Pneumocystis carinii* pneumonia	Cytomegalovirus infections
Hairy leukoplakia	Cryptococcal meningitis	Disseminated *Mycobacterium avium-intracellulare* infection
Herpes zoster	*Toxoplasma* encephalitis	Progressive multifocal leukoencephalopathy
Pulmonary tuberculosis	Kaposi's sarcoma	Dementia
Pneumococcal infections	Lymphoma	Wasting
Chronic pelvic inflammatory disease		
Carcinoma of the cervix		

FIGURE 422–2. Time line of AIDS-related complications.

Antiretroviral Therapy (see Ch. 421)

Antiretroviral therapy is currently in its infancy. Only one approved treatment is available—zidovudine (previously known as azidothymidine or AZT). Fortunately, zidovudine has shown significant antiretroviral and clinical activity across a spectrum of persons with HIV infection.

Zidovudine has also demonstrated clinical efficacy in the treatment of patients with severe ARC and AIDS. This efficacy is defined as both a prolongation in survival and an improvement in quality of life as assessed by increased Karnofsky performance status, weight gain, neurocognitive functioning, and fewer opportunistic infections. Zidovudine may also increase platelet counts in HIV-associated idiopathic thrombocytopenic purpura and improve the dermatologic and rheumatologic manifestations associated with HIV.

The optimal dosing schedule for zidovudine remains to be defined (see Ch. 421). A dose of 100 mg orally five times per day is currently recommended, but the best schedule and lowest effective dosage are uncertain. Persons with HIV-associated neurologic disease may benefit from a higher dose of 200 mg orally five times daily.

Zidovudine may cause significant toxicity in persons with HIV infection, predominantly involving suppression of erythropoiesis and myelopoiesis. The occurrence of toxicity is clearly related to the stage of HIV infection, pretreatment hemoglobin and neutrophil counts, and zidovudine dosage. Nonhematologic toxicities may include nausea, headaches, alterations in mental status, myositis, fevers, rash, hepatitis, and seizures.

All persons with HIV infection and a CD4 lymphocyte count of less than 500 per cubic millimeter should receive zidovudine (Table 422–2). If an individual's CD4 lymphocyte count is greater than 500 per cubic millimeter, his or her CD4 lymphocyte count should be repeated at intervals of 6 months to closely monitor

the need for zidovudine. It is also likely that the therapeutic efficacy of zidovudine may be demonstrated in HIV-infected persons with greater than 500 CD4 lymphocytes per cubic millimeter in the future, and consequently the threshold value of CD4 lymphocytes may be altered. Once zidovudine is begun, complete blood counts and chemistries should be followed every other week for 2 months, then monthly thereafter provided that these parameters remain stable. The management of zidovudine-related toxicity can be very challenging (Table 422–3). Anemia may be managed through dosage reduction, transfusions, or the administration of erythropoietin. Zidovudine-associated neutropenia is generally well tolerated down to absolute neutrophil counts of 500 per cubic millimeter and may respond to dosage reduction or the administration of granulocyte colony stimulating factors when necessary. As a general therapeutic principle, most clinicians attempt to maintain patients on zidovudine whenever possible without interruptions. Concern about frequent discontinuations of therapy originates in the observations of increases in p24 antigen levels and virus culture positivity in patients who have recently discontinued zidovudine. CD4 lymphocyte counts in persons with pretreatment counts greater than 200 per cubic millimeter receiving zidovudine are followed at least every 6 months owing to the need for initiation of PCP prophylaxis when counts fall below 200 per cubic millimeter. In persons with pretreatment counts of less than 200 per cubic millimeter on zidovudine and PCP prophylaxis, the follow-up of CD4 lymphocyte counts adds little to therapeutic decisions, given the lack of currently available therapeutic alternatives.

Zidovudine-resistant HIV isolates were recently identified from persons with ARC or AIDS who had received prolonged zidovudine treatment. However, there were no clinical or laboratory correlations with the isolation of resistant virus. The clinical significance of zidovudine-resistant isolates, the effect of disease stage on the frequency of resistant isolates, and the ramifications

TABLE 422–1. INITIAL EVALUATION OF THE HIV-INFECTED PATIENT

Medical history with special attention to:
  Duration of HIV infection (timing and geography of high-risk sexual or needle-sharing activity, transfusion history, history of mononucleosis syndrome)
  Previous evaluations
  HIV-related symptoms and complications (fatigue, weight loss, fevers, chills, night sweats, diarrhea, dementia, thrush, herpes zoster, hairy leukoplakia, AIDS manifestations)
  Sexually transmitted diseases history (syphilis, herpes simplex, hepatitis B, gonorrhea, chlamydia)
  Previous tuberculosis testing or exposure
  Previous residential and travel history
  Medication history and allergies
Physical examination with special attention to:
  Skin (seborrhea, psoriasis, folliculitis, Kaposi's sarcoma)
  Lymphatics (extrainguinal lymphadenopathy)
  Oropharynx (thrush, hairy leukoplakia, ulcerations, Kaposi's sarcoma)
  Genitalia (ulcerations, Kaposi's sarcoma, penile discharge, epididymitis)
  Rectum (ulcerations, condylomata, hemorrhoids, fistulas, abscesses, prostatitis, Kaposi's sarcoma)
  Neurologic (peripheral neuropathy, dementia, myelopathy, focal central nervous system lesions)
Laboratory examination
  Complete blood count with differential (leukopenia, thrombocytopenia, anemia)
  Electrolytes with kidney and liver chemistries (chronic hepatitis, renal insufficiency, Addison's disease)
  Lymphocyte subset analysis (number and percentage of CD4 lymphocytes)
  VDRL
  PPD
Vaccinations
  Pneumovax
  Influenza

for the initiation of zidovudine treatment remain to be determined. Many other drugs to treat HIV infection are in the process of laboratory or clinical development (see Ch. 421).

Access and entry into HIV treatment trials are important issues for patients and health care providers. Participation is increasingly available through both academic and private medical centers. Many persons with HIV infection are well informed regarding their illness and potential treatments, and access to new agents is an extremely important issue in their health care. The efficient entry of interested patients into well-designed clinical trials serves to advance the development of improved treatment most rapidly.

Persons with HIV infection not enrolled in clinical trials may choose to pursue complementary or alternative treatments to zidovudine. Such treatments, it is hoped, are not to the exclusion of zidovudine. Given the recognition that many of these treatments are of unproven benefit but also of little potential harm to patients, most AIDS clinicians accept their patients' desires to pursue complementary treatments.

TREATMENT OF HIV-RELATED COMPLICATIONS

All patients with progressive HIV infection can be anticipated to have a series of complications due to their immune compromise. These complications can be broadly categorized as early or late (Fig. 422–2). Treatment may be preventive in patients identified as high risk for a given complication, or it may begin after the complication has occurred.

TABLE 422–2. THERAPEUTIC DECISIONS IN HIV INFECTION

CD4 Count (per mm³)	Recommendation
>500	Follow CD4 count every 3–6 months
≤500, >200	Begin zidovudine, follow CD4 count every 3–6 months
≤200	Begin zidovudine and PCP prophylaxis

TABLE 422–3. SUGGESTED SCHEME FOR THE MANAGEMENT OF ZIDOVUDINE-ASSOCIATED HEMATOLOGIC TOXICITY

Anemia defined by symptoms or hemoglobin ≤ 8 grams/dl
  Reduce zidovudine dose to 100 mg PO q8h
  Transfuse as needed
  Erythropoietin
  Alternative antiretroviral agent
Neutropenia
  ANC* > 750/mm³
    Maintain zidovudine dosage
  ANC 500–750/mm³
    Follow neutrophil count closely
    Maintain zidovudine dose if ANC stable
    Reduce zidovudine dose to 100 mg PO q8h if ANC falling
  ANC < 500/mm³
    Hold zidovudine
    Alternative antiretroviral agent

*ANC = Absolute neutrophil count.

Preventive Treatment

The most common AIDS-defining complication in persons with HIV infection is PCP. Persons with CD4 lymphocyte counts less than 200 per cubic millimeter, CD4 percentage less than 20 per cent, early symptoms and signs of HIV infection, and a previous history of PCP are at highest risk for the development of PCP. Consequently, PCP prophylaxis is now recommended for these patients. Currently a variety of prophylactic regimens are available; each offers relative advantages and disadvantages (Table 422–4). Direct comparative clinical trials are underway and should clarify the merits of different prophylactic regimens, especially when combined with zidovudine.

Preventive treatment is being explored for tuberculosis, toxoplasmosis, and candidiasis. All HIV-infected persons with a positive PPD should receive 1 year of isoniazid. They may also be tested for the presence of *Toxoplasma* antibody; clinical trials are evaluating the role of suppressive treatment for persons previously infected with *Toxoplasma*. Finally, antifungal agents such as clotrimazole, ketoconazole, and fluconazole may be given in a preventive fashion to avoid oropharyngeal candidiasis.

Acute and Chronic Treatment

Many of the complications of HIV infection are infectious illnesses caused by opportunistic pathogens. Three principles are important in prescribing treatment for complicating infections: The infections are frequently widely disseminated at the time of diagnosis, the host immune response is minimal, and without chronic suppressive therapy many infections relapse. Chronic therapy is important for many bacterial, protozoal, fungal, and viral infections. As the number of infectious complications increases, the complexity of an individual's chronic suppressive treatment increases. With the improved recognition of infectious complications, the improved treatment options for these complications, and the use of survival-prolonging antiretroviral drugs such as zidovudine, many persons with AIDS are now developing multiple chronic infections necessitating lifelong suppression.

Neoplasms are also common complications of progressive HIV infection. Although the incidence of Kaposi's sarcoma has de-

TABLE 422–4. PROPHYLACTIC REGIMENS FOR *PNEUMOCYSTIS CARINII* PNEUMONIA

	Advantages	Disadvantages
Sulfamethoxazole-trimethoprim	Low cost Systemic	Hematologic toxicity Fever Cutaneous reactions
Dapsone	Systemic	Hematologic toxicity Hepatic toxicity Fever Cutaneous reactions
Aerosolized pentamidine	Topical	High cost Bronchospasm Upper lobe or extra-pulmonary *Pneumocystis*

TABLE 422–5. EVALUATION OF THE FEBRILE PATIENT WITH HIV INFECTION

A. History
1. Duration, severity, and pattern of fever
2. Localizing symptoms (headache, visual changes, central nervous system abnormalities, pharyngitis, odynophagia, cough, chest pain, abdominal pain, changes in bowel habits or stools, urinary tract symptoms, skin abnormalities, or changes in lymph nodes)
3. Previous febrile episodes and associated causes
4. CD4 lymphocyte counts
B. Physical examination
1. Vital signs
2. Special emphasis
   a. Eye—retinitis, papilledema
   b. Oropharynx—thrush, ulcerations, Kaposi's sarcoma
   c. Lungs—physical findings of pneumonia
   d. Abdomen—hepatobiliary disease, gastroenteritis, colitis
   e. Genitalia—prostatitis, sexually transmitted diseases
   f. Rectum—ulcerations, abscesses
   g. Skin—ulcerations, abscesses
   h. Central nervous system—nuchal rigidity, focal abnormalities
C. Laboratory studies
1. General
   a. Complete blood count with differential
   b. Blood cultures
      Routine bacterial
      Lysis/centrifugation tubes—fungi, mycobacteria
   c. Serum cryptococcal titer
   d. Urinalysis
2. Respiratory symptoms
   a. Chest radiograph
   b. Arterial blood gas
   c. Sputum induction with special stains
   d. Bronchoscopy
3. Central nervous system abnormalities
   a. Head computed tomography or magnetic resonance scanning
   b. Lumbar puncture

creased, it remains a frequent complication of AIDS. Isolated lesions are usually not treated, and locally symptomatic disease may respond to radiation therapy. When disseminated cutaneous or visceral disease is present, interferon-α or combination chemotherapy may be useful. Non-Hodgkin's lymphomas may occur in persons with AIDS and may be treated with traditional chemotherapy and/or radiation therapy. Unfortunately, the use of chemotherapy may prohibit the concomitant prescription of zidovudine owing to combined myelosuppression.

The neurologic complications of HIV infection are also relatively common. Among the most problematic are HIV-associated peripheral neuropathy and dementia. The neurocognitive and behavioral abnormalities may respond to antiretroviral therapy with zidovudine, especially in high doses. The treatment of HIV-associated peripheral neuropathy is more difficult and may respond only to symptomatic treatment such as amitriptyline.

As the longevity of persons with AIDS increases, the number of complications also increases. Given the need for chronic suppressive treatment, one person with AIDS may be receiving many oral, intravenous, and aerosolized medications. This plethora of drugs forces the clinician to be keenly aware of drug interactions and also raises difficult issues of patient compliance and pharmaceutical costs.

Evaluation of the Febrile Patient

The most common reason for an unscheduled clinic visit of a person with HIV infection is the development of fever. The clinician must begin the evaluation with a careful history (Table 422–5). Important elements of fever include its severity (low grade versus hectic), duration, and pattern. The discovery of localizing symptoms (headache, visual changes, central nervous system abnormalities, pharyngitis, odynophagia, cough, chest pain, abdominal pain, changes in bowel habits or stools, urinary tract symptoms, skin abnormalities, or changes in lymph nodes) is very useful in identifying a fever source. The history of previous febrile episodes and associated causes is essential. Patients may frequently offer insightful hypotheses about the etiology of their fever. Finally, recent CD4 counts may be helpful in grossly assessing the likelihood of an opportunistic infection. For exam-

ple, a person with a recent CD4 lymphocyte count of less than 250 per cubic millimeter is clearly at risk for an opportunistic infection. Conversely, a person with a recent CD4 lymphocyte count greater than 250 per cubic millimeter is less likely to have an opportunistic infection.

A careful physical examination begins with vital signs. Obviously the temperature is important in a febrile patient, but pulse, blood pressure, and especially respirations need close attention. In patients complaining of dyspnea, it is frequently useful to stress the patient by walking or climbing stairs and observe the respiratory response. On physical examination, special emphasis should be placed upon the eye, oropharynx, lungs, abdomen, genitalia, rectum, skin, and central nervous system.

Laboratory studies should be tailored to the significant historical and physical findings. In general, blood counts, blood cultures including the use of lysis/centrifugation tubes for the isolation of fungi and mycobacteria, and serum cryptococcal antigen titers are useful tests when no specific etiology for the fever is apparent. For the patient with respiratory symptoms, a chest radiograph and arterial blood gas measurement are important. Remember that the most common radiographic appearance of PCP is a normal chest radiograph, although other radiographic appearances of PCP (upper lobe disease, unilateral or nodular infiltrates) may be found. Sputum induction with the use of rapid special stains for microorganisms can be performed immediately in the clinic. In some centers, the use of sputum induction with stains employing monoclonal antibodies against *P. carinii* can detect greater than 90 per cent of cases of proven PCP. Bronchoscopy can be performed if necessary in patients with a nondiagnostic sputum examination. In patients with headaches or central nervous system abnormalities, imaging of the brain with computed tomography or magnetic resonance scanning and lumbar puncture is essential.

The evaluation and treatment of febrile patients may frequently be accomplished on an outpatient basis. Many opportunistic infections including PCP, cryptococcal meningitis, *Toxoplasma* encephalitis, and cytomegalovirus retinitis can be treated on an outpatient basis. However, important elements of outpatient care must include a medically stable, compliant, and well-informed patient with easy access to the health care provider, the availability of personal care providers within the home, and home health care agencies to provide nursing, pharmaceutical, and technical care when necessary. Potentially home-based care can be beneficial to both patients and the health care system. Patients may be more comfortable and have an increased sense of control at home. Tremendous cost savings may also be realized through home-based care, and limited resources such as hospital beds may be reserved for the most acutely ill patients.

COUNSELING AND PSYCHOSOCIAL ISSUES

The proper recognition of the complex psychosocial issues in the care of persons with HIV infection offers the clinician an opportunity to truly excel in providing patient care. As a biologic process, HIV infection is simply a chronic viral infection resulting in progressive immunologic impairment. However, the person with HIV infection faces daily problems owing to the powerful psychological and social responses that accompany the diagnosis. Frequently persons with HIV infection may have been rejected by other health care providers, and the clinician must begin with an attitude of compassion, tolerance, and patience. The successful clinician caring for persons with HIV infection must adopt a comprehensive approach to patient care.

Counseling

Counseling for persons with HIV infection begins with a description of the biologic processes relevant to transmission and natural history. As a general principle, the clinician should not assume that patients are already familiar with these issues and should begin with a basic discussion. Modes of HIV transmission should be frankly discussed, with ample opportunity for patient-initiated questions. Prevention must be encouraged through safer sex measures, the avoidance of needle sharing, needle cleansing, and certain methods of birth control (Table 422–6). Frequently discussions of prevention are most productive when the patient

TABLE 422-6. MEASURES TO PREVENT HIV TRANSMISSION

Means of Transmission	Preventive Measures
Sexual contact	Use of condoms; use of spermicidal foams containing nonoxynol-9; limiting the number of sexual partners; informing sexual partners; no exchange of body fluids
Shared needles	No sharing of needles; cleaning needles with bleach; needle exchanges; education of health care workers about avoiding needle sticks
Blood or blood products	Screening of all donated blood and blood products for the presence of HIV antibody; heat treatment of clotting factors
Perinatal transmission	Certain means of birth control
Breast milk	Bottle feeding

is accompanied by his or her sexual partner, friends, or family. Prevention can be a successful means of interrupting HIV transmission. The homosexual community has engaged in an active program of self-education regarding prevention of HIV infection, and both indirect and direct evidence strongly suggest a decreased incidence of new HIV infections. Reaching intravenous drug users with educational campaigns presents a much greater challenge, but modest effects in decreasing the incidence of new HIV infections have been realized in areas where intense efforts are concentrated. Counseling about prevention is the most important intervention that can be offered until a vaccine or truly effective treatment becomes available.

The natural history of HIV infection should be reviewed with all HIV-infected persons. Explanation of the need for regular medical follow-up and the potential symptoms of HIV infection and its complications serve to improve their care. Persons with HIV infection may be well educated with regard to their medical illness, treatment, and prognosis. These patients frequently request an increased level of self-participation in their medical care. Although this desire for increased self-control may be perceived as threatening to the clinician, significant benefits can be gained by allowing this participation. Persons with HIV infection must be viewed within the context of young persons diagnosed with a chronic and perhaps ultimately fatal viral illness for which the therapeutic options are of limited benefit. In many respects, they have very little control over their illness. However, to the extent that any sense of control can be encouraged, a patient's anxiety level will be reduced. The successful sharing of control with patients requires a mature and understanding clinician who is not threatened by his or her patient's independence.

Psychological Issues

A proper consideration of the psychological issues of HIV infection begins with the understanding of risk behaviors. The issues of sexuality, intravenous drug use, transfusions, and parenthood must be acknowledged and accepted. Frequently these issues have resulted in important personality traits that antedate the development of HIV infection and continue to resurface during its course. They may lead to feelings of guilt, low self-esteem, isolation, mistrust, and discrimination which need to be addressed. Each risk category and each individual has a different mix of these feelings. In addition, the clinician must not allow his or her own reaction to risk behaviors to interfere with the provision of patient care.

Certainly an awareness of one's own HIV infection and its prognosis can lead to anxiety. Anxiety is a very common finding among persons with HIV infection across risk group categories and disease stages. Additional anxiety can result from concerns about sexuality; sharing the knowledge of one's infection with others and the potential for negative reactions; the loss of one's job, appearance, material possessions, and significant others; fear of the unknown; and loss of control in the waning stages of one's illness. Anxiety may lead to the difficulties with substance abuse commonly seen in persons with HIV infection. Alleviating anxiety may be accomplished by involving the patient actively in his or her own care, through frequent clinic visits, and through participation in peer support groups.

Once an individual is diagnosed with AIDS and the attendant recognition of AIDS as a terminal illness follows, a curious psychological paradox may occur for both the person with AIDS and his or her health care provider. Naturally persons with AIDS become bereaved as they recognize the finite period of their lives. They must develop personal priorities that incorporate the prognosis of AIDS. Preparing for death involves the difficult issues of the aggressiveness of health care interventions including cardiopulmonary resuscitation, writing a will, assigning durable power of attorney, identifying primary home care providers, and decisions about burial or cremation. However, persons with AIDS need a hopeful approach to the immediate demands of their health care whenever possible. Hope can be maintained by focusing on short-term health care goals and helping persons with AIDS to focus on short-term personal goals. In addition, currently available treatments for AIDS on both a practicing and research basis provide some opportunity of hope for a more prolonged survival with an improved quality of life. The navigation of this paradox may be very difficult for both persons with AIDS and health care providers, and the balance may tip in excessively depressed or hopeful directions. The use of community-based support groups may be helpful in maintaining this balance, and occasionally psychiatric consultation is necessary. Health care providers should also recognize that they may face their own fears about mortality as they aid their patients.

Clinicians must also investigate the social supports available to their patients. Significant issues include interpersonal support (lovers, spouses, family, and friends), insurance information (availability of coverage, limits of coverage, the ability to extend health insurance coverage beyond the period of employment, home care benefits, disability and life insurance), employment, and housing. Each of these issues may impact tremendously on the life of a person with HIV infection or AIDS. The contributions of a social worker may be invaluable in these areas.

SUMMARY

For the clinician caring for HIV-infected persons, both HIV infection and AIDS have become chronic illnesses to be managed over a period of years. The potential therapeutic interventions are rapidly increasing and have thus far contributed significantly to the improved quantity and quality of life for persons with HIV infection and AIDS. The clinician also has the opportunity to become involved with the complex social and psychological responses to HIV infection. In the future, all must hope for continued improvements in the treatment of HIV infection and for a more educated and enlightened response from society.

PART XXII
DISEASES CAUSED BY PROTOZOA AND METAZOA

423 Introduction to Protozoan and Helminthic Diseases

Adel A. F. Mahmoud

Human infections with parasitic protozoa and helminths account for a major proportion of the diseases caused by infectious agents. The magnitude of these infections is staggering; malaria infects 600 million, and ascariasis and trichuriasis 1 billion each, and 600 million are estimated to be infected with either schistosomiasis or filariasis. In spite of some worldwide efforts to control the spread and consequences of these infections, the associated morbidity and mortality have not been appreciably reduced. Furthermore, in the developed countries, infection with protozoa and helminths is being seen with increasing frequency in immigrants and is also among the more important causes of disease in the growing number of patients with depressed immune responses. Exciting developments have recently been reported concerning our understanding of the host-parasite relationship and the introduction of new and safe wide-spectrum chemotherapeutic agents.

BIOLOGY OF PARASITIC PROTOZOA AND HELMINTHS

This group of infectious agents belongs to the animal kingdom, unlike bacteria, viruses, or fungi. Such distinction led to restricting the term "parasite" to include only protozoa and helminths, whereas it should include all infectious agents because of their specialized dependent mode of life. The host-parasite relationship in protozoan and helminthic infections is complex because of the distinctive biologic features of the organisms. Although protozoa are unicellular pathogens and are mainly microscopic in size, they are far larger than viruses and bacteria. Protozoa multiply within mammalian hosts, as do viruses, bacteria, and fungi. Infection, therefore, can be initiated by a relatively small inoculum of organisms, which then multiply within the host and reach the numbers that cause disease.

By contrast, helminths are multicellular organisms with well-developed organ structures. They vary in size from 1 cm to approximately 10 meters. Unlike other infectious agents, helminths do not multiply within mammalian hosts. Re-exposure is, therefore, necessary to increase the number of helminths in a host. This distinguishing feature has important clinical significance, as disease in most helminthiasis is closely related to intensity of infection. For example, anemia results from hookworm infection only if the individual is harboring a significant worm load or there are other reasons for nutritional deficiencies. In rare circumstances, such as strongyloidiasis in the immunosuppressed, the worm can increase its population through an autoinfection cycle. This leads to life-threatening infection that necessitates aggressive medical attention.

Eosinophilia, when present, is a useful clinical manifestation of worm infections that migrate in host tissues. Worms that reside exclusively in body cavities, such as adult cestodes in the lumen of small intestines, are not associated with eosinophilia. Increased eosinophil counts may be observed in peripheral blood or affected tissues of infected individuals. Specific chemotherapy is usually followed by an increase in cell count before it subsides to normal levels. Eosinophilia in helminthic infections may be related to their ability to kill multicellular organisms. Because of the large size of most invading worms, killing of these targets by eosinophils occurs extracellularly and is mediated by a combination of oxidative and nonoxidative mechanisms.

Parasitic protozoa and helminths have developed elaborate mechanisms for evasion of host-protective responses. One of the best studied is antigenic variation noted in African trypanosomiasis. Parasitemia in infected individuals declines with the development of a protective antibody response but is followed by the emergence of a new parasite variable antigen; the organisms are therefore capable of avoiding the host response and increasing their numbers. The trypanosomes are capable of expressing at least 100 different variable antigens, allowing a long chronic course of infection. The organisms contain individual genes for all the different variable glycoproteins, but only one is expressed at a time. The multiplicity of trypanosome variable glycoprotein genes and of mechanisms for introducing mutations into them illustrates the complexity and sophistication of these pathogens.

The constantly changing nature of infectious disease is best illustrated in parasitic protozoan and helminthic infections. For example, new human pathogens such as *Isospora* and *Cryptosporidium* species have been appreciated only recently as causes of diarrheal illness, particularly in the immunosuppressed. These new developments add to difficulties in the treatment and control of parasitic protozoa and helminths. Recently, new chemotherapeutic agents have been developed, such as praziquantel and ivermectin, which are safe and effective broad-spectrum antihelminthics. However, the ever-spreading resistance of the parasites causing malaria and their mosquito vectors to most available compounds is imposing a considerable challenge to clinicians and public health specialists.

APPROACH TO THE PATIENT WITH PROTOZOAN OR HELMINTHIC INFECTION

Since most of the clinical manifestations of protozoan and helminthic diseases are not specific or pathognomonic, a high degree of suspicion is essential. The simple question "Where have you been?" and knowledge of the general geographic distribution of parasitic protozoa and helminths often save exhaustive and costly diagnostic workups and may spare human lives. Furthermore, inquiry into the immune status of individual patients, other drug therapies, or other diseases may be helpful in establishing the diagnosis of an opportunistic protozoan or helminthic infection.

The next phase in attempting to reach correct diagnosis involves interpretation of the presenting symptoms and signs. Peripheral blood eosinophilia remains an important and early indication of infections with tissue-invading worms. Definitive diagnosis in most cases requires isolation and identification of the specific pathogen. Since the number of cases seen by any single laboratory in North America is limited, expertise is required for correct identification that may not be available to many practicing physicians. Serologic testing for evidence of exposure to specific protozoa or helminths is currently available in many clinical or state laboratories or by consultation with the Centers for Disease Control. Although positive serologic results do not usually differentiate between past or present exposure, they are particularly helpful to physicians practicing outside areas endemic to these infectious diseases.

Centers for Disease Control: HHS Publication No. (CDC) 90–8280. Health Information for International Travel, Atlanta, Georgia, 1990, 164 pp. *A review of the geographic distribution of worldwide infections, updated yearly. It also contains the most recent recommendations for prophylaxis.*

Drugs for parasitic infections. Med Lett Drugs Ther 32:23, 1990. *A review of antiparasitic drugs published and updated annually. It includes dose, availability, and alternative choices.*

Mahmoud AAF: Parasitic protozoa and helminths: Biological and immunological challenges. Science 246:1015, 1989. *A selected review of some of the unique biologic, immunologic, and molecular aspects of malaria and schistosomes that accounts for the ability of these organisms to invade and establish themselves as parasites in humans.*

Warren KS, Mahmoud AAF (eds.): Tropical and Geographical Medicine, 2nd ed. New York, McGraw-Hill, 1990. *Detailed description of the biology and molecular understanding of protozoa and helminths and the diseases they cause in individuals and in populations.*

424 Malaria

Donald J. Krogstad

DEFINITION. Malaria is a disease characterized by recurrent fever and chills associated with the synchronous lysis of parasitized red blood cells. Its name is derived from the belief of the ancient Romans that malaria was caused by the bad air of the marshes surrounding Rome.

ETIOLOGY. Malaria is produced by intraerythrocytic parasites of the genus *Plasmodium*. Four plasmodia produce malaria in humans: *Plasmodium falciparum, Plasmodium vivax, Plasmodium ovale,* and *Plasmodium malariae*. The severity and characteristic manifestations of the disease are governed by the infecting species, the magnitude of the parasitemia, and the cytokines released as a result of the infection.

INCIDENCE, PREVALENCE, AND RESURGENCE. Incidence. Although precise data are difficult to obtain, malaria is unquestionably one of the most common infectious diseases. At least 200 to 300 million cases of malaria occur each year, with 2 to 3 million deaths. Most deaths are due to *P. falciparum* infection and occur among children less than 5 years old in sub-Saharan Africa. One of the major unanswered questions about malaria is how plasmodia produce repetitive infections without stimulating an effective (protective) immune response.

Prevalence. The prevalence of malaria varies widely; it may reach 10 per cent or more in hyperendemic areas. Thus its impact on the health of the developing world is enormous.

Resurgence. The major factors responsible for the resurgence of malaria are drug resistances: (1) the widespread resistance of the anopheline vector to economical insecticides such as chlorophenothane (DDT) and (2) the increasing prevalence of chloroquine resistance in *P. falciparum*, which is now endemic in South America, Southeast Asia, and Africa.

LIFE CYCLE AND EPIDEMIOLOGY. Life Cycle. The life cycle can be viewed as beginning with synchronous asexual replication of the erythrocytic stage of the parasite (Fig. 424–1; see Color Plate 11*A* to *D*). During the asexual erythrocytic cycle, the parasites mature from rings to trophozoites to schizonts, which ultimately rupture the red cell and release merozoites that enter uninfected red cells via receptors such as Duffy factor in *P. vivax*; the cycle is then repeated. By contrast, some erythrocytic parasites mature to sexual forms (gametocytes) that are ingested by the female anopheline mosquito. Within the mosquito intermediate host, male and female gametocytes mature to gametes, fuse to form an ookinete that matures to a zygote and ultimately produces the sporozoites that are infectious for humans. When an infected mosquito bites a human, sporozoites travel via the bloodstream to the liver, where they enter hepatocytes and mature to tissue schizonts, which release merozoites that are infectious for red cells and produce the asexual erythrocytic cycle. Two of the four species that infect humans (*P. vivax* and *P. ovale*) produce dormant (hypnozoite) forms in the liver,

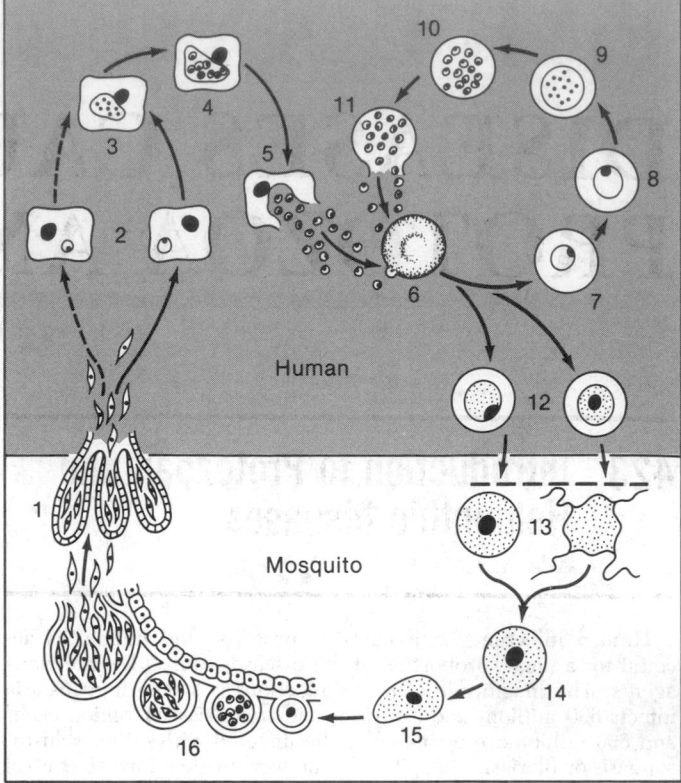

FIGURE 424–1. Life cycle of the malaria parasite. The lower and upper halves of the diagram indicate the anopheline mosquito and human parts of the cycle, respectively. Sporozoites from the salivary gland of a female *Anopheles* mosquito are injected under the skin (1). They then travel through the bloodstream to the liver (2) and mature within hepatocytes to tissue *schizonts* (4). Up to 30,000 parasites are then released into the bloodstream as *merozoites* (5) and produce symptomatic infection as they invade and destroy red blood cells. However, some parasites remain dormant in the liver as *hypnozoites (2, dashed lines from 1 to 3)*. These are the parasites that cause relapsing malaria (in *P. vivax* or *P. ovale* infection). Once within the bloodstream, merozoites (5) invade red cells (6) and mature to the *ring* (7,8), *trophozoite* (9), and *schizont* (10) asexual stages. Schizonts lyse their host red cells as they mature and release the next generation of merozoites (11), which invade previously uninfected red cells. Within the red cell some parasites differentiate to sexual forms (male and female *gametocytes*) (12). When taken up by a female *Anopheles* mosquito, the gametocytes mature to *male* and *female gametes*, which produce *zygotes* (14). The zygote invades the gut of the mosquito (15) and develops into an *oocyst* (16). Mature oocysts produce *sporozoites*, which migrate to the salivary gland of the mosquito (1) and repeat the cycle. The dashed line between 12 and 13 indicates that absence of the mosquito vector prevents natural transmission via this cycle. Infection by the injection of contaminated blood bypasses this constraint and permits transmission among intravenous drug addicts or to recipients of blood transfusions. (Reproduced with permission from Krogstad DJ: Blood and tissue protozoa. *In* Schaecter M, Medoff G, Schlessinger D [eds.]: Mechanisms of Microbial Diseases. © 1989, the Williams & Wilkins Company, Baltimore.)

which mature 6 to 11 months or more after the initial infection and thus produce relapsing malaria.

Two characteristics of the life cycle are essential for the long-term survival of the parasite: multiplicity of replication and antigenic variability. *Multiplicity of replication* is apparent at each stage of the life cycle. The mature asexual erythrocytic schizont releases 8 to 32 merozoites when it ruptures its host red cell; up to 10,000 sporozoites result from one zygote; and 10,000 to 30,000 merozoites are released from one tissue (exoerythrocytic) schizont in the liver. This multiplicity of replication provides a redundancy that protects the parasite against losses from both immune and nonimmune host factors. *Antigenic variability* is associated with the morphologic changes that occur during the parasite's life cycle and similarly protects the parasite against the host immune response. For example, antibodies against sporozoites are ineffective against the asexual erythrocytic stages of the infection. Similarly, immune responses directed against asexual erythrocytic stages have no effect against the sexual (gametocyte) stages of the parasite. In addition, antigenic variation exists among strains of the same species. These observations are critically relevant to the development of a malaria vaccine (see below).

Epidemiology. The epidemiology of malaria is determined by the distributions of the anopheline mosquito vectors required for natural transmission and of the infected human reservoir. Both factors are present in endemic areas throughout the tropics. Important determinants of transmission include the vector population (vectors such as the *Anopheles gambiae* complex in Africa are more efficient), temperature (elevated temperatures shorten the life of the vector and hasten the maturation of the parasite within the vector), and control programs (which reduce both the vector population and the prevalence of human infection).

Competent mosquito vectors are present in the United States (*A. albimanus* in the east and *A. freeborni* in the west). Transmission in the United States is limited by the absence of infected humans, but natural mosquito-borne transmission can and does occur with the importation of infected humans (e.g., the return of soldiers after their exposure in endemic areas). Mosquito-borne transmission (*introduced malaria*) occurred in the United States after World War II, the Korean War, the Vietnam War, and, most recently, the arrival of refugees from Southeast Asia.

PATHOGENESIS. Species-Dependent Factors. Malaria is a multifactorial disease that can be explained in part, but not completely, by the magnitude of the parasitemia. *Plasmodium falciparum* is the most lethal parasite because it can invade red cells of any age and can thus produce unrestricted parasitemias involving 10^6 or more parasitized red cells per cubic millimeter of blood (≥ 20 per cent of circulating red cells). Conversely, *P. vivax* and *P. ovale,* which invade only young red cells, are limited to parasitemias of 25,000 or less per cubic millimeter, and *P. malariae,* which invades only older red cells, is limited to parasitemias of 10,000 or less per cubic millimeter.

The Host Immune Response. Because millions of people experience repetitive episodes of malaria throughout their lives in the tropics, the immune response to natural infection is inadequate by definition. Thus the term *semi-immune,* rather than immune, is used for residents of malaria-endemic areas. The reasons for the inadequate host immune response are only partially clear and are likely to be central to the development of a successful vaccine. For example, most exposed persons make antibodies directed against the repetitive epitope or epitopes on the surface of the sporozoite, and antibodies to asexual stages have been shown to reduce the magnitude of the parasitemia in children. However, cell-mediated immune responses are less frequent and may be essential for effective immunity. At least two factors have been identified that may be relevant to the poor cell-mediated response to sporozoite antigen: (1) The sites that determine the cell-mediated response are in the hypervariable region of the molecule, and (2) the ability to produce a cell-mediated response may be restricted by the individual's human leukocyte antigen (HLA) haplotype (immune restriction).

Peripheral Sequestration of Parasitized Red Cells. With maturation, red cells containing *P. falciparum* parasites develop knobs that contain histidine-rich proteins. In vivo, these knobs adhere to endothelial cells in the peripheral microvasculature via proteins such as thrombospondin, ICAM-1, or CD36. This phenomenon has at least two consequences: (1) It enhances the microvascular obstruction and pathology produced by the parasite, and (2) it removes mature *P. falciparum* parasites from the circulation, so that only early asexual erythrocytic stages, such as rings, are seen on peripheral blood smears.

Cytokines in the Pathogenesis of Malaria. Recent studies suggest that the release of cytokines in malaria is a central factor in the pathogenesis of the disease. Cytokines that have been shown to be important include tumor necrosis factor–α (TNF–α). Serum levels of TNF–α are elevated in severe *P. falciparum* infection and correlate with complications such as cerebral malaria and death, although a direct cause-and-effect relationship has not been established. Interferon-γ (IFN-γ) has antiparasitic activity against the exoerythrocytic stages of the parasite in the liver. However, neither TNF-α nor IFN-γ has been shown to inhibit the replication of asexual erythrocytic stages of the parasite in vitro.

PATHOLOGY. The pathology of severe malaria is that of a microvascular disease involving the brain, lung, and kidney.

Postmortem examination in fatal *P. falciparum* infection demonstrates parasitized red cells in the capillaries of the brain and other affected organs. In severe cases, acute tubular necrosis may be present, and the liver, spleen, and other sites in the reticuloendothelial system may be filled with dark malarial pigment from the phagocytosis of parasitized red cells. This predominantly microvascular pathology is consistent with the importance of sequestration and cytokine release in the pathogenesis of severe *P. falciparum* malaria (see above). By contrast, the other malarias that infect humans produce lower parasitemias, do not sequester, and are rarely fatal.

CLINICAL MANIFESTATIONS. Fever and Chills. Most patients with malaria present with recurrent fever and chills (at 48-hour intervals for *P. vivax* and *P. ovale* and at 72-hour intervals for *P. malariae*). By contrast, patients with *P. falciparum* infection typically have irregular fever and chills and rarely present with a regular 48-hour cycle of symptoms despite the 48-hour cycle of the parasite.

Coma. Coma (cerebral malaria) is the most feared complication of *P. falciparum* infection and has a substantial fatality rate. Although it has been attributed to the blockage of capillaries with parasitized red cells, both hypoglycemia and the effects of cytokines such as TNF-α are important factors. Hypoglycemia in *P. falciparum* malaria may have at least three causes: (1) the release of insulin from the pancreatic β cell by quinine or quinidine during treatment, (2) glucose consumption by the massive numbers of parasites present in the patient, and (3) depletion of liver glycogen stores in persons who have not eaten for several days before seeking medical care because they were ill with malaria. Hypoglycemia is particularly important to consider because it is treatable. Although the effects of TNF-α undoubtedly contribute to cerebral malaria, it is difficult to separate them from the magnitude of the parasitemia because the concentration of TNF-α and the magnitude of the parasitemia correlate with each other.

Renal Failure. Patients with massive parasitemias may have dark urine from the free hemoglobin produced by hemolysis (blackwater fever) and may later develop renal failure. Although hemolysis alone should not produce renal failure, some degree of renal impairment is typical in such patients. In most instances, the patients recover uneventfully; however, acute renal failure may occur with a time course similar to that of other causes of acute tubular necrosis.

Pulmonary Edema. This complication also occurs in patients with high *P. falciparum* parasitemias (≥ 5 per cent of circulating red cells). Hemodynamic measurements indicate that this is a noncardiogenic form of pulmonary edema with normal pulmonary arterial and capillary pressures. These findings and the association with high TNF-α levels suggest that the pathogenesis of this pulmonary edema may be similar to that of bacterial septicemia.

Gastrointestinal Manifestations. Diarrhea is common among children with *P. falciparum* infection. Although the pathogenesis of this complication is unclear, postmortem studies of children with diarrhea demonstrate parasitized red cells in the microvasculature of the intestine.

DIAGNOSIS. Giemsa-Stained Thick and Thin Smears. The most direct way to diagnose malaria is to prepare and examine Giemsa-stained thick or thin smears using oil immersion magnification ($\times 1000$). Giemsa's stain is preferable to Wright's stain, especially for persons with *P. vivax* or *P. ovale* infection, because the Schüffner's dots characteristic of those infections are often not visible with Wright's stain. Thick smears are more sensitive than thin smears because the red cells have been lysed. As a result, approximately 10 times as much blood can be examined per field and thus per unit of time. However, because the red cells have been lysed, it is not possible to determine the effect of the parasite on red cell size or the position of the parasite within the red cell on a thick smear (Table 424–1). Therefore, persons without previous experience in reading thick smears should consider using thin smears to identify the infecting parasite or parasites. A common mistake is to require characteristic gametocytes for a diagnosis of *P. falciparum* infection. Because gametocytes require longer to develop than asexual parasites (7 to 10 days versus 2 days), they are usually not present in the peripheral blood when nonimmune tourists or expatriates first become symptomatic. Conversely, gametocytes are frequently present in

TABLE 424–1. MALARIA PARASITES THAT INFECT HUMANS

	Parasitemia (per μl blood)	Complications
P. falciparum	$\geq 10^6$	Coma (cerebral malaria) Hypoglycemia Pulmonary edema, renal failure Anemia
P. vivax	25,000	Late (2–3 mo) splenic rupture
P. ovale	25,000	—
P. malariae	10,000	Immune complex nephrotic syndrome

	Morphology		
	Red Blood Cell Size	Schüffner's Dots	Stages
P. falciparum	No RBC enlargement	Absent	Rings, occasionally gametocytes
P. vivax	Enlarged host RBC	Present	All forms
P. ovale	Enlarged host RBC	Absent	All forms
P. malariae	No RBC enlargement	Present	All forms

	Relapse from Hypnozoites	Antimalarial Resistance
P. falciparum	No	Chloroquine and pyrimethamine-sulfadoxine
P. vivax	Yes	Possibly chloroquine
P. ovale	Yes	None known
P. malariae	No	None known

RBC = red blood cell

the blood of semi-immune residents of endemic areas with few or no symptoms or asexual parasites. A second common mistake is to assume that the patient can have only one kind of parasite: Approximately 5 per cent of persons with malaria have more than one type of parasite.

Fluorescent Staining with Acridine Orange. Fluorescence microscopy is one of two new techniques for detecting malaria parasites in peripheral blood specimens. This technique takes advantage of the fact that parasitized red cells are less dense than unparasitized red cells. A finger stick specimen is taken into a capillary tube prepared with acridine orange (to stain the nucleic acid in the parasite) and an anticoagulant. After centrifugation, parasitized red cells are found at the top of the red cell layer just below the buffy coat. Experienced investigators can examine a blood specimen in 30 to 40 seconds (less time than necessary to examine a thick or thin smear).

DNA Probes. Several investigators have developed *Plasmodium* and species-specific (e.g., *P. falciparum*–specific) DNA probes that can detect 40 to 100 parasites per microliter of blood (similar to the 1 to 10 parasites per microliter threshold of the thick smear). Problems that remain to be solved in the application of this technology include the development of signal systems as effective as ^{32}P that are not radioactive and the role, if any, of the polymerase chain reaction in enhancing the sensitivity of the assay under field conditions.

Serology (Antibody Testing). Testing for antibodies to plasmodia is of limited value. In endemic areas, most persons have antibody titers from previous infections whether or not they were infected recently. In addition, 3 to 4 weeks may be required to develop a diagnostic rise in antibody titer, whereas the decision to treat must be made in the first few hours of evaluation. However, serology may be of value retrospectively in nonimmune persons (expatriate tourists) who have been treated empirically for malaria without a microscopic diagnosis. For example, a high titer of antibodies against *P. vivax* suggests that the patient has had a recent *P. vivax* infection and should receive primaquine if it has not been given previously (see the section on treatment, below).

PREVENTION. The acquisition of malaria by exposed nonimmune persons may be prevented by taking antimalarials prospectively (chemoprophylaxis); by using insect repellents and otherwise reducing contact with the anopheline vector; and possibly, in the future, by a malaria vaccine (immunoprophylaxis).

Chemoprophylaxis. Drugs used for chemoprophylaxis should be safe because they are given to healthy persons for long periods. They should also have long serum half-lives so that they can be given infrequently. On the basis of these criteria, chloroquine is an excellent drug for chemoprophylaxis in areas without chloroquine-resistant *P. falciparum* (Table 424–2). It is the only chemoprophylactic agent safe for pregnant women and does not produce retinal toxicity at the doses used for antimalarial chemoprophylaxis. Unfortunately, chloroquine-resistant strains of *P. falciparum* are now established in Southeast Asia, South America, and Africa. For areas with chloroquine-resistant *P. falciparum*, mefloquine is now the recommended chemoprophylactic agent, although resistance to mefloquine is developing in Southeast Asia. Doxycycline is an alternative, with the advantage that it also reduces the frequency of traveler's diarrhea. The disadvantages of doxycycline include the need to take it daily, photosensitivity reactions, and vaginitis. Because of hypersensitivity reactions to pyrimethamine-sulfadoxine (Fansidar) and both agranulocytosis and hepatitis with amodiaquine, neither of these agents is recommended for chemoprophylaxis.

Vector Control. Because of widespread drug resistance in *P. falciparum*, increasing emphasis is placed on reducing exposure to the anopheline vector, especially in hyperendemic areas such as Africa. Strategies that are successful and should be considered include DEET *(N,N'*-diethyl toluamide)–containing insect repellents and insecticide (pyrethrin)–impregnated bed nets. DDT is no longer effective in most regions of the world because of widespread resistance.

Immunoprophylaxis—Development of a Malaria Vaccine. Although a malaria vaccine is not available, it is hoped that this goal will ultimately be achievable. Because the three major parasite stages in humans are antigenically distinct, a successful vaccine will likely need to contain at least three parasite antigens (sporozoite, merozoite, and gametocyte). A vaccine need not be 100 per cent effective to be valuable. For example, a vaccine that requires boosting could be quite effective because of the repetitive exposure to natural infection in endemic areas. In addition, a vaccine that limits the magnitude of the parasitemia could have a marked effect on survival even if it had no effect on the incidence of infection, because severe morbidity and death are associated with high parasitemias.

TREATMENT. Successful treatment of patients with malaria depends primarily on effective antimalarial drugs. However, it is also dependent on ancillary measures as diverse as the infusion of glucose and exchange transfusion. Monitoring of the blood glucose level is important because hypoglycemia is a common cause of coma and because both quinine and quinidine stimulate the release of insulin directly from the pancreatic β cell. Steroids are contraindicated in cerebral malaria because they prolong the duration of coma.

The treatment of chloroquine-susceptible malaria (*P. vivax, P. ovale,* or *P. malariae* malaria and chloroquine-susceptible *P. falciparum* malaria) is satisfactory (Table 424–3) because chloroquine is a safe and effective antimalarial. However, the treatment of chloroquine-resistant *P. falciparum* malaria is unsatisfactory. Potential choices include quinidine, quinine, and mefloquine. For comatose patients, intravenous quinidine may be the safest treatment. With the measurement of serum quinidine levels (2.0 to 5.0 μg per milliliter is usually adequate; ≥6 μg per milliliter is potentially toxic) and cardiac monitoring (for a QT interval greater than 0.6 second or QRS widening beyond 25 per cent of baseline) during intravenous infusion, the risk of quinidine cardiovascular toxicity is low. Although pyrimethamine-sulfadoxine

TABLE 424–2. CHEMOPROPHYLAXIS OF MALARIA*

For Areas without Chloroquine-Resistant *Plasmodium falciparum*:

Chloroquine phosphate (Aralen)	500 mg/wk (300 mg chloroquine base) during exposure and for 4 wk after leaving the endemic area

For Areas with Chloroquine-Resistant *Plasmodium falciparum*:

Mefloquine (Lariam)	250 mg/wk during exposure and for 4 wk after leaving the endemic area
Doxycycline	100 mg/d during exposure and for 4 wk after leaving the endemic area

*Updated recommendations on malaria chemoprophylaxis may be obtained 24 hours a day, 7 days a week, through the Centers for Disease Control (CDC) Hot Line at (404) 639-1610.

TABLE 424–3. TREATMENT OF MALARIA

P. vivax, _P. ovale_, _P. malariae_, and Chloroquine-Susceptible _P. falciparum_:

For patients unable to take oral medications:

IM chloroquine: 2.5 mg/kg IM q 4 hr or 3.5 mg/kg q 6 hr (total dose not to exceed 25 mg/kg base)

IV chloroquine: 10 mg/kg base over 4 hr, followed by 5 mg/kg base q 12 hr (given in a 2-hr infusion; total dose not to exceed 25 mg/kg base)

For patients able to take oral medications:

PO chloroquine: 10 mg/kg = 600-mg base, followed by an additional 300-mg base after 6 hr and 300-mg base again on days 2 and 3

Chloroquine-Resistant _P. falciparum_:

For patients unable to take oral medications:

IV quinidine: 6.25 mg/kg quinidine base (10 mg/kg quinidine gluconate) IV over 1 to 2 hr, followed by a constant infusion of 0.0125 mg/kg quinidine base (0.02 mg/kg quinidine gluconate) IV per minute until the parasitemia is < 1% or oral treatment is tolerated

For patients able to take oral medications:

PO quinine*: 650 mg quinine sulfate (540 mg quinine base) q 8 hr until significant improvement, or for 10 d

PO mefloquine: 750 mg as a single oral dose

PO pyrimethamine + sulfadoxine: 3 tablets (75 mg pyrimethamine plus 1500 mg sulfadoxine) as a single dose

To Prevent Relapse in _P. vivax_ or _P. ovale_ Infection:

PO primaquine†: 15 mg primaquine base (26.3 mg primaquine phosphate) daily × 14 d

---

*A number of investigators recommend tetracycline (250 mg PO q 6 hr for 7 to 10 days), pyrimethamine plus sulfadiazine or sulfisoxazole (25 mg twice daily plus 500 mg q 6 hr PO for 5 days), or 3 tablets of pyrimethamine-sulfadoxine (total of 75 plus 1500 mg PO once) in addition to oral quinine. These regimens have not been shown to be more effective than quinine alone.

†To prevent potentially severe hemolysis, patients should be tested for glucose-6-phosphate dehydrogenase deficiency prior to treatment with primaquine.

IM = Intramuscular; IV = intravenous.

(Fansidar) has been used for treatment, it is now controversial because of the increasing prevalence of resistance in areas of chloroquine resistance.

Patients with _P. vivax_ or _P. ovale_ infection should be tested for glucose-6-phosphate dehydrogenase deficiency before treatment with primaquine, which is used to eradicate persistent hypnozoites in the liver so that relapse may be prevented.

PROGNOSIS. Virtually all patients with _P. vivax_, _P. ovale_, or _P. malariae_ infection respond well to chloroquine and make an uneventful recovery. Although chloroquine-resistant strains of _P. vivax_ have been reported from Indonesia, these reports have not yet been confirmed. For patients with _P. falciparum_ infection, the quantitative parasite count is the best predictor of the outcome. Patients with 5 per cent or greater parasitemia (≥250,000 parasites per microliter of blood) are at increased risk of severe and complicated malaria, including death. In addition to standard antimalarial treatment (outlined above), such patients should be considered for more heroic measures, such as exchange transfusion, if they do not improve within the first 12 to 24 hours of treatment.

Canfield CJ, Chongsuphajaisiddhi T, Danis M, et al.: Severe and complicated malaria. Trans R Soc Trop Med Hyg 89 (Suppl 2):1, 1990. _A comprehensive review of the pathogenesis and treatment of severe falciparum malaria._

Good MF, Pombo D, Quakyi IA, et al.: Human T-cell recognition of the circumsporozoite protein of _Plasmodium falciparum:_ Immunodominant T-cell domains map to the polymorphic regions of the molecule. Proc Natl Acad Sci USA 85:1199, 1988. _Evidence that the determinants of T cell reactivity are in hypervariable regions of the circumsporozoite protein._

Grau GE, Taylor TE, Molyneux ME, et al.: Tumor necrosis factor and disease severity in children with falciparum malaria. N Engl J Med 320:1586, 1989. _Serum levels of TNF are increased in children with severe falciparum malaria._

Krogstad DJ, Gluzman IY, Klye DE, et al.: Efflux of chloroquine from _Plasmodium falciparum:_ Mechanism of chloroquine resistance. Science 238:1283, 1987. _The basis of chloroquine resistance is rapid efflux of the drug from the resistant parasite._

Miller KD, Greenberg AE, Campbell CC: Treatment of severe malaria in the United States with a continuous infusion of quinidine gluconate and exchange transfusion. N Engl J Med 321:65, 1989. _Efficacy and safety of the continuous intravenous infusion of quinidine._

Miller LH, Howard RJ, Carter R, et al.: Research toward malaria vaccines. Science 234:1249, 1986. _A review of the rationale for a vaccine and of the problems that will need to be addressed in producing a vaccine._

Udeinya IJ, Schmidt JA, Aikawa M, et al.: Falciparum malaria–infected erythrocytes specifically bind to cultured human endothelial cells. Science 213:555, 1981. _Knobs on falciparum-infected cells bind to endothelial cells and thus explain the sequestration of red cells with mature falciparum parasites._

White NJ, Warrell DA, Chanthavanich P, et al.: Severe hypoglycemia and hyperinsulinemia in falciparum malaria. N Engl J Med 309:61, 1983. _Hypoglycemia may result from quinine or quinidine treatment, which releases insulin from the pancreatic β cell._

425 African Trypanosomiasis (Sleeping Sickness)

Thomas C. Quinn

DEFINITION. Known widely as sleeping sickness, African trypanosomiasis is an acute and chronic disease caused by _Trypanosoma brucei_. The parasites are transmitted to humans through the bite of tsetse flies located in regions of Africa between 15 degrees north and 15 degrees south latitude. In humans, there are two distinct forms of the disease, East African trypanosomiasis caused by _T. brucei rhodesiense_ and West African trypanosomiasis caused by _T. brucei gambiense_. Although there is some clinical overlap, East African trypanosomiasis primarily causes an acute febrile illness with myocarditis and meningoencephalitis that is rapidly fatal if not treated, while West African trypanosomiasis is characterized as a chronic debilitating disease with mental deterioration and physical wasting (Table 425–1). A closely related variant, _T. brucei brucei_, is noninfectious for humans, but causes a chronic wasting illness in cattle, called nagana, which has a considerable indirect effect on human nutrition in sub-Saharan Africa.

ETIOLOGY AND LIFE CYCLE. Trypanosomes are motile hemoflagellates with a single undulating membrane that passes along the length of the parasite, terminating in an anterior flagellum (Color Plate 11_E_). Located anteriorly is a kinetoplast, an organelle containing topologically interlocked circular DNA molecules and mitochondria. In the peripheral blood of humans, trypanosomes vary in length from 10 to 40 μm. Both short stumpy and long slender forms can be present in a patient at the same time. The different variants of _T. brucei_ cannot be distinguished morphologically but can be identified by differences in pathogenicity for certain animals, as well as in biochemical

TABLE 425–1. A COMPARISON OF GAMBIAN AND RHODESIAN SLEEPING SICKNESS

	Gambian (West African)	Rhodesian (East African)
Etiologic agent	_Trypanosoma brucei gambiense_	_Trypanosoma brucei rhodesiense_
Vector	_Glossina palpalis_ or _tachinoides_ (riverine tsetse)	_Glossina morsitans_ (savanna tsetse)
Distribution	West and Central Africa	East Africa
Reservoir	Humans (domestic animals)	Wild game
Course of infection	Slow (months–years)	Rapid (<1 yr)
Clinical features		
Lymphadenopathy	+ + (Winterbottom's sign)	±
Myocarditis, heart failure	−	+ +
Neurologic symptoms	+ +	+
Disseminated intravascular coagulation	−	+
Parasitemia	Low	High

requirements, electrophoretic pattern of component enzymes, and DNA hybridization.

T. brucei is transmitted by the tsetse fly *Glossina*, within which it undergoes several developmental changes. During the bite of an infected host, trypanosomes are ingested and within the insect midgut rapidly differentiate into procyclic forms with loss of their dense surface coat, composed of variant surface glycoprotein. After 2 to 3 weeks of multiplication within the midgut the procyclic trypanosomes migrate to the insect's salivary glands, where they change morphologically into epimastigotes. These forms further undergo multiplication and ultimately differentiate into metacyclic trypanosomes that are coated with characteristic variant surface glycoprotein and are infectious to mammalian hosts. When a new host is bitten by the tsetse fly, the trypanosomes present in the salivary glands are injected into the connective tissue and blood. Within the human host they divide by binary fission and undergo antigen variation, a process by which they continually change their surface glycoproteins and evade the immune system of the host. With the bite of another tsetse fly, ingestion of the parasite occurs, and the life cycle of the organism is completed (Fig. 425–1). Mechanical transmission can theoretically also occur via blood transfusion or by interrupted biting of a tsetse fly feeding on an infectious person and directly thereafter biting an uninfected individual.

EPIDEMIOLOGY. It is estimated that African trypanosomiasis infects more than 20,000 Africans annually and that approximately 50 million people live at risk of acquiring trypanosomiasis because of the presence of the disease and its vector. Approximately 4 million square miles in Africa remain unpopulated because of the presence of *T. brucei brucei* infection, which results in the loss of domestic and wild animals, including cattle, waterbuck, bushbuck, and buffalo.

T. b. gambiense occurs primarily in the west and central regions of sub-Saharan Africa. Although it primarily infects humans, there may be animal reservoirs, such as pigs, dogs, and sheep. Gambian sleeping sickness is spread mainly by three species of tsetse fly, *Glossina palpalis*, *G. tachinoides*, and *G. fuscipes*. Distribution of these flies includes shaded areas along rivers and streams, where the conditions of temperature, darkness, and moisture are optimum.

T. b. rhodesiense differs from *T. b. gambiense* in that it is primarily a parasite of wild game, with humans serving only as occasional hosts. The geographic distribution of *T. b. rhodesiense*

is primarily East Africa from Ethiopia and eastern Uganda south to Zambia and Botswana. Rhodesian sleeping sickness is spread by tsetse flies of the *G. morsitans* group, including *G. pallidipes* and *G. swynnertoni*. These flies can survive in the open savanna, and Rhodesian sleeping sickness usually occurs among individuals visiting or traveling through an endemic area. Consequently, hunters, fishermen, and tourists are at risk, exposing themselves to vectors that usually feed on wild animals.

Imported African trypanosomiasis is a rare disease, with only 15 cases diagnosed in Americans since 1967. Most of these cases were among Americans who had been on safari in East Africa for a very brief period. Nearly all of these cases were initially misdiagnosed because of the unfamiliarity of American physicians with this disease. With an increase in international travel, 20,000 Americans are now estimated to visit endemic areas yearly, and approximately 10,000 aliens enter the United States each year from countries in Africa where the infection is endemic.

PATHOGENESIS AND PATHOLOGY. Following the bite of the tsetse fly, trypanosomes accumulate in the connective tissue, where they multiply to produce a local chancre (trypanoma). The organisms subsequently spread through the lymphatics, resulting in enlargement of lymph nodes secondary to reactive plasma cell and macrophage infiltration. The trypanosomes eventually disseminate to the circulatory system, where the parasitemia usually remains at low intensity and the organisms multiply by binary fission.

The host immune response plays an integral role in the pathogenesis of African sleeping sickness, although the exact nature of the immunopathogenic reactions has not been clearly defined. Trypanosomes survive by periodically altering their surface antigenic coat, avoiding successful eradication by the host. One organism can produce multiple antigenic variants (100 or more), each genetically determined and selected by the host antibody response. Consequently trypanosomes occur in the peripheral blood of infected individuals in waves, with each parasite wave consisting of a serologically distinct organism.

Tissue damage is induced by either toxin production or immune complex reaction with release of proteolytic enzymes. Immune complexes consisting of variant antigens of the organism and complement-fixing antibodies have been demonstrated in both the circulation and the target organs of infected patients. The production of autoantibodies is a prominent feature, and they are frequently directed against antigen components of red cells, brain, and heart. Anemia secondary to autoimmune hemolysis can be severe, resulting in anoxia and further tissue destruction. Thus the host-parasite interaction can result in generalized febrile episodes, lymphadenopathy, and myocardial and pericardial inflammation, along with anemia, thrombocytopenia, disseminated intravascular coagulation, and renal disease primarily during the acute stage of the disease.

During this period of circulatory dissemination, trypanosomes localize in the small vessels of the central nervous system (CNS). Pathologic changes in the CNS are most prominent in chronic cases of Gambian sleeping sickness. The meninges are thickened and infiltrated with lymphocytes, plasma cells, and morular cells. Morular cells are modified plasma cells (up to 20 mm in diameter) with large granular inclusions that have been shown to consist of immunoglobulin. These cells may play an important role in the local production of immunoglobulin M (IgM) in the cerebrospinal fluid. Edema, hemorrhages, and granulomatous lesions are frequently present, along with thrombosis as a result of endoarteritis and with neuronal degeneration.

African trypanosomes appear to induce a state of B cell polyclonal activation caused either by interference with host T cell control of antibody production or by a B cell mitogen released by the parasite. Polyclonal hypergammaglobulinemia, with very high levels of IgM, is commonly seen. High levels of nonspecific heterophile antibody, rheumatoid factor, and autoantibodies are also produced.

CLINICAL FEATURES. The signs and symptoms of sleeping sickness differ according to the infecting organism (Table 425–1). Rhodesian sleeping sickness, due to *T. b. rhodesiense*, causes a rapid progressive disease often resulting in cardiac failure and acute neurologic manifestations. Gambian sleeping sickness, caused by *T. b. gambiense*, is typically a more chronic illness with primarily neurologic features. However, this difference is not absolute; in some cases Gambian sleeping sickness can

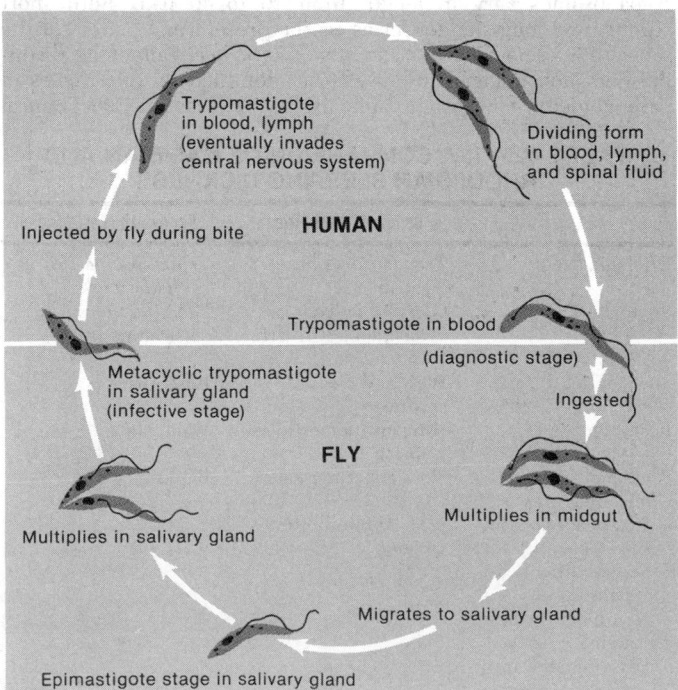

FIGURE 425–1. Life cycle of *Trypanosoma (Trypanozoon) brucei*, *T. (T.) B. gambiense*, and *T. (T.) b. rhodesiense*.

Gambian Sleeping Sickness. Within several days following the bite by an infected tsetse fly, a trypanosomal nodule or chancre develops, typically on the exposed parts of the body. Within a week the lesion becomes a hard, painful nodule surrounded by erythema and swelling, which persists for 1 to 2 weeks. After this incubation period, clinical features develop after systemic, lymphatic, and circulatory invasion of the trypanosomes. Fever, headache, dizziness, and weakness occur in the majority of these patients. Febrile episodes may last 1 to 6 days, alternating with afebrile periods. Lymphadenopathy with prominent supraclavicular and posterior cervical enlargement is seen in more than 80 per cent of infected individuals. Known as Winterbottom's sign, these enlarged lymph nodes are usually discrete, rubbery, and painless. Moderate splenomegaly may occur, and urticaria and erythematous rashes have also been observed. Electrocardiograms are often abnormal, but clinical signs of heart disease are unusual.

Six months to several years after the first appearance of symptoms, the clinical features of this early hemolymphatic stage progress to a late meningoencephalitic stage. Behavioral and personality changes are often the first signs of CNS involvement. Later, more florid psychological changes may occur, with hallucinations and delusions. Reversion of sleep rhythm is characteristic, with drowsiness during the day, a feature from which the disease derives its name. Other nervous symptoms include tremor, most characteristically of the face and lips, and hyperesthesia, causing some patients to avoid common practices such as closing (Kerandel's sign) or locking doors (key sign). Without treatment, the patient's level of consciousness progressively deteriorates until he or she finally lapses into stupor. Alterations in thermoregulation may lead to hypothermia or hyperthermia, and progressive neurologic alterations lead to convulsions, chorea, and athetosis. The cerebrospinal fluid shows an increase in cells and protein, much of which is IgM. Free immunoglobulin light chains may be present. Most of the cells are lymphocytes, but a few are plasma cells and morula cells. Trypanosomes may also be evident within the cerebrospinal fluid.

Rhodesian Sleeping Sickness. This disease is more acute than Gambian sleeping sickness, and symptoms usually occur a few days after the victim has been bitten by the tsetse fly. Alternating periods of high fever, malaise, and headache, followed by several days of well-being, are often misinterpreted as acute malaria infection. Lymphadenopathy is not prominent in this variety of the disease, and Winterbottom's sign is usually absent. Tachycardia with arrhythmias and extrasystoles is common. Anemia, thrombocytopenia, and disseminated intravascular coagulation are usually evident within the first several weeks of infection. Liver enzyme values are often elevated, and electrocardiograms are abnormal, usually reflecting underlying myocarditis. Neurologic features are similar to those described for Gambian sleeping sickness, but they occur much earlier and with more rapid deterioration. Without treatment the disease may result in death within a matter of weeks to months, without clear distinction into an early and late phase, as described for Gambian trypanosomiasis.

DIAGNOSIS. Although a presumptive diagnosis of trypanosomiasis is based on clinical suspicion, history of travel to areas where this disease is endemic, and tsetse fly exposure, confirmation of the diagnosis is based solely on the demonstration of trypanosomes. These organisms may be found in the blood (Color Plate 11E), bone marrow, centrifuged cerebrospinal fluid, lymph node aspirates, and scrapings from the chancre. Giemsa's or Wright's stain of the buffy coat of centrifuged heparinized blood make identification easier, since the trypanosomes are often concentrated in the buffy coat. In patients with Gambian sleeping sickness, in which trypanosomes are found less frequently in the blood, concentration methods such as ion exchange chromatography, diethylaminoethyl (DEAE) filtration, culture, or animal inoculation should be used.

All patients should have a lumbar puncture prior to and following therapy to determine whether CNS involvement is present. Documentation of CNS involvement is imperative, since suramin, a drug effective against the hemolymphatic stage of *T. brucei*, does not penetrate the spinal fluid. CNS disease is manifested by pleocytosis and elevation of spinal fluid total

protein and IgM levels. Trypanosomes can be found in most patients, provided that the cerebrospinal fluid is examined immediately after collection and that clean glassware is used. For those patients in whom trypanosomes cannot be found, measurement of the cerebrospinal fluid IgM is often of great diagnostic help. A high cerebrospinal fluid IgM value and a modest increase in total protein are almost pathognomonic of sleeping sickness.

Several immunodiagnostic tests have been developed for African trypanosomiasis, including an indirect hemagglutination test, indirect fluorescent antibody test, and enzyme-linked immunosorbent assay (ELISA), that are useful for epidemiologic surveys. A simple direct agglutination test for stained trypanosomes performed on cards (CATT) has been developed and is commercially available. However, at present, no serologic test provides sufficient definitive information for treatment of a patient without demonstration of the organism.

TREATMENT. Suramin* is the drug of choice for the early hemolymphatic stage of both *T. b. gambiense* and *T. b. rhodesiense* infections before CNS invasion has occurred. Suramin does not cross the blood-brain barrier in increased amounts, and it will not cure the disease once CNS invasion has occurred. The dose is 20 mg per kilogram of body weight given intravenously up to a maximum single dose of 1 gram. Suramin is freshly prepared as a 10 per cent aqueous solution. Intramuscular injection is not advised because of local irritation and pain. Suramin binds to plasma proteins and may persist in the circulation at low concentrations for as long as 3 months. A test dose of 200 mg is given initially; if no adverse side effects are noted, then full doses of the drug may be given on days 1, 3, 7, 14, and 21. A single course for an adult is usually 5 grams; it should not exceed 7 grams.

Suramin is a toxic drug that may result in idiosyncratic reactions in some individuals (1 in 20,000). The drug is excreted entirely by the kidneys; renal damage may result because of deposition of the drug in the renal tubules. The urine should be examined prior to administration of each dose of suramin, and if proteinuria or casts are present, treatment should be stopped. Other side effects include a papular eruption, photophobia, arthralgias, peripheral neuritis, fever, and agranulocytosis.

Pentamidine isethionate* is an alternative drug for the treatment of early hemolymphatic African trypanosomiasis, but it is much less active against *T. rhodesiense* than is suramin. The dose is 4 mg per kilogram of body weight; it is given every other day by intramuscular injection for a total of 10 injections. Pentamidine is also ineffective in the treatment of CNS trypanosomiasis.

The arsenical melarsoprol* (Mel B) is the treatment of choice for both Gambian and Rhodesian sleeping sickness once involvement of the CNS has occurred. The drug is given in three courses of 3 days each. The recommended dosage is 2.0 to 3.6 mg per kilogram per day given intravenously in three divided doses for 3 days, followed 1 week later by 3.6 mg per kilogram per day in three divided doses for 3 days. This latter course is then repeated 10 to 21 days later. Melarsoprol is a highly toxic drug and should be administered with great care. If signs of arsenical toxicity occur, the drug should be discontinued.

The most important side effects involve the CNS. A reactive encephalopathy, probably due to release of trypanosomal antigens, may occur early in the course of treatment, and its incidence has been reported to be as high as 18 per cent. It may develop very rapidly or insidiously, and its mortality is about 50 per cent. Clinical indications of reactive encephalopathy include high fever, headache, tremor, seizures, and finally coma. It has been suggested that corticosteroids protect patients from melarsoprol encephalopathy, but this assertion has not been clearly documented. Alternative drugs for CNS involvement include tryparsamide, melarsonyl potassium (Mel W), and nitrofurazone. These drugs appear either to be more toxic than Mel B or less effective in the treatment of CNS disease. Difluoromethylornithine (eflornithine, DFMO), a specific, irreversible inhibitor of polyamine biosynthesis, has been shown to be curative in animal models inoculated with *Trypanosoma* species. In a preliminary open field trial, 20 patients, 18 of whom had CNS infection with *T. b.*

---

*Available from the Centers for Disease Control, Atlanta, GA.

gambiense, had a clinical response with parasitic clearance of the CSF. The recommended dosage is 400 mg per kilogram per day given intravenously in four divided doses for 2 weeks, followed by 300 mg per kilogram per day given orally in four doses for 30 days. Frequent side effects include diarrhea and anemia. Further studies are under way to define optimal treatment regimens, and its efficacy in *T. b. rhodesiense* has not been determined. Regular follow-up with clinical examination and lumbar puncture is necessary for all patients for at least 1 year after treatment.

PROGNOSIS. Untreated African sleeping sickness is almost invariably fatal. Many patients with early Gambian sleeping sickness may remain relatively well for months to years without treatment, but once CNS involvement has occurred, death is inevitable unless treatment is given. Death frequently results from pneumonia in Gambian sleeping sickness and from heart failure in Rhodesian sleeping sickness. Treatment with suramin in the early phase of sleeping sickness results in a cure rate of over 90 per cent. A few patients may subsequently develop CNS involvement and require further treatment. Mel B achieves a parasitologic cure in at least 90 per cent of cases of advanced disease, and many patients may recover completely. Unfortunately, some patients are left with irreversible neurologic damage. Approximately 5 per cent of patients may die during the course of Mel B therapy.

CONTROL AND PROPHYLAXIS. Measures to prevent and control African trypanosomiasis can be instituted at three different levels: surveillance and treatment, chemoprophylaxis, and vector control. Surveillance with treatment is necessary to reduce the human reservoir of infection, particularly in areas where epidemics have occurred in the past. Pentamidine has been successfully used as a chemoprophylactic in Gambian sleeping sickness when given as a single intramuscular injection of 4 mg per kilogram every 3 to 6 months. However, the drug is generally not recommended for mass use, and it appears to be ineffective against Rhodesian trypanosomiasis.

Vector control requires destruction of tsetse fly habitats by selective clearing of vegetation and spraying with insecticides, which are effective only temporarily. Because of the wide range of the tsetse fly, these vector control measures are not economically feasible except when it is necessary to break transmission in epidemics. For individual protection, avoidance of contact with infected tsetse flies is best achieved by the use of repellents and protective clothing.

A vaccine is not currently available because of the occurrence of antigenic variation. However, the potential for development of a vaccine has increased with the progress in cultivation of *T. brucei* in vitro and analysis of the chemical structure of its variant antigens.

Donelson JE, Rice-Ficht AC: Molecular biology of trypanosome antigenic variation. Microbiol Rev 49:107, 1985. *A review of the genetic control of host-parasite interaction in trypanosomiasis.*

Jennings FW: Future prospects for the chemotherapy of human trypanosomiasis. Combination chemotherapy and African trypanosomiasis. Trans R Soc Trop Med Hyg 84:618, 1990. *A review of the different drug regimens for treatment of trypanosomiasis and discussion of their advantages and toxicities.*

Kirchhoff LV: Agents of African trypanosomiasis (sleeping sickness). *In* Mandel GL, Douglas RJ, Bennett JE (eds.): Principles and Practice of Infectious Disease, 3rd ed. New York, John Wiley & Sons, 1990, pp 2085–2090. *An excellent chapter on the biology and clinical features of African trypanosomiasis.*

Molyneux DH: Selective primary health care: Strategies for control of disease in the developing world: VIII. African trypanosomiasis. Rev Infect Dis 5:945, 1983. *A review of the various chemotherapeutic, vector, and environmental control measures for sleeping sickness.*

Pepin J, Milord F, Guer C, Schechter PJ: Difluoromethylornithine for arseno-resistant *Trypanosoma brucei gambiense* sleeping sickness. Lancet 2:1431, 1987. *Successful use of this less toxic drug (DFMO) in the treatment of T. gambiense.*

Poltera AA: Pathology of human African trypanosomiasis with reference to experimental African trypanosomiasis and infections of the central nervous system. Br Med Bull 41:169, 1985. *A review of the clinical and pathologic findings of CNS disease in both human and animal models infected with African trypanosomiasis.*

Van Nieuwenhove S, Schechter PJ, DeClercq J, et al.: Treatment of gambiense sleeping sickness in the Sudan with oral DFMO, an inhibitor of ornithine decarboxylase; first field trial. Trans R Soc Trop Med Hyg 79:692, 1985. *A successful clinical treatment trial of 20 patients with chronic Gambian trypanosomiasis with DFMO, a new nontoxic trypanosomicidal drug.*

World Health Organization: Epidemiology and control of African trypanosomiasis. Report of a WHO Expert Committee. WHO Tech Rep Ser 739:36, 1986. *An excellent review on the topic of African trypanosomiasis.*

426 American Trypanosomiasis (Chagas' Disease)

Franklin A. Neva

DEFINITION. Chagas' disease, resulting from infection with the protozoan parasite *Trypanosoma cruzi*, is named after the Brazilian physician Carlos Chagas, who discovered the parasite. Distinction should be made between infection caused by the parasite, as manifested by positive serologic findings, and clinical disease. Chronic disease manifestations develop years after initial infection in the form of chronic cardiomyopathy with conduction defects or with dysfunction of the esophagus or colon (mega syndromes).

LIFE CYCLE OF THE ETIOLOGIC AGENT. The causative agent, *T. cruzi*, is usually transmitted as a zoonosis. Various species of blood-sucking reduviids become infected when they take a blood meal from animals or humans who have circulating parasites, trypomastigotes, in the blood. The ingested parasites transform into epimastogotes and multiply in the midgut of the insect vector, where they later transform once again into metacyclic trypomastigotes in the hindgut of the bug. When the infected bug takes a subsequent blood meal, it frequently defecates during or after feeding, so that the infective metacyclic forms are deposited on the skin. Transmission to a second vertebrate host occurs when the feeding puncture site or a mucous membrane is inadvertently contaminated with infective bug feces. The parasites can penetrate a variety of host cell types, within which they transform into intracellular amastigote forms. In contrast to certain other intracellular organisms, amastigotes of *T. cruzi* are not enclosed in phagolysosomes. They multiply in the cytoplasm, elongate, transform into motile trypomastigotes, and rupture out of the cells. Liberated organisms penetrate new cells or are carried into the bloodstream to initiate further cycles of multiplication, preferentially in muscle cells, or are ingested by new vectors to maintain the cycle (Fig. 426–1).

Asymptomatic infected individuals with low-level parasitemia can transmit *T. cruzi* via blood transfusion. Another route of transmission of the parasite is congenital infection.

EPIDEMIOLOGY. *T. cruzi* and its arthropod vectors are widely distributed from the southern United States through Mexico and Central America into South America down to central Argentina and Chile. The parasite is restricted to the Western Hemisphere. In most countries where it occurs, the parasite cycle is sylvatic; i.e., it takes place in wild animals and vector bugs that associate with them. Human contact with sylvatic vectors is sporadic and accidental. A peridomestic cycle occurs under conditions in which infected animals, such as opposums and rats, live close to human habitations, and vector bugs may invade houses to seek a blood meal. Certain species of triatomine bugs, such as *Triatoma infestans*, *Rhodnius prolixus*, and *Panstrongylus megistus*, have a great propensity to invade, live, and breed in houses if suitable microenvironments are present. Cracks and holes in adobe mud huts or in crude wooden walls, thatched roofs, and household rubble provide ideal hiding and breeding places for the bugs, which venture out at night to feed upon sleeping inhabitants. Under these conditions *T. cruzi* is transmitted from person to person—a domiciliary cycle—and Chagas' disease becomes a public health problem. Thus, human trypanosomiasis in Latin America is primarily an infection of poor people living in substandard housing in rural areas.

The prevalence of antibodies to the parasite in human populations varies widely in different countries, as well as within regions of a country. A recent nationwide survey in Brazil found about 10 per cent of the rural population to be infected. It is not unusual for up to half of all inhabitants in selected villages to be antibody positive. Countries with the highest incidence of both infection and disease due to *T. cruzi* include Brazil, Argentina, Chile, Bolivia, and Venezuela. It is estimated that in all of the Americas a total of 15 million people are infected. In many Latin American countries, positive serologic findings for *T. cruzi* constitute a social stigma; a lower socioeconomic background is implied, and employers are reluctant to hire someone who may later develop chronic Chagas' disease.

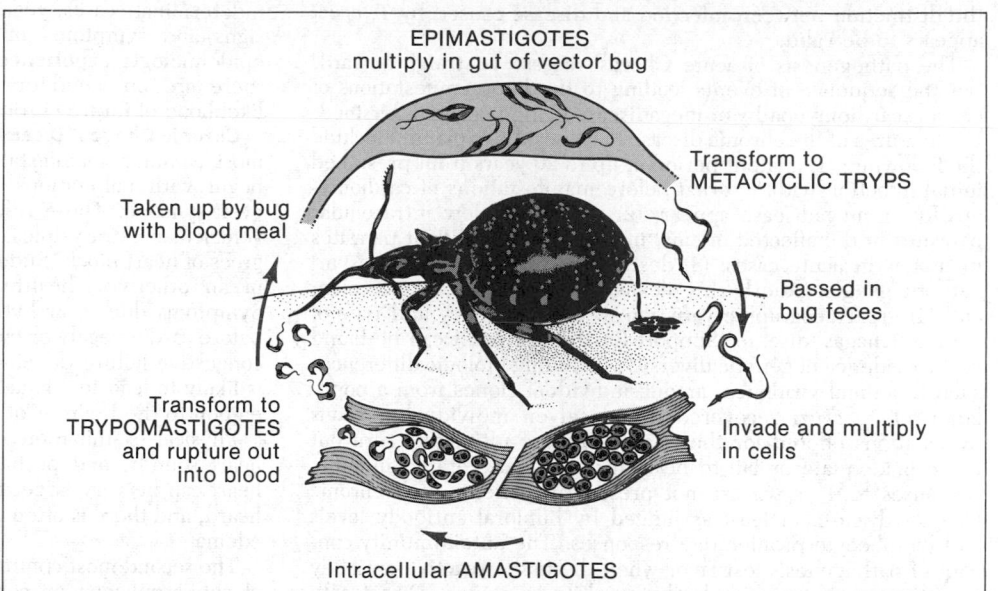

EPIMASTIGOTES
multiply in gut of vector bug

Transform to
METACYCLIC TRYPS

Taken up by bug
with blood meal

Passed in
bug feces

Transform to
TRYPOMASTIGOTES
and rupture out
into blood

Invade and multiply
in cells

Intracellular AMASTIGOTES

FIGURE 426–1. Life cycle of *Trypanosoma cruzi.*

Considerable geographic variation exists in both the prevalence and the type of chronic disease manifestations. In Brazil, for example, cardiomyopathy and megadisease are common, and often a patient has both types of involvement. However, chagasic megaesophagus and megacolon are virtually unknown in Venezuela, Colombia, and Panama, whereas cardiomyopathy is relatively high, moderate, and low in prevalence, respectively. In general, the frequency of cardiac disease in Central America and Mexico in seropositive persons is low, even though rates of seropositivity may be substantial. Also in these countries heart disease tends to develop later in life than in Brazil.

The situation regarding Chagas' disease in the United States is interesting because only four autochthonous acute cases have been recognized despite the presence of *T. cruzi* in vector bugs as well as in animal reservoirs. The lack of transmission of *T. cruzi* to humans in this country is probably due to preference of the vectors for sylvatic habitats and their tendency to defecate late after feeding. Yet in some areas of the West, bites from aggressive and abundant reduviid bugs can be a source of annoyance to, and allergic reactions in, suburbanites and outdoorspeople. Because of increased Hispanic immigration in recent years, sporadic cases of chronic Chagas' disease will probably be encountered in the United States.

PATHOLOGY AND PATHOGENESIS. In *acute Chagas' disease*, a local inflammatory lesion called a chagoma may develop at the site of entry of the parasite. Histologically, the chagoma shows mononuclear cell infiltration, interstitial edema, and intracellular aggregates of amastigotes in cells of the subcutaneous tissue and muscle. Other pathologic changes in the acute disease are known only for the severe cases that come to autopsy, since the great majority of cases are subclinical and self-limiting. Biopsy specimens from enlarged lymph nodes show hyperplasia, and amastigotes may be present in reticular cells. Skeletal muscle tissue from muscle biopsies have shown organisms and focal inflammation. In acute cases that have a fatal outcome there is invariably myocarditis with an enlarged heart. Microscopically, there is degeneration of cardiac muscle fibers and prominent but patchy areas of inflammation with nests of amastigotes in the muscles. The brain and meninges may also be parasitized in acute Chagas' disease. Virtually all organs and cell types can be invaded by *T. cruzi.*

The organs primarily affected in *chronic Chagas' disease* are the heart and certain hollow viscera, such as the esophagus and colon. Surprisingly, the intracellular *T. cruzi* usually cannot be found in the affected organs, or a few may be demonstrable after protracted search of many tissue sections. The heart in those patients with chronic disease who die suddenly, presumably of ventricular arrhythmias or heart block, may be normal in size or only moderately enlarged. Other patients with chronic chagasic cardiomyopathy develop cardiomegaly and die of intractable failure. The hearts are both hypertrophied and dilated, with thinning, especially at the apex to form a characteristic apical aneurysm. Mural thrombi, with subsequent embolization of the lungs and peripheral organs, are frequently seen. The coronary arteries are generally normal.

Microscopic findings in the heart are not specific, consisting of focal mononuclear cell infiltrates, hypertrophy of cardiac fibers with patchy areas of necrosis, variable fibrosis, and edema. The components of the conduction system of the heart most often involved by inflammatory changes are the sinoatrial and atrioventricular nodes, as well as the right branch and left anterior branches of the bundle of His. Andrade's detailed studies of these pathologic changes indicated that they correlated well with electrocardiographic (ECG) changes during life but were diffusely scattered without specific localization to the conducting system.

When either the esophagus or the colon is affected in chronic Chagas' disease, the gross appearance is of dilatation and hypertrophy of the affected organ. The microscopic pathologic changes are disappointingly similar to those in the heart, again with no or very few organisms. However, myenteric ganglion cells are strikingly reduced in number. This type of parasympathetic denervation may also be found in other hollow viscera, such as duodenum, ureters, or biliary tree.

The significant pathology of *congenital Chagas' disease* is chronic placentitis, with inflammatory changes and focal necrosis in the chorionic villi. Amastigotes of *T. cruzi* are present in the lesions. The presence of lesions and organisms in the placenta may be associated with abortion, stillbirth, or acute disease in the fetus. However, pregnancy may result in a normal fetus, even though placental lesions are present.

The extent and clinical significance of pathologic changes in those individuals with antibodies to *T. cruzi* but without evidence of disease, i.e., the *indeterminate form*, are not yet clear. Such indeterminate cases may have significantly reduced numbers of esophageal or colonic ganglion cells. It has been claimed that endocardial biopsy specimens from indeterminate cases have recognizable pathologic changes. In addition, in some indeterminate cases there is a chronic low level of parasitemia. Therefore, one point of view is that everyone with positive serologic findings has a continuing subclinical disease process that will become manifested with time. On the other hand, even in those areas where chronic Chagas' disease is common, one half or more of those with a positive serology will die of causes other than Chagas' disease. In most Latin American countries, where endemicity is much lower, a positive serologic finding constitutes a relatively small risk factor for later chronic disease. Until better information on this issue becomes available and, more important, until the pathogenesis of chronic Chagas' disease is unraveled, the distinction between infection and disease caused by *T. cruzi* appears to be valid.

The pathogenesis of acute Chagas' disease is straightforward, but the sequence of events leading to the late manifestations of chronic cardiomyopathy or megadisease is still poorly understood. Key features of the chronic disease that must be explained include the following: (1) a latent period of up to 20 years from presumed initial infection with *T. cruzi* before manifestations of cardiomyopathy or megadisease appear; (2) no or very few intracellular parasites in the affected organs, in contrast to abundant parasites in tissues in acute cases; (3) destruction of autonomic parasympathetic ganglia (Auerbach's plexus) of the esophagus and colon; and (4) great geographic variation in the frequency and type of chronic Chagas' disease. Support for the last point can be found in the evidence of genetic diversity, including biologic differences such as animal virulence, among individual clones from a population of *T. cruzi* recovered from a given individual. Various explanations offered for the chronic disease ultimately turn out to be inadequate or fail to be confirmed. Exaggerated immune responses to *T. cruzi* are not present in patients with chronic Chagas' disease, at least as judged by humoral antibody levels and lymphocyte proliferative responses. The autoimmunity concept of pathogenesis lost favor when the tissue reactive antibody in patients was found to be heterophile in nature. Direct cell-mediated cytotoxicity to heart muscle has also been proposed as a mechanism for the chronic disease. An even more complicated type of autoimmune response involving anti-idiotypic antibodies as T cell antigens, as well as differential responses in antigen presentation, has also been proposed to explain chronic Chagas' disease. But a unifying concept of pathogenesis for chronic Chagas' disease is still lacking.

Some insight into the host-parasite balance that exists in individuals chronically infected with *T. cruzi* is provided by observations on the influence of intercurrent infections or interventions affecting the immune status. One such experience concerns the development of acute disease observed in a number of recipients of heart transplants for chagasic cardiomyopathy, presumably because of the heavy immunosuppression required. On the other hand, although the experience is still early, there are no reports that human immunodeficiency virus (HIV) infection precipitates either acute or chronic manifestations of Chagas' disease.

CLINICAL PRESENTATION. In endemic areas, first exposure to *T. cruzi* generally is subclinical and goes unnoticed. When those initially exposed do develop clinical manifestations, the disease is an acute systemic infection. Chronic Chagas' disease, in contrast, evolves as a later sequel with specific organ involvement and no systemic features.

Acute Chagas' Disease. Although acute Chagas' disease is most commonly seen in children, it can occur at any age, depending upon the nature of exposure to the causative organism. The incubation period under natural conditions cannot be established accurately but is probably at least a week. A local area of erythema and induration (chagoma) may develop in the skin at the site of parasite entry. When infection takes place via the conjunctival route, as it frequently does, the local periorbital swelling is referred to as Romaña's sign. The chagoma is often accompanied by regional adenopathy and persists for several weeks. Other signs of acute Chagas' disease include fever, generalized lymphadenopathy, hepatosplenomegaly, and transient skin rashes.

Myocarditis, accompanied by tachycardia and nonspecific ECG changes, can occur in the acute stage. Meningoencephalitis is another serious complication, particularly in very young patients. Fatal outcome in acute Chagas' disease is rare, but when it does occur, it is due to myocarditis and congestive failure or to meningoencephalitis.

Signs and symptoms of acute disease gradually subside within a few weeks to several months even without treatment. Trypanosomes, which have been demonstrable by direct microscopy in the peripheral blood during the acute phase, become more difficult to find and then disappear. The patient then enters the *indeterminate phase*, which is characterized by the presence of antibodies to *T. cruzi* and often also by the presence of low-level parasitemia in the blood demonstrable only by special sensitive methods. This state of apparent complete recovery with positive serologic findings may continue indefinitely without further evidence of disease or sequelae. However, a variable proportion of indeterminate cases, years to a decade or more later, will develop signs and symptoms of chronic Chagas' disease. Except for epidemiologic experience from a particular geographic region, there are no laboratory or clinical indicators to predict the likelihood of future chronic disease.

Chronic Chagas' Disease. Cardiac signs and symptoms are the most common manifestations of chronic disease and are apt to begin with palpitations, dizziness, precordial discomfort, and even syncope. These reflect a variety of arrhythmias, including ventricular extrasystoles, bouts of tachycardia, and various degrees of heart block. Sudden death due to ventricular tachycardia in an otherwise healthy young adult is not at all unusual. Symptoms due to arrhythmias may be present for a long time before cardiomegaly or evidence of cardiac failure appears. When congestive failure develops, it is predominantly right sided and is likely to lead to a fatal outcome within a few years. Peripheral emboli to the brain or other organs are frequent.

Physical examination reveals only an irregular pulse, distant heart sounds, and perhaps a gallop rhythm. With failure, the heart can be very large, functional regurgitant murmurs may be heard, and there is often congestive hepatomegaly and peripheral edema.

The second most common chronic manifestation is megadisease of the esophagus or colon, most frequently the former. The symptoms are indistinguishable from those of idiopathic achalasia and include dysphagia, feeling of fullness after eating or drinking only small amounts, chest pain, and regurgitation. Aspiration with secondary pneumonia is a common complication in advanced cases, as are weight loss and cachexia. Salivary gland hypertrophy secondary to hypersalivation is sometimes seen. Esophageal cancer is reported to be more frequent in patients with chagasic megaesophagus, as with idiopathic achalasia.

Patients with chagasic megacolon suffer from chronic constipation and abdominal pain. Volvulus, obstruction, and perforation of the bowel may occur. An astonishing history of going several weeks between bowel movements can be obtained from some patients with severe megacolon. Megaesophagus and megacolon may both be present in the same patient, and cardiomyopathy can occur with either form of megadisease.

DIAGNOSIS. For both acute and chronic Chagas' disease, a history of possible exposure to *T. cruzi* should be sought. Usual tourist travel to endemic areas is not likely to provide sufficient exposure to infected vectors. Blood transfusion from a chronically infected donor can be a source of infection.

For *acute Chagas' disease* direct microscopic examination of anticoagulated blood or a buffy coat preparation for motile trypanosomes is the most important procedure. Organisms are more difficult to find on stained thin or thick blood films, but the morphology of organisms seen on direct microscopy should be confirmed in a stained preparation. Red cells may be lysed, using 0.083 per cent NH_4Cl to concentrate parasites by centrifugation. If parasites cannot be found in the peripheral blood and acute disease is still suspected, blood can be cultured on NNN (Novy, MacNeal, and Nicolle's medium) or other suitable media. Inoculation of mice with patient's blood may sometimes result in recovery of the parasite. Biopsy of an enlarged lymph node or of skeletal muscle for culture and/or histologic examination is another possibility.

The most sensitive technique for recovery of trypanosomes from the blood is a procedure referred to as xenodiagnosis. It is basically a form of blood culture using the insect vector, by allowing up to 40 normal, laboratory-reared reduviid bugs to feed directly upon the patient or on the patient's blood through a membrane. Circulating parasites ingested by the bugs multiply in the gut and can be detected when the intestinal contents are examined 30 days later. Under experimental conditions, polymerase chain reaction techniques to demonstrate low levels of parasitemia appear promising, but no simple and specific methods are yet available for routine use.

Serologic testing is generally not needed for the diagnosis of acute disease. Parasite-specific immunoglobulin M (IgM) antibodies detected by immunofluorescence or direct agglutination do not become positive until 20 to 40 days after the onset of symptoms. In certain situations this delayed antibody response permits the demonstration of seroconversion. Other laboratory tests often show nonspecific changes, such as a lymphocytic leukocytosis, elevated sedimentation rate, or transient electrocardiographic abnormalities. Reversible cardiomegaly and even pericardial effusion may occur.

The diagnosis of *chronic Chagas' disease* requires demonstration of antibodies to *T. cruzi* in the presence of the characteristic cardiac abnormalities and/or megadisease. Thus, except for the positive serologic findings, the diagnosis relies heavily upon clinical judgment in excluding other causes of heart disease or gastrointestinal dysfunction. A positive xenodiagnosis is strongly suggestive, but not in itself diagnostic, of chronic disease, since patients in the indeterminate phase may have low-level parasitemia. A variety of assays for specific antibody are available, and generally the results of different tests are comparable. However, there are cross-reactions in some tests with sera from patients with leishmaniasis or syphilis, for example. Therefore, in individual cases it may be very helpful to confirm the presence of antibody to specific antigens of *T. cruzi* with more sophisticated tests, such as immunoblots.

Symptomatic heart involvement in the chronic disease is manifested by characteristic ECG abnormalities, often without cardiomegaly. The most common of these is complete right bundle branch block. Other frequent ECG findings are left anterior hemiblock, ventricular extrasystoles, and even complete heart block. If heart failure is present, radiographs and echocardiograms will show generalized cardiomegaly with a reduced ejection fraction (Fig. 426–2).

Chagasic megaesophagus in the early stages shows only delayed emptying and minimal dilatation on studies after a barium swallow. With more advanced disease, retention of swallowed material and eosophageal dilatation are progressively increased. Manometric studies show spasm of the esophageal sphincter and uncoordinated peristaltic movements. Endoscopy should be performed to rule out malignant disease. However, all of these findings are indistinguishable from idiopathic achalasia. Barium enema with air contrast shows the dilated colon with impaired peristalsis, but other causes of colonic obstruction must be ruled out.

DIFFERENTIAL DIAGNOSIS. When acute Chagas' disease is symptomatic and severe, it can resemble a variety of acute systemic infections. Romaña's sign must be distinguished from other causes of unilateral orbital edema, such as the reaction to an insect bite, trauma, or orbital cellulitis.

Congenital infections are virtually indistinguishable from congenital toxoplasmosis, cytomegalic inclusion disease, and syphilis.

Various cardiomyopathies, such as postpartum, alcoholic, and endomyocardial fibrosis, can resemble chronic Chagas' heart disease. Endocardial biopsy is of dubious diagnostic value because of the nonspecific pathologic changes in chagasic cardiomyopathy; it might, however, identify other causes of heart disease. The characteristic heart murmurs of rheumatic valvular disease are helpful in differentiating this entity from chagasic cardiomyopa-

thy. The value of positive serologic findings for *T. cruzi* in the differential diagnosis of both heart and megadisease will depend upon the background prevalence of antibodies in the general population.

TREATMENT. Two drugs with reasonable antitrypanosomal activity are currently in use for the treatment of Chagas' disease. One of these is a nitrofuran derivative, nifurtimox (Lampit, Bayer 2502), which has been extensively evaluated. Nifurtimox* is the only drug available in the United States for treatment of Chagas' disease; it is used in a dose of 8 to 12 mg per kilogram per day. The second drug, benznidazole (Radinil, Roche 7-1051), is a nitroimidazole derivative that appears to be equal to nifurtimox in efficacy, although there is less experience with its use. The exact mechanism of antitrypanosomal action of both of these drugs is not known.

There is now considerable evidence that if patients with acute Chagas' disease are treated with either nifurtimox or benznidazole, the likelihood of future chronic disease is reduced. Many patients treated in the acute phase never develop antibodies to *T. cruzi*, or do so only transiently. From this observation, plus the fact that xenodiagnosis in such treated patients often does not indicate parasites, it is assumed that parasites can be eliminated and the patient cured if treated in the acute stage. However, nifurtimox is not uniformly effective in producing these results, and parasite strains from certain geographic areas (Brazil) appear to be less responsive to treatment than do strains from other countries (Argentina and Chile).

The frequency of side effects from both nifurtimox and benznidazole is high, and since they are administered for 60 to 90 days, drug toxicity is a serious problem. The most common adverse effect with nifurtimox is gastrointestinal intolerance, with anorexia, nausea, vomiting, and abdominal pain. Neurologic symptoms include restlessness, insomnia, disorientation, paresthesias, polyneuritis, and even seizures. Skin rashes can also occur. Peripheral neuropathy and bone marrow suppression have been reported with benznidazole. These side effects subside when the dosage of the drugs is reduced or treatment is stopped.

Since these drugs have shown effectiveness in treatment of acute Chagas' disease, some Latin American physicians are also treating chronic and indeterminate cases. There is no evidence that the established pathologic changes of chronic Chagas' disease can be reversed by nifurtimox or benznidazole therapy. The question of whether drug treatment in the indeterminate case, i.e., the asymptomatic patient with positive serologic findings, would prevent development of later chronic disease is controversial. Although it would not be easy, the issue ideally could be settled by a controlled, long-term prospective study. Some data

---

*An investigational drug that must be obtained from the Centers for Disease Control Drug Service (404-639-3356).

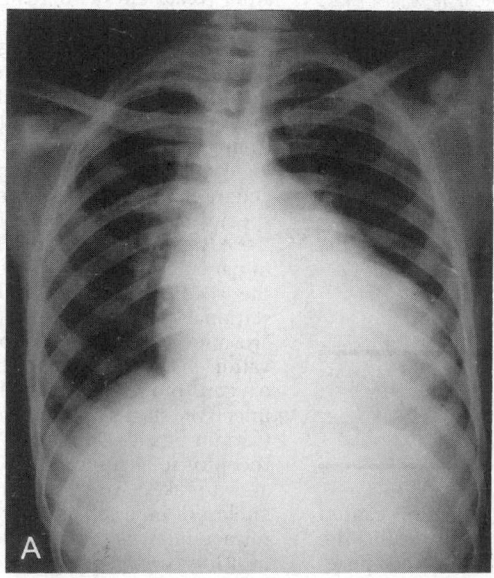
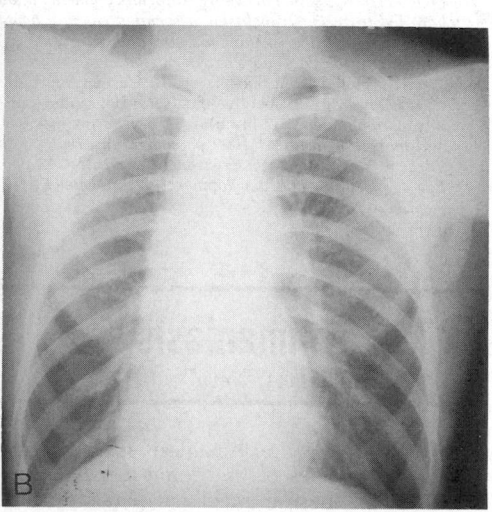

FIGURE 426–2. *A*, Cardiac silhouette in a patient with chronic chagasic cardiomyopathy and heart failure. *B*, Chest radiograph showing a widened mediastinum due to a greatly dilated megaesophagus of chronic Chagas' disease.

suggest that low-level parasitemia, as assessed by xenodiagnosis, can be reduced or eliminated after treatment with antitrypanosomal drugs, including allopurinol. But such studies require critical confirmation to establish their ultimate influence on the development of chronic disease, as well as risk versus benefit evaluation.

The treatment of patients with established chronic heart disease is supportive. Patients with frequent ventricular premature beats can benefit from antiarrhythmic drugs such as amiodarone. Cardiac pacemakers may prolong survival of those with complete heart block. The congestive failure of chagasic cardiomyopathy is disappointingly refractory to the usual cardiotropic drugs.

More options are open for the management and treatment of megadisease. In the early stages of megaesophagus, pneumatic dilatation of the sphincter is probably more effective than bougienage. For more advanced cases, various surgical procedures involving myotomy of the sphincter or partial resection are necessary. Early stages of megacolon can be managed by manipulation of diet and use of laxatives and occasional enemas. Sometimes resection of an aperistaltic section of the colon can be done in more severe cases.

PREVENTION. Chagas' disease could be eliminated as a serious health problem for the rural poor of Latin America by adequate housing and education. But stark socioeconomic realities dictate another approach to control. This consists mainly of the use of residual insecticides directed at domiciliary vectors. The use of benzene hexachloride (BHC), sprayed once or twice a year, has been very effective when used systematically.

Serologic testing in blood banks to avoid the use of seropositive donors is carried out in endemic areas. Another precaution is to add 1:4000 gentian violet to blood 24 hours before use to kill trypanosomes that may be present. With the recent occurrence of several transfusion-associated cases of acute Chagas' disease in North America, the question of serologic screening of blood donors has been raised for areas of the country with large Latin American populations. The development of vaccines is still in the research stage.

American Trypanosomiasis Research. PAHO Scientific Publication 318, 1975. *Proceedings of an international symposium with useful reviews on all aspects of the subject, including the vector bugs and control of the disease.*

Amorin DS, Manco JC, Gallo L Jr, et al.: Chagas' disease as an experimental model for studies of cardiac autonomic function in man. Mayo Clinic Proc (Suppl) 57:48, 1982. *A careful evaluation of cardiac autonomic function (changes in heart rate after vagal blockade with atropine and after Valsalva maneuver and hand grip exercise) that indicates that some individuals infected with T. cruzi, but without overt signs of heart disease, show evidence of cardiac autonomic denervation. There are many references to previous similar studies by the first author.*

Dias JCP: The indeterminate form of human chronic Chagas' disease. A clinical epidemiological review. Rev Soc Bras Med Trop 22:147, 1989. *A well-balanced review in English by a Brazilian expert. It documents the important point that infection with T. cruzi does not invariably progress to chronic disease.*

Dvorak J, Gibson C, Maekelt A: A bibliography on Chagas' disease (1968–1984). Washington, D.C., National Institutes of Health, Pan American Health Organization and World Health Organization, 1985. *This Medlars-based computer-processed bibliography is a complete listing of references on an annual basis, by author and subject for the period indicated. For real students of the subject!*

Kirchhoff LV: Is *Trypanosoma cruzi* a new threat to our blood supply? Ann Intern Med 111:773, 1989. *This short editorial comments upon the circumstances that have led to recent transfusion-associated cases of acute Chagas' disease in the United States. The arguments for and problems associated with serologic screening of blood donors are discussed.*

Maguire JH, Hoff R, Sherlock I, et al.: Cardiac morbidity and mortality due to Chagas' disease: Prospective electrocardiographic study of a Brazilian community. Circulation 75:1140, 1987. *A 6-year prospective study of ECG changes and mortality in about 1000 people in an area of Brazil endemic to Chagas' disease. Antibodies to T. cruzi were present in 42 per cent of the population. Excess mortality and development of abnormal ECGs were clearly related to positive serology.*

427 Leishmaniasis

Franklin A. Neva

DEFINITION. Leishmaniasis is a protozoan infection caused by various species of the genus *Leishmania*. Paradoxically, the host cells for these intracellular parasites are mononuclear phagocytes, cells that normally destroy microorganisms. In nature the infection is usually a zoonosis, with transmission of the parasite by sandflies to wild or domestic animals, especially rodents and canines, with humans as incidental hosts.

Human leishmanial infections can result in three main forms of disease, sometimes with dual manifestations in the same patient. The *visceral* form (kala-azar) is a systemic disease with parasites in the reticuloendothelial system, characterized by hepatosplenomegaly, fever, weight loss, leukopenia, and ultimately death if the disease is untreated. The *cutaneous* disease is generally manifested by one or more indolent ulcers, but a wide spectrum of skin involvement can occur. When parasites from skin lesions sometimes metastasize to produce later destructive lesions of the oronasopharynx, the result is *mucocutaneous* leishmaniasis. Although parasite species are the main determinant for the form of disease, clinical manifestations and outcome are also dependent upon the immune response of the host.

ETIOLOGY. *Leishmania* exist in two morphologic forms, a motile flagellate, or *promastigote*, and a smaller, nonmotile intracellular form, the *amastigote*. Promastigotes are found in the sandfly vector as well as in cultures, both habitats requiring temperatures of about 22 to 26°C. Also called *Leishman-Donovan* or *LD bodies* after their describers, amastigotes are the form of parasite found in humans or other vertebrate hosts. In addition to a nucleus, these 2 by 5 μm round or oval bodies contain a characteristic rodlike structure of extranuclear DNA, the *kinetoplast*, a useful structure in morphologic identification and differentiation from other intracellular organisms.

In the infected animal, leishmania are found only in monocytes and macrophages, where they multiply by binary fission. An appropriate sandfly vector becomes infected by ingesting organisms during a blood meal from tissue juice or cells in the skin or blood. In the gut of the sandfly, the parasites transform to promastigotes and multiply as spindle-shaped flagellates 15 to 26 μm long and 2 to 3 μm wide. In vectors ultimately capable of transmitting the parasite, promastigotes tend to migrate into the pharynx and buccal cavity. At least 7 days are needed before the sandfly becomes infective. The actual mechanism by which infective promastigotes are transferred to a new vertebrate host is not clear—possibly by regurgitation into the bite wound during a blood meal or perhaps even by being rubbed into abrasions after a successful swat. Once inoculated, the promastigotes are taken up by macrophages; they transform into amastigotes and begin to multiply. A vasoactive factor in sandfly salivary glands that enhances parasite infectivity has been described. Amastigotes that rupture from infected macrophages are taken up by adjacent cells; some infected cells may be transported to distant sites via the blood or lymphatics.

Classification of *Leishmania* is based primarily upon patterns of parasite isoenzymes separated by electrophoresis and immunologic reactions of surface and parasite-soluble (EF or excretion factor) antigens with monoclonal and polyclonal antisera. Additional taxonomic criteria include hybridization of kinetoplast DNA after treatment with restriction endonucleases and the type of disease produced in experimental animals. For example, *L. donovani* produces a progressive disease in hamsters similar to human visceral disease, and strains of *L. major* produce cutaneous ulcers in BALB/c mice with later visceralization and death. The most meaningful classification of *Leishmania* will probably come from correlating biochemical and immunologic results with biologic characteristics of the organisms. Table 427–1 summarizes geographic distribution and usual clinical features of the main species of *Leishmania*.

PARASITE-HOST INTERACTION. Some of the early events in parasite-macrophage interaction are easier to understand since the recent finding with *L. major* that only organisms in the stationary growth phase, both in culture and in the sandfly vector, are infective. Log-phase promastigotes are readily lysed by activation of complement in fresh serum and are susceptible to the oxygen burst of macrophages when ingested. Stationary, or infective, stages are more resistant to both of these host defenses. Certain ligands on macrophage membranes, such as CR3 and the receptor for mannose-fucose, are involved in parasite attachment and uptake. After ingestion by macrophages, leishmania are enclosed in a phagocytic vacuole. In contrast to some other intracellular organisms, leishmania not only survive but also multiply within phagolysosomes into which lysosomal enzymes

TABLE 427–1. GEOGRAPHIC DISTRIBUTION AND CLINICAL DISEASE CAUSED BY DIFFERENT SPECIES OF *LEISHMANIA*

Species	Geographic Distribution	Clinical Manifestations
L. mexicana complex (*L. m. mexicana, L. m. amazonensis, L. m. venezuelensis,* ? others)	New World—from southern U.S. through Central America, northern and central South America, Dominican Republic	Cutaneous ulcers; small proportion of patients may develop diffuse cutaneous (DCL) or mucocutaneous (MCL) leishmaniasis
L. braziliensis complex (*L. b. braziliensis, L. b. panamensis, L. b. guyanesis, L. b. peruviana*)	New World—from Central America through various parts of South America, including Brazil, Venezuela, Bolivia, Peru to northern Argentina	Cutaneous ulcers; some cases may later develop MCL (probably more likely if cutaneous lesion not treated adequately)
L. major	Northern Africa, Middle East, Central Africa, and southern Asia	Cutaneous ulcers
L. tropica	Middle East and southern Asia	Cutaneous ulcers and chronic relapsing cutaneous disease (recidivans form); rarely kala-azar
L. aethiopica	Ethiopia	Cutaneous ulcers, rarely DCL
L. donovani	Old World—East Africa and south of Sahara, southern Asia, including India and Iran	Visceral leishmaniasis; small proportion may develop post–kala-azar dermal leishmaniasis
L. infantum (? separate species)	Old World—North Africa and southern Europe	Visceral leishmaniasis; rarely cutaneous
L. chagasi (? separate species)	New World—foci in several areas of Brazil, Venezuela, Honduras, and Colombia, and isolated cases elsewhere in Central and South America	Visceral leishmaniasis; also nonulcerative cutaneous

*DCL = Diffuse cutaneous leishmaniasis; MCL = mucocutaneous leishmaniasis.

are discharged. The parasite is probably protected from this enzyme assault by the presence of abundant membrane-bound acid phosphatase. Leishmanial parasites within macrophages in vitro can be destroyed by activating cells or exposure to certain lymphokines, such as interferon-γ.

The variation in temperature sensitivity of various species of leishmania is a critical factor that determines clinical expression of the disease. For example, *L. donovani* can survive and multiply in macrophages at higher temperatures than can cutaneous strains. Among isolates causing cutaneous disease in the Americas, most members of the *L. mexicana* complex are inhibited to a greater extent at 37°C than are strains of the *L. braziliensis* complex. These differences in temperature tolerance probably explain why some varieties of cutaneous leishmaniasis can be treated successfully by local heat.

IMMUNOLOGY. The pattern of humoral and cell-mediated immune responses that normally develops during or after leishmanial infection varies with the clinical form of disease. Serum antibody can be demonstrated by a variety of tests, usually indirect immunofluorescence assay (IFA) or enzyme-linked immunosorbent assay (ELISA), in patients with established visceral or cutaneous leishmaniasis. Cell-mediated immunity in leishmaniasis can be evaluated by a delayed hypersensitivity skin test (leishmanin or Montenegro test) or by lymphocyte proliferation to leishmanial antigen. Positive skin test results and lymphocyte proliferation are normally present in patients with cutaneous disease, but only after recovery or effective treatment in patients with visceral disease. Cell-mediated immunity is absent or suppressed during active visceral infections.

Resistance to leishmaniasis is best correlated with the presence of cell-mediated immunity. Its absence in visceral disease has already been noted, and it is dramatically demonstrated in a rare form of disease called *diffuse cutaneous leishmaniasis* (DCL). In patients with DCL, not only is there specific anergy to the skin test but also parasites are very abundant in lesions, lymphocytes are scanty, lesions do not ulcerate, and response to chemotherapy is poor. Antigen-specific suppressor cells have been demonstrated in DCL. In contrast, a normal immune response in cutaneous leishmaniasis is generally associated with lesions that ulcerate and show relatively few parasites but abundant lymphocytes and even giant cells, plus a positive skin test. This relationship of immune response to clinical forms of disease in leishmaniasis is similar to that in leprosy (see Ch. 334).

VISCERAL LEISHMANIASIS (Kala-Azar)

EPIDEMIOLOGY. The visceral form of leishmaniasis, caused by *L. donovani* and related organisms, has worldwide distribution. Certain regions continue to be endemic areas of this disease. These include the following: northeastern India, especially Assam

and Bihar states; Kenya, Sudan, and Ethiopia in eastern Africa; northeastern China; the shores of the Caspian Sea and Iran in southern Asia; the countries of Europe, North Africa, and the Middle East surrounding the Mediterranean; and northeastern Brazil. In addition to these macrofoci, smaller foci occur outside these areas. In the Western Hemisphere, for example, visceral leishmaniasis is sporadically seen in southern Brazil, Paraguay, and northern Argentina, as well as in the vicinity of Belém at the mouth of the Amazon. In addition, there are foci of transmission in Venezuela, Colombia, and Honduras. Isolated cases occur in other Central American countries and Mexico.

With such a wide geographic distribution of the disease, it is not surprising that different species of phlebotomine flies are involved in the various regions. What is surprising is that the causative organisms from these widely separated regions are relatively uniform in their properties. The organisms causing visceral leishmaniasis in the Mediterranean region (*L. infantum*) and those in the Americas (*L. chagasi*) are very similar to one another, but sufficiently different from *L. donovani* to be considered separate species. *L. chagasi* was probably introduced to the New World by explorers or their dogs.

FACTORS AFFECTING TRANSMISSION. A common transmission cycle for *L. donovani* that takes place close to people involves dogs as reservoir hosts and sandfly vectors that will also feed on humans. The domestic dog, as well as wild canines such as the fox, develop a chronic systemic disease very similar to that of humans when infected with *L. donovani*. But an additional unique feature of leishmanial infection in canines is the frequent presence of organisms in the skin, including the nose and ears, which are favorite feeding sites of sandflies. An epidemiologic cycle of the parasite involving wild foxes, domestic dogs, and humans via the vector *Lutzomyia longipalpis* has been documented in northeastern Brazil. The domestic dog has also been incriminated as an important reservoir host for visceral leishmaniasis of the Mediterranean region and in certain areas of China.

Rodents are the likely reservoir in the Sudan, and the activity of the vector, *Phlebotomus orientalis*, is high in clumps of acacia woodland near villages. In Kenya, transmission of disease is associated with termite hills, which serve as resting places for the vector, *P. martini*, and around which village men gather in the evening. However, the animal reservoir in Kenya has not been identified. In some regions such as northeastern India, humans appear to be their own reservoir, and several factors serve to facilitate person-to-person transmission. The vector, *P. argentipes*, has a preference for human blood. The parasite is found in circulating monocytes in Indian cases of kala-azar more frequently than usual. Dermal lesions that develop after the initial disease in Indian patients may be an additional source of parasites for the vector.

The past few decades have seen a resurgence of visceral leishmaniasis in regions where it had disappeared after the widespread use of chlorophenothane (DDT) for malaria control. Phlebotomine populations were greatly reduced around houses, but zoonotic transmission was not affected. When the use of residual insecticides was discontinued, transmission to people was re-established. This has occurred in the countries around the Mediterranean, with an epidemic reported in western Italy.

Outbreaks of visceral leishmaniasis have often followed famine, wars, and civil or political disturbances resulting in malnutrition and mass migration of people. It is not known whether this is due to greater exposure to infected vectors, defective immune response, reactivation of latent infection, or a combination of these and other factors.

PATHOLOGY. The organs mainly affected are the liver, spleen, bone marrow, and elements of the reticuloendothelial system in diverse sites. These organs and tissues hypertrophy, with the increased cells made up of parasitized macrophages and histiocytes, but with little or no lymphocytic response. Generalized enlargement of lymph nodes is not a consistent finding (see below), but hyperplasia of lymphoid tissue in the nasopharynx and in the Peyer's patches of the gut is common. Endothelial proliferation occurs in certain organs as within septa of pulmonary alveoli and in renal glomeruli.

The spleen is enlarged, sometimes to tremendous size, but is firm and has a thick capsule. Although the splenic pulp is friable and there may be infarcts, the nature and chronic course of the enlargement make the spleen relatively resistant to tears from an aspirating needle. Enlargement of the liver is due to hyperplasia of the Kupffer cells, which are packed with amastigotes. Only rarely are parenchymal cells of the liver parasitized. There may be focal granulomas and some fibrosis in the liver in chronic untreated cases.

The bone marrow is infiltrated with parasitized macrophages, a process that may later impair red and white cell production. The enlarged spleen undoubtedly also contributes to the anemia and leukopenia. There is a striking polyclonal B cell activation that results in high immunoglobulin G (IgG) and total serum protein values. Some organs, most notably the kidneys, may show pathologic changes secondary to deposition of immune complexes.

CLINICAL FEATURES. The incubation period is long, generally 1 to 3 months, but it may be as short as 10 to 14 days. There are well-documented instances of activation of latent infection several years after exposure to the parasite, under conditions of immunosuppression. The onset is usually insidious and difficult to date, especially among people who regard intermittent fevers and lassitude as normal. Fever, accompanied by sweating, weakness, and weight loss, gradually becomes noticeable. These symptoms, perhaps including nonproductive cough and abdominal discomfort produced by an enlarging liver and spleen, may continue for months with the patient still up and about. In some patients the course of disease is more rapid, with high temperature and chills, simulating typhoid fever or acute brucellosis. The most prominent physical findings are fever, splenomegaly, and cachexia, which is especially evident in the thorax and shoulder girdle (Fig. 427–1). Although the fever pattern can be variable, ultimately it often exhibits characteristic twice-daily elevations to 38 to 40°C for some time. Generalized adenopathy is common in patients from some geographic areas, but it is seldom striking. In light-skinned patients, hyperpigmentation of the skin may be noted; the term *kala-azar* is Hindi for black sickness. Splenic enlargement can be extreme in this disease, often reaching the iliac fossa, and the organ is firm and nontender. Some otherwise typical cases may involve only modest hepatosplenomegaly.

COURSE AND COMPLICATIONS. There is increasing evidence from skin test and serologic surveys, as well as prospective epidemiologic studies, that asymptomatic and subclinical infections with spontaneous recovery are more common than is overt disease. Poor nutritional state is a critical predisposing factor. When infection becomes clinically apparent, manifestations of systemic disease include fever, weight loss, fatigue, and anemia. Subcutaneous edema, ascites, and other evidence of hypoalbuminemia may develop. Bleeding from the nose or gums can

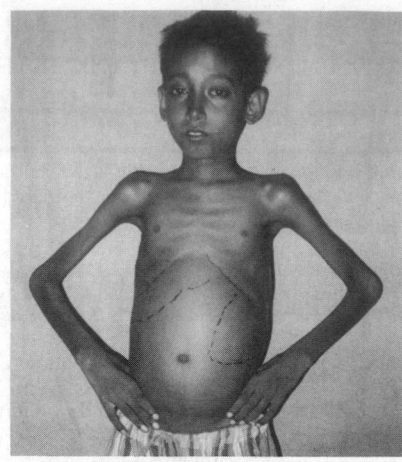

FIGURE 427–1. Indian patient with kala-azar. Note wasting of thorax and shoulder girdle and hepatosplenomegaly as outlined.

occur. Finally, after an illness that may be as short as a few months or as long as a year, the patient becomes emaciated and exhausted. In the great majority of instances, death is due to intercurrent infections such as pneumonia, tuberculosis, dysentery, and gangrenous stomatitis. Advanced cases are particularly susceptible because of leukopenia and undoubted impairment of cell-mediated immunologic function, although specific mechanisms have not been defined. Another cause of death is massive gastrointestinal bleeding.

SKIN LESIONS ASSOCIATED WITH KALA-AZAR. In the early stages of visceral leishmaniasis, small nodules in the skin containing parasites have been described at or near the inoculation site. There are scattered reports of the demonstration of parasites even in apparently normal skin. A somewhat more common type of cutaneous lesion, although variable by geographic location, is post–kala-azar dermal leishmaniasis (PKDL). This is the development in some patients, weeks or months after recovery from disease, of papular or nodular lesions containing many parasites. Depigmentation of the skin resembling vitiligo may occur as a sequel to PKDL. The presence of chronic, nonulcerative, papular lesions, often located on the face of children and young adults, has been described from endemic areas for kala-azar in Honduras. Although these patients had no history of kala-azar, *L. chagasi* was cultured from the lesions. No systemic evidence of disease or consistent immunologic abnormalities are demonstrable in cases of PKDL or the atypical cutaneous disease.

SPECIFIC LABORATORY DIAGNOSIS. Since other clinical states may mimic certain features of visceral leishmaniasis, demonstration of the parasite, preferably by culture, is essential before treatment is undertaken. In addition, presence or absence of the parasite can be used to monitor response to treatment. Organisms are most readily recovered by aspiration from bone marrow, spleen (see Color Plate 11F), liver, lymph nodes, or blood. Material obtained is:

1. Used to make smears and slides stained with Giemsa or other Romanovsky stains for examination under oil immersion for amastigotes. Although bone marrow aspiration is usually the method of choice, splenic aspiration can be done if the spleen is readily palpable, if prothrombin and bleeding times are normal, and if proper technique is used (see Chulay and Bryceson for details).

2. Inoculated into appropriate culture media.

3. Inoculated into hamsters, but 3 to 4 months may be required before organisms are found in their liver or spleen, so this method is not very practical.

Immunologic Tests. By the time patients with visceral leishmaniasis come to clinical attention, they invariably have readily demonstrable antileishmanial serum antibodies. For this, the ELISA test using promastigotes as antigen is probably the most practical; it can be read visually if necessary and is applicable for testing large numbers of sera, including specimens eluted from filter paper. The IFA test employing either amastigotes or promastigotes as antigen has been used, as has direct agglutination of fixed promastigotes. In certain areas of Latin America, there may be cross-reactions with sera from people infected with *Trypanosoma cruzi.* The leishmanin skin test for delayed hypersensitivity is negative in cases of active visceral leishmaniasis but becomes positive after recovery.

Laboratory Findings. Most of the laboratory abnormalities involve the hematopoietic system. Leukopenia, with absolute reductions in neutrophils and eosinophils and a relative increase in lymphocytes and monocytes, is characteristic. In one series the total white cell count was below 4000 in 90 per cent of cases by 1 month after onset of symptoms, and it frequently may be around 2000. Thrombocytopenia is also present, and the erythrocyte sedimentation rate is increased. A moderately severe normocytic and normochromic anemia, unless complicated by blood loss or deficiency states, is very common, caused by increased red cell destruction. In late stages of the disease prothrombin, bleeding, and clotting times are prolonged.

Total serum proteins are increased to levels of 9 to 10 grams per deciliter, virtually all IgG, because of polyclonal B cell activation. Serum albumin levels, especially in advanced cases, are normal or low. The striking hyperglobulinemia is the basis for the old recommended diagnostic tests, such as the formol-gel test and Chopra reaction, before specific serodiagnosis was available. Evidence for circulating immune complexes, based upon C1q binding in the serum, is readily demonstrable. Liver function tests show only mild abnormalities, if any.

DIFFERENTIAL DIAGNOSIS. Chronic malaria in endemic regions may present some problems in differential diagnosis. In malaria-immune individuals, the presence of malaria parasites in the blood does not rule out the additional diagnosis of leishmaniasis. Conversely, an enlarged spleen is hardly enough on which to base the diagnosis. Tropical splenomegaly syndrome (an exaggerated immune response to malaria) could easily be confused with the clinical picture of visceral leishmaniasis. Several different forms of schistosomiasis may also mimic visceral leishmaniasis: the acute disease with fever and hepatosplenomegaly, the severe chronic variety with Symmers' fibrosis and portal hypertension, and chronic relapsing enteric fever that can be a complication of schistosomiasis. Other diseases that may resemble kala-azar include lymphoma, cirrhosis of the liver with hypersplenism, miliary tuberculosis, brucellosis, typhoid fever, and subacute bacterial endocarditis.

TREATMENT. The drug of choice for treatment has been and remains pentavalent antimony (Sb), even with novel approaches to possible use of other drugs. The Sb preparation available in the United States* and some European countries is sodium stibogluconate (Pentostam), a preparation containing 100 mg of Sb per milliliter. The dose is 20 mg per kilogram of body weight, given daily by intramuscular or intravenous injection, not exceeding 1000 mg of Sb per day. Another pentavalent Sb preparation used in Latin America, meglumine antimonate (Glucantime), is virtually identical but contains a slightly lower concentration of Sb per milliliter. The total dose required for cure varies in different parts of the world; Mediterranean kala-azar generally responds to 10 or 15 doses, whereas the disease in Kenya requires 30 injections, and up to 30 per cent of cases may still relapse within 6 months. Pentavalent Sb is relatively nontoxic in comparison to trivalent Sb, except for local pain at the injection site when given intramuscularly. Other side effects are cumulative with dose and include arthralgias, weakness, nausea, vomiting, slight elevation of liver enzyme values, and nonspecific T wave changes if electrocardiograms are obtained.

Response to treatment is not dramatic and may not be apparent for several weeks. Useful indicators to follow are temperature, spleen size, hemoglobin, and white blood cell count. Weekly splenic aspirates were used by one group, with "cure" defined as two successively negative aspirates a week apart. Since relapse may occur up to a year after apparent cure, monthly follow-up for 6 months and then follow-up after a year are recommended.

Primary unresponsiveness to Sb, that is, little or no improvement during or after the first course, occurs in up to 10 per cent of cases. Actual resistance of the parasite to Sb has been difficult to document in humans; therefore, lack of response may reflect

*From Centers for Disease Control, 404-329-3670, 8:00 A.M. to 4:39 P.M. EST Monday through Friday; 404-329-2888, evenings, weekends, and holidays.

ineffective immune mechanisms of the host. Allopurinol combined with Sb is reported to be of benefit in some unresponsive patients. Pentamidine is a second-line drug. The dosage of pentamidine† is 4 mg per kilogram given intramuscularly three times weekly for 10 doses, but severe pain at the injection site is common, and sterile abscess formation can occur. Additional systemic side effects of anorexia, nausea, abdominal pain, hypotension, and development of diabetes in 10 per cent of patients make the decision to use pentamidine a difficult one. Another second-line drug, amphotericin B, must be given intravenously on alternate days at 1 mg per kilogram each time over many weeks to achieve the recommended total dose of 1.5 to 2.0 grams. This drug regularly produces chills, fever, and nausea with each dose and a cumulative reduction of hemoglobin and renal function. New approaches to treatment include incorporation of drugs in liposomes for more efficient uptake by macrophages and use of interferon-γ combined with Sb.

Supportive treatment can be very important, especially in the malnourished and debilitated. These patients are prone to develop complicating bacterial infections for which proper treatment must be instituted. Fluid and electrolyte imbalance must be corrected, and hemorrhagic complications may require blood transfusion. Good nursing care, attention to oral hygiene, adequate diet, and correction of nutritional deficiencies are, of course, desirable.

PREVENTION. Since the epidemiology of kala-azar varies among different geographic areas, the local conditions responsible for transmission must be understood to implement preventive measures. Where sandflies are in or around houses, vector control with insecticides is appropriate. If an animal reservoir such as the domestic dog is involved, destruction of infected dogs, especially strays, can be instituted. If focal sites of infected flies are known, they can be destroyed or avoided. Personal protection by wearing protective clothing in the evenings, using insect repellents, and sleeping under fine mesh netting is applicable under some circumstances.

CUTANEOUS LEISHMANIASIS OF THE OLD WORLD (Oriental Sore) AND NEW WORLD (Including Mucocutaneous or Espundia)

EPIDEMIOLOGY. Although basically the same disease, there are differences in epidemiology and clinical course in cutaneous leishmaniasis of the Old and New Worlds. In the Mediterranean basin, Middle East, and southern Asia, the disease tends to be clinically more benign and occurs in semiarid and desert climates; transmission can become established in villages and cities. Cutaneous leishmaniasis in the Americas is acquired by workers in the jungle or by farmers and their families living at its edges. The New World disease sometimes produces later metastatic and destructive lesions of the mucous membranes.

The epidemiology of cutaneous leishmaniasis is best understood in southern Russia, Iran, and Middle Eastern countries where infected desert rodents (*Rhombomys opimus* and *Psammomys obesus*) live in burrows with phlebotomine vectors (often *Phlebotomus papatasii*). People are infected with *L. major* when they invade this environment to establish settlements or excavate archaeologic ruins. If settlements are established, the parasite may adapt to a new transmission cycle with dogs and humans as reservoirs and an urban sandfly such as *P. sergenti* as vector. Parasite species from such locations are often identified as *L. tropica.* The commonness of typical face scars in adults in Iran, Afghanistan, Syria, and Iraq indicates the high frequency of cutaneous leishmaniasis in these countries.

The epidemiology of cutaneous leishmaniasis in West Africa and the sub-Sahara belt is less clear. Human cases are sporadic, with a rural transmission cycle, and the parasite species is often *L. major.* In Ethiopia and Kenya, however, the animal reservoir is often the hyrax (*Procavia*), the vector is *Phlebotomus longipes*, and the parasite species is *L. aethiopica.*

In the Americas, cutaneous leishmaniasis occurs from Texas to northern Argentina (see Color Plate 10C), with only Chile free of the disease. Except for some areas of Peru, where the domestic

†Available from Centers for Disease Control, Atlanta, GA.

dog is a reservoir, New World cutaneous leishmaniasis is a forest or jungle zoonosis, with forest rodents or sloths serving as animal reservoirs. Western Hemisphere sandfly vectors are now classified as members of the genus *Lutzomyia*.

The organism in Texas (10 human cases), Mexico, and northern Central America is mainly *Leishmania m. mexicana*. Members of the *L. braziliensis* complex are predominant in the remainder of Central America, Panama, and northern South America. This species complex also extends into Brazil, Bolivia, and tropical regions of Peru, with complex ecologic combinations of jungle animal reservoirs and sandfly vectors. Yet within the major distribution of a group, there may be isolated pockets of a second species complex, such as *L. b. braziliensis* in Belize, where *L. mexicana* predominates, or *L. mexicana* on the Atlantic coast of Panama, and *L. m. amazonensis* in many sites of central Brazil. Additional members of the two major complexes, or even new species, are likely to be described as newer methods of taxonomy are applied.

PATHOLOGY. The earliest changes at the site of inoculation have not been described. Established lesions show a large accumulation of macrophages containing amastigotes, with variable numbers of lymphocytes and plasma cells. There may be focal accumulations of polymorphonuclear cells, especially in areas of necrosis, but the exact mechanism for ulceration of the epithelium is not clear. With time, numbers of parasites diminish and the lesion heals. In other instances the lesion persists and a granulomatous histologic reaction is seen, including multinucleated giant cells. This is the type of pathology seen in *chronic relapsing cutaneous leishmaniasis*, also known as the *lupoid* or *recidivans* form. Delayed skin test reactivity to leishmanial antigen is present in normally healing and recidivans leishmaniasis.

The unusual complication known as diffuse cutaneous leishmaniasis (DCL), associated with anergy to leishmanial antigen, has a different histologic picture. DCL lesions show a heavy infiltrate of foamy or vacuolated macrophages containing large numbers of amastigotes with only scant numbers of lymphocytes. Moreover, the overlying epithelium is not ulcerated.

The lesions of mucocutaneous leishmaniasis (espundia) represent the metastatic spread of organisms via the bloodstream to mucous membranes of the nose, mouth, and upper pharyngeal tissues. The histology is a confusing mixture of granulomatous inflammatory cell reaction with necrosis, fibrosis, and often response to secondary bacterial infection. Organisms are usually scanty. Tissue destruction can involve cartilage with perforation of the nasal septum, loss of much of the nose and palate, and even involvement of the larynx.

CLINICAL MANIFESTATIONS. The lesion begins as a small erythematous papule on exposed areas, often the face or extremities, within 2 to 8 weeks after infection. The papule develops a tiny vesicle that opens and oozes some serous fluid and enlarges to form an ulcer with firm, raised, and reddened edges. The ulcer can remain relatively dry with a central crust (dry form) or may ooze (wet form). Lesions can be single or multiple; small satellite papules may occur at the edge of a larger lesion. Subcutaneous nodules in a centripetal alignment from an ulcer may develop (sporotrichoid form). Cutaneous leishmanial lesions generally heal spontaneously, but the process can take a few months to a year or more. The result is a depressed, depigmented scar. *Recidivans* or *lupoid leishmaniasis* may sometimes develop months or years after healing of a primary lesion and may persist for years. This lesion exhibits central healing with nonulcerative papules developing in the periphery or center of the scar. Regional adenopathy may or may not occur with cutaneous leishmaniasis; this finding is not helpful in differential diagnosis.

COMPLICATIONS. Metastatic spread of parasites and development of destructive naso-oropharyngeal lesions is a serious later sequel to cutaneous disease. This mucous membrane involvement occurs almost exclusively in the Western Hemisphere and is said to be associated primarily with *L. braziliensis* infections. Mucocutaneous disease due to *L. mexicana amazonensis* does occur, so until more data correlating parasite type with clinical disease are available, this complication can also be related to geographic region as well as to parasite species. Thus, mucocutaneous leishmaniasis is most common in central Brazil and adjacent portions of Bolivia, Peru, and Ecuador, and is relatively uncommon in Panama and Central America. Mucosal involvement generally does not become manifest until the initial skin lesion has healed, even many years later, and presumably is more likely to occur if there has been no or inadequate treatment of the original ulcer.

Earliest signs and symptoms of mucosal disease commonly involve the nose, with epistaxis and obstruction. Perforation of the nasal septum is common, or the upper lip may be involved. The process can destroy cartilaginous structures of the nose and palate and extend to the larynx. Death may result from aspiration pneumonia or suffocation. Distinction should be made between the mucuous membrane involvement that occurs as direct extension from a facial lesion, as in Ethiopia, and the late metastatic form seen in South America.

DCL is a rare complication that offers insight into immunity to leishmaniasis because it features antigen-specific anergy and cell-mediated immunosuppression. DCL seems to occur more commonly in certain countries (Dominican Republic, Venezuela, Mexico, and Ethiopia) and in the Americas is caused by organisms belonging to the *L. mexicana* complex. The disease begins with one or only a few nodular lesions that do not ulcerate but go on to metastasize to other cutaneous sites, primarily the face and extensor surfaces of the limbs. The subcutaneous nonulcerative nodular lesions are not associated with fever or other systemic symptoms and do not involve visceral organs. The appearance, distribution, and chronic nature of DCL have often led to the erroneous diagnosis of lepromatous leprosy (Fig. 427–2). No mortality is associated with DCL, but disfigurement and ulceration secondary to trauma at pressure points lead to chronic morbidity, since this disease is notoriously unresponsive to the usual antileishmanial drugs.

DIAGNOSIS. Leishmaniasis can be suspected in anyone who develops one or more chronic ulcers on exposed areas of skin after recently visiting or working at archaeologic sites in the Middle East, at Mayan ruins, or in jungle or rural areas of Latin America. Ideally, diagnosis should be confirmed by culture of the organism in NNN (Novy, MacNeal, and Nicolle's medium) or other appropriate media from a biopsy or aspirated specimen obtained from the edge of the lesion. Culture is the most sensitive method for detection of organisms. Excisional or punch biopsy offers an additional advantage of providing a portion of the specimen for histopathologic examination and routine bacteriologic, fungal, and acid-fast cultures in cases in which a wider differential diagnosis is required. Appropriate impression smears can also be made and stained from biopsy material, whether culture is possible or not. If biopsy is not possible because of circumstances or location of the lesion, scrapings from a slit made in involved skin or from the debrided base of an ulcer can be cultured or stained for organisms. The characteristic amastigotes

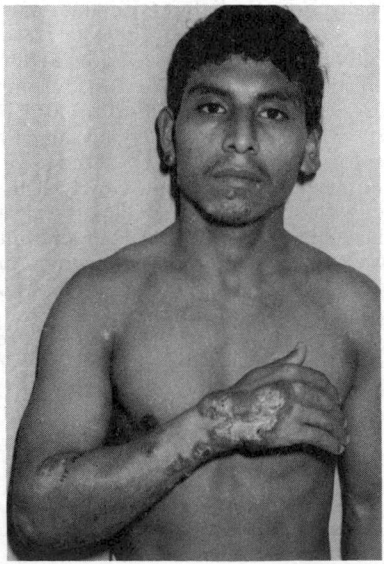

FIGURE 427–2. Patient with diffuse cutaneous leishmaniasis of 5 years' duration. Note nonulcerative lesions of chin, ear lobes, right arm, and hand.

in lesions appear larger and are more easily recognized in smears than in tissue sections. A recent technique that may permit direct and rapid diagnosis, as well as species differentiation of leishmania, is blotting with radiolabeled DNA probes. The numbers of parasites present and ease of culture vary with the strain, but the concentration of parasites in lesions tends to diminish with time as healing occurs, and they are also reduced if the ulcer is secondarily infected with bacteria. It is usually more difficult to culture or demonstrate organisms in lesions of mucocutaneous disease.

A positive leishmanin skin test and serum antibody can usually be demonstrated in patients by the time a cutaneous lesion has ulcerated. These tests remain positive in mucocutaneous disease. Serologic tests are not very useful in diagnosis because antibody levels are low. It must also be remembered that positive skin and serologic tests can reflect a previous rather than a current leishmanial infection.

Cutaneous leishmaniasis must be differentiated from the following conditions, with decreasing likelihood of occurrence: nonspecific tropical or traumatic ulcers due to bacterial infection or stasis; fungal infections, especially sporotrichosis and blastomycosis; mycobacterial infections such as *Mycobacterium marinum* and *tuberculosis;* syphilis and other treponematoses of the skin; sarcoidosis; and neoplastic ulcers. Mucocutaneous leishmaniasis is especially likely to mimic infection with *Paracoccidiodes brasiliensis*, histoplasmosis, Wegener's disease, midline granuloma, or rhinoscleroma.

TREATMENT. As described earlier for visceral leishmaniasis, the standard and recommended treatment for cutaneous leishmaniasis is pentavalent Sb, available in the United States as Pentostam.* The dose is 15 to 20 mg of Sb per kilogram by intramuscular or intravenous injection, not exceeding 1000 mg per dose. The drug is given daily for 15 to 20 days. Modest elevation of liver enzymes and/or mild, nonspecific ST or T wave electrocardiographic changes may occur during therapy, especially after six or eight doses. These changes are generally not associated with symptoms, but it may be prudent to monitor them.

Old World cutaneous leishmaniasis, especially in patients from the Middle East, often heals spontaneously within 6 months. Since leishmaniasis in this region does not metastasize to mucosal tissues, treatment may justifiably be withheld if the lesion is not extensive and appears to be healing.

In contrast, if the infection is known or suspected to originate from an endemic area of mucocutaneous disease, some authorities recommend longer (20 to 30 days) or multiple-course therapy. However, healing of the lesion is the ultimate clinical criterion for successful treatment.

Regardless of the infecting species of parasite, it is not unusual for cutaneous leishmanial lesions to require a second course of Sb treatment. Two weeks of rest and clinical observation are generally allowed between courses of treatment. Although different strains of leishmania can vary in their susceptibility to Sb, there is no evidence of drug resistance. Yet the circumstances required to eliminate the organisms from a lesion are not fully understood, and probably a normal immunologic response on the part of the host is required.

Amphotericin B is indicated in cases in which antimonials have failed to control the disease. Side effects are common and can be severe. The effective total dose is lower than for many systemic mycoses, with a total dose of 1.5 to 2.0 grams for a 60-kg adult often being sufficient.

A number of other drugs with varying degrees of antileishmanial activity may be useful in treatment under certain circumstances. Ketoconazole,† in a daily dose of 400 or 600‡ mg, may be effective against certain species of parasites but must be given for 4 weeks. Other orally administered drugs, such as rifampin or metronidazole, have been touted on the basis of limited or uncontrolled trials, but they are clearly inferior to Sb. Innovative approaches to therapy are under way with liposome-encapsulated compounds and even topically applied drugs containing paromomycin; their ultimate usefulness remains to be established.

*Available from Centers for Disease Control, Atlanta, GA.
†This use is not listed in the manufacturer's directive.
‡Exceeds the dose recommended by the manufacturer.

The application of local heat (40° to 41°C) for 25 hours or more over a period of 4 or 5 days may be effective for lesions caused by the *L. mexicana* complex organisms.

PREVENTION. Transmission of leishmaniasis in cities can be prevented by control of sandfly populations with insecticides or destruction of breeding sites. Where reservoirs and vectors are sylvatic, other measures must be employed, such as insect repellents and use of protective clothing over exposed parts of the body. Vaccines should theoretically be effective, since immunity to second episodes of cutaneous disease does exist. However, the effectiveness of immunization with either viable or killed organisms has been difficult to evaluate.

Badero R, Jones TC, Carvalho EM, et al.: New perspectives on a subclinical form of visceral leishmaniasis. J Infect Dis 154:1003, 1986. *A prospective epidemiologic study in Brazil that documents a feature of kala-azar long suspected—namely, that subclinical infection is common and some infected individuals recover spontaneously.*

Chulay JD, Bryceson ADM: Quantitation of amastigotes of *L. donovani* in smears of splenic aspirates from patients with visceral leishmaniasis. Am J Trop Med Hyg 32:475, 1983. *This reference outlines a way to follow patients for response to treatment, including details of their technique for splenic aspiration.*

Marsden PD: Mucosal leishmaniasis ("espundia" Escomel, 1911). Trans R Soc Trop Med Hyg 80:859, 1986. *An excellent review of the clinical aspects of the subject by a real student of the disease. The paper is thoroughly referenced.*

Ponce C, Ponce E, Morrison A, et al.: *Leishmania donovani chagasi:* New clinical variant of cutaneous leishmaniasis in Honduras. Lancet 337:67, 1991. *A description of a benign skin disease in endemic areas for kala-azar, caused by the same organism that produces visceral disease.*

Sacks DL: Metacyclogenesis in leishmania promastigotes (minireview). Exp Parasitol 69:100, 1989. *A short review of the immunologic and biochemical events that occur and confer infectivity to leishmanial parasites as they grow in culture and in the gut of the sandfly vector.*

Sacks DL, Lal SL, Shrivastava SN, et al.: An analysis of T cell responsiveness in Indian kala-azar. J Immunol 138:908, 1987. *Documentation of the antigen-specific T cell unresponsiveness in Indian kala-azar patients during active disease.*

Velasco D, Savarino SJ, Walton BC, et al.: Diffuse cutaneous leishmaniasis in Mexico. Am J Trop Med Hyg 41:280, 1989. *Although this paper concerns an unusual complication of cutaneous leishmaniasis, it stimulates thinking about the factors involved in pathogenesis of this disorder.*

428 Toxoplasmosis

Henry Masur

Toxoplasmosis is a common disease of birds and mammals caused by the protozoan *Toxoplasma gondii*. The name *T. gondii* is derived from the Greek word *toxon*, meaning arc, and from the North African rodent *gondi*, in which the organism was first recognized. *T. gondii* currently infects over 500 million humans around the world. This obligate intracellar protozoan can proliferate readily and cause clinically important disease in individuals with normal or abnormal immune function. A clear distinction must be kept in mind between *T. gondii* infection, which is defined by the presence of viable organisms in a patient, and toxoplasmosis, a relatively uncommon occurrence that indicates an active disease process.

THE PROTOZOA. Three forms exist in the life cycle of *T. gondii*: the *cyst*, the *trophozoite (tachyzoite)*, and the *oocyst*. The trophozoite has an arc or oval form and is about 3 to 7 μm in size. It is an obligate intracellular form that proliferates in acute infection. Trophozoites can enter cytoplasmic vacuoles in any nucleated mammalian cell. They divide by endodyogeny, an asexual process whereby two daughter cells are formed within one parent cell. Division continues until the cell ruptures, releasing trophozoites to infect adjacent cells. As the host develops immunity, trophozoite proliferation slows.

Toxoplasma cysts are 10 to 200 μm forms that contain several thousand very slowly dividing organisms; these appear to develop within host cells. Cysts can be seen in any tissue, but they are most common in brain, skeletal muscle, and cardiac muscle. Cysts are more resistant to environmental conditions than are trophozoites and remain viable after exposure to digestive enzymes.

Oocysts are 10 to 12 μm oval forms that exist uniquely in the intestinal mucosa of cats. Toxoplasma released from cysts or oocysts in the cat intestine enter epithelial cells, where they proliferate and then mature by gametogony into microgametocytes or macrogametocytes. A zygote is formed by the union of the gametocytes; this zygote matures in 1 to 4 days into an oocyst. Large quantities of oocytes (up to 10 million per day) are excreted by the cat for 1 to 3 weeks, beginning 3 to 5 days after ingestion of the Toxoplasma cysts or oocysts. Cats also get a concurrent systemic infection. Oocysts are not infectious until they undergo sporogony outside the body, a process that requires 1 to 21 days, depending on environmental conditions. Oocysts are quite hardy: They can exist outside the body for at least a year in warm, moist soil.

EPIDEMIOLOGY. Toxoplasma infection is a worldwide zoonosis. Natural infection occurs by ingestion of cysts or oocysts and by transplacental transmission. In nature the cycle of infection is probably maintained by cats, birds, and small mammals. Primary human infection usually occurs by accidental ingestion of infected cat feces or by consumption of inadequately cooked meat. The relative importance of these primary routes probably depends on the amount of rare meat consumed, hygienic practices, climate, and the proximity of a feline population. When cats consume infected animals or inadequately cooked meat scraps, they become infected and excrete oocysts. Children are particularly likely to come into contact with contaminated cat feces when playing in sand or to inhale aerosolized dried feces under dusty conditions. Cockroaches and flies have also been shown to transfer oocysts to uncovered food.

In North America and Western Europe, where many cats are confined to the home and eat only processed foods, and where food is usually covered and refrigerated, the consumption of rare meat is probably of greater epidemiologic importance than contact with cats or insects. Pork and lamb are more likely to contain cysts than is beef. If meat is not cooked to 60°C, or frozen to −20°C (a temperature not reliably reached by most commercial freezers), the cysts may be infective.

Toxoplasma has been transmitted rarely by needle stick accidents involving laboratory workers, by accidental inoculation during autopsy procedures, by transfusion of infected blood products, and by transplantation of an infected heart or kidney. A few immunodeficient patients (particularly some with acquired immunodeficiency syndrome [AIDS]) have parasitemia, and persistent parasitemia for a year has been described in an apparently healthy individual.

Secondary Toxoplasma infection can occur by transplacental transmission. Such transmission occurs only if an immunocompetent mother acquires Toxoplasma infection during the pregnancy or perhaps during the few months prior to conception. Some women with human immunodeficiency virus (HIV) infection can probably have persistent parasitemias that reflect reactivation of latent infection and that can be persistent over many months or several years. It is only this unique group of women who could have more than one pregnancy complicated by congenital toxoplasmosis. The frequency of congenital toxoplasmosis is thus dependent on the frequency with which women of childbearing age acquire Toxoplasma infection. In the United States and Europe, 0.5 to 1 per cent of women show high or rising antitoxoplasma titers during pregnancy. The likelihood of transmission increases progressively during successive trimesters of pregnancy, from 17 to 65 per cent.

The frequency of Toxoplasma infection in any population depends on a variety of sociologic, economic, and environmental factors. Among both men and women, there is increasing prevalence of positive serologic results with increasing age. In the United States fewer than 1 per cent of infants have congenital Toxoplasma infection; the incidence rises abruptly during the teenage years; and from age 15 to 50 years, there is an increase of approximately 1 per cent per year. Thus, about 20 to 70 per cent of adults in this country have positive serologic tests for Toxoplasma infection, the precise number depending on the specific population studied. Individuals in cold, arid, or mountainous regions tend to have a lower frequency than do those in tropical areas. There are isolated communities that have little or no Toxoplasma infection. The regional variations cannot all be explained on the basis of meat-eating habits, the presence of felines, or climatic extremes.

PATHOGENESIS AND PATHOLOGY. Toxoplasma organisms are liberated from cysts or oocysts in the gastrointestinal tract, where they multiply in the mucosal cells. Trophozoites then disseminate via the bloodstream or lymphatics to infect any nucleated host cell. Multiplication of the trophozoites within host cell vacuoles does not appear to disturb host cell function until the dividing organisms cause the cell to rupture. As adjacent cells are infected and they are themselves ruptured, progressive tissue necrosis occurs and an inflammatory response is elicited. The inflammatory response typically consists of mononuclear cells, a few polymorphonuclear cells, and edema. How extensive the tissue necrosis and dissemination become depends on the effectiveness of both humoral and cellular immune mechanisms. Although any organ can be involved, small foci of infection are most often established in lymph nodes, skeletal muscle, myocardium, and brain. Even after effective immunologic response, the organisms are not eradicated; a few cysts form in these organs as early as the first week of infection and remain dormant for the lifetime of the host unless host immunity is diminished, in which case active proliferation of the organisms can again cause substantial local disease and dissemination. In some patients, primary infection can be associated with widely disseminated disease, since most of these patients have defects in cell-mediated immune mechanisms.

The histopathologic changes in lymph nodes are so characteristic that they are virtually diagnostic even in the absence of a visualized or cultivated organism. The lymph node shows reactive follicular hyperplasia with irregular clusters of epithelioid histiocytes. Trophozoites or cysts are rarely seen in lymph nodes, although promptly performed cultures grow the organism in many cases.

When other organs are involved, the pathologic findings can vary from a few isolated cysts to a marked inflammatory response associated with extensive necrosis. In skeletal muscle or brain, an isolated cyst can be found unassociated with any inflammatory response or with any clinical manifestations of organ dysfunction; this response is most often seen in chronic latent infection without active disease. In patients with disseminated disease, however, the heart, brain, liver, spleen, kidney, pancreas, or other organs can manifest an intense inflammatory response surrounding areas of necrosis that can vary greatly in size. The inflammatory response consists of lymphocytes, plasma cells, and monocytes in association with edema. Perivascular mononuclear inflammatory changes are often seen contiguous to the necrotic areas. Intracellular and extracellular trophozoites are usually found in the periphery of the lesion rather than in the necrotic center; these trophozoites can be very difficult to distinguish from inflammatory debris.

The central nervous system may contain single or multiple necrotic lesions with margins of mononuclear cells. Periaqueductal and periventricular necrosis in congenital infection may lead to obstruction of the aqueduct of Sylvius or the foramen of Monro, resulting in obstructive hydrocephalus. The necrotic areas may ultimately calcify. In the eye, single or multiple necrotic lesions in the retina are the first manifestations of Toxoplasma infection. Mononuclear cell infiltrates are seen in association with cysts or trophozoites. Granulomatous inflammation occurs secondary to the necrotizing retinitis. The disease involves the posterior chamber almost exclusively and may be complicated by iridocyclitis, glaucoma, or cataracts.

In immunocompetent patients, primary Toxoplasma infection is associated with both a humoral and a cellular immune response. Antibodies (both IgG and IgM) against various Toxoplasma antigens can be detected in the blood. These specific antibodies have roles in producing extracellular killing of organisms (in conjunction with alternate complement pathway) and in promoting intracellular killing when opsonized organisms are ingested by mononuclear phagocytes. Subsequently, lymphocytes become responsive to Toxoplasma antigens and produce lymphokines. These lymphokines, especially interferon-γ and interleukin 2, which are secreted by antigen-sensitized CD4-positive (helper) T cells, enable mononuclear phagocytes to inhibit Toxoplasma replication and to kill the intracellular organisms. Even immunocompetent individuals are not able to eliminate all Toxoplasma organisms from the body; cysts characteristically form in brain and muscle and remain viable for the lifetime of the host. With the exception of those in the retina, these cysts do not cause disease unless host immune function is altered.

CLINICAL MANIFESTATIONS. *Acquired Toxoplasmosis in the Immunocompetent Individual.* The vast majority of individuals who are infected with *T. gondii* after birth have no apparent clinical symptoms. In the small number of individuals with a symptomatic illness, lymphadenopathy (90 per cent), fever (40 per cent), and malaise (40 per cent) are the common manifestations. The lymphadenopathy is classically symmetric in the posterior auricular, anterior cervical, or posterior cervical chains. Generalized lymphadenopathy or localized unilateral enlargement or enlargement of a solitary node can also be seen. The nodes are characteristically rubbery and nontender. Splenomegaly occurs in about 30 per cent of patients. Fever is usually low grade, but on occasion can be high, rapidly fluctuating, and prolonged. Fatigue can be a prominent feature. A minority of patients have a sore throat, maculopapular rash, myalgias, arthralgias, urticaria, or headache. The sore throat presents as hyperemia rather than as an exudative pharyngitis. For most patients with clinically apparent disease, toxoplasmosis is self-limiting over a period of several weeks. Toxoplasmosis can, however, be a prolonged, severely debilitating disorder that may prevent the patient from working for many weeks or months. The lymph nodes may fluctuate in size during the recovery period.

In immunocompetent adults, specific organ involvement can lead to clinically significant disease involving the lungs, myocardium, pericardium, liver, skin, and skeletal muscle. These manifestations may dominate the clinical picture. Glomerulonephritis has been reported. Death due to toxoplasmosis in immunocompetent individuals is extremely rare.

Laboratory evaluation reveals a normal leukocyte count with a slight lymphocytosis or monocytosis. When atypical lymphocytes are present, they are found only in small numbers. The hemoglobin is usually normal, although a Coombs-negative hemolytic anemia has occasionally been reported. Serum transaminase levels are rarely elevated to more than twice normal. The chest radiograph is usually normal; hilar adenopathy is unusual. On the electrocardiogram ST and T wave abnormalities may be seen if myocarditis is present.

Ocular Involvement in the Immunocompetent Individual. *Toxoplasma* has been estimated to cause 20 to 35 per cent of cases of retinochoroiditis in children and adults. This ocular disease is almost always a consequence of congenital infection; there are very few well-documented cases of eye disease caused by infection acquired after birth.

Symptoms of retinochoroiditis are usually noted initially during the second or third decade of life. Symptoms and the degree of vision loss depend on the location and the extent of retinal involvement. Patients may complain of blurred vision, scotomas, pain, or epiphora. Strabismus may be an early sign in children. The lesions appear acutely as white or yellow cotton-like patches that have indistinct, elevated margins. Inflammatory exudate in the vitreous may obscure visualization of the fundus. As the lesions age, they become atrophic with whitish-gray plaques, more distinct borders, and black spots of choroidal pigment. Lesions may be peripheral, but characteristically they occur near the posterior pole of the retina. They are usually multiple and vary in age, but single lesions do occur. Panuveitis and papillitis with optic atrophy can occur. Exclusively anterior uveitis has never been proved to be caused by *Toxoplasma*.

Patients with *Toxoplasma* retinochoroiditis have an unpredictable clinical course. Episodes of active disease may occur once or many times but usually stop after the age of 40. Recurrent episodes are often associated with progressive loss of vision.

Toxoplasmosis in the Immunodeficient Patient. Toxoplasmosis can occur as a disseminated disease in patients with immunodeficiencies. In most cases, it probably represents reactivation of latent infection rather than primary infection. The disease occurs with particular frequency in patients with AIDS but is also seen occasionally in patients with hematologic malignant conditions (particularly Hodgkin's disease) and organ transplants. The clinical manifestations are variable. Fever, hepatosplenomegaly, pneumonitis, maculopapular rash, myositis, myocarditis, meningoencephalitis, and central nervous system mass lesions may be seen. The lymphadenopathy characteristic of acquired disease in the immunocompetent patient is often absent. This syndrome is usually fulminant and rapidly fatal. It is very difficult to distinguish from numerous other infectious and noninfectious processes that can present in a similar fashion. The most common manifestation, particularly in patients with AIDS, is central nervous system involvement with fever, headache, confusion progressing to coma, focal neurologic signs, and seizures. The cerebrospinal fluid shows nonspecific changes that usually include pleocytosis and moderately increased protein and normal glucose content. Computed tomography usually shows one or more lesions that are contrast enhancing in a ring or nodular pattern.

Toxoplasmosis has been serologically associated with progressive polymyositis. It is unclear whether the association reflects the etiology of the muscular disorder or whether the disorder activates *Toxoplasma* infection. A few patients with polymyositis and high antitoxoplasma antibody titers have responded symptomatically to antitoxoplasma therapy.

Congenital Disease. Congenital toxoplasmosis is the result of acute infection acquired by the mother just before or during gestation. These *Toxoplasma* infections in the mother are usually asymptomatic, as is *Toxoplasma* infection acquired by other immunocompetent hosts, and thus there is nothing to warn the mother or her physician unless serologic testing is routinely performed. The likelihood that the fetus will become infected and the severity of the congenital infection are largely dependent on when during the gestation the infection is acquired. When the infection occurs late during gestation or involves very few organisms, the infant will probably have no immediate clinical manifestations but will have positive humoral and cellular immune responses to *Toxoplasma*. Cysts of *Toxoplasma* organisms persist in the retina, brain, myocardium, and/or skeletal muscle for the infant's lifetime. If the infant remains immunocompetent during its lifetime, the subsequent clinical manifestations that might occur are retinochoroiditis, which usually flares during the second or third decade of life; seizures; and mild retardation. In infants who are infected early during gestation or with large inocula, the clinical sequelae can be severe. Spontaneous abortion, stillbirth, and prematurity may result. The infant may be born with microphthalmia, microcephaly, seizures, cerebral calcifications, bilateral retinochoroiditis, rash, lymphadenopathy, pneumonitis, fever, or hepatosplenomegaly, which can result in severe incapacity. If the cerebral inflammatory response involves the aqueduct of Sylvius, hydrocephalus may result. Clinical manifestations of these complications may be apparent at birth or may become obvious several months later when the infant fails to reach normal milestones.

DIAGNOSIS. The diagnosis of toxoplasmosis can be based on serologic tests, lymph node histology, the demonstration of trophozoites in body tissues or fluids, or isolation of *T. gondii* from certain sites. Which diagnostic test is most appropriate depends on the clinical situation.

Serology. Measurement of antitoxoplasma antibody titers is the most commonly employed mechanism for diagnosing toxoplasmosis. The *Sabin-Feldman dye test*, which uses live *T. gondii*, is the most sensitive and specific serologic test but is only available at a few centers. The Sabin-Feldman dye test and the indirect fluorescent antibody (IFA-IgG) test give comparable titers that measure IgG antibodies. Titers begin to rise 1 to 2 weeks after infection and reach a peak after 2 to 8 weeks that is almost always 1:1000 or higher. Titers drift down slowly over several years and persist at low levels (1:16 to 1:64) for the patient's lifetime. The height of the initial peak does not correlate with severity of clinical disease. IFA-IgG titers are positive at stable low levels in adults with reactivated ocular disease and in most immunocompetent patients with disseminated toxoplasmosis. Titers in infants may be elevated because of passively transferred maternal antibodies. Sequential studies over 4 to 6 months must be performed to determine whether the infant's titers are rising, suggesting that the infected infant is producing antibody, or whether they are falling (usually by 50 per cent per month) and attributable to passively transferred maternal antibodies.

Tests for IgM antibody (IgM fluorescent antibody or double-sandwich enzyme-linked immunosorbent assay [ELISA] techniques) are particularly useful for establishing recent *Toxoplasma* infection because titers appear early (as early as 5 days after infection) and disappear within several months. IgM tests have not been carefully standardized; the significance of specific titers needs to be evaluated by the laboratory performing the test. IgM titer elevations are recognized in 80 per cent of immunocompetent individuals with acute disease and in infants with congenital disease, but they are not elevated in adults with reactivated ocular disease or in most immunoincompetent individuals with disseminated toxoplasmosis.

The indirect hemagglutination (IHA) test as performed in most laboratories measures antibodies that increase very late in the course of infection (and persist for years). Thus the test is a poor screening device for identification of pregnant women who have acquired Toxoplasma infection early during gestation and who might otherwise have elected abortion. The IHA tests that are available in commercial kits are often poorly standardized and difficult to interpret.

False-positive results are not known to occur with the Sabin-Feldman dye test. The IFA-IgG and IgM-IFA tests may produce false-positive results if antinuclear antibody is present. Rheumatoid factor can also cause false-positive IgM-IFA titers.

In general, acute acquired toxoplasmosis is suggested serologically by the Sabin-Feldman dye test or IFA-IgG titers of 1:1000 or higher and proved convincingly by the documentation of elevated IgM-IFA or IgM-ELISA titers or by the documentation of a two-tube (or greater) titer rise in the Sabin-Feldman dye test, IFA-IgG test, and perhaps the IHA test. Thus, a pregnant woman with stable IFA-IgG titers below 1:1024 is presumed to have chronic, latent infection acquired prior to conception. A stable IFA-IgG titer of 1:1024 or higher may represent recent infection, acquired during pregnancy, and the woman should thus be assessed by other techniques such as the IFA-IgM. Serial IFA-IgG titers that rise by two tubes or more would confirm very recent acquisition of Toxoplasma infection. Congenital toxoplasmosis in infants is documented by demonstrating elevated complement fixation or IgM-IFA titers or by showing that the Sabin-Feldman dye test or IFA titers are stable or rising over 4 to 6 months. Ocular toxoplasmosis or toxoplasmosis in the immunoincompetent host cannot be diagnosed with certainty by antibody testing. A negative Sabin-Feldman dye test result or IFA-IgG test titer (<1:4) excludes Toxoplasma as a cause of the ocular disease in the immunocompetent patient. In immunosuppressed patients, serology is not highly useful. Since most cases of toxoplasmosis in this population appear to represent reactivation of latent infection, seropositive individuals are much more likely to develop Toxoplasma disease than are seronegative individuals. A typical serologic pattern for a patient with Hodgkin's disease or AIDS and active cerebral toxoplasmosis would be a stable IFA-IgG titer of 1:16 to 1:256 and a negative IgM-IFA. Cerebral toxoplasmosis has probably occurred in a few seronegative AIDS patients, however. The host may not produce specific antibody in some such cases either because of inadequate humoral response to primary infection or because of deficiencies in antibody production despite chronic, latent infection.

Isolation of the Organism. T. gondii can be isolated from leukocytes, body fluids, or tissue by direct inoculation of the specimens subcutaneously or intraperitoneally into mice. The mice are then examined periodically for the presence of antibody to Toxoplasma, for the presence of trophozoites in the peritoneum, or for the presence of cysts in the brain. Isolation can also be performed by tissue culture. The isolation of the Toxoplasma organisms from leukocytes or body fluids is convincing evidence of acute infection, although parasitemia persisting for a year has been described, especially in immunodeficient patients. The isolation of Toxoplasma organisms from tissue does not provide convincing evidence of acute infection because a tissue cyst may have been present for many years and may be irrelevant to the active disease process. Isolation of Toxoplasma organisms requires several weeks to carry out.

Histologic Diagnosis. The histologic findings in the lymph nodes of patients with acute toxoplasmosis, described earlier, are so characteristic as to be diagnostic. The inflammatory reaction in other tissues is much less specific. In nonlymphoid tissue, free or intracellular tachyzoites must be demonstrated for the diagnosis of toxoplasmosis to be established. The demonstration of Toxoplasma cysts proves that the patient was infected by T.

gondii at some time in the past but does not document that the current clinical disease is related. Histologic diagnosis is the preferred technique for patients with urgent clinical syndromes, especially immunoincompetent patients with cerebral mass lesions. The diagnosis of cerebral toxoplasmosis can be established by assessing empiric response to a 2-week course of pyrimethamine (Daraprim) and sulfadiazine, especially in patients with HIV infection and circulating CD4+ lymphocyte counts below 200 per cubic millimeter. A guided needle biopsy (if such a procedure is technically feasible) is preferable when there is considerable diagnostic uncertainty, i.e., in most patients without HIV infection.

DIFFERENTIAL DIAGNOSIS. The differential diagnosis of a patient with lymphadenopathy includes lymphoma, Hodgkin's disease, AIDS, sarcoidosis, mycobacterial disease, cytomegalovirus disease, mononucleosis, brucellosis, tularemia, cat scratch disease, and many other infectious processes. Toxoplasmosis can be distinguished from mononucleosis by the absence of atypical lymphocytosis, exudative pharyngitis, increased serum transaminase levels, and heterophile antibodies. Appropriate serologic tests, cultures, and lymph node biopsies are necessary to distinguish the other processes. Toxoplasmosis in immunosuppressed patients may mimic other disseminated infections. The central nervous system mass lesions need to be distinguished by biopsy from neoplastic or other infectious processes in non-AIDS patients; an empiric trial of therapy is probably sufficient diagnostically if response is prompt in patients with HIV infection and low CD4+ lymphocyte counts.

Toxoplasma retinochoroiditis needs to be distinguished on the basis of lesion morphology, serology, and appropriate cultures from cytomegalovirus, herpes, tuberculosis, histoplasmosis, syphilis, and sarcoidosis. Congenital toxoplasmosis must be distinguished from cytomegalovirus disease, syphilis, herpes simplex infection, rubella, erythroblastosis fetalis, and bacterial sepsis.

THERAPY. The need and duration of therapy depend on the clinical setting. Most immunocompetent adults with lymphadenopathic disease do not need specific antitoxoplasma therapy. Patients with severe or prolonged constitutional symptoms, patients with specific organ dysfunction, immunoincompetent patients, and probably patients infected by direct inoculation (laboratory workers and transfusion recipients) merit treatment. Treatment for patients with retinochoroiditis or for pregnant patients is more controversial.

A combination of pyrimethamine and sulfadiazine is effective in inhibiting the replication of trophozoites. There are no drugs that will kill trophozoites or eradicate the cyst form. Pyrimethamine can only be given orally. In adults an initial dose of 75 mg is given, followed by 25 mg daily. Infants should be given 1 mg per kilogram for 3 days, followed by 0.5 mg per kilogram per day. Sulfadiazine, 1.0 to 1.5 grams orally every 6 hours, is the adult dose. Infants should receive 100 mg per kilogram per day. Triple sulfonamides (sulfamerazine, sulfamethazine, and sulfadiazine) can be substituted for sulfadiazine, but sulfisoxazole (Gantrisin) is ineffective. Good urine flow should be maintained by adequate fluid intake to prevent crystalluria. Since sulfa drugs and pyrimethamine inhibit folate synthesis, folinic acid (leucovorin), 5 to 10 mg, should be administered two to three times weekly to reduce bone marrow toxicity. Platelet counts and white blood cell counts should be monitored at least twice weekly during therapy. Pyrimethamine is a potential teratogen and is not desirable to use in pregnant women.

Evaluation of the effectiveness of sulfadiazine and pyrimethamine therapy in immunocompetent patients has been limited by the marked variability in clinical course and the frequency of spontaneous improvement. There is considerable anecdotal experience, however, that specific therapy can shorten the symptomatic period of fever and fatigue (although not the lymphadenopathy) in immunocompetent patients with acquired disease and is probably effective in hastening the resolution of serious organ dysfunction. Often a 4- to 6-week course of therapy is given and then the clinical situation re-evaluated. In Toxoplasma retinochoroiditis, primary therapy should be directed at controlling the hypersensitivity response with anti-inflammatory drugs such as corticosteroids if the lesions are extensive or central. Pyrimethamine and sulfadiazine should be used to prevent local proliferation of the organisms and potential dissemination during periods when corticosteroids are given.

Sulfadiazine and pyrimethamine have been effective in immunosuppressed patients with disseminated disease in controlling systemic symptoms and specific organ dysfunction. For AIDS patients, some authorities advocate the use of higher daily doses of pyrimethamine (50 to 100 mg) in conjunction with sulfadiazine, but the benefits of these higher doses have not been established. Long-term therapy should be strongly considered for the duration of immunosuppression; for AIDS patients, therapy should probably be continued for life. Some authorities recommend reduced dosages for long-term suppression in AIDS patients after the initial lesion resolves radiologically, but whether such reduced doses are equally effective as full doses is uncertain. Bone marrow toxicity and skin rash are major management problems in many of these patients, particularly those with AIDS or those treated with antineoplastic chemotherapy.

In pregnant women who plan to complete their pregnancy despite the acquisition of *Toxoplasma* infection during gestation, pyrimethamine has been used despite its teratogenic potential. There is some evidence that sulfadiazine alone may be effective therapy. In Europe spiramycin* has been used, but its efficacy has not been clearly established. Congenital toxoplasmosis should be treated aggressively, whether or not the infant is symptomatic, because organism proliferation can continue after birth. Antitoxoplasma therapy does not reverse damage that has already occurred.

For patients who cannot tolerate sulfadiazine and pyrimethamine, there are several promising alternatives. For AIDS patients, the combination of intravenous clindamycin (2.4 grams per day) plus pyrimethamine appears to be quite efficacious but associated with considerable toxicity. Other promising regimens being assessed include oral clindamycin plus pyrimethamine; newer macrolides, such as azithromycin or clarithromycin or roxithromycin, either alone or in combination with pyrimethamine; and the new hydroxynaphthoquinone 566C80.

PREVENTION. Effective prevention should be directed against minimizing consumption of undercooked meat or exposure to oocyst-infected cat feces. Pet cats should be kept in the house and should not be fed raw meat or have access to wild rodents or birds. Susceptible individuals or pregnant women who are seronegative should avoid sandboxes or moist soil where outdoor cats may defecate.

Congenital toxoplasmosis can be largely avoided if pregnant women follow the aforementioned precautions carefully. Serologic testing at the time of the mother's first prenatal examination and again at 16 to 18 weeks of gestation permits recognition of mothers who have acquired toxoplasmosis early in pregnancy and allows consideration of therapeutic abortion.

Brooks RG, McCabe RE, Remington JS: Role of serology in the diagnosis of toxoplasmic lymphadenopathy. Rev Infect Dis 9:1055, 1987. *Serologic results in 92 cases of toxoplasma lymphadenopathy diagnosed by lymph node biopsy.*

Daffos F, Forestier F, Capella-Pavlovsky, et al.: Prenatal management of 746 pregnancies at risk for congenital toxoplasmosis. N Engl J Med 318:271, 1988. *Prenatal diagnosis, maternal therapy, and postnatal follow-up for a large series of women are reviewed.*

Leport C, Raffi F, Matheron S, et al.: Treatment of central nervous system toxoplasmosis with pyrimethamine/sulfadiazine combination in 35 patients with the acquired immunodeficiency syndrome. Efficacy of long term continuous therapy. Am J Med 84:94, 1988. *Detailed information about the efficacy and toxicities of treatment with sulfadiazine-pyrimethamine.*

McCabe RE, Brooks RG, Dorgman RF, et al.: Clinical spectrum in 107 cases of toxoplasmic lymphadenopathy. Rev Infect Dis 9:754, 1987. *Extensive compilation of clinical data from lymph node biopsy–proven cases with 14 illustrative case reports.*

Schlaegel TF: Ocular Toxoplasmosis and Pars Planitis. New York, Grune and Stratton, 1978. *A comprehensive survey of the history, epidemiology, clinical features, and laboratory aspects of ocular toxoplasmosis.*

*Spiramycin is available from the National Center for Orphan Drugs and Rare Diseases (703–522–2590) in Virginia and (1–800–336–4797) in Washington, D.C.

429 Cryptosporidiosis
Rosemary Soave

Cryptosporidiosis is a gastrointestinal infection characterized by watery diarrhea, abdominal cramps, malabsorption, and weight loss. It is usually a severe, unrelenting illness in immunocompromised patients, particularly those with the acquired immunodeficiency syndrome (AIDS), and a self-limited disease in the immunologically normal host. It is caused by the coccidian protozoan *Cryptosporidium*, long associated with disease in animals. In 1981–82, identification of *Cryptosporidium* in 47 AIDS patients with severe enteritis brought the protozoan to the attention of the medical community. As more physicians have looked for this parasite, the number of reported cases of cryptosporidiosis has continued to rise, and it has come to be recognized as an important public health problem worldwide. There is currently no known effective therapy.

THE PROTOZOAN. *Cryptosporidium* (which means "hidden spore") belongs to the class Sporozoa and the suborder Eimeriorina, or true coccidia. Other pathogens of humans in this group include *Toxoplasma gondii, Isospora belli,* and *Sarcocystis* species. Although many species within the genus *Cryptosporidium* have been described, recent cross-transmission experiments suggest that little or no host specificity exists. Because the number of cryptosporidial species is not known, the organism is commonly referred to as *Cryptosporidium* sp.

The 4- to 5-μm, spherical, acid-fast *Cryptosporidium* oocyst is the environmentally resistant form of the parasite that is identified in fecal specimens (Fig. 429–1). Sporulated (mature) oocysts contain four elliptical (2 to 4 × 6 to 8 μm), flat, aflagellar but motile sporozoites that are released (excystation) in the host intestinal tract upon dissolution of the oocyst's outer wall. Sporozoites implant on the host mucosal epithelium and undergo asexual and sexual development within a parasitophorous vacuole. The parasite-host cell relationship is unique in that the parasite is intracellular, i.e., enveloped by a host cell membrane, but extracytoplasmic. Sporozoites develop into trophozoites and subsequently undergo asexual multiplication (merogony), formation of macrogametes and microgametes (gametogony), fertilization, and oocyst formation. Newly formed oocysts that are expelled in the feces are immediately infective. The ability of *Cryptosporidium* to develop completely within one host (monoxenous life cycle) imparts a tremendous potential for reinfection and may contribute to the refractory nature of the illness that is seen in *Cryptosporidium*-infected AIDS patients.

EPIDEMIOLOGY. Although more than 40 reports of cryptosporidial infection have emanated from at least 35 countries spanning 6 continents, the true prevalence of cryptosporidiosis in either immunocompetent or immunocompromised hosts is unknown. These surveys of selected populations have revealed infection rates ranging from 0.6 to 20 per cent in the developed world and 4 to 32 per cent in the developing world. Available reports indicate that *Cryptosporidium* is ubiquitous and a major cause of diarrhea worldwide. They also suggest that higher infection rates are associated with young age (<2 years); warm, wet weather; and overcrowding. In addition, several studies have revealed higher than expected rates of seropositivity, suggesting that active or recent cryptosporidial infection may be common in the general population. As of 1986, the Centers for Disease Control estimated that 3 to 4 per cent of AIDS patients had cryptosporidiosis. In recent studies conducted at the National Institutes of Health and The Johns Hopkins Hospital, approximately 16 per cent of AIDS patients with diarrhea were found to be infected. By contrast, more than 50 per cent of AIDS patients

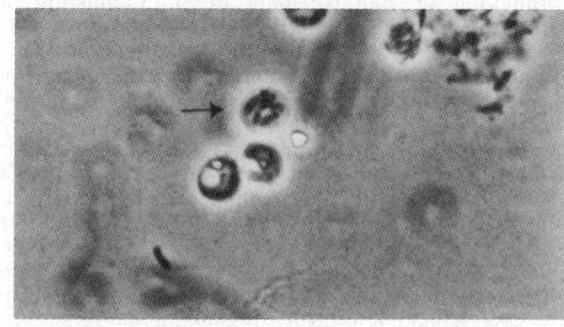

FIGURE 429–1. Wet mount of human stool showing three cryptosporidial oocysts and sporozoites (*arrow*) (×630).

in Haiti and parts of Africa have cryptosporidiosis. Asymptomatic carriage of the parasite has been documented in immunocompetent and immunocompromised subjects, but the frequency with which it occurs and its significance have yet to be determined.

Transmission of *Cryptosporidium* between humans and domestic animals has been well documented, and it is likely that both serve as reservoirs of the disease. For humans, however, spread from person to person and via contaminated water may be more common than zoonotic transmission. Spread of the parasite via sexual contact or aerosolization has been suggested but not confirmed. Person-to-person transmission has been implicated in day care center outbreaks, clusters of infection among contacts of index cases, and nosocomial spread of infection among patients and health care workers. Contaminated water appears to be responsible for infection in travelers and swimmers, and in at least four major community outbreaks in the United States and two in the United Kingdom. *Cryptosporidium* oocysts have been found in surface and drinking waters, as well as in sewage effluent samples from different geographic regions of the United States. Like *Giardia lamblia*, the environmentally resistant *Cryptosporidium* oocyst is not affected by the chlorine concentrations used to decontaminate drinking water. Infectivity of *Cryptosporidium* appears to be destroyed by freeze-drying; a 30-minute exposure to temperatures above 60°C or under −20°C; or treatment with 50 per cent ammonia, full-strength bleach, or 10 per cent formalin for 30 minutes.

PATHOLOGY AND PATHOGENESIS. *Cryptosporidium* has been found in the pharynx, esophagus, stomach, duodenum, jejunum, ileum, appendix, colon, rectum, gallbladder, pancreas, bile, and pancreatic ducts, as well as within colonic submucosal vessels of infected immunocompromised (primarily AIDS) patients. The parasite has also been detected in sputum, tracheal aspirates, bronchoalveolar lavage, and lung tissue of a small number of immunocompromised patients with gastrointestinal cryptosporidiosis. Light microscopic evaluation of Giemsa-stained or hematoxylin-eosin–stained *Cryptosporidium*-infected tissue reveals small, spherical, basophilic structures along the epithelial cell brush border. Ultrastructural studies reveal the entire spectrum of endogenous stages of the organism adherent to the enterocyte surface and enveloped by a membrane, believed to be derived from the host cell. Histologic changes are nonspecific and minimal, resembling those described for giardiasis, i.e., villous atrophy, crypt elongation, and minimal subjacent inflammatory infiltrates of the lamina propria. By contrast, marked histologic changes ranging from acute inflammation to gangrenous necrosis of the gallbladder and biliary duct epithelium have been described for patients with cryptosporidial cholangitis or cholecystitis.

The pathogenic mechanisms by which *Cryptosporidium* causes enteritis are unknown. The secretory nature of the diarrhea and the presence of malabsorption suggest that an enterotoxin-mediated mechanism and/or physical destruction of the brush border may be operative.

CLINICAL MANIFESTATIONS. The spectrum of cryptosporidial infection ranges from asymptomatic infection to fulminant diarrhea. Cryptosporidiosis is characterized by watery diarrhea, cramping abdominal pain (often exacerbated by food ingestion), weight loss, and flatulence. Nausea, vomiting, anorexia, myalgias, and malaise may also be present. Fever, leukocytosis, and eosinophilia are not common. Fecal examination reveals cryptosporidial oocysts and mucus, but no leukocytes or blood. Vitamin B_{12}, xylose, and fat malabsorption has been documented. Radiographic abnormalities are nonspecific and include prominent mucosal folds, intestinal wall thickening, small bowel dilatation, and disordered motility.

The incubation period for human cryptosporidiosis appears to be between 2 and 14 days. The severity and course of the illness are determined by host immunocompetence. In the immunologically normal host, infection is often explosive in onset and lasts an average of 10 to 14 days. Clearance of the parasite from stool lags behind clinical resolution by 2 to 3 weeks, thus creating problems for infection control. Although self-limited, symptoms are often severe enough to justify therapeutic intervention, were it available. Infection in AIDS patients often begins insidiously and escalates in severity as the underlying immune defect be-

comes more profound. Frequent (6 to 25), voluminous (1 to 25 liters) daily bowel movements, profound weight loss, and stool oocyst shedding often persist for months.

Biliary cryptosporidiosis has been documented only in immunocompromised patients. Because invasive procedures that may not be justified in the absence of treatment options are a prerequisite for definitive diagnosis, the incidence of this complication is not known. Most patients with biliary cryptosporidiosis have classic signs of cholangitis, including severe right upper quadrant pain, nausea, and vomiting. Serum levels of alkaline phosphatase and γ-glutamyl transpeptidase are elevated, but serum bilirubin and transaminase levels are normal. Radiographic evaluation may reveal a dilated gallbladder, thickened gallbladder wall, and dilated bile ducts with luminal irregularities. Patients undergoing endoscopic retrograde cholangiopancreatography (ERCP) are often found to have cryptosporidia studding the surface epithelium and in the bile. In certain instances, cholecystectomy or endoscopic papillotomy has resulted in transient improvement of both symptoms and laboratory abnormalities.

DIAGNOSIS. The diagnosis of cryptosporidial enteritis is based on identification of the oocyst form of the parasite in fecal specimens. Since 1981, various staining techniques for detecting oocysts have been popularized, including several modifications of the acid-fast stain (Kinyoun, Ziehl-Neelsen), the fluorescent auramine-rhodamine stain, and the periodic acid–Schiff (PAS) and carbol fuchsin–negative stains. With the acid-fast stain, acid-fast (red) oocysts may be easily distinguished from yeast that are similar in size and shape but are not acid fast (they stain green). The sensitivity, specificity, and relative merits of the various staining methods have not been determined. Most recently, a method for detecting cryptosporidial oocysts that uses a fluorescein-labeled immunoglobulin (IgG) monoclonal antibody was made available commercially (Meridien Diagnostics, Cincinnati, OH). This method appears to be more sensitive and specific than other currently available techniques, and its role in the clinical laboratory is currently being investigated. Since the pattern of fecal oocyst shedding in human cryptosporidiosis has not been determined, and the sensitivity of the various methodologies is also not known, the optimal number of negative stool specimens required to confirm the absence of cryptosporidia has yet to be defined. Stool concentration techniques do not appear to be necessary for routine diagnosis but are most useful in detecting oocysts in follow-up specimens, asymptomatic contacts, or environmental samples.

Although the sensitivity and specificity of stool examination compared with small intestinal biopsy have not been determined, stool examination appears to be more sensitive. In addition to being invasive and costly, intestinal biopsies may be falsely negative owing to autolysis during processing and sampling difficulties related to the parasite's patchy distribution and the paucity of inflammatory changes to guide the endoscopist.

Anticryptosporidial IgG and IgM have been detected in both immunocompetent persons and patients with AIDS by immunofluorescent assay (IFA) and enzyme-linked immunosorbent (ELISA) assay. Antibody titers rise within 6 to 8 weeks after the onset of infection and decline within 1 year. Immunocompetent hosts generally have higher titers. The IgM response is often absent or minimal in patients with AIDS. Serologic studies are not useful in the diagnosis of acute cryptosporidiosis but do have a role in defining the epidemiology of the disease.

TREATMENT. In contrast to all the other opportunistic infections of AIDS patients, there is currently no known effective therapy for cryptosporidiosis. Identification of potentially active agents has been severely hampered by the absence of an asymptomatic, small-animal model of the chronic disease and by an inability to cultivate the organism in vitro. Investigational therapy has not been given to the immunocompetent host with cryptosporidial enteritis because illness in these patients is usually self-limited. Persons receiving corticosteroids or cytotoxic agents may be successfully managed by discontinuation of the immunosuppressive drugs.

Because of the severe nature of the illness in AIDS patients with cryptosporidiosis, a vast array of antidiarrheal, antimicrobial, and immunomodulating agents have been administered in an unprecedented manner with few preclinical data to support their use. Early anecdotal reports of success using the antitoxoplasma macrolide spiramycin led to two controlled studies with this agent. A placebo-controlled clinical trial of oral spiramycin in 54 AIDS patients with cryptosporidiosis failed to show any difference between placebo and drug. Subsequent pharmacokinetic studies suggested that this may have been due to suboptimal drug absorption. As a result, the intravenous form of spiramycin is being evaluated in a single-blind placebo-controlled trial. In a recently concluded study, the benzeneacetonitrile derivative diclazuril, known for its activity against the animal pathogen *Eimeria*, was found to have some promise as an anticryptosporidial agent. Since lack of absorption appeared to be a significant problem, future trials employing a more absorbable congener of diclazuril are being planned. Anecdotal reports of amelioration of cryptosporidial infection with paromomycin are also being verified. α-Difluoromethylornithine, an irreversible ornithine decarboxylase inhibitor that is active against a number of protozoa, has been found to be moderately efficacious against *Cryptosporidium*, but toxicity (bone marrow suppression and gastrointestinal irritation) has limited its use.

The mechanisms by which the immunocompetent host successfully deals with cryptosporidial infection are poorly understood but appear to include both intact T cell– and B cell–mediated immunity. Novel attempts at modulating immune function in *Cryptosporidium*-infected patients centered on the use of immune bovine colostrum, bovine milk globulins, and bovine transfer factor have provided interesting and promising results that require further investigation.

In the absence of any proven effective therapy for cryptosporidiosis, careful management of fluid and electrolyte balance is of paramount importance. All classes of nonspecific antidiarrheal agents, including the long-acting, parenterally administered somatostatin analogue octreotide acetate, may be useful, when used in trial-and-error fashion, for individual patients. However, their safety in *Cryptosporidium*-infected patients is not known. Total parenteral nutrition often provides major benefits, but its use is controversial owing to the need for an invasive procedure and its high cost.

Crawford FG, Vermund SH: Human cryptosporidiosis. CRC Crit Rev Microbiol 16:113, 1988. *This exhaustive review covers all aspects of cryptosporidiosis in humans.*

Fayer R, Ungar BLP: *Cryptosporidium* spp. and cryptosporidiosis. Microbiol Rev 50:458, 1986. *This thoroughly referenced review emphasizes the biologic and veterinary aspects of Cryptosporidium.*

Jokipii L, Jokipii AM: Timing of symptoms and oocyst excretion in human cryptosporidiosis excretion in human cryptosporidiosis. N Engl J Med 315:1643, 1986. *A clinical and parasitologic study of 68 immunocompetent patients with cryptosporidiosis in Finland.*

Soave R: Treatment strategies for cryptosporidiosis. Ann NY Acad Sci 616:442, 1990. *A thoroughly referenced up-to-date review of the approaches to treating cryptosporidiosis.*

430 Giardiasis

David P. Stevens

DEFINITION. Giardiasis is an infection of the small intestine caused by the flagellated protozoan *Giardia lamblia*. When symptomatic, it results in diarrhea, malabsorption, and weight loss.

ETIOLOGY. The organism exists in two forms: the motile, flagellated, pear-shaped trophozoite, 12 to 15 μm in length, or the smaller, tough-walled oval cyst. Trophozoites either attach to the microvilli of the intestinal epithelium or move about in the unstirred layer of mucus just above the epithelial surface. The trophozoites, carried caudally by peristalsis, eventually encyst and pass into the environment. The cyst is resistant to many environmental stresses, including concentrations of chlorine normally found in treated municipal water supplies. It is ingested eventually by a subsequent host. Excystation occurs in the acid environment of the stomach, and infection is again established in the small intestine.

EPIDEMIOLOGY. Giardiasis is present in all climates. It spreads by two routes: water-borne infection, particularly in contaminated community water supplies, and direct person-to-

person transmission. Dozens of epidemics have been described in the United States consequent to breakdown of community water filtration systems. Epidemics in day care centers for children and among promiscuous male homosexuals indicate that direct person-to-person spread can occur. Household contacts must be tested for infection, even if they are asymptomatic.

A role for animal reservoirs of infection has been suggested by the demonstration of *Giardia*-infected beaver upstream from communities where outbreaks of human infection have occurred. It is likely that both beaver and dogs carry *Giardia* species infectious for humans. Campers must be particularly mindful of the risk of drinking untreated water, no matter how pristine the water source. The American Rockies are areas of particularly high risk.

Giardia is a frequent source of diarrhea in travelers returning from endemic areas. Twenty-three per cent of North American travelers returning from Leningrad have been shown to have giardiasis. The incubation period is 7 to 21 days. Typically, the infected traveler develops symptoms several weeks after returning home, and on this basis the infection may be distinguished from that caused by toxigenic *Escherichia coli* and other forms of infectious traveler's diarrhea with shorter incubation periods.

PATHOGENICITY. Jejunal mucosal biopsies from infected persons range in appearance from normal to marked subtotal mucosal atrophy with submucosal inflammatory cell infiltration, reduced villus height, and elongated crypts. Electron microscopic observation of epithelial cells beneath overlying adherent trophozoites shows deformation and blunting of the individual microvilli.

CLINICAL MANIFESTATIONS. *Giardia* infection is frequently asymptomatic. In those persons who are ill, disease ranges from mild diarrhea to severe, debilitating malabsorption and weight loss. Reversible lactase deficiency as well as malabsorption of fat and vitamin B_{12} has been documented. The majority of symptoms result from malabsorption and include abdominal distention, cramps, nausea, flatulence, borborygmi, and frequent loose, bulky, foul, and urgent stools. Fever and chills may be present. Blood or mucus in the stool is *not* typical of giardiasis. Upper gastrointestinal symptoms such as nausea and epigastric pain may distinguish giardiasis from infectious disorders of the colon. Although the infection is frequently self-limited, many persons have a prolonged, indolent illness with waxing and waning symptoms and progressive weight loss.

DIAGNOSIS. The diagnosis is established by demonstration of cysts or trophozoites in stools or of trophozoites in small bowel contents. Because excretion of the organism in stool is episodic and its demonstration elusive, at least three stool specimens should be examined before a negative conclusion is drawn. If no organisms are seen, the small bowel contents may be sampled. This can be achieved by aspiration or passage of a string that will absorb sufficient jejunal fluid for examination. Microscopic examination of a wet preparation of jejunal contents usually reveals motile organisms in the infected person. Small bowel biopsy may be reserved for situations in which these measures are unsuccessful. The small bowel roentgenogram usually shows an edematous mucosa, but this finding is nonspecific. Hematologic values are normal. Eosinophilia should not be expected, since this is a finding associated with infections by worms, not protozoa.

TREATMENT. All infected persons should be treated. There is occasional justification for a trial of therapy in the patient with typical signs and symptoms of giardiasis but in whom efforts to demonstrate the organism fail. Therapy is achieved with quinacrine hydrochloride, 100 mg three times per day for 10 days. When this drug is contraindicated, metronidazole,* 250 mg three times per day for 7 days, is an alternative. Treatment with either drug may be unsuccessful in 5 to 20 per cent of patients, requiring a second course of therapy.

Stevens DP: Selective primary health care: Strategies for control of disease in the developing world: XIX. Giardiasis. Rev Infect Dis 7:530, 1985. *A review of epidemiologic, clinical, and therapeutic aspects of giardiasis.*

Stevens DP: Giardiasis: Host-pathogen biology. Rev Infect Dis 4:851, 1982. *A detailed review of the sparse knowledge available on the pathogenesis of this infection.*

*This use is not listed in the manufacturer's directive but is recommended by the Centers for Disease Control.

431 Amebiasis

Jonathan I. Ravdin

Human amebiasis is due to infection with the enteric protozoan *Entamoeba histolytica*. This parasite infects 10 per cent of the world's population, with the disease burden highest in poor, developing areas. To manage patients with amebiasis appropriately, physicians must have knowledge of the biology of the organism, risk factors for infection, mechanisms of disease, pathogenesis and host immunity, the presenting manifestations of the invasive syndromes, the correct diagnostic approach, alternative therapeutic drug regimens, and strategies for prevention of infection.

BIOLOGY OF *E. HISTOLYTICA* AND EPIDEMIOLOGY. Infection results from ingestion of the fecally excreted acid-resistant cyst form. Excystation occurs in the small bowel, leading to colonization of the colon with *E. histolytica* trophozoites. Transmission of infection results from fecal contamination of water or food or direct fecal-oral contact because of poor hygiene or anal-oral sexual practices. Epidemiologic and molecular biology studies indicate that there are distinct pathogenic and nonpathogenic strains. Infection with the latter does not result in systemic invasive disease or antigenic exposure. Approximately 10 per cent of those with pathogenic infection present clinically with invasive amebiasis, although all manifest a serum antibody response. The relative frequency of pathogenic and nonpathogenic infection varies, depending on geographic area. Regions of the world with a high incidence of invasive amebiasis include Mexico, parts of South America, Western and South Africa, the Indian subcontinent, the Middle East, and Southeast Asia. High-risk groups in the United States include sexually promiscuous male homosexuals, the institutionalized mentally retarded population, and travelers or emigrants from areas of high prevalence (especially Mexican-Americans). Groups that, when infected, can experience an increased severity of invasive amebiasis are the very young (under age 2 years), pregnant women, malnourished individuals, and patients on corticosteroids.

PATHOGENESIS AND HOST IMMUNITY. *E. histolytica* trophozoites cause disease by sequentially adhering to colonic mucus, disrupting mucosal barriers with proteolytic enzymes, and producing contact-dependent lysis of host cells, including responding inflammatory cells. Trophozoite adherence to colonic mucins is mediated by a galactose-binding surface protein; attachment by this protein is the first step in the amebic lysis of human cells. Tissue destruction is enhanced following parasite lysis of responding polymorphonuclear leukocytes, owing to release of toxic neutrophil components. Intestinal infection with nonpathogenic *E. histolytica* usually clears within 8 to 12 months without evidence of a specific immune response. Cure of invasive amebiasis is associated with resistance to recurrent disease, but not necessarily immunity to asymptomatic intestinal infection. Protective immunity is apparently mediated by development of an amebicidal cell-mediated immune response with lymphokine-activated macrophages and a CD8 subset of cytotoxic lymphocytes serving as effector cells. It is unclear whether the serum or secretory antiamebic antibody response that develops after pathogenic infection has any protective role. Acute amebiasis is associated with the occurrence of antigen-specific suppression of cell-mediated responses to *E. histolytica*, facilitating parasite survival in tissues.

CLINICAL DISEASE SYNDROMES. The disease syndromes caused by *E. histolytica* are summarized in Table 431–1. It is unknown whether health is impaired by asymptomatic infection with nonpathogenic *E. histolytica;* unfortunately, there is as yet no clinically applicable means to differentiate between pathogenic and nonpathogenic infection. Occasionally, infected patients present with nonspecific gastrointestinal complaints, such as bloating and cramps, without evidence of invasive colitis. Amebic rectocolitis is characterized by the subacute onset of bloody diarrhea over days, abdominal tenderness, weight loss, and fever in only one third of cases. Fulminant colitis with perforation is uncom-

TABLE 431–1. CLINICAL SYNDROMES ASSOCIATED WITH *E. HISTOLYTICA* INFECTION

Intestinal Disease
Asymptomatic infection
Symptomatic noninvasive infection
Acute rectocolitis (dysentery)
Fulminant colitis with perforation
Toxic megacolon
Chronic nondysenteric colitis
Ameboma

Extraintestinal Disease
Liver abscess
Liver abscess complicated by:
  Peritonitis
  Empyema
  Pericarditis
Lung abscess
Brain abscess
Genitourinary disease

Reproduced with permission from Mandell GL, Douglas RG Jr, Bennett JE (eds.): Principles and Practices of Infectious Diseases. 3rd ed. New York, Churchill Livingstone, 1989.

mon; patients are in a toxic state, are acutely ill, and have a rigid, tender abdomen. Toxic megacolon is an unusual complication that is associated with the inappropriate use of corticosteroids when amebic colitis is mistaken for idiopathic inflammatory bowel disease. Chronic nondysenteric amebic colitis can manifest with years of intermittent bloody diarrhea, a syndrome symptomatically indistinguishable from ulcerative colitis. Ameboma is a rare segmental form of chronic amebic colitis that is more common in the cecum and ascending colon and presents as a tender abdominal mass that can be confused with colonic carcinoma.

Extraintestinal disease consists mainly of amebic liver abscess, which can occur up to 5 months after intestinal infection. Two types of presentation have been observed. One is an acute presentation of fewer than 10 days' duration that consists of high fever and marked right upper quadrant tenderness. Alternatively, with more than 10 days of symptoms, pain and weight loss predominate, with fever being less frequent. Fewer than a third of patients have concurrent diarrhea. Extension of an amebic liver abscess into the peritoneum or pericardium is more likely with a left lobe abscess and results in a very acute clinical presentation. Disease can extend to the pleura, causing empyema, and, less likely, can disseminate hematogenously to the lung and brain.

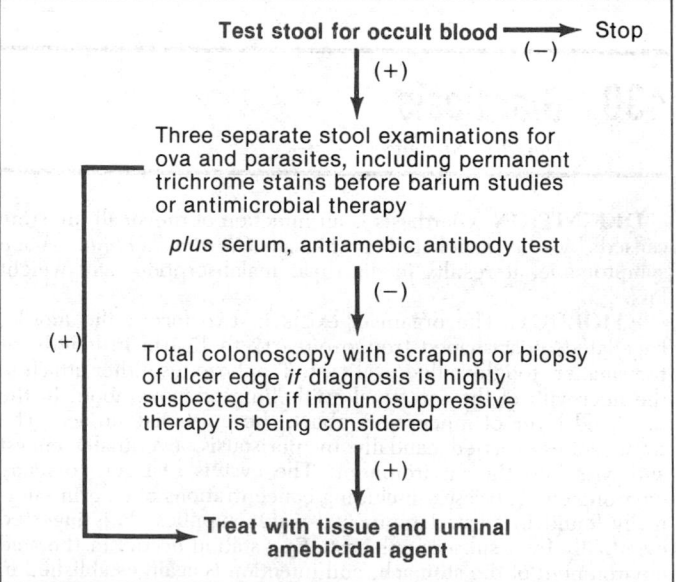

FIGURE 431–1. Diagnostic evaluation for acute amebic rectocolitis in a patient with suggestive epidemiology and clinical manifestations. (Reproduced with permission from Kass EH, Platt R [eds.]: Current Therapy in Infectious Disease—3. Philadelphia, B. C. Decker, 1990.)

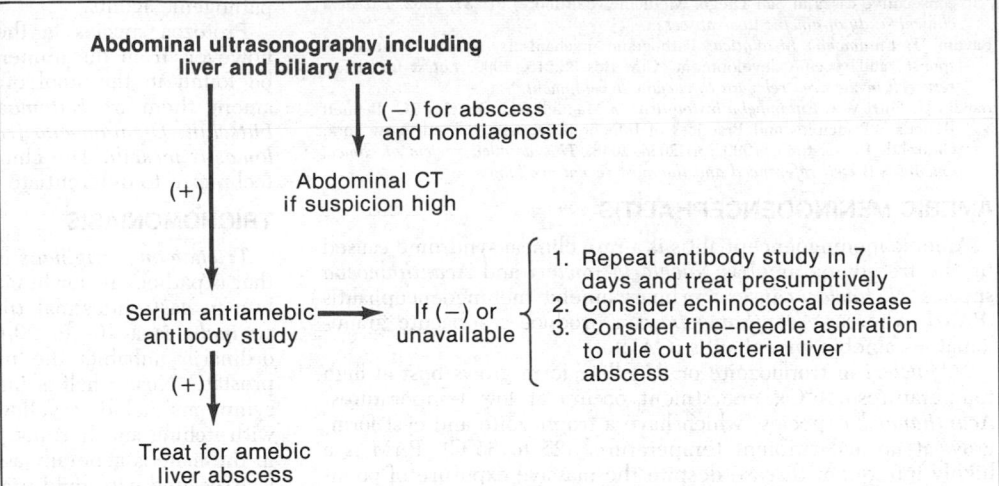

FIGURE 431–2. Diagnostic evaluation for amebic liver abscess in a patient with suggestive epidemiology and clinical manifestations. (Reproduced with permission from Kass EH, Platt R [eds.]: Current Therapy in Infectious Disease—3. Philadelphia, B. C. Decker, 1990.)

DIFFERENTIAL DIAGNOSIS AND WORKUP. Algorithms for the diagnosis of amebic colitis and liver abscess are provided in Figures 431–1 and 431–2, respectively. The differential diagnosis of acute amebic colitis includes infection due to *Shigella*, *Campylobacter*, *Salmonella*, *Yersinia*, and invasive *E. coli* species or to *Clostridium difficile* toxin-mediated disease. Amebiasis is one cause of inflammatory colitis in which fecal leukocytes may be absent, owing to the ability of trophozoites to lyse human neutrophils. Unfortunately, the diagnosis of intestinal amebiasis still rests upon the morphologic identification of trophozoites in fecal specimens (see Color Plate 11*H*). At least three stool samples are necessary to reach a 90 per cent yield; samples should be refrigerated or placed in fixative if they cannot be processed immediately. Laboratories in the United States frequently falsely identify fecal leukocytes as trophozoites; careful study with skilled microscopy is necessary. Serology for antiamebic antibodies is positive in more than 85 per cent of patients with amebic colitis and is very helpful. Interpretation of results can be difficult in highly endemic areas, where up to 25 per cent of the population is seropositive owing to the persistence of serum antibodies for years after pathogenic *E. histolytica* infection. Endoscopy with biopsies of the ulcer edge is diagnostic in 90 per cent of cases; this is helpful if a rapid diagnosis is needed, if serology results are nondiagnostic, or to differentiate amebiasis from idiopathic inflammatory bowel disease.

The key study in the diagnosis of amebic liver abscess is abdominal ultrasonography, a rapid, noninvasive procedure that should differentiate between biliary tract disease and a cavity in the liver. The differential diagnosis can then be narrowed to amebic liver abscess, pyogenic bacterial abscess, echinococcal cyst, and hepatoma. Attention to epidemiologic risk factors and detection of serum antiamebic antibodies are usually sufficient to establish the diagnosis, with the caveat that serology may be negative in patients with fewer than 7 days of symptoms. However, if concern exists regarding a bacterial abscess and a serologic study is not immediately available, then a "skinny-needle" aspiration, guided by ultrasonography, or computed tomography, can be performed. This procedure is diagnostic of bacterial abscess; aspiration of an amebic abscess normally yields a yellow proteinaceous fluid without white blood cells or amebas. The trophozoites are found in tissue at the periphery of the liver lesion.

THERAPY. Regimens for the treatment of amebiasis are summarized in Table 431–2. Therapy usually requires a tissue-active agent followed by a drug effective in the bowel lumen. In pregnant women, the use of nonabsorbable agents (paromomycin) or the judicious use of metronidazole is advisable. It is controversial whether therapy is necessary for asymptomatic *E. histolytica* intestinal infection without evidence of tissue invasion; however, this may be advisable in areas where pathogenic infection is likely or reinfection is not expected. Careful follow-up of stool examination is necessary, as all available agents are incompletely effective in eradicating intestinal infection. Patients with amebic liver abscess respond gradually with decreased pain and fever after 3 to 5 days of therapy. A small minority do not respond at all within 3 days or have a very large abscess that appears close to rupture; needle aspiration is indicated in such patients. After aspiration, continued therapy with metronidazole alone should be adequate. There is no evidence that the addition of other therapeutic agents is necessary. Although fewer than 20 per cent of patients with liver abscess have trophozoites found in their stool, follow-up with a luminally active agent is advisable.

PREVENTION. *E. histolytica* infection can be prevented by the availability of clean water, adequate sanitation, and avoidance of sexual practices or living conditions that facilitate direct fecal-oral contamination. Boiling is the only reliable way of killing cysts; halide solutions are not reliable. In endemic areas, uncooked foods such as salads and vegetables should be avoided. No vaccine or acceptable form of chemoprophylaxis is available; however, current research on the pathogenesis of amebiasis and the host immune response has led to the identification of multiple *E. histolytica* antigens that are candidates for vaccine development.

Healy GR: Diagnostic techniques for stool samples. *In* Ravdin JI, (ed.): Amebiasis: Human Infection by *Entamoeba histolytica*. New York, Churchill Livingstone, 1988, pp 106–119. *A recent authoritative review of the diagnosis of amebiasis using fecal specimens; the text contains more than 50 chapters on all aspects of* E. histolytica *infection.*

Katzenstein D, Rickerson V, Braude A: New concepts of amebic liver abscess derived from hepatic imaging, serodiagnosis, and hepatic enzymes in 67

TABLE 431–2. THERAPEUTIC REGIMENS FOR TREATMENT OF AMEBIASIS*

Cyst Passers
Diloxanide furoate, 500 mg tid × 10 days, or
Paromomycin, 30 mg/kg/day in 3 divided doses × 5–10 days, or
Tetracycline, 250 mg qid × 10 days, then diiodohydroxyquin, 650 mg tid × 20 days

Invasive Rectocolitis
Metronidazole, 750 mg tid × 5–10 days
  or 2.4 grams qd × 2–3 days
  or 50 mg/kg × 1 dose
  plus diloxanide furoate or paromomycin or
Dehydroemetine, 1–1.5 mg/kg/day × 5 days plus diloxanide furoate or paromomycin

Liver Abscess
Metronidazole, 750 tid × 5–10 days or 2.4 mg qd × 1–2 days plus diloxanide fuorate or paromomycin or
Dehydroemetine, 1–1.5 mg/kg/day × 5 days plus diloxanide furoate or paromomycin or
Chloroquine (base), 600 mg qd × 2 days, 300 mg base qd × 2–3 weeks (can be added to other regimens)

*All dosages are for oral administrtion except dehydroemetine, which is given intramuscularly; metronidazole can be used intravenously.

Adapted with permission from Mandell GL, Douglas RG Jr, Bennett JE (eds.): Principles and Practices of Infectious Diseases. 3rd ed. New York, Churchill Livingstone, 1989.

consecutive cases in San Diego. Medicine (Baltimore) 61:237, 1982. *Excellent clinical study of amebic liver abscess.*

Ravdin JI: *Entamoeba histolytica:* Pathogenic mechanisms, human immune response, and vaccine development. Clin Res 38:215, 1990. *Latest update on research in the area relevant to vaccine development.*

Ravdin JI, Petri WA: *Entamoeba histolytica. In* Mandell GL, Douglas RG, Bennett JE (eds.): Principles and Practices of Infectious Disease. 3rd ed. New York, Churchill Livingstone, 1990, pp 2036–2048. *This detailed review of clinical amebiasis is well referenced and the most recent available.*

AMEBIC MENINGOENCEPHALITIS

Amebic meningoencephalitis is a rare clinical syndrome caused by the free-living amebas *Naegleria fowleri* and *Acanthamoeba* species. *N. fowleri* causes a primary amebic meningoencephalitis (PAM), whereas *Acanthamoeba* can produce a subacute granulomatous amebic encephalitis (GAE).

N. fowleri in trophozoite or flagellate form grows best at high temperatures (46°C); encystment occurs at low temperatures. *Acanthamoeba* species, which have a trophozoite and cyst form, grow at normal ambient temperatures (25 to 35°C). PAM is a highly infrequent disease despite the massive exposure of populations to warm fresh water. GAE is usually restricted to immunosuppressed populations, such as those with acquired immunodeficiency syndrome (AIDS) or those with organ transplants. *N. fowleri* enters the central nervous system by penetrating the nasal mucosa and cribriform plate and is highly cytolytic. GAE probably results from hematogenous dissemination and can be distinguished from PAM by the presence of cysts in tissue.

PAM is characterized by the abrupt onset of headache, fever, and meningismus, with rapid development of focal neurologic findings, including olfactory loss. A neutrophilic cerebrospinal fluid (CSF) pleocytosis is frequently associated with increased CSF protein and hypoglycorrhachia. A negative CSF Gram stain result, India ink preparation, culture for bacteria, and cryptococcal antigen study in a patient with acute meningitis who has a history of exposure to fresh water suggests the need to examine the CSF for motile trophozoites (10 to 30 μm), a finding that is diagnostic. In contrast, GAE manifests subacutely over weeks with focal central nervous system signs, headache, fever, and depressed mental status and is often complicated by seizures. The presence of *Acanthamoeba* organisms in a nodular or ulcerative skin lesion is helpful; study of the CSF usually reveals a nonspecific lymphocytosis with abnormally elevated protein levels. A brain biopsy is necessary to differentiate GAE from toxoplasmosis, pyogenic brain abscess, and other causes of focal central nervous system disease.

There is no treatment known to be efficacious for PAM or GAE. Treatment with systemic and intrathecal amphotericin B was associated with survival in two patients with PAM. *Acanthamoeba* organisms are usually susceptible in vitro to ketoconazole, miconazole, 5-flucytosine, and pentamidine. After determination of susceptibility of the patient's isolate in vitro, the above agents and amphotericin B can be considered. These are rare disorders, and the risk of PAM from diving or waterskiing in warm fresh water cannot be quantified. Opportunistic infections other than those caused by *Acanthamoeba* are much more frequent in immunosuppressed patients.

Petri WA, Ravdin JI: Free Living Amebas. *In* Mandell GL, Douglas RG, Bennett ED (eds.): Principles and Practices of Infectious Diseases. 3rd ed. New York, Churchill Livingstone, 1990, pp 2049–2055. *This is an up-to-date, well-referenced review of disease caused by free-living amebas.*

432 Other Protozoan Diseases

David P. Stevens

The human host provides an ever changing environment for protozoan infections. With the increasing prevalence of immunodeficiency, caused by either immunosuppressant drugs or the acquired immunodeficiency syndrome (AIDS), protozoan infections that were previously considered rare or exotic are now observed more frequently. With this changing epidemiologic setting, additional protozoa will play the opportunist's role as pathogenic agents.

Protozoa species in these settings should be distinguished, however, from the numerous nonpathogenic protozoa that may be found in the stool of apparently healthy persons. Notable among them are *Entamoeba coli, Endolimax nana, Iodamoeba bütschlii, Dientamoeba fragilis, Trichomonas hominis,* and *Chilomastix mesnili.* The clinician must rely on a skilled laboratory technician to differentiate these agents from pathogenic species.

TRICHOMONIASIS

Trichomonas vaginalis is the only species of the trichomonads that is pathogenic for humans. *T. tenax* and *T. hominis* infect the human gastrointestinal tract but are harmless commensals. *T. vaginalis* is a 10- to 20-μm motile, flagellated organism that ordinarily inhabits the urethra, urinary bladder, vagina, and prostate. Nearly half of infections are asymptomatic. Recognized symptoms include a yellow, creamy vaginal discharge associated with itching and burning. Dysuria may be prominent. Infection in the male is generally asymptomatic. Occasionally, however, it is associated with mild urethral burning of brief duration.

Diagnosis is made microscopically by identification of the organism in a wet preparation of the exudate. Long-term complications are unrecognized in otherwise healthy persons. Treatment of both partners is advised for this sexually transmitted disease. Treatment with a single 2-gram dose of metronidazole is as effective as metronidazole, 250 mg three times daily for 7 days. It is frequently associated with side effects of nausea, a metallic taste, or alcohol intolerance.

Lossick JG: Sexually transmitted vaginitis. Urol Clin North Am 11:141, 1984. *An authoritative clinical report for further detailed study.*

BALANTIDIASIS

Balantidium coli is a large, motile, oval ciliate, some 5 to 10 times the size of an erythrocyte. The trophozoite form resides as a facultative anaerobe in the colon. The great majority of infections in humans are noninvasive, asymptomatic, and self-limited. Infrequently a cause of disease, this protozoan can penetrate the colonic mucosa with formation of deep ulcers. Illness consists of dysentery, usually bloody, often with resulting dehydration and prostration. Complications include colonic perforation at the site of the ulcers. Infection may extend to mesenteric lymph nodes and, less commonly, the appendix and terminal ileum. Isolated reports of infection of the vagina, liver, lung, and pleura have documented that extraintestinal migration of the organism is rare.

Balantidia infect numerous nonhuman reservoirs, particularly swine. It is said that 80 per cent of pigs in England carry this organism. The relevance of various other animal reservoirs, such as rats, to human infection is debated. The importance of porcine infections to human disease is borne out, however, by the documented high incidence of balantidiasis in communities where swine and humans live together closely, e.g., in New Guinea, Micronesia, Peru, and southern Russia. Poor nutrition and debilitating illness seem to predispose to symptomatic balantidiasis. Person-to-person spread probably occurs in settings where crowding and poor hygiene exist.

Ingestion of *Balantidium* cysts—resistant to drying and other environmental stresses—leads to infection in the susceptible host. Excystation occurs at an unknown location in the gastrointestinal tract, and multiplication occurs in the colon. Encystation occurs in the distal colon or after expulsion into the environment.

The diagnosis is confirmed by microscopic demonstration of trophozoites in fresh wet preparations of liquid stool or scrapings of colonic ulcers. Cysts are less frequently observed in stool, and concentration techniques are usually required. Differentiation from amebiasis and idiopathic ulcerative colitis must always be considered.

Therapy is reserved for the patient with symptomatic infection and consists of tetracycline, 500 mg four times daily for 10 days. Metronidazole, 250 mg four times daily for 7 days, is probably effective and may serve as alternative therapy when tetracycline is not tolerated.

Knight R: Giardiasis, isosporiasis, and balantidiasis. Clin Gastroenterol 7:31, 1978. *There are few useful clinical reviews on balantidiasis; this is the best of the lot.*

BABESIOSIS

Babesiosis is an uncommon febrile illness spread by the northern deer tick, *Ixodes dammini*. Babesiosis and Lyme disease are both spread by this same vector and are found most frequently in Massachusetts—including the off-shore islands—portions of New Jersey, New York, Maryland, Minnesota, and Wisconsin. The illness typically includes fever, malaise, headache, chills, weakness, arthralgias, and nausea. Splenomegaly is uncommon. There is no rash. Parasitemia is demonstrated by observation of typical intraerythrocytic forms. Confirmation of elevated convalescent antibody titers to the infectious organism, *Babesia microti*, may be obtained through the Centers for Disease Control. Contaminated blood transfusions have been implicated as the cause of a few rare cases. Infection is usually self-limited but may be severe in splenectomized patients. Therapy with quinine sulfate, 650 mg every 6 hours, combined with clindamycin, 300 mg every 6 hours, given intravenously, has been successful in severely ill patients.

Ruebush TK, Cassady PB, Marsh HJ, et al.: Human babesiosis on Nantucket Island. Ann Intern Med 86:6, 1977. *This report summarizes well the clinical aspects of this infection.*

SARCOSPORIDIOSIS

Infections with *Sarcocystis hominis* (previously designated *Isospora hominis*) may be associated with abdominal pain, diarrhea, and nausea. The human is the definitive host, with sexual reproduction taking place in the small intestine; cattle are the intermediate host, where the sarcocyst resides in skeletal or cardiac muscle with little or no reaction. While infection in humans is relatively common in areas of the world where undercooked beef is ingested, the definition of the precise role of this agent in human disease remains clouded by its frequent coincidence with other pathogenic agents.

Beaver PC, Gadgil RK, Morera P: Sarcocysts in man: A review and report of five cases. Am J Trop Med Hyg 28:810, 1979. *This reference provides a good starting point into the available clinical literature.*

433 Cestode Infections

Charles H. King

Humans are infected by a number of different cestodes of the phylum Platyhelminthes (flatworms). The species most commonly causing human infection are summarized in Table 433–1.

One key to understanding the broad spectrum of cestode-associated disease is to recall that tapeworm parasites divide their life cycle between two or more different animal hosts. The first, or *intermediate,* host is typically an insect or herbivorous vertebrate that ingests parasite eggs in fecally contaminated food or water. The tapeworm eggs hatch into invasive oncospheres in this primary host's intestinal tract and then migrate into the host viscera or muscles to develop into immature cystic forms, called cysticerci or cysticercoids (for Cyclophyllidea cestodes such as *Taenia* and *Hymenolepis*), or procercoid larvae (for Pseudophyllidea cestodes such as *Diphyllobothrium*). For the latter parasite group, the procercoid forms become infectious for humans if they are consumed by a second intermediate host (usually a fish or reptile) and become plerocercoid cysts.

The *definitive* host for a tapeworm species is a carnivorous or omnivorous mammal that acquires infection by consuming larval cysts in the uncooked tissues of an intermediate host. Upon exposure to stomach acid and bile salts in the digestive tract, larvae excyst and develop into mature tapeworms within the intestinal lumen. Adult tapeworms contain two sections: a *scolex* (or head), used to adhere to the wall of the intestine, and a *strobila,* or tapelike chain of developing segments called proglottides. The hermaphroditic segments produce large numbers of fertile, infectious parasite eggs that reach the environment either free or enclosed within segments in the host's feces.

In general, humans serve as *either* definitive *or* intermediate hosts for a given cestode species. For example, we are strictly definitive hosts for the tapeworms *Diphyllobothrium latum* (the "fish" tapeworm) and *Taenia saginata* (the "beef" tapeworm). These adult tapeworms do not enter the tissues of the human body and cause only minimal clinical symptoms. In contrast, we are solely intermediate hosts for *Echinococcus granulosus* (hydatid cyst disease), *E. multilocularis* (alveolar cyst disease), *T. multiceps* (coenurosis), and *Spirometra* species. In the human body, these parasites develop as larval cysts and cause significant, symptomatic tissue damage.

There are two exceptions to this rule. First, patients with *T. solium* infection may be infected with larval cysts (cysticercosis), adult tapeworms ("pork" tapeworm), or both. Second, in the case of the dwarf tapeworm, *Hymenolepis nana,* complete egg-to-tapeworm development can take place within a single human host. *H. nana* can thus be transmitted directly from person to person, and internal autoinfection may substantially increase the tapeworm burden of an infected individual. For all other cestode infections, increases in parasite burden occur only by means of continued exposure to egg-contaminated or larvae-infested foods and water.

INTESTINAL CESTODE (TAPEWORM) INFECTIONS

Diphyllobothrium latum

D. latum tapeworms are the largest parasites that infect humans, ranging up to 10 meters in length. Infection is acquired by ingestion of parasite cysts in the tissues of smoked or uncooked freshwater fish (e.g., as sushi, sashimi, or ceviche). Tapeworms develop to maturity within 3 to 6 weeks after exposure and may survive for up to 20 years. Infection is prevalent (up to 2 per cent of local residents) in many parts of the world; endemic foci are found in lake or delta regions of Scandinavia, the U.S.S.R., Japan, Europe, Chile, and North America. Contamination of freshwater bodies by raw sewage increases the risk for *D. latum* infection, but stable transmission may also occur owing to local infection of alternate definitive hosts, such as foxes, wolves, minks, and bears.

TABLE 433–1. COMMON HUMAN CESTODE INFECTIONS

Species	Infective Stage for Humans	Common Name	Pathology	Therapy
Diphyllobothrium latum	Adult	Fish tapeworm	Pernicious anemia	Niclosamide or Praziquantel
Hymenolepis nana	Adult	Dwarf tapeworm	Rarely symptomatic	
Taenia saginata	Adult	Beef tapeworm	Rarely symptomatic	
Taenia solium	Adult	Pork tapeworm	Rarely symptomatic	
	Larva	Cysticercosis	Brain and tissue cysts	Albendazole* Praziquantel Surgery
Echinococcus granulosus	Larva	Hydatid cyst disease	Solitary tissue cysts	Surgery Albendazole*
Echinococcus multilocularis	Larva	Alveolar cyst disease	Multilocular cysts	Surgery Albendazole*
Taenia multiceps	Larva	Bladderworm, coenurosis	Brain and eye cysts	Surgery
Spirometra mansonoides	Larva	Sparganosis	Subcutaneous larvae	Surgery

*This drug has not been approved by the Food and Drug Adminstration at the time of publication.

CLINICAL MANIFESTATIONS. For most patients, *D. latum* infection produces few, if any, symptoms. These are typically limited to nonspecific complaints of weakness, dizziness, craving for salt, diarrhea, and intermittent abdominal discomfort. Occasional patients may experience vomiting, severe abdominal pain, and weight loss. In cases of multiple infection, biliary or intestinal obstruction may occur. One to 2 per cent of patients with *D. latum* infection develop significant vitamin B$_{12}$ deficiency, resulting in megaloblastic anemia and/or neurologic disease. Folate deficiency may also occur. Vitamin B$_{12}$ deficiency is a product of extensive vitamin uptake by the worm as well as worm-induced interference with gastrointestinal uptake by the host (despite normal gastric acidity and intrinsic factor production). Vitamin B$_{12}$ deficiency is most common among older patients and is more likely to occur in patients with low dietary intake of vitamins, multiple tapeworms, or a tapeworm in the proximal jejunum. In the debilitated host, nervous system complications can be quite extensive and can range from peripheral neuropathy to the syndrome of severe combined degeneration (see Ch. 244).

DIAGNOSIS. The diagnosis of *D. latum* infection is made by stool examination for characteristic operculated eggs that are 65 by 45 µm. Recovery of proglottides is infrequent owing to segment degeneration during intestinal transit.

TREATMENT. Treatment is with niclosamide or praziquantel, as summarized in Table 433–2. Severe vitamin B$_{12}$ deficiency can be rapidly treated by parenteral vitamin injections.

PREVENTION. Fish tapeworm infection is prevented by avoiding consumption of raw, smoked, or salted fish from endemic areas. Parasite cysts may be killed by cooking (above 56°C for 5 minutes) or by freezing (-20°C for 24 hours). Control of human sewage and frequent screening of high-risk populations help to eliminate the human reservoir (but not the zoonotic reservoirs) of infection.

Hymenolepis nana

H. nana, or dwarf tapeworm, is found frequently in warm, dry climates and is prevalent in Southern and Eastern Europe, Asia, Africa, Central and South America, and Australia. It is the only human tapeworm that does not require an intermediate host. In the small intestine, hatching eggs release oncospheres that penetrate the villi of the mucosa. Four to 5 days later, the developed cysticercoid ruptures out of the villus and a parasite scolex attaches to the lining of the ileum, maturing in 10 to 12 days. Mature worms are small, measuring 25 to 40 mm long by 1 mm wide. Autoinfection can occur internally, i.e., within the small bowel, or externally, via the fecal-oral route, resulting in heavy infection. With time, however, a regulatory immunity to infection may develop, so that *H. nana* infection can be spontaneously cleared. Intensive infection is more common in institutionalized, malnourished, or immunodeficient individuals.

CLINICAL MANIFESTATIONS. The clinical manifestations of *H. nana* vary with intensity and may include diarrhea, anorexia, abdominal pain, and pallor. A statistical association with phlyctenular keratoconjunctivitis has been observed and has been tentatively ascribed to the immune response to infection.

DIAGNOSIS. The diagnosis of *H. nana* infection is made by stool examination for eggs of 30 to 47 µm that have a characteristic double membrane. Proglottides are usually not seen in the stool.

TREATMENT. Treatment is with niclosamide or praziquantel, as outlined in Table 433–2. In comparison to the treatment of other tapeworm infections, longer courses of niclosamide and higher doses of praziquantel are recommended for the therapy of *H. nana* infection because of the relative resistance of larval cysticercoids to drug therapy. Because of the potential for late emergence of worms from viable cysticercoids remaining in the ileum, heavily infected individuals should be retested for infection and retreated 10 to 14 days after initial therapy.

PREVENTION. Because *H. nana* is easily transmitted from person to person, sanitation and hand washing are essential to control this parasite. Mass chemotherapy may also be used to suppress endemic transmission, particularly within closed institutions.

Taenia saginata

T. saginata, or beef tapeworm infection, is widespread in cattle-breeding areas of the world. Endemic foci (defined as prevalence greater than 10 per cent) are found in the southern U.S.S.R., in the Near East, and in central and eastern Africa. Infection is less common in other parts of the world but is found at prevalence rates of 0.1 to 5 per cent in Europe, Southeast Asia, and South America. Infection is acquired by the consumption of cysticerci in the muscle tissue of infected cattle. The consumption of dishes such as steak tartare, "bleu" or rare steak, and undercooked shish kebabs is associated with infection in North American travelers to endemic areas.

CLINICAL MANIFESTATIONS. *T. saginata* infection may cause nonspecific complaints of weakness and mild abdominal discomfort in a minority (one third) of patients. Because *T. saginata* proglottides are motile, they may cause acute abdominal symptoms by migrating into and obstructing the appendix or the pancreatic and biliary ducts. A psychologically distressing feature of infection (and often the first symptom reported by the patient) occurs when motile proglottides migrate out of the anus onto skin or clothing or when they are observed moving in the feces.

DIAGNOSIS. The diagnosis of taeniasis is most readily established by stool examination and perianal inspection for parasite proglottides and eggs. It is not possible, however, to distinguish *T. saginata* eggs from those of *T. solium* morphologically, and the definitive diagnosis of *T. saginata* infection requires pathologic examination of proglottid features or DNA hybridization studies. In practice, because patients with *T. solium* are at risk for self-infection with cysticercosis (see below), and because medical therapy for taeniasis is both safe and highly effective, treatment of an undetermined *Taenia* species infection should not be delayed pending speciation of the infecting tapeworm.

TREATMENT. Treatment of beef tapeworm infection is with praziquantel or niclosamide, as outlined in Table 433–2. Both medications are highly effective in eliminating infection, and no special preparation or purgation is required. After therapy, the parasite scolex is digested within the gastrointestinal tract before it is passed in the feces. Although with the highly effective medications currently in use one no longer needs to collect the scolex to be assured that the parasite head has been expelled, digestive destruction of the head limits our ability to establish a species-specific clinical diagnosis for individual *Taenia* infections.

TABLE 433–2. THERAPY FOR INTESTINAL CESTODE (TAPEWORM) INFECTION

	Niclosamide	Praziquantel
Dosage		
Adults	2 grams (4 tablets)	10–20 mg/kg for all age groups
Children > 34 kg	1.5 grams (3 tablets)	(25 mg/kg for *H. nana*)
Children 11–34 kg	1 gram (2 tablets)	
Administration	For most tapeworm species, taken as a single dose; tablets must be thoroughly chewed before swallowing to obtain complete therapeutic effect; a 7-day course of drugs is used for *H. nana*, with reduced pediatric doses on days 2–7	Taken as a single dose for all species; may repeat after 7 days for heavy *H. nana* infections
Side effects	Nausea, vomiting, abdominal pain, diarrhea, drowsiness, dizziness, headache, pruritus	Mild but frequent, including dizziness, myalgias, nausea, vomiting, diarrhea, abdominal pain
Pregnancy	No known mutagenic effects; considered safe if indicated; because of risk of cysticercosis by autoinfection in *T. solium* tapeworm infection, therapy should not be delayed	

PREVENTION. *T. saginata* infection is prevented by avoidance of foods containing undercooked or raw beef. As for the fish tapeworm, cooking to 56°C for 5 minutes or freezing at −20°C for 7 to 10 days destroys the infective larvae. Because humans are the sole reservoir for infection, effective sanitation and periodic treatment of those in contact with cattle can have a significant impact on transmission.

Taenia solium

T. solium, also known as pork tapeworm, causes human infection in two different forms. Individuals who consume undercooked pork containing intermediate parasite cysts will develop intestinal *T. solium* tapeworms. Individuals who consume parasite eggs may develop intermediate parasite cysts within the tissues of the body. (This condition, called *cysticercosis,* is described in more detail in the section on tissue cestode infections.) Autoinfection, most likely via the fecal-oral route, is possible, and a single patient may harbor both adult tapeworm and tissue cysticerci. *T. solium* infection is prevalent in Mexico, Central and South America, Africa, Southern Europe, Southeast Asia, and the Philippines. Most infections seen in the United States and Canada are found in immigrants from these endemic foci.

CLINICAL MANIFESTATIONS. *T. solium* tapeworms are relatively short (3 meters) but may survive for several decades once established in the human jejunum. Generally, tapeworm infections with *T. solium* produce minimal or no symptoms, being limited to mild, nonspecific abdominal complaints. Unlike *T. saginata* proglottides, the segments of *T. solium* are nonmotile and are unlikely to cause obstruction.

DIAGNOSIS. The diagnosis of intestinal infection with *T. solium* tapeworm is made by examination of the stool for eggs and proglottides. Since the eggs are morphologically indistinguishable from those of *T. saginata,* study of the proglottid or head of the tapeworms is required for species identification. Stool samples and proglottides should be handled with care because of the risk of acquiring cysticercosis by accidental ingestion of *T. solium* eggs.

TREATMENT. *T. solium* tapeworm infection is treated with either niclosamide or praziquantel, as outlined in Table 433–2. Once diagnosis is established, therapy should be instituted as soon as possible because of the risk of autoinfection with cysticercosis. Therapy for cysticercosis is substantially longer and more intensive than that for intestinal infection and is described in detail in the section on tissue cestode infections.

PREVENTION. Individuals may avoid *T. solium* tapeworm infection by avoiding foods containing raw or undercooked pork. Meat inspection and improvements in pork-raising practices have successfully reduced transmission in some areas. In endemic areas, periodic chemotherapy of human populations may reduce the reservoir of egg production and reduce pork infestation.

Other Intestinal Cestodes

Other tapeworms that occasionally infect humans include the dog tapeworm *Dipylidium caninum* and the rodent tapeworm *Hymenolepis diminuta*. These are most common in children and are acquired by inadvertently ingesting the intermediate larval forms of these parasites in the bodies of fleas or other insects. Usually, *D. caninum* and *H. diminuta* infections produce minimal symptoms. Diagnosis is established by stool examination, and infections are readily treated with standard doses of niclosamide or praziquantel.

TISSUE CESTODE (CYST) INFECTION

Echinococcosis

Human echinococcosis causes significant morbidity and mortality in livestock-raising regions in all parts of the world. The causative agents of "hydatid" and "alveolar" cyst disease in humans are the intermediate larval forms of the tapeworms *Echinococcus granulosus* and *E. multilocularis,* respectively.

Like other cestodes, *Echinococcus* tapeworms have both intermediate and definitive hosts. For *Echinococcus* species, dogs and other canines are the definitive hosts. Tapeworm-infected animals pass eggs in their feces, which contaminate the local environment. Contamination of grazing areas and foodstuffs results in egg ingestion by intermediate hosts, e.g., humans, sheep, goats, camels, and horses for *E. granulosus* and mice or other small rodents for *E. multilocularis*. Life cycle transmission is completed when the definitive carnivore host consumes meat or offal of the intermediate host that contains hydatid or alveolar cysts. Protoscolices within the cysts mature in the lumen of the canine gut to become adult, egg-bearing tapeworms. Because the cysts of *Echinococcus* contain a germinal layer that can produce multiple internal "daughter" cysts by asexual budding, an individual dog may develop infection with dozens of tapeworms after consumption of a single large cyst. Once the tapeworms mature, a heavily infected dog may contaminate 10 or more hectares of ground with infectious eggs in the space of a week.

In most areas of the world, burial practices make humans a "dead-end" host for *Echinococcus*, i.e., human infection does not perpetuate transmission in the local ecosystem. Nevertheless, the "inadvertent" hydatid cyst disease caused by *E. granulosus* and the more aggressive alveolar cyst disease caused by *E. multilocularis* are severe or even fatal illnesses for a significant minority of infected individuals.

EPIDEMIOLOGY. *E. granulosus* is common in livestock-raising areas of both developed and developing countries. Sheep- and goat-herding populations that keep dogs as pets or work animals are at highest risk for hydatid cyst disease. Until recently, hydatid disease was common in Australia, New Zealand, Argentina, Chile, Ireland, Scotland, the Basque country, the Mediterranean basin, and throughout middle Europe. Currently, the area with the highest prevalence in the world is the Turkana and Samburu regions of northwestern Kenya, where domestic and feral transmission of *E. granulosus* is perpetuated among nomadic farmers by poor hygienic practices. Occasional hydatid disease transmission is also found in central Asia, Mexico, the United States, and South America.

Alveolar cyst disease due to *E. multilocularis* is usually transmitted by wild animals, e.g., foxes and bush dogs, and is found in the arctic regions of the United States, Canada, and the U.S.S.R.

CLINICAL MANIFESTATIONS. Human disease caused by *Echinococcus* species results from bloodborne invasion of the liver (50 to 70 per cent of patients), lungs (20 to 30 per cent), or other organs by developing parasite oncospheres. As these mature, they grow within tissues by concentric enlargement (*E. granulosus*) or by extension through adjacent host tissues (*E. multilocularis*). At any given time, most infected individuals are asymptomatic, and it may take 5 to 20 years for a cyst to grow to sufficient size (3 to 15 cm) to cause symptoms. When present, symptoms and findings refer to the anatomic site of involvement and derive from local inflammation, secondary bacterial infection, obstruction, or local mass effect. In hydatid cyst disease, the growing cyst becomes surrounded by a fibrous capsule formed by host immune reaction. Within this primary unilocular cyst, multiple daughter cysts, each containing an infective protoscolex, develop by asexual budding of the germinal layer. In alveolar cyst disease, the parasite cyst is not well separated from surrounding tissues, and lateral budding and malignancy-like growth (including distal metastasis of daughter cysts) may occur.

Patients with symptomatic hydatid liver cysts may complain of abdominal discomfort or mass in the right upper quadrant. Cyst leakage into the peritoneal cavity or pleural space may be associated with fever, urticaria, or a severe anaphylactoid reaction. Invasion of the biliary system often leads to the passage of daughter cysts into the common bile duct, with clinical and chemical evidence of intermittent obstruction resembling choledocholithiasis. Individuals with symptomatic hydatid involvement of the lungs present with cough, hemoptysis, and pleurisy. Spontaneous rupture of the cyst may lead to intrathoracic spread or to evacuation of daughter cysts via the bronchus. At either lung or liver sites, bacterial superinfection may cause an acute presentation with symptoms of sepsis. Hydatid involvement of the brain is marked by slow-onset mass effect, hydrocephalus, and often seizures. Cysts of the bone frequently fail to form a discrete capsule but rather cause local erosion of the cortex, resulting in pathologic fracture.

Symptomatic alveolar cyst disease most frequently refers to liver involvement and manifests as vague, mild upper quadrant and epigastric pain. Signs of hepatomegaly or obstructive jaundice may be present. Occasionally, metastatic lesions in the lung or brain are the first to cause symptoms by local inflammation or mass effect.

DIAGNOSIS. Laboratory evaluation may show marked eosinophilia, but this finding is inconstant (30 per cent prevalence). In hydatid cyst disease, radiographic and ultrasonographic studies typically show characteristic large, avascular cysts containing internal structures consistent with daughter cysts. Detection of mural calcification strongly favors the diagnosis of hydatid cyst. The differential diagnosis includes hemangioma, metastatic carcinoma, and remote bacterial or amebic liver abscess. Confirmatory evidence of infection may be obtained by serology (sensitivity of 60 to 90 per cent, depending on the test used). Serologic testing is available commercially or from the Centers for Disease Control, Atlanta, GA (through local state health departments). Until recently, it has not been recommended to perform closed aspiration on the cyst for diagnosis, as cyst leakage has the potential to initiate a severe allergic reaction and may result in the metastatic spread of daughter cysts. However, a recent clinical series has reported successful computed tomography (CT)–guided thin-needle aspiration of hydatid cysts for diagnosis. This procedure, when followed by immediate instillation of ethanol to kill viable protoscoleces, was associated with minimal side effects and was followed by apparent regression of cysts on CT scans. Further trials of this simplified approach to diagnosis and therapy appear warranted.

With alveolar cyst disease due to *E. multilocularis*, the organism's appearance on radiographic and sonographic imaging often mimics that of hepatic carcinoma. A definitive diagnosis may require either angiography or open biopsy at surgery. Precautions must be taken to prevent metastatic dissemination of daughter cysts at the time of surgery.

TREATMENT. Stable, asymptomatic, calcified cysts do not require specific therapy but should be monitored by serial imaging over several years to ensure a benign resolution. When technically feasible, expanding, symptomatic, or infected cysts are best removed in toto at surgery, with care taken to isolate and kill the cyst with hypertonic saline (25 to 30 gm per deciliter) or other cidal agents (such as iodophor, ethanol, or 10 per cent formalin) prior to excision, to avoid secondary spread or parasite cysts. Surgical resection should include careful closure of biliary and enteric fistulas and extensive postoperative drainage of the cyst bed to prevent fluid accumulation and secondary bacterial infection. Alveolar cyst disease may require wide resection, i.e., total lobectomy of liver or lung, to remove all cyst material.

In many cases, symptomatic echinococcal cysts are not amenable to resection. In such cases, oral drug therapy with the anthelminthics, either long-term mebendazole (40 mg per kilogram of body weight per day in three divided doses for 6 to 12 months) or albendazole* (200 mg twice a day for one to eight periods of 28 days each, separated by drug-free rest intervals of 14 to 28 days), has been recommended for cure or palliation. Cure rates, particularly for difficult cases with recurrent or extrahepatic/extrapulmonary cysts, have been low (less than 33 per cent), although a majority of patients show some improvement. Because the efficacy of drug therapy is limited, a combined medical-surgical approach should be individualized for each patient.

PREVENTION. The transmission of echinococcal disease has been prevented by regular praziquantel treatment of tapeworm-infected dogs in endemic areas. This approach, used in New Zealand and other endemic areas, has markedly reduced the prevalence of hydatid cyst disease in these areas over the past three decades. Related emphasis has been put on isolated butchering of livestock hosts to reduce transmission to working and feral dogs. Currently, human transmission is most common in the least-developed areas of the world, where veterinary practices are limited or nonexistent and butchering is done in the home environment. Research is focusing on means to identify infected populations rapidly and on finding the most effective ways to treat feral vectors.

---

*This drug has not been approved by the Food and Drug Administration at the time of publication. In the United States, compassionate use may be available through Smith Kline & French Laboratories, Philadelphia, PA.

Cysticercosis

Cysticercosis represents human tissue infection with the intermediate cyst forms of the pork tapeworm *T. solium*. Cysticercosis is acquired by ingestion of *T. solium* eggs in contaminated foods. Infection prevalence is approximately 1 to 10 per cent in endemic areas of Latin America, India, Asia, Indonesia, and parts of Africa. Because of its potentially life-threatening complications, cysticercosis has greater clinical significance than does intestinal *T. solium* tapeworm infection, particularly if cyst disease involves the central nervous system, the eyes, the heart, or other vital organs.

CLINICAL MANIFESTATIONS. The clinical manifestations of cysticercosis depend on the location and number of infecting cysts. Cysticerci are bladder-like, fluid-filled cysts containing an invaginated protoscolex. They are often surrounded by a dense fibrous capsule of host origin. In infected humans, cysticerci are usually multiple, 0.5 to 2 cm in size, and distributed widely throughout the body. Many patients have minimal, if any, symptoms of infection. However, symptomatic *neurocysticercosis* (i.e., cerebral cysticercosis, eye or spinal cord involvement) requires medical attention. This syndrome has an estimated mortality of up to 50 per cent, and any neurologic, cognitive, or personality disorder in an individual from an endemic area should be considered a possible manifestation of undiagnosed neurocysticercosis. In the past decade, diagnosis of this condition has been facilitated by the advent of CT scanning and magnetic resonance imaging (MRI), both of which are highly sensitive in detecting central nervous system cysticerci. Patients with central nervous system involvement have an average of 10 cysts distributed throughout the brain and spinal cord. These cysts may be in different stages of development, with symptoms commonly arising when older cysts begin to die, lose osmoregulation, and release antigenic material to provoke significant host inflammatory response.

In practice, neurocysticercosis may be divided into six discrete syndromes for management. In the *acute invasive* stage of cysticercosis, immediately after infection, the patient may experience fevers, headache, and myalgias associated with significant peripheral eosinophilia. Heavy infection at this stage may result in a clinical picture of "cysticercal encephalitis" associated with coma and rapid deterioration. This presentation should be treated aggressively with antiparasitic agents and anti-inflammatory drugs. After cysticerci become established, *parenchymal central nervous system cysticercosis* (50 per cent of cases) is associated with seizures, intellectual impairment, and personality changes. Compression due to swelling or inflammation around the cysts may result in focal deficits, signs of cerebral edema, and/or hydrocephalus. Seizures may be focal (jacksonian), referring to the specific cortical locus of involvement, or may be generalized. *Subarachnoid cysticercosis* (30 per cent of cases) is frequently associated with obstruction of cerebrospinal fluid (CSF) flow. Intracranial hypertension may manifest as vomiting, headache, and visual disturbances. Sensorial changes may include apathy, amnesia, dementia, hallucination, and emotional disturbance. Like other forms of basilar meningitis, pericysticercal inflammation at the base of the brain may cause obstruction or vasculitis of the cerebral arteries, leading to intermittent ischemia or stroke. *Intraventricular cysticercosis* (15 per cent of cases) is, because of its location, the most difficult to diagnose and treat. Symptomatic cysts are most frequent in the fourth ventricle, where they cause outflow obstruction and increased intracranial pressure without localizing signs. An aggressive variant of ventricular neurocysticercosis, called racemose cysticercosis, frequently involves the basal cisterns. This form of cysticercosis has been noted most often in young women and involves multiple, rapidly spreading cysts in the cerebrum and around the base of the brain. Whereas symptoms due to isolated cysts may remit, racemose cysticercosis usually has a progressive, deteriorating course if therapy is not given. Those with *spinal cysticercosis* may present with cord compression, radiculopathy, transverse myelitis, or signs of meningitis, depending on the location of involvement. *Ocular cysticercosis* is a distinct syndrome that manifests as eye pain, scotomata, and decreasing vision due to iridocyclitis, clouding of the vitreous, and retinal inflammation or detachment.

DIAGNOSIS. A definitive diagnosis of cysticercosis requires examination of biopsy material obtained from a tissue cyst. However, a presumptive diagnosis may be made on the basis of a history of residence in an endemic area, the presence of characteristic radiographic findings on plain films (calcified cysts in soft tissues) or scans (multiple, low-density, enhanced, and unenhanced lesions on CT or MRI), and suggestive laboratory findings. Infection with *T. solium* tapeworm is present in about 25 per cent of neurocysticercosis cases. In neurocysticercosis, examination of the cerebrospinal fluid may show hypoglycorrhachia, elevated total protein levels, and lymphocytic and eosinophilic pleocytosis (5 to 500 cells per microliter). Serum and CSF enzyme-linked immunosorbent assay (ELISA) and Western blot testing for specific immunoglobulin M (IgM) and immunoglobulin G (IgG) anticysticercal antibodies have a sensitivity of 75 to 100 per cent. These tests are available through commercial laboratories or from the Centers for Disease Control, Atlanta, GA (samples should be sent through state health departments). It should be noted, however, that antiparasite antibodies may persist long after infection, and a positive IgG serology merely indicates prior *Taenia* exposure, not necessarily active disease. The differential diagnosis of neurocysticercosis includes tumor, hydatid cyst disease, vasculitis, and chronic fungal and mycobacterial infection.

TREATMENT. Given the high prevalence of cysticercosis in some areas of the world, it is evident that most cysticerci do not cause significant symptoms. For *symptomatic* cysts outside the central nervous system, the optimal therapy is surgical removal, as this ensures complete elimination of the cyst. In the case of symptomatic neurocysticercosis, which carries an associated mortality of up to 50 per cent, therapy is definitely indicated, but surgery may be risky or technically unfeasible. An alternative approach to the control of some forms of neurocysticercosis has been demonstrated in recent clinical studies: Drug therapy with either praziquantel (50 mg per kilogram per day in three divided doses for 14 to 30 days) or albendazole* (15 mg per kilogram per day for 30 days) has been associated with alleviation of symptoms and regression of cyst size and number in patients with viable (nonenhancing) cysts in the cerebral parenchyma. However, drug therapy has provided only limited improvement in patients with arachnoiditis and no improvement in patients with intraventricular cysts. For these latter presentations, the treatment of choice remains surgery and/or palliation with shunting, anticonvulsants, and anti-inflammatory agents. It should be noted that in about 20 per cent of treated cases, the initiation of drug therapy is associated with a severely symptomatic, increased inflammatory response at the site of the cyst. This inflammation may be controlled with corticosteroids, but corticosteroids are not recommended for routine use in all patients, as they may significantly alter the pharmacokinetics of the anthelminthics used to treat infection. Follow-up tomographic scanning should be repeated 3 months after the cessation of therapy to ensure adequate response. If necessary, a repeat course of drug therapy with the alternate agent may be given to improve response. Because parasite-induced ocular inflammation does not respond well to systemic anti-inflammatory agents, patients with cysticercosis of the eye (20 per cent of cases of neurocysticercosis) should not receive drug therapy until the eye disease has been controlled surgically.

PREVENTION. As discussed earlier, the prevention of *T. solium* transmission requires control of human tapeworm infections, careful personal hygiene, and a high level of community sanitation.

Coenurosis

A different, but more rare, form of tissue cysticercosis may be caused by larval stages of the dog tapeworms *T. multiceps* and *T. serialis*. Lesions tend to be solitary and are distinguished pathologically from *T. solium* cysticerci on biopsy. Ocular involvement is common, and surgical resection is currently the only effective mode of therapy.

Sparganosis

Sparganosis is a tissue cestode infection caused by the plerocercoid larval stages of *Spirometra* species tapeworms of cats and other carnivores. Humans may become infected by ingestion of

---

*This drug has not been approved by the Food and Drug Administration at the time of publication.

infected water fleas (*Cyclops*), by ingestion of uncooked meat from infected animals (reptiles, birds, or mammals), or by cutaneous exposure (e.g., via traditional skin or eye poultices) to uncooked, infected meat. Usually, the larva encysts within the intestinal submucosa or skin. In some cases, however, parasites may invade the eye or central nervous system and cause significant inflammatory pathology at the site of encystment. Occasionally, proliferation into surrounding tissues occurs by lateral budding of the parasite (termed *sparganum proliferum*). The treatment of choice for sparganosis is ethanol injection and/or surgical removal, as limited experience with medical anthelminthic therapy has shown no beneficial effect.

Bia FJ, Barry M: Parasitic infections of the central nervous system. Neurol Clin 4:171, 1986. *Explores the range of parasite infections of the brain and their differential diagnosis.*

Davis A, Dixon H, Pawlowski Z: Multicentre clinical trials of benzimidazole carbamates in human cystic echinococcosis (phase 2). Bull WHO 68 67:503, 1989. *Up-to-date review of experience in multicenter trials of medical therapy for hydatid and alveolar cyst disease.*

Del Brutto OH, Sotelo J: Neurocysticercosis: An update. Rev Infect Dis 10:1075, 1988. *Extensive review of the diagnosis and treatment of this varied and complex disease. Contains a useful flow diagram on therapy for neurocysticercosis.*

Filice C, Di Perri G, Strosselli M, et al.: Parasitologic findings in percutaneous drainage of human hydatid liver cysts. J Infect Dis 161:1290, 1990. *Description of a small series of patients undergoing CT-guided diagnosis and treatment of hydatid cyst disease.*

Flisser A, Reid A, Garcia-Zepeda E, et al.: Specific detection of *Taenia saginata* eggs by DNA hybridization. Lancet 2:1429, 1988. *Description of a promising technique for species-specific diagnosis of* Taenia *infections from stool samples.*

King CH, Mahmoud AAF: Drugs five years later: Praziquantel. Ann Intern Med 110:290, 1989. *A summary of new data on the anthelminthic agent praziquantel since its release in the United States. Includes a listing of doses recommended for cestode therapy; with references.*

Pau A, Perria C, Turtas S, et al.: Long-term follow-up of the surgical treatment of intracranial coenurosis. Br J Neurosurg 4:39, 1990. *Recent review of treatment of this rare cestode infection.*

Pawlowski ZS: Cestodiases: Taeniasis, cysticercosis, diphyllobothriasis, hymenolepiasis and others. *In* Warren KS, Mahmoud AAF (eds.): Tropical and Geographical Medicine. 2nd ed. New York, McGraw-Hill, 1990, pp 490–504. *A detailed and current review of cestode infections (excluding Echinococcus species).*

Schantz PM, Okelo GBA: Echinococcosis (hydatidosis). *In* Warren KS, Mahmoud AAF (eds.): Tropical and Geographical Medicine. 2nd ed. New York, McGraw-Hill, 1990, pp 505–518. *Up-to-date review of human infection with Echinococcus species. Useful for hydatid disease as well as less common E. multilocularis and E. vogeli infections.*

Sotelo J, Escobedo F, Penagos P: Albendazole vs praziquantel for therapy for neurocysticercosis. A controlled trial. Arch Neurol 45:532, 1988. *A small head-to-head comparison of these two agents. Overall results were comparable (76 versus 73 per cent) for the two drugs in terms of cyst regression. A later study by the same group favors albendazole therapy, but flaws in study design make its analysis and conclusions unconvincing.*

Teitelbaum GP, Otto RJ, Lin M, et al.: MR imaging of neurocysticercosis. AJR 153:857, 1990. *Important description of a noninvasive modality for diagnosing parenchymal and ventricular neurocysticercosis.*

---

434 Schistosomiasis *(Bilharziasis)*

Adel A. F. Mahmoud

DEFINITION. Schistosomiasis, a chronic worm infection, affects more than 200 million people in the world; several hundred million more live in endemic areas and are at risk of exposure to the parasites. In view of its prevalence and the morbidity it causes, schistosomiasis ranks among the most important public health problems of tropical and subtropical areas. The schistosomes are blood flukes that parasitize the venous channels of the definitive human host; infection is transmitted via freshwater snails. Humans may be infected by one of five species: *Schistosoma haematobium*, *S. mansoni*, *S. japonicum*, *S. intercalatum*, or *S. mekongi*. Each species is endemic in specific geographic areas of the world; infection in humans may result in defined clinical syndromes. Other species that occasionally infect humans include *S. bovis*, *S. matthei*, and some avian schistosomes. In many parts of the world, enhanced agricultural productivity involving water conservation schemes is an economic necessity.

Inadvertently, these projects create ideal breeding places for the snail intermediate host, thus increasing prevalence of schistosomiasis in the population and possibly causing its spread to new areas. Currently, schistosomiasis is endemic in various areas of Africa, Asia, South America, and the Caribbean islands. In the United States, there are approximately 400,000 infected individuals; these include Puerto Ricans, and immigrants or travelers who have been exposed while in endemic areas. Because of the absence of susceptible snails, the life cycle of the schistosomes cannot be established in this country.

ETIOLOGY. The schistosomes differ from other trematodes that infect humans in having separate sexes. The species of schistosomes that infect humans share some common features, although they are morphologically distinctive. Each worm has two suckers (anterior and ventral), and the bifurcate intestinal ceca unite posteriorly. The larger male (0.6 to 2.2 cm × 2 to 4 mm) has a ventral gynecophoric canal in which the female is held during copulation. The slender female worm (1.2 to 2.6 cm × 1 to 2 mm) has a rounded body with pointed ends.

Adult schistosome worms parasitize defined sites of the venous vasculature of humans. *Schistosoma haematobium* worms inhabit the venous plexus around the lower end of the ureters and the urinary bladder, whereas *S. mansoni*, *S. japonicum*, *S. intercalatum*, and *S. mekongi* are located in the mesenteric veins. Sexual maturity of female worms requires the presence of living mature males; when ready to deposit eggs, the worms move against the bloodstream toward the small venous radicles. The female schistosomes deposit ova singly or in bunches, depending on the species of the parasite, and retreat in the direction of blood flow. Egg deposition has been estimated at 300 per day for female *S. haematobium* and *S. mansoni* worms and 3000 per day for *S. japonicum*. The ova of each species have characteristic morphologic features, which are of diagnostic importance. Once deposited in the host, eggs attempt to penetrate the venous capillaries and escape to the bladder or intestinal lumen; enzymatic secretions are thought to aid egg migration. The proportion of ova escaping from infected individuals varies in each species and also may depend on the extent of pathology and state of resistance in the host. Eggs that fail to reach the lumen of urinary tract or gut are trapped in these organs or may be carried by portal blood to the liver; these ova result in inflammatory and immunopathologic changes that are a major cause of disease in schistosomiasis.

The schistosome eggs, upon deposition by female worms, contain immature miracidia; they take approximately 10 to 12 days to develop while migrating through the host tissues. Once mature, miracidia have a mean lifespan of 11 to 12 days. Promiscuous urination and defecation by infected individuals result in dissemination of the parasite eggs in the environment. In fresh water the schistosome ova hatch within a few hours. Miracidia escape head first and swim, usually near the surface of water; they remain infective to the snail intermediate host for approximately 8 hours. On encountering the specific snail, the miracidia penetrate its tissues and undergo tremendous asexual multiplication and transformation into hundreds of cercariae. Schistosome infection of snails causes varying degrees of pathology in their liver and sexual organs and reduces their lifespan. Development of schistosomes inside the snail takes approximately 4 to 6 weeks, but it varies with the species of the parasite and mollusc and with changes in environmental conditions. Cercariae, the infective forms to humans, emerge from the snails under specific conditions of light and temperature; they are elongate with a pear-shaped body and a long forked tail and measure approximately 400 to 600 μm in length. They can survive in fresh water for almost 72 hours but lose their infectivity considerably within the first 24 hours. Cercariae attach to skin of mammalian hosts by their oral or ventral suckers. Burrowing of the skin is helped by vertical vibratory movements of their bodies and secretions of the cephalic penetration glands; the process is usually completed within a few minutes. During penetration, the cercariae shake off their tails and change into the next stage of the life cycle, the schistosomula, which lie in tunnels in the stratum corneum parallel to the skin surface. Schistosomula are covered by a heptalaminar membrane (instead of the trilaminar cercarial membrane) and can no longer survive in fresh water. They are thought to remain in the skin for 1 to 3 days before migrating to the lungs, finally reaching the liver in 2 to 4 weeks. In the intrahepatic portal system, the worms complete the major digestive and sexual stages of their development. Adult worms start their migration to their final habitat in 2 weeks and mate; viable eggs can be seen in the excreta 5 to 9 weeks after cercarial penetration.

The mean lifespan of adult schistosome worms inside the human host is not exactly known. Several individual case reports indicate that worms may live 20 to 30 years. This, however, represents extreme cases, as examination of infected individuals who migrate to nonendemic areas indicates that the mean lifespan of the worms is in the range of 3 to 10 years.

EPIDEMIOLOGY. The endemicity of schistosomiasis in any specific area is dependent upon the unsanitary disposal of urine and feces, the presence of suitable snail hosts, and human exposure to cercaria-infected bodies of water. Furthermore, the epidemiology of schistosomiasis is complex because of the existence of several stages of the life cycle of the parasite and the multitude of factors affecting each. Since adult schistosomes, like many parasitic worms, do not multiply in the human body, a close correlation obtains between worm load and fecal or urinary egg counts; estimates of intensity of infection can therefore be obtained by ova-enumerating procedures. Quantifying worm loads is important epidemiologically as well as for the individual patient, as it determines the potential of participation in transmission of schistosomiasis and predicts, to a large extent, the risk of morbidity and pathologic outcome.

In endemic areas, schistosomiasis prevalence and intensity show characteristic association with age. Schistosomiasis is acquired early in childhood; prevalence and intensity gradually increase to a peak in the second decade of life. In older individuals, a modest reduction of prevalence may be seen along with a sharp fall in intensity of infection. The marked drop in intensity in adults may be due to a decrease in their water-related activities. Development of immunity may also explain the age-related decrease in intensity. Intensity of infection in endemic communities shows another characteristic feature: Most infected individuals harbor low worm loads, and only a small proportion acquire heavy infection. The underlying mechanism of this clustering of heavy infection in schistosomiasis is not known but may be due to varying degrees of susceptibility and/or response of humans to the parasites.

Observations in endemic areas suggest that the schistosomiasis transmission rate is slow. Several ecologic as well as host factors help maintain this slow rate. For example, the prevalence of schistosomal infection in the snail intermediate host is usually low, ranging between 0.6 and 2 per cent. Cercarial dispersion in water bodies is considerable; cercariae appear in significant numbers only during certain hours of the day and lose their infectivity shortly thereafter. Once within the human host, no more than 40 per cent of cercariae mature into adult worms. In addition, attempts to measure incidence rates in endemic areas have confirmed the relatively slow rate of transmission, ranging from 2 to 4 per cent per year.

In some areas, the endemicity of schistosomiasis may be maintained by animal reservoirs; this is especially the case with *S. japonicum*, which infects dogs and cows. Although both *S. haematobium* and *S. mansoni* can infect primates and rodents, the role of these animals as reservoirs does not seem to be epidemiologically important.

PATHOGENESIS. Schistosomiasis is initiated by cercarial penetration of skin; inside the host three maturational forms of the parasite evolve: schistosomula, adults, and eggs. These stages are associated with morphologic, biochemical, and antigenic changes of the worm, which add to the complexity of the host-parasite relationship. Disease caused by schistosomiasis occurs mainly in those with high egg counts. This relationship, however, is not exact, as the roles of other factors such as genetic background and immunologic modulatory mechanisms are now being elucidated.

Three distinct disease syndromes caused by schistosomiasis have been described; each corresponds roughly to a stage in the parasite development in the host. Cercarial dermatitis, or swimmer's itch, may be seen in infections with human schistosomes but is more common when avian or other nonhuman cercariae penetrate the skin. Swimmer's itch caused by nonhuman schistosomes is commonly seen in the North Central United States, where some lakes are infected. The condition has also been reported in subjects exposed to *S. mansoni* or *S. haematobium* but rarely after exposure to *S. japonicum*. Primary exposure to these larvae results in either no reaction or immediate pruritic macular rash. On repeated exposures, sensitization occurs, and a more pronounced papular eruption develops with erythema, edema, and pruritus. Histopathologically, edema, round cell infiltrate, and eosinophilia can be seen in the dermis and epidermis. Although the mechanism of this reaction is not known, it is probably due to the host response to dying larvae and the subsequent development of humoral and cellular immunity.

Acute schistosomiasis, or Katayama fever, is a serum sickness–like syndrome that occurs 3 to 9 weeks after infection. This period coincides with the onset of egg production and its associated increase in antigenic challenge to the host. Clinically significant acute schistosomiasis occurs more often with *S. japonicum* infections but has also been reported with the other species. It is seen in previously unexposed individuals; the severity of symptoms and signs correlates with intensity of infection. Very little is known of the mechanism of this syndrome; it manifests itself as fever, abdominal pain, and headache with hepatosplenomegaly and eosinophilia. Elevations of serum immunoglobulin (Ig)G, IgM, IgE, and specific antischistosomal antibodies have also been observed, leading to the suggestion that the syndrome is a form of immune complex disease.

The basic pathologic lesion in chronic schistosomiasis is the egg granuloma. Although the schistosomes do not multiply in the definitive host, they continually produce eggs; some of these are trapped in the tissues. Enzymes and antigens are subsequently released from the eggs to facilitate their migration out of the body. These parasite products sensitize the host lymphocytes, which migrate to areas of egg deposition and recruit other cells through the secretion of lymphokines, and a compact cellular infiltrate "granuloma" is formed. Several cell types are prominent in the schistosome egg granuloma: lymphocytes, macrophages, eosinophils, and fibroblasts. The size of these granulomas and the resulting fibrosis lead to most of the chronic fibro-obstructive lesions in schistosomiasis. In *S. haematobium* infection, granulomas at the lower end of the ureters impede urine flow and cause hydroureter and hydronephrosis. In infections with other schistosome species, granulomas in the intestinal wall are associated with the abdominal manifestations of the disease, and those in the liver result in presinusoidal obstruction of portal blood flow, portal hypertension, splenomegaly, and esophageal varices. Less commonly, eggs may be carried to almost any organ or tissue in the body, eliciting granuloma formation and its pathologic sequelae. The size of the granulomatous response represents a delicate balance between sensitizing and modulating mechanisms. In chronic schistosomiasis, granulomas spontaneously modulate—i.e., their size decreases significantly—which may result in slowing the progression of disease manifestations. Modulation has been shown to be mediated by several arms of the host's immune system, including serum antibodies, anti-idiotypic antibodies, immune complexes, suppressor lymphocytes, and macrophages. Functionally, granulomas serve to destroy the parasite eggs. Among the cells constituting the granulomatous response, eosinophils play a key role in egg destruction.

The immune response of individuals with schistosomiasis includes humoral as well as cellular components. The degree and extent of these responses provide the balance between asymptomatic infection and disease manifestations. Furthermore, mechanisms that control the host immune response, such as genetic background, have been demonstrated to influence the extent of granuloma formation and consequently disease. The host immune response to schistosome antigens also is inversely related to intensity of infection; impaired responses are seen only in those with heavy worm loads. Whether the defect in immunity is a cause or consequence of infection is not yet clear. Another aspect of the host's immune response in schistosomiasis relates to the development of peripheral blood as well as tissue eosinophilia. Schistosomiasis, similar to other worm infections with tissue phases, results in a significant increase of peripheral blood eosinophils, especially during the acute phase of infection. Later, in the chronic stage, the eosinophil count may not be significantly elevated. Eosinophils are seen in subcutaneous tissues around the entry points of cercariae, and they constitute approximately 50 per cent of the cells in egg granulomas. Eosinophils have been shown to play a central role in host defenses against the invading

stage of the parasite (schistosomula) and the phase (ova) retained in the tissues.

Acquired immunity to schistosomiasis may explain the drop in intensity of infection observed in older individuals in endemic areas. This phenomenon may be explained equally by the differences in patterns of contact with infected waters and by changes in the rate of egg production by adult worms. Studies in vitro have demonstrated that several human cells—eosinophils, neutrophils, basophils, monocytes, cytotoxic T lymphocytes and platelets—may alone or in combination with complement components or antischistosomal antibodies damage the larvae of the parasite. The biologic relevance of these observations in humans is not yet clear.

MANAGEMENT. Diagnosis of schistosomiasis must be based on the clinical presentation, positive geographic history, and finding the parasite eggs in the excreta or biopsy material. Quantification of infection and assessment of viability of the eggs are important procedures not only for planning therapy but also for prognostic evaluation. For physicians practicing in nonendemic areas, e.g., North America, most infected individuals present with the early acute and nonspecific features of the infection. Eosinophilia and serologic evidence of exposure to schistosome infection are two particularly helpful laboratory findings. Safe chemotherapeutic antischistosomal agents are now available and provide high cure rates (e.g., praziquantel). Appropriate management of individuals with schistosomiasis must take into consideration the extent of disease and intensity of infection. Antischistosomal therapy, if given early during the course of disease, may lead to reversal of pathologic lesions. In late cases, chemotherapeutic measures may be useful only in preventing further damage from the presence of the parasite.

CONTROL. The intimate relationship between humans and bodies of fresh water in their environment leads to schistosomiasis endemicity. In addition, the lack of precise knowledge of the epidemiology of infection and disease has hampered efforts for its control. Several developments, such as single-dose oral chemotherapeutic agents and better appreciation of transmission dynamics, have led to a clearer definition of strategies for control of schistosomiasis. Ideally, eradication of infection should be the target, but this is impossible to achieve with the currently available tools and the economic and social structure of the endemic areas. Research toward antischistosome vaccine is progressing, but not to the extent of contemplating human trials soon. A more realistic approach is based on control of disease and reduction of transmission. The most cost-effective measure currently advocated is targeted chemotherapy, combined with focal mollusciciding if needed. Because of the specific features of infection dynamics, treated individuals persist with low egg counts for a few years. In addition, health education, attempts at raising socioeconomic standards, providing privies, and abandoning obsolete agricultural practices offer means for achieving progress in containing this infection.

Those traveling to endemic areas should be given proper advice. There are virtually no safe freshwater bodies in most of the areas endemic for schistosomiasis. Avoiding contact with these water sources is strongly recommended.

Capron A, Dessaint JP, Capron M, et al.: Immunity to schistosomes. Progress toward vaccine. Science 238:1065, 1987. *A detailed description of evidence in vitro and components of protective effector mechanisms against schistosomiasis.*

Chapman PJ, Wilkinson PR, Davidson RN: Acute schistosomiasis (Katayama fever) among British air crew. Br Med J 297:1101, 1988. *A description of the acute clinical, parasitologic, and laboratory findings in 10 British subjects who swam in fresh water in Ghana. The article emphasizes the nonspecific nature of the clinical presentation. Peripheral blood eosinophilia and enzyme-linked immunosorbent assay (ELISA) were most helpful in establishing the diagnosis.*

King CH, Mahmoud AAF: Drugs five years later: Praziquantel. Ann Intern Med 110:290, 1989. *A review of the clinical applications of praziquantel as a safe, oral, broad-spectrum antihelminth.*

Mahmoud AAF (ed.): Clinical Tropical Medicine and Communicable Diseases. Vol. 2: Schistosomiasis. London, Bailliere's Tindall, 1987. *A concise review of the biology, immunology, and clinical features of human schistosomiasis written by physicians and scientists.*

Mahmoud AAF: Strategies for vaccine development: Schistosomiasis. Ann NY Acad Sci 589:136, 1989. *A summary of the available protective monoclonal antibodies and purified schistosome antigens with promise as vaccines.*

Mahmoud AAF, Arap Siongok TK, Ouma J, et al.: Effect of targeted mass treatment on intensity of infection and morbidity in schistosomiasis mansoni. Lancet

1:849, 1983. *Evaluation of the clinical and parasitologic effects of targeting chemotherapy to those with hepatosplenomegaly and heavy infection.*

Mahmoud AAF, Warren KS, Peters PA: A role for the eosinophil in acquired resistance to *Schistosoma mansoni* infection as determined by antieosinophil serum. J Exp Med 142:805, 1975. *Demonstration of the in vivo protective function of eosinophils in animals with schistosomiasis.*

World Health Organization: Atlas of the Global Distribution of Schistosomiasis. Geneva, World Health Organization, Parasitic Diseases Programme, 1987. *Detailed information on the geographic distribution of the different schistosome infections in humans.*

World Health Organization: The Control of Schistosomiasis. Technical Report Series 728, pp 1–113, World Health Organization, Geneva, Switzerland, 1985. *An up-to-date examination of the epidemiology, morbidity, and methods of control of schistosomiasis. The report also includes a summary of control programs in endemic areas and an outline for a strategy of morbidity control.*

SCHISTOSOMIASIS HAEMATOBIA (Urinary Bilharziasis)

S. haematobium infection is endemic in Africa and some parts of the Middle East; it is highly prevalent in the Nile Valley and extends along the Mediterranean coast of the continent. In West Africa it is more widely disseminated than *S. mansoni*; its distribution in East and South Africa is patchy. In Southwest Asia the endemic area includes most countries of the Middle East and Arabian peninsula. Clinically, infection with *S. haematobium* is the most significant of the human schistosome infections because symptoms such as hematuria and dysuria occur early and affect approximately two thirds of infected individuals. In endemic areas, extensive hydroureter and hydronephrosis can be demonstrated in a considerable proportion of infected children; the natural history of these lesions and the course of disease in adults have not been clearly defined.

Adult male *S. haematobium* worms are distinguished by their finely tuberculate surface and by the presence of four to five large testes. The ovaries are found in the posterior half of the female body and contain 20 to 30 eggs. Mature *S. haematobium* eggs measure approximately 143×50 μm and are spindle shaped with a rounded anterior end and a conical posterior end that tapers to a terminal delicate spine. Eggs are mainly found in urine of infected individuals but may occasionally be seen in stools or rectal biopsy material. The main intermediate hosts of *S. haematobium* in North Africa and the Middle East are freshwater snails of the genus *Bulinus*; in Africa south of the Sahara they belong to the subgenus *Physopsis*.

PATHOLOGY AND CLINICAL MANIFESTATIONS. In the urinary bladder, the formation of egg granulomas leads to hyperemia, tubercles, ulcers, and polyps; as healing proceeds, sandy patches and scarring may be seen. Obstructive uropathy is the main functional disturbance caused by schistosomiasis haematobia. Other urinary tract disorders, such as bacteriuria, calculi, and bladder cancer, have been epidemiologically associated with *S. haematobium* infection, but no causal relationship has yet been confirmed. Ova of *S. haematobium* have occasionally been found in the lungs with subsequent focal pulmonary arteritis and diffuse hypertensive arteriolar changes; chronic cor pulmonale may occur in these patients.

Swimmer's itch and acute schistosomiasis have rarely been described in *S. haematobium* infection. By contrast, symptoms related to the urinary tract, including dysuria, hematuria, or frequency, occur in a large proportion of infected individuals. Hematuria is characteristically terminal, but with extensive ulceration the whole stream of urine may be bloody, along with passage of clots. In late cases, symptoms related to secondary infection of the urinary tract, severe obstructive uropathy, or neoplasia may appear. Urine examination reveals proteinuria and hematuria; both signs are closely related to intensity of infection. An association between *S. haematobium* infection and bacteremia, mainly caused by *Salmonella* organisms, has been reported. Renal function may be compromised in patients with obstructive uropathy. Cytoscopic examination shows some degree of pathology in almost all infected individuals, the most common being hyperemia near the ureteral openings and the bladder trigone. Sandy patches, tubercles, ulcers, and polyps are less frequently seen. Radiographically, bladder calcification is a characteristic feature of urinary schistosomiasis; it is found in approximately 50 to 80 per cent of infected individuals. Other pathologic lesions are also frequently seen in 40 to 60 per cent of patients, including obstructive uropathy, hydroureter, hydronephrosis, and filling defects in the bladder and ureters. Ultrasonographic examination of the urinary tract confirms the bladder lesions and their obstructive sequelae.

DIAGNOSIS. Urine examination for *S. haematobium* eggs can be performed by direct or concentration methods. Excretion of the parasite eggs is maximal around mid-day, when samples should optimally be obtained. Diagnosis and quantification of infection can be achieved by filtering 10 ml of urine through a Nuclepore membrane. Examination of more than one urine sample may be necessary to establish the diagnosis; rectal biopsy may be done in suspected cases with negative urine results. Serology may be needed to diagnose early or light infection. Once *S. haematobium* infection is diagnosed, assessment of urinary tract pathology by ultrasonography is recommended. In addition, care must be taken in some endemic areas for early detection of bladder cancer by appropriate cytologic and histologic examinations.

TREATMENT. See Management of Schistosomiasis, below.

King CH, Lombardi G, Lombardi C, et al.: Chemotherapy based control of schistosomiasis haematobia. II. Metrifonate vs. praziquantel control of infection associated morbidity. Am J Trop Med Hyg 42:587, 1990. *The article presents data on long-term effects of metrifonate and praziquantel on the clinical as well as ultrasonographic manifestations of* S. haematobium *infection in school-aged children.*

Mott KE, Dixon H, Osei-Tutu E, et al.: Relation between intensity of *Schistosoma haematobium* infection and clinical hematuria and proteinuria. Lancet 1:1005, 1983. *Correlation of proteinuria and hematuria with counts of* S. haematobium *eggs in urine.*

Warren KS, Mahmoud AAF, Muruka JF, et al.: Schistosomiasis haematobia in Coast Province, Kenya. Am J Trop Med Hyg 28:864, 1979. *Correlation of morbidity, with egg counts in schistosomiasis haematobia; even in lightly infected children disease manifestations are significant.*

Wilkins A, Gilles H: Schistosomiasis haematobia. *In* Mahmoud AAF (ed.): Clinical Tropical Medicine and Communicable Diseases. Vol. 2: Schistosomiasis. London, Bailliere's Tindall, 1987, pp 333–348. *A comprehensive review of the epidemiology, pathology, and clinical features of schistosomiasis haematobia based on wide experience in Africa.*

SCHISTOSOMIASIS MANSONI (Intestinal or Hepatosplenic Bilharziasis)

Infection with *S. mansoni* is endemic in Africa, the Middle East, South America, and some Caribbean islands. The distribution of schistosomiasis mansoni in Africa overlaps with that of schistosomiasis haematobia. In Southwest Asia, it occurs in Yemen and Saudi Arabia. *S. mansoni* is sporadically distributed all over the northern part of South America and is endemic in several Caribbean countries and islands and in many parts of Puerto Rico.

Adult male *S. mansoni* worms have a grossly tuberculate surface and usually contain seven small testes. In the female, the ovary occupies the anterior half of its body, with a short uterus containing one to four ova. Mature eggs measure 155×66 μm and are oval with a lateral, long spine. The intermediate snail hosts of *S. mansoni* are species of the genus *Biomphalaria* in Africa and *Australorbis tropicorbis* in the Americas.

PATHOLOGY AND CLINICAL MANIFESTATIONS. Acute schistosomiasis mansoni is the most common early presentation encountered by physicians in North America. Symptoms appear between 3 and 7 weeks after exposure and include fever, anorexia, abdominal pain, and headache. Less often, diarrhea, nausea, and vomiting may occur. Hepatosplenomegaly, eosinophilia, and increased serum immunoglobulins are the main clinical signs. Most of these manifestations correlate significantly with intensity of infection as evaluated by stool egg counts.

Schistosoma mansoni eggs are primarily deposited in the small veins around the large intestine; some of the eggs may be trapped in the gut wall or break loose into the portal circulation to be carried to the small intrahepatic portal venules. On examination, the intestinal mucosa appears red and granular with pinpoint elevations surrounded by hyperemic zones. There may be minute hemorrhages and ulcerations. Sessile and pedunculated polyps, mainly in the rectosigmoid area, have been reported in Egyptians infected with *S. mansoni*, but not in persons from other endemic areas. Pathologic examination of the liver in lightly infected individuals shows schistosome eggs with and without granulomas and mild portal inflammation. In advanced cases, the typical picture of Symmers' fibrosis is seen; the eggs are concentrated in and around large portal tracts with marked fibrosis and obstructive portal venous lesions. The lobular arrangement of liver parenchyma and its function are usually maintained. However, these structural changes lead to marked alteration of hepatic hemodynamics, such as obstruction of portal blood flow through the liver and increase in number and size of intrahepatic arterial branches, thus shifting the blood flow through the liver from mainly portal to arterial sources. Portal hypertension leads to congestive splenomegaly and formation of portosystemic venous shunts at the lower end of the esophagus and other sites. In these patients, schistosome eggs may find their way to the pulmonary circulation, bypassing the obstructed portal blood flow. In the lungs, granulomas form around the trapped eggs, leading to arteriolar fibrosis and pulmonary hypertension.

Nervous system involvement in schistosomiasis mansoni is rare; the main clinical presentation, as in schistosomiasis haematobia, is transverse myelitis. The preferential involvement of the spinal cord may be due to the anatomic location of adult worms. The underlying pathologic lesions are usually granulomas forming around eggs in the spinal cord.

Infection with *S. mansoni* does not have characteristic or specific symptomatology. Early symptoms of acute schistosomiasis, as described earlier, are all nonspecific in nature. This is particularly the case in travelers who are accidentally exposed to infection in endemic areas. In chronic schistosomiasis mansoni, infected individuals have a slightly higher incidence of crampy abdominal pain (21 to 48 per cent) and bloody diarrhea (4 to 28 per cent) than do matched uninfected controls from the same endemic area. Other frequently mentioned nonspecific symptoms and signs, such as weakness, inability to work, or diarrhea, have not been convincingly demonstrated in any controlled studies. Significant enlargement of the liver is seen in 4 to 11 per cent of infected subjects, and splenomegaly occurs in 3 to 7 per cent. Patients with schistosomal hepatosplenomegaly present with a unique form of liver disease. The pathophysiologic changes are based on alteration of hemodynamics, fibrosis of large portal tracts, and very little derangement of liver function. Enlargement of the liver usually occurs in the left lobe, but later, in the course of infection and particularly in adults, uniform hepatomegaly may be seen. Ultrasonographic examination of the liver shows evidence of specific patterns of fibrosis, which distinguishes this syndrome from other causes of hepatomegaly. Simultaneously, gross enlargement of the spleen may occur; the organ is characteristically rubbery hard. Laboratory examination may show indications of anemia and a low degree of eosinophilia but no changes in liver function test results until late in the course of disease. Total serum proteins are usually normal, but gamma globulin increases are common. An association between schistosomal hepatosplenomegaly and hepatitis B antigen and antibody presence has been described, but its pathophysiologic significance is not clear. Although hepatosplenomegaly usually occurs in heavily infected individuals, other underlying mechanisms may be involved. An association between human leukocyte antigen (HLA) haplotypes and schistosomal hepatosplenomegaly has been demonstrated. In patients with pure schistosomal fibrosis uncomplicated by cirrhosis or viral hepatitis, liver function is preserved for a long time. These individuals often present clinically with an episode of hematemesis caused by rupture of esophageal varices without prior complaints. Bleeding may recur several times while the liver parenchyma maintains its normal functions. Finally, however, symptoms and signs of liver cell failure ensue, along with the development of stigmata of chronic liver disease and ascites.

Several less defined clinical syndromes have been associated with schistosomiasis mansoni. Formation of antigen-antibody complexes and their deposition in the kidney glomeruli have been demonstrated in infected laboratory animals as well as in individuals with chronic schistosomiasis mansoni. However, the prevalence of this syndrome and the rate at which it occurs in schistosomiasis are unknown, since proteinuria and nephrotic syndrome are not particularly prevalent in schistosomiasis-endemic areas. Cor pulmonale in schistosomiasis is a better defined disease entity, although its incidence is not known. It usually occurs in patients with advanced hepatosplenic schistosomiasis mansoni or japonica because of the development of collateral circulation. In *S. haematobium*–infected individuals, the anatomic location of adult worms may help eggs reach the systemic circulation directly and become trapped in the pulmonary arterioles. Patients with schistosomal pulmonary hypertension present clinically with symptoms and signs similar to those in cor pulmonale of other causes. Aneurysmal dilation of the pulmonary artery and its branches, along with right ventricular hypertrophy, may occur.

DIAGNOSIS. Stool examination for the characteristic *S. mansoni* eggs is the definitive diagnostic procedure. Because assessing intensity of infection is essential, quantitative techniques are recommended. The Kato thick smear method involves examination of sieved 50-mg stool samples placed on glass slides and spead under a cellophane cover slip presoaked in 50 per cent glycerol. The slides should be left at least 24 hours to allow for clearing of fecal material; the embryo within the ovum also clears, but the characteristic shape of the eggshell is retained. Rectal biopsy or serologic testing may be used for diagnosis of stool-negative cases, particularly in lightly infected individuals.

TREATMENT. See Management of Schistosomiasis, below.

Abdel-Salam E, Abdel Khalik A, Abdel-Meguid A, et al.: Association of HLA class I antigens (A1, B5, B8, and CW2) with disease manifestations and infection in human schistosomiasis mansoni in Egypt. Tissue Antigens 27:142, 1986. *A large-scale, population-based study of association between certain HLA haplotypes and hepatosplenomegaly due to schistosomiasis mansoni.*

Mahmoud AAF, Abdel Wahab MF: Schistosomiasis. *In* Warren KS, Mahmoud AAF (eds.): Tropical and Geographical Medicine. 2nd ed. New York, McGraw-Hill, 1990, pp 458–473. *Detailed description of the clinical manifestations of S. mansoni infection and its characteristic features in ultrasonographic examination of the liver.*

Prata A: Schistosomiasis mansoni in Brazil. *In* Mahmoud AAF (ed.): Clinical Tropical Medicine and Communicable Diseases. Vol. 2: Schistosomiasis. London, Bailliere's Tindall, 1987, pp 349–369. *A review of the clinical features as seen in an endemic area, with emphasis on diagnostic methods.*

SCHISTOSOMIASIS JAPONICA

On the main Asian continent, schistosomiasis japonica is prevalent in some parts of China, Thailand, Laos, Cambodia, and Malaysia. It is also endemic in Taiwan, Japan, the Philippines, and Celebes. This schistosome species characteristically infects humans and domestic animals such as cats, dogs, and cattle, thus providing reservoir hosts that may contribute to its endemicity in certain areas of the Far East.

Adult *S. japonicum* male worms have a nontuberculate surface and seven medium-sized testes. The ovary occupies the middle part of the body of female worms and contains 50 to 100 ova. *S. japonicum* eggs are found in stools of infected individuals; they measure 89 × 67 μm and are oval or rounded with a lateral short, sometimes curved spine. The intermediate hosts for *S. japonicum* are snails of the genus *Oncomelania*.

PATHOLOGY AND CLINICAL MANIFESTATIONS. Cercarial dermatitis is not a prominent feature of schistosomiasis japonica. Katayama fever, or acute schistosomiasis, was named after the district in Japan endemic for *S. japonicum* infections. Symptoms usually begin 5 to 7 weeks after infection and are similar to those associated with schistosomiasis mansoni. The clinical features usually subside in a few days but may last for several months, and fatalities have been reported. The chronic manifestations of schistosomiasis japonica are related to ova deposited in the intestines and liver; adult worms produce 10 times more eggs than those of *S. mansoni*. These ova are laid in aggregates and remain so in the intestinal wall or when carried to the liver by the portal blood flow. In addition, *S. japonicum* eggs differ from those of *S. mansoni* in their tendency to calcify in tissues. Schistosomiasis japonica granulomas vary in size tremendously and tend to show signs of necrosis.

Individuals with chronic schistosomiasis japonica may present with no symptoms or several nonspecific complaints. Controlled surveys in endemic areas have shown no particular increase in complaints of weakness, abdominal pain, or diarrhea in infected individuals. Clinical signs of hepatosplenomegaly are more frequently seen in infected than in uninfected individuals, but they are not uniformly correlated with intensity of infection. Severe hepatosplenic disease caused by schistosomiasis japonica may be seen in endemic areas, but its prevalence and relationship to intensity of infection and other complicating factors are unknown.

Cerebral schistosomiasis japonica is a unique syndrome reportedly occurring in 2 to 4 per cent of infected individuals in the endemic countries. *S. japonicum* infection of the central nervous system preferentially affects the brain. The lesions consist of large aggregates of eggs in the cerebral venous system, but adult worms have never been found in the brain. Cerebral schistosomiasis japonica presents clinically early in the course of the infection; the most frequent manifestation is focal jacksonian epilepsy; less commonly, generalized encephalitis may be the presenting feature.

DIAGNOSIS. Stool examination for S. japonicum eggs is the only reliable diagnostic procedure. The Kato thick smear technique provides both diagnosis and quantitative assessment of infection. Rectal biopsy or serologic testing may be used in individuals with light infections, particularly when a less common manifestation, such as cerebral schistosomiasis, is encountered.

TREATMENT. See Management of Schistosomiasis, below.

Olveda RM, Domingo EO: Schistosomiasis japonica. In Mahmoud AAF (ed.): Clinical Tropical Medicine and Communicable Diseases. Vol. 2: Schistosomiasis. London, Bailliere's Tindall, 1987, pp 397–417. *Description of epidemiology, clinical features, and diagnostic methods. The article is based on wide experience with schistosomiasis japonica in the Philippines.*

Warren KS, Su DL, Xu CY, et al.: Morbidity in schistosomiasis japonica in relation to intensity of infection; study of 2 royal brigades in Anhui Province, China. N Engl J Med, 309:1533, 1983.

OTHER HUMAN SCHISTOSOMES

Endemic foci for S. intercalatum are found in Central and West Africa. Adult worms inhabit the mesenteric blood vessels, and terminal spine eggs are seen in stools of infected individuals. Symptoms usually ascribed to this species of schistosome include abdominal pain, diarrhea, and blood in stools. Diagnosis is based on positive geographic history and finding parasite ova upon fecal examination.

S. mekongi is the most recent schistosome species to be described as a cause of infection and disease in humans. The parasite is endemic in some parts of the mainland of Southeast Asia. Adult worm and eggs are similar to those of S. japonicum; ova of S. mekongi are, however, smaller. In symptomatic patients, a syndrome not unlike that due to S. japonicum has been observed. It includes abdominal pain, diarrhea, and heptosplenomegaly. Diagnosis is established by fecal examination for parasite ova.

Hofstetter M, Nash TE, Cheever AW, et al.: Infection with *Schistosoma mekongi* in Southeast Asian refugees. J Infect Dis 144:420, 1981. *Description of clinical and parasitologic features of schistosomiasis mekongi.*

MANAGEMENT OF SCHISTOSOMIASIS

Chemotherapy is the major antischistosome strategy for eradication of parasites in infected individuals and for reducing incidence, intensity, and morbidity in populations of endemic areas. The current drug of choice is praziquantel, a pyrazinoisoquinoline derivative that is effective against all species of schistosomes that infect humans. Praziquantel has several advantages as the chemotherapeutic agent of choice, including oral administration, low incidence of toxicity and side effects, and marked antiparasitic activity. The recommended dose of praziquantel for treatment of infections with S. haematobium, S. intercalatum, or S. mansoni is 40 mg per kilogram of body weight administered once. For S. japonicum infection, it is recommended to administer 30 mg per kilogram twice in 1 day, and for S. mekongi, 20 mg per kilogram three times in one day. These dosages have been shown to result in parasitologic cure in approximately 80 per cent of treated individuals and in a highly significant reduction of intensity of infection. Side effects of praziquantel are rare, usually mild, and self-limiting. These include abdominal pain, headache, dizziness, and skin rashes.

The effect of antischistosome chemotherapeutic agents on disease manifestations is variable. It is dependent on the duration of infection and extent of disease. Treatment is expected to result in reversal of pathology, e.g., hematuria and hepatosplenomegaly, in infected children. By contrast, adults with established fibro-obstructive disease in the liver and urinary tract may not show significant clinical improvement following chemotherapy. Other therapeutic or surgical methods may therefore be necessary to correct the anatomic lesions. Furthermore, medical management of the chronic sequelae of schistosomiasis, such as liver fibrosis, portal hypertension, and esophageal varices, should be conducted according to established practices and taking into consideration

the unique pathophysiologic characteristics of disease due to schistosomiasis.

Mahmoud AAF: Praziquantel for the treatment of helminthic infections. Adv Intern Med 32:193, 1987. *A summary of the known anthelminthic effects of praziquantel in experimental animals and humans.*

435 Hermaphroditic Flukes

S. K. K. Seah

The hermaphroditic flukes are unlike the *Schistosoma* flukes in that they have male and female organs in the same worm and self-fertilize. The ones that are of medical importance are (1) flukes that parasitize the biliary tract, i.e., *Clonorchis sinensis, Opisthorchis viverrini, Opisthorchis felineus, Fasciola hepatica, Dicrocoelium dendriticum,* and *Metorchis conjunctus;* (2) flukes that parasitize the intestinal lumen, i.e., *Fasciolopsis buski, Heterophyes heterophyes, Echinostoma ilocanum, Gastrodiscoides hominis,* and *Metagonimus yokogawai;* (3) flukes that parasitize the lung, i.e., *Paragonimus westermani* and other species; and (4) the mesocercarial stage of *Alaria americana,* which causes generalized systemic infection.

The more important of these flukes, such as *Clonorchis* and *Opisthorchis,* affect many millions of people in Asia and Eastern Europe. All of these flukes parasitize other mammals, and some of them, such as *Fasciola hepatica,* are of major importance in veterinary medicine. Although most of these flukes have limited geographic distribution, with the migration of people around the world, human infections are often seen in nonendemic areas.

The hermaphroditic flukes are leaflike, nonsegmented, and bilaterally symmetric, ranging in size from a few millimeters to several centimeters. On one end is the anterior or oral sucker, and just behind it is the ventral sucker or acetabulum. The acetabulum acts as a holdfast to the epithelial tissue of the final host.

Eggs appear in bile and stool or, in the case of the lung fluke, in sputum and stool. The eggs are operculated. Some are fully embryonated when passed; others may require time for embryonation. The embryonated egg contains the first-stage larva, or miracidium. After hatching in fresh water, the miracidium penetrates, or is ingested by, a suitable first intermediate host, a snail. In the snail, the miracidium develops into thousands of cercariae, which are released into the water. The cercariae attach themselves to or penetrate the second intermediate hosts, which, depending on the flukes, may be freshwater fish, crustaceans, frogs, or aquatic plants. The final definitive hosts (humans or animals) acquire the infection by ingesting encysted metacercariae.

Infection by digenetic or hermaphroditic trematodes is treated by the broad-spectrum anthelminthic praziquantel. Personal prevention of infection includes eating only well-cooked fish or crustaceans and avoiding raw watercress in endemic areas. Community prevention consists of cleaning up the environment and preventing infection of the intermediate hosts.

Seah SKK: Digenetic trematodes. Clin Gastroenterol 7:98, 1978. *A good review of all the hermaphroditic flukes.*

HEPATIC HERMAPHRODITIC FLUKES

Clonorchiasis (*Clonorchis sinensis*)

This infection is very common in the Far East, especially southern China, Taiwan, Hong Kong, Japan, and Korea, where raw or undercooked fish has long been considered a delicacy. *Opisthorchis* is almost identical to *Clonorchis* in its morphology, epidemiology, and clinical manifestations. Opisthorchiasis is very common in Thailand, Laos, the Philippines, and Eastern Europe. In some areas, virtually the whole population is infected. Even infants are infected, as they are fed chopped raw fish as a dietary supplement. More than 40 species of freshwater fish, mainly the carp and salmon group, harbor metacercariae.

Clonorchis sinensis has a very long lifespan (probably up to 50 years), and this parasitic infection will likely remain important in endemic areas for many years. Clonorchiasis occurs in all parts of the world where there are Asian immigrants. Many hundreds of thousands of Southeast Asian refugees and other Asian immigrants have come to North America in recent years, and surveys show that a large percentage of these have asymptomatic liver fluke infection.

After the contaminated fish is ingested, the metacercariae excyst in the duodenum. Most of the larval flukes ascend the biliary tree directly, but some may pass via the portal circulation to the liver. During maturation of the fluke, marked desquamation of the biliary epithelium takes place. The fluke matures in 2 to 3 weeks and begins to lay eggs. Flukes prefer to reside in the second-order bile ducts, but in heavy infection they are found throughout the biliary system, including the gallbladder, and sometimes in the pancreatic duct. Adult flukes are grayish-brown and 15 mm by 3 mm. They feed on secretions of the bile duct mucosa. They cause low-grade inflammatory changes in the biliary tree, proliferation of the biliary epithelium, and progressive portal fibrosis. As a rule, there is no parenchymal damage, and cirrhosis does not result from uncomplicated clonorchiasis.

CLINICAL MANIFESTATIONS. Acute clonorchiasis occurs 1 to 3 weeks after the ingestion of encysted metacercariae. The condition is only rarely diagnosed and is a flulike illness. Fever, chills, abdominal pain, diarrhea, tender hepatomegaly, and mild jaundice may be present. The white cell count is elevated, and there is marked eosinophilia. The serum alkaline phosphatase, aspartate aminotransferase (AST) (SGOT), alanine aminotransferase (ALT) (SGPT), and bilirubin levels are elevated. The clinical presentation is often confused with acute viral hepatitis, which is even more common in these tropical endemic areas. Acute clonorchiasis is therefore rarely recognized. The ova of *C. sinensis* appear in the stool or bile 3 or 4 weeks after ingestion of the metacercariae. The history of eating raw fish in the endemic area and the eosinophilia should suggest the diagnosis.

The majority of people with the ova of *C. sinensis* in their stool have no symptoms even when heavily infected. It is impossible to predict who will develop the complications of chronic clonorchiasis. A small percentage of infected individuals will develop the symptoms of chronic clonorchiasis, which include inflammation, infection, stones, obstruction, and neoplastic changes in the biliary tree. Acute suppurative cholangitis is a serious febrile illness often associated with hypoglycemia and *Escherichia coli* bacteremia. The biliary system is blocked by numerous flukes and becomes secondarily infected. The condition carries a high mortality rate. Recurrent pyogenic cholangitis is a recurrent febrile illness associated with clonorchiasis and intrahepatic bile duct calculi. During surgical operation or autopsy, *Clonorchis* flukes are not consistently found, as in the case of acute suppurative cholangitis. With recurrent pyogenic cholangitis, cirrhosis may eventually develop. The flukes occasionally block the pancreatic ducts and induce pancreatitis. Cholangiocarcinoma is a late complication of chronic clonorchiasis. Clonorchiasis has no causal relation to hepatocellular cancer.

DIAGNOSIS. The diagnosis is made by finding the characteristic light bulb–shaped, operculated eggs in the stool or duodenal aspirate. The eggs average 29 μm by 16 μm. Unfortunately, the *C. sinensis* egg is almost identical to those of *Opisthorcis, Heterophyes,* and *Metagonimus.* To be absolutely certain of the diagnosis, one must examine the adult fluke. However, geographic distribution may help in separating *Clonorchis* from *Opisthorcis.* In a patient with abdominal or other symptoms and *C. sinensis* eggs in the stool, it is often difficult to decide if the complaint is due to clonorchiasis. It is often necessary to eliminate other current illnesses before attributing the symptoms to clonorchiasis. As a rule, in uncomplicated established clonorchiasis, there is no eosinophilia, elevation of sedimentation rate, anemia, or abnormal liver function test results, and radioisotope scan and ultrasonography (B scan) of the liver are normal.

In acute clonorchiasis, leukocytosis, marked eosinophilia, and abnormal liver function test results are present. This condition must be distinguished from hepatic amebiasis and visceral larva migrans. In the former, eosinophilia is absent and serology for amebiasis is positive. In the latter, the serology for toxocariasis is positive. The presence of the flukes provokes irregular antibody response, and a large variety of serologic and skin tests are available in some centers. However, these are not sufficiently specific and sensitive for clinical use.

TREATMENT. Praziquantel has revolutionized the treatment of this condition. The recommended dose is 75 mg per kilogram of body weight, divided in three doses on the same day (this dose of praziquantel exceeds the manufacturer's recommendation). This drug is very well tolerated, and no long-term toxicity has been shown. At the dose recommended, some gastrointestinal disturbance and transient headaches may occur. Because this drug is safe, it is recommended that all cases of clonorchiasis, symptomatic or not, be treated. The cure rate of a single-day treatment is almost 100 per cent. Stool should be checked for ova of the fluke 1 month, 6 months, and 1 year after treatment. Retreatment may be necessary. In parts of the endemic areas, mass treatment is showing encouraging results by reducing the prevalence of this infection.

The treatment of complications such as calculi, suppurative cholangitis, recurrent pyogenic cholangitis, and pancreatitis is both medical and surgical. Conservative treatment consists of broad-spectrum antibiotics and intravenous fluids. If this is not effective, a permanent and adequate drainage procedure, such as choledochoduodenostomy, is required. A course of praziquantel should be given when the patient is able to swallow the tablets.

PREVENTION. In endemic areas, freshwater fish should be well cooked before being eaten. In hyperendemic areas, where a large proportion of the population is infected, mass chemotherapy with a single dose of praziquantel (40 to 50 mg per kilogram of body weight at bed time) is recommended. The local people should be educated regarding how this infection is acquired and should change the habit of eating raw fish.

Opisthorchiasis (*Opisthorchis viverrini* and *felineus*)

Opisthorchis felineus is common in Eastern and Central Europe, India, Japan, and the Philippines. *O. viverrini* is common in Thailand, Laos, and Kampuchea. In parts of Thailand and the U.S.S.R., the infection rate is as high as 90 per cent of the population. Many animals, especially cats, are natural reservoirs. The life cycle, mode of transmission, pathology, clinical manifestations, treatment, and prevention are similar to those of *Clonorchis sinensis.* Cholangiocarcinoma can also result from chronic opisthorchiasis.

Dicroceliasis

Dicrocoelium dendriticum is a lancet-shaped fluke, measuring 10 mm by 2 mm, that normally lives in the biliary tree of sheep, cattle, and other herbivores. The operculated eggs are passed in the feces and are ingested by land snails. Cercariae are released in slime balls shed by the snails, which act as the first intermediate host. The slime is ingested by ants, the second intermediate host. Herbivores become infected by eating the ants. Very rarely, true human infection occurs when such ants are ingested. Less rarely, spurious infection in humans occurs when raw infected liver is eaten. This infection is seen in Europe, the Mediterranean basin, and Asia. The maturing flukes move from the biliary vasculature into the biliary tree and gallbladder and may give rise to symptoms of abdominal pain and vomiting. The diagnosis is made by finding the characteristic ova in the stool. Praziquantel, given in a dose similar to that for clonorchiasis, is the treatment of choice.

Fascioliasis (*Fasciola hepatica*)

Fasciola hepatica is a common parasite in the biliary tract of sheep and cattle, but it may also infect all types of mammals, including humans. It has worldwide distribution in sheep and is prevalent in low, wet pastures, where suitable species of snails are present. The cercariae, discharged from the snails, attach themselves to water plants and encyst as metacercariae. Humans are infected mainly as a result of eating watercress and other aquatic plants gathered in these pastures. In the duodenum, the immature fluke penetrates the mucosa, enters the abdominal cavity, and through some unexplained hepatotropism penetrates Glisson's capsule. The immature flukes migrate throughout the liver for some weeks until they reach the biliary tract, where they mature in about 2 months. The fluke is 3.0 cm by 1.3 cm, and the eggs are large, ovoid, and operculated, measuring 140 μm by 75 μm.

CLINICAL MANIFESTATIONS. *Acute Fascioliasis.* Invasion and maturation occur during the first 3 months after ingestion of the metacercariae. The immature flukes produce small necrotic foci along the migration paths. There may be no significant symptoms, or there may be abdominal pain, hepatomegaly, fever, vomiting, and jaundice. Leukocytosis and marked eosinophilia are present, but *F. hepatica* eggs are not found in the stool at this stage.

Established Infection. The mature flukes now produce metabolites that irritate the biliary passages, resulting in hyperplasia. Obstruction and dilation of the biliary passage and cholecystitis may occur. There may be abdominal pain, hepatomegaly, recurrent urticaria, jaundice, irregular fever, diarrhea, and weight loss. Anemia from blood loss can be severe. The obstruction and irritation may produce thickening of the biliary tree, atrophy of the hepatic cells, and biliary cirrhosis. Cholelithiasis is common. A relationship between fascioliasis and biliary cancer is not proved.

Extrabiliary Fascioliasis. Ingestion of raw sheep and goat liver containing young flukes causes the condition called halzoun (suffocation). This pharyngeal fascioliasis is due to the lodgment of flukes in the upper respiratory and digestive tracts. Inflammation and edema may lead to dysphagia, dyspnea, and even asphyxiation. Cutaneous fascioliasis, usually in the upper abdomen, manifests as migratory nodules that are 2 to 5 cm. Rarely, the flukes may be found in the lung, peritoneum, muscles, eye, and brain.

DIAGNOSIS. In acute infection, the diagnosis is made in an endemic area by a high index of suspicion and the clinical triad of fever, hepatomegaly, and marked eosinophilia. A history of ingestion of wild watercress supports the diagnosis. At this stage, the stool does not contain eggs. Serologic tests, such as complement fixation, are helpful. In chronic infection, the stool contains the characteristic large, operculated eggs (140 μm × 75 μm). Duodenal and biliary aspirate provides a higher yield than does fecal examination. Liver function test results reflect the degree of hepatic cellular damage and biliary obstruction. Intravenous or percutaneous cholangiography, B scan, and magnetic resonance imaging (MRI) scan may show filling defects. The diagnosis is often made during surgical operation for biliary disease. The diagnosis of halzoun in an endemic area is made by the history of ingestion of raw liver and the finding of a pharyngeal mass.

TREATMENT. Praziquantel is effective, and the dosage is 75 mg per kilogram of body weight divided into three doses per day for 2 days. Ectopic flukes are removed surgically. Prevention consists of not eating raw watercress and raw sheep and goat liver in the endemic areas.

Fasciola gigantica

This large fluke is a liver parasite of herbivorous animals and occasionally of humans in Asia and Africa. The life cycle, mode of infection, clinical manifestations, and treatment are similar to those of *F. hepatica.*

Bunnag D, Harinasuta T: Trematode infections excluding schistosomiasis. *In* Gilles HM (ed.): Recent Advances in Tropical Medicine. No. 1. Edinburgh, Churchill Livingstone, 1984, pp 223–227. *A good review especially of opisthorchiasis.*

Gibson JB, Sun T: Clonorchiasis. *In* Marcial-Rojas RA (ed.): Pathology of Protozoal and Helminthic Diseases. Baltimore, The Williams & Wilkins Company, 1977, pp 546–566. *Profusely illustrated; very good on all aspects, especially on epidemiology and pathology as seen in Hong Kong.*

Schwartz DA: Cholangiocarcinoma associated with liver fluke infections: A preventable source of morbidity in Asian immigrants. Am J Gastroenterol 81:76, 1986. *Emphasizes the importance of early diagnosis and treatment of all liver fluke infections in the prevention of bile duct cancer in the high-risk group.*

LUNG HERMAPHRODITIC FLUKES (Paragonimiasis)

Paragonimiasis is due to infection with the adult *Paragonimus westermani* and other species. As a rule, the infection is in the lung, where the flukes are encapsulated in the parenchyma. The disease is also called pulmonary diastomiasis, endemic hemoptysis, and Oriental lung fluke disease. Human paragonimiasis occurs most commonly in the Far East, especially central China, Japan, Korea, Vietnam, Thailand, and the Philippines. It also occurs in the Indian subcontinent, Central and South America, and West Africa. In addition to *P. westermani*, more than 30 species may affect humans. Most of these flukes are parasites of mammals, especially of the cat family, foxes, dogs, cattle, and pigs.

The adult flukes live singly or in pairs encapsulated in the cystic spaces in the lung. They are ovoid, plump, and leaflike and measure about 1.0 cm by 0.5 cm by 0.4 cm. Oval, yellowish-brown, operculated ova (90 μm × 55 μm) are coughed up and expelled in the sputum or are swallowed and passed in the feces. The flukes have a lifespan of 5 to 6 years. In fresh water, the miracidia escape from the ova and penetrate the first intermediate host, a suitable snail. After several weeks, the cercariae emerge and penetrate the second intermediate host, the crayfish or crab. Humans or animals acquire the infection by eating raw meat or viscera of the freshwater crustacean. In Korea and West Africa, fresh crab juice is used as a home remedy in the treatment of measles. In the duodenum the metacercariae excyst, enter the abdominal cavity, migrate through the diaphragm into the pleural space, and end up in the lung parenchyma, where they mature and begin to lay eggs about 2 months after ingestion of the crayfish. This circuitous route of migration explains the extrapulmonary cysts of *Paragonimus.*

PATHOLOGY. The migratory larval flukes tunnel into the lung at the periphery. This condition is accompanied by an inflammatory reaction with many eosinophils. They finally encyst with a fibrous tissue wall. The cyst may communicate with a bronchus and may often be secondarily infected with abscess formation. The death of the fluke is followed by calcification. Flukes in the abdominal cavity may cause abscess and adhesion and intestinal ulceration, resulting in bloody diarrhea with mucus and ova. In the brain, the temporal and occipital lobes are the favored sites of eosinophilic granulomas containing flukes or ova. Lodgment of the flukes in the spinal cord causes transverse myelitis. Adult flukes have been found in other organs.

CLINICAL MANIFESTATIONS. In the rare case of acute paragonimiasis, there may be fever, chills, and chest pain. The symptoms and physical signs are indistinguishable from those of bronchopneumonia. As a rule, the onset is insidious, and the symptoms are those of chronic bronchitis and bronchiectasis. Cough, especially in the morning, that is productive of thick, gelatinous, blood-tinged sputum, is the most prominent symptom. Exertional dyspnea and night sweats are common. Frank hemoptysis often occurs after a paroxysm of coughing. Chest pain and pleural effusion may be present, and clubbing of the fingers may occur. The most characteristic finding is persistent moist, coarse rales over the area of involvement. Chest radiographs early in the disease show patchy, cloudy infiltrations, but later dense, nodular opacities or ring shadows indicate the site of the cysts. Pleural thickening and calcification may be seen late in the disease.

Abdominal paragonimiasis occurs when the flukes localize in the abdomen. The symptoms are nonspecific dull ache, tenderness, and diarrhea, which may be bloody and accompanied by mucus. An abdominal mass with lung disease in a patient from an endemic area should raise suspicion of this disorder. On rare occasions, the fluke localizes in the brain, resulting in a seizure disorder similar to cysticercosis. There may be pareses of varying degrees and optic atrophy with papilledema. The cerebrospinal fluid shows a raised protein concentration, and eosinophils are present. Children with cerebral paragonimiasis are usually mentally retarded. Subcutaneous localization of the fluke results in abscess formation.

DIAGNOSIS. The diagnosis rests mainly on finding ova in the sputum and stool. The differential diagnoses based on the chest radiographs are bronchopneumonia, bronchiectasis, tuberculosis, tumor, and the rarer fungal infections. In practice, the most important differential diagnosis is tuberculosis. Active tuberculosis and paragonimiasis often are present in the same individual from the endemic area.

Abdominal paragonimiasis must be differentiated from intestinal parasitic and nonparasitic infections and other intra-abdominal disorders. The finding of ova in the stool does not necessarily indicate abdominal paragonimiasis. The cerebral presentation must be differentiated from other causes of seizure disorder, space-occupying leisons, cysticercosis, hydatid disease, and meningoencephalitides.

Moderate eosinophilia is usual in early cases, but in established cases there may be no abnormal hematologic findings. As with other helminthic infections, serologic testing is not useful.

TREATMENT. Praziquantel is the treatment of choice. The dosage is 75 mg per kilogram of body weight divided into three doses daily for 2 days. Paragonimiasis of the central nervous system requires surgery. Praziquantel should be given before surgery. Subcutaneous flukes should also be surgically removed.

PREVENTION. In theory, prevention is simple. Freshwater crustaceans must be well cooked before eating, and hands and utensils should be thoroughly washed after contact with raw crabs and crayfish. However, in endemic areas it is difficult to persuade people to relinquish long-established cooking and eating habits and the use of raw crab juice for medicinal purposes.

Chung CH: Human paragonimiasis. *In* Marcial-Rojas RA (ed.): Pathology of Protozoal and Helminthic Diseases. Baltimore, The Williams & Wilkins Company, 1971, pp 504–535. *Profusely illustrated and very detailed description of the pathologic changes in this condition.*

Higashi K, Aoki H, Tatebayashi K, et al.: Cerebral paragonimiasis. J Neurosurg 33:515, 1971.

Monson MH, Koenig JW, Sach R: Successful treatment with praziquantel of six patients infected with the African lung fluke *Paragonimus uterobilateralis.* Am J Trop Med Hyg 32:371, 1983. *Describes the use of this drug in the West African species of Paragonimus.*

INTESTINAL HERMAPHRODITIC FLUKES

Fasciolopsiasis (*Fasciolopsis buski*)

Fasciolopsis buski is the largest intestinal fluke and is normally a parasite of pigs. Human infection is widespread in southern China, Southeast Asia, and the Indian subcontinent. The eggs are passed in the feces, and the miracidia are released and penetrate a snail. The cercariae encyst as metacercariae on edible water plants. Often the edible plants are peeled to remove the "skin," and the metacercariae are swallowed in the process. The larvae attach themselves to the upper small intestine, where they mature in about 4 weeks. The adult fluke measures about 3.0 cm by 1.2 cm.

CLINICAL MANIFESTATIONS. Many light infections are asymptomatic, but heavy loads of flukes produce symptoms, especially in children. The worm load may be up to several thousand. The flukes attach themselves to the duodenal and jejunal mucosa and produce symptoms by trauma, obstruction, and toxin production. Abdominal pain, gastrointestinal hemorrhage, diarrhea, and intestinal obstruction may occur. In severe cases, edema of the face, trunk, and legs, as well as ascites, may be present.

DIAGNOSIS. This rests on finding the large ova (135 μm $\times$ 80 μm) or on recovering the characteristic adult flukes in the stool. Difficulty may be encountered in distinguishing the ova of *F. hepatica* and *F. buski.* Eosinophilia is common and may exceed 50 per cent of the white cell count. In some centers, serologic and skin tests are available, but these are not sensitive and specific. Facial edema may require differentiation of fasciolopsiasis from trichinosis or the nephrotic syndrome.

TREATMENT. Praziquantel is the treatment of choice. The dosage is 75 mg per kilogram of body weight divided into three doses per day for 2 days. Personal prevention consists of avoidance of eating raw aquatic plants in endemic areas. Community prevention consists of eradicating the snails with molluscacides, public education, and prevention of fecal contamination of ponds.

Other Intestinal Hermaphroditic Flukes

Heterophyes heterophyes and *Metagonimus yokogawai* are small flukes that are acquired by eating raw or undercooked fish that contain the metacercariae. The former is found in Egypt, Tunisia, southern China, India, and the Philippines, and the latter in the Far East and Indonesia. The adult fluke is 2 to 3 mm long and attaches itself to the intestinal mucosa. Usually, the infection is light, and there are few symptoms. Very rarely, the eggs gain access to the circulation and may be found in the organs. As a rule, the eggs are passed in the stool; they closely resemble *Clonorchis* eggs. Infection by both flukes can be treated with praziquantel. Differentiation of the two species requires examination of the adult flukes by experts. Many species of the genus *Echinostoma* infect humans in the Far East, but they rarely produce symptoms. *Gastrodiscoides hominis* occurs in India and Malaysia and may cause diarrhea. In western Canada,

the eggs of *Metorchis conjunctus,* which are somewhat similar to those of *Clonorchis,* are occasionally found in the stools of humans who eat raw fish. If treatment is required, praziquantel (75 mg per kilogram of body weight in three divided doses for 1 day) is the treatment of choice.

Alaria americana is an intestinal trematode of carnivores, such as the fox, wolf, lynx, or skunk. Two cases of human infection by the mesocercariae of this fluke have been reported in Ontario. The mesocercaria is a stage of development between the cercaria and the metacercaria. The cercariae emerging from the snail penetrate tadpoles. As the tadpole grows into a frog, the mesocercariae tend to concentrate in the hind legs. When the frog is eaten by a carnivore, the mesocercariae develop into metacercariae and adult flukes in the lung and the gut, respectively. When humans, who are not the normal host, eat the frog, the mesocercariae migrate all over the body. In the first reported case, the mesocarcaria was surgically removed from the retina of the eye. The second case was a fatal systemic infection manifested by severe respiratory distress, coma, coagulation abnormality, and vasculitis. At autopsy, mesocercariae were found in all organs. The diagnosis is made by biopsy of affected organs. No effective treatment is known, although praziquantel may be useful.

Faust EC, Beaver PC, Jung RC: Intestinal flukes. *In* Faust EC, Beaver PC, Jung RC: Animal Agents and Vectors of Human Disease. 4th ed. Philadelphia, Lea & Febiger, 1975, pp 134–141. *A good reference for the less important parasites. Emphasis is on the parasitology, life cycles, and morphology.*

Fernandes BJ, Cooper JD, Cullen JB, et al.: Systemic infection with *Alaria americana* (Trematoda). Can Med Assoc J 115:1111, 1976. *The first report of generalized infection with mesocercariae of this fluke. Good description of the clinical course and autopsy findings.*

436 Nematode Infections

James W. Kazura

Nematodes (phylum Nematoda), or roundworms, include a vast number of species of free-living and parasitic helminths of plants and animals. These multicellular organisms differ markedly from unicellular bacteria and protozoa in that they have well-differentiated organ systems with specialized nervous, muscular, gastrointestinal, and reproductive functions. Parasitic nematodes are nonsegmented worms varying in length from several millimeters to approximately 2 meters. Nematodes have four larval stages and adult worms of both sexes. With the exception of *Strongyloides* and a few other helminths of medical importance, larval forms are produced after mating of sexually mature adult parasites, which by themselves are incapable of multiplying in the mammalian host. The inability of adult worms to replicate has important implications for the propensity of this class of organism to establish an infection and cause disease. Unlike the situation pertaining to bacterial, viral, or protozoan infections, casual or a low degree of exposure to infective stages of helminthic parasites generally does not result in patent infection or pathologic manifestations. Repeated or intense exposure to a large number of infective larvae is required for establishment of infection and development of disease.

Nematode infections are endemic in both temperate and tropical climates. They are transmitted either by the fecal-oral route or by inoculation of infective larvae into the skin, primarily by blood-feeding intermediate insect vectors. The prevalence of infection is greatest in circumstances conducive to the development and transmission of infective forms of the parasites, i.e., overcrowded, perennially warm geographic areas with poor sanitation, such as in many less developed countries of Africa, Asia, and Latin America and economically poor areas of North America and Europe.

The epidemiology of human nematode (as well as trematode and cestode) infections has several unique features. The infection in an endemic area has a negative binomial distribution, i.e., the majority of individuals in an endemic area have low parasite burdens and a small number harbor relatively high burdens.

Persons in the latter group have the greatest significance from an epidemiologic perspective in that they contribute most substantially to transmission and are most likely to develop pathologic manifestations. This characteristic implies that transmission in an endemic area may be decreased or interrupted by reduction of the parasite burden in a small proportion of the population. In addition, because total worm load correlates directly with the propensity to develop disease, treatment of lightly infected persons may not be indicated or may be unnecessary, especially if the available chemotherapy has major side effects.

Nematode infections of medical importance may be broadly classified into those in which the route of infection, larval migration, and disease manifestations are primarily gastrointestinal and those that affect other tissues. The former group includes hookworms (Ancylostoma duodenale, Necator americanus), the roundworm Ascaris lumbricoides, the pinworm Enterobius vermicularis, and the whipworm Trichuris trichiuria. Animal intestinal nematodes such as Trichostrongylus and Anisakis species also occasionally infect and cause disease in humans. Trichinella spiralis, Strongyloides stercoralis, and Angiostrongylus cantonensis infect humans by the oral route, but disease manifestations are due primarily to migration in other tissues. Tissue-invasive nematodes include lymphatic filariae (Wuchereria bancrofti, Brugia malayi, and B. timori), skin-dwelling Onchocerca volvulus and Loa loa, and the guinea worm, Dracunculus medinensis.

Anderson RM, May RM: Helminthic infections of humans: Mathematical models, population dynamics, and control. Adv Parasitol 24:1, 1985. An excellent discussion of the relationship of the biology of parasitic helminthic infections to their epidemiology and control strategies.

INTESTINAL NEMATODES

These infections include hookworm disease, ascariasis, enterobiasis, trichuriasis, and rarely animal nematodiases. They are prevalent in temperate and tropical areas of the world, especially those that are overcrowded and have poor sanitation. Intestinal nematode infections have little morbidity in most cases and are easily treated with mebendazole.

Hookworm Disease

ETIOLOGY AND EPIDEMIOLOGY. The major hookworms that infect humans are Ancylostoma duodenale and Necator americanus. A. ceylonicum infection is less common and occurs primarily in the South Pacific. Animal hookworms such as A. braziliense and Uncinaria stenocephala do not undergo full development in incidentally exposed humans. Infection occurs when exposed skin maintains contact for several minutes with soil contaminated with parasite eggs containing viable larvae. Larvae penetrate the skin and subsequently migrate to and mature in the lungs. The parasites then break into the air spaces, ascend the trachea, and are swallowed. Adult worms mature in the upper small intestine and attach to the mucosa by their buccal capsules. Female worms release more than 10,000 eggs per day, which are passed in the stools and deposited in the soil. The prepatent period (duration of time between infection and passing of eggs in the feces) is 40 to 105 days. Adult hookworms have a lifespan of 2 to 5 years.

Hookworms infect over 1 billion persons worldwide. The highest prevalences of infection (80 to 100 per cent) occur in tropical and less developed countries, where environmental and socioeconomic conditions are especially favorable to transmission. These include warm, moist soil; lack of public sewage disposal systems; and the habit of walking barefoot. The higher prevalence of hookworm infection in children than adults results from more frequent exposure of skin to larvae in soil among children. As is the case in other intestinal nematode infections, acquired resistance is minimal or does not develop at all as a consequence of previous infection.

PATHOGENESIS AND CLINICAL MANIFESTATIONS. Hookworm disease is due primarily to gastrointestinal blood loss and attendant iron deficiency anemia. The latter correlates directly with the total worm burden. Adult worms attached to the mucosa of the upper small intestine digest ingested blood as well as cause focal bleeding mediated by helminth-derived proteases. A. duodenale is estimated to cause a blood loss of 0.3 ml per day

per worm; N. americanus induces loss of approximately 0.03 ml per day. Nutritional deficiencies secondary to coexisting conditions that result in low iron stores (e.g., malabsorption, insufficient dietary intake in children, and multiparous women) contribute significantly to morbidity. Hypoproteinemia has been reported in children with hookworm disease in less developed countries. This complication is most likely due to coexisting malnutrition rather than gastrointestinal disease caused by hookworm infestation per se. Abdominal signs or symptoms are not caused by hookworm infection.

Pruritus at the site of larval skin penetration ("ground itch") occurs occasionally. In the case of primary exposure, local itching and erythematous papules lasting 1 week develop. More intense pruritus, vesiculation, and edema of 2 to 3 weeks' duration may occur after repeated exposure to infective larvae. Migration of hookworm larvae through the lungs rarely causes pulmonary symptoms.

DIAGNOSIS. Hookworm infection is diagnosed by identification of the characteristic round eggs containing convoluted larvae. Direct smears of freshly passed stool using the Kato or other techniques are satisfactory for the diagnosis of moderately to heavily infected cases (more than 400 eggs per gram).

TREATMENT AND PREVENTION. Mebendazole, administered orally at a dosage of 100 mg twice daily for 3 days, is the treatment of choice. Iron supplementation should be included if the degree of anemia and complicating illnesses warrant it. Administration of mebendazole to pregnant women should be delayed until after delivery. Light infections (feces with fewer than 400 eggs per gram) do not cause blood loss sufficient to induce iron deficiency. Therefore, in the absence of the complicating factors discussed above, individuals with such infections do not require anthelminthic chemotherapy. The ideal method for preventing hookworm infection is improvement of hygienic conditions. Use of footwear, especially by children, is currently the only practical means of avoiding infection.

Ascariasis

ETIOLOGY AND EPIDEMIOLOGY. Ascaris lumbricoides are roundworms 2 to 3 cm in length that reside in the lumen of the jejunum and in the mid-ileum. Infection occurs by the oral route when soil containing embryonated eggs is ingested. Larvae are released from eggs in the small intestine, penetrate the gut, and migrate to the liver and then lungs via the blood or lymphatic circulation. Following maturation in the lungs over a 4-week period, the parasites ascend the respiratory tract and are swallowed. Adult worms reach sexual maturity (i.e., female worms release eggs that are detectable in feces) approximately 60 days after infection.

Ascariasis affects approximately one quarter of the world's population and is likely the most prevalent helminthiasis of humans. Infection is common in Africa, Asia, and Latin America, especially in areas of high population density and unhygienic conditions. The use of human feces as fertilizer, defecation in soil, and hand-to-mouth contact with contaminated soil are major factors that contribute to the spread of Ascaris. The ability of Ascaris eggs to remain viable in harsh environmental conditions (embryonated eggs remain infectious after exposure to freezing temperatures and desiccation for several weeks) also facilitates transmission.

PATHOGENESIS AND CLINICAL MANIFESTATIONS. Disease caused by A. lumbricoides is infrequent and generally correlates with the intensity of infection. The majority of infected individuals are asymptomatic.

Symptomatic cases can be divided into two broad categories based on the phase of infection and site of pathology, i.e., pulmonary or gastrointestinal tract. Pulmonary disease is caused by the migration of larvae in the small vessels of the lung and their subsequent rupture into alveoli. Tissue damage is thought to be due to the host immune response, which includes production of immunoglobulin E (IgE) and eosinophilia. Transient pulmonary infiltrates, fever, cough, dyspnea, and eosinophilia lasting 1 to several weeks are the major clinical manifestations. This complex of symptoms and signs is frequently seasonal and coincidental with environmental changes that favor development of infective-stage larvae in eggs (e.g., spring rains that follow cold and dry periods). Intestinal signs and symptoms are due either to obstruction caused by the presence of an exceptionally large number of parasites in the small intestine or to migration of adult worms to unusual sites, such as the biliary tree or pancreatic duct. Intestinal obstruction almost always occurs in children less than 6 years old. The onset is sudden and characterized by colicky abdominal pain and vomiting. Heavily infected children are also prone to biliary disease or pancreatitis secondary to lodging of *Ascaris* in the ducts draining these organs. A malabsorption syndrome characterized by steatorrhea and low vitamin A levels has been reported in Latin American children with ascariasis.

DIAGNOSIS. Intestinal infection is diagnosed by the presence of the typical oval, thick-shelled *Ascaris* eggs in thick smears of fecal specimens. The existence of adult worms in pancreatic or biliary ducts should be suspected in children who have high egg outputs in conjunction with jaundice or pancreatitis. Pulmonary ascariasis cannot be diagnosed on the basis of identification of ova in feces because adult worms have not yet matured and reached the intestinal tract. Biopsy of the lung is unlikely to demonstrate larvae and is not recommended.

TREATMENT AND PREVENTION. Uncomplicated intestinal ascariasis is treated with mebendazole (100 mg orally twice per day for 3 days). Children with heavy infections or those with biliary tract obstruction should be given piperazine (50 to 75 mg per kilogram of body weight per day for 2 days), which causes neuromuscular paralysis of the worms and expulsion of intact helminths. No specific treatment is recommended for pulmonary ascariasis because the condition is self-limited.

The major means of preventing *Ascaris* infection is improvement of hygienic and socioeconomic conditions. Mass chemotherapy has been successful in reducing worm loads, but frequent retreatments are required.

Enterobiasis

Enterobius vermicularis or pinworm infection is cosmopolitan in its distribution. It is especially common in overcrowded settings and spreads rapidly in conditions in which person-to-person contact is frequent, such as in institutions for children.

Infection occurs by the fecal-oral route. Embryonated eggs carried on the fingernails, bed clothing, or bedding are ingested and hatch in the upper small intestine. Larvae subsequently pass distally and develop in the large bowel into adult parasites measuring 2 to 5 mm in length. Female worms migrate nightly out of the rectum and deposit large numbers of ova (11,000 per worm) in the perianal and perineal areas. Larvae in the deposited eggs become infective within several hours of exposure to ambient oxygen. Infectivity is usually maintained for 1 to 2 days.

The vast majority of pinworm infections are asymptomatic or associated with perianal pruritus and consequent sleep deprivation. *E. vermicularis* is a rare cause of appendicitis and, when the adult worms follow an aberrant path of migration, vulvovaginitis, urethritis, or peritonitis.

The diagnosis of pinworm infection is easily made by identification of ova on a piece of cellophane tape applied to the perirectal area in the morning. *E. vermicularis* eggs are oval and slightly flattened on one side. It is unusual to find eggs in feces or adult worms in the perianal area. Repeated examinations may be necessary.

Treatment is by administration of a single dose of mebendazole (100 mg one time) to affected individuals as well as close associates, such as family members. Several treatments may be required (every 3 to 4 months) if exposure continues, such as in institutional settings. Although personal cleanliness is recommended as a means of limiting transmission of enterobiasis, there is no clear-cut demonstration that it prevents infection.

Trichuriasis

Trichuris trichiura or whipworm infection is similar to pinworm infection in that it is limited to the gastrointestinal tract and does not have a tissue migratory phase. Eggs containing infective larvae mature in warm, moist soil over a 2-week period. Ingested eggs hatch in the small bowel and subsequently develop in epithelial cells of the cecum and ascending colon into adult worms that are 40 mm in length. The body of the parasite protrudes into the colonic lumen. Its anterior portion has a whiplike shape.

As is the case with most intestinal nematode infections, trichuriasis is most common in overcrowded areas with poor sanitation.

The estimated prevalence worldwide is 800 million, with approximately 2 million cases in the southern United States. Children are more frequently infected than adults and also more likely to have higher worm burdens.

Adults with trichuriasis are usually asymptomatic. In children with heavy infections (more than 10,000 eggs per gram of feces), a syndrome of dysentery, growth retardation, and rectal prolapse has been described. The pathologic manifestations include infiltrates of eosinophils and neutrophils accompanied by epithelial denudation. Complicating diseases such as shigellosis and amebiasis may contribute to this condition in children.

Whipworm infection is diagnosed by identification of football-shaped eggs in direct smears of fecal specimens. Mebendazole at the same dosage indicated for ascariasis is satisfactory treatment.

Other Animal Nematodiases

Humans may serve as paratenic hosts for several nematodes that ordinarily parasitize the intestine of other mammals. Able to complete their life cycle in their natural hosts, these helminths are incapable of doing so in humans and display aberrant immigration patterns in both intestinal and nonintestinal tissues.

Several species of the genus *Trichostrongylus* infect both humans and domestic ruminants. The infection is found widely in the Middle and Far East and Australia. Ova are passed in the stool of ruminants and hatch in the soil. Humans are incidentally infected when larvae are ingested with leafy vegetables. The adult worms live in the intestines and suck small amounts of blood; heavy infections result in anemia. Diagnosis is made by identifying ova, which resemble those of hookworm, in the stool. Treatment is with thiabendazole, 25 mg per kilogram of body weight twice a day for 2 days.

Anisakis is an intestinal nematode of marine mammals. Several species of saltwater fish are intermediate hosts. Human infection occurs when raw fish is eaten. The larvae of both *Anisakis* and *Phocanemia decipiens* have been implicated. Most cases have been reported in Japan or Western Europe, particularly Scandinavia. The larvae invade the wall of the small intestine or stomach, causing pain and, rarely, intestinal obstruction or perforation. Gastric anisakiasis can be diagnosed endoscopically and treated by removal of the worms. Intestinal anisakiasis often resembles an acute abdomen, leading to laparotomy. Thiabendazole, 25 mg per kilogram twice a day for 3 days, may be given if surgical intervention is not required. Infection is prevented by cooking or freezing fish prior to eating.

Capillaria philippinensis infection has been reported from the Philippines and Thailand. This nematode is thought to parasitize birds, with fish and crustaceans serving as intermediate hosts. Humans are infected by eating the raw intermediate hosts. The ingested larvae mature and live in the crypts of the small intestine, where they reproduce. The result is often a heavy infection; up to 40,000 adult worms have been recovered at one autopsy. The clinical syndrome includes severe malabsorption and protein-losing enteropathy. The diagnosis is made by finding eggs or larvae in the stool; an intradermal test is also available. The treatment of choice is mebendazole, 200 mg twice a day for 20 days; an alternative is thiabendazole, 25 mg per kilogram daily for 30 days. Supportive care, such as fluid and electrolyte replacement and a high-protein diet, is also important.

Gnathostoma spinigerum is an intestinal nematode of dogs and cats; fish are intermediate hosts. The infection is endemic in rodents in the Far East and Thailand. Human infection has also been reported in South America. Infective larvae are ingested by humans in raw or undercooked fish. The larvae do not complete their life cycle in humans but migrate through the body. The most frequent site is subcutaneous tissues, where larvae are found in eosinophilic granulomas. A few weeks after infection, pruritic or painful subcutaneous nodules and swellings appear. These may be migratory and develop into abscesses. In central nervous system gnathostomiasis, hemorrhagic tracts may be found in the brain. Fever, vomiting, and abdominal pain occur a few days after ingestion of larvae. Paralysis of the extremities, encephalitis, and subarachnoid hemorrhage have been reported. Eye involvement with uveitis and orbital cellulitis represents a third variety.

Peripheral eosinophilia is usual in cutaneous gnathostomiasis; the diagnosis may be established by biopsy. In central nervous system infection, blood eosinophilia is an inconstant feature, but eosinophils are present in the cerebrospinal fluid, as in the case of angiostrongyliasis. Treatment of subcutaneous lesions consists of surgical removal. For central nervous system infection, mebendazole, 200 mg every 3 hours for 6 days, may be given. The infection may be prevented by cooking fish thoroughly before eating.

Several nematodes that ordinarily parasitize the intestine of monkeys occasionally infect humans. *Oesophagostomum* has been reported from Africa, Asia, and Brazil; it is responsible for the formation of granulomas in the intestinal wall. *Ternidens diminutus* is sometimes found in the human colon in Africa and Asia; a heavy infection may cause anemia. *Physaloptera mordens*, also reported from Africa, may attach itself to the esophagus, stomach, or small intestine of humans. The definitive host of *Lagochilascaris minor* is unknown. About 30 human cases have been reported from Central and South America, usually with worms invading the soft tissues of the neck and throat and sinuses.

Khuroo MS, Zargar SA, Mahajan R: Sonographic appearances in biliary ascariasis. Gastroenterology 93:267, 1987. *A discussion of the ultrasound appearance of this unusual but clinically important aspect of ascariasis.*

Pawlowski ZS: Ascariasis: Host-pathogen biology. Rev Infect Dis 4:806, 1982. *Reviews the basic biology and host interactions of* Ascaris.

Schad GH, Banwell JG: Hookworms. *In* Warren KS, Mahmoud AAF (eds.): Tropical and Geographical Medicine. New York, McGraw-Hill, 1990. *A general review of biology, clinical aspects, and epidemiology of hookworm infection. Synthesizes a large amount of confusing literature.*

Schultz MG: Ascariasis: Nutritional implications. Rev Infect Dis 4:815, 1982. *Reviews the basic biology and host interactions of* Ascaris.

Smith JW, Wootten R: Anisakis and anisakiasis. Adv Parasitol 16:93, 1978. *An exceptionally complete review.*

TOXOCARIASIS

DEFINITION. Visceral larva migrans (VLM) and ocular larva migrans (OLM) are caused by ingestion and subsequent development and migration of embryonated eggs of the canine roundworm *Toxocara canis*. Roundworms of cats (*T. cati*) and raccoons (*Baylisascaris procyonis*) also rarely cause VLM.

ETIOLOGY. In its normal canine host, *T. canis*, ingested embryonated eggs follow a route of migration similar to that described for *Ascaris*, i.e., larvae penetrate the small intestinal mucosa, migrate to the lungs, are reswallowed, and develop into adult worms in the small intestine; the adult worms lodge there and release eggs that are passed in the feces. When embryonated *T. canis* eggs are ingested by humans, larvae also migrate throughout the body (lung, liver, brain, muscles, and occasionally eyes) but fail to complete development to the adult stage. Tissue necrosis secondary to penetrating larvae and associated host inflammatory reactions, such as eosinophil-rich granulomas, are the underlying cause of disease.

EPIDEMIOLOGY. Toxocariasis is endemic in both temperate and tropical areas of the world. The vast majority of symptomatic cases occur in young children. This age group is most likely to be infected by virtue of frequent and intimate handling of dogs (especially newborn puppies that may be hyperinfected), playing in areas where dogs and cats defecate (e.g., public sandboxes), and the habit of geophagia. The potential of exposure to embryonated eggs is high in that *T. canis* infection is common in dogs (a 20 per cent infection rate in dogs in the United States).

CLINICAL MANIFESTATIONS. The vast majority of children who ingest *T. canis* eggs are asymptomatic. VLM is the most common clinically defined entity attributable to *T. canis*. It is most frequent in children less than 5 years old (there are no published series of adults with VLM) and is characterized by fever less than 39°C; pulmonary symptoms, including wheezing and cough; and, less frequently, pain in the right upper quadrant. These symptoms have a gradual onset and resolve over 4 to 8 weeks. Physical signs include wheezing and hepatomegaly in about one quarter of cases. Larvae less commonly migrate to the brain and heart and cause focal neurologic defects and heart failure.

OLM has an incidence approximately one-tenth that of VLM and affects children older than 8 to 10 years. Visual disturbances due to VLM are not distinguishable from other causes of focal intraretinal granulomas or space-occupying lesions, such as tuberculosis and retinoblastoma. *T. canis* larvae may migrate intraretinally and produce transient and recurrent impairment of vision.

DIAGNOSIS AND TREATMENT. VLM is diagnosed on the basis of suspicion of ingestion of *T. canis* eggs in a child with the symptoms described above. Eosinophilia, elevated erythrocyte sedimentation rate, and generalized hypergammaglobulinemia are also consistent with the diagnosis. Biopsy to document the presence of larvae is insensitive and not recommended. An enzyme-linked immunosorbent assay (ELISA) for measurement of anti-*Toxocara* antibodies is helpful if elevated immunoglobulin M (IgM) antibodies and a rise in titer between acute and convalescent phases are documented. Most cases of VLM are not life threatening and are self-limited. Treatment is therefore not required. In persons with severe pulmonary, cardiac, or neurologic involvement and high-grade eosinophilia (more than 10,000 per cubic millimeter of blood), albendazole (200 mg twice daily for 10 to 20 days) and corticosteroids may be used with the aim of reducing symptoms and shortening the course of the illness. No controlled studies, however, demonstrate the efficacy of this approach.

OLM represents a diagnostic dilemma in that it must be distinguished from intraretinal neoplasms and infections. Expert ophthalmologic consultation is necessary. Computerized tomography and fluorescein angiography are helpful in diagnosis. Elevated anti-*Toxocara* antibody titers in aqueous fluid relative to serum values are consistent with OLM. It is unclear if administration of anthelminthics is useful for the treatment of OLM.

VLM and OLM may be prevented by periodic deworming of dogs, especially puppies, and limiting their defecation in public places.

Glickman LT, Schantz PM, Cypess RH: Epidemiologic characteristics and clinical findings in patients with serologically proven toxocariasis. Trans R Soc Trop Med Hyg 73:254, 1979. *An excellent description of the major clinical manifestations of toxocariasis.*

CUTANEOUS LARVA MIGRANS

Animal hookworms, most frequently the dog parasite *Ancylostoma braziliense* and less commonly *Uncinaria stenocephala* and *Bunostomum phlebotomum*, are the major etiologic agents of cutaneous larva migrans, or creeping eruption. *Ancylostoma duodenale*, *Necator americanus*, and *Strongyloides stercoralis* may produce a similar syndrome during the phase of infection that involves penetration of the skin.

The disease occurs when skin comes into direct and prolonged contact with hookworm larvae contained in the feces of dogs, cats, or humans. Moist areas visited by animals, such as vegetation near beaches and exposed soil covered by porches, are common sites in which humans may be infected. Cutaneous larva migrans in the United States is most prevalent in southern coastal regions.

Clinical manifestations result from penetration and migration of larvae in the epidermal-dermal junction of the skin. Within several hours of contact with exposed skin, the patient notes pruritus and development of raised erythematous serpiginous lesions. The lesions migrate approximately 1 cm per day and evolve into bullae. Multiple lesions may appear if large areas of the body have been exposed, as in sunbathing. The extremities are the most common area of the body affected.

Creeping eruption may be treated by topical application of thiabendazole oral suspension. This may be prepared by trituration of a 500-mg tablet in 5 grams of petroleum jelly. If untreated, cutaneous larva migrans is self-limited, with resolution of signs and symptoms in several weeks to 2 months.

ANGIOSTRONGYLIASIS

Angiostrongylus cantonensis is a cause of eosinophilic meningitis in Asia and the South Pacific. Small numbers of cases have also been reported in Cuba and Africa. *Angiostrongylus costaricensis* is a rare cause of gastrointestinal bleeding. The nematode is limited in its distribution to Central and South America. Humans are infected with these rodent (primarily rat) nematodes following ingestion of poorly cooked or raw intermediate mollusc hosts, such as snails, slugs, and prawns. Fresh vegetables may also be contaminated with infective larvae and serve as a vehicle of infection.

In the case of *A. cantonensis* infection, ingested infective larvae penetrate the gut wall and migrate to small vessels of the meninges and, less commonly, the spinal cord and eye. An intense local inflammatory reaction ensues within 1 week. Fever, meningismus, and headache develop in association with eosinophilic pleocytosis of the cerebrospinal fluid. Strabismus, paresthesias, and vomiting have been observed in a minority of cases. Diagnosis is based on a history of ingesting potentially contaminated foodstuffs and the presence of eosinophils in cerebrospinal fluid. Larvae are usually not found in cerebrospinal fluid. Other less common causes of eosinophilic meningitis of infectious etiology include *Trichinella spiralis, Taenia solium, Toxocara canis, Gnathostoma spinigerum,* and *Paragonimus westermani.* Symptomatic *A. cantonensis* infection resolves over a 2-week period. The value of administering specific anthelminthic therapy or corticosteroids has not been established.

A. costaricensis larvae penetrate the mucosa of the terminal ileum, appendix, and ascending colon. The larvae subsequently develop into adult worms in the local lymphatics and mesenteric arterioles. Eggs released by the female worms elicit multiple eosinophil-rich granulomatous reactions that cause edematous, thickened bowel and necrosis (secondary to mesenteric blood vessel obstruction). Clinical presentations typically include right-sided abdominal pain, vomiting, and fever. Abnormal laboratory findings include leukocytosis with eosinophilia (at least 10 per cent, with a white cell count greater than 10,000 per cubic millimeter). Parasite larvae and eggs are not present in stools. A palpable mass secondary to granulomatous lesions may be present and cause intestinal obstruction. Less frequently, gastrointestinal bleeding is the principal manifestation. Treatment is surgical. There is no demonstrated benefit of specific anthelminthic chemotherapy.

Koo J, Pien F, Kliks MM: *Angiostrongylus (Parastrongylus) eosinophilic meningitis.* Rev Infect Dis 10:1155, 1988. *An excellent discussion of the biology of the helminth and the clinical manifestations of human infection.*

Silvera CT, Ghali VS, Heimann J, et al.: Angiostrongyliasis: A rare cause of gastrointestinal hemorrhage. Am J Gastroenteral 84:329, 1988. *A case report of* A. costaricensis *infection and excellent discussion of clinical manifestations of this uncommon infection.*

TRICHINOSIS

DEFINITION. Infection of humans by *Trichinella spiralis* occurs when viable infective larvae are eaten in undercooked pork or other meats. The majority of infected individuals are asymptomatic. Clinical manifestations in heavily infected persons include diarrhea, myalgias, fever, and, less commonly, myocarditis and neurologic disease. Trichinosis occurs in all areas of the world, including the Arctic and temperate regions. The incidence of trichinosis in the United States has decreased markedly over the past several decades.

ETIOLOGY. Infection is initiated by ingestion of infective larvae encysted in striated muscle. Excystment occurs in the acid-pepsin environment of the stomach, and parasites develop into sexually mature adult worms in the upper to middle small intestine of the human host. Completion of the enteric phase of the parasite life cycle takes about 1 week, with adult worms remaining viable and productive of larval offspring for an additional 3 to 5 weeks. The systemic phase commences 1 week after infection, when larvae released by female worms migrate through blood vessels and lymphatics and invade multiple organ systems. Mature third-stage larvae develop in host-derived nurse cells in striated skeletal and cardiac muscle, where they become encysted and remain viable for years. As is the case with most helminthiases, the severity of symptoms is related to the total parasite load. Because adult worms are incapable of reproducing themselves, the number of infective larvae ingested is the most important determinant of worm load (i.e., number of larvae that invade muscle and other tissues).

EPIDEMIOLOGY. *T. spiralis* infection is enzootic in omnivorous and carnivorous animal populations, including rats, bears, and aquatic mammals of the Arctic. The nematode is introduced into domestic animals such as pigs and horses by feeding them garbage containing carcasses of these animals, most commonly rats. Human infection usually occurs in two settings: first, when undercooked or smoked pork products or beef contaminated with nematodes are eaten, and second, when flesh of poorly cooked wild game, such as bear or boar meat, is ingested. An important source of infection in Alaskan and Canadian Arctic native populations is uncooked walrus meat.

The annual incidence of human trichinosis in the United States has decreased from more than 450 in 1947–1949 to fewer than 56 between 1982 and 1986. This decline is primarily due to fewer cases related to ingestion of commercial pork products. Recent cases in the United States occur in point-source outbreaks associated with ingestion of game or noncommercial pork products.

PATHOGENESIS AND CLINICAL MANIFESTATIONS. Tissue-invasive *T. spiralis* larvae elicit an eosinophilic granulomatous reaction that may result in significant end-organ tissue damage and dysfunction. Skeletal muscle is the most frequent site involved. Myocardial damage, pulmonary infiltration, and focal neurologic damage secondary to invasion by larvae are seen in only the most heavily infected persons. The systemic phase of infection usually occurs 2 to 3 weeks after ingestion of infective larvae and may last for 2 months. Clinical manifestations typically include myalgias (especially of the gastrocnemius and masseter), periorbital edema, and fever. Myocardial damage may manifest as heart failure or dysrhythmias.

The enteric phase of infection may also cause gastrointestinal signs and symptoms, such as diarrhea and abdominal cramps. These typically occur within 1 week of eating contaminated meat and last less than 2 weeks. Reports from the Canadian Arctic suggest that the *T. spiralis* larvae that infect walrus meat may cause diarrhea of 1 to 3 months' duration in the absence of myalgias or other signs of larval invasion of deeper tissues.

DIAGNOSIS. A diagnosis of trichinosis should be considered in individuals with generalized myalgias and eosinophilia (more than 600 eosinophils per cubic millimeter). Serologic testing for *T. spiralis* antibodies is available at the Centers for Disease Control. Elevation of IgM antibodies or a more than fourfold rise in titer between acute and convalescent phases of infection is helpful in diagnosis. The levels of creatine phosphate kinase and of serum immunoglobulins and the erythrocyte sedimentation rate are also increased for several weeks after infection. Muscle biopsy (e.g., of the gastrocnemius) may demonstrate larvae, although their absence does not exclude the diagnosis. Most important to consider in the differential diagnosis of trichinosis are the eosinophilia-myalgia syndrome associated with L-tryptophan and idiopathic hypereosinophilic syndrome.

TREATMENT AND PREVENTION. If patients present at a time when adult parasites are in the intestine (i.e., during the initial 1 to 2 weeks after infection, when gastrointestinal symptoms are prominent), thiabendazole is recommended at a dosage of 25 mg per kilogram of body weight twice a day for 1 week. Larvae in muscle are not killed by this drug, and treatment is primarily symptomatic with antipyretics and analgesics. Although there are too few recent cases to establish clearly a possible beneficial effect of corticosteroids, they may be useful to diminish the severity of inflammation when signs of myocarditis, neurologic disease (e.g., seizures, focal weakness), or pulmonary insufficiency develop. *T. spiralis* infection is prevented by killing larvae in meat products. This is achieved by heating to 80.5°C. Freezing, smoking, or exposure to microwave does not reliably kill the helminth.

Bailey TM, Schantz PM: Trends in the incidence and transmission patterns of trichinosis in humans in the United States. Comparisons of the periods 1975–1981 and 1982–1986. Rev Infect Dis 12:5, 1990. *A comprehensive review of the epidemiology of trichinosis.*

MacLean JD, Viallet J, Law C, et al.: Trichinosis in the Canadian Arctic: Report of five outbreaks and a new clinical syndrome. J Infect Dis 160:513, 1989. *Excellent description of severe gastrointestinal manifestations of* T. spiralis *in a population in which the prevalence of trichinosis is among the highest in the world.*

STRONGYLOIDIASIS

DEFINITION. *Strongyloides stercoralis* infection is endemic in warm climates worldwide, including the southern United States. In immunologically normal individuals, infection is usually asymptomatic or causes gastrointestinal dysfunction, manifest as abdominal pain, bloating, or bleeding. Persons who have deficient cell-mediated immunity are permissive for development of an autoinfective and hyperinfective life cycle of the nematode that markedly increases the total worm load. Life-threatening acute pulmonary disease and organ dysfunction due to dissemination of larvae to aberrant sites such as the brain, pancreas, and kidneys may result in immunocompromised hosts.

ETIOLOGY. *S. stercoralis* infection occurs when skin contacts free-living filariform larvae in the soil. After penetrating the skin, the parasite embolizes to the small vessels of the lungs via the venous circulation. Rhabditiform larvae then break into the alveolar spaces, ascend the respiratory tree, and are swallowed. Further development to adult worms occurs in the duodenum and upper jejunum, where egg-laying parasites live in the mucosa and submucosa. Rhabditiform larvae are released from eggs and are passed from the body in stools. Infective filariform larvae develop in the soil by two alternative means, either by direct transformation from rhabditiform larvae or indirectly from free-living intermediate forms.

Several unusual features of the life cycle of *S. stercoralis* are critical to understanding how this parasitic nematode causes life-threatening disease. First, unlike the vast majority of human helminthic parasites, adult worms are only of the female sex and reproduce parthogenetically in the gastrointestinal tract. The total worm burden in the host may therefore be greatly expanded in the absence of repeated exposure to infective larvae in the environment. Second, rhabditiform larvae may develop into infective filariform larvae in the gastrointestinal tract as well as after passage in feces, as described above. Occurrence of the former process in immunocompromised hosts allows autoinfection, whereby larvae pass directly through the bowel (internal autoinfection) or perianal skin (external autoinfection) to reinitiate migration and development in the lungs. When this event is frequent, a hyperinfection syndrome ensues. Disseminated strongyloidiasis refers to a situation of hyperinfection in which the organisms also migrate to and cause pathology in organs not usually traversed by larvae, such as those of the central nervous system.

EPIDEMIOLOGY. *S. stercoralis* infection is endemic in Africa, Asia, Latin America, and areas of Eastern and Southern Europe. Prevalence rates based on examinations of stools for rhabditiform larvae vary from more than 40 per cent in areas of sub-Saharan Africa to 1 to 7 per cent in rural Eastern Europe. In the United States, the infection is endemic in rural Appalachia and other parts of the South. Prevalences range from 0.4 to 3 per cent in the United States. Refugees from Asia have a higher prevalence of infection than do indigenous Americans. Surveys of homosexual men conducted before 1980 indicate a frequency of infection of 3.9 per cent. It is likely that most studies of prevalence underestimate infection because they are based on examination of a single stool specimen, which is less sensitive than multiple examinations performed over days or weeks.

Strongyloidiasis is especially common in overcrowded situations in which sanitation and personal hygiene are poor, such as in institutions for retarded children and camps for prisoners of war. An unusually high frequency of *S. stercoralis* infection has also been reported in persons with asymptomatic human T cell lymphotropic virus (HTLV)–I infection.

PATHOGENESIS. Adult worms and larvae penetrating the upper small bowel cause an enteritis characterized histopathologically by eosinophil and mononuclear cell infiltration of the lamina propria. Edema and mucosal atrophy are present on gross examination. Ulcerative lesions with hemorrhages are present in the most severe cases. Filariform larvae in the lungs elicit an inflammatory response in the alveoli consisting of mononuclear cells and eosinophils. In hyperinfection syndrome, these may coalesce and result in alveolar hemorrhage.

Autoinfection leading to exceptionally high worm loads (hyperinfection) and disseminated strongyloidiasis occur in persons with deficient cell-mediated immunity. Groups at risk include persons who are chronically taking corticosteroids, renal transplant recipients, patients with Hodgkin's disease and other lymphomas, and leukemic patients. Because *S. stercoralis* may persist and remain asymptomatic for decades after exposure (e.g., in military veterans who were imprisoned in the South Pacific during World War II), it is important to keep in mind that a change in immune status may convert a previously asymptomatic infection to hyperinfection. Surprisingly, there is no clear-cut evidence that persons with acquired immunodeficiency syndrome (AIDS) have a propensity to develop disseminated strongyloidiasis, despite a higher frequency of infection in homosexual men.

CLINICAL MANIFESTATIONS. More than 50 per cent of immunocompetent infected persons are asymptomatic. The frequency of clinical manifestations among infected immunocompromised subjects is not known.

Signs and symptoms of *S. stercoralis* infection are attributable to the presence of adult worms in the upper gastrointestinal tract and larval invasion and attendant host pathologic responses in the lung, skin, and aberrant sites of migration, such as the brain, eyes, pancreas, and kidney. Immunocompetent individuals rarely develop signs or symptoms attributable to larval migration outside the gut.

Gastrointestinal disease usually manifests as abdominal bloating, vague epigastric pain, and diarrhea with nausea. Symptoms are exacerbated by eating. Hematochezia and melena occur in fewer than 20 per cent of subjects with intestinal strongyloidiasis. Major causes of morbidity related to *S. stercoralis* infection of the intestine are paralytic ileus, small bowel obstruction, and a malabsorption syndrome.

Pulmonary signs and symptoms in immunocompromised persons with hyperinfection syndrome are similar to those seen in the adult respiratory distress syndrome, i.e., acute onset of dyspnea, productive cough, and hemoptysis. These are accompanied by fever, tachypnea, hypoxemia, and respiratory alkalosis. *Strongyloides* larvae may also invade the central nervous system, pancreas, eye, and so on and cause signs and symptoms attributable to tissue destruction in these sites.

Dermatologic manifestations include self-limited creeping eruption and, more commonly, larva currens. The latter is due to migration of filariform larvae produced by a process of external autoinfection as described above. The larvae elicit serpiginous erythematous papules and occasionally urticaria around the buttocks, upper thigh, and lower abdomen. The lesions migrate approximately 10 cm per hour. Larva currens has been noted among former prisoners of war in the South Pacific.

DIAGNOSIS. The unequivocal diagnosis of *S. stercoralis* infection is dependent on identification of larvae in host tissues or gastrointestinal and pulmonary secretions. The existence of filariform larvae in stools implies an active autoinfection.

Intestinal strongyloidiasis is most easily diagnosed by identification of parasites in direct smears of freshly passed stools. Rhabditiform larvae are 225 to 380 μm in length. Repeated examinations and concentration of stools increase the sensitivity of this method from approximately 25 to 80 per cent. Examination of fluid obtained by duodenal aspiration or passage of a swallowed string into the upper small bowel may also be used if stool examinations are negative. Serologic tests are sensitive but not generally available. The differential diagnosis of intestinal *S. stercoralis* infection includes sprue, peptic ulcer, regional enteritis, and ulcerative colitis.

Hyperinfection syndrome and disseminated strongyloidiasis are diagnosed by identification of filariform larvae (500 to 600 μm in length) in gastrointestinal secretions, as described above, or in pulmonary tissues, secretions, or washings, such as those obtained by bronchoalveolar lavage or in sputum. Larvae have also been recovered from cerebrospinal fluid, peritoneal washings, kidneys, urine, skin, and brains of immunocompromised persons.

Accompanying laboratory abnormalities frequently include eosinophilia. However, eosinophilia may not develop in immunocompromised hosts. Lack of eosinophilia is therefore not helpful in excluding strongyloidiasis in the differential diagnosis. The differential diagnosis of hyperinfection and disseminated strongyloidiasis includes overwhelming bacterial or fungal sepsis.

COMPLICATIONS. Disseminated strongyloidiasis is frequently accompanied by fungal or bacterial sepsis. Gram-negative enterococcal and polymicrobial septicemia has been observed. These infections likely result from translocation of gut organisms by migrating larvae.

TREATMENT. Uncomplicated intestinal strongyloidiasis should be treated with thiabendazole (25 mg per kilogram of body weight twice daily for 2 days with a maximum of 3 grams per day). Parasitologic cure rates are greater than 90 per cent. Thiabendazole at the same daily dosage should be given to immunocompromised patients with hyperinfection syndrome (i.e., pulmonary disease) or disseminated disease. The drug should be continued for a minimum of 5 to 7 days, although 1 to 2 weeks may be required if organ dysfunction and larval recovery persist. Symptomatic improvement and failure to detect larvae in gastrointestinal secretions or other sites are indicative of cure. Corticosteroids and other immunosuppressive agents should be discontinued when possible.

PREVENTION. Infection is preventable by avoiding skin contact with contaminated soil. Immunocompromised patients in endemic areas should be advised to avoid walking barefoot. Persons residing in endemic areas who are to become immunosuppressed (e.g., for renal transplantation) should have their stools examined three times for the presence of larvae, and they should be treated if the examination is positive. Because infected individuals may be incorrectly categorized as uninfected by this test, it is suggested by some authorities that prophylactic thiabendazole (25 mg per kilogram of body weight daily for 2 days) be given in the month preceding iatrogenic immunosuppression. Positive serology for *S. stercoralis* is also an indication for thiabendazole administration prior to immunosuppression.

Cook GC: *Strongyloides stercoralis* hyperinfection syndrome: How often is it missed? Q J Med 64:625, 1987. *Discusses in detail the differential diagnosis and pitfalls in diagnosis of strongyloidiasis in the immunocompromised host.*

Neva FA: Biology and immunology of human strongyloidiasis. J Infect Dis 153:397, 1987. *An overview of the biology of* Strongyloides stercoralis *and utility of serodiagnostic tests.*

DeVault GA Jr, King JW, Rohr MS, et al.: Opportunistic infection with *Strongyloides stercoralis* in renal transplantation. Rev Infect Dis 12:653, 1990. *Excellent discussion of clinical presentation and management of hyperinfection in immunocompromised hosts.*

Genta RM: Global prevalence of strongyloidiasis: Critical review with epidemiologic insights into the prevention of disseminated disease. Rev Infect Dis 11:755, 1989. *Well-balanced synthesis of the validity of multiple epidemiologic surveys of strongyloidiasis in the United States and other areas of the world.*

437 Filariasis

437.1 INTRODUCTION

Eric A. Ottesen

Eight filarial parasites commonly infect humans (Table 437–1), but three are responsible for most of the pathology associated with these infections. These are the lymphatic dwelling filariae *Wuchereria bancrofti* and *Brugia malayi* and the subcutaneous filarid *Onchocerca volvulus.*

All eight species are transmitted by biting arthropods (Table 437–1) and go through complex life cycles that include a slow maturation phase of 3 to 18 months from the time infective larvae are introduced by the vector until the adult worms mature and reside in the lymph nodes, subcutaneous tissue, or body cavities. The offspring of these adults (microfilariae) are 200 to 300 μm long and 5 to 7 μm wide. They either circulate in the blood or migrate through the skin, awaiting ingestion by the appropriate arthropod in which they develop over 1 to 2 weeks to infective forms capable of initiating this life cycle again. Adult worms are long lived (probably up to 15 years), while microfilariae probably live about 6 months. Patent infection is generally not established unless exposure to infective larvae is intense and prolonged, and manifestations of disease usually develop slowly.

Diagnosis can be extremely difficult because in endemic populations it relies almost exclusively on parasitologic techniques to demonstrate microfilariae in the blood or tissue, and at present, there are no completely satisfactory methods for making a definitive diagnosis in states of "amicrofilaremic filariasis" (before or after the microfilaremic state). When microfilariae circulate in the blood, they do so with or without a distinct periodicity (Table 437–1). Some are garbed in sheaths while others are sheathless. These two features, as well as other more subtle morphologic distinctions, are helpful diagnostically. Microfilariae can be identified either by direct observation of Giemsa-stained blood smears or, more sensitively, by concentration techniques using Knott's method (examination of centrifuged sediment after mixing 1 ml of blood with 9 ml of 2 per cent formalin) or membrane filtration of 1 ml or more of blood through a 3-μm or 5-μm pore Nuclepore membrane filter. Skin microfilariae are best sought by performing skin snips either as described in Ch. 437.4 or using a corneal-scleral biopsy punch. Antibody detection, although helpful in certain situations, is generally nondiagnostic because it cannot differentiate current from past infection or exposure and because of antigenic cross-reactivity between the filariae and other helminth parasites.

Diethylcarbamazine (DEC)* has been the single mainstay of treatment for all filarial infections since the late 1940's; however, it shows variable effectiveness for the different conditions. The new drug ivermectin,† because of greater efficacy and fewer side effects, has replaced DEC as the drug of choice for onchocerciasis; it is currently under evaluation for use in lymphatic and other filariases. Suramin,† although extremely toxic, is also used for onchocerciasis.

Filariasis. Ciba Found Symp: 127:305, 1987. *A multiauthored compendium of the current forefronts of understanding in most aspects of the filarial diseases.*

Greene BM: Onchocerciasis. *In* Warren KS, Mahmoud AA (eds.): Tropical and Geographic Medicine. 2nd ed. New York, McGraw-Hill, 1990, pp 429–439. *Detailed clinical, parasitologic, and epidemiologic discussion of onchocercal infection and the new developments in its treatment and control.*

Ottesen EA: The filariases and tropical eosinophilia. *In* Warren KS, Mahmoud AA (eds.): Tropical and Geographical Medicine. 2nd ed. New York, McGraw-Hill, 1990, pp 407–429. *Detailed clinical, parasitologic, and epidemiologic discussion of filarial disease.*

---

*Not commercially available in the United States but may be obtained in special circumstances from Lederle Laboratories, Pearl River, NY.

†Available from the Centers for Disease Control, Parasitic Disease Drug Service, Atlanta, GA.

437.2 LYMPHATIC FILARIASIS

Eric A. Ottesen

ETIOLOGY. There are three lymphatic-dwelling filarial parasites of humans, *Wuchereria bancrofti*, *Brugia malayi*, and *Brugia timori*. Adult worms are threadlike in form (2 to 10 cm

TABLE 437–1. THE COMMON FILARIAL PARASITES OF HUMANS

Species	Distribution	Vector	Primary Pathology	Microfilariae Primary Location	Periodicity	Presence of Sheath
Wuchereria bancrofti	Tropics worldwide	Mosquitoes	Lymphatic, pulmonary	Blood, hydrocele fluid	Nocturnal, subperiodic	+
Brugia malayi	Southeast Asia	Mosquitoes	Lymphatic, pulmonary	Blood	Nocturnal, subperiodic	+
Brugia timori	Indonesia	Mosquitoes	Lymphatic	Blood	Nocturnal	+
Onchocerca volvulus	Africa; Central and South America	Black fly	Skin, eye, lymphatic	Skin, eye	None or minimal	−
Loa loa	Africa	Horse fly	Allergic	Blood	Diurnal	+
Mansonella perstans	Africa; South America	Midge	? Allergic	Blood	None	−
Mansonella streptocerca	Africa	Midge	Skin	Skin	None	−
Mansonella ozzardi	Central and South America	Midge	Vague	Blood	None	−

long by less than 0.4 cm wide) and usually reside in the lymph nodes or afferent lymphatic channels. The female worms produce large numbers of microfilariae (200 to 300 μm long), which circulate in the peripheral blood awaiting ingestion by mosquito intermediate hosts, which are necessary to continue the parasite's life cycle. After about 2 weeks in these mosquitoes, the microfilariae develop into infective third-stage larvae (L_3's). When infected mosquitoes feed, these L_3's leave the mosquito mouth parts and come to rest on the surface of the host's skin. Only if they manage to penetrate the skin through the puncture at the site of the bite can transmission be successful; after a further developmental period lasting as long as 4 to 12 months, adult worms can again be found in the lymphatic tissues, where they mate and produce another generation of microfilariae. The adult parasites may remain viable in the human host for decades.

EPIDEMIOLOGY. For *W. bancrofti*, humans are the only definitive host and thus the natural reservoir for infection. Indeed, considerable experimental effort to establish the parasite in a wide variety of mammalian hosts has met with minimal success. *W. bancrofti* is found throughout the tropics and subtropics, including areas of South America and the Caribbean, Africa, Asia, and the Pacific. Two forms of the parasite are distinguished by the periodicity of their circulating microfilariae. Nocturnally periodic forms have microfilariae detectable in peripheral blood primarily at night, whereas in the subperiodic forms the microfilariae are usually present in the blood at all hours but with maximal levels often in the late afternoon. Generally, subperiodic bancroftian filariasis is found only in the Pacific islands east of 160 degrees E longitude (including New Caledonia, Fiji, Samoa, Ellis and Cook Islands, Society Islands, and the Marquesas); elsewhere *W. bancrofti* is nocturnally periodic. The natural vectors are *Culex fatigans* in urban settings and usually anopheline or aedean mosquitoes in rural areas.

The distribution of brugian filariasis is much more restricted, being limited primarily to parts of Malaysia, Indonesia, India, China, Korea, the Philippines, and Japan. Again, there are both nocturnally periodic and subperiodic forms of the parasite. The former is more common and is transmitted in coastal rice fields primarily by mansonian and anopheline mosquitoes; mansonian mosquitoes, found in swamp forests, are the major vectors of the subperiodic form. Unlike *W. bancrofti*, *B. malayi* can be a natural infection of cats and can be established in a number of laboratory animals. *B. timori* has been described from only two Indonesian islands.

PATHOLOGY. Most of the pathology of bancroftian and brugian filariasis is initiated in the lymphatics. Although details of the pathogenesis are lacking, the progression of pathologic changes is clear. Damaged lymphatics lead first to reversible lymphedema and then to chronic obstructive changes (elephantiasis) in the limbs, breasts, or genitalia, or to chyluria. The location of lymphatic damage determines the site and type of pathology expressed.

Adult worms, residing in the afferent approaches or cortical sinuses of the lymph nodes, induce local reactions by undefined mechanisms that result in dilatation of the lymphatics and hypertrophy of the vessel walls. Endothelial and connective tissue proliferation leads to polypoid growths that protrude into the lymphatic lumen, but even while the vessels remain patent, normal lymphatic function is not ensured. Indeed, lymphangiographic studies have clearly documented the development of a characteristic tortuosity of the lymph vessels with loss of valvular function and backflow of lymph leading to lymph stasis and lymphedema even during this "preobliterative phase."

Because of a still undefined interplay between the host immune system and the parasite, local inflammatory and granulomatous reactions subsequently develop around the adult worms, with infiltration of plasma cells, eosinophils, and giant cells. Fibrosis occurs, and the fragmented parasites are either completely resorbed or partially calcified. Lymphatic obstruction develops, and associated endophlebitis may further complicate the lymphatic obstruction. Although there is subsequent formation of collateral lymphatics and some recanalization of obstructed vessels, lymphatic function remains compromised. Repeated infection with increasing host response to the parasite leads to the chronic changes of advanced elephantiasis.

CLINICAL MANIFESTATIONS. Though previously not well recognized, a major distinction exists between the clinical presentation of lymphatic filariasis in individuals native to the endemic regions (whose exposures have been lifelong) and that of those entering such areas and meeting the infection for the first time. In these latter (e.g., long-term visitors, military personnel, settlers) the most common presentations are localized inflammatory reactions, especially adenolymphangitis, and evidence of immediate hypersensitivity responses to the parasites (i.e., urticaria, eosinophilia, and immunoglobulin E [IgE] elevations). Only rarely do such individuals present with the contrasting set of findings characteristic of the infection in those native to the endemic areas, i.e., asymptomatic microfilaremia, "filarial fevers," lymphatic obstruction, and, less commonly, the tropical pulmonary eosinophilia syndrome (Ch. 437.3).

Patients manifesting asymptomatic microfilaremia rarely come to the physician's attention except through an incidental finding of microfilariae in the peripheral blood smear during mass surveys in endemic regions, or when blood eosinophilia leads to a diagnostic evaluation for filariasis. Such asymptomatic persons appear to be clinically unaffected by the parasites. Though unproven, it is likely that in some of these individuals the infections clear spontaneously, whereas the infections of others subsequently progress and become symptomatic, but what determines such clinical changes is unclear.

"Filarial fevers" are acute febrile episodes characterized by high temperature (often with shaking chills), lymphatic inflammation (i.e., lymphadenitis and lymphangitis), and transient local edema. They occur as often as 6 to 10 times per year in affected persons and usually last 3 to 7 days before subsiding spontaneously. The factors that initiate these episodes are unknown, but they are definitely parasite related. The lymphangitis characteristically develops in a retrograde fashion, extending peripherally *from* the draining node where the adult parasites reside. Regional nodes are enlarged and painful, and the entire lymphatic tract often becomes indurated and inflamed. Concomitant local thrombophlebitis is common. In brugian filariasis especially, a single local abscess may form along the inflamed lymphatic and subsequently rupture to the surface, leaving a characteristic scar. Neither the lymphatic inflammation nor the characteristic abscesses appear to be bacterially induced. Such lymphadenitis and lymphangitis occur in the upper and lower extremities with both bancroftian and brugian filariasis, but involvement of the genital lymphatics is almost exclusively a feature of *W. bancrofti* infection. Thus, acute *bancrofti* episodes may also involve funiculitis, epididymitis, scrotal pain, and tenderness. Patients with filarial fevers may be microfilaremic but more often are not.

As lymphatic damage progresses, the edema and anatomic distortion that were initially transient develop into the permanent changes of elephantiasis. Pitting edema yields to brawny edema, and both thickening of subcutaneous tissue and hyperkeratosis develop. Fissuring of the skin develops along with nodular and papillomatous hyperplastic changes. Superinfection (especially with the dermatophytes) becomes a problem. In addition, in bancroftian filariasis, obstructed genital lymphatics may lead to scrotal lymphedema or hydrocele, whereas obstruction of the retroperitoneal lymphatics can increase hydrostatic pressure in the renal lymphatics, causing their rupture into the renal pelvis or tubules and leading to chyluria. Characteristically, chyluria is intermittent, sometimes lasting for days or weeks before abating spontaneously and then recurring; often it is most prominent in the morning, after the patient first arises.

DIAGNOSIS. Definitive diagnosis of filariasis can be made only by the demonstration of parasites, either adult worms associated with the lymphatics (rarely observed) or microfilariae in the blood, hydrocele fluid, or chylous urine. These fluids can be examined directly (20 cu mm on a slide with or without red blood cell lysis), after concentration of the parasites by centrifugation in 2 per cent formalin (Knott's technique), or after filtration through a membrane (3- to 5-μm Nuclepore) filter. The time of blood collection should take into account the parasite's possible nocturnal periodicity.

Because many persons with filariasis (especially those with chronic pathology) are not microfilaremic, diagnosis must often be made clinically. The differential diagnosis is broad but in the acute episodes primarily includes thrombophlebitis, infection, and trauma. The edema and other lymphatic obstructive changes associated with chronic filariasis must be distinguished from the manifestations of congestive heart failure, malignant disease, trauma, postsurgical scarring, and a number of less common congenital and idiopathic abnormalities of the lymphatic system. The many disorders associated with serum immunoglobulin E (IgE) and blood eosinophil elevations must be considered in evaluating asymptomatic filarial infections. Several specific points may help in this differential diagnosis: (1) Exposure to filariae must be prolonged or intense (for at least several months) before persons become infected; (2) the physical finding or history of *retrograde* lymphangitis can often aid in distinguishing filarial from bacterial lymphangitis; (3) although lymphadenopathy is characteristic of filariasis, alone it is never diagnostic; (4) lymphangiographic patterns of elephantiasis and chyluria are well defined, so that even though not always diagnostic, lymphangiography is sometimes useful in distinguishing filarial from congenital or neoplastic lymphatic abnormalities; (5) although total serum IgE and blood eosinophil levels are often elevated in filarial infections, they cannot distinguish filarial from other helminth infections except in the case of the tropical eosinophilia syndrome (see Ch. 437.3); and (6) because most residents of endemic regions have been immunologically "sensitized" to filarial antigens through years of bites by infected mosquitoes and because filarial antigens cross-react extensively with those of other nematode parasites, positive results in the numerous serologic and skin tests that have been developed are of little diagnostic value *except* in those individuals who are not native to endemic areas.

TREATMENT. Available chemotherapy for lymphatic filariasis is both limited and inadequate. Diethylcarbamazine* (DEC, 6 mg per kilogram per day given in single or divided doses for 2 to 3 weeks) rapidly kills microfilariae in vivo, but its effect on adult parasites is less dramatic. Thus, following treatment with DEC, although the blood is temporarily free of microfilariae, the infection itself has often not been terminated, and several courses of DEC or long-term intermittent treatment with low doses of DEC are often required to kill the adult parasites. Early trials with ivermectin† in bancroftian and brugian filariasis indicate excellent effectiveness in clearing microfilaremia after a single oral dose, but its effects on adult parasites and its optimal dosing schedules are still under study.

Side effects of DEC treatment, although not so frequent or severe as those seen in onchocerciasis, can be troublesome, especially in brugian filariasis. These include fever, chills, headache, dizziness, nausea, vomiting, and arthralgias, all usually occurring in the first 24 to 36 hours. Both the likelihood of developing such reactions and the degree of their severity are directly related to the number of circulating microfilariae. Thus, the side effects of DEC administration at these dosage levels are due not to direct drug toxicity but to allergic or immunologic responses of the host to dying parasites. To avoid these reactions in highly parasitemic persons, one can initiate treatment with very small doses of DEC or premedicate the patients with steroids, as suggested for onchocerciasis (see Ch. 437.4). A very few patients may also develop filarial fever episodes with lymphangitis and lymphadenitis in the first days after DEC treatment. All of these side effects occur early in treatment and generally subside even with continued administration of the drug.

Severe chronic lymphatic damage has recently been shown to have a surprising degree of reversibility. All such affected patients should receive long-term low-dose DEC (to eradicate persistent or new filarial infections) and diligent attention to local care of the lymphedematous extremity through limb elevation, use of special massage techniques and elastic stockings, and prevention of superficial bacterial and fungal infection. More severely affected patients may benefit remarkably from surgical decompression of the lymphatic system through "nodovenous shunt" surgery followed by excision of redundant tissue. Hydroceles can be repeatedly drained or managed surgically. Chyluria also can sometimes be corrected surgically, but, interestingly, many cases have been reported in which diagnostic lymphangiography itself appears to have terminated the leak of chyle into the urine, probably as a result of its sclerosing effects.

PREVENTION. DEC kills developing preadult forms of many filarial species, and its value as a prophylactic agent in humans (10 mg per kilogram on 2 consecutive days each month) has recently been established. In addition, for public health programs DEC has been used successfully as a protective measure to reduce infection rates in selected populations. Because of its microfilaricidal effects, small doses administered intermittently (or even as an additive to common table salt) to all residents of an endemic region‡ (e.g., 3 mg per kilogram monthly) reduce the number of bloodborne microfilariae in the community to levels so low that successful transmission of the infection by mosquitoes cannot occur. Other approaches to filariasis control designed to eradicate the mosquito vectors have also proved effective for the short term but have been difficult to sustain.

Filariasis. Ciba Found Symp 127:305 1987. *A multiauthored compendium of the current forefronts of understanding in most aspects of the filarial diseases.*

Ottesen EA: Efficacy of diethylcarbamazine in eradicating infection with lymphatic-dwelling filariae in humans. Rev Infect Dis 7:341, 1985. *A thorough review of observations from the literature, finally concluding that the more DEC administered (preferably over an extended period), the greater the likelihood that lymphatic filarial infections will be eradicated.*

Ottesen EA: Filariasis now. Am J Trop Med Hyg 41(Suppl):9, 1989. *A review of recent advances in our understanding of the immunopathogenesis, diagnosis, and treatment of lymphatic filarial infections.*

World Health Organization: Lymphatic pathology and immunopathology in filariasis: Report of the twelfth meeting of the scientific working group on filariasis. TDR/FIL-SWG(12)/85.3, 1986, p 33. *A report available through WHO that summarizes the most recent advances in understanding the pathogenesis and optimal management of the consequences of filaria-induced lymphatic obstruction.*

---

‡This use is not listed in the manufacturer's directive.

437.3 TROPICAL EOSINOPHILIA

Eric A. Ottesen

Tropical eosinophilia is a syndrome of acute and chronic lung disease first defined in the 1940's but not generally recognized as being of filarial etiology until the 1960's. Its main clinical features are a history of residence in a filaria-endemic region; paroxysmal cough and wheezing, which generally occur at night; scanty sputum production; occasional weight loss, low-grade fever, and adenopathy; and extreme blood eosinophilia (>3000 per microliter). It is more common in men than in women. Chest roentgenograms can be normal but generally show increased bronchovascular markings, diffuse interstitial lesions, or mottled opacities primarily involving the mid and lower lung fields. Tests of pulmonary function almost always indicate restrictive abnormalities and usually obstructive defects as well. The association of the syndrome with filarial infection was first recognized by finding very high levels of antifilarial antibody in these patients and by noting the favorable response to treatment with antifilarial drugs (now diethylcarbamazine* [DEC], 6 to 10 mg per kilogram per day for 3 to 4 weeks). Later, several reports described microfilariae or their degenerating remnants in lung biopsy specimens. Most recently, extremely high levels of total serum IgE (usually 10,000 to 100,000 ng per milliliter) have been found in these patients, and an appreciable fraction of this IgE has been shown to be directed against filarial antigens.

Because of these and other findings, tropical eosinophilia is now considered a form of "occult filariasis" in which host immunologic hyperresponsiveness to the parasite results in such rapid clearance of microfilariae from the blood that this stage of the parasite is essentially never detectable. Generally, this microfilarial clearance takes place in the lungs, and the clinical symptoms appear to result largely from the allergic and inflammatory reactions elicited by the cleared parasites. In some subjects, however, trapping of the microfilariae occurs predominantly in

---

*Not commercially available in the United States but may be obtained in special circumstances from Lederle Laboratories, Pearl River, NY.

†Available in the United States from the Centers for Disease Control, Atlanta, GA.

---

*Not commercially available in the United States but may be obtained in special circumstances from Lederle Laboratories, Pearl River, NY.

other organs of the reticuloendothelial system (liver, spleen, lymph nodes), and in these persons the major clinical manifestations are those resulting from hepatomegaly, splenomegaly, or lymphadenopathy. It has been postulated that infection with nonhuman filarial parasites is the major cause of tropical eosinophilia. Almost certainly, however, the syndrome is caused not by an "abnormal parasite" but rather by an abnormal host response to those same parasites (*Wuchereria bancrofti* and *Brugia malayi*) that commonly cause lymphatic filariasis (see Ch. 437.2). In this respect, tropical eosinophilia may be similar to another pulmonary eosinophilic disorder, allergic bronchopulmonary aspergillosis, both in its clinical expression and in its pathogenesis (see Ch. 406).

Diagnosis depends primarily on distinguishing tropical eosinophilia from the other important eosinophilic syndromes with pulmonary involvement, namely, Löffler's syndrome, chronic eosinophilic pneumonia, allergic aspergillosis, certain vasculitic syndromes, the idiopathic hypereosinophilia syndrome, drug allergies, and some helminth infections. Although there is no one clinical or laboratory criterion that will distinguish tropical eosinophilia from these other conditions, a history of residence in the tropics, high levels of specific filarial antibodies, and a response to DEC therapy are the most helpful differential points. Within 3 to 7 days after initiation of DEC, there is almost always marked improvement or disappearance of symptoms. Resolution may not be complete, however, and relapse may occur months to years later and require retreatment. DEC will not, of course, reverse permanent pulmonary damage (primarily an interstitial fibrosis), which frequently develops prior to successful diagnosis and treatment of the disorder.

Pinkston P, Vijayan VK, Nutman TB, et al.: Tropical pulmonary eosinophilia: Characterization of the lower respiratory tract inflammation and its response to therapy. J Clin Invest 80:216,1987. *Clinical and bronchoalveolar lavage studies probing the pathologic and immunopathologic mechanisms of the pulmonary pathology in this disorder.*

Rom WN, Vijayan VK, Cornelius MJ, et al.: Persistent lower respiratory tract inflammation associated with interstitial lung disease in patients with tropical pulmonary eosinophilia following conventional treatment with diethylcarbamazine. Am Rev Respir Dis 142:1088, 1990. *Bronchoalveolar lavage evidence that despite 3 weeks of DEC treatment (6 mg per kilogram per day), there was a persistent low-grade eosinophilic alveolitis in most patients 6 to 36 months after treatment; the recommendation for alternative treatment regimens is made.*

437.4 ONCHOCERCIASIS (River Blindness)

Bruce M. Greene

Onchocerciasis is a disease, most commonly manifest by skin and ocular damage, resulting from chronic infection with the filarial parasite *Onchocerca volvulus*.

ETIOLOGY. Onchocerciasis is a vector-borne disease, transmitted from person to person by the bite of the black fly, *Simulium* species. The female black fly ingests microfilariae from the skin of an infected person while taking a blood meal. Within the vector, microfilariae develop into infective larvae over a period of 6 to 8 days, and these larvae are transmitted to another person when the fly bites again. Over a period of several months, the larvae undergo a series of transformations leading to the development of adult worms that coil up into spherical bundles located in the subcutaneous tissues and deeper fascial planes. After a prepatent period of 9 to 18 months, the adult male and female worms reproduce sexually to yield millions of microfilariae that migrate through the skin and ocular tissues.

Microfilariae are highly motile, are unsheathed, and measure 210 to 320 μm in length and 6 to 9 μm in width. Infective larvae measure approximately 600 μm in length and in the human host undergo a molt to stage 4 larvae after a period of several days. Adult female worms are 23 to 70 cm in length, while the males are 3 to 6 cm long and weigh only 1 per cent as much as the female.

The lifespan of the adult worm in humans is known not to exceed 18 years, and the average survival is probably 8 to 10 years.

PREVALENCE AND EPIDEMIOLOGY. *Onchocerca volvulus* infects an estimated 20 to 40 million persons, principally in equatorial Africa in a broad belt extending from the Atlantic coast on the west to the Red Sea and Indian Ocean on the east. In the Western Hemisphere, the major focus is in Guatemala, on the Pacific slope of the Sierra Madre. Additional foci exist in Yemen, southwestern Saudi Arabia, southern Mexico, Venezuela, and northwestern Brazil, Colombia, and Ecuador.

Endemicity of *O. volvulus* in human populations is dependent upon habitation of fly-infested areas by sufficient, but not excessive, numbers of people who are exposed to human-biting flies during daily activities such as farming, fishing, bathing and washing, and water collection. Black flies deposit eggs on vegetation, rocks, sticks, and debris in freely flowing streams and rivers, and these develop into larvae and pupae that attach to vegetation and continuously filter the water to obtain oxygen and nutrients. Because of the dependency of the fly on waterways for reproduction, flies concentrate around streams and rivers. As a result, infection in human populations and disease tend to be similarly distributed; hence the term *river blindness*. The vector usually flies only a few kilometers from waterways but may fly as many as 20.

Approximately 1 to 4 per cent of infected persons become blind, and onchocerciasis ranks as the fourth leading cause of blindness in humans. In hyperendemic areas, more than one half of adults become blind. A much higher percentage of persons develop skin disease and/or some ocular involvement. Because blindness or serious ocular involvement, or severe debility resulting from skin disease, typically occurs during the third and fourth decades of life, the impact of the disease on the community is particularly devastating, frequently incapacitating the heads of households.

PATHOLOGY AND PATHOGENESIS. The disease affects primarily the skin, lymph nodes, and ocular tissues. In the skin, histopathology reflects a low-grade chronic inflammatory process. The end stage shows loss of elastic fibers, atrophy, and fibrosis. The onchocercomata, which are fibrous subcutaneous nodules containing adult worms, show a rim of chronic inflammation with fibrosis and extensive capillary infiltration surrounding the worms themselves. Lymph nodes show chronic inflammatory changes and, in some cases, fibrosis and atrophy. In the eye, neovascularization and scarring of the cornea lead to loss of transparency and blindness. The remainder of the eye is frequently involved by a chronic nongranulomatous inflammatory process that leads to anterior uveitis and associated chronic complications, chorioretinitis with damage to the retinal pigment epithelium, and optic atrophy.

The basis for the pathologic changes of onchocerciasis is believed to be the host reaction to chronic infestation with microfilariae. A multiplicity of factors appears to contribute to the pathologic changes; these include toxic or tissue-altering products of host granulocytes and lymphoid cells, which are reacting to the parasite, and perhaps products of the microfilariae themselves.

CLINICAL MANIFESTATIONS. The earliest signs of infection include pruritus and intermittent papular rash with some thickening of the skin, which may be localized to one area of the body, and conjunctivitis. In nonresidents of endemic areas, who are usually lightly infected, these are frequently the only manifestations. Onchocercomata are firm, 0.5- to 3-cm subcutaneous nodules that are nontender and freely movable if not attached to periosteum. These frequently occur in clusters that can be disfiguring. Common locations include the skin overlying bony prominences, including the superior iliac crests, the coccyx, the greater trochanter of the femur, the bony thorax, and the scalp and head region. With chronic infection, permanent skin changes occur, including loss of elasticity, a chronic, scaling hyperkeratotic maculopapular pruritic rash with mottled hypopigmentation or hyperpigmentation, and, finally, atrophy, leading in some cases to areas of breakdown with the risk of superinfection. Chronic skin manifestations are unpredictably punctuated by transient episodes of localized rash, erythema, and edema. In Central America the dermal manifestations are most prominent around the head and neck, while in Africa they more commonly involve the trunk, buttocks, and lower extremities. Lymph node involvement is usually manifested by enlargement, particularly in the inguinal and femoral regions, and in some cases by secondary obstructive changes in the groin region or in an extremity. Early ocular manifestations include punctate keratitis and anterior uveitis. Chronic changes include sclerosing keratitis, chorioretinitis (which leads to progressive constriction of visual fields), optic atrophy, and complications due to persistent anterior uveitis, including meiosis, pupillary distortion, and glaucoma. In general, the severity of disease correlates with intensity and duration of infection.

DIAGNOSIS. The diagnosis can be made clinically by the presence of onchocercomata, typical skin changes, or eye findings of onchocerciasis, including microfilariae in the cornea or anterior chamber in otherwise normal-appearing eyes. The diagnosis is confirmed by finding microfilariae of *O. volvulus* in the skin of the patient. This is done by biopsy, using a corneoscleral biopsy instrument or a razor blade, to yield approximately 1 to 2 mg of skin, including superficial dermis. The skin is weighed and incubated in tissue culture medium or saline, and the microfilariae that emerge are counted after a 3-hour or overnight incubation. These must be distinguished from the smaller *Mansonella streptocerca* microfilariae. The skin-snipping technique has the inherent advantage of providing a measure of intensity of infection, with fewer than 10 microfilariae per milligram of skin constituting a light infection and greater than 100, a heavy infection. For greatest reliability, four to six biopsies are done in different areas, including the hips, calves, and shoulders. Although elevated titers of antifilarial antibodies may support the diagnosis of onchocerciasis, a definitive immunodiagnostic technique has not yet been developed.

TREATMENT. Ivermectin,* a newly developed semisynthetic macrocyclic lactone, is now the drug of choice to treat onchocerciasis. The dosage is 150 μg per kilogram, given in a single dose on an empty stomach, once every year or every 6 months. The retreatment interval depends upon parasite burden, disease severity, and rapidity of recurrence of symptoms. Nonresidents of endemic countries often require more than once-a-year treatment because of rapid recurrence of pruritus in these hyperreactive individuals. Ivermectin should not be given to pregnant women, individuals with a serious central nervous system disorder or an acute illness, children less than 5 years of age or 15 kg in weight, and mothers who are nursing children within a week of delivery. Ivermectin causes killing of microfilariae but does not kill adult worms effectively. Therefore, retreatment is necessary over a period of years.

Diethylcarbamazine citrate† (DEC) was previously the standard drug used to treat onchocerciasis. Although well tolerated in uninfected persons, DEC frequently causes complications and side effects when given to individuals infected with *O. volvulus;* these complications appear to result in part from the massive killing of microfilariae that occurs over a few days after initiation of DEC therapy. This results in fever, intense pruritus, lymph node pain and swelling, prostration, hypotension, and arthralgias. In the eye, a worsening of ocular inflammation occurs transiently, and permanent sight-threatening lesions may occur in the posterior segment of the eye. In an effort to minimize these complications, patients should be given corticosteroids (e.g., prednisone 40 to 60 mg per day) starting the day before initiation of DEC therapy and continuing for 4 to 7 days as needed. DEC therapy should be started with a test dose of 25 to 50 mg and then increased to 4 mg per kilogram per day to complete a 10-day course. Because of the superior safety and tolerability of ivermectin, DEC should be reserved for persons who cannot be treated with ivermectin. Suramin, although it does kill adult worms, should *not* be used except in rare circumstances, as it is toxic and impractical.

Removal of nodules containing adult worms in the head region is indicated because of the increased risk of ocular involvement. Other palpable nodules should also be removed if feasible.

PROGNOSIS. With treatment, the early ocular and cutaneous changes are reversible, but for persons living in an endemic area, therapy must be given repeatedly, since neither DEC nor ivermectin is curative of the infection, and reinfection usually occurs continuously. The atrophic skin changes, sclerosing keratitis, and disease in the posterior segment of the eye are not helped by therapy.

PREVENTION. There is no proven chemoprophylaxis. Vector control is difficult and expensive but has achieved remarkable success in some areas of Africa. Protective clothing, insect repellents, and avoidance of areas harboring the vector are useful measures for visitors to endemic areas.

Anderson J, Fuglsang H, Hamilton PJS, et al.: Studies on onchocerciasis in the United Cameroon Republic: II. Comparison of onchocerciasis in rain-forest and sudan-savanna. Trans R Soc Trop Med Hyg 68:209, 1974. *Detailed analysis of clinical manifestations with comparison of forest and savanna types of disease.*

Greene BM, Dukuly ZD, Muñoz B, et al.: A comparison of 6, 12, and 24 monthly dosing with ivermectin for treatment of onchocerciasis. J Infect Dis 163:376, 1991. *Retreatment at 6-month, as opposed to yearly, intervals may provide an advantage in the first 1 to 2 years, but very little thereafter.*

Greene BM, Taylor HR, Cupp EW, et al.: Comparison of ivermectin and diethylcarbamazine in the treatment of onchocerciasis. N Engl J Med 313:133, 1985. *Shows that ivermectin is better tolerated, more effective, and safer than diethylcarbamazine.*

WHO Expert Committee on Onchocerciasis: Third Report. Technical Report Series No. 752. Geneva, World Health Organization, 1987. *Comprehensive summary of the disease and its distribution and impact.*

437.5 LOIASIS

Eric A. Ottesen

Loa loa is indigenous only to the rain forest belt of western and central Africa. Mature female parasites, about twice the size of the males, are 50 to 70 mm long and 0.5 mm wide. They live wandering through the subcutaneous tissue in humans, usually attracting attention only when they cross the eye subconjunctivally. The sheathed microfilariae produced by these females circulate with a diurnal periodicity that peaks at about noon.

Clinical loiasis presents in two primary forms, one more common among individuals native to endemic regions and the other more common in visitors to these areas who acquire infection. Among the natives, loiasis is often entirely asymptomatic until an adult worm appears moving across the eye or blood examination reveals microfilaremia. Such individuals may also have occasional episodes of Calabar swellings. These are characteristic localized areas of erythema and angioedema (up to 5 to 10 cm in diameter) that occur primarily on the extremities and last 1 to 3 days before regressing spontaneously. These swellings appear to be a hypersensitivity reaction to the adult worm, whose presence can also be detected in some patients by either a subcutaneous crawling sensation or the appearance of a fine vermiform hive in the skin. When the inflammation extends to nearby joints or peripheral nerves, corresponding symptoms may develop. Rarely, nephropathy (probably immune complex mediated) and encephalopathy have been reported.

The major difference between this presentation and that seen in outsiders who acquire infection is the greater predominance of allergic or hyperreactive symptoms in the latter. Episodes of angioedema are likely to be more frequent and debilitating, and patients are much less likely to have microfilariae in the blood. In addition, they often present with extensive blood eosinophilia (30 to 60 per cent of an elevated total leukocyte count), much like patients with tropical eosinophilia (Ch. 437.3). Diagnosis in these patients often cannot be made parasitologically and must be based on the characteristic history, clinical presentation, blood eosinophilia, and elevated filarial antibody titers. If untreated, a small (but undefined) percentage of such patients develops severe cardiomyopathy, presumably secondary to the hypereosinophilia elicited by the infection.

Treatment is with diethylcarbamazine* ([DEC], 6 to 10 mg per kilogram per day for 2 to 3 weeks). The drug is extremely effective against microfilariae but less so against adult worms, so that multiple courses of treatment are often necessary before there is complete resolution of signs and symptoms. In cases of

---

*Available in the United States from the Centers for Disease Control, Atlanta, GA.

†Available in the United States from Lederle Laboratories, Pearl River, NY.

*Available in the United States from Lederle Laboratories, Pearl River, NY.

heavy microfilaremia (greater than several hundred microfilariae per milliliter of blood), allergic and other inflammatory side effects of treatment may be so severe that a regimen of 0.5 to 1.0 mg per kilogram DEC per dose (with or without simultaneous steroids) is safer for initiating treatment. DEC is effective in preventing loiasis when taken in prophylactic doses of 300 mg weekly.

Klion AD, Massougbodji A, Sadeler BC, et al.: Loiasis in endemic and non-endemic populations: Immunologically-mediated differences in clinical presentation. J Infect Dis, in press. *A clinical and immunological study contrasting the presentations of* Loa loa *infection in patients who have lived their entire lives in the endemic areas and patients who acquired their infections while visiting these areas.*

Nutman TB, Miller KD, Mulligan M, et al.: Diethylcarbamazine prophylaxis for human loiasis: Results of a double-blind study. N Engl J Med 319:752, 1988. *A placebo-controlled study in Peace Corps volunteers showing clearly that clinical loiasis can be prevented by weekly DEC in long-term visitors to endemic countries.*

437.6 DRACUNCULIASIS

Donald R. Hopkins

Dracunculiasis, or guinea worm disease, is caused by infection with the parasite *Dracunculus medinensis.* It occurs in the Indian subcontinent and Africa, where up to 5 million persons living in rural areas are thought to be affected annually and more than 100 million persons are at risk of infection.

Diagnosis of patent infections is easy. The thin adult female worms, each up to 1 meter long, emerge directly through the skin, usually of the lower leg, ankle, or foot. The worms emerge 10 to 14 months after victims have drunk water containing infected *Cyclops,* a barely visible crustacean that serves as the parasite's intermediate host. When persons harboring such emerging worms enter a stagnant source of drinking water, such as a step well or pond, larvae are released into the water, where some are ingested by *Cyclops.* When humans drink water containing *Cyclops* with infective larvae, the larvae penetrate the intestinal or stomach wall, mature, and mate, after which the male worms die.

The adult worms emerge slowly, over a period of weeks or months. Emergence may be preceded by generalized allergic symptoms and is usually accompanied by a blister that ruptures to form an ulcer at the site of emergence. Some worms present first as a serpentine cord just beneath the skin or at the center of an abscess. No immunity develops, so persons in endemic areas are infected year after year.

The great social and economic significance of dracunculiasis, which rarely is fatal, derives from the fact that emergence of the worm is very painful and is often associated with swelling, local arthritis, and secondary infection. Thus, victims are often unable to farm or sometimes even walk for weeks or months. Over half of the adults in a village may be crippled at the same time, and the seasonal infection tends to occur precisely when villagers need to harvest or plant their crops. School attendance is also affected.

Treatment is difficult because anthelminthics such as thiabendazole or metronidazole only marginally reduce the duration of emergence and associated pain. Aspirin can help relieve the pain. Emerging worms are best rolled around a small stick as their predecessors have been for centuries, care being taken not to break the worm (which would exacerbate the inflammation). Some worms can be removed surgically. Victims should be immunized against tetanus, which is sometimes caused by secondary infection of the ulcer around the emerging worm. Persons at risk should be taught to boil their drinking water or filter it through a cloth and to avoid entering sources of drinking water when the infection is patent.

Since the most effective intervention against this infection is to provide safe drinking water, efforts began during the International Drinking Water Supply and Sanitation Decade (1981–1990) to provide safe water to dracunculiasis-endemic areas as a priority and thereby eliminate the disease. By the end of 1990, India had reduced its reported dracunculiasis cases by 90 per cent, Pakistan had almost eliminated the disease altogether, and most of the remaining major endemic countries had begun programs to eradicate the disease by 1995.

Hopkins DR, Ruiz-Tiben E: Dracunculiasis Eradication: Target 1995. Am J Trop Med Hyg 43:296–300, 1990. *A recent review of all aspects pertaining to control and eradication of dracunculiasis.*

Muller R: *Dracunculus* and dracunculiasis. *In* Dawes B (ed.): Advances in Parasitology. Vol 9. New York, Academic Press, 1971, pp 73–151. *A thorough consideration of the parasite's biology, life cycle, and the disease it produces.*

437.7 OTHER FILARIAL INFECTIONS

Eric A. Ottesen

PERSTANS FILARIASIS

Mansonella perstans (formerly *Dipetalonema perstans, Acanthocheilonema perstans*) is distributed in a broad belt across the center of Africa and in northeast South America. Adult worms, up to 70 to 80 mm long, reside in the body cavities (pleural, peritoneal, and pericardial) and in the mesentery, perirenal, and retroperitoneal tissues. Microfilariae are liberated *unsheathed* from the females and circulate in the blood without regular periodicity.

M. perstans infection was long thought to be asymptomatic, because up to 90 per cent of individuals with the parasite appeared to have no difficulty with it. Subsequent studies, however, indicate clearly that *M. perstans* is capable of inducing a variety of symptoms, including angioedematous swellings much like the Calabar swellings of loiasis; fever; headache; pain in bursae and/or joint synovia, in serous cavities, or over the liver; neurologic or psychological symptoms; and extreme exhaustion. There is some evidence that symptoms are more prominent in outsiders coming to endemic regions, but in all series at least a quarter of the patients were asymptomatic despite persistent microfilaremia.

Treatment with diethylcarbamazine* ([DEC], 5 to 6 mg per kilogram per day for 2 to 3 weeks) is often ineffective, with multiple courses usually necessary to achieve cure. When the parasites are eliminated, however, patients characteristically lose their symptoms (no matter how vague), lose their eosinophilia, and regain a sense of well-being.

Adolph PE, Kagan IG, McQuay RM: Diagnosis and treatment of *Acanthocheilonema perstans* filariasis. Am J Trop Med Hyg 11:76, 1962. *Results from a series of patients observed in the United States after returning from missionary work in Africa.*

Clarke V deV, Harwin RM, MacDonald DF, et al.: Filariasis: *Dipetalonema perstans* infections in Rhodesia. Cent Afr J Med 17:1, 1971. *Discussion of the clinical expression of* M. perstans *filariasis in Africans and Europeans living in East Africa.*

STREPTOCERCIASIS

Mansonella streptocerca is transmitted by midges, especially *Culicoides grahami.* It occurs in the tropical forest belt of Africa from Ghana to Zaire. The adult worms are subcutaneous, especially over the torso; and the microfilariae, which have characteristic shepherd's-crook tails, are found in the skin (see Ch. 437.4 for skin-snipping technique).

Infection is usually symptomless, but the adult worms may produce hypopigmented macules (to be distinguished from leprosy), and the microfilariae occasionally cause itching papular rashes similar to those of onchocerciasis. Both adult worms and microfilariae are killed by diethylcarbamazine* (e.g., 7 to 10 days of treatment at 6 mg per kilogram per day).

Meyers WM, Connor DH, et al.: Human streptocerciasis: A clinicopathologic study of 40 Africans (Zairians) including identification of the adult filaria. Am J Trop Med Hyg 21:528, 1972. *Covers the clinical aspects and gives references to other aspects.*

MANSONELLA OZZARDI INFECTION

M. ozzardi is restricted in distribution to Central and South America and certain islands of the Caribbean. Adult worms have

---

*Not commercially available in the United States but may be obtained in special circumstances from Lederle Laboratories, Pearl River, NY.

been recovered in humans only twice, both times from the peritoneal cavity. *Unsheathed* microfilariae circulate in the blood with little or no periodicity.

Many investigators consider these parasites to be nonpathogenic, but in one of the fullest clinical studies of an affected population it was asserted that the major clinical presentation is severe articular pain or dysfunction, especially in the arms and shoulders. Headache, fever, pulmonary symptoms, adenopathy, hepatomegaly, and pruritic skin eruptions also occurred in a small number of patients with a frequency greater than that in nonparasitized individuals in the same population. Diethylcarbamazine* has little or no effect on this infection, but a single case report suggests that ivermectin† is effective therapy.

Marinkelle CJ, German E: Mansonelliasis in the comisaria del Vaupes of Colombia. Trop Geogr Med 22:101, 1970. *A very complete and interesting account of clinical manifestations ascribed to* M. ozzardi *infections in South American Indians.*

Nutman TB, Nash TE, Ottesen EA: Ivermectin in the successful treatment of a patient with *Mansonella ozzardi* infection. J Infect Dis 156:662, 1987. *A single case report presenting clinical and immunologic evidence for the effectiveness of ivermectin (140 μg per kilogram given once) in an* M. ozzardi *infection.*

HUMAN DIROFILARIASIS

Dirofilaria species are filarial parasites mostly of dogs, cats, and raccoons that sometimes infect humans but almost never fully develop to complete their life cycles in this abnormal host. The distribution of cases is worldwide and reflects the distribution of the parasites in animals.

Two general types of clinical presentation predominate. Pulmonary dirofilariasis, caused by the dog heartworm *D. immitis*, usually presents as an asymptomatic solitary pulmonary nodule but occasionally with chest pain, cough, or hemoptysis. Microscopically there is local eosinophilia and granuloma formation accompanied by infarction and thrombosis around an impacted, immature worm. The second common clinical presentation is that of a subcutaneous nodule found anywhere on the body (or within the eye) that results usually from infection with the subcutaneous dwelling filarids of dogs (*D. repens*) or raccoons (*D. tenuis*) but occasionally from infection with *D. immitis*. Local lesions again are granulomatous and eosinophilic and are sometimes accompanied by bacterial superinfection.

Definitive diagnosis and treatment most often result from the same surgical (excisional) procedure. Blood eosinophilia is not a regular finding in these patients nor are detectable antifilarial antibodies. Furthermore, since the worms are usually incompletely developed, microfilaremia occurs only in the rarest of circumstances. These "abnormal" parasite infections do not respond to DEC, and their treatment is primarily surgical.

Dissanaike AS: Zoonotic aspects of filarial infections in man. Bull WHO 57:349, 1979. *A scholarly, readable discussion of the human's interaction with zoonotic filarial infections.*

---

*Not commercially available in the United States but may be obtained in special circumstances from Lederle Laboratories, Pearl River, NY.

†Available in the United States from the Centers for Disease Control, Atlanta, GA.

---

438 Arthropods and Leeches

William L. Krinsky

ARTHROPODS AS AGENTS OF DISEASE

Disease associated directly with arthropods results from toxins, or allergic responses to the organisms or their products when humans are exposed by bites or stings, simple contact, or invasion through the skin or natural orifices. Arthropods most often involved in these types of exposure are listed in Table 438–1.

Physicians usually become aware of insects and their relatives (spiders, mites, ticks, scorpions, millipedes, and centipedes) when patients present with skin lesions caused by arthropods, when infestations of the creatures themselves are seen, when

TABLE 438–1. ARTHROPODS CAUSING HUMAN PATHOLOGY

Human Exposure	Arthropod	Antigens or Toxins
Bites	Insects (lice, bedbugs, and other true bugs; fleas; flies including mosquitoes, black flies, biting midges, sandflies, horse and deer flies, stable flies, tsetse flies, keds; ants)	Salivary secretions, venoms
	Arachnids (chigger and other rodent and bird mites; ticks; spiders)	
	Centipedes	
Stings	Insects (some ants, wasps, and bees)	Venoms
	Arachnids (scorpions)	
Invasion	Insects (fly larvae, *Tunga* fleas)	Salivary secretions, excretions
	Arachnids (scabies mites)	
Simple contact	Insects (caterpillars, pupae, or adults of moths and butterflies; blister and some rove beetles)	Setae, spines, secretions (venoms) and excretions
	Arachnids (stored product mites)	
	Millipedes	

foreign bodies extracted from skin or sense organs are identified as arthropods, or when respiratory symptoms develop in response to arthropods or their products. Dermatoses associated with arthropods and human infestations with arthropods (e.g., lice, mites, fly larvae) are discussed in detail in this chapter. Arthropods as vectors are mentioned here; detailed discussions of arthropod-borne pathogens may be found elsewhere in this book.

Alexander JO: Arthropods and Human Skin. Berlin, Springer-Verlag, 1984. *This is the first comprehensive text devoted to dermatologic problems associated with arthropods.*

Harwood RF, James MT: Entomology in Human and Animal Health. 7th ed. New York, The Macmillan Company, 1979. *This is a comprehensive textbook that provides detailed references to the diverse arthropod-associated problems discussed here.*

Biting Arthropods

Louse Infestations (**Pediculosis**)

Pediculosis is infestation of the body with lice. The observation of louse eggs (nits) cemented to hairs of the scalp or lice themselves confirms the diagnosis of head louse (*Pediculus capitis*) infestation. Nits (or lice) attached to the seams of clothing (often in undergarments) indicate the presence of body lice (*P. humanus*), and nits or lice attached to pubic hairs indicate a pubic (crab) louse (*Phthirus pubis*) infestation.

The eggs are pearly yellow-white and opaque, elongate-oval, about 0.8 mm long and 0.3 mm wide, and are attached singly to each hair or clothing fiber. After hatching, the nits appear translucent and opalescent. Although nits may be numerous, usually not more than 10 to 20 lice are associated with infested persons. The head louse egg is cemented on a hair about 1 mm above the scalp surface.

Head and body lice are very similar in appearance. Adult head lice are 2.5 to 3.5 mm long, and adult body lice are 3.0 to 4.5 mm long. Each immature and adult head and body louse has three pairs of about equal-sized legs bearing claws for gripping hairs or fibers. Adult pubic lice, somewhat crablike in appearance, are 1 to 2 mm long, about as broad, grayish-white or yellowish-brown, and they have forelegs narrower than the other pairs. All immature lice (three stages in each species) resemble their respective adults except in size, and all immature lice and adults are obligate bloodsucking ectoparasites. The body louse is the only known natural vector of the pathogens of louse-borne typhus, trench fever, and louse-borne relapsing fever.

Head lice and their nits are found most frequently in the hair over the postauricular and occipital regions. Body lice are usually seen in clothing, with nits in the seams and creases in areas that contact the body. Crab lice and nits are found on hairs in the pubic and perianal regions, sometimes on hairs on the thighs and abdomen, less commonly on axillary hairs, beard, mustache, eyebrows, and eyelashes, and rarely on the scalp. Pubic infestations are found only in postpubertal individuals.

The skin lesions produced by the bites of lice are erythematous papules that may be accompanied by urticaria or lymphadenopathy. Extensive erythema and pruritus result from hypersensitivity to louse saliva. Crab lice typically induce nonpruritic small gray-blue macules (0.3 to 1.0 cm in diameter) with irregular borders (maculae ceruleae) that may persist for months. The lesions produced by any of the species may be covered with hair matted with eggs, dried serous secretions, and dark louse excrement. The latter, seen on the body or in underclothing, should trigger a search for lice. Excoriations from scratching disguise bite lesions and may lead to impetigo or to furuncular or eczematous lesions. The possibility of louse infestation should be considered when pyoderma is seen. The combination of lichenification and pigmentation in chronically infested individuals is called vagabond's disease (morbus vagabondus). A nondescript macular or papular erythematous rash on the trunk may be the presenting sign for an undiscovered head louse infestation. Postauricular and posterior cervical lymphadenopathy in the absence of other node enlargement should suggest head lice. Body louse infestation may be differentiated from scabies by the absence of lesions on the hands and feet and the common occurrence of lesions in the intrascapular region. The differential diagnosis of louse-induced dermatitis from various mite-induced lesions or non–arthropod-associated dermatoses is made by finding nits or lice.

Treatment for lice includes shampoos, creams, and lotions containing insecticides. The most often used preparations contain lindane (γ benzene hexachloride) or pyrethrins with piperonyl butoxide. Malathion and permethrin, a synthetic pyrethrin, are being used more frequently because of their apparent ovicidal effect. One effective treatment for head lice or pubic lice is a 4-minute shampoo of the affected areas with about 25 ml of 1 per cent lindane shampoo. This may not be ovicidal; therefore, the treatment may be repeated 7 to 10 days later if lice or new nits are seen. Patients infested with body lice may apply lindane (1 per cent) lotion or cream to affected areas. This should be thoroughly washed off 6 to 8 hours later. Lindane should be used with caution on infants, children, and pregnant women. Infested clothing and linen should be washed in hot water (60°C) for 20 minutes or dry cleaned.

After being treated, lice and nits can be removed with a metal comb with teeth 0.1 mm apart. Moisture or oil rinses may make removal easier. Mechanical removal is recommended for facial pubic louse infestations.

Prevention of recurrence involves treatment of infested human contacts and materials (fomites). Pillow cases, hats, scarves, and other items should be washed or cleaned. Infested combs and brushes should be cleaned and boiled or soaked for 1 hour in lindane shampoo or Lysol (2 per cent). Head and body lice survive only about 3 days (10 days maximum) away from the body. Sexual partners of persons with pubic lice should be treated, and bedding, towels, and clothing should be washed or dry cleaned. Pubic lice do not survive longer than 24 hours away from a body. Transmission via toilet seats is unlikely. Fumigation after any louse infestation is unnecessary, but vacuuming is helpful to remove stray lice and shed hairs with affixed nits.

Arnold HL, Odom RB, James WD: Andrews' Diseases of the Skin. 8th ed. Philadelphia, W. B. Saunders Company, 1990, pp 512–515. *This text has excellent photographs of nits, lice, and skin lesions seen in pediculosis.*

Raber IM: Pediculosis cilaris. *In* Parish LC, Nutting WB, Schwartzman RM (eds.): Cutaneous Infestations of Man and Animal. New York, Praeger, 1983, pp 138–143. *This is a lucid description of the clinical aspects and treatment of pubic louse infestation of the eyelashes.*

Witkowski JA, Parish LC: Pediculosis. *In* Parish LC, Nutting WB, Schwartzman RM (eds.): Cutaneous Infestations of Man and Animal. New York, Praeger, 1983, pp 125–137. *A concise, well-documented discussion of clinical louse infestations.*

Flea Bites

Most fleas, unlike lice, do not infest the body. The common flea species that suck blood from humans visit the body for a few minutes to hours, during which time feeding occurs. As in louse infestations, flea bites generally cause pruritus. Each bite lesion is an erythematous papule with a hemorrhagic punctum. Sensitization of an individual to flea saliva may result in papular urticaria (common in affected children), bullous eruptions, or erythema multiforme–type lesions. Bites are usually multiple and irregularly grouped. Bites in adults appear as widespread papules that become lichenified or as grouped papules overlying erythema or edema. Persons entering a previously infested room that has been vacant for weeks or months often suffer from multiple bites on the ankles and legs as hungry fleas emerge from pupal cocoons in floor crevices, debris, or carpeting. As with louse bites, excoriated lesions may become infected and furuncular.

Flea eggs are usually laid off the host, and larvae live off the host, feeding on organic debris. Adults reach their hosts by jumping. Flea species that most often bite humans are the cat flea (*Ctenocephalides felis*), the dog flea (*C. canis*), and somewhat less commonly the so-called human flea (*Pulex irritans*). Occasionally, household infestations with fleas may arise from abandoned wild animal nests built near houses.

Treatment of flea bites is symptomatic and involves the use of antipruritic and anti-inflammatory creams or lotions or oral antihistamines. Secondary infections may require antibiotic therapy. Infested pets should be treated with specific insecticides. Floors, carpets, upholstered furnishings, and pets' sleeping quarters should be sprayed or dusted with insecticides to kill larval, pupal, and adult fleas. A thorough cleaning, including vacuuming, of infested premises should eliminate the insects. Because fleas at all stages can live for weeks or months, a repeat insecticide application may be necessary.

Persons may protect themselves from fleas with repellents containing diethyl metatoluamide. Wild animal (especially rodent) fleas that feed on humans may transmit the bacilli of plague or tularemia, as well as the less virulent rickettsia of murine (flea-borne) typhus. Less common pathogens transmitted by accidental ingestion of fleas (mostly by children) are the dwarf tapeworm *Hymenolepis diminuta* and the dog tapeworm *Dipylidium caninum*.

Bagnall B, Rook A: Arthropods and the skin. *In* Rook A (ed.): Recent Advances in Dermatology. No. 4. Edinburgh, Churchill Livingstone, 1977. *This review includes information about the ecology of fleas and pathogenesis and clinical features of infestations.*

Smit FGAM: Siphonaptera (fleas). *In* Smith KGV (ed.): Insects and Other Arthropods of Medical Importance. London, British Museum (Natural History), 1973. *This is a careful overview of the medical importance of fleas.*

Bedbugs and Kissing Bugs

Bedbugs (Cimicidae) are flat, mahogany-brown, wingless insects (5 to 7 mm long). Most species are bloodsucking ectoparasites of birds and bats. Two species (*Cimex lectularius* and *C. hemipterus*) feed almost exclusively on humans; the former is cosmopolitan; the latter has a tropical distribution. Both species cause irritating, pruritic bite lesions in sensitized individuals. The bugs become engorged with blood in 3 to 15 minutes and feed only at night or in subdued light. They hide in crevices of bedding, beds, floors, and furnishings and in wood and paper trash accumulations during the day. The bites are often seen in short linear groups and vary from small urticarial lesions to large erythematous papules or bullae. The lesions are often excoriated, and eczematous reactions and pyoderma may be seen. Hypersensitivity reactions may include asthma, generalized urticaria, and arthralgia. While some affected persons complain of being awakened at night, most are troubled by the lesions on arising in the morning. Treatment is symptomatic. Prevention includes removal of debris that harbors the bugs, use of insecticides in crevices and cleaning of infested furnishings.

Triatomine kissing bugs (Reduviidae) that suck blood from a diversity of hosts are found in the New World subtropics and tropics and in Asia. Most of these cone-nosed bugs (8 to 38 mm long) are tan, brown, or black, with yellow or red spots around the dorsal edge of the abdomen. The bugs feed rapidly at night. Sensitive individuals may develop papular lesions, small vesicles, or, in the extreme, large urticarial or hemorrhagic nodular to bullous lesions. Generalized anaphylactoid reactions, including shock and angioneurotic and laryngeal edema, have occurred. Kissing bugs may feed anywhere on the body. Domesticated species in the tropics are found most often in thatched houses or those with mud floors. In the southwestern United States, a species (*Triatoma protracta*) living in wood rat nests in desert areas occasionally invades homes. Treatment of bites or allergic reactions is symptomatic. In Central and South America, these insects are vectors of Chagas' disease trypanosomes.

Crissey JT: Bedbugs—an old problem with a new dimension. Int J Dermatol 20:411, 1981. *This review article discusses bedbug biology and the possible role of these bugs in human disease.*

Ryckman RE: Host reactions to bug bites (Hemiptera, Homoptera): A literature review and annotated bibliography. Parts I, II. Calif Vector Views 26, Nos. 1–2, 1979. *This is an excellent source of specific references about all bugs that prey on humans.*

Mosquitoes and Other Bloodsucking Flies

Mosquitoes (Culicidae) are found worldwide, breeding wherever there is stagnant water. While biting, a female mosquito (3 to 6 mm long) induces a pruritic wheal that becomes an erythematous papule. In sensitive persons, bullous lesions, cellulitis, or hemorrhagic necrotic reactions may follow the bites. Systemic anaphylactic reactions are rare. The most serious medical problems associated with mosquitoes relate to their transmission of the agents of yellow fever, dengue, arboviral encephalitides, malaria, and filariasis.

Biting midges (Ceratopogonidae), also called "punkies" or "no-see-ums" because of their minute size (most are 0.6 to 2 mm long), give a painful bite. The resulting erythematous punctiform lesions may become papular and pruritic. Vesicles may develop that ooze fluid for days. These midges, especially *Culicoides* species, bite mostly on exposed parts of the body and may be pestiferous in sandy seashore or marshy areas where they breed. Biting occurs mostly at dawn or dusk.

Black flies (Simuliidae), also called buffalo gnats, are small (1 to 5 mm long), humpbacked, tan to black insects that breed only in running water. They are troublesome bloodsuckers in northern temperate regions. The bites may become hemorrhagic papules that ooze blood for hours. These lesions may be painful and cause recurrent pruritus. Lymphadenopathy is common in sensitive individuals, who may develop localized edema. Cephalalgia, fever, and nausea may occur following large numbers of bites. Black fly species found at high elevations in Central and South America and along rivers in Africa transmit *Onchocerca volvulus*, the etiologic agent of river blindness.

Phlebotomine sandflies (Psychodidae) are delicate, small (2 to 3 mm long), hairy flies found mainly in subtropical and tropical areas. Various species are abundant in rain forests in the New World and in arid areas in the Mediterranean region and Asia. Biting occurs at night or in subdued light. The bites may be painful, occur usually on the extremities, and cause pruritus and elevated pale urticarial lesions that become papular. Vesicular or bullous lesions may occur. Phlebotomine flies are vectors of sandfly (pappataci) fever, bartonellosis, and leishmaniasis.

Other flies that may attack humans and cause painful bites are horse and deer flies (Tabanidae), stable flies, and tsetse flies. Tsetse flies, found only in Africa, transmit the trypanosomes of African sleeping sickness.

Treatment of any of these fly bites is symptomatic and includes the use of topical corticosteroids and oral antihistamines to reduce itching. Personal protection from biting flies involves the use of screen enclosures, headnets, and insect repellents. Protective clothing and open mesh jackets impregnated with repellents are effective.

Allen JR: Mosquitoes and other biting flies. *In* Parish LC, Nutting WB, Schwartzman RM (eds.): Cutaneous Infestations of Man and Animal. New York, Praeger, 1983, pp 344–355. *This is a concise, clearly presented review of the pathogenesis and clinical aspects of fly bites.*

Chiggers and Other Biting Mites

Chiggers are the larvae (six-legged stage) of trombiculid (itch or harvest) mites. These larvae (0.15 to 0.40 mm long) are white to yellow or orange-red and are found on many vertebrates.

Human infestation occurs following contact with grassy or shrubby vegetation inhabited by the mites. First exposure may not produce dermatitis or may produce only slightly irritating, transient erythematous macules or papules (1 to 2 mm). The more commonly seen skin reactions to chigger feeding are extremely pruritic, papular, papulovesicular or papulourticarial lesions (4 to 20 mm) that persist with burning and itching for days to weeks. The lesions may fade and flatten or become hemorrhagic, purpuric, or vesicular. Diagnosis is dependent upon morphology and distribution of lesions, exposure history, and observation of the mites. Engorging chiggers may be apparent as minute reddish blebs embedded in hair follicles. The mites most often attach to skin covered by clothing, especially near belts, straps, or elastic bindings. Scrub itch mites of Asia and South Pacific Islands usually do not cause dermatitis, but they are vectors of scrub typhus rickettsiae.

Other mites that bite humans, but that are rarely recovered from the lesions they cause, are pyemotid (straw, hay, or grain itch) mites, cheyletoid (cat or dog fur and predatory) mites, and dermanyssid (chicken, red, house mouse, tropical rat, fowl, and rodent) mites. All of these mites are extremely small (about 0.4 to 1 mm long), and depending on the species, the six-legged larvae or eight-legged nymphs and adults may attack humans. The resulting skin lesions may be extremely variable.

The differential diagnosis of mite-induced dermatitis depends on associating the patient with a source of mites. Sources include wild and domestic animals, agricultural commodities, dried floral arrangements, infested furniture, and, in chigger-associated cases, particular outdoor habitats.

Treatment of dermatitis associated with biting mites is symptomatic. Antipruritic lotions and creams or oral antihistamines are useful. Secondary infections may require antibiotic therapy. Rare allergic reactions, including edema and asthma, require emergency treatment.

Prevention of recurrences is dependent on destruction or fumigation of the mite source. Personal repellents (containing sulfur or diethyltoluamide) are helpful in preventing chigger infestation, although avoidance of infested areas is the best prevention. *Rickettsia tsutsugamushi* is the only pathogen of major medical importance specifically associated with mite transmission. *R. akari*, the etiologic agent of rickettsialpox, is transmitted by the house mouse mite.

Krinsky WL: Dermatoses associated with the bites of mites and ticks (Arthropoda: Acari). Int J Dermatol 22:75, 1983. *This review includes a list of mites causing human dermatitis and discusses clinical findings.*

Parkhurst HJ: Trombidiosis (infestation with chiggers). Arch Dermatol Syphilol 35:1011, 1937. *This is an extensive review of the biology and clinical importance of chiggers.*

Tick Bites and Tick Paralysis

Ticks, like mites, are arachnids that have six-legged larvae and eight-legged nymphs and adults. Ticks, found worldwide, are grouped in two major families, soft ticks (Argasidae) and hard ticks (Ixodidae). The former, which have rugose integuments, are associated with restricted habitats, such as rodent burrows and bird nests, and rarely feed on humans. When they do, most attach for only a matter of minutes and produce maculate, erythematous lesions (6 to 30 mm in diameter). Some species in Africa cause extensive ecchymosis; pain, pruritus, edema, ulceration, and necrotic lesions have also been observed. The pajaroello (talaja) tick (*Ornithodoros coriaceus*), found in Mexico, California, and Oregon, is known to produce hemorrhagic, painful lesions. Soft ticks are of primary medical importance as vectors of the borreliae of relapsing fevers.

Hard ticks have smooth, hard, shiny integuments and are found on a diversity of animals and in grass and forests. Ticks carried on dogs, cats, or other animals sometimes drop off and attach to humans. Hard ticks remain embedded in the skin for days while becoming engorged with blood and usually do not cause pain or discomfort. Engorging ticks, mistakenly identified as pedunculated moles or warts, are usually noticed only by chance observation. Typical tick bite lesions are small indurations with peripheral erythema. Unusual manifestations of hard tick bites include various forms of nonspecific dermatitis, acrodermatitis chronica atrophicans, necrotic ulcers, and alopecia. Most hard ticks attach, feed, drop off, and are never noticed. Nodular lesions that may persist for years at the sites of bites must be differentiated from malignant conditions, such as lymphomas. Hard ticks are vectors of the etiologic agents of various arboviral hemorrhagic fevers and encephalitides, several kinds of tick-borne typhus (including Rocky Mountain spotted fever), tularemia, babesiosis, ehrlichiosis, and Lyme disease. An engorging tick itself may induce tick paralysis (discussed below).

Attached soft ticks may be easily removed by gentle traction with a forceps. Hard ticks require strong constant traction. Use of heat, flames, or caustic substances is ill advised and may cause unnecessary damage to the patient. Hard ticks, embedded in sensitive sites, such as the ear canal or genitals, may be covered with petrolatum. The ticks then detach within about 2 hours and can be gently removed. Complete extraction of the mouthparts lessens the chance of secondary infection. Persistent nodules that cause discomfort should be surgically excised.

Tick paralysis is an unusual form of ascending flaccid paralysis that occurs while a tick is attached to the body. Mostly children (especially girls) are affected. Tick paralysis in humans has been associated with only a small number of hard tick species in North America, Europe, South Africa, and Australia. Most cases have been caused by female wood ticks, the Rocky Mountain wood tick (*Dermacentor andersoni*) in western North America and the common dog tick (*D. variabilis*) in eastern North America. Although nonspecific numbness or irritability may occur before the onset of paralysis, the initial consistent sign is *weakness in the legs*. Leg tendon reflexes are reduced or absent, and Romberg's sign is often present. Sensory changes are rarely noted. Blood counts and lumbar puncture usually give no indication of the disease. Complete paralysis of the extremities may occur within a few days after a tick attaches. If the cause is unrecognized, paralysis usually progresses, causing speech dysfunction, dysphagia, and ultimately death from aspiration or respiratory paralysis. If a tick is found, removal usually results in reversal of paralysis with a return to normal function in hours to weeks, depending on the severity of the neurologic deficit. The patient should be examined for other ticks, with special attention to concealed areas, such as the scalp, ear canals, axillae, popliteal fossae, anus, and genitals. Even after all ticks are removed, death may occur in patients who exhibit bulbar or respiratory paralysis.

The clinical presentation of tick paralysis may suggest poliomyelitis, Guillain-Barré syndrome, diphtheritic polyneuropathy, transverse myelitis, botulism, or other acutely developing neuropathies. The specific etiologic agent of *Dermacentor* tick paralysis is unknown.

Prevention of tick bites and tick paralysis includes avoidance of tick-infested habitats. Individuals and their pets who enter such habitats should be thoroughly examined for ticks. Personal measures that may prevent ticks from reaching the skin include wearing long-sleeved shirts and long pants, tucking pants legs into socks, and using chemical repellents.

Gothe R, Kunze K, Hoogstraal H: The mechanisms of pathogenicity in the tick paralyses. J Med Entomol 16:357, 1979. *This review lists the tick species that have been associated with paralysis, general clinical aspects, and experimental observations.*

Krinsky WL: Dermatoses associated with the bites of mites and ticks (Arthropoda: Acari). Int J Dermatol 22:75, 1983. *This is a review of skin lesions caused by acarines and epidemiologic and clinical factors helpful in diagnosis.*

Spider Bites

All spiders are eight-legged arachnids that use venom to immobilize their prey. Relatively few species have mouthparts (chelicerae) large and strong enough to inject venom into human skin. Among the better known spiders that cause moderate to severe reactions in humans are the widows (*Latrodectus* species) of the Old and New World, brown spiders (*Loxosceles* species) of the Americas and southern Africa, wandering spiders (*Phoneutria* species) in South America, species of *Chiracanthium* in both hemispheres, and funnel web spiders (*Atrax* species) in Australia.

The black widow (shoe button) spider (*Latrodectus mactans*) female may bite if its web is disturbed. Its abdomen is 6 mm wide and 9 to 13 mm long and is shiny black with a reddish hourglass marking or less well defined markings on the underside. The spider lives in sheltered, dark, dry places, such as in garages and in old stone walls and outhouses. The bite, which may not be felt, may become slightly swollen and appear as two erythematous puncture marks. Within a few hours, a bitten person develops intense muscle pains and commonly a tightening feeling in the chest. Abdominal (boardlike) rigidity and waves of excruciating cramping pain are characteristic. Respiratory distress, nausea, vomiting, profuse perspiration, headache, vertigo, paresthesias of the extremities, and hyperactive reflexes are common. Speech difficulty and visual dysfunction may occur. In untreated adults, the pathologic effects of the venom usually disappear within 2 to 3 days. Death from cardiac or respiratory arrest occurs mostly in very young children and elderly or hypertensive persons.

The differential diagnosis requires consideration of various abdominal and vascular crises, such as perforated ulcer, acute appendicitis or pancreatitis, cholelithiasis, nephrolithiasis, splenic, renal, or mesenteric embolism, volvulus, porphyria, tetanus, and strychnine and lead poisoning. The generalized muscle pain, the lack of abdominal tenderness, and the peripheral sensory changes help to differentiate the widow spider bite.

Treatment with muscle relaxants temporarily relieves muscle pains. A specific antivenin available from Merck Sharp and Dohme is effective against all *Latrodectus* venom and neutralizes the effects of the venom. Because the antivenin is derived from horses, horse serum sensitivity testing is required before the antivenin is administered.

The brown (violin or fiddleback) spiders, including *Loxosceles reclusa* (brown recluse) and *L. laeta* of the western hemisphere, are also secretive, living in secluded places in houses and nesting in clothing, and they may bite when disturbed. They are 10 to 15 mm long and have a dark violin-shaped mark on the brown to gray cephalothorax. Their bites are most often recognized when a serious condition, *necrotic arachnidism*, is the result. The sometimes painful lesion that develops 2 to 6 hours after a bite is a bulla or pustule surrounded by concentric rings of ischemia and erythema. Within 24 to 48 hours, the lesion becomes cyanotic, and a central necrotic area begins to form. This area may slowly expand (up to 20 cm) over days to weeks. The resulting ulcer may not heal for weeks or months. Systemic reactions to the bite include fever, chills, edema, nausea, vomiting, dizziness, myalgias, and arthralgias; morbilliform and petechial eruptions may occur within 48 hours of the bite. A fatal complication, most often seen in children, is *intravascular hemolysis*, followed by hemoglobinuria and acute renal failure.

Treatment of necrotizing lesions is mainly symptomatic and may include antibiotic therapy for secondary infection. Dapsone is effective in promoting healing.

Lucas S: Spiders in Brazil. Toxicon 26:759, 1988. *This review describes the most venomous species in Brazil and their habitats and behavior, as well as clinical aspects of envenomation, epidemiology, and prevention.*

Southcott RV: Arachnidism and allied syndromes in the Australian region. Rec Adelaide Child Hosp 1:99, 1976. *This detailed review treats basic biology and clinical aspects of arachnid bites and infestations and is relevant to much of the world's fauna.*

Wong RC, Hughes SE, Voorhees JJ: Spider bites. Arch Dermatol 123:98, 1987. *This detailed review gives accounts of the most venomous North American spiders and discusses recent approaches to diagnosis and treatment.*

Centipede Bites

Centipedes are multilegged, elongated (up to 30 cm) arthropods with one pair of legs on each body segment. The first pair of legs is modified as poison claws that are used to inject venom into prey. Centipedes, which shun the light and are found under rocks and forest litter, rarely bite. The characteristic bite lesion has two punctate hemorrhages in the center of an erythematous swelling. Centipede bites may cause severe (fiery) local pain that may be followed by inflammation, edema, and superficial necrosis. Systemic reactions may include headache, dizziness, and vomiting. The transient effects of a bite may be accompanied by irregular pulse, muscle spasm, or lymphadenopathy. In general, centipede bites cause no long-term pathologic effects.

Southcott RV: Arachnidism and allied syndromes in the Australian region. Rec Adelaide Child Hosp 1:99, 1976. *This includes a careful review (pp 174–177) of clinical aspects of centipede bites and some case histories.*

Stinging Arthropods

Bee, Wasp, and Ant Stings

Bees, wasps, and ants (order Hymenoptera) are insects that include solitary and social species. Females have an egg-lay-

tube (ovipositor) that has been modified as a sting that secretes venom from abdominal glands. Social bees include honeybees and bumblebees, which all have two pairs of membranous wings and are stocky, hairy, and often yellow and black or brown. The honeybee (*Apis mellifera*) and its close relatives are found worldwide and often are responsible for human sting reactions. The honeybee has a barbed sting that becomes embedded in skin, and as the bee tries to escape, it leaves its venom apparatus and other abdominal organs and soon perishes. Vespid wasps (yellow jackets, hornets, paper wasps) are smooth insects, sleeker than bees and often yellow and black or with combinations of yellow, red, brown, or black. These wasps make the paper nests found in trees, under eaves of houses, or underground. Honeybees and bumblebees may sting when disturbed while seeking nectar or pollen at flowers. Vespid wasps may become pestiferous around food, being especially attracted to sweet or fermented liquids, fruit, fish, and meats. Mutillid wasps (velvet ants, cow killers), which are hairy and wingless, sometimes sting persons in sandy, arid environments.

Human reactions to stings usually include intense local pain, followed by the appearance of a red punctum surrounded by a blanched area and erythema. A wheal forms and the swelling and erythema, accompanied by pruritus, may last for a few hours. Multiple stings, especially on the face, may cause extensive edema, multiple vesicles, bullae, or purpura. Treatment includes gentle removal of the sting by scraping with a sharp blade (in cases of honeybee envenomation), application of ice, and topical hydrocortisone or oral antihistamines. Severe and sometimes fatal allergic reactions to stings of bees and wasps that occur in sensitized individuals are discussed in Ch. 248.

Ants (Formicidae) of some species can sting, causing severe pain. Two groups of New World stinging ants are the fire ants (*Solenopsis* species) and harvester ants (*Pogonomyrmex* species). These ants build ground nests that protrude as large mounds. An ant may grip the skin with its mandibles and then insert its sting. The ant may pivot and sting many times. This behavior, compounded by the common occurrence of mass attacks, leads to a clustering of lesions. The usual reaction to the sting is fiery, sharp pain, followed by a wheal and flare response. A clear vesicle appears that becomes pustular after about 24 hours. This sterile pustule may persist for 3 to 10 days and dry as a crust that sloughs, leaving a macule, scar, or fibrous nodule. Systemic reactions such as dizziness, nausea, vomiting, profuse perspiration, cyanosis, and asthma occur in allergic individuals but may also be seen in cases of multiple stings. Symptomatic treatment of local reactions is similar to that for bee and wasp stings.

Harwood RF, James MT: Venoms, defense secretions, and allergens of arthropods. *In* Entomology in Human and Animal Health. 7th ed. New York, The Macmillan Company, 1979. *This is a review of the biology and clinical importance of stinging Hymenoptera.*

Paull BR: Imported fire ant allergy. Perspectives on diagnosis and treatment. Postgrad Med 76:155, 1984. *A well-illustrated review of the distribution and clinical aspects of fire ant stings.*

Scorpion Stings

Scorpions are mostly subtropical and tropical arachnids that have a pair of lobster-like claws (pedipalps) anteriorly and a curved spine posteriorly that is an outlet for the proteinaceous venom produced by a pair of venom glands. Scorpions are nocturnal predators that sting quickly and repeatedly when disturbed in their hiding places under rocks, lumber, and vegetation or in shoes, bedding, or clothing left on the ground. In the United States, one scorpion species, *Centruroides sculpturatus*, of about 40 native species causes severe pathologic effects in humans. This small (about 6 cm long), straw-colored species is found only in Arizona. The arid regions that extend from North Africa to India are inhabited by the most abundant and dangerous scorpions.

The nature and severity of human reactions to scorpion stings are not consistent with the size, appearance, or aggressiveness of different species. Intense and immediate pain at the site of a sting is common to all cases. When a mildly toxic scorpion such as *C. vittatus*, a common southern United States species, is involved, the pain may be followed by local swelling and perhaps skin discoloration, regional lymphadenopathy, pruritus, or paresthesias, and less commonly by nausea and vomiting. These reactions are transient, lasting for minutes to as long as 24 hours.

The more toxic species cause local pain but little or no skin response, and systemic effects are usually noted within a few minutes to 24 hours after the sting. Symptoms may include anxiety, drowsiness, syncope, increased salivation, lacrimation, perspiration, diminished vision, photophobia, numbness and sluggishness of the tongue, vomiting, diarrhea or involuntary defecation and micturition, priapism, muscular fibrillations or spasms, and convulsions. Clinical signs may include hypotension or hypertension, irregular pulse, tachycardia and arrhythmias, irregular respiration, rapid shifts in body temperature, oliguria or polyuria, and hemiplegia. Laboratory tests may reveal hyperglycemia, glycosuria, serum glutamic-oxaloacetic transaminase (SGOT) increase, hematuria, and melena. Pathologic changes that may lead to death include myocarditis, pulmonary edema, and shock. Respiratory paralysis is the usual immediate cause of death. In the most toxic cases, death may occur within minutes of the sting or not for over 40 hours later, but most deaths occur in 2 to 20 hours after the sting. The mortality is highest in children. Close monitoring of affected patients is important because sudden relapses, often involving acute respiratory distress, may occur after a patient's condition seems to have stabilized.

The most important treatment for moderate to very toxic stings is administration of an antivenin. Antivenin to *C. sculpturatus* is available in Arizona from the Antivenom Production Laboratory, Arizona State University, Tempe, Arizona 85281 (602-965-6443 or 602-965-1457) and Poison Control in Phoenix (602-253-3334). Antivenins against other species are available from laboratories in Mexico, Brazil, Europe, Africa, and Asia. In India, where antivenin is not available, acute pulmonary edema and hypertension have been successfully treated with vasodilators, such as prazosin hydrochloride.

Early treatment of stings may include cooling of the sting site for up to 2 hours and use of a local anesthetic. Oxygen administration or artificial respiration, sodium phenobarbital injection, and parenteral solutions, including blood plasma, may be needed to treat respiratory distress, convulsions, and shock, respectively. Calcium gluconate (10 ml of 10 per cent solution) given as a slow intravenous injection reduces muscle spasms. In the United States, morphine and meperidine are contraindicated because they enhance the toxic effects of *C. sculpturatus* venom. Morphine and barbiturates are not recommended for treatment of any scorpion stings because these drugs inhibit the bulbar respiratory centers.

Personal protection includes wearing heavy gloves and boots when reaching into hidden areas in which scorpions may hide. Shaking out shoes and other materials left on the ground before using them is essential. Removal of litter from around houses, sealing cracks in foundations, and selective use of pesticides are helpful means of preventing scorpions from inhabiting houses and gardens.

Chippaux JP, Goyffon M: Producers of antivenomous sera. Toxicon 21:739, 1983. *Addresses of antivenom suppliers are listed in this article by type of venomous animal and continent.*

Keegan HL: Scorpions of Medical Importance. Jackson, University of Mississippi Press, 1980. *This book reviews scorpion morphology, taxonomy, biology, and geographic distribution, as well as clinical aspects and prevention of scorpion envenomation.*

Invasive Arthropods

Scabies

The scabies mite (*Sarcoptes scabiei*), unlike the other mites discussed, burrows into the skin and, because it reproduces on humans, can maintain a continuous infestation. Fertile female mites burrow into the skin and lay their eggs as they tunnel. Immature stages (larvae and nymphs) move out to the surface and enter hair follicles. Further development and mating take place near the skin surface. The mite burrows are slightly raised, curved, or tortuous gray lines, 5 to 15 mm long, and at the end of each is a female, a minute pearly bleb. The burrows are restricted to the horny layer of the skin and occur most often in the sides of the fingers, the interdigital webs, flexor surfaces of the wrists, elbows, skin around the nipples, and penis. Other lesions, including erythematous papules, lichenified patches, and pustules, which occur in sites other than the burrows, may be seen on the abdomen, thighs, and buttocks. In infants and young children, burrows may occur in the palms and soles, and papular lesions may be seen on the scalp, face, and neck.

Intense pruritus begins from 2 to 6 weeks after first exposure to the mite. Definitive diagnosis of the lesions is often difficult because of excoriations. In very clean individuals, few lesions may be present, and burrows may not be clearly visible. Generalized urticarial papules may result from previous treatment with fluorinated corticosteroids. Some patients have pruritic inflammatory nodules (≤12 mm in diameter) that occur on covered skin, especially the axillae, abdomen, scrotum, and penis. A severe form of scabies most often seen in immunologically compromised persons is called *crusted scabies* (originally called Norwegian scabies). As the name implies, warty plaques occur frequently on the hands and feet, and extensive scaling covers the scalp to the trunk or below. Horny debris collects under the fingernails, which are usually distorted and thickened. Pruritus, erythema, and lymphadenopathy may occur.

Diagnosis of any scabies infestation depends on observation of a mite in skin scrapings of a burrow or in situ, by gently raising the top of a burrow with a sterile needle and looking with a magnifier. In most scabies cases, only 10 to 15 mites are present on the body. In crusted scabies, large numbers of mites are present. To obtain a scraping of a burrow, an area suspected of infestation is scraped with a scalpel blade. The scraped material is examined at 50 to 100 times magnification. The movements of a living mite may be observed if the material is placed on a slide without any mounting media. Otherwise, the scraping may be cleared in potassium hydroxide (20 per cent) or suspended in mineral oil under a coverslip on the slide. The adult female mite is about 300 to 400 μm long, oval, with the dorsum convex and venter flattened. It has four pairs of legs, two pairs directed anteriorly and two posteriorly. Each anterior leg ends in an unjointed stalk with a distensible thin-walled sac at its tip; each posterior leg ends in a long, thick bristle. The size of the mite egg is about 100 × 150 μm.

Scabies lesions initially may be diagnosed as those of other skin conditions, e.g., neurodermatitis, dermatitis herpetiformis, lichen planus, and various other kinds of mite-associated dermatitis, such as that caused by *Cheyletiella* fur mites. The distribution of lesions and observation of the mite rule out these other diagnoses. Secondary infections appearing as pyoderma are common, and nephrogenic strains of streptococci infecting the lesions may cause acute glomerulonephritis.

Treatment of uncomplicated scabies involves application of one of various acaricides. Permethrin (5 per cent in dermal cream) in a single-dose regimen has recently been used with success. Lindane (1 per cent) cream or lotion is often used in a manner similar to that suggested for pediculosis, namely, an 8- to 12-hour treatment for adults, followed by thorough washing. Use of lindane on infants and pregnant women is discouraged. Pruritus and dermatitis may persist for days after adequate treatment. Antipruritic medications are often prescribed.

Transmission occurs during contact with infested persons or with clothing recently worn by such persons. Transmission between bed partners is common and does not require body contact. All household and intimate contacts should be treated to prevent recurrence or continued transmission. The female mite survives for only 2 to 3 days away from a host; therefore, as with louse infestations, fumigation of premises is unnecessary. Clothing, especially undergarments, bedding, and towels should be laundered in hot water.

Scabies mites infesting domestic animals, including dogs and cats, occasionally cause dermatitis in humans, but the lesions are usually limited to the areas that contact the animals. These mites are usually not recovered from humans.

Green MS: Epidemiology of scabies. Epidemiol Rev 11:126, 1989. *This article reviews clinical and epidemiologic aspects of scabies.*

Mellanby K: Scabies. Middlesex, England, E. W. Classey (1943), 1972. *This classic work, available in this reprinted form, is a comprehensive review of the basic biology, clinical evolution, and treatment of scabies.*

Myiasis and Tungiasis

Myiasis is the infestation of living vertebrate tissue by fly larvae. Many flies (order Diptera) that normally deposit eggs or larvae on carrion, manure, or decaying organic matter sometimes deposit their immature stages in open wounds or infected human tissues. These include blow flies, also called greenbottle or bluebottle flies (Calliphoridae), flesh flies (Sarcophagidae), and house flies (Muscidae). The larvae of some of these flies are attracted to draining infections or to clothing stained with urine or feces. The larvae crawl into lesions or natural orifices when an infected person sleeps on the ground or is otherwise exposed to flies. Individuals immobilized because of physical illness or old age who have such open lesions or infections, and especially those who are living in poor sanitary conditions, are particularly susceptible. Urogenital myiasis may cause dysuria, hematuria, and pyuria.

Some fly larvae invade intact skin of domestic animals or humans; species in this group include the human bot fly (*Dermatobia hominis*) found in Central and South America, the African tumbu fly *Cordylobia anthropophaga*, and some species of *Wohlfahrtia* that have a predilection for the tender skin of infants.

Fly larvae that live in food, e.g., vinegar flies (Drosophilidae) and cheese skippers (Piophilidae), are sometimes accidentally ingested and may cause gastrointestinal discomfort.

Wound or dermal myiasis often results in furuncular lesions, and an infested individual notices a swelling and feels pain or movement under the skin where the larvae are feeding on tissue fluids. Careful observation of the top of a lesion enables one to see two dark respiratory openings (spiracles) through which the larva breathes. Treatment consists of gentle compression of the swelling and removal of the larva with a forceps. A local anesthetic may be helpful because recurved spines may hold the larva tightly under the skin. Topical antibiotics are used to control or prevent secondary infections. Removal of larvae that crawl into sensory openings or urogenital and anal orifices may require irrigation or surgical intervention. Intestinal myiasis is usually self-limited, ceasing when the larvae are passed in the stool. Dermal myiasis of most kinds, if untreated, progresses until the mature larvae back out of the skin and drop to the ground to pupate. The physical and emotional distress caused by the presence of living larvae can be prevented if a physician considers the possibility of such an infestation and removes the larvae early in the infestation. Warble fly larvae, which normally migrate from the legs of cattle through the body to the back, in human infestations also migrate dorsally and, unless they reach a cutaneous exit site, may cause extensive tissue damage that leads to chronic illness or death.

Prevention of myiasis requires frequent changing of dressings on wounds and use of screening.

Tungiasis is the infestation of vertebrate, including human, skin by the female flea *Tunga penetrans* (chigoe, jigger, or sand flea). This flea occurs in sandy soil in subtropical and tropical regions of the Americas, the West Indies, and Africa. It usually feeds between the toes, under a toenail, or in the sole of the foot and becomes embedded as it gorges on blood. The flea, which remains embedded permanently, may cause irritation, pain, or pruritus, and the resulting swelling is often pustular. Secondary skin infections and tetanus are complications of infestations, and autoamputation of digits in Africans is apparently caused by inflammatory reactions to the flea.

Treatment of tungiasis includes removal of the flea with a sterile needle or blade, tetanus vaccination, and application of topical antibiotics. Personal protection against *T. penetrans* includes wearing footwear and using insect repellent. Sleeping above the ground surface usually prevents the flea from reaching the body.

Brothers W, Heckmann R: Tungiasis (*Tunga penetrans*) in Utah. J Parasitol 65:782, 1979. *This note succinctly describes the clinical problem and gives references to cases.*

Harwood RB, James MT: Myiasis. *In* Entomology in Human and Animal Health. New York, The Macmillan Company, 1979. *This is a thorough review of different clinical forms of myiasis.*

Arthropods and Contact Dermatitis

Various species of nonbiting mites found in stored products may cause dermatitis when they contact human skin. These microscopic foodstuff mites (Acaridae, Glycyphagidae) are found in commodities, including grains, cereals, seeds, bulbs, dried herbs, copra, dried vegetables, cured meats, mushrooms, humus, cheese, and animal and plant material used for stuffing furniture, pillows, and mattresses. Dried fruit mites (Carpoglyphidae) are found not only in dried fruits but also in jams, jellies, spoiled fruit, wine, caramel, flour, and dried milk products. The skin reactions to these mites vary, but pruritic diffuse erythema with urticarial wheals or erythematous papular eruptions are common. Laborers in granaries, food-processing plants, and commercial kitchens and dockworkers are most susceptible.

Another form of pruritic dermatitis is caused by contact with various caterpillars, pupae, adults, and some egg masses of moths and butterflies (order Lepidoptera). Urticating setae and spines on these life forms may cause mechanical irritation of the skin or may have toxic effects. Contact with setae, spines, or hairs may cause intense stinging or fiery pain, followed by the formation of wheals, local edema, erythema, and pruritus. Less common reactions include lymphadenopathy, cephalalgia, shocklike symptoms, or convulsions.

Treatment of dermatitis caused by foodstuff and dried fruit mites or lepidopteran spines or setae is symptomatic. Antipruritic substances, including antihistamines, corticosteroids, and anesthetics, have been used. Commodities containing mites must be fumigated or destroyed. Spines or setae of lepidopterans may be removed from the skin with fine forceps. Use of protective clothing and thorough washing of exposed materials help prevent continuation of these forms of dermatitis.

A third form of contact dermatitis results from vesicants produced by blister beetles (Meloidae) and some rove beetles (Staphylinidae). Cantharidin, first isolated from the meloid called the Spanish fly, is found in all species of blister beetles. Contact with this substance causes mild to severe vesicular dermatitis.

Similar lesions, which usually follow a burning sensation and tanning of the skin, result from contact with millipedes. Some species of these herbivorous myriapods exude a fluid from pores along the length of the body. Secretions from the aforementioned beetles or millipedes cause burning pain and conjunctivitis if they are rubbed into the eyes.

Treatment of toxic dermatitis associated with beetles or millipedes includes rapid washing of the skin or eyes, if affected, and use of local anesthetics. The dermal reactions caused by contact with mites, lepidopterans, beetles, and millipedes are usually transitory and do not have long-lasting effects.

Harwood RB, James MT: Vesicating Coleoptera. In Entomology in Human and Animal Health. New York, The Macmillan Company, 1979, pp 441–443. This section discusses the nature of vesicant chemicals from beetles and reviews clinical cases.

Radford AJ: Millipede burns in man. Trop Geogr Med 27:279, 1975. Geographic distribution, toxicology, pathogenesis, clinical features, and treatment of millipede envenomation are carefully reviewed.

Southcott RV: Lepidoptera and skin infestation. In Parish LC, Nutting WB, Schwartzman RM (eds.): Cutaneous Infestations of Man and Animal. New York, Praeger, 1983, pp 304–343. This chapter gives a comprehensive review of worldwide lepidopterism, including pathogenesis and clinical presentations.

PENTASTOMIASIS (Linguatuliasis)

Pentastomiasis is infestation with pentastomids, little-known invertebrates called tongue worms, which have been variously classified as arthropods or helminths. These bloodsucking endoparasites are found as adults in the lungs of reptiles and birds or in the nasal cavity of carnivores, especially cats and dogs. Herbivores are normal intermediate hosts, but humans and other mammals can be dead-end aberrant hosts for the larvae. Ingested eggs hatch, and the larvae burrow through the intestine and migrate to diverse tissues, where they molt several times and become encysted as third-stage larvae.

Human infestations have occurred in Europe, Africa, and North, Central, and South America. Two species account for most cases, Armillifer armillatus, found in pythons and other vipers in tropical Africa, and Linguatula serrata, found in canids in Europe and the Near and Middle East.

Infection occurs by accidental ingestion of tongue worm eggs contaminating food or drink, by ingestion of eggs picked up on fingers from handling infected snakes or lizards, or by ingestion of improperly cooked or raw reptiles. The third-stage larvae (20 to 25 mm long) encysted in fibrous capsules occur most often in the liver and are rarely noted except incidentally at autopsy or as calcified cysts (3 to 6 mm in diameter) on radiographic examination. Rarely, a mass of cysts in the intestinal wall may cause obstruction. Cysts compressing vital structures such as bile ducts or bronchi may lead to infections or obstructions.

Linguatuliasis, the direct infection of humans with third-stage larvae of Linguatula species, occurs most often in Lebanese people who eat raw or inadequately cooked liver or lymph nodes of goats and sheep. The ingested larvae migrate to the nasopharynx from the stomach. These larvae (5 to 10 mm long) cause Halzoun's syndrome, characterized by paroxysmal coughing, sneezing, and nasal and lacrimal discharge, accompanied by pain and itching in the throat. Other symptoms may include hoarseness, dyspnea, dysphagia, and vomiting. Submaxillary and cervical lymph nodes may be enlarged. Recovery in most cases is spontaneous in 7 to 10 days; however, death from asphyxiation due to tonsillar edema has been reported. A similar syndrome seen in Sudan, Turkey, and Greece is called Marrara's syndrome.

Prevention of pentastomiasis includes proper cooking of exotic foods such as herbivore organs and reptiles, improved hygiene of persons handling reptiles, and ingestion only of clean water and thoroughly washed raw vegetables.

Drabick JJ: Pentastomiasis. Rev Infect Dis 9:1087, 1987. This review discusses biology, parasitology, clinical manifestations, pathology, diagnosis, treatment, and epidemiology.

Herzog U, Marty P, Zak F: Pentastomiasis: Case report of an acute abdominal emergency. Acta Trop 42:261, 1985. This report reviews clinical and epidemiologic information.

LEECHES AS AGENTS OF DISEASE (Hirudiniasis)

Leeches of medical importance are bloodsucking annelid worms. Each has a ventral anterior or posterior sucker. The former encloses teeth that cut through the skin after the leech attaches. Feeding occurs within a half-hour or more.

The leeches most often feeding on humans are aquatic (freshwater) species of Hirudo, the cosmopolitan medicinal leeches; Limnatis, the nasal leeches found from the Canary Islands east through Europe, Africa, and Asia; Dinobdella, found in Asia; and terrestrial species of Haemadipsa, found in Asia, Indonesia, Australia, Pacific Islands, and Central and South America. Humans are subject to attack by large leeches in tropical rain forests or to infestation with aquatic species while wading or swimming.

Wounds produced by leeches often go unnoticed, except for the oozing blood or prolonged bleeding caused by an anticoagulant, hirudin. Pruritus is common at bite sites, and although leeches are not known to transmit any human pathogens, secondary infections may occur. Immature aquatic leeches may be ingested with water and infest the upper respiratory and digestive tracts or may invade the mouth, nose, eyes, vagina, urethra, or anus of swimmers.

Attachment of leeches to the nasal passages may cause epistaxis. Attachment to the larynx may cause hoarseness, dyspnea, and hemoptysis, and attachment to the pharynx or esophagus may cause dysphagia and hematemesis. Hemorrhaging from leech infestations may be so severe, especially in children, that anemia occurs, leading to death.

Techniques used for removing leeches from the respiratory and digestive tracts include a steady pull on the specimen with a forceps or hemostat or narcotizing the leech with a spray of 5 per cent cocaine hydrochloride before removal. In genitourinary infestations, irrigation with a strong salt solution may cause the leeches to detach. A leech attached to skin or respiratory or digestive tract surfaces may be induced to release its grip by holding it in a hemostat and touching the exposed part of the worm with a small flame or other cauterant.

Prevention of attack by aquatic and land leeches includes use of protective clothing and of insect repellents. Repellents applied to boots, trouser legs, and exposed skin are quite effective, but, because they are water soluble, must be reapplied every few hours in wet tropical regions where leeches are commonly found.

Keegan HL, Radke MG, Murphy DA: Nasal leech infestation in man. Am J Trop Med Hyg 19:1029, 1970. This paper discusses two cases and reviews other clinical reports and treatment.

439 Snake Bites

Jay P. Sanford

EPIDEMIOLOGY. Of the nearly 3500 species of snakes, fewer than one tenth are venomous. The poisonous varieties belong to five families (Table 439–1). Throughout the world, snake bites are estimated to account for 30,000 to 40,000 deaths annually. The largest number occur in Burma (Russell's viper) and Brazil (*Bothrops jararaca*). In the United States, the number of snake bites is estimated at 8000 per year. Twenty to 60 per cent of the bites by venomous snakes in the United States result in little or no envenomation (poisoning). Most bites occur in the states bordering on the Gulf of Mexico. Despite the large number of bites with envenomation, fewer than 15 deaths occur, and almost all of these are due to rattlesnake bites. This low case fatality ratio reflects the virtual absence of members of the families Elapidae and Hydrophidae in the United States.

Coral snakes, eastern and western varieties, are found in southern and western states (North Carolina, South Carolina, Georgia, Florida, Alabama, Mississippi, Louisiana, Arkansas, Texas, New Mexico, and Arizona). Their fangs are short and permanently erect. They envenomate through chewing movements. Since they are nocturnal and shy, they rarely bite humans.

The pit vipers (Crotalidae) are identified by a small depression between the eyes and nostrils. Their fangs are long and hinged, folding back when the mouth is closed and erect when open. Upon contact, venom is expressed by muscular contraction. The pit vipers are generally aggressive. The eastern (*Crotalus adamanteus*) and western (*C. atrox*) diamondback rattlesnakes are the largest and most dangerous in the United States. Their distribution includes the aforementioned states plus California, Nevada, and Oklahoma. Cottonmouths (*Agkistrodon piscivorus*), or water moccasins, are found along streams in the southern and southeastern states. They may inflict facial bites when disturbed while resting on tree branches. Contrary to lore, they can bite under water. Copperheads (*A. contortrix*), or highland moccasins, have a geographic distribution similar to that of the cottonmouths. Their bite is painful but rarely fatal.

PATHOGENESIS. Snake venoms are probably the most complex of all poisons. Because of the heterogeneous composition and multiplicity of effects, snake venoms cannot be classified simply as neurotoxic, cardiotoxic, myotoxic, or hematotoxic on the basis of the snake family (Table 439–2).

Venoms from Elapidae and Hydrophidae snakes contain basic polypeptides that produce presynaptic and/or postsynaptic neuromuscular block with resultant flaccid paralysis, including respiratory paralysis. Cobra cardiotoxin, an additional basic polypeptide, depolarizes cell membranes of skeletal, cardiac, and smooth muscles, thus contributing to paralysis. Venom of the South American rattlesnake (*Crotalus durissus*) contains an acidic protein with nondepolarizing curare-like neuromuscular blocking effects. Viperatoxin isolated from the Palestine viper causes a

TABLE 439–1. VENOMOUS SNAKES OF THE WORLD

Family	Common Varieties	Geographic Distribution
Crotalidae	Pit vipers (rattlesnakes, water moccasins, copperheads), fer-de-lance, bushmaster	Americas, Asia
Elapidae	Cobras, kraits, mambas, coral snakes, death adder	Worldwide except Europe
Columbridae	Boomslangs, bird snakes	Africa
Hydrophidae	Sea snakes	Indo-Pacific waters
Viperidae	True vipers (Russell's viper), puff adder	Worldwide except Americas

TABLE 439–2. BIOCHEMISTRY OF SNAKE VENOMS

Toxins	Family	Mechanism of Injury/Death
Neurotoxin (basic polypeptide)	Elapidae, Hydrophidae, South American rattlesnake (*Crotalus durissus terrificus*), Palestine viper (*Vipera palestinae*)	Respiratory paralysis
Cardiotoxin	Elapidae	Cardiovascular depression
Enzymes Phospholipase A 5-Nucleotidase Phosphodiesterase Deoxyribonuclease II Ribonuclease Adenosine-triphosphatase Nucleotide pyrophosphatase Exopeptidase Hyaluronidase L-Amino acid oxidase	Elapidae, Hydrophidae, Crotalidae, Viperidae (Absent in spitting cobra)	Hemolysis
Proteases	Crotalidae, Viperidae	Hypotension due to release
Acetylcholinesterase	Elapidae (absent in spitting cobra, mamba, coral snake)	
Alkaline phosphatase		
Acid phosphatase		

peripheral nerve conduction block. A variety of enzymes, mostly hydrolases and phospholipase A, are present in most venoms. Bradykinin is released from bradykininogen by most crotalid and viperid venoms but not by Elapidae except the king cobra (*Ophiophagus hannah*). The venom of a single snake seldom contains all of the toxins. The composition and potency of venom are highly variable and differ not only among species but even among individual snakes.

SYMPTOMS AND SIGNS. *Pit Viper Envenomation.* In the United States, most victims reach a physician within 15 minutes to 3 hours. At that time, it is essential to determine whether or not envenomation has occurred and, if it has occurred, to determine the severity; this has important therapeutic implications. The clinical effects are summarized in Table 439–3. The most important early findings of envenomation are swelling at the bite, usually occurring within 10 minutes, and pain, although pain may be absent. Mild envenomation is characterized by local edema (1 to 5 inches in diameter) and pain without systemic symptoms or signs. With moderate envenomation, local findings are more extensive—edema of 6 to 12 inches in diameter. Systemic findings occur: weakness, sweating, nausea, faintness, dizziness, ecchymoses, and tender regional lymph nodes. With severe envenomation, systemic involvement includes tachycardia; tachypnea; hypothermia; hypotension; ecchymoses; paresthesias of the scalp and finger and toe tips; and muscle fasciculations. With very severe envenomation, gingival bleeding, hematemesis, hematuria, melena, oliguria, and coma occur.

Over the first 12 hours, the skin develops a tense, discolored appearance and bullae, which may be either serous or hemorrhagic.

Coral Snake Envenomation. The bite wound usually resembles scratch marks and is somewhat painful, but there is little or no edema. The onset of systemic manifestations is usually delayed 1 to 6 hours. Paresthesias around the bite may occur within several hours. Systemic symptoms may include weakness, apprehension, giddiness, nausea, vomiting, excess salivation, and even a sense of euphoria. Bulbar and cranial nerve paralysis may develop with ptosis, diplopia, papillary dilation, excess salivation, dysphagia, dysphonia, and respiratory failure. Paralysis may last 6 to 14 days, and muscular strength may not be fully regained for 6 to 8 weeks.

LABORATORY FINDINGS. Proteolytic enzymes in venoms not only produce tissue damage but also have a marked effect on coagulation, thrombin-like activity being most prominent. Within the first few hours, there is a drop in platelets owing to local consumption (occasionally to fewer than 10,000 per milliliter), a decrease in fibrinogen, and an increase in fibrin degradation products. Striking increases in prothrombin time and partial thromboplastin time occur with severe envenomation. Erythrocytes show a peculiar "burring," indicating membrane damage, and drops in hematocrit and hemoglobin concentration occur.

With pit viper envenomation, baseline laboratory tests should include complete blood count, platelet count, prothrombin time, partial thromboplastin time, bleeding time, urinalysis, and serum electrolytes. Blood should be obtained for typing and crossmatching. In patients with envenomation of moderate or greater severity, arterial blood gas determinations and an electrocardiogram are indicated. Hematologic studies should be repeated every 4 to 6 hours for the first day or until the coagulopathy has stabilized. With coral snake envenomation, repetitive coagulation studies are not indicated.

TREATMENT. *First Aid.* The initial goal of first aid is to minimize systemic absorption of the toxin. This is accomplished by restraining the patient to minimize muscular activity, application of compressive dressings, and transport to the hospital with as little effort exerted by the patient as circumstances permit. With neurotoxic venoms, absorption may result in respiratory arrest, for which resuscitation is essential. Respiratory paralysis may develop within 15 minutes following cobra bites. The snake should be killed if this can be done quickly and safely and taken along with the patient to allow accurate identification; this may obviate unnecessary therapy. The dead snake must be handled with care, since the head of an apparently dead snake can deliver a venomous bite for up to an hour after being severed. The potential value of incision and suction is less than the risks, which include delay in antivenin (antivenom) administration. The site of the bite should be wiped but not incised. Incisions can aggravate bleeding; damage nerves and tendons; introduce infection, especially with mouth suction; and delay healing. An absorption-delaying compressive bandage, preferably crepe (not a tourniquet) should immediately be applied firmly, as for a sprain, over the bite site and up the entire limb. The affected part should be immobilized (splinted) promptly. If available, an inflatable splint provides both compression and immobilization. The patient should be promptly transported to the nearest medical treatment facility. The compressive bandage should not be released during transit. The affected area should not be placed in ice. Cryotherapy results in greater tissue damage with the potential for necessitating amputation.

Hospital Care. On admission it is important to determine, if possible, if the bite was inflicted by a pit viper—specifically, rattlesnake, moccasin, or copperhead—or a coral snake and whether envenomation has occurred. The mainstay of therapy is physiologic monitoring in an intensive care unit and, for rattlesnake bites with envenomation, antivenin, which is a horse serum product; hence it has a high potential of causing serum sickness later. There are two antivenins: one polyvalent for North American pit vipers and another for eastern coral snakes. Water moccasin and copperhead bites can be managed without antivenin, avoiding immediate anaphylactic reactions and later serum sickness. With rattlesnake bites, for minor envenomation, anti-

venin is not indicated. For more serious rattlesnake envenomation, antivenin should be administered. For mild envenomation, three to five ampules of antivenin should be diluted (10 ml each) and then added to 500 ml of intravenous fluid. Skin or conjunctival sensitivity tests are unreliable in predicting early reactions to antivenin. Treatment should not be delayed 20 to 30 minutes to await results. All patients given antivenin should be regarded as likely to have a reaction; the incidence ranges from 3 to 54 per cent. Epinephrine should be available in a syringe before the infusion is started. At the first sign of anaphylactoid reaction, bronchospasm, hypotension, or angioedema, the infusion should be stopped and 0.5 ml of 1:1000 epinephrine injected intramuscularly. This is almost always effective, and the antivenin infusion can be restarted. A history of allergy to horse serum contraindicates antivenin unless the risk of death from envenomation is high and the patient is pretreated with epinephrine. The 500 ml should be given intravenously over 60 minutes. If the amount is adequate, the swelling will not progress and paresthesias will decrease. If progression occurs, the dose should be repeated. For moderate envenomation 5 to 10 vials, for severe envenomation 10 to 20 vials, and for very severe envenomation up to 40 vials (400 ml) may be required. In one series, the average dose required for adults with severe bites was 16 vials. Larger doses are required for bites in children and for those involving the fingers. Antivenin neutralizes both the local and the systemic effects of the venom.

In coral snake bites, if any symptoms or signs develop within the first several hours, 3 to 5 vials of antivenin (*Micrurus fulvius*) should be given intravenously. Even in the absence of symptoms, patients should be observed in the hospital for approximately 48 hours because onset of symptoms may be delayed and insidious. If neurotoxic signs appear (Table 439–3) an edrophonium test should be done: atropine sulfate (0.6 mg) given by slow intravenous infusion, followed by edrophonium chloride (10 mg) given intravenously over 2 minutes. If improvement occurs, neostigmine methylsulfate should be administered (beginning with 25 µg per kilogram of body weight per hour) by continuous infusion.

Antibiotics are usually recommended. Bacteriologic cultures of rattlesnake venom and fangs show growth from over 90 per cent. Aerobic gram-negative bacilli (*Enterobacter* sp., *Pseudomonas* sp., and *Citrobacter* sp.) and histotoxic clostridia (*Clostridum perfringens*) are the predominant isolates. On the basis of the microbiologic results, administration of one of the newer beta-lactam antibiotics—piperacillin, ceftazidime, or carbenicillin clavulanate—is most appropriate. A tetanus toxoid booster is recommended.

In the severely envenomated patient, concurrent supportive measures include the management of shock and of respiratory and renal failure. Glucocorticoids have been recommended, but a controlled trial of prednisone therapy helped neither local nor systemic effects of viperine poisoning. Despite the hypofibrinogenemia and increase in fibrin degradation products, heparin is not of benefit.

Decompressive fasciotomy is indicated only if edema within closed muscular compartments is inadequately controlled, compartmental pressures are 30 mm Hg or higher, and arterial blood supply is compromised. From the end of the first to the third week, the majority of patients will develop serum sickness, the prevalence approximating 1 per cent per milliliter of horse serum administered. Steroids are useful for treatment of serum sickness reactions.

TABLE 439–3. PIT VIPER ENVENOMATION: SYMPTOMS AND SIGNS (PERCENTAGE)

Local		Systemic						
		Generalized		*Hematologic*		*Neuromuscular*		
Fang marks	100	Weakness	70	Thrombocytopenia	42	Paresthesia of scalp, fingertips	63
Edema	74	Tachycardia	60	Increased clotting time	37	Faintness, dizziness	57
Pain	65	Hypotension	54	Decreased hemoglobin	37	Paresthesias of affected part	57
Vesicles	40	Sweating	43	Burring of RBC	18	Fasciculations	41
Necrosis	27	Nausea/vomiting	42	Thrombocytosis	16		
		Hypothermia	42	Bleeding	15		
		Tachypnea	40				
		Regional adenopathy	40				

Data from Russell FE: Snake venom poisoning in the United States. Annu Rev Med 31:247, 1980.

PROGNOSIS. If adequate antivenin has been administered intravenously, mortality is virtually nil. If cryotherapy has been avoided, amputation or serious resultant deformities are uncommon.

BITES CAUSED BY SNAKES NOT FOUND IN THE UNITED STATES

VIPER (VIPERIDAE) BITES. Bites by Russell's viper are the leading cause of fatal snake bite in Pakistan, India, Bangladesh, Sri Lanka, Burma, and Thailand. They are an occupational hazard of rice farmers. Up to 70 per cent of the protein content of the venom is phospholipase A2, which can induce hemolysis, rhabdomyolysis, presynaptic neurotoxicity, and shock. Geographic variation in clinical manifestations is striking. The most common systemic signs are those of neurotoxicity; external ophthalmoplegia, ptosis, difficulty in opening the mouth ("pseudotrismus"), and inability to protrude the tongue are observed. Symptoms include drowsiness, headache, vomiting, and abdominal pain. Incoagulable blood commonly leads to spontaneous hemorrhage, often massive. Generalized muscle tenderness, myoglobinuria, and oliguria also are common. In some countries, viper bite envenomation is the most common cause of acute renal failure. Management requires intensive supportive therapy and specific antivenin. Antivenin is most effective when administered within 4 hours, 400 to 500 ml often being required. Adequate doses restore blood coagulability but do not reverse shock, nephrotoxicity, or myotoxic signs. Causes of death include shock; pituitary, intracranial, and gastrointestinal hemorrhage; and tubular or renal cortical necrosis. Individuals who recover often show clinical or laboratory evidence of hypopituitarism.

COBRA (ELAPIDAE) BITES. Bites are almost invariably painful. Local necrosis is often preceded by bullae, which may not develop for 2 to 4 days after the bite. Neurotoxic symptoms may appear as early as 3 minutes after a bite, with onset rare after 6 hours. Respiratory paralysis may occur within 15 minutes. Responses to intravenous edrophonium chloride (administered as above) usually occur. The effectiveness of cobra antivenin is inconsistent. Maintenance of adequate ventilation is essential. In survivors, neurotoxic manifestations usually resolve within a week.

Burch JM, Agarwal R, Mattox KL, et al.: The treatment of crotalid envenomation without antivenin. J Trauma 28:35, 1988. *A report of 81 patients managed by close physiologic monitoring in an intensive care unit without antivenin or surgical therapy. Excellent results were obtained.*

Curry SC, Kraner JC, Kunkel DB, et al.: Noninvasive vascular studies in management of rattlesnake envenomations to extremities. Ann Emerg Med 14:1081, 1985. *Provides details for monitoring, using noninvasive arterial studies. All but 1 of 25 patients received antivenin, and none underwent early surgical decompression.*

Malasit P, Warrell DA, Chanthavanich P, et al.: Prediction, prevention and mechanism of early (anaphylactic) antivenom reactions in victims of snake bites. Br Med J 292:17, 1986. *A study demonstrating the futility of intradermal and conjunctival tests for hypersensitivity.*

Minton SA: Neurotoxic snake envenoming. Semin Neurol 10:52, 1990. *An excellent brief summary of clinical manifestations.*

Russell FE: Snake venom poisoning in the United States. Annu Rev Med 31:247, 1980. *An excellent general review by one of the foremost authorities on the subject in the United States. An excellent source of clinical features.*

Stewart RM, Page CP, Schwesinger WH, et al.: Antivenin and fasciotomy debridement in the treatment of the severe rattlesnake bite. Am J Surg 158:543, 1989. *An experimental study in rabbits showing superior survival and preservation of muscle function in animals treated with antivenin alone.*

Tun-Pe, Phillips RE, Warrell DA, et al.: Acute and chronic pituitary failure resembling Sheehan's syndrome following bites by Russell's viper in Burma. Lancet 2:763, 1987. *A study of 33 patients; of 24 survivors, 46 per cent had evidence of pituitary insufficiency.*

Warrell DA: Snake venoms in science and clinical medicine. 1. Russell's viper: Biology, venom and treatment of bites. Trans R Soc Trop Med Hyg 83:732, 1989. *If you are going to read only one paper, select this one. A thorough, succinct review with good bibliography.*

Warrell DA, Looareesuwan S, Theakston RGD, et al: Randomized comparative trial of three monospecific antivenoms for bites by the Malayan pit viper (Calloselasma rhodostoma) in southern Thailand: Clinical and laboratory correlations. Am J Trop Med Hyg 35:1235, 1986. *The authors' clinical observations are very helpful in understanding management and complications.*

Watt G, Meade BD, Theakston RDG, et al.: Comparison of tensilon and antivenom for the treatment of cobra-bite paralysis. Trans R Soc Trop Med Hyg 83:570, 1989. *Results of a double-blind study of edrophonium versus placebo and a study of antivenin.*

440 Venomous and Poisonous* Marine Animals

John Williamson

The story of the effects of venomous and poisonous marine creatures on humankind dates from antiquity, but their scientific study remains relatively neglected. The animals are found in greatest variety and profusion in warmer tropical and subtropical waters—the very seas that attract human activities. Communities dependent on the seas as a food source or as a tourist attraction are typically foremost in studying the subject. Current research is being conducted in Australia, French Polynesia, Japan, China, Southeast Asia, Greece, India, Russia, and the United States (including Hawaii). Although the subject has emerged from the realm of folklore, lack of objectivity still exists. *Human injury by venomous marine creatures results from accidental or intentional human interference with the animal or its territory.*

TAXONOMIC CLASSIFICATION

Taxonomic classification has been customary but is of limited practical value to those responsible for treatment and prevention of marine envenomation. The animals listed in Table 440–1 have accounted for the majority of human deaths and a significant number of the poisonings and injuries that are documented to date.

ANIMALS CAUSING HUMAN FATALITIES

Table 440–1 lists marine invertebrates and vertebrates that have caused fatalities by envenomation and animals responsible for fatal poisonings in humans.

Box Jellyfish

The northern Australian box jellyfish (*Chironex fleckeri*) and the Phillipines' closely related *Chiropsolmus quadrigatus* have been responsible for 80 documented human deaths since 1884; many more fatalities remain unconfirmed. Found only in tropical West Indo-Pacific waters, they are true jellyfish, carrying up to 60 extendable tentacles. These tentacles bear a vast number of nematocysts (stinging capsules, including microbasic mastigophores) that discharge massively when a person blunders into them and becomes entangled. The animals are difficult to see under natural conditions. This massive envenomation produces rapid systemic venom delivery that is enhanced by struggling, and collapse occurs within minutes in serious cases. Seventy per cent of fatalities occur in women and children (small body mass and hairless skin). The venom of *Chironex fleckeri* at least is a high

---

*The currently held view is that the administration of venoms requires mechanical penetration, whereas the term *poison* implies oral ingestion. The term *toxins* (here marine zootoxins) refers to both venoms and poisons.

TABLE 440–1. MARINE ANIMALS CAUSING HUMAN FATALITIES

I. From Envenomation
  A. Invertebrates
    1. Box jellyfish (*Chironex fleckeri, Chiropsolmus quadrigatus*)
    2. Blue-ringed octopuses (Family Octopodidae)
    3. Portuguese man-of-war (Bluebottle) (*Physalia* ssp.—Atlantic Ocean only)
    4. Venomous cone shells (Family Conidae)
  B. Vertebrates
    1. Venomous sea snakes (Family Hydrophidae)
    2. Scorpionfishes, including stonefishes (Family Scorpaenidae)
    3. Stingrays (Order Rajiformes)
    4. Catfish (Suborder Siluroidei)
II. From Poisoning
  A. Ciguatoxic fishes
  B. Tetrodotoxic fishes
  C. Shellfish
  D. Sea turtles
  E. Viscera of whales, porpoises, polar bears, walruses, seals

molecular weight protein mixture containing "lethal" and dermatonecrotic factors. Death in massive envenomations is by myocardial systolic standstill. Respiratory depression also can occur. Intravenous verapamil (dose titrated) may revert the myocardial effects.

The densely adherent tentacles produce whip wheals with a diagnostic ladder pattern on the envenomated skin. Treatment is immediate resuscitation on the beach, vinegar dousing, compressive bandaging, and injection of the specific antivenom, intravenously if possible, in a dosage large enough to be effective. The antivenom is sheep antiserum; therefore, appropriate precautions are necessary.

Blue-Ringed Octopus

At least two species (*Hapalochlaena maculosa* and *H. lunulata*) have produced morbidity and mortality. The venom is located in the salivary glands and is injected by a bite that may be painless. The salivary toxin contains tetrodotoxin (M.W. 319), a unique biologic material also found in the flesh of puffer fish (see below). It inhibits action potentials (Fig. 440–1) by specific blockade of sodium ion transport. Clinically, the danger is respiratory failure and hypoxia. Airway protection and expired air resuscitation are lifesaving. There is no antivenom. First aid is as for snakebite (see Ch. 439) and must include early compression-immobilization bandaging.

Portuguese Man-of-War (Bluebottle)

This is the world's best known jellyfish and probably the most common source of human stings. Thousands of stings occur annually the world over, usually during the summer months. *Physalia* exists in at least two different forms, an Atlantic (large, two long tentacles) and a Pacific (smaller, single long tentacle) form. The Atlantic form has caused human death (at least five in the United States the past 3 years). No fatalities from the Pacific form are yet known. Sting pain is immediate and severe. The sting pattern is a linear white beaded wheal. Allergic reactions to the protein-mix venom are possible. Mechanisms of death are unknown. The uncommon death usually occurs within minutes. Vinegar dousing for *Physalia* stings remains controversial. Ice packs are recommended for analgesia. Compression-immobilization bandaging is not recommended. There is no antivenom. Regional lymphadenopathy and vomiting may occur. *Physalia* occurs in numbers, or "navies"; hence stings among swimmers and divers are usually multiple.

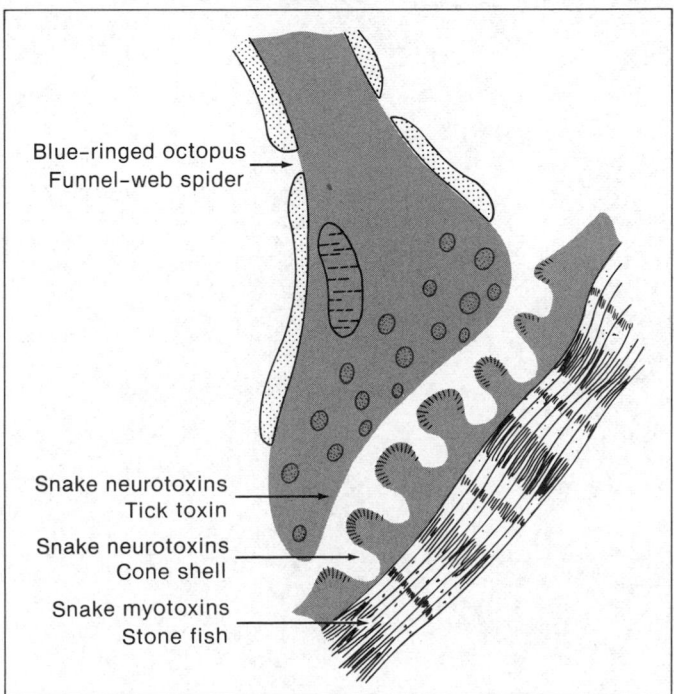

FIGURE 440–1. Scheme of a somatic neuromuscular junction, showing sites of action of a number of animal toxins. (Courtesy of Dr. V. Callanan, Townsville, North Queensland, Australia.)

Venomous Cone Shells

There are 37 cases of cone shell envenomation in the literature, 8 of them fatalities. Seven species of cone shells are considered dangerous. The injected venom produces postsynaptic neuromuscular blockade (Fig. 440–1) and thus death from hypoxia (respiratory failure). On-the-spot airway protection and expired air resuscitation are lifesaving. No antivenom exists. First aid is as for snakebite and must include compression-immobilization bandaging.

Venomous Sea Snakes

Apart from the predominance of these snakes in warmer waters, the proven lethality of several species, and the availability of an antivenom that is effective against all sea snake venoms (*Enhydrina schistosa* antivenom—Melbourne and Bombay), the subject of sea snakebite can be considered as for land snakebite. Early application of compression-immobilization bandages to the bite site is crucial first aid treatment for sea (and most terrestrial) snakebites.

Scorpionfishes and Stonefishes

Deaths from zebrafish stings have been documented. No firm record of a fatality from stonefish (*Synanceja*) stings has been located in Australia, where these stings are not uncommon. In this group of animals dorsal spines inject the venom. The ensuing pain is devastating, with intense local tissue swelling and discoloration. Immersion of the envenomated part in hot water offers partial pain relief. Medical management is for pain relief (conduction anesthesia), prevention of wound infection, tetanus immunization and, in the case of stonefish stings, specific antivenom injection, with appropriate precautions. Tourniquets or compressive bandages should not be used.

Catfish and Stingrays

Despite their ubiquity, catfish rarely cause human death. Stingrays certainly do! Documented deaths are all associated with barb penetration of the chest or abdomen. The deposited venom is powerfully tissue necrosing. No antivenom is available. All such wounds should be referred to early and sophisticated medical assessment. Pieces of the brittle stingray spines may break off in wounds, necessitating radiography and perhaps careful exploration with the patient under anesthesia, prior to local wound debridement.

Ciguatera (Poisoning by Fish in the Tropics)

This poisoning occurs in all tropical and subtropical seas and is a major public health and economic problem in the Pacific. About 1500 cases of ciguatera poisoning occur annually in the South Pacific alone. Deaths have occurred. The search for a simple chemical test of fish flesh to reveal the presence of ciguatoxin is proceeding. Symptoms are gastrointestinal (nausea, abdominal pain, vomiting, and diarrhea) and peripheral neurologic (paresthesias, especially circumoral and intraoral, dental discomfort, and a classic confusion of peripheral temperature sense; that is, hot and cold are confused). A generalized skin itch that is potentiated by alcohol consumption occurs.

Ciguatoxin is believed to be passed along in the food chain. One source may be a dinoflagellate, *Gambierdiscus toxicus*. Treatment is symptomatic. Symptoms may persist for months. Following a serendipitous clinical observation, recent use of intravenous mannitol for acute ciguatoxin poisoning (1 gm per kilogram of body weight administered over 30 minutes) is encouraging; the mechanism of mannitol's action in this setting is unclear (molecular scavenger?). The precise chemical structure of ciguatoxin remains uncertain.

Tetrodotoxic Fishes

These include toad fish and puffer fish. Ingestion of the toxin in the fish flesh produces symptoms and signs characteristic of tetrodotoxin's action potential blockade (Fig. 440–1), viz.: numbness, motor weakness, ataxia, and respiratory failure. Tetrodotoxin is one of the most toxic of known poisons and is the active component in blue-ringed octopus envenomation (see above).

There is no specific antidote, so management of a patient is symptomatic.

Shellfish Poisoning

Paralytic shellfish poisoning is due to the ingestion of saxitoxin and is associated with a fatality rate of about 8.5 per cent. This condition should be distinguished from the gastrointestinal and the allergic types of shellfish poisoning. Like ciguatoxin (see above), saxitoxin is thought to originate in dinoflagellate organisms, at the beginning of the marine food chain. Treatment is symptomatic. No specific antidote is known.

Whales, Porpoises, Polar Bears, Walruses, and Seals

Poisoning results from the ingestion of the viscera of these animals, notably liver or kidneys. The intoxication from such organs of polar bears, walruses, and seals is believed to be due to hypervitaminosis A.

SOME NONFATAL ENVENOMATIONS (Table 440–1)

Numerous, sometimes serious, nonfatal envenomations continue to occur from true jellyfish (Class Scyphozoa), including *Carybdeid medusae* (notably *Carukia barnesi*—"*Irukandji*"), and the "hydroids" (Class Hydrozoa), including the Pacific *Physalia* species (bluebottle, or Portuguese man-of-war; see above), sea nettle (*Chrysaora quinquecirrha*), mauve stinger (*Pelagia noctiluca*), moon jellyfish (*Aurelia aurita*), and *Gononemus*. Others have included corals and anemones (Class Anthozoa) and toxic sponges (Class Demospongiae).

A vast array of marine animals continue to be involved in less serious human envenomations, accompanied by symptoms ranging from mild local pain and itching to serious allergic manifestations. Certain management principles are becoming established.

1. Household vinegar inactivates undischarged nematocysts of several medically significant species of jellyfish (*Irukandji, Carybdia tamoya, C. rastoni,* and *Chironex*). Vinegar does nothing for the pre-existing pain of these stings.

2. In general, ethyl alcohol should not be applied to serious marine stings.

3. Nematocyst inhibition appears to be a "species-specific" phenomenon.

4. Allergic phenomena can play a significant role in some marine envenomations, such as jellyfish stings and toxic sponge contacts. Susceptible patients are those with a history of atopy.

5. Immediate pain relief continues as a major research goal. Local cooling (ice) helps in some jellyfish stings.

6. Serum-specific immunoglobulins (especially immunoglobulin G [IgG]) are detectable in stung patients, assist in sting identification, and may persist for years.

Burnett JW, Calton GJ: Jellyfish envenomation syndromes updated. Ann Emerg Med 16:1000, 1987.

Burnett JW, Calton GJ, Fenner PJ, et al.: Serological diagnosis of jellyfish envenomations. J Comp Biochem Physiol 91C:79, 1988. *Authoritative and to the point.*

Burnett JW, Othman IB, Endean R, et al.: Verapamil potentiation of *Chironex* (box-jellyfish) antivenom. Toxicon 28:242, 1990. *The advancing front in therapy.*

Fenner PJ, Williamson JA, Skinner RA: Fatal and non-fatal stingray envenomation. Med J Aust 151:621, 1989. *The situation at present.*

King GK: Acute analgesic and cosmetic benefits of box-jellyfish antivenom. Med J Aust 154:365, 1991. *Illustrates the short- and long-term value of appropriate Chironex antivenom administration.*

Martin CJ, Audley I: Cardiac failure following *Irukandji* envenomation. Med J Aust 153:164, 1990. *A serious new syndrome in the Indo-Pacific; with references.*

Sutherland SK: Australian Animal Toxins. 2nd ed. Melbourne, Australia, Oxford University Press, 1990. *This detailed and profusely illustrated work is a hallmark in the subject of animal envenomation and poisoning, both marine and terrestrial. The definitive work on snake and spider bite management.*

Williamson J: Ciguatera and mannitol: A successful treatment. Med J Aust 153:306, 1990. *The use of mannitol in acute ciguatoxin poisoning.*

Williamson J, Fenner P, Burnett J: The Marine Stinger Book. 4th ed. Brisbane, Surf Life Saving Association of Australia, Queensland State Centre, 1991. *A concise illustrated account of the subject.*

PART XXIII
NEUROLOGY

SECTION ONE / PRINCIPLES OF CLINICAL NEUROLOGIC DIAGNOSIS

441 Clinical Study of the Patient

441.1 APPROACH TO THE PATIENT

Fred Plum and Jerome B. Posner

The great, continuing triumphs of genetic, cellular, and molecular biology that have marked the past 20 years have added greatly to our understanding of neurologic-neuromuscular function and the etiology and mechanisms of neurologic diseases. At last count, more than 95 distinct genetic disorders of the nervous system have been assigned to specific chromosomal or mitochondrial loci. In 39 of these, the particular enzymatic abnormality has been delineated, and hardly a month passes without new discoveries in this realm. Efforts to transfer missing genes to deficient hosts have been started, and functionally effective nerve cell transplants have been placed successfully in the human brain in efforts to correct parkinsonism. These triumphs presage entirely new and potentially remarkable approaches to future neurologic therapy.

Despite these advances, the fundamental challenge in successfully diagnosing and treating patients with neurologic symptoms or disease remains in (1) understanding the genesis of their complaints, (2) parsimoniously but effectively utilizing laboratory aids to rule in or out the presence of structural-chemical disease, and (3) managing them with full recognition that the individual physician still represents the most important component in improving the health and spirits of another, suffering human being. This section particularly addresses the third principle.

The evaluation of patients whose complaints potentially implicate the nervous system challenges the physician on several levels. At the outset, patients often arrive frightened at the prospect of neurologic disease. They are afraid of pain, often disturbed by the threat of visible crippling, and terrified of chronic disorders such as Alzheimer's and other degenerative diseases. Often they use misleading or incorrect terminology to describe their symptoms, and some repress critical information because they fear its implications. Another issue is the ambiguity of many neurologic complaints. Ultimately, all symptoms of whatever origin are neurologic, since they necessarily require abnormal stimulation of either peripheral or central nervous pathways to make themselves felt. Separating primary neurologic symptoms from those reflecting trouble in other bodily organs represents only a first small step down the diagnostic trail. Even seemingly direct neurologic complaints such as headache, nausea, dizziness, tinnitus, fatigue, and generalized weakness are as likely to signal the presence of an emotional disorder as a somatic neurologic abnormality, and the distinction often evades laboratory investigation. To assign the basis of such complaints accurately requires that the physician know why *this* symptom occurred in *this* patient at *this* particular time. To reach such answers often takes time and repeated questioning, but until the physician fully understands these matters he or she can neither treat present disability nor anticipate future developments.

Even more important than separating emotional from somatic

neurologic complaints is recognizing the urgency for prompt diagnosis and treatment of serious neurologic disorders. If nerve cells die they cannot regenerate or be repaired. Furthermore, the older the patient, the less likely the brain is able to substitute a new, learned function for one damaged or destroyed by disease. The guiding principle in treating neurologic illness is that the more rapidly the doctor can reach an accurate diagnosis, the more likely he or she is to prevent progression and reduce future disability. The mandate is clear: In seriously and acutely ill patients with neurologic abnormalities, life- or brain-threatening complications must be treated immediately even while proceeding with diagnostic procedures that may take much longer to complete. By contrast, patients whose diseases lack quick and specific remedies (e.g., most psychosomatic disorders, degenerative diseases, or residua of severe trauma) usually need far more from the doctor than the local pharmacy can supply.

Several important maxims apply to all treatment situations: Protect the brain first, no matter what successive steps must follow; relieve pain even while proceeding with diagnosis; and give reassurance, hope, and explanation at every step along the way. In order to plan long-term management effectively and economically, try to construct an accurate prognosis as early as possible. In acute, self-limited illnesses, such as meningococcal meningitis or most cases of acute inflammatory polyneuritis, for example, one usually can predict the probable outcome within a few days of onset. One even knows for most such patients the difference in convalescent time required before they return to their former occupations. With diseases with intermediate outcomes, such as multiple sclerosis, full recovery is less certain and the risk of relapse or chronic disability requires the physician to appraise all aspects of the patient's life in order to give proper guidance. At the worst extreme are patients who become severely aphasic and hemiplegic from stroke or demented from Alzheimer's disease. They may never recover independence, and their proper early management often requires that one guide families through major social and financial readjustments in planning for the future. How the doctor manages such complexities determines his or her effectiveness as a physician.

441.2 CLINICAL DIAGNOSIS

Fred Plum and Jerome B. Posner

A logical approach to neurologic problems yields high clinical dividends in accuracy of diagnosis and selection of appropriate therapy. The following imperatives outline a widely used strategy.

Focus strongly on the relevant history, weighing the biologic implications of the patient's symptoms in order to link such descriptions to known neuroanatomic and physiologic perturbations. Vague symptoms can sometimes reflect educational problems or mental decline in the patient. Alternatively, they may hint at a distressed psyche more than a diseased soma. By contrast, perturbations of specific sensory, motor, or language pathways often produce symptoms that almost immediately hint at the general nature of "where and what" the neurologic abnormality may be.

Pay attention to chronology. The identification of remote, temporary sensorimotor or visual symptoms in a 35 year old who now, several years later, develops an "acute" paraparesis suggests an exacerbating and remitting disorder such as multiple sclerosis rather than a new spinal neoplasm. Conversely, a several-year history of sharply episodic, brief experiences of depersonalization accompanied by automatic behavioral activity in a patient with a recently developing unilateral headache suggests temporal lobe seizures heralding the recent expansion of an intracranial mass lesion rather than the onset of a migraine syndrome late in life.

Try to place the origin of symptoms and signs on at least a crude neuroanatomic map. Taken together, do the findings fit a common-sense interpretation? Do they suggest disease in a single anatomic locus or do they reflect dysfunction affecting several different anatomic areas? Do they suggest a system disorder (e.g., motor neuron disease or neuromuscular disease) rather than a focal structural lesion, e.g., a single spinal neoplasm producing focal lower motor neuron changes at one level accompanied by upper motor neuron abnormalities below that level?

Are the symptoms and signs consistent with known physical disorders? For example, chronic weakness and fatigue lasting more than 6 months unaccompanied by physical or laboratory abnormalities suggest chronic anxiety-depression rather than structural disease or systemic metabolic dysfunction. Beware, however; some diseases affecting the nervous system move so slowly that their early symptoms and signs may not be readily localizable. A corollary to not overdiagnosing somatic disorders is that it is equally important not to jump to conclusions regarding psychiatric diagnoses unless other findings by history or physical or projective tests support such conclusions. For example, low-grade astrocytomas of the frontal lobe may produce new-onset behavioral abnormalities long before they cause focal abnormalities on the neurologic examination or unequivocal alterations in magnetic resonance images.

Form etiologic hypotheses logically, apply common sense, and consider the common before the rare. Age, previous symptoms, epidemiologic frequency, gender in X-linked diseases (e.g., muscular dystrophy or adult-onset optic atrophy) as well as personal changes in the home and workplace all can contribute important elements that must be weighed in the evaluation.

Reach ultimate diagnoses deliberately, basing conclusions on their capacity to satisfy known principles of anatomy, perturbed neurologic function, and disease mechanisms. Avoid undue efforts to fit collections of signs and symptoms into inexact syndromes. Physicians who too rapidly attempt to match selected symptoms and signs into an iteratively constructed diagnosis often find it difficult to surrender prematurely made conclusions. A more open mind, aware that early working diagnoses are necessarily probablistic, is in a better position to modify preliminary hypotheses in order to meet unexpected changes as they evolve in the clinical course or the laboratory findings. Lastly and importantly, order tests sparingly, armed with knowledge of what each procedure can or cannot provide and how it specifically may help to diagnose or confirm the particular patient's problem.

441.3　THE NEUROLOGIC HISTORY

Jerome B. Posner

The neurologic history usually supplies a greater proportion of the diagnostically relevant information than does either a medical history or the neurologic examination. Many neurologic diseases (e.g., migraine and, often, epilepsy) are not accompanied by abnormal physical or laboratory findings, and in these instances the physician must depend solely on the history to reach an appropriate diagnosis. Even when the patient suffers from a neurologic disease marked by physical signs and/or laboratory abnormalities, the history usually supplies about 80 per cent of the total diagnostic information. Furthermore, because neurologic abnormalities affect such important functions as thinking, moving, and feeling, it is unusual to have significant abnormal signs that have not been reflected in symptoms. (Exceptions occur in

demented patients and those with lesions of the nondominant parietal lobe, characterized by denial of disability. In these instances, abnormal behavior may be recognized by family and friends.) Thus, findings on examination not recognized by the patient or family are likely to be irrelevant or even misleading. By contrast, symptoms complained of by the patient, such as mild weakness or alterations of sensation, are probably significant even if too subtle to be detected by the examination. Because patients so keenly appreciate neurologic symptoms, a meticulous history often allows a physician to localize the disease anatomically and to understand its pathophysiology even before he begins the physical examination.

Taking the neurologic history usually occupies the majority of time spent in an initial visit with a patient suffering a neurologic disorder. At the completion of the history, the physician should be able either to make a definite diagnosis or to formulate three or four hypotheses which can be tested by the physical and laboratory examinations. To reach this goal, the experienced physician gradually develops a targeted approach, similar to that which follows.

BE INTERESTED AND SUPPORTIVE. Try not only to gain diagnostic information but also to learn enough about the patient's psychologic and social background to establish a satisfactory doctor-patient relationship. Diagnostic information is often lost when the patient does not volunteer symptoms that he believes would not interest the physician or that are too intimate to tell to an "unsympathetic stranger." Such information is more readily forthcoming if the physician demonstrates interest, reassurance, and support.

BE ALERT TO NONVERBAL CUES. What the patient does is often as important as what he or she says. The patient's overall appearance and demeanor, tone of voice, or tendency to sigh or shed a tear in discussing what appear to be relatively trivial symptoms may be important clues to an underlying depression or severe anxiety over those symptoms.

REQUIRE PRECISION. Do not accept jargon or names of diseases from the patient. Jargon terms such as "dizziness" or diagnostic appellations such as "sinus headache" require an exact definition.

MAINTAIN A BALANCE BETWEEN LISTENING AND ASKING. Elicit the history in the patient's own words and, whenever possible, allow the patient to tell the story without interruption. Excessive interruptions imply impatience or disinterest and may lead to the exclusion of vital information. However, the physician must ask direct questions to encourage relevance, achieve precision, and place each symptom in its correct context. If the information is not volunteered, the physician must ask about the intensity and frequency of the complained symptoms, their duration, events and factors that precipitate or relieve them, and any other symptoms associated in time with the patient's major complaint.

FORM HYPOTHESES. Do not be a passive recipient of the patient's story. While taking the history, one must sift and distill the information in order to retain the relevant and discard the irrelevant. Concurrently, one must form hypotheses about the nature of symptoms as they are presented and test those hypotheses by asking pertinent questions. Hypotheses are tested and refined during the course of taking the history, so that by the end the physician has three or four potential diagnoses to guide the physical and laboratory examinations. The best hypotheses are broad explanations of the patient's symptoms in anatomic and/or pathophysiologic terms, which are gradually refined into etiologic terms as the history develops. Hypotheses should give preference to illnesses that are probable (i.e., common diseases are more likely than rare diseases), serious (e.g., brain tumors should be considered before tension headache), treatable (e.g., spinal cord meningioma and vitamin B_{12} deficiency should be ruled out before making a diagnosis of multiple sclerosis), and novel (some patients have rare diseases, and these should not be forgotten).

ALWAYS TAKE A COMPLETE HISTORY. Even if the diagnosis seems clear from the chief complaint and the present illness, elicit other aspects of the patient's history in order to rule in or out other physical or psychologic disabilities that could contribute to the patient's discomfort. In particular, inquire about the patient's mood (e.g., is he depressed or suicidal?), his usual daily activities (and whether the illness interferes with them), his sexual activities, the nature of psychologic and physical support at home, and his or her view of the illness and its effects.

END BY SUMMARIZING. At the end of the history, summarize the history as you understand it, asking the patient if the summary is correct and if anything has been overlooked.

OBTAIN FURTHER HISTORY FROM THE PATIENT'S FAMILY AND FRIENDS. If the history appears incomplete, and particularly if part of the illness involves changes in mental state or episodic unconsciousness, ask family, friends, and colleagues to supply missing elements, giving their views on how the signs and symptoms affect the patient's daily life.

441.4 THE NEUROLOGIC EXAMINATION

Fred Plum

Several texts contain detailed techniques of bedside neurologic examinations. In most clinical circumstances, however, an understanding of a few fundamental principles about the nervous system plus the mastering of a brief but systematically thorough approach to the examination can give reliable and effective answers. The secret is to learn well an approach that covers the main elements of nervous system function and to be familiar with ways to seek out more exhaustive evaluations if and when the history or examination suggests special abnormalities. Under all circumstances, however, the details of how one examines the patient should be geared to evaluating clinical hypotheses derived from the history.

An effective neurologic examination proceeds from general to specific in its principles and rostral to caudal in its anatomy. The examination checks on the integrity of major functions but avoids details that do not relate to the complaints of most patients. In awake and talking patients, begin to evaluate mental status and language as they give their histories. Apply at least a brief mental examination on everyone, but be gentle and understanding: "How has your memory been? Can I just check a couple of points with you?" Check orientation. Examine memory for recent events, for public figures, and for three unrelated words after a 5-minute interval. Review the capacity to handle abstractions (boy—dwarf, small tree—bush, proverbs). Provide a problem in simple arithmetic (the number of nickels in $1.35). Check serial sevens. Have the patient repeat five numbers or the spelling of "world" backwards. Be patient and remember that anxiety can compromise the performance of even a normally good mind, but if in doubt, perform a minimental status evaluation (see Table 450–3). Have the patient stand and walk; bear in mind that the nervous system is the organ of communication and behavior, and that one learns most about human beings by watching them attempt natural tasks. To detect apraxia (see Ch. 449) watch the patient at least partially dress and undress; remark on alertness-dullness; hyperactivity-apathy; adventitious movement–akinesia; visible deformities, asymmetries, or weaknesses in functional tasks; hypertrophies-atrophies; cutaneous abnormalities (pox, birthmarks, café au lait spots, pigmented or hair spots over spinal defects); a straight, flat, or crooked spine. Learn to observe constantly and closely, comparing what you see with what you already have encountered in thousands of people living everyday lives. Wise physicians gain experience not only from their patients but from the everyday world in which they live.

Examine cranial functions. Palpate the skull and test the neck gently for suppleness and length. Then examine the following in every patient: vision, the optic fundi, pupillary activity, ocular movements, corneal reflexes, jaw movement, facial movement, hearing, swallowing, speaking, and breathing. One can omit examinations of smell, taste, facial sensation, labyrinthine-vestibular activity, sternocleidomastoid function, or detailed tongue movements unless symptoms suggest the involvement of these areas. Examine in everyone the extremities and trunk for hypertrophy or atrophy, size, gross strength, muscle tonus, adventitious movements (e.g., tremors, fasciculations, tics), coordination (rhythmic movements and point-to-point tests), and reflexes. If the patient has no sensory symptoms, he or she is unlikely to have abnormal sensory signs. Nevertheless, check the distal extremities briefly for the threshold perception of vibration and

pin prick. Examine the plantar responses. Evaluate autonomic and sphincter functions as part of the general medical examination. Get in the habit of examining the neck over the carotid arteries for bruits that may herald partial stenoses. Above all, be systematic and consistent in the approach and *do not jump at diagnosis until all the evidence is in.* Doctors tend to make diagnoses quickly and surrender wrong ones reluctantly. By contrast, they view even partial unknowns as challenging problems. Try to choose the latter approach until matters become certain.

USE OF LABORATORY TESTS. Advances in laboratory methods during recent years have remarkably increased the accuracy of diagnosis and physiologic evaluations. At the same time, excessive technology raises the costs of medical care unnecessarily. More than anything else, the physician's ordering practices influence this aspect of health care costs. The doctor must recognize the precise advantages for both positive and negative knowledge that derive from each test, then gear his or her ordering to hypotheses gained from the history and whatever additional clues come from the neurologic examination. For example, when managing an adult with recent onset of headache, the results of a computed tomographic scan, whether normal or abnormal, commonly help management and provide the patient with great reassurance. However, to repeat scans unnecessarily or to order irrelevant tests just for the sake of "a complete workup" wastes the time and resources of all concerned.

De Jong RN: The Neurologic Examination. New York, Harper and Row, 1979. *The standard, detailed text describing the bedside evaluation of patients.*

Landau WM: Strategy, tactics and accuracy in neurological evaluation. Ann Neurol 27:86, 1990. *A master clinician expounds his approach.*

441.5 NEUROLOGIC DIAGNOSTIC PROCEDURES

Jonathan D. Victor

LUMBAR PUNCTURE

Sampling the cerebrospinal fluid (CSF) is indispensable in diagnosing infections of the central nervous system and needs to be performed on an emergency basis when bacterial meningitis is suspected. Table 441–1 lists other indications for lumbar puncture, as well as major contraindications.

ELECTRODIAGNOSTIC STUDIES

Examinations performed in the clinical neurophysiology laboratory are best viewed as extensions of the bedside neurologic examination. The neurologic examination, fundamentally, is a series of observations of the patient's response to a traditional set of standard stimuli. The techniques of clinical neurophysiology allow one to detail the responses with a greater temporal reso-

TABLE 441–1. COMMON INDICATIONS AND CONTRAINDICATIONS FOR LUMBAR PUNCTURE

Diagnostic indications
  Known or suspected meningitis and encephalitis
    Acute: bacterial, viral
    Subacute: tuberculous, syphilitic, fungal, neoplastic
    Chronic: syphilitic, granulomatous, neoplastic
  Intracranial or intraspinal hemorrhage, if CT or MRI is not available
  Multiple sclerosis
  Acute polyneuropathy
  Suspected benign intracranial hypertension (pseudotumor), if CT or MRI is negative
Therapeutic indications
  Intrathecal administration of antimicrobial or chemotherapeutic agents
  CSF drainage in benign intracranial hypertension or communicating hydrocephalus
Contraindications
  Intracranial hypertension due to mass lesion or obstructive hydrocephalus
  Bleeding diathesis
  Local skin or epidural infections

lution, to demonstrate the activity of single cells and cell populations that underlie the responses, and to quantify the observations.

It is important to remember that neurophysiologic tests are not etiologic tests. They do not replace the basic neurologic paradigm of reasoning from localization to possible etiologies but rather add to the precision and sensitivity with which functional pathology can be defined.

Electroencephalography

The electroencephalogram (EEG) is a record of the spontaneous electrical activity of the brain as recorded on the scalp. The clinical EEG is typically recorded from 8 to 16 pairs of electrodes (called "derivations"). The "international 10-20" system of electrode placement provides coverage of the scalp at standard locations denoted by the letters F (frontal), C (central), P (parietal), T (temporal), and O (occipital) with subscripts (odd for left-sided placements, even for right-sided placements, and "z" for midline placements).

Recorded in this fashion, electrical potentials due to normal brain activity have a typical amplitude of 30 to 100 μV and an irregular wavelike variation in time (Fig. 441–1A). The main generators of the EEG are thought to be postsynaptic potentials, with the largest contribution arising from pyramidal cells in cortical layer III. The minute amplitude of the EEG compared with the ECG is a consequence of two facts: The normal ECG is generated by cells that are synchronously activated and geometrically aligned, whereas the normal EEG is generated by cells that are asynchronously activated and, in general, not geometrically aligned. Thus, the EEG is a composite record of fluctuating correlations between the activities of many populations of cells.

Ongoing EEG activity, called the *background,* is described in terms of frequency ranges: less than 3.5 Hz (delta), 4 to 7.5 Hz (theta), 8 to 13 Hz (alpha), and greater than 13.5 Hz (beta). In awake but relaxed normal adults, the background consists primarily of alpha activity in occipital and parietal areas and beta activity in central and frontal areas. Variations in this pattern occur as a function of age (particularly in the first years of life)

and behavioral state (e.g., vigilant versus relaxed versus drowsy versus asleep; eyes open versus eyes closed).

EEG ABNORMALITIES. EEG abnormalities can be divided into two categories: alterations in the background activity and paroxysmal activity. Global abnormalities in the EEG background are seen in diffuse brain dysfunction associated with developmental delay, metabolic disturbances, infections, and degenerative diseases. EEG background abnormalities are never specific enough to establish a diagnosis. For example, the "burst-suppression" pattern illustrated in Figure 441–1B may be seen in severe anoxic brain injury as well as in coma due to barbiturates. Several encephalopathies, however, have characteristic EEG features that suggest a diagnosis. For example, an excess of beta activity suggests intoxication with barbiturates, benzodiazepines, and related drugs. Triphasic slow waves (Fig. 441–1C) are typical of metabolic encephalopathies, particularly those due to hepatic and renal dysfunction. Creutzfeldt-Jakob disease and subacute sclerosing panencephalitis have characteristic EEG signatures, consisting of background alterations along with periodic paroxysmal discharges (see below).

Psychiatric illness is not associated with prominent changes in the EEG. Thus, a normal EEG helps to distinguish pseudodementia from dementia and psychogenic unresponsiveness from neurologic disease.

Thalamocortical connections play a major role in establishing the normal EEG background. Thus, although brain stem and diencephalic activity is not directly registered in the EEG, structural lesions of the brain stem may cause diffuse changes in background activity via their effect on thalamocortical relays.

The EEG is an adjunctive test in the determination of brain death. An active EEG readily distinguishes de-efferented or locked-in states (such as severe Guillain-Barré syndrome and basal pontine infarction) from cortical inactivity (see Ch. 445). Electrocerebral silence, however, does not necessarily imply brain death, since it may be produced by reversible conditions such as barbiturate intoxication and hypothermia.

Focal or lateralized abnormalities in the EEG background imply similarly localized disturbances in brain function and thus suggest the presence of underlying structural lesions. CT and MRI imaging have largely supplanted the EEG as a localizing technique. An important exception is herpes simplex encephalitis,

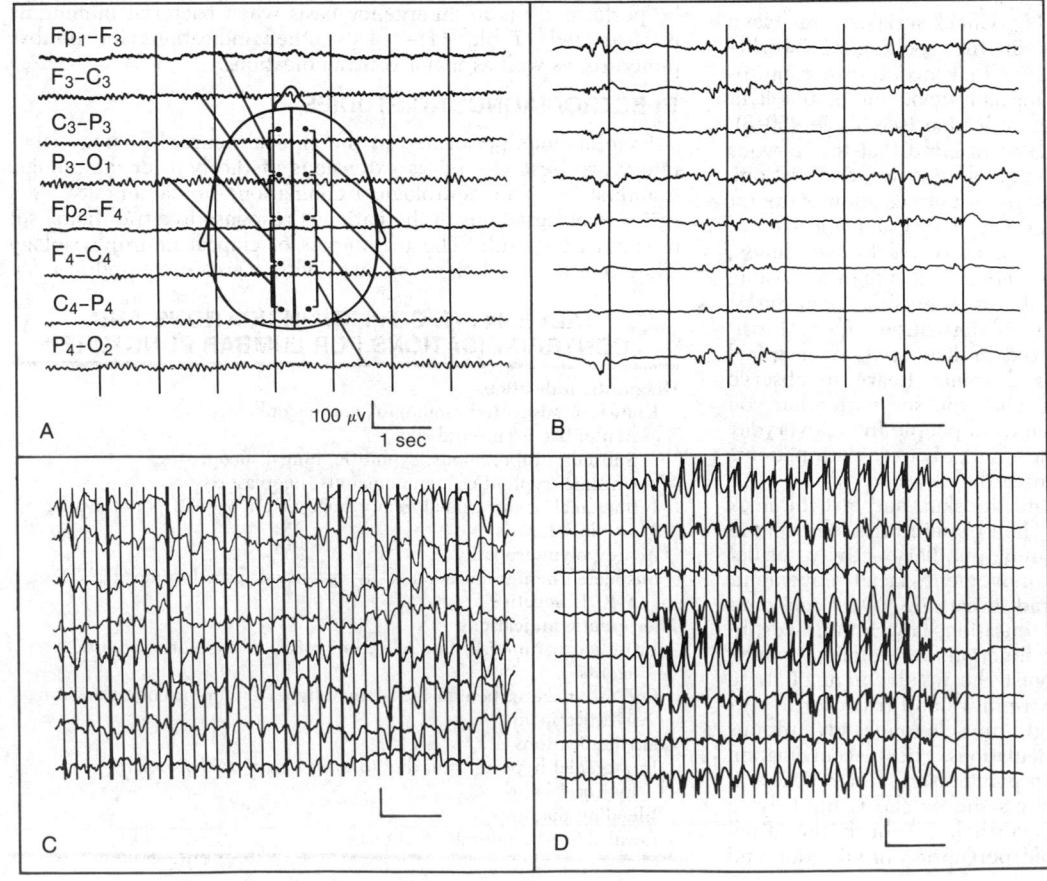

FIGURE 441–1. Normal and abnormal EEG's. *A,* The EEG of a normal alert adult. *B,* Burst-suppression, a pattern seen in severe cerebral dysfunction. *C,* Triphasic slow waves, seen in metabolic encephalopathies. *D,* A brief spike-and-wave seizure. In each record, the top four tracings are from parasagittal left-sided bipolar electrode placements (Fp$_1$–F$_3$, F$_3$–C$_3$, C$_3$–P$_3$, P$_3$–O$_1$); the lower four tracings are from the corresponding right-sided placements (Fp$_2$–F$_4$, F$_4$–C$_4$, C$_4$–P$_4$, P$_4$–O$_2$). The scale represents 1 sec and 100 μV. Note the reduced vertical scale in *D.*

which may produce focal abnormalities in temporal leads before imaging techniques demonstrate structural changes.

Paroxysmal EEG activity ("spikes" and "sharp waves") reflects pathologic synchronization of neurons. As such, this finding implies a brain region with epileptogenic potential. Spikes and sharp waves commonly appear in the EEG records of epilepsy patients during the interictal period. Along with routine clinical information, the location and character of EEG paroxysms and their relationship to the background help to classify the epileptic disorder, guide rational anticonvulsant therapy, and assist prognosis. Some patients with epilepsy may not show paroxysmal activity on a routine EEG, either because the focus is infrequently active or because it is too small or too deep to be evident in scalp recordings. The diagnostic yield of the EEG can be increased by *activation procedures*, such as hyperventilation and photic stimulation, by prolonged ambulatory monitoring, or through the use of special recording sites, including nasopharyngeal leads, anterior temporal leads, and surgically placed subdural and depth electrodes.

During a seizure, paroxysmal EEG activity becomes continuous and rhythmic and replaces normal background activity (see Ch. 483). In partial seizures with secondary generalization, paroxysmal activity begins in one brain region and spreads to uninvolved regions. The EEG identifies a focal onset of seizures more accurately than clinical observation alone. In primary generalized seizures, paroxysmal EEG activity is bilateral at onset. An example is shown in Figure 441–1D.

Whether focal or generalized, seizures with motor manifestations are unlikely to be subtle clinical events. However, sensory seizures, psychomotor seizures, and other forms of seizures without major motor manifestations may require an EEG for identification and diagnosis.

Evoked Potentials

External stimuli evoke changes in the ongoing electrical activity of the brain that may be extracted from scalp recordings by signal-averaging techniques. The three modality-specific evoked potentials discussed below form the bulk of clinical practice.

VISUAL EVOKED POTENTIALS (VEP). The VEP is commonly elicited by stimulating the retina with repetitive reversals of black-and-white checkerboard patterns. The most robust component is an occiput-positive wave several microvolts in amplitude, occurring approximately 100 msec after pattern reversal. Termed the P-100, its cellular origins include a mixture of excitatory and inhibitory synaptic signals. The VEP is recorded separately for each eye. Interocular differences in P-100 latency imply prechiasmal conduction abnormalities, and bilateral delay in the P-100 latency implies bilateral conduction defects in the visual system. Since VEP's measure central response time rather than visual resolution, they may be abnormal in patients with normal visual acuity and visual fields. VEP's are particularly useful in identifying unsuspected optic nerve or cerebral abnormalities in patients whose clinical signs point to disease affecting the brain stem or spinal cord. Demonstration of such multifocal lesions in the appropriate setting fortifies the clinical diagnosis of multiple sclerosis. Delayed optic nerve conduction may also be due to compressive lesions (e.g., pituitary tumor), metabolic disorders (e.g., vitamin B_{12} deficiency), and other neurodegenerative diseases (e.g., olivopontocerebellar atrophy). In infants and patients who cannot cooperate with behavioral tests, VEP's elicited by a graded series of stimuli provide a measure of visual resolution and contrast sensitivity.

BRAIN STEM AUDITORY EVOKED POTENTIALS (BAEP). The BAEP is commonly elicited by brief clicks presented to one ear while random noise is presented to the other ear. The normal response, recorded by an electrode at the ear referenced to the vertex, consists of a series of submicrovolt waves at approximately 1-msec intervals. Wave I is generated at the distal end of the eighth nerve, wave III is generated along auditory pathways at the level of the superior olive, and wave V is generated at the level of the inferior colliculus. BAEP abnormalities commonly accompany mass lesions in the cerebellopontine angle and intraparenchymal brain stem lesions affecting the auditory pathways. Since the BAEP shows a stereotyped maturational pattern in the first 2 years of life, it is a valuable means of assessing the developmentally delayed or at-risk neonate.

BAEP's elicited by a sequence of increasingly intense click stimuli provide a measure of auditory threshold in infants and patients who cannot cooperate with behavioral tests. In the appropriate clinical setting, absence of BAEP potentials rostral to wave II accompanied by still-remaining peripherally generated potentials supports the diagnosis of brain death.

SOMATOSENSORY EVOKED POTENTIALS (SEP). An SEP may be elicited by brief electrical stimulation delivered to any of several sensory nerves and dermatomes, but median, peroneal, and posterior tibial nerves are most commonly used. Scalp electrodes placed over somatosensory areas record submicrovolt potentials, and the spinal cord volley and peripheral nerve action potential often can be recorded by appropriately placed electrodes. With median nerve stimulation, potentials generated at medullary and midbrain-thalamic levels can be identified. Compressive, demyelinating, or metabolic disturbances affecting central sensory pathways delay centrally generated potentials but not potentials generated prior to entry to the spinal cord. Upper- and lower-extremity SEP's, in conjunction with nerve conduction studies and EMG, can help to identify radiculopathies and plexopathies.

OTHER PHYSIOLOGIC MEASURES OF BRAIN ACTIVITY. The limitations of the EEG have motivated many approaches to provide functional images of the brain with better spatial resolution. Two of these techniques deserve mention here.

Positron emission tomography (PET) is an isotopic, computed tomographic method for imaging regional cerebral blood flow and metabolism. It provides a spatial resolution of somewhat better than 1 cm. In normal subjects, PET has identified local brain regions activated by specific sensory, motor, and cognitive tasks. In vegetative and demented patients, PET demonstrates characteristic global patterns of metabolic derangements. In patients with epilepsy, PET may demonstrate focal metabolic abnormalities even when structural changes are not apparent. At present, the main limitations of PET are the high doses of radioisotope required, its relatively poor temporal resolution, and its high cost.

Magnetoencephalography (MEG), the recording of magnetic fields generated by intracranial current loops, achieves a higher spatial resolution than the EEG because magnetic fields are virtually unaffected by the volume-conduction effects that distort the brain's electrostatic fields. Since MEG retains excellent temporal resolution, it adds to the ability of electrical recordings to localize the generators of evoked potentials and epileptic spikes. Unfortunately, the minute size of the brain's magnetic fields and the costly and cumbersome nature of present-day detectors limit MEG to investigational use.

Nerve Conduction Studies and Electromyography

NERVE CONDUCTION STUDIES. Many motor and sensory peripheral nerves can be stimulated percutaneously at one or more points along their length. The induced electrical activity of muscles can be recorded with surface electrodes or with appropriately inserted needle electrodes. The *conduction velocity* of motor nerves can be calculated from the difference in latency of the motor response evoked by stimulation at two or more points along their length. Conduction velocity in sensory nerves can be determined by recording sensory nerve action potentials elicited by electrical stimulation at proximal or distal sites.

The function of nerve roots and segments of peripheral nerves that lie too close to the spinal cord to be studied directly may be assayed by the F-response and H-reflex. The *F-response* describes a muscle action potential that results from antidromic conduction of a volley along a motor nerve to the anterior horn cell body and back again to muscle. The *H-reflex*, a muscle response that represents the electrical equivalent of the monosynaptic stretch reflex, is elicited by stimulating sensory fibers in the corresponding peripheral afferent nerve. Under normal circumstances, it is readily recorded only in the soleus after stimulation of the tibial nerve. It thus serves to test the S1 root only.

Compound nerve action potentials are elicited by electrical stimulation of a peripheral nerve and are recorded by electrodes placed at a second site along the nerve. The response is dominated by the larger and more rapidly conducting myelinated nerve fibers. Accordingly, demyelinating neuropathies characteristically slow the conduction velocities. By contrast, axonal neuropathies, in which individual cell bodies or axons fail, decrease the amplitude of evoked motor and sensory responses but preserve normal conduction velocities until all of the largest myelinated fibers are affected.

Routine clinical tests cannot readily assess the function of unmyelinated fibers. Percutaneous microneurographic recording from single nerve fibers in the intact peripheral nerve represents an investigational approach to study unmyelinated and small myelinated fibers.

Electromyography (EMG) is performed by inserting a needle electrode into the muscle. At rest, a normal muscle with normal innervation remains electrically silent. With denervation, spontaneous activity occurs, consisting predominantly of fibrillation potentials and positive sharp waves. Fasciculation potentials, representing synchronous firing of entire motor units, occur mainly in anterior horn cell disorders and mechanical disturbances affecting motor nerve roots and may result in fasciculations that visibly dimple the overlying skin. Fibrillation potentials, representing electrical activity of single muscle fibers, and positive sharp waves occur predominantly in neurogenic lesions but can also be seen in dystrophies and inflammatory myopathies.

After the muscle's resting activity is observed, the patient is asked to gradually contract the muscle. This permits observation of individual motor units and their pattern of *recruitment*. In myopathies, degeneration of muscle fibers leads to a decrease in the size of motor units: Voluntary contraction recruits a normal number of units but with small amplitude and short duration. In denervated muscle, voluntary activity recruits a decreased number of units. With chronic denervation, collateral sprouting by remaining motoneurons leads to residual motor units of abnormally large amplitude and duration. Myotonic discharges, abnormal repetitive discharges that vary in amplitude and frequency, are seen in a variety of specific myopathies.

Table 441–2 summarizes how nerve conduction studies and EMG distinguish myopathies from neuropathies and indicate whether a neuropathy is demyelinating or axonal. Note that radiculopathies are distinguished from polyneuropathies on the basis of the distribution of the affected nerves and muscles rather than the findings in the affected areas. Detailed analysis of EMG activity may also help define central disturbances of motor control.

TABLE 441–2. TYPICAL ELECTROPHYSIOLOGIC FEATURES OF NEUROPATHIES AND MYOPATHIES

	Nerve Conduction Velocity	F-response	H-reflex	Electromyography
Inflammatory myopathy or dystrophy	Normal	Normal	Normal	Fibrillations; positive sharp waves; small motor units
Metabolic myopathy	Normal	Normal	Normal	Small motor units
Axonal neuropathy	Normal	Normal	Normal	Fibrillations; positive sharp waves; fasciculations; large motor units with distal predominance
Demyelinating neuropathy	Slowed diffusely	Delayed or absent diffusely	Delayed or absent	Normal motor units
Radiculopathy	Normal	Delayed or absent in damaged root	Delayed or absent if S1 is involved	Fibrillations; positive sharp waves; fasciculations; large motor units if chronic
Motoneuron disease	Normal	Normal	Normal	Fibrillations; positive sharp waves; fasciculations; large motor units diffusely

NEUROMUSCULAR TRANSMISSION STUDIES. Diseases of the neuromuscular junction are identified by the presence of abnormal neuromuscular transmission in the setting of otherwise normal nerve conduction studies. At the normal neuromuscular junction, the amount of acetylcholine released exceeds severalfold the requirements for activating the muscle. Repetitive action potentials cause a mild decrement in acetylcholine release, but the safety factor prevents a decrement in the postsynaptic response. In myasthenia gravis, immunologic blockade reduces the safety factor of the postsynaptic receptors. As a result, repetitive stimulation of a motor nerve elicits a rapid diminution of the evoked muscle action potential, paralleling the decreasing amounts of acetylcholine released. In botulism and Eaton-Lambert syndrome, repetitive stimulation overcomes a presynaptic blockade and produces a gradual increase in the size of the evoked muscle action potential.

Pathologic reductions in the safety factor magnify the normal variability of the time interval between nerve action potential and depolarization of the postsynaptic fiber. This increased variability, or "jitter," can be assayed by simultaneously recording two muscle fibers in the same motor unit with single-fiber EMG electrodes. The jitter study is a more sensitive test of defective neuromuscular transmission than repetitive stimulation.

Aminoff MJ (ed.): Electrodiagnosis in Clinical Neurology, 2nd ed. New York, Churchill Livingstone, 1986. *Comprehensive introduction to EEG, EP, EMG, and other modalities.*

Chiappa KH: Evoked Potentials in Clinical Medicine. New York, Raven Press, 1983. *Emphasis on practical matters and interpretation.*

Kimura J: Electrodiagnosis in Diseases of Nerve and Muscle: Principles and Practice, 2nd ed. Philadelphia, F. A. Davis, 1989. *A standard reference.*

Niedermeyer E, Lopes da Silva F: Electroencephalography: Basic Principles, Clinical Applications, and Related Fields, 2nd ed. Baltimore, Urban and Schwartzenberg, 1987. *Encyclopedic, authoritative.*

Regan D: Human Brain Electrophysiology. New York, Elsevier, 1989. *Encyclopedic, emphasis on fundamentals and evoked potentials.*

Spehlmann R: EEG Primer. New York, Elsevier, 1981. *Clear and concise.*

Spehlmann R: Evoked Potential Primer. New York, Elsevier, 1985. *Clear and concise.*

441.6 RADIOLOGIC IMAGING TECHNIQUES

Michael Deck

Neurologic patient care has improved dramatically in the last 20 years because of a revolution in imaging techniques such as computed tomography (CT) introduced in 1972, magnetic resonance imaging (MRI) in the late 1970's, and positron emission tomography (PET) and single-proton emission computed tomography (SPECT), which have been the subject of increasing interest over the last 10 years. Improvements in ultrasound equipment with digital processing of the image and superimposed Doppler imaging have facilitated the diagnosis of intracranial cerebrovascular disease in adults as well as brain damage in neonates. Magnetic resonance spectroscopy (MRS), currently being evaluated, measures various aspects of regional brain metabolism that may complement the findings of PET and SPECT.

Interventional radiology of the brain also has developed to the point that it is now possible to place microcatheters directly into the feeding arteries of arteriovenous malformations or arteriovenous fistulas, so as to treat the lesion with rapidly polymerizing glues such as N-butyl-cyanoacrylate, with platinum microcoils, or with detachable liquid-filled microballoons. Similarly, balloon dilatation techniques can now be used to treat intracranial arterial stenosis due to atheroma and intracranial vasospasm resulting from subarachnoid hemorrhage.

THE SKULL AND BRAIN

PLAIN RADIOGRAPHY. Plain radiographs of the skull are routinely taken in frontal, lateral, and half-axial projections. Such films are useful principally in the initial evaluation of head trauma, in which demonstration of fractures of the vault and base may influence subsequent management. Depressed bone fragments may require elevation, and involvement of the paranasal sinuses or mastoid air cells may result in meningitis, requiring prophylactic antibiotics. Most skull radiographs are taken for medicolegal reasons. Their diagnostic and prognostic value is limited because of poor correlation with injury of the underlying brain, a condition that is much better demonstrated by CT or MRI.

CT and MRI have supplanted plain radiographs in the evaluation of intracranial mass lesions such as tumors, hematomas, and infarcts, as well as in the detection of optic foramen enlargement due to tumors and bony sclerosis due to meningiomas. Tumors and inflammatory lesions of the paranasal sinuses and abnormalities of the craniovertebral junction also are demonstrated better by CT or MRI than plain radiography.

COMPUTED TOMOGRAPHY (COMPUTED AXIAL TOMOGRAPHY, CAT). CT employs an x-ray source with a tightly collimated beam passing through the anatomic area under study. An array of x-ray detectors numbering from 520 to 4800 measure the radiation absorbed by the organs targeted by the x-ray beam during a 360-degree rotation lasting 1 to 6 seconds. The analogue output from each detector is digitized and then computed to calculate a coefficient of absorption for each "pixel" in the field, using a mathematical process called filtered backprojection. The resulting computed image is displayed on a cathode-ray tube monitor that may be viewed directly or photographed onto transparent film. CT images from current equipment demonstrate anatomic structures in the skull and brain with high spatial resolution. Fresh hemorrhages within either the brain or the subarachnoid, subdural, or epidural spaces can be identified because of the greater x-ray attenuation of clotted blood. Areas of calcification may have similar appearances but are usually more irregular and have a higher attenuation value. Many CT examinations employ contrast enhancement with intravenous iodinated material to demonstrate normal vascular structures as well as the abnormal endothelial permeability that accompanies certain types of tumors and inflammatory processes.

Although contrast enhancement can add critical information in many CT examinations of the brain, the material also carries a small risk of adverse anaphylactic reactions. The general population has about a 1 in 10,000 chance of serious anaphylactic reaction and a 1 in 40,000 chance of death. These dangers increase fourfold in patients with previous allergic history to iodinated contrast material, iodine, or shellfish. The risk may be reduced by administering an antihistamine drug immediately before or 50 mg of prednisone orally 24, 12, and 6 hours before the injection. Special techniques can be used to improve the resolution of CT and generate physiologic data. These include the following:

1. Coronal projections to image the floor of the skull, the sella turcica, and the petrous bones.

2. Image reformatting to generate coronal or sagittal images from multiple axial images. The technique, which depends on absolute immobilization of the patient, produces good resolution but results in greater amounts of radiation to the brain and potentially the eye. Three-dimensional reformatting may be useful for displaying surfaces and contours and is increasingly utilized by craniofacial surgeons to evaluate facial trauma and congenital anomalies.

3. Ultrathin sections of 1.5 mm or less to examine areas requiring high detail, such as the sella turcica, orbits, and petrous bones.

4. Bone targeting, which employs a special reconstruction algorithm to define fine anatomy such as the ossicles and osseous labyrinth of the petrous bone.

5. Dynamic scanning achieved by performing rapid sequence scans after rapidly injecting a bolus of contrast agent. The subsequent contrast enhancement and washout can help to differentiate an aneurysm or arteriovenous malformation from a vascular tumor.

6. CT cisternography and myelography performed by injecting water-soluble nonionic contrast material (iohexol or iopamidol) into the subarachnoid space and running the contrast material to scan the area of suspected abnormality. This technique may help to delineate tumors of the sella region, the foramen magnum, and the spinal canal. It may also be used to investigate CSF rhinorrhea and CSF dynamics in hydrocephalic patients.

MAGNETIC RESONANCE IMAGING (MRI, NUCLEAR MAGNETIC RESONANCE IMAGING). MRI, a rapidly developing technology, has replaced CT as the examination of choice for most neurologic conditions. Nuclear magnetic resonance occurs when hydrogen atoms or certain other elements with an odd number of nuclear particles, such as sodium or phosphorus, are placed in an intense magnetic field varying between 3,000 and 15,000 gauss (0.3 to 1.5 tesla). The nuclei behave like small magnets and align themselves in the field. When stimulated by a pulse of radioenergy of a specific frequency (the Larmor frequency), determined by the intensity of the main magnetic field, the nuclei flip off axis. While in this energized state, the nuclei spin in phase as they subsequently relax into their original alignment with the main magnetic field, thereby emitting a small radiofrequency signal. The image is generated by a number of such magnetic resonance signals, transformed by a computer using techniques similar to those employed in CT. The resulting images demonstrate a high contrast between various tissues due largely to differences in the rate at which magnetized nuclei in tissues of different chemical composition resume their original state (T1 and T2).

The intensity of the MR image may be measured on the viewing console using a movable cursor similar to that on a CT scanner. Using standard "spin-echo" imaging sequences, a short T1 relaxation time (e.g., fat) results in high intensity (bright) while a long T1 relaxation time (e.g., cerebrospinal fluid) results in low signal intensity. Conversely, a short T2 relaxation time (fat) results in a low signal intensity and a long T2 relaxation time (CSF) results in a high signal intensity.

Thus the appearance of fat, brain, and CSF on a T1-weighted spin echo (TE 30, TR 500) reverses on a T2-weighted spin echo (TE 80, TR 2000). The concentration of protons also affects intensity, as it is the signal from the proton that is being measured. Other factors affecting the signal intensity include flow, magnetic susceptibility, paramagnetic effects, and the static field strength of the device.

MR images may be obtained in axial, coronal, sagittal, or oblique planes simply by changing the switching of the instrument's several magnetizing coils. Paramagnetic contrast agents developed for use with magnetic resonance imaging contain unique elements such as gadolinium that, because of the large number of unpaired electrons in their outer shells, have a marked effect on the T1, or spin-lattice relaxation time, of protons. Gadolinium chelated to DTPA is used in a manner similar to iodinated contrast media in CT to define areas of increased vascularity and/or capillary permeability. Recently, methods have been developed to quantify pulsatile and nonpulsatile flow of blood within the arteries and veins. The resulting images have a resolution similar to those of intravenous digital subtraction angiography techniques. Other methods permit quantitation of the flow of CSF through the aqueduct and posterior fossa in various disease entities such as aqueduct stenosis, communicating hydrocephalus, and transtentorial brain herniation.

MRI is contraindicated for patients who harbor cardiac pacemakers or ferrous foreign bodies such as shrapnel. Intracranial aneurysm clips provide a relative contraindication unless made from nonmagnetic titanium or stainless steel.

The presence of metal prostheses, spinal rods, certain metallic dental implants, and metallic cranioplastic prostheses may produce interfering artifacts but carry no risk of injury to the patient.

CEREBRAL ANGIOGRAPHY. Most cerebral angiograms are performed with an intra-arterial catheter inserted over a guide wire into the femoral artery and passed upward to the aortic arch or into the carotid or vertebral arteries. Although cerebral angiography is a relatively safe procedure in experienced hands, complications, such as arterial damage, emboli to the brain, and contrast neurotoxicity, occur in 1 to 2 per cent of procedures. New, less toxic non-ionic contrast agents are now replacing traditional ionic contrast materials, and the use of smaller catheters facilitates performing the examination on outpatients.

Arterial digital subtraction angiography (DSA) uses computerized imaging enhancement to improve the contrast of the injected contrast agent and lower the dose required.

Intravenous DSA is performed using similar equipment and rapid injections of contrast material into a peripheral vein or the right atrium. The procedure may be performed as an outpatient procedure for demonstrating the aortic arch and great vessels in the neck, as well as the intracranial cerebral arteries and veins. Intravenous DSA is not satisfactory for demonstrating small

TABLE 441–3. IMAGING MODALITY OF CHOICE IN DISEASES OF THE CNS

	CT	CT+C	MRI	MRI+Gd
Brain				
Gliomas	+	++	+++	++++
Metastases	+	+++	+++	++++
Meningiomas	+	+++	++	++++
Lymphoma	+	++	+++	++++
Postoperative tumor recurrence and radiation necrosis	+	++	++	++++
Hematomas	+++	–	++++	–
Subarachnoid hemorrhage	+++	–	+	–
Aneurysm and arteriovenous malformation	+	++	+++	–
Head trauma	+++	–	+++	–
Infarcts	++	+	+++	++
Abscess	+	++	+++	++++
AIDS	+	+++	+++	++++
Multiple sclerosis	–	+	++++	++++
Hydrocephalus/atrophy	++	++	++++	–
Congenital anomalies	+	+	++++	–
Sellar tumors	+	++	++++	+++
Posterior fossa				
Acoustic neurinomas	+	++	++++	+++
Meningiomas	+	+++	+++	++++
Epidermoid tumors	+	+	++++	–
Cholesterol granuloma	+	+	++++	–
Basilar artery aneurysm	+	++	++++	–
Arachnoid cysts				
Craniovertebral junction	+	+	++++	–
Intra-axial gliomas	+	++	++++	+++
Cerebellar tumors	+	+++	+++	++++
Spine				
Trauma	+++	–	+++	–
Degenerative disc disease	+++	–	++++	–
Postoperative disc disease	++	+++	+++	++++
Metastatic bone disease	++	–	++++	+++
Arteriovenous malformation of the cord	–	+	+++	+++

CT = Computed tomography; C = contrast enhancement; MRI = magnetic resonance imaging; Gd = gadolinium enhancement; – = no additional value.

aneurysms of the circle of Willis or intracranial arterial abnormalities such as occlusions from emboli or vasculitis. Its rate of complications is about the same as that of arterial angiography.

THE SPINE

RADIOGRAPHY (PLAIN FILMS). *Conventional radiography of the spine* demonstrates bony abnormalities such as degenerative disc disease, primary and metastatic tumors, and fractures of the vertebral bodies. Plain radiographs are the best method for demonstrating osteophytes in the neural foramina in the cervical, thoracic, and lumbar spine. Plain films should be obtained prior to myelography, CT, or MRI to identify segmentation anomalies at the thoracolumbar and lumbosacral junctions.

COMPUTED TOMOGRAPHY. CT of the spine demonstrates abnormalities of the spinal cord, meninges, vertebral bodies, and intervertebral articulations as well as those affecting paravertebral and prevertebral soft tissues. CT supplemented with intravenous contrast enhancement may be used to demonstrate vascular tumors of the spinal cord and meninges and can be valuable in distinguishing recurrent herniation of lumbar intervertebral discs from postsurgical scarring.

Postmyelogram CT or CT with intrathecal contrast improves delineation of subtle nerve root displacement due to posterolateral herniation of the intervertebral discs and associated osteophytes. It is also useful in demonstrating cysts and hydromyelia of the spinal cord, conditions in which CT may detect entry of contrast agent into the cavity 12 to 24 hours after intrathecal injection.

MAGNETIC RESONANCE IMAGING. MRI of the spine has replaced CT as the examination of choice because it gives better resolution of the spinal cord, subarachnoid space, and vertebral anatomy and clearly depicts the intervertebral discs, showing the state of hydration of the nucleus pulposus and the condition of the annulus with usually clear and unequivocal demonstration of any rupture of the annulus.

MRI of the spine with enhancement by Gd-DTPA defines spinal cord tumors and inflammatory processes of the meninges and differentiates recurrent disc herniation from postoperative scar tissue.

MYELOGRAPHY. Myelography is the most sensitive examination for demonstrating intradural mass lesions and can be helpful when an MRI is equivocal or shows multilevel disc disease without a predominant level of pathology. Iodinated water-soluble non-ionic contrast agent (iohexol, iopamidol) is introduced by lumbar puncture or if indicated by lateral cervical puncture (C1–C2). The contrast is hyperbaric and flows by gravity. By tilting the patient on a radiographic table, the contrast may be manipulated under fluoroscopic control from the lumbosacral region to the base of the skull.

Complications of myelography are rare, and the study is often performed as an outpatient procedure. Nevertheless, neurotoxic and other complications rarely can occur. They include injury to nerve roots by the lumbar puncture needle; subarachnoid, subdural, or epidural bleeding; infection; and aggravation of spinal cord compression by mass lesions due to changes of pressure in the subarachnoid space.

IMAGING TECHNIQUES IN SPECIFIC DISEASE CATEGORIES (Table 441–3)

Tumors of the Cerebral Hemispheres

GLIOMAS (Fig. 441–2). Gliomas are demonstrated better with MRI than with CT because the superior sensitivity of MRI to slight changes in water content produces a focal area of hyperintensity on T2-weighted images. Tumors adjacent to the skull are seen better on MRI because of the absence of bone artifact. Differentiation of tumor from peritumoral edema may be obvious or difficult depending on the tumor margin but is improved with Gd-DTPA enhancement, which may demonstrate the areas of blood-brain barrier disruption or hypervascularity. Pre-gadolinium T1-weighted images may demonstrate hyperintensity due to hemorrhage into the tumor.

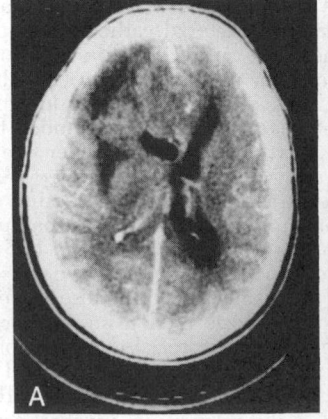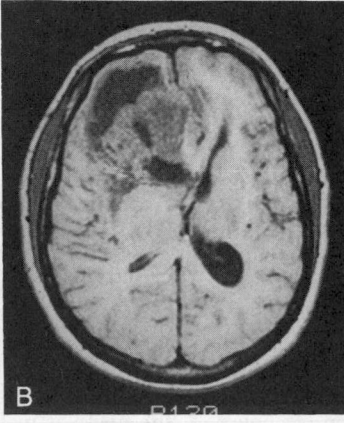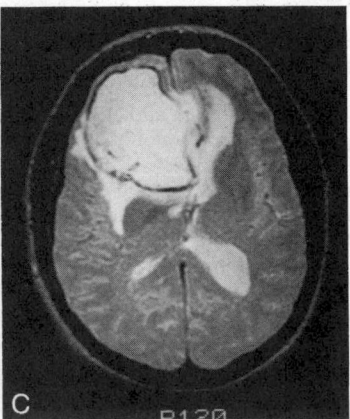

FIGURE 441–2. Right frontal glioblastoma multiforme. *A*, CT axial section with iodinated contrast enhancement. *B*, MRI axial section, 500/30 SE (T1-weighted). *C*, MRI axial section, 2000/80 SE (T2-weighted).

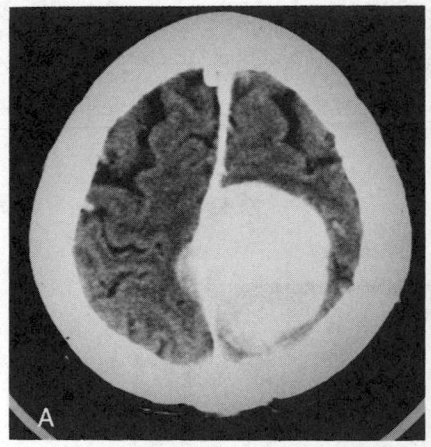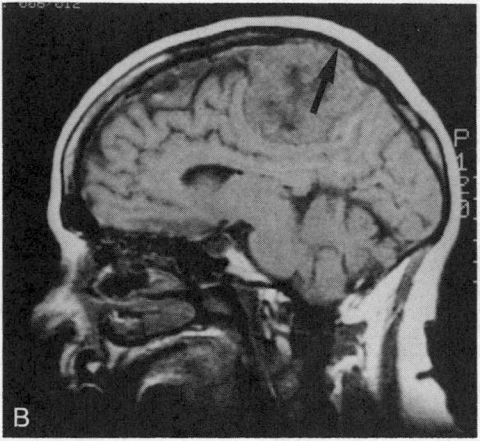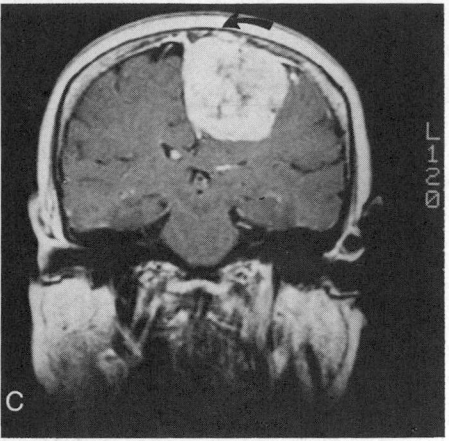

FIGURE 441–3. Left parietal parasagittal meningioma. *A,* CT axial section with iodinated contrast enhancement. *B,* MRI sagittal 500/30 SE section demonstrates invasion of the superior sagittal sinus *(arrow).* *C,* MRI coronal 500/30 SE section after intravenous administration of gadopentetate dimeglumine demonstrates intense enhancement of the tumor, dural extension, and invasion of the superior sagittal sinus *(arrow).*

METASTASES. Metastases usually show better by MRI than by contrast-enhanced CT. Occasionally metastases may be missed on a regular MRI or contrast-enhanced CT but image clearly on a postcontrast MRI. Since gadolinium-enhanced MRI is the superior examination, it should be performed when metastases are suspected or when evaluating "extent of disease."

Multiple metastases may resemble other disease processes such as *Toxoplasma* abscesses or even the active stage of multiple sclerosis. An accurate history is always required and sometimes even a biopsy.

MENINGIOMAS (Fig. 441–3). Meningiomas are usually well demonstrated on contrast-enhanced CT but if small they may be difficult to identify on MRI without contrast. Almost all meningiomas, however, exhibit intense homogeneous gadolinium enhancement; visualization, particularly of the components adjacent to the inner table of the skull, may be superior. MRI scans in multiple planes increase the examiner's confidence of the extracerebral location of these tumors.

Postoperatively, enhanced MRI is superior to enhanced CT for demonstrating residual tumor, invasion of the venous sinuses, and surgical scar formation.

LYMPHOMAS. Primary and secondary lymphoma of brain is shown better by MRI than CT, although the changes may sometimes resemble meningiomas or gliomas, thus requiring a biopsy for ultimate diagnosis. Patients with AIDS may simultaneously harbor lymphoma and *Toxoplasma* granulomas that cannot be differentiated by MRI except as part of evaluating the response to anti-*Toxoplasma* therapy.

TUMOR STATUS. Postoperative evaluation of tumor recurrence and radiation necrosis may be difficult with either CT or MRI if only a single examination is available. Contrast enhancement on CT and MRI may persist for several months after surgery, and radiation therapy may open the blood-brain barrier to contrast agent in such a way as to result in a deteriorating appearance of associated images. Chronic postradiation changes with demyelination of white matter are detected better on MRI than on CT. True radiation necrosis may be indistinguishable from recurrent tumor by either enhanced MRI or CT, but positron emission tomography (PET) utilizing fluorodeoxyglucose as a measure of regional cerebral metabolic rate typically demonstrates hypoactivity in areas of radionecrosis and hyperactivity in recurrent tumor. Some gliomas, however, may have low metabolic activity due to cystic components or a low grade of malignancy so that differentiation is not absolutely certain.

Other Brain Lesions

HEMATOMAS AND HEMORRHAGE. CT plays an important role in the diagnosis of intracranial hemorrhage (Fig. 441–4) and is routinely performed as an emergency procedure following recent severe head injury or stroke. Acute hemorrhages appear as areas of increased density depending on the anatomic location (spherical or irregular if intracerebral, lentiform if chronic subdural, and concavo-convex if acute subdural or epidural). The CT-recorded increased density of clot fades so that by 10 to 14 days after bleeding occurs the area may be isodense relative to brain but has a thin rim of contrast enhancement. Subacute subdural hematomas (Fig. 441–5) are frequently visualized better after contrast because of enhancement of the adjacent brain surface. Subsequently the aging clot, although unchanged in size, becomes hypodense, approaching the density of the CSF.

Intracranial hemorrhages cause complex changes with resultingly rapid dramatic changes of MRI signal intensity during the first 4 days. Accordingly the appearance of such bleeding depends upon time of onset, source (arterial or venous), location (subarachnoid, subdural, intraparenchymal), and whether or not rehemorrhage occurs. Other factors affecting MRI reliability include the pulse sequences used and the field strength of the magnet.

An acute hemorrhage in any location is isointense or slightly hyperintense on T1-weighted spin-echo images but is hyperintense or heterogeneous on T2-weighted spin-echo techniques. At this stage such hemorrhage resembles an acute infarct, tumor, or abscess/granuloma, but the presence of blood may be inferred by a gradient-echo scan that accentuates the magnetic susceptibility effect of the iron in hemoglobin.

During the first 24 hours after clot formation oxyhemoglobin in the intact red cells changes to deoxyhemoglobin and methemoglobin, resulting in a decreased signal intensity on the T2-weighted spin-echo images.

Between 3 and 6 days after clot formation there is lysis of red cells with accumulation of extracellular deoxyhemoglobin and methemoglobin that results in a shortening of the T1 relaxation time, leading to increased signal intensity on T1-weighted spin-echo images.

After about 5 days, when red cell lysis is complete, there is complete conversion of deoxyhemoglobin to methemoglobin, resulting in a marked decrease in T1 relaxation time and an increase in the T2 relaxation time. This produces high signal intensity on T1- and T2-weighted spin-echo images, the unmistakable hallmark of hemorrhage. This appearance remains for 30 to 40 days, after which the T1 hyperintensity gradually decreases. Finally, the aging hemorrhage approaches the signal intensity of CSF, but the margin may remain hypointense (dark) owing to the paramagnetic effect of hemosiderin in the surrounding macrophages, resulting in a "tattoo" at the site of hemorrhage.

Because of these complex changes, CT is often easier to interpret during the first 48 hours after a hemorrhage. If gradient-echo techniques are used, however, it appears that MRI may be more sensitive than CT during this time, although fresh hemorrhage may be indistinguishable from old hemorrhage or areas of abnormal brain mineralization.

ANEURYSMS AND ARTERIOVENOUS MALFORMATIONS. Aneurysms and arteriovenous malformations may be

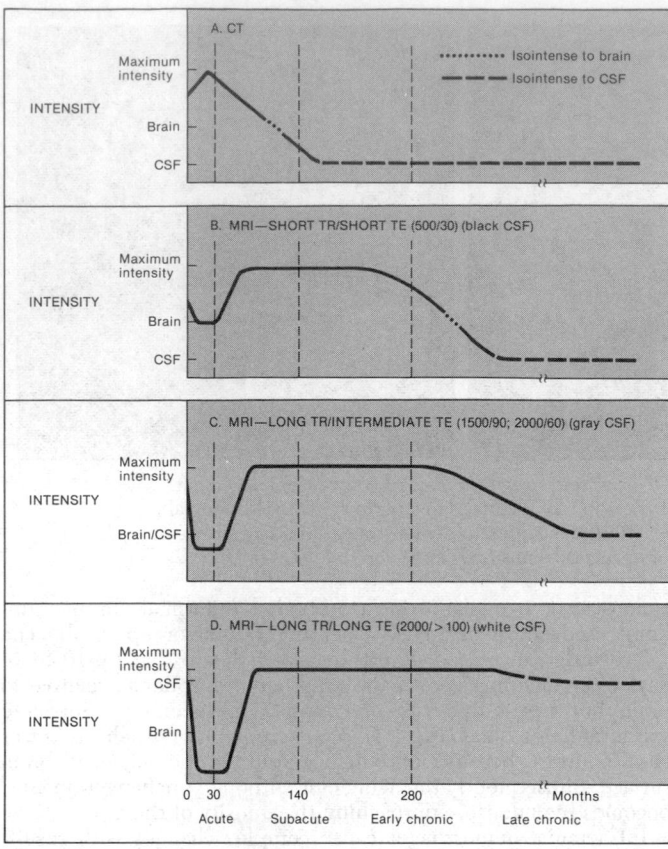

FIGURE 441–4. Appearance of hemorrhage on computed tomography (CT) and magnetic resonance imaging (MRI) with different techniques over time.

HEAD TRAUMA. Following significant head trauma, conventional radiographs of the skull are obtained to detect fractures of the skull vault and associated fractures of the facial bones and cervical spine. Particular attention to the upper cervical spine is required in the elderly patient because of the possibility of a fractured odontoid process or a "bamboo" fracture of a spine affected by ankylosing spondylitis.

CT is the best examination for demonstrating acute brain

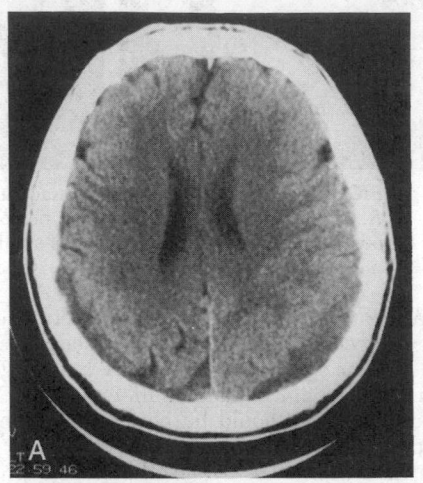

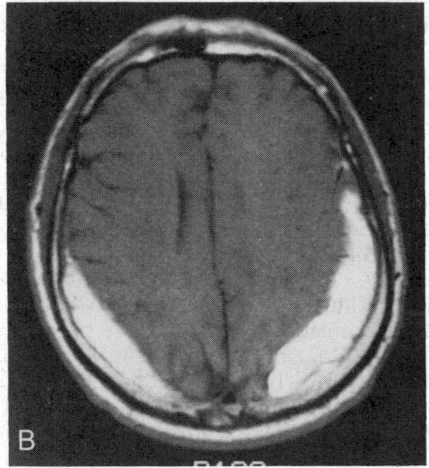

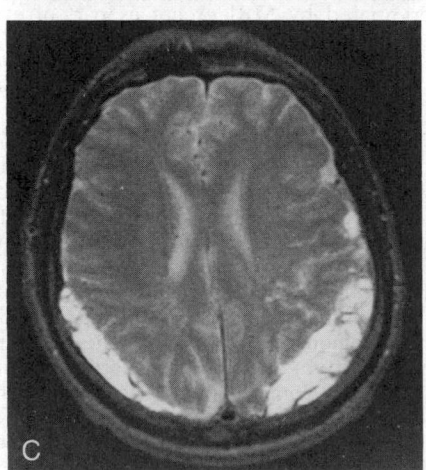

FIGURE 441–5. Bilateral subacute subdural hematomas. *A*, CT axial section shows low-attenuation biparietal extracerebral collections. *B*, MRI axial 500/30 SE section reveals biparietal hyperintense collections. *C*, MRI axial 2000/40 SE section demonstrates hyperintense collections with heterogeneous centers due to fibrous bands in the clot.

diagnosed by CT because of curvilinear calcifications, contrast enhancement of the lumen, and mass effect. MRI is superior to CT, however, because the rapidly flowing blood in the lumen of the aneurysm or the nidus of a malformation results in a "signal void." Aneurysms as small as 3 mm may be detected, and surrounding hemorrhage in the brain is readily identified. Giant aneurysms greater than 1 cm in diameter may have turbulent flow, leading to heterogeneous signal intensity with an appearance similar to that of mural thrombosis.

Subarachnoid hemorrhage, usually due to rupture of an aneurysm, is better shown on CT than on MRI because of the effects of CSF on clot formation, deoxyhemoglobin accumulation, and resolution of the hemorrhage (Fig. 441–6). *In suspicious cases, however, subarachnoid hemorrhage should never be excluded unless a lumbar puncture is normal.*

Cerebral arteriography remains essential to demonstrate the precise anatomy of the aneurysm neck, to exclude multiple aneurysms, and to demonstrate flow patterns and anatomic anomalies of the circle of Willis prior to surgical or endovascular intervention.

Most arteriovenous and venous malformations can be differentiated on MRI, but cerebral arteriography is required to differentiate a venous malformation from a small "high-flow" arteriovenous malformation and also to demonstrate the dural component of an arteriovenous malformation.

Cavernous hemangiomas, small benign tumors that can arise in the cerebral hemispheres, cerebellum, or brain stem, cause gradual neurologic deterioration owing to small recurrent hemorrhages. On CT they appear as hyperdense masses with variable contrast enhancement. On MRI they produce a pathognomonic appearance with heterogeneous hyperintensity on T1-weighted spin-echo and a dark rim on T2-weighted images. A cerebral arteriogram may be normal except for a faint homogeneous stain without a mass effect.

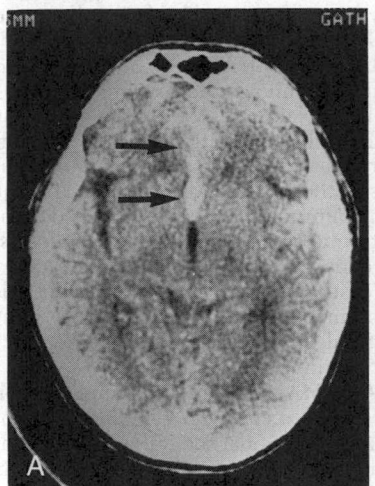 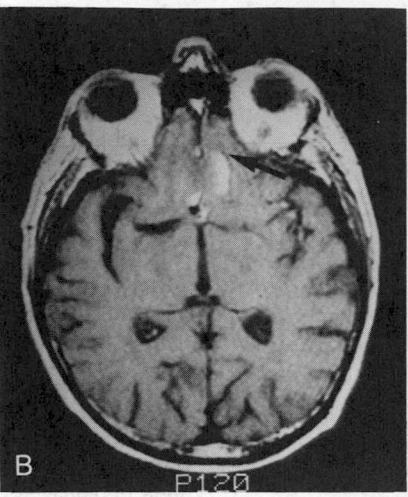 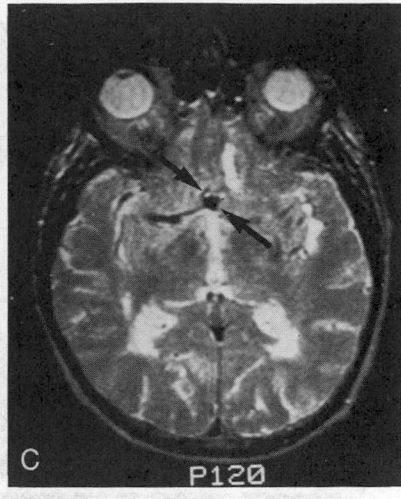

FIGURE 441–6. Subarachnoid hemorrhage due to rupture of anterior communicating artery aneurysm. *A,* CT axial section demonstrates hyperdense blood in the interhemispheric fissure *(arrows). B,* MRI axial 500/30 SE section demonstrates hyperintense blood along the olfactory groove *(arrow). C,* MRI axial 2000/80 SE section (T2-weighted) scan demonstrates the aneurysm of the anterior communicating artery *(arrows).*

contusions or intracranial hemorrhages during the first 48 hours. Later MRI is superior for imaging small hemorrhagic collections revealing cerebral contusions, and axonal shearing injuries.

CEREBRAL INFARCTS (Fig. 441–7). CT is currently the imaging modality of choice in acute stroke. Any degree of significant hemorrhage can be detected, permitting an early decision for use of anticoagulants.

MRI, however, demonstrates changes in the brain parenchyma earlier and also is superior for detecting thrombosis of the carotid artery or intracerebral arteries. Venous sinus occlusion leading to infarction also is demonstrated better with MRI.

An acute infarct appears as an area of hyperintensity on T2-weighted spin-echo images within 4 hours after onset of stroke; CT images may remain normal for the first 12 to 24 hours. After 4 days, areas of contrast enhancement may be detected with CT or even better with MRI owing to the development of pial and subpial collateral arteries and capillaries. Old infarcts with areas of focal brain atrophy or "encephalomalacia" are seen better with MRI than CT, and areas of old hemorrhage are also demonstrated.

In elderly patients with hypertension or arteriosclerosis and in patients with vasculitis such as lupus erythematosus, foci of hyperintensity on T2-weighted images often appear in the hemispheres or cerebellum, even though the CT remains normal.

INFLAMMATORY BRAIN LESIONS. CT and MRI demonstrate inflammatory changes due to herpes simplex encephalitis, progressive multifocal leukoencephalopathy, and cytomegalovirus infection because of brain edema, mass effect, and occasionally

contrast enhancement. MRI is superior to CT for demonstrating multiple granulomas such as those that affect AIDS victims (Fig. 441–8); the use of gadolinium enhancement increases their detectability. Unfortunately, it is not always possible by either CT or MRI to differentiate concurrent inflammatory lesions such as *Toxoplasma* granulomas from tuberculomas or from neoplasms such as primary lymphomas.

MRI with gadolinium enhancement is superior to CT for demonstrating acute and chronic meningitis as well as subdural and epidural empyemas. Intracerebral abscesses are demonstrated equally well with contrast-enhanced MRI and contrast-enhanced CT, but abscesses adjacent to the ethmoid sinuses and petrous temporal bones may be demonstrated best on coronal MRI images with contrast enhancement.

MULTIPLE SCLEROSIS AND WHITE MATTER DISEASE. MRI is much better than CT for detecting hyperintense areas of demyelination due to multiple sclerosis (Fig. 441–9). Contrast enhancement after Gd-DTPA differentiates acute plaques from old healed lesions. Lesions are identified by MRI in about 80 per cent of patients with multiple sclerosis, whereas CT demonstrates lesions in only 25 per cent of such patients.

Focal hyperintensities similar to those of multiple sclerosis are seen frequently in elderly patients and are usually due to ischemic demyelination or to multiple small infarcts. Similar lesions also can follow radiation therapy, Lyme disease, and, occasionally, severe recurrent migraine headaches. Small disseminated metastases may have a similar appearance.

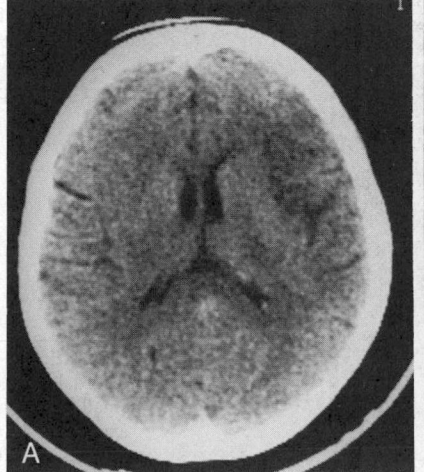 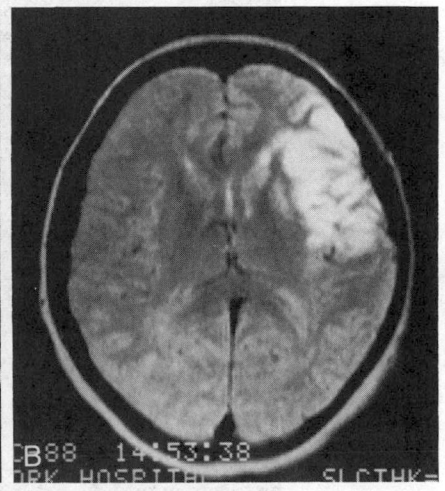

FIGURE 441–7. Acute left frontal infarct. *A,* CT axial section at 24 hours demonstrates a vague area of decreased attenuation of the left frontal lobe. *B,* MRI axial 2000/30 SE section reveals a very hyperintense area of the left frontal lobe with involvement of the cerebral cortex and adjacent basal ganglia due to a partial occlusion of the middle cerebral artery.

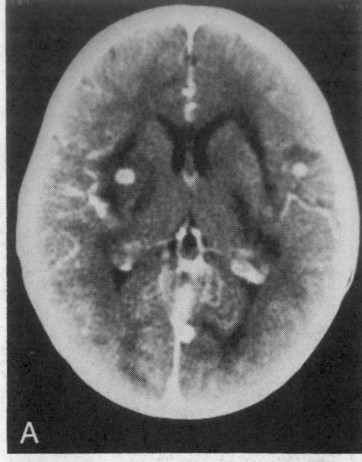
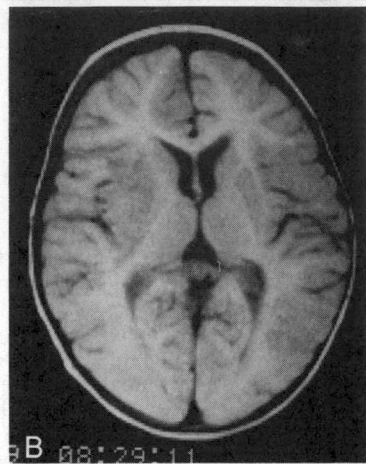
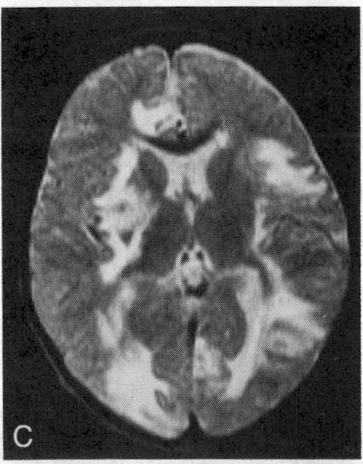
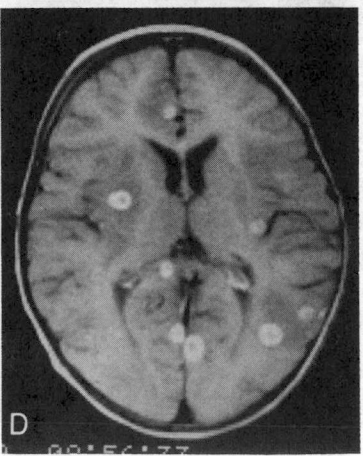

HYDROCEPHALUS AND ATROPHY. Both hydrocephalus and atrophy are associated with loss of brain volume and increased volume of CSF. Hydrocephalus results from obstruction to the flow of CSF from the site of production (the choroid plexus of the lateral third and fourth ventricles) to the site of absorption at the cranial and spinal arachnoid granulations. Rarely, overproduction of CSF has been claimed to be due to a papilloma of the choroid plexus. MRI is the examination of choice for differentiating hydrocephalus from atrophy and for determining whether the site of obstruction is at the foramen of Monro or the aqueduct of Sylvius. MRI with gadolinium enhancement should be performed to detect small infiltrating tumors or chronic meningitis.

In the presence of large cerebral tumors, chronic aqueduct stenosis, or colloid cysts obstructing the third ventricle, caudal herniation of the brain stem through the tentorium may be demonstrated on sagittal MRI images and may precede the usual clinical signs of that condition.

CONGENITAL ANOMALIES. MRI is superior for demonstrating and understanding certain developmental anomalies of the brain. The multiplanar coronal sagittal and axial images make structural changes more apparent, and MRI better distinguishes areas of damaged or injured brain following perinatal anoxia.

SELLAR TUMORS. MRI is superior to CT in delineating tumors of the pituitary glands (Fig. 441–10), the suprasellar region, and the optic chiasm. Contrast enhancement is essential in CT studies of this region and is increasingly used with MRI examination.

MR images in the sagittal and coronal planes demonstrate the normal pituitary gland, including the hyperintense posterior pituitary. Microadenomas are detected reliably using thin-section T1-weighted spin-echo sequences in the coronal plane. They show up as hypointense nodules with mass effect, resulting in displacement of the pituitary stalk, upward bulging of the diaphragma sellae, and erosion of the adjacent sellar floor. Large adenomas extending into the suprasellar cisterns may displace the optic nerves and chiasm superiorly and the cavernous internal carotid arteries laterally. Cerebral arteriograms no longer are required to exclude an aneurysm.

Analysis of the signal intensity (on T2-weighted images) separates solid fibrous adenomas from soft or cystic ones. Craniopharyngiomas and meningiomas may be differentiated from each other by their suprasellar location, tissue characteristics, and enhancement pattern after administration of gadolinium. The precise location of adjacent cranial nerves and cerebral arteries may be identified, aiding the preoperative planning and surgical removal of the tumor.

POSTERIOR FOSSA LESIONS. MRI is superior to CT for all posterior fossa studies because of its multiplanar capabilities, absence of bone artifacts, and superior contrast detection between gray and white matter and CSF. Tumors arising outside the cerebellum and brain stem provide a clearly differentiated image from primary intra-axial tumors. Tumors arising in the skull base and clivus are detected because of the normal high signal intensity of fat-containing bone marrow. The MRI examination should be modified for the posterior fossa to include high-resolution coronal and axial images with T1-weighted spin echo. Gadolinium enhancement is increasingly employed to demonstrate the total extent of meningiomas and to rule out additional tumors.

Acoustic Neurinomas. These benign tumors usually originate from the superior vestibular division of the eighth cranial nerve

FIGURE 441–8. Multiple tuberculous granulomas in a child with AIDS. *A*, Axial CT section with iodinated contrast enhancement reveals scattered small, dense nodules. *B*, MRI axial 500/30 SE section is normal. *C*, MRI axial 2000/80 section demonstrates multiple areas of "brain edema." *D*, MRI axial 500/30 SE section after gadopentetate dimeglumine administration reveals multiple small "ring-enhancing" lesions. The appearance is similar to that of *Toxoplasma* abscesses and metastases.

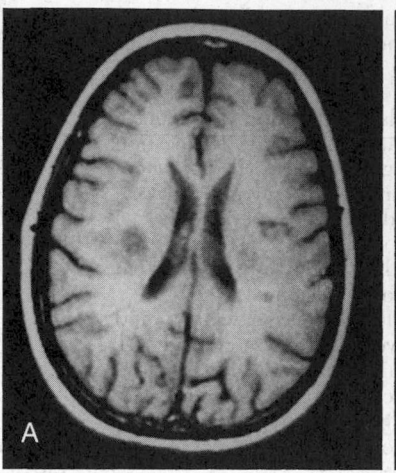
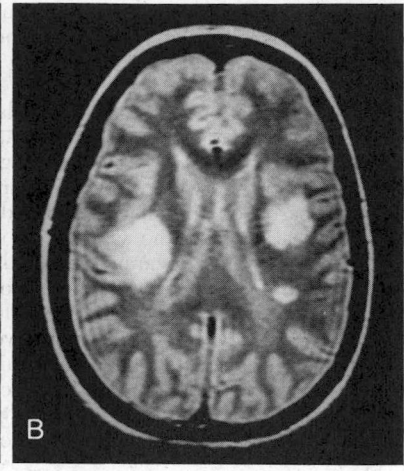

FIGURE 441–9. Multiple sclerosis. *A*, MRI axial 500/30 SE section reveals several areas of low signal intensity due to plaques of demyelination. *B*, MRI axial 2000/40 SE (proton-density) section demonstrates that the areas of demyelination are more numerous and larger.

in the internal auditory canal of the petrous temporal bone. They cause sensorineural hearing loss and vertigo, symptoms that can be caused by tumors as small in diameter as 5 mm or less or as large as 4 cm, a size at which they can distort and compress the brain stem and produce secondary hydrocephalus.

MRI demonstrates acoustic neurinomas as slightly hypointense or isointense masses in the internal auditory canal with extension into the adjacent cerebellopontine angle cistern. On T2-weighted images the tumor becomes hyperintense but may be obscured by the hyperintensity of the surrounding CSF. The separate divisions of the seventh and eighth cranial nerves are visible on the contralateral side. Such tumors show marked enhancement after gadolinium administration. Acoustic neurinomas can be bilateral in 5 per cent of patients, most of whom suffer from neurofibromatosis type 2.

Meningiomas of the Posterior Fossa. Meningiomas can grow anywhere in the posterior fossa. Those in the cerebellopontine angle appear similar to acoustic neurinomas but rarely extend into the internal auditory canal. Meningiomas frequently have a "beaklike" extension along the dura that is never seen with acoustic neurinomas. Gadolinium enhancement is necessary to visualize the dural beak. Meningiomas may infiltrate and obstruct the adjacent venous sinuses, resulting in a loss of signal void. Such sinus-contained tumors show up well on postcontrast images.

Epidermoid Tumors. These interesting tumors consist of glittering white folds of epidermal tissue surrounded by CSF. The tumors produce a mass effect and insinuate themselves into the basal cisterns, wrapping around blood vessels and cranial nerves. On CT the lesions appear as fluid densities, sometimes resembling an arachnoid cyst. Epidermoid tumors show no contrast enhancement.

MRI demonstrates the full extent of the tumor, and subtle

changes in signal intensity on T2-weighted spin-echo images usually clearly differentiate the growth from surrounding CSF. Considerable deformity of the brain stem can occur before abnormal neurologic signs develop.

Cholesterol Granulomas of the Petrous Apex. These unusual lesions are of uncertain etiology but often contain brown fluid with cholesterol crystals, thought to be the result of an inflammatory response to hemorrhage into infected petrous apical air cells. The clinical effects are usually due to compression of adjacent cranial nerves V, VI, VII, or VIII.

Basilar Artery Aneurysms. Both saccular and fusiform aneurysms may be difficult to diagnose using CT in the axial plane. Diagnosis is straightforward on MRI because of the characteristic signal void of the lumen and the clear anatomic localization. The lumen, however, may be heterogeneous owing to turbulent slow flow resembling extensive thrombosis.

Arachnoid Cysts. Primary arachnoid cysts of the posterior fossa occur in the prepontine cistern, cerebellopontine angle, and cisterna magna. On MRI they demonstrate a signal intensity identical to that of CSF. The associated mass effect of the cyst usually differentiates it from an enlarged cisterna magna.

Craniovertebral Junction. MRI is superior to CT for demonstrating basilar impression, whether due to congenital anomalies at the craniovertebral junction or to soft bone collapse such as occurs in Paget's disease or osteogenesis imperfecta. Brain stem compression caused by atlantoaxial subluxation due to rheumatoid arthritis or trauma is also well shown. Abnormal cerebellar tonsils due to Chiari I malformation or the Arnold-Chiari malformation are easily detected.

Intra-axial Posterior Fossa Tumors. Intracranial tumors of the brain stem such as gliomas, ependymomas, cavernous hemangiomas, and metastases often present with progressive unilateral or bilateral cranial nerve palsies similar to those caused by

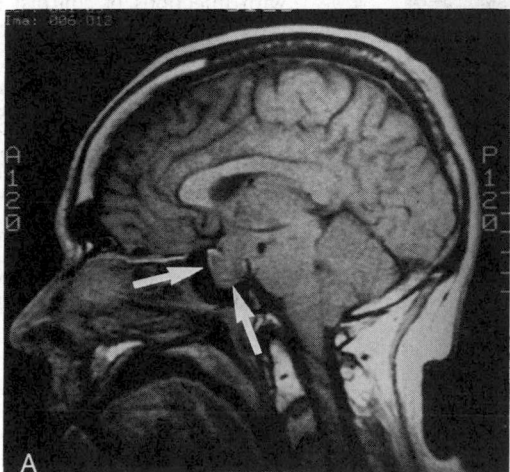
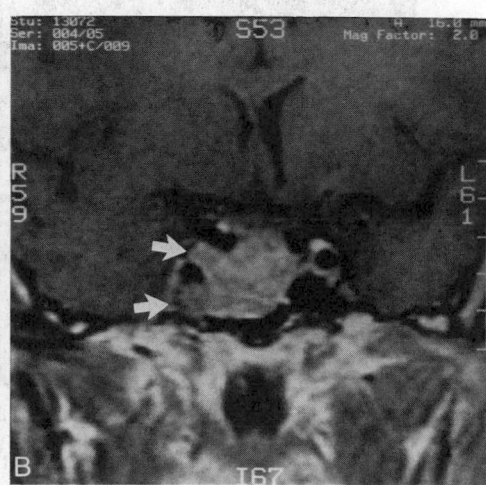

FIGURE 441–10. Pituitary adenoma. *A*, MRI 500/30 SE sagittal section demonstrates enlargement of the sella (*arrows*), with an isodense mass extending from the sella to occupy the interpeduncular cistern and the anterior half of the third ventricle. *B*, MRI 500/30 SE coronal section after gadopentetate dimeglumine administration. The tumor is enhanced and extends into the right cavernous sinus (*arrows*) as well as to the suprasellar cistern.

extracranial tumors. Imaging techniques are crucial in the diagnosis and usually determine treatment such as radiation or chemotherapy, as surgical biopsy may have a high complication rate.

MRI examination with multiple planes, multiple sequences, and contrast enhancement demonstrates the intra-axial location and extent of the mass with a high degree of confidence. Differentiation between a glioma and ependymoma may be possible based on the sharply defined edge of an ependymoma and its location near the ventricular surface. Metastases of the brain stem vary in appearance depending upon the site of origin and may be mistaken for granulomas or lymphoma.

CEREBELLAR TUMORS. Medulloblastomas as well as solid and cystic astrocytomas are usually well demonstrated with CT or MRI with contrast enhancement. Hemangioblastomas, often cystic, are better shown on MRI with contrast enhancement. The upper spinal cord should be included in the study, since the area may contain additional hemangioblastomas.

The Spine

TRAUMA. Conventional radiographs are performed initially to demonstrate fracture and dislocation. Following a neck injury radiographs of the cervical spine are usually taken in flexion and extension to detect instability due to ligamentous injury after midposition views with a collar have revealed normal alignment and an intact odontoid process. CT is helpful in demonstrating fractures of the neural arch and articular facets as well as transverse fractures of the vertebral body and post-traumatic disc herniations that may result in cord nerve root compression. If spinal cord injury is evident clinically, MRI examination may be used to elucidate the cause, such as hematomyelia or epidural hematoma, and may assist in the decision for conservative or surgical management.

DEGENERATIVE DISC DISEASE. Plain radiographs should be taken to demonstrate the vertebrae and disc spaces. Views in flexion and extension are often helpful in showing instability at the intervertebral articulation.

MRI is the study of choice for demonstrating degeneration or prolapse of the discs (Fig. 441–11). Images are obtained in the sagittal plane and in the oblique axial planes through the intervertebral discs using various T1- or T2-weighted spin-echo sequences or gradient-echo techniques. Disc prolapse is identified and the annular deficit is usually clearly seen. Spinal stenosis, if present, is easily identified, and spinal cord or cauda equina compression may be detected.

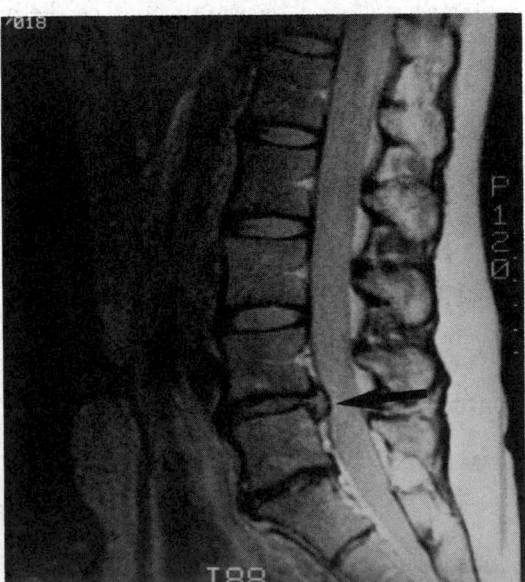

FIGURE 441–11. Herniation of a lumbar intervertebral disc. MRI 1500/30 SE sagittal section reveals a midline posterior prolapse of the nucleus pulposus of the L4/5 intervertebral disc (arrow) with an obvious dehiscence of the annulus fibrosis.

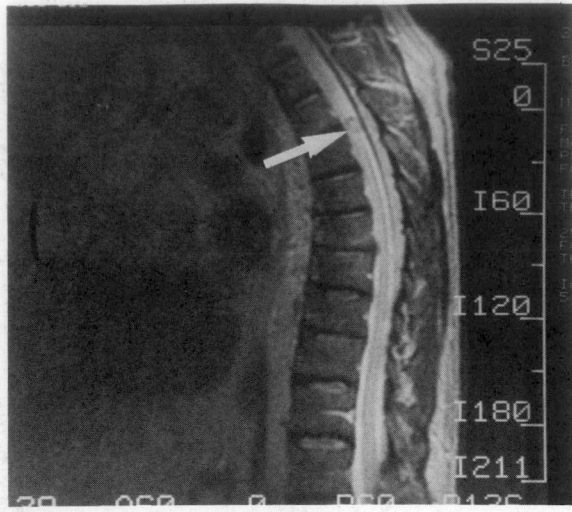

FIGURE 441–12. Thoracic neurofibroma. MRI 2000/80 SE sagittal section demonstrates an ovoid tumor (arrow) overlying the thoracic spinal cord.

In the cervical region, spinal stenosis with instability of the intervertebral joints may lead to cystic changes in the spinal cord that are easily seen on MRI.

In the postoperative patient with recurrent symptoms, MRI with gadolinium enhancement is necessary to differentiate recurrent disc prolapse from postoperative scarring in the epidural space.

If MR images are degraded by implanted metallic clips or patient motion, a CT examination of the area may be used in the postoperative patient. Intravenous iodinated contrast is used to differentiate enhancing epidural scars from recurrent disc disease.

PRIMARY TUMORS, HYDROMYELIA, AND DEMYELINATING DISORDERS OF THE SPINAL CORD. MRI is the study of choice (Fig. 441–12). Gadolinium enhancement is required to demonstrate areas of increased vascularity in the spinal cord due to inflammatory and neoplastic processes. In cases of an apparent hydromyelia, small intramedullary tumors with extensive associated cysts may be overlooked on nonenhanced studies. Meningeal metastases either from systemic cancer or from central nervous system tumors show enhancement after gadolinium on MRI.

METASTATIC BONE DISEASE. MRI is the most accurate technique for detecting osseous metastases and epidural masses that may result in cord or cauda equina compression. The approach is replacing emergency myelography and is usually sufficient to direct radiotherapy to the appropriate areas. MRI or CT may be used to direct needle biopsies of suspected metastases of the vertebrae.

ARTERIOVENOUS MALFORMATIONS OF THE SPINAL CORD. Although large arteriovenous malformations may be identified on MRI or MR angiography, myelography is necessary to identify small malformations. Selective spinal arteriography with injections of contrast into multiple intercostal and lumbar arteries is required to identify the precise feeding artery and nidus of the malformation.

Brant-Zawadski M, Norman D (eds.): Magnetic Resonance Imaging of the Central Nervous System. New York, Raven Press, 1987. *An up-to-date atlas of MRI demonstrating the classic appearances of a variety of brain lesions.*

Huk WJ, Gademann G, Friedmann G: Magnetic Resonance Imaging of Central Nervous System Diseases. Berlin, Springer-Verlag, 1990.

Newton TH, Potts DG (eds.): Advanced Imaging Techniques: Modern Neuroradiology. Vol. 2. San Anselmo, Calif., Clavedel Press, 1983. *Contains, among other useful information, an excellent description of the physics and techniques of various imaging modalities written for nonphysicians.*

Stark DD, Bradley WG (eds.): Magnetic Resonance Imaging. St. Louis, CV Mosby, 1988. *A comprehensive text containing detailed technical and clinical descriptions of MRI.*

442 Neurologic Problems Associated with Aging

Fred Plum

Persons older than 60 years are predisposed to several specific neurologic diseases discussed elsewhere in this section (Table 442–1). In addition, aging-related changes in the peripheral and central nervous systems produce worrisome symptoms in a far larger number. The process of aging importantly affects neurologic structures governing mood, intellectual processing, skilled movement, and the perceptions mediated by the special senses (Table 442–2). Symptoms of mild autonomic insufficiency, including constipation, nocturia, relative insomnia, sexual inadequacy, mild orthostatic hypotension, and increased susceptibility to hypothermia, affect many, if not most, persons more than 70 years of age. Almost half of those who survive beyond age 85 develop signs and symptoms of clinically diagnosable Alzheimer's disease, stroke, or both. Not surprisingly, many of the remainder become apprehensive about developing these conditions. Furthermore, many drugs employed to ameliorate symptoms in various body systems also can cause brain dysfunction in the elderly. These considerations can make difficult the problem of distinguishing benign neurologic symptoms from those related to disease (Table 442–3).

Many, perhaps most, persons living beyond age 70 have at least some recent memory loss, many have lost their life-long regular occupations, and few have developed active social, recreational, or athletic diversions to fill their time. Despite even television's lulling immanence, many become anxious and some depressed. Severe depression affects more than 15 per cent of those older than 65 years, striking men more than women. Antidepressant medication often is effective but may be tolerated only at doses substantially lower than those indicated for younger persons. Chapter 451 discusses this problem at greater length.

No effective treatment for organic memory loss has appeared, but that due to anxiety or inattention may be helped by counseling or referral to appropriately concerned lay or religious associations. The merely anxious do best with reassurance; benzodiazepines or other tranquilizers seldom provide enduring benefit and sometimes make matters worse. Physiologic sleep in the elderly becomes less satisfying; deep, stage 4 sleep disappears and the remainder becomes more fitful and less lengthy. Furthermore, natural circadian rhythms intensify their effects, increasing the urge to postprandial drowsiness. A postlunch siesta can minimize or prevent the latter, heading off embarrassment and the appearance of senility that surround those who uncontrollably doze off at meetings or social gatherings. Otherwise, reassurance is all that is needed to alleviate concern about reduced ability to sleep. Sedative use for sleep problems in the elderly is almost never helpful and sometimes harmful. For the already addicted, it may be impossible to discontinue such drugs. Otherwise their use should be confined briefly to emergencies or travel that extends beyond more than four to six time zones. In such instances, one can use one-half the smallest available (0.125 mg) triazolam tablet, i.e., a dose of approximately 0.060 mg, which usually brings at least brief sleep with no or minimal toxic side effects.

Postural and musculoskeletal problems abound in the elderly.

TABLE 442–1. NEUROLOGIC DISORDERS ESPECIALLY RELATED TO AGING

Alzheimer's disease and related dementias
Cerebrovascular disease
"Idiopathic" degenerative disorders
 Parkinson's disease
 Senile tremor and allied movement disorders
 Motor neuron diseases
 Late-life ataxias
Spinal arthropathies with nerve root or spinal cord entrapment
Cranial arteritis
Herpes zoster
"Idiopathic" peripheral neuropathy
Drop attacks and falls

TABLE 442–2. AGING CHANGES IN THE NERVOUS SYSTEM (65 TO 80 YEARS)

Brain shrinks and neuron counts decrease
 Frontal lobe (30%)
 Temporal lobe (45%)
 Basal ganglia (30%)
Cerebral blood flow and metabolism eventually decline
Speed of central and peripheral neural processing slows
Autonomic and muscle stretch reflexes lose sensitivity
Central and peripheral cholinergic systems decay
Olfactory, visual, and auditory-vestibular systems deteriorate
Susceptibility increases to degenerative, vascular, and immune-mediated disorders

Joint and muscle-tendon pain sometimes can be difficult to separate from nerve root pain. Except for hip and knee replacements, however, few patients benefit from surgical treatment. Most of the symptoms derive from longstanding wear and tear on joints and tendons, but changes in basal ganglia, postural reflexes, and perceptual functions contribute. Even in the absence of true parkinsonism, standing and walking become more stooped; the restless, normal, spontaneous muscular activity that characterizes more youthful life disappears; and physiologic tremor intensifies. Inadvertent falls become an increasing risk. The skeletal muscles lose their tone, reflex speeds slow down, and strength declines. All these changes reduce the sense of well-being but can be ameliorated somewhat by postural education and exercise. Even walking with briskly swinging arms can reduce discomfort and improve the sense of vigor. More extensive muscular activity must be appropriately individualized.

Chronic feelings of dizziness, "spaciness," or giddiness plague the elderly. True vertigo is uncommon (see Ch. 453), but slowed or reduced baroceptor reflexes frequently induce brief orthostatic dysequilibrium. Similarly, contradictions among visual, labyrinthine-vestibular, and proprioceptive perceptions develop and often generate a sense of giddiness or unsteadiness during standing or walking. Extending the head and looking skyward while walking or standing accentuates the contradictions between visual and proprioceptive signals, making matters worse. Among the very old, extremes of head extension (e.g., women leaning backward to the hairdresser's sink, men painting the ceiling) can induce true vertigo, which may derive from vertebral artery compression. All but the last of the above symptoms can be minimized by careful explanation, since anxiety plays a role in every case. No drugs help the symptoms and many worsen them. Maneuvers that induce true vertigo should be specifically advised against.

Population surveys indicate that symptom-producing high-pitched, ringing tinnitus affects about 25 per cent of all persons aged over 60, probably reflecting gradual high-tone hearing loss. Only rarely is this distressing, and there is no effective treatment. The finding of progressive nerve deafness deserves referral to an otologist or neurologist. Most serious visual impairment in the elderly stems from cataracts, glaucoma, or macular degeneration (see Ch. 511 to 513). Once these conditions are excluded or treated by ophthalmologic evaluation, the physician can deal with nonspecific symptoms of visual fatigue or intermittent impairment of acuity by reassurance and common sense.

A variety of medications cause unwanted neurotoxic side effects in the elderly, including depression of mood, delirium, dyssomnia, and incoordination. Many produce side effects even at

TABLE 442–3. COMMON NONSPECIFIC SYMPTOMS OF NEUROLOGIC AGING

1. Recent memory loss
2. Depression or hopelessness
3. Insomnia-fatigue
4. Postural unsteadiness, giddiness, "spaciness," vertigo
5. Hearing difficulty—tinnitus, high-tone deafness, nerve deafness
6. Dimmed vision—cataracts, glaucoma, macular degeneration, presbyopia
7. Nocturia and/or incontinence
8. Vulnerability to drugs

TABLE 442–4. POTENTIAL NEUROTOXIC DRUG REACTIONS IN THE ELDERLY, MOSTLY DOSE-RELATED

Analgesics	
Aspirin (large doses)	Tinnitus, confusion
Nonsteroidal anti-inflammatory drugs	Confusion, aseptic meningitis
Opiates	Increased vulnerability to known effects
Anticholinergics	
Includes many agents employed for gastric difficulties (e.g., metoclopramide, atropine), urinary frequency, or parkinsonism; also tricyclic antidepressants and several tranquilizers	Confusion, hallucinations, glaucoma, urinary retention, constipation, hypothermia
Antihypertensives	Postural hypotension, erect giddiness, falls
Anticonvulsants	
Carbamazepine; phenytoin	Lethargic confusion; ataxia, mild confusion
Benzodiazepines	Depression, amnesia, confusion, drowsiness, falls
Cimetidine and other H₂ blockers	Confusion
Corticosteroids	Delirium
Digitalis	Confusion, hallucinations
Dopaminergic agents	
Levodopa	Dyskinesias, postural hypotension, confusion
Bromocriptine	

dosages and measured drug levels that lie within the "therapeutic ranges." Table 442–4 lists major pharmacal offenders, which should be prescribed cautiously.

The neurologic examination in healthy elderly patients reflects the inevitable decay that sooner or later affects nearly all neurologic systems. In addition, three fourths of those who live beyond 70 years have a major disorder of at least one other bodily system which reduces their sense of well-being. Nearly all have at least some difficulty with recent memory compared with their younger years. Nevertheless, "normal" old persons retain sufficient cognitive and verbal activity to perform bedside mental status examinations at a normal level. Old-age changes in station, gait, mood, and neuromuscular functions have been mentioned above. As many as half of the very old have difficulty converging the eyes, and a substantial fraction show functionally unimportant limitations of conjugate upgaze. Pupillary miosis is common. As the skeletal muscles weaken, interosseous atrophy gradually, unavoidably affects the hands and feet. The capacity to perform rapid skilled movements slows, and many persons develop a mild, non-parkinsonian tremor of the head or hands. Deep-tendon reflexes decline in amplitude and Achilles tendon jerks often disappear. Extensor plantar responses are *not* a normal finding. In asymptomatic patients, however, they sometimes can reflect benign osteoarthritic spinal cord encroachment rather than serious brain or spinal cord dysfunction. Perception of pain, touch, and proprioceptive sensation remain essentially intact in normal elderly persons, but most have reduced vibratory perception in the distal lower extremities. A few develop peripheral neuropathy demonstrable more in the lower than the upper extremities and characterized chiefly by annoying paresthesias and a degree of proprioceptive impairment. Such patients should be evaluated for metabolic disorders or possible nerve root compression, but for most the cause remains unknown and the treatment is symptomatic.

Creasey H, Rapoport SI: The aging human brain. Arch Neurol 17:2–10, 1985. *Succinctly summarizes morphologic and chemical changes in the aging brain. Despite these, brain blood flow, metabolic rate, and "crystallized" intelligence frequently remain within normal limits because of the plasticity of the organ.*

Hale WE, Perkins LL, May FE, et al.: Symptom prevalence in the elderly. An evaluation of age, sex, disease and medication use. J Am Geriatr Soc 34:333–340, 1986. *Among 1927 women and 1140 men over age 65 years, nocturia affected 80 per cent, over 20 per cent had tinnitus, more than 15 per cent had dizziness or "spaciness," and 7 per cent (men) to 14 per cent (women) had frequent headaches.*

Hazzard WR, Andres R, Bierman EL, Blass JP (eds.): Principles of Geriatric Medicine and Gerontology, 2nd ed. New York, McGraw-Hill, 1990. *Part 3, Section 1 provides a good background to the neurobiology of the aging brain and the specific diseases that affect the central and peripheral nervous systems.*

Katzman R, Terry R: The Neurology of Aging. Philadelphia, F. A. Davis, 1983. *An excellent small monograph concentrating especially on principles of age-related symptoms, with less attention to specific disorders.*

SECTION TWO / DISORDERS OF CEREBRAL FUNCTION

443 Disturbances of Consciousness and Arousal

Fred Plum

DEFINITIONS AND MECHANISMS OF ALTERED CONSCIOUSNESS

Consciousness is a brain-generated psychological state expressed in two dimensions: wakefulness and the self-aware cognition of past events and future anticipations which accompanies the normal wakeful state. Disease or dysfunction that impairs this combination usually causes readily identifiable conditions as defined in Table 443–1. Occasionally, however, either certain forms of neurologic damage or the presence of a severe psychiatric disorder can mimic an unconscious state. A later section discusses these potentially deceptive conditions.

Impaired consciousness can be *sustained*, i.e., prolonged for periods lasting for hours or more, or *brief*, with the lapse enduring for no more than a few seconds to an hour or so. The longer the duration of an abnormal state of consciousness, the more likely it is to reflect structural damage to the brain rather than a transient alteration in its function. Sustained alterations of consciousness are discussed in Ch. 444. Brief loss of consciousness is considered in Ch. 446.

The normal capacity to awaken and direct attention depends upon ontogenetically primitive arousal mechanisms lodged within or in close association with the ascending reticular activating system (ARAS). The ARAS consists of a loosely organized, fairly dense column of neurons which extends forward along the brain's central core from approximately the upper third of the pons to the deep reaches of the hypothalamus and the thalamus. The system includes cholinergic, adrenergic, and serotonergic fibers as well as others employing still undefined neurotransmitters. The self-aware, cognitive aspects of consciousness depend largely on the interconnected neural networks of the cerebral hemispheres, including their cortical mantles and their extensive interconnections with the thalamus, basal ganglia, and cerebellum. Normal conscious behavior depends on the continuous,

TABLE 443–1. STATES OF ALTERED CONSCIOUSNESS OR UNRESPONSIVENESS

Coma: A state of unarousable unresponsiveness; even strong exteroceptive stimuli fail to elicit recognizable psychological responses.

Stupor: Spontaneous unarousability interruptable only by vigorous, direct external stimulation.

Hypersomnia, pathologic drowsiness, obtundation: Terms applied to an increase above the patient's normal sleep/wake ratio, often accompanied during wakefulness by reduced attention and interest in the environment.

Delirium: An acute or subacute reduction in awareness, attention, orientation, and perception ("clouding of consciousness"), usually fluctuating and accompanied by abnormal sleep/wake patterns and often psychomotor disturbances.

Syncope: Brief loss of consciousness due to global failure of cerebrovascular perfusion.

Dementia: A sustained or permanent multidimensional or global decline in cognitive functions.

Vegetative state: A sustained, complete loss of cognition, with wake/sleep cycles and other autonomic functions remaining relatively intact. The condition can either follow acute, severe bilateral cerebral damage or develop gradually as the end stage of a progressive dementia.

Locked-in state: Preservation of intellectual activity accompanied by severe or total incapacity to express voluntary responses due to damage to or dysfunction of descending motor pathways in the brain or peripheral motor nerves. Most, but not all, such patients can use vertical eye movements to signal by code.

effective interaction between these cerebral systems and the subcortical activating mechanisms.

Impaired consciousness can be partial or complete, acute or chronic. By definition, acute disturbances of consciousness always include at least some change of the normal wake-sleep cycle toward a reduction in alertness and attention. These reductions often are accompanied by diffuse impairments of normal cognitive activity, reflecting a close interdependence between cortical and cognitive mechanisms and the ascending activating systems. Accordingly, acute lesions that affect either the ascending system or diffusely impair large amounts of the cortex reduce the level of consciousness. Since its anatomic subcortical cross-sectional area is small, yet the system projects diffusely to the cortex and subcortical structures, acute damage to or depression of the ARAS carries a high risk of blocking cortical arousal. By contrast, any given region of cortex feeds back to only a limited subcortical area so that disease or dysfunction at the cerebral level usually must impair extensive areas of cerebral activity bilaterally to cause stupor or coma. The tempo of the damage also is important. With disease that gradually affects either the cortex or the ascending activating mechanisms alone, arousal mechanisms tend to adapt so rapidly that wakefulness never is altogether lost. Accordingly, slowly advancing, diffuse cerebral disease causes a multifaceted dementia rather than the clouded consciousness with fluctuating or reduced arousal that results from acute disturbances. Among subcortical reticular structures, the posterior hypothalamus is essentially the only locus where a chronic lesion produces a permanent loss or severe reduction of the capacity to reawaken.

444 Sustained Impairments of Consciousness

Fred Plum

Three classes of neurologic disorders may produce sustained impairment of consciousness. These include (1) supratentorial mass or destructive lesions that either secondarily compress or directly destroy deep midline thalamic-hypothalamic activating structures, (2) posterior fossa mass or destructive lesions that compress or destroy the brain stem's upper pontine–mesence-

phalic reticular formation, and (3) metabolic-diffuse abnormalities that acutely or subacutely impair the functions of the two cerebral hemispheres, the brain stem, or both. Metabolic abnormalities especially tend to affect both cerebral and ascending arousal mechanisms concurrently. Table 444–1 enumerates the more common specific causes of stupor and coma according to these mechanisms.

PATHOPHYSIOLOGY AND CATEGORICAL DIAGNOSIS OF DELIRIUM, STUPOR, AND COMA

INTRACRANIAL MASS LESIONS. Intracranial mass and destructive lesions that immediately or eventually impair consciousness can arise either above or below the tentorium, the fibrous structure that divides the diencephalon and forebrain from the brain stem. Whether such lesions are supra- or subtentorial in location, their effects and outcome depend on (1) the geographic anatomy of the abnormality, (2) its size and rate of enlargement, and (3) any reactive changes it causes in surrounding brain. These reactive changes include tissue edema and vasodilatation as well as proliferative inflammatory and glial responses. Their volume and effect can be as dangerous as the primary lesion itself, since they can triple the size of the primary lesion. Such severe reactions are especially prominent in and around malignant neoplasms, acute infarctions, hemorrhages, or abscesses. Since the skull is inexpansible, all enlarging masses eventually cause intracranial shifts and compressions that endanger the vitality of adjacent and remote brain areas.

As mass lesions form and enlarge within the cranial cavity, local intracranial compliance declines, cerebrospinal fluid flow and absorption are impeded, and the intracranial pressure rises, first within tissues adjacent to the abnormality and then more generally. If the process is not interrupted, intracranial distortion and pressure eventually increase sufficiently to impede the blood supply in areas of compressed tissue. When this occurs, arteriolar resistance intermittently fails, leading to temporary increases in intracranial blood volume which produce brief but potentially dangerous episodes of greatly increased intracranial pressure, called *pressure waves*.

As could be expected, functional neurologic abnormalities accompanying the above pathophysiologic changes occur earliest in regions in and adjacent to the primary lesion, then gradually affect more remote brain areas made vulnerable by being compressed against unyielding edges of bone or dura. Particularly at risk of this complication are structures that become squeezed against the falx cerebri or herniate into the restricted apertures of the tentorial notch or foramen magnum, thereby impacting areas critical to consciousness and even survival (Fig. 444–1).

TABLE 444–1. THE COMMON CAUSES OF STUPOR AND COMA

Supratentorial lesions (causing secondary upper brain stem dysfunction)
  Cerebral hemorrhage
  Large cerebral infarction
  Subdural hematoma
  Epidural hematoma
  Brain tumor
  Brain abscess (rare)
Subtentorial lesions (compressing or destroying the rostral reticular formation)
  Pontine or cerebellar hemorrhage
  Brain stem infarction
  Brain stem or cerebellar tumor
  Cerebellar abscess
Metabolic and diffuse lesions (see also Table 444–5)
  Exogenous poison
  Infections
    Meningitis
    Encephalitis
  Concussion and postictal states
  Anoxia or ischemia
  Hypoglycemia
  Ionic and electrolyte disorders
  Endogenous toxin due to organ failure or deficiency
  Nutritional deficiency
Psychogenic unresponsiveness

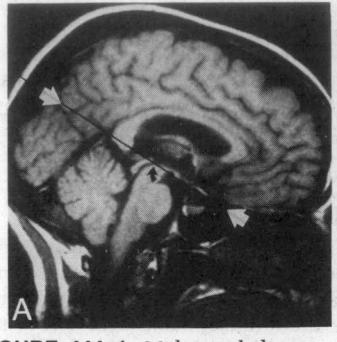
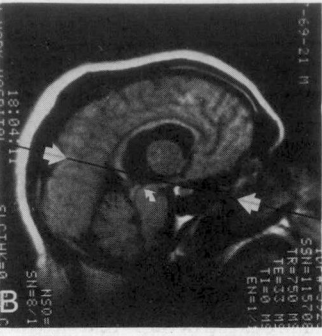
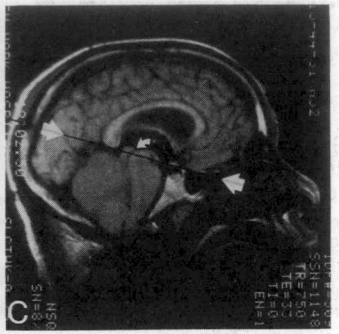
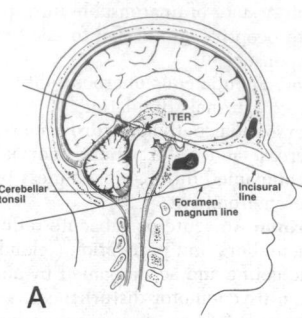

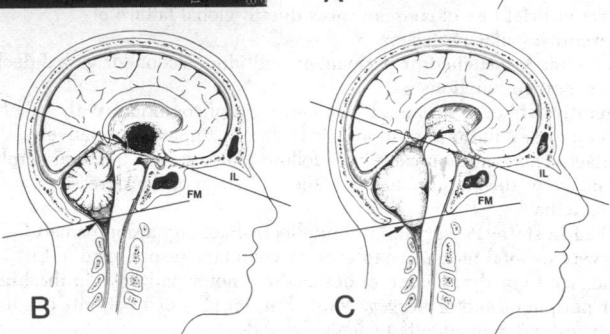

FIGURE 444–1. Midsagittal diagrams and magnetic resonance images of a normal adult brain compared with downward and upward transtentorial herniation as well as foramen magnum herniation. A, Normal 45-year-old male brain. The incisural line (IL) defines the plane of the tentorial opening, which extends from the junction between the vein of Galen and the cerebral venous straight sinus posteriorly to the anterior clinoid process. The iter, i.e., the rostral opening of the aqueduct of Sylvius (*black curved arrow*) lies on or within 2 mm of the IL. The cerebellar tonsils remain well above the foramen magnum (FM). B, Downward transtentorial herniation due to a chronic colloid cyst lying in the third ventricle of a 52-year-old man (dark round shadow on diagram). The curved white arrow on the MRI scan points to the aqueduct, posterior thalamus, and mesencephalon, which are displaced 8 mm caudally of the IL. The cerebellar tonsils are visible at the level of the foramen magnum. C, Upward tentorial plus foramen magnum herniation has occurred secondary to a cerebellar lymphoma in a 32-year-old man with HIV-I infection. The cerebellum is enlarged. The iter (*black curved arrow*) and the rostral mesencephalon have herniated 6 mm above the IL, and the brain stem is flattened against the base of the skull. The cerebellar tonsils have herniated into the foramen magnum.

SUPRATENTORIAL MASS LESIONS CAUSING COMA.
Enlarging supratentorial lesions that affect the cerebral hemispheres or diencephalon most often produce stupor or coma by shifting brain tissue either horizontally across the midline or caudally toward the tentorium. Either way, the process compresses and displaces the diencephalon, producing distinctive clinical features (Table 444–2). Localizing symptoms such as frontal headache, focal seizures, or other changes consistent with unilateral hemispheric disease almost always appear first, followed, as the lesion enlarges, by the development of altered consciousness. In keeping with this sequence, most patients demonstrate a combination of *focal* hemispheric signs, e.g., sensorimotor abnormalities, aphasia, or visual field defects, followed by signs of *diffuse* supratentorial dysfunction, consisting of nonfocal headache, reduced attention, confusion, and somnolence. If untreated, the process eventually produces stupor and evidence of bilateral corticospinal tract dysfunction reflecting secondary distortion and compression of the opposite hemisphere and the deep-lying diencephalon. Decerebrate responses to noxious stimuli emerge in these circumstances as late and dangerous events.

Some supratentorial masses can arise and enlarge in neurologically silent areas such as the frontal lobes or the subdural space. In such instances, signs and symptoms of diffuse cerebral dysfunction and increased intracranial pressure can predominate, consisting of papilledema, confusion, apathy, or hypersomnolence (see Ch. 447). In either event, computed tomography (CT) or magnetic resonance (MR) images of coma-causing supratentorial

masses disclose a large, space-occupying lesion, characteristically associated with evidence of displacement of adjacent tissues caudally, across the midline, or both. An important negative finding is that, unless the brain already has begun to herniate into the tentorial notch, no clinical evidence of brain stem dysfunction can be found; pupillary and oculovestibular reflexes remain intact, and decerebrate motor responses develop only as a late sign.

Stupor or coma with supratentorial lesions implies that the deeply located diencephalon is already compressed or distorted, threatening the advent of potentially irreversible midbrain compression. Such impaction-herniation begins either with downward displacement of the diencephalon (central herniation) or with the uncus of the temporal lobe squeezing against the midbrain in the tentorial notch (uncal herniation). Either way, characteristic syndromes evolve (Table 444–3). With impending *central* herniation, stupor becomes gradually deeper, and patients sigh, yawn, or develop periodic breathing. The pupils shrink to 1 to 2 mm

TABLE 444–2. CHARACTERISTICS OF SUPRATENTORIAL LESIONS LEADING TO COMA

Initiating symptoms usually cerebral-focal: aphasia; focal seizures; contralateral hemiparesis, sensory change, or neglect; frontal lobe behavioral changes; headache.

Dysfunction moves rostral to caudal: e.g., focal motor → bilateral motor → altered level of arousal.

Abnormal signs usually confined to a single or adjacent anatomic level (not diffuse).

Brain stem functions spared unless herniation develops.

TABLE 444–3. SIGNS OF INCIPIENT DOWNWARD HERNIATION

	Central	Uncal
Arousal	Impaired early, before other signs	Impaired late, usually with other signs
Breathing	Sighs, yawns, sometimes Cheyne-Stokes respirations	No early change
Pupils	First small reactive (hypothalamus), then one or both approach midposition	Ipsilateral pupil dilates, followed by somatic third nerve paralysis
Oculocephalic responses	Initially sluggish, later tonic conjugate	Unilateral third nerve paralysis
Motor signs	Early hemiparesis opposite to hemispheric lesion followed by ipsilateral motor paresis and extensor plantar response	Motor signs late, sometimes ipsilateral to lesion

in diameter, reflecting hypothalamic dysfunction, but retain their light reflexes. Later, one or both pupils may ominously dilate. Loss of forebrain inhibition on the brain stem results in the development of brisk oculomotor reflexes (see Ch. 453). Until mesencephalic insufficiency develops, oculovestibular reflex responses (cold caloric test) are marked by tonic deviation of the eyes toward the stimulated side. Bilateral dysfunction develops in corticospinal motor pathways, causing hyperactive deep tendon reflexes, spasticity, extensor plantar responses, and, eventually, decerebrate or decorticate reflex posturing, worse on the body side contralateral to the brain mass.

With *uncal* herniation, signs generally resemble the above except that as the uncus slides over the tentorial edge, it may compress the third nerve ahead of it before the diencephalon is squeezed (Table 444–3). Shortly afterward, somatic oculomotor functions of the third nerve usually deteriorate, and the involved eye turns outward. If the herniating process continues, the opposite third nerve becomes involved, and other mesencephalic functions begin to fail. Effective treatment of impending diencephalic-midbrain compression-herniation must be initiated before these late signs of deterioration appear.

SUBTENTORIAL MASS OR DESTRUCTIVE LESIONS CAUSING COMA. Subtentorial mass or destructive lesions cause stupor or coma if they directly damage or compress the ascending activating systems that arise from the paramedian rostral pontine tegmentum and mesencephalon. Since such coma-causing abnormalities almost always affect adjacent neuro-ophthalmologic centers, they often produce tell-tale neurologic signs that pinpoint the anatomy of damage (Table 444–4).

Subtentorial lesions that cause coma by directly injuring the upper brain stem (e.g., infarcts or hemorrhages) usually produce coma from the outset. The pupils are always abnormal, owing to dysfunction or destruction of pontine sympathetic pathways, third nerve nuclei, or their fibers. Dysconjugate eye movements are common, as are nystagmus, bizarrely or independently moving eyes, ocular bobbing, or rotating ocular deviation. Unilateral facial anesthesia involving both the brow and lower face, absent caloric responses to either side, and conjugate eye deviation toward the paralyzed arm and leg all suggest a subtentorial lesion. The combination of flaccidity in the arms and flexor responses in the legs signifies pontine-midbrain damage. CT scans in such cases reveal cerebellar or pontine hemorrhage as well as expanding cerebellar hematomas, neoplasms, or, sometimes, infarctions. MR produces even better images of the cerebellum and brain stem, readily identifying even small areas of infarction or other damage.

Compressive lesions of the posterior fossa, such as hemorrhages, abscesses, or tumors of the cerebellum or fourth ventricle, rarely cause coma until late in their course, at which time they may cause the mesencephalon to herniate upward through the tentorial notch or force the cerebellar tonsils to impact downward into the foramen magnum. These developments produce deepening stupor, failure of upward gaze, unequal or fixed pupils, and irregularly irregular breathing patterns. In such instances, occipital headache, nystagmus, diplopia, nausea, vomiting, cranial nerve signs, and ataxia usually precede unconsciousness. The circumstances call for immediate treatment consisting of shrinking the brain and, in most instances, surgical decompression of the lateral cerebral ventricles.

METABOLIC AND DIFFUSE BRAIN DISTURBANCES CAUSING STUPOR AND COMA. Definition. The term *metabolic* or *diffuse encephalopathy* describes the behavioral state produced by a group of brain-affecting disorders that impair predominantly the organ's higher functions and usually pursue a temporary, reversible course. They all produce clouding of consciousness, characterized by impaired attention, difficulty in concentration, reduced intellectual capacity, and altered sleep-wake patterns (Table 444–5). Metabolic encephalopathy is a major comorbidity factor in a variety of serious medical and surgical illnesses, and its effects complicate patient management both in and out of hospital. Especially susceptible to metabolic encephalopathy are patients who are critically ill from systemic disease or major surgery as well as the aged. If one includes examples of the toxic effects of abused and therapeutic drugs, the metabolic encephalopathies make up the largest category of illnesses causing confusion, stupor, or coma.

Disorders or drugs affecting several neurochemical and neuropharmacologic systems can cause a metabolic encephalopathy. Prominent examples are those with anticholinergic and sedative effects. Other common causes include a number of inflammatory or infectious illnesses, physiologic disturbances such as epilepsy or complicated migraine, diffuse brain trauma, and disseminated structural lesions such as certain forms of cancer or cerebral thromboembolism. Diffuse, acute or subacute, bilateral, multilevel cerebral and subcerebral dysfunction that almost always spares pupillary reactivity is the hallmark of metabolic encephalopathy and is a combination only rarely produced by structural brain disease.

Terminology. Classic neurologic thinking has employed the term *delirium* or *acute toxic psychosis* for the more blatantly agitated and severely disoriented, hallucinatory-delusional forms of metabolic encephalopathy. Quieter, less severe disturbances have been termed *acute* or *subacute confusional states*. This chapter often employs these terms as being more descriptively informative than the usage adopted by the American Psychiatric Association's Diagnostic Manual, which applies the term *delirium* to all examples of acquired confusion, agitation, disorientation, or hallucinations occurring in the setting of structural or known neurochemical brain disease.

Clinical Features. The clinical evaluation of confused or delirious states attempts first to determine whether observed changes in consciousness are due to metabolic rather than structural brain disease or psychiatric dysfunction. One then proceeds to define the particular metabolic or structural defects and treat them. Evaluations of the history, the pattern of impaired consciousness, motor activity, and autonomic activity help answer the first question, whereas the general physical examination, evaluation of pulmonary ventilation, and laboratory tests assist with the second (Table 444–6). The history is especially important and should inquire into previous systemic medical illnesses, psychiatric history, access to potentially intoxicating drugs or alcohol, and recent changes in behavior.

State of Consciousness and Mental Content. Disorders of attention are the earliest sign and the hallmark of metabolic brain disease. Some patients act quietly perplexed, preoccupied, and unable to concentrate sufficiently to deal with significant stimuli in the environment. Others appear hypervigilant and distractible, picking at the bedclothes and attending briefly to each new environmental stimulus no matter how trivial or irrelevant. Still others lose contact with the environment, becoming completely preoccupied and often frightened by vivid fragmentary hallucinations or delusions. Early attentional deficits may be subtle and easily mistaken for normal, slightly odd behavior. Soon, however, other symptoms emerge, including emotional lability, insomnia or drowsiness, and often vivid nightmares. As delirium worsens, some patients express the fear of "going crazy." Others lie quietly or sleep when left alone. None reads for substance or attends with any interest to the surrounding world. With more severe metabolic disturbances, patients become drowsy and finally stuporous or comatose. The prevailing affect depends partly on the nature of the illness and partly on how rapidly it develops. Remarkably, previous personality often has surprisingly little influence on delirious behavior. Rapidly developing metabolic abnormalities are more likely to produce agitation or stupor than are those that evolve more slowly.

Disturbances in cognition consistently accompany altered alertness and awareness, causing difficulties with immediate recall and the ability to abstract. Normal subjects readily recall and repeat six or seven digits forward and five or six backward and

TABLE 444–4. TELLTALE SIGNS OF PRIMARY SUBTENTORIAL LESIONS CAUSING COMA

Onset of coma often sudden
Symptoms of brain stem dysfunction may precede coma
Localizing brain stem signs always present
    Caloric responses disconjugate or absent
    Pupil(s) abnormal: pinpoint (pons), fixed (midbrain), irregular and/or unequal (midbrain-pontine)
    Often "bizarre" signs: ocular bobbing, ataxic breathing, etc.
    Often signs of cerebellar or bilateral motor dysfunction

TABLE 444–5. COMMON CAUSES OF METABOLIC OR DIFFUSE BRAIN DYSFUNCTION CAUSING DELIRIUM OR COMA

I. Exogenous poisons
  A. Alcohol–sedative drug abuse, acute or chronic, immediate or withdrawal
  B. Acid poisons or poisons with acidic breakdown products:
  Paraldehyde
  Methyl alcohol
  Ethylene glycol
  C. Psychotropic drugs, acute or chronic:
  Opiates and their congeners
  Cocaine
  Amphetamines
  Tricyclic antidepressants and anticholinergic drugs
  Lithium
  Phenothiazines
  LSD-mescaline
  Monoamine oxidase inhibitors
  D. Other drugs:
  Anticonvulsants
  Steroids
  Cardiac glycosides
  Cimetidine
  Salicylates
II. Mixed metabolic encephalopathy
  Age + drugs + intensive care unit + postoperative state + fracture, etc.
III. Deprivation of oxygen, substrate, or metabolic cofactors
  A. Hypoxia (interference with oxygen supply to the entire brain; cerebral blood flow normal)
    1. Decreased oxygen tension (usually $PaO_2 < 35$ mm Hg) and content of blood: pulmonary disease, alveolar hypoventilation, decreased atmospheric oxygen tension (e.g., high altitude)
    2. Decreased oxygen content of blood—normal tension:
    Anemia (Hb < 40% normal)
    Carbon monoxide poisoning
    Methemoglobinemia
  B. Ischemia (diffuse or widespread multifocal interference with blood supply to brain)
    1. Decreased cerebral blood flow resulting from decreased cardiac output:
    Hemorrhagic or septic shock
    Stokes-Adams syndrome, cardiac arrest, cardiac arrhythmias
    Myocardial infarction
    Aortic stenosis
    Pulmonary embolism
    2. Decreased cerebral blood flow resulting from decreased systemic peripheral resistance:
    Syncope: orthostatic, vasovagal
    Carotid sinus hypersensitivity
    Hypovolemia
    3. Decreased cerebral blood flow due to generalized or multifocal increase in cerebrovascular resistance:
    Hyperventilation syndrome
    Increased blood viscosity (polycythemia, cryo- and macroglobulinemia, sickle cell anemia)
    Bacterial meningitis and encephalitis
    Subarachnoid hemorrhage

    4. Decreased local cerebral blood flow due to widespread small vessel occlusion or tissue necrosis:
    Disseminated intravascular coagulation
    Systemic lupus erythematosus
    Subacute bacterial endocarditis
    Cardiopulmonary bypass
    Small emboli (fat, fibrin, platelets)
    Acute viral encephalitis
    5. Alterations of blood flow due to failure of autoregulation:
    Hypertensive encephalopathy
  C. Hypoglycemia:
  Hyperinsulinism: exogenous; endogenous
  D. Cofactor deficiency:
  Thiamine (Wernicke's encephalopathy)
  Pyridoxine
  Vitamin B_{12}
IV. Diseases of organs other than brain
  A. Nonendocrine organs:
  Liver (hepatic coma)
  Kidney (uremic coma)
  Lung (CO_2 narcosis)
  B. Hyper- and/or hypofunction of endocrine organs:
  Panhypopituitarism
  Thyroid (myxedema-thyrotoxicosis)
  Parathyroid (hyper- and hypocalcemia)
  Adrenal (Addison's disease, Cushing's disease)
  C. Other systemic diseases:
  Diabetes
  Cancer and its treatments
  Porphyria
  Sepsis
V. Abnormalities of fluid, ionic, or acid-base environment of CNS
  A. Water and sodium (hyper- and hyponatremia; hypo- and hyperosmolality)
  B. Acidosis (metabolic and respiratory)
  C. Calcium (hyper- and hypocalcemia)
VI. Disordered temperature regulation
  A. Hypothermia
  B. Heat stroke, fever, malignant neuroleptic syndrome
VII. Infections or inflammation of CNS
  A. Leptomeningitis
  B. Encephalitis
  C. Acute "toxic" encephalopathy
  D. Parainfectious encephalomyelitis
  E. Cerebral vasculitis
  F. Subarachnoid hemorrhage
VIII. Miscellaneous diseases of uncertain pathophysiology
  A. Seizures and postictal states
  B. Concussion

can identify the common denominator between such pairs as an apple and an orange or a fly and a tree; confused patients cannot. But the examiner must be cautious; innate intelligence and education also determine cognitive abilities. Unless the physician already knows the patient, it may be difficult to attribute mild mental changes to a metabolic defect. Loss of memory for recent

TABLE 444–6. CHARACTERISTICS OF METABOLIC ENCEPHALOPATHY

Confusion, lethargy, delirium often precede or replace coma
Motor signs, if present, usually symmetric
Bilateral asterixis, myoclonus appear
Pupillary reactions usually preserved; tonic calorics often present
Sensory abnormalities usually absent
Hypothermia common
Abnormal signs reflect incomplete brain dysfunction at multiple anatomical levels

events and disorientation for time are hallmarks of organic brain disease. Orientation to place and time should be specifically tested by asking the date and year, the day of the week, and the present location.

Perceptual errors, e.g., mistaking the physician for someone else, as well as illusions and hallucinations, are more serious symptoms. Hallucinations are common and usually animate. They frighten and agitate some patients, but others tolerate them quietly and must be asked about their presence. Delirious hallucinations or delusions may be visual, auditory, or tactile, alone or in combination; rarely are they systematic. By contrast, schizophrenic delusions or hallucinations are usually systematic in pattern and consist almost exclusively of endogenous auditory perceptions.

Characteristically, the mental status examination fluctuates in metabolic encephalopathy, with patients out of contact one moment and lucid the next. Such intervals appear unpredictably and last for minutes or hours. Delirious patients typically become more disoriented at night and in unfamiliar surroundings. The presence of restraints, intermittent background noise, and unfamiliar activity accentuates their confusion.

Motor Activity. Bilateral tremor, asterixis, and multifocal myoclonus are hallmarks of metabolic brain disease. The *tremor* ranges from fine to coarse, is irregular at a rate of about eight to ten per second, and involves the distal more than proximal parts of the extremities. Fine tremor usually disappears at complete rest and is best brought out in the fingers of the outstretched hands. Coarse tremor such as accompanies certain drug withdrawals or intoxications may be so heavy that it shakes the bed.

Asterixis describes an abnormal, irregular, distal involuntary jerking movement, best elicited with arms outstretched, hands pronated, and fingers extended. Severe examples border on myoclonus. Asterixis is encountered rarely, and then unilaterally, in patients with structural brain disease.

Multifocal myoclonus consists of sudden nonrhythmic, nonpatterned coarse jerks affecting resting groups of muscles. The movements most often affect the face and shoulders but can occur anywhere in the body. They are accentuated by voluntary or passive movement. Multifocal myoclonus occurs most frequently in uremia, in hypercarbic-anoxic encephalopathy, with penicillin or lithium overdose, and in association with the progressive dementia of Creutzfeldt-Jakob disease (see Ch. 478).

Psychomotor activity in delirium can range from extremes of picking at the bedcovers, sustained restlessness, and thrashing about to total immobility. Increased psychomotor activity is typical of acute deliria such as delirium tremens and other drug withdrawal states. More commonly, toxic confusional states are marked by lethargy, drowsiness, and general bradykinesia. Some acutely delirious patients alternate over a few hours between psychomotor overactivity and quiet apathy. Others may be unwilling or unable to stay in bed. They pace the halls, move constantly, and often shout vulgarities or aggressive threats. Unless restrained, many confused patients fall in trying to walk or during efforts to climb out of bed.

Speech is often abnormal. Patients with increased psychomotor behavior often speak rapidly, muttering or slurring speech into an incomprehensible jumble. Bradykinetic patients may speak slowly, monotonously, and so softly as to be barely heard.

Seizures, hyperactive stretch reflexes, and *signs of mild focal brain dysfunction* frequently accompany severe metabolic brain disease, especially after alcohol-sedative withdrawal. The seizures are usually generalized and the motor abnormalities usually symmetric. Nevertheless, focal paresis and focal seizures occasionally occur, especially with hypoglycemia, hepatic encephalopathy, or postanoxic encephalopathy.

Autonomic Activity. *Pupillary light reactions are preserved in metabolic coma with rare exceptions, and their absence requires a specific search for a pre-existing or acute structural lesion.* Nevertheless, a few exceptions exist; the ingestion of drugs possessing an anticholinergic action can paralyze the pupils transiently in either mid-position or dilation. Also, exposure to severe anoxia or asphyxia can produce fixed mid-position or dilated pupils. If sustained, these imply irreversible brain stem damage. In general, the pupils usually remain symmetric in metabolic brain disease, but are often asymmetric and sometimes fixed in patients comatose from structural brain disease.

Hypothermia is common in sedative intoxication as well as with hypoglycemia and myxedema. *Hyperthermia* with profuse perspiration and tachycardia accompanies most agitated deliria and is especially common with delirium tremens. Hyperthermia without perspiration suggests anticholinergic drug ingestion, infection, heat stroke, or the malignant neuroleptic syndrome that sometimes develops with neuroleptics or anesthetic drugs. Less severe, unexplained hyperthermia can reflect idiosyncrasy to a variety of widely used drugs, including salicylates.

Laboratory Tests. The causes of metabolic coma are legion. In many instances the history (e.g., of drug abuse, systemic disease, exposure to toxins) immediately suggests the cause. When this is uncertain, tests listed in Table 444–7 should be performed immediately to establish the presence of life-threatening metabolic defects. Unless strong evidence indicates a specific metabolic or infectious process causing the delirium, diagnostic CT or MR brain imaging is desirable. Imaging shows no immediately pertinent abnormalities in metabolic encephalopathy, although

TABLE 444–7. LABORATORY EVALUATION OF METABOLIC BRAIN DISEASE

Test	Reason for Test
Immediate	
Glucose	Hypoglycemia, hyperosmolar coma
Na$^+$	Osmolar abnormalities
Ca^{++}	Hyper- or hypocalcemia
BUN	Uremia
Arterial blood pH, PCO_2, PO_2	Acidosis, alkalosis, hypoxia
Lumbar puncture	Infection, hemorrhage, meningeal carcinomatosis
Later	
Liver function tests	Hepatic coma
Sedative drug levels	Overdose
Blood and CSF culture	Sepsis, encephalitis, meningitis
Full electrolytes, including Mg^{++}	Electrolyte imbalance
Coagulation profile	Intravascular coagulation
EEG	Seizure disorder

one can detect pre-existing abnormalities such as chronic subdural hematoma or previous brain damage, the effects of which can mimic or accentuate metabolic delirium.

PSYCHIATRIC DISORDERS. Psychiatric disorders capable of producing the behavioral appearance of impaired consciousness include delirious stages of acute schizophrenic or manic attacks, the nearly total withdrawal of severe depression or certain forms of catatonia, and the pseudocoma of hysteria and malingering (Table 444–8). Especially in the early stages of such disorders, distinction from physiologic alterations of consciousness sometimes can be difficult. Psychiatric amnesia is the most common pseudo-organic symptom and the most readily diagnosed. One should suspect psychiatric amnesia especially when the experience covers sharply delineated periods of time, has an abrupt onset and offset with total amnesia in the middle, is nonprogressive in nature, and relates either to experiences that provoked severe anxiety or to potentially punishable behavior. Catatonic withdrawal states or psychotic deliria in psychiatric illness sometimes can be difficult to differentiate from those of metabolic origin, but applying the guidelines given in Table 444–9 usually provides the answers. As a general rule, however, if the patient's cooperation can be elicited to obtain satisfactory answers, recent memory and cognitive functions usually turn out to be preserved in the functional psychoses. Hallucinations are auditory rather than visual or tactile, and neither asterixis nor multifocal myoclonus occurs. Patients with extreme anxiety may hyperventilate, producing respiratory alkalosis, a diffusely slow electroencephalogram, and sometimes tetany. Otherwise, physical and laboratory evaluations in psychogenically altered consciousness remain normal.

TABLE 444–8. PSYCHIATRIC STATES RESEMBLING ACUTE IMPAIRMENT OF CONSCIOUSNESS

1. **Catatonic states.** Uncommon conditions occurring in either schizophrenic or severe depressive illness which may resemble organic stupor. Mutism, bilateral motor resistance, hypokinesia, and even rigidity are common. Absent are pathologic reflexes, as well as abnormal brain images, EEG's, and laboratory chemical tests.
2. **Acute psychotic deliria.** Uncommon. Involves adult patients of any age, more frequently those older than 50 years. The state can arise with either affective or schizophrenic disorders. Agitation, fear, and hypermobility are prominent. Auditory or visual hallucinations occur, not necessarily paranoid but usually systematized. Fast, coarse tremor can be present and tends to last longer than drug-alcohol withdrawal tremors. Verbal responses, when elicitable, usually reflect orientation for time and place, but distractibility or muteness often limits more detailed mental testing. Pathologic reflexes are lacking. EEG and laboratory chemical tests remain normal in the absence of medical complications. The condition can be difficult to diagnose, but an agitated delirium that lasts longer than 2 weeks almost always reflects psychiatric disease.
3. **Hysteria-malingering.** Unarousable unresponsiveness, usually of brief duration, unaccompanied by physiologic abnormalities and often associated with obviously factitious responses to stimulation.

TABLE 444–9. ORGANIC AND FUNCTIONAL PSYCHOSES COMPARED

Variable	Organic	Functional
Onset	Usually > 30 years	Usually < 40 years
Family history	Usually negative	Often abnormal psychiatrically
Immediate history	Drugs, alcohol, acute medical or neurologic illness	No established medical or neurologic features
Psychology of history	Psychologically coherent	Psychologically incoherent
	Agitation, tremor, noisiness, inattention	Same
Major (psychotic) symptoms		
Orientation and memory	Abnormal	Normal if answers obtained
Delusions or hallucinations	Visual, sometimes olfactory or auditory; nonsystematic (chaotic)	Mainly auditory; systematic: tell a story
Mood	Fearful or apathetic; delusions often regarded as unwanted	Consistent with psychotic symptoms
Coma or akinetic (catatonic) state	Systemic and/or neurologic signs present; EEG abnormal	Neurologic signs absent; EEG normal
Fever, leukocytosis	Signs of medical illness often present	Absent (except malignant hyperthermia or catatonia)
Alcohol-drug intoxication or withdrawal	Often present	Absent
Clinical or EEG seizures	Often present	Absent

Patients with hysterical pseudocoma have normal somatic neurologic examinations. Breathing is eupneic or voluntarily hyperpneik. Most such patients lie supine and quietly unresponsive, with limbs remaining either flaccid or resisting movement in unpredictable patterns. Eyelids usually are closed, actively resist opening, and may spontaneously flutter. Furthermore, the eyelids are incapable of the slow closure that follows passive raising of the lids of patients with physiologic coma. The pupils in psychiatric unresponsiveness are briskly responsive or, if cycloplegics have been self-instilled, widely dilated. Oculocephalic responses are unpredictable, but if the diagnosis is doubtful, irrigating the tympanum with 50 ml of cold water produces physiologic nystagmus rather than the tonic eye deviation or absent responses shown by comatose patients with structural or metabolic disease. Sometimes, the eyes may deviate toward the bed when the patient is turned to one side.

Occasionally, psychiatric pseudodelirium or unresponsiveness can be superimposed on underlying physical illness. An example is the patient hospitalized with a severe medical or neurologic illness who becomes so anxious that he or she is unable to cope and withdraws psychologically to the point of unresponsiveness. In such doubtful instances, slow infusions of small amounts of sodium amobarbital (Amytal interview) may allow the physician to establish contact and rapport with the patient. Since the drug may similarly awaken patients rendered unconscious by continuous focal seizures, close clinical observation and, if possible, an EEG are best done before the test.

ACUTE CENTRAL NERVOUS SYSTEM POISONING. Table 444–10 lists the most frequent acute neurotoxic poisonings in the United States, gives their principal signs of toxicity, and outlines their treatment. To find descriptions of poisons not included in this section, especially chronic neurotoxic agents, the reader should consult the textbooks listed in the references. Almost all drugs in overdose amounts are likely to be mixed with intoxicating amounts of alcohol, thereby making their clinical signs more difficult to appraise. Nevertheless, clinical appraisal must be used to diagnose the specific agent causing several of these reaction patterns, since chemical tests are in many instances either unavailable or impractically slow. When any doubt exists, one should keep admission serum samples for possible later analysis. With most of the drugs, tolerance develops to chronic ingestion and individuals may react differently to similar doses. Accordingly, blood levels and size of the dose are unreliable guides to the potential depth of coma or other complications. The mixing of agents adds to the unreliability. Only the opiates and some of the sedatives create an immediate risk of death; concurrent alcohol ingestion enhances both these risks. Opiate poisoning is discussed in greater detail in Ch. 15.

Pathogenesis. All sedative drugs depress the central nervous system, although not equally on a gram-molecular weight basis, and not to the same degree so far as different central structures are concerned. The duration of action varies widely and depends largely on how the particular drug is detoxified or eliminated. The benzodiazepines, short-acting barbiturates, pentobarbital, secobarbital, and amobarbital are detoxified by the liver, as is methaqualone. They exert their maximal effects promptly after being absorbed and, even in huge doses, seldom cause neurologic depression lasting longer than 3 to 5 days. Barbital and phenobarbital are partially detoxified by the liver and partially excreted in the urine. Severe poisoning with the latter agent can cause coma lasting 10 to 14 days. Glutethimide, nowadays seldom used, has a short duration of action comparable to that of secobarbital, but it is poorly absorbed from the gut and may degenerate into more long-lasting neurotoxic metabolites. Meprobamate has an intermediate duration of effect lasting for days. Bromide rarely causes full coma, but, once it reaches high levels, it replaces chloride in the blood and tissues and persists for weeks to cause symptoms without further ingestion.

Although the sedatives have few important effects outside the nervous system, barbiturates, glutethimide, and meprobamate in toxic doses tend to produce hypotension. Glutethimide possesses anticholinergic properties and is the only sedative that predictably produces light-fixed pupils in only moderately heavy anesthetic doses.

A withdrawal syndrome consisting of tremulousness, agitation, and sometimes delirium and convulsions can develop after prompt withdrawal from chronic exposure to any of the hypnotic sedatives. Convulsions are a particular problem after withdrawal from barbiturates, meprobamate, and methaqualone.

Clinical Manifestations. Stupor or coma caused by depressant drug poisoning usually presents the characteristic picture of acute general anesthesia. The depression of the central nervous system tends to be bilateral and symmetric and the drug affects simultaneously many levels, including the spinal cord. Respiratory and circulatory controlling mechanisms in the lower brain stem are affected only with very high doses or not at all, and, except with glutethimide or extremely large doses of barbiturates, the pupillary light reflexes are preserved. Early in the course of acute poisoning, patients can demonstrate muscular hypertonus or even spasticity as the result of uneven depression of different neurologic levels. Within a short time, usually an hour or less, flaccidity supervenes, and the stretch reflexes tend to disappear. Even moderate degrees of drug depression can depress or block the oculovestibular reflexes.

As mentioned, blood levels are a poor index to the depth of coma. Generally speaking, however, blood levels of short-acting barbiturates of more than 2.5 mg per deciliter and phenobarbital blood levels of more than 12 mg per deciliter are associated with very deep coma to the level at which apnea and hypotension become management problems. Apnea rarely supervenes with the benzodiazepines, even at very high doses.

Diagnosis. The combination of acutely occurring unresponsiveness, with preserved or sluggish pupillary reactions, absent oculovestibular reactions, motor areflexia, hypothermia, and relative depression of respiration and circulation is clinically diagnostic of sedative-anesthetic drug poisoning. Only infarction or hemorrhage of the pons resembles this clinical state, and with lesions of the pons the pupils are usually small or pinpoint, the stretch reflexes are generally preserved or hyperactive, and the plantar responses are extensor. Specific chemical tests detect barbiturates, glutethimide, meprobamate, methaqualone, and bromides in blood or urine, and can be done as emergency measures.

TABLE 444–10. COMMON DRUG POISONINGS, SIGNS OF TOXICITY, AND TREATMENT

Drug	Signs and Symptoms		Diagnostic Test	Treatment
	Mild	*Severe*		
Opiates				
Heroin Morphine Meperidine Methadone Hydromorphone Oxycodone Levorphanol	"Nodding" drowsiness, small pupils, urinary retention, slow and shallow breathing; skin scars and subcutaneous abscesses; duration 4–6 hours; with methadone, duration to 24 hours	Coma; pinpoint pupils, slow irregular respiration or apnea, hypotension, hypothermia, pulmonary edema	Response to naloxone Urine	Naloxone, 0.4 mg intravenously or intramuscularly; repeat at 15-minute intervals if patient responds and gradually increase intervals; repeat in 3 hours if necessary; if no response by second dose, suspect another cause; treat shock; find and detect infection
Depressants				
Alcohol Barbiturates Chloral hydrate Glutethimide (Doriden) Meprobamate (Equanil)	Confusion, rousable drowsiness, delirium, ataxia, nystagmus, dysarthria, analgesia to stimuli	Stupor to coma; pupils reactive, usually constricted; oculovestibular response absent; motor tonus initially briefly hyperactive, then flaccid; respiration and blood pressure depressed; hypothermia; with glutethimide, pupils moderately dilated, can be fixed; with meprobamate, withdrawal seizures common; with methaqualone, coma, occasional convulsions, tachycardia, cardiac failure, bleeding tendency	Blood, urine, breath Blood Blood Blood	Intubate, ventilate, lavage; drainage position; antimicrobials; keep mean blood pressure >90 mm Hg and urine output >300 ml per hour; avoid analeptics; hemodialyze severe phenobarbital poisoning
Methaqualone (Quaalude, Sopor, Mandrax)	Hallucinations, agitation, motor hyperactivity, myoclonus, tonic spasms		Blood	As above; diuresis of little help
Benzodiazepines (Librium, Valium, Tranxene, Ativan, Dalmane, etc.) Ethchlorvynol (Placidyl)	Usually taken with another sedative if poisoning is attempted	Coma seldom severe if drug taken alone	Blood	As above; diuresis of little help
Stimulants				
Amphetamines Methylphenidate	Hyperactive, aggressive, sometimes paranoid, repetitive behavior, dilated pupils, tremor, hyperactive reflexes; hyperthermia, tachycardia, arrhythmia Acute torsion dystonia	Agitated, assaultive and paranoid excitement; occasionally convulsions; hypothermia; circulatory collapse	Blood	Chlorpromazine
Cocaine	Similar but less prominent than above; less paranoid, often euphoric	Twitching; irregular breathing, tachycardia, arrhythmia, occasionally convulsions	Blood, urine	Diazepam plus specific symptomatic
Psychedelics (LSD), mescaline, psilocybin, phencyclidine (PCP, angel dust)	Confused, disoriented, perceptual distortions, distractable, withdrawn or eruptive, leading to accidents or violence; wide-eyed, dilated pupils; restless, hyperreflexic; less often, hypertension or tachycardia	Panic		Reassure; diazepam satisfactory; avoid phenothiazines
Scopolamine-atropine (knockout drops, Transderm delirium)	Agitated or confused, visual hallucinations, dilated pupils, flushed and dry skin	Florid toxic disoriented delirium, visual hallucinations; later, amnesia, fever, dilated fixed pupils, hot flushed dry skin, urinary retention		Reassure; sedate lightly, (1) avoid phenothiazines; (2) do not leave alone

Table continued on following page

TABLE 444-10. COMMON DRUG POISONINGS, SIGNS OF TOXICITY, AND TREATMENT *Continued*

Drug	Signs and Symptoms		Diagnostic Test	Treatment
	Mild	*Severe*		
Antidepressants				
Tricyclics (Tofranil, Elavil, Desipramine, etc.)	Restlessness, drowsiness, tachycardia, ataxia, sweating	Agitation, vomiting, hyperpyrexia, sweating, muscle dystonia, convulsions, tachycardia or arrhythmia	Blood	Symptomatic; gastric lavage Intensive care, anticonvulsants, and antiarrhythmics for severe cases
MAO inhibitors (Parnate, Nardil, Eutonyl, etc.)	Hypertensive crises, agitation, drowsiness, ataxia	Hypotension; headache; chest pain; agitation; coma, seizures and shock	Clinical	Symptomatic; gastric lavage
Neuroleptics (phenothiazines, butyrophenones, etc.)	Acute dystonia, somnolence, hypotension	Coma; convulsions (rare); arrhythmias; hypotension	Blood	Anticholinergics; diphenhydramine; symptomatic; gastric lavage
Lithium	Mild lethargy	Sustention-intention tremor, lethargy; muteness with appearance of distraction; coma; multifocal seizures; slow or fluctuating course	Blood	Hydrate if mild; hemodialyze for delirium, coma, or convulsions
Acid-forming intoxicants				
Methanol (formic); ethylene glycol (oxalic and hippuric); other organic alcohols	Inebriation with hyperpnea	All produce progressive hyperventilation, drunkenness, stupor, eventually convulsions and death. Early blindness with methanol	Blood shows increasingly severe anion-gap acidosis	Inhibit hepatic alcohol dehydrogenase by giving alcohol until acidosis controlled; treat acidosis vigorously
Salicylate				
Aspirin	Tinnitus, dyspnea	Older persons: confusional state or toxic delirium leading to stupor, convulsions, coma	Blood salicylate > 60 mg/dl	Alkaline diuresis

CLINICAL EVALUATION OF DELIRIUM, STUPOR, OR COMA

The immediate step consists of assuring vital cardiorespiratory systems and protecting against further damage to the central nervous system. Once these measures are taken, the keys to diagnosis, specific treatment, and prognosis lie in carefully examining the patient, systematically seeking the answers to a few central questions:

Is the process neurogenic or psychogenic in origin?

If neurogenic, is (are) the lesion(s) supratentorial, subtentorial, focal, or multifocal-diffuse?

Once the immediate cause of loss of consciousness is under control, is the appropriate treatment medical or surgical?

If the illness is nonstructural, is it exogenously toxic or endogenously metabolic, already maximal (e.g., postanoxic, postintoxicant), or progressive; is it worsening or improving?

Which immediate treatment best halts the pathologic process and sustains the patient?

DIFFERENTIAL HISTORY. If sudden unconsciousness is not an expected consequence of an already known illness, witnesses to the onset provide the most helpful immediate information. Was the onset gradual or abrupt? Was it preceded by headache and, if so, of what location and duration? Was paralysis or seizure activity observed? Were antecedent or prodromal symptoms noted? Did the onset occur in a circumstance or geographic area in which drugs, trauma, or foul play could be suspected? What medications might the patient have taken? Beyond these immediacies, what has been the patient's physical and mental health for the past few days, weeks, or months?

PHYSICAL AND NEUROLOGIC EXAMINATION. In cases of deep unresponsiveness, one first carries out steps 1 to 5 described below under Emergency Management, then proceeds with the physical examination. Under urgent circumstances, the physician should be able to conduct a highly focused, pertinent physical and neurologic examination on patients in coma in less than 5 minutes. This includes appraising cardiopulmonary status

as indicated above and systematically carrying out the main features of the examination outlined in Table 444–11. In the course of the above, trauma or seizures make themselves evident. In patients with coma of unknown cause, clues should be sought to drug exposure, as well as to past serious medical or psychiatric problems. Companions should be asked about recent neurologic function and dysfunction.

For patients presenting with less severe impairments, i.e., acute-subacute confusion, delirium, or hypersomnolence, the examiner can take a more deliberate approach. Usually, a detailed history can precede the exigencies of stabilizing vital functions and a thorough organ-by-organ physical examination can be conducted. Either way, by the end of the initial examination, the findings should begin to indicate which of the four major causes of coma, as listed in Table 444–1, is responsible for the patient's acute problem. At that juncture, one can move toward obtaining supplementary or reinforcing laboratory tests as indicated below.

LABORATORY STUDIES. Unless the acutely obtained clinical findings make the diagnosis and appropriate treatment immediately obvious, blood should be drawn for laboratory tests listed in Table 444–7. Lumbar puncture is best deferred until after a contrast-enhanced brain CT or an MRI is obtained, so long as the images can be obtained promptly as an emergency procedure. If imaging is not available and the findings suggest acute, treatable meningitis or encephalitis, the physician has no choice but to proceed cautiously with lumbar puncture, using a No. 20 or 22 needle. The EEG (see Ch. 441) is diagnostically indispensable for detecting delirious states caused by continuously recurring partial complex seizures. A normal EEG rules out organic causes of acute unresponsiveness.

EMERGENCY MANAGEMENT OF COMA. Faced with acute coma of uncertain origin, one must treat the patient first, even as the history and initial diagnostic tests are being applied. Certain measures apply to the care of all patients:

1. *Assure an adequate airway and oxygenation.* Immediately check and clean out the upper airway. If the patient is deeply

TABLE 444–11. THE NEUROLOGIC EXAMINATION IN COMA

1. Guarantee vital functions as indicated in text.
2. Feel the scalp for hematomas (overlying fracture lines); be sure the neck is not fractured; test *gently* for stiff neck.
3. Test language. Test arousability by words, loud sounds, noxious stimuli. If vocalizations occur, check quickly for appropriate phrases, actual words, and presence or absence of aphasia.
4. Do a neuro-ophthalmologic examination.
   Funduscopy (if difficult can be deferred until patient is stabilized)
   Papilledema? (increased intracranial or venous sinus pressure)
   Hemorrhages (subarachnoid hemorrhage; hypertensive encephalopathy; diabetes; hypoxic-hypercarbic encephalopathy)
   Pupils
   Light reaction. Use bright flashlight and, if necessary, magnifying glass to be certain. Absence means potentially fatally deep sedative poisoning or acute or chronic structural brain stem damage (e.g., tabetic pupils).
   Equality. 15% of normals have mild anisocoria but new or >2 mm dilation means parasympathetic (third nerve) palsy.
   Extraocular movements. Absence acutely means deep drug poisoning, severe brain stem damage, Wernicke's encephalopathy, polyneuropathy, or botulism.
   Dysconjugate at rest means an acute third, fourth, or sixth nerve palsy or internuclear ophthalmoplegia. Tonic conjugate deviation toward a paralytic arm and leg means forebrain seizures or a contralateral pontine destructive lesion; away from the paralytic arm and leg means forebrain gaze paralysis.
   Spontaneous eye movements. In coma patients, nystagmus, bobbing, independently moving eyes all mean brain stem damage.
   Oculocephalic (away from direction of head turning) or oculovestibular (toward cold caloric irrigation) responses. Absence of responses means drugs or severe brain stem disease; dysconjugate responses with equal pupils mean internuclear ophthalmoplegia, with unequal pupils mean third nerve disease.
5. Examine the motor systems.
   Strength
   Unilateral weakness or motionlessness of arm and leg means contralateral supraspinal upper motor neuron lesion, most often cerebral; if of arm, leg, and face, contralateral cerebral lesion. Occasionally arm and leg weakness can reflect contralateral brain stem lesion.
   All four extremities weak or motionless implies metabolic disease; less likely is brain stem disease (tone and reflexes increased) or peripheral disease (tone and reflexes decreased).
   Attempt to elicit reflex posturing
   Arm flexed, leg extended—contralateral deep cerebral-thalamic lesion
   Arm and leg extended—thalamic or mesencephalic lesion
   Arms extended and legs flexed or flaccid—pontine lesion
   Legs flexed, arms flaccid—pontomedullary or spinal lesion
   Compare side-to-side reflexes and examine plantar responses.
6. Seek seizure activity or abnormal movements. (1) Generalized? (2) Focal? (3) Multifocal? (4) Myoclonic?
   Control 1 immediately, 2 and 3 deliberately; if 4, treat underlying disease.
   Acute tremor, asterixis, multifocal myoclonus—seek metabolic cause.
7. Inspect breathing.
   Regular hyperpnea: metabolic acidosis; pulmonary infarction; congestive failure or alveolar infiltration; sepsis; salicylism; hepatic coma
   Cyclically irregular (Cheyne-Stokes): low cardiac output plus bilateral cerebral or upper brain stem dysfunction
   Irregularly irregular gasping, slow or weak: lower brain stem dysfunction (including hypoglycemia, drug effects), less often peripheral ventilatory paralysis
8. Proceed with laboratory tests and emergency management as described in text.

unresponsive, insert an endotracheal airway, but first give 1 mg of atropine intravenously to guard against hypoxigenic vagal-induced asystole. Be sure that no neck fracture exists before extending the head for intubation. Auscultate both lung bases to assure that the lower airway is open. Ventilate if necessary and keep arterial PaO_2 greater than 80 mm Hg and $PaCO_2$ 30 to 35 mm Hg. To empty the stomach in comatose patients suspected of acute orally ingested drug poisoning, initiate lavage only after the cuffed airway tube is in place.

2. *Maintain circulation.* Insert venous line(s) and start Ringer's lactate solution. Determine and maintain a satisfactory cardiac rate and rhythm. Avoid overhydration but keep mean blood pressure at 80 to 90 mm Hg, using dopamine if necessary. In poisoning cases maintain urine flow at 300 ml or more per hour. In any patient during the early stages of coma, check electrolytes acutely and at 12-hour intervals thereafter.

3. *Draw blood for emergency laboratory analysis.* Give IV Narcan to protect against opiate intoxication and 50 mg thiamine to prevent accentuation of Wernicke's encephalopathy.

4. *Give glucose.* If hypoglycemia is a possible diagnosis, give 50 ml of 50 per cent glucose. Draw blood first in order not to lose evidence for the diagnosis. The glucose does not appreciably intensify serum hyperosmolality.

5. *Stop generalized motor seizures.* Repetitive convulsions can result from either cerebral structural lesions, pre-existing epileptic disorders, or acquired metabolic-diffuse encephalopathies. In either event, status epilepticus can cause coma and within a short period of time produces irreversible brain damage as well. Start treatment with intravenous diazepam. Give 5 to 10 mg or more, if necessary, at a rate of 1 to 2 mg per minute, keeping a ventilator available to treat depressed breathing. As soon as convulsions stop, give between 500 and 1000 mg of phenytoin intravenously at a rate of less than 50 mg per minute. If seizures continue, give more diazepam or resort to barbiturate general anesthesia. Repetitive focal seizures and myoclonus are less damaging to brain than are generalized convulsions, and their continuation does not require the use of general anesthesia.

6. *Restore blood acid-base and osmolar balance.* Extremes of either acidosis or alkalosis usually reflect profound metabolic problems, severe circulatory insufficiency, the postictal state (muscular lactic acidosis), or hyperadrenocorticism. Since severe metabolic acidosis can precipitate cardiovascular irregularity and alkalosis depresses breathing, they should be corrected. Extreme hypo- and hyperosmolality are equally dangerous to brain and should be corrected, the first by withholding fluids (except water by mouth) and stopping diuretics and the second by administering fluids (and insulin for hyperglycemia). Beware of too rapid reversal. Osmotic delays across the blood-brain barrier during treatment can lead to large fluid shifts in or out of the brain. Also, too rapid correction of hyponatremia can produce central pontine myelinolysis (Ch. 456). A reasonable goal in treating osmolal shifts is to correct blood by about 0.5 mOsm per hour.

7. *Treat infection.* Several kinds of infection can cause or intensify delirium and coma. Obtain nose, throat, blood, and wound cultures, and perform lumbar puncture if indicated. With any sign of infection, begin antimicrobial treatment after obtaining the cultures cited above, based on either the results of smears or the most probable clinically suggested organism.

8. *Treat extreme body temperatures.* Hyperthermia above 40°C or hypothermia below 34°C should be brought to within 3°C of normal.

9. *Consider specific antidotes.* Many, if not most, patients admitted to emergency rooms in coma have taken an overdose of drugs, often in combination. For narcotic overdose, give 0.4 mg of naloxone intravenously every 5 minutes until the subject awakens. If the subject may be an addict, dilute the dose in 10 ml of saline and give slowly, trying to minimize withdrawal phenomena. Remember that naloxone's duration of action of 2 to 3 hours is shorter than that of several narcotics, and the dose may require repeating. Analeptics of any kind are contraindicated.

Recently, flumazenil, a benzodiazepine antagonist, has been found useful in treating patients with benzodiazepine overdose, with or without concurrent ingestion of other depressant drugs. Length of unresponsiveness was shortened, and complications were reduced. The agent has not yet been released for use in the United States.

10. *Control agitation,* avoiding barbiturates but employing diazepam or haloperidol as necessary.

11. *Prevent complications.* If possible, keep unconscious patients semiprone in the drainage position and change their position from side to side, but never place them fully supine. In most instances, treat potential pulmonary infection with a broad-spectrum antibiotic. Poisoned patients and many with head injuries are unconscious for only a few days, and the risk of

emergence of drug-resistant bacterial infections is less of a concern than is pneumonia caused by already aspirated material. It is wise to protect the corneas against abrasions, using ophthalmic ointment and, if necessary, taping the lids shut.

RECOVERY AND PROGNOSIS. Patients recovering from coma require close medical supervision. Severe pneumonitis can develop as late as 3 to 4 days after recovery. If antimicrobial drugs were started during coma, they are best continued for at least 48 hours after it ends. Permanent physical sequelae are rare. Among 356 of our own cases of sedative drug overdose, residual brain injury was observed only once (in a patient who suffered an acute cardiac arrest). Peripheral nerve injuries from pressure developed in 6 subjects, and 14 subjects had pressure skin lesions leaving scars. There were no other physical residua.

Convalescent management varies according to the patient's underlying psychiatric disorder and attitudes. Suicide attempts are never accidents, and reports of near-fatal ingestion caused by misunderstanding the dose or forgetting previous doses carry little validity. The expert opinion of a psychiatrist should be sought before deciding whether to release or to institutionalize a patient. The immediate prognosis is good, but there is a high incidence of recurrent attempts over the years.

PROGNOSIS IN SEVERE BRAIN DAMAGE

An important part of the physician's responsibility includes forecasting the outcome of illness. Modern medical advances currently save many lives that only a few years ago would have been lost to severe disease or trauma. Unfortunately, however, when severe brain dysfunction accompanies acute illness, these advances create the risk that if the cerebrum fails to recover, vigorous treatment may be followed by an unwanted outcome. According to Harris polls, most persons in the United States prefer death to a life of severe, permanent neurologic disability and often express this view in the form of a living will. Several empirically based guidelines can help the physician's decisions in such instances by predicting with a high degree of certainty between good and very poor neurologic outcomes following illnesses causing severe brain damage or coma.

Nontraumatic Coma

The outcome from medical coma depends upon (a) its cause, and (b), excepting only depressant drug poisoning, the initial

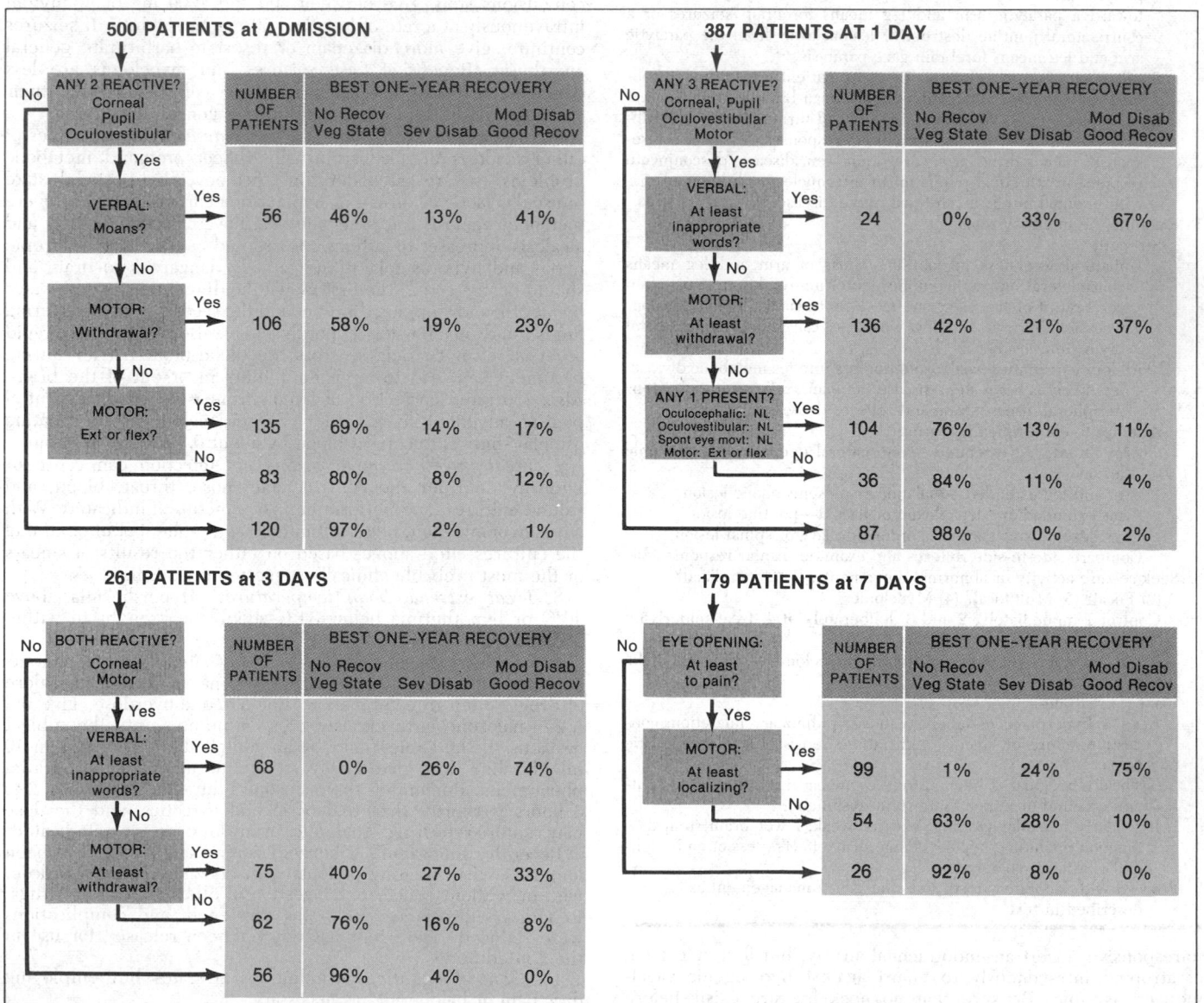

FIGURE 444–2. The best 1-year outcome for 500 optimally treated patients in coma from nontraumatic causes. For each time period following onset, the diagram correlates the degree of recovery with clinical signs observed at that point. Although the diagrams describe actual events in a specific population, the numbers in most instances are sufficiently large to provide a basis for estimating prognosis among similarly affected patients in the future. (From Levy DE, Bates D, Caronna JJ, et al.: Prognosis in nontraumatic coma. Ann Intern Med 94:293, 1981, with permission.)

severity and extent of neurologic damage as revealed by clinical neurologic signs obtained within the first few days of illness.

Depressant drug poisoning, no matter how deep the coma, reflects a state of general anesthesia. Barring severe complications, almost all patients with drug intoxication who reach medical attention recover completely. This favorable prognosis applies even when coma is so profound that normal brain stem reflexes and the EEG temporarily disappear. Since most comas of unknown origin leading to emergency house calls or emergency room visits are due to drug ingestion, such initially undiagnosed patients should receive maximal treatment unless direct evidence points to severe structural brain damage and the use of drugs by ingestion or for therapy has been ruled out.

Aside from drug poisoning, the acute or subacute development in the course of medical illness of loss of consciousness lasting more than a few hours carries a poor prognosis, with only about 15 per cent of patients making a good recovery. The major problem in making early treatment decisions lies in discriminating between patients who have a chance of reaching a good outcome and those whose chances of neurologic recovery are extremely small. In making such early decisions, clinical signs of abnormal forebrain and/or upper brain stem function have been found to be the most powerful available discriminating indicators. The nature of the underlying illness and age have secondary influences but do not modify importantly the accuracy of early signs in distinguishing between probably good and poor outcomes. No laboratory determinants have been found to predict outcome accurately.

The clinical tests most valuable for estimating the capacity for recovery after medical coma are identical to those used in making the initial diagnosis and in following the later course of the patient in coma. In most instances, early functional changes evolve so rapidly that one cannot reliably estimate the outcome of coma within the first minutes to hours, a time when improvement often occurs. After about 6 hours, however, so long as the patient has not received heavy doses of sedative drugs or alcohol, certain neurologic findings begin to correlate increasingly with the potential for neurologic recovery or otherwise. By the end of the first day, clinical signs accurately predict about two thirds of the patients who actually will do well. With each successive day, the signs develop greater predictive power. When considered appropriate to the patient's expressed wishes, treatment can be adjusted accordingly.

Figure 444–2 provides a series of algorithms that describe the actual outcome of 500 patients in coma from medical illness (mostly cardiac arrest) related to their neurologic findings at 6 hours and on days 1, 3, and 7 following onset. The charts disclose that signs of brain stem dysfunction (absent pupillary or corneal responses, imperfect or absent oculocephalic responses, or abnormal motor responses to stimulation) worsened the prognosis and, in combination, indicated a nearly hopeless outlook when they persisted beyond the third day.

Following an acute diffuse brain injury such as follows cardiac arrest, a few patients become immediately vegetative following the ictus and remain so as the days pass into weeks. Most who fail to speak until after the end of the second week are left with prominent intellectual defects, especially in recent and anterograde memory, even if sensorimotor activities return to normal. Persistence of coma or the vegetative state in an adult for more than 4 weeks almost never is associated with later complete recovery and the longer the mindless state lasts, the greater the chance of permanent disability. Care must be taken in such instances to rule out a locked-in state (see Table 443–1).

Traumatic Coma

Coma following head injury has a statistically better outcome than that associated with medical illness. About 50 per cent of patients in coma from head injury die, many instantly. Acute treatment may somewhat improve the outcome of those who reach hospital. Recovery in traumatic cases is closely linked to age: the younger the better. As with medical coma, severely abnormal neuro-ophthalmologic signs reflecting brain stem dysfunction imply a poor prognosis, with approximately 90 per cent of such patients either dying or remaining in near-vegetative states.

Dreisbach RH, Robinson WO: Handbook of Poisoning, 11th ed. Norwalk, CT, Appleton and Lange, 1987. *Succinct and handy, an excellent quick source to consult in emergencies, especially for poisoning in children.*

Feldmann E, Gandy SE, Becker R, et al.: MRI demonstrates descending transtentorial herniation. Neurology 38:697, 1988. *Sagittal images of brain demonstrate the physical basis of the herniation syndromes described in this text.*

Gilman AG, Rall TW, Nies AS, Taylor P (eds.): Goodman and Gilman's The Pharmacological Basis of Therapeutics, 8th ed. New York, Pergamon, 1990. *The "bible" of pharmacology and associated toxicology addresses major drug poisonings in authoritative chapters.*

Goetz CG: Neurotoxins in Clinical Practice. New York, SP Medical and Scientific, 1985. *A useful guide, classified by agent and syndrome, to all forms of exogenous toxins affecting the nervous system.*

Plum F: Coma and related global disturbances of the human conscious state. *In* Jones EG, Peters A (eds.): Cerebral Cortex. Vol. 9, Altered Cortical States. New York, Plenum Press, 1991. *A recent chapter describing current advances in pathophysiology.*

Plum F, Posner JB: Diagnosis of Stupor and Coma, 3rd ed., rev. Philadelphia, F. A. Davis, 1982. *Provides more discussion of the material described in this chapter.*

445 Brain Death
Fred Plum

Modern resuscitative devices can maintain the functions of the heart, lungs, and visceral organs for hours or days after the life-maintaining centers of the brain stem tissue have stopped functioning. The economic waste of this hopeless condition, as well as the increasing success of organ transplant programs, has led countries worldwide to adopt the principle that death of the person occurs when either the brain or the heart irreversibly fails in its functions. In the United States the time of brain death has been accepted as the time of the person's death in legal terms. Many states accept the brain death concept by statute, and in no state has the principle failed to meet legal challenge. The Presidential Commission set as the criterion for brain death the "irreversible cessation of all functions of the entire brain, including the brain stem." Guidelines for the practical application of these principles are listed in Table 445–1. One of the supplementary criteria often is particularly desirable when making decisions at 6 hours to facilitate organ transplant.

Certain points in the diagnosis of brain death must be emphasized. *Recoverable drug depressant poisoning can in all ways resemble brain death and must be explicitly ruled out.* In any doubtful case, any evidence of EEG activity or of reflex activity of the brain stem means that the brain is not dead and contravenes immediate discontinuation of life support. However, purely spinal reflex activity can persist after brain death, including reflexes of the limbs and even some remarkably complex movements, including flexion of the trunk and raising of outstretched arms.

TABLE 445–1. CRITERIA FOR DIAGNOSIS OF BRAIN DEATH

1. **Nature and duration of coma must be known**
   a. Known structural disease or irreversible systemic metabolic cause
   b. No chance of drug intoxication or hypothermia; no paralyzing or potentially anesthetizing drugs recently given for treatment
   c. Body temperature must be above 34°C
   d. Six-hour observation of no brain function is sufficient in cases of known structural cause when no drug or alcohol is involved in causation or treatment; otherwise, 12 hours plus negative drug screen required
2. **Absence of cerebral and brain stem function**
   a. No behavioral or reflex response to noxious stimuli above foramen magnum level
   b. Fixed pupils
   c. No oculovestibular response to 50 ml ice water calorics
   d. Apneic off ventilator with oxygenation for 10 minutes
   e. Systemic circulation may be intact
   f. Purely spinal reflexes may be retained
3. **Supplementary (optional) criteria**
   a. EEG isoelectric for 30 minutes at maximal gain
   b. Brain stem–evoked responses reflect absent function in vital brain stem structures
   c. No cerebral circulation present on angiographic examination

It is recommended that physicians faced with applying and acting upon the diagnosis of brain death familiarize themselves with the additional pertinent material listed in the references and whenever possible obtain confirmation with an experienced consultant.

Abrams MB, et al.: Deciding to Forego Life-Sustaining Treatment. A Report on the Ethical, Medical, and Legal Issues in Treatment Decisions. President's Commission for the Study of Ethical Problems in Medicine and Biomedical and Behavioral Research. Washington, D.C., United States Government Printing Office, March, 1983. *A long and thoughtful report on the problems associated with the terminally ill and the neurologically hopelessly damaged patient.*

Barber J, et al.: Guidelines for the determination of death: Report of the medical consultants on the diagnosis of death to the President's Commission for the Study of Ethical Problems in Medicine and Biomedical and Behavioral Research. Neurology 32:395, 1982. *The detailed report describing that cardiac death and brain death are equivalent and giving criteria for each.*

Council on Scientific Affairs and Council on Ethical and Judicial Affairs: Persistent vegetative state and the decision to withdraw or withhold life support. JAMA 263:426, 1990. *The article provides criteria for the diagnosis of permanent unconsciousness and summarizes the data that support their reliability.*

Levy DE, Caronna JJ, Singer BH, et al.: Predicting outcome from hypoxic-ischemic coma. JAMA 253:1420, 1985. *Prospective correlations were obtained between early neurologic signs and eventual course in 210 patients, mostly with cardiac arrest. By 72 hours, signs accurately selected between good or poor eventual outcome in over 75 per cent of patients.*

446 Brief Loss of Consciousness

Fred Plum

Brief loss of consciousness (BLOC), defined as loss of self-awareness lasting from a few minutes to as much as an hour, is a relatively common symptom. If one excludes conditions readily diagnosed by circumstances or history such as acute traumatic concussion, a known recurrent minor seizure disorder, or accidental insulin-induced hypoglycemia, most such cases are due to causes listed in Table 446–1. As the table indicates, *syncope*, defined as brief unconsciousness due to a temporary, critical reduction of cerebral blood flow, is by far the most common cause of BLOC. With any of the conditions, however, reliable observations of the attack itself often are unavailable. Under such circumstances, a careful history and physical examination, including any possible information gained from witnesses, generally give more diagnostic information than any other approach.

Certain immediate guidelines aid in differential diagnosis. Patients under age 50 years with no previous history of cardiac disease, seizures, antihypoglycemic medication, or drug-alcohol abuse almost all turn out to have either benign syncope or a disorder undiagnosable from available evidence. Such patients rarely require an evaluation more elaborate than a careful history and physical examination plus standard blood counts and blood chemistry determinations. For those over age 40, an electrocar-

TABLE 446–1. PRINCIPAL CAUSES AND APPROXIMATE FREQUENCIES OF BRIEF LOSS OF CONSCIOUSNESS OF UNKNOWN ORIGIN

Syncope	
Primarily neurogenic-vasodepressor	55%
Primarily cardiogenic	10%
Central Nervous System	<10%
First seizure	
Cerebral vascular insufficiency	
Subarachnoid hemorrhage	
Intracranial pressure waves	
Drugs-Metabolic	<10%
Alcohol-sedative blackouts	
Narcotic overdose	
Hypoglycemia—exogenous or endogenous	
Antihypertensive drugs	
Diagnosis Unknown	15–20%

diogram (ECG) should be obtained. Computed tomography and electroencephalographic examinations are not cost-effective in the absence of abnormal neurologic symptoms or signs.

446.1 SYNCOPE

ETIOLOGY AND INITIAL CONSIDERATIONS. A brief dysfunction of vasodepressor cardiovascular reflexes causes most syncope. Less frequent causes include primary cardiovascular disease or the drugs employed to treat it, primary or secondary orthostatic hypotension, and, rarely, cerebral arterial vascular disease. Seizure disorders or psychiatric episodes represent possibly confusing conditions when only a retrospective history can be obtained. Acute, severe vertiginous attacks sometimes can induce secondary, reflex syncope. Hysterical unresponsiveness, although not uncommon, cannot be diagnosed reliably in retrospect. Diagnostic signs of such attacks are given in Table 446–2.

Among patients over age 50 with no historical or physical features suggesting cardiac, neurologic, or systemic illness, benign syncope remains the most common cause of unexplained BLOC. Nevertheless, most authorities recommend at least 24 hours of prolonged ECG monitoring in such instances. In Kapoor's study of 433 mostly older patients (mean age, 56 years) with presumed syncope, prolonged ECG recording independently provided important diagnostic information in approximately 20 per cent.

MECHANISMS OF SYNCOPE. Unconsciousness results when generalized cerebral blood flow declines to approximately 40 per cent of normal. Such a drop usually reflects a fall in cardiac output by half or more, and a fall in mean erect arterial blood pressure to below 40 to 50 mm Hg. Given this principle, it comes as no surprise that posture contributes importantly to the event. Syncope of any cause is far more common in the sitting or standing position than during recumbency. Indeed, recumbent syncope must be regarded as reflecting either serious cardiovascular disease or neurologic disease until proved otherwise.

Pathophysiologic changes in several bodily systems, acting alone or together, can cause the changes in global cerebral blood flow necessary to induce syncope. These include (1) temporarily or permanently abnormal neural reflexes acting on an otherwise normal cardiovascular system; this category includes the most common causes of fainting in persons who have no history of serious cardiovascular disease; (2) abnormal intrinsic cardiovascular function, including especially disease of the conduction system predisposing to malignant arrhythmias; (3) impaired right heart filling secondary to functionally increased resistance to venous return; (4) acute or subacute loss of blood volume; (5) increased resistance of cervical or intracranial arterial vascular beds; (6) subacute or chronic autonomic insufficiency producing severe orthostatic hypotension. Table 446–3 lists subcategories of these disorders which are discussed more fully in the following paragraphs.

Neurogenic Mechanisms in Normal and Abnormal Cardiovascular Control. Sympathetic and parasympathetic influences on the cardiovascular system normally act in a finely tuned and balanced manner to slow the heart (vagal) and regulate the degree of constriction of the large venous capacitance vessels of the trunk and extremities (sympathetic outflow). Imbalance, be it a reflection of paralysis or excessive activity in either system, can perturb heart rhythm and rate, slacken venomotor tone, and lead to either reduced left ventricle output, reduced right heart filling, or the two combined. Depending on the degree of blood pressure

TABLE 446–2. SIGNS OF PSYCHOGENIC PSEUDOSYNCOPE

Lids close actively, may flutter, and often resist examiner's attempt to open them.
Breathing: eupnea or acute hyperventilation.
Pupils responsive or dilated (self-administered cycloplegic).
Oculocephalic responses unpredictable; calorics produce quick nystagmus.
Motor responses unpredictable, often bizarre and self-protecting.
No pathologic reflexes. EEG normal in awake patient.

I. Mainly impaired right heart filling
   A. Reflex abnormalities
      1. Vasodepressor ("vasovagal"): capacitance veins dilated, cardiac rate normal or slow
         a. Psychophysiologic (limbic) stimuli, including hyperventilation
         b. Visceral reflex (micturition, pain, gastrointestinal dilatation, acute labyrinthine vertigo)
         c. Carotid baroreceptor sensitivity
      2. Primary or secondary autonomic insufficiency (Ch. 452)
   B. Hypovolemia: hemorrhage, acute salt-water loss, protein loss, enteropathy, burns
   C. Mechanically impaired right heart return: Valsalva maneuver, tussive excess, abrupt chest compression; term pregnancy; pulmonary embolism; pericardial tamponade
II. Globally impaired cardiac output
   A. Reflex abnormalities
      1. Vagal sinus arrest
         a. Psychophysiologic (rare)
         b. Visceral stimulation: glossopharyngeal neuralgia, swallow syncope, direct tracheal stimulation, dilatation of hollow viscus
         c. Carotid baroreceptor sensitivity
   B. Intrinsic cardiac disease (with or without reflex enhancement) (Table 446–4).
III. Primary cerebral ischemia (uncommon)
   A. Multivessel cervical arterial obstructive disease
   B. Transient acute increase in intracranial pressure (plateau waves)
   C. Basilar migraine (rare in adults)
   D. Vertebral-basilar TIA's (rare)

---

fall and the patient's age and posture, hypoperfusion sufficient to produce vagal reflex syncope can require as much as 30 seconds or more to evolve or can be so abrupt as to produce immediate unconsciousness. To produce primary cardiac syncope, sinus bradycardia in most healthy persons must fall below about 30 to 35 beats per minute in order to cause functionally important cerebral blood flow changes; asystole for longer than 3 to 5 seconds usually causes fainting in the erect position at any age. Higher rate and shorter duration thresholds apply to older patients and those with diseased hearts. Atrioventricular arrest, however, is extremely uncommon in persons with healthy hearts, possible exceptions being overtrained athletes and rare "hypervagal" subjects undergoing severe psychophysiologic threats.

PHYSIOLOGIC REFLEX (VASOVAGAL) SYNCOPE. Most functionally benign syncope stems from reduced right heart filling resulting from venomotor failure and dilatation of the capacitance veins of the splanchnic-innervated abdominal cavity and the lower extremities. Relaxation of arterial resistance vessels plays a lesser role. Since gravitational factors contribute importantly to the impaired venous return, fainting caused by impaired right heart filling always occurs in the erect or, occasionally, sitting position.

Acute vasodepressor syncope is the most common cause of fainting and typically is marked by a diphasic course. During an initial brief period of apprehension and anxiety, heart rate, blood pressure, total systemic resistance, and cardiac output all may increase. This initial sequence, however, often is lacking. The vasodepressor phase follows, during which heart rate slows and blood pressure falls, cardiac output declines, and the cerebral blood flow eventually drops. Both sympathetic and parasympathetic abnormalities are involved, since atropine prevents the bradycardia but not the depressor response. Symptoms of palpitation, salivation, and anxiety characteristically mark the first phase, whereas progressive sensations of lightheadedness, giddiness, abdominal sinking sensations, nausea, urinary urgency, and finally "gray-out" or faintness accompany the vasodepressor component. Occasionally the reflex suppression of sympathetic tone comes so rapidly that the affected subject topples like a log. Rarely, with a severe attack of vasodepressor syncope, as with other forms of profound reduction of cardiac output and cerebral ischemia, brief tonic convulsive movements result (convulsive syncope).

During vasodepressor syncope, subjects appear pale (but not dead-white or cyanotic), and the accompanying parasympathetic hyperactivity characteristically induces piloerection and sweating. Since cardiac action continues, awareness and normal cardiovascular reflexes usually return promptly once the subject becomes supine. Vomiting or explosive diarrhea may follow. Occasionally, emotionally generated dysautonomic influences on the heart can be so profound as to induce arrhythmia. Engel and others have speculated that this mechanism can cause sudden death associated with sudden grief or fright.

Fainting is more likely in circumstances of emotional perturbation, in hungry subjects, after a heavy, alcohol-supplemented meal, in a warm, moist environment, and after prolonged standing. A few individuals give a history of lifelong susceptibility to fainting attacks. Rarely, one gets a history suggesting predisposition to vasodepressor syncope based on an autosomal dominant trait, with family members in several generations having been susceptible to recurrent vasodepressor attacks.

Visceral reflex syncope acts via the same medullospinal pathways as the examples cited above. A sense of faintness or even complete syncope can follow immediately after any of the following: emptying a full bladder from the standing position (*micturition syncope*), acute visceral pain (as occurs with a suddenly distended gut or an abrupt joint or ligament injury), an attack of severe vertigo (as occurs with Ménière's disease), or a migraine attack.

Carotid sinus syncope type 2 describes a severe vasodepressor response to carotid sinus massage. The condition is seldom a practical consideration except with neoplasms of the neck that directly irritate afferent glossopharyngeal fibers.

The diagnosis of vasodepressor syncope is made largely by history; rarely are the events medically witnessed. Among young persons who lack histories or physical findings of neurologic or cardiovascular disease, treatment is symptomatic. When impending sensations of faintness threaten, persons should be promptly placed in the supine position. Placing the head far forward in a sitting position is usually ineffective because it fails to empty the enlarged pool of blood located in the muscles and veins of the lower extremities. Subjects who have fainted should be mobilized slowly, because the reflex abnormality occasionally can persist for as long as 2 hours. Prophylactic treatment has little value except when fainting occurs in response to a disease or injury that requires attention. Occasionally, overtrained athletes with chronically slow hearts and a history of syncope during exertion are helped by a regimen of reduced training combined with oral anticholinergic agents.

SYNCOPE DUE PRIMARILY TO CARDIAC CAUSES. Pathologic reflex (vagovagal attacks) result primarily from failure of left heart output associated with reflexly induced changes in the cardiac rhythm, including nodal or sinus arrest, atrioventricular asystole, atrioventricular block, sinoatrial block, and ventricular arrhythmias. Usually these are accompanied by relatively minor vasodepressor changes in the peripheral vasculature, implying a lesser sympathetic abnormality. Most patients with vagovagal attacks belong to the older population and have associated heart disease, resulting in abnormally intense cardiac responses to a relatively normal degree of increased parasympathetic stimulation or sympathetic inhibition. Vagal bradycardia or arrest occasionally is induced by sudden emotional stimuli, but more commonly follows acute noxious or abnormal visceral stimulation. Severe bradycardia or arrest especially accompanies glossopharyngeal neuralgia, swallowing in patients with mechanical esophageal lesions, sudden painful dilatations of a hollow viscus, prostatic manipulation, tracheal stimulation, or visceral wounds. *Carotid sinus syncope type 1* is a rare phenomenon in which massage or pressure of the sinus induces transient asystole.

Cardiac syncope almost always reflects serious heart disease. As already noted, to cause syncope, cardiac output must fall by at least half. In the absence of severe heart disease, this rarely occurs from primary alterations in cardiac rhythm or myocardial strength. Given a normal heart, neither bradycardia above 30 beats per minute nor tachycardia up to 200 beats per minute causes syncope in the supine or seated position so long as functioning vasomotor reflexes remain. Analyses of large series of patients show serious associated cardiac risk factors, including those listed in Table 446–4. In the case of patients over 40 years of age or those showing such risk factors, prolonged (Holter) monitoring of cardiac activity is indicated. In the absence of specific predisposing abnormalities discovered by history, physi-

TABLE 446–4. CARDIOVASCULAR ABNORMALITIES FREQUENTLY ASSOCIATED WITH SYNCOPAL ATTACKS

Myocardial infarction	Ventricular tachycardia
Aortic stenosis	Sick sinus syndrome
Severe cardiomyopathy	Complete heart block
Severe hypertension	Asystole ($> \pm 3$ sec erect, ± 8 sec supine)
Pulmonary embolism	
Pulmonary hypertension	Bradycardia <44/min
Dissecting aortic aneurysm	Tachycardia >160–180/min
Pacemaker malfunction	

cal examination, and such ECG monitoring, additional studies such as direct electrophysiologic studies of the heart, cardiac catheterization, coronary or cerebral angiography, brain CT scanning, and electroencephalography seldom add helpful information. Management of cardiac syncope depends upon the nature of the underlying heart disease, although affected persons should be considered for pacemaker insertion.

OTHER CAUSES OF FAINTING. Orthostatic Hypotension. Acute orthostatic hypotension occasionally can occur in normal persons after acute blood loss, e.g., cryptic gastrointestinal hemorrhage, or following prolonged standing as with soldiers at parade rest in a hot sun; affected subjects undergo a sudden collapse of sympathetic reflex tone. Recurrent symptoms of syncope or faintness accompanying the erect position usually can be traced to the presence of the chronic use of diuretics and vasodepressor drugs or to neurologic disorders involving the peripheral or central nervous system. Chronic hypovolemia, such as occurs in the elderly cardiac or systemically ill patient, also predisposes to syncope, especially following periods of bed rest or prolonged sitting. Increased age as well as many drugs accentuate tendencies to orthostatic hypotension. The latter include most antihypertensive agents and many of the antidepressants, phenothiazines, and sedatives. Neurogenic causes of autonomic insufficiency are discussed in Ch. 452.

Orthostatic hypotension sufficient to cause cerebral symptoms can occur either rapidly upon standing or develop insidiously over seconds or minutes. Although symptoms of faintness and giddiness predominate, some patients lack such prodromal warnings, presumably because of the absence of strong efferent parasympathetic activity. Sometimes when chronically ill patients sit for long periods or stand, they become confused or tremulous without the usual sensations of faintness or collapse. Diagnosis comes from observing an acute or progressive decline in the mean blood pressure of more than 10 to 15 mm Hg in the erect position. Autonomic insufficiency can be inferred by observing an unchanging pulse rate despite the hypotension, and confirmed by tilt-table tests or by identifying other autonomic impairment. The simplest way to evaluate sympathetic tone at the bedside is to take the pulse while the supine patient performs a vigorous Valsalva maneuver for a matter of 30 seconds or so. The normal response consists of a palpable post-Valsalva slowing of pulse and a 10 to 30 mm Hg rise in mean blood pressure.

Treatment of orthostatic hypotension depends upon the cause. Symptomatic treatment requires eliminating drugs that cause hypotension, searching for and correcting causes of blood volume depletion, and applying elastic stockings to the lower extremities. When other measures fail, an increased salt intake and, subsequently, administering the salt-retaining steroid fludrocortisone, 0.3 to 0.8 mg per day in divided doses, can be cautiously initiated. The chronic use of vasopressor agents seldom helps. Just as vasomotor reflexes can be deconditioned by excess bed rest, they can be at least partially reconditioned by erect activity. Every effort should be made to keep susceptible patients up and walking.

Mechanically Impaired Right Heart Filling. In patients with congestive heart disease or cardiopulmonary failure, a strong *Valsalva maneuver* or sustained coughing (*tussive syncope*) raises intrathoracic pressure sufficiently to impede venous return and induce syncope. *Term pregnancy* causing compression of abdominal veins can occasionally induce a similar, posturally related effect. *Pulmonary embolism* and *acute cardiac tamponade*, due most often to subpericardial aortic dissection, act similarly to reduce the right heart filling and critically reduce cardiac output.

Recurrent symptoms of chronic hypovolemia are common in the chronically ill, especially in cardiac patients, the elderly, and those kept at bed rest for sustained periods (in whom baroceptor reflexes also become blunted). Syncope is a risk in all these groups, especially with prolonged motionless sitting.

Cerebral Vascular Disease. Intrinsic cerebral vascular diseases only rarely cause episodes of brief loss of consciousness. Although syncopal episodes might be expected on anatomic grounds as part of the symptom complex associated with vertebral-basilar insufficiency, such is rarely the case. Several reports describing symptoms in large numbers of patients with vertebral-basilar insufficiency do not mention a single example, nor have we encountered such in the extensive New York Hospital experience. By contrast, brief periods of confusion or even unconsciousness do occasionally mark the course of patients with severe stenosis or occlusion of one or both internal carotid arteries; they may or may not show concurrent narrowing of the vertebrobasilar system. In a few such patients, pulse and blood pressure have been monitored through the attacks, which are marked by brief unresponsiveness associated with transient amnesia but no seizures or EEG changes. Surgical removal of carotid stenoses have helped some, but not all, affected patients. Presumably the spells reflect transient, global blood flow reductions to the cerebral hemispheres associated with hemodynamic insufficiency in cervical arterial circulations.

446.2 NONSYNCOPAL CAUSES OF BRIEF ALTERATIONS OF CONSCIOUSNESS

HYPERVENTILATION. The disorder is mechanistically closely related to syncope in that a globally reduced cerebral blood flow gives rise to sensations of giddiness, faintness, and other distress. Full unconsciousness rarely occurs without some additional abnormal maneuver. The abnormal state is most often part of an anxiety response and often is accompanied by sensations of suffocation, pressure on the chest, and a sense of being unable to obtain the satisfaction of a lung-filling deep breath. Extreme or prolonged hyperventilation can produce feelings of unreality with anxiety bordering on panic.

In healthy subjects, only a modest increase in respiratory rate and depth is required to drop Pa_{CO_2} levels promptly to 25 mm Hg or less; once a new steady state develops, little more than the normal level of breathing is sufficient to match bodily CO_2 production and maintain hypocapnia. Casual inspection may show no more than a respiratory rate of 16 to 18 per minute, interrupted perhaps by occasional sighs. Hypocapnia induces cerebral vasoconstriction. This reduces the amount of oxygen delivered to the brain and is the presumed basis of the accompanying sensations.

Symptoms and signs include feelings of unreality, difficulty in concentrating, and several hard-to-explain sensory complaints, such as unilateral or bilateral chest pain or paresthesias involving the body and extremities. Symptoms of facial twitching, carpal spasm, and perioral paresthesias are more easily understood as part of alkalotic tetany.

Diagnosis is easy when otherwise structurally healthy patients complain of the aforementioned symptoms in settings of anxiety or dyspnea but necessarily is conjectural when made in retrospect. Some patients can reproduce their symptoms by voluntarily overbreathing and the maneuver can be helpful in guiding treatment. Most often the symptoms are observed as part of a larger pattern of anxiety and must be treated accordingly.

Hyperventilation occasionally precipitates syncope under special circumstances. Children sometimes voluntarily hyperventilate, then perform a vigorous Valsalva maneuver to induce syncope (fainting lark). Athletes may repeat a similar sequence in contests such as weight lifting or squat jumps. More dangerous is a pattern wherein underwater swimmers hyperventilate before diving, then exhaust their oxygen reserves before producing sufficient carbon dioxide to produce dyspnea. The ensuing cerebral hypoxia can induce fatal submersion syncope.

SEIZURE DISORDERS. Seizure disorders, discussed fully in Ch. 483, produce a diagnostic problem under four principal circumstances:

1. *Rapid, profound syncope* may induce a single brief tonic seizure or series of clonic twitches as a result of abrupt cerebral ischemia (*convulsive syncope*). The response is more likely when the subject has made maximal efforts to stand or sit despite premonitory symptoms. Differential diagnosis rests on identifying the following as more consistent with syncope than epilepsy: the attendant psychologic circumstances and physical appearance, the associated medical conditions and body position, the brief quality of the seizure, rapid recovery, and the presence of a normal neurologic examination and interictal EEG.

2. *Akinetic seizures* consist of attacks of suddenly falling or pitching to the ground, starting in early childhood. Similar episodes occur in the supine position and are marked by unresponsiveness accompanied by generalized muscular hypotonia or brief body spasm. Diagnosis rests on the typical history, the age of onset, and the presence of an abnormal EEG. *Absence (petit mal) seizures* rarely provide a diagnostic problem, since children with petit mal, although out of contact, neither fall nor turn pale and usually have no memory of the episode. The EEG is abnormal and frequently diagnostic.

3. *Partial complex (psychomotor) seizures* sometimes include brief behavioral automatisms in which the subject recalls only being out of contact and may retrospectively consider himself to have suffered a state of unconsciousness. Usually the presence of a characteristic, self-recognized aura or set of incipient symptoms indicates the diagnosis. Falling to the ground rarely occurs unless a generalized seizure develops. Witnessed attacks and the abnormal EEG usually are typical.

4. *Postictal unresponsiveness* from grand mal attacks produces unconsciousness lasting minutes, the duration usually depending on the severity of the preceding convulsion. Diagnosis is a problem only if the seizure was unwitnessed, in which case the state may look like concussion or profound fainting. Even so, the postictal state is marked initially by flushing (cyanosis), giving way to pallor, hyperpnea, and deep unresponsiveness, none of which occurs in syncope.

HYPOGLYCEMIA (see Ch. 219). Hypoglycemia, usually caused by excess exogenous insulin, less often by insulin secreted from endogenous tissues, can produce a variety of relatively brief episodes of neurologic dysfunction. These can consist, variably, of brief confusional episodes, seizures of a variety of types, narcolepsy-like syndromes, and focal or tetraparetic weakness with or without coma but not resembling syncope. Diagnosis depends on suspicion plus the detection of blood sugars of less than 30 to 40 mg per deciliter during an attack.

DRUG OR ALCOHOL BLACKOUTS. Drug or alcohol blackouts consist of episodes of such severe intoxication that they anesthetize memory for the event, leaving the subject with an episode of focal amnesia. Many are accompanied by "passing out," consisting of deep, barely arousable sleep.

CONCUSSION-POSTCONCUSSION AMNESIA. Variable periods of memory loss for immediate subsequent events can follow brief periods of concussive unconsciousness. The usual question is whether an intrinsic malady caused the fall or whether the fall represented the whole illness. Only diagnostic diligence can solve the issue.

ACUTE INTRACRANIAL HYPERTENSION. Plateau waves, associated with this condition, can produce brief episodes of loss of consciousness that resemble syncope, as described above. Occasionally, such brief unconsciousness may accompany the onset of acute subarachnoid hemorrhage. The unconscious episode, which is syncopal in its abruptness and often accompanied by either a tonic extensor spasm or brief clonic jerks, is most often due to an acute cardiac arrhythmia or asystole accompanying the onset of bleeding. Cerebral hemorrhage with intraventricular rupture can produce similar events.

DROP SPELLS. As discussed in Chapter 454, these are poorly understood attacks affecting older persons. The legs suddenly and unexplainedly give way, and the women fall, often injuring themselves but experiencing no observed interruption of consciousness. The cause is unknown.

CONVERSION REACTIONS OR MALINGERING (PSEUDOSYNCOPE). Hysterical or other forms of psychogenic unresponsiveness are almost impossible to diagnose in retrospect. If such a condition occurs during the physical examination, the diagnosis can be reached by the absence of physiologic abnormality and the presence of additional, often bizarre features (see Table 446–2). Most subjects awaken with gentle but firm confrontation. A few do so only when advised that psychiatric admission lies in store. Mutilating stimuli are neither justified nor often successful in proving the diagnosis.

Aminoff MJ, Scheinman MM, Griffin JC, Herre JM: Electrocerebral accompaniments of syncope associated with malignant ventricular arrhythmias. Ann Intern Med 108:791, 1988. *Ten of 17 episodes of syncope caused by electrically induced ventricular tachycardia or arrhythmia had accompanying tonic seizures or irregular muscular twitching. The results illustrate the high incidence of convulsive syncope.*

Engel GL: Psychological stress, vasodepressor (vasovagal) syncope and sudden death. Ann Intern Med 89:403, 1978. *Must reading for the internist by one of the pioneers in understanding of both the physiology and emotion of cardiovascular responses.*

Evans DW, Lum LC: Hyperventilation: An important cause of pseudoangina. Lancet 1:155, 1977. *A clinical article, emphasizing the often misleading symptoms of the disorder.*

Kapoor WN: Evaluation and outcome of patients with syncope. Medicine 69:160, 1990. *Among 433 medically studied patients with a median age of 61, one quarter had a cardiac cause. In another 40 per cent exact cause was uncertain but their findings resembled those of the remaining one third who were concluded to have noncardiac causes.*

Mandis AS, Linzer M, Salem D, Estes NA: Syncope. Current diagnostic evaluation and management. Ann Intern Med 112:850, 1990. *A comprehensive review of the problem identifying rare as well as common causes and emphasizing laboratory evaluations, especially of cardiovascular mechanisms.*

Savage DD, Corwin L, McGee DL, et al.: Epidemiologic features of isolated syncope: The Framingham Study. Stroke 16:626, 1985. *In a population of 5209 men and women aged 30 to 62 years and then followed for a mean of 26 years, 3.3 per cent developed syncope without evidence for concurrent cardiovascular or neurologic disease. Such isolated syncope was not associated with any subsequent increased incidence of stroke, cardiovascular disease, or early mortality compared with the remainder of the cohort.*

Yanagihara T, Klass DW, Piepgras DG, Houser OW: Brief loss of consciousness in bilateral carotid occlusive vascular disease. Arch Neurol 46:858, 1989. *Briefly describes three cases and reviews this uncommon disorder.*

447 Sleep and Its Disorders

Anthony Kales

Humans spend at least one third of their lives asleep, yet physiologists little understand the specific biologic events that explain why we need sleep and what mechanisms underlie sleep's sense of joyous reward. Certain empiric features, however, provide useful guides to the evaluation and management of most of the sleep complaints that arise in standard clinical practice.

PHYSIOLOGY OF SLEEP. Natural sleep-wake rhythms cycle at about 25 hours rather than coinciding with the solar 24-hour schedule. As a result, many persons depend on external cues to keep their diurnal cycle "on time." The normal diurnal clock resists natural changes in its pattern by more than about 1 hour per day, which explains the sleep irregularities that often accompany adaptation to new time zones or switches in work shifts.

Individuals differ considerably in their natural sleep patterns. Normal adults can average as little as 4 to as much as 11 hours of sleep per day. Most adults in nontropical areas are comfortable with 6.5 to 8 hours daily, taken in a single period. Children and adolescents sleep more than adults, and young adults more than older ones. Normal sleep consists of a series of behaviorally and electroencephalographically (EEG) defined cycles, including neurophysiologically active periods accompanied by rapid eye movements, called REM sleep, interspersed with four progressively deeper, quieter sleep stages graded 1 to 4 on the basis of increasingly slow EEG patterns. Stages 3 and 4 (deep) sleep gradually lessens with age and usually disappears after age 55.

SLEEP DISORDERS. Both functional and organic disorders can perturb sleep. Insomnia, the most common of the sleep disorders, most often reflects psychological disturbances; hypersomnia can have similar origins but often reflects organic dysfunction of the brain. The parasomnias, including sleep walking, night terrors, and nightmares, similarly most often have a func-

TABLE 447-1. GUIDELINES FOR TAKING A SLEEP HISTORY

Define the specific sleep problem.
Assess the clinical course of the condition.
Distinguish among sleep disorders.
Reassess previous diagnoses.
Evaluate 24-hour sleep/wakefulness patterns.
Question the bed partner.
Determine the presence of other sleep disorders.
Obtain a family history of sleep disorders.
Evaluate the impact of the sleep disorder.

tional basis. They usually have benign associations in childhood but often reflect psychopathology in adolescents and adults. By contrast, narcolepsy and sleep apnea are exclusively of organic origin, the first being a chronic genetically related disorder and, the second occurring predominantly in middle-aged men and associated with obesity and cardiovascular problems. Accordingly, the first step in evaluating a sleep complaint is to obtain a thorough history (Table 447-1).

Sleep complaints are common at all ages and range widely in their nature and biologic importance, a natural variation that sometimes makes it difficult for the physician to distinguish trivial from serious problems and to appraise their medical importance.

INSOMNIA

Insomnia is by far the most common sleep complaint, affecting as many as one fifth of all patients who consult general physicians. Short-term insomnia often results from stressful life events or the recent onset of medical disorders. Chronic, severe insomnia, by contrast, often becomes a central complaint and the focus of distress and is perceived by the patient as a distinct disorder itself.

CLINICAL FEATURES. Most patients with chronic insomnia report difficulty in falling asleep, either alone or in combination with difficulty in staying asleep or early final awakening. Compared with normal sleepers, insomniacs feel worse in the morning than late at night and arise feeling sleepy, groggy, physically and mentally tired, depressed, worried, tense, anxious, and irritable. Characteristically, these symptoms persist during the day and contribute to feelings of depression, hopelessness, and fears of losing self-control. As bed time approaches, they become even more tense, anxious, and ruminative about health, death, work, and personal problems. Many such persons show autonomic hyperactivity evidenced by increased heart rate, muscle tension, increased body temperature, and peripheral vasoconstriction.

ETIOLOGY. Acute or short-term insomnia can be associated with a variety of situational (work-related, interpersonal, or financial difficulties) or medical problems including ascent to high altitudes, pain, cardiopulmonary disorders, thyrotoxicosis, or the febrile prodromes to influenza. Drugs of a variety of kinds, including caffeine, cigarettes, alcohol, steroids, amphetamines and other stimulants, energizing antidepressants, central adrenergic blockers, and bronchodilators, can impair both falling asleep and staying asleep.

Notwithstanding the above possible causes, psychological distress is the most common cause of chronic insomnia. Patients with longstanding sleep difficulties show less than adequate coping mechanisms to stressful life events. Many display specific personality patterns characterized by chronic anxiety, rumination, neurotic depression, inhibition of emotions, and an inability to discharge anger outwardly. They generally handle external stress and conflicts by internalizing their emotions, generating a combination of emotional arousal and autonomic activation. This state of hyperarousal leads to difficulty in initiating sleep, whether at the beginning of the sleep period or when returning to sleep following nocturnal or other awakenings. Fear of sleeplessness further intensifies the emotional arousal, thus insidiously conditioning and perpetuating insomnia.

DIAGNOSIS. Evaluation of transient or situational insomnia focuses on identifying the stressful factors and providing reassurance about those that interfere with restful sleep. When addressing chronic insomnia, the evaluation should include a complete history that assesses various sleep, drug, medical, and emotional factors (Table 447-1). It is important to assess sleep/wakefulness patterns on a 24-hour basis, particularly in the elderly. Widespread insomnia affecting this age group results in their ingesting a high proportion of all the sedatives prescribed in this country.

In taking the general medical and drug history, conditions and medications that are known to be associated with disturbed sleep should be identified. Although *sleep apnea* and *nocturnal myoclonus* only rarely serve as causes for the primary complaint of insomnia, symptoms of these disorders should stimulate a detailed inquiry, including obtaining information from the bed partner. Most importantly, underlying emotional factors contributing to chronic sleep difficulty must be identified.

MANAGEMENT. The successful and effective treatment of chronic insomnia usually requires attention to several factors, including general measures for improving sleep hygiene and lifestyle; supportive, insight-oriented, or behavioral psychotherapeutic techniques; adjunctive use of hypnotic medication; or use of antidepressant medication.

Measures for improving sleep hygiene and lifestyle include regularizing the patient's schedule; emphasizing that the bedroom should be the handmaiden of rest and sleep rather than of conflict and worry; and improving the sleep environment by minimizing noise and disruptions. Providing a gradually increasing daily activity and exercise program has been shown to increase early night slow-wave sleep.

Allowing for modest variation, times to retire and awaken should be regularized. In counseling the insomniac, it is helpful to explain how anxiety participates in the vicious circle that exacerbates and maintains the condition. Patients can be taught to reduce stress and anxiety by managing emotions more effectively through pertinent stress management techniques (Table 447-2). Most patients with severe, chronic insomnia require psychotherapy.

Benzodiazepine hypnotics have largely replaced other drugs in the adjunctive pharmacologic treatment of insomnia, primarily owing to their greater margin of safety and degree of effectiveness. Five benzodiazepines are marketed currently as hypnotics: flurazepam, temazepam, triazolam, quazepam, and estazolam; the last has been recently introduced, and significant data are lacking regarding its safety, particularly in terms of long-term use, drug dependence, and withdrawal issues. In adults, for the long-term adjunctive drug treatment of chronic insomnia, intermittent use of flurazepam, 15 mg, and quazepam, 15 mg, is recommended. These agents maintain their efficacy very well with continued use and produce few adverse reactions, and their intermittent use minimizes the occurrence of daytime sedation. In the elderly, or when a mild, short-term hypnotic effect is desired, temazepam, 15 mg, may be used. Triazolam is not recommended because of frequent and severe adverse reactions, including the following:

TABLE 447-2. GENERAL MEASURES IN TREATING INSOMNIA (STRESS- AND DRUG-INDUCED DISTURBANCES)

Recommendation	Implementation
Manage stress properly	Recognize association between stressful events and sleeplessness.
	Ventilate conflicts and anger to avoid internalization.
	Be tolerant of occasional sleeplessness.
	Avoid rumination over sleep difficulty.
	Relaxation exercise may be helpful.
Avoid drug-induced sleep disturbances	Minimize use of caffeine, cigarettes, stimulants, and other medications.
	Recognize that alcohol may cause fragmentation of sleep.
	Be aware of hyperexcitability states (early morning insomnia and daytime anxiety) caused by hypnotics with a short half-life.
	Recognize sleep disturbances following drug withdrawal.

hyperexcitability states (early morning insomnia and daytime anxiety) and cognitive impairment (memory impairment/amnesia, confusion, delusions, hallucinations, and delirium), both occurring during drug administration; and withdrawal difficulties (rebound insomnia) following drug termination. These serious safety concerns and the lack of efficacy of the recommended starting dose (0.25 mg) result in a very narrow benefit-to-risk ratio for triazolam.

When depression contributes a major factor to insomnia, antidepressants with sedative side effects, such as tricyclics, are generally indicated. Neuroleptics with sedative effects are preferred for psychotic patients who have insomnia.

PARASOMNIAS: SLEEPWALKING, NIGHT TERRORS, AND NIGHTMARES

These conditions are common. About 15 per cent of children, for example, have had at least one sleepwalking episode, and 1 to 3 per cent report night terrors. Nightmares are a current problem for approximately 5 per cent of the general population and a past problem for another 5 per cent.

CLINICAL FEATURES. Sleepwalking (somnambulism) occurs in episodes lasting for several minutes. During this period, patients generally have blank expressions, behave as if they are indifferent to the environment, and exhibit low levels of awareness and reactivity, manifested by clumsiness and purposeless activity. They rarely recall the events upon awakening. Night terror episodes have the additional and often dramatic characteristics of extreme vocalization and movement, excessive autonomic discharges, and panic. Sleepwalking and night terrors appear to fall along a pathophysiologic continuum and share many clinical and physiologic similarities (Table 447–3).

Nightmares are most often associated with fears of attack, falling, or death, and in many patients the nightly themes recur. Nightmares occur during REM sleep and may take place at any time during the night but are more likely during the late night when REM sleep periods increase in length. Patients typically report considerable sleep disruption and have vivid recall of the dream content, characteristics that easily differentiate nightmares from the more dramatic but forgotten night terrors.

ETIOLOGY. Genetic, developmental, organic, and psychological factors have been proposed as causing parasomnias. Maturational components are implicit in their frequent onset in childhood and termination by late adolescence. Febrile episodes and brain tumors occasionally have been implicated but are rare causes. Somnambulism-like episodes also have been pharmacologically induced by lithium, high doses of neuroleptic drugs, and triazolam. Furthermore, withdrawal of certain drug treatments, resulting in an increase in REM sleep (REM rebound), may be associated with a temporary increase in the intensity of dreaming and the possible occurrence of nightmares.

Psychological abnormalities seldom accompany early childhood parasomnias. When the disorders begin in late childhood or adolescence, however, they often persist into adulthood, usually associated with significant psychopathology.

DIAGNOSIS. Sleepwalking or night terror–like activity that begins in middle or old age should prompt the physician to rule out brain tumor or other cerebral disorders, including sedative intoxication. Night terrors should be differentiated from temporal lobe epilepsy, which, however, rarely expresses itself during sleep. Most "sleepwalking" in elderly persons reflects episodes of confusion and nocturnal wandering rather than a parasomnia. A careful drug history is important in the evaluation of persons who have nightmares. This is because administration or withdrawal of certain drugs, including alcohol, induces marked

TABLE 447–3. CLINICAL CHARACTERISTICS OF SLEEPWALKING AND NIGHT TERRORS

Episodes early in the night when stages 3 and 4 of sleep predominate
Confusion on awakening and minimal recall of event
High risk of injury
Often a family history of sleepwalking or night terrors
Onset usually in childhood or early adolescence
Usually outgrown by late adolescence
Psychopathology suspected with adult onset
Some elderly patients have central nervous system pathology

TABLE 447–4. INDICATIONS FOR SLEEP LABORATORY RECORDING

Always
  Sleep apnea

Sometimes
  Narcolepsy

Infrequent
  Insomnia
  Nocturnal myoclonus
  Parasomnias

changes in the frequency, intensity, and disturbing content of dreaming. Many patients are unaware of such connections.

Adult patients with chronic parasomnias commonly show serious psychopathology deserving psychiatric consultation. It is important to differentiate night terrors, and particularly sleepwalking, from hysterical dissociative phenomena such as amnesia, fugue states, and multiple personalities. Most patients experiencing the latter conditions demonstrate complex and purposeful behaviors and describe longer episodes that may last as long as several hours compared with the minutes-long duration of parasomniac sleepwalking.

Sleep laboratory recordings are seldom useful in evaluating parasomnias (Table 447–4), an exception being when nocturnal epilepsy is strongly suspected.

MANAGEMENT. The most important consideration in managing episodic sleepwalking or night terrors is protection from injury. Attempts to interrupt the episodes should be avoided, since intervention often confuses and frightens the patient even more. Minimizing children's exposure to potentially traumatic experiences, such as terrifying movies and television programs or frightening bedtime stories, can help to reduce the frequency of nightmares. Parents should be counseled and reassured that affected children usually outgrow the conditions by late adolescence, if not sooner. Drugs such as diazepam and flurazepam that suppress stages 3 and 4 sleep may be prescribed as adjuncts to psychotherapy for adults who experience night terrors or sleepwalking. Psychotropic medication is not recommended in children. Depression, especially in men with nightmares, deserves special attention because these persons may be at higher risk for suicide. Overtly psychotic behavior associated with nightmares is best treated with neuroleptic drugs.

NARCOLEPSY

Narcolepsy is a serious clinical problem that usually begins before age 25 years and persists throughout life. The estimated incidence is about one person per thousand population, with men and women equally affected.

CLINICAL FEATURES. Narcolepsy is characterized by excessive daytime sleepiness and irresistible sleep attacks that usually occur in conjunction with one or more of three auxiliary symptoms: cataplexy, sleep paralysis, and hypnagogic hallucinations. The sleep attacks may last from a few seconds to half an hour and may be precipitated by sedentary, monotonous activity of any kind, including driving, sitting in lectures, or even eating meals. Excessive daytime sleepiness and sleep attacks usually usher in the disease, with the auxiliary symptoms appearing several years later.

About three fourths of narcolepsy patients have *cataplexy*, a brief and sudden loss of muscle control without loss of consciousness. The severity of cataplectic attacks ranges from light knee buckling or drooping of the jaw to complete collapse. Episodes are precipitated by strong emotions such as fear, surprise, laughter, or anger.

Sleep paralysis and *hypnagogic hallucinations* describe short (a minute or less) episodes that occur during the transition between wakefulness and sleep. Sleep paralysis consists of a transient experience of being unable to move any muscle (breathing persists). Hypnagogic hallucinations are vivid hallucinatory perceptions (usually visual or auditory) that appear particularly while drifting into sleep. About half of narcoleptic patients complain of disturbed nocturnal sleep, which may be a direct

TABLE 447–5. DIFFERENTIAL DIAGNOSIS OF SLEEP APNEA AND NARCOLEPSY

	Sleep Apnea	Narcolepsy
Age of onset	Middle age	Adolescence
Sex distribution	Predominantly male	Equal sex distribution
Daytime sleepiness	+ +	+ +
Sleep attacks	+ +	+ + +
Auxiliary symptoms	– –	+ + +
Snoring/snorting	+ + +	– –
Nocturnal breath cessation	+ + +	– –
Disturbed nocturnal sleep	+ + +	+ +
Associated medical conditions (hypertension, obesity, etc.)	+ +	– –
Family history	+	+ + +
Adverse psychosocial consequences	+ + +	+ + +

effect of the disorder or due to the use of stimulant medication to control daytime sleep, or both.

ETIOLOGY. Family studies showing a 10 to 50 per cent incidence of affected first-degree relatives and a high incidence of HLA concordance imply a strong genetic predisposition. The pattern must be multifactorial, however, since monozygotic twins have a high rate of discordance. The sleep attacks and other manifestations of the auxiliary symptoms of narcolepsy appear to be closely related to aberrations in the neurophysiologic mechanisms of REM sleep, since REM sleep ushers in a large proportion of narcoleptic sleep patterns, in contrast to those of normals, in whom the first REM period occurs after about 70 to 90 minutes of nonrapid eye movement (NREM) sleep.

Many narcoleptics show a high level of psychopathology that is a secondary reaction to the disorder, resulting in considerable psychosocial disturbances that need to be addressed.

DIAGNOSIS. Usually, the history is typical. Passing consideration should be given to hysteria (rarely expressed as brief, episodic hypersomnia), seizures (characterized by automatisms but not brief sleep states), or true neuropathologic hypersomnia (sleep episodes last longer). Narcolepsy must be differentiated from sleep apnea (Table 447–5). A history of cataplexy and the other auxiliary symptoms make the diagnosis certain. In questionable instances, especially in the absence of cataplexy, multiple daytime nap recordings may detect sleep-onset REM periods and/or extremely short sleep latencies in narcoleptics. A sleep latency of less than 5 minutes on at least two of five 20-minute opportunities to sleep between 10:00 A.M. and 6:00 P.M. strengthens the diagnosis.

MANAGEMENT. Therapy begins nonpharmacologically by prescribing therapeutic naps to enhance alertness for daytime tasks. Patients should be warned about the potential dangers of driving or other activities requiring full alertness and muscle control. Physicians should check with their local department of motor vehicles regarding the legal responsibility for reporting narcolepsy. One must advise and educate patients gently but honestly that this is a frequently misunderstood chronic disorder. All concerned must learn that narcolepsy is a physical illness and not under voluntary control.

Pharmacotherapy involves separate treatments for the sleep attacks and cataplexy. Methylphenidate is the preferred drug for treating sleep attacks because of its prompt onset of action and relatively few side effects. Other potential agents include amphetamines, modafinil, mazindol, and selegiline.

Imipramine and other nonsedating antidepressants can be helpful in preventing cataplexy; the drugs also alleviate sleep paralysis but have little effect on the sleep attacks. Imipramine acts rapidly and requires a lower dose than when treating depression. Stimulants and antidepressants can be combined for patients who require treatment for both sleep attacks and auxiliary symptoms. Because this combination may produce serious side effects such as hypertension, careful titration and monitoring are necessary.

SLEEP APNEA

This disorder affects men more than women and is often associated with obesity and hypertension. The clinical diagnosis of sleep apnea syndrome includes quantification of the number of apneic events, the degree of associated oxygen desaturation, and the patient's total clinical picture. Apneas are characterized as central (i.e., neurogenic), obstructive (peripheral), or mixed. In central apnea, an uncommon condition related to central nervous system disorders, breathing efforts cease or become minimal, whereas in obstructive apnea, the most common form of sleep apnea, respiratory efforts persist and even become unusually prominent but are rendered ineffective by upper airway blockage. Sleep apnea also can occur as a late manifestation of chronic peripheral neuromuscular diseases, including myotonic muscular dystrophy and motor neuron disorders.

CLINICAL FEATURES. Patients with obstructive sleep apnea characteristically provide a history of excessive daytime sleepiness, sleep attacks, and repetitive nocturnal breath cessations followed by brief arousals (probably related to choking or hypercapnia); breathing resumes accompanied by loud snoring and gasping sounds. The disorder usually has its onset before the age of 40.

In most patients, the bed partner or roommate observes episodes of breath cessation followed by snorting and gasping. Some patients become self-aware of nighttime choking experiences. Excessive body movements during sleep, diaphoresis, secondary enuresis, early morning headaches, and sexual impotence may occur.

Most patients with symptomatic obstructive sleep apnea have at least moderate systemic hypertension and obesity. The hypoxia and carbon dioxide retention associated with the nocturnal apneic events eventually can induce polycythemia, pulmonary hypertension, cardiomegaly, right-sided heart failure, and persistent cardiac dysrhythmias as well as cognitive impairment, psychological distress, and psychosocial disruption.

ETIOLOGY. Multiple factors in addition to obesity can contribute to the etiology of sleep apnea, including inherent predisposition, hypothyroidism, and a menopausal lessening of the respiratory stimulating effects of progestational hormones. Clinical inspection usually detects no anatomic abnormalities of the upper airway. Nevertheless, smaller pharyngeal areas have been demonstrated in some cases. Chronic vasomotor and nasal obstruction may increase the frequency of apneic episodes in others. Alcohol ingestion, smoking bronchitis, and sleep deprivation can increase the number and severity of sleep apneic events.

DIAGNOSIS. Thorough assessment of suspected sleep apnea begins with a complete sleep history (see Table 447–1). When a patient reports excessive daytime sleepiness, sleep attacks, or unusual snoring or gasping sounds during sleep, families or roommates should be questioned about severe snoring or interrupted breathing. A complete medical history and a physical examination with otorhinolaryngologic evaluation should follow, as well as measurements of hematocrit, chest radiography, electrocardiography, and 24-hour ECG monitoring. A family history

TABLE 447–6. TREATMENT OF SLEEP APNEA

Method	Response	Disadvantages
Mild apnea		
Weight loss	Delayed and limited	None
Pharmacologic (protriptyline, medroxyprogesterone)	Limited and inconsistent	Side effects
Moderate/severe apnea		
Continuous positive air pressure	Effective initially Long-term efficacy uncertain	Compliance (?) Mechanical problems Discomfort
Dental appliance	60%–80% effective Long-term efficacy not determined	Discomfort and compliance (?) Cannot use with full dentures
Uvulopalatopharyngoplasty	50% effective Delayed relapse	Possible operative morbidity Irreversible
Tracheostomy	100% effective	Operative and postoperative morbidity

of loud snoring or excessive daytime sleepiness provides an important clinical clue. The patient's psychosocial and vocational functioning should be assessed. Ultimately, the clinician depends on the result of a sleep laboratory evaluation with recording of respiration and ear oximetry (Table 447–4) to confirm the diagnosis and its severity.

MANAGEMENT. Treatment options depend upon severity, specific type of apneic events, and level of daytime functioning (Table 447–6). Steps should be taken to improve underlying medical illnesses or complications such as congestive heart failure, chronic reversible respiratory disorders, and metabolic abnormalities that could impair upper airway functioning. Drugs that depress the central ventilatory drive, such as sedative/hypnotics, barbiturates, narcotics, sedating analgesics, and alcohol, should be avoided.

Severe cases of sleep apnea syndrome can interfere with many aspects of normal life. While initiating treatment, physicians should counsel the patient, his family, and, if appropriate, his employer that the excessive daytime sleepiness and associated symptoms are beyond volitional control and are likely to improve. Patients who fail to improve with dietary and conservative drug efforts should receive the advice of an experienced consultant before embarking on surgical therapy.

Kales A, Kales JD: Evaluation and Treatment of Insomnia. New York, Oxford University Press, 1984. *An excellent, comprehensive monograph on the subject.*

Kales A, Soldatos CR, Kales JD: Sleep disorders: Insomnia, sleepwalking, night terrors, nightmares and enuresis. Ann Intern Med 106:582–592, 1987. *A very useful and clear clinical description of the various sleep disorders.*

Kales A, Vela-Bueno A, Kales JD: Sleep disorders: Sleep apnea and narcolepsy. Ann Intern Med 106:434–443, 1987. *A very useful clinical description of these sleep disorders.*

Parkes JD: Sleep and Its Disorders. Philadelphia, W. B. Saunders Company, 1985. *An excellent, detailed textbook on the subject.*

Roth B: Narcolepsy and Hypersomnia. Revised and edited by R. Broughton. Basel, S. Karger, 1980. *A comprehensive monograph on this important disorder.*

448 Diagnosis of Regional Cerebral Dysfunction

Antonio R. Damasio

Localizing the site of neurologic dysfunction based on clinical signs and symptoms is a crucial step in the assessment of neurologic diseases. Although advanced and noninvasive neuroimaging techniques localize many brain lesions, the abnormalities associated with some diseases often elude all but research-level imaging procedures. For instance, in most degenerative diseases, the regional anatomic defect can be defined only on the basis of clinical signs. The diagnosis of most epileptogenic foci, a key element in the therapeutic management of epileptic patients, is another example.

Figure 448–1 diagrams the regional neuroanatomy of the adult human brain. The accuracy of regional clinical diagnosis depends on numerous factors. First, elementary motor and sensory disorders, which are related to dysfunction in motor and sensory pathways and in primary motor and sensory cortices, can be detected earlier than disorders of language or thinking, which result from dysfunction in association cortices. The localization of the underlying lesions is generally more precise in the former than in the latter. This difference reflects the fine anatomic and functional modularity of the primary sensory and motor systems and the fact that cognitive processes depend on far more complex and distributed anatomic systems. Furthermore, the neural substrate for integrative processes is prone to vary individually, different individuals having different endowments for specific abilities. For instance, language or visuospatial skills are linked to a variety of genetic and epigenetic factors and are influenced by age, educational background, and even gender. Second, the pathologic type of lesion and its rate of development influence the rate of appearance and the extent of symptoms. Most infarcts cause their damage rapidly and lead to an abrupt onset of signs followed by at least some improvement. By contrast, most intracranial tumors generate symptoms gradually and the brain adapts to the tumor enlargement. Some slow-growing meningiomas can reach the size of a plum before they cause detectable dysfunction, while small brain metastases from a carcinoma elsewhere in the body may cause major symptoms rapidly. Thirdly, the mass effect and the edema that accompany large infarcts and some tumors may cause a shift of brain structures and thereby compress remote and otherwise intact areas of the brain against the rigid frame of the skull and dural meninges. Compression can generate false localizing signs and lead to impairment in attention, motivation, and wakefulness which can, in turn, mask or aggravate other symptoms (see Ch. 446).

OCCIPITAL LOBES

The occipital cortices are solely dedicated to visual processing. Information from both lateral geniculate nuclei arrives in each primary visual cortex (Brodmann's area 17); these cortices occupy the superior and inferior banks of the calcarine fissure (see also Ch. 454.2). This region contains a retinotopic projection of visual information. The inferior visual field maps onto the superior calcarine cortex and vice versa; the right visual field maps into the left calcarine region and conversely for the left visual field; the central part of the retina projects onto the caudal part of the calcarine region, at the occipital pole, while progressively more peripheral sectors of the retina project to more anterior sectors of the calcarine region. Beyond area 17, visual information is widely distributed by a large number of functionally distinct regions, located within the association cortices of Brodmann's areas 18 and 19. The main goals of these parallel processing units are (1) to generate representations of the form, volumetric shape, texture, movement, color, and spatial location of stimuli in the external world, and (2) to serve as the distributed storage sites for the records of visual perception that become committed to memory and are later used in the processes of visual recall, recognition, imagetic thinking, and dreaming.

Damage to the calcarine cortices (Table 448–1) or to the optic radiations as they approach the calcarine region, causes varied field defects for form vision (hemianopias or quadrantanopias) depending on the region affected (e.g., damage to the left superior calcarine region causes a right inferior quadrantanopia; damage to an entire calcarine region leads to a hemianopia). When damage is confined to inferior occipital cortices but spares the calcarine regions, patients may develop achromatopsia, a disturbance of color perception without compromise of form vision (damage to the left side causes right hemiachromatopsia and vice versa). Damage to left occipital cortices and underlying periventricular white matter combined with destruction of the interhemispheric visual pathways, often causes a disorder of reading without concomitant impairment of writing (alexia without agraphia). This may be accompanied by an impairment of color naming without impairment of color perception (color anomia). Bilateral damage to inferior visual association cortices causes agnosia, a selective impairment of visual recognition (see Ch. 449). However, lesions that extensively involve the right occipital cortices (inferior *and* superior) can cause agnosia for unique faces and places, and lesions that involve left occipital cortices (inferior *and* superior) can cause agnosia for manipulable objects. Bilateral damage to superior visual association cortices leads to disturbances of visual attention (visual disorientation or simultanagnosia) and stereo vision (astereopsis). Visual disorientation can also result from bilateral superior parietal lesions, as a component of Balint syndrome (see Parietal Lobe, below). Lesions that involve the lateral occipital cortices about their middle tier can cause defects of motion perception. Infarctions in the territory of one or both posterior cerebral arteries are the most common cause of pathology in the occipital lobes.

TEMPORAL LOBE

The temporal lobes contain structures necessary for visual and auditory perception, language, memory, and affect. The most characteristic signs of temporal lobe damage are impairments of memory, which can be caused by lesions of either side, and impairments of language, usually related to dominant hemisphere lesions (see Ch. 449). The cortical structures related to vision are located in the inferior and lateral aspects of the lobe (part of area 37, areas 20 and 21). They are higher-order association cortices that receive information from the occipital association cortices. The inferior component of the geniculocalcarine pathway (Meyer's loop) courses in the depth of the temporal lobe (see Ch. 453).

The primary auditory cortices (areas 41 and 42) are located in the first temporal gyrus at the end of the most complex chain of subcortical processing stations of any sensory portal of the brain. Their purpose is the representation of acoustic frequencies and intensities for a large range of pitched and unpitched sounds (speech, music, environmental noises) so as to permit their recognition and spatial localization. The record of those representations is contained in the auditory association cortices which surround the primary cortices bilaterally, in the superior temporal gyrus (largely area 22). Although the auditory input from the contralateral ear prevails functionally over the ipsilateral input, each cortex receives information from both ears, so unilateral temporal lesions never cause deafness.

The medial temporal lobes contain cortical and subcortical structures of the limbic system, e.g., the entorhinal cortex (area 28) located in the anterior part of the parahippocampal gyrus; the hippocampal formation; and the amygdala. These highly inter-

connected structures are privy to information emanating from all sensory cortices as well as the diencephalon, and they project back to both. They correlate perceptual inputs, ongoing verbal and nonverbal thought operations, and the status of the internal milieu. This correlation is indispensable for memory, affective experience, and emotional expression. Lesions of this region severely compromise those functions.

The temporal lobes can be compromised by numerous pathologic processes (Table 448–2). Epileptogenic scars and intracranial tumors are common; head injury often damages anterior temporal structures, and herpes simplex encephalitis has a predilection for the region; the highest and earliest concentration of cytoskeletal pathology in Alzheimer's disease is in entorhinal cortex and hippocampus; the hippocampus is selectively vulnerable to anoxia. Patients with temporal epileptogenic lesions experience a variety of affective, sensory, and visceral disturbances and exhibit emotional and motor disturbances that can appear before or during a seizure. In some patients, more subtle but longer-lasting behavioral changes develop between seizures. Tables 448–3 and 448–4 list the major ictal and interictal symptoms. Although violent behavior is often blamed on temporal lobe dysfunction, the evidence indicates that temporal lobe epilepsy should not be regarded as a medical explanation for criminal aggression. Bilateral removal of this region in animals causes the Klüver-Bucy

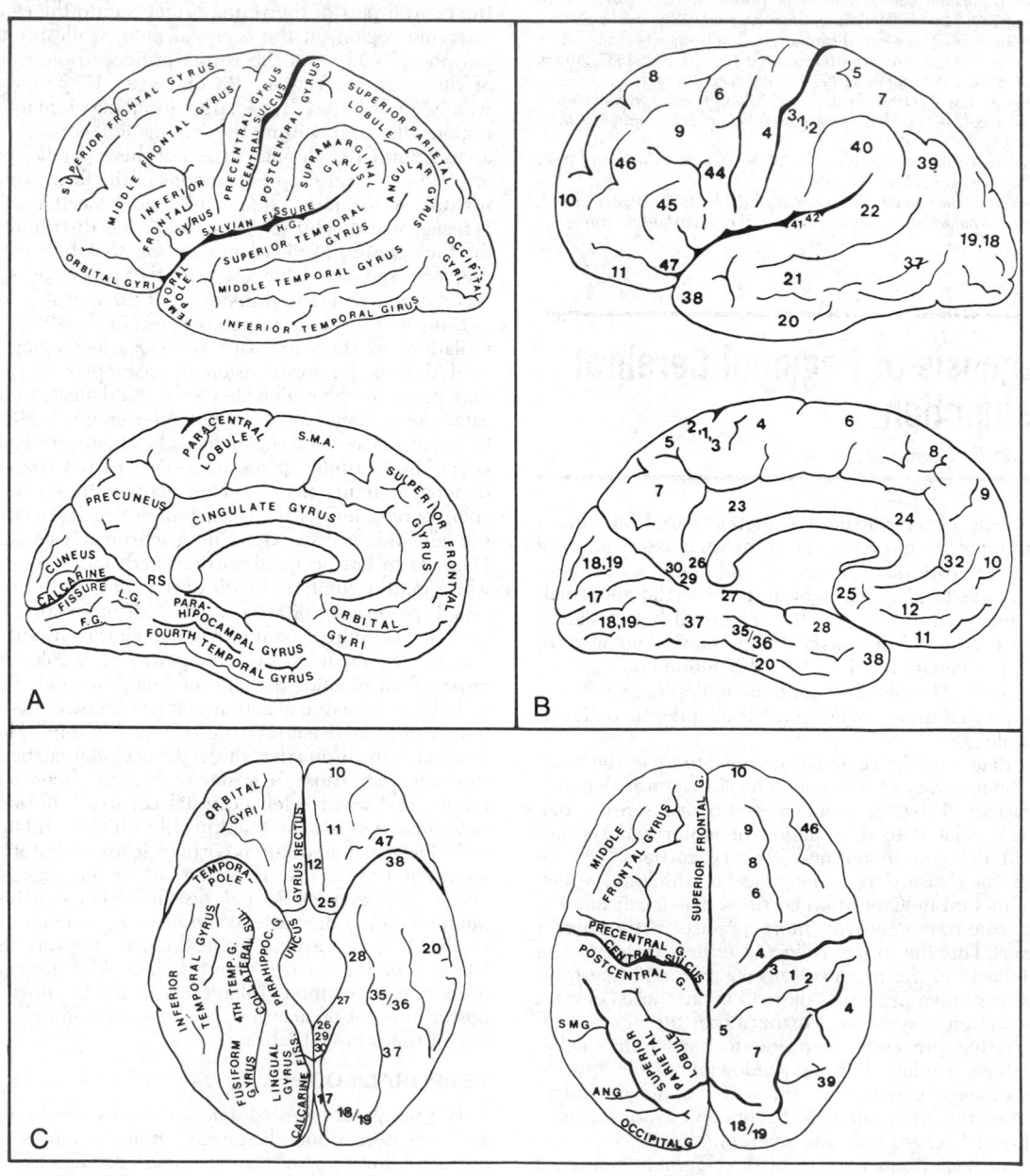

FIGURE 448–1. The principal gyri, sulci, and Brodmann's cytoarchitectonic areas of the human brain. *A,* Gyri and sulci in lateral *(top)* and mesial *(bottom)* view. *B,* Brodmann's areas in lateral *(top)* and mesial *(bottom)* view. *C,* Gyri, sulci, and Brodmann's areas in orbital *(left)* and superior *(right)* view.

TABLE 448–1. CHARACTERISTIC MANIFESTATIONS OF OCCIPITAL LOBE DAMAGE

Sign	Qualification	Lesion
Hemiachromatopsia	Right or left field (whole hemifield affected)	Left or right inferior mesial cortex and white matter
Pure alexia	Noted anywhere in intact field	Left inferior cortex and white matter (including outflow of callosum)
Color anomia	Seen only in left visual field in combination with right hemianopia	Left inferior and mesial
Visual agnosia	Noted anywhere in intact field	Usually bilateral inferior (but right occipital may involve faces and places and left occipital may involve manipulable objects)
Visual disorientation	Noted anywhere in intact field	Bilateral superior
Astereopsis	Noted anywhere in intact field	Bilateral superior
Impaired movement detection	Noted anywhere in intact field	Bilateral superior

syndrome, a disorder characterized by indiscriminate sexual behavior, excessive orality, and placidity. The full syndrome rarely develops in humans, but some components are often noted in patients with extensive bilateral temporal damage caused by herpes simplex encephalitis and the dementias of degenerative or post-traumatic etiologies.

PARIETAL LOBE

The anterior aspect of the parietal lobe contains the postcentral gyrus where Brodmann's areas 3, 1, and 2 receive somatosensory information obtained from nerve terminals in the contralateral half of the body (the projections are somatotopically organized with the largest share given to the phonatory apparatus and hand). These cortices are interlocked with the primary motor cortex in the precentral gyrus (area 4), and project to the superior parietal lobules (area 5 and 7), and inferior parietal lobules (areas 39 and 40, respectively, the angular and supramarginal gyri). A second source of somatic sensation is area S2, located in the upper bank of Sylvian fissure, which receives bilateral information and distributes it to ipsilateral parietal cortices. These cortices generate representations of the perceiver's body and of three-dimensional stimuli as apprehended by somatosensory processing and interweave such representations with appropriate motor programs as well as pertinent visual and auditory information.

Damage to the hand projection sector of the postcentral somatosensory cortex in either hemisphere impairs the ability to recognize form (astereognosia), scale, texture, and weight of objects in the contralateral hand. (The thresholds for touch, pain, vibration, and temperature are generally not disturbed.)

TABLE 448–2. MANIFESTATIONS OF TEMPORAL LOBE DAMAGE

	Unilateral	Bilateral
Posterolateral	Aphasia* Pure-word deafness* Amusia†	Global auditory agnosia (includes aphasia, amusia, and agnosia for environmental sounds)
Medial	Verbal* or nonverbal memory impairment Complex seizures	Amnesia
Anterolateral and inferior	Anomia* Nonverbal memory impairment Visual agnosia Complex seizures	Amnesia

*Usually left hemisphere
†Right hemisphere only

TABLE 448–3. ICTAL MANIFESTATIONS OF TEMPORAL LOBE EPILEPTIC FOCI

Medial Basal Structures	Lateral Structures
Olfactory hallucinations Memory disturbances (dejà vu or jamais vu); forced thinking, dreamy state	Language impairment; hissing, roaring or clicking hallucinations; vertigo

Epigastric distress
Blank staring
Repetitive somatic automatisms

Damage to the dominant or nondominant inferior parietal lobule causes diverse manifestations. The dominant somatosensory cortex develops dynamic representations of (a) the body and of its movements (especially those of the hand and phonatory apparatus) and (b) the shapes of objects located within arm's reach (in so-called intrapersonal space). Dysfunction in the area of the dominant angular gyrus disrupts reading and writing, planning and execution of representational hand movements in specific contexts (apraxia), arithmetic skills (acalculia), finger recognition (finger agnosia), right-left orientation and the ability to copy drawings, diagrams, and execute three dimensional constructions (constructional apraxia). Dysfunction in the dominant supramarginal gyrus is mainly associated with aphasia (Table 448–5).

The nondominant parietal cortices hold a dynamic representation of extrapersonal space (the space beyond arm's reach) based on somatosensory, visual, and auditory cues. *Both* hemispaces are represented in this region. The attentional survey of external sensory events and projected movements in both hemispaces also depend on this nondominant region, damage to which leads to complex defects in spatial processing. The defects are especially pronounced in the hemispace opposite the lesion and cause the commonly encountered neglect syndrome. Not only is the left hemispace inappropriately attended but the left side of the body itself may be neglected and left hemiplegia or hemisensory loss may be ignored or actively denied (anosognosia). The ability to negotiate a route without hitting obstacles placed to the left side of the body, the skill to follow a previously known and automated route (in a house or town), and the capacity to learn a new route are all compromised by nondominant inferior parietal lesions. So is constructional ability, which is far more disturbed than with equivalent lesions on the dominant side. Unlike their counterparts with left-sided lesions, patients with such nondominant injuries show little concern for their condition and often offer an indifferent affect. An adequate rehabilitation program must take into account this reduced motivation. When these structures are affected on the right side together with the right nearby auditory cortices (as a result of extensive cerebrovascular damage affecting the nondominant middle cerebral artery territory), patients may become acutely confused.

Bilateral damage confined to superior parietal lobules causes ocular apraxia (the inability to direct gaze voluntarily toward new visual stimuli appearing in the periphery of the visual field), bilateral optic ataxia (the inability to generate precise contralateral hand movements toward an outbound target under visual guidance), and an impairment of visual attention, a breakdown in the ability to apprehend the visual panorama in a coherent, seamless manner (this is known as visual disorientation or simultanagnosia). The combination of ocular apraxia, optic ataxia, and visual disorientation constitutes the Balint syndrome. Common causes are bilateral infarctions in the border zone between the posterior and

TABLE 448–4. INTERICTAL TRAITS OF PATIENTS WITH TEMPORAL LOBE EPILEPTIC FOCI

Lack of humor
Sadness
Obsessiveness
Metaphysical preoccupation
Hyposexuality
Dependence

TABLE 448–5. MANIFESTATIONS OF PARIETAL LOBE DAMAGE

Superior parietal lobule	Bilateral damage causes Balint syndrome. Unilateral damage causes mainly optic ataxia and transient abnormalities of pursuit eye movements.
Inferior parietal lobule — left	Aphasia; alexia; agraphia; acalculia; constructional apraxia; right/left disorientation; finger agnosia
Inferior parietal lobule — right	Neglect; anosognosia; inappropriate affect
Post-Rolandic cortices	Subjective alterations in somatic sensation. Astereognosia

middle cerebral artery territories and bilateral metastases. Unilateral damage to the superior parietal lobule causes optic ataxia and defective pursuit eye movements.

FRONTAL LOBES

The human frontal cortices encompass nearly half of the entire cortical mantle and include a large number of diverse anatomic fields. Their operations assist with movement control; general problem solving; decision making; planning; generation of willful responses; regulation of social behaviors, emotion, affect, and autonomic function; and regulation of language and thought processes. Understanding of the correspondence between structure and function is less advanced for frontal cortices than for other cerebral regions. Furthermore, impairments of the functions outlined above are less easy to detect in clinical and laboratory settings than in real life.

The motor sector of the frontal lobe (the precentral and premotor cortices) is located mainly in the lateral frontal surface but spills into the mesial surface as well. The precentral cortex (area 4 or M1) contains a somatotopic representation of contralateral body movements in which the phonatory apparatus and hand are accorded the largest share. It is the principal target of re-entrant projections from cerebellum and motor thalamus. The premotor region (area 6) is part of a network for motor programming, and it receives re-entrant projections from basal ganglia as well as projections from the posterior sensory cortices. It integrates incoming movement-related information for final transmission to the corticospinal tract. Part of the nearby area 8, known as the frontal eye field, controls voluntary eye movements (seizures originating in this area cause the eyes to *deviate away from the lesion;* damage by an infarction makes the eyes deviate *toward the lesion*). The mesial aspect of area 6 contains the supplementary motor area (SMA or M2). The SMA is anatomically contiguous with the rest of the premotor cortex but constitutes a functionally separate region. (It contains a whole body map in its relatively small cortical surface.) Damage to area 4 causes varied degrees of focal paralysis in the contralateral side of the body or face (involvement of corticospinal projections in corona radiata or internal capsule causes less focal paralysis). Damage to the lateral aspect of area 6 causes impairments of motor learning and execution as well as transient forms of neglect, while involvement of the SMA leads to mutism and contralateral akinesia. Infarctions and parasagittal tumors in this region often compromise part of both SMA and the nearby cingulate gyrus (area 24) located immediately beneath the cingulate sulcus. The cingulate is a limbic cortex and its acute damage also causes akinesia, mutism, transient neglect, and an impairment of motivation (abulia). Tumors impinging in this region may cause speech arrest and seizures characterized by vocalization and may trigger involuntary movement synergies involving contralateral limbs and trunk. Motor symptoms of frontal lobe lesions are presented in Table 448–6.

The frontal lobes also contain limbic cortices in the posterior orbital surface. Involvement of this region is associated with disturbances of social behavior. These include inability to recognize the social value of real-life situations and an inability to plan future social actions appropriately. On occasion, especially with large lesions, patients may exhibit inappropriate demeanor (facetiousness). During the acute phase of frontal limbic damage patients are generally akinetic and inattentive and may exhibit inappropriate behavior regarding their sphincters. They may urinate or defecate in public although sphincter function per se is preserved.

Areas 44 and 45 on the dominant side are known as Broca's area. Their damage causes aphasia (see Ch. 449). Damage to the nondominant side of this area alters the prosodic qualities of speech. The most anterior regions of the frontal lobe accommodate the prefrontal cortices (areas 46, 9, 10, 11, 12), damage to which impairs decision making and planning, reduces creativity, and alters the regulation of affect and emotion. With permanent damage, the magnitude of the deficit relates directly to the bilaterality or unilaterality of the lesion, the size of the lesion, and the previous intellectual caliber and occupation of the patient. Relatively small unilateral lesions produce minor impairments that are difficult to detect and tend to recover. Large bilateral prefrontal lesions, however, although they leave motor, perceptual, and language functions intact, are incompatible with maintaining a socially adapted, fully self-conscious and creative personality. The defects are most noticeable in patients who undergo bilateral prefrontal ablations for the treatment of large midline brain tumors. Even then, however, the impairments can be better sensed by appraising social and occupational behavior than by neuropsychologic tests, most of which may be passed flawlessly.

The frontal lobes are especially vulnerable to closed head injury resulting in many of the signs described above as well as in the formation of cortical scar tissue and the appearance of seizures. The lateral sectors are frequently compromised by infarctions and meningiomas. The mesial sector is often struck by infarctions or hemorrhages, mostly as a consequence of ruptured anterior communicating or anterior cerebral artery aneurysms. Meningiomas arising in the falx are another common cause of damage. The posterior orbital sector is often involved by herpes simplex encephalitis, by hemorrhages from ruptured anterior circulation aneurysms, and by meningiomas arising in the sphenoid and ethmoid regions. The brunt of the effects of normal-pressure hydrocephalus reflect damage to the frontal white matter. Finally, all prefrontal cortices are markedly involved in Pick's disease, and both prefrontal and frontal limbic cortices are involved to some extent in Alzheimer's disease. When involvement of frontal lobe structures is caused by large tumors, especially by malignant gliomas which often arise in the white matter of one hemisphere but traverse the corpus callosum to involve the other, patients exhibit the florid disturbances outlined above and also impairments of attention and balance (see Ch. 454), along with primitive reflexes (grasp reflex, Gegenhalten or paratonia, echopraxia).

TABLE 448–6. MOTOR SYMPTOMS OF FRONTAL LOBE DISEASE*

	Structural Damage	Seizure
Precentral gyrus	Focal distal weakness, maximal in lower face, hand, less often foot; increased reflexes, mild spasticity, Babinski sign	Jacksonian: focal onset on face, thumb, foot. "March" toward proximal limb and trunk.
Corona radiata or internal capsule	Hemiplegia; increased spasticity	
Premotor (lateral)	Ocular ipsiversion; paratonic resistance to passive motion; grasping; hypokinesia; optic ataxia, aphasia	Adversive: ocular contraversion.
Premotor (mesial)	Mutism	Involuntary synergies (elevated arm and leg, body turning); speech arrest and/or vocalization

*All arise contralateral to the brain lesion.

Bear DM, Fedio P: Quantitative analysis of interictal behavior in temporal lobe epilepsy. Arch Neurol 34:454, 1977. *An effort to quantify the personality traits of epileptics.*

Damasio H, Damasio AR: Lesion Analysis in Neuropsychology. New York, Oxford University Press, 1989. *A method to study the anatomic location of cerebral lesions, and a review of advances in neuropsychology.*

Eslinger PJ, Damasio AR: Severe disturbance of higher cognition after bilateral frontal lobe ablation. Neurology 35:1731, 1985. *An example of the extreme dissociation of behavior caused by frontal lobe damage. The lesions prompted a variety of socially unacceptable behaviors but did not interfere with language or memory. The intelligence quotient remained superior.*

Gazzaniga M, Le Doux J: The Integrated Mind. New York, Plenum Press, 1978. *A brief and lucid survey of the integration of higher functions and of the role the cerebral commissures play in it.*

Heilman K, Valenstein E (eds.): Clinical Neuropsychology. Oxford, Oxford University Press, 1985. *A multiauthored collection of essays on major aspects of neuropsychology.*

Hier DB, Mondlock J, Caplan LR: Behavioral abnormalities after right hemisphere stroke. Neurology 33:337, 1983. *An analysis of a large series of patients with damage to the right parietal lobe.*

Mesulam M-M: (ed.): Principles of Behavioral Neurology. Philadelphia: F. A. Davis Co., 1985, pp. 125–168. *Another collection of comprehensive reviews on neuropsychology.*

Penfield W, Jasper W: Epilepsy and the Functional Anatomy of the Human Brain. Boston, Little, Brown, and Company, 1954. *The classic monograph on what epilepsy and the electrical stimulation of the cerebral cortex tell us about the neural substrates of higher brain function.*

449 Disturbances of Memory and Language

Antonio R. Damasio

The concerted operation of multiple but relatively specific cortical systems is the basis for the most complex human abilities: the acquisition and categorization of knowledge (learning and memory), the translation of knowledge in a verbal code (language), the manipulation of nonverbal and verbal knowledge in thought processes, the ability to select responses and solve problems (decision-making, planning, creativity), and the reflection upon ongoing cognitive activities in the perspective of one's autobiography (self-consciousness). These functions presume the normal operations of attention (the ability to concentrate willfully on a specific mental content to the exclusion of others) as well as motivation (the affective impetus to sustain a given mental activity or action).

MEMORY AND ITS IMPAIRMENTS

Memory is the ability to make a record of perceptions of the external world, usually combined with perceptions of the perceiver's body and movements. Memory also encompasses the ability to store concepts derived from the categorization of those records and to manipulate the records internally for recall and recognition. The terms "learning" and "memory" are used almost interchangeably, although learning should be used only to denote "memory acquisition."

Unless the process of consolidation takes over, the memory of objects or events that we perceive is retained only briefly (less than 60 seconds). The material held during that period is said to be in *short-term memory* or *immediate memory* (Table 449–1). (Immediate memory is preserved in most amnesias.) If those materials are to be recorded into permanent or *long-term memory*, an active physiologic process must start promptly. The process of consolidation takes time, and recently acquired memories are more vulnerable to decay than those that have been

TABLE 449–1. TYPES OF MEMORY

Factual (declarative)
Skill (procedural)

Short-term (immediate)—less than 60 seconds
Long-term—more than 60 seconds

Recent

Remote

held long and internally rehearsed. Newer memories are known as *recent* memories, and older memories as *remote*.

Memory for unique faces, objects, or events is often termed *episodic* (e.g., the memory of a personal friend or a favorite landscape), whereas memory for classes of objects or events is usually known as *generic* or *semantic* (e.g., the knowledge that allows us to categorize a car as a transport vehicle, a dog as an animal, or a given locale as urban or rural). Episodic and semantic memories pertain to factual knowledge and are known as *declarative*. Declarative memory contrasts with *procedural* memory, which is based on skills rather than facts and refers to actions rather than to the knowledge necessary to acquire those actions. Dancing, the playing of instruments, typing, and swimming are examples of *procedural* memory. Procedural memory is spared in most amnesias.

MEMORY MECHANISMS. The thesaurus of facts and rules acquired in a lifetime is stored in the association cortices of every lobe of both hemispheres. Memories are dynamically and flexibly distributed in overlapping neuron ensembles linked by patterned, highly specific, and hierarchically organized corticocortical and commissural connections. Access to single-modality memories depends on association cortices near the primary sensory cortex that conveyed the information in the first place (the impaired access or partial destruction of those cortices causes an *agnosia*—Table 449–2). Access to memories of polymodal events depends on cortices farther away from sensory sources. Finally, access to unique and complex polymodal episodes depends on inferior and anterolateral temporal cortices (impaired access or partial damage to such cortices causes *amnesia*).

The ability to lock sensory events into neural structures to form a permanent record depends on the normal operation of the hippocampal system, the basal forebrain, and the diencephalon, as well as several brain stem nuclei. The elucidation of the respective roles of these components is imperfect, but it appears that the hippocampus, which is informed about relationships between components of an event via connections from the higher-order association cortices, binds and stabilizes information according to its appropriate temporal and spatial links. The stabilization appears to involve molecular and cellular changes during long-term potentiation. Through the interconnected amygdala the hippocampus also influences basal forebrain, diencephalon, and brain stem nuclei. The basal forebrain and brain stem, in turn, provide the cerebral cortex with neurochemical inputs that probably also contribute to stabilize records at the cellular level (acetylcholine from the nucleus basalis of Meynert in the basal forebrain, noradrenaline from the locus coeruleus in the brain stem, and other, still ill-defined mediators and modulators). The hippocampal interconnections with the diencephalon sample the status of the internal milieu at the time of a given sensory experience, informing on the value of a particular stimulus or event in the context of instinctual goals. Finally, the ascending brain stem reticular formation contributes importantly because

TABLE 449–2. DISTINGUISHING AMNESIA FROM OTHER IMPAIRMENTS

Agnosia	Impaired recognition of stimuli presented in one sensory channel (e.g., object, face, voice, melody) that cannot be explained by defective perception.
Anomia	Impaired retrieval of the name for a stimulus (e.g., object or face) that is otherwise properly perceived and properly recognized.
Amnesia	A pervasive impairment of the ability to recall and recognize unique events and unique stimuli. The defect is independent of the sensory channel used to probe memory (e.g., given a unique person, *neither* the face *nor* the voice is recognizable).
Aphasia	A pervasive impairment of linguistic processing; (e.g., structure of sentences; assembly of phonemes in a word; retrieval of words from the lexicon).
Dysarthria	Defective articulation of speech sounds without compromise of linguistic processing. When the articulation breakdown is complete, the term *anarthria* applies.

most learning presumes attention and arousal. The neural structures and systems involving the acquisition of procedural memories are different: After bilateral destruction to hippocampus and basal forebrain, most motor skills remain intact and new motor skills can be learned. The motor and sensory cortices generate those memories and so do the cerebellum, the neostriatum, and the motor nuclei of the thalamus. A discussion of the molecular and cellular changes related to memory is outside the scope of this chapter.

MEMORY DISORDERS. Table 449–3 lists several terms that are helpful in describing and classifying the amnesias. The terms *anterograde* and *retrograde* are especially important. Anterograde designates the time compartment *since* the amnesia began. Retrograde refers to the time compartment *prior* to the onset of amnesia and to information previously acquired that may not be retrievable in recall or recognition. Retrograde amnesia can be as short as hours or days, as is often the case in post-traumatic situations, or may extend back years or even decades, as in Korsakoff's amnesia or the amnesias that follow herpes simplex encephalitis.

Some middle-aged and elderly persons have an increasing but isolated difficulty in recalling proper names and recent events of limited importance. This "benign forgetfulness" is not a predictor of the progressive dementias and is best treated with prompt and vigorous reassurance. The most frequent causes of incapacitating memory loss are the degenerative dementias, head injury, cerebrovascular disease, encephalitis, brain anoxia and ischemia, and nutritional impairment (Table 449–4).

A major part of our knowledge about the critical contribution to memory of the hippocampal formation and its input and output stations came from a single, well-studied patient who underwent *bilateral medial temporal lobe resection* to treat epilepsy. He became severely amnesic postoperatively and has remained unable to learn factual memories to this day. His severe anterograde amnesia contrasts with a largely spared retrograde memory and with preserved generic memories and procedural learning. The amnesias caused by *postanoxic encephalopathy,* in which anterograde memory is heavily involved, also are caused by hippocampal damage in which the CA1 sector is selectively damaged. Together with the evidence that specific areas of the entorhinal cortex and subiculum are damaged in amnesic patients with *Alzheimer's disease,* these findings underscore the importance of hippocampus in memory (see Ch. 450). *Herpes simplex encephalitis* commonly damages the hippocampal region bilaterally, but it involves other anterolateral and inferior regions of the temporal cortices. Such patients suffer not only an anterograde memory defect but also a severe retrograde amnesia that can span virtually their entire lives, especially when the right hippocampal area is heavily involved. Bilateral damage to hippocampus can also be caused by infarctions in the territory of the posterior cerebral arteries. Infarctions in the area of the basal forebrain (septal nuclei, nucleus accumbens, nucleus basalis of Meynert) due to ruptured aneurysms in the anterior circulation are also associated with amnesia. Both anterograde and retrograde memory are involved, but unlike temporal lobe amnesia, the defect is mild, tends to improve, and appropriate cueing helps recall. *Head injury* is another major cause of amnesia. Even modest head trauma results in transient dysfunction of the hippocampus and diencephalon. *Korsakoff's*

TABLE 449–3. TYPES OF AMNESIA

Retrograde	Amnesia for information learned before the onset of illness
Anterograde	Amnesia for information that presented itself after onset of illness
Global	Information cannot be retrieved through *any* sensory channel
Modality-specific	Same as associative agnosia; information cannot be retrieved through the affected channel, e.g., vision
Permanent	
Stable	Example: postencephalitic
Progressive	Example: Alzheimer's disease
Transient	Examples: transient global amnesia, post-traumatic amnesia

TABLE 449–4. ETIOLOGIES OF AMNESIA

Alzheimer's disease and other degenerative dementias
Head injury
Herpes simplex encephalitis
Ruptured anterior circulation aneurysms with infarction in basal forebrain
Infarctions in other memory-related systems, e.g., medial thalamic nuclei; temporal cortices
Anoxic/ischemic encephalopathy
Wernicke-Korsakoff encephalopathy
Psychogenic amnesia

syndrome is a severe amnesia that compromises both anterograde and retrograde memories and is accompanied by confabulation and lack of insight. It is caused by attacks of severe thiamine deficiency, generally in the setting of alcoholism, and often accompanies or follows acute Wernicke encephalopathy (see Ch. 456), or delirium tremens (see Ch. 14), although it can occur whenever thiamine-free calories are the mainstay of nutrition. Thiamine deficiency results in bilateral damage to diencephalic structures, including the dorsal medial nucleus of the thalamus and the hypothalamic mamillary bodies. The consistent presence of these lesions in Korsakoff's amnesia established the diencephalon as a crucial component of the memory-related network.

Transient global amnesia (TGA) is a self-limited memory impairment during which the patient can identify himself but is unable to recall events preceding the episode and generally cannot recognize places. Patients with TGA remain attentive, have normal language and reasoning, and are generally distressed by their disorientation. They tend to ask repeatedly where they are, what they have been up to, and what is going on. Most TGA episodes last about 4 or 5 hours (but may be shorter or longer), and the disorientation gradually clears. The attacks leave no residual impairment and are generally nonrecurrent. Status epilepticus with complex partial or petit mal seizures may mimic TGA but can be distinguished because patients with seizures are generally noninquisitive and inattentive. Most TGA attacks occur in middle-aged or older persons and presumably reflect transient vascular insufficiency affecting memory-related areas in the temporal lobe or thalamus.

Psychogenic amnesia is generally greatest for emotionally important events and may erase circumscribed epochs of the past while leaving intact epochs immediately preceding or following the amnesic period. It may include disorientation to self. Questions such as "Who am I?" or "What is my name?", unless uttered during delirium or a seizure, raise the possibility of a psychogenic process. Psychogenic amnesia must be distinguished from emotional upheaval (which often impairs attention and produces inconsistent performance in psychological testing), from depression (which may reduce communication to monosyllables), and from organic amnesias (in which emotionally reinforced material tends to be recalled better than neutral events, and disorientation is worst for time, less for place and persons, and never for self).

Treatment. Patients with acute post-traumatic amnesia tend to recover spontaneously. The same is true of amnesia caused by overmedication or delirium. Memory loss caused by depression (pseudodementia) has a good prognosis when psychological and psychiatric treatment is effective. A less fortunate prognosis accompanies amnesia following prolonged post-traumatic coma. When coma lasts more than 2 or 3 weeks, most patients over 25 years old tend not to recover from the memory loss. Patients with amnesia due to herpes encephalitis recover only when the lesions are mostly or solely unilateral and even those persons retain substantial impairments. In most amnesias the recovery is inversely proportional to the initial severity and is constrained by the extent and placement of lesions. The bulk of improvement usually takes place within the first year after onset, especially within the first 6 months. Neuroactive peptides, neurotransmitter precursors, neurotransmitters, and special dietary agents have no proven usefulness in chronic organic amnesia.

AGNOSIA. Agnosia is the inability to recognize a previously familiar sensory stimulus despite the integrity of elementary perception of the stimulus and the absence of defects of intelligence, motivation, or attention. It is "a percept stripped of its meaning." The disorder is a form of monomodal amnesia, a disability that prevents a perceived stimulus from triggering pertinent, previously acquired information whose evocation would reveal its identity. Agnosia results from dysfunction of association cortices of the affected sensory modality, which contain records of purely modal processing. *Visual agnosia* is the most frequent example. It consists of the failure to recognize familiar faces (prosopagnosia) or objects (visual object agnosia), despite the ability to describe their physical structures, copy them, or recognize the stimulus by sound (prosopagnosics can recognize the possessor of a face by voice). The phenomenon is generally associated with bilateral occipitotemporal lesions, although visual object agnosia can be caused by *left* unilateral lesions of the occipital lobe, and *right* unilateral lesions reduce the efficiency of face recognition.

LANGUAGE AND ITS DISORDERS

Verbal languages are arbitrary symbolic codes in which words stand for properties of external stimuli, actions, and relationships, as well as for the intellectual and emotional reactions that such stimuli evoke in the perceiver. The normal brain acquires and stores a dictionary of such words in at least one language, a lexicon, and develops a highly automated process of two-way translation between the mechanism to reconstruct word representations and the mechanism to reconstruct nonverbal representations of objects, actions, or concepts. The process of language comprehension is the translation of sentences (structured sequences of words) into sequences of approximate nonverbal counterparts whose ongoing manipulation is known as thought. Nouns, verbs, or adjectives have fairly direct referential nonverbal equivalents. On the contrary, functor words (conjunctions, prepositions and adverbs, verb endings) refer to abstract relationships. Functors, together with word order, are the key to the grammatical organization of sentences (syntax) and their nonverbal counterparts in thought. The formulation of speech or writing is the rendering of a nonverbal thought process in a syntactic frame filled with appropriate lexical elements. The lexical and syntactic operations of language depend on phonemic and graphemic devices, which can enact correspondences between sounds, their visual representations, and the articulatory patterns that permit their sensorimotor implementation in phonetic utterances or writing. Oral verbal expression also depends on word stress and the intonational contour of sentences, i.e., the fundamental frequency of the sounds in an utterance as well as the durational elements of speech. The term *prosody* subsumes the latter qualities of verbal expression.

NEURAL SUBSTRATES OF LANGUAGE. Verbal language is characteristically human, and its experimental study is restricted to human beings. Considerable knowledge has been gathered about the neural substrates of language from the cognitive and neuroanatomic study of patients with acquired impairments caused by focal brain lesions (aphasias). Most such studies have relied largely on postmortem, computed tomography, and magnetic resonance imaging analysis, although more recent evaluations have been conducted using positron emission tomography (PET). Electrical stimulation of different regions of the cerebrum during surgery for seizures or motor disorders also has provided information on the neural representation of language. The preoperative precaution of pharmacologically inactivating part of the hemispheres with the intracarotid injection of a barbiturate (Amytal) has also contributed important clues. A salient finding, first noted more than a century ago and thoroughly confirmed since, is that the left hemisphere of more than 95 per cent of individuals is especially adroit at language processing. In left language–dominant persons all aspects of language depend largely on left-hemisphere processing, with the partial exception of some aspects of prosody. Handedness is an imperfect but clinically useful indicator of language dominance. In almost all right-handed persons the left hemisphere is dominant for language, and its damage in key areas leads to severe aphasia. Most left-handed and ambidextrous persons (about 70 per cent) are also left language–dominant, although they may have additional language representation in the right hemisphere. About one third of left-handers have either bilateral language representation or right-hemisphere language representation. Such persons are at a disadvantage in that lesions of either side can cause aphasia, although the disability tends to be less severe and to improve. Even extreme right-handed individuals with full language domi-

nance in the left hemisphere possess some language representation in the opposite hemisphere (especially for nouns and verbs; adjectives are poorly represented and functor words probably not at all). The right hemisphere of such a person has little access to speech output and little syntactic capability. It has been suggested that gender is an important variable in language representation, but the available data do not permit conclusive statements. Certainly both men and women can develop aphasia with similar signs and following similar lesions. Language representation is definitely different in children, however. Most children who suffer severe brain lesions up to age 5 or 6 years can recover from aphasia and continue to develop language to nearly normal levels. Left-hemisphere lesions sustained later, especially after puberty, have the same consequences as for adults.

Some asymmetric abilities of the cerebral hemispheres have been related to neuroanatomic asymmetries. The left planum temporale, the area of association cortex located immediately behind the transverse gyrus (the primary auditory cortex), is far larger than the right in about 70 per cent of individuals. The sizable difference is visible on gross inspection and in the microscopic cytoarchitectonic structure of the area. In the same individuals, the left sylvian fissure is longer on the left than on the right so as to accompany the larger extent of the posterior temporal region, and more horizontally placed so as to accommodate a more voluminous left lower parietal lobule (supramarginal gyrus and angular gyrus). Fetuses show these anatomic symmetries as early as the sixteenth week of gestation, and the changes can be identified by MRI as well as in the vascular patterns of cerebral angiographies.

Language depends on a wide network of cortical and subcortical processing units, and its knowledge and operations are distributed within key cortical regions (see Fig. 448–1). The principal set of language areas is located around the left sylvian fissure (the perisylvian language region). In its posterior aspect lies Wernicke's area (the posterior auditory association cortex, or Brodmann's area 22; it includes the planum temporale and the posterior portion of the first temporal gyrus). Immediately below and behind lies area 37, the lateral aspect of which, in the posterior sector of the second and third temporal gyri, is committed to language. Above and behind the sylvian fissure lie the supramarginal gyrus (area 40) and the angular gyrus (area 39). In the anterior aspect of the perisylvian region in the inferior and posterior aspect of the frontal operculum lie areas 44 and 45, also known as Broca's area. Between sit the motor and sensory regions associated with sensory motor phonatory representations. Also contributing to the language network are components of the basal ganglia (especially in the head of the caudate nucleus and parts of the putamen), some thalamic nuclei, the supplementary motor areas (especially the one on the left), and the anterior cingulate gyri.

THE APHASIAS. Aphasia (or dysphasia) is a disturbance of the comprehension or formulation of verbal messages caused by newly acquired brain disease. Although developments in cognitive science have led to a linguistic-based approach to aphasia, Geschwind's diagnosis of aphasic disorders in terms of the comprehension of language, the fluency of output, and the ability to repeat sentences remains clinically useful because of the strong relationship between these traits and the anatomic sites of the underlying lesions. Table 449–5 summarizes the important clinical clues.

Damage to the posterior sector of the left superior temporal gyrus and its surround causes *Wernicke aphasia*. Patients speak fluently, with normal melodic contour, and even a normal syntactic frame. However, they select wrong words (semantic paraphasias), so the intelligibility of their otherwise well-formed verbal messages may be low (jargon aphasia). Likewise, their comprehension of verbal message is poor because of their inability to translate words into nonverbal meanings. Wernicke aphasics with severe comprehension defects may develop paranoid reactions and become homicidal or suicidal. Wernicke aphasia must be distinguished from *auditory agnosia*, the inability to recognize objects or actions by the characteristic sounds they made (due to bilateral lesions in auditory cortex), and *pure word deafness*, an agnosia restricted to words which allows patients to recognize nonspeech sounds and to produce normal speech (owing to

TABLE 449–5. DIAGNOSTIC POINTERS TO THE MOST FREQUENT APHASIA TYPES

	Speech	Comprehension	Repetition	Other Signs	Localization
Broca	Nonfluent; effortful	+	−	Right hemiparesis worse in arm; aware of defect; frustrated	Lower posterior frontal
Wernicke	Abundant; fluent; well articulated	−	−	Often none; may be euphoric and/or paranoid	Posterior and superior temporal
Conduction	Fluent with some articulatory defects	+	−	Often none; cortical sensory loss in right arm	Usually supramarginal gyrus; may extend to insula and primary auditory cortex
Global	Scant; nonfluent	−	−	Right hemiparesis worse in arm; may present *without* hemiparesis	With hemiparesis: massive perisylvian lesion; without hemiparesis: separate Broca and Wernicke area damage
Transcortical motor	Nonfluent; explosive	+	+		Anterior or superior to Broca area
Transcortical sensory	Scant; fluent	−	+		Surrounding Wernicke area, posteriorly or inferiorly
Atypical ("basal ganglia")	Fluent dysarthric	−	−/+	Right hemiparesis worse in arm	Head of caudate; anterior limb of capsule
Atypical ("thalamus")	Fluent	−	+	Attentional and memory defects in acute phase	Anterolateral thalamus

+ = Intact or largely preserved
− = Impaired

dominant lesions undercutting the auditory cortex). It is also different from the logorrhea of manic states, the logical thought derailment of schizophrenia, and the rare verbal salads of chronic schizophrenics.

Posterior lesions outside the Wernicke area produce more restricted disturbances. Lesions of the supramarginal gyrus give rise to *conduction aphasia,* a disorder in which the patient speaks fluently, has relatively preserved comprehension, but makes sound substitution errors (phonemic paraphasias). The major impairment of repetition stands out among these comparatively milder defects. Other strategically placed lesions of the posterior dominant hemisphere selectively compromise reading or writing. Alexia (inability to comprehend written language while retaining relatively normal vision) without concomitant writing impairment results when a lesion destroys the left visual cortex and, in addition, involves the outflow of the splenium of the corpus callosum. This placement cuts off projections that otherwise connect the unaffected right visual cortex to language areas of the left. Despite their inability to comprehend the written word, patients with "pure" alexia can speak and write normally, in contrast to those with a combination of *alexia with agraphia* (impairment of writing despite normal motor function of the hand), in whom both reading and writing are compromised. In its pure form the abnormality is rare and follows lesions of the left angular gyrus. More frequently alexia and agraphia are accompaniments of Wernicke aphasia.

Broca aphasia is characterized by nonfluent, effortful, melodically flat speech, often shorn of functor words and marred by poor word order. The syntactic defect far outweighs the lexical impairment. Comprehension is well preserved in conversation. Broca aphasia must be distinguished from dysarthria, a disorder of speech articulation that does not impair the linguistic structure of communication. Many Broca aphasics are mute in the first hours or days after the onset of the disorder and only gradually develop the characteristic verbal signs. The intent to communicate, however poorly, is rarely in question. The lesion compromises Broca's area and adjacent cortical and subcortical territories. Because of patterns of vascular supply, many such patients also suffer a contralateral hemiparesis. Apraxia is added when the lesion involves the adjacent premotor cortex. Aphasia caused by lesions confined to Broca's area has a comparatively good prognosis.

Global aphasia consists of a severe loss of all aspects of language operation. Acutely, patients are often mute and have a right hemiplegia. The paucity of speech may become chronic, the patient being able neither to comprehend nor to produce language (except in the form of expletives or brief phrases). Despite rehabilitation efforts, the prognosis is poor, and patients often become depressed and listless, more so than Wernicke aphasics.

As indicated in Table 449–5, two possible localizations can be associated with global aphasia.

With all the aphasias described above, patients are unable to repeat long sentences after the examiner. With some language defects, however, repetition is preserved. The dissociation between intact repetition and disturbed comprehension or speech output implies that Wernicke and Broca regions, as well as their interconnections, must be intact and that the causative lesions may lie near but outside those areas. There are two frequently encountered aphasias of this type: *transcortical motor* and *transcortical sensory* (Table 449–5).

Mutism accompanies a variety of conditions. It may describe the initial state of patients who evolve into Broca or global aphasia but produce no speech at all acutely. It may describe patients with bilateral premotor lesions who often remain chronically mute. Mutism has been applied to the paroxysmal speech arrest caused by seizures arising out of the supplementary motor or Broca areas, generally as an irritative response to an overlying tumor, and to the absence of speech in acute psychoses. Prominent mutism affects patients with lesions of the dominant-sided supplementary motor area and/or nearby cingulate, who not only do not speak but show no inclination to communicate through facial expression or gestures. Those patients also are generally motionless and when they recover do not exhibit aphasic symptoms. Mutism is not *anarthria,* a severe impairment of articulation that prevents speech but allows both the vivid expression of the intent to communicate and the frustration of not being able to do so (anarthria is caused by bulbar or pseudobulbar defects and can be confirmed by the presence of other signs of nuclear and supranuclear paralysis of lingual–vocal cord functions). Nor is mutism the same as *aphonia,* in which the phonatory apparatus is locally inoperative for mechanical or psychogenic reasons.

Some aphasias can be caused by infarcts in the dominant basal ganglia, especially when they involve the head of the caudate and the anterior limb of the internal capsule, and by infarcts in anterolateral nuclei of the dominant thalamus. Their appearance indicates that subcortical structures contribute to language processing, probably by assisting cortical units. The basal ganglia aphasias most often show a combination of fluent, dysarthric speech accompanied by impaired auditory comprehension and a right hemiparesis. The thalamic aphasias resemble transcortical sensory aphasia.

Although seizures or transient vascular insufficiency can cause brief language disturbances, the development of a selective disturbance in language that lasts more than a few hours always reflects a structural and focal lesion. The most common causes are infarction and hemorrhage in the distribution of a major cortical artery branch. Less frequent causes are head trauma and space-occupying lesions.

Damasio H: Neuroimaging contributions to the understanding of aphasia. *In* Boller F, Grafman J (eds.): Handbook of Neuropsychology, Vol. 2. Amsterdam, Elsevier, 1989, pp. 3–46. *A description of different aphasia types and their localization.*

Damasio AR: Time-locked multiregional retroactivation: A systems level proposal for the neural substrates of recall and recognition. Cognition 33:25–62, 1989. *A testable and nontraditional model of neural systems underlying memory in humans.*

Damasio AR, Tranel D, Damasio H: Amnesia caused by herpes simplex encephalitis, infarctions in basal forebrain, Alzheimer's disease, and anoxia. *In* Squire L (ed.): Handbook of Neuropsychology, Vol. 3. Amsterdam, Elsevier, 1989, pp. 149–166. *A review of the profiles and anatomic correlates of the amnesias.*

Damasio AR, Tranel D, Damasio H: Face agnosia and the neural substrates of memory. Annu Rev Neurosci 13:89–109, 1990. *A discussion of the cognitive and neuropsychological aspects of this intriguing phenomenon, with information applicable to the understanding of memory.*

Dudai Y: The neurobiology of memory: Concepts, findings, trends. Oxford, Oxford University Press, 1989. *A comprehensive review of the neuroscience of memory.*

Geschwind N: Disconnection syndromes in animals and man. Brain 88:237, 585, 1965. *A seminal discussion on the anatomic basis of memory.*

Ojemann GA, Creutzfeldt OD: Language in humans and animals: Contribution of brain stimulation and recording. *In* Plum F, Mountcastle VB, et al. (eds.): Handbook of Physiology, Section 1: The nervous system. Vol. V, Higher functions of the brain, Part 2. Bethesda, MD, American Physiological Society, 1987, pp. 675–699. *Electrical stimulation and recording from the cerebral cortex provide clues to the neural basis of language.*

Raichle ME: Exploring the mind with dynamic imaging. Semin Neurosci 2:307–315, 1990. *A review of recent findings on language based on PET research.*

Scoville WB, Milner B: Loss of recent memory after bilateral hippocampal lesions. J Neurol Neurosurg Psychiatry 20:11, 1957. *Removal of the uncus and underlying amygdaloid complex resulted in little behavioral change. When the hippocampus was removed bilaterally, memory loss ensued.*

Victor M, Adams RD, Collins GH: The Wernicke-Korsakoff Syndrome and Related Neurologic Disorders Due to Alcoholism and Malnutrition, 2nd ed. Philadelphia, F. A. Davis Company, 1989. *The classic monograph on the subject provides evidence for the role of the diencephalon in memory.*

450 Alzheimer's Disease and Related Dementias

Antonio R. Damasio

Introduction

The term *dementia* describes a pervasive decline in a number of crucial functions resulting in the loss of personal and social independence in a previously competent individual. Although a defect in memory is often the core impairment in dementia, the term applies only to patients who have additional impairments in intellect as reflected by defective problem-solving, decision-making, and judgment. Those impairments are usually accompanied by disturbances in language and spatial orientation. Isolated defects in memory (amnesia) or in language (aphasia) do not qualify for the diagnosis of dementia even when their severity curtails normal behavior. The term *dementia* also does not apply to mentally retarded individuals who have never become intellectually competent (the term *amentia* may be used instead) and should not be applied to disturbances of attention, regardless of how profound they may be, for which the terms *confusional state* or *delirium* should be reserved.

From a physiopathologic standpoint, dementia occurs when several of the cerebral systems that support learning, memory, decision-making, and language are rendered dysfunctional by *any* neurologic disease process. Dementia can be a stable state when the disease is self-limited (such as may follow brain damage from cardiac arrest or result from multiple cerebral lesions following head trauma). In most instances, however, the dementia develops insidiously, as a result of diseases such as Alzheimer's or communicating hydrocephalus. Although the term *dementia* is equally appropriate for either stable or evolving mental decline, in practice dementia generally denotes a progressive condition of gradual and often slow course.

Table 450–1 lists the most frequent causes of progressive dementia. Dementia has never been a rare occurrence but of late its frequency has been rising steeply. In part, this may reflect public and physician awareness of the condition, but far more important is the remarkable rise of longevity in the indus-

TABLE 450–1. THE MOST FREQUENT CAUSES OF PROGRESSIVE DEMENTIA

Alzheimer's disease
Other degenerative diseases, e.g., Pick's, Parkinson's, Huntington's; progressive supranuclear palsy
Multiple cerebral infarcts
Chronic drug use
Depression
Intracranial mass lesions
Communicating hydrocephalus
Endocrine and metabolic disorders
CNS infections, e.g., HIV opportunistic, syphilis, Creutzfeldt-Jakob disease

trialized world. Progress in medicine and the environment over the past four decades has extended life expectancy by about 15 years, dramatically increasing the incidence of late-life neurologic diseases, with degenerative diseases and especially Alzheimer's disease topping the list. Some recent studies have claimed that as many as 50 per cent of individuals over the age of 80 develop Alzheimer's disease. Even assuming some exaggeration in those predictions, the impact of this disease in medicine and society cannot be overemphasized. Furthermore, all dementia is not Alzheimer's dementia: Many patients so affected have conditions that are partially or completely reversible (Table 450–2). The diagnosis of dementia must be rigorously made, followed by an attempt to uncover its probable etiology.

Diagnosing Dementia

The imperative first step lies in establishing that there is indeed a decline in cognitive and behavioral capacities indicative of underlying neurologic disease. Many normal older individuals inappropriately sense that their mental abilities are diminishing. It is equally important to reassure such persons about the benign nature of their complaints as to make a diagnosis of dementia in those who suffer it. Forgetfulness, especially of proper names, is common at any age and is accentuated by anxiety, fatigue, and depression in late life. Benign forgetting, however, is accompanied neither by amnesia for recent social and personal events nor by impaired judgment and decision-making (although depression may severely impair decision-making and planning). A probing history and interview, together with a normal neurologic examination, can rapidly exclude the possibility of dementia. In addition, brief tests such as the Minimental Status Examination or the Iowa Battery for the Detection of Mental Decline offer simple measures of psychological ability that can be used to reassure the concerned patient (Table 450–3 and references).

If the brief examinations and detection tests suggest that dementia exists, the next step is to establish a premorbid baseline, something that the patient may be unable to provide and may depend on testimony from a reliable relative or escort. What is the patient's education and cultural background? What have been his or her professional and social achievements? Whenever possible, specific information should be sought about years of education, degrees achieved, professional positions, and the judgment of colleagues, friends, and relatives.

The examination should evaluate the following: (1) orientation, (2) attention, (3) social appropriateness, (4) affect, (5) memory, and (6) language. Most of these emerge almost automatically as the evaluation proceeds. What is the patient's attitude toward the examiner? Is he or she cooperative? Socially appropriate? Attentive and able to communicate verbally? Oriented to time and place? Can the patient relate recent public and personal

TABLE 450–2. TREATABLE CAUSES OF DEMENTIA

Inappropriate or excessive use of medications or alcohol
Resectable intracranial tumors
Subdural hematomas
Depression
Communicating hydrocephalus
Endocrine and metabolic disorders, e.g., hypothyroidism, vitamin B_{12} deficiency
CNS infections

TABLE 450–3. OUTLINE OF MINIMENTAL STATUS EXAMINATION*

Test	Score
What is the year, season, date, day, month?	5
Where are you: state, county, town, place, floor?	5
Name three objects: State slowly and have patient repeat (repeat until patient learns all three)	3
Do reverse serial 7's (five steps) or spell "WORLD" backwards	5
Ask for the three unrelated objects above	3
Name from inspection a pencil, a watch	2
Have patient repeat "No if's, and's, or but's"	1
Follow a three-stage command (1 pt each) ("Take a paper in your hand, fold it, and put it on the floor.")	3
Read and obey, "Close your eyes."	1
Write a simple sentence	1
Copy intersecting pentagons	1

*Reprinted by permission from Folstein MF, Folstein SE, McHugh PR: Minimental state. A practical method for grading the cognitive state for the clinician. J Psychiatr Res 12:189, 1975. The authors found that out of a possible total score of 30, mean score for dementia was 9.7, depression with cognitive impairment was 19.0, and uncomplicated affective depression was 27.6.

events (the accuracy of the latter corroborated by an escort)? Patients with early Alzheimer's disease tend to be cooperative, socially appropriate, and attentive, but their recent memory clearly shows a decline. Patients with dementia due to brain tumors, CNS infections, or hydrocephalus are more often distractible, less appropriate, and careless of appearances.

Some traditional mental status tests such as the recall of three unrelated words at 5 minutes, the reverse spelling of WORLD, or the backwards subtraction of serial 7's, can give helpful hints but are not reliable. Many nondemented patients with aphasia, amnesia, parietal lobe dysfunction, or mere emotional distraction can fail such tests; conversely some patients with early dementia can pass them. The popular Minimental Status Examination fares better (Table 450–3).

A formal neuropsychological evaluation conducted by a trained neuropsychologist offers the most reliable means to diagnose the presence and severity of dementia. Such evaluations quantify intellectual and problem-solving ability, memory, speech and language, perception, attention and concentration, and personality. Many of the standardized tests, such as the Wechsler Adult Intelligence Scale—Revised, the Wechsler Memory Scale—Revised, and the Benton Visual Retention Test, permit a level of diagnostic precision that cannot be approximated by bedside evaluations or screening batteries. Formal neuropsychological examination is especially useful in distinguishing dementia from depression.

Differential Diagnosis

There are more than 50 possible causes of dementia, but many are rare and the most frequent, Alzheimer's disease, has a fairly distinctive profile. Nonetheless, only histologic analysis of brain tissue at autopsy offers an absolute confirmation of Alzheimer's disease, so that clinical diagnosis remains one of exclusion. Because some of the less frequent causes of dementia can be treated and occasionally may mimic Alzheimer's disease, it is important to rule them in or out. The distinction depends largely on the results of a small group of critical tests (Table 450–4).

ALZHEIMER'S DISEASE

PATHOGENESIS AND MANIFESTATIONS. Alzheimer's disease is caused by a progressive and selective degeneration of neuron populations in the entorhinal cortex, the hippocampus, the high-order association cortices of the temporal, frontal, and parietal regions, and some subcortical nuclei in the basal forebrain (septal nuclei and nucleus basalis) and brain stem (locus coeruleus). The neuronal damage and the attending loss of synaptic density disable several neuronal networks essential to learning and retrieval of memories. By itself, the cortical component of the damage would explain the prominent memory defects of Alzheimer patients. In addition, however, damage to cholinergic neurons in the basal forebrain results in a loss of delivery of acetylcholine to the cerebral cortex, whereas damage to the brain

stem's locus coeruleus precludes the delivery of norepinephrine to the cerebral cortex. Those neurochemical defects are likely to worsen, if not independently explain, many of the behavioral changes seen in Alzheimer patients. At autopsy, the brains of Alzheimer patients are atrophied, especially in the regions where most neurons die. Characteristically, the motor and primary sensory cortices remain unaffected, as do the basal ganglia and cerebellum. Histologically, the diseased neurons show up as containing cytoplasmic neurofibrillary tangles composed of paired helical filaments visible with stains such as Congo red and thioflavin S. The most prominent anatomic change, however, consists of prominent amyloid plaques containing degenerated neuronal fragments, all surrounding a small, dense core of amyloid material. The neuropathologic diagnosis of Alzheimer's disease, however, depends not only on the presence of neurofibrillary tangles and neuritic plaques but also on their anatomic distribution and quantity. Neurofibrillary tangles are present in other diseases, including the dementia that follows repeated boxing injuries. Indeed, neuritic plaques are present in the brains of normal aged persons, only the number of abnormalities being different from the Alzheimer brain. Such findings lead some investigators to believe that Alzheimer's dementia may represent an accelerated form of brain aging rather than a conventional disease.

In about 25 per cent of cases of Alzheimer's disease, the history reveals a relative affected by the disease, and in some rare families the disease can start early (fifth or sixth decade) and affect the offspring in an autosomal dominant pattern. Also, patients with trisomy 21 (Down syndrome) invariably develop the neuropathologic changes of Alzheimer's disease in their third or fourth decades. These findings have stimulated a major effort to identify a chromosomal defect responsible for the condition, but to date no such linkage has been found. The search for toxins, infectious agents, and nutritional or environmental factors has been equally disappointing.

Clinically, Alzheimer's disease is characterized by a relentless impairment of memory and decision-making that generally begins insidiously and can progress for a decade or longer. Most Alzheimer's disease starts after age 60 and the incidence increases with each decade thereafter. Analyses show a greater incidence in women, some of which may reflect their increased longevity compared to men. In most patients the gradual impairment of memory dominates the early clinical picture. They fail to learn new recent events, both public and personal. A defect in recognition of previously known familiar places or situations is often an inaugural sign. As time passes, the impairments worsen. Despite preserving their speech, their motor performances, and their social graces, patients are not able to retain employment and sooner or later become unable to cope with the activities of daily living. A loss of affective resonance is common, which relatives may describe as shallowness or lack of interest. Unwise decisions regarding property or investments are often made during these early stages of the disease, especially if a protective family member is not available to intervene. Signs of poor judgment and a deterioration of social relationships commonly ensue.

Sometimes Alzheimer's disease takes other forms of onset (Table 450–5). Some patients become suspicious of friends, employers, or spouse, developing paranoid ideas, especially during the evening and night hours. They may awaken in the middle of the night disoriented to place and time and behaving in acute psychotic fashion. In another variant, language may be especially compromised. In those instances memory for words

TABLE 450–4. USEFUL TESTS IN THE EVALUATION OF DEMENTIA

Brain computed tomography or magnetic resonance imaging
Neuropsychological evaluation
Complete blood count and erythrocyte sedimentation rate, serologic test for syphilis
Metabolic screen (SMA 12–16)
Serum thyroxine, vitamin B$_{12}$ level
Chest radiograph
Cerebrospinal fluid analysis: cells, protein
Electroencephalography

TABLE 450–5. VARIETIES OF ALZHEIMER'S DISEASE ONSET

Amnesic form	Gradual decline for episodic learning and deficient episodic recall.
Psychiatric form	Delusional ideation, especially severe during the night, dominates the presentation.
Aphasic form	A severe anomia of gradual onset precedes other aspects of mental decline by at least 2 years.

suffers the most, with patients displaying a remarkable anomia that precludes naming of specific objects and people. Finally, the disease occasionally begins by compromising visual attention. Patients report an inability to perceive simultaneously more than one object in the visual field and become unable to orient themselves along previously familiar routes. Whatever the variants, however, a pervasive impairment of memory eventually sets in. In striking contrast to the intellectual decay, motor performance (strength, coordination) remains preserved in most cases during the first years of the disease. Some patients with Alzheimer's disease can even learn *new* motor skills despite their otherwise ravaged ability to retain new factual information. (Nevertheless, rare exceptions exist. A patient has recently been described with left hemiplegia and dementia whose autopsy revealed neuropathologic changes entirely characteristic of Alzheimer's disease.)

Despite the fact that Alzheimer's disease is the most common cause of dementia and that rich neurochemical and neuropathologic characterizations are now available for the disease, no reliable antemortem marker exists for the diagnosis. Accordingly, diagnosis must be formulated in terms of probability, based on the identification of a typical profile and the exclusion of other potentially similar conditions.

A detailed diagnostic codification for Alzheimer's disease is listed in the references. In order to diagnose probable Alzheimer's disease, one must (1) document the dementia by neuropsychological tests revealing scores significantly below the range commensurate with the patient's age and educational level; (2) verify that impairment of memory is a critical component; and (3) verify that the onset of dementia was not sudden or rapidly progressive. A diagnosis of Alzheimer's disease should not be entertained if early in the presentation (1) there are motor signs such as hemiparesis or gait disorder (but see exception above); (2) there is loss of somatic sensation; (3) there is a visual field defect; and (4) seizures have occurred. The EEG should be normal early in the course of the disease, although as the disease progresses it may reveal a nonspecific pattern of slowing. The cerebrospinal fluid should also be normal, containing no cells and either a normal or mildly elevated protein level. CT or MR may be normal early in the course or reveal enlargement of sulci. The enlargement can become quite pronounced in late stages of the disease but is generally more symmetric and severe than in Pick's disease (see below). Positron emission tomography has revealed a consistent pattern of diminished metabolic activity in the temporoparietal regions.

MANAGEMENT. There is no cure for Alzheimer's disease, and no drug tried so far can alter the progress of the disease.

Tacrine (tetrahydroaminoacridine) exerts a modest central cholinesterase inhibition effect and has been found to produce limited improvement in selective mental status tests in patients with Alzheimer's disease. Thus far, at least, beneficial effects have been demonstrated for activities of daily living. Liver toxicity is a risk and must be guarded against.

There are numerous nonpharmacologic ways in which caregivers can ameliorate the manifestations or consequences of Alzheimer's disease and reduce the heavy burdens of caretaking that fall on families. During early stages of the disease, when patients can remain at home, strategically placed cue cards around the house can help patients orient themselves and carry on tasks relating to their self-care. Variations of such a strategy also can help patients cope with nondemanding social activities. An emphasis on tasks that require motor skills (music playing, dancing, card playing, typing, drawing) can help to make the days more pleasurable to the patient and less frustrating to caretakers.

Appropriate drugs help to cope with bouts of anxiety, depression, or paranoid ideation that some patients show. Drugs also can be used to regulate the sleep cycle and avoid nighttime waking and "sundowning." Reduction of environmental stresses and random sensory stimuli can yield surprisingly good results in this regard. Eventually a decision may be needed regarding nursing home placement and the securing of appropriate medical care in such a setting. The Alzheimer's Disease and Related Disorders Association has chapters in every state which can guide physicians and patients to services dedicated to these patients. The references also contain a valuable guide to management. A comprehensive discussion of the diagnosis and prognosis of the disease, as well as of the limited knowledge currently available about it, probably constitutes the greatest help a physician can render to relatives.

DISTINGUISHING ALZHEIMER'S DISEASE FROM OTHER DEMENTIAS

Treatable Dementias

INAPPROPRIATE OR EXCESSIVE USE OF MEDICATIONS. This is perhaps the most frequent and most amenable to correction. Naturally, it can coexist with Alzheimer's disease, but it is important to determine that it is not the cause of dementia when the diagnosis of Alzheimer's disease is entertained in a patient who is taking target drugs. Cough suppressants, barbiturates, benzodiazepines, tricyclic antidepressants, monoamine oxidase inhibitors, anticholinergics, and digitalis are the common offenders. The combination of some of these drugs with alcohol in an elderly and frail individual can easily mimic Alzheimer's disease.

DEPRESSION. This should always be considered in the differential diagnosis because it can present as mental decline, in which case it is known as masked depression or pseudodementia. As noted, expert psychological testing is the key to the diagnosis. A number of neuropsychological tests are capable of discriminating depression from Alzheimer's disease with high specificity. The Benton Visual Retention Test, for example, is passed by nearly all patients who are eventually diagnosed as having pseudodementia, whereas patients who are eventually confirmed to have Alzheimer-type dementia fail or perform at the borderline level. Antidepressant medication, psychotherapy, and, if needed, electroconvulsive therapy can effectively solve the problem.

BRAIN TUMORS AND SUBDURAL HEMATOMAS. Tumors that involve structures of the limbic system, e.g., meningiomas that compress frontal lobe structures or gliomas that infiltrate the white matter of frontal and temporal cortices, often present as dementia. Distractibility, bradykinesia, and apathy dominate the clinical picture and a CT or MR scan easily confirms the suspicion. In most instances, meningiomas can be resected with success. The elderly are prone to develop subdural hematomas after relatively minor, and thus easily forgettable, head injuries. Such hematomas, especially when bilateral, can lead to dementia, often with little in the way of a telltale history. CT or MRI is diagnostic.

COMMUNICATING HYDROCEPHALUS. Communicating hydrocephalus of the so-called normal-pressure variety is another late-life condition easily detected by brain imaging. The lateral ventricles and the third ventricle are enlarged, the sulci may be effaced, and the sampling of cerebrospinal fluid pressure in a routine lumbar puncture may fail to reveal an elevation because the pressure waves that pound the ventricular walls are intermittent. Not uncommonly the past history reveals a significant neurologic antecedent such as bacterial meningitis, subarachnoid hemorrhage, or severe head injury. The dementia is probably due to pervasive dysfunction in white matter pathways surrounding the ventricles. The clinical picture is dominated by impaired attention and flatness of emotional expression and always includes a gait disorder and urinary incontinence, neither of which affects early Alzheimer's patients. The gait disorder consists of a loss of the automatic motor patterns that are normally engaged in walking (apraxia) combined with a broad-based ataxia. An intraventricular shunt may reverse the symptoms in selected patients.

OTHER CAUSES. Endocrine and metabolic disorders, especially hypothyroidism and vitamin B_{12} deficiency, also cause dementia. They are easily detectable and largely correctable. Syphilis and fungal infections can cause reversible dementias. In the appropriate setting syphilis is an especially important diagnostic consideration. Many other dementias exist that can be reversed upon correcting the conditions to which they are secondary. Chronic liver disease, chronic lung disease, and uremia are obvious examples.

Nontreatable Forms of Dementia

PICK'S DISEASE. In spite of its low frequency, the number of Pick's disease cases appears to be rising. This is a degenerative condition characterized by a markedly asymmetric loss of neurons in the frontal and anterior temporal regions. In some cases, the involvement is virtually unilateral and may be largely confined to either the temporal or frontal lobe (hence the term *lobar atrophy*). An intriguing preponderance for involvement of the left hemisphere has been noted. Histologic analysis reveals loss of cortical neurons in the atrophied areas. Two signs that assist with the microscopic diagnosis are the presence of Pick's neurons (pale, swollen neurons that fail to take conventional stains and are thus achromatic) and Pick's bodies (a silver-staining cytoplasmic inclusion easily distinguishable from a neurofibrillary tangle). Pick's neurons are more commonly found in the frontal region, whereas Pick's bodies are virtually found only in the temporal region. Neurofibrillary tangles and neuritic plaques are not a histologic feature of the disease.

Pick's disease has two prevalent profiles. Both usually begin in the sixth or seventh decade and affect women more frequently than men. In one profile, the patient has a gradual mental decline not unlike that seen in Alzheimer's disease but in which impairments of judgment, decision-making, and affect predominate over the recent memory defect. Social appropriateness deteriorates more rapidly than learning and memory. Not uncommonly, these patients make unwise business decisions and if they live alone they may care little about their appearance. Eventually, memory impairment sets in. This profile correlates with preponderant involvement of the frontal lobe. In the other prevalent profile, patients begin by complaining of a problem with name finding. Few specific names for objects or people can be produced, although speech articulation, syntactic processing, memory, and judgment may be intact. In most instances, within 2 to 5 years, memory and judgment begin to decline. The anatomic correlate is involvement of the *left* temporal lobe. Incidentally, Pick's original description was of the latter profile, although the former has become the textbook standard.

The left temporal form of Pick's brings into the discussion an elusive entity known as *progressive aphasia without dementia*. The pattern observed in some of the patients resembles Pick's disease, but the language disorder has remained the most prominent or sole symptom. It is possible that these cases are examples of Pick's disease in which involvement beyond the left temporal cortices is minimal or delayed. Other evidence suggests that the condition reflects either a variant of Alzheimer's disease or a nonspecific spongiform degeneration. The diagnosis of Pick's disease in the early stages is hazardous, although after about 2 years of evolution the clinical profile becomes suggestive. By then, state-of-the-art CT or MR should provide evidence of asymmetric lobar atrophy.

PARKINSON'S DISEASE. Dementia complicates a mounting number of cases of idiopathic parkinsonism. From a clinical standpoint it is important to ensure that the mental decline is not due to the effects of anticholinergic medication or to the multifarious cognitive changes induced by levodopa. Histologic study of brain tissue of demented patients with Parkinson's disease has shown in many but not all instances abundant neurofibrillary tangles and neuritic plaques identical to those encountered in Alzheimer's disease.

HUNTINGTON'S DISEASE. Patients with Huntington's disease are prone to a host of cognitive and behavioral changes (see Ch. 461). Depression and psychotic states are part of the clinical picture. They may precede chorea and dystonia and persist into the later stages, producing a high suicide rate. Measurable mental decline is often found as the disease progresses. Distractibility and slowness of cognitive processing hallmark the presentation.

The dementia is best explained by extensive cortical dysfunction secondary to neuron loss in the basal ganglia, especially in the caudate.

MULTIPLE VASCULAR LESIONS. A variety of conditions resulting in multiple strokes, large and small, can cause dementia. The following should be considered:

1. Multiple small infarcts (multiple infarct dementia), occurring at different points in the history and involving cortical or subcortical gray matter, especially in the territories of middle cerebral and anterior cerebral arteries. The history and physical examination of such patients invariably reveal systemic hypertension, diabetes, signs of widespread vascular disease, or a combination of the above. The age range is similar to that during which degenerative diseases strike, but a careful history and neurologic examination disclose distinctive clues. For instance, the development of the dementia is stepwise, punctuated by datable events. The patient, family, or relatives can describe specific events during which disturbances of speech, orientation, or motor impairment developed, often followed by some recovery. In short, the mental decline is cumulative but not really gradual. Naturally, if the information source does not have proper insight, or if the events occurred a long time before, there is the risk of smoothing out the history profile and misleading the examiner. Helpful clues under such circumstances are the finding of focal motor defects, especially weakness, ataxia, or urinary incontinence. Alzheimer's disease shows none of these abnormalities during its early clinical course.

2. Multiple demyelinating lesions occurring in the surround of a blood vessel are revealed by MRI in the subcortical white matter. This puzzling condition, sometimes called Binswanger's disease or subcortical arteriosclerotic encephalopathy, can have a dementia profile indistinguishable from that of Alzheimer's disease. Most affected patients are hypertensive, however, although the condition has been described in normotensive individuals. Both CT and MRI reveal enlargement of the lateral ventricles disproportionate to the enlargement of the cortical sulci. MRI also reveals an abundance of periventricular lucencies, which show up as white on T2-weighted images. It should be noted that similar lucencies can be seen in normal older individuals but generally without ventricular enlargement of the same magnitude.

3. Multiple infarcts caused by vasculitis such as congophilic angiopathy, isolated angiitis of the central nervous system, and systemic lupus erythematosus. These are all rare conditions that present in a far more severe and dramatic way than degenerative diseases, multiple infarct dementia, or Binswanger's disease. Such patients usually become acutely ill and are more likely to be admitted to an inpatient service than to remain ambulatory patients. The severity of the condition usually is paralleled by a relatively rapid course compared to the longer time scale of most of the other dementias discussed above. Other clues help the diagnosis. For instance, congophilic angiopathy causes medium to large *hemorrhagic* infarctions. Congophilic angiopathy often coexists with Alzheimer's disease for reasons that are not clear. Lupus is rare in the elderly, and the signs of systemic involvement are diagnostic. Isolated angiitis is more elusive, but the severity and rapidity of the course help the diagnosis.

CENTRAL NERVOUS SYSTEM INFECTIONS. Until recently, the most frequent form of nontreatable infectious dementia has been the transmissible form of Creutzfeldt-Jakob disease, a spongiform encephalopathy (see Ch. 478.6). This rapidly evolving dementia is hallmarked by defects in attention, visual perception, and motor coordination. Once the disease is established, myoclonus is a consistent sign and can be easily evoked by a sudden unexpected noise (startle myoclonus). Myoclonus occurs, albeit infrequently, in advanced stages of Alzheimer's disease but is otherwise uncommon. Triphasic waves in the EEG support the diagnosis. The cerebrospinal fluid is normal. Over the past decade, immune suppression in the setting of HIV infection has become the most common infectious cause of dementia. In some cases the dementia is due to direct HIV involvement of the cerebral parenchyma; in others it is caused by opportunistic infections.

Cummings JL, Benson DF: Dementia: A Clinical Approach. Boston, Butterworths, 1983. *A monograph that discusses the differential diagnosis of the dementias.*

Eagger SA, Levy R, Sahakian BJ: Tacrine in Alzheimer's disease. Lancet 337:989–992, 1991.

Eslinger P, Damasio AR, Benton A, Van Allen M: Neuropsychological detection of abnormal mental decline in older persons. JAMA 253:670–674, 1985. *A brief neuropsychological test for the screening of early dementia.*

Folstein MF, Folstein SE, McHugh PR: Minimental state. A practical method for grading the cognitive state for the clinician. J Psychiatr Res 12:189, 1975. *The authors found that out of a possible total score of 30, mean score for dementia was 9.7, depression with cognitive impairment was 19.0, and uncomplicated affective depression was 27.6.*

Katzman R, Terry R: The Neurology of Aging. Philadelphia, F. A. Davis, 1983. *A discussion on aspects of the many needs of the aging patient, including conditions that must be differentiated from dementia.*

Mace NL, Rabin PV: The 36-hour Day. A Family Guide to Caring for Persons with Alzheimer's Disease, Related Dementing Illnesses, and Memory Loss in Later Life. Baltimore, Johns Hopkins University Press, 1981. *An invaluable book for families and friends of the affected.*

McKhann G, Drachman D, Folstein M, et al.: Clinical diagnosis of Alzheimer's disease. Report of the NINCDS-ADRDA Work Group under the auspices of Department of Health and Human Services Task Force on Alzheimer's disease. Neurology 34:939–944, 1984. *A codification of criteria for the diagnosis of Alzheimer's disease.*

Van Hoesen GW, Damasio AR: Neural correlates of cognitive impairment in Alzheimer's disease. *In* Plum F (ed.): Handbook of Physiology: Higher Functions of the Nervous System. Bethesda, MD, American Physiological Society, 1987, pp. 871–898. *A review of the neuropsychological and neurobiologic characteristics of the disease.*

451 Psychiatric Disorders in Medical Practice

Gary J. Tucker

Perhaps of most concern to the nonpsychiatric physician is the process of psychiatric diagnosis. When does the wide range of human behavior become a pathologic process needing intervention and when is it a variation of normal response to life events? Lacking clear laboratory tests, precise anatomic dysfunctions, or specific pathologic findings, the diagnostic process in psychiatry has followed traditional medical practice for such conditions, i.e., to delineate syndromes and to categorize patterns of symptomatology. However, these syndromes and categories until recently have been broad, often regional, and idiosyncratic. A massive revision of diagnostic practice in psychiatry occurred in 1980 with the publication by the American Psychiatric Association of the third edition of the *Diagnostic and Statistical Manual of Mental Disorders (DSM III)*, now revised. The key components of this nomenclature represent diagnostic criteria that are descriptive and data based, and they require that the clinician view psychiatric disorders from a number of different aspects or axes. The specific symptoms not only include those that must be present but also identify explicit symptoms that must be excluded before a diagnosis can be made. For example, to make the diagnosis of "schizophrenia," one must exclude depressive illness. The clinician must also stipulate the role of biologic, characterologic, and sociologic factors that affect the illness in terms of five axes. Axis I is the specific syndrome, such as schizophrenia, affective disorder, etc. Axis II includes specific personality disorders such as antisocial, dependent, and specific developmental disorders, language disorders, reading disorders, etc. Axis III consists of contributing physical disorders and medical conditions. Axis IV consists of psychosocial stressors. Axis V designates the highest level of adaptive functioning the patient manifested in the past year. All of these axes add to the diagnostic description of the patient and are important in understanding and treating the specific condition. For example, a 50-year-old lawyer with a major depression may be described as follows: Axis I—major depression; Axis II—obsessive personality; Axis III—diabetes, hypertension; Axis IV—marital discord; Axis V—good social and work functioning.

At various times most people experience anxiety, depression, sleep disturbance, and/or somatic preoccupation. In most cases such symptoms are transient, and the precipitants to such symptoms are often evident—an upcoming examination, a new job, marriage, divorce, work or family problems. In these instances the physician has no difficulty in reassuring the patient that the symptoms are transient and situational. However, when these symptoms persist and/or when they occur in situations that have no clear precipitants, they should become of concern to the physician. In order to classify someone as having a psychiatric illness, one must consider the following factors: (1) Do the signs and symptoms fit a psychiatric diagnosis? For example, when patients say they are sad or depressed, do they meet the diagnostic criteria for a diagnosis of depression or dysthymic disorder (see Tables 451–7 and 451–9)? (2) Is there a family history of similar symptoms? Many psychiatric illnesses tend to have a genetic or familial basis. (3) Is the longitudinal pattern of the symptoms consistent with the natural history of a psychiatric disorder? Emotional symptoms associated with specific situations are usually classified as reactions to the situation (see grief reactions); they do not usually become psychiatric disorders. (4) Are the symptoms incapacitating? All persons have enduring patterns of relating, perceiving, and reacting to others. These constitute various components of a person's personality and may take the form of such patterns as obsessive, passive, or antisocial personality traits. When such characteristics interfere with the individual's ability to function, however, the condition is regarded as a personality disorder, named for the predominant personality characteristic. (5) Do delusions and hallucinations exist? Delusions and hallucinations in the absence of other medical causes always indicate major psychiatric illness. Although illusory phenomena can often occur at times of tiredness, intoxication, fever, etc., their occurrence in clear states of consciousness should alert one to the presence of major psychiatric illness.

The proper delineation of psychiatric disorders from normal emotional reactions rests on a careful history, a mental status evaluation, and a knowledge of psychiatric syndromes. If the findings of the history and mental status evaluation do not fit into any of the known psychiatric syndromes, the physician should reserve judgment and follow the patient. In many cases, the symptoms neither persist nor return and all can be reassured. If the symptoms continue, one may recognize a clear psychiatric syndrome. With all persistent emotional and behavioral symptoms, however, the physician must first rule out systemic medical disorders.

DIFFERENTIATING PSYCHIATRIC DISORDERS FROM MEDICAL DISORDERS

While it has always been evident that the central nervous system mediates behavior, there has been a reluctance to look at major psychiatric illnesses as disorders of the central nervous system. However, as biologic studies of psychiatric patients progress and specific psychopharmacologic agents are found to affect behavior, it becomes increasingly evident that psychiatric disorders are disorders of central nervous system functioning. This awareness includes recognition that the central nervous system has a limited number of ways of responding to stress. For example, hallucinations can arise from psychological causes, from toxins in the blood, from head trauma, from seizure disorders, and from fever. With such potentially diverse etiologies, it is imperative that the physician seek clues to differentiate the causes of the behavior change (Table 451–1).

Many clues in the history can suggest something other than an intrinsic psychiatric illness as a cause of abnormal behavior. Most patients with psychiatric illnesses have had psychiatric symptoms or reveal seeds of the current disturbance in their histories. When a patient presents with a good premorbid social history, a good work history, a warm and supportive family, and well-preserved personality, one should seek nonpsychiatric factors to

TABLE 451–1. CLUES TO NONPSYCHIATRIC DISORDERS AFFECTING BEHAVIOR

1. The signs and symptoms do not fit into an established psychiatric diagnostic category.
2. There is no prior psychiatric history or symptoms.
3. The patient demonstrates an abrupt change in behavior or personality.
4. Signs and symptoms fluctuate rapidly.
5. The condition does not respond to treatment.

explain the behavior change. Many physicians tend erroneously to view behavior changes only in a psychological framework. Abrupt changes in behavior, personality, mood, or ability to function should be evaluated for possible organic causes. As indicated, most decompensating patients with psychiatric illness describe similar, albeit less severe, symptoms in the past. To give an example: A 60-year-old man who has been formal and proper his entire life but abruptly becomes bawdy and flirtatious is probably not experiencing the onset of a major psychiatric illness but rather is showing personality changes associated with a new disturbance of the central nervous system, such as brain tumor, vascular disease, endocrine abnormality, or drug reaction. Rapid fluctuations in mental status also suggest a new disturbance rather than a psychiatric disorder. Patients with psychiatric disease occasionally are delusional and hallucinating in the morning but free of these symptoms the same evening (or vice versa). By contrast, the resolution of the delusions and hallucinations associated with schizophrenia typically requires days to weeks. Similarly, motor behavior does not change rapidly in psychiatric illness. Patients with encephalopathies, by contrast, often have a "motor drivenness" with episodic desires to move about, to get up and walk. This restlessness is particularly prominent in delirious states. Lastly, and perhaps most subtly, when a patient does not respond to the usual interventions one should suspect the possibility of an incorrect diagnosis. For example, when a patient with hallucinations and delusions has been treated unsuccessfully with adequate doses of neuroleptic medications for an appropriate period of time with no change in the symptoms, one should consider the possibility of a disorder other than schizophrenia. These simple guidelines often alert the clinician to multiple diagnostic possibilities.

Goodwin D, Guze S: Psychiatric Diagnosis, 4th ed. New York, Oxford University Press, 1989. *An excellent overall text on descriptive psychiatry and the basis for diagnostic groupings.*

Lishman W: Organic Psychiatry, 2nd ed. Oxford, Blackwell, 1987. *A comprehensive description of neurologic and medical complications of behavioral disorders.*

Pincus J, Tucker G: Behavioral Neurology, 3rd ed. New York, Oxford University Press, 1985. *This monograph discusses differential diagnosis and behavioral aspects of neurologic disease as well as neurologic aspects of psychiatric disorders.*

Schiffer RB, Klein RF, Sider RC: The Medical Evaluation of Psychiatric Patients, New York, Plenum Press, 1989. *A detailed explication of the comorbidity of medical illnesses and behavioral symptoms.*

Spitzer RL (ed.): Diagnostic and Statistical Manual of Mental Disorders, 3rd ed., rev. Washington, D.C., American Psychiatric Association, 1987. *A useful, widely accepted outline of diagnostic features of the gamut of psychiatric disorders.*

SCHIZOPHRENIC DISORDERS

Schizophrenia and some forms of affective disorders comprise the major psychotic illnesses. (Psychosis is defined as the presence of hallucinations and/or delusions.) Kraepelin, a noted German psychiatrist, observed that among hospitalized psychotic patients there were two longitudinal patterns. The first seemed to be characterized by exacerbations and remissions in mood and cognitive functioning which he labeled "manic-depressive illness," and the second was characterized by a chronic psychotic course with its onset in youth and deteriorating social function, which he labeled "dementia praecox" (a dementing illness of young people). In 1911 Eugene Bleuler, a Swiss psychiatrist, changed the name of dementia praecox to "schizophrenia." He described the central features of schizophrenia as a psychotic process manifested by disturbed thinking, changes in the emotional responsiveness of the patient, and a preoccupation with their own inner life, or autism. By schizophrenia he did not mean a "split personality" but more a splitting of psychological functions. While some functions, such as the ability to communicate, were often impaired, others, such as memory and mathematical abilities, were sustained. In essence, this early concept remains a good definition of the schizophrenic process.

Schizophrenia most often has its onset in late adolescence. The course of the illness is usually marked by a decline in psychosocial functioning, with a tendency for the patient to become downwardly mobile in social class. The introduction of neuroleptics in 1954 brought about some improvement in the treatment of these patients, but the observations of Kraepelin of an ultimate deteriorating course still hold true. Current treatment aims toward shorter hospitalizations for schizophrenics with more vigorous attempts to retain the patient in a community setting. Physicians encounter two principal groups of schizophrenic patients, one with an acute florid psychotic illness and the other suffering chronic illness with less florid symptoms. The care of these two groups differs in that the acute management is simple, whereas the care and rehabilitation of the chronic patient can be extremely difficult. The nationally pursued process of "deinstitutionalization" has thrust this latter patient population into our everyday world.

DIAGNOSTIC CRITERIA AND CLINICAL SIGNS AND SYMPTOMS. Table 451–2 lists the clinical symptoms of schizophrenia. Note the emphasis on hallucinations and delusions. The ones cited are typical of schizophrenia, although similar hallucinations and delusions can occur in affective disorders and organic conditions; however, the course of these later illnesses is different. A study by Cloninger et al. (1985) demonstrates the importance of the presence of delusions and hallucinations in the diagnosis of schizophrenia. They found that the greater the number of delusions and hallucinations present, particularly persecutory delusions, delusions of control, firmly fixed mood incongruent delusions, and auditory hallucinations, the more likely was the person to progress to a chronic psychotic condition. Other prominent symptoms of schizophrenia are the presence of incoherence and the inability of the patient to communicate with others in a logical and goal-directed fashion. As an example of the speech of a schizophrenic, the patient may respond as follows when asked why he was brought to the hospital: "You are a Nazi; God sent me to save the world; I have a lovely apartment; your eyes are blue."

The stipulation that these criteria must last for a 6-month period (demonstrating a deterioration from a previous level of functioning) defines a more chronic population (Table 451–3). When the duration of symptoms is shorter than 6 months, it is inadvisable to use the diagnosis of schizophrenia. This allows the clinician to withhold judgment and encourages a search for other disorders. This is particularly important with the first episode of psychotic illness, in that it is difficult to differentiate an acute manic episode from an acute schizophrenic episode. Psychotic episodes due to toxic drug reactions, sleep deprivation, and medical causes invariably last less than 6 months (Table 451–4).

In the past many subtypes of schizophrenia have been described, but their predictive validity has been poor except for catatonia and paranoia. Catatonic symptoms include either markedly retarded motor behavior (often to the point of no voluntary movement, the patient retaining any posture into which he is passively placed) or markedly agitated motor behavior. The importance of a catatonic diagnosis, in either the retarded or the agitated form, has retained some validity in conferring a better

TABLE 451–2. SCHIZOPHRENIA*

A. Characterized by psychotic symptoms during the active phase of illness. One of the major symptom categories below must be present for at least 1 week (or less if symptoms respond to treatment):
 1. Two of the following:
   a. Delusions
   b. Prominent hallucinations (throughout the day for several days or several times a week for several weeks; each hallucinatory experience is not limited to a few brief moments)
   c. Incoherence of speech or marked loosening of verbal associations
   d. Catatonic behavior
   e. Flat or grossly inappropriate affect
 2. Bizarre delusions (i.e., involving a phenomenon that the individual's subculture would regard as totally implausible, e.g., thoughts being broadcast out loud, being controlled by a dead person)
 3. Prominent hallucinations of a voice keeping up a running commentary on the individual's behavior or thoughts, or two or more voices conversing with each other

B. During the course of the disturbance, a decrease in functioning in such areas as work, social relations, and self-care.

C. Major depressive or manic syndrome and medical conditions ruled out.

D. Continuous psychiatric symptoms for at least 6 months.

*Modified from American Psychiatric Association: Diagnostic and Statistical Manual of Mental Disorders, 3rd ed., rev. Washington, DC, APA, 1987. Used with permission.

1. Marked social isolation or withdrawal
2. Marked impairment in role functioning as wage-earner, student, or homemaker
3. Markedly peculiar behavior (e.g., collecting garbage, talking to self in public, hoarding food)
4. Marked impairment in personal hygiene and grooming
5. Blunted, flat, or inappropriate affect
6. Digressive, vague, overelaborate, or circumstantial speech; poverty of speech; or poverty of content of speech
7. Odd beliefs or magical thinking, e.g., superstitiousness, belief in clairvoyance, telepathy, "sixth sense," "others can feel my feelings," overvalued ideas, ideas of reference
8. Unusual perceptual experiences, e.g., recurrent illusions, sensing the presence of a force or person not actually present
9. Marked lack of initiative, interests, or energy

*Modified from American Psychiatric Association: Diagnostic and Statistical Manual of Mental Disorders, 3rd ed., rev. Washington, DC, APA, 1987. Used with permission.

prognosis, but there is also evidence that catatonia may be more related to affective disorders than to schizophrenia. The paranoid forms of schizophrenia also show some unique features in that the paranoid delusions are often the only major symptoms and they tend to remain stable over time.

EPIDEMIOLOGY. The prevalence of schizophrenia in the general population is about 1 per cent for lifetime risk, or about an 0.5 in 1000 incidence of recorded or treated cases per year in the United States. The schizophrenic syndrome has a similar worldwide incidence, the only cultural difference being that prognosis for recovery seems better in rural environments than in urban settings. The prevalence rate is eight times higher in the lower than in the higher socioeconomic classes. Since the parents of schizophrenics have a social class distribution similar to that of the general population, the lower position of the patients appears to be a result of the illness rather than the cause of it.

Since the highest incidence of schizophrenia is in younger people, whose illness often becomes chronic, the number of cases is constantly increasing. Seventy per cent of schizophrenics become ill between ages 15 and 35, and the illness affects males slightly more than females. Peak onset in males lies between 15 and 24 years and in females between 25 and 34 years. There are slight ethnic differences, with a higher incidence in Scandinavian countries and in nonwhites. The chronicity of the illness presents an enormous cost. A recent study notes that although schizophrenia affects only one-twelfth as many persons as does myocardial infarction, the cost is six times as great.

PATHOPHYSIOLOGY. The pathophysiology of schizophrenia is unknown, nor has an anatomic origin of the symptoms been determined. Nevertheless, a number of conditions (including trauma, seizure disorders, and Huntington's disease) can produce schizophrenia-like hallucinations and delusions. Many authors have reported a higher than normal incidence of nonlocalizing neurologic abnormalities in schizophrenia, changes that are not present in other psychiatric conditions. These include defects in stereognosis, graphesthesia, and various skilled motor activities. Minor vestibular system defects, usually consisting of a reduction in the nystagmus response unrelated to medication use, have been noted in schizophrenic patients. Deficits in smooth-pursuit

eye movements during pendulum tracking have been reported in schizophrenia as well as in other psychoses. Other evidence of organic damage, including EEG abnormalities, is tantalizingly frequent.

Twenty-five per cent of hospitalized schizophrenic patients show abnormally slow EEG tracings using standard recording techniques; with more complex instrumentation the incidence rises as high as 80 per cent. Since the development of pneumoencephalography, reports of gross anatomic cerebral changes in subgroups of schizophrenic patients have been frequent. With the rapid developments of computed tomography (CT), magnetic resonance imaging (MRI), and more dynamic measures such as single photon emission (SPECT) and positron emission tomography (PET), these reports have been more consistent and refined. CT and MRI studies have both shown lateral ventricle and third ventricle enlargement, widened cortical sulci, cerebellar atrophy, cerebral asymmetry, and decreased brain density consistently in many, but not all, studies in subgroups of schizophrenic patients. Not all of these changes occur in the same subgroups. Although it is not yet clear what the implications of these findings are, there have been correlative studies of these abnormalities with increased cognitive disturbance, poorer premorbid adjustment, and longer duration of illness. However, as with most new techniques, there is great variation of the instruments and methodologies used in these studies as well as the definitions of the populations. As more standardization of the techniques and diagnostic criteria occur, there should be greater consistency of findings. Using the more dynamic measures, changes have been reported in the cerebral blood flow in the anterior frontal regions, the temporal cortex, and the globus pallidus, as well as decreased D2 receptor sites in schizophrenics. Neuropsychological testing shows a great deal of overlap between the findings in patients with clear-cut organic disease and those with schizophrenia to the point where the tests often fail to distinguish between the two conditions.

Most of the above-described dysfunctions imply an abnormality in the functional integration of sensory and cognitive information in schizophrenia.

Strong evidence implicates a genetic factor in schizophrenia to a degree that 10 to 15 per cent of the offspring of a schizophrenic parent are at risk for the disease. Furthermore, the coincidence of schizophrenia in monozygotic twins is roughly 60 per cent. Additional evidence for a genetic factor comes from studies of children of schizophrenic parents, who are raised by either their natural or adoptive, nonschizophrenic parents: The chance of developing the disease is identical, regardless of the developmental environment. While genetic factors are evident in the transmission of schizophrenia, the family has been implicated in other ways in its development. Previous theories relate to the "schizophrenogenic mother," but little scientific documentation has been provided. A more likely hypothesis of family interaction was developed by Leff and others, who noted that certain family environments had a great deal of "expressed emotion." In these families with much highly charged emotional interaction, schizophrenic patients seemed to do very poorly. Those environments that were less stimulating emotionally allowed the schizophrenic to function better. Hogarty et al. discuss these familial factors more extensively.

Additional indirect evidence for biologic mechanisms in schizophrenia derives from pharmacologic studies: (1) Most of the neuroleptic drugs effective in controlling schizophrenic symptoms act as dopamine blockers in the central nervous system. (2) Many psychoactive drugs such as mescaline and amphetamines are dopaminergic and also have the potential for creating psychotic reactions. Further suggestions of altered dopamine metabolism in schizophrenic patients come from the inconsistent findings of both elevated and reduced levels of homovanillic acid, its major metabolite in the CSF and urine. As yet, most of these biologic findings, as well as the results of parallel animal studies, are too inconsistent or incomplete to permit unifying hypotheses.

PROGNOSIS AND TREATMENT. Prognosis in schizophrenia is poor and specific therapy lacking. Over a 25- to 30-year period, approximately one third of cases show some recovery or remission, and the remainder either have major residual symptoms or are still hospitalized. The major treatment is neuroleptic medication.

TABLE 451–4. USUAL SYMPTOMATIC PATTERNS OF PSYCHOTIC DISORDERS

	Acute Schizophrenia	Mania	Major Depression	Delirium
Delusions	+ + + +	+ + + +	+ + +	+ +
Hallucinations	+ + + +	+ +	+ +	+ + +
Disorientation/confusion	0	0	0	+ + + +
Incoherent speech	+ + + +	+ + +	0	+ + + +
Depressed mood	+	0	+ + + +	+
Grandiosity	+ +	+ + + +	0	0

Table 451–5 lists the drugs most commonly used in the treatment of schizophrenia. The goal of treatment is to decrease as many of the symptoms as possible. As long as hallucinations, delusions, and disorganized thinking persist, the accepted practice is to increase the dose of medication until reaching a maximum decrease in symptoms. The response is usually achieved in a period of 2 to 3 weeks, with decreases in hallucination and thought disorder and a variable response of delusions. The most frequent limiting factor is the appearance of extrapyramidal side effects, the most common of which are dystonia, akathisia (restlessness), and parkinsonism. These occur most commonly in the first 2 to 4 months of drug use.

There is little difference in efficacy in the neuroleptics (Table 451–5), and lack of efficacy usually reflects too low a dose. If, however, no response occurs to a phenothiazine-type drug (e.g., chlorpromazine), one usually changes to another class of neuroleptics, such as a butyrophenone (haloperidol) or a thioxanthene. The physician should become familiar with one drug from each of these classes of neuroleptics for acute and maintenance use. The major long-term hazard in the use of these medications is tardive dyskinesia.

Tardive dyskinesia is a syndrome of involuntary movements, usually choreoathetoid, that may affect the mouth, lips, tongue, extremities, or trunk. Although usually associated with use of neuroleptics for 6 months or more, tardive dyskinesia can occur with shorter administration. Patients on neuroleptics should be periodically evaluated for these abnormal movements. A frequent early sign consists of vermicular movements of the tongue. Anticholinergic drugs do not help this condition. The symptoms may decrease with an increase of the medication, but such improvement usually is only temporary and may lead to a vicious circle of worsening chorea and increased drug dosages. The cause of tardive dyskinesia is not known, but it is believed to represent the development of dopaminergic hypersensitivity. Although no effective treatment has been found, in many instances gradually decreasing the dose of neuroleptics induces a slow remission of the symptoms (see also Ch. 462).

Despite the above conditions, the use of neuroleptics is effective, and the drugs should be used to help the patient function with as few symptoms as possible despite the potential side effects. Removing schizophrenic patients from medication greatly increases the chances of hospitalization within the following 6 months. This lag represents a major problem in that most patients immediately feel and do better without the medications. As a result, families and patients often fail to associate the cessation of medication with the subsequent relapse.

In spite of the fact that typical neuroleptics are the treatment of choice for schizophrenia, they are not a panacea and there are alternative or adjunctive agents that the clinician may consider. At this stage these agents should be regarded as novel. They include medications such as anticonvulsants, benzodiazepines, calcium channel blockers, and monoamine agonists and antagonists. Additionally, the recent FDA approval of clozapine (Clozaril), an atypical antipsychotic with potent serotonergic, adrenergic, and histaminergic blocking activity and relatively weak

TABLE 451–5. DRUGS COMMONLY USED FOR TREATMENT OF SCHIZOPHRENIA*

	Daily Dosage Range (mg)
Phenothiazines	
Chlorpromazine (Thorazine)	300–1500
Thioridazine (Mellaril)	150–800
Perphenazine (Trilafon)	8–64
Trifluoperazine (Stelazine)	4–60
Fluphenazine (Prolixin)†	2–20
Butyrophenones	
Haloperidol (Haldol)†	2–40
Thioxanthenes	
Thiothixene (Navane)	6–60

*Owing to untoward extrapyramidal reactions, one often needs to administer these drugs along with such drugs as benztropine mesylate (Cogentin), trihexyphenidyl HCl (Artane), diphenhydramine HCl (Benadryl).

†Comes in two injectable slow-release forms that can be given every 10 days to 3 weeks.

TABLE 451–6. DRUGS USED IN ACUTELY AGITATED STATES

Drug	Dose*	24-hr Maximum
Haloperidol (Haldol)	5–10 mg every 1–2 hr I.M. or P.O.	50 mg
Thiothixene (Navane)	5–10 mg every 2–4 hr I.M. or P.O.	40 mg
Lorazepam (Ativan)	0.5–1.0 mg every 1–2 hr I.M. or P.O.	10 mg

*Doses should be 50 to 75 per cent reduced in the elderly or medically ill.

and equivalent D_1 and D_2 dopamine-blocking activity, represents a significant advance in the treatment of schizophrenia. It should be reserved for those patients with treatment-resistant illness, those who are unable to tolerate good trials of neuroleptics due to side effects, or those with tardive dyskinesia. The fact that there is a cumulative incidence of agranulocytosis of 2 per cent after a year of treatment with clozapine necessitates weekly CBC monitoring of patients treated with this medication. It has minimal risk for producing extrapyramidal symptoms (EPS), probably does not cause tardive dyskinesia, and is reported to be efficacious in 30 per cent of treatment-resistant schizophrenics.

Most criteria for judging prognosis in schizophrenia are related to short-term outcome and can be summarized by saying that the more acute and florid the early symptoms or, as some have phrased it, the more the patient has "positive" symptoms (delusions, hallucinations, agitation, and depressive symptoms), the more likely he is to recover from the acute episode. The more insidious the onset and the more lacking in emotional display (negative symptoms), the worse the short- and long-term prognoses. The natural history of the illness (even in treated patients) seems to be of two major types: (1) an episodic, relapsing course with each episode resulting in a lower level of psychosocial functioning; and (2) a gradual, slow decline in functional ability. Both courses eventually result in a progressive loss of psychosocial capacities (see Table 451–3). Recent treatment efforts in schizophrenia have taken a rehabilitative, or psychoeducational, approach in which the family is educated about the problems of schizophrenia and issues of living are openly dealt with.

ACUTE USE OF NEUROLEPTIC MEDICATION. Neuroleptic drugs are also useful for patients who are markedly agitated with or without delusions and hallucinations (Table 451–6). They also help to control agitated states associated with organic delirium and dementia. In elderly patients and in those with delirium and/or dementia, the doses should be much lower until the patient's reaction is ascertained. Since acutely agitated psychotic patients respond to lorazepam as well as to neuroleptics, the initial use of benzodiazepines is probably safer in cases in which the source of the agitation is not known and in manic states for which long-term neuroleptic medication is not planned.

Andreasen N (ed.): Brain Imaging: Applications in Psychiatry. Washington, D.C., American Psychiatric Press, 1989. *A comprehensive review of CT, MRI, SPECT, PET, and EEG investigations of behavioral disorders.*

Cloninger C, Martin R, Guze S, et al.: Diagnosis and prognosis in schizophrenia. Arch Gen Psychiatry 42:15–25, 1985. *An excellent study of the implications of symptoms for prognosis in schizophrenia.*

Hogarty G, Anderson C, Reiss A, et al.: Family psychoeducation, social skills training, and maintained chemotherapy in the aftercare treatment of schizophrenia. Arch Gen Psychiatry 43:633–642, 1986. *A convincing review and study of the role of psychosocial factors in the treatment of schizophrenia.*

Kaplan H, Saddock B: Comprehensive Textbook of Psychiatry, 5th ed. Baltimore, Williams & Wilkins, 1989. *An excellent and detailed overview of all aspects of schizophrenia.*

Schulz C, Tamminga C: Schizophrenia: A Scientific Focus. New York, Oxford Press, 1989. *A comprehensive review of current knowledge about schizophrenia.*

Strauss J, Carpenter W: Schizophrenia. New York, Plenum Press, 1981. *A comprehensive presentation of major aspects of schizophrenic disorders.*

AFFECTIVE DISORDERS

A difficulty in clinical psychiatric diagnosis is that similar terms are used to describe feeling states that differ greatly in degree and sometimes in kind. Such is the case with the term *depression*. In common use the meaning may extend from a description of a brief pang of regret to profound feelings of futility and suicidal despair. At what point along this spectrum does one label the condition "illness"? When does normal grief become pathologic? This section discusses these questions.

Many have attempted to classify depressive illnesses based on *symptomatology*, e.g., psychotic versus neurotic; *supposed etiology*, e.g., endogenous versus reactive; or *age*, e.g., childhood, involutional. None of these distinctions has resisted careful investigation. The most recent characterization of depressive illness has been simplified into *bipolar disorders*, identifying wide swings of mood; *major depressive illness*, marked by severe depressive symptoms but without manic swings; and two milder forms, *cyclothymic disorder* and *dysthymic disorder* (formerly called depressive neurosis). These latter two terms describe milder forms of bipolar disorders and depression that fall short of the specific diagnostic criteria for the more serious disorders.

Symptoms of depression also are classified by the company they keep. The psychiatric condition alone would be classified as a primary affective disorder, but when symptoms of affective disorders accompany medical conditions, they are termed secondary affective disorders. Marked depressive symptoms have been noted with various endocrine disorders, tumors, seizure disorders, vitamin deficiencies, and particular neurologic disorders such as multiple sclerosis, Parkinson's disease, and stroke. Depressive symptoms also can be associated with drugs used to treat medical conditions. In at least some instances, the consistency of the symptoms may reflect the fact that similar neurotransmitter systems are altered in both the primary and secondary affective disturbances.

Major Depression

The symptomatology and diagnostic criteria for major depression are listed in Table 451–7. Although many patients have single episodes of major depressive illness, the condition also can be repetitive, and this recurrent condition is frequently called unipolar depressive illness. Fifty per cent of patients with a single episode of major depression eventually have another depressive episode.

The key features of major depression are a markedly gloomy mood in which there is a loss of interest in life, a lack of pleasure in almost all activities, and a general feeling of hopelessness and worthlessness. The illness takes the form of a cognitive change in which the patient seemingly looks at the world with "black glasses," and everything thought about or accomplished is minimized or negated: The wealthy and successful career person talks about his or her impending financial doom and general lack of accomplishment in life; the gifted artist dismisses his creations as trivial. When vegetative functions (sleep, appetite, psychomotor activity) are markedly impaired and a complete loss of pleasure accompanies almost all activities with no reactions to pleasurable stimuli, we often add the term *melancholia*.

Depressive symptoms range in severity from mild mood swings to severe delusions about self-worth, accomplishments, and the future. The "blackness" of the presentation in the depressed

TABLE 451–7. MAJOR DEPRESSIVE EPISODE*

A. At least five of the following symptoms have been present during the same 2-week period; at least one of the symptoms was either 1 or 2 below and not related to a physical condition. These symptoms can be subjective reports or reported by others and must occur nearly every day.
   1. Depressed mood most of the day (e.g., the patient feels "down" or "low")
   2. Loss of interest or pleasure in all or almost all activities
   3. Significant weight loss or weight gain when not dieting or binge-eating (e.g., more than 5 per cent of body weight in a month), or decrease or increase in appetite
   4. Insomnia or hypersomnia
   5. Psychomotor agitation or retardation
   6. Fatigue or loss of energy
   7. Feelings of worthlessness or excessive or inappropriate guilt (which may be delusional)
   8. Diminished ability to think or concentrate, or indecisiveness
   9. Thoughts that he or she would be better off dead, or suicidal ideation, nearly every day; a suicide attempt
B. 1. An organic etiology has been ruled out
   2. Not a normal reaction to the loss of a loved one
C. Not superimposed on schizophrenia

*Modified from American Psychiatric Association: Diagnostic and Statistical Manual of Mental Disorders, 3rd ed., rev. Washington, DC, APA, 1987. Used with permission.

patient is most often accompanied by severe motor retardation with profound sleep and appetite disturbance and suicidal ideation. Nevertheless, some severe depressions can present in a highly anxious, agitated state. The history of previous episodes (either manic or depressive) aids in the diagnosis.

Affective Disorders in the Elderly

The increasing precision of psychiatric diagnosis has made it evident that at the two ends of life, i.e., childhood and aging, the psychopathology of affective disorders is less distinct than during the years between. Elderly patients may have many dysphoric symptoms but not meet the precise diagnostic criteria for major affective disorder. Diagnosis in the elderly is also complicated by two factors: (1) the behavioral and cognitive changes caused by the aging of the central nervous system (although, other than minor memory impairments, the presence of cognitive impairments should make one consider a more comprehensive workup for dementia), and (2) the presence of other medical illnesses and their attendant medications.

The most common psychiatric symptoms in community populations of older adults are those of depression (15 per cent), hypochondriasis (14 per cent), suspiciousness (17 per cent), and persecutory ideation (4 per cent). As many as one third complain of difficulty in falling asleep, awakening during the night, or being sleepy during the day. All these symptom rates increase for the institutionalized elderly. By contrast, cases fulfilling the specific diagnoses of major depression, dysthymia, and schizophrenia occur at a much lower rate than in younger populations.

Although the aged patient may not meet full diagnostic criteria for affective disturbance, persistent symptomatology nevertheless deserves a trial of cautious pharmacologic intervention. This is particularly true when one looks at elderly patients who have cognitive impairments. Community samples of aged populations show about a 4 to 5 per cent prevalence of severe cognitive impairment. The figure may not entirely reflect degenerative brain disease, however, since the biologic changes that occur with affective illness also can cause cognitive impairments detected by both neuropsychological testing and clinical neurologic examination. This is true in younger populations as well. The abnormalities can include not only problems with memory and orientation, but signs of minor neurologic impairment as well; all may clear after a trial of antidepressive medication. The term "pseudodementia" has been used for these potentially treatable cognitive changes in elderly affectively disordered patients.

DIAGNOSIS. The diagnosis is made on clinical grounds as discussed above. Many tests to aid the diagnosis of depression have been introduced, including the dexamethasone suppression test (DST), the thyroid-stimulating hormone (TSH) response (see below), and many measures of disturbed sleep function such as rapid eye movement (REM) latency. Unfortunately, none has proved to be diagnostically reliable or specific for affective disorder. In diagnosing depression, the interview is central.

EPIDEMIOLOGY. The sex distribution of major depression is almost two-to-one female to male. The peak incidence for women is 35 to 45 years, whereas the age pattern is less clear for men. There may also be an increased incidence in women in their early 50's. The prevalence is about 3.2 per 100 males and about 4.5 to 9.3 per 100 females. Incidence is 82 to 201 new cases per 100,000 for men and 247 to 598 new cases per 100,000 for women. The mean duration of first attack of an untreated depressive illness is about 13 months. The episodes, if they recur, are likely to be similar in nature and respond to treatment in a similar fashion. As with bipolar illness, alcoholism is a frequent complication of depressive illness, particularly when it has a recurring course.

Patients in primary care clinics (5 to 10 per cent) and on medical inpatient services (15 per cent) show an increased prevalence of depression.

PATHOPHYSIOLOGY. Pathophysiologic theories of affective disorders have developed along three major lines: (1) endocrine studies; (2) neurotransmitters; and (3) electrophysiologic studies. Depressed patients frequently have elevated levels of cortical steroids in the blood and urine and at least half fail to suppress cortisol secretion after dexamethasone administration. Thyroid-stimulating hormone (TSH) response to thyrotropin-releasing hormone also has been found to be aberrant in many depressed patients, even though their blood T_3 and T_4 levels are normal. Growth hormone, prolactin, gonadal hormones, CRF, and melatonin have all been shown to have diminished responses in subgroups of affective disorders. Although none of these findings is specific for any type of depressive illness or consistent in all depressive illnesses, they nevertheless suggest the presence of pituitary-hypothalamic dysfunction in affective disorders.

Studies of neurotransmitters in depression have been stimulated largely by the success of pharmacologic agents used to treat affective disorders. Many of the tricyclic compounds and the MAO inhibitors effective in the treatment of depression increase the availability of catecholamines and indolamines in the central nervous system. L-Dopa, used to treat Parkinson's disease, is a major catecholamine (dopamine) precursor and may in itself induce mania. These and other observations have given rise to the catecholamine-indolamine hypothesis of depression. The theory postulates that a certain level of amines and/or receptor sensitivity to catecholamines functions to generate a normal mood. Receptor insensitivity, a depletion of amines, or a decrease in their synthesis or storage leads to depression. Conversely, if the amines are in excess or the receptors are hypersensitive, mania may develop. Recently, the acetylcholine system has also been implicated in affective disorders, a "balance" between adrenergic and cholinergic function being postulated as necessary for the stabilization of mood. Neither theory, however, is entirely satisfactory, since it has been found that the tricyclic drugs affect many receptor systems and that their main action may be one of changing or regulating the sensitivity of the receptor rather than acting directly as neurotransmitters. Furthermore, newer drugs that have antidepressant effects do not affect these transmitter systems. One study, for example, has found that the anticonvulsant carbamazepine favorably affects the course of certain patients with bipolar illness.

Electrophysiologic studies on affective illness have concentrated on changes in sleep functions, especially the presence of changes in the REM sleep pattern during episodes of active illness. A subgroup of patients with affective disorder shows a shortened REM latency. Furthermore, analyses of circadian rhythms provide increasing evidence for autumn and winter precipitation of some bipolar disorders, with depressive illnesses apparently related to diminished ambient light in winter climates. The change has been correlated with alterations of melatonin metabolism.

TREATMENT. In most cases the physician is presented with someone who seems mildly sad and self-deprecating, with perhaps slight sleep and appetite disturbances. In such patients an attempt at counseling about the events in their lives and helping delineate appropriate priorities and activities, along with prescriptions for adequate exercise, diet, rest, and general health measures, may suffice. When symptoms become more marked, particularly when they disturb sleep and appetite, and the person becomes unable to perform work, school, or household tasks, one should consider adding antidepressant medication to the above regimen (Table 451–8). If the mild symptoms have been present for a number of years, a trial of medication may be in order. With prominent depressive symptomatology hospitalization may be necessary, the major indication being to prevent suicide (15 per cent of patients with major affective disorders commit suicide). As discussed in a later section, it is a wise step in medicine to ask all patients with depression of mood, apathetic fatigue, or ill-defined somatic symptoms if they have ever considered the situation sufficiently unbearable that suicide becomes an option.

The approach and response to drug therapy in depression vary considerably among both physicians and patients. Perhaps the best prediction of a favorable response is if a blood relative has responded well to a similar agent. In patients who present primarily with insomnia and marked vegetative disturbances as well as some agitation, amitriptyline (or nortriptyline) is somewhat more sedating, particularly if given at bedtime. Imipramine (or desipramine) is less sedating and often avoids the drowsiness that amitriptyline causes. After initial CBC, liver profiles, and in older patients an ECG, it is best to start these medications in single

TABLE 451–8. ANTIDEPRESSANT DRUGS

Dose	Daily Dosage Range (mg)*	Anticholinergic Effects
Tricyclics		
Imipramine (Tofranil)	50–150	+ +
Amitriptyline (Elavil)	50–150	+ + +
Nortriptyline (Aventyl)	50–150	+ +
Desipramine (Norpramin, Pertofrane)	50–150	+
Doxepin (Sinequan)	150	+ +
Tetracyclic		
Maprotiline (Ludiomil)	50–225	+
Other		
Fluoxetine (Prozac)	20–80	0
Buproprion (Wellbutrin)	300–450	0
Trazodone (Desyrel)	150–600	0
MAOI's†		
Phenelzine (Nardil)	15–90	+ +
Tranylcypromine (Parnate)	20–30	+ +

*In most cases the dose should be reduced 30 to 50 per cent in the elderly and medically ill.
†Monoamine oxidase inhibitors.

doses at bedtime. An initial starting dose of 50 mg may be rapidly increased every several days until a total dosage of 150 mg per night is reached. As stated earlier, with elderly patients all psychotropic drugs should be used cautiously, and doses of antidepressants should be decreased by 30 to 50 per cent from the above. For example, one would start an elderly patient on 10 or 25 mg of an antidepressant such as amitriptyline (nortriptyline) at bedtime or even every other night. For prolonged treatment the elderly may often respond to smaller doses (10 to 75 mg). However, if after 6 weeks the elderly patient has not responded to doses as high as 75 mg and there are no marked side effects, doses can be slowly increased. In the normal adult without medical illness, if there is no response to 150 mg per day within 6 weeks, then the dosage can often be increased to as much as 200 to 300 mg (this is beyond manufacturers' guidelines). It is wise, however, to obtain the counsel of a specialist prior to using these doses. If there is still no response one could switch to another tricyclic or immediately to an MAOI. Blood level measurements are available for most of the tricyclic antidepressants, although their main usefulness is to indicate that the person is taking and absorbing the drug. Only nortriptyline has had an effective therapeutic window (50 to 140 ng per milliliter) established.

It is useful to caution patients that the antidepressants do not produce an immediate response, although if given at bedtime they may improve sleeping immediately. Also, the prominent anticholinergic side effects and hypotension are often a bother, and patients should be forewarned. Some of the supposed side effects of the medication are also accompaniments of the depressive illness, and patients, if questioned, may reveal that they have had many of the symptoms prior to taking the medication. Several of the new antidepressants, fluoxetine and buproprion, have entirely different actions and have succeeded when traditional medications have failed. One must recognize that the tricyclics have a quinidine-like effect and have been used to treat some cardiac arrhythmias.

For patients who fail to respond to tricyclic antidepressants, psychiatric consultation is critical. However, some have found it useful to add 0.25 µg per day of triiodothyronine (T_3) to the tricyclic dosage, particularly in female patients. Also, the addition of lithium to tricyclic regimens has been found to have a marked augmenting effect on the response to antidepressant tricyclics (neither of the above is in FDA-approved use).

The monoamine oxidase inhibitors (MAOI's) have enjoyed a return to usage recently with the introduction of fluoxetine and buproprion. They had been underutilized in the United States owing to their tendency to cause hypertensive crises following the ingestion of foods containing tyramine. However, for patients not responding to tricyclic medications or those with atypical depressions marked predominantly by anxiety symptoms, they are quite effective. Patients can be started on MAOI drugs immediately following tricyclic cessation. The reverse, however, does not hold, and patients stopping an MAOI drug must wait 7 to 14 days before starting a tricyclic antidepressant. If dietary restrictions are followed and sympathetic amine medications are avoided, MAOI's are usually safe, their major side effects being hypotension and insomnia. They have milder anticholinergic effects and often are easier to tolerate than the tricyclic antidepressants, but the specific side effects and indications for use are still being delineated.

In older patients, in those who fail to respond to pharmacotherapeutic interventions, and in those with complicated medical conditions which the drugs might adversely affect, electroconvulsive therapy (ECT) is probably the safest treatment. Whereas 60 per cent of most affective disturbances respond to pharmacotherapy, close to 80 per cent improve after ECT. There are few contraindications: When ECT is administered in association with modern anesthetic techniques, the morbidity is reduced to that of the anesthesia alone. With careful monitoring, even patients with recent cerebral or myocardial insults can be treated with ECT.

PROGNOSIS. Antidepressant drugs should be continued for 6 to 20 weeks after patients become free of symptoms. More prolonged treatment is desirable for those who have had recurrent episodes. Many patients have been maintained for years on tricyclic antidepressants and MAOI's without major impairment. Nevertheless, in spite of the best treatment, between 15 and 20 per cent of depressives go on to a chronic course. Most patients with a single episode continue to function well and, in fact, often tend to use the depressive episode as a chance to reorient and reorganize their lives and proceed to function better than they had previously.

Dysthymic Disorder (Depressive Neurosis)

DEFINITION. The symptoms consist of a depressed mood of longstanding duration with a severity less intense than in a major depressive disorder. These patients often seem to have situational reasons for their illness. Many present primarily with physical complaints to physicians. Substance and drug abuse, as well as personality profiles that involve dependency and obsessional symptomatology, are often part of the clinical picture. The diagnostic criteria are outlined in Table 451–9.

EPIDEMIOLOGY. As this condition is treated in many settings, the epidemiologic distribution is difficult to determine. One estimate of prevalence is 60 per 1000. Women predominate and familial patterns have not been established.

PATHOPHYSIOLOGY. There is evidence that various personality conflicts and situational precipitants are related to these conditions more than to the other affective disorders.

TREATMENT. Many types of short-term psychotherapy have been effective in treating these conditions. Patients who respond poorly to psychotherapy often benefit from antidepressant medication.

GRIEF REACTIONS

Physicians often find it emotionally difficult to deal with the relatives of patients who have died or been seriously injured, yet such contacts provide important preventive medicine. Grief should be looked upon as a biologic process with psychological roots. Issues of loss and attachment are extremely prominent in bereavement. In normal bereavement 50 per cent of persons experience depressed mood, sleep disturbances, and crying lasting anywhere from 2 to 6 months. Furthermore, many grief reactions resolve only slowly over a number of years. This is particularly true in older persons who have lost spouses of many years' duration.

During bereaved states general health deteriorates, and there is often an increase in serious illness. A decrease in lymphocyte responses in husbands during mourning has been described. Some persons lose contact with reality and blame themselves, constantly asking, "Why did this happen?" Others even have difficulty in accepting that the person is dead. Anger and withdrawal can prevail. Some survivors, particularly when the death was violent, experience stress responses similar to those of combat veterans, who in addition to the symptoms related above may have frequent and often violent intrusive mental images.

These normal reactions can blur into a more serious state with intense and prolonged symptoms lasting 6 months or more. Some survivors undergo a delayed response, functioning well immediately after the event but experiencing later symptoms of bereavement, often precipitated by the death of another person or the anniversary of the death of the loved one. Others can develop hypochondriacal symptoms resembling those of the deceased. Panic attacks and depressive illness may develop also in prolonged grief reactions.

The prevention and treatment of grief reactions can often be undertaken by the physician in his normal contact with the bereaved survivor. Lindeman has outlined several valid principles: (1) Allow the patient to share his feelings about the death of the relative. The physician can be extremely helpful in discussing the normal process of grief and the reactions that people experience. (2) Review the relationships of the deceased with the important people in their lives. (3) Help grieving persons to accept their feelings and fears about things such as their ability to cope, their fears about "going crazy," anger, etc. (4) Discuss with the bereaved how they are adapting to the stress and what modes they are using to cope. (5) Attempt to formulate the future relationships between the bereaved and others in their lives. (6) Find new persons with whom the bereaved can develop relationships.

While the above matters can only be touched on in the acute situation, they often can be dealt with over time. Even the gathering of information about these areas is often seen as useful by the patient. If the condition progresses to an abnormal degree, the use of medications for the appropriate conditions, e.g., affective disturbance or panic disorder, is indicated. The use of mild sedation and hypnotics at the acute stage is also useful. Support groups have been organized to deal with both the normal and excessive processes of grieving and appear to be useful.

SUICIDAL BEHAVIOR

About 75 per cent of patients who actually commit suicide will have seen a physician within the previous 6 months. Most practicing physicians encounter half a dozen potentially suicidal patients per year, among whom 10 to 12 actually do away with themselves over the ensuing years. The figures illustrate how important it is for the physician to detect various clues. Suicide is higher in patients with psychiatric problems, with the highest incidence occurring in those with affective disorders or alcoholism or those who are in the early post-hospital phase of schizophrenic disorders. Suicidal behavior is not specific to any one major psychiatric disturbance. For example, about the same percentage of schizophrenic patients commit suicide as do patients with major depression. Suicidal behavior occurs across a spectrum of mental illness, and a good argument can be made that it should be treated as a distinct problem separate from the major psychiatric disorders. Effective pharmacologic treatments for depression and schizophrenia have been available since the 1950's, yet there is no evidence that these treatments have reduced the suicidality of either population. Therapy that may be pertinent in reducing suicidality includes techniques to enhance one's social supports,

---

TABLE 451–9. DYSTHYMIA*

A. At least 2 years (1 year for children and adolescents) during which there has been depressed mood most of the day, more days than not (either by subjective account, e.g., feels "down" or "low," or is observed by others to look sad or depressed) and at least two of the following:
  1. Poor appetite or overeating
  2. Insomnia or hypersomnia
  3. Low energy or fatigue
  4. Low self-esteem
  5. Poor concentration or difficulty making decisions
  6. Pessimism
B. During that 2-year period the patient is never without the above symptoms for more than 2 months at a time.
C. No clear evidence of a major depressive episode during the first 2 years of the disturbance.
D. Has never had a manic episode.
E. No psychotic symptoms and symptoms not the residual phase of schizophrenia.
F. Not sustained by a specific organic factor or substance, e.g., prolonged administration of an antihypertensive medication.

*Modified from American Psychiatric Association: Diagnostic and Statistical Manual of Mental Disorders, 3rd ed., rev. Washington, DC, APA, 1987. Used with permission.

development of problem-solving and other coping skills, and treatments designed to reduce alcohol use, especially during periods of stress. Pharmacologic interventions aimed specifically at suicidal behavior, interventions that, for the most part, involve manipulation of the serotonergic system, are now being investigated.

The typical patient who makes a suicide attempt is a white female, 20 to 40 years of age, who ingests pills, usually after an interpersonal conflict. By contrast, the typical successful suicide victim is a white male, 45 years of age or older, often separated, widowed, or divorced, who lives alone and may be unemployed or retired. Patients who commit suicide suffer a high incidence of poor physical health, medical care within the past 6 months, and evidence of some psychiatric disturbance. Many have a previous history of suicide attempts or threats.

Doctors often feel more awkward than their patients in discussing suicidal thoughts or intent. It must be done understandingly, but almost all seriously ill adults should be asked gently if they have had thoughts about death or suicide. Comments patients make about feeling they would be "better off dead" or "people would be better off without me" should be taken seriously. Preoccupations with funerals, cemetery lots, and the buying of weapons should make one suspicious. Any patient who presents with vague complaints should be asked about his or her emotional state. If any indication of suicidal intent is forthcoming, one must immediately evaluate its seriousness, inquiring about the following: (1) Has the person considered actual suicide? If so, what plans have been made and how specifically? The more specific, the more worrisome. (2) What other psychopathology exists? Is the patient agitated, seriously depressed, etc.? (3) What precipitating stresses exist? (4) Are there people in the environment whom the person trusts and who could help? (5) Will the person agree to work with you and contact you if his suicidal feelings intensify? (6) If no reassurance comes from the patient or relatives that the situation can be managed at home, hospitalization may be necessary.

An even more difficult evaluation is how to treat those who have made a recent unsuccessful suicide attempt. After a suicide attempt there often is a brief period of days to weeks of lightening of the depressive mood, after which strong self-destructive feelings reappear. The more lethal the risk (i.e., the higher was the potential risk of death in the initial suicide attempt), the more determined should be the effort to provide psychiatric treatment, preferably in a hospital. If patients express an explicit intent to die, often stated with determination and conviction, there is no question about the necessity for hospitalization.

Most patients after suicide attempts should have a psychiatric consultation, but sometimes this may not be possible and the nonpsychiatric physician must assess the suicidal potential. Part of the evaluation of the patient can also serve as the initial formation of a doctor-patient relationship. If they have a supportive environment and will keep contact, some of these patients can be managed as outpatients. Physicians should be aware of writing potentially lethal prescriptions for patients who may have suicidal tendencies. For example, for a routine dosage schedule of tricyclic antidepressants (150 mg per day), even a week's supply provides a potentially lethal overdose.

SUICIDE IN ADOLESCENTS. Nine to 18 per cent of children and adolescents have made suicide attempts. This astoundingly high figure correlates with turmoil in the family as well as disturbed parent/child interactions. There are also significant correlations with substance abuse, depressive illness, and conduct disorders in children and adolescents as well as histories of physical and sexual abuse. Many of these children and adolescents had threatened suicide previously. Many have done poorly in school and have records of chronically aggressive behavior. One of the most difficult questions which faces the psychiatrist is whether to hospitalize an adolescent at risk for suicide. The answer relates primarily to the severity of the suicidal behavior and the patient's intent to "be dead." Interestingly, in adolescents, it also relates to the presence of assaultive behavior in that the hostility toward self can also be directed against others. The environmental supports available to see someone through a depressive episode also mitigate the need for hospitalization. It is extremely important in treating the adolescent to provide some

form of individual counseling, usually centered around coping skills and cognitive therapy as well to work with the environmental support system or the patient's family. Pharmacologic treatment is quite effective for affective illness in adolescents.

SUICIDE AND AGING. Age groups over age 70 years have a higher suicide rate, with single males at the peak. Some of the risk factors are unemployment, isolation, poor health, pain, feelings of being rejected, history of mental illness, and previous suicide attempts. A history of alcoholism is a high comorbid factor within suicidal behavior. Many elderly pursue indirect suicide by stopping eating or necessary medications. Electroconvulsive therapy is often the most effective form of treatment for suicidal behavior in geriatrics.

Bipolar Disorders

Bipolar disorders (previously called manic-depressive disorders) are probably the most homogeneous diagnostic grouping in psychiatry, as they consist of a marked change in mood that varies from major depressive episodes (as discussed) (see Table 451–7) to significant manic episodes as defined below. There is usually a return to normal behavior between episodes. There is little difficulty in recognizing the illness if one looks at the longitudinal course. However, if patients are examined only briefly, at a particular moment in time, manic excitement can be confused with schizophrenic psychosis. The depressive phase of bipolar illness can also be misconstrued as a catatonic state.

DIAGNOSTIC CRITERIA AND CLINICAL SIGNS AND SYMPTOMS. The manic phase of the illness is characterized by an expansive euphoric mood in which grandiose plans and ideas predominate. It is important to be aware that despite this expansiveness and grandiosity, patients who are frustrated or disagreed with can often become quite irritable and at times aggressive. The major diagnostic criteria are listed in Table 451–10. The patient can be psychotic in the manic phase, with delusions and hallucinations that are consistent with the grandiosity; however, persecutory delusions, feelings of being controlled, etc., can also be present. At times it is difficult to distinguish an excited schizophrenic patient from a manic one. As already stated, one must examine the longitudinal course of the illness, either until the occurrence of a depressive episode or a deteriorating course after remission of the acute symptom, in order to diagnose a schizophrenic process. In all instances, it is crucial to rule out organic factors.

The average age of onset of bipolar disorder is about 30 years, but about 20 per cent of patients have an onset below the age of 20. In females, the onset of the condition seems to have a bimodal distribution, with one peak falling between 20 and 30 years and the other between 40 and 50 years. The peak age of onset of schizophrenia is much younger, but the age of onset of bipolar

TABLE 451–10. MANIC EPISODE*

A. A distinct period (lasting at least 1 week) when mood was abnormally and persistently elevated, expansive, or irritable.
B. During the period of mood disturbance, at least three of the following symptoms have been present to a significant degree:
  1. Inflated self-esteem (grandiosity, which may be delusional)
  2. Decreased need for sleep, e.g., feels rested after only 3 hours of sleep
  3. More talkative than usual or pressure to keep talking
  4. Flight of ideas or subjective experience that thoughts are racing
  5. Distractibility, i.e., attention too easily drawn to unimportant or irrelevant external stimuli
  6. Increase in activity (either socially, at work, or sexually) or physical restlessness
  7. Excessive involvement in activities that have a high potential for painful consequences which is not recognized, e.g., buying sprees, sexual indiscretions, foolish business investments, reckless driving
C. The episode of mood disturbance was sufficiently severe to cause marked impairment in occupational functioning, usual social activities, or relationships with others.
D. At no time during the disturbance have there been delusions or hallucinations for as long as 2 weeks in the absence of prominent mood symptoms (i.e., before the mood symptoms developed or after they have remitted), which would be more indicative of schizophrenia.

*Modified from American Psychiatric Association: Diagnostic and Statistical Manual of Mental Disorders, 3rd ed., rev. Washington, DC, APA, 1987. Used with permission.

illness overlaps enough so that the differential diagnosis of a psychotic illness in a young person is difficult and may change as the clinical picture evolves over time. Almost half the patients with bipolar disorders have at least two to three episodes of illness, and as many as one third experience seven or more episodes of illness once the pattern has started. Each episode of illness, whether it is a manic or a depressive phase, can last from 4 to 13 months; some of these go on to chronicity and some are over much sooner. The course of the illness, however, has been modified significantly with the advent of lithium therapy, especially with respect to diminishing both the severity and the frequency of the episodes. The shorter durations are usually related to the effectiveness of the treatment. Although some patients rapidly alternate between extremes over 2 to 4 days, most episodes have a longer duration and, frequently, after a manic phase there can be a subsequent depressive phase. Chronicity, again as opposed to schizophrenia, is not a major problem with manic-depressive illness, being cited as low as 1 per cent in some studies. Mortality with bipolar illness averages between two and two and one-half times the expected rate for that age; suicide occurs in about 8 to 10 per cent.

EPIDEMIOLOGY. The lifetime risk for developing bipolar illness ranges from 0.6 to 0.9 per cent of the population. The incidence per hundred thousand per year in men is from 9 to 15 new cases and for women from 7.4 to 32 new cases. The risk increases with a family history of bipolar illness. The exact mechanism of the genetic transmission in bipolar illness is uncertain but suggests autosomal dominance with incomplete penetration. There is a 72 per cent concordance in monozygotic twins and a 19 per cent concordance in same-sex dizygotic twins. Both the course of illness and the response to treatment are similar among blood relatives. In one well-studied Amish family, the abnormal gene has been identified on chromosome 11. Other families with equally strong genetic patterns, however, have not possessed this particular chromosomal alteration.

PATHOPHYSIOLOGY. Most of what is known about the pathophysiology of bipolar illness is similar to what is known about the biology of the major depressive disorders.

DIAGNOSIS AND TREATMENT. The treatment of bipolar disorders has three distinct aspects: the manic episode, the major depressive episode, and long-term maintenance therapy. Prior to any specific therapy, an adequate medical workup is necessary in order to be certain that the patient suffers from a primary affective illness. The patient in an acute manic state is delusional, grandiose, and hyperactive and in this condition looks similar to any patient with psychosis. If this is the first episode, one cannot differentiate this state phenomenologically from the first episode of schizophrenia or a psychosis due to physical illness. The major differential diagnosis of the first episode rests on a careful history, family history, and physical and laboratory examination (see Table 451–3). The past history and the nature of onset of the illness are important, as noted previously. Furthermore, most psychiatric disorders have a familial pattern. A psychiatrist should be involved in the evaluation of patients who present with their first psychotic episode.

The treatment of the acute manic phase is usually undertaken in the hospital, as it is imperative to protect the patient from his own misdeeds, e.g., spending inordinate amounts of money, making embarrassing speeches, etc. If the family is supportive, however, and feels it can control the situation, treatment can be started outside of the hospital. Lithium is not useful for the acute management of mania and if the patient is severely agitated, sedation is necessary. Neuroleptics are not used in the long-term treatment of bipolar illness, but the use of benzodiazepines, particularly lorazepam, effectively controls most acute manic states (see Table 451–6). If the agitation is marked and not controlled with medication, one should obtain psychiatric consultation to consider using ECT to control the manic excitement. Manic excitement creates a medical emergency in which patients can die from exhaustion.

Although most general physicians treat acute mania rarely, the use of lithium is something they may encounter more often. Lithium effectively prevents relapses in over 60 per cent of bipolar illnesses. The drug is slightly more effective in preventing manic relapses than the depressive episodes, and its most specific use seems to be in preventing manic recurrences. Nevertheless, its use should be considered with any repetitive affective disturbance.

Prior to the beginning of lithium therapy, a CBC, urinalysis, electrolytes, creatinine, BUN, thyroid studies, and a baseline ECG and EEG should be obtained. Chronic medical illnesses, especially renal insufficiency, can contraindicate use of the agent. Lithium has a half-life of 24 to 36 hours, and it takes at least 4 days to achieve a steady state. The specific therapeutic effectiveness is not evident until at least 4 to 10 days after institution of therapy. Consequently, lithium is not a good medication for the acutely agitated or manic patient but should be started early in anticipation of maintenance use. It is necessary to monitor the serum level of lithium, adequate levels for acute illness being in the range of 0.8 to 1.4 mEq per liter. For maintenance therapy, satisfactory responses accompany blood levels of 0.4 mEq per liter. Dose and blood level, however, should be titrated against clinical effectiveness for each patient. Once maintenance levels are reached patients usually can be maintained for long periods with minimal contact. Doses usually are given twice daily, as absorption from the gastrointestinal tract is rapid and the drug peaks in the serum within 1 to 2 hours. Serum lithium levels of more than 2 mEq per liter are highly dangerous and represent a medical emergency requiring immediate hospitalization and, sometimes, hemodialysis. Of most concern with regard to side effects in the long-term use of lithium is the development of mild leukocytosis, hypothyroidism, diabetes insipidus, and, occasionally, renal tubular damage. While these long-term side effects are not trivial, they are uncommon and must be weighed against the propensity of untreated patients to be chronically hospitalized. For patients who do not respond to lithium therapy or cannot tolerate it, increasingly encouraging reports describe the effective use of carbamazepine and other anticonvulsants in treating bipolar conditions.

The depressive phase of bipolar illness is treated the same as any major depressive disorder, as outlined previously.

Patients with bipolar disorders are often reluctant to continue with their medications, particularly lithium, as they feel it inhibits them, decreases their energy, or even affects their creativity. Consequently, a good deal of discussion about these issues is pertinent for the patient and especially for the family. The enlistment and assistance of the family of the patient with bipolar disorder are important. During either acute mania or severe depressive reactions, verbal interventions are often difficult, and it is useful simply to repeat some major reassuring statements—that they are a patient, that they are going to get better, and that this is not their normal state. While the role of precipitants is not clear in the onset of bipolar illness, it is important for patients to remain in treatment, and this can often be accomplished by helping them understand what situations seem to be stressful in their lives. Family and marital counseling often is useful.

PROGNOSIS. The more episodes a patient has had, the more likely he is to have another. Nevertheless, if one takes as indices of outcome successful marital and occupational adjustment, approximately two thirds of patients do well. About 15 per cent have some improvement, and the remainder do poorly. While manic or depressive episodes may cause much acute social disruption, including job loss and marital strife, the wide spacing of episodes often spares long-term social decay. Patients with bipolar disease usually function normally between episodes. Accordingly, a major goal of treatment is to protect the patient during episodes so as to minimize social disruption. Nevertheless, while the prognosis is not as devastating as in schizophrenia, it is still fraught with a significant amount of periodic and, sometimes, long-term functional disability.

Busse E, Blazer D: Geriatric Psychiatry. Washington, D.C., American Psychiatric Press, 1989. *An excellent and comprehensive review of geriatric psychiatry.*

Conte H, Plutchik R, Wild K, et al.: Combined psychotherapy and pharmacotherapy for depression. Arch Gen Psychiatry 43:471–480, 1986. *A good review of treatment of unipolar depression.*

Hodgkinson S, Sherrington R, Gurling H, et al.: Molecular genetic evidence for heterogeneity in manic depression. Nature 325:805, 1987. *Study of three large Icelandic kindreds indicates that although a single autosomal dominant allele predisposes to bipolar illness, linkage analysis does not incriminate the abnormal gene locus on chromosome 11. Genetic heterogeneity appears to underlie the expression of the manic-depressive phenotype.*

Katon W, Roy-Burne P: Antidepressants in the medically ill. Clin Chem 34:829–836, 1980. *A useful and necessary article for treating depressed medical patients.*

Michels R (ed.): Psychiatry. Philadelphia, J.B. Lippincott Company, 1985. *Excellent and detailed overview of affective disorders, especially with respect to treatment.*

Parkes CM, Weise RS: Recovery from Bereavement. New York, Basic Books, 1983. *Excellent summary of treatment of grief.*

Pfeffer CR: Clinical perspectives on treatment of suicidal behavior among children and adolescents. Psychiatr Ann 20:143–153, 1990. *An excellent general article on the management of suicidal behavior in children, adolescents, applicable to adults as well.*

Post RM, Ballenger J: Neurobiology of Mood Disorders. Baltimore, Williams & Wilkins, 1984. *A comprehensive overview of biologic and pharmacologic aspects of affective disorders.*

Shucter S, Zisook S.: Treatment of spousal bereavement. Psychiatr Ann 16:295–308, 1986. *An excellent discussion of treatment of bereavement.*

Simons A, Murphy G, Levine J, et al.: Cognitive therapy and pharmacotherapy for depression. Arch Gen Psychiatry 43:43–50, 1986. *A study of the use of cognitive therapy in depression.*

ANXIETY DISORDERS

Anxiety is the most ubiquitous psychiatric symptom. It occurs as part of most major psychiatric syndromes, particularly depressive ones, and represents several semidistinct entities. Anxiety also accompanies at least some aspects of most normal lives, and it can be an effective stimulus to improved performance. The performance curve follows an inverted U: A little anxiety can improve performance, performance then plateaus as the anxiety increases, and eventually too much anxiety causes a decrease in the ability to function. Currently, anxiety disorders are divided into two major categories: (1) panic disorders, which are episodic, "attack-like" symptoms; and (2) generalized anxiety disorder, which is a persistent state of anxiety.

Most patients with anxiety symptoms, including those with panic disorder, consult a general physician first. Such patients, who are extremely high users of medical services, usually complain vaguely that "something is wrong." A retrospective study of 55 patients with panic disorder referred for psychiatric consultation from primary care physicians revealed that 89 per cent initially presented with one or two somatic complaints and, in most, somatic misdiagnoses continued for months or years. The most frequent symptom patterns were (1) cardiac (chest pains, tachycardia, irregular heartbeat); (2) gastrointestinal (epigastric distress); and (3) neurologic (headache, dizziness/vertigo, syncope, or paresthesias). In a random survey of 195 patients in a primary care practice screened with structured interviews, 13 per cent met DSM-III criteria for panic disorder.

DIAGNOSTIC CRITERIA AND CLINICAL SIGNS AND SYMPTOMS. A panic attack produces a distinct symptomatic event. There is a precipitous sensation of feelings of fear, impending doom, or imminent death, accompanied by a potential host of physical symptoms (Table 451–11). Affected patients often complain of the physical symptoms in an agitated state. These circumstances differ markedly from chronic anxiety states, in which symptoms are more gradual and do not create life-threatening fears. Generalized anxiety disorder is a pervasive feeling of anxiety or "nervousness" that lacks the attack-like characteristics of panic disorder. The symptoms of generalized anxiety disorders are mainly muscle tension, autonomic hyperactivity, and apprehensive hypervigilant behavior.

A strong association links agoraphobia and panic attacks. Agoraphobia is defined as a morbid fear and avoidance of being alone or being in public places, resulting in a marked restriction of travel, often to the point of becoming housebound. In many cases the agoraphobia is secondary to panic attacks: The patient restricts activities for fear of having a panic attack and thereby develops an agoraphobic profile. Consequently, one looks for the presence of panic attacks or panic attack–like symptoms in patients with agoraphobia, as they often respond to the same treatment given for panic attacks. Simple phobias, e.g., fear of flying, heights, snakes, respond better to behavioral management than to drug treatment and are usually associated with generalized anxiety rather than panic-like episodes.

EPIDEMIOLOGY. Recent epidemiologic studies of panic disorder have noted a prevalence rate of 0.4 to 1.2 per 100. The rates are highest in persons aged 25 to 44 years and in the separated and divorced. The rates are lowest in persons over the age of 64 and bear no relationship to race or education. For agoraphobia the prevalence rates are between 2.5 and 5.8 per 100. There is a marked prevalence for women (two to four times that of men), with an age range of 18 to 64 years. The rates for generalized anxiety disorder range from 2.5 to 6.4 per 100, again slightly more common in young women. Genetic studies have shown that monozygotic twins have higher concordance for anxiety disorders than do dizygotic twins when the proband has panic disorder but not when he has a generalized anxiety disorder.

PATHOPHYSIOLOGY. Panic attacks can be precipitated in susceptible patients by sodium lactate infusions, caffeine (P.O.), CO_2 inhalation, yohimbine (P.O.), isoproterenol (I.V.), and benzodiazepine receptor antagonists. All of these agents interact with the noradrenergic system and particularly the locus coeruleus system, which contains most of the brain's noradrenergic cell bodies. Recent studies of cerebral blood flow and metabolism in patients with panic disorder show asymmetric changes in the parahippocampal region.

TREATMENT. There are two major treatments available for panic attacks, one pharmacologic, the other psychological. The key to treatment is the establishment of a supportive relationship with the patient. Affected patients are often frightened, concerned about "going crazy" and/or dying, and somewhat ashamed of the symptoms. It is useful for the physician immediately to reassure the patient by clarifying that what he experiences is part of a well-known illness that causes these feelings. It is often useful to educate patients with appropriate reading material.

Well-controlled studies have demonstrated the effective treatment of panic attacks with tricyclic antidepressants (particularly imipramine), MAOI's (particularly phenelzine), and the benzodiazepines (particularly alprazolam). The doses and treatment pattern of the tricyclics and the MAOI's are similar to those used for affective disorders, and the dose of alprazolam is usually between 4 and 6 mg per day.* At times the β-blocking agents offer relief, but they are not as dramatic and effective as the antidepressants and alprazolam. The doses of the antidepressants may need to be somewhat higher for these conditions than for affective disorders (tricyclics are usually used in the range of 150 to 300 mg; the MAOI's in the range of 60 mg or more per day— both higher than manufacturers' guidelines). Pharmacologic treatment should last for 6 months to 1 year after response, with the drugs then gradually tapered. β-Blocking agents can be useful for treating the tachycardia and palpitations associated with panic attacks. β Blockers can also be used to decrease the cardiac symptoms associated with tricyclic use, which is often reassuring to the patient.

The treatment of generalized anxiety disorders has less clear guidelines. Although benzodiazepines and psychological interventions are commonly emphasized, their benefit is more difficult to evaluate. A patient on benzodiazepines for 6 to 12 months may experience withdrawal symptoms on cessation of medication.

TABLE 451–11. PANIC DISORDER*

A. At some time during the disturbance, one or more panic attacks (discrete periods of intense discomfort or fear).

B. Either four attacks within a 4-week period, or one or more attacks were followed by a period of persistent fear of having another attack.

C. At least four of the following symptoms during the attacks:
  1. Shortness of breath (dyspnea) or smothering sensations
  2. Choking sensation
  3. Palpitations or accelerated heart rate (tachycardia)
  4. Chest pain or discomfort
  5. Sweating
  6. Dizziness, unsteady feelings, or faintness
  7. Nausea or abdominal distress
  8. Depersonalization or derealization
  9. Numbness or tingling sensations (paresthesias)
  10. Flushes (hot flashes) or chills
  11. Trembling or shaking
  12. Fear of dying
  13. Fear of going crazy or of doing something uncontrolled

D. An organic etiology (e.g., amphetamine or caffeine intoxication, hyperthyroidism) has been ruled out.

*Modified from American Psychiatric Association: Diagnostic and Statistical Manual of Mental Disorders, 3rd ed., rev. Washington, DC, APA, 1987. Used with permission.

*Exceeds manufacturer's recommended dosage.

Furthermore, one must be concerned and cautious about the addicting potential of the benzodiazepines and to some extent the tricyclics. Consequently, the treatment of generalized anxiety disorders should rely heavily on counseling, relaxation techniques, behavioral modification, exercise, etc., rather than on prolonged pharmacologic interventions.

Certain medical conditions can simulate panic attacks and must be excluded. These include arrhythmias, angina, respiratory illnesses, asthma, obstructive pulmonary disease, various endocrine disturbances (hyperthyroidism, pheochromocytoma), seizure disorders, vertiginous conditions, and pharmacologic stimulants and caffeine. Withdrawal syndromes can simulate panic-like states, particularly withdrawal from central nervous system depressants (e.g., barbiturates and, occasionally, benzodiazepines). Medical conditions that are often noted in patients with severe panic attacks include episodic hypertensive episodes, peptic ulcer disorder, and mitral valve prolapse.

Sequelae of the Vietnam conflict caused considerable interest on *post-traumatic stress disorders*. The basic differentiation of post-traumatic stress disorder from generalized anxiety disorder is the presence of a clear antecedent that is recognizable as potentially causing symptoms of distress in almost anyone. Another major characteristic of post-traumatic stress disorder is the feeling of re-experiencing the trauma, through either recurring or intrusive recollections, dreams, or sudden feelings that the event is about to recur. Patients often exhibit a lack of emotional responsiveness or involvement with the world after the trauma. Other symptoms may include hyperalertness, "startle responses," sleep disturbance, guilt, and memory and concentration difficulties. Affected persons may avoid activities that could evoke recollections of the traumatic event. While medications are sometimes useful for acute symptoms (especially if accompanied by panic attacks or depressive symptoms), the major treatment of post-traumatic stress is psychotherapeutic, particularly group sessions. At times narcosynthesis has been used successfully.

PROGNOSIS IN ANXIETY DISORDERS. The ubiquity of anxiety symptoms and the blurring of panic disorder into generalized anxiety or chronic anxiety and phobic states, as well as a strong association with depressive illness, make a prognosis difficult to establish. In general, panic disorder may run a limited course with episodic patterns; long periods of remission can intervene with no symptomatology at all. Only about one quarter of patients with panic disorder are treated, implying a high incidence of spontaneous remission in cases that do not come to medical attention. Nevertheless, many patients become housebound for a significant part of their lives. Follow-up studies of 5 to 20 years' duration show that about 50 to 60 per cent of the patients recovered or were much improved. Drug abuse and alcoholism are potentially serious complications.

Katon W, et al.: Chest pain: Relationships of psychiatric illness to coronary arteriographic results. Am J Med 84:1–9, 1988. *An excellent overview of the relation between anxiety and somatic symptoms.*

Klerman G (ed.): Update on anxiety and panic disorders. J Clinic Psychiatry, Supplement to Vol. 47, 1986. *This whole issue is an up-to-date review of all aspects of anxiety disorders, diagnosis, treatment, and research.*

Roy-Burne P, Katon W: An update of treatment of anxiety disorders. Hosp Commun Psychiatry 38:835–843, 1987. *A complete update of treatment.*

Sonnenberg S, Blank A, Talbott J: The Trauma of War. Washington DC, American Psychiatric Press, 1985. *A good review of current knowledge on post-traumatic stress disorder.*

SOMATIZATION DISORDERS

Somatization disorders consist of psychologically engendered symptoms suggesting organ dysfunction for which associated physical or laboratory dysfunction is either absent or trivial in relation to the degree of complaint. If physicians can find no clear biologic mechanism for a set of symptoms because they are too vague, diffuse, or disparate (or even anatomically impossible) and the symptoms could fulfill some purpose in the patient's life (e.g., would help to avoid some area of responsibility, deny failure, evoke increased attention by the family or others, etc.), they should have a high index of suspicion of a purely psychological disorder. However, these patients should not be treated lightly. Many vague symptoms arise early in organic disease, and patients must be examined carefully, supported, and followed. For example, among one group of 85 patients diagnosed as hysterical, 42 were given a diagnosis 10 years later of an organic

TABLE 451–12. COMMON FEATURES IN THE HISTORIES OF PATIENTS WITH SOMATIZATION SYMPTOMS

1. Developmental histories of gross neglect, child abuse, and/or sexual abuse
2. Unstable adult relationships characterized by multiple divorces and often physical violence
3. Past family histories of alcoholism
4. A past history of alcohol abuse prior to the start of somatization
5. Past history of substance abuse
6. A positive review of systems on medical history
7. A polysurgery history
8. A history of litigious relationships with authority figures
9. Past history of psychiatric illness
10. Modeling of pain behavior in their families as ways of solving problems and coping with intimate relationships

disease that could have explained their initial symptoms. In a similar manner patients with unfounded symptoms should also be evaluated for major depression and panic disorder, as those conditions can present primarily with somatic complaints. Patients who tend to present with somatization often have histories that are characterized by disturbed interpersonal relations and emotional disruptions (Table 451–12).

Diverse disorders can present with medically unfounded somatic symptoms, including such disparate conditions as somatization disorder (Briquet's syndrome), hypochondriasis, conversion disorder (hysteria), psychogenic pain disorders, factitious disorders, and malingering. What ties these conditions together are the following characteristics: (1) symptoms that suggest a physical disorder; (2) no demonstrable clinical signs or clear physiologic mechanism evident; (3) some evidence that the symptoms may be associated with psychological factors; (4) symptoms that do not seem to be under voluntary control (except in malingering and factitious disorder).

Somatization disorder, or Briquet's syndrome, has been studied in most detail and is a condition manifested by frequent and recurrent multiple somatic complaints, usually beginning before the age of 30.

DIAGNOSTIC CRITERIA AND CLINICAL SIGNS AND SYMPTOMS. If one looks at the diagnostic criteria for somatization disorder, the number and variety of somatic symptoms are impressive (Table 451–13). It is also evident from the range of these symptoms that patients meeting these criteria have all types of somatic symptoms, from conversion reactions to pain syndromes; it is the number of symptoms over time and their persistence that are important diagnostically. While the minor symptoms may seem common to everyone, they are reported

TABLE 451–13. SOMATIZATION DISORDER*

A. Many physical complaints or a belief that he or she has been sickly, for several years beginning before the age of 30.
B. At least 13 symptoms from the following list:
1. *Gastrointestinal symptoms*, e.g., vomiting (other than during pregnancy), abdominal pain (other than when menstruating), nausea (other than motion sickness), bloating (gassy), diarrhea, intolerance of (gets sick on) several different foods
2. *Pain symptoms* such as pain in extremities, back pain, joint pain, pain during urination, other pain (other than headaches)
3. *Cardiopulmonary symptoms*, e.g., shortness of breath when not exerting oneself, palpitations, chest pain, dizziness
4. *Conversion symptoms*, e.g., amnesia, difficulty swallowing, loss of voice, deafness, double vision, blurred vision, blindness, fainting or loss of consciousness, seizure or convulsion, trouble walking, paralysis or muscle weakness, urinary retention or difficulty urinating
5. *Psychosexual symptoms*, e.g., burning sensation in sexual organs or rectum (other than during intercourse), sexual indifference, pain during intercourse, impotence
6. *Female reproductive symptoms*, e.g., painful menstruation, irregular menstrual periods, excessive menstrual bleeding, vomiting throughout pregnancy

*Modified from American Psychiatric Association: Diagnostic and Statistical Manual of Mental Disorders, 3rd ed., rev. Washington, DC, APA, 1987. Used with permission.

with such vigor and intensity that the physician almost feels obligated to investigate them. This constellation of symptoms was described in 1859 by Briquet and has been confirmed over and over again, most convincingly in a series of studies by Guze in the early 1960's.

EPIDEMIOLOGY. The syndrome occurs mostly in females. About 1 per cent of the population is estimated to suffer from somatization disorder. The condition runs in families, but in males it correlates significantly with the occurrence of sociopathy and alcoholism rather than somatic symptoms.

PATHOPHYSIOLOGY. The condition is marked by an empiric collection of symptoms, the exact etiology and pathophysiology of which are not understood. Most patients come from a low education level and lack sophistication; however, there are many exceptions to this characterization. Most explanations have been sociologic and psychological and center on the somatization as a signal of personal distress. Consequently the behavior is often interpreted as a way to obtain help from caregivers or as a mechanism of obtaining social supports and, perhaps, manipulating relationships. It has also been postulated to represent a cognitive style whereby somatic symptoms are used in place of emotional expression.

TREATMENT. These patients are difficult to treat. Perhaps the most important factor should be the attempt to rule out depressive and panic disorders, as there is a high correlation of depressive symptomatology with many of these conditions. Patients with somatization disorders can make the physician feel that there is an urgent need to intervene; however, this temptation should be resisted. Careful evaluation of the history is extremely important for, as is evident, most of them do not respond to treatment. It is not that these patients enjoy their pain but that they are seeking other things, e.g., attention, relief from other problems. Perhaps the most important thing the physician can convey to patients is that they will neither seriously worsen nor die, and although the physician may not know the cause of the complaint he is willing to see them through the illness episode. In fact, it is almost paradoxic that by scheduling these patients for frequent regular visits the physician often not only saves time but may decrease the patient's need to develop symptoms in order to be seen. After one becomes certain of the diagnosis and of the absence of a pathologic process, the diagnostic workup should be kept to a minimum, as the more the physician investigates the more the patient becomes convinced that something is wrong. There is a tendency to dispense medications to these patients, and one of the complications is not only addiction but such a confusion and plethora of drugs that they become a cause of untoward symptoms. The major goal of treatment should be to keep to a minimum the medical and surgical interventions. A general attempt should be made to substitute inquiry into the patient's life as opposed to procedures. A helpful attitude on the part of the physician is that he is more interested in maintaining the relationship than in curing the symptoms and that a successful outcome is the reduction in the number of physicians the patient sees and medications prescribed.

In summary, treatment of these difficult patients should include (1) recognizing the disorder; (2) listening to the patient to determine what has been helpful or harmful in the past; (3) defining a clear contract for continued supervision with no assurances for dramatic cure (or attempts at dramatic intervention beyond what the symptoms warrant). The scheduling of visits can be based on the frequency of visits over the past 2- to 3-month period; (4) empathizing with patients about their suffering, avoiding statements such as "It's all in your head" or "There is nothing wrong with you"; (5) openly discussing the risks of too much medical intervention and avoiding opiates and benzodiazepines owing to their potential for abuse. Tests should be ordered on the basis of objective symptoms, not just complaints; and (6) expecting a long-term relationship with slow improvement.

PROGNOSIS. Somatization disorders are more a way of life than a discrete episodic illness. The patient maintains a propensity for expression of emotional need or distress with somatic symptoms. While the episodes may wax and wane, it is clear that these patients are wedded to the medical establishment.

Other Conditions Associated with Somatic Symptoms

Somatization disorder has been extensively studied, but there are other conditions that are similar to somatization disorder that can be confusing to the physician. Although the term *hysteria* has been dropped from official use and such conditions are now termed *conversion reactions*, such patients present commonly to physicians and make up about 1 per cent of a neurologist's practice. The predominant disturbance in conversion disorder is a loss or alteration in physical functioning suggesting a physical disorder. Often the loss or distortion of neurologic function is not fully explained by any known disease process as determined by physical and laboratory examination. Much of what has been covered with regard to somatization disorder is true of hysterical conditions. These patients do not necessarily have histrionic personalities (overly dramatic, attention seeking, shallow manipulative relationships, etc.). They do have physical complaints, but when examined closely their symptoms conform more to a psychological than a physiologic reaction.

Hypochondriasis is often simple to recognize in that the patient presents with a belief that a disease is present for which diagnosis and treatment are necessary. The complaints are more circumscribed, with often minute examination and description of bodily functions to the physician. As the physician talks to the patient he becomes increasingly aware that the patient is more concerned about the belief of illness than the discomfort from symptoms. In fact, the symptoms are not especially distressing or painful. This is in marked contrast to the patient with chronic pain whose pain is often out of proportion to the physical findings.

In patients with chronic pain, the continuation of the pain often allows the avoidance of activities in the patient's life or the obtaining of emotional or financial support from others. Affected patients frequently have histories of addiction, seeing many physicians, and undergoing multiple surgical procedures.

The genesis of many of the above conditions lies at an involuntary level in that the symptoms and the motivation for them are not in the control of the patient. Two conditions, factitious disorder and malingering, are voluntarily controlled by the patient. These patients, often described as having *Munchausen's syndrome*, induce illnesses in themselves, e.g., fevers (by injection), dermatitis, blood disease (anemia), or seizures. Affected patients are often associated with the health professions, and one can discern no clear goal or gain from their behavior. They frequently are peripatetic, traveling from hospital to hospital. When a factitious disorder is diagnosed, these patients should be confronted openly as to their behavior and what treatment (as some may be necessary) will be provided and not provided. In true malingering, the goal of the illness behavior is often evident (or evident after extensive inquiry), and the condition is usually less a chronic than a factitious disorder. In most cases we see partial malingering, in which an individual exaggerates symptoms of a real disease or attributes a voluntarily induced disability to an accident or injury. In both these conditions there is a tendency to be angry with the patient, but it is best to confront him about the situation in a nonjudgmental rather than an angry manner. Particularly when compensation issues surround the case, treatment is pointless until any legal questions or damage awards are settled.

Katon W, Egan K, Miller D: Chronic pain: Lifetime psychiatric diagnosis and family history. Am J Psychiatry 142:1156–1160, 1985. *An interesting study of the relationship between pain syndromes and psychiatric problems.*

Lipsitt P: Medical and psychologic characteristics of "crocks." Psychiatry Med 1:15–25, 1970. *Still one of the best discussions of the management of patients with many somatic complaints.*

Marsden CD: Hysteria—A neurologist's view. Psychol Med 16:277–288, 1986. *An excellent review of hysteria.*

Quill T: Somatization disorder. JAMA 254:3075–3079, 1985. *A good discussion of the physician's role in the treatment of patients with somatic disorder.*

Ries R, Balcon J, Katon W: The medical abuser: Differential diagnosis and management. J Fam Pract 3:257–265, 1981. *Good differential diagnosis of somatic complaints.*

Slater E, Glithero E: A followup of patients diagnosed as suffering from "hysteria." J Psychosomatic Res 9:9–13, 1965. *A classic article discussing the potential hazards in the diagnosis of hysteria.*

Smith R, Mouson RA, Ray DC: Psychiatric consultation in somatization disorders. N Engl J Med 314:1407–1413, 1986. *Emphasizes the importance of diagnosis of somatization.*

SECTION THREE/PATHOPHYSIOLOGY AND MANAGEMENT OF MAJOR NEUROLOGIC SYMPTOMS

452 Autonomic Disorders and Their Management

Clifford B. Saper

The autonomic nervous system consists of collections of nerve cell bodies (ganglia) associated with the cranial and spinal nerves that innervate all of the internal organs and contribute to the regulation of their function. Disorders of the autonomic nervous system are of great importance to internal medicine, as they can present as disorders of virtually any organ system in the body. Furthermore, the central regulation of autonomic response is closely tied to neuroendocrine control, and both are often involved by central disorders. Aspects of neuroendocrine disease are discussed in Ch. 209, 211 to 215, and 229. This chapter focuses on disorders of the autonomic nervous system (Table 452–1) and discusses them in the overall context of diseases affecting basic integrative functions of the nervous system.

DISORDERS OF PERIPHERAL AUTONOMIC FUNCTION

Organization of Peripheral Autonomic Regulation

The peripheral autonomic nervous system consists of three main divisions. The *parasympathetic* division includes the outflow from the cranial nerves and the low lumbar and sacral spinal cord. The cholinergic preganglionic fibers synapse upon cholinergic ganglion cells that are located in or near the tissues that are innervated. The *sympathetic* division comprises the autonomic outflow from the thoracic and high lumbar segments of the spinal cord. Cholinergic preganglionic fibers end in paravertebral or prevertebral ganglia upon noradrenergic or in some

cases cholinergic ganglion cells and also innervate the adrenal medulla. Postganglionic fibers may travel a considerable distance with various peripheral nerves to innervate their target tissues. The *enteric* nervous system includes neurons, many cholinergic, that are intrinsic to the wall of the gut. These neurons form an independent network that is loosely under the control of the other two divisions of the autonomic nervous system. Neurons in all three divisions of the autonomic nervous system commonly employ a wide variety of peptide neuromodulators. Under specific physiologic conditions, these peptides may enhance or suppress the activity induced by the primary neurotransmitter. In some cases, different functions in a peripheral tissue may be subserved by different transmitters released by the same set of neurons (e.g., in the salivary gland, parasympathetically mediated secretion is caused by acetylcholine, but the concomitant vasodilatation is due to vasoactive intestinal peptide).

Knowledge about the different neurotransmitter and receptor types associated with the peripheral autonomic nervous system has resulted in the availability of a wide range of drugs to modify autonomic responses. Some key autonomic drugs and their clinical uses are listed in Table 452–2. These are covered in detail in clinical pharmacology texts.

Pandysautonomias

ACUTE PANDYSAUTONOMIA. Widespread failure of the autonomic nervous system may evolve acutely or subacutely as part of a parainfectious inflammatory polyneuropathy (of the Guillain-Barré type). In rare cases, the autonomic neuropathy predominates. In most patients, however, the autonomic changes are easily overlooked, as the clinical course is dominated by motor paralysis. In severe cases, once the patient is intubated and artificially ventilated, the autonomic neuropathy becomes the chief life-threatening complication. Wide swings in blood

TABLE 452–1. DISORDERS OF THE AUTONOMIC NERVOUS SYSTEM

Peripheral Autonomic Disorders	Genitourinary disorders
Pandysautonomias	Incontinence
Acute pandysautonomia	Urinary retention
Tetanus	Spastic bladder
Chronic autonomic neuropathy	Impotence
Familial dysautonomia	**Disorders of Central Autonomic Integration**
Idiopathic autonomic insufficiency (Shy-Drager	Emotional disorders
syndrome)	Panic disorder
Regional dysautonomia	Psychosomatic illness
Horner's syndrome	Cardiac arrhythmias
Paraspinal tumors	Thermoregulatory disorders
Somatosympathetic dysreflexia	Poikilothermia
Reflex sympathetic dystrophy (causalgia)	Paroxysmal hypothermia
Disorders of specific autonomic functions	Hyperthermia and fever
Pupillary disorders	Malignant hyperthermia
Horner's syndrome	Feeding disorders
Oculomotor paresis	Hyperphagia and obesity
Cardiovascular disorders	Hypophagia and inanition
Glossopharyngeal neuralgia	Disorders of fluid and electrolyte regulation
Carotid sinus hypersensitivity	Hypernatremia, hyperosmolality, and absence of thirst
Sweating disorders	Hyperdipsia, hyponatremia, and water intoxication
Hyperhidrosis	Paroxysmal hyponatremia
Anhidrosis	Central reproductive disorders
Gastrointestinal disorders	Arousal disorders
Disorders of motility	Hypersomnolence
Vomiting	Insomnia

TABLE 452–2. SYSTEMIC EFFECTS OF SOME COMMONLY USED AUTONOMIC DRUGS

Receptor Type	Drug Type (Example)	Tissue	Effect
Muscarinic cholinergic	Antagonist (atropine)	Pupil	Mydriasis
		Salivary gland	Dry mouth
		Bronchi	Dilation
		Heart	Tachycardia
		Gut	Decreased motility and secretion
α-Adrenergic	Antagonist (phenoxybenzamine)	Blood vessels	Vasodilation
α_1-Adrenergic	Agonist (phenylephrine)	Blood vessels	Vasoconstriction
	Antagonist (prazocin)	Blood vessels	Vasodilation
α_2-Adrenergic	Agonist (clonidine)	Blood vessels	Vasoconstriction
β-Adrenergic	Agonist (isoproterenol)	Heart	Increased rate and contractility
β_1-Adrenergic	Antagonist (metoprolol)	Heart	Decreased rate and contractility
β_2-Adrenergic	Agonist (terbutaline)	Bronchi	Dilation

pressure and heart rate occur but usually reverse themselves in a few minutes. Generally, putting the patient into the Trendelenberg position is sufficient to maintain cerebral perfusion during hypotensive periods. Cardiac arrhythmias of all types may occur, presumably as a result of the instability of autonomic innervation of the cardiac conducting system. These must be treated gingerly, as the underlying conduction abnormality may change very rapidly.

TETANUS. A similar subacute pandysautonomia is also seen in severe cases of tetanus. Tetanus toxin, elaborated by *Clostridium tetani* organisms in an infected wound, is transported by autonomic as well as motor axons back to the spinal cord, where it is taken up by and inactivates the terminals of inhibitory interneurons. Treatment of the motor manifestations of tetanus by paralyzing and sedating the patient does little to abate the autonomic storm. Up to 40 per cent of patients with tetanus in an intensive care environment may suffer cardiac arrest as a result of arrhythmias. They are generally easily resuscitated with standard measures.

CHRONIC AUTONOMIC NEUROPATHY. The axons of the peripheral autonomic nervous system generally are of small caliber and poorly myelinated or unmyelinated. Certain polyneuropathies that have a predilection for small-diameter axons can result in autonomic changes. *Amyloid neuropathy,* for example, often includes a major autonomic component that may present as a gastrointestinal motility disorder or orthostatic hypotension. Similarly, *diabetic neuropathy,* although it is often dominated by sensory or motor complaints, may cause widespread autonomic failure. The neuropathy of *acute intermittent porphyria* and certain toxic agents, such as *Vacar* (a rat poison), may have a prominent autonomic component. Acute poisoning with *organophosphate insecticides* that block acetylcholinesterase results in a hypercholinergic state, including miosis and cardiac slowing, that lasts for several days. The neuropathy that follows several weeks later usually does not have a strong autonomic component. Other peripheral neuropathies that may have an autonomic component are listed in Table 452–3.

CHRONIC DYSAUTONOMIA. Recessively inherited *familial dysautonomia* of the Riley-Day type is most commonly seen in

TABLE 452–3. PERIPHERAL NEUROPATHIES THAT MAY HAVE AN AUTONOMIC COMPONENT

Autonomic symptoms often prominent	Arsenic
	Mercury
Guillain-Barré syndrome	Organic solvents
Amyloid neuropathy	Acrylamide
Diabetic neuropathy	Vasculitis
Acute intermittent porphyria	Systemic lupus erythematosus
Vacar (rat poison)	Rheumatoid arthritis
Autonomic symptoms may occur	Mixed connective tissue disease
Renal failure	Thiamine deficiency
Toxic neuropathies	Leprosy
Vinca alkaloids	Charcot-Marie-Tooth disease
Perhexiline maleate	Fabry's disease
Thallium	

Ashkenazi Jewish children. Symptoms referable to the autonomic nervous system and relative indifference to pain are present from birth.

Idiopathic autonomic insufficiency of the *Shy-Drager* type may develop as a chronic degenerative condition in middle age or late adult life. The presenting complaint is often orthostatic hypotension, but signs or symptoms of pupillary, gastrointestinal, genitourinary, sweating, or other autonomic abnormalities are elicited on history and physical examination. A summary of tests of the autonomic nervous system is presented in Table 452–4. Idiopathic autonomic insufficiency is part of a spectrum of disorders, ranging from isolated orthostatic hypotension, with or without parkinsonian features, to *multisystem atrophy* with evidence of cerebellar and extrapyramidal involvement. At autopsy, degenerative changes may be seen in the autonomic ganglia as well as in the preganglionic cell groups in the medulla and the spinal cord. Additional cell loss is seen in other affected areas in multisystem atrophy.

Idiopathic autonomic insufficiency is distinguished from nonneurologic causes of orthostatic hypotension by the lack of compensatory tachycardia, indicating impairment of either the peripheral or central components of the baroreceptor reflex. Severe autonomic neuropathy affecting the glossopharyngeal or vagus nerves may also impair the baroreceptor response but is typically associated with other evidence of sensory or motor neuropathy. Other cardiovascular signs include loss of sinus arrhythmia and absence of normal overshoot in the diastolic blood pressure during phase IV of the Valsalva maneuver. An abnormally accentuated blood pressure response to intravenous infusion of norepinephrine is consistent with widespread denervation supersensitivity.

Pupils are often small and poorly responsive to light. Pharmacologic testing (Table 452–4) can determine whether the deficit is central or peripheral. Sweating impairment also may be either of central or peripheral origin. Absence of axon reflex sweating indicates a peripheral lesion. Gastrointestinal impairment may include diarrhea, constipation, incontinence, or abdominal pains. There may also be urinary hesitancy, urgency, or incontinence or impotence in men.

Orthostatic hypotension is generally the most disabling aspect of autonomic degeneration. Indomethacin may be effective in selected patients. Other patients require elastic stockings or even entire lower body suits to reduce blood pooling in the lower extremities during standing. Treatment with mineralocorticoids, such as fludrocortisone, can expand intravascular blood volume and cause elevation of blood pressure in all positions. In such patients, the head of the bed should be elevated in recumbency to minimize hypertensive effects on the brain. Occasionally, oral sympathomimetic agents, such as ephedrine, or monoamine oxidase inhibitors are employed. The latter must be used with caution, as the ingestion of vasoactive amines present in many common foods, including certain wines, cheeses, pickled foods, and smoked meats, can cause severe hypertension.

When idiopathic autonomic insufficiency is associated with a multisystem neurologic degenerative disease, it may be accompanied by ataxia, rigidity, bradykinesia, tremors, weakness, or other neurologic disturbances.

The segmental organization of the sympathetic nervous system can result in regional disturbances of function. The most common of these is caused by injury to the cranial sympathetic innervation arising from the superior cervical ganglion, or *Horner's syndrome*. Miosis, ptosis, and anhydrosis may occur if the ascending sympathetic fibers are injured below the level at which they enter the skull with the internal carotid artery. Damage to sympathetic fibers along the course of the intracranial carotid artery produces only oculosympathetic paresis (Raeder's syndrome). Unfortunately, this difference is only of marginal value clinically, as the Horner's syndrome produced by extracranial lesions is often incomplete. Lesions of the central descending sympathoexcitatory pathway, running through the lateral portions of the brain stem from the hypothalamus to the spinal cord, may produce a central Horner's syndrome, in which there is miosis and ptosis as well as loss of sweating over the entire ipsilateral body. Postganglionic Horner's syndrome can be differentiated from preganglionic or central lesions by pharmacologic testing (Table 452–4). The most common cause of Horner's syndrome is atherosclerotic disease affecting the vasa nervorum originating in the carotid artery. However, Horner's syndrome may also be seen when an intrathoracic or cervical tumor involves the sympathetic chain. Hence, evaluation of Horner's syndrome should include radiographic or magnetic resonance examination of the pulmonary apices and paracervical area.

Paraspinal tumors at lower levels along the sympathetic chain may cause loss of sweating over the involved dermatomes. This deficit can be appreciated by running the handle of a tuning fork down the skin in the paraspinal region. The smooth movement is interrupted by the dry skin at the level of the lesion. Occasionally, compression of a midthoracic spinal root, which carries visceral sensory fibers, by a disc or tumor may present as abdominal pain.

Stimulation of pain fibers at any level results in both local (spino-spinal) and generalized (spino-bulbo-spinal) *somatosympathetic reflex responses*, including sweating, vasoconstriction, and pupillodilatation. In patients with a pre-existing spinal cord transection, a noxious stimulus below the level of the transection may produce only local sympathetic reflex responses. Hence it is important in the paraplegic patient to investigate asymmetric sympathetic responses for a local lesion that might cause pain in an intact individual.

Following injury to peripheral nerves, aberrant regeneration may result in *reflex sympathetic dystrophy*. It is believed that the sympathetic efferent fibers form excitatory synapses along the course of damaged peripheral sensory nerves. Normally innocuous sensory stimulation, such as covering the affected limb with a sheet or with clothing, may cause excruciating burning pain, associated with variable autonomic changes. Atrophic changes in the skin and bone may reflect abnormal sympathetic innervation or disuse. Relief can sometimes be obtained with guanethidine or phenoxybenzamine. If regional sympathetic block alleviates pain, removal of the affected ganglion can produce permanent relief.

Disorders of Specific Autonomic Functions

PUPILS. Anisocoria, asymmetry of pupillary size, may reflect a deficit of sympathetic innervation of the smaller pupil (causing miosis) or parasympathetic innervation of the larger one (causing mydriasis). As both the oculosympathetic and oculomotor (parasympathetic) innervations participate in lid elevation, ptosis if present generally indicates the abnormal eye. Anisocoria may be longstanding and of little clinical significance, but pupillary asymmetry of recent onset should be evaluated by a neurologist. Impairment of sympathetic innervation of the iris (pupillodilator) muscle is not always accompanied by ptosis or a sweating deficit (Horner's syndrome). The pupilloconstrictor fibers travel in the dorsomedial part of the oculomotor nerve, where they may be selectively affected by temporal lobe herniation or by an aneurysm of the posterior communicating artery. Pharmacologic testing may aid in the identification of the pupillary abnormality (Table 452–4). The most common cause of a large pupil is instillation of atropinic eye drops or application of a scopolamine patch near the face (to prevent motion sickness); the pharmacologically dilated pupil does not respond even to strong solutions of pilocarpine. Another common cause of a large, poorly reactive pupil is *Adie's syndrome*, an idiopathic condition involving degeneration of the ciliary ganglion. The pupil usually shows sector paralysis and constriction with accommodation, and it dilates and responds to light after a period in complete darkness. The abnormal pupil responds briskly to 0.1 per cent pilocarpine (Table 452–4), and there is concomitant loss of tendon reflexes in most cases.

CARDIOVASCULAR. The baroreceptor reflex is an important protective response, causing bradycardia and peripheral vasodilatation to counteract an acute increase in blood pressure, or the

TABLE 452–4. TESTS OF AUTONOMIC FUNCTION*

Test	Interpretation
Pupillary responses	
4% cocaine	Pupillodilatation indicates release of normal catecholamine stores.
1% hydroxyamphetamine	
1% phenylephrine	Pupillodilatation indicates denervation supersensitivity.
0.1% epinephrine	
0.1% pilocarpine	Pupilloconstriction indicates denervation supersensitivity.
2.5% methacholine	
Sweating responses	
Thermal sweating	Regional absence of sweating indicates sympathetic cholinergic denervation.
Galvanic skin response	Increased conductivity under mild stress indicates normal adrenergic innervation.
1:1000 pilocarpine	Intradermal injection causes axon reflex sweating.
1:10,000 acetylcholine	
Axon reflex	
1:1000 histamine	Intradermal injection normally causes wheal and flare.
Cardiovascular responses	
Orthostatic challenge	Pulse normally increases and diastolic blood pressure falls <15 mm Hg.
Carotid sinus massage	Normally causes fall in blood pressure and heart rate.
R-R interval	Normally increases during inspiration (sinus arrhythmia).
Valsalva maneuver	Longest to shortest R-R interval ratio normally is ≥ 1.4.
Cold pressor test	Immersing hand in ice water normally increases blood pressure and heart rate.
Plasma catecholamines	Normally increase response to standing or stress.
Norepinephrine infusion 0.05 µg/kg/min	Diastolic blood pressure increase ≥ 20 mm Hg indicates supersensitivity.
Genitourinary, rectal responses	
Cremasteric reflex	Stroking skin of thigh normally causes testicular retraction.
Anal wink reflex	Scratching perianal skin normally causes anal sphincter contraction.
Bulbocavernosus reflex	Squeezing glans penis or clitoris normally causes anal contraction.

*For details see McLeod and Tuck, 1987.

reverse response during hypotension. The afferent fibers for the response run in the glossopharyngeal (carotid sinus) and vagus (aortic depressor) nerves, while the efferent response includes both parasympathetic and sympathetic components. Injury to the glossopharyngeal or carotid sinus nerves in the neck (often by a tumor) can cause episodic attacks of hypotension and bradycardia, which often present as syncope. In most cases, there is an associated pain or paresthesia in the cutaneous distribution of the glossopharyngeal nerve (in the external auditory meatus or the pharynx), known as *glossopharyngeal neuralgia*. The situation is analogous to tic doloreaux, in which there are intermittent volleys of firing in the affected nerve. Atropine or a transvenous pacemaker may prevent the bradycardia associated with the attacks, but loss of vasoconstrictor tone sometimes results in symptomatic hypotension despite these maneuvers. Anticonvulsants, particularly phenytoin and carbamazepine, may prevent the attacks.

Carotid sinus syncope (see Ch. 446) is a condition seen most commonly in elderly individuals with carotid atherosclerosis. Even mild pressure over the carotid bulb, such as a tight shirt collar, can produce a full-blown carotid sinus response, resulting in syncope. The diagnosis is made by gently compressing the carotid artery below the angle of the jaw while the electrocardiogram (ECG) is monitored. Facilities for cardiac resuscitation must be immediately available, as the compression may result in sinus arrest. Vigorous massage should be avoided, as it may dislodge an embolus, resulting in a transient or even permanent neurologic deficit. Treatment of carotid sinus hypersensitivity is the same as that for glossopharyngeal neuralgia.

SWEATING. Human sweat glands are innervated by both noradrenergic sympathetic fibers (mediating emotional responses) and cholinergic sympathetic fibers (thermal sweating). Certain somatosympathetic reflexes can produce generalized or regional sweating, in response to innocuous or noxious somatosensory stimuli. *Paroxysmal localized hyperhidrosis* is a rare condition that probably represents an exaggeration of normal somatosympathetic reflexes. Generalized hyperhidrosis, particularly involving the hands and the soles of the feet, is most likely a normal variant. Drugs directed at interrupting α-adrenergic transmission (phenoxybenzamine, clonidine) have been useful in some cases of localized hyperhidrosis. In extreme cases, regional sympathectomy has been performed.

Idiopathic anhydrosis may be segmental or generalized. This rare condition is sometimes associated with Adie's syndrome (Ross syndrome), but in other cases there are no other signs of autonomic impairment. In some cases the impairment is preganglionic and in others postganglionic, as judged by the axon reflex sweating response (Table 452–4). In most recorded patients, the deficits have been stable and did not go on to involve other autonomic functions.

GASTROINTESTINAL. Disorders of intestinal motility, which may be due to damage to the parasympathetic innervation of the gut or to dysfunction of the enteric nervous system itself, are discussed in Chapter 100. Specific abnormalities of esophageal contraction and colonic tone have been noted in patients suffering from depression and may predict response to antidepressant medication.

Vomiting is a neurally mediated gastrointestinal reflex that is coordinated by neurons in the medullary reticular formation. Chemical emetic agents such as certain narcotics or dopaminergic agonists act at the area postrema, a chemosensory zone on the fourth ventricular surface of the medulla, to elicit the vomiting reflex. Local dopaminergic connections are thought to mediate the response, and antidopaminergic drugs such as prochlorperazine may act at the level of the area postrema to suppress vomiting. Intractable vomiting without any gastrointestinal abnormalities has been reported in certain patients with tumors involving the medullary cell groups controlling vomiting or their connections. Treatment of the tumor with steroids and radiation therapy generally results in improvement.

GENITOURINARY. The urinary bladder is composed of interlacing smooth muscle fibers of the detrusor covered by an internal mucous membrane and an outer serosa. The detrusor is innervated by parasympathetic neurons whose preganglionic cell bodies are located in the intermediolateral column at the second through fourth sacral segments. Parasympathetic fibers travel through the pelvic plexus and nerve. Additional motor neurons located in the ventral horn at the same levels constitute Onuf's nucleus. Their axons run through the pelvic nerve to innervate striated accessory muscles of micturition (including the external urethral sphincter) in the pelvic floor. Neurons of Onuf's nucleus are strikingly preserved in motor neuron disease but are lost along with autonomic preganglionic cells in idiopathic autonomic insufficiency. The internal sphincter at the bladder neck is innervated via the hypogastric nerve by sympathetic prevertebral pelvic ganglia whose preganglionic innervation arises from the intermediolateral column at the T12–L1 level.

During bladder filling the intravesical pressure remains relatively constant as a result of sympathetically mediated relaxation of the detrusor muscle and inhibition of parasympathetic tone in response to bladder stretch sensation. Bladder relaxation during filling and subsequent coordination of micturition are under the control of Barrington's nucleus, located in the floor of the fourth ventricle at the pontine level. Brain stem control of micturition is, in turn, under voluntary regulation by areas within the cerebral sensory and motor cortex lying along the medial wall of the cerebral hemisphere. When bladder fullness is sensed and the environmental conditions are appropriate, micturition is initiated by Barrington's nucleus, under forebrain control. There is a fall in external sphincter pressure, resulting in reflex relaxation of the internal sphincter and contraction of the bladder.

Forebrain impairment results in loss of voluntary control of micturition but does not otherwise affect the complex sensory and motor program that results in normal voiding. Incontinence in such patients can be managed by using adult diapers or external urinary collection devices without risk of frequent urinary tract infections or damage to the upper urinary tract. Injury to the bulbospinal pathway from Barrington's nucleus to the sacral intermediolateral column, however, causes major disruption of coordinated bladder function. Acutely following spinal cord injury there is a period of spinal shock, during which the bladder does not undergo reflex contraction as it fills. The bladder may overfill, overstretching the muscular wall, and elevation of bladder pressure above 40 mm H_2O can result in hydronephrosis. Such patients require urinary catheterization to prevent vesical and renal damage.

One to 2 weeks following injury, spinal reflex control of the bladder returns. Some patients can induce reflex bladder emptying by somatosensory stimulation, such as stroking the skin over the thigh. The spastic bladder reflexively contracts at a lower volume and, because detrusor action is not coordinated with sphincter opening, rarely empties completely. Postvoid residual urine in excess of 25 to 50 ml is an important sign of impairment of supraspinal pathways controlling the bladder. Injury to sensory nerves supplying the bladder also may cause overfilling and incomplete emptying, indicating the importance of sensory feedback in bladder control. Patients with significant postvoid residual urine are at increased risk for urinary tract infections, but bladder overfilling with elevated pressures may ultimately be a greater problem. It is important to monitor bladder pressure in such patients with cystometrography. Elevations in pressure above 40 mm H_2O may require continuous or intermittent catheterization to prevent damage to the upper urinary tract.

Pharmacologic intervention, aimed at augmenting or suppressing autonomic motor responses of the bladder or internal sphincter, cannot reconstitute the coordinated control of the different components of the lower urinary tract. Bethanacol, a cholinergic agonist, is used to augment bladder contraction to improve emptying. It is most effective in combination with an α-adrenergic blocker, such as phenoxybenzamine or prazocin, that simultaneously reduces pressure of the internal sphincter. Baclofen may be used to decrease spastic contraction of the external sphincter. Drugs that have atropinic properties, including a surprising variety of antiarrhythmic, antihistamine, neuroleptic, and antidepressant medications, may inhibit bladder contraction, resulting in overfilling and urinary retention (Table 452–5).

Erectile function in males is under parasympathetic control by the same sacral levels as the urinary system. Sensory afferent fibers travel via the pudendal nerve, while parasympathetic motor fibers run in the pelvic nerve. Sympathetic innervation via the

TABLE 452–5. SOME COMMONLY PRESCRIBED DRUGS THAT MAY IMPAIR URINARY FUNCTION

Antiarrhythmics	Chlorpromazine	Dopa/carbidopa
Atropine	Antidepressants	Bromocriptine
Diisopyramide	Amitriptyline	Benztropine
Antihistamines	Imipramine	Trihexiphenidyl
Diphenhydramine	Antiparkinsonian agents	Antispasmodics
Neuroleptics	Amantadine	Baclofen
Haloperidol		

hypogastric nerve contracts the seminal vesicles during ejaculation and closes the bladder neck to prevent retrograde emission. Although supraspinal influences are of great importance, reflex erection and ejaculation can occur in patients after spinal injury. Neurogenic impotence can result either from damage to descending pathways relaying forebrain influence from the hypothalamus to the sacral preganglionic neurons or from injury to the sensory or parasympathetic motor innervation of the penis. A variety of drugs that block either parasympathetic or sympathetic function can interfere with erectile function (Table 452–6). As erections normally occur several times nightly during periods of rapid eye movement sleep, it is possible to document organic disorders of erection by measuring penile tumescence overnight. Disorders of male sexual dysfunction are considered in Ch. 222.

DISORDERS OF INTEGRATIVE CONTROL OF THE AUTONOMIC NERVOUS SYSTEM

ORGANIZATION OF CENTRAL AUTONOMIC AND ENDOCRINE REGULATION. The autonomic nervous system is under three levels of central control. The *preganglionic* neurons located in the medulla and the spinal cord provide the final common pathway for central autonomic control. Each of these neurons integrates the inputs from many sources, including afferents from higher levels of the nervous system and local reflex responses. A series of *brain stem and spinal* cell groups coordinates *reflex control* of the autonomic nervous system. These nuclei receive cranial (parasympathetic) and spinal (sympathetic) afferent information and control a variety of important reflexes (e.g., swallowing, maintaining blood pressure, initiation of voiding). Both the preganglionic neurons and the brain stem reflex neurons are under the control of *forebrain integrative* cell groups that coordinate autonomic function with behavior and with endocrine control.

The hypothalamus is the most important area for integration of behavior with autonomic responses and with neuroendocrine control of the anterior and posterior pituitary glands (Fig. 452–1). Because the hypothalamus consists of tightly packed, interwoven pathways and cell groups, it is unusual for an injury to involve selectively a single functional system. Nevertheless, considerable progress has been made in determining the anatomic substrates for specific integrative functions, and disorders of these systems are occasionally encountered (Table 452–7). In addition, autonomic dysfunction is a frequent concomitant of emotional disorders.

Emotional Disorders

Portions of the insular and cingulate areas of the cerebral cortex and the amygdala are believed to regulate autonomic responses to emotional stress. In healthy individuals, stress can induce sympathetic responses, such as pupillodilatation, dry mouth, and increases in blood pressure. In patients with *panic disorder* (see Ch. 451), such autonomic responses can become overwhelming and convince the patient that there is a serious organic problem.

TABLE 452–6. SOME COMMONLY PRESCRIBED DRUGS THAT MAY IMPAIR ERECTILE FUNCTION

Drugs causing impotence		Drugs causing priapism
Parasympatholytics	Propranolol	Chlorpromazine
Atropine	Prazocin	Thioridazine
Amitriptyline	Vasodilators	Trazadone
Sympatholytics	Hydralazine	Prazocin
Methyldopa	Diuretics	Dopa/carbidopa
Guanethidine	Hydrochlorothiazide	
Clonidine	Antihistaminergic	
	Cimetidine	

PET studies show increased metabolism in the structures of the medial temporal lobe and the insular cortex during panic attacks. After eliminating the possibility of pheochromocytoma (see Ch. 229), anxiolytic or antidepressant drugs are usually found helpful.

In some individuals under chronic emotional stress, a variety of syndromes are seen implicating autonomic control of the internal organs. While *psychosomatic illness* is often thought to be nonorganic and may respond to psychotherapeutic drugs, there is considerable evidence that some organic disorders that are seen in anxious patients also may be caused by autonomic dysregulation. For example, swallowing disorders often represent abnormal control of peristalsis. Erosive gastritis and even frank ulceration may occur as a result of autonomic dysfunction. Perhaps the most serious problems are encountered in patients with pre-existing cardiac abnormalities, who may have cardiac arrhythmias under stressful conditions. Retrospective studies of victims of sudden death due to lethal ventricular arrhythmias indicate a much higher incidence of behavioral stress in the period preceding the attack. The protective effect of β-adrenergic blockers against sudden death in the post–myocardial infarction patient may be due in part to the reduction in such arrhythmias.

Thermoregulatory Disorders

Thermoresponsive neurons in the medial preoptic area monitor brain temperature and activate autonomic, endocrine, and somatomotor responses to match body temperature to a set-point, which is normally 37°C in humans. Control of body temperature requires shifting blood flow between deep and superficial vascular beds and regulating conservation of body fluids (increased urination in the cold, increased sweating in the heat). Hence, thermoregulation is tightly linked to control of blood pressure, volume, and electrolyte composition, which are also regulated by neurons around the anteroventral tip of the third ventricle (see below).

Poikilothermia, defined as a fluctuation in body temperature of more than 2°C with changes in ambient temperature, is the most common disorder of heat regulation in humans. Lesions in the posterior hypothalamus or midbrain result in severe damage to the hypothalamic pathways for autonomic as well as behavioral thermoregulation. Relative poikilothermia can also result from metabolic disorders such as sedative drug ingestion, hypoglycemia, or hypothyroidism, and in a mild form is often seen in old age. Such patients are dangerously susceptible to lowered environmental temperature. Conversely, patients with relative poikilothermia or those taking anticholinergic drugs that prevent thermal sweating may experience dangerously elevated body temperatures during periods of hot weather. *Heat stroke*, in which body temperature may exceed 42°C, is often fatal and requires prompt treatment by cooling the patient in an ice bath and expanding body fluids. Death is often a result of ventricular arrhythmia (see also Ch. 532).

PAROXYSMAL HYPOTHERMIA. Occasional patients are encountered who suffer episodic attacks during which they thermoregulate in a nearly normal fashion but around a lowered set-point. During an attack, a body temperature of 32°C or lower is maintained for a period of several days to 2 weeks. Attacks occur up to several times per year and may be accompanied by fatigue, malaise, somnolence, hypoventilation, hypotension, cardiac arrhythmias, lacrimation, ataxia, and asterixis. During the attacks, the patient may behaviorally thermoregulate to maintain the lowered set-point. In some patients, the serum sodium may decrease in tandem with the body temperature, to levels of 110 mEq per liter or even lower. Attacks subside spontaneously and are followed by heat conservation measures to bring body temperature up to the normal set-point. Nearly all such patients have evidence of injury to the preoptic area of the hypothalamus. Paroxysmal hypothermia is sometimes seen in patients with agenesis of the corpus callosum, most likely because the corpus callosum and the preoptic area are both embryologic derivatives of the lamina terminalis, which fails to form normally. Anticonvulsants have been prescribed to alleviate attacks but have rarely been effective.

HYPERTHERMIA AND FEVER. During an immune re-

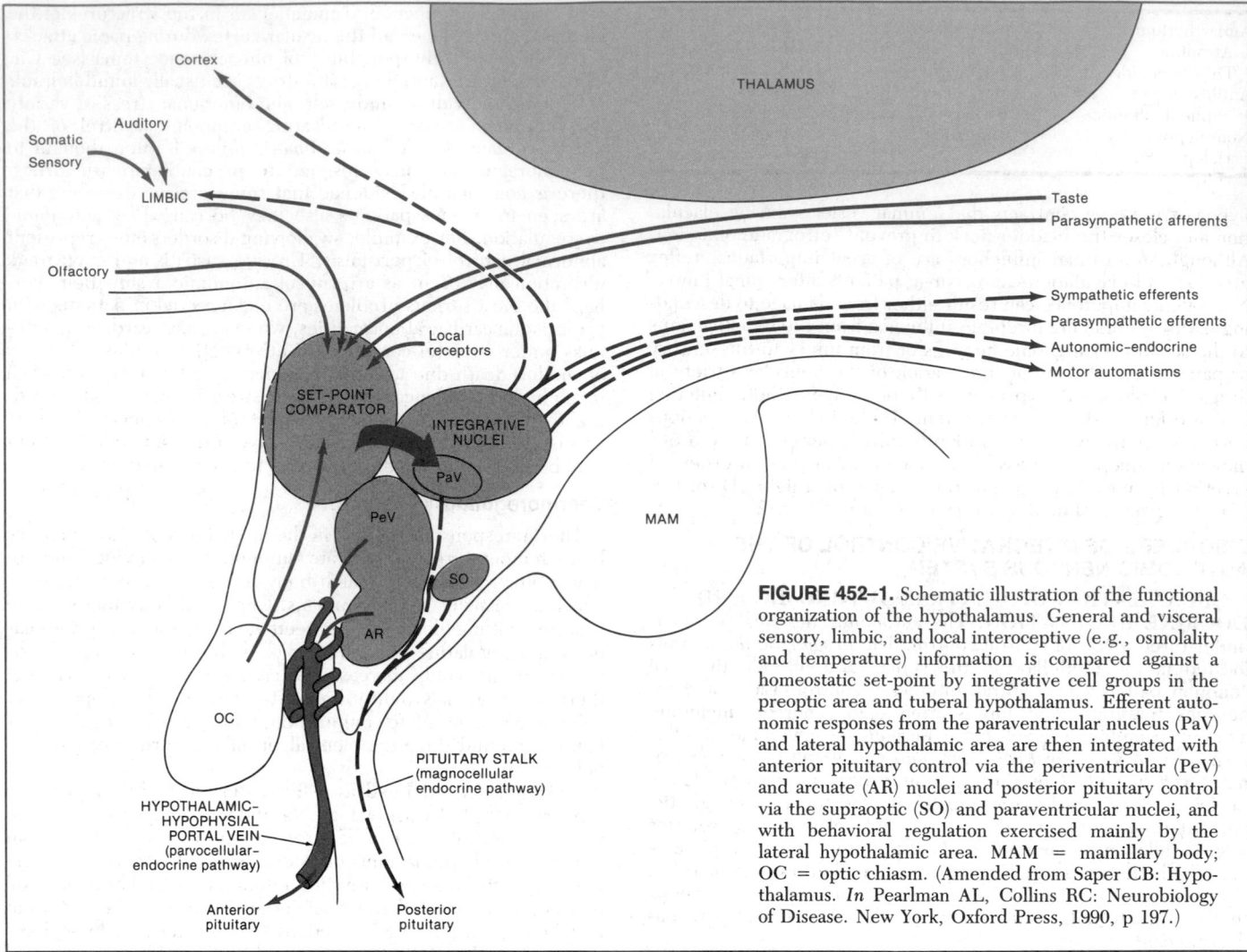

FIGURE 452–1. Schematic illustration of the functional organization of the hypothalamus. General and visceral sensory, limbic, and local interoceptive (e.g., osmolality and temperature) information is compared against a homeostatic set-point by integrative cell groups in the preoptic area and tuberal hypothalamus. Efferent autonomic responses from the paraventricular nucleus (PaV) and lateral hypothalamic area are then integrated with anterior pituitary control via the periventricular (PeV) and arcuate (AR) nuclei and posterior pituitary control via the supraoptic (SO) and paraventricular nuclei, and with behavioral regulation exercised mainly by the lateral hypothalamic area. MAM = mamillary body; OC = optic chiasm. (Amended from Saper CB: Hypothalamus. *In* Pearlman AL, Collins RC: Neurobiology of Disease. New York, Oxford Press, 1990, p 197.)

sponse, macrophages release cytokines, such as interleukin-1 and tumor necrosis factor, that act on neurons or glial cells at the organum vasculosum of the lamina terminalis, a vascular structure outside the blood-brain barrier that sits in the anteroventral tip of the third ventricle, to cause a febrile response. Prostaglandins are a critical mediator for producing fever and some of the endocrine and metabolic changes that accompany it. Fever, an upward resetting of the thermoregulatory set-point, is achieved by normal heat conservation mechanisms, including shivering and behavioral thermoregulation. Drugs that inhibit the generation of prostaglandins are the mainstay of treatment of fever, but there is considerable debate on the wisdom of treating low-grade fever (<38.5°C) during an infectious illness. An elevated body temperature may improve the function of certain immune cells while impairing the defenses of invading microorganisms.

Any physical injury to the brain that allows the entry of macrophages or activates microglial cells to produce cytokines induces a febrile response as well. Hence, fever may be seen after head trauma, intracranial surgery, or cerebral hemorrhage or infarction. Central neurogenic fever is often proposed as a mechanism for fever of unknown origin, but careful investigation generally demonstrates that most if not all of these cases are normal cerebral responses to cytokine generation by immune cells or tumors.

Malignant hyperthermia can occur in patients who have been exposed to certain drugs. During induction of anesthesia, partic-

TABLE 452–7. REGIONAL HYPOTHALAMIC SYNDROMES

Region	Normally Regulates	Disorders
Preoptic	Blood volume, pressure, and electrolytes	Paroxysmal hyponatremia
		Essential hypernatremia
	Thermoregulation	Paroxysmal hypothermia
Tuberal	Gastrointestinal tract and feeding	Hyperphagia (ventromedial lesions)
		Hypophagia (lateral lesions)
	Reproduction	Hypogonadism
	Emotions	Rage responses
Posterior	Arousal	Hypersomnolence
	Descending autonomic and motor pathways	Poikilothermia

ularly with halothane and succinylcholine, certain patients sustain sudden massive muscle contractions accompanied by a rapid rise in body temperature to 42°C or greater. The response is believed to be due to the anesthetic's causing the release of calcium stores from the sarcoplasmic reticulum. Circulatory and respiratory collapse and death can ensue unless immediate treatment with intravenous dantrolene and supportive measures are instituted. A similar picture of muscular rigidity and elevated body temperature can occasionally be seen following treatment with neuroleptic drugs. The pathogenesis of the *neuroleptic malignant syndrome* is not understood, but such patients can sometimes be improved by administering dopaminergic agonists such as bromocriptine.

Feeding Disorders

To provide a constant supply of substrate for energy metabolism, it is necessary to balance bodily requirements against the daily intake of nutrients and body stores of glycogen, fat, and protein. To accomplish this task, the hypothalamus monitors blood glucose, fatty acids, and perhaps other nutrients and attempts to match blood glucose to a set-point. Body weight, which is regulated within a rather narrow range in most people, is also thought to be matched to a set-point, but this is clearly secondary to the immediate need for metabolic substrate. The neural mechanisms regulating energy metabolism and feeding are mainly coordinated in the region of the ventromedial nucleus of the hypothalamus and the nearby paraventricular nucleus. The control of feeding is closely related to autonomic control of the gastrointestinal system.

HYPERPHAGIA AND OBESITY. Lesions in the region of the ventromedial nucleus of the hypothalamus can result in massive overeating and obesity. Experimental studies indicate that overeating is largely in response to parasympathetically mediated hyperinsulinemia, causing a chronically lowered blood glucose. Transection of the vagus nerve below the diaphragm corrects insulin secretion and overeating. Hence, hypothalamic hyperphagia is mainly a disorder of autonomic control of the pancreas, with a resultant attempt to defend the blood glucose set-point.

The *Klein-Levin syndrome* is a poorly understood disorder in which patients, typically adolescent boys, have episodic attacks of somnolence, often sleeping up to 20 hours per day. When awake, they appear dull and often confused and consume enormous quantities of food. Attacks may last up to 2 weeks and can recur several times per year. Pathologic verification of the site of the lesion in typical cases is lacking, but a similar syndrome may be seen acutely in encephalitis involving the hypothalamus.

The *Prader-Willi syndrome* is a congenital disorder due to a deletion in chromosome 15, which includes mental retardation, hypogonadism, and hyperphagia, often with massive obesity. The cause of the overeating is not known.

HYPOPHAGIA AND INANITION. Large lesions in the region of the lateral hypothalamic area, at the level of the ventromedial nucleus, result in aphagia, which may recover to hypophagia and regulation around a new, lower body weight set-point. Such lesions, which must be bilateral, are usually devastating, and selective impairment of eating on this basis has rarely been reported in adults. More often, patients with hypothalamic damage and inanition are somnolent and show a variety of endocrine abnormalities. There is no evidence for injury to the hypothalamus in anorexia nervosa.

Children may demonstrate a quite different response to congenital hypothalamic tumors or malformations. In the diencephalic syndrome of infancy, there is profound emaciation, despite good feeding and linear growth. The affected children are often exceptionally good-natured. The difference from adults with similarly placed tumors probably reflects the capacity for plasticity and formation of new neuronal connections during development.

Central Disorders of Fluid and Electrolyte Regulation

The medial preoptic area, around the anteroventral tip of the third ventricle, plays a critical role in regulating blood pressure, volume, and electrolyte composition. Endocrine control (mineralocorticoids and especially vasopressin), autonomic regulation (control of blood flow in different vascular beds, innervation of sweat glands and kidney, especially the juxtaglomerular apparatus controlling renin release), and behavioral response (drinking) all play important roles in this process. Disorders of the release of vasopressin, by neurons whose cell bodies are located in the supraoptic and paraventricular nuclei, are discussed in Ch. 75 and 214. Coordinated central disorders of fluid regulation are rare.

HYPERNATREMIA, HYPEROSMOLALITY, ABSENCE OF THIRST. Neurogenic hypernatremia is a rare disorder marked by impairment of the normal responses to osmolar stimuli. Hence, there is a deficit in vasopressin response to increased sodium and osmolality and an absence or relative deficiency of thirst. Vasopressin response to hypovolemia may be maintained, and there is preservation of habitual drinking of water (often related to meals) which may be sufficient to maintain serum osmolality under normal conditions. During hot weather, when there is increased loss of water through evaporation of sweat, patients often fail to increase their water consumption adequately and may suffer attacks of fatigue, fever, muscle cramps and tenderness, and even myoglobinuria (associated with hypokalemia). With serum sodium in excess of 180 mEq per liter, patients may experience confusion or even become stuporous, and some may die.

The hypothalamic injury giving rise to essential hypernatremia has been accurately localized in only a few cases but in all of these seems to involve the preoptic area in the region of the anteroventral third ventricle. Treatment consists of training the patient to drink adequate amounts of fluids, particularly during hot weather. Spironolactone, chlorpropamide, and thiazide diuretics have been used to reduce serum sodium and increase potassium. During an attack of severe hypernatremia, when it becomes necessary to provide intravenous fluid and potassium supplementation, it is important not to reduce serum sodium by more than 20 mEq per liter per day. More rapid correction has been associated with central pontine myelinolysis, which may leave the patient quadriplegic.

HYPERDIPSIA, HYPONATREMIA, AND WATER INTOXICATION. Excessive water drinking in the absence of either hypovolemia or serum hyperosmolality is termed primary hyperdipsia and must be distinguished from the compensatory hyperdipsias of diabetes insipidus, diabetes mellitus, and polyuric renal failure. In the absence of inappropriate vasopressin secretion, symptoms of water intoxication, such as stupor, delirium, or convulsions, are infrequent. Most severe hyperdipsia occurs in persons who have psychiatric disturbances. We have seen only one case of primary hyperdipsia, in a patient who had suffered an attack of encephalitis involving the hypothalamus during childhood.

PAROXYSMAL HYPONATREMIA. Many of the patients with paroxysmal hypothermia (see above) suffer simultaneous hyponatremia, which may be sufficiently severe (serum sodium <110 mEq per liter) to cause symptoms of confusion or even convulsions. The serum sodium is regulated around the reduced set-point but may respond to fluid restriction.

Central Reproductive Disorders

Reproductive hormonal control, behavior, and the associated autonomic responses are controlled by poorly defined mechanisms in the medial basal hypothalamus overlying the pituitary stalk. To the extent that it relies upon control of blood flow in specific vascular beds, the autonomic regulation of sexual function must be coordinated with control of body temperature and fluid balance. The change in body temperature that accompanies ovulation and the fluid shifts seen in the perimenstrual period in women are examples of this integration.

Reproductive endocrine disorders are covered in Ch. 213 and 224. Male erectile function, which is dependent upon sacral parasympathetic innervation of the penis, may be affected by diseases of the peripheral autonomic nervous system (see above) as well as psychogenic factors acting at the level of the forebrain. Diagnosis and treatment of male sexual dysfunction are discussed in Ch. 222.

Arousal Disorders

The function of the autonomic nervous system is to augment the activity of various organ systems to deal with perturbations of internal homeostasis. Of all the body's organs, the single most important one to activate during an external threat is the brain. The ascending activating system, running from the brain stem reticular formation to the diencephalon, increases the responsiveness of the forebrain to external stimuli and may be considered a cerebral component of the autonomic system. Ch. 443, 444, and 446 describe the details of altered states of consciousness. We discuss here briefly disorders associated with lesions of the ascending arousal system. Sleep disorders are discussed in Ch. 447.

HYPERSOMNOLENCE. Following lesions of the ascending activating system at the level of the rostral brain stem, there is typically impairment of level of consciousness acutely. After a few weeks, the forebrain recovers spontaneous wake-sleep cycles. Prolonged sleeplike stupor lasting longer than a few weeks is seen only when lesions involve the posterior diencephalon. It is not clear whether this continued somnolence results from injury to the thalamus, to the hypothalamus, or to the connections of these structures. Methylphenidate, amphetamine, and bromocriptine have been used in these patients, with some anecdotal reports of success.

INSOMNIA. Sleep is an active process, requiring the participation of hypnogenic influences arising from the lower brain stem and serotoninergic neurons in the midbrain raphe. We have seen one patient in whom destruction of the medulla, below the level of the ascending activating system, resulted in a chronically wakeful state. Lesions of the preoptic area may also cause a decrease in sleep, but this may be secondary to the deficit in thermoregulation.

Peripheral Autonomic Disorders

Krane RJ, Goldstein I, Saenz de Tejada I: Impotence. N Engl J Med 321:1648–1659, 1989. *A thorough review of the physiology and pathophysiology of erectile function.*

McGuire EJ: The innervation and function of the lower urinary tract. J Neurosurg 65:278, 1986. *A thoughtful review of the physiology and pathophysiology of micturition.*

McLeod JG, Tuck RR: Disorders of the autonomic nervous system: Part 1. Pathophysiology and clinical features. Ann Neurol 21:419, 1987. *A recent review of autonomic physiology and pathophysiology.*

McLeod JG, Tuck RR: Disorders of the autonomic nervous system: Part 2. Investigation and treatment. Ann Neurol 21:519, 1987. *A guide to pharmacologic testing and treatment of autonomic dysfunction.*

Schwartzmann RJ, McLellan TL: Reflex sympathetic dystrophy. A review. Arch Neurol 44:555, 1987. *A review of the pathophysiology and clinical aspects of reflex sympathetic dystrophy.*

Central Autonomic Disorders

Greenberg HS, Rocher LL, Clavin DB, et al.: Episodic hyperhidrosis, hypothermia, and agenesis of the corpus callosum. Neurology 33:1122, 1983. *A review of paroxysmal hypothermia.*

Loewy AD, Spyer KM: Central Regulation of Autonomic Functions. New York, Oxford Press, 1990. *A comprehensive series of reviews on the central components of the autonomic nervous system.*

Plum F, Posner JB: The Diagnosis of Stupor and Coma, 3rd ed., rev. Philadelphia, F. A. Davis, 1982. *A comprehensive review of mechanisms of arousal and evaluation of neurologic impairments in comatose patients.*

Plum F, van Uitert R: Non-endocrine diseases and disorders of the hypothalamus. Res Publ Assoc Res Nerv Ment Dis 56:415, 1977. *A comprehensive review of the integrative disorders of autonomic function.*

Saper CB: Hypothalamus. In Pearlman AL, Collins RC: Neurobiology of Disease. New York, Oxford Press, 1990, p 197. *A review of hypothalamic regulation of integrated functions and their disorders.*

Talman WT: Cardiovascular regulation and lesions of the central nervous system. Ann Neurol 18:1, 1985. *A review of central control of the circulation and the effects of nervous system lesions on cardiac arrhythmias and blood pressure control.*

453 The Special Senses
Robert W. Baloh

453.1 SMELL AND TASTE

Approximately 2 million American adults suffer from disorders of taste and smell, yet there is relatively little information available on how to evaluate or treat these patients. These disorders have been neglected because they are seldom fatal and, unlike abnormalites of vision and hearing, are not considered serious handicaps. Chemosensory disorders, however, often reduce the enjoyment and quality of life and are important to patients who suffer from them. Disorders of taste interfere with digestion because taste stimulants alter salivary and pancreatic flow, gastric contractions, and intestinal motility. Smell also contributes to the anticipation and ingestion of food, since much of what we taste derives from olfactory stimulation during ingestion and chewing. The inability to detect noxious tastes and odors can result in food or gas poisoning, particularly in elderly subjects. In the extreme, chemosensory disorders can lead to overwhelming stress, anorexia, and depression.

DEFINITIONS. Disorders of taste and smell are defined as follows: *Ageusia*, absence of taste; *hypogeusia*, diminished sensitivity of taste; *dysgeusia*, distortion of normal taste; *anosmia*, absence of smell; *hyposmia*, diminished sensitivity of smell; and *dysosmia*, distortion of normal smell. *Hypergeusia* and *hyperosmia* (increased sensitivity of taste and smell) also occur, but little is known about their cause or significance.

ANATOMY. The sensory receptor for taste, the taste bud, is made up of approximately 50 cells arranged to form a pear-shaped organ. The life span of these cells is about 10 days, and they are constantly being renewed from dividing epithelial cells surrounding the bud. Taste buds are located on the tongue, soft palate, pharynx, larynx, epiglottis, uvula, and the upper one third of the esophagus. The taste buds located on the anterior two thirds of the tongue and on the palate are innervated by the seventh cranial nerve. The ninth cranial nerve innervates the posterior one third of the tongue and the folds or clefts on the lateral border of the tongue. The ninth and tenth nerves innervate taste buds in the pharynx. Afferent signals from the taste buds project to the nucleus of the solitary tract in the medulla and then via a series of relays to the thalamus and postcentral somatosensory cerebral cortex. Free nerve endings of the fifth cranial nerve are found on the tongue and in the oral cavity, and lesions involving these pathways also can alter taste perception.

Olfactory receptors lie in a roughly dime-sized area of specialized pigmented epithelium that arches along the superior aspect of each side of the nasal mucosa. Specialized bipolar sensory cells in this region thrust short receptor hairs into the overlying mucosa to detect aromatic molecules as they dissolve. As with taste buds, the specialized receptor portion of the bipolar neuron undergoes continuous renewal, turning over approximately every 30 days. Thin axons of the bipolar neurons course through small holes in the cribriform plate of the ethmoid bone to form connections in the overlying olfactory bulb on the ventral surface of the frontal lobe. From here second- and third-order neurons project directly and indirectly to the prepiriform cortex and parts of the amygdaloid complex of both sides of the brain, representing the primary olfactory cortex.

PATHOPHYSIOLOGY OF CHEMOSENSORY DISORDERS. Disorders of taste and smell can be divided into local, systemic, and neurologic (Table 453–1). The taste buds and the specialized receptor portion of the bipolar olfactory cells are constantly being renewed, and the process of renewal can be affected by nutritional, metabolic, and hormonal states, therapeutic radiation, drugs, and age. For example, with interruption of mitosis by antiproliferative agents, a return of normal taste

TABLE 453–1. COMMON CAUSES OF LOSS OF TASTE AND SMELL

	Taste	Smell
Local	Radiation therapy	Allergic rhinitis, sinusitis, nasal polyposis, bronchial asthma
Systemic	Cancer, renal failure, hepatic failure, nutritional deficiency (B_{12}, zinc), Cushing syndrome, hypothyroidism, diabetes mellitus, infection (influenza), drugs (antirheumatic and antiproliferative)	Renal failure, hepatic failure, nutritional deficiency (B_{12}), Cushing syndrome, hypothyroidism, diabetes mellitus, infection (viral hepatitis, influenza), drugs (nasal sprays, antibiotics)
Neurologic	Bell's palsy, familial dysautonomia, multiple sclerosis	Head trauma, multiple sclerosis, Parkinson's disease, frontal tumor

function takes a minimum of 10 days, while a return to normal olfactory function takes more than 30 days. Numerous local conditions such as colds and allergies, chronic sinusitis, and nasal polyposis can influence the sense of smell by restricting airway patency. Accidental blows to the head can shear the fine axons of the bipolar olfactory neurons, resulting in loss of smell. Lesions of the fifth, seventh (*chorda tympani*), and ninth cranial nerves can lead to disordered taste sensation. Olfactory and gustatory disturbances can serve as important diagnostic signs for focal neurologic lesions (e.g., frontal lobe tumors). Hallucinations of smell and taste occur with epileptogenic lesions affecting the mesial temporal lobe and insular region, respectively. Finally, olfactory disturbances and hallucinations occur with a number of psychiatric illnesses (particularly depressive illness and schizophrenia).

EXAMINATION OF TASTE AND SMELL. Olfaction can be tested grossly at the bedside with a few easily recognized odors such as coffee, chocolate, and the roselike aroma of the compound phenylethyl alcohol. (Avoid nasal irritants.) Each nostril is tested separately to determine whether the problem is unilateral or bilateral. More detailed testing can be obtained in specialized clinics in which a variety of qualitatively distinct substances that span a number of established odor classes are presented with a forced-choice paradigm. Gustatory sensation is typically tested with weak solutions of sugar, salt, and acetic acid, or vinegar. The patient must keep his tongue protruded and respond to questions either by nodding the head or pointing to names of the tastes written on cards. The protruding tongue is dried and a drop of test solution is applied to the lateral border of each side. The anterior two thirds and posterior one third of the tongue should be tested separately.

COMMON CAUSES OF LOSS OF SMELL AND TASTE. The most frequently encountered causes of loss of smell are local obstructive disease, viral infections, head injuries that sever the neurons crossing through the cribriform plate, and normal aging. Patients can lose their sense of smell not only from chronic allergies and sinusitis but also from the nasal sprays and drops that they use to treat these conditions. The most common cause of loss of the sense of taste is drug ingestion, particularly antirheumatic and antiproliferative drugs and drugs containing sulfhydryl groups in their molecular structure, such as penicillamine and captopril. Patients with poor dental hygiene commonly complain of distortions of taste. Many of the systemic disorders listed in Table 453–1 probably have their effect by decreasing the rate of turnover of sensory receptors on the tongue and olfactory epithelia. Disturbances of smell and taste in malnourished patients have been attributed to specific deficiencies in vitamins and minerals, such as zinc. However, it is possible that the loss of protein and calorie intake impairs the functioning of taste buds and olfactory cells in the same manner that it impairs the regeneration of intestinal epithelia. Viral illnesses such as influenza and viral hepatitis produce disorders of both taste and smell. The loss of olfactory sensation after viral illnesses may be due to scarring of the subepithelial tissue and the replacement of olfactory epithelium with respiratory epithelium. Multifocal neurologic disorders such as multiple sclerosis can affect the central olfactory and gustatory pathways at multiple levels, and therefore abnormalities of taste and smell are common in such patients. Treatment, other than avoiding drugs known to affect taste or smell, is unsatisfactory.

Estrem SA, Renner G: Disorders of smell and taste. Otolaryngol Clin North Am 20:133, 1987. *Concise clinical review.*

Schiffman SS: Taste and smell in disease. N Engl J Med 308:1275, 1337, 1983. *A well-referenced two-part short review.*

Taste and smell disorders: parts 1 and 2. Ear Nose Throat J 68:286, 291, 297, 316, 331, 352, 354, 362, 373, 386, 393, 398, 1989. *Two issues devoted to diagnosis and management.*

453.2 NEURO-OPHTHALMOLOGY

The mechanistic understanding of vision impairment along with disturbances of pupillary and oculomotor control lies close to the heart of diagnosing neurologic disorders. Diseases of the eye itself are further considered in Part XXIV.

VISION

One of the most difficult diagnostic problems is vision loss that cannot be explained by obvious abnormalities of the eye. In order to properly evaluate such a patient the examining physician must be familiar with the anatomy and physiology of the afferent visual system. The afferent visual pathways cross at right angles to the major ascending sensory and descending motor systems of the cerebral hemispheres and in their anterior portion are intimately related to the vascular and bony structures at the base of the brain. Not surprisingly, localization of lesions within the afferent visual pathways has great localizing value in neurologic diagnosis.

DEFINITIONS. *Amblyopia* refers to dimness or partial loss of vision, *amaurosis* to blindness. *Scotomas* are areas of relative or complete vision loss isolated within a comparatively better total field of vision for the particular eye. Involvement of the macular area or its projections produces *central scotomas*. Scotomas that lie near the macular visual area are sometimes called *paracentral*, whereas those that extend into macular vision from the more peripheral field may be termed *cecocentral*.

Visual field defects impairing half or nearly half of a field are termed *hemianopic*. Those affecting less than this extent are called *partial field defects*, often with the additional designation of *quadrantic* or *altitudinal* (superior or inferior), depending on the abnormality. A vision defect that affects similar points of the right or left half-field in both eyes is called *homonymous*; identical areas of involvement from the two eyes are termed *congruent*.

ANATOMY OF THE VISUAL PATHWAYS. Light entering the eye falls on the retinal rods and cones, which transduce the stimulus into neural impulses to be transmitted to the brain. The distribution of visual function across the retina takes a pattern of concentric zones increasing in sensitivity toward the center, the fovea. The fovea consists of a "rod-free" central grouping of approximately 100,000 slender cones. The ganglion cells subserving these cones send their axons directly to the temporal aspect of the optic disk, forming the papillomacular bundle. Axons originating from ganglion cells in the temporal retina must curve above and below the papillomacular bundle, forming dense arcuate bands.

The arteries supplying the optic nerve and retina both derive from branches of the ophthalmic artery. The central retinal artery approaches the eye along each optic nerve and pierces the inferior aspect of the dural sheath about 1 cm behind the globe to enter the center of the nerve. The artery emerges in the fundus at the center of the nerve head, from which it nourishes most of the retina by superior, medial, inferior, and lateral branches. Anastomotic branches derived from the choroidal and posterior ciliary arteries supply the nerve head itself and the macular region. Venous drainage from the retina and nerve head flows primarily via the central retinal vein, whose course of exit from the eye parallels that of the entry of the artery. The venous anatomy explains why inflammatory lesions of or adjacent to the optic nerve head cause venous distention and ipsilateral papilledema (optic neuritis), whereas inflammation lying posterior to the point where the vein leaves the nerve produces only visual loss without swelling of the nerve head (retrobulbar neuritis).

What each eye "sees" is termed its visual field (Fig. 453–1). The nasal side of the left eye and the temporal side of the right eye see the left side of the world, and the upper half of each retina sees the lower half of the world. Behind the eye, the optic nerve passes through the optic foramen and sphenoid bone to reach the optic chiasm. In the chiasm, nerves from the nasal half of each retina decussate and join the fibers from the temporal half of the contralateral retina. From the chiasm, the optic tracts pass around the cerebral peduncles to reach the lateral geniculate ganglia of either side. At the level of the geniculus, fibers serving corresponding points in each retinal half visual field lie adjacent to each other, and this proximity is maintained in the subsequent relay to the calcarine cortex. The geniculocalcarine radiation initially fans out into superolateral and inferolateral projections, the latter passing around the lateral ventricle and for a short distance into the temporal lobe (Meyer's loop) before turning posteriorly to head for the striate cortex of the occipital lobe. At the occipital pole, the striate cortex (Area 17) lies along the superior and inferior bands of the calcarine fissure, with macular

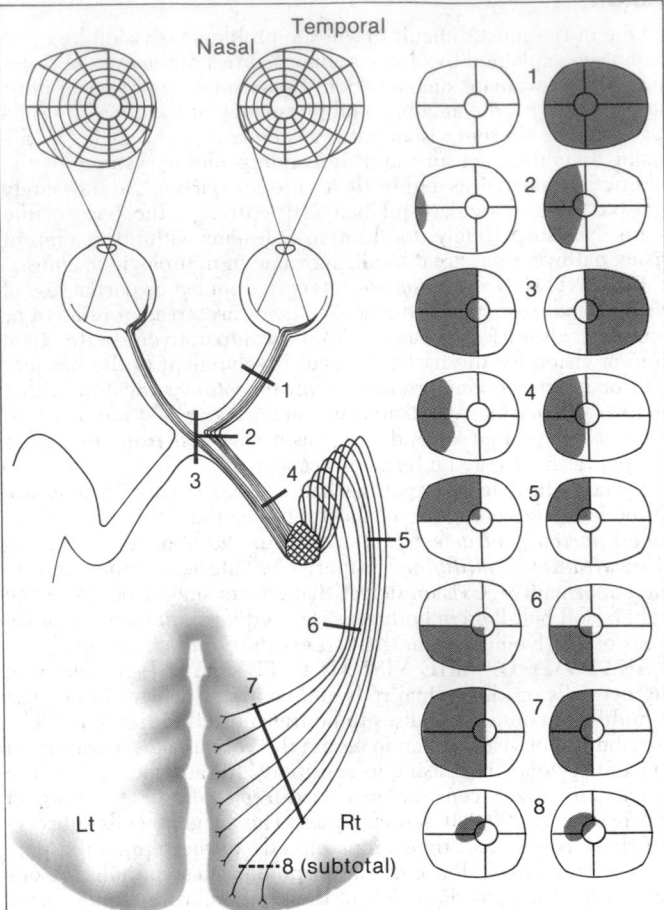

FIGURE 453–1. Visual fields that accompany damage to the visual pathways. 1. Optic nerve: Unilateral amaurosis. 2. Lateral optic chiasm: Grossly incongruous, incomplete (contralateral) homonymous hemianopia. 3. Central optic chiasm: Bitemporal hemianopia. 4. Optic tract: Incongruous, incomplete homonymous hemianopia. 5. Temporal (Meyer's) loop of optic radiation: Congruous partial or complete (contralateral) homonymous superior quadrantanopia. 6. Parietal (superior) projection of the optic radiation: Congruous partial or complete homonymous inferior quadrantanopia. 7. Complete parieto-occipital interruption of optic radiation. Complete congruous homonymous hemianopia with psychophysical shift of foveal point often sparing central vision, giving "macular sparing." 8. Incomplete damage to visual cortex: Congruous homonymous scotomas, usually encroaching at least acutely on central vision.

fibers projecting most posteriorly to the occipital pole and more peripheral retinal projections lying more anteriorly. Each occipital pole "sees" the opposite half of the world. Fibers serving the superior retinal quadrants project to the superior bank of the calcarine fissure, and those from the inferior quadrants project to the inferior bank. The macular field is represented strictly unilaterally.

LOCALIZATION OF LESIONS WITHIN THE VISUAL PATHWAYS. Monocular vision loss is due to a lesion of one eye or its retina or optic nerve. Binocular visual loss, on the other hand, can result from disease located anywhere in the visual pathways from the retinae to the occipital poles. Lesions involving or compressing the optic chiasm produce nonhomonymous visual abnormalities that affect the unilateral visual fields incongruously (e.g., the bitemporal hemianopia illustrated by Lesion 3 in Fig. 453–1). Optic tract abnormalities are comparatively rare but produce characteristic visual changes. The fibers serving identical points in the homonymous half fields do not fully commingle in the anterior optic tract, so lesions encroaching on this structure produce incongruous and usually incomplete homonymous hemianopias. Lesions of the geniculate ganglia, visual radiations, or visual cortex produce congruent hemianopic field defects that may go unrecognized unless the hemianopia intrudes on macular vision. Bilateral damage to the visual radiations or optic cortex

produces cortical blindness. Postgeniculate amaurosis can be differentiated from pregeniculate amaurosis by (1) a normal funduscopic appearance, (2) intact direct and consensual pupillary light reactions, and (3) the presence of anatomically appropriate lesions by brain imaging.

EXAMINATION OF THE AFFERENT VISUAL SYSTEM. Visual function for neurologic purposes consists of "best corrected visual activity." If the visual acuity is not normal, then it must be determined whether acuity can be improved with lenses or at least with the use of a pinhole. Patients with uncorrected myopia or presbyopia correct vision to nearly normal by gazing at the test chart through a pinhole in a card held immediately over the eye. The tiny aperture overcomes any aberration created by failure of the lens to accommodate. The normal reference is a recognition of letters at an idealized 20 feet, and acuity charts are designed with even larger letters that normally are recognized at proportionally greater distances. Thus, if one reads at 20 feet letters no better than those normally perceived at 40 feet, vision is recorded as 20/40. Small visual charts that are easily carried in the physician's case permit quick and fairly accurate bedside appraisals of acuity. Finger counting is a reasonable approximation of an acuity of 20/200, and the greatest distance at which this can be accomplished should be recorded.

Visual fields can be tested at the bedside by confrontation, and rough estimates of their integrity can be made even in patients with reduced alertness. The fields should be tested individually for each eye, since the pattern of visual field defects can provide important localizing information. A quick screen of the visual fields can be made by having the patient fixate on the examiner's nose and identify the number of fingers flashed in each of the four visual field quadrants. With practice and a cooperative subject, accurate confrontation fields can be obtained that outline even scotomas. The examiner should place the test object (e.g., a red match head) midway between his eye and the patient's eye and test the patient's unilateral visual field against his own. Ophthalmoscopic examination permits direct visualization of the cornea, lens, vitreous, retina, and optic disk. Ophthalmologists routinely dilate the pupil to examine the optic fundus, but this step should be avoided in acutely ill patients or those suspected of neurologic diseases until one is certain that an intrinsic pupillary abnormality will not be important in reaching a diagnosis or in following the patient's course. Corneal, lenticular, or vitreous opacities large enough to produce visual symptoms almost always can be detected with the ophthalmoscope.

COMMON CAUSES OF VISUAL LOSS. (See also Ch. 510 and 513.) *Eye.* The cause of monocular vision loss due to ocular and retinal lesions often can be detected with ophthalmoscopic examination or with measurement of intraocular pressure. *Glaucoma* caused by impaired absorption of the aqueous humor results in a high intraocular pressure that usually produces gradual visual loss, "halos" seen around illuminated lamps, and, often, pain and redness in the affected eye. Infrequently, rapid vision loss can occur with few premonitory symptoms. Diagnosis comes from the tonometric measurement of a high intraocular pressure and may be suspected by palpating an abnormally firm globe and observing a deep, pale optic cup and attenuated blood vessels. *Retinal tears and detachments* give rise to unilateral distortions of the visual image such as sudden angulations or curves of objects containing straight lines (metamorphopsia). *Hemorrhages* into the vitreous humor or unilateral *infections* or *inflammatory lesions* of the retina can produce scotomas that in all ways resemble those resulting from primary disease of the central visual pathway.

Binocular vision loss due to retinal disease in younger subjects is usually due to *heredodegenerative conditions*. Vascular diseases, diabetes, idiopathic (senile) macular degeneration, and bilateral retinal detachments are causes in older age groups. In the *pigmentary retinal degenerations* visual loss begins peripherally and proceeds centrally, and often very slowly, before acuity (central vision) is impaired. By contrast, *macular degenerations* impair central vision early in their course. Most of the retinal degenerations produce characteristic and recognizable ophthalmoscopic appearances. With pigmentary degenerations the visual fields shrink progressively in size. With macular degenerations, on the other hand, the fields show noncongruent central scotomas.

Optic Nerve. Acute or subacute monocular vision loss due to optic nerve disease is most commonly produced by demyelinating disorders, vascular obstruction, or neoplasm. Demyelinating disease of the nerve head (*optic neuritis* or *papillitis*) produces papilledema along with loss of central vision in the affected eye only; subjectively unrecognized scotomas sometimes may be found in the other eye. Demyelination in the optic nerve behind where the retinal vein emerges (*retrobulbar neuritis*) initially leaves a normal-looking disk but a central or paracentral scotoma. With chronic demyelinating disorders the optic disk becomes pale and atrophic. More than 50 per cent of patients who initially present with optic neuritis or retrobulbar neuritis go on to develop typical symptoms and signs of multiple sclerosis. Vascular lesions produce either total amaurosis or a sector field defect consistent with an intraocular arterial occlusion (*ischemic optic neuropathy*). The common causes of transient monocular vision loss and their differential features are listed in Table 453–2. *Tumors* invading the optic nerve or space-occupying lesions compressing it anywhere between the orbit and the chiasm cause gradually decreasing central vision (intrinsic or far advanced lesions) or a sector defect of the peripheral visual field. With such chronic lesions the affected optic nerve becomes visibly atrophic.

Acute binocular vision loss due to bilateral optic nerve disease is most often caused by demyelinating disease and less frequently by optic nerve or retinal vascular disease or by toxic or nutritional optic neuropathies. In younger persons and those lacking a clear history of toxic exposures demyelinating lesions overwhelmingly predominate (optic neuritis). Symptoms are of abrupt or subacute onset with visual blurring or loss of acuity, which may progress rapidly to blindness within hours or days. There may be pain about the eyes, particularly on eye movement.

Papilledema resulting from increased intracranial pressure occasionally causes vision loss under one of three circumstances: (1) Acute transient episodes of amaurosis lasting a few seconds and attributable to acute increases in intracranial pressure (plateau waves) that interfere with retinal venous drainage into the cavernous sinus or with vascular irrigation of the occipital lobe; (2) acute bilateral sustained amaurosis following abrupt surgical relief of longstanding, severely increased, intracranial pressure (a rare cause); (3) progressive loss of peripheral vision with longstanding, severe papilledema, presumably owing to pressure atrophy of the most peripherally lying fibers in the tightly sheathed optic nerve. Table 453–3 gives the main differential points between papilledema and optic neuritis. Subacute or chronic binocular vision loss due to optic nerve disease results mainly from *toxic nutritional* causes and the *inherited optic atrophies*. The latter sometimes accompany spinocerebellar degeneration or selectively affect the optic nerves in both juveniles and adults (Leber's forms). With either cause visual loss is moderate or severe and primarily or initially affects central vision; ophthalmoscopy shows mild to moderate primary optic atrophy.

TABLE 453–2. COMMON CAUSES OF TRANSIENT MONOCULAR VISION LOSS

Category (Typical Duration)	Causes	Differential Features
Thromboembolism (1–5 min)	Atherosclerosis	Other atherosclerotic vascular disease, associated crossed hemiparesis, angiography (carotid atheromata)
	Cardiac	Valvular disease, mural thrombi, atrial fibrillation, recent MI
	Blood dyscrasia	Blood tests + for sickle cell anemia, macroglobulinemia, multiple myeloma, polycythemia, etc.
Vasospasm (5–30 min)	Migraine	Ipsilateral headache, other classic aura, and family history
Vascular compression (few sec)	Papilledema	Precipitated by position change, Valsalva maneuver, or pressure waves
	Tumor	Associated slowly progressive monocular visual loss
Vasculitis (1–5 min)	Temporal arteritis	Associated headache, polymyalgia rheumatica, palpable temporal artery, elevated sedimentation rate

TABLE 453–3. DIFFERENTIATION OF OPTIC NEURITIS FROM PAPILLEDEMA

	Optic Neuritis	Papilledema
Central-cecocentral vision loss	Present	Absent
Distribution	Usually unilateral	Usually bilateral
Ocular pain on movement	Present	Absent
Direct light reflex	± Reduced	Intact
CT or MRI scan of head	Normal	Often abnormal
Visual evoked responses	Abnormal	Normal
Lumbar puncture pressure	Normal	Elevated

Chiasm and Optic Tract. Patients with lesions of the optic chiasm and optic tract are often unaware of visual impairment until the deficit encroaches on central vision in one or both eyes. Intrinsic or extrinsic neoplasms and parachiasmal arterial aneurysms are the most common lesions in this location. *Gliomas* that arise in the chiasm are rare in adulthood but, when they occur, impair central vision early. Extrinsic space-occupying lesions compressing the chiasm can arise from the superior, lateral, or inferior aspect and include *dysgerminomas, craniopharyngiomas, pituitary adenomas, meningiomas* arising from the sphenoid bones, and large *aneurysms* of the carotid artery. The diagnosis rests on finding the characteristic visual field abnormalities (bitemporal hemianopsia for chiasm and incongruous homonymous hemianopsia for optic tract lesions) and identifying the specific lesion with computed tomography (CT) or magnetic resonance imaging (MRI). Pituitary apoplexy (due to acute hemorrhage into the gland, occurring most frequently in patients with unrecognized pituitary adenomas) can result in sudden vision loss. Prompt neurosurgical intervention under steroid coverage is required for most patients.

Visual Radiations and Occipital Cortex. Lesions involving the postgeniculate visual pathways most often result from *vascular damage, traumatic injuries, neoplasms* or, rarely, *inflammatory* or *degenerative disorders* involving the cerebral white matter. Their localization can be deduced by the resulting visual field defects (see Fig. 453–1). Vascular disease of the occipital lobes is the most common cause of homonymous visual field defects in the middle-aged and elderly population. Typically, the onset of such field defects is associated with other signs and symptoms of transient ischemic episodes in the vertebrobasilar distribution. Bilateral damage to the visual radiations or occipital cortex produces *cortical blindness*. Most often, there are other signs of vascular disease including focal neurologic findings. *Anton's syndrome* refers to cortical blindness with denial of visual defect. Affected patients not only deny the fact that they are blind but confabulate details of their visual environment from memory. Autopsy studies reveal lesions of the medial, temporal, and parietal lobes as well as the calcarine cortex. *Tumors* are rarely confined to the limits of the occipital lobes; therefore neurologic deficits with occipital tumors are rarely only visual.

PUPILLARY CONTROL

The neuromechanisms that control pupil size and reactivity are complex, yet they can be evaluated by simple clinical procedures. The diameter of the pupil is determined by the antagonistic actions of the iris sphincter and dilator muscles with the latter playing a minor role. If the sphincter muscle is severed or ruptured it does not retract toward one quadrant but rather continues to function except in the altered segment. Therefore, the pupillary response can be evaluated even in the presence of significant damage to the iris.

DEFINITIONS. A difference in the size of the pupils is called *anisocoria*. *Mydriasis* refers to a dilated pupil while *miosis* refers to a constricted pupil. *Hippus* refers to a pupil that is constantly changing in size (a physiologic phenomenon that has no pathologic significance). *Light-near dissociation* refers to a pupil that responds to accommodation but not to light. An *afferent pupil* is a pupil that responds poorly, or not at all, to direct light but has a normal consensual response when a light is shined in the opposite eye.

ANATOMY AND LOCALIZATION OF LESIONS WITHIN PUPILLARY PATHWAYS. The size of the pupil is governed by tonic balance between sympathetic and parasympathetic inner-vation of the muscles of the iris. Sympathetic stimulation dilates the pupil, and parasympathetic stimulation constricts it. In the normal resting state, light entering the eye provides the major stimulus governing the size of the pupil (Fig. 453–2). Light activates the retinal rods and cones with maximal sensitivity in the macular area. The optic nerve fibers follow the crossed and uncrossed visual pathways to the pregeniculate portion of the optic tracts, where the receptor fibers for light diverge to the pretectal nucleus located at the midbrain diencephalic junction. Interneurons project from this nucleus to the Edinger-Westphal nuclei atop the midbrain third nerve complex of either side. From that point paired parasympathetic efferents leave the midbrain with the third nerves to travel in the interpeduncular space across the petroclinoid ligament and edge of the tentorium, where, after traversing the cavernous sinus, they enter the superior orbital fissure. In the orbit the parasympathetic efferents synapse in the ciliary ganglion from which short ciliary nerves enter the eye to reach the pupillary muscles.

Lesions of the retina or optic nerve result in an ipsilateral afferent pupillary defect. Pretectal lesions commonly produce light-near dissociation; i.e., the pupils respond to accommodation but not to light. Damage to a third nerve or its parasympathetic postganglionic fibers results in a dilated pupil that does not respond to direct or consensual stimulation.

The principal sympathetic control of the pupil originates in the ventral lateral hypothalamus (first-order neuron) from which fibers descend ipsilaterally to the lower brain stem tegmentum and thence to the cervical cord, where they lie superficially and synapse with the preganglionic neurons in the intermedial lateral column of the upper three thoracic segments. Preganglionic fibers (second-order neurons) emerge with the ventral roots of C8, T1, and T2 and ascend in the neck to synapse in the superior cervical ganglion adjacent to the base of the skull. Postganglionic (third-order neurons) pupillary fibers accompany the internal carotid artery through the skull, leaving it to follow the ophthalmic branch of the trigeminal nerve to reach the pupillodilator muscle of the eye.

Sympathetic paralysis of the eye with ptosis and miosis (Horner's syndrome) can result from lesions anywhere along the course of the pathway described above. Topical diagnosis is made best by identifying associated signs in the brain stem or neck or along the carotid artery.

EXAMINATION OF THE PUPIL. The pupillary response to light should be examined in a dimly lighted room, in which case the pupils are in a semidilated state. First, the size and symmetry of the pupils are assessed by shining a dim light onto the face from below so that both pupils are seen simultaneously in the indirect illumination. To test light reactivity, gaze is directed at a distant object and first one and then the other pupil is illuminated with a very bright light source. If a pupil reacts poorly to direct light, it is observed as the opposite eye is illuminated (consensual response). Pupils that react poorly to light should be tested for activity to the near reflex. This is done by first having the patient gaze at a distant object and then quickly fixate on his fingertip just in front of his nose.

COMMON CAUSES OF PUPILLARY ABNORMALITIES. The differential features for distinguishing between several common causes of a dilated pupil are illustrated in the logic tree shown in Figure 453–3. With so-called benign pupillary dilatation or *physiologic anisocoria* there is a lifelong difference in the size of the two pupils with normal reflex reactions; the disparity remains constant during constriction and dilatation. Lesions compressing or damaging the tectal region interrupt the afferent light reflex bilaterally to produce dilated (>5 mm) and light-fixed pupils (e.g., Lesion 2, Fig. 453–2). Pupillary constriction on accommodation is preserved until late stages. Tumors of the pineal gland (e.g., dysgerminomas) and *localized infarctions* are the most common lesions in this location. *Adie's tonic pupil* is a medium-to-large (3 to 6 mm) pupil that constricts little or not at all to light and slowly to accommodation but constricts with the instillation of dilute pilocarpine (0.125 per cent). The abnormal pupil is associated with diminished or absent deep tendon reflexes in the extremities. The condition usually affects one eye (occasionally both), is more common in women 25 to 45 years of age, and carries no serious implications. Its cause is unknown. Unexplained unilateral or bilateral dilated pupil as an isolated finding can result from the *accidental or intentional instillation of mydriatics*. The recent widespread use of transdermal scopolamine has increased the problem. Failure of the pupil to constrict promptly with pilocarpine (1 per cent) gives the diagnosis if the history is unclear. Interruption of the emerging third nerve in the ventral midbrain or along the proximal part of its course produces a mid-dilated pupil 6 to 7 mm in diameter. Important causes of compression of the third nerve in this region are *aneurysms, neoplasia,* and *brain herniation* due to increased intracranial pressure. In nearly all cases the pupillary involvement is associated with other signs of third nerve involvement, as

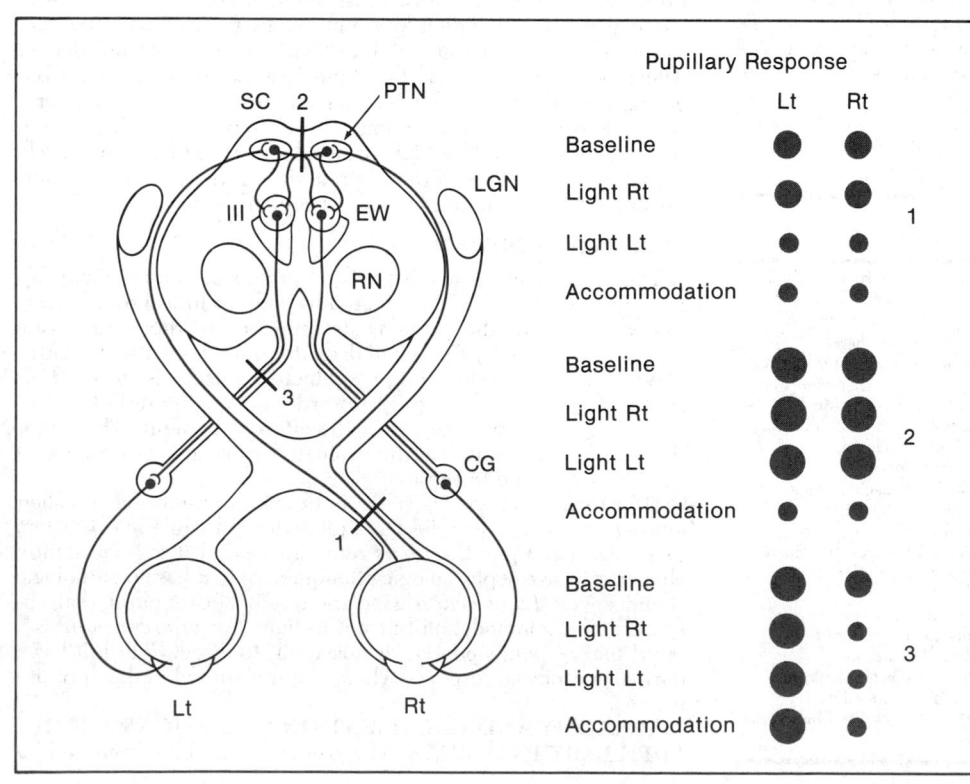

FIGURE 453–2. Pupillary responses associated with lesions of the (1) optic nerve, (2) pretectum, and (3) oculomotor nerve. SC = Superior colliculus; PTN = pretectal nucleus; EW = Edinger-Westphal nucleus; LGN = lateral geniculate nucleus; RN = red nucleus; CG = ciliary ganglion.

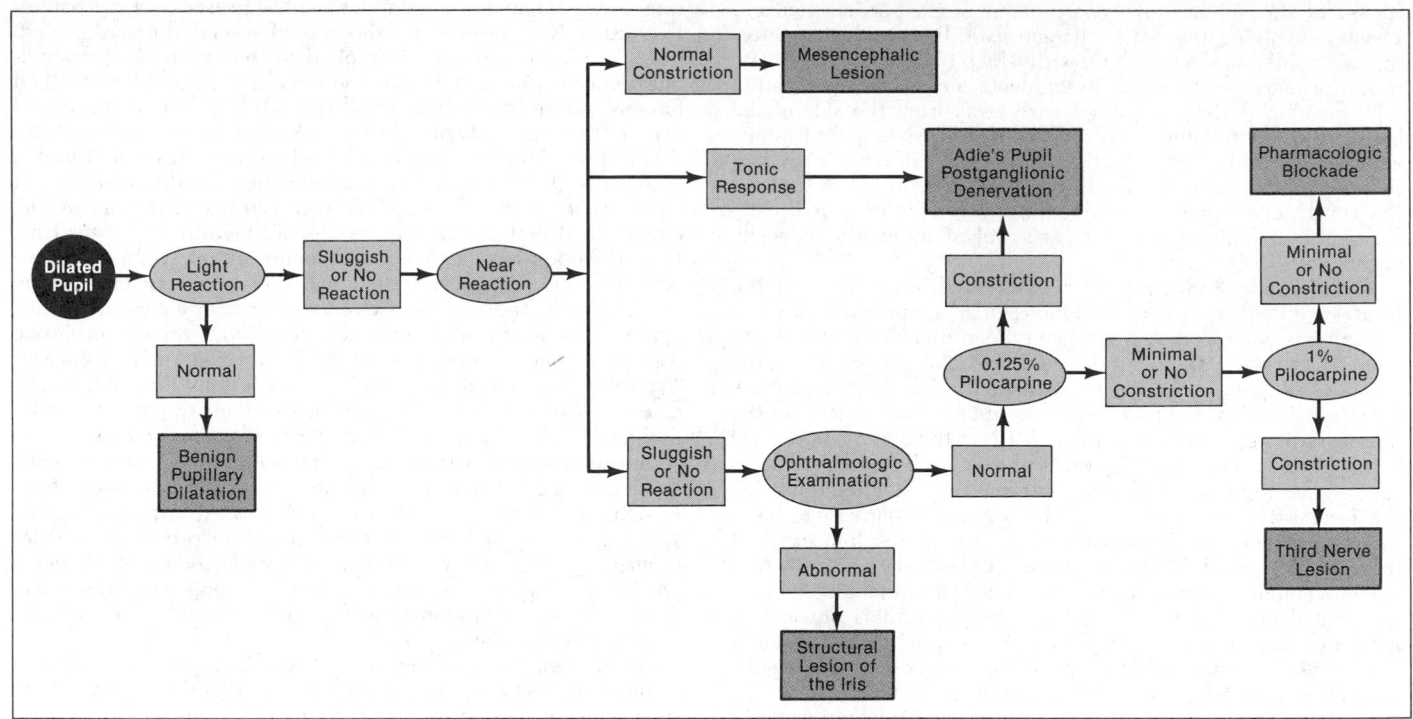

FIGURE 453–3. Evaluation of a dilated pupil.

described in the section below dealing with localization of lesions in oculomotor pathways. Rarely, compressive lesions such as a posterior communicating artery aneurysm can present with an isolated dilated pupil.

As noted above, the causes of *Horner's syndrome* are numerous because of the long course of sympathetic innervation to the eye. It is unlikely that a patient with a central nervous system lesion will present with an isolated Horner syndrome. The most common lesions producing Horner syndrome involve the ascending second-order neuron in the neck or the extracranial postganglionic neuron; *malignant tumors in the apex of the lung* are by far the most common. *Argyll Robertson pupils* are small (1 to 2 mm), unequal, irregular, and fixed to light; they constrict to accommodation. Their principal cause is tertiary neurosyphilis, although partial Argyll Robertson changes occur with diabetes and certain of the autonomic neuropathies.

OCULOMOTOR CONTROL

Abnormal eye movements can result from disturbances at several levels. Disconjugate eye movements result from lesions of the individual ocular muscles, the myoneural junctions, the oculomotor nerves and their three paired nuclei in the brain stem, and the internuclear medial longitudinal fasciculus (MLF) that yokes the eyes in parallel movements. Supranuclear lesions typically produce disorders of conjugate gaze (gaze palsies).

DEFINITIONS. The term *strabismus* describes an involuntary deviation of the eye from its normal physiologic position. *Nonparalytic strabismus* is due to an intrinsic imbalance of ocular muscle tone and is usually congenital. *Paralytic strabismus* results from defects in ocular muscle innervation. Strabismus is called *comitant* when the relationship between the two ocular axes remains constant in all directions of gaze, *noncomitant* when they change, and *latent* when the imbalance is brought out only by covering one eye to prevent fixation. Latent strabismus can become *manifest* during great fatigue or in association with high fever in systemic illness. Congenital comitant strabismus present at birth or soon thereafter carries with it the strong risk that if uncorrected the subject will suppress vision in the nondominant eye during the developmental period when it usually forms its connections with the visual cortex. The result is unilateral, permanent reduction of vision in the nondominant eye (*amblyopia ex anopia*). Strabismus beginning after binocular fusion has developed does not lead to permanent visual loss. *Nystagmus* is an involuntary rhythmic oscillation of the eyes that usually has clearly defined fast and slow components. By convention, the direction of the fast component defines the direction of nystagmus. Physiologic nystagmus refers to nystagmus that occurs in normal subjects, while pathologic nystagmus implies an underlying abnormality. *Physiologic nystagmus* may be vestibular induced (rotational or caloric), visual induced (optokinetic), or end point (occurring on extreme lateral gaze). *Pathologic nystagmus* may be spontaneous (present in the primary position with the patient seated), positional (induced by change in head position), or gaze evoked (induced by change in eye position).

ANATOMY AND LOCALIZATION OF LESIONS WITHIN THE OCULOMOTOR PATHWAYS. *Nuclear and Internuclear Pathways.* The abducens nerve supplies the lateral rectus muscle. Selective involvement of the abducens nerve anywhere along its pathway leads to isolated weakness of abduction of the affected eye. Destruction of the abducens nucleus in the brain stem leads to a conjugate gaze paralysis (ipsilateral) because, in addition to oculomotor neurons, the nucleus contains interneurons destined for the contralateral medial rectus nucleus. The trochlear nucleus supplies the contralateral superior oblique muscle which intorts the eye and moves it down. Patients with superior oblique weakness note an increase in diplopia with head tilt toward the side of weakness and often tilt the head in the opposite direction. At rest there is slight upward deviation of the involved eye and downward movement is impaired when the affected eye is turned in. The third cranial nerve supplies the remaining ocular muscles. Involvement of the third nerve nucleus in the midbrain always produces at least some bilateral oculomotor weakness; the superior rectus division of the nucleus supplies the contralateral superior rectus muscle (all other divisions supply ipsilateral muscles). Peripheral third nerve paralysis can result from lesions damaging the structure anywhere from its origin in the ventral midbrain to where it enters the orbit via the superior orbital fissure. Depending on its completeness, a third nerve palsy produces a widely dilated pupil, severe ptosis, and an externally deviated eye held in position by the unopposed contraction of the lateral rectus muscle. In such conditions, the continued trochlear action reveals itself by intorsion of the eye when the subject attempts to look down and in.

The MLF interconnects the abducens nucleus in the pons with the contralateral oculomotor nuclear complex in the midbrain. It terminates cephalad in the interstitial nucleus in the rostral midbrain and can be traced as far caudad as the thoracocervical region of the spinal cord (coordinating nuchal-ocular control). Lesions involving the MLF characteristically produce an internuclear ophthalmoplegia (INO) with which the eyes are conjugate in the primary position but disconjugate on lateral gaze. With a fully developed INO on lateral gaze away from the side of the lesion the contralateral eye abducts and shows nystagmus, whereas the ipsilateral adducting eye partially or completely fails to move nasally because of failure of ascending impulses to reach the third nerve nucleus. Adduction for convergence is usually relatively maintained. Upbeat gaze-evoked nystagmus typically occurs with INO.

Supranuclear Pathways. The pathway descending from the frontal eye fields in the frontal lobe regulates rapid voluntary eye movements (*saccades*). A signal from the frontal eye field activates a burst of firing in the contralateral horizontal gaze center in the paramedian pontine reticular formation. This high frequency burst (or pulse) of neuronal firing is transmitted directly to the nearby sixth nerve nucleus and via MLF to the contralateral third nerve nucleus. For voluntary vertical gaze both frontal eye fields send signals to the vertical gaze center in the pretectum (probably the interstitial nucleus of the MLF). Acute lesions involving a frontal eye field (e.g., hemorrhage or infarction) result in transient (24 to 72 hours) inability to direct the eyes contralaterally. Vertical eye movements are not affected by unilateral frontal lobe lesions. Bilateral damage to the frontal eye fields or their descending pathways may produce the inability to move the eyes voluntarily (horizontal or vertical) despite preserved reflex eye movements, a condition called *oculomotor apraxia.* Lesions involving the horizontal-gaze center in the pons produce an ipsilateral paralysis of conjugate gaze and tonic deviation of the eyes to the contralateral hemiorbit. Lesions of the pretectum selectively impair vertical gaze with the vertical up-gaze center being slightly rostral and dorsal to the vertical down-gaze center.

Pathways descending from the parieto-occipital region of the two hemispheres subserve slow visual tracking or *smooth pursuit movements.* The exact location of these descending pathways is not completely known, but there are strong projections to the ipsilateral superior colliculus and ipsilateral pons. The cerebellar flocculus is also a critical relay station for smooth pursuit pathways. Lesions of the parieto-occipital region, pons, and cerebellum impair smooth pursuit and optokinetic slow phases when the target moves ipsilateral to the lesion. The *convergence* center is located in the rostral-dorsal midbrain near the vertical-gaze center. Lesions in this region typically impair convergence and voluntary vertical gaze (particularly up-gaze). Pathways for cortical control of convergence have not been identified. The fourth supranuclear oculomotor control system, the *vestibulo-ocular reflex,* and its examination are discussed below.

EXAMINATION OF EYE MOVEMENTS. Fixation and gaze holding are tested by having the patient look center, right, left, up, and down. Each position should be held steady and unwavering with the observer documenting carefully abnormal movements or ocular disconjugacies. Each supranuclear oculomotor control system is examined separately. *Saccades* are tested by having the patient fixate alternately on two targets such as the examiner's finger and nose; the speed and accuracy are noted. *Smooth pursuit* is tested by slowly moving a target back and forth and up and down and observing the patient's ability to produce smooth tracking movements. It the target velocity is low (less than 30 degrees per second) normal subjects should be able to pursue without requiring catch-up saccades. *Convergence* is tested by having the patient follow a target moving from far to near. The degree of normal convergence varies considerably and depends on the cooperation of the patient. A clear sign that the patient is attempting to converge is simultaneous pupillary constriction.

COMMON CAUSES OF ABNORMAL OCULOMOTOR CONTROL. Strabismus. The flow chart in Figure 453–4 outlines the logic for determining the common causes of strabismus. A comitant strabismus present since childhood is usually a benign *congenital disorder.* As noted earlier, latent congenital strabismus can become manifest in adulthood in association with a systemic illness. An acquired skew deviation (vertical displacement of the ocular axes) can result from any number of lesions involving the

brain stem and has little localizing value. Noncomitant strabismus can result from restrictive disease of the orbit or from abnormal muscle or oculomotor nerve function. The presence of mechanical restriction is confirmed by the use of forced duction testing. (After a topical anesthetic is applied to the eye the ophthalmologist grasps the muscle insertion with a large blunt-toothed forceps and identifies mechanical restriction.) Common causes of *orbital restrictive disease* include dysthyroid ophthalmopathy, orbital pseudotumor, trauma, and orbital mass lesions. Variable strabismus that increases with fatigue suggests the likelihood of *myasthenia gravis.* A Tensilon test can usually confirm the diagnosis. If both restrictive disease and myasthenia gravis have been excluded most patients with noncomitant strabismus have processes affecting the oculomotor nuclei, their fascicles, or the cranial nerves themselves. Common causes of an *isolated third nerve palsy* in an adult include aneurysm, vascular occlusive disease (including diabetes mellitus), trauma, and neoplasm. Typically, but not always, third nerve lesions due to vascular disease spare the pupil. Vascular disease and trauma are by far the most common causes of *isolated trochlear nerve palsies.* The abducens nerve is particularly vulnerable to isolated traumatic involvement because of its long pathway outside the brain stem. Lesions at distant sites that produce increased intracranial pressure can lead to abducens nerve dysfunction producing a "false localizing sign." Other common causes of *isolated sixth nerve palsies* are vascular disease, trauma, and neoplasm. About one fourth of cases with cranial nerve palsies (third, fourth or sixth nerves) remain undiagnosed.

Internuclear Ophthalmoplegia (INO). INO may be unilateral or bilateral, partial or complete, depending on the location of the lesion and the degree of damage to the MLF. *Demyelinating* and small *vascular lesions* are the most common cause of unilateral INO unaccompanied by other ocular palsies or brain-stem signs. Larger brain-stem lesions that damage one or more oculomotor nuclei plus the MLF often produce bizarre combinations of disconjugate eye movements coupled with nuclear oculomotor palsies. Myasthenia gravis can produce an ophthalmoparesis resembling INO owing to the greater involvement of the medial rectus compared to the lateral rectus. Demyelinating diseases are by far the most common causes of bilateral INO involvement.

Disorders of Conjugate Gaze. As noted earlier, infarction of the frontal cortex results in transient contralateral gaze paresis. Tumors and infarction of the paramedian pontine reticular formation produce ipsilateral horizontal gaze paralysis. With the so-called locked-in syndrome (secondary to basilar artery thrombosis) voluntary horizontal eye movements are absent; the patient's only remaining motor functions are vertical eye and lid movements. Lesions of the pretectum typically affect only vertical eye movements, although the descending pathways from the frontal eye fields to the horizontal gaze centers in the pons can also be affected. With the *dorsal midbrain syndrome* (Parinaud syndrome) patients present with a conjugate up-gaze paresis. When they attempt to make upward saccades they develop convergence retraction nystagmus. As noted earlier, impaired convergence and light-near dissociation of the pupillary reflexes are also part of the syndrome. The most common causes of the dorsal midbrain syndrome include tumors of the pineal gland (dysgerminomas), aqueductal stenosis, and localized infarction.

Nystagmus. Spontaneous nystagmus can be congenital or acquired. *Congenital nystagmus* typically has a high frequency and variable wave form (occasionally pendular) and is highly fixation-dependent. It is usually not associated with a structural brain lesion. The lifelong history confirms the diagnosis. Spontaneous nystagmus due to a *peripheral vestibular* lesion (i.e., in the labyrinth or vestibular nerve) usually has combined horizontal and torsional components and is strongly inhibited with fixation (Table 453–4). Acquired persistent spontaneous nystagmus that is not inhibited by fixation indicates a lesion in the brain stem and/or cerebellum (*central vestibular*). The latter is often purely vertical or horizontal, since the vertical and horizontal vestibulo-ocular pathways separate beginning at the vestibular nuclei. Spontaneous *downbeat nystagmus* is commonly seen with lesions of the medulla or cervicomedullary junction (e.g., Arnold-Chiari malformation).

Gaze-evoked nystagmus is always in the direction of gaze and is usually present with and without fixation. It is most commonly

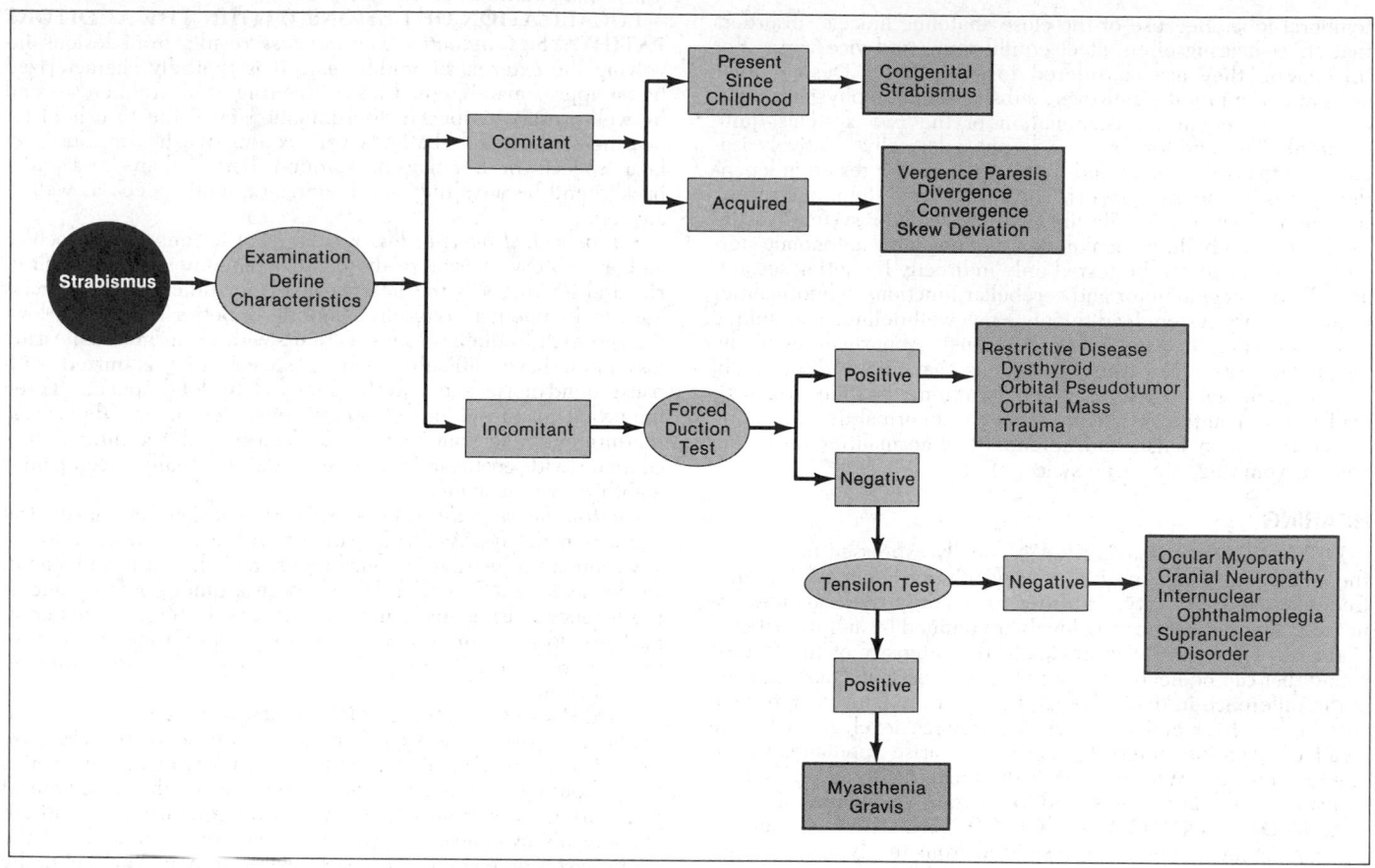

FIGURE 453–4. Diagnostic approach to strabismus.

produced by ingestion of *drugs* such as phenobarbital, phenytoin, alcohol, and diazepam. It can also occur in patients with such varied conditions as myasthenia gravis, multiple sclerosis, and cerebellar atrophy. Asymmetric horizontal gaze-evoked nystagmus indicates a structural brain-stem or cerebellar lesion (particularly at the cerebellopontine angle) with the lesion usually being on the side of the larger amplitude nystagmus. *Rebound nystagmus* is a type of gaze-evoked nystagmus that either disappears or reverses direction as the eccentric gaze position is held. When the eyes are returned to the primary position nystagmus occurs in the direction of the return saccade. Rebound nystagmus occurs in patients with cerebellar atrophy and focal structural lesions of the cerebellum; it is the only variety of nystagmus thought to be specific for cerebellar involvement. *Disconjugate gaze-evoked nystagmus* most commonly results from lesions of the MLF (see above), but it can also occur with other lesions of the brain stem involving the oculomotor nuclei. Positional nystagmus is discussed on page 2110.

TABLE 453–4. KEY DISTINGUISHING FEATURES OF PERIPHERAL AND CENTRAL TYPES OF SPONTANEOUS AND POSITIONAL NYSTAGMUS

Type of Nystagmus	Peripheral (End Organ and Nerve)	Central (Brain Stem and Cerebellum)
Spontaneous	Unidirectional, fast phase away from lesion, combined horizontal torsional, inhibited with fixation	Bidirectional or unidirectional; often pure horizontal, vertical, or torsional; *not* inhibited with fixation
Static positional	Direction-fixed or direction-changing, inhibited with fixation	Direction fixed or direction-changing, *not* inhibited with fixation
Paroxysmal positional	Vertical-torsional, occasionally horizontal-torsional, vertigo prominent, fatigability, latency	Often pure vertical, vertigo less prominent, no latency, nonfatigable

Other Ocular Oscillations. *Ocular bobbing* consists of a fast conjugate downward eye movement followed by a slow return to the primary position. The phenomenon accompanies severe displacement or destruction of the pons or, much less often, metabolic CNS depression. *Ocular myoclonus* consists of continuous rhythmic pendular oscillations, most often vertical, with a rate of 2 to 5 beats per second. Often it accompanies palatal myoclonus and has a similar pathogenesis. *Square wave jerks* and *ocular flutter* consist of brief, intermittent, horizontal oscillations (saccades) arising from the primary gaze position. These types of ocular oscillation are most commonly seen with cerebellar disease but can also accompany more diffuse central nervous system disorders. *Opsoclonus* consists of rapid, chaotic, conjugate, repetitive, saccadic eye movements (dancing eyes). One type of opsoclonus accompanies cerebellar dysfunction, but the most chaotic varieties are associated with brain-stem encephalitis or the remote effects of systemic neoplasm, especially neuroblastoma in children. *Ocular dysmetria* refers to over- and undershooting of saccadic eye movements often followed by multiple attempts at refixation. It reflects cerebellar dysfunction.

Burde RM, Savino PJ, Trobe JD: Clinical Decisions in Neuro-ophthalmology. St. Louis, The C. V. Mosby Company, 1985. *Liberal use of flow charts to help the clinician answer the question, "Given the symptom and signs, what is the disease?"*

Glaser JS: Neuro-ophthalmology, 2nd ed. Hagerstown, MD, Harper & Row, 1990. *An excellent one-volume didactic introductory text.*

Leigh RJ, Zee DS: The Neurology of Eye Movement, 2nd ed. Philadelphia, F. A. Davis Company, 1991. *An up-to-date monograph that gives the clinical and physiologic details of modern investigations on ocular control.*

453.3 HEARING AND EQUILIBRIUM

The neural pathways subserving hearing and those most important for equilibrium and spatial orientation are anatomically proximate in much of their course from their end organs in the inner ear to their termination in the superior portion of the temporal lobe. Because of the close anatomic linkage, disorders that affect hearing often affect equilibrium, and vice versa. For this reason they are considered together here. Despite their anatomic propinquity, however, substantial pathophysiologic differences make clinical examination of the two systems quite different. The auditory system is physiologically relatively isolated, so that its function and dysfunction can be tested independently of other neural systems. The vestibular system, in contrast, has many close physiologic links with the motor system (particularly the cerebellum, oculomotor system, and autonomic nervous system) and can be tested only indirectly by noting secondary effects on oculomotor and cerebellar functions. Abnormalities of the auditory system lead to only a few well-defined and unique symptoms (i.e., hearing loss or tinnitus). Abnormalities of the vestibular system can cause symptoms that mimic disorders of the other neural structures. Such symptoms include dizziness, ocular abnormalities (nystagmus), motor abnormalities (including ataxia or sudden falls), and autonomic abnormalities (including nausea, vomiting, and even syncope).

HEARING

DEFINITIONS. *Hearing loss* is usually expressed in terms of the ability to hear *pure tones*, which are defined by their frequency and intensity. In order to quantify the magnitude of hearing loss, normal hearing levels are defined by an international standard. These levels approximate the intensity of the faintest sound that can be heard by normal ears. A patient's hearing level is the difference in decibels (dB) between the faintest pure tone that he can hear and the normal reference level given by the standard. *Tinnitus* refers to noises that arise spontaneously in one or both ears. With *diplacusis* the tonal quality of a pure tone is distorted so that it may sound like a complex mixture of tones.

ANATOMY AND PHYSIOLOGY OF HEARING. In normal hearing, sound waves are transmitted from the tympanic membrane via the three ossicles of the air-filled middle ear (air conduction) to the oval window and the basilar membrane of the fluid-sealed cochlea. The ossicles serve to increase the gain from the tympanum to oval window about 18-fold, compensating for the loss that sound waves moving from air to fluid would otherwise suffer. In the absence of this system, sound may reach the cochlea by vibration of the temporal bone (bone conduction) but with much less efficiency (approximately 60 dB loss). Hair cells lying along the cochlear basilar membrane detect the vibratory movement of that membrane and transduce vibration into nerve impulses. The nerve impulses are relayed via nerve cells that synapse at the base of hair cells and have their bodies in the spiral ganglion to the cochlear nucleus of the ipsilateral pontine tegmentum. The spiral cochlea mechanically analyzes the frequency content of sound. For high-frequency tones, only sensory cells in the basilar region are activated, whereas for low-frequency tones all or nearly all sensory cells are activated. Therefore, with lesions of the cochlea and its afferent nerve the hearing levels for different frequencies are usually unequal, typically resulting in better hearing sensitivity for low-frequency than for high-frequency tones. Within the brain stem, auditory signals ascend from the ventral and dorsal cochlear nuclei to reach the superior olivary nuclei of both sides. Thus nervous system lesions central to the cochlear nucleus do not cause monaural hearing loss, and, conversely, unilateral central lesions do not cause deafness. From these structures the pathway projects by way of the lateral lemnisci to the inferior colliculi. Each inferior colliculus transmits to the other and to its ipsilateral medial geniculate body, which in turn sends the final projection to the transverse auditory gyrus lying in the superior portion of the ipsilateral temporal lobe.

The normal ear can detect sound frequencies ranging between 20 and 20,000 hertz (Hz); the upper range drops off fairly rapidly with advancing age. The ear is most sensitive between 500 and 4000 Hz, which roughly corresponds to the frequency range most important for understanding speech. The hearing level in this range has several practical implications in terms of the degree of handicap and the potential for useful correction with amplification. A 30 to 40 dB hearing level in the speech range would impair normal conversation, whereas an 80 dB hearing level

would make everyday auditory communication almost impossible (the social definition of deafness).

LOCALIZATION OF LESIONS WITHIN THE AUDITORY PATHWAYS. *Conductive hearing loss* results from lesions involving the external or middle ear. It is typically characterized by an approximately equal loss of hearing at all frequencies and by well-preserved speech discrimination once the threshold for hearing is exceeded. Patients with conductive hearing loss can hear speech in a noisy background better than in a quiet background because they can understand loud speech as well as anyone.

Sensorineural hearing loss results from lesions of the cochlea and/or auditory division of the eighth cranial nerve. With sensorineural hearing loss the hearing levels for different frequencies are usually unequal, typically resulting in better hearing for low- than for high-frequency tones. Patients with sensorineural hearing loss often have difficulty hearing speech that is mixed with background noise and may be annoyed by loud speech. Three important manifestations of sensorineural lesions are diplacusis, recruitment, and tone decay. Diplacusis and recruitment are common with cochlear lesions; tone decay usually accompanies eighth nerve involvement.

Central hearing disorders result from lesions of the central auditory pathways. As a rule patients with central lesions do not have impaired hearing for pure tones, and they can understand speech as long as it is clearly spoken in a quiet environment. If the listener's task is made more difficult with the introduction of background noise or competing messages, performance deteriorates more markedly in patients with central lesions than in normal subjects.

EXAMINATION OF HEARING. **Bedside Test.** A quick test for hearing loss in the speech range is to observe the response to spoken commands at different intensities (whisper, conversation, shouting). Tuning fork tests permit a rough assessment of the hearing level for pure tones of known frequency. The clinician can use his own hearing level as a reference standard. In the Rinne test, nerve conduction is compared to bone conduction by holding a tuning fork (preferably 512 Hz) against the mastoid process until the sound can no longer be heard. It is then placed 1 inch from the ear and in normal subjects can be heard about twice as long by air as by bone. If bone conduction is better than air conduction, the hearing loss is conductive, but care must be taken to assure that the bone conduction is not heard in the normal ear. In the Weber test, the tuning fork is placed on the patient's forehead or upper teeth. Normally this sound is referred to the center of the head. If it is referred to the side of unilateral hearing loss, the hearing loss is conductive; if it is referred away from the side of unilateral hearing loss, the loss is sensorineural. The Weber test is often unreliable in conductive hearing loss because the patient cannot accept the fact that he hears better in what he knows to be the diseased ear.

Audiometry. *Pure tone testing* is the nucleus of most auditory examinations. Pure tones at selected frequencies are presented via either earphones (air conduction) or a vibrator pressed against the mastoid portion of the temporal bone (bone conduction), and the minimal level that the subject can hear is determined for each frequency. Two speech tests are routinely used. The *speech reception threshold* (SRT) is the intensity at which the patient can correctly repeat 50 per cent of the words presented. The SRT is a test of hearing sensitivity for speech and should reflect the hearing level for pure tones in the speech range. The *speech discrimination test* is a measure of the patient's ability to understand speech when it is presented at a level that is easily heard. In patients with eighth nerve lesions speech discriminations can be severely reduced, even when pure tone thresholds are normal or nearly normal, whereas in patients with cochlear lesions discrimination tends to be proportional to the magnitude of hearing loss.

Recruitment is usually measured by the alternating binaural loudness balance (ABLB) test (if the hearing loss is unilateral). This test compares the loudness for tones of varied intensities as perceived by the pathologic ear and the normal ear. Recruitment is present if smaller increases in stimulus intensity are required in the poorer ear than in the better ear to maintain equal loudness. Otologists employ a variety of special tests to evaluate hearing loss, including tone decay, distorted speech testing and dichotic stimulation, acoustic impedance, tympanometry, and stapedius muscle contraction. The text by DeWeese and Saunders gives details.

Brain stem auditory evoked responses (BAER) can be recorded from scalp electrodes at 0 to 10 msec (early), 10 to 50 msec (middle), and 50 to 500 msec (late) following a click stimulus. The early potentials reflect electrical activity at the cochlea, eighth cranial nerve, and brain stem; the later potentials reflect cortical activity. Computer averaging of the responses to 1000 to 2000 clicks separates the evoked potential from background noise. Early evoked responses may be used to estimate the magnitude of hearing loss and to differentiate among cochlea, eighth nerve, and brain-stem lesions.

CAUSES OF HEARING LOSS. **Conductive Hearing Loss.** The logic for identifying common causes of hearing loss is shown in Figure 453–5. The history, examination, and audiometry usually provide the key differential features. The most common cause of conductive hearing loss is *impacted cerumen* in the external canal. This benign condition is usually first noticed after bathing or swimming when a droplet of water closes the remaining tiny passageway. The most common serious cause of conductive hearing loss is inflammation of the middle ear, *otitis media,* either infected (suppurative) or noninfective (serous). Fluid accumulates in the middle ear, impairing the conduction of airborne sound. Since the air cavity of the middle ear is in direct connection with the mastoid air cells, infection can spread through the mastoid bone and, occasionally, into the intracranial cavity. Chronic otitis media with perforation of the tympanic membrane can result in an invasion of the middle ear and other pneumatized areas of the temporal bone by keratonizing squamous epithelium (*cholesteatoma*). Cholesteatomas can produce erosion of the ossicles and bony labyrinth, resulting in a mixed conductive-sensorineural hearing loss. *Otosclerosis* commonly produces progressive conductive hearing loss by immobilizing the stapes with new bone growth in front of and below the oval window. The hearing loss is typically conductive, although in some persons the cochlea may be invaded by foci of otosclerotic bone, producing an additional sensorineural hearing loss. Otosclerosis usually stabilizes when the hearing level reaches 50 to 60 dB and rarely progresses to deafness. Other common causes of conductive hearing loss include trauma, congenital malformations of the external and middle ear, and glomus body tumors.

Sensorineural Hearing Loss. Genetically determined deafness, usually from hair cell aplasia or deterioration, may be present at birth or may develop in adulthood. The diagnosis of *hereditary deafness* rests on the finding of a positive family history. In many instances the inheritance is through a recessive gene or a dominant gene with low penetrance, making it difficult to determine the genetic nature of the disorder. *Intrauterine factors* resulting in congenital hearing loss include infection (especially rubella);

toxic, metabolic, and endocrine disorders; and anoxia associated with Rh incompatibility and difficult deliveries.

Acute unilateral deafness usually has a cochlear basis. *Bacterial or viral infections* of the labyrinth, *head trauma* with fracture or hemorrhage into the cochlea, or *vascular occlusion* of a terminal branch of the anterior inferior cerebellar artery all can damage extensively the cochlea and its hair cells. An acute idiopathic, often reversible, unilateral hearing loss strikes young adults and is presumed to reflect an isolated viral infection of the cochlea and auditory nerve terminals. Sudden unilateral hearing loss often associated with vertigo and tinnitus can result from a *perilymphatic fistula.* Such fistulae may be congenital or may follow stapes surgery or head trauma. *Drugs* cause acute and subacute bilateral hearing impairment. Salicylates, furosemide, and ethacrynic acid have the potential to produce transient deafness when taken in high doses. More toxic to the cochlea are aminoglycoside antibiotics (gentamicin, tobramycin, amikacin, kanamycin, streptomycin, and neomycin). These agents can destroy cochlear hair cells in direct relation to their serum concentrations. Some antineoplastic chemotherapeutic agents, particularly cisplatin, cause severe ototoxicity.

Subacute relapsing cochlear deafness occurs with *Meniere syndrome,* a condition associated with fluctuating hearing loss and tinnitus, recurrent episodes of abrupt and often severe vertigo, and a sensation of fullness or pressure in the ear. Recurrent endolymphatic hypertension (hydrops) is believed to cause the episodes. Pathologically, the endolymphatic sac is dilated, and the hair cells become atrophic. The resulting deafness is subtle and reversible in the early stages but subsequently becomes permanent and is characterized by diplacusis and loudness recruitment. The disorder is usually unilateral, but in about 20 to 40 per cent of patients bilateral involvement occurs.

The gradual, progressive, bilateral hearing loss commonly associated with advancing age is called *presbycusis.* Presbycusis is not a distinct disease entity but rather represents multiple effects of aging on the auditory system. It may include conductive and central dysfunction, although the most consistent effect of aging is on the sensory cells and neurons of the cochlea. The typical audiogram of presbycusis is a symmetric high-frequency hearing loss gradually sloping downward with increasing frequency. The most consistent pathology associated with presbycusis is degeneration of sensory cells and nerve fibers at the base of the cochlea. The recurrent trauma of *noise-induced hearing loss* affects approximately the same cochlear region and is almost as common, particularly among those with exposure to loud explosive or industrial noises. Loud, blaring, modern music has become a recent offender. The loss almost always begins at 4000 Hz and does not affect speech discrimination until late in the

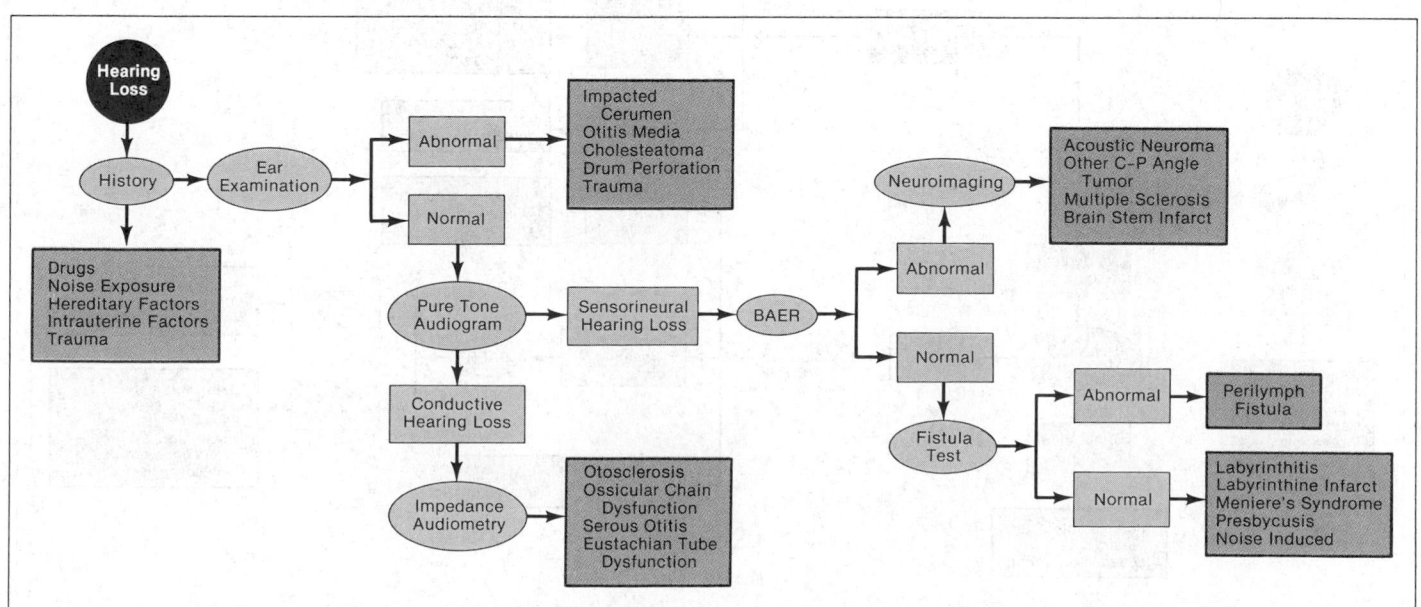

FIGURE 453–5. Evaluation of hearing loss.

disease process. With only brief exposure to loud noise (hours to days) there may be only a temporary threshold shift, but with continued exposure permanent injury begins. The duration and intensity of exposure determine the degree of permanent injury.

Hearing loss from direct damage to the acoustic nerve in the petrous canal occasionally results from infection within or trauma to the surrounding bone; severe deafness of abrupt onset marks the event and is usually associated with acute vertigo due to concurrent vestibular nerve injury. Progressive unilateral hearing loss that arises insidiously and worsens by almost imperceptible degrees is characteristic of benign neoplasms of the cerebellopontine angle, such as *acoustic neuromas*. In about 10 per cent of cases the hearing loss can be acute, apparently owing to either hemorrhage into the tumor or compression of the labyrinthine vasculature.

Central Hearing Loss. Central hearing loss is unilateral only if it results from damage to the pontine cochlear nuclei on one side of the brain stem. Such can occur with *ischemic infarction* of the lateral brain stem (e.g., occlusion of the anterior inferior cerebellar artery), a plaque of *multiple sclerosis*, or, rarely, invasion or compression of the lateral pons by a *neoplasm* or *hematoma*. Bilateral *degeneration* of the cochlear nuclei accompanies some of the rare recessive inherited disorders of childhood. As noted, clinically important unilateral hearing loss never results from neurologic disease arising rostrad to the cochlear nucleus. Although bilateral hearing loss could, in theory, result from bilateral destruction of central hearing pathways, in practice this is rare since involvement of neighboring structures in brain stem or hemisphere would usually produce overwhelming neurologic disability.

TREATMENT OF HEARING LOSS. If an underlying disorder has not yet destroyed the auditory system and can be ameliorated medically or surgically, hearing may be improved or preserved. Most patients with otosclerosis respond to stapedectomy. Closure of a perilymph fistula may improve hearing. Antibiotic and decongestive treatment of otitis media should prevent permanent hearing loss. A low-salt diet and diuretics are effective in selective cases of Meniere syndrome, particularly if episodes are precipitated by premenstrual water retention. The surgical treatment of Meniere syndrome is still controversial. Hearing aids amplify sound, usually with the goal of making speech intelligible. Patients with conductive hearing loss require

simple amplification, but those with sensorineural hearing loss often need frequency-selective amplification in order to make hearing aids useful. Recent advances in acoustic technology have markedly improved the outlook for the latter. Monitoring audiograms in patients with exposure to noise or ototoxic drugs is critical for prevention of permanent hearing loss.

TINNITUS. The flow chart in Figure 453–6 outlines the logic for determining the common causes of tinnitus. A careful history should be taken to identify common offending drugs (Table 453–5). With *objective tinnitus* the patient hears a sound arising external to the auditory system, a sound that can usually be heard by the examiner with a stethoscope. Objective tinnitus usually has benign causes such as noise from temporomandibular joints, opening of eustachian tubes, or repetitive muscle contractions. Sometimes, in a quiet room, the patient can hear the pulsatile flow in the carotid artery or a continuous hum of normal venous outflow through the jugular vein. The latter can be obliterated by compression of the jugular vein or extreme lateral rotation of the neck. Pathologic objective tinnitus occurs when patients hear turbulent flow in vascular anomalies or tumors (e.g., glomus jugulare tumor). Objective tinnitus may also be an early sign of increased intracranial pressure. Such tinnitus, which is usually overshadowed by other neurologic abnormalities, can be obliterated by pressure over the jugular vein. It probably arises from turbulent flow through compressed venous structures at the base of the brain.

Subjective tinnitus can arise from sites anywhere in the auditory system. The sounds most frequently complained of are metallic ringing, buzzing, blowing, roaring, or, less often, bizarre clanging, popping, or nonrhythmic beating. Tinnitus heard as a faint, moderately high-pitched, metallic ring can be observed by almost anyone who concentrates attention on auditory events in a quiet room. Sustained louder tinnitus accompanied by audiometric evidence of deafness occurs in association with both conductive and sensorineural hearing loss. Tinnitus observed with otosclerosis tends to have a roaring or hissing quality, while that associated with Meniere syndrome often produces sounds that vary widely in intensity with time and quality, sometimes including roaring or clanging. Tinnitus with other cochlear or auditory nerve lesions tends to be higher pitched and ringing in quality. Audiometric and brain stem–evoked response testing can help distinguish between lesions involving the conducting apparatus, the cochlea, and the auditory nerve.

Tinnitus without observable deafness appears sporadically and

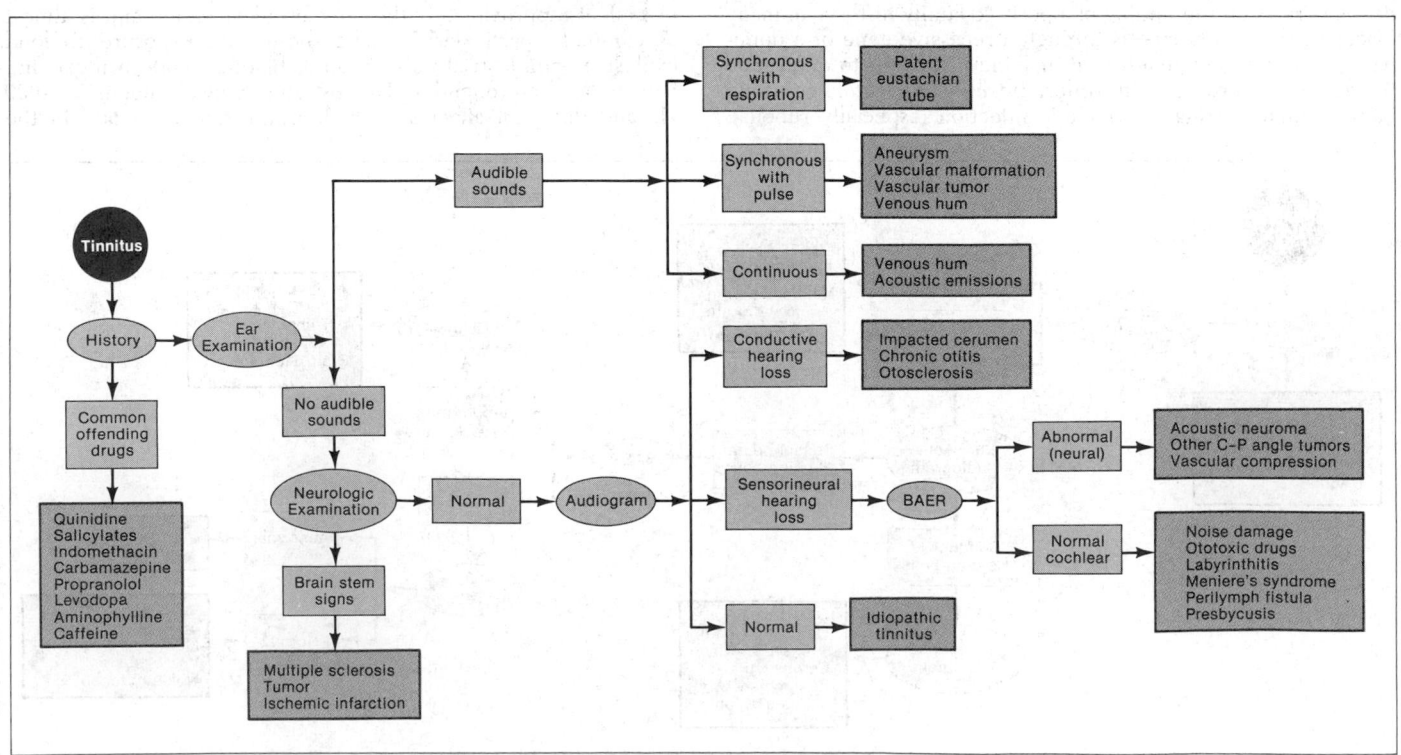

FIGURE 453–6. Evaluation of tinnitus.

TABLE 453–5. DRUGS COMMONLY ASSOCIATED WITH TINNITUS

Quinidine	Propranolol
Salicylates	Levodopa
Indomethacin	Aminophylline
Carbamazepine	Caffeine

for variable lengths of time in many persons without other evidence of an ongoing pathologic process. In many instances one suspects that the auditory experience is no more than an anxious preoccupation with normal auditory physiology.

TREATMENT OF TINNITUS. Most patients with tinnitus can be helped by detailed interview together with the relevant examination and laboratory investigations followed by reassurance where this can be given. Often exacerbating factors such as chronic anxiety and depression can be identified. In patients with hearing loss and tinnitus a hearing aid may improve communication in two ways, as amplification of ambient sound may effectively mask the tinnitus. This mechanism probably explains the frequent observation that removal of cerumen from the external auditory canal to improve ambient hearing also improves tinnitus. Also, when cerumen is attached to the tympanic membrane, tinnitus may result from local mechanical effects on the conductive system. For patients who find their tinnitus most obtrusive when trying to sleep, a bedside FM clock radio tuned between stations can provide an effective masking sound that will switch itself off after the patient falls asleep. A careful drug history should be taken, and a drug-free trial period should be considered when possible. Some patients who notice that caffeine, alcohol, or nicotine exacerbates their tinnitus experience significant relief when these drugs are discontinued.

Surgical treatment of tinnitus has been disappointing. Even when a lesion can be localized to the inner ear or cochlear nerve, removing these structures often has little effect on the tinnitus. A single exception to the generally dismal record of surgical treatment of tinnitus is complete cure of objective tinnitus after surgical correction of a vascular malformation or tumor in the mastoid.

EQUILIBRIUM—VESTIBULAR SYSTEM

DEFINITIONS. *Vertigo* is a subtype of dizziness in which there is an illusion of movement, most commonly rotation. *Physiologic vertigo* occurs in normal subjects when there is a mismatch among the vestibular, visual, and somatosensory systems induced by some external stimulus. The most common example is coming to a sudden stop after several whirling turns. The vestibular signals arising from the semicircular canals are in conflict with the visual signals that indicate a stable surround. *Pathologic vertigo* occurs when there is an imbalance in the vestibular system caused by a lesion within the vestibular pathways anywhere from the inner ear to the cerebral cortex. *Oscillopsia* refers to an illusion of oscillation of the environment.

ANATOMY AND PHYSIOLOGY OF THE VESTIBULAR SYSTEM. The paired vestibular end organs lie within the temporal bones next to the cochlea. Each organ consists of three semicircular canals that detect angular acceleration and two otolith structures, the utricle and saccule, that detect linear acceleration (including gravitational). Like the cochlea, these organs possess hair cells that act as force transducers, converting the forces associated with head acceleration into afferent nerve impulses. The hair cells of the three semicircular canals, each of which is oriented at right angles to the others, are concentrated in the crista, where they are embedded in a gelatinous mass called the cupula. Movement of the head causes the endolymph to flow either toward or away from the cupula, bending the hair cells and, depending on the direction of endolymphatic movements, either exciting or inhibiting the afferent nerve firing. Since the afferent nerves arising from the semicircular canals are tonically active, the baseline activity can be increased or decreased depending on the direction of hair cell bending. Furthermore, the two sets of semicircular canals are approximately mirror images of each other, so that rotational movement of the head that excites one canal inhibits the analogous canal on the opposite side. The hair cells of the utricle and saccule are concentrated in an area called the macule. The macule of the

utricle lies approximately in the plane of the horizontal canal and the macule of the saccule is approximately in the plane of the anterior canal. The hair cells are embedded in a membrane that contains calcium carbonate crystals or otoliths; the density of otoliths is considerably greater than that of the endolymph. Linear accelerations of the head combine with the linear acceleration of gravity to distort the otolith membrane, thereby bending the underlying hair cells and modulating the activity of the afferent nerve terminals at the base of the hair cells.

The afferent vestibular nerves have their cell bodies in Scarpa's ganglion. The nerve fibers travel in the vestibular portion of the eighth cranial nerve contiguous to the acoustic portion. Fibers from different receptor organs terminate in different vestibular nuclei at the pontomedullary junction. There are also direct connections with many portions of the cerebellum, the greatest respresentation being in the flocculonocular lobe, the so-called vestibular cerebellum. Efferent fibers from the brain stem travel through the vestibular nucleus to reach hair cells of the semicircular canals and macules. Efferent fibers are inhibitory in nature and, like the efferent fibers of the cochlea, may function to enhance inputs to which the brain attends. From the vestibular nuclei second-order neurons make important connections to the vestibular nuclei of the other side, to the cerebellum, to motor neurons of the spinal cord, to autonomic nuclei in the brain stem, and, most importantly for the examining clinician, to the nuclei of the oculomotor system. Fibers from the vestibular nuclei also ascend through the brain stem and thalamus to reach the cerebral cortex bilaterally. The exact site of cortical representation is unclear. Clinical evidence points to both superior temporal and inferior parietal lobes as likely sites.

LOCALIZATION OF LESIONS WITHIN THE VESTIBULAR PATHWAYS. Vertigo can be caused by either the peripheral or central vestibular apparatus. In general, peripheral vertigo is more severe, is more likely to be associated with hearing loss and tinnitus, and often leads to nausea and vomiting. Nystagmus associated with peripheral vertigo is usually inhibited by visual fixation. Central vertigo is generally less severe than peripheral vertigo and is often associated with other signs of central nervous system disease. The nystagmus of central vertigo is not inhibited by visual fixation and frequently is prominent when vertigo is mild or absent.

EXAMINATION OF THE VESTIBULAR SYSTEM. Most vestibular problems presenting to the physician are episodic, and often there are neither symptoms nor signs when the physician examines the patient. The history, therefore, can become paramount for identifying vestibular dysfunction. The history should attempt to distinguish vertigo (the illusion of movement in space) from light-headedness (presyncope), ataxia (disequilibrium of the body without true movement in space), and psychogenic symptoms (the feeling of dissociation or, sometimes, dysequilibrium). If the history is not clear, bedside provocative tests to mimic the symptom may assist in making a pathophysiologic diagnosis. Hyperventilation, which lowers the $PaCO_2$ and decreases cerebral blood flow, causes a light-headed sensation associated with syncope. Ask the patient to hyperventilate maximally for 1 to 3 minutes to cause light-headedness. If the episode mimics the patient's symptoms it suggests that anxiety and hyperventilation may be playing an important role. In addition, during the course of hyperventilation the patient may suffer dry mouth, chest tightness, and paresthesias, which he may recognize as part of his spontaneous attacks, thus helping in diagnosis.

Bedside tests of vestibulospinal function are often insensitive because most patients can use vision and proprioceptive signals to compensate for any vestibular loss. Patients with acute unilateral peripheral vestibular lesions may past point or fall toward the side of the lesion, but within a few days balance returns to normal. Patients with bilateral peripheral vestibular loss have more difficulty compensating and usually show some imbalance on the Romberg and tandem walking tests, particularly with eyes closed.

The vestibulo-ocular reflex can be tested at the bedside by inducing physiologic nystagmus and searching for pathologic nystagmus. In an alert human, rotating the head back and forth in the horizontal plane induces compensatory horizontal eye movements that are dependent on both the smooth pursuit and vestibular systems. Because of the combined visual and vestibular input, a patient with complete loss of vestibular function and normal pursuit may still have normal compensatory eye movements on this test. The doll's-eye test is a useful bedside test of vestibular function in a comatose patient, however, since such patients cannot generate pursuit or corrective fast components. In this setting slow conjugate compensatory eye movements indicate normally functioning vestibulo-ocular pathways. Since the vestibulo-ocular reflex has a much higher frequency range than the smooth pursuit system, a qualitative bedside test of vestibular function can be made by having the patient shake his head back and forth at frequencies above 1 Hz while reading a standard visual acuity chart. A decrease in visual acuity of more than one line compared to testing with the head still indicates an abnormal vestibulo-ocular reflex.

The caloric test uses a nonphysiologic stimulus to induce endolymphatic flow in the horizontal semicircular canal and horizontal nystagmus by creating a temperature gradient from one side of the canal to the other. With a cold caloric stimulus the column of endolymph nearest the middle ear falls because of its increased density. This causes the cupula to deviate away from the utricle (ampullofugal flow) and produces horizontal nystagmus with the fast phase directed away from the stimulated ear. A warm stimulus produces the opposite effect causing ampullopedal endolymph flow and nystagmus directed toward the stimulated ear (mnemonic: COWS—cold opposite, warm same). Because of its ready availability ice water (approximately 0° C) is usually used for bedside caloric testing. To bring the horizontal canal into the vertical plane the patient lies in the supine position with head tilted 30 degrees forward. Infusion of 10 ml of ice water induces a burst of nystagmus usually lasting from 1 to 3 minutes. A comatose patient shows only a slow tonic deviation toward the side of stimulation. Greater than a 20 per cent asymmetry in nystagmus duration suggests a lesion on the side of the decreased response. This should always be confirmed, however, with standard bithermal caloric testing and electronystagmography (see below).

Examination for pathologic vestibular nystagmus should include a search for spontaneous and positional nystagmus (see Table 453–4). Since vestibular nystagmus secondary to peripheral vestibular lesions is inhibited with fixation, the yield is increased by impairing fixation (such as with +30 lenses, Frenzel glasses). Two general types of positional nystagmus can be identified on the basis of nystagmus regularity: static and paroxysmal. One induces static positional nystagmus by slowly placing the patient into the supine, then right lateral, and then left lateral position. This type of positional nystagmus persists as long as the position is held. Since direction-changing and direction-fixed static positional nystagmus occur with both peripheral and central vestibular lesions, their presence indicates only a dysfunction somewhere in the vestibular system. As with spontaneous nystagmus, however, lack of suppression with fixation and signs of associated brain-stem dysfunction suggest a central lesion.

Paroxysmal positional nystagmus is induced, after a brief delay, by a rapid change from erect sitting to supine head-hanging left, center, or right position (the so-called Hallpike maneuver). It is initially high in frequency but dissipates rapidly (within 30 seconds to 1 minute). The most common variety of paroxysmal positional nystagmus, benign positional nystagmus, usually has a 3 to 10 second latency before onset and rarely lasts longer than 30 seconds. The nystagmus is always torsional with fast phase directed upward (i.e., toward the forehead). It is usually prominent in only one head-hanging position, and a burst of nystagmus in the reverse direction occurs when the patient reassumes the sitting position. Another key feature is that the severe vertigo and nystagmus that the patient experiences with the initial positioning rapidly disappear with repeated positioning (fatigability). Benign positional nystagmus is a sign of vestibular end-organ disease (probably damage to the posterior semicircular canal, see p. 2111).

Electronystagmography (ENG) is a technique for recording eye movements that allows precise quantification of both physiologic and pathologic nystagmus. A standard ENG test battery includes (1) tests of visual ocular control (saccades, smooth pursuit, and optokinetic nystagmus); (2) a careful search for pathologic nystagmus with fixation and with eyes open in darkness; and (3) measurement of induced physiologic nystagmus (caloric and rotational). ENG can be helpful in identifying a vestibular lesion and localizing it within the peripheral and central pathways.

EVALUATING THE "DIZZY" PATIENT. The history is key, since it determines the type of dizziness (vertigo, light-headedness, feeling of dissociation, disequilibrium), associated symptoms (neurologic, audiologic, cardiac, psychiatric), precipitating factors (position change, trauma, stress, drug ingestion), and predisposing illness (systemic viral infection, cardiac disease, cerebrovascular disease). Features that distinguish between vestibular and nonvestibular types of dizziness are summarized in Table 453–6. The examination should include complete neurologic, head and neck, and cardiac assessments. When focal neurologic signs are found, neuroimaging usually leads to a specific diagnosis. When vertigo is present without focal neurologic symptoms or signs, audiometry and electronystagmography aid in localizing the lesion to the labyrinth or eighth nerve. Patients with hyperventilation syndrome and/or acute anxiety should be identified after the history and examination so that needless tests are not obtained. A detailed cardiac evaluation (including Holter monitoring) often identifies the cause of episodic presyncopal light-headedness.

COMMON CAUSES OF VERTIGO. The logic for identifying common causes of vertigo is shown in Figure 453–7.

Physiologic Vertigo. Physiologic vertigo includes common disorders such as *motion sickness*, *space sickness*, and *height vertigo*. In these conditions vertigo (defined as an illusion of movement) is minimal or absent while autonomic symptoms predominate. With height vertigo, patients often experience acute anxiety and panic reaction. Subjects with motion sickness and space sickness typically develop perspiration, nausea, vomiting, increased salivation, yawning, and generalized malaise. Gastric motility is reduced and digestion impaired. Even the sight or smell of food is distressing. Hyperventilation is a common sign, and the resulting hypocapnia leads to changes in blood volume, with pooling in the lower parts of the body predisposing to postural hypotension and syncope. An unusual variant of motion sickness continues when the subject returns to stationary conditions after prolonged exposure to motion. Typically, affected patients report that they feel the persistent rocking sensation of a boat long after returning to solid ground. Rarely, the syndrome can last for months to years after exposure to motion and can even be incapacitating. The cause is unknown.

Physiologic vertigo can often be suppressed by supplying sensory cues that help to match the signals originating from different sensory systems. Thus, motion sickness, which is exacerbated by sitting in a closed space or reading (giving the visual system the miscue that the environment is stationary), may be improved by looking out at the environment and watching it move. Height vertigo, caused by a mismatch between sensation of normal body sway and lack of its visual detection, can often be relieved either by sitting or by visually fixating a nearby stationary object.

TABLE 453–6. DISTINGUISHING BETWEEN VESTIBULAR AND NONVESTIBULAR TYPES OF DIZZINESS

	Vestibular	Nonvestibular
Common descriptive terms	Spinning (environment moves), merry-go-round, drunkenness, tilting, motion sickness, off-balance	Light-headed, floating, dissociated from body, swimming, giddy, spinning inside (environment stationary)
Course	Episodic	Constant
Common precipitating factors	Head movements, position change	Stress, hyperventilation, cardiac arrhythmia, situations
Common associated symptoms	Nausea, vomiting, unsteadiness, tinnitus, hearing loss, impaired vision, oscillopsia	Perspiration, pallor, paresthesias, palpitations, syncope, difficulty concentrating, tension headache

Reprinted with permission from Baloh RW, Honrubia V: Clinical Neurophysiology of the Vestibular System, 2nd ed. Philadelphia, F. A. Davis Company, 1990.

Benign Positional Vertigo (BPV). BPV is by far the most common cause of pathologic vertigo. Patients with this condition develop brief episodes of vertigo (less than 1 min) with position change, typically when turning over in bed, getting in and out of bed, bending over and straightening up, or extending the neck to look up. BPV can result from *head injury, viral labyrinthitis,* and *vascular occlusion,* or it may occur as an isolated symptom of unknown cause (in about 50 per cent of cases). The latter is particularly common in the elderly. This syndrome is important to recognize, since, in the vast majority of patients, the symptoms spontaneously remit within 6 months of onset. It does commonly recur, however. The diagnosis rests on finding characteristic fatigable paroxysmal positional nystagmus after a rapid change from the sitting to head-hanging position (described on p. 2110). The pathophysiology of BPV is not established, but some investigators have postulated that debris from the utricular macule may become attached to the cupula of the posterior semicircular canal and artificially stimulate that canal when it is in the dependent position. Consistent with this theory, the burst of paroxysmal positional nystagmus is in the plane of the posterior canal of the "down ear," and the positional nystagmus disappears after the ampullary nerve has been surgically resected from the posterior canal on the diseased side. If the history and physical findings are typical, no further evaluation is necessary. If the history or findings are atypical, the condition must be distinguished from other causes of positional vertigo that may occur with tumors or infarcts of the posterior fossa. Typical BPV is not associated with such conditions. The treatment for most patients is simple reassurance. Since the vertigo can be extinguished by fatigue, many patients find that exercises involving repetitive position changes that initially produced the vertigo provide prolonged relief.

Acute Peripheral Vestibulopathy ("Acute Labyrinthitis"). One of the most common clinical neurologic syndromes at any age is the acute onset of vertigo, nausea, and vomiting lasting for several days and not associated with auditory or neurologic symptoms. Most affected patients gradually improve over 1 to 2 weeks, but some develop recurrent episodes. A large percentage report an upper respiratory tract illness 1 to 2 weeks prior to the onset of vertigo. This syndrome occasionally occurs in epidemics (epidemic vertigo), may affect several members of the same family, and more often erupts in the spring and early summer. All of these factors suggest a viral origin, but attempts to isolate an agent have been unsuccessful, except for occasional findings of a herpes zoster infection. Pathologic studies showing atrophy of one or more vestibular nerve trunks, with or without atrophy of their associated sense organs, are evidence of a vestibular nerve site and, probably, viral etiology for many patients with this syndrome (*viral neurolabyrinthitis*). In some patients attacks of acute vestibulopathy (usually less severe) recur over many months or years. There is no way of predicting whether a person who suffers a first attack will have repetitive attacks.

Meniere Syndrome. The typical clinical features of Meniere syndrome are described on page 2107. This disorder accounts for about 10 per cent of all patients with vertigo. The diagnosis is based on documenting episodic severe attacks accompanied by tinnitus, ear fullness, and fluctuating hearing levels on audiometric testing.

Post-traumatic Vertigo. Vertigo, hearing loss, and tinnitus often follow a blow to the head that does not result in temporal bone fracture, the so-called *labyrinthine concussion.* Although they are protected by a bony capsule, the delicate labyrinthine membranes are susceptible to blunt trauma. Blows to the occipital or mastoid region are particularly likely to produce labyrinthine damage. *Transverse fractures* of the temporal bone typically pass through the vestibule of the inner ear, tearing the membranous labyrinth and lacerating the vestibular and cochlear nerves. Complete loss of vestibular and cochlear function is the usual sequela, and the facial nerve is interrupted in approximately 50 per cent of cases. Examination of the ear often reveals hemotympanum, but bleeding from the ear seldom occurs, since the tympanic membrane usually remains intact. As noted above, *benign positional vertigo* is also a common sequela of head trauma. *Fistulae* of the oval and round windows can result from impact noise, deep-water diving, severe physical exertion, or blunt head injury without skull fracture. The mechanism of the rupture is a sudden negative or positive pressure change in the middle ear or a sudden increase in cerebrospinal fluid pressure transmitted to the inner ear via the cochlear aqueduct and internal auditory canal. Clinically, the rupture leads to the sudden onset of vertigo or hearing loss, or both. Surgical exploration of the middle ear is warranted when there is a clear relationship between the onset of vertigo or hearing loss, or both, and the onset of severe exertion, barometric change, head injury or impact noise.

Postconcussion Syndrome. The so-called postconcussion syndrome refers to a vague dizziness (rarely vertigo) associated with anxiety, difficulty in concentrating, headache, and photophobia induced by a head injury resulting in concussion. Occasionally, similar, less pronounced symptoms are associated with mild head injury judged to be trivial at the time. The cause is unknown, but animal studies indicate that small multifocal brain lesions (petechiae) commonly occur after concussive brain injury.

Other Peripheral Causes of Vertigo. Vertigo can be associated with *chronic bacterial otomastoiditis,* either from direct invasion of the inner ear by the bacteria or by erosion of the labyrinth by a cholesteatoma. Radiographic studies of the temporal bone readily identify these disorders. Just as *otosclerosis* can result in sensorineural hearing loss it can also produce vertigo by involving the bony labyrinth. The typical audiometric findings of a combined conductive and sensorineural hearing loss should suggest this diagnosis. Several *drugs* that damage the auditory system (see p. 2107), such as the aminoglycosides, may also damage the vestibular labyrinth. The patient may suffer acute vertigo, either along with or independent of hearing loss and tinnitus, if the

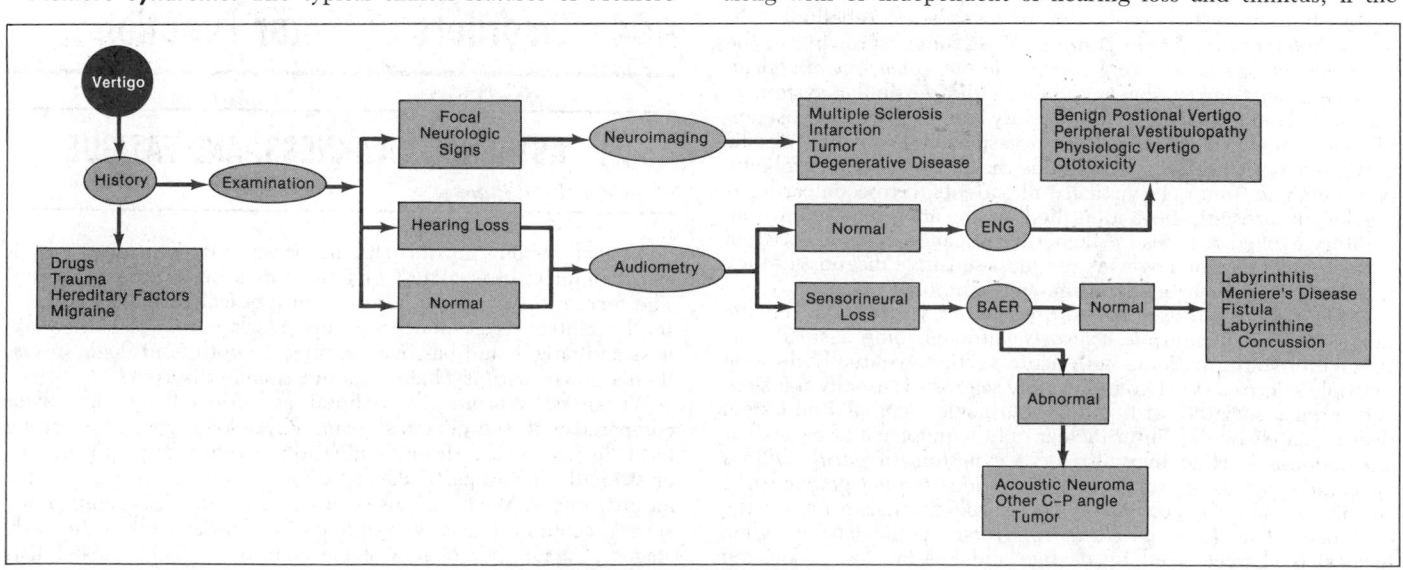

FIGURE 453–7. Evaluation of vertigo.

toxic effect is asymmetric. More often there is a progressive symmetric loss of vestibular function leading to imbalance but not vertigo. Unfortunately, many patients being treated with ototoxic drugs are initially bedridden and unaware of the vestibular impairment until they recover from their acute illness and try to walk. Then they discover that they are unsteady on their feet and that the environment tends to jiggle in front of their eyes (*oscillopsia*). Younger patients adapt after weeks to the labyrinthine failure; older ones may be left permanently disabled. Usually there is no nystagmus (because of the symmetric involvement), but the patient is ataxic. Caloric and rotational tests during electronystagmography can document impairment or absence of vestibular function. The best treatment is prevention. If the drug is discontinued early during the course of symptoms the disorder may stabilize or improve.

Vascular Insufficiency. Vertebrobasilar insufficiency is a common cause of vertigo in the elderly (see also Ch. 469). Whether the vertigo originates from ischemia of the labyrinth, brain stem, or both structures is not always clear, since the blood supply to the labyrinth, eighth cranial nerve, and vestibular nuclei originate from the same source, the basilar vertebral circulation. Vertigo with *vertebrobasilar insufficiency* is abrupt in onset, usually lasting several minutes, and is frequently associated with nausea and vomiting. Associated symptoms resulting from ischemia in the remaining territory supplied by the posterior circulation include visual illusions and hallucinations, drop attack and weakness, visceral sensations, visual field defects, diplopia, and headache. These symptoms occur in episodes either in combination with the vertigo or alone. Vertigo may be an isolated initial symptom of vertebrobasilar ischemia, but repeated episodes of vertigo without other symptoms should suggest another diagnosis. Vertebrobasilar insufficiency usually is caused by atherosclerosis of the subclavian, vertebral, and basilar arteries. Occasionally, episodes of vertebrobasilar insufficiency are precipitated by postural hypotension, Stokes-Adams attacks, or mechanical compression from cervical spondylosis. Diagnostic studies including CT scans are usually normal, since the vascular insufficiency is transient and function returns to normal between episodes. Angiography can be helpful in confirming the diagnosis but carries a risk and rarely leads to definitive therapy.

Vertigo is a common symptom associated with *infarction of the lateral brain stem or cerebellum*, or both. The diagnosis usually is clear, based on the characteristic acute history and pattern of associated symptoms and neurologic findings. Occasionally cerebellar infarction or hemorrhage presents with severe vertigo, vomiting, and ataxia without associated brain-stem symptoms and signs that might suggest the erroneous diagnosis of acute peripheral vestibular disorder. The key differential point is the finding of clear cerebellar signs (extremity and gait ataxia) and gaze-evoked nystagmus. Such patients must be watched carefully for several days, since they may develop progressive brain-stem dysfunction owing to compression by a swollen cerebellum.

Cerebellopontine-Angle Tumors. Most tumors growing in the cerebellopontine angle (e.g., *acoustic neuroma, meningioma, epidermal cyst*) grow slowly, allowing the vestibular system to accommodate so that they produce a vague sensation of disequilibrium rather than acute vertigo. Occasionally, however, episodic vertigo or positional vertigo heralds the presence of a cerebellopontine-angle tumor. In virtually all patients, retrocochlear hearing loss is present, best identified by an abnormal brain-stem auditory evoked response. Magnetic resonance imaging (MRI) of the cerebellopontine angles is the most sensitive diagnostic study for identifying a cerebellopontine-angle tumor.

Other Central Causes of Vertigo. Acute vertigo may be the first symptom of *multiple sclerosis*, although only a small percentage of young patients with acute vertigo eventually develop multiple sclerosis. Vertigo in multiple sclerosis is usually transient and often associated with other neurologic signs of brain stem disease, in particular, internuclear ophthalmoplegia or cerebellar dysfunction. Vertigo may also be a symptom of *parainfectious encephalomyelitis* or, rarely, *parainfectious cranial polyneuritis*. In this instance the accompanying neurologic signs establish the diagnosis. The *Ramsay Hunt syndrome* (geniculate ganglion herpes) is characterized by vertigo and hearing loss associated with facial paralysis and, sometimes, pain in the ear. The typical

lesions of herpes zoster, which may follow the appearance of neurologic signs, are found in the external auditory canal and, sometimes, over the palate. Rarely is herpes zoster responsible for vertigo in the absence of the full-blown syndrome. *Granulomatous meningitis* or *leptomeningeal metastasis* and cerebral or systemic *vasculitis* may involve the eighth nerve, producing vertigo as an early symptom. In these disorders cerebrospinal fluid analysis usually suggests the diagnosis. Patients suffering from *temporal lobe epilepsy* occasionally experience vertigo as the aura. Vertigo in the absence of other neurologic signs or symptoms is never caused by epilepsy or other diseases of the cerebral hemispheres.

TREATMENT OF VERTIGO. Treatment of vertigo can be divided into two general categories: specific and symptomatic. Specific therapies include antibiotics for bacterial or syphilitic labyrinthitis, anticoagulants for vertebrobasilar insufficiency, and surgery for acoustic neuroma. When possible, treatment should be directed at the underlying disorder. In most cases, however, symptomatic treatment is either combined with specific therapy or is the only one available (e.g., with acute peripheral vestibulopathy). Many different classes of drugs have been found to have antivertiginous properties, and in most instances the exact mechanism of action is uncertain. All of these agents produce potentially unpleasant side effects, and the decision on which drug or combination to use is based on their known complications and on the severity and duration of the vertigo. An episode of prolonged, severe vertigo is one of the most distressing symptoms that one can experience. Affected patients prefer to lie still with eyes closed in a quiet, dark room. Antivertiginous drugs with sedation such as phenergan (25 mg four times daily [q.i.d.]) or diazepam (5 mg q.i.d.) may be helpful. Prochlorperazine suppositories (25 mg) may stop vomiting. In more chronic vertiginous disorders, when the patient is trying to carry on normal activity, less sedating antivertiginous medications such as meclizine (25 mg q.i.d.) or transdermal scopolamine (0.5 mg every 3 days) may provide relief. Transdermal scopolamine has also been shown to prevent motion sickness. To be most effective, the patch must be in place several hours before exposure to motion. Scopolamine should be used cautiously in elderly subjects because it tends to produce confusion, memory loss, and even hallucinations.

Baloh RW: Dizziness, Hearing Loss and Tinnitus: The Essentials of Neurotology. Philadelphia, F. A. Davis Company, 1984. *More details in a similar format.*
Baloh RW, Honrubia V: Clinical Neurophysiology of the Vestibular System, 2nd ed. Philadelphia, F. A. Davis Company, 1990. *Monograph reviewing basic and clinical aspects of vestibular function.*
DeWeese DD, Saunders WH: Textbook of Otolaryngology, 6th ed. St. Louis, The C. V. Mosby Company, 1982. *A good text with chapters on hearing loss, tinnitus, dizziness, and vertigo.*
Hazell JWP: Tinnitus I, II and III. J Otolaryngol 19:1, 6, 11, 1990. *Up-to-date clinical review.*

454 Disorders of Motor Function

454.1 ASTHENIA, WEAKNESS, AND FATIGUE
Fred Plum

As many as one fifth of patients presenting to primary physicians complain of weakness or fatigue as a prominent symptom. The term *asthenia* finds more use in medical than lay parlance. Its descriptive usage nonspecifically overlaps that of both weakness and fatigue and has been applied to both neurologic (myasthenia gravis) and psychiatric (neurasthenia) disorders.

Weakness is arbitrarily defined as reduced muscle power compared with the person's norm. Physiologic weakness can be focal, in which case the individual often refers to a specific loss of strength during particular acts, e.g., walking, lifting, playing an instrument. Weakness also can be generalized, accompanying several acute or subacute systemic disorders as well as the early stages of a number of neurologic conditions. Table 454–1 lists levels of disease that may result in more or less specific weakness.

TABLE 454–1. CAUSES OF ACUTE OR SUBACUTE WEAKNESS

Condition	Examples or Mechanisms
Joint or muscle injury-inflammation	Movement of the part induces pain.
Primary muscle disease	Genetically transmitted muscle or mitochondrial disorders; inflammatory or granulomatous myopathies; corticosteroid administration
Neuromuscular junction	Myasthenia gravis; Lambert-Eaton myasthenic syndrome
Peripheral motor or sensorimotor pathways (lower motor neuron)	Damage to peripheral motor nerves, spinal motor roots, anterior horn cells
	N.B.: Dysfunction of proprioceptive sensory pathways can produce the illusion of weakness secondary to impaired position sense.
Corticospinal pathways (upper motor neuron)	Disease or injury to the system anywhere from above the anterior horn cell to frontal lobe motor areas
Basal ganglia	Hypokinesia, slow starting, and weakness in parkinsonism
Cerebellum	Sense of incomplete strength with neocerebellar damage
Hysterical or pretended weakness	Signs inconsistent with specific physiologic failure

Table 454–2 defines several particular acute or subacute disorders that may cause generalized weakness. Beyond these classes of specifically identifiable disorders, however, most chronic weakness unaccompanied by diagnosable neurologic or appropriate medical conditions is more likely to have a psychiatric than a neurologic genesis.

Fatigue, as employed in medical terms, describes a reduction in performance due to an experienced deterioration in capacity. Fatigue can be local or general, acute or chronic, and, depending on circumstance, the sense of exhaustion may follow, accompany, or precede attempts at either motor or intellectual effort. Most short-term fatigue lasting for minutes to as much as a few weeks in duration can be traced to recognized antecedents, such as acute systemic illness, severe emotional perturbation, or intense effort of either a physical or intellectual nature. Recurrent, rapidly developing fatigue involving local or generalized striated muscle is typical of myasthenia gravis or, less often, the metabolic myopathies (see Ch. 498). Multiple sclerosis and Parkinson's disease characteristically are accompanied by chronic feelings of fatigue, usually worse at the end than at the beginning of the day. Still-cryptic processes such as tuberculosis, systemic cancer, subacute endocarditis, collagen vascular disease, and certain endocrinopathies represent less frequent causes. Subacute, disabling fatigue also can accompany early HIV involvement of the brain, but that condition also causes recognizable abnormalities in cognitive capacities.

As a group, subacutely or chronically fatigued patients compared with nonexhausted controls have not shown higher long-term antibody titers against Epstein-Barr virus, Lyme borreliosis,

TABLE 454–2. MEDICAL-NEUROLOGIC ILLNESSES COMMONLY ASSOCIATED WITH ACUTE-SUBACUTE GENERALIZED WEAKNESS OR FATIGUE

Systemic	Neurologic
Acute bacterial-viral infections	Myasthenia gravis
Thyrotoxicosis	Early polyneuropathy
Post–myocardial infarction	Multiple sclerosis
Addison's disease	Parkinsonism
Disseminated malignancy	Postconcussion syndrome
Anticancer chemotherapy	Sustained drug use
Acute hepatitis; acute Epstein-Barr virus or Lyme disease	
Severe anemia	

or other organisms. A condition defining "chronic fatigue of recent onset" with a duration of greater than 6 months but less than 1 year and accompanied by objectively verified signs of low-grade fever, painful lymph nodes, and nonexudative pharyngitis recently has been set aside as a distinct syndrome deserving of complex medical evaluation. Such studies as exist to date, however, find few relevant physical or laboratory abnormalities in most chronically fatigued patients. Furthermore, little evidence has been advanced that the physical signs cited above identify any specific somatic illness that might respond to medicinal measures.

All well-analyzed studies of patients with chronic debilitating fatigue emphasize the frequency of the symptoms (up to 25 per cent or more of primary care patients), the lack of identifiable medical abnormalities, and a high incidence of psychiatric disorder. Symptoms of chronic anxiety, personality disorders, or depression have been identified in as many as 80 per cent of such cohorts. The condition frequently includes somatoform complaints unaccompanied by physical or laboratory abnormalities as well as expressions of autonomic dysfunction including breathlessness, palpitations, tachycardia, constipation-diarrhea, sexual impairment, inappropriate sweating, and unsatisfactory sleep patterns. Prospective and retrospective studies in these patients consistently have identified significantly more manifestations of depression, somatic anxiety, and emotional maladjustment than were expressed by nonfatigued controls chosen from patients with neuromuscular disease or recovering from known viral illnesses. No satisfactorily evaluated treatment program has been forthcoming for persons with chronic fatigue. Most patients with somatoform disorders of this kind have sustained better outcomes when "floated" by physicians providing repeated reassurances at short intervals than by psychiatrists attempting intense psychotherapy. Advisory psychiatric consultation, as well as modest doses of tricyclic antidepressants for some, have at times been found to reduce an otherwise high rate of incapacitating somatoform complaints.

Holmes GP, Kaplan JE, Gantz NM, et al.: Chronic fatigue syndrome: A working case definition. Ann Intern Med 108:387, 1988. *Definition of a syndrome in search of a medical cause.*

Kroenke K, Wood DR, Mangelsdorff AD, et al.: Chronic fatigue in primary care. Prevalence, patient characteristics and outcome. JAMA 260:929–934, 1988. *Among 1159 consecutive outpatients in primary care clinics, 24 per cent described chronic fatigue as a major problem. Screening psychometric instruments identified depression, somatic anxiety, or both among 80 per cent of fatigued patients versus 12 per cent of controls.*

Rowland LP: Weakness: The syndromes caused by weak muscles. *In* Rowland LP (ed.): Merritt's Textbook of Neurology, 8th ed. Philadelphia, Lea and Febiger, 1989, pp 50–54. *A systematic explanation of patterns of weakness accompanying disease entities ranging from muscle to brain.*

Smith GR, Monson RA, Ray DC: Psychiatric consultation in somatization disorder. A randomized controlled study. N Engl J Med 314:1407–1413, 1986. *Psychiatric consultation offering suggestions on management to primary physicians reduced quarterly health care charges in the treatment groups by 49 to 53 per cent.*

454.2 ATAXIA AND RELATED GAIT DISORDERS

Fred Plum

Any neurologic illness that affects sensorimotor functions in the lower extremities can interfere with the coordinated act of walking. Accordingly, an introductory analysis of the differential features of certain gait abnormalities may prove helpful in diagnosis. Other chapters provide descriptions of the specific abnormalities that characterize parkinsonism, chorea, athetosis, spastic paraparesis, and various forms of poly- and mononeuritic motor weakness.

ATAXIA. Ataxia is a failure of muscular coordination expressed as irregularity or awkwardness of movement. Common usage has applied the term most often to an unsteadiness of walking, but the same principles apply to disturbances in coordinated movements affecting the upper extremities, the speech mechanisms, or even the eye movements. In the literal sense, ataxia can result from any abnormality in motor function, whether induced by faulty peripheral sensory mechanisms or by disturbances of descending corticospinal, basal ganglion, or cerebellar control.

Most often the analysis of ataxia as a diagnostic problem lies in distinguishing disturbances in proprioceptive control from those caused by weakness, cerebellar-vestibular abnormalities, or the influence of toxic drugs.

PROPRIOCEPTIVE (SENSORY) ATAXIA. Proprioceptive ataxia can result from abnormalities anywhere along the afferent pathway from peripheral nerve, dorsal root, dorsal spinal funiculus, or, less often, the brain stem lemniscal system or the sensory projection from the thalamus to the parietal lobe cortex. The functional defect results from an impaired perception of the location of the body part combined with relatively preserved strength in the member. Afferent peripheral nerve, dorsal root, and spinal lesions are most often caused by inflammatory-demyelinating neuropathy, diabetic neuropathy, syphilitic tabes dorsalis, or meningomyelopathy, as well as any of several inherited forms of spinocerebellar degeneration (see Ch. 463). Cobalamin (B$_{12}$) deficiency involves both the peripheral nerve and the dorsal column of the cord, whereas multiple sclerosis and compressive cord diseases affect the cord alone.

Nerve or root lesions cause a bilateral defect that characteristically (1) affects the lower more than the upper extremities; (2) involves position sense as much as or more than vibratory sensation; (3) shows absent or greatly reduced deep tendon reflexes; and (4) produces a broad-based, weaving gait that with severe sensory loss becomes lurching, sometimes leg flinging, or pounding, and is worse in the dark (rombergism). Spinal dorsal column lesions produce similar symptoms except that position loss may be more profound, the signs may be less equally symmetric, the tendon reflexes can be preserved, and pathologic reflexes may be present if the abnormality also involves the descending corticospinal tract. By contrast, spinal cord compression tends to impair vibration sensation more than position. Brain stem lemniscal involvement resembles spinal impairment but is seldom bilateral; position sense loss may outstrip vibratory impairment. Patients with peripheral or spinal sensory ataxia are subjectively well aware of their deficits. They are also aware that their lack of coordination is not due to "dizziness," which distinguishes them from patients with vestibular disorders. Parietal or thalamoparietal proprioceptive impairment produces an ataxia that is usually unilateral and (1) affects the contralateral upper extremity as severely as the lower, (2) impairs position sense disproportionately more than vibration, and (3) may go partially unrecognized or be denied by the patient (anosognosia).

CEREBELLAR ATAXIA. The motor abnormality associated with cerebellar lesions depends on the localization of the abnormality in the cerebellum and whether or not adjacent or related neural structures are involved. Thus midline, lateral-hemispheric, and cerebellar outflow lesions tend to produce somewhat distinct syndromes. These differences become blurred when cerebellar tumors compress the adjacent brain stem to produce additional dysfunction or when diseases such as disseminated sclerosis or spinocerebellar degeneration affect neurologic structures that lie remote from the cerebellum.

Spinocerebellar disorders produce a predominantly sensory ataxia superimposed on which is a variable degree of cerebellar dyssynergia, depending on the extent of specific cerebellar inflow and outflow pathway involvement.

Midline cerebellar dysfunction results principally from degenerative (nutritional-alcoholic) or neoplastic (e.g., medulloblastoma, hemangioblastoma, metastasis) disease. The gait is characteristic with legs thrust widely apart and extended, the arms extended in compensatory balance, and walking accomplished by short steps. Affected patients usually look at the ground for additional sensory stabilization and turn en bloc. With extension into the anterior midline cerebellum, stretch reflexes become hyperactive. In the early stages of the illness, the upper extremities and cranial nerves can be affected little or not at all, even in the presence of substantial lower extremity ataxia. As the disorder advances, rhythmic truncal titubation appears, as can difficulty in rhythmic movements of the upper extremities and, eventually, even nystagmus. Posterior midline space-occupying lesions may add retropulsion (see below) to this symptom complex.

Lateral cerebellar hemispheric abnormalities produce ipsilateral hypotonia and incoordination of the limbs, an irregular

swaying gait and a tendency to drift toward the side of the lesion. The feet are spread apart, although not so broadly as with midline lesions, and patients characteristically cannot manage close-footed tandem walking. Rombergism is absent, but, as with all ataxias, distorted vision or closing the eyes accentuates the patient's unsteadiness. Rhythmic movements and point-to-point tests are impaired in both the upper and lower extremities. If classic intention tremor appears, it implies that the abnormality includes the outflow from the dentate nucleus or its projection through the superior cerebellar peduncle to the red nucleus of the midbrain.

DRUNKENNESS. Drunkenness, whether due to alcohol or depressant drug intoxication, results mainly from bilateral labyrinthine-vestibular dysfunction and is accompanied by sensations of both vertigo and dizziness. Few patients with cerebellar disease suffer as much incapacity as the reeling, lurching, twisting, and falling inebriate. Lesser degrees of intoxication produce unsteadiness, a tottering, cautious gait with the feet placed moderately widely apart, clumsiness, dysarthria, and nystagmus in all directions.

VESTIBULAR ATAXIA. Chronic unilateral impairment of the vestibulosensory system can occur with lesions anywhere along the peripheral eighth nerve pathway from labyrinth to brain stem. Patients with such abnormalities tend to drift toward the side of impairment and then quickly correct the deviation in the opposite direction. Turning accentuates their unsteadiness and induces missteps. Bilateral damage or degeneration of the vestibular nuclei in the brain stem results in a narrow-based ataxia with poor compensating movements in the limbs. Patients may drift or fall to either side, and some show a tendency to retropulsion and falling backward. Patients with vestibular dysfunction depend heavily on visual proprioception, so closing the eyes accentuates the gait disorder.

SPASTIC ATAXIA. Combined abnormalities of the spinal dorsal columns and cortical spinal tracts produce a characteristic broad-based tottering and sometimes pounding gait with the knees held high but the legs moving stiffly. The condition occurs with demyelinating diseases and other intrinsic spinal disorders such as vascular malformations, cobalamin deficiency, arachnoiditis, and, occasionally, neoplasms.

FRONTAL LOBE GAIT DISORDERS. Patients with frontal lobe disease can suffer any of several gait disorders, depending upon the anatomic distribution of the lesions. Unilateral injury to the foot-leg area of the somatosensory cortex produces a focal monoparesis, whereas bilateral motor-premotor damage results in a relatively narrow-based, stiff-legged impairment, sometimes with scissoring of the legs. More anteriorly placed premotor and prefrontal abnormalities arise in association with deep bilateral tumors, multiple cerebral infarctions, or communicating, "low pressure" hydrocephalus. The ensuing ataxia consists of a severe difficulty in initiating walking or otherwise using the lower extremities so long as the patient is in the erect position. The feet appear glued to the floor (magnet reaction), and attempts to walk often consist of short shuffles or even hops, before the legs get moving. Walking, once (or if) it begins, proceeds as a halting and broad-based movement made easier by guidance or support. Advanced cases tend to retropulse or fall backward, even from a sitting position. At least some dementia almost always accompanies the gait disorder.

Patients with frontal ataxia of this type show a considerably greater ability to move their legs when lying supine than when standing. Examination of the lower extremities discloses an increased paratonic resistance to passive movements coupled with bilateral plantar grasp responses, extensor thrust responses, and usually accentuated tendon reflexes. These reflex abnormalities and physiologic dysfunctions best explain the difficulty in movement.

HEMIPARESIS. Both pyramidal-corticospinal and extrapyramidal motor disorders may have a hemiparetic pattern, potentially confusing their early differentiation. Severe spastic hemiplegia from damage to the corticospinal tract or the full-blown stooped, festinating, semishuffling gait of parkinsonism is so well known and readily recognized as to require no discussion. In their initial stages, both pyramidal and extrapyramidal disorders produce mild or inconstant weakness, a susceptibility to easy fatigue in the affected member, and a sense of stiffness. Both corticospinal hemiparesis and parkinsonian hemiparesis incipiently produce a gait disorder marked by a slack arm and a reduction of automatic accessory movements on the affected side, a tendency to scuff the toe, and a measure of bodily akinesia. Both may result in an increase in muscular resistance to passive stretch on the involved side. The following points help in differential diagnosis. Patients with early pyramidal tract dysfunction tend to have unilaterally increased reflexes on the affected side. When walking, they flex the wrist and fingers, circumduct the lower extremity, and hold the foot in an equinovarus position. Patients with early hemiparetic parkinsonism, on the other hand, tend to have greater facial and bodily hypokinesia, to stoop, to have difficulty in performing two independent motor acts simultaneously, and to show at least some mild cogwheel resistance on rotary movements of the elbow or wrist. They extend the affected wrist and step the weak foot forward rather than circumducting it. The foot itself is held in simple varus position. The deep tendon reflexes may or may not be slightly asymmetric.

GAIT DISTURBANCES IN THE ELDERLY. Any of several specific visual, somatosensory, or motor diseases may impair walking in elderly persons. Less easily classified but fairly typical walking difficulties include a tendency to walk with slow, short, mincing, and unsteady steps (marche à petits pas). Fairly common is a stooped position coupled with a moderately broad-based, unsteady gait, sometimes associated with computed tomographic evidence of a chronic communicating hydrocephalus (see Ch. 486).

RETROPULSION. A tendency to step backward from the standing position or to fall backward while sitting can be a symptom of several serious, acquired midline abnormalities of the brain. The physiology is poorly understood. The abnormality accompanies midline tumors of the posterior cerebellum as well as degenerative disorders affecting the central vestibular mechanisms bilaterally, and has been reported in association with bilateral lesions affecting the sides of the third ventricle, the basal ganglia, and the frontal lobes. Occasionally the abnormality is associated with large, unilateral frontal lobe neoplasms that produce an increase in intracranial pressure and intracranial shift. Retropulsion of posterior fossa origin is especially dangerous, as it often comes on suddenly and is accompanied by a loss of the normal postural protective mechanisms that guard against injury during falling.

HYSTERICAL GAIT. Hysteria can mimic a variety of hemiparetic, steppage, or ataxic gait disorders. With a hemiparetic type, the pattern usually reveals its genesis by an atypical dragging behind of the affected leg during a series of hops or supported steps. The most obviously factitious hysterical disorder is a lurching, irregularly based, sometimes bent-forward walk in which the patient grasps any object in reach for support and reels from side to side inconsistently. Such patients may sink to the floor, but almost never endure an unsupported, self-injuring fall. Other than the examination of gait, the neurologic examination is normal in these patients. Signs of altered muscular tonus or abnormal reflexes are absent, and the bizarre movements not only differ from the expected pattern of sensory or cerebellar dysfunction but often change from examination to examination.

Garcin R: Coordination of voluntary movement and the ataxias. *In* Vinken PJ, Bruyn GW, Garcin R (eds.): Handbook of Clinical Neurology, Vol 1, Disturbances of Nervous Function. Amsterdam, North Holland, 1969, pp 293, 309. *A detailed and thoughtful exposition of clinical and physiologic principles.*
Keane JR: Hysterical gait disorders: 60 cases. Neurology 39:586, 1989. *A lively and perceptive evaluation of the problem finds that dystonia and chorea are most likely to be overlooked, and that prompt diagnosis leads to the best outcomes.*

454.3 EPISODIC LOSS OF MOTOR FUNCTION

Jerome B. Posner

Sometimes patients, especially in their older years, report episodic loss of motor function affecting one or more extremities unilaterally or bilaterally. The motor loss is brief in duration and is followed quickly by a return to normal. When the legs are affected bilaterally, the patient, if erect, falls (drop attacks). Episodic loss of motor function can be caused by several pathophysiologic abnormalities. Because the symptoms are episodic,

TABLE 454–3. CAUSES OF FALLING IN THE ELDERLY

Drop Attacks	Other Causes
Cryptogenic (see text)	Generalized weakness
Cardiac arrhythmias	Orthostatic hypotension
Transient cerebral ischemia	Sedative drugs
Cataplexy (Ch. 447)	Visual loss
Plateau waves (Ch. 486)	Gait disorders (Ch. 454.2)
Vestibular failure	
Seizures	
Psychogenic	

most such persons are normal by the time the physician sees them, so preliminary diagnosis depends on obtaining an accurate description of the event. The paragraphs below describe some causes of episodic loss of motor function.

DROP ATTACKS AND FALLS

The most perplexing diagnostic problem associated with episodic loss of motor function is the so-called drop attack (Table 454–3). A drop attack is a falling spell that occurs without warning and is not accompanied by changes in sensorium or by other neurologic symptomatology. In a classic drop attack, the patient, usually elderly, does not lose consciousness, has not tripped or otherwise lost his balance, and is able to resume normal activity immediately or shortly following the fall. Affected persons suffer no accompanying neurologic signs but sometimes fall with sufficient suddenness and force to cause injury. The attacks are more common in women and can occur episodically for months or years without the development of other nervous system disease. Although the falls sometimes produce injury, most drop attacks have a benign prognosis, either responding to treatment when a cause can be identified or resolving spontaneously when no cause is identified. The stroke rate and overall survival of elderly patients with drop attack are no different from those of age-matched controls. The pathophysiology of drop attacks is poorly understood. Abnormal tonic, long-loop, posture-controlling reflexes to extensor muscles have been postulated, but the mechanism lacks proof. In most elderly patients, a specific cause is never identified (cryptogenic drop attacks). When a cause is identified, cardiac arrhythmia or cerebral ischemia is usually the offender.

Transient cerebral ischemia produces bilateral leg weakness when motor pathways are involved bilaterally but only rarely causes sudden collapse. Bilateral weakness is likely only when the ischemia occurs in the distribution of either the anterior spinal or the vertebrobasilar arterial system. Episodic spinal cord ischemia is usually accompanied by sensory as well as motor symptoms, and with vertebrobasilar ischemia, most patients suffer other signs of brain stem ischemia as well (see Ch. 469).

Cataplexy, the sudden loss of motor tone without paralysis or change in consciousness, is an occasional cause of drop attacks. The fall to the ground is usually slower than with the classic drop attacks, and the patient rarely hurts himself (Ch. 447). Cataplexy can occur in young adults as part of the narcoleptic-cataplectic disorder (Ch. 447). Otherwise, cataplexy occasionally occurs as an isolated symptom of the sudden rises of intracranial pressure (*plateau waves*) that sometimes accompany brain tumors or hydrocephalus (Ch. 486). Because there are important connections between the vestibular system and pathways controlling muscle tone, sudden *labyrinthine-vestibular failure* such as occurs in Meniere's disease can cause drop attacks. Such episodes are almost always accompanied by vertigo and usually by nausea and vomiting as well. *Akinetic or myoclonic seizures* causing drop attacks are common in childhood but rare in adults. However, drop attacks occasionally have been reported in adults which appear to be epileptic in origin and respond to anticonvulsant drugs.

Falls in the elderly are extremely common, annually affecting one third of elderly persons living at home and as many as half of the residents in nursing homes. Ten to 20 per cent of these falls result in body-damaging injury. A minority of falls in the elderly are due to drop attacks (Table 454–3). Careful evaluation often detects previously unrecognized medical problems, the

TABLE 454–4. CAUSES OF TRANSIENT FOCAL MOTOR PARALYSIS

Transient carotid or basilar ischemia
Nonconvulsive seizures
Complicated migraine
Plateau waves (rare)

identification of which, although not always preventing future falls, substantially decreases future emergency hospitalizations.

DIAGNOSIS. The first task is to determine whether the patient was truly unconscious at any time during the episode. If so, the first diagnosis should be syncope, and the diagnostic evaluation is directed toward that disorder (see Ch. 446.1). If the patient was conscious throughout the episode and the disorder cannot be attributed to tripping or loss of balance, the physician should probe carefully for accompanying symptoms or signs that may help to localize the cause. Back pain, lower extremity paresthesias or sensory loss, or sudden changes in bladder or bowel function accompanying the drop attacks suggest spinal cord dysfunction. Headache, diplopia, and dysarthria accompanying the attack suggest brain stem dysfunction, probably caused by vertebrobasilar arterial insufficiency. Tinnitus or vertigo suggests a vestibular disorder. Severe headache, particularly if accompanied by nausea and vomiting, suggests plateau waves from increased intracranial pressure.

Magnetic resonance imaging (MRI) can rule out brain tumor or hydrocephalus (plateau waves). In the absence of demonstrated syncope or a cause of increased intracranial pressure, the most serious potential diagnoses are cardiac arrhythmias and vertebrobasilar transient ischemic attacks. These diagnoses require appropriate laboratory evaluation.

OTHER TRANSIENT PARALYSES

Episodic loss of motor function in one or more extremities can be a perplexing problem (Table 454–4). Affected patients may complain of sudden or rapid loss of motor function involving an arm or a leg or both, with or without associated sensory symptoms, but without abnormal motor movements of either the arm or the leg. The most common cause is transient cerebral ischemia in the distribution of the internal carotid artery (see Ch. 469). All patients suffering episodic loss of motor function on one side of the body should be considered to be suffering from transient ischemic attacks until proven otherwise. In transient ischemic attacks and the much less frequent plateau waves of increased intracranial pressure, there is usually sudden loss of motor function lasting 5 to 15 minutes and, in the instance of plateau waves, often an accompanying headache and sometimes some clouding of consciousness. With atonic seizures and migraine, the onset of motor dysfunction is usually, but not always, slower, but it, too, persists for 5 to 20 minutes. The motor weakness in late-life migraine may or may not be accompanied by a contralateral headache that appears as the paralysis disappears.

MRI can identify intracranial abnormalities while noninvasive ultrasonography or angiography can detect carotid vascular lesions. Electroencephalography may assist in the diagnosis of a seizure disorder, but the EEG is often normal between episodes. A past or family history of migraine assists in the diagnosis of late-life migraine. Therapeutic trials directed successively at treatment of the several causes of these episodic attacks sometimes help in reaching a definitive diagnosis.

Fisher CM: Late-life migraine accompaniments as a cause of unexplained transient ischemic attacks. Can J Neurol Sci 7:9, 1980. *A classic paper describing neurologic abnormalities, including episodic paralyses in patients with late-life migraine.*

Meissner I, Wiebers DO, Swanson JW, et al.: The natural history of drop attacks. Neurology 36:1029, 1986. *A comprehensive analysis of 108 mostly elderly patients with drop attacks, defining the diagnostic approach, treatment, and prognosis.*

Rubenstein LZ, Robbins AS, Josephson KR, et al.: The value of assessing falls in an elderly population. A randomized clinical trial. Ann Intern Med 113:308–316, 1990. *A randomized clinical trial of the prophylactic value of assessing nursing home patients who fall.*

455 Disorders of Sensation

Jerome B. Posner

455.1 MAJOR SENSORY SYMPTOMS

An organism perceives its environment through its sensory systems. When a sensory system is disordered, sensation may be diminished, increased, or distorted. Table 455–1 lists definitions for major sensory abnormalities.

Anatomy and Physiology of Sensory Pathways

Two major sensory pathways subserve exteroception (cutaneous sensation) and conscious proprioception. The first pathway subserves the sensations of pain, temperature, and crude touch. The receptors are naked nerve endings (nociceptors and thermoreceptors) connected either to small (5μ), thinly myelinated, "A delta" fibers, which conduct at about 35 meters per second, or to unmyelinated "C" fibers (1 to 2 μ), which conduct at about 0.5 meter per second. (This dual set of fibers explains the phenomenon of "double pain." A noxious stimulus elicits first a sharp, pricking, well-localized pain mediated by the more rapidly conducting fibers, and the C fibers mediate a burning, poorly localized, exceedingly unpleasant "second pain.") Those sensory fibers, all of which have their cell borders in the dorsal root ganglia, enter the spinal cord and synapse in the dorsal horn. The ascending (second order) pain pathways cross the spinal cord and divide into two groups: the neospinothalamic tract, which is believed to subserve the perception of intensity and localization of pain, temperature, and crude touch, and the phylogenetically older paleospinothalamic tract, which is believed to subserve the arousal and emotional components of pain. The axons of the neospinothalamic tract arise from the dorsal horn, cross the anterior commissure, and ascend in the anterolateral quadrant of the spinal cord. The axons terminate in the ventral basal complex of the thalamus, principally within the ventral posterolateral nucleus (VPL) ipsilateral to the side of their ascent. The thalamic terminations of these fibers coincide to a large extent with those of the dorsal column. Third-order neurons from the thalamus project to somatosensory area 1 (sensorimotor cortex), with the same somatotopic localization as other sensory modalities. Lesions at the brain stem or thalamic level often lead to chronic so-called "thalamic pain." The paleospinothalamic tract, whose cells of origin in the dorsal horn receive C-fiber input, also crosses in the anterior commissure and ascends in the spinal cord closely applied to but more ventral than the neospinothalamic tract. Many of the fibers of the paleospinothalamic tract send collaterals to the reticular formation of the brain stem.

The second system subserving the functions of light touch, position sense, and tactile localization begins as encapsulated terminals (mechanoreceptors) connected to larger myelinated fibers. These large fibers enter the spinal cord via the dorsal root ganglion, lying in a position medial to the smaller fibers that subserve pain and temperature. Most of the large fibers ascend without synapsing in the posterior and to a lesser extent lateral columns of the spinal cord to reach the gracile and cuneate nuclei in the low brain stem. Second-order neuron fibers then decussate and ascend in the medial lemniscus to reach the contralateral ventral posterolateral thalamus. Third-order neurons projected

TABLE 455–1. MAJOR SENSORY SYMPTOMS DEFINED

Hypesthesia, anesthesia: reduction or loss of cutaneous touch sensation
Hypalgesia, analgesia: reduction or loss of cutaneous pain sensation
Hyperesthesia: lowered sensory threshold to cutaneous touch
Hyperalgesia: lowered cutaneous threshold to noxious stimuli
Hyperpathia: elevated threshold to noxious stimuli with accentuated discomfort above the threshold
Paresthesias: spontaneously arising exteroceptive sensation (e.g., pins and needles sensations, burning sensations)
Dysesthesias: unpleasant distortion of innocuous afferent stimuli
Allodynia: the perception of an ordinarily nonpainful stimulus as painful or excruciating

from the thalamus terminate in the cerebral cortex, predominantly in the sensorimotor strip surrounding the Rolandic fissure. Lesions of this system lead to loss of sense of position of the limbs and body in space, inability to localize tactile stimuli or to distinguish between one and two closely placed stimuli (two-point discrimination), and inability to describe accurately the size, shape, and texture of objects (stereoanesthesia). Subcortical lesions of the system also cause loss of the ability to recognize vibratory sensation (pallesthesia).

The two major exteroceptive systems are anatomically separated through much of their course, particularly in the spinal cord, and they differ physiologically as a result of fiber size. Thus, lesions at different sites in the nervous system and lesions of different physiologic natures cause unique sensory syndromes that assist in localizing the site and nature of the disorder. A discussion of the principles of pain management can be found in Ch. 26.

Localization of Sensory Disorders

PERIPHERAL NERVES. Sensory perception begins when a physical or chemical stimulus alters the activity of a *sensory receptor* in such a way that the stimulus is transduced into an electrical potential (receptor potential). Many diseases of peripheral nerves affect both large and small fibers, leading to a diminution of all sensory modalities to approximately equal degree. In some disorders of peripheral nerves, however, small or large fibers can be involved preferentially, leading to a "dissociated sensory loss." When small fibers are predominantly affected, pain and temperature sensation are involved out of proportion to light touch, vibration, and position sense. Spontaneous pain and burning dysesthetic sensations are common and often provide the presenting complaints. Because autonomic fibers are also small, trophic changes in skin and joints may accompany such a small-fiber peripheral neuropathy, but because motor fibers and the afferent portion of the stretch reflex are subserved by large fibers, these functions may be relatively preserved despite sometimes profound loss of pain and temperature sensation. Such selective small fiber damage is sometimes encountered in diabetes and is common in some of the hereditary neuropathies as well as in toxic-nutritional neuropathies (Ch. 499 and 500).

Large fiber damage, more common in demyelinating neuropathies, is characterized by profound loss of localizing touch and proprioception, with relative preservation of crude touch, pain, and temperature sensation. Paresthesias are common. The deep tendon reflexes are lost because of damage to large afferent fibers from muscle, and there is usually weakness as well.

The diagnosis of a peripheral neuropathy (see Ch. 495 to 502) involving sensory fibers is established by the distribution of the sensory loss, which may be in the distribution of a single nerve, multiple individual nerves, or a symmetric distal stocking-and-glove distribution. Polyneuropathies are distributed distally because longer axons are more vulnerable to disease than shorter ones. In general, mononeuropathies are caused by local disease (e.g., compression entrapment), mononeuritis multiplex by vascular disorders (e.g., polyarteritis), and polyneuropathies by immunologic or metabolic disorders (e.g., demyelinating-inflammatory neuropathy, diabetes, uremia, nutritional neuropathy).

SPINAL CORD. True dissociation of sensory loss is more common in spinal cord disorders than in those originating in peripheral nerves or roots. Lesions of the posterolateral columns produce profound loss of position and vibration sense with normal crude touch, pain, and temperature sensation. Usually corticospinal tracts are involved as well as sensory pathways, and thus many such patients often have hyperactive reflexes and extensor plantar responses. Lesions of the spinothalamic tract or of crossing fibers from the posterior horn to the spinothalamic tract cause loss of pain and temperature sense with preservation of vibration, position, and localizing touch. Such dissociated sensory loss is common in syringomyelia and may occur with infarction of the anterior portion of the spinal cord from occlusion of the anterior spinal artery. In both of these disorders, motor function may be relatively well preserved. When only one side of the spinal cord is involved, one finds loss of proprioceptive sensation on the ipsilateral side and loss of pain and temperature sensation on the contralateral side, both below the level of the lesion. There is

usually a small band of decreased sensation to all modalities resulting from damage to the posterior horn at the level of the lesion. This so-called Brown-Séquard syndrome is sometimes seen with tumors either compressing or invading the spinal cord and is a common presenting syndrome in radiation myelopathy. Lesions of the spinal cord are rarely confused with those of peripheral nerves, even when the latter show dissociated sensory loss, because the sensory loss in spinal cord lesions is usually proximal as well as distal and restricted to those segments below the spinal cord level damaged. Thus, by the time a polyneuropathy causes substantial sensory loss above the knees, nerve fibers supplying the fingertip are usually involved as well, whereas with a thoracic spinal cord lesion the arms are always spared. Furthermore, motor signs of upper motor neuron disease, particularly extensor plantar responses, usually correctly identify the central nature of a spinal cord disorder rather than pointing to a peripheral disturbance.

BRAIN STEM. In the lower brain stem, spinothalamic and proprioceptive pathways remain separated, lateral lesions of the medulla causing loss of pain and temperature sensation on the ipsilateral side of the face (a result of damage to the descending root of the trigeminal nerve) and the contralateral side of the body. This sensory abnormality is usually accompanied by other signs of lateral medullary damage (Wallenberg's syndrome) and spares proprioceptive pathways. Higher in the brain stem, as the two pathways converge in their route toward the thalamus, damage causes contralateral sensory loss to all modalities, usually accompanied by cranial nerve palsies, ataxia (from the cerebellar outflow), and motor weakness.

CEREBRUM. In the thalamus, damage to the ventral posterolateral nucleus causes decreased sensation of all modalities on the contralateral side of the body and face. Sensory loss is often accompanied by dysesthesias. A *thalamic syndrome* often appears 4 to 6 weeks after acute thalamic damage and has been attributed to denervation hypersensitivity of sensory neurons in the midbrain reticular formation. The patient develops spontaneous pain in the distribution of the sensory loss, usually associated with a dysesthetic response to touch and a hyperresponsiveness to pinprick once threshold is exceeded. The thalamic syndrome is rare but causes a particularly unpleasant pain intractable to most therapeutic endeavors. Conversely, surgical lesions of the intralaminar nuclei, which receive fibers from the paleospinothalamic tract, often decrease pain without affecting sensory thresholds.

Lindblom U, Ochoa JL: Somatosensory function and dysfunction. *In* Asbury AK, McKhann GM, McDonald WI (eds.): Diseases of the Nervous System, 2nd ed. Philadelphia, WB Saunders, 1991, in press.

455.2 HEADACHE AND OTHER HEAD PAIN

Headache ranks ninth among the causes of visits to physicians and is a major source both of time lost from work and of medical diagnostic procedures. The frequency of disabling headache is explained in part by the rich nerve supply to the head (including afferent nerve fibers from trigeminal, glossopharyngeal, vagus, and upper three cervical nerves) and in part by the psychological significance of head pain, causing anxiety about even modest discomfort, whereas a pain of equal severity elsewhere in the body might be ignored. Head pain can result from distortion, stretching, inflammation, or destruction of pain-sensitive nerve endings as a result of intra- or extracranial disease in the distribution of any of the aforementioned nerves. However, most head pain arises from extracerebral structures and carries a benign prognosis. The physician's twofold task is first to distinguish the very much more common, benign head pain from rarer but more serious causes and then to administer appropriate treatment. The diagnosis can usually be established by history and physical findings alone; skull radiographs, computed tomographic (CT) and magnetic resonance (MR) images, and other diagnostic tests are seldom required. Table 455–2 is a simplified classification of the pathogenesis of head pain; the overwhelming majority of

TABLE 455–2. PATHOPHYSIOLOGIC CLASSIFICATION OF HEADACHE

Vascular Headache
  Migraine headache
    Classic migraine
    Common migraine
    Complicated migraine
    Variant migraine
  Cluster headache
    Episodic cluster
    "Chronic" cluster
    Chronic paroxysmal hemicrania
  Miscellaneous vascular headaches
    Carotidynia
    Hypertension
    Orgasmic, exertional, and
      cough headache
    Hangover
    Toxins and drugs
    Occlusive vascular disease

Cranial Neuralgias

Tension Headache
  Common tension headache
  Depressive equivalent
  Conversion reaction
  Temporomandibular joint
    dysfunction
  Atypical facial pain

Traction-Inflammation Headache
  Cranial arteritis
  Increased or decreased
    intracranial pressure
  Extracranial structural lesions
  Pituitary tumors

Extracranial Structural Lesions
  Paranasal sinusitis and tumors
  Dental infections
  Otitis
  Ocular lesions
  Pituitary tumors
  Cervical osteoarthritis

headaches are either migraine or so-called tension headaches, with both abnormalities frequently playing a role in a given individual. Other forms of headache are much less common.

Migraine and Other Vascular Headaches

The term *vascular headache* applies to a group of clinical syndromes of unknown etiology in which the final step in pathogenesis of the pain appears to be dilatation of one or more branches of the carotid artery, leading to stimulation of nerve endings supplying that artery. There may be a release of noxious substances by either the arterial wall or nerve endings, causing a substantially lowered pain threshold. Such substances as serotonin, substance P, bradykinin, histamine, and prostaglandins alone or in combination have all been implicated in the pathogenesis of vascular headache. Most vascular headaches are unilateral, often but not always throbbing, and recurrent over months or years. Individual headaches are precipitated in some by identifiable environmental, dietary, or psychological factors. During the course of a vascular headache, the involved arteries may be tender to the touch, and pain may be relieved temporarily by compression of the carotid artery, only to return with increased intensity when compression is released. Most vascular headaches can be relieved by prompt administration of ergotamine; recurrent headaches can often be prevented by one of several prophylactic drugs (see below). So-called common migraine may affect as many as 25 per cent of the population. Other vascular headache syndromes are less common, but each has distinctive clinical findings.

CLASSIC MIGRAINE

Classic migraine is distinguished by well-defined symptoms of neurologic dysfunction that precede or, less often, accompany the headache. Neurologic symptoms are usually visual, consisting of bright flashing lights (scintillation or fortification scotomata) beginning in the center of a homonymous visual half-field and radiating over 10 to 30 minutes outward toward the periphery. Less commonly, the visual abnormalities are monocular (retinal) or consist of hemianoptic loss of vision in place of or following the scintillating scotomata. Other neurologic disturbances that can occur in classic migraine include unilateral paresthesias, usually involving the hand and perioral area, aphasia, hemiparesis, and hemisensory defects. An uncommon variant named *basilar artery migraine* occurs predominantly in children and adolescents and is characterized by vertigo, ataxia, and diplopia, along with hemiparesis or hemisensory changes. Rarely, confusion, stupor, or even coma may develop. Neurologic symptoms of classic migraine usually last no longer than 30 minutes and generally clear before the headache phase begins. However, in some instances neurologic signs may persist for hours or, rarely, for days, throughout and even beyond the headache phase of the illness.

The pathogenesis of the neurologic dysfunction is not fully understood. Measurements of regional cerebral blood flow during episodes of classic migraine have shown a wave of focal hyperemia followed by abnormally low flow spreading from posterior to anterior over the cerebral cortex. The flow reduction may be sufficient to cause the neurologic symptoms and, rarely, cerebral infarction. In most cases, however, the reduced cerebral blood flow is insufficient to account for the neurologic symptoms. One explanation is that there may be a wave of physiologic "spreading" depression that spreads across the cortex, accounting for both the neurologic symptoms and the changes in blood flow. Changes in brain blood flow do not accompany common migraine, even though the headache phase of the illness is similar. Thus, it is likely that if "spreading depression" is the cause of the neurologic symptoms of migraine, it is only one of several precipitating factors that may produce the headache.

The syndrome of classic migraine has four parts: (1) The *prodromal phase* occurs in a minority of patients and consists of an alteration of mood, often occurring for 24 or more hours before the headache. Patients may complain of increased hunger or thirst, drowsiness, euphoria, or depression. In some patients, known precipitants such as red wine commonly induce an attack. (2) The second phase consists of the *neurologic symptoms* described above. The neurologic symptoms may occur without subsequent headache (termed migraine equivalent), particularly in older people. (3) The third phase usually begins as the neurologic symptoms clear and characteristically consists of a unilateral throbbing frontotemporal *headache* on the side opposite the neurologic symptoms. The headache is frequently accompanied by nausea, photophobia, vomiting, diarrhea, phonophobia (noise intolerance), and a general feeling of being unwell. The headache commonly lasts 4 to 6 hours but may persist for 1 or more days. If the headache is prolonged, it may change into a dull, aching, bilateral pain extending back into the neck and shoulders. The headache phase is often terminated either by vomiting or by a period of sleep. (4) The *postheadache* phase is characterized by a feeling of exhaustion, tenderness of the scalp at the site of the headache, and recurrence of headache on sudden head movement.

The diagnosis of classic migraine is made by history; physical findings are absent, and laboratory evaluation is not helpful. When the attacks are atypical, particularly when neurologic disability is severe or prolonged, CT or MR imaging may be required to rule out structural lesions of the brain. However, such instances are rare. The treatment of classic migraine is similar to that of common migraine (see below), except that classic migraine attacks usually occur no more than four or five times a year and rarely more than once a month.

COMMON MIGRAINE

Common migraine is similar to classic migraine except that neurologic symptoms are absent. Many patients with classic migraine also have episodes of common migraine. Common migraine is characterized by recurrent headaches, often severe, frequently beginning unilaterally, and usually associated with malaise, nausea and/or vomiting, and photophobia. The disorder often begins in childhood, affects women more often than men, and runs in families (70 per cent of patients give a family history). Identifiable factors that often precipitate individual headaches are holidays and weekends, menstrual periods, foods (especially red wine, chocolate, nuts, and aged cheese), environmental stimuli (such as bright sunlight, too much sleep, and undue emotional stress or resentment). Medical conditions and their treatment may also precipitate attacks. Vasodilators such as nitroglycerin and antihypertensives and serotonin releasers such as reserpine, as well as estrogens and oral contraceptives, have been reported to cause migraine attacks in susceptible individuals. The diagnosis of common migraine is usually made by the history. Important historical points that help distinguish migraine from the equally common tension headaches (see below) include their unilaterality, their association with nausea or vomiting, the tendency of migraine to awaken one from sleep, a positive family history, and a positive response to ergot preparations. When the diagnosis is in doubt, treatment of the patient for common migraine often clarifies the issue.

TREATMENT. The best treatment for migraine is prevention.

The patient should avoid known precipitating factors. Medications known to cause migraine should be withdrawn if others can be substituted. Foods commonly implicated may also be withdrawn and, if withdrawal is effective, replaced one at a time to determine the specific precipitant. The patient should attempt to avoid undue stress or fatigue and not to sleep excessively on weekends. If these methods fail and severe headaches occur frequently (once a week or more), pharmacologic prophylaxis is indicated. Several agents have been reported effective in the prophylaxis of migraine, but not every patient responds to each agent. Perhaps the safest and most effective class of drugs are the β-adrenergic blockers, particularly propranolol. The drug is begun at a dose of 80 mg a day in divided doses and increased as tolerated until headaches are controlled. Recent reports suggest that calcium channel blockers such as verapamil* (80 mg three to four times daily) sometimes are effective. Amitriptyline* in gradually increasing doses from 25 to 125 mg daily may be useful if the above drugs fail. Methysergide, a serotonin antagonist, is effective at a dose of 2 mg three to four times daily. Methysergide must be employed cautiously because it can cause serious side effects, including vascular insufficiency, retroperitoneal or pleural fibrosis, and fibrotic thickening of heart valves. The side effects can be minimized by gradually withdrawing the drug for 1 month after every 4 to 6 months of treatment.

Acute attacks, if mild, often respond to analgesic agents and bedrest. More severe attacks are best treated by ergot preparations such as ergotamine tartrate. The drug, given parenterally, is sufficiently effective (85 to 90 per cent) to be useful as a diagnostic test. Oral ergot 1 to 2 mg given at the onset of a headache is effective in about 50 per cent of patients. However, during the headache, absorption of the oral form of the drug is often poor, and better results can be achieved with sublingual or rectal preparations. The best nonparenteral results are generally achieved by the insertion of half of a 2-mg ergotamine rectal suppository. The side effects of *ergotism* (muscle pain, vasoconstriction, mottled skin, peripheral gangrene, multifocal encephalopathy) make it unwise to treat frequent migraine headaches in this way, and one should switch to prophylaxis if the headaches occur more than once a week. For patients who present to emergency rooms with very severe headaches, intravenous phenothiazines (e.g., prochlorperazine 10 mg IV or chlorpromazine 10 mg IV) have proved to be superior to narcotics, as has droperidol, 0.5 cc IM.

MIGRAINE VARIANTS

Several migraine syndromes differ sufficiently from classic and common migraine to earn separate names. *Ophthalmoplegic migraine* is the name given when an ocular motor palsy develops during the course of a severe migraine attack. Ophthalmoplegic migraine usually begins in childhood and is characterized by unilateral pupillary dilatation, ptosis, and paralysis of ocular muscles occurring 12 to 24 hours *after* the beginning of an attack of severe migraine. The ophthalmoplegia usually clears within hours to days but frequently recurs. Angiography may be required to rule out a carotid aneurysm. *Hemiplegic migraine* is a familial syndrome in which aphasia, confusion, and hemiparesis or hemiplegia precede or more often accompany the migraine attack. Repetitive episodes alternating from side to side may occur over many years. *Complicated migraine* is a term applied to attacks of migraine prodromes in which the focal neurologic defects may last for the entire headache attack and may even leave permanent residua. The few available anatomic studies of such patients have shown ischemic brain infarction involving the functionally impaired region.

CLUSTER HEADACHE

Cluster headaches are short-lived attacks of severe, acute, and intense unilateral head pain that occur in clusters lasting several weeks, only to disappear for months or years. The disorder affects men much more than women and usually begins between the third and sixth decades. Clusters characteristically occur in the spring and fall and last 3 to 8 weeks. The individual headaches occur one to several times a day, particularly at night, awakening the victim from sleep. They frequently have a clock-setting

---

*This use is not listed in the manufacturer's directive.

predictability. Each attack, which lasts 30 minutes to 2 hours, is characterized by rapid onset of a knife-like pain in the nostril or behind the eye which spreads to involve the forehead. During the attack, the ipsilateral nostril may water and the eye tear. In about 20 per cent of instances, homolateral Horner's syndrome develops. During the course of the headache, the patient is usually unable to lie still (the opposite of the situation with migraine) and restlessly paces the floor. The pain may be so severe that the patient bangs his head against the wall or threatens suicide. The headache disappears as abruptly as it arises, usually leaving no residua. Unlike the patient with migraine, the patient with cluster headaches does not feel systemically ill, and there is no nausea, vomiting, or sense of exhaustion when the headache ceases. During the time when clusters are occurring (but not between) alcohol invariably induces an attack. When the headaches occur frequently, Horner's syndrome may outlast the head pain.

The pathogenesis of cluster headache is unknown, although it is believed to be a vascular headache related to migraine. The diagnosis is established by the characteristic history. Treatment of an acute attack is usually not worthwhile, since by the time the patient absorbs the analgesic agents the attack is over. In some patients the headache rapidly responds to oxygen inhalation. Several drugs prevent attacks of cluster headache. Ergotamine tartrate given prophylactically in a dose of 1 mg four times a day, or 2 mg at bedtime if the attacks are all nocturnal, is often effective. The drug should be withdrawn every seventh day to prevent the symptoms of ergotism and to see if the cluster has ceased. Methysergide 2 mg three to four times daily is also often effective; since the cluster rarely lasts more than 8 weeks, the drug can be discontinued and therefore is safe. Prednisone 40 mg daily in divided doses may also work and can be added to methysergide if the former is only partially effective. Lithium carbonate in daily doses of 0.9 to 1.5 grams sometimes works.

CLUSTER VARIANTS

Several variants of cluster headache should be recognized by the physician, since their treatment may be different. The most striking is *chronic paroxysmal hemicrania*, a rare disorder consisting of painful episodes similar to cluster headaches that appear many times a day and recur unremittingly for years. There may be as many as 10 to 20 headaches daily, each lasting 10 to 30 minutes. Indomethacin* orally in doses of 75 to 150 mg daily has relieved all subjects. A cluster variant characterized by daily cluster headache without remission, multiple brief jabs of pain in the head, and a background of continuous unilateral headache of variable severity exacerbated by exertion has recently been described and is said to respond to indomethacin in most instances. Patients who did not respond to indomethacin did so to tricyclic antidepressants.

OTHER VASCULAR HEADACHES

Several vascular headache variants deserve mention so that the physician may recognize them as benign and treat them appropriately. Included are *orgasmic headaches*, several short-lived bilateral throbbing headaches occurring in either sex and appearing abruptly at orgasm. The attack can be differentiated from subarachnoid hemorrhage because the headache usually disappears within minutes to an hour or more and may recur repetitively. Usually the illness is self-limited, but if not it may respond to 1 mg of ergot given an hour before sexual activity. *Exertional headache* occurs, as the name implies, during active exercise. Like orgasmic headaches, these are usually bilateral and throbbing, and may last several hours. They respond well to indomethacin. Vascular headaches have been reported to follow minor *trauma* to the carotid artery in the neck and to *carotid endarterectomy*. These headaches are unilateral, recurrent, and severe and usually respond to prophylaxis with propranolol. *Carotidynia* is the name given to spontaneous vascular headaches associated with unilateral anterior neck pain and/or carotid tenderness. They usually respond to the same treatment as vascular headaches. When attacks of carotid pain and/or headache recur, the diagnosis

---

*This use is not listed in the manufacturer's directive.

is not difficult, but the first attack must be distinguished from a spontaneous dissection of the carotid artery and may require intravenous angiography for diagnosis.

Hangover headache is part of a larger syndrome, usually including premature awakening from an evening of overindulging and often accompanied by a fine tremor of the extremities and mild gastric distress or nausea, mental dulling, and mild incoordination. The pathogenesis is related to alcohol withdrawal, dehydration, and the toxic effect of various congeners found with different intoxicants. *Nitrites* can induce pulsating headache and, occasionally, facial flushing, most often after the ingestion of processed foods ("hot dog" headache). *Monosodium glutamate* has been blamed for the "Chinese restaurant syndrome," characterized by postprandial headache, tight sensations about the face and head, and, less often, giddiness and diarrhea.

Cough headache is, as the name implies, sudden and often severe headache related to cough. The headache may last only seconds or may persist minutes to hours after a single cough or a coughing paroxysm. In some patients, cough headache is a symptom of an intracranial mass lesion. Most patients, however, do not have underlying structural disease; in these patients the disorder is probably similar to exertional and orgasmic headaches and has a vascular origin. *"Ice pick"* headaches are brief (1 to 2 seconds), sharp focal head pains occurring at unpredictable intervals and at different areas of the head. They do not indicate intracranial disease. *Thunderclap* headaches are sudden, severe, "exploding" pains that involve the entire head and resolve slowly over hours. Although these headaches may indicate an unruptured cerebral aneurysm, most are without pathologic significance. A severe thunderclap headache probably deserves evaluation with CT or MR to look for a cerebral aneurysm. In some patients angiography may be indicated.

Hypertensive headaches occur only in patients with very severe or episodic hypertension. They are characterized by early-morning, usually throbbing, occipital headache that responds to the treatment of the hypertension.

Tension Headaches

Tension headaches are characterized by a steady, nonpulsatile, unilateral, or bilateral aching pain, beginning in the occipital, frontal, or temporal regions. The headaches are also called "muscle contraction headaches" because they are frequently accompanied by tight and tender muscles at the site of most severe pain. They are probably the most common cause of headache in the adult. Tension headaches are recurrent, often present every day, and usually begin in early afternoon or evening, with a dull occipital or frontal pain that may spread to grip the entire head "in a vise." Unique among headaches, the pain may be constantly present for days, weeks, or months and is often associated with tenderness in the posterior cervical, temporalis, or masseter muscles. The pain may be quite severe, but patients rarely complain of nausea, vomiting, or malaise, although modest dizziness, blurring of vision, and sometimes tinnitus may occur. These headaches are more frequent in women, in individuals who are tense and anxious, and in those whose work or posture requires sustained contraction of posterior cervical, frontal, or temporal muscles. The symptoms of common migraine and tension headaches overlap, and many patients suffer from both. The distinguishing features favoring tension headaches include pressure or tightness, which is worst at the back of the neck, increased severity of pain as the day progresses, and pain that is preceded by or associated with anxiety-producing situations. Tension headaches are less commonly unilateral than migraine and less commonly associated with nausea and vomiting. They seldom awaken the patient from sleep and do not respond to ergot preparations.

The pathogenesis of tension headaches is unknown. Electromyographic investigation shows no sustained muscle contraction in the tender muscles, nor are there changes in blood flow to the muscles to suggest the presence of ischemia. In many respects muscle pain and tenderness in tension headaches resemble the fibromyalgia syndrome. Some have suggested that the pathogenesis of both is the accumulation of substances in the muscles which sensitize nociceptive nerve endings. Because decreased pain perception thresholds have been identified in patients with chronic tension headaches, others have suggested that the process is a central one.

TREATMENT. The first step in treatment is to identify causal factors. If these include abnormalities of posture leading to sustained muscle contraction, they should be corrected. Many patients with tension headache, particularly chronic ones, are depressed and respond to treatment with antidepressant agents such as amitriptyline. Others are tense and anxious and respond to anti-anxiety agents such as diazepam. This drug, in a dose of 15 to 20 mg a day for 2 to 3 weeks, is often effective as a diagnostic test. The relief of chronic headache establishes the diagnosis for the physician and helps to convince the patient that tension and anxiety are playing a major role in the headache. In addition, these drugs frequently break up a cycle of anxiety–muscle tension–anxiety, so that a short course may give prolonged relief. Addiction, however, is a potential complication of chronic use.

An individual headache may be treated with aspirin. This drug is probably more useful for tension headaches than acetaminophen because of its anti-prostaglandin properties. Vasoactive agents used for the treatment of migraine have no role in this disorder unless vascular headaches are concomitantly present. Some clinics report that biofeedback treatments effectively relieve muscle contraction and thus the headache. For sharply localized, painful areas present at the site of headache, injection with local anesthetics may transiently relieve the headaches. Sometimes massage has a similar effect.

TENSION HEADACHE VARIANT

Several rather characteristic headache syndromes of unknown cause may have muscle contraction and psychological tension as part of their pathogenesis. The syndrome most clearly related to muscle contraction headache is the so-called temporomandibular joint syndrome. Patients complain of unilateral or bilateral head pain, usually in the temporal region and in the jaw, often radiating into the ear. The pain is often associated with tenderness of the masseter and temporalis muscles and may be exacerbated by chewing. Accompanying symptoms often include limitation of full movement at the temporomandibular joint when opening the jaw, bruxism, and malocclusion. The disorder sometimes responds to dental manipulation, particularly use of a mouth guard during sleep that prevents bruxism. However, for most patients analgesics and anxiolytic agents effectively treat muscle-contraction head pain. *Post-traumatic headaches* are dull, generalized, aching head pains that follow head injury. The injury is often mild. The patient suffering the "post-traumatic syndrome" complains of headache often coupled with unsteadiness, giddiness, difficulty concentrating, insomnia, and fatigue. Contrary to popular belief, the syndrome is not more common in patients seeking compensation for the injury. It often persists for months or years. Treatment, like that of muscle contraction headaches, consists of psychological support and reassurance and the use of mild analgesics and sometimes anxiolytic agents. Patients should be encouraged to return to work as soon as possible and to try to live a normal life despite the symptoms. The disorder can blend into *depressive headache*, a chronic generalized headache, usually vaguely described, sometimes associated with giddiness and unsteadiness, that occurs as a frequent and sometimes predominant manifestation of depression. The headache may have muscle contraction and tension as its pathogenesis or may be a *somatic delusion* in a severely depressed patient. In either event, the treatment of choice is an antidepressant drug.

ATYPICAL FACIAL PAIN

Atypical facial pain or atypical facial neuralgia is a term used to describe a syndrome characterized by steady aching facial pain, usually unilateral, localized to the lower part of the orbit, maxillary area, and sometimes the jaw. The pain begins without a known precipitating episode and may last for hours to days. It may spread to involve the head or neck, and muscles of the jaw and neck are often tender. Sometimes autonomic symptoms including sweating, flushing, rhinorrhea, and pallor are present. The disorder usually affects women, often in early middle age. Patients affected with the disorder are tense, anxious, and often chronically depressed. The pathogenesis of the illness is unknown. The autonomic changes have led some to suggest that the syndrome is a migraine variant, and the muscle tenderness and depression have led others to suggest that it be classified with musculoskeletal tension pain. Patients suffering from atypical facial pain should be examined carefully for local pathology of the eyes, nose, teeth, sinuses, and pharynx, but such is rarely found. Careful psychological evaluation often reveals a masked depression. Treatment is usually unsatisfactory. Analgesic agents are usually not helpful, and patients respond poorly to psychotherapy. In some patients, ergot preparations or propranolol is effective, suggesting a vascular pathogenesis for the face pain. Others respond to physical methods such as massage and biofeedback. Antidepressants sometimes help. It is important to recognize that the syndrome is not caused by structural disease and that patients require no invasive diagnostic or therapeutic procedures. Dental extraction does more harm than good. This disorder should not be confused with trigeminal neuralgia, discussed below; carbamazepine is ineffective.

Head Pain Due to Traction or Inflammation

CRANIAL ARTERITIS

This condition receives detailed consideration in Ch. 267 but deserves mention here as an important cause of headache in the elderly. The illness almost always appears after age 60 and usually later. It usually begins with unilateral or bilateral temporal, occipital, or fronto-occipital head pain of variable intensity, often coupled with tenderness of the painful areas. Many patients have pain in the jaw muscles, making chewing uncomfortable. Nodules occasionally are palpable on affected vessels. The great risk is occlusion of retinal arteries secondary to untreated inflammation. Diagnosis depends on suspicion and usually on the presence of an elevated erythrocyte sedimentation rate. Diagnosis should be confirmed by arterial biopsy because definitive steroid treatment, once started, often must be maintained for many months. Since migraine, vascular headaches, and depressive headaches also can have their onset in the elderly, a confirmed diagnosis is essential.

MENINGITIS AND SUBARACHNOID HEMORRHAGE

Acute and subacute meningitis cause headache by inflammation of the pain-sensitive meninges surrounding the brain. The headache is usually generalized, throbbing, and very severe. It may be rapid or gradual in onset, and by the time it is fully developed is associated with nuchal rigidity. The diagnosis is established by lumbar puncture. In patients suspected of harboring an intracranial mass lesion, MR scan of the brain should be performed first and lumbar puncture deferred, unless the physician suspects that the patient is suffering from acute bacterial meningitis, in which case lumbar puncture must be done immediately. In *subarachnoid hemorrhage*, the initial sudden headache is caused by alteration of intracranial pressure. This headache is succeeded by a chronic persistent headache, often accompanied by nuchal rigidity that results from inflammation of the meninges caused by the blood. In a patient suspected of having suffered a subarachnoid hemorrhage, a CT scan should be performed first. The presence of extravascular blood establishes the diagnosis and obviates the need for lumbar puncture, which may exacerbate the bleeding by altering intracranial dynamics. The absence of identifiable hemorrhage on CT scan, however, does not rule out a small subarachnoid hemorrhage, and lumbar puncture then must be performed to establish or rule out the diagnosis definitively.

ALTERATIONS OF INTRACRANIAL PRESSURE

Headache from altered intracranial pressure is caused by compression or traction of pain-sensitive vascular and neural structures over the apex and base of the brain. In the instance of *intracranial hypotension*, the loss of spinal fluid decreases the buoyancy of the brain so that the organ descends when the upright position is assumed, exerting traction on structures at its apex and compression on structures at its base. (In rare instances, the small bridging veins that enter the sagittal sinus may rupture and cause subdural hematomas.) In *intracranial hypertension*, the source of pain is probably compression of vascular and neural structures at the base of the brain by tumor or edematous brain.

INTRACRANIAL HYPERTENSION. Increased intracranial pressure per se does not lead to headache unless pain-sensitive

structures are distorted. Many patients with high intracranial pressure from brain tumors, jugular venous obstruction, hydrocephalus, or pseudotumor cerebri do not suffer headache. If headache is present, it may be mild or severe, throbbing or steady, localized or generalized. When localized, it usually overlies the site of the lesion, but posterior fossa lesions may cause bifrontal headache. The headache is characteristically at its worst early in the morning, although, unlike cluster headache, it usually does not awaken the patient from sleep. It is exacerbated by stooping, coughing, moving the head suddenly, or straining at stool. Many patients prefer to sleep in the sitting position. The headache is rarely continuously intense. Transient rises of intracranial pressure called plateau waves (see Ch. 486) sometimes cause 5 to 20 minutes of severe headache accompanied by nausea, vomiting, or other neurologic signs. These episodes are commonly precipitated by assuming the upright posture but can also be precipitated by coughing, sneezing, or straining.

The treatment of headache related to increased intracranial pressure is the treatment of the underlying disease. Mild analgesics produce temporary relief; narcotic analgesics should not be used because of their tendency to produce respiratory depression and further raise the pressure in neurologically compromised individuals.

INTRACRANIAL HYPOTENSION (see Ch. 486) **AND LUMBAR PUNCTURE HEADACHE.** Intracranial hypotension usually follows a lumbar puncture and is due to continued leakage of cerebrospinal fluid through a rent in the dural sheath. The syndrome develops 12 hours to several days after the lumbar puncture and is characterized by headache on assuming the upright position. There is no evidence that a period of recumbency after a lumbar puncture prevents subsequent development of the headache. The headache usually begins as a dull ache in the posterior cervical area, radiating laterally toward the shoulders and cephalad toward the frontal area. It persists, often growing more severe, as long as the patient remains upright, and when most severe it may be associated with perspiration, nausea, and vomiting. Persistent headache of intracranial hypotension can lead to diplopia, probably a result of traction on the abducens nerves. The diagnosis of post–lumbar puncture headache is made by history; spontaneous intracranial hypotension is suspected by the history of positional headache and confirmed by low (<30 mm H₂O) or even negative CSF pressure on attempted lumbar puncture. The fluid is usually normal, but there may be an elevated protein concentration if the needle has entered a subdural or epidural fluid collection. Analgesics relieve the mildest headaches; the most severe ones can be controlled only by assuming the recumbent position. The headaches usually clear within a few days to a few weeks; in rare instances, surgical repair of the torn dura is necessary.

Extracranial Structural Causes of Headache

NASAL AND SINUS HEADACHE

Although acute or chronic inflammation and neoplasms of the paranasal sinuses can cause headache, most patients who have been physician- or self-diagnosed as having sinus headaches are in fact suffering from either vascular or tension headache. Most true paranasal sinus headaches result from acute inflammation causing pain localized over the involved sinus and associated with stigmata of acute infection, including fever, swelling, and tenderness over the sinus and engorgement of the turbinates, ostia, nasofrontal ducts, and superior nasal spaces. Most of the discomfort comes from the ostia, which are many times more sensitive than the poorly innervated walls of the sinuses. Typically, "sinus" headache commences in the morning (frontal) or early afternoon (maxillary) and subsides in the early or late evening. The pain is dull and aching, is made worse by changing head position, and is seldom associated with nausea and vomiting. Sinus headache is best treated with decongestants and analgesics. Persistent purulent discharges should be cultured and appropriate antimicrobial drugs employed. Chronic suppurative disease in the frontal, ethmoid, and sphenoid sinuses, or in the mastoid air cells, may result in osteomyelitis and inflammation of adjacent cranial tissues. Headache persisting after surgical drainage of the diseased sinus is evidence for extradural and possibly subdural infection. More chronic inflammation and neoplasms, particularly when they occur in the sphenoid sinus, may not be accompanied by the usual physical signs of sinusitis. In such instances, sinus radiographs or MR scan may be required to establish the diagnosis.

DENTAL PAIN

Noxious stimuli in a tooth usually evoke local toothache, but severe dental pain can be extremely difficult to localize. Afferent fibers from the teeth are contained in the second and third divisions of the trigeminal nerve, and tooth pain can be referred to areas of the head supplied by these nerves. More commonly, in association with toothache, tooth extraction, or a tender, diseased tooth, distant tissues exhibit surface hyperalgesia, tenderness, and vasomotor reactions, such as tender eyeballs, reddening of the conjunctivae, and tenderness of the auricular and temporal tissues. Because of secondary muscle contraction, other sites of tenderness and pain may be noted behind the ears, behind the lower border of the mastoid process, and in the muscles of the occiput, neck, and shoulders. The upper teeth frequently hurt in association with disease of the nasal and paranasal structures. Occasionally, in coronary insufficiency, pain is experienced in the lower jaw. One should beware of ascribing bizarre pains in and around the jaws to a dental origin unless unequivocal acute inflammatory dental lesions are present. Dental extraction rarely ameliorates neuralgias or atypical facial pain. However, hysterical or delusional face pain is often attributed by the patient to prior dental work. Headache should not be attributed to a diseased tooth unless the injection of procaine into the tissues about the suspected tooth greatly reduces the intensity of, or eliminates, such headache.

AURAL PAIN

Severe pain in the vicinity of the ear can be caused by disease of the teeth, acute tonsillitis, inflammatory and neoplastic disease of the larynx and nasopharynx, temporomandibular joint disorders, tumors, inflammation in the posterior fossa, and disease of the cervical spine and its soft tissues. Pain in the ear is also associated with vascular headaches, atypical facial pain, and herpes zoster of the fifth and seventh cranial nerves and, rarely, the glossopharyngeal nerve. True glossopharyngeal neuralgia causes severe pain radiating from the tonsil into the ear. It has the usual timing feature of "tic" (see Cranial Neuralgias, below).

Primary ear disease is an infrequent but important source of headache, because it almost always indicates inflammation or destructive disease. Acute otitis media (purulent or nonpurulent), furunculosis of the ear canal, traumatic rupture of the tympanum, and fracture of the anterior wall of the bony canal all cause pain in the ear associated with tenderness of adjacent skeletal muscles. Osteomyelitis of the mastoid bone may be associated with inflammation of the nearby periosteum as well as of dura and adjacent tissues (epidural abscess)—both sources of pain in or behind the ear. Pain in this region also accompanies tumors of the acoustic nerve and inflammation and thrombosis of the lateral sinus.

EYE PAIN AND HEADACHE

Errors of *refraction* (hypermetropia, astigmatism, anomalies of accommodation), disturbances of ocular muscle equilibrium, and glaucoma are universally described as causing headache, but most such headaches are probably tension headaches rather than truly related to "eye strain." Refractive errors are also said to give origin to such other symptoms as aching of the eyes, "sandy" feeling in the eyes, pulling sensations in and about the orbit, and conjunctival congestion. Headache is mild in degree and usually starts around and over the eyes and subsequently radiates to the occiput and back of the head.

The pain of *glaucoma* at first remains localized in the eyeball, then extends along the rim of the orbit and, finally, throughout most of the area supplied by the ophthalmic division of the trigeminal nerve. Nausea and vomiting sometimes accompany such headaches, which can become prostratingly severe if not treated promptly.

With inflammation of the iris and ciliary body, light may cause intense pain in the eye and adjacent areas because of movement of the inflamed iris. When the iris is immobilized, pain is allayed.

PITUITARY PAIN

Headache caused by pituitary tumors is the result of compression and distortion of pain-sensitive structures at the base of the skull, particularly the diaphragma sella. Pain is generally referred to the frontal or temporal regions bilaterally and may on occasion be referred to the vertex or occipital regions. Because the pain is not related to intracranial pressure, it does not have the same temporal characteristics of most brain tumor headaches and instead can occur at any time and is frequently chronic and unremitting. The diagnosis can be established by endocrine examination and by an MRI of the pituitary fossa employing 1-mm cuts. Acute headache occurring with known pituitary lesions (*pituitary apoplexy*) usually results from infarction or hemorrhage into the tumor. Sudden expansion of the tumor may compromise the overlying optic chiasm, leading to visual loss, or invade the laterally lying cavernous sinus, producing ocular palsies. Pituitary apoplexy should be treated surgically by emergency drainage of the hemorrhagic or infarcted material.

NECK PAIN

Osteoarthritis of the zygapophyseal joints of the upper cervical spine is an occasional cause of perplexing headache. The pain is generally constant, aching, and perceived in the upper cervical and occipital areas. It may radiate to the vertex of the head or even the orbit. At times, vertex or orbital pain is more severe than occipital and neck pain, leading to confusion in diagnosis. The pain probably results from entrapment of the C3 root by overgrowth of the C2 zygapophyseal joint. A syndrome of unilateral upper nuchal and occipital pain accompanied by ipsilateral numbness of the tongue occurring on sudden turning of the head is probably explained by compression of the second cervical root in the atlanto-occipital space. Such acute pain can be prevented by restricting neck movement with a cervical collar. Upper cervical nerve blocks relieve more chronic pain and are useful diagnostically as well as therapeutically. A few reports suggest that severe headache and neck pain affecting young male weight lifters (weight-lifter's headache) may result from pull or tear of cervical ligaments during the strain of exertion.

Cranial Neuralgias

The term cranial neuralgias refers to several distinctive head pains that appear to result from sudden and excessive discharge from the involved nerve. The best-known cranial neuralgia is trigeminal neuralgia. The concept of cranial neuralgias has been expanded to include the chronic burning pain that frequently follows herpes zoster infection of the nerve. Some also include atypical facial pain and temporomandibular joint syndrome under the cranial neuralgias, but these probably have tension or vascular disturbances as their pathogenesis and in this chapter are included under those headings.

TRIGEMINAL NEURALGIA. Trigeminal neuralgia (tic douloureux) is characterized by sudden, lightning-like paroxysms of pain in the distribution of one or more divisions of the trigeminal nerve. Most trigeminal neuralgia is caused by compression of the trigeminal nerve by arteries or veins of the posterior fossa. In some patients there is no identifiable structural disease. Occasionally trigeminal neuralgia may be a symptom of a gasserian ganglion tumor, multiple sclerosis, or a brain-stem infarct involving the descending root of the trigeminal nerve.

The history is diagnostic. The pain occurs as brief, lightning-like stabs, frequently precipitated by touching a trigger zone around the lips or the buccal cavity. At times, talking, eating, or brushing the teeth serves as a trigger. The pains rarely last longer than seconds, and each burst is followed by a refractory period of several seconds to a minute in which no further pain can be precipitated. The pains, however, often occur in clusters so that the patient may report somewhat erroneously that each pain lasts for hours. The pain is limited to one or more divisions of the trigeminal nerve, usually the second, or third, or both. Spontaneous remissions and exacerbations are common, the exacerbations tending to occur in spring and fall. Between paroxysms of pain, the patient is asymptomatic. Tic pain rarely occurs at night. In idiopathic trigeminal neuralgia, the neurologic examination is entirely normal. In symptomatic trigeminal neuralgia, there may be sensory changes in the distribution of the trigeminal nerve, and such a finding should prompt a careful search for structural disease of the nervous system.

Carbamazepine is the drug of choice for the treatment of trigeminal neuralgia. The anticonvulsant drug is given in doses varying from 400 to 800 mg a day, but because of its sedative properties the initial dose is 100 mg twice daily, gradually increased to the required maintenance dose. No more than 1200 mg should be taken daily. The drug is not an analgesic and is only effective for specific kinds of pain such as trigeminal neuralgia, glossopharyngeal neuralgia, and the lightning pains of tabes dorsalis. Side effects include dizziness, sedation and, rarely, aplastic anemia. Phenytoin* in doses of 400 mg a day is also effective in trigeminal neuralgia but less so than carbamazepine. Occasionally the two drugs appear to be synergistic. Baclofen* 60 to 80 mg daily has also been found to be a useful agent. If medical treatment fails, surgical intervention is necessary.

The most popular operations consist of lesioning of the gasserian ganglion (either by radiofrequency or glycerol injections) and posterior fossa craniotomy to relieve the compression of the trigeminal nerve by vascular structures. Gasserian ganglion lesions can be made under local anesthesia, are generally effective initially, but have a high relapse rate. Posterior fossa craniotomy is as effective as gasserian ganglion lesions and appears to have a lower relapse rate. The purpose of both operations is to relieve pain with little or no loss of sensation, thus preventing the dreaded complications of anesthesia dolorosa. Either of these operations is preferable to section of the nerve root proximal to the ganglion. However, that operation affords permanent relief. If surgery on the ganglion is contemplated, a prior test of local anesthesia of the ganglion or the peripheral branches of the nerve is desirable because some patients find the sensory loss less tolerable than the pain itself.

GLOSSOPHARYNGEAL NEURALGIA. Glossopharyngeal neuralgia is characterized by pain similar to that of trigeminal neuralgia but in the distribution of the glossopharyngeal and vagus nerves. The trigger zone is usually in the tonsil or posterior pharynx, and the pain spreads toward the angle of the jaw and the ear. Occasional patients suffer cardiac slowing or arrest during these attacks as a result of the intense afferent discharge over the glossopharyngeal nerve. Carbamazepine is often effective, but if it fails, glossopharyngeal nerve roots are sectioned in the posterior fossa. Symptomatic glossopharyngeal neuralgia is occasionally the presenting complaint of a tonsillar tumor, and careful examination of the pharynx and tonsillar fossa must be carried out.

OTHER NEURALGIAS. Similar but much rarer disorders than trigeminal or glossopharyngeal neuralgia have been reported to involve the greater occipital nerve and the nervus intermedius portion of the facial nerve. The clinical features and treatment of these rare disorders are similar to those for trigeminal neuralgia.

Diagnostic Evaluation

Headache is an extremely common disorder, and the excessive application of expensive and highly technical laboratory procedures to the diagnosis and management of benign head pain has been a substantial cause of unnecessary medical costs. Set against this truism is the fact that in some instances a timely MRI or lumbar puncture can give life-saving information about an otherwise undiagnosable problem. Given these antitheses, the following principles may help in the management of the individual patient:

1. Patients with chronic classic or common migraine or with chronic tension headache rarely require more than a careful history and examination. Even when the unilateral prodromes and headache of longstanding, classic migraine consistently affect the same side, the incidence of associated intracranial lesions remains so low that scans are unnecessary and arteriography unjustified.

2. Headaches that are of recent origin or progression deserve investigation. This principle especially applies to headaches that have a consistently focal distribution, follow trauma, or begin after the age of 30 years. MRI is more sensitive than CT.

3. The EEG is almost never useful in the diagnosis of diseases causing headache and can be omitted. Skull radiographs are useful in diagnosing headache only (a) when searching for abnormalities involving the base of the brain such as sellar and suprasellar lesions or (b) immediately following head trauma. CT scans have discriminating capacities superior to those of plain films and, when available, make radiographs unnecessary.

4. Diagnostic lumbar puncture should be performed with any acute headache that (a) is accompanied by fever or (b) is explosive or the most severe headache ever suffered (a history typical of acute subarachnoid hemorrhage—but see thunderclap headache, p. 2120). Lumbar puncture should, if possible, be deferred until after CT scanning with other forms of acute headache, especially if stiff neck but no fever is present. (This combination may indicate partial herniation of cerebellar tonsils into the foramen magnum secondary to an intracranial mass lesion.)

5. Now that CT and MRI are widely available, radioisotopic brain scanning rarely if ever adds useful information and is expensively superfluous.

Bonica JJ: The Management of Pain, 2nd ed. Philadelphia, Lea and Febiger, 1990. *A two-volume multiauthored encyclopedia of the causes of pain and its management. Individual chapters describe anatomy, physiology, pathology, and pain disorders affecting head, neck, back, and the remainder of the body. Everything you wanted to know about pain and more.*

Cady RK, Wendt JK, Kirchner JR, et al.: Treatment of acute migraine with subcutaneous sumatriptan. JAMA 265:2831, 1991. *A first North American report on a potentially favorable drug for migraine.*

Diamond S (ed.): Headache. Med Clin North Am 75:521, 1991. *The latest monograph on all aspects of the problem.*

Mathew NT (ed.): Headache. Philadelphia, W.B. Saunders Company, 1990, Vol. 8, No. 4. *A multiauthored monograph describing pathophysiology, diagnosis, and management of headaches and other head pain.*

455.3 SOME SPECIFIC PAIN SYNDROMES

Some chronic painful disorders are associated with a specific constellation of signs and symptoms which establishes them as identifiable pain syndromes. Those most commonly encountered in clinical practice include the *neuropathic pain* disorders of diabetic polyneuropathy (see Ch. 498), sympathetically maintained pain, postherpetic neuralgia, phantom limb pain, and the *non-neuropathic pain* syndromes, fibromyalgia and myofascial pain. Taken together, these syndromes cause chronic, usually unremitting pain that is often disabling and difficult and frustrating to treat.

SYMPATHETICALLY MAINTAINED PAIN. This term applies to severe pain, usually burning in quality and associated with autonomic changes including swelling, vasomotor instability, and abnormalities of sweating. The pain syndrome usually follows an injury, often minor, to an extremity. If the injury has involved a peripheral nerve, particularly the sciatic or median nerve, the syndrome is called *causalgia.* If the injury does not involve a peripheral nerve, if there has been no trauma, or if the syndrome follows a visceral illness (e.g., myocardial infarction), the term applied is *reflex sympathetic dystrophy.* (Older and outmoded terms include post-traumatic painful osteoporosis, Sudek's atrophy, post-traumatic spreading neuralgia, minor causalgia, and shoulder-hand syndrome.) The exact pathophysiology of the disorder is unknown, but, as the name implies, abnormal activity of the sympathetic nervous system plays an important role in both the pain and the autonomic symptoms.

The disorder is characterized by severe and continuous pain exacerbated by emotional stress and is usually associated with severe hyperpathia so that moving or touching the limb is often intolerable. At first the pain is localized to the site of injury or the distribution of the nerve injured, but with time it spreads to involve the entire extremity. Spread to other areas of the body sometimes occurs. Along with the pain go vasomotor changes including vasodilatation (warm and dry skin) or vasoconstriction (cyanosis, cool skin). Other autonomic changes may include edema and either hypo- or hyperhidrosis; trophic changes of the skin, subcutaneous tissues, muscles, and bone (osteoporosis) also occur. The entire symptom complex rarely affects any one patient,

---

*This use is not listed in the manufacturer's directive.

and one sign or symptom usually predominates. Untreated, the disorder can lead to muscle atrophy, fixation of joints, and a useless extremity. The diagnosis is largely a clinical one but can be supported by laboratory tests that document autonomic instability or trophic changes including increased uptake in involved bones on radionuclide bone scan, bone atrophy or plain radiographs, and temperature abnormalities on thermography.

The earlier the treatment, the more effective it is likely to be. Treatment is directed at blocking sympathetic outflow to the involved site while stimulating and mobilizing the painful site. To that end, a combination of repetitive sympathetic ganglionic blocks with lidocaine and vigorous physical therapy is used. In addition, sympatholytic agents (e.g., phenoxybenzamine up to 120 mg a day in divided doses) and short courses of corticosteroids have been reported to be effective. How often these techniques afford permanent relief is unknown, and many patients fail to respond. In refractory patients pharmacologic agents directed at neuropathic pain, including tricyclic antidepressants (e.g., amitriptyline, 50 to 150 mg at bedtime), anticonvulsants (e.g., carbamazepine, 600 to 800 mg a day in divided doses), and oral local anesthetics (e.g., mexiletine 300 mg three times a day) can be tried. The disorder is often difficult and frustrating to treat, and in such cases the physician is advised to consider referral to a multidisciplinary pain clinic.

POSTHERPETIC NEURALGIA. Postherpetic neuralgia refers to severe and prolonged burning pain with occasional lightning-like stabs in the involved dermatome after an attack of herpes zoster. Severe postherpetic neuralgia is usually a disease of elderly patients and, like most chronic pain, is exacerbated by emotional upset and relieved to some degree by distraction. Touching the involved area sometimes exacerbates the pain. Treatment of postherpetic neuralgia is not entirely satisfactory. The initial treatment should be directed toward stimulating the painful area. In some patients brisk rubbing applied repeatedly with a terrycloth towel or stimulation of the dermatome with a cutaneous electrical stimulator often brings relief which long outlasts the stimulus and is occasionally permanent.

Most patients, however, require multimodality therapy, which includes not only stimulation of the area but physical therapy, psychological support, and pharmacologic treatment. The application of topical pharmacologic agents, such as lidocaine, sometimes gives temporary relief, and anecdotal evidence claims that topical application of capsaicin is useful. Lancinating pains, which are usually a minor component, usually respond to anticonvulsants (e.g., carbamazepine, 400 to 600 mg a day in divided doses), but anticonvulsants do not affect the continuous pain. The latter may be treated by tricyclic antidepressants or mexiletine (see above); neuroleptics (e.g., fluphenazine 1 to 3 mg daily) may also be helpful. When these conservative approaches fail, one should consider either anesthetic approaches with subcutaneous local injection or sympathetic blockade. The only surgical approach that has proved at all useful is the dorsal root entry zone lesion. Adrenocorticosteroids and acyclovir, both of which may diminish pain in the acute stage, have little or no effect on the development of postherpetic neuralgia. In many patients, the disease runs its course and, after a year or two, disappears spontaneously.

The pharmacologic approach is the same as that described for the neuropathic pains above and includes tricyclic antidepressants, anticonvulsants, neuroleptics, and sometimes sympathetic blockade. Referral to a multidisciplinary pain center may be helpful.

PHANTOM LIMB PAIN. Phantom limb pain is a chronic and severe pain appearing to be localized in an amputated or totally denervated limb. All patients suffer phantom sensations after amputation and as many as 60 to 70 per cent suffer significant pain, especially if there has been severe preamputation pain. The pain is frequently similar to that suffered before amputation, or at times it may resemble muscle pain with the phantom seeming to be in a cramped or uncomfortable position. In most instances, the pain lessens and disappears with time, but sometimes it becomes a chronic and severe problem. Therapy is difficult. A search should be made for painful neuromas, but these are an uncommon cause, and even if small neuromas are found and removed, the pain is not usually relieved. Surgical procedures directed at the central nervous system are often not helpful. The pain may be triggered by touching the amputation stump, and eventually even touching healthy areas may trigger pain. Phantom pain is sometimes permanently abolished by cutaneous stimulation, either rubbing or electrical stimulation, or by repeated anesthetic blocks of peripheral nerves proximal to the stump. The pharmacologic approach is the same as that described for the neuropathic pains above and includes tricyclic antidepressants, anticonvulsants, neuroleptics, and sometimes sympathetic blockade. Referral to a multidisciplinary pain center may be helpful.

FIBROMYALGIA AND MYOFASCIAL PAIN. Fibromyalgia (also called fibrositis) is characterized by widespread or generalized musculoskeletal pain associated with morning stiffness, disturbed sleep and fatigue (nonrestorative sleep) and at times by vague complaints of a feeling of swelling or paresthesias. On examination, *tender points* can be found at multiple sites over muscles and ligaments, particularly at the upper borders of the trapezius, supraspinatus, and upper gluteal area and below the lateral epicondyle of the elbow and the medial epicondyle of the femur. The disorder usually occurs in middle-aged women and is often associated with anxiety and depression. Tension headaches and irritable bowel syndrome are common in these patients and may have a similar pathogenesis.

The myofascial pain syndrome refers to chronic pain in a regional distribution associated with trigger point(s). *Trigger points* are tender, sometimes hardened areas in a muscle which, when palpated, reproduce the distribution of the spontaneous pain. When injected with a local anesthetic, both the local and referred pain are relieved.

The pathophysiology of these syndromes is poorly understood. Some observers have reported microscopic changes at trigger points (so-called fibrous nodules), suggesting that a tonic contraction of muscle has led to structural changes. Others have suggested that release of noxious substances, such as lactic acid, potassium, or kinins from chronically contracted muscles, may be responsible for the pain and tenderness associated with the syndromes.

Treatment is often difficult and frustrating. In some patients, mild analgesic drugs, heat, and massage yield temporary or long-term relief. In patients with trigger points (myofascial pain), massage or even injection of trigger points with local anesthetics may give relief. Biofeedback, with the patient trying consciously to relax contracted muscle recorded by surface EMG, has been reported to be useful. Antidepressants are modestly effective and produce at least a short-term remission in about 20 per cent of patients. For most patients, a combination of the above physical methods with investigation and treatment of associated psychological disorders is necessary if long-term relief is to be achieved.

Bonica JJ: The Management of Pain, 2nd ed. Philadelphia, Lea and Febiger, 1990. *A two-volume multiauthored encyclopedia of the causes of pain and its management. Individual chapters describe each of the pain syndromes mentioned in this section.*

Fricton JR, Awad EA (eds.): Myofascial Pain and Fibromyalgia. Advances in Pain Research and Therapy. Volume 17. New York, Raven Press, 1990. *A comprehensive analysis of the pathophysiology, diagnosis, and treatment of fibromyalgia and myofascial pain.*

Payne R: Neuropathic pain syndromes, with special reference to causalgia and reflex sympathetic dystrophy. Clin Pain 2:59, 1986. *A thorough review of the pathogenesis and management of a perplexing pain problem.*

Thompson JM: Tension myalgia as a diagnosis at the Mayo Clinic and its relationship to fibrositis, fibromyalgia, and myofascial pain syndrome. Mayo Clin Proc 65:1237–1248, 1990. *Outlines specific criteria for various forms of this disorder and appropriate approaches to treatment.*

SECTION FOUR / ALCOHOL AND NUTRITIONAL COMPLICATIONS

456 Nutritional Disorders of the Nervous System

Ivan Diamond

The neurologic effects of either general or specific nutritional deprivations are common worldwide (Table 456–1). In the developed countries of Western Europe and North America, many of these disorders are observed most frequently in association with chronic alcohol abuse. Other major causes include food faddism; chronic starvation such as can occur with cancer, infantile malnutrition, or psychiatric illness; intestinal malabsorption; and the complicated postoperative state. The conditions are relatively common, especially in large public hospitals that serve the underprivileged. More important, they often go undiagnosed. One recent study, for example, determined that only 20 per cent of patients found at autopsy to have Wernicke's encephalopathy had their condition correctly diagnosed and treated during life.

Although conditions such as Wernicke's encephalopathy can develop in as little as a few weeks after an acute illness such as hyperemesis gravidarum, most nutritional syndromes among alcoholics develop only following prolonged severe abuse with years of proportional semistarvation. Binge drinkers who eat well between bouts of intoxication seldom suffer neurologic complications. Genetic predisposition also may contribute to neurologic vulnerability. Ch. 201 and 204 more extensively discuss nutritional requirements and the systemic effects of their deprivation.

THE WERNICKE-KORSAKOFF SYNDROME

Wernicke's Encephalopathy

This acute disorder occurs most commonly in chronic alcoholics but also can accompany the other conditions listed in Table 456–2. This is the only alcohol-related neurologic disorder that can be corrected by a specific vitamin—thiamine.

CLINICAL MANIFESTATIONS. A clinical triad of ophthalmoplegia, ataxia, and global confusion is characteristic, although the condition should be suspected and treated in any chronically malnourished subject suffering from a confusional state of recent onset. Affected patients may complain of double vision or difficulty with balance. There is almost always horizontal nystagmus on lateral gaze. Vertical nystagmus, usually on upward gaze, occurs in about 50 per cent of cases. Bilateral, often asymmetric, lateral rectus palsies are characteristic and may develop rapidly. Defects in conjugate gaze are common. Bilateral ptosis and total external or an apparent internuclear ophthalmoplegia occur rarely. Light-fixed pupils should suggest an alternate or additional diagnosis.

Virtually all patients have an ataxic gait due to cerebellar involvement. This can vary widely in severity. Peripheral neuropathy and vestibular dysfunction frequently complicate Wernicke's encephalopathy. Intention tremor is less common, and speech disturbances are rare.

Most patients have an acute confusional state characterized by inattention, disorientation, and sleepiness. Stupor or coma occurs but is rare. Sometimes patients may be hyperactive and agitated (alcohol withdrawal, see Ch. 14), but most are apathetic, indifferent, and amnesic.

Associated physical abnormalities related to chronic alcoholism or poor nutrition are often present (see Ch. 118). Tachycardia and orthostatic hypotension are common. Hypothermia occurs less frequently; any fever should prompt a search for concomitant infection. Patients with Wernicke's encephalopathy do not develop beriberi heart disease (see Ch. 204).

PATHOLOGY. The major lesions occur in the periventricular regions of the diencephalon, mid-brain, and brain stem and in the superior vermis of the cerebellum; they may consist of areas of demyelination and glial proliferation. Microglia are prominent in acute lesions and fibrous astrocytes in older ones. Acute lesions show capillary dilation with occasional petechial hemorrhages. In experimental animals, defects in serotonergic transmission can be demonstrated in affected areas.

TREATMENT. Thiamine is specific. Because intestinal absorption is impaired in malnourished alcoholics, thiamine (50 to 100 mg) is given parenterally before starting infusions. Glucose administered prior to giving thiamine can precipitate or worsen the encephalopathy. Recovery begins promptly. Ophthalmoplegia and gaze palsies often begin to resolve during the first day. Nystagmus, gait ataxia, and confusion may improve within days to weeks, although many patients are left with residual nystagmus or gait ataxia. Nearly all patients with Wernicke's encephalopathy recover from the global confusional state, but many are left with a residual disorder of memory—Korsakoff's amnestic syndrome.

TABLE 456–1. MAJOR ACQUIRED NUTRITIONAL SYNDROMES AFFECTING THE NERVOUS SYSTEM

Vitamin A (carotene)	Night blindness, possibly pseudotumor in children
Vitamin B	
B_1 (thiamine)	Peripheral neuropathy, Wernicke-Korsakoff syndrome
	Possibly amblyopia, cerebellar degeneration, cerebral atrophy
B_2 group	
Panthothenic acid	Possibly burning feet syndrome
Nicotinic acid	Pellagra, polyneuropathy, spastic ataxia, amblyopia, psychosis-dementia
Riboflavin	Possibly burning feet syndrome, amblyopia
B_6 (pyridoxine)	Convulsions in B_6-deprived babies and older children, possibly peripheral neuropathy
B_{12} (cyanocobalamin)	Combined systems disease, peripheral neuropathy, dementia
Folic acid	Impaired peripheral nerve function, possibly neuropathy and encephalopathy
Vitamin C (ascorbic acid)	Retinal and occasionally cerebral hemorrhages
Vitamin E (α-tocopherol)	Peripheral neuropathy and cerebellar degeneration
Starvation	Possibly developmental neurologic defects in infants

TABLE 456–2. CONDITIONS PREDISPOSING TO WERNICKE'S ENCEPHALOPATHY

Chronic alcoholism
Starvation
Persistent vomiting
Hyperemesis gravidarum
Gastric malignancy
Gastritis
Intestinal obstruction
Digitalis intoxication
Systemic diseases
Malignancy
Hepatic failure
Disseminated tuberculosis
Uremia
Iatrogenic
Inadequate parenteral nutrition
Chronic hemodialysis

Korsakoff's Syndrome

CLINICAL MANIFESTATIONS (see also Ch. 452). There is a characteristic defect in forming new memories (anterograde amnesia) and in summoning previously established memories (retrograde amnesia). Patients are usually disoriented for place and time. Immediate recall is intact, but patients are unable to remember the same items several minutes later. Unhesitating confabulation often occurs early in the course. Other aspects of cognitive function, including arousal, language, praxis, and judgment, are spared.

PATHOLOGY. The findings are of active or remote Wernicke's encephalopathy. Damage to the dorsal medial nucleus of the thalamus probably accounts for the memory deficits.

TREATMENT. Patients with Korsakoff's syndrome should be given thiamine to treat coexistent Wernicke's encephalopathy and to prevent progression of the amnesia. About 20 per cent of patients recover completely, but more than half show little or no change. Improvement may take 1 to 3 months to be recognizable.

METABOLIC CONSIDERATIONS. Thiamine (vitamin B_1) in human tissues is derived entirely from dietary sources, is absorbed in the small intestine (see Ch. 204), and is transported into the brain by a saturable, energy-dependent transport system. Alcohol inhibits thiamine absorption. A series of reactions produces phosphorylated thiamine derivatives, and thiamine pyrophosphate (TPP) is a required co-enzyme for pyruvate dehydrogenase, α-ketoglutarate dehydrogenase, branched-chain α-keto acid dehydrogenase, and transketolase. The affinity of transketolase for TPP appears reduced in Wernicke's encephalopathy. Individuals with this enzyme abnormality are at greater risk to develop functional thiamine deficiency when dietary levels are compromised, as in alcoholism.

The confusional state and oculomotor disturbances seen in Wernicke's encephalopathy respond to thiamine treatment, and it is said that recovery may proceed during thiamine therapy whether or not alcohol consumption continues. However, calorie-containing ethanol appears to be an important contributing factor to the neurologic deficits. Calorie-deprived prisoners of war who developed Wernicke's encephalopathy rarely exhibited the irreversible amnestic syndrome. Moreover, nystagmus, ataxia, and the memory deficits often fail to improve after thiamine therapy, indicating that some areas of the brain have become irreversibly damaged. Serotonin deficiency may play a role in the memory disorder, but the molecular metabolic defect that precedes tissue damage in Wernicke's encephalopathy and Korsakoff's amnestic syndrome is not known.

ALCOHOLIC CEREBRAL ATROPHY

Many chronic alcoholics develop cerebral atrophy that increases with age and that can be visualized on computed tomographic (CT) scans of the brain. There is usually symmetric enlargement of the lateral ventricles and an increase in the size of cerebral sulci and the width of interhemispheric and sylvian fissures. The abnormalities may lessen if drinking is discontinued. Many chronic alcoholics also show deficiencies on psychometric examination. The CT scan abnormalities, however, correlate poorly with such specific cognitive defects. The specific mechanisms of these cerebral abnormalities are not known.

ALCOHOLIC-NUTRITIONAL NEUROPATHY

CLINICAL MANIFESTATIONS. Polyneuropathy is common among alcoholic patients. The most typical complaints are weakness, pain, and paresthesias in the hands and especially the feet. Symptoms usually begin insidiously in the legs and progress proximally and symmetrically. Abnormal motor and sensory signs develop concomitantly. Patients may complain of burning pain and heat sensations on the plantar surfaces of the feet and aching pain in the calves. Dysesthesias can become so severe that light touch and deep pressure are intensely unpleasant. Burning pain made worse by contact can interfere with walking despite adequate strength.

On examination, muscle weakness and wasting are usually more prominent distally, affecting legs more than arms and never the latter exclusively. The muscles may feel tender to pressure. Weakness can be so severe that contractures develop at the ankles and knees. Sensory abnormalities usually involve all modalities, but especially the pain and temperature modalities early in the course, and are more prominent distally. The deep tendon reflexes are usually absent to diminished in a distal to proximal distribution. Even asymptomatic patients often show mild sensory loss in the feet and absent Achilles tendon reflexes.

Involvement of the vagus nerve and thoracoabdominal sympathetic chain occurs rarely and can produce hoarseness, dysphagia, vocal cord paralysis, and hypotension. Cerebrospinal fluid protein levels are usually normal.

PATHOPHYSIOLOGY AND TREATMENT. The classic pathologic findings in alcoholic neuropathy are axonal degeneration and demyelination. Alcoholic-nutritional neuropathy, since it first affects smaller sensory fibers, is characterized by axonal degeneration, with electromyographic signs of denervation and normal nerve conduction velocities often present at an early stage. Later, additional nutritional change may result in slow nerve-conduction velocities.

A specific vitamin deficiency has not been identified in alcoholic neuropathy. Treatment consists of a balanced diet with supplemental B vitamins. Recovery is slow and often incomplete. Several weeks may be needed for motor improvement to begin, and it may take a year before patients with marked weakness begin to walk.

ACUTE AND CHRONIC ALCOHOLIC MYOPATHY

ACUTE MYOPATHY. This is a dramatic and life-threatening condition that develops in chronic alcoholics during prolonged heavy drinking. Symptoms begin abruptly with pain, cramps, tenderness, weakness, and swelling of the legs. Muscle involvement may be generalized or confined to one limb. Creatine phosphokinase activity in blood is elevated, and muscle biopsy shows acute rhabdomyolysis. Myoglobinuria often occurs and may lead to acute renal failure, hyperkalemia, and death. Electromyography usually shows evidence of a primary myopathy (see Ch. 441.5). Recovery usually follows days to weeks of abstinence, occasionally leaving residual proximal muscle weakness in its wake.

CHRONIC MYOPATHY. This is a chronic, painless disorder of proximal muscle weakness and atrophy that occurs rarely in alcoholics and develops only after excessive drinking. It can be mild or severe. Muscles of the pelvic girdle and thighs are involved most frequently; weakness of shoulder girdle muscles is less common. Alcoholic myopathy and cardiomyopathy (Ch. 50) often develop concurrently. Improvement usually occurs within 2 to 3 months after ethanol withdrawal. A coexistent peripheral neuropathy may contribute to the weakness.

ALCOHOLIC CEREBELLAR DEGENERATION

Cerebellar cortical degeneration occurs frequently in chronic alcoholics and in several presumably nutritional disorders in underdeveloped countries. About half the patients have an associated peripheral neuropathy. Men are affected more often than women. Most patients give a history of episodic binge drinking superimposed on heavy consumption extending over many years. Some complain of progressive unsteadiness and difficulty in walking, but these more insidiously developing symptoms often reflect a superimposed peripheral neuropathy that may clear with treatment. Abnormalities of gait and station are the most common findings. Initially, unsteadiness occurs during rapid turns, and tandem walking is difficult or impossible. Gradually, the feet become more widely based, walking becomes hesitant, and truncal ataxia is added. Ataxia of the legs may be demonstrable on heel to shin tests, but nystagmus, dysarthria, and tremor are rare. Often the syndrome develops abruptly or rapidly over several weeks and then remains stable. Sometimes the disorder evolves more slowly, with exacerbation following a binge or during an intercurrent illness. The most prominent pathologic abnormality is degeneration of the neurons of the anterior and superior cerebellar vermis with loss of Purkinje cells. CT or magnetic resonance (MR) images confirm cerebellar vermis atrophy. Abstinence, dietary treatment, and supplemental B vitamins may produce moderate improvement in the gait ataxia as peripheral neuropathy resolves.

NUTRITIONAL AMBLYOPIA

The condition involves retrobulbar neuritis affecting maculopapillary fibers, caused by a nutritional deficiency and encountered primarily in alcoholics. Patients complain of dim or blurred vision that evolves gradually over weeks to months. Decreased visual acuity occurs in one or both eyes, accompanied by bilateral symmetric central or centrocecal scotomas. Peripheral visual fields are usually unaffected, and funduscopic examination is normal. Treatment consists of abstinence, diet, and supplemental B vitamins. The extent of recovery varies inversely with the severity of impairment before therapy.

CENTRAL PONTINE MYELINOLYSIS

Central pontine myelinolysis (CPM) is a rare disorder that affects alcoholics primarily but also occurs in children and adults with severe electrolyte disorders, liver disease, malnutrition, anorexia, burns, cancer, Addison's disease, sepsis, and Wilson's disease.

PATHOPHYSIOLOGY, SIGNS, AND SYMPTOMS. The signs and symptoms relate closely to the pathologic change, which consists of a varying extent of symmetric focal myelin destruction involving the basal central pons, with similar lesions occasionally affecting extrapontine areas (Fig. 456–1). There is no associated inflammation or nerve cell destruction, and the lesions appear to be reversible with time and proper nutritional and fluid balance.

Typically, CPM evolves within days or weeks in severely ill patients. Almost always, the condition follows by 1 to 3 days a period of profound hyponatremia followed by rapid osmolal correction of greater than 20 mEq per liter. Mental symptoms often are prominent and consist of clouded consciousness or exacerbation of pre-existing delirium. Reflecting interruption of corticospinal pathways in the pons, a flaccid or spastic quadriparesis ensues, accompanied in many instances by bulbar difficulties of speaking and swallowing. Some patients develop a supranuclear ophthalmoplegia, and the mortality is high. Reflecting the sparing of the pontine tegmentum, sensory abnormalities usually fail to develop. The characteristic story has recently led to the diagnosis of many cases during life, confirmed by abnormalities on CT or MRI scan. Some patients recover; others remain tetraplegic. Treatment consists of meticulous maintenance of electrolytes, especially sodium balance and adequate nutrition.

MARCHIAFAVA-BIGNAMI DISEASE

This is a rare disorder consisting of symmetric demyelination of the corpus callosum and adjacent white matter. The lesions can be imaged by CT scan. The disorder affects mainly middle-aged men, severely addicted to various kinds of alcoholic beverages. Patients may have a progressive dementia accompanied by agitation or apathy, hallucinations, and emotional disorders until seizures, stupor, and coma supervene. Clinical findings such as rooting and sucking responses, grasp reflexes, paratonic rigidity, incontinence, and a slow hesitant gait suggest bilateral frontal

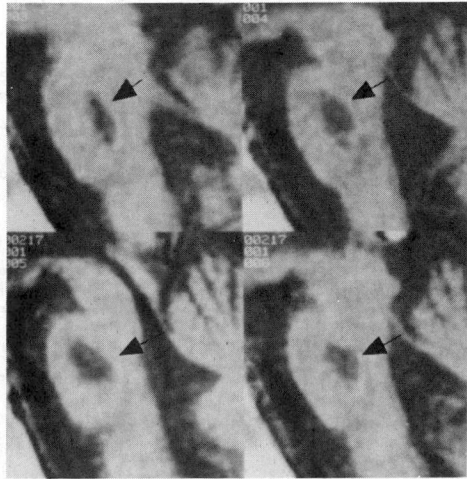

FIGURE 456–1. Central pontine myelinolysis. Magnetic resonance images were obtained in the sagittal plane using a "T₁-weighted" pulse sequence. An area of decreased signal is seen in the pons (*arrows*). (Photographs courtesy of Drs. Michael E. Charness and Robert L. DeLaPaz.)

lobe involvement. Recovery is rare, and the specific etiology is unknown.

VITAMIN E DEFICIENCY

Vitamin E deficiency is a complication of intestinal malabsorption in patients with chronic steatorrhea often due to cholestatic liver disease or cystic fibrosis (see Ch. 64). Patients with vitamin E deficiency develop a slowly progressive, distinctive neurologic syndrome with areflexia, cerebellar ataxia, ophthalmoplegia, pigmentary retinopathy, loss of vibratory sensation, and muscle weakness. Neurologic signs usually begin in childhood or adolescence with a loss of deep tendon reflexes followed by mild reduction in vibratory sensation; position sense is less affected, and pain and temperature sensation may be normal. Babinski signs are variable. A progressive external ophthalmoplegia is commonly associated with limitation of upward gaze. There may be impaired visual acuity and night vision because of pigmentary retinopathy. Muscle weakness and atrophy are often late complications, affecting muscles diffusely, distally, or in a proximal myopathic distribution. Untreated patients can become severely disabled. Vitamin E deficiency probably is responsible for the similar neurologic syndrome that develops in abetalipoproteinemia (see Ch. 463).

Vitamin E is an antioxidant that appears to protect unsaturated fatty acids of membrane phospholipids from oxidative degradation. The major pathologic findings in vitamin E deficiency are axonal degeneration of peripheral nerves and dorsal columns, reduced numbers of large myelinated fibers in peripheral nerves, and breakdown of the outer rod segments of the retina. Deposition of lipopigment, perhaps due to polymerization of peroxidized fatty acids, occurs in selected neurons and nonneural tissue. Similar neurologic abnormalities have been produced in animals with experimental vitamin E deficiency.

Serum vitamin E levels are low, particularly when related to serum lipids or cholesterol. Neurophysiologic studies usually show evidence of an axonal neuropathy with abnormal sensory nerve conduction velocities or amplitudes, and abnormal H-reflexes. Motor nerve conduction is altered less often or less severely, but evidence of denervation may be found in the tongue and somatic muscles. Central somatosensory conduction is often delayed, consistent with posterior column axonal degeneration. Electroretinograms and visual evoked potentials are abnormal according to the severity of the neurologic findings.

Treatment with vitamin E often improves the neurologic condition, but high oral doses or parenteral administration may be necessary. Early treatment of unaffected children with cholestasis probably prevents the neurologic complications of vitamin E deficiency (Ch. 204).

COBALAMIN (VITAMIN B₁₂) DEFICIENCY

Cobalamin (vitamin B₁₂) deficiency causes subacute degeneration of white matter in the dorsal and lateral columns of the spinal cord, peripheral nerves, optic discs, and cerebral hemispheres. The neurologic findings usually accompany a macrocytic (pernicious) anemia, but anemia need not be present. Hematologic and pathophysiologic considerations of cobalamin deficiency and details of treatment are discussed in Ch. 204.

CLINICAL MANIFESTATIONS. Neurologic symptoms develop in most patients with long untreated pernicious anemia, especially those in whom anemia has been masked by folate ingestion. Occasional examples can occur with cobalamin deficiency due to intestinal malabsorption, gastrectomy, or inadequate diet. Patients first complain of paresthesias in the hands or legs, such as tingling, numbness, and "pins and needles" sensations. Stiffness and weakness of the legs with unsteadiness in walking may be bothersome, particularly in the dark. Neurologic symptoms progress relentlessly if untreated; ataxia and stiffness eventually are followed by paraplegia and dysfunction of bowel and bladder. Psychological symptoms are frequent and include apathy and depression, irritability and paranoid tendencies, nocturnal confusion, and dementia. Intellectual deterioration does not usually develop in the absence of other neurologic signs. Failing vision with central scotomas occurs rarely.

Initially, one may find few objective changes despite complaints of paresthesias. Later, symmetric distal impairment of vibratory sensation occurs, usually first in the legs but eventually reaching the trunk and arms. Position sense is affected less prominently, although Romberg's test may be positive. The earliest changes are those of a peripheral neuropathy. The patellar and Achilles tendon reflexes are diminished or absent, and there may be decreased perception of touch, pain, and temperature in the feet and ankles. In the intermediate advanced case, one finds symmetric weakness in the legs associated with spasticity, clonus at the knees and ankles, increased or decreased deep tendon reflexes, and extensor plantar responses. Tingling distal paresthesias may follow flexion of the neck (Lhermitte's sign). Recent studies attributing a wide variety of vague neuropsychiatric difficulties to cobalamin deficiency in the absence of either reduced serum B_{12} levels or abnormal Schilling tests remain to be verified by independent, controlled studies.

PATHOLOGY. The most prominent findings are in the peripheral nerves and dorsal and lateral columns of the spinal cord. Fragmentation and spongy degeneration of myelin usually begin in the lower cervical and upper thoracic regions; in untreated patients the disease progresses up and down the spinal cord and reaches into the ventral columns. Myelin sheaths and axons are destroyed, and wallerian degeneration is found in the spinal cord funiculi. Cerebral white matter is affected late. Peripheral nerves may show distal degeneration.

DIAGNOSIS AND PATHOPHYSIOLOGY. Serum vitamin B_{12} levels are low and appear to correlate with the severity of the neurologic findings. The cerebrospinal fluid (CSF) protein concentration may be increased slightly. Neurologic disorders that can be confused with cobalamin deficiency include multiple sclerosis, cervical spondylosis, spinal cord tumors, and syphilitic meningomyelitis. A virtually identical syndrome has been reported after chronic abuse of nitrous oxide.

PATHOGENESIS. The molecular pathogenesis of the neurologic lesion in cobalamin deficiency is unknown. Cobalamin exists in different forms, some of which are required for at least two enzymes: N-5-methyltetrahydrofolate homocysteine methyltransferase, which catalyzes the synthesis of methionine and regeneration of tetrahydrofolate, and methylmalonyl-CoA mutase, which generates succinyl-CoA. Cobalamin deficiency produces elevated serum levels of homocyteine and methylmalonic acid. Prolonged exposure to nitrous oxide, which produces a neurologic disorder resembling combined system disease, also inhibits methionine synthesis.

TREATMENT. Intramuscular administration of cobalamin is the only treatment for cobalamin deficiency due to pernicious anemia or other malabsorptive states. Therapy should be started immediately and continued throughout the patient's lifetime. Early neurologic changes can be rapidly and completely reversed if treatment with cobalamin is begun promptly within the first few weeks or months of symptoms. If the neurologic manifestations have reached the stage of spinal cord dysfunction, therapy will halt progression, but improvement cannot be guaranteed.

Blass JP: Vitamin and nutritional deficiencies. In Siegel GJ, Agranoff BW, Albers RW, Molinoff PB (eds.): Basic Neurochemistry. 4th ed. New York, Raven Press, 1989. *A clear discussion of the basic neurochemistry of the vitamins.*

Charness ME, Simon RP, Greenberg D: Ethanol and the nervous system. N Engl J Med 321:442, 1989. *A scholarly review with many references.*

Diamond I: Alcohol neurotoxicity. In Asbury AK, McKhann GM, McDonald WI (eds.): Diseases of the Nervous System. 2nd ed. Philadelphia, W. B. Saunders Company, 1992. *A comprehensive discussion of recent advances and the pathophysiology of alcohol-related neurologic disorders. A helpful bibliography.*

Harper CG, Giles M, Finlay-Jones R: Clinical signs in the Wernicke-Korsakoff complex: A retrospective analysis of 131 cases diagnosed at necropsy. J Neurol Neurosurg Psychiatry 49:341, 1986. *In this large series from Australia, correct antemortem diagnosis was reached in only 20 per cent of cases; most of the missed cases lacked ophthalmoplegia.*

Lindenbaum J, Mealton EB, Savage DG, et al.: Neuropsychiatric disorders caused by cobalamin deficiency in the absence of anemia or macrocytosis. N Engl J Med 318:1720, 1989. *A recent report of 141 patients suggesting that neurologic symptoms occur commonly without anemia and that measurement of serum methylmalonic acid and total homocyteine is useful in the diagnosis.*

Satya-Murti S, Howard L, Krohel G, et al.: The spectrum of neurologic disorders from vitamin E deficiency. Neurology 36:917, 1986. *A recent study of nine patients with more variable features. A helpful bibliography.*

Sterns RH, Riggs JE, Schochet SS: Osmotic demyelination syndrome following correction of hyponatremia. N Engl J Med 314:1535, 1986. *A recent report of eight patients and a review of the literature suggests that to avoid myelinolysis serum sodium should be raised by less than 12 mmol per liter per day.*

SECTION FIVE / THE EXTRAPYRAMIDAL DISORDERS

Joseph Jankovic

457 Introduction

The term *extrapyramidal* refers to the anatomic and functional characteristics that distinguish the basal ganglia–regulated motor system from the pyramidal (corticospinal) and cerebellar systems. Extrapyramidal movement disorders are divided descriptively into *hypokinesias*, characterized by poverty and slowness of movement; *hyperkinesias*, manifested by abnormal involuntary movements; and miscellaneous motor disturbances (Table 457–1). Before discussing the clinical, pathophysiologic, and therapeutic aspects of the different movement disorders, it is important to review the anatomic and functional organization of the basal ganglia.

FUNCTIONAL AND NEUROCHEMICAL ANATOMY OF THE BASAL GANGLIA

The six paired nuclei that constitute the basal ganglia include the caudate nucleus, putamen, globus pallidus (or pallidum), nucleus accumbens, subthalamic nucleus, and substantia nigra (Fig. 457–1). The caudate nucleus and putamen, although separated by the internal capsule, share cytoarchitechtonic, chemical, and physiologic properties; they are often referred to as the *corpus striatum*, neostriatum, or simply striatum. The striatum is a highly inhomogeneous structure composed of subregions

TABLE 457–1. MOVEMENT DISORDERS

Hypokinesias	Hyperkinesias	Miscellaneous
Parkinsonism	Tremor	Ataxia
Hypomimia	Dystonia	Gait disorders
Dysarthria	Chorea	Hyperekplexia
Sialorrhea	Athetosis	Hemifacial spasm
Micrographia	Ballism	Myokymia
Shuffling gait	Tics	Stiff-person syndrome
Other signs of	Myoclonus	Psychogenic
bradykinesia	Stereotypy	
and rigidity	Akathisia	
	Restless legs	
	Paroxysmal dyskinesias	

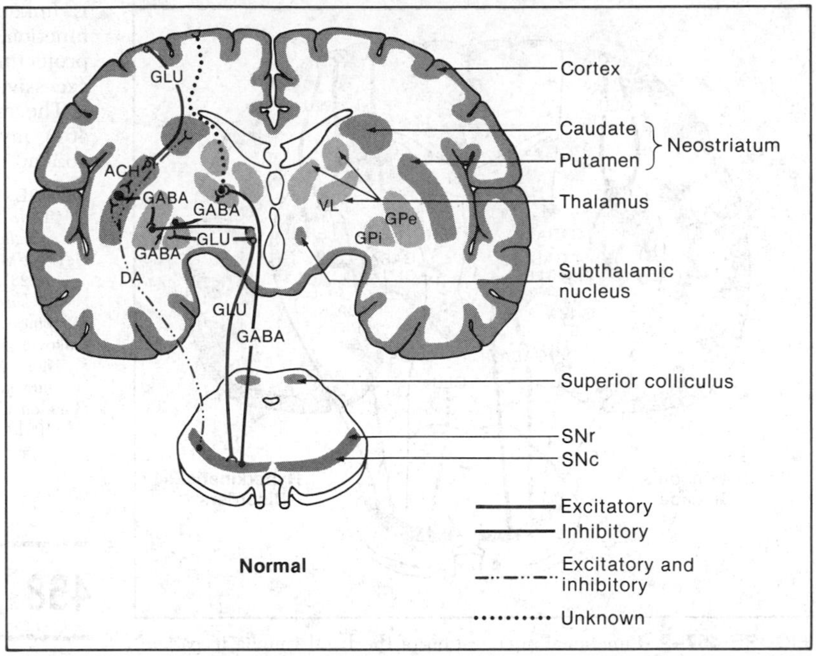

FIGURE 457–1. Anatomy of the basal ganglia and their connections. ACH = acetylcholine; GABA = γ-aminobutyric acid; GLU = glutamate; GP = globus pallidum (e = external, i = internal); DA = dopamine; SN = substantia nigra (c = compacta, r = reticulata); VL = ventrolateral.

termed striosomes and matrix. The limbic system provides major input to the striosomes, whereas neocortical areas primarily project to the matrix. Although the internal capsule separates the internal segment of the globus pallidus (GPi) and the pars reticulata of the substantia nigra (SNr), evidence suggests that these nuclei should be regarded as a single functional structure. The term *lenticular nucleus* refers to the putamen and globus pallidus combined because of their lenslike shape.

Recent anatomic and physiologic data suggest a complex organization of the basal ganglia and related structures (Fig. 457–1). According to this schema, the sensorimotor, association, and limbic cortical areas provide anatomically and functionally segregated inputs to the dorsal (the caudate and putamen) and ventral (nucleus accumbens, not shown) striatum. The somatosensory, motor, and premotor cortical areas project mainly to the putamen, while the posterior parietal and temporal and frontal association cortical areas project largely to the caudate and nucleus accumbens. The anatomy is consistent with the concept that the putamen is primarily concerned with motor function and the caudate is more involved with emotional and cognitive processes. The corticostriatal afferents are mediated by the excitatory neurotransmitter glutamic acid. The other major striatal afferents originate in the substantia nigra pars compacta (SNc), which provides major dopaminergic inhibitory input to the basal ganglia via the nigrostriatal pathway. Other inhibitory inputs to the striatum arise from the brain stem raphe nuclei (serotonergic) and from the locus ceruleus neurons (noradrenergic). The striatum is composed largely of cholinergic neurons, and some excitatory cholinergic projections to the striatum originate in the midline intralaminar thalamic nuclei.

The striatal nuclei project somatotopically to the external segment of the globus pallidus (GPe) and the GPi-SNr complex. The striatal efferents utilize the inhibitory neurotransmitter γ-aminobutyric acid (GABA). The subthalamic nucleus (STN) regulates the output of the basal ganglia to the thalamus by modulating the inhibitory GABAergic afferents from the GPe and the excitatory glutamatergic efferent projections to the GPi-SNr complex. The efferent inhibitory GABAergic projections from the GPi terminate in the thalamus. The thalamic nuclei in turn project to the supplementary motor area of the cortex and the primary motor cortex.

MOVEMENT DISORDERS

Single-cell recordings in behaving animals and other physiologic studies have demonstrated that one of the primary roles of the basal ganglia is to scale the movement amplitude and velocity rather than to initiate movements. Besides their critical role in the execution of movement, the basal ganglia also seem to be involved in the preparation for movement.

In addition to impaired voluntary movements, dysfunction in the basal ganglia can also cause a variety of abnormal involuntary movements. Correlations between the various types of abnormal movements and sites of experimental and pathologic lesions have provided helpful insights into and better understanding of the function of the basal ganglia. The remainder of this section is organized according to the major categories of movement disorders into hypokinetic (parkinsonian), hyperkinetic, and miscellaneous movement disorders (Table 457–1).

HYPOKINESIAS (PARKINSONIAN DISORDERS)

Bradykinesia is manifested clinically by slowness of automatic and spontaneous movements and impaired ability to initiate voluntary movements (akinesia). This typical parkinsonian symptom presumably results from loss of the inhibitory dopamine input to the striatum and hypoactivity of the GPe neurons. This, in turn, causes functional disinhibition (excitation) of the STN, inducing an increase of neuronal activity in the GPi, thereby raising the tonic inhibitory output from the basal ganglia (GPi) to the thalamus and to the cortical projection areas (Fig. 457–2). The altered activity in the "motor" circuit is manifested by increased movement time, which becomes particularly prolonged when a parkinsonian subject performs sequential movements.

Rigidity, another cardinal sign of parkinsonism, is demonstrated clinically by increased resistance against passive movement of a body part, usually associated with the "cogwheel" phenomenon. A parkinsonian patient perceives rigidity as a feeling of joint stiffness and muscle tightness. The pathophysiologic mechanisms of rigidity have been attributed to pallidal disinhibition resulting in increased suprasegmental activation of normal spinal reflex mechanisms.

Postural instability due to loss of righting reflexes can cause propulsion (tendency to fall forward) and retropulsion (tendency to fall backward). It is one of the most disabling symptoms of Parkinson's disease. The mechanism of postural instability is unknown, but it has been attributed primarily to involvement of the pallidum. Other hypokinetic manifestations are listed in Table 457–1.

HYPERKINESIAS (ABNORMAL INVOLUNTARY MOVEMENTS)

Tremor is a rhythmic oscillatory movement produced by alternating or synchronous contractions of opposing muscle groups. Tremors are divided into rest or action tremors; the latter are further subdivided into postural or contraction tremors (e.g.,

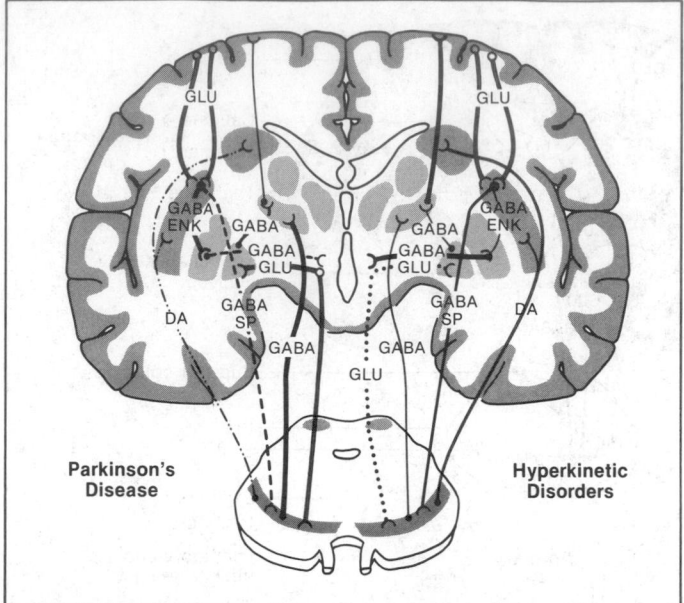

FIGURE 457–2. Functional organization of the basal ganglia in parkinsonian disorders and hyperkinetic movement disorders. ACH = acetylcholine; GABA = γ-aminobutyric acid; GLU = glutamate; DA = dopamine; ENK = enkephalin; SP = substance P.

arms outstretched in front of the body or in a "wing-beating" position) and kinetic or intention tremors (e.g., during target-directed movement, such as the finger-to-nose maneuver). *Rest tremor,* usually asymmetric at onset, is the typical tremor of Parkinson's disease. When it involves the hands, it causes a supinating-pronating oscillatory (pill-rolling) movement at approximately 4- to 6-Hz frequency. Parkinsonian tremor also often involves the legs, feet, lips, tongue, chin, and voice but almost never affects the head or neck. *Postural tremor,* with frequency ranging between 4 and 12 Hz, is most typically seen in patients with essential tremor. *Kinetic (intention) tremors* are slow and more irregular movements with a rate of 1.5 to 3 Hz. Kinetic tremors usually indicate an abnormality of the cerebellum or its outflow pathways (the dentate nucleus, the superior cerebellar peduncle, and contralateral red nucleus).

Dystonia is produced by involuntary, sustained (tonic) or spasmodic (rapid or clonic), patterned, and repetitive muscle contractions, frequently causing twisting (e.g., torticollis), flexing or extending (e.g., writer's cramp, retrocollis), and squeezing (e.g., blepharospasm, writer's cramp) movements or abnormal postures. Dystonia is usually constant but occurs in some cases only during particular activities. Examples of task-specific dystonias include writer's or typist's cramp and inversion of a foot while running. As dystonia progresses, the involuntary contractions also appear at rest. A characteristic feature of dystonia is that the spasms lessen in intensity with "sensory tricks," such as touching one side of the face to maintain a primary position, thus counteracting involuntary torticollis. Dystonia can fluctuate in intensity and is exacerbated by stress, fatigue, activity, or a change in posture. It subsides during sleep, relaxation, and hypnosis. These features and the bizarre nature of dystonic patterns sometimes are wrongly attributed to psychogenic causes. About half of patients with dystonia have a coexistent postural tremor, identical to essential tremor. The anatomic substrate for dystonia is unknown. Clinicopathologic studies of patients with secondary dystonias most often implicate the putamen and the rostral brain stem in its genesis.

Chorea consists of continuous, abrupt, rapid, brief, flowing, unsustained, irregular, and random jerklike movements. Choreic patients frequently mask the abnormal movements by voluntary semipurposeful activities. A characteristic feature of chorea is the inability to maintain voluntary sustained contraction. Examples include an inability to sustain manual grip or tongue protrusion and the dropping of objects. Muscle stretch reflexes are usually

"hung up" and "pendular." Affected patients typically have a peculiar, irregular, and dancelike gait. The pathogenesis of chorea is unknown. Some findings point to abnormalities in caudate function. A selective loss of the GABA-enkephalin striatal neurons projecting to the GPe, found in Huntington's disease, results in excessive inhibition of STN neurons.

The movement disorders of athetosis (Ch. 461), ballism (Ch. 461), myoclonus (Ch. 462), tics (Ch. 462), and stereotypies (Ch. 462) are discussed in later chapters of this section.

Albin RL, Young AB, Penney JB: The functional anatomy of basal ganglia disorders. TINS 12:366, 1989. *An excellent review of current understanding of the basal ganglia connections in the normal and diseased brain.*

DeLong MR: Primate models of movement disorders of basal ganglia origin. TINS 13:281, 1990. *A review of the MPTP model of parkinsonism used in the study of basal ganglia circuitry. Hyperactivity of the STN is associated with bradykinesia, and a chemical lesion in the STN reduces this cardinal sign.*

Jankovic J, Tolosa E (eds.): Parkinson's Disease and Movement Disorders. Baltimore-Munich, Urban and Schwarzenberg, 1988. *A comprehensive review of hypokinetic, hyperkinetic, and miscellaneous movement disorders.*

Marsden CD, Fahn S: Movement Disorders 3. London, Butterworths Scientific, 1991. *A comprehensive review of different movement disorders by recognized experts.*

458 Parkinsonism

Parkinsonism is a clinical syndrome dominated by four cardinal signs: tremor at rest, bradykinesia, rigidity, and postural instability. Less prominent manifestations concern the mood and intellect, oculomotor control, autonomic function, and the sensory system (Table 458–1). The average age at onset is 55 years, with about 1 per cent of persons 60 years of age or older having the disease. Men are affected more frequently than women by a ratio of 3:2. At least two major subtypes of Parkinson's disease (PD) have been identified: One subtype is characterized by tremor as the dominant parkinsonian feature, and the other is dominated by postural instability and gait difficulty (PIGD). The *tremor subtype* of PD is associated with relatively normal mental status, earlier age at onset, and slower progression of the disease than is the *PIGD subtype,* which shows more bradykinesia, dementia, and a more rapidly progressive course.

Resting tremor and bradykinesia are the most typical parkinsonian signs and are virtually synonymous with the diagnosis. Bradykinesia accounts for most of the associated parkinsonian symptoms and signs: general slowing down of movements and of activities of daily living; lack of facial expression (hypomimia or masked facies); staring expression due to decreased frequency of blinking; impaired swallowing, which causes drooling; hypokinetic and hypophonic dysarthria; monotonous speech; small handwriting (micrographia); difficulties with repetitive and simultaneous movements; difficulty in arising from chair and turning

TABLE 458–1. NONMOTOR DISTURBANCE IN PARKINSON'S DISEASE

Neurobehavioral Abnormalities in Parkinson's Disease
  Personality changes (apathy, lack of confidence, fearfulness, anxiety, emotional lability and inflexibility, social withdrawal, dependency)
  Dementia (tip-of-the-tongue phenomenon [partial anomia], spatial disorientation, paranoia, psychosis, hallucinations)
  Bradyphrenia (slow thought processes, loss of concentration, difficulty with concept formation)
  Depression
  Sleep disturbance
  Sexual dysfunction
  Psychiatric side effects of therapy

Other Nonmotor Manifestations of Parkinson's Disease
  Autonomic dysfunction (orthostatic hypotension, respiratory dysregulation, flushing, "drenching sweats," constipation, sphincter and sexual dysfunction)
  Sensory symptoms (paresthesias, pains, akathisia; visual, olfactory, and vestibular dysfunction)
  Seborrhea, pedal edema, fatigue, weight loss

over in bed; shuffling gait with short steps; decreased arm swing and other automatic movements; and start hesitation and freezing. Freezing, manifested by sudden and often unpredictable inability to move, is one of the most disabling of all parkinsonian symptoms.

Several disorders other than PD can cause at least part of the parkinsonian syndrome (Table 458–2). Non-PD parkinsonian disorders can be distinguished clinically from PD by the presence of atypical findings, absence or paucity of tremor, and poor response to levodopa. The last feature may be partly explained by the fact that postsynaptic dopamine receptors are preserved in PD, but they are decreased in the other parkinsonian syndromes.

PARKINSON'S DISEASE

Pathogenesis

The most typical pathologic hallmarks of PD are (1) neuronal loss with depigmentation of the substantia nigra (SN) and (2) Lewy bodies, which are eosinophilic cytoplasmic inclusions in neurons consisting of aggregates of normal filaments. These abnormalities are most prominent in the ventrolateral region of the SN that projects to the putamen. At least an 80 per cent loss of dopaminergic neurons in the substantia nigra and the same degree of dopamine depletion in the striatum must appear before clinical symptoms of PD become evident.

Motor symptoms of PD result chiefly from degeneration of the nigrostriatal pathway, causing a deficiency of dopamine in the putamen and, to a lesser degree, the caudate nucleus. The cognitive deficits and some neurobehavioral symptoms have been attributed to degeneration of the dopaminergic mesocortical and mesolimbic pathways, and the associated autonomic dysfunction may be partly caused by dopamine depletion in the hypothalamus. Besides dopamine deficiency, impairment of the other neurotransmitters may be responsible for some of the associated findings. For example, degeneration of the noradrenergic locus ceruleus may contribute to the "freezing" phenomenon and to depression. Degeneration of the cholinergic nucleus basalis probably relates to the dementia that eventually affects about a third of all PD patients.

Although several hypotheses are currently being investigated, the etiology of PD is still unknown. Genetic factors may increase its risk, but the contribution is more complex than simple mendelian inheritance. The "environmental" hypothesis of PD is primarily based on the observation that the meperidine analogue 1-methyl-4-phenyl-1,2,3,6-tetrahydropyridine (MPTP), originally used by heroin addicts, causes parkinsonism in humans and in animals. MPTP must be oxidized to a pyridine MPP+ to be neurotoxic, and antioxidants such as deprenyl (a selective monoamine oxidase [MAO]–B inhibitor) prevent MPTP-induced experimental parkinsonism. As a result, it has been postulated that some environmental MPTP-like toxin might be responsible for human PD. An alternative hypothesis is that an endogenous toxin, such as dopamine, damages susceptible neurons. During the process of oxidative deamination, dopamine generates hydroxyl radicals and hydrogen peroxide, which, in the presence of iron deposits in the brain, could lead to lipid peroxidation and neurotoxicity, possibly by interfering with mitochondrial oxidative metabolism. Observed abnormalities in mitochondrial complex I activity have stimulated renewed interest in the role of genetic susceptibility in PD.

Treatment

The finding that deprenyl prevents MPTP-induced parkinsonism has stimulated interest in antioxidative therapy as a means of retarding the progression of PD. Some studies have found that deprenyl slows the development of motor disability and the rate of disease progression when used in the early stages of PD. These findings, if confirmed, suggest the possibility of favorably altering the natural course of the disease.

In addition to its possible protective effect, deprenyl may provide moderate symptomatic relief. After starting deprenyl, many patients report improvement in their energy level and bradykinetic symptoms. The effect may be due to deprenyl's ability to increase striatal concentrations of dopamine by blocking its metabolism by MAO. The addition of one of the anticholinergic drugs, such as trihexyphenidyl, may provide additional symptomatic relief, particularly in younger patients and patients in whom tremor predominates. Associated depression, present in many parkinsonian patients, can be treated with tricyclic antidepressants, such as amitriptyline or nortriptyline. Because the anticholinergics, including the tricyclics, can produce undesirable psychological symptoms as well as side effects, such as dry mouth, blurring of vision, and urinary hesitancy, amantadine may offer a useful alternative, particularly in elderly patients. Amantadine, however, while helpful in controlling both tremor and bradykinesia, can also cause adverse effects, including livedo reticularis, ankle edema, exacerbation of congestive heart failure, and mild anticholinergic side effects.

Many neurologists favor employing combinations of deprenyl, the anticholinergics, and amantadine until they no longer provide a satisfactory control of parkinsonian symptoms. At that point, in socially or occupationally disabled patients, levodopa combined with carbidopa, a peripheral dopa decarboxylase inhibitor, is added to the antiparkinsonian regimen. The starting dosage of carbidopa/levodopa is 25 mg/100 mg twice daily, to be gradually increased over 3 weeks to three times per day. The dosage is then adjusted, depending on the severity of symptoms and occupational demands. Some patients require as much as 25/250 four or five times daily; others tolerate no more than 25/100 four times daily. Although levodopa can suppress tremor, it is most useful in controlling bradykinesia and rigidity. Postural instability may be ameliorated by levodopa in early stages, but dopaminergic therapy is usually ineffective later on. Levodopa is contraindicated in patients with diagnosed melanoma and should be used with caution in those with prominent psychosis or dementia, peptic ulcer disease, and cardiac arrhythmias.

About 15 per cent of parkinsonian patients fail to improve with levodopa. Most of these nonresponders probably suffer from a form of postsynaptic parkinsonism rather than PD. A failure to respond to levodopa should also suggest the possibility of a wrong diagnosis, a drug interaction (concomitant use of dopamine receptor blocking agents, such as antipsychotic and antiemetic drugs), and pharmacokinetic reasons, such as insufficient dosage, slow stomach emptying, and competition for absorption in the small intestine and at the blood-brain barrier by amino acids in protein meals. In any event, almost all patients who initially improve lose their response to levodopa sometime between 3 and 8 years after onset.

TABLE 458–2. CAUSES OF THE PARKINSON SYNDROME

I. **Primary (Idiopathic) Parkinsonism**
   Parkinson's disease
   Juvenile parkinsonism
II. **Secondary (Acquired, Symptomatic) Parkinsonism**
   Infectious: postencephalitic, slow virus
   Drugs: neuroleptics (antipsychotic, antiemetic drugs),
      reserpine, tetrabenazine, α-methyldopa, lithium, flunarizine,
      cinnarizine
   Toxins: MPTP, CO, Mn, Hg, CS_2, methanol, ethanol
   Vascular: multi-infarct, hypotension shock
   Trauma: pugilistic encephalopathy
   Other: parathyroid abnormalities, hypothyroidism, hepatocerebral
      degeneration, brain tumor, normal-pressure hydrocephalus,
      syringomesencephalia
III. **Heredodegenerative Parkinsonism**
   Autosomal dominant Lewy body disease
   Huntington's disease
   Wilson's disease
   Hallervorden-Spatz disease
   Olivopontocerebellar and spinocerebellar degenerations
   Familial basal ganglia calcification
   Familial parkinsonism with peripheral neuropathy
   Neuroacanthocytosis
IV. **Multiple-System Degenerations (Parkinsonism-Plus)**
   Progressive supranuclear palsy
   Shy-Drager syndrome
   Striatonigral degeneration
   Parkinsonism-dementia-ALS complex
   Corticobasal ganglionic degeneration
   Alzheimer's disease
   Hemiatrophy-parkinsonism

The two primary reasons why PD patients lose their response to levodopa are (1) natural progression of the disease and (2) development of complications as a result of chronic levodopa therapy. Although nonneuronal elements may participate in the conversion of levodopa to dopamine, the surviving striatal dopaminergic terminals are primarily responsible for this process. With progression of the disease and accompanying cellular degeneration, this capacity for conversion of levodopa to dopamine is lost, and the patient develops motor fluctuations and symptomatic deterioration.

The most challenging problem in the management of PD is the treatment of levodopa complications. Side effects caused by peripheral dopamine (and dopamine stimulation of the medullary vomiting center, which is not protected by the blood-brain barrier) include gastrointestinal symptoms, tachycardia, and orthostatic hypotension. The most common central side effects of levodopa therapy include psychiatric problems, dyskinesias (seen in about 80 per cent of patients after 3 years of therapy), and clinical fluctuations (seen in about 50 per cent of patients after 5 years of therapy). The most common form of clinical fluctuation is the wearing-off effect, characterized by end-of-dose deterioration and recurrence of parkinsonian symptoms as a result of shorter (sometimes only 1 to 2 hours) duration of benefit after a given dose of levodopa. Slow-release preparations of levodopa (e.g., Sinemet CR, Madopar CR) have been shown to prolong the plasma (and presumably brain) levels and may be useful in the treatment, and possibly prevention, of motor fluctuations. Deprenyl can also prolong the duration of benefit from each levodopa dose.

Because the onset of levodopa-induced complications seems to be related to the duration of levodopa therapy, some authorities delay initiating levodopa therapy until the patient's symptoms begin to interfere with normal activities. Once levodopa treatment is initiated, the dose should be maintained as low as possible (Fig. 458–1). Therefore, instead of increasing the dosage of levodopa, dopamine agonists such as bromocriptine or pergolide should be introduced early in the course of anti-PD therapy. These drugs directly activate the dopamine receptors. Initially, dopamine agonists were used primarily as adjunctive therapy in patients with levodopa-induced fluctuations. The role of dopamine agonists in the treatment of PD has broadened, however, and these agents are now recommended in the early phases of

therapy in an attempt to delay or reduce the risk of levodopa side effects. In experimental studies, pergolide has been shown to exert its dopaminergic effects on both D_1 and D_2 receptors without presynaptic dopamine, and it may improve parkinsonian symptoms even before levodopa is given. Some authorities, therefore, give pergolide as the first dopaminergic drug. However, as symptoms increase, dopamine agonists must be combined with levodopa. The starting dosage for bromocriptine is 1.25 mg twice a day and for pergolide, 0.05 mg twice a day. The dosage should be increased slowly to prevent gastrointestinal, psychiatric, autonomic, and other side effects. The side effects of dopamine agonists are similar to those of levodopa, although dopamine agonists may produce hallucinations, delusions, and other psychiatric symptoms more often than does levodopa. They also can cause erythromelalgia manifested by painful erythema of the legs, which is not usually seen with levodopa. Other motor and nonmotor symptoms of PD may require more specific therapy.

Surgical treatment of PD remains of unproven long-term value, although stereotaxic thalamotomy is occasionally employed in an attempt to ameliorate disabling tremor. Surgical transplantation of autologous adrenal medulla or fetal substantia nigra into the striatum remains under investigation.

As with all progressive, disabling diseases, psychological support of patients and family offers important help. Patients should be encouraged to learn about their disease (by reading educational material provided by the national and local support organizations) and to be physically and socially active.

SECONDARY PARKINSONISM

POSTENCEPHALITIC PARKINSONISM. Many individuals who survived the acute febrile illness and encephalopathy during the pandemics of encephalitis lethargica (von Economo's encephalitis) between 1919 and 1926 later developed a variety of movement disorders, including parkinsonism. The postencephalitic syndrome was also manifested by hemiparesis, involuntary ocular deviations (oculogyric crises), dystonia, chorea, tics, and behavioral problems. Postencephalitic parkinsonism has a slower progression and is more sensitive to levodopa therapy. Although the virus or viruses responsible for encephalitis lethargica were never isolated, infections caused by coxsackie, Japanese B, and western equine encephalitis viruses have since been identified as being complicated by parkinsonism.

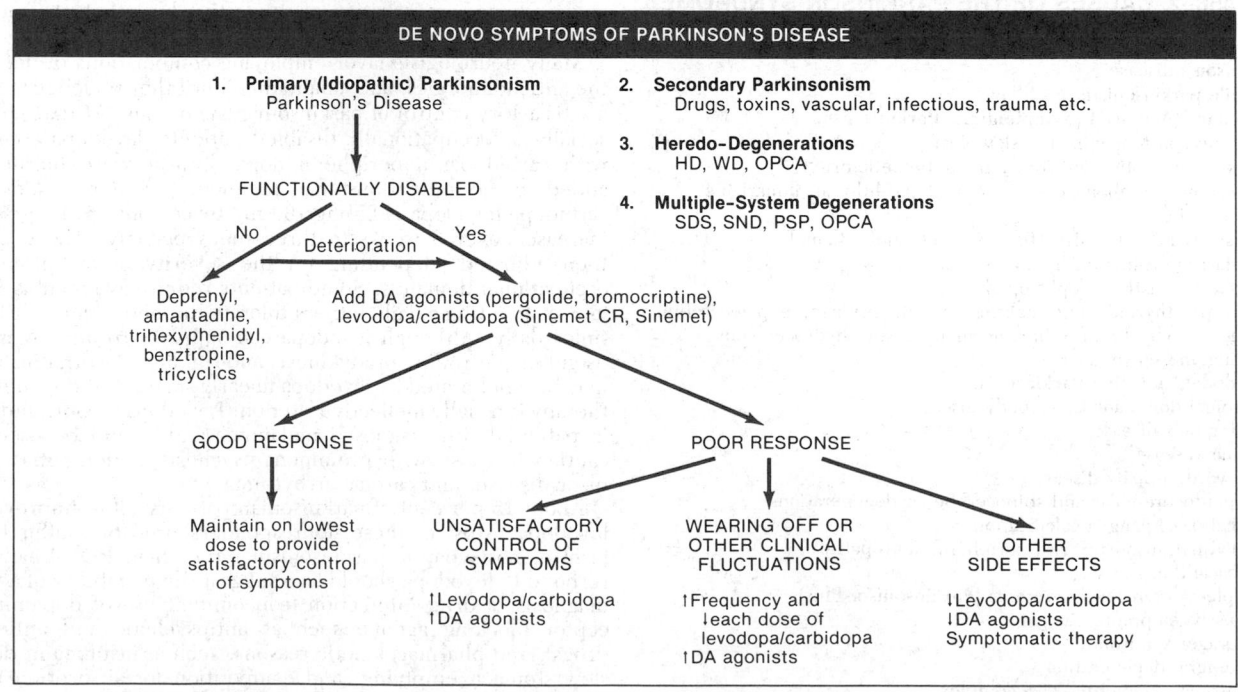

FIGURE 458–1. Diagrammatic representation of therapeutic approach to patients with parkinsonism. DA = dopamine; HD = Huntington's disease; OPCA = olivopontocerebellar atrophy; PSP = progressive supranuclear palsy; SDS = Shy = Drager syndrome; Sinement CR = controlled = release levodopa/carbidopa; SND = striatonigral degeneration; WD = Wilson's disease.

DRUG-INDUCED PARKINSONISM. After PD, drugs that deplete dopamine stores or block dopamine receptors are the most common causes of parkinsonian findings. Drugs that deplete the presynaptic stores of dopamine, such as reserpine and tetrabenazine (an investigational drug not available for general use in North America), and drugs that block the dopamine receptors, such as antipsychotic and antiemetic agents, can cause a parkinsonian syndrome clinically indistinguishable from idiopathic parkinsonism (PD). The same drugs can also cause a variety of other movement disorders, such as akathisia, dystonic reactions, and various tardive syndromes (e.g., tardive stereotypy, tardive dystonia, and tardive akathisia).

VASCULAR PARKINSONISM. Cerebrovascular disease accounts for only a small proportion of parkinsonism. Single strokes rarely cause parkinsonian findings, although multiple small infarctions involving the striatum can produce the syndrome. Brain imaging is helpful in the diagnosis. One form of vascular parkinsonism is the so-called "lower body parkinsonism," manifested chiefly by gait disturbance with short steps, "freezing," and difficulties with turning. (Chronic communicating, "low-pressure" hydrocephalus causes a similar clinical picture.) Patients with vascular parkinsonism may have dementia, hyperactive reflexes, and urinary incontinence, but tremor is rare. Levodopa therapy usually fails, probably because ischemia damages the striatal postsynaptic receptors. The diagnosis is suggested by these atypical findings in patients with a history of stroke risk factors.

HEREDODEGENERATIVE PARKINSONISM

Very few parkinsonian patients have a family history suggesting a specific pattern of inheritance. With such a history, the differential diagnosis should include one of the heredodegenerative disorders (Table 458–2).

HALLERVORDEN-SPATZ DISEASE. This rare condition is manifested by childhood or adult-onset progressive dementia, bradykinesia, rigidity, and spasticity, variously combined with dystonia, choreoathetosis, ataxia, seizures, amyotrophy, and retinitis pigmentosa. Most reported cases have suggested an autosomal recessive inheritance. Neuropathologically, iron accumulates in the globus pallidus (GP) and SN, accompanied by axonal swelling and neuronal degeneration in the basal ganglia, corticospinal tract, and cerebellum. Cysteine, found to be increased in the GP, possibly chelates iron, causing a generation of free radicals and subsequent neuronal degeneration.

FAMILIAL BASAL GANGLIA CALCIFICATIONS. Calcium may accumulate in the basal ganglia in association with hypoparathyroidism or as a result of a familial disorder, sometimes referred to as Fahr's disease. Affected patients exhibit parkinsonism, chorea, dementia, and palilalia. Brain imaging may detect basal ganglia calcification in clinically unaffected relatives.

OLIVOPONTOCEREBELLAR AND SPINOCEREBELLAR DEGENERATIONS. The combination of parkinsonism and cerebellar ataxia characterizes olivopontocerebellar degeneration or atrophy (OPCA), a heterogeneous group of neurodegenerative disorders most often inherited in an autosomal dominant pattern, but occasionally occurring sporadically. In addition to the parkinsonism-ataxia complex, patients with OPCA often exhibit marked dysarthria, neuro-ophthalmologic signs, and a variable degree of upper and lower motor neuron signs (see Ch. 465).

MULTIPLE-SYSTEM DEGENERATIONS (PARKINSONISM-PLUS)

Approximately 10 to 15 per cent of all patients with parkinsonian findings have a more widespread disorder classified clinically as "parkinsonism-plus syndrome" and pathologically as a "multiple-system degeneration." In addition to parkinsonism, such patients suffer from additional findings that may include supranuclear ophthalmoparesis (progressive supranuclear palsy), dysautonomia (Shy-Drager syndrome), ataxia (OPCA), laryngeal stridor (striatonigral degeneration), apraxia and alien hand (corticobasal degeneration), dementia (Alzheimer's disease with parkinsonism and diffuse Lewy body disease), and a combination of dementia and motor neuron disease (parkinsonism–dementia–amyotrophic lateral sclerosis [ALS] complex). The etiology for all forms of this syndrome is unknown.

PROGRESSIVE SUPRANUCLEAR PALSY. Progressive supranuclear palsy (PSP) is the most common of the parkinsonism-plus syndromes, accounting for about 8 per cent of all parkinsonian patients evaluated in a PD clinic. PSP has its onset in the seventh decade, about 10 years after the usual onset of PD. Initial symptoms consist of a gradual onset of postural instability, unsteady gait, and supranuclear vertical ophthalmoparesis, first expressed by impairment of downward gaze. Later, upward and then lateral conjugate gaze also become impaired, but until the advanced stage, the external ophthalmoparesis can be overcome by labyrinthine stimulation via the oculocephalic maneuver. Patients with PSP often exhibit axial rigidity, nuchal dystonia, and a rigid-dystonic facial expression with deep nasolabial folds (in contrast to the flattened facies seen in patients with PD). Mild to moderate dementia is a late sign; tremor almost never occurs. Neither the hypokinetic rigidity nor the other changes respond to antiparkinsonian drugs. The poor response to these drugs is partly explained by the loss of postsynaptic D_2 receptors.

Pathologically, PSP is characterized by selective neuronal loss and gliosis affecting the midbrain tegmentum and tectum, the internal segment of the globus pallidus (GPi), the subthalamic nucleus (STN), the vestibular and dentate nuclei, the basal nucleus of Meynert, and the pedunculopontine nucleus. Neurofibrillary tangles, somewhat different from those in Alzheimer's disease, and granulovacuolar degeneration involve nerve cells in these areas.

SHY-DRAGER SYNDROME. When patients with atypical parkinsonism (usually without tremor) complain of orthostatic light-headedness, incontinence, sexual impotence, and other autonomic symptoms, the diagnosis of Shy-Drager syndrome should be considered (see Ch. 452).

Cedarbaum JM: Pharmacokinetic and pharmacodynamic considerations in management of motor response fluctuations in Parkinson's disease. Neurol Clin 8:31, 1990. *A review of the pharmacology of levodopa, deprenyl, and dopamine agonists.*

Jankovic J: Parkinsonism plus syndromes. Movement Disord 4:S95, 1989. *A survey of most of the secondary forms of parkinsonism.*

Jankovic J: Clinical aspects of Parkinson's disease. In Marsden CD, Fahn S (eds.): New Trends in the Treatment of Parkinson's Disease. Carbforth, England, Parthenon Publishing, 1990, pp 51–73 *A review of the pathophysiologic mechanisms of parkinsonian signs and symptoms.*

Jankovic J, McDermott M, Carter J, et al.: Variable expression of Parkinson's disease: An analysis of the DATATOP database. Neurology 40:1529, 1990. *An analysis of clinical correlates in 800 patients in early stages of PD, not yet treated with dopaminergic drugs.*

Marsden CD: Parkinson's disease. Lancet 1:948, 1990. *A critical review of the current knowledge about the pathogenesis and therapeutics of PD.*

459 Tremors

ESSENTIAL TREMOR

Essential tremor is the most common type of symptomatic tremor, affecting about 0.5 per cent of the American population. The tremor is inherited in an autosomal dominant pattern with high penetrance. Affected patients lack the hypokinetic features and rigidity of Parkinson's disease (PD), discussed in the preceding chapter. Essential tremor typically produces flexion-extension oscillation of the hands at the wrists or adduction-abduction movements of the fingers when arms are outstretched in front of the body. Although frequently referred to as "benign essential tremor," it may be disabling, often causing spilling of liquids and interfering with handwriting. Essential tremor also frequently involves the head and voice, which helps to differentiate it from parkinsonian tremor. Another useful distinguishing feature is the occurrence of essential tremor during maintenance of posture; parkinsonian tremor is usually present when the affected body part is at relative rest. Parkinsonian patients, however, often exhibit postural tremor, and patients with essential tremor may have tremor at rest, suggesting an overlap between PD and essential tremor.

The frequency of essential tremor ranges from 4 to 12 Hz, and the oscillation may be produced by either alternating or synchronous contractions of antagonistic muscles. Some forms occur only during a specific activity, such as writing or holding an object in a particular position. Such *focal task-specific tremors* may be associated with task-specific dystonias ("occupational cramps") or with generalized essential tremor and dystonia. Nearly half of all patients with essential tremor show evidence of an associated dystonia. The nature of the link is unknown.

Essential tremor has many variants, including isolated head, voice, tongue, facial, and chin tremors and orthostatic tremor. Although considered a variant of essential tremor, orthostatic tremor usually does not respond to propranolol; clonazepam, however, provides satisfactory control in most patients. Focal tremor may be rarely induced by trauma to the affected body part. This peripherally induced tremor is often associated with focal dystonia and reflex sympathetic dystrophy.

β-Adrenergic blocking drugs (e.g., propranolol at 80 to 240 mg per day) are the most effective agents in the treatment of essential tremor. Modest doses of alcohol also reduce the tremor in most instances, but this is an impractical approach to treatment. Other occasionally useful drugs include primidone (starting dosage is 25 mg at bedtime; the daily dosage can be gradually increased to 750 mg per day), lorazepam, and alprazolam. Patients with a disabling essential tremor that does not respond satisfactorily to medications sometimes improve with local injections of botulinum toxin. Thalamotomy is used as a last resort.

Hubble JP, Busenbark KL, Koller WC: Essential tremor. Clin Neuropharmacol 12:453, 1989. *A comprehensive review of physiology, pharmacology, and clinical aspects of tremors.*

Lou J-S, Jankovic J: Essential tremor: Clinical correlates in 350 patients. Neurology 41:234, 1991. *A comprehensive analysis of clinical features of a large cohort of patients with essential tremor.*

Rosenbaum F, Jankovic J: Focal task-specific tremor and dystonia: Categorization of occupational movement disorders. Neurology 38:522, 1988. *A review of 28 patients with dystonia, tremor, or a combination present only during specific activities, such as writing or typing.*

Tasker RR: Tremor of parkinsonism and stereotactic thalamotomy. Mayo Clin Proc 62:736, 1987. *A review of current experience with surgical treatment of tremors.*

460 Dystonias

DEFINITION

Dystonia may be defined as a syndrome dominated by involuntary, sustained (tonic) or spasmodic (rapid or clonic), patterned, and repetitive muscle contractions, frequently causing twisting (e.g., torticollis), flexing or extending (e.g., writer's cramp, retrocollis), and squeezing (e.g., blepharospasm) movements or abnormal postures. Dystonia is frequently associated with other movement disorders, particularly tremor, myoclonus, and parkinsonism. About 1 of 3000 people is diagnosed as having dystonia, but the true prevalence is probably much higher.

CLASSIFICATION

Dystonia may vary in severity, and it may progress as follows: task-specific (occurring only during a specific activity, such as writing or typing) → action (present only during, not necessarily specific, activity) → overflow (involving adjacent muscles) → at rest (present even during rest) → fixed postures (joint contractures). Dystonia is exacerbated by stress, fatigue, activity, or a change in posture and is relieved by sleep, relaxation, hypnosis, and a variety of sensory tricks. While the vast majority of dystonias are continual, some occur paroxysmally and some have marked diurnal variations (Fig. 460–1). Partly because of fluctuations in severity, sometimes influenced by the emotional state of the patient, dystonia is often mistakenly attributed to psychogenic causes.

Dystonia can be classified according to its *distribution* as focal, segmental, multifocal, generalized, or unilateral (hemidystonia). Most childhood-onset dystonias begin focally, usually in one foot; other body parts become involved later, eventually resulting in generalized dystonia. In contrast, adult-onset dystonias tend to remain focal or segmental. Examples of focal dystonia include blepharospasm, oromandibular dystonia, torticollis, spasmodic dysphonia, and occupational (e.g., writer's, typist's, pianist's)

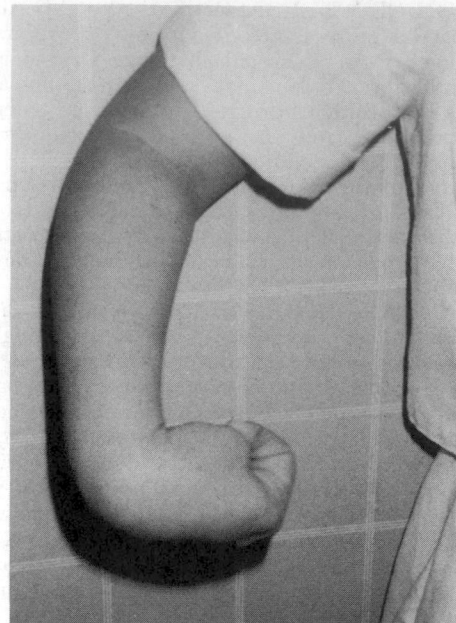

FIGURE 460–1. Focal dystonia of the distal right arm.

cramps (Fig. 460–1). Blepharospasm is categorized as a *focal* dystonia when it occurs alone (essential blepharospasm). However, blepharospasm is often associated with dystonic movements in the adjacent facial, oromandibular, laryngeal, and neck muscles. This *segmental dystonia* is sometimes referred to as Meige's syndrome, but the term *"cranial-cervical dystonia"* is more descriptive.

The most common form of dystonia is *cervical dystonia* (Table 460–1). According to the position of the head, cervical dystonia can be categorized as torticollis, laterocollis, anterocollis, retrocollis, or a combination of these abnormal postures. There is a 3:2 female preponderance, and the onset is usually in the fifth decade. Local pain is reported by about half the patients, and radiculopathy complicates cervical dystonia in about 20 per cent. Half of all patients with cervical dystonia have an associated head-neck tremor. The tremor can be dystonic, seen only when the patient attempts to keep the head straight; essential, in which case the tremor persists irrespective of the position of the head; or a combination of dystonic and essential. About half the patients report a movement disorder such as tremor or dystonia in family members. The etiology of most cervical dystonias is unknown. In 15 per cent of cases, however, cervical dystonia can be attributed to either local trauma or an exposure to neuroleptic drugs.

PATHOGENESIS

The pathoanatomy of dystonia is unknown, but studies suggest a predominant involvement of the basal ganglia, particularly the putamen, and the brain stem. Brain imaging and autopsy examinations usually yield normal findings. Electrophysiologic studies suggest increased excitatory drive from the basal ganglia to brain stem interneurons. Postmortem biochemical analyses have found evidence of enhanced noradrenergic transmission in the rostral brain stem. Some cases of dystonia appear to be caused or triggered by peripheral nerve or root injury.

TABLE 460–1. DISTRIBUTION OF DYSTONIA

Distribution	N*
Cervical	326
Blepharospasm and oromandibular dystonia	228
Generalized	169
Blepharospasm	109
Focal (distal)	79
Spasmodic dysphonia	67
Hemidystonia	51
Oromandibular dystonia	48

*N = 1000 at Baylor College of Medicine.

PRIMARY DYSTONIA

This category accounts for 85 per cent of cases. Primary dystonias with onset in childhood have been previously termed *dystonia musculorum deformans*. Childhood-onset dystonias are often inherited, usually in an autosomal dominant pattern; about half of adult-onset cases seem to have a genetic basis. Other members of the family may have only partial manifestations, such as club foot, scoliosis, torticollis, writer's cramp, bruxism, or essential tremor. Genetic dystonia seems to have a higher prevalence among Ashkenazi Jews, but both Jewish and non-Jewish dystonias have been linked to a marker in the q32–q34 region of chromosome 9. An X-linked dystonia has been recently described in Filipino families.

SECONDARY DYSTONIA

Occasionally, a specific, and potentially treatable, cause of dystonia can be identified (Fig. 460–1). One of the most important examples is *Wilson's disease*. Neurologic symptoms represent the first manifestations in about 50 per cent of patients with this autosomal recessive disorder, appearing during their second or third decade. Changes usually consist of a gradual onset of dysarthria; drooling; dementia; clumsiness, often affecting handwriting; postural tremors; gait disturbance; and various forms of dystonia affecting distal and proximal body parts. Dystonia of facial and bulbar muscles is responsible for the dysarthria and drooling as well as the typical fixed pseudo-smile (risus sardonicus), inspiratory noises, and dysphagia. Other motor abnormalities include parkinsonism, cerebellar findings, a wing-beating proximal tremor, and other movement disorders. All patients with neurologic findings have a Kayser-Fleischer ring, a greenish-brown copper infiltration of the cornea near the scleral junction. Further details are given in Ch. 192.

Tardive dystonia is a persistent form of dystonia caused by exposure to dopamine receptor blocking drugs, such as major tranquilizers (e.g., chlorpromazine, thioridazine, fluphenazine, thiothixene, haloperidol, loxapine, amoxapine) and certain antiemetics (e.g., prochlorperazine, metoclopramide) (Fig. 460–2). Curiously, levodopa can also cause intermittent dystonia (and focal dystonia may be the presenting symptom of Parkinson's

disease). In all drug-induced dystonias, the offending drug should be withdrawn or the dosage reduced whenever possible. In contrast to focal, segmental, or generalized dystonia, hemidystonia is associated with an identifiable etiology in a majority of cases. These etiologies include subcortical infarction, arteriovenous malformation, abscess, tumor, and other lesions, some of which can be treated surgically. There are many other causes of secondary dystonia, but only a few are amenable to therapy.

TREATMENT

The treatment of most dystonias consists of supportive therapy (e.g., relaxation techniques, prostheses), medications, botulinum toxin injections, and surgery. The anticholinergic drugs are sometimes beneficial. Trihexyphenidyl, the most frequently used anticholinergic, must be started in low doses and slowly increased to tolerance, perhaps up to 60 mg per day. Some children can tolerate such high doses, but anticholinergic side effects usually limit adult tolerance to 20 to 25 mg daily or less. In advanced cases, dopamine-depleting and dopamine receptor blocking drugs may be added. Muscle relaxants (e.g., diazepam or lorazepam), baclofen, and carbamazepine sometimes provide benefit. About 10 per cent of patients with childhood or adolescence dystonia improve with use of levodopa. Diurnal fluctuations with exacerbation of the movement disorder toward the end of each day are typical in this form of dystonia. In patients with refractory focal dystonia and, less often, segmental dystonia, injection of the paralysis-inducing botulinum A toxin (Botox) into the contracting muscles provides effective, albeit temporary, relief. Such approaches are best left to those with experience in this treatment.

Patients who are socially and occupationally disabled by dystonia despite optimal medical therapy, including botulinum toxin, sometimes can be helped surgically. Surgical procedures include orbicularis myectomy for blepharospasm, cervical rhizotomy for neck dystonia, and thalamotomy for hemidystonia or generalized (predominantly distal) dystonia. Such procedures are effective in a majority of patients but have both potentially serious complications and high rates of symptom recurrence, making them a last resort.

Fahn S, Marsden CD, Calne DB: Dystonia 2. Advances in Neurology, Vol. 50. New York, Raven Press, 1988. *A series of papers presented at a symposium on dystonia, summarizing current knowledge about all aspects of this disorder.*

Fletcher NA, Harding AE, Marsden CD: A genetic study of idiopathic torsion dystonia in the United Kingdom. Brain 113:379, 1990. *A review of inheritance in dystonic families in England suggests that 85 per cent are inherited in an autosomal dominant pattern with 40 per cent penetrance.*

Jankovic J, Brin M: Therapeutic applications of botulinum toxin. N Engl J Med, April 25, 1991. *A critical review of studies using botulinum toxin in different dystonic and other disorders.*

Jankovic J, Leder S, Warner D, Schwartz K: Cervical dystonia. Clinical findings and associated movement disorders. Neurology, in press. *Largest reported series of patients with cervical dystonia (torticollis).*

Nygaard TG, Marsden CD, Fahn S: Dopa-responsive dystonia: Long-term treatment response and prognosis. Neurology 41:174, 1991. *A comprehensive review of a potentially treatable dystonia that affects up to 10 per cent of children with dystonia.*

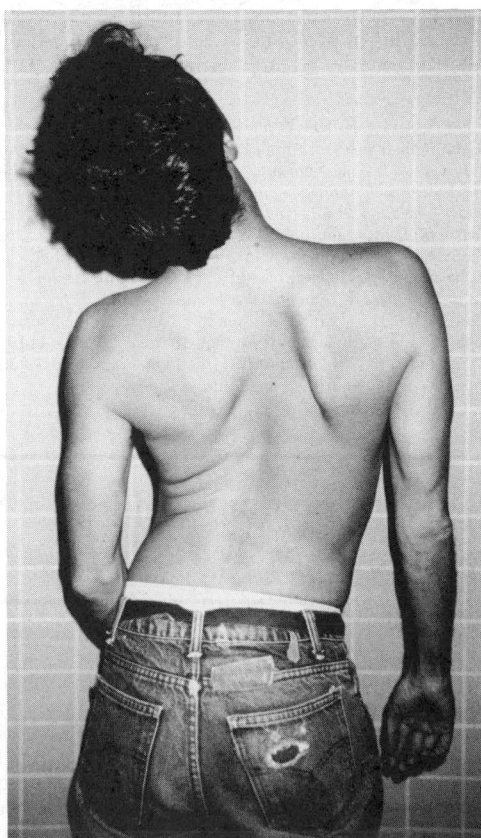

FIGURE 460–2. Truncal dystonia in a manic-depressive patient with tardive dystonia secondary to a variety of antipsychotic drugs.

461 Choreas, Athetosis, and Ballism

HUNTINGTON'S DISEASE

Huntington's disease (HD), an autosomal dominant disorder with complete penetrance, is the most common form of hereditary chorea. Besides chorea, the other two components of the HD triad are a decline in cognitive functioning leading to dementia and various emotional and psychiatric disturbances. A major milestone in HD research has been the identification of a gene marker on chromosome 4. Treatment, however, remains as ineffective as it was in 1872, when George Huntington first described the disease. The estimated prevalence of HD in the United States is 4 to 8 per 100,000 people. Although about 10 per cent of HD cases begin before age 20, the peak age at onset is in the fourth and fifth decades. Juvenile HD often first manifests with progressive parkinsonism, dementia, and seizures. In contrast, adult HD often starts with the insidious onset of clumsiness and adventitious, fidgety, random, brief movements. Initially, these purposeless movements may be incorporated into and masked by normal intentional acts, delaying the recognition of chorea. Chorea often begins distally, but as the disease progresses, it becomes generalized and can interrupt voluntary movements. Characteristically, patients with HD have difficulty in maintaining tongue protrusion or a steady grip, and their gait is often irregular, hesitant, unsteady, and dancelike. Other motor symptoms include dysarthria, dysphagia, and postural instability.

Neurobehavioral symptoms may precede motor changes and usually consist of personality changes, apathy, social withdrawal, agitation, impulsiveness, depression, mania, paranoia, delusions, hostility, hallucinations, or psychosis. Cognitive changes are manifested chiefly by loss of recent memory and impaired judgment. Progressive motor dysfunction, dementia, and incontinence eventually lead to institutionalization and death from aspiration, infection, and poor nutrition. The duration of illness from onset to death is about 15 years for adult HD and 8 to 10 years for the juvenile variant.

Postmortem changes in HD brains include neuronal loss and gliosis in the cortex and the striatum, particularly the caudate nucleus. Chorea seems to be primarily related to the loss of striatal neurons projecting to the lateral globus pallidus (GPe), whereas rigid-akinetic symptoms correlate with the additional loss of striatal neurons projecting to the medial globus pallidus (GPi). Loss of medium-sized spiny neurons, which normally constitute 80 per cent of all striatal neurons, is associated with a marked decrease in γ-aminobutyric acid (GABA) synthesis. There is also a decline in acetylcholine activity, presumably resulting from a degeneration of cholinergic striatal interneurons. The neuropeptides are markedly altered in HD: Levels of substance P, cholecystokinin, and metenkephalin are decreased, but somatostatin, thyrotropin-releasing hormone, neurotensin, and neuropeptide Y levels are increased. The number of dopamine, acetylcholine, and serotonin receptors is decreased in the striatum.

Reliable clinical diagnosis depends on the combination of chorea, emotional disturbances, progressive dementia, and a family history suggestive of autosomal dominant inheritance. Because spontaneous mutations are rare, lack of family history raises questions of paternity or misdiagnosis. The correct diagnosis of HD is supported by evidence of caudate atrophy on neuroimaging studies and hypometabolism in the basal ganglia by positron-emission scanning with fluoro-2-deoxyglucose. A specific marker for HD has been identified on the short arm of chromosome 4, making genetic diagnosis likely in the future.

Treatment is symptomatic only. The psychosis may improve with neuroleptics, such as haloperidol, pimozide, fluphenazine, and thioridazine, but these drugs can induce tardive dyskinesia and other adverse effects and should be used only if absolutely needed to control symptoms. Monoamine-depleting drugs, such as reserpine (0.25 mg to 8 mg per day) and tetrabenazine (an investigational drug not available for general use in North America), may relieve chorea, do not cause tardive dyskinesia, and may be as effective as the dopamine-blocking drugs. Unfortunately, these drugs can cause or exacerbate depression, sedation, akathisia, and parkinsonism. Anxiolytics and antidepressants may also be useful in some patients with psychiatric problems associated with HD. Genetic aspects of HD should be discussed openly with the patients to provide them and their relatives with nondirective counseling.

OTHER CHOREIC DISORDERS

Besides HD, other genetically transmitted choreas include *benign hereditary chorea*, a nonprogressive chorea with childhood onset, and *paroxysmal choreoathetoses. Senile chorea* is a rare symptom complex in which chorea begins after age 60 and is unaccompanied by the neurobehavioral symptoms or family history of HD. Some patients have been reported to have pathologic changes identical to those of HD; others have had predominant degeneration of the putamen rather than the caudate. *Neuroacanthocytosis*, also referred to as "chorea-acantho-

cytosis," usually presents in the third or fourth decade of life with a combination of self-mutilation manifested by lip and tongue biting, generalized chorea, lingual dystonia, and motor and phonic tics. Other features include seizures, amyotrophy, areflexia, and elevated levels of serum creatine phosphokinase. Wet blood or Wright-stained fast-dry smears reveal more than 15 per cent of red blood cells as acanthocytes. Neuroimaging usually demonstrates caudate atrophy. The condition may have a pattern of autosomal recessive inheritance but its genetics are still unclear. *Sydenham's chorea*, now an uncommon disorder, has an autoimmune basis, most often appearing as a consequence of infection with group A streptococcus. Unlike arthritis and carditis, which occur soon after such infection, chorea and various neurobehavioral symptoms may be delayed for 6 months or longer. Chorea appearing during pregnancy (chorea gravidarum), with use of birth control pills, or during the course of systemic lupus erythematosus probably has a similar pathogenesis.

ATHETOSIS

Athetosis is a slow form of chorea characterized by twisting, writhing movements. It most often accompanies static encephalopathy due to cerebral palsy, kernicterus, prematurity, glutaric aciduria, poststroke hemiplegia, and other causes of early life brain damage. In some cases, the movement disorder becomes progressive after decades of no apparent change. Athetosis usually does not respond to pharmacologic therapy.

BALLISM

Ballism is a form of forceful, flinging, high-amplitude, coarse chorea. Because the involuntary movement usually affects only one side of the body, the term hemiballism is used. The movement disorder is often preceded by hemiparesis associated with a hemorrhagic or ischemic stroke involving the contralateral subthalamic nucleus (STN) or adjacent structures. Less common causes of hemiballism include abscess, arteriovenous malformation, cerebral trauma, hyperosmotic hyperglycemia, tumor, and multiple sclerosis. Lesions produced by these pathologic processes usually involve the STN, but hemiballism has been described in patients with lesions outside the STN. Dopamine-blocking and -depleting drugs, used in the treatment of chorea, are beneficial in most patients with hemiballism, but the disorder usually subsides spontaneously in a matter of several weeks. Occasional examples of prolonged disabling and medically intractable hemiballism can be treated with contralateral thalamotomy or pallidectomy.

Albin RL, Reiner A, Anderson KD, et al.: Striatal and nigral neuron subpopulations in rigid Huntington's disease: Implications for the functional anatomy of chorea and rigidity-akinesia. Ann Neurol 27:357, 1990. *Using neuropeptide immunochemistry, the investigators conclude that chorea correlates with damage to the striatal projections to GPe, whereas parkinsonian signs observed in some HD patients result from additional damage in the projections to the GPi.*

Dewey RB, Jankovic J: Hemiballism-hemichorea: Clinical and pharmacologic findings in 21 patients. Arch Neurol 46:862, 1989. *Clinical and brain imaging correlations in a series of patients with hemiballism, hemichorea, or both.*

Hardie RJ, Pullon HWH, Harding AE, et al.: Neuroacanthocytosis. A clinical, haematological and pathological study of 19 cases. Brain 114:13, 1991. *A detailed description of patients with this frequently unrecognized and clinically heterogeneous neurologic-hematologic disorder.*

462 Tics, Myoclonus, and Stereotypies

TICS

Tics describe involuntary, abrupt, sudden, isolated, brief movements (*motor tics*); sounds produced by nose, mouth, or throat (*vocal/phonic tics*); or sensations (*sensory tics*). Motor tics may be simple (e.g., eye blinking, nose twitching, head jerking) or complex (e.g., repetitive touching, jumping, kicking, pelvic gyrations). Similarly, vocal/phonic tics may be simple (e.g., throat clearing, grunting, sniffing) or complex (e.g., echolalia, palilalia, coprolalia). Characteristics of tics include suppressibility, increase with stress and excitement, decrease with distraction and concentration, suggestibility, waxing and waning, and possible persistence during sleep.

The most common cause of tics is the *Gilles de la Tourette's syndrome*, an autosomal dominant disorder dominated by tics and a variety of behavioral manifestations. Transient tics of childhood and persistent simple tics probably represent fragmentary forms of Tourette's syndrome. The following criteria are required for diagnosis: (1) Both multiple motor and one or more phonic tics must be present at some time during the illness, although not necessarily concurrently; (2) the tics occur many times a day, nearly every day or intermittently through a period of more than a year; (3) the anatomic location, number, frequency, complexity, type, and severity of tics change over time; (4) onset is before age 21; and (5) involuntary movements and noises cannot be explained by other medical conditions. Because of the fluctuating, heterogeneous, and often bizarre manifestations of Tourette's syndrome, affected patients frequently have their illness misdiagnosed by physicians and are mistreated by schoolmates, teachers, co-workers, and strangers.

Epidemiologic studies suggest that Tourette's syndrome is mostly a genetic disorder, occurring commonly and with penetrance approaching 100 per cent, particularly in males. In addition, some cases are nongenetic and may be triggered or caused by neuroleptics, carbon monoxide poisoning, head trauma, viral encephalitis, cocaine abuse, or opiate withdrawal. Many patients with Tourette's syndrome suffer from obsessive-compulsive disorder and have problems with attention and learning. Sleep disorders are common and include parasomnias, bedwetting, and interruption of sleep by tics.

Therapy requires individual attention. Since most patients experience waxing and waning of symptoms and a generally favorable natural course, reassurance and behavioral therapy may be sufficient in mild cases. Drugs usually are indicated when tics cause physical discomfort or social embarrassment. Judicious use of dopamine receptor blocking drugs, such as fluphenazine, pimozide, and haloperidol, often reduces the frequency and severity of tics and may ameliorate impulsive and aggressive behavior. These drugs, however, cause sedation, depression, and weight gain. Furthermore, tardive dyskinesia is a potentially serious complication of chronic neuroleptic therapy. Clonazepam, clonidine, fluoxetine, and clomipramine seem to be particularly helpful in the treatment of obsessive-compulsive disorder and other behavioral problems frequently associated with Tourette's syndrome.

MYOCLONUS

Myoclonus describes a jerklike movement produced by a sudden, rapid, and brief contraction (positive myoclonus) or a muscle inhibition (negative myoclonus). Myoclonus may be focal, multifocal, segmental, or generalized. *Segmental myoclonus* usually involves either the branchial structures, innervated by the lower cranial nerves and upper cervical nerve roots, or other body parts innervated by the spinal roots and nerves; it consists of rhythmic (1 to 3 Hz) contractions caused by a lesion of the brain stem or spinal cord. *Palatal myoclonus* results from acute or chronic lesions involving the anatomic triangle linking dentate, red, and inferior olivary nuclei. *Generalized myoclonus* is believed to reflect discharges arising from the brain stem reticular formation and is categorized as physiologic, essential, epileptic, or symptomatic. Two forms of myoclonus are associated with sleep: physiologic sleep myoclonus, occurring normally during initial phases of sleep, and nocturnal myoclonus, now called *"periodic movements of sleep,"* often associated with *"restless legs syndrome"* as well as with abnormal involuntary movements while the person is awake.

Causes of myoclonus include acute and prolonged hypoxia and ischemia; various metabolic, infectious, and toxic factors; and exposure to neuroleptic drugs (tardive myoclonus). Myoclonus can be associated with familial chorea and dystonia and with many neurodegenerative disorders, including parkinsonism, progressive myoclonus epilepsy, and a variety of rare heredodegenerative disorders. Multifocal myoclonus often develops in the late stages of Creutzfeldt-Jakob disease and, less frequently, Alzheimer's disease.

The specific physiologic and pharmacologic pathogeneses of myoclonus are unknown; clinical studies suggest an abnormality in the brain stem reticular formation. Clonazepam, lorazepam,

TABLE 462–1. NEUROLEPTIC-INDUCED MOVEMENT DISORDERS

Acute-Transient	Chronic-Persistent
Dystonic reaction	Tardive stereotypy
Action tremor	Tardive chorea
Parkinsonism	Tardive dystonia
Akathisia	Tardive akathisia
Neuroleptic malignant syndrome	Tardive tics
	Tardive myoclonus
	Tardive tremor

valproate, carbamazepine, and 5-hydroxytryptophan have been reported to have antimyoclonic activity. Clonazepam, at a dosage of 1 to 9 mg per day, is the drug of first choice, but the development of adverse effects, such as drowsiness, ataxia, and sexual dysfunction, often limits its usefulness.

STEREOTYPIES

The term "stereotypy" describes a continuous or intermittent, involuntary, coordinated, patterned, repetitive, rhythmic, purposeless, but seemingly purposeful and ritualistic movement. Stereotypies may be simple (e.g., chewing movement, foot tapping, body rocking) or complex (e.g., complicated rituals, sitting down and arising from a chair). They can be volitionally suppressed. The stereotypic behavior displayed by some animals when placed in restraining environments has been used as an experimental model of hyperkinetic movement disorders. Stereotypies can accompany a variety of human behavioral disorders, such as anxiety, obsessive-compulsive disorders, Tourette's syndrome, schizophrenia, akathisia, autism, and mental retardation. Stereotypies and self-stimulatory or self-injurious behavior constitute the most recognizable symptoms in mentally retarded and autistic patients.

Tardive dyskinesia, a persistent movement disorder caused by exposure to dopamine receptor blocking drugs, is one of the most common causes of stereotypies. Many other tardive movement disorders can result from the use of dopamine receptor blocking drugs (neuroleptics) (Table 462–1). The term "akathisia" describes the combination of stereotypy and a sensory component, such as an inner feeling of restlessness. Akathisia, whether due to neuroleptics, Parkinson's disease, or other causes, is sometimes confused with the syndrome of *restless legs*. Both disorders are characterized by stereotypic movements and motor restlessness, but patients with restless legs complain more of paresthesias, particularly a creeping or crawling sensation in the legs associated with an irresistible urge to keep the limbs in motion. The restless legs syndrome is often worse at night, causing insomnia, and it may be associated with periodic movements of sleep. Elderly women appear to be at particularly high risk for tardive dyskinesia. The use of high doses and depot injections of neuroleptics carries an increased risk of tardive dyskinesia. The mechanism of the disorder is poorly understood but is believed to result from the development of supersensitive dopamine receptors caused by chronic neuroleptic blockade. Prevention is the best treatment for the drug-induced movement disorders. Whenever possible, drugs other than the neuroleptics should be used for psychiatric or gastrointestinal problems. When no alternative exists, the dosage and duration of exposure should be kept at a minimum. Spontaneous remissions of tardive dyskinesia occasionally follow withdrawal of the offending agent. Dopamine-depleting drugs, such as reserpine and tetrabenazine, are the most effective drugs in the symptomatic treatment of tardive dyskinesia.

Jankovic J: Stereotypies. *In* Marsden CD, Fahn S (eds.): Movement Disorders 3. London, Butterworths, 1991. *A review of animal and clinical studies of stereotypic disorders.*

Kurlan R: Tourette's syndrome: Current concepts. Neurology 39:1625, 1989. *A critical review of current knowledge about the motor and behavioral aspects of Tourette's syndrome.*

Miller LG, Jankovic J: Drug-induced dyskinesias. *In* Appel SH (ed.): Current Neurology. Vol 10. Chicago, Year Book Medical Publishers, 1990, pp 321–355. *A comprehensive review of tardive dyskinesia and related disorders.*

Patel VM, Jankovic J: Myoclonus. *In* Appel SH (ed.): Current Neurology. Vol 8. Chicago, Year Book Medical Publishers, 1988, pp 109–156. *A comprehensive review of the classification, physiology, and pharmacology of myoclonus.*

SECTION SIX / DEGENERATIVE DISEASES OF THE NERVOUS SYSTEM

Robert B. Layzer

The term "degenerative diseases" refers to a varied assortment of central nervous system disorders characterized by gradual and progressive loss of neural tissue. This section deals with several degenerative diseases of unknown cause: the hereditary ataxias, paraplegias, and amyotrophies; the phakomatoses; syringomyelia; and amyotrophic lateral sclerosis. Several important diseases are discussed in other chapters concerned with dementia, extrapyramidal diseases, and autonomic disorders. Some degenerative diseases are difficult to classify because they involve multiple anatomic locations; these *multisystem atrophies* have arbitrarily been assigned to the chapters that deal with their principal symptom (see Table 463–1).

463 Hereditary Cerebellar Ataxias and Related Disorders

The symptoms of hereditary ataxia may be intermittent or progressive. *Intermittent or periodic ataxia* occurs in children with a variety of recessively inherited biochemical disorders, such as aminoacidurias and disorders of pyruvate metabolism. A rare, autosomal dominant disease known as hereditary periodic ataxia is characterized by attacks of vertigo, nystagmus, ataxia, and dysarthria, lasting several hours; it responds to prophylactic treatment with acetazolamide.

Progressive ataxia occurs in children with known biochemical disorders such as abetalipoproteinemia and some of the lipidoses, but most diseases in this category are of unknown etiology. Those that begin before age 20, including Friedreich's ataxia and ataxia-telangiectasia, are usually inherited in an autosomal recessive fashion, while most adult-onset types are autosomal dominant.

FRIEDREICH'S ATAXIA

This autosomal recessive disease, with a carrier frequency of nearly 1 in 100 and a prevalence of 2 in 100,000, is probably the most common type of hereditary ataxia. The biochemical mechanism is unknown, but the abnormal gene has been mapped to the short arm of chromosome 9.

PATHOLOGY. At autopsy the spinal cord is atrophic. There is loss of nerve cells in the dorsal root ganglia and Clarke's columns, and "dying-back" degeneration of nerve fibers in the dorsal columns, pyramidal tracts, spinocerebellar tracts, and peripheral nerves. Minor changes are present in the brain stem

and cerebellum. The heart shows chronic interstitial fibrosis and ventricular hypertrophy.

CLINICAL MANIFESTATIONS. Progressive ataxia of gait usually begins in childhood or adolescence and within a few years is accompanied by loss of deep reflexes, limb ataxia, Babinski signs, and cerebellar dysarthria. The ability to walk is lost about 15 years after onset. Most patients eventually exhibit scoliosis, pronounced impairment of vibration and position sense in the lower extremities, and pes cavus. Some develop wasting of distal limb muscles, a stocking-glove deficit of superficial sensation, nystagmus, deafness, or optic atrophy. Intellect remains normal. A hypertrophic cardiomyopathy is present in most patients and often leads to supraventricular arrhythmias; heart failure is probably the major cause of death. Insulin-dependent diabetes mellitus develops in 10 to 20 per cent of patients. The mean age at death is 37 years.

DIAGNOSIS. Sensory nerve action potentials are small or absent. Electromyography may show signs of denervation in distal limb muscles, but motor nerve conduction velocities are normal. The cerebrospinal fluid is normal except for mild elevation of the protein content in a few cases. Computed tomographic (CT) brain scans may show mild cerebellar atrophy late in the disease. Electrocardiography often shows inverted T waves, right- or left-axis deviation, and right or left ventricular hypertrophy; conduction disturbances are uncommon.

DIFFERENTIAL DIAGNOSIS. The constellation of progressive ataxia, areflexia, Babinski signs, and onset before age 25 is usually diagnostic. However, a similar picture can occur in vitamin B_{12} deficiency and in vitamin E deficiency (including abetalipoproteinemia). True Friedreich's ataxia is sometimes confused with a less common autosomal recessive type of early-onset progressive ataxia, in which the tendon reflexes are preserved; in the latter syndrome, optic atrophy, scoliosis, and electrocardiographic abnormalities are rare.

ATAXIA-TELANGIECTASIA

Ataxia-telangiectasia is an autosomal recessive, multisystem disease affecting the skin, nervous system, and immune system. Its prevalence has been estimated at 1 to 2 per 100,000. The gene mutation has been localized to the long arm of chromosome 11. Although the precise biochemical defect is not known, it appears to involve defective DNA repair, with an increased frequency of chromosomal breakage and translocations. The main neuropathologic abnormality is a severe loss of neurons in the cerebellar cortex, dentate nuclei, and inferior olives. The level of α-fetoprotein in the blood is elevated in nearly all cases.

Beginning at a few years of age, affected children show progressive cerebellar ataxia and incoordination, choreoathetosis, and a peculiar incoordination of head and eye movements known as oculomotor apraxia. Some develop opsoclonus. Later, fine venous telangiectases appear on the conjunctivae, ears, face, and

TABLE 463–1. THE MULTISYSTEM ATROPHIES

Disease	Heredity	Principal Feature	Associated Features	Chapter
Shy-Drager syndrome	Sporadic	Autonomic insufficiency	Parkinsonism, cerebellar ataxia, dysphagia, laryngeal stridor, amyotrophy	452
Progressive supranuclear palsy	Sporadic	Ophthalmoplegia, especially vertical	Gait ataxia, axial dystonia, parkinsonism, pseudobulbar palsy, dementia	460
Kearns-Sayre syndrome	Sporadic	Ptosis and ophthalmoplegia	Short stature, cerebellar ataxia, retinal degeneration, heart block, deafness, mitochondrial myopathy, mental deficiency, Babinski signs	504
Hereditary ataxias, adult type	Autosomal dominant	Cerebellar ataxia	Ophthalmoplegia, dementia, parkinsonism, dystonia, optic atrophy, retinal degeneration, dysphagia, amyotrophy	463

skin creases. The thymus gland and lymph nodes are underdeveloped, and serum immunoglobulin A (IgA) levels are usually low; the resulting impairment of immunity leads to repeated bacterial infections in the respiratory tract. An axonal polyneuropathy appears late in the disease. Lymphoreticular malignancies and other forms of cancer develop in 10 to 20 per cent of patients. Most patients die of infection or neoplasm in the second or third decade of life.

ADULT-ONSET CEREBELLAR ATAXIA

Hereditary ataxia starting in adult life is nearly always an autosomal dominant disorder with multiple neurologic manifestations, among which cerebellar signs are prominent. The classification of these diseases is difficult because the clinical features vary greatly even within the same family, and there is no agreement with regard to how many genetically distinct diseases exist in this category. In southern England, cases of this type are about one-tenth as numerous as cases of Friedreich's ataxia. Brain enzymes related to cholinergic synaptic transmission have been reported to be present in reduced amount.

PATHOLOGY. Many cases have the pathologic features of olivopontocerebellar atrophy, with loss of neurons in the inferior olives and pontine nuclei (which provide major afferent pathways to the cerebellum), as well as degeneration of the spinocerebellar tracts, corticospinal tracts, and posterior columns. Neuronal degeneration is sometimes found in the cerebellar cortex, dentate nucleus, basal ganglia, midbrain, cerebral cortex, and spinal cord, including the anterior horns. The pathology, however, is as variable as the clinical findings, even within a given family. In cases of Azorean origin (Machado-Joseph disease), the cerebellar cortex and olives are spared.

CLINICAL MANIFESTATIONS. The age of onset, though quite variable, is usually between 20 and 50. Cerebellar ataxia of gait, dysarthria, and incoordination of the limbs usually dominate the clinical picture, so that the ability to walk is lost within 15 years. The other manifestations are extremely variable. Babinski signs and increased reflexes are commonly present, and some patients have spastic weakness in the legs. Vibration and position sense are sometimes lost as the disease advances, and the reflexes may disappear as the primary sensory neurons degenerate. Extrapyramidal findings may include impassive facies, cogwheel rigidity, chorea, athetosis, dystonia, and facial dyskinesia. Many patients have supranuclear oculomotor disorders such as lid retraction, ptosis, nystagmus, slow eye movements, and gaze paresis, especially upgaze. Optic atrophy, with pale discs, is common. Personality change or dementia, muscle wasting and fasciculation in the tongue and distal extremities, and bulbar symptoms of dysphagia or hoarseness are other common manifestations. Death occurs approximately 20 years after onset, at an average age of 57.

Pigmentary degeneration of the retina, beginning in the macula, is an early and constant feature in some families, suggesting that these cases may be genetically distinct. A few families seem to have a "pure" cerebellar syndrome beginning in the seventh decade of life. There is much controversy about the status of Machado-Joseph disease, which affects mainly people of Portuguese and Azorean descent. Although the range of clinical manifestations in these patients is similar to that of patients who have typical olivopontocerebellar atrophy, the pathologic features are said to be distinct because the inferior olives are spared. However, only a few cases have come to autopsy.

DIAGNOSIS. CT or magnetic resonance (MR) images may show atrophy of the cerebellar folia and pons, with enlargement of the fourth ventricle and pontine cisterns. The cerebrospinal fluid is usually normal. Sensory nerve action potentials are small or absent in patients with absent reflexes; in patients with preserved reflexes, somatosensory evoked potentials may be abnormal.

DIFFERENTIAL DIAGNOSIS. Nonhereditary cases of late-onset cerebellar degeneration are at least as common as the hereditary kind. Some are associated with alcoholism or a visceral malignancy, but in many, no apparent cause can be established. These patients' cerebellar symptoms tend to begin between the ages of 40 and 60 and may be accompanied by dementia, extrapyramidal signs, or Babinski signs. Some cases of this kind have the pathologic features of olivopontocerebellar atrophy, but

whether there is any genetic link to the autosomal dominant ataxias is unclear. It should be noted that patients presenting with ataxia may later develop the typical signs of progressive supranuclear palsy or one of the other multisystem atrophies listed in Table 463–1.

Harding AE: The Hereditary Ataxias and Related Disorders. Edinburgh, Churchill Livingstone, 1984. *A detailed review of the hereditary cerebellar ataxias and spastic paraplegias, including the author's own study of several hundred patients and family members. A modern classic.*

464 Hereditary Spastic Paraplegias

This is a diverse group of uncommon diseases whose main symptom is an insidiously beginning, progressive spasticity of the lower extremities. Families with "pure" hereditary spastic paraplegia (Strümpell's disease) are the most numerous, but many rare variants have been reported in which spasticity is associated with other neurologic, ocular, or cutaneous manifestations, overlapping with the spinocerebellar degenerations. The prevalence of these diseases is not well established. Harding found 29 families with hereditary spastic paraplegia in southern England, compared with 11 families of autosomal dominant late-onset cerebellar ataxia. Rare examples of *primary lateral sclerosis*, although sporadic in incidence, may belong to this class.

PATHOLOGY. In the pure form, the spinal cord shows degeneration of the lateral corticospinal tracts and posterior columns, most severe in the thoracic region. Less often there is minor degeneration of the spinocerebellar tracts, anterior corticospinal tracts, anterior horn cells, and cortical Betz cells. The dorsal root ganglia, posterior roots, and peripheral nerves are normal, suggesting that the dorsal column degeneration is caused by "dying-back" of the central processes of the sensory neurons.

CLINICAL MANIFESTATIONS. Most patients with pure hereditary spastic paraplegia continue to walk for many years and have a normal lifespan. Many cases begin in infancy with delayed walking, but the onset can be as late as the seventh decade. Spasticity of the legs and a stiff, slow gait are the main symptoms. Affected persons walk on their toes, trip easily, and are unable to run. About one fourth have pes cavus. The legs are spastic with hyperactive reflexes, clonus, and Babinski signs, while the arms are usually normal. Later the legs may become weak, the arms may show increased reflexes, and distal muscle wasting may develop, especially in the hands. Vibration and position sense may become impaired in the legs, and many patients develop urinary frequency, urgency, and precipitancy, although sexual function remains normal. Most patients become unable to walk sometime in the sixth or seventh decade.

DIAGNOSIS. The cerebrospinal fluid is normal. Electromyography may show denervation in the distal limb muscles, but the sensory nerve action potentials are preserved, even in patients showing decreased vibration and position sense. Somatosensory evoked potentials, however, are consistently small or unobtainable, reflecting a degeneration of dorsal column fibers.

DIFFERENTIAL DIAGNOSIS. Hereditary spastic paraplegia must be distinguished from nonhereditary causes of slowly progressive myelopathy such as cervical spondylosis, intraspinal tumor, arteriovenous malformation of the spinal cord, multiple sclerosis, amyotrophic lateral sclerosis, and myelopathy associated with human T cell lymphotropic virus 1 (HTLV-1 tropical spastic paraparesis, Ch. 478.3). Magnetic resonance (MR) imaging has simplified the diagnosis of many of these conditions.

Harding AE: The Hereditary Ataxias and Related Disorders. Edinburgh, Churchill Livingstone, 1984. *A detailed review of the hereditary cerebellar ataxias and spastic paraplegias, including the author's own study of several hundred patients and family members. A modern classic.*

465 Hereditary and Acquired Intrinsic Motor Neuron Diseases

Degenerative diseases of several kinds can attack the large motor neurons of the spinal cord or the brain to produce selective impairment of muscle strength or motor skill. Those of childhood are largely hereditary, while the major adult disorder, amyotrophic lateral sclerosis, is nearly always sporadic, with few clues illuminating either its etiology or molecular pathogenesis. Table 465–1 lists the major disorders in this category, and the references provide greater detail on the many subtypes.

HEREDITARY AMYOTROPHIES

Hereditary spinal muscular atrophy is a syndrome of progressive muscular weakness and atrophy resulting from selective degeneration of the motor neurons of the spinal cord. A comparable disorder of the lower brain stem nuclei produces progressive bulbar palsy. Many different clinical syndromes have been delineated based on the age of onset, the pattern of muscular weakness, the rate of progression, and the mode of inheritance. Using this approach, at least 15 separate genetic disorders can be recognized. Pearn (1980) has estimated that 1 in 40 Caucasians carries a gene for spinal muscular atrophy. No consistent biochemical defect is known, although hexosaminidase deficiency has been identified in a few cases.

PATHOLOGY. At the time of postmortem examination in the spinal cases, the anterior horns show gliosis and loss of large neurons, and many of the remaining motor neurons are undergoing degeneration. The ventral roots are atrophic owing to loss of myelinated nerve fibers. Similar changes are observed in the motor nuclei of the brain stem in bulbar cases.

In the well-developed infantile and childhood types, microscopic examination of the skeletal muscles using histochemical techniques shows large groups of round, atrophic muscle fibers and large groups of hypertrophied fibers staining uniformly as either type 1 or type 2. These features reflect the continuing process of denervation and reinnervation. However, at an early stage of infantile spinal muscular atrophy the only finding may be uniform atrophy of all muscle fibers, with preservation of the normal "checkerboard" fiber-type pattern. In slowly progressive cases of juvenile or adult onset, atrophic muscle fibers are found mainly in small groups; most muscle fibers are of normal size but are arranged in groups of uniform fiber type. After many years some muscle fibers show secondary myopathic changes, such as internal nuclei, splitting, or degeneration.

ACUTE INFANTILE SPINAL MUSCULAR ATROPHY

Werdnig-Hoffmann disease is a fatal, early infantile form of spinal and bulbar muscular atrophy that appears to be a single genetic entity. Inherited as an autosomal recessive trait, it is one

TABLE 465–1. THE MAJOR INTRINSIC MOTOR NEURON DISEASES

Hereditary
Spinal muscular atrophy
  Type I. Acute, infantile (Werdnig-Hoffmann disease)
  Type II. Late infantile and childhood type
  Type III. Juvenile and adult types
  Familial amyotrophic lateral sclerosis (ALS)
Acquired
Acute: anterior poliomyelitis
Chronic:
  ALS alone
  Anterior horn cell degeneration associated with spinocerebellar
    degeneration, Shy-Drager syndrome, parkinsonism, Creutzfeldt-
    Jakob disease
  Remote neoplasms, other
  Primary lateral sclerosis (rare)

of the most common fatal hereditary diseases of childhood, with an annual incidence of 1 in 20,000 live births and a carrier frequency in the general population of about 1 in 80. The abnormal gene is located on the long arm of chromosome 5.

In at least one third of the cases, there is a prenatal onset, with reduced fetal movements, weakness at birth, or congenital joint deformities. In the remainder of cases, the disease becomes apparent in the first 2 or 3 months of life. There is progressive, flaccid weakness of the trunk and limbs, with severe hypotonia, poor head control, and diminished movements of the limbs, more severe in the proximal muscles. Weakness of the intercostal muscles causes retraction of the chest during inspiration; the cry is weak, and coughing is ineffective. Bulbar weakness causes difficulty in sucking and swallowing. The tendon reflexes are usually absent. Death occurs before 3 years of age; 50 per cent of the patients die in the first 7 months of life and 95 per cent in the first 18 months.

The serum creatine kinase activity and the cerebrospinal fluid are normal. Electromyography shows reduced activation of motor unit potentials, many of which are of increased size, duration, and complexity. Fibrillations may be present, and in the majority of cases there is a spontaneous, regular discharge of motor unit potentials at a frequency of 5 to 15 Hz. It is important to distinguish this disease from treatable disorders such as infant botulism and chronic inflammatory polyneuropathy. The former is identified by repetitive nerve stimulation tests showing abnormal neuromuscular transmission and the latter, by abnormalities of nerve conduction and increased protein levels in the cerebrospinal fluid.

PROGRESSIVE MUSCULAR ATROPHY IN CHILDREN

Proximal Type. Clinically, this is a rather diverse disorder, but most cases are now thought to be caused by a single autosomal recessive gene, located on the long arm of chromosome 5, near or at the locus for Werdnig-Hoffmann disease. The incidence of this syndrome is 1 in 24,000 live births, and the carrier rate is approximately 1 in 90. A milder, autosomal dominant form is also known.

Weakness starts any time from birth to 8 years of age, usually before 1 year of age. The weakness affects the trunk and limbs and initially is more severe in proximal muscles. The limb muscles become atrophic, the tendon reflexes are lost, and joint contractures may develop. Fasciculations are not prominent but may be apparent in the fingers, producing a fine, irregular tremor. The face and jaws may be weak, and the tongue may be atrophic and show fasciculation.

Children with early onset may never be able to walk and often develop severe scoliosis, limb deformities, and respiratory insufficiency. Many eventually die of pulmonary infection, but some very weak patients survive into adult life, the progress of the disease apparently having arrested early in childhood. Children with a later onset of weakness tend to have a milder course, with slowly progressive proximal weakness, increased lumbar lordosis, and a waddling gait. Those with autosomal recessive inheritance rarely walk after age 20, while those with the rare autosomal dominant form may still be walking in middle age.

Serum creatine kinase activity may be mildly or moderately increased in patients with slowly progressive weakness, apparently because of secondary myopathic changes in muscle. The cerebrospinal fluid is normal. Electromyography shows the typical changes of chronic denervation and reinnervation as well as fibrillations and fasciculations, serving to distinguish these patients from similar patients with muscular dystrophy. Spontaneous, regular discharges of single motor unit potentials, like those found in infants with Werdnig-Hoffmann disease, are seen in children whose weakness began before age 2, but not in those with onset later in childhood.

Many of these children benefit from active and passive physical therapy and the judicious use of lightweight braces. Special attention should be given to spinal support to counteract scoliosis. Later in childhood, surgical immobilization of the spine may be indicated.

Distal Type. This category includes both dominant and recessive disorders and accounts for about 10 per cent of all cases of spinal muscular atrophy. Distal limb weakness and muscle wasting, more severe in the lower extremities, usually begins in early childhood and tends to be mild and slowly progressive. Three quarters of the patients have pes cavus, and, except for the absence of sensory deficits, the disorder is often clinically indistinguishable from Charcot-Marie-Tooth disease. However, patients with spinal muscular atrophy have normal conduction in motor and sensory nerves. A rare scapuloperoneal type, with autosomal recessive inheritance, is characterized by distal leg weakness and scapular winging, starting in infancy; there may also be bulbar symptoms such as laryngeal stridor.

Bulbar Type. The Fazio-Londe syndrome is a rare, fatal disorder of young children characterized by degeneration of the motor neurons of the brain stem resulting in progressive paralysis of the face, throat, larynx, and tongue and sometimes the ocular and jaw muscles. The cases have occurred sporadically or among siblings, suggesting autosomal recessive inheritance.

SPINAL MUSCULAR ATROPHY OF ADOLESCENT OR ADULT ONSET

Patients with late-onset spinal muscular atrophy have slowly progressive muscular weakness and usually continue to walk for two or three decades or more. Although much less common than the infantile and childhood types, the adult types include at least four clinical and eight genetic categories.

Proximal Type. These patients resemble patients with muscular dystrophy, and clinical examination may offer few clues to the neurogenic character of the proximal weakness. Fasciculations and muscle cramps are usually not prominent, and the serum creatine kinase activity may be substantially increased. To add to the confusion, males with onset of symptoms in their teens may have large calves. Some patients eventually develop mild bulbar symptoms, such as dysphagia. Electromyography serves to establish the neurogenic nature of the disorder, and muscle biopsy is rarely needed. Families with autosomal dominant and autosomal recessive inheritance have been described. A distinctive X-linked recessive variety, known as bulbospinal neuronopathy, is associated with gynecomastia and dysphagia.

Scapuloperoneal and Facioscapulohumeral Types. Both myopathic and neurogenic scapuloperoneal syndromes are known, and several varieties begin in the second or third decade of life. Autosomal dominant, autosomal recessive, and X-linked recessive forms have been described. The common feature of these disorders is progressive atrophy and weakness of the shoulder girdle and lower leg muscles, though weakness eventually may spread to the other limb muscles. Electromyography and muscle biopsy can distinguish the anterior horn cell diseases from the muscular dystrophies, but the prognosis is similar in both groups. A few families have an autosomal dominant form of spinal muscular atrophy resembling facioscapulohumeral muscular dystrophy.

Distal Type. This is usually a childhood disorder, but there are a few families with distal amyotrophy beginning in the third or fourth decade of life, inherited as an autosomal dominant trait. Some familial as well as adult cases exhibit onset in middle age and such a slow progression as never to be incapacitating, even in old age.

AMYOTROPHIC LATERAL SCLEROSIS

Amyotrophic lateral sclerosis (ALS) is a fatal degenerative disease of the central nervous system characterized by slowly progressive paralysis of the voluntary muscles. The French neurologist Charcot gave a detailed clinical and pathologic description in 1865. Little substantive knowledge about the cause and treatment of the disorder has been added since.

INCIDENCE. The annual incidence is about 1 case per 100,000 population, the prevalence being 4 to 6 cases per 100,000. Geographical pockets of much higher incidence in Guam, the Kii peninsula of Japan, and western New Guinea suggest possible, still unknown, exogenous causes. Ninety-five per cent of cases in the United States are sporadic, but a few families have several members with the typical clinical picture of sporadic ALS arising in an autosomal dominant pattern. Males are affected slightly more often than females. Although the disease can appear as early as the third decade of life, most cases begin after the age of 40, and the incidence increases with age into the eighth decade.

PATHOLOGY. Degeneration of the motor neurons of the spinal cord and lower brain stem is marked by extensive cell loss and astrocytic gliosis. Swellings containing neurofilaments are often found on axons close to their cell bodies. As the Betz cells and large pyramidal neurons of the motor cortex disappear, the corticospinal tracts degenerate, leaving gliosis in the lateral columns of the spinal cord. The ventral spinal roots are depleted of large myelinated nerve fibers, but surviving axons develop distal sprouts that reinnervate some muscle fibers, so that skeletal muscle histopathology shows both muscle fiber atrophy and fiber-type grouping.

ETIOLOGY. Few clues exist to the cause of ALS. Some authors regard the disease as a manifestation of premature aging or a deficiency of a neurotrophic factor. Other speculations include toxic exposure to minerals such as lead or aluminum, deficiency of calcium or magnesium, infection by an unidentified virus, and autoimmunity. Benign paraproteinemia has been encountered in a small proportion of patients, and antiganglioside antibodies have been found in the serum in a majority of the cases, but the significance of these findings is unclear.

CLINICAL MANIFESTATIONS. The major symptom consists of slowly progressive muscle weakness involving the limbs, trunk, breathing muscles, throat, and tongue. Most patients have a mixture of lower and upper motor neuron symptoms, although either may predominate. The former include muscle weakness, wasting, fasciculations, and cramps; the latter include stiffness and slowness of movement, slow and clumsy speech, and explosive release of laughter and crying (pseudobulbar palsy). The ocular muscles are not affected except in patients who survive long times after bulbar paralysis has begun. No impairment affects bladder, bowel, or sexual function. The stretch reflexes are diminished in severely denervated muscles, but more often signs of lower motor neuron weakness are combined with brisk reflexes, a finding nearly specific to ALS. Babinski signs are often present. Sensation is normal except for an expected diminution of vibration sense in the feet in older patients, and mental function is nearly always normal.

The onset is insidious, and initial symptoms may be confined to a single limb (especially the distal muscles), both limbs on one side, or to lower cranial nerves. Gradually, however, the patchy and asymmetric weakness becomes widespread, and the patient becomes unable to walk, dress, or feed himself or herself. There is loss of weight because of muscle atrophy and impaired swallowing; the speech becomes unintelligible; choking interferes with eating and sleeping; and breathing becomes difficult even at rest. Death occurs from pulmonary infection and insufficiency. The average survival is 3 years after onset of symptoms, but a few patients live for 10 years or longer in a severely debilitated state.

DIAGNOSIS. Because there are no specific laboratory tests, the diagnosis is based principally on clinical criteria. The disease to be diagnosed as ALS should have a relentlessly progressive, gradual course; lower motor neuron signs should exist at widely separate levels of the nervous system, or upper motor neuron signs should be found well above the level of the lower motor neuron signs; and no conflicting findings such as sensory loss, incontinence, or ocular weakness should be present. The cerebrospinal fluid is normal except for a mild elevation of protein concentration in some cases. Computed tomography (CT) and magnetic resonance (MR) imaging of the brain and spinal cord are unrevealing. Electromyography shows active and chronic denervation in multiple muscles of the brain stem, upper and lower extremities, and trunk; motor nerve conduction velocity is normal or slightly reduced, and sensory nerve conduction is normal. Serum creatine kinase activity is normal or moderately increased.

DIFFERENTIAL DIAGNOSIS. Although ALS is nearly always fatal, a few patients stop deteriorating or even recover normal strength, but such cases are extremely rare. Other motor neuron disorders, treatable myelopathies and neuropathies, and even thyrotoxic myopathy must be distinguished from ALS (see Table 465–2).

TREATMENT. With a disease as grim as ALS, the physician must be careful to avoid premature misdiagnosis. Once the diagnosis is certain, however, some explanation must be given to the patient and the family. This requires considerable tact and gentleness; often it is best to convey the information gradually

TABLE 465–2. DIFFERENTIAL DIAGNOSIS OF AMYOTROPHIC LATERAL SCLEROSIS

Disease	Distinguishing Features
Benign fasciculations	No weakness, atrophy, or electromyographic (EMG) abnormality
Motor neuron diseases	
*Lead or mercury toxicity	Increased lead or mercury levels
Benign focal amyotrophy	Onset in youth, strictly focal, no upper motor neuron signs
Postpolio progressive muscular atrophy	Slow course, no upper motor neuron signs
Subacute motor neuronopathy in lymphoma	Plateau in few months, later improvement
*ALS in lung cancer or B cell dyscrasia	Improves on treatment of tumor
Hereditary spinal muscular atrophy	Symmetric, slow course, no upper motor neuron signs
*Thyrotoxic myopathy with fasciculations	Myopathic EMG
*Compressive myelopathy due to cervical spondylosis or extramedullary tumor	Sensory symptoms, no lower motor neuron signs in legs, cord compression on MRI or myelography
*Immune-mediated multifocal motor neuropathy	Multifocal nerve conduction block, very high antiganglioside antibody titers

*Treatable conditions

on successive visits, allowing the relentless progression of weakness to speak for itself.

No medication has been shown to be beneficial, and physical therapy does not delay the neuromuscular deterioration. Quack remedies surface periodically; for their own protection, patients who wish to try experimental forms of treatment should be referred to a reputable academic center.

Patients with impaired gait may benefit from using a cane or a walker, and patients who suffer from severe dysphagia without other disabling symptoms can be offered nasogastric tube feeding or a gastrostomy. The most difficult medical question, however, involves the therapeutic role of artificial ventilation. Most patients, understanding the hopeless prognosis, prefer not to be kept alive artificially in a state of total paralysis, unable to communicate except with eye movements. Nevertheless, some patients have survived for several years in this fashion, living at home with the help of a devoted and intelligent family. It is important to discuss these issues when patients are in the early stages of respiratory involvement, so that they can make decisions in advance about whether or not to accept emergency resuscitation during a respiratory crisis.

PRIMARY LATERAL SCLEROSIS

Primary lateral sclerosis (PLS) describes a relatively rare condition characterized by painless, insidiously beginning, and gradually progressing spastic weakness that involves first the lower limbs but that in some instances ascends the neuraxis to affect the upper extremities. Rarely, pseudobulbar palsy adds its limitations to the woes of quadriplegia. In most instances, the disease begins in middle or late life with a duration that occasionally lasts no more than a year but most often persists for well over a decade before complications or intercurrent illness causes death. Typically, neurologic examinations show a relatively symmetric spastic paraparesis or quadriparesis with heightened deep tendon reflexes and extensor plantar responses but no hint of sensory abnormality. Neither clinical nor electrical studies detect evidence of skeletal muscular denervation in PLS. Similarly, central nervous system imaging procedures disclose no relevant abnormalities involving either brain or spinal cord. The cerebrospinal fluid remains unremarkable, and appropriate tests fail to disclose HIV, HTLV, or other inflammatory processes. Autopsy examinations, performed in a number of cases, have revealed ascending bilateral demyelination of the thoracolumbar corticospinal tracts extending to levels anywhere from the lower cord up to and including the cerebral peduncles. Cerebral degeneration has not

been noted. The cause of PLS is not known, but sporadically arising familial spastic paraplegia cannot be excluded in cases selectively involving the lower extremities. No specific treatment exists, although baclofen may bring modest relief of stiffness.

Brzustowicz LM, Lehner T, Castilla LH, et al.: Genetic mapping of chronic childhood onset spinal muscular atrophy to chromosome 5q 11.2–13.3. Nature 344:540, 1990. *Evidence that the infantile and childhood types of spinal muscular atrophy are allelic disorders of a single gene.*

Dubowitz V: Muscle Disorders in Childhood. London, W.B. Saunders Company, 1978, pp 146–90. *A rich compendium of clinical observations on the spinal muscular atrophies, by a leading neuromuscular expert. Superb illustrations.*

Mitsumoto H, Hanson MR, Chad DA: Amyotrophic lateral sclerosis. Recent advances in pathogenesis and therapeutic trials. Arch Neurol 45:189, 1988. *An extensive review of putative variants and possible mechanisms or treatment for this devastating disorder; 336 references.*

Siddique T, Figlewicz DA, Pericak-Vance MA, et al.: Linkage of a gene causing familial amyotrophic lateral sclerosis to chromosome 21 and evidence of genetic-locus heterogeneity. N Engl J Med 324:1381, 1991. *Twenty-three kindreds with this rare condition were evaluated by polymorphic markers for possible specific chromosome markers. Positive linkage to chromosome 21 was found in about half, adding a crucial suggestion relating to cellular susceptibility in this devastating illness.*

Tandan R, Bradley WG: Amyotrophic lateral sclerosis: Part 1. Clinical features, pathology, and ethical issues in management. Part 2. Etiopathogenesis. Ann Neurol 18:271, 419, 1985. *A recent review of research and treatment, with an important discussion of the ethical issues involved in the use of respirators.*

Younger DS, Chou S, Hayes AP, et al.: Primary lateral sclerosis. A clinical diagnosis reemerges. Arch Neurol 45:1304, 1988.

466 Syringomyelia

Syringomyelia is a disorder of the spinal cord and, often, the lower brain stem, characterized by slowly progressive enlargement of a fluid-filled cyst (syrinx) within the cord or medulla. Most cases are congenital in origin, related to maldevelopment of the cervicomedullary junction; others are caused by arachnoiditis, intraspinal tumor, or trauma. A prevalence of 8.4 cases per 100,000 has been suggested.

PATHOLOGY. In congenital cases, the cyst is thought to represent an enormously dilated remnant of the fetal central canal, which usually does not communicate with the fourth ventricle. It is lined by glial tissue, and in places by remnants of ependyma, and contains clear fluid identical to cerebrospinal fluid. Extending from the high cervical level or medulla to the thoracic or lumbar cord, the cyst varies in shape and size at different levels and is variably associated with damage to the anterior horns, crossing spinothalamic fibers, and lateral columns. Most patients have a Chiari type of congenital cerebellar malformation, in which the flattened ectopic tonsils descend caudally and press against the dorsal aspect of the upper cervical cord so as to obstruct both the exit foramina of the fourth ventricle and the subarachnoid space at the foramen magnum.

Acquired syringomyelia may result from basal arachnoiditis, obstructing the cerebrospinal fluid pathways around the foramen magnum, or may develop in a segment of the cord rendered abnormal by an intramedullary tumor, spinal arachnoiditis, or severe traumatic injury. In nontumor cases the cavity is lined only by glia, whereas in tumor cases the cyst wall may contain both tumor and glial cells. The cyst fluid may have an increased protein concentration in post-traumatic and tumor cases.

PATHOGENESIS. The mechanism of cyst formation and expansion is poorly understood. In congenital syringomyelia the cavity probably originates before birth as a dilatation of the primitive central canal. Enlargement of the cyst is somehow related to obstruction of the subarachnoid space at the cervicomedullary junction by the ectopic cerebellar tonsils, causing a pressure gradient between the cyst and the subarachnoid space, especially during straining, coughing, or sneezing. The mechanism may be similar in cases of basal arachnoiditis. In patients with spinal arachnoiditis, the cyst may originate in an area of ischemic myelomalacia, and in cases associated with tumor or severe injury there is cystic degeneration of the spinal cord before the syrinx starts to expand. Why the cyst continues to enlarge in these noncommunicating cases is hard to understand, since there is no apparent pressure gradient between the cyst and the subarachnoid space. Obstruction of cerebrospinal fluid circulation due to spinal arachnoiditis may be an important factor.

CLINICAL MANIFESTATIONS. The classic clinical picture of congenital syringomyelia is of a slowly progressive, asymmetric, destructive process in the central portion of the cervical and thoracic spinal cord, damaging the anterior horn cells, the crossing spinothalamic tract fibers, and the lateral corticospinal tracts. This causes muscle weakness and wasting in the hands and arms; scoliosis owing to denervation of paraspinal muscles; loss of arm reflexes; spastic weakness of the lower extremities; and a *dissociated sensory loss* with impaired perception of pain and temperature in the neck, arms, and upper trunk and preserved light touch perception and proprioception. Some patients experience a deep, aching pain in the neck or arms. Symptoms usually begin between 25 and 40 years of age and advance relentlessly for decades, although one third of the patients have long periods of stability. The deficits may worsen suddenly after a fall or after coughing or sneezing. Ten per cent of patients develop a painless arthropathy (Charcot joint) of the shoulder, elbow, or hand. Extension into the medulla may cause nystagmus, dysphagia, or wasting of the tongue, and some patients have hydrocephalus or cerebellar signs related to an associated Chiari malformation.

The manifestations of acquired syringomyelia depend on the segment of the spinal cord affected. Posttraumatic syringomyelia, developing in paraplegic or quadriplegic patients months or years after the injury, is revealed by weakness and sensory impairment rising craniad from the transected level. The cases associated with arachnoiditis following previous purulent meningitis, subarachnoid hemorrhage, surgery, trauma, or spinal anesthesia tend to involve the thoracic and lower cervical segments. Syringes associated with intramedullary spinal cord tumor extend for variable distances rostrad or caudad to the tumor.

DIAGNOSIS. Myelography, once widely employed, has been rendered largely obsolete by magnetic resonance (MR) imaging, which is both safer and more informative. Such images outline the size and extent of the cavity as well as the presence of cerebellar ectopia, arachnoiditis, or an intraspinal tumor (Fig. 466–1). Electromyography reveals active and chronic denervation in wasted upper extremity muscles, but sensory nerve conduction is normal in the analgesic hand, since the lesion is located proximal to the dorsal root ganglia. The cerebrospinal fluid is normal except for a raised protein content in cases associated with tumor or arachnoiditis.

TREATMENT. Various surgical procedures have been devised in the hope of arresting the neurologic deterioration, but none has been reliably successful. For congenital syringomyelia associated with cerebellar ectopia, it is often sufficient to perform a posterior decompression of the foramen magnum, ensuring that

the fourth ventricle communicates with the subarachnoid space. Acquired syringomyelia is usually treated by decompressing the cyst via a syringoarachnoid, syringopleural, or syringoperitoneal shunt. It has not been satisfactorily established that the outcome of any of these procedures is superior to the natural history of the disease. Several neurosurgical reports, however, suggest that these operations often reduce chronic pain and arrest the progression of neurologic symptoms, especially if performed before severe neurologic disability develops.

Anderson NE, Willoughby EW, Wrightson P: The natural history and the influence of surgical treatment in syringomyelia. Acta Neurol Scand 71:472, 1985. *A thoughtful critique of the uncertain role of surgical treatment for syringomyelia.*

467 The Phakomatoses

The phakomatoses, or neurocutaneous syndromes, are congenital disorders characterized by disordered growth of ectodermal tissues, producing distinctive skin lesions and malformations or tumors of the nervous system. More than 20 syndromes have been described, the most important of which are neurofibromatosis 1 and 2, tuberous sclerosis, and Sturge-Weber disease.

NEUROFIBROMATOSIS 1 (von Recklinghausen's Disease)

Neurofibromatosis 1 is characterized by multiple café au lait spots on the skin, multiple peripheral nerve tumors, and a variety of other dysplastic abnormalities of the skin, nervous system, bones, endocrine organs, and blood vessels. It is one of the most common genetic diseases, occurring approximately once in every 3000 births and present in about 30 persons per 10,000 population. It is inherited as an autosomal dominant trait, but 40 to 60 per cent of cases are clinically sporadic. Even allowing for the difficulty of detecting the trait in mild cases, there seems to be a remarkably high mutation rate, on the order of 10^{-4} per locus per generation. The gene has been mapped to a large region (about 13 kilobases) of the long arm of chromosome 17.

PATHOLOGY. The peripheral nerve tumors are of two types, schwannomas and neurofibromas, the latter derived from both Schwann cells and perineural fibroblasts. Neurofibromas of sensory nerve twigs produce the distinctive subcutaneous nodules; in peripheral nerve trunks the tumor appears as a fusiform enlargement or plexiform neuroma. Schwannomas arise in cranial and spinal nerve roots and also in peripheral nerve trunks. Both types of tumor occasionally become malignant. The brain may show disordered architecture, hamartomas, gliomas, and meningiomas.

CLINICAL MANIFESTATIONS. Some manifestations are congenital, but most appear gradually during childhood and adult life. Café au lait spots become larger and more numerous with age; the majority of patients eventually have more than six spots greater than 1.5 cm in diameter. Other skin lesions include freckles (axillary freckles being specific to this disease); soft, pedunculated, cutaneous neurofibromas; and firm, subcutaneous neurofibromas.

Plexiform neurofibromas may grow to lemon or even melon size, leading to grotesque overgrowth of soft tissues and bone in a limb or around the orbit. Enlarging nerve trunk tumors may cause pain and impairment of motor and sensory function; intraspinal nerve root tumors do the same and also compress the spinal cord. Gliomas of the optic nerve and chiasm are the most frequent intracranial tumor; they usually behave in an indolent fashion as hamartomas do. A hamartoma of the hypothalamus may cause precocious puberty.

About 10 per cent of children are mentally deficient, and about 10 per cent develop seizures, half in association with an intracranial tumor. Kyphoscoliosis, dysplasia of the skull, bowed legs, and other bone abnormalities are common. Pheochromocytoma occurs in about 5 per cent of patients, usually in adult life, and hypertension may result from renal artery dysplasia.

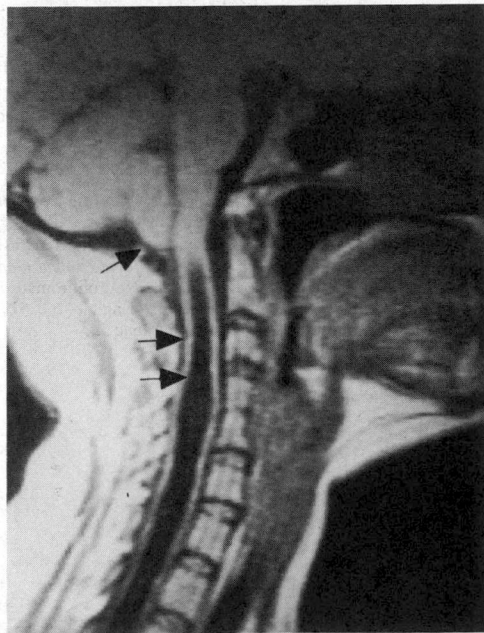

FIGURE 466–1. Magnetic resonance image of upper spine and foramen magnum in a patient with syringomyelia and a small Chiari I malformation (*single arrow*). The syrinx appears as a dark central area in the cervical and thoracic spinal cord (*double arrows*).

DIAGNOSIS. The diagnosis of neurofibromatosis is usually evident on clinical grounds, but biopsy of a neurofibroma can be diagnostic in otherwise cryptic cases. Spinal nerve root tumors often have a dumbbell shape, with intraspinal and extraspinal components; these are most readily identified on magnetic resonance (MR) imaging. For diagnosis of intracranial tumors and hamartomas either computed tomographic (CT) or MR images are suitable.

TREATMENT. Most patients live a normal life with few or no symptoms. Small cutaneous or subcutaneous neurofibromas can be removed if they are painful or frequently irritated, but large plexiform neurofibromas should usually be left alone. A few become malignant with continued invasion and fatal outcome. Asymptomatic peripheral nerve trunk schwannomas can sometimes be removed safely by an experienced surgeon. Intraspinal and intracranial schwannomas are approached in the usual surgical fashion. Optic nerve gliomas are generally treated with radiation, but it is not clear whether this improves the outcome.

NEUROFIBROMATOSIS 2

Often called central neurofibromatosis, this rare disease is characterized by the occurrence of bilateral acoustic neuromas and often other intracranial tumors, such as meningiomas and ependymomas. A few café au lait spots are present in 42 per cent of cases. Inherited as an autosomal dominant trait, the disease has a prevalence of 0.1 per 100,000. The responsible gene has been assigned to the long arm of chromosome 22. Family members at risk for the disease should be screened regularly with hearing tests and brain stem auditory evoked responses.

TUBEROUS SCLEROSIS

The typical clinical triad of tuberous sclerosis consists of mental deficiency, epilepsy, and a characteristic facial eruption known as adenoma sebaceum. The disease is inherited as an autosomal dominant trait, but about 80 per cent of the cases are sporadic, owing to new mutations. The incidence is about 3 cases per 100,000 births, the prevalence is about 10 per 100,000 population, and the mutation rate is 10.5×10^{-6} per gene per generation. Recently, the gene has been mapped to the long arm of chromosome 11.

PATHOLOGY. The facial papules of adenoma sebaceum are angiofibromas. The cerebral hemispheres contain multiple hamartomas or tubers, which give the disease its name; these are characterized by disordered architecture, proliferating and abnormal astrocytes, and deposits of calcium. Occasionally a subependymal nodule forms a giant cell astrocytoma, obstructing the foramen of Monro. The common retinal hamartomas are also probably of glial origin. Visceral lesions include multiple rhabdomyomas of the heart, multiple angiomyolipomas of the kidneys, and cystic transformation of the lungs by proliferating fibrous, muscular, and vascular tissue.

CLINICAL MANIFESTATIONS. Mental deficiency may be mild or severe, but one third of affected individuals have normal or even superior intelligence. Seizures occur in 80 per cent of cases, usually starting before the age of 5, and are often difficult to control with medication. In infants the seizures often take the form of infantile spasms; these children tend to be more severely impaired mentally. Occasionally, diagnosis escapes attention until late adolescence or adult life, when investigation of a seizure disorder of new onset turns up subtle skin lesions or multiple retinal or intracranial hamartomas.

Nearly all patients have distinctive skin lesions. Hypopigmented spots are present from the time of birth in nearly 100 per cent of patients; they are more numerous on the trunk and are easier to see with a Wood lamp. The next most common is adenoma sebaceum, a papular, salmon-colored eruption on the center of the face, especially in the nasolabial folds. It usually appears around 4 years of age and becomes more prominent after puberty. Leathery "shagreen" patches over the lower back and fibromas of the nailbeds affect perhaps 40 per cent of patients.

Retinal hamartomas are present in about half the patients. About 30 per cent of patients have cardiac rhabdomyomas, which sometimes cause arrhythmia or congestive heart failure. Renal tumors occur in two thirds of patients and are usually asymptomatic, though pain and bleeding can occur. Cystic disease of the lungs, an uncommon complication, mainly affects women over the age of 20; the symptoms include pneumothorax, dyspnea, cyanosis, and cor pulmonale.

DIAGNOSIS. Calcified cerebral lesions and subependymal nodules are well seen on brain CT, but uncalcified cortical tubers may show up better with MRI. Adenoma sebaceum, ungual fibromas, and hypopigmented spots are diagnostically specific, but retinal hamartomas also occur in neurofibromatosis. In 85 per cent of patients the electroencephalogram (EEG) is abnormal, most often showing epileptiform activity.

Treatment is confined to symptomatic control of the epilepsy and to surgical therapy of the occasional hamartoma that undergoes gliomatous changes and enlarges to produce symptoms.

STURGE-WEBER SYNDROME

The Sturge-Weber syndrome is a nonhereditary, congenital disorder of facial and cerebral blood vessels characterized by a facial angioma (port-wine stain), seizures, and mental deficiency. The condition involves a defect of embryonic development, with persistence of a vascular plexus in the cephalic portion of the neural tube. The incidence is about 5 in 100,000 births.

The facial angioma is usually unilateral but may extend to the other side and conforms largely but not strictly to trigeminal nerve subdivisions. There may be cavernous angiomas of the tongue, gums, or mouth, and choroidal angiomas may cause congenital glaucoma. An angioma of the occipital and parietal leptomeninges accompanies the facial nevus on the same side, and the underlying cerebral hemisphere is atrophic, with degenerative changes and deposits of iron and calcium in the superficial layers of the cerebral cortex. The cortical calcifications and atrophy are easily seen on brain CT. Neurologic symptoms develop in infancy or early childhood, consisting of focal or generalized seizures. Half of the children become mentally impaired, and one third develop a hemiparesis. When seizures are difficult to control with medication, early surgical removal of the affected part of the brain may improve control and prevent intellectual deterioration.

Gomez MR (ed.): Tuberous Sclerosis. New York, Raven Press, 1979. *A compilation of the Mayo Clinic experience, with excellent illustrations of the skin and retinal lesions.*

Riccardi VM: Medical progress. Von Recklinghausen neurofibromatosis. N Engl J Med 305: 1617, 1981. *A good review of the multiform clinical manifestations.*

Wertelecki W, Rouleau GA, Superneau DW, et al.: Neurofibromatosis 2: Clinical and DNA linkage studies of a large kindred. N Engl J Med 319: 278, 1988. *Includes evidence assigning the gene to chromosome 22.*

SECTION SEVEN / CEREBROVASCULAR DISEASES

William A. Pulsinelli and David E. Levy

468 Cerebrovascular Diseases— Principles

The family of cerebrovascular diseases can be classified according to whether they affect the brain's vascular supply either focally or diffusely (Fig. 468–1). The generic term *stroke* has come to signify the abrupt impairment of brain function caused by a variety of pathologic changes involving one (focal) or several (multifocal) intracranial or extracranial blood vessels. Approximately 80 per cent of all strokes are caused by too little blood flow (ischemic stroke), and the remaining 20 per cent are nearly equally divided between hemorrhage into brain tissue (parenchymatous hemorrhage) or the surrounding subarachnoid space (subarachnoid hemorrhage). In contrast, diseases that affect the heart or the systemic circulation cause generalized hypoperfusion and diffuse brain dysfunction or injury. Ischemic stroke and the hypoperfusion syndromes affecting the brain share much pathophysiology, and therefore both processes are considered together in Ch. 469; hemorrhagic stroke is addressed in Ch. 470.

Often cited as the third most frequent cause of death in the developed countries, stroke imposes an even greater impact on society in terms of the visible disability it causes. Many stroke victims survive for years with major impairments of speech, intellect, and motor or sensory function. Unlike survivors of myocardial infarction, who may be able to engage in most nonstrenuous activities, stroke victims often have difficulty with everyday acts like dressing, eating, walking, and communicating.

EPIDEMIOLOGY

The annual incidence and death rates for stroke have showed a steady decline in the United States throughout the twentieth century and for most European countries and Japan since approximately 1960. In the United States, a 1 per cent per year decrease in the annual mortality rate from stroke recorded since 1915 accelerated in the early 1970's to approximately 5 per cent per year. A recent analysis of a representative U.S. population indicates that the stroke incidence has stabilized at approximately 0.5 to 1.0 per 1000 population. Incidence rates in most European countries are only slightly higher (1.5 per 1000), but several Eastern European countries and Japan have rates of 3 per 1000, for unexplained reasons. At these current rates, stroke remains the third leading cause of medically related deaths and, after Alzheimer's disease, the most frequent cause of neurologic morbidity in developed countries.

Several other important facts about stroke incidence have emerged: a higher incidence and death rate for stroke among blacks than whites in the United States; approximately similar rates in men and women, in contrast to the male predominance for myocardial infarction; and importantly, a strikingly higher incidence (20 to 30 per 1000) for those over the age of 75. The last fact takes on particular significance in view of the aging population in North America, Europe, and parts of Asia.

CEREBROVASCULAR ANATOMY

Since most strokes are caused by abnormalities within the cerebral circulation, some understanding of cerebrovascular anatomy helps in arriving at the correct diagnosis and determining the underlying pathogenesis and prognosis. For example, symptoms that signal selective involvement of cortical blood vessels suggest cerebral emboli rather than atherothrombosis; clinical changes that cannot be attributed to a specific vascular territory may have causes other than a stroke; and transient ischemia of the vertebrobasilar system carries a better prognosis than does that of the carotid artery circulation.

The brain is supplied by four major arteries: the left and right internal carotid and vertebral arteries (Fig. 468–2). The left common carotid artery arises from the aortic arch, but the other vessels originate from branches of the aorta; the right common carotid artery stems from the innominate artery, and the left and right vertebral arteries take off from their respective subclavian arteries.

INTERNAL CAROTID ARTERIES. Each common carotid artery bifurcates in the majority of individuals just below the angle of the jaw and approximately at the level of the thyroid cartilage into an internal and external carotid artery (Fig. 468–2). The *internal carotid artery (ICA)* usually lies posterior and somewhat medial to the *external carotid artery* as the former ascends to the cranial vault. The ICA enters the cranium through the foramen lacerum and travels a short distance within the petrous portion of the temporal bone. It then enters the cavernous

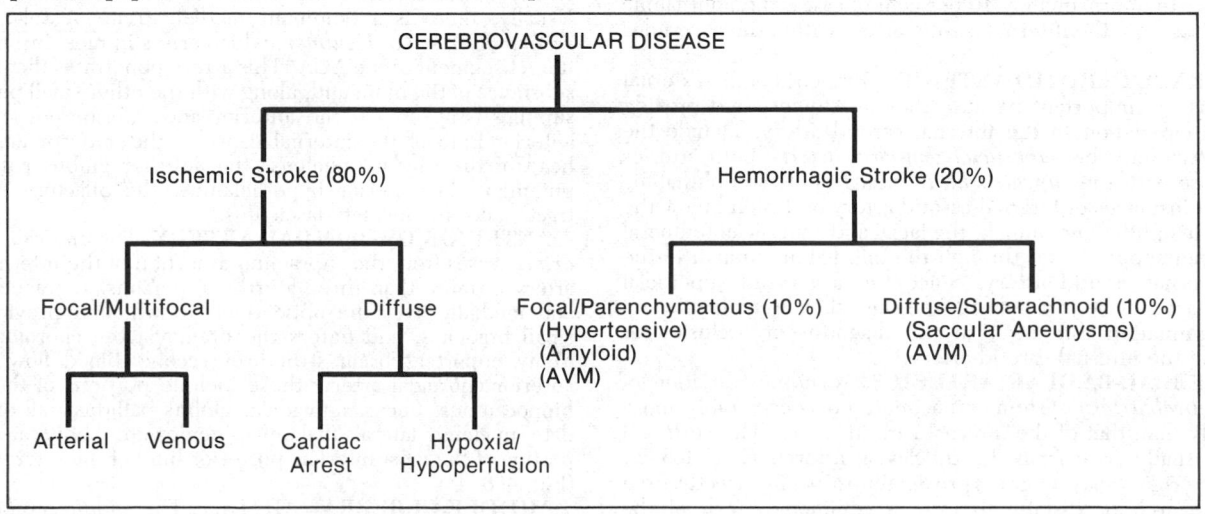

FIGURE 468–1. Classification of cerebrovascular disease.

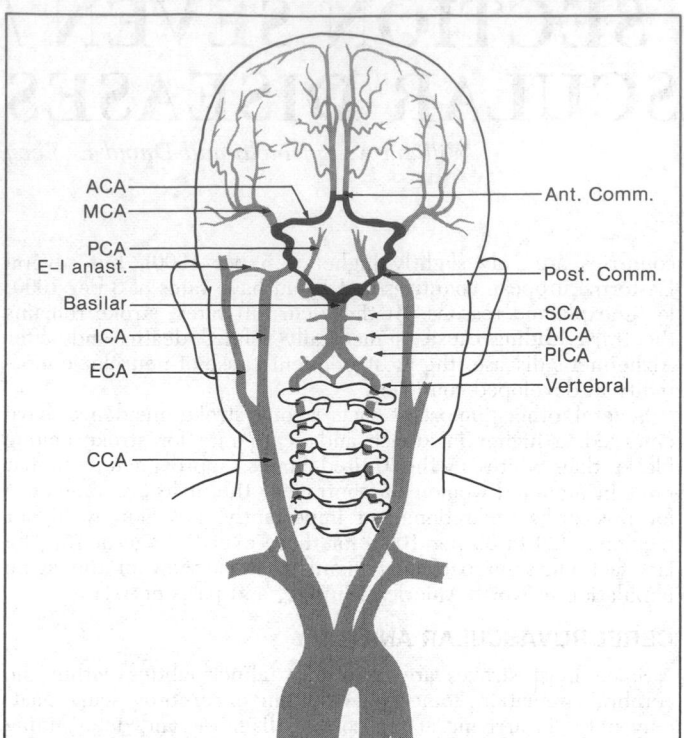

FIGURE 468–2. Extracranial and intracranial arterial supply to brain. Vessels forming the circle of Willis are highlighted in dark red. Abbreviations for intracranial and extracranial arteries are as follows: ACA = anterior cerebral artery; MCA = middle cerebral artery; PCA = posterior cerebral artery; E-I Anast = extracranial-intracranial anastomosis; ICA = internal carotid artery; ECA = external carotid artery; CCA = common carotid artery; Ant. Comm. = anterior communicating artery; Post. Comm. = posterior communicating artery; SCA = superior cerebellar artery; AICA = anterior inferior cerebellar artery; PICA = posterior inferior cerebellar artery. (Modified from Lord R: Surgery of Occlusive Cerebrovascular Disease. St. Louis, C.V. Mosby Company, 1986; with permission.)

sinus before penetrating the dura and ascends above the clinoid processes to divide into the *anterior* and *middle cerebral arteries.* The portion of the internal carotid artery that lies between the cavernous sinus and the supraclinoid process forms an **S** shape and is sometimes referred to as the carotid syphon by neuroradiologists. The internal carotid artery gives off no branches in the neck and a few nutritive branches within the petrous bone, and then at the supraclinoid level, the *ophthalmic, posterior communicating,* and *anterior choroidal arteries* usually arise in that order. In approximately 10 per cent of cases, the ophthalmic artery arises from the internal carotid artery within the cavernous sinus.

EXTERNAL CAROTID ARTERIES. Branches of the external carotid artery, important because they anastomose and provide collateral circulation to the internal carotid artery, include the *facial artery* and the *superficial temporal artery.* Both arteries anastomose with the *supratrochlear* branches of the ophthalmic artery. In instances of internal carotid artery occlusion below the level of the ophthalmic branch, the facial and superficial temporal arteries can supply blood through the ophthalmic branch to the distal internal carotid artery. Since the facial and superficial temporal arteries lie just beneath the skin, they are palpable and their examination can assist in the diagnosis of occlusion or stenosis of the internal carotid artery.

VERTEBRAL-BASILAR ARTERIES. Anatomic variation of the *vertebral artery* system is encountered considerably more frequently than that of the internal carotid artery. The vertebral arteries usually arise from the subclavian arteries (Fig. 468–2), but their origins may migrate proximally to begin directly from the aortic arch or distally to form a common branch of the thyrocervical trunk. The vertebral arteries enter the foramen of

the sixth cervical vertebra or, much less commonly, at the fourth, fifth, or seventh cervical vertebral level. The vertebral arteries ascend through the transverse foramina and exit at C1, where they turn 90 degrees posteriorly to pass behind the atlantoaxial joint before penetrating the dura and entering the cranial cavity through the foramen magnum. The portion of the vertebral artery that loops behind the atlantoaxial joint is prone to mechanical trauma, and rotation of the head to approximately 60 degrees may cause arterial narrowing and reduce blood flow to the ipsilateral vertebral artery.

Intracranially, the vertebral arteries lie lateral to the medulla oblongata and then course ventrally and medially, where they unite at the medullopontine junction to form the *basilar artery.* The basilar artery bifurcates at the pontomesencephalic junction into the *posterior cerebral arteries.*

In up to 20 per cent of persons, the right or left vertebral artery terminates before reaching the basilar artery, leaving the latter to be supplied inferiorly by a single vessel. Intracranial branches of the vertebral arteries include medial branches, which unite to form the *anterior spinal artery,* and lateral branches to the dorsolateral medulla and posterior cerebellum, called the *posterior inferior cerebellar arteries.*

CIRCLE OF WILLIS. The *circle of Willis* (Fig. 468–2) is formed by the union at the base of the brain of both anterior cerebral arteries via the *anterior communicating artery* and the middle cerebral arteries with the posterior cerebral arteries on each side via the *posterior communicating arteries* (Fig. 468–2). Anomalies of the circle of Willis occur frequently; in large autopsy series of normal individuals, more than half showed an incomplete circle of Willis. The most common sites for such abnormalities, which usually present as hypoplasia or atresia, are the posterior communicating arteries (22 per cent) and the anterior cerebral arteries (10 per cent).

ANTERIOR CEREBRAL ARTERY. The *anterior cerebral arteries* (ACA) pass medially above the optic chiasm and head rostrally toward the interhemispheric fissure, where they arc caudally to lie just dorsal to the corpus callosum (Fig. 468–3). In approximately 10 per cent of normal individuals, the A1 segment of the ACA (the portion between the middle cerebral and anterior communicating arteries) is atretic or absent, leaving its distal portion to be supplied by the opposite ACA via the anterior communicating artery. Branches of the ACA supply the frontal poles, the entire superior surfaces of the cerebral hemispheres where their distal branches anastomose with those of the middle cerebral artery, and all of the medial surfaces of both cerebral hemispheres with the exception of the calcarine cortex. Cortical areas served by the ACA include the motor and sensory cortex of the legs and feet, the supplementary motor cortex, and the presumed cortical micturition center lying in the paracentral lobule (Figs. 468–3 and 468–4).

The A1 and A2 segments (the portion between the anterior communicating artery and the genu of the corpus callosum) give off many small branches that penetrate the anterior perforated substance of the brain. These small penetrating branches include all of the *anterior* and some of the *medial lenticulostriate* arteries. Usually, there is a dominant medial striate vessel called the *recurrent artery of Heubner,* which arises in most instances from the A1 segment of the ACA. This artery penetrates the perforated substance of the brain and, along with the other small perforators, supplies (Fig. 468–4) the anterior and inferior portions of the anterior limb of the internal capsule, the anterior and inferior head of the caudate nucleus, the anterior globus pallidus and putamen, the anterior hypothalamus, the olfactory bulbs and tracts, and the uncinate fasciculus.

ANTERIOR CHOROIDAL ARTERY. The *anterior choroidal artery* arises from the supraclinoid portion of the internal carotid artery in more than three fourths of persons. It travels caudally and medially over the optic tract, to which it provides a few small branches, and enters the brain via the choroidal fissure. Many important brain structures receive blood flow from the anterior choroidal artery; these include portions of the anterior hippocampus, uncus, amygdala, globus pallidus, tail of the caudate nucleus, lateral thalamus, geniculate body, and a large portion of the most inferior, posterior limb of the internal capsule (Fig. 468–4).

MIDDLE CEREBRAL ARTERY. The *middle cerebral artery* (MCA) provides flow to most of the lateral surface of the cerebral

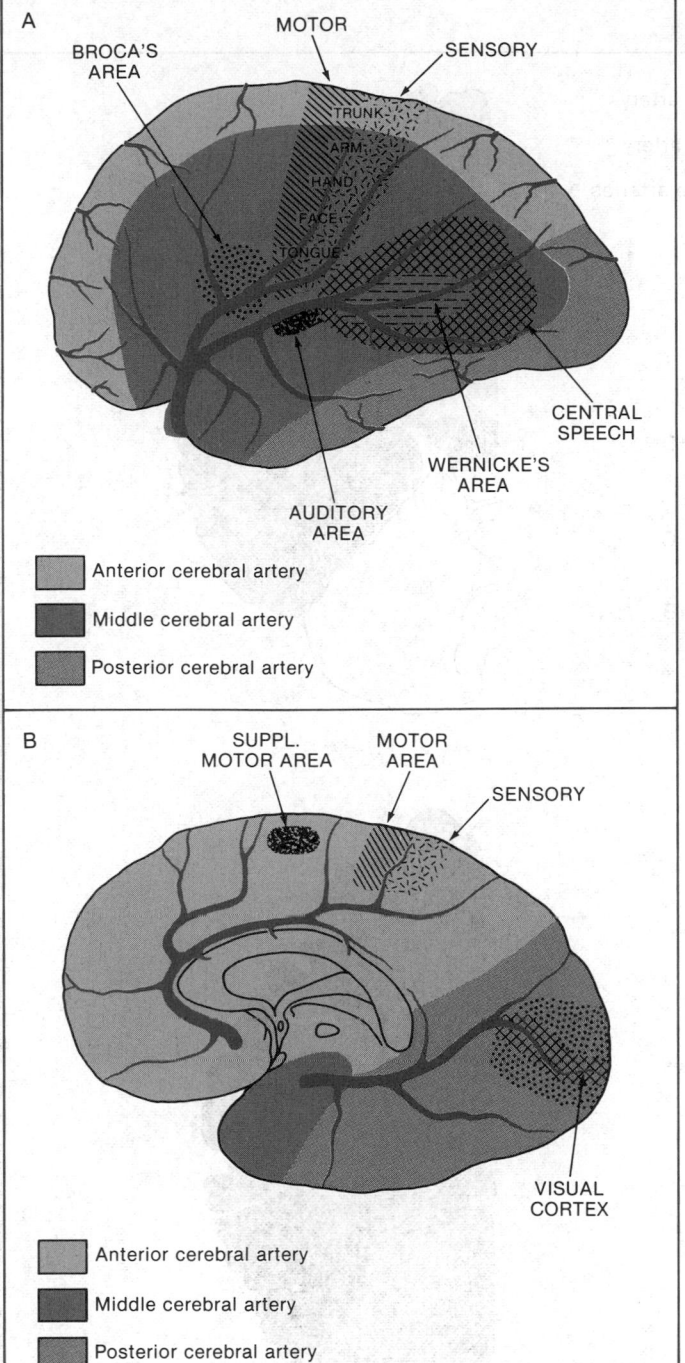

FIGURE 468–3. Lateral (A) and medial (B) views of the cerebral hemisphere showing the surface distributions of the anterior, middle, and posterior cerebral arteries.

hemispheres and is the vessel most frequently involved in ischemic stroke (Figs. 468–3 and 468–4). As the main MCA trunk passes laterally towards the sylvian fissure, it gives rise to some of the *medial* and all of the *lateral lenticulostriate* arteries. These arteries irrigate (Fig. 468–4) the putamen, the head and body of the caudate nucleus, the lateral globus pallidus, the full vertical extent of the anterior limb of the internal capsule, and a superior portion of the posterior limb of the internal capsule. The middle cerebral artery extends into the sylvian fissure, where it branches into several smaller arteries grouped into a superior division, which feeds the cortical surface above the fissure, and an inferior division, which supplies the cortical surface of the temporal lobe. The territory of the MCA includes the major motor and sensory areas of the cortex, the areas for contraversive eye and head movement, the optic radiations, auditory sensory cortex, and, in the dominant hemisphere, the motor and sensory areas for language.

POSTERIOR CEREBRAL ARTERY. Blood flow to both *posterior cerebral arteries* (PCA) is derived primarily from the basilar artery (70 per cent of the time) and from the internal carotid arteries (10 per cent of the time). In the remaining 20 per cent, one PCA is supplied by the internal carotid artery and the other by the basilar artery. The PCA pass dorsal to the third cranial nerves and across the cerebral peduncles and then ascend upward along the medial edge of the tentorium, where they branch into anterior and posterior divisions. The anterior division (Figs. 468–3 and 468–4) supplies the inferior surface of the temporal lobe, where its terminal branches anastomose with branches of the MCA. The posterior division supplies the occipital lobe, where its terminal branches anastomose with both the ACA and the MCA. In its most proximal course along the base of the brain, the PCA gives off several groups of penetrating arteries commonly referred to as the thalamogeniculate, the thalamoperforating, and the posterior choroidal arteries. The red nucleus, the substantia nigra, medial parts of the cerebral peduncles, the nuclei of the thalamus, the hippocampus, and the posterior hypothalamus all receive blood from these penetrating branches (Fig. 468–4).

BRAIN STEM BLOOD FLOW. At all rostrocaudal levels of the brain stem, the ventral medial portion is supplied by short paramedian vessels; the ventrolateral portion by short circumferential branches from the vertebral or basilar arteries; and the dorsolateral portion and cerebellum by long circumferential branches, which include the *posterior inferior cerebellar* arteries, which arise from the vertebral arteries, and the *anterior inferior* and *superior cerebellar* arteries, which arise from the basilar artery (Fig. 468–5A and B).

The pyramids, the inferior olives and medial lemnisci, the medial longitudinal fasciculi, and the emerging fibers of the hypoglossal nerve (Fig. 468–5A) derive blood from the vertebral arteries. Longer branches from the vertebral arteries and posterior inferior cerebellar arteries supply the spinothalamic tracts, the vestibular nuclei, the sensory nuclei of the fifth cranial nerve, the descending fibers of the sympathetic nervous system, the restiform body, and the emerging fibers of the vagus and glossopharyngeal nerves. The most cephalad and dorsal segment of the medulla includes the vestibular and cochlear nuclei, which, along with the posterior portion of the cerebellum, receive flow from the posterior inferior cerebellar artery.

The basilar artery gives rise to perforating branches as it spans the ventral midline pons and midbrain (Fig. 468–5B). These short perpendicular branches distribute blood to the paramedian structures, including the corticospinal tracts, the pontine reticular nuclei, the medial lemnisci, the medial longitudinal fasciculi, and the pontine reticular nuclei. The *anterior inferior cerebellar artery* feeds blood to the lateral pons, including the emerging seventh and eighth cranial nerves, the trigeminal nerve root, the vestibular and cochlear nuclei, and the spinothalamic tracts. It also branches to the most dorsal and lateral of these structures on its dorsal course toward the cerebellum.

At the midbrain level, the basilar artery lies in the midline in the peduncular fossa. Short branches pass laterally and dorsally to both sides to supply the cerebral peduncles, the emerging fibers of the third nerve, medial portions of the red nuclei, the medial longitudinal fasciculus, the oculomotor nuclei, and the midbrain reticulum. The superior cerebellar arteries contribute to the dorsal midbrain supply, including that of the colliculi and the superior portion of the cerebellum on each side.

VENOUS DRAINAGE. The veins in the brain, unlike those in many other parts of the body, do not accompany the arteries (Fig. 468–6). Cortical veins drain into the superior sagittal sinus, which runs posteriorly between the cerebral hemispheres. Deeper structures drain into the inferior sagittal sinus and great cerebral vein (of Galen), which join at the straight sinus. The straight sinus runs posteriorly along the attachment of the falx cerebri and tentorium and joins the superior sagittal sinus at the torcular Herophili, from which the two transverse sinuses arise. Each transverse sinus passes laterally toward the petrosal bone, to become the sigmoid sinus, which exits the skull into the internal jugular vein. Each cavernous sinus communicates with its contralateral twin and surrounds the ipsilateral carotid artery; both drain posteriorly into the petrosal sinuses, which in turn drain into the sigmoid sinus.

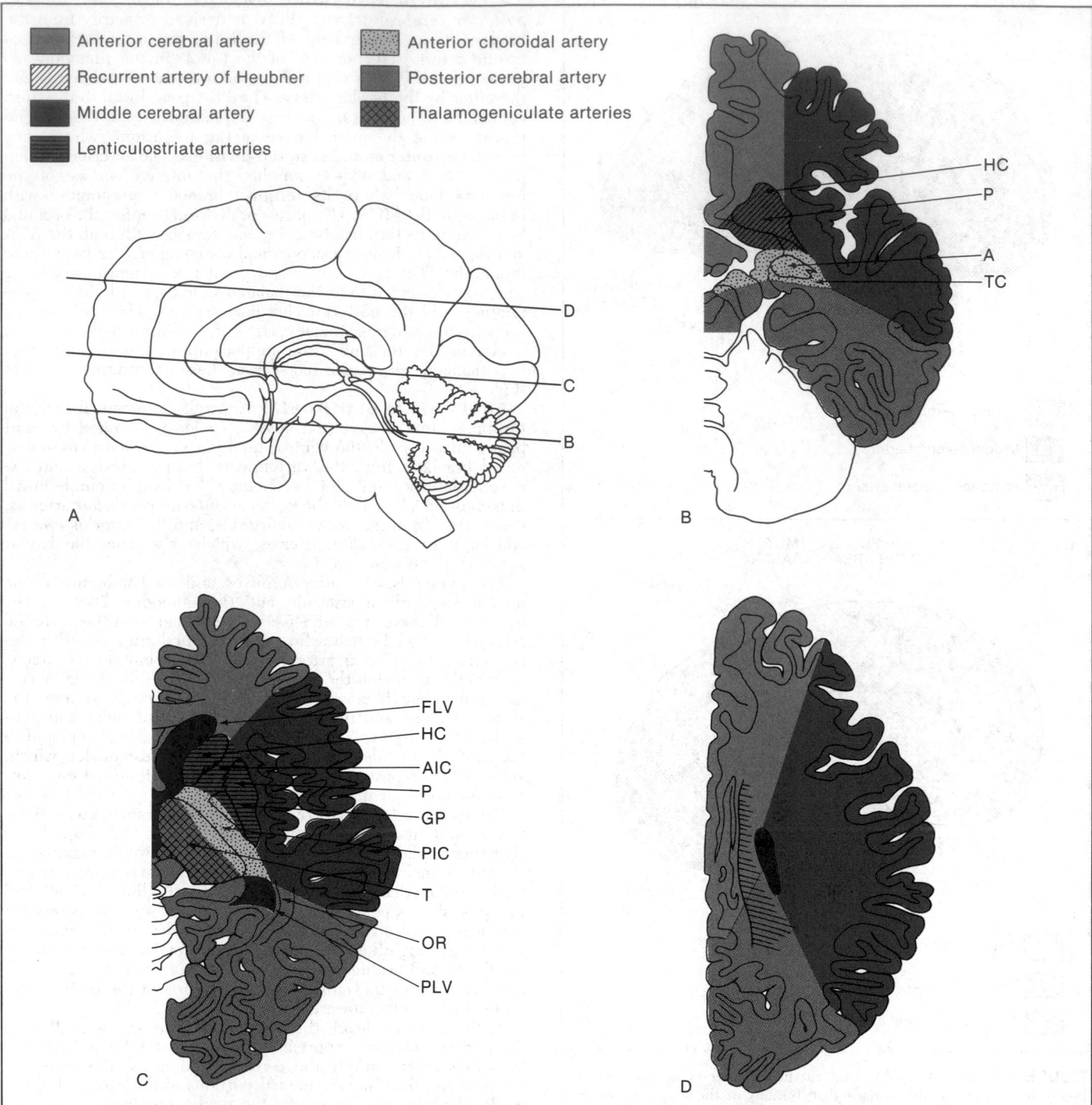

FIGURE 468–4. Arterial supply of deep brain structures. *A*, Sagittal view of the brain showing the computed tomographic (CT) planes through which views B,C, and D were taken. *B*, CT plane through the head of the caudate nucleus (HC), putamen (P), amygdala (A), tail of the caudate nucleus (TC), hypothalamus, temporal lobe, midbrain, and cerebellum. *C*, CT plane through the frontal horn of the lateral ventricle (FLV), head of the caudate nucleus (HC), anterior and posterior limbs of the internal capsule (AIC, PIC), putamen (P), globus pallidus (GP), thalamus (T), optic radiations (OR), and posterior horn of the lateral ventricle (PLV). *D*, CT plane through the centrum semiovale. (Modified from De Armond S, Fuso M, Dewey M: Structure of the Human Brain. New York, Oxford Press, 1989; with permission.)

NORMAL PHYSIOLOGY

CEREBRAL METABOLISM AND BLOOD FLOW. The brain performs no mechanical work; nevertheless, the energy demands to support normal electrophysiologic brain activity in conscious humans equal, on a per weight basis, those of metabolically active tissues like the heart and kidney. The energy demands necessary to drive membrane ion pumps, to synthesize, store, and release neurotransmitters, and to maintain tissue structure are met almost entirely by the aerobic metabolism of glucose to CO_2 and H_2O. The normal, conscious human consumes approximately 160 μmoles of O_2 and 30 μmoles of glucose per 100 grams of brain each minute (Table 468–1).

Approximately 10 per cent of available blood glucose is extracted and phosphorylated by the brain in a single pass, yet only 80 per cent of this glucose is used to generate energy. The 5:1 ratio of O_2 versus glucose consumption (Table 468–1) indicates

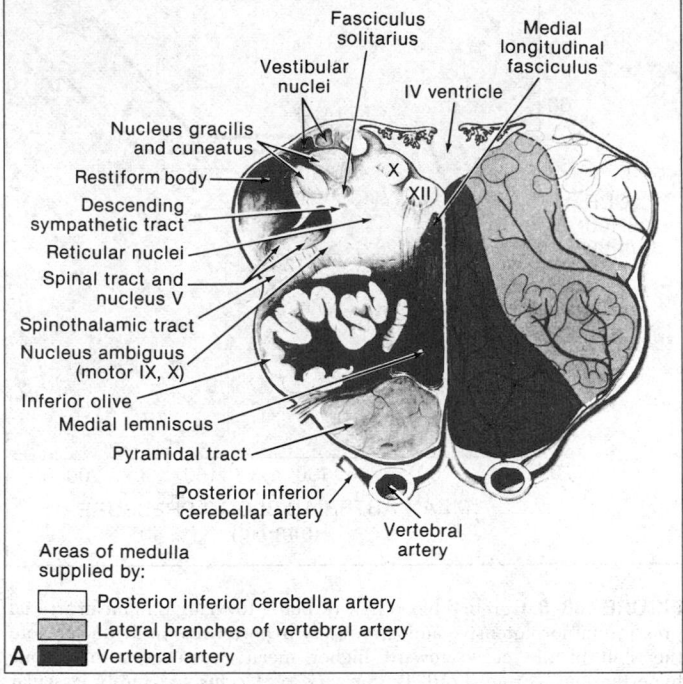

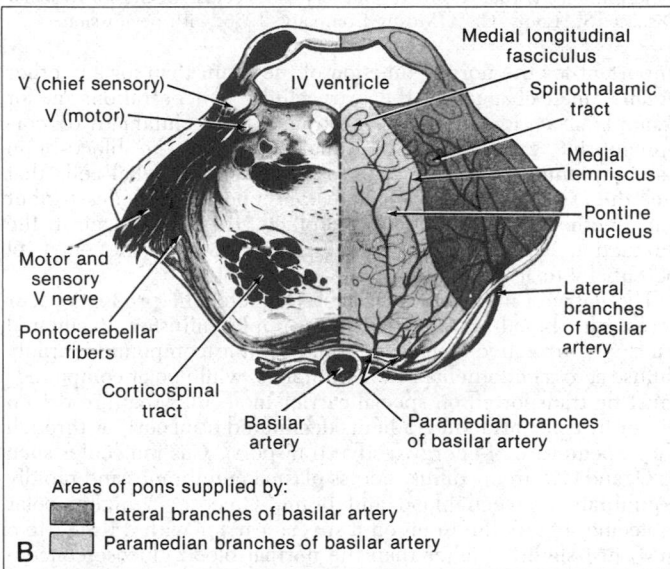

FIGURE 468–5. *A*, Cross-section of the medulla oblongata at the level of the hypoglossal nuclei (XII). Short branches of the vertebral and anterior spinal arteries supply the medial medulla. Longer circumferential branches, including the posterior inferior cerebellar artery, supply the lateral portions of the medulla. *B*, Cross-section of the mid-pons. The medial portion receives the blood supply from short, perforating basilar artery branches. More laterally, the blood supply comes from lateral basilar artery branches.

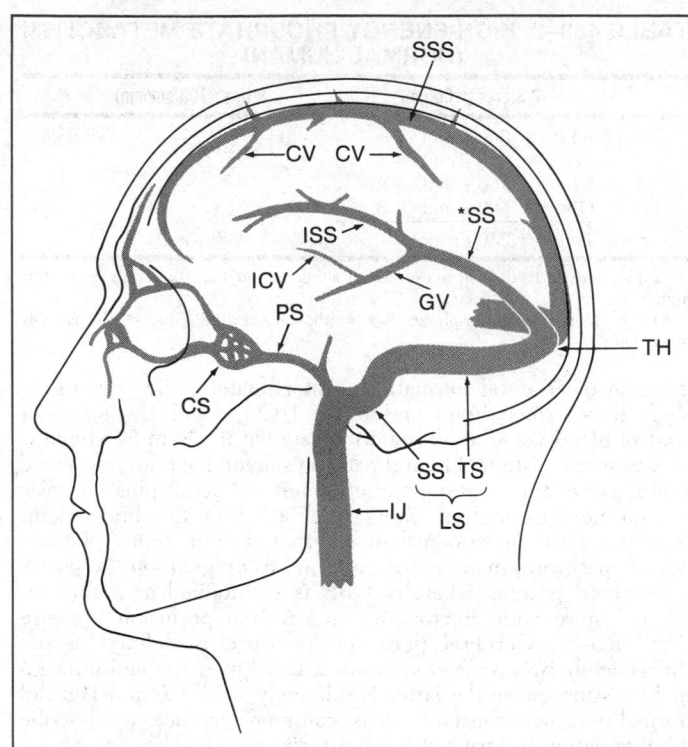

FIGURE 468–6. Venous drainage of intracranial structures. SSS = superior sagittal sinus; CV = cortical veins; ISS = inferior sagittal sinus; ICV = internal cerebral vein; GV = great vein of Galen; *SS = straight sinus; TH = torcular Herophili; PS = petrosal sinus; CS = cavernous sinus; TS = transverse sinus; SS = sigmoid sinus; LS = lateral sinus; IJ = internal jugular vein. (Amended with permission from Gates P, Barnett H, Mohr J, et al. [eds.]: Stroke: Pathophysiology, Diagnosis and Management. New York, Churchill Livingstone, 1986.)

μmoles of O_2 and 260 μmoles of glucose to 100 grams of brain each minute (see Table 468–1). These values exceed the brain's normal consumption rates of O_2 and glucose by factors of approximately 2 and 9, respectively, suggesting modest reserves of these molecules in the blood vascular compartment. In fact, the blood vascular reserves for both O_2 and glucose must be small, since changes of synaptic activity related to, for example, the normal acts of speaking or listening are tightly *coupled*, both temporally and spatially, to a proportional increase in CBF. As a consequence, the anatomic segregation of the brain's functional activities results in an ever-changing mosaic of regional metabolic/blood flow values that reflect moment-to-moment changes in electrophysiologic activity.

The coupling of CBF to regional synaptic activity and thereby to local metabolic activity represents only one of several important mechanisms regulating normal CBF. Changes in the respiratory rate or volume, which lead to even mild hypercapnia or hypocapnia, respectively dilate or constrict cerebral resistance vessels, so that CBF shows a linear relationship to Pa_{CO_2} (Fig. 468–7). This normal physiologic response to Pa_{CO_2} is exploited clinically to treat cerebral herniation syndromes. Mechanical hyperventilation to a Pa_{CO_2} of 20 to 25 mm Hg reduces CBF by approximately 40 to 45 per cent and normal adult cerebral blood volume from 50 ml to approximately 35 ml. While seemingly small, this 15 ml of additional intracranial volume is sufficient to retard the pro-

that approximately 20 per cent of glucose carbons are not oxidized. Approximately 10 to 15 per cent of glucose is metabolized to lactate, which may be lost to the circulation; the remainder is used for the synthesis of neurotransmitters, fats, and, to a small degree, proteins. Each mole of glucose metabolized by the brain through glycolysis and the mitochondrial respiratory chain therefore yields approximately 30 moles of ATP instead of the expected 38.

Unlike muscle or other tissues, the brain stores few glucose, glycogen, or other high-energy phosphate (ATP, phosphocreatine) reserves (Table 468–2) but instead relies on a sizable and well-regulated blood flow to satisfy its immediate needs for energy. Cerebral blood flow (CBF) averages 60 ml per 100 grams of brain per minute in the normal, conscious human; in the absence of such flow, the brain has sufficient high-energy stores to support normal metabolic needs for only a few minutes. At normal arterial O_2 tensions and blood glucose concentrations, CBF delivers 350

TABLE 468–1. METABOLIC ACTIVITY (NORMAL CONSCIOUS HUMAN)

	Consumed	Supplied
	(/100 gm brain/min)	
CBF	60 ml	—
O_2	156 μmol	350 μmol
Glucose	33 μmol	260 μmol

CBF = cerebral blood flow.

TABLE 468–2. HIGH-ENERGY PHOSPHATE METABOLISM (NORMAL HUMAN)

~ P Stores (/100 gm)*	~P Use (/100 gm/min)
ATP = 300 μmol	
PCr = 400 μmol	
Glu = 150 μmol (×2)	
Gly = 500 μmol (×3)	
Total = 2500 μmol	800 μmol

*Values are derived from anesthetized subjects and may therefore be slightly higher than in awake subjects.

ATP = adenosine triphosphate; PCr = phosphocreatine; Gluc = glucose; Gly = glycine.

gression of cerebral herniation. Unfortunately, the response is short lived, since brain and blood HCO_3^- and H^+ ions that control blood vessel tone re-equilibrate within 30 to 60 minutes.

A complex system of neural pathways involving both peripheral sympathetic and parasympathetic nerve fibers, plus intrinsic central nervous system fibers originating in the brain stem, regulates CBF in response to external stimuli. Some of these neural pathways may participate in *autoregulation*, a poorly understood process whereby CBF is maintained at a constant level despite wide fluctuations in cerebral perfusion pressure (Fig. 468–8). Cerebral perfusion pressure is defined as the difference between mean systemic arterial pressure and intracranial pressure; since the latter is relatively small (10 mm Hg) and normally nearly constant, it is common practice to describe autoregulation in terms of mean arterial pressure.

Autoregulation has both upper and lower limits (Fig. 468–8); at mean arterial pressures above 150 mm Hg, blood flow increases and capillary pressure rises, while at mean arterial pressures below 50 mm Hg, CBF falls. Increased capillary pressure in hypertensive patients may be a factor in intracerebral hemorrhage and hypertensive encephalopathy. In patients with chronic hypertension, the upper and lower autoregulatory limits are shifted toward higher systemic pressures (Fig. 468–8). Consequently, rapid therapeutic reduction of blood pressure to apparently normal levels carries with it the potential for further lowering of cerebral blood flow in hypertensive patients with ongoing cerebral ischemia. Chronic treatment with antihypertensive agents causes a readjustment of the autoregulatory curve toward more normal values.

BLOOD-BRAIN BARRIER. Regulation within narrow limits of the extracellular ionic and molecular composition is more

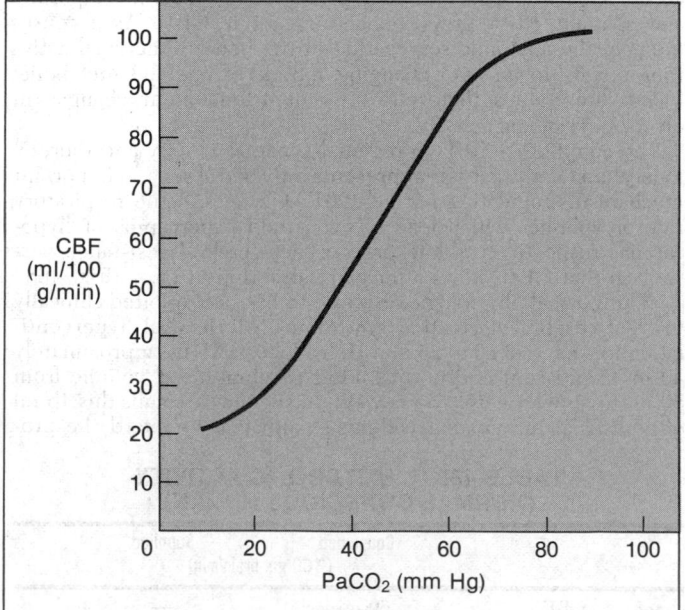

FIGURE 468–7. Cerebral blood flow response to changes in the arterial CO_2 tension. (From Lord R: Surgery of Occlusive Cerebrovascular Disease. St. Louis, C. V. Mosby Company, 1986; with permission.)

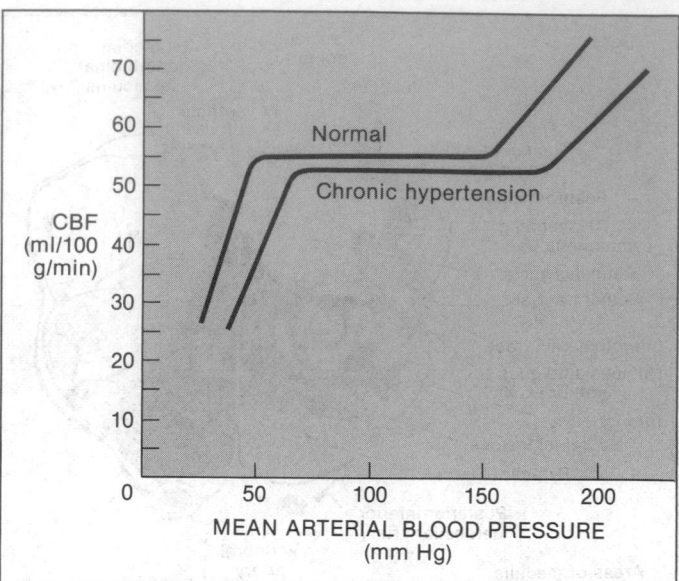

FIGURE 468–8. Cerebral blood flow response to changes in mean arterial pressure in normotensive and chronically hypertensive individuals. Note the shift of the curve toward higher mean pressures with chronic hypertension. (From Lord R: Surgery of Occlusive Cerebrovascular Disease. St. Louis, C. V. Mosby Company, 1986; with permission.)

important for the normal function of the brain than for any other organ. Small changes in the extracellular concentrations of, for example, Na^+ ions or the neurotransmitters glutamate or norepinephrine greatly alter neuronal function. The blood-brain barrier, composed anatomically of unique endothelial cells that lack the usual transendothelial channels and that seamlessly abut one another (tight junctions), protects the brain against the fluctuating composition of blood and minimizes the entry of potentially toxic compounds.

The entry of nutrients and egress of metabolic products occur across the blood-brain barrier via simple diffusion, facilitated transport, or active transport. Lipid-soluble compounds rapidly diffuse across endothelial cell membranes, while polar compounds must be transported on special carrier molecules that are driven either by concentration gradients (facilitated transport) or through the expenditure of energy (active transport). Gas molecules such as O_2 and CO_2 freely diffuse across plasma membranes and rapidly equilibrate between blood and brain. Glucose, a highly polar molecule, enters the brain on a special carrier with a Km (7 to 8 mM) just slightly higher than the normal blood glucose concentration. The rate of brain glucose transport is normally two to three times faster than the metabolism of glucose, but since glucose uptake depends so highly on its concentration, a reduction of blood sugar to one-third the normal amount, caused by either ischemia or hypoglycemia, may compromise normal metabolism (Table 468–3).

PATHOPHYSIOLOGY/PATHOLOGY OF CEREBRAL ISCHEMIA

The pathophysiologic consequences of failed O_2 and glucose delivery to the brain encompass a cascade of events that vary qualitatively and quantitatively with the severity of the ischemic insult. The severity of cerebral ischemia, defined as the degree and duration of blood flow loss, largely determines whether the brain suffers only temporary dysfunction, irreversible injury to a few highly vulnerable neurons (selective ischemic necrosis), or

TABLE 468–3. HUMAN HYPOXIC-ISCHEMIC THRESHOLD VALUES

	Pa$_{O_2}$ (mm Hg)	CBF (ml/100 gm/min)	Blood Glucose (mg/dl)
Normal	90	60	80
Stupor	30–40	20–30	25–30
Coma	20–30	15–20	20–25
Brain injury	<20	<15	<20

TYPES OF CEREBRAL HYPOXIA-ISCHEMIA. Cerebral hypoxia-ischemia can be conveniently divided on the basis of clinical criteria into focal or multifocal ischemia from vascular occlusion, global ischemia from complete failure of cardiovascular pumping, and diffuse hypoperfusion-hypoxia caused by respiratory disease or reduced perfusion pressure. *Focal cerebral ischemia*, resulting most frequently from embolic or thrombotic occlusion of extracranial or intracranial blood vessels, variably reduces blood flow within the involved vascular territory. Blood flow to the central zone of the ischemic vascular bed usually is severely reduced but rarely reaches zero because of partial filling from collateral blood vessels. In the transition zones between normally perfused tissue and the severely ischemic central core, blood flow is moderately reduced. This rim of moderately ischemic tissue has been called the "ischemic penumbra," and although brain cells in this region remain viable longer than do those in the ischemic core, they too will die if left deprived of adequate blood flow.

Focal cerebral ischemia sufficient to cause clinical signs or symptoms and lasting only 15 to 30 minutes causes irreversible injury to specific, highly vulnerable neurons. If the ischemia lasts an hour or longer, infarction of part or all of the involved vascular territory is inevitable. Clinical evidence of permanent brain injury from such ischemia may or may not be detectable, depending upon the region and the amount of brain tissue involved (see Ch. 469).

Global cerebral ischemia, typically caused by cardiac asystole or ventricular fibrillation, reduces blood flow to zero throughout all of the brain. Global ischemia lasting more than 5 to 10 minutes is usually incompatible with recovery of consciousness in normothermic individuals. Brain damage from more transient global ischemia, uncomplicated by periods of prolonged hypotension or hyperglycemia, is limited to specific populations of highly vulnerable neurons. This "selective ischemic necrosis" of neurons involves, for example, the CA1 pyramidal neurons of hippocampus, the cerebellar Purkinje cells, and the pyramidal neurons in neocortical layers 3, 5, and 6 (Table 468–4). While selective ischemic necrosis of neurons is typical of transient global ischemia, such injury may also accompany prolonged hypoxemia, carbon monoxide poisoning, and focal cerebral ischemia of brief duration. Cardiac resuscitation complicated by prolonged hypotension or hyperglycemia may cause cerebral infarction, particularly in border zones that lie between the terminal branches of major arterial supplies.

Diffuse cerebral hypoxia, uncomplicated by cerebral ischemia, is limited to conditions of mild to moderate hypoxemia, since myocardial contractility and blood pressure fall with severe hypoxemia. As a consequence, pure cerebral hypoxia causes cerebral dysfunction but not irreversible brain injury. Individuals with pure cerebral hypoxia from altitude sickness, pulmonary disease, or severe anemia present with confusion, cognitive impairment, and lethargy; the onset of coma signals cardiovascular compromise and imminent brain damage. With relatively *acute* changes in arterial oxygen tension from normal to a Pa_{O_2} of 40 mm Hg (see Table 468–3) or with a fall in the hemoglobin concentration below 7 grams per deciliter, compensatory increases of cerebral blood flow become inadequate, and clinical signs and symptoms of cerebral hypoxia develop. Chronic exposure to such low oxygen or hemoglobin levels invokes other poorly defined compensatory mechanisms, which allow near-normal cerebral function. The climbers of Mount Everest, having slowly acclimatized to breathing ambient air, developed only minor impairments of short-term memory and motor function despite having arterial oxygen tensions of 28 mm Hg.

NEUROPATHOLOGY OF CEREBRAL ISCHEMIA. Ischemic injury to the brain can be classified on the basis of cytopathologic criteria into four types. Cerebral *autolysis*, most frequently seen in brain-dead patients preserved on mechanical ventilators for several days, reflects complete and permanent loss of blood flow accompanied by enzymatic autodigestion of the tissue.

Cerebral *infarction*, usually caused by focal vascular occlusion, is characterized histopathologically by necrosis of neurons, glia, and, in some areas, endothelial cells. Microscopically, neurons within the infarct appear eosinophilic, are shrunken, and have pyknotic nuclei. The histologic appearance of cerebral infarction differs from that of autolysis. Such differences probably reflect the permanent and complete loss of blood flow and the early release of lysosomal proteolytic enzymes in the autolytic tissue. Cerebral infarcts are frequently described as pale (anemic) despite the fact that microscopically most of them harbor extravasated red blood cells. Ischemic infarcts that show gross petechial hemorrhages are termed "hemorrhagic infarctions." The hemorrhagic areas lie most often along border zones of partially perfused tissue and occur most frequently with transient embolic occlusion followed by reperfusion of the infarcted vascular bed. Presumably, exposure of the necrotic tissue to the full pressure head of arterial blood leads to hemorrhage.

Transient arrest of the cerebral circulation (global ischemia) for periods of a few minutes causes *selective ischemic necrosis of neurons* (see Table 468–4) that are highly vulnerable to ischemia for unexplained reasons. Microscopically, these neurons evolve through several stages of "eosinophilic or ischemic cell change" and eventually appear shrunken and eosinophilic, containing darkly staining, pyknotic nuclei. Although such injury may be limited to only a small percentage of the total neuronal population, profound neurologic deficits manifested as cognitive impairment and/or movement disorders can be associated.

The time required for histologic changes to reach their maximum in areas of cerebral infarction differs markedly from the time course of injury encountered in selective ischemic necrosis of neurons. Infarction usually requires only a few hours before histologic stains sharply outline the distinct margins between living and dying neurons and glia. By contrast, selective ischemic necrosis of neurons evolves more slowly and sometimes requires several days or more to mature fully. For example, pyramidal neurons in the CA1 zone of the hippocampus remain histologically normal for 24 hours following cardiac arrest and require 48 hours or more before all of the cells that are destined to die show signs of irreversible injury. This delayed onset and the slow progression of injury following transient cerebral ischemia have important implications for potential therapies that may be initiated even after the onset of the ischemic insult.

Another distinctive neuropathologic lesion due to ischemia is *demyelination* of the central hemispheric white matter. Such injury is usually the consequence of carbon monoxide poisoning or other prolonged periods of moderately severe hypoxemia or cerebral hypoperfusion. Within these lesions, nerve cell axons are demyelinated, and there is generalized loss of oligodendroglial cells.

MOLECULAR MECHANISMS. In severely ischemic tissue—for example, the central ischemic vascular bed of an occluded MCA—energy-rich compounds remain sufficient to maintain normal function for only seconds, and glycogen, glucose, phosphocreatine, and ATP become depleted in a few minutes (see Table 468–2). Soon thereafter, the tissue begins to lose structural integrity. With the failure of energy-dependent membrane pumps, neuronal and glial cell membranes depolarize and allow the influx of Na^+ and Ca^{2+} ions and the efflux of K^+ ions. Elevated intracellular Ca^{2+} and other second messengers activate lipases and proteases, which in turn release membrane-bound free fatty acids and denature proteins. Depolarization of presynaptic terminals releases abnormally high concentrations of excitatory and inhibitory neurotransmitters, which may further exacerbate injury. If blood flow is restored in 15 to 30 minutes and no other complicating variables, such as hyperglycemia, are involved, most of these events are reversible, and only neurons selectively vulnerable to ischemia will die. If ischemia lasts hours

---

TABLE 468–4. ORDER OF DECREASING NEURONAL VULNERABILITY TO ANOXIA

Hippocampus
    CA1, CA4 > CA3 > granule cells
Cerebellum
    Purkinje > stellate and basket > granule > Golgi cells
Striatum
    Small and medium-sized > large neurons
Neocortex
    Layers 3,5,6 > layers 2,4

or more, cerebral infarction develops. What distinguishes ischemia-sensitive from ischemia-resistant neurons, why some of these neurons die rapidly, whereas others require days, and why glial cells are generally more resistant than neurons to ischemia remain challenging questions for basic research.

In contrast to the rapid cascade of events caused by severe ischemia, moderate ischemia triggers poorly defined mechanisms that sacrifice electrophysiologic activity to preserve brain structure, at least temporarily. Acute reduction of blood flow below one-half that of normal exceeds the capacity of compensatory mechanisms, such as increased O_2 and glucose extraction, to maintain normal synaptic function. The electroencephalogram (EEG) slows, and if ischemia is diffuse, the patient becomes confused, lethargic, or stuporous. The molecular mechanisms that suppress normal synaptic activity in the face of moderately compromised blood flow are unknown. Depletion of whole tissue energy reserves is not an explanation, since these remain normal, partly as a consequence of the decreased energy demand normally used to maintain membrane ion pumps and EEG activity. Some theorize that microregional reduction of the extracellular ATP concentration in the vicinity of the presynaptic terminals relieves the normal blockade of K^+ ion movement through ATP-sensitive K^+ channels and thereby hyperpolarizes the presynaptic membrane so as to inhibit synaptic transmission. With slightly greater ischemia, all synaptic activity ceases and the EEG becomes isoelectric. This too occurs with only partial depletion of high-energy stores, indicating that generalized energy failure cannot account for this early loss of synaptic activity. Prompt recovery of blood flow restores full function and structural integrity to the tissue. If moderate ischemia persists for several hours, however, irreversible injury will develop, probably as a consequence of compromised calcium homeostasis. Tissues with partial depletion of ATP and partial loss of calcium homeostasis may benefit from pharmacologic therapies that reduce calcium movement through voltage-dependent and neurotransmitter-dependent ion channels.

CEREBRAL EDEMA. Pathologic increases in the water content of the brain (edema) accompany all types of ischemic and hemorrhagic stroke. Brain swelling and raised intracranial pressure are proportionally related to the volume of the accumulated water; in many instances, they can cause neurologic deterioration and death by transtentorial herniation. Cerebral edema and herniation represent the immediate cause of death in one third of all ischemic and three quarters of all hemorrhagic strokes.

Brain edema is categorized on the basis of pathophysiologic and anatomic criteria as intracellular, interstitial, or periventricular. Intracellular edema, also called cytotoxic edema, represents an accumulation of intracellular osmoles and water causing cell swelling at the expense of the interstitial brain volume. Intracellular edema develops rapidly in ischemic brain tissue as energy-dependent membrane ion pumps fail and Na^+ ions and osmotically bound water derived from interstitial and the blood vascular compartment enter the cell. Cell swelling occurs predominantly in astrocytes, but neurons, oligodendroglial cells, and endothelial cells also are involved to a lesser degree. The osmolality of ischemic brain increases acutely from 310 mOsm to approximately 350 mOsm; 20 of these mOsm represent influx of ions, primarily Na^+. The identity of the remaining particles is unknown (idiogenic osmoles). The intracellular accumulation of water increases from a normal value of approximately 79 per cent to 81 per cent of brain weight. This 1 to 2 per cent increase in the volume of brain is insufficient in most instances to cause cerebral herniation. If cerebral circulation is re-established before permanent brain injury develops, intracellular brain edema resolves within a matter of hours without permanent sequelae.

Interstitial brain edema, also called vasogenic edema, is caused by the movement of large molecules and water from plasma into the interstitial spaces of the brain. Ischemia-induced damage to the endothelial cells making up the blood-brain barrier allows macromolecules such as plasma proteins to enter the interstitial space, carrying with them osmotically bound water. The bulk of this plasma filtrate accumulates preferentially in the interstitial spaces of the white matter. Interstitial brain edema that accompanies cerebral infarction progressively worsens for 3 to 4 days after a stroke. Fluid accumulation within the vicinity of damaged

endothelial cells and the zone of infarction can raise the local water content of brain by as much as 10 per cent. Such large volume increases can easily lead to transtentorial herniation and death.

Periventricular edema reflects the obstruction of cerebrospinal fluid (CSF) outflow pathways, the accumulation of CSF, and the transependymal movement of CSF into the white matter surrounding the periventricular regions. Such edema can be caused by intracerebral and subarachnoid hemorrhage if it interferes with CSF outflow pathways.

Barnett HJ, Stein BM, Mohr JP, et al. (eds.): Stroke: Pathophysiology, Diagnosis and Management. New York, Churchill Livingstone, 1986. *A comprehensive two-volume overview of all aspects of ischemic and hemorrhagic stroke.*

Caplan LR, Stein RW: Stroke: A Clinical Approach. Boston, Butterworths, 1986. *A pragmatic description of the diagnosis and treatment of stroke.*

Plum F, Pulsinelli WA: Cerebral metabolism in hypoxic-ischemic brain injury. In Asbury AK, McKann GM, McDonald IW (eds.): Diseases of the Nervous System. 2nd ed. Philadelphia, W.B. Saunders Company, 1992. *A contemporary review of the pathogenesis of ischemic injury to brain.*

Siesjo BK, Bengtsson F: Calcium fluxes, calcium antagonists, and calcium-related pathology in brain ischemia, hypoglycemia and spreading depression: A unifying hypothesis. J Cereb Blood Flow Metab 9:127, 1989. *A contemporary review of calcium homeostasis and the pathogenesis of calcium-related mechanisms in cerebral ischemia.*

West JB: Tolerance to severe hypoxia: Lessons from Mt. Everest. Acta Anaesth Scand 34(Suppl 94):18, 1990. *A description by the expedition leader of respiratory physiology and the effects of sustained hypoxemia during the ascent of Mt. Everest.*

469 Ischemic Cerebrovascular Disease

469.1 FOCAL ISCHEMIA

CLASSIFICATION

The clinical manifestations of focal ischemic stroke result from interference with blood circulation to the brain; the precise signs and symptoms depend on the region deprived of flow. For any brain region, however, focal ischemia can be classified into categories that have important pathologic and management implications.

STROKE VERSUS TRANSIENT ISCHEMIC ATTACK (TIA). *Stroke* is defined as a neurologic deficit lasting more than 24 hours caused by reduced blood flow in a particular artery supplying the brain. The usual pathologic outcome is infarction in the ischemic portion of the brain. A *transient ischemic attack,* or *TIA,* by contrast, is defined arbitrarily as a similar neurologic deficit lasting less than 24 hours. Originally, the time limit for transient neurologic deficits due to ischemia was less than 1 hour, but the definition was subsequently expanded to encompass events lasting up to 24 hours. Most TIA's resolve within an hour; thus once a deficit has lasted longer than an hour, it is likely to be classified as a presumptive stroke and is often associated with permanent brain injury. Computed tomographic (CT) brain scans frequently show cerebral infarction in areas affected by "TIA's" lasting longer than several hours. The relevant clinical distinction between a TIA and a stroke is whether the ischemia has caused brain damage (infarction or selective ischemic necrosis). Since no clear temporal threshold separates the two, decisions concerning the initiation of therapy and its type are unavoidably vague.

STABLE VERSUS UNSTABLE STROKES. Patients with *unstable strokes* are identifiable by either improvement or deterioration of their signs or symptoms. Deciding whether a stroke is unstable may be difficult, since in theory all strokes require some period to reach a stable maximum or minimum. The decision depends on an accurate history, on the interval between onset of symptoms and the first examination, and, later, on the frequency and duration of observation. Two thirds of patients with anterior circulation strokes and a higher number of those with vertebrobasilar strokes who are examined within a few hours of onset fluctuate in their signs and symptoms during the first week.

The identification of patients with worsening signs and symptoms, frequently referred to as *progressing stroke* or *stroke in evolution,* is particularly important, since if the cause can be identified, treatment to limit brain damage may be possible. The pathogenesis of progression may involve one or a combination of factors. Clot propagation has been suggested, but little direct evidence supports this conclusion. Other equally, if not more important, causes for progressing stroke include compromise of cardiac output due to myocardial ischemia, cardiac arrhythmias, and congestive heart failure. Systemic hypotension and increased blood viscosity can adversely affect the course of acute cerebral ischemia, as can associated pneumogenic hypoxemia or systemic electrolyte imbalance. Progression of cerebral edema, which usually maximizes by 3 to 4 days, contributes to neurologic deterioration with large strokes but not with smaller ones. Bleeding into the infarct affects as many as 40 per cent of patients but seldom causes new symptoms.

COMPLETE VERSUS INCOMPLETE STROKES. An important distinction is that made between a *complete* and an *incomplete stroke.* The terms refer to whether the affected vascular territory has been completely involved; if not, more brain remains at risk of additional focal ischemia, making treatment an urgent matter. The clinical distinction between complete and incomplete strokes can be difficult, especially soon after onset. As a practical matter, the distinction between a complete and incomplete stroke is often based on the severity of functional loss, for example, hemiplegia versus hemiparesis.

CLINICAL MANIFESTATIONS AND VASCULAR SYNDROMES
(Table 469–1)

INTERNAL CAROTID ARTERY. The carotid artery bifurcation and origin of the internal carotid artery provide the most frequent sites for atherothrombosis of cerebral blood vessels. Symptoms from such severe stenoses closely resemble those caused by middle cerebral artery disease (see below). Flow through the ophthalmic artery is often affected sufficiently to produce *transient monocular blindness* (also called amaurosis fugax). Severe bilateral internal carotid artery stenosis can sometimes cause cerebral hemispheric hypoperfusion and symptoms in *border zones* between the major vascular territories. Anterior circulation TIA's more frequently herald the presence of internal carotid artery disease than of intracranial atherosclerosis. Similarly, acute headache ipsilateral to an acutely ischemic hemi-

TABLE 469–1. CLINICAL MANIFESTATIONS OF ISCHEMIC STROKE

Occluded Blood Vessel*	Clinical Manifestations
ICA	Ipsilateral blindness (variable)
	MCA syndrome (see below)
MCA	Contralateral hemiparesis, sensory loss (arm, face worst)
	Expressive aphasia (dominant) or anosognosia and spatial disorientation (nondominant)
	Contralateral inferior quadrantanopsia
ACA	Contralateral hemiparesis, sensory loss (leg worst)
PCA	Contralateral homonymous hemianopsia or superior quadrantanopsia
	Memory impairment
Basilar apex	Bilateral blindness
	Amnesia
Basilar artery	Contralateral hemiparesis, sensory loss
	Ipsilateral bulbar and/or cerebellar signs
Vertebral artery and/or PICA	Ipsilateral loss of facial sensation, ataxia
	Contralateral hemiparesis, sensory loss
Superior cerebellar artery	Gait ataxia, nausea, dizziness, headache progressing to ipsilateral hemiataxia, dysarthria, gaze paresis
	Contralateral hemiparesis, somnolence

*ICA = internal carotid artery; MCA = middle cerebral artery; ACA = anterior cerebral artery; PCA = posterior cerebral artery; PICA = posterior inferior cerebellar artery.

sphere more frequently signals occlusion of the internal carotid artery than of the intracranial vessels.

ANTERIOR CEREBRAL ARTERY. Occlusion of one anterior cerebral artery (ACA) distal to the anterior communicating artery produces motor and cortical sensory symptoms in the contralateral leg and, less often, proximal arm. Other manifestations of ACA occlusion include gait ataxia and sometimes urinary incontinence from damage to the parasagittal frontal lobe. Language disturbances, manifested as decreased spontaneous speech, may accompany generalized depression of psychomotor activity. ACA occlusion does not typically cause paralysis of both legs, an acute syndrome more likely related to spinal cord disease or occlusion of the superior sagittal sinus, which drains the medial surfaces of both cerebral hemispheres.

ANTERIOR CHOROIDAL ARTERY. Brain image analyses suggest a clinical syndrome associated with occlusion of this vessel. Affected patients suffer a hemiparesis involving the face, arm, and leg; variable hemisensory loss; and in some instances hemianopsia from optic tract ischemia. The syndrome is difficult to distinguish from middle cerebral artery (MCA) ischemia.

MIDDLE CEREBRAL ARTERY. Most ischemic strokes involve part or all of the territory of the MCA, with emboli from the heart or extracranial carotid arteries accounting for most cases. Emboli may occlude the main stem of the MCA but more frequently produce distal occlusions of either the superior or the inferior branch. Occlusion of the superior branch causes weakness and sensory loss that are greatest in the face and arm; vision is spared, but an inferior quadrantanopsia may rarely coexist. Hemianopsias reported with MCA infarction more likely reflect hemineglect than true blindness, since deeply penetrating MCA branches supply only the dorsal, parietal half of the optic radiations. Voluntary gaze away from the side of the lesion may be impaired, but full-range oculocephalic or oculovestibular reflexes remain (Ch. 453.3). In the dominant hemisphere, the deficit includes an expressive (Broca's) aphasia with impaired fluency, naming, and writing, but relatively preserved comprehension. In the nondominant hemisphere, unilateral neglect, anosognosia (unawareness of the deficit), and spatial disorientation may be detected.

Occlusion of the inferior branches of the MCA infrequently produces sensory loss, most notably of integrated sensations, such as perception of shapes (stereognosis). In the dominant hemisphere, occlusion of the inferior division of the MCA causes receptive (Wernicke's) aphasia, with fluent speech characterized by jargon and paraphasias; comprehension, naming, reading, and writing are often abnormal.

The so-called deep MCA syndrome may occur from selective occlusion of the MCA main stem, causing ischemia in the territory of the lenticulostriate vessels but sparing the superior and inferior MCA branches. Collateral filling of the distal MCA cortical branches prevents cortical injury, but since the lenticulostriates are end-arteries, infarction of the deep MCA territory evolves. Alternatively, the lenticulostriates may be occluded by local atherosclerotic or hypertensive vascular disease. Patients with occlusion of the lenticulostriate arteries develop internal capsular infarction accompanied by hemiparesis or hemiplegia without visual, language, or sensory disturbances.

Proximal occlusions of the MCA may affect both superior and inferior branches as well as perforating branches to the internal capsule, optic radiations, and basal ganglia, thus resulting in contralateral hemiplegia, hemianesthesia, dense homonymous hemianopsia, and global aphasia with dominant or anosognosia with nondominant hemisphere involvement.

POSTERIOR CEREBRAL ARTERY. Occlusion of the posterior cerebral artery (PCA) distal to its penetrating branches most frequently causes complete contralateral loss of vision or a superior or inferior quadrantanopsia, depending upon whether the lower or the upper calcarine arteries are affected individually. Central (macular) vision may be spared owing to collateral supply from the MCA. If only the calcarine cortex is involved, the patient is usually aware of the vision loss, but denial of unilateral or bilateral blindness can ensue if one or both adjacent parietal cortices are affected (Ch. 449). Difficulty in reading (dyslexia) and performing calculations (dyscalculia) may follow ischemia of the dominant PCA territory.

Proximal occlusion of the PCA causes ischemia of penetrating branches (thalamogeniculate, thalamoperforating, posterior choroidal) to thalamic and limbic structures. The results are hemisensory disturbances that may chronically change to intractable pain on the defective side (thalamic pain). Memory dysfunction may result, especially with bilateral occlusions. With involvement of the subthalamic nucleus, wild, uncontrolled, flailing limb movements called hemiballism may develop (Ch. 461).

VERTEBRAL AND BASILAR ARTERIES. Focal brain stem ischemia produces a group of so-called "crossed syndromes" in which contralateral (pyramidal, spinothalamic, dorsal column) long-tract abnormalities (e.g., hemiparesis or hemisensory deficit) are accompanied by signs of ipsilateral cerebellar or brain stem nuclear dysfunction (e.g., ataxia, lower motor neuron facial weakness, third cranial nerve paresis). Occlusion of a vertebral artery and interference with flow through the ipsilateral *posterior inferior cerebellar artery* cause the *lateral medullary syndrome*, consisting of severe vertigo, nausea, vomiting, nystagmus, ipsilateral ataxia, and ipsilateral Horner's syndrome. There is an ipsilateral loss of facial pain and temperature sense and a contralateral loss of the same sensory modalities in trunk and limb. Discrete lesions in the distribution of the *anterior inferior cerebellar artery* are less common.

The *superior cerebellar artery* supplies most of the cerebellar cortex. Occlusion of this vessel is the most common cause of *cerebellar infarction*, characterized initially by gait ataxia, headache, nausea, vomiting, dizziness, ipsilateral clumsiness, and dysarthria. Subsequent brain swelling may induce ipsilateral gaze paresis and/or nystagmus toward the side of the infarction; ipsilateral facial weakness is sometimes seen. With further progression, lethargy and stupor deepen, and contralateral hemiparesis sometimes develops. Cerebellar edema formation can obstruct the fourth ventricle, producing hydrocephalus, and can result in herniation of the cerebellum either upward across the tentorium or downward through the foramen magnum (see Fig. 444–7).

Vertebrobasilar ischemia often produces multifocal lesions, scattered on both sides and along a considerable longitudinal extent of the brain stem. Except for cerebellar infarction and the lateral medullary syndrome, the clinical syndromes of discrete lesions are thus seldom seen in pure form. *Vertebrobasilar ischemia (VBI)* manifests with various combinations of symptoms such as dizziness (usually vertigo), diplopia, facial weakness, ataxia, and long-tract signs. Distinguishing mild VBI from more banal causes of dizziness can be difficult; the solution lies in identifying other, more specific symptoms or signs of parenchymal brain stem disease. Rarely does the person with VBI present with "dizziness" in the absence of other brain stem signs or symptoms.

Basilar artery occlusion produces massive deficits. The *locked-in state* is one possible consequence; in this condition, paralysis of the limbs and most of the bulbar muscles means that the patient can communicate only by moving the eyes or eyelids to command. Normal intelligence can often be demonstrated through codes involving eye movements. *Occlusion of the basilar apex* (or *top-of-the basilar*) is usually caused by emboli that lodge at the junction between the basilar artery and the two PCA's. The condition produces an initial reduction in arousal followed by blindness and amnesia (from interruption of flow into the PCA's) and abnormalities of vertical gaze and pupillary reactivity (from tegmental damage).

DIAGNOSIS

HISTORY. The history should emphasize the precise onset of the clinical deficit and the course since onset (stable or unstable). Preceding TIA's are more likely to be associated with an ischemic than a hemorrhagic stroke. Headache more often occurs with hemorrhage and embolus than with atherothrombotic ischemic stroke. The possibility of other diagnoses (e.g., hypoglycemia or seizures) should be considered. A thorough search for vascular disease risk factors (see below) should be made in the initial evaluation, since their presence will strengthen the likelihood of an ischemic stroke and influence eventual management.

PHYSICAL EXAMINATION. The neurologic examination serves to localize the lesion site, but the general medical examination more frequently provides clues to pathogenesis. Specific attention should be given to the cardiovascular examination and to evidence of hematologic disease. The arterial blood pressure in both arms, cardiac rhythm, and other cardiac abnormalities, such as murmurs or opening snaps, should be carefully recorded. The vascular examination should include gentle palpation and auscultation (with a bell-type stethoscope) of the carotid arteries in the neck and sometimes also orbital auscultation. Ophthalmoscopy can detect retinal cholesterol or platelet-fibrin emboli as well as evidence of chronic hypertensive or diabetic disease. The presence of retinal hypertensive changes can indicate that hypertension has been chronic rather than transiently stroke associated. Except with posterior circulation insufficiency or previous strokes, loss of consciousness or confusion should prompt consideration of other diagnoses.

LABORATORY EXAMINATION. *Hematologic Tests.* These include a complete blood count and platelet count (to evaluate for polycythemia, thrombocytosis, bacterial endocarditis, and severe anemia); blood for glucose, prothrombin time, and partial thromboplastin time; and a lipid profile. In the elderly, determination of the erythrocyte sedimentation rate should be performed urgently to exclude giant cell arteritis; in the young, the presence of antiphospholipid antibodies helps to identify immune-related disease processes predisposing to stroke. Other blood tests (e.g., protein C, protein S, measurements of viscosity or platelet function, and tests for collagen vascular diseases) may be indicated in younger patients without other obvious causes for their strokes. The rising incidence of syphilis in urban areas makes a serum VDRL desirable. Tests of renal function and serum electrolyte measurements help to establish systemic illnesses as well as the milieu in which subsequent diagnostic tests (e.g., contrast injection) and treatments might be offered.

Cardiovascular Examination. All stroke patients require a standard 12-lead electrocardiogram (ECG) and rhythm strip at admission to exclude acute myocardial ischemia and arrhythmias. Authorities disagree over whether one should search with echocardiography for a cardiogenic source of emboli in acute focal stroke, since the yield is low in patients who have no history or physical evidence of cardiac disease. Our practice is to employ two-dimensional echocardiography or, less often, transesophageal echocardiography in patients with focal stroke who are (1) young; (2) have no detectable atherothrombosis of the appropriate extracranial vessel, regardless of age; and (3) have no detectable risk factors, including polycythemia or oral contraceptive use. In suitable patients, *stress testing* during convalescence may be recommended to evaluate possible ischemic cardiovascular disease.

Brain Imaging. Although routine blood, urine, and ECG analyses are obtained immediately upon hospital admission, brain imaging is the most important differential diagnostic test to identify other causes of focal neurologic dysfunction, such as neoplasms or subdural hematomas, and to distinguish ischemic from hemorrhagic stroke. CT scanning, the most commonly used imaging technique, has limitations that must be considered. CT cannot always detect cerebral infarction; the size, location, and age of the lesion affect the lesion's visibility. Infarcts less than 5 mm in diameter often escape detection, especially within the brain stem, where bone artifact may interfere with resolution. Further, only about 5 per cent are visible on CT scan within the first 12 hours; detection increases to approximately 50 per cent between 24 and 48 hours and approximately 90 per cent by the end of 1 week.

Infarcts appear as hypodense areas on non–contrast-enhanced CT scans with increasingly well demarcated margins as edema peaks between 3 and 5 days (Fig. 469–1). Contrast-enhancing agents carry a small risk of neurotoxicity, and they may normalize the CT density of an otherwise small hypodense infarct, making the infarct less visible. Accordingly, one should use contrast-enhancing agents during the acute phase of the ischemic stroke only to seek out a mass lesion and only after a noncontrast scan has been obtained.

CT scans immediately delineate primary cerebral hemorrhage, but hemorrhagic conversions of an ischemic infarct usually develop only after 1 to 2 days (Fig. 469–1), and a few continue to appear for up to 4 weeks.

Magnetic resonance imaging (MRI) is more sensitive than CT

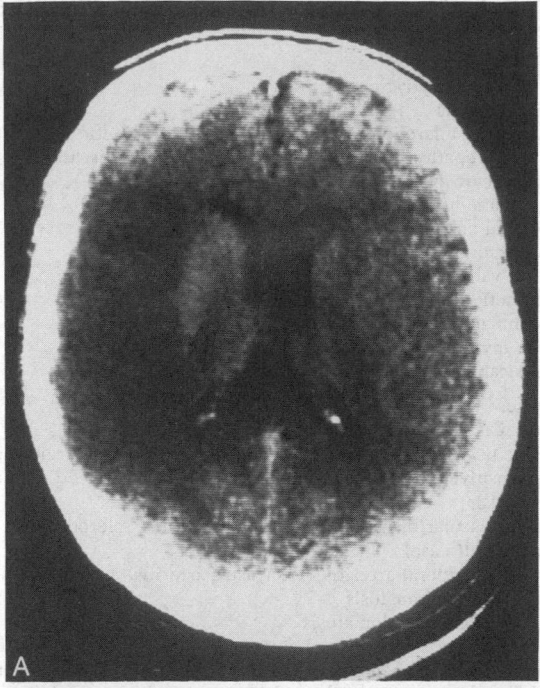

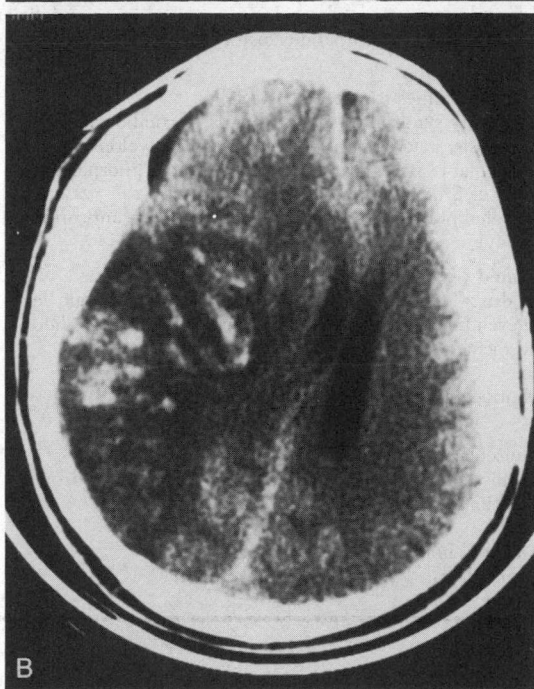

FIGURE 469–1. Right middle cerebral artery distribution infarctions shown on computed tomography (CT) at 24 hours. In *A*, hypodensity on the left side of the figure represents an ischemic infarction; in *B*, inhomogeneous areas of increased density interspersed with decreased density and mass effect on the left side of the figure represent a hemorrhagic infarction. This inhomogeneity distinguishes hemorrhagic infarction from primary brain hemorrhage (compare with Fig. 470–3).

to changes in tissue structure and may provide a more accurate and earlier measure of cerebral infarction. MRI, however, is more costly, and, with the present equipment, requires more time to perform than CT; in addition, the need to exclude ferromagnetic materials from the MRI suite, as well as the difficulty in monitoring patients in the scanner, makes MRI unsuitable for many acutely ill patients. If the diagnosis remains in doubt, MRI may be used after the acute phase to verify infarction.

Lumbar Puncture. Lumbar puncture (LP) is no longer widely used in routine stroke diagnosis because noninvasive CT or MRI detects cerebral hemorrhage and anticoagulation begun within 6 hours after a lumbar puncture risks causing a spinal epidural hematoma. An LP is important, however, in diagnosing neurosyphilis or meningitis, as, for example, in patients with acute stiff neck who show no blood on brain imaging. If an LP is to be done in those suspected of having had a stroke, it should be preceded by funduscopic examination and brain imaging if possible to rule out raised intracranial pressure.

Noninvasive Cerebrovascular Examination. Several noninvasive techniques help to evaluate the cerebrovascular supply. Indirect tests that examine blood flow in the periorbital or orbital circulation include *Doppler sonography* and *quantitative oculopneumoplethysmography* (OPG). Periorbital Doppler sonography measures the amplitude of pulsations and the direction of blood flow in the periorbital arteries. Normally, blood flows from the intracranial vault to the skin surface. In severe internal carotid artery disease, blood flow reversal can be detected by Doppler sonography. Quantitative OPG measures the systolic blood pressure and amplitude of pulsations in the ophthalmic artery. Internal carotid artery stenosis is detected by comparing the values between the eyes or the eye and the systemic systolic blood pressure. Both Doppler sonography and OPG do not easily distinguish between severe stenosis and occlusion of the internal carotid artery, and neither technique readily detects a less than 60 per cent stenosis of the artery.

Direct examination of the common, internal, and external carotid arteries is best achieved with *duplex ultrasonography*. Duplex ultrasonography consists of B-mode ultrasonography, which produces a real-time image of the carotid vessels and a range-gaited pulsed Doppler that is visually guided by the B-mode image to measure the frequency shift associated with increased blood velocity through a stenotic lumen. The combination of the precise location of the Doppler frequency signal and the B-mode image provides the most accurate noninvasive method for analyzing disease of the extracranial circulation. Limitations of the technique include (1) access to only the portion of the carotid circulation that lies between the clavicles and the mandible (in approximately 10 per cent of patients, the carotid bifurcation lies above the angle of the jaw, making ultrasonography difficult or impossible); (2) absorption of sound waves by calcium within a mural plaque, which may "shadow" and obscure a plaque on a distal vessel wall; and (3) echolucency of acute thrombi, which can be indistinguishable from flowing blood.

The direction and velocity of blood flow in the intracranial blood vessels originating from the circle of Willis may be examined with low-frequency *pulsed transcranial Doppler*, a technique still being evaluated for its usefulness as a diagnostic tool. The intracranial blood vessels can also be examined on reconstructed CT or MRI images. A still experimental technique involves the imaging of flowing blood using *magnetic resonance angiography*. The procedure produces images of the extracranial and intracranial blood vessels, as well as atherosclerotic abnormalities of the carotid bifurcation; some aneurysms can also be detected. Several different software programs are currently being evaluated, and the procedure remains investigational.

Cerebral Angiography. Intracranial and extracranial *cerebral angiography* of elderly patients prone to ischemic stroke carries a 2 to 4 per cent risk of producing a reversible neurologic deficit and a 0.5 to 1.0 per cent risk of permanent neurologic deficits or death. Accordingly, angiography should be reserved for specific indications in which it may reveal abnormalities amenable to therapy. Examples include a search for fibromuscular dysplasia, arterial dissection, or cranial arteritis or a preparation for cerebrovascular surgery. *Digital subtraction arteriography* permits use of smaller amounts of intravascular contrast material and may thus be of lower risk, especially in patients with marginal renal or cardiac function. *Digital subtraction venous angiography* is no longer widely used because of its unreliability in detecting plaque ulcerations and in differentiating carotid stenosis from complete occlusion.

Other Techniques. Methods for measuring CBF are still largely investigational; they include *positron emission tomographic (PET)* methods, usually using radiolabeled water or carbon dioxide; *single-photon emission computed tomography (SPECT);* and radiolabeled and stable *xenon* inhalation techniques.

DIFFERENTIAL DIAGNOSIS OF ISCHEMIC STROKES AND TIA'S

The clinical diagnosis of ischemic or hemorrhagic stroke relies primarily on the clinician's understanding of brain function and pathology. Deficits that evolve over weeks are usually caused by a brain mass, either *primary or metastatic brain tumor* or *brain abscess. Subdural hematoma* should be distinguishable from stroke by the hematoma's more prolonged course and its combination of diffuse and focal dysfunction.

TIA's may be confused with classic or complicated *migraine,* the former being associated with scintillating scotomata and the latter with hemiparesis or other focal deficits; some of the underlying pathophysiology may be ischemic for both TIA's and migraine, but evidence is accumulating that nonischemic electrical disturbances (spreading depression) are involved in the pathophysiology of migraine.

Seizures can be confused with TIA's. Most such seizures produce motor activity or positive sensory phenomena, whereas most strokes and TIA's produce weakness and sensory loss, but seizures can sometimes produce these "negative" symptoms. The postictal state following (unobserved) seizures is even more likely to imitate an ischemic deficit. Serial observations usually permit the rapid differential diagnosis of stroke versus seizure, but prompt differentiation may be difficult and may interfere with early stroke treatment. As with migraine, stroke and seizure can coexist: A small proportion of strokes (about 10 per cent), especially embolic strokes, are associated at onset with seizures.

Hemorrhagic stroke often enters the differential diagnosis for ischemic stroke. Although the anatomic locations of the two may differ, with hemorrhage seldom involving a discrete vascular territory, clinical differentiation can be uncertain, making CT scan necessary. Other illnesses included in the differential diagnosis of vertebrobasilar ischemia include, as mentioned above, nonspecific dizziness, Ménière's disease, or peripheral vestibulopathy.

CAUSES AND PATHOGENESIS (Table 469–2)

ATHEROSCLEROSIS. Atherosclerosis of extracranial and intracranial arteries accounts for approximately two thirds of all ischemic strokes and an even greater proportion of those affecting patients over the age of 60. Atherosclerosis causes strokes either by *in situ stenosis* or *occlusion* or by *embolization* of plaque material to distal cerebral vessels. In either case, the clinical and pathologic effects depend on the adequacy of collateral circulation to the affected vascular territory. It is not uncommon for unilateral or, more rarely, bilateral occlusion of the internal carotid artery to develop without neurologic symptoms, especially if the stenosis or occlusion develops slowly. In instances of marked stenosis or occlusion of extracranial arteries that is combined with intracranial atherosclerosis, cerebral perfusion occasionally can relate closely to small changes in perfusion pressure. One effect can be a worsening stroke deficit associated with orthostatic blood pressure changes that would otherwise be considered normal.

The more common effect of atherosclerosis is that a plateletfibrin embolus detaches from a plaque and floats distally, where it occludes a smaller branch. Such emboli are likely to produce symptoms, since the more distal the occlusion, the less likely can collateral filling prevent damage. In these cases of artery-toartery embolization, the embolus usually emanates from a plaque at the bifurcation of the common carotid artery or at the point where the vertebral arteries originate from the subclavian arteries.

EMBOLI OF CARDIAC ORIGIN. Cerebral emboli of a cardiac source may account for up to one third of all ischemic strokes. Thrombus formation and the release of thromboemboli from the heart are promoted by arrhythmias and structural abnormalities of the heart valves and chambers.

Mural Thrombi. Mural thrombi typically form under areas of dyskinetic myocardium damaged by *myocardial infarction.* As many as 35 per cent of patients with recent anterior wall infarction harbor mural thrombi, and if not anticoagulated, nearly 40 per cent of these embolize systemically within 4 months after the myocardial infarction. *Cardiomyopathies* can also predispose to mural thrombi and embolization. They are defined as diseases of

TABLE 469–2. CAUSES OF ISCHEMIC STROKES

Atherosclerosis

Emboli of Cardiac Origin
 Mural thrombus
  Myocardial infarction (anterior wall septum, akinetic segment)
  Cardiomyopathy (infectious, idiopathic, Chagas' disease)
 Valvular heart disease
  Rheumatic heart disease
  Bacterial endocarditis
  Nonbacterial endocarditis (carcinoma, Libman-Sacks)
  Mitral valve prolapse
  Prosthetic valve
 Arrhythmia (atrial fibrillation)
 Cardiac myxoma
 Paradoxical emboli

Vasculitides
 Primary CNS vasculitis
 Systemic necrotizing vasculitis (polyarteritis nodosa, allergic angiitis)
 Hypersensitivity vasculitis (serum sickness, drug-induced, cutaneous vasculitis)
 Collagen vascular diseases (rheumatoid arthritis, scleroderma, Sjögren's disease)
 Giant cell (temporal arteritis, Takayasu's arteritis)
 Wegener's granulomatosis
 Lymphomatoid granulomatosis
 Behçet's disease
 Infectious vasculitis (neurovascular syphilis, Lyme disease, bacterial and fungal meningitis, tuberculosis, acquired immunodeficiency syndrome [AIDS], ophthalmic zoster, hepatitis B)

Hematologic Disorders
 Hemoglobinopathies (sickle cell, HbSC)
 Hyperviscosity syndromes (polycythemia, thrombocytosis, leukocytosis, macroglobulinemia, multiple myeloma)
 Hypercoagulable states (carcinoma, pregnancy, puerperium)
 Protein C or S deficiency
 Antiphospholipid antibodies (lupus anticoagulant, anticardiolipin antibody)

Drug Related
 "Street drugs" (cocaine, "crack," amphetamines, lysergic acid, phencyclidine, methylphenidate, sympathomimetics, heroin, pentazocine)
 Alcohol
 Oral contraceptives

Other
 Fibromuscular dysplasia
 Arterial dissection (trauma, spontaneous, Marfan's syndrome)
 Homocystinuria
 Migraine
 Subarachnoid hemorrhage/vasospasm
 Other emboli (fat, bone marrow, air emboli)
 Moyamoya

the myocardium of variable, often unknown, cause and usually are characterized by cardiac enlargement, systemic embolism, and conduction abnormalities or arrhythmias. In one study, systemic emboli were found in approximately 15 per cent of patients with congestive or dilated cardiomyopathy, a subgroup of the condition that is usually caused by alcohol abuse or viral infections. Patients who also had atrial fibrillation had a higher incidence of embolism (33 per cent) than did those without (14 per cent). As a note of therapeutic importance, none of the cardiomyopathy patients on anticoagulation had systemic emboli.

Valvular Heart Disease. Although less common than previously, *rheumatic heart disease* often gives rise to systemic embolization. In one series, 20 to 25 per cent of patients with mitral stenosis developed systemic emboli, although most had coexisting atrial fibrillation.

Acute or subacute *infective endocarditis* produces vegetations on heart valves, debris that can embolize into the cerebral circulation. Many emboli are relatively small, but those associated with endocarditis caused by staphylococcus, fungi, or yeast often are large enough to occlude proximal intracranial arteries. In autopsy series, systemic emboli are found in as many as 30 per cent of patients with infective endocarditis. Prompt recognition of the heart lesion based on the presence of fever, a murmur, petechiae, and other characteristics, such as Osler's nodes and Roth spots, in patients with underlying valvular disease or intravenous drug use should prompt blood cultures and treatment with antibiotics to reduce the risk of embolism. Anticoagulation is not effective and may even increase the risk of parenchymal bleeding. Infective endocarditis is associated with other forms of cerebrovascular disease, including cerebral hemorrhage, subarachnoid hemorrhage, and mycotic aneurysm, as well as cerebral abscess.

Embolization from heart valves also occurs in *nonbacterial endocarditis (NBTE)*, in which predominantly platelet-fibrin vegetations form on the heart valves and then embolize into the systemic circulation. NBTE occurs commonly in association with cancer of the stomach, prostate, ovary, pancreas, and lung. In one autopsy series of patients with NBTE, cerebral emboli were found in one third. Clinically, diffuse encephalopathy as well as focal stroke is observed; associated disseminated intravascular coagulation accompanies about 20 per cent of cases.

Libman-Sacks (atypical verrucous) endocarditis is associated with systemic lupus erythematosus. In this condition, soft, friable vegetations form on the leaflets of any of the heart valves, not just the tricuspid valve, as believed earlier. Systemic (and cerebral) emboli are rare.

Mitral valve prolapse describes a billowing of the mitral leaflets into the left atrium during systole. Although usually asymptomatic, some patients experience palpitations or chest pain. The diagnosis is suggested by auscultatory and echocardiographic criteria, but normal standards are uncertain, making the true incidence of the condition unknown; it is estimated to be 6 to 10 per cent in healthy, young women. In part because of different diagnostic criteria, the role of mitral valve prolapse in cerebral embolism remains controversial: Several analyses of strokes in young adults suggest a disproportionately high representation of patients with mitral valve prolapse, but others indexed on patients with mitral valve prolapse suggest that systemic embolism is infrequent. In one of these latter studies, however, the risk of cerebral embolism was 5 to 10 per cent. Coexisting infective endocarditis or arrhythmia contributes to cerebral embolism.

Prosthetic heart valves carry a high risk of systemic (including cerebral) embolism, mechanical heart valves having a higher risk than biologic valves (e.g., porcine). The overall risk of embolism is roughly equivalent in anticoagulated patients with mechanical valves and in nonanticoagulated patients with biologic valves: 1 to 3 per cent per year for aortic prostheses, and 3 to 5 per cent per year for mitral substitutions.

Arrhythmias. *Atrial fibrillation,* with or without valvular disease, strongly increases the risk of embolic ischemic stroke, especially in patients over the age of 60. In one large series, the risk of ischemic stroke was 6 to 7 per cent per year. The risk is highest shortly after development of atrial fibrillation: Up to one third of emboli occur in the first month. Embolism can also accompany therapeutic cardioversion. About 35 per cent of patients with nonvalvular atrial fibrillation sooner or later will have an ischemic stroke. In some, embolism underlies the stroke; in others, the fault lies in coexisting intrinsic cerebrovascular disease associated with coronary artery disease. Even thyrotoxic, nonvalvular atrial fibrillation is associated with a 10 to 12 per cent risk of stroke. The one group without a strikingly increased risk is patients with lone atrial fibrillation, meaning those without other clinical evidence of cardiopulmonary disease.

Cardiac Myxoma. Cardiac tumors are uncommon, occurring in about 0.05 per cent of autopsies. *Myxomas* account for about 35 per cent of all intracardiac tumors but are the ones most likely to embolize, from either overlying thrombus or the tumor itself. In one series, about one quarter of patients with autopsy-proven cardiac myxomas had clinical evidence of strokes. Aneurysms and intracranial hemorrhage were also reported. The coexistence of hemolytic anemia due to red blood cell trauma and lysis sometimes suggests a cardiac tumor, but firm diagnosis requires echocardiography or angiography.

Paradoxical Emboli. Emboli of venous origin have long been known to cross a patent foramen ovale into the systemic circulation. Recent evidence employing bubble echocardiography found that 40 per cent of stroke patients under age 55 with a normal cardiac evaluation by history, examination, and ECG had a patent foramen ovale detected by bubble echocardiography.

VASCULITIDES. A group of disorders classified as vasculitides cause focal or multifocal cerebral ischemia through inflammation and necrosis of extracranial and/or intracranial blood vessels. The pathogenesis of vascular inflammation differs among these disorders, but all involve, to some degree, deposition of humoral and cellular immune complexes and infiltration of polymorphonuclear and mononuclear cells in blood vessel walls. In most cases, the cause of the inflammatory response is unknown, but in others, infection, a postinfectious or neoplastic process, or a hypersensitivity immune reaction triggers the inflammation.

Segmental inflammation of cerebral blood vessels causes cerebral ischemia acutely at the site of involvement through platelet aggregation and/or clot formation or chronically through fibrinoid necrosis, which narrows the vessel lumen. Central nervous system (CNS) vasculitis, although a rare cause of stroke, is itself not uncommon and should enter the differential diagnosis whenever a young patient presents with a stroke or a patient of any age presents with a diffuse encephalopathy.

Symptoms of CNS vasculitis include cognitive disturbances, headache, and seizures (encephalopathy), which occur more frequently than with focal neurologic dysfunction. The differentiation from other causes of encephalopathy depends on the angiographic appearance of a "beadlike" segmental narrowing of cerebral blood vessels and/or the finding of characteristic inflammatory histopathology in leptomeningeal and cortical biopsy specimens. Cerebral angiograms may appear normal in 20 to 30 per cent of histologically positive cases of cerebral vasculitis. In addition, because of the segmental or "skip" nature of the inflammatory response, the histopathology may go undetected in the presence of a positive angiogram.

The diagnosis of CNS vasculitis is aided by the presence or absence of peripheral nervous system or systemic organ involvement and by identifying the underlying cause of the inflammation. Primary CNS vasculitis, Behçet's disease, Takayasu's arteritis, and temporal arteritis are notable for their infrequent involvement or noninvolvement of the peripheral nervous system. By contrast, the hypersensitivity and systemic necrotizing vasculitides frequently produce polyneuropathies.

Primary CNS arteritis, giant cell arteritis, and vasculitis associated with certain CNS infections deserve specific attention, since these may present initially or solely with neurologic signs and symptoms.

Primary CNS Arteritis. Primary arteritis of the CNS, also called granulomatous arteritis of the CNS, causes headache and other encephalopathic-like symptoms in young or middle-aged individuals. The course is usually insidiously progressive but may wax and wane for periods of several months. It is a diagnosis of exclusion.

Giant Cell Vasculitis. *Temporal arteritis* and *Takayasu's arteritis* are characterized by a granulomatous vasculitis of medium-sized and large arteries. Temporal arteritis affects predominantly patients over the age of 60, causing constitutional symptoms such as fever, malaise, weight loss, and headache. In half of the patients, symptoms consistent with polymyalgia rheumatica may coexist, including jaw, neck, and facial pain, as well as morning stiffness. Tenderness and pain over the temporal arteries and an elevated erythrocyte sedimentation rate are frequently, but not always, present. Biopsy of the superficial temporal artery provides the definitive diagnosis. Because of the segmental nature of the vasculitis, serial sections should be examined. Even then, typical features of fever, malaise, tender scalp vessels, and a grossly elevated sedimentation rate dictate the early initiation of corticosteroid therapy because of the high risk of acute ischemic blindness. A *dramatic* response to therapy is semidiagnostic.

Takayasu's arteritis affects primarily young women and involves mainly the aortic arch, the large brachiocephalic arteries derived from the arch, and the abdominal aorta. Mononuclear infiltrates and fibrous proliferation produce progressive narrowing of the lumen of these vessels, causing reduced flow into the upper extremities (hence the name "pulseless disease") and cerebral ischemia. Although initially diagnosed in Japanese women, in recent years its recognition in Western countries has led to more frequent diagnosis.

Infectious Vasculitis. Bacterial, fungal, and viral infections can induce CNS vasculitis and cerebral ischemia (Table 469-2). Neurosyphilis and its meningovascular complications have increased considerably in recent years (see Ch. 472) and should be considered in patients with atypical or unexplained cerebrovascular disease.

HEMATOLOGIC ABNORMALITIES. *Hemoglobinopathy.* Among the hemoglobinopathies, *sickle cell disease* is by far the most common cause of stroke. In sickle cell disease, a single substitution of the amino acid valine for glutamate at the sixth position of the β-globin molecule causes the mutant molecule HbSS to become highly insoluble and polymerize under deoxygenated conditions. The polymerization alters the erythrocyte's shape ("sickling") and decreases the cell's deformability, leading to increased blood viscosity, microvascular sludging, and microvascular infarction. Sickle cell disease also causes hyperplasia of fibrous tissue and muscle cells of the vascular intima, leading to stenosis and occlusion of some medium-sized to large cerebral arteries.

Ischemic stroke occurs in approximately 15 per cent of patients with HbSS and in a much smaller percentage of those with sickle cell trait (HbSA) or HbSC. At normal arterial oxygen saturations of 95 to 100 per cent in HbSS, some sickling is present, and at 65 per cent, i.e., just slightly lower than normal venous oxygen saturation, approximately 75 per cent of erythrocytes sickle. Ischemic stroke arises most frequently in children, whereas hemorrhagic stroke is more common in adults with HbSS; subarachnoid hemorrhage in patients with sickle cell disease is frequently the result of a ruptured saccular aneurysm.

Small changes in oxygen tension, dehydration, acidosis, or infection can precipitate sickle cell crisis and stroke. Cerebral angiography causes an increased risk for patients with sickle cell disease. In instances when such angiography is necessary to evaluate the source of intracerebral hemorrhage, the level of HbSS should be reduced to less than 20 per cent through transfusions.

Hyperviscosity Syndrome. Cerebral blood flow is inversely related to blood viscosity. The latter is directly proportional to the number of circulating red and white blood cells, the aggregation state, the number of platelets, and the plasma protein concentration. Blood flow is inversely proportional to the deformability of erythrocytes and blood velocity (shear rate). Patients with the hyperviscosity syndrome can present either with focal neurologic dysfunction or, more frequently, with diffuse or multifocal signs or symptoms, including headache, visual disturbances, cognitive impairment, and seizures.

Cellular hyperviscosity, associated with *polycythemia, thrombocytosis,* or *leukocytosis* of any cause, can reduce CBF below threshold levels for cerebral dysfunction and injury. Hematocrits above 50 per cent, white cell counts greater than 150,000 per microliter, and platelet counts in excess of 1 million per microliter increase the risk of stroke.

Elevated plasma protein concentrations caused by *macroglobulinemia* or *multiple myeloma* elevate plasma viscosity and increase stroke risk. Approximately 25 per cent of patients with macroglobulinemia experience some form of cerebral ischemia, and a lesser number of patients with multiple myeloma experience the hyperviscosity syndrome. Of the various forms of multiple myeloma, those with a predominance of immunoglobulin A (IgA) most frequently develop a hyperviscosity syndrome because this particular molecule is likely to form high molecular weight polymers.

Hypercoagulable States. Cancer, particularly the adenocarcinomas, pregnancy, and the puerperium have all been associated with a "hypercoagulable state" that predisposes to arterial and venous thrombosis. Despite the fact that any one of several abnormalities, including elevations of fibrinogen levels, alterations of partial thromboplastin or prothrombin times, and platelet aggregation, occurs in the hypercoagulable state, no tests have been devised to diagnose it specifically.

Protein C or S Deficiency. Proteins C and S are two naturally occurring anticoagulants synthesized in the liver via vitamin K–dependent mechanisms. Deficiencies of either are rare, dominantly inherited, and expressed phenotypically by incomplete penetrance. Homozygotes develop serious and frequently fatal clotting abnormalities at birth, while heterozygotes may show no signs of hypercoagulability. Proteins C and S act in concert to inactivate the activated coagulating Factors V and VIII; protein

C also triggers the endogenous fibrinolytic pathways. Deficiencies in either are associated with ischemic vascular disease. Because of incomplete penetrance, the occurrence of thrombosis and stroke in the adult is extremely rare.

Antiphospholipid Antibodies. A strong epidemiologic association links a group of antiphospholipid antibodies to cerebral ischemia manifested clinically as atypical migraine, TIA, recurrent strokes, or ischemic encephalopathy. These antibodies bind to membrane phospholipids and include anticardiolipin antibody, the lupus anticoagulant, and antibodies causing a false-positive VDRL. The pathogenetic relationship between the antibodies and enhanced cerebral thrombosis is unknown. The syndrome may manifest at any age but usually affects patients less than 50 years old. Antiphospholipid antibodies often accompany collagen vascular disease, especially systemic lupus erythematosus, as well as valvular heart disease. Circulating titers of phospholipid antibodies correlate poorly with either the incidence or the severity of cerebral ischemia.

DRUG-RELATED CAUSES OF STROKE. An extensive list of "street" drugs (Table 469–2) has been associated with stroke, reflecting as much the social patterns of drug abuse as the unique properties of the drugs themselves. The sharing of nonsterile needles to inject many of these drugs intravenously (e.g., heroin, cocaine) may precipitate infectious processes (bacterial endocarditis, hepatitis B, mycotic aneurysms) that lead to strokes. Several of the drugs are potent vasoconstrictors and may initiate cerebral vasospasm. Others have been associated with cerebral vasculitis caused either by immune responses to the primary drug or by hypersensitivity to contaminating adulterants. The intravenous injection of oral medications (pentazocine [Talwin], methylphenidate [Ritalin]) that have been crushed and suspended in water for intravenous injection can cause cerebral microemboli from particles of talc and cellulose used as ingredients in the pills. These particles are thought to be trapped by pulmonary arterioles, causing local arteritis and later arteriovenous shunts that allow the microemboli to reach the CNS.

Over-the-counter cold remedies and nasal decongestants containing sympathomimetics such as ephedrine, phenylpropanolamine, and phenoxazoline have been associated with ischemic stroke. Cases have been reported following the prolonged use of oral cold medications as well as in patients who chronically overuse nasal decongestants.

The risk of ischemic and hemorrhagic stroke is increased from 4- to 13-fold among users of high-dose estrogen contraceptives. The coexistence of hypertension, prolonged use of the pill, smoking, a previous history of migraine, and age exceeding 35 years seems to enhance the risk of contraceptive-related stroke. A clear association between stroke and the newer low-dose estrogen contraceptives has not been established.

OTHER CAUSES OF STROKE. *Fibromuscular dysplasia* (or hyperplasia) describes areas of segmental nonatherosclerotic arterial narrowing, usually caused by fibroplasia and smooth muscle proliferation, that alternate with rings of medial thinning. The condition affects the carotid and vertebral arteries, usually at the level of the second cervical vertebra rather than at the origin of the vessels; it also affects the renal arteries and is associated, therefore, with hypertension. Fibromuscular dysplasia predominates in women and occurs, on the average, in the sixth decade of life. The condition is uncommon: In one angiographic series, fibromuscular dysplasia was identified in fewer than 1 per cent of vessels studied. It produces ischemic stroke both by the hemodynamic effects of stenosis and by thromboembolism. The condition is also associated with aneurysm formation and with arterial dissection. Angiography usually enables one to make the diagnosis, although flow studies with MRI may prove increasingly useful. Because of its rarity, there is little information about treatment.

A *dissecting aortic aneurysm,* although uncommon, can occlude major branches of the aorta supplying the cranial circulation and produce ischemic strokes. Chest, back, or abdominal pain accompanying the stroke and differences in palpable pulses or in blood pressure in the limbs suggest the diagnosis. Emergency angiography is needed to confirm it.

Extracranial *dissections of the carotid artery* are increasingly recognized. Many follow relatively trivial trauma (e.g., pharyngeal injury with blunt objects in children and neck torsion, sometimes from chiropractic manipulation, in adults). Some are associated with fibromuscular dysplasia, others with a variety of childhood conditions, including Ehlers-Danlos and Marfan's syndromes as well as tuberous sclerosis. Pathologically, intraluminal blood enters the subintimal or medial vascular planes, and the lumen becomes progressively narrowed and thrombosed. Carotid artery dissections can sometimes be recognized clinically by intense ipsilateral pain. Angiography may be needed for diagnosis, but MRI is sometimes sufficient.

Homocystinuria is characterized by dislocated ocular lenses, bone deformities, a marfanoid appearance, mental retardation, accelerated atherosclerosis, and arterial or venous thromboses. Several different genetic defects can cause homocystinuria, but the most frequent is a deficiency of the enzyme cystathionine β-synthase. The pathogenesis of accelerated atherosclerosis and enhanced thrombosis associated with homocystinuria is unknown, but approximately one third of affected individuals have one or more strokes by the age of 15 years. In some studies, heterozygous homocystinuria has been reported in as many as one quarter of young persons who have suffered strokes. Treatment with pyridoxine or folic acid may limit disease progression.

Reactive vascular narrowing (*vasospasm*) causes ischemic strokes in two settings. One causes substantial disability in *subarachnoid hemorrhage* (Ch. 470.1). Vasospasm also presumably explains ischemic strokes seen in a small number of patients with *migraine* headaches. Migraineurs develop ischemic strokes, either in conjunction with migraine (in which case they appear to result from a prolonged migraine attack) or remote from the attack (in which case more traditional stroke mechanisms, such as atherosclerosis, are likely to be responsible).

Fat emboli typically occur several days after trauma and fracture of the long bones. Although focal ischemic strokes may occur, more typically the condition manifests with seizures and a diffuse encephalopathy consistent with disseminated embolization. Associated findings include petechiae and fat emboli visible on funduscopic examination. Fat globules may be identified in urine or CSF.

Air emboli can occur with open heart surgery, in patients with pneumothorax, or in divers who ascend too rapidly to the surface. Like fat emboli, air emboli cause altered mental status and seizures, but the changes are maximal immediately after the embolization. Segmental areas of pallor may be observed on the tongue, and there may be marbling of the skin and air emboli seen on funduscopic examination. When caused by sudden decompression, the condition is treated in a decompression chamber.

Moyamoya disease is a rare condition that is most common among the Japanese, in whom it has been reported to affect fewer than 0.1 per 100,000 of the general population. A "definite" diagnosis requires demonstration of bilateral terminal internal carotid artery occlusion that involves the origins of the MCA and ACA and an abnormal vascular network at the base of the brain that is believed to provide collateral circulation. The abnormal collateral channels appear on angiograms as a "smoky haze," hence the Japanese term "moyamoya." The cause of the vascular occlusion is unknown, but it occurs most commonly in children (peak incidence at age 6 years), in whom it may be associated with ischemic stroke; in adults, it more commonly causes hemorrhage. The diagnosis requires that no known predisposing cause exist, but a similar angiographic picture is seen occasionally with acute tonsillitis, atherosclerosis, meningitis, cancer, trauma, and radiotherapy.

A condition in which the walls of small arteries are thickened and disorganized, referred to by some as lipohyalinosis, was originally believed to underlie small, subcortical brain infarcts called *lacunes*. The condition was thought to be related to hypertension and to require management that differed from that for more conventional strokes. Lacunes were initially described as being associated with a restricted number of characteristic syndromes (e.g., pure motor stroke), but over the years, progressively more clinical syndromes have been attributed to lacunes. Moreover, traditional causes of stroke, including diabetes and hyperlipidemia, have appeared in these patients with almost the same frequency as in those with nonlacunar, ischemic stroke. Perhaps as a result, treatment recommendations, which initially differed for lacunar strokes, now parallel those for nonlacunar strokes.

PREVENTION AND TREATMENT OF STROKE

Currently, there are several promising but no proven therapies for acute ischemic stroke. Even when effective treatments become available, the physician's opportunity to deliver medical care and the utility of a particular pharmacotherapy will be hampered by time constraints; the evolution of irreversible brain damage occurs within 2 to 3 hours of focal vascular occlusion (see Ch. 468). Such considerations place a premium on preventing stroke.

The reduction of stroke risk factors, through therapy for hypertension, diabetes mellitus, smoking, atherosclerosis, and cardiac arrhythmias (Table 469–3) is largely responsible for the marked decline in the incidence of stroke over the past 30 to 40 years. Unfortunately, the effectiveness of stroke prevention is not well appreciated by either the medical or the lay community. Untreated or poorly treated hypertensives, diabetics, and smokers continue to enter the hospital with acute stroke.

Risk Factors and Primary Prevention Therapies

Stroke risk factors have been determined on the basis of mathematical abstractions of epidemiologic data that imply an association or a cause-effect relationship. This section categorizes such risk factors as *definite* or *presumed* and indicates whether they are related to *genetic* and *lifestyle* factors or to *disease processes*. Treatable risk factors are emphasized, and the expected outcome of such prophylactic therapy is presented.

DEFINITE GENETIC AND LIFESTYLE RISK FACTORS. *Hypertension.* This is the most powerful risk factor for stroke. Even within relatively "normal" ranges of blood pressure, the risk of stroke increases by approximately 50 per cent for every 5 mm Hg increase in diastolic pressure throughout the range of 70 to 110 mm Hg. All components of blood pressure (systolic, diastolic, mean) correlate with the incidence of stroke, and the elevation of the systolic pressure is probably a direct cause of stroke that is independent of the secondary complications of hypertension, such as atherosclerosis or arterial rigidity. The risk of stroke is approximately four times greater in patients with definite hypertension (160/95 mm Hg) than in normotensive individuals and is twofold higher in so-called borderline hypertensive individuals. Antihypertensive therapy that lowers the diastolic pressure by as little as 6 mm Hg reduces stroke risk by nearly one quarter in as little as 2 to 3 years. Data from the Framingham Study indicate that the control of hypertension is equally beneficial in reducing stroke risk in the eighth and ninth decades of life as at earlier ages.

Smoking. Smoking increases stroke risk twofold to fourfold. Those who stop smoking substantially reduce their risk of stroke over a period of 2 to 5 years, but their level of risk may not return completely to that of nonsmokers.

Age, Gender, and Race. Age, gender, and race are all unalterable risk factors for stroke, but they may signal treatable disease processes. The incidence of stroke approximately doubles with each decade between ages 45 and 85. Unlike cardiovascular ischemia, in which the incidence in men is approximately three times that in women, stroke occurs only 1.3 times more often in men than in women. The stroke risk in U.S. blacks is approximately 1.3 times that of whites. Some of the differences may be related to environmental or lifestyle factors, since southeastern blacks have a higher stroke rate than do northern ones. Similarly, the high incidence of stroke in the Japanese is not seen in their kindred living in Hawaii.

TABLE 469–3. PREVENTION OF STROKE

Treat hypertension and diabetes mellitus
Stop smoking
Limit alcohol intake
Control diet and obesity
Thoughtful use of oral contraceptives
Anticoagulants for atrial fibrillation and selected acute myocardial infarctions
Antiplatelet agents for carotid/vertebrobasilar atherosclerosis
Endarterectomy for symptomatic carotid artery atherosclerosis of 70–99%

POSSIBLE GENETIC AND LIFESTYLE RISK FACTORS.
Cholesterol, Lipids, Diet, and Obesity. Several dietary factors and obesity may play a role in stroke incidence, but the evidence is inconclusive. Diet and obesity may predispose toward diabetes mellitus and cardiovascular disease, and such patients have a higher chance of dying of stroke than do age-matched controls. Despite the incontrovertible relationship between elevated blood cholesterol and lipids and coronary artery disease, no conclusive evidence currently links lipid abnormalities to stroke. Nevertheless, most authorities strongly advise stroke-prone patients to lower elevated cholesterol and triglyceride levels. Because of the relationships that link obesity with diabetes mellitus, elevated blood pressure, and lipid abnormalities, weight control also is recommended for stroke-prone patients.

Alcohol. Moderate alcohol consumption relates inversely to the incidence of atherosclerosis and coronary artery disease, and a similar reduction of stroke risk with moderate alcohol consumption has also been suggested but not proved. By contrast, binge drinking may increase the incidence of both hemorrhagic and ischemic stroke, especially when combined with cigarette smoking. Much of the latter risk may be attributable to a combination of hemoconcentration and hypertension associated with heavy alcohol consumption.

Oral Contraceptives. Although formerly available high-dose estrogen oral contraceptives were related to stroke, the association is less clear for current preparations. Nevertheless, the combination of oral contraceptives with other risk factors, such as migraine, smoking, hypertension, and age greater than 35 years, may act in combination to raise stroke risk, and many recommend against oral contraceptives in such circumstances.

DEFINITE DISEASE-RELATED RISK FACTORS. *Heart Disease.* Rheumatic valvular disease plus atrial fibrillation increases the risk of stroke 17-fold. Chronic or paroxysmal atrial fibrillation without lesions of the heart valves is associated with a fivefold increase in the risk of stroke. Chronic anticoagulation with warfarin is recommended for most fibrillators, especially those with a history of prior embolism, the presence of a left atrial thrombus on two-dimensional echocardiography, or the coexistence of dilated or hypertrophic cardiomyopathy or of thyrotoxic heart disease, as well as prior to direct-current (DC) conversion. Asymptomatic individuals over the age of 60 may be considered for anticoagulation on an individual basis. Preliminary data from a U.S. study indicated that treatment of chronic atrial fibrillation with warfarin or aspirin reduced the risk of embolic stroke by approximately 80 per cent; other studies indicate that only warfarin confers such benefits. Furthermore, low-dose warfarin with a target prothrombin time ratio that is 1.2 to 1.5 times the control value conferred protection similar to that conferred by conventional warfarin therapy. Valvular disease related to bacterial or nonbacterial endocarditis, myxomatous degeneration of the mitral valve or other diseases causing mitral valve prolapse, mitroannular calcification, and prosthetic heart valve replacements all predispose toward cerebral emboli.

Myocardial infarction involving the anterior wall or septum is associated with a mural thrombus in up to one third of patients, and of these, approximately 15 per cent will suffer a cerebral embolus within a 2-year interval. Acute anticoagulation therapy with heparin, with later conversion to warfarin therapy, is recommended for patients with myocardial infarction involving the anterior or septal wall or in patients with an intramural thrombus detected by two-dimensional echocardiography. Anticoagulation should continue until the two-dimensional echocardiogram indicates resolution of the thrombus. Such therapy reduces the incidence of stroke by approximately one half.

Stroke and TIA. The occurrence of an initial stroke is a powerful predictor of recurrent stroke. Patients between the ages of 45 and 65 years have a 10- to 20-fold increased risk of having a recurrent versus an initial stroke. The comparative risk drops to eightfold for those over the age of 65. The apparent decrease in the incidence of recurrent stroke with age reflects the marked increase in the incidence of an initial stroke in patients over the age of 65. The annual stroke risk following a TIA is 5 per cent per year, which declines to 3 per cent after 3 years. After the occurrence of amaurosis fugax, the annual risk of stroke is 1 to 2 per cent.

Strong evidence derived from meta-analyses supports the use of prophylactic aspirin to protect against strokes in patients with prior strokes or TIA's. Similarly prophylactic antiplatelet therapy with ticlopidine has also been shown to protect against such secondary events. A decision to use antiplatelet or anticoagulant therapy in patients with prior strokes must take into account both the individual patient's risk of further functional loss and the risks of treatment.

Asymptomatic Carotid Stenosis. Individuals with asymptomatic carotid stenosis or carotid bruits have approximately a 1.5- to 2-fold increase in the risk of stroke compared with the general population. Cerebral infarction in this population, however, occurs as frequently in a vascular territory different from the stenotic artery as in the involved one. Asymptomatic carotid stenosis or bruit is a marker of cerebrovascular disease and signals an increased risk of stroke, but not necessarily one in the territory of the involved vessel. No large, randomized, placebo-controlled trial has determined the efficacy of prophylactic antiplatelet therapy in patients with asymptomatic carotid stenosis or bruits.

Other Diseases. Diabetes mellitus is a risk factor independent of hypertension and is associated with an approximate threefold increase in the risk of stroke. No present data indicate that normalization of the blood sugar level reduces the incidence of stroke. Polycythemia, sickle cell disease, migraine, CNS vasculitis, and several infectious diseases all somewhat increase the risk of stroke.

ASPIRIN TREATMENT FOR THE PREVENTION OF STROKE

Although prophylactic aspirin therapy in a healthy population of U.S. physicians reduced the incidence of myocardial infarction, no change occurred in the incidence of ischemic stroke, and a slight increase was detected in the incidence of hemorrhagic stroke. Antiplatelet agents cannot be recommended for stroke prophylaxis in healthy individuals.

SURGICAL TREATMENT FOR THE PREVENTION OF STROKE. The role of *prophylactic surgery* in the prevention of ischemic stroke is highly controversial. A multi-institutional, randomized trial of an external carotid artery–middle cerebral artery anastomosis showed no benefit, and the procedure has been largely abandoned. *Carotid endarterectomy,* designed to remove stenotic plaques from diseased carotid arteries, was developed in the mid 1960's, and from 1971 until about 1984 the number of such operations steadily increased, despite controversy concerning its efficacy. Several multicenter trials in North America are currently examining the indications and efficacy of carotid endarterectomy versus medical therapy in symptomatic and asymptomatic carotid stenosis. Preliminary results from one study indicate that endarterectomy significantly reduces ipsilateral stroke in patients with recent symptoms of ischemia and angiographically proven 70 to 99 per cent ipsilateral carotid artery stenosis. Only patients with a 50 per cent or greater 5-year life expectancy were entered in the study. The procedure is not appropriate for vertebrobasilar disease (Table 469–4). Although *angioplasty* is used widely for coronary artery disease, its utility for cerebrovascular atherosclerosis has not been established.

Surgery for *subclavian steal* is almost never indicated. This steal is a radiographic finding associated with occlusion or severe stenosis of a proximal subclavian artery, resulting in retrograde flow in the ipsilateral vertebral artery. The finding is only rarely associated with symptoms of vertebrobasilar ischemia when the ipsilateral arm is exercised; in most cases, it is merely a radiographic curiosity.

Management and Treatment of Acute Stroke

Patients clinically diagnosed as having an *acute ischemic stroke* should be admitted to the hospital unless the deficit has existed for several days and is stable. The initial history and physical

TABLE 469–4. GUIDELINES FOR CAROTID ENDARTERECTOMY

1. Recent ischemic symptoms (TIA, minor stroke)
2. Angiographically proven ipsilateral stenosis (70–99%)
3. Surgical risk ≤ 5%
4. Five-year cardiovascular life expectancy > 50%

examination emphasize the rapid diagnosis of ischemic cerebral ischemia (TIA or stroke) and the exclusion of seizures, hypoglycemia, tumor, and other alternative diagnoses. As already noted, a normal CT scan within the first several hours is consistent with an ischemic stroke. Admission is also advised for patients with *new-onset TIA's* or those in whom TIA's are occurring with markedly increasing frequency or severity (*crescendo TIA's*).

GENERAL MANAGEMENT. Once admitted, stroke patients should be maintained for at least 24 hours at bed rest to avoid postural hypotension. Since autoregulation (see Ch. 468) is usually ineffective in areas of ischemic brain, CBF will decline if systemic blood pressure falls because of postural changes or volume restriction. Hypertension, if present, should be treated, but with limited, stepwise reductions in blood pressure, for the same reason. If patients have bulbar dysfunction affecting chewing or swallowing, mouth feedings should be avoided to reduce the chance of aspiration. Virtually all patients should have intravenous catheters placed to facilitate urgent treatments. If oral feedings are restricted for prolonged periods, supplementation with intravenous thiamine becomes important to prevent Wernicke's disease; eventually, hyperalimentation or feeding by nasogastric or gastrostomy tube may be needed.

In the early days of an ischemic stroke, passive range-of-motion exercises to the affected limbs can help retain mobility and prevent contractures. Later, more intensive rehabilitation individualized to improve gait, speech, dexterity, and ability to manage activities of daily living is important. Patients often benefit from brief, intensive rehabilitation in specialized hospitals before being sent home. All patients at bed rest should be encouraged to flex and extend their ankles periodically to reduce the chances of deep venous thrombosis, and all should also take occasional deep breaths to combat atelectasis.

PHARMACOTHERAPY (Table 469–5). No pharmacologic therapy has been proved effective for acute ischemic stroke. Nonetheless, several agents are used, depending on the underlying pathophysiology. Intravenous *heparin* is frequently begun on an acute basis for progressing or incomplete stroke, but as already noted, results are difficult to determine. One recent, controlled study, for example, failed to demonstrate any effectiveness of modest heparinization when used in patients with stable, incomplete strokes. An important point is that none of the studies of heparin have examined the effect of beginning within the first hours after stroke onset, so that poor study design may have masked detection of any benefit. A current multicenter trial in North America of heparinoid therapy in acute stroke may provide better guidelines.

Despite underlying bleeding into the blood vessel wall, patients with vascular dissections are often treated with heparin in an effort to maintain patency of the vascular lumen and limit the likelihood of embolism; no proof of efficacy exists. Patients with lacunar strokes were previously considered not to benefit from heparin, but that view has been modified in recent years, possibly as the distinction from larger strokes has blurred.

Patients whose strokes are attributed to emboli of cardiac origin are sometimes treated acutely with heparin. As noted below, chronic oral anticoagulation is usually started concurrently, but debate surrounds the use of heparin until oral anticoagulation takes effect. Some advocate heparin because of concern about early re-embolization and the possibility that warfarin (Coumadin) sometimes enhances coagulability during the first 6 to 8 hours of therapy; others worry about the risks of hemorrhage into the initial stroke. It seems clear that the risk of bleeding is greater

TABLE 469–5. PHARMACOTHERAPY

Prophylactic
  Antiplatelet: aspirin, nonsteroidal anti-inflammatory drugs (NSAID's), ticlopidine
  Anticoagulant (for emboli of cardiac origin, some TIA's): Coumadin or other warfarin derivatives
Acute Treatment
  Anticoagulant (progressing stroke, some emboli): heparin
  Calcium channel blockers (vasospasm with subarachnoid hemorrhage): nimodipine
  Unproven agents or therapies: thrombolytics, antioxidants, glutamate/ aspartate antagonists, possibly hypothermia
No Value: corticosteroids

for larger infarcts; a reasonable course is to withhold heparin from these patients and reserve it for those with smaller strokes. Heparin is generally not given to patients with bacterial endocarditis in whom embolization to the brain has occurred, since evidence suggests an increased risk of bleeding in such cases. Although not intended to reduce cerebral ischemia, low-dose heparin or heparinoids should be used in contraindication-free immobile patients to reduce the chance of peripheral thrombophlebitis.

As noted, *warfarin* anticoagulation is sometimes begun in patients with acute embolic strokes to prevent subsequent embolic strokes. The rationale is that therapeutic anticoagulation will not be achieved for several days after stroke onset, thereby reducing the risk of bleeding into the embolic infarct. This strategy is most useful in patients with large embolic infarctions, in whom the risk of secondary bleeding is greatest.

Patients with stable, complete strokes or those admitted with new-onset or crescendo TIA's are often placed on *aspirin* prophylactically at admission. It is advisable to observe these patients in the hospital for several days, however, until the situation has stabilized. When heparin might be initiated in response to subsequent deterioration, it may be wiser to use shorter-acting antiplatelet medications like nonsteroidal anti-inflammatory drugs (*NSAID's*, e.g., indomethacin or ibuprofen). Such agents share many of aspirin's antiplatelet actions, but unlike aspirin, which permanently inactivates platelet cyclo-oxygenase, NSAID's remain active only while in the bloodstream. Consequently, if necessary, heparin can be started and the NSAID held, thereby avoiding concomitant use of an anticoagulant and antiplatelet agent.

Because of their success in the treatment of myocardial infarction, *fibrinolytic agents*, such as tissue plasminogen activator (t-PA), are currently being tested in the management of acute stroke. Early evidence suggests that the rate of intracranial bleeding may be somewhat increased. Undoubtedly, some such hemorrhages simply reflect conversion of an ischemic to a hemorrhagic infarction without accompanying clinical worsening, an event known to occur in conventionally treated ischemic strokes. Symptomatic parenchymal hematomas develop in only 3 to 5 per cent of patients if fibrinolytic agents are given within 1 to 3 hours of stroke onset; this risk may be acceptable if benefit is established. Striking clinical improvement has been reported in some patients, but double-blind, randomized studies are only just beginning.

Several recent studies have shown that the calcium channel blocker *nimodipine,* 30 mg by mouth every 6 hours, favorably but modestly affects long-term neurologic outcome in ischemic stroke. The benefit has not been seen in all studies, however, and the drug's mechanisms remain unclear.

A trial of the opiate antagonist naloxone showed no benefit. Corticosteroid administration has no benefit in acute ischemic stroke and may be harmful. Experimental studies of acute stroke suggest that antioxidants and inhibitors of excitatory amino acid neurotransmitters may have promise, but neither class of agent has been tested clinically. Ultimately, stroke treatment may employ several of these modalities.

OUTCOME AND REHABILITATION

About 10 to 15 per cent of patients with ischemic stroke will die, some because of brain swelling or neurologic dysfunction directly related to the stroke (e.g., impaired respiration with medullary infarctions) but most because of systemic complications, such as myocardial infarction, pulmonary embolism, and pneumonia. Several studies show an association of stroke with subendocardial necrosis. Most large population studies report that about one fifth of patients surviving stroke require long-term institutionalization and one third to one half of the remaining are left with various disabilities. Most functional recovery takes place during the first 3 months, but some continued slow improvement is possible.

Probably because of overlapping risk factors, the leading cause of death in patients who survive the initial stroke is myocardial infarction, underscoring the importance of cardiac evaluation. Patients who have had one stroke are at increased risk of having additional ones, particularly those whose strokes are attributed to emboli of cardiac origin.

VENOUS STROKE

Although considerably less common than arterial cerebrovascular disease, venous occlusions can cause massive damage and death. As with ischemic strokes from arterial disease, the primary mechanism of brain damage is reduction in capillary blood flow, in this instance because of increased outflow resistance. Back-transmission of high pressure into the capillary bed usually results in early brain swelling from edema and superimposes a potentially severe degree of hemorrhagic infarction in subcortical white matter.

The most dangerous form of venous disease arises when the superior sagittal sinus is occluded, but obstruction of a transverse sinus or one of the major veins over the cerebral convexity (e.g., vein of Labbé) can also produce significant damage. Venous occlusions occur most commonly in association with coagulopathies, often in the puerperal period or in patients with disseminated cancer, and sometimes as a result of contiguous disease, such as infection or cancer. The transverse sinus can be occluded as a consequence of inner ear infections, producing a once common condition called otitic hydrocephalus.

With *superior sagittal sinus obstruction*, veins draining into the sinus from the superior and medial surfaces of both cerebral convexities are commonly obstructed, and thus in its early stages, the condition can result in bilateral weakness and sensory changes in the legs. This bilaterality should alert the clinician to the possibility of sinus thrombosis. Brain swelling and bilateral involvement can produce lethargy or stupor early in the course. Seizures occur more often with venous than with arterial occlusion, possibly because of the irritating effect of parenchymal blood on the cortex.

The differential diagnosis of venous obstruction can include traditional arterial strokes but more often extends to diffuse processes such as herpes simplex encephalitis and meningitis. Diagnosis of the disease depends on the recognition of impaired venous flow. Increasingly, this is detected by loss of flow artifact on MRI. On contrast CT scans, a nonenhanced triangular area surrounded by contrast in the posterior sinus (the empty "delta" sign) should suggest the diagnosis. Since MRI is not infallible, angiography is still the definitive way to make the diagnosis, but attention must be directed to films showing the venous phase.

The management of venous sinus thrombosis increasingly relies on the use of heparin anticoagulation, even in the presence of superimposed parenchymal hemorrhage. Venous occlusions are serious and often fatal, but acute anticoagulation started as soon as the diagnosis is recognized appears to lessen substantially the morbidity and mortality of the condition. Anticonvulsants should be used as needed to control seizures and limit concomitant increases in CBF that might otherwise aggravate brain swelling and bleeding. Without aggressive treatment, venous strokes can be very serious. Nonanticoagulated superior sagittal sinus occlusion that is not complicated by infection carries a mortality rate of 25 to 40 per cent. Uncontrolled series suggest that early heparin therapy can reduce the mortality and morbidity by more than half.

469.2 DIFFUSE ISCHEMIA

Brief diffuse cerebral ischemia causes syncope without any permanent sequelae (Ch. 443). Prolonged diffuse ischemia, by contrast, has devastating consequences. The most common cause is cardiac asystole or other forms of overwhelmingly severe cardiopulmonary failure. Aortic dissection and global hypoxia or carbon monoxide poisoning can cause a similar picture.

Diffuse hypoxia-ischemia typically kills neurons in the hippocampus, cerebellar Purkinje cells, the striatum, and cortical layers 3, 4, and 6. Clinically, it results in unconsciousness: coma followed in many instances by a chronic vegetative state. If patients do not regain consciousness within a few days, the

prognosis for return of independent function becomes very poor. Early absence of pupillary light reflexes, corneal reflexes, and reflex eye movements also predicts a poor outcome. Patients lacking all of these responses even within the first day of hypoxic-ischemic coma have less than a 5 per cent chance of resuming independent activities within 1 year (see Ch. 443). Even if consciousness is regained, such patients often suffer long-term impairment of memory and sometimes a variety of sensorimotor syndromes consistent with lesions in a boundary zone distribution. One such abnormality produces weakness and sensory changes that are greatest in the proximal arm, the cortical representation of which lies between the territories of the ACA and MCA.

Other than prompt and aggressive efforts to restore cardiovascular circulation, no treatments have been found to help patients who are comatose after cardiac arrest. A randomized, multi-institutional trial of barbiturates was without benefit, and corticosteroids may even be harmful. In young patients hypoxic because of drowning, evidence suggests that hypothermia may prolong resistance to ischemic damage, but therapeutic hypothermia in adults can induce cardiac arrhythmias and has not yet been tested. Chronically unconscious patients have not been shown to benefit from either physical or electrical stimulation programs.

Antiplatelet Trialists' Collaboration: Secondary prevention of vascular disease by prolonged antiplatelet treatment. Br Med J 296:320, 1988. *A meta-analysis of 31 randomized trials concluding that aspirin reduces stroke risk by 22 per cent.*

Barnett HJ, Stein BM, Mohr JP, et al. (eds.): Stroke: Pathophysiology, Diagnosis and Management. New York, Churchill Livingstone. 1986. *A comprehensive review of the diagnosis and management of ischemic and hemorrhagic stroke.*

The Boston Area Anticoagulation Trial for Atrial Fibrillation: The effect of low-dose warfarin on the risk of stroke in patients with nonrheumatic atrial fibrillation. N Engl J Med 323:1505, 1990. *A multi-institutional study showing the striking effectiveness of low-dose warfarin in preventing stroke in patients with non-rheumatic atrial fibrillation.*

Classification of Cerebrovascular Diseases III. Special Report from the National Institute of Neurological Disorders and Stroke. Stroke 21:637, 1990. *A contemporary classification of stroke with brief descriptions of each category.*

Collins R, Peto R, MacMahon S, et al.: Blood pressure, stroke, and coronary heart disease, Part 2. Short-term reductions in blood pressure: Overview of randomised drug trials in their epidemiological context. Lancet 335:827, 1990. *A meta-analysis showing a strong association between even modest hypertension and stroke and striking benefits from blood pressure management.*

Del Zoppo GJ: Thrombolytic therapy in cerebrovascular disease. Stroke 19:1174, 1988. *A comprehensive review of animal and human studies of thrombolytics published up to 1988.*

Editorial: Left ventricular thrombosis and stroke following myocardial infarction. Lancet 335:759, 1990. *A brief summary of recommended anticoagulation therapy to reduce embolic stroke after myocardial infarction.*

Haas WK, Easton DJ, Adams HP Jr, et al.: A randomized trial comparing ticlopidine hydrochloride with aspirin for the prevention of stroke in high-risk patients. N Engl J Med 321:501, 1989. *A multicenter trial showing a significant but small advantage of ticlopidine over aspirin.*

Hachinski V, Norris JW: The Acute Stroke. Philadelphia, FA Davis, 1985. *A comprehensive review of the diagnosis and treatment of ischemic stroke.*

Pulsinelli WA, Jacewicz M, Buchan AM: Hypoxic-ischemic disorders in stroke. *In* Johnston MD, McDonald R, Young AB (eds.): Scientific Basis of Neurologic Drug Therapy. Philadelphia, FA Davis, 1992. *Contemporary review of the pharmacologic treatment of ischemic stroke.*

Recommendations on Stroke Prevention, Diagnosis, and Therapy: Special Report from the World Health Organization. Stroke 20:1407, 1989. *A contemporary review of stroke risk factors and their prevention.*

Sandercock P: Recent developments in the diagnosis and management of patients with transient ischemic attacks and minor ischemic strokes. Q J Med 78:101, 1991. *A review of current diagnosis and management of transient ischemic attacks and stroke.*

Stroke Prevention in Atrial Fibrillation Study: Preliminary report of the Stroke Prevention in Atrial Fibrillation Study. N Engl J Med 322:863, 1990. *Preliminary report of a multi-institutional study emphasizing the importance of warfarin or, at least in the nonelderly, aspirin to prevent stroke in atrial fibrillation.*

470 Hemorrhagic Cerebrovascular Disease

Approximately 20 per cent of all strokes consist of intracranial hemorrhages, half into the subarachnoid space and the remainder within the brain itself. The acute rise in intracranial pressure

TABLE 470–1. CAUSES OF SPONTANEOUS INTRACRANIAL HEMORRHAGE

1. Arterial aneurysms
   a. "Berry" aneurysm
   b. Fusiform aneurysm
   c. Mycotic aneurysm
   d. Aneurysm with vasculitis
2. Cerebrovascular malformations
3. Hypertensive-atherosclerotic hemorrhage
4. Hemorrhage into brain tumor
5. Systemic bleeding diatheses
6. Hemorrhage with vasculopathies
7. Hemorrhage with intracranial venous infarction

from arterial rupture causes loss of consciousness in approximately half the patients, and many of these die of cerebral herniation (see Ch. 443). However, since hemorrhage into the subarachnoid space or brain parenchyma causes less tissue injury than does ischemia, patients who survive often show a remarkable recovery.

Like ischemic stroke, hemorrhagic stroke can be thought of as diffuse (subarachnoid and/or intraventricular) or focal (intraparenchymal). Subarachnoid hemorrhage (SAH) is caused by rupture of surface arteries (aneurysms, vascular malformations, head trauma), with blood usually limited to the cerebrospinal fluid (CSF) space between the pial and arachnoid membranes (Table 470–1). Intracerebral hemorrhage is most frequently caused by the rupture of arteries lying deeply within the brain substance (hypertensive hemorrhage, vascular malformations, head trauma), but in some instances the force of blood from ruptured surface arteries may penetrate the brain parenchyma. Blood within the cerebral ventricles results either from reflux of subarachnoid blood through the fourth ventricular foramina or by extension from a site of intraparenchymal hemorrhage.

470.1 ANEURYSMAL SUBARACHNOID HEMORRHAGE

EPIDEMIOLOGY

Rupture of a saccular or "berry" aneurysm causes approximately 80 per cent of all SAH's, 5 per cent are caused by mycotic aneurysm rupture, and an even smaller percentage reflects bleeding from atherosclerotic, neoplastic, or dissecting cerebral aneurysms. The incidence of aneurysmal SAH is approximately 10 per 100,000 population, with 80 per cent of these occurring in persons 40 to 65 years old, 15 per cent in those 20 to 40 years old, and 5 per cent in those below 20 years of age. Women are slightly more likely than men (3:2) to suffer rupture of a cerebral aneurysm, especially during pregnancy.

ETIOLOGY AND PATHOGENESIS

SACCULAR ANEURYSMS. The pathogenesis of saccular aneurysms reflects a combination of congenital, acquired, and hereditary factors. Congenital defects in the muscle and elastic tissue of the arterial media, seen at autopsy in 80 per cent of normal vessels of the circle of Willis, gradually deteriorate as they are exposed over time to the hemodynamic stresses of pulsatile blood flow. These defects lead to microaneurysmal dilatations (<2 mm) of the circle of Willis arteries in 15 to 20 per cent of the population. Larger (>5 mm) aneurysms are found in 5 per cent of the population. These larger, potentially symptomatic saccular aneurysms are characteristically distributed at the arterial bifurcations, 80 per cent being located in the anterior, carotid artery–derived, arterial circulation and the rest lying along the bifurcation of the vertebrobasilar arteries (Fig. 470–1).

The remarkably high incidence of wall defects in the media of normal vessels, the high frequency of incidental microaneurysms, and the tendency for aneurysms to enlarge with time and rupture when they exceed 1 cm in diameter imply that both congenital and acquired factors influence the pathogenesis of rupture. On the other hand, the relative rarity of SAH suggests that other factors, possibly genetic, may predispose to aneurysm formation. A modest incidence of familial saccular aneurysms as well as their

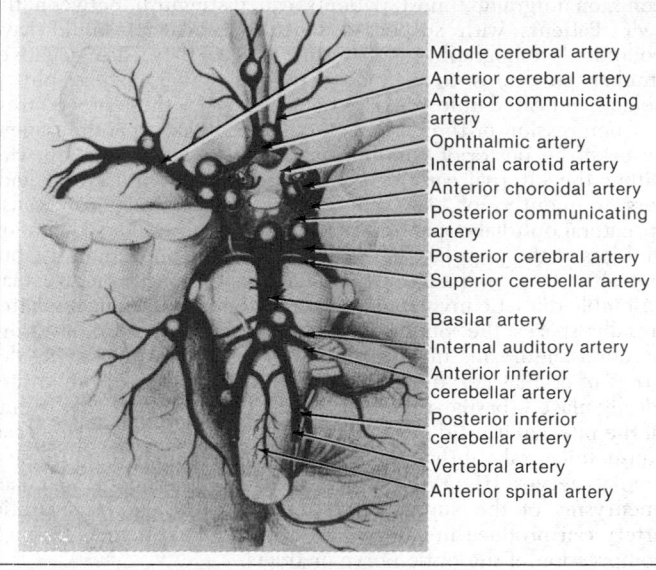

FIGURE 470–1. The common sites for berry aneurysms to develop at the bifurcation of arteries on the undersurface of the brain.

association with polycystic kidney disease, Ehlers-Danlos syndrome, and other connective tissue disorders implicates hereditary factors. Although hypertension per se is not a significant risk factor for aneurysmal SAH, aneurysms have been known to rupture under conditions associated with a sudden rise in blood pressure, including extremes of emotional excitement and physical exertion such as coitus and athletic events.

FUSIFORM ANEURYSMS. Fusiform or ectatic aneurysms acquire their name from the spindle-shaped dilatation and elongation that occur in large arteries at the site of arteriosclerotic narrowing. These aneurysms develop most frequently in the basilar artery but may also affect the internal, middle, and anterior cerebral arteries of individuals with widespread arteriosclerosis and hypertension. They rarely rupture and are difficult to treat when they do because their shape and stiff walls preclude easy surgical clipping. Progressive dilatation and the tortuous elongation of the vessel cause neurologic dysfunction most frequently by compressing surrounding structures. Typically, ectatic aneurysms of the basilar artery compress cranial nerves V, VII, and VIII, causing facial pain, hemifacial spasm, and hearing loss with vertigo, respectively. Fusiform aneurysms may imitate the features of cerebellopontine angle tumors, or they may mimic pituitary and suprasellar mass lesions. The underlying arteriosclerotic disease may cause ischemic stroke either through occlusion of the vessel or by producing cerebral embolism from a clot formed within the aneurysm. Rarely, ectasia of the basilar artery causes communicating hydrocephalus by interfering with normal CSF outflow at the level of the third ventricle.

MYCOTIC ANEURYSMS. Mycotic cerebral aneurysms are caused by septic degeneration of arterial wall muscle and elastic tissue. In contrast to saccular and fusiform aneurysms, which are located primarily in large arteries at the base of the brain, mycotic aneurysms form in more distal cerebral arteries at the point where small septic cardiogenic emboli lodge. They are frequently multiple and can be found in either the anterior or the posterior cerebral circulation.

CLINICAL PRESENTATION

Prodromal signs and symptoms caused by compression of surrounding brain structures, by warning or "sentinel" leaks, or by embolization of the aneurysmal clot to distal arteries frequently precede the catastrophic rupture of saccular aneurysms. Focal headaches may signal compression of pain-sensitive structures from an expanding aneurysm, in which case the headache is usually progressive, or by "sentinel" leaks that cause sudden, focal head pain. Such sentinel headaches are frequently severe and may be accompanied by nausea or vomiting or may cause meningeal irritation. Despite the similarity of these headaches to common migraine, most patients can distinguish between the two. Patients with suspected sentinel headache should have computed tomographic (CT) scans and, if these are negative, lumbar punctures to exclude active bleeding; angiography is seldom indicated unless SAH is documented by these procedures.

Compression of the oculomotor nerve by an expanding aneurysm of the posterior communicating artery at its junction with either the internal carotid or the posterior cerebral artery and, less frequently, of the superior cerebellar artery can cause ipsilateral ophthalmoparesis, ptosis, and later pupillary dilatation and loss of the pupillary light reflex. Orbital pain frequently, but not always, accompanies these signs. The clinical picture may resemble diabetic involvement of cranial nerve III, but the latter usually spares the pupil. Other compression syndromes from cerebral aneurysms include amnesia combined with varying degrees of cranial nerve III paresis and quadriparesis from strategically placed, basilar-tip aneurysms. Giant (>2.5 cm) aneurysms of the internal carotid artery lying within the cavernous sinus can cause unilateral ophthalmoplegia and orbital pain by compressing cranial nerves III, IV, VI, and the first division of V. Giant aneurysms of the supraclinoid portion of the internal carotid artery can produce unilateral vision loss or field defects through compression of the optic nerve or tracts.

Rupture of saccular aneurysms into the subarachnoid space seldom is associated with focal signs or symptoms. Nearly half of patients so affected lose consciousness, at least transiently, as intracranial pressure exceeds cerebral perfusion pressure. Approximately 10 per cent of patients remain in coma for several days, depending upon the location of the aneurysm and the amount of bleeding. Patients who remain conscious and those who awaken from coma commonly recall the sudden onset as producing the "most excruciating headache" of their life. Rupture of an intracranial aneurysm in the absence of headache is rare, and some reported cases probably reflect amnesia for the event.

In addition to the frequent change in the level of consciousness, acute SAH causes meningeal irritation, nuchal rigidity, and photophobia, symptoms that may require several hours to develop. Subhyaloid retinal hemorrhages occur in 20 to 30 per cent of patients as a result of increased intracranial pressure, raised retinal venous pressure, and dissection of blood along the optic nerve sheath. Blood pressure is frequently elevated, and body temperature usually rises, particularly during the early days after bleeding as blood products produce a chemical meningitis. Focal neurologic dysfunction is not a prominent feature of SAH unless there is associated compression by the aneurysm of surrounding brain structures, the jet of blood dissects directly into a clinically relevant brain region, or vasospasm occurs as a complication (see below).

LABORATORY EXAMINATION

Serum electrolytes should be measured at the time of admission to serve as a baseline for detecting later hyponatremia. A complete blood count, including platelets and clotting times, should be obtained to evaluate possible infection or hematologic or clotting abnormalities. The electrocardiogram (ECG) may show various abnormalities, including heightened T waves, shortened PR intervals, peaked or inverted T waves, and increased U waves. These ECG abnormalities and subsequent arrhythmias have been attributed to multifocal myocardial necrosis caused by elevated levels of circulating catecholamines.

CT scans reveal subarachnoid blood within the basal cisterns in about three quarters of patients within 48 hours of bleeding. Magnetic resonance (MR) images have a lower index of accuracy. Detection of intracranial blood on the CT scan, however, becomes more difficult with time as blood and its breakdown products become isodense. Blood localized to the basal cisterns, the sylvian fissure, or the intrahemispheric fissure more frequently indicates rupture of a saccular aneurysm, while blood lying over the convexities or within the superficial parenchyma of the brain is more consistent with either the rupture of an arteriovenous malformation or a mycotic aneurysm. The amount and location of blood within the subarachnoid space relate directly to an aneurysm's location and the likelihood of subsequent vasospasm. Importantly, an early CT scan also allows a baseline evaluation

of ventricular size to compare against later hydrocephalus caused by hemogenic obstruction of CSF outflow pathways. A contrast-enhanced CT scan may aid in the identification of an arteriovenous malformation and some large (>1.0 cm) aneurysms but should be obtained only after a noncontrast study has been completed, since contrast agents may obscure detection of subarachnoid blood.

If the CT scan fails to show blood, a lumbar puncture is diagnostic. To avoid puncture of the venous plexus lying on the anterior wall of the spinal canal, the spinal needle should be advanced slowly, with frequent removal of the trocar to detect first entry of the subarachnoid space. A traumatic lumbar puncture usually can be distinguished from SAH by the failure of the latter to show a decrease in the red blood cell (RBC) count between the first and last tubes of CSF (Table 470–2). In addition, in the presence of bloody fluid, one of the CSF samples should be centrifuged immediately and the supernate examined for the presence of xanthochromia by visual inspection and testing the fluid with a benzidene (Hemoccult) stick. Red blood cells in the spinal canal begin to lyse within 2 to 3 hours, and the centrifuged supernate will then appear pink. Later (10 hours) as the hemoglobin is converted to bilirubin, the fluid develops a yellow tinge (xanthochromia). The CSF pressure is usually elevated and may remain so for many days. Spinal fluid samples taken within the first 24 hours often show a white blood cell (WBC) count consistent with the normal circulating WBC-RBC ratio (ca. 1:1000); later samples contain increased polymorphonuclear and mononuclear cells secondary to chemical meningitis caused by breakdown products of subarachnoid blood. The CSF blood glucose level is usually normal early, but as chemical meningitis develops, the level may decrease, but rarely to less than 40 mg per deciliter. The protein content of the CSF is usually elevated, consistent with contamination by blood (1 mg per deciliter of protein for every 1000 RBC's).

Cerebral angiography remains the definitive study to detect the source of SAH. In instances in which the diagnosis of aneurysmal SAH is certain, the timing and need for a cerebral angiogram should be determined by surgical considerations (see below). When diagnostic doubt exists, the angiogram should be performed immediately. Since as many as one third of patients with aneurysmal SAH harbor multiple cerebral aneurysms, both carotid and both vertebral arteries should be examined. It is interesting that among patients with multiple cerebral aneurysms, almost half have identically placed aneurysms in the left and right circulation, so-called mirror aneurysms. Cerebral angiography fails to detect the source of bleeding in 10 to 20 per cent of cases. Such patients are thought to have a better prognosis, with only a 1 to 2 per cent chance of recurrent SAH. Failure to detect the source of bleeding may result from obliteration of an aneurysm through clotting; because bleeding was caused by rupture of a small, superficial venous angioma; or when hemorrhage has occurred from a spinal cord aneurysm or arteriovenous malformation (AVM). The presence of back pain or spinal cord symptoms at onset should prompt a search for a spinal source of hemorrhage. Repeat cerebral angiography is indicated 3 to 4 weeks later when the initial angiogram is negative and no other clues to the bleeding site can be found.

Cerebral angiography is recommended immediately in patients who have septic endocarditis and SAH to search for possible mycotic aneurysms. Since 25 per cent of patients with subacute bacterial endocarditis and evidence of systemic embolism harbor one or more cerebral mycotic aneurysms, they should also undergo cerebral angiography.

LATE MEDICAL AND NEUROLOGIC COMPLICATIONS

The medical complications of SAH include cardiac myonecrosis and arrhythmias attributed to abnormal levels of circulating

TABLE 470–2. "TRAUMATIC TAP" OR SUBARACHNOID HEMORRHAGE?

	"Traumatic Tap"	Spontaneous Subarachnoid Bleed
Xanthochromia	Absent	Onset: 4–6 hr Duration: approximately 6 wk
Red cell count (serial tubes)	Decreasing	Constant
Blood clot formation	Rapid	Slower

epinephrine. Symptomatic hyponatremia may also develop from the inappropriate secretion of antidiuretic hormone.

Late neurologic complications include *rebleeding* from the same aneurysm, cerebral *vasospasm* and its ischemic consequences, *hydrocephalus* caused by blockage of CSF outflow pathways, and occasionally *seizures*. Aneurysmal rerupture is suggested by new headache or neurologic worsening but can be diagnosed firmly only if a repeat CT scan or lumbar puncture shows the presence of new blood in the subarachnoid space. Approximately one third of patients with aneurysmal SAH rebleed during the first month, the incidence being highest during the first 2 weeks after the initial bleed. Patients with an unclipped aneurysm who survive their initial bleed for more than 1 month have a 2 to 3 per cent yearly risk of rebleeding.

Cerebral vasospasm as diagnosed by cerebral angiography is defined as an abnormal narrowing of cerebral arteries. Vasospasm has been reported in up to 75 per cent of patients with SAH, half of whom develop strokelike neurologic signs and symptoms. The peak onset for cerebral vasospasm is between days 3 and 14, but the complication can develop as late as 3 weeks after SAH. Arteries forming the circle of Willis and their major branches are the initial site of involvement, with more distal arteries becoming involved later. The amount and location of blood detected within the basal cisterns on CT scans correlate with the incidence and location of cerebral vasospasm.

The molecular mechanisms causing cerebral vasospasm are unknown but probably involve release of vasoactive amines and polypeptides, which pathologically influence vascular smooth muscle contraction. Vasospastic vessels show medial necrosis within the first few weeks, and later medial atrophy, subendothelial fibrosis, and intimal thickening.

Communicating hydrocephalus may develop as early as the first or second week after SAH. Patients with more extensive bleeding are more likely to develop the complication, but its incidence correlates with the amount of blood on CT images less clearly than does the development of vasospasm. Red blood cells and their breakdown products cause hydrocephalus by obstruction of CSF outflow pathways both at the level of the fourth ventricle and through the pacchionian granulations lining the venous sinuses. Seldom does communicating hydrocephalus require surgical treatment early after SAH.

Seizures are infrequent but can complicate SAH. The presence of seizures usually signals cortical damage either from bleeding into the neocortex or from ischemic necrosis.

TREATMENT

SACCULAR ANEURYSMS. The definitive therapy for a ruptured saccular aneurysm consists of surgical clipping of the aneurysm to prevent rebleeding. Medical therapy aims to reduce the risk of rebleeding and cerebral vasospasm and to prevent other medical complications before and after surgical intervention. Patients should be kept quiet at bed rest, with the administration of appropriate analgesics for the treatment of headache and gentle sedation. Stool softeners minimize straining with subsequently increased intracranial pressure. Hypertension should be treated, but not aggressively, since some of the elevated pressure may represent normal compensatory mechanisms to maintain cerebral perfusion pressure in the face of increased intracranial pressure or cerebral arterial narrowing. Systolic pressures in the range of 160 to 170 mm Hg and diastolic pressures in the range of 90 to 100 mm Hg are acceptable. The voltage-regulated calcium channel antagonist nimodipine should be given orally in a dosage of 60 mg every 4 hours for 21 days. Although it does not reduce the frequency of vasospasm, nimodipine lowers by one third the incidence of cerebral infarction in patients suffering SAH and cerebral vasospasm.

The effects of cerebral vasospasm can also be partly overcome by raising cerebral perfusion pressure through plasma volume expansion and pressor agents, usually phenylephrine or dopamine. Such measures, however, may raise the risk of rebleeding and should be undertaken only in patients with surgically clipped saccular aneurysms.

Efforts to reduce the incidence of rebleeding with ε-aminocaproic acid, an inhibitor of fibrinolysis, have been successful. Such therapy is not recommended for routine use, since it increases the incidence of vasospasm, cerebral infarction, and subsequent hydrocephalus.

TABLE 470–3. HUNT CLASSIFICATION OF PATIENT'S CONDITION

Grade	Condition
0	Unruptured aneurysm
1	Asymptomatic or minimal headache and slight nuchal rigidity
1A	No acute meningeal or brain reaction but with fixed neurologic deficit
2	Moderate to severe headache, nuchal rigidity; no neurologic deficit other than cranial nerve palsy
3	Drowsiness, confusion, or mild focal deficit
4	Stupor, moderate to severe hemiparesis, possible early decerebrate rigidity and vegetative disturbances
5	Deep coma, decerebrate rigidity, and moribund appearance

The optimal time to clip a ruptured saccular aneurysm remains controversial. An increasingly accepted approach is to operate either within the first 3 days or after days 10 to 14. The logic relates to the timing of intrinsic rebleeding and the onset of cerebral vasospasm. Since the incidence of aneurysmal rebleeding is highest during the first 2 weeks after SAH and the mortality associated with each bleed approaches 40 to 50 percent, the aneurysm should be clipped as soon as possible. Nevertheless, undertaking aneurysmal surgery in the presence of active vasospasm has been associated consistently with poor neurologic outcomes. As a result, most surgeons avoid operating during days 3 to 10, when maximal cerebral vasospasm is likely. Patients in Hunt's grade 1 to 3 (Table 470–3) should, if possible, have their aneurysms clipped prior to 3 days if the cerebral angiogram shows little or no evidence of cerebral vasospasm. In patients whose aneurysm is clipped early, preliminary studies suggest that lysing blood clots in the basal cisterns with locally applied fibrinolytic drugs, followed by washing the blood out, may reduce subsequent vasospasm. Aneurysmal clipping should be delayed until 10 to 14 days after the last documented SAH in patients who present to hospital later than 3 days, who have active vasospasm on early cerebral angiograms, or who fall initially into a poor clinical grade (Hunt 4 and 5). In instances of delayed surgical intervention, most authorities recommend repeating the cerebral angiogram prior to surgery to rule out the continued presence of vasospasm. Some neurosurgeons also recommend postoperative angiograms to verify proper clip placement and obliteration of the aneurysm.

MYCOTIC ANEURYSMS. Unruptured mycotic aneurysms should be treated with antibiotics appropriate for the infecting organism and followed angiographically. Single aneurysms and those in surgically accessible areas should be considered for prompt surgical clipping.

PROGNOSIS

The mortality rate from aneurysmal SAH is 50 to 60 per cent after 1 year. Almost half such patients die before reaching the hospital, and most of the remaining die during the first month. An equally high mortality accompanies each episode of rebleeding. Approximately 25 per cent of survivors have persistent neurologic deficits.

Unruptured cerebral aneurysms detected incidentally during cerebral angiography bleed at a yearly rate of 1 to 3 per cent. Aneurysm size is strongly associated with the likelihood of rupture, so that saccular aneurysms less than 5 mm should be followed carefully, aneurysms between 5 and 10 mm may be considered for surgical clipping, and those greater than 10 mm should be clipped at the earliest convenience. The experience of the surgical team critically affects decisions and outcome concerning such treatment.

470.2 HEMORRHAGE FROM VASCULAR MALFORMATIONS

CLASSIFICATION AND EPIDEMIOLOGY

Congenital vascular malformations of the brain and spinal cord fall into five categories according to vessel size and type. *Venous angiomas*, the most common cerebrovascular malformations, are composed entirely of veins and usually lie close to the brain's surface. Hemorrhage from a venous angioma is uncommon and rarely fatal. Nevertheless, these lesions have gained considerable attention, since they are readily detected by CT scans. They seldom produce seizures and headaches. A cerebral *varix* is a single dilated vein and very rarely causes clinical symptoms.

Telangiectasias are uncommon vascular anomalies composed of tangles of small, capillary-like vessels. They are usually located deep in the brain (diencephalon, brain stem, cerebellum) and rarely produce symptoms. Because of their strategic location, hemorrhage from these small vessels can occasionally be fatal.

Cavernous angiomas are large sinusoidal channels served by large feeding arteries and veins. Many of the channels thrombose, and the remainder have very low blood flow, which makes their visualization on angiograms difficult. They are readily detected by CT scan and rarely bleed, but they may cause headaches and seizures.

The most common symptomatic vascular anomaly is the *arteriovenous malformation* (AVM). AVM's are composed of tangles of arteries connected directly to veins without intervening capillaries. The resulting vessels are thin walled owing to poorly developed elastic and muscle tissue within the media. The large arteries, which feed the AVM, usually show hypertrophy of the media and thickening of the endothelium. Brain tissue is usually absent from the AVM but when present is nonfunctional. AVM's can be located anywhere in the brain and can produce headaches, seizures, focal neurologic deficits, or intracranial hemorrhage. Intracranial hemorrhage from vascular malformations accounts for 1 per cent of all strokes and 10 per cent of all SAH's. The prevalence of AVM's among the general population is uncertain, but autopsy studies of unselected patients indicate that 4 to 5 per cent harbor some form of vascular malformation, of which only 10 to 15 per cent produce symptoms. Familial cases of AVM's are rare, indicating that the problem reflects sporadic abnormalities in embryologic development.

CLINICAL PRESENTATION

Most AVM's manifest with intracranial hemorrhage, a lower proportion causing seizures or progressive neurologic disability as first symptoms. The initial hemorrhage tends to occur during the second through fourth decades, with the risk of rebleeding averaging approximately 6 to 7 per cent the first year, 2 per cent after 5 years, and 1 to 2 per cent thereafter. The decline in the incidence of rebleeding with time may reflect the spontaneous thrombosis of arterial feeders. The initial and subsequent hemorrhages are associated with a 10 per cent chance of death. If the rebleed rate of 1 to 2 per cent is maintained for life, the young individual who presents with a hemorrhagic AVM faces a 50 to 60 per cent chance of an incapacitating or fatal repeat hemorrhage during a normal lifespan.

AVM's may bleed into the subarachnoid space, into the brain parenchyma, or into the ventricular system. Focal neurologic signs and symptoms depend upon the severity of the bleed and the extent to which brain parenchyma has been destroyed. Bleeding into the subarachnoid space is usually less severe than with saccular aneurysms, and blood tends to localize over the cerebral convexities rather than in the basal cisterns. The incidence of cerebral vasospasm with AVM hemorrhage appears less than for aneurysm SAH, perhaps because less blood accumulates around the large arteries at the base of the brain. No explanation has been provided for the observation that small AVM's (<2.5 cm) tend to bleed more frequently than do large AVM's (>5 cm).

Approximately one third of patients who harbor an AVM present with seizures, of which about half have a focal onset. Focal neurologic deficits independent of seizures also develop, resulting from vascular thrombosis and brain tissue hypoperfusion caused by either vascular compression or a "steal" syndrome. Shunting of blood through arteriovenous fistulas may draw blood away from normal brain tissue, causing hypoperfusion and dysfunction of the brain proximal to the AVM. With treatment of the AVM, either through surgical resection or by embolization of the feeding arteries, some of these focal neurologic signs may improve or disappear. Approximately 10 per cent of patients with AVM's have a history of headache, the location of which seldom coincides with the site of the AVM. Some AVM-associated headaches closely resemble migraine, but unlike migraine, most AVM-associated headaches rarely alternate between the two sides of the head.

LABORATORY EXAMINATION

The laboratory evaluation for intracranial hemorrhage from an AVM is similar to that described for aneurysmal SAH. A CT scan with contrast is diagnostic in approximately 85 per cent of patients. MR images are equally, if not more, effective in diagnosis. Angiography remains the definitive test to identify the AVM and delineate its feeding arteries and draining veins. Since approximately 10 per cent of AVM's are associated with saccular aneurysms, four-vessel angiography is indicated even if the AVM is defined by unilateral carotid injection. In addition, extracranial or contralateral arteries occasionally supply intracranial AVM's and should be considered in the angiographic evaluation.

TREATMENT

Uncertainties concerning the natural history of unruptured AVM's, as well as the efficacy and complications associated with newer forms of interventional therapy, make it difficult to define a simple set of guiding therapeutic principles. Generally speaking, unruptured AVM's that manifest with either seizures or headache may be treated conservatively, especially in patients older than 55 to 60 years. In such patients, hypertension should be controlled, platelet antiaggregating agents and anticoagulants avoided, and anticonvulsants given to control the seizures.

Interventional therapeutic options include surgical resection of the AVM, embolization of the feeding arteries, or radiation-induced thrombosis. Various considerations, including age, the degree of neurologic dysfunction, and location of the AVM, must be considered when choosing treatment. The present custom is to treat younger patients (<55 years) more aggressively, resecting surgically accessible AVM's, since removal of the AVM and *all* its arterial feeders is curative. In older patients or if the AVM lies in language-vulnerable areas or deep in the brain, use of focused gamma x-rays or proton beam radiation is safer but only effective in lesions less than 3 cm in diameter. Embolization of the feeding arteries is rarely recommended as the sole interventional therapy, since such an approach totally obliterates the arterial feeders in only about 40 per cent of cases. Arterial embolization is frequently used in conjunction with either surgery or focused radiation therapy.

470.3 FOCAL CEREBRAL HEMORRHAGE

Focal hemorrhage occurs spontaneously in three common settings: hypertension, ruptured AVM's, and amyloid (or congophilic) angiopathy. Additional contributing causes are excessive anticoagulation, systemic bleeding diatheses, and trauma.

EPIDEMIOLOGY

In the United States, primary intracerebral hemorrhage occurs with an incidence of about 12 per 100,000 population, a rate similar to that for SAH but only 10 per cent that for ischemic stroke. Age-adjusted rates for men are about 50 per cent higher than for women, and rates for blacks are over twice those for whites. As with ischemic stroke, the incidence appears to be declining; excluding hemorrhage associated with anticoagulation, the rate in Rochester, Minnesota, fell from about 15 per 100,000 in 1945 to 5 per 100,000 in the early 1970's. Hypertension has declined in frequency during the same period, but no conclusive data link the two trends.

PATHOLOGY

The pathologic picture of primary intracerebral hemorrhage typically consists of a large confluent area of blood that clots and then weeks later begins slowly to be phagocytosed; after several months, the only residuum may be a small, collapsed cavity lined by hemosiderin-containing macrophages. Although hemorrhages may destroy brain tissue locally, histologic examination suggests that displacement of normal brain tissue and dissection along fiber tracts account for much of the pathology. Consequently, hemorrhage may be less destructive of brain tissue than is ischemic infarction.

In hypertensive persons at least, active bleeding probably occurs over a very short time; radiolabeled red cells injected intravenously in patients more than 2 hours after initial symptoms do not appear to leak into brain. This observation suggests that the source of bleeding is rapidly compressed, in part by extravascular blood, and that delayed clinical worsening in patients with primary hemorrhage is related to mechanisms such as brain swelling and not to continued bleeding.

PATHOGENESIS

Hypertension can produce hemorrhages throughout the brain, but usually they occur in four locations: external capsule-putamen, internal capsule-thalamus, central pons, and cerebellum (Fig. 470–2). A smaller number arise throughout the subcortical white matter. Bleeding in such instances is believed to result from rupture of microaneurysms in small, intracerebral arteries (50 to 150 μm in diameter). The pathology of the microaneurysms includes replacement of normal lining endothelium, media, and elastic tissue with fibrous tissue and fat. Similar changes can lead to necrotic vascular degeneration, which, along with microaneurysms, predisposes to hemorrhage. A strong relationship links microaneurysms to hypertension; in one autopsy series, microaneurysms were found in 46 of 100 hypertensive brains and in 85 per cent of hypertensive persons with hemorrhages, but in only 7 of 100 normotensive brains.

Amyloid (or congophilic) angiopathy is a pathologic diagnosis, increasingly encountered in the elderly. Unrelated to generalized amyloidosis and occasionally hereditary, the condition often appears in the brains of patients with Alzheimer's disease and has been associated with nonhypertensive hemorrhage. It is rare in patients under age 55. Amyloid deposits, chemically related to those in Alzheimer plaques, are seen in the media and adventitia of medium- and small-sized arteries. In contrast to hypertensive hemorrhages, bleeding in amyloid angiopathy most often occurs in the lobar subcortical white matter (Fig. 470–2). Multiple small hemorrhages may be associated with the condition.

Anticoagulation, fibrinolysis, and other hematologic abnormalities can be associated with intracerebral hemorrhages. Warfarin anticoagulation has been implicated in about 10 per cent of primary intracerebral hemorrhages. With the less aggressive programs of low-dose warfarin anticoagulation (target prothrombin time ratio of 1.2 to 1.5) now used for peripheral venous disease and to prevent arterial embolism, the rate of intracranial bleeding in one recent study had fallen to under 1 per cent with 2 years of treatment. Data from large-scale studies of fibrinolysis (e.g., tissue plasminogen activator, t-PA) in acute myocardial infarction indicate that at a total t-PA dose no greater than 100

mg, the rate of symptomatic intracerebral hemorrhage is only about 0.5 per cent (although in one small series, it was 5 per cent); at higher doses of 150 mg, the rate rises to about 1.5 per cent. Cerebral hemorrhages occur in *leukemia, polycythemia, hemophilia,* and other clotting abnormalities, and they also occur in patients using *amphetamines* and *cocaine.*

Although *trauma* causes intracerebral (as well as subarachnoid) hemorrhage, the diagnosis is usually aided by the history as well as by coexistent external signs of trauma, SAH, and, on CT scan, multifocal, inhomogeneous hemorrhages and areas of decreased density (see Ch. 487).

CLINICAL PRESENTATION

Large cerebral hemorrhages usually produce catastrophic, acute syndromes. The onset is often associated with physical (or emotional) activity; onset during sleep is rare. Common early features include alterations in consciousness, headache, nausea, and vomiting. Although uncommon, seizures occur, possibly reflecting cortical irritation by blood. With the increasing ability to recognize less dramatic hemorrhages by using CT and MRI, neurologists now realize that hemorrhages can also produce less severe dysfunction that may be indistinguishable clinically from ischemic stroke. Clinical evolution over hours is common and usually attributed to secondary brain swelling.

The clinician should be able to recognize common hemorrhagic syndromes (Table 470–4) to anticipate dangerous brain swelling and provide appropriate medical and supportive management. Hypertensive hemorrhages typically occur deep within the cerebral (or cerebellar) hemispheres, producing several well-described syndromes. In the following paragraphs, percentages indicate the approximate contribution of each specific syndrome to all primary intracerebral hemorrhages.

PUTAMINAL HEMORRHAGE (35 TO 50 PER CENT). Patients with massive putaminal hemorrhages (Fig. 470–3) become lethargic or comatose within minutes to hours of onset and concurrently develop contralateral weakness (including face) and a contralateral hemianopsia and gaze paresis (with eyes deviated toward the hemorrhage). For unknown reasons, some patients develop an ipsilateral gaze palsy (with the eyes deviated toward the paretic limbs). Brain stem reflexes remain intact, and the gaze paresis can be overcome with oculovestibular stimulation. A contralateral sensory deficit is often detectable. Pupillary size may be normal initially, but as the upper brain stem is compressed, pupils first constrict and then dilate, and limb posturing develops. Although some patients display their maximal deficit at onset, the majority progress over the first several hours.

THALAMIC HEMORRHAGE (10 TO 15 PER CENT). Some patients with thalamic hemorrhages lose consciousness early in the clinical course, but those who are awake often experience contralateral hemiparesis, sensory changes, and homonymous hemianopsia (the last often clearing quickly). A contralateral gaze palsy (as with putaminal hemorrhage) is occasionally present. Some patients develop fixed downward ocular deviation, presumably from compression of the adjacent midbrain tectum. Pupillary reactions to light are usually preserved, although pupils are often small, reflecting hypothalamic sympathetic disturbances.

PONTINE HEMORRHAGE (10 TO 15 PER CENT). Traditional teaching held that coma always accompanied the onset of pontine hemorrhage, but refined imaging shows that with smaller hemorrhages this is not always the case. In the comatose patient, small, reactive pupils are common, oculovestibular responses are lost early, and vomiting often occurs at onset. Patients usually have quadriplegia and bilateral extensor posturing. If facial weakness is present, it commonly has characteristics of a lower motor neuron weakness. Ocular bobbing is sometimes reported.

CEREBELLAR HEMORRHAGE (10 TO 30 PER CENT). Because cerebellar hemorrhage initially spares the brain stem, consciousness is usually preserved in the early stages. Occipital headache is usually the first symptom, followed by unsteady gait, clumsiness, nausea, and vomiting, which may be severe and repetitive. Motor weakness is seldom prominent at onset, but with progression and brain stem compression, contralateral hemiparesis and caloric-resistant ipsilateral gaze paresis help to localize the lesion to the posterior fossa. Pupillary reactions are usually

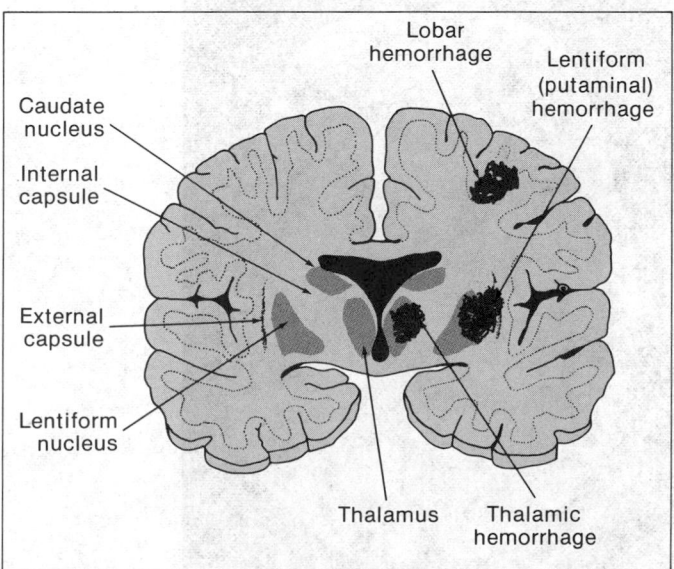

FIGURE 470–2. A coronal section through the cerebral hemispheres illustrating thalamic, putaminal, and lobar subcortical hemorrhages.

TABLE 470–4. CLINICAL FEATURES OF COMMON HYPERTENSIVE HEMORRHAGES

Clinical	Site of Hemorrhage			
	Putaminal	*Thalamic*	*Pontine*	*Cerebellar*
Unconsciousness	Later	Later	Early	Late
Hemiparesis	Yes	Yes	Quadriparesis	Late
Sensory change	Yes	Yes	Yes	Late
Hemianopic	Yes	Yes	No	No
Pupils:				
Size	Normal	Small	Small	Normal
Reaction	Yes	Yes or no	Yes or no	Yes
Gaze paresis:				
Side	Contralateral Sometimes ipsilateral	Contralateral	Ipsilateral	Ipsilateral
Response to calorics	Yes	Yes	No	Yes or no
Downward eye deviation	No	Yes	No	No
Ocular bobbing	No	No	Sometimes	Sometimes
Gait lost	No	No	Yes	Yes
Vomiting	Occasional	Occasional	Often	Severe

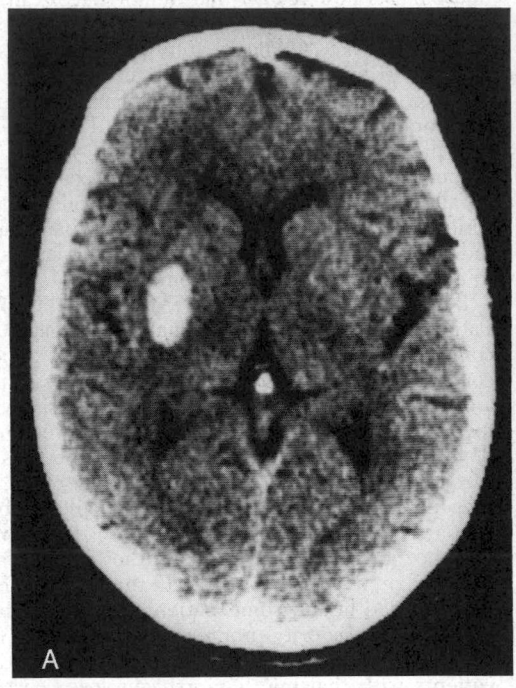

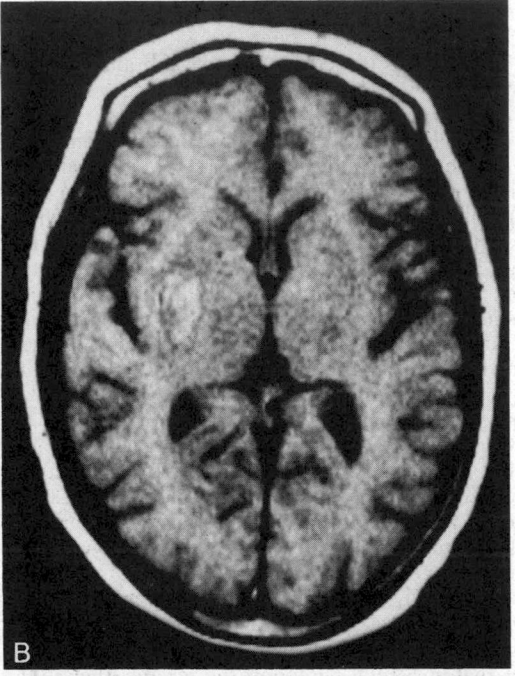

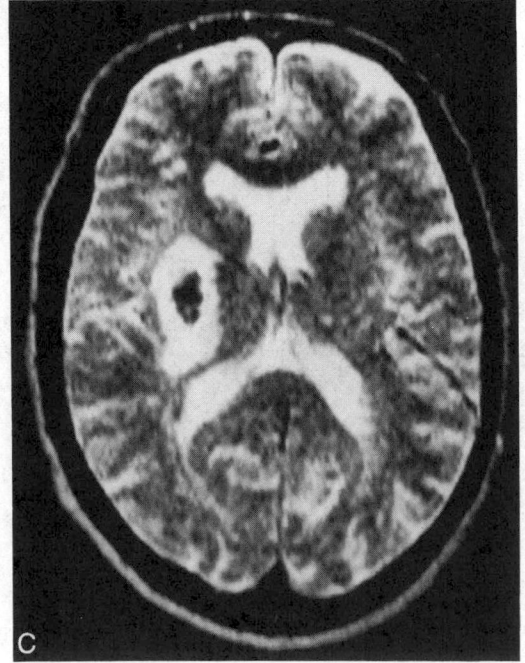

FIGURE 470–3. Hypertensive putaminal hemorrhage shown on CT at 24 hours (A), T₁-weighted magnetic resonance image (MRI) at 72 hours (B), and T₂-weighted MRI at 72 hours (C). Uniform hyperdensity on CT distinguishes primary hemorrhage from hemorrhagic and nonhemorrhagic infarction (compare with Fig. 469–1). The relative, though mild, hyperintensity on the T₁-weighted MRI image distinguishes hemorrhage from the hypointensity of nonhemorrhagic infarction; T₁-weighted MRI scans within 24 hours (not available for this patient) typically display more marked hyperintensity than at 72 hours. The core of the hematoma appears hypointense on the T₂-weighted MRI scan at 72 hours; T₂-weighted MRI scans within 12 hours (not available) typically show hyperintensity of greater degree than do concurrent T₁-weighted images. The rim of hyperintensity in C probably represents edema fluid. (Reproduced with permission from Zimmerman RD, Hier L, Snow R, et al.: Acute intracranial hemorrhage: Interval changes on sequential MR scans at 0.5 tesla. AJNR 9:47–57, 1988. © 1988, American Society of Neuroradiology.)

preserved. Further deterioration in arousal can result from several sources: extension into or compression of the brain stem, herniation of cerebellar tissue downward through the foramen magnum or upward across the tentorium, or hydrocephalus caused by obstruction of CSF flow into or out of the fourth ventricle. Prompt recognition and treatment of cerebellar hemorrhage before this stage can be life saving.

LOBAR CEREBRAL HEMORRHAGES. Lobar hemorrhages typically occur with amyloid angiopathy. The clinical presentation depends on the actual location of the hemorrhage, but there are some common features. Most patients are elderly; headache, nausea, and vomiting probably occur with about the same frequency but less intensity as in deep, hypertensive hemorrhages. Coma and seizures are less common, possibly because the bulk of the hemorrhage is in subcortical white matter.

LABORATORY EXAMINATION

Noncontrast CT scans demonstrate areas of hemorrhage as zones of increased density and rule out infarction (Fig. 470–3). Spontaneous hemorrhages typically display homogeneous areas of increased density and a mass effect, whereas hemorrhagic infarctions are characterized by areas of increased density (blood) interspersed with areas of decreased density (infarction). CT does not always distinguish reliably between a primary intraparenchymal hemorrhage and a hematoma resulting from a ruptured aneurysm. Similarly, some primary intracerebral hemorrhages dissect into the ventricular or subarachnoid system, inducing secondary intraventricular hemorrhage or SAH.

The MRI picture of hemorrhage depends on the precise sequence used and the age of the hemorrhage. At present, the advantages and disadvantages of MRI in this condition remain incompletely described, particularly in the early hours after onset. One known advantage of MRI is its ability to detect small hemorrhages, especially in the brain stem. Cerebral angiography is seldom used to evaluate acute hemorrhages, except those attributed to mycotic aneurysm being considered for surgical intervention.

TREATMENT

The management of acute parenchymal hemorrhage is supportive, but vigilance for transtentorial or foramen magnum herniation must be exercised, particularly with cerebellar hemorrhages. Herniation is initially treated with hyperventilation (which takes advantage of the vasoconstricting effect of hypocapnia; see Ch. 468) and osmotic agents (e.g., mannitol), but both of these interventions lose effectiveness with time. Corticosteroids have not been effective in treating brain edema from cerebral hemorrhage, and since they carry added risks (e.g., immunologic compromise, gastrointestinal hemorrhage), they are not advocated.

Direct surgical evacuation of acute spontaneous cerebral hemorrhage seldom is justified, occasional cerebellar hemorrhages providing a possible exception. What few comparative studies are available suggest that acute surgical evacuation of hematomas from the cerebral hemispheres does not substantially improve mortality and considerably increases the risk of severe residual neurologic disability if the patient survives. Cerebellar hemorrhages require surgical attention only if they are followed by signs indicating secondary brain stem compression. In such instances, lateral ventricular shunting appears to produce results as good as or better (fewer neurologic residua) than surgical removal of hematomas. Large lesions greater than 3 cm in diameter that continue to cause brain stem dysfunction after the shunt is placed occasionally benefit from clot evacuation.

As with ischemic strokes, blood pressure should not be lowered precipitously in patients with acute cerebral hemorrhage, since parenchymal blood and edema formation are likely to compress the tissue vascular bed and increase vascular resistance; an abrupt and steep reduction in systemic blood pressure could lower perfusion pressure below the critical threshold, thereby superimposing ischemic on hemorrhagic damage.

PROGNOSIS

The prognosis for patients with intraparenchymal hemorrhage is surprisingly good if they survive the acute illness, but mortality is higher (30 to 40 per cent) than in ischemic stroke (10 to 20 per

cent). As with ischemic stroke, recent studies show that about one fifth of patients surviving hemorrhage require institutionalization; in contrast to ischemic stroke, however, most of the remaining survivors achieve a good status or complete recovery. Age and large hemorrhage size are associated with a worse prognosis, and prognosis after extensive brain stem hemorrhage is guarded. In contrast to SAH, the risk of recurrent hemorrhage is relatively low, the exception being that AVM's can rebleed at rates approaching 2 per cent per year within the first several years of the initial bleed.

PROPHYLAXIS

Epidemiologic data strongly suggest that control of hypertension reduces the risk of hypertensive intraparenchymal hemorrhage. Careful control of anticoagulation and avoidance of other agents known to be associated with hemorrhage (e.g., amphetamines) should reduce the risk of hemorrhage. At present, there is no way to control the risk of bleeding from amyloid angiopathy.

470.4 HYPERTENSIVE ENCEPHALOPATHY

Hypertensive encephalopathy is a syndrome that accompanies markedly elevated blood pressures. Clinically, the disorder is characterized by symptoms of increased intracranial pressure (headache, nausea, vomiting, visual blurring) and of focal neurologic dysfunction, along with seizures and progressive stupor and coma. Retinal changes characteristic of severe hypertension are common and often include hemorrhages or papilledema, but arteriolar narrowing may be the only abnormality.

The cause of neurologic dysfunction is not clearly established. One theory, largely discounted, was based on observed retinal vasospasm and hypothesized that similar intracerebral vasospasm caused focal ischemia and resultant neurologic dysfunction. More recent evidence rests on the observation that with severe hypertension the upper limit of cerebral arterial autoregulation is exceeded, and blood flow rises passively with further increases in systemic blood pressure. Coincident with this inability to maintain constant blood flow, progressively higher pressures are transmitted into the capillary system, causing movement of plasma and even some cellular elements from blood into surrounding brain tissue. Resulting local and diffuse edema is postulated to cause the focal and diffuse neurologic changes.

Uremia uncomplicated by hypertension can produce a similar clinical picture, but this is easily excluded by determining the blood urea nitrogen (BUN) or creatinine values. Other complications of hypertension to be considered in the differential diagnosis include hemorrhagic and ischemic stroke, but in these conditions, focal signs predominate, whereas in hypertensive encephalopathy they are accompanied by prominent signs of diffuse dysfunction. Increased intracranial pressure from obstructive hydrocephalus, brain tumor, or subdural hematoma, particularly if pressure is transmitted into the fourth ventricle, can elevate blood pressure and slow the pulse (Cushing's sign). Usually, the absence of retinal changes suggesting chronic hypertension and the presence of signs reflecting the underlying neurologic diagnosis differentiate such neurogenic hypertension from hypertensive encephalopathy.

Hypertensive encephalopathy is a medical emergency. Treatment should be directed to acute, deliberate lowering of blood pressure (e.g., with intravenous nitroprusside), avoiding hypotensive or even normal levels. In most patients with chronic hypertension, the upper and lower limits of autoregulation are shifted upward, and if systemic pressure is lowered below the lower limit of the patient's intrinsic autoregulation (which can rise as high as 120 mm Hg), cerebral ischemia can result. When associated with pregnancy (eclampsia), hypertensive encephalopathy usually responds well to prompt delivery of the fetus. Hypercapnia, by dilating cerebral blood vessels, can exacerbate the effects of hypertensive encephalopathy, and seizures also are associated with further increases in cerebral blood flow and capillary pressure. Both should be avoided by controlled ventilation, when required, and anticonvulsants such as intravenous diazepam, 10 to 20 mg given slowly in repeated doses as needed to control seizures, and followed by phenytoin or carbamazepine.

With prompt treatment, the prospect is excellent for full recovery from the immediate episode. Long-term management requires close supervision of and compliance with an effective antihypertension program.

Biller J, Godersky JC, Adams HP Jr: Management of aneurysmal subarachnoid hemorrhage. Stroke 19:1300, 1988. *A review of practice to 1988, at which time antifibrinolytics, now seldom used, were still advocated and calcium channel blockers were achieving acceptance.*

Brown RD Jr, Wiebers DO, Forbes G, et al.: The natural history of unruptured intracranial arteriovenous malformations. J Neurosurg 68:352, 1988. *A follow-up study of 168 patients to define the natural history of clinically unruptured intracranial AVM's.*

Dias MS, Sekhar LN: Intracranial hemorrhage from aneurysms and arteriovenous malformations during pregnancy and the puerperium. Neurosurgery 27:855, 1991. *A review article discussing the risks and medical and surgical management of intracerebral hemorrhage in pregnant women.*

Gilbert JJ, Vinters HV: Cerebral amyloid angiopathy: Incidence and complications in the aging brain. I. Cerebral hemorrhage. Stroke 14:915, 1983. *Eleven patients with fatal cerebral hemorrhage and amyloid angiopathy.*

Juvela S, Heiskanen O, Potanen A, et al.: The treatment of spontaneous intracerebral hemorrhage: A prospective randomized trial of surgical and conservative treatment. J Neurosurg 70:755, 1989. *A randomized trial of 52 patients with brain hemorrhage showing that while surgery saves lives, it does not improve function.*

Kassell NF, Torner JC, Haley EC, et al.: The International Cooperative Study on the timing of aneurysm surgery. Part I: Overall management results. J Neurosurg 73:18, 1990. *This manuscript summarizes the results of the International Cooperative Study on saccular aneurysms and documents the status of medical management in the 1980's.*

Kassell NF, Torner JC, Jane JA, et al.: The International Cooperative Study on the timing of aneurysm surgery. Part 2: Surgical results. J Neurosurg 73:37, 1990. *This manuscript describes 3521 patients with ruptured saccular aneurysms who came from 68 centers. It presents a contemporary discussion of the diagnosis of SAH, prevention of rebleeding, vasospasm, and early versus late surgical intervention.*

Mendelow AD: Spontaneous intracerebral hemorrhage. J Neurol Neurosurg Psychiatry 54:193, 1991. *An editorial reviewing current diagnosis and management of intracerebral hemorrhage.*

Vermeulen M, van Gijn J: The diagnosis of subarachnoid haemorrhage. J Neurol Neurosurg Psychiatry 53:365, 1990. *A review justifying the use of CT instead of lumbar puncture to diagnose SAH and the interpretation of CSF in patients with a negative CT.*

SECTION EIGHT / INFECTIONS AND INFLAMMATORY DISORDERS OF THE NERVOUS SYSTEM

Roger P. Simon

471 Parameningeal Infections

Parameningeal central nervous system infections include those that affect brain parenchyma directly (brain abscess), those that produce suppuration in potential spaces covering the brain and spinal cord (epidural abscess and subdural empyema), those that produce occlusion of the contiguous venous sinuses and cerebral veins (cerebral venous sinus thrombosis), and remote infectious processes (bacterial endocarditis and sepsis) that result in diffuse, multifactorial involvement of the central nervous system.

BRAIN ABSCESS

Brain abscess is an uncommon disorder, accounting for only 2 per cent of intracranial masses. Abscesses produce localized, circumscribed central nervous system infections that manifest clinically as an expanding mass lesion, with symptoms and findings similar to those of other space-occupying lesions, such as brain tumors. Brain abscesses, however, often progress more rapidly than tumors and more frequently produce meningeal involvement.

ETIOLOGY. Infections resulting in brain abscess originate or extend from extracerebral locations. Although the most frequent predisposing factors have changed over the past decades and vary with the given hospital's population and referral base, the most common (Table 471-1) are bloodborne metastases from unknown sources and from lung or heart, direct extension from parameningeal sites (otitis, cranial osteomyelitis, sinusitis), recent or remote head trauma or neurosurgical procedures, and infections associated with cyanotic congenital heart disease. Bloodborne infections seed the brain via hematogenous spread and produce abscesses in brain regions in proportion to the blood flow; accordingly, parietal lobe abscesses predominate. Extension of infection from otitis and mastoiditis involves contiguous brain regions of the temporal lobe and cerebellum, whereas abscesses resulting from sinusitis affect contiguous brain regions of the frontal and temporal lobes. Currently, the most common cause of brain abscess in many urban hospitals is toxoplasmosis occurring in immunodeficiency states due to co-infection with the human immunodeficiency virus (HIV).

PATHOLOGY. On the basis of findings of clinical and experimental research, most brain abscesses evolve over a number of stages, beginning with vascular seeding of brain parenchyma, producing early cerebritis during the first 1 to 3 days. Inflammatory infiltrates of polymorphonuclear cells, lymphocytes, and plasma cells follow within 24 hours. By 3 days, the surrounding area shows a marked increase in perivascular inflammation. The late cerebritis phase develops approximately 4 to 9 days after infection, during which time the center becomes necrotic, containing a mixture of debris and inflammatory cells. Neovascularity is maximal at this time. Early reactive astrocytes surround the zone of cerebritis and proceed to early capsule formation between approximately 10 and 13 days. At this time, the necrotic center shrinks slightly, and a well-developed fibroblast layer evolves. The late capsule stage continues to evolve between 14 days and 5 weeks, with continual shrinking of the necrotic center and a relative decrease in the inflammatory cells. The capsule thickens as reactive astrocytes proliferate.

BACTERIOLOGY. The pathogenic organisms vary considerably, depending on the clinical circumstances. *Staphylococcus aureus* is the most common isolate in trauma-related cases. In patients with HIV-associated disease, *Toxoplasma* is the most common offending organism and bacterial abscesses are rare. Among other abscesses, the most commonly isolated pathogens are anaerobic organisms, but aerobic and microaerobic streptococci, *Staphlycoccus aureus*, *Bacteroides*, *Proteus*, and other gram-negative bacilli may also be found (Table 471-1). *Actinomyces*, *Nocardia*, and *Candida* are less frequent offenders. Infection is often polymicrobial. Culture-negative abscesses from surgical specimens occur in 30 per cent of antibiotic-treated patients and in 5 per cent of patients operated on before antibiotic administration.

CLINICAL PRESENTATION. Signs of infection may be

TABLE 471–1. SUMMARY OF UCSF CASES ACCORDING TO TIME PERIODS

	1970–1974	1975–1980	1981–1986	Total
Number of Cases	22(%)	33(%)	47(%)	102(%)
Etiology				
Local infection	2(9)	4(12)	13(28)	19(19)
Cardiac	6(27)	6(18)	5(11)	17(17)
Surgery	1(4)	7(2)	8(17)	16(16)
Trauma	2(9)	1(3)	6(13)	9(9)
Pulmonary	4(18)	4(12)	1(2)	9(9)
Immunocom- promise	2(9)	2(6)	2(4)	6(6)
Other	1(4)	4(12)	0(0)	5(5)
Unknown	4(18)	4(12)	13(28)	21(21)
Organisms				
Aerobic	16(73)	27(82)	34(72)	77(75)
Anaerobic	5(23)	8(24)	7(15)	20(20)
Multiple	5(23)	8(24)	7(15)	20(20)
None cultured	6(27)	6(18)	14(30)	26(25)
Deaths	9(41)	3(9)	2(4)	14(14)

Adapted with permission from Mampalam TJ, Rosenblum ML: Trends in the management of bacterial brain abscesses: A review of 102 cases over 17 years. Neurosurgery 23:451–457, 1988.

minimal or absent. Almost half of affected patients maintain a normal body temperature, and fewer than a third show a peripheral white cell count above 11,000 per microliter. Neck stiffness is rare in the absence of increased intracranial pressure.

Otherwise, the presenting features resemble those of any expanding intracranial mass (Table 471–2). A headache of recent onset is the most common symptom, representing distortion or irritation of pain-sensitive structures within the cranial vault, especially those of the great venous sinuses and the dura about the base of the brain. If the process continues untreated, isolated headache will increase in severity and become accompanied by focal signs followed by obtundation and coma. Hemiparesis and aphasia represent involvement of motor and language brain regions. Lethargy progressing to stupor occurs especially with frontal abscesses or with mass effect compressing the contralateral hemisphere or rostral brain stem. Seizures may occur with abscesses involving the cortical gray matter. The period of evolution may be as brief as many hours or as long as many days to weeks with more indolent organisms.

CEREBROSPINAL FLUID EXAMINATION. Cerebrospinal fluid (CSF) examination is not useful in diagnosing brain abscess, since the findings range from normal to those of purulent meningitis, depending on the walling off of the brain abscess or its closeness to CSF compartments (Table 471–3). More important, since abscesses often expand rapidly, lumbar puncture may precipitate or aggravate impending transtentorial herniation. If possible, the procedure should be deferred until after brain images are obtained, which may eliminate the value of CSF analysis.

NEUROIMAGING. Computed tomography (CT) and magnetic

TABLE 471–2. BRAIN ABSCESS: PRESENTING FEATURES IN 43 CASES

Headache	72%
Lethargy	71%
Fever	60%
Nuchal rigidity	49%
Nausea, vomiting	35%
Seizures	35%
Ocular palsy	27%
Confusion	26%
Visual disturbance	21%
Weakness	21%
Dysarthria	12%
Stupor	12%
Papilledema	10%
Dysphasia	9%
Hemiparesis	9%
Dizziness	7%

Reproduced with permission from Chan CH, Johnson JD, Hofstetter M, et al.: Brain abscess, a study of 45 consecutive cases. Medicine 65:415–431, 1986.

resonance imaging (MRI) are the laboratory studies of choice for diagnosing brain abscesses and monitoring their response to therapy. MRI may be especially useful for posterior fossa abscesses, as it provides an artifact-free view of the brain stem and cerebellum. In addition, MRI with intravenous gadolinium contrast is superior in demonstrating cerebritis, surrounding edema, and the extent of mass effect.

The evolution of the abscess can be estimated radiologically. In the early cerebritis stage, images reveal a low-density lesion with partial ring enhancement. In the late cerebritis and early capsule stage, well-formed ring-enhancing lesions are seen. The ring enhancement is typically thin walled and uniform, with subtle medial thinning adjacent to the ventricular system. Thick, nonuniform, or nodular enhancement should raise suspicion of an alternative etiology. Delayed scans show diffusion of contrast material into the lucent center, with gradual development of a homogeneous appearance. In the late capsule stage, well-formed ring enhancement may be seen with no delayed diffusion of contrast. Other ring-enhancing lesions that may mimic the image of brain abscess include primary and metastatic tumor, a resolving infarct or hematoma, and, rarely, demyelinating disease.

TREATMENT. Pyogenic brain abscess may be treated with antibiotic therapy alone or antibiotics combined with surgical aspiration or excision. Needle aspiration may be performed stereotactically with CT guidance while the patient is under local anesthesia; excision requires craniotomy. Aspiration offers the advantage of identifying the infecting organism. Initial surgical therapy may be preferred when significant mass effect is present, when the abscess adjoins the ventricular surface (raising the possibility of catastrophic rupture into the ventricular system), when abscesses arise in the posterior fossa (with the potential of brain stem compression), or when abscesses reach a large size (greater than 3 cm diameter) or become refractory to medical therapy. Medical therapy alone is indicated for surgically inaccessible, multiple abscesses (seen in 10 per cent of patients) or abscesses in the early cerebritis stage. With medical therapy alone, the causal organism is not identified, and antibiotic coverage directed toward the most likely organisms (streptococci and anaerobes) is needed. A suggested regimen includes penicillin G, 4 million units given intravenously (IV) every 4 hours, and metronidazole, 15 mg per kilogram IV over 1 hour, followed by 7.5 mg per kilogram given IV or orally every 6 hours. If staphylococcal infection is suspected (e.g., a history of trauma or intravenous drug abuse), oxacillin or nafcillin should be added at a dosage of 3 grams IV every 6 hours. Concomitant corticosteroid therapy may attenuate edema surrounding abscesses.

With medical therapy alone, the resolution of abscesses can be

TABLE 471–3. SUMMARY OF LUMBAR FLUID CHANGES ASSOCIATED WITH BRAIN ABSCESS*

		Number of Patients	Per Cent
Pressure			
<200 mm		38	38
200–300 mm		35	35
>300 mm		26	26
	Total	99	
White cells per mm³			
<5		61	29
5–100		81	38
>100		71	33
	Total	213	
Protein mg per dl			
<50		26	24
50–100		38	35
>100		44	41
	Total	108	
Glucose mg per dl			
>40		89	79
<40		23	21
	Total	112	

*Most of these data were obtained before brain imaging was widely available.

Reproduced with permission from Fishman RA: Cerebrospinal Fluid in Diseases of the Nervous System. Philadelphia, W. B. Saunders Company, 1980, p 264.

followed by serial CT or MRI. Antibiotics must be continued until the abscess cavity resolves completely. A failure to demonstrate abscess shrinkage in 4 weeks constitutes an antibiotic failure; a surgical procedure should then be performed. Of note is that the ring enhancement may persist after clinical and CSF normalization. Treatment durations are approximately 4 weeks for surgically treated patients and 6 weeks for unoperated on patients.

Abscesses associated with HIV infection are assumed to be due to *Toxoplasma gondii*. The diagnosis is confirmed by response to empiric treatment with daily doses of sulfadiazine, 12 to 15 mg per kilogram, given orally, and pyrimethamine, 25 to 50 mg, given orally. An alternate regimen is pyrimethamine given orally and clindamycin, 900 to 1200 mg IV every 6 hours (or 600 mg orally every 6 hours) for patients allergic to sulfa drugs.

PROGNOSIS. The current mortality rate is 5 to 15 per cent, depending on locale and the nature of pre-existing illness. Outcome also correlates inversely with the abscess size and the degree of neurologic dysfunction at presentation. Age, cause, number of abscesses, or corticosteroid use does not affect outcome.

SPINAL EPIDURAL ABSCESS

Infection within the epidural space about the spinal cord is an uncommon but readily diagnosable and treatable cause of paralysis and death. Its incidence is 0.5 to 1.0 per 10,000 hospital admissions in the United States, but the frequency is substantially increased in the intravenous drug–using population.

CLINICAL PRESENTATION. Patients are usually systemically ill with fever (to 38° to 39°C) in virtually all acutely evolving cases and in the majority of those with a subacute evolution. The initial feature is acute or subacute back pain, with focal percussion tenderness being virtually universal; stiff neck and headache are common. As the infection progresses, over hours, days, or weeks, radicular pain occurs, the site varying with the location of the abscess. Accordingly, this radicular component can be mistaken for sciatica, a visceral abdominal process, chest wall pain, or cervical disc disease. If the condition is unrecognized at this stage, the symptoms rapidly evolve, over a few hours to a few days, to produce weakness and finally paralysis at the spinal level dictated by the site of the infection. This characteristic progression from focal pain and tenderness to pain with radicular signs or symptoms evolving to pain with signs of weakness or paralysis below the level of the lesion is highly typical of an expanding epidural process. In this clinical setting, spinal epidural abscess should be assumed, systemic antibiotics begun, and urgent neuroradiologic confirmatory diagnostic procedures pursued.

The differential diagnosis includes compressive and inflammatory processes involving the spinal cord (transverse myelitis, intervertebral disc herniation, metastatic tumor), which can usually be differentiated clinically by the absence of systemic infection. Transverse myelitis, however, may be associated with fever; the most useful differential feature is its rapid evolution to maximum deficit within 24 to 48 hours or less. Other infectious processes that may have back or neck pain or tenderness as a notable feature must be excluded as well (bacterial meningitis, perinephric abscess, disc space infection, bacterial endocarditis). *Spinal subdural empyema* produces a similar but rare syndrome that often cannot be differentiated clinically from epidural abscess.

ETIOLOGY. Although a specific source cannot always be identified, infections of the epidural space originate from contiguous spread or via hematogenous routes from a distant source. Cutaneous sites of infection are the most common remote sources, especially in intravenous drug users. Abdominal, respiratory tract, and urinary sources are also common. Osteomyelitis may be a cause by either direct extension or hematogenous spread, especially when associated with sepsis. Contiguous spread of infection occurs, most commonly from psoas abscesses, decubitus ulceration, perinephric and retropharyngeal abscesses, surgical sites, or epidurally placed catheters. Whether or not venous spread can occur from pelvic infections via Batson's plexus of spinal veins remains unsettled. Minor back trauma has been implicated in producing a cutaneous hematoma near the spine, which is subsequently seeded via hematogenous sources.

PATHOPHYSIOLOGY. The anatomy of the epidural space dictates the location of the abscess, the frequency of epidural infections being proportional to the volume of the epidural space. Because the size of the intravertebral canal remains relatively constant while the circumference of the spinal cord changes, this is maximal in the thoracic region, next largest in the lumbar region, and least at the cervical spine enlargement. Further, as the dura about the cord is adherent to the vertebral columns anteriorly, the potential epidural space lies posteriorly, as do most epidural abscesses. Anteriorly situated abscesses can occur from contiguous spread of osteomyelitis but represent less than a fifth of all epidural abscesses. Since no anatomic barriers separate spinal segments in the epidural space, such abscesses usually extend over three to five or more vertebral segments.

As the epidural space is not confined rostrocaudally, there is no clear abscess cavity or focal mass to provide a situation of simple compression for spinal cord compromise in epidural abscess. Clinical signs often are substantially greater than would have been predicted from the anatomic extent of pus or granulation tissue found at surgical exploration. Further, in many instances, no frank compression is found on postmortem examination. The spinal cord dysfunction then is likely to be multifactorial, involving toxic processes secondary to inflammation, as well as venous thrombosis, thrombophlebitis, ischemia, and edema. The lack of a clear compressive etiology has important implications for treatment.

BACTERIOLOGY. Causative organisms can be identified by culture or Gram stain from pus obtained at exploration (90 per cent of cases), blood cultures (60 to 70 per cent of cases), or CSF (20 per cent of cases). *Staphylococcus aureus* accounts for most infections, followed by streptococci and gram-negative anaerobes. Tuberculous abscesses remain common, representing as many as 25 per cent of cases in high-risk populations.

DIAGNOSIS. CSF examination is often performed because of associated fever and meningeal signs. The fluid usually is nonspecifically abnormal, containing normal glucose levels, a moderately elevated protein content (400 to 500 mg per milliliter), and a lymphocytic pleocytosis (22 to 150 per cubic millimeter). Spinal fluid cultures yield organisms in about 25 per cent of cases. Almost 90 per cent of patients show a peripheral blood leukocytosis.

Plain spine radiographs, with attention to the area of percussion tenderness, may show osteomyelitis/discitis, a compression fracture, or a paravertebral mass. MRI is considered the study of choice for the evaluation of a suspected epidural abscess because of its ability to demonstrate the craniocaudal extent of the extradural soft tissue mass, associated mass effect upon the cord or cauda equina, and potential signal abnormalities within the discs and vertebral body marrow. The additional advantage, if any, of an intravenous gadolinium contrast agent has not been defined. If MRI is unavailable or technically impossible, CT with myelography usually provides adequate information.

TREATMENT. The disease is fatal in the absence of antibiotic therapy. Unless culture and sensitivities dictate otherwise, penicillinase-resistant penicillin (nafcillin, 12 grams per day, or oxacillin, 12 grams per day) with an aminoglycoside (gentamicin, 5 mg per kilogram per day) should be started empirically as antistaphylococcal treatment for presumed bacterial infection. For confirmed *Staphlyococcus aureus* abscesses, penicillinase-resistant penicillin can be used alone, but many authorities add rifampin (300 mg every 12 hours) because of its ability to penetrate the abscess cavity. Therapy should be continued intravenously for 3 to 4 weeks in the absence of osteomyelitis and 6 to 8 weeks with associated osteomyelitis. Surgical decompression was once felt to be mandatory, but early diagnosis by CT or MRI, as well as the absence of clearly compressive lesions at surgery and postmortem examination, has revised the treatment approach. Many examples demonstrate that medical therapy alone can be curative, particularly in instances in which diagnosis can be established prior to neurologic abnormalities, associated medical complications exist that increase the surgical risk, and complete paraplegia (or quadriplegia) has been present for more than 48 hours. Needle aspiration of the abscess or laminectomy should be performed to determine the causative organism when blood cultures are negative. Medical management of cervical epidural abscesses requires close neurologic evaluation because of the small space available to the abscess and the potential for quadriparesis.

PROGNOSIS. The chances of partial or complete recovery relate inversely to the amount of neurologic dysfunction at the time of diagnosis. Patients with abnormalities limited to pain recover without deficit. Approximately half the patients with some weakness have complete resolution, and nearly half the patients with paralysis of less than 36 hours' duration show some recovery of motor function. In tuberculous epidural abscess, recovery of motor function has been reported even after paralysis lasting for weeks.

VENOUS SINUS THROMBOSIS SECONDARY TO INFECTION

Thrombosis of cerebral veins or sinuses may be of idiopathic origin (Ch. 469), may occur in the setting of hematologic disorders or coagulation abnormalities (Ch. 155), or may result from local or contiguous infectious processes. The last-named syndromes are dealt with here.

Venous drainage from the brain begins with venules and veins that drain into the great venous sinuses. The venous sinus system itself lacks valves, permitting retrograde propagation of clots or infections emanating from structures such as those located in the central portion of the face or the middle ear.

Septic Cavernous Sinus Thrombosis

The cavernous sinuses comprise the most caudal dural venous chambers at the skull base. The paired structures lie on either side of the pituitary fossa, immediately above the midline sphenoid sinus. The cavernous sinus encloses the "cavernous portion" of the internal carotid artery; the third, fourth, and sixth cranial nerves en route to the apex of the orbit; and the ophthalmic and maxillary branches of the trigeminal nerve, which supply sensation to the forehead, periocular regions, cornea, and malar area of the face. Septic cavernous sinus thrombosis most commonly results from extension of infections involving the neighboring sphenoid and ethmoid sinuses, the central portion of the face, or the pharynx or tonsils.

Presenting symptoms are headache and/or lateralized facial pain, followed in a few days to weeks by fever, and involvement of the orbit, producing proptosis and chemosis secondary to obstruction of the ophthalmic vein. Paralysis of oculomotor nerves follows rapidly. Sensory dysfunction in the first and second divisions of the trigeminal nerve and a decrease in the corneal reflex are less obvious. Further involvement of the contiguous orbital contents follows, with mild papilledema and decreased visual acuity, sometimes progressing to blindness. Extension to the opposite cavernous sinus or to other intracranial sinuses with cerebral infarction, or increased intracranial pressure secondary to impaired venous drainage can result in stupor, coma, and death.

The differential diagnosis includes carotid cavernous sinus fistula (diagnosed by ocular bruit and an afebrile state); idiopathic granulomatous involvement of the cavernous sinus (the Tolosa-Hunt syndrome) or orbit (orbital pseudotumor, diagnosed by relative sparing of the orbital contents); and orbital cellulitis (infection localized to the orbit but sparing the structures of the cavernous sinus). Some overlap often occurs between involvement of these contiguous structures of the orbit and involvement of the cavernous sinus.

The CSF is abnormal in almost all cases, sometimes with a profile resembling that of purulent meningitis or parameningeal infection.

The most common causative organism is *Staphyloccocus aureus*, with streptococci and pneumococci being less common; anaerobic infection has been reported. Radiologic evaluation includes sinus imaging, with attention to the sphenoid and ethmoid sinuses. MRI (with and without intravenous contrast) can often demonstrate venous thrombosis by illustrating the lack of the normal "flow void" within vascular structures. Cranial CT scans, employed with or without intravenous contrast material, are seldom helpful. Cerebral angiography is usually unnecessary but may demonstrate extrinsic narrowing of the intracavernous portion of the internal carotid artery.

Treatment relies on early diagnosis and consists of the prompt drainage of infected paranasal sinuses as well as specific antistaphylococcal agents, such as nafcillin or oxacillin, given intravenously. Heparin anticoagulation may reduce morbidity from associated brain ischemia, but this treatment remains controversial in cases involving infection.

Lateral Sinus Thrombosis

Septic thrombosis of the lateral sinus results from acute or chronic infections of the middle ear. The symptoms consist of ear pain followed by headache, nausea, vomiting, and vertigo, evolving over several weeks. On examination, most patients are febrile. An abnormality on otologic examination is nearly invariable; mastoid swelling may be seen. Sixth cranial nerve palsies can occur, but other focal neurologic signs are rare. Papilledema occurs in half the cases, and elevated CSF pressure is present in most, especially with occlusion of the right lateral sinus (which is the major venous conduit from the superior sagittal sinus). CSF contents are usually normal, although parameningeal inflammatory profile may be seen.

Treatment includes intravenous antibiotics to cover staphylococci and anerobes (nafcillin or oxacillin with penicillin or metronidazole). Surgical drainage (mastoidectomy) may be required. Increased intracranial pressure seldom needs direct treatment unless visual fields show progressive constriction. The outcome is usually favorable.

Septic Sagittal Sinus Thrombosis

This uncommon condition occurs as a consequence of purulent meningitis, infections of the ethmoid or maxillary sinuses spreading via venous channels, compound infected skull fractures, or, rarely, neurosurgical wound infections. Symptoms include manifestations of elevated intracranial pressure (headache, nausea, and vomiting) that evolve rapidly to stupor and coma. Seizures and hemiparesis may result from cortical infarction. The rate of progression, severity of symptoms, and prognosis are all related to the location of thrombosis involving the sinus. When only the anterior third of the sinus is obstructed, symptoms are less intense and evolve more slowly. If or when the thrombosis progresses to involve the middle and posterior thirds of the sinus, deterioration progresses more rapidly and outlook for recovery declines.

CSF abnormalities accompany well over half the cases. The opening pressure is increased in proportion to the extent of the sagittal sinus involvement, and a pleocytosis usually reflects the association of a meningeal or parameningeal process.

Radiologically, septic sagittal sinus thrombosis may be excluded by visualization of the normal sagittal sinus during the venous phase of cerebral angiography. Contrast-enhanced CT scanning may reveal a contrast void lying at the junction of the transverse and sagittal sinuses (the region of the torcula); this so-called "delta sign" represents an intraluminal clot surrounded by contrast material. An appropriately programmed MRI scan will demonstrate an abnormal increase in signal intensity (absent flow void) within the affected venous sinus.

Intravenous antibiotics should be directed at organisms recovered from the meningeal process or the parameningeal site. *Staphyloccocus aureus*, β-hemolytic streptococci, pneumococci, and *Klebsiella* are the most common organisms. Initial antibiotic treatment should include nafcillin and an aminoglycoside. Associated paranasal sinusitis should be drained surgically. Heparin use in septic venous thrombosis is controversial, as the mortality rate (resulting from cerebral infarction) still approaches 8 per cent. Experience with noninfected sinus thrombosis has shown that heparin therapy substantially reduces morbidity-mortality, even when CT scans show evidence of hemorrhagic infarction (Ch. 469).

NEUROLOGIC COMPLICATIONS OF INFECTIOUS ENDOCARDITIS

Neurologic complications occur in one third of patients with bacterial endocarditis and triple the general mortality rate of the disease. Most such complications derive from valvular vegetations. Cerebral (but not systemic) emboli are more common from mitral valve endocarditis, for reasons unknown. The time of embolization during the course of endocarditis depends upon the virulence of the organism and whether it produces acute or subacute disease. With acute endocarditis (predominantly staphylococci or enterococci), embolization occurs early, often during the first week, while in subacute disease (predominantly viridans group streptococci or enterococci) emboli occur over the full course of treatment and occasionally after treatment is completed. Emboli lodge in the peripheral branches of the middle cerebral artery, in most cases with resultant hemiparesis. Focal seizures may result.

Whether or not warfarin anticoagulation decreases the risk of embolization remains a controversial issue. This therapy was administered in an earlier period to decrease platelet fibrin vegetations that sequestered the bacteria away from the body's defenses. Current evidence suggests a high rate of hemorrhagic intracerebral complications from warfarin anticoagulation in native valve endocarditis, but not in prosthetic valve endocarditis. Mechanisms to explain the difference remain unknown. Nevertheless, most authorities believe that patients already receiving chronic anticoagulation at the time of diagnosis of endocarditis should be maintained on such therapy.

Mycotic aneurysms complicate endocarditis in 2 to 10 per cent of cases and are more common in acute than subacute disease. The middle cerebral artery is most commonly involved, with the aneurysms being located distally in the vessel, differentiating them from congenital berry aneurysms. The process by which the aneurysmal dilatation occurs remains in dispute, although embolization of infectious vegetations is accepted as the inciting event. Aneurysmal rupture results in 80 per cent mortality, and early diagnosis is therefore important. Whom to subject to angiography is uncertain. However, clinical or radiologic evidence of cerebral or other embolization defines the high-risk group. Other suggested indications for angiography include severe headache (presumably the result of aneurysmal leakage). When an unruptured aneurysm is identified by angiography, it may resolve with antibiotic therapy alone. Accordingly, following such patients with serial angiograms is indicated, as surgical therapy requires excision of the infected portion of the artery. Patients with proximal mycotic aneurysms have a greater risk of perioperative stroke than do those with distal involvement.

Small brain abscesses may complicate the course of endocarditis, but macroscopic abscesses are rare. Most occur in the setting of acute, rather than subacute, endocarditis. Multiple microabscesses, however, can result in a diffuse encephalopathy similar to that seen in sepsis. Such lesions may escape detection on CT scanning and are not amenable to surgical drainage. Antibiotic treatment of the primary disease is indicated.

A CSF pleocytosis occurs in 70 per cent of patients with neurologic complications, but in an unknown number of patients in whom the central nervous system is clinically spared. The CSF profile may be that of a purulent meningitis (polymorphonuclear predominance, elevated protein level, and low glucose level) or that of a parameningeal infection (lymphocytic predominance, modest protein elevation, and normal glucose level). A hemorrhagic component may be seen. Purulent CSF is associated with signs of meningeal irritation and infection with a virulent organism producing an acute endocarditis.

SUBDURAL EMPYEMA

Empyema refers to infection in a preformed space, in this case that separating the dura and arachnoid. Subdural empyema is responsible for one fifth of localized intracranial infections and results from direct extension from infected paranasal sinuses or, less frequently, untreated chronic otitis. Unilateral empyema is most common, as the falx prevents passage across the midline, but bilateral and/or multiple concurrent empyemas occur. Cortical venous thrombosis or brain abscess develops in approximately one fourth of cases; purulent meningitis is a less common accompaniment.

Symptoms initially reflect those of chronic otitis or sinusitis, upon which lateralized headache (a universal feature), fever, and obtundation become superimposed. Vomiting, meningeal signs, and focal neurologic abnormalities (hemiparesis or seizures) usually follow. If the disease remains untreated, obtundation progresses, and the septic mass and swollen underlying brain soon lead to venous thrombosis or death from herniation. The major differential diagnosis is that of meningitis. Nuchal rigidity and obtundation occur in both, but papilledema and lateralizing deficits are more common in empyema. Lumbar puncture, if obtained because of the suspicion of meningitis, reveals an elevated intracranial pressure accompanied by an increased protein content and a polymorphonuclear pleocytosis with usually a normal glucose concentration in the CSF. Either CT or MRI can be diagnostic of empyema, showing an extra-axial, crescent-shaped mass with an enhancing rim lying just below the inner table of the skull over one or both hemispheres. MRI better detects underlying parenchymal edema.

Treatment requires both surgical drainage of the empyema cavity and high-dose intravenous antibiotics directed toward organisms found at the time of craniotomy. The bacteriology of subdural empyemas is similar to that of sinusitis and cerebral abscess, discussed above. Anticonvulsants should be administered prophylactically, as seizures are common.

If cortical infarction from venous thrombosis does not occur, the prognosis is surprisingly favorable, although chronic epilepsy results in one third of patients.

CRANIAL EPIDURAL ABSCESS

Infections of the epidural space coexist most often with subdural empyema and less frequently with chronic sinusitis or otitis alone. Symptoms and signs are headache and fever with focal neurologic abnormalities due to the coexistent subdural empyema or brain abscess. The diagnosis is made with MRI or contrast-enhanced CT scan (which demonstrate an enhancing lenticular lesion in the epidural space), and the abscess is treated by surgical drainage followed by systemic antibiotics. In uncomplicated cases, the prognosis is excellent.

MALIGNANT EXTERNAL OTITIS

This necrotizing osteitis occurs in elderly patients with diabetes. The associated organism, *Pseudomonas aeruginosa*, is a normal flora of the external ear. In this case, it produces an external otitis that fails to respect normal anatomic boundaries. The result consists of a rapidly evolving syndrome of ear pain, facial swelling, osteomyelitis, and purulent meningitis accompanied by multiple cranial nerve palsies. Urgent treatment with antipseudomonal penicillin (mezlocillin) or a third-generation cephalosporin (ceftazidime) and tobramycin, as well as surgical debridement and drainage, is essential. The mortality rate is high.

Brain Abscess

Haimes AB, Zimmerman RD, Morgello S, et al.: MR imaging of brain abscesses. AJR 152:1073, 1989. *Reviews MRI of brain abscesses and its differential diagnosis.*

Mampalam TJ, Rosenblum ML: Trends in the management of bacterial brain abscesses: A review of 102 cases over 17 years. Neurosurgery 23:451, 1988. *A recent review from a referral center with attention to the issue of corticosteroid therapy.*

Maniglia AJ, Goodwin WJ, Arnold JE, et al.: Intracranial abscesses secondary to nasal, sinus, and orbital infections in adults and children. Arch Otolaryngol Head Neck Surg 115:1424, 1989. *Association of sinus disease with brain abscesses is reviewed.*

Patel KS, Marks PV: Management of focal intracranial infections: Is medical treatment better than surgery? J Neurol Neurosurg Psychiatry 53:472, 1990. *Discussion of the issue of nonsurgical management.*

Spinal Epidural Abscess

Danner RL, Hartman BJ: Update on spinal epidural abscess: 35 cases and review of the literature. Rev Infect Dis 9:265, 1987. *An up-to-date review of all aspects.*

Del-Curling O Jr, Gower DJ, McWhorter JM: Changing concepts in spinal epidural abscess: A report of 29 cases. Neurosurgery 27:185, 1990. *A recent neurosurgical series.*

Lasker BR, Harter DH: Cervical epidural abscess. Neurology 37:1747, 1987. *Specific problems of cervical abscesses are reviewed and anatomic considerations are addressed.*

Leys D, Lesoin F, Viaud C, et al.: Decreased morbidity from acute bacterial spinal epidural abscesses using computed tomography and nonsurgical treatment in selected patients. Ann Neurol 17:350, 1985. *The issue of nonsurgical treatment is introduced.*

Venous Sinus Thrombosis Secondary to Infection

Southwick FS, Richardson EP, Swartz MN: Septic thrombosis of the dural venous sinuses. Medicine 65:82, 1986. *Complete review of all aspects.*

Neurologic Complications of Infectious Endocarditis

Davenport J, Hart RG: Prosthetic valve endocarditis 1976–1987. Antibiotics, anticoagulation, and stroke. Stroke 21:993, 1990. *Anticoagulation in prosthetic valve endocarditis is readdressed.*

Pruitt AA, Rubin RH, Karchmer AW, et al.: Neurologic complications of bacterial endocarditis. Medicine 57:329, 1978. *Major review of all aspects from a single referral center.*

Subdural Empyema

Kaufman DM, Miller MH, Steigbigel NH: Subdural empyema: Analysis of 17 recent cases and review of the literature. Medicine 54:485, 1975. *A complete discussion of clinical features from patients at a single center.*

Pathak A, Sharma BS, Mathuriya SN, et al.: Controversies in the management of subdural empyema. A study of 41 cases with review of literature. Acta Neurochir 102:25, 1990. *A recent large series and literature review.*

Weingarten K, Zimmerman RD, Becker RD, et al.: Subdural and epidural empyemas: MR imaging. AJR 152:615, 1989. *MRI is described.*

Cranial Epidural Abscess

Silverberg AL, DiNubile MJ: Subdural empyema and cranial epidural abscess. Med Clin North Am 69:361, 1985. *Reviews the topic.*

Malignant External Otitis

Johnson MP, Ramphal R: Malignant external otitis: Report on therapy with ceftazidime and review of therapy and prognosis. Rev Infect Dis 12:173, 1990. *A recent review of clinical and therapeutic aspects.*

472 Neurosyphilis

The resurgence of primary and secondary syphilis (now estimated to be 14.7 cases per 100,000) first occurred among promiscuous homosexual males but has more recently spread to heterosexual contacts via prostitutes. If untreated, approximately 7 per cent of patients with primary syphilis infection will develop some form of symptomatic neurosyphilis.

PATHOPHYSIOLOGY. Each of the neurologic manifestations of syphilis results from a chronic, insidious meningeal inflammatory process occurring as a reaction to treponemal invasion of the central nervous system (CNS). An inflammatory response in the cerebrospinal fluid (CSF) occurs in 34 per cent of asymptomatic persons with syphilis, with the CSF abnormalities peaking at 13 to 18 months after the primary infection. This CNS invasion dictates the risk of future symptomatic and asymptomatic neurosyphilis, which amounts to approximately 30 per cent following a primary infection but falls to 1 per cent or less if CSF examination is normal 5 years after the primary infection (Merritt, 1946).

CLINICAL SYNDROMES. The clinical manifestations of neurosyphilis are conventionally divided into acute syphilitic meningitis, cerebrovascular syphilis, syphilitic dementia (general paresis), and tabes dorsalis. These entities, however, form an overlapping spectrum. For instance, paresis and tabes may coexist (taboparesis). After primary infection, these clinical subtypes of neurosyphilis follow a predictable time course (Fig. 472–1) based on the evolution of the meningeal inflammatory process. Why this inflammatory process becomes symptomatic at a particular stage in a particular patient is unknown. Symptomatic syphilitic meningitis is the earliest manifestation of nervous system syphilis, often occurring coincident with a secondary rash. The meningeal inflammation later extends to involve the cerebral blood vessels and, when symptomatic, results in cerebrovascular neurosyphilis (usually seen within the first 5 years following primary infection). The so-called parenchymal forms of neurosyphilis (paresis and tabes) occur after a more protracted interval. Syphilitic meningitis and cerebrovascular syphilis, the earlier forms, are therefore the most frequently observed manifestations of neurosyphilis in the present epidemic.

Acute Syphilitic Meningitis. Symptomatic meningeal syphilis occurs during the first months to a year or two after the primary infection, with 10 per cent of cases occurring coincident with a secondary rash. The course is subacute. Headache is common, and asymmetric cranial nerve abnormalities are prominent (especially those involving auditory function, facial strength, eye movements, and vision, this last being secondary to unilateral or bilateral optic papillitis). Patients are afebrile; meningeal signs are often present, and some patients become confused. The CSF shows a lymphocytic pleocytosis. Accurate diagnosis is important, as relatively mild symptoms may resolve spontaneously without treatment, leaving the patient at risk for progression to the fixed deficits associated with the later forms of neurosyphilis.

Cerebrovascular Syphilis. As the meningeal inflammatory process progresses, a diffuse vasculitis evolves, compromising the cerebral arteries traversing the subarachnoid space and producing a subacute encephalopathy with ischemia-caused focal features. Associated symptoms include confusion, personality change, and intellectual decline, usually followed by the emergence of focal deficits resulting from occlusion of specific vessels. Arteries in the middle cerebral artery distribution are most often involved, but any cerebral or spinal vascular bed may be affected alone or in combination, the condition often evolving over a period of several hours or days. The resulting syndrome is distinct from thromboembolic stroke because of the associated encephalopathy, the multifocal pattern, and the subacute time course.

Diagnosis is confirmed by finding an inflammatory spinal fluid with a positive serology; angiography is unnecessary, but if performed demonstrates vasculitis of medium-sized arteries. Areas of ischemia observed on computed tomography (CT) or magnetic resonance imaging (MRI) in association with the characteristic CSF suggest the diagnosis. These ischemic areas most often arise in the deep cerebral white matter and follow the distribution of the lenticulostriate branches of the middle cerebral artery.

Syphilitic Dementia. Dementia paralytica, or general paresis of the insane, is the diffuse meningoencephalitic form of neurosyphilis. Affected patients usually present 10 to 20 (range, 3 to 30) years after the primary infection. General paresis affects men four to seven times more frequently than women, perhaps because the infectivity of *Treponema pallidum* declines during pregnancy.

Syphilitic dementia produces notoriously nonspecific symptoms, the pattern of which can be mimicked by almost any organic brain syndrome. The colorful descriptions of grandiose delusional states and psychosis are well known but were uncommon even in the prepenicillin era. Then, as now, a simple dementing illness predominated. Tremors of the hands, tongue, and lips, resulting in disordered handwriting and dysarthria, were classically described as characteristic; modern experience is insufficient to confirm the observations.

Several features help to differentiate paresis from other causes of dementia. Syphilitic dementia has a relatively early onset, most commonly beginning between ages 30 and 50, and it progresses rapidly if untreated, being fatal within months to a few years. An inflammatory CSF is always found, and the blood and CSF syphilis serologies are always positive.

Tabes Dorsalis. The term describes a myeloneuropathy that characteristically occurs 10 to 20 years after primary infection (range, 5 to 50 years). A sensory neuropathy results, with the primary lesions affecting either the proximal dorsal root entry zones or the dorsal root ganglia. As with paresis, a marked male predominance (7:1) was noted in the prepenicillin era.

The classic triad of symptoms includes lightning pains, sensory ataxia, and urinary disturbance. The triad of most common and earliest signs is that of pupillary abnormalities, lower extremity areflexia, and the Romberg sign. Lightning pains are transient, agonizing, shooting pains described as being "like the twanging of a single fiddle string," which are most common in the legs but which may affect any region of the body. Characteristic is an early loss of vibration and position sense attributed to secondary degeneration of the posterior columns of the spinal cord. The proprioceptive impairment engenders a wide-based, unsteady gait that is exacerbated by elimination of visual input (eye closure): the Romberg sign. Bladder hypotonia with overflow incontinence results from deafferentation of the lower sacral sensory nerve roots. Rectal incontinence is uncommon; genital sensory and autonomic impairment eventually results in impotence. Peripheral autonomic impairment often develops and, along with loss of peripheral nociceptive afferent fibers, is responsible for the development of trophic (Charcot) joint deformities and distal extremity ulcers. The sensory impairment is responsible for the loss of deep tendon reflexes.

Of the pupillary abnormalities, half have the classic Argyll Robertson pattern, being small, irregular, and bilaterally reacting

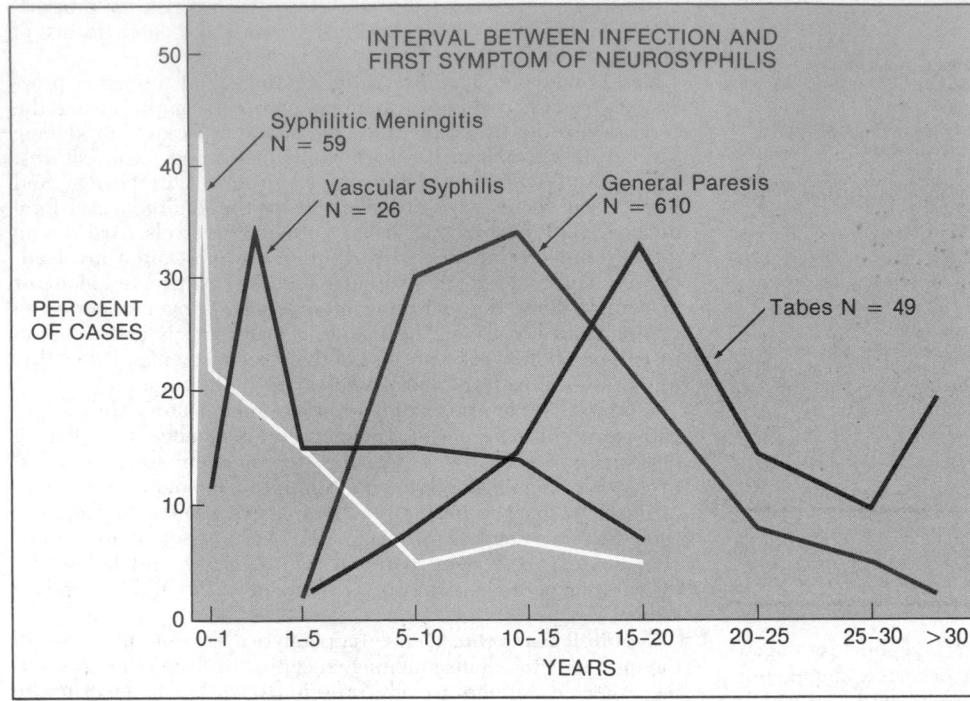

INTERVAL BETWEEN INFECTION AND
FIRST SYMPTOM OF NEUROSYPHILIS

PER CENT OF CASES

Syphilitic Meningitis N = 59
Vascular Syphilis N = 26
General Paresis N = 610
Tabes N = 49

YEARS

FIGURE 472–1. Interval between primary and symptomatic neurosyphilis by type (meningeal, vascular, paresis, tabes), abstracted from the literature and presented as per cent of total cases within type. (Reproduced with permission from Simon RP: Neurosyphilis. Arch Neurol 42:606–613, 1985.)

poorly to light but constricting briskly to accommodation (the phenomenon of light-near dissociation). Other pupillary abnormalities in tabes include unilateral mydriatic pupils with loss of pupillary light reflex.

CEREBROSPINAL FLUID EXAMINATION. A chronic, insidious inflammatory response within the CSF (Table 472–1) accompanies each of the clinical syndromes of neurosyphilis and provides the ultimate diagnostic test establishing the presence of active neurosyphilis and/or its response to therapy. The absence of a CSF inflammatory response excludes a diagnosis of active neurosyphilis and therefore precludes a clinical response to antibiotic therapy. As with any chronic meningitis, the γ globulin portion of the protein content is commonly elevated, and oligoclonal bands may be present.

Active neurosyphilis causes an abnormal CSF. The possibility of a negative serology in neurosyphilis is difficult to ascertain from the classic literature because of the relatively insensitive Wasserman test and the unrecognized inclusion of nonsyphilitic syndromes of cerebrovascular disease and viral meningitis. When the clinical diagnosis was characteristic, however, only rare cases showed a negative CSF serology (even with the Wasserman reaction): In 100 paretic patients reported by Merritt (1946), the CSF Wasserman test was positive in every case. Wilson also reported universal CSF positivity in 77 cases of paresis. Theoretically, a negative CSF VDRL might occur in the presence of severe immunosuppression, as a prozone phenomenon, or, in an

early case, as a manifestation of the CSF inflammatory response preceding seropositivity. This last situation may explain occasional recent reports of false-negative results or delayed conversions in early meningeal syndromes.

The role of the more sensitive treponemal test (fluorescent treponemal antibody [FTA]) in diagnosing CNS syphilis remains uncertain because of a high false-positive response and decreased sensitivity (75 per cent); without supporting clinical or laboratory data, the diagnostic value of a reactive CSF FTA is unknown. An additional confirmatory test is to inject CSF into rabbit testes; a reactive testicular swelling and recovery of spirochetes prove treponemal infectivity.

TREATMENT. Since neurosyphilis of all clinical types is associated with a CSF inflammatory response, the CSF cell count provides the ultimate monitor of the effectiveness of therapy. Normalization of the spinal fluid is the required endpoint of antibiotic therapy. Once the CSF remains normal for 2 years, relapses fail to occur.

Penicillin is the drug of choice. Various regimens from 12 to 24 mU per day have been suggested, but it is not clear that the higher doses alter the clinical outcome. Intramuscular benzathine penicillin usually results in undetectable levels in CSF and accordingly should not be used for treatment of neurosyphilis. Spirocheticidal levels (0.03 IU per milliliter, 0.018 μg per milliliter) in CSF are exceeded with 12 million units of IV penicillin daily in four divided doses. Some regimens include probenecid

TABLE 472–1. MODERN EXAMPLES OF CSF FINDINGS IN VARIOUS NEUROSYPHILITIC SYNDROMES

Syndrome	OP	WBC	Glu	Prot	Gamma Globulin*	VDRL	
						Blood	*CSF*
Meningitis	170	154 (94% L)	29	95		1:64	1:4
Cerebrovascular	192	58 (87% L)	41	119	IgG index .93	1:512	1:16
Paresis		220	49	305	IgG index 1.99	1:128	1:8
Tabes (active)		62		140		1:16	1:28
Tabes (inactive)		2	76	43		1:16	1:2

*Normal IgG index = 0.23 to 0.64.

OP = Opening pressure; WBC = white blood cells; Glu = glucose; Prot = protein; VDRL = Venereal Disease Research Laboratory; CSF = cerebrospinal fluid; L = lymphocytes; IgG = immunoglobulin G.

TABLE 472–2. CSF RESPONSE TO PENICILLIN TREATMENT*

	Admission	Day 7	Day 21	6 Mo
Opening pressure, mm CSF	120	—	—	Normal
Cells/cu mm	207 (94% L)	100 (100% L)	24 (100% L)	0
Glucose, mg/dl	51	66	54	66
Protein, mg/dl	50 (14.4% gamma globulin)	38	48	34
Serology (VDRL)				
CSF	1:2	1:1	—	—
Blood	1:64	1:64	1:64	1:64

*Meningovascular syphilis treated with aqueous penicillin G, 24 million units daily for 21 days; data from Holmes MD, Brant-Zawadski MM, Simon RP: Clinical manifestations of meningovascular syphilis. Neurology 34:553–556, 1984.

to increase concentrations in CSF by decreasing reabsorption of penicillin through the choroid plexus. Probenecid, however, also decreases parenchymal penicillin concentrations by competing for uptake at membrane transport sites.

The optimal duration of penicillin treatment for neurosyphilis is uncertain. Complete normalization of CSF is uncommon during the usual 2- to 3-week course of intravenous treatment, but the spinal fluid continues to return to normal over the next weeks to months (Table 472–2). Proof of adequate treatment requires a normalized cell count and a falling protein content at 6 months.

HUMAN IMMUNODEFICIENCY VIRUS (HIV) INFECTION IN NEUROSYPHILIS. Neurosyphilis and HIV-associated disease may coexist, both being consequences of sexual promiscuity. It has been recently suggested that syphilis is an opportunistic infection in HIV disease, and that in such patients syphilis follows an atypical, penicillin-resistant, aggressive course. However, syphilitic syndromes described in these patients are not different in either time course or clinical presentation from those in the pre-AIDS era. Further, the apparent "penicillin resistance" may represent coexistent HIV-induced CSF pleocytosis that is not altered by penicillin therapy. In addition, the occasional recovery of treponemes following penicillin treatment for syphilis in HIV–co-infected patients was similarly observed in the pre-AIDS era. Antibody production to syphilis by plasma cells is impaired with progressive immunosuppression, however, which has resulted in a loss of FTA reactivity in 10 per cent of a San Francisco cohort. Accordingly, a decline in the immune capacity

of patients with HIV infection does occur late in this disease, but its association with any continued activity nervous system syphilis in such patients remains speculative.

The principles of treating neurosyphilis in HIV–co-infected patients are similar to those used in patients without the retrovirus disease; intravenous penicillin should be used in spirocheticidal doses, and the spinal fluid should be monitored as an index of therapy. As noted, when the inflammatory response is due partly to syphilis and partly to HIV infection, only a portion of the pleocytosis will disappear, leaving a new plateau level of CSF cellularity. The Centers for Disease Control (CDC) recommends that patients co-infected with HIV and syphilis for more than 1 year should have an examination of their CSF, whether or not they have neurologic symptoms.

CDC: Recommendations for diagnosing and treating syphilis in HIV-infected patients. MMWR 37:600, 1988. *Current recommendations.*

Jordan KG: Modern neurosyphilis—a critical analysis. West J Med 149:47, 1988. *Review and critique of diagnostic, clinical, and laboratory criteria for neurosyphilis with and without HIV co-infection.*

Merritt HH, Adams RD, Solomon HC: Neurosyphilis. 2nd ed. New York, Oxford University Press, 1946. *The classic descriptive work of the prepenicillin era.*

Musher DM, Hamill RJ, Baughn RE: Syphilis in the presence of human immunodeficiency virus infection. Ann Intern Med 113:872–881, 1990, *A critique of the association between syphilis and HIV infection.*

Simon RP: Neurosyphilis. Arch Neurol 42:606, 1985. *A review of the clinical syndromes, CSF, and serologic diagnostic criteria.*

Wilson SAK: Neurology. Vol 1. London, E. Arnold Company, 1940, pp 455–459. *Extensive single-author experience with neurosyphilis in the prepenicillin era.*

SECTION NINE / VIRAL INFECTIONS OF THE NERVOUS SYSTEM

473 Introduction

Richard W. Price

Agents belonging to nearly all the major groups of animal viruses can infect the central nervous system. The spectrum ranges from the large, complex DNA herpesviruses to small, relatively simple viruses with DNA or RNA genomes, such as the papovaviruses and retroviruses. Also included are agents not yet fully characterized that cause the spongiform encephalopathies in which the nature of "transmissible material" remains uncertain. As a result, neurologic manifestations of viral infections can be almost equally diverse, extending from the typical acute febrile encephalitides to chronic progressive disorders that clinically resemble degenerative neurologic diseases.

In most cases, particularly in those infections presenting as acute encephalitis, nervous system involvement is an uncommon complication of a relatively common systemic infection. In adaptive terms, extension of infection to the central nervous system is "accidental" and may even preclude survival of the virus and its transmission to a new host. For example, the polioviruses cause enteric infections in which replication in the gut and fecaloral transmission determine the essential survival and transmission of the organism; extension of infection to anterior horn cells of the spinal cord devastates the host but does not contribute to the "life cycle" of the virus. By contrast, the neurotropic herpesviruses, including herpes simplex virus type 1, are exquisitely adapted to cause latent and reactivated infection within the peripheral nervous system; in this case, the sensory neuron is the reservoir for latent virus, and reactivated virus exploits axoplasmic transport to reinfect the epithelium and consequently induce local shedding of virus. However, even in the case of the herpesviruses, central nervous system complications, such as acute herpes encephalitis, are "accidental" and not essential in the organism's adaptive strategy. Rabies illustrates an illness in which central nervous system infection plays a central role in the life cycle of the virus: Involvement of the brain produces "rabid," biting behavior that actually contributes to virus transmission.

Viruses can enter the nervous system along a number of avenues. Transport up peripheral nerves can allow direct passage from epithelium or viscera to the central nervous system, and once virus enters the brain, similar intraneural passage by axoplasmic transport can facilitate further spread. It has been demonstrated that a number of viruses are transported along nerve processes by both orthograde and retrograde axoplasmic transport systems. This mode of transport allows rapid passage over long distances and also provides an avenue that is protected from immunologic interference. Many, if not most, viruses, however, enter the brain via hematogenous dissemination, with passage across the vascular endothelium. As a general rule, agents that travel over neural routes tend to produce initially focal neurologic symptoms and signs, while those that disseminate hematogenously cause more diffuse clinical changes. Exceptions exist, however. One lies in the selective vulnerability of particular nervous system structures or cells to infection with particular agents. Focal or multifocal disease can also follow general hematogenous dissemination in a random seeding of brain regions. Many viruses preferably infect the meninges rather than the brain, gaining access via the choroid plexus.

While within the nervous system a number of viruses appear not to discriminate among neurons, glial, or endothelial cells, others choose selective targets. Such selectivity is probably determined to a great extent by cell-surface molecules, principally glycoproteins, that serve as receptors for viruses and determine the character of attachment and subsequent entry into cells. Different cell types may also vary in their capacity to support virus-directed metabolism and replication.

The character of virus-cell interactions can assume a number of courses: *abortive infection* results in little or no change in the cell and no virus replication; *acute productive/lytic infection* is characterized by a full replication cycle with production of progeny and subsequent cell death; *chronic productive infection* may allow prolonged release of progeny virus without cell death; in *latent infection*, the viral genome resides in the cell, either integrated into the host genome or as a separate genomic fragment with little or no gene transcription or translation but retention of the capacity to reactivate subsequently; *transforming infection* results in increased and characteristically abnormal cell proliferation, usually in the absence of virus replication; *defective infection* may result in nonproductive infection or production of incomplete particles, yet cause varying degrees of cell alteration and viral antigen expression.

Diagnostic approaches to viral diseases depend on the clinical setting and specific agents involved. Available methods of diagnosis include serologic assessment of host-antibody responses in serum or cerebrospinal fluid, direct identification of virus in brain or cerebrospinal fluid using viral isolation techniques or methods that identify viral antigens or nucleic acid, and histologic examination of infected tissue for pathognomonic reactions (e.g., formation of inclusion bodies or other specific cell changes).

In the past, limitations of treatment made specific virologic diagnosis either largely an academic exercise or important principally for epidemiologic purposes. Efforts to combat viral disease consisted exclusively of prevention through active, or at times passive, immunization. These time-honored methods still predominate, and the prevention of poliomyelitis remains a landmark of biomedical research. In the past two decades, however, antiviral chemotherapy has become a practical reality. Effective therapy is now available for neurotropic herpesviruses and for human immunodeficiency virus, and the promise exists not only for more effective treatments for infection by these groups of viruses but also for the development of chemotherapeutic agents that will act selectively against several other important viruses causing neurologic diseases.

Johnson RT: Viral Infections of the Nervous System. New York, Raven Press, 1982. *Although now outdated in certain details, this remains an excellent introduction to the general principles of viral infection of the nervous system.*

474 Acute Viral Meningitis and Encephalitis

Richard W. Price

DEFINITIONS. The terms *viral meningitis* and *viral encephalitis* refer to infections of the leptomeninges and brain parenchyma, respectively. When the spinal cord is involved along with the brain, the term *viral encephalomyelitis* may be used. When both meninges and brain parenchyma appear to be involved, *viral meningoencephalitis* sometimes is employed, although viral encephalitis is almost always accompanied by meningeal inflammation. The nonspecific term *aseptic meningitis* refers to an inflammatory process of the meninges accompanied by a predominantly mononuclear cell pleocytosis and not caused by pyogenic bacterial infection. Although viral infections are the most common cause of aseptic meningitis, infections by other types of organisms, as well as chemical irritation of the meninges and reactions to certain medications, can cause a similar clinical picture and cerebrospinal fluid profile. Most viral meningitides are benign, self-limiting processes with a low acute morbidity and only rare long-term sequelae. While viral encephalitides are also often benign, they more often result in significant morbidity and mortality.

Acute central nervous system infections caused by a variety of viruses are appropriately considered together because their clinical aspects are largely indistinguishable. Viral infections causing more distinct neurologic symptoms and signs are considered separately in subsequent sections.

ETIOLOGIES. Many viruses can cause acute encephalitis or meningitis (Table 474–1). Table 474–2 indicates the most common virus groups and the syndromes they produce.

Enteroviruses are small, nonenveloped RNA viruses of the picornavirus family with numerous serotypes, over 50 of which have been associated with meningitis or encephalitis. This family includes members of the coxsackie A and B, echovirus, and newer enterovirus groups, as well as the three poliovirus subtypes (see Ch. 475).

The arboviruses include agents of several families that are transmitted by mosquitoes or ticks. More than 15 different arboviruses have been associated with encephalitis in varied geographic areas of the world. In the United States, the five most important are eastern and western equine encephalitis, St. Louis encephalitis, California encephalitis (with most cases involving the LaCross subtype), and Colorado tick fever. Less common within the continental states are Venezuelan equine encephalitis and Powassan encephalitis.

Herpes simplex virus type 1 causes severe encephalitis, but usually with characteristical focal features, while herpes simplex virus type 2 causes aseptic meningitis in association with primary or secondary genital herpes (see Ch. 476). Lymphocytic choriomeningitis (LCM) virus, an arenavirus, is a sporadic cause of meningitis and occasionally encephalitis. Aseptic meningitis has now been recognized as a complication of acute infection by the retrovirus causing the acquired immunodeficiency syndrome (AIDS; see Part XXI). Adenoviruses are respiratory viruses that only rarely cause meningitis or severe childhood encephalitis.

The acute neurologic disease associated with measles, vaccinia, and rubella infections in most cases represents postinfectious encephalomyelitis (see Ch. 479). This may also be true of the encephalitis that has occasionally been reported with influenza and parainfluenza virus infections.

EPIDEMIOLOGY. Viral meningitis and encephalitis are relatively common disorders. In one study in Rochester, Minnesota, for example, the incidence of aseptic meningitis was nearly 11 per 100,000 person-years, while that of viral encephalitis was more than 7 per 100,000 person-years. This finding was compared with a rate of 8.6 episodes of bacterial meningitis. A relatively low mortality rate in this study (3.8 per cent) may have reflected the inclusion of milder cases and the predominance of the LaCross type of viral encephalitis. In other epidemiologic settings, the mortality is considerably greater. In general, a specific etiologic diagnosis is identified in only about 10 to 15 per cent of cases of meningitis and encephalitis in the United States.

TABLE 474-1. VIRUSES ASSOCIATED WITH ACUTE CENTRAL NERVOUS SYSTEM INFECTIONS IN THE UNITED STATES

RNA Viruses
Picornaviruses (enteroviruses)
  Polioviruses
  Coxsackieviruses, groups A and B
  Echoviruses
  Enteroviruses
Togaviruses
Eastern equine encephalitis*
Western equine encephalitis*
St. Louis encephalitis*
Powassan*
Tick-borne encephalitis
Rubella
Bunyavirus
  California encephalitis* (includes LaCross subtype)
Orbivirus
  Colorado tick fever*
Arenavirus
  Lymphocytic choriomeningitis
Rhabdovirus
  Rabies
Myxoviruses and paramyxoviruses
  Influenza
  Parainfluenza
  Mumps
  Measles
Retroviruses
  Human immunodeficiency virus type 1

DNA Viruses
Herpesviruses
  Herpes simplex, types 1 and 2
  Varicella zoster
  Epstein-Barr
  Cytomegalovirus
Adenoviruses

*Arthropod-borne viruses (arboviruses).

Each of the viruses causing central nervous system infection has its own epidemiologic pattern. Because of the predominance of enteroviruses and arboviruses, the overall incidence of viral meningitis and encephalitis peaks in the late summer. Enterovirus epidemics in temperate climates characteristically take place in the summer, with transmission occurring by the fecal-hand-oral route, often involving young children, with rapid spread in family or social groups. The geographic and seasonal incidence of arbovirus infection relates to the life cycle of arthropod vectors and animal reservoirs (Ch. 389) and their contact with humans. Eastern equine encephalitis virus is limited largely to the Atlantic and Gulf coasts, while western equine encephalitis virus is confined to the western two thirds of the country, with the highest incidence in the middle states. The latter virus causes many more human infections than does the eastern virus, but only 1 in 100 of those infected develops encephalitis. St. Louis encephalitis virus causes disease in both rural and urban areas over a large part of the United States. In the rural areas, the virus has the same pattern as western encephalitis virus, but in urban areas more explosive outbreaks can occur. In recent years, the LaCross subtype of the California encephalitis virus has been related to encephalitis every year over a wide geographic area of

TABLE 474-2. RELATIVE FREQUENCY OF MENINGITIS AND ENCEPHALITIS OF KNOWN VIRAL ETIOLOGY

Viral Agent	Viral Meningitis (%)	Viral Encephalitis (%)
Enteroviruses	83	23
Arboviruses	2	30
Mumps	7	2
Herpes simplex	4	27
Varicella	1	8
Measles	1	<1

Reproduced with permission from Jubelt B: Enterovirus and mumps virus infections of the nervous system. Neurol Clin 2:187, 1984.

the eastern United States, particularly in the midwestern states, with disease confined largely to children. Colorado tick fever occurs in the Rocky Mountain area; about 18 per cent of infected patients develop meningitis, but encephalitis is rare. Venezuelan encephalitis has spread into Florida and the southwestern states and, in most of those infected, produces an influenza-like illness, but about 3 per cent develop acute meningitis or encephalitis. Powassan virus is a rare cause of encephalitis in Canada and along the northern border of the United States.

Lymphocytic choriomeningitis virus is the major zoonotic virus causing meningitis and encephalitis. Humans acquire the infection by contact with dust or food contaminated by excreta of the common house mouse. Human disease is more common in winter, when the natural host tends to move indoors. Lymphocytic choriomeningitis virus has also been found in hamsters, and human infections have been traced to laboratory and pet hamsters.

Mumps virus spreads by the respiratory route, with infection occurring throughout the year but increasing in incidence during the spring. Although mumps virus infects the two sexes equally, males develop meningitis three times more frequently than females.

PATHOGENESIS. Events leading up to the development of the acute viral encephalitides and meningitides can be divided into three stages. The first involves exposure of an external body surface to the virus, usually with local replication of the "inoculum." In the case of enteroviruses, the infecting virus is contained in body fluids or excreta from infected persons and transferred by direct contact or within contaminated environmental materials, while the arboviruses are introduced by an arthropod bite. The next stage involves systemic viremia and amplification of virus in visceral organs; a secondary viremia may then lead to invasion of and replication within the nervous system or meninges. With the exception of rabies virus, the neurotropic herpesviruses, and perhaps the polioviruses, agents that cause acute viral encephalitis or meningitis reach the nervous system hematogenously. This factor accounts for the widespread distribution of cerebral dysfunction associated with most of the encephalitides.

In viral encephalitis, infection of neurons, glial cells, and even vascular endothelium leads to cell dysfunction and sometimes cell death. Inflammatory responses follow, and lymphocytes and macrophages first line the blood vessels and then migrate into the parenchyma. Clinical symptoms and signs depend on the distribution of infection and on both the direct effect of the virus and the secondary inflammatory reactions in the tissue. The relative contribution of direct viral infection or secondary host reactions to the genesis of brain dysfunction varies, depending on the particular infecting virus. The remarkable degree of recovery in many patients suggests that secondary immune responses often play an important role in producing symptoms.

CLINICAL MANIFESTATIONS. The systemic accompaniments of most acute viral encephalitides and meningitides are similar but depend on the particular virus. Often central nervous system manifestations are preceded or accompanied by fever, malaise or myalgia, gastrointestinal disturbance, respiratory symptoms, or rash. These are followed in viral meningitis by the development of headache, photophobia, stiff neck, and other signs of meningeal irritation, usually with an intensity milder than that of bacterial meningitis.

When encephalitis is present, evidence of diffuse or, less commonly, focal brain dysfunction accompanies or overshadows the signs of meningeal irritation. Patients characteristically exhibit altered attention and consciousness, ranging from confusion to lethargy or coma. Motor function may also be abnormal, with weakness, altered tone, or incoordination, reflecting affliction of the cortex, basal ganglia, or cerebellum in varying degree. In severe cases, generalized or focal seizures may occur, and their control may be difficult. Some patients exhibit myoclonus or tremor. Hypothalamic involvement may lead to hyperthermia or hypothermia, autonomic dysfunction with vasomotor instability, or diabetes insipidus. Abnormalities of ocular motility, swallowing, or other cranial nerve functions are uncommon. Similarly, spinal cord infection is usually less conspicuous but can result in flaccid weakness, with acute loss of reflexes in the most severe cases. Focal symptoms other than seizures are usually minor and overshadowed by generalized brain dysfunction, but in some patients hemiparesis, visual disturbance, or sensory loss may be prominent. Such focal abnormalities are particularly characteristic of herpes encephalitis (see Ch. 476).

The time course of acute viral meningitis and encephalitis is variable. The onset may occur within a matter of hours or may evolve more slowly over a few days. Usually, maximum deficit appears within 1 to 4 days.

LABORATORY FINDINGS. Examination of the cerebrospinal fluid is essential. The presence of 10 to 1000 mononuclear cells per cubic millimeter is characteristic. On occasion, early examination may show acellular fluid or predominance of polymorphonuclear leukocytes, but the typical mononuclear pleocytosis soon evolves. The pressure may be elevated, while the glucose level is characteristically normal or only modestly reduced. The protein content is usually elevated (50 to 100 mg per deciliter) and may exhibit increased immunoglobulin concentration and the presence of oligoclonal bands. An increased protein content and number of cells may persist for weeks and perhaps months after convalescence, and the oligoclonal bands can be detected for an even longer period.

Systemic laboratory findings may vary, depending on the etiologic agent. Generally, the white blood cell count is not elevated, but either elevations or depressions can be seen, usually with a lymphocytic predominance. Involvement of salivary glands or pancreas in mumps may elevate the serum amylase level.

Neurodiagnostic tests usually reveal nonspecific abnormalities, with notable exception in the case of herpes simplex encephalitis (see Ch. 476). The electroencephalogram characteristically exhibits generalized slowing, but focal sharp-wave or spike activity can occur in association with seizures. Computed tomography (CT) and magnetic resonance imaging (MRI) are usually normal early in the course of the nonherpetic viral encephalitides, but focal edema and contrast enhancement may appear in the more severe cases. The greatest value of these neuroimaging procedures lies in excluding alternative diagnoses.

DIAGNOSIS. With a few exceptions, the neurologic and laboratory findings accompanying the acute viral meningoencephalitides are insufficiently distinct to allow an etiologic diagnosis, and it may even be difficult to distinguish these disorders from a number of nonviral diseases. The epidemiologic setting (e.g., time of year, exposure to insects, the local community) and accompanying systemic manifestations may be helpful in presumptive virologic diagnoses. Thus, involvement of the nervous system by mumps virus is usually suspected from associated clinical parotitis or pancreatitis, although the neurologic disease can be the sole or presenting clinical manifestation; conversely, a certain history of previous mumps eliminates this diagnostic possibility. Several enterovirus infections produce a rash, which usually accompanies the onset of fever and persists for 4 to 10 days. In infections by coxsackievirus A5, 9, and 16 and echovirus 4, 6, 9, 16, and 30, the rash is typically maculopapular and nonpruritic and may be confined to the face and trunk or may involve extremities, including the palms and soles. Echovirus 9 infections can cause a petechial rash resembling meningococcemia. Herpangina, characterized by grayish vesicular lesions on the tonsillar fossae, soft palate, and uvula, can accompany group A coxsackie infection. In coxsackievirus A16 and, rarely, other group A serotype infections, a vesicular rash may involve hands, feet, and oropharynx. As discussed below, the encephalitis related to Epstein-Barr virus occurs in the setting of acute mononucleosis, and the principally postinfectious encephalitides related to measles and varicella follow overt systemic diseases with characteristic rashes.

Because no specific treatment exists for acute viral meningitis and encephalitis (except herpes), and their signs and symptoms are often nonspecific, exclusion of other diagnoses becomes important. Potentially confusing are partially treated bacterial meningitis; rickettsial infections; Lyme disease; meningitis caused by a variety of nonpyogenic organisms, including *Mycobacterium tuberculosis* and *Cryptococcus neoformans* and other fungi; meningeal or parameningeal bacterial infections; brain abscess; subacute bacterial endocarditis; and the cerebral vasculitides. Among noninfectious causes, trimethoprim-sulfamethoxazole, nonsteroidal analgesics, OKT3 antibody given for immunosuppression,

intravenous immunoglobulin, and certain other drugs may occasionally cause a sterile meningeal reaction. Without a cerebrospinal fluid examination, the differential diagnosis becomes even broader, encompassing additional toxic and vascular diseases. Most alternative diagnoses can be suspected or eliminated by the cerebrospinal fluid profile or by appropriate brain imaging.

Despite the absence of effective treatment, specific virologic diagnosis is useful both for prognosis in the individual patient and for epidemiologic implications for the populations at risk. Diagnosis usually relies on serology, although direct detection of the organism in the cerebrospinal fluid, blood, or stool may also be achieved in some cases. Selection of tests and their interpretation depend upon the particular organism. Almost all acute viral syndromes occur in the setting of a first encounter with the agent, which then results in lasting immunity. In these cases, seroconversion documented by a fourfold or greater rise in antibody titers between acute and convalescent sera is a principal means of diagnosis. A notable exception is herpes simplex encephalitis, in which antibody titers must be more cautiously interpreted (Ch. 476). Attempts at direct viral isolation are of limited value in clinical management and must be tailored to the suspected agent. Arboviruses and enteroviruses can be isolated from the blood but are seldom recoverable at the time of clinically evident meningitis or encephalitis. During the acute disease, coxsackieviruses and echoviruses are most readily isolated from stool or cerebrospinal fluid and, in some cases, throat washings. Lymphocytic choriomeningitis virus can be isolated from blood or cerebrospinal fluid. Mumps virus may be isolated from saliva, throat washings, or cerebrospinal fluid. Type 2 herpes simplex virus may also be cultured from the cerebrospinal fluid or identified in genital lesions.

TREATMENT. Treatment of acute viral encephalitis and meningitis (except herpes) is directed at symptom relief, supportive care, and preventing and managing complications. Strict isolation is not essential, although when enteroviral infection is suspected, precautions in handling of stools and the practice of careful hand washing should be instituted. Those with measles, chickenpox, rubella, or mumps virus infections should observe the usual precautions of isolation from susceptible individuals. Arboviruses are not characteristically spread from person to person but require an intermediate insect vector.

The headache and fever of meningitis can usually be managed with judicious doses of acetaminophen. Severe hyperthermia (>40°C) may require vigorous therapy, but modest temperature elevations may serve as a natural defense mechanism and are best left untreated.

Patients with severe encephalitis often become comatose. Since, however, some may achieve remarkable recovery, vigorous support and avoidance of complications are essential. Meticulous care in an intensive care unit setting with respiratory and nutritional support is therefore usually justified.

Although seizures sometimes complicate encephalitis, prophylactic anticonvulsants are not routinely recommended. If seizures develop, they can usually be managed with phenytoin and phenobarbital. If status epilepticus ensues, appropriate vigorous therapy should be instituted to prevent secondary brain injury and attendant hypoxia (Ch. 483). Similarly, secondary bacterial infections should be sought and promptly treated.

Modest increases in intracranial pressure can be treated with mannitol or glycerol, but this is usually only of short-term benefit. Steroids should probably generally be avoided in the treatment of encephalitis because of their inhibitory effects on host immune responses, but they may be required for control of intracranial hypertension in some patients.

PROGNOSIS. Full recovery from viral meningitis usually occurs within 1 to 2 weeks of onset, although some patients describe fatigue, light-headedness, and asthenia persisting for months.

The prognosis of encephalitis is dependent on the etiologic agent. Arbovirus encephalitides have variable mortality rates; that with eastern equine encephalitis is approximately 50 per cent; with St. Louis, 10 per cent; with western equine, 10 per cent; with Venezuelan equine, 1 per cent; and with California, less than 0.5 per cent. The mortality rates for western equine encephalitis are greater in children under 1 year of age, and for St. Louis encephalitis they are greater in the elderly. Nonfatal encephalitis caused by eastern, western, and St. Louis viruses leaves a relatively high rate of neurologic sequelae. Encephalitis associated with mumps or LCM virus is very rarely associated with death, and sequelae are infrequent. Hydrocephalus has been reported as a late sequela of mumps meningitis and encephalitis in children.

Chonmaitree T, Baldwin CD, Lucia HL: Role of the virology laboratory in diagnosis and management of patients with central nervous system disease. Clin Microbiol Rev 2:1, 1989. *A review of laboratory procedures used in the diagnosis of acute viral diseases of the central nervous system.*

Evans AS: Viral Infections of Humans: Epidemiology and Control. 3rd ed. New York, Plenum Publishing Corporation, 1989. *A useful text dealing with the epidemiology of viral infections; contains individual chapters dealing with the major groups, including the arboviruses, enteroviruses, and herpesviruses.*

Johnson RT: Viral Infections of the Nervous System. New York, Raven Press, 1982. *A comprehensive monograph reviewing the pathogenesis, epidemiology, and clinical features of central nervous system viral infections.*

Jubelt B: Enterovirus and mumps virus infections of the nervous system. Neurol Clin 2:187, 1984. *A useful review of the pathogenetic and clinical aspects of enterovirus and mumps virus infections.*

Jubelt B, Miller JR: Viral infections. *In* Merritt's Textbook of Neurology. Philadelphia, Lea & Febiger, 1989. *An excellent general review with a useful bibliography of "classic" and recent articles on individual infections.*

Nicolosi A, Hauser WA, Beghi E, et al.: Epidemiology of central nervous system infections in Olmstead County, Minnesota, 1950–1981. J Infect Dis 154:399, 1986. *Provides incidence figures for viral meningitis and encephalitis.*

Rennels MB: Arthropod-borne virus infections of the central nervous system. Neurol Clin 2:241, 1984. *A review of the major epidemic arbovirus infections in the United States.*

Whitley RJ: Viral encephalitis. N Engl J Med 323:242, 1990. *A recent review that emphasizes herpes encephalitis management and differential diagnosis.*

475 Poliomyelitis
Richard W. Price

DEFINITIONS. Poliomyelitis (acute anterior poliomyelitis, infantile paralysis) is an acute illness caused by the three strains of poliovirus. The disease selectively destroys the motor neurons of the spinal cord and brain stem to cause flaccid asymmetric weakness. Until recently one of the most feared of all human infectious diseases, poliomyelitis is now almost entirely preventable by vaccination.

ETIOLOGY. The three antigenically different strains of poliovirus (types 1, 2, and 3) are classified in the genus *Enterovirus* within the family Picornaviridae. These are small (approximately 270 nm), roughly spherical particles with icosahedral symmetry containing a single-stranded RNA core and are surrounded by a protein capsid. Lacking a lipid envelope, the polioviruses are resistant to lipid solvents and stable at low pH.

INCIDENCE, PREVALENCE, AND EPIDEMIOLOGY. In the United States, the number of cases of paralytic poliomyelitis, which averaged 21,000 per year over the 5 years before the introduction of vaccines, has now fallen to just a few cases yearly. However, in less advanced regions of the world, polioviruses remain endemic, and paralytic polio continues to occur, with a seasonal incidence of infection in temperate zones but a more even distribution throughout the year in tropical areas. Poliovirus is acquired by the oral route and subsequently replicates in the oropharynx and lower gastrointestinal tract. It may be secreted for a week or two in saliva and for more prolonged periods in feces, which provides the major avenue of host-to-host transmission. Spread of polioviruses is greatly influenced by standards of hygiene, and greatest dissemination occurs within families or other crowded circumstances.

Paralysis is an unusual complication of poliovirus infection. During an epidemic, 95 per cent of infections are asymptomatic and only 1 to 2 per cent result in neurologic symptoms and signs; the remaining 4 to 8 per cent of affected individuals suffer nonspecific (minor) illness. Where poliovirus is endemic and among children during epidemics, the incidence of neurologic manifestations is even lower. A number of factors increase the incidence of paralytic disease, including advancing age, recent hard exercise, tonsillectomy, and pregnancy. Immunity to each of the three types of poliovirus is lifelong, but infection with one strain does not necessarily protect against subsequent infection

by another. In the United States, poliomyelitis due to live-attenuated strains is as common as disease related to wild-type virus.

PATHOGENESIS AND PATHOLOGY. Polioviruses selectively infect certain neuronal populations, inducing highly stereotyped pathology, and in this manner contrast with most of the viruses causing acute encephalitis or meningitis.

The poliovirus invades the nervous system only after prior systemic replication. An initial alimentary phase with local replication in the intestinal mucosa and spread to the local lymphatics is followed by a viremic phase, which results in seeding of the nervous system. Once within the central nervous system, poliovirus may disseminate along neural pathways, attacking principally motor neurons of the spinal cord and lower brain stem, the brain stem reticular formation, and, to a lesser extent, the precentral gyrus. Convalescent poliomyelitis is characterized by loss of motor neurons and denervation atrophy of their associated skeletal muscles.

CLINICAL MANIFESTATIONS. The incubation period from virus exposure to the neurologic phase characteristically lasts between 4 and 10 days but may be prolonged to 4 to 5 weeks. The major illness usually begins with fever and malaise and is followed within hours by generalized headache, vomiting, and within another day by the development of neck and back stiffness. Patients at this time often are drowsy but on arousal are irritable and apprehensive. Progression may stop at this point, making the illness indistinguishable from other enterovirus meningitides. When paralysis develops, it usually begins on the second to fifth day after the onset of headache. Weakness, however, may be among the initial symptoms or, rarely, especially in children, may be delayed for 7 to 10 days. Children generally exhibit less intense systemic symptoms than do adults, who characteristically appear acutely ill and are tremulous, flushed, and agitated. Their muscles are often sensitive and stiff.

Poliomyelitis preferentially damages the larger somatic motor neurons. In all but the most severe cases, the involvement tends to include the lumbar segments to a greater degree than the cervical, and the spinal cord more than the brain stem. The damage and consequent paralyses are usually asymmetric, weakness characteristically being more proximal than distal, and in mild cases affecting parts of muscles rather than the entire muscle or the distribution of a single motor root. The asymmetry may be such that one member is rendered useless yet the contralateral one is spared entirely. About 50 per cent develop acute urinary retention. The trunk musculature is least commonly affected. The affected muscles are flaccid, and the deep tendon reflexes may be absent. Atrophy develops rapidly, usually beginning within a week in paralyzed muscles and progressing over the ensuing weeks. Once it starts, progression of the motor deficit for more than 3 to 5 days is rare.

About 10 to 15 per cent of cases affect the lower brain stem motor nuclei. Involvement of the ninth and tenth cranial nerve nuclei leads to paralysis of pharyngeal and laryngeal musculature, with resultant difficulty in phonation and swallowing. Parts of the facial muscles can be involved, either unilaterally or bilaterally. Less often, the tongue and muscles of mastication are partially paralyzed. External oculomotor weakness occurs only rarely and never permanently. The pupils are spared. Direct involvement of the brain stem reticular formation can disrupt breathing and swallowing and can produce serious disturbances in cardiovascular control. Poliomyelitis seldom causes permanent functional paralysis of the bulbar muscles, probably because of the relatively small size of the motor units served by brain stem nuclei and because overwhelming disease in these critical segments usually kills the patient.

DIAGNOSIS AND DIFFERENTIAL DIAGNOSIS. Because of its rarity in the United States, poliomyelitis may present diagnostic difficulties. In its early phases, it may be difficult to differentiate from other acute meningitides, and when paralysis ensues, a major differential diagnosis is with the Guillain-Barré syndrome and other predominantly motor polyneuropathies. However, for practical purposes, no other acute disease produces headaches, stiff neck, fever, and asymmetric flaccid paralysis without sensory loss coupled with an increase in white blood cells in the cerebrospinal fluid (CSF). Diagnosis may be more difficult if these major findings are equivocal or lacking. The CSF rarely shows a persistence of significant pleocytosis in polyneuritis, and CSF protein levels above 100 mg per milliliter are frequent. Acute intermittent porphyria may cause an illness similar to that of postinfectious polyneuropathy. At times, acute transverse myelitis may be confused with poliomyelitis, but in the former a sensory and motor level at the appropriate spinal cord segment usually serves to separate an inflammatory cord transection from diffuse anterior horn cell involvement. Both epidemic neuromyasthenia (Iceland disease) and pleurodynia (Bornholm's disease) may be confused with mild attacks of poliomyelitis. The epidemiologic setting, the lack of CSF abnormalities, and the absence of clear motor paralysis serve to distinguish these entities. In rare cases, infection with other enteroviruses can produce a paralytic illness resembling mild paralytic poliomyelitis. Both coxsackievirus and echoviruses have been reported to cause encephalitides with prominent (but not extensive) motor neuron symptoms and signs. Diagnosis can be established by isolation of virus from blood or CSF or by serologic evidence of acute poliovirus infection. In cases related to vaccine strains, viral isolates can be distinguished in the laboratory.

TREATMENT. There is no specific treatment, but supportive care can be important in reducing suffering during the acute attack, in maintaining vital functions to ensure survival, and perhaps in modifying the overall outcome and disability. Important measures include preventing contractures, maintaining airway and cardiovascular stability, and preventing excessive calcium mobilization and bed sores.

PROGNOSIS. Death in poliomyelitis is usually the result of bulbar involvement and is attributable to respiratory and cardiovascular impairments. Death rates are higher in adolescents and adults than in children. Mortality also varies with individual epidemics and has been considerably reduced with modern management of respiratory insufficiency. Patients who survive an episode of acute paralytic poliomyelitis usually recover considerable motor function. Generally, motor improvement begins within the first weeks after onset, and 60 per cent of eventual recovery is achieved by 3 months and 80 per cent by 6 months. The degree of permanent paralysis cannot be assessed accurately until 2 to 3 months have passed.

The Postpolio Syndrome. A number of patients with previous poliomyelitis develop further functional deterioration later in life. In some this relates simply to musculoskeletal decompensation or other factors but does not involve new weakness. However, in others there is a true loss of strength; the condition in these patients has been referred to as postpoliomyelitis progressive muscular atrophy (PPMA). This disorder is characterized by progressive weakness beginning 30 or more years after an attack of poliomyelitis. Clinicians in the United States are now much more likely to see this late complication of poliomyelitis than the initial paralytic disease. Most commonly, it presents as a late-life progression of weakness in already affected muscles, or, less often, in muscles previously thought to be normal. This weakness is often accompanied by fasciculations, and there may be additional atrophy. Muscle biopsy shows type grouping consistent with active denervation-reinnervation. Overall, the prognosis is generally good, with only slow progression of further weakness, which may plateau and rarely leads to a severe increase in disability or to death. This development must be distinguished from motor neuron disease of a more malignant variety (Ch. 465), which has also been described many years after acute poliomyelitis but appears to be much less common than the more gradual and benign syndrome of PPMA.

PREVENTION. Poliomyelitis can be prevented by either live-attenuated or killed polio vaccines. These are now given routinely in Western cultures, although the practice of immunization has relaxed as the threat of developing paralytic poliomyelitis has become less conspicuous. If this trend is not reversed, a resurgence of the disease can be expected. An important consequence of accurate diagnosis of poliomyelitis is the prompt institution of local vaccination programs for communities at risk, including subcultures in which vaccination is avoided for religious or other reasons.

Dalakas MC, Elder G, Hallett M: A long-term follow-up of patients with postpoliomyelitis neuromuscular symptoms. N Engl J Med 314:959, 1986. *Describes the clinical and laboratory features of late-onset weakness in patients suffering poliomyelitis earlier in life.*
Price RW, Plum F: Poliomyelitis. In Vinken PJ, Bruyn GW (eds.): Handbook of Clinical Neurology. Vol. 32, Part I. Amsterdam, Elsevier North-Holland, 1978. *A general review of clinical and biologic aspects of poliomyelitis.*
Wyatt HV: Incubation of poliomyelitis as calculated from the time of entry into the central nervous system via the peripheral nerve pathways. J Infect Dis 12:547, 1990. *Discusses the pathogenesis of poliomyelitis, hypothesizing that axoplasmic transport of virus over motor nerves provides the major portal of entry into the central nervous system and explains the tropism for anterior horn cells.*

476 Herpesvirus Infections of the Nervous System

Richard W. Price

Three of the six human herpesviruses (see also Ch. 371 to 375) share an essential "neurotropism" in their adaptation for survival and transmission. Herpes simplex virus types 1 and 2 (HSV-1 and HSV-2) and varicella zoster virus all establish in sensory ganglion neurons a latent infection that can subsequently reactivate to release progeny virus into the territory of the ganglion's epithelial innervation. The major complications of these infections in adults include adult-type herpes simplex encephalitis caused by HSV-1; aseptic meningitis, radiculitis, and sacral autonomic insufficiency caused by HSV-2; and encephalitis, myelitis, radiculopathy, and vasculitis complicating herpes zoster. Prompt diagnosis of infections by these viruses is important, since they are now amenable to selective antiviral drug therapy. Two of the remaining human herpesviruses, Epstein-Barr virus and cytomegalovirus, although largely lymphotropic, can also cause neurologic disease in the setting of systemic illness.

476.1 HERPES SIMPLEX ENCEPHALITIS (HSE)

Adult-type HSE is a sporadic disease with a severe morbidity and high mortality. Both HSV-1 and HSV-2 are capable of causing encephalitis, but type 1 by far predominates. In contrast, HSV-2 accounts for the great majority of neonatal herpetic encephalitis, which is not considered here.

EPIDEMIOLOGY AND PATHOGENESIS. Although the most common identified cause of severe, sporadic viral encephalitis in the United States, HSE is nonetheless uncommon. The disease afflicts persons of all postneonatal ages, with peaks of incidence in late childhood and middle age. It occurs with approximately equal frequency throughout the year, and case-to-case transmission does not occur. Immunosuppression plays no apparent role.

HSV-1 is a ubiquitous organism; more than 90 per cent of adults exhibit serologic evidence of exposure, and most harbor latent ganglionic infection. Recurrent cold sores resulting from viral reactivation occur in perhaps one fourth of adults. Although HSE may occur as a primary infection, it likely more often results from reactivated virus or perhaps from reinfection by a new strain of virus.

The characteristic gross and microscopic pathology of herpetic infection, particularly its anatomic localization, distinguishes HSE from other encephalitides. Although often asymmetric, the disease is usually bilateral and afflicts the medial temporal and inferior frontal lobes and related "limbic" structures, including the hippocampus, amygdaloid nuclei, olfactory cortex, insula, and cingulate gyrus. Necrosis with petechial hemorrhage is so intense that the disease was once called *acute necrotizing encephalitis*. Microscopically, hemorrhagic necrosis with mononuclear inflammation characterizes involved areas, with neurons and glia often containing Cowdry type A intranuclear inclusions during the acute phase of infection. The gray matter is affected predominantly, but infection extends into the white matter as well.

CLINICAL MANIFESTATIONS. HSE most commonly presents as an abruptly beginning subacute illness causing local and diffuse cerebral dysfunction. Typically, patients are febrile, although in as many as 10 per cent fever may be absent, and thus herpes encephalitis warrants consideration even in afebrile patients who present with an acutely altered mental status. Severe headache, focal or generalized convulsions, and alterations in behavior and consciousness are the most prominent symptoms. Common symptoms including disorientation, delusions, agitation, personality changes, or dysphasia sometimes lead erroneously to psychiatric referral. Motor paralyses are present in fewer than half of affected individuals.

DIAGNOSIS. Evaluation of suspected HSE has been an area of controversy, principally related to the issue of diagnostic brain biopsy. Among the arguments for brain biopsy are that (1) it is the most sensitive and accurate diagnostic method, contrasting with the insensitivity and difficulty in early interpretation of serologic studies and neurodiagnostic procedures; and (2) this procedure results in identification of alternative diagnoses, some of which respond to specific treatment. Arguments against brain biopsy relate to its potential short- and long-term sequelae, the benignity of empiric therapy, and the improved sensitivity and accuracy of magnetic resonance imaging (MRI) compared with earlier diagnostic methods. Important issues regarding management also relate to the facilities, expertise, and experience available to the patient at the admitting hospital. This author feels that, all in all, in most instances patients are appropriately managed without biopsy and that the combination of clinical and laboratory features warrants an approach utilizing empiric therapy with persistent pursuit of alternative diagnoses.

The most important step in management involves prompt recognition of HSE as a diagnostic possibility and rapid institution of acyclovir therapy. Among the important neurodiagnostic evaluations in patients suspected of having HSE are MRI, cerebrospinal fluid (CSF) analysis, and electroencephalography. While computed tomographic (CT) scanning is surprisingly insensitive in detecting early HSE, with two fifths or more patients having normal scans, MRI, at least on the basis of anecdotal experience, more often detects characteristic abnormalities. The latter include virtually pathognomonic increased signal, particularly on T_2-weighted sequences, in the same regions showing pathology at autopsy: the medial temporal lobes, inferior frontal regions, insulae, and cingulate gyri, often bilateral (Fig. 476–1). The MRI also allows more sensitive detection of alternative diagnoses, such as brain abscess, vasculitis, or demyelination. Some patients are so ill or agitated that MRI may not be possible; in these patients, biopsy might be needed.

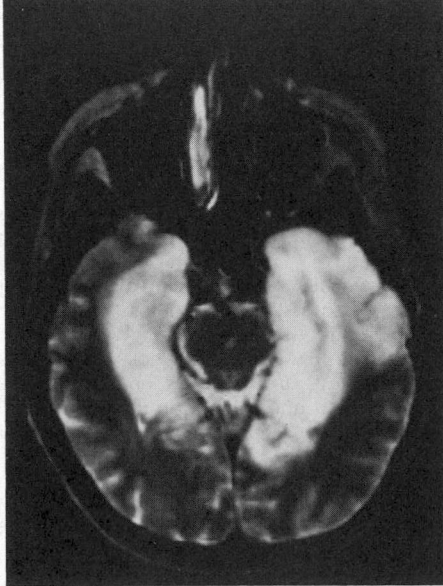

FIGURE 476–1. MRI scan of a 54-year-old woman with herpes simplex encephalitis who presented with fever, dysphasia, and confusion. The T_2-weighted image shows increased signal in both medial temporal lobes, with more extensive involvement on the left (right side of figure).

CSF examination is also important in detecting evidence of virus infection. Most patients exhibit a mononuclear pleocytosis with 50 or more leukocytes per cubic millimeter, although fewer or even a normal number of cells may be noted. The protein content is usually mildly elevated, and the glucose level is normal or only mildly reduced. Like MRI, cerebrospinal fluid analysis may also be useful in establishing alternative diagnoses, such as bacterial or fungal infection. In more than three fourths of patients, the electroencephalogram exhibits focal abnormalities, most often showing spike and slow-wave or sharp-wave patterns over the involved temporal lobes.

Attempts at isolating HSV-1 from CSF rarely succeed. Newer methods of diagnosis seeking detection of viral antigens (by enzyme-linked immunoassay) or nucleic acid (by polymerase chain reaction gene amplification) are under development. Isolation of the virus from the oropharynx is useless, since no relationship exists between symptomatic or asymptomatic viral shedding at such peripheral sites and brain infection. HSV-1 is often reactivated by other neurologic diseases eliciting fever, creating a source of false-positive serologic responses in patients suffering from nonherpetic encephalitis or meningitis.

In contrast to the epidemic encephalitides, in which documentation of seroconversion provides a major method of diagnosis, in HSE serologic testing is often inconclusive. This is particularly true at the onset, when prompt diagnostic decisions are critical. Even during convalescence, analyses of blood and CSF antibody titers can give false-negative or false-positive results.

TREATMENT. The introduction of antiviral therapy has greatly improved the outcome of HSE. This was first demonstrated with vidarabine, and even greater benefit has been shown with acyclovir, which has become the treatment of choice. HSE is treated by an intravenous infusion of 10 mg per kilogram given over a 1-hour period every 8 hours for 10 days. The therapeutic efficacy of acyclovir is restricted to the herpesviruses by virtue of the drug's selective interaction with two virus-coded enzymes, thymidine kinase and DNA polymerase; acyclovir is thus not a broad-spectrum antiviral. Because acyclovir is excreted principally by the kidney, caution must be exercised in patients with renal impairment. Side effects of acyclovir are generally few, although neurotoxicity rarely occurs, manifested as altered consciousness, tremors, hallucinations, and seizures. Other aspects of care also require meticulous attention. Optimally, patients with HSE should be managed in the intensive care setting of a tertiary referral center.

PROGNOSIS. Both age and initial neurologic status significantly influence the prognosis in HSE; even with antiviral therapy, patients who are comatose when first treated often fare poorly. Extensive infection and brain damage are present in most of these patients as a result of a more fulminant illness and, sometimes, a delay in beginning therapy. Many patients, however, particularly those younger than 30 years old who are neurologically intact when treatment begins, recover normal or nearly normal function. Patients with minor neurologic deficits may survive without severe long-term sequelae and return to normal function if diagnosis is made and specific treatment is instituted early in the course. In a few patients, and despite antiviral treatment, HSE can relapse within a few weeks after the acute disease, resulting in severe sequelae. The pathogenesis of such relapses is unknown.

476.2 NEUROLOGIC COMPLICATIONS OF GENITAL HERPES

Genital herpes, most often caused by HSV-2, may be complicated by local or radicular pain, aseptic meningitis, autonomic (bowel, bladder, and sexual) dysfunction, and rarely myelitis. These complications are more common in association with primary genital herpes but may occur with recurrent disease as well. Prodromal neuritic symptoms commonly precede recurrences and may involve the buttock, the groin, or, less commonly, the lower extremities.

Aseptic meningitis and autonomic dysfunction may occur either independently or together. Meningitic symptoms are associated with primary genital herpes in about one fourth of patients, but only a minority require hospitalization. Its course is benign, usually clearing in 4 to 10 days without residua. The CSF profile is typical of an aseptic meningitis, with a mononuclear pleocytosis, mild protein elevation, and normal, or occasionally reduced, glucose level. When the history clearly implicates an epidemiologic and temporal relationship with genital herpes and the CSF findings are those of a typical mononuclear profile, a clinical diagnosis can usually be made. Specific diagnosis can often be established by isolation of HSV-2 at lumbar puncture.

Urinary retention, constipation, and sexual impotence in association with genital herpes are less common than meningitis. Symptoms and signs of a sacral sensory radiculopathy sometimes accompany the autonomic changes. The pathophysiology of this disorder is uncertain, but direct herpetic infection of nervous system structures is likely. Fortunately, autonomic dysfunction is reversible, and patients can be assured that their symptoms will probably clear. Although unusual, these autonomic symptoms can recur. It is important to consider and pursue the diagnosis of HSV-2 infection in patients who present with isolated bladder, bowel, or sexual dysfunction. It is critical not to make an inappropriate diagnosis of spinal neoplasm or, especially, early multiple sclerosis. When there is a clear history of genital herpes, the cause of autonomic dysfunction is usually readily established clinically. Inspection and viral culture of genital lesions, plus accompanying antibody titers, which may appear and rise slowly only in primary HSV-2 infection, provide additional help.

In adults, HSV-2 only rarely produces adult-type herpes encephalitis indistinguishable from that caused by HSV-1. Transverse myelopathy due to HSV-2 is very rare.

Epithelial HSV-2 primary infections and recurrences can be treated with acyclovir, but the effect on the neurologic complications of genital herpes is uncertain. In the absence of adequate data, it appears appropriate to give acyclovir for neurologic complications of primary genital herpes.

In patients with frequent recurrent attacks of genital herpes, early, self-initiated treatment of recurrent lesions with oral acyclovir has been advocated, beginning therapy at the onset of prodromal symptoms. This approach is probably appropriate for the rare patient with recurrent herpetic meningitis.

476.3 NEUROLOGIC COMPLICATIONS OF VARICELLA ZOSTER VIRUS INFECTIONS

Herpes zoster (HZ) (shingles, zona) is a dermatomal cutaneous infection caused by reactivation of the varicella zoster virus that normally lies latent in sensory ganglia following an early attack of varicella. In addition to its cutaneous manifestations, zoster is accompanied by neuritic symptoms and may be complicated by an array of neurologic sequelae. The varicella zoster virus is distantly related to HSV, sharing only minor antigen cross-reactivity.

INCIDENCE AND EPIDEMIOLOGY. HZ is a common disorder, with an annual incidence estimated at 3.4 cases per 1000 persons. Unlike varicella, HZ occurs throughout the year, with neither significant clustering of cases nor seasonal or yearly preponderance. Case exposure in HZ is rarely identified. Two factors, age and immunosuppression, significantly influence its incidence. The disease is uncommon in childhood, relatively constant in those between 20 and 50 years of age (approximately 2.5 cases per 1000 annually), and thereafter doubles its incidence in those between the ages of 50 and 60 and redoubles it in those between age 80 and 90. Immunosuppression due to systemic disease (in particular, Hodgkin's disease and other lymphoreticular malignancies), cytotoxic drugs, corticosteroids, radiation therapy, or infection by human immunodeficiency virus (HIV) predisposes. In some cases, a history of neoplasm, radiation exposure, or physical injury in the proximity of the dorsal root ganglion or nerve is elicited.

Age is an important factor also in the development of postherpetic neuralgia, which develops almost exclusively in persons older than 50 years of age. The incidence of postherpetic pain varies, ranging between 15 and 75 per cent, depending on clinical definition of the syndrome and selection of patients. Immunosuppression predisposes to spread of virus beyond the ganglion-nerve-dermatome unit into the central nervous system or systemically.

PATHOGENESIS AND PATHOLOGY. Once the reactivation of latent varicella zoster virus occurs, it characteristically spreads within the sensory ganglion and travels centrifugally over the peripheral nerve processes of this ganglion, eventually seeding the skin with the resultant dermatomal vesicular rash.

Cell-mediated defenses rather than humoral immunity are critically involved in protecting the host during HZ. Pathologically, acutely infected dorsal root ganglia and nerve show the presence of a mononuclear inflammatory response, neuronal degeneration with intranuclear Cowdry type A inclusion bodies, and similar infection of surrounding satellite cells. The peripheral nerve may contain parallel changes. In more severe cases, dorsal root ganglia above and below the primarily affected ganglion also show active herpetic infection.

CLINICAL MANIFESTATIONS. Prodromal sensory symptoms include dermatomal pain, itching, or paresthesias, which often antecede by several days the eruption of the segmental rash. The early pain of zoster may be confused with other types of neuropathic or visceral pain. The most frequently involved dermatomes are those extending from the third thoracic to the second lumbar segments and the first (ophthalmic) division of the trigeminal nerve. The rash itself initially consists of erythematous macules that vesiculate over 12 to 24 hours. Normally the vesicular fluid pustulates within 72 hours; in a week the pustules begin to dry, and crusting takes place by 10 to 12 days. The crusts, in turn, fall off in 2 to 3 weeks. In the immunocompromised host, this time course may be protracted. In uncomplicated cases, the rash heals with a variable degree of superficial scarring, at times leaving areas of hyperpigmentation or depigmentation, which may be anesthetic. More severe cases may leave denervation of a large segment of the dermatome.

Zoster can affect any of several of the cranial nerves. The ophthalmic division of the trigeminal nerve is the most commonly affected, and the condition may be complicated by spread to orbital structures, resulting in acute and long-term ocular sequelae. Spread of cutaneous rash along the bridge of the nose to its tip should be taken as a signal of impending ocular infection, prompting early ophthalmologic consultation. Facial palsy, with or without accompanying loss of taste on the anterior two thirds of the tongue, may accompany either otic zoster (Ramsay Hunt syndrome), with rash confined to a segment of the auricle, or the second and third cervical dermatone (cervical collar zoster). Occasionally, infection of the ninth and tenth or fifth cranial nerve may antecede facial weakness. As with other motor syndromes (see below), weakness is often delayed for a variable period after the rash. Eighth nerve dysfunction with sensorineural hearing loss or vertigo occurs in the same setting as facial palsy but with less frequency. HZ may rarely cause facial palsy in the absence of rash (*zoster sine herpete*). Zoster of the ninth and tenth cranial nerves is unusual and may be overlooked without a careful search for the pharyngeal rash or ipsilateral laryngeal or pharyngeal palsy.

HZ of the extremities or trunk can also be complicated by segmental motor weakness, the motor loss usually corresponding to the involved cutaneous dermatome. Weakness characteristically develops from a few days to 2 weeks after the onset of the rash, and longer delays are rare. Its onset is characteristically abrupt, occurring over hours or 1 or 2 days, with little or no subsequent deterioration. Weakness abates or disappears in about 85 per cent of cases.

Myelitis of variable extent is a less common complication of HZ and results from direct viral invasion of the spinal cord, perhaps augmented by local inflammatory responses. It occurs most commonly in the immunosuppressed person and, like motor paresis, is characteristically delayed after the onset of the rash. The most common manifestation is bladder dysfunction. Other signs include mild or transient asymmetric reflexes, lower extremity weakness, and sensory disturbance. Severe myelopathy can produce a partial Brown-Séquard syndrome or total cord transection. Characteristically, involvement lies at the same spinal cord segment as the rash but may ascend to a higher level. Spinal MRI or myelography may be needed to rule out coexisting epidural tumor.

At least three types of brain involvement may complicate zoster: diffuse encephalitis, focal parenchymal infection, and vasculitis. Headache, stiff neck, and mild diffuse encephalitis often accompany acute HZ but are difficult to distinguish from the effects of fever, sepsis, narcotic analgesics, and other underlying medical problems. Most such patients recover. In more severe diffuse encephalitis, chances for recovery may also be good if other complications of the disease do not intervene. The clinical picture is that of an acute or subacute delirium accompanied by cerebrospinal fluid pleocytosis with few focal features.

Focal varicella zoster virus encephalitis is a rare complication in immunosuppressed patients that can resemble progressive multifocal leukoencephalopathy. The onset may be temporally remote from the cutaneous rash. The cerebral lesions involve principally the white matter. Brain biopsy is required for diagnosis, allowing identification of Cowdry type A inclusions or of varicella zoster virus antigens or nuclei acids.

Cerebral vasculitis is probably the most common serious postzoster central nervous system complication. Affected patients usually develop delayed contralateral hemiplegic strokes following ophthalmic division zoster owing to inflammation or occlusion of the internal carotid artery and its major branches ipsilateral to the rash. The delay between the rash and the onset of cerebral dysfunction varies from none to as much as 6 months, with a mean interval of 7 weeks. A more widespread cerebral vasculitis following zoster in other locations has also been reported. The pathogenesis is still incompletely understood, but the characteristic involvement of local vessels innervated by the infected ganglion, in conjunction with reports suggesting the presence of viral nucleocapsids and viral antigens within vessels, suggests that the arteries are directly infected. Additional contributions may be made by secondary local inflammatory responses and thrombosis, leading to vascular occlusion or distal embolization. Arteriographic evidence of vasculitis or occlusions in the involved vessels and the clinical setting usually allow diagnosis.

DIAGNOSIS. The clinical diagnosis of HZ is seldom difficult. The dermatomal distribution and the evolution of the vesicular rash are characteristic, and only rarely does herpes simplex infection assume a similar pattern and confuse the diagnosis. Difficulty, however, may occur early in the disease, when pain or other sensory symptoms precede the rash. The rare case of zoster sine herpete may require additional methods of diagnosis, and, in cases with an occult rash, a careful search is necessary. When there is a question of the diagnosis, a Tzanck test examining lesion scrapings, a direct culture, or immunohistochemical identification of infected cells can provide specific identification of varicella zoster virus. Serology may also be helpful, although the commonly used complement fixation test can cross-react between HSV and varicella zoster virus.

THERAPY. The goals are to relieve the acute segmental infection, to curtail spread of infection either systemically or to other areas of the nervous system, and to prevent postherpetic neuralgia. The means available consist of using antiviral drugs to interrupt viral replication and perhaps corticosteroids to modify local inflammatory responses. Treatment of individual patients must take into account their background risk for particular complications.

Since involvement of the ophthalmic division of the trigeminal nerve risks spreading to orbital structures, such infections should receive early antiviral treatment. Systemic antiviral therapy should also be used for immunosuppressed patients, who are more susceptible to severe disseminated infection. In young patients with normal immune function, there is usually no requirement for specific therapy because zoster is usually mild with swift recovery and no residua. Older nonimmunosuppressed persons are susceptible to postherpetic neuralgia; two controlled studies of such individuals have suggested that a brief course of corticosteroids may reduce the subsequent incidence of pain without untoward complications. A reasonable course begins with a daily dose of 60 mg of prednisone (or the equivalent glucocorticoid) in four individual doses with rapid tapering so that patients are off medication within 7 to 10 days. Whether the addition of acyclovir to the corticosteroids is helpful has not been evaluated.

The antiviral treatment of choice for HZ is acyclovir. The nucleoside can abort the rash and prevent systemic spread when administered promptly by the intravenous route. The recommended intravenous dosages vary from 5 to 10* mg per kilogram infused every 8 hours for 5 days. More recently, the use of oral acyclovir has been suggested at a dosage of 800 mg* every 4 hours with omission of the nighttime dose, particularly in individuals who are not at marked risk of developing viral complications.

Intravenous acyclovir is indicated for patients in whom varicella zoster virus infection progresses to cause myelitis or encephalitis, although delay in institution reduces its overall effect. No satisfactory data indicate whether either acyclovir or steroids improve the outcome of HZ-associated motor weakness. Similarly, there is no proven effective treatment for zoster-associated cerebral vasculitis. Postherpetic neuralgia is discussed in Ch. 455.

476.4 NEUROLOGIC COMPLICATIONS OF CYTOMEGALOVIRUS AND EPSTEIN-BARR VIRUS INFECTIONS

Both human cytomegalovirus and Epstein-Barr virus infections can cause neurologic disease. While in children cytomegalovirus is an important and relatively common cause of congenital neurologic deficit, central and peripheral nervous system infections in adults occur almost exclusively in the setting of immunosuppression. Central nervous system complications of Epstein-Barr virus infections occur in the setting of acute mononucleosis. Both viruses have been implicated in triggering the Guillain-Barré syndrome.

Cytomegalovirus encephalitis and, less commonly, meningoencephalitis or myelitis have been reported as opportunistic infections in adults suffering from impaired cell-mediated immunity. Earlier these complications were reported most commonly in patients undergoing organ transplantation, but more recently their occurrence has been noted principally in association with acquired immunodeficiency syndrome (AIDS). The clinical features of cytomegalovirus brain infection have been imprecisely characterized, but the major symptoms and signs appear to reflect diffuse brain dysfunction with concomitantly impaired levels of attention and cognition, paralleling the symptomatology of a metabolic encephalopathy. At times, focal deficits (e.g., hemiparesis) or seizures are superimposed. Pathologically, infection of the brain by this virus is marked by scattered microglial nodules, some of which contain typical cytomegalovirus intranuclear inclusions. As many as one fourth of autopsied AIDS patients have neuropathologic evidence of central nervous system cytomegalovirus infection, although in most the infection appears to be mild, and indeed its contribution to symptoms is uncertain. Some patients may exhibit ventricular subependymal abnormalities or small abscess-like lesions on MRI.

More recently, the role of cytomegalovirus in causing severe ascending polyradiculopathy has been delineated. This syndrome is usually characterized by the subacute evolution of severe, painful polyradiculopathy that begins with sacral or lumbar sensory, motor, and autonomic dysfunction and is accompanied by CSF pleocytosis with nearly diagnostic polymorphonuclear cell predominance.

The diagnosis of cytomegalovirus encephalitis is difficult. Most AIDS patients, particularly homosexual men, have circulating antibody to the virus, and in many it can be isolated from urine or blood, yet they do not suffer nervous system infection. For this reason, serologic evaluation and systemic virus isolation are not particularly helpful in diagnosis; rather, one must rely on clinical suspicion. Cytomegalovirus polyradiculopathy can be diagnosed by the CSF findings, including the prominence of neutrophils and the isolation of virus. Recently, the antiviral nucleoside ganciclovir been found effective in treating certain

---

*Exceeds manufacturer's recommended dosage.

manifestations of cytomegalovirus infection, including particularly the retinopathy that sometimes complicates AIDS. No information is yet available regarding the drug's efficacy in central nervous system infections caused by human cytomegalovirus, but individual case reports suggest that ganciclovir may be helpful in patients with cytomegalovirus polyradiculopathy.

The neurologic complications of Epstein-Barr virus infection range from symptoms of headache, photophobia, weakness, and fatigue, which occur relatively frequently in infectious mononucleosis, to more serious, but uncommon, complications that have been described principally in the context of individual case reports. These include encephalitis, meningoencephalitis, Guillain-Barré syndrome, Bell's palsy, acute cerebellar ataxia, and transverse myelitis. It is likely that most of these neurologic complications result from immune-mediated injury rather than direct viral infection.

Bale JF Jr: Human cytomegalovirus infection and disorders of the nervous system. Arch Neurol 41:310, 1984. *A general review of the nervous system complications of human cytomegalovirus, including both congenital and adult infections.*

Corey L, Spear PG: Infections with herpes simplex viruses. N Engl J Med 314:749, 1986. *A review of the clinical spectrum and treatment of HSV infections.*

Esiri MM: Herpes simplex encephalitis. An immunohistochemical study of the distribution of viral antigen within the brain. J Neurol Sci 54:209, 1982. *An excellent paper outlining the topography of HSV infection in brain, using immunohistochemistry.*

Hilt DC, Buchholz D, Krumholz A, et al.: Herpes zoster ophthalmicus and delayed contralateral hemiparesis caused by cerebral angiitis: Diagnosis and management approaches. Ann Neurol 14:543, 1983. *A report of four cases and review of the literature related to herpes zoster–associated cerebral angiitis.*

Horten B, Price RW, Jimenez D: Multifocal varicella-zoster virus leukoencephalitis temporally remote from herpes zoster. Ann Neurol 9:251, 1981. *A report of two immunosuppressed patients with multifocal varicella zoster virus encephalitis.*

Jemsek J, Greenberg SB, Taber L, et al.: Herpes zoster–associated encephalitis: Clinicopathologic report of 12 cases and review of the literature. Medicine 62:81, 1983. *A review of encephalitis complicating HZ.*

Miller RG, Storey JR, Greco CM: Ganciclovir in the treatment of progressive AIDS-related polyradiculopathy. Neurology 40:569, 1990. *Describes the clinical and therapeutic aspects of cytomegalovirus polyradiculopathy in AIDS patients.*

Price RW: Neurobiology of human herpesvirus infections. CRC Crit Rev Clin Neurobiol 2:61, 1986. *A general review of the pathophysiology of neurotropic herpesvirus infections and their neurologic complications.*

Whitley RJ: Viral encephalitis. N Engl J Med 323:242, 1990. *A review emphasizing HSE and favoring the role of brain biopsy.*

477 Rabies

Richard W. Price

DEFINITION. Rabies is a viral infection with nearly worldwide distribution that affects principally wild and domestic animals but also involves humans, resulting in a devastating, almost invariably fatal encephalitis.

ETIOLOGY, PATHOGENESIS, AND PATHOLOGY. Rabies virus is a bullet-shaped, enveloped, single-strand RNA virus classified in the rhabdovirus family and *Lyssavirus* genus. It has particular neurotropic properties, and unlike many of the other viruses causing acute encephalitis, it appears to require central nervous system infection as an essential part of its "life cycle."

Viral transmission to both animals and humans characteristically results from the bite of a rabid animal, although cases of transmission by aerosol in the laboratory or in a bat cave and by transplanted infected corneal tissue have also been recorded. Once the virus breaches the protective epithelium, it reaches the central nervous system via peripheral nerves, exploiting retrograde axoplasmic transport. The interval between the bite and the onset of disease is variable, ranging from days to a year or more, but in most cases lasting 1 to 2 months. This delay may relate to amplification of the virus in peripheral tissues, particularly skeletal muscle, before it gains access to the central nervous system over motor and sensory nerves. During this delay, the virus can be eliminated by host immune mechanisms; indeed, it is this delay that affords an opportunity for prophylactic postexposure immunization after the rabid bite. Evidence suggests a

possible role for the nicotinic acetylcholine receptor and the neuromuscular junction in the concentration and access of rabies virus to the central nervous system. Once virus enters peripheral and central nervous system pathways, immune defenses are unlikely to be able to suppress further replication and spread of infection, which includes axoplasmic transport and perhaps transsynaptic transmission.

The central nervous system, in turn, is involved in the subsequent transmission of the virus by infected animals in two essential ways: (1) Infection of certain brain regions underlies the characteristic behavioral changes in the rabid animal, leading to increased biting activity; (2) antegrade transport of the virus to salivary glands leads to virus shedding. In concert, these two aspects of infection ensure transmission and survival of the virus in the wild. They also have practical diagnostic implications for the human disease. The characteristic altered behavior in humans often results in a distinct clinical picture distinguishing rabies from other viral encephalitides. Antegrade virus transport also affords a means of diagnosing rabies by isolation from saliva or immunohistochemical staining of infected cutaneous nerves innervating hair follicles.

Pathologic findings are variable and include both nonspecific and specific abnormalities. Perhaps most remarkable is the frequent apparent discrepancy between the degree of pathologic change, particularly neuronal loss, and the severe antemortem clinical state. Nonspecific changes include perivascular mononuclear infiltrates and microglial response, although inflammation may be scant in relation to the widespread distribution of infected cells detected immunohistochemically. Similarly, neuronal destruction is less prominent than the abundance of viral antigen, which is located principally in neurons but also in astrocytes. More specific changes include the presence of Negri bodies, eosinophilic neuronal intracytoplasmic inclusion composed of viral nucleoprotein. At autopsy, infection is usually widespread in the brain, but with prominent involvement of the brain stem and spinal cord and also involvement of the hippocampus, basal ganglia, cortex, and other structures. The relation of virus infection of neurons and the attendant inflammatory reaction to the clinical manifestations remains incompletely understood. Rabies virus infection of neurons may alter their membrane properties or synaptic transmission. Whatever the means by which infection perturbs neuronal function, patients eventually manifest widespread brain dysfunction that terminally impairs respiratory and autonomic control.

EPIDEMIOLOGY. The epidemiology of rabies varies in different parts of the world, falling into two patterns. In *sylvatic rabies*, infection is maintained in wildlife reservoirs. Thus, in the United States, rabies is endemic in the striped skunk in the central states, in the raccoon in the southeastern and mid-Atlantic states, and in the red fox in northern New York and adjacent regions of Canada; bat rabies has a wide geographic range. A similar pattern holds in other developed nations, where human rabies is rare and more often results from direct contact with wildlife than from secondary transmission to the domestic dog or cat and then to humans. This pattern contrasts with the one in much of Asia, Africa, and South America, where *urban rabies* is maintained as an epizootic infection in the domestic dog and human disease is far more common.

CLINICAL MANIFESTATIONS. After the silent incubation period, clinical rabies frequently begins with a prodromal phase, which may include nonspecific symptoms of malaise, fever, and headache but also more specific local symptoms related to the site of the original bite. These include itching, paresthesias, or other sensations beginning in the area of the healed wound and then spreading to a wider region and eventually involving the whole limb or side of the body.

Within a few days, the full-blown illness begins, taking one of two forms—encephalitic (*furious*) or paralytic (*dumb*) rabies—perhaps depending on the source and strain of the infecting virus. In its initial phase, encephalitic rabies is often distinguished from other viral infections by irritability of the patient and hyperactivity of a number of automatic reflexes. Periods of calm lucidity may alternate with confusion and seeming intense anxiety precipitated by internal or external stimuli. Hydrophobia, with reflexive intense contraction of the diaphragm and accessory respiratory and other muscles, is induced upon attempts to drink or even at the sight of water. Similarly, blowing or fanning air on the chest may induce intense laryngeal, pharyngeal, or other muscle spasms (aerophobia). High fever persists throughout the illness.

Paralytic rabies is less common and more readily misdiagnosed. Patients present with weakness, usually beginning in the bitten extremity and spreading to involve all four limbs and the facial muscles. Early in the course, both consciousness and sensory function are spared. Helpful signs include myoedema and pilo-erection, and fever is also present. As the disease progresses, it may converge with the encephalitic form, accompanied by some of the same irritative phenomena. Both forms evolve into lethargy and coma, with prominent alterations of respiratory and cardio-vascular function. Tachycardia may precede bradycardia with ectopic rhythms, and the breathing pattern becomes irregular with cluster or periodic respirations. Patients succumb to respi-ratory failure or cardiovascular collapse within a mean interval of 4 days from onset, although patients may survive as long as 3 weeks or more. Intensive supportive care may extend survival longer; in three clinically unusual cases, patients with partial vaccine-induced immunity have been reported to survive with intensive care. However, additional experience with vigorous support has not duplicated this overall effect on long-term sur-vival.

DIAGNOSIS. Rabies is usually suspected on the basis of a history of animal bite or other exposure, although in as many as one third of cases no such history is obtained. Definitive ante-mortem diagnosis is established by immunohistochemical iden-tification of rabies virus antigen in hair follicle nerve endings of biopsied skin, usually obtained from the nape of the neck. Isolation of virus from saliva or the presence of antirabies anti-bodies in blood in the absence of vaccination or in the cerebro-spinal fluid may also be used to establish diagnosis. Postmortem diagnosis is usually made by histologic or immunohistochemical examination of the brain.

The differential diagnosis depends on the clinical presentation and the epidemiologic setting. In the case of paralytic rabies, diagnosis is most often confused with the Guillain-Barré syn-drome, poliomyelitis, or other neuropathies or myelopathies, while the encephalitic form must be differentiated from other viral and infectious encephalitides, tetanus, and toxic encepha-lopathies. In regions where vaccine is prepared using neural tissue (still the practice in many regions of the world with the highest rates of rabies), allergic encephalomyelitis remains a principal differential diagnosis.

TREATMENT AND PREVENTION. Unfortunately, estab-lished central nervous system disease remains essentially untreat-able. Disease prevention relies on public health measures to reduce animal reservoirs and on postexposure immune prophy-laxis to abort viral penetration of the central nervous system after a rabid bite or other contact. Although clinical rabies is a rare disease in most developed countries such as the United States, the decision to administer active prophylaxis remains a relatively common clinical issue. The physician first determines the type of possible exposure; an open wound or disrupted mucous mem-brane exposed to saliva may warrant postexposure prophylaxis, whereas contact of saliva with intact skin may not. The first step in management is to administer prompt local wound care, thor-oughly washing with soap or iodine. The epidemiologic setting is important in determining the likelihood that the biting animal might be rabid and often requires consultation with local health authorities to ascertain which animals carry rabies in the geo-graphic setting. In the absence of previous vaccination, both passive (rabies immune globulin of human origin) and active (human diploid cell vaccine) immunizations are administered, whereas individuals with previous vaccination (e.g., laboratory workers) required only active vaccine. Fortunately, such tissue culture–derived vaccines are safe, with a very low incidence of major adverse reactions, in contrast to earlier nerve tissue–derived vaccines.

Baer GM, Bridbord K, Hui FW, et al. (eds.): Research towards rabies prevention. Rev Infect Dis (Suppl) 10:S5773, 1988. *A compendium of brief papers presented at a symposium dealing with various aspects of rabies, particularly strategies for prevention, but covering a broad range of related tissues.*
Centers for Disease Control: Rabies surveillance, United States, 1988. MMWR 38:1, 1989. *Reviews the animal and human epidemiology of rabies in the United States over the past four decades, providing a guide to risk after animal exposure.*
Fishbein DB, Baer GM: Animal rabies: Implications for diagnosis and human treatment. Ann Intern Med 109:935, 1988. *An editorial outlining current recommendations for prophylaxis and treatment as well as future prospects for control of animal and human infection.*
Hemachudha T: Rabies. *In* McKendall RR (ed.): Viral Disease. Elsevier Science Publishing Company, New York, 1989, pp 383–404. *A recent comprehensive review written from the perspective of a neurologist who has personal experi-ence with clinical rabies.*
Immunization Practices Advisory Committee: Rabies prevention—United States, 1984. MMWR 33:393, 407, 1984. *U.S. guidelines on prevention of rabies by vaccination.*
Kaplan C, Turner GS, Warrell DA: Rabies: The Facts. Oxford, England, Oxford University Press, 1986. *A brief, highly readable monograph.*

478 Slow Virus Infections of the Nervous System

478.1 INTRODUCTION

Richard W. Price

The term *slow infections* was first applied by Bjorn Sigurdsson to a group of transmissible diseases of sheep characterized by an incubation period and course measured in months or years rather than hours or days, as in typical acute viral or bacterial infections. Subsequently, several human diseases sharing these characteris-tics have been described. Although often considered together because of their chronic nature, these disorders are in fact heterogeneous with respect to their clinical manifestations, neu-ropathology, etiology, and pathogenesis. Although in some in-stances the infections are accompanied by inflammatory pathol-ogy, in several, symptoms and signs typical of the acute encephalitides are absent, and both clinically and pathologically they resemble degenerative or hereditary diseases of the nervous system. Two of the sheep diseases upon which Sigurdsson based his concept of slow infections, *visna* and *scrapie*, have subse-quently proved to have human counterparts. Visna is caused by a retrovirus and somewhat resembles the nervous system infec-tions caused by the human immunodeficiency virus type 1 (HIV-1) responsible for acquired immunodeficiency syndrome (AIDS) and tropical spastic paraparesis caused by human T cell lympho-tropic virus type I (HTLV-I), while scrapie closely parallels Creutzfeldt-Jakob disease and kuru.

The agents causing the slow infections are taxonomically diverse, as are the mechanisms by which they maintain chronic progressive infection and cause clinical symptomatology (Table 478–1). Thus, HIV is an RNA-containing retrovirus that codes for a DNA intermediary that can integrate into the host genome and persist for the life of the cell; progressive multifocal leuko-

TABLE 478–1. HUMAN SLOW VIRUS INFECTIONS OF THE CENTRAL NERVOUS SYSTEM

Disease	Etiologic Agent	
	Name	*Classification*
AIDS dementia com-plex	Human immunodefi-ciency virus type 1	Retrovirus (RNA)
Tropical spastic para-paresis	Human T cell lympho-tropic virus type 1	Retrovirus (RNA)
Progressive multifocal leukoencephalopathy	JC virus	Papovavirus (DNA)
Subacute sclerosing panencephalitis	Measles virus	Paramyxovirus (RNA)
Progressive rubella panencephalitis	Rubella virus	Togavirus (RNA)
Creutzfeldt-Jakob syn-drome, Gerstmann-Sträussler-Scheinker disease, kuru	—	Spongiform encepha-lopathy agents (cod-ing material uncer-tain), prions

encephalopathy is caused by a small, nonenveloped DNA-containing papovavirus; subacute sclerosing panencephalitis is due to the enveloped RNA measles virus; and Creutzfeldt-Jakob disease is caused by an agent that has not yet been definitively identified but may consist of a modified cell protein only (see Ch. 478.6). Contributions of host immune responses to the development and symptomatology of these diseases are similarly varied. In the case of progressive multifocal leukoencephalopathy, a conventional virus that circulates commonly in the human community and is ordinarily associated with little, if any, disease causes devastating central nervous system infection in the presence of depressed host cell–mediated immunity. HIV-1 causes profound systemic disease by virtue of its predilection for infecting the helper-inducer (T4) subset of lymphocytes, with the resultant systemic immunosuppression perhaps playing a role in the subsequent development of progressive brain disease by this same virus. The pathogenesis of myelopathy caused by HTLV-I most likely significantly involves immunopathologic mechanisms. Subacute sclerosing panencephalitis appears to result from defective replication in the brain of a once-common conventional virus and is accompanied by an exuberant but ineffective antibody response. In the case of Creutzfeldt-Jakob disease, immunosuppression plays no role in the development or progression of the disease, and indeed there is little evidence that the host recognizes the infectious agent as foreign.

The diversity of the agents causing these slow infections, along with their variable cell and tissue tropism, host susceptibility, and pathologic reactions, has led to speculation that viruses may play a role in several of the common neurodegenerative disorders, including multiple sclerosis, amyotrophic lateral sclerosis, parkinsonism, and Alzheimer's disease. To date, however, no direct evidence for such an infectious cause of any of these disorders has been identified.

Johnson RT: Viral Infections of the Nervous System. New York, Raven Press, 1982.
  Contains sections dealing with the general background as well as the specific slow virus infections of the nervous system.

478.2 HUMAN IMMUNODEFICIENCY VIRUS INFECTION AND THE AIDS DEMENTIA COMPLEX

Richard W. Price

DEFINITION. Among the common neurologic complications of human immunodeficiency virus type 1 (HIV-1) infection (see Ch. 414) is the *AIDS dementia complex*, which appears to relate pathogenetically in an elemental way to the AIDS virus itself rather than to secondary opportunistic infection. The nomenclature for this "subcortical" dementing syndrome is still in a state of flux, and several alternative terms have been used, including AIDS dementia, subacute encephalitis, HIV dementia, and HIV encephalopathy. Recently, the World Health Organization proposed new terminology, using the term *HIV-1–associated cognitive/motor complex* to encompass the full constellation of features and with subcategories referring to patients with predominantly cognitive (*HIV-1–associated dementia*) or myelopathic (*HIV-1–associated myelopathy*) presentations. The term *HIV-1–associated minor cognitive/motor disorder* was introduced to designate patients with mild symptoms and signs and only minimal functional impairment of work or activities of daily living. In this section, we continue to use the earlier AIDS dementia complex terminology.

Although this condition may relate to HIV-1 itself, and in some patients appears to be caused by productive HIV-1 infection within the CNS, it is important to distinguish the AIDS dementia complex, which refers to a clinical syndrome, from HIV-1 brain infection, a pathobiologic process. Although the syndrome and the infective process overlap, they are not equivalent.

CLINICAL MANIFESTATIONS. The AIDS dementia complex is characterized by a triad of cognitive, motor, and behavioral dysfunction. Patients' earliest symptoms usually consist of diffi-

culties with concentration and memory. They complain of losing track of their train of thought or conversations and find that they need to keep lists to maintain their daily schedules. Many complain of "slowness" in thinking. Complex tasks at work or in the home, such as balancing the checkbook or reconciling other personal financial affairs, become increasingly difficult and take longer to complete.

Despite these complaints, early in the evolution of the illness, bedside screening or mental status testing may yield results within the normal range, although characteristically patients are slower and less facile than previously. With advancing disease, patients perform poorly on tasks requiring concentration and attention, such as word and digit reversals and serial subtraction. Eventually, a larger array of mental status tests are abnormal, and psychomotor slowing is more prominent.

Symptoms of motor dysfunction usually are less prominent than those of intellectual impairment. However, motor abnormalities, including, particularly, slowing of rapid successive and alternating movements of the extremities and eyes, are almost always noted on examination. Abnormal reflexes are common, with generalized hyperreflexia (in the absence of concomitant neuropathy) along with release signs such as snout or glabellar responses. With disease progression, symptomatic difficulty with balance or incoordination may be evident; patients may drop things more frequently or become slower and less precise with hand activities, including writing. Similarly, gait incoordination may result in more frequent tripping or falling or in a perceived need to exercise new care in walking. In more advanced disease, ataxia and, subsequently, leg weakness limit ambulation. Patients with early or predominating spastic-ataxic gait are usually shown to have vacuolar myelopathy pathologically (see below). Bladder and bowel incontinence is common in the late stages of the disease.

Psychological depression appears to be surprisingly infrequent in these patients, despite the prominence of psychomotor slowing. Patients appear uninterested and lack initiative but are not dysphoric. In a minority, a more agitated organic psychosis with manic features may be the presenting or predominant aspect of the illness.

In those with a severe progressive course, the end stage of the AIDS dementia complex is nearly vegetative; patients lie in bed with a vacant stare and with paraparesis or quadriparesis and incontinence. They may be mute or exhibit an extraordinary delay in making brief verbal responses. Unless intercurrent illness develops, the level of arousal is usually preserved.

DIAGNOSIS AND DIFFERENTIAL DIAGNOSIS. Diagnosis relies on identifying the characteristic clinical features of the AIDS dementia complex and excluding other conditions. No single laboratory test establishes the presence of the syndrome. In those with milder forms, perhaps the major difficulty is in distinguishing true cognitive impairment from the effects of fatigue and systemic illness or from psychiatric conditions, including anxiety and depression. The history is critical in establishing functional decline, and an observant friend or family member may be particularly helpful in judging change in performance. Neuropsychological testing can be helpful in providing objective evidence of characteristic impairment of attention and motor speed but must be interpreted, taking into account the patient's background, including age and education, as well as confounding conditions such as substance abuse, previous head trauma, and the effects of various medications. Formal neuropsychological studies are also useful for quantitatively following the patient's progression or response to treatment.

In those with more severe disease, the differential diagnosis most commonly centers on distinction from the other neurologic complications noted in HIV-1–infected patients (see Ch. 414) or, less commonly, from dementing or myelopathic neurologic disease observed in the normal population. Both neuroimaging procedures and cerebrospinal fluid (CSF) examination are essential aspects of evaluation, although principally to eliminate other conditions rather than to establish a diagnosis of the AIDS dementia complex. Computed tomography (CT) and magnetic resonance imaging (MRI) detect the nearly universal finding of cerebral atrophy with widened cortical sulci and enlarged ventricles. In some patients, MRI also shows patchy or diffuse signal changes in the hemispheric white matter and, less commonly, the basal ganglia or thalamus.

Routine CSF analysis is not specifically diagnostic, and findings may be indistinguishable from those in asymptomatic HIV-1–infected patients, with variable elevation of protein content or mononuclear cells. Elevations of CSF neopterin and β_2-microglobulin levels have been reported to correlate with the presence and severity of the AIDS dementia complex, but these markers of immune activation are also increased in central nervous system opportunistic infections and are therefore not specific. Unfortunately, HIV-1 isolation from the CSF is not diagnostically helpful, since the virus can also be cultured from asymptomatic seropositive subjects. The p24 core protein is seldom detected by immunoassay in the CSF of patients with milder clinical disease.

EPIDEMIOLOGY. The frequency of the AIDS dementia complex increases as the systemic effects of HIV-1 infection and resultant immunosuppression worsen. This complication is rare in patients who are otherwise entirely asymptomatic but begins to become more frequent in those manifesting constitutional symptoms (fever, weight loss, malaise). Its prevalence increases further as the helper (CD4+) blood lymphocyte counts fall and opportunistic infections develop, so that preterminally the majority of AIDS patients may manifest this neurologic syndrome. However, precise prevalence figures are not available, and, indeed, with the introduction of antiviral treatment, the epidemiologic pattern of this neurologic disease may be changing. In general, milder forms of the AIDS dementia complex, with a static or indolently progressive course, are more common in patients with preserved immune function (CF4+ lymphocyte counts above 200 per cubic millimeter), while the progressive and more severe forms characteristically develop in patients with advanced immunosuppression. In addition, although there is a general parallel between the onset and severity of this neurologic condition and the onset and severity of systemic complications, wide individual variability exists; at one extreme, the clinician encounters patients with little or no systemic disease but with severe AIDS dementia complex, while at the other end of the spectrum are patients with repeated episodes of opportunistic infection who remain neurologically preserved.

PATHOLOGY AND PATHOGENESIS. The neuropathologic findings in patients with the AIDS dementia complex include at least three "subsets" of major abnormalities: (1) central gliosis and white matter pallor, (2) multinucleated cell encephalitis, and (3) vacuolar myelopathy. In general, these findings correlate with the clinical severity. Central gliosis and white matter pallor are almost universal findings and, in isolation, are the major abnormality in patients with milder AIDS dementia complex. Rarely, they are the only abnormalities in patients with even more severe clinical symptoms and signs. Virologic studies to date have usually failed to detect evidence of productive HIV-1 brain infection in this subgroup of patients.

Multinucleated cell encephalitis is characterized by the presence of perivascular and, at times, parenchymal cell reactions that include macrophages and microglial cells along with multinucleated cells derived from fusion of these two cell types. These multinucleated cells are infected by HIV-1, and, indeed, the cell fusion likely results from interaction of the viral glycoproteins gp120 and gp41 with the CD4 cell receptor. Multinucleated cell encephalitis is thus properly referred to as *HIV-1 encephalitis* and is noted in patients with more severe and progressive AIDS dementia complex.

Vacuolar myelopathy, while defined pathologically, can also often be distinguished clinically on the basis of the predominant myelopathic symptoms and signs. Patients with this condition usually present with spastic-ataxic gait difficulty but with proportionally little sensory disturbance and usually no definable sensory "level." Histologically, the disorder closely resembles subacute combined spinal cord degeneration accompanying vitamin B_{12} deficiency. Its pathogenesis is uncertain, and results conflict regarding the role of direct spinal cord HIV-1 infection, although clearly it is independent of the type of productive infection that produces multinucleated giant cells.

The pathogenesis of the neurologic injury underlying the AIDS dementia complex has been difficult to unravel from a number of aspects. Since the major "functional elements" of the brain, i.e., the neurons, oligodendrocytes, and astrocytes, do not appear to be infected, it remains uncertain how these cells are damaged. In both the gliosis-pallor and the vacuolar myelopathy subsets, overt HIV-1 brain infection is absent or undetectable, and even

in multinucleated cell encephalitis the magnitude of neurologic dysfunction often appears to exceed the distribution and extent of productive infection. Speculation has centered on possible indirect mechanisms of injury involving toxic molecules of either viral (e.g., gp120) or cellular (e.g., cytokines elaborated by infected cells or by uninfected cells responding to infection) origin. It is also possible that nonproductive infection of glia or even neurons might lead to cell dysfunction without virus replication as a result of restricted viral genome transcription or translation. Whatever the mechanisms, however, HIV-1 infection, either of brain or of systemic organs, appears to be the *prime mover* in the pathogenesis of the AIDS dementia complex and thus the major target of therapy.

TREATMENT AND PROGNOSIS. Several reports now suggest that zidovudine (also azidothymidine, or AZT) relieves, at least partially, the symptoms and signs of the AIDS dementia complex. Therapeutic effect has been documented by improvement in neuropsychological test performance in two placebo-controlled trials (one in adults and the other in children with AIDS). Dose recommendations remain uncertain, but in the absence of precise information, conventional dosage (100 mg every 4 hours while the patient awake) is advised. Limitations of treatment most often relate to hematologic toxicity, but noninflammatory myopathy has also been reported (see Ch. 414). In patients whose neurologic condition deteriorates on these doses, the clinician may attempt to increase the dose, although toxicity is more likely. Additional antiretroviral drugs are currently being assessed with respect to their effect on this condition.

Symptomatic management is also important. In the subset of patients who present with mania, lithium or neuroleptics may be helpful. However, these patients may be unusually susceptible to the side effects of neuroleptics and other psychotropic drugs, and thus treatment should be cautious and begin with low doses.

Navia BA, Cho ES, Petito CK, et al.: The AIDS dementia complex: II. Neuropathology. Ann Neurol 19;525, 1986. Navia BA, Jordan BD, Price RW: The AIDS dementia complex: I. Clinical features. Ann Neurol 19:517, 1986. *Companion articles describing the clinical and pathologic features of the AIDS dementia complex.*

Price RW, Brew B, Sidtis J, et al.: The brain in AIDS: Central nervous system HIV-1 infection and the AIDS dementia complex. Science 239:586, 1988. *A review discussing the pathogenesis of the AIDS dementia complex.*

Sidtis JJ, Price RW: Early HIV-1 infection and the AIDS dementia complex. Neurology 40:323, 1990. *A review of the issue of the AIDS dementia complex in asymptomatic HIV-1 seropositive individuals.*

478.3 HUMAN T CELL LYMPHOTROPIC VIRUS TYPE I–ASSOCIATED MYELOPATHY AND TROPICAL SPASTIC PARAPARESIS

Richard W. Price

DEFINITION. Human T cell lymphotropic virus type I (HTLV-I) was the first human retrovirus to be identified in the laboratory and the second, after human immunodeficiency virus type 1 (HIV-1), to be etiologically implicated in neurologic disease. This connection was made when a survey in Martinique discovered that nearly 60 per cent of patients with tropical spastic paraparesis (TSP) were seropositive for HTLV-I. A similar serologic association was soon established in other tropical areas, and, concomitantly, Japanese workers implicated this virus in the etiology of a myelopathy occurring principally in the Kyushu district; because this is not a tropical region, they proposed the name HTLV-I–associated myelopathy (HAM). Although the two conditions were first considered to be clinically distinct, subsequent comparison of the clinical and laboratory features suggests that the tropical and Japanese conditions are, in fact, the same disease, and the combined term HAM/TSP has been advocated.

ETIOLOGY AND EPIDEMIOLOGY. HTLV-I is a genomically complex virus classified among the oncogenic retroviruses. Although infection is most often asymptomatic, the virus has been implicated in acute T cell lymphoma/leukemia (ATLL) as well as HAM/TSP. In Japan it is estimated that myelopathy develops in about 1 in every 2000 infected carriers and ATLL in perhaps 1 in 10,000 carriers, and the two conditions rarely coexist. Infection is widely prevalent in much of the Caribbean, in certain parts of South Africa, South India, Colombia, Peru, and the Seychelles Islands, as well as Japan. In the United States, endemic infection is found principally in certain parts of the Southeast, chiefly among blacks; however, the influx of Caribbean and other migrants, as well as perhaps transfusion-related transmission, has resulted in more widespread sporadic dispersion. Both HAM/TSP and ATLL follow this same geographic pattern. Infection is thought to be transmitted sexually from males to females, in breast milk, and by transfusion, the last factor having led to serologic blood donor screening. Although some preliminary observations suggested that multiple sclerosis might be associated with this retrovirus, numerous subsequent studies have failed to substantiate such a connection.

HAM/TSP usually afflicts individuals between 20 and 65 years old and most commonly begins between ages 35 and 45 years. For those infected early in life, this implies a very prolonged incubation period. In patients infected by transfused blood, however, the incubation period is as short as 5 or 6 months. Otherwise, most cases are sporadic, although there is an occasional familial incidence. The variability in disease expression among those infected has led to the suggestion that host factors, including histocompatibility immune response genes, might be cofactors in the development of HAM/TSP.

CLINICAL MANIFESTATIONS. The salient feature of HAM/TSP is spastic paraparesis or paraplegia. Typically, the onset is gradual, with steady disease progression over months to years and a tendency in many instances to stabilize later on. Occasionally, the disorder begins more abruptly and has a more irregular course. Patients almost universally exhibit spastic legs; bladder and bowel disturbance is present in more than three quarters, while only about half have position or vibratory sensory impairment. Low back stiffness and pain are common. The gait may at times appear ataxic, and probably fewer than one tenth of affected persons have symptoms of neurologic dysfunction outside the spinal cord. Optic atrophy, nerve deafness, peripheral neuropathy, a clinical picture of pseudo–amyotrophic lateral sclerosis with anterior horn cell disease, and polymyositis have all been noted. Patients may also have systemic findings involving the lung (lymphocytic alveolitis), skin, and eyes (cotton-wool spots).

Characteristic cerebrospinal fluid (CSF) findings include oligoclonal immunoglobulin bands and intrathecal synthesis of anti–HTLV-I antibodies. The CSF cell count may be normal or show a mild lymphocytic pleocytosis; lymphocytes with flower-like nuclear changes similar to those seen in ATLL may be present. About half of patients have abnormal signal in the cerebral white matter detected by magnetic resonance imaging (MRI), indicating subclinical involvement.

The diagnosis of TSP/HAM relies principally on the identification of the clinical manifestations and documentation of viral infection; CSF abnormalities, including the high level of antibodies to the virus, are also helpful. Because of the high rate of asymptomatic HTLV-I infection, other neurologic conditions are likely to develop in seropositive patients, and thus the diagnosis requires more than simply ascertaining the presence of antibodies in a patient with spinal cord or other neurologic abnormalities. In addition, current serologic screening methods may not discriminate between HTLV-I and the related retrovirus, human T cell lymphotropic virus type II (HTLV-II), which has not yet been clearly implicated in causing neurologic disease; additional testing with Western blot or direct characterization of viral isolates can be used to discriminate between the two viruses.

PATHOLOGY AND PATHOGENESIS. Neuropathologically, in the spinal cord the corticospinal tracts are most severely affected, although abnormalities are usually more widely distributed. Perivascular inflammation involving lymphocytes, macrophages, and plasma cells, along with fibrosis, is notable. Gliosis is prominent, with loss of myelin and, frequently, axons as well. While scattered perivascular inflammation is also present in the brain, parenchymal changes are usually minimal or absent. Immunologic studies show activation of major histocompatibility class I antigens in association with the inflammatory and gliotic responses.

Although HTLV-I antigens have been noted in at least one case, most other attempts to identify infected cells have been negative, indicating that productive infection is minimal. This observation, along with the prominence of inflammation and the therapeutic response to corticosteroids and other immunosuppressive measures, suggests that immunopathologic processes are significantly involved in the genesis of spinal cord injury. HTLV-I infection is associated with a state of immune activation with circulating activated T cells. Whether the neurologic injury relates to immune reactions to HTLV-I antigens and consequent "innocent bystander" injury of adjacent neural tissue or to true autoimmunity with activation of immune responses against self-antigens is uncertain.

TREATMENT AND PROGNOSIS. Immunosuppression using corticosteroids, plasma exchange, or other measures has been reported, principally by the Japanese, to alleviate TSP/HAM, although remission may not be well sustained. Antiviral therapy (with zidovudine or newer antiretroviral drugs used for AIDS) has not yet been assessed in TSP/HAM. As noted above, the course and outcome are variable. Usually the disease becomes disabling, but not directly life limiting; thus supportive measures are of paramount important, as in other spinal cord diseases.

Jacobson S, Shida H, McFarlin DE, et al.: Circulating CD8 + cytotoxic T lymphocytes specific for HTLV-I pX in patients with HTLV-I associated neurological disease. Nature 348:245, 1990. *The cytotoxic lymphocytes were identified in HTLV-I–infected patients with neurologic manifestations of the disease but not in seropositive individuals who lacked neurologic involvement. HTLV-I–specific cytotoxic lymphocytes may contribute to the neurologic manifestations of the disease.*

Roman GC, Vernant J-C, Osame M (eds.): HTLV-I and the Nervous System. Proceedings of an international meeting organized by the Departments of Neurology of Texas Tech University and La Meynard Hospital, April 15–16, 1988, Fort-de-France, Martinique, French Antilles. New York, Alan R. Liss, 1989. *Contains reviews of the clinical, epidemiologic, and biologic aspects of TSP/HAM.*

478.4 SUBACUTE SCLEROSING PANENCEPHALITIS AND PROGRESSIVE RUBELLA PANENCEPHALITIS

Richard W. Price

Subacute sclerosing panencephalitis (SSPE), a "slow" infection caused by measles virus, usually affects children, but its onset can extend into young adulthood. Patients usually have a history of measles within the first 2 years of life, and it is speculated that such early host exposure allows emergence of persistent defective virus replication. Fortunately, its incidence has markedly decreased in recent years.

Clinically, SSPE usually begins with cognitive and behavioral changes; progresses to include motor dysfunction with prominent myoclonus, choreoathetosis, dystonia, and rigidity; and usually pursues a progressive course with steady deterioration over 1 to 3 years to eventual rigid quadriparesis and a vegetative state. The condition is more common in a rural setting and affects males more often than females. The electroencephalogram (EEG) reveals periodic complexes with synchronous bursts of two to three per second slow waves, recurring at 5- to 8-second intervals. The cerebrospinal fluid (CSF) is characterized by a high immunoglobulin concentration, oligoclonal bands, and abundant intrathecal synthesis of antibody to measles virus antigens. Serum measles antibody titers are also high. These findings are usually sufficiently characteristic for diagnosis, but brain biopsy may be needed for definitive diagnosis in some cases. The distinct pathology of SSPE includes gliosis, loss of myelin, and perivascular infiltrates of lymphocytes and plasma cells in white and gray matter. Intranuclear inclusions containing viral nucleocapsids are noted in both neurons and glia.

Measles virus may also cause a subacute encephalitis in the immunocompromised host. The prominence of cognitive and motor dysfunction in these patients resembles SSPE, but the clinical setting, its subacute onset and more rapid evolution, and the presence of seizures rather than myoclonus are distinctive. Brain pathology includes abundant intranuclear inclusions, but inflammation is minimal, and neither serum nor CSF antibody titers against measles virus are high. For this reason, brain biopsy is usually needed for diagnosis.

Progressive rubella panencephalitis is a rare disorder resembling SSPE but caused by rubella virus and developing as a complication of either the congenital rubella syndrome or, more typically, childhood rubella. A hiatus of years separates early infection from the onset of neurologic deterioration, which is characterized by behavioral changes, intellectual decline, ataxia, spasticity, and sometimes seizures. Myoclonus is not a prominent feature, as it is in SSPE. Serology or viral isolation from brain or peripheral blood lymphocytes confirms the etiology.

With the advent of widespread measles and rubella immunization, these disorders have been all but eliminated in the United States, although SSPE still occurs in less advanced parts of the world. There is no known treatment.

Graves M: Subacute sclerosing panencephalitis. Neurol Clin 2:267, 1984. *A thorough general review of SSPE.*

Wolinsky JS: Subacute sclerosing panencephalitis, progressive rubella panencephalitis, and multifocal leukoencephalopathy. *In* Waksman B (ed.): Immunologic Mechanisms in Neurologic and Psychiatric Disease. New York, Raven Press, 1990, pp 259–268. *A recent review of the pathogenesis of SSPE and subacute rubella encephalitis.*

478.5 PROGRESSIVE MULTIFOCAL LEUKOENCEPHALOPATHY

Richard W. Price

DEFINITION. Progressive multifocal leukoencephalopathy (PML) is an opportunistic viral infection of the central nervous system caused by a papovavirus, JC virus. Initially described in patients with a variety of underlying disorders accompanied by impaired T lymphocyte/macrophage–mediated immune defenses, it now most frequently occurs in patients with advanced human immunodeficiency virus type 1 (HIV-1) infection. It is one of the AIDS-defining opportunistic conditions. As the name implies, it is a disorder that affects principally the white matter of the brain, usually encompassing more than one lesion and pursuing an inexorably progressive course.

ETIOLOGY AND EPIDEMIOLOGY. Two factors are important in the development of PML: exposure to JC virus in the past and suppression of T cell–related immune defenses against the virus. With respect to the former, JC virus has a virtually worldwide distribution, and the majority of the population exhibits serologic evidence of exposure by the teenage years. Primary infection is benign, and, indeed, disease accompanying initial exposure has not been clearly defined. PML appears to result almost always from reactivation of latent JC virus infection rather than from recent exposure. The virus is thus innocent, except under circumstances in which the host's T lymphocyte–directed immunity is impaired and rendered unable to suppress JC virus reactivation and subsequent continued replication and spread. Recent studies indicate that JC virus infection in PML patients is not confined to the brain but also involves peripheral blood mononuclear cells, probably chiefly B lymphocytes.

While the incidence of PML has increased with the AIDS epidemic to complicate perhaps 2 to 5 per cent of cases, it may also complicate organ transplantation, lymphoreticular and hematologic malignancies (particularly in the context of cytoreductive chemotherapy), autoimmune disorders, and other immunosuppressed states associated with T lymphocyte dysfunction.

CLINICAL MANIFESTATIONS AND DIAGNOSIS. PML is characterized by the gradual onset and usually steady progression of focal neurologic dysfunction, usually involving the cerebral hemispheres. Thus, patients may present with homonymous visual field disturbance, hemiparesis, hemisensory disturbance, aphasia, apraxia, or other "cortical" dysfunction, depending on the location of the demyelinating focus. Posterior fossa abnormalities with cerebellar dysfunction or signs of brain stem involvement are less common. Most often the patient is otherwise well, without constitutional symptoms (e.g., fever, malaise), and consciousness is preserved. Headache or seizures are unusual, occurring in 10 per cent or fewer of patients.

Diagnosis is often suspected on the basis of the underlying condition (e.g., AIDS) and the clinical presentation of focal neurologic deficit. Neuroimaging is helpful in demonstrating loss of white matter rather than an expanding mass (as, for example, in toxoplasmosis or primary central nervous system lymphoma). Computed tomographic (CT) scanning is less sensitive than magnetic resonance imaging (MRI), both with respect to detecting multiple lesions and in distinguishing white matter localization, most commonly adjacent to the cerebral cortex. Characteristically, contrast enhancement is absent. Although MRI in the AIDS dementia complex may show multifocal abnormalities in the white matter that superficially resemble those of PML, patients with AIDS dementia complex usually do not have focal neurologic symptoms and signs.

Cerebrospinal fluid (CSF) is usually acellular, with normal or only mild elevation of protein content. Serologic studies usually document the presence of serum antibodies against JC virus, but this is of very limited diagnostic utility, since antibody titers are indistinguishable from those of the normal population and do not rise with the onset or progression of the disease. CSF JC virus antibodies are usually not detected. Culture of the virus from CSF or blood is very difficult, requiring specialized techniques, and thus is not useful for diagnosis. Identification of viral nucleic acid in the CSF, blood, or urine using in situ hybridization or the polymerase chain reaction is currently being explored, but the sensitivity and specificity of these methods have yet to be defined. For these reasons, brain biopsy is still necessary for definitive diagnosis. The distinct histologic abnormalities usually permit diagnosis on routinely processed and stained tissue, but immunohistochemical identification of JC antigens or in situ hybridization to identify viral nucleic acid may also be useful.

PATHOLOGY AND PATHOGENESIS. The pathology of PML provides an example of the selective effects of a virus on different cell populations within the brain. Thus, the major macroscopic finding of demyelination results from the progressive productive-lytic infection of oligodendrocytes. Infection of these cells is marked by enlargement of the nucleus by a nucleocapsid-filled inclusion. Lesions begin as microscopic centers of infection, which then spread concentrically outward; oligodendrocytes are lost in the center, and their nuclei are swollen, with inclusions at the periphery. Since myelin is composed of the elaborated cytoplasmic membranes of these cells, their lysis results in the characteristic demyelination; in mild lesions, axons are relatively spared, while in more severe, coalescent foci, frank cavitation may result. Macroscopic pathology consists of multiple foci of enlarging demyelinating "plaques." Astrocytes undergo marked alteration, with formation of bizarre nuclei resembling transformed cells, but without apparent real malignant potential. Neurons, on the other hand, are spared. Inflammation is usually minimal, but in perhaps 15 per cent of cases, perivascular mononuclear infiltrates may be more conspicuous.

TREATMENT AND PROGNOSIS. There is no established treatment for PML. Earlier anecdotes of response to cytosine arabinoside have not been confirmed by more recent observations. Spontaneous remissions have been reported, including two in patients with AIDS.

Berger JR, Kaszovitz B, Post MJD, et al.: Progressive multifocal leukoencephalopathy associated with human immunodeficiency virus infection: A review of the literature with a report of sixteen cases. Ann Intern Med 107:78, 1987. *A review of AIDS-associated PML.*

Houff SA, Major EO, Katz DA, et al.: Involvement of JC virus–infected mononuclear cells from the bone marrow and spleen in the pathogenesis of progressive multifocal leukoencephalopathy. N Engl J Med 318:301, 1988. *A report emphasizing the presence of systemic JC virus infection in PML.*

Walker DL: Progressive multifocal leukoencephalopathy: An opportunistic viral infection of the central nervous system. *In* Vinken PJ, Bruyn GW, Klawans HL (eds.): Handbook of Clinical Neurology. Vol. 34: Infections of the Nervous System, Part II. Amsterdam, Elsevier North-Holland, 1978. *A comprehensive review from the pre-AIDS era that emphasizes the virologic and clinical aspects of PML.*

478.6 CREUTZFELDT-JAKOB DISEASE

Paul E. Bendheim

DEFINITION. Creutzfeldt-Jakob disease (CJD) is a subacute central nervous system disorder characterized by a progressive dementia, myoclonus, and distinctive electroencephalographic and neuropathologic findings. Although uncommon, it is the most prevalent of the human subacute spongiform encephalopathies—fatal diseases caused by transmissible pathogens of uncertain type. Accumulating research data indicate that these disorders are probably unique in regard to their etiologic agents.

ETIOLOGY. CJD is closely related to kuru, scrapie, and a rare, inherited human disease termed the Gerstmann-Sträussler-Scheinker syndrome (GSS). *Scrapie* is a spongiform encephalopathy of sheep and goats experimentally transmissible to other animal species. The scrapie agent is not known to cause disease in humans. *Kuru* is a disease previously endemic among the Fore people inhabiting an area in the eastern highlands of Papua New Guinea. Cerebellar dysfunction, dementia, and progression to death within 2 years were typical. Women and children were affected much more frequently than men. Circumstantial evidence indicates that the kuru agent was transmitted through the ritual handling of affected tissues, especially brain, from deceased relatives. This cultural practice was discontinued, and the incidence of kuru has decreased dramatically since 1959. Brain tissues from patients dying of kuru were inoculated into the brains of chimpanzees, which, after a prolonged incubation period, developed a similar disease. Subsequently, the neuropathology of kuru and that of CJD as well as GSS were noted to be similar, and experimental transmission studies using CJD-affected or GSS-affected brain were undertaken successfully, eventually in a wide range of laboratory animals.

The CJD, GSS, kuru, and animal spongiform encephalopathy agents are unlike any known virus or other well-characterized transmissible pathogen. This has resulted in the terms *slow virus, virino,* and *prion* being used interchangeably with "agent" to refer to them. Prion proteins (PrP) in humans and animals are closely related, with the locus of the PrP genes in hereditary GSS lying on the short arm of chromosome 20. Current knowledge favors a direct role for abnormal PrP variants in the pathogenesis of both hereditary GSS and acquired CJD. The scrapie and CJD agents provoke no inflammatory response or specific antibody production. They are resistant to chemical and physical treatments that inactivate most viruses, including heat, formaldehyde, nuclease digestion, and ultraviolet and ionizing radiation. The agents can be inactivated by procedures that denature proteins. Unique fibrillar structures are observed in electron micrographs of samples prepared from brain tissue of individuals with CJD. They resemble the abnormal fibrils that accumulate in scrapie-affected animals and represent an aggregated form of the CJD protein.

INCIDENCE AND EPIDEMIOLOGY. On a worldwide basis, the incidence of CJD is one case per million population. This incidence peaks in the fifth through seventh decades, although cases have been documented as early as the second decade. The sexes are equally affected. Approximately 250 deaths occur in the United States each year. Higher rates have been noted in Israel among Libyan-born Jews and in circumscribed areas of Czechoslovakia and Chile.

CJD usually occurs sporadically in middle-aged adults without known exposure. A family history is evident in 8 per cent of patients and suggests common exposure or a genetic susceptibility. Several reports document iatrogenic human-to-human transmission via cornea transplants and via the reuse of stereotaxic electroencephalographic (EEG) electrodes that had unknowingly been previously implanted in a patient with CJD. Several cases have resulted from the use of dura mater allografts. Additional clusters of cases suggesting neurosurgical transmission have been reported. In the past 6 years, CJD has been diagnosed in 12 individuals in four countries who had received human pituitary gland growth hormone replacement therapy. It seems apparent that certain lots of the cadaveric hormone preparation were contaminated with the CJD agent. Incubation periods were between 4 and 21 years, emphasizing the astonishingly long incubation times of the spongiform encephalopathies. Additional cases may yet appear, since more than 10,000 patients worldwide received this form of human growth hormone prior to its discontinuation in 1985.

Worldwide, the incidence of CJD is the same in countries with endemic sheep scrapie as it is in those without scrapie, indicating that there is no apparent transmission to humans from this animal

reservoir. In the past 5 years, a major outbreak of a new veterinary disease, bovine spongiform encephalopathy (BSE), or *mad cow disease,* has appeared in Great Britain. BSE has not occurred in the United States. BSE appears to have had its origin in the use of food supplements contaminated with the sheep scrapie agent. Although unlikely, it is too early in the BSE epidemic in Great Britain to determine if the passage of the scrapie agent through cattle poses any increased risk to humans. Nevertheless, British authorities have taken measures to prevent human consumption of contaminated beef.

PATHOLOGY. The pathologic findings in CJD are limited to the central nervous system, although the transmissible agent can be detected in many organs. Cortical neuronal depletion, marked reactive astrocytosis, intracellular vacuolar or spongiform change, and the absence of inflammation are the major features. Amyloid fibrils and plaques occur in virtually all cases.

CLINICAL MANIFESTATIONS. Vague psychiatric or behavioral symptoms suggesting a personality change often herald the onset of CJD, but within a few weeks or months a relentlessly progressive dementia becomes evident. Myoclonus is usually present and often prominent at some time during the course. Deterioration is usually rapid, and 90 per cent of victims die within 1 year. CJD patients are afebrile and have normal blood and cerebrospinal fluid profiles. In the late stages, the EEG in at least 75 per cent of cases shows a diffusely slow background with superimposed complexes, which may or may not be associated with myoclonus.

The dementia can be accompanied by signs of involvement of any part of the central nervous system. Most patients develop signs of cerebellar and pyramidal tract dysfunction as the disease advances. Visual disturbances, extrapyramidal signs, and various dysphasias often occur. The terminal stage is marked by decorticate and decerebrate postures, stupor, and coma. Massive myoclonic responses to auditory or other sensory stimuli may create the false impression that the patient is alert and responsive.

Subtypes of CJD based on distinctive clinical presentations have been delineated. The optic type features visual disturbances, usually cortical blindness. The dyskinetic form has prominent extrapyramidal signs, while the ataxic variant resembles kuru with its marked cerebellar involvement. GSS is an autosomal dominant genetically transmitted form of CJD with slower progression and signs of spinocerebellar ataxia. A specific mutation in the gene that codes for the CJD precursor protein has been found in some patients with this familial form of CJD. This mutation results in a protein with leucine substituted for proline at PrP codon 102, a step that promotes its aggregation into the characteristic brain amyloid.

DIAGNOSIS. The diagnosis of CJD should be considered when a relatively rapidly progressive dementia develops in an adolescent or adult patient with normal spinal fluid. The presence of myoclonus or the characteristic EEG recording is strongly supportive, but often either or both are absent in early stages. All treatable diseases that can cause dementia need to be specifically tested for before a presumptive diagnosis of CJD or another untreatable dementia is made. Neither brain imaging nor laboratory evaluations are useful in diagnosis. Brain biopsy has been the usual method to establish definitive diagnosis. Research level, two-dimensional electrophoresis, however, has also provided accurate diagnosis in an increasing number of cases. In early cases, psychological depression, the AIDS dementia complex, and a number of rare dementias, including collagen vascular diseases and paraneoplastic limbic encephalitis, must be considered. Rarely, lithium toxicity can present with a clinical picture and EEG pattern resembling those of CJD. Discontinuation of the drug results in improvement within a few weeks.

Alzheimer's disease (see Ch. 450), the most common neurodegenerative dementia, usually has a more protracted course, without either the myoclonus or the typical EEG of CJD. Amyloid deposition in the brain is a pathologic hallmark of both Alzheimer's disease and CJD, but the amyloid proteins deposited in these two diseases are structurally unrelated. The development of specific antibodies for both these amyloid proteins allows rapid immunologic differentiation between CJD and Alzheimer's disease if a brain biopsy or postmortem examination is done.

TREATMENT AND PROGNOSIS. No effective treatment is available, and the disease appears to be uniformly fatal.

PREVENTION. Although CJD can be transmitted, the risk to health care workers and others having contact with patients is no higher than that to the general population. Isolation of patients is not indicated, but certain guidelines should be followed. Hospital workers should wear gloves when handling tissues, blood, and spinal fluid. Accidental skin contact with possibly contaminated fluids or materials should be followed by washing with 1N sodium hydroxide or a 1:10 dilution of 5 per cent household chlorine bleach (sodium hypochlorite). All laboratory samples should be clearly marked and needles disposed of properly. The agent can be inactivated on contaminated surfaces using a 1:10 dilution of bleach for 1 hour. Surgical and pathologic instruments should be steam autoclaved for 1 hour at 132°C. No organs, tissues, or tissue products from patients with CJD or with any ill-defined neurologic disease should be used for transplantation or replacement therapy.

Bock G, Marsh J (eds.): Novel infectious agents and the central nervous system. Ciba Foundation Symposium 135. Chichester, United Kingdom, Wiley-Interscience Publications, 1988. *A monograph from an international symposium* with chapters on epidemiologic, pathologic, and research aspects of CJD and scrapie.

Brown P, Cathala F, Castaigne P, et al.: Creutzfeldt-Jakob disease: Clinical analysis of a consecutive series of 230 neuropathologically verified cases. Ann Neurol 20:597, 1986. *Clinical features are detailed in this large series of documented cases.*

Harrington MG, Merril CR, Asher DM, Gajdusek DC: Abnormal proteins in the cerebrospinal fluid of patients with Creutzfeld-Jakob disease. N Engl J Med 315:279, 1986. *The original report showing that CJD, but not other dementias, is associated with specific abnormalities in CSF proteins.*

Prusiner SB: Molecular biology of prion disease. Science 252:1515, 1991. *A thorough summary of the epidemioloy in animals and humans of this still mysterious infectious disease plus a description of the molecular biology and genetics of sporadic and inherited forms of CJD.*

Rosenberg RN, White CL III, Brown P, et al.: Precautions in handling tissues, fluids, and other contaminated materials from patients with documented or suspected Creutzfeldt-Jakob disease. Ann Neurol 19:75, 1986. *Safety guidelines for health care workers and specific decontamination protocols for surgical and pathologic instruments.*

SECTION TEN / NEUROLOGIC DISORDERS ASSOCIATED WITH ALTERED IMMUNITY OR UNEXPLAINED HOST-PARASITE ALTERATIONS

Jerry S. Wolinsky

479 Central Nervous System Complications of Viral Infections and Vaccines

Central nervous system (CNS) symptoms and signs arising in the course of systemic infections usually reflect direct CNS invasion by the inciting organism. Less frequently, systemic infections, especially viral infections, or the administration of certain vaccines give rise to CNS abnormalities that do not appear to depend on direct invasion of the brain but rather reflect presumed autoimmune or toxic mechanisms. Several reasonably distinct patterns of involvement have been delineated. Two of these, *acute disseminated encephalomyelitis* and *acute hemorrhagic encephalomyelitis*, appear to be mediated by immune mechanisms and have a peripheral nervous system counterpart, *acute inflammatory polyneuropathy*, or the *Guillain-Barré syndrome*. The remainder, *Reye syndrome, acute toxic encephalopathy*, and *acute cerebellar ataxia of childhood*, are likely to be toxic in origin.

ACUTE DISSEMINATED ENCEPHALOMYELITIS (ADE)

DEFINITION. Acute disseminated encephalomyelitis (*parainfectious* or *postinfectious encephalomyelitis, acute demyelinating encephalitis, immune-mediated encephalomyelitis*) is an acute disease of the CNS that most commonly occurs in association with viral infections or as a complication of vaccination. Involvement of brain and spinal cord is usually widespread but may be limited clinically to discrete areas such as the optic nerves, as in optic neuritis or papillitis, or to a single spinal cord level, as in acute transverse myelitis.

ETIOLOGY AND PATHOGENESIS. Table 479–1 lists principal factors predisposing to ADE. The neurologic complications usually occur 6 to 10 days after the appearance of the exanthem or onset of other specific symptoms. However, ADE can occur prior to or concomitantly with systemic symptoms of infection. Characteristically, ADE begins 10 days to 3 weeks after initiation of the vaccination regimen. Perhaps the most easily understood form of ADE is that which followed vaccination against rabies with (now obsolete) inactivated inoculum of fixed rabies virus propagated in animal brain. These early vaccines were contaminated with CNS proteins, including the antigens associated with myelin. Both complement-fixing antibody and specific lymphocyte blast transformation responses to crude and purified CNS antigens have been measured in blood of patients receiving rabies vaccine, and the responses were highest in those whose vaccination was complicated by ADE; the incidence of neuroparalytic accidents was reported to be as high as 1:600 to 1:6000 persons. Current rabies vaccines derived from virus grown in human diploid cells appear to be essentially free of neural complications (Ch. 477).

A compelling analogy links rabies vaccine–related ADE to the animal experimental disorder *experimental allergic encephalo-*

TABLE 479–1. PRINCIPAL CONDITIONS PREDISPOSING TO ACUTE DISSEMINATED ENCEPHALOMYELITIS

Infections	
Measles	*Mycoplasma pneumoniae*
Varicella zoster	Respiratory agents
Influenza	Epstein-Barr
Rubella	
Vaccines: smallpox, measles, rabies (Semple vaccine)	

myelitis (EAE). In EAE, brain homogenates, highly purified myelin components, or peptides containing the encephalogenic sequences of myelin basic protein (MBP) or proteolipid protein (PLP) can induce an acute CNS perivascular inflammatory and demyelinative reaction that is histologically identical to ADE. In affected animals, clinical disease begins 10 to 14 days after sensitization and is associated with both humoral and cellular immune responses directed against the inciting CNS antigen. Furthermore, EAE can be adoptively transferred to naive animals by T lymphocytes, suggesting that this cell type is of primary importance in the pathogenesis.

The occurrence of ADE following viral infections is more difficult to understand. Encephalitis is relatively frequent following measles (1:1000 cases), but there is little evidence to implicate invasion of the CNS by measles virus as an obligate prerequisite. Theoretical data support the possible importance of sequence similarities between measles virus and other viral antigens and CNS proteins such as MBP and PLP. Very early in the course of measles ADE, specific blast transformation responses to MBP are apparent in the lymphocytes of children, and measurable quantities of MBP are released into the cerebrospinal fluid (CSF). These findings support the hypothesis that acute measles transiently alters the immune system, which in some persons results in a breakdown of tolerance to CNS antigens. Despite the usual absence of CNS symptoms, this process appears to occur frequently, as reflected by a high incidence of abnormal-appearing electroencephalograms (EEG's). Both EEG abnormalities and clinical ADE can occur after vaccination with live-attenuated measles virus but at a markedly lower frequency, with ADE arising in about 1:1,000,000 vaccinated persons.

INCIDENCE. Valid incidence figures for ADE are difficult to derive. Encephalitis complicates about 1:1000 cases of measles. ADE following vaccination for smallpox is only of historical interest but occurred in the United States with a reported incidence of 2.9 per million primary vaccinations. ADE following other childhood viral illnesses or vaccinations is uncommon. Most adult cases of ADE have no identifiable antecedents.

PATHOLOGY. Neuropathologic change consists of perivenular infiltration by lymphocytic and mononuclear cells and variable amounts of primary demyelination extending in centripetal manner from involved vessels of the white matter. The axons are relatively spared. This primary lesion can occur throughout the neuraxis but tends to be most prominent in the centrum semiovale of the cerebrum and in the pontine white matter. The brain may appear somewhat swollen or grossly normal. Repair occurs through remyelination. In certain cases, large, confluent demyelination can take on a superficial resemblance to the plaques of multiple sclerosis, differing primarily in that all lesions reflect a similar time of onset.

CLINICAL MANIFESTATIONS. The clinical disorder can resemble almost any of the acute encephalitides. In adults, neurologic symptoms often first suggest the illness. With the childhood exanthemata, CNS symptoms usually begin about 5 days after the onset of the rash (range 0 to 24 days, with rare examples of ADE preceding the rash). The course of the preceding illness is in no way atypical for patients who subsequently develop ADE. Fever or recrudescence of fever is nearly universal. Headache, with or without meningismus, and lethargy occur in 20 to 80 per cent of cases. In about half of the cases, one or more generalized seizures occur. Usually the onset of altered consciousness is abrupt, occurring within a few hours, but CNS symptoms sometimes evolve over several days. Stupor, delirium, or coma develops in severe cases. Multifocal motor and sensory deficits of varied severity are common and often asymmetric.

The EEG is abnormal in appearance, with widespread slowing of background rhythms. The CSF in children almost invariably shows a modest mononuclear pleocytosis of 20 to 200 cells per cubic millimeter and occasionally higher. The fluid contains a slight elevation of protein content, a normal glucose level, and a raised myelin basic protein level. After several days, magnetic resonance imaging (MRI) characteristically defines scattered white matter lesions, at least some of which enhance with paramagnetic agents during the acute phases of the disease.

The duration of active CNS disease varies from days to weeks, often with a protracted convalescence. The overall mortality is about 20 per cent. About 90 per cent of survivors recover completely or nearly completely, although severe residual deficits can occur.

DIAGNOSIS. Diagnosis in ADE is by exclusion. First, encephalitis, meningitis, or meningoencephalitis must be excluded as a direct effect of a virus or other infectious agent. In the setting of a recent exanthematous illness or vaccination, ADE is more readily implied. However, in pathologic series of clinically diagnosed ADE occurring in the course of mass vaccination programs, postmortem examination proved the majority of patients to have had other illnesses, including potentially treatable CNS infections. Differentiation of an initial severe episode of multiple sclerosis can be challenging, even with MRI help, but subsequent recurrences eventually make the proper diagnosis clear.

TREATMENT. Treatment consists of supportive care, including the use of anticonvulsants and, when necessary, intensive care monitoring. Although sometimes employed clinically, neither corticosteroids nor other immunosuppressive drugs have proved beneficial.

ACUTE HEMORRHAGIC LEUKOENCEPHALITIS

Acute hemorrhagic leukoencephalitis is a fulminant and fatal syndrome believed to have an immunopathogenesis similar to that of ADE. Typically, the illness arises either spontaneously or following an uneventful upper respiratory illness. Sudden headache precedes the neurologic symptoms, which include seizures and rapid progression from lethargy to coma in a matter of a few hours to several days. Major focal neurologic abnormalities are common and may suggest lateralized cerebral involvement. Systemic signs and symptoms include fever and marked peripheral leukocytosis. The accompanying CSF pleocytosis usually shows a preponderance of polymorphonuclear cells and sometimes evidence of minor degrees of hemorrhage into the subarachnoid space. More than 80 per cent of all recognized cases of acute hemorrhagic leukoencephalitis are fatal, although these findings may be biased by selective reports of postmortem studies. The brain is usually swollen, and examination shows bilateral but asymmetric abnormalities, with petechial hemorrhages scattered throughout the white matter. Microscopic lesions consist of features reminiscent of hyperimmune forms of EAE. The clinical differential diagnosis includes ADE and acute viral encephalitis, especially herpes simplex encephalitis (see Ch. 476.1). Computed tomography (CT) or MRI may be diagnostically helpful in selected cases. Therapy is supportive.

Griffin DE: Monophasic autoimmune inflammatory diseases of the CNS and PNS. Res Publ Assoc Res Nerv Ment Dis 68:91, 1990. *A review of recent advances in unraveling parainfectious nervous system disease.*

Kesselring J, Miller DH, Robb SA, et al.: Acute disseminated encephalomyelitis—MRI findings and the distinction from multiple sclerosis. Brain 113:291, 1990.

480 Reye Syndrome

DEFINITION. Reye syndrome is a well-delineated biphasic disease in which one of several common viral illnesses is followed by an acute and sometimes fatal encephalopathy associated with fatty infiltration and dysfunction of the liver.

ETIOLOGY AND PATHOGENESIS. Reye syndrome most commonly occurs following influenza A, influenza B, herpes varicella zoster, and, to a lesser extent, several other common virus infections. Many other common viral illnesses have been implicated, each at a much lower frequency. Little evidence links the precipitating viral infection directly to either the CNS or hepatic involvement. A toxic origin is proposed for both types of involvement. The hepatic dysfunction appears to be the primary error and the direct result of a mitochondrial disturbance that causes secondary metabolic derangements, including hyperammonemia, lactic acidemia, and elevated levels of serum free fatty acids. These metabolic derangements have been implicated in the pathogenesis of the brain swelling and increased intracranial pressure that dominate the clinical course of severe cases. What causes the mitochondrial impairment remains to be clarified. Epidemiologic evidence suggests that aspirin plays a potentiating role in the pathogenesis of this syndrome.

INCIDENCE. Reye syndrome occurs most commonly among children between 1 and 15 years of age but has been reported in adolescents and is increasingly recognized in adults. Inner city black infants may be especially at risk for the disease. Prospectively derived incidence figures for the most susceptible age groups are as high as 6.2 per 100,000 children.

PATHOLOGY. The liver shows a noninflammatory, panlobular, hepatocellular accumulation of lipid droplets and both histochemical and ultrastructural evidence of inflammation. At postmortem examination, swelling of astrocytic foot processes and ultrastructural changes in mitochondria similar to those seen in hepatic mitochondria may be found in the greatly swollen brain.

CLINICAL MANIFESTATIONS AND COURSE. Reye syndrome is a biphasic disorder. As symptoms of the initial viral illness begin to wane or clear, the dramatic features begin, usually with intractable vomiting associated with lethargy or delirium. Early diagnosis is confirmed by the findings of nonicteric hepatic dysfunction, an elevated arterial blood ammonia level, and serum transaminase levels that exceed three times normal levels. Hepatic enlargement is present in about one half of the cases. Children under 1 year of age often show hypoglycemia. Signs of CNS deterioration include the development of generalized seizures, deepening obtundation, and transtentorial herniation. The CSF is under increased pressure but is acellular, with otherwise normal constituents.

DIAGNOSIS. Diagnosis rests on the clinical findings and appropriate biochemical abnormalities. Liver biopsy usually is not necessary. Central nervous system infection, inborn errors of metabolism, such as ornithine transcarbamylase deficiency and systemic carnitine deficiency, and the presence of known hepatotoxins, including valproate, salicylates, and paracetamol, among others, must be actively excluded. A childhood syndrome, distinguishable from Reye syndrome only by the absence of hepatic involvement and a high incidence of acute convulsions, can follow both banal viral infections and vaccination.

TREATMENT. Affected patients require intensive care monitoring until the course of the disease is well established. Hypoglycemia and electrolyte abnormalities must be corrected. Many authorities suggest hydration with solutions of high glucose content. Appropriate measures should be taken to monitor intracranial pressure continuously in the more severely affected cases, as judicious control of intracranial hypertension contributes to a favorable outcome. Mortality is about 10 per cent.

Ede RJ, Williams R: Reye's syndrome in adults. Br Med J 296:517, 1988. *Although uncommon, such cases do occur and need management different from that for children.*

Pranzatelli MR, DeVivo DC: Pharmacology of Reye syndrome. Clin Neuropharmacol 10:96, 1987. *A comprehensive review including detailed recommendations for medical management.*

481 Neurologic Complications in the Immunologically Compromised Host

Modern treatment of several previously fatal conditions in many instances leads to an immunocompromised state that is associated with opportunistic infections of the CNS. Such treatments include transplantation for organ failure, chemotherapy and radiotherapy of malignancies, and immunosuppressive treatment of autoimmune diseases. The epidemic emergence of the acquired immunodeficiency syndrome (AIDS) also has been associated with a marked increase in the number of unusual CNS infections likely to be encountered in routine practice.

CNS INFECTIONS IN TRANSPLANT RECIPIENTS. Renal transplantation is now commonplace, and bone marrow, cardiac, and other organ transplantations are performed with increasing effectiveness. Hospital-acquired bacterial species predominate in early infections in transplant recipients. Immunosuppression, especially lethal irradiation used in the preparation for marrow transplantation from nonidentical donors, almost predictably gives rise to reactivation of herpesviruses: first herpes simplex viruses types 1 and 2 (HSV), then herpes varicella zoster virus (HVZ), and finally cytomegalovirus (CMV). The systemic manifestations of each can be overwhelming, but symptomatic CNS dissemination has so far been remarkably infrequent. However, encephalitis or meningitis can complicate either HSV or HVZ infections. Also, while EEG, CT, or MRI findings evolve as anticipated in the intact host, the CSF pleocytosis is often absent, especially in patients with severe leukopenia. CNS involvement by CMV has been pathologically documented in transplant patients but has not been associated with a recognizable clinical syndrome and at present appears to be asymptomatic. The availability of effective antiviral chemotherapy now makes it imperative to attempt early diagnosis in cases of suspected HSV or HVZ meningoencephalitis (see Ch. 473).

Transplant patients are at greatest risk of infection by opportunistic agents after the second month of the transplant. They remain at risk while they are on most immunosuppressive regimens, if they are azotemic, and when there are ongoing graft-versus-host or chronic rejection reactions. *Listeria monocytogenes*, *Cryptococcus neoformans*, and *Aspergillus fumigatus* account for the overwhelming majority of infections. *Toxoplasma gondii*, *Candida* species, *Nocardia asteroides*, the rhinocerebral phycomycoses, and *Coccidioides immitis* are less frequently encountered.

The acute or subacute development of fever in the transplant patient should suggest *Listeria* meningitis even in the absence of meningeal signs. The CSF has the characteristics of a purulent meningitis, although occasionally patients with *Listeria* infection have misleading mononuclear pleocytosis (see Ch. 301). Otherwise unexplained headache of acute or chronic duration, even in the absence of a febrile response or confusion, should suggest the possibility of cryptococcal meningitis. A mononuclear pleocytosis with or without a low glucose content is the characteristic CSF finding (see Ch. 403). India ink preparations can provide immediate confirmation of diagnosis, and tests for cryptococcus antigen can be more helpful than direct culture of the organism from the CSF. Since both listerial and cryptococcal meningitis represent some of the most frequently encountered and more manageable infections that affect the immunocompromised host, careful attention must be given to symptoms that suggest infection of the CNS.

Aspergillus fumigatus infections of the CNS usually are manifested as acute fulminant disease with seizures, obtundation, and, frequently, apoplectic onset of focal neurologic deficits. The propensity of *Aspergillus* to invade and destroy blood vessels underlies the frequent strokelike appearance of infected patients. Low-density lesions with ill-defined, poorly contrast-enhancing borders may be seen on CT, but diagnosis depends on brain biopsy in the absence of systemic disease. Current diagnostic and therapeutic approaches to this CNS infection are inadequate (see Ch. 406).

CNS INFECTION IN PATIENTS WITH LYMPHOMA, LEUKEMIA, OR CHRONIC IMMUNOSUPPRESSIVE THERAPY. Splenectomy, often used in the staging of Hodgkin's disease, places patients at increased risk for conventional bacterial infections that may be complicated by meningitis. In community-acquired infections, *Haemophilus influenzae* and *Streptococcus pneumoniae* species predominate. Metastatic spread from various systemic sites by a wide spectrum of bacterial organisms is a continual threat for all immunosuppressed patients. The usual signs and symptoms of CNS infection can be obscured by the anti-inflammatory effect of therapy. The use of chronic immunosuppressive therapy for leukemia, lymphoma, or presumed autoimmune disorders can be complicated by *Listeria monocytogenes* in a manner similar to that described for transplant patients. The emergence of listerial meningitis often follows an increase in the intensity of the immunosuppressive regimen.

Cryptococcal meningitis and *Aspergillus* meningoencephalitis are significant sources of morbidity for this group of patients. Their clinical appearances parallel those seen in organ transplant patients. Segmental zoster, occasionally with dissemination, is a well-recognized problem among these patients, and CNS toxoplasmosis is occasionally encountered. Of special interest is *progressive multifocal leukoencephalopathy* (PML) (Ch. 478.5), which may account for up to 10 per cent of all CNS infections in this patient group. Progressive deterioration in mental status and the evolution of focal neurologic deficits in the absence of

meningismus or CSF abnormalities characterize the clinical symptomatology of PML. Serial CT scans are usually diagnostic, but the recent observation that some patients with CNS infections by HVZ can have a clinical course similar to that of PML must be considered because HVZ is potentially responsive to antiviral chemotherapy.

Conti DJ, Rubin RH: Infection of the central nervous system in organ transplant recipients. Neurol Clin 6:241, 1988. *A comprehensive review of an extensive experience with opportunistic CNS infections.*

SECTION ELEVEN / THE DEMYELINATING DISEASES

482 The Demyelinating Diseases
Donald H. Silberberg

The demyelinating diseases affect myelin to a greater extent than other nervous system components. This section discusses disorders that primarily affect central nervous system (CNS) myelin; the demyelinating peripheral neuropathies are discussed in Ch. 497. A few disorders, such as the neurologic complications of vitamin B_{12} deficiency and some of the leukodystrophies, affect both central and peripheral myelin.

Since central myelin is an extension of the oligodendrocyte, which manufactures the myelin sheath, most demyelinating diseases include alterations in or disappearance of this glial cell. An oligodendrocyte process wraps around a segment of an axon in a concentric fashion to form myelin. One oligodendrocyte sends processes to as many as 20 or 30 axons within a surrounding area of several millimeters, myelinating axon segments of 1 mm or less on each fiber. The most active synthesis of myelin starts in utero and continues for the first 2 years of life; subsequently, slower synthesis continues until the adult CNS is achieved.

Each tightly compacted layer of mature myelin is a bimolecular lipid leaflet between parallel layers of hydrated protein, which is in close apposition to the polar groups of the lipid molecules. The lipids, which constitute about 75 per cent of the dry weight of myelin, include cerebroside, phospholipids, and cholesterol. Proteins include the distinctive molecule, myelin basic protein (the antigen capable of eliciting experimental allergic encephalomyelitis in experimental animals), myelin-associated glycoprotein, proteolipid proteins, and many others detectable by electrophoretic separation but not yet well characterized. Turnover of the components of mature myelin continues at a slower rate than the rate during development. Both developing and mature forms of myelin are readily susceptible to injury by many diseases.

CLASSIFICATION. Definitive classification awaits an understanding of the causes of these disorders. Failing that, a mixed temporal-etiologic-descriptive classification must serve as the scaffold. A useful distinction is to separate what seem to be acquired disorders from those that are errors in development (Table 482–1). Multiple sclerosis will be discussed first, since it is by far the most common of these problems.

MULTIPLE SCLEROSIS

DEFINITION. Multiple sclerosis (MS) is a disorder of unknown etiology, defined by its clinical characteristics and by typical scattered areas of brain, optic nerve, and spinal cord demyelination. Clinical diagnosis requires evidence on neurologic examination of two or more CNS white matter lesions, preferably with at least a month's interval between symptoms, in a patient of the appropriate age, in whom evidence is lacking of any other explanation for the signs and symptoms. MS usually produces its

first clinical symptoms in those between ages 15 and 50 years. Occasional cases occur beyond these extremes, but the average age of onset is 33. Most patients recover clinically to some extent from individual bouts of demyelination, producing the classic remitting and exacerbating course of the early disease. Except for autopsy findings, currently available laboratory data may support the clinical diagnosis but cannot be used to define MS.

ETIOLOGY. The cause of MS remains unknown. The tissue response has features of an immunopathologic process, with perivenular mononuclear cell infiltration and absence of any overt histopathologic evidence of an infection. Two other lines of evidence point to either an immunologic cause or immunologic participation in the MS process: (1) the frequent elevation of cerebrospinal fluid (CSF) gamma globulin levels and the common oligoclonal pattern in the gamma globulin region on CSF electrophoresis, apparently synthesized by plasma cells in areas of demyelination, and (2) changes in the proportion of lymphocyte subclasses in the peripheral blood, CSF, and brain lesions. These changes are, however, nonspecific and may be the consequence of demyelination induced by some other disease mechanism, rather than the cause of the demyelination.

TABLE 482–1. DISORDERS SELECTIVELY AFFECTING MYELIN

I. **Demyelinating diseases (acquired destruction of preformed myelin)**
  A. Multiple sclerosis
    1. Uniphasic events presumably related to multiple sclerosis
      a. Optic neuritis
      b. Acute transverse myelopathy
  B. Parainfectious disorders
    1. Acute disseminated encephalomyelitis
    2. Acute hemorrhagic leukoencephalopathy
  C. Viral infections
    1. Progressive multifocal leukoencephalopathy
    2. Subacute sclerosing panencephalitis
  D. Nutritional disorders
    1. Combined systems disease (vitamin B_{12} deficiency)
    2. Demyelination of the corpus callosum (Marchiafava-Bignami disease)
    3. Central pontine myelinolysis
  E. Anoxic-ischemic sequelae
    1. Delayed postanoxic cerebral demyelination
    2. Progressive subcortical ischemic encephalopathy
II. **Dysmyelinating diseases (developmental failure to form or maintain myelin)**
  A. The leukocystrophies
    1. Metachromatic leukodystrophy
    2. Sudanophilic (Pelizaeus-Merzbacher disease)
    3. Globoid cell (Krabbe's disease)
    4. Adrenoleukodystrophy (Schilder's disease)
    5. Others (e.g., Alexander's, Canavan's, Seitelberger's disease)
  B. Aminoacidurias (e.g., phenylketonuria)
  C. Neonatal hypothyroidism

Epidemiologic studies suggest an infectious etiology. Perhaps the best evidence for this is the outbreak of MS that occurred in the Faroe Islands during the 20 years following the start of World War II. The Faroes were occupied by British troops during the war. No cases of MS had occurred prior to the occupation. The sudden appearance of MS starting several years after the arrival of the troops strongly suggests the presence of an infectious agent. The geographic areas where MS is prevalent are farther from the equator, suggesting the presence of an environmental factor, presumably an infectious agent. Efforts continue without confirmed success to recover a virus from MS tissues. MS is among the diseases with a strong linkage to certain human leukocytic antigen (HLA) haplotypes. The particular haplotype varies from one population group to another. In North America, haplotypes Dw2 and DR2, D locus markers, are found in about 65 per cent of MS patients, compared with 15 per cent of control subjects. Recent work suggests linkage to T cell receptor genes as well. Additional evidence for an immunogenetic component in the etiology of MS is the increase in frequency of MS among close relatives and the fact that MS is rare among Asians, even after emigration to the United States. A possible synthesis is that MS is an unusual consequence of infection by a common virus, or any of several viruses, with subsequent immunologic alterations in genetically susceptible individuals.

INCIDENCE AND PREVALENCE. The prevalence of MS in the northern United States and Canada and in northern Europe is at least 60 per 100,000 population, perhaps higher, based on recent data from Rochester, Minnesota. The risk is somewhat higher for women. MS is almost unknown among Asians and African blacks. There is little evidence for changing incidence or prevalence, except where population patterns are undergoing changes as the result of immigration.

EPIDEMIOLOGY. MS is more common farther from the equator in North America, in Europe, and in Australia and New Zealand. Regional population figures are punctuated by many reports of clusters of cases in a small area, such as particular cantons in Switzerland.

Many of the population studies were done before the availability of HLA typing, so that some of the observed regional differences may prove to have a genetic basis. MS occurs in both members of about 50 per cent of monozygous twin pairs when the disease has been identified in one. This finding supports the concept that genetic susceptibility may increase the chances of developing MS but is not sufficient to cause it and may not be required for its development.

PATHOLOGY. The lesions of MS consist of scattered areas of dissolution of CNS myelin, within which the axons remain intact. The border between histologically normal myelin and myelin dissolution is often sharp or may shade from normal to thinning before bare axons occur. Some areas show only partial myelin destruction. Lesions range in size from 1 mm to several centimeters in diameter and occur throughout the brain, optic nerves (which are central tracts of white matter), and spinal cord. Although plaques may occur anywhere within CNS myelin, predilections involve the optic nerves, periventricular regions within the cerebrum, and cervical spinal cord. Most plaques occur near blood vessels.

Oligodendrocytes disappear from within plaques initially. Subsequently, immature oligodendrocytes appear as attempts to remyelinate occur. However, remyelination is not nearly so complete as to explain the remissions of neurologic dysfunction that characterize MS. Astrocytes proliferate, forming the scar that lent the term "sclerosis" to multiple sclerosis. One always finds many more plaques at autopsy than could have been suspected on the basis of the clinical history and examination. Similarly, the sensitivity and resolution provided by magnetic resonance imaging (MRI) often reveal clinically unsuspected plaques. The acute lesion of MS may produce considerable edema, visible as cord swelling on myelography or as optic nerve enlargement on imaging studies. Occasionally, typical plaques of MS are found in previously asymptomatic individuals at autopsy.

B lymphocytes appear to synthesize much of the excess of gamma globulin that is found in and around plaques and in CSF. These plasma cells occur throughout affected tissue and persist in large numbers throughout a patient's lifetime, correlating with the observation that once CSF gamma globulin elevation appears, it persists. It is not known whether plasma cells and other mononuclear cells precede, accompany, or follow myelin and oligodendrocyte destruction.

LABORATORY ABNORMALITIES. *Cerebrospinal Fluid.* Increased CSF gamma globulin synthesis occurs in 80 to 90 per cent of MS patients, more commonly after the first year following the onset of symptoms. Normal CSF gamma globulin is less than 13 per cent of total CSF protein by most testing methods. The gamma globulin is mostly immunoglobulin (Ig) G but often contains IgA and IgM as well. Separate discrete "oligoclonal" bands are seen in the gamma region on agarose or polyacrylamide gel electrophoresis in about 90 per cent of patients, including some with normal IgG quantitation. These abnormalities are helpful when other causes of the phenomenon are excluded; these include CNS syphilis, subacute sclerosing panencephalitis, chronic meningitis, and any disease associated with a peripheral blood paraproteinemia, such as human T cell lymphotropic virus I (HTLV-I) infection. Other CSF abnormalities in MS can include elevation in total protein, usually to no more than 100 mg per deciliter, and an increase in the number of mononuclear white cells, usually to 5 to 15 per cubic millimeter, rarely to more than 50 per cubic millimeter. Myelin destruction releases myelin basic protein (MBP) into the CSF, which can be detected by radioimmunoassay. The amount present correlates wtih disease activity and lesion size and location; none is detectable normally, or during quiescent periods in MS patients. MBP levels rise in association with acute attacks or rapid progression. This serves as an index of disease activity but is not specific to MS. Myelin destruction from any other cause, such as acute infarction, causes a similar elevation of MBP.

Alterations in the ratio of subclasses of peripheral blood and of CSF lymphocytes occur at the time of acute exacerbations. These changes, which may indicate abnormalities of immunoregulation, are currently of investigative interest only.

Neurophysiologic Function Studies. The presence of myelin enhances the propagation of the nerve impulse along the axon. Loss of myelin, from any cause, slows conduction velocity. This alteration in conduction velocity can be measured by timing the appearance of an evoked potential (visual, auditory, or somatosensory) after an appropriate stimulus. Measurement of the latency of the visual evoked response (VER) is used most widely (Ch. 441.5). The normal latency from stimulus to VER in most laboratories is less than 102 to 105 milliseconds. A prolonged latency indicates an abnormality in the visual system, most commonly within the optic nerve in patients with MS. An abnormality of the visual, auditory, or somatosensory evoked response is used to detect dysfunction (prolonged conduction velocity) either as an objective measurement of what has already been detected clinically or for detection of a presumed subclinical abnormality.

CT and MRI Scans. Hypodense areas seen with the computed tomographic (CT) scan reflect the presence of lesions in various stages, ranging from inflammation with edema to various degrees of demyelination. Edema, which may resemble a mass lesion, often occurs acutely. During this stage, leakage of intravenously injected iodinated contrast material into the lesion area reflects abnormal leakage of the blood-brain barrier. Atrophy is seen in instances of severe demyelination.

MRI provides a much more sensitive method for detecting abnormalities in MS, and often reveals many more areas of hyperintensity on T$_2$-weighted images than were suspected clinically. The use of intravenously injected paramagnetic agents, such as gadolinium, permits detection of alterations in the blood-brain barrier with MRI, which occur with new activity in a particular area. The abnormalities detected by CSF examination, by neurophysiologic testing, and by imaging are not specific for MS (see Role of Laboratory Aids, below).

CLINICAL MANIFESTATIONS. *Onset.* The random distribution of MS lesions leads to a variety of initial symptoms and signs, alone or in combination. Further, it must be kept in mind that lesions occur in clinically silent areas of CNS white matter so that the first lesion that announces itself clinically may not be the first that has occurred in an individual. Common initial problems include weakness of one or more extremities, unilateral vision loss (optic neuritis), incoordination, and paresthesias (Table 482–2). Urinary frequency, incontinence, hesitancy, or retention;

TABLE 482–2. FIRST SYMPTOMS OF MULTIPLE SCLEROSIS IN 937 PATIENTS*

Symptom	Per Cent†
Weakness	48
Paresthesias	31
Vision loss	25
Incoordination	15
Vertigo	6
Sphincter impairment	6

*Combined series of Carter et al.: Res Publ Assoc Nerv Ment Dis 28:471, 1950; Poser CM: Recent advances in multiple sclerosis. Med Clin North Am 56:1343, 1972; and McAlpine et al.: Multiple Sclerosis: A Reappraisal. 2nd ed. Edinburgh, Churchill Livingstone, 1972.

†Many patients experience more than one symptom at onset.

vertigo; hearing loss; facial, extremity, or truncal pain; dysarthria; and changes in intellectual function occur less commonly initially. Weakness most often affects the lower extremities and may produce a range of dysfunction from slight fatigability to paraparesis. The arm and hand may be involved alone or with the legs. Patients who develop paraparesis often develop urinary urgency and constipation. Incoordination as the result of cerebellar lesions, or loss of position sense, may occur independently of weakness and often leads to gait impairment or to tremor-like, clumsy movements of the arms and hands. Paresthesias range from the spontaneous perception of vague pins-and-needles discomfort, or girdle-like pressures, to the pain of classic trigeminal neuralgia. Loss of perception of vibration and position at the ankle and toes is common; loss of pain and touch perception is less frequent. Impairment of two-point discrimination over the palmar surface of the fingertips often accompanies cervical cord lesions.

Vision loss can vary in degree from slight blurring with a small central scotoma, slight decrease in acuity, and a slight impairment of color perception to no light perception. The patient often reports acute pain on eye movement. Other visual symptoms include blurring secondary to nystagmus on primary gaze, or explicit perception of nystagmus as spontaneous movement of objects (oscillopsia). Diplopia often occurs as the result of involvement of the pontine white matter. Horizontal nystagmus of the abducting eye on lateral gaze with paresis of the adducting eye, termed *internuclear ophthalmoplegia*, is common. It is often unilateral at first and is due to lesions involving the median longitudinal fasciculus in the pons. In rare instances, extensive midline lesions lead to alterations of consciousness.

The speed of onset of symptoms varies from minutes to days, and in patients with a chronic progressive course, symptoms may appear to increase gradually over many months. The timing of recovery (remission) varies enormously but usually occurs over the course of 2 to 8 weeks following an acute bout.

Clinical Course. At least 70 per cent of patients improve in the days to months following their initial bout, the degree ranging from slight to virtual disappearance of the neurologic dysfunction. Whether or not a particular patient will improve, and to what extent, is as unpredictable as whether or not more lesions will occur and when. Overall, about three fourths of patients experience exacerbations and remissions early in their course. In many, however, as time goes by, the recovery from individual bouts decreases, disability results from accumulated failures to improve, and the course becomes chronically progressive.

About 30 per cent of patients develop successive disabilities without remission, often with long periods of clinical stability between periods of deterioration. This chronic progressive course occurs more commonly in patients experiencing their first neurologic manifestations after age 45. Patients whose disease onset has occurred at an older age seem to compress the course of events and often develop the same degree of dysfunction within a few years that takes decades to occur in a patient whose onset has occurred at a younger age.

Most patients experience additional difficulties at some time after their initial symptoms; subsequent acute bouts or chronic progression may produce signs and symptoms in any combination. Several generalizations are of interest but help little when counseling the individual. Ten years after onset, about 50 per cent of

patients are still able to carry out their household and/or employment responsibilities. Twenty years after onset about 25 per cent have these capacities. However, a fortunate few patients never develop significant disabilities, whereas others are bedridden within months after onset. One of the major psychological burdens borne by patients with MS is the uncertainty about their future. Most neurologists find it useful to emphasize the hopeful possibilities, allowing the patient's course to reveal its own manner of progression.

The average interval from clinical onset to death is 35 years; 75 per cent are living 25 years after diagnosis. Premature death is usually due to bacterial infection resulting from urinary retention, decubiti, or inability to handle pulmonary secretions. Rarely, primary respiratory failure from lower medullary lesions spells the terminal event.

Factors Possibly Affecting the Clinical Course. Elevation of body temperature by as little as 0.5°C noticeably reduces neurologic function transiently in some patients, particularly those with recent disease activity. Reduction in visual acuity, incoordination or weakness, and sensory or bladder dysfunction can be affected. This is the result of slowed axonal conduction induced by heating, and the alterations disappear within hours of regaining normal body temperature. This contributes to the fact that many patients' conditions worsen concomitantly with an intercurrent infection. However, it is likely that immunologic changes induced by infection are responsible, since the temperature effect is a transient one. Patients should be instructed to rest and respond to respiratory infections with more care than they might otherwise exercise and to use aspirin to reduce fever.

Pregnancy makes neither exacerbations nor progression of MS more likely. Decisions regarding childbearing should be made on the basis of the patient's overall situation, rather than on the basis of this concern alone.

DIAGNOSIS. Despite the availability of increasingly complex laboratory aids, MS remains fundamentally a clinical diagnosis (Table 482–3). Physical signs on examination providing solid evidence for two or more lesions of central white matter occurring at least a month apart in a patient between age 10 and the early 50's, in the absence of any other possible etiology, are required. If the evidence for a second lesion is history or a laboratory abnormality alone, the diagnosis should be considered possible or probable, rather than clinically definite MS. The differential diagnosis includes cervical cord compression resulting from tumor or cervical spondylosis; cerebral, cerebellar, brain stem, and pituitary tumors; familial spinocerebellar degenerations; acute systemic lupus erythematosus (SLE); sarcoidosis; brain stem atherosclerotic cerebrovascular disease; vitamin B_{12} deficiency; chronic barbiturate or other intoxications; and psychogenic disturbances (Table 482–4).

If all of the patient's signs can be attributed to a lesion in a single area of the nervous system, the working assumption must be that one is not dealing with MS. In patients with a persistent headache, seizures, persistent and progressive unifocal signs, or

TABLE 482–3. SCHUMACHER PANEL CRITERIA FOR DIAGNOSIS OF (CLINICALLY DEFINITE) MULTIPLE SCLEROSIS

1. Neurologic examination must reveal objective abnormalities that can be attributed to dysfunction of the central nervous system.
2. Examination or case history must supply evidence that two or more parts of the central nervous system are involved.
3. Evidence of central nervous disease must reflect predominant involvement of white matter, that is, long-tract damage.
4. Involvement of the neuraxis must have followed one of two time patterns:
   a. Two or more episodes of worsening, each lasting at least 24 hours and each at least a month apart.
   b. Slow or stepwise progression of signs and symptoms over at least 6 months.
5. At onset the patient must be between 10 and 50 years old.
6. A physician competent in clinical neurology should decide that the patient's condition could not better be attributed to another disease.

Reprinted with permission from Schumacher G, Beebe G, Kibler R, et al.: Problems of experimental trials of therapy in multiple sclerosis: Report by the panel on the evaluation of experimental trials of therapy in multiple sclerosis. Ann NY Acad Sci 122:552–568, 1965.

TABLE 482–4. DIFFERENTIAL DIAGNOSIS OF MULTIPLE SCLEROSIS

Multifocal, CNS, relapsing and remitting course
Systemic lupus erythematosus, periarteritis nodosa
Primary CNS granulomatous angiitis
Sarcoidosis
Meningovascular syphilis
Atherosclerotic cerebrovascular disease, particularly vertebrobasilar distribution
Sjögren's syndrome
Drug intoxication
Lyme disease
Behçet's disease

Multifocal, CNS, progressive course
Familial or sporadic spinocerebellar degenerations
B_{12} deficiency myelopathy (subacute combined degeneration), optic neuropathy, cerebral dysfunction, and/or peripheral neuropathy
HTLV-I myelopathy

Single site, relapsing and remitting course
Brain tumors, particularly posterior fossa
Spinal cord tumor
Sarcoidosis
Arteriovenous malformation

Single site, progressive course
Brain, spinal cord tumors
Cervical spondylosis
Thoracic herniated intervertebral disc
Arnold-Chiari malformation
Paraspinous abscess
HTLV-I myelopathy
Human immunodeficiency virus (HIV) myelopathy
Idiopathic transverse myelopathy

papilledema (without a central scotoma), MRI is the most sensitive screening procedure. MRI examination of the spinal canal often obviates myelography to exclude cervical mass lesions.

Spinocerebellar degenerative diseases differ from MS by having associated abnormalities (such as the areflexia commonly seen with Friedreich's ataxia); by progressing slowly within a given neuroanatomic system, such as the cerebellum and its connections; and by exhibiting an abnormal family history. However, MS occurs more commonly in first-degree relatives of patients with MS, so that family history alone is not sufficient to make the distinction. Neurologic presentation of SLE in young women can be distinguished by appropriate immunologic testing. The neurologic manifestations of B_{12} deficiency may precede the peripheral red blood cell abnormalities by several years; the deficiency is detected by the serum B_{12} level, Schilling test, and methylmalonic acid levels. The correct diagnosis of brain stem arterial disease in patients in their 50's can sometimes be difficult; absence of CSF abnormalities associated with MS helps, as does the fact that all the abnormalities can be localized to a small anatomic area. The clinician's suspicion of chronic drug intoxication, often accompanied by nystagmus and ataxia, may be substantiated by appropriate blood levels or other evidence of disturbed behavior.

The total absence of objective neurologic signs at any time, together with apparent weakness or sensory loss or symptom patterns that fail to conform to known neuroanatomic systems, raises the suspicion of psychogenic illness. However, one must be wary, for many patients with urinary retention, urgency, or incontinence; ataxia; or vague sensory symptoms occurring in the early stages of MS have had their condition misdiagnosed as psychoneurotic. MRI, evoked response, or CSF abnormalities help exclude purely psychogenic disturbances but must not be overinterpreted.

Role of Laboratory Aids. The rational use of laboratory abnormalities requires an awareness of their limitations. Elevation of the CSF gamma globulin or the appearance of an oligoclonal pattern within the gamma region on electrophoresis is not specific for MS, although the non-MS causes can usually be readily excluded. However, these abnormalities fail to appear in 10 to 20 per cent of patients with clinically definite MS. Further, many patients who experience a single episode of neurologic abnormality, such as optic neuritis or transverse myelopathy, may

exhibit CSF gamma globulin abnormalities but do not develop a second clinically visible lesion after long follow-up. Thus it is not appropriate to make the diagnosis of MS with a first neurologic attack, even when one encounters CSF gamma globulin abnormalities.

Similarly, although evoked potential abnormalities serve to suggest the possibility of a lesion in that part of the CNS tested, the nonspecific nature of the electrophysiologic alterations makes it unwise to base a diagnosis on such data. A patient with paraparesis and prolonged latency of the VER may have MS but could possibly have two tumors, pernicious anemia, systemic vasculitis, or a spinal cord tumor plus an uncorrected refractive error. Similarly, multiple lesions detected via MRI may reflect many other multifocal disease processes. Despite these cautions, the discovery of CSF abnormalities commonly associated with MS, evoked potential evidence of a second lesion, and/or multiple lesions on MRI help greatly to focus on MS as a possible or probable diagnosis.

TREATMENT. Management of MS requires a combination of an understanding of the personal problems posed by an unpredictable disorder of unknown etiology; an awareness of the measures available to alleviate spasticity, urinary incontinence, and other dysfunctions; and a skeptical approach to "definitive" treatments that are proposed to alter the course of the illness. The fact that over 70 per cent of patients experience spontaneous improvement following an acute bout makes evaluation of proposed treatment difficult, time consuming, and expensive. Nevertheless, carefully conducted controlled trials are the only means for deciding whether or not an agent helps patients with MS. Testimonial-style reports should not be accepted as evidence until a controlled study has confirmed the findings. At present, no method for prevention of MS is known.

Dealing with patients affected by a chronic, sometimes disabling disease for which there is no specific treatment is frustrating to many physicians. Patients with MS often report that they must help alleviate their physician's depression by denying problems. Most patients respond well to an explanation of the disease, a discussion of those things that can be done, and assurance that vigorous research is under way to develop better treatment.

Acute bouts of neurologic dysfunction may be treated with short-term administration of corticosteroids. There is evidence that administration of adrenocorticotropic hormone (ACTH) for 10 to 14 days somewhat shortens exacerbations, although the ACTH (or other corticosteroid) does not alter the long-term course of MS. From 40 to 80 units of ACTH per day may be used; prednisone, 40 to 60 mg per day, or equivalent doses of other oral corticosteroids are often employed as alternatives. The period of treatment should not exceed 3 or 4 weeks, with appropriate precautions to avoid steroid complications. It must be emphasized that there is no evidence that corticosteroids (or any other agent) modify the MS pathogenic process. Beneficial effects are most probably due to anti-edema and anti-inflammatory effects. Many responsible clinicians choose not to treat patients in this manner, believing that minimal evidence favors steroid use.

Over 45 substances or other treatments are currently being evaluated in clinical trials, ranging from immunomodulators, such as interferons, to monoclonal antibodies directed at specific T lymphocyte subsets; none can be recommended at present.

Physical therapy plays an important role in several aspects of patient management, including developing alternative muscle strengths, preventing contractures, improving daily living, and providing supportive psychotherapy. Immersion in a cool bath or swimming pool improves neurologic function transiently by lowering body temperature and improving axonal conduction. Occupational therapy is often a key to the patient's adjustment to MS.

The chronic fatigue often associated with MS often responds to amantadine, 200 to 300 mg per day. Spasticity and flexor spasms can be alleviated with baclofen or with diazepam, which inhibits central synaptic transmission. Individual responses vary sufficiently that one must start with very low doses and increase slowly if needed. Many patients depend on spasticity for support while walking, so that removal of this aid or induction of weakness or drowsiness as temporary side effects limits treatment. Occasionally, leg contractures occur despite physical therapy and require orthopedic surgical relief for ease of handling the patient.

Bladder dysfunction is usually the result of incomplete emptying, accumulation of residual urine, and overflow frequency or incontinence and infection. Rational treatment requires careful urologic evaluation, often including urodynamic studies, to plan appropriate pharmacologic therapy. Uninhibited bladder contraction leading to urinary frequency or incontinence may be alleviated by controlling infection and restricting fluid intake prior to trips or several hours before sleep. Imipramine, oxybutynin chloride, or propantheline may help patients who cannot initiate urination or cannot fully empty their bladder. Attempts to void at fixed intervals and the Credé maneuver often help. If catheterization becomes necessary, many individuals can learn self-catheterization to avoid the complications of an indwelling catheter. Long-term urinary bacterial suppressant therapy is helpful in minimizing infection in patients carrying residual urine. The possibility of an ascending urinary tract infection must be sought and treated appropriately in any patient with recurrent cystitis.

Constipation usually responds to stool softeners and laxatives. Many patients must be reassured that no harm arises from the lack of a daily bowel movement.

Painful paresthesias and dysesthesias may occur and fortunately are usually transient. Carbamazepine, diazepam, or phenytoin usually provides relief. Prevention of decubiti in the paraplegic or desensitized patient requires constant vigilance.

Specific psychiatric support is often needed to aid patients and their families. The incidence of marital breakup, changes in roles within the family, and financial problems is exceeded only by the frequency of frustration over the unpredictability of MS. The physician often must call on a range of associates, including social workers, community agency workers, and psychiatrists, to help these patients cope.

Brown FR, Beebe GW, Kurtzke JF, et al.: The design of clinical studies to assess therapeutic efficacy in multiple sclerosis. Neurology 29:1, 1979. *A thorough review of the many factors that must be taken into consideration in designing a study to determine whether or not a proposed treatment benefits patients with MS.*

Gonzalez-Scarano F, Grossman RI, Galetta S, et al.: Multiple sclerosis disease activity correlates with gadolinium-enhanced MRI. Ann Neurol 21:300, 1987.

Kurtzke JF, Hyllested K: Multiple sclerosis in the Faroe Islands: I. Clinical and epidemiological features. Ann Neurol 5:6, 1979. *A lucid description of the remarkable, seemingly limited epidemic of MS in the Faroe Islands.*

McDonald WI, Silberberg DH (eds.): Multiple Sclerosis. London, Butterworths, 1986.

Poser C, Presthus J, Horstal O: Clinical characteristics of autopsy-proved multiple sclerosis. Neurology 16:791, 1966. *A valuable analysis of the presentation and signs and symptoms that developed among a large series of patients in whom MS was proved by autopsy.*

Poser S, Raun E, Wikstrom J, et al.: Pregnancy, oral contraceptives, and multiple sclerosis. Acta Neurol Scand 59:108, 1979. *The largest study of the possible effect of pregnancy or oral contraceptives on the course of MS; this study shows no relationship.*

Prineas J, Kwon E, Goldenberg P, et al.: Multiple sclerosis. Oligodendrocyte proliferation and differentiation in fresh lesions. Lab Invest 61:489, 1989. *One of a series of elegant descriptions of the tissue alterations produced by MS.*

MULTIPLE SCLEROSIS VARIANTS

Neuromyelitis Optica (Devic's Disease)

Neuromyelitis optica describes a syndrome characterized by the occurrence of partial or complete transverse myelopathy and optic neuritis. Loss of vision and paraplegia may occur in either disorder, and days or weeks may elapse between the onsets of the two symptom complexes. It is best considered a syndrome, in that it may occur as the result of MS, acute disseminated encephalomyelitis, SLE, or sarcoidosis. When this symptom complex occurs in the course of MS, its clinical and pathologic features are indistinguishable from those of MS.

Diffuse Sclerosis, Transitional Sclerosis

These terms describe a group of progressive neurologic disorders occurring primarily in young patients who manifest severe neurologic deficits of various types with progressive visual and mental deterioration. These are pathologists' terms, which were first used in the late nineteenth century. Schilder described three cases of what came to be known as Schilder's cerebral sclerosis, or Schilder's disease. It is likely that three separate conditions have been included as Schilder's disease and that this eponymic designation should be discarded. Some cases represent the result of severe confluent extensions of large lesions of MS. Some represent white matter disease of known viral origin, such as subacute sclerosing panencephalitis and progressive multifocal leukoencephalitis (see Ch. 478). A third group includes the leukodystrophies (see later discussion). It is probable that adrenoleukodystrophy was the disorder identified by Schilder in one of his early cases.

Possibly Related Monophasic Disorders

ACUTE DISSEMINATED ENCEPHALOMYELITIS. This disorder is discussed in Ch. 481. It can be noted here that an episode of acute disseminated encephalomyelitis can closely resemble an attack of MS. Distinction may be impossible until sufficient time has elapsed to determine whether or not a second bout occurs. The distinction between acute disseminated encephalomyelitis and MS is blurred by the occurrence of typical exacerbations in the course of MS, concomitant with intercurrent viral infection.

OPTIC NEURITIS. Optic neuritis denotes partial or complete loss of vision in one or both eyes, attributable to one or more optic nerve lesions of unknown etiology. If a cause is known, it is more precise to describe, for example, syphilitic optic neuropathy or optic neuritis or neuropathy secondary to MS. Retrobulbar neuritis describes a lesion in the posterior two thirds of the optic nerve. The term papillitis indicates a lesion in the anterior portion of the optic nerve, leading to an ophthalmoscopic appearance indistinguishable from that of acute papilledema but differing from the papilledema of increased intracranial pressure by being associated with reduction of visual acuity early in its course. The vision loss usually, but not always, affects macular vision, with appearance of a central scotoma and a reduction in color perception. Pain on eye movement is frequent during the first few days of the event. Unless the patient has papillitis, ophthalmoscopic examination is normal for the first 2 to 3 weeks, after which disc pallor with loss of small vessels on the disc or more severe atrophy may develop.

Vision loss occurs over the course of hours to several days and almost always recovers to some degree within several weeks. Blindness as the result of the optic nerve demyelination of MS rarely occurs. Optic neuritis can occur as the presenting sign of MS (see Table 482–2) or at any time during the course of the disease. Practically all MS patients exhibit optic nerve demyelination at autopsy, which underlies the usefulness of the VER. Approximately 60 per cent of patients who develop idiopathic optic neuritis go on to develop the clinical manifestations of MS. The presence of CSF or MRI abnormalities associated with MS makes this course somewhat more likely but does not have firm predictive value; MS may develop in the absence of initial laboratory abnormalities, and conversely, no further clinical signs may occur despite CSF or MRI findings.

The illnesses that can mimic idiopathic optic neuritis include optic nerve compression on any basis, neurosyphilis, ischemic optic neuropathy (in older patients), pernicious anemia, Leber's optic atrophy (which is hereditary), tobacco-alcohol amblyopia, and chronic papilledema with optic atrophy and vision loss, associated with prolonged increased intracranial pressure.

LEUKODYSTROPHIES

The leukodystrophies are diseases of dysmyelination, rather than demyelination, in that the normal formation of myelin is interfered with by a genetically determined biochemical defect. The classification of leukodystrophies is based on their histopathology. A biochemical defect is known for several, but they remain relatively rare, incurable disorders, affecting individuals from the first months of life to the 20's.

Metachromatic Leukodystrophy

This, the most common of the leukodystrophies, describes diffuse dysmyelination, usually starting in the first 10 years of life. It produces personality changes leading to dementia, convulsions, cranial nerve abnormalities, and finally severe spasticity or rigidity. Death usually occurs in from 2 to 4 years, although longer survival is reported. Juvenile and adult-onset cases have been reported.

The appearance of metachromatic material (staining red with toluidine blue) in the urinary sediment and in peripheral nerves usually allows diagnosis during life. The metachromatic material also collects in the liver, gallbladder, kidneys, and spleen. The CSF protein is usually elevated above 100 mg per deciliter.

Metachromatic leukodystrophy is usually inherited as an autosomal recessive trait. The pathogenesis of the widespread loss of normal myelin is accumulation of sulfatides in glial cells, in Schwann cells, within myelin lamellae, and in the cytoplasm of some nerve cells. The underlying biochemical defect is abnormally low activity of arylsulfatase A, an enzyme in the system that normally reduces the concentration of cerebroside sulfate. An effort to prevent disease progression by bone marrow transplantation appears to have succeeded.

Sudanophilic Leukodystrophy

This subset includes a heterogeneous group of diseases that have in common only the fact that extensive CSF myelin destruction occurs, associated with products of myelin breakdown, cholesterol esters that stain bright red with the usual fat stains. This staining quality distinguishes these diseases from the metachromatic leukodystrophies. These pathologic characteristics are found in aminoacidurias, adrenoleukodystrophy, and Pelizaeus-Merzbacher disease.

ADRENOLEUKODYSTROPHY. This disorder causes diffuse and multifocal dysmyelination, and adrenocortical insufficiency. The X-linked form, occurring exclusively in males, is associated with a defective gene in the Xq28 region, leading to impairment of the degradation of very long chain fatty acids. The onset occurs most often in childhood but has been reported in adults, with a progression of symptoms similar to those of metachromatic leukodystrophy. CSF protein is elevated in most patients. Endocrine testing reveals primary adrenal failure. Instances of adrenal failure alone have been reported in relatives of patients with adrenoleukodystrophy, and paraparesis has been observed in female carriers.

Pathologic examination reveals widespread changes in CNS myelin and peripheral nerve demyelination, with numerous lipid lamellar inclusions throughout the tissue. An effort to prevent disease progression by bone marrow transplantation appears to have been successful.

PELIZAEUS-MERZBACHER DISEASE. This rare leukodystrophy affects males primarily, is inherited as an X-linked recessive trait, and starts in early infancy. It progresses slowly, producing extensive, diffuse, symmetric disturbances of myelin staining associated with gliosis within the cerebrum and cerebellum. The peripheral nervous system is not affected. The underlying biochemical defect is unknown. No treatment is available.

Globoid Cell Leukodystrophy (Krabbe's Disease)

This disease affects infants in the first 2 to 3 months of life, initially producing irritability and unexplained episodes of crying, sensitivity to light and noise, and failure to achieve developmental milestones. During the second year, these children become opisthotonic, developing myoclonic jerks, atypical seizures, and optic atrophy. Rare instances occur in late infancy or in adulthood.

Neuropathologic examination reveals marked loss of myelin throughout the brain with the presence of round or oval mononuclear cells the size of large glia or as large, irregular multinucleated cells. These globoid cells contain galactocerebroside (galactosyl ceramide), which accumulates in abnormal quantities. The disorder probably is transmitted as an autosomal recessive trait. No treatment is known.

Spongy Degeneration of White Matter

Many disorders can produce the pathologic changes leading to this label, including aminoacidurias and other metabolic disturbances. Instances affecting infants in whom no underlying metabolic defect is apparent are called Canavan's disease, with spastic paraplegia, severe mental retardation, optic atrophy, enlargement of the head, and death occurring by 18 months. Spongiform degeneration is also produced by exposure to large amounts of hexachlorophene in infancy and by Creutzfeldt-Jakob disease in adults (see Ch. 478.6).

Aubourg P, Blanche S, Jambaque I, et al.: Reversal of early neurologic and neuroradiologic manifestations of X-linked adrenoleukodystrophy by bone marrow transplantation. N Engl J Med 322:1860, 1990.

Krivit W, Shapiro E, Kennedy W, et al.: Treatment of late infantile metachromatic leukodystrophy by bone marrow transplantation. N Engl J Med 322:28, 1990.

Moser HW, Moser AB, Singh I, et al.: Adrenoleucodystrophy: Survey of 303 cases, biochemistry, diagnosis and therapy. Ann Neurol 16:628, 1984.

Seitelberger F: Pelizaeus-Merzbacher's disease. In Vinken P, Bruyn G (eds.): Handbook of Clinical Neurology. Vol 10. Amsterdam, North-Holland, 1970, p 150. An excellent review of this and related degenerative diseases of myelin.

THE SYNDROME OF ACUTE TRANSVERSE MYELITIS

CLINICAL DESCRIPTION. Acute transverse myelitis or myelopathy describes the rapid onset of paraparesis or paraplegia as the result of spinal cord dysfunction. The term transverse myelitis has a slightly more specific meaning, referring to acute transverse myelopathy of unknown etiology. The onset of weakness is often preceded by abrupt or rapidly developing, localized back pain or radicular pain, often in the thoracic region. This is followed by paresthesias of the toes and feet and rapidly ascending sensory loss and weakness. Urinary and fecal incontinence is common. The speed of progression varies from minutes, as with an infarction, to steady or stepwise progression over several days, as often occurs with compression due to a tumor or as a result of MS. It is often difficult to separate the patient who has developed an idiopathic transverse myelopathy from the one who has a detectable and often treatable underlying cause. Presentation of the syndrome of acute spinal cord dysfunction demands immediate and careful consideration of the differential diagnosis so as to undertake appropriate treatment if warranted.

DIFFERENTIAL DIAGNOSIS. Table 482–5 lists disorders that produce an acute or subacute transverse myelopathy with varying degrees of frequency.

Bacterial infections of the spinal cord and its surrounding spaces are considered in Ch. 471. HTLV-I myelopathy is considered in Ch. 478.3.

Viral infection of the spinal cord occurs with direct extension by the varicella (herpes) zoster or other viruses. Alternately, spinal cord inflammation and demyelination may follow a viral infection, such as measles or other common viruses, either as an isolated phenomenon or as part of the more widespread acute disseminated encephalomyelitis.

Spinal cord compression from metastatic tumor may present acutely, even though the tumor has been present for a longer time. Centrally *herniating intervertebral discs* may lead to acute cord compression with or without local pain. In each instance, myelography is usually required for diagnosis, although CT scans or MRI may be sufficient. Trauma often leads to an acute transverse myelopathy in what is usually an obvious setting.

Rapidly progressing myelopathy in a previously healthy person should always raise the question of *spontaneous epidural, subdural, or intraparenchymal bleeding*, as may occur from an arteriovenous malformation, or as a complication of anticoagulation or blood dyscrasia. CT or MR imaging visualizes the blood. Surgical decompression is often appropriate. Other vascular

TABLE 482–5. ACUTE OR SUBACUTE TRANSVERSE MYELOPATHY

Associated with infection
  Bacterial
  Spinal epidural abscess
  Intramedullary abscess
  Viral, e.g., herpes zoster
  Postviral, e.g., rubella with disseminated encephalomyelitis

Compression
  Tumor, especially metastatic
  Trauma
  Herniated intervertebral disc

Vascular
  Acute extradural, subdural, or parenchymal hemorrhage
  Dissecting aortic aneurysm
  Arteritis
  Lupus erythematosus

Idiopathic

causes of transverse myelopathy include interruption of spinal cord blood supply by dissecting aortic aneurysm or traumatic aortic rupture. Inflammatory disorders affecting blood vessels, such as disseminated lupus erythematosus or giant cell arteritis, may produce an acute myelopathy.

Subacute myelopathy is a common manifestation of MS, either as a first clinical manifestation or in a patient with previous clinical evidence of the disorder. Motor dysfunction is usually much more prominent than sensory loss, and complete cord transection syndrome only rarely occurs. When a patient with isolated transverse myelopathy has CSF oligoclonal bands, abnormal visual or brain stem auditory evoked response values, or MRI evidence of multiple lesions, one must suspect MS. However, the probability has not yet been established, and it is not appropriate to consider that combination with a single clinical event as having established the diagnosis of MS (see Table 482–2).

In many instances, no identifiable cause of acute transverse myelopathy is found even at autopsy, although some will prove to have an occult arteriovenous malformation or unsuspected MS. The degree of acute neurologic impairment among patients with the idiopathic syndrome ranges from partial to complete; the speed of onset ranges from hours to days. Patients who progress acutely to total paralysis are less likely to improve than those whose impairments develop over several days or longer. Idiopathic acute transverse myelopathy may leave a patient paraplegic regardless of treatment or may lead to complete or nearly complete recovery, probably depending on the degree of necrosis that occurs initially.

LABORATORY AIDS. An imaging procedure is essential in the evaluation of acute transverse myelopathy. Increasingly sensitive CT and MRI techniques are beginning to replace myelography. The CSF examination is usually obtained as part of or following the appropriate imaging procedure and is often essential.

PATHOLOGY. Idiopathic acute transverse myelopathy is associated with destruction of neurons, glia, and tracts at the level involved. A range of inflammatory cells have been seen acutely. Invasion by macrophages with subsequent cord atrophy and hypertrophy, and adhesion of the meninges to the spinal cord occur and sometimes lead to spinal block. The pathology of instances secondary to known causes depends on the disorder in question.

TREATMENT. Time is of the essence. Treatment may halt progression but may not restore function already lost. Diagnostic studies must be undertaken on an emergency basis, and when cord compression is present, surgical decompression and treatment with antibiotics or with corticosteroids are needed quickly. In idiopathic transverse myelopathy, MS, or cord compression, corticosteroids may reduce edema and lead to earlier restitution of function, although the effect on long-term outcome is problematic. Treatment of specific recognized etiologies is covered elsewhere. Urinary retention must be treated symptomatically with intermittent catheterization. Fecal impaction must be prevented. Patients with cervical lesions may require ventilatory assistance.

Berman M, Feldman S, Alter M, et al.: Acute transverse myelitis: Incidence and etiological considerations. Neurology 31:966, 1981. *A retrospective study of a well-defined population.*

Ropper AH, Poskanzer DC: The prognosis of acute and subacute transverse myelopathy based on early signs and symptoms. Ann Neurol 4:51, 1978. *Reviews the experience of a large general hospital with an excellent description of the clinical findings and follow-up.*

SECTION TWELVE / THE EPILEPSIES

483 The Epilepsies

Jerome Engel, Jr.

DEFINITION AND PREVALENCE. Epilepsy is the term applied to a group of disorders, sometimes called *the epilepsies,* that are characterized by the behavioral consequences of recurrent, spontaneous, transient paroxysms of abnormal brain activity. The epileptic attack or seizure, the common denominator of all of these conditions, may appear as impaired consciousness, involuntary movement, autonomic disturbance, or psychic or sensory experiences.

Epileptic disorders most commonly begin in early childhood but can appear at any time. Approximately 0.5 per cent of the United States population suffers from active seizures. It is estimated that 1 in 10 persons will experience at least one epileptic seizure during his or her lifetime. Prevalence is greater in areas of the world that have a higher incidence of brain injury due to high rates of infection, poor perinatal care, and frequent head trauma.

PATHOGENESIS. Most investigators believe that the fundamental abnormality in all epileptic conditions lies in the cerebral cortex, including the limbic cortex (hippocampus). In chronic epilepsy, the recurrent neuronal paroxysms that underlie ictal (seizure) events are transient expressions of a more permanently physiologically disordered cortex. Even though seizures themselves are intermittent, the physiologic abnormality persists throughout the interictal (between seizures) period.

An epileptogenic cortex in the interictal state is characterized by the appearance of brief, high-amplitude electrical discharges that usually can be recorded from the scalp by *electroencephalography (EEG).* The typical interictal EEG discharge consists of a sharp negative transient followed by a slower wave, referred to as a *spike-and-wave complex.* Studies in animals indicate that the EEG spike-and-wave complex reflects the summation of highly synchronized abnormal neuronal membrane potentials: large paroxysmal depolarization shifts followed by prolonged after-hyperpolarizations. The depolarization shift results in enhanced neuronal excitation, while the after-hyperpolarization represents inhibition that may prevent ictal development. These abnormal membrane events reflect inherent pathologic properties of individual epileptic neurons as well as disturbances in interconnections of neuronal aggregates. However, the fundamental mechanisms that underlie spontaneous recurrent seizures in the various forms of chronic human epilepsy remain unknown.

Whatever the precise mechanism, ictal symptoms in human seizures reflect the functions of the cortex from which they arise, and the symptoms may gradually progress as the local discharge spreads to adjacent areas. Propagation to distant brain areas can proceed along fiber tracts to produce additional symptoms. With widespread or bilateral involvement, consciousness is impaired and generalized tonic-clonic convulsions can occur. *Partial seizures* are seizures initiated in only part of the cerebral cortex. They can, but do not always, spread to involve larger areas of the brain. *Generalized seizures* are seizures that begin bilaterally from the start, presumably as a result of synchronizing afferent influences from brain stem and diencephalon acting on diffusely epileptogenic cortex or on widespread, multiple cortical epileptogenic foci. This condition has been referred to as *corticoreticular epilepsy.*

Seizures stop not merely as a result of neuronal exhaustion but also because of self-activating inhibitory mechanisms. These events can depress neuronal function after a seizure, producing prominent postictal symptoms. Generalized convulsions and partial seizures with impaired consciousness are followed by diffuse EEG suppression and periods of confusion and fatigue that can last minutes to hours. Partial seizures may also be followed by transient, localized EEG suppression and focal neurologic deficits, known as *Todd's paralysis*, that reflect postictal dysfunction of cortical structures involved in the ictal event.

ETIOLOGY. Epileptic seizures can be a natural reaction to physiologic stress or transient systemic injury *(reactive seizures)*, or they can indicate an epileptic disorder. This disorder can reflect intrinsic, nonprogressive, and presumably hereditary cerebral disturbances, with seizures as the only manifestation of abnormal brain function *(primary epilepsies)*, or can be symptomatic of some known pathologic process affecting the brain *(secondary epilepsies)* (Table 483–1). Several factors often exist in the same patient, and commonly the combination of a cerebral insult and a genetic predisposition determines the appearance of epileptic seizures. Systemic illness or trauma may uncover a latent epileptic condition.

Genetic Factors. Genetic factors may contribute to the development of epilepsy in three ways: (1) An individual may inherit a low threshold for seizures; (2) genetic traits underlie certain specific primary epileptic conditions; and (3) many inherited diseases of the brain are associated with structural disturbances that produce seizures.

A number of poorly understood genetic factors determine the susceptibility of individual brains to the development of generalized convulsions. Under certain circumstances a single isolated generalized convulsion can occur as a reaction to insults such as sleep deprivation, alcohol or sedative drug withdrawal, use of convulsant drugs, fever, and acute head trauma. Recurrent generalized convulsions may also be induced by reversible infectious, toxic, or metabolic processes and are limited to the period of systemic illness. Occurrence of such reactive seizures generally indicates an inherited lowered threshold for seizures and not a chronic epileptic condition. The most commonly encountered reactive seizures are the *benign febrile convulsions* of infancy and early childhood. Persons with lowered convulsive thresholds are also more likely to develop chronic recurrent seizures of all types if irreversible brain injury occurs for other reasons.

Inherited primary epilepsies account for 30 per cent of chronic epileptic disorders. Autosomal dominant genetic traits have been identified as the basis of characteristic EEG patterns that underlie the generalized *petit mal epilepsy* and partial *sylvian epilepsy*, but not all individuals with these EEG traits have seizures. Primary epilepsies are relatively benign, and most remit spontaneously in adolescence or early adulthood.

Secondary epilepsies are most often due to acquired factors; however, inherited neurologic diseases can also produce brain lesions that give rise to chronic recurrent epileptic seizures. These include inborn errors of metabolism, such as phenylketonuria and the lipoidoses; other degenerative diseases, not only those that affect gray matter, such as the progressive myoclonus epilepsies, but also the leukodystrophies; and syndromes such as tuberous sclerosis and neurofibromatosis that are associated with the development of cerebral ectopic or alien tissue.

Acquired Factors. Congenital lesions due to prenatal and perinatal injuries are commonly encountered in epileptic patients.

Minor focal lesions that can give rise to partial seizures include microgyria, porencephalic cysts, areas of calcification, and atrophy. More severe trauma, anoxia, and infections such as toxoplasmosis, cytomegalic inclusion disease, rubella, herpes, and syphilis also can produce diffuse cerebral damage and secondary generalized seizure disorders.

Head trauma with cicatrix formation is an important cause of epileptic seizures. Chronic recurrent seizures occur in 30 per cent of patients with acute hematomas, 15 per cent of those with depressed skull fractures, and 5 per cent of those hospitalized for severe closed head trauma. Epilepsy is rare, however, after head trauma without loss of consciousness. Seizures occurring at the time of injury (contact seizures) or within the first week thereafter do not necessarily herald development of a recurrent epileptic disorder. Chronic posttraumatic seizures usually have a delayed onset, most often beginning 6 to 12 months following injury and occasionally starting even many years later.

Infectious processes involving the brain and its coverings can produce acute and chronic seizures. As with trauma, generalized seizures during active meningitis and encephalitis may not indicate a recurrent epileptic condition. Recurrent generalized and partial seizures occur with slow virus infections and are common late sequelae when adhesions or scars result from purulent meningitis, fungal infections, or destructive viral processes such as herpes simplex encephalitis. Partial seizures may be the first sign of focal bacterial encephalitis or abscess formation, lesions especially likely to produce chronic epilepsy. Tuberculomas and parasitic infestations, particularly cysticercosis and schistosomiasis, are common causes of partial seizures in some developing countries and because of increased international travel are sometimes found outside their endemic areas.

About half of all *brain tumors* located in the anterior and middle cranial fossae produce epileptic symptoms. Partial seizures are common with *Sturge-Weber syndrome* and often result from small cryptogenic hamartomas, ectopias, and angiomas.

Cerebrovascular diseases produce seizures in many ways. Partial seizures are rare during acute strokes and usually reflect embolic events with bleeding into the cortex rather than thrombosis. Completed strokes, however, often produce scar tissue that can become epileptogenic months or years later. Such a process is presumed to be the most common cause of unexplained recurrent partial seizures in the elderly. Partial and generalized seizures are early symptoms of cerebral venous thrombosis, cerebral arteritis, and hypertensive encephalopathy (now rare). Partial seizures often occur with arteriovenous malformations (AVM's), and small cortical hemorrhages of any cause can produce refractory partial seizures or focal myoclonic jerks.

Systemic toxic and metabolic disturbances, both exogenous and endogenous, as well as *ionic imbalance*, such as hyponatremia, can cause reactive generalized convulsions, which occasionally can lead to status epilepticus with subsequent brain damage or death. Toxic or metabolic disturbances may occasionally cause partial seizures when superimposed on unsuspected focal cerebral

TABLE 483–1. CAUSES OF EPILEPSY

Type of Disorder	Genetic Factors	Acquired Factors
Reactive seizures (transient reaction to stress or insult, not epilepsy)	Lowered threshold	Physiologic stress Sleep deprivation Alcohol or sedative drug withdrawal Convulsant drugs Fever Acute head trauma Toxic, metabolic, and infectious processes
Primary epilepsy (without structural lesions, usually benign)	Genetic trait	Little or none
Secondary epilepsy (with structural lesions and associated neurologic disturbances)	Lowered threshold Inherited diseases associated with epilepsy: Inborn errors of metabolism Degenerative diseases Ectopic or alien tissue	Congenital lesion Head trauma Infections Cerebrovascular diseases Brain tumors Systemic toxic and metabolic disorder Hippocampal sclerosis Miscellaneous disorders

lesions from old head injuries. These occur most commonly in alcohol and drug abusers who are undergoing withdrawal. Hyperosmolar conditions such as nonketotic hyperglycemia and uremia may also give rise to partial seizures, presumably because of brain shrinkage that tears bridging vessels and produces small areas of hemorrhage into the cortex.

Miscellaneous disorders that can cause seizures include systemic diseases that give rise to cerebral pathology, such as the collagen vascular diseases and blood dyscrasias; and cerebral gray matter degenerative diseases, such as allergic encephalopathies and, very rarely, the presenile and senile dementias. Demyelinating diseases occasionally produce lesions adjacent to cortex that cause epileptic attacks: seizures occur in 3 per cent of patients with multiple sclerosis.

Hippocampal sclerosis, consisting of largely unilateral neuronal loss often accompanied by astrocytic proliferation in the hippocampus and adjacent limbic structures, is found in over half the patients who have undergone temporal lobe resection for complex partial seizures. This may be the most common pathologic finding in epilepsy and, in some cases, could be both the cause and the result of seizures. Prolonged convulsive seizures are known to produce cell loss in the hippocampus, the neocortex, and the cerebellum. Some authorities believe that prolonged convulsions (lasting more than 30 minutes), such as those that occasionally accompany fever in infancy or childhood exanthems, can produce mesial temporal sclerosis and that this lesion becomes epileptogenic later in life. In any event, this form of epileptic brain damage suggests that in some situations epilepsy itself becomes a cause of progressive symptoms. For this reason, convulsive seizures should be controlled as promptly as possible.

CLINICAL MANIFESTATIONS AND CLASSIFICATION. Classification of *epileptic seizures* is based on their clinical manifestations (Table 483–2). Partial seizures are more likely than generalized seizures to be associated with a localized cerebral lesion that could represent a curable cause of epilepsy. When a treatable underlying cause is not present, the choice of antiepileptic drugs is usually determined by the seizure type. Specific *epileptic syndromes* have also been defined on the basis of seizure manifestations and other clinical features (Table 483–3). Although the pathophysiologic mechanisms are unknown for most, diagnosis of an epileptic syndrome usually has important therapeutic and prognostic implications.

Partial Seizures. Although the expression of partial seizures depends on the areas of cerebral cortex that are involved, the precise anatomic origin of specific seizures cannot always be accurately inferred from ictal symptoms, since functional localization within the brain remains inexact. Moreover, epileptic

TABLE 483–2. CLASSIFICATION OF EPILEPTIC SEIZURES*

Partial seizures (focal, local)
  Simple partial seizures
    With motor signs
    With somatosensory or special sensory symptoms
    With autonomic symptoms or signs
    With psychic symptoms
  Complex partial seizures
    Simple partial onset followed by impairment of consciousness
    With impairment of consciousness at onset
  Partial seizures evolving to generalized tonic-clonic convulsions
    (secondarily generalized)

Generalized seizures (convulsive or nonconvulsive)
  Nonconvulsive seizures
    Absence seizures
    Atypical absence seizures
    Myoclonic seizures
    Atonic seizures
  Convulsive seizures
    Tonic-clonic seizures
    Tonic seizures
    Clonic seizures

Unclassified epileptic seizures

*Modified from Commission on Classification and Terminology of the International League Against Epilepsy: Epilepsia 22:489, 1981.

TABLE 483–3. SOME DISTINCTIVE EPILEPTIC SYNDROMES

Type of Disorder	Partial	Generalized
Reactive seizures		Febrile convulsions
Primary epilepsy	Sylvian epilepsy	Petit mal epilepsies
		Juvenile myoclonic epilepsy
Secondary epilepsy	Temporal lobe epilepsy	Lennox-Gastaut syndrome
	Epilepsia partialis continua	Progressive myoclonus epilepsies
		West's syndrome

manifestations may reflect dysfunction produced by propagation away from the primary focus as much as or more than from the area where the lesion lies.

Partial seizures are classified as simple when consciousness is preserved. *Simple partial seizures* reflect an ictal discharge that is localized within one hemisphere and can take many forms (Table 483–4).

Motor symptoms begin with clonic or tonic movements of a discrete body part. Areas of the body with large representation in the motor cortex, such as the face and hand, are involved most frequently. When spread occurs in an orderly fashion along the precentral gyrus, clonic motor symptoms can progress (e.g., from thumb or face), which is termed a *jacksonian march*. More commonly, however, ictal discharges in frontal cortex activate multiple muscle groups to produce complex versive movements, such as turning of the head, eyes, or body to one side and posturing with one or more extremities. Other simple motor manifestations include speech arrest or vocalizations when language areas are involved; eye or lid twitching, which is most often initiated from the frontal or occipital cortex; and inappropriate laughter unassociated with humor (*gelastic epilepsy*). Simple partial clonic or tonic motor seizures can be followed by a transient *Todd's paralysis* of involved muscles, which rarely persists longer than 48 hours.

Sensory symptoms occur with lesions in or connected to primary sensory cortex. Thus, localized paresthesias or numbness, unformed luminous visions, unpleasant olfactory and gustatory sensations, vertigo, and sounds can result from lesions of appropriate cortical areas. Postictal negative sensory phenomena, such as blindness and anesthesia, may occasionally occur.

Autonomic symptoms often are due to ictal involvement of limbic structures in the mesial temporal and frontal lobes that project to the hypothalamus and brain stem. They commonly consist of feelings of epigastric rising or distress, nausea, or vague light-headedness. In other autonomic seizures, ictal signs and symptoms such as pallor, flushing, sweating, piloerection, pupillary dilatation, cardiac arrhythmia, and incontinence may be apparent.

TABLE 483–4. SIGNS AND SYMPTOMS OF SIMPLE PARTIAL SEIZURES

Motor
  Focal without march
  Focal with march (jacksonian)
  Versive
  Postural
  Phonatory

Sensory
  Somatosensory
  Special sensory (visual, auditory, olfactory, gustatory, vertiginous)

Autonomic
  Any autonomic sign or symptom

Psychic
  Dysphasic
  Dysmnesic (e.g., déjà vu)
  Cognitive (e.g., dreamy state)
  Affective (e.g., fear, anger)
  Illusions
  Structured delusions

Psychic symptoms can accompany ictal discharges in limbic and association cortex and can mimic features of psychiatric disorders. These include dysmnesic symptoms, such as feelings of familiarity (déjà vu) and unfamiliarity (jamais vu) and forced thinking; cognitive disturbances, such as dreamy states, depersonalization, and time distortion; affective symptoms, such as fear and rage, which often are associated with appropriate autonomic changes, depression, and, on rare occasions, elation; illusions, such as multiple images (polyopsia) or distortions of size (micropsia and macropsia); and hallucinations consisting of stereotyped mixed sensory experiences, such as visions of well-formed, recognizable faces or specific scenes accompanied by voices that can be understood, familiar smells, and emotional responses. Persistent psychic symptoms in epileptic patients may also be postictal.

Simple partial seizures are usually brief and do not interfere with daily living unless they occur frequently or evolve into other types of attacks. Simple partial seizures without obvious motor manifestations may be referred to as *auras* when the patient perceives them as a warning of impending, more noticeable epileptic symptoms. Patients who complain only of simple partial seizures may report having many seizures a week or many a day, with each lasting a few seconds.

Partial seizures are classified as complex when they impair consciousness. Approximately 40 per cent of patients with epilepsy experience *complex partial seizures* with impaired consciousness ranging from amnesia for the ictal event to behavioral unresponsiveness. Complex partial seizures usually reflect bilateral ictal involvement of limbic structures, particularly the hippocampus, amygdala, and their connections. The seizure may begin with impaired consciousness from the start or evolve from a simple partial event (aura). Because complex partial seizures most often originate in mesial temporal limbic areas, autonomic auras are common. Complex partial seizures preceded by olfactory auras are called *uncinate fits*. Such attacks may be more consistently associated with brain tumors than are other types of seizures.

The term complex partial seizure is not synonymous with *temporal lobe, psychomotor,* and *limbic seizures.* These latter designations have more specific anatomic implications and may involve ictal symptoms resulting from unilateral activation of mesial temporal limbic structures without impaired consciousness. Some atypical complex partial seizures, on the other hand, may not reflect primary activation of the limbic system. The typical complex partial seizure (temporal lobe or psychomotor attack) begins with a stare at the time consciousness is impaired and purposeless movements called *automatisms*. Oroalimentary automatisms, such as chewing, swallowing, sucking, and lip smacking, are most common and presumably reflect amygdala involvement. Other examples of automatisms include verbal utterances of sounds or words; gestural movements, such as fumbling, posturing, and picking at clothing; expressions of emotion; and ambulation. Ongoing activities such as washing dishes or even driving a car may continue automatically. Patients may undress, run, respond to commands, and demonstrate a variety of complicated automatisms that indicate a residual ability to relate to the environment despite the ictal state. In some types of complex partial seizures, patients can display irregular thrashing movements of the extremities, scream, fall, or exhibit bizarre behavior that can be difficult to differentiate from hysteria.

Complex partial seizures usually last from a few seconds to a few minutes and are followed by confusion as well as amnesia for the ictal event, although most patients remember an aura. Postictal anterograde amnesia and automatisms are common, and aphasia often occurs when seizures begin in the dominant hemisphere. In cases of unusually prolonged or recurrent complex partial seizures, postictal anterograde memory disturbance can persist for hours or days.

Complex partial seizures and postictal symptoms can severely disrupt daily life. While it is not uncommon for patients to have many complex partial seizures a week and several auras a day, even one or two seizures a year may prevent them from driving a car or destroy a chosen career.

Both simple and complex partial seizures can evolve into *secondarily generalized tonic-clonic convulsions.* Most patients with partial seizures experience at least some secondarily generalized seizures, but generalization usually occurs infrequently and is more easily controlled by drugs than are partial ictal symptoms. Some patients, particularly those with lesions in the frontal lobes, have partial seizures that always generalize secondarily. When such secondarily generalized partial seizures begin in a silent area of the brain, their partial origin may be overlooked by both the patient and observers. When neither ictal symptoms nor signs provide a clue that a seizure is secondarily generalized, postictal focal or lateralizing signs and symptoms, such as reflex asymmetry, focal weakness, or aphasia, may indicate a partial seizure disorder. Differentiation from true generalized convulsions in these cases helps to identify potentially progressive or treatable focal lesions.

Partial Syndromes. *Sylvian* or *rolandic epilepsy* (benign partial epilepsy of childhood with centrotemporal spikes) is a familial disorder that can afflict as many as 20 per cent of children with seizures. It is characterized by nocturnal generalized convulsions and simple partial seizures that occur during the day. Typically, the partial seizures begin with perioral or lingual paresthesias, although other sensory or motor symptoms may occur, especially involving the face. The EEG demonstrates centrotemporal interictal spikes that may be unilateral or bilaterally independent. Associated neurologic deficits are lacking, and the seizures respond well to medication. The disorder almost always disappears during adolescence.

Temporal lobe (psychomotor, limbic) epilepsy is the most common chronic epileptic syndrome and may account for 40 per cent of adult epilepsies. The underlying lesion characteristically involves mesial temporal limbic structures and is most often hippocampal sclerosis. The syndrome can also be caused by lesions elsewhere that produce ictal discharges that preferentially propagate to mesial temporal structures. Patients experience auras and typical complex partial seizures, as described earlier. They may also have memory deficits and psychiatric symptoms and usually exhibit unilateral or independent bilateral anterior temporal EEG spikes. Seizures in this disorder can be difficult to control medically but may be abolished by surgical resection.

Continuous partial epilepsy (epilepsia partialis continua) also is often unresponsive to medication. This disorder occurs in adults after severe cerebral injury, such as anoxia or stroke, and occasionally with brain tumors. It can also begin in young children with a rare unilateral chronic cerebral inflammatory disorder of unknown cause (*Rasmussen's syndrome*). The continuous focal motor seizures usually reflect widespread or multiple rather than single lesions that usually are not amenable to localized surgical resection. Seizures can be abolished by large resections, such as hemispherectomy, and this procedure may be indicated in some children who already have hemiatrophy and hemiparesis.

Generalized Seizures. *Absences* are brief losses of consciousness that can be of two types. Both begin almost exclusively in childhood and take the form of a blank stare, which can also be associated with mild clonic movements of eyelids and face, more generalized jerks, alterations in motor tone, and simple automatisms. *Petit mal absences* affect about 10 per cent of epileptic children, last less than 10 seconds, and begin and end abruptly without preictal or postictal EEG or clinical disturbances. *Atypical absences* also occur in about 10 per cent of epileptic children, can last longer than 10 seconds, and produce some degree of postictal confusion. Petit mal and atypical absences must not be confused with each other or with complex partial seizures consisting only of brief lapses of consciousness, since cause, prognosis, and treatment differ for the three seizure types.

Absences can occur spontaneously hundreds of times a day. Petit mal absences respond well to appropriate medications, tend to disappear during adolescence, and are rarely disabling. Atypical absences may be refractory to therapy and can disrupt normal function. Children with atypical absences, however, are usually hampered more by other seizures and by neurologic and mental deficits.

Myoclonic seizures are single, rapidly recurrent, bilaterally synchronous shock-like jerks of the face, trunk, and extremities that are not associated with loss of consciousness. In most patients with myoclonic seizures, these events cluster shortly after waking or when falling asleep. A single myoclonic jerk that occurs while a person is falling asleep, however, is a normal physiologic event. A prolonged attack can terminate in a generalized tonic-clonic convulsion. Myoclonic seizures occur in certain rare benign genetic epileptic disorders of the primary generalized type, such as *juvenile myoclonic epilepsy (impulsive petit mal)*, and respond well to drug therapy.

In contrast to myoclonic seizures, there are many other types of myoclonic jerks that are not generalized and should not be considered epileptic. These include the following: asymmetric or sporadic jerks (involving first one area of the body and then another) that are spontaneous or induced by movement or sensory stimulation and that result from anoxic, toxic, and metabolic disturbances; similar events associated with the *progressive myoclonus epilepsies*, due to lesions of the diencephalon, brain stem, and cerebellar nuclei; regular rhythmic *palatal myoclonus* and *segmental myoclonus* that are caused, respectively, by medullary and spinal cord lesions; and *benign familial (essential) myoclonus* of unknown origin.

Tonic-clonic (grand mal) convulsions occur at least once in 80 per cent of epileptic patients and can be the expression of reactive seizures, partial seizures that secondarily generalize, or a generalized epileptic disorder. Convulsions that are not secondarily generalized from partial seizures never have auras, although patients may occasionally recognize nonspecific affective changes or experience a flurry of bilaterally synchronous myoclonic jerks some hours before a seizure occurs. The typical generalized convulsion begins with a sudden cry accompanied by loss of consciousness, falling, and bilateral tonic extensor rigidity of the trunk and extremities. After several seconds of rigidity, recurrent synchronous clonic muscular contractions ensue for 1 or 2 minutes, until the seizure ends, leaving the patient flaccid and unconscious. Cyanosis results from breath-holding during the tonic phase, and autonomic hyperactivity is prominent. The blood pressure increases abruptly, the body temperature rises, and patients salivate and may have urinary and fecal incontinence. Often they bite their tongue and the inside of their mouth. Occasionally, generalized convulsive attacks consist of either tonic or clonic activity alone.

Postictal depression can last many minutes, occasionally hours, and rarely a day or more. During this period, patients gradually regain consciousness but feel exhausted, frequently complain of headache, and wish to sleep. A few remain disoriented for some time. Focal or lateralized postictal symptoms do not occur following true generalized tonic-clonic convulsions.

Grand mal convulsions rarely occur more than a few times a year in primary generalized epileptic disorders but can occur daily in severe secondary generalized disorders. In both situations, however, the attacks tend to respond well to antiepileptic drugs.

Atonic seizures (drop attacks) begin almost exclusively in childhood and usually reflect diffuse lesions of the brain. The ictal episode consists of a sudden, extremely brief loss of tone. In its simplest form, the child's head drops for a second or less. More severe forms cause tone to disappear in the entire body, leading to collapse, sometimes with serious injuries, such as concussion, broken bones, and lost teeth. Atonic seizures occur many times a day and are refractory to drug therapy but do respond to corpus callosotomy; they can be the most debilitating ictal manifestation of secondary generalized epilepsies. Brief *tonic seizures* and myoclonic jerks also cause drop attacks in this patient population.

Generalized Syndromes. One or more *febrile convulsions* occur in 3 to 4 per cent of otherwise healthy children between the ages of 6 months and 5 years and consist of brief tonic-clonic reactive generalized seizures. Although febrile convulsions can be recurrent, the syndrome is benign. It is not considered an epileptic disorder, and treatment is usually not necessary. A genetic basis is certain but poorly defined. Affected children outgrow their vulnerability between 3 and 5 years of age, although 5 per cent develop seizures without fever later. Features that would discount the diagnosis of benign febrile convulsions are the following: seizures lasting longer than 10 minutes, focal abnormalities during or after the seizure, or an abnormal neurologic or mental status examination result. In such instances, an underlying neurologic disorder is likely and treatment is required.

The *petit mal epilepsies* are inherited conditions that account for 10 per cent of childhood epilepsies. Several varieties are recognized, depending on the age of onset, frequency of EEG spike-and-wave discharges, and occurrence of myoclonic seizures. Infrequent grand mal seizures can occur in all forms, or they may occur alone. They are characterized by frequent petit mal absences in an otherwise neurologically normal child. Response to appropriate medication is usually excellent, especially when onset is in early childhood. These disorders often remit in adolescence; juvenile-onset or myoclonic seizures tend to worsen the prognosis.

Juvenile myoclonic epilepsy is another common inherited epileptic condition. It begins in middle to late childhood with bilaterally synchronous myoclonic seizures. The paroxysms can be completely controlled with appropriate medication, and there are no other associated disturbances. The condition should not be confused with the myoclonic disorders characterized by sporadic, often stimulus-sensitive, myoclonic jerks, such as postanoxic myoclonus and the progressive myoclonus epilepsies. These last-mentioned sporadic myoclonic events are not epileptic, are extremely difficult to treat, and are usually associated with other evidence of diffuse cerebral injury.

The *Lennox-Gastaut syndrome* describes a nonspecific epileptic condition of children suffering from diffuse or multiple lesions of the brain. Although patients with the Lennox-Gastaut syndrome can have absences, convulsions, and myoclonic jerks identical to the primary generalized type, usually they also have or develop additional neurologic impairment, mental subnormality, and multiple seizure types, including drop attacks. Seizures associated with the Lennox-Gastaut syndrome and other secondary generalized epileptic disorders are difficult to control. The patients often are severely handicapped by the frequent attacks as well as other static or progressive interictal neurologic deficits.

The *progressive myoclonus epilepsies* constitute a group of familial cerebral degenerative disorders that affect both cortical and subcortical gray matter, leading to progressive neurologic deficits, dementia, sporadic multifocal myoclonic jerks, and secondary tonic-clonic convulsions. Whereas the epileptic seizures respond well to medication, patients are severely disabled by the nonepileptic sporadic myoclonus and other handicaps. The course may be rapid, with severe neurologic and mental impairment (*Lafora type*); intermediate (*Unverricht-Lundborg type*); or relatively slow, with little mental impairment or EEG disturbance (*Ramsay Hunt syndrome*, which is associated with cerebellar disturbances and may be considered a separate entity). A benign familial myoclonic syndrome (*essential myoclonus*) without epileptic seizures has an excellent prognosis and responds readily to treatment.

Unclassified Seizures. Certain *neonatal seizures* and *infantile spasms* (seen in *West's syndrome*) reflect severe diffuse disturbances of brain function from a variety of causes. These events are age dependent and have not been adequately classified as epilepsy, and some may be of subcortical origin. It is important to note here only that the underlying cerebral dysfunction often results in chronic secondary epileptic conditions later in life, usually the *Lennox-Gastaut syndrome*.

Patterns of Seizure Occurrence. Appreciation for precipitating factors and temporal patterns of certain epileptic seizures can influence approaches to management. In some of the primary generalized epileptic disorders, seizures may be induced by specific sensory stimuli, most commonly flashing light (*photosensitive epilepsy*). Reading, video games, music, and other specific complex stimuli may activate seizures in patients with rarer forms of primary and secondary *reflex epilepsy*. The seizures themselves range from brief absences through synchronous myoclonic jerking to partial seizures and occasional generalized convulsions. *Hyperventilation* is a potent activator of petit mal absence seizures and sometimes will precipitate other types of ictal events as well. Emotional stress, drowsiness, sleep deprivation, and withdrawal from alcohol and sedative drugs are well-established precipitants of partial and generalized convulsive seizures in patients with chronic epilepsy. Some patients have seizures that occur only at night or only during the day. Others exhibit regular cycles of seizures over days or months or patterns of seizure clusters followed by prolonged seizure-free periods. The term *catamenial epilepsy* is used when seizures regularly recur in women around the menstrual period. Women with all forms of epileptic disorders commonly experience more frequent seizures at this time of the month, and seizures may worsen or disappear during pregnancy. *Status epilepticus* refers to a condition of rapidly recurrent epileptic seizures or continuous ictal symptoms. The latter occur with continuous partial epilepsy and also in a form of *absence status (spike wave stupor)*, which is discussed further on. Of the rapidly recurrent forms, generalized convulsive status epilepticus is a life-threatening situation demanding immediate treatment, and complex partial status epilepticus requires prompt intervention.

Complex partial status epilepticus is a rare condition of rapidly recurring seizures characterized by a fluctuating level of consciousness, automatic behavior, and ictal EEG discharges recorded over the temporal lobe. The condition may be confused clinically with a psychosis or metabolic disturbance and must be included in the differential diagnosis of altered states of consciousness; failure to treat it promptly can be followed by prolonged memory deficits.

Absence status, or *spike wave stupor*, consists of a continuous state of dulled mentation, which is often of a subtle nature. Eye blinking and other associated movements can occur, and there is a characteristic EEG pattern of diffuse spike-and-wave discharges. The condition occurs fairly often in patients with atypical absences and is also seen with a juvenile form of primary generalized petit mal epilepsy. A rare type of absence status of unknown cause also affects older adults with no previous history of epilepsy. Absence status is not a medical emergency, since no secondary brain damage occurs. The benign and adult forms respond well to antiepileptic drugs, but atypical absence status associated with diffuse lesions of the brain may be extremely difficult to control.

Major motor status epilepticus exists when generalized tonic-clonic convulsions recur so frequently that consciousness is not regained between them. This condition can occur with the generalized disorders but is more commonly a result of partial seizures that secondarily generalize. In the latter instance, the partial onset often is not recognized because of the severity of the attacks. Toxic and metabolic disturbances, including drug and alcohol withdrawal, can precipitate major motor status epilepticus in epileptic patients as well as in nonepileptic individuals with genetically low seizure thresholds. Major motor status epilepticus can also be a presenting symptom of acute intracranial hemorrhage and infections, as well as brain tumors and other focal processes, especially in the frontal lobes. Major motor status epilepticus is a life-threatening situation demanding immediate treatment.

DIAGNOSIS. Diagnosis in epilepsy involves searching for treatable causes when possible and recognizing epileptic conditions that indicate a specific prognosis and therapy. When a treatable cause of epilepsy is not revealed, management of the seizures is determined by correct diagnosis of the type of epileptic disorder.

History. The history is overwhelmingly important. The patient's description of any auras should be recorded as well as the ictal behavioral changes observed by others. The occurrence of an aura or any focal signs at onset, during progression, or in the postictal period indicates a partial rather than a generalized seizure disorder. If more than one type of seizure occurs, each should be described separately. Often patients will report several seizure types, which after careful questioning are revealed to be variations of the same ictal phenomenon and not evidence of multiple lesions. For instance, when auras are not followed by further symptoms, they may be recognized as one event, while the same aura that spreads to become a complex partial seizure may be reported as another phenomenon. If on occasion there is evolution to a secondarily generalized seizure without postictal recall of the aura, a careful description of the initial ictal events by an observer will often verify that the generalized convulsion is a manifestation of the same epileptogenic lesion. When patients report only seizures that are generalized from the start, an attempt should be made to determine whether convulsive and nonconvulsive ictal manifestations resemble those of benign genetic disorders, generalized disorders caused by diffuse or multiple brain lesions, or secondarily generalized partial seizures caused by a focal lesion. Clues to differential diagnosis derive from the circumstances and age of the patient at onset of seizures and how they may have changed with time or treatment. If the patient has been treated previously, it is important to know what drugs have been used and the specifics of their therapeutic and toxic effects.

The history can provide crucial etiologic information. In chil-

dren, patterns of early development may delineate the difference between a progressive degenerative disorder and a static lesion. There may be evidence of specific predisposing factors, such as perinatal injury, intracranial infections, or reactions to immunizations. A history of a prolonged childhood convulsion preceding the onset of complex partial seizures raises the possibility that hippocampal sclerosis is the cause of the subsequent chronic epileptic disorder. In older patients there may be hints of cerebrovascular disease or metastatic cancer. Prior head trauma is usually relevant only if it resulted in loss of consciousness. A specific injurious event, such as a fall, may be mistakenly interpreted as having generated traumatic epilepsy when it actually represented the first seizure.

The family history can reveal important genetic factors. The existence of relatives with similar seizures or other neurologic symptoms suggests a specific primary epileptic disorder. A family history of individuals with isolated seizures or varied epileptic conditions may indicate the inheritance of a lowered threshold for seizures.

The psychosocial history can give important clues to diagnosis and indicate the need for more specific evaluations. Patients with benign inherited epileptic disorders usually have normal school and work histories and no evidence of mental disturbance. A history of specific cognitive deficits suggests a focal lesion, while more generalized mental impairment suggests a diffuse abnormality. When the latter is progressive, more detailed laboratory, EEG, and psychometric examinations can determine whether the patient has an underlying degenerative disease, increasing dysfunction because of recurrent seizures, or toxic symptoms of overmedication.

Physical Examination. A careful physical examination can reveal evidence of systemic diseases responsible for seizures as well as stigmata of tuberous sclerosis, neurofibromatosis, hemangiomas, and other predisposing congenital disorders. Asymmetry (hemiatrophy) in the size of hands, feet, and face may indicate a longstanding abnormality in one cerebral hemisphere. Clumsiness, posturing, and hyperreflexia or a more marked diffuse impairment suggests a secondary rather than a primary generalized seizure disorder. Focal neurologic and mental status disturbances support a diagnosis of partial epilepsy. Poor attention span in patients on drug therapy may indicate side effects of medication rather than structural lesions. Increasing degrees of fixed neurologic and mental impairment confer a poor prognosis for both seizure control and psychosocial adaptation.

Many patients can be observed during a seizure. Status epilepticus usually lasts until hospitalization, absences can be provoked by hyperventilation, reflex seizures are easily induced (it is unwise to attempt to induce tonic-clonic convulsions), and spontaneous seizures may occur in the examining room. The initial manifestations and early development should be noted. Consciousness should be assessed by repeating a phrase to determine whether the patient can recall it after the seizure is over. Even if the seizure appears to be generalized at the start, postictal examination of neurologic and mental status may reveal focal deficits that indicate that a partial seizure has occurred.

Laboratory Studies. Epilepsy provides no diagnostic hematologic or chemical laboratory tracers, but such tests can help to diagnose underlying disease processes that give rise to seizures. One or more generalized epileptic attacks can mildly increase protein content and white cell count in the cerebrospinal fluid for 24 to 48 hours. Although up to 100 white cells per cubic millimeter have been reported after major motor status epilepticus, a lumbar puncture revealing more than 10 white cells per cubic millimeter should initiate a search for an intracranial inflammatory process. Complete blood count, liver function tests, blood urea nitrogen, and urinalysis are necessary in all patients about to begin antiepileptic drug therapy to establish a baseline for evaluating possible subsequent toxic side effects.

Structural Imaging. Magnetic resonance imaging (MRI) is preferred to x-ray computed tomography (XCT) unless a disorder associated with small calcified lesions is suspected. Structural imaging is necessary for adolescents and adults with the recent onset of seizures but may be avoided in younger children when history and other examinations indicate a primary generalized disorder or a nonprogressive lesion. Cerebral angiography should

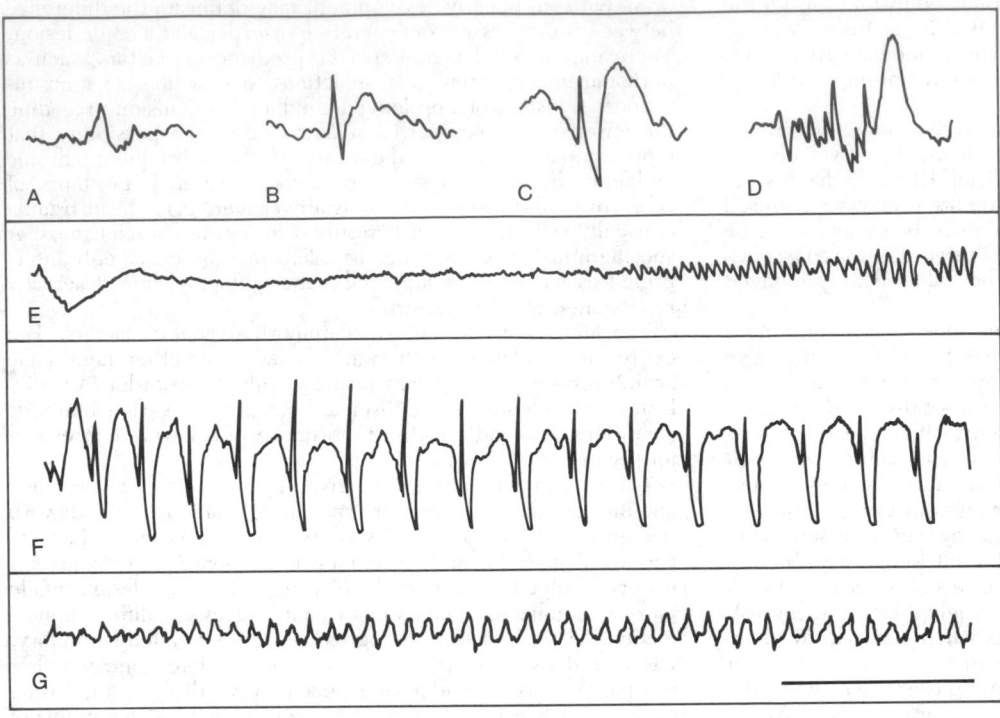

FIGURE 483–1. Examples illustrate waveforms of typical interictal electroencephalographic (EEG) transients and ictal EEG discharges. *A,* Interictal sharp wave. *B, C,* Interictal spike-and-wave complexes. *D,* Interictal poly-spike-and-wave complex. *E,* Recruiting rhythm typical of generalized convulsion onsets. *F,* Repetitive spike-and-wave discharges typical of absence seizures. *G,* Rhythmic pattern seen with temporal lobe seizures. Line at the bottom right of the figure represents 1 second.

be confined to cases in which surgery is considered or a primary vascular disorder is suspected.

Psychometric Studies. Psychometric testing, including standard tests of attention, performance and verbal IQ, memory, language, and personality, can help verify the existence of a focal or diffuse brain disturbance. When there is concern that mental function is changing, serial testing can document the effects of disease or therapy. An astute psychometrician should also be able to offer advice for improving psychosocial adaptation.

Electroencephalography. The EEG is the most useful diagnostic laboratory test for epilepsy. However, overinterpretation of the EEG often generates an unwarranted diagnosis of epilepsy. A number of spike-like EEG events can be normal, and 2 per cent of the nonepileptic population may have abnormal, epileptiform spike-and-wave complexes on their EEG's but never develop seizures. Conversely, 20 per cent of patients with epilepsy do not demonstrate epileptic abnormalities on a routine interictal EEG. Whereas an EEG can help verify a clinical diagnosis of epilepsy, interictal epileptiform EEG abnormalities alone should be considered neither necessary nor sufficient information for arriving at this diagnosis. If a seizure occurs in the EEG laboratory, the association of an ictal EEG pattern with observed clinical behavior makes possible a definitive diagnosis.

The pattern of interictal EEG abnormalities may help determine the type of epileptic disorder (Figs. 483–1 and 483–2). Focal spike-and-wave discharges or slow waves indicate a partial

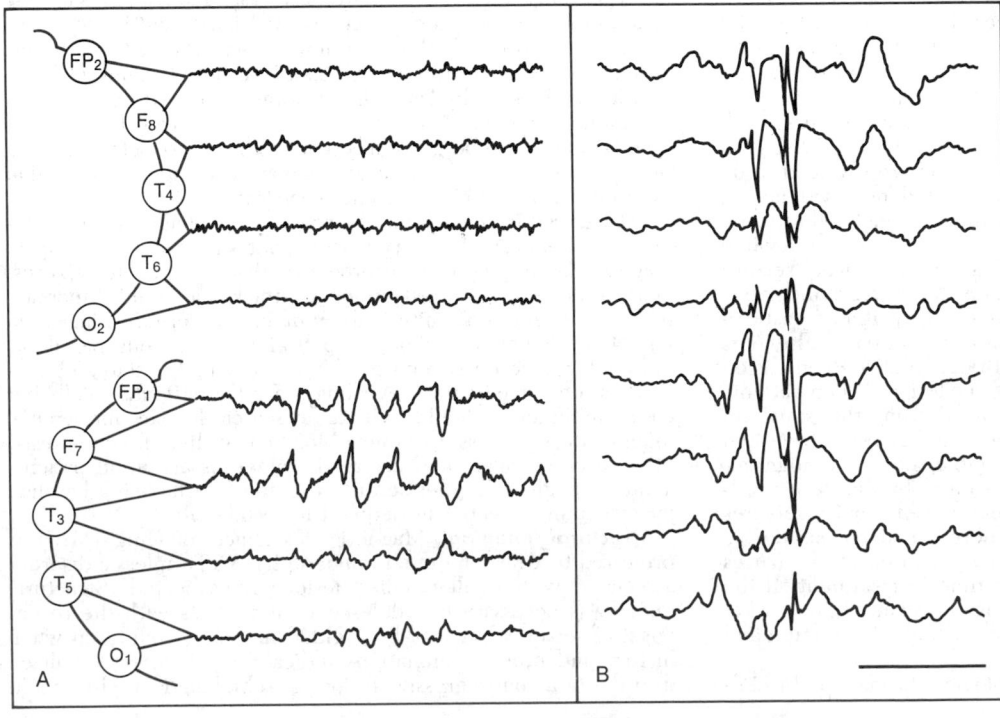

FIGURE 483–2. Examples illustrate the spatial distribution of typical focal (*A*) and generalized (*B*) epileptiform EEG discharges. *A,* Left anterior temporal spikes, sharp waves, and slowing. *B,* Generalized, frontally predominant, spike-and-wave burst. Line at the bottom right of the figure represents 1 second.

epileptic disorder. A diagnosis of benign sylvian epilepsy can be confirmed by the occurrence of characteristic centrotemporal spikes. While bilaterally synchronous EEG discharges can be seen with focal lesions (*secondary bilateral synchrony*), especially in the frontal lobes, such activity more often indicates a generalized epileptic disorder. Baseline nonepileptiform EEG abnormalities suggest a secondary epileptic disorder, although antiepileptic drugs can produce mild, diffuse EEG slowing.

Typical petit mal absences are associated with symmetric, synchronous, and regular *three-per-second* (or faster) *spike-and-wave* discharges that begin and end abruptly without postictal EEG changes. This EEG pattern is usually easily distinguished from the *slow and irregular spike-and-wave* discharges (2.5 per second or less) seen in the Lennox-Gastaut syndrome.

Activation procedures used in the EEG laboratory include hyperventilation for absences, photic stimulation for photosensitive epilepsy, and sleep. But there are major pitfalls: Hyperventilation in children and some normal adults can induce high-amplitude slowing resembling spike-and-wave discharges; photomyogenic responses of facial muscles to photic stimulation can occur in normal individuals and during drug and alcohol withdrawal and should not be considered evidence of epilepsy; a number of normal sharp transients that occur during sleep and on arousal often are misinterpreted as epileptic spikes.

Nonstandard techniques, available in some laboratories, may offer additional diagnostic advantages. Recordings from sphenoidal electrodes can clarify interictal EEG spike patterns originating in mesial temporal structures, but the same information often can be obtained more easily from ear lobe or lower temporal scalp electrodes. Special epilepsy centers throughout the country offer prolonged EEG telemetry and television monitoring to provide a precise electroclinical description of habitual seizures when diagnosis is in doubt. Ambulatory EEG monitoring is also useful, particularly to quantify ictal events that have already been characterized.

A repeat EEG may be indicated to determine whether behavioral deterioration is due to an increase in subclinical seizure activity, an increase in drug side effects, or a progressive underlying lesion. If necessary, long-term EEG recordings combined with frequent antiepileptic drug level determinations can improve medical management by allowing dose schedules to be tailored to individual patients' needs.

DIFFERENTIAL DIAGNOSIS. The diagnosis of epilepsy should be made only on firm clinical evidence. Such a diagnosis can have irreversible psychosocial effects resulting in the loss of a driver's license, a job, independence, and self-esteem. Consequently, a physician often does more harm by making an unjustified diagnosis than by reserving judgment until the nature of the disorder has declared itself adequately. When doubt exists, injury can be minimized by warning the patient to avoid the conditions that might have precipitated the event and to be aware of potentially dangerous situations, should another event occur. Systemic, neurologic, and behavioral disturbances can give rise to episodic events that might be mistaken for epileptic seizures (Table 483–5).

Systemic Disturbances. *Syncope* is the most common systemic disturbance confused with epilepsy (Ch. 443). Syncope can be associated with convulsive movements in susceptible individuals (*convulsive syncope*) but should still be treated as syncope, not as epilepsy. Because cardiac syncope can cause a convulsion, while seizures may be associated with cardiac arrhythmias, diagnostic monitoring in at-risk patients with blackout spells should ideally include both electrocardiographic (ECG) and EEG recordings.

Neurologic Disturbances. Transient ischemic attacks must be considered when intermittent neurologic symptoms occur in older patients. Prodromal migraine symptoms, particularly with basilar migraine, can resemble symptoms of epileptic seizures, and the distinction between migraine and epilepsy is not always completely clear. All-night polysomnography may be necessary to distinguish dyssomnias from nocturnal epileptic events. Although some forms of paroxysmal dyskinesia can be successfully treated with antiepileptic medication, they are not epileptic disorders.

Behavioral Disturbances. *Psychogenic seizures* (sometimes referred to as *pseudoseizures*) may be manifested in ways that have psychological significance. They may consist of pelvic thrusting and alternate thrashing of the limbs or may involve motor

symptoms that do not fit with known anatomic spread patterns but they only rarely result in injury to the patient, despite risk. Nevertheless, it is usually impossible to make this diagnosis definitively from a description or even from observation of the seizure. Virtually any paroxysmal behavior, no matter how bizarre, could be an epileptic event. The diagnosis of psychogenic seizures can be made with some confidence, however, when ictal events are suggestive for the reasons just stated, EEG recordings are normal, antiepileptic medication is ineffective, and evidence of secondary gain is obtained during psychiatric interview. EEG telemetry and video monitoring of ictal events can help in this differential diagnosis. Clear EEG changes or an elevated postictal serum prolactin level can confirm the occurrence of an epileptic convulsion, but their absence does not necessarily rule out this possibility; simple partial ictal events usually have no EEG correlates that can be recorded from the scalp and only rarely elevate the serum prolactin level. Repeated bilaterally synchronous myoclonic jerks unassociated with loss of consciousness can be mistaken for psychogenic events. Even if a definite diagnosis of a psychogenic seizure disorder can be made, many such patients have epileptic seizures as well. When psychogenic seizures and epileptic seizures coexist, EEG and video monitoring can help to differentiate the two types and provide a basis for independently assessing the results of psychiatric and medical treatment.

Episodic dyscontrol is a poorly defined entity consisting of intermittent periods of inappropriately violent, occasionally destructive behavior. Confusion with epilepsy is compounded by the fact that some patients with this syndrome have epileptic seizures as well. If the episodic behavior lasts only several minutes, is uncharacteristic of the patient's interictal personality, and there is amnesia for the event with appropriate remorse afterward, this could conceivably reflect an epileptic disturbance. Although ictal EEG recordings have not supported this contention, an occasional patient with episodic dyscontrol may be helped by antiepileptic medication. Organized and directed violence is not seen during the epileptic seizures described earlier, and epilepsy is never the cause of premeditated criminal acts.

TABLE 483–5. NONEPILEPTIC EPISODIC DISORDERS

Systemic
Syncope
Breath-holding spells
Hyperventilation syndrome
Alcoholic blackouts
Intermittent porphyria
Hypoglycemia
Pheochromocytoma
Tetanus
Psychomimetic drugs

Neurologic
Trasient ischemic attacks
Vertebral basilar insufficiency
Transient global amnesia
Migraine
Narcolepsy
Hypersomnia (e.g., Kleine-Levin syndrome, sleep apnea)
Dyssomnias (e.g., sleep walking, bed wetting, night terrors)
Paroxysmal vertigo
Trigeminal neuralgia
Gilles de la Tourette's syndrome
Extrapyramidal disorders (e.g., hemiballism, chorea, athetosis)
Paroxysmal dyskinesias
Hemifacial spasms
Startle disease (hyperekplexia)
Myoclonic disorders

Behavioral
Psychogenic seizures
Attentional deficits
Episodic dyscontrol
Obsessive-compulsive behavior
Dissociative states (e.g., psychogenic fugue)
Panic attacks
Schizophrenia

TABLE 483–6. PHARMACOLOGIC DATA FOR THE COMMONLY USED ANTIEPILEPTIC DRUGS (ORAL ADMINISTRATION)

Drug	Seizure Type	Adult Dose (mg/kg/d)	Therapeutic Range (µg/ml)	Half-life (hr)	Peak Time (hr)	Daily Doses
Carbamazepine (Tegretol)	P, GC	15–25	8–12	12	2–6	4
Phenytoin (Dilantin)	P, GC	3–8	10–30	24	3–12	2
Primidone (Mysoline)†	P, GC	10–20	5–15	12	2–4	4
Phenobarbital	P, GC	2–4	15–40	96	6–18	1
Clorazepate (Tranxene)	P, GC	0.7–1.0	1–2*	30*	1*	2
Ethosuximide (Zarontin)	A	10–30	40–100	40	2–3	2
Clonazepam (Klonopin)	A, M	0.03–0.3	0.01–0.05	30	1–2	2
Methsuximide (Celontin)	P, A	10–25	20–40*	40*	<3	2
Valproate (Depakene)	All	15–60	50–100	14	1–4	4
Divalproex sodium (Depakote)	All	15–60	50–100	14	3–5	4

*For derived metabolite.
†Substantial antiepileptic effect is also obtained from derived phenobarbital.
P = partial; GC = generalized convulsive; A = absence; M = myoclonus.
Modified with permission from Engel J Jr: Seizures and Epilepsy. Philadelphia, F.A. Davis, 1989.

Some epileptic symptoms can be confused with behavioral disturbances. Frequently occurring absences in children can be mistaken for attentional deficits, learning disabilities, and disciplinary problems, but the EEG should provide the correct diagnosis. Certain simple partial seizures with sensory or psychic symptoms may be interpreted as schizophrenic hallucinations. Epileptic hallucinations usually are more stereotyped and more likely to have visual components than are psychotic hallucinations. Rarely, dissociative states may represent continuous epileptic seizures or prolonged periods of postictal confusion.

TREATMENT. Treatable causes of epileptic seizures include intracerebral lesions that can be surgically removed and toxic, metabolic, infectious, and vascular diseases that require medical management. A treatable cause cannot be found in most patients with chronic recurrent seizures, however, and the objective of therapy is then to maximize useful function, ideally by complete eradication of seizures without introduction of unwanted side effects. Adequate control is usually possible with appropriate pharmacologic, surgical, and psychosocial management. However, only about half of patients treated for chronic epilepsy can expect to become seizure free indefinitely.

Pharmacologic Therapy. Although many antiepileptic drugs are available, it is prudent to become familiar with and use the few that are most effective for each of the various seizure types (Table 483–6). Pharmacologic therapy is based on obtaining an accurate diagnosis of seizure type or epileptic syndrome, selecting the single most appropriate drug for that diagnosis (monotherapy), and correlating measurements of drug levels in the serum with patient reports to adjust dosages and dose schedules for the best control and fewest side effects. The best control does not necessarily mean the greatest reduction in seizure frequency. In certain patients, the disability caused by some continued seizures may be less than limitations induced by therapy. For example, the occurrence of a few absences a day for a child is preferable to an alternative of no seizures on a dose of medication that produces continuous sedation and impairs school performance. Similarly, aggressive therapy is not justified for a patient with refractory epilepsy when high drug levels exacerbate existing physical and mental handicaps without producing a worthwhile improvement in the seizure pattern.

Pharmacokinetic Principles. Dose planning for individual antiepileptic drugs depends on pharmacokinetic factors that determine the amount of available drug in the blood. The therapeutic ranges for individual antiepileptic drugs refer to the ranges of steady-state levels of each drug that by trial and error have been most effective in controlling seizures with minimal or no side effects. Average or approximate pharmacokinetic variables for the commonly used antiepileptic drugs appear in Table 483–6.

The proper dose schedule for a newly introduced drug depends on balancing the need for rapid control of seizures against the avoidance of side effects. If a patient has been warned about the possible occurrence of another seizure and takes appropriate precautions, it usually is not necessary to build a drug level rapidly at the risk of producing severe toxicity. It is more important that the patient accept the drug of first choice. Patients

can be encouraged to remain on medication by beginning a drug regimen slowly, taking the medication with meals when nausea is anticipated, using higher doses at bedtime when sedation is anticipated, and reducing doses transiently when untoward side effects occur. Most unpleasant dose-related side effects are temporary, and an appropriate regimen eventually can be instituted. A loading dose can be given practically for some drugs (phenytoin and phenobarbital) when the risk of repeated seizures requires therapeutic levels to be achieved rapidly despite side effects. A loading dose of 1.5 (rather than 2) times the calculated total daily dose may be an adequate compromise between obtaining rapid seizure control and producing minimal side effects if the planned maintenance schedule is begun less than one half-life after the loading dose.

Although a maintenance steady-state level of a drug can be achieved with an interdose interval of approximately one half-life time, in this situation drug levels will fall below the protective range if a single dose is missed. However, a dose schedule that requires a drug to be taken too frequently may be inconvenient and reduce compliance. An interdose interval of 0.5 half-life, which amounts to one to four times a day for the commonly used medications, is usually recommended. Failure to achieve a therapeutic drug level using recommended dose schedules most commonly reflects noncompliance by the patient but also may result from aberrant absorption and metabolism, and dose schedules must then be determined individually from measurements of serum drug levels.

The recommended therapeutic range for a given drug is based on average measures. One should use these values as a guide rather than a goal; therapeutic drug levels in individual patients may be well above or below the average. Once an effective maintenance schedule has been achieved, determinations of serum drug levels, always drawn at the same time after a given dose, provide a reliable long-term record of steady-state conditions. Such measurements are useful when recurrent seizures or side effects result from decreases or increases in available drug (Table 483–7).

Enzyme Induction and Inhibition. Enzyme induction by the

TABLE 483–7. INDICATIONS FOR SERUM ANTIEPILEPTIC DRUG LEVELS

To establish individual therapeutic range
  Initiation of treatment while seizures remain uncontrolled

To identify altered pharmacokinetics
  Loss of seizure control or appearance of toxic symptoms
  Addition of second antiepileptic drug or change in drug regimen
  Questionable change in drug efficacy during:
    Intercurrent illness
    Multiple drug therapy
    Altered physiologic state, such as pregnancy or puberty
  Unexplained behavioral or neurologic symptoms that might be evidence of toxicity

To document compliance

liver is a common reason for the late appearance of subtherapeutic serum drug levels after an effective maintenance schedule has been achieved. If seizures recur following a period of control, owing to enzyme induction, the dose of the initial anticonvulsant should be increased gradually to the desired blood level or to toxicity rather than immediately adding a new drug. The latter may merely enhance enzyme induction and further decrease serum drug levels. Addition of a second drug can also inhibit liver enzymes and cause toxic effects owing to increased levels of the first drug. If it is necessary to add a second anticonvulsant, serum levels of both agents require checking to ensure that adequate but not toxic levels of both have been attained. In general, if the first drug recommended for treatment has no effect on seizure control despite adequate serum levels or achieves control only at the expense of severe toxicity, it is best to replace it with a second drug. Gradual withdrawal of the first drug may induce a temporary exacerbation of seizure frequency, which does not necessarily indicate that the second drug is ineffective. Occasionally, the use of more than one drug becomes unavoidable, particularly when patients have more than one type of seizure.

Selection of Antiepileptic Drugs. Preferred Agents. While specific types of seizures respond to specific drugs (Table 483–8), many factors determine the choice of the best single drug for an individual patient. The trend today is to treat generalized convulsive and partial seizures first with either carbamazepine or phenytoin. While both drugs offer the same protection, phenytoin use is associated with a high incidence of disturbing cosmetic side effects.

Primidone and phenobarbital are also used for convulsive and partial seizures. They are less effective than carbamazepine and phenytoin, but phenobarbital is the least expensive of the available antiepileptic drugs and has the fewest dangerous side effects. Sedation is common but may not be a problem at lower doses and may subside over time even at higher doses. Furthermore, both carbamazepine and phenytoin can dull mentation at high doses. Phenobarbital commonly causes hyperkinetic activity and other undesirable behavioral disturbances in children. Most epileptologists now generally prefer carbamazepine for this age group. Phenobarbital should not be given to patients with depressive tendencies. It can exacerbate psychological depression and is the most common instrument of suicide in the epileptic population.

Valproate suppresses generalized seizures and is also occasionally effective against partial seizures as well. Consequently, the drug may be used to treat generalized convulsions even when they secondarily generalize from a partial seizure. Although valproate has few sedative and adverse cognitive side effects compared with other antiepileptic drugs and does not produce the cosmetic side effects associated with phenytoin, it has been associated with serious idiosyncratic hepatotoxicity. Most fatal hepatic dysfunction, however, has been encountered in small children on multiple drugs and is not a realistic concern in patients over the age of 10 who are on monotherapy. The enteric-coated form (divalproex sodium) is usually preferred to reduce the incidence of gastrointestinal side effects. Valproate increases serum levels of barbiturates, which can result in inadvertent sedation or even coma.

Ethosuximide and valproate are the drugs of choice for absence seizures. Since valproate is effective against generalized convul-

TABLE 483–8. THERAPEUTIC CLASSIFICATION OF EPILEPTIC SEIZURES

Seizure Type	Preferred Drugs
Partial seizures and generalized convulsions	Carbamazepine Phenytoin Phenobarbital Primidone Valproate
Absences	Ethosuximide Valproate Clonazepam
Myoclonus	Clonazepam Valproate

sions, it is used when absences and generalized convulsions coexist. It is also recommended by many in disorders such as petit mal epilepsy in which generalized convulsions might occur, even if they have not appeared by the time therapy is instituted. Valproate is the drug of choice for mixed seizure disorders and for juvenile myoclonic epilepsy because of its broad spectrum of action. It is also widely used for other types of generalized seizures.

The drugs of choice for nonepileptic forms of myoclonus are the benzodiazepine clonazepam, and valproate. Benzodiazepines tend to lose their effectiveness with time as tolerance develops. In progressive myoclonus epilepsy, in which myoclonic jerks and seizures are both present, valproate may be the best hope for control with monotherapy. If this is unsuccessful, clonazepam plus carbamazepine or phenytoin may be required. Clonazepam and valproate given together may interact to make seizures worse and produce unpleasant side effects.

If epileptic seizures do not respond to first-line antiepileptic medications, patients should be referred to specialized epilepsy centers for management. Additional medications that might be effective as primary epileptic drugs, or as adjunctive therapy, include clorazepate for partial and convulsive seizures, clonazepam for absences, and methsuximide for absence, atonic, and partial seizures. Acetazolamide can be a useful adjunctive medication when given from 10 days premenstrually through the end of menses to ameliorate catamenial accentuation of seizures.

Side Effects. Almost all antiepileptic drugs potentially produce undesirable side effects, and physicians should consult the *Physicians' Desk Reference* or a current textbook before first use. Common dose-related side effects of carbamazepine and the hydantoins include nausea, dizziness, diplopia, and ataxia. Sedation, impaired mentation, and hyperactivity occur most often with the barbiturates and benzodiazepines. These symptoms may abate with time. Drug-induced folic acid deficiencies may reach symptomatic levels in some patients and require vitamin supplements. Idiosyncratic side effects that usually affect skin, blood, liver, and kidneys are potentially more serious. When a new drug is introduced, complete blood counts and appropriate blood chemistry analyses should be obtained every 4 weeks for several months and then monitored every 3 to 12 months as long as therapy continues. Leukopenia with counts as low as 3000 per cubic millimeter with carbamazepine does not necessarily indicate impending agranulocytosis, but a neutrophil count of less than 1000 per cubic millimeter is cause for concern. Serum alkaline phosphatase levels are often elevated with antiepileptic drug use, but this finding alone does not indicate a hepatotoxic reaction. Mild pruritus may be treated medically. Evidence of blood dyscrasias, liver or kidney damage, or more serious skin rash requires prompt discontinuation of medication and referral to the proper specialist. Cosmetic side effects commonly associated with phenytoin include hirsutism, gingival hyperplasia, and coarsening of features; weight gain and alopecia are occasionally seen with valproate therapy. Carbamazepine can cause water retention and is not used for patients at risk for congestive heart failure. A paradoxical increase in seizure frequency may result from elevated drug levels, particularly with phenytoin, and can cause seizures to recur after a period of control.

Special Considerations. *Pregnancy* presents particular problems for women with epilepsy. Serum drug levels can fall as a result of noncompliance and increased elimination, so frequent drug level determinations are recommended. A decreased serum drug level need not be corrected, however, unless it is accompanied by an exacerbation of seizures. First-time convulsions in the third trimester usually indicate eclampsia. If required, short-term administration of appropriate antiepileptic agents poses little or no risk to the fetus at this point and should be used instead of the still common practice of therapy with magnesium sulfate. The risk of major and minor malformations in children born of mothers on antiepileptic medication is approximately twice that of untreated epileptic mothers, but this difference may be due to the severity of the disorder as well as to the teratogenic effects of these drugs. Valproate is believed to produce neural tube defects, and a teratogenic effect of trimethadione has also been well established; consequently, they are not recommended during the first trimester of pregnancy. Polypharmacy and unnecessarily high drug levels also increase the potential for problems during this period. Otherwise, there is no evidence that one antiepileptic medication is any worse than another during pregnancy. There is little to be gained from discontinuing effective medication once pregnancy has been determined, especially after the first trimester has been completed. The risk to mother and fetus from seizures may be greater than the risk from drugs. Hemorrhagic disease of the newborn occurs with the mother's use of phenobarbital and phenytoin and can be treated with vitamin K. Maternal drug levels can cause sedation and withdrawal in the newborn, but only rarely do they present a problem for breastfed infants.

Age is a factor that must be taken into account when planning pharmacotherapy. The rate of metabolism is slower, renal clearance is decreased, and protein binding is less in neonates and the elderly than in children and adults. Consequently, the half-life of drugs is longer and the percentage of free drug is greater for a given serum concentration at the extremes of age. In children, however, the metabolic rate is higher than in adults, and the half-life of drugs may be shorter, requiring more frequent doses to achieve a steady-state level. The risk of fatal hepatic dysfunction with valproate may be as high as 1 in 500 for children under the age of 2 who are on polytherapy. Elderly patients at risk for congestive heart failure should not be treated with carbamazepine, which can cause water retention. Barbiturates and, to a lesser extent, benzodiazepines, produce reversible hyperkinetic and aggressive behaviors in children as well as confusion, agitation, and depression in the elderly.

Surgical Therapy. *Resective surgery* has proved safe and beneficial and can cure a chronic epileptic condition when all else fails. At present, it is a greatly underutilized therapeutic modality. Most surgical facilities will consider epileptic patients potential candidates for resective surgical therapy if (1) a partial seizure disorder has been documented, (2) seizures continue at a frequency that seriously interferes with daily living despite adequate levels of appropriate antiepileptic medication, and (3) there is not substantial interictal mental retardation or psychosis. Patients with complex partial seizures of temporal lobe origin are ideal candidates for surgery. Worthwhile improvement occurs in over 85 per cent of such patients, and as many as two thirds may become seizure free after anterior temporal lobectomy. Local resection of an extratemporal focal epileptogenic lesion is also possible if the area of cortex can be identified precisely and removed safely. A history of generalized convulsions, a focus in the dominant hemisphere, or the presence of bilateral independent temporal spike foci on EEG does not contraindicate surgery.

Section of the corpus callosum has been particularly effective in controlling otherwise intractable drop attacks, and patients with other secondary generalized and partial seizure patterns have experienced improvement from this operation. While *hemispherectomy* is the most effective surgical procedure for epilepsy, it is justified only for children who have severely incapacitating unilateral seizures and hemiparesis with a useless hand.

Other Therapeutic Measures. Patients with some types of seizures may benefit from special management. Reflex seizures induced by specific stimuli can be treated by avoiding the stimuli. For example, epileptic photosensitivity can be abolished by patching one eye or wearing colored glasses, and desensitization is possible for many forms of reflex seizures. Spread of some simple partial seizures may be aborted by strong or painful sensory stimulation administered at onset. When seizures occur only at specific times of the day, medications can be adjusted to ensure maximum levels at those times, and daily schedules can be altered so that the patient is home or in a safe environment when at risk.

Patients with all types of seizures should remain active and maintain daily habits that ensure regular meals, adequate sleep, and a reduction in unnecessary stress. Alcohol or sedative drugs can be taken sparingly, but excessive use can provoke seizures during withdrawal. Patients who have seizures associated with an alteration in consciousness, particularly those that occur without warning, should be counseled to avoid hazardous situations: They should not swim alone, should shower rather than bathe, should not climb to unprotected heights, and should not operate potentially dangerous power-driven machines, including automobiles.

Emergency Treatment. First aid for a generalized tonic-clonic convulsion consists of protecting the patient from self-injury. Clothing should be loosened, sharp objects removed from the area, and the patient's head cushioned from impact. Hard objects or fingers must not be inserted into the patient's mouth—patients do not choke on their own tongues. When the seizure is over, turn the patient's head to drain oral secretions. Have someone stay with the patient during the postictal period until full consciousness has returned. It is not necessary to call an ambulance unless the patient has never had a seizure before, the seizure lasts longer than 10 minutes, another attack occurs before consciousness is regained, or there is evidence of injury, respiratory distress, or pregnancy. Patients should not be forcibly restrained during complex partial seizures but should be protected from surrounding hazards until ictal and postictal symptoms cease and they can care for themselves.

Status Epilepticus. The various forms of status epilepticus require specialized approaches to treatment. *Major motor status epilepticus* is a medical emergency requiring immediate intervention to prevent permanent brain damage or death. A recommended approach is given in Table 483–9. As soon as the airway is secured, a quick neurologic examination should be performed to appraise critical forebrain and brain stem functions. There may be evidence of an acute intracerebral lesion with herniation or other life-threatening conditions. Because the effects of diazepam are short lived, it should be administered simultaneously with a longer acting antiepileptic drug. Phenytoin usually is preferred, since it produces no sedative effects. This allows the patient to regain consciousness when seizures are terminated and facilitates neurologic evaluation. If seizures persist after the institution of appropriate therapy, high intravenous doses of phenobarbital or general anesthesia with short-acting barbiturates are recommended. When intubation and ventilation are necessary, the progress of treatment should be monitored closely with EEG

TABLE 483–9. MANAGEMENT OF CONVULSIVE STATUS EPILEPTICUS

Treatment Goal	Cumulative Time Since Arrival in Emergency Room
Restore homeostasis	0–15 min
Airway, blood pressure, nasal O_2; record ECG; intubate only if necessary	
Administer 50 ml 50% glucose and 100 mg thiamine IV	
Start isotonic saline slow drip IV	
Stop convulsive seizures	
Diazepam, 0.25 mg/kg IV up to 20 mg (<5 mg/min), followed immediately by phenytoin, 18 mg/kg IV (<50 mg/min); monitor blood pressure and ECG; repeat 7 mg/kg if necessary	
or	
Lorazepam, 0.1 mg/kg IV (<2 mg/min), with subsequent medication determined by serum drug levels or, if necessary, phenytoin IV as above	15–60 min
If seizures persist:	
Intubate; EEG should be used at this point	60–120 min
Phenobarbital, 20 mg/kg IV (<100 mg/min)	
If seizures persist:	
General anesthesia with short-acting barbiturates (e.g., pentobarbital, 5 mg/kg, then 1–3 mg/kg/hr); adjust dose to obtain burst suppression pattern on EEG without depressing blood pressure severely, and titrate to keep patient seizure-free	
Use additional anticonvulsants as necessary	After 2–3 hr
Obtain anticonvulsant blood levels	
Diagnostic evaluation (do concurrently with above)	
History, examination, urinalysis for toxic screen	

Modified with permission from Engel J Jr: Seizures and Epilepsy. Philadelphia, F.A. Davis, 1989.

recordings. Once status has been controlled, maintenance drug therapy is instituted. The most common cause of major motor status epilepticus is a sudden reduction or discontinuation of antiepileptic drugs in patients with known seizure disorders.

Absence status epilepticus can be aborted early by ethosuximide or valproate. Once under way, however, it is treated with intravenous diazepam followed by valproate, because parenteral preparations of antiabsence drugs are not available. An adult form of absence status, without previous history, and postictal absence-like status respond to the protocol outlined in Table 483–9. Complex partial status should be treated as aggressively as generalized convulsive status. Neither absence status nor complex partial status is life threatening, however, and general anesthesia may not be necessary. Both absence and complex partial status can be mistaken for psychiatric disturbances until EEG recordings demonstrate their typical ictal patterns. Simple partial status epilepticus (continuous partial epilepsy) may be effectively treated with intravenous diazepam or lorazepam followed by phenytoin, but this is not a medical emergency and usually does not warrant more aggressive measures.

Psychosocial Considerations. To some extent, psychosocial disturbances among epileptics are situational. Because most seizures occur spontaneously and unpredictably, many patients spend their lives anticipating inappropriate behavior, embarrassment, or serious injury. Epileptics are frequently unable to find work if they admit to a seizure disorder, so that their opportunities for rewarding social relationships are reduced. In most states, patients with seizures that impair consciousness are not allowed to drive. These factors contribute to a higher incidence of depression and suicide among epileptics than in the general population.

Although the evidence is controversial, aberrant personality traits, affective disorders, and psychoses, including late paranoid schizophrenia, have been reported to be more common among patients with epilepsy, particularly those with complex partial seizures of limbic origin. It is unclear to what extent these disturbances result from the underlying pathologic lesions or specific seizure activity, how much can be attributed to the effect of long-term antiepileptic drug therapy, and how much relates to

limitations imposed on daily living and the stigma of being epileptic.

Only about one in four patients with uncontrolled epilepsy is handicapped by seizures alone. The others have physical, intellectual, and/or psychiatric disabilities that disrupt their daily lives. Epileptic seizures, perhaps more than any other neurologic symptom, are modified by internal and external influences that are under the control of the patient and other persons. For these reasons, treatment of the epileptic patient requires more than manipulation of anticonvulsant drugs, and outcome depends upon more than just seizure control. The physician must come to know the patient and the patient's family, their psychological interactions, and their social situation. Furthermore, improving psychosocial adaptation itself often leads to a reduction in seizure frequency. To provide the comprehensive care required by patients with seizure disorders, the physician must attend to the patient as well as to the neurologic disorder. The doctor must be friend as well as therapist.

Engel J Jr: Seizures and Epilepsy. Philadelphia, F. A. Davis, 1989. *A thorough overview of the field of epileptology and an introduction to the literature.*
Engel J Jr (ed.): Surgical Treatment of the Epilepsies. New York, Raven Press, 1987. *A comprehensive presentation of modern surgical therapy for epilepsy.*
Epilepsy Abstracts 1947–present. Published now by Excerpta Medica, *this monthly journal contains abstracts of all epilepsy-related papers and is an easy introduction to the literature on any subject.*
Levy RH, Dreifuss FE, Mattson RH, et al. (eds.): Antiepileptic Drugs. 3rd ed. New York, Raven Press, 1989. *A multiauthored compendium of recent concepts of pharmacologic therapy for epilepsy.*
Penfield W, Jasper H: Epilepsy and the Functional Anatomy of the Brain. Boston, Little, Brown and Company, 1954. *A classic by pioneers of modern epileptology; describes epileptic phenomena and applications of clinical data to the understanding of normal brain functions.*
Porter RJ: Epilepsy: 100 Elementary Principles. 2nd ed. Philadelphia, W. B. Saunders Company, 1989. *A small volume of clinical pearls.*
Roger J, Dravet C, Bureau M, et al.: Epileptic Syndromes in Infancy, Childhood and Adolescence. London, John Libbey Eurotext, Ltd., 1985. *Detailed descriptions of the currently recognized epileptic syndromes.*

SECTION THIRTEEN / INTRACRANIAL TUMORS AND STATES OF ALTERED INTRACRANIAL PRESSURE

484 Intracranial Tumors: General Considerations

Nicholas A. Vick

Approximately 14,000 new cases of primary brain tumors are treated each year in the United States. Metastases of the brain are even more frequent and contribute considerably to suffering and death from systemic cancer. The diversity of brain tumors makes it important to attend to what is characteristic about each histologic type, since attention to biologic specificity crucially guides present therapy and almost certainly will advance future understanding of these lesions and their treatment.

The classification of brain tumors is a subject often beset with confusing terminology, understood only by the knowledgeable. This text employs a simpler approach, classifying brain tumors into *metastatic, primary extra-axial,* and *primary intra-axial*

(Table 484–1). These categories include all of the primary brain tumors listed in the World Health Organization classification (Table 484–2), adds pituitary and metastatic tumors, and is obviously simple. Moreover, it follows practical clinical thinking. This chapter deals with the general biology, clinical features, and treatment of brain tumors as an overall problem. The following

TABLE 484–1. THE COMMON BRAIN TUMORS IN ADULTS WITH PERCENTAGE INCIDENCE BY CATEGORY*

Metastatic	Primary Extra-axial	Primary Intra-axial
Lung (37)	Meningioma (80)	Glioblastoma (47)
Breast (19)	Acoustic neuroma (10)	Anaplastic astrocytoma (24)
Melanoma (16)	Pituitary adenoma (7)	Astrocytoma (15)
Colorectum (9)	Other (3)	Oligodendroglioma (5)
Kidney (8)		Lymphoma (2)
Other (11)		Other (7)

*These figures, given in parentheses, can be extremely variable from one center to another, depending on referral pattern. They are given here as general estimates based upon many published series.

TABLE 484–2. WORLD HEALTH ORGANIZATION CLASSIFICATION OF BRAIN TUMORS*

A. Astrocytic tumors
  1. Astrocytoma
     a. Fibrillary
     b. Protoplasmic
     c. Gemistocytic
  2. Pilocytic astrocytoma
  3. Subependymal giant cell astrocytoma (ventricular tumor or tuberous sclerosis)
  4. Astroblastoma
  5. Anaplastic (malignant) astrocytoma
B. Oligodendroglial tumors
  1. Oligodendroglioma
  2. Mixed oligoastrocytoma
  3. Anaplastic (malignant) oligodendroglioma
C. Ependymal and choroid plexus tumors
  1. Ependymoma
     Variants:
     a. Myxopapillary ependymoma
     b. Papillary ependymoma
     c. Subependymoma
  2. Anaplastic (malignant) ependymoma
  3. Choroid plexus papilloma
  4. Anaplastic (malignant) choroid plexus papilloma
D. Pineal cell tumor
  1. Pineocytoma (pinealocytoma)
  2. Pineoblastoma (pinealoblastoma)
E. Neuronal tumors
  1. Gangliocytoma
  2. Ganglioglioma
  3. Ganglioneuroblastoma
  4. Anaplastic (malignant) gangliocytoma and ganglioglioma
  5. Neuroblastoma
F. Poorly differentiated and embryonal tumours
  1. Glioblastoma
     Variants:
     a. Glioblastoma with sarcomatous component (mixed glioblastoma and sarcoma)
     b. Giant cell glioblastoma
  2. Medulloblastoma
     Variants:
     a. Desmoplastic medulloblastoma
     b. Medullomyoblastoma
  3. Medulloepithelioma
  4. Primitive polar spongioblastoma
  5. Gliomatosis cerebri

*This is one of several formal schemes that are based on neuropathologic criteria. Metastasis is not considered, and one can get no sense of a given tumor as a *clinical* problem, as suggested by the simple classification in Table 484–1.

chapter describes the particular behavior of the most important subtypes in accordance with the outline of Table 484–1.

"Is it benign or malignant?" is invariably the first question patients, families, and physicians ask when confronted with a diagnosis of brain tumor. About a third of primary brain tumors can be called benign. Meningiomas and acoustic neuromas are good examples, since they grow relatively slowly, often can be removed completely, and do not recur after such a removal.

Nevertheless, the concept of malignancy in the central nervous system has a different meaning from that which applies to systemic cancers. For one thing, the term "malignant" has nothing to do with metastasis out of the central nervous system, which is extraordinarily rare. It has, however, everything to do with anatomic location and the possibility of complete surgical removal. If a meningioma is so positioned that it cannot be completely removed, such as at the base of the brain, it is likely to kill the patient eventually, even though it may possess only indolent growth characteristics. Unless a tumor can be completely excised to the last cell, all intracranial neoplasms are potentially malignant in that they may recur, and often do.

INITIAL EVALUATION

SYMPTOMS AND SIGNS. Brain tumors present clinically in two patterns, not necessarily mutually exclusive. One pattern consists of nonfocal symptoms of *increased intracranial pressure*, such as headaches, nausea, vomiting, confusion, and lethargy. The other consists of symptoms or signs of *focal brain dysfunction*, such as hemianopia, hemiparesis, selected cranial nerve palsies, or focal motor seizures (Table 484–3). Such signs of focal brain dysfunction may have convincing localizing value even before an image of the brain is made by computed tomography (CT) or magnetic resonance imaging (MRI). Some tumors that arise in neurologically "silent" areas, such as the parietal or frontal association cortices, may produce only minor symptoms of headache, confusion, behavioral change, or, eventually, a seizure, despite growing to a considerable size. These symptoms may not indicate at all what part of the brain is affected or may lead to a localizing diagnosis only in the hands of a neurologically experienced consultant. Although the capacity to reach early diagnosis by CT or MRI has greatly reduced the numbers of patients in whom symptoms of increased intracranial pressure represent initial complaints, examples still remain, especially in association with fast-growing tumors and in children. The latter are particularly likely to have tumors in the posterior fossa that tend to obstruct spinal fluid pathways earlier than do supratentorial tumors. As implied, the tempo with which a brain tumor grows also influences the presenting symptoms. Despite the fixed space of the skull (once infantile sutures have closed), the human brain possesses a remarkable capacity to make room for a slowly growing tumor (Fig. 484–1). Because of this, and even allowing for the relative rapidity of growth of aggressive brain tumors such as glioblastomas, the rule is that the patient usually appears better clinically than might be expected from the degree of abnormality seen on CT or MRI scan.

DIFFERENTIAL DIAGNOSIS. Patients who present with symptoms and signs of increased intracranial pressure or a first convulsive seizure need to be hospitalized. Diagnosis and treatment measures must be started at once; it is a waste of time and may be unsafe to wait. On the other hand, those who present with focal neurologic impairment and who do not have symptoms of increased intracranial pressure may reasonably be evaluated in the outpatient setting for other conditions that are often considerations in the differential diagnosis of brain tumor (Table 484–4). The tempo of evolution of symptoms and signs of focal neurologic impairment, much more than their severity, governs urgency of evaluation. The tempo also strongly influences diagnostic considerations. Although an occasional brain tumor may manifest with such rapid onset of hemiparesis or aphasia that a stroke is mimicked, most do not. Further, most strokes do not evolve over several weeks, though some may do so. Associated aspects of the history, such as recent head trauma, previous episodes of reversible neurologic impairment, or recent infection and fever, should direct attention to diagnostic alternatives such as subdural hematoma, multiple sclerosis, or cerebral abscess. Simply stated, it is the careful history, not the neurologic examination, that usually points to the alternative diagnoses.

IMAGING AND OTHER DIAGNOSTIC PROCEDURES

Brain imaging by MRI or CT scans is an indispensable component of the modern diagnosis of brain tumors. Only seldom, however, are such images sufficient to offer tissue diagnoses, since one type of tumor can look like another or even resemble nonneoplastic mass lesions, such as brain abscesses, fungal infections, parasitic invasions, demyelinating diseases, and even strokes. For definitive diagnosis and adequate treatment planning, one must obtain a tissue diagnosis whenever possible. This can be made either by direct surgical biopsy or, in the case of some nonneoplastic conditions, by judging CT or MRI responses to particular therapies.

MRI is almost always superior to CT scanning in providing diagnostic information for all types of intracranial mass lesions. Several features account for this superiority. MRI resolution is slightly better, but, more important, discrimination between tissue components is greater. Furthermore, MRI outlines posterior fossa structures and tumors with a clarity that CT cannot achieve because of x-ray distortions due to the bony structure of that region. In several types of tumor, particularly the low-grade gliomas, MRI may show extensive brain infiltration in cases that fail to produce any image abnormality on CT or, at most, a vague low density. It should be noted that although either MRI or CT should be used with contrast enhancement in cases of suspected

TABLE 484–3. FOCAL CLINICAL MANIFESTATIONS OF BRAIN TUMORS

Frontal Lobe	**Corpus Callosum**	**Sella/Optic Nerve/Pituitary**
Generalized seizures	Dementia (anterior)	Endocrinopathy
Focal motor seizures (contralateral)	Behavioral changes (posterior)	Bitemporal hemianopia
Expressive aphasia (dominant side)	Asymptomatic (mid)	Monocular visual defects
Behavioral changes		
Dementia		
Gait disorders, incontinence		
Parietal Lobe	**Basal Ganglia**	**Pons/Medulla**
Receptive aphasia (dominant side)	Hemiparesis (contralateral)	Cranial nerve dysfunction
Spatial disorientation (nondominant side)	Movement disorders very rare	Ataxia, nystagmus
Cortical sensory dysfunction (contralateral)		Weakness, sensory loss
Hemianopia (contralateral)		Spasticity
Temporal Lobe	**Thalamus**	**Cerebellopontine Angle**
Complex partial (psychomotor) seizures	Sensory loss (contralateral)	Deafness (ipsilateral)
Generalized seizures	Behavioral changes	Loss of facial sensation (ipsilateral)
Behavioral changes	Language disorder (dominant side)	Facial weakness (ipsilateral)
Olfactory and complex visual auras		Ataxia
Occipital Lobe	**Midbrain/Pineal**	**Cerebellum**
Hemianopia (contralateral)	Paresis of vertical eye movements	Ataxia (ipsilateral)
Visual disturbances (unformed)	Pupillary abnormalities	Nystagmus
	Precocious puberty (boys)	

brain tumor, the passage of such contrast agents beyond the blood-brain barrier into the tissue does not necessarily imply the presence of a histologically malignant tumor. For example, although malignant gliomas almost always show contrast enhancement, so do meningiomas, which are entirely benign if they can be fully removed surgically.

It is now generally understood that a CT scan done without contrast enhancement is of little value in the diagnosis of brain tumors or other mass lesions. While it is true that hemorrhage, calcifications, hydrocephalus, and shift can be well seen on a noncontrast CT scan, the interpretation of even these conditions is tentative because each can have an underlying causative structural abnormality such as a brain tumor, which may fail to appear on a noncontrast CT study. Allergy to CT dye is rare and readily manageable. Currently available nonionic CT dyes have an extremely low incidence of side effects. There is little risk that currently used CT dyes will cause renal dysfunction in normally hydrated patients who are not known to have kidney disease.

MRI initially provided two types of images, designated T$_1$ and

T_2. For brain tumors, the former generally showed a well-demarcated area of low density and the latter, bright whiteness that encompassed a more extensive region owing to the signal of the surrounding brain edema (Fig. 484–2). With the availability for general usage in 1988 of *gadolinium contrast for MRI*, a new set of criteria of usage and differential diagnostic considerations in brain imaging have quickly evolved (Table 484–5). T$_1$ gadolinium imaging is the most precise way to image a brain tumor, and often patients can be followed with that type of study alone. Such an approach is easier for patients because it reduces the length of time otherwise spent on T$_2$ scanning. Now and then, T$_2$ images are useful. For example, T$_2$ images, besides showing the extent of edema, also delineate the demyelinating effects of radiation upon white matter.

Cerebral angiography has become seldom used in the diagnosis of brain tumors. In a few circumstances, however, neurosurgeons, in preparation for surgery, require a more precise knowledge of the pattern and position of blood vessels that can be obtained only by angiography. The procedure is also used to embolize certain tumors, such as highly vascular meningiomas, or to study cerebral dominance by injection of sodium amytal into the carotid artery (the Wada test) in left-handed individuals who are to have surgery near language areas. Cerebral dominance in such persons is quite variable; preoperative determination of cerebral localization helps surgeons to plan the extent of surgery and avoid postoperative language deficits.

Examination of the *spinal fluid* has virtually been abandoned in the diagnosis of brain tumors. Several exceptions exist, however. One is that the patient may be thought to have an inflammatory disorder mimicking a brain tumor. Another is that a patient initially believed to have a brain tumor because of clinical symptoms and signs of increased intracranial pressure has negative MRI scans and needs the diagnosis of benign intracranial hypertension established (see Ch. 486). In addition, spinal fluid cytology may be useful for determining instances of malignant meningitis secondary to metastatic neoplasms, in association with spinal spread of medulloblastoma in some children and in identifying primary lymphomas of the brain in cases in which MRI changes are ambiguous.

TABLE 484–4. THE MAIN DIFFERENTIAL DIAGNOSES OF BRAIN TUMORS

Hematomas, especially in tumors that have a tendency to bleed, such as melanoma
Abscesses, including fungal
Granulomas
Parasitic infections, such as cysticercosis
Vascular malformations, especially those without arteriovenous shunts
Solitary large plaques of multiple sclerosis
Seldom, progressive strokes

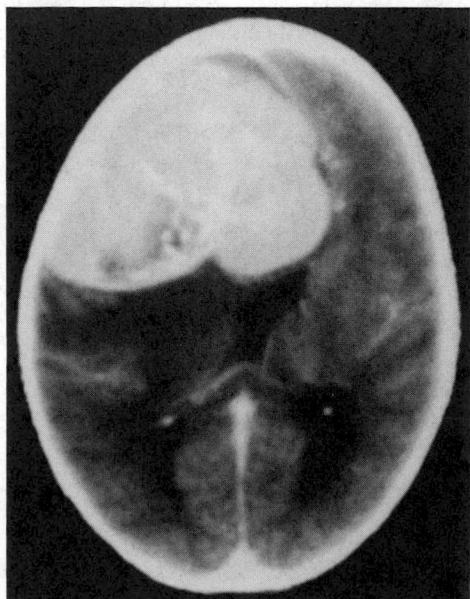

FIGURE 484–1. CT scan with contrast of a meningioma in a patient who presented with mild cognitive deficits, illustrative of the size a slow-growing tumor can attain in the brain. The tumor was completely resected.

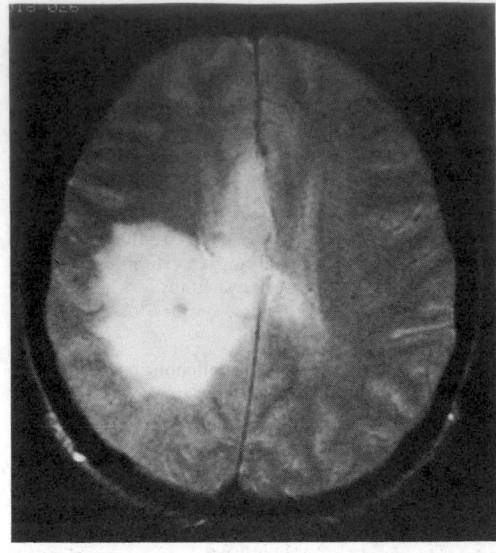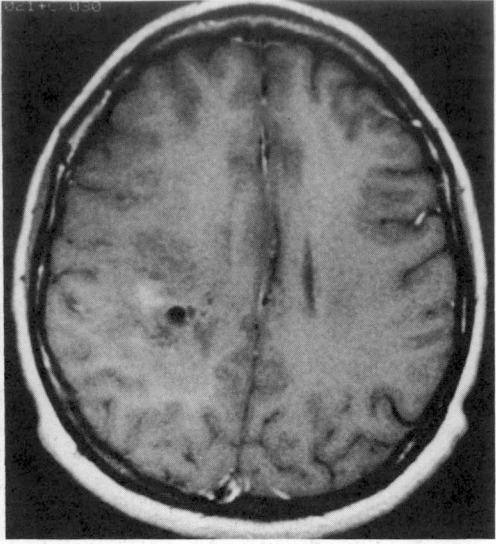

FIGURE 484–2. Low-grade astrocytoma as imaged by MRI. On the left, T_2-weighted image; on the right, T_1-weighted image, gadolinium contrast with minimal enhancement. The images are typical of this tumor, which is being detected with increasing frequency in seizure patients by MRI. Many are invisible on CT scans.

The electroencephalogram (EEG) has virtually no role in the diagnosis of brain tumors, although the procedure is sometimes useful in managing seizures in brain tumor patients. Furthermore, depth electrode studies as well as intraoperative monitoring can be of great importance in identifying and removing epileptogenic areas associated with certain tumors (see Ch. 483). The details of the EEG do not assist in the selection of anticonvulsant drugs in brain tumor patients.

Positron emission tomography (PET) is able to quantify biochemical functions, such as oxygen and glucose utilization, within tumors as well as normal brain tissue. PET scanning is a powerful research tool of limited availability for routine clinical purposes. Its actual spatial resolution is practically and theoretically inferior to that of both CT and MRI. It can differentiate radiation-induced brain injury and necrosis from recurrent tumor, which neither CT nor MRI can do. It is not an imaging tool for high-volume, regular clinical purposes.

TABLE 484–5. T₁ GADOLINIUM MRI CHARACTERISTICS OF BRAIN TUMORS

Metastases	These are remarkably variable (see Fig. 485–1). Some enhance brightly and solidly with gadolinium. Others are in ring configuration. Many are invisible with contrast CT.
Acoustic Neuromas	These are invariably intensely contrasted by gadolinium, even more reliably than by CT.
Meningiomas	Same as for acoustic neuromas.
Pituitary Adenomas	These always enhance less than the normal pituitary gland. MRI is superior in every way to CT, especially when thin slices and magnified views are ordered.
Glioblastoma	These are almost always in ring configuration (see Fig. 485–2).
Anaplastic Astrocytomas	These are sometimes solidly bright; they are often patchy, may be noncontrasting, and may look like low-grade astrocytoma.
Low-grade Astrocytomas	These do not enhance (see Fig. 485–2). They are often invisible by CT or are imaged only as vague low density.
Oligodendrogliomas	These generally do not enhance unless anaplastic and are often invisible on CT unless they are calcified.
Primary Brain Lymphomas	These usually exhibit homogeneous enhancement and are smoothly rounded. Periventricular location is common. They are multiple in about a fourth of cases. This lesion does not often look like glioblastoma but is easily mistaken for metastases if multiple.

TREATMENT

PREOPERATIVE CONSIDERATIONS AND MEDICAL MANAGEMENT. In almost every instance when a brain tumor is suspected on the basis of the combined results of history, physical findings, and imaging studies, the *first consideration is its surgical resectability*. There are exceptions, such as cases of multiple brain metastases in a patient with known systemic cancer. Patients with single brain metastases, defined by MRI, may be candidates for surgical resection of the metastasis, depending on their systemic medical status. It is unproductive to embark upon an extensive systemic evaluation in the search for an unknown primary cancer in patients with a single resectable presumed brain metastasis. If a primary tumor is not quickly revealed by a careful medical evaluation, with special attention to skin (for melanoma), breasts, and lungs, the pathologic diagnosis of the brain tumor will need to be disclosed by resection or, if unresectable owing to its position, by biopsy.

While small meningiomas or acoustic neuromas usually do not require treatment to reduce intracranial pressure, in the majority of brain tumor patients it is appropriate to start *dexamethasone* promptly. The purpose is to reduce intracranial pressure, which accompanies the majority of brain tumors, and to relieve neurologic symptoms caused by peritumoral brain edema (Fig. 484–3). No other steroid has ever been shown to be superior to dexamethasone for the reduction of peritumoral brain edema. The

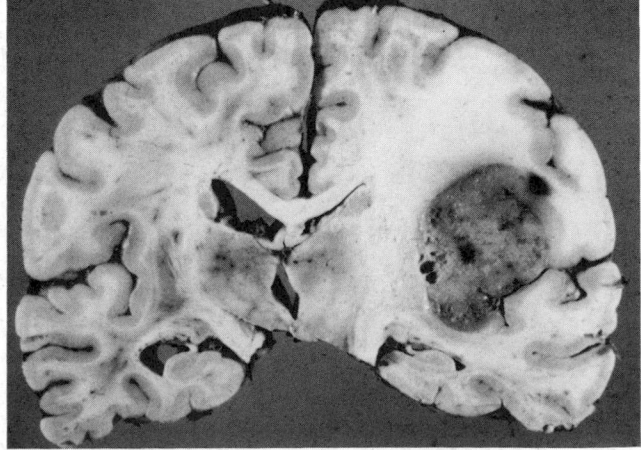

FIGURE 484–3. Gross coronal pathologic specimen of a solitary metastasis from a non–small cell lung carcinoma to the right cerebral hemisphere. The tumor is well circumscribed. It causes marked edema that greatly expands the cerebral white matter. Metastatic tumors such as this can often be surgically resected.

drug's long biologic half-life and steady action upon the brain have made it the steroid of choice for treating patients with brain tumors. It should be started with an immediate oral dose of 24 or 48 mg, followed with 8 or 12 mg twice daily. It is well absorbed by mouth, and its action by that route is almost as rapid as when given intravenously. Dexamethasone need not be given more than twice a day, since its biologic half-life is so long. Breakfast and dinner are convenient times; the presence of food in the stomach precludes the need for antacids. H_2 blockers should be given only if the patient has a prior history of peptic ulcer disease. If focal neurologic symptoms are due to peritumoral vasogenic edema, dexamethasone will induce improvement within 48 hours and usually sooner. If there is no benefit, the neurologic symptoms are likely to be due to damage of the brain tissue by the tumor and not to edema.

Edema associated with brain tumors is due chiefly to abnormally fenestrated endothelium in the tumor, which permits excess flow of fluid from capillaries into the growth. Normally, solutes are transported through capillaries into brain by dissolving in and diffusing through the cerebral endothelium, a phenomenon dependent on lipid solubility and molecular size. Endothelial cells also possess some facilitated or carrier-mediated processes that are stereospecific, saturable, and independent of lipid solubility and molecular size. In brain tumors, these selective properties of the blood-brain barrier are overwhelmed by increased bulk flow and hydraulic conductivity through the defective endothelium. The result is vasogenic edema, and it is this reaction that dexamethasone so greatly reduces.

In instances of extreme intracranial pressure, the speed and action of dexamethasone are not sufficient to reduce the brain swelling quickly enough to prevent complications. In such instances, hyperosmotic solutions of *mannitol* must be given. The usual dosage is 0.5 to 2.0 gm per kilogram given intravenously over 15 minutes, followed by additional boluses of 25 gm as needed. The osmotic action of mannitol occurs within minutes. Clinical improvement may be dramatic. It is unusual for preoperative brain tumor patients to decompensate so severely from increased intracranial pressure that intubation becomes necessary. Nevertheless, this does occur. In such cases the Pa_{CO_2} must be decreased by passive hyperventilation to approximately 25 mm Hg. The effect constricts the cerebral vasculature and promptly induces a major reduction of intracranial pressure, which can be life saving.

About 20 per cent of brain tumor patients develop *seizures* some time in their lives, even if they do not have seizures at the time of diagnosis. It is conventional and probably effective to treat all patients with supratentorial tumors with anticonvulsants before surgery. Most patients with acoustic neuromas or other posterior fossa tumors have a low probability of convulsive seizures and do not need such drugs. Phenytoin is the best initial drug because it can be administered either intravenously or orally, unlike either carbamazepine or valproic acid, which can be used only orally. An intravenous drug is especially useful for continuation during the perioperative period. If required, patients may be switched easily to alternative oral drugs later. Phenytoin should be started orally, giving 1000 mg over 12 hours, or intravenously, with 1000 mg given over 1 hour. Thereafter, the usual dosage is 300 to 400 mg daily, administered in one dose or split between breakfast and dinner, along with dexamethasone. Periodic blood levels need to be checked to adjust the dosage to ensure concentrations of 10 to 20 μg per milliliter.

SURGERY. Although complete excision of a brain tumor is the ultimate goal in every case, this is not always possible. Even potentially curable tumors, such as meningiomas or acoustic neuromas, may reside in positions that make complete resection technically impossible. Malignant gliomas lack microscopic boundaries, even though they may appear by imaging studies to have well-defined limits. How much surgical success can be achieved with these tumors depends on several factors, including the tumor's proximity to cognitively indispensable areas, the skill and experience of the neurosurgeon, and, to a degree, the general health of the patient and preoperative level of neurologic function. The combination of current standards of neurosurgical anesthesia, the capacity to control intracranial pressure, and the recent addition of lasers to other operative tools such as the operating microscope have greatly increased the surgeon's capacity for well-chosen radical resection. Correspondingly, the relative risks of

surgery have become less age dependent than was previously the case. The greatest surgical risk is to neurologic function and the fear of unacceptable postoperative neurologic deficits. For this reason, radical operations upon tumors involving language areas, sensorimotor regions, the basal ganglia, corpus callosum, and brain stem are generally avoided. However, partial removal in these areas by specialized stereotaxic methods may be surprisingly effective. MRI facilitates such surgery by showing that the tumor has pushed aside functionally critical brain structures and that a macroscopic tumor edge can be delineated. As for the extent of surgery itself, it has been repeatedly shown that resection of the maximal possible amount of tumor consistent with functional preservation provides patients with better neurologic function and longer lives.

A number of patients have tumors that cannot be even partially resected because they invade language-related or other functionally indispensable areas of the brain. Most such lesions are intra-axial tumors, such as the gliomas. While current imaging techniques may produce a seemingly characteristic picture highly suggestive of a particular histologic diagnosis, effective treatment planning demands a tissue diagnosis. The only possible exception to this rule consists of certain brain stem tumors that are technically too dangerous on which to perform a biopsy. In some hands, even these may be approached by the method of MRI-guided stereotaxic biopsy, a technique that has considerably improved the opportunity to make unequivocal tissue diagnoses before treatment, regardless of the brain region. Most such stereotaxically guided biopsies are performed upon the cerebral hemispheres. The tissue specimens are small, but they are almost invariably adequate to establish a diagnosis. Morbidity, chiefly hemorrhage, occurs in about 2 per cent of cases. Patients usually need to remain in the hospital for less than 48 hours. Open biopsies of brain tumors are rarely justifiable. If the skull and dura are to be opened, the surgeon should be prepared to do a gross total resection or, at least, a major removal of as much tumor as is consonant with preservation of neurologic function.

The postoperative management of neurosurgical patients is now a relatively standard matter best left to specialized intensive care units. Deep leg vein thrombophlebitis leading to pulmonary embolism is a recurrent problem, only partially helped by prophylactic application of compression boots. Close observation and early passive exercises and mobilization are imperative. The staff must monitor and maintain anticonvulsant levels to prevent postoperative seizures. Dexamethasone should be administered at adequate levels for at least 5 days to minimize the further development of surgically induced brain edema. The drug can be tapered thereafter.

RADIOTHERAPY. All forms of external beam radiation, whether γ photons emitted from ^{60}Co sources or x-rays generated from linear accelerators, act similarly. They produce fast-moving electrons and free radicals in biologic tissue that interrupt chemical bonds between DNA base pairs. Affected cells either die or become so altered that their mitotic rate is greatly diminished. Radiotherapy is given in small daily fractions to build to a total dose. It appears safer and more effective to do this than to give larger fractions over shorter periods. Hyperfractionation, defined as two (or more) doses during a day, does not seem to be worthwhile. Therapeutic brain irradiation with particulate radiation such as neutrons has been attempted experimentally at facilities with cyclotrons. Such densely ionizing radiation, however, dissipates its energy in short path lengths, causes more damage in biologic media, and has shown no therapeutic advantage over γ photons or x-rays. Interstitial (implanted) radiotherapy (brachytherapy) is being tried and is of considerable interest. It is usually given in the form of $^{125}I_3$ or $^{192}Ir_4$ in "seeds" with placement by stereotaxic techniques. This method permits localized high-dosage radiation with sharp edges and sparing of the adjacent brain. Considerable controversy exists about the actual utility of such interstitial radiotherapy, but it can be effective in well-selected patients. The intense localized radiation of this technique, however, sometimes causes coagulative necrosis of the tumor being treated. This necrosis may create an additional mass, which can produce a dangerous degree of increased intracranial pressure, sometimes requiring further surgery for relief.

The *complications of radiotherapy* are usually said to be

infrequent, perhaps 2 to 5 per cent of cases. These figures, however, are unrealistically low if one includes effects on long-term survivors. They reflect the fact that most irradiated patients with brain tumor die before brain injury appears. Postradiation neurologic damage is unusual before a year after treatment and may not become apparent for several years. About 30 per cent of patients with glioblastomas who receive radiotherapy develop neurologic impairment with disturbed mobility and dementia if they live for twice the predicted survival time for their particular type of tumor. Another 30 per cent remain ambulatory but are unemployable owing to impairment of memory function. In these patients, while no evidence of tumor recurrence can be found by imaging studies, characteristic demyelinative changes of the white matter of the brain are evident. Dementia is a considerable problem in children who survive radiotherapy for medulloblastoma. This problem occurs because about 50 per cent survive treatment for 5 years. Such consequences emphasize the validity of waiting with radiotherapy for patients with low-grade astrocytomas and oligodendrogliomas until the progression of disease is unequivocal. Most of them will survive 5 to 10 years after the time of diagnosis, and there is little evidence to document that radiotherapy prolongs their survival.

Except in the few instances in which the process creates a surgically resectable necrotic mass, no useful treatment exists for postradiation neurologic damage. Clinical progression is the rule, though some patients stabilize with a restricted degree of impairment and do not become grossly impaired. Occasional individuals have episodic worsening that evolves in a strokelike pattern. Dexamethasone or anticoagulation or both have been found useful in some instances. The pathophysiology of these strokelike events is thought to be due to obliterative changes of small blood vessels induced by radiation, a process that may be independent of the demyelinating effects reflecting selective damage of oligodendrocytes. Neither CT nor MRI scanning definitively differentiates tumor recurrence from radiation necrosis of the brain. As noted earlier, PET can, since necrotic masses have very low glucose utilization compared with recurrent tumor.

Despite its limitations, external beam radiotherapy has proven value in controlling the growth of malignant gliomas and metastatic brain tumors. It doubles median survival time for both types of tumors. Radiation therapy, however, has little, if any, value for recurrent meningiomas and acoustic neuromas. These are almost invariably better handled by reoperation. Primary brain lymphomas are so responsive to radiotherapy that many neurologists and radiotherapists continue to use it alone despite the fact that chemotherapy may prove to provide superior initial treatment. It has already been mentioned that solitary brain metastases are best managed by surgical resection.

Radiotherapy is being studied to see whether, in fact, it actually adds to the survival of the latter group of patients. Strategies to limit the distribution of radiation to the tumor area and to increase dosage to the tumor itself are rational, as are efforts to enhance the radiation sensitivity of tumor compared with the surrounding brain. Neither approach has succeeded as yet.

CHEMOTHERAPY. Chemotherapy for brain tumors has had a disappointing record. The reasons are many, but inadequacy of drug delivery, tumor cell heterogeneity, and inherent resistance are among the important ones. Almost all efforts have been directed toward the primary brain tumors, especially the gliomas. Metastatic brain tumors regularly occur while systemic metastases are responding to chemotherapy. The alkylating agents have been the most useful drugs, although their bone marrow toxicity has been a limitation. BCNU (bischloroethylnitrosurea), the most frequently used drug, remains the most effective single agent available to treat the malignant astrocytomas. The combination of procarbazine, CCNU (cyclohexylchloroethylnitrosourea), and vincristine is the most effective multidrug regimen for the malignant astrocytomas, and it is probably superior to BCNU. It has an unusually beneficial effect against oligodendrogliomas. Overall, however, no more than 10 per cent of patients with malignant gliomas have meaningful and durable responses to chemotherapy, whether it is given immediately after radiotherapy (when its effect is especially hard to assess) or at the time of recurrence. Efforts to improve response to chemotherapy by delivering drugs through the carotid artery have not been successful. BCNU,

usually given intravenously, has intolerable toxicity when given by the intra-arterial route. Cisplatin is being studied for possible utility as an intra-arterial drug in highly selected patients.

The pharmacokinetics of drugs used in brain tumor chemotherapy are not well understood. Knowledge about their ability to gain adequate concentration within the tumors is minimal, and almost nothing is known about chemosensitivity. There have been efforts to explore these issues in animal models; the athymic (nude) mouse has been used extensively with human glioblastoma xenografts, but the observations in this model have proved to be overpredictive when tried clinically. Nonetheless, occasional remarkable responses to chemotherapy do occur in patients with glioblastomas or anaplastic astrocytomas, and as mentioned, oligodendrogliomas may be particularly responsive. The relative infrequency of ependymomas and other uncommon gliomas has left uncertain the efficacy of chemotherapy in their outcomes. Among other primary intra-axial brain tumors, primary brain lymphoma has a reasonably good response rate. The drugs used are those given regularly for systemic lymphoma. Patients with primary brain lymphoma do better with chemotherapy added than with radiotherapy alone. On average, 3- to 4-year survivals can now be expected.

Several additional forms of medical treatment for brain tumors have been attempted experimentally. These include slow release of BCNU from implanted biodegradable polymers and the administration of interferons, other biologic response modifiers, and radionuclides coupled with monoclonal antibodies. None have met with appreciable success to date. In all probability, much new biologic knowledge, such as the sequential genetic events that influence the malignant transformation and progression of brain tumors, will be required before new medical treatments become practical realities.

485 Specific Types of Brain Tumors and Their Management

Nicholas A. Vick

METASTATIC TUMORS

All systemic cancers are capable of metastasizing to the intracranial contents and skull, though some do so more readily than others. The most frequent are lung, breast, and melanoma. This is not surprising, since they are among the most common cancers. In many instances, brain metastases produce symptoms before the primary tumor is suspected. Furthermore, the primary cancer may not be found without considerable effort.

Patterns of metastasis to the nervous system have some variability, but none are truly characteristic. Non–small cell carcinoma of the lung and renal carcinoma tend to be associated with single metastases, whereas small cell carcinoma of the lung, breast carcinoma, and melanoma often generate multiple secondary deposits. The metastases may be miliary in melanoma. T_1 gadolinium magnetic resonance imaging (MRI) scans are critical in the imaging of brain metastases (Fig. 485–1). *Multiple metastases* may be revealed with this method, while T_2 MRI and contrast computed tomography (CT) may show only one or, in rare instances, none. For multiple metastases, whole-brain irradiation is the best form of treatment as long as the patient's systemic condition indicates a potential for high-quality survival. Patients with widespread systemic metastasis who are unlikely to survive more than a few months are best treated with dexamethasone alone.

The major benefit of aggressive surgery in patients with a *single brain metastasis* is for the quality of life that remains. Studies of evaluation of performance are compelling. Some of the best outcomes are in patients who present with non–small cell lung carcinoma and no other metastasis except for a single one in the brain ("solitary" brain metastasis) if both tumors are removed surgically. In patients with little, but potentially controllable, systemic tumor burden, the resection of a single metastasis is often worthwhile. However, no difference in mortality

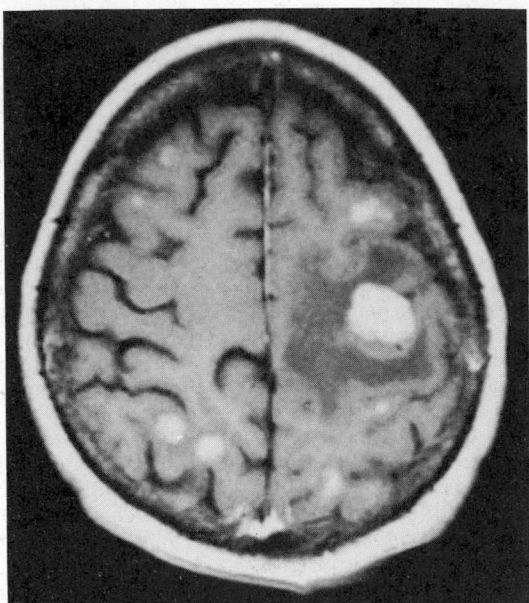

FIGURE 485–1. MRI scan, T_1 gadolinium, of multiple metastases from breast carcinoma. The tumors were not visible on CT, even after giving a contrast agent.

TABLE 485–1. METASTATIC BRAIN TUMORS

These tumors affect 10% of cancer patients (and still another 20% have dural meningeal involvement).

At least 50% are multiple.

If solitary (the only metastatic lesion in the body), surgery clearly provides best results in most cases. Surgery may be the best approach even if other metastases are present in patients in good condition.

Radiotherapy is useful palliation but not curative. Long-term survivors may have consequential side effects such as dementia.

at 2 years distinguishes patients who have been operated on from those who receive radiotherapy alone. This is because most patients with systemic metastases die of their systemic illness and not their brain metastasis.

Metastases to the dura and meninges are more common than generally recognized. Meningeal carcinomatosis manifests with headache, cranial nerve palsies, and stiff neck. These symptoms are due to the presence of tumor cells within the spinal fluid and to small deposits on the meninges around cranial nerves, at the base of the brain, and upon spinal roots. The diagnosis of meningeal carcinomatosis is made by cytologic examination of large-volume spinal fluid specimens. As many as three or more spinal taps may be needed to find the tell-tale cells in some cases. The spinal fluid protein level is generally elevated, and the glucose concentration may be low. The latter changes are sufficiently characteristic, in the absence of evidence of infection, to suggest the diagnosis. T_1 gadolinium MRI scanning may image the small deposits in the meninges. They are especially evident in the cauda equina even in the absence of clinical symptoms referable to lumbosacral nerve roots. The treatment of meningeal carcinomatosis includes irradiation of the brain and spinal cord, which usually provides benefit but rarely long remission. In patients with limited systemic metastases, intrathecal chemotherapy with methotrexate through an Ommaya reservoir is appropriate; occasional patients respond impressively. Most do not, however, and the effective treatment of meningeal carcinomatosis remains a difficult problem. In the future, the still experimental treatment of meningeal carcinomatosis with isotope-emitting radionuclides coupled to monoclonal antibodies may replace intrathecal chemotherapy.

Table 485–1 lists some key features of metastatic brain tumors.

PRIMARY EXTRA-AXIAL TUMORS

Meningiomas, acoustic neuromas, and pituitary adenomas are the most frequent in this group, which, by definition, are tumors that are not of the brain itself but of its coverings, the cranial nerves, and the adjacent structures. The primary extra-axial tumors differ from tumors of the brain in many ways. They are not of neuroectodermal origin, they are histologically unrelated, and most are truly benign, since they can be excised completely and cured. They exert effects upon the brain by pressure and only occasionally by actual invasion.

Meningiomas, which are growths of the fibroblast-like cells of the dura and arachnoid villi, account for about 15 per cent of all primary brain tumors. They occur more often in women. The biologic explanation is unknown, but the finding has stimulated interest in the presence of estrogen receptors in these tumors. Only a few causative factors are known. Meningiomas may occur

many years after radiation delivered to the head, in which setting they may be multiple. A relationship to head trauma has never been convincingly documented. Some examples follow a familial pattern. Such cases, as well as most apparently sporadic examples, are associated with a loss of a portion of chromosome 22.

Most meningiomas arise as solitary tumors in certain characteristic sites, such as over the cerebral convexities, attached to the sagittal sinus or at the base of the brain, attached to the dura of the sphenoid sinus, the olfactory grooves, or the region of the sella. In some of these areas, they may be difficult to remove completely without excessive risk and may recur slowly but repeatedly. Many meningiomas grow so slowly that serial CT or MRI images suggest no enlargement over many years. It is this slow growth that at times permits the brain to accommodate them with relatively modest symptoms even when the tumors are remarkably large (see Fig. 484–1). Many are detected incidentally. Small, asymptomatic meningiomas are often best watched by imaging studies at intervals; in the elderly, even large, asymptomatic ones may not require surgery.

Most *acoustic neuromas* consist of distinctive growths of Schwann cells (schwannoma) of the eighth cranial nerve. Almost all are unilateral and not apparently familial. Bilateral acoustic neuromas, which have a different tissue type, are rare, familial, and diagnostic of neurofibromatosis II. This autosomal dominant condition occurs with nearly 100 per cent penetrance in successive generations and derives from a gene deletion on chromosome 22.

Typically either form of acoustic neuroma grows on the nerve into a round mass just as the nerve emerges from the acoustic canal into the cerebellopontine angle. Some such tumors produce symptoms when they are extraordinarily small and confined within the canal. Others may go unsuspected until they grow to rather large size, filling the cerebellopontine angle and compressing the brain stem. Acoustic neuromas greatly surpass in frequency any other tumor of cranial nerves. Partial or complete nerve deafness is characteristic and is the usual presenting symptom. As acoustic neuromas gradually grow, they sequentially affect the fifth and then the seventh cranial nerves on the same side. When large, they cause cerebellar ataxia on the same side and, ultimately, symptoms of brain stem dysfunction. MRI scans accurately detect even very small acoustic neuromas. All patients who develop hearing loss in the middle years of life should be considered to have an acoustic neuroma until proved otherwise. Audiometry alone is suggestive but not diagnostic; caloric tests of labyrinthine function almost always show abnormalities, but the most efficient physiologic study is the auditory evoked response. Current microsurgical techniques yield remarkably good results, usually preserving the seventh nerve and, occasionally, preserving hearing as well.

Pituitary Adenomas

According to the hormones they produce, these tumors may cause endocrine symptoms, such as hypothyroidism, amenorrhea, galactorrhea, infertility, acromegaly, or Cushing's syndrome (Ch. 161). Null cell adenomas may manifest with the symptoms of hypopituitarism. With the exception of these hormonal impairments, early symptoms, if any, are usually limited to nonspecific headaches. As pituitary adenomas enlarge, they erode the sella turcica and extend above it to compress the optic nerves, eventually causing bitemporal visual field defects. Rare hemorrhages into large pituitary tumors can cause pituitary apoplexy, producing a characteristic syndrome that requires emergency decompression to preserve vision. Progressive headaches are usually the only warning of this catastrophic event.

Current endocrinologic and MRI techniques greatly facilitate the diagnosis of pituitary tumors, especially if 1-mm cuts and magnified views through the sella are obtained. Medical treatment with bromocriptine may be effective but is slow in yielding results. Its value can be determined by careful endocrinologic follow-up. The drug must be continued indefinitely. Only surgical removal can produce a cure. The safety and efficiency of transsphenoidal pituitary surgery warrant its consideration in all patients, including those with microadenomas that are confined to the sella and larger tumors that, in the past, could be approached only by a subfrontal craniotomy. Radiotherapy may be required in occasional patients who have large and incompletely removed macroadenomas.

Less common primary extra-axial tumors include *craniopharyngiomas*, related *suprasellar epidermoid cysts*, and *Rathke cleft cysts*. Although they reflect congenital abnormalities of the brain and most frequently become symptomatic in childhood, as many as one third can first appear in adult life, some as late as the sixth decade. In adults, craniopharyngiomas may compress the frontal lobes and are an infrequent cause of dementia. As a group, such tumors are almost always benign and surgically curable if they can be separated from adjacent parasellar structures, optic nerves, and hypothalamus. Pineal region tumors include *pineocytomas* and *pineoblastomas* derived from pineal parenchymal cells, as well as *teratomas* and *germinomas*. These two groups appear with about equal frequency, all having the capacity to be biologically aggressive, making them difficult to manage surgically. Characteristic symptoms and signs include increased intracranial pressure, paresis of upward gaze, pupillary dysfunction, convergence nystagmus, and hydrocephalus due to obstruction of cerebrospinal fluid outflow pathways. Precocious puberty occurs in young males, the result of destruction of the pineal by germinomas. The true pineal tumors may cause delayed puberty. Intracranial *chordomas*, tumors of residual notochordal tissue, are rare and usually arise within the skull at the base of the brain, on the clivus. They are regionally invasive and rarely can be controlled even with aggressive surgery and radiotherapy. *Lipomas* of the skull occur chiefly in midline structures, especially over the corpus callosum. *Arachnoid cysts* can arise anywhere on the surface of the brain; some grow to remarkable size. Most arachnoid cysts are incidental, cause no symptoms, and are best left alone. Their infrequency, as well as that of the other extra-axial tumors mentioned, stands in contrast to the frequency and clinical importance of meningiomas and acoustic neuromas (see Table 484–1).

PRIMARY INTRA-AXIAL TUMORS

This group comprises mainly tumors of the glioma family, including astrocytomas, oligodendrogliomas, ependymomas, medulloblastomas, less common neuroectodermal tumors, and primary brain lymphoma. They possess in common the quality of direct, invasive involvement of the substance of the brain, making them rarely curable by surgical excision owing to the difficulty or impossibility of defining their microscopic borders. Accordingly, gliomas are fundamentally malignant, although some may behave in an indolent manner.

Astrocytomas are the most common of the gliomas. Their cause is unknown, familial examples constituting only 1 per cent of cases. Astrocytomas have occurred as a late consequence of radiation to the head or skull. The most aggressive variant, *glioblastoma multiforme*, accounts for more than 50 per cent of all primary brain tumors. Glioblastoma (astrocytoma IV) is distinguished pathologically from the less aggressive *anaplastic astrocytoma* (astrocytoma II/III) on histopathologic grounds, and the two have important clinical differences. Glioblastoma is more common, is more characteristic of older age groups, and has a median survival time of less than 1 year even with aggressive treatment with surgery, radiotherapy, and chemotherapy. By contrast, patients with anaplastic astrocytoma have a median survival time of slightly more than 2 years. Age is an important variable for both of these tumors: The younger the patient, the better the prognosis. Glioblastoma in children, for example, has

a median survival of more than 2 years. In adults, men are affected more often than women. Anaplastic astrocytomas and glioblastoma occur in multicentric locations in about 5 per cent of cases. In these instances, they may be mistaken for multiple cerebral metastases or for primary brain lymphoma on imaging studies.

Glioblastomas and anaplastic astrocytomas produce a similar clinical picture, and CT or MRI images may be somewhat alike (Fig. 485–2). In most instances, the onset is relatively rapid and heralded by seizures, headaches, and focal neurologic deficits. A minority of patients with these tumors have relevant histories of seizures with onset years before; one assumes that such malignant growths evolve from long-existing, low-grade astrocytomas. Sequential genetic alterations occur in astrocytomas as they become more aggressive. Tissue culture studies show that a high proportion of glioblastomas have increased numbers of chromosome 7 and rearrangements or losses of chromosomes 9p, 10, 17p, and 22. A lower incidence of these abnormalities can be detected in anaplastic astrocytomas. These genomic changes may relate to the presence of an abnormal and possibly unique receptor to epidermal growth factor that is expressed on glioblastoma cells.

Low-grade astrocytomas can pursue a highly variable course, and many of them do not progress to malignancy. Indeed, some are extremely indolent in their growth, so that the median survival time of patients with low-grade astrocytomas is a full 7 years from the time of diagnosis. This prognosis means little in individual cases, however, because the course of these tumors is, as noted before, highly variable. In some patients, low-grade astrocytomas transform to glioblastoma within a few years, whereas other astrocytomas can remain indolent for 10 years or more. Many low-grade astrocytomas will have spread too extensively before diagnosis can be made to allow surgical resection (see Fig. 484–2). By contrast, smaller, favorably situated ones sometimes can be totally removed and the patient apparently cured. Paradoxically, astrocytomas associated with large cysts have a much better prognosis. This favorable circumstance occurs most often in the cerebellum in children and young adults but also in the cerebral hemispheres.

Low-grade astrocytomas, with or without cysts, are invariably solitary, though they may extend into several contiguous brain structures. Some may involve large adjacent areas of frontal and temporal lobe in one hemisphere. Others invade the brain stem, usually producing devastating symptoms and signs in children but sometimes pursuing a surprisingly indolent course in adults. Brain stem astrocytomas cannot be operated upon except in rare instances when they are exophytic. Most infiltrate the brain stem and enlarge it. In a similar way, optic nerve astrocytomas, an uncommon cause of vision loss that affects chiefly children, enlarge the optic nerves and may erode the optic foramina. They grow slowly, are sometimes associated with neurofibromatosis,

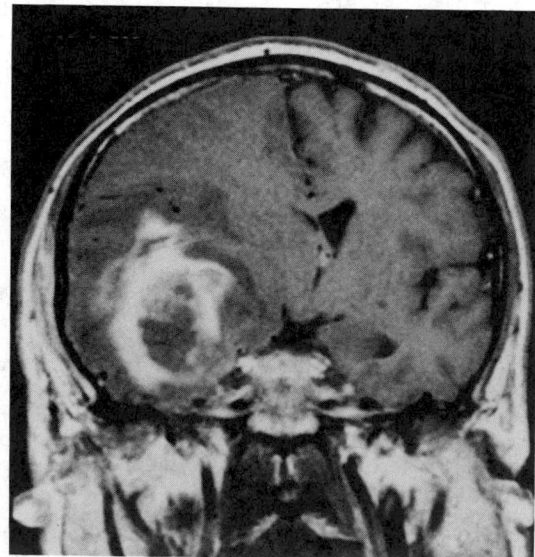

FIGURE 485–2. MRI scan, T_1 gadolinium enhanced, of a temporal lobe glioblastoma, showing typical ring configuration of contrast with central necrosis and marked mass effect.

and are often best left untreated until MRI scanning documents unequivocal tumor growth or vision declines. What to do at that point is controversial. Many authorities withhold radiation treatment for low-grade astrocytomas, at least until all other approaches fail and for as long as the quality of life can be maintained. Two important reasons support this position. One is that little well-controlled evidence indicates that radiation greatly shrinks these tumors, eradicates them, slows their growth, or prevents their conversion into malignant astrocytomas. The other, as already remarked upon, is that radiation damages the normal brain, producing selective neuronal injury, areas of radiation necrosis, or both.

Oligodendrogliomas are the most "benign" of the gliomas, although some develop anaplastic features. Their clinical manifestations usually are indistinguishable from those of low-grade astrocytomas. Seizures are an important early symptom. Oligodendrogliomas occur chiefly in the cerebral hemispheres and especially in the frontal lobes. Many contain flecks of calcium, demonstrable by brain imaging. Complete surgical resection is the therapeutic goal but often cannot be realized because of the size and location of the tumors. Despite their slow growth, most oligodendrogliomas respond well to chemotherapy. As many as 80 per cent improve with a regimen that combines procarbazine, CCNU, and vincristine. This response to chemotherapy seems to be superior to that observed with radiotherapy alone. Oligodendroglioma is the primary intra-axial tumor most likely to bleed spontaneously. In addition, anaplastic oligodendrogliomas tend to spread through the spinal fluid to the meninges. A few of these tumors eventually become so anaplastic that they histologically and clinically resemble glioblastomas.

Medulloblastomas occur chiefly in the region of the fourth ventricle and affect principally children and young adults. They cause characteristic symptoms of cerebellar and brain stem dysfunction. In children, aggressive surgery and radiotherapy yield a 5-year survival of 50 per cent, but many children treated in this manner suffer serious, permanent postradiation intellectual deficits. Several reports indicate that chemotherapy with cyclophosphamide and vincristine improves survival, and other drugs are being tried.

Medulloblastoma is characterized by an amplification of the *c-myc* oncogene and abnormalities of chromosome 17. Medulloblastomas arising in the cerebral hemispheres resemble, or may be the same as, *primitive neuroectodermal tumors* (PNET). These tumors are radiosensitive, like medulloblastomas of the fourth ventricle and cerebellum, and at times respond temporarily to aggressive chemotherapy.

Gangliogliomas are composed of neoplastic astrocytes and abundant dysmorphic neoplastic neurons. They occur chiefly in the temporal lobes of children and young adults, have an unusually slow growth rate, and may have a good prognosis even when untreated. Some are associated with tuberous sclerosis.

Primary brain lymphoma is increasing in frequency among both the acquired immunodeficiency syndrome (AIDS) and, for unknown reasons, the non-AIDS populations. These growths involve the brain diffusely, producing infiltrating and often multicentric tumors that tend to lie deep in the brain and adjacent to ventricular surfaces. Almost all of these tumors are B cell derived; the eye is the only other extranodal site that is regularly involved concomitantly. Only rare patients go on to develop systemic lymphoma, and that occurs late in the disease. Primary brain lymphoma is fundamentally unresectable. It responds temporarily to radiotherapy but is rarely cured. Steroids are an important component of treatment; dexamethasone is uniquely chemotherapeutic for this tumor. Median survivals of 3 years can now be expected with the addition of multidrug chemotherapy to radiotherapy.

Rare intra-axial brain tumors include *choroid plexus papillomas* and *carcinomas*, which are even less common than the benign but troublesome *colloid cysts* of the third ventricle. The last-mentioned lesion may cause hydrocephalus by blocking the outflow of cerebrospinal fluid from the lateral ventricle. *Capillary hemangioblastomas* arise in the cerebellum and elsewhere. They are sometimes associated with an autosomal dominant inherited disorder that includes retinal angiomatosis as well as cysts and tumors of the pancreas, kidneys, and adrenals (von Hippel syndrome). Some of these cerebellar capillary hemangioblastomas secrete erythropoietin and cause polycythemia.

Vascular malformations of the brain are more frequent and important than the above-named rare brain tumors and often can be mistaken for gliomas. They frequently manifest with nonhemorrhagic symptoms such as seizures. They sometimes resemble brain tumors in appearance on CT or MRI, and a distressing number, especially of the capillary variety (which lack large arteriovenous shunts), cannot be imaged by cerebral angiography. Many of these abnormalities lie in the brain stem and thalamus; because they are indistinguishable from brain tumors on even the best imaging studies, they may undergo biopsy as a diagnostic step, with devastating results. Vascular malformations of the brain involving large-caliber vessels are readily diagnosed by CT or MRI even without cerebral angiography.

Abscesses and *granulomas* of the brain cannot usually be distinguished from tumors by CT or MRI alone. If systemic evaluations fail to suggest a proper diagnosis, reliable management demands that biopsy be used. Even in the non-AIDS population, surprising alternatives to the clinical and radiologic diagnosis of a brain tumor are regularly revealed by biopsy. In many instances, potentially tragic errors of management can be avoided by taking a direct approach and studying the tissue of the intracranial lesion.

Fadul C, Wood J, Thaler H, et al.: Morbidity and mortality of craniotomy for excision of supratentorial gliomas. Neurology 38:1374, 1988. *A recent paper that documents convincingly the safety and efficacy of aggressive surgery for gliomas.*

Marks JE: Radiation treatment of brain tumors: Concepts and strategies. Crit Rev Neurobiol 5:93, 1989. *A short, clear, practical review.*

Patchell RA, Tibbs PA, Walsh JW, et al.: A randomized trial of surgery in the treatment of single metastasis to the brain. N Engl J Med 322:494, 1990. *An important paper, not only for its conclusion, which clearly supports surgery for a single metastasis, but also because it is an example of what careful clinical trials in neuro-oncology can achieve. Jerome Posner's editorial comments on this paper, and on metastasis in general, are in the same issue and are masterful.*

Russell DS, Rubinstein LJ: Pathology of Tumours of the Nervous System. 5th ed. Baltimore, The Williams & Wilkins Company, 1989. *The definitive text, indispensable, scholarly, complete, and beautifully redone by Professor Rubinstein just before his death in 1989.*

Shapiro WR: Brain tumors. Semin Oncol 13:1, 1986. *An issue devoted to the subject with wide-ranging and excellent review articles.*

Stewart DJ: The role of chemotherapy in the treatment of gliomas in adults. Cancer Treat Rev 16:129, 1989. *A comprehensive review with an exhaustive list of references.*

Vick NA, Bigner DD (eds.): Neuro-oncology. Neurol Clin 3:4, 1985. *A collection of excellent reviews of the important topics in the field, both clinical and in the basic sciences.*

486 Disorders of Intracranial Pressure

Nicholas A. Vick and David A. Rottenberg

INTRACRANIAL HYPERTENSION

GENERAL PRINCIPLES. Cerebrospinal fluid (CSF) pressure in excess of 250 mm CSF is usually a manifestation of serious underlying neurologic disease. Intracranial hypertension is most often associated with rapidly expanding mass lesions, CSF outflow obstruction, or cerebral venous congestion; however, a variety of systemic and central nervous system disorders may be accompanied by an increase in intracranial pressure (ICP) (Table 486–1). Lumbar CSF pressure may not accurately reflect ICP. In patients with intracranial mass lesions and brain herniation, lumbar CSF pressure may be normal or even low despite grossly elevated supratentorial CSF pressure. Kinking of the aqueduct of Sylvius by adjacent mass lesions, diencephalic–temporal lobe transtentorial herniation, or cerebellar compression of the fourth ventricle, with or without accompanying descent of the cerebellar tonsils into the foramen magnum, each can impede the free transmission of CSF into the lumbar subarachnoid space.

Headache is the principal symptom associated with intracranial hypertension. Headache is produced by traction on pain-sensitive

TABLE 486–1. PATHOGENESIS OF INCREASED INTRACRANIAL PRESSURE

Perturbation	Proximate Cause	Clinical Example
Increased dural sinus venous pressure	Sinus compression or occlusion	Sagittal sinus thrombosis Otitic hydrocephalus Brain tumors
	Increased sinus blood flow	CO_2 retention Arteriovenous malformation
	Increased peripheral venous pressure	Internal jugular vein occlusion Superior vena cava syndrome Congestive heart failure
Increased CSF outflow resistance	Ventricular outflow obstruction Obliteration of the cisternal and/or convexity subarachnoid space	Brain tumors Aqueductal stenosis Meningitis Extradural or subdural masses
	Plugging of the arachnoid villi	Cerebral masses or edema Subarachnoid hemorrhage Infectious polyneuritis Spinal cord tumors
Increased rate of CSF formation	Increased choroidal CSF formation Increased extrachoroidal CSF formation	Choroid plexus papilloma Hypo-osmolality Cerebral edema
Unknown	Increased cerebral volume Increased sagittal sinus pressure Increased CSF outflow resistance	Benign intracranial hypertension

cerebral blood vessels or dura mater lying at the base or, less often, the vertex of the brain. Focal neurologic signs reflect the presence of impending herniation with intermittent vascular compression, midline shift, or axial distortion of the brain stem (see Ch. 443). In the absence of such shifts, increased ICP alone may be asymptomatic. *Papilledema* is the most reliable sign of ICP; but in many patients with increased ICP, it fails to develop. Moreover, in some patients with benign intracranial hypertension, papilledema develops and then subsides spontaneously, although CSF pressure remains pathologically elevated. Papilledema is not synonymous with increased ICP. Ocular hypotony, bilateral optic neuritis, orbital venous stasis, retrobulbar tumors, granulomatous inflammation, or cystic lesions of the optic nerve sheath may produce inflammatory changes in the optic disc indistinguishable from the papilledema caused by the absence of intracranial hypertension. Most papilledema caused by intracranial hypertension, however, is bilateral, whereas most of these other causes affect only one eye at a time. Retinal venous pulsations, when present, imply that CSF pressure is normal or not significantly elevated, but their absence is not helpful diagnostically. Patients with increased ICP, often complain of worsening symptoms, particularly headache, in the morning, perhaps because plateau waves (spontaneous elevations of ICP) occur more commonly during sleep.

The initial treatment of any patient with increased ICP whose neurologic status is deteriorating is aimed at reducing the volume of the intracranial contents in an attempt to prevent brain damage (Table 486–2). If ICP approaches the systolic blood pressure, the cerebral perfusion pressure decreases and irreversible ischemia may develop. Some believe that head elevation and fluid restriction are useful; furosemide, barbiturates, antihypertensives, and muscle relaxants are often used. Almost always, ICP is not the actual cause of the patient's distress; the definitive treatment of intracranial hypertension is ultimately determined by the nature of the underlying pathologic process.

TABLE 486–2. EMERGENCY TREATMENT OF IMPENDING HERNIATION IN ACUTELY DECOMPENSATING PATIENTS

Therapy	Dosage or Procedure	Onset (Duration) of Action
Hyperventilation	Lower Pa_{CO_2} to 25 to 30 mm Hg	Seconds (minutes)
Osmotherapy	Mannitol, 0.5 to 2.0 gm/kg intravenously over 15 minutes, followed by 25 gm as needed	Minutes (hours)
Corticosteroids	Dexamethasone, 50 mg intravenous push, followed by 50 mg daily in divided doses	Hours (days)

Benign Intracranial Hypertension

Benign intracranial hypertension is a syndrome of increased ICP unaccompanied by localizing neurologic signs, intracranial mass lesion, or CSF outflow obstruction in an alert, otherwise healthy-looking patient. These patients are almost always obese and considerably more often women. Benign intracranial hypertension (also called pseudotumor cerebri, serous meningitis, or otitic hydrocephalus) may be associated with a variety of systemic and iatrogenic disorders (Table 486–3). The cause is usually unknown. Chronically increased ICP may give rise to the "empty sella syndrome," which refers to a radiographically globular enlargement of the sella turcica, an incompetent diaphragma sellae, and a compressed but functioning pituitary.

The diagnosis of benign intracranial hypertension is one of exclusion. Intracranial masses (tumors, hematomas, infections) and CSF outflow obstruction must be excluded by computed tomography (CT) or magnetic resonance imaging (MRI). Cerebral angiography is occasionally necessary to rule out dural venous

TABLE 486–3. SYSTEMIC AND IATROGENIC DISORDERS ASSOCIATED WITH BENIGN INTRACRANIAL HYPERTENSION

Commonly Prescribed Drugs
Nalidixic acid
Nitrofurantoin
Phenytoin
Sulfonamides
Tetracycline
Vitamin A

Endocrine and Metabolic Disorders
Addison's disease
Cushing's syndrome
Hypoparathyroidism
Levothyroxine therapy
Menarche, pregnancy, oral contraceptives
Obesity and irregular menses
Steroid therapy/withdrawal

Hematologic Disorders
Cryoglobulinemia
Iron deficiency anemia

Miscellaneous Disorders
Dural venous sinus obstruction/thrombosis
Head trauma
Internal jugular vein ligation
Lupus erythematosus
Middle ear disease

sinus or cortical venous thrombosis. Lumbar puncture, which is usually deferred until CT or MRI has revealed a normal or small ventricular system, is required to confirm the diagnosis. Lumbar spinal fluid pressure is elevated, frequently above 300 mm CSF, but the composition of the fluid is normal; the protein content is usually in the low normal range, below 20 mg per deciliter.

PATHOPHYSIOLOGY. In most cases, the causal mechanism is unknown. Chronically elevated ICP necessarily implies an increase in dural sinus venous pressure, an increase in CSF outflow resistance, an increase in the rate of CSF formation (if it ever really occurs), or some combination of these factors. One or more of these mechanisms must elevate the CSF pressure. Pathogenetic hypotheses that postulate an increase in brain bulk consequent on an increase in cerebral blood volume or in brain water content (interstitial brain edema) do not provide an adequate explanation. The constancy of obesity, often extreme, has suggested the possibility of a disorder of the hypothalamus. But no data have emerged to support this idea. Despite decades of knowledge of the association with obesity, the link remains completely obscure. The strikingly greater incidence in women than in men (4:1) is also unexplained but surely important in some way.

CLINICAL MANIFESTATIONS. Most patients complain of headache. Other common early symptoms include nausea and vomiting, visual disturbances (blurring, obscuration of vision, scotomata), retro-ocular pain, diplopia, tinnitus, and vertigo. Bilateral papilledema, the cardinal feature, is almost invariably present and may be associated with peripapillary retinal hemorrhages, exudates, or both. Vision loss, the only serious complication of benign intracranial hypertension, may occur either early or late in the course of the disease but is seen less than feared. Transient obscurations of vision do not predict subsequent failure of vision. Characteristically, visual field testing reveals enlarged blind spots. Generalized constriction of the peripheral isopters and inferior nasal quadrantanopsia are less frequently observed, as are central and paracentral scotomata. Diplopia, caused by unilateral or bilateral abducens palsy, may develop as a false localizing sign. The remainder of the neurologic examination is always normal. It is important to distinguish pseudopapilledema—an anomalous elevation of the optic disc—from true papilledema, which is prima facie evidence of increased ICP. Anomalous elevation of the disc, which may be associated with identifiable hyaline bodies (drusen), should suggest the diagnosis of retinitis pigmentosa.

In some instances, benign intracranial hypertension is a self-limited disease in which CSF pressure returns to normal as clinical symptoms remit over several months. However, clinical improvement is not always accompanied by a reduction in CSF pressure, and there is a vexing subgroup of patients whose pressure remains persistently elevated after neurologic signs and symptoms have resolved. The course of such cases implies that clinical symptoms may be independent of the absolute magnitude of CSF pressure and that chronically raised ICP may be totally asymptomatic. In addition, despite persistently elevated CSF pressure, patients do not become hydrocephalic. The ventricular system remains small, or no larger than normal. This finding suggests that whatever mechanism "resets" CSF pressure above normal does not predispose to the development of communicating hydrocephalus and that the two conditions are biologically unrelated.

TREATMENT. Unfortunately, no convincing evidence exists that any of the frequently recommended treatment modalities are regularly efficacious. The high rate of spontaneous remission complicates the evaluation of various therapies. At present, four general approaches to symptomatic treatment are used: (1) repeated lumbar puncture, (2) pharmacologic treatment, (3) ventriculosystemic or lumboperitoneal shunting, and (4) incision of the optic nerve sheath.

Frequent (such as alternate day), large-volume lumbar punctures may provide relief of symptoms and document the occurrence of remission. Either it is beneficial or remission occurs independently during the period of treatment. Corticosteroids and diuretics have been the mainstay of medical treatment, and both are effective; or, again, the disease remits during the period of treatment. Dexamethasone, furosemide, and acetazolamide are often tried. CSF shunting procedures are not without risk, and their long-term efficacy remains to be established. Incision of the optic nerve sheath for the relief of papilledema and vision loss is heroic and fortunately performed infrequently. Now and then, it is done because lumbar punctures, steroids, diuretics, and ventriculosystemic or lumboperitoneal shunting have failed in the rare patient with vision loss.

HYDROCEPHALUS

Hydrocephalus refers to the net accumulation of CSF within the cerebral ventricles and their consequent enlargement. Although acute obstructive hydrocephalus usually produces a sudden increase in intraventricular pressure, CSF pressure is frequently normal (or low) in patients with chronic hydrocephalus. It is customary to distinguish between "noncommunicating" and "communicating" hydrocephalus; the former is produced by lesions that obstruct the intracerebral CSF circulation at or proximal to the foramina of Luschka and Magendie, the latter by obstruction of the basal cisterns or convexity subarachnoid space in such a way that the ventricular system communicates with the spinal subarachnoid space but CSF cannot drain through the arachnoid villi into the superior sagittal sinus. Since both "noncommunicating" and "communicating" types of hydrocephalus are obstructive and both are treated by shunts, the distinction really has less meaning than that usually ascribed to it. Perhaps the important distinction should be between obstructive and nonobstructive hydrocephalus. Ventricular dilatation associated with severe cerebral atrophy, sometimes called "hydrocephalus ex vacuo," is the best example of nonobstructive hydrocephalus. It is so different from obstructive hydrocephalus that it is misleading to use the term hydrocephalus except in the setting of obstruction.

DIAGNOSIS. Hydrocephalus is easily diagnosed by CT or MRI. The diagnosis must take into account the increase in ventricular volume that accompanies normal aging and the presence or absence of cerebral atrophy. Enlargement of the temporal horns and an inability to visualize the sylvian and interhemispheric fissures or cerebral sulci, plus the presence of periventricular lucencies (CT) or periventricular hyperintensity (MRI), favor the diagnosis of hydrocephalus. A normal or small fourth ventricle in the presence of enlarged lateral and third ventricles suggests aqueductal stenosis.

ACUTE VERSUS CHRONIC HYDROCEPHALUS. Sudden, complete ventricular outflow obstruction leads to acute hydrocephalus, coma, and, if untreated, death; partial obstruction is more common and only moderately less dangerous (Table 486–4). Chronic hydrocephalus in the adult is most often caused by aqueductal stenosis or the complications of subarachnoid hemorrhage. Other reported causes and associations are listed in Table 486–4. In many instances, the cause of symptomatic chronic hydrocephalus ("normal-pressure hydrocephalus") cannot be determined. Unequivocally asymptomatic hydrocephalus may be found in approximately 4 per cent of patients over the age of 60 who consult a neurologist for assorted neurologic complaints and who undergo CT scanning.

CLINICAL MANIFESTATIONS. The patient with acute ob-

TABLE 486–4. CAUSES OF HYDROCEPHALUS

Acute
Cerebellar hemorrhage/infarction
Colloid cyst of the third ventricle
Exudative meningitis
Head trauma
Intracranial tumor/hematoma
Spontaneous subarachnoid hemorrhage
Viral encephalitis

Chronic
Aqueductal stenosis
Ectasia and elongation of the basilar artery (rare)
Granulomatous meningitis
Head trauma
Hindbrain malformations
Meningeal carcinomatosis
Brain and spinal cord tumors
Spontaneous subarachnoid hemorrhage
Syringomyelia

TABLE 486–5. CAUSES OF ABNORMALLY LOW (0–50 mm) CSF PRESSURE

Dehydration-hypovolemia
Cranial-intraspinal CSF block
Post–CNS surgery
CSF fistula
Post–LP drainage
Spontaneous-idiopathic; dural nerve sheath tear

structive hydrocephalus may have severe headache, lethargy, signs of increased ICP, papilledema, abducens palsy, and signs of the causative lesion. Hyperactive reflex and bilateral extensor plantar responses are almost invariably present. Ventricular CSF pressure is markedly increased, but if CSF pathways are blocked, this increase may not be transmitted to the lumbar subarachnoid space. Patients with chronic communicating hydrocephalus, including normal-pressure hydrocephalus, have a progressive dementia characterized by forgetfulness and psychomotor retardation, an unsteady gait, and urinary incontinence. Bilateral pyramidal and extrapyramidal signs may be present. Some patients have an overtly parkinsonian disorder. The lumbar CSF pressure is usually normal or nearly normal in range, although overnight recording of ventricular CSF pressure may reveal intermittent waves of elevated pressure.

TREATMENT. Acute hydrocephalus responds dramatically to ventricular drainage and CSF diversion. Treatment of the primary lesion is the treatment of choice, although temporary ventricular decompression or ventriculosystemic shunt may be necessary in some cases. Ventricular shunting has also been used for patients with chronic communicating hydrocephalus. Unfortunately, not all patients respond, or response may be delayed for weeks or months; moreover, there are no reliable clinical or neuroradiologic predictors of shunt response. Recent onset and mild dementia remain better predictors than does isotope cisternography. Absence of cerebral atrophy and temporary improvement after lumbar puncture seem to correlate with benefit from a shunt operation.

INTRACRANIAL HYPOTENSION

CSF pressure measured at a lumbar puncture site, with the patient in the lateral decubitus position, normally ranges from 70 to 200 mm CSF (5 to 15 mm Hg). Low or zero lumbar CSF pressure can be recorded under several circumstances, as indicated in Table 486–5. Symptoms of the first two or three circumstances on that list are likely to be dominated by the underlying illnesses. The remainder of the circumstances tend to cause a consistent syndrome characterized by severe, throbbing frontal and occipital headache, which usually appears within 30 seconds after the patient assumes an erect posture and which subsides completely upon the patient's lying flat. Associated complaints may include dizziness, nausea, stiff neck, photophobia, and, rarely, diplopia due to an associated abducens nerve palsy. The disorder often arises 3 to 21 days after lumbar puncture. The pathogenesis is similar to that of lumbar puncture headache (p. 2121).

Rare cases of CSF hypotension may occur spontaneously, producing, in previously healthy persons, symptoms similar to those already described. The onset can be acute or subacute and is occasionally precipitated by mild trauma, such as a fall on the buttocks or a casual bump to the head. The cause usually remains unknown, although spontaneous rupture of a dural nerve sheath has been postulated. Diagnosis can be difficult, since spontaneous pressure in the lumbar subarachnoid space can be zero, giving the false impression of missing the thecal sac. Treatment is symptomatic; spontaneous recovery usually requires days to a few weeks. When post–lumbar puncture symptoms are persistent, disabling, or both, an epidural "blood patch" may be indicated. The actual need for blood patches is far less than the frequency with which the procedure is done by worried physicians for impatient sufferers of post–lumbar puncture headache. This procedure involves the injection of 10 ml of the patient's own blood into the epidural space to seal a presumed dural leak. Rarely, in very long-lasting cases, surgical exploration has exposed the dural leak, which must be sutured.

Ahlskog JE, O'Neill BP: Pseudotumor cerebri. Ann Intern Med 97:249, 1982. A critical review of the clinical syndrome. The section on patient management is excellent.

Bell WE, Joynt RJ, Sahs AL: Low spinal fluid pressure syndromes. Neurology 10:512, 1960. A detailed clinical account of the neurologic manifestations of intracranial hypotension. A classic.

Corbett JJ, Savino PJ, Thompson HS, et al.: Visual loss in pseudotumor cerebri. Arch Neurol 39:461, 1982. This paper provides a detailed and definitive discussion of the only serious complication, vision loss.

Lyons HK, Meyer FB: Cerebrospinal fluid physiology and the management of increased intracranial pressure. Mayo Clin Proc 65:684, 1990. A superb review with excellent references.

Petersen RC, Bahram M, Laws ER Jr: Surgical treatment of idiopathic hydrocephalus in elderly patients. Neurology 35:307, 1985. A clinically oriented review of the indications for, risks of, and benefits to be expected from the surgical treatment of normal-pressure hydrocephalus.

Ropper AH, Kennedy SK: Neurological and Neurosurgical Intensive Care. 2nd ed. Rockville Md., Aspen Publishers Inc, 1988. Chapter 3 is a brief but excellent resource, with 129 well-chosen references, on all aspects of the treatment of intracranial hypertension.

SECTION FOURTEEN / INJURY TO THE HEAD AND SPINAL CORD

Lawrence F. Marshall

487 Head Injury

GENERAL CONSIDERATIONS

Head injury is a major public health problem. Not only is traumatic brain injury responsible for more than 50,000 deaths each year in the United States, but a veritable epidemic of less severe injuries results in long-term morbidity because of intellectual and behavioral changes. Although severe head injury is mainly a disease of the young, with its greatest frequency occurring between the ages of 15 and 30 years, it spares no age or socioeconomic group. Missile injuries, particularly gunshot wounds that penetrate the skull and brain, are more frequent in urban regions of economic and social decay but are far from confined to such areas.

Head injury includes a spectrum of pathologic changes with varying degrees of severity. Underlying almost all nonpenetrating brain trauma is diffuse axonal injury, a condition in which axons are either sheared at the time of impact or degenerate soon after because of irreversible traumatic or ischemic damage to the fibers. Superimposed upon such white matter changes are contusions, which represent hemorrhage mixed into the tissue, and hematomas, more focal collections of blood. Hematomas can occur on the external surface of the dura (extradural hematoma), under the dura and over the underlying brain (subdural hematoma), or within the substance of the brain (intraparenchymal hematoma). In mild and moderate head injury the frequency of surgical hematomas is low. As the degree of neurologic injury increases, however, the severity of diffuse axonal injury rises in almost direct proportion, as does the frequency of intracranial hematomas. Most severe head injuries are characterized by a mixture of pathologic changes consisting of a combination of contusion, diffuse axonal injury, and, in approximately 40 per cent of the cases, hematomas of a size needing surgical attention.

MECHANISM OF BRAIN DAMAGE

Damage to the brain as a result of traumatic injury occurs through a variety of dynamic processes. The impact, in addition to causing immediately variable degrees of abnormality, sets into motion a series of events which, if left uninterrupted, may result in much more severe changes in the tissues and even death. The last 15 years have made it increasingly apparent that primary damage to the brain that at first seems moderate and compatible with a good recovery in many cases may give way to the later development of intracranial hematoma or ischemic brain damage as a result of shock and/or hypoxia.

PRIMARY DAMAGE

Primary traumatic damage to the brain can be separated into three basic processes: (1) diffuse axonal injury (DAI), (2) brain contusion, and (3) intracranial hematoma. DAI always occurs in severe head injury and has a predilection for the brain stem, corpus callosum, and deep white matter. Experimental studies suggest that minor degrees of DAI probably occur in patients who suffer only a *concussion*, i.e., a transient loss of consciousness usually associated with no or minimal residua. With more severe head trauma, the number of areas and the severity of DAI increase proportionately. Some patients with almost immediately fatal injury have shown white matter injuries that completely interrupted long sensorimotor pathways at the cervicomedullary junction.

Brain contusions as shown in Figure 487–1 are common. Traumatic contusions can occur throughout the brain but are more frequent on the cortical surface and in the superficial white matter. Contusions vary in size from less than 2 to 3 ml to much larger lesions. Such areas of tissue injury are important for several reasons. First, they represent areas of at least partially irreversible damage to the brain. Depending on the size and location of the contusions, the consequences can range from undetectable to a dense hemiplegia or aphasia. Second, contusions may act as mass

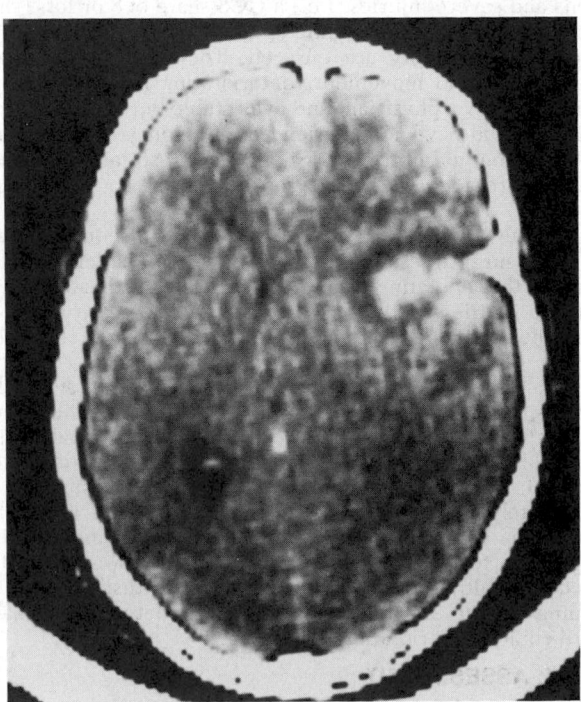

FIGURE 487–1. Brain contusion.

lesions because of the development of secondary edema in the surrounding tissues. Such mixtures of edema and hemorrhagic tissue may enlarge, progressively causing brain displacement and distortion.

The third type of primary injury to the brain, which can develop within hours or days following injury, is intracranial hemorrhage, resulting in epidural, subdural, or intraparenchymal hematomas.

Epidural hematomas usually result from moderate impact injuries. A baseball striking the head, an assault producing only a transient loss of consciousness, or a fall from a horse are typical precipitating events. Extradural hematomas characteristically follow fractures of the temporal bone associated with laceration of the middle meningeal artery. In some instances, the epidural hemorrhage may follow a fracture tearing one of the major draining venous sinuses of the brain. The clinical course of epidural hematoma is classically described as one of a transient loss of consciousness, followed by a period of lucidity and then a rather abrupt deterioration. Actually, this sequence occurs in only a minority of patients: Some lose consciousness immediately following impact, whereas others deteriorate abruptly without a history of initial loss of consciousness.

In the apparently minimally injured patient brought to an emergency room following an ostensibly minor head injury, skull radiographs considerably assist in triage. The absence of a skull fracture makes a hematoma sufficiently unlikely so that, with the exception of the elderly, it is usually safe to send the patient home. Elderly patients, who sometimes develop delayed, venous hematomas, or those with fractures should have computed tomography (CT) scans before being discharged. Such persons should be hospitalized for close observation if the neurologic examination is abnormal or if consciousness is altered in any way. The early detection of extradural hemorrhages is of utmost importance because most affected patients do not initially have irreversible brain damage.

Subdural hematomas are divided into three subgroups: acute, subacute, and chronic. An *acute subdural hematoma* almost always signifies severe brain injury and is associated with significant DAI and contusions in approximately 80 per cent of patients. Most patients with acute subdural hematomas are unconscious from impact, and half die. Nevertheless, approximately 20 per cent develop a more or less isolated subdural hematoma that can expand and cause abrupt deterioration. Recent studies have demonstrated that early surgery for acute subdural hematomas improves outcome, particularly in patients who show little other associated injury to the brain. The frequency of subdural hematomas increases with age, presumably because age-associated brain atrophy more readily allows the expansion of such venous bleedings. Most subdural hematomas are caused by laceration of the bridging veins that drain blood from the surface of the brain into the major sinuses or by laceration of cortical veins in the region of the sylvian fissure. Acute subdural hematomas are especially likely following assaults, falls (particularly in the elderly or in the alcoholic), and motor vehicle accidents when the head is decelerated suddenly on impact.

Subacute subdural hematomas consist of blood clots that underlie the dura on the surface of the brain, developing from 48 hours to 1 week following injury. Some must arise within a few hours of impact but do not reach a sufficient size to cause either depression of consciousness or a focal neurologic deficit. Patients with subacute subdural hematomas are usually older than age 50, occasionally have been taking anticoagulants, and usually have less serious head injuries than those with acute subdural hematomas. Only a small percentage are in coma when first seen and, if the hematoma is diagnosed promptly following its onset, most enjoy a good outcome.

Chronic subdural hematomas have distinct qualities. They usually occur between 1 and 6 weeks following injury, often bilaterally. Many follow trivial injuries, such as striking the head on a door, with no associated loss of consciousness. Indeed, affected patients often forget the inciting event. Patients with chronic subdural hematomas characteristically come from older age groups and many suffer from chronic illnesses, including alcoholism and dementia. Headache, worse in the morning, hypersomnolence or confusion, mild focal weakness, difficulty writing, and unsteadiness are common complaints. Chronic subdural hematomas, because of age-related shrinkage of the brain, may reach a substantial size in excess of 100 cc before the patient seeks medical attention. The mechanisms of this enlargement are poorly understood. Partly, they may be secondary to the development of an overlying capillary membrane which bleeds intermittently into the clot. In addition, tears in the arachnoid membrane may allow one-way entry of CSF from the subarachnoid space. The treatment is relatively straightforward. Some resolve spontaneously. For larger clots, a twist drill hole and puncture of the dura suffice for many patients. Many surgeons leave a drain in the subdural space to allow gravity drainage for 24 to 48 hours following evacuation of the clot. In some instances, particularly if CT scanning reveals an area of increased density, two burr holes are placed to allow irrigation of the subdural space. Craniotomy should be avoided if possible in elderly debilitated patients.

The third type of intracranial hematoma is the *intraparenchymal hemorrhage*, sometimes called intracerebral hemorrhage. These may vary in size from 1 to 100 ml, but they are usually considered for surgical drainage only when they exceed 15 to 20 ml. Intraparenchymal hemorrhages are usually caused by vascular disruption at the time of impact but may be exacerbated by arterial hypertension or coagulation disturbances, especially in alcoholic patients. Since hematomas generally enlarge by approximately 40 per cent during the first 24 hours after injury, those detected on a first CT scan but not operated on should be rescanned within 16 to 24 hours.

PREHOSPITAL CARE AND INITIAL RESUSCITATION

Head injuries often occur under circumstances that traumatize other organ systems as well. Fractures of the long bones and injuries to the chest and abdomen are common, particularly as a result of motor vehicle accidents or pedestrian-vehicle interactions. Until recently, concerns about secondary insults such as shock and hypoxia arose primarily among the more severely injured. Present evidence, however, indicates that even moderate levels of hypotension can convert a reversible brain injury to one with ischemic brain damage. Accordingly, immediate and adequate restitution of blood pressure and intravascular fluid volume and the institution of early steps to prevent or treat hypoxia represent essential preventive measures.

Utilization of the Glasgow Coma Scale (GCS) shown in Table 487–1 provides a simple and reproducible means for serially assessing the head-injured patient. This examination, which assesses the patient's ability to respond to pain, to speak, and to

TABLE 487–1. GLASGOW COMA SCALE

The Glasgow Coma Scale is a practical means of monitoring changes in level of consciousness, based upon eye opening and verbal and motor responses. The responsiveness of the patient can be expressed by summation of the figures. The lowest score is 3, the highest is 15.

Eyes open	Spontaneously (eyes open does not imply awareness)	4
	To speech (any speech, not necessarily a command)	3
	To pain (should not use supraorbital pressure for pain stimulus)	2
	Never	1
Best verbal response	Oriented (to time, person, place)	5
	Confused speech (disoriented)	4
	Inappropriate (swearing, yelling)	3
	Incomprehensible sounds (moaning, groaning)	2
	None	1
Best motor response	Obeys commands	6
	Localizes pain (deliberate or purposeful movement)	5
	Withdrawal (moves away from stimulus)	4
	Abnormal flexion (decortication)	3
	Extension (decerebration)	2
	None (flaccidity)	1
	Total Score	_____

open his or her eyes, when performed in concert with examination of the pupils, serves as an excellent field guide to the severity of injury. All four limbs must be tested for responsiveness either to verbal command or to pain in order not to overlook focal neurologic deficits, such as hemiparesis, paraparesis, or quadriparesis. Changes in pupillary responsiveness suggest brain stem compression, which must be detected early and dealt with promptly if treatment is to be successful.

Patients who cannot follow commands, do not open their eyes to noxious stimuli, and fail to utter words or comprehensible sounds are considered in coma (GCS score of 8 or less) and require early assurance of a secured airway. The frequency of shock and hypoxia increases in proportion to the severity of injury. Hypoxia occurs in approximately one third of all severe head injuries, and significant pulmonary shunting affects more than half. Because of these changes, early controlled intubation, often at the scene of the injury, is highly recommended for severe head injuries. Search for sources of hemorrhage is essential and should include the less obvious ones such as scalp lacerations and pelvic fractures. If such cannot be found, neurogenic hypotension should be suspected. Fluid resuscitation should begin at the scene, with recognition of the difficulties in administering large amounts of fluid under these conditions. Current evidence suggests that even with modern paramedic systems shock often receives inadequate treatment in the field and that newer strategies, utilizing hypertonic saline or pressor agents, may be required. Table 487–2 demonstrates the influence of shock on outcome in 699 head injury cases treated at four neurosurgical head injury centers. As noted, the presence of hypotension at outset almost doubled the mortality suffered by the entire cohort.

Once the airway has been secured and fluid resuscitation initiated, stabilization of the cervical spine and transport become the next priorities. In general, the neck should be placed in a neutral position. However, if the patient is awake and chooses to hold the neck in an unusual position, it should not be forced to the neutral position. Some patients with cervical spine fractures but no neurologic deficit have been made quadriplegic by ill-advised attempts to straighten the neck.

Upon arrival at the hospital the priorities of maintaining airway and circulation remain uppermost. Adequate oxygenation with a PaO_2 above 80 and moderate hyperventilation to $PaCO_2$ of 27 to 30 mm Hg to control brain swelling are initial objectives. A mean systolic blood pressure of at least 100 mm Hg is mandatory.

CT SCANNING

The availability of rapid-sequence CT scanning has revolutionized the care of the head injured. Patients with focal neurologic deficits and severe injuries, i.e., a GCS score of 8 or less, should receive immediate CT scanning as soon as a secured airway and hemodynamic stability are ensured. To minimize the risks of transportation and movement, deteriorating patients should be accompanied by a physician, and even stable but seriously injured patients should have an experienced emergency room or trauma nurse present at all times. Supervised respiratory assistance should assure adequate ventilation during transport and during the scan.

The results of CT scans heavily influence subsequent management. If a surgical lesion is demonstrated, the patient should be taken to the operating room immediately. Otherwise severe traumatic injuries are best treated in intensive care units, with lesser injuries being handled in units that provide close observation.

Several findings on the CT scan, other than intracranial hematomas, merit close attention and forewarn of possible deterioration. Compression or absence of the mesencephalic cistern augurs a high risk of intracranial hypertension and death, even in patients whose clinical examination at the time suggests only a moderately severe injury. Unilateral or bilateral hemispheric swelling almost always predicts the likelihood of dangerous intracranial hypertension. In patients showing such swelling or those who have multiple areas of hemorrhagic contusion, repeat CT scanning within 24 hours is essential to detect abnormalities before clinical deterioration takes place.

SERIAL ASSESSMENT

Close observation, with particular attention to the development of tachypnea and bradycardia, is important. Table 487–3 lists the

TABLE 487–2. OUTCOME RELATED TO SECONDARY INSULT AT TIME OF ARRIVAL AT HOSPITAL FOR MUTUALLY EXCLUSIVE INSULTS

Secondary Insults	Number of Patients	Per Cent of Total Patients	Outcome Percentages		
			Good–Moderate	*Severe–Vegetative*	*Dead*
Total cases	699	100.0	42.9	20.5	36.6
Neither	456	65.2	51.1	21.9	27.0
Hypoxia	78	11.2	44.9	21.8	33.3
Hypotension	113	16.2	23.7	14.2	60.1
Both	52	7.4	5.8	19.2	75.0

Hypoxia = Pao_2 <60 mm Hg; hypotension = SBP <90 mm Hg.

signs that portend potential intracranial catastrophe. An increase in systolic blood pressure of 15 mm Hg or more or a decline in heart rate of 15 beats per minute often gives the first hints of the development of an intracranial mass lesion.

Tachypnea holds particular importance. Respiratory rates over 20 per minute are abnormal in patients over 15 years of age and imply the development of pulmonary edema or infection. Similarly, increasing headache is often present but overlooked; it may reflect a rising intracranial pressure. The use of continuous flow sheets in an intermediate care setting or in a neurologic observation unit assists in monitoring the course and detecting subtle changes in vital signs.

THE INTENSIVE CARE MANAGEMENT OF THE SEVERELY HEAD INJURED

The overriding objective in the care of the severely head injured is to prevent further insults to the traumatized brain. The situation requires meticulous attention to detail and continuous vigilance to detect and counteract deterioration in hemodynamic, pulmonary, and neurologic function. The brain's vulnerability to secondary injury extends beyond shock and hypoxia. Fever increases the metabolic rate of the tissue by approximately 13 per cent for each degree Celsius, a demand that the already injured brain may not be able to meet. Seizures are a major threat—they increase tissue energy requirements and trigger a rise of up to 400 per cent in cerebral blood flow, accentuating any existing increase in the intracranial pressure.

The objectives in the critical care of head injury shown in Table 487–4 illustrate an approach that includes both the avoidance of systemic insults to the brain and the treatment of intracranial hypertension. Elevations of intracranial pressure above the normal of 15 mm Hg accompany most severe head injuries, and much evidence suggests that they contribute directly to further tissue damage if left untreated. Compression of the mesencephalic cistern, usually readily detected by CT scans and generally referred to as "diffuse swelling," is frequent in patients with even moderately severe injuries. Since mortality in such cases can be reduced from approximately 85 to 35 per cent with early and rapid intervention for intracranial hypertension, most academic neurosurgical centers record the intracranial pressure (ICP) continuously so as to treat intracranial hypertension whenever it develops. Several available techniques are discussed in the references to this chapter.

ICP monitoring should not be initiated in patients with coagulation disturbances. Patients in whom multiple contusions can be detected by a first CT scan can be assumed to have a trauma-related coagulopathy that will correct itself within a few hours, after which a ventricular cannula can be inserted.

The treatment of *traumatic intracranial hypertension* is central to the intensive care of the critically brain-injured patient. The cornerstone of management is to deliver moderate hyperventilation, maintaining a $Paco_2$ in the 27 to 32 mm Hg range so as to obtain moderate intracerebral arterial vasoconstriction. Levels of more extreme hyperventilation may be counterproductive by producing excessive vasoconstriction. The head should be maintained in a neutral position because turning it to the right or left may introduce venous obstruction and a rise in ICP. Also, the head should be elevated to not more than 30 degrees. Intravascular volume must be maintained using balanced salt solutions. Dextrose and water should be avoided. Head trauma often induces salt retention initially so that half-normal saline may be

TABLE 487–3. SIGNS OF POTENTIAL INTRACRANIAL CATASTROPHE AND WHAT THEY MAY SIGNIFY

Signs	Changes	Implications
Respiration	Rate >20	Pulmonary edema or pneumonitis
Pulse	Change >10/min and/or heart rate <60	Each may indicate elevated ICP with transtentorial herniation
Blood pressure	Change in systolic >15 mm Hg and/or widening pulse pressure	
Headache*	Is it increasing?	Often indicates increased ICP
Pupils	Enlargement Asymmetry Irregular shape (oval) Decrease in reactivity Change from preresuscitation	Transtentorial herniation until proven otherwise
Motor	Decrease of 1 point on GCS New focal deficit	Increased mass effect New hemorrhage Recurrent hemorrhage
Level of consciousness	Abrupt decrease	Increased ICP Seizures Hypotension
	Transient	Seizures Hypoxia
	Progressive decrease	Rehemorrhage Brain stem involvement Septicemia Electrolyte imbalance Vasospasm Hydrocephalus

*All changes except headache may occur in both awake and unconscious patients. GCS = Glasgow coma scale; ICP = intracranial pressure.

TABLE 487-4. ICU MANAGEMENT OF SEVERE HEAD INJURY AND INTRACRANIAL HYPERTENSION

1. Head elevated 30 degrees and in neutral plane
2. Intubation with controlled ventilation to an arterial $PaCO_2$ of 27–30 mm Hg
3. Good pulmonary toilet
4. Maintain fluid balance with 0.5 normal saline
5. Maintain systolic arterial pressure between 100 and 160 mm Hg
6. Maintain cerebral perfusion pressure >70 mm Hg (CPP = MAP − ICP)
7. Adequate sedation
8. Muscle relaxants prn (must use sedation concurrently)
9. Maintain normothermia
10. Adequate anticonvulsant therapy
11. Ventricular drainage for intracranial hypertension
12. Mannitol, 0.25 mg/kg, if No. 11 fails or is not available
13. Hypnotic for elevated ICP in patients with diffuse or hemispheric swelling

most useful to meet fluid needs. Since hyperglycemia exacerbates ischemic brain injury in experimental animals and there is an important component of ischemia in many patients suffering head injury, it appears wise to avoid glucose infusions.

Muscle relaxants with vecuronium or other short-acting agents may be helpful in controlling ICP, but should not be used without adequate sedation. Morphine sulfate by continuous infusion of 2 to 8 mg per hour is the least complicated and most effective regimen. Details of ventricular drainage and other specialized techniques for controlling dangerous levels of intracranial pressure are discussed in the references to this chapter.

Anticonvulsants have a limited but important use in acute traumatic head injury. Temkin et al. found that phenytoin given for the first 7 days after injury reduced the incidence of post-traumatic epilepsy during that period, but no study has shown a protective effect when medication was continued beyond the first week.

THE LONG-TERM CONSEQUENCES OF SEVERE HEAD INJURY

Severe head injury causes serious long-term intellectual and behavioral impairment. Most such patients suffer from residual difficulties in recent memory, abstract thinking, and the rapidity of information processing. Depression, fatigue, and impetuosity accentuate these cognitive deficits. By contrast, long-term deficits of motor function are relatively uncommon and considerably less socioeconomically important. Many rehabilitation programs have been developed to assist the severely head injured in the management of these problems. Therapies tailored to individual needs often favorably influence the long-term outcome and can be cost-effective if appropriate objectives are defined early and the program is appropriately structured. Counseling of the family is essential. Divorce, suicide, and spouse abuse are common eventualities but can be reduced in frequency by early intervention.

MINOR HEAD INJURY

Minor head injury is defined as including a GCS score of 13 to 15 following emergency room or hospital admission combined with a return to a normal level of consciousness within 24 hours. Most but not all such patients have normal CT scans. Patients suffering minor head injuries characteristically experience early post-traumatic problems with recent memory, concentration, and abstract thinking. In most patients such problems subside within the first 1 to 3 months following minor injury, although approximately 15 per cent are left with cognitive deficits that, although improved, do not completely remit. Age is a specific risk factor, and many elderly persons develop chronic dizziness and disequilibrium after even minor trauma. Such symptoms are classified as a *post-traumatic or postconcussive syndrome*. Past medical opinion has regarded such symptoms as psychogenic or prompted by hopes for secondary gain. Recent evidence fails to support such associations and indicates that a small percentage of patients suffer modest but permanent residual cognitive impairment.

Many patients with minor head injuries suffer transiently from insomnia, depression, and headache. Early support and reassur-ance from the physician often improve these symptoms. If headache persists for more than 60 to 90 days, propranolol, 30 to 60 mg in three divided doses, may bring relief.

MODERATE HEAD INJURY

Patients who have not been rendered comatose by their injuries but have a depressed level of consciousness for several hours or days following injury are classified as having suffered moderate head injuries. These patients have GCS scores of 9 to 12. Such patients almost always suffer measurable cognitive and behavioral difficulties over the long term. Nevertheless, many eventually return to gainful employment. Even so, the potential for social disruption is high, and traits of impetuousness and heightened irritability often create socioeconomic problems. Depression is frequent and may respond to tricyclic antidepressants. Intervention, using a variety of psychological services including social workers and psychiatrists, has a more favorable impact if carried out early rather than after the problems have overwhelmed the patient and family.

Cooper P (ed.): Head Injury, 2nd ed. Baltimore, Williams & Wilkins, 1987. *A modern definitive discussion of head injury.*
Levin HS, Eisenberg HM, Benton AL: *In* Levin HS (ed.): Mild Head Injury. New York, Oxford University Press, 1989. *A comprehensive review of the sequelae of minor and moderate brain injury.*
Marshall SB, Marshall LF, Vos H, Chesnut R: Neuroscience Critical Care: Pathophysiology and Patient Management. Philadelphia, W. B. Saunders Co., 1990. *Particular emphasis on assessment of the neurologically impaired patient, modern neuroradiology, and intensive care.*
Stein SC, Ross SE: The value of computed tomographic scans in patients with low-risk head injuries. J Neurosurg 26:638, 1990. *Incidence of CT abnormalities in the patient with minor head injury.*

488 Spinal Cord Injury

The cervical spine sacrifices bony mass in order to allow tremendous flexibility and rotatory capacity. In contrast, the lumbar spine is ideally designed for its major function of weight bearing. Modern modes of transport and recreation have made the spine and its encased spinal cord particularly vulnerable to injury. Fortunately, most injuries to the spinal column do not result in spinal cord injury, but there are still approximately 35 spinal cord injuries per million Americans each year. In addition to the neurologic deficit that such injuries can produce, they often result in persistent and severe pain and, if not treated properly, bony deformity. The mortality rate of spinal cord injury has fallen to less than 5 per cent, so that long-term survival is now the rule. Associated with this, however, are tremendous costs stemming from medical treatment, lost occupations, and the need for life-long medical and emotional support systems for many paraplegics and nearly all quadriplegics.

NATURE OF THE INJURY

About half of all serious spinal injuries affect the cervical level, with nearly 50 per cent of such cases becoming quadriplegic. Next most frequent is high thoracic cord damage, with the remainder distributed variously at lower spinal levels. Three major abnormalities damage the tissue: destruction from either direct trauma, e.g., gunshot wounds, or secondary bone displacement; compression by displaced or broken bones; and ischemia due to compression or laceration of spinal arteries. Postinjury edema of both spinal soft tissues and the cord itself accentuates these changes. Reversal or prevention of such post-traumatic alterations may explain the beneficial effects of methylprednisolone mentioned below.

Spinal cord injuries can be categorized as complete or incomplete. Acute, complete injuries most often produce acute *spinal shock*, with loss of all sensorimotor functions including flaccidity and loss of reflexes at and below the level of injury. A few such cases may show sustained priapism. Less severe injuries can produce a *central cord syndrome* resulting from ischemia or hematomas of the cervical cord (Fig. 488–1), resulting in a syringomyelia-like clinical syndrome characterized by weakness in the distal upper extremities combined with impaired or lost pain and temperature sensations in the arms but sparing of touch and often of all functions below the cervical cord level. The upper extremity weakness generally improves in such cases. Other patterns of cord injury may produce an anterior spinal artery syndrome (see Ch. 493) or can result in partial hemisection, producing distal weakness and proprioceptive loss ipsilateral to the cord damage accompanied by contralateral pain and temperature impairment.

EMERGENCY MANAGEMENT

For the physician and internist, the most important elements in treating traumatic spinal cord injury arise at the scene of the accident or within the first few hours of arrival at the hospital. After that time, effective management increasingly depends on experienced neurosurgeons or orthopedists, supplemented if at all possible by the resources of a tertiary care center equipped to meet the needs of acute paraplegic or quadriplegic injuries.

At the site of injury three major concerns are paramount: maintenance of ventilation, protection against shock, and neck immobilization to prevent further spinal cord damage.

Damage to high thoracic or cervical spinal levels creates the immediate risk of ventilatory failure due to acute paralysis of intercostal-abdominal muscles, loss of diaphragmatic activity, or both. Untoward movement of the neck in such patients risks converting a partial injury to a complete one, making nasotracheal intubation preferable to standard orotracheal intubation. Tracheostomy or cricothyroidotomy should be avoided if possible because these procedures often put pressure on the vertebral column.

Severe hypotension often follows cervical injury because the lesion interrupts the descending sympathetic pathways; bradycardia characteristically accompanies the low blood pressure. Such neurogenic hypotension can be distinguished from hypovolemic shock by the tachycardia of the latter. In either case, the legs should be elevated gently to improve venous return and fluids delivered in amounts sufficient to counter both the traumatic and neurogenic aspects of the problem. It is not widely realized that severe hypotension during the early minutes or hours after injury is itself a potential cause of spinal cord damage.

The neck and spine should be immobilized as gently as possible at the injury site, using a carrying board, sandbags and adhesive tape, or a Philadelphia collar. Soft collars are ineffective. The head is best maintained in a neutral position but should not be forced into such an attitude lest the maneuver induce further spinal cord damage.

Recent controlled studies indicate that giving large doses of methylprednisolone within 8 hours of the onset of trauma appears to reduce the degree of eventual neurologic dysfunction in acute traumatic paraplegia. Dose levels used in the study trial included immediate intravenous administrations of 30 mg per kilogram of body weight of the steroid followed by continuous infusion of 5.4 mg per kilogram per hour for the next 23 hours. Treatment begun more than 8 hours after injury was not helpful.

HOSPITAL CARE

The medical care of spinal cord injuries is a specialty unto itself. Such patients often are critically ill owing to a combination of systemic injuries, blood and fluid loss, various fractures, and infections. Considerable expertise is required for the accurate interpretation of spinal radiographs. Patients with cervical fracture-dislocations usually are placed in strong traction prior to administering definitive surgical repair. Usually, the latter step is deferred until patients regain a stable medical course. Injuries to the thoracic or lumbar level provide an exception to this principle; since traction has little benefit, open surgery, when indicated, usually is carried out earlier.

Medical management of spinal injuries emphasizes the guiding principles of trauma care. Rotating beds reduce the risk of decubitus erosions, meticulous chest physiotherapy and pulmonary toilet can minimize lung complications, and cardiovascular as well as fluid-electrolyte stability requires continuous attention. Pneumatic antiembolism stockings, vigorous fluid replacement, and early mobilization have reduced the frequency of deep venous thromboses in such patients by one third. Anticoagulants should be considered for severely immobilized patients who do not require early surgery. Nearly all patients with traumatic cord injury require prolonged urinary bladder catheterization. Meticulous effort to prevent infection should be applied from the start and, whenever staff experience permits, indwelling catheters should be replaced by intermittent catheterization at 4- to 6-hour intervals. Acidification of the urine with vitamin C or cranberry juice helps to reduce the incidence of infection.

Trauma patients require heavy nutrition to feed the demands of wound healing and the efforts of rehabilitation. For those who cannot eat, enteral solutions sufficient to meet caloric need can be started within 3 to 4 days after injury. Every effort should be given to supplying appetizing food and vitamins subsequently.

Autonomic dysfunction complicates the convalescence of more than half of patients who suffer severe spinal cord injuries above the midthoracic level. Disconnected distal autonomic pathways can induce a variety of troublesome phenomena, including systemic hypertension, reflex sweating, skin flushing, headache, and painful flexor spasms of the lower extremities. Bladder distention and infection are frequent factors producing such reflex dysautonomia and require urgent treatment. Diazepam, in small doses initially, and baclofen given chronically may be useful for the treatment of reflex spasms. Some centers have successfully employed the continuous intrathecal administration of baclofen by an indwelling pump to prevent disabling reflex spasms of this type.

PHYSICAL AND OCCUPATIONAL THERAPY AND REHABILITATION

Almost all patients with spinal cord injury require prolonged postacute care. Those with complete transections have suffered a devastating injury with life-long functional and psychiatric con-

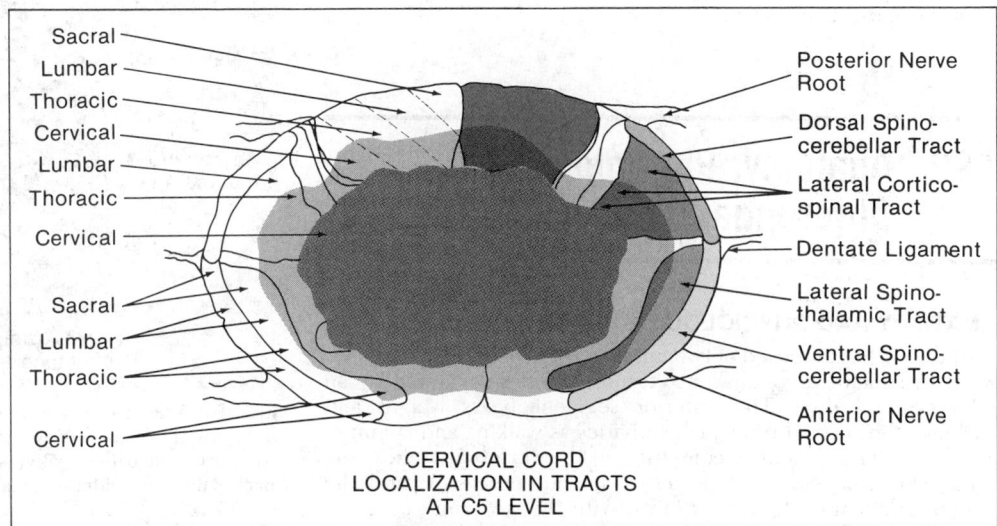

FIGURE 488–1. Diagrammatic description of the spinal pathways at the lower cervical level showing the usual distribution of the contusion-hemorrhage that causes a central cord syndrome.

Sacral
Lumbar
Thoracic
Cervical
Lumbar
Thoracic
Cervical
Sacral
Lumbar
Thoracic
Cervical

Posterior Nerve Root
Dorsal Spinocerebellar Tract
Lateral Corticospinal Tract
Dentate Ligament
Lateral Spinothalamic Tract
Ventral Spinocerebellar Tract
Anterior Nerve Root

CERVICAL CORD
LOCALIZATION IN TRACTS
AT C5 LEVEL

sequences. Early physical and emotional therapy is critical in minimizing these effects. Early range of motion prevents contractures, diminishes the risk of venous thrombosis, protects the skin, and boosts morale. A comprehensive and individualized management plan is essential. Patients and family members must be counseled in detail about probable changes in lifestyle. All of these features are best carried out in experienced rehabilitation centers that can provide assistance in home modification, driver retraining, and vocational rehabilitation. Depression following an initial period of denial occurs in almost all patients and may be masked by jocularity. If the rehabilitation team moves quickly to provide emotional as well as physical management, many patients with spinal cord injury can return to a competitive place in modern society. Most of the injured do best if a single physician organizes the long-term aspects of urinary tract management, skin care, sexual problems, and emotional-vocational needs.

Bracken MB, Shepard MJ, Hellenbrand KG, et al.: A randomized, controlled trial of methylprednisolone or naloxone in the treatment of acute spinal cord injury. N Engl J Med 322:1405, 1990. *The first study to clearly demonstrate the efficacy of pharmacologic treatment for spinal cord injury.*

Cooper PR: Management of posttraumatic spinal instability. *In* Neurosurgical Topics. Park Ridge, IL, American Association of Neurological Surgeons, 1990. *Detailed, step-by-step management of spinal cord injury.*

Marshall LF, Knowlton S, Garfin SR, et al.: Deterioration following spinal cord injury. A multicenter study. J Neurosurg 66:400, 1987. *A demonstration that most patients have an identifiable cause of deterioration.*

Temkin NR, Dikmen SS, Wilensky AJ, et al.: A randomized, double-blind study of phenytoin for the prevention of post-traumatic seizures. N Engl J Med 323:497, 1990. *Four hundred and four patients with serious head trauma were randomly assigned to treatment with phenytoin or placebo within 24 hours of injury; significant reduction in seizure incidence (p < 0.001) occurred only between drug loading time and day 7.*

SECTION FIFTEEN / MECHANICAL LESIONS OF THE SPINE AND RELATED STRUCTURES

Jerome B. Posner

The vertebral column, its contents (spinal cord, exiting nerve roots) and surrounding structure (spinal ligaments, paraspinous muscles) are responsible for some of the most common afflictions of man. Neck and/or back pain originating from these structures affects almost every individual at some time of life. Each year 4 per cent of Americans suffer an episode of low back pain. The disorder ranks next to alcoholism as the leading cause of time lost from work. More than 200,000 spinal operations are performed in the United States annually.

Most back and neck pain is transient and neither life-threatening nor associated with obvious pathologic abnormalities. However, in the few patients who suffer from serious structural disease of the spine or spinal cord, severe neurologic abnormalities may develop which, unless correctly diagnosed and treated, may lead to paralysis, sensory loss, and incontinence. Because the pathophysiology of most neck and back pain is poorly understood, the physician often encounters patients in whom he can neither make a certain diagnosis nor prescribe rational therapy. From this vast group he must cull the small number of patients suffering potentially remediable structural disease of the spine so that appropriate treatment can be instituted before permanent neurologic damage occurs.

489 Anatomy, Physiology, and Differential Diagnosis

ANATOMY AND PHYSIOLOGY OF THE SPINE

The spine is composed of two functional segments. The *anterior segment* contains two adjacent vertebral bodies separated by an intervertebral disc. The anterior segment bears weight and cushions the spine during such activities as walking and running. The posterior segment is composed of the vertebral arches, the transverse processes, the posterior spinous processes, and the paired articulations known as *facets* with the facet joint between

them. The *posterior segment* is non–weight-bearing but protects the contained spinal cord and nerve roots and allows the spine to move in extension and rotation. The midcervical and lower lumbar levels are particularly mobile, making them susceptible to mechanical disorders such as osteoarthritis and herniated discs (see Ch. 490). Several ligaments offer the spine passive support and paravertebral muscles support the spine actively by voluntary and reflex contraction.

Only parts of the spine are pain-sensitive (Fig. 489–1). The *periosteum* of the vertebral body is pain-sensitive so that compression fractures are at least initially painful. The *intervertebral disc* is probably not pain-sensitive. However, if the disc bulges and compresses the outer layers of the annulus fibrosus or the posterior longitudinal ligament, pain may result even if the nerve root is not involved. Posteriorly, the synovium-lined *facet joints* are pain-sensitive and may be an important source of neck and back pain, although the intraspinal ligaments holding the poste-

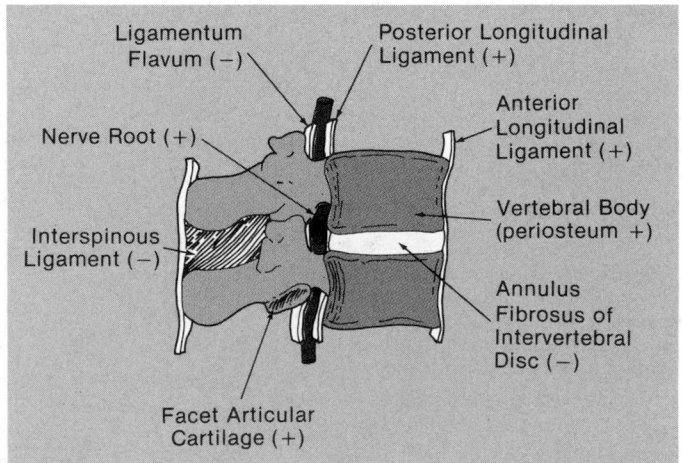

FIGURE 489–1. Pain-sensitive structures of the spine. This lateral view indicates the pain-sensitive structures with a plus sign (+) and those structures not pain-sensitive with a minus sign (−). (From Posner JB: Back pain and epidural spinal cord compression. Med Clin North Am 71:185–205, 1987.)

rior elements are not. Most of the pain-sensitive structures are innervated by the recurrent meningeal or sinuvertebral nerves, a branch of each spinal nerve that arises just distal to the dorsal root ganglion and re-enters the spinal canal through the intervertebral foramen. The sinuvertebral nerves also receive fibers from neighboring grey rami or directly from thoracic sympathetic ganglia. *Sympathetic nerves* contain sensory fibers and probably play a role in the transmission of pain. The *paravertebral muscles* surrounding and supporting the spine are also pain-sensitive, particularly when overstretched or in spasm. These muscles are probably the most common source of both acute and chronic neck and back pain (myofascial pain syndromes). The pain-sensitive *nerve root* usually occupies only a small portion of the intervertebral foramen through which it exits the spinal canal. When the spine is extended (i.e., hyperlordotic posture), the intervertebral foramen becomes smaller, potentially impinging on the nerve root and leading to overlap of the facet joints, giving potential irritation of pain-sensitive synovial membranes. Thus, pain in patients with intervertebral disc or facet joint disease may be exacerbated by extension and relieved somewhat by flexion of the spine. Additionally, hyperlordosis, a common postural abnormality, sometimes leads to chronic low back pain; most back exercises aim at developing a flat or slightly flexed, but not hyperlordotic, lumbar spine.

The spinal cord and its attached motor, sensory, and autonomic nerve roots are the primary occupants of the spinal canal. The spinal cord itself extends in the adult from the first cervical to the first lumbar vertebral body, and the spinal roots continue in the subarachnoid space to the second sacral vertebra. The caudal portion of the spinal cord is called the *conus medullaris*, and the bunched lumbar and sacral roots that exit below the cord are the *cauda equina*.

Within the canal several processes can compress or deform the spinal cord and its roots. The resulting signs and symptoms depend on the location of the abnormality, its speed of development, and whether it affects the nerve roots or the spinal cord alone. In the cervical spine, the spinal cord and vertebral segments lie at approximately the same level; thus, the C5 vertebral body marks the C5 spinal segment and emerging nerve roots are virtually horizontal. The more caudad spinal cord segments and vertebral segments move out of alignment so that thoracic spinal cord segments gradually become two to three levels higher than the corresponding vertebral segments (e.g., T8 vertebral body marks the T11 thoracic segment). Most of the lumbar and sacral cord is found between T10 and L1 lumbar segments. As a result, the nerve roots travel a descending pathway in the subarachnoid space before exiting via the vertebral foramen. In addition, because there is a C8 spinal segment and no C8 vertebral body, cervical spine nerve roots exit above the vertebral body with the same number (e.g., the C4 root exits between C3 and C4). Thus, a herniated C4–C5 disc may compress the C5 or C6 root but not the C4 root.

In the thoracic and lumbar spine, nerve roots leave the intervertebral foramen above the disc (e.g., the L4 root exits between L4 and L5 and the S1 root between L5 and S1) so that a herniated disc between L4–L5 vertebral bodies usually compresses the L5 nerve root; a herniated disc between L5 and S1 usually compresses the S1 root (Fig. 489–2). If the disc protrudes medially (less common than laterally protruding discs), an L4–L5 disc may compress sacral roots rather than the L5 lumbar root. Only if the disc completely extrudes into the vertebral canal does an L4–L5 disc compress the L4 root.

The size of the vertebral canal relative to the spinal cord varies from level to level and among persons. There is generally more space in the lumbar and cervical areas than in the thoracic area. Thus, herniated thoracic discs (uncommon) are more likely to cause myelopathy than cervical or lumbar herniations. In some individuals the spinal canal is congenitally small (spinal stenosis). Disc herniation or osteoarthritis is more likely to cause myelopathy in these individuals than in those with capacious canals.

TYPES OF PAIN

The cardinal symptom of lesions of the spine or its contents is pain. The type and location of pain often help substantially in diagnosis.

LOCAL PAIN. Local pain results from the irritation of nerve

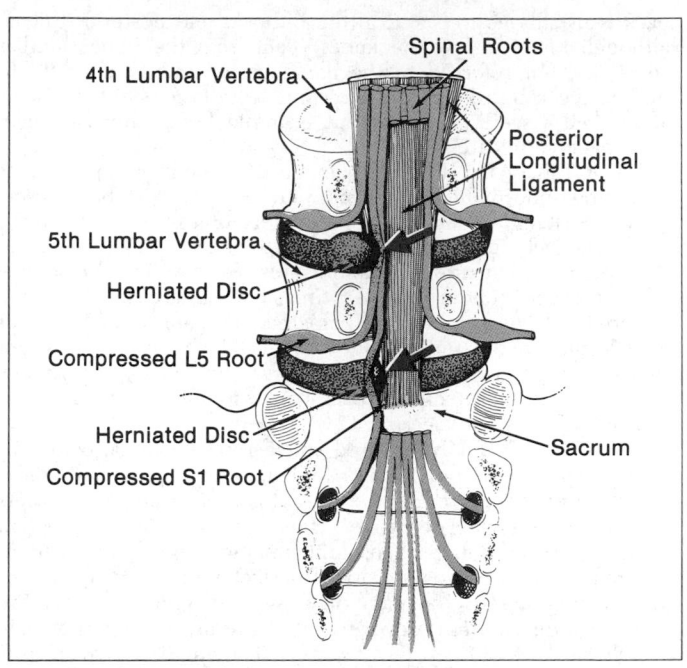

FIGURE 489–2. Nerve root compression by herniated disc. The figure illustrates that the posterior longitudinal ligament tapers as it reaches the lower lumbar area, leaving a weakened area laterally allowing disc herniation. An L4–L5 disc is shown lateral to the L5 root, displacing it medially; a herniated disc between L5 and S1 displaces the root laterally. (From Posner JB: Back pain and epidural spinal cord compression. Med Clin North Am 71:185–205, 1987.)

endings at the site of the pathologic process. Metastatic tumors and osteoporotic collapse of a vertebral body cause pain at the site of the lesion by irritation of nerve endings in the periosteum surrounding the vertebral body. Metastatic tumors involving the vertebral body that do not distort the periosteum are usually painless. Intervertebral discs cause local pain when they compress nerve endings in the anulus fibrosus or posterior longitudinal ligament. Local pain is usually steady and aching but may be intermittent, occurring particularly when the involved structure is moved. Local pain is usually associated with tenderness to palpation or percussion. The site of local pain is diagnostically helpful. Most spine pain from mechanical causes (e.g., herniated disc) occurs either in the neck or low back, since these structures are most mobile and more subject to injury. However, tumors often strike the thoracic area, and osteoporotic vertebral collapse often affects the structurally weaker thoracic vertebral bodies.

The *character* of the local pain is helpful diagnostically. Pain caused by lumbar muscle or ligamentous strain or by herniated disc usually disappears when the patient lies recumbent. Herniated lumbar disc pain is often exacerbated by sitting and relieved by standing or walking. The pain of spinal stenosis, on the contrary, is often absent when lying or sitting and occurs only when the patient walks. Vertebral metastases with or without epidural spinal cord compression cause pain that is often more prominent when lying and sometimes is relieved by sitting up; many patients with spinal cord compression elect to sleep in a sitting position. Even if pain is absent in the lying position, movement such as turning over in bed or arising may be particularly painful.

REFERRED PAIN. Referred pain arises from deep somatic or visceral structures and is perceived at a distant area within the same spinal segment but not necessarily in dermatomal distribution (radicular pain, see below). In many instances, the distribution is sclerotomal or myotomal. Referred pain, like local pain, has a deep aching quality and is often associated with tenderness of subcutaneous tissues and muscles at the site of referral. Maneuvers that affect local pain usually have the same effect on referred pain. Pain referred from pathologic abnormalities of the cervical spine often is either just medial to the scapula or over the lateral aspect of the arm; pain referred from the low back is usually appreciated in the buttocks and posterior thighs, although rarely below the knees. Pain from the upper lumbar spine is often referred to the flank, groin, and anterior thigh. Pain also can be referred to the spine from lesions of thoracic or abdominal viscera, a prominent example being the back pain from pancreatic carcinoma.

MUSCLE PAIN. Muscle pain occurs when an injury to or structural abnormality of the spine induces paravertebral muscle spasm. Sustained contraction of paravertebral muscles gives rise to chronic aching pain, usually felt lateral to the midline of the neck or back. Palpation of painful muscles may reveal evidence of spasm and tenderness. At times, when areas of extreme sensitivity (trigger points) are palpated, the pain may be felt not only locally in the muscle but also may be referred to distant structures. Trigger points define myofascial pain syndromes, common causes of neck and back pain without structural abnormalities of the spine (see p. 2124).

RADICULAR PAIN. Injured spinal roots or spinal cord produce, respectively, radicular or funicular pain. Radicular pain is the prominent symptom of nerve root compression. Nerve roots are not usually pain-sensitive. However, chronic compression leads to edema and, perhaps, inflammation and demyelination; the root then becomes sensitive to stretching or compression. When compressed, the pain may be experienced only in the cutaneous distribution (dermatome) of the involved root or may be felt locally and deep in muscles that it supplies. Root pain is usually least severe in positions that minimize compression and most severe in positions that compress or stretch the root. Root pain is usually exacerbated by increasing intraspinal pressure by coughing, sneezing, and straining.

FUNICULAR PAIN. Funicular pain is caused by compression of the long tracts of the spinal cord. Funicular pain is less sharp than radicular pain and is often described as a cold, unpleasant sensation in the extremity. Its distribution is more diffuse than that of radicular pain but like root pain is usually exacerbated by movements that stretch the cord (neck flexion, straight leg raising) or that increase intraspinal pressure.

In addition to pain, chronic compression of nerve roots can produce paresthesias, sensory loss, weakness, atrophy, and hyporeflexia in root-supplied areas, thus localizing the lesion. Knowing the myotomal and dermatomal distribution of spinal roots (Table 489–1) often allows one not only to localize the lesion but also to suggest its etiologic diagnosis: Involvement of a single root is more likely to occur with intervertebral disc herniation (Ch. 490), whereas multiple root dysfunction is likely to be caused by tumor or chronic inflammation. However, myotomal and dermatomal localization must be utilized cautiously. In the first place, not every body obeys the standard maps. Also, contiguous dermatomes overlap, and the apparent size of a dermatome can vary between examinations, depending on central nervous system excitability. Nevertheless, the localizing diagnosis of root lesions is usually accurate.

The clinical signs of spinal cord compression depend on the speed with which the compression develops, the transverse and longitudinal site of the lesion, and the vulnerability of the individual spinal fibers. The spinal cord accommodates considerably to gradually developing compression (e.g., from meningiomas); such disorders can cause the gradual onset of painless paraparesis or paraplegia. Because of this accommodation, subsequent decompression, even when patients are severely paraparetic, often leads to complete resolution of neurologic symptoms. On the other hand, rapidly developing lesions such as epidural hematomas, acute midline herniated discs, or epidural spinal cord compression from metastatic tumor are usually painful and cause rapidly developing neurologic signs that respond poorly to therapy once severe paraparesis has developed.

The site of compression in the transverse plane may determine clinical signs, particularly when the compression develops slowly. For example, laterally located lesions compressing one side of the spinal cord may cause the Brown-Séquard syndrome (ipsilateral hemiparesis, vibration and position sense loss, with contralateral pain and temperature loss); compression of the posterior portion of the cord may cause bilateral position and vibratory loss, with preservation of pain and temperature sensation and of

TABLE 489–1. DIAGNOSIS OF NERVE ROOT LESIONS

	C2–C3	C5	C6	C7	C8	Nerve T1
Pain	Back of head, lateral face, behind ear (occasionally vertex or orbit)	Medial scapula, lateral border of arm	Lateral forearm, thumb and index finger	Posterior arm, lateral hand, midforearm, and medial scapula	Medial forearm and hand	Deep aching in shoulder and axilla to olecranon
Sensory loss	Posterior scalp, pinna, lateral face	Lateral border of upper arm	Lateral forearm, including thumb	Mid-forearm and middle finger	Medial forearm and little finger	Axilla down to olecranon
Reflex loss	None	Biceps	Supinator	Triceps	Finger stretch	None
Motor deficit	None	Deltoid, supraspinatus, infraspinatus, rhomboids	Biceps, brachioradialis, brachialis (pronators and supinators of forearm)	Latissimus dorsi, pectoralis major, triceps, wrist extensors, wrist flexors	Finger flexors, finger extensors, flexor carpi ulnaris (thenar muscles in some patients)	*All* small hand muscles (in some thenar muscles via C8)
Some causative lesions	Tumor, injury	Brachial neuritis, cervical disc or spondylosis, upper plexus injury	Cervical disc or spondylosis	Cervical disc or spondylosis	Pancoast tumor, rare in disc lesions or spondylosis, metastatic tumor, thoracic outlet syndrome	Pancoast tumor, cervical rib, outlet syndromes, metastatic carcinoma in deep cervical nodes
Autonomic changes	Gustatory sweating					Horner's syndrome

motor power. However, most lesions twist the cord as they compress it and also interfere with the vascular supply to sites beyond the compression. Accordingly, one can depend only in a general way on the neurologic signs to evaluate the exact transverse site of compression. The longitudinal location of the lesion is more important. Cervical lesions cause quadriplegia, thoracic lesions, paraplegia; and upper lumbar lesions, normal motor function with bowel and bladder dysfunction and extensor plantar responses (conus medullaris syndrome). Lesions below the first lumbar vertebral body compress the cauda equina, causing loss of bowel and bladder function with lower motor neuron leg weakness and normal plantar reflexes.

Certain spinal tracts appear to be more vulnerable to compression than others. The corticospinal tracts and posterior columns are particularly vulnerable, the spinothalamic tracts and descending autonomic fibers less so. As a result, weakness, spasticity, and reflex hyperactivity tend to be the earliest signs of spinal cord compression, with paresthesias and vibratory and position sense loss occurring soon thereafter. Loss of pain and temperature sensation and of bladder and bowel function usually occurs late in the course of spinal cord compression. The spinocerebellar pathways are also sensitive to compression, and at times ataxia mimicking cerebellar disease may be the only sign of spinal cord compression.

APPROACH TO THE PATIENT

Most mechanical lesions of the spine and its contents begin with pain and only later produce other signs of neurologic dysfunction. There are many potential causes of neck or back pain. One survey listed over 100 causes (Table 489–2). The task for the physician is to separate those patients with potentially serious disease from those with more common, if unknown, causes of back pain who need only reassurance, sometimes coupled with bed rest, analgesics, and physical therapy.

HISTORY. The diagnostic evaluation begins with the history. Get a complete description of the pain. Most spine pain begins acutely or subacutely and often follows, by minutes to hours, some unaccustomed physical activity, particularly lifting or bending. Patients may awaken stiff and sore the morning after unusual exercise or may develop acute back pain on arising in the morning, without any obvious precipitating event. Most neck pain begins as a stiff neck, often on awakening, without a history of unusual activity. In many patients, neck or low back pain recurs episodically over many years. Most neck or back pain is dull and aching in quality, exacerbated by movement and relieved by rest. Pain that is present when the patient is immobile and cannot be relieved by positional manipulation should lead the physician to consider a more serious disorder (e.g., tumor or extruded disc). *Radicular pain,* particularly if accompanied by paresthesias or loss of sensation, indicates mechanical compression of the nerve root supplying that dermatome and implies identifiable structural disease (e.g., herniated disc). *Referred pain* does not imply compression of a root.

A history of serious systemic illness may suggest disease of vertebral bodies. Carcinoma of the breast or thyroid may cause back pain from bony metastases years after the primary tumor has been successfully treated. Previous systemic infection may lead to delayed onset of vertebral osteomyelitis or epidural abscess. A family history may also give clues to the etiology of back pain. Neurofibromas causing neck or back pain by compression of nerve root or the spinal cord may be associated with neurofibromatosis. Rheumatoid arthritis and ankylosing spondylitis are causes of familial back pain.

EXAMINATION. A careful general physical examination may reveal evidence of systemic disease such as cancer or infection. Urinary tract infections, pelvic disease, abdominal aneurysms, and other intra-abdominal or intrathoracic processes sometimes cause back pain by impinging on vertebral bodies or paravertebral structures. Special attention should be paid to mobility of the spine and paravertebral structures. Most patients who complain of a stiff neck have some limitation of movement of the cervical spine, but if gradual movement of the cervical spine causes intense pain, if pain on neck flexion is referred to the thoracic or lumbar area, or if neck flexion causes paresthesias radiating into the arms, legs, or back (Lhermitte's sign), spinal cord compression should be suspected. Most low back pain not caused by a herniated disc is exacerbated by flexion and relieved by lying down. The paravertebral muscles are often in spasm, are tender

TABLE 489–1. DIAGNOSIS OF NERVE ROOT LESIONS *Continued*

Roots T4	T10	L2	L3	L4	L5	S1	S2–S4
Anterior chest and/or upper back	Midback and/or anterior abdomen	Across thigh	Across thigh	Down to medial malleolus	Back of thigh, lateral calf, dorsum of foot	Back of thigh, back of calf, lateral foot	Buttocks, genitalia, back of thigh
Usually none (upper back and chest at nipple level)	Usually none (mid-back and abdomen at umbilicus level)	Often none	Often none	Medial leg	Dorsum of foot	Behind lateral malleolus	Buttocks, genitalia
None	Decreased abdominal reflex	None	Adductor reflex	Knee jerk	None	Ankle jerk	Bulbocavernosus
Not discernible	None	Hip flexion, adduction of thigh	Knee extension, adduction of thigh	Inversion of foot	Dorsiflexion of toes and foot (latter L4 also)	Plantar flexion and eversion of foot	Bladder and bowel
Intravertebral or paravertebral tumor, herpes zoster	Intravertebral and paravertebral tumor, herpes zoster	Neurofibroma, meningioma, neoplastic disease; disc lesions very rare except at L4 < 5 per cent			Disc lesions, metastatic malignancy, neurofibromas, meningioma		Tumor, midline disc
Chest wall, piloerection, hyperhidrosis, unilateral gynecomastia, galactorrhea	Chest wall, piloerection, hyperhidrosis, retrograde ejaculation	Alterations in temperature and color of all or parts of the leg or thigh					Incontinence, impotence, urinary retention

TABLE 489–2. SOME CAUSES OF BACK PAIN

Common Causes
Degenerative disorders
  Osteoarthritis, facet syndrome
  Herniated disc
  Spinal stenosis
  Nerve root entrapment
Muscle dysfunction
  Spasms, fatigue, fibromyalgia, and myofascial pain
Psychosomatic (e.g., stress, conversion reaction, tension states)
Trauma
  Lumbar strain (acute or chronic)

Less Common Causes
Congenital disorders
  Facet tropism (asymmetry)
  Transitional vertebra
  Spondylolysis and spondylolisthesis
Infections (e.g., disc space infection, tuberculosis, epidural and
  subdural abscess, herpes zoster, meningitis, sacroiliac joint
  infection)
Inflammatory diseases (e.g., ankylosing spondylitis, arachnoiditis,
  rheumatoid arthritis)
Metabolic disorders (e.g., osteoporosis, gout, diabetic neuropathy,
  Paget's disease)
Postoperative (e.g., sequelae of scar formation, arachnoiditis)
Scoliosis (e.g., idiopathic, postparalytic, aging)
Trauma
  Lumbosacral, sacroiliac strain
  Compression fracture (vertebral body or transverse process)
Dislocation or subluxation
Tumors
  Benign bone and neural tumors (e.g., neurinoma, ependymoma,
    meningioma, osteoid osteoma, hemangioma, osteoblastoma)
  Malignant bone and neural tumors
    Primary (e.g., multiple myeloma, osteosarcoma)
    Secondary (metastases)
Visceral disease (e.g., visceral inflammation, female pelvic pathology,
  retroperitoneal pathology, aortic aneurysm, prostatic disease)

to palpation, and straighten the normally lordotic lumbar spine. Almost any severe low back pain, particularly if it radiates into a lower extremity, can increase when the extended leg is raised from the bed (straight leg raising sign). However, pain referred to the contralateral back or leg when the non-painful leg is raised (crossed straight leg raising) implies root compression. Forced extension of the hip (reverse straight leg raising) can elicit pain from upper lumbar root disease (L4 and above). Point tenderness over a spinous process raises the suspicion of involvement of the vertebra by either tumor or infection.

The neurologic examination is important. Sensory loss, reflex diminution, and weakness all suggest neurologic disease that requires further evaluation. The distribution of abnormalities localizes the lesion. Remember, however, that patients in severe pain may be reluctant to move the painful part, making normal muscles appear weak. Likewise, guarding can affect deep tendon reflexes, either increasing or decreasing them with respect to the normal side. Repeating the neurologic examination after pain has been relieved by analgesics usually clarifies whether or not there is neurologic dysfunction. Clear and reproducible neurologic signs, particularly sensory loss in a dermatomal distribution or a diminished stretch reflex, imply root compression.

Careful examination can reveal inconsistencies (e.g., leg pain on straight leg raising that appears when the patient is recumbent but not when sitting) that suggest a psychological rather than a physiologic basis.

LABORATORY AIDS TO INVESTIGATION. For most patients with back or neck pain, laboratory tests are neither required nor helpful. Plain radiographs of the spine rarely reveal relevant, clinically unsuspected findings, and more sensitive tests (e.g., CT and MR) often identify abnormalities such as herniated discs in asymptomatic as well as in symptomatic patients. Radiographic examination of neck or back should be undertaken only when the history and examination suggest specific findings (e.g., fracture or dislocation). If the clinical examination points to other signifi-cant disease of the neck or back (e.g., herniated disc) and if pain does not respond to conservative measures in a few weeks, the physician should proceed directly to MR imaging, which can identify all elements of the spinal column and its contents in multiple planes. Patients suspected of harboring tumors, infection, or vascular disease should be imaged without delay.

The only abnormalities not easily identified by MR are subluxations of vertebral bodies with movement. Flexion and extension plain radiographs of the neck or back settle that issue. Images of the neck and back must be interpreted with caution, since degenerative disc changes are frequently found in asymptomatic patients and increase with age. MR imaging, even though more expensive than CT and *radionuclide bone scan,* is so much more sensitive that it will probably replace these tests. Invasive tests, such as *myelograms, spinal angiography,* and *discography,* should be performed only in those special few instances when surgery is planned and MR does not give adequate information.

A committee of the American Academy of Neurology has determined that "based on the present medical literature, infrared *thermography* [does not] provide sufficiently reliable . . . [diagnostic] information . . . to accept it . . . for . . . neck or back pain and/or . . . radiculopathy. . . ."

Electromyography and nerve conduction studies, particularly using H and F responses, can help identify the presence and site of proximal sensory and motor root damage and anterior horn cell dysfunction. *Somatosensory evoked potentials* can be recorded along the spinal cord or in the brain after a peripheral nerve is stimulated and can sometimes identify the approximate site of a spinal cord lesion (see Ch. 441.2).

ANESTHETIC BLOCKS. Injections of local anesthesia into sites that are potential sources of neck or back pain sometimes aid diagnosis. Injection of facet joints may relieve both local and referred pain arising from osteoarthritis of those joints (see *facet syndrome,* p. 2236). Injection of trigger points may aid in the diagnosis of *myofascial back pain* (see p. 2124). Similarly, injections into and around the sacroiliac joint or intraspinal lesions may aid in diagnosis. Repetitive injections occasionally provide prolonged relief.

MANAGEMENT OF THE PATIENT WITH NECK AND BACK PAIN. If no clinical findings suggest serious structural disease of the spine, nerve roots, or spinal cord, patients should be treated as if they suffered from an acute neck or back strain, without further diagnostic evaluation. Because most patients recover within a few weeks without specific therapy, it is difficult to assess various therapeutic regimens. For severe pain, the best treatment probably consists of 2 to 3 days of bed rest on a firmly supported mattress in the position most comfortable. The best position for low back pain is usually semi-Fowler's position (head slightly elevated with pillows under the knees). For neck pain use a cervical pillow that maintains the normal lordotic curve rather than flexes the neck as regular pillows do. A soft cervical collar may be as effective in immobilizing the neck as bed rest. Bed rest may be combined with analgesic agents (usually aspirin or acetaminophen) and with local heat. Patients should be encouraged to stay recumbent, except to go to the toilet, until pain diminishes. As pain subsides, patients should gradually ambulate and start strengthening exercises for the paravertebral muscles of the neck and back, to prevent recurrence of pain. Other treatment modalities, including physical therapy, traction, procaine or saline injection into trigger points, transcutaneous stimulation, and spinal manipulation, are not more efficacious than the regimen described above. One recent study suggests that chiropractic manipulation of the back produces more rapid and prolonged relief of nonsciatic low back pain than does physical therapy with or without manipulation. Manipulation of the neck is potentially dangerous, however, because it can occlude the vertebral arteries as they enter the skull.

Using standard therapy, 70 to 80 per cent of patients become free of pain and able to return to full activity within a 4-week period. During the period of bed rest, repeated physical and neurologic examinations are unwise, since vigorous movement of the neck, back, and extremities can exacerbate pain and delay improvement. A small minority of patients continue to have chronic pain, and they, along with those whose initial examination has suggested more serious disease, need further evaluation.

The management of specific causes of nerve root and spinal cord compression, such as a herniated disc, is detailed in the chapters that follow.

Bonica JJ: Management of Pain, 2nd ed. Philadelphia, Lea and Febiger, 1990. *Excellent and detailed chapters on pain in the neck (Ch. 47) and in the low back (Ch. 71 and 72) which deal with management as well as diagnosis.*

Frymoyer JW: Back pain and sciatica. N Engl J Med 318:291–300, 1988. *A medical progress article reviewing acute and chronic low back pain.*

Reed TW, Dwyer S, Browne W, et al.: Low back pain and mechanical origin: Randomized comparison of chiropractic and hospital out-patient treatment. Br Med J 30:1431–1437, 1990. *A report sure to elicit continuing controversy on the medical management of low back pain.*

490 Intervertebral Disc Disease

HERNIATED DISC. Herniated intervertebral discs are the most common cause of neck or low back pain associated with a clearly defined structural abnormality. Lumbar and cervical strain and myofascial pain syndromes (see Ch. 489) are more common but not marked by clear pathologic abnormalities. Between each two vertebral bodies is a fibrocartilaginous intervertebral disc. The disc consists of a soft inner nucleus pulposus (a remnant of the notochord) surrounded by thicker fibrous tissue (the anulus fibrosus). The nucleus pulposus is gelatinous in structure and acts as a shock absorber between adjacent vertebral bodies. With advancing age, the nucleus loses fluid, volume, and resiliency, and the entire disc structure becomes more susceptible to trauma and compression. Tears develop in the anulus fibrosus as a result of repeated minor trauma, and eventually, if the tears become large enough, a portion of the soft nucleus pulposus herniates through the anulus. Asymptomatic herniation may occur into the center of the vertebral bodies bordering the disc (Schmorl's nodules). When, however, disc material herniates into the vertebral canal, it can compress nerve endings and nerve roots, causing pain and other symptoms. Generally, the disc herniates lateral to the posterior longitudinal ligament, thus compressing spinal roots as they enter the intervertebral foramen. Occasionally the disc herniates more centrally, compressing either the spinal cord in the cervical or thoracic area or the cauda equina in the lumbar area. The term *herniated disc* refers to a disc that maintains continuity with the nucleus pulposus; extruded disc refers to a fragment within the spinal canal that has lost continuity with the disc itself. The signs and symptoms of herniated discs are caused by compression of either nerve roots or the spinal cord. The specific signs and symptoms depend in part on whether the predominant compression is spinal cord or nerve root, and in part on the level at which the neural structures are compressed (see Ch. 489). The most common sites of disc herniation are in the lumbar area, between L4 and L5 and between L5 and S1, compressing the L5 and S1 roots, respectively. L3–L4 herniations are less common. In the cervical area, the common herniations occur between C5 and C6 (C6 root) and, especially, C6 and C7 (C7 root). Less commonly, herniations appear between C3 and C4, C4 and C5, and C7 and T1. Thoracic disc herniations are less common but can cause severe myelopathy because the thoracic area is the narrowest of the entire vertebral canal and the cord has a relatively poor vascular system, making it vulnerable to ischemic compression. Although clinical localization in diagnosis of disc disease is usually quite accurate, at times an extruded disc fragment may be large enough to affect several roots, or may migrate from the disc space in which it herniated, to cause signs at a distance.

The most common symptom of a herniated disc is pain. Local pain is felt as a dull aching in the neck or back, with an associated stiffness of those structures, frequently occurring episodically in response to minor trauma (or no discernible trauma at all) months or years prior to the development of radicular pain. The exact pathogenesis of the local pain in disc disease is not known, but some believe that it results from compression of the sinuvertebral nerve, a recurrent branch of the nerve root that supplies the dura mater. Radicular pain may occasionally be the first sign of disc disease but is far more likely to follow repeated bouts of local pain. Radicular pain is generally sudden in onset, often following minor trauma such as a twist, turn, or unusual bend. Radicular pain is perceived as sharp and well localized and may radiate from the back along the entire distribution of the involved root or affect only a portion of the root. Both local pain and radicular pain have the characteristics of being exacerbated by activity and relieved by rest.

With cervical disc herniation, most patients hold their necks stiffly and resist passive movement. Lateral bending either to or away from the side of the herniated disc frequently exacerbates both the local and radicular pain. The patient may be more comfortable with his neck slightly flexed but is usually comfortable only in the recumbent position. Patients with lumbar disc disease are most comfortable lying, most uncomfortable sitting, and a little less uncomfortable standing. The back is held stiffly, so that the normal lumbar lordotic curve is no longer apparent, and pain is usually exacerbated by extension of the back. Slow forward bending sometimes relieves the pain. Muscle spasm is prominent with both cervical and lumbar disc disease. Raising the intraspinal pressure, as by coughing, sneezing, or straining, increases the pain sharply. Stretching the compressed root also aggravates the pain. In the upper extremities, extending the arm and laterally flexing the neck away from the extended arm often reproduces radicular pain. In the lower extremities, raising the extended leg with the patient in the recumbent position frequently reproduces the pain of an L5 or S1 radiculopathy and, if the spontaneous pain is reproduced by raising the contralateral leg (crossed straight leg raising), the sign is very suggestive of herniated disc disease. Symptoms of L4 radiculopathy can often be reproduced by extending the hip (stretching the femoral nerve) when the patient is lying in the prone position. Often tenderness is present along the entire distribution of the nerve(s) supplied by the compressed root as well as in muscles supplied by the root. In patients with cervical disc disease, palpation or light percussion of the brachial plexus in the supraclavicular fossa or axilla often causes pain. In patients with lumbar disc disease, palpation over the femoral nerve (L4) in the groin or over the sciatic nerve (L5–S1) in the calf, thigh, or buttocks often causes severe pain. Occasionally tenderness in the calf (the posterior tibial nerve) is so striking as to suggest that the patient is suffering from thrombophlebitis rather than disc herniation. Other neurologic signs that commonly accompany disc disease include paresthesias and sensory loss in the distribution of the involved root and motor weakness in the myotome supplied by that root. The most important single sign is a diminished or absent reflex, giving objectively verifiable evidence of neurologic disease.

If an intervertebral disc herniates medially rather than laterally, it may spare the root and involve the spinal cord directly. When this occurs, there may be little or no pain or pain in a bilateral radicular distribution. Sometimes the pain is felt at a site far distant from the disc herniation as a result of compression of long sensory tracts in the spinal cord (funicular pain). The signs and symptoms of cord involvement are the same as those of compression of the spinal cord by other mass lesions. In contradistinction to diseases that arise within the spinal cord, compressive lesions tend to spare bladder and bowel function until late. (The exception is when the compression occurs either at the conus medullaris or in the cauda equina.)

The diagnosis of herniated disc is deduced from the characteristic clinical symptoms and findings. In many patients with radiculopathy, findings are minimal and the history must establish the diagnosis. When the patient complains of back pain, with or without a radicular component, but has no motor, sensory, or reflex changes to suggest the site of a radiculopathy, the differential diagnosis includes pain arising from pain-sensitive nerve endings in the muscles, ligaments, and joints of the vertebral bodies and the paravertebral structures. These structures must be examined carefully to determine which of them is responsible. MRI is helpful (see Ch. 489).

There is controversy about the management of herniated discs. Most physicians believe that the first step is bed rest. Some investigators have reported that adrenocorticosteroids, either taken orally or injected into the epidural space, may hasten resolution of pain and other symptoms. No controlled studies support this recommendation. Steroids injected into the epidural or subarachnoid space are contraindicated and may produce severe inflammatory reactions. Surgery is indicated when (1) bed rest fails, and the patient is incapacitated by severe, intractable pain; (2) a centrally placed lumbar disc compresses the cauda equina, producing urinary dysfunction; (3) motor weakness (e.g., foot drop) is severe and gets worse on bed rest; or (4) acute cervical or thoracic discs cause substantial myelopathy. Myelography may be performed before surgical extirpation to localize the site of disc herniation and to determine whether other disc lesions or tumors are present as well, but in many cases MRI suffices. The best operation removes the involved disc, leaving as much bone as possible intact. Fusion of the lumbar spine is rarely necessary. Lumbar disc operations are done posteriorly via a laminotomy. Cervical disc operations may be done either posteriorly to decompress the cord or anteriorly across the neck to remove the disc without disturbing posterior bony elements. The surgical approach for myelopathy should probably be anterior if the disc is in the cervical area and lateral if the disc is in the thoracic area.

Disc dissolution by the injection of the enzyme chymopapain directly into a lumbar disc space has received enthusiastic support from some centers and, in the best hands, appears as effective as surgery. Occasional, serious anaphylactic reactions can occur and the procedure's role remains uncertain. Percutaneous aspiration of disc material is usually safe and often effective in relieving root compression without a laminotomy.

SPONDYLOSIS. Spondylosis is a term applied to chronic degenerative disease of intervertebral discs associated with reactive changes in the adjacent vertebral bodies. Spondylotic changes in the neck and low back increase with age and are almost invariably present in the elderly. Spondylosis is usually asymptomatic except when the reactive tissue compresses a nerve root or the spinal cord. When this occurs, the signs and symptoms are similar to those of herniated disc disease, but the onset is less abrupt and the treatment often more difficult. In both the cervical and lumbar areas, spondylosis is more likely to produce spinal cord or cauda equina symptoms if the sagittal diameter of the spinal canal is congenitally narrow.

Cervical Spondylosis. Most patients suffer either radiculopathy or myelopathy, but not both. Pain is common but usually less acute and severe than with herniated discs. Even muscle spasm may be absent. However, the vertebral degenerative changes in the neck lead to limitation of movement in all directions. The classic picture of cervical spondylotic myelopathy is one of little or no pain but slowly developing weakness, atrophy, and fasciculations in the upper extremities, particularly the small muscles of the hand, accompanied by spastic paraparesis with decreased proprioception in the legs. At first the findings may suggest a diagnosis of amyotrophic lateral sclerosis. However, in cervical spondylosis there are sensory changes, particularly vibration loss in the lower extremities, and in amyotrophic lateral sclerosis fasciculations extend to innervated areas beyond the cervical level. The differential diagnosis also includes other compressive lesions of root and spinal cord as well as chronic multiple sclerosis. The diagnosis of cervical spondylitic myelopathy is established with MRI, which accurately delineates the size of the cervical canal and the site of spinal cord and/or root compression.

The natural history of cervical myelopathy and radiculopathy is not well established. Many patients experience long periods of pain relief and remission or stabilization of neurologic symptoms, making it difficult to evaluate the effect of a particular treatment. Many physicians prefer, once having established the diagnosis, to begin with conservative treatment with a brief period of bed rest accompanied by cervical traction and stabilization of the neck with a soft collar. If collar and traction are successful, they should be continued. However, if the patient develops progressive neurologic signs in the face of conservative treatment, surgical therapy is indicated. Most neurosurgeons believe that if the spinal cord compression occurs at one or two segments, anterior removal of the disc material with spinal fusion is the preferred course. If more than a few segments are involved, laminectomy with foraminotomy is preferred.

In some patients with cervical spondylosis (or with congenital narrowing of the cervical spinal canal, or both), neurologic symptoms are exacerbated by exercise, with pain, numbness, and weakness appearing when a particular extremity is exercised. The pathogenesis is thought to be compression of the spinal cord so severe that the blood supply to the area cannot increase during its activity, leading to ischemia of cord and root structures (pseudoclaudication).

LUMBAR SPONDYLOSIS. Most of the considerations described above apply. The symptoms of lumbar spondylosis are similar to those of herniated disc, often occurring at multiple levels. One outstanding difference is the frequent presence of *pseudoclaudication* from cauda equina compression in patients with spinal stenosis due to either spondylosis or congenital narrowing. Typically, symptoms and signs are evoked or accentuated by walking and include pain, paresthesias, and weakness in the lower extremities. All of the symptoms may disappear when the patient ceases walking, even though he remains in the standing position. At times, however, the symptoms may be exacerbated by prolonged standing and relieved only by sitting or lying down. Pseudoclaudication of the cauda equina may be distinguished from intermittent vascular claudication in several ways. In vascular disease, the pulses in the lower extremities are usually absent or become absent as exercise begins. Also, the symptoms are usually reproducible and stereotypic, i.e., the patient can predict the exact distance he can walk at a given speed before symptoms develop. Symptoms of cauda equina pseudoclaudication are less stereotypic, so that on some days patients can walk much longer distances than on others. The reason for this variability is not known. In patients with pseudoclaudication, the narrowed lumbar canal is easily measured by MRI. With severe lumbar stenosis, conservative treatment usually fails, and decompressive laminectomy is the treatment of choice.

OTHER CAUSES OF BACK AND NECK PAIN. Several common pathophysiologically poorly understood disorders that produce pain in the back or neck can be confused with intravertebral disc disease or cervical or lumbar spondylosis. These include pain arising in lumbosacral, sacroiliac, or zygapophyseal joints that results from muscle spasm or muscle tension and the fibromyalgia and the myofascial pain syndromes (see p. 2124). These disorders usually cause chronic aching local pain that, when severe, may be referred to distant sites. Typical radicular pain never occurs. As a group, the diagnosis is usually suspected by finding tenderness at a specific muscle site or limitation of motion in a specific joint. The diagnosis is supported by a lidocaine block, which should completely relieve the pain if the presumptive diagnosis is correct.

The *facet syndrome* is believed to result from osteoarthritis or trauma of the zygapophyseal joints or their synovial membranes. In the low back it is characterized by pain in the back, buttocks, and thighs. It is often relieved by flexion and aggravated by extension of the spine and frequently accentuated by rest and relieved by movement. Characteristically the area is stiff and painful in the morning and improves somewhat as the day wears on. There is tenderness to palpation of the joint. Anesthetic blocks of the joint relieve both the local and referred pain. Similar chronic pain may have its origin in the lumbosacral or sacroiliac joints.

Musculoskeletal pain is also a common but poorly understood cause of low back and probably neck pain. In patients with painful muscle spasm the normal lordotic curve is usually straightened and tight, and tender muscles can be palpated by the examiner. Local anesthetic blocks, followed by gentle mobilization, usually relieve the spasm and the pain. Prolonged contraction of muscles, such as results from sustained posture or psychological stress, may produce similar pain and tenderness. Fibromyalgia and myofascial pain syndromes often affect the neck and back, as noted above and on p. 2124.

491 Neoplasms of the Spinal Canal

Neoplastic growths that cause nerve root or spinal cord compression can be paravertebral, extradural, intradural, or intramedullary (Fig. 491–1). Most of those causing spinal cord compression are extradural and metastatic. Most extradural neoplasms originate in the vertebral body surrounding the spinal cord and

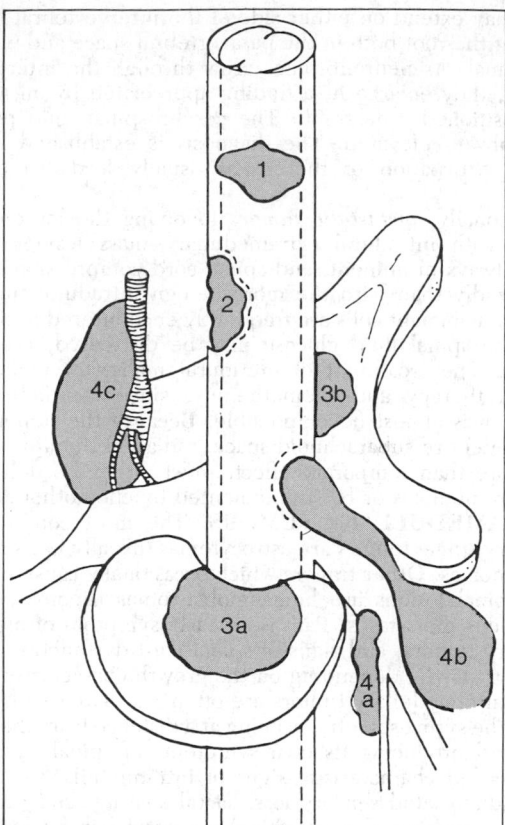

FIGURE 491–1. Pathophysiology of myelopathy caused by neoplasms. 1, The tumor may arise in or metastasize hematogenously to the substance of the spinal cord (intramedullary). 2, The tumor may be extraparenchymal but intradural. 3, The tumor may be extradural, extending either from the vertebral body (3a) or from a spinous process (3b), and cause symptoms by compressing the spinal cord. 4, The tumor may originate in or spread to the paravertebral space and produce its symptoms either by (4a) invading nerve roots, (4b) invading the epidural or subdural space through the intervertebral foramen, or (4c) compressing radicular arteries to cause spinal cord ischemia. (From Andreoli TE, Carpenter CCJ, Plum F, Smith LH Jr (eds.): Cecil Essentials of Medicine. Philadelphia, W. B. Saunders Company, 1986.)

compress spinal roots or cord without invading them. Most intradural neoplasms also cause symptoms by compressing spinal roots or cord without invading, but unlike extradural neoplasms the majority are benign and slow growing. Intramedullary neoplasms cause symptoms both by invading and by compressing spinal structures; the tumors may be either benign or malignant.

PARAVERTEBRAL TUMORS. Neoplastic lesions that begin in or metastasize to the paravertebral space often cause serious and perplexing neurologic problems. The tumor may extend longitudinally within the paravertebral space, progressively compressing or invading nerve roots. At times, such tumors grow through an intervertebral foramen and compress not only the nerve root but also the spinal cord. Rarely, spinal cord symptoms may be caused by paravertebral tumors compromising radicular arteries that supply the spinal cord. If the tumor is more lateral than the immediate paravertebral space, the brachial, lumbar, or sacral plexus may be compressed, causing symptoms similar to those of root compression but with a different pattern of sensory and motor loss. The symptoms of extravertebral tumor begin insidiously with severe, unremitting pain, often with a burning quality and usually localized just lateral to the spine, radiating in a bandlike pattern in the distribution of the involved dermatome(s). If the lesion involves abdominal or thoracic roots, motor and sensory changes are usually not appreciated by either the patient or the examiner. Autonomic changes may be a prominent or the only neurologic sign. Hyperhidrosis occurring in a band coinciding with the site of the pain strongly suggests the diagnosis. When the tumor involves cervical or lumbar roots, the pain may be soon followed by numbness in fingertips or toes, with accompanying weakness and reflex diminution, depending on the roots

involved. Autonomic changes, including anhidrosis or hyperhidrosis, may affect the arm or leg. Horner's syndrome or diaphragmatic paralysis often accompanies cervical or upper thoracic paravertebral tumors. The diagnosis is best established by MR scan of the level suggested by the clinical findings. The scans can also determine whether the lesion has grown through the intervertebral foramen or has eroded vertebral bodies.

The differential diagnosis of paravertebral tumor includes disorders that cause paravertebral pain with or without compression of nerve roots. *Myofascial pain syndromes* cause low back or neck paravertebral pain with referred pain into arms or legs. On examination there is often marked tenderness of muscles and, sometimes, trigger points identified by either their hardness to palpation or their ability to reproduce symptoms when compressed. Relief of pain in these instances can be produced by injecting the trigger point with saline solution or a local anesthetic. Temporary relief of pain after such injection does not imply that structural disease is absent; the trigger points may be a reaction to spinal or nerve root disease. In myofascial syndromes, autonomic, sensory, or motor changes are never present. Disease of kidneys and other viscera lying in the retroperitoneal space may cause pain similar to that of paravertebral tumors, but the pain usually does not radiate and is not associated with autonomic, motor, or sensory changes. Percussion of the involved viscera reproduces the pain that is described as a dull ache rather than a neurogenic burning pain. Spontaneous or induced *entrapment neuropathies* not caused by tumor occasionally mimic the symptoms of paravertebral tumor. Chronic pain after a thoracotomy (*post-thoracotomy pain*) probably results from entrapment of nerve roots at the time of surgery, perhaps with neuroma formation. The pain characteristically appears shortly after surgery and may be unremitting for many years. Motor, sensory, or autonomic changes are rare. The pain can sometimes be relieved by paravertebral anesthetic blocks.

The management of paravertebral masses depends on the diagnosis. In patients known to have cancer, particularly lymphomas or carcinomas of the breast or lung, the tumor can be assumed to be metastatic and should be treated with radiation therapy and, if available, chemotherapy. If the patient has no history of cancer, a biopsy is required and, depending on the site of the lesion, resection may be attempted both to establish a diagnosis and to decompress the nerve roots. Once the diagnosis is established by biopsy, further therapy such as radiation or chemotherapy may be indicated.

EXTRADURAL TUMORS. Extradural neoplasms compress spinal roots and cord in one of three ways. Either they arise in vertebrae surrounding the spinal cord and grow into the epidural space or they arise in the paravertebral space and grow through the intervertebral foramen to compress the cord laterally. Rarely, tumors may arise in the epidural space itself, without involving either vertebral or paravertebral structures. Most extradural neoplasms are metastatic (e.g., carcinomas of the breast, lung, prostate, or kidney). Some extradural neoplasms arise de novo in the vertebral bodies (e.g., chordoma, osteogenic sarcoma, myeloma, chondrosarcoma). A minority of extradural neoplasms are benign (e.g., osteoma, osteoid osteoma, angioma). Because extradural neoplasms usually destroy bone before producing spinal cord compression, local pain is the first symptom and may precede either radicular pain or other symptoms of spinal cord compression by weeks or months, depending on the rate of growth of the tumor. Rarely, extradural neoplasms may be painless and the first symptoms may be spinal cord dysfunction. As with other causes of spinal cord compression, extradural neoplasms cause symptoms first distally and later proximally. Thus, even thoracic and cervical neoplasms generally cause weakness and numbness in the legs before trunk and upper extremity muscles are involved. The diagnosis of extradural spinal cord compression must be suspected by the history of pain followed by signs and symptoms of spinal cord dysfunction and confirmed by radiographic study. In about 85 per cent of patients suffering from extradural spinal cord compression, there are bone lesions at the site of compression on plain radiographs. In those few patients with negative plain radiographs, radionuclide bone scan, CT, or MR scan may demonstrate a bone lesion. MRI usually also establishes the site and degree of spinal cord compression, often obviating the need for an invasive myelogram.

The differential diagnosis of extradural neoplasms includes inflammatory disease of bone and epidural abscess (e.g., vertebral tuberculosis, bacterial osteomyelitis), acute or subacute epidural hematomas, herniated intervertebral discs, spondylosis, and, very rarely, extramedullary hematopoiesis (in patients with severe and chronic anemias) or epidural lipomatosis (in patients on chronic steroid therapy). MRI often distinguishes those from tumor, but sometimes definitive diagnosis requires biopsy of the lesion either via decompressive laminectomy or by percutaneous needle biopsy.

The treatment of extradural neoplasms depends on the cause. Most neoplasms that cause extradural spinal cord compression are malignant and progress rapidly. Once spinal cord symptoms begin, paraplegia may develop in hours to days. Paraplegia is usually irreversible, whereas treatment often can correct mild to moderate spinal cord dysfunction. Thus, early diagnosis and effective emergency treatment of extradural spinal cord compression are mandatory. The treatment of patients known to be suffering from cancer who develop signs and symptoms of spinal cord compression from extradural metastases is radiation therapy. Therapy should begin with corticosteroids (dexamethasone, 16 to 100 mg daily) to decrease spinal cord edema, followed immediately by radiation therapy. If effective chemotherapeutic agents are available, they should be used in conjunction with steroids and radiation therapy for the treatment of metastatic or primary malignant tumors of the extradural space. In patients not known to be suffering from a primary cancer, metastatic disease is the most common cause of extradural spinal cord compression, but in these instances a definitive diagnosis must be made by biopsy. Such patients should begin corticosteroid therapy followed by surgery with removal of as much tumor as possible for both diagnostic and therapeutic purposes. If a malignant neoplasm is encountered at operation, radiation therapy should be begun as soon after the surgery as is practical. In a few patients in whom radiation therapy and chemotherapy are ineffective, resection of the vertebral body involved by tumor may delay the development of paraplegia. In some patients with extradural tumors and destruction of the vertebral body, subluxation may compress the cord and may be relieved by surgery. Benign extradural tumors require surgery.

INTRADURAL EXTRAMEDULLARY TUMORS. Most intradural tumors are benign. Meningiomas and neurofibromas are the two most common types. Teratomas, arachnoid cysts, and lipomas are less common. *Meningioma* occurs in middle-aged and elderly women, predominantly in the thoracic region of the spinal cord. Another common site is at the foramen magnum. Meningiomas are benign, slow growing, and usually located on the posterior aspect of the spinal cord. Pain is the first symptom in the majority of patients, but in about 25 per cent the meningioma is painless, the first symptoms being those of spinal cord compression. Because they are often located on the posterior aspect of the cord, paresthesias and sensory changes beginning distally in the lower extremities are a frequent early symptom and are often mistaken for peripheral neuropathy. As the disease progresses, however, corticospinal tract signs betray the spinal origin. Even when spinal cord signs and symptoms are obvious, the lack of pain may lead one to suspect a degenerative or demyelinating disease such as multiple sclerosis rather than a neoplasm. MRI usually settles the issue when contrast enhancement is used. Many meningiomas have a density similar to that of normal brain and spinal cord, making them difficult to identify on noncontrast MRI, but they all intensely contrast-enhance, making identification easy. The treatment of spinal cord compression from meningiomas is surgical removal. Because the tumor grows so slowly and the cord has an opportunity to adapt to compression, even patients with severe neurologic disability often make a full recovery after the lesion is removed.

The second common cause of intradural spinal cord compression is *neurofibroma.* Because these tumors usually arise from the dorsal root, radicular pain is often the first symptom, preceding signs of spinal cord compression by months or years. When spinal cord compression develops, it progresses slowly. Some patients with spinal neurofibroma suffer from neurofibromatosis. That diagnosis may be suspected either by a positive family history or by the cutaneous stigmata of the disease. A neurofibroma may extend on either side of the intervertebral foramen, involving the root both in the paravertebral space and within the spinal canal. As neurofibromas grow through the intervertebral foramen, they enlarge it, a finding appreciated by an appropriately positioned radiograph. The cerebrospinal fluid protein is almost always elevated. The diagnosis is established by MRI. Surgical extirpation of the lesion usually leads to complete recovery.

Occasionally, *metastatic tumors* involving the leptomeninges present with intradural extramedullary mass lesions. Pain is almost always prominent, and spinal cord compression develops more rapidly than with the more benign intradural tumors. In addition, malignant cells are frequently encountered in the spinal fluid. The spinal fluid glucose may be decreased, the protein elevated. The treatment of intradural malignant neoplasms is radiation therapy and chemotherapy, since complete surgical extirpation is almost never possible. Because the tumor usually seeds the entire subarachnoid space, radiation therapy, if it is to have more than temporary effect, must either be delivered to the entire neuraxis or be supplemented by chemotherapy.

INTRAMEDULLARY TUMORS. The most common intramedullary spinal tumors are astrocytomas (usually low grade) and ependymomas. Other tumors which occasionally cause intramedullary spinal lesions are hemangioblastomas, lipomas, and hematogenous metastases. Pain is an early symptom of most intramedullary tumors, and signs of spinal cord dysfunction progress rapidly or slowly, depending on the growth characteristics of the tumor. Intramedullary tumors are often associated with syringomyelia, the syrinx sometimes being at a distance from the primary tumor and producing its own symptoms of spinal dysfunction. The so-called characteristic signs of intramedullary spinal cord lesions (dissociated sensory loss, sacral sparing, and early onset of bladder and bowel dysfunction) are not reliable enough clinically to distinguish intramedullary from extramedullary lesions; that diagnosis is established by MRI. In some patients with longstanding benign intramedullary lesions, plain radiographs of the spine may show widening of the spinal canal and erosion of the pedicles. The differential diagnosis of intramedullary tumors includes intramedullary abscesses and syringomyelia without tumor. A definitive diagnosis is established by biopsy. Successful surgical removal of intramedullary tumors is possible, particularly with ependymomas and hemangioblastomas and sometimes with gliomas as well. Highly skilled and experienced surgeons are necessary for tumors to be removed without increasing neurologic symptoms. If the tumor cannot be totally excised, postoperative radiation therapy often delays recurrence.

Ependymomas have a predilection to involve the lower end of the spinal cord and the filum terminale. An unusual symptom sometimes produced by such tumors is hydrocephalus with headache, papilledema, and enlarged cerebral ventricles. The pathogenesis of the hydrocephalus is believed to be the plugging of pacchionian granulations by protein exuded from the tumor into the spinal fluid.

Byrne TN, Waxman SG (eds.): Spinal Cord Compression. Philadelphia, F.A. Davis, 1990. *Specific chapters cover non-neoplastic as well as neoplastic causes of spinal cord compression and noncompressive myelopathies simulating spinal cord compression.*

492 Inflammatory Diseases Compressing the Spinal Canal

Inflammatory diseases that compress nerve roots and spinal cord can be extradural, intradural, or intramedullary. Extradural inflammatory lesions include vertebral tuberculosis or bacterial osteomyelitis with extradural extension and primary extradural bacterial abscesses. These entities are discussed in Ch. 471. Intradural but extramedullary inflammatory diseases include bacterial, fungal, and parasitic meningitis, inflammatory disease of the leptomeninges of unknown cause such as sarcoidosis or Behçet's syndrome, and reactions to foreign substances such as myelographic contrast material, spinal anesthetics, or steroids. Occasionally, leptomeningeal infiltration with tumor or subarachnoid hemorrhage causes an inflammatory response of the leptomeninges that mimics subacute or chronic infection. All of these inflammatory intradural lesions can lead to spinal arachnoiditis. *Spinal arachnoiditis* is characterized by neck and back pain and by radicular pain in the distribution of the roots involved in the inflammatory process. Dysfunction of multiple roots, particularly in the lumbosacral area, is common; occasional patients go on to develop signs of spinal cord dysfunction (often caused by syrinx formation), which may progress to paraplegia. The diagnosis of spinal arachnoiditis is established by myelography. A myelogram reveals spotty and irregular collections of contrast material with impairment of the flow through the subarachnoid space. Sometimes there is a complete block to the passage of the myelographic contrast material. The spinal fluid may contain an increased cellular response and a decreased glucose concentration. The protein concentration is usually elevated. Sometimes a specific infectious organism can be identified either by microscopic examination or by culture. There is no therapy for spinal arachnoiditis unless a specific treatment-sensitive infective agent is identified.

Intramedullary infectious processes include bacterial and parasitic abscesses and acute transverse myelitis. These entities are discussed under the appropriate chapter headings.

Byrne TN, Waxman SG (eds): Spinal Cord Compression. Philadelphia, F.A. Davis Co., 1990. *Chapters discuss vascular and inflammatory causes of spinal cord compression and noncompressive myelopathies mimicking spinal cord compression.*

Caplan LR, Norohna AB, Amico LL: Syringomyelia and arachnoiditis. J Neurol Neurosurg Psychiatry 53:106–113, 1990. *A recent well-referenced discussion of chronic arachnoiditis and its sequelae.*

493 Vascular Disorders Compressing the Spinal Canal

Extradural, intradural, and intramedullary vascular disorders all can cause spinal cord compression. The most common and serious extradural vascular disease is *spinal epidural hematoma*. Hemorrhage into the spinal epidural space may occur spontaneously or be associated with trauma, a bleeding diathesis, or a vascular malformation. It is particularly common in patients being treated with anticoagulants. It may occasionally follow lumbar puncture, particularly in patients with bleeding abnormalities. Hemorrhage usually arises from the epidural venous plexus and tends to collect over the dorsum of the spinal cord covering several segments. The clinical picture is characterized by the sudden onset of severe localized back pain and the rapid development of spinal cord dysfunction, often leading to complete paraplegia in several hours. If the patient has a known bleeding disorder, the clinical diagnosis is easily established. In patients without known bleeding or clotting disorders, the differential diagnosis includes acute epidural abscess and acute transverse myelopathy. Although occasional patients recover from paraparesis related to epidural spinal cord compression spontaneously, the majority require emergency surgical evacuation if neurologic function is to be preserved. The more rapidly the paralysis develops and the longer the delay in decompression, the less likely is the patient to recover.

Intradural but extramedullary vascular lesions are usually caused by hemorrhage from *vascular malformations* on the surface of the spinal cord. *Spinal subarachnoid hemorrhage* is characterized by the sudden onset of back pain, often with a radicular component with or without the development of signs of spinal cord compression. Lumbar puncture reveals evidence of subarachnoid hemorrhage with red cells, xanthochromic spinal fluid, and usually an elevated protein concentration. In the absence of spinal cord signs, the differential diagnosis includes spontaneous intracerebral subarachnoid hemorrhage.

Vascular malformations also may lie within the substance of the spinal cord where they can give rise to intramedullary hemorrhage (hematomyelia) as well as subarachnoid hemorrhage. The sudden development of partial or complete transverse myelopathy is the most common onset. If blood leaks into the subarachnoid space, pain in the neck and back and other signs of meningeal irritation occur.

Arteriovenous malformations may also compress the spinal cord or give rise to hemodynamic changes that result in spinal ischemia. In such cases, distortion and compression of the cord by enlarged, abnormal vessels occur only gradually, producing slowly progressive symptoms of spinal cord dysfunction. Exacerbation of symptoms may accompany menstrual periods or pregnancy.

Complete or partial recovery of function can follow episodes of spinal cord ischemia or even small hemorrhages. The unchanging localization of the attacks and the prominence of pain help differentiate arteriovenous malformations from other recurrent neurologic disorders such as multiple sclerosis. Rarely, a bruit may be heard by auscultation over the site of the malformation. MRI identifies most hemorrhages and vascular malformations, but angiography with regional catheterization of radicular vessels is necessary to identify feeding vessels as a preliminary step to surgical treatment. Advances in microsurgery have increased the chances for satisfactory removal of these lesions. Embolization of the malformation or ligation of feeding arteries has been performed when the abnormality cannot be removed surgically.

Barnwell SL, Dowd CF, Davis RL, et al.: Cryptic vascular malformations of the spinal cord: Diagnosis by magnetic resonance imaging and outcome of surgery. J Neurosurg 72:403–407, 1990. *Description of a clinical entity usually not diagnosed before the advent of MRI.*

Gueguen B, Merland JJ, Riche MC, Rey A: Vascular malformations of the spinal cord. Neurology 37:969–979, 1987. *A good description of the anatomy and approach to treatment of these disorders.*

Mattle H, Sieb JP, Rohner M, Mumenthaler M: Nontraumatic spinal epidural and subdural hematomas. Neurology 37:1351–1356, 1987. *A recent paper with good references to the previous literature.*

494 Congenital Anomalies of the Craniovertebral Junction, Spine, and Spinal Cord

Congenital anomalies of the spine are common and are often encountered on radiographs of patients suffering from neck or low back pain. Some congenital anomalies such as *spina bifida occulta* can be considered variants of normal and are probably never responsible in and of themselves for low back pain. Others such as the *Klippel-Feil syndrome* (congenital fusion of two or more cervical vertebrae) are not responsible for neck pain or other neurologic symptoms except when associated with coexisting congenital anomalies of the central nervous system. Congenital abnormalities of the spine that are common and usually asymptomatic but that must be considered potential causes of neck or back pain include *facet tropism* (misalignment of the facets on the two sides of the corresponding vertebral body; several authorities believe that this increases rotational stress on the facet joints and may cause back pain); *transitional vertebrae*, such as in sacralization to a lumbar vertebra or lumbarization of a sacral vertebra (these alter spinal mechanics and result in instability and stress, sometimes producing back pain); and *spondylolisthesis* (forward slipping of one vertebral body onto another caused by a defect between the articular facets). A third group of congenital anomalies of the spine consists of those that are likely to cause not only neck or back pain but also neurologic disability. These include *basilar impression*, which is often associated with *Arnold-Chiari malformation* (see later discussion). Severe spinal *scoliosis* or *kyphosis*, congenital *stenosis* of the lumbar or cervical spinal canal, anterior and lateral spinal *meningoceles*, and *diastematomyelia* are other causes of back pain and neurologic disability. Diastematomyelia is a bony abnormality that divides the spinal canal, leading to duplication of the spinal cord. It is usually associated with evidence of spina bifida on plain radiographs, and sometimes the bony septum can be identified as well. Patients who become symptomatic in adulthood almost always have some cutaneous abnormality, especially hypertrichosis over the sacral area. The disorder may be associated with other congenital abnormalities of the central nervous system as well.

ARNOLD-CHIARI MALFORMATION

INFANTILE FORM. The Arnold-Chiari malformation is characterized by downward displacement of the cerebellum through the foramen magnum of the skull and by similar caudal elongation of the medulla. The infantile form is commonly associated with other midline defects such as spina bifida and meningocele, hydrocephalus caused by aqueductal or fourth ventricular obstruction, and other congenital malformations of the brain and cord. The infantile form of the Arnold-Chiari malformation usually occurs because of hydrocephalus in the early months of life, with evidence of spina bifida or frank paraparesis resulting from meningomyelocele. Therapy is directed toward surgical relief of the hydrocephalus with a ventricular shunting procedure and repair of the meningomyelocele. Prognosis is poor for patients with extensive defects.

ADULT FORM. The malformation may be asymptomatic until adult life, when the patient gradually develops symptoms and signs of dysfunction of the cerebellum, lower cranial nerves, pyramidal tracts, and posterior columns. Posterior cranial displacement may occur with coughing or straining. Downbeat nystagmus is characteristic. At times the initial signs may be those of hydrocephalus secondary to obstruction of the cerebrospinal fluid pathways or to coexisting syringomyelia of the cervical spinal cord and medulla (see Ch. 466). Commonly there is radiographic evidence of fusion of the cervical vertebrae, platybasia, or basilar impression, but MR scan establishes the diagnosis even when there are no coexisting bony abnormalities. The Arnold-Chiari malformation in adults may simulate syndromes produced by tumors near the foramen magnum or by multiple sclerosis. Surgical enlargement of the foramen magnum and decompression of the cervicomedullary junction benefit selected cases.

BASILAR IMPRESSION AND PLATYBASIA

Basilar impression refers to abnormal invagination of the cervical spine into the base of the posterior fossa of the skull. The diagnosis is made from sagittal MR reconstructions or lateral roentgenograms of the skull which show excessive protrusion of the tip of the odontoid process of the axis above Chamberlain's line, i.e., a line drawn from the back of the hard palate to the posterior margin of the foramen magnum. *Platybasia* refers to flattening of the base of the skull, wherein lateral roentgenograms of the skull reveal flattening of the angle between the orbital plates of the anterior fossa and the clivus, the sloping anterior floor of the posterior fossa. The abnormality by itself has no clinical significance.

These malformations are usually developmental in origin, and there may be hereditary transmission. Occasionally, basilar impression may result from metabolic bone diseases such as rickets, osteitis deformans, osteomalacia, osteogenesis imperfecta, or fibrous dysplasia. Minor degrees of deformity of the base of the skull give rise to no symptoms. The neck appears shortened, and its movements may be limited. With more severe invagination, there may be signs of impaired function of the cerebellum, lower cranial nerves, pyramidal tracts, and posterior columns. Syringomyelia and syringobulbia may be present. Increased intracranial pressure may develop owing to obstruction of the foramina of the fourth ventricle and the basal cisterns. The clinical manifestations must be differentiated from those caused by neoplasms in the region of the foramen magnum and multiple sclerosis. When neurologic signs are progressive, surgical decompression of the posterior fossa and upper cervical cord may be indicated.

Vinken PJ, Bruyn GW, Klawans HL, Myrianthopoulos NC (eds.): Handbook of Clinical Neurology. Volume 50, Malformations. New York, Elsevier Science Publishers, 1987. *A recent comprehensive review of congenital malformations of the brain and spine.*

SECTION SIXTEEN / DISEASES OF THE PERIPHERAL NERVOUS SYSTEM

Herbert H. Schaumburg

495 Introduction and Basic Terminology

The structure and function of the peripheral nervous system (PNS) appear deceptively simple when compared with the central nervous system (CNS). Actually, however, PNS diseases represent a potentially confusing jumble of conditions whose only common thread appears to be PNS dysfunction. Thus, while the anatomic diagnosis of peripheral neuropathy is readily established in nearly 100 per cent of cases by symptoms and signs, the correct cause is determined in less than one half of cases except in a few special centers. Recent clinical and experimental studies propose a simple, anatomic classification of most PNS disorders, suggesting that a working knowledge of the common peripheral neuropathies can be easily mastered. Since common diseases (diabetes or malignancy) produce more than one type of anatomic reaction in the PNS and most physicians are "etiology oriented," this chapter is organized according to individual diseases, stressing their common anatomic and pathophysiologic features whenever possible.

Certain terms associated with peripheral nerve disease have, by common usage, acquired set connotations. These include:

Radiculopathy. This term designates a selective abnormality of the dorsal (sensory) or ventral (motor) nerve root between the point where it joins the spinal cord or brain stem and the more distal point where the two roots fuse to form the peripheral nerve.

Neuropathy (peripheral neuropathy). This is the usual term for any disorder of peripheral nerves and replaces the term *peripheral neuritis*.

Polyneuropathy (symmetric polyneuropathy). This designates a generalized process resulting in widespread and symmetric effects on the peripheral nervous system.

Focal or multifocal neuropathy (mononeuropathy, mononeuropathy multiplex). These terms indicate local involvement of one or more individual peripheral nerves.

Dysesthesia. This term, like paresthesia, is poorly defined; it is commonly used to describe an unpleasant sensation produced by an ordinarily painless stimulus.

Paresthesia. This term indicates a spontaneous aberrant sensation such as pins and needles or tingling.

Hypoesthesia. This term refers to diminished sensation.

Hyperesthesia. This condition is an excessive response to sensory stimulus, even when the sensory threshold is elevated.

496 Anatomic Classification of Neuropathy

SYMMETRICAL GENERALIZED NEUROPATHY (Polyneuropathy)

DISTAL AXONOPATHY (DYING-BACK NEUROPATHY). This is the most common morphologic reaction of the peripheral nervous system (PNS) to toxins and underlies many metabolic and hereditary neuropathies.

The pathologic features include initial degeneration of the distal ends of large and long axons; the myelin sheath breaks down concomitantly with axonal disintegration. Axonal degeneration appears to advance slowly proximally toward the nerve cell body. Schwann cells and their connective tissue tubes remain in distal nerves, facilitating appropriate peripheral regeneration (Fig. 496–1).

Many prominent clinical phenomena closely correlate with the morphologic profile. Gradual onset reflects chronic metabolic disease or prolonged intoxication, stocking-glove sensorimotor loss reflects distal axonal degeneration in long nerves (sciatic, ulnar), normal cerebrospinal fluid (CSF) protein reflects the sparing of proximal sited nerve roots, and slow recovery corresponds to the indolent rate of axonal repair.

MYELINOPATHY. The term myelinopathy, when applied to the PNS, refers to conditions in which the lesion primarily affects myelin or the myelinating (Schwann) cell. Acute inflammatory demyelinating polyradiculoneuropathy (AIDP) is the only frequently encountered disease that primarily affects PNS myelin. It is likely that the demyelination of spinal roots and nerves in this disorder results from an immune system–mediated attack on PNS myelin.

The cardinal pathologic features, depicted in Figure 496–2, include primary destruction of the myelin sheath with the axon usually left intact. Demyelination initially affects multiple sites in nerves. The Schwann cell subsequently divides and rapidly remyelinates the axon to restore function.

TABLE 496–1. CLASSIFICATION OF PERIPHERAL NEUROPATHY

Symmetric generalized polyneuropathy
  Distal axonopathy (associated with drugs, industrial chemicals, metabolic diseases, deficiency syndromes)
  Myelinopathy (AIDP, CIDP associated with diphtheria, genetic leukodystrophies)
  Neuronopathy (associated with motor neuron diseases, herpes zoster neuronitis, carcinomatous sensory neuronopathy)

Focal and multifocal neuropathies (mononeuropathy)
  Ischemia (vasculopathy)
  Trauma
  Infiltration (granulomatous, malignancy)

Many prominent clinical findings correlate with the morphologic profile. Onset is rapid and recovery (once commenced) occurs steadily, reflecting the speed of demyelination and ease of remyelination. Initial changes may be distal or proximal or may affect cranial nerves. Generalized weakness and reflex loss are dominant features, reflecting the vulnerability of long myelinated fibers, and the CSF protein is usually elevated because inflammation in spinal roots results in leakage of protein into the surrounding subarachnoid space.

NEURONOPATHY. This term denotes conditions in which the initial morphologic changes occur in the neuron cell body. If the changes are intense, the affected neuron dies and permanent total motor or sensory dysfunction in the affected segment follows. The neuronopathies are a heterogeneous, poorly understood group of conditions and include many disorders of motor, sensory, and autonomic neurons. Infectious neuronopathies include familiar conditions such as poliomyelitis (motor neuronopathy) and herpes zoster ganglionitis (sensory neuronopathy). Some hereditary and toxic neuropathies probably are best conceptualized as neuronopathies. In general, a diffuse peripheral nerve disorder that is exclusively motor or sensory and that is characterized by little or no recovery should suggest the possibility of a primarily neuronal disorder.

An outline of the classification of peripheral neuropathy is provided in Table 496–1.

FOCAL AND MULTIFOCAL NEUROPATHIES (Mononeuropathy)

These conditions are characterized by dysfunction of an isolated peripheral nerve. Usually both motor and sensory symptoms are present. Trauma is the most common cause of monofocal neuropathy. Instances of nontraumatic focal neuropathies may pose

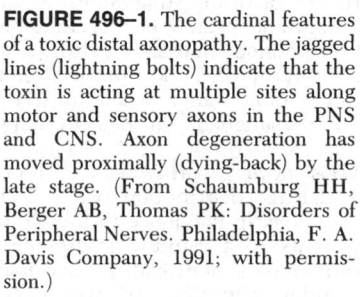

FIGURE 496–1. The cardinal features of a toxic distal axonopathy. The jagged lines (lightning bolts) indicate that the toxin is acting at multiple sites along motor and sensory axons in the PNS and CNS. Axon degeneration has moved proximally (dying-back) by the late stage. (From Schaumburg HH, Berger AB, Thomas PK: Disorders of Peripheral Nerves. Philadelphia, F. A. Davis Company, 1991; with permission.)

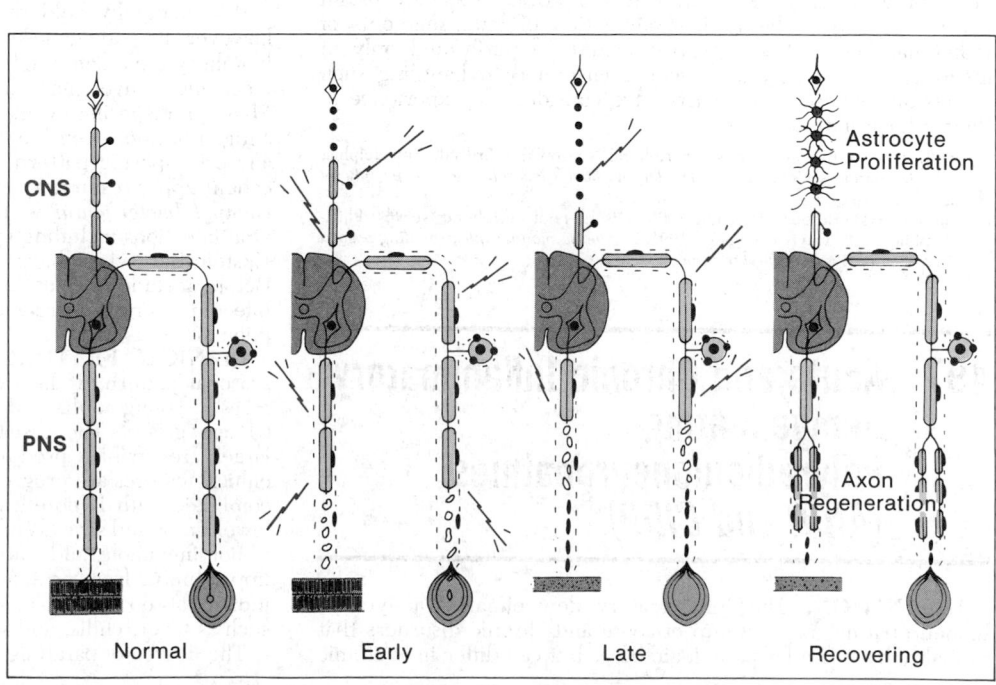

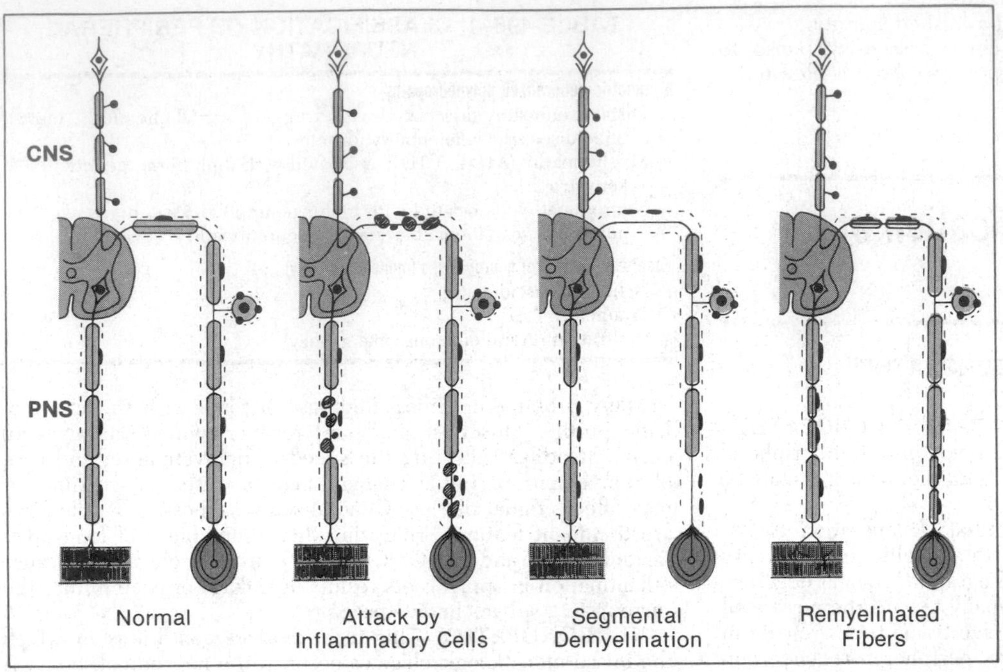

FIGURE 496-2. The cardinal pathologic features of an inflammatory myelinopathy. Axons are spared as is CNS myelin. After the attack, the remaining Schwann cells divide and remyelinate the denuded segments of axons. (From Schaumburg HH, Berger AB, Thomas PK: Disorders of Peripheral Nerves. Philadelphia, F. A. Davis Company, 1991; with permission.)

Normal   Attack by Inflammatory Cells   Segmental Demyelination   Remyelinated Fibers

formidable diagnostic problems and usually require extensive evaluation for the underlying cause (ischemia, infiltration by tumor, amyloid, leprosy, among others).

DIAGNOSIS. Nerve conduction studies performed by an expert in neuromuscular disease are the initial diagnostic procedures (see Ch. 441). They are critical in determining the presence of neuropathy, whether suggested by clinical features or subclinical. Nerve conduction studies also establish the location of focal peripheral nerve lesions such as carpal tunnel or other entrapments. Also, they usually indicate whether a symmetric polyneuropathy is axonal or demyelinating, a crucial first step in diagnosis.

Nerve biopsy may be useful in identifying the cause of multiple mononeuropathy syndromes (amyloidosis, sarcoidosis, leprosy, and vasculitis). Conditions readily diagnosed on clinical grounds, such as diabetic neuropathy and AIDP, do not require biopsy. Biopsy is seldom helpful in distal axonopathies, since most display similar nonspecific findings.

Either the sural nerve at the ankle or the radial nerve at the wrist may be sampled under anesthesia. Tissue should be processed for routine histopathologic study, electron microscopy, and nerve fiber teasing. The latter technique is especially useful because it allows the rapid examination of long segments of individual fibers. Nerve biopsy should be performed only in institutions served by a surgeon accustomed to handling such tissues and whose pathologists have considerable experience in their interpretation.

Dyck PJ, Thomas PK, et al. (eds.): Peripheral Neuropathy, 3rd ed. Philadelphia, W. B. Saunders Company, 1991. *The authoritative reference on peripheral nerve disease.*

Schaumburg HH, Berger AB, Thomas PK: Disorders of Peripheral Nerves. Philadelphia, F. A. Davis Company, 1991. *A concise monograph providing a good introduction to this complex subject.*

497 Acute and Chronic Inflammatory Demyelinating Polyradiculoneuropathies (AIDP and CIDP)

DEFINITION. The inflammatory demyelinating polyradiculoneuropathies are a group of acute and chronic disorders that probably have similar pathologic bases but can differ in anatomic sites and temporal profile. The most common is AIDP (Guillain-Barré syndrome), a rapidly evolving paralytic illness of unknown origin. Its salient morphologic feature is widespread inflammatory peripheral nervous system (PNS) demyelination, presumably secondary to a hypersensitivity reaction. The other, less common, form of inflammatory neuropathy is chronic inflammatory demyelinating polyneuropathy (CIDP). AIDP is the most common acute paralytic illness in young adults and almost the only form of inflammatory polyneuropathy encountered in general medical practice.

PATHOLOGY, PATHOGENESIS, AND PREDISPOSING FACTORS. Inflammatory cell infiltration (lymphocytes and plasma cells) followed by segmental demyelination is the hallmark of AIDP. Axons are relatively spared and blood vessels are normal. These reactions are most pronounced in spinal roots, limb girdle plexuses, and proximal nerve trunks; less intense changes are also present in distal nerves and autonomic ganglia. There is virtually no inflammatory change in the central nervous system (CNS). Within 2 to 3 weeks of the onset of acute demyelination, Schwann cell proliferation occurs as a prelude to remyelination and recovery.

It is generally held that AIDP is an autoimmune disorder; however, its pathogenesis is unclear. There is evidence for both lymphocyte-mediated delayed hypersensitivity and for a humoral mechanism involving antibodies to peripheral nerve myelin. Many predisposing events have been implicated, but a common antigen has not been identified, and HLA studies fail to disclose any predisposing pattern. Sixty per cent of cases have an antecedent upper respiratory infection or gastrointestinal illness (e.g., *Campylobacter jejuni*) within 1 month of onset. A host of common viral infections including infectious mononucleosis, hepatitis, and Epstein-Barr virus have been implicated. Other predisposing factors include vaccination against rabies and swine flu, HIV infection, surgery, pregnancy, and malignancy (especially lymphoma).

CLINICAL FEATURES. AIDP occurs worldwide in a nonseasonal pattern. It has a bimodal age distribution, with most cases in young adults and a lesser peak in incidence in the 45 to 64 age group. The disease consists of a rapidly progressive, largely reversible, predominantly motor neuropathy. Cardinal clinical features are progressive and usually symmetric weakness, combined with hyporeflexia. Weakness usually begins in distal lower limbs and spreads upward (ascending paralysis); this pattern is not inevitable and patients may have weakness of proximal upper limbs, face, or even extraocular muscles. Most weakened individuals do not appear systemically ill, and constitutional signs such as fever, chills, and weight loss are unusual.

The degree of paralysis varies from a mild footdrop to extreme weakness of all extremities and of the face. Severe involvement may lead to flaccid quadriplegia with inability to breathe, swallow, speak, or close the eyes. Limb weakness is generally symmetric and early muscle atrophy mild. Tendon reflexes usually disappear.

The presence of facial weakness helps to distinguish AIDP from most other neuropathies, apart from those related to sarcoidosis. Rarely, limb ataxia, paralysis of eye movements, and diffuse hyporeflexia may be the sole manifestations. Central nervous system involvement is not part of this illness. Increased intracranial pressure and papilledema rarely occur late.

Sensory symptoms, usually distal paresthesias, are present in most cases and rarely persist or progress (in contrast to weakness). Mild impairment of distal position and vibration sensation and slight loss of pinprick sensation over the toes are common.

Autonomic dysfunction accompanies most cases. Relative tachycardia is universal. Orthostatic hypotension and hypertension are frequent, difficult to treat, and can complicate the management of patients with respiratory compromise. Death can occur suddenly following unexplained fluctuations in blood pressure or cardiac dysrhythmias.

Cerebrospinal fluid (CSF) and electrodiagnostic studies are helpful. The CSF protein concentration is usually normal during the first 3 days of illness; it then steadily rises and may exceed 500 mg per deciliter. The CSF protein level may remain elevated even after recovery is under way. Mononuclear cells, usually less than 10 per cubic millimeter, are present in as many as half the cases.

At the commencement of illness, distal motor nerve conduction may be normal. Presumably, in such cases the disease process is confined to spinal roots and proximal nerves. If the demyelination affects distal nerves as well, slowing of motor conduction, characteristic of segmental demyelination, occurs. Analysis of the F response, a measurement of proximal motor conduction, can be useful in early diagnosis of patients who display normal distal motor conduction.

Differential diagnosis is not difficult, especially since the decline of poliomyelitis and diphtheria in North America. Hypokalemia, tick paralysis, botulism, acute myelitis, and cervical spine fracture should be ruled out rapidly.

COURSE AND PROGNOSIS. Rapid progression of weakness is characteristic of AIDP. Paralysis is maximal by 1 week in more than half, by 3 weeks in 80 per cent, and by 1 month in 90 per cent. In the other patients, weakness may progress for variable intervals up to 8 weeks.

Recovery usually begins 2 to 4 weeks after progression ceases. The pattern is variable, normally proceeding at a steady pace. Within 6 months 85 per cent of patients are ambulatory. Occasionally, individuals experience more rapid recovery and are able to return to work within 2 months following quadriparesis. Rare cases show little or no improvement.

Most patients eventually recover but one out of 20 dies and more than half suffer residual peripheral nervous system damage, with one sixth remaining handicapped by weakness. Some initial features help in predicting the eventual outcome. Older patients and those with electrodiagnostic evidence of axonal compromise do less well than individuals who experience only mild distal extremity weakness and subsequently improve within weeks of the first signs.

TREATMENT. Early and accurate diagnosis is crucial since plasmapheresis, the accepted therapy, when administered within the first 2 weeks shortens the clinical course and reduces morbidity. A continuous-flow regimen of 200 to 250 cc per kilogram is given within 2 weeks. Patients suspected of having AIDP must be admitted to the hospital even if involvement is minimal, since neuropathy may evolve rapidly and unpredictably. In general, they should be admitted to a unit where respiratory care is available, and remain until their condition stabilizes or improves. Tidal volume, oxygen saturation, vital capacity, blood pressure, and ability to cough and swallow should be closely monitored, since they can change without warning.

If a need for mechanical ventilation is anticipated (as determined by the degree of respiratory effort, the vital capacity, and the blood gases), it should be instituted early without waiting for decompensation.

Autonomic dysfunction may produce pupillary disturbances, neuroendocrine disturbance, peripheral pooling of blood, poor venous return, cardiac arrhythmias, and low cardiac output. Beat

to beat (R-R) variation of the heart rate during normal and deep breathing is a reliable index. Pharmacologic manipulation of blood pressure in AIDP patients is perilous and should be avoided unless absolutely necessary.

Some patients are unable to swallow or to gag. Feeding should be done through a small nasogastric tube. The patient should be sitting when food is given and for 30 to 60 minutes thereafter to minimize the risk of aspiration.

If patients with AIDP can be carried through the acute stage of progressive paralysis (usually 2 to 3 weeks), strength will gradually return. Since most patients achieve good recovery after months of weakness, the importance of fastidious supportive care in the acute stage cannot be overstressed. Glucocorticoids are contraindicated.

CHRONIC INFLAMMATORY DEMYELINATING POLYNEUROPATHY

DEFINITION, PATHOLOGY, AND PATHOGENESIS. Affected individuals initially have an illness similar to AIDP (although usually with a more gradual onset) but subsequently undergo either a chronic relapsing or progressive course. The salient histologic features of both chronic forms are similar to those of AIDP. Segmental demyelination, "onion bulb" formations areas of thickened nerves due to repeated demyelination-remyelination, and lymphocytic infiltration are prominent findings.

CLINICAL FEATURES. The progressive form is more common and, except for cases associated with HIV, there is rarely a clear temporal relationship to antecedent infections. The cardinal symptoms and signs reflect predominant motor involvement: weakness of the extremities, intercostal muscles, and lower cranial nerves. Sensory complaints are almost as common as weakness, and objective signs of sensory loss are more frequent in the chronic disorders than in AIDP. Hyporeflexia or areflexia occur in almost all cases.

The development and course of illness are the salient features that distinguish between the progressive and relapsing variants. Each has a protracted onset and an indolent progression.

The progressive form usually proceeds in stepwise fashion but may be gradual. If untreated, the condition may become disabling or fatal; the prognosis is uncertain. The course of the relapsing form may vary considerably in interval between episodes and rate and degree of recovery. With treatment, improvement is generally good between episodes. Life-threatening episodes with respiratory insufficiency are more common early in the illness.

The CSF protein level is elevated at some stage of the illness in almost every case. Slowed nerve conduction in both motor and sensory nerves is characteristic, although not always present. Nerve conduction studies can be extremely helpful in diagnosis, especially in the progressive form. The histologic picture is characteristic for these disorders. The differential diagnosis of the relapsing form is seldom a problem after several episodes have occurred. The differential diagnosis of the progressive disorder is sometimes extremely difficult. Unless nerve conduction studies display characteristic changes, it may be indistinguishable from a chronic axonopathy.

TREATMENT. Glucocorticoids are sometimes efficacious in treating chronic polyneuropathy, in contrast to the acute form. Human immune globulin therapy is gaining acceptance as a first-line treatment; it appears especially effective in HIV-associated cases. Plasma exchange may produce dramatic improvement in the relapsing form and is sometimes effective in the progressive disorder. It offers a useful alternative for individuals who cannot tolerate long-term corticosteroids or other immunosuppressive therapy.

McCombe PA, Pollard JD, McLeod JG: Chronic inflammatory demyelinating polyneuropathy. Brain 110:1617, 1987. *A detailed review of the clinical and therapeutic issues of the disorders.*

McKhann GM: Guillain-Barré syndrome: Clinical and therapeutic observations. Ann Neurol 27(Suppl 1):S13, 1990. *A timely review that thoughtfully analyzes the role of plasmapheresis and other therapies in AIDP.*

Ropper AH, Eelco FM, Wijdicks MD, Truax BT: Guillain-Barré Syndrome. Philadelphia, F. A. Davis Company, 1991. *A comprehensive monograph discussing the disorder.*

498 Diabetic and Other Endocrine Neuropathies

THE DIABETIC NEUROPATHIES

A variety of peripheral nerve disorders may occur in diabetes mellitus. Diabetic neuropathies may be classified as either mononeuropathies or symmetric polyneuropathies, but mixed syndromes often occur. For instance, an individual with symmetric sensory polyneuropathy may develop acute third-nerve palsy (a mononeuropathy). See Table 498–1.

Symmetric Polyneuropathy

PATHOLOGY. The experimental animal model of diabetic neuropathy exhibits only nerve conduction abnormalities without degeneration of nerve fibers; therefore, the early fundamental, pathologic diabetic changes in peripheral nerve are unclear. Previous human histopathologic studies were described in individuals with chronic neuropathy; nerves from biopsy or autopsy displayed a mixture of axonal loss and segmental demyelination. These observations suggested that axonal loss was primary and reflected an underlying metabolic disorder and that segmental demyelination was secondary to focal axonal change. Clearly fiber loss is the predominant change in chronic cases, restricting potential recovery. Postmortem histopathologic studies of long segments of nerves of diabetics indicate a multifocal pattern of fiber loss along nerves, suggesting that ischemia has a role in the symmetric neuropathies. Microangiopathic changes in the vasa nervorum are prominent in such nerve tissue. Sural nerve biopsies of diabetics contain abundant endoneurial capillary changes that include reduplicated basement lamina, closed lumens, and increased numbers of endothelial nuclei. These abnormalities appeared to correlate with degree of nerve fiber loss.

PATHOGENESIS. The clinical features of symmetric polyneuropathy, which often selectively involve particular fiber types, favor a metabolic basis. Elevated levels of neurotoxic ketones have been sought but not found. Distal axonopathy may be one of the mechanisms operating in individuals with the common progressive distal symmetric sensory neuropathy. No valid animal models are currently available to test this hypothesis.

Confounding a metabolic explanation is the inconsistent relationship of severity of neuropathy to control of blood glucose. There are many instances of "well-controlled" patients who develop severe sensorimotor neuropathy and others with "poor control" who have no evidence of neuropathy. The balance of recent evidence favors the notion that hyperglycemia is an important determinant of diabetic neuropathy and improved glycemic control is beneficial for nerve function.

Glycemic control does help two types of symmetric diabetic neuropathy. One affects the newly diagnosed, insulin-dependent diabetic whose nerve conduction velocity and distal sensation loss improve following institution of therapy. The other occurs in individuals with acute painful neuropathy associated with rapid weight loss (diabetic neuropathic cachexia) in whom institution of glycemic control is followed by weight gain and recovery from neuropathy.

Among the proposed biochemical mechanisms underlying diabetic neuropathy, accumulation of nerve sorbitol and depletion

TABLE 498–1. CLASSIFICATION OF DIABETIC NEUROPATHIES

Symmetric polyneuropathies
  Distal primary sensory neuropathy
  Autonomic neuropathy
  Rapidly reversible neuropathy

Mononeuropathy and multiple mononeuropathies
  Cranial neuropathies
  Focal nerve lesions (other than cranial)
  Proximal painful lower limb neuropathy (diabetic amyotrophy)

TABLE 498–2. SYMMETRIC DIABETIC POLYNEUROPATHY SYNDROMES

Distal sensory neuropathy
Autonomic neuropathy
Symmetric proximal lower limb neuropathy
Rapidly reversible neuropathy

of nerve myoinositol have received most attention. Sorbitol accumulates in the lens of the eye, alters the state of hydration, and may, by this mechanism, lead to cataract formation. Sorbitol also accumulates in nerve, but not in sufficient quantities to lead to osmotic damage unless it is confined to a particular cell compartment. Controlled clinical trials of aldose reductase inhibitors (the enzyme responsible for sorbitol accumulation) have been inconclusive.

Myoinositol is a cyclic hexitol normally present in nerve and is a precursor of membrane polyphosphoinositides that may regulate the patencies of ion channels. Nerve myoinositol concentration is reduced in experimental diabetes but is normal in human nerve biospy specimens. Although the addition of small quantities of myoinositol to the diet of animals with experimental diabetes may prevent reduction in nerve conduction velocity, the administration of dietary inositol to humans with diabetic neuropathy has little beneficial effect.

It is suggested that prolonged hyperglycemia may induce nonenzymatic glycosylation of vessel membrane protein. These membrane changes possibly account for progressive alteration of both endoneurial capillary wall and the endoneurial matrix, producing ischemic change in multiple levels of nerve.

CLINICAL FEATURES. See Table 498–2. *Distal Sensory Polyneuropathy.* This is the most common type of diabetic peripheral nerve disorder, estimated to be present in about 40 per cent of individuals with diabetes of 25 years' duration. It is present in less than 10 per cent of patients at the time of diagnosis (which it may antedate) and is uncommon in children.

Neuropathy may be asymptomatic, with abnormal signs first detectable on routine examination, or there may be a variety of symptoms. There appear to be three consistent patterns:

1. A "large-fiber" pattern with paresthesias in legs, absent ankle jerks, and impaired senses of light touch, vibration, and position in the lower limbs. Slight distal weakness is common and the hands may become involved.

2. A "small-fiber" pattern with dull aching pain and impaired cutaneous pain, touch, and temperature sensations. Position and vibration sense, deep tendon reflexes, and strength are usually spared. Autonomic nervous system dysfunction may accompany this variant.

3. A rare "pseudotabetic" pattern associated with long-term diabetes. Severe reduction of cutaneous and deep senses permits ulceration of the feet and distal joint deformity. Romberg's sign is present, tendon reflexes are absent in the legs, and hypotension and Argyll Robertson pupils may be observed.

The course is variable in sensory neuropathy. Most often it fluctuates and then plateaus. The pseudotabetic variety of the illness has an especially bad prognosis. Electrodiagnostic tests usually reveal changes in sensory conduction and variable alteration in motor conduction. The cerebrospinal fluid protein is usually elevated, sometimes to a very high level.

There is no specific treatment. Simple analgesics rarely help the severe pain that accompanies sensory neuropathy. Trial treatment with phenytoin, carbamazepine, phenothiazine, and tricyclic antidepressants is advocated. Persons with pain and temperature insensitivity of hands and feet are vulnerable to injuries that potentially can cascade into ulceration, cellulitis, lymphangitis, osteomyelitis, and osteolysis. Similar abnormalities are seen in syphilitic tabes, leprosy, inherited amyloidosis, and other inherited and acquired neuropathies, with the aforementioned sensory loss. The goal in treatment is to prevent the onset of tissue damage or, when it has occurred, to promote healing and prevent further damage. Persons with loss of pain and temperature sensation should not engage in most forms of manual labor or perform potentially bruising tasks with the hands and feet. Repeated inspection of hands and feet is necessary. If any bruise or ulcer appears, weight bearing or rough use should be stopped until healing occurs. Shoes should be wide and well constructed, with the insides inspected to remove retained objects or nails. Patients should soak the feet in lukewarm water for 15 minutes twice daily and cover them lightly with petrolatum lotion to retain moisture in the softened skin.

Autonomic Neuropathy. Diabetic autonomic neuropathy generally is associated with symmetric sensory neuropathy and occasionally predominates. Autonomic involvement can be asymptomatic or cause incapacitating disability. Three types of dysfunction are prominent: gastrointestinal, cardiovascular, and genitourinary. The common gastrointestinal disturbances are gastroparesis, episodic nocturnal diarrhea, and colonic dilatation. Gastroparesis is often asymptomatic; it is best identified by radiographic or nuclear scans that demonstrate delayed emptying. Cardiovascular manifestations include impaired vasomotor reflexes (postural hypotension), elevated heart rate, and loss of respiratory sinus arrhythmia. Genitourinary disturbances are especially distressing and include disordered micturition with large residual volume, retrograde ejaculation, and impotence. Impotence is sometimes the initial manifestation of autonomic neuropathy. It usually steadily worsens and rarely, if ever, is reversed by control of hyperglycemia, the use of testosterone, or penile implants.

Treatment of autonomic disturbances is difficult. Gastroparesis secondary to vagal denervation can be treated with either neostigmine or metoclopramide. Diabetic diarrhea may be helped by codeine phosphate or diphenoxylate, but not all cases respond favorably. A single 250-mg dose of tetracycline, if given at the outset, sometimes aborts the attack. Simple cases of postural hypotension may be helped by support stockings. More severe cases may require supplemental sodium in the diet plus sodium-retaining steroids.

Symmetric Proximal Lower Extremity Motor Neuropathy. This syndrome is most common in elderly diabetics but may appear at any age and occasionally heralds the onset of the metabolic disorder. Initial symptoms of low back and thigh pain are followed by slowly progressive weakness and atrophy of thigh and gluteal muscles. Loss of patellar reflexes is universal, but sensation is strikingly spared. Recovery is variable.

Rapidly Reversible Neuropathy. Newly diagnosed untreated diabetics may display asymptomatic slowing of nerve conduction velocity. This slowing is rapidly reversed by lowering blood sugar concentration to normal levels. It seems unlikely that this phenomenon is associated with structural breakdown in peripheral nerve fibers; it is not known whether such individuals are at greater risk of developing persistent symptomatic neuropathy.

MONONEUROPATHY AND MULTIPLE MONONEUROPATHY

PATHOLOGY AND PATHOGENESIS. It is believed that isolated peripheral nerve lesions in diabetics have a vascular basis. Several clinical facts support this notion: They have an abrupt onset, often recover spontaneously, and are most common in the elderly. Three careful autopsy studies, two of oculomotor palsy and one of femoral neuropathy, have demonstrated focal vascular lesions within the area of nerve damage.

CLINICAL FEATURES. See Table 498–3. *Cranial Nerve Lesions.* Isolated or multiple palsies of extraocular muscle nerves or lower cranial nerves may be the first indication of diabetes in asymptomatic older adults. The third nerve is most frequently affected. Onset is usually abrupt and is associated with an intense, retro-orbital aching sensation. Sparing of the pupillomotor fibers in diabetic third-nerve palsy helps distinguish this condition from lesions that compress the nerve, such as aneurysm. Satisfactory recovery of nerve function usually occurs within several weeks.

Focal Limb Lesions. Almost every isolated peripheral nerve can be affected by diabetic mononeuropathy. Lesions of the ulnar, radial, sciatic, peroneal, tibial, and lateral cutaneous nerves of

TABLE 498–3. DIABETIC MONONEUROPATHY AND MULTIPLE MONONEUROPATHY

Cranial nerve lesions
Focal limb lesions
Truncal neuropathy
Asymmetric proximal lower extremity motor neuropathy

the thigh are especially common. Diabetic nerves are especially vulnerable to compression, and lesions frequently appear at such sites. Onset is abrupt and usually painful. Recovery is usually good in distally sited lesions and less satisfactory if the lesions are proximal. Treatment includes physical therapy and use of appropriate orthotic devices.

Truncal Neuropathy. The syndrome of acute unilateral pain in the distribution of one or more thoracic nerves occurs in older individuals and can appear in any diabetic state. Pain is often intense, poorly localized, and associated with hypersensitivity and loss of pain sense. Recovery over a 2-year period is usual.

Asymmetric Proximal Lower Extremity Motor Neuropathy. This syndrome usually appears after middle age, in the setting of substantial recent weight loss. Cardinal findings include rapidly progressive, painful, asymmetric weakness of thigh muscles, loss of knee jerks, and few sensory abnormalities. The spinal fluid protein level is usually elevated, and weakness is usually bilateral, differentiating the condition from acute nerve root disease. Recovery is gradual. There is considerable variation in the clinical features, and many patients display distal weakness as well. Treatment includes major analgesics for relief of the self-limited pain, and physical therapy.

OTHER ENDOCRINE NEUROPATHIES

Hypothyroidism is associated with both mononeuropathy and symmetric polyneuropathy. Clumsiness and limb ataxia of uncertain origin are common, probably due to cerebellar disease. Thyroid replacement therapy ameliorates the carpal and tarsal tunnel syndromes as well as the diffuse symmetric neuropathy.

Acromegaly produces entrapment neuropathies at wrist and elbow and a distal symmetric polyneuropathy. Proximal weakness occurs independently of the peripheral neuropathies and may make the clinical profile confusing. The carpal tunnel syndrome presumably results from compression by acral soft-tissue hyperplasia and osteoarthritis. Improvement follows removal of the pituitary tumor; surgery of the carpal ligament is seldom necessary. Symmetric polyneuropathy usually occurs late in the illness; it bears no relationship to plasma levels of growth hormone. No studies have been made on the effect of removal of the pituitary adenoma on neuropathy.

Aminoff MJ (ed.): Neurology and General Medicine. New York, Churchill Livingstone, 1989. *An excellent encyclopedic text covering the neurology of systemic diseases.*

Asbury AK: Understanding diabetic neuropathy. N Engl J Med 319:577, 1988. *A thoughtful summary of pathogenetic theories and treatment strategies for diabetic neuropathy.*

Dyck PJ, Thomas PK, Asbury AK, et al.: Diabetic Neuropathy. Philadelphia, W. B. Saunders Company, 1986. *A book that covers all aspects of diabetic neuropathy.*

499 Hereditary Neuropathies

Hereditary neuropathies represent a group of slowly progressive disorders characterized by the type of inheritance, their natural history, and the population of neurons involved. Predominant involvement of lower motor neurons (progressive muscular atrophy) is called *inherited motor neuropathy*; involvement of sensory neurons is *hereditary sensory neuropathy* (HSN); involvement of both motor and sensory neurons is *hereditary motor and sensory neuropathy* (HMSN); and involvement of autonomic neurons is *dysautonomia*.

Expression of clinical symptoms varies widely from patient to patient, and functional disability is frequently less than might be expected from the neurologic signs. Certain of these disorders (HMSN types I and II) are common and account for many cases of cryptogenic neuropathy. The number of correct diagnoses increases considerably when the patient's asymptomatic relatives are examined clinically and by nerve conduction studies.

TABLE 499–1. THE HEREDITARY MOTOR AND SENSORY NEUROPATHIES (HMSN)

Nomenclature	Heredity	Clinical Features	Pathology and Pathogenesis
HMSN type 1 (peroneal muscle atrophy; hypertrophic form of Charcot-Marie-Tooth disease)	Autosomal dominant	Common; many mild cases; childhood onset; slow progression; predominantly motor; deformed feet (pes cavus); extreme distal lower limb atrophy; very slow motor nerve conduction	Possibly a distal axonopathy but much segmental demyelination and remyelination ("onion bulbs"); nerves may be enlarged
HMSN type II (neuronal form of Charcot-Marie-Tooth disease or peroneal muscle atrophy)	Autosomal dominant	Less common than type I; onset in second decade; nerve conduction almost normal; otherwise, identical to type I	Possibly a motor and sensory neuronopathy syndrome; loss of fibers; little remyelination (no "onion bulbs")
HMSN type III (Déjérine-Sottas disease)	Autosomal recessive	Rare; infantile onset; short stature, scoliosis, pes cavus; steady progression to severe disability; very slow nerve conduction	Few studies; enlarged nerves; many "onion bulbs"; pathogenesis unclear

HEREDITARY MOTOR AND SENSORY NEUROPATHY

These disorders, previously described by various eponyms (Charcot-Marie-Tooth disease, Déjérine-Sottas disease) are now numerically subdivided into types I, II, and III. Table 499–1 outlines their salient features.

DISORDERS OF PERIPHERAL SENSORY NEURONS

Patients with disorders of peripheral sensory neurons characteristically suffer from pain, cutaneous injury from lack of sensation, unsteady movement from kinesthetic sensory loss, or combinations of these conditions. Frequently they also have autonomic dysfunction. The nature of these symptoms and the associated sensory loss correspond reasonably well with the populations of fibers affected. Thus patients with loss of pain and temperature sensation and with autonomic impairment have degeneration mostly of unmyelinated and small myelinated fibers, whereas patients with loss of touch-pressure sensation have degeneration of large myelinated fibers of cutaneous nerves. In advanced disease this selectivity of involvement by fiber size tends to be lost.

HEREDITARY SENSORY NEUROPATHY, TYPE I. Hereditary sensory neuropathy, type I, is a dominantly inherited sensory radicular neuropathy. It has been variously termed perforating ulcers of the feet, mutilating acropathy, acrodystrophic neuropathy, and hereditary sensory radicular neuropathy. The severity varies widely. Sensory loss is usually more severe over the feet and legs than in the hands and forearms, and some patients have lancinating pains. Pain and temperature sensation are affected more than touch-pressure sensation. Nerve conduction of motor fibers is usually normal, as is life expectancy in most cases. Late in the disorder, perforating ulcers of the foot may develop, especially in patients with poor foot care.

HEREDITARY SENSORY NEUROPATHY, TYPE II. This is a recessively inherited disorder, also called congenital sensory neuropathy, that usually manifests itself in infancy or childhood with a mutilating acropathy characterized by paronychia, whitlows, ulcers of the fingers and plantar surfaces of the feet, and, frequently, unrecognized fractures of the extremities. Sensory loss affects all types of cutaneous and sometimes kinesthetic sensation and is most marked distally in all four limbs. Tendon reflexes are usually absent.

HEREDITARY SENSORY NEUROPATHY, TYPE III (Dysautonomia of Riley-Day). Familial dysautonomia is a recessively inherited disorder of Jewish infants and children. It affects peripheral autonomic neurons, peripheral sensory neurons, peripheral motor neurons, and probably other central nervous system neurons. Characteristics are onset in infancy, poor feeding, repeated episodes of vomiting and pulmonary infections, autonomic disturbances, and premature death. Autonomic abnormalities include defective lacrimation, defective temperature control, skin blotching, excessive perspiration, hypertension, and postural hypotension. There is insensitivity to pain, areflexia,

corneal insensitivity, and absence of the fungiform papillae of the tongue. An abnormality of nerve growth factor is postulated.

Dyck PJ, Thomas PK (eds.): Peripheral Neuropathy, 3rd ed. Philadelphia, W. B. Saunders Company, 1991. *A large, multiauthored reference text.*
Schaumberg HH, Berger AB, Thomas PK: Disorders of Peripheral Nerves, 2nd ed. Philadelphia, F. A. Davis Company, 1991. *A succinct, clearly expressed, comprehensive monograph.*

500 Toxic Neuropathies

UREMIA

DEFINITION AND ETIOLOGY. Uremic polyneuropathy can be associated with chronic renal insufficiency of any type. The cause is unknown. It is believed that uremic neuropathy is related to dialyzable toxins or metabolites normally excreted by the kidneys. The responsible agent has a molecular weight exceeding that of urea or creatinine.

PATHOLOGY. Axonal degeneration is characteristic of this disorder, and the distribution suggests that it is a distal axonopathy. The nature of the axonal change is nonspecific.

CLINICAL FEATURES. Initially, sensory symptoms predominate, with especially frequent tingling paresthesias of the leg. Occasionally a "burning foot" or "restless leg" syndrome accompanies uremic polyneuropathy. Muscle cramps in the distal extremities are common. Diminished sensation in distal limbs is the most consistent feature, usually in combination with hyporeflexia and moderate weakness.

Uremic neuropathy has an insidious onset, and subclinical cases are common. Most cases progress over several months to reach a plateau despite worsening of the renal state. The prognosis of untreated uremic neuropathy is poor.

TREATMENT. Successful renal transplantation both prevents

TABLE 500–1. PHARMACEUTICAL AGENTS ASSOCIATED WITH GENERALIZED NEUROPATHY

Chloramphenicol	Nucleosides (ddC, ddI)
Dapsone*	Nitrofurantoin*
Disulfiram	Nitrous oxide
Ethionamide	Phenytoin
Gold	Platinum (cis-platin)†
Glutethimide	Pyridoxine†
Hydralazine	Sodium cyanate
Isoniazid†	Taxol
Metronidazole-misonidazole	Thalidomide†
	Vincristine

*Predominantly motor.
†Predominantly sensory.

TABLE 500-2. AGENTS CAUSING SYMPTOMS ASSOCIATED WITH TOXIC NEUROPATHY

Acrylamide (truncal ataxia)
Allyl chloride
Arsenic (sensory, brown skin, Mees' lines)
Buckthorn toxin
Carbon disulfide
Cyanide
Dimethylaminopropionitrile (urinary complaints)
Biologic toxin in diphtheritic neuropathy (pharyngeal neuropathy)
Ethylene oxide
n-Hexane
Lead (wrist drop, abdominal colic)
Lucel-7 (cataracts)
Mercury
Methyl bromide
Organophosphates (cholinergic symptoms, delayed onset of neuropathy)
Thallium (pain, alopecia, Mees' lines)
Trichloroethylene (facial numbness)
Vacor

and reverses uremic polyneuropathy. Patients with mild cases display prompt relief of paresthesias and a steady return of strength. Recovery is more prolonged in advanced cases and is not always complete. Chronic hemodialysis is less helpful and often ineffective in reversing the neuropathy.

PHARMACEUTICAL AGENTS

GENERAL. New pharmaceutical agents are constantly being implicated on clinical-epidemiologic grounds as causes of peripheral neuropathy. Except for isoniazid, pyridoxine, and vincristine, few careful experimental studies of these substances have been conducted. Since following prolonged use most of the offending agents produce an insidious-onset distal axonopathy, little in the clinical diagnostic profile helps to identify the specific offending agent. The most important diagnostic factor in these disorders is a meticulous history of drug use. Table 500-1 lists pharmaceutical agents that are associated with generalized neuropathy. Treatment consists of withdrawing the drug if symptoms are prominent or progressive.

OCCUPATIONAL, BIOLOGIC, AND ENVIRONMENTAL AGENTS

GENERAL. Many potentially toxic chemicals are deployed in the work place and general environment, and several have been implicated as causes of peripheral neuropathy, usually of the distal axonopathy type. Since the various agents result in similar clinical syndromes, a careful occupational and environmental history is often the most important clue for diagnosis. The various agents are listed in Table 500-2, with prominent clinical features included in parentheses. *Buckthorn* and *diphtheritic neuropathies*, which are demyelinating conditions, are the sole examples of diseases in which biologic toxins are consistently associated with neuropathy. Diphtheria is further discussed in Ch. 306.

Spencer PS, Schaumburg HH: Experimental and Clinical Neurotoxicology. Baltimore, Williams & Wilkins, 1980. *A multiauthored comprehensive text with special emphasis on the peripheral nervous system.*

501 Miscellaneous Disease-Specific Neuropathies

NEUROPATHY ASSOCIATED WITH MALIGNANCY AND DYSPROTEINEMIA

Direct compression of nerves by metastatic tumors occurs within the spinal canal or invertebral foramina and behind tight fascial sheaths. Bronchogenic, renal, prostatic, and breast carcinomas are especially prone to such metastases. The direct and nonmetastatic neurologic effects of cancer are described in Ch. 162.

TABLE 501-1. FAMILIAL AMYLOID POLYNEUROPATHIES

Type	Source of Amyloid
I (Portuguese)	met/val 30 TTR substitution
II (Indiana)	ser/ile 84 TTR substitution
III (Van Allen)	Variant apolipoprotein A1
IV (Finnish)	Not yet established
Other forms	
Jewish	ile/phe 33 TTR substitution
Appalachian	ala/thr 60 TTR substitution
German	tyr/ser 77 TTR substitution

Met = methionine; val = valine; ser = serine; ile = isoleucine; phe = phenylalanine; ala = alanine; thr = threonine; tyr = tyrosine.
From Schaumburg HH, Berger AB, Thomas PK: Disorders of Peripheral Nerves. Philadelphia, F. A. Davis Company, 1991; with permission.)

Polyneuropathy is more common in multiple myeloma than in most other malignancies; furthermore, subclinical neuropathy appears to be frequent. Recent evidence has demonstrated that the benign gammopathies are also associated with polyneuropathy; some resemble motor neuron disease.

AMYLOID NEUROPATHY

Extracellular deposition of the fibrous protein amyloid is associated with peripheral neuropathy in both hereditary (nonimmunoglobulin-derived) amyloidosis and nonhereditary (immunoglobulin-derived) amyloidosis.

Seven different forms of familial amyloid polyneuropathy are currently recognized (Table 501-1), characterized by their clinical features and, except in two types, by a specific genetic mutation in the transthyretin (prealbumin) gene. The variant transthyretin (TTR) proteins have different amino acid substitutions; for example, in type I the variant TTR results from substitution of methionine for valine at position 30 in the molecule.

Hereditary amyloidosis is frequent only in endemic regions such as Portugal and Japan. In the Portuguese variety, which is inherited as an autosomal-dominant trait, the disorder usually begins in the third, fourth, or fifth decade and affects predominantly small sensory and autonomic fibers. Lumbosacral dermatomes show a syringomyelia-like loss of pain and thermal discrimination with preservation of touch-pressure sensation. Loss of potency in the male, postural hypotension, and bladder and bowel incontinence are common in advanced stages. The disorder tends to progress over a decade or so. Biopsied sural nerves show an endoneurial reduction in unmyelinated and small myelinated fibers with nodular deposits of amyloid among the nerve trunks.

Nonhereditary amyloidosis may be divided into primary and secondary varieties. The peripheral neuropathy of primary amyloidosis also affects the distal aspects of the lower extremities more than the upper and includes small fibers as much as or more than larger ones. When typical symptoms of neuropathy are associated with enlargement of the heart, nephropathy, and enlargement of the tongue, the diagnosis of primary amyloidosis should be strongly suspected and can be confirmed by histologic examination of rectal mucosa, kidney, carpal ligament, muscle, gingiva, nerve, or bone marrow. No effective treatment for the neuropathy is available.

Patients with multiple myeloma who develop a symmetric carpal tunnel syndrome should be investigated for systemic amyloidosis.

NEUROPATHY ASSOCIATED WITH NECROTIZING ANGIITIS AND RHEUMATOID ARTHRITIS

No fewer than nine disorders are associated with vasculitis and ischemic neuropathy. These include polyarteritis nodosa, rheumatoid arthritis, systemic lupus erythematosus (SLE), hypersensitivity angiitis, allergic granulomatosis (Churg-Strauss syndrome), Sjögren's syndrome, Wegener's granulomatosis, cranial arteritis (temporal arteritis), and nonsystemic vasculitic neuropathy.

Only polyarteritis nodosa, rheumatoid arthritis, and lupus erythematosus are encountered with any frequency in clinical practice. Although the fundamental expression of these conditions varies considerably, they all produce similar clinical and pathologic syndromes of ischemic mononeuritis multiplex. The pathogenesis of nerve fiber destruction in each condition presumably relates to focal ischemia from arteriolar occlusion. The clinical features are similar to those depicted for the mononeuropathies associated with diabetes (see Ch. 498).

Rheumatoid arthritis, in addition to producing a vascular mononeuropathy, may also cause entrapment neuropathy (reflecting prolonged immobilized postures and nerve compression by articular deformity) and a chronic symmetric sensory neuropathy. This latter disorder develops with long-term rheumatoid arthritis and is characterized by mild, distal, symmetric sensory loss. Although frequently painful, the condition is generally benign and improves spontaneously. Corticosteroid treatment is not indicated.

Neuropathy can accompany a variety of systemic illnesses other than those described in this chapter. Table 501-2 lists some of the more common conditions, and the text by Aminoff gives further details.

BELL'S PALSY (Idiopathic Facial Paralysis)

PATHOLOGY AND PATHOGENESIS. Neither the pathology nor the pathogenesis of this common illness is known. It is likely that mild cases with rapid recovery represent segmental demyelination and that axonal degeneration occurs in instances with prolonged dysfunction.

CLINICAL FEATURES. Idiopathic unilateral facial paralysis may develop rapidly within a few hours or evolve over 1 or 2 days and is often accompanied by pain behind the ipsilateral ear and excess tearing. Numbness of the face is a common complaint but inevitably refers to a proprioceptive sensation that accompanies weakness. Global facial muscle weakness is the hallmark of this condition. Hyperacusis, diminished lacrimation, and abnormal taste sensation are present to variable degrees. Untreated, 80 to 85 per cent of all patients with Bell's palsy recover completely or almost so. In a smaller number, persistent facial weakness ensues. Rarely, motor recovery fails completely. Aberrant regeneration is frequent. There may be embarrassing synkinetic movements (chewing producing eye winking) or excessive lacrimation.

Patients who are going to recover completely usually begin to show improvement during the first 2 weeks, while those destined to have permanent residual disability show no changes in status for 3 or more months. Except when paralysis is incomplete, there is little in the acute clinical profile to indicate prognosis. In patients who have complete paralysis from the onset, reliance must be placed on careful observation and electrodiagnostic tests of nerve excitability (performed at about 1 week after the onset).

Most authorities recommend treatment with prednisone, 1 mg per kilogram daily in two divided doses for 4 days, with dosage tapered to a total of 5 mg per day within 10 days. It is claimed that prednisone therapy should be instituted as soon as possible if it is to have an effect in decreasing residual paralysis and synkinetic movements. In any event, pain usually subsides promptly. Residual severe facial paralysis has a distressing cosmetic effect. Hypoglossal-facial nerve anastomosis will restore facial tone and is the operation of choice.

Hemifacial spasm, irregular clonic contractions of one side of the face, may be a temporary or permanent consequence of Bell's palsy. More commonly, hemifacial spasm develops without antecedent cause. In such cases, facial nerve compression by posterior fossa lesions (e.g., aberrant arterial loops, acoustic nerve tumors, aneurysms) may be present. Therapeutic choices include carbamazepine, botulinum toxin injection into the orbicularis oculi, and microsurgical nerve root decompression.

TABLE 501–2. OTHER MEDICAL CONDITIONS ASSOCIATED WITH NEUROPATHY

Herpes zoster (see Ch. 476.3)
Leprosy (see Ch. 334)
Sarcoidosis (see Ch. 67)
Human immunodeficiency virus (HIV) (see Ch. 414)
Lyme borreliosis (see Ch. 343)
Alcoholism, nutritional deficiency, malabsorption (see Ch. 456)

ACUTE BRACHIAL NEURITIS (Idiopathic Brachial Plexus Neuropathy)

Brachial neuritis is a syndrome wherein abrupt shoulder and neck pain is followed by a disabling upper limb weakness in a healthy individual.

PATHOLOGY AND PATHOGENESIS. There have been no thorough pathologic examinations of this condition, and the pathogenesis is unknown. Biopsy of cutaneous nerves has revealed nonspecific axonal degeneration. In most cases there is no common antecedent illness, immunization, or toxic exposure; some cases follow surgical procedures. The clinical profile is identical to that in certain serum vaccine paralyses, and a common immunologic basis has been suggested.

CLINICAL FEATURES. The condition arises as an acute, painful, and usually monophasic illness characterized by brachial plexus dysfunction. It is especially common in males aged 18 to 40. A cardinal feature is sudden severe shoulder girdle–scapular pain, occasionally extending into the arm or hand. The pain persists for a few days to a week and then subsides concomitantly with or shortly after the appearance of weakness, although it sometimes persists for several weeks. The serratus anterior is the single most commonly affected muscle. Distal weakness occurs less frequently. Rarely, the entire arm and ipsilateral diaphragm are affected. Uncommonly, weakness may appear in the other arm. Tendon reflexes are diminished in the involved extremity, but sensory loss is slight or negligible, being most commonly found at the apex of the shoulder. Involvement is usually restricted to muscles innervated by the brachial plexus. Weakness and atrophy of involved muscles lasts for months in many cases, but total recovery occurs in 90 per cent within 2 or 3 years. Treatment consists of physical therapy and orthotic devices to prevent joint damage. Corticosteroid therapy has no demonstrated value. There are occasional recurrences.

TRIGEMINAL NEUROPATHY

Rare cases are encountered of a slowly progressive bilateral sensory loss confined to the territory of the trigeminal nerve. This may lead to tissue destruction, particularly around the nostrils, as a result of repeated picking and scratching. High-level trichloroethylene exposure may cause this syndrome. Sjögren's syndrome, systemic sclerosis, and trigeminal neurilemomas should be excluded. Some cases have been found at autopsy to have infiltration of the trigeminal ganglion with amyloid. The explanation for other cases is obscure.

ACUTE PANDYSAUTONOMIA

Acute autonomic neuropathy is a poorly understood, rare condition. Pathologic studies are unavailable. The onset and time course are abrupt and progression is steady. Principal symptoms include postural hypotension, cramping abdominal pain, and varying amounts of diarrhea and constipation. Hypotension may be so severe that the patient cannot sit up without losing consciousness. Affected subjects reportedly improve with time, but few long-term follow-up studies are available.

Aminoff MJ (ed.): Neurology and General Medicine. New York, Churchill Livingstone, 1989.
Dyck PJ, Thomas PK (eds.): Peripheral Neuropathy, 3rd ed. Philadelphia, W. B. Saunders Company, 1991.
Halperin JJ, Luft BJ, Volkman DJ, et al: Lyme neuroborreliosis. Peripheral nervous system manifestations. Brain 113:1207, 1990. *A recent review of the many forms this disorder can take.*
Kelley JJ: Peripheral neuropathies associated with monoclonal proteins. A clinical review. Muscle Nerve 8:138, 1985. *A clear overview of this heterogeneous group of disorders.*
Moore PM, Cupps T: Neurological complications of vasculitis. Ann Neurol 14:155, 1983. *A comprehensive review of the protean neurologic complications of these disorders, especially the neuropathies.*

502 Acute Physical Injury and Chronic Compression-Entrapment Neuropathies

ACUTE PHYSICAL INJURY. The results of recent experimental studies suggest a simple classification for acute nerve injury in which the clinical features, including prognosis, closely

TABLE 502–1. TYPES OF NERVE INJURY

Type	Anatomic Lesion	Clinical Features	Course and Prognosis
Class 1	Either (A) transient conduction block due to ischemia or (B) demyelination	(A) Mild sensory loss and weakness (ischemic type) from transient abnormal posture (legs crossed) (B) Prolonged compression (Saturday night palsy) with paralysis and moderate sensory loss below site of lesion	(A) Rapid complete recovery (B) Gradual (lasting weeks) complete recovery
Class 2	Axonal interruption; connective tissue intact	Closed crush and percussion injury; loss of motor, sensory, and autonomic function below site of lesion; surgical exploration not indicated	Very slow recovery; prognosis best with distal lesions
Class 3	Transection of axons and connective tissue sheaths	Severe stretch injuries (heavy blows, motorcycle accidents) or penetrating wounds; total loss of all motor, sensory, and autonomic function; surgical intervention indicated for penetrating wounds	Little recovery even with surgical repair; poor prognosis

approximate the nature of the acute injury. Basically there are three different types (classes 1 through 3). In mild injury (class 1) axonal integrity is maintained but myelin may be damaged. In more severe injury (class 2) axonal continuity is lost but the connective tissue framework of the nerve is maintained. In the most severe injuries (class 3), nerve fibers and connective tissue are damaged to varying degrees. Table 502–1 depicts the types of nerve injury and their corresponding anatomic and clinical features.

COMPRESSION-ENTRAPMENT NEUROPATHY. The pathophysiologic features of chronic compressions and entrapment are still debated. It is widely believed that demyelination initially occurs and, if the condition persists, axonal destruction may follow. Several clinical forms are common, including carpal tunnel syndrome, ulnar palsy, and meralgia paresthetica (Table 502–2).

CARPAL TUNNEL SYNDROME. The median nerve becomes compressed at the wrist as it passes deep within the tissue to the flexor retinaculum. The usual symptoms include numbness, tingling, and burning sensations in hand and fingers. Pain sometimes radiates up the forearm as far as the elbow or even as high as the shoulder or root of the neck. These sensations are occasionally restricted to the radial fingers but may affect all digits. Pain and paresthesias are most prominent at night and often wake the patient from sleep. They may be relieved by shaking the hand. The hand tends to feel numb and useless on waking in the morning, but these sensations subside after brief use. The symptoms may recur following use or when the patient is sitting with the hands immobile. Such symptoms may persist for many years without objective signs of median nerve damage. In other patients, weakness of the thumb muscles develops in association with atrophy of the lateral aspect of the thenar eminence. Sensory loss may appear over the tips of the fingers. Occasionally, patients have motor symptoms of median nerve deficit in the hand without paresthesias, or motor and sensory signs may be discovered incidentally in the absence of symptoms, particularly in older individuals.

Most cases of carpal tunnel compression occur in middle-aged and often obese females. In younger women it is commonly

TABLE 502–2. COMPRESSION-ENTRAPMENT NEUROPATHIES

Common
Carpal tunnel
Ulnar palsy (cubital tunnel)
Lateral femoral cutaneous nerve of the thigh (meralgia paresthetica)
Rare
Cervical rib–thoracic outlet
Tarsal tunnel (tibial nerve at ankle)
Morton's neuroma (plantar nerve in anterior foot)

associated with excessive use of the hands, and it may develop in males after unaccustomed use of the hands, such as in housepainting. The disorder may be caused by tenosynovitis at the wrist, by involvement of the wrist joint in rheumatoid arthritis, or as a consequence of osteoarthritis of the carpus, perhaps in relation to an old fracture. Other predisposing causes are pregnancy, myxedema, acromegaly, infiltration of the transverse carpal ligament in primary amyloidosis, and chronic hemodialysis treatments. Diagnosis is based on clinical symptoms, Tinel's sign over the median nerve in the tunnel, and demonstration of slowed conduction at the wrist by motor nerve velocity studies. Individuals with muscle weakness and wasting or prominent sensory loss should undergo decompression of the nerve by section of the transverse carpal ligament. In patients with paresthesias alone or when the cause is probably tenosynovitis at the wrist, a reduction in hand activity may be sufficient to allow the symptoms to subside. Injection into the carpal tunnel of a long-acting corticosteroid preparation sometimes gives temporary relief, as does splinting of the wrist to reduce movement. When troublesome symptoms persist, decompression is advisable.

For most patients with paresthesias, symptoms are relieved by decompression. Sensory impairment and cutaneous hyperesthesia, however, may persist postoperatively, and there may not be recovery after prolonged denervation of the thenar muscles.

ULNAR PALSY. The ulnar nerve may be injured at the elbow, especially in persons with a shallow ulnar groove, those who rest their weight on their elbows excessively, and those who are cachectic and lie in bed. Injury may occur years following a previously malunited supracondylar fracture of the humerus with bony overgrowth (*tardive ulnar palsy*). Contrary to the findings in the carpal tunnel syndrome, muscle weakness and atrophy characteristically predominate over sensory symptoms and signs. Patients notice atrophy of the first dorsal interosseous muscle or difficulty in performing fine manipulation. There may be numbness of the small finger, the contiguous half of the proximal and middle phalanges of the ring finger, and the ulnar border of the hand. Treatment in mild cases consists of prevention of further injury. A doughnut cushion for the elbow may be helpful. Mobilizing and transplanting the nerve to a position in front of the medial epicondyle sometimes prevents further progression.

LATERAL CUTANEOUS NERVE OF THE THIGH. *Meralgia paresthetica* is an entrapment neuropathy resulting from compression of this nerve as it passes under the inguinal ligament. Although the case often remains unexplained, obese persons wearing tight girdles, individuals with gun belts, and those with pendulous abdomens are especially prone to develop numbness or burning sensations over the lateral thigh. Sometimes prolonged standing or walking provokes the symptoms. Weight reduction may help, and in many cases the condition subsides spontaneously. Surgical decompression is rarely necessary.

CERVICAL RIB AND THORACIC OUTLET SYNDROME.
Rarely, angulation of the brachial plexus over an abnormal rib or fibrous band can damage its lower fibers and lead to gradually progressive weakness and wasting of the small hand muscles. Numbness and pain may occur along the inner border of the forearm and hand. Surgical removal of the rib or fibrous band sometimes abolishes pain and paresthesias, but the small muscles of the hand often fail to recover strength. The overwhelming majority of individuals with paresthesias of the fingers prove to have either root compression from a cervical disc or carpal tunnel syndrome, not cervical rib or thoracic outlet.

Dawson D, Hallett M, Millender L: Entrapment Neuropathies, 2nd ed. Boston, Little, Brown and Co., 1990. *An extensive, excellently illustrated text covering all diagnostic and therapeutic aspects of these common disorders.*
Sunderland S: The anatomy and physiology of nerve injury. Muscle Nerve 13:771, 1990. *A concise review of the salient features of nerve injury.*

SECTION SEVENTEEN / DISEASES OF MUSCLE (MYOPATHIES) AND NEUROMUSCULAR JUNCTION

Andrew G. Engel

503 General Approach to Muscle Diseases

Muscle diseases are caused by derangements in the structure or function of the muscle fiber or in the innervation, blood supply, or connective tissue elements of muscle. A myopathy is a muscle disease not related to a demonstrable alteration in the innervation of muscle. Disorders that affect the innervation of muscle are considered in Ch. 495 through 502. Ch. 504 through 508 consider the myopathies. Ch. 509 deals with diseases of the neuromuscular junction. To facilitate the understanding of muscle diseases, this chapter begins with a brief overview of the structure and function of muscle.

BASIC STRUCTURE AND FUNCTION OF MUSCLE

Each voluntary muscle contains myriad muscle fibers. A small proportion of the fibers is confined to muscle spindles and innervated by γ or β motor neurons and by sensory neurons. These intrafusal fibers function as mechanoreceptors and participate in regulating the motor tone. Most muscle fibers are extrafusal and are innervated by α motor neurons. A *motor unit* consists of one α motor neuron and all muscle fibers innervated by that neuron. The peripheral axon of the motor neuron extends into muscle, where it divides into terminal branches that reach the neuromuscular junction on individual fibers. The number of motor units per muscle and the number of muscle fibers per motor unit vary from muscle to muscle. In general, motor units are smaller in small muscles subserving delicate movements (e.g., the external ocular, facial, and intrinsic hand muscles) than in large muscles maintaining posture or exerting strong force (e.g., biceps or quadriceps). The territory of a motor unit is a cylinder of the same length as the fibers and with a diameter that extends over a few millimeters. Muscle fibers belonging to different motor units intermingle with each other, so that the territories of individual motor units overlap. Many physiologic, biochemical, histochemical, and morphologic features of the muscle fibers are regulated by their innervation. Consequently, all muscle fibers in a motor unit share similar properties or are of the same type. Three major muscle-fiber (and motor-unit) types can be recognized: Type I, slow-twitch, fatigue-resistant fibers, high in oxidative enzymes but low in glycolytic enzymes; Type IIB, fast-twitch fatigable fibers, high in glycolytic enzymes and low in oxidative enzymes; and Type IIA, intermediate-twitch, fatigue-resistant fibers, high in glycolytic enzymes and with an intermediate content of oxidative enzymes. The myofibrillar ATPase, also different in the three fiber types, provides a convenient histochemical marker. In most human muscles the three fiber types occur in about equal proportions. Because the motor unit territories overlap, the fiber types intermingle randomly.

The muscle fibers of an adult are about 50 μm in diameter. Each fiber contains multiple subsarcolemmal nuclei. The myofibrils, which account for most of the fiber volume, are associated with mitochondria, glycogen granules, transverse (T) tubules, and sarcoplasmic reticulum (SR). The myofibrils, 0.5 to 1.0 μm wide, consist of repeating units, or sarcomeres, limited by Z disks. The latter anchor 1-μm-long thin filaments that extend from each Z disk toward the center of the sarcomere. The thin filaments interdigitate with 1.6-μm-long thick filaments in the central region (A-band) of the sarcomere. That part of the sarcomere which contains only thin filaments is referred to as the I band. It is the sarcomeres of adjacent myofibrils lying in register that give the striated appearance to the muscle fiber. The thin filaments are composed of actin, troponin, and tropomyosin. The thick filaments are made up nearly entirely of regularly arrayed myosin molecules. The head of each myosin molecule projects laterally from the thick filament and can serve as a cross-bridge between myosin and actin. The T-tubules are inward extensions of the muscle fiber surface membrane and propagate the action potential into the depth of the fiber. The SR abuts on the T-tubules and partially envelops individual myofibrils. In the resting state the SR sequesters calcium into its lumen by means of an ATPase and thereby maintains a very low calcium concentration (about 10^{-7} M) around the myofilaments.

When the T-tubules are depolarized by an action potential, voltage sensors embedded in their wall open calcium release channels positioned on the abutting SR surfaces and calcium escapes from the SR into the myofilament space. The released calcium binds to troponin on the thin filaments, which then acts on tropomyosin to allow repeated binding of the myosin cross-bridges to actin. Each binding is associated with a conformational change in the cross-bridge that exerts a force on the thin filament toward the center of the sarcomere. The cross-bridge cycle requires adenosine triphosphate (ATP), which is split by an ATPase on the cross-bridge. If ATP is depleted, the cross-bridges remain attached to the thin filaments and the muscle becomes stiff, as in rigor mortis. When ATP is available, the unloaded fiber shortens, the thin filaments are propelled into the A-band, and the Z disks are pulled closer together in every sarcomere. The active state subsides with calcium reuptake by the SR; interaction between actin and the cross-bridges ceases and relaxation sets in.

THE DIAGNOSIS OF MUSCLE DISEASES

The diagnosis of a muscle disease rests on a tripod: the clinical data, the electromyogram (EMG), and the muscle biopsy. None of the three approaches is entirely adequate by itself, but their combined use yields the correct diagnosis in a very high proportion of cases. Examples of disorders that are similar by clinical criteria but require muscle biopsy and EMG for accurate diagnosis are polymyositis, limb-girdle dystrophy, and adult acid maltase deficiency; distal muscular dystrophies, progressive muscular atrophy, and the slow-channel myasthenic syndrome; benign congenital myopathies, mitochondrial myopathies, and childhood or juvenile spinal muscular atrophies.

CLINICAL DATA. _The Genetic History._ This is relevant to diagnosis as well as counseling in the muscular dystrophies, congenital myopathies, and inherited metabolic myopathies. A negative family history, however, does not exclude autosomal recessive inheritance, an incompletely penetrant autosomal-dominant gene in one parent, or a new mutation. In autosomal dominant disorders (e.g., myotonic and facioscapulohumeral dystrophy or the familial periodic paralyses) a negative family history needs to be validated by examination of both parents. The clinical examination or biochemical tests may help in detecting heterozygotes in autosomal-recessive or X-linked recessive diseases. In Duchenne and Becker dystrophy, carrier detection and prenatal diagnosis are facilitated by dystrophin and DNA analysis.

The History of the Illness. **Age at Onset, Duration, and Rate of Progression of Symptoms.** Most benign congenital myopathies, congenital muscular dystrophy, congenital myasthenic syndromes, a number of inherited metabolic myopathies, and the acute form of spinal muscular atrophy present in infancy. Duchenne dystrophy usually presents in early childhood. Many inherited myopathies, inherited anterior horn cell diseases, and most hereditary peripheral neuropathies present in childhood or early adult life. Limb-girdle, Becker, and facioscapulohumeral dystrophy usually present in adolescence; myotonic, oculopharyngeal, limb-girdle, and distal dystrophies can present in adult life. Dermatomyositis and scleroderma can begin in childhood or adult life; pure polymyositis is unusual before adolescence; and inclusion body myositis seldom presents before the fifth decade.

Muscle weakness evolving over a few hours suggests an exogenous intoxication (e.g., organophosphorus or barium poisoning), periodic paralysis, or rhabdomyolysis. An abrupt onset of symptoms also can occur in myasthenia gravis or with other defects of neuromuscular transmission. Acute muscle weakness appearing during or after recovery from a Reye syndrome–like metabolic crisis suggests an enzyme defect in organic acid metabolism associated with secondary carnitine deficiency. Weakness evolving over a few days to a few weeks can occur in acute postinfectious polyneuropathy (Guillain-Barré syndrome), toxic neuropathies, and acute dermatomyositis. A subacute evolution, over a period of weeks to months, is seen in motor neuron disease; some metabolic myopathies, such as corticosteroid-induced or thyrotoxic myopathy; late-onset nemaline myopathy; and most cases of dermatomyositis and idiopathic polymyositis. A slow evolution over a number of years is typical of most dystrophies but can also occur in the inflammatory myopathies, such as inclusion body myositis, and in motor neuron disease.

Effects of Exercise, Rest After Exercise, Diet, and Temperature. Weakness appearing or increasing during exercise suggests a defect of neuromuscular transmission or in muscle energy metabolism. Weakness that decreases with exercise but increases during rest after exercise is typical of the periodic paralyses. Depending on the type of periodic paralysis, alterations in sodium, potassium, and carbohydrate intake can improve or exacerbate the symptoms. Fasting or a high-fat diet may provoke or worsen symptoms in patients with defects of fatty acid oxidation. Exposure to cold worsens myotonia and can provoke weakness in periodic paralysis and paramyotonia congenita. Exposure to heat can increase neuromuscular transmission defects.

Symptoms in Muscle Diseases. Relatively few symptoms are associated with diverse muscle diseases: weakness, decrease of muscle bulk, increased fatigability, muscle pain, cramps, stiffness, and discoloration of the urine caused by myoglobinuria. The cardinal symptom is muscle weakness, but patients often describe its consequences instead of speaking of weakness. Patients complaining of cramps sometimes suffer from contractures or tetany. The term _stiffness_ is used to describe a variety of conditions, such as the stiff-man syndrome, neuromyotonia, and myotonia.

Muscle Weakness. Vague complaints, such as constant fatigue and exhaustion, or weakness of all muscles of uncertain duration

in a patient who can carry out the tasks of everyday living suggest functional weakness. Patients with organic and evolving muscle weakness can always specify the tasks that they cannot do at present but could do a year, a month, or a few weeks before the examination.

Weakness of the cranial, cervical, torso, and limb muscles presents stereotypically. Weakness of muscles supplied by cranial nerves causes drooping of the eyelids (ptosis, third cranial nerve); double vision (diplopia, third, fourth, and sixth cranial nerves); failure of the eyelids to close at night, altered facial expression, difficulty in whistling or sucking from a straw (seventh cranial nerve); inability to close the jaw, difficulty in chewing hard food (fifth cranial nerve); difficulty in pronouncing words (dysarthria), hypernasal voice, nasal regurgitation of liquids, and difficulty in swallowing (dysphagia) (tenth and twelfth cranial nerves). Weakness of the cervical muscles is shown by difficulty in lifting the head from a pillow or holding the head erect, and weakness of the truncal muscles by difficulty in rolling over in bed or sitting up from the supine position. Weakness of the arm muscles is related as difficulty in holding the arms overhead, lifting heavy objects, or using the hands for motor tasks. Weakness of the pelvic girdle and of the proximal lower extremity muscles is reflected by difficulty in rising from sitting or squatting, climbing stairs, and stepping in or out of the bathtub. Weakness of the distal lower extremity may cause flopping of the feet or difficulty in rising on the toes.

Other Symptoms. In evaluating _abnormal fatigability_, it is important to define the duration and intensity of exercise that provokes it. Even mild exercise can induce fatigue in patients with defects of neuromuscular transmission or with mitochondrial myopathies that involve an electron transport complex. Brief periods of intense, anaerobic exercise precipitate fatigue in patients with glycolytic enzyme defects, but sustained exercise is required to induce fatigue in carnitine palmityltransferase deficiency.

Muscle pain (myalgia) at rest can occur in some of the inflammatory myopathies (especially dermatomyositis and the eosinophilia-myalgia syndrome), during acute viral infections, in polymyalgia rheumatica, myxedema, myotonic disorders, and necrotizing vasculitis, during attacks of myoglobinuria, and in neuropathies associated with vitamin-B$_1$ deficiency, arsenic intoxication, and alcoholism. _Muscle pain during and after exercise_ is experienced when the energy supply to muscle is restricted, as with defects in glycolysis or fatty acid oxidation, AMP deaminase deficiency, ischemia (as in intermittent claudication, scleroderma, and amyloidosis involving muscle), or in normal subjects after unusually strenuous exercise.

Muscle cramps last from seconds to minutes, are associated with high-frequency (up to 150 Hz) discharges of the motor units, and can be initiated by strong contractions and stopped by stretching the muscle. They occur with dehydration, azotemia, hyponatremia, myxedema, in partially denervated muscles, and sometimes in normal individuals without known cause.

Muscle contractures are electrically silent, last from a few to more than 30 minutes, occur only in patients with glycolytic enzyme defects, are provoked only by exercise, and involve only those muscles that had been exercised.

The facial and carpopedal spasms of _tetany_ occur with hypocalcemia or hypomagnesemia and are associated with high-frequency (up to 300 Hz) axonal discharges. High-frequency electrical discharges also occur in muscle in the _stiff-man syndrome_, _neuromyotonia_, and _myotonia_, arising in the spinal cord, the peripheral nerves, and in the muscle fiber surface membrane, respectively.

In _myotonic disorders_ mechanical or electrical stimuli applied to any region of the muscle fiber surface membrane elicit repetitive spike discharges that wax and wane in amplitude and frequency. Mechanical deformation of the membrane during contraction acts as positive feedback, again depolarizing the membrane. This electrical activity, which is independent of the anatomic arrangement of the fibers in the motor unit, causes tetanic contraction of the individual fibers. The symptoms are stiffness, difficulty in relaxing muscles after a strong contraction, being muscle-bound at the beginning of exercise, and improvement with continued exercise.

Myoglobinuria follows the excessive release of myoglobin from muscle during a period of rapid muscle fiber destruction (rhabdomyolysis). Weakness, muscle pain, and malaise are associated features.

The Clinical Examination. Inspection. This can reveal muscle atrophy, hypertrophy, contractures, winging of the scapulas, fasciculations (twitching of portions of muscles at rest caused by single contractions of motor units), myokymia (fine undulating movements of muscles associated with sustained abnormal motor-unit activity). The examiner also notes the patient's stance and gait, ability to walk on toes and heels, hop on one foot, and rise from sitting, squatting, or lying supine.

Inspection provides information on the distribution of weakness, which is then confirmed by detailed manual muscle testing. For example, weakness of the pelvic girdle muscles causes a waddling gait; if there is also weakness of the back extensor muscles, the gait is also lordotic with hyperextension of the upper torso. Muscle atrophy consistently predicts muscle weakness, but not all weak muscles are atrophic, and muscle atrophy can be masked by obesity. Muscle hypertrophy not from voluntary exercise is common in myotonia congenita; it also occurs in the course of Duchenne and Becker and—less commonly—of limb-girdle dystrophy. Hypertrophy may appear with chronic partial denervation, acid maltase deficiency, the permanent myopathy of periodic paralysis, myxedema, sarcoidosis, amyloidosis, and cysticercosis. The nonspecific term *pseudohypertrophy* refers to enlargement of a weak muscle.

Manual Muscle Testing. This part of the examination requires knowledge of the origin, insertion, action, and innervation of the muscles tested, a consistent technique, and a generally accepted rating scale. A commonly used scale is that adopted by the British Medical Research Council: 5, normal power; 4, active movement against gravity and resistance; 3, active movement against gravity; 2, active movement with gravity eliminated; 1, trace contraction; 0, no contraction. Experienced examiners further differentiate among slight, mild, and moderate weakness within Grade 4. The results are recorded and used for following the patient's clinical course.

The distribution of the weakness can help in formulating the clinical diagnosis, as shown by the following examples. Weakness greater in proximal than distal muscles suggests a myopathy rather than a neuropathy. Predominantly distal muscle weakness suggests a neuropathy but can also occur in myotonic and other distal dystrophies and inclusion body myositis. Selective involvement of some muscles with sparing of others is more likely to occur in dystrophy than in inflammatory muscle disease, but it can also occur in such diverse entities as adult acid maltase deficiency, focal myositis, or the slow-channel myasthenic syndrome. The external-ocular and other cranial muscles can be affected by the Guillain-Barré syndrome, neuromuscular transmission defects, some mitochondrial myopathies, oculopharyngeal dystrophy, and myotubular myopathy. Diffuse, symmetric weakness of multiple cranial muscles with ptosis but with sparing of the ocular movements suggests myotonic dystrophy. Motor neuron disease can affect the bulbar muscles but spares the external ocular muscles except rarely in terminal stages. Selective weakness of the triceps, wrist extensor, finger extensor, iliopsoas, hamstring, anterior tibial, and peroneal muscles, with relative sparing of other muscles, suggests upper motor neuron involvement.

Other Findings. *Action myotonia* is observed as an inability to open the fist or the eyes promptly after closing them tightly for a few seconds. *Percussion myotonia* appears as a local postpercussion contraction followed by abnormally slow relaxation. It can best be observed in the tongue, deltoid, thenar, and extensor digitorum communis muscles. A local swelling appearing for a few seconds at the site of percussion is not myotonia but *myoedema*, seen in myxedema and emaciation.

The *deep tendon reflexes* are diminished in proportion to the weakness in most myopathies; an early loss of tendon reflexes is observed in neurogenic diseases of muscle, inclusion body myositis, the Lambert-Eaton myasthenic syndrome, and in a number of benign congenital myopathies. Slow relaxation of the reflexes is typical of myxedema.

A complete *examination of the nervous system* is also relevant to the evaluation of muscle weakness. Table 503–1 lists clinical guidelines that differentiate nerve from muscle disease. Peripheral neuropathy, ataxia, neurosensory hearing loss, myoclonus, fluctuating neurologic deficits, and mental deterioration can be associated with mitochondrial myopathies.

Recognition of the *signs or symptoms of an associated illness* can point to the cause of the myopathy. Examples are collagen-vascular diseases, sarcoidosis, amyloidosis, the endocrine myopathies, and the mitochondrial myopathies with multisystem involvement. *Involvement of organs or tissues other than muscle* provides further diagnostic clues. For example, cardiomyopathy can be associated with myotonic dystrophy, Emery-Dreifuss dystrophy, certain types of periodic paralysis, thymomatous myasthenia gravis, familial limb-girdle myasthenia, and late-onset nemaline myopathy. Cardiomyopathy and/or hepatic enlargement can occur in sarcoidosis and in the myopathies associated with deficiencies of acid maltase, debranching enzyme, carnitine, acyl-CoA dehydrogenase, and of a mitochondrial electron transport complex.

Serum Enzymes of Muscle Origin. The serum creatine kinase (CK) level is elevated in many muscle diseases. The enzyme is released into serum from injured skeletal or cardiac muscle. CK is a dimer of muscle-specific (M) and brain-specific (B) monomers, and the different CK isoenzymes can be distinguished by electrophoretic analysis. Mature muscle contains predominantly the MM isoenzyme, whereas in mature cardiac muscle the MB form predominates. Accordingly, abnormal CK release from muscle increases mostly the MM isoenzyme, whereas CK release from heart increases the MB form in serum. Injured muscle releases other enzymes, such as aldolase, lactate dehydrogenase, and aspartate aminotransferase, but the increases are less marked and can derive from other tissues, such as the liver and erythrocytes. The serum CK level is a sensitive index of muscle fiber injury in a myopathy; it also can increase slightly or modestly in motor neuron disease, chronic peripheral neuropathies, after severe voluntary exertion, or following a convulsion.

ELECTROMYOGRAPHY (EMG). This test consists of the analysis of spontaneous, evoked, and voluntarily generated potentials from nerve and muscle. The procedure is useful in distinguishing between broad categories of disease, such as myopathy versus neuropathy, or demyelinating versus axonal neuropathy. In some instances the types of electrical potentials and the pattern of abnormality suggest a disease category, such as an inflammatory myopathy, a myotonic disorder, or a storage myopathy. A progressive decrease of the amplitude of the compound muscle action potential evoked by low-frequency repetitive nerve stimulation (decremental response) is observed with defects of neuromuscular transmission. Sequential assessment of an EMG abnormality can provide useful information of the distribution, degree of activity, and progression of a disease. For example, persistent fibrillation potentials in polymyositis reflect continuing disease activity; the decremental response can be used to monitor the course of myasthenia gravis; and alterations in nerve conduction velocities are a guide to the progression of peripheral neuropathies. Further details of the usefulness of EMG are given in Ch. 441.2, 496, and 509.

THE MUSCLE BIOPSY. Biopsy specimens are used for light microscopic, ultrastructural, and biochemical studies. In most

TABLE 503–1. CLINICAL CLUES DIFFERENTIATING MUSCLE FROM NERVE DISEASE

	Myopathy	Neuropathy-Neuronopathy
Distribution	Mainly proximal and symmetric	Distal if symmetric; nerve or root distribution if mono- or multifocal
Atrophy	Late and mild	Early and prominent
Onset	Usually gradual	Often rapid
Fasciculations	Absent	Sometimes present
Reflexes	Lost late	Lost early
Tenderness	Diffuse in myositis	Focal in nerve or root disease
Cramps	Rare	Common
Sensory loss	Absent	Often present
Muscle enzymes	Usually elevated	Usually not or slightly elevated

instances, light microscopic observations with enzyme histochemical studies are sufficient for diagnosis.

Muscles showing mild to moderate weakness are biopsied. Strong muscles may not show diagnostic pathologic change, and in more severely affected muscles excessive amounts of connective tissue may obscure the basic pathologic process. Muscles that have been injected (as is often the case for the deltoid) or recently examined by EMG are unsuitable for diagnosis.

Light Microscopy. The following pathologic alterations can be recognized in conventional paraffin sections of muscle: excessive variation in muscle fiber diameter; isolated or grouped atrophic fibers; target formations; increase in the number of internally located nuclei; focal loss of cross-striations; loss of myofibrillar markings; cytoplasmic inclusions; vacuolar change; fiber necrosis and phagocytosis; inflammatory exudates; invasion of non-necrotic fibers by mononuclear cells; regenerating fibers; ring fibers (caused by aberrant myofibrils); and proliferation of connective tissue elements. Histochemical studies of fresh-frozen sections reveal the dimensions of the muscle fibers in the native state; the distribution and abundance of mitochondria, lipid, and glycogen in the muscle fibers; myofibrillar integrity; increased lysosomal activity; the presence or absence of certain enzymes (phosphorylase, phosphofructokinase, cytochrome *c* oxidase, AMP deaminase); the histochemical profiles of the muscle fibers; and the distribution of the histochemical fiber types.

Neurogenic alterations in muscle consist of the appearance of atrophic fibers, singly or in groups of varying size; target formations; and grouping of histochemical fiber types caused by reinnervation of previously denervated fibers by collateral nerve sprouts. Central nuclei, loss of cross-striations, and hypertrophy and degeneration of nondenervated fibers also can occur in partially denervated muscle. Further details of muscle biopsy changes can be found in Dubowitz's monograph on the subject.

Electron Microscopy. This is primarily a research tool used in studying previously unrecognized syndromes and diseases of neuromuscular transmission or in analyzing mechanisms of muscle fiber injury. However, in some instances electron microscopy does have a role in diagnosis (e.g., in identifying the filamentous inclusions in inclusion body myositis or in revealing capillary microtubular inclusions and necrosis in dermatomyositis when inflammation and perifascicular atrophy are absent).

Biochemical Studies. These are essential for defining the biochemical basis of those metabolic myopathies in which the clinical or histologic data suggest a defect in carbohydrate, lipid, or mitochondrial metabolism. The direct measurement of the glycogen and carnitine content of muscle, assays of enzymes associated with glycolysis or fatty acid oxidation, determination of various aspects of mitochondrial respiration, analysis of cytochrome spectra, and a search for mitochondrial DNA deletions are examples of procedures currently used in the diagnosis of metabolic myopathies.

Dubowitz V: Muscle Biopsy: A Practical Approach. Philadelphia, Baillière Tindall, 1985. *A well-illustrated guide to the processing and interpretation of the muscle biopsy specimen.*

Engel AG, Banker BQ (eds.): Myology. New York, McGraw-Hill Book Company, 1986. *A multiauthored book on the anatomy, physiology, and biochemistry of skeletal muscle, the approach to muscle diseases, and the clinical aspects of muscle diseases.*

Walton J (ed.): Disorders of Voluntary Muscle. 5th ed. New York, Churchill-Livingstone, 1988. *A popular, multiauthored book with excellent chapters on the basic science and clinical aspects of muscle diseases.*

504 Muscular Dystrophies

DEFINITION AND BASIC CONCEPTS. Muscular dystrophies are inherited myopathies of unknown etiology associated with progressive muscle weakness, destruction and regeneration of the muscle fibers, and eventual replacement of the muscle fibers by fibrous and fatty connective tissue. There is no accumulation of metabolic storage material in the muscle fibers. Ultrastructural studies in Duchenne dystrophy indicate that breakdown of the muscle fiber plasma membrane is an early abnormality in the course of muscle fiber destruction. The lesions are conditioned by a deficiency of dystrophin, a 400-kilodalton cytoskeletal protein that represents the primary product of the Duchenne/Becker gene. The membrane lesions result in the influx of calcium-rich extracellular fluid and complement components into the fiber, activation of intracellular proteases and complement, and, eventually, removal of the necrotic fiber by macrophages. It is not yet known whether membrane lesions initiate muscle fiber destruction in the other dystrophies. Recognition of the molecular basis of the other dystrophies awaits the identification of the primary product of the dystrophic genes.

The current classification of the muscular dystrophies is based on the mode of inheritance, age of onset and rate of progression, distribution of the involved muscles, and associated findings in muscle or other organs. This is not entirely satisfactory because some cases cannot be fitted into currently recognized groups, and some dystrophies, such as the limb-girdle, distal, and facioscapulohumeral types, are heterogeneous by clinical, pathologic, or genetic criteria. A classification of the muscular dystrophies based on the categories used by Gardner-Medwin (1980) is shown in Table 504–1. A more precise classification awaits the chromosomal assignment and mapping of the loci of dystrophic genes (thus far accomplished in Duchenne, Becker, facioscapulohumeral, and myotonic dystrophy) and the availability of probes that can identify the presence of a given dystrophic gene in a given patient.

DUCHENNE DYSTROPHY. This is a lethal, X-linked recessive disorder of childhood. The abnormal gene is positioned on band Xp21 of the X chromosome. In over 65 per cent of patients deletions have been detected in dystrophin gene which prevent the formation of translatable mRNA; and in nearly all patients immunoblotting or immunostaining shows complete absence of dystrophin from muscle. The incidence is close to 1 in 3300 male births, the mutation rate being about 1 in 10,000. The disease is present at birth, becomes symptomatic during early childhood, leads to failure of ambulation near the end of the first decade, and terminates fatally near the end of the second decade. Early symptoms are developmental delays, difficulty in running or climbing stairs, frequent falls, and enlargement of the calves. Initially the weakness is more proximal than distal. Except for the sternocleidomastoids, the cranial muscles and the external

TABLE 504–1. CLASSIFICATION OF THE MUSCULAR DYSTROPHIES

X-linked Recessive Dystrophies
Duchenne dystrophy
Becker dystrophy
Emery-Dreifuss dystrophy with joint contractures and atrial paralysis
  ? Scapuloperoneal syndrome variant
  ? Rigid-spine syndrome variant

Autosomal-recessive Dystrophies
Autosomal-recessive childhood (limb-girdle) muscular dystrophy
Scapulohumeral (limb-girdle) muscular dystrophy
Autosomal-recessive distal muscular dystrophy
  With necrotizing features
  With rimmed vacuoles
Congenital muscular dystrophy
  Without cerebral abnormalities*
? Autosomal-recessive rigid-spine syndrome

Autosomal-dominant Dystrophies
Facioscapulohumeral dystrophy
  With inflammatory changes in muscle
  With cochlear hearing loss and retinal telangiectasis
Autosomal-dominant scapuloperoneal dystrophy (? related to facioscapulohumeral dystrophy)
Dominantly inherited adult-onset limb-girdle dystrophy*†
Oculopharyngeal dystrophy
Myotonic dystrophy
Autosomal-dominant distal dystrophy
  With onset in upper limbs (Welander type)
  With onset in lower limbs

*Variable clinical phenotypes suggest genetic heterogeneity.
†X-linked dominant form may also exist.

anal sphincter are spared. The proximal deep tendon reflexes disappear in about half the cases by the age of 10. Joint contractures, caused by uneven weakness of agonist and antagonist muscles, appear in the majority of patients between 6 and 10 years of age. After ambulation is lost, all muscles decrease in size and paraspinal muscle weakness causes progressive kyphoscoliosis. Weakness of the respiratory muscles can be detected after the age of 10, but the diaphragm is relatively spared. Carbon dioxide retention and anoxemia occur terminally with respiratory infections. Pure respiratory failure without infection can also occur and is an irreversible terminal event. The heart is affected with scarring of the posterobasal portion of the left ventricle, producing tall right precordial R waves and deep left precordial Q waves in the electrocardiogram in 90 per cent of the patients. Clinically significant cardiomyopathy is uncommon and in only 10 per cent of cases is death related to cardiac dysfunction. Central nervous system involvement is indicated by lower than average intelligence and mild cerebral atrophy.

Infrequently, Duchenne dystrophy manifests in females who have Turner's (XO) or Turner's mosaic (X/XX or X/XX/XXX) syndrome, a structurally abnormal X chromosome, or an X-autosomal translocation. In a few female heterozygotes, the disease manifests because of incomplete inactivation of the maternal X chromosome.

BECKER DYSTROPHY. The disorder has an incidence of about 1 per 20,000 male births. The gene locus is the same as for Duchenne dystrophy, but the mutations do not prevent the formation of translatable mRNA, so that a dystrophin molecule smaller or larger than normal in size and/or reduced in amount is produced. The manifestations of the two diseases are also similar, but Becker dystrophy begins later and evolves more slowly. In Becker dystrophy the mean ages for onset of symptoms, becoming chair-bound, and death are 12, 30, and 42 years, respectively. All patients show marked enlargement of the calves until the terminal stage. The serum creatine kinase (CK) level is markedly elevated in preclinical and clinical stages of the disease but begins to decline after the age of 20. Contractures develop at the wheelchair stage. Only some patients show electrocardiographic abnormalities, and only a minority are mentally retarded. The disease usually can be distinguished from Duchenne dystrophy by its more benign course. Immunoblot analysis of dystrophin extracted from muscle reliably distinguishes between Becker and Duchenne dystrophy, as well as between sporadic cases of Becker and limb-girdle dystrophy.

X-LINKED MUSCULAR DYSTROPHY WITH EARLY JOINT CONTRACTURES AND CARDIOMYOPATHY (EMERY-DREIFUSS DYSTROPHY). The disease presents in childhood, progresses slowly, and involves distal or proximal muscles in the lower extremities and proximal muscles in the upper extremities. There is no muscle hypertrophy. The serum CK is moderately elevated. Contractures of the knees, elbows, and cervical and dorsolumbar spine appear early in the disease. Atrial conduction defects and paralysis, requiring treatment by pacemaker, appear later. The disorder has been referred to as Emery-Dreifuss dystrophy and as X-linked scapuloperoneal myopathy, the distinction depending only on whether the proximal or distal muscles are affected in the lower limbs. The lack of muscle hypertrophy, early contractures, slow progression, relatively low serum CK, and overt cardiac involvement distinguish this disease from Duchenne dystrophy; all these features but the slow progression differentiate it from Becker dystrophy. When cardiomyopathy cannot be detected or the pedigree of X-linked inheritance is not established, the disease can be difficult to distinguish from the rigid-spine syndrome or other heterogeneous scapuloperoneal syndromes.

LIMB-GIRDLE SYNDROMES. The term *limb-girdle dystrophy* was applied by Walton and Nattrass in 1954 to a group of 18 patients (11 males and 7 females). The shoulder girdle was first affected in 13 cases (Erb type) and the pelvic girdle in 5 (Leyden-Möbius type). The face was spared. The onset was in the second decade in 7 patients and later in the others. Severe disability appeared over the next 20 years. An autosomal-recessive inheritance was postulated, although in one family the inheritance appeared to be autosomal dominant. Subsequently, a number of incompletely defined disorders were called limb-girdle dystro-

phy. The following diseases now appear to be reasonably distinct entities.

Childhood Muscular Dystrophy of Autosomal-Recessive Inheritance. This disease presents in the first or second decade, progresses slowly, and involves pelvic and pectoral girdle muscles without muscle hypertrophy. The serum CK level is moderately elevated (up to tenfold). Ambulation is lost near the end of the second decade. Cardiac abnormalities are absent. More severe variants, with muscle hypertrophy and death before the age of 20, have been described in inbred Amish and Tunisian kinships.

Scapulohumeral Muscular Dystrophy of Autosomal-Recessive Inheritance. Phenotypically this entity resembles that described by Erb in 1884. The onset is usually in the second decade. The shoulder girdle is initially affected; weakness then slowly extends to the pelvic girdle and to distal limb muscles. Facial muscles are spared. There is no muscle hypertrophy. The serum CK is moderately elevated at the onset but decreases with progression of the disease.

Adult-Onset Limb-Girdle Dystrophy of Dominant Inheritance. This is a rare condition with onset from the second through the sixth decade of life. It begins proximally and remains restricted to limb-girdle muscles. The serum CK level is normal or elevated. In some families there are rimmed vacuoles in the muscle fibers. In some kindreds the expression of the disease is restricted to either males or to females. Thus, this disease is also heterogeneous.

The Differential Diagnosis of Limb-Girdle Syndromes. All patients with limb-girdle syndromes need to be further investigated by EMG and muscle biopsy. Only a minority have a pedigree consistent with autosomal-recessive or -dominant inheritance and can be fitted into one of the above clinically distinct syndromes. The differential diagnosis in these patients includes inherited metabolic myopathies (e.g., acid maltase deficiency or a lipid storage myopathy); morphologically distinct congenital myopathies or their late-onset variants (e.g., nemaline, central core, and myotubular myopathies); or progressive muscular atrophy. In sporadic cases of a limb-girdle syndrome the differential diagnosis includes the same diseases, and also inflammatory myopathies (polymyositis, inclusion body myositis, or sarcoidosis confined to muscle); endocrine myopathies, sporadic Duchenne dystrophy, Duchenne dystrophy manifesting in female carriers, sporadic Becker dystrophy, and sporadic Emery-Dreifuss dystrophy before the appearance of joint contractures or cardiomyopathy.

FACIOSCAPULOHUMERAL DYSTROPHY. The inheritance is autosomal dominant with high penetrance and variable expression. The gene resides at the tip of chromosone 4. The disease presents in childhood or adult life. It involves the facial muscles early and then descends to the scapular fixators, the muscles of the upper arm, and the anterior leg muscles. Early signs include failure to bury the eyelashes, an expressionless face, pouting lips, winging of the scapulas when the arms are raised, and an inward-sloping anterior axillary fold. The rate of progression and the extent to which pelvic girdle, forearm, and lower torso muscles are eventually affected vary considerably between and within families. There is no muscle hypertrophy; joint contractures are uncommon; and the serum CK level is normal or shows mild elevation. A number of variants have been described. In some families a conspicuous inflammatory reaction appears in affected muscles, but the course of the illness is unaltered by corticosteroid therapy. In other families an associated sensorineural hearing loss occurs, with or without retinal telangiectasis and progressive painless blindness (Coats syndrome). The differential diagnosis includes progressive muscular atrophy, congenital myopathies (e.g., nemaline, central core, and myotubular myopathy), mitochondrial myopathies, sporadic cases of Emery-Dreifuss dystrophy before the appearance of joint contractures or cardiomyopathy, the scapuloperoneal syndrome, the slow-channel myasthenic syndrome, and polymyositis.

MYOTONIC DYSTROPHY. Transmission is by dominant inheritance with high penetrance and variable expressivity. The gene resides on the proximal long arm of chromosome 19 and shows close linkage to the gene encoding the muscle isoform of creatine kinase. The incidence is about 1 in 7500 births. A typical distribution of the weakness, myotonia, and multisystem abnormalities characterizes the disease.

Myotonic dystrophy presents in childhood or adult life; the

mean age at onset is 19 years. Myotonic symptoms either precede or accompany the muscle weakness. As the disease evolves, the myotonia diminishes in those muscles severely affected by the dystrophic process. Distal limb, levator palpebrae, masticatory, facial, cervical, pharyngeal, laryngeal, and upper esophagus muscles are commonly affected. External ophthalmoplegia is rare. Weakness can also appear in the proximal limb and respiratory muscles. The latter, when severe, results in alveolar hypoventilation, hypercapnia, arterial oxygen unsaturation, and increasing somnolence. Action myotonia is commonly observed in facial, lid elevator, and hand muscles; percussion myotonia is usually found in tongue, thenar, finger extensor, and selected proximal limb muscles.

A congenital form of myotonic dystrophy can occur in infants born to affected mothers. The onset is at birth with hypotonia, respiratory distress, and cranial muscle weakness. Myotonic phenomena, absent at birth, appear later in childhood. Motor development is delayed and mental retardation common.

Myotonic dystrophy produces systemic abnormalities including frontal baldness, subcapsular cataracts, testicular atrophy and ovarian dysfunction in adult life, extrathyroidal hypometabolism, end-organ unresponsiveness to insulin, mental changes, and hypercatabolism of IgG. Cardiac conduction defects are common and can cause sudden death. Gastrointestinal smooth muscle involvement results in reduced lower esophageal and gastric motility and dilatation of segments of the colon. Some patients have bouts of diarrhea alternating with constipation and colicky abdominal pain. Less frequent manifestations are pigmentary retinal degeneration and cranial anomalies (hyperostosis cranii, small sella turcica, large paranasal sinuses, and prognathism).

The pathologic alterations in the affected muscles are relatively distinct. These consist of very large muscle fibers with numerous central nuclei, sarcoplasmic masses, ring fibers, and variable type 1 fiber atrophy. Necrotic fibers are uncommon, which may explain why the serum CK level is normal or only slightly elevated.

DISTAL DYSTROPHIES. A number of genetically distinct entities has been recognized. An *autosomal-dominant type*, initially described in a large Scandinavian kinship by Welander, presents between the fourth and sixth decades with selective weakness and atrophy of the forearm extensor and intrinsic hand muscles and then involves the anterior leg and small foot muscles. In patients homozygous for the dominant gene, the onset is earlier and proximal muscles are also affected. In other non-Scandinavian kinships with late onset and dominant inheritance, the disease first involves the lower extremities. The serum CK level is normal or slightly increased. Two varieties of *autosomal-recessive distal muscular dystrophies* have been described. In both there is a juvenile onset and the lower limbs are affected before the upper. In one type there is frequent fiber necrosis and regeneration and the serum CK level is markedly increased. In the other type the muscle fibers harbor rimmed vacuoles and the serum CK level is only slightly increased.

The differential diagnosis of the distal muscular dystrophies includes myotonic dystrophy, inclusion body myositis, debranching enzyme deficiency, distal mitochondrial myopathy, distal chronic spinal muscular atrophy, and the neuronal form of peroneal muscular atrophy.

OCULOPHARYNGEAL MUSCULAR DYSTROPHY. The disease, inherited as an autosomal dominant, presents in the fifth or sixth decade with progressive ptosis and dysphagia. Later, all external ocular and other voluntary muscles may become affected. Death usually results from starvation or aspiration pneumonia. The serum CK level is normal or slightly increased. Muscle biopsy discloses intranuclear tubular filaments and rimmed vacuoles in the muscle fibers. This syndrome needs to be distinguished from mitochondrial myopathies that involve the external ocular muscles with or without affecting facial and limb muscles, and with or without multisystem features. In the mitochondrial myopathies, as discussed below, the age of onset and mode of inheritance are variable, and the muscle biopsy displays ragged red fibers.

SCAPULOPERONEAL SYNDROMES. These are heterogeneous disorders identified by the distribution of the affected muscles. An X-linked recessive form of scapuloperoneal myopathy with early joint contractures which also involves the spine and produces late cardiac atrial paralysis is essentially identical with Emery-Dreifuss dystrophy. An autosomal-dominant scapulo-peroneal myopathy resembles facioscapulohumeral dystrophy except that the face is spared. Other autosomal-dominant forms of the scapuloperoneal syndrome are associated with chronic anterior horn cell disease (Stark-Kaeser syndrome) or with a hypertrophic sensorimotor neuropathy (Davidenkow syndrome).

THE RIGID-SPINE SYNDROME. This is also a heterogeneous disorder in which muscle contractures involve the spine as well as other joints. The X-linked recessive form with cardiomyopathy and scapuloperoneal weakness appears to be identical with Emery-Dreifuss dystrophy. An autosomal-dominant form presenting with proximal muscle weakness in the first decade is also recognized. In most cases the disease is sporadic, begins in the first decade, and results in widespread muscle weakness and atrophy during the second decade.

CONGENITAL DYSTROPHIES. These present at birth with weakness and hypotonia, with or without multiple joint contractures. Most cases are sporadic; in some families several siblings are affected, suggesting autosomal-recessive inheritance. The weakness involves limb, torso, cervical, and sometimes the facial muscles. The serum CK level is normal or elevated. The subsequent course is one of slow or rapid progression, or the weakness increases only slightly during early childhood and then remains unchanged. The differential diagnosis includes Duchenne or autosomal-recessive limb-girdle dystrophy presenting at birth, morphologically distinct congenital myopathies, and acute infantile spinal muscular atrophy. The Fukuyama form of congenital dystrophy is associated with mental retardation, seizures, developmental abnormalities in the central nervous system, a progressive course, and death by the age of 10. The inheritance is autosomal recessive.

TREATMENT OF THE MUSCULAR DYSTROPHIES. There is no specific treatment of any of the muscular dystrophies. Physical therapy to prevent contractures, orthoses, and corrective orthopedic surgery can be used to improve the quality of life in some stages. The cardiac conduction defects in Emery-Dreifuss dystrophy and myotonic dystrophy may require treatment by pacemaker. The myotonia in myotonic dystrophy is rarely a clinical problem but can be treated with phenytoin (0.3 to 0.6 gram daily) or by quinine (0.3 to 1.5 grams daily).

Preventive treatment consists of prenatal diagnosis in families with known pedigrees, carrier detection, and genetic counseling. Some Duchenne carriers are recognized by immunostaining muscle for dystrophin, which may show scattered dystrophin-negative fibers. In some Becker carriers dystrophin of abnormal size or amount is detected by immunoblotting. Close to 65 per cent of Duchenne or Becker carriers and fetuses at risk can be identified by DNA analysis using cDNA probes or the polymerase chain reaction; carriers not identified this way may still be detected in families with known carriers by linkage analysis. In myotonic dystrophy, DNA markers closely linked to the locus of the disease allow prenatal diagnosis and detection of presymptomatic cases in 90 per cent of families.

Engel AG, Banker BQ (eds.): Myology. New York, McGraw-Hill Book Company, 1986. *An excellent, comprehensive description of the muscular dystrophies authored by multiple experts.*

Gardner-Medwin D: Clinical features and classification of the muscular dystrophies. Br Med Bull 36:109, 1980. *A revision of the classification proposed by Walton and Nattrass. Also contains concise and accurate summaries of the major clinical features of the different muscular dystrophies.*

Harper PS: Myotonic Dystrophy. Philadelphia, W.B. Saunders Company, 1979. *A modern classic—thorough in coverage, thoughtful in analysis, and written in a lively style.*

Kunkel LM, Hoffman EP: Duchenne/Becker muscular dystrophy. Br Med Bull 45:630, 1989. *A concise overview of current knowledge of the gene defective in Duchenne and Becker dystrophy, an account of normal and abnormal dystrophin, and a guide to newly available diagnostic tools.*

Miyoshi K, Kawai H, Iwasa M, et al.: Autosomal-recessive distal muscular dystrophy as a new type of progressive muscular dystrophy. Brain 109:31, 1986. *A well-documented study and a good review of the different types of distal muscular dystrophies.*

Shaw DJ, Harper PS: Myotonic dystrophy: Developments in molecular genetics. Br Med Bull 45:745, 1990. *Summary of recent progress in mapping the myotonic dystrophy gene and the application of this work to disease prediction.*

Wijmenga C, Frants RR, Brouwer OF, et al.: Location of facioscapulohumeral muscular dystrophy gene on chromosome 4. Lancet 336:651, 1990. *An important first step to cloning the gene and identifying its product.*

505 Morphologically Distinct Congenital Myopathies

DEFINITIONS AND BASIC CONCEPTS. The diseases in this group are characterized by the following features:

• The course is nonprogressive or relatively nonprogressive. The prognosis is generally benign except in reducing body myopathy and in the X-linked form of myotubular myopathy.

• A distinct pattern of inheritance is observed in some diseases (e.g., central core disease, nemaline myopathy); others are genetically heterogeneous (e.g., myotubular myopathy).

• Muscle weakness is present at birth or appears in early childhood. It is proximal or diffuse and may or may not involve the cranial muscles.

• The muscle bulk is normal or reduced. There is no muscle hypertrophy.

• The deep tendon reflexes are reduced or absent in most cases.

• Skeletal abnormalities related to the weakness, such as a high-arched palate, kyphoscoliosis, dislocated hips, and pes cavus, are common.

• The serum CK level is normal, except in some older patients with myotubular or sarcotubular myopathy.

• The EMG is normal or suggests a myopathy. Spontaneous electrical activity is absent in all cases, except for fibrillation potentials and myotonic discharges in some cases of myotubular myopathy.

• Each disease has one or more distinguishing, but not specific, morphologic features. Type I fiber preponderance and small type I fibers occur in most disorders.

Central Core Disease. The disease is transmitted by autosomal-dominant inheritance. The cranial muscles are usually not affected. The core formations can be central or peripheral, extend through the length of the fiber, are devoid of mitochondria, and may show focal myofibrillar degeneration. T-tubules, SR profiles, and glycogen are decreased in the cores.

Nemaline (Rod) Myopathy. An autosomal-dominant inheritance with variable expressivity has been demonstrated in some families. Facial, masticatory, oropharyngeal, neck flexor, respiratory, and proximal and distal limb muscles are typically affected. An oval face, micrognathia, and malocclusion are common. The disease is most severe in the first few years of life because of feeding difficulty and respiratory infections. Subsequently, some increase in strength takes place, and the clinical course remains stable. The nemaline bodies represent a replicative anomaly of the Z disk.

Myotubular (Centronuclear) Myopathy. X-linked recessive, autosomal-recessive, and autosomal-dominant forms of the disease have been described. The X-linked type is associated with severe respiratory muscle weakness and leads to death in early infancy. The autosomal-dominant form is relatively mild and may not present until adult life. External ocular, facial, oropharyngeal, and neck muscles are often affected. In each disorder the muscle fibers contain rows of central nuclei surrounded by cytoplasmic material, reminiscent of maturing myotubes. Type I fiber atrophy and type II fiber hypertrophy are common associated features.

Multicore Disease. The onset occurs in the first few months of life. Weakness is greater in proximal than distal muscles and in the upper than lower extremities. Ptosis as well as weakness of external ocular, facial, and neck muscles can occur. The inheritance is autosomal recessive with rare families manifesting heterozygotes or autosomal dominant with marked variation in penetrance. Individual muscle fibers contain myriad small core formations devoid of mitochondria.

Congenital Fiber Type Disproportion. The disease may occur in successive generations, suggesting an autosomal-dominant inheritance. Weakness is usually present at birth and tends to improve after the age of 2 years. Muscle contractures, skeletal deformities, and short stature are common. There is type I fiber atrophy and type II fiber hypertrophy with or without type I fiber predominance.

Other Morphologically Distinct Congenital Diseases. These less frequently encountered entities are identified by their morphologic abnormalities in muscle: fingerprint body myopathy, sarcotubular myopathy, reducing body myopathy, trilaminar myopathy, myopathy with focal lysis of the myofibrils in type I fibers, and spheroid body myopathy.

Late-Onset Variants. Adult-onset cases of central core disease, nemaline myopathy, myotubular myopathy, and multicore disease also exist. In some of these cases mild disease probably has been present since birth but is recognized only after additional progression in adult life or when discovery of an affected younger relative prompts investigation of other family members.

Two other forms of late-onset nemaline myopathy are noteworthy. One is sporadic, evolves subacutely or chronically, affects the proximal limb and torso but not the cranial muscles, and may cause death from respiratory failure. The CK level is normal. In some cases there is an associated monoclonal gammopathy. The EMG shows myopathic changes and fibrillation potentials. Histologically, there is progressive accumulation of nemaline rods and progressive atrophy of rod-containing fibers. Another late-onset form occurs in a familial setting, is associated with cardiomyopathy, and can result in sudden death.

Banker BQ: The congenital myopathies. *In* Engel AG, Banker BQ (eds.): Myology. New York, McGraw-Hill Book Company, 1986, pp 1527–1581. *A comprehensive, well-illustrated review. It raises numerous unanswered questions about etiology and nosology.*

506 Inflammatory Myopathies

DEFINITION AND CLASSIFICATION. Inflammatory myopathies represent a heterogeneous group of disorders. Most inflammatory myopathies are diffuse in distribution, but some are focal, affecting circumscribed regions in single or multiple muscles. Some are caused by or related to bacterial, parasitic, or viral infections. In most other inflammatory myopathies the etiology is undetermined, but an autoimmune etiology is suspected, and in inclusion body myositis both an autoimmune and a viral etiology have been postulated. A classification of the inflammatory myopathies is shown in Table 506–1. This section focuses on selected aspects of the idiopathic inflammatory myopathies not covered in other chapters.

Myopathies Related to Retrovirus infections. These can appear early or late in the course of immunodeficiency virus (HIV) infections. The most common form is HIV-associated polymyositis, which presents early in the infection and is mediated by T cells. Necrotizing myopathy without inflammation, or myopathies with nemaline rods or giant cells, necrotizing vasculitis, focal myositis in the form of pseudothrombophlebitis, and recurrent myoglobinuria without other predisposing factors can also occur. Attempts to immunolocalize HIV antigens in muscle fibers have consistently failed, and the manner in which the HIV virus induces myopathies is unclear. Zidovudine, an agent for treatment of the HIV infection, itself may induce a toxic mitochondrial myopathy that can coexist with the myopathy related to the HIV infection.

Human T-cell leukemia virus type I (HTLV-I), an agent associated with chronic spastic paraparesis, also can be associated with polymyositis, but the virus has not been shown to infect muscle fibers.

Autoimmunity in Idiopathic Inflammatory Myopathies. An autoimmune etiology in inflammatory myopathies has been inferred from one or more of the following observations: (1) The myopathy is associated with another identifiable autoimmune disease (e.g., systemic lupus erythematosus or rheumatoid arthritis). (2) Laboratory tests suggest an altered immune state (e.g., increased serum gamma globulins, decreased total hemolytic complement in serum, and positive tests for antibodies against native DNA, other nuclear or cytoplasmic antigens, or rheumatoid factor). (3) A predominantly mononuclear inflammatory exudate in muscle. (4) There is evidence of focal invasion and destruction of muscle fibers by antigen-specific cytotoxic T

TABLE 506–1. CLASSIFICATION OF INFLAMMATORY MYOPATHIES

Infections

Parasitic: toxoplasmosis, sarcosporidiosis, African trypanosomiasis, American trypanosomiasis, cysticercosis *(Taenia solium)*, trichinellosis

Bacterial: pyomyositis, septic myositis, gas gangrene *(Clostridium welchii)*, leprous myositis

Spirochetal: Lyme disease *(Borrelia burgdorferi)*

Viral: acute myositis following influenza or other viral infections, retrovirus-related myopathies (HIV, HTLV-I)

Idiopathic, autoimmune origin suspected

Pure polymyositis

Dermatomyositis

Inclusion body myositis

Scleroderma involving muscle

Inflammatory myopathy associated with another autoimmune disease (systemic lupus erythematosus, rheumatoid arthritis, Sjögren's syndrome, rheumatic fever, overlap syndromes, chronic graft-versus-host disease, polyarteritis nodosa)

Sarcoidosis involving muscle

Inflammatory myopathies with eosinophilia

    Eosinophilic polymyositis

    Localized eosinophilic myositis

    Eosinophilic perimyositis

    Diffuse fasciitis with eosinophilia

    Eosinophilia-myalgia induced by L-tryptophan preparations

Focal myositis

    Focal proliferative myositis

    Localized nodular myositis

        Pseudothrombophlebitis of a calf muscle

    Orbital myositis

Polymyalgia rheumatica*

Other inflammatory myopathies

    Localized myositis ossificans

    Generalized myositis ossificans

*There are no inflammatory changes in muscle.

---

cells. (5) The diseases respond to corticosteroids or other immunosuppressants. The first criterion, if fulfilled, represents strong, but indirect, evidence for an autoimmune origin of the myopathy. Laboratory tests suggesting an altered immune state are positive in a proportion of patients with dermatomyositis and in polymyositis. A mononuclear inflammatory exudate also can occur in some genetically determined muscle diseases (e.g., Duchenne or facioscapulohumeral dystrophy). Inclusion body myositis, in which an inflammatory exudate is often prominent, most cases of scleroderma, and some cases of pure polymyositis and dermatomyositis do not respond to immunosuppressants. Further, neither the factors that initiate self-sensitization nor the sensitizing antigen have been defined in any of the major inflammatory myopathies (idiopathic polymyositis, inclusion body myositis, dermatomyositis, and scleroderma). None has been transferred to an experimental animal.

Inclusion Body Myositis. This entity differs from the other idiopathic inflammatory myopathies in several respects. Clinically, it is not usually associated with another autoimmune disease and responds poorly to corticosteroids or other immunosuppressants. Most patients are older than 50, and there is male predominance. The disease evolves slowly, affecting the lower limbs first, involving both proximal and distal muscles, and resulting in selectively severe weakness and atrophy of the quadriceps. Facial, cervical, and pharyngeal muscles are spared. There is an early loss of deep tendon reflexes from the affected limbs. The serum CK level is mildly elevated or normal. The EMG indicates myopathic changes and abnormal electrical irritability, as in dermatomyositis or polymyositis, but there may be additional neurogenic features, such as an increase in the amplitude of motor unit potentials or mild slowing of nerve conduction velocities. Affected muscles show a typical pattern of histologic change: rimmed vacuoles in a significant proportion of the fibers; eosinophilic intranuclear and cytoplasmic inclusions in a few fibers; small groups of atrophic fibers without type grouping; and an endomysial and a lesser perivascular inflammatory exudate. The exudate is enriched in cytotoxic T cells that focally surround,

invade, and destroy non-necrotic fibers. Necrotic fibers also occur but are less common than in polymyositis. Ultrastructural studies show that the rimmed vacuoles contain myeloid structures and other cytoplasmic degradation products and that the inclusions consist of microtubular filaments resembling paramyxovirus nucleocapsids. The differential diagnosis of inclusion body myositis includes motor neuron disease, distal and other muscular dystrophies, peripheral neuropathies, and pure polymyositis. The diagnosis is usually clarified by a careful study of the muscle biopsy.

Differences Between Dermatomyositis and Pure Polymyositis. Dermatomyositis and pure polymyositis resemble each other in the predominantly proximal distribution of the muscle weakness, a mononuclear inflammatory exudate in muscle, myopathic changes and spontaneous electrical activity in the EMG, and responsiveness to corticosteroid therapy. Consequently, they are often treated as a single entity in evaluating their etiology, natural history, and therapy. However, several aspects of dermatomyositis differentiate it from pure polymyositis: (1) The characteristic rash of dermatomyositis is lacking in pure polymyositis. (2) Capillary injury and necrosis are early and constant findings in dermatomyositis. Many of the injured capillaries react to the membrane attack complex of complement, whereas other vessels are found to be occluded by platelet thrombi or to harbor microtubular inclusions. (3) Muscle fibers at the periphery of the fascicles undergo selective degeneration and atrophy. (4) The inflammatory exudate is concentrated at perimysial and perivascular sites and is enriched in B cells and helper T cells. (5) There is no evidence for T-cell–mediated cytotoxicity directed against the muscle fibers. These findings suggest that a humoral response against vascular elements plays an important role in the pathogenesis of dermatomyositis.

By contrast, in pure polymyositis there is no capillary necrosis or loss. The inflammatory exudate contains fewer B cells and helper T cells than in dermatomyositis, and B cells are virtually absent from the endomysium. There are focal invasion and destruction of non-necrotic muscle fibers by antigen-specific cytotoxic T cells accompanied by macrophages indicating cell-mediated cytotoxicity directed against the muscle fiber. Necrosis of isolated fibers also occurs. These findings suggest that a component of the muscle fiber surface membrane is a target of the immune effector response.

Differences Between Scleroderma and the Other Major Inflammatory Myopathies. In scleroderma, the serum CK level is either normal or only slightly elevated, spontaneous electrical activity is often absent from the EMG, and necrotic fibers are uncommon. The pathologic changes are those of fibrosis and inflammation involving the perimysium and the perimysial blood vessels. The inflammatory cells at these sites are predominantly T cells and macrophages. The findings suggest a cell-mediated immune response against a perimysial and/or vascular component in muscle.

Eosinophilia-Myalgia Related to L-Tryptophan Preparations. This syndrome appeared in 1989 in patients consuming L-tryptophan preparations. The features consisted of eosinophilia ($>10^9$ per liter), marked myalgias, fasciitis, and often a peripheral neuropathy. Interstitial pneumonitis, myocarditis, and encephalopathy occurred in some subjects. An autoimmune pathogenesis was implicated by onset or progression of the syndrome after withdrawal of the L-tryptophan preparation, inflammatory cells in the affected tissues, and responsiveness to immunotherapy in some cases. The pathologic substrate is an interstitial inflammation associated with an occlusive microangiopathy and fibroplasia. Thus far the triggering factor appears to be a contaminant of L-tryptophan produced by a single manufacturer, but the chance remains that this may not be the only source. Patients should be advised against L-tryptophan ingestion, at least until the matter is settled completely.

Myositis Ossificans. The *localized form* appears as a tender swelling after trauma to a muscle. After a few months this becomes hard and ossified. Therapy consists of excision. The *generalized form* represents an autosomal-dominant disease with variable expressivity that begins in childhood, involves many muscles, and causes progressive rigidity of body parts. The initial lesions appear in fascia and dermis and are associated with inflammation, local hemorrhage, and connective tissue proliferation. Cartilage and bone formation occur at a later stage. Other congenital malformations (microdactyly of the great toe, exostoses, absence of upper incisors or of ear lobules, and hypogenitalism) are found in most patients. There is no effective therapy.

Banker BQ: Other inflammatory myopathies. *In* Engel AG, Banker BQ (eds.): Myology. New York, McGraw-Hill Book Company, 1986, pp 1501–1524. *A well-illustrated review of the myopathies associated with eosinophilia, focal myositis, orbital myositis, and myositis ossificans.*

Dalakas MC, Illa I, Pezeshkpour GH, et al.: Mitochondrial myopathy caused by long-term zidovudine therapy. N Engl J Med 322:1098, 1990. *Excellent histologic analysis of the drug-induced mitochondrial myopathy, which is distinct from but can coexist with an HIV-related T-cell–mediated myopathy.*

Emslie-Smith A, Engel AG: Microvascular changes in early and advanced adult dermatomyositis. A quantitative study. Ann Neurol 27:343, 1990. *Presents evidence that the muscle microvasculature is an early and specific target of the disease process in dermatomyositis and highlights the differences between dermatomyositis and other inflammatory myopathies.*

Engel AG, Arahata K: Mononuclear cells in myopathies: Quantitation of functionally distinct subsets, recognition of antigen-specific cell mediated cytotoxicity in some diseases, and implications for the pathogenesis of the different inflammatory myopathies. Hum Pathol 17:704, 1986. *Describes antigen-specific T-cell–mediated cytotoxicity against the muscle fiber in polymyositis and inclusion body myositis, but not in dermatomyositis or scleroderma.*

Lotz B, Engel AG, Nishino H, et al.: Inclusion body myositis. Observations in 40 patients. Brain 112:727, 1989. *A summary of the clinical and morphologic features and a guide to the diagnosis of the disease.*

Martin RW, Duffy J, Engel AG, et al.: Eosinophilia myalgia syndrome associated with L-tryptophan ingestion: Clinical features and aspects of pathophysiology. Ann Intern Med 113:124, 1990. *A detailed account of the clinical and pathologic features of the syndrome in 20 patients.*

Simpson DM, Bender AN: Human immunodeficiency virus–associated myopathy. Ann Neurol 24:79, 1988. *A good description of several types of HIV-related myopathies.*

507 Metabolic Myopathies

GLYCOGEN STORAGE DISEASES. These are described in detail in Ch. 169. When muscle is involved, glycogen-filled vacuoles appear in the fibers; the glycogen excess can vary from slight to marked, and definitive diagnosis requires demonstration of a specific enzyme deficiency. Of the several glycogenoses, only glucose-6-phosphate dehydrogenase and liver phosphorylase deficiencies fail to affect muscle. All glycogenoses that affect muscle are transmitted as autosomal-recessive traits except phosphoglycerate kinase deficiency, which is X-linked recessive.

Acid Alpha-1,4-Glucosidase (Lysosomal Acid Maltase) Deficiency. The gene encoding the enzyme is mapped to chromosome 17. Various mutations affecting the synthesis, phosphorylation, and maturation of the enzyme have now been identified. Three major clinical variants exist. The *infantile type* presents in early infancy with generalized and rapidly progressive weakness and heart, tongue, and liver enlargement. There is widespread and marked glycogen excess in tissues, including lower motor neurons. Death occurs from cardiorespiratory failure before the age of 2 years. The *childhood type* presents in infancy or early childhood as a myopathy. Weakness is more proximal than distal, and there may be calf enlargement simulating muscular dystrophy. Glycogen excess is less marked and confined to muscle. Death occurs before age 20 of respiratory failure. The *adult type* presents between the second and seventh decade of life, either with slowly progressive limb muscle weakness that mimics limb-girdle dystrophy or polymyositis or with insidiously developing ventilatory insufficiency leading to respiratory failure. In all three types the serum CK level is increased, but to less than 10 times normal. The EMG in affected muscles shows myopathic changes and excessive abnormal electrical irritability, including myotonic discharges (but there is no clinical myotonia). The muscle biopsy demonstrates a vacuolar myopathy with high glycogen content and acid-phosphatase reactivity in the vacuoles, an appearance that otherwise occurs only in chloroquine myopathy and a rare cardioskeletal lysosomal storage disorder without acid maltase deficiency.

Debranching Enzyme Deficiency. A disabling myopathy affecting both proximal and distal muscles can appear in childhood or (more commonly) in adult life. Often there is a history of a protuberant abdomen and hypoglycemic episodes in childhood, along with muscle fatigue on exertion. Persistent hepatomegaly and biventricular cardiac hypertrophy are found in most cases. There is a diminished glycemic response to epinephrine and glucagon and an impaired rise of lactic acid after ischemic exercise. The EMG shows myopathic changes and abnormal electrical irritability in affected muscles.

Branching Enzyme Deficiency. The disease presents in infancy with progressive hepatosplenomegaly and failure to thrive. The abnormal starchlike glycogen, which resists diastase digestion, induces nodular cirrhosis and liver failure. Death occurs in early infancy from liver or heart failure. Muscle weakness is variable; if present, the tongue is severely affected.

Phosphorylase b Kinase (PBK) Deficiency. This syndrome shows marked clinical and genetic heterogeneity. Cardiac PBK deficiency is a fatal disease of infancy. An autosomal recessive form presents in childhood with weakness or hepatomegaly that improves with age; PBK is deficient in muscle, liver, and erythrocytes. An X-linked recessive disease presents in children with asymptomatic hepatomegaly or mild hypoglycemia; PBK is deficient in liver and erythrocytes. Another form of PBK deficiency which is restricted to muscle presents with exercise intolerance and myoglobinuria or a late-onset myopathy simulating muscular dystrophy.

Glycolytic Enzyme Defects: Myophosphorylase, Phosphofructokinase (PFK), Phosphoglycerate Kinase (PGK), Phosphoglycerate Mutase (PGM), and Lactate Dehydrogenase (LDH) Deficiencies. The common features are muscle cramps and periodic myoglobinuria on strenuous exertion since childhood; easy fatigability; a venous lactate level that fails to rise after ischemic exercise in myophosphorylase and PFK deficiencies, and fails to rise or rises by less than 100 per cent in PGK, PGM, and LDH deficiencies. Muscle cramps are prominent. They are caused by electrically silent contractures and are not associated with ATP depletion; their mechanism is not understood. The muscle glycogen excess is slight to modest. Permanent muscle weakness and atrophy are also slight, but they may increase with age. Fatal infantile variants have been identified in myophosphorylase and PFK deficiency. In PFK deficiency hyperuricemia and gout occur in some cases, and there is mild hemolytic disease caused by a partial erythrocyte enzyme defect. PGK mutations result in severe hemolytic anemia and neurologic deficits but no myopathy, or produce a myopathy with only the features described above.

DISORDERS OF FATTY ACID METABOLISM. Long-chain fatty acids taken up by muscle are utilized for energy metabolism or incorporated into triglycerides and stored as lipid droplets. Long-chain fatty acids entering the catabolic pathway are esterified with coenzyme A (CoA) to form acyl-CoAs. These react with carnitine to form acylcarnitines in a reaction catalyzed by carnitine palmityltransferase I, an enzyme positioned on the inner surface of the outer mitochondrial membrane. The acylcarnitines are transported through the inner mitochondrial membrane by a carnitine-acylcarnitine translocase and are then reconverted to acyl-CoAs by carnitine palmityltransferase II on the inner surface of the inner mitochondrial membrane. The acyl-CoAs undergo repeated cycles of β-oxidation, generating acetyl-CoAs that enter the citric acid cycle or form ketone bodies. The inner mitochondrial membrane is impermeable to long-chain fatty acids, CoA, and acyl-CoAs. Consequently, carnitine, carnitine-acyltransferases, and carnitine-acylcarnitine translocase jointly regulate the oxidation of fatty acids and modulate the intramitochondrial CoA/acyl-CoA ratio. Excessive intramitochondrial accumulation of an acyl-CoA compound leads to its conversion to a corresponding acylcarnitine. The acylcarnitine so formed leaves the mitochondrion via the translocase, diffuses out from the cell, and is preferentially excreted by the kidney. If this process continues, the muscle and body carnitine stores become depleted.

Derangements in fatty acid oxidation produce a variety of syndromes that affect muscle and other organs. The possible consequences include one or more of the following: intermittent energy shortage in muscle causing *rhabdomyolysis* and *myoglobinuria*; intramitochondrial acyl-CoA excess and CoA deficiency, secondary carnitine depletion, and inhibition of multiple mitochondrial enzyme systems (these events trigger a *Reye syndrome–like metabolic crisis* associated with hypoglycemia, acute fatty infiltration of the liver, hyperammonemia, marked release

TABLE 507–1. LIPID STORAGE MYOPATHIES ASSOCIATED WITH CARNITINE DEFICIENCY

Primary muscle or systemic carnitine deficiency
Organic acidurias with acyl-CoA dehydrogenase deficiencies*
  Long-chain acyl-CoA dehydrogenase deficiency
  Medium-chain acyl-CoA dehydrogenase deficiency
  Short-chain acyl-CoA dehydrogenase deficiency
  Multiple acyl-CoA dehydrogenase deficiency
  Long-chain 3-hydroxyacyl-CoA dehydrogenase deficiency
  Short-chain 3-hydroxyacyl-CoA dehydrogenase deficiency
Organic acidurias with defects in branched-chain amino acid metabolism*
  Isovaleryl-CoA dehydrogenase deficiency†
  Propionyl-CoA carboxylase deficiency
  Methylmalonyl-CoA mutase deficiency
  β-hydroxy-β-methylglutaric-CoA lyase deficiency
Defects in mitochondrial respiratory chain or energy utilization‡
  Block at NADH-coenzyme Q reductase (Complex I deficiency)
  Mitochondrial ATPase deficiency (Complex V deficiency)
Miscellaneous disorders‡
  Idiopathic Reye syndrome
  Valproate therapy
  Renal Fanconi syndrome
  Cirrhosis with cachexia

*Associated with secondary carnitine deficiency.
†This enzyme is also an acyl-CoA dehydrogenase.
‡Only some patients become carnitine deficient.

of enzymes from muscle and liver into serum, and encephalopathy); and triglyceride accumulation in muscle producing a *lipid-storage myopathy.* Many carnitine-deficiency syndromes are secondary to another metabolic defect in fatty acid oxidation, branched-chain amino acid metabolism, or the respiratory chain. A lipid storage myopathy can be caused by primary carnitine deficiency or by another defect of fatty acid oxidation with or without secondary carnitine deficiency (Table 507–1).

Carnitine Palmityltransferase Deficiency. The normal enzyme is a long-chain carnitine acyltransferase. The inheritance is autosomal recessive with reduced penetrance in women. The symptoms consist of muscle aching, fatigability, and periodic myoglobinuria on sustained exertion, especially if combined with fasting and exposure to cold. There are no symptoms between attacks, and the muscle lipid content is normal or only slightly increased. The mutant enzyme is not diminished in amount but is abnormally sensitive to inhibition by its own product and substrate, which explains why symptoms appear only when fatty acid metabolism is stressed and why little or no lipid accumulates in muscle.

Acyl-CoA Dehydrogenase Deficiencies. Deficiencies of the long-chain, medium-chain, and short-chain specific enzymes, and in the factors that transfer electrons from multiple acyl-CoA dehydrogenases to coenzyme Q (multiple acyl-CoA dehydrogenase deficiency), have been identified. Each syndrome causes secondary carnitine depletion, a lipid storage myopathy, and organic aciduria. The urinary organic acid and acylcarnitine profiles reflect the site of the metabolic block. *Short-chain acyl-CoA dehydrogenase deficiency* is associated with adult-onset lipid storage myopathy. Ketogenesis is not impaired and there are no metabolic crises. The other acyl-CoA dehydrogenase deficiencies produce intermittent metabolic crises resembling Reye syndrome. *Long-chain acyl-CoA dehydrogenase deficiency* usually has a neonatal onset and is associated with hepatomegaly and cardiomyopathy. *Medium-chain acyl-CoA dehydrogenase deficiency* presents in the first or second year of life with a metabolic crisis. Between attacks the patients are well or have mild weakness, easy fatigability, and mild hepatomegaly. *Multiple acyl-CoA dehydrogenase deficiencies* are genetically and biochemically heterogeneous. Severe neonatal forms with cardiomyopathy and milder late-onset cases have been described. Some cases respond to riboflavin therapy. The acyl-CoA dehydrogenase deficiencies are treated with a low-fat, high-carbohydrate diet and L-carnitine supplements (2 to 4 grams daily in adults and 100 mg per kilogram daily in infants and children). Crises can be prevented by avoiding fasting and maintaining alimentation at all times, especially during febrile illnesses. The crises are treated by intravenous therapy to correct the hypoglycemia and electrolyte abnormalities, and by L-carnitine, initially 100 mg per kilogram and then 25 mg per kilogram every 4 hours.

Primary Carnitine Deficiency Syndromes. Primary systemic carnitine deficiency is an autosomal recessive disease due to impaired carnitine transport in muscle, heart, kidney, and fibroblasts. A renal carnitine leak caused by the transport defect results in further tissue carnitine depletion. The disease is associated with cardiomyopathy, weakness, and episodes of hypoketotic hypoglycemic encephalopathy; it responds to carnitine replacement therapy. A myopathic form of primary carnitine deficiency also exists and may respond to prednisone therapy.

Other Lipid Storage Myopathies. Autosomal-recessive and -dominant lipid storage myopathies associated with lifelong weakness, myalgias, and electrical myotonia, but without carnitine deficiency, have been described. *Chanarin's disease* is a rare autosomal recessive condition with congenital ichthyosis, steatorrhea, and lipid storage in muscle fibers, hepatocytes, gastrointestinal epithelial cells, epidermal cells, monocytes, myelocytes, and fibroblasts.

MITOCHONDRIAL MYOPATHIES. These disorders are defined by a specific biochemical and/or a nonspecific morphologic abnormality in muscle mitochondria. The biochemical defects involve mitochondrial enzymes encoded by nuclear or mitochondrial DNA transmitted by, respectively, mendelian or vertical maternal inheritance. In many mitochondrial myopathies a substantial proportion of the muscle fibers appears ragged red in the trichrome stain. These fibers harbor accumulations of functionally defective mitochondria that are often large, contain abnormal cristae and various inclusions, and fail to react for cytochrome *c* oxidase. A current classification of mitochondrial myopathies is shown in Table 507–2.

From a clinical standpoint, in many mitochondrial myopathies there is slowly progressive weakness of limb and/or external ocular and other cranial muscles, abnormal fatigability on sustained exertion, and lactacidemia on exertion or even at rest. Some mitochondrial disorders affect multiple organs or systems, and the myopathy is but one facet of a multisystem disease.

Myopathies with Defective Energy Conservation. Luft syndrome is a hypermetabolic myopathy. Thyroid function studies exclude hyperthyroidism, but the basal metabolic rate is markedly elevated. The few patients observed to date had heat intolerance, hyperphagia, diaphoresis, polydipsia without polyuria, and progressive weakness since childhood. Oxidative phosphorylation was uncoupled, possibly because of abnormal recycling of calcium between the mitochondria and the cytosol.

TABLE 507–2. CLASSIFICATION OF MITOCHONDRIAL MYOPATHIES

Biochemically distinct disorders
  Defective energy conservation
    Hypermetabolic myopathy (Luft syndrome)
    Mitochondrial ATPase deficiency
  Impaired substrate utilization or transport
    Acyl-CoA dehydrogenase deficiencies
    Carnitine palmityltransferase deficiency
    Primary and secondary carnitine deficiency syndromes
    Defects in the pyruvate dehydrogenase complex
  Defects in the mitochondrial respiratory chain
    Coenzyme Q deficiency
    Complex I (NADH-coenzyme Q oxidoreductase) deficiency
    Complex II (succinate-coenzyme Q oxidoreductase) deficiency
    Complex III (coenzyme Q-cytochrome *c* oxidoreductase) deficiency
    Complex IV (cytochrome *c* oxidase) deficiency
      Fatal infantile type
      Benign infantile type
      Benign with external ophthalmoplegia
      Necrotizing encephalomyopathy (Leigh's syndrome)
      Trichopoliodystrophy (Menkes' disease)
Clinically distinct syndromes caused by mitochondrial DNA mutations
  Progressive external ophthalmoplegia with mitochondrial myopathy
  Kearns-Sayre syndrome (retinitis pigmentosa, heart block, external ophthalmoplegia plus other features)
  Myoclonus, generalized seizures, cerebellar syndrome, lactacidemia, plus other features (MERF)
  Encephalopathy with strokelike episodes and lactacidemia, plus other features (MELAS)
Recognizable only by morphologic criteria

Mitochondrial ATPase deficiency is a multisystem disease that presents in childhood. It produces muscle weakness associated with a myopathy and peripheral neuropathy, high-tone hearing loss, frequent vomiting, increased spinal fluid protein, basal ganglia calcifications, retinopathy, ataxia, and dementia. Secondary carnitine deficiency and lipid storage in muscle can also occur. A point mutation of mitochondrial DNA affecting subunit 6 of complex V has been observed in one pedigree.

Impaired Substrate Utilization Caused by Transport or Enzyme Defects. These disorders include the primary carnitine deficiencies, acyl-CoA dehydrogenase deficiencies, carnitine palmityltransferase deficiency (all dealt with above), and *defects in the pyruvate dehydrogenase complex*. The latter are associated with various neurologic syndromes that include movement disorders, ataxia, neuropathy, subacute necrotizing encephalomyelopathy (Leigh's syndrome), and fatal infantile lactic acidosis. The muscle biopsy shows ragged red fibers, lipid excess, or denervation atrophy.

Defects in the Mitochondrial Respiratory Chain. The mitochondrial respiratory chain includes four distinct enzyme complexes and also coenzyme Q and cytochrome *c*. The components are attached to the inner mitochondrial membrane and carry reducing equivalents from reduced nicotinamide adenine dinucleotide (NADH), flavin adenine dinucleotide ($FADH_2$), and electron-transferring flavoprotein (ETF) to molecular oxygen. A fifth complex, an ATPase, uses released energy to phosphorylate ADP to ATP in a tightly coupled process. Mitochondrial ATPase deficiency was discussed above. Defects in the electron transport complexes are associated with marked clinical, biochemical, and genetic heterogeneity. The reasons for this are that each complex is composed of multiple subunits, different subunits of a given complex are encoded by different genes, some subunits of a given complex are encoded by mitochondrial rather than nuclear DNA, some subunits are tissue specific, and some subunits are developmentally regulated. Mitochondrial DNA (mtDNA) can undergo point, deletion, or duplication mutations. With homoplasmic mutations, a single population of mutant mtDNA appears in all cells and produces a single clinical syndrome. With heteroplasmic mutations, normal and mutant forms of mtDNa coexist in the same cell, and subsequent cell replication leads to uneven segregation of normal and mutant DNA. The phenotypic expression depends on the proportion of mutant to normal mtDNA in cells of a given tissue, as well as tissue dependence on oxidative metabolism and the severity of the oxidation-phosphorylation defect.

Coenzyme Q Deficiency. A deficiency of mitochondrial coenzyme Q has been associated with a familial syndrome of marked lipid and mitochondrial excess in muscle, severe lactacidemia, intermittent myoglobinuria, progressive muscle weakness, cognitive deficits, cerebellar ataxia, and seizures. The activities of complex I, II, III, and IV and cellular cytochrome levels were normal.

Complex I (NADH-Coenzyme Q Oxidoreductase) Deficiency. Most of these begin in childhood and allow survival to adult life. Either muscular or central nervous system manifestations dominate the clinical picture. In the former group the findings include muscle weakness, exercise intolerance, exertional lactacidemia, and ragged red fibers in muscle. Headaches, progressive visual loss, hemiparesis, dysphasia, dementia, dystonia, and cerebral atrophy affect the latter group. A fatal infantile form also exists.

Complex III (Coenzyme Q–Cytochrome *c* Oxidoreductase) Deficiency. These also begin in childhood or adult life. Muscle weakness, exercise intolerance, exertional lactacidemia, and ragged red fibers are constant findings. Some patients also have external ophthalmoplegia and/or dementia, myoclonus, ataxia, pyramidal signs, and loss of proprioception. The muscle symptoms in one patient were improved by treatment with menadione and vitamin C, agents that can function as electron transfer mediators instead of complex III.

Complex IV (Cytochrome *c* Oxidase) Deficiency. Several syndromes are associated with this defect. A *fatal infantile mitochondrial myopathy* presents at birth or shortly thereafter with weakness, hypotonia, and lactacidemia. Renal Fanconi syndrome *or* cardiomyopathy *or* liver enlargement can be associated with the fatal infantile syndrome. Muscle contains large accumulations of mitochondria, lipid, and glycogen. The phenotypic variability is attributed to the existence of tissue-specific subunits of complex IV. A *benign infantile myopathy* with reversible complex IV deficiency presents neonatally with profound weakness of all but the ocular muscles, hepatomegaly, macroglossia, and severe lactacidemia. Spontaneous improvement begins after 6 months, and only mild weakness persists into later life. Complex IV deficiency in muscle, liver, and brain also has been described in some cases of *necrotizing encephalomyelopathy* (Leigh's syndrome) and *trichopoliodystrophy* (Menkes' disease).

Progressive External Ophthalmoplegia with Mitchondrial Myopathy. In addition to the external ocular muscles, the disorder can affect other cranial, truncal, and limb muscles. More than half of the cases are sporadic and stem from a heteroplasmic mtDNA deletion arising in the maternal ovum or in early fetal life.

Kearns-Sayre Syndrome. The disease presents in childhood. Nearly all cases are sporadic, and are caused by large heteroplasmic mtDNA deletions arising in the maternal ovum or in early fetal life. Dominantly inherited nuclear DNA mutations affecting mtDNA have also been observed. The rate of progression, severity, and system involvement vary from case to case. The original description in 1958 was that of retinitis pigmentosa, heart block, and external ophthalmoplegia. Subsequently ataxia, hearing loss, short stature, and increased spinal fluid protein were noted in more than half of the cases. Muscle weakness, mental changes, pyramidal signs, hypogonadism, and diabetes occur in less than half of the cases. Serum and spinal fluid lactate and pyruvate levels are increased, and the muscle fibers contain morphologically abnormal mitochondria. The presence of heart block requires treatment by pacemaker.

Myoclonus, Generalized Seizures, Cerebellar Syndrome, Mitochondrial Myopathy, and Lactacidemia. The syndrome presents in childhood or adult life. A maternally inherited heteroplasmic point mutation of mtDNA involving transfer RNA has been observed in several pedigrees. Short stature, dementia, hearing loss, and optic atrophy are frequent; spasticity, central hypoventilation, endocrinopathies, and peripheral neuropathy occur less often.

Mitochondrial Myopathy, Encephalopathy, Lactacidemia, and Strokelike Episodes (MELAS). The main distinction between this syndrome and the preceding one is the occurrence in adolescence or young adulthood of strokelike episodes associated with intermittent vomiting. Brain imaging during the acute episodes discloses areas of encephalomalacia not in the territories of the main blood vessels. Other associated features include short stature, seizures, hearing loss, progressive dementia, macular degeneration, and calcification of the basal ganglia. Early development is normal, and the family history is often positive. MELAS is caused by a heteroplasmic mtDNA point mutation involving transfer RNA.

ENDOCRINE MYOPATHIES. Muscle weakness can be a symptom of any endocrine disorder. The serum CK level is normal, except in myxedema and in uremic hyperparathyroidism. The EMG is normal or myopathic without spontaneous electrical activity. The histologic alterations in muscle are often nonspecific, such as type II fiber atrophy, focal increases and decreases in mitochondria, and focal myofibrillar degeneration. Fiber necrosis and regeneration and connective tissue proliferation are uncommon.

Glucocorticoid-Induced Myopathy. Muscle weakness commonly occurs in Cushing's syndrome and in patients receiving relatively high doses of glucocorticoids. Fluorinated drugs (dexamethasone, triamcinolone) are more pathogenic than nonfluorinated ones (prednisone). Considerable variation exists in the minimal dosage that induces myopathy. However, daily treatment for 3 months with 60 mg prednisone in divided doses induces some weakness in nearly all patients. Women are more susceptible than men, and divided daily doses are more pathogenic than single or alternate daily doses. The onset is usually insidious but occasionally sudden with diffuse myalgias. The weakness is more proximal than distal and affects the lower more than the upper limbs. Hip and ankle flexors are selectively severely affected. The cranial muscles are spared. The serum CK level remains normal. The biochemical basis of the disease is poorly understood. Reduced protein synthesis, accelerated protein degradation, and enhanced lysosomal protease activity all may contribute. Therapy consists of reducing the steroid dosage to the lowest possible level. Muscle strength returns to normal within 1 to 4 months after therapy is stopped.

Adrenal Insufficiency. Weakness is a typical feature, closely related to derangements in fluid and electrolyte balance and possibly to the associated hypotension. Joint contractures, especially of the knees and not related to muscle weakness, may also occur. Hyperkalemia in chronic adrenal insufficiency can be a cause of secondary periodic paralysis (discussed below).

Thyrotoxic Myopathy. Both acute and chronic forms have been described. The acute form, seldom seen, appears during a thyroid storm and is associated with bulbar weakness. Some patients have responded to anticholinesterases and may have had acute myasthenia gravis beginning during thyrotoxicosis. The chronic form appears in 80 per cent of untreated cases of hyperthyroidism. The hyperthyroid state can be mild and of long duration or present for only a few weeks before the onset of the weakness. Weakness is predominantly proximal, less often both proximal and distal. The deep tendon reflexes are hyperactive or normal. The serum CK level remains normal. The EMG shows myopathic motor unit potentials but never fibrillation potentials.

Graves' ophthalmopathy is described in Ch. 216. Thyrotoxic periodic paralysis is considered below.

Hypothyroid Myopathy. Muscle aching, cramps, slow relaxation of the reflexes, ridging of the muscles on percussion (myoedema), and an increase of the serum CK level are common findings in myxedema. Muscle enlargement and limb-girdle weakness occur only occasionally. The Debré-Semelaigne syndrome consists of muscle hypertrophy, weakness, and slow movements in the cretinous child. The same features and painful spasms in hypothyroid adults constitute Hoffmann's syndrome.

Muscle Symptoms in Hyperparathyroidism and Osteomalacia. Parathormone and biologically active forms of vitamin D are important regulators of calcium metabolism and the serum calcium level. Vitamin D also affects calcium metabolism, protein synthesis, ATP stores, and force generation in muscle. Furthermore, conditions that lead to osteomalacia (vitamin D deficiency, renal tubular acidosis, or chronic renal failure) are associated with secondary hyperparathyroidism. Proximal muscle weakness, fatigability, and muscle pain and tenderness, usually with bone pain and tenderness, can occur in primary and secondary hyperparathyroidism and in osteomalacia.

A more malignant syndrome can appear in uremic hyperparathyroidism. Here, metastatic calcification of the media and proliferation of the intima of small blood vessels produce skin and visceral infarcts and a necrotizing myopathy with marked elevation of serum enzymes and myoglobinuria.

Muscle Symptoms in Hypoparathyroidism. The typical neuromuscular symptom is tetany. This is considered in Ch. 235.

Acromegaly and Hypopituitarism. Acromegaly initially causes muscle hypertrophy, particularly if the disorder begins before growth ceases. Later generalized weakness and atrophy develop. Muscle biopsies can show segmental muscle fiber degeneration, type I or type II fiber atrophy, or no pathologic change. The serum CK level remains normal. A hypertrophic distal neuropathy and nerve entrapment are common in acromegaly.

Hypopituitarism in children causes dwarfism and poor muscle development. Pituitary failure in adults results in weakness and fatigability with little muscle atrophy. The weakness itself may reflect the combined influence of thyroid, adrenal, and growth hormone deficiencies.

THE PERIODIC PARALYSES (PP). These disorders occur as either inherited (primary) or acquired (secondary) illnesses and can be further classified according to measurable alterations in the serum potassium level during attacks (Table 507–3). The primary types are transmitted by autosomal-dominant inheritance, but nearly a third of the cases arise sporadically. It is important to realize that in the primary forms the serum potassium decreases or increases but may still remain within the normal range during attacks and is normal or low-normal between attacks. By contrast, in secondary PP caused by potassium wastage or retention the serum potassium is always markedly reduced or elevated during and even between attacks.

In each type of PP the propagation of the muscle fiber action potential fails during an attack. Recent studies indicate the presence of distinct abnormalities in the sodium channel of the muscle fiber plasma membrane in the primary periodic paralyses

TABLE 507–3. CLASSIFICATION OF THE PERIODIC PARALYSES

Primary
  Hypokalemic
  Normokalemic
  Hyperkalemic
    without myotonia
    with myotonia
    with paramyotonia
  With cardiac arrhythmia (hyper-, hypo-, or normokalemic)
Secondary
  Hypokalemic
    Thyrotoxic
    Urinary potassium wastage
    Gastrointestinal potassium wastage
    Barium intoxication
  Hyperkalemic
    Renal insufficiency
    Adrenal insufficiency

that tend to reduce the resting membrane potential. The action potential mechanism fails during the attack because of diverse abnormalities residing in the voltage-sensitive sodium channel.

The different types of periodic paralysis share several common features: (1) The paralytic attacks last from less than an hour to as long as several days. (2) The weakness can be localized or generalized. (3) The deep tendon reflexes diminish and then disappear during attacks. (4) The muscle fibers become inexcitable to direct or indirect electrical stimulation during the attacks. (5) The generalized attacks begin proximally and spread distally. Respiratory and cranial muscles tend to be spared except in the most severe attacks. (6) Rest after exercise provokes weakness in the muscles that had been exercised. Continued mild exercise aborts attacks. (7) Exercise followed by rest of a single muscle can induce weakness of that muscle without any detectable change in the potassium level in the systemic circulation. (8) Exposure to cold can provoke weakness in the primary forms of the disease. (9) Complete recovery occurs after initial attacks. (10) In the primary disorders permanent weakness and a persistent vacuolar myopathy can develop after repeated attacks. Despite these similarities, the different forms of PP differ in their response to sodium, potassium, or carbohydrate loading, as well as their pattern of urinary electrolyte excretions during attacks, and in some of their clinical features.

Primary Hypokalemic Periodic Paralysis. The attacks begin in the first or second decade, increase in frequency during early adult life, and become less frequent or cease during the fourth or fifth decade. When attacks recur daily, the patient is weakest in the morning and becomes stronger as the day passes. High dietary sodium or carbohydrate intake as well as excitement provokes or exacerbates the episodes. Major attacks are associated with urinary retention of sodium, potassium, chloride, and water. The diagnosis is supported by a positive family history and a decrease in serum potassium during an attack. An abnormally low serum potassium level between attacks suggests secondary rather than primary PP. In diagnosing sporadic cases one must exclude potassium wastage and thyrotoxicosis. The oral or intravenous administration of glucose, 2 grams per kilogram of body weight, combined with 10 to 20 units of insulin given subcutaneously, may provoke an attack within 2 to 3 hours. Depression of the serum potassium during the attack and a favorable response to 2.5 to 7.5 grams of potassium chloride (KCl) given orally must be demonstrated. Provocative tests must never be done in patients already hypokalemic, and potassium chloride must not be given to patients unless they have adequate renal or adrenal reserve.

Thyrotoxic Periodic Paralysis. This disease resembles primary hypokalemic PP in the changes in serum and urinary electrolytes that accompany the attacks and in the response to glucose, insulin, potassium, and rest after exercise. However, 95 per cent of the cases are sporadic, the male to female ratio is six to one, most cases occur among Asians, the onset is usually in adult life, and correction of the hyperthyroidism prevents further attacks.

Barium-Induced Periodic Paralysis. The accidental ingestion of absorbable barium salts such as barium carbonate induces hemorrhagic gastroenteritis, hypertension, cardiac arrhythmias, convulsions, hypokalemia, and muscle paralysis. Barium blocks potassium channels and thereby reduces potassium efflux from muscle; potassium uptake by muscle, mediated by the sodium-potassium pump, continues, and hypokalemia results.

Periodic Paralysis Secondary to Urinary or Gastrointestinal Potassium Loss. The differential diagnosis of hypokalemia resulting from urinary or gastrointestinal potassium depletion is discussed in Ch. 74. Paralytic attacks do not occur unless the serum potassium falls below 3 mEq per liter, and during the attacks the serum potassium decreases even further. Other neuromuscular complications of severe potassium depletion include a necrotizing myopathy, myoglobinuria, and latent or manifest tetany.

Primary Hyperkalemic Periodic Paralysis. The attacks begin in the first or second decade. They are often brief but can last up to several days. Between attacks the serum potassium is normal or slightly lower than normal. During major attacks potassium moves out from muscle. The serum potassium increases but may not exceed the normal range, and the urinary potassium excretion increases. Myotonic, paramyotonic, and nonmyotonic forms of hyperkalemic PP can be distinguished. In *myotonic hyperkalemic PP* myotonia can be detected in facial, tongue, finger extensor, and thenar muscles between attacks. In *paramyotonic hyperkalemic PP* exposure to cold causes widespread and severe myotonia, and exercise in the cold is followed by prolonged weakness not reversed by rewarming. Paralytic attacks are provoked by orally administered KCl, 50 to 100 mg per kilogram, given in an unsweetened solution in the fasting state. The test is contraindicated in subjects already hyperkalemic or those without adequate renal or adrenal reserve. Paramyotonia congenita without hyperkalemic PP is discussed in the next chapter.

Secondary Hyperkalemic Periodic Paralysis. This can occur when the serum potassium level exceeds 7 mEq per liter. The usual cause is renal or adrenal insufficiency, but hyperkalemia from exposure to spironolactone and during attacks of malaria also have caused paralytic attacks. The diagnosis is suggested by the presence of a very high serum potassium level during attacks, persistent hyperkalemia between attacks, and the associated primary disorder.

Primary Normokalemic Periodic Paralysis. There are no consistent changes in the serum potassium during the attacks. The existence of the disease has been questioned because some patients are sensitive to potassium salts. The observations suggest that normokalemic PP is a heterogeneous entity.

Primary Periodic Paralysis with Cardiac Arrhythmia. Affected patients suffer from PP and tachyarrhythmias that can cause sudden death. The cardiac symptoms are provoked or worsened by hypokalemia and digitalis; are refractory to disopyramide phosphate, propranolol, or phenytoin; but may respond to imipramine. Dysmorphic features, such as short stature, clinodactyly, and microcephaly can also occur. The PP has been clearly related to hyperkalemia in some patients, but hypokalemic and normokalemic PP were diagnosed in others.

Therapy of the Periodic Paralyses. In all forms of primary PP, acetazolamide, from 250 mg to 2 grams daily, can prevent attacks or decrease their frequency. The metabolic acidosis induced by the drug may prevent sodium channel inactivation by small depolarizations. Prolonged exposure to the drug promotes the formation of renal calculi.

The treatment of attacks of *primary hypokalemic PP* consists of giving 2 to 10 grams of oral KCl. Preventive therapy includes acetazolamide, a low-carbohydrate and relatively low-sodium (2.3 grams per day) diet, and 2.5 grams of KCl taken orally three times daily. *Thyrotoxic PP* is treated by antithyroid therapy, KCl supplements, and a low-carbohydrate, low-sodium diet. Acetazolamide is ineffective.

In *primary hyperkalemic PP* one treats the acute attacks with 2 grams per kilogram of glucose by mouth and 15 to 20 units of crystalline insulin subcutaneously. The inhalation of 1.3 mg metaproterenol every 15 minutes for three doses, or of 0.18 mg albuterol repeated once after 10 minutes, has aborted acute attacks. Preventive treatment consists of acetazolamide or thiazide diuretics and frequent high-carbohydrate meals. Tocainide, 300 to 400 mg three to four times daily, prevents cold-induced

stiffness and weakness in paramyotonic hyperkalemic PP. The drug acts by blocking sodium channels in muscle.

The periodic paralyses caused by excessive wastage or retention of potassium are treated by correcting existing electrolyte abnormalities and, if possible, removing the existing cause. In acute barium poisoning, 10 ml of a 10 per cent solution of sodium sulfate is administered intravenously every 30 minutes until symptoms subside.

NUTRITIONAL AND TOXIC MYOPATHIES. Diffuse muscle atrophy and weakness associated with type II fiber atrophy are commonly observed in malnourished or cachectic patients. The muscle weakness in nutritional osteomalacia has been attributed partly to disuse and partly to malnutrition.

Vitamin E Deficiency. This has now been implicated in progressive gait and limb ataxia, sensorimotor neuropathy, extraocular muscle paresis, and a myopathy in which giant abnormal lysosomes accumulate in muscle. The cause is a malabsorption syndrome, as detailed in Ch. 102 and 456. High doses of vitamin E may be of benefit.

Myopathy in Alcoholism. An acute necrotizing myopathy associated with myoglobinuria occurs in chronic alcoholics after a bout of drinking. Hypokalemia caused by sweating, vomiting, diarrhea, and renal wastage may act as a precipitating factor. The hypokalemia may be followed by hyperkalemia as myoglobinuria and renal failure develop. A subacute alcoholic myopathy with proximal muscle weakness and elevation of the serum CK level may also exist. If so, it is usually associated with a chronic neuropathy.

Chloroquine Myopathy. The side effects of the drug include macular and corneal degeneration, peripheral neuropathy, and myopathy. Muscle weakness appears when the daily dosage is 500 mg for a year or longer. Pathologically, the condition produces a vacuolar myopathy and constitutes a prototype for myopathies due to an excited autophagic mechanism.

Emetine Myopathy. Emetine, an ipecac alkaloid, is used to treat amebiasis. Side effects include cardiotoxicity and muscle weakness. A reversible myopathy involving proximal limb muscles has been observed in patients with feeding disorders who abuse ipecac to induce vomiting and in alcoholics receiving emetine for aversion therapy. The pathologic findings include focal destruction of mitochondria and focal myofibrillar degeneration.

Other Toxic Myopathies. *Epsilon amino-caproic acid,* an inhibitor of fibrinolyis and of clot dissolution, infrequently causes myalgias, myonecrosis, and myoglobinuria. *Colchicine* in customary doses induces a vacuolar myopathy in patients with gout and renal insufficiency who attain elevated plasma drug levels. The antiarrhythmic agent *amiodarone* can induce an autophagic myopathy and a peripheral neuropathy. *Lovastatin,* an inhibitor of mevalonic acid and cholesterol biosynthesis, causes a necrotizing myopathy with or without myoglobinuria in less than 0.5 per cent of patients. Concomitant therapy with immunosuppressants increases the risk of myopathy. *Isoretinoic acid,* a vitamin A analogue for treating acne, infrequently causes myalgias, elevation of the serum creatine kinase, and reversible muscle damage. *Cocaine* abuse can result in a necrotizing myopathy and myoglobinuria. The myopathy induced by *zidovudine* is considered in Ch. 506.

MALIGNANT HYPERTHERMIA. This is an autosomal dominant disorder in which exposure to inhalation anesthetics (halothane, methoxyflurane, enflurane) or succinylcholine triggers an uncontrolled release of calcium from the sarcoplasmic reticulum (SR) into the myofilament space. The high intracellular calcium level activates phosphorylase kinase, saturates troponin, and overloads mitochondria with calcium. These events cause accelerated glycolysis, ATP consumption, uncontrolled muscle contraction, uncoupling of oxidative phosphorylation, and excessive production of heat, lactate, and carbon dioxide. The basic abnormality is a mutation involving the calcium release channel of the SR. The gene that encodes for the calcium release channel and causes the disease has been mapped to region q13.1 of chromosome 19. A similar syndrome also can occur in myotonic disorders, Duchenne dystrophy, branchial hypertrophic myopathy, central core disease, and a congenital myopathy with dysmorphic features. It is not yet known what proportion of patients with these disorders is at risk.

Warning signs of the attack include tachypnea, tachycardia,

increased carbon dioxide production, cyanosis, rising temperature, rigidity, sweating, and unstable blood pressure. Failure to obtain muscle relaxation with adequate doses of succinylcholine represents an early warning sign. Subsequently, body temperature rises rapidly (up to 1° C every 5 minutes), followed by a rapidly evolving lactic acidosis, respiratory acidosis from carbon dioxide overproduction, muscle rigidity, hyperkalemia, variable alterations in the serum calcium, and muscle fiber breakdown reflected by very high serum CK levels, myoglobinemia, and myoglobinuria.

Therapy of the acute syndrome consists of body cooling, hydration, sodium bicarbonate infusion, mechanical hyperventilation, and diuretics to maintain urine flow. More specific treatment consists of dantrolene, a medication that blocks excitation-contraction coupling between the T-tubules and the SR. The drug is given intravenously, 1 to 2 mg per kilogram, which may be repeated every 5 minutes to a total of 10 mg per kilogram. The mortality remains high. Screening of relatives of patients for the metabolic defect is important. Seventy per cent of those at risk have increased serum CK activity. If well standardized, an in vitro halothane contracture test on fresh muscle can also predict susceptibility. Preventive treatment of individuals at risk consists of dantrolene, 4 to 8 mg per kilogram per day in four divided doses for 1 to 2 days prior to surgery and, if possible, alternative methods of anesthesia.

Other Hyperthermic States. Two other syndromes are associated with hyperthermia, autonomic instability, abnormal muscle rigidity, and myoglobinuria. The *malignant neuroleptic syndrome* occurs in less than 1 per cent of all patients exposed to neuroleptics, and especially in young men. It evolves over 1 to 3 days and lasts 5 to 10 days after drug withdrawal. The mortality is about 25 per cent. A nearly identical *hyperthermic syndrome in Parkinson's disease* is precipitated by abrupt withdrawal of antiparkinson medications. The same treatment as in malignant hyperthermia, including the use of dantrolene up to 10 mg per kilogram per day, is beneficial in both disorders.

MYOGLOBINURIA. The clinical syndrome of myoglobinuria is associated with brown discoloration of urine by myoglobin and metmyoglobin. Myoglobin, a 17,000-molecular-weight protein with a prosthetic heme group, is present in muscle at a concentration of 1 gram per kilogram. It has a lower renal excretory threshold than hemoglobin. Small amounts of myoglobin not sufficient to discolor urine are excreted in various necrotizing myopathies. The visible discoloration of urine by myoglobin indicates both massive and acute muscle destruction (rhabdomyolysis) and warns of impending renal damage. The pigment has to be distinguished from hemoglobin and porphyrins. If there is no hemoglobinemia or hematuria, a positive benzidine test strongly suggests myoglobinuria. However, myoglobinuria itself can induce microhematuria, and certain identification of myoglobin must be made specifically. The immunoprecipitation assay has the virtue of being simple and quantitative but is so sensitive that it detects the pigment in the absence of overt myoglobinuria.

Muscle pain, swelling, and weakness precede overt myoglobinuria by a few hours. In addition to myoglobin, phosphate, potassium, creatine, and muscle enzymes are released into the circulation. The heme pigment in the glomerular filtrate and casts in the tubules cause proteinuria, hematuria, and tubular necrosis. Renal failure is more likely if there are also hypotension, acidosis, and hypovolemia. With increasing renal insufficiency, hyperphosphatemia, hypocalcemia, tetany, and life-threatening hyperkalemia appear. Death results from renal or respiratory failure. Otherwise, the myoglobinuria and proteinuria disappear in 3 to 5 days. The marked hyperenzymemia decreases gradually, and muscle strength returns relatively slowly after major attacks. EMG abnormalities, and especially fibrillation potentials, can persist for several months.

Myoglobinuria can have many causes: metabolic, infectious, toxic, ischemic and/or traumatic, secondary to another myopathy, and idiopathic. It is likely that many of the so-called idiopathic cases have a metabolic or infectious etiology.

Myoglobinuria Caused by a Metabolic Disturbance. The common denominator is impaired substrate utilization for energy metabolism, or a critical substrate deficiency in the face of excessive demands for energy. Most diseases in this group were considered earlier in this chapter. Deficiencies of phosphorylase kinase, myophosphorylase, phosphofructokinase, phosphoglycer-

ate mutase, phosphoglycerate kinase, and lactate dehydrogenase block anaerobic glycolysis; coenzyme Q and succinate dehydrogenase deficiencies interfere with oxidative phosphorylaton; and carnitine palmityltransferase deficiency impairs fatty acid oxidation when it is most needed. Substrate deficiency in the face of excessive demands and derangements of muscle metabolism account for the myoglobinuria associated with malignant hyperthermia, the malignant neuroleptic syndrome, and the abrupt withdrawal of antiparkinson drugs. Substrate deficiency may also account for the myoglobinuria that occurs after severe exercise in untrained individuals, as in military recruits.

Almost any severe metabolic insult can cause myoglobinuria. These include carbon dioxide poisoning, extreme hypoglycemia, severe hypokalemia, hypernatremia, or water intoxication.

Myoglobinuria with Infections. This can occur after influenza A, herpes simplex, Epstein-Barr, and coxsackievirus infections and early in the course of HIV infection. The precise mechanism of the rhabdomyolysis is not understood. Myoglobinuria also occurs with bacterial infections accompanied by high fever and sepsis, and with muscle gangrene caused by clostridial infection.

Toxic Myoglobinuria. The myoglobinuria associated with alcoholism was considered above. Intoxication with barbiturates, amphetamine, cocaine, and other narcotics, especially if associated with agitation or coma, can produce myoglobinuria. Myoglobinuria occurring with lovastatin, epsilon-amino-caproic acid, or amiodarone was discussed earlier in this chapter. The toxin of the Malayan sea snake, *Enhydrina schistosa*, induces myalgias, trismus, flaccid paralysis, and myoglobinuria.

Ischemic and Traumatic Myoglobinuria. Massive ischemia of muscle from any cause (e.g., major vessel occlusions, angiopathy in uremic hyperparathyroidism), crush injuries, or prolonged pressure on dependent muscles in the immobile comatose patient can induce myoglobinuria. Localized ischemic necrosis of muscle and sometimes myoglobinuria occur in severe forms of the anterior tibial syndrome.

Myoglobinuria Secondary to Other Myopathies. Myoglobinuria has been observed infrequently in acute dermatomyositis (where the cause is probably ischemia), systemic lupus erythematosus, and muscular dystrophies.

Treatment. The acute episode is treated by rest, maintenance of adequate urine flow by hydration and diuretics, and alkalinization of the urine with sodium bicarbonate. Other measures consist of treatment of the renal insufficiency as required and removal of the offending cause if possible.

Engel AG, Banker BQ: Myology. New York, McGraw-Hill Book Company, 1986. *Chapters by DiMauro and Bresolin, DiMauro and Papadimitron, Engel, Gronert, Morgan-Hughes, Penn, Ruff, and Victor provide detailed reviews of several of the metabolic myopathies.*

Fontaine B, Khurana TS, Hoffman EP, et al.: Hyperkalemic periodic paralysis and the adult muscle sodium channel α-subunit gene. Science 250:1000, 1990. *A linkage analysis study indicating that a mutation in the sodium channel α-subunit gene accounts for the myotonic form of primary hyperkalemic periodic paralysis.*

Goto Y, Nonaka I, Horai S: A mutation in the tRNA$^{Leu(UUR)}$ gene associated with the MELAS subgroup of mitochondrial myopathies. Nature 348:651, 1990. *Clear evidence that MELAS, like MERRF and the Kearns-Sayre syndrome, is caused by a mitochondrial DNA mutation.*

Lehamn-Horn F, Küther G, Ricker K, et al.: Adynamia episodica hereditaria with myotonia: A non-inactivating sodium current and the effect of extracellular pH. Muscle Nerve 10:363, 1987. *This paper presents cogent reasons for recognizing three forms of hyperkalemic periodic paralysis and discusses aspects of the pathophysiology.*

McLennan DH, Duff C, Zorzato F, et al.: Ryanodine receptor gene is a candidate for predisposition to malignant hyperthermia. Nature 343:559, 1990. *Provides evidence that a mutation in the gene encoding the sarcoplasmic reticulum calcium release channel (which is a receptor for ryanodine) predisposes to malignant hyperthermia.*

Moxley RT, Ricker K, Kingston WJ, et al.: Potassium uptake in muscle during paramyotonic weakness. Neurology 39:952, 1989. *Presents clinical and physiologic criteria for distinguishing pure paramyotonia congenita from myotonic hyperkalemic periodic paralysis.*

Ogasahara S, Engel AG, Frens D, Mack D: Muscle coenzyme Q deficiency in familial mitochondrial myopathy. Proc Natl Acad Sci USA 86:2379, 1989. *The first report of selective and severe human coenzyme Q deficiency and its clinical and metabolic consequences.*

Roth D, Alarcon FJ, Fernandez JA, et al.: Acute rhabdomyolysis associated with cocaine intoxication. N Engl J Med 319:673, 1988. *Cocaine intoxication can cause acute myoglobinuria associated with renal failure, hepatic dysfunction, disseminated intravascular coagulation, and a high mortality.*

Shoffner JM, Wallace DC: Oxidative phosphorylation diseases. Disorders of two genomes. Adv Hum Genet 19:27, 1990. *An excellent overview of the genetic, biochemical, clinical, and therapeutic aspects of mitochondrial disorders affecting oxidative phosphorylation.*

Tein I, DeVivo DC, Bierman F, et al.: Impaired skin fibroblast carnitine uptake in primary carnitine deficiency manifested by childhood carnitine-responsive cardiomyopathy. Pediatr Res 28:247, 1990. *A description of the varied manifestations of primary systemic carnitine deficiency and the response to replacement therapy.*

508 Miscellaneous Myopathies

INFILTRATIVE MYOPATHIES. Systemic Amyloid Myopathy. The most common neurologic complication in various types of amyloidosis is a predominantly sensory-autonomic neuropathy. Amyloid deposition in muscle is frequent, but the muscle involvement is usually subclinical. Occasionally amyloidosis presents or is associated with an overt myopathy characterized by muscle enlargement, macroglossia, stiffness, exertional muscle pain, and proximal or diffuse weakness. Electromyography shows myopathic features in proximal muscles with or without changes of neuropathy distally. The amyloid deposits, identified by their metachromasia and affinity for Congo red stain, appear between and around the mural elements of the small vessels and extend into the interstitial spaces, where they tightly surround individual muscle fibers.

Hypertrophic Branchial Myopathy. This sporadic illness presents between the second and fourth decades of life and is restricted to muscles that derive from the embryonic branchial cleft. The disease evolves with slowly progressive, asymmetric, bilateral enlargement of temporalis, masseter, and pterygoid muscles. Weakness is minimal or absent. The swelling itself is painless but may lead to pain with jaw opening. The EMG and muscle biopsy show nonspecific myopathic alterations in the affected muscles. There is no satisfactory treatment. When chewing is impaired, partial excision of the enlarged muscles has proved beneficial.

SYNDROMES ASSOCIATED WITH ABNORMAL MUSCLE ACTIVITY. These can be caused by (1) abnormal neural activity in the central nervous system (e.g., dystonia, tetanus, stiff-man syndrome); (2) abnormal excitability of the peripheral nervous system (neuromyotonia, tetany, cramps); (3) abnormal excitability of the muscle fiber surface membrane (myotonic disorders); (4) a defect within the muscle fiber resulting in abnormal mechanical activity (e.g., malignant hyperthermia, contractures without electrical activity, and slow relaxation of electrically silent muscle fibers). Dystonia, tetanus, and tetany are considered in Ch. 235, 310, and 460. The remaining entities were discussed earlier in this section or will be discussed below.

Stiff-Man Syndrome. This is a disease of adult life affecting men more frequently than women. Initially intermittent spasms of axial and limb muscles are followed by continuous stiffness that immobilizes the patient. Agonist and antagonist muscles are simultaneously affected, preventing voluntary movement. The EMG shows constant firing of normal motor unit potentials in the stiff muscles. There are no signs of cerebral or spinal cord disease. Spinal anesthesia relieves the spasms. The disease is frequently associated with organ-specific autoimmune diseases, and especially insulin-dependent diabetes mellitus. Autoantibodies are detected in at least 60 per cent of patients against glutamic acid decarboxylase, the enzyme that converts glutamic acid to the inhibitory neurotransmitter gamma-aminobutyric acid (GABA). In tissue sections the autoantibodies bind to GABA-ergic neurons and pancreatic islet β cells. These findings suggest that the disease is caused by immune-mediated impairment of GABA-ergic inhibitory pathways. Relatively high doses of diazepam or baclofen, which increase GABA-mediated central inhibition, and clonidine, which prevents norepinephrine release from nerve terminals, may improve or relieve the symptoms.

Neuromyotonia. This can be generalized or focal. *Generalized neuromyotonia* is sporadic or familial. Some of the familial cases are associated with a peripheral neuropathy; some of the sporadic cases have an intrathoracic malignancy. Abnormal impulses arising in peripheral motor axons produce continuous muscle fiber activity that persists even during sleep. Depending on the site of origin in the axon, the abnormal activity is abolished by proximal nerve block or block of neuromuscular transmission. The EMG shows very high frequency (150 to 300 Hz) recurring bursts of motor unit potentials. The involuntary activation of multiple motor units causes stiffness and delayed relaxation of the affected muscles and continuous, small, undulating movements of the overlying skin (*myokymia*). Phenytoin or carbamazepine may inhibit the abnormal discharges and relieve the symptoms.

Similar high-frequency and rhythmically recurring bursts of motor unit potentials occur in *facial myokymia* seen with demyelinating or other lesions of the brain stem.

Focal neuromyotonia can occur following peripheral nerve lesions, but here the firing rate is slower (30 to 60 Hz). The delayed relaxation of an affected muscle after a willed contraction mimics action myotonia.

A benign syndrome of *muscle cramps, fasciculations, and myokymia* associated with low-frequency bursts of motor unit potentials also occurs and may incorrectly suggest the diagnosis of early motor neuron disease.

A syndrome associated with *myokymia, hyperhydrosis, mental symptoms, thymoma, and anti-acetylcholine receptor antibodies* but without symptoms of myasthenia gravis has been recently described.

Schwartz-Jampel Syndrome. This is an autosomal-recessive disease that begins in early childhood. It is characterized by chondrodystrophy, bone and joint deformities, short stature, a doleful facial expression with blepharospasm, hypertrichosis, muscle stiffness, and muscle hypertrophy or atrophy. There is delayed muscle relaxation suggesting myotonia. The EMG, however, shows high-frequency repetitive discharges, not myotonic discharges. Muscle biopsy reveals neurogenic and myogenic features.

Myotonia Congenita. Autosomal-dominant (Thomsen's disease) and autosomal-recessive forms are recognized. Both are benign and associated with diffuse muscle hypertrophy and diffuse action, percussion, and electrical myotonia. Cold increases the myotonia, and sustained exercise improves it. The membrane defect consists of a markedly reduced chloride conductance. Quinine, 0.3 to 1.5 grams daily, or phenytoin, 0.3 to 0.6 gram daily, relieves the myotonia.

Paramyotonia Congenita. This autosomal-dominant disease resembles myotonic hyperkalemic periodic paralysis. There are pure cases, however, in which potassium loading does not induce weakness. The myotonia is worsened rather than improved by exercise. Exercise in the cold causes prolonged electrically silent stiffness and weakness not relieved by rewarming. Although the membrane shows an abnormal increase in sodium conductance on cooling, this fails to explain the prolonged stiffness induced by cooling. Tocainide, 300 to 400 mg three to four times daily, prevents the cold-induced symptoms.

Slow Relaxation of Electrically Silent Muscle Fibers. This is a rare disease in which there is impaired muscle relaxation that is rapidly worsened by exercise. The slowly relaxing fibers are electrically silent. The defect lies within the calcium-pump ATPase of the sarcoplasmic reticulum.

Rippling Muscles. This is a benign and dominantly inherited disorder presenting in late childhood or adult life. Sporadic cases also occur. Local compression of a muscle evokes myoedema. This is replaced by a longitudinal depression parallel to the long axis of the muscle which then moves to the periphery of the muscle in 10 to 20 seconds in a wave that resembles the plucking of a chromatic scale on a harp. The response to percussion superficially resembles myotonia, but the rippling muscles are electrically silent. Mild muscle pain, stiffness at the beginning of exercise, and mild elevation of the serum CK level are associated features.

Auger RG, Daube JR, Gomez MR, et al.: Hereditary form of sustained muscle activity of peripheral nerve origin causing myokymia and muscle stiffness. Ann Neurol 15:13, 1984. *An excellent discussion of the differential diagnosis of neuromyotonias and related syndromes.*

Halbach M, Höberg V, Freund H-J: Neuromuscular, autonomic and central cholinergic hyperactivity associated with thymoma and acetylcholine receptor antibody. J Neurol 234:433, 1987. *The authors postulate that in this unique disorder anti-acetylcholine receptor antibodies facilitate rather than inhibit cholinergic action.*

Ii K, Hizawa K, Nunomura S, et al.: Systemic amyloid myopathy. Acta Neuropathol (Berl) 64:114, 1984. *A clear clinical and pathologic description and review of the relevant literature.*

Karpati G, Charuk J, Carpenter S, et al.: Myopathy caused by a deficiency of Ca^{2+}-ATPase in sarcoplasmic reticulum (Brody's disease). Ann Neurol 20:38, 1986. *Provides an explanation for the slow relaxation of electrically silent muscle fibers.*

Mancall EL, Patel AN, Hirschhorn AM: Hypertrophic branchial myopathy. Neurology 24:1166, 1974. *A classic account of a neglected myopathy.*

Ricker K, Moxley RT, Rohkamm R: Rippling muscle disease. Arch Neurol 46:405, 1989. *A good description of an uncommon disease and a review of the literature.*

Rüdel R, Lehmann-Horn F: Membrane changes in cells from myotonia patients. Physiol Rev 65:310, 1985. *An up-to-date account of the clinical features and membrane abnormalities in the myotonic syndromes.*

Solimena M, Folli F, Aparisi R, et al.: Autoantibodies to GABA-ergic neurons and pancreatic beta cells in stiff-man syndrome. N Engl J Med 322:1555, 1990. *The report provides strong evidence that stiff-man syndrome is an organ-specific autoimmune disease and describes useful diagnostic tests.*

509 Disorders of Neuromuscular Transmission

DEFINITION AND BASIC CONCEPTS. Disorders of neuromuscular transmission can be acquired or inherited and are associated with abnormal weakness and fatigability on exertion. In each disorder the safety margin of neuromuscular transmission is compromised by one or more specific mechanisms. The following paragraphs provide a brief review of the anatomic and physiologic aspects of neuromuscular transmission.

The motor end-plate consists of a nerve terminal separated from the postsynaptic region by the synaptic space. Acetylcholine (ACh) is stored in quantal packets (6,000 to 10,000 molecules per packet) in synaptic vesicles in the nerve terminal. The vesicles release ACh into the synaptic space by exocytosis. The postsynaptic region has junctional folds containing on their terminal expansions acetylcholine receptor (AChR) molecules packed at a density of about 10^4 sites per square micrometer. The binding of two ACh molecules to an AChR molecule opens the AChR ion channel. After the ion channel closes, ACh dissociates from AChR. Acetylcholinesterase (AChE) is distributed throughout the basal lamina of the synaptic space at a density of about 2,500 sites per square micrometer.

In the resting state single ACh quanta are randomly released into the synaptic space. The high local ACh concentration saturates all nearby AChE sites so that most ACh molecules can reach postsynaptic AChR's. The AChR packing density is so high that ACh needs to diffuse only 0.3 μm along the top and 0.3 μm down along the junctional folds before it meets all the AChR it can saturate. The resultant resting depolarizations of the muscle fiber are known as miniature end-plate potentials (MEPP's). The MEPP amplitude depends on the number of ACh molecules in the quantum, the number of available AChR's, the geometry of the synaptic space, and the average depolarization generated by the opening of an AChR ion channel. When ACh dissociates from AChR it is hydrolyzed by AChE to choline and acetate. Choline is taken up by the nerve terminal and is reutilized for ACh synthesis.

Depolarization of the nerve terminal by nerve impulse opens voltage-sensitive calcium channels in the presynaptic membrane. The calcium influx increases the probability of synaptic vesicle exocytosis. The exocytosis occurs adjacent to active zones in the presynaptic membrane. The voltage-sensitive calcium channels are represented by regularly arrayed large membrane particles in the active zones.

The quanta released by a nerve impulse generate an end-plate potential (EPP), the amplitude of which depends on the MEPP amplitude and the number of quanta (m) released by the nerve impulse. The value of m depends on the probability of release

(p) and the number of quanta readily available for release (n) according to the relationship $m = np$. *The safety margin of neuromuscular transmission is defined as the difference between the actual EPP amplitude and the EPP amplitude required to trigger the muscle fiber action potential.*

Repetitive stimulation results in a frequency-dependent depression of the EPP amplitude and of the safety margin to a certain plateau. The decrease is mainly due to a decrease in n. Repetitive stimulation also can facilitate transmitter release by increasing p, or n, or both. The temporal profiles of the opposing processes are such that (1) a defect of neuromuscular transmission is most readily detected by a train of five to ten stimuli delivered at a low (2 to 3 Hz) frequency; (2) tetanic stimulation results in transient improvement and then a worsening of the defect.

Table 509–1 shows a classification of currently recognized defects of neuromuscular transmission. Botulism is described in Ch. 309, the others in this chapter.

MYASTHENIA GRAVIS (MG). This is an acquired autoimmune disorder in which pathogenic autoantibodies induce AChR deficiency at the motor end-plate. The safety margin of neuromuscular transmission is compromised by the small amplitude of the MEPP and consequently of the EPP. Circulating AChR antibodies are present in 80 to 90 per cent of the cases, and IgG and complement components are deposited on the postsynaptic membrane. AChR deficiency results from complement-mediated lysis of the junctional folds, accelerated internalization and destruction of AChR cross-linked by antibody (modulation), and, to a lesser extent, by antibodies blocking the binding of ACh to AChR.

Clinical Features. The incidence is two to five per year per million and the prevalence 13 to 64 per million. The female to male ratio is six to four. The disease may present at any age, but the incidence in females peaks in the third decade and in males in the sixth or seventh decade.

The disease can involve either the external ocular muscles selectively or the general voluntary muscle system. The symptoms may fluctuate from hour to hour, day to day, or over longer periods. They are provoked or worsened by exertion, exposure to extremes of temperature, viral or other infections, menses, and excitement. Ocular muscle involvement is usually bilateral, asymmetric, and typically associated with ptosis and diplopia. Weakness of other muscles innervated by cranial nerves results in loss of facial expression, everted lips, a smile that resembles a snarl, jaw drop, nasal regurgitation of liquids, choking on foods and secretions, and a slurred, hypernasal speech of a reduced volume. Abnormal fatigability of the limb muscles causes difficulty in combing the hair, lifting objects repeatedly, climbing stairs, walking, and running. Depending on the severity of the disease, dyspnea appears on moderate or mild exertion or is present even at rest. The abnormal fatigability can be demonstrated by asking the patient to look up without closing the eyes for a minute, to count loudly from one to one hundred, to hold the arms abducted to the horizontal position for a minute, or to perform repeated

TABLE 509–1. CLASSIFICATION OF DISORDERS OF NEUROMUSCULAR TRANSMISSION

Autoimmune
  Myasthenia gravis
  Lambert-Eaton myasthenic syndrome
Congenital
  Familial infantile myasthenia*
  End-plate acetylcholinesterase deficiency*
  Slow-channel syndrome†
  End-plate AChR deficiency*
  High-conductance fast-channel syndrome*
  Paucity of synaptic vesicles and reduced quantal release‡
  Putative abnormality of ACh-AChr interaction‡
Toxic
  Botulism
  Drug-induced
  Pesticide poisoning

*Autosomal-recessive inheritance
†Autosomal-dominant inheritance
‡Autosomal-recessive inheritance suspected

deep knee-bends. The deep tendon reflexes are normally active even in weak muscles. Atrophy of masseter, temporal, facial, or tongue muscles, and less often of other muscles, occurs in about 15 per cent of patients.

Initially, the symptoms are purely ocular in 40 per cent, are generalized in 40 per cent, and involve only the extremities in 10 per cent and only the bulbar or bulbar and eye muscles in another 10 per cent. Subsequently, the weakness can spread from ocular to facial to lower bulbar muscles and then to torso and limb muscles, but the sequence may vary. Proximal limb muscles are affected more than distal ones. In the most advanced cases the weakness is universal. By the end of the first year, the ocular muscles are affected in nearly all patients. The symptoms remain ocular in only 16 per cent. In nearly 90 per cent of those in whom the disease becomes generalized, this occurs within the first year after the onset. Progression is most rapid within the first 3 years, and more than half of the deaths caused by MG occur in that period. Spontaneous remissions lasting from weeks to years can occur. Long remissions are uncommon, and most remissions occur during the first 3 years.

Two thirds of patients with MG have thymic hyperplasia and 10 to 15 per cent have thymoma. A few with thymoma also develop myocarditis or giant cell myositis. In about 10 per cent the MG is associated with another autoimmune disease, such as hyperthyroidism, polymyositis, systemic lupus erythematosus, Sjögren's syndrome, rheumatoid arthritis, ulcerative colitis, pemphigus, sarcoidosis, pernicious anemia, and Lambert-Eaton myasthenic syndrome.

A clinical classification of MG, originally proposed by Osserman, is based on the distribution and severity of symptoms: group 1, ocular; group 2A, mild generalized; group 2B, moderately severe generalized; group 3, acute fulminating; group 4, late severe. Another classification, proposed by Vincent and Newsom-Davis, is according to the age of onset and the presence or absence of thymoma: Type 1, MG with thymoma: The disease is usually severe and the AChR antibody level is high; there is no association either with sex or with HLA antigen. Type 2, no thymoma, onset before age 40: The AChR antibody level is intermediate; there is female preponderance and an increased association with HLA-A1, HLA-B8, and HLA-DRw3 antigens (HLA-B12 in Japan). Type 3, no thymoma, onset after age 40: The AChR antibody level tends to be low; there is male preponderance and increased association with HLA-A3, HLA-B7, or HLA-DRw2 antigens (HLA-A10 in Japan). Striated muscle antibodies are found in 90 per cent, 5 per cent, and 45 per cent, respectively, in the three types. The association with other autoimmune diseases is highest in Type 3 and lowest in Type 1. Both classifications are discussed further in the Engel chapters cited in the references.

Transient Neonatal MG. Circulating AChR antibodies can be detected in most infants born to myasthenic mothers, but only 12 per cent of such children develop MG, usually during the first few hours of life. The findings are feeble cry, feeding and respiratory difficulty, general or facial weakness, and ptosis. The mean duration is 18 days. There is no relation between the severity of MG in mother and infant. The disease is caused by the transfer of AChR antibodies or immunocytes from mother to infant, or perhaps fetal AChR damaged by maternal antibodies triggers a transient immune response in the infant.

Diagnosis. This is based on the characteristic history, physical examination, anticholinesterase tests, and laboratory studies. The latter include EMG studies, tests for AChR antibodies, and in selected cases, microelectrode studies in vitro of neuromuscular transmission and ultrastructural and cytochemical studies of the end-plate.

Anticholinesterase Tests. Edrophonium given intravenously acts within a few seconds, and its effects last for a few minutes. One to 2 mg of the drug is injected intravenously over 15 seconds. If there is no response in 30 seconds, an additional 8 to 9 mg is injected. The evaluation of the response requires objective assessment of one or more signs, such as degree of ptosis, range of ocular movements, and the force of the hand grip. Possible cholinergic side effects of the drug include fasciculations, flushing, lacrimation, abdominal cramps, nausea, vomiting, and diarrhea. The drug must be given cautiously to patients with cardiac disease, for it may cause sinus bradycardia, atrioventricular block, and, rarely, cardiac arrest. Atropine is used to reverse toxicity. Intramuscular neostigmine, 0.5 to 1.0 mg, acts maximally in about 30 minutes, and its effects last up to 2 hours, allowing a more leisurely evaluation of changes in clinical status.

Electromyography. Supramaximal stimulation of a motor nerve at 2 to 3 Hz results in a 10 per cent or greater decrement of the amplitude of the evoked compound muscle action potential from the first to the fifth response. The test is positive in nearly all patients, provided that two or more distal and two or more proximal muscles are examined. The decrement is caused by a normally occurring decrease in the number of quanta released from the nerve terminal, and hence in the amplitude of the EPP, at the beginning of low-frequency stimulation. In MG the EPP amplitude is already reduced by the AChR deficiency, and the additional decrease during stimulation results in blocking of transmission at an increasing number of end-plates. Single-fiber EMG compares the timing of action potentials between pairs of closely adjacent muscle fibers in the same motor unit during a willed contraction. In MG the low amplitude and relatively long rise time of the EPP cause abnormally long interpotential intervals and intermittent blocking of action potential generation at some fibers.

Serologic Tests. The usual AChR antibody test measures the binding of antibody to AChR labeled with radioactive α-bungarotoxin. The toxin itself is attached irreversibly to the ACh binding site of AChR. The antibody binding test is positive in nearly all patients with moderately severe or acute severe MG, in 80 per cent with mild generalized MG, in 50 per cent with ocular MG, but in only 25 per cent of those in remission. In a few patients only antibodies that block the binding of ACh to AChR can be detected. The antibody titer correlates only loosely with disease severity but in individual patients a greater than 50 per cent decrease in titer for more than 12 months is nearly always associated with sustained clinical improvement. Striated muscle antibodies also occur in MG patients. Their role remains unknown but they often are associated with thymoma.

Other Diagnostic Studies. Immune complexes can be localized at the MG end-plate in cryostat sections even when circulating AChR antibodies cannot be detected. C3 localization is technically the easiest and most convenient way to confirm the suspected diagnosis. Electrophysiologic studies of neuromuscular transmission in vitro can distinguish between atypical cases of MG, the Lambert-Eaton myasthenic syndrome, and some of the congenital myasthenic syndromes.

Differential Diagnosis. This includes neurasthenia, oculopharyngeal dystrophy, mitochondrial myopathies involving the external ocular and/or other cranial and limb muscles, intracranial mass lesions compressing cranial nerves, drug-induced myasthenic syndromes, and other disorders of neuromuscular transmission listed in the table. Neurasthenia is recognized by giving way on muscle testing and the lack of objective clinical and laboratory findings. In myopathies involving the ocular muscles, the weakness does not fluctuate, diplopia is seldom a symptom, the muscle biopsy may show distinct morphologic abnormalities, and pharmacologic and laboratory tests for MG are negative. Drug-induced and other myasthenic syndromes are considered below.

Therapy. Anticholinesterases, alternate-day prednisone treatment, azathioprine, thymectomy, and plasmapheresis are currently used to treat MG. Anticholinesterases are useful in all clinical forms of the disease. Pyridostigmine bromide (Mestinon) (60-mg tablets) acts for 3 to 4 hours, and neostigmine bromide (15-mg tablets) for 2 to 3 hours. The former drug has fewer muscarinic side effects and is therefore more widely used. One half to four tablets of pyridostigmine bromide are given every 4 hours in the daytime. This medication is also available in 180-mg "time-span" tablets for use at bedtime and as a syrup for children and patients requiring nasogastric feeding. If troublesome muscarinic side effects occur, these can be treated with 0.4 to 0.6 mg atropine given orally two or three times daily. Postoperatively or in critically ill patients intramuscularly injectable pyridostigmine bromide (the dose is one thirtieth of the oral dose) and neostigmine methylsulfate (the dose is one fifteenth of the oral dose) can be used.

Progressive weakness despite increasing amounts of anticholinesterases signals the onset of a myasthenic or cholinergic crisis.

Cholinergic crises are associated with muscarinic effects, such as abdominal cramps, nausea, vomiting, diarrhea, miosis, lacrimation, increased bronchial secretions, diaphoresis, and bradycardia. In a myasthenic crisis the muscarinic effects are not conspicuous, and 2 mg edrophonium given intravenously improves rather than worsens the weakness. In practice, however, the two types of crises often are difficult to distinguish, and overmedication of a myasthenic crisis can convert it into a cholinergic crisis. Therefore, patients who have increasing difficulty with respiration, feeding, or handling secretions and who are not responding to relatively high doses of anticholinesterases are best treated by drug withdrawal, tracheal intubation or tracheostomy, support with respirator, and intravenous feeding. Refractoriness to drug therapy usually disappears after a few days.

In patients with generalized disease not responding adequately to modest doses of anticholinesterases, other forms of therapy must be employed. Thymectomy increases the remission rate and improves the clinical course of MG. Although controlled clinical studies of thymectomy according to age, sex, and severity of disease have never been carried out, there is general agreement that the best response occurs in young women with hyperplastic thymus glands and high antibody titer. Thymoma represents an absolute indication for thymectomy because the tumor is often locally invasive. Computed tomography of the mediastinum is a sensitive screening test, but it can give false-positive results.

Alternate-day prednisone treatment induces remission or significantly improves the disease in more than half the patients. The treatment is relatively safe provided that one institutes the usual precautions for patients taking corticosteroid therapy. With an average dose of 70 mg on alternate days, the average time for significant improvement is 5 months. After the improvement reaches a plateau the dose must be lowered gradually over several months to establish the minimum maintenance dose.

Azathioprine in doses of 150 to 200 mg per day also induces remissions or measurable improvement in more than half the treated patients. The minimum time for improvement is 3 months. Surveillance to detect side effects (pancytopenia, leukopenia, serious infection, and hepatocellular injury) must be maintained during therapy.

Plasmapheresis is indicated in severe generalized or fulminating MG refractory to other forms of treatment. Daily exchanges of 2 liters of plasma result in objective improvement and lower the AChR antibody titer in a few days. Plasmapheresis, however, is expensive and does not confer greater long-term protection than immunosuppressants alone.

LAMBERT-EATON MYASTHENIC SYNDROME. This is an acquired autoimmune disease in which pathogenic autoantibodies cause a deficiency of voltage-sensitive calcium channels at the motor nerve terminal. This deficiency restricts calcium ingress into the terminal when it is depolarized by nerve impulse and thereby reduces the probability of quantal release. Among patients over 40 years, 70 per cent of males and 30 per cent of females have an associated carcinoma, usually a small-cell carcinoma of the lung. The syndrome may predate tumor detection by up to 3 years. In one third of patients the syndrome is non-neoplastic and occurs at any age. In these cases there is an association with other autoimmune disorders, HLA-B8 and DRw3 antigens, and organ-specific autoantibodies.

Patients have weakness and fatigability of proximal limb and torso muscles with relative sparing of extraocular and bulbar muscles. The lower limbs are more severely involved than the upper ones. On maximal voluntary contraction the force produced by a weak muscle increases for a few seconds and then again decreases. The tendon reflexes are hypoactive or absent in most patients. Autonomic manifestations (dry mouth, impotence, decreased sweating, orthostatic hypotension, or altered pupillary reflexes) occur in one half of the patients.

On EMG, the amplitude of the compound muscle action potential evoked by a single nerve stimulus from rested muscle is abnormally small. Repetitive stimulation at 2 Hz induces a further decrement, but stimulation at frequencies higher than 10 Hz or voluntary exercise for a brief period markedly facilitates the response so that the evoked potential attains normal amplitude.

Anticholinesterases are only slightly effective. Guanidine hydrochloride (10 mg per kilogram per day) or 3,4-diaminopyridine (1 mg per kilogram per day) increases quantal release from the nerve terminal and relieves the symptoms. However, the former drug has severe toxic side effects, and the latter is not yet available in clinical practice. Optimal treatment of non-neoplastic cases consists of modest doses of alternate-day prednisone and 2 mg per kilogram per day of azathioprine.

CONGENITAL MYASTHENIC SYNDROMES. *Familial Infantile Myasthenia.* This is an autosomal-recessive disorder characterized by fluctuating ophthalmoparesis since birth, feeding difficulty during early infancy, weakness after exercise, and attacks of apnea precipitated by crying, vomiting, or fever. The symptoms tend to improve with age. A decremental EMG response is present in muscles weak when examined. Weakness can be induced in some, but not all, muscles by exercise or repetitive stimulation at 10 Hz for a few minutes. Unlike in autoimmune MG, the postsynaptic region is intact and there is no AChR deficiency. The MEPP amplitude is normal in rested muscle but decreases to abnormally low values after 10-Hz stimulation for a few minutes. This suggests a presynaptic defect in ACh resynthesis or in ACh packaging into synaptic vesicles. Weakness, when present, responds to small or modest doses of anticholinesterases. Parenteral anticholinesterase therapy is indicated in crises. Parents of young patients must be taught to use a hand-assisted ventilatory device and to inject appropriate doses of neostigmine intramuscularly during crises.

Congenital End-Plate Acetylcholinesterase Deficiency. Sporadic and familial cases in males and females have been observed to date. Severe weakness refractory to anticholinesterases and a decremental EMG response are present in all voluntary muscles from birth. There is total absence of AChE from all end-plates. ACh-AChR interaction and the duration of the EPP are prolonged, so that a single stimulus applied to a motor nerve evokes two or more compound muscle action potentials. The motor nerve terminals are small and contain a reduced number of releasable ACh quanta. AChR is preserved or reduced at the end-plate. The AChR loss, if present, is caused by degenerative changes in the junctional folds, which can be accounted for by the ACh excess, but this in itself is mild because ACh release is also reduced. The safety margin of neuromuscular transmission is compromised by lack of releasable ACh quanta and by AChR deficiency.

Slow-Channel Syndrome. This is an autosomal-dominant disorder with high penetrance and variable expressivity. It presents in infancy or later life with selective weakness, fatigability, and atrophy of cervical, shoulder girdle, and forearm muscles. There is variable involvement of extraocular, other cranial, truncal, or limb muscles. The tendon reflexes are normal or hypoactive. Anticholinesterases are usually ineffective. A decremental EMG response appears in clinically affected muscles. The basic abnormality is slow closure of the AChR ion channel. This prolongs the duration of the EPP, causes a stimulus-linked repetitive compound action potential in all muscles, and allows abnormal accumulation of calcium in the postsynaptic region. The calcium excess results in destruction of the junctional folds, loss of AChR, and myopathic changes near the end-plates. The safety margin of neuromuscular transmission is compromised by the AChR deficiency and the altered end-plate geometry.

Congenital End-Plate AChR Deficiency. This is an autosomal-recessive disorder that presents during infancy. The symptoms and electrophysiologic abnormalities resemble those in autoimmune MG and respond to anticholinesterases. Circulating AChR antibodies are absent, and no immune complexes are found at the end-plate. The cause has not been established. It could stem from decreased synthesis, impaired membrane insertion or accelerated degradation of AChR, or abnormal ACh-AChR interaction.

Other Congenital Myasthenic Syndromes. These were recently recognized by in vitro electrophysiologic and ultrastructural analysis. In the *high-conductance fast-channel syndrome*, the conductance of the AChR ion channel is abnormally high but its open time is reduced. The disease is familial and is associated with mild fatigable weakness of ocular and limb muscles since birth. In another syndrome with *paucity of synaptic vesicles and reduced quantal release*, neuromuscular transmission is compromised by a decrease in m, which is due to a decrease in n. The disease presents in the neonatal period, involves all muscles, is moderately severe, and is partially responsive to anticholinesterase medications. In a syndrome caused by a *putative abnormality of ACh-AChR interaction*, the MEPP amplitude is markedly reduced without AChR deficiency, synaptic vesicles are of normal size, and analysis of ACh-induced current noise suggests abnormal interaction of ACh with AChR. The disorder presents in the neonatal period, is severely disabling, and responds poorly to anticholinesterase medications.

DRUG-INDUCED MYASTHENIC SYNDROMES. These are uncommon in clinical practice. Tetracycline, polymyxin and aminoglycoside antibiotics, antiarrhythmic agents (procainamide, quinidine), β-adrenergic blockers (propranolol, timolol), phenothiazines, lithium, trimethaphan, methoxyflurane, and magnesium given parenterally or in cathartics reduce the safety margin of neuromuscular transmission. However, overt myasthenic symptoms do not usually appear unless an overdose of the drug is administered or the renal or hepatic elimination of the drug is impaired. The same drugs and inhalation anesthetic agents also can potentiate neuromuscular blocking agents used during surgical procedures and both may worsen or unmask pre-existing disorders of neuromuscular transmission. Calcium channel blocking drugs can worsen the transmission defect in the Lambert-Eaton myasthenic syndrome.

Succinylcholine, a depolarizing blocking drug, is used to induce muscle relaxation during anesthesia. A single dose of the drug sufficient to cause transient apnea is eliminated by plasma pseudocholinesterase in 2 to 10 minutes. In approximately 1 of 2500 patients receiving the drug, prolonged apnea occurs and persists up to several hours. Most of these patients have an autosomal-recessive abnormality of the plasma pseudocholinesterase. In some genetic variants the plasma pseudocholinesterase activity is abnormally low; in others the enzyme shows increased sensitivity to inhibition by dibucaine.

PESTICIDE POISONING. Poisoning with pesticides containing long-acting anticholinesterases causes ACh accumulation at central, muscarinic, and nicotinic cholinergic synapses. The intoxication is associated with alterations in sensorium, severe muscarinic effects, and muscle weakness from desensitization of AChR at the neuromuscular junction. Therapy consists of respiratory support, large doses of atropine (2 to 4 mg intramuscularly and repeated as necessary) and pralidoxime (1 gram intravenously, repeated in 20 minutes if necessary).

Engel AG, Banker BQ (eds.): Myology. New York, McGraw-Hill Book Company, 1986. *Chapters by Engel and Magelby ably discuss the detailed anatomy, physiology, and clinical dimensions of neuromuscular transmission.*

Engel AG, Walls T, Nagel A, et al.: Newly recognized congenital myasthenic syndromes. Prog Brain Res 84:125–137, 1990. *An account of the clinical, morphologic, and electrophysiologic aspects of recently recognized congenital myasthenic syndromes.*

Grob D, Brunner NG, Namba T: The natural course of myasthenia gravis and effect of therapeutic measures. Ann NY Acad Sci 377:652, 1981. *A model clinical study.*

Nelson TC, Burritt MF: Pesticide poisoning, succinylcholine-induced apnea and pseudocholinesterase. Mayo Clin Proc 61:750, 1986. *A good description of pesticide poisoning and the different pseudocholinesterase deficiencies.*

Swift TR: Disorders of neuromuscular transmission other than myasthenia gravis. Muscle Nerve 4:334, 1981. *A thorough review of drug-induced myasthenic syndromes.*

Vincent A, Lang B, Newsom-Davis J: Autoimmunity to the voltage-gated calcium channel underlies the Lambert-Eaton myasthenic syndrome, a paraneoplastic disorder. Trends Neurosci 12:496, 1989. *A readable overview of the autoimmune etiology and immunopathology of the disease.*

Because many systemic diseases affect the eyes, ophthalmoscopy is a necessary skill for the physician. The pupil of the eye is a window opening onto the arterioles and venules of the retina, the optic disc, and the pigmented tissues of the fundus. Ch. 453 describes the autonomic and somatic motor disorders of ocular control and reviews the clinically important anatomy of the visual pathways.

The discussion that follows highlights the interrelationship between ocular and systemic disease, beginning with a discussion of visual loss, then a brief review of the two common ophthalmic disorders—cataract and glaucoma, before turning to ocular entities and ocular manifestations of medical disorders likely to present to nonophthalmic physicians.

510 Visual Loss

Visual loss may be either transient (see Ch. 453) or permanent, with most of the potential causes capable of producing either one. A major purpose of the ophthalmologic examination is to establish the etiology of visual loss. Except when it reflects a structural alteration in the eye, as in high myopia, the need for refractive correction is considered a variant of normal, not a disease process. Furthermore, when evaluating a patient for reduced vision, only the best-corrected acuity should be considered. Uncorrected acuity is of little interest in assessing the pathophysiology of eye disorders.

Many conditions can cause visual loss (Table 510–1). Normal visual development in an infant requires formed images on the retina and intact visual pathways in the rest of the brain. A neonatal eye with a dense opacity of the media such as a mature cataract (see below) does not develop useful vision unless the opacity is removed soon after birth and any resulting large refractive error is corrected quickly. Visual development proceeds through critical stages; any interruption of these stages during

TABLE 510–1. DIFFERENTIAL DIAGNOSIS OF VISUAL LOSS

Opacities of the media	Corneal opacities (leukomas, edema, dystrophy) or irregularity; anterior chamber blood or inflammation; cataract; vitreous opacities
Chorioretinal disease	Macular and other retinal degenerations; retinal detachment; toxic, vascular, and traumatic retinopathies; infectious and inflammatory chorioretinitis; retinal tumors
Optic nerve disease	Glaucoma, other optic neuropathies (inflammatory, toxic, traumatic, vascular, hereditary); compressive and infiltrative neuropathy; optic nerve tumors
Visual pathway disorders	Vascular, inflammatory, infectious, degenerative, developmental, neoplastic
Amblyopia	Strabismic, nutritional deprivation, anisometropic, ametropic, idiopathic
Psychogenic	

early childhood can permanently prevent the normal capacity for processing visual information even if the causative condition is treated later on. If both eyes are involved, the development of nystagmus (rhythmic to-and-fro movements of the eye) at about 3 or 4 months of age signals that this critical period has been exceeded.

Normal adult levels of visual acuity can be measured electrophysiologically by 6 months of age, but the neural connections that permit fine visual processing become permanently established only later in childhood. During the first few years of life, strabismus—misalignment of the visual axes of the two eyes—may result in suppression of central vision in one eye. Such visual loss in an eye that appears anatomically normal is termed amblyopia. A large, uncorrected refractive error—ametropia—or a major difference in the refractive error in the two eyes—anisometropia—may also lead to amblyopia. (The term *amblyopia* is also sometimes applied to processes in which the ophthalmoscopic signs are subtle, e.g., toxic-nutritional amblyopia.) Strabismic amblyopia is potentially reversible until 6 to 10 years of age, when the neural processing networks for vision become fixed for life. With this final step in visual development, the visual system achieves adult inflexibility, and misalignment of the visual axes results in permanent diplopia rather than suppression.

Careful ophthalmic examination and appropriate testing should allow classification of reduced vision into one of the categories listed (Table 510–1): opacities of the media, chorioretinal disease, optic nerve disease, visual pathway disorders, amblyopia, or psychogenic visual loss. Two or more processes may affect the same eye.

PSYCHOGENIC VISUAL LOSS

Visual loss not attributable to an organic process is termed psychogenic. Alternative designations are functional, nonorganic, nonphysiologic, hysterical, and malingering. The last two are best avoided. Hysteria suggests to some a sexual bias and must be considered a psychiatric, not an ophthalmologic, diagnosis; malingering imputes motives that are difficult to prove. Functional visual loss, the usage currently preferred by some authorities, is potentially confusing because *functional amblyopia* refers to those forms of amblyopia in which the process is potentially reversible with treatment (strabismic, ametropic, and anisometropic). In these instances there is presumably an underlying physiologic alteration in the visual system itself.

Psychogenic visual loss is not necessarily a diagnosis of exclusion. Certain patterns of visual loss cannot represent organic disease. Concentric constriction of visual fields is a common finding in nonphysiologic visual loss but also occurs with advanced glaucoma and retinitis pigmentosa and after bilateral occipital infarctions. Failure of the visual field to expand to an appropriate stimulus with increased testing distance—tubular fields—is, however, diagnostic of psychogenic visual loss. Similarly, patients who claim to be completely blind in one eye but who have normal pupillary reactions, full stereopsis, and normal ipsilateral visual evoked responses must have a nonphysiologic component to their visual loss. Other testing techniques also may result in normal subjective responses from a supposedly blind eye.

Most cases of psychogenic visual loss occur in the setting of minor psychological reactions rather than major psychiatric disorders. Sometimes both organic and nonorganic components coexist. Unless the visual loss prevents the patient from working or attending school, simple reassurance and careful follow-up with treatment of intercurrent organic abnormalities constitute appropriate management, and spontaneous improvement occurs.

Isenberg SJ: The Eye in Infancy. Chicago, Year Book Medical Publishers, 1989. *This monograph contains discussions of visual development and amblyopia.*

Thompson HS: Functional visual loss. Am J Ophthalmol 100:209, 1985. *An experienced clinician offers an approach to the problem.*

Jaffe NS, Jaffe MS, Jaffe GF: Cataract Surgery and Its Complications, 5th ed. St. Louis, The C. V. Mosby Company, 1990. *This profusely illustrated monograph addresses most of the issues of modern cataract surgery and includes extensive references.*

511 Cataract

A cataract is an opacity of the lens that produces painless, gradual loss of vision. Cataracts are described according to their location—nuclear (deep in the lens), cortical (more superficial), and subcapsular (immediately beneath the capsule). Cataracts are classified as immature, mature, or hypermature. An immature cataract has some clear cortex; a mature cataract is totally opaque—the pupil appears white (leukokoria). A hypermature cataract has liquefied cortex that leaks through the capsule and may excite destructive inflammation. Immature cataracts are usually removed for visual reasons. A mature or hypermature cataract in an eye with potentially useful vision should be removed to prevent irreversible damage.

ETIOLOGY. Congenital cataracts are a feature of rubella embryopathy and often are associated with other congenital malformations. Acquired cataracts may result from trauma, radiation, or metabolic disorder. Several examples of colorful cataracts have diagnostic, but little visual, significance. In Wilson's disease, orange copper deposits may appear on the anterior capsule—the sunflower cataract. Chlorpromazine administration may result in a brown or white dusting on the anterior lens surface. Red, green, and blue opacities in the lenticular cortex characterize myotonic dystrophy, but are occasionally encountered in its absence.

Hypocalcemia may be cataractogenic. Cataracts occur in disorders of carbohydrate metabolism: hypoglycemia, galactosemia, and diabetes mellitus. Diabetics do not necessarily have an increased incidence of cataracts, but theirs progress rapidly, perhaps because of variations in lens hydration.

Systemic corticosteroids promote formation of posterior subcapsular cataracts. Because of the path light takes through the lens, posterior subcapsular cataracts reduce vision more than similar, eccentric opacities. Central posterior opacities get in the way of light, especially when the pupil is small, as in bright light or with close work. Difficulties with driving and reading are often the first complaints.

Most cataracts have no known etiology. The common nuclear sclerotic cataract, or senile cataract, is often familial, but no specific factors have been proven to accelerate or retard its development.

TREATMENT. The treatment for cataract is surgical removal. With the exception of mature and hypermature cataracts and of immature cataracts that have swollen sufficiently to threaten to precipitate angle-closure glaucoma, most cataracts are removed for visual reasons. Considerations in planning cataract extraction are the patient's visual needs, the potential for improvement, and the risks of surgery. A person who drives requires surgery when the better eye is worse than 20/40, the legal minimum for a driver's license in most states. By contrast, an elderly patient with 20/200 vision and limited visual needs may be happy without intervention. Care must be taken to identify intercurrent ocular disease; removal of the lens of an eye with advanced glaucoma or macular degeneration does not improve vision.

The risk of cataract surgery itself is small. Despite the possibility of intraocular hemorrhage, postoperative infection, corneal decompensation, or problems with wound healing, the chances for a good visual outcome are excellent. Even successful cataract surgery, however, increases the likelihood of subsequent retinal detachment, and a small percentage of eyes postoperatively develop prolonged cystoid macular edema with reduced acuity.

General anesthesia constitutes a major portion of the risk. Cataract surgery, however, can usually be performed under local anesthesia, and this should be considered the method of choice in medically fragile patients.

512 Glaucoma

Glaucoma comprises a group of disorders in which elevated intraocular pressure damages the optic nerve. The major types of glaucoma are open-angle, angle-closure, congenital, and secondary.

The dynamics of aqueous humor control intraocular pressure. The aqueous humor is derived from blood by a process of secretion and ultrafiltration in the ciliary body. Aqueous humor then passes from the posterior chamber through the pupil to fill the anterior chamber, the space between the back of the cornea and the plane of the iris and pupil. The aqueous humor is reabsorbed through the trabecular meshwork, located in the angle between the cornea and the iris, to enter Schlemm's canal, which connects with the venous system (Fig. 512–1).

OPEN-ANGLE GLAUCOMA

In chronic open-angle glaucoma, the most common type, a block in aqueous humor reabsorption exists at the level of the trabecular meshwork. Intraocular pressure rises above its normal maximum of 21 mm Hg and gradually destroys axons and supporting tissue on the optic disc.

The prevalence of open-angle glaucoma varies with the population studied and the diagnostic criteria employed. A conservative estimate of unequivocal glaucoma in American and European adults is 0.5 per cent. Patients with increased intraocular pressure without signs of optic nerve damage are considered to have *ocular hypertension*. Treatment of ocular hypertension may be initiated if the pressure exceeds 30 mmHg.

Open-angle glaucoma is ordinarily asymptomatic until well advanced. Only rarely does the elevated intraocular pressure cause corneal edema, with the attendant perception of halos around lights. Pain is not characteristic of open-angle glaucoma. Initially only the peripheral visual field is lost; visual acuity remains normal until late in the course of the disease. Diagnosis is made by measurement of intraocular pressure, examination of the optic disc, and testing of the visual fields. Gonioscopy, the visualization of the angle structures under high magnifications with special contact lenses, can distinguish an angle-closure from an open-angle mechanism.

The treatment of open-angle glaucoma is primarily medical. Topical administration of parasympathomimetics (pilocarpine and carbachol), β-adrenergic blockers (timolol, betaxolol, and levobunolol), and sympathomimetics (epinephrine and dipivefrin) decreases intraocular pressure. When these medications—individually and in combination—are ineffective in arresting progressive disc damage and visual field loss, topical indirect parasympathomimetics (echothiophate) and systemic carbonic anhydrase inhibitors (acetazolamide and methazolamide) may be prescribed.

If maximum tolerated medical therapy fails to halt progression, surgery is indicated. *Laser trabeculoplasty* opens aqueous outflow channels by burning the surface of the trabecular meshwork. If all else fails, a surgical fistula can be created between the anterior chamber and the subconjunctival space, allowing direct absorption of aqueous humor by subconjunctival and episcleral vessels.

The management of open-angle glaucoma depends upon early recognition, careful follow-up, and patient compliance with therapeutic regimens. Routine measurement of intraocular pressures *(tonometry)* at general physical examinations is often advocated, but careful ophthalmoscopy with referral of patients whose central excavation ("cup") exceeds one third of the disc's area may be an equally effective screen.

ANGLE-CLOSURE GLAUCOMA

Angle-closure glaucoma develops when the normal path of aqueous flow is interrupted in an eye with a shallow anterior

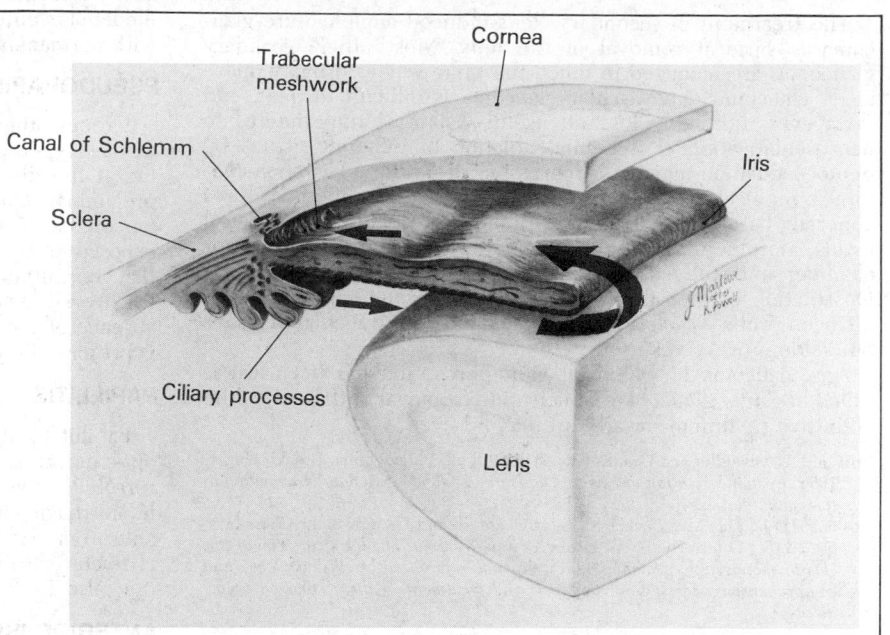

FIGURE 512-1. Circulation of aqueous humor in the normal eye. Aqueous is produced in the ciliary body and its processes, fills the posterior chamber (which also contains the lens), passes through the pupil (*large arrow*), and is reabsorbed through the trabecular meshwork into the canal of Schlemm.

chamber, the consequence of a structurally anomalous anterior segment. Intraocular pressure is normal until resistance to aqueous flow through the pupil—pupillary block—bows the iris forward to obstruct the resorptive surfaces in the angle. The pressure then rises precipitously, often to above 50 mm Hg (Fig. 512-2).

Acute angle-closure glaucoma is generally monocular. The eye is red and painful and the pupil is about 6 mm and fixed. Vision is decreased. The patient is diaphoretic, nauseated, and often vomits.

Typical angle-closure glaucoma is easy to recognize. Occasionally, chronic or subacute angle-closure mimics open-angle glaucoma. Gonioscopy then distinguishes between the two mechanisms. The elderly do not necessarily develop the full set of clinical signs and symptoms. Always consider angle-closure glaucoma in patients with a fixed, mid-dilated pupil and decreased vision.

Angle-closure can be precipitated in predisposed eyes by dilating the pupils. The risk of pharmacologic dilation is assessed by noting the depth of the anterior chamber. Eyes with shallow anterior chambers are at risk for angle-closure. This distinction is not always easy to observe, and even an experienced ophthal-

mologist sometimes cannot determine whether an angle will close with dilation. The risk of dilation increases with age, and everyone over the age of 50 whose anterior chamber is less than full depth should be considered to have the potential for angle-closure. This does not mean that most patients should not be dilated, but rather that dilation should be performed with a short-acting mydriatic agent such as tropicamide or hydroxyamphetamine, and the patient observed until the mydriatic begins to wear off.

A nonophthalmologist should probably not routinely dilate adult outpatients. Children and in-patients may be dilated if there is no other contraindication such as recent head trauma, an iris-fixated intraocular lens, or impending general anesthesia. With these exceptions, the diagnostic benefits of dilation outweigh the risk of precipitating angle-closure. Should angle-closure glaucoma develop, it can be recognized and promptly treated.

An acute angle-closure attack creates an emergency. Initial management consists of administration of parenteral acetazolamide, oral glycerol, isosorbide (in diabetics) or intravenous mannitol, plus topical pilocarpine and a β-adrenergic antagonist. Once the attack has been broken, the anatomic predisposition can be circumvented by connecting the posterior and anterior chamber through the peripheral iris, either with a laser—*laser iridotomy*—or by surgical iridectomy. The anterior segment abnormality that underlies angle-closure glaucoma is bilateral, and prophylactic surgery on the other eye is usually indicated.

CONGENITAL GLAUCOMA

Congenital glaucoma is an open-angle glaucoma that results from dysgenesis of the angle structures. Increased intraocular pressure enlarges the immature eye (*buphthalmos*); a corneal diameter greater than 12 mm suggests congenital glaucoma. Progressive corneal enlargement disrupts the deeper layers of the cornea, with resulting corneal edema and loss of transparency. The cornea of a child with advanced congenital glaucoma is enlarged, with a ground-glass translucency.

Treatment of congenital glaucoma is both surgical and medical. The condition is fortunately rare, as the prognosis for preservation of vision is only fair.

SECONDARY GLAUCOMA

Secondary glaucoma develops as the consequence of another ocular disease. Examples of secondary glaucomas are angle-closure glaucoma precipitated by intumescence of the lens, glaucoma developing as a result of formation of new vessels in the angle, and glaucoma in a chronically inflamed eye. Severe blunt trauma to the eye damages angle structures, predisposing to the subsequent development of open-angle glaucoma.

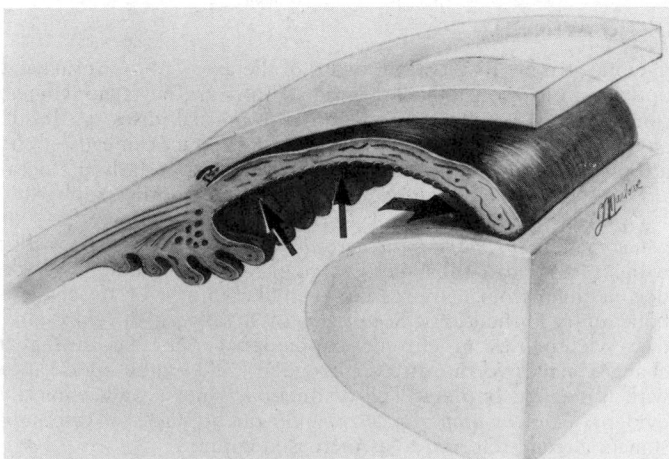

FIGURE 512-2. Angle-closure glaucoma. Owing to an anatomic anomaly in the anterior segment of the eye, the aqueous becomes trapped behind the pupil, bowing the iris forward (iris bombé) to cover the trabecular meshwork, which lies in the angle between the iris and the cornea.

The treatment of secondary, lens-induced angle-closure glaucoma is surgical removal of the lens. Most other secondary glaucomas are managed in much the same way as primary open-angle glaucoma. Neovascular glaucoma is difficult to treat, and most eyes ultimately lose all useful vision. If the stimulus to neovascularization is ischemia, ablation of ischemic tissues by photocoagulation may halt progression. If neovascularization continues, medical control becomes ineffective. Filtering procedures generally fail because exuberant tissue growth closes the surgical fistula, a problem that may be avoided by connecting the anterior chamber and the subconjunctival space with a plastic valve. Destruction of the ciliary body by an externally applied liquid nitrogen probe—*cyclocryotherapy*—controls intraocular pressure but seldom preserves useful vision.

Any glaucoma in which all light perception has been lost is called *absolute glaucoma*. Enucleation (removal of the eye) is the definitive treatment for a blind, painful eye.

Epstein DL: Chandler and Grant's Glaucoma, 3rd ed. Philadelphia, Lea & Febiger, 1986. *Epstein's revision of this text adds an excellent section on examination of the eye in glaucoma.*

Hoskins HD Jr, Kass MA: Becker-Shaffer's Diagnosis and Therapy of the Glaucomas, 6th ed. St. Louis, The C. V. Mosby Company, 1989. *The latest revision of this classic monograph provides an extensively referenced, well-illustrated, and comprehensive overview of diagnosis and treatment of these common ocular diseases.*

513 Disc Swelling and Optic Atrophy

The optic disc marks the transition from retina to optic nerve. The central retinal artery and vein pass through the disc and bifurcate on its surface. There is considerable normal variation in the disc's ophthalmoscopic appearance. A central excavation or cup occupies a variable portion of its substance; vessels are often seen curving over the edge of this cup.

Over one million axons originate in the ganglion cells of the retina and pass through each optic disc. Although these axons are nearly transparent, a bright ophthalmoscope will visualize fine reflective striations on the disc's surface and the immediately surrounding retina. Disc swelling can be a consequence of ischemia, infarction, infiltration, or local changes in tissue pressures (Table 513–1).

PAPILLEDEMA (See Color Plate 13B)

Disc swelling from increased intracranial pressure is termed papilledema. The swelling reflects primarily accumulation of axoplasm in and around the disc, appearing ophthalmoscopically as a protrusion of the disc, most obvious just adjacent to its normal borders. With rapid increases in intracranial pressure, the veins become engorged and hemorrhages may appear on the disc and adjacent retina.

TABLE 513–1. CAUSES OF DISC SWELLING

Increased intracranial pressure (papilledema)	Compressive optic neuropathy Graves' disease
Inflammatory optic neuropathy (papillitis)	Sphenoid wing meningioma Vasculopathies
Infiltrative optic neuropathy Sarcoidosis	Anterior ischemic optic neuropathy
Leukemia and other malignancies	Central retinal vein occlusion Malignant hypertension
Optic nerve tumors Angioma	Toxic-metabolic optic neuropathy Idiopathic
Optic nerve meningioma	Pseudopapilledema
Childhood optic nerve glioma	Optic disc drusen
Malignant optic nerve glioma	Hyperopia
Metastatic carcinoma	Other anomalies

Papilledema is usually bilateral but may be asymmetric. Visual acuity remains normal in acute papilledema. Long-standing papilledema eventually leads to secondary optic atrophy, sometimes with permanent loss of vision (see below).

PSEUDOPAPILLEDEMA

Various other disc appearances may be confused with papilledema. Hyperopic (farsighted) eyes are small, with axonal crowding at the disc. Drusen, depositions of hyaline material in the prelaminar optic nerve, can produce swollen discs in young persons (see Color Plate 13D). In time, the buried drusen become exposed and are visible ophthalmoscopically as refractile bodies that resemble rock crystals. Such anomalous discs are often discovered incidentally. One clue to their nature is the frequent absence of the physiologic cup, for in true papilledema the cup is preserved until the disc swelling is far advanced.

PAPILLITIS

Papillitis indicates an anterior inflammatory or demyelinating optic neuritis. In many instances the disc appears normal—*retrobulbar neuritis*. In papillitis, the disc is swollen and may be hemorrhagic, an appearance ophthalmoscopically indistinguishable from papilledema. Unlike papilledema, however, acuity is characteristically reduced, and the condition is usually unilateral. (See also Tables 452.2 and 452.3.)

ANTERIOR ISCHEMIC OPTIC NEUROPATHY

Papillitis is largely a disease of the young. In older persons, acute disc swelling and loss of vision suggest infarction—anterior ischemic optic neuropathy. Often only the superior or inferior half of the disc is involved, with consequent loss of function in the inferior or superior visual field. Most instances of ischemic optic neuropathy are idiopathic, but the disorder may be the initial manifestation of giant cell or temporal arteritis, a disease of the elderly described in Ch. 267.

OTHER CAUSES OF DISC SWELLING

Bilateral disc swelling may accompany severe hypertension. The relative roles of local vascular changes and of increased intracranial pressure in the pathogenesis are uncertain. Markedly decreased intraocular pressure, encountered after ocular surgery or injury, also produces disc swelling, and the disc may swell acutely during an attack of angle-closure glaucoma. Disc swelling is also a feature of some toxic and hereditary optic neuropathies.

Compression causes disc swelling only when the nerve is constricted. This occurs in some patients with the orbitopathy of Graves' disease (Ch. 516), pseudotumor of the orbit (Ch. 516), and sphenoid wing meningioma. Intrinsic tumors of the optic nerve, the most common being glioma and meningioma, may present as disc swelling and visual loss. Infiltration of the optic nerve heads is also encountered in leukemia, metastatic carcinoma, and sarcoid.

OPTIC ATROPHY

Optic atrophy results from death of the axons in the retina and optic nerve. Disc pallor and optic atrophy are not synonymous; some temporal pallor is a feature of normal discs. A lesion anywhere from the retina through the optic tract can cause optic atrophy. Lesions behind the lateral geniculate in early life occasionally cause trans-synaptic degeneration and optic atrophy.

Optic atrophy may be classified as primary, secondary, or glaucomatous. *Primary optic atrophy* refers to progressive pallor without loss of disc substance, a sign of retrograde or anterograde degeneration from compression, vascular injury, or toxic metabolic injury to the axons. *Secondary optic atrophy* develops after disc swelling, as in chronic papilledema. Vascular and glial changes may give the disc an irregular, milky gray appearance with ill-defined borders. The distinction is not always clinically evident. *Glaucomatous optic atrophy* denotes loss of disc substance, already referred to as increased cupping.

Optic atrophy is difficult to recognize in young children, in whom the discs may have a pale appearance normally. In adults with nuclear sclerotic cataracts, pallor may be masked by the lens acting as a yellow filter. The diagnosis of optic atrophy should not be made unless there is evidence of alteration in visual function: decreased acuity or field—or, in infants, nystagmus.

Ultimately, optic atrophy is not a clinical finding but a pathologic entity. In retinitis pigmentosa there is a primary dystrophy of the rods and cones. The ganglion cells remain intact, but secondary vascular and gliotic changes produce a waxy pallor of the disc, but not a true optic atrophy, since the axons are preserved.

LEBER'S HEREDITARY OPTIC NEURORETINOPATHY (LEBER'S DISEASE)

This disorder, sometimes called Leber's optic atrophy (see Color Plate 13C), produces acute or subacute visual loss in men around the age of 20 years. Women are much less often affected, with onset at age 30 or above. Initially the discs appear swollen because of opacification of the peripapillary nerve fiber layer, but the swelling does not represent edema, since fluorescein angiography demonstrates only telangiectatic vessels that do not leak dye. With time central vision is lost in both eyes, and optic atrophy evolves. Although no effective treatment exists, vision occasionally improves spontaneously. The disorder is transmitted via an abnormality in maternal mitochondrial DNA, explaining the sex-linked heredity. Most cases can be diagnosed by study of mitochondrial DNA from peripheral leukocytes.

Miller NR: Walsh and Hoyt's Clinical Neuro-Ophthalmology, 4th ed. Baltimore, Williams & Wilkins Company, 1982, Vol 1, pp 175–271, 311–317, 329–342. *The pages cited contain a comprehensive review of the entities discussed here.*
Singh G, Lott MT, Wallace DC: A mitochondrial DNA mutation as a cause of Leber's hereditary optic neuropathy. N Engl J Med 320:1300, 1989. *Describes the genetic analysis that identifies a point mutation in three families with Leber's disease.*

514 Uveitis

Uveitis denotes inflammation of the uveal tract—the iris, ciliary body, and choroid. There are two major clinical types, anterior and posterior (Table 514–1). Anterior uveitis, also known as *iritis* or *iridocyclitis*, has as its hallmark cells in the anterior chamber. Curiously, it is the rare case of iritis that displays any recognizable iris abnormality. Posterior uveitis may take the form of *chorioretinitis*. The choroid and retina are so intimately connected that it is difficult to have inflammation of one without the other.

Acute anterior uveitis presents with congestion of the eye, often in a perilimbal distribution described as ciliary flush. Frequently, the eye is painful, vision reduced, and the pupil small and poorly reactive. The diagnosis is confirmed on slit lamp examination by the presence of free cells in the aqueous humor, visible as bright points as the slit beam passes through the anterior chamber. In more severe inflammation, *keratitic precipitates*, cellular aggregates on the back of the cornea, appear.

Anterior uveitis may be a manifestation of a systemic inflammatory disease such as sarcoid, an infection such as syphilis or

TABLE 514–1. DISEASES ASSOCIATED WITH UVEITIS

	Infectious	Other
Anterior (iridocyclitis)	Herpes zoster *Herpesvirus hominis* Hansen's disease	Ankylosing spondylitis Rheumatoid arthritis Reiter's syndrome
Posterior (chorioretinitis)	Toxoplasmosis Toxocariasis Histoplasmosis Measles	
Both anterior and posterior	Syphilis Coccidioidomycosis Onchocerciasis Brucellosis	Sarcoid Behçet's syndrome Vogt-Koyanagi-Harada syndrome Inflammatory bowel disease

tuberculosis, or idiopathic. In some instances inflammation may be marked, with large, oily keratitic precipitates, a variant termed *granulomatous iritis*.

UVEITIS AND ARTHRITIS

Juvenile rheumatoid arthritis (see Ch. 258) and ankylosing spondylitis (see Ch. 259) are especially apt to be associated with uveitis. Young men with this disorder may have recurrent episodes that respond to standard treatments (see below). A majority are HLA-B27 positive. By contrast, the uveitis accompanying juvenile rheumatoid arthritis is chronic and may initially be subclinical. Young women with the pauciarticular form of juvenile rheumatoid arthritis who develop uveitis often have white and quiet eyes. With time, however, adhesions, called posterior synechiae, form between the iris and lens, potentially causing secondary pupillary block glaucoma or occlusion of the pupil. The inflammation may lead to cataract formation and ectopic calcification in the corneal epithelium—band keratopathy. Physicians treating seronegative pauciarticular arthritis should schedule slit lamp and dilated examinations several times a year. Posterior synechiae are visible with a hand light after instillation of mydriatics, as the pupil does not fully dilate and develops an irregular, scalloped border.

REITER'S SYNDROME

The triad of arthritis, urethritis, and conjunctivitis suggests Reiter's syndrome (see Ch. 259). This develops most often in men between the ages of 20 and 40 as a nonbacterial urethritis followed by polyarthritis and ocular inflammation. The initial ocular manifestation is usually a mucopurulent conjunctivitis, followed in many cases by an anterior uveitis. Keratitis and episcleritis also occur. As in ankylosing spondylitis, with which it shares similarities, HLA-B27 is often positive.

BEHÇET'S SYNDROME

Uveitis (or retinitis) is a cardinal feature of Behçet's syndrome (see Ch. 269). In some cases a characteristic layer of white cells forms in the lower portion of the anterior chamber (*hypopyon*). In other patients the primary ocular manifestation is a retinal vasculitis and vitritis. Rarer neuro-ophthalmic manifestations such as cranial nerve palsies or homonymous hemianopias are part of a wider central nervous system involvement.

UVEOMENINGITIS—THE VOGT-KOYANAGI-HARADA SYNDROME

Another systemic disease with characteristic ocular inflammation is uveomeningitis (the Vogt-Koyanagi-Harada syndrome). This disease affects the uvea, retina, meninges, and skin and is more common in Asians. Manifestations include meningeal signs, alopecia, poliosis, vitiligo, tinnitus, and dysacousis. There may be an anterior or a posterior uveitis with exudative retinal detachment.

MALIGNANCY MASQUERADING AS UVEITIS

A steroid-responsive exudative process simulating uveitis can occur in adults over the age of 40 as part of a lymphoreticular neoplasia (variously called reticulum cell sarcoma, histiocytic sarcoma, or—when the brain is involved—primary CNS lymphoma). Diagnosis may be made from the cytology of a vitreous aspirate. Radiation treatment has palliative value.

An apparent iritis developing during a course of treatment for leukemia may represent infiltration of the anterior segment. Diagnosis and therapy are similar to those for reticulum cell sarcoma.

TREATMENT

The treatment of uveitis consists largely of topical or, when the inflammation is prolonged or severe, systemic immunosuppression. Prednisolone or dexamethasone topically, or prednisone orally, is the preferred drug. Cytotoxic immunosuppressive agents are sometimes used in chronic, intractable uveitis. Topical administration of mydriatic-cycloplegics in anterior uveitis reduces discomfort and retards posterior synechiae formation.

Dinning WJ: Systemic Inflammatory Disease and the Eye. Bristol, Wright, 1987. *Describes the medical and ophthalmologic findings in a variety of systemic disorders.*

Kanski JJ: Uveitis: A Colour Manual of Diagnosis and Treatment. London, Butterworths, 1987. *Briefly considers and illustrates many entities.*

Nussenblatt RB, Palestine AG: Uveitis: Fundamentals and Clinical Practice. Chicago, Year Book Medical Publishers, 1989. *Contains chapters on Vogt-Koyanagi-Harada syndrome and other unusual uveitides.*

Rosenthal AR: Ocular manifestations of leukemia: A review. Ophthalmology 90:899, 1983. *This paper covers the retinal, orbital, optic nerve, and uveal manifestations of leukemia.*

Smith RE, Nozik RA: Uveitis: A Clinical Approach to Diagnosis and Management. Baltimore, Williams & Wilkins, 1989. *After a practically oriented discussion of uveitis in general, Smith and Nozik address both clinical syndromes and diagnostic entities, offering specific therapeutic recommendations.*

515 Ocular Infections

Ocular infections (or inflammations) are most sensibly grouped according to their locations. The most common superficial infection is a *blepharoconjunctivitis* or, more simply, *conjunctivitis*. Infection of the lacrimal gland is a *dacryoadenitis;* infection of the lacrimal drainage system, a *dacryocystitis*. Corneal involvement is called *keratitis*. Uveitis, scleritis, and episcleritis, which are seldom infectious, are discussed elsewhere (see Ch. 514, 518). Infection or inflammation inside the eye is an *endophthalmitis*. An infectious *vitritis* is a form of endophthalmitis. Some *chorioretinitis* is infectious. *Panophthalmitis* refers to infection that extends through the sclera or cornea and involves adjacent orbital tissues.

CONJUNCTIVITIS

The etiologies for the conjunctivitides include allergic, viral, bacterial, chlamydial, and chemical. Mild acute viral conjunctivitis, with a watery discharge and lids that are sealed closed upon awakening, usually requires only symptomatic treatment—warm or cool compresses and a topical vasoconstrictor to whiten the eye. Antibiotics have no clear efficacy. Any severe or chronic conjunctivitis should be managed by an ophthalmologist.

GONOCOCCAL CONJUNCTIVITIS. Purulent conjunctivitis is usually bacterial and amenable to antibiotics. An important variety is gonococcal conjunctivitis, a disease of the newborn (*gonococcal ophthalmia neonatorum*) and of sexually active adults. The eye is markedly inflamed with a copious discharge and swollen lids, a picture described as hyperpurulent conjunctivitis.

The discharge should be Gram stained and cultured on Thayer-Martin medium. Treatment consists of parenteral antibiotics and saline lavage of ocular secretions. Because of the emergence of penicillinase-producing strains, use of a β-lactamase–resistant cephalosporin such as ceftriaxone may be warranted. Untreated gonococcal infection can penetrate the intact eye and destroy it; treatment should be immediately initiated if there is a reasonable suspicion of the diagnosis.

CHLAMYDIAL CONJUNCTIVITIS. In some parts of the world, chronic chlamydial conjunctivitis leads to conjunctival scarring and corneal vascularization, a disease known as *trachoma*. The resulting blindness is an important international public health problem. In developed countries, chlamydial infection manifests as a subacute conjunctivitis, frequently with associated urethritis. Although a keratitis may be present, severe corneal damage does not ensue. Chlamydial conjunctivitis, also called *inclusion blennorrhea* because of the cytoplasmic inclusions found in Giemsa-stained conjunctival scrapings, is difficult to eradicate in adults unless treated with systemic tetracycline or erythromycin.

HERPETIC KERATITIS (See Color Plate 13A)

Viral keratitis is a common and potentially serious consequence of infection with herpes simplex. The corneal involvement may be recognized by the characteristic *dendrite*, a branching epithelial ulcer. Topical antiviral agents promote healing but recurrence is frequent with increasing risk of corneal stromal involvement and scarring. Topical steroids activate epithelial herpes infections and should not be used without ophthalmologic consultation. Herpes zoster also can produce an acute dendritic keratitis.

CORNEAL ULCERS

Bacterial and fungal infections of the cornea are a serious threat to vision. Corneal ulcers tend to develop in the context of ocular trauma or contact lens wear, after surgery, or with pre-existing corneal disease. Corneal ulceration appears as an area of white, gray, or yellow infiltrate that stains with fluorescein. Such patients should be referred promptly to an ophthalmologist for evaluation and treatment with topical antibiotics and other measures.

ENDOPHTHALMITIS

Infection inside the eye most often follows accidental or surgical perforation of the eye. Epidemics have occurred following use of contaminated solutions in intraocular surgery. Only rarely do infections elsewhere metastasize to the eye.

Bacterial endophthalmitis must be treated aggressively if there is to be any chance of preserving vision. When the infection is recognized, cultures and smears are taken from the anterior chamber and vitreous cavity by aspiration, and a course of intravitreal and, sometimes, systemic, topical, and periocular antibiotics is begun. The choice of antibiotics depends on what organisms, if any, are found on the Gram stain. Surgical vitrectomy may be warranted.

***CANDIDA* ENDOPHTHALMITIS.** *Candida albicans* is the most prevalent organism causing metastatic (endogenous) endophthalmitis. Fungemia after prolonged use of intravenous catheters or parenteral drug abuse results in colonization of the eye, with multiple white, fluffy chorioretinal infiltrates. These often involve the macula, reducing central vision. Careful direct ophthalmoscopy through a dilated pupil is indicated in patients at risk. Most *Candida* endophthalmitis requires systemic or intravitreal administration of antifungal agents, although spontaneous resolution has been observed.

INFECTIOUS CHORIORETINITIS

CONGENITAL TOXOPLASMOSIS (see Color Plate 13*H*). A common type of infectious chorioretinitis is *toxoplasmosis*, acquired in utero. This protozoan parasite can remain dormant in large, pigmented chorioretinal scars for many years and then become active, with white infiltration at the border of the scar and an overlying vitritis. If a previously uninvolved macula is threatened, treatment with pyrimethamine and sulfa or with clindamycin may be indicated.

CYTOMEGALOVIRUS CHORIORETINITIS (see Color Plate 14*G*). Cytomegalovirus chorioretinitis appears in immunosuppressed hosts as a discrete area of white or yellow retinal opacification with associated hemorrhage and vascular sheathing. The ophthalmoscopic picture resembles that of a branch retinal vein occlusion (see Ch. 519), but in this instance, one eye often has multiple foci, and there is a tendency for bilaterality.

Diagnosis can be made clinically and by culture of throat and urine. Dosages of immunosuppressive drugs should be reduced, if possible. The efficacy of treatment with antiviral agents is being actively evaluated.

OTHER INFECTIOUS CHORIORETINITIDES. Syphilis and tuberculosis are now rarely encountered as chorioretinitis. Herpes simplex retinitis resembles that of cytomegalovirus. Cryptococcal meningitis may have an associated chorioretinitis. Focal chorioretinitis can accompany subacute sclerosing panencephalitis (Ch. 478).

Darrell RD (ed.): Viral Diseases of the Eye. Philadelphia, Lea & Febiger, 1985. *Individual chapters on herpesvirus, cytomegalovirus, and measles, among others.*

Elliott AJ: Endophthalmitis in systemic disease: A review of *Candida albicans* endophthalmitis. Semin Ophthalmol 2:229, 1987. *While Elliott concludes that systemic therapy is necessary, some clinicians report successful management of intravitreal infection with vitrectomy and intravitreal amphotericin B alone (see Brod RD, Flynn HW Jr, Clarkson JG, et al.: Endogenous* Candida *endophthalmitis: Management without intravenous amphotericin B. Ophthalmology 97:666, 1990.)*

Stern GA, Engel HM, Driebe WT Jr: The treatment of postoperative endophthalmitis: Results of differing approaches to treatment. Ophthalmology 96:62, 1989. *Reviews 26 cases and makes therapeutic recommendations for bacterial endophthalmitis.*

Tabbara KF, Hyndiuk RA: Infections of the Eye. Boston, Little, Brown and Company, 1986. *Forty-three chapters cover most known infectious entities.*

Wilhelmus KR: Bacterial corneal ulcers. Int Ophthalmol Clin 24:1, 1984. *This practical clinical review can serve as a manual of diagnosis and management.*

516 Orbital Disease and Tumors

GRAVES' ORBITOPATHY

The orbitopathy of Graves' disease consists of inflammation and infiltration of orbital tissues, with characteristic enlargement and scarring of the extraocular muscles. The varied clinical manifestations include lid retraction, exophthalmos, and limitation of eye movement.

Graves' orbitopathy frequently develops in persons previously treated for hyperthyroidism. When the orbitopathy first appears, the patient may be hyperthyroid, euthyroid, or hypothyroid. A classic Graves' orbitopathy in the absence of a demonstrable thyroid abnormality, even to sophisticated testing, is referred to as *ophthalmic Graves' disease.* Coronal computed tomography demonstrating enlarged ocular muscles is probably the most sensitive diagnostic maneuver.

Graves' orbitopathy is the most frequent cause of both unilateral and bilateral exophthalmos. Retraction of the upper lid to expose sclera above the cornea exaggerates the appearance of exophthalmos and predisposes to a major complication, corneal exposure. Tethering of the eye by fibrotic muscles produces a mechanical ophthalmoplegia. Movement up and out is often restricted; pure loss of abduction mimicking sixth nerve palsy occurs. Ophthalmoplegia is not necessarily accompanied by exophthalmos.

Enlargement of the ocular muscles at the apex of the orbit may lead to another major complication of Graves' orbitopathy—compressive optic neuropathy. Severe exposure or major visual loss from compressive optic neuropathy is an indication for treatment. Systemic steroids reduce exophthalmos and relieve optic nerve compression temporarily. Surgical decompression of the orbit by one of several routes is one definitive therapy; orbital irradiation is also used. Direct surgery on the ocular muscles relieves diplopia and permanent lid retraction.

INFLAMMATORY PSEUDOTUMOR OF THE ORBIT

Orbital pseudotumor is an idiopathic inflammation that falls within the spectrum of lymphoproliferative disorders. Its clinical manifestations are pain, exophthalmos, and limitation of eye movement. There may also be erythema and swelling of the lids. Orbital pseudotumors can mimic orbital infection, true tumors, or the orbitopathy of Graves' disease. The major site of inflammation is muscle (myositis), nerve (perineuritis), sclera (scleritis), or lacrimal gland (dacryoadenitis).

If the inflammation is posterior to the orbital apex in the walls of the cavernous sinus, the painful ophthalmoplegia that results is called the *Tolosa-Hunt syndrome.* Orbital pseudotumor merges pathologically and clinically with orbital lymphoma, which in turn merges with systemic lymphoma.

Initial evaluation of a patient with clinical signs and symptoms of orbital pseudotumor includes orbital ultrasonography and computed tomography. A trial of high-dose systemic corticosteroids is usually indicated prior to biopsy. Orbital biopsy is not a trivial undertaking and should be reserved for steroid-unresponsive or recurrent processes. Some histologically benign infiltrations do not respond to corticosteroids. Biopsy in such cases reveals fibrous tissue—*sclerosing pseudotumor.* Occasionally, a patient with a histologically benign pseudotumor subsequently develops a systemic lymphoma.

A necrotizing vasculitis, Wegener's granulomatosis, must also be included in the differential diagnosis of orbital pseudotumor, especially when the inflammation is bilateral. Most cases of Wegener's granulomatosis involve contiguous sinus structures, but local ocular forms of the disease have been reported. The combination of progressive proptosis and sinus disease also sug-gests orbital aspergillosis, especially in residents of warmer climates.

RHABDOMYOSARCOMA

Rhabdomysarcoma is the most common malignant tumor of the orbit during the first decade of life and occurs during the second and third decades. The initial presentation is usually ptosis with lid infiltration and proptosis. Progression may be extremely rapid, the clinical picture mimicking trauma or cellulitis. Biopsy and prompt treatment with irradiation and chemotherapy result in a high percentage of survival, although vision in the eye on the side of the tumor is seldom preserved.

OTHER ORBITAL TUMORS

The variety of primary, secondary, and metastatic tumors in the orbit is large. Most present with exophthalmos, visual loss, and limitation of eye movement. High degrees of malignancy are rare with meningiomas, gliomas, hemangiomas/lymphangiomas, and dermoids. Carcinomas of the lacrimal or meibomian glands represent a serious threat to life, and some cases require the most distressing of all ophthalmologic surgery—*exenteration,* removal of the orbital contents. Carcinoma from contiguous sinuses invades the orbit, and breast carcinoma is especially likely to metastasize to the orbit.

Char DH: Thyroid Eye Disease. Baltimore, Williams & Wilkins, 1985. *Char reviews his subject comprehensively and recommends treatment emphasizing short-term steroids and high-voltage radiotherapy.*

Goldberg RA, Rootman J, Cline RA: Tumors metastatic to the orbit: A changing picture. Surv Ophthalmol 35:1, 1990. *An orbital tumor was the presenting sign of cancer in 42 per cent of cases. In women breast was the most common primary, followed by carcinoid; in men prostate, then melanoma and renal cell carcinoma.*

Kennerdell JS, Dresner SC: The nonspecific orbital inflammatory syndromes. Surv Ophthalmol 29:93, 1984.

Mauriello JA Jr, Flanagan JC: Management of orbital inflammatory disease. A protocol. Surv Ophthalmol 29:104, 1984. *Consecutive papers that provide an overview of pseudotumor of the orbit.*

517 Intraocular Tumors

RETINOBLASTOMA

Retinoblastoma, a malignancy of the retina, is the most common intraocular tumor of childhood (and one of the more common tumors at any site). One third are bilateral. About 6 per cent of retinoblastomas are inherited as an autosomal dominant disease; half of these are bilateral. Ninety per cent of retinoblastomas are discovered before the age of three.

MALIGNANT MELANOMA

Primary melanomas develop in the conjunctiva, iris, ciliary body, or choroid; skin melanomas have a predilection for metastasis to the eye and orbit. Malignant melanomas of the choroid are the most common primary intraocular tumor of adulthood. Most occur in middle-aged Caucasians.

The prognosis of malignant melanoma of the choroid depends upon size, cytology, and the presence or absence of extrascleral extension. Choroidal malignant melanomas often metastasize to the liver.

The differential diagnosis of a pigmented intraocular mass includes benign choroidal nevus, senile disciform macular degeneration (also known as central exudative hemorrhagic retinopathy), peripheral exudative hemorrhagic chorioretinopathy, choroidal hemangioma, and hypertrophy or hyperplasia of the retinal pigment epithelium. Many eyes have been removed because of the suspicion of malignant melanoma when the pathology revealed a benign condition.

Enucleation is the traditional treatment for malignant melanoma of the choroid. Other approaches include photocoagulation, radiotherapy, and local resection. Many pigmented choroidal tumors can be followed safely without intervention, especially when they are found incidentally in the seeing eyes of elderly patients.

METASTATIC CARCINOMA TO THE EYE

Once considered rare, metastatic cancer has become the most common ocular malignancy of adulthood, its incidence exceeding that of choroidal melanoma. Most are carcinomas invading the choroid (see Color Plate 13E), the most common coming from the breast. Next in frequency are carcinomas of the lung, followed by kidney, gastrointestinal tract, testis, and prostate. With lung or renal carcinoma, the primary site may be inapparent at the time the metastasis is detected.

If tumor is identified elsewhere, removal of the eye is seldom indicated. Enucleation should be performed only if the eye is completely blind and painful, as palliative radiotherapy or chemotherapy may preserve vision.

Char DH: Clinical Ocular Oncology. New York, Churchill Livingstone, 1989. *Extensively referenced and illustrated, this monograph provides an overview of ocular oncology.*

Yanoff M, Fine BS: Ocular Pathology: A Text and Atlas, 3rd ed. Philadelphia, Harper Medical, 1989. *A comprehensive textbook with clinicopathologic correlations.*

518 Episcleritis, Scleritis, and the Dry Eye

To a neurologist, the eye is an anterior extension of the brain; to a rheumatologist, the eye is a joint. Medicine and ophthalmology come together in the diagnosis and management of rheumatoid and connective tissue disorders. Uveal manifestations are discussed in Ch. 514; the toxicity of drugs used in treatment in Ch. 520; and the retinal changes in Ch. 519.

EPISCLERITIS AND SCLERITIS

Inflammation of the collagenous shell of the eye is either superficial (*episcleritis*) or deep (*scleritis*). The transparent, avascular cornea is continuous with the opaque, vascular sclera and may be secondarily involved.

Episcleritis resembles a localized conjunctivitis. The inflammation is deeper, however, and the dilated vessels do not always blanch with topically applied phenylephrine 2.5 per cent, as in a pure conjunctivitis. Episcleritis usually is self-limited (although it may be recurrent) and does not permanently damage the eye. Most episcleritis is idiopathic, but it may be encountered in rheumatoid arthritis, polyarteritis nodosa, Wegener's granulomatosis, systemic lupus erythematosus, dermatomyositis, progressive systemic sclerosis, and relapsing polychondritis.

Scleritis is more likely than episcleritis to accompany a systemic disease, although the list of associations is about the same for the two disorders. Any portion of the sclera may be affected. The diagnosis is especially difficult with posterior scleritis, which may present as ocular pain or as an exudative retinal detachment. Anterior scleritis often consists of a prolonged, indolent inflammation with eventual permanent structural alteration of tissues. Pain may be prominent and severe.

Initially in scleritis the inflammation is localized and may be nodular or diffuse. With prolonged inflammation, scleral thinning results in a localized bluish discoloration as the underlying choroid becomes visible. Scleral necrosis with perforation is possible; this is especially frequent in rheumatoid arthritis. The adjacent cornea may melt away.

Management of scleritis is difficult. Local steroid injections may predispose to perforation. Systemic corticosteroids and other antirheumatic drugs are useful in some patients. The ocular process often closely parallels the activity of the underlying disease, and the best approach is systemic therapy.

KERATOCONJUNCTIVITIS SICCA

Corneal inflammation as the result of drying is referred to as *keratoconjunctivitis sicca*. Keratoconjunctivitis sicca, a dry mouth (xerostomia), and a connective tissue disorder constitute *Sjögren's syndrome*. The underlying pathophysiology appears to be an autoimmune reaction affecting the lacrimal and salivary glands. Sjögren's syndrome is common in patients with rheumatoid arthritis, especially middle-aged women. Complaints of burning, irritation, or excessive secretions suggest a dry eye but are notoriously nonspecific.

Diagnosis depends upon demonstration of tear hyposecretion (usually by decreased wetting of a strip of litmus or filter paper placed between the lower lid and the eye in the inferior cul-de-sac) accompanied by corneal and conjunctival epithelial damage. Once epithelial cells start to slough, the corneal surface will take up fluorescein instilled into the conjunctival sac. Devitalized cells that have not yet been sloughed stain with rose bengal, making this dye an even more sensitive test for keratitis sicca.

Treatment consists of tear replacement and reduction of tear turnover. Various preparations of artificial tears are available. Other therapeutic maneuvers include occlusion of the lacrimal puncta to reduce tear outflow and placement of contact lenses, moisture chambers, or goggles over the eyes to decrease evaporation. Such measures are reserved for severe keratitis.

Baum J: Clinical manifestations of dry eye states. Trans Ophthalmol Soc UK 104:415, 1985. *Outlines the clinical and laboratory signs and associations. Other papers in the same issue are relevant.*

Benson WE: Posterior scleritis. Surv Ophthalmol 32:1, 1988. *Discusses the clinical manifestations of both posterior and other forms of scleritis.*

519 Ocular Vascular Disease

SYSTEMIC HYPERTENSION AND ARTERIOSCLEROSIS

Although the retinal vascular abnormalities in hypertension are nonspecific and variable, they can be important diagnostically and therapeutically. The effects of blood pressure on the retinal vessels depend upon both its absolute level and duration. Although essential hypertension is a disease of arterioles, the retinal vascular bed lacks sympathetic innervation, and the fundus changes must be considered secondary.

Arteriolar narrowing is the commonest hypertensive change and the most difficult to differentiate as abnormal. The normal ratio of the diameters of the arteriolar and venous blood columns is 2:3 or 3:4. A decrease in this ratio can best be appreciated in the smaller branches away from the disc.

Other findings include microaneurysms, hemorrhages, lipid deposits, and edema. Retinal and disc edema usually follows a rapid increase in systemic blood pressure. Disc edema defines the entity *malignant hypertension*. By contrast, opacification (or sclerosis) of the vessel walls—described ophthalmoscopically as copper or silver wiring—accompanies longstanding hypertension.

Thickening of the arteriolar wall explains arteriovenous nicking and venous dilation distal to the crossing. Cotton-wool spots are signs of local ischemia; hemorrhages and hard exudates reflect vascular leakage. Microaneurysms indicate irreversible structural alterations in the capillary beds. Retinal vascular occlusions (see below) and ischemic optic neuropathy are potential consequences of hypertensive vascular changes.

The only pure arteriosclerotic funduscopic change is atheroma of the retinal arterioles. These are seen as yellow-white plaques in the central retinal artery or its first branches, where the arteries still have an internal elastic lamina. The plaques must be differentiated from calcific or lipid emboli, which are usually smaller or more peripheral. Hypertension accelerates atherosclerosis, but atherosclerosis does not require hypertension.

DIABETIC RETINOPATHY (see Color Plate 14E and F)

Diabetic retinopathy, the most common of the vascular retinopathies, shares many features with hypertensive retinopathy. The pathophysiologic defect in diabetic retinopathy appears to lie at the level of the retinal capillaries. Progressive degeneration of the capillary walls results in leakage (hemorrhages and exudates), diffuse and focal expansion (microaneurysms), and closure of small vessels. The ischemic retina in the focal areas of nonperfusion elaborates factors stimulating new vessel and fibrous ingrowth. (A similar retinopathy can follow radiotherapy given as part of the treatment for head and neck cancers, which damages the capillary wall cells.)

Diabetic retinopathy is classified as *background* or *proliferative*. Background retinopathy is further subdivided into *simple background*—with microaneurysms, dot/blot hemorrhages, and hard exudates—and a *preproliferative* form. In preproliferative background retinopathy there is beading of veins, cotton-wool spots, and many hemorrhages. Also characteristic is intraretinal new vessel pathology, so-called *intraretinal microvascular anomalies*.

In proliferative retinopathy, neovascularization appears on the disc and elsewhere, especially along the major vascular arcades. There may be fibrovascular proliferation and vitreous hemorrhages. Proliferative diabetic retinopathy confers a poor visual prognosis.

Background retinopathy alone reduces visual acuity when there is edema or exudation in the macula. More new cases of blindness result from background retinopathy with macular edema than from proliferative retinopathy, because the former is much more prevalent. Background retinopathy with macular edema is common in type 2 diabetics over age 50.

TREATMENT. Good diabetic control appears to retard the progression of retinopathy. Ablation of ischemic retina by panretinal photocoagulation helps preserve central vision in patients with early proliferative retinopathy, making this the current treatment of choice. Advanced proliferative retinopathy may require major intraocular surgery—*vitrectomy*. In such cases the visual prognosis is guarded but an estimated 50 to 75 per cent of operated patients experience some visual improvement.

OTHER VASCULAR RETINOPATHIES (See Color Plate 14)

SYSTEMIC LUPUS ERYTHEMATOSUS. The retinopathy is common but nonspecific; the most frequent findings are retinal hemorrhages and cotton-wool spots. Cotton-wool spots are not exudations but, rather, localized areas of axoplasmic stasis caused by ischemia, which may indicate active vasculitis. Patients with lupus often also have hypertensive retinopathy. Central nervous system involvement may be associated with optic and chiasmal neuropathy, papilledema, ocular motor cranial nerve palsies, hemianopias, and a migraine-like syndrome.

HEMATOLOGIC DISEASE. Anemia and thrombocytopenia predispose to retinal and subconjunctival hemorrhages. When these are the result of leukemia, the hemorrhages often have a white center—the classic but nonspecific *Roth spot*. Roth spots also are encountered in subacute bacterial endocarditis (see Color Plate 14*B*) and other conditions.

Leukemia can cause hyperviscosity retinopathy, characterized by venous tortuosity and dilation, retinal hemorrhages, and vascular occlusions. A chronically elevated leukocyte count also predisposes to capillary drop out and microaneurysm formation, but proliferative retinopathy is rare. Other causes of hyperviscosity retinopathy are Waldenström's macroglobulinemia, multiple myeloma, polycythemia, and sickle cell anemia. In extreme cases sludging of blood in the veins is visible ophthalmoscopically.

PERIPHERAL RETINAL NEOVASCULARIZATION. Diabetic retinopathy affects largely the posterior pole of the eye. The retinopathy of prematurity (retrolental fibroplasia) and sickle cell disease have their major impact on the peripheral retina.

The ocular and systemic manifestations of sickling hemoglobinopathies correlate poorly. In patients with sickle cell anemia, proliferative retinopathy is rare. Peripheral neovascularization is more common in sickle cell hemoglobin C disease (SC) and sickle cell thalassemia (S-thal). Patients with sickle cell trait usually have no ocular symptoms, although hypoxia encountered at high altitudes may precipiatate hemorrhages and vascular occlusions.

The ocular findings in sickle hemoglobinopathies include small, dark red, comma-shaped conjunctival vascular segments, best seen on the inferior bulbar conjunctiva after instillation of a topical vasoconstrictor. Ischemic infarction of iris segments is also observed. In addition to the "sea fan" peripheral neovascularization, other characteristic retinal findings include hemorrhages that have a salmon pink coloration from hemoglobin breakdown products and black chorioretinal scars with irregular borders in the equatorial periphery.

About one fifth of proliferative sickle retinopathy regresses spontaneously. The rest, if untreated, progress to retinal detachment and vitreous hemorrhage. Treatment consists of photocoagulation or trans-scleral cryotherapy or diathermy.

RETINAL VASCULAR OCCLUSIONS

CENTRAL RETINAL ARTERY OCCLUSION (CRAO) (see Color Plate 14*C*). The central retinal artery is a branch of the ophthalmic artery, in turn a branch of the internal carotid artery. Occlusion of the central retinal artery causes sudden, usually nearly complete, visual loss in one eye. Ophthalmoscopy reveals arteriolar narrowing and vascular stasis (most obvious as segmentation of the venous blood column—"boxcar" pattern).

Within hours the infarcted superficial layers of the retina lose their normal transparency to assume a milky white translucency. Because the thin retina over the fovea receives its oxygen from the underlying choroid, this region retains its normal reddish pink color. This contrasts with surrounding tissue, producing an appearance described as a cherry red macula. (A similar appearance is encountered in certain lipid storage diseases, in which abnormal metabolic products partially opacify the ganglion cell layer.)

Eventually arterial flow is restored, the edema resolves, and the fundus appearance returns to near normal. The disc, which is initially normal because it derives its blood supply from the surrounding choroid, gradually becomes pale and atrophic. After several weeks it is difficult to distinguish a central retinal artery occlusion from other causes of primary optic atrophy.

Acute central retinal artery occulsion is an emergency. Rarely, prompt action may dislodge an embolus and restore circulation in time to prevent retinal death and thus preserve vision. For a nonophthalmologist this action consists of firm, intermittent pressure on the globe with the heel of the hand to alternately raise and lower intraocular pressure. Ophthalmologists use other measures: retrobulbar injection of anesthetic and anterior chamber paracentesis to lower the pressure in the ocular vascular bed. Seldom does treatment save vision.

In some persons, portions of the retina are supplied by vessels arising from the choroidal circulation, and such areas may be spared if the central retinal artery alone is occluded. Most eyes with CRAO are deprived of useful vision.

CRAO's are the result of emboli (atheromatous, myxomatous, and material from diseased or artificial heart valves), of local small vessel disease, or of carotid occlusion. A CRAO is sometimes the initial sign of giant cell arteritis or polyarteritis nodosa. CRAO has been reported in patients with sickle cell trait after trauma or other stress.

BRANCH RETINAL ARTERY OCCLUSION (BRAO) (see Color Plate 14*D*). Branch arterial occlusions present as sudden loss of vision in a sector of the field affected. Ophthalmoscopically one observes a wedge-shaped area of infarcted retina spreading outward from an arteriolar bifurcation. Branch retinal artery occlusions are almost always embolic in origin. By far the most common source of emboli in older adults is the ipsilateral carotid artery. In children and young adults, migraine, coagulation abnormalities, increased intraocular pressure, and oral contraceptives may predispose to vascular occlusions.

CENTRAL RETINAL VEIN OCCLUSION (CRVO) (see Color Plate 14*H*). The dramatic ophthalmoscopic findings of dilated, tortuous veins, extensive retinal hemorrhages, and disc swelling in one eye have classically been called a central retinal vein occlusion. Actually there is evidence that such *hemorrhagic retinopathy* is the consequence of both arterial ischemia and venous disease.

A CRVO presents as sudden unilateral visual loss in older adults, but unlike a CRAO, a CRVO is not an emergency, as there is no accepted immediate therapy. There are also no specific accompanying diseases, although hypertension and diabetes are loosely associated, and hypercoagulable states must be considered.

Visual prognosis varies. In the fully developed form usually encountered in older persons, vision is poor and generally remains so. Panretinal photocoagulation may decrease the risk of subsequent neovascular glaucoma. A less severe ophthalmoscopic picture is encountered in younger patients. Acuity in such *partial central retinal vein occlusion* or *venous stasis retinopathy* is only slightly reduced, and the visual prognosis is good. Ischemic oculopathy after carotid occlusion produces a similar retinopathy; retinal arterial pressures measured by ophthalmodynamometry or oculopneumoplethysmography are low in such cases.

BRANCH RETINAL VEIN OCCLUSIONS. Patients with branch vein occlusions complain of blurred vision. In the fundus, hemorrhages and cotton-wool spots spread out in a wedge from an arteriovenous crossing. As in CRVO, there are few specific systemic associations. Neovascular glaucoma is rare, but vision may be persistently reduced by macular edema. Branch retinal vein occlusion must be distinguished from viral retinitis (see Ch. 515).

Catalano RA, Tanenbaum HL, Majerovics A, et al.: White centered retinal hemorrhages in diabetic retinopathy. Ophthalmology 94:388–392, 1987. *This paper considers the differential diagnosis of Roth spots and reports their common appearance in diabetic retinopathy.*

Hall S, Buettner H, Luthra HS: Occlusive retinal vascular disease in systemic lupus erythematosus. J Rheumatol 11:846, 1984. *Two cases with large retinal vessel occlusion.*

Kearns TP: Differential diagnosis of central retinal vein obstruction. Ophthalmology 90:475, 1983. *This paper is one of four in the same issue that describes the work-up, differential diagnosis, and management of CRVO.*

Little HL, Jack RL, Patz A, et al.: Diabetic Retinopathy. New York, Thieme-Stratton Inc., 1983. *A collection of 31 position papers on various aspects of diabetic retinopathy.*

McCrary JA III: Venous stasis retinopathy of stenotic or occlusive carotid origin. J Clin Neuro Ophthalmol 9:195, 1989. *Reviews the findings and differential diagnosis.*

520 The Eye and Medications

DRUGS WITH OCULAR SIDE EFFECTS

ANTICHOLINERGICS. A variety of systemic drugs have ocular side effects. Any medication with anticholinergic properties can dilate the pupil and diminish accommodation (the ability to focus at close range). The possibility of angle-closure is the basis for the caution that such medications are contraindicated in glaucoma. Patients on therapy for open-angle glaucoma are at little risk, as mydriasis will not usually affect intraocular pressure. If the patient has known angle-closure, previous iris surgery all but eliminates the danger of dilation. Only when there is a potential for angle-closure are such drugs contraindicated, and this is usually unrecognized. Of the systemic anticholinergic drugs, only transdermal scopolamine can dilate and fix pupils and paralyze accommodation, even in young persons.

CORTICOSTEROIDS. Prolonged administration of systemic dosages of corticosteroids often leads to the formation of posterior subcapsular cataracts. Topical corticosteroids increase intraocular pressure in genetically predisposed persons. Topical steroids also activate herpes simplex keratitis and should be administered only under the supervision of an ophthalmologist.

QUININE AND CHLOROQUINE. Quinine may cause acute blindness, with narrowing of the retinal arterioles. An overdose increases the probability of toxic effects, but rare persons are sensitive even to therapeutic doses. Other symptoms of quinine toxicity include dizziness, tinnitus, and hearing loss. Central vision may improve, with persistent constriction of peripheral field and evolution of optic atrophy.

The synthetic antimalarials chloroquine and hydroxychloroquine have a specific retinal toxicity. This usually appears only after prolonged administration in doses exceeding 250 mg per day for chloroquine and 400 mg per day for hydroxychloroquine. Reduced visual acuity is the usual initial symptom, the parafoveal retina being most affected. Chloroquine binds to pigmented tissues, exerting a toxic effect on the retinal epithelium with loss of pigmentation in a target-like or bull's-eye pattern around the fovea. Discontinuation of the drug may result in improvement, but if the process is moderately advanced, visual loss may be progressive.

Chloroquine, hydroxychloroquine, and a variety of other drugs including the antiarrhythmic amiodarone cause whorl-like corneal epithelial deposits that are usually asymptomatic. Such deposits disappear after discontinuation of the drug.

THIORIDAZINE. Phenothiazines are potentially toxic to retina and retinal pigment epithelium, producing a coarse pigmentary degeneration. Of those now in common use, only thioridazine has clinically significant toxicity, and then only with dosages exceeding 1 gram per day for prolonged periods.

ETHAMBUTOL. Various drugs have been implicated in optic neuropathies. Only with ethambutol is the incidence of such side effects high enough that monitoring is considered mandatory. The physician administering ethambutol should perform monthly checks of acuity and color vision, especially when dosages exceed 15 mg per kilogram.

AMIODARONE. Amiodarone represents a class of drugs having the property of cationic amphiphilia. Amiodarone binds to polar lipids and accumulates within lysosomes, producing whorl-like depositions of pigment in the corneal epithelium which resemble the keratopathy of Fabry's disease (see Ch. 173). Amiodarone keratopathy seldom causes symptoms, but instances of disc swelling and visual loss resembling ischemic optic neuropathy have been reported. The visual effects of amiodarone papillopathy must be balanced against the risk of cardiac arrhythmia in deciding whether to decrease the dosage.

OCULOCUTANEOUS DISORDERS

A variety of related disorders (including erythema multiforme, Stevens-Johnson syndrome, and toxic epidermal necrolysis, or Lyell's syndrome) arise as idiosyncratic responses to drugs or infections. Their ocular manifestations are a bullous conjunctival eruption followed by a cicatricial conjunctivitis. Adhesions may obliterate the conjunctival sacs and prevent the normal production and distribution of tears. A severe dry eye may be the most disabling sequela.

Early treatment with topical steroids (and perhaps antibiotics to prevent secondary infection) sometimes limits damage. Sweeping the conjunctival fornices several times a day with a sterile glass rod inhibits adhesions.

SYSTEMIC SIDE EFFECTS OF TOPICAL OCULAR MEDICATIONS (Table 520–1)

Medications in solution are easily absorbed from the nasal mucosa, and systemic side effects are more likely with drops than ointments. Dilation of the pupil with 10 per cent phenylephrine solution can precipitate hypertension; topical epinephrine may increase ventricular extrasystoles, and timolol maleate can cause bronchospasm in asthmatics.

Topical anticholinergics such as atropine, scopolamine, and cyclopentolate may contribute to confusional states in the elderly.

TABLE 520–1. SYSTEMIC SIDE EFFECTS OF TOPICAL OCULAR HYPOTENSIVES

β-Blockers (timolol, betaxolol, levobunolol)
  Bronchospasm
  Bradycardia/hypotension
  Light-headedness/depression/fatigue
  Neuromuscular blockade in myasthenia gravis
Miotics
  Pilocarpine
    Brow ache (usually transient)
    Cholinergic overdose
  Echothiophate
    Prolonged action of succinylcholine or procaine
Sympathomimetics (epinephrine, dipivefrin)
  Tachycardia
  Atrial and ventricular arrhythmias
  Hypertension
  Headache

Cyclopentolate is occasionally a cause of acute hallucinations and even psychosis in the young. Pilocarpine, used in large doses in the treatment of acute angle-closure glaucoma, has resulted in cholinergic overdose—nausea, vomiting, salivation, and gastrointestinal cramps. As these are also symptoms of the angle-closure attack itself, such toxicity may not be immediately recognized, leading to continued administration and cardiovascular collapse.

Echothiophate iodide, an organophosphate used in the treatment of some forms of childhood strabismus and of open-angle glaucoma, predisposes to cholinergic crisis, mimicking an acute surgical abdomen. Also, patients receiving echothiophate have impaired metabolism of succinylcholine. Use of succinylcholine during the induction of general anesthesia in a patient receiving echothiophate has caused death.

Drug information inserts for tranquilizers, bronchodilators, vasoconstrictors, and other medications that alter autonomic nervous system function often include a caution against their use in glaucoma. Such warnings generally refer to the potential for precipitating angle-closure glaucoma by pupillary dilation and do not apply to most patients being treated for glaucoma (see Ch. 512). The actual risk affects persons with narrow angles, who would be unlikely to carry the diagnosis of glaucoma, as a determination of the potential for angle-closure should have been made by the examining ophthalmologist.

CARBONIC ANHYDRASE INHIBITORS

Acetazolamide and methazolamide inhibit aqueous production and are used systemically to reduce intraocular pressure when topical medications are inadequate. Most patients experience paresthesias; their absence is thought by some to indicate noncompliance. Carbonic anhydrase inhibitors also induce a systemic acidosis, with a syndrome of malaise and anorexia, depression, and weight loss that responds to concurrent administration of sodium bicarbonate and may rarely cause blood dyscrasias. Acetazolamide increases the incidence of urolithiasis. The combination of a carbonic anhydrase inhibitor and a thiazide diuretic depletes body potassium. Carbonic anhydrase inhibitors should not be given to people with known allergy to sulfonamides.

Everitt DE, Avorn J: Systemic effects of medications used to treat glaucoma. Ann Intern Med 112:120, 1990. *This brief review addresses internists.*

Fraunfelder FT, Meyer SM: Drug-Induced Ocular Side Effects and Drug Interactions, 3rd ed. Philadelphia, Lea & Febiger, 1989. *A compendium based on the experience of the National Registry of Drug-Induced Side Effects and the literature.*

Grant WM: Toxicology of the Eye, 3rd ed. Springfield, IL, Charles C Thomas, 1986. *An enormous review with component parts that are coherent and readable.*

Imperia PS, Lazarus HM, Lass JH: Ocular complications of systemic cancer chemotherapy. Surv Ophthalmol 34:209, 1989. *Tables and text elucidate the article's title.*

PART XXV
SKIN DISEASES
Frank Parker

521 Introduction

An understanding of how the skin functions in health and disease is relevant to every physician for several reasons: First, the skin is the interface with our environment and serves many functions crucial to survival, such as protection against the elements and thermoregulation. Second, the psychological roles the skin and its appendages, the hair, and nails, play in our appearance cannot be overestimated. Third, skin problems are exceedingly common, as some 30 per cent of Americans have dermatologic conditions requiring a physician's care, and indeed patients expect their physician to have a working knowledge of cutaneous disorders. Ten common skin problems constitute 76 per cent of the burden of skin disease as established by population survey (Table 521–1). Fourth, the skin can be readily examined and biopsied and frequently provides evidence of internal disease. The trained examiner recognizes certain apparently insignificant skin findings as subtle signs of life-threatening disease.

Chapter 522 reviews the functions subserved by the skin and the local variations in skin structures which help to explain the localization of certain disease processes to specific areas. Chapter 523 discusses the examination of the skin and presents an approach to diagnosing skin diseases based upon clinical morphology. Nine major disease groupings are described, and the common dermatologic conditions and their etiologies are discussed (Ch. 525). Chapter 524 contains a guide to general principles of therapy. Chapter 525 describes skin diseases of general medical importance as well as specific therapy for each disease.

Arnold HL, Odom RB, James WP: Andrews' Diseases of the Skin. Philadelphia, W.B. Saunders Company, 1990. *An up-to-date text covering cogent aspects of clinical dermatology.*

Callen JP: Cutaneous Aspects of Internal Disease. Chicago, Year Book Medical Publisher, 1981. *Discussions of skin disorders that confront the clinician which have underlying systemic disorders. Discussion of the pathogenesis of these disorders is provided by a number of contributing authorities.*

Fitzpatrick TB, Eisen AZ, Wolff K, et al.: Dermatology in General Medicine. New York, McGraw-Hill Book Company, 1987. *A detailed and well-illustrated textbook covering all aspects of dermatology. Two volumes.*

Hurwitz SH: Clinical Pediatric Dermatology. Philadelphia, W. B. Saunders Company, 1981. *A well-written and well-illustrated book of dermatology of children and adolescents.*

Lookingbill DP, Marks JG: Principles of Dermatology. Philadelphia, W. B. Saunders Company, 1985. *A concise, well-illustrated textbook covering major topics in general dermatology.*

Rook A, Wilkinson DS, Ebling FJG, et al.: Textbook of Dermatology. Oxford, Blackwell Scientific Publication, 1986. *This three-volume multiauthored text covers every aspect of dermatology in great detail. It is well written and referenced.*

522 The Structure and Function of Skin

The skin serves a variety of functions crucial to survival and health. In general, the functions may be correlated with specific properties of epidermal or dermal regions. The epidermis differentiates to form anucleate cornified cells that act as a relatively impermeable protective barrier to the outward loss of body fluids and the inward penetration of various substances and microorganisms. These lamellae of cornified surface cells together with the brown pigment melanin also play an important role in protecting against the carcinogenic effects of ultraviolet radiation. Two components of the dermis, the unique circulatory system and the specialized cutaneous appendages, the sweat glands, play a vital role in the body's thermoregulation. Finally, the skin is important immunologically. Both the epidermis (Langerhans' cells) and dermis (epidermodermal junction structures) are sites at which a number of immunologic reactions occur that can give rise to unique inflammatory skin diseases.

ANATOMIC CONSIDERATIONS

The skin is composed of two mutually dependent layers: the outer *epidermis* and inner *dermis*, both cushioned on the fat-containing subcutaneous tissue, the *panniculus adiposus* (Figs. 522–1 and 522–2).

EPIDERMIS. The stratified cellular epidermis contains two main zones of cells (keratinocytes), an inner region of viable cells, the *stratum germinativum*, and an outer layer of anucleate cells known as the *stratum corneum*, or horny layer. Three strata of cells are recognized in the germinativum: the *basal, spinous,* and *granular* layers, each representing progressive stages of differentiation and keratinization of the epidermal cells as they evolve into the dead, tightly packed stratum corneum cells on the skin surface.

The epidermis is derived from the mitotic division of the basal cells resting on the basement membrane (*basal lamina*), with the daughter cells moving outward to the surface, where they become polyhedral as they synthesize increasing quantities of intracellular insoluble protein, keratin. These *stratum spinosum cells* attach to one another mechanically by desmosomes, complex modifications of the cellular membranes that impart a spinous or quill-like appearance to the cells. Desmosomes play a crucial role in maintaining the adherence of the epidermal cells to one another.

TABLE 521–1. PREVALENCE OF COMMON DERMATOLOGIC DISEASE IN THE UNITED STATES*

	Rate per 1000	Numbers (in 1000's)
Fungus infections	81.1	15,733
Tinea pedis	38.7	7509
Tinea unguium	21.8	4232
Tinea versicolor	8.4	1623
Tinea cruris	6.7	1301
Acne vulgaris	68.1	13,217
Cystic acne	1.9	375
Acne scars	1.7	321
Seborrheic dermatitis	28.2	5476
Verruca vulgaris	8.5	1684
Folliculitis	8.0	1553
Atopic dermatitis	6.9	1332
Lichen simplex chronicus	4.5	882
Hand eczema	1.6	311
Dyshidrotic eczema	2.1	405
Psoriasis	5.5	1070
Vitiligo	4.9	957
Herpes simplex	4.2	824

*Persons 1 to 74 years of age—noninstitutionalized.
Reprinted from the chapter by Dr. Marie-Louise Johnson in the 17th edition of the Cecil Textbook of Medicine, with her permission.

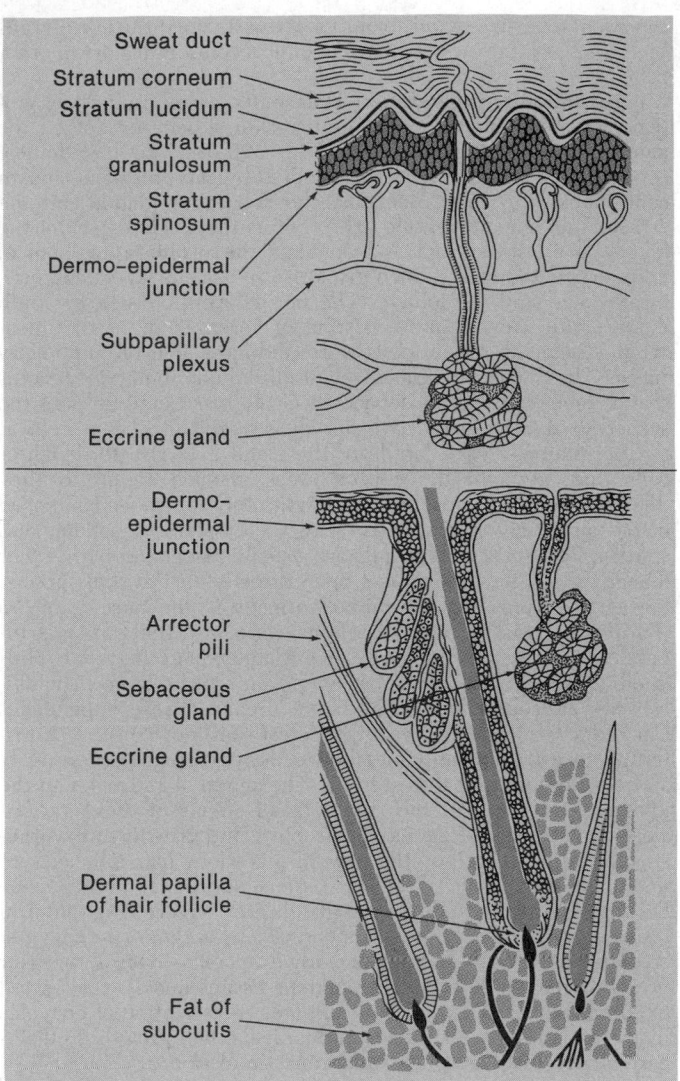

FIGURE 522–1. Structure of the skin. (Adapted from the 17th edition of the Cecil Textbook of Medicine with the permission of Dr. Marie-Louise Johnson.)

With further outward displacement the differentiating cells of the spinous layer become flattened, and refractile keratohyalin granules appear in the cytoplasm, accounting for the designation of *granular layer* that rests just below the stratum corneum.

The transformation from viable granular cells to anucleate, nonviable cornified cells is abrupt. The cornified layer consists of up to 25 layers of tightly packed, highly flattened horny cells.

The differentiation of the epidermal cells involves the formation of fibrous proteins known as *keratin*. The process of maturation of the epidermis (cornification) is complete in the stratum corneum, yielding cells with mature keratin, namely, a system of filaments embedded in a continuous matrix (which is probably derived from the keratohyalin granules) within a thickened cell membrane. The stratum corneum limits the rate of passage of ions and molecules into and out of the skin.

The basal layer of epidermis has a permanent population of germinal cells whose progeny undergo the specific pattern of differentiation just described. The new keratinocytes require about 14 days to evolve into stratum granulosum cells and another 14 days to reach the surface of the stratum corneum and be shed. Proper control of proliferation of basal cells and their subsequent orderly differentiation into keratinized stratum corneum cells produces the smooth, pliable surface of the skin. Alterations in the homeostatic state of cell division, defects in differentiation, or changes in exfoliation from the surface can lead to irregularities in the skin surface, characterized as roughening, scaling, and hyperkeratosis (accumulation of excessive layers of stratum corneum).

Two other cell types are found in the epidermis, the *melanocyte*

and the *Langerhans' cell*. Both are dendritic cells with cytoplasmic arms that stretch out to contact the keratinocytes in their vicinity. The melanocytes are pigment (melanin)-producing cells that are arrayed in the basal epidermal layer and hair follicles, whereas the Langerhans' cells are usually found in the suprabasal layers of the epidermis, and at times in the dermis. Each dendritic cell has a different origin and function.

Melanocytes evolve in the neural crest of the embryo and migrate to the skin in early embryonic life. These cells synthesize brown, red, and yellow melanin pigments that give us our distinctive skin coloration. Melanocytes contain distinctive submicroscopic organelles (melanosomes) within which melanin is synthesized. A specific enzyme, tyrosinase, found within the melanosome, oxidizes tyrosine to dihydroxyphenylalanine (DOPA) and then to DOPA quinone. Additional nonenzymatic oxidation and polymerization occur to form the final product, melanin. Two kinds of melanin are recognized: eumelanin (brown-black biochrome) and phaeomelanin (yellow-red biochrome that contains large quantities of cysteine). The genetic make-up of the individual determines which melanin is produced, thus providing the various colors and hues of our skin and hair. Once the melanosomes are fully melanized, the resulting melanin granules are transported out the dendritic processes of the melanocyte and transferred into the adjacent epidermal cells (or into hair in the case of hair follicles).

Langerhans' cells, derived from bone marrow, contain a unique submicroscopic racket-shaped organelle (Birbeck granule) and are now recognized as playing a major immunologic role in the skin (Fig. 522–2). They contain surface receptors for immunoglobulins,

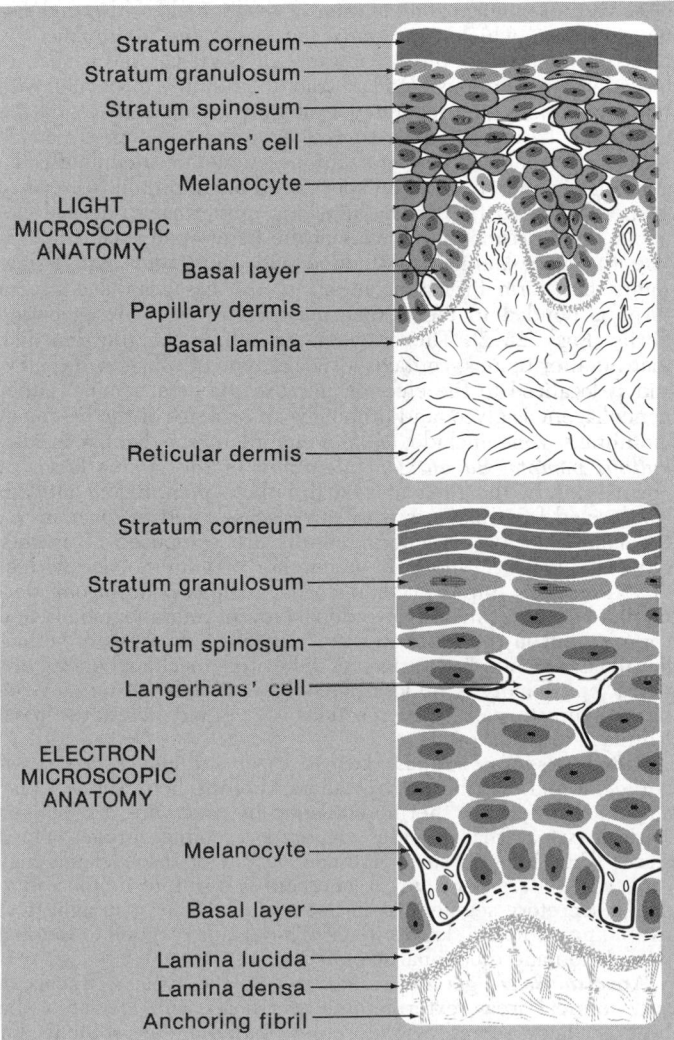

FIGURE 522–2. Diagrammatic representation of the light microscopic and electron microscopic anatomy of the skin.

complement, and Ia-antigens and are able to capture external antigenic materials that contact the skin and to circulate to draining lymph nodes and there induce specific sensitization of immunocompetent T cells. Langerhans' cells thus play a central role in delayed hypersensitivity reactions of the skin (allergic contact dermatitis).

DERMIS. Beneath the epidermis is the principal mass of the skin, the dermis, which is a tough, resilient tissue with viscoelastic properties. It consists of a three-dimensional matrix of loose connective tissue composed of fibrous proteins (collagen and elastin) embedded in an amorphous ground substance (glycosaminoglycans). At the microscopic level the collagen fibers resemble an irregular meshwork oriented somewhat parallel to the epidermis. Coarse elastic fibers are entwined in the collagenous fibers, being particularly abundant over the face and neck. This fibrous and elastic matrix serves as a scaffolding within which networks of blood vessels, nerves, and lymphatics intertwine and the epidermal appendages, sweat glands, and pilosebaceous units rest.

Dermoepidermal Junction. The structures situated at the interface between the epidermis and dermis constitute an anatomic functional unit of complex membranes and lamellae laced by divergent types of filaments that together serve to support the epidermis, weld the epidermis to the dermis, and act as a filter to the transfer of materials and inflammatory or neoplastic cells across the junction zone. At the level of light microscopy, this boundary zone is seen as an undulating pattern of rete ridges (downward finger-like or ridge-like extensions of the epidermis) and dermal papillae (upward projections of the dermis into the epidermis) (Fig. 522–2). Periodic acid–Schiff (PAS) staining discloses a thin uniform zone of intense reaction along this undulating junction, which represents the basement membrane. By electron microscopy the membrane (or basal lamina) is seen to be a dense continuous fibrillar structure running in parallel with the undulations but separated from the dermal surfaces of the epidermal basal cells by a thin clear amorphous space (lamina lucida). Several substructural fibrous elements, including collagen, elastic microfibrils, and specialized anchoring fibrils, course perpendicular to the lamina attaching epidermal to dermal elements. The plasma membranes of the basal epidermal cells that face the basal lamina are studded with numerous hemidesmosomes that form firm attachments to the basal lamina; this, in turn, is bonded to the dermal connective tissue by anchoring fibrils (Fig. 522–2). The basement membrane in the skin, like that in other tissues, contains a special type of collagen (Type IV) and is localized to the electron microscopic basal lamina. Other noncollagenous glyco- and proteoglycan proteins of the basement membrane zone include *laminin* (found in the lamina lucida), *bullous pemphigoid antigen* (identified in the lamina lucida of normal skin by their reactivity with bullous pemphigoid antibodies derived from patients with this disease), and *fibronectins* (in the lamina lucida). Anchoring fibrils are composed of another type of collagen (Type VII). A number of immunologically mediated diseases (lupus erythematosus, bullous pemphigoid, dermatitis herpetiformis) involve deposition of immunoglobulin and complement in the junction zone, causing inflammatory vesiculobullous reactions; a variety of inherited mechanobullous diseases (epidermolysis bullosa) also cause serious blistering reactions owing to pathologic reactions above and below the basal lamina.

Cutaneous Appendages. Two to three million *eccrine sweat glands*, found distributed over all parts of the body surface, play an important part in thermoregulation by producing a hypotonic solution (sweat) that provides evaporative cooling in times of heat stress (Fig. 522–1). The combined output of these glands may exceed 1.5 liters per hour. Each gland is a simple tubule with a coiled secretory segment deep in the dermis and a straight duct extending up to the skin's surface. The glands respond to thermal stimulation and emotional stress.

Apocrine sweat glands are localized to the axillae, circumanal and perineal areas, external auditory canals, and areolae of the breasts. They secrete viscid, milky material that accounts for axillary odor when bacteria degrade the secretion. Apocrine secretion occurs with both adrenergic and cholinergic stimulation. The exact function of these sweat glands is unclear, but they may represent a vestige of our evolutionary past, since the odoriferous secretions function as cutaneous chemical communicators in other primates.

Pilosebaceous Appendages. Hair units, or pilosebaceous appendages, are found over the entire skin surface except on the palms, soles, and glans penis (Fig. 522–1). The hair follicle consists of the hair shaft surrounded by an epithelial sheath continuous with the epidermis, the sebaceous gland, and the arrector pili smooth muscle. The bulb is the thickest part of the follicle at its lower end and contains the proliferating pool of undifferentiated cells, which gives rise to various layers comprising the hair and the follicle. The proliferating cells in the bulb differentiate into a hair consisting of keratinized, hard, imbricated, flattened cortex cells surrounding a central medullary space. The sebaceous glands are multilobular holocrine glands that connect into the pilosebaceous canal (hair canal) through the sebaceous duct. Germinative undifferentiated sebaceous cells at the periphery of each lobule of the gland give rise to daughter cells that move to the central areas of each acinus as they differentiate and form sebum (a complex oily substance composed of tri- and diglycerides, fatty acids, wax esters, squalene, and sterols). The sebaceous glands are usually associated with a hair follicle, although some glands open directly on the skin surface. Sebaceous glands are also found normally in the buccal mucosa (Fordyce's spots), around the female areola (Montgomery's tubercles), on the prepuce (Tyson's glands), and in the eyelids (meibomian glands). The sebaceous glands and certain hair follicles are androgen-dependent target organs. These appendages can reduce testosterone to dihydrotestosterone, convert testosterone to estradiol, and metabolize dehydroepiandrosterone to androstenedione and testosterone. The action of androgen on the pilosebaceous units is the sum total of effects of these various weak and strong androgens. Sebaceous gland growth and synthesis of sebum, as well as the growth of various hair follicles, are under the control of androgens. Various androgens produced by the testes, ovaries, and adrenal glands are converted to dihydrotestosterone (DHT) in these appendages by action of an enzyme, 5α-reductase. DHT combines with a specific cytosol receptor protein found in androgen-dependent tissues and is transported to chromosomal DNA where it initiates transcription of enzymes that stimulate sebaceous gland and follicular hair growth. Follicles particularly responsive to androgen stimulation are found over the frontal and vertex areas of scalp, beard, chest, axillae, and upper and lower pubic triangles.

The rate at which hair grows and the size of the hair shaft are modulated in some hair follicles by androgens. Hair follicles are formed in early embryonic life, and no more develop after birth. Males and females have approximately the same number of hair follicles distributed over the body, but the degree of hairiness depends on two distinct features of hair growth—the *hair cycle* and the *hair pattern.* Hair growth consists of recurring cycles of growth (anagen phase), regression (catagen phase), and resting (telogen phase). Throughout telogen the resting hair lies high in the follicle, where it forms a stubby hair bulb that is easily shed. When anagen begins there is a burst of mitotic activity and the follicle grows downward to reconstitute a new hair bulb. The hair bulb cells divide rapidly and keratinize to form a new hair shaft that dislodges the old resting club telogen hair. With a hand lens a fallen or plucked hair can be identified by inspection as having been resting (telogen, root of the hair is a rounded fine bulb) or actively growing (anagen, elongated root with fine white sheath). Catagen is the brief respite when mitosis ceases and the hair follicle pulls upward in the dermis as the hair shaft evolves into a telogen club hair. In the adult scalp 85 per cent of the hairs are in anagen at any given time, 14 per cent in telogen, and 1 per cent in catagen. Considerable variation in timing of the cycle occurs from one region of the body to another, and the length of anagen determines the length of hairs. Thus, short hairs are found on the arms and eyebrows with relatively short anagen periods (few months), while long anagen periods are seen in the scalp (up to 6 years).

Hair cycles also vary with the second important feature of hair growth, namely, hair pattern or the type of hair growing in each follicle. Two types of hairs are seen: vellus hair (fine, soft, short, nonpigmented, and common on "nonhairy" areas of the body) and terminal hair (coarse, long, pigmented, and found on hairy areas of the body).

PLATE 13 EYE DISEASES

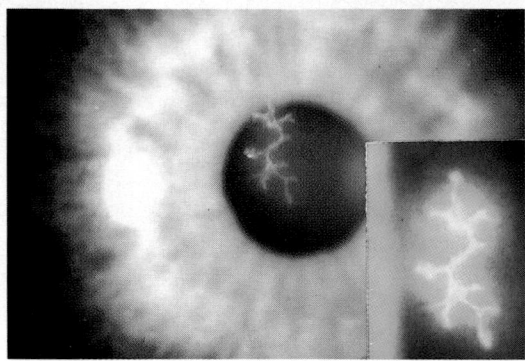

A, Herpes simplex corneal epithelial keratitis in diffuse light and *(inset)* in light passed through a cobalt blue filter after fluorescein staining.

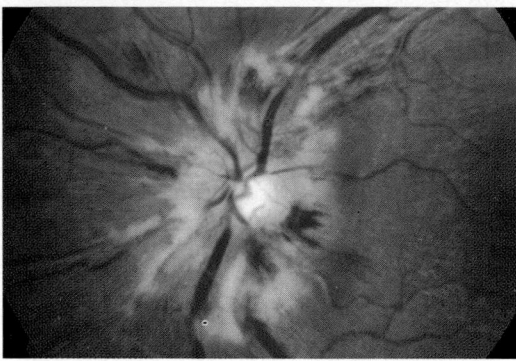

B, Papilledema in a young person. Note disc swelling, hemorrhages, and exudates, with preservation of the physiologic cup.

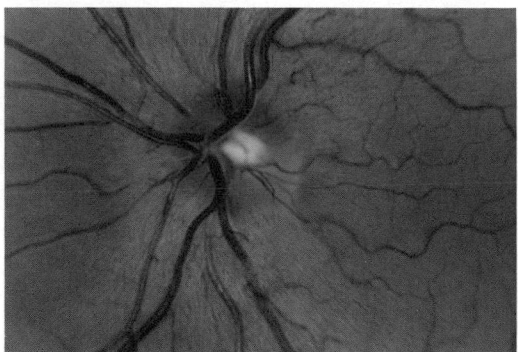

C, Disc in acute Leber's hereditary optic neuropathy. The disc tissue appears hyperemic, with peripapillary telangiectasia and opacification of the nerve fiber layer. Fluorescein angiography revealed no dye leakage.

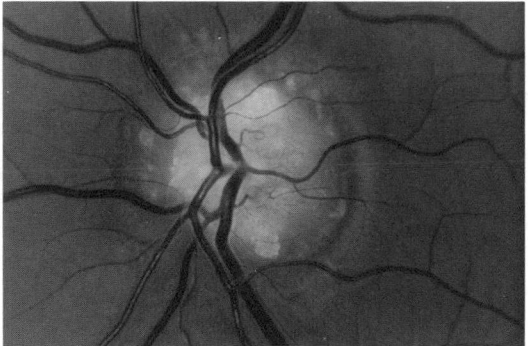

D, Optic disc drusen (also called hyaline bodies). Although obvious here, these calcified excrescences may be difficult to see in young persons, in whom the disc elevation they produce is mistaken for papilledema. (Also, they should be distinguished from retinal drusen—see *F* below.)

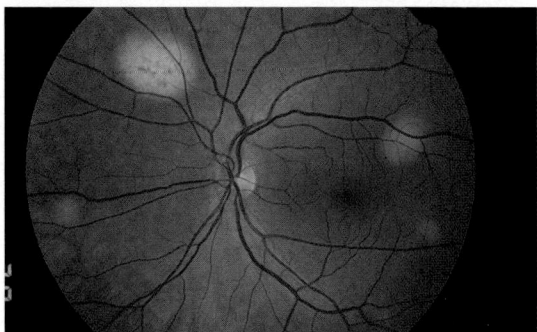

E, Multiple white choroidal metastases in a man with lung carcinoma.

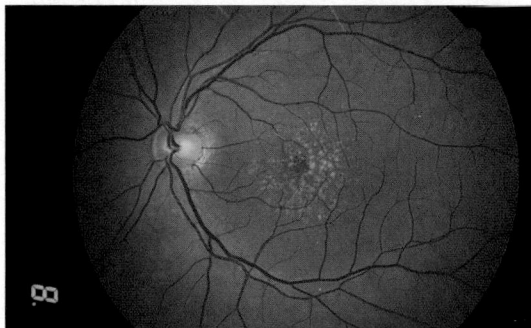

F, Retinal drusen. Multiple small white dots in the macula that represent abnormal accumulations in the retinal pigment epithelium basement (Bruch's) membrane. Such drusen are often precursors to visual loss from senile macular degeneration. (These should be distinguished from optic disc drusen—see *D* above.)

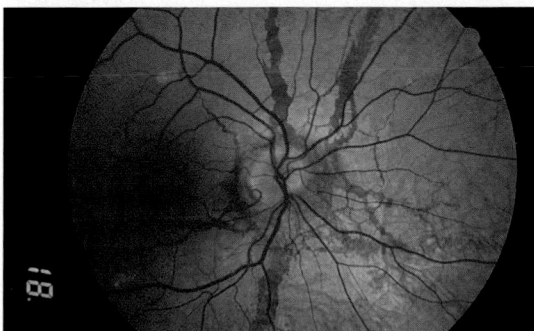

G, Angioid streaks in pseudoxanthoma elasticum. Breaks in the retinal pigment epithelium basement (Bruch's) membrane radial and circumferential to the disc indicate an underlying defect in elastic tissue formation.

Photographs taken by Mr. Harry Kachadoorian, C.R.A., University of Massachusetts Medical School, Worcester, Massachusetts.

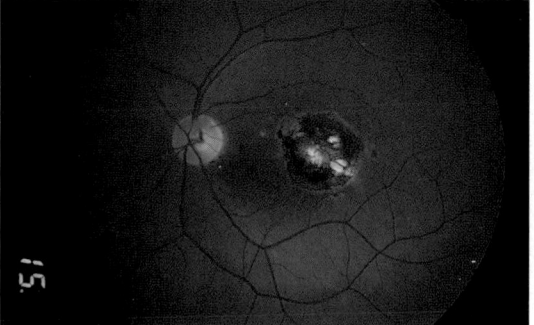

H, Macular chorioretinal scar. The appearance is typical of congenital toxoplasmosis, although other causes of chorioretinitis are included in the differential diagnosis.

PLATE 14 EYE DISEASES

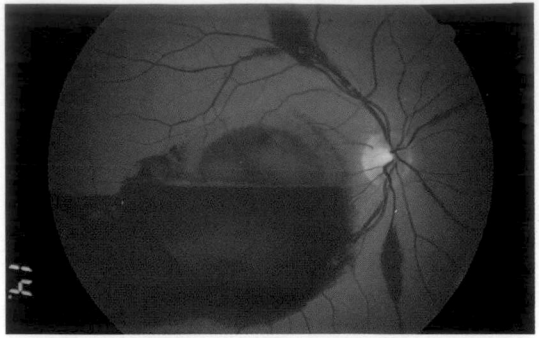

A, Preretinal (subhyaloid) hemorrhage. This occurred after a difficult intubation in an asthmatic woman with a previously normal eye examination. Similar findings are seen as a manifestation of diabetic retinopathy and in association with subarachnoid hemorrhage. The blood forms a meniscus with the patient in the upright position.

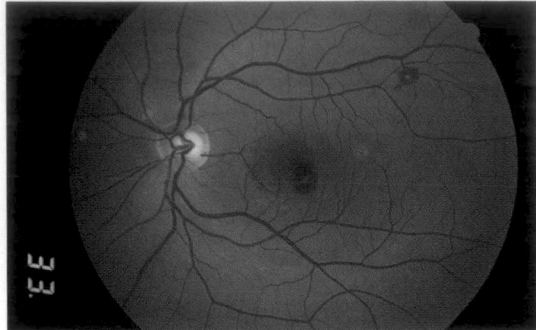

B, Roth spots. Multiple white centered hemorrhages in a man with recurrent subacute bacterial endocarditis. White centered hemorrhages are also seen with leukemia and diabetes. The small white scars are probably the residua of previous episodes.

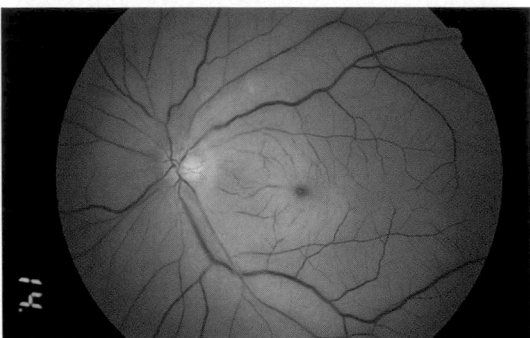

C, Central retinal artery occlusion. The retina is diffusely pale, lending a prominence to the normal coloration of the central fovea, often described as a cherry red spot.

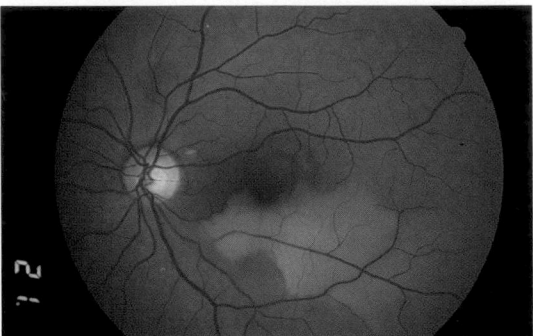

D, Inferior branch retinal artery occlusion. A pie-shaped sector of pale, infarcted retina extends from the embolic occlusion at the first branch of the arteriole of the inferior temporal arcade.

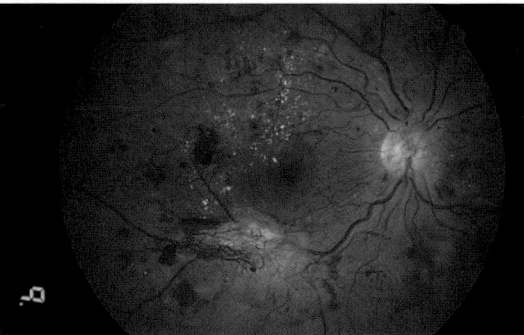

E, Proliferative diabetic retinopathy. Multiple hemorrhages, exudates, and new vessels are visible, with chorioretinal striae extending toward an area of fibrovascular proliferation along the inferior temporal arcade.

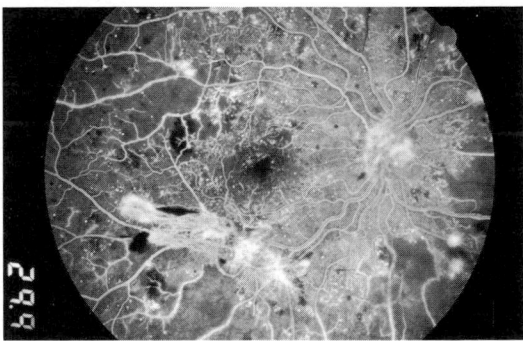

F, Fluorescein angiogram of the same fundus pictured in E. The new vessels, especially at the disc and the area of fibrovascular proliferation, are seen to leak fluorescein. Many of the "dot hemorrhages" are revealed as microaneurysms that fill with dye.

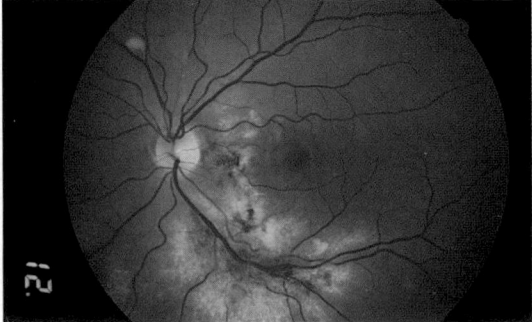

G, Cytomegalovirus retinitis in a patient with AIDS. There is a sector of retinal necrosis and hemorrhages along the inferior temporal arcade.

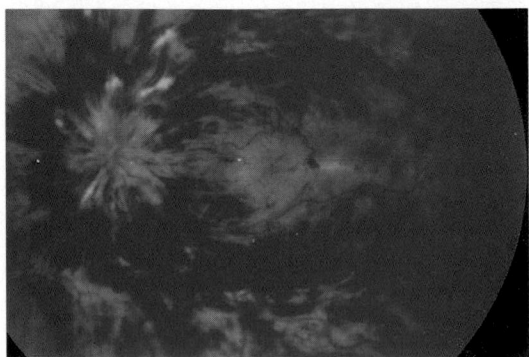

H, Central retinal vein occlusion. The disc is swollen with diffuse retinal hemorrhages and cotton-wool spots.

Photographs taken by Mr. Harry Kachadoorian, C.R.A., University of Massachusetts Medical School, Worcester, Massachusetts.

PLATE 15 SKIN DISEASES

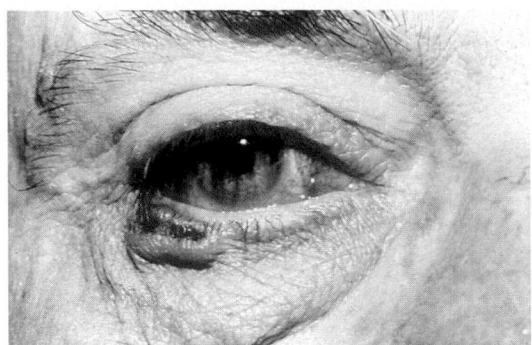

A, Basal cell cancer. Tumor with rolled, opalescent borders and central "rodent" ulcer.

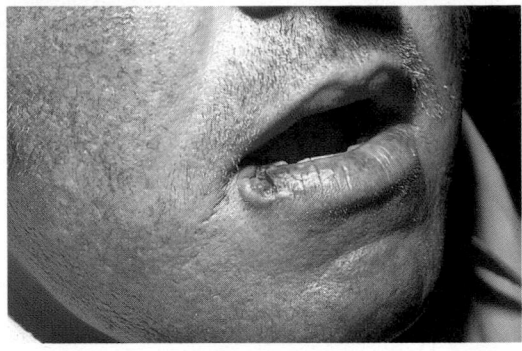

B, Squamous cell cancer. Firm nodule with eroded surface on the lower lip.

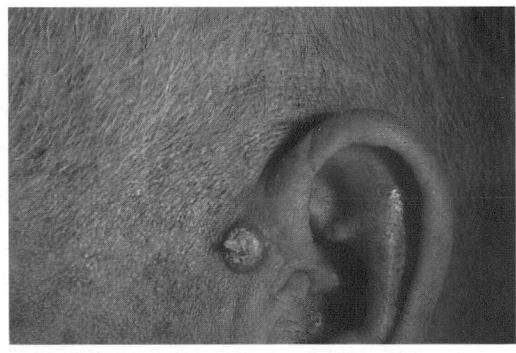

C, Cutaneous horn. Keratotic horn evolving from red nodule at base. These commonly are squamous cell cancers.

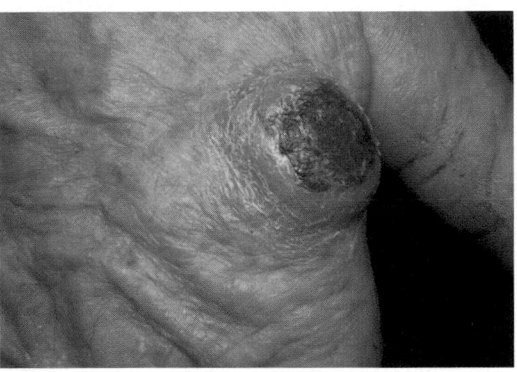

D, Keratoacanthoma. Large nodular lesion with central keratotic crater.

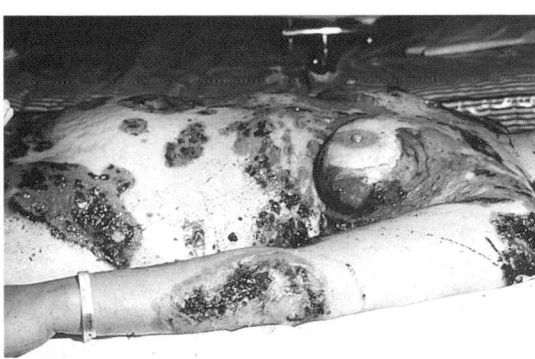

E, Pemphigus vulgaris. Intraepidermal bullae are easily ruptured, leaving superficial crusted erosions with thin shreds of blister roof along the edges. Careful examination reveals some intact blisters (primary lesions) below the breast.

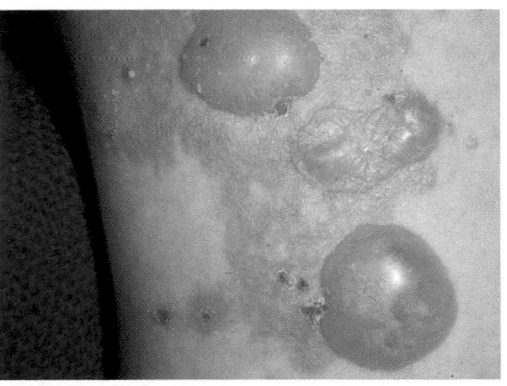

F, Bullous pemphigoid. Tense subepidermal bullae on an erythematous base.

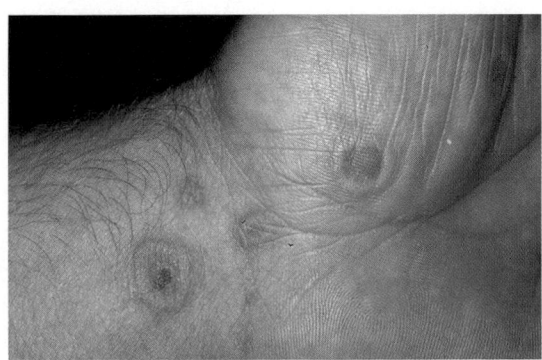

G, Erythema multiforme. Target or "bull's-eye" annular lesions with central vesicles and bullae.

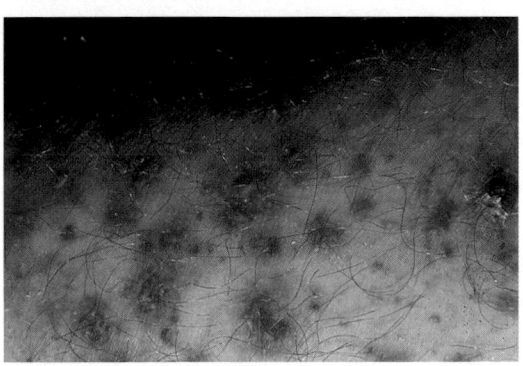

H, Palpable purpura. Leukocytoclastic vasculitis commonly causes raised purpuric and ulcerated lesions on legs.

PLATE 16 SKIN DISEASES

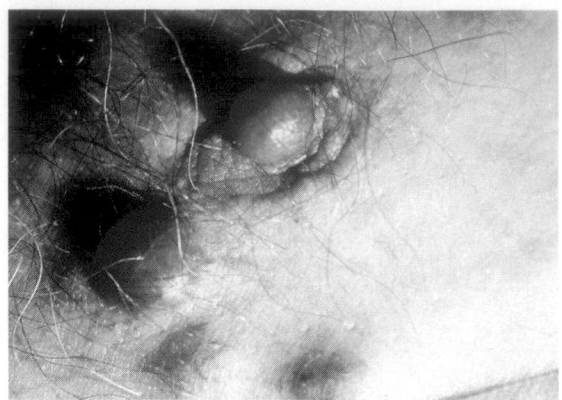

A, Skin metastases. Firm, hard, red nodules.

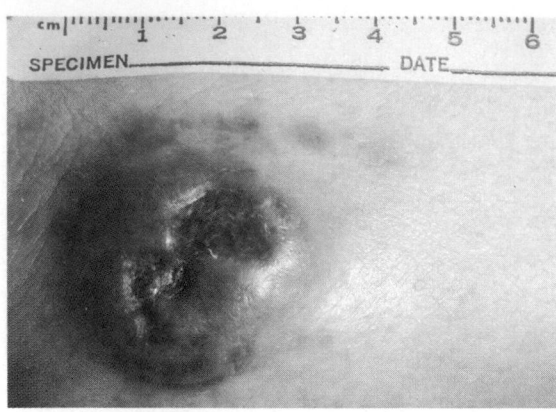

B, Mycosis fungoides, tumor stage.

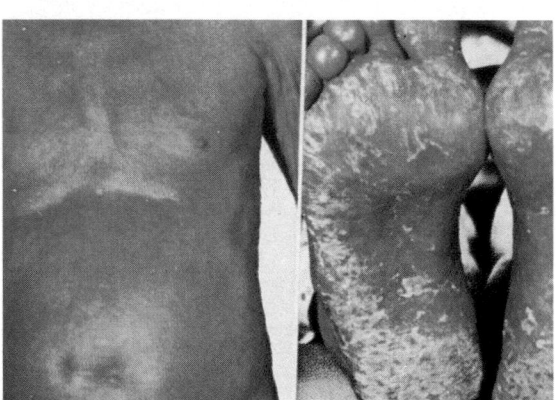

C, Sézary syndrome, exfoliative dermatitis stage.

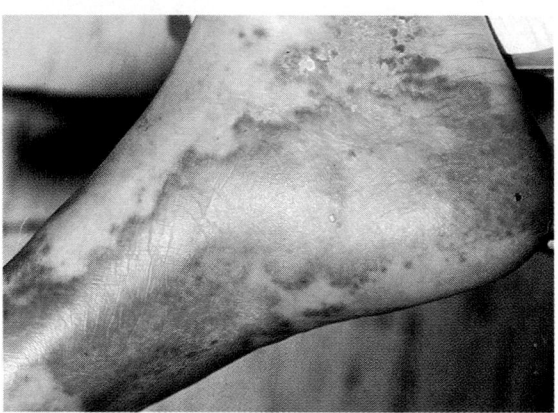

D, Classic Kaposi's sarcoma.

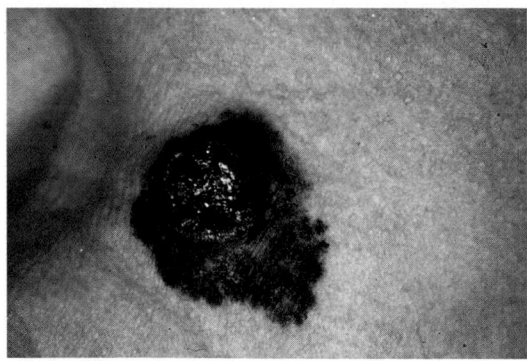

E, Malignant melanoma. Darkly pigmented, nodular lesion with irregular outline, irregular shades of dark pigmentation, and irregular surface configuration.

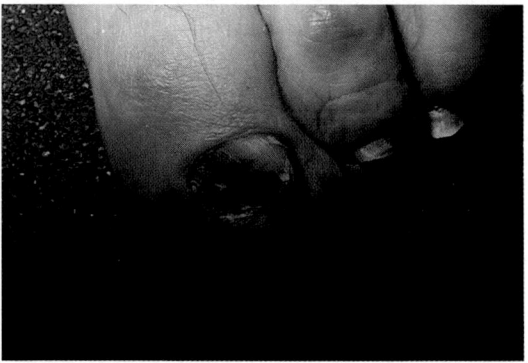

F, Subungual melanoma. Dark blue-black pigment within nail bed, with irregular dark pigment on the tip of the great toe.

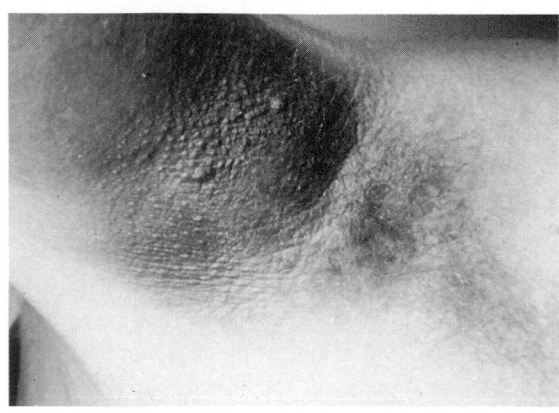

G, Acanthosis nigricans. Axillary lesion.

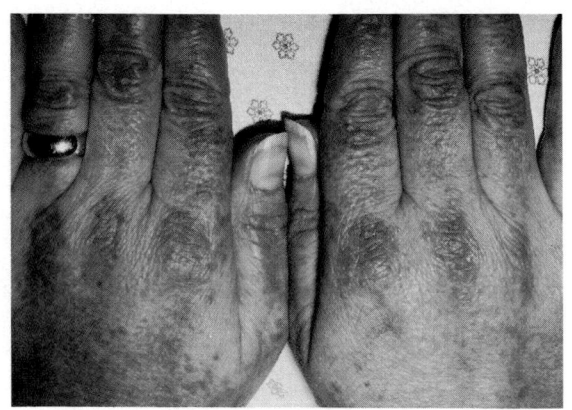

H, Dermatomyositis. Gottron's papules over the knuckles.

The dramatic changes in both hair cycle and hair pattern which occur at puberty are selectively mediated by either testosterone or dihydrotestosterone. The characteristic increase in hairiness at puberty is not the result of formation of new follicles. Rather, the increased hairiness results from the conversion of vellus hair follicles to large terminal follicles. In the axillae and lower pubic triangle this conversion is mediated by testosterone and androstenedione. In other regions such as the beard, chest, upper pubic triangle, nostrils, and external ears, this conversion is mediated by dihydrotestosterone. Paradoxically, DHT also mediates the reverse process, namely, the miniaturization of large terminal follicles into vellus hairs. Such physiologic miniaturization occurs with the reshaping of the frontal hairline from a straight line to an M-shaped configuration at puberty. This occurs in all men and in the majority of women.

Maternal androgens ensure full development and function of sebaceous glands at birth. The vernix caseosa covering the neonate is mostly sebum. Normally sebaceous glands atrophy after birth, until puberty, when androgens again stimulate their activity. Acne is often one of the earliest signs of puberty. Disorders of androgen excess in adult women (e.g., polycystic ovary syndrome) are also associated with increased sebaceous activity and acne. Estrogens in large amounts decrease gland size and secretion.

FUNCTIONS OF THE SKIN

PROTECTION. Several structures in the skin, including the stratum corneum, melanin, cutaneous nerves, and the dermal connective tissue, provide protective functions of importance to our survival. The skin protects against the loss of essential fluids, the entrance of toxic agents and microorganisms, and damage from ultraviolet radiation, mechanical shearing forces, and extreme environmental temperatures.

The *stratum corneum* serves as a low-permeability barrier that not only retards water loss from the inner epidermal hydrated layers, but also shields against damage from the environment. The barrier properties of the horny layer are of practical importance from several points of view: First, excessive drying or inflammatory reactions in the skin (e.g., eczema) lead to roughness and scaling as the normally compact layers of horny cells are disrupted. This leads to increased transepidermal water loss and, if extensive areas of the horny layer are disrupted (as in generalized exfoliative dermatitis, erythroderma, or burns), the total water loss can contribute to fluid and electrolyte imbalance. Second, with breaks in the horny layer, external substances more readily gain entrance to the underlying epidermis. Thus, various chemical substances, including medications placed on injured skin, have a greater opportunity for systemic absorption or a greater propensity to act as haptens or antigens, increasing the possibility of allergic contact dermatitis. This is a particularly common event when neosporin is used topically on chronically inflamed skin (such as in areas of stasis dermatitis or otitis externa), leading to superimposed allergic contact dermatitis. Third, the disruption of the barrier increases the chance of colonization of pathologic bacteria in the skin, especially in the presence of tissue fluid exudates, which serve as excellent culture media. Fourth, percutaneous absorption of various topical medications used in treating skin conditions, such as topical steroids, can be enhanced by hydrating the stratum corneum with the use of occlusive plastic wraps.

The stratum corneum not only serves as a barrier to the invasion of various bacteria, it also harbors a number of aerobic and anaerobic resident organisms (i.e., *Staphylococcus epidermidis*, diphtheroids, *Proprionibacterium acnes*, and *Pityrosporon*). Breaks in the stratum corneum, poor hygiene, and excessive humidity with maceration (especially in intertriginous areas) all contribute to cutaneous infections such as impetigo, erysipelas, folliculitis, furunculosis, and ecthyma.

A second structural component that provides protection is the *melanocyte*, which produces melanin pigment. Melanin is a large polymer that has the unique capability of absorbing light over the broad range of 200- to 2400-nm wave lengths. It serves as an excellent screen against the untoward effects of solar ultraviolet radiation, such as aging and wrinkling of the skin and the development of cutaneous neoplasms. The importance of melanin is dramatically illustrated by the high incidence of skin cancers

in sun-exposed areas of the body, particularly in light-skinned, blue-eyed, easily sunburned individuals and in albinos. Ultraviolet light exposure also causes aging and wrinkling of the skin. Neither sex nor race affects the number of melanocytes in the epidermis. Negroid skin contains the same number of melanocytes as Caucasian skin, but the pigmentation is more intense as a result of the synthesis of more melanin that is dispersed throughout the melanocytes and adjacent keratinocytes. Accordingly, black skin is much less likely to form skin cancers, and it ages more slowly than white skin.

A third structural component in the skin which plays a part in protection is the dermal *nerves*. Nerve endings are extensively distributed in the skin in two general morphologic types: free nerve endings and specialized endings (Pacini's and Meissner's corpuscles), which mediate many sensations including pain, pressure, and itch. Pain is important to our survival, since we pull away from the source of pain and avert further injury. Loss of sensation (e.g., diabetic neuropathy) may result in deep traumatic ulcers (trophic ulcers) without the patient's awareness of them. Damage to the dermatomal nerves (e.g., herpes zoster) may result in prolonged burning pain and hypesthesias (postherpetic neuralgia).

Itch is another important sensation mediated by cutaneous nerves. It is the most common symptom in dermatology and may occur in conjunction with a number of dermatologic diseases or without clinically evident skin disease (pruritus) (Tables 522–1 and 522–2). Itch and pain are carried on unmyelinated C fibers found in the upper portion of the dermis of the skin, mucous membranes, and cornea. The afferent C fibers enter the dorsal horn of the spinal cord, synapse, cross the midline, and ascend the spinothalamic tracts to the thalamus. Then the impulse proceeds to the sensory area of the postcentral gyrus of the cortex. Cutting the spinothalamic tract, as in an anterolateral hemichordotomy, abolishes pain and itch. A variety of peripheral mediators stimulate the C fibers and induce itching. These include histamine, trypsin, proteases, peptides (bradykinin, vasoactive intestinal peptide, substance P—all potent histamine releasers), and bile salts. Prostaglandins are modulators of pruritus rather than primary mediators, lowering the threshold to itching evoked by both histamine and pain. Central modulators of pruritus, such as systemic morphine, cause itch while relieving pain by acting on central opiate receptors.

Generalized itching in the absence of primary skin disease (pruritus) may be an important sign of internal disease (Table 522–2). Such diverse conditions as uremia, cholestatic biliary disease, lymphoma and myeloproliferative diseases, thyrotoxicosis, diabetes, carcinoma, iron deficiency anemia, and psychiatric disorders may cause severe pruritus. An important cause of pruritus is psychic stress. Some patients with psychogenic pruritus believe the itching is caused by invisible parasites in the skin. Such patients scratch until excoriations and prurigo papules (thickened papular areas of skin due to constant rubbing) evolve in areas that the patient can readily reach (extremities, scalp, upper back). Dry skin (xerosis) is a common cause of itching in older individuals. Certain drugs (aspirin, opiates) can cause itching without a visible rash. Patients with polycythemia vera display a unique type of pruritus, namely, itching triggered by sudden changes in temperature, especially as the patient emerges from a warm bath. The itch is prickly in nature and lasts minutes to hours.

The tough, viscoelastic properties imparted to the skin by the

TABLE 522–1. SKIN DISEASES ASSOCIATED WITH ITCHING

Xerosis (dry skin)
Insect infestations (scabies, pediculosis, insect bites)
Dermatitis (atopic, contact, nummular) including poison ivy contact
Drugs (opiates, aspirin, quinidine)
Lichen planus
Urticaria
Dermatitis herpetiformis (burning itch)
Sunburn
Fiber glass dermatitis

TABLE 522–2. PRURITUS ASSOCIATED WITH SYSTEMIC DISEASE

Systemic Disease	Postulated Etiology
Uremia	Secondary hyperparathyroidism, high skin calcium concentration, proliferation of mast cells, xerosis

Obstructive biliary disease
  Primary biliary cirrhosis
  Cholestatic hepatitis secondary to drugs (chlorpropamide)
  Intrahepatic cholestasis of pregnancy
  Extrahepatic biliary obstruction
	High concentrations of bile salts in skin

Hematologic and myeloproliferative disorders	Unknown
Lymphoma including Hodgkin's disease	
Mycosis fungoides	
Polycythemia vera	
Iron deficiency anemia	

Endocrine disorders
  Thyrotoxicosis
  Hypothyroidism
  Diabetes
	Unknown

Carcinoid	Serotonin
Visceral malignancies Breast, stomach, lung	Unknown

Psychiatric disorders
  Stress
  Delusions of parasitosis
	Unknown

Neurologic disorders
  Multiple sclerosis (paroxysmal itching)
  Notalgia paresthetica—local itch of back, medial shaft scapula (local neuropathy)
  Brain abscess
  CNS infarct
	Unknown

fibrous proteins (collagen and elastin) and amorphous ground substance that make up the dermis provide protection from shearing forces applied to the skin. The viscous and elastic properties of the ground substance allow it to resist compression and accept molding, thus serving to reduce point pressure on more sensitive skin structures.

THERMOREGULATION. Thermoregulation is subserved concomitantly by the cutaneous vasculature and the sweat glands. A massive network of interconnecting musculocutaneous arteries and venules, as well as capillaries, arteriovenous shunts, and small venules, plays a crucial role in the maintenance of body temperature (Fig. 522–1). The major fraction of the blood volume of the skin is contained in the large venous plexus, in which the blood moves with low velocity close to the surface, enabling maximal dissipation of heat. Equally important in thermoregulation is the formation of eccrine sweat, which provides cooling by evaporation from the skin's surface. For every gram of water that is evaporated from the skin, 580 calories of heat are lost.

Blood flow through the skin is 10 to 20 times that required to supply needed metabolites and oxygen. Under basal conditions 8.5 per cent, or 450 ml per minute of the total blood flow, passes through the skin, the control of flow being primarily by the sympathetic nervous system (via epinephrine and norepinephrine). Blood flow can increase up to 3.5 liters per minute with exercise in a warm environment. Because the heat conductivity and specific heat of blood are high, large amounts of heat can be dissipated through the skin. Both central (hypothalamic heating) and peripheral thermoreceptors stimulate sweating via the sympathetic nervous system, but in the case of sweat glands, acetylcholine is the postganglionic transmitter. Increase in body core temperature is the strongest stimulus for inducing sweating, whereas peripheral (cutaneous) thermoreceptors are only one tenth as effective in eliciting perspiration.

Response to cold begins when blood cooler than normal passes to the hypothalamus, which then elicits both heat conservation and heat production mechanisms. The sympathetics are excited, constricting cutaneous blood vessels and thereby reducing the transfer of heat to the body surface. Impulses from the hypothalamus also activate the motor center for shivering, which increases heat production by as much as 50 per cent. Conversely, when blood warmer than normal passes to the hypothalamus, the central heat production mechanism becomes inoperative, and cutaneous blood vessels dilate, allowing blood to accumulate near the skin surface and heat to be lost by conduction and convection. Vasodilatation also occurs reflexly through direct warming of the skin surface (in warm environments). In addition, stimulation of the hypothalamus produces sweating and increases evaporative heat loss. With periodic exposure to heat or to heat and work stresses (i.e., daily 1- or 2-hour exposures for 10 to 14 days), the secretory capacity of the eccrine sweat glands is enhanced (i.e., acclimatization).

One example of the crucial role of cutaneous vasculature in thermoregulation and in cardiovascular homeostasis is widespread inflammatory conditions of the skin causing *erythroderma*. In such diseases as generalized dermatitis, psoriasis, drug reactions, and underlying lymphomas, the inflammatory response in the skin can cause generalized cutaneous vasodilatation with diversion of 10 to 20 per cent of cardiac output through the skin. Central blood volume may be decreased. To maintain blood pressure, cardiac output must increase and in older individuals with impaired cardiac reserve high-output failure may occur in association with tremendous loss of body heat with wide swings in temperature and shivering.

THE SKIN AS AN ENDOCRINE ORGAN. Many metabolic activities of the skin are under hormonal regulation to the extent that the skin is recognized as an important hormone end organ. Indeed, not only do sebaceous glands and certain hair follicles respond readily to androgens, but they are capable of many diverse steroid transformations, as described above.

Dihydrotestosterone causes sebaceous glands to enlarge at puberty, the growth of certain hair (male sexual hair of the beard, chest, upper pubic triangle, nose, and ears), and the growth and development of the external genitalia. Antiandrogens, drugs that block the conversion of testosterone to DHT, do this by competitively inhibiting either 5α-reductase or the cytosol receptor protein for DHT. Drugs such as cimetidine and spironolactone have antiandrogenic activity and have been used to treat acne and hirsutism. In addition, thyroid hormones can regulate hair growth and alter the texture of the skin (fine, sparse hair and smooth, soft skin in hyperthyroidism; coarse hair and cool, rough, thick skin in hypothyroidism). Further, hormones affect melanin pigment formation, melanocyte-stimulating hormone, and estrogen-stimulating skin pigmentation.

THE SKIN AS AN IMMUNOLOGIC ORGAN. The epidermis and the dermoepidermal junctional area serve as active participants in immunologic reactions. The skin is composed of immunologically important cells including keratinocytes, Langerhans' cells, and melanocytes as well as immunologic structures such as the lamina lucida and basal lamina that are involved in a variety of bullous reactions of the skin.

Epidermal Immunologically Important Cells. Perhaps the most important immunologic cell in the epidermis is the Langerhans cell, comprising 2 to 5 per cent of the total epidermal cell population. Langerhans' cells play a role in a number of immunologic reactions, including macrophage–T cell interaction, T and B lymphocyte interactions, graft-versus-host (GVH) reactions, and skin graft rejection. The Langerhans cell synthesizes and expresses Ia antigens (Class II antigens, immune response gene–associated antigens) that are crucial in processing and presenting allergens to sensitized T lymphocytes critical in the elicitation of delayed hypersensitivity contact dermatitis. Lymphokines, made by the Langerhans cells during these immunologic reactions, augment and enhance these processes and also contribute to the accompanying inflammatory response.

Keratinocytes also play a role in immunologic responses by expressing Ia antigens on their surfaces in such conditions as GVH reaction, mycosis fungoides, allergic contact dermatitis, lichen planus, and tuberculoid leprosy. In these conditions the keratinocytes make lymphokines, particularly interleukin 1 (ETAF, epidermal cell thymocyte factor), which provides a second signal supplementing macrophages (Langerhans' cells) in mitogen- and antigen-induced T cell activation. In addition, epidermal cells make other cytokines such as prostaglandin E$_2$ and leukotrienes that participate in inflammatory reactions in the skin. Keratinocytes are the immunologic target in the pemphigus group of diseases where circulating autoantibodies against intercellular antigen of the epidermis and mucous membrane epithelium initiate intraepidermal acantholytic bullae.

The Dermoepidermal Junction as an Immunologic Structure. A variety of inflammatory diseases often characterized by bullous reactions seem to be mediated by immunoreactants, including IgG, IgA, and IgM, and complement deposition along the dermoepidermal junctional area. The anatomic site of blister formation correlates with the position of deposition of these immunoreactants. The antigens in several diseases have been isolated and partially characterized. The use of immunofluorescent techniques at the light microscopic and especially the ultrastructural level has been very helpful in more precisely diagnosing these bullous conditions. These are summarized in Table 522–3, along with immunofluorescent skin findings in connective tissue diseases.

INFLAMMATORY REACTIONS IN THE SKIN AND WOUND HEALING.

Cutaneous inflammation reflects the sum of the effects of biologic products of cells (mast cells, infiltrating neutrophils, monocytes/macrophages, lymphocytes) as well as the effects of the products of the complement system, membrane-derived arachidonic acid metabolic pathways (prostaglandins and leukotrienes) and the Hageman factor–dependent pathways of coagulation, fibrinolysis, and kinin generation. Early phases of wound healing also encompass many of these reactions.

Cutaneous Inflammation. A variety of pathophysiologic reactions initiate inflammation, including infectious, immunologic, and toxic processes that affect the epidermis or dermis, or both. Mast cells in the skin not only function as the sentinel cells in immediate-type hypersensitivity reactions but also as major effector cells in inflammatory reactions releasing (1) histamine, prostaglandin D$_2$, and leukotrienes, which cause vascular dilatation and increased permeability, redness, swelling, pain, and itch; (2) chemotactic factors for eosinophils and neutrophils; (3) proteases that interact with the complement, kinin, and fibrinolytic pathways; and (4) heparin, which may play a role in local angiogenesis. Degranulation of mast cells occurs in response to various antigens that cross-link IgE on the mast cell surface

(immediate hypersensitivity reactions), to by-products of complement activation C3a and C5a (as occurs in leukocytoclastic vasculitides), as well as to radiocontrast media, aspirin, insect venom, and various physical stimuli. Circulating peripheral blood cells infiltrate local tissue sites in response to chemotactic factors released by mast cells and other infiltrating cells. Basophils release histamine and chemotactic substances, such as those involved in allergic contact reactions, bullous pemphigoid, erythema multiforme, and inflammatory responses. Neutrophils release myeloperoxidase, acid hydrolases, and neutral proteases that are active against microbes and cause tissue destruction (dermatitis herpetiformis, psoriasis, leukocytoclastic vasculitis, and bacterial infections of the skin). Eosinophils release major basic protein and peroxidase (allergic drug reactions in the skin, bullous pemphigoid). Lymphocytes release lymphokines that modulate immunologic and inflammatory responses (lichen planus, lupus erythematosus, allergic contact dermatitis, tuberculoid leprosy). Monocytes and macrophages engulf foreign proteins and microorganisms (granulomatous reactions in the skin such as sarcoidosis, deep fungus and acid-fast bacilli infections, and cutaneous foreign body responses). In addition, both classic and alternate complement pathways release products that induce mast cell degranulation and induce inflammation. (The activation of the system seems to play a role in inflammatory reactions in hereditary complement deficiencies causing lupus erythematosus–like syndromes or pyodermas, as well as necrotizing vasculitis.)

Wound Healing in the Skin. Healing proceeds temporally in three phases: substrate, proliferative, and remodeling. The initial substrate phase, encompassing the first 3 to 4 days after wounding, is so named because the cellular and other interactions lead to preparation for subsequent events. During this phase vascular and inflammatory components prevail (vascular clotting in the severed vessels; leukocyte and macrophage chemotaxis into the area to ingest bacteria, debride the wound, and degrade collagen). The proliferative phase (10 to 14 days after wounding) results in regeneration of epidermis, neoangiogenesis, and proliferation of fibroblasts with increased collagen synthesis and closure of the skin defect. The final remodeling phase takes place over 6 to 12 months, during which time a more stable form of collagen is laid

TABLE 522–3. IMMUNOFLUORESCENT CUTANEOUS FINDINGS IN IMMUNOLOGICALLY MEDIATED SKIN DISEASE

Diseases	Biopsy Findings of Direct Immunofluorescence Immunoreactants (DIF)	Ultrastructural Localization of Immunoreactants	Site of Blister Formation on Routine Light Microscopic Pathology	Serum Findings: Indirect Immunofluorescence (IIF)
Bullous Diseases				
Pemphigus (all forms)	Deposits of IgG intercellular areas between keratinocytes	Between keratinocytes	Suprabasilar in pemphigus vulgaris; substratum corneum in pemphigus foliaceus	IgG antibodies to intracellular areas of keratinocytes in 95% of patients
Bullous pemphigoid	IgG and/or complement (C) in basement membrane zone (BMZ)	Lamina lucida and hemidesmosomes—upper part lucida and sub-basal cells	Subepidermal	IgG Ab to BMZ in 70%
Cicatricial pemphigoid	IgG and/or C in BMZ	Lamina lucida	Subepidermal	IgG antibodies to BMZ in 10%
Herpes gestationis	Complement in BMZ—occasionally IgG	Lamina lucida—close to lamina densa	Subepidermal—sub-basal cell—above lamina densa	IgG antibodies to BMZ in 20% (HG factor in 25%)
Dermatitis herpetiformis	IgA and C in dermal papillae (granular deposits)	Granular IgA associated with microfibril bundles in dermal papilla	Subepidermal in dermal papillae—papillar dermal microabscesses	No circulating antibodies
Epidermolysis bullosa acquisita	IgG in BMZ	Sublamina densa amorphous granular deposits	Subepidermal	No circulating antibodies
Linear IgA bullous dermatosis in childhood	IgA and complement in linear deposition in BMZ	—	Subepidermal	No circulating antibodies
Connective Tissue Diseases				
Bullous SLE	IgG, IgM, and complement in BMZ in involved and normal skin—linear homogeneous	Just beneath lamina densa (basal lamina)	Subepidermal	No circulating antibodies to BMZ; ANA found in 90%
Discoid LE	IgG, other Ig, and C in lesional skin at BMZ	—	—	No circulating antibodies to BMZ; ANA titers normal
Systemic LE	IgG band at BMZ in normal skin (over 90% in sun-exposed areas)	—	—	Elevated ANA titers
Systemic sclerosis	Nucleolar IgG	—	Epidermal thinning and increased dermal collagen	ANA, speckled, 85%, centromere + in CREST syndrome
MCTD	IgG/IgM in BMZ in some patients; nuclear IgG in epidermis	—	—	Speckled ANA and ENA (extractable nuclear antigens)
Dermatomyositis	Negative	—	—	ANA often normal range

down to form a scar of progressively increasing tensile strength. In some instances so much collagen is deposited in the healing wound that an elevated *hypertrophic scar* (red, raised scar within the boundaries of the original wound) or keloid (scar tissue extending beyond the boundaries of the original injury into surrounding normal tissue) is produced. Keloids, which occur most commonly over the anterior chest, upper back, and deltoid regions, rarely regress, and they recur after excision. Fibroblasts from keloid areas synthesize collagen at significantly greater rates than normal skin, even in tissue culture.

THE COSMETIC IMPORTANCE OF SKIN. With age virtually all the structures and functions of the skin change. Environmental insults, especially chronic sun exposure, cause far greater damage to the skin than time itself. Sun exposure over a lifetime, especially in fair-skinned, easily sunburned individuals, accelerates the aging process, resulting in thin, wrinkled skin in exposed areas. The major age changes in gross appearance of skin include roughness, wrinkling, laxity, uneven pigmentation, and a variety of benign and malignant proliferative lesions.

Changes with aging at the structural, physiologic, and biochemical levels are as follows: (1) A decrease in epidermal turnover rate of approximately 50 per cent occurs between the third and seventh decades. Concurrent loss of dermal elastic and collagen fibers accounts for the paper-thin, transparent quality of aged skin and the easy rupture of dermal vessels. Further, with age there is increasing cross-linkage of collagen and elastin, making the dermis more rigid and therefore less able to withstand shearing forces. Aged skin, when "tented up," only slowly returns to its original form, whereas young skin readily snaps back. (2) Sun-damaged aged skin shows microscopic collagen damage. Dermal collagen is replaced by amorphous basophilic staining material. This condition, termed *elastosis*, results in deep wrinkling and furrowing, especially over the face and back of the neck, and yellow papules and nodules in a reticular pattern on the face. (3) Decreases in the number of functioning sebaceous and sweat glands contribute to the dryness of aged skin and to impaired thermoregulation in aged persons. (4) Reduction in the vascular network in the skin surrounding hair bulbs and eccrine and sebaceous glands may be responsible for the atrophy of these appendages with age. (5) A 50 per cent reduction in the number of Langerhans' cells may account in part for the age-associated decrease in immune responsiveness and allergic contact dermatitis reactions in the elderly. (6) Loss of enzymatically active melanocytes (10 to 20 per cent per decade) causes irregular pigmentation of the skin and graying of the hair. (7) Gradual reduction occurs in the number of body hairs, especially in the scalp, axillary, and pubic regions (related in part to decreased androgen production). (8) Linear growth of nails also decreases by 30 to 50 per cent between early and late adulthood. Often nails become brittle and thickened. (9) A number of proliferative growths are associated with aging skin, including skin tags (acrochordon), cherry angiomata, seborrheic keratosis, lentigines, and sebaceous hyperplasia.

523 Examination of the Skin and an Approach to Diagnosing Skin Diseases

General considerations in history taking and physical examination:

THE DERMATOLOGIC HISTORY

A proper history includes the following: where the patient's skin condition first appeared; what it looked like and what symptoms, if any, were associated with it initially; how the skin disease progressed and changed and what has been done to treat the condition (by the patient or by other physicians).

A careful review of the systemic medications (both proprietary and prescribed) that the patient is taking is in order. The relationship of the onset of the skin rash to the use of systemic internal medications is particularly crucial in evaluating the possibility of a drug reaction.

A history of atopic diseases or skin cancer and a careful family history of skin problems help to alert the physician to genetic and familial aspects of dermatosis.

If contact dermatitis is suspected, a detailed work and hobby history can identify exposure to allergens or irritants, for instance by noting the waxing of the skin condition in relation to time on the job and waning during time away from work, such as weekends and vacations. Environmental exposure to the elements such as sun, cold, and heat may be important in provoking skin reactions. Also, when dealing with possible infectious and parasitic processes of the skin, it is useful to determine whether family members or sexual partners are similarly affected.

Psychological stress, although seldom a sole cause of cutaneous conditions, can exacerbate many dermatoses (e.g., acne, psoriasis, seborrhea, atopic eczema).

THE PHYSICAL EXAMINATION

Dermatology is a visual specialty, and because the identification of skin lesions is a crucial aspect of dermatologic diagnosis the examiner's eye and a magnifying lens are the most important tools. Good lighting is essential, either daylight or fluorescent light simulating daylight. At times side lighting in a darkened room is also useful for detecting minimally raised or depressed lesions.

The skin should be examined from head to toe in a systematic manner, so that all regions of the integument, including the nails and the mucous membranes, are evaluated. It is not unusual for the informed and observant physician to find some significant skin lesion, such as a basal cell carcinoma or even a melanoma, of which the patient is unaware. The general assessment of the entire skin, then, allows the examiner to determine the pattern of the skin problem before focusing on specific lesions. Distribution of the skin problem may follow neural (as in a dermatome) or vascular patterns (as in livedo reticularis). In addition, factors related to the patient's general medical condition can also be discerned in the skin by noting signs of aging, pigmentation, trauma, nutrition, and hygiene. Color changes related to underlying systemic conditions (e.g., jaundice with hepatobiliary conditions, cyanosis with various cardiopulmonary diseases, diffuse hyperpigmentation with Addison's disease, paleness with anemia) are important to the assessment.

In each region of the body the physical examination includes three maneuvers: (1) *Observation* for color or surface changes. It is extremely important when observing skin lesions to use an alcohol sponge to wipe off cosmetics or any oil or foreign material that might be present on the skin. (2) *Touch or light stroking* to perceive texture changes, warmth, and moisture. Smoothness or roughness of the skin depends on such things as normal keratinization, proper hydration of the stratum corneum, and normal cutaneous blood flow. (3) *Palpation* to determine the consistency and pliability of the skin by stretching the integument between the fingers. Plasticity depends on the normal structure and function of dermal connective tissue and ground substance.

Because there are many hundreds of dermatoses, a logical process of elimination is required to narrow the possibilities, first to specific groups of diseases and finally to one condition. Such a diagnostic approach is based on specific morphologic descriptions of the skin lesions that the physician sees and feels, together with an appropriate history and laboratory tests. Three steps are involved in this systematic approach. First, the entire skin is examined for primary and secondary skin lesions that allow the examiner to place the patient in one of nine diagnostic groups (the second step) (Table 523-1). Many skin conditions are found in each group, but all of the conditions in a given group manifest the same primary and secondary lesions. The third step involves differentiating the one disease the patient has from the others in the group. This is done by looking for several specific features, such as the distribution of skin lesions, any unusual shapes of the lesions or arrangement of several lesions (annular, serpiginous, dermatomal), color of the lesion including dominant hue and the color pattern, and the surface characteristics (particularly the appearance of scales or verrucous or vegetative changes).

STEP 1: DESCRIPTION OF PRIMARY AND SECONDARY SKIN LESIONS.

STEP 1: DESCRIPTION OF PRIMARY AND SECONDARY SKIN LESIONS. Primary skin lesions are uncomplicated lesions that represent the initial pathologic change, uninfluenced by secondary alterations such as infection, trauma, or therapy. Secondary skin lesions are changes that occur as consequences of progression of the disease or scratching or infection of the primary lesions (Fig. 523–1). Most of the primary changes can also, at times, occur as secondary manifestations; for example, pustules may appear as primary lesions of folliculitis or as secondary lesions when scaling, itching lesions are scratched and infected. The trick is to recognize any single primary skin lesion as the initial change characteristic of the disease.

The terminology used to describe primary and secondary skin changes is the basic language of dermatology, the means by which one can accurately describe skin diseases to a colleague. If this terminology is not used correctly it will be difficult to arrive at the precise diagnosis of skin diseases. Each descriptive word is not only a short account of what is seen on the surface of the skin but also relays specific information about processes within the skin. A diagrammatic representation and description of primary and secondary skin lesions are presented in Figure 523–2.

STEP 2: ASSIGNMENT OF THE LESION TO A MAJOR GROUP OF DISEASES. Each disease within a given group shares the same primary and secondary skin lesions. Some diseases have overlapping traits so they may be assigned to more than one group. An arbitrary grouping that has proved to be of practical value is listed below and is used later in this chapter to discuss specific diseases within each group (Table 523–1).

STEP 3: NARROWING THE POSSIBILITIES TO THE EXACT DIAGNOSIS. Of great importance is the distribution of the skin disease, for many conditions have typical patterns or affect specific regions. For example, psoriasis commonly affects extensor surfaces and atopic eczema flexor areas of the extremities (Fig. 523–2). Photoreactions are confined to parts of the body exposed to sunlight. Involvement of the palms and soles is seen in erythema multiforme, secondary syphilis, psoriasis, and eczema. Contact dermatitis to exogenous allergens or irritants often presents with unusual patterns and distributions corresponding to the areas where the offending material came in contact with the skin. The best way to examine for distribution is to step away from the patient and view from a few feet away.

Another important clue in differentiating diseases in a given group is to consider the shape of the individual lesions and the arrangement of several lesions in relation to each other. A *linear* arrangement of lesions may indicate a contact reaction to an exogenous substance brushing across the skin, a pathologic process involving a vascular or lymphatic vessel, or a cutaneous nevus (Fig. 523–2). *Zosteriform* refers to lesions arranged along the cutaneous distribution of a spinal nerve. It is thus bandlike and unilateral and denotes herpes zoster and, occasionally, metastatic carcinoma of the breast or the dermatomal hemangiomatous growths of Sturge-Weber syndrome. *Annular* lesions are circular with normal skin in the center. Annular macules are observed in drug eruptions, secondary syphilis, and lupus erythematosus. Resolving hives may leave annular configurations. Annular lesions with scale suggest dermatophytosis or pityriasis rosea. *Iris* lesions are a special type of annular lesion in which an erythematous annular macule or papule develops a second red ring or a purplish papule or vesicle in the center (target or bull's-eye lesion). Iris lesions are seen in erythema multiforme. *Arciform* lesions form partial circles or arcs and may be seen in dermatophyte infections. *Polycyclic* patterns evolve when numerous annular lesions enlarge and run together. *Serpiginous* (snakelike, undulating, linear) patterns are seen in creeping eruptions and in psoriasis. *Herpetiform* refers to a grouping of lesions such as occurs in herpes simplex or dermatitis herpetiformis.

Other physical features are important in diagnosing skin diseases: Dry, lichenified lesions suggest a chronic state of a disease, whereas wet, weeping, macerated lesions suggest acute reactions. Abscesses are soft and fluctuant, whereas nodules are usually firm. Redness caused by dilatation of superficial blood vessels blanches with pressure, whereas erythema caused by extravasated blood as occurs in petechiae and purpuric lesions does not blanch. Hues of brown to black usually indicate melanin, although some drugs (e.g., tetracycline) cause brown-black pigmentation in the skin. The variation in color from melanin is related to the depth of the pigment in the skin—the deeper the pigment the more blue-black the color.

DIAGNOSTIC TESTS AND AIDS IN EXAMINATION OF THE SKIN

Certain technical, clinical, and laboratory aids and procedures, when combined with the history and physical examination, are indispensable in arriving at the correct diagnosis.

VISUAL AIDS. *Magnification.* Certain diagnostic findings are revealed by magnification of the skin lesions, for example, the follicular plugging seen in discoid lupus erythematosus, or fine telangiectasias in the pearly, opalescent borders of basal cell cancers.

Transillumination. Oblique lighting in a darkened room can be useful in detecting slight degrees of elevation or depression of lesions as well as fine wrinkling or atrophy of the epidermis. In addition, the application of a penlight directly to nodular lesions in a dark room may give clues as to the density and make-up of

TABLE 523–1. MAJOR GROUPS OF DERMATOLOGIC DISEASES BASED ON THE CLINICAL MORPHOLOGY OF THE SKIN CONDITION

Group	Clinical Morphology	Examples of Diseases in the Group
Eczema or dermatitis	Macules (erythema), papules, vesicles, lichenification, fine scaling, excoriations, crusting	Contact dermatitis, atopic dermatitis, stasis dermatitis, photodermatitis, scabies, dermatophytoses, exfoliative dermatitis, candidiasis
Maculopapular eruptions	Macules, erythema, papules	Viral exanthems, drug reactions, verruca vulgaris, Kawasaki's disease, vasculitic and purpuric eruptions
Papulosquamous dermatoses	Papules, plaques, erythema with unique scales	Psoriasis, Reiter's syndrome, pityriasis rosea, lichen planus, seborrheic dermatitis, ichthyosis, secondary syphilis, mycosis fungoides, parapsoriasis
Vesiculobullous diseases	Vesicles, bullae, erythema	Herpes simplex and zoster, hand-foot-and-mouth disease, insect bites, bullous impetigo, scalded skin syndrome, pemphigus, pemphigoid, dermatitis herpetiformis, porphyria cutanea tarda, erythema multiforme
Pustular diseases	Pustules, cysts, erythema	Acne vulgaris and rosacea, pustular psoriasis, folliculitis, gonococcemia
Urticaria, persistent figurate erythemas, cellulitis	Wheals and figurate, raised erythema, scaling	Urticaria, erythema annulare centrifugum, erysipelas, necrotizing fasciitis
Nodular lesions	Nodules and tumors, some associated with erosions and ulceration	Benign and malignant tumors—basal cell cancer, squamous cell cancer, rheumatoid nodules, xanthomas
Telangiectasias, atrophic, scarring, ulcerative diseases	Atrophic, sclerotic telangiectasias and ulcerative changes	Connective tissue diseases, radiation dermatitis, lichen sclerosus et atrophicus, vascular insufficiency (arterial and venous), pyoderma gangrenosum
Hyper- and hypomelanosis	Increased and decreased melanin deposition in skin	Acanthosis nigricans, café au lait spots, vitiligo, tuberous sclerosis, xeroderma pigmentosum, chloasma, freckles

such lesions. Cystic lesions allow transmission of some light, whereas nodules composed of cellular infiltrates do not.

Diascopy. Firm pressure with a microscope slide against skin lesions differentiates erythema of capillary dilatation from that of extravasated blood. Sarcoidosis, tuberculosis, and other granulomatous inflammatory reactions in the skin are suggested if diascopy of the lesions shows a characteristic "apple-jelly" or glassy, fawn-colored appearance.

Long-wave Ultraviolet or Wood's Light Examination. Long-wave ultraviolet light (UVA) (360 nm) is useful in evaluating several conditions of the skin. Wood's light is of great help in estimating subtle variations in pigmentation. It exaggerates the differences in the degree of pigmentation when the skin is examined with the lamp in a dark room. Melanin is a universal absorber of UV light, so decreased melanin shows more reflection (light color) and increased melanin less reflection (darker color).

Pigment in the epidermis is exaggerated with UVA light, but that in the dermis is not, so a reasonable guess as to the site of melanin in the skin can be made. Wood's light may be the only means of recognizing the hypomelanotic ash leaf–shaped macules in tuberous sclerosis. The extent of vitiligo and melanotic nevi (which appear darker than surrounding normal skin) can also be determined. Some superficial fungal infections of the scalp fluoresce blue-green; erythrasma, a superficial intertriginous bacterial infection that produces a porphyrin, fluoresces a brilliant coral red; *Pseudomonas* infections may give off yellow-green color under a Wood's light.

CLINICAL TESTS. Patch Tests. Patch testing is used to validate a diagnosis of allergic contact sensitization and to identify the causative allergen. Since the entire skin of sensitized humans is allergic, the test reproduces the dermatitis in one small area where the allergen is applied, usually on the back. The suspected allergen is applied to the skin, occluded, and left in place 48 hours. A positive test reproduces an eczematous response at the

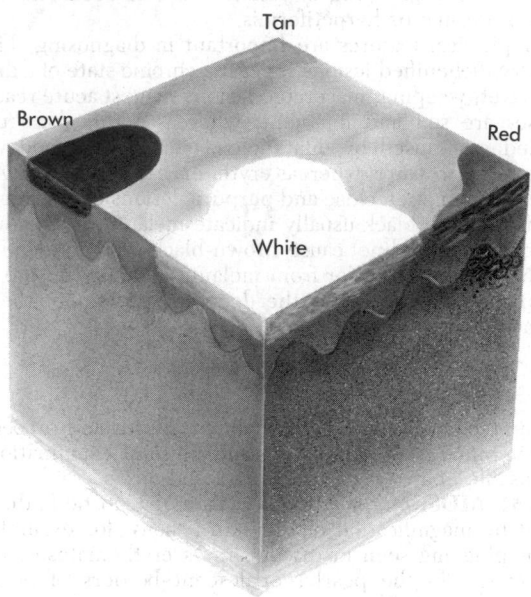

MACULE
A circumscribed color change

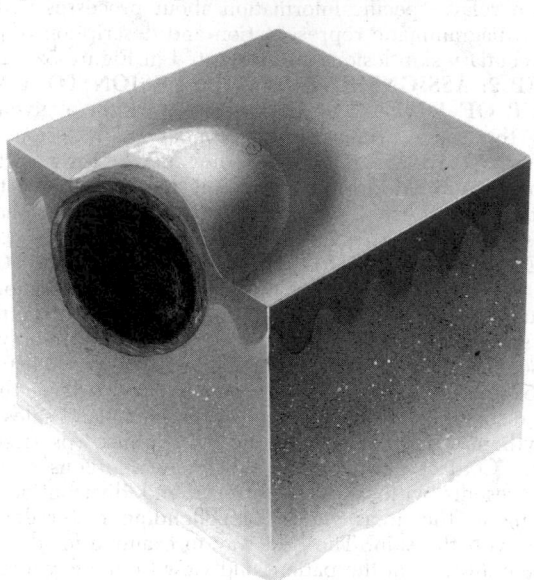

CYST
Semi-solid sac
Resilient

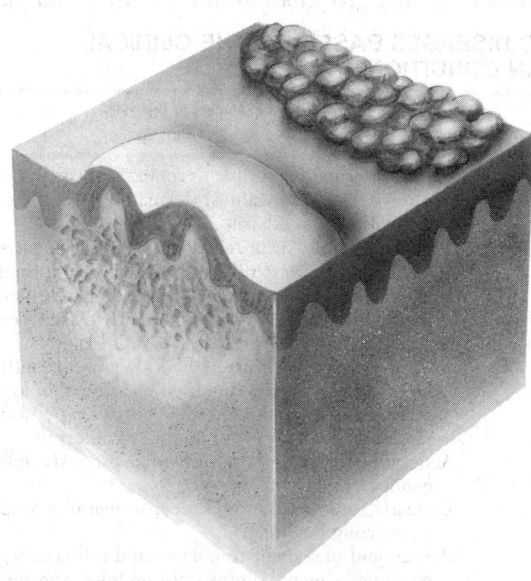

PAPULE
A solid elevation 1 cm or less
skin colored or not

PLAQUE
Raised, circumscribed,
extensive

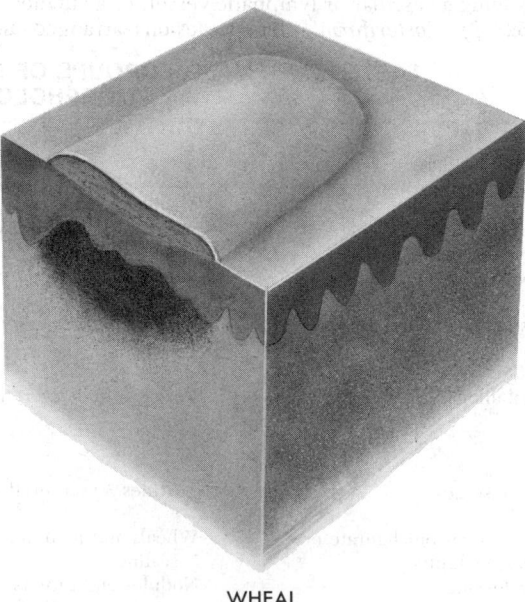

WHEAL
Evanescent
Edematous
Erythematous

FIGURE 523–1. Lesions of the skin. (From the 17th edition of the Cecil Textbook of Medicine, with the permission of Dr. Marie-Louise Johnson.)

test site from 48 hours up to a week after the test. The latter is a delayed hypersensitivity reaction. Considerable experience is required to accurately perform and interpret patch tests. *Photo-patch testing* is performed to detect photocontact allergy. Suspected photoallergens are placed on the skin in two sets. One set of allergens is irradiated with appropriate wavelengths of light after the patches are in place on the skin 24 hours; the second set of the same photoallergens is kept covered to serve as controls. Photoallergens cause an erythematous reaction that will be evident 24 hours after exposure to light.

Physical Contact Testing. *Darier's sign* is the development of an urticarial and flare reaction after vigorously rubbing cutaneous mast cell (urticaria pigmentosa) lesions of the skin. The rubbing degranulates the mast cells, releasing histamine.

Nikolsky's sign demonstrates disadherence of the epidermal cells to one another. Pushing, rubbing, or rotating normal skin near bullous lesions causes the epidermis to be dislodged, leaving a moist, glistening defect. This sign is present in various forms of pemphigus and in toxic epidermal necrolysis.

The *Koebner phenomenon* occurs in certain skin diseases that tend to evolve new skin lesions after traumatic injury in areas of apparently normal skin. Thus, psoriasis may evolve within surgical scars and after sunburn or in the wake of a drug reaction involving the skin. Lichen planus may also exhibit this phenomenon.

Pathergy, the development of pustular and ulcerative lesions

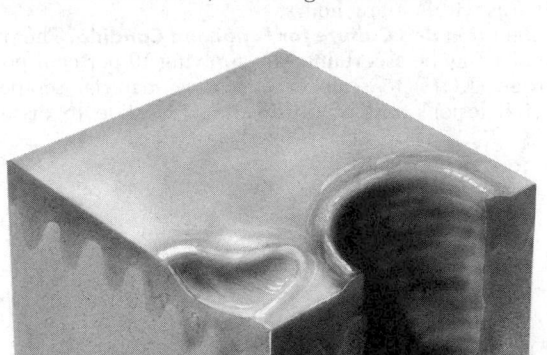

EROSION
Superficial denudation

ULCER
Defect penetrates dermis

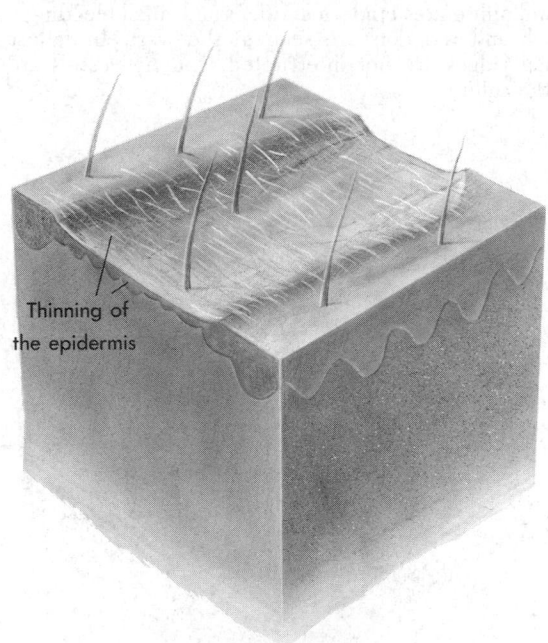

Thinning of the epidermis

ATROPHY

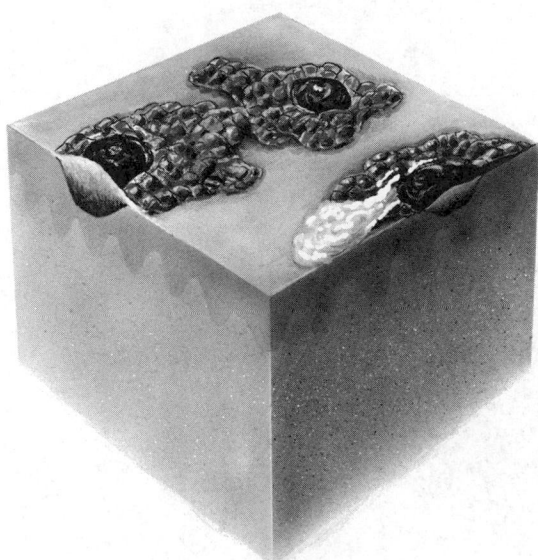

CRUST
Coagulated blood elements

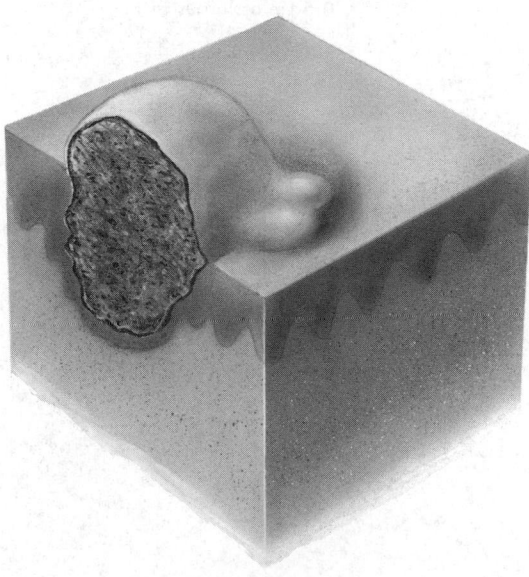

PUSTULE
Fluid-filled sac with neutrophils

FIGURE 523–1 *Continued*

Illustration continued on following page

at the site of needle puncture, is suggestive of Behçet's syndrome and pyoderma gangrenosum.

Hair-pull examination is done to assess hair loss in the scalp. It is often useful to pull vigorously on scalp hairs to (1) determine whether there is an increased number of falling hairs (normally only one or two can be removed with a tug of a group of hairs between the thumb and forefinger); (2) ascertain the ratio of anagen to telogen hairs; and (3) examine the hairs under a microscope for various congenital malformations of the shaft. Normally 10 to 15 per cent of scalp hairs are in telogen, whereas in telogen effluvium the percentage is greatly increased.

Paring Hyperkeratotic Lesions to Differentiate Warts from Calluses. After the hyperkeratosis is pared away, the wart displaces and obliterates epidermal ridges and small bleeding points, and black and red dots are seen in the wart. In calluses the epidermal ridges are not interrupted, and no vessels are seen within the callus.

LABORATORY PROCEDURES. *Gram's Stain and Cultures.*
Gram's stain for bacteria and bacteriologic cultures are extremely important when the primary lesion is a pustule or furuncle or appears to be impetigo. When an unusual cutaneous infection is considered in an immunosuppressed patient, a skin biopsy specimen can be minced or ground in a sterile mortar and cultured for aerobic and anaerobic bacteria, including typical and atypical mycobacteria, deep fungi, and *Candida*. A more rapid method of screening for infectious agents in a skin infection in immunosuppressed patients (often the first sign of septicemia in such patients is pustules, nodules, or ulcerative lesions) is to perform frozen sections on a skin biopsy specimen taken from the lesion and to obtain Gram's stains, acid-fast bacterial stains, and PAS stains (to identify fungal and yeast elements). This may provide a diagnosis within a few hours.

Examination and Culture for Fungi and Candida. The presence of mycelia may be ascertained by applying 10 per cent potassium hydroxide (KOH) to scale or exudative material scraped from suspected lesions and briefly heating the slide to dissolve the

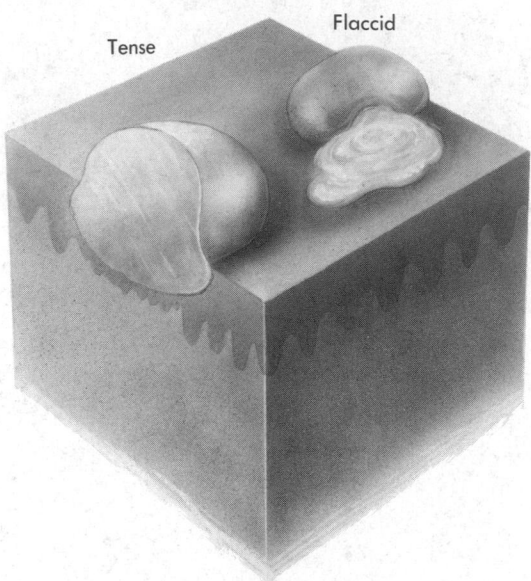

BULLAE
Fluid-filled
0.5 cm or larger

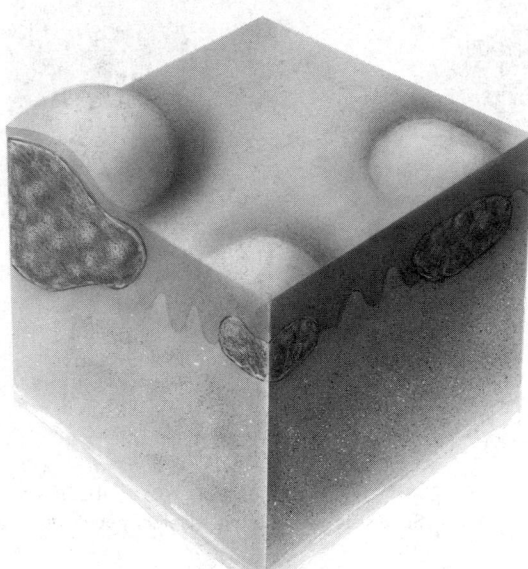

NODULE
Solid deeper lesion

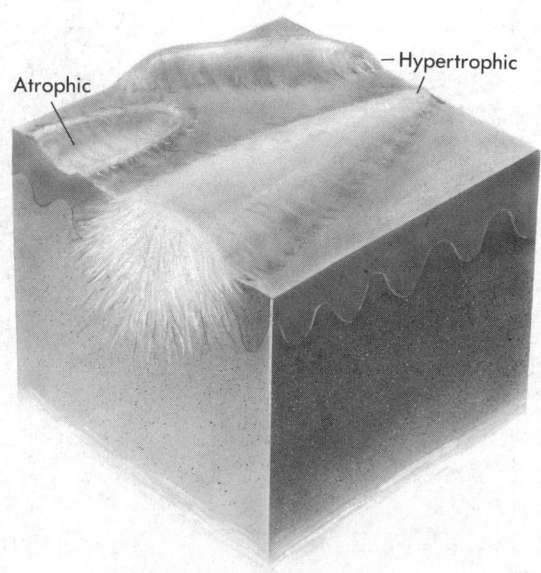

SCAR
FIGURE 523–1 *Continued*

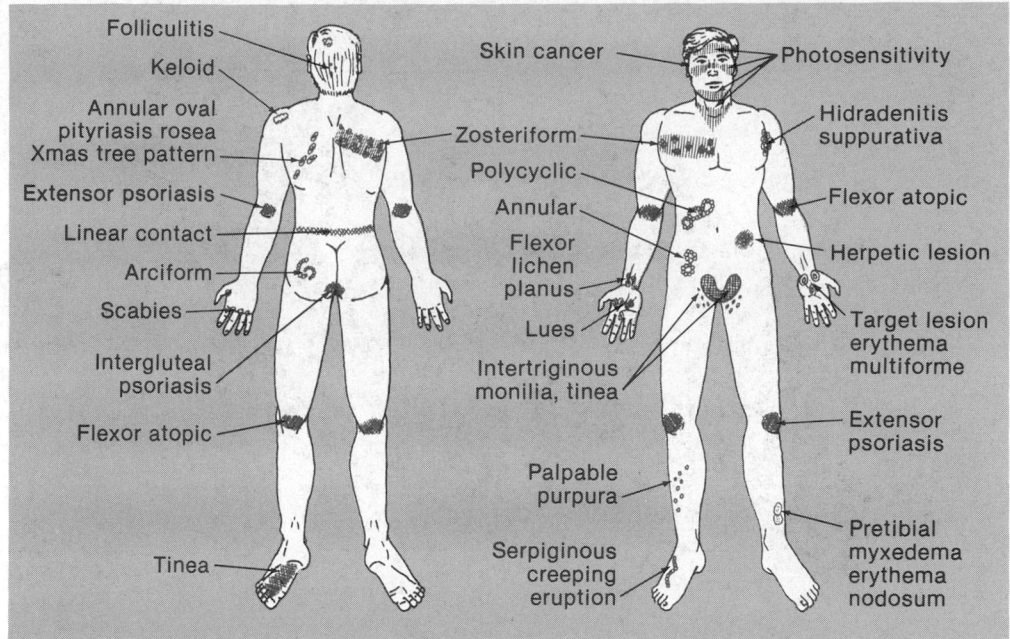

FIGURE 523–2. Configurational and regional diagnostic aids for the diagnosis of primary and secondary skin lesions.

keratin. Hyphal elements can be observed by direct microscopic examination (Fig. 523–3). Dermatophyte hyphae appear as long, branching, refractile, walled structures; *Candida* appears as shorter, linear hyphae in association with budding yeast forms (see Fig. 523–2); tinea versicolor is seen as round yeast forms with short, club-shaped hyphae (so-called spaghetti and meatballs

pattern) (see Fig. 525–4). KOH examination of skin scrapings is mandatory to rule out tinea. A classic dictum is "if the skin lesion is scaly, scrape it."

Tzanck Smear. The microscopic examination of cells from the base of vesicles reveals the presence of giant epithelial cells and multinucleated giant cells in herpes simplex, herpes zoster, and

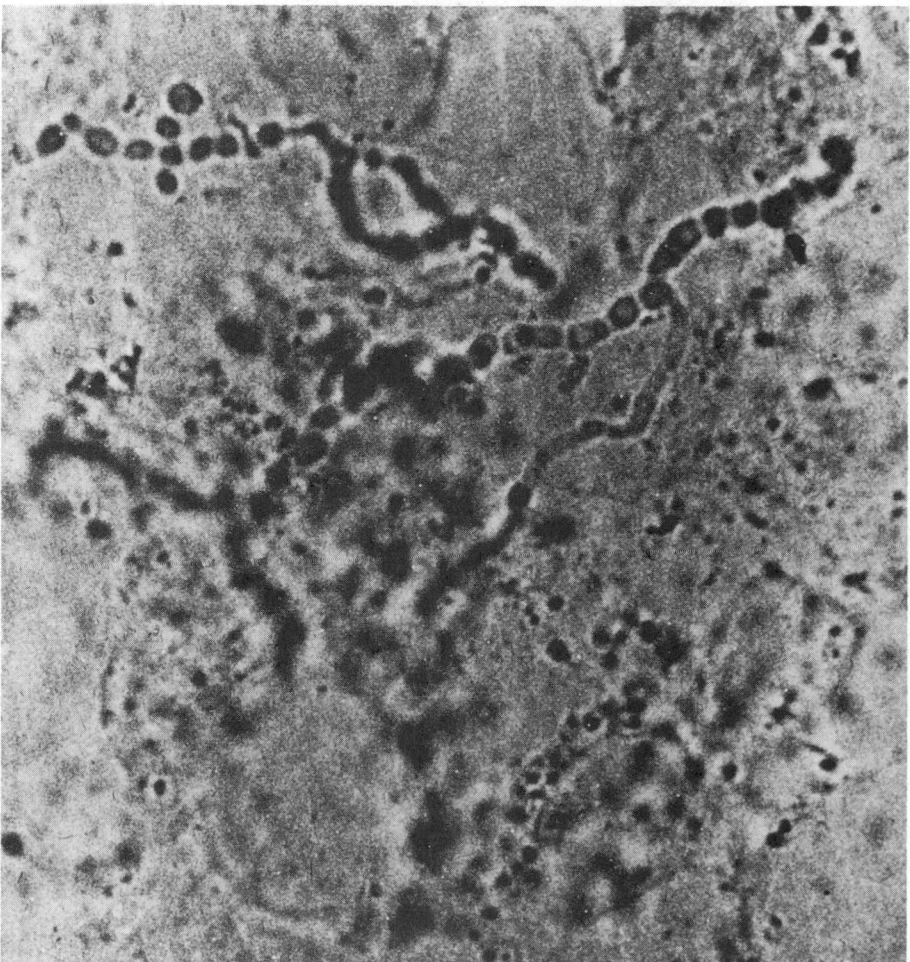

FIGURE 523–3. KOH preparation of mycelial hyphae, high power. (From the 17th edition of the Cecil Textbook of Medicine, with the permission of Dr. Marie-Louise Johnson.)

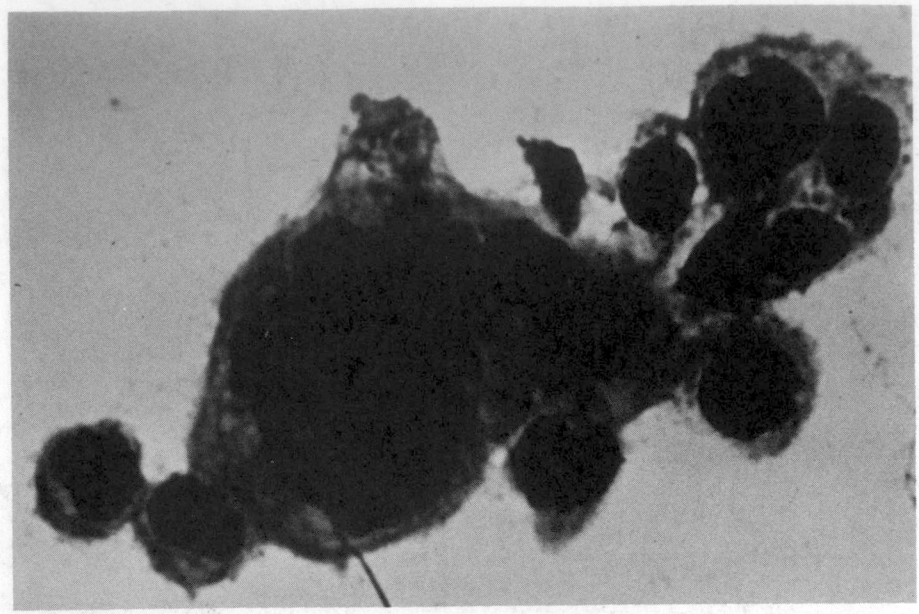

FIGURE 523–4. Positive Tzanck smear, herpes simplex. (From the 17th edition of the Cecil Textbook of Medicine, with the permission of Dr. Marie-Louise Johnson.)

varicella. Material is obtained from the base of a vesicle by gentle scraping with a scalpel and is spread on a glass slide and stained with Giemsa's or Wright's stain for the examination (Fig. 523–4).

Skin Biopsy. Lesions characteristic of the eruption (primary lesions) should be biopsied. Lesions altered by scratching, infection, crusting, or lichenification are not likely to provide useful information.

Clinical indications for biopsy include lesions thought to be malignant; lesions that fail to heal, increase in size, bleed easily, or ulcerate spontaneously; tumors or growths of uncertain nature; and many inflammatory conditions, especially those for which the diagnosis is uncertain.

Four types of biopsies can be performed. The choice of technique determines the size and shape of the specimen obtained (Fig. 523–5). The procedure selected should secure the tissue most likely to contain the pathologic alterations and leave the smallest cosmetic defect. For the most complete histopathologic assessment an *elliptical, full-thickness excision* is best because, in one procedure, the entire lesion is removed and secured for diagnosis and the remaining defect is easily sutured. The excisional biopsy technique is indicated when malignant melanoma is suspected or when a lesion is deep in skin or subcutaneous tissue and its orientation in surrounding tissue is relevant for diagnosis. A second procedure is the *paramedian incisional biopsy,* in which a thin but deep elliptical section is taken through the center of the lesion including normal skin at each end. This is especially useful in diagnosing large keratoacanthomas. A third biopsy method is the *shave,* or *parallel incision,* in which Xylocaine is injected locally under the lesion to lift it above the skin surface, and a scalpel (the knife horizontal to the skin surface) is used to "shave" off the protruding part of the skin and lesion. This technique is useful for diagnosing malignant and benign tumors when subsequent treatment by curettage and electrodesiccation is anticipated. It should never be used when melanoma is suspected, because the specimen obtained is too superficial for adequate histologic grading. Shave biopsy is convenient for removing superficial benign tumors such as seborrheic keratoses or skin tags. The fourth technique, *punch biopsy,* utilizes a tubular blade to cut out a circular plug of skin by slightly rotating and pushing the cutting edge deep into the dermis. The specimen is clipped off at its base with scissors, and the defect can be readily closed with sutures. Punch biopsies are used to diagnose inflammatory diseases and tumors.

If at first a skin biopsy does not provide an answer and there is a diagnostic dilemma, it is necessary and appropriate to rebiopsy. It is useful to give the pathologist adequate clinical history so that the specimen may be properly interpreted.

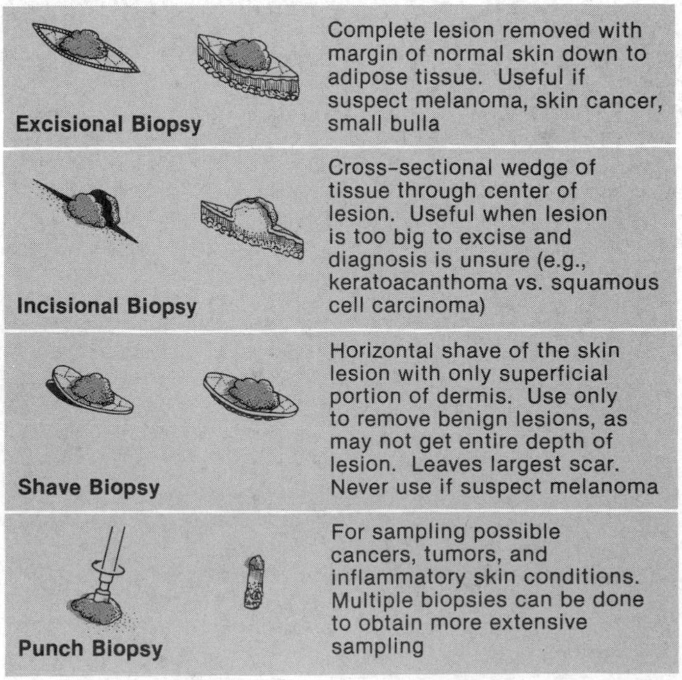

Excisional Biopsy	Complete lesion removed with margin of normal skin down to adipose tissue. Useful if suspect melanoma, skin cancer, small bulla
Incisional Biopsy	Cross-sectional wedge of tissue through center of lesion. Useful when lesion is too big to excise and diagnosis is unsure (e.g., keratoacanthoma vs. squamous cell carcinoma)
Shave Biopsy	Horizontal shave of the skin lesion with only superficial portion of dermis. Use only to remove benign lesions, as may not get entire depth of lesion. Leaves largest scar. Never use if suspect melanoma
Punch Biopsy	For sampling possible cancers, tumors, and inflammatory skin conditions. Multiple biopsies can be done to obtain more extensive sampling

FIGURE 523–5. Methods of skin biopsy.

524 Principles of Therapy

GENERAL CONSIDERATIONS

The skin is uniquely susceptible to topical as well as systemic forms of therapy. Significant progress has been made in controlling and curing some infectious and inflammatory skin diseases, although the pathogenesis of many skin conditions remains unknown, and only palliative and supportive therapies are available.

The goals of therapy are to define and remove the cause of the disorder, restore the structural and functional integrity of the skin, and relieve symptoms. Relief of such symptoms as itching, pain, or cosmetic disfigurement is an important goal. Damaged skin needs protection, as its barrier function is impaired. This can be assured with dressings and by minimizing scratching and avoiding abrasive clothing and soaps or chemicals. Removal of debris, such as excessive scale, hyperkeratoses, crusts, and infection, is also a crucial goal of therapy if the skin is to heal. Topical and systemic medications, dressings, and other treatments can alter skin temperature and blood flow and thus favorably affect the metabolism of the skin.

Some topical and systemic forms of therapy that have proven beneficial are discussed in this chapter.

TOPICAL MODES OF THERAPY

SOAKS AND WET DRESSINGS. The use of water, with or without various additives, can provide many benefits to the skin, including soothing comfort, antipruritic effects, and increased rate of epidermal healing with hydration and debridement of crusts, dead skin, and bacteria.

Baths. When the area of involvement is too large to apply compresses, a bath is useful. Baths with whirlpool action are particularly useful for debridement of large or deep ulcers. Medicated baths can evenly distribute soothing antipruritic and anti-inflammatory agents to widespread lesions. Starch and oatmeal complexes are commercially available in forms suitable for tub baths. Tar bath preparations are available for use in conjunction with ultraviolet light treatments. Bath oil prevents drying by leaving a thin film of emollient on the skin. The tub should be one-half full, and the soak should last no longer than 20 to 30 minutes, to avoid maceration. Warm baths cause vasodilation and may increase itching; cool baths constrict vessels and usually sooth pruritus. The best time to apply lubricants is immediately after the bath so that they may hold water in the hydrated stratum corneum.

Wet Dressings. Water and medication can be applied to the skin with dressings (finely woven cotton, linen, or gauze) soaked in solution. As water evaporates, the skin is cooled and pruritus is soothed. For maximal benefit from evaporation, the dressing should be no more than a few layers thick and should be dipped in the solution and reapplied to the area of treated skin every few minutes for 15 to 30 minutes several times a day. Wet compresses, especially with frequent changes, provide gentle debridement, the cleansing resulting from transfer of crusts, scales, and cutaneous debris to the compress. If the compresses are permitted to dry (wet to dry compresses) and to become adherent, the debriding effect is greater and can even damage the skin. The dressing may need to be remoistened in place to facilitate removal. Wet compresses also leach water-binding proteins from the stratum corneum and epidermis, causing drying, a desirable effect for moist, oozing and weeping lesions. Wet compresses are therefore useful in treating acute vesicular, bullous, oozing or weeping conditions as well as crusty, swollen, and infected skin. There are two types of wet dressings, open or unoccluded and closed or occluded.

The *open wet dressing* is applied directly to the skin, leaving the dressing exposed to the air. The fluid is allowed to evaporate, providing a cooling, antipruritic effect. Frequent reapplication of the compresses debrides exudate, crust, and bacterial contamination and dries out the skin, rapidly decreasing oozing and weeping.

Closed wet dressings, in which the moist fabric dressings are applied to the skin and covered with an impervious material such as plastic, oil cloth, or Saran wrap, may be useful when some degree of maceration and heat retention is required. For example, if there is excessive keratin of the palms or soles or when an early abscess needs heat to help localize the infection, this form of dressing may be appropriate. Closed dressings are less frequently used than open dressings.

Dry dressings protect the skin, hold medications against the skin, keep clothing and sheets from rubbing, and keep dirt and air away. Such dressings also prevent patients from scratching and rubbing. In the case of neurodermatitis or stasis dermatitis, they are often left in place for several days. Soft casts or castlike boots (e.g., Unna boot) serve the same purposes.

The medication most commonly added to baths and dressings is aluminum acetate, which serves to coagulate bacterial and serum protein. As a 5 per cent preparation it is known as Burow's solution, and it must be further diluted for use. Burow's solution can be readily made by dissolving tablets or powder packets in

appropriate amounts of water. (One tablet or packet in 500 ml = 1:20 concentration.) Potassium permanganate and silver nitrate are occasionally added to soak solutions for their antimicrobial properties, but they stain the skin, may be absorbed if used over large raw areas of skin, and may burn the skin if used in high concentrations. The question is often raised about the use of antimicrobial agents in wet dressings, but the quantities needed for adequate concentration in the dressing would make their use exceedingly inefficient and wasteful.

"Occlusive dressings" are being used with increasing frequency in the treatment of acute wounds and chronic venous, diabetic, and pressure ulcers. A variety of dressings is available including *films* (e.g., Op-Site, AcuDerm), *nontransparent adhesive hydrocolloids* (e.g., DUODERM), and *semitransparent nonadhesive hydrogels* (e.g., VIGILON), all of which enhance wound healing.

TOPICAL MEDICATIONS. Topical medications are the mainstay of dermatologic therapy. In general, topical medications consist of two major agents, the active ingredient or specific medication and the vehicle or base in which the active material is dissolved. Both are important in treating skin conditions.

Bases or Vehicles. Bases come in a variety of forms. *Powders* promote dryness by absorbing evaporative moisture. They are used to reduce moisture, maceration, and friction in intertriginous areas. Powders may be inert chemicals (corn starch, talcum), or they may contain medications. *Lotions* are suspensions of insoluble powders in water. As water on the skin surface evaporates, it cools, creating a feeling of dryness and leaving a uniform film of powder on the surface. The addition of alcohol increases the cooling effect. *Creams* are emulsions of oil in water (more water than oil). They seem to vanish into the skin because water evaporates and the residual oil is spread thinly and imperceptibly over the skin. *Ointments* consist of oils with variable smaller amounts of water added in suspension. They have a pleasant lubricating effect on dry or diseased skin, but they may also give a greasy feeling to the skin and clothing. Oils in bases give a softening effect to the skin by forming an occlusive layer that traps water and retards evaporation through the stratum corneum. Thus, ointments with large amouts of oil in them give a more sustained, softening effect to the skin than creams or lotions. In fact, ointments with large percentages of inert oil in them may be occlusive and thereby retain heat, increase pruritus, and increase percutaneous absorption of added active ingredients. The more occlusive ointments should not be used on oozing or infected areas, as the resulting occlusion and warmth may increase bacterial growth. *Pastes* are mixtures of powder and ointment (e.g., zinc oxide paste). *Sprays*, another form of base, are Freon-propelled aerosols.

Bases thus represent a spectrum of varying amounts of water and oil in emulsion. At one end of the spectrum are lotions with less than 5 or 10 per cent oil in water; creams are composed of relatively more oil dispersed in water, but water is still the continuous phase. As the oil-water ratio reverses and oil becomes the continuous phase, the preparation, considered an ointment, is more lubricating, leaving a noticeable greasy film on the skin. At the far end of the spectrum is inert mineral oil or petrolatum.

Selection of a base or emollient depends on the condition being treated and the needs of the patient. A powder in water, such as calamine lotion, permits evaporation and cooling with some drying. Lotions are useful for pruritic, oozing reactions. Petrolatum, by contrast, retains heat and promotes hydration and even maceration of the stratum corneum. Ointments are used most often on dry, scaling conditions in which endogenous hydration of the stratum corneum is defective. Between these two extremes there is a spectrum of possibilities that permit some cooling but add lubrication. Choice depends on the needs of and cosmetic acceptance by the patient.

Active Agents—Specific Agents. Having made a judgment about the base or vehicle required, the physician makes a separate selection of active ingredients to be added.

Topical steroids have revolutionized the practice of dermatology, providing effective local anti-inflammatory and antipruritic effects. Topical steroids have two basic anti-inflammatory actions. First, they cause immediate and profound constriction of cutaneous blood vessels. This is believed to prevent mobilization of polymorphonuclear leukocytes and monocytes into the reaction site. Second, they directly interfere with the inflammatory activities of cells that are already present (e.g., mast cells). Corticosteroids used in topical preparations are intrinsically active without need for further metabolism; this accounts for their rapid effect on cutaneous blood vessels as manifested by blanching of the skin. Therapeutic action is also rapid. Topical steroids slow the mitotic rate of fibroblasts, decreasing collagen synthesis, and possibly enhance collagen catabolism. They further interfere with phagocytosis and the skin's ability to fight off bacterial, viral, and fungal infections. Topical corticosteroids that are effective in treating skin diseases all have the basic hydrocortisone structure. A 1 per cent concentration of hydrocortisone ointment or cream continues to serve as a norm for comparing potency of subsequently modified topical steroids. By fluorinating hydrocortisone or adding acetonide, the potency of the steroid is greatly enhanced. Occlusion increases the efficacy of most topical steroids. Topical corticosteroid preparations may be classified in a general way as of low, intermediate, or high potency (Table 524–1). The potency corresponds closely to the degree of anti-inflammatory effectiveness as well as to the incidence and severity of associated side effects. Although some corticosteroids (particularly fluorinated compounds) are more topically active than others, the potency of a preparation is also related to the concentration of active drug in the vehicle and to the nature of the vehicle in which the steroid is mixed. Since corticosteroids are poorly soluble in most vehicles, many preparations deliver only a fraction of the drug to target cells. Of the various types of vehicles used in steroid preparations, ointments are the most efficient by virtue of the excellent solubility of steroids in ointments and because the occlusive nature of ointments increases stratum corneum permeability. Second in order of efficiency is acetone-alcohol gel, whereas creams and lotions are less useful. Some examples of topical steroids and their grouping according to potency are listed in Table 524–1.

The adverse effects of topical steroids relate almost exclusively to the intermediate and high-potency compounds. Epidermal and dermal atrophy can be a pronounced effect; decreased collagen synthesis and reduced stromal support for dermal blood vessels lead to telangiectasia, purpura, and striae. These are especially likely to occur in intertriginous "occluded" areas of the skin and on the face. Fluorinated steroids can cause a perioral scaling, papular and pustular dermatitis (perioral dermatitis), or facial redness, telangiectasia, and acne rosacea–like eruption. Potent topical steroids applied for prolonged periods around the eyes can occasionally cause glaucoma and even cataracts. Topical steroids can predispose to or worsen skin infections such as folliculitis, tinea, and candidiasis. Systemic absorption of potent topical steroids may lower plasma cortisol levels when they are used with occlusion over as little as 20 per cent of the body, but this is unusual.

The combined characteristics of drug potency and vehicle type should be used to advantage in treatment. Intermediate-potency steroids are useful in most dermatologic conditions. Ointments are useful for thickened skin or for dry, exposed areas where creams or gel preparations rapidly evaporate. Low-potency steroids are used to treat the face and the thin and occluded skin of the groin and genital area. Lotions and gels are best for hairy

TABLE 524–1. POTENCY RANKING OF SOME COMMONLY USED TOPICAL STEROIDS

Potency	Generic Name	Clinical Applications
High	Fluocinonide 0.05%; betamethasone dipropionate 0.05%; halcinonide 0.1%	Recalcitrant psoriasis; discoid lupus erythematosus; recalcitrant lichen planus
Intermediate	Triamcinolone acetonide 0.1%; betamethasone valerate (cream) 0.1%; fluocinolone acetonide 0.01%	Dermatitis—allergic contact, atopic; psoriasis; neurodermatitis
Low	Desonide 0.05%; hydrocortisone 1.0% or 2.5%	Intertrigo; pruritus ani; seborrheic dermatitis

TABLE 524–2. GUIDELINES FOR SELECTING TOPICAL STEROIDS

Location or Type of Lesion	Suggested Potency of Steroid	Suggested Vehicle
Areas of Body		
Trunk, arms, legs	Intermediate or low	Ointment or cream
Palms, soles	Intermediate or high	Ointment
Scalp	Intermediate or low	Lotion, gel, aerosol
Intertriginous areas	Low	Cream, lotion
Face	Low	Cream, lotion
Area around eyes	Low	Cream or ophthalmic preparation
Ears	Intermediate or low	Cream, gel or lotion
Types of Lesion		
Dry, scaling, fissuring, lichenified lesion	Intermediate	Ointment
Thickened, hyperkeratotic skin patches	High	Ointment
Oozing, weeping lesions	Intermediate	Lotion, cream
Ulcerative lesions.	Do not use topical steroids	

areas. High-potency steroid preparations should not be used to treat most dermatologic conditions. Their use is primarily reserved for areas of skin that have been substantially thickened by disease, such as dense plaques of psoriasis or chronic dermatitis. There is a substantial risk of local side effects with these high-potency steroids, and the onset of these effects is more rapid than with less potent drugs. Table 524–2 gives some guidelines for selecting the steroid potency and vehicle most useful in various areas of the body.

Topical steroids are usually applied once or twice a day. The stratum corneum acts as a reservoir and continues to release topical steroid into the skin after the initial application. Chronic dermatoses become less responsive after prolonged use of topical steroids. This phenomenon is referred to as *tachyphylaxis*. Changing to another topical steroid often overcomes this phenomenon.

Intralesional corticosteroids are used to shrink inflammatory acne cysts and hypertrophic scars and keloids. They are occasionally injected into unresponsive, localized dermatoses such as alopecia areata, granuloma annulare, discoid lupus erythematosus, psoriasis, and lichen simplex chronicus. Several types of steroids are used for this purpose, varying in their duration of action. Triamcinolone acetonide is the most widely used, and its maximal duration of action is 4 to 6 weeks. Triamcinolone hexacetonide is longer acting (6 to 8 weeks); injectables of shorter duration (2 to 4 weeks) include Celestone and Decadron. The steroids should be diluted to less than 5 mg per milliliter to avoid the risk of causing significant skin atrophy. Since intralesional steroid preparations are crystalline and dissolve in the tissues very slowly over weeks to months, great care is necessary in using low concentrations and in shaking the diluted material just prior to injecting into the dermis to avoid the often disfiguring side effects of atrophy that can occur if precipitates settle in the solution.

Topical Antibiotics. These are used to help suppress bacteria in erosions or superficial infections and occasionally in chronic leg ulcers. Silver sulfadiazine preparations are particularly useful as an adjunct to currently accepted principles of burn wound care. The commonly used topical antibiotics are bacitracin, neomycin, clindamycin phosphate, erythromycin, and tetracycline hydrochloride. The latter three are used to treat acne vulgaris. All topical antibiotics have the potential to sensitize, but neomycin is particularly prone to do so, especially after long-term use on chronic stasis dermatitis and leg ulcers. Mupirocin, a new topical antibiotic ointment, is particularly useful in treating staphylococcal and streptococcal infections of the skin; when used three times a day for a week it eliminates 87 per cent of skin pathogens and may decrease nasal staphylococcus carriers.

Topical Antifungal Agents. Antifungals are used to treat localized infections by superficial dermatophytes, *Candida*, and tinea versicolor. Topical broad-spectrum antifungal preparations effective against all of these organisms include clotrimazole, econazole, and miconazole creams and lotions used two times a day. Topical agents useful against dermatophytes but not *Candida* include haloprogin and Tinactin. Over-the-counter preparations, perhaps less effective against dermatophytes, are undecylenic acid and Verdefam. No topical preparations are useful against nail infections with these fungal organisms. Nystatin creams, oral suspensions, and vaginal tablets are effective against *Candida* infections in various areas of the body. Ketoconazole is a broad-spectrum imidazole antifungal agent highly effective against dermatophytes, *Candida*, and tinea versicolor. It is available in cream and oral forms.

Tars and Anthralin. Crude coal tar is often applied directly to the skin to treat psoriasis. Tars increase the effectiveness of ultraviolet light and reduce the accelerated mitotic rate of keratinocytes in psoriasis. Tars are often incorporated into shampoos for control of seborrheic dermatitis and in bath oils for use in psoriasis.

Anthralin is a synthetic coal tar derivative that is used in the treatment of psoriasis. Both tar and anthralin cause staining of clothing and skin. They can also be irritating. Anthralin must be started at the lowest concentrations (0.1 per cent) and initially left on the skin for short periods of time (0.5 hour) to avoid irritation.

Antiparasitic Topical Medications. Antiparasitics are employed for the treatment of pediculosis capitis, pediculosis pubis, and scabies. The lice of pediculosis corporis live in the seams of clothes and bedding. These must be disinfected by washing or dry cleaning. One per cent gamma benzene hexachloride (lindane), cromatiton, and pyrethrin compounds (RID) all are useful in treating pediculosis and scabies. Lindane is not suggested for children less than 6 years of age or for pregnant or lactating women.

Sunscreens. Sunscreens help protect the skin from the acute and chronic effects of UV radiation. They are rated by their sun protective factor (SPF). The SPF, which ranges from 3 to 50, is the factor by which the product extends the period of exposure to reach the sunburn reaction that would have taken place without the sunscreen. The action of topical photoprotectives is to reduce penetration of photoactive nonionizing radiation. Such protection can be achieved by either absorbing or reflecting the radiation. No sunscreen enhances tanning. Rather, if partial block is achieved, it permits melanin production relative to the radiation transmitted and the inherent capacity of the partially protected skin to respond. Most sunscreens are less effective in blocking UVA (320 to 400 nm) than UVB (290 to 320 nm). Para-aminobenzoic acid and its esters protect the skin from UVB and allow UVA to pass. Other non-PABA chemical sunscreens such as benzophenones and cinnamates are also useful against UVB and, to some extent, UVA. If protection against UVA is required, a sunscreen containing benzophenones or anthranilate compounds should be sought. For complete protection or total blockade of UVB and UVA, physical sunscreens containing titanium dioxide, zinc oxide, or iron oxide are available as heavy creams or pastes that reflect ultraviolet light.

SYSTEMIC MODES OF THERAPY FOR DERMATOLOGIC CONDITIONS

ANTIHISTAMINES. By occupying histamine-receptor sites on various cell membranes, antihistamines interfere with one or more of the actions of histamine. Their most specific use is in the control of allergic disorders mediated by histamine, such as urticaria, angioedema, and allergic rhinitis. Non–histamine-induced itching is also suppressed by antihistamines by virtue of their sedative, soporific side effects. Antihistamines are of two major classes, the classic H_1 blockers and the newer H_2 blockers, which also decrease gastric acid secretion. H_1 blockers have three problems: (1) They don't block all the effects of histamine. (2) They provide only limited protection against anaphylaxis because mediators other than histamine are involved in this reaction. (3) They are not selective in their effects (i.e., they also have anticholinergic and sedative effects). Antihistamines (H_1 blockers) can be arranged into several groups depending on their molecular configurations (Table 524–3).

An effective agent for a given patient may be selected from one group or from a combination of groups, but its effects are

TABLE 524–3. ANTIHISTAMINES ARRANGED ACCORDING TO THEIR MOLECULAR CONFIGURATIONS

Antihistamine Group	Generic Name (Proprietary Name)
H_1 receptor antagonists	
Ethanolamines	Diphenhydramine (Benadryl)
	Bromodiphenhydramine (Ambenyl)
	Clemastine (Tavist)
Piperidines	Cyproheptadine (Periactin)
	Azatadine (Optimine)
Phenothiazines	Promethazine (Phenergan)
	Trimeprazine (Temaril)
Alkylamines	Chlorpheniramine (Chlortrimeton)
	Dexchlorpheniramine (Dimetane)
Ethylenediamines	Tripelennamine (Pyribenzamine, PBZ)
	Pyrilamine (Neoantergan)
Piperazines	Hydroxyzine (Atarax)
	Meclizine (Bonamine)
Miscellaneous H_1 receptor antagonists	
Tricyclic compounds	Doxepin (Sinequan)
H_2 receptor antagonists	Cimetidine (Tagamet)
	Ranitidine (Zantac)

unlikely to be enhanced by combining antihistamines within a given group. If response to one antihistamine is minimal, another from a different group should be added or substituted. Evidence that blood vessels in human skin have H_2 as well as H_1 receptors has led to the evaluation of H_2-receptor antagonists such as cimetidine in combination with an H_1 antagonist, and the combination has proved to be effective in the treatment of some cases of chronic urticaria otherwise unresponsive to H_1 antagonists.

Antihistamines should be started in moderate doses until sufficient improvement occurs or until troublesome side effects develop. Generally, they are administered three or four times a day. Low doses should be given to elderly patients, as they are unusually sensitive to central nervous system side effects such as confusion, dizziness, and syncope, as well as to urinary retention, dry mouth, and blurred vision. In children, paradoxically, antihistamines may induce hyperactivity.

SYSTEMIC STEROIDS. Systemic steroids are used for a number of dermatologic conditions, but they have several drawbacks: (1) Prolonged administration leads to adrenal suppression and susceptibility to infection. (2) Many diseases such as psoriasis and atopic dermatitis may worsen after steroid withdrawal. (3) Safer and simpler therapy is available for most common dermatoses. Systemic corticosteroids are used in three types of situations. First, patients severely ill with life-threatening diseases known to be responsive to corticosteroids (anaphylactic reactions, extensive erythema multiforme, acute exfoliative dermatitis, pemphigus vulgaris) are initially given high doses—80 to 100 mg daily. Second, patients with conditions that are acute and severe but self-limited are treated with steroids to control or suppress the condition during a predicted period of activity. Examples include widespread poison ivy dermatitis, extensive sunburn, and acute generalized urticaria of known cause. Intermediate doses of 60 to 80 mg of prednisone daily are used initially and then tapered over 1 to 2 weeks. Third, steroids are used for patients with chronic dermatologic conditions that, because of periodic exacerbations, intermittently require low doses (15 to 20 mg) of prednisone together with supportive topical therapy. Examples include flares of chronic atopic dermatitis, pemphigoid, and some connective tissue diseases.

SYSTEMIC ANTIFUNGAL AGENTS. Two systemic agents are available for superficial fungal infections: griseofulvin and ketoconazole. *Griseofulvin* is active against dermatophytes but not against tinea versicolor or *Candida*. It is fungistatic, entering the horny layer of the skin via the sweat and the nails by incorporation into the keratinizing cells at the nail matrix. The entire nail must grow out with the griseofulvin incorporated into it before tinea at the distal end of the nail is affected. It is for this reason that griseofulvin must be given for many months before dermatophytic infections of the toenails are cleared. Less time is required for infections of fingernails and glabrous skin.

TABLE 524–4. SUGGESTED DOSAGE AND LENGTH OF TREATMENT WITH GRISEOFULVIN FOR DERMATOPHYTE INFECTIONS

Region of Dermatophyte Infection	Dose of Griseofulvin Ultrafine	Length of Treatment
Extensive or resistant tinea corporis	500 mg b.i.d.	30 days
Tinea pedis	500 mg b.i.d.	2–4 months
Onychomycosis		
fingernails	500 mg b.i.d.	4–6 months
toenails	500 mg b.i.d.	12–18 months, but frequently cannot clear toenail involvement
Tinea capitis	500 mg b.i.d.	4–6 weeks

Griseofulvin is the treatment of choice for tinea capitis, onychomycosis, and tinea corporis too extensive for topical therapy and for superficial fungal infections in immunosuppressed patients (Table 524–4).

Ketoconazole, a broad-spectrum imidazole antifungal agent, is effective against dermatophytes and, unlike griseofulvin, also against tinea versicolor and *Candida*. Several instances of anaphylactic reactions to ketoconazole have been recorded, as well as fatal hepatocellular toxicity, so ketoconazole should be used only for extensive cutaneous or systemic *Candida* infections and extensive dermatophyte infections unresponsive to griseofulvin. Liver enzyme levels should be determined before starting treatment and monitored at monthly intervals during treatment.

RETINOIDS. Retinoids are derivatives of natural vitamin A compounds. Two retinoids, isotretinoin and etretinate, are available for use in the treatment of dermatologic conditions. Retinoids decrease epidermal cell proliferation and keratinization and inhibit sebaceous gland activity. Etretinate has been found to be useful in severe psoriasis, especially the erythrodermic and pustular forms, as well as in several forms of ichthyosis. Isotretinoin has proved to be especially useful in severe cystic acne, often inducing prolonged remissions for several years after the drug is given for the usual 3- to 4-month course. The retinoids have many side effects, including cheilitis, conjunctivitis, dryness and fragility of skin, congenital malformations (heart defects, hydrocephalus, microtia), osteophytic growths on the vertebrae, epiphyseal closure in growing youngsters, corneal opacities, night blindness, and elevations of very low density and low density lipoproteins.

SYSTEMIC GOLD SALTS. Chrysotherapy has been useful in the treatment of autoimmune bullous disease, particularly pemphigus vulgaris. Intramuscular compounds have been used in the same manner as in rheumatoid arthritis. Remissions with a mean duration of 21 months or longer have been obtained in some patients with these bullous diseases. Generally a total dose of 400 to 600 mg of gold must be given before bullae respond.

SYSTEMIC ANTIBIOTICS. These are frequently used to treat cutaneous bacterial infections and conditions aggravated by bacterial overgrowth such as acne vulgaris, acne rosacea, and acute dermatitis. Because most bacterial infections of the skin involve *Staphylococcus aureus* or *Streptococcus pyogenes* (erysipelas, cellulitis, folliculitis, furunculosis, carbunculosis), the penicillins, cephalosporins, and erythromycins are commonly used in treating these conditions. In addition, erythromycin and tetracyclines are effective in controlling acne vulgaris and acne rosacea. Trimethoprim-sulfamethoxazole is used for pyodermas in patients allergic to penicillin, for pyodermas caused by methicillin-resistant *S. aureus*, as an alternative therapy for gonorrhea, and occasionally for the treatment of acne vulgaris. The sulfone antibiotic dapsone is occasionally used successfully in treating noninfectious diseases such as dermatitis herpetiformis, pyoderma gangrenosum, and leukocytoclastic cutaneous vasculitis. How dapsone brings about improvement in these conditions is not known.

ANTIMALARIALS. Chloroquine, hydroxychloroquine, and quinacrine are beneficial for cutaneous lupus erythematosus, polymorphic light eruption, solar urticaria, and porphyria cutanea tarda. Antimalarials bind DNA, inhibit the LE cell phenomenon and antinuclear antibody reactions, block chemotaxis, and antag-

onize histaminic responses, all of which may be related to the therapeutic effects on the diseases mentioned above. Cutaneous and mucous membrane pigmentation, nausea, diarrhea, and cycloplegia are common toxic effects, but retinopathy is the adverse reaction of greatest concern. Quinacrine does not cause retinopathy.

SYSTEMIC ANTIVIRAL AGENTS. Acyclovir and vidarabine are used for treating herpes simplex and zoster skin and systemic infections. These drugs can be given intravenously, and acyclovir is also administered orally. Intravenous acyclovir is used in severe primary genital herpes simplex, in neonatal herpes simplex, and in cutaneous herpes simplex and zoster infections in immunosuppressed patients. Oral acyclovir is also effective in primary and recurrent genital herpes simplex and eczema herpeticum. The usual oral dose is 200 mg five times a day for 5 to 10 days; IV acyclovir is usually given at a dose of 15 mg per kilogram per day. Oral acyclovir is also effective in herpes zoster infections, but higher doses are required—800 mg 5 times a day orally for 10 days. Acyclovir is activated to acyclovir monophosphate by herpes simplex virus–coded thymidine kinase; the monophosphate is further phosphorylated to acyclovir triphosphate, which inhibits viral DNA synthesis. This antiviral agent is thus selectively activated only by virus-infected cells with little disruption of host cellular metabolism. This accounts for the low incidence of side effects. Acyclovir ointment is also available for mild primary genital and labial infections and for localized, chronic cutaneous lesions in immunosuppressed patients.

SYSTEMIC CYTOSTATIC DRUGS. Cytotoxic drugs such as methotrexate, cyclophosphamide, azathioprine, and hydroxyurea are used in a number of skin conditions when they cannot be controlled by more conventional means. Thus, psoriasis, when it is generalized, severe, and life-ruining, may be treated with modest doses of methotrexate, azathioprine, or hydroxyurea; life-threatening bullous diseases such as pemphigus vulgaris are occasionally treated with these agents as an alternative to high doses of corticosteroids.

ULTRAVIOLET LIGHT AS A THERAPEUTIC AGENT. UV phototherapy is used primarily in patients with psoriasis and vitiligo, but it may also help patients with nummular and atopic eczema, pityriasis rosea, the pruritus of uremia, and mycosis fungoides. UV light units are available in two wavelength ranges, UVB (the sunburn range of 280 to 320 nm) and UVA (long wavelength spectrum of 320 to 400 nm). The use of topical tar preparations, which "photosensitize" the skin to UVB wavelengths, adds to the effectiveness of treatment (the so-called Goeckerman regimen). This method used over many weeks to months is highly effective in controlling psoriasis.

UVA light units are employed by dermatologists (and also commercial suntan centers) to cause tanning rather than burning. The ability of UVA to evoke a sunburn is 1000 times less than that of UVB. The primary use of UVA is in the treatment of severe, extensive psoriasis and vitiligo, for which it is used in combination with topical or oral psoralen, a drug that binds to DNA in the skin and sensitizes it to the effects of UVA. The combination of psoralen with UVA light is called PUVA. The long-term side effects of PUVA therapy are unknown, although it seems to induce squamous and basal cell cutaneous carcinomas. The unprotected cornea and retina can be damaged by UV light, especially PUVA. Stringent guidelines for protecting the eyes, such as wearing special protective eye glasses for 24 to 48 hours after taking the psoralens as well as regular eye examinations, must be observed.

Shelley WB, Shelley GD: Advanced Dermatologic Therapy. Philadelphia, W.B. Saunders Company, 1987.

525 Skin Diseases of General Importance

In Chapter 523, an approach to diagnosing skin diseases was discussed in which the specific morphologic descriptions of primary and secondary skin lesions are used to place the condition into one of nine large diagnostic groups. These nine groups, encompassing the majority of skin diseases, are listed in Table 523–1. In this chapter, some of the diseases in each of these groups are discussed, providing the clinician with a differential diagnosis of conditions within each group. As stressed in Ch. 523, the differential diagnosis within each major group depends on such things as variations in distribution; specific location and symmetry of lesions; and shape, arrangement, color, and texture of lesions.

THE ECZEMAS (DERMATITIS)

The term *eczema* is derived from the Greek word that means "to boil out," a reference to the fact that eczematous reactions may be vesicular and oozing. Eczematous dermatitis is an inflammatory response of the skin to multiple exogenous and endogenous agents, although often the etiology is not clear. Eczemas are defined by their clinical appearance and are subdivided either by their pattern of distribution or by etiologic factors (when known). Many eczematous processes are related to immunologic reactions (Table 525–1).

The term *eczema* or *eczematous dermatitis* is applied to eruptions characterized histologically by epidermal intercellular edema, termed *spongiosis*. Eczemas can be acute, with marked spongiosis causing red papules and vesicles and oozing, weeping, and crusting, or they may be chronic, with redness, scaling, fissuring, and especially lichenification. Indeed, both acute and chronic forms of eczema may be seen in the same patient, with the acute reaction progressing to oozing and crusting; with

continued pruritus, the patient's rubbing and scratching converts the eczema to the chronic, dry, lichenified form. The hallmarks, then, of all types of eczematous dermatitis are (1) marked pruritus and (2) varying degrees of erythema along with papules, vesicles, fine scaling, or lichenification.

A number of the eczematous processes are listed in Table 525–1, along with some useful diagnostic findings that help to differentiate one from another. Histology of various types of eczemas is the same; skin biopsies identify a lesion as an eczematous reaction, but it does not differentiate among the various types of eczema.

CONTACT DERMATITIS. Contact dermatitis is the best understood cause of eczematous reactions and potentially the most correctable. For any eczematous rash, the clinician should first determine whether it could be a contact reaction. If the cause can be identified, avoidance of the offending substance will be curative. There are two types of contact dermatitis, *irritant* and *allergic*. Irritant contact dermatitis is produced by substances that simply irritate or have a direct toxic effect on the skin, such as acids, alkalis, solvents, and detergents; no immunologic process is involved. Allergic contact dermatitis, on the other hand, is a delayed-type hypersensitivity reaction that occurs in response to a wide variety of allergens commonly found in the environment. The allergens consist of small molecular weight substances that act as haptens and bind to proteinaceous components of the skin to form the sensitizing antigen. The antigen is processed by

TABLE 525–1. ECZEMATOUS DERMATITIS SKIN ERUPTIONS

Clinical Type	Etiology or Suspected Cause	Distinctive Diagnostic Findings
Eczemas with Known Causes		
Contact dermatitis		
Irritant contact	Chemical agents that have direct toxic effects on skin	Contact precedes rash by hours to days
Allergic contact	Chemical agents that elicit type IV delayed hypersensitivity reaction on skin	Contact precedes rash by 2 or more days; in both instances site and configuration of eczema reaction conforms to site of contact with exogenous substances (plants, medicaments, cosmetics, metals); patch tests
Photodermatitis	Ultraviolet light exposure plus topical or systemic substances induce type IV delayed hypersensitivity	Eczematous reaction in sun-exposed areas of skin with sharp "cut off" borders, i.e., face, ears, V of neck, dorsum of hands, extensor surfaces of arms
Eczematous drug-induced reaction	Drugs such as penicillin taken internally	Generalized eczema reaction evolves after taking medications (usually 10 or more days after first beginning drug; sooner if previously exposed) and clears with stopping drugs
Dermatophyte and *Candida* eczematous reactions	Dermatophytes and *Candida* induce eczematous inflammatory reaction	Dermatophyte or yeast found in scales or exudate
Infectious eczematoid dermatitis	Products from draining infected skin areas induce eczema reaction—linear infections, leg ulcers	Occurs near site of infection or other draining lesion; clears with treatment of infection
Dermatophytid	Hypersensitivity reaction occurring on distant areas of skin in response to products from fungal infection of other areas of skin	Often vesicular eruption of palms or fingers with dermatophyte infection of feet
Autosensitization	Hypersensitivity reaction to cutaneous or bacterial antigens released from area of acute dermatitis	Generalized dermatitis following localized acute dermatitis
Xerotic eczema or eczema craquelé	Dry skin or xerosis	Can lead to redness and fissuring of skin that appear as cracks in dried mud
Eczemas with Unknown or Unclear Etiologies		
Atopic eczema	Hereditary disposition in association with familial tendency for asthma and allergic rhinitis	Eczematous reaction often localized to face, neck, antecubital, and popliteal areas
Stasis dermatitis	Chronic venous insufficiency	Associated with varicosities, leg edema, hyperpigmentation, and ulcers
Lichen simplex chronicus (neurodermatitis)	Repeated scratching leads to eczema	Lichenified patches in areas within reach of fingers (nape of neck, lower legs)
Nummular eczema	Dry skin, underlying infections	Coin-shaped patches on extensor areas of extremities and trunk
Seborrheic dermatitis	Occurs in areas of high concentrations of sebaceous glands; may be related to intrinsic yeast in skin (*Pityrosporon ovale*)	Inflammatory, yellow, greasy, scaling patches on scalp, retroauricular areas, eyebrows, nasolabial fold, and presternal areas
Dyshidrotic eczema	Emotional stress—unrelated to disturbances in sweating	Pruritic vesicles on palms, soles
Nonspecific eczematous dermatitis	No obvious cause—diagnosis of exclusion after above eczemas ruled out	Acute and chronic eczema patches anywhere on body; severe itching

Langerhans' cells in the epidermis (see Ch. 521), which then present the antigen to T lymphocytes to elicit sensitization. Sensitization to the allergen requires 10 to 14 days to develop after the first encounter; subsequent exposure to the allergen elicits the eczematous response in 1 to 7 days (delayed hypersensitivity).

The onset of irritant reactions after exposure to the topical substance is variable. Skin damage is evident within hours after contact with a strong irritant. Weaker irritants may require multiple applications and days or weeks before the development of the eczema (e.g., housewife's eczema of the hands due to chronic exposure to water and detergents). Contact dermatitis accounts for more than 50 per cent of all occupational illnesses (excluding injury). In the industrial setting, approximately 70 per cent is irritant and 30 per cent allergic contact dermatitis.

Both irritant and allergic contact eczemas are initially confined to sites of contact, and therefore unique patterns of distribution and configuration suggest contact dermatitis as well as provide clues to the contactant. Thus, allergic reactions to plants, such as poison oak or ivy, appear as linear, red, papular and vesicular streaks where the plant brushes across the skin. Allergies to metals (especially nickel) cause eczematous reactions under rings or watchbands or on the lobes of ears (earrings). Dermatitis under a ring may also stem from trapped water and irritating soap residues.

The most common allergens causing allergic contact dermatitis are pentadecylcatechol (allergen in poison oak, ivy, and sumac as well as in cashews, mangos, and ginkgo trees), paraphenylenediamine (a substance in hair dyes which cross-reacts with benzocaine and hydrochlorothiazide), nickel, mercaptobenzothiazol and thiuram (components in rubber), and ethylenediamine (a preservative in many medications and also found in industrial dyes and insecticides). Other common sources of contactants include topical medications (neomycin, anesthetics such as benzocaine, topical antihistamines), preservatives (ethylenediamine, merthiolate, parabens), vehicles (propylene glycol), and cosmetics (fragrances, preservatives, paraphenylenediamines). It is obvious that a detailed history of the patient's occupation, hobbies, habits, clothing, cosmetics, and medications applied to the skin is necessary to find the contactant. Careful detective work on the part of the physician and the patient often brings to light the etiologic factor. One must not overlook the possibility that a topical medicine is perpetuating or exacerbating a pre-existing dermatitis.

There is no standard testing method available for diagnosing irritant contact dermatitis. For allergic contact eczema, the causative agent can be identified by patch tests, but these must be properly performed and interpreted by trained dermatologists.

Therapy of contact dermatitis is avoidance of the irritant or allergen if possible. This may require a change in lifestyle or occupation. Sometimes protective clothing is curative. Barrier creams are of little benefit. Acute, severe generalized contact dermatitis is treated with a short (10- to 14-day) course of systemic steroids and wet dressings or baths. Milder eczematous reactions respond to topical steroids and systemic antihistamines.

PHOTODERMATITIS. A variety of skin reactions, termed photosensitivity reactions, may occur in response to exposure to ultraviolet light. Some appear as eczematous reactions, so-called photoallergic dermatitis, which may occur in response to topical as well as systemic substances in the presence of UV light. The distribution of the eczematous eruption in light-exposed areas is an important feature in the differential diagnosis, with the cheeks, nose, forehead, and tips of ears as sites of predilection. The backs of hands and forearms are also frequently involved and, of course, the history of exposure to UV light prior to the onset of the reaction is important in identifying light sensitivity (see Fig. 523–2).

Photoallergic dermatitis is immunologic. Absorption of a specific wavelength of ultraviolet light by a topical substance or a systemic drug (which is deposited in the skin from the cutaneous circulation) causes chemical conversion of the substance or drug to a hapten that binds cutaneous proteins to become a complete antigen capable of eliciting a type IV delayed hypersensitivity reaction similar to an allergic contact dermatitis reaction. Photoallergic reactions appear only where the UV light hits the skin,

even though the systemic drug or topical photoallergen is present in the skin all over the body; i.e., the reaction depends on UV light hitting the skin with the allergen in it. Long wavelength UVA light is usually responsible for these reactions. UVA light penetrates window glass (UVB light is blocked by glass), so the reaction often occurs even though the patient remains indoors. Such drugs as thiazides and phenothiazines can cause photoeczematous reactions; a number of topically applied substances, such as methylcoumarin, musk ambrette, halogenated salicylanilids, and topical sunscreening agents, can cause a similar reaction. Photopatch testing can identify substances in materials causing these reactions. Avoidance of the offending material is often curative. Oral or topical steroids relieve the inflammatory reaction.

ATOPIC DERMATITIS. This chronic, eczematous condition of the skin is often associated with a personal or family history of atopic disease (asthma, allergic rhinitis, and atopic eczema). Pruritus is a prominent symptom, and the consequent scratching and rubbing lead to lichenification, most typically in the antecubital and popliteal flexural areas. The eczema usually manifests itself after the first few months of life, appearing on the face and extensor areas of the extremities as acute and subacute, red, vesicular and oozing dermatitis. Many cases resolve spontaneously by puberty only to recur in adolescence and adulthood as a chronic dermatitis with scaling, dryness, and lichenification over the face, neck, upper chest, and characteristically the antecubital and popliteal fossae (flexural dermatitis). Atopics have a readily identifiable facies with diffuse erythema, perioral pallor, and a redundant crease or fold below the lower eyelids (Dennie-Morgan fold). The palms often have an increased number of skin markings, noticeable as fine cross-hatched lines. Stroking the skin in atopic dermatitis causes a white line, or dermatographism, probably due to dermal edema and vasoconstriction.

The exact cause of atopic dermatitis is not known, but a number of immunologic and pharmacologic abnormalities are seen in association with the skin condition. For example, IgE reaginic antibodies are increased in 80 per cent of atopic patients, especially those with extensive skin disease (and such patients respond to many antigens applied by skin prick testing), but these antibodies seem to play no definitive role in *causing* atopic eczema. Avoiding antigens to which these patients react by scratch test does not improve the eczema. Patients with atopic eczema also have depressed cell-mediated immunity, with deficient T suppressor cells. This may account for the overproduction of IgE, resulting in unusual susceptibility to cutaneous herpes simplex, vaccina, molluscum contagiosum, and wart infections. Neutrophil and monocyte chemotaxis is reduced during exacerbations of eczema, explaining the frequent staphylococcal skin infections in these patients. Treatment with oral antibiotics to reduce staphylococcal flora (or overt staphylococcal infections such as folliculitis, furuncles, or cellulitis) often results in marked improvement in the eczema.

Atopic individuals are often tense, resentful, aggressive, and restless, but it is not clear whether this is a basic characteristic of the diathesis or the result of living with chronic, unremitting itching and skin inflammation. Whether these personality traits are primary or secondary, the physician must help the patient meet the stresses of life.

Keratoconjunctivitis and stellate anterior subcapsular cataracts are associated with atopic eczema, particularly in patients with extensive skin changes. The conjunctivitis and keratitis usually start in childhood. The cataracts may also begin at a young age and form rapidly, often by age 20. Keratoconus is seen in 25 per cent of atopics.

The treatment of atopic dermatitis is the same as for other eczematous eruptions and includes topical steroids, emollients, and systemic antihistamines. In some children (less than 2 years of age) food allergy can cause atopic dermatitis, but dietary factors remain controversial. Skin tests or RAST tests help identify which foods may be responsible. Positive results must be confirmed with controlled food challenges and elimination diets. Allergic immediate skin testing and desensitization have been of little value in atopic dermatitis.

Skin irritation must be avoided by wearing soft cotton clothing. Counseling, psychotherapy, and stress reduction may sometimes be helpful. Patients often worsen during the autumn and winter seasons when decreased humidity in homes associated with the use of central heating causes increased skin dryness and itching. The frequent use of emollients is the best treatment for skin dryness, especially immediately after bathing when the skin is hydrated. Topical corticosteroids are the most important means of controlling the inflammatory response, and the least potent forms should be utilized, usually in an ointment base. Systemic steroids should be used only in short courses to overcome exacerbations not controlled by topical steroids.

STASIS DERMATITIS. This is an eczematous eruption of the lower legs secondary to peripheral venous insufficiency. Venous incompetence causes increased hydrostatic pressure and capillary damage with extravasation of red blood cells and serum. These conditions seem to trigger an inflammatory, brawny, edematous, red, and hyperpigmented petechial scaling or weeping reaction, usually around the medial malleolus or distal one third of the lower leg. Secondary allergic contact dermatitis frequently complicates this problem when neomycin is used chronically to treat accompanying stasis ulcers. The cornerstone of managing stasis dermatitis is prevention of venous stasis and edema with the use of supportive hose while the patient is ambulatory. Weight reduction is helpful in obese patients. The eczema is treated with topical steroids and wet compresses when oozing and crusting are present. Occasionally chronic stasis dermatitis, when secondarily infected, can undergo exacerbation with spread of the acute inflammation to distant areas of the body, a condition known as *autosensitization dermatitis*. These secondary eczematous patches evolve on the face, neck, and extensor areas of the extremities. Control is achieved with topical steroids (occasionally oral steroids if the reaction is severe) and antibiotics to control the cutaneous infection.

NUMMULAR ECZEMATOUS DERMATITIS. This condition is defined by coin-shaped patches predominantly on the extensor surfaces of the arms and legs, but the trunk is often involved as well. Lesions appear as patches of minute vesicles and papules that spread to become scaling and thickened, occasionally clearing in the center so that they may resemble superficial fungal infections. Mild to severe pruritus accompanies the eczematous patches. Although the cause is unknown, many factors acting alone or in combination may play a role. Dry skin is a frequent accompaniment, and the disease reaches a peak in the winter months. Irritating substances such as wool and soap and frequent bathing may also contribute to the condition. The combination of topical steroids (usually of intermediate potency), 3 per cent crude coal tar, and ultraviolet light treatments is helpful in controlling this form of eczema. The condition tends to persist with remissions and recurrences.

LICHEN SIMPLEX CHRONICUS. Also known as neurodermatitis, this is a chronic, pruritic, lichenified eczematous eruption that results from constant scratching. Pruritus often precedes the scratching, and rubbing induces lichenification, initiating a vicious circle of itch-scratch-itch. In most patients it is a nervous habit. Patches of neurodermatitis commonly are found on the nape of the neck, lower legs, groin, or other regions of the body within easy reach of the hands. Occasionally constant scratching results in scaling, thickened, excoriated papules and nodules (prurigo nodularis). Treatment consists of explaining to the patient the cause and the need to stop rubbing. Topical steroids and antihistamines may also be helpful, and steroids injected into the lesion will break the itching cycle more successfully than topically applied steroids.

SEBORRHEIC DERMATITIS. Seborrheic dermatitis is characterized by erythematous, eczematous patches with yellow, greasy scales localized to hairy areas and regions of the skin with high concentrations of sebaceous glands, especially the middle of the face, nasolabial folds, eyebrows, ear canals, retroauricular folds, and presternal areas. Dandruff is scaling of the scalp without inflammation. In severe cases the axillae and groin regions can also be involved. Seborrheic dermatitis may appear in infants until about 6 months of age ("cradle cap"); after that it does not appear until after puberty. Patients with neurologic disorders, such as Parkinson's disease or stroke, may have a dramatic flare of their seborrhea. Although the precise cause of seborrhea is unknown, the exacerbations associated with emotional stress and neurologic disease suggest a role of the central nervous system. Some studies suggest that the condition is related to excessive growth of yeast organisms (*Pityrosporum*) on the skin. It is sometimes difficult to differentiate seborrhea from psoriasis when the latter is localized to the scalp, ears, and face.

Antiseborrheic shampoos containing tar, sulfur, salicylic acid, selenium sulfide, or zinc pyrithione are the most useful form of treatment. The shampoo should be used daily, rubbed into the scalp and left on for 5 minutes before rinsing. Inflammatory seborrhea that does not respond to shampoos alone will benefit from a topical steroid lotion or gel in hairy areas and hydrocortisone cream for facial glabrous skin. Continual use of shampoo and topical steroids is required to control this chronic dermatitis. The use of topical or oral antiyeast medication, ketoconazole, may be of help in controlling seborrhea in some patients.

XEROTIC ECZEMA AND ECZEMA CRAQUELÉ. These conditions are characterized by chapping and symptomatic dryness that may lead to visible fissuring through the stratum corneum, giving criss-crossing cracks that resemble dried mud. Such changes occur most commonly in winter, and they respond to the frequent use of emollients and/or hydrocortisone ointments.

HAND ECZEMA. Hand eczema is most common in housewives, cooks, food handlers, and medical personnel. The most common etiologic factors are constant exposure to mild primary irritants (soap, water), frequent hand washing, atopy, and nummular dermatitis. Allergic contact dermatitis may be another cause. *Dyshidrotic eczema* (pompholyx), a relatively noninflammatory, recurrent, pruritic, vesicular eruption of the palms and soles of unknown etiology, differs from other hand eczemas in that the primary involvement is on the palm instead of the dorsum of the hands. The term *dyshidrotic eczema* suggests malfunction of the sweat ducts, but this is a misnomer. Pompholyx, from the Greek meaning bubble, is a more apt term. Emotional stress tends to be a trigger. Vesicles on the palms can also represent *dermatophytid*, an allergic reaction to a dermatophyte infection on the feet. If potassium hydroxide (KOH) examination of the feet is positive, treatment of the fungus will clear up the palmar reaction as well.

Treatment of hand dermatitis involves avoidance of primary irritants such as soap, solvents, detergents, and frequent exposure to water. The use of cotton gloves with rubber gloves over them is useful in protecting the hands in water. Topical steroids and emollients are also beneficial, and potent topical steroids are often required.

EXFOLIATIVE DERMATITIS (ERYTHRODERMA). Total body cutaneous erythema, edema, scaling, and fissuring may occur as an idiopathic entity without preceding dermatologic or systemic disease, or it may be the result of a variety of cutaneous diseases (atopic or contact dermatitis, psoriasis, seborrheic dermatitis, autosensitization, pityriasis rubra pilaris) or systemic disorders (mycosis fungoides, lymphomas, leukemias) as well as a reaction to a number of drugs (antibiotics, barbiturates, antiepileptic agents, gold) (Fig. 525–1). Other organ systems are affected by the general erythroderma and changes in the stratum corneum barrier function. For example, the diffuse redness and warmth of the skin reflect vasodilation and increased blood flow through the immense cutaneous vasculature. Blood flow may be increased 100-fold in erythroderma, and 5 to 8 per cent of the total cardiac output may be directed to the dilated, inflamed, cutaneous vasculature. This has two consequences. First, a compensatory increase in cardiac output occurs. In older individuals with underlying cardiac disease, heart failure may ensue. The second consequence is defective thermoregulation. Increased heat loss leads to decreased core temperature, shivering, and swings in temperature. When high-output failure occurs and/or thermoregulation is impaired, oral steroids decrease the cutaneous inflammation and correct the abnormalities. In less acute situations total body applications of topical steroids with plastic sauna suit occlusion reverse the erythroderma.

FUNGAL INFECTIONS OF THE SKIN. Fungal infections may be confused with eczematous conditions. These infections include dermatophytosis, candidiasis, and tinea versicolor. *Dermatophytes* are a homogeneous group of fungi that live on the keratin of the stratum corneum, nails, and hair and frequently provoke an inflammatory reaction in the skin with pruritus, redness, scaling, and vesiculation. Three genera of dermatophytes cause these infections: *Trichophyton*, *Microsporum*, and *Epidermophyton*. Dermatophytosis of the trunk (tinea corporis) can be caused by several species (*T. rubrum* and *T. mentagrophytes* are

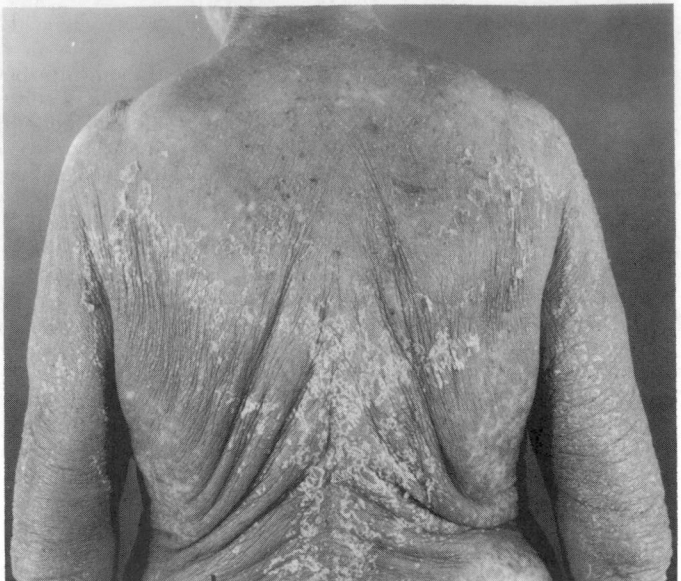

FIGURE 525–1. Exfoliative erythroderma. (From the 17th edition of the Cecil Textbook of Medicine, with permission of Dr. Marie-Louise Johnson.)

most common), resulting in annular inflamed patches with elevated scaling and, at times, vesicular borders with a tendency for central clearing. The eruption may be widespread and may mimic nummular eczema. Very extensive, red, scaling lesions with elevated serpiginous borders may occur in diabetic and immunosuppressed patients. The usual ringworm of the scalp appears as scaling areas of hair loss with black dots indicating breakage of hair shafts. Most infections are now due to *T. tonsurans* or *M. canis*. The latter agent may fluoresce under Wood's light, but this should not be used for diagnosis. Rather, examination with KOH preparations and cultures for fungi should be performed (using plucked hairs and scales from the affected areas in the scalp). Tinea cruris infection in the groin appears as red patches with elevated serpiginous and scaling borders. The scrotum is seldom involved. Erythrasma is still another type of intertriginous erythema caused by a *Corynebacterium* infection. It appears as velvety red patches with fine scale which, under Wood's light examination, fluoresce a diagnostic coral pink color. Erythromycin clears this infection. Tinea of the feet (pedis) and hands (manus) often present together. Infections of the feet appear in three forms: (1) interdigital maceration, scaling, and fissuring (*T. rubrum* and *T. mentagrophytes*); (2) diffuse, dry, scaling and mild erythema of the plantar surface, often extending onto the sides of the feet in a "moccasin" distribution, occasionally associated with dry scaling of one palm ("two foot–one hand syndrome"); (3) vesiculopustular lesions on the insteps of the feet. Involvement of the nails—onychomycosis—often accompanies hand and foot dermatophytosis.

Candidiasis, particularly involvement by *C. albicans* (Fig. 525–2), causes inflammatory skin reactions. Intertriginous moniliasis occurs in the groin, perineum, gluteal folds, inframammary areas, axillae, and digital webs. Typically, the folds become macerated and erythematous with small satellite papules and erosions around the periphery of the main lesion. Obesity, diabetes, and use of antibiotics may play a role in *Candida* infection. Chronic mucocutaneous candidiasis is a rare condition characterized by superficial *Candida* infection of the skin, nails, and oral and genital mucosal surfaces complicating a variety of systemic immunodeficiencies (see Ch. 405). *Tinea versicolor*, a common superficial fungus infection caused by *Pityrosporon orbiculare*, is identified by scaling, red to brown or white, oval patches over the neck, trunk, and upper arms. As the name versicolor implies, the lesions vary in color (Fig. 525–3). During the summer months when the skin is exposed to ultraviolet light, the lesions appear hypopigmented, as the infection prevents the involved skin from forming pigment. Examination of the lesion with KOH reveals budding yeast forms and club-shaped hyphae (Fig. 525–4).

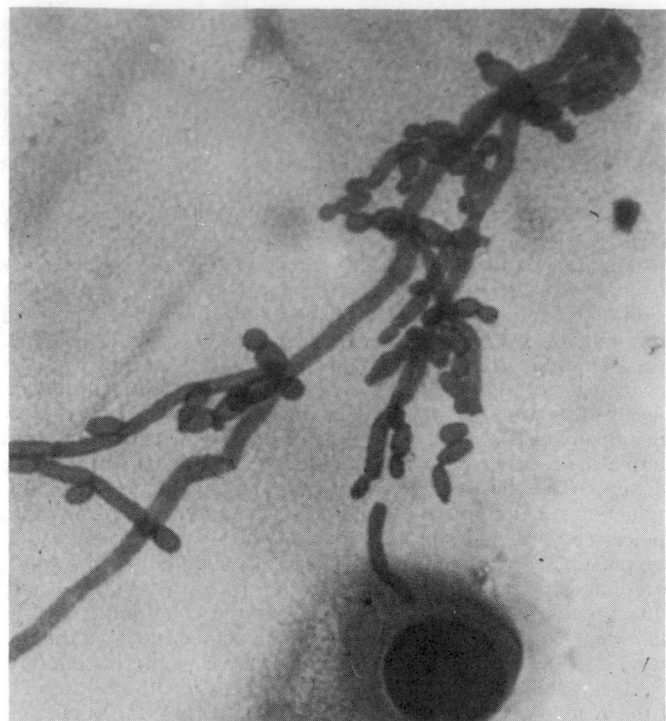

FIGURE 525–2. *Candida albicans.* (From the 17th edition of the Cecil Textbook of Medicine, with the permission of Dr. Marie-Louise Johnson.)

Treatment of fungal infections of the skin can be accomplished with topical or systemic agents. If the dermatophytic or candidal glabrous skin infection is localized, econazole, miconazole, clotrimazole, and ciclopirox creams, ointments, and lotions are effective when applied two to three times a day for 3 to 4 weeks. Tinea versicolor also responds to these agents, but selenium sulfide antidandruff shampoo is less expensive and also effective. Application of the shampoo to the involved areas of skin for 10

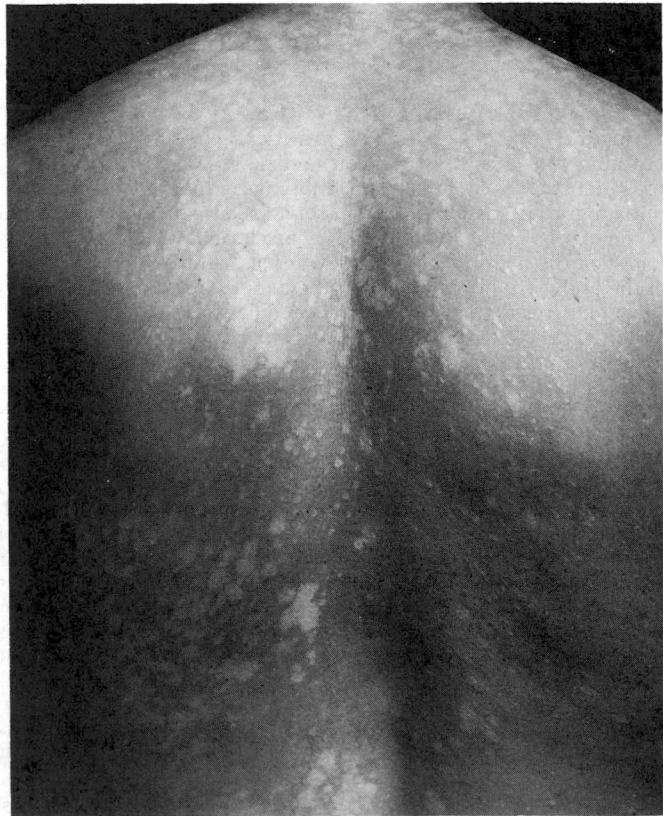

FIGURE 525–3. Tinea versicolor. (From the 17th edition of the Cecil Textbook of Medicine, with the permission of Dr. Marie-Louise Johnson.)

minutes each night for 3 to 4 weeks will clear the disease, although the hypopigmentation will not resolve until the patient is exposed to the sun. Regular shampooing with selenium sulfide reduces reinfection rates. Widespread fungal lesions, or those resistant to topical therapy, may require systemic agents. Griseofulvin is an effective, safe agent and the treatment of choice for dermatophyte infections, but it is not effective for *Candida* infections. The drug must be given for varying periods of time, depending on the site of infection. The micronized form (Ultrafine, U/F) seems to be most consistently effective. Approximately 10 mg per kilogram per day is used in children and 1 gram per day in adults (see Table 524–4).

Ketoconazole is a second oral medication useful for dermatophytes, but it is also effective in *Candida* infections. Because ketoconazole occasionally causes severe liver damage, it should not be used initially for dermatophyte infections. It is useful in mucocutaneous candidiasis at a dose of 200 to 400 mg per day in adults. Because of its toxicity, liver function tests should be performed every 2 to 4 weeks.

MACULOPAPULAR SKIN DISEASES

The rashes included in this group represent diverse cutaneous and systemic conditions characterized by widespread erythematous macules and papules. Some of the conditions also have associated petechiae or purpura (Table 525–2).

VIRAL EXANTHEMS. Because many *viral exanthems* are maculopapular, this group of skin diseases is often termed morbilliform, or measles-like. The clinical appearance of virus-induced erythema is not specific for a given etiologic agent; other signs and symptoms help to suggest a particular viral agent. Most viral exanthems are preceded by a prodrome of fever and constitutional symptoms. A history of previous exposure to infected individuals may be obtained. Incubation times vary from days to weeks depending on the virus. Drug history may also be important, especially with infectious mononucleosis, in which only 3 per cent of patients have a maculopapular or petechial eruption, but with the administration of ampicillin the frequency approaches 100 per cent. In measles (rubeola) and rubella, the erythematous macules and papules begin on the face and spread to the trunk and extremities, fading with desquamation in 6 days in rubeola and on the third day in rubella. The rashes associated with enterovirus infection are most commonly rubella-like but occasionally are purpuric. Exanthem subitum (roseola infantum) displays fleeting, discrete, red papules surrounded by a whitish halo that begins on the trunk and then evolves on the neck. Erythema infectiosum (fifth disease) is an alarming-appearing red, "slapped cheek" rash over the face with reticulate maculopapular lesions on the extremities that clear in 3 to 6 days. Mucous membranes are sometimes involved. In rubella, red spots occur on the soft palate. In measles, Koplik's spots, tiny gray-white papules on an erythematous base, are found on the buccal mucosa opposite the molars. An erythematous, maculopapular rash that begins peripherally on the palms and soles and spreads to the trunk, often with a petechial component, is seen in *atypical measles*. This is a hypersensitivity reaction to wild measles virus in a partially immune host (one who has been vaccinated with killed measles virus).

SCARLETINIFORM ERUPTIONS. Scarlet fever, *Kawasaki's syndrome*, and *toxic shock syndrome* also present with erythematous macular and papular eruptions. Group A streptococcal pharyngitis or tonsillitis with a strain producing erythrogenic toxin initiates a confluent, papular eruption with sandpaper texture that begins on the neck and upper chest and evolves over the abdomen and extremities. The face is flushed, and circumoral pallor is prominent. Extensive desquamation occurs in 4 to 5 days. Punctate redness of the palate is seen in scarlet fever along with strawberry tongue.

Kawasaki's syndrome, a condition of unknown cause, displays a morbilliform or scarletiniform eruption more prominent on the trunk than on the face. Most distinctive are magenta red discolorations of the palms and soles associated with indurative edema of the hands and feet. The skin and extremity changes occur within 3 to 4 days of the onset of fever, along with mucous membrane inflammatory changes consisting of conjunctivitis and strawberry tongue. Palm, sole, and fingertip desquamation occurs 10 to 18 days after the onset of fever. Asymmetric lymphadenopathy, especially in the cervical area, is seen in 75 per cent of patients—hence the name *mucocutaneous lymph node syndrome*. This is a disease of young children and occasionally young adults, and 1 to 2 per cent of these individuals develop coronary aneurysms or myocardial infarction, sometimes fatal.

Toxic shock syndrome is a serious condition arising from toxins elaborated by *Staphylococcus aureus* infections, often in menstruating women using tampons but also in patients with postsurgical infections. The rash is an erythematous, macular, diffuse eruption that blanches readily with pressure followed by desquamation of the affected skin, in association with fever, strawberry tongue, hypotension, vomiting, and renal insufficiency. The rash often spares the skin where clothing fits tightly with pressure on the skin, e.g., waistline where underwear elastic and belt press tightly.

DRUG REACTIONS. The most common forms taken by drug eruptions are hives and morbilliform rashes (Fig. 525–5). The erythematous macules and papules that often become confluent usually begin within a week of initiating the drug. Unfortunately,

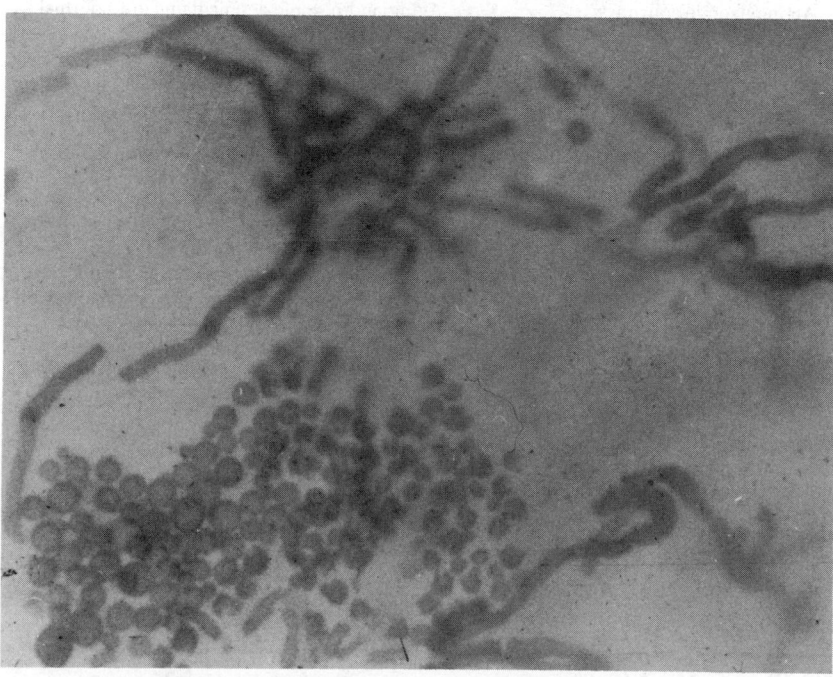

FIGURE 525–4. *Pityrosporon orbiculare.* (From the 17th edition of the Cecil Textbook of Medicine, with the permission of Dr. Marie-Louise Johnson.)

there are no laboratory tests to identify a responsible drug, so heavy reliance must be placed on the history. Often patients are taking several drugs. In trying to select the offending medication from the list, two variables to consider are (1) the temporal relationship between the initiation of the drug and the rash and (2) the odds that a given drug is likely to cause an eruption. Drugs most likely to cause maculopapular eruptions include trimethoprim-sulfamethoxazole, penicillin G, semisynthetic penicillins, ampicillin, quinidine, gentamicin sulfate, and blood products. Itching is common with drug reactions, and fever may occur. It is difficult to differentiate the maculopapular drug rash from viral exanthems except that viral prodromata and viral mucous membrane lesions are lacking in drug rashes (see section on drug reactions at the end of this chapter).

Verruca vulgaris and *molluscum contagiosum* are two examples of viral infections confined to the skin which elicit unique papular lesions. Wart papilloma virus induces various forms of warts: *common warts*, dome-shaped papules with corrugated, hyperkeratotic surfaces; *flat warts*, slightly raised, smooth, flat-topped papules often on the hands and face; *plantar warts*, painful papules on the soles of the feet covered by a thick callus with black puncta within the lesion; *condylomata acuminata*, or veneral warts, soft, moist, sessile, pedunculated and verrucous papules involving the perianal and genital areas. *Molluscum*

contagiosum is caused by a DNA poxvirus that infects epidermal cells to induce smooth, dome-shaped, translucent papules with a central umbilication from which a cheesy core can be expressed. These lesions occur most commonly on the trunk, face, and genitals. The treatment of warts relies on a variety of nonspecific destructive techniques, including liquid nitrogen cryotherapy, salicylic and lactic acid combinations, cantharidin, and podophyllin. Molluscum contagiosum lesions are removed by curettage of the central core, liquid nitrogen freezing, or cantharidin application for short periods of time (30 to 60 minutes).

Purpuric maculopapular skin lesions should cause the physician to consider a different group of conditions (Table 525–2). Purpura, because it represents extravasation of red blood cells outside the cutaneous vessels, cannot be blanched as erythema can. Purpura can be classified as nonpalpable (macular) and palpable (papular). Nonpalpable purpura results from bleeding into the skin without associated inflammation of the vessels and indicates either a bleeding diathesis or blood vessel fragility. Nonpalpable purpura can be *petechial* (macules less than 3 mm) or *ecchymotic* (macules larger than 3 mm). Thrombocytopenia causes petechiae, whereas abnormalities in the blood-clotting cascade commonly cause ecchymoses. Necrotic ecchymoses are found when thrombi form in dermal vessels, leading to infarction and hemorrhage as in disseminated intravascular coagulation (DIC). Palpable purpura results from inflammatory damage to cutaneous blood vessels, the inflammation causing elevated lesions as in vasculitis (see Color Plate 15H).

TABLE 525–2. SOME MACULAR AND PAPULAR SKIN CONDITIONS

Clinical Condition	Etiology	Distinctive Diagnostic Features
Nonpetechial or Nonpurpuric		
Viral exanthem	Hematologic dissemination of virus to skin where vascular response is elicited	Rubella, rubeola—begin on face; mucous membranes often involved—Koplik's spots; palate petechiae rash preceded by fever and prodromata
Scarlet fever	*Streptococcus* erythrogenic toxin	Sore throat preceding rash; bright erythema that feels like sand paper; desquamates; strawberry tongue
Kawasaki's disease	Unknown	Morbilliform or scarletiniform rash; red palms and soles; desquamation of hands and feet 10 to 18 days after fever
Toxic shock syndrome	*Staphylococcus aureus* toxin	Diffuse, maculopapular rash sparing areas where clothing presses on skin; associated with strawberry tongue, fever, vomiting, and renal insufficiency
Drug eruptions	Drugs	Often rash begins proximally and proceeds distally—legs involved last; no prodromata
Verruca vulgaris	Papillomavirus	Corrugated, hyperkeratotic papule
Molluscum contagiosum	Poxvirus	Smooth, dome-shaped, translucent papules with central umbilication
Petechial or Purpuric Component		
Nonpalpable Purpura		
Thrombocytopenic and blood clotting abnormalities	Thrombocytopenia	Petechiae and ecchymoses in dependent areas
Actinic (senile) purpura	Aging and chronic actinic damage to dermal collagen	Flat ecchymoses, usually on arms
Steroids	Thin dermis by decreasing dermal collagen	Flat ecchymoses on arms, legs
Amyloidosis of skin	Infiltration of dermal vessels by amyloid makes them more fragile	Petechiae and purpura with or without waxy papules around eyes; can be precipitated by trauma, including pinching ("pinch" purpura)
Ehlers-Danlos syndrome	Several variants, all with defects in collagen formation leading to decreased support and increased fragility of cutaneous blood vessels	Easy bruising of skin and joint hyperelasticity
Shamberg's disease	Capillaritis of dermal vessels—usually unknown cause, occasionally due to drugs	Hyperpigmentation with petechiae superimposed, usually on legs
Hypergammaglobulinemic purpura	Hypergammaglobulinemia of variety of causes associated with immune complex damage to blood vessels	Purpura and petechiae on lower legs
Disseminated intravascular coagulation	Intravascular clotting causes thrombosis in blood vessels with subsequent purpura and skin necrosis; induced by infections, malignancies	Hemorrhagic and purpuric star-shaped ecchymoses with skin necrosis and deep hemorrhagic crusts
Infections Causing Purpura		
Meningococcemia, disseminated gonococcemia, Rocky Mountain spotted fever, subacute bacterial endocarditis	Direct invasions of blood vessels by infective organisms or hypersensitivity vascular damage to vessels—Shwartzman reaction or immune complex reactions	Varying forms of petechiae and purpura in skin and mucous membranes
Palpable Purpura		
Vasculitis	Immune complex disease	Palpable purpuric lesions, ulcers on legs can be seen with drugs, infections, collagen vascular disease and underlying malignancies

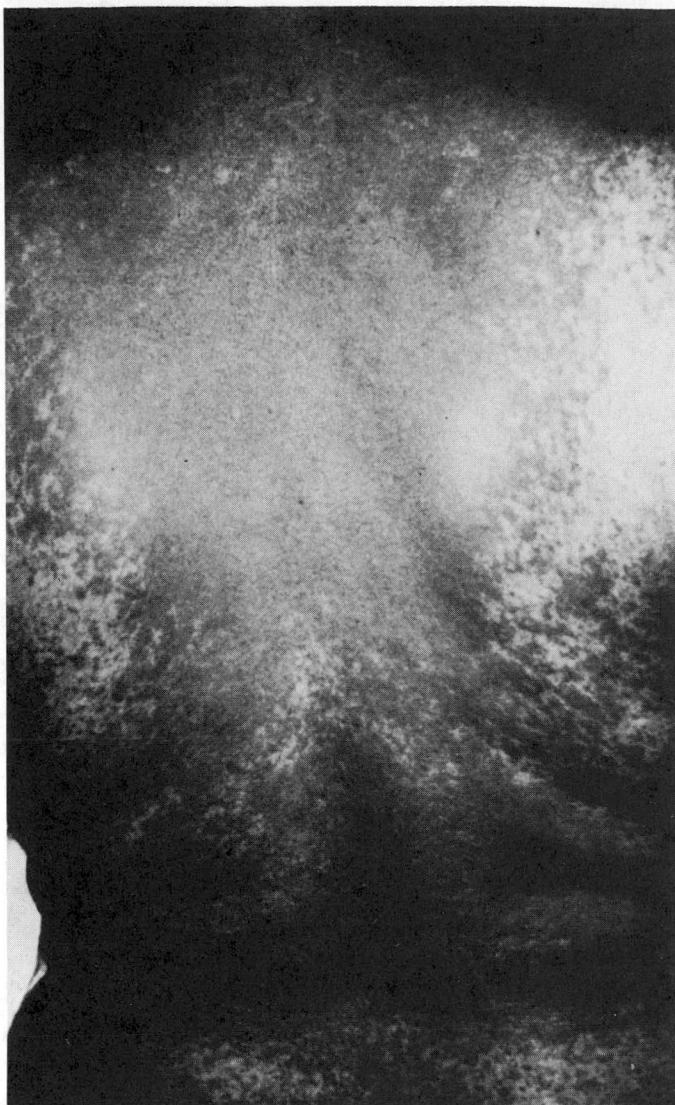

FIGURE 525–5. Drug eruption. (From the 17th edition of the Cecil Textbook of Medicine, with permission of Dr. Marie-Louise Johnson.)

NONPALPABLE PURPURAS. Nonpalpable purpuras include thrombocytopenic conditions, senile or actinic purpura, blood clotting abnormalities, Schamberg's disease, hypergammaglobulinemic conditions, and disseminated intravascular coagulation. *Actinic (senile) purpura* is a common problem in older individuals, the result of increased vessel fragility reflecting dermal connective tissue damage from chronic sun exposure and aging. Minor trauma induces ecchymoses, usually on the dorsum of the hands and forearms. The skin in these areas is thin and fragile. Topically or systemically administered steroids can induce similar purpura. Other causes of vascular fragility of the skin include *amyloidosis* and the *Ehlers-Danlos* syndrome. *Schamberg's disease*, or *pigmented purpuric dermatitis*, is an idiopathic capillaritis that causes petechial lesions of the lower legs (occasionally the arms and trunk) in association with hyperpigmentation. The lesions have the appearance of cayenne pepper. Occasionally Schamberg's disease is secondary to a drug reaction. Petechiae and purpura also occur in *hypergammaglobulinemic purpura*, a syndrome characterized by episodes of fever and arthralgias, which appear to be the result of immune complex–mediated damage to small blood vessels. *Disseminated intravascular coagulation* (DIC) refers to uncontrolled clotting within blood vessels with the formation of diffuse thrombosis. The skin is frequently involved with hemorrhage, ecchymosis, and infarction. DIC occurs in association with bacterial sepsis (particularly meningococcemia), as a postviral or poststreptococcal infection phenomenon (*purpura fulminans*), or in conjunction with malignancies such as prostatic carcinoma and acute myelocytic leukemia. The most distinctive hemorrhagic skin lesions are stellate (star-shaped) purpuric ecchymoses with necrotic centers. The center of the lesion is dark gray, indicative of necrosis and impending slough. Petechiae are seen, and hemorrhagic bullae, acral cyanosis, mucosal bleeding, and prolonged bleeding from wound sites can occur. Patients may be systemically ill with fever, shock, and renal failure.

A variety of infectious diseases cause cutaneous petechiae, purpura, or ecchymoses. Already mentioned is *meningococcemia*, in which the organisms produce acute vasculitis or local Shwartzman-like reactions with erythematous macules, petechiae, purpura, and ecchymosis on the trunk and legs. These may become confluent, often with central necrosis. Patients with acute meningococcemia are ill with fever, malaise, headache, meningeal signs, and hypotension. The skin lesions of *disseminated gonococcemia* begin as tiny red papules and petechiae and then evolve into painful purpuric pustules and vesicles scattered on the distal extremities. Fever, polyarthritis, or monoarticular arthritis may be present. The rash of *Rocky Mountain spotted fever* appears between the second and sixth day of the illness, initially as small, erythematous macules that blanch on pressure but then evolving into petechiae, purpura, and ecchymoses. The rash first occurs on the acral areas and then spreads to the extremities and trunk. Small areas of necrosis may occur on the fingers, toes, and ear lobes. Fever, severe headache, toxicity, confusion, and myalgias commonly occur. *Infective endocarditis* is associated with petechial and purpuric skin lesions. Petechiae appear in crops in the conjunctivae, buccal mucosa, upper chest, and extremities. Splinter hemorrhages (linear, red to brown streaks under the fingernails or toenails); Osler nodes (2- to 15-mm, tender, red nodules on the pads of the fingers and toes); and Janeway lesions (small, painless plaques and palpable, purpuric nodules on the palms or soles) may be seen. The skin lesions are related to immune complex vasculitis or septic emboli.

PALPABLE PURPURAS. *Vasculitis* and *necrotizing angiitis* are terms used in disorders in which there is segmental inflammation in the blood vessel wall with accumulation of neutrophils and fibrinoid necrosis. The vascular reaction is mediated by immune complexes. Papules with purpura result from extravasation of blood from the damaged vessels. Although all sizes of blood vessels may be affected, the vasculitis in the skin involves venules. If the process is extensive or if large vessels are involved, skin necrosis and ulceration may occur. Depending upon the size of the blood vessels affected, at least five types of vasculitis may involve the skin. The size and type of vessels in the skin, in turn, determine the kind of morphologic lesion (Table 525–3).

In general, as the vasculitis involves progressively larger and more deeply situated vessels, the skin lesions become more nodular, with larger ulcerative or gangrenous processes. The term *granulomatous vasculitis* refers to angiitis associated with a histiocytic proliferation that also involves necrotizing granulomas in the connective tissue of multiple organs, causing rhinorrhea, sinusitis, cough, arthralgias, and ocular and neurologic symptoms (Churg-Strauss vasculitis).

Necrotizing leukocytoclastic vasculitis can occur in a variety of settings including (1) sepsis, (2) connective tissue disease—especially systemic lupus erythematosus and rheumatoid arthritis, (3) cryoglobulinemia, (4) drug reactions, and, occasionally, (5) underlying carcinomas, lymphomas, or leukemias. In many instances no apparent cause is found.

Circulating immune complexes have been demonstrated in patients with necrotizing angiitis. Immunoglobulins and complement are found in the affected vessel wall by direct immunofluorescence. The immune complexes lodge in the small vessel walls and activate the complement system, forming the anaphylatoxins C3a and C5a, which recruit neutrophils that induce inflammatory and necrotic damage to the vessel with accompanying fragmented nuclei of the neutrophils (so-called nuclear dust).

Several syndromes are associated with leukocytoclastic vasculitis, depending on the organ systems affected. *Henoch-Schönlein syndrome* occurs most often in children, frequently preceded by an upper respiratory infection and accompanied by arthralgias, abdominal pain, and renal vasculitis. IgA is usually found along with complement in the involved vessels on direct immunofluorescence. *Hypocomplementemic vasculitis* is characterized by urticaria-like lesions, arthritis, and low serum complement. IgG and C3 are present in vessels taken from early skin lesions. Facial and laryngeal edema may also occur. A third form consists of purpura, arthralgia, weakness, and *mixed cryoglobulinemia* (mixed cryoglobulins contain IgG and IgM with anti-IgG or rheumatoid factor activity), which may be idiopathic or occasionally associated with systemic lupus erythematosus, infectious mononucleosis, lymphomas, or primary biliary cirrhosis.

If the vasculitis is idiopathic and cutaneous, the skin responds to prednisone (60 to 80 mg per day) or dapsone (100 to 150 mg per day). Systemic vasculitides may require prednisone and cyclophosphamide (2 mg per kilogram per day).

Necrotizing cutaneous vasculitis may occur in association with *hepatitis B* and in patients with *intestinal bypass surgery* for morbid obesity or in patients with jejunal diverticula or other gastrointestinal conditions characterized by bacterial overgrowth. An *arthritis-dermatitis syndrome* with intestinal bypass surgery may occur with polyarthritis and palpable purpura or purpuric nodules and pustules on the trunk, legs, feet, and arms. Antigenic components of the intestinal bacterial overgrowth lead to the formation of cryoprotein immune complexes that deposit in the skin and joints, causing a hypersensitivity vasculitis and nondeforming arthritis. Antibiotics such as chloramphenicol, sulfamethoxazole-trimethoprim, tetracycline, and metronidazole have been reported to improve the condition.

PAPULOSQUAMOUS SKIN DISEASES

Unique scales are the common characteristic of diseases in this group. *Squamous* refers to scaling that represents thickened stratum corneum and thus implies an abnormal keratinization process. The lesions, in addition to being scaly, are characterized by sharply demarcated, red to violaceous papules and plaques that result from thickening of the epidermis and/or underlying dermal inflammation.

The papulosquamous disorders have diverse etiologies and include psoriasis, Reiter's syndrome, pityriasis rosea, lichen planus, pityriasis rubra pilaris, secondary syphilis, mycosis fungoides, and ichthyosiform eruptions (Table 525–4).

PSORIASIS. Psoriasis is a genetically determined, chronic epidermal proliferative disease of unpredictable course. Onset is most frequent in early adult life, but it may begin at any age. Once the disease becomes manifest, it may remain localized to a few areas or may cause intermittent or continuous generalized disease.

The lesions appear as erythematous papules and plaques surmounted by silvery, thick scales that resemble mica (micaceous) and that are easily removed and may accumulate in the patient's clothing or bed (Fig. 525–6). In intertriginous areas maceration prevents scales from accumulating, but the lesions remain red and sharply defined. Classically, lesions are distributed symmetrically over areas of bony prominence such as elbows and knees. They also commonly occur on the trunk and scalp and in the intergluteal cleft. The latter two areas are frequently overlooked.

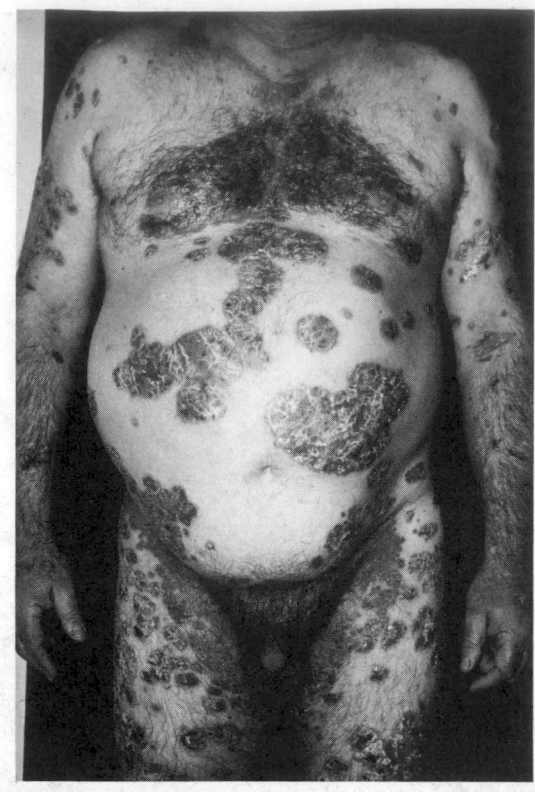

FIGURE 525–6. Psoriasis. (From the 17th edition of the Cecil Textbook of Medicine, with the permission of Dr. Marie-Louise Johnson.)

Palms and soles may be involved, with diffuse redness, scaling, and, at times, pustular lesions. Nail involvement occurs in up to 50 per cent of patients. The nails may be pitted with small ice pick–like depressions on the surface of the nail plate. Onycholysis can also occur, in which a plaque of psoriasis in the distal nail bed causes a red-brown discoloration that is reminiscent of an oil stain under the nail. Another helpful diagnostic feature is the Koebner phenomenon, in which intense trauma to the skin induces new skin lesions. Thus, scratches or surgical incisions elicit linear papulosquamous lesions that should alert the physician to the diagnosis. This may also explain the high incidence of psoriasis on the elbows and knees. Other aggravating factors include streptococcal infections, emotional stress, overuse of alcohol, and drugs, including lithium and beta blockers. Several common variants of psoriasis may also be seen: (1) *guttate psoriasis*, in which numerous, small papular lesions with silvery scales evolve suddenly over the body, often 1 to 3 weeks following streptococcal pharyngitis; (2) *inverse psoriasis*, in which plaques evolve in intertriginous areas and thus lack the typical silver scale because of maceration and moisture; (3) *pustular psoriasis*, a form

TABLE 525–3. TYPES OF VASCULITIS AND ASSOCIATED SKIN LESIONS

Type of Vasculitis	Blood Vessels Involved	Type of Skin Lesion
Leukocytoclastic or hypersensitivity angiitis: Henoch-Schönlein purpura, cryoglobulinemia, hypocomplementemic vasculitis	Dermal capillaries, venules, and occasional small muscular arteries in internal organs	Purpuric papules, hemorrhagic bullae, cutaneous infarcts
Rheumatic vasculitis: systemic lupus erythematosus; rheumatoid vasculitis	Dermal capillaries, venules, and small muscular arteries in internal organs	Purpuric papules; ulcerative nodules; splinter hemorrhages; periungual telangiectasia and infarcts
Granulomatous vasculitis		
Churg and Strauss allergic granulomatous angiitis	Dermal small and larger muscular arteries and medium muscular arteries in subcutaneous tissue and other organs	Erythematous, purpuric, and ulcerated nodules, plaques, and purpura
Wegener's granulomatosis	Small venules, arterioles of dermis, and small muscular arteries	Ulcerative nodules; peripheral gangrene
Periarteritis: classic type limited to skin and muscle	Small and medium muscular arteries in deep dermis, subcutaneous tissue, and muscle	Deep subcutaneous nodules with ulceration; livedo reticularis; ecchymoses
Giant cell arteritis: temporal arteritis, polymyalgia rheumatica, Takayasu's disease	Medium muscular arteries and larger arteries	Skin necrosis over scalp

of the disease in which superficial pustules occur in one of three presentations—pustules studding typical plaques; pustules confined to the palms and soles; and a rare generalized eruption in which pustules evolve abruptly on large areas of erythematous skin accompanied by fever and leukocytosis; (4) *erythroderma*—occasionally the psoriasis can become generalized to involve erythema and scaling of the entire integument. This may occur secondary to a general Koebner phenomenon with overvigorous therapy, a drug reaction, or withdrawal of oral steroids; (5) *psoriatic arthritis*—arthritis may accompany psoriasis in 10 to 15 per cent of cases.

At times Reiter's syndrome may be confused with psoriasis. The skin lesions of the two disorders are indistinguishable clinically and histologically. In Reiter's syndrome pustular and hyperkeratotic papules and plaques commonly occur on the palms and soles (keratoderma blenorrhagica) and scaling, red patches evolve encircling the glans penis and within the groin (balanitis circinata). The presence of asymptomatic erosions on the tongue and buccal mucosa, urethritis, iritis or conjunctivitis, arthritis, and occasionally diarrhea should suggest the diagnosis.

The pathogenesis of psoriasis is unknown, but it appears to be a multifactorial disease in patients who are genetically predisposed. There is an increased prevalence of psoriasis in individuals with HLA antigens BW17, B13, and BW37. Thirty per cent of patients have a family history of disease. The basic alteration represents an accelerated cell cycle in an increased number of dividing cells, culminating in rapid epidermal cell proliferation. Cellular turnover is increased sevenfold, and the transit time from the basal layer to the top of the stratum corneum is 3 or 4 days rather than the usual 28 days. This rapid turnover of keratinocytes alters keratinization, resulting in thickened epidermis (seen as papules and plaques) and parakeratotic stratum corneum (silvery scales). The basic mechanism underlying this benign proliferative reaction is unknown.

The goal of therapy is to decrease epidermal proliferation and underlying dermal inflammation. There is no curative agent for psoriasis, and treatment suppresses the condition only as long as it is administered. Three types of topical therapies are employed: (1) topical steroids, usually with intermediate and strong potency agents administered once or twice a day; (2) topical tars and anthralin preparations, often used once a day in combination with topical steroids; (3) ultraviolet light, either UVB with tar or UVA with oral psoralens (see Ch. 524).

Two systemic types of therapy are available, but because of their side effects these should be reserved for severe widespread disease that is unresponsive to topical measures: (1) antimetabolites or antimitotic agents, including methotrexate, azathioprine, and hydroxyurea. The most commonly used is methotrexate in low doses, usually given on a weekly basis. Because these agents affect bone marrow and liver (in the case of methotrexate), complete blood counts and liver function tests should be performed regularly, together with intermittent liver biopsies. (2) Etretinate, a retinoid, is particularly useful in pustular and erythrodermic forms of psoriasis. Careful monitoring of blood counts, plasma triglycerides, and liver function is required, and avoidance of pregnancy during the use of this drug is mandatory.

PITYRIASIS ROSEA. Oval or round, tannish pink or salmon colored, scaling papules and plaques appear rapidly over the

TABLE 525–4. PAPULOSQUAMOUS SKIN DISEASES

Disease	Appearance of Lesion	Distribution	Mucous Membrane Involvement	Other Features
Psoriasis	Erythematous plaques with silvery, mica-like scales, usually nonpruritic	Anywhere: scalp, knees, elbows, intergluteal cleft favored; symmetric	None	Koebner phenomenon, nail involvement, arthritis
Reiter's syndrome	Erythematous, silvery scaled plaques; hyperkeratotic papules of palms and soles (keratoderma blennorrhagicum)	Similar to psoriasis	Frequent: mouth, genitals; balanitis circinata	Nail involvement, arthritis, urethritis, conjunctivitis, iritis
Pityriasis rosea	Tannish pink, oval papules and plaques with delicate collarette scale; may or may not be pruritic	Rash preceded by herald patch, Christmas tree pattern on trunk; spares face, extremities	None	May be associated with upper respiratory infection; drugs may cause similar rash
Secondary syphilis	Ham red or copper colored scaling papules and plaques, sometimes annular	Generalized: palms and soles often involved	Mucous patches, often white or red; condyloma warts of anal area	Condylomata in genital area; serologic test for syphilis positive
Lichen planus	Violaceous polygonal, flat-topped papules with white scale or Wickham's striae. May be hyperkeratotic, annular, or bullous lesions; pruritic	Often on wrists and ankles, but can be generalized; Koebner reaction	Frequent reticulated white patches or erosive lesions in mouth or genital areas	Occasionally involves nails; drugs can cause similar reaction
Pityriasis rubra pilaris	Red, scaling plaques and patches with follicular horny excretions, especially on dorsum of hands and fingers; diffuse, yellow hyperkeratoses of palms and soles	Often diffuse, rough scaling erythema involving entire body with islands of normal skin	Occasionally lacy white plaques in mouth	Remits spontaneously in 2–4 years; nail changes as in psoriasis
Pityriasis lichenoides et varioliformis acuta (Mucha-Habermann disease)	Red, discrete, palpable papules that vesiculate and then become hemorrhagic, crust, scale, and leave a scar	Scattered lesions over trunk and extremities	May resemble leukocytoclastic vasculitis	May resolve in a few months or persist for years
Pityriasis lichenoides et varioliformis chronica (chronic parapsoriasis)	Guttate to larger, red, slightly scaling papules and plaques; nonpruritic	Usually on trunk	Some forms may represent early stages of mycosis fungoides	Responds to UVB light treatments
Mycosis fungoides	Persistent, pruritic, red, thickened plaques with fine scales as seen in eczema, or thick mica-like scales suggestive of psoriasis; may ulcerate	Scattered asymmetrically over trunk, extremities; girdle area often first area involved	Neoplastic T-cell lymphoma	May show islands of normal skin within red areas
Ichthyosis	A variety of syndromes with variation in scaling skin; fine, light scales to large, thick, coarse, verrucous scales that resemble fish skin; hyperkeratosis of palms and soles	Variable distribution but can involve flexural or extensor surfaces of extremities or trunk	Autosomal dominant, recessive, and X-linked recessive conditions	See Table 525–5

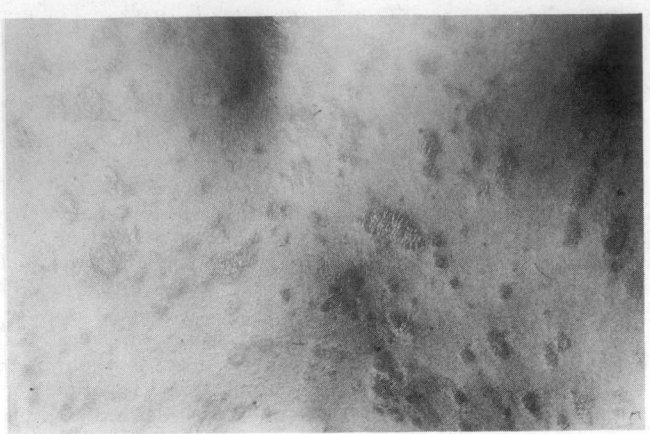

FIGURE 525–7. Pityriasis rosea. (From the 17th edition of the Cecil Textbook of Medicine, with the permission of Dr. Marie-Louise Johnson.)

trunk, neck, upper arms, and legs (Fig. 525–7). Several features of this self-limited papulosquamous condition are unique. First, the generalized eruption is preceded by a single lesion, termed the "herald patch," that is commonly misdiagnosed as "ringworm." The herald patch can occur anywhere but often appears on the neck or lower trunk area and precedes the general rash by several days to a week. Second, the oval patches have an unusual fine, white scale located near the border of the plaques, forming a collarette. Third, the lesions follow skin cleavage lines, in a pattern likened to a Christmas tree. Last, the condition spontaneously involutes in 1 to 2 months. Recurrences are rare. Itching occasionally is a prominent symptom.

Pityriasis rosea occasionally is preceded by a mild upper respiratory infection, and its greatest incidence is in the winter months, suggesting a viral etiology. However, the disease does not occur endemically and is not transmitted person to person.

Such conditions as tinea corporis and guttate psoriasis may be considered in the differential diagnosis, but two possibilities should always be entertained: drug eruption and secondary syphilis. If the rash persists longer than 2 or 3 months or generalizes to involve the trunk, extremities, and especially the face, a drug reaction should be considered. Such medications as gold compounds, barbiturates, captopril, clonidine, and tripelennamide can cause such a rash. Secondary syphilis should be suspected and a serologic test obtained if the rash involves palms and soles and if fever, coryza, or mucous membrane erosions (socalled mucous patches) are present.

Treatment of pityriasis rosea is usually not necessary, although topical corticosteroids and antihistamines may relieve itching and decrease erythema. Ultraviolet light (UVB), given as three to five treatments eliciting a mild erythema reaction, often clears the rash.

LICHEN PLANUS. This idiopathic, pruritic, inflammatory condition of the skin is included in the papulosquamous group of diseases because the primary lesion is a unique papule. The papules are flat topped (planus) and polygonal in configuration (i.e., the sides conform to normal fine skin folds) and have a lilac or purple hue. They may have visible scales on their surface, but more characteristic are subtle, fine white dots or white reticulated lines (Wickham's striae) surmounting the shiny, flat tops (resembling the appearance of a lichen). Wickham's striae are more visible under a hand lens after the application of a drop of mineral oil to the surface of the papule. The Koebner phenomenon occurs

in lichen planus, so linear streaks of papules at the sites of skin trauma may be noted.

Although lichen planus can occur anywhere on the body, typical locations are the ankles, wrists, mouth, and genitalia. There may be only a few papules or innumerable ones in a generalized distribution. Mucous membranes are commonly involved, the lesions appearing most frequently as asymptomatic white streaks in a reticulated pattern on the buccal mucosa, tongue, gums, or lips. At times blisters and erosions are superimposed (erosive lichen planus), causing severe discomfort. Lichen planus involving the male genitalia may appear as violaceous annular lesions. Rarely, lichen planus may appear as violaceous annular and polycyclic lesions on the legs and arms, or as hyperkeratotic, follicular, scarring alopecia. All lichen planus lesions leave residual hyperpigmented macules in their wake.

The etiology of lichen planus is not known, but two conditions may mimic lichen planus skin lesions and thus offer clues to an immune etiology. Certain drugs such as thiazides, phenothiazines, gold, quinidine, and antimalarials can cause lichen planus–like, generalized eruptions. Second, some patients with graft-versus-host disease also develop a skin reaction that closely resembles lichen planus. The eruption can evolve into the usual chronic graft-versus-host sequelae of diffuse dermal sclerosis, cicatricial alopecia, reticulated pigmentation, and ulceration.

Lichen planus tends to be a chronic condition lasting for months to years. Perhaps two thirds of patients experience spontaneous resolution in 1 to 2 years. In general, the more acute, intense, and widespread the eruption, the more likely it is that an early remission may occur.

Treatment is nonspecific and often unsuccessful. Topical steroids help suppress the inflammatory reaction and itching. Severe oral lichen planus may respond to etretinate.

PITYRIASIS RUBRA PILARIS. This idiopathic papulosquamous and keratotic disease has an uncertain and often chronic course. The condition can appear in a familial form (autosomal dominant) with onset in infancy or childhood or as an acquired disease evolving during the fourth to sixth decades. In either form the following features help in diagnosis: (1) diffuse salmon color of involved skin with sharply bordered residual areas of normal skin (so-called island sparing), (2) waxy, yellow keratoderma of palms and soles similar to carnauba wax, and (3) erythematous hyperkeratotic papules on the dorsal surfaces of the proximal portions of the phalanges. The condition remits spontaneously in 2 to 4 years in 80 per cent of patients. Differentiation from psoriasis may be difficult. The cause of this disease is unknown, although low serum levels of retinol-binding protein have been found. High doses of vitamin A have been reported to help the condition, as has etretinate.

PITYRIASIS LICHENOIDES ET VARIOLIFORMIS ACUTA (MUCHA-HABERMANN DISEASE OR PLEVA). This unusual condition of unknown cause usually begins as widely scattered, red papules that may be purpuric and/or vesicular. Although not initially papulosquamous, the lesions evolve into scaling, eroded, and crusted papules that leave depressed scars in their wake. Lesions develop in crops, often in association with malaise and fever, and persist for months or years. Acute lesions show a lymphocytic vasculitis. No therapy is effective, although tetracycline, systemic corticosteroids, and cytotoxic agents may give short-lived remissions.

ICHTHYOSIS. A variety of inherited and acquired conditions cause rough, dry skin with retained scale simulating fish skin. On close inspection there may be fine scales with keratin-plugged follicles or large, polyhedral, loosely adherent scales.

A number of inherited ichthyosis conditions are recognized (Table 525–5), the most common being *ichthyosis vulgaris*, a dominant trait in which the cells of the stratum corneum are

TABLE 525–5. ICHTHYOSIFORM DERMATOSES

	Inheritance	Onset	Distribution	Clinical Associations	Kinetics
Lamellar ichthyosis	Autosomal recessive	Birth	Body, palms, soles	Ectropion	Increased
Epidermolytic hyperkeratosis	Autosomal dominant	Birth	Predominant flexural involvement	Blisters	Increased
X-linked ichthyosis (steroid sulfatase deficiency)	X-linked	Birth	Trunk	Corneal opacities	Normal
Ichthyosis vulgaris	Autosomal dominant	Childhood	Spares flexural areas	Atopy	Normal

Reprinted from the chapter by Dr. Marie-Louise Johnson in the 17th edition of the Cecil Textbook of Medicine, with her permission.

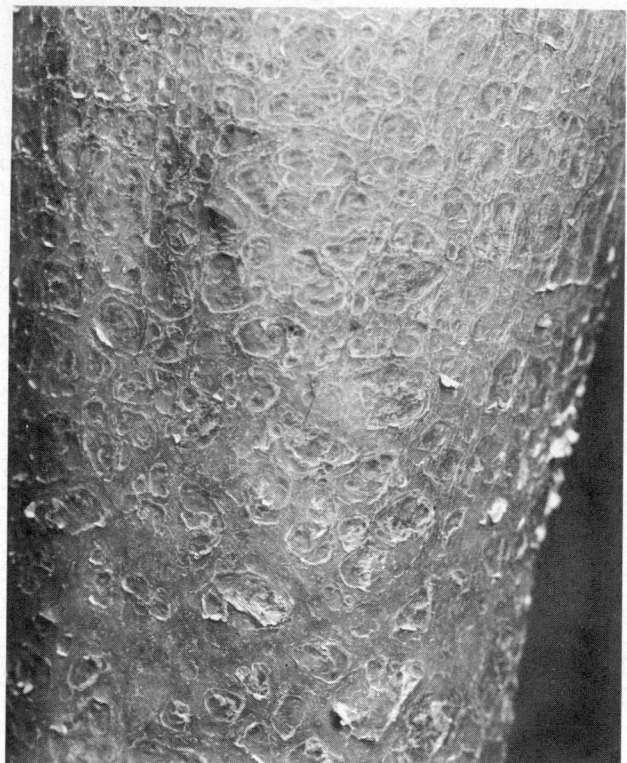

FIGURE 525–8. Ichthyosis. (From the 17th edition of the Cecil Textbook of Medicine, with the permission of Dr. Marie-Louise Johnson.)

retained, forming fishlike or reptilian scales on the extensor surfaces of the extremities (Fig. 525–8). Other forms of ichthyosis such as *lamellar* and *epidermolytic hyperkeratoses* may be associated with considerable erythema and blistering of the skin. Lamellar ichthyosis may be present at birth (collodion baby). A deficiency of steroid sulfatase has been found in association with *X-linked ichthyosis*. Mothers of such babies often have a prolonged labor, as steroid sulfatase appears to play an important role in the parturition process.

Emollients and keratolytic agents (propylene glycol, salicylic acid, lactic acid) are often useful in softening the skin. In severe ichthyosis oral retinoids, such as 13-*cis*-retinoic acid and etretinate, have been beneficial.

VESICULOBULLOUS DISEASES

Vesicles and bullae, when intact, are readily recognized primary skin lesions. Crusts or superficial erosions are secondary lesions that lead one to suspect a preceding fluid-filled primary lesion. The etiology of blistering disease includes bacterial and viral infections, contact dermatitis, and autoimmune and metabolic diseases. The pathogenesis of the blister formation is often helpful in understanding its anatomic location: Blisters occur either within the epidermis (intraepidermal) or at the dermoepidermal junction (subepidermal) (Table 525–6).

Intraepidermal vesicles or bullae usually contain clear fluid (but may become filled with purulent material secondarily) and have very thin roofs, so they are flaccid in appearance and are easily broken. At times the blisters are difficult to recognize, and only erosions, crusts, or the thin shreds of the epidermal blister roofs remain. Subepidermal blisters, on the other hand, have an epidermal roof and are tense and remain intact. Hemorrhagic fluid is common in subepidermal blisters because of their location close to dermal capillaries.

Biopsy of early vesicles or blisters is imperative in diagnosis. Immunofluorescence studies on biopsy material may differentiate certain immunologically mediated diseases. Pathologic studies are most informative when performed early, before therapy has been initiated.

INTRAEPIDERMAL VESICULOBULLOUS DISEASES. Pathologic processes involved in epidermal blister formation include spongiosis, primary cell damage, and acantholysis. Spongiosis, a common form of blister formation in eczematous proc-

esses, represents edema between cells of the prickle layer and liquefaction of cells, which gradually increases the size of the fluid spaces. Primary epidermal cell damage with fluid accumulation is seen in viral infections and friction damage. Blisters may also occur when cellular desmosomal attachments and intercellular cementing substances are immunologically or chemically altered, causing dyshesion referred to as acantholysis (pemphigus).

Bullous impetigo, a subcorneal infection of the skin with staphylococcal and/or streptococcal organisms, causes large, fragile, clear or cloudy bullae that form thin, honey-yellow crusts and a delicate collarette-like remnant of blister roof after the blisters rupture. Autoinoculation results in satellite lesions. The superficial epidermal blistering is caused by the toxic effects of an epidermal toxin elaborated by certain strains of these bacterial organisms.

A more serious variant of bullous impetigo is *staphylococcal scalded skin syndrome,* usually affecting infants and characterized by the formation of rapidly progressive, painful, erythematous patches in which large flaccid bullae evolve and shed as large sheets of skin, leaving a denuded, scalded-appearing surface. With only slight trauma the skin readily slides off, much like wet wallpaper slides off a wall (Nikolsky's sign—see Ch. 523). In contrast to localized bullous impetigo in which the *Staphylococcus aureus* may be recovered in the skin lesions, the bullae of scalded skin syndrome are sterile, although a staphylococcal infection may be found in the conjunctiva, nose, or pharynx. The widespread intraepidermal blistering results from an epidermal toxin elaborated by specific strains of *Staphylococcus* and hematogenously carried to the skin. These are penicillinase-resistant strains of *Staphylococcus* and therefore require methicillin-type antibiotics.

A somewhat similar condition, *toxic epidermal necrolysis* (TEN), occurs in adults, often secondary to drugs (e.g., ampicillin, allopurinol) and occasionally to *Staphylococcus* infections in an immunosuppressed patient. TEN is a reaction to a variety of antigenic materials that cause a suprabasilar split in the epidermis with necrosis of much of the overlying epidermis. Because of the more extensive destruction of epidermis and barrier stratum corneum layer (as opposed to staphylococcal scalded skin syndrome, in which the split is subcorneal), TEN is often fatal and, when extensive, should be treated as a widespread burn would be cared for. TEN also often involves the mucous membranes and therefore may be confused with Stevens-Johnson syndrome (see below).

Viral infections of the skin may cause vesicles and bullae by virtue of direct infection of the keratinocytes and the destructive effect on the cells. Vesicles caused by viruses often display two important characteristics: (1) they tend to occur in groups on an indurated erythematous base, and (2) they often take on an umbilicated appearance.

Herpes simplex is caused by two strains of DNA *Herpesvirus* (type 1, which commonly causes infections above the waist, and type 2, which most frequently is responsible for those in the genital region). Primary infections, gingivostomatitis, and vulvovaginitis, are extensive vesicular eruptions that quickly become necrotic, leaving painful, purulent erosions. The herpesvirus is highly contagious, spread by direct contact with infected individuals. The virus penetrates the epidermal cells, undergoes replicative cycles, and eventually lyses the host cell membrane. The virus is neuropathic, traveling up cutaneous nerves to dorsal nerve root sensory or autonomic ganglia, where it resides in a nonreplicative state. Reactivation of the replicative cycle triggers recurrence, and the virus spreads back down the nerve to induce grouped, umbilicated vesicles on an indurated, red base in areas of the skin innervated by the infected ganglia. Periods of latency vary, and recurrences have a shorter course than primary infections (1 to 2 weeks versus 3 weeks). A number of factors seem to induce recurrences, including fever, ultraviolet light, physical trauma, menstruation, and emotional stress. Recurrences are most common on the lips and face (herpes labialis), genital regions (herpes genitalis), and fingers (herpetic whitlow). *Eczema herpeticum* is a generalized herpes simplex skin infection in areas of atopic dermatitis. Recurrent herpes infections are contagious from the time the vesicular lesions develop to the time the vesicles re-epithelialize. Between attacks there is little chance of causing infection, although perhaps 1 or 2 per cent of individuals may be chronically shedding the virus in the saliva or genital excretions (women may also have active herpes simplex infections of the cervix and be unaware of them).

A complication of herpes simplex infection, *erythema multiforme*, is a hypersensitivity skin and mucous membrane reaction that evolves 1 to 2 weeks following herpetic recurrences as a result of an immune complex reaction to the herpes antigen. Herpes infection is only one etiologic stimulus leading to erythema multiforme (see below).

Diagnosis of herpes infections (including zoster and varicella) is made with a Tzanck preparation of material taken from the roof of vesicles. The contents are smeared onto a slide and stained with Wright's or Giemsa's stain to reveal multinucleated giant cells (see Ch. 523).

Acyclovir administered orally and intravenously is the most frequently used form of therapy for primary and recurrent forms of herpes (see Ch. 371 and Fig. 523–4).

Varicella infection, when initially encountered, causes chickenpox, a generalized pruritic eruption with widespread, delicate vesicles on an erythematous base which have been likened to a dew drop on a rose petal. They often become umbilicated, hemorrhagic, and pustular and may leave scars. Chickenpox lesions occur predominantly on the trunk but also involve the head, extremities, and mucous membranes of the mouth and conjunctiva. Successive crops of lesions evolve for a week. *Herpes zoster* is a recrudescence of latent varicella virus in persons who previously had varicella. It appears as grouped, umbilicated, and, at times, hemorrhagic vesicles and pustules on an erythematous base situated unilaterally along the distribution of cranial or spinal nerves. Frequently several immediately adjacent dermatomes are involved. Bilateral involvement is rare. Zoster is frequently associated with a prodrome of severe radicular pain in the involved areas. A common useful sign in making the diagnosis is hypesthesia of the dermatomal areas—the patient often bitterly complains that the rubbing of clothing on the area is intolerable. Most patients with herpes zoster are over 50 years of age, and cancer patients (especially those with lymphomas such as Hodgkin's disease) are particularly prone to this infection. In such patients or in immunocompromised individuals, cutaneous dissemination from the original dermatome may occur, as well as visceral involvement of liver, lung, and central nervous system. Postherpetic neuralgia is common in individuals over 50. Treatment of herpes zoster is usually symptomatic with Burow's compresses, analgesics, and acyclovir, especially in immunocompromised patients (800 mg five times per day orally for 10 days).

Insect bites including flea and fire ant bites may also induce

TABLE 525–6. VESICULOBULLOUS DISEASES

Location of Blister in Skin	Etiology if Known	Important Physical Findings	Other Facts of Note in History of Laboratory Results
Intraepidermal Blisters			
Bacterial infectious processes			
Bullous impetigo (subcorneal)	Staph toxin	Large, fragile, clear or cloudy bullae that break to leave honey-yellow crusts on face, neck, extremities; erythematous areas that slough as superficial blisters	An initial site may be followed by multiple pruritic autoinoculated sites
Staph scalded skin syndrome—upper epidermal blisters	Staph toxin		
Viral infections			
Herpes simplex, eczema vaccination, herpes zoster varicella (ballooning degeneration)	Direct cell damage	Grouped umbilicated vesicles on erythematous base anywhere on body; diffuse umbilicated vesicles in sites of atopic eczema; unilateral grouped umbilicated, clear or hemorrhagic vesicles in dermatomal distribution	Frequently recurrent; respond to acyclovir
Insect bites	Insect toxins or proteases, delayed hypersensitivity	Papules, bullae—pruritic	Associated with radicular pain and hypesthesia of involved dermatome; respond to acyclovir
Eczema–acute contact (spongiosis)	Type IV hypersensitivity or irritant	Vesiculobullous lesions on red base; often form unusual patterns of contact with substances	
Autoimmune diseases			
a) Pemphigus vulgaris and vegetans (suprabasilar split)	a) Autoimmune interepidermal cell IgG and C3	a) Superficial, flaccid bullae that readily rupture, leaving nonhealing erosions over the body that can cause death; Nikolsky's sign prominent	a) 100% of patients develop mucous membrane blisters, erosions
b) Pemphigus foliaceus and erythematosus (subcorneal split)	b) Autoimmune IgG and/or C3 between cells in upper epidermis	b) Superficial blisters crusting, oozing over scalp and face in seborrhea distribution or butterfly-like rash	b) Seldom see mucous membrane involvement
c) Hailey-Hailey disease (suprabasilar split)	c) Genetically inherited—dominant	c) Superficial erosive blisters, vesicles, pustules in flexural areas of body	c) No mouth lesions
Subepidermal Blisters			
Autoimmune or immunologic			
Bullous pemphigoid	C3 in lamina lucida	Tense bullae on normal or erythematous skin	
Herpes gestationis	C3 in basement membrane zone	Erythematous plaques, tense vesicles, and pruritic bullae that evolve first on abdomen and then on extremities; often polycyclic	Develops during 2nd or 3rd trimester of pregnancy—clears with delivery; increased fetal wastage
Erythema multiforme	Hypersensitivity reaction in blood vessels of dermis to number of antigens—immune complexes seen	Multiforme lesions of red urticaria, papules and target lesions on extremities, palms	Can involve mouth, eyes (Stevens-Johnson syndrome)
Cicatricial pemphigoid	Subepidermal IgG linear in basement membrane zone	Scarring blisters in the mucous membrane; 25% have blisters on skin	Causes blindness; stenosis of urethra, anal areas
Dermatitis herpetiformis (vesicles in dermal papillae)	Immunologic deposition of IgA in dermal papillae	Grouped, symmetrically distributed vesicles and urticarial papules on scalp, scapulae, buttocks, elbows, knees	Intense burning, itch; high incidence of asymptomatic celiac sprue
Metabolic			
Porphyria cutanea tarda	Metabolic defect in porphyrin metabolism	Tense bullae that leave scars in sun-exposed areas; bullae induced by sun, trauma	May also see facial hirsutism and hyperpigmentation
Bullous disease of renal disease	Unknown	Bullae usually in extremities	
Bullous disease in diabetics	Unknown	Large bulla on acral areas	
Mechanicobullous diseases			
Epidermolysis bullosa (split above, below, and within dermal-epidermal zone)	Variety of inherited conditions	Tense blisters that erode and scar, especially in recessively inherited forms; can lead to severe scars covering digits	Severe forms may involve mouth, esophagus
Epidermolysis bullosa acquista (blister below lamina densa)	Linear IgG and C3 deposits below lamina densa	Tense blisters that lead to scars and milia in pressure and trauma sites on hands, feet; scarring mucous membrane lesions also occur	Circulating antibody to sublamina densa antigen found

vesicles or bullae, a response to injected toxins or foreign chemicals or proteins in the bite or an allergic reaction to them.

Several unusual conditions, the *pemphigus diseases*, cause blistering in the epidermis by virtue of the process of acantholysis. Nikolsky's sign is commonly present in these conditions. *Pemphigus vulgaris* (see Color Plate 15E) and a variant, *pemphigus vegetans*, which heals with hypertrophic, "vegetative" surfaces, are acquired autoimmune diseases of the skin and mucous membrane. The superficial bullae, evolving just above the basal layer, readily rupture, leaving denuded, bleeding, weeping and crusted erosions over the body which do not heal. The oral mucosa is almost always involved and is frequently the presenting site. The painful erosions characteristically spill over the vermilion border of the lips and onto the skin. Lesions of the skin occur anywhere but often in pressure and friction areas. The blisters arise on normal-appearing skin. The usual course of untreated pemphigus vulgaris is slow progression with extensive denudation, leading to fluid and electrolyte imbalance, sepsis, and death. Pain from mouth lesions prevents adequate food intake. Skin biopsy of early vesicles should be obtained for routine histologic examination. The edge of a bulla, including adjacent normal skin, should be examined by direct immunofluorescence to make the diagnosis. Immunofluorescence shows deposits of immunoglobulins (usually IgG) and/or C3 in the intercellular spaces around keratinocytes (see Table 522–3). Antibodies to the intercellular areas of the epidermis are found in the serum of patients with pemphigus vulgaris. High doses of systemic steroids (100 to 200 mg of prednisone per day) over prolonged periods usually control the disease. Methotrexate and other cytotoxic agents are useful as steroid-sparing agents. Treatment with intramuscular gold is often successful, occasionally inducing long-term remissions (Ch. 524).

Pemphigus foliaceus is a less severe disease in which the acantholytic separation within the epidermis is in the upper portion of the prickle layer. *Pemphigus erythematosus* may be a localized variant of pemphigus foliaceus presenting with superficial blisters, erosions, and crusting and oozing over the scalp and face in a seborrheic dermatitis–like rash or often simulating the butterfly rash of systemic lupus erythematosus. Mucous membrane involvement in pemphigus foliaceus and pemphigus erythematosus is unusual, and lower doses of systemic steroids generally control these conditions. Immunofluorescent studies on skin from the edge of lesions reveal immunoglobulin and/or C3 in the intercellular areas of the upper portions of the epidermis.

Familial benign pemphigus, or Hailey-Hailey disease, is a dominantly inherited disorder with suprabasal cell acantholysis, the groups of bullae arising on erythematous skin in the flexural areas (neck, axillae, groin). Spreading erosions display vesicles and pustules at the borders with a moist, granular center. Warm weather and superficial bacterial infections seem to cause flares with spontaneous exacerbations and remissions continuing for years. Familial benign pemphigus differs from other forms of pemphigus in its genetic pattern, absence of mouth lesions, benign course, and absence of intercellular antibodies. Antibiotics, both topical and systemic, may improve acute flares of the disease.

DERMAL-EPIDERMAL VESICULOBULLOUS DISEASES. Separation of the epidermis from the dermis occurs in a variety of bullous diseases resulting from autoimmune and immunologic reactions, metabolic disturbances, and a number of inherited mechanicobullous conditions (Table 525–6).

Bullous pemphigoid (see Color Plate 15F), a disease of the elderly, is an autoimmune disorder in which tense, large blisters occur on normal or erythematous skin, often in the groin, axillae, and flexural areas. Nikolsky's sign is not present, and only one third of patients have oral blisters. Healing usually occurs in some blisters without scarring while new lesions evolve. Itching may be severe or absent. Skin biopsy specimens display a subepidermal blister through the lamina lucida (at the electron microscopic level), and direct immunofluorescence reveals deposition of the IgG immunoglobulin and complement. Circulating antibodies to the lamina lucida zone are found in 70 per cent of patients (see Table 522–3). The prognosis is good, and the disease usually subsides after months or years. Widespread bullae require therapy with 40 to 60 mg of oral prednisone per day and occasionally with immunosuppressive agents.

Another subepidermal blistering disease, *herpes gestationis*, is a rare autoimmune condition that occurs during pregnancy and the postpartum period. The name of the disease is misleading, for it is not associated with *Herpesvirus* infection. The blisters develop at any time throughout the course of pregnancy, although they most often begin during the second and third trimesters and subside a few weeks post partum. Some patients may experience transient flares or recurrences with each menstrual period or following the use of oral contraceptives. There are recurrences with subsequent pregnancies. Herpes gestationis is a pruritic condition with numerous tense vesicles arising on both normal-appearing and erythematous areas of skin. Arcuate and polycyclic red plaques with peripheral blistering are seen. The lesions first appear on the abdomen and then spread to involve the entire integument. Skin biopsy findings are indistinguishable from those of bullous pemphigoid by light microscopy, and examination of perilesional skin by direct immunofluorescence reveals C3 and less often an IgG linear band just below the epidermis. There is associated fetal mortality as high as 30 per cent, and there is also an increased rate of premature live births. Transient vesiculobullous lesions may infrequently occur in some otherwise healthy infants of affected mothers. Occasionally the patients' intractable pruritus and extensive bullae respond to high-potency topical steroid ointments and diphenhydramine, but most patients require oral prednisone (20 to 60 mg daily) throughout pregnancy with intermittent tapering.

Cicatricial pemphigoid (benign mucosal pemphigoid), another subepidermal blistering disease, has a predilection for mucous membranes, especially the conjunctiva where it causes scarring that leads to synblepharon and blindness. Subepidermal blisters also occur on the skin in one quarter of patients. Subepidermal IgG staining is seen on direct immunofluorescence, but circulating immunoglobulin antibodies are infrequently found. Therapy is unsatisfactory, although dapsone and gold may slow this chronic and progressive condition. Ophthalmologic care should be sought for the eye involvement.

Dermatitis herpetiformis is a chronic, intensely pruritic, vesicular disease that is identified by the bilaterally symmetric (herpetiform) grouping of papules, urticarial plaques, and vesicles over the elbows, knees, buttocks, low back, scapular areas, and scalp. The itching often has a burning quality. The blisters occur just below the epidermis, where collections of neutrophils are found in the dermal papillae. Direct immunofluorescence testing of perilesional normal-appearing skin reveals granular deposits of IgA at the tips of the dermal papillae. Approximately 75 per cent of patients have an associated gluten-sensitive enteropathy that is usually asymptomatic. A gluten-free diet strictly followed for at least 12 months causes remissions or significantly reduces the required dose of dapsone or sulfapyridine, either of which promptly clears the disease. The rash recurs when therapy is stopped.

Erythema multiforme (see Color Plate 15G) is an immunologic reaction in the skin and mucous membranes often mediated by circulating immune complexes that evolve in response to a number of antigenic stimuli (infections, drugs, connective tissue disease). As the name implies, the skin reaction is characterized by a variety of lesions, namely, erythematous plaques, blisters, and target or bull's-eye lesions. The mucous membranes of the mouth and eye may also be involved, and this is referred to as *Stevens-Johnson syndrome.* Typically the cutaneous lesions favor the extremities (often the palms) and are symmetric. Target lesions are diagnostic and are recognized by a central, dark purple area or a blister surrounded by a pale, edematous, round zone, surrounded in turn by a peripheral rim of erythema. In Stevens-Johnson syndrome the skin disease is more widespread, with blisters and painful erosions in the mouth and eyes. The patients look and feel ill with fever, prostration, and difficulty in eating. Histologically, subepidermal separation is found in the blistering center of the target lesion, and when early lesions are biopsied, immunofluorescence reveals immunoglobulin and complement in the walls of the small dermal blood vessels; the inflammation and bullae form in response to vascular damage and leaking. In one half of cases no etiology is found for the reaction, but a cause should be sought in all cases, especially drugs (penicillins, barbiturates, phenytoin [Dilantin], and sulfonamides) and infections (herpes simplex, *Streptococcus*, *Mycoplasma pneumoniae*). Recurrent herpes simplex infection is the most common cause of recurrent erythema multiforme. It is not clear whether medical therapy favorably alters the course of idiopathic erythema multiforme, although treatment of a precipitating infection seems appropriate and acyclovir may prevent recurrences of herpes-associated erythema multiforme. Stopping suspected drugs is also imperative. The value of systemic steroids in erythema multiforme and Stevens-Johnson syndrome is controversial. In addition, IV fluids may be required in patients with severe oral involvement, and topical anesthetics (viscous Xylocaine) may help to decrease mouth discomfort.

An example of a bullous disease caused by a metabolic disorder is *porphyria*. Porphyria is a group of disorders characterized by abnormalities in the heme biosynthetic pathway, resulting in the excessive accumulation of various porphyrins (see Ch. 191). In several types of porphyria light reacts with photosensitizing porphyrins in the circulation and skin to cause both acute and chronic alterations in the integument. The onset of photosensitivity in childhood and severe scarring, hair loss, and discolored red teeth are recognized findings in the very rare *congenital erythropoietic porphyria*. Adult porphyrias causing skin changes are, at times, more subtle. Photodistributed skin fragility, with bullae and erosions that leave scars over the dorsum of the hands, forearms, and face, is a frequently missed sign of *porphyria cutanea tarda* (a familial or acquired deficiency in the enzyme uroporphyrinogen decarboxylase). Urinary uroporphyrins and coproporphyrins are markedly elevated, causing the urine to appear dark brown and fluoresce an orange-red color under Wood's light. Both sun exposure and mild trauma to the skin induce subepidermal bullae that leave scars (Fig. 525–9). Facial hair, predominantly on the temples and lateral cheeks, mottled facial pigmentation, and, at times, diffuse scleroderma-like changes on the face and neck also occur. Porphyria cutanea tarda is worsened by alcohol and birth control pills. There seems to be an associated iron overload syndrome with elevated liver stores and serum iron. The treatment of choice is phlebotomy to reduce hepatic iron. When used carefully, antimalarials are also effective.

Other metabolic bullous diseases are those seen with chronic renal disease and diabetes mellitus. Subepidermal bullae occasionally occur in association with hemodialysis in chronic renal

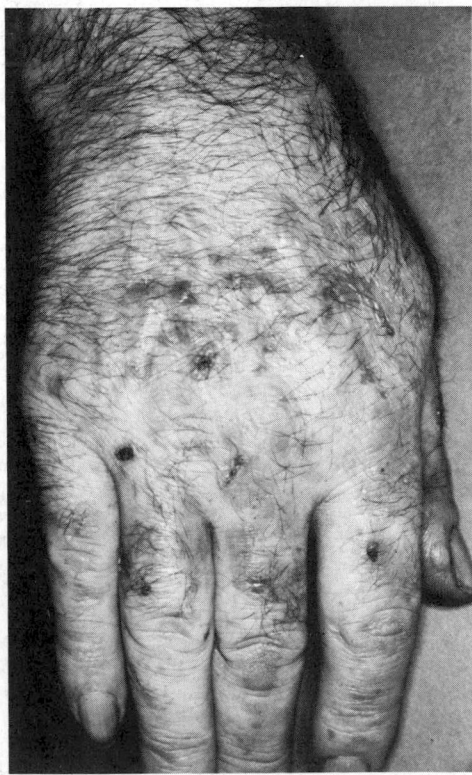

FIGURE 525–9. Porphyria cutanea tarda. (From the 17th edition of the Cecil Textbook of Medicine, with the permission of Dr. Marie-Louise Johnson.)

failure. The bullae are found on light-exposed areas, primarily the dorsa of hands, and may be worsened by sunlight. A few such patients have elevated uro- and coproporphyrins, suggesting that porphyria cutanea tarda is unmasked by dialysis, but most patients have had no alterations in porphyrin metabolism. These latter patients with *bullous dermatosis of hemodialysis* have scarring, tense, asymptomatic bullae without surrounding erythema. High doses of furosemide have also been reported to produce a bullous eruption on light-exposed skin of patients on hemodialysis. *Bullosis diabeticorum* appears as tense, bullous lesions on a noninflammatory base, usually localized to the lower extremities. These are related to trauma in diabetic patients with small vessel disease. A "pseudoporphyria" syndrome with skin changes identical to those seen in porphyria but without abnormalities in porphyrin metabolism is also being recognized with increasing frequency in patients receiving nonsteroidal anti-inflammatory drugs.

The last group of subepidermal bullous diseases is the *mechanobullous conditions*, a variety of inherited defects in various structures found within and above the dermal-epidermal junction (*epidermolysis bullosa*). Blisters, erosions, ulcers, and varying degrees of scarring result from minor trauma to the skin. The forms vary by inheritance pattern, level of blister formation, and degree of scarring. Scars and milia at sites of repeated trauma are more common in the recessive dystrophic variants (anchoring fibrils are missing in these epidermolysis bullosa dystrophica patients). In severe forms the mouth and esophagus are involved, adhesions cover the digits, and growth is retarded. The more serious forms appear at birth, whereas milder types occur later in life. No therapy is available except in the severe dystrophic form in which two thirds of patients may be helped by phenytoin (Dilantin), which decreases the excess production of collagenase found in this condition.

An acquired type of epidermolysis bullosa (EB), *EB acquisita* (EBA), has recently been recognized. EBA occurs in adult life and is easily confused with EB dystrophica and/or bullous pemphigoid. It presents with bullous lesions and skin fragility to minor trauma over pressure points and on the hands and feet, which heal with wrinkled scars and milia (yellow-white inclusion cysts). Oral lesions as well as extensive esophageal, laryngeal, and ocular scarring, features of cicatricial pemphigoid, may also be seen. The blisters occur below the lamina densa zone, where linear deposits of IgG and complement react with an EBA autoantigen. Circulating antibodies to this sublamina densa antigen are found in many patients. No satisfactory therapy is available.

PUSTULAR DISEASES OF THE SKIN

Pustules usually bring to mind infection, but not all pustular dermatoses are caused by pathogenic microorganisms. Pustular conditions often occur in association with erythematous papules, cysts, and nodules and may open to form crusts (Table 525–7).

NONINFECTIOUS PUSTULAR SKIN DISEASES. *Acne* is the most common pustular condition of the skin. It is an inflammatory disorder affecting pilosebaceous units and hence is usually found over the face and upper trunk where the greatest concentration of these skin appendages is found. Several factors play a pathogenic role in acne as individuals enter puberty: (1) androgenic stimulation of the sebaceous glands and increased sebum production (see Ch. 522); (2) abnormal keratinization and impaction in the pilosebaceous canal (comedones) causing obstruction to sebum flow; (3) proliferation of anaerobic bacteria, *Propionibacterium acnes*, which predispose to rupture of the pilosebaceous unit with extravasation into the surrounding dermis, resulting in sterile, inflammatory papules, pustules, and cysts. The inflammatory lesions lead to disfiguring scarring. Therapy of acne is usually successful in controlling the disease until the patient "grows out" of this condition. Treatment is directed at correcting the three major factors that seem to cause acne. Thus, topical agents that remove comedones such as benzoyl peroxide and topical vitamin A preparations are particularly effective because their action allows sebum to flow freely onto the surface of the skin. Topical and oral antibiotics (tetracycline and erythromycin) are indicated in patients with inflammatory papules and pustules. Last, decreasing sebum production has beneficial effects, and oral 13-*cis*-retinoic acid decreases sebaceous gland size and sebum production. This drug should be used primarily for severe cystic

TABLE 525–7. PUSTULAR DISEASES OF THE SKIN

Name of Skin Condition	Etiology	Important Physical Findings	Other Facts of Note in History or Laboratory Results
Noninfectious Pustular Diseases of the Skin			
Acne	Androgens; follicular orifice keratinization problem; *Propionibacterium acnes*	Open and closed comedones; red papules, pustules, cysts; scarring of face and upper trunk	Rule out acneiform eruptions such as caused by drugs, greasy cosmetics, endocrinologic abnormalities
Rosacea	Unknown	Red papules, pustules on background of erythema, telangiectasia; central face flushing is a common problem; rhinophyma; eye involvement	Seen in patients usually older than those with acne
Perioral dermatitis	May be caused by potent topical steroids; variant acne	Perioral and periorbital red scaling patches, papules, and pustules	
Pustular psoriasis	Variant of psoriasis	Sterile pustules localized to palms and soles or generalized over body	Patient is toxic with fever, leukocytosis; can die of generalized form
Miliaria pustulosa	Occlusion of sweat glands in hot environment	Discrete red papules or pustules with red base over trunk, especially back	
Infectious Pustular Diseases of the Skin			
Localized to the skin			
Folliculitis, carbuncles, furuncles	*Staphylococcus aureus* invasion of hair follicles	Discrete pustules with red base with centrally placed hairs on buttocks, thighs, beard, scalp	Gram's stain, culture
Candidiasis	*Candida* organisms	Satellite pustules around beefy red patches in moist intertriginous areas	KOH preparation; culture
Hot tub folliculitis	*Pseudomonas aeruginosa*	Widely scattered, pruritic pustules with red base over trunk and extremities	Gram's stain, culture; folliculitis resolves spontaneously in 10-14 days; *Pseudomonas* contaminates hot tubs, whirlpools, and swimming pools
Dermatophytes-kerion	Dermatophyte	Boggy patch with pustules in scalp	KOH, culture
Tinea barbae	Dermatophyte	Pustular inflammatory reaction in beard area	
Systemic infectious (septicemias)			
Bacterial septicemia (gonococcal, streptococcal, fungal—*Candida*)	Gonococcus	Purpuric pustules—acral lesions in gonococcus; *Staphylococcus aureus; Candida*	Associated with arthritis in gonoccoccus; patients usually ill

acne. The clinician should recognize that other factors may play a role in exacerbating acne, including oil-based cosmetics and drugs (androgenic hormones, antiepileptics [phenytoin], high-progestin birth control pills, systemic corticosteroids, when taken in high doses, and iodide- and bromide-containing agents). Occasionally endocrinologic conditions characterized by excess androgen secretion may cause acne, i.e., polycystic ovarian disease, adrenal or ovarian tumors.

Rosacea is a chronic inflammatory disorder affecting the blood vessels and pilosebaceous units of the face in middle-aged individuals. Patients with rosacea have papules and pustules superimposed on diffuse erythema and telangiectasia over the central portion of the face. An important component of the patients'

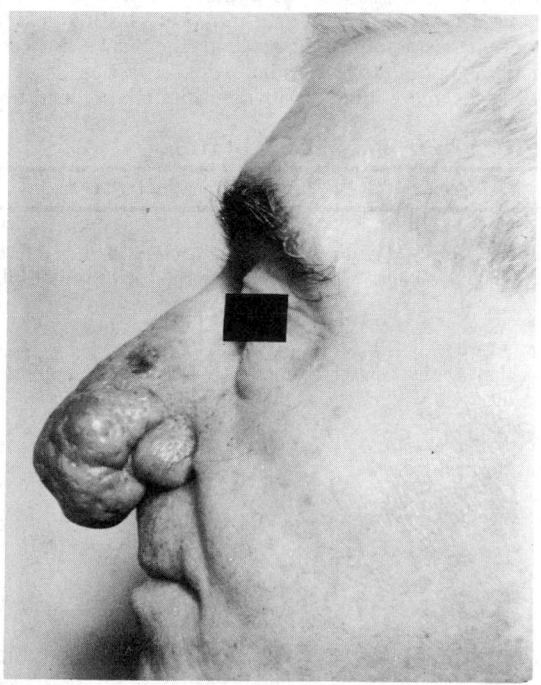

FIGURE 525–10. Rhinophyma. (From the 17th edition of the Cecil Textbook of Medicine, with the permission of Dr. Marie-Louise Johnson.)

history is easy flushing and blushing of the face, and this is often accentuated when alcohol, caffeine-containing, or hot spicy foods are ingested. Hyperplasia of the sebaceous glands, connective tissue, and vascular bed of the nose sometimes causes *rhinophyma* or a large, red, bulbous nose (Fig. 525–10). Ocular complications occur in a small but significant number of rosacea patients; these include blepharitis, chalazion, conjunctivitis, and keratitis. Progressive keratitis can lead to scarring and blindness. Rosacea and the eye complications are usually dramatically responsive to tetracycline, but the antibiotic must be continued for life (at the lowest dose that suppresses the condition) because rosacea recurs when therapy is interrupted. High-potency topical corticosteroid preparations may induce or aggravate pre-existing rosacea and should not be used for long periods of time on the face.

Perioral dermatitis, as the name suggests, is a conspicuous affliction consisting of red papules, pustules, and fine scaling erythema in a concentric oval about the mouth, sparing the skin immediately adjacent to the lips. Perioral dermatitis is probably a variant of rosacea or acne, and is most often seen in women between 18 and 40 years of age. Tetracycline is the mainstay of therapy, usually requiring 250 mg twice a day for 6 to 8 weeks.

Hidradenitis suppurativa is a chronic suppurative and scarring problem of the apocrine glands appearing as tense, draining lesions with retracted scars in the axillae and anogenital regions (Fig. 525–11).

Psoriasis can occasionally present in a pustular form, either localized to the palms and soles or as a generalized, total body reaction associated with fever and leukocytosis.

Miliaria, or heat rash, represents an inflammatory reaction caused by occlusion of sweat ducts with extravasation of their contents into the surrounding tissue. Occlusion of the duct at the level of the epidermal granular layer results in *miliaria rubra* (discrete, small, red papules), especially on the trunk and back. The presence of discrete lesions not associated with hair follicles suggests the diagnosis. In more deeply situated occlusion of the duct, *miliaria pustulosa,* or pustules with surrounding erythema, is seen. In the ambulatory patient miliaria results from exposure to a hot, humid environment, while in bedridden patients fever, sweating, and occlusion of the skin on bed sheets are predisposing factors. The problem usually remits with cooling and ventilation of the patient's skin.

INFECTIOUS CAUSES OF SKIN PUSTULES. *Folliculitis,* a *Staphylococcus aureus* infection of the hair follicle, appears as pustules with a red rim with hair emanating from the center of

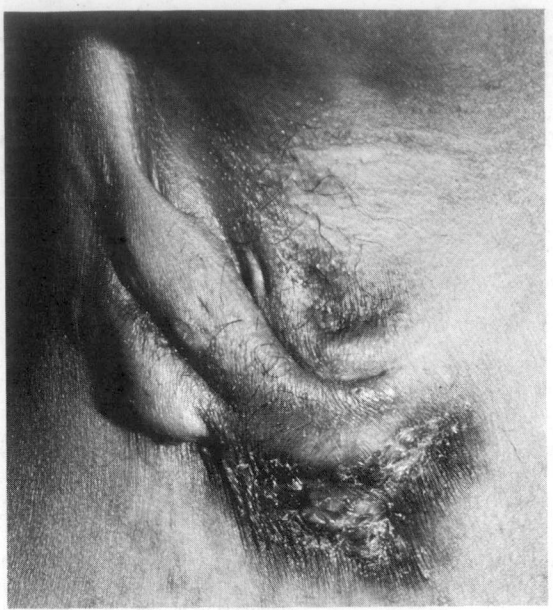

FIGURE 525–11. Hidradenitis suppurativa, axilla. (From the 17th edition of the Cecil Textbook of Medicine, with the permission of Dr. Marie-Louise Johnson.)

the pustule. Folliculitis typically occurs in hairy regions where clothing rubs (buttocks, thighs) or on the face. The key to diagnosis is finding a central hair in the pustule. Occasionally the follicular infection can extend more deeply to form a larger, red, fluctuant nodule that "points" to drain pus from one (furuncle) or more follicles (carbuncle). Systemic antibiotics such as erythromycin or dicloxacillin usually clear extensive infections; topical antiseptic cleansers such as povidone-iodine or chlorhexidine can resolve mild folliculitis and may be useful in preventing recurrences.

Candidiasis appears as beefy red patches in intertriginous, moist areas characteristically surrounded by satellite pustules. Paronychia, a painful red swelling in the periungual regions of the finger, may also drain pus in which *Candida* can be found with a KOH preparation. Topical agents such as clotrimazole and miconazole are used two or three times a day. These must be used for many weeks before the infection is cleared.

Hot tub folliculitis is a generalized, pruritic folliculitis caused by *Pseudomonas aeruginosa* that is acquired in hot tubs, whirlpools, or swimming pools contaminated by this organism. It usually begins 6 hours to 5 days after hot tub soaking and affects many people using the facility. It appears as a vesicular and then pustular eruption over the trunk, buttocks, legs, and arms but spares the head and neck. *Pseudomonas* can often be cultured from fresh pustules. In most instances the folliculitis resolves within 7 to 10 days without specific treatment. The tubs and pools implicated in causing this type of folliculitis should be cultured for *Pseudomonas* and disinfected.

Dermatophytes can, at times, infect hair follicles and result in pustules, particularly in the beard (tinea barbae) and scalp (kerions). These are readily confused with a bacterial folliculitis. Kerions appear as indurated, boggy, inflammatory plaques studded with pustules. These intense inflammatory reactions to superficial dermatophytes (especially *T. verrucosum*) respond to griseofulvin therapy, although a short course of oral corticosteroids is also useful.

Deep fungal infections such as *blastomycosis, sporotrichosis,* and *coccidioidomycosis* may cause pustules, as well as verrucous, ulcerative papules and nodules. Sporotrichosis characteristically spreads up cutaneous lymphatics and appears as nodular, pustular lesions in a linear distribution.

SYSTEMIC INFECTIONS CAUSING PUSTULES ON THE SKIN. A variety of septicemias including gonococcemia, staphylococcal septicemia, and *Candida* septicemia (in immunosuppressed patients) cause pustular lesions associated with purpura.

URTICARIA, PERSISTENT FIGURATE ERYTHEMAS, CELLULITIS

This group of skin lesions is of disparate appearance and etiology. The common feature is a raised edematous, red plaque with a sharply demarcated border (Table 525–8).

URTICARIAL REACTIONS. Urticaria, the most common condition in this group, appears as wheals, transient erythematous and edematous swellings of the dermis caused by local increase in permeability of capillaries and small venules. This increased permeability results from histamine and other chemical substances released from cutaneous mast cells by Type I IgE hypersensitivity reactions, as well as by nonimmunologic mechanisms (see Ch. 245). Certain agents such as aspirin, opiates, and some foods degranulate mast cells directly without an allergic mechanism. Other urticarial reactions are immunologically mediated by such allergens as infections (viral, i.e., hepatitis, sinus and tooth infections), infestations (systemic parasites), drugs, pollens, and injections (blood products, vaccinations). Other hives are caused by physical modalities: light (solar urticaria), cold (cold urticaria), heat or exercise (cholinergic urticaria), or pressure or rubbing of the skin (dermatographism). Hives are transient, any given lesion lasting less than 24 hours, although new hives may continuously evolve. Acute urticaria (i.e., lasting less than 6 weeks) often results from drugs and the cause is frequently identified. The etiology of chronic urticaria (lasting longer than 6 to 8 weeks) is more difficult to identify. Hives covering large

TABLE 525–8. URTICARIA, PERSISTENT FIGURATE ERYTHEMAS, CELLULITIS

Skin Condition	Etiology	Important Physical Findings	Other Facts of Note
Urticaria-like Reactions			
Urticaria	Drugs, foods, infections, physical modalities (heat, cold, light)	Transient, red wheals that usually stay in one area of skin less than 6–8 hours	Occasionally chronic sinus infection or apical tooth abscess can be silent cause
Erythema marginatum	Associated with rheumatic fever	Transient annular lesions	Associated with carditis
Urticaria pigmentosa	Abnormal accumulation of mast cells	Pigmented papules of skin; Darier's sign present	In adult, mast cells may infiltrate lymph nodes, liver, spleen, GI tract
Figurate Erythemas			
Erythema annulare centrifugum	Occasionally an "id" reaction to tinea infection elsewhere on the body	Annular lesions with red border and trailing scale; persist for many days or months	May mimic ringworm
Erythema chronicum migrans	Part of Lyme disease caused by bite of tick and spirochete infection	One or more slowly expanding annular lesions	Arthritis, cardiac problems, Bell's palsy often part of Lyme disease
Cellulitis			
Erysipelas	Streptococcal infection of dermis	Erythematous, warm, painful area with sharply demarcated border	Responds readily to penicillin
Necrotizing fasciitis	Mixed, aerobic, and anaerobic infection in fascial plane	Deep red, painful cellulitis that causes purpura and then tissue necrosis; moves rapidly	Seen in immunosuppressed patients and diabetics

areas and producing deep tissue swelling are termed *angioedema*. This condition can involve the tongue and throat and threaten to close off the airway. In such patients a careful history about medications (including over-the-counter drugs, especially cold tablets or medications containing aspirin) should be elicited. Infections such as "silent" sinusitis or apical abscess of teeth must be looked for. In addition, physical types of urticaria should be considered: *cholinergic* urticaria is characterized by evanescent multiple, small wheals surrounded by a wide pink flare induced by heat and exercise; *solar* urticaria by large plaques in sun-exposed areas; *cold* urticaria by wheals that evolve with exposure to cold. Urticaria accompanied by fever and arthralgias occurs in serum sickness reactions and in the prodromata of viral hepatitis. Occasionally urticaria occurs in conjunction with internal conditions such as malignancies or connective tissue diseases. Hereditary angioedema, an autosomal dominant disorder, causes recurrent urticaria, angioedema, intestinal colic, and life-threatening laryngeal edema.

If the cause for the urticaria cannot be found or avoided, symptomatic control is achieved with antihistamines or oral steroids. Acute angioedema or laryngeal edema requires rapid systemic treatment with epinephrine and diphenhydramine (see Ch. 245).

Other urticaria-like skin lesions include *erythema multiforme* (see above); *juvenile rheumatoid arthritis skin lesions*—small, 2- to 3-mm, salmon-colored hives that last only a few hours appearing with fever spikes; *erythema marginatum*—lesions found in 10 per cent of patients with acute rheumatic fever (Ch. 298). *Urticaria pigmentosa* (mastocytosis), a disease caused by increased accumulations of mast cells in the skin and at times in lymph nodes, liver, spleen, bones, and gastrointestinal tract (see Ch. 252), presents with multiple tan to brown, papular spots that urticate when rubbed (Darier's sign) owing to the release of histamine from the mast cells. A skin biopsy specimen stained with Giemsa's stain will readily identify increased numbers of mast cells in the dermis. When the lesions in the skin develop in early childhood, the condition is usually limited to skin and the lesions resolve by puberty, leaving only hyperpigmented macules. If the skin lesions evolve in adulthood there is a greater chance for mast cell infiltration of the organ systems noted above, and the skin lesions persist. Symptoms and findings in mastocytosis depend on the organ systems involved and the release of various vasoactive substances contained in the increased masses of mast cells. Hepatosplenomegaly, lymphadenopathy, and bone pain may occur secondary to infiltrates. Patients may experience flushing, palpitations, headache, syncope, hypotension, abdominal pain, and diarrhea, all related to histamine and prostaglandin release from the mast cells.

FIGURATE ERYTHEMAS. This is a group of uncommon conditions characterized by annular, polycyclic, and geographic erythematous skin lesions. These conditions, in contrast to the urticarial reactions, persist for many days or even years, moving slowly or rapidly over the skin surface (hence, the term sometimes used for these reactions—persistent figurate erythema).

The most common of these diseases, *erythema annulare centrifugum*, appears as one or more annular lesions with an elevated erythematous border and a fine scale on the inner aspect of the border (trailing scale).

Erythema chronicum migrans is the unique annular skin lesion found in Lyme disease caused by a spirochete inoculated by infected tick bites (see Ch. 343 and Color Plate 10A).

CELLULITIS. Although superficially resembling urticaria, these inflammatory infections of the dermis are readily distinguished from hives by their persistent, slowly enlarging nature as well as their pain and warmth. Group A streptococci and *Staphylococcus aureus* are the organisms most commonly responsible. *Erysipelas* is sometimes identified separately from cellulitis. It displays a sharply demarcated painful border and an "orange-peel" epidermal surface. Group A *Streptococcus* is the usual cause. Patients usually feel ill and are febrile. Cellulitis on the lower legs in adults may develop from fissures between the toes from tinea pedis. Systemic antibiotics, erythromycin, dicloxacillin, or the cephalosporins are the drugs most commonly used.

Necrotizing fasciitis is a special form of cellulitis involving the deep fascial structures underlying the skin. Rapidly evolving in enclosed fascial spaces, usually in diabetics or immunosuppressed patients, these infections are caused by a mixture of aerobic and

anaerobic gram-negative organisms and must be diagnosed early by deep fascial biopsy and treated immediately with a broad spectrum of antibiotics and surgical debridement.

NODULES AND TUMORS OF THE SKIN

Nodular and tumorous lesions of the skin may evolve within the epidermis or the dermis and subcutaneous tissue, arising in various skin appendages and structures, including melanocytes. Such nodular lesions may represent benign or malignant growths, infiltrative or inflammatory reactions. In many instances the structures giving rise to the nodule reflect the colors of these structures; i.e., vascular lesions appear red to purple, whereas lesions involving melanocytes appear pigmented.

In general, epidermal nodules are recognized by localized thickening of the epidermis or corneum with hyperkeratosis or scale. Dermal or subcutaneous nodules appear as lumps, often with no alteration in the overlying epidermis.

Of primary concern in every patient with a nodule is whether it is benign or malignant. This is not always easy to discern, and therefore skin nodules and tumors often must be biopsied. Some clinical generalizations can be made in distinguishing benign from malignant tumors (Table 525–9).

Common nodular lesions of the skin are listed in Table 525–10.

NONPIGMENTED NODULES—BENIGN. *Warts* are benign epidermal growths caused by papilloma viruses (see above, under Maculopapular lesions).

Sebaceous hyperplasia occurs as papular and occasionally nodular lesions on the faces of individuals past 50 years of age. This proliferation of sebaceous glands surrounding a hair follicle appears as groups of yellow papules evolving in an annular configuration with a central pore. Sebaceous hyperplasia is sometimes clinically difficult to differentiate from basal cell cancers, although the yellow discoloration and central pore may help. At times skin biopsy may be necessary. No treatment is generally required.

Keratoacanthomas (see Color Plate 15D), or self-healing epitheliomas, are rapidly growing neoplasms of epidermal keratinocytes that are biologically benign. These lesions resolve spontaneously, leaving a scar. Keratoacanthomas are usually found on sun-exposed areas and begin as flesh-colored papules that rapidly grow over a period of 6 weeks, evolving a central keratin-filled crater. The lesions remain for 6 to 8 weeks and then subside. Such lesions are best excised because they leave unsightly scars and are difficult to differentiate from squamous cell cancer, even histologically.

Epidermal inclusion cysts appear as flesh-colored, firm nodules in the skin, particularly over the scalp and trunk. A helpful diagnostic sign is a central enlarged pore where the epidermis has invaginated to form the cyst. If the central pore is patent, slight squeezing will express white, cheesy, foul-smelling keratin and sebum. If the cyst is bothersome it can be excised.

Lipomas are more deeply situated than epidermal inclusion cysts; although they can feel firm and even rubbery, like a cyst, they usually are multilobulated and softer in consistency. If the diagnosis is in doubt and especially if the lesion is firm, a biopsy is indicated. Lipomas may be multiple, and familial multiple epidermal cysts and lipomas, fibromas, and osteomas associated with intestinal polyps are recognized as Gardner's syndrome.

Neurofibromas, focal proliferations of neural tissue within the dermis, may present in two forms: (1) soft, flesh-colored, pro-

TABLE 525–9. CLINICAL FEATURES HELPFUL IN DISTINGUISHING BENIGN FROM MALIGNANT TUMORS

Clinical Feature	Benign	Malignant
Configuration	Symmetric, sharp borders	Asymmetric, irregular borders
Rate of growth	Slow	Slow or rapid
Friability	No friability	Often friable
Bleeding or ulceration	Seldom bleed or ulcerate	Often bleed and ulcerate
Consistency	Firm or soft	Usually firm to hard
Color	Uniform color and pigmentation	Irregularity of color and pigmentation

TABLE 525–10. NODULAR LESIONS OF THE SKIN

Lesion	Appearance	Distribution	Etiology	Other Factors
Nonpigmented Nodules–Benign				
Warts	Skin-colored, corrugated hyperkeratotic surface	Anywhere on body	Papillomavirus	Appearance may vary, depending on location of wart; i.e., plantar warts are flat with callus on surface; condylomata acuminata are soft, moist, cauliflower-like nodules
Sebaceous hyperplasia	Yellow, papular nodules around hair follicles	Face	Benign hyperplasia of sebaceous glands	
Keratoacanthoma	Rapidly growing nodule with keratin-filled central crater	Sun-exposed areas	Benign hyperplasia of keratinocytes	Resolves spontaneously leaving scars
Epidermal inclusion cyst	Flesh-colored, firm nodules with rubbery consistency and enlarged pore on surface	Often scalp, face, trunk	Epidermally lined cysts	Occasionally becomes secondarily infected
Lipoma	Multilobulated, firm nodule with normal overlying epidermis	Extremities, trunk	Benign localized hypertrophy of adipose tissue	
Neurofibroma	Soft, flesh-colored, protruding nodules that can be invaginated deeper into skin—buttonhole sign	Extremities, trunk	Hyperplasia of neural tissue in dermis	Can be associated with von Recklinghausen's disease and café au lait spots and axillary freckling
Nonpigmented Nodules—Malignant				
Basal cell carcinoma	Opalescent, waxy nodule often with ulceration	Sun-exposed areas, 97% face, neck, arms	Ultraviolet light and genetics play a role	Locally invasive—seldom metastasizes
Squamous cell cancer	Hard, smooth or verrucous nodules that often show hyperkeratinization	Sun-exposed areas	Ultraviolet light and genetics play a role	May be metastatic, especially those on lower lip
Pigmented Nodules—Benign				
Seborrheic keratosis	Light brown to black verrucous lesions with stuck-on appearance	Face, trunk	Seen in older people	Individual lesions of uniform color
Dermatofibroma	Firm dermal papules and nodules with overlying brown hyperpigmentation; dimple sign—dimpling of epidermis with pinching of skin	Usually legs	Trauma, insect bites induce dermal fibrosis	Can be flesh-colored or red
Nevi	Uniformly pigmented, flat to nodular symmetrically shaped lesions	Anywhere on body	Accumulation of benign pigmented nevus cells	Itching nevi or changes in color, size, or configuration are danger signs of melanoma
Pigmented Nodules—Malignant				
Melanoma	Flat to nodular, pigmented lesions with asymmetry of growth, irregular borders, variegation of pigmentation, and diameter greater than 6 mm	Anywhere on body	Probably ultraviolet light exposure; genetic predisposition	Itching may be early sign of melanoma; melanoma can arise from pre-existing nevi
Vascular Tumors of Skin				
Hemangiomas	Flat to nodular, red, blue, purple, soft lesions	Anywhere on body	Proliferation of blood vessels of dermis	Strawberry hemangiomas usually regress; port-wine stains persist
Pyogenic granuloma	Bright red nodules that readily bleed	Extremities, hands, fingers	Proliferation of blood vessels following trauma	
Kaposi's sarcoma	Red, purple, brown papules and plaques	Legs, neck, trunk	Cytomegalovirus, AIDS	Seen most often with AIDS or immunosuppression
Inflammatory Nodules of Skin				
Erythema nodosum	Multiple, red, painful nodules; do not ulcerate; involute leaving bruises	Pretibial areas	Hypersensitivity reaction in subcutaneous fat	Number of antigenetic stimuli: drugs, infections, intestinal inflammatory disease
Subcutaneous fat necrosis	Red nodules, tender	Lower legs, thighs	Fat necrosis secondary to release of pancreatic lipase	Pancreatitis, pancreatitic cancer
Rheumatoid nodules	Nonpainful, firm nodules	Elbows, knees, fingers	Unknown	Rheumatoid arthritic changes with high rheumatoid factor titer
Nodules Associated with Metabolic Conditions				
Xanthomas	Nontender, firm, yellow to red papules and nodules	Elbows, knees, Achilles tendons	Hyperlipoproteinemias	Xanthomas related to genetic disorder of lipoprotein metabolism (primary) or secondary to underlying diseases

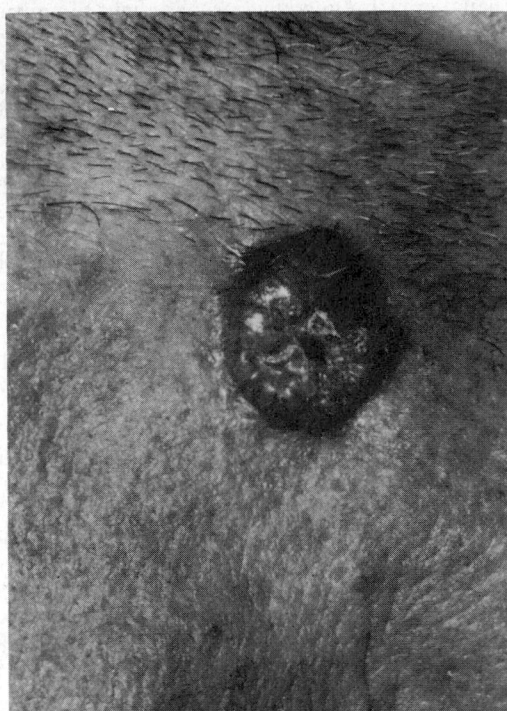

FIGURE 525–12. Basal cell epithelioma. (From the 17th edition of the Cecil Textbook of Medicine, with the permission of Dr. Marie-Louise Johnson.)

truding nodules that, on compression, can be invaginated into what feels like a defect in the skin (buttonhole sign), and (2) deep, firm, dermal or subcutaneous nodules. Neurofibromas may be solitary, but when they are multiple *von Recklinghausen's disease* should be considered, especially when café au lait spots (light brown macules) and axillary freckling are seen.

NONPIGMENTED NODULES—MALIGNANT. Malignant tumors of the epidermis—*basal cell* and *squamous cell carcinomas*—are related to the amount and intensity of electromagnetic radiation, including ultraviolet light and x-radiation, the skin has received over a lifetime. Such cancers are therefore found most commonly on sun-exposed areas, especially the face, neck, arms, and hands. The cancers are more common in patients living in southern latitudes of the northern hemisphere and in Australia in those with light complexions who sunburn easily, and especially in patients whose occupations keep them outdoors. In addition, these epidermal cancers are more common in immunosuppressed patients, attesting to the importance of the immune surveillance system in cancer etiology. A personal or family history of skin cancer should always make the physician more alert to the possibility of cancer.

Basal cell carcinoma (see Color Plate 15A) is a malignancy arising from the basal cells of the epidermis. These tumors rarely metastasize, but they have considerable potential for extensive, local destruction. Four clinical forms should be recognized: (1) The *nodular* type, the most common, appears as a pearly or opalescent, irregularly shaped papule or nodule with a central depression or crater; telangiectasias and a rolled, waxy border are often in evidence. When ulceration and crusting occur, it is referred to as a rodent ulcer (Fig. 525–12). Many times the raised, waxy border is subtle and is observed more readily by stretching the skin. (2) *Superficial* basal cell carcinoma is recognized as a red, slightly scaling, eczematous plaque that may be slightly eroded and crusted. Careful examination reveals a thread-like, pearly, rolled edge. This is an easily overlooked neoplasm, frequently confused with psoriasis or eczematous patches, so that a high index of suspicion, along with skin biopsy, is needed to make the diagnosis. (3) *Pigmented* basal cell carcinoma appears as a blue-black nodule or plaque with a pearly, opalescent sheen as seen in other basal cell cancers. Melanocytes are not histologically involved in these cancers, merely stimulated to make more pigment, and the prognosis of these pigmented forms is the same as for other basal cell cancers. (4) *Scarring* or *sclerosing* basal cell cancers present as atrophic, white, sometimes slightly eroded

or crusted plaques with telangiectasia. This is the most difficult form to cure because of its indistinct borders. The diagnosis of basal cell carcinoma should be confirmed by biopsy. Treatment depends on the location of the lesion, the morphologic type, the size of the tumor, and whether it is primary or recurrent. Treatment modalities include curettage and electrodesiccation, scalpel excision, radiotherapy, and cryotherapy. When these are selected properly each modality has a cure rate of greater than 90 per cent. A specialized form of excision using careful histologic orientation and detailed mapping of the extent of the tumor is the Mohs surgical technique. This tedious form of surgery is used for recurrent basal cell cancers, sclerosing basal cell cancers, and large primary basal cell cancers in regions in which recurrences are likely (particularly in the nasolabial folds and the periorbital and immediate preauricular areas).

Squamous cell carcinoma (see Color Plate 15B), a malignant neoplasm of the keratinocytes, is a less common but more aggressive type of cancer than basal cell cancer. Squamous cell carcinoma is locally invasive and has the potential to metastasize. It occurs primarily on the head and neck, upper extremities, and trunk, presenting as firm, red, smooth or verrucous nodules. Hyperkeratoses may be prominent, and indeed "cutaneous horns" are often squamous cell carcinomas (see Color Plate 15C). The cancers also display increased friability, ulceration, and crusting (Fig. 525–13). *Bowen's disease* is a squamous cell cancer in situ, appearing as red, scaling, crusted, sharply demarcated plaques. Squamous cell cancer in situ on the penis in uncircumcised males evolves as velvety red patches on the glans and foreskin (erythroplasia of Queyrat). Bowen's disease and erythroplasia are banal, easily overlooked conditions that can metastasize if not diagnosed early. *Actinic keratoses*, precancerous lesions of atypical keratinocytes, appear as red, ill-marginated macules and papules with yellow-brown, adherent scales in sun-damaged skin. They may evolve into squamous cell cancers. Any lesion suspected of being a squamous cell cancer should be biopsied. Excision is the treatment of choice in squamous cell cancers. Actinic keratoses are treated with liquid nitrogen freezing or, if numerous, with topical 5-fluorouracil applied as 1 or 5 per cent cream or solution over 2- to 4-week period.

PIGMENTED NODULES—BENIGN. *Seborrheic keratoses* are neoplasms of the epidermal cells that appear on the face and trunk in middle age. These 2-mm to 5-cm, elevated, tan to brown or occasionally black, round to oval lesions have a verrucous or crumbly, greasy surface and a stuck-on appearance. No therapy is necessary unless they are of cosmetic concern, and then liquid nitrogen cryotherapy or curettage is an effective means of removal.

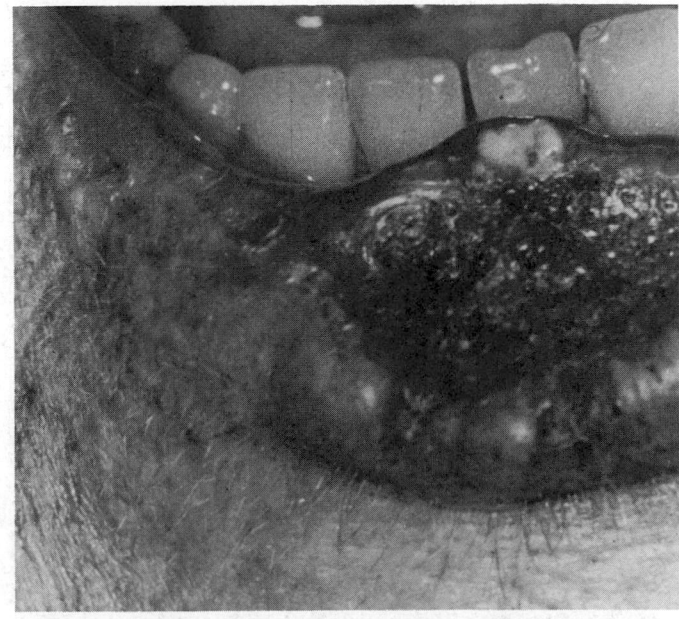

FIGURE 525–13. Squamous cell carcinoma. (From the 17th edition of the Cecil Textbook of Medicine, with the permission of Dr. Marie-Louise Johnson.)

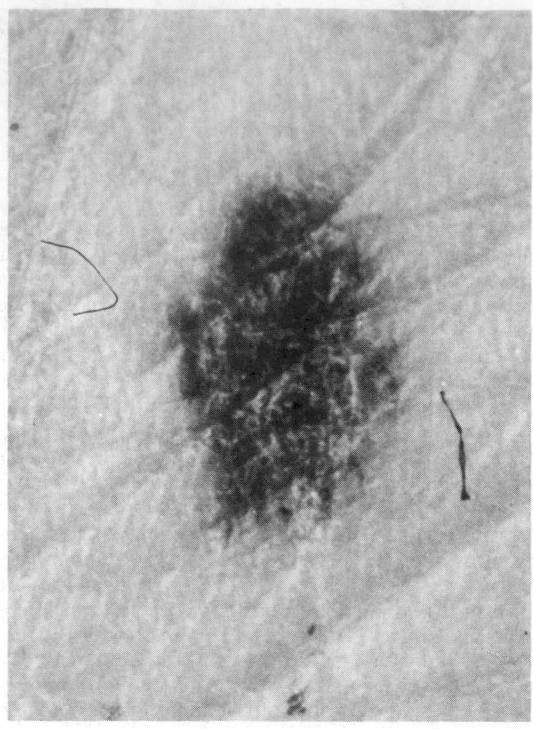

FIGURE 525–14. Junctional nevus. (From the 17th edition of the Cecil Textbook of Medicine, with the permission of Dr. Marie-Louise Johnson.)

Dermatofibromas are areas of focal dermal fibrosis accompanied by overlying epidermal thickening and hyperpigmentation, appearing clinically as brown papules or nodules. A useful diagnostic test is the "dimple sign," in which pinching the lesion results in central dimpling of the overlying epidermis. Some dermatofibromas are dark brown in color and occasionally raise the concern of melanoma, but the fibromas are symmetric and uniform in color. The lesions occur frequently on the lower extremities and less often on the arms, and they may be multiple. Although therapy is usually not required, simple excision can be done.

Nevi, or *moles,* are benign accumulations of pigment-forming nevus cells. They may be congenital or acquired, and most nevi evolve before age 35, appearing sometime after the first year of life. There are three forms, representing various stages of biologic evolution and growth: *Junctional nevi* are light to brown macular lesions (Fig. 525–14). *Compound nevi* have flat, junctional portions along with brown papules with a smooth or rough surface; these evolve from junctional nevi in older children and young adults. Later, *intradermal nevi* evolve from the compound nevi as flesh-colored to brown papules or sessile growths (Fig. 525–15). Although nevi vary in appearance and color, individually they are uniform in color, symmetric in their growth and configuration, and usually less than 6 mm in diameter. Occasionally nevi darken in color or may itch, and new nevi may develop during pregnancy, but symptomatic nevi that change should be regarded suspiciously.

PIGMENTED NODULES—MALIGNANT. Malignant melanoma (see Color Plate 16*E* and *F*) is the cutaneous neoplasm of melanocytes and nevus cells. Four important clinical features are useful in recognizing malignant melanoma, the so-called A-B-C-D's of diagnosis:

A = Asymmetry of the lesion is due to irregular, random growth of the malignant cells associated with irregular surface topography and papules and nodules.

B = Borders of the tumors are irregular with notching and pigment "spilling" out beyond the edges.

C = Color variegation consists of browns, blacks, blues, and even shades of red and white. The variations in color represent different depths of invasion of pigment cells along with inflammatory reaction and immunologic response to the malignant cells.

D = Diameter or size of melanomas tends to be greater than 6 mm before they are recognized.

Several clinical forms or presentations of melanoma can be identified, each of these forms demonstrating the above characteristics. *Lentigo maligna melanoma* is a slowly evolving, multicolored lesion on the head and neck. It is preceded by lentigo maligna (in situ melanoma), which extends peripherally and is an unevenly pigmented, dark brown to black macule that can grow to a size of 5 to 7 cm over a period of many years before nodules develop, signifying dermal invasion (Fig. 525–16). *Superficial spreading melanoma* may occur on any area of the body, appearing as irregularly pigmented lesions with papules, nodules, and notched borders (Fig. 525–17). Invasion into the dermis occurs more rapidly than in lentigo maligna melanoma. *Nodular melanoma* appears as a rapidly growing, blue-black, smooth or eroded nodule (Fig. 525–18). It invades dermis early in its evolution, so it is less likely to be diagnosed in a premetastatic stage. *Acral lentiginous melanoma* occurs on the palms, soles, and digits. It evolves as an irregular, enlarging, variegate-colored, brown to black growth similar to lentigo maligna melanoma but more aggressive in its propensity for dermal invasion early in its course. Only minor degrees of papular elevation may be associated with deep invasion.

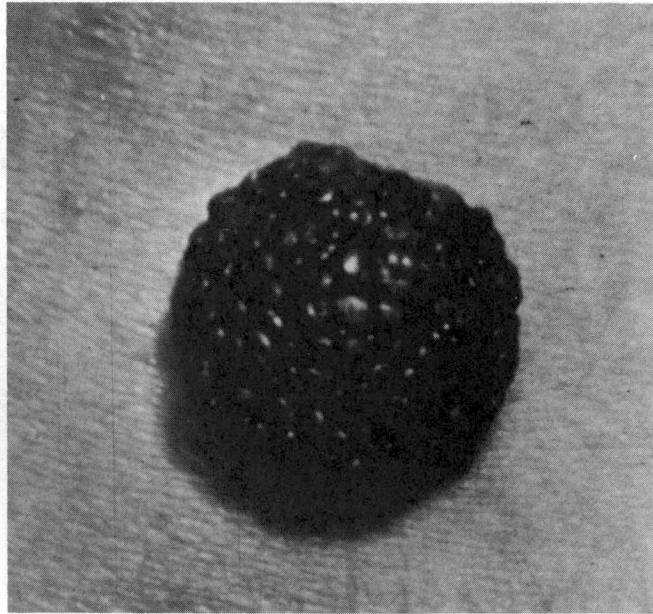

FIGURE 525–15. Intradermal nevus. (From the 17th edition of the Cecil Textbook of Medicine, with the permission of Dr. Marie-Louise Johnson.)

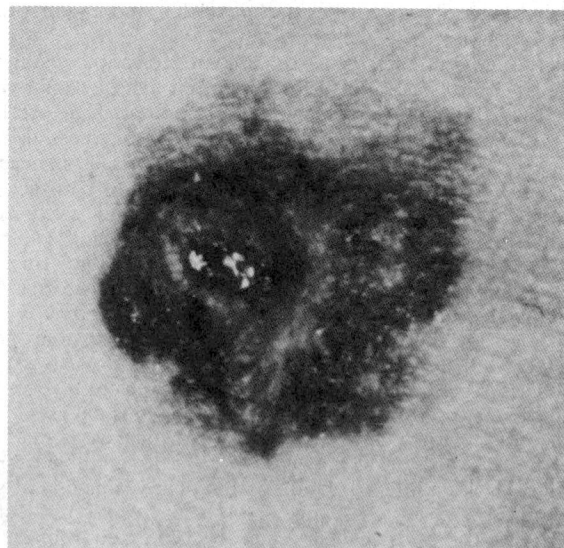

FIGURE 525–16. Lentigo maligna. (From the 17th edition of the Cecil Textbook of Medicine, with the permission of Dr. Marie-Louise Johnson.)

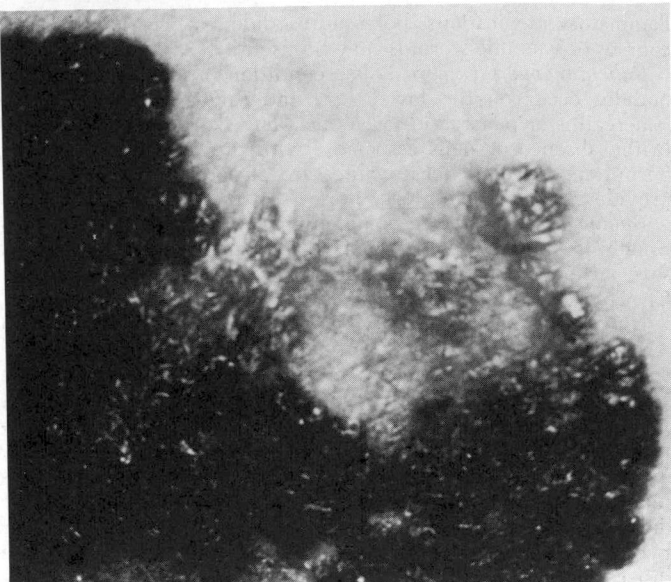

FIGURE 525–17. Superficial spreading melanoma. (From the 17th edition of the Cecil Textbook of Medicine, with the permission of Dr. Marie-Louise Johnson.)

One third of melanomas may arise from existing nevi, so that a change in size, shape, and color or itching of a pigmented lesion (a common symptom in melanomas) should be carefully investigated. Early diagnosis is the key to survival of patients with melanoma. The deeper the malignant cells invade the dermis, the more likely is metastasis. The depth of dermal invasion can be microscopically measured from the granular cell layer in the epidermis to the deepest penetration of melanoma cells into the dermis. If the melanoma is thin (< 0.76 mm), there is a virtually 100 per cent cure rate. If the depth is greater than 1.6 mm, only a 20 to 30 per cent 5-year survival is seen.

Any suspicious pigmented lesion must be biopsied, preferably by excision. Definitive, wide surgical excision should be undertaken only after confirmation of melanoma is established histologically. In large lesions such as lentigo maligna, it is acceptable to do incisional biopsy prior to definitive therapy. Suspicious pigmented lesions should never be shave-biopsied or shave-excised, nor should they be electrocauterized. Full-thickness tissue through the lesion is required for diagnostic and prognostic evaluation.

The precise cause of melanoma is unknown, but sunlight and heredity have been suggested as risk factors. The occurrence of melanoma has been increasing during the past few decades. Familial occurrence of malignant melanoma is seen in families with the *dysplastic nevus syndrome*. Numerous atypical, haphaz-ardly colored, red-brown nevi with irregular borders are found over the trunk, extremities, and scalp. Biopsy of these atypical nevi reveals disordered melanocytic proliferation. The nevi may have an increased risk of developing melanoma, although the melanomas can also arise from normal skin in these individuals. Close clinical follow-up and excision of suspicious nevi are important.

VASCULAR TUMORS OF THE SKIN. *Hemangiomas,* benign proliferations of dermal vessels, appear as red, blue, or purple, flat to papular and nodular lesions present at or soon after birth. Their appearance depends upon the number, size, and depth of the proliferating vessels. Thus, capillary angiomas are composed of small, superficial vessels causing *nevus flammeus* and *strawberry hemangiomas. Cavernous hemangiomas* are made up of larger and deeper vessels. Cavernous and strawberry angiomas often enlarge at an alarming rate over the first year or two and then usually involute by age nine or ten. Cavernous hemangiomas are less likely to resolve and at times may be deeply situated, large lesions that, when located in strategic locations (around the eye and mouth), may require systemic steroids that, in some instances, shrink these tumors. Platelet consumption by large cavernous hemangiomas may occur in the *Kasabach-Merritt syndrome*. Ordinarily no therapy is required for hemangiomas; watchful waiting allows the lesions to resolve spontaneously, the cosmetic result usually being superior to that obtained by therapeutic intervention. When large hemangiomas ulcerate, bleed, or impinge on vital structures or functions (e.g., around the ears, eyes, nose, mouth), oral steroids given over short periods of time in the dose of 1 to 2 mg per kilogram body weight shrink the tumor temporarily while awaiting the natural involution.

Pyogenic granuloma, a bright red, raspberry-like growth that can reach a centimeter in size, is friable and bleeds easily when traumatized. These lesions occur most often on arms, legs, fingers, and hands. They enlarge rapidly within weeks but have no malignant potential; they represent capillary hemangiomatous proliferation and occur following injury or surgery. The term *pyogenic* is a misnomer, as no infectious process is involved. These lesions are treated with excision, curettage and electrocauterization, or cryotherapy. Occasionally amelanotic melanoma may present as a pyogenic granuloma, so pathologic examination of pyogenic granulomas should be performed.

Kaposi's sarcoma (see Color Plate 16D) is a rare neoplasm of multifocal origin which presents as red-purple to blue-brown macules, plaques, and nodules of the skin and other organs. The cutaneous lesions may be firm or compressible, solitary or numerous, and may even appear initially as a dusky stain, especially about the toes.

These round-cell and spindle-cell sarcomas are also found in viscera and until their association with AIDS was recognized, seemed to occur predominantly in older men, leading to their demise. In Europe and North America, where Kaposi's sarcoma is more frequently seen among Jews and those of Mediterranean descent, the lesions commonly affect the lower extremities, are indolent, and often are associated with chronic lymphedema, indicating tumor infiltration of the lymphatics. Men are affected 10 to 15 times more often than women, are usually in their seventh decade, and have an average survival time of approximately 10 years. The incidence of such Kaposi's sarcoma reported for the United States is less than 0.1 per 100,000 population and fewer than 0.02 per cent of all malignancies.

In tropical Africa, however, there is an endemic belt at an altitude of 1200 to 1500 meters where the disease accounts for 3 to 9 per cent of all malignancies, afflicting the black population while sparing white people and Indians. It has a peak incidence in the first decade, with most patients less than 20 years of age, and with survival of less than 3 years. Visceral rather than cutaneous involvement and marked lymphadenopathy are the predominant clinical signs in these African children, who exhibit a unique form of Kaposi's sarcoma found in no other population.

The selective geographic distribution of the lymphadenopathic type of Kaposi's sarcoma is remarkably similar to that of Burkitt's lymphoma. With electron microscopic studies that affirm an association between cytomegalovirus and Kaposi's sarcoma, another parallel is made with Burkitt's lymphoma, the malignancy so closely linked to the Epstein-Barr virus. In the acquiring of Kaposi's sarcoma, therefore, it would seem that infectious agents

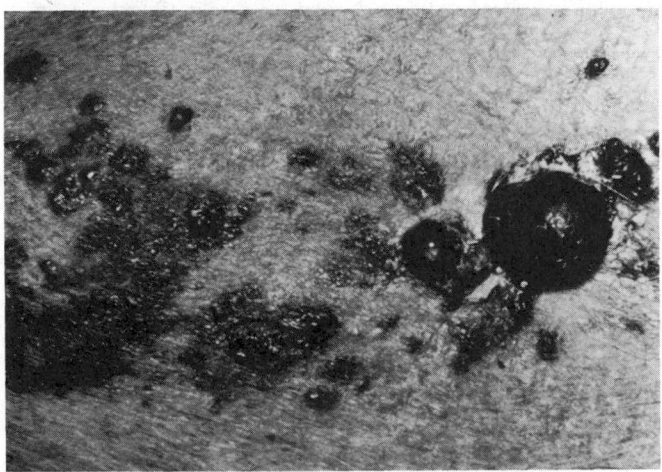

FIGURE 525–18. Nodular melanoma. (From the 17th edition of the Cecil Textbook of Medicine, with the permission of Dr. Marie-Louise Johnson.)

and immune status are of significance, as well as genetic and environmental factors. Kaposi's sarcoma has been observed to complicate systemic lupus erythematosus being treated with immunosuppression and to appear along with tumors of lympho-reticular origin in the immunosuppressed recipients of renal transplants. It is known to coexist with other primary malignancies. However, its appearance as an aggressive lethal tumor in the young male homosexual is the stunning observation of grave concern. Those affected have a mean age in the fourth decade. Their skin lesions are generalized in distribution and are smaller, softer, and lighter in color than the classic firm, indurated lesions of the legs. Mucous membrane tumors or symptomatic visceral or lung lesions may appear before the hemorrhagic sarcomas of the skin. Average survival time from onset of the disease is less than 2 years.

Such fulminant Kaposi's sarcoma appears alone or with *Pneumocystis carinii* pneumonia and other opportunistic infections in increasing numbers in male homosexuals and drug abusers. A small painless red nodule of the skin, easily overlooked, can signal a profoundly compromised immune state and grave prognosis (see Ch. 417 and Color Plate 12*D*).

INFLAMMATORY NODULES OF THE SKIN. *Erythema nodosum* is an inflammatory reaction in subcutaneous fat which represents a hypersensitivity response to a number of antigenic stimuli. These well-localized, multiple, tender, red, deep nodules, 1 to 5 cm in size, usually develop bilaterally over the pretibial areas. They eventually involute, leaving yellow-purple bruises. Ulceration does not occur. Immunoglobulin and complement deposition has been found in deep blood vessels in early lesions, and in some patients circulating immune complexes have been detected. The localization of the painful nodules to the lower legs may be related to hemodynamic factors. Although no cause can be found in many patients, the following etiologic factors have been identified: drugs (especially oral contraceptives), pregnancy, inflammatory bowel disease, sarcoidosis, streptococcal infection, *Yersinia* enterocolitis, deep fungus infections, and tuberculosis. If the etiology cannot be identified and eliminated, symptomatic therapy with aspirin, nonsteroidal anti-inflammatory medications, potassium iodide, or occasionally short courses of systemic steroids may be useful.

Subcutaneous fat necrosis is a condition in which tender, red nodules occur on the lower legs and thighs in patients with pancreatitis or pancreatic carcinoma. The skin lesions may occur in the absence of signs associated with the internal carcinoma. Serum amylase and lipase values are elevated, and skin biopsy provides diagnostic findings.

Rheumatoid nodules are subcutaneous inflammatory lesions usually found over elbows, knees, and fingers in patients with severe rheumatoid arthritis and high rheumatoid factor titer (see Ch. 258).

NODULES ASSOCIATED WITH METABOLIC DISEASES AND MISCELLANEOUS CONDITIONS. *Xanthomas* are focal collections of lipid-containing histiocytes in the dermis and tendon sheaths which appear as yellowish papules (eruptive xanthomas), plaques (xanthelasma), nodules (xanthoma tuberosum), and xanthomas in tendons and tendon sheaths (xanthoma tendinosum). Xanthomas often arise in association with inherited hyperlipoproteinemias (see Ch. 172) or in a variety of underlying metabolic diseases that alter lipoprotein metabolism, such as diabetes, hypothyroidism, cholestatic liver disease, pancreatitis, and renal disease, and in reaction to some drugs (e.g., 13-*cis*-retinoic acid). Xanthelasma usually develops in the absence of hyperlipidemia, although hypercholesterolemia (and increased low density lipoproteins) may be present.

Patients with gout occasionally deposit sodium urate in the skin, forming firm, hard papules and nodules (tophi) that may discharge whitish crystals in the pinnae of the ears and periauricular areas.

ATROPHIC SKIN CONDITIONS WITH SCARRING, INDURATION, ULCERATION, AND TELANGIECTASIAS

Connective tissue diseases are the most common conditions that lead to this spectrum of cutaneous changes.

SCARRING. *Lupus erythematosus* may be localized to the skin (discoid lupus) or present as a systemic condition (see Ch. 261) (Table 525–11). Discoid lupus skin lesions appear as red plaques with white, cohesive scales that often are accentuated in the follicular openings (follicular plugging). The plaques eventu-

TABLE 525–11. ATROPHIC SKIN CONDITIONS WITH SCARRING, INDURATION, ULCERATION, AND TELANGIECTASIAS

Condition	Etiology	Important Physical Findings	Other Facts of Note
Connective Tissue Diseases			
Discoid lupus	Autoimmune conditions	Plaques with atrophic centers, erythematous and telangiectatic borders; follicular plugging prominent	May rarely be associated with systemic LE
Systemic lupus	Unknown	Erythematous, scaling, telangiectatic rash in sun-exposed areas; butterfly configuration on face; periungual telangiectasias	Antinuclear antibodies plus arthritis and serositis
Dermatomyositis	Unknown	Heliotrope of eyelids; Gottron's papules on knuckles, poikilodermatous changes on face, V of neck, elbows	Proximal muscle weakness; occasionally associated with underlying cancer
Morphea	Unknown	Localized patches of induration with erythematous borders	Seldom related to systemic sclerosis
Progressive systemic sclerosis	Unknown	Hidebound, indurated, tight skin over acral areas and face; periungual and matlike telangiectasias; ulceration of fingertips	Raynaud's phenomenon common; lungs, heart, GI tract may also be involved
Lichen sclerosus et atrophicus	Unknown	Porcelain white, indurated plaques commonly on genitalia but may occur on trunk; follicular plugging may be seen	
Cutaneous Ulcers of Extremities			
Venous and arterial insufficiency	Impairment of vascular flow	Arterial insufficiency causes ulcers; gangrene acrally with associated claudication; venous ulcers usually around malleoli in association with stasis dermatitis	Lower leg and foot edema common in venous insufficiency
Hemoglobinopathies	Poor oxygenation of tissue	Sickle cell anemia and other hemoglobinopathies can cause ulcerations on lower third of leg	
Pyoderma gangrenosum	Hypersensitivity reaction	Deep, necrotic ulcer with undermined violaceous borders, usually on the legs	Associated with ulcerative colitis, rheumatoid arthritis, dysproteinemia
Ecthyma gangrenosum	*Pseudomonas* septicemia	Ulcers with erythematous borders, usually in body folds	Often early sign of *Pseudomonas* septicemia
Genital Ulcers			
Venereal diseases			
Herpes	*Herpesvirus hominis*	Grouped vesicles that leave superficial erosions	
Syphilis	*Treponema pallidum*	Superficial, indurated, painless ulcer	VDRL may or may not be positive
Chancroid	*Haemophilus ducreyi*	Multiple, soft, painful ulcers with undermined edges	
Lymphogranuloma venereum	*Chlamydia trachomatis*	Transient, painless skin ulcer—inguinal bubo	
Granuloma inguinale	*Donovania granulomatis*	Nodules that erode with granulation tissue ulcer	
Behçet's disease	Autoimmune disease	Multiple shallow genital ulcers in association with oral aphthae and iritis	Erythema nodosum, arthritis, and CNS symptoms also seen

ally atrophy, with depression and scarring along with hypopigmentation in the center of the lesions and a hyperpigmented rim. The lesions usually occur in sun-exposed areas and, when they involve the scalp, cause scarring alopecia. Systemic lupus erythematosus presents as an erythematous rash with a violaceous hue, accentuated in sun-exposed areas, especially the malar area, producing a butterfly configuration. Telangiectasias may also be prominent, and, at times, fine scaling is seen. Occasionally bullae, erosions, and ulcers also occur. Periungual telangiectasia is a prominent finding in systemic lupus as well as in other connective tissue diseases. Subacute lupus is a form in which psoriasiform skin patches are found on the face and trunk. Skin biopsy for both routine and direct immunofluorescence pathologic examination is useful in confirming the diagnosis (see Table 522–3).

Dermatomyositis (see Ch. 268 and Color Plate 16*H*) findings include violaceous edema of eyelids (heliotrope), flat-topped papules over the knuckles (Gottron's papules), and reticulated patches of hyper- and hypopigmentation, erythema, and telangiectasia (poikiloderma) found on the V of the neck, face, elbows, and knees.

X-radiation can cause chronic skin changes of atrophy, telangiectasias, irregular pigmentation, and eventually ulceration. Within these areas malignant changes may later appear.

DERMAL INDURATIONS (SCLEROSIS). *Scleroderma* is a condition in which excessive collagen is found in the dermis (see Ch. 262). *Morphea* is localized scleroderma confined to the skin, whereas *systemic scleroderma*, or *progressive systemic sclerosis*, is a more extensive form in which fibrosis diffusely involves the skin as well as internal organs (see Ch. 262). Morphea lesions are asymptomatic, oval to irregular, whitish, firm, thickened patches with an erythematous border. The plaques are most often found on the trunk. The thickened skin in progressive systemic sclerosis is not sharply demarcated, but rather causes indurated, "hidebound" tight skin over the fingers, toes, and extremities (acrosclerosis). Thickening of the facial skin causes smoothness and loss of wrinkles except for furrowing around the mouth. Ulcerations followed by pitted scars occur on the fingertips. Telangiectasia may be prominent, appearing as periungual telangiectasias and multiple, small punctate macules on the face and hands (matlike telangiectasia). A variant of systemic scleroderma, the *CREST syndrome*, displays extensive telangiectasias over face and hands. Patients with *hereditary hemorrhagic telangiectasia* also display telangiectasia, particularly around the mouth and nose and on the fingers, as well as vascular malformations in the gastrointestinal tract and, at times, the lung. No cutaneous induration is found in this condition.

Lichen sclerosus et atrophicus may be confused with morphea, presenting as porcelain white, atrophic, indurated plaques most commonly on the vulva or on the male genitalia (balanitis xerotica obliterans). At times it occurs as scattered patches on the trunk. Purpuric areas may also be seen within the lesions.

Myxedema may cause a doughy thickening of the skin from deposition of glycosaminoglycans in the dermis. This may be localized to the pretibial areas (pretibial myxedema) as firm, nonpitting plaques and nodules with accentuation of the follicular orifices giving a peau d'orange appearance.

CUTANEOUS ULCERS. Primary skin ulcers are caused by a wide variety of etiologies and conditions. The location of the ulcers, the symptoms associated with them, and the rapidity of their appearance are important clues in diagnosing their various etiologies.

Ulcers of the extremities are frequently associated with vascular disease. Sudden pain associated with numbness of an extremity and ulceration suggest arterial occlusion. Ulceration of digits associated with a purplish red color with dependency and pallor when the extremity is elevated suggests arteriosclerotic peripheral vascular disease. Brawny edema, brown discoloration, and dermatitis over the lower legs in association with ulcers around the malleoli are seen with venous insufficiency. Sickle cell anemia causes ulcerations in the lower third of the leg. Areas of pressure and trauma, particularly on the foot, in patients with peripheral neuropathy, are susceptible to neurotrophic ulcers (mal perforant), as in diabetes and leprosy. The skin around the ulcer is anesthetic and calloused. Pressure sores or decubitus ulcers occur in immobilized debilitated patients. Shearing forces, friction, moisture, and pressure contribute to the development of these sores. The sacral and coccygeal areas, ischial tuberosities, and greater trochanters are favored sites. The best treatment of

pressure sores is prevention by frequently moving immobilized patients, keeping the skin clean, and using air mattresses.

An unusual and dramatic ulcerative condition, *pyoderma gangrenosum*, often begins as an inflammatory nodule or pustule resembling a furuncle which breaks down, ulcerates, and gradually enlarges peripherally. Fully developed, the lesions are moderately deep, red, necrotic ulcers with undermined, violaceous, edematous borders. These lesions, which typically evolve on the lower legs, are postulated to represent a Shwartzman-like hypersensitivity reaction to a number of underlying internal conditions, including chronic ulcerative colitis, regional ileitis, rheumatoid arthritis, dysproteinemias, and occasionally leukemia or lymphoma. In over one half of the cases no etiology is identified.

Ecthyma gangrenosum is characterized by ulcerative lesions, often in the body folds (anogenital and axillary areas), in immunosuppressed patients with *Pseudomonas* septicemia. The painless lesions begin as hemorrhagic bullous patches that become necrotic and ulcerate and are surrounded by considerable erythema with a central gray to black eschar. *Pseudomonas* can be cultured from these skin lesions.

Ulcerations on the genitalia are suggestive of venereal disease, including herpes simplex (multiple grouped vesicles and erosions), syphilis (indurated, painless, round ulcer with a clean base), chancroid (single or multiple, soft, painful, purulent ulcers with undermined erythematous edges), lymphogranuloma venereum (transient, painless skin ulcer with associated inguinal buboadenopathy), and granuloma inguinale (small nodules on genitalia which erode and become filled with velvety red granulation).

Multiple genital ulcers also occur in *Behçet's syndrome* in association with oral ulcers and ocular disease (iridocyclitis). Erythema nodosum, arthritis, and neurologic and intestinal involvement may also occur. The oral and genital ulcers are small, painful aphthae. Occasionally sterile pustules and ulcers at the site of minor trauma such as blood sampling can occur (pathergy) (see Ch. 269).

Geometric, bizarre-shaped, angular ulcers are characteristic of a self-inflicted, factitial cause.

HYPER- AND HYPOPIGMENTATION OF THE SKIN

Disorders of melanin pigmentation can be classified as hypomelanoses (decreased or absent epidermal melanin) or hypermelanoses (increased epidermal or dermal melanin). Hyper- and hypomelanosis can be further subdivided into localized or generalized (total body) alterations of pigmentation (Table 525–12).

Hyperpigmentary Conditions

LOCALIZED PIGMENTARY CONDITIONS. *Freckles* (ephelides) are light brown-red macules found in sun-exposed areas which are caused by increased melanin production in normal numbers of melanocytes. These occur in fair-complexioned individuals with red or sandy hair. Ultraviolet radiation increases melanin production in these lesions.

Lentigines are also hyperpigmented macules, but they occur because of increased numbers of melanocytes in the basal layer of the epidermis. Two types are recognized: (1) *lentigo simplex*, which occurs in early life and is congenital, and (2) *actinic lentigines*, which are acquired in middle age and are related to sun damage over the face, arms, and dorsum of the hands. Actinic lentigines are sometimes difficult to distinguish from early lentigo maligna on the face, but actinic lentigines have no malignant potential. The *multiple lentigines syndrome* is a rare, dominantly inherited condition characterized by hundreds of *Lentigines* on the trunk, head, extremities, palms, and soles, and it is associated with Electrocardiographic abnormalities, Ocular hypertelorism, Pulmonary stenosis, Abnormal genitalia, Retarded growth, and Deafness (thus the acronym LEOPARD syndrome). Another dominantly inherited condition is *Peutz-Jeghers syndrome*, distinctive for its numerous lentigines occurring around the mouth, eyes, hands, and feet in association with gastrointestinal polyps, gastrointestinal hemorrhage, and occasionally malignant degeneration of the polyps.

Melasma (chloasma) of the face usually affects women, and in this instance the melanocytes produce more melanin than normal in response to hormonal factors (occurs during pregnancy or while on birth control pills) in association with ultraviolet radiation. This type of pigmentation occurs symmetrically over the malar eminences, forehead, and upper lip (Fig. 525–19). The lesions may fade with delivery but often persist and are accentuated when birth control pills are used. Hydroquinone, a bleaching agent (2 to 4 per cent creams), may help reduce the pigmentation but many authorities believe these are of no value and that they may worsen the problem. Sunscreens are also useful.

Postinflammatory hyperpigmentation is the term given to macular pigmentation following inflammatory skin diseases (lichen planus typically causes brown to blue pigmentation).

Café au lait spots are light brown (coffee-with-cream hue) macules that occur on the trunk and extremities in neurofibromatosis (Fig. 525–20). Six or more such lesions, each greater than 1.5 cm in diameter, are diagnostic for this dominantly inherited disease. Axillary freckling, discrete neurofibromas (Fig. 525–21), and large plexiform neurofibromas along with bony abnormalities combine to make this a disfiguring condition. Ten per cent of the normal population have isolated café au lait spots. In *Albright's disease* (polyostotic fibrous dysplasia) three or four large, irregularly shaped (so-called "coast-of-Maine" configuration), hyperpigmented macules are usually found unilaterally distributed on the buttocks or cervical area.

Xeroderma pigmentosum is a rare, heterogeneous group of diseases with hereditary deficiencies of enzyme systems in the skin that repair ultraviolet-induced damage to keratinocyte and melanocyte DNA. This inability to maintain the integrity of DNA leads to extreme sun sensitivity and multiple freckles over the face, lips, conjunctivae, and extremities which evolve into varia-

bly sized pigmented patches interspersed with hypopigmented areas. Keratoses, keratoacanthomas, basal and squamous cell cancers, and malignant melanomas evolve and frequently lead to early death. This entity should be thought of whenever one finds otherwise unexplained extreme sensitivity to the sun or excessive freckling in youngsters. This disease can be subtle in its initial presentation, and total avoidance of the sun from early life may prevent subsequent fatal skin cancers.

GENERALIZED HYPERPIGMENTATION. Diffuse brown hyperpigmentation is a feature of *Addison's disease* with accentuation of the pigment in body folds (palmar creases), pressure points (knuckles, elbows), and gingival mucous membrane. A similar type of diffuse hyperpigmentation is seen following adrenalectomy in patients with Cushing's disease due to a pituitary tumor, as well as in patients with pancreatic and lung carcinomas. In all of these instances the generalized hypermelanosis results from overproduction of melanocyte-stimulating hormone (MSH) and adrenocorticotropic hormone (ACTH). These trophic hormones share common amino acid sequences. Both MSH and ACTH secretions are increased in Addison's disease as a result of diminished output of cortisol by the adrenals. Oat cell cancers of the lung and pancreatic carcinomas have been found to excrete increased amounts of MSH, thus causing similar hyperpigmentation. Melanocyte MSH receptors bind MSH, which stimulates intracellular cyclic AMP, and this, in turn, increases tyrosinase activity and pigment formation in melanocytes.

A number of drugs can cause Addisonian-like hypermelanosis including busulfan, cyclophosphamide, and nitrogen mustard. Blue-gray pigmentation may occur either diffusely or in localized patches following use of chlorpromazine, minocycline, and antimalarial drugs. In addition, inorganic trivalent arsenicals (found in insecticides and contaminated water) may also produce a

TABLE 525–12. HYPER- AND HYPOPIGMENTATION OF THE SKIN

	Etiology	Important Physical Findings	Other Facts of Note
Hyperpigmentation			
Localized			
Freckles	Increased melanin synthesis in skin	Light brown macules on sun-exposed areas	UV light accentuates
Lentigines	May be congenital or related to chronic sun exposure	Flat, light brown, uniformly pigmented lesions	No malignant potential
Melasma	Hormonal changes (pregnancy, birth control pills) plus sunlight	Irregular, flat, light brown areas on malar areas, cheeks, forehead	May fade after delivery or coming off birth control pills
Café au lait spots	Dominantly inherited pigmented lesion	Single to multiple coffee-with-cream-colored macules; may be associated with neurofibromatosis	Six or more such lesions suggest neurofibromatosis
Generalized			
Addison's disease	Increased MSH, ACTH	Diffuse hyperpigmentation with accentuation in body folds, palmar creases	Similar pigmentation with lung cancer; Cushing's disease with pituitary tumor
Hemochromatosis	Deposition of iron in skin and increased melanin in skin	Metallic gray-brown hyperpigmentation	
Chronic arsenic exposure	Stimulation of melanin synthesis in skin	Generalized hyperpigmentation studded with small depigmented macules	Keratosis on palms and soles
Hypopigmentation			
Localized			
Vitiligo	Immunologically mediated loss of melanocytes	Symmetrically distributed depigmented macules around body orifices and over bony prominences	In small percentage of cases associated with pernicious anemia, diabetes, thyroiditis, hyperthyroidism, Addison's disease
Piebaldism	Failure of melanocytes to migrate to skin in embryologic development	White forelock and depigmented patch—midline forehead, thorax	
Pityriasis alba	Dry skin	Pink, oval hypopigmented patches that often scale on face, trunk	Often accompanies atopic eczema, dry skin
Tuberous sclerosis	Dominantly inherited condition	Ash leaf–shaped, white macules on trunk, extremities; often present at birth	Associated with adenoma sebaceum, tuberous sclerosis
Generalized			
Oculocutaneous albinism	Autosomal recessive traits with variable degrees of tyrosinase insufficiency	White skin, hair; no pigment in fundi oculi; translucent irides	Nystagmus and eye problems common
Phenylketonuria	Deficiency of enzyme converting phenylalanine to tyrosine, so decreased precursor for melanin synthesis	Generalized depigmentation of hair, skin, eye color	Severe mental developmental defects if not diagnosed early and treated with special diet

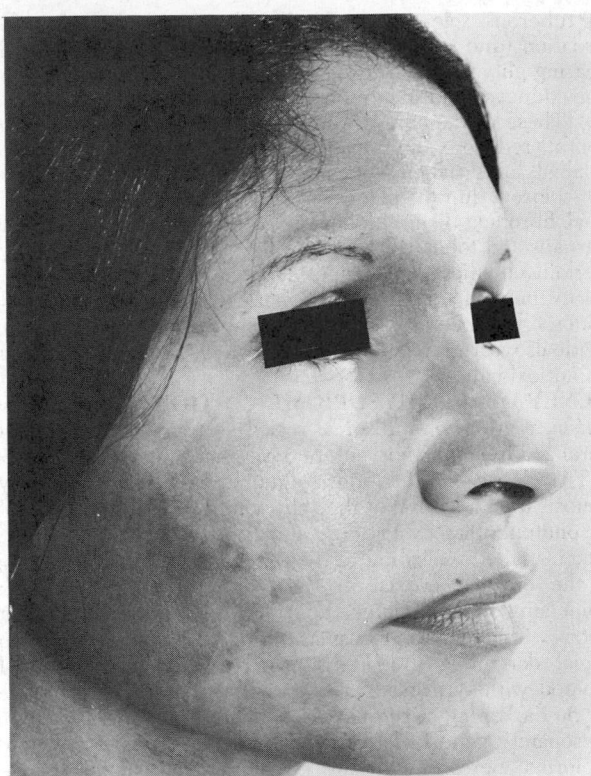

FIGURE 525–19. Melasma. (From the 17th edition of the Cecil Textbook of Medicine, with the permission of Dr. Marie-Louise Johnson.)

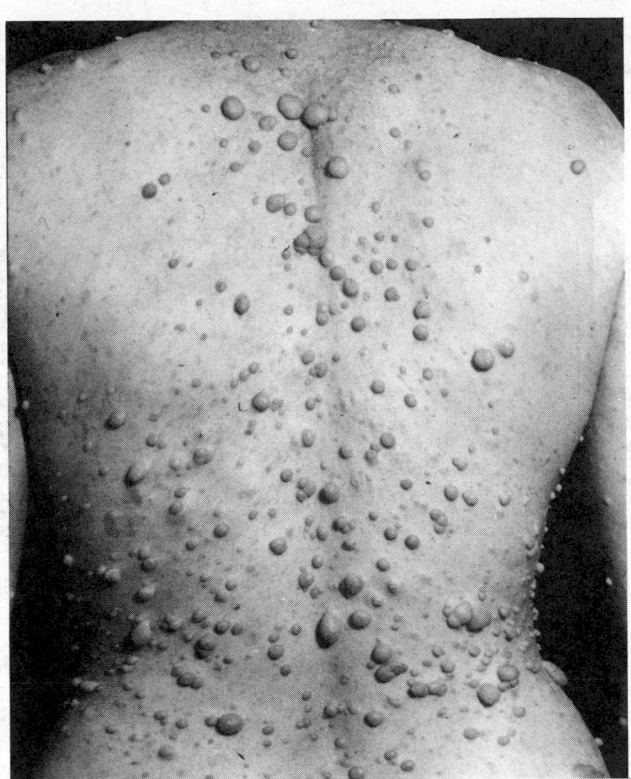

FIGURE 525–21. Neurofibromatosis—von Recklinghausen's disease. (From the 17th edition of the Cecil Textbook of Medicine, with the permission of Dr. Marie-Louise Johnson.)

generalized brown pigmentation, but in this instance the hypermelanosis is studded with small, scattered, depigmented macules (likened to rain drops on a dusty road) and punctate keratoses on the palms and soles. *Hemochromatosis* causes a metallic gray-brown, generalized hyperpigmentation resulting from the combination of increased pigment formation in the skin and iron deposition.

Hypopigmentary Conditions

LOCALIZED PIGMENTARY CHANGES. *Vitiligo,* a circumscribed hypomelanosis of progressively enlarging amelanotic macules in a symmetric distribution around body orifices and over bony prominences (knees, elbows, hands), is familial in 36 per cent of cases. In one third of cases some spontaneous repigmentation occurs, particularly in sun-exposed areas. White hairs are common in the vitiliginous areas. Although most patients with vitiligo are healthy, there is an increased association with certain autoimmune conditions such as thyroiditis, hyperthyroidism, Addison's disease, pernicious anemia, and diabetes mellitus. Melanocytes are absent from the vitiliginous macules. Circulating complement-binding antimelanocyte antibodies have been found in some vitiligo patients. The use of PUVA may give some repigmentation, but it may require 200 or more such treatments.

Piebaldism is a local hypopigmentary condition representing an autosomal dominant hypomelanosis on the extremities, anterior surface of the thorax, and especially over the midline of the forehead and central scalp. A white forelock is typical. The hypomelanosis stems from the lack of normal migration of the melanocytes to these regions during embryologic development.

Waardenburg's syndrome, another autosomal dominant condition, may be confused with piebaldism, as a white forelock is seen, but other abnormalities are also found at birth, including perceptive deafness, heterochromia, and hypertelorism.

A common localized form of hypopigmentation, *pityriasis alba,* appears as slightly pink and hypopigmented, oval to round patches with mild, fine scaling. These occur on the cheeks of children, but they may also be found on the trunk, mimicking the hypopigmented, scaling patches seen in tinea versicolor (a KOH examination of the scales may be necessary to differentiate these two conditions). Pityriasis alba is most frequently seen in atopic dermatitis patients.

Tuberous sclerosis, an autosomal dominant condition, displays white macules in 98 per cent of cases. These depigmented macules characteristically are found on the trunk or buttocks in an oval or mountain ash–leaf configuration (Fig. 525–22). The presence of three or more of these macules is strongly suggestive of tuberous sclerosis, and because the hypomelanotic patches are

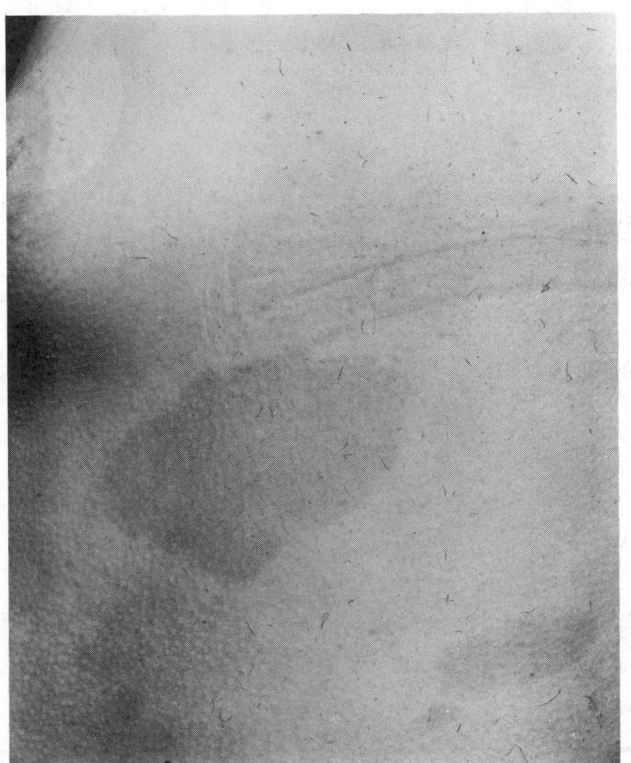

FIGURE 525–20. Café au lait spot. (From the 17th edition of the Cecil Textbook of Medicine, with the permission of Dr. Marie-Louise Johnson.)

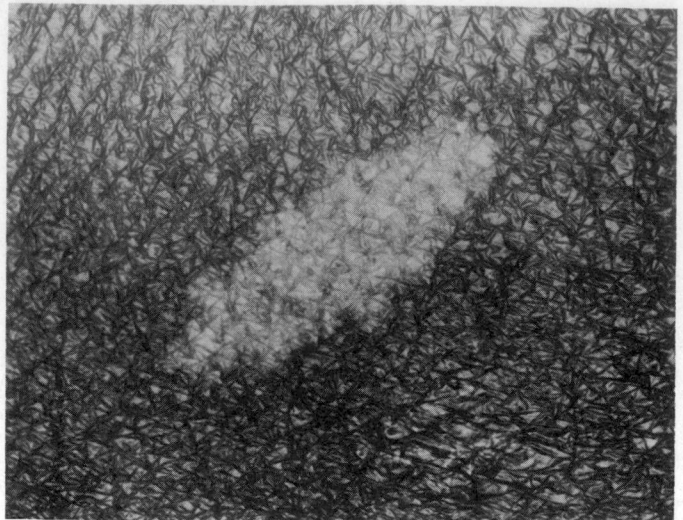

FIGURE 525–22. Tuberous sclerosis ash leaf. (From the 17th edition of the Cecil Textbook of Medicine, with the permission of Dr. Marie-Louise Johnson.)

present at birth, they represent one of the earliest signs of the condition. Examination with Wood's light is often useful in visualizing the lesions, which histologically contain melanocytes with decreased numbers of melanosomes. Newborns with unexplained seizures or mental retardation should be screened with a Wood's light for the presence of the white spots. CT brain scans are also useful in defining the tumorous dysplasia. Patients with tuberous sclerosis (epiloia) suffer from seizures, mental retardation (due to hamartomatous gliomas), phakomas (yellow-appearing gliomatous tumors of the retina), bilateral hamartomas of the kidneys, and a number of hamartomatous tumors of the skin. These cutaneous lesions include *adenoma sebaceum* (smooth, red to yellow papules over the butterfly area and nasolabial folds which appear by age four), shagreen patches (flesh-colored, lumpy plaques over the lumbosacral area), and ungual fibromas (firm, pink papules in the periungual areas of fingernails and toenails).

Certain chemicals, particularly phenol derivatives, when applied to the skin, may cause permanent depigmentation. Hypomelanosis has been observed on the hands of black-skinned individuals wearing rubber gloves in which hydroquinone is used as an antioxidant.

GENERALIZED HYPOPIGMENTATION. *Oculocutaneous albinism,* a group of autosomal recessive traits, is recognized by generalized hypomelanosis of the skin, hair, and eyes (Table 525–13). The classic constellation of findings includes marked hypomelanosis or amelanosis of the skin, white or faintly yellow-blond hair, photophobia, nystagmus, and translucent irides. Albinism can be classified according to the presence or absence of tyrosinase, the enzyme crucial in the synthesis of eumelanin and pheomelanin. Normal plucked hair bulbs darken when incubated in vitro with tyrosine; tyrosinase-positive albinos display some minimal darkening (but not normal) of the hair bulb when incubated with tyrosinase, whereas tyrosinase-negative patients show no darkening of the hair bulb. These two types of albinism have separate gene loci. Although melanogenesis is deficient in both forms, persons with the tyrosinase-positive form develop some pigmented nevi and less eye damage than tyrosinase-negative albinos. Persons with *phenylketonuria* have diffuse hypopigmentation, with light hair and blue eyes. This is an autosomal recessive disorder in which the enzyme that converts

TABLE 525–13. ALBINISM

	Inheritance	Frequency	Skin Color	Pigmented Nevi Freckles	Hair	Eyes Color	Red Reflex
Oculocutaneous Albinism							
Tyrosinase-negative	AR*	1 in 34,000	pink/wte	none	white	gray-blue	present
Tyrosinase-positive	AR	blk: 1 in 15,000 wte: 1 in 40,000	wte-cream	present	wte-yellow red: darkens	blue-yellow brown	present but may be absent in dark races
Yellow-mutant	AR	rare—Amish, Polish, German-American; blacks (American, Ceylonese, African)	wte at birth, slgt tan pos	present	wte-birth red/yellow 6 mos	blue at birth: darkens	present
Hermansky-Pudlak syndrome	AR	rare—cases from Puerto Rico; Southern Holland; Madras	cream-lgt normal	present	wte-red dk brown	blue-gray to brown	wte—present blk—absent
Cross-McKusick-Breen syndrome (oculocerebral hypopigmentation syndrome)	AR	extremely rare—3 in Amish family	pink/wte	present	wte-lt yel	gray-blue	?, cataracts
Chédiak-Higashi syndrome	AR	rare in most countries; none in blacks	pink/wte	present	blond-dk brown-steel gray	blue to brown	present but diminishes with time
Oculocutaneous Albinoidism	AD†		pink/wte	?	wte blond	blue	present
Ocular Albinism							
Vogt	X-linked	uncommon	normal	present	normal	blue	
Forsius-Eriksson	X-linked	less common	normal	present	normal	blue	
Autosomal recessive	AR	10 families	normal	present	normal	blue	present

*AR = Autosomal recessive.
†AD = Autosomal dominant.
Reprinted from the chapter by Dr. Marie-Louise Johnson in the 17th edition of the Cecil Textbook of Medicine, with her permission.

phenylalanine to tyrosine is deficient. Consequently, melanin synthesis is decreased (see Ch. 177).

REGIONAL DIAGNOSIS OF SKIN DISEASES— COMMONLY ENCOUNTERED PROBLEMS BY ANATOMIC REGION

Many skin diseases have a predilection for certain areas or regions of the body, often related to variations in the structure and function of the integument (Table 525–14).

Disorders of the Nails

The nail is a plate of hard keratin synthesized from an invagination of the epidermis. The proximal nail fold houses the matrix of the nail where basal cells rapidly proliferate and differentiate into the nail plate, which grows over the nail bed. Nails grow continuously throughout life. The average fingernail grows 0.5 to 1.2 mm per week, whereas toenails grow at one half to one third this rate. It takes a fingernail about 5.5 months and the toenails 12 to 18 months to regrow from the matrix, although rate of growth slows as the individual gets older. Defects in nail formation go by various terms useful in describing nail disorders:

1. *Brittleness*—easy breaking of nail tips
2. *Leukonychia*—white discoloration of nails
3. *Striations*—longitudinal ridges running parallel or perpendicular to the length of the nail
4. *Onycholysis*—separation of the nail plate from the bed
5. *Onychogryphosis*—hypertrophy and thickening of the nail
6. *Onychomycosis*—dystrophy, destruction of the nail due to yeast and fungal infections
7. *Pitting*—discrete pitlike depressions in the nail surface
8. *Koilonychia*—spoon-shaped deformity of the nails (concave nail with everted edges)
9. *Pterygium formation*—growth of cuticle onto the nail plate.

SKIN DISEASES INVOLVING NAILS. Nail changes in *psoriasis* have been described above. Fingernails are more frequently involved than toenails. Fungal infection must be ruled out.

Therapy of psoriatic nail changes is not satisfactory, although topical tar and steroid preparations may be of some help.

In 10 per cent of *lichen planus* patients, accentuated longitudinal nail ridging occurs as well as pterygium formation resulting from destructive focal scarring of the matrix. Early treatment with oral steroids is indicated to arrest the cicatricial course.

Nail pitting frequently occurs in *alopecia areata* along with onycholysis. The nail is susceptible to deformities when *eczematous* processes involve the periungual regions and matrix. *Atopic eczema* and other eczematous entities may cause pitting, transverse striations, and onycholysis.

Onychomycosis, or fungal infections of the nail, may be caused by dermatophyte (tinea unguium) or candidal infections. Infection of toenails is more frequent than fingernails, but all nails may be involved. The nail plate is discolored (cloudy, yellowish or brown), thickened, crumbly, and onycholytic with accumulation of debris under the nail. White superficial onychomycosis appears as white patches in the toenail plate due to organisms growing on the surface barely penetrating the nail. Scrapings reveal hyphae upon KOH examination. An unusual condition, *chronic mucocutaneous candidiasis*, is caused by widespread *Candida albicans* infection leading to diffuse white thickening of all nails.

Topical antifungal therapy is ineffective, so oral griseofulvin is given for dermatophyte infection until the nails appear clear. Ketoconazole (200 mg daily) is an alternative should griseofulvin fail or when *Candida* is the causative agent. Oral therapy requires 4 to 6 months for fingernails and 12 to 16 months for toenails. In older individuals toenail problems may never be eradicated because the nails grow so slowly. Residual fungal spores in the patient's shoes and environment are no doubt responsible for the high frequency of recurrence, and for this reason topical antifungal powders may be helpful in long-term prophylaxis.

Paronychia, or painful, red swelling of the nail fold, is usually caused by *Candida albicans*. At times a small abscess or purulent discharge is seen. This infection usually occurs in hands constantly exposed to a wet environment (bartenders, janitors). Therapy

TABLE 525–13. ALBINISM *Continued*

	Eyes				Hair Bulb Incubation (Tyrosine)	Defect	Melanosome Maturation by Stage	Complications or Associated Problems
Nystagmus	Photophobia	Visual Acuity	Pigment in Fundus	Other				
marked	severe	legally blind	none	—	negative	no tyrosinase	I-unmelanized II	skin malignancy basal cell ca squamous cell ca
present but less	present but variable	severe defect in children; may improve with age	none; some with age	pigment cartwheel pupil, limbus	positive	no access of enzyme to tyrosine	I, II, some III, rare IV	skin malignancy basal cell ca squamous cell ca
present but variable	present but variable	marked defect; may improve with age	none; some with age	pigment cartwheel effect	neg to pos ?	unknown ? pheomelanogenesis	I, II, III	unknown
present but variable	present, may be severe	normal or slight decrease	none; some with age	may have pigment cartwheel	positive	pleiotropic effect— single gene mutation	I, II, III	storage-pool defect platelets; ceroid-like material in RE system, oral mucosa, urine
marked	—	blind	?, cataracts	?, cataracts	weakly positive	decreased melanocytes	I, II, III, IV	oligophrenia, athetosis, severe mental retardation
absent or slight	absent or slight	normal or slight decrease	some; increase with age	normal for cartwheel effect	positive	giant melanosomes, lethal defect in leukocytes	I, II, III, IV	infections; hematologic and neurologic abnormalities; lymphoreticular malignancy
no	no	normal or slight decrease	punctate		positive	unknown	unknown	none
present	severe	marked decrease	reduced		positive			
latent	absent or slight	color blind			positive			
present	severe	marked decrease			positive			

TABLE 525–14. REGIONAL DERMATOLOGY

Region of Skin	Type of Skin Group	Disease Process
Scalp	Papulosquamous and ecze-matous	Psoriasis, seborrheic dermatitis, tinea capitis, eczema (atopic, contact)
	Pustular	Folliculitis, kerion
	Nodular	Nevi, seborrheic keratosis, pilar cysts, verruca
	Atrophic and telangiectatic	Connective tissue disease, scleroderma, discoid LE
Face	Pustular	Acne, rosacea, folliculitis, tinea
	Papulosquamous and ecze-matous	Psoriasis, seborrheic dermatitis, contact dermatitis (cosmetics), atopic dermatitis, impetigo, lupus erythematosus, photodermatitis
	Vesicular	Herpes zoster and herpes simplex, insect bites
	Nodular	Basal cell cancers, squamous cell cancers, melanomas, keratoacanthomas, nevi, actinic keratosis, tuberous xanthomas
Trunk	Papulosquamous and ecze-matous	Psoriasis, atopic and contact eczema, tinea versicolor, pityriasis rosacea, scabies
	Vesiculobullous	Pemphigus, bullous pemphigoid
	Maculopapular	Secondary syphilis, drug reaction, viral exanthems
	Nodular	Nevi, seborrheic keratosis, lipoma, basal cell cancer, keloid, neurofibroma, angiomas, melanoma
	Pustular	Acne
	Urticarial	Hives
Arms and forearms	Eczematous and papulo-squamous	Contact dermatitis—plants; atopic dermatitis, lichen planus
	Nodular	Nevi, warts, seborrheic keratosis, actinic keratosis
	Atrophic telangiectasia	Scleroderma, dermatomyositis
Legs	Eczematous and papulo-squamous	Contact dermatitis, stasis dermatitis, atopic dermatitis, psoriasis, lichen planus
	Nodular	Erythema nodosum, dermatofibromas, nevi, melanoma, Kaposi's sarcoma, lipoma
	Maculopapular	Vasculitis, Schamberg's disease, actinic purpura, pretibial myxedema
	Atrophic, telangiectatic, and ulcerative	Scleroderma, dermatostasis ulcers, arterial insufficiency
Genitalia and groin	Eczematous and papulo-squamous	Contact dermatitis, seborrheic dermatitis, scabies, pediculosis pubis, psoriasis, Reiter's syndrome, erythrasma, tinea, candidiasis, lichen planus, intertrigo, lichen simplex chronicus
	Vesiculobullous	Herpes simplex, Stevens-Johnson syndrome
	Ulcerative and atrophic	Syphilis, chancroid, lymphopathia venerum, Behçet's syndrome
	Nodular	Verrucae vulgaris, erythroplasia of Queyrat, squamous cell cancer, sebaceous cyst, molluscum contagiosum
	Pustular	Hidradenitis suppurativa
Hands	Eczematous and papulo-squamous	Allergic contact and irritant contact dermatitis, dyshidrosis, pyoderma, tinea, dermatophytids, scabies, atopic dermatitis, secondary syphilis
	Vesiculobullous, pustular	Erythema multiforme, hand-foot-and-mouth disease, porphyria cutanea tarda, psoriasis
	Nodular	Warts, squamous cell cancer, actinic keratosis, keratoacanthoma, pyogenic granuloma, granuloma annulare, synovial cysts
	Hypopigmented	Vitiligo
	Atrophic-telangiectatic	Scleroderma, dermatomyositis
Feet	Eczematous and papulo-squamous	Contact dermatitis, atopic dermatitis, tinea, psoriasis, lichen planus
	Vesiculobullous	Tinea, epidermolysis bullosa, erythema multiforme
	Nodules	Verruca, corn, nevus
	Atrophic-telangiectatic	Scleroderma

consists of avoidance of water and the use of antifungal solutions two or three times a day for a month or two.

EXOGENOUS FACTORS CAUSING NAIL CHANGES. Cosmetics, trauma, and occupational influences can all cause nail deformities. Nail hardeners, enamel removers, and stick-on nails all may cause reactions including onycholysis, subungual hyperkeratoses, paronychia, and contact dermatitis around the nails. Nail manipulation, biting, and tight-fitting shoes may induce nail injury. A variety of systemic drugs may induce color changes or other alterations in the nails (e.g., chronic arsenic ingestion causes transverse white lines—Mees' lines; antimalarials, blue-brown coloration; minocycline, variable brown discoloration).

NAIL DISTURBANCES IN SYSTEMIC DISEASES. *Splinter hemorrhages* result from the extravasation of blood from longitudinally oriented vessels of the nail bed. Although often thought to be associated with bacterial endocarditis, they are much more commonly associated with trauma to the nails. *Beau's lines* are commonly associated with systemic disease, but they are nonspecific, appearing as transverse depressions across the nail plates of all nails following any severe disability that temporarily interferes with nail growth, including systemic infections, myocardial infarction, and use of chemotherapeutic agents. *Longitudinal pigmented bands* occur most often in response to trauma or a nevus located in the matrix, but in white individuals a melanoma must be ruled out. *Yellow nail syndrome* exhibits yellow thickening of all the nails with absence of the lunula and variable degrees of onycholysis in association with a number of pulmonary conditions such as bronchiectasis, pleural effusion, and chronic obstructive pulmonary disease. Lymphedema of the extremities may be a third component of the syndrome. *Clubbing* of the nails (increased bilateral curvature of the nails with enlargement of the soft connective tissue of the distal phalanges resulting in the flattening of the obtuse angle formed by the proximal end of the nail and the digit) occurs most often with respiratory ailments, including bronchiectasis, lung abscess, and pulmonary neoplasms. Cardiovascular disease and chronic gastrointestinal diseases (ulcerative colitis, sprue) are also associated with clubbing. When clubbing is found with bone pain and proliferative periostitis, it is termed *hypertrophic osteoarthropathy,* and the condition is most often associated with bronchogenic squamous cell carcinoma. *Nail-patella syndrome* is a dominantly inherited condition affecting both mesodermal and ectodermal structures which causes defective growth of nails (often the nails are missing) in association with hypoplasia or absence of the patellae and enlarged, palpable iliac horns. *Hereditary ectodermal dysplasia* appears in two forms, hidrotic and anhidrotic. The teeth and hair are involved similarly in both (anodontia, hypodontia, and peg-shaped teeth in association with soft, downy, scant hair in the scalp and eyebrows), but in the hidrotic form sweat gland function is normal and the nails are small, thickened, and longitudinally striated.

TUMORS OF THE NAIL. A variety of benign tumors occur around the nail unit. These include *periungual fibromas, myxoid cysts,* and *subungual exostoses.* Surgical removal of the benign tumors is the only certain means of cure.

The main malignant tumor involving the nails is *melanoma,* which appears as a pigmented area at the base of the nail or as a longitudinal pigmented streak in the nail. Nevi can give the same appearance, and biopsy of the lesion in the matrix is the only absolute way of making a diagnosis.

Disorders of the Mucous Membranes

Any abnormality of color, texture, or appearance of the mucous membranes should be investigated. Malignant changes should be suspected in infiltrated or ulcerated lesions and a biopsy performed.

ULCERATIVE AND BULLOUS LESIONS. *Acute ulcerative* lesions may be caused by trauma (from jagged teeth or ill-fitting dentures); bacterial infections such as acute necrotizing ulcerative gingostomatitis (Vincent's angina; infection with *Borrelia vincentii* and fusiform bacilli which cause punched-out ulcers in the interdental papillae and gingival inflammation); infections with *Staphylococcus* and gram-negative organisms in patients receiving chemotherapy; viral infections such as primary herpetic gingivostomatitis with small vesicles that rupture leaving shallow, discrete ulcers anywhere in the mouth; infectious mononucleosis, which frequently causes exudative tonsillitis and aphthous ulcers of the buccal and labial mucosae; a coxsackievirus infection termed herpangina which results in vesicles that rupture, leaving 1- to 2-mm ulcers with a grayish base over the pharynx; *Candida* infections causing white pseudomembranous lesions; drug reactions that can elicit oral ulcerations (salicylates, barbiturates, antiepileptic drugs, and particularly drugs used for chemotherapy such as methotrexate, actinomycin-D, and daunorubicin, which are extremely toxic to mucosal epithelium).

Chronic oral ulcerations are most frequently caused by bullous diseases (pemphigus, cicatricial pemphigoid, bullous pemphigoid—see above). Both discoid and systemic lupus erythematosus may have associated mouth lesions with central depressed erosions and elevated keratotic borders. Reiter's syndrome may include superficial erythematous erosions anywhere in the oral cavity. Any chronic, localized, erosive lesion in the mouth should be viewed with concern as a possible carcinoma.

Recurrent ulcerative conditions of the mouth are most commonly aphthous stomatitis or herpes simplex stomatitis. *Aphthous stomatitis* is manifested by multiple punched-out ulcers on the buccal and labial mucosae that may be grouped, simulating herpes. A severe form of aphthous stomatitis (periadenitis mucosa necrotica recurrens) with large, deep, recurrent painful ulcers may involve any area of the mouth. An immunologic reaction to intrinsic mouth bacteria may play a role in aphthous ulcers, as tetracycline suspension mouthwashes may reduce the duration, size, and pain of the oral ulcers.

Recurrent *herpes simplex* of the oral mucosa is unusual but should be differentiated from aphthous stomatitis by Tzanck preparation and herpes cultures. Another recurrent condition is Behçet's syndrome (see above). Erythema multiforme may present as an acute, recurrent, erosive stomatitis in association with target lesions of the skin.

WHITE PATCHES. Thrush (*Candida albicans* infection of the oral epithelium) appears as curdy white membranes that can be scraped away, leaving an inflamed base. It is most common in newborns and in immunosuppressed adults and is a common presenting symptom in AIDS, especially in Africa. KOH examination of material scraped from the white patch is diagnostic. Clotrimazole troches dissolved in the mouth twice a day are very successful in clearing such infections. The white oral lesions of lichen planus have been mentioned above. Leukoplakia is discussed in Ch. 95.

GLOSSITIS AND DISEASES AFFECTING THE TONGUE. Two common clinical varieties of glossitis (see Ch. 95) are geographic tongue and black hairy tongue. *Geographic tongue* is a recurrent condition characterized by loss of filiform papillae on the dorsum of the tongue. Typically, a white margin of desquamating epithelium surrounds a central, red, atrophic area. Lesions often migrate across the surface of the tongue, giving a maplike appearance. The lesions may be uncomfortable but are often asymptomatic. The cause is unknown, and no treatment is available. *Black hairy tongue* is a condition recognized by elongated black or brown filiform papillae that grow on the posterior tongue and extend toward the tip. The condition is seen in patients using systemic antibiotics and in those who smoke or chew tobacco and have poor oral hygiene, allowing an overgrowth of pigment-producing bacteria. Gentle brushing of the involved area with a soft tooth brush and hydrogen peroxide several times a day may be of some value.

Strawberry tongue is the name applied to the white exudative glossitis with prominent red papillae poking through the exudate. After several days the tongue becomes beefy red. Typically a strawberry tongue is found in scarlet fever, Kawasaki's disease, and toxic shock syndrome.

Atrophy of the filiform papillae occurs as a response to iron-deficiency anemia and vitamin B_{12} and folate deficiency.

Glossodynia, or burning tongue syndrome, occurs in elderly women and is usually a psychological condition without mucosal abnormalities. Occasionally glossitis or stomatitis occurs as a result of irritant reactions to chewing gum, mouthwashes, and dentifrices.

CARCINOMA OF THE MUCOUS MEMBRANES. Squamous cell carcinoma is the most common oral malignancy, and its incidence increases with age (see Ch. 95). The sites of origin in order of decreasing frequency are the tongue, lower lip, oropharynx, floor of the mouth, gingiva, buccal mucosa, and hard

palate. Predisposing factors include use of all forms of tobacco (especially smokeless) and alcohol. AIDS patients may develop Kaposi's sarcoma on the palate, and such patients have an increased number of squamous cell cancers, especially on the tongue. Premalignant and malignant mucous membrane cancers are usually painless and appear most commonly as red, erythroplastic lesions in two distinct forms. The first is a granular, red, velvety lesion with either stippled or patchy areas of (white) keratin within or peripheral to the lesion. The second appears as a smooth, nongranular lesion, primarily red, with minimal or no keratosis. Leukoplakia or white lesions may also be precancerous, but only 4 per cent of leukoplakias develop into cancer. Less than 5 per cent of patients have attendant bleeding, ulceration, or induration with early cancers. It is incumbent upon the practitioner finding such red or white lesions to remove irritants that might cause keratoses; if the lesions do not resolve over a 2- to 4-week period, they should be biopsied.

DISEASES OF THE LIPS. Irritant or allergic contact cheilitis with redness, scaling, and fissuring can result from topical medications (lip salves), cosmetics (lipsticks), mouthwashes and dentifrices, and various dental materials. A careful history may establish the probable cause, which must be confirmed by patch testing.

Angular cheilitis, or *perlèche*, is an acute or chronic inflammation of the skin and contiguous labial mucous membrane at the angles of the mouth. Causative factors include poorly fitting dentures that permit saliva to accumulate at the angles of the mouth, riboflavin and iron deficiencies, and *Candida* infections.

Actinic cheilitis is a dry, scaling premalignant reaction, often with white, leukoplakic plaques most pronounced on the lower lip, in individuals chronically exposed to ultraviolet light.

Alterations of Hair Growth

The evaluation of patients with alopecia or hirsutism requires a detailed history, physical examination, and, at times, laboratory and biopsy examination. Important points in the history include age of onset, medications taken, recent emotional or physical stress, diet, grooming techniques, and family history of baldness or hair disorders.

HAIR LOSS (ALOPECIA)

In the growth phase, scalp hair grows about 10 to 15 mm every month. Physical, chemical, and emotional events cause fluctuations in hair growth and if severe enough may stop growth entirely. The physical examination is important in noting the pattern of hair loss and whether or not scarring is present. Nonscarring alopecia may be a temporary phenomenon, whereas scarring is indicative of permanent hair loss.

NONSCARRING ALOPECIA. *Localized Alopecia.* Alopecia areata is characterized by well-circumscribed, round or oval patches of nonscarring hair loss, usually over the scalp or in the beard, eyebrows, or eyelashes. Erythema may be present early in the course of the patches. Characteristically the periphery of patches of hair loss is studded with "exclamation point hairs," so named because these hairs are fractured, with tapered shafts resembling punctuation marks. Histologic features of this disease include small dystrophic hair follicles and a lymphocytic infiltrate around the hair bulbs. Occasionally all the scalp hair is lost (alopecia totalis), and all the body hair may fall out (alopecia universalis). Alopecia areata has a variable, unpredictable course. Most patients regrow hair within a few months, but one fourth of individuals experience recurrences. The more extensive the alopecia, the poorer the prognosis. Alopecia involving the occipital region or eyebrows, lashes, and nasal hairs portends a poor prognosis. Alopecia areata may be an autoimmune disease and is occasionally associated with Hashimoto's thyroiditis and pernicious anemia. Topical, intralesional, and systemic steroids give variable benefits. Recent modes of therapy include induction of allergic or irritant contact dermatitis (1 per cent anthralin, or topical dinitrochlorobenzene), photochemotherapy with PUVA, and topical minoxidil.

Tinea capitis is most likely to be confused with alopecia areata. However, tinea infection appears as one or more patches of hair loss with mild scaling and erythema and broken hair shafts leaving residual black stumps (black dot ringworm). Although Wood's light examination causes hairs to fluoresce bright green with *Microsporum audouini* and *M. canis* infections, these are now rare causes of tinea capitis; rather, nonfluorescing *Trichophyton tonsurans* is the usual etiology. Griseofulvin is the drug of choice in treating these infections.

Trichotillomania refers to traumatic, self-induced alopecia and results from compulsive twisting and rubbing, which causes breaking and epilation of the hair shafts. The scalp is usually affected, less often the eyebrows and lashes. If the patient can be given insight into the nature of the condition it is self-limited, but when more severe emotional problems underlie the trichotillomania, referral for psychiatric evaluation should be considered.

Women who develop hair thinning at the margins of the scalp may be using excessive traction or other traumatic hair styling techniques (*traction alopecia*). Traction from overtight hair curling such as corn rowing and the use of hot combs to straighten hair leads to progressive hair thinning and even scarring.

Hair loss is sometimes seen in the scalp of patients with *secondary syphilis.* The hair loss is spotty, often "moth-eaten" in appearance.

Androgenic alopecia, or male pattern baldness, involves the frontal, vertex, and upper occipital regions of the scalp while sparing the posterior and lateral margins. The process may begin at any age after puberty, with temporal recession of hair usually noted first. There is no actual loss of hair but rather the conversion of thick terminal hairs to fine, unpigmented, poorly seen vellus hairs. Common baldness is genetically predetermined and androgen dependent. Males who are castrated prepubertally or men born with low testosterone production, as in Klinefelter's syndrome, do not become bald, regardless of their genetic predisposition to balding. Women may also show balding, but it is milder with only diffuse thinning. However, women with elevated androgen levels, as occur in masculinizing disorders, have baldness in a pattern similar to that in men. Topical minoxidil may slow androgenic hair loss. Surgical techniques such as hair transplants (plugs of hair-bearing areas from the sides of the scalp placed in the thinned frontal and crown areas) or scalp reduction may be useful in some patients.

Diffuse or Generalized Alopecia.
Stress alopecia, or *telogen effluvium,* is a transient, reversible, diffuse hair loss of scalp hair that results from alterations in the normal hair cycle. Normally 80 to 85 per cent of scalp hair follicles are in the growing anagen stage, while 15 to 20 per cent are in the resting (telogen) stage of growth (Ch. 522). Severe emotional and physiologic stress (high fever, systemic illness, major surgery with general anesthesia, crash diet) and certain drugs (heparin, coumarin, allopurinol, amphetamines, β-blocking agents, lithium, probenecid, thiouracil) may cause growing anagen hairs to convert prematurely to resting telogen hairs, which are subsequently shed. Pregnancy and oral contraceptives cause hairs to grow continually, rather than cycling at programmed times to telogen. After childbirth or discontinuation of oral contraceptives, anagen follicles "catch up" by simultaneously entering telogen, and shedding follows 2 to 4 months later. If the stress resolves, the hair regrows in 4 to 6 months. Diffuse hair loss may not be noticeable until there is greater than 50 per cent scalp hair loss. The patient may become aware of increased hair shedding (greater than 125 to 150 hairs per day) without thinning. Gentle pulling of the hair verifies the degree of shedding; if more than five hairs come out when a dozen are grasped, excessive shedding is present. All the hair bulbs that come out are telogen (i.e., a white bulb at the end of the shaft instead of an elongate white sheath as seen in anagen hairs).

Toxic alopecia, or *anagen effluvium,* occurs if hair growth is disrupted during anagen. The newly synthesized hair shaft is weakened and the hair breaks readily. Thinning may be extreme, occurring within a few weeks of an insult, involving all 80 per cent of follicles in anagen on the scalp. Chemotherapeutic agents, especially doxorubicin and related agents, exert their effect on rapidly growing cells in the hair bulb and commonly cause anagen hair damage in cancer patients receiving chemotherapy. Radiotherapy to the scalp area does the same thing. *Retinoids* and *hypervitaminosis A* cause hair loss owing to their interference with keratinization.

Diffuse hair loss over the scalp occurs in *hypothyroidism,* associated with hair that is dry and brittle. Nutritional deficiency (essential fatty acid, biotin, zinc, iron deficiency anemia) also causes diffuse alopecia.

Seborrheic dermatitis, with erythema and yellow, greasy scales throughout the scalp, may also be associated with mild, diffuse hair loss. Treatment of the seborrhea with tar shampoos and topical steroids to control the inflammatory response reverses the hair loss.

Diffuse scalp hair loss also occurs because of *hair shaft weakness,* either acquired (due to braiding, permanent wave solutions, or excessive heat when drying or straightening hair) or resulting from congenital hair shaft weakness. Patients with congenital hair shaft weakness have sparse fine or wiry hair from early childhood. A few of the more common conditions that can be identified with the naked eye, hand lens, or microscope include short beaded hair—monilethrix; twisted hair—pili torti; banded hair—low sulfur hair syndrome; and trichorrhexis nodosa—multiple hair shaft fractures.

SCARRING ALOPECIA.
Scarring alopecias display atrophy of the scalp and absence of hair follicles. These cicatricial areas of hair loss can be the result of a variety of pathologic processes that permanently destroy the hair follicles.

Localized Scarring Alopecia. *Systemic lupus erythematosus* causes diffuse, nonscarring alopecia of the scalp in 20 per cent of patients, along with short, broken (lupus) hairs in the frontal margin, whereas *discoid lupus erythematosus* causes oval scarring areas of alopecia. Typical plaques have an active erythematous margin, white atrophic center, and telangiectasias and keratin-filled follicles.

Morphea, when it involves the scalp, causes firm, hairless, ivory colored, indurated lesions. At times morphea takes on linear patterns that simulate saber wound (en coup de sabre).

Aplasia cutis is a developmental, rectilinear defect in skin formation anywhere on the scalp but usually on the vertex in the newborn.

A number of *physical injuries* such as mechanical trauma, burns, and radiodermatitis may also cause local scarring alopecias.

Nonlocalized Scarring Alopecia. *Lichen planus* may cause diffuse, patchy scarring alopecia (*lichen planopilaris*). Typical lichen planus lesions are often found in other areas of the body. Biopsy of the affected areas may help in the diagnosis.

Poorly understood conditions of the scalp, *pseudopelade* and *folliculitis decalvans* cause oval, scarred, bald areas that are often multiple and may coalesce to form large, irregular, noninflammatory plaques, most often on the vertex. Pseudopelade may be the result of a variety of entities, including lupus erythematosus, lichen planus, or scleroderma. Folliculitis decalvans is characterized by follicular inflammation that leads to destruction of follicles and permanent alopecia. Small follicular pustules are usually seen.

HIRSUTISM (EXCESSIVE HAIR GROWTH)

Excessive hair growth, usually a complaint of females, may be due to either endocrinologic or nonendocrinologic conditions. When women are affected in those areas of the body which normally develop hair as a secondary sex characteristic in males, their hirsutism generally reflects treatable endocrinopathy, as it is these follicles that are responsive to high concentrations of testosterone and are capable of converting various androgens to dihydrotestosterone (Ch. 522).

NONENDOCRINE HIRSUTISM.
Ethnic or *racial hirsutism* is characterized by excessive hair growth on the upper lip, beard area, chest, nipples, or lower abdomen in women without menstrual abnormalities or masculinization. Type of hair, rate of hair growth, and distribution of hair over the body differ among the races, relating to variations in the sensitivity of follicles to circulating androgens. A male pattern of hirsutism is more common in females whose ancestors came from the southern parts of Europe. Orientals and American Indians have less body hair. If endocrinologic abnormalities are not found (serum testosterone, dehydroepiandrosterone, and androstenedione are normal), bleaching or shaving may be sufficient to make the hair less noticeable. Electrolysis permanently destroys hair follicles but is time consuming and costly. Spironolactone,* which has antian-

---

*This use is not listed in the manufacturer's directive.

drogenic properties (200 mg per day), used for a period of 12 months is also useful in decreasing hair growth.

Certain *drugs* may also increase hair growth. Androgenic or steroidal medications, such as anabolic steroids, corticosteroids, and contraceptives, may cause increased hair growth in the beard, chest, and groin areas. Drugs such as phenytoin, phenothiazines, cyclosporine, and minoxidil cause excess hair in both men and women anywhere on the body.

Porphyria cutanea tarda causes increased hairiness of the face, especially on the temples and pinnae of the ears. Treatment of the condition results in decrease of hair growth.

ENDOCRINE HIRSUTISM. A distinction must be made between hirsutism caused by increased androgen production with and without virilization. In general, virilization is a sign of markedly elevated androgens derived from the adrenal glands or ovaries, especially adrenogenital syndrome, congenital adrenal hyperplasia, Cushing's disease or syndrome, Stein-Leventhal syndrome (polycystic ovarian syndrome), and occasionally malignant adrenal or ovarian tumors. Any woman with hirsutism and accompanying virilization should be tested for excess cortisol and androgen production.

Simple or *idiopathic hirsutism* is the designation given to those hirsute women in whom a specific etiologic diagnosis cannot be made and in whom normal or slightly elevated adrenal or ovarian androgens are found. The cause may be slightly increased production and metabolism of androgens or increased sensitivity of hair follicles to normal levels of androgens. Such patients have been successfully treated with cyclically administered birth control pills or with spironolactone.

PHOTOSENSITIVITY AND OTHER REACTIONS TO LIGHT

Certain wavelengths of light are capable of inducing a number of undesirable cutaneous reactions, including sunburn, skin aging, carcinogenesis, and a variety of photosensitivity reactions.

Clinically, photorelated conditions occur in a typical distribution of light-exposed areas, which should make the diagnosis of light-related reactions apparent (see Fig. 523–2). Thus, maximal changes occur over the forehead, malar eminences, bridge of the nose, and pinnae of the ears, with sparing of the upper lip (shaded by the nose), periorbital areas, and submental region. The V of the neck, dorsum of the hands, and forearms are often involved, with a sharp demarcation where clothing and watch bands cover the skin. In addition, light must be suspected from historical evidence. Seasonal recurrences are seen, especially in the spring or early summer. The evoked reaction may be to light alone, to light in association with exogenous substances (taken internally, such as drugs or externally applied materials), or to abnormal metabolites as in porphyria.

The incidence of photoreactions depends on a number of factors such as the amount of light reaching the earth's surface, season of the year, latitude and weather conditions, and thickness of the ozone layer, as well as topographic features of the environment. There are some useful climatologic and environmental factors to keep in mind which have bearing on the amount of sunlight hitting the skin. For example, 50 per cent of the daily ultraviolet light is emitted between 11 A.M. and 2 P.M., so avoiding exposure to sunlight during this time may be useful in minimizing photoreactions. Sitting in the shade does not protect against UV exposure, because 50 per cent of the ambient ultraviolet light is received; 90 per cent of ultraviolet light penetrates clouds, so one can get sunburns even in the shade and on cloudy days.

Electromagnetic radiation (EMG) from the sun has been arbitrarily classified into spectral regions measured in nanometers, ranging from short cosmic rays to long radiowaves. The solar spectrum that commonly affects human skin is in the ultraviolet light range (290 to 400 nm), which is subdivided into three bands designated as UVC (shorter than 290 nm), UVB (290 to 320 nm), and UVA, or long-wave ultraviolet light (320 to 400 nm). UVC does not reach the earth, being absorbed by ozone; UVB, or the sunburn spectrum, causes burning, tanning, aging, and carcinogenic changes in the skin. UVA is melanogenic and erythrogenic, but the amount of energy required to produce these effects is 1000 times greater than UVB. UVA causes skin reactions through window glass, and these wavelengths are often responsible for photoreactions in which chemical photosensitizers and UV radiation interact to cause inflammatory skin reactions.

The amount of UV light reaching various levels of the skin depends on wavelength. The longer wavelengths penetrate deeper into the dermis. Thus, depending on the wavelength of light and depth of penetration, the reactions may involve absorption by cellular DNA, RNA, and cutaneous proteins (keratin, collagen, etc.).

Direct Photo Effects on the Skin

ACUTE EFFECTS. Sunburning and tanning are common acute reactions to sun exposure and are attributed primarily to UVB light, although prolonged exposure to UVA can produce mild burn and marked hyperpigmentation. The sunburn reaction is a complex inflammatory process causing dyskeratotic cells, spongiosis, vacuolation of keratinocytes, and edema from capillary leakage, 12 to 24 hours after exposure to light. Occasionally, in addition to redness and pain, blisters may evolve. Prostaglandins may play a role in the burn reaction, as they are found in increased quantities in UV sunburned skin, and aspirin or indomethacin, prostaglandin synthesis inhibitors, can reduce the burn.

Three to four days after a sunburn, new melanin pigment is formed. Several cellular and molecular changes occur in the skin after each sunburn reaction which, if repeated, may lead to the chronic effects of UV light. A few days after UV light burning, epidermal mitosis and hyperplasia occur and DNA, RNA, and proteins in the skin are damaged.

CHRONIC EFFECTS. Degenerative changes of the skin consisting of wrinkling, telangiectasias, and keratoses are the long-term effects of chronic exposure to UV light. A furrowed and leathery condition of the skin may develop along with yellow papules and plaques due to solar degeneration of the dermal collagen, especially in fair-skinned individuals. These changes are caused by both UVB and UVA radiation. Such changes can be minimized by daily topical applications of effective sunscreens (see Ch. 524).

A number of malignant and premalignant skin lesions are associated with chronic sun exposure, including actinic keratoses, keratoacanthomas, basal cell and squamous cell carcinomas, and probably melanomas (see above).

Indirect Photo Effects on the Skin

Photoreactions that occur when systemic or topical chemicals induce photosensitivity or when there is an underlying immunologic, biochemical, or genetic abnormality that predisposes to sun sensitivity are considered indirect reactions; i.e., the sun alone does not cause photoreactions.

EXOGENOUS FACTORS CAUSING PHOTOSENSITIVITY. Chemical agents either taken systemically or placed topically on the skin can cause one of two general types of photoreactions: phototoxic and photoallergic. In these photosensitivity reactions, the absorption spectrum of a given drug, substance, or chemical is maximal at a certain wavelength of light that induces molecular changes in the exogenous material, which, in turn, initiates the cutaneous reaction. In most of the drug or chemical photosensitivity reactions, the wavelengths that evoke abnormal reactions are in the 320 to 400 nm (UVA) region. The reactions include acute, abnormal sunburn responses and eczematous and urticarial reactions.

Phototoxic reactions are those nonimmunologic cutaneous responses that occur in most individuals when enough light energy of a specific wavelength is absorbed by an appropriate concentration of drug or chemical in the skin. Free radicals are generated in the photosensitizer which damage cell membranes and lysosomes, inducing an exaggerated sunburn reaction, with intense redness, swelling, pain, and occasionally blistering. Most phototoxic agents absorb UVB light.

Photoallergic reactions to topical chemicals or internal drugs represent an acquired, altered response to light which involves immunologic mechanisms. Absorption of specific wavelengths of light by chemicals or drugs causes changes in their chemical configuration so that these substances become haptens that bind to proteins in the skin to become a complete antigen capable of eliciting a type IV delayed hypersensitivity immunologic response. The clinical manifestations of such photoallergic reactions

TABLE 525–15. CHARACTERISTICS OF PHOTOTOXIC AND PHOTOALLERGIC REACTIONS OF THE SKIN

Reaction	Phototoxic	Photoallergic
Clinical changes	Prolonged sunburn	Eczema or urticaria
Relative incidence	All people receiving chemical and exposed to appropriate wavelength of light	Few individuals exposed to chemical and appropriate wavelength of light
Concentration of drug necessary for reactions	High	Low
Reaction possible on first exposure	Yes	No
Incubation period necessary after first exposure	No	Yes
"Flares" at distant, previously involved sites possible	No	Yes
Cross-reaction to structural related agents	No	Frequent
Immunologic mechanism involved	No	Yes—type IV delayed hypersensitivity

are usually eczematous in nature (occasionally urticarial), evolving 24 hours after exposure to the sun in sun-exposed areas of the skin. The action spectrum is generally long-range UVA light, and less energy is required to elicit the reaction than for the production of phototoxic reactions.

Table 525–15 summarizes the differences between phototoxic and photoallergic reactions.

SYSTEMIC PHOTOSENSITIZERS. Drugs may cause either phototoxic or photoallergic reactions. Table 525–16 lists some of the drugs and chemicals that may induce photosensitivities and the type of reaction and action spectrum thought to induce them.

TOPICAL AGENTS CAUSING PHOTOSENSITIVITY. Most topical photosensitizing agents respond to the UVA action spectrum. Drugs and chemicals that induce *phototoxic contact reactions* include coal tar derivatives, topical drugs (phenothiazines, sulfonamides), dyes (eosins, methylene blue), and plant derivatives (furocoumarins). The photosensitive properties of coal tar

TABLE 525–16. SYSTEMIC PHOTOSENSITIZERS

Name	Type of Photoreaction	Action Spectrum (nm)
Sulfonamides	Phototoxic and photoallergic	290–320
Sulfonylureas (tolbutamide, chlorpropamide)	Phototoxic	290–360
Chlorothiazides	Phototoxic and photoallergic	290–320 320–400
Phenothiazines	Phototoxic, urticaria eruption, gray-blue hyperpigmentation	290–400
Antibiotics (tetracyclines, griseofulvin, nalidixic acid)	Phototoxic and photoallergic bullae	320–400
Furocoumarins (psoralens)	Phototoxic	
Nonsteroidal anti-inflammatory agents	Phototoxic and photoallergic	Unknown
Anticancer drugs (DTIC, fluorouracil, methotrexate, vinblastine)	Phototoxic	Unknown
Estrogens, progestins, and other drugs	Phototoxic, melasma	?290–320
Chlordiazepoxide (Librium)	Photoallergic	290–360
Cyclamates	Phototoxic and photoallergic	290–360
Quinidine, quinine	Photoallergic	320–400

derivatives and furocoumarins (psoralens) are utilized in treating certain skin diseases with ultraviolet light.

When plants, vegetables, or fruits containing a phototoxic chemical cause phototoxicity, the reaction is referred to as a *phytophotodermatitis.* Photocontact dermatitis develops with contact with plants in the Umbelliferae family, such as figs, cow parsnip, fennel, parsley, parsnip, and gas plant. Phytophotodermatitis also occurs in individuals exposed to Persian limes and celery. Such reactions are caused by furocoumarin compounds found in the plant which readily penetrate the epidermis. Two things are needed for initiation of phytophotodermatitis: (1) contact with a sensitizing furocoumarin and (2) subsequent exposure to UV radiation greater than 320 nm. Phytophotodermatitis may take on unique clinical forms: (1) berloque dermatitis presents as streaky erythema followed by hyperpigmentation in areas where perfumes containing oil of Bergamot (a psoralen) are applied to the skin (e.g., on the neck); (2) criss-cross linear streaks of erythema, vesicles, and bullae that heal with hyperpigmentation where meadow grass or other related plants rub on the skin; (3) oil of the rind of a Persian lime causes erythema and pigmentation on the hands of bartenders.

Photoallergic contact dermatitis, a form of delayed allergic hypersensitivity, evolves in some individuals after exposure to such chemicals as fragrances (methylcoumarin and musk ambrette), halogenated salicylanilides, sunscreens, and blankophores, or optical whitening agents, used in laundry soaps and bleaches. These photoallergic responses appear as eczematous reactions. A number of perfumes (after-shave lotions, colognes, etc.) contain musk ambrette, a synthetic fragrance fixative that causes a photoeczematous reaction over the face and hands. Paradoxically, sunscreening agents containing PABA esters and cinnamates that readily absorb UV light may cause eczematous photoallergic reactions. A small number of individuals have persistent chronic eczematous dermatitis after all exposure to the photosensitizing agent has ceased—so-called persistent light reactivity. Such patients may be so photosensitive that they react to artificial fluorescent light.

Identifying the cause of contact photoallergic reactions can be done with photopatch testing (Ch. 523). Treatment of photocontact sensitivity obviously begins by eliminating the photosensitizing agent and minimizing sunlight exposure (avoiding sun and use of sunscreens). Topical and, at times, oral steroids may be needed to decrease the cutaneous inflammatory response.

ENDOGENOUS CONDITIONS ASSOCIATED WITH PHOTOSENSITIVITY. Certain immunologic, biochemical, and genetic diseases display photoreactions as a prominent feature.

Immunologic diseases with photosensitivity include connective tissue conditions such as lupus erythematosus, both discoid and systemic, and solar urticaria. Solar urticaria, hives with itching and burning, evolves within minutes of sunlight exposure and lasts an hour or more. The inciting wavelength of light differs among patients.

Biochemical conditions associated with photosensitivity include two forms of porphyria: porphyria cutanea tarda and erythropoietic protoporphyria. These are discussed above (see Vesiculobullous Diseases).

Pellagra, once a common disease, especially in the southeastern United States, is caused by an inadequate diet and a deficiency of nicotinic acid. It is still seen occasionally with alcoholism, poor dietary intake in the elderly, and malabsorption. The carcinoid syndrome may also be associated with pellagra because tryptophan, the precursor of nicotinic acid, is diverted to serotonin production by the tumor. A scaly dermatitis on sun-exposed parts of the skin, especially on the face, the neck, and the back of the hands, is seen in association with diarrhea and dementia (the three D's). Low serum vitamin levels establish the diagnosis of this condition, and dietary replacement clears the skin and other signs of the disease.

Other Photosensitivity Conditions

A condition known as *polymorphous light eruption* (PML) presents with a variety of skin lesions, including eczematous patches, red to violaceous papules or plaques, and urticarial lesions over the face, the nape and V of the neck, and the back of the hands. The rash characteristically arises hours to days after sun exposure. The onset is frequently in early summer with some degree of resistance being acquired with continued sun exposure. Recurrences each spring and summer are common, and the eruption remits during the winter. The disease may begin at any age, but it is most frequent during the first half of life. The etiology is unknown, and its diagnosis is one of excluding other photosensitivity conditions.

PML may respond to the use of sunscreens with an SPF of 15 and, if elicited by UVA light, sunscreens with benzophenone or anthranilate to improve protection against the UVA spectrum. If sunscreens fail, the induction of tolerance by tanning with PUVA or UVB light or a short course of antimalarial agents or oral steroids may occasionally be needed.

Actinic reticuloid is another form of persistent photodermatitis of unknown etiology which occurs in middle-aged males and causes a most distressing photoreaction of red papules and pruritic eczematous patches. Both UVB and UVA appear to play a role. PUVA chemotherapy may help control the condition.

DERMATOLOGIC MANIFESTATIONS IN THE IMMUNOCOMPROMISED HOST

Immunosuppression causes an increase in benign and malignant skin growths as well as a variety of infections in the skin (see Ch. 287). Cutaneous neoplasms such as squamous cell and basal cell carcinomas occur with a much higher frequency than would be expected. Transplant patients have an estimated risk of skin cancer that is 7.1 times greater than normal. Most patients have multiple skin cancers.

Any skin lesion, no matter how innocuous, should be carefully evaluated in the immunosuppressed host. The gross morphology of infections is so frequently modified by the altered inflammatory response in the immunocompromised patient that early skin biopsies are essential for diagnosis. The array of potential pathogens is imposing in these patients, and even common infectious processes are greatly modified or obscured by immunocompromising illness. Skin infections are common, accounting for 22 to 33 per cent of infections in immunosuppressed patients.

Microbial involvement of the skin and subcutaneous tissue can be grouped into two major categories in immunocompromised patients: (1) *primary skin infections* that are typical of those occurring in nonimmunocompromised hosts, widespread involvement with infectious agents that commonly cause localized skin infection, and primary skin infections from opportunistic agents that rarely cause skin infection in normal patients; and (2) *disseminated systemic infections* metastatic to the skin from a noncutaneous portal of entry.

PRIMARY SKIN INFECTIONS. Typical primary skin infections, including group A streptococcal and *Staphylococcus aureus* cellulitis, are frequent, although more unusual causes of cellulitis in granulocytopenic patients must also be considered (*Pseudomonas,* anaerobic bacteria). Skin biopsy of the cellulitic areas for Gram's stain and culture is often helpful.

Unusually widespread, primary cutaneous infections by viruses and skin dermatophytes are also common. Warts caused by papillomavirus may be numerous, disfiguring, and difficult to remove. Malignant transformation has been documented in such warts in immunosuppressed individuals. Herpes simplex infections may present as chronic, large, ulcerated lesions persisting for weeks to months (herpes phagedena, especially in the genital areas), and there may be internal dissemination from cutaneous sites. Reactivation of herpes zoster infections is common in immunocompromised hosts, with systemic dissemination. Widespread dermatophyte infections of the skin appear as scaling, red patches that provide a portal of entry for bacterial infection.

Unusual opportunistic primary skin infections with atypical *Mycobacterium, Aspergillus, Rhizopus,* and *Candida* organisms cause cellulitis-like reactions that form a central pustule and eschar. Skin biopsy of such lesions with a portion of the biopsy processed by frozen section and specially stained for AFB and fungi may identify the pathologic organisms rapidly.

DISSEMINATED INFECTION METASTATIC TO THE SKIN. Hematogenous dissemination of infection to the skin from distant primary sites frequently occurs in patients with impaired host defenses. Three groups of organisms are responsible for this:

TABLE 525–17. CUTANEOUS DRUG REACTIONS

Type of Skin Reaction	Drugs Likely to Cause Skin Reaction
Eczematous (allergic contact reaction)	Antihistamines, neomycin, formaldehyde, sulfonamides
Photodermatitis	
Phototoxic	Chlorpromazine, psoralens, demeclocycline, doxycycline
Photoallergic	Promethazine, griseofulvin, Diuril, hypoglycemic drugs
Exfoliative dermatitis	Carbamazepine, hydantoins, nitrofurantoin, isoniazid, gold, allopurinol, phenothiazines
Maculopapular eruption (exanthematous)	Penicillin, sulfonamides, hypoglycemic drugs, phenothiazines, allopurinol, phenytoin, quinine, gold salts, captopril, meprobamate
Papulosquamous reactions Psoriasiform, lichen planus, pityriasis rosea–like	Beta blockers, lithium (psoriasiform), thiazides, gold, phenothiazines, quinidine, antimalarials (lichen planus–like); gold (PR-like); others—practolol, dapsone, ethambutol, furosemide
Vesiculobullous reactions	Azapropazone, captopril, clonidine, furosemide, gold, psoralens, barbiturates, phenytoin, Hydrodiuril, penicillamine
Toxic epidermal necrolysis	Acetazolamide, allopurinol, barbiturates, carbamazepines, gold, hydantoin, nitrofurantoin, pentazocine, tetracycline, quinidine
Pustular—acneiform reactions	Androgen hormones, corticosteroids, iodides, bromides, hydantoin, lithium
Urticaria and erythemas	
Urticaria	May occur with anaphylaxis; penicillin, xenogenic sera, cephalosporins, sulfonamides, barbiturates, hydralazine, phenylbutazone, hydantoin, quinidine, x-ray contrast media
Erythema multiforme	Sulfonamides, hydantoin, barbiturates, penicillin, carbamazepines, allopurinol, amikacin, phenothiazides
Nodular lesions	
Erythema nodosum	Birth control pills, sulfonamides, diuretics, gold, clonidine, propranolol, furosemide, opiates, penicillin
Vasculitis reaction	Allopurinol, barbiturates, carbamazepine, chlorothiazide, cimetidine, gold, indomethacin, hydantoin, piperazine, sulfonamides
Telangiectatic and LE reactions	Procainamide, hydralazine, phenytoin, penicillamine, trimethadione, methyldopa, carbamazepine, griseofulvin, nalidixic acid, oral contraceptives, propranolol
Pigmentary reaction	Anticonvulsants, antimalarials, antitumor agents (bleomycin, busulfan, cyclophosphamide, doxorubicin, melphalan), oral contraceptives, corticotropin, tetracyclines, phenothiazines, amiodarone
Other cutaneous reactions	
Fixed drug reactions	Phenolphthalein, barbiturates, gold, sulfonamides, meprobamate, penicillin, tetracyclines, analgesics
Alopecia	Alkylating agents, antimetabolites, heparin, coumarin, hydantoin, accutane, gold, nitrofurantoin, propranolol, colchicine, allopurinol
Hypertrichosis	Anabolic agents, diazoxide, minoxidil, phenytoin

(1) *Pseudomonas* and other gram-negative bacilli; (2) endemic systemic mycoses (*Histoplasma, Coccidioides*); and (3) opportunistic fungi (*Aspergillus, Candida,* Mucoraceae). The range of cutaneous clinical presentations of these infections is varied and mimicked by all of these infections, namely (a) *vesicles and bullae* that become hemorrhagic, (b) *gangrenous cellulitis* with necrotic ulcerations, and (c) widespread, red, warm, fluctuant *nodules* with pustules and purpura. Prompt biopsy of these lesions with frozen sections stained for bacterial and hyphal elements may provide rapid diagnosis.

CUTANEOUS DRUG REACTIONS

Rashes are among the most common adverse reactions to drugs and occur in 2 to 3 per cent of hospitalized patients. Any drug can potentially produce a rash, and over-the-counter preparations should be considered when defining drug reactions.

The causes of adverse drug reactions are multiple, including *toxic* (too much drug is given or degradation of the drug is slow owing to an underlying disease or action of another drug), *idiosyncratic* (unanticipated side effects), and *allergic* reactions. Because tests for drug allergy are not available, it is often difficult to be sure one is dealing with an allergic reaction. However, a hypersensitivity reaction can be suspected when (1) rechallenge or re-exposure to small amounts of the drug elicits the same response, (2) the reaction appears following several days to weeks of administration of the drug, (3) the reaction occurs when the patient is exposed to a structurally similar drug, and (4) the clinical response does not resemble the general pharmacologic effects of the drug.

Some of the most common drugs causing skin reactions in hospitalized patients are amoxicillin, trimethoprim-sulfamethoxazole, ampicillin, penicillin G, allopurinol, dipyrone, gentamicin sulfate, mefruside, nitrazepam, and barbiturates. Drugs least likely to cause allergic skin reactions include digoxin, antacids, promethazine, acetaminophen, nitroglycerin, aminophylline, propranolol, antihistamines, cromolyn, and emollient laxatives.

Table 525–17 lists the various morphologic types of drug reactions and some of the drugs capable of inducing each reaction.

Fixed drug eruptions are unique reactions that appear in the same area of the skin each time the responsible drug is administered. These appear as macular, eczematous, or even bullous, pink to dark red patches occurring as few or many lesions. When the drug is stopped the lesions fade, leaving postinflammatory hyperpigmentation. The lesions return in the same place within a few hours of taking the drug again.

Nonsteroidal anti-inflammatory drugs are being used with increasing frequency and may cause cutaneous reactions including vesiculobullous photosensitivity reactions, serum sickness, erythroderma, fixed drug reactions, and toxic epidermal necrolysis.

The treatment of drug reactions is discontinuation of the suspected agent. Often the patient is taking many drugs, and generally once a drug reaction is suspected all nonessential drugs should be stopped and appropriate substitutes used for the necessary medications. An asymptomatic eruption may require no therapy, or a mild reaction with pruritus may be controlled with topical steroid applications and antihistamines. In severe conditions such as exfoliative dermatitis, oral steroids are often indicated. Most drug eruptions resolve in 1 to 2 weeks after withdrawal of the drug, but some reactions take months to clear. While an occasional reaction may be fatal (e.g., toxic epidermal necrolysis), patients with drug eruptions usually have an excellent prognosis.

PART XXVI

OCCUPATIONAL AND ENVIRONMENTAL MEDICINE

526 Principles of Occupational Medicine

Charles E. Becker

Occupational medicine is concerned with the physical and emotional safety and health of workers. It encompasses issues of public concern, particularly the quality of air and water, the degree of environmental pollution, and the complex mosaic of legal, economic, social, and ethical questions that are raised whenever human action produces human disorders.

Among the 100 million workers in the United States today, approximately 100,000 deaths per year are attributed to the workplace. Yet there are only 10,000 physicians whose self-determined primary specialty is occupational medicine, and only 500 of these have subspecialty board certification. Primary care internists, family physicians, and emergency physicians constitute the "front line" for identification of work-related disorders. Therefore, they must learn to target the medical history and to recognize classic signs and symptoms of occupational and environmental disorders.

Occupational medicine deals almost exclusively with diagnosis and prevention, not treatment. The diagnosis of an occupational disease may be difficult, since occupational diseases (1) may simulate many other disorders, (2) often lack unique pathology, and (3) may be marked by a long latency period between exposure and the manifestation of the disease.

Problems from chemical contamination do not always remain exclusively in the workplace; they may extend into the community: polychlorinated biphenyls (PCB's) in Japan; dioxin in Seveso, Italy; radiation exposure at Three Mile Island; mercury contamination in Minamata Bay; lead pollution in cities and around smelting plants; and nervous system, liver, and reproductive toxicity from chlordecone (Kepone) in Virginia. These events give rise to important political, social, and economic considerations that emphasize the need for specialized training in occupational medicine.

Competency in occupational medicine is best acquired from a base of general training in internal medicine, with extended knowledge and experience in epidemiology, industrial hygiene, biostatistics, and toxicology. The relationship between workplace-environmental exposure and disease centers on four basic concepts: recognition, prevention, exacerbation, and latent manifestation. Workplace-associated diseases are presumed to be preventable when recognized and fully understood. Since the signs and symptoms of occupational diseases may be identical to those of many other diseases, a high level of suspicion is required for the recognition that allows prevention. Rather than causing an illness, occupational environmental conditions may, in fact, exacerbate or compound a pre-existing condition. For example, a patient with toxicity from aminoglycoside antibiotics may have additional otologic injury from loud noises occurring at work. Although some environmental and occupational diseases become manifest acutely, many have a long latency period and may extend from the workplace into the family or society and thus present important considerations in diagnostic and preventive strategies (e.g., asbestos exposure).

In occupational medicine there are four basic categories of hazard: physical, biologic, psychological, and chemical. Physical hazards may include vibration, heat, noise, radiation, and trauma. Occupational injuries account for approximately 14,000 deaths, 245 million lost work days, and $25 billion in direct and indirect costs annually in the United States. Biologic hazards include the well-known occupational risks of hepatitis, human immunodeficiency virus (HIV) infection, or tuberculosis. Psychological hazards of stress and work-shift changes are complex and will be discussed subsequently. Chemical hazards involve exposure to solvents, dusts, vapors, and gases. It is important here to distinguish between toxicity and hazard. *Toxicity* is the inherent capability of a material to cause injury to a living cell. *Hazard* is the chance of a resultant injury from use of such a material in a given setting. Asbestos, for example, is a useful fire retardant construction material with known basic toxicity that may become hazardous only during repair or demolition work or fire, which may cause its release into the air.

In occupational medicine one is also concerned with the difference between exposure and dose. Exposure is determined by surveillance of the environment with the knowledge that a toxic agent has had the potential of being delivered into the body. For example, environmental measurements of lead can provide an index of exposure. These environmental measurements are often made by experts called industrial hygienists. Dose, however, can be assessed only by biologic monitoring of blood, urine, and hair and by indices of enzyme systems that may be affected. In the case of lead, the total dose delivered is dependent on the amount that is respirable and the amount absorbed from the gastrointestinal tract. Figure 526–1 depicts the complex interactions in the field of occupational medicine.

This chapter outlines some of the basic concepts and a few selected disorders encompassed in occupational medicine. Other chapters in this section describe at length occupational diseases of the lung (Ch. 527) and of the skin (Ch. 529) and a variety of chemical and physical sources of injury. Some chapters in other parts of the book contain useful information related to the discipline: toxic nephropathies (Ch. 80), epidemiology of cancer (Ch. 158), painful back and painful shoulders (Ch. 274 and 275), and neuropathies associated with the workplace (Ch. 533).

THE OCCUPATIONAL-ENVIRONMENTAL HISTORY

Key elements of an occupational and environmental history should be added to the data base collected on all patients. In every problem-oriented assessment of a current illness, individual problem lists should include such questions concerning the occupational health history: Are symptoms associated with work, or do they improve during vacations and weekends? Are other workers similarly affected? Is there or has there been direct exposure to dust, fumes, and chemicals? Have there been work-related injuries? Is periodic testing and medical surveillance or routine industrial hygiene sampling of the workplace performed?

A careful work history should include a chronologic list of all previous jobs with a reasonably detailed description of the work site, the scope of a typical work day, and such pertinent factors as protective equipment, ventilation, and pre-employment examinations.

A specific listing of the total number of days missed on each job and the reasons for the absences may be useful. Has a worker compensation claim been filed in the past? Does the worker perform additional jobs, i.e., is he or she moonlighting? A patient may not relate work to health, so the physician should obtain initially, on each examination, specific answers to common occupational problems, such as the following: Have you ever been exposed to loud noises, excessive vibration, or heat? Do you work with asbestos? Have you been exposed to radioactive chemicals? Have you had previous chemical exposure? During the military, what were your duties? Recent "right-to-know" legislation often allows workers to receive a written description of their chemical exposures, which the physician can help interpret.

The environmental health history should include information about industries located in the neighborhood, exposure to hazardous waste or toxic spills, jobs of the spouse, degree of air pollution, and types of hobbies and recreational activities that also may contribute to health-related problems, such as painting, sculpturing, welding, or woodworking.

In addition, it may be important to elicit a description of home insulation or heating as well as exposure to cleaning agents and insecticides. Special questions should be directed toward unique workplace problems, such as working hours and job schedule (Do these affect your sleep pattern? Are you bored on the job?). The reproductive history is essential: the number of miscarriages, children, stillbirths, previous pregnancies; difficulty in conceiving; and changes in libido and menses.

SIGNS AND SYMPTOMS OF OCCUPATIONAL AND ENVIRONMENTAL DISORDERS. Because occupational and environmental diseases have a long latency and may be synergistic with other causes of disease, the clinician should always consider that the signs and symptoms may be caused by occupational or environmental conditions. Sometimes it may be useful to identify all the signs and symptoms that could be associated with disease caused by the environment or the workplace. Knowledge of exposure to certain substances may implicate or suggest the cause: chlorinated hydrocarbons and acne; arsenic and thallium and alopecia; solvent exposure and anosmia; chlorinated hydrocarbons and arrhythmias; and aniline dyes and bladder or other cancers.

Reproductive hazards, noise-induced hearing abnormalities, work-shift changes, and ergonomics are discussed as important occupational entities not covered specifically by other chapters in this section.

REPRODUCTIVE HAZARDS

Seven per cent of all newborns in the United States have birth defects, approximately 70 per cent of which are of unknown cause. The relationship between exposure to environmental and occupational agents and consequent development of male and female reproductive abnormalities is an area of intense study and interest. Animal studies have demonstrated the transmission to subsequent generations of chemically induced abnormalities of sperm and at a rate determined by mendelian principles. These observations have sparked interest in predicting and thereby preventing reproductive hazards from environmental agents. Short-term bioassays for mutagenesis, such as the Ames test, have been used to screen agents to predict reproductive outcome. These relatively inexpensive and rapid initial screening tests of chemicals can be performed in animals or bacteria. Agents encountered in the environment or the workplace can clearly cause reproductive hazards, e.g., testicular toxicity of dibromochloropropane (DBCP) recognized in California chemical workers. Male workers with sterility suffered no systemic illness and were working in an environment that was alleged to be safe. Previous laboratory tests in animals had suggested reproductive hazards from this chemical. The controversy surrounding this event sparked great interest in this subject. To date, the following environmental and occupational agents have been shown to cause adverse reproductive effects in men: anesthetic gases, carbon disulfide, diethylstilbestrol, toluene diamine, ethylene dibromide, chlordecone, and ionizing radiation. A much stronger data base is required to assess environmental effects on pregnancy outcome, spontaneous abortion, and stillbirth.

NOISE-INDUCED HEARING LOSS

More than 5 million people in the United States have noise-induced hearing loss. This most common form of hearing loss is associated with damage to, and loss of, hair cells in the organ of Corti. Early or moderately advanced noise-induced hearing loss is associated with normal hearing in the low frequencies but gradually increasing loss of hearing at higher frequencies (with a maximum of 3, 4, or 6 kHz). There may be some return toward normal function at 8 kHz. The audiometric shape of this curve is not pathognomonic because other otologic disorders (e.g., that caused by aminoglycoside antibiotic therapy) can result in an identical audiogram. Some of the hearing loss attributed to aging (presbycusis) may be due to the nearly ubiquitous noise pollution in modern society. Epidemiologic studies suggest that aging individuals in a nonindustrialized society have much better hearing preservation than older Americans. Major individual differences in susceptibility to noise-induced hearing loss occur. Men are much more susceptible to noise-induced hearing loss than women. Smoking and lack of skin pigmentation may also be risk factors for noise-induced hearing loss. Hearing impairment from occupational and environmental factors is a major and entirely preventable public health problem.

WORK-SHIFT CHANGES

Twenty per cent of American workers work evenings or nights. In some industries, such as automobile production, petrol chemicals, and textile manufacturing, shift workers number nearly 50 per cent. There is growing evidence to suggest clinically significant health effects from shift work on health care workers who work many hours without sleep. Twenty per cent of workers are unable to tolerate shift work, tolerance for which also diminishes with increasing age. Daily physiologic variations known as circadian rhythms are distorted by shift work, which in turn alters the quality of sleep and causes important disturbances of the gastrointestinal tract and other organs. Diabetes mellitus and epilepsy may be aggravated by shift work, and the risk of accidents

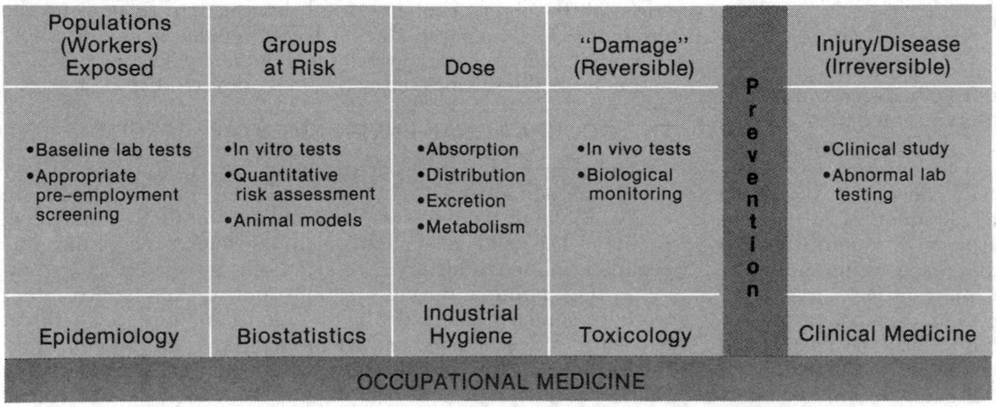

Populations (Workers) Exposed	Groups at Risk	Dose	"Damage" (Reversible)	Prevention	Injury/Disease (Irreversible)
• Baseline lab tests • Appropriate pre-employment screening	• In vitro tests • Quantitative risk assessment • Animal models	• Absorption • Distribution • Excretion • Metabolism	• In vivo tests • Biological monitoring		• Clinical study • Abnormal lab testing
Epidemiology	Biostatistics	Industrial Hygiene	Toxicology		Clinical Medicine
OCCUPATIONAL MEDICINE					

FIGURE 526–1. Multidisciplinary approach to occupational (environmental) medicine.

may be increased. Shift workers tend to have an increased number of subjective health complaints in general and may have enhanced risk factors complicating management of other medical disorders.

ERGONOMICS

Ergonomics is the interface of a worker with his or her work station, machine, or work environment. This interface may create physical and psychological stresses that present as common diseases to internists. Physical factors may include repetitive motion disorders, back injuries, and musculoskeletal problems. Psychological factors involve attention span, memory, vigilance, and behavior. They may play an important role in safety in the workplace and are often called *human error*. Ergonometric problems may progress from chronic discomfort of aches and pains to temporary disabling conditions, such as sprains, strains, tendinitis, and fibromyositis syndromes. These syndromes ultimately lead to long-term disabilities—nerve entrapment, chronic back pain, and musculoskeletal disorders. Careful history taking will suggest an ergonometric problem that frequently involves highly repetitive, monotonous work or fast-paced production jobs. Sometimes extremely sedentary work, such as word processing or microscopic inspection, may also cause a disability. It may be essential to make a visit to the plant to observe the work station in order to assist the patient in resolving an ergonometric problem. Reducing physical and psychological stresses may have beneficial effects that seem out of proportion to the magnitude of the changes in the work practice.

CONCLUSIONS

Strictly speaking, all diseases that are not genetic in origin are "environmental." Even genetic disorders are not totally endogenous, since they most frequently alter the ability of the host to accommodate to the environment. Broadly conceived, even the infectious diseases and nutritional disorders are environmental in origin. In practice, however, the term *environmental medicine* is used in a much more restrictive sense to reflect the chemical and physical hazards to which an individual is exposed and the injuries that may result from that exposure. Occupational medicine is that subset of environmental medicine directly concerned with the hazards of the workplace. The following chapters describe in greater detail some of the specific hazards and injuries incident to modern occupations. The topics selected cannot be inclusive, since the boundaries of occupational and environmental medicine are indistinct, merging into the traditional domains of internal medicine, epidemiology, toxicology, surgery, orthopedics, and many other clinical and basic science disciplines.

Ladou J: Current Occupational Medicine: Diagnosis and Treatment. Los Altos, Calif., Lange Medical Publications, 1990. *A full review of key occupational topics.*

Morgan WK, Seaton A: Occupational Lung Diseases. 2nd ed. Philadelphia, W.B. Saunders Company, 1984. *Useful, conservative approach with easy readings for occupational lung disease.*

Olsen K: Poisoning and Drug Overdose. Appleton-Lange, 1990. *A useful, up-to-date reference on acute and chronic chemical exposure.*

Proctor N, Hughes J, Hathaway GJ: Chemical Hazards of the Workplace. 3rd ed. Norwalk, Conn., Van Nostrand Reinhold, 1991. *Updated classic reference on workplace exposure.*

Rosenstock A, Cullen M: Clinical Occupational Medicine. Philadelphia, W.B. Saunders Company, 1986. *Useful, inexpensive guide to common occupational health problems.*

Selikoff I: The role of the internist in occupational medicine. Am J Indust Med 8:95, 1985. *An elder statesman of occupational medicine puts everything in perspective.*

527 Occupational Pulmonary Disorders

Dean Sheppard

The lung is the major interface between the human and the external environment. As such, the lungs and airways have evolved an elaborate system to filter out the myriad of potentially toxic particles and gases present in inspired air in order to protect the delicate gas-exchanging apparatus of the alveolar surface. This system is remarkably durable. The irritant gases and approximately 2 mg of dust inhaled daily by urban dwellers generally have no effect on lung function. Even the high concentrations of dust, irritants, and carcinogens present in cigarette smoke, inhaled daily for periods of 50 years or more, fail to cause disease in most smokers. Given the continuing contact between the lungs and the environment, however, it is not surprising that the lungs are the most common site of serious environmentally induced disease. Environmental pollutants are generally present in highest concentration at sites of industrial use or production. Thus, environmentally induced lung disease usually results from occupational exposure.

The major determinants of disease in a given individual are the toxicity of the material inhaled, the dose and duration of exposure (including the duration of lung retention, which may be several years for some inhaled particles), and the individual's host defenses. One would like to be able to identify host factors that predispose to the development of occupational disease in order to advise individuals at risk to avoid particular occupations, but unfortunately this is rarely possible. A few notable exceptions are the increased susceptibility of cigarette smokers to asbestos-induced carcinoma of the lung and the increased susceptibility of atopic individuals to some types of occupational asthma. In general, a more fruitful approach to the prevention of occupational lung disease is protection of all workers from exposures that can be anticipated to cause disease in any. This approach is most likely to be effective if it includes a significant margin of safety, limiting exposures to levels considerably less than the exposure anticipated to cause disease. These principles underlie the workplace exposure standards promulgated by the American Council of Government Industrial Hygienists and more recently by the U.S. Occupational Safety and Health Administration. However, the standard-setting process is a slow one, and in the absence of adequate data, the assessments of disease probability on which they are based are necessarily subjective. Furthermore, as new data emerge, standards need to be continually revised, but this process too can take many years. Keeping these shortcomings in mind, physicians cannot assume that a given occupational exposure is not responsible for causing a disease, even if the exposure level was below the current standard.

Even if workplace standards could be set instantaneously with the emergence of new scientific data, individual practicing physicians would still play a critical role in the identification and ultimate prevention of occupational lung disease. Onset of occupational disease is often delayed long after exposure (e.g., up to 60 years for mesothelioma caused by asbestos exposure). Furthermore, the first cases of an occupational disease are rarely recognized as being caused by work exposure, especially when the disease is a common one, such as asthma or carcinoma of the lung. Thousands of new chemicals are introduced into the workplace each year without systematic screening for their ability to cause disease. Therefore, new causes of occupational lung disease will undoubtedly continue to emerge. Identification of these new causes of lung disease and prevention of additional cases will continue to be the responsibility of practicing physicians.

Even when adequate workplace standards exist, they are hard to enforce, especially for workers who are self-employed or who work in small shops. Under these circumstances the identification of an individual worker with an occupationally induced lung disease can be the first indication of unsafe working conditions. Thus, a diagnosis of occupational lung disease necessitates a report to the appropriate public health agency and a thorough investigation of the workplace to identify additional cases and prevent future ones.

The lung responds to injury in a limited number of ways. Virtually any type of lung disorder can be caused by an occupational exposure. The specific type of disorder is determined by the site of deposition of the responsible agent, the dose and duration of exposure, the susceptibility of specific lung cells to the agent's toxic effects, and the nature of the interaction between the agent and local host defense mechanisms.

Gases are deposited in the respiratory system based on their water solubility. Water-soluble gases, such as ammonia and sulfur dioxide, are nearly entirely removed from inspired air by the aqueous layer lining the nose, oropharynx, and upper airways. These gases thus are most likely to cause disease in the airways. Relatively water-insoluble gases, such as nitrogen dioxide and phosgene, bypass the upper airways and injure the distal airways and alveoli. In contrast, particles are deposited based on size or, more accurately, on "aerodynamic diameter," which means that a particle is deposited out of a moving airstream in the same fashion as would be a perfect sphere of that diameter. During quiet breathing through the nose, essentially all particles with aerodynamic diameters in excess of 10 μm are deposited on the nasal mucosa. During strenuous exercise, however, because of increased airflow and mouth breathing, up to 20 per cent of particles between 10 and 20 μm in diameter are deposited within the airways. Particles between 3 and 10 μm in diameter can be deposited throughout the tracheobronchial tree. More central deposition is favored by high inspiratory flow rates, by airway obstruction, and by the presence of increased quantities of mucus. Particles between 0.1 and 3 μm in diameter can also be deposited in the airways but are preferentially deposited within the alveoli. Smaller particles are mainly exhaled. A fiber is also deposited on the basis of aerodynamic diameter and not length. This explains why fibers up to 25 μm long are often deposited in alveoli.

GENERAL APPROACH TO A PATIENT WITH SUSPECTED OCCUPATIONAL LUNG DISEASE

HISTORY. A thorough occupational history is the most important step in diagnosing any occupationally induced disease. The history must go beyond the patient's present job to a complete list of each job done throughout the patient's lifetime. Job titles often are not helpful. Rather, a detailed description of what the patient actually did and what materials he or she worked with should be elicited. The relationship of the patient's work site to other associated jobs is important, as is the use and adequacy of exhaust ventilation and personal protective devices. For instance, one electrician could develop asbestosis from working near insulators in the holds of ships, while another electrician working outdoors on new-building construction might have no significant asbestos exposure. The presence or absence of special work clothes, lockers, and showers should be noted, since hazardous materials (e.g., asbestos) brought home by workers who have worked in their street clothes can cause disease in family members. Hobbies should also be described in detail; hazardous exposures in home workshops can cause disease (e.g., asthma from exposure to isocyanate varnishes). Each job and hobby should be recorded in chronologic order to ensure that all working years are accounted for. The temporal relationship between symptoms and exposure can also be important. This is especially true for disease with acute symptomatic exacerbations, such as occupational asthma and hypersensitivity pneumonitis. In all cases, it is important to determine that symptoms did not precede exposure. Because of the high prevalence of cigarette smoking, the important toxic effects of cigarette smoke itself on the lungs, and the possible interactions between smoking and occupational exposures, a careful quantitative smoking history is also important. Finally, it is important to seek out historical information that would suggest a nonoccupational cause for the patient's lung disease. For instance, a history of uveitis and parotid enlargement might suggest that sarcoidosis rather than asbestos exposure was responsible for a given patient's interstitial lung disease.

ROENTGENOGRAPHIC TECHNIQUES. Chest roentgenographs are important in the evaluation of patients suspected of having parenchymal lung disease and in detecting pleural abnormalities in workers exposed to asbestos. They can also be useful in surveillance of workers in hazardous occupations to detect subclinical abnormalities. For standardization of epidemiologic surveys, roentgenographic abnormalities should be characterized by trained and certified readers using the International Labor Office (ILO) classification system. In this system small parenchymal opacities are described by shape (irregular or rounded) and size. Profusion (the concentration of opacities) is scored on a 12-point scale (0/−, 0/0, 0/1, up to 3/3, 3/+). Large parenchymal opacities and the extent and width of pleural thickening are also quantified. This scoring system allows the clinician to make a

reasonable assessment of prognosis in individual patients. Computed tomography (CT) is more sensitive and specific than standard chest radiographs in detecting pleural abnormalities. Nonetheless, this technique is seldom necessary in symptomatic individuals, and its expense does not justify its use in screening. Similarly, although CT may be more sensitive than standard radiographs in detecting parenchymal infiltrates, the clinical significance of infiltrates detected by CT only is uncertain. Roentgenographs are not useful in evaluating patients with suspected occupational airway diseases.

PULMONARY FUNCTION TESTS. Tests of static lung function are important in evaluating patients suspected of having occupationally induced interstitial lung diseases or those with dyspnea of undetermined etiology. When these tests are abnormal, they provide information about the pattern and extent of lung dysfunction. Tests of static lung function do not provide information about the *cause* of lung dysfunction (occupational or not) or about dynamic abnormalities (e.g., bronchospasm or decreased pulmonary vascular reserve). Thus, for instance, many, if not most, patients with occupational asthma will have normal screening pulmonary function tests between symptomatic episodes. Special studies such as bronchial provocation tests (see below) may be required before a diagnosis of occupational lung disease can be excluded. An additional problem of tests of static lung function is the wide range of normal values seen among healthy individuals. For example, if an individual worker starts with a vital capacity near the upper limit of normal (120 per cent of predicted), his or her vital capacity would need to fall by one third (to 80 per cent of predicted) before it would be considered abnormal. If, as is often the case, a single measurement is made after many years of employment and a vital capacity of 90 per cent of predicted is recorded, a significant occupationally induced loss of lung function could easily be overlooked. To avoid this problem, serial measurements of lung function should be performed on the same equipment for surveillance of workers in occupations suspected of causing occupational lung disease. Accelerated rates of decline of lung function can thus be detected before the test results deviate from the predicted normal range.

In addition to tests of static lung function, pulmonary exercise testing can provide important information for the evaluation of any patient with unexplained dyspnea. This test can distinguish between cardiovascular and pulmonary limitations to exercise and can identify pulmonary vascular dysfunction (as occurs with interstitial fibrosis) in some patients with normal static lung function. In addition, exercise limitation can be measured and compared with the patient's actual job requirements.

EVALUATION OF THE JOB SITE. In the clinical evaluation of a worker suspected of having any occupationally induced disorder, it is important to inspect and monitor his or her workplace. It is essential to do so if a diagnosis of an occupationally induced disorder has been established. Inspections usually require the assistance of a trained industrial hygienist who may be employed by the worker's company, the worker's compensation insurance company, a state or federal agency (e.g., the Occupational Safety and Health Administration), or a specialized occupational health clinic. In addition to a visual walk-through inspection and direct observation of each of the worker's job tasks (and adjacent workers' tasks), an inspection should include air sampling for agents suspected of being released by the work processes involved. Even if for some reason air sampling cannot be obtained, direct site inspection can provide important clues to the occupational etiology of a worker's disease. For example, a maintenance worker with asthma may be found to be working in a warehouse in which toluene di-isocyanate is used in manufacturing.

Morgan WKC, Seaton A: Occupational Lung Disease. 2nd ed. Philadelphia, W. B. Saunders Company, 1984. *A reasonably priced, up-to-date textbook.*
Parkes WR: Occupational Lung Disorders. 2nd ed. London, Butterworths, 1982. *A detailed and very well-referenced textbook by a single author.*
Rom WN (ed.): Environmental and Occupational Medicine. Boston, Little, Brown & Company, 1983. *A comprehensive review of occupational medicine with excellent introductory chapters covering issues of assessment and control of workplace hazards and broad coverage of individual exposures and diseases.*

AIRWAY DISORDERS

Occupational Asthma

Occupational asthma is defined as asthma that occurs in a previously healthy individual as a result of occupational exposure.

TABLE 527–1. COMMON CAUSES OF OCCUPATIONAL ASTHMA

Agents	Occupational Exposure
Low Molecular Weight Chemicals	
Isocyanates	Plastics, varnishing, spray painting, foundries
Anhydrides: phthalic, trimellitic, tetrachlorophthalic	Plastics, epoxy resins
Soldering fluxes	Electronics, aluminum plants
Metal salts: platinum, chromium, nickel	Metal plating, refining, tanning
Wood dusts: red cedar, redwood, zebrawood	Sawmills, carpentry
Complex Organic Materials	
Plant dusts: grain, coffee bean, castor bean	Grain handlers, bakers, agricultural workers
Laboratory animals	Laboratory workers, animal handlers
Shellfish: crab, prawn, oyster	Shellfish processors
Biologic enzymes	Detergents, pharmaceuticals, chemical industry

This is usually distinguished from an exacerbation of pre-existing asthma on the basis of pre-employment history. Work-induced exacerbations of pre-existing asthma are also an important cause of morbidity and may qualify the affected worker for worker's compensation. Asthma is a common disease (affecting 3 to 6 per cent of the U.S. population), but most patients with mild disease can function normally under most circumstances (Ch. 57). Thus, virtually every occupation includes a significant number of workers with asthma. Patients with asthma are extremely sensitive to bronchoconstrictor stimuli and may develop symptomatic attacks from exposure to occupational irritants (e.g., low concentrations of sulfur dioxide gas) that have no effect on their nonasthmatic coworkers. In this circumstance, although the worker's asthma may have antedated occupational exposure, management would be the same as for patients with true occupational asthma, including application for compensation and job retraining if these are required to avoid further exposure.

CAUSATIVE AGENTS. Well over 100 causative agents are now recognized, and the list continues to grow (Table 527–1). This list can be roughly divided into highly reactive low molecular weight chemicals (such as toluene di-isocyanate and trimellitic anhydride) that share the ability to cause acute airway injury and complex organic materials such as animal dander and grain dust. Since asthma is common and usually of unknown cause, the occupational etiology of asthma is often missed. In addition, thousands of new chemicals are introduced into the workplace each year, but it takes many years for any association between exposure to a chemical and induction of asthma to be recognized. Finally, many workers are simultaneously exposed to dozens or even hundreds of different chemicals, so determining the single one responsible for causing asthma is often difficult. For all these reasons, a diagnosis of occupational asthma must often be considered on the basis of clinical characteristics even if a worker is not exposed to any agent already known to cause asthma. On the other hand, if it can be determined that a worker with asthma of recent onset *is* exposed to an agent known to commonly cause asthma (for instance, toluene di-isocyanate, grain dust, and western red cedar dust cause asthma in approximately 5 per cent of exposed workers), this information should increase the suspicion that the worker's asthma is occupationally induced.

PATHOPHYSIOLOGY. Organic materials such as animal excreta, green coffee beans, and shellfish extracts probably serve as antigens and cause asthma primarily as a result of repeated immediate hypersensitivity responses in the airways. Some of these agents (e.g., animal excreta) are most likely to affect individuals with a previously demonstrated predisposition to atopy. Most of the low molecular weight chemicals that cause asthma are too small to serve as antigens by themselves. These chemicals could trigger immediate hypersensitivity responses by combining with tissue proteins or by altering tissue proteins to create new antigenic determinants. Some of these agents (e.g., toluene di-isocyanate) can cause acute airway injury and inflammation in the absence of immune sensitization. Asthma appears to be more common in workers exposed to repeated accidental spills, suggesting that this acute airway injury may contribute to the development of asthma.

CLINICAL MANIFESTATIONS. *Cough* is the most common initial manifestation of occupational asthma. This is often preceded by symptoms of *rhinitis*, which is associated with asthma in up to 70 per cent of affected workers. Intermittent *chest tightness, dyspnea,* and *wheezing* may be present initially or develop weeks to months after the onset of cough and rhinitis. Initially, these symptoms occur with a distinctive temporal relationship to work exposure. The three most common temporal patterns are an immediate response characterized by short-lived symptoms occurring at the time of work exposure, a late response characterized by symptoms that begin 4 to 12 hours after exposure, and a dual response that combines elements of the first two (Fig. 527–1). Unfortunately, the immediate response—the pattern most commonly recognized as due to work exposure—is the least common. Furthermore, workers who experience dual responses are much more likely to notice the late response than the immediate one, because the late response is usually longer in duration and more difficult to treat. Thus, a typical history of occupational asthma would include symptoms that are most prominent in the evening or at night. Initially, improvement in these symptoms during weekends and vacations is the most important clue to their occupational origin. Eventually, however, as the worker's asthma becomes more severe, any temporal relationship with work may disappear, and an affected worker may complain of persistent asthma indistinguishable from asthma of any other etiology.

Symptoms of occupational asthma can develop at any time after the onset of employment but usually appear after months to years of exposure to the responsible agent. When the diagnosis is suspected soon after the onset of symptoms and further exposure to the responsible agent is prevented, most affected workers gradually improve. Workers who are diagnosed after several years of symptomatic asthma, however, or who continue to be exposed after the diagnosis has been established can develop

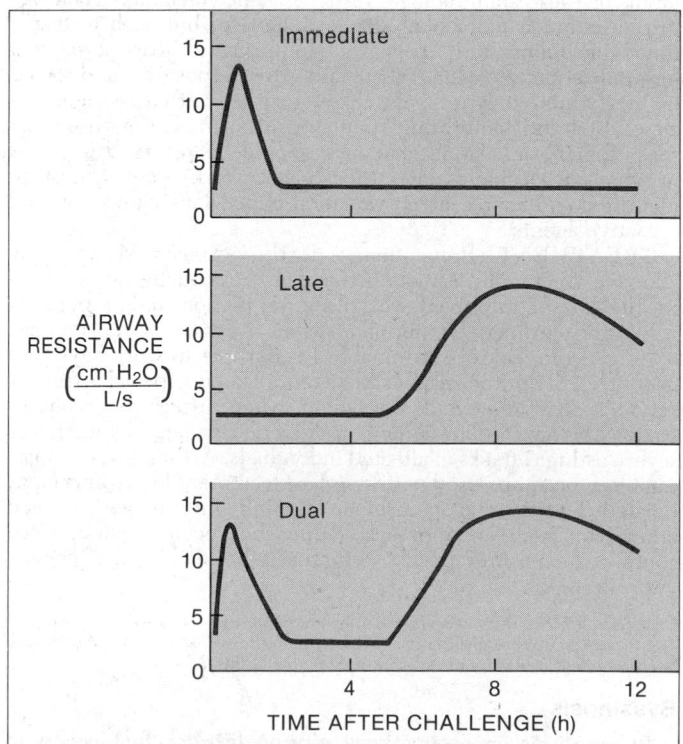

FIGURE 527–1. Temporal patterns of bronchoconstriction (as indicated by increases in airway resistance) after exposure to agents responsible for causing occupational asthma. Delayed responses that can begin from 4 to 12 hours after exposure tend to be more prolonged than immediate responses and thus often cause more prominent symptoms. (Reprinted by permission of the Western Journal of Medicine, from Sheppard D: Occupational asthma. West J Med 137:480, 1982.)

asthma that may persist for years (and perhaps indefinitely) even if further exposure ceases.

DIAGNOSIS. As noted above, a history of new-onset rhinitis, cough, chest tightness, dyspnea, and/or wheezing in a previously healthy worker is essential. Screening pulmonary function test results are usually normal between symptomatic episodes but may reveal reversible (or fixed) airway obstruction. Measurement of spirometry (forced expiratory volume in 1 second [FEV_1] and forced vital capacity [FVC]) before and after a work shift may reveal a more than 10 per cent decrease, but this test is insensitive because of inconsistent exposures over a single work shift and varied temporal patterns of response. If the worker is still actively employed, repeated measurements of peak expiratory flow can be performed and symptoms recorded at 2-hour intervals over a 2-week period that should ideally include at least two weekends. This method is sensitive to intermittent airway obstruction and provides information on the temporal relationship between obstruction and exposure. A 20 per cent difference between the best and worst values of peak flow during any 24-hour period is abnormal. If symptoms are recorded but peak flow does not vary, an explanation for the symptoms other than asthma should be sought.

A single measurement of nonspecific airway responsiveness (e.g., by methacholine or histamine challenge) can confirm a diagnosis of asthma but does not provide information about the occupational etiology. Furthermore, nonspecific airway responsiveness can be normal in workers with occupational asthma, especially during periods of minimal exposure to the responsible agent. Demonstration of a dramatic *increase* in airway responsiveness in association with work exposure does provide strong supportive evidence of an occupational etiology.

Skin testing and/or measurement of specific immunoglobulin E (IgE) antibody can be useful for selected causes of occupational asthma. These include animal exposures, green coffee beans, platinum salts, and trimellitic anhydride. For most causes of occupational asthma, however, the responsible antigens have not been sufficiently well characterized to allow definitive interpretation of these immunologic tests. Specific inhalation challenge testing is much more likely to be definitive, but such testing is time consuming and expensive, requiring at least 2 days of hospitalization to evaluate sham and actual exposures, and should be performed only in specialized centers with experience in generating and monitoring simulated exposures. For these reasons, specific inhalation challenge should be reserved for cases in which a specific agent rather than a work process must be identified and for research evaluation of previously unrecognized causative agents.

TREATMENT. Prevention of further exposure is the only effective treatment. Although this can occasionally be achieved by the use of improved workplace ventilation and/or personal respiratory protective equipment when exposure is intermittent, often affected workers are unable to continue to work anywhere in the vicinity of the responsible agent. This is especially true for vapors such as toluene di-isocyanate, where exposure to concentrations below the lower limit of detection (<1 ppb) can trigger severe asthma attacks in affected individuals. Asthmatic symptoms can often be suppressed with standard treatment for asthma (e.g., inhaled β-adrenergic agonists and theophylline) or with inhaled cromolyn. Such an approach cannot be recommended, since continued exposure appears to increase the likelihood of persistent asthma.

Chan Yeung M: A clinician's approach to determine the diagnosis, prognosis, and therapy of occupational asthma. Med Clin North Am 74:811, 1990. *A practical, up-to-date review by the leading investigator in this field.*

Byssinosis

Byssinosis is an occupational airway disorder that occurs in workers exposed to dust generated during the handling of crude cotton, hemp, or flax. This disorder differs from other forms of occupational asthma in that symptoms of chest tightness and dyspnea are most prominent during the initial work shift following a weekend or vacation and tend to diminish over the course of each work week. Although the dust component responsible for these symptoms has not been definitively identified, contaminants

such as bacterial endotoxins may play a prominent role. Steam cleaning crude cotton before it is carded and engineering controls to reduce airborne dust concentrations can both markedly reduce the incidence of acute symptoms. Long-term chronic exposure to cotton dust also appears to cause productive cough and accelerated loss of lung function in some workers.

Holt PG: Current trends in research on the etiology and pathogenesis of byssinosis. Am J Ind Med 12:711, 1987.
Mundie TG, Ainsworth SK: Etiopathogenic mechanisms of bronchoconstriction in byssinosis: A review. Am Rev Respir Dis 133:1181, 1986.

Industrial Bronchitis

Workers in a number of dusty industries have an increased prevalence of chronic daily productive cough. This effect of occupational dust exposure has been most clearly demonstrated in workers exposed to coal, grain, and cotton dusts. A similar increased prevalence of productive cough has been reported in workers chronically exposed to high concentrations of sulfur dioxide gas in smelters and paper pulp mills and in welders who are chronically exposed to a variety of irritant gases. The high prevalence of cigarette smoking among industrial workers and the potent effect of smoking in causing bronchitis often make establishing an occupational cause of bronchitis difficult. Each of the exposures noted above has been reported to cause bronchitis even in nonsmokers. In the absence of smoking, lung function is usually normal in workers with industrial bronchitis. Nonetheless, the prospective demonstration of accelerated loss of lung function in grain workers and data demonstrating a high prevalence of airway obstruction in cotton workers suggest that these exposures can cause chronic airflow limitation.

PARENCHYMAL LUNG DISORDERS

Disorders Caused by Inorganic Dusts

SILICOSIS

DEFINITION. Silicosis is the parenchymal lung disease caused by inhalation of particles of crystalline silicon dioxide (SiO_2). Free silicon dioxide is usually encountered in nature as quartz. Other crystalline forms, cristobalite and tridymite, are most often encountered in industry as by-products produced when amorphous silicates are heated to high temperature. More complex silicates such as asbestos, talc, and kaolin, cause clinically distinct pulmonary responses and will be discussed separately.

OCCUPATIONAL EXPOSURE. Silicon dioxide is widely deposited through the rock that makes up the earth's surface. Industrial activities that involve cutting, polishing, or shearing rock are thus all potential sources of respirable silica. These include mining, tunneling, quarrying, and stone cutting. Industrial uses of sand, which is largely composed of quartz, can lead to exposure to high concentrations of respirable silica, especially the use of sand for abrasive blasting. Sand is also widely used in foundry work, glass blowing, and pottery making.

PATHOLOGY AND PATHOGENESIS. Three different forms of silicosis are roughly related to the intensity of exposure to respirable silica. *Chronic silicosis* is defined as radiographic abnormalities that are first noted 15 years or more after the onset of exposure. *Accelerated silicosis* resembles the chronic disease but occurs 5 to 15 years after the onset of exposure to high concentrations of silica. *Acute silicosis* occurs within 5 years of the onset of exposure, is virtually always caused by massive exposure, and is clinically and pathologically quite different from the other two forms.

Chronic silicosis is characterized by small nodules that may be diffusely distributed or present primarily in the upper lobes (Fig. 527–2). Nodules are also present in hilar lymph nodes. The nodules have an acellular core composed of concentric swirls of hyalinized collagen and are surrounded by a cellular capsule containing macrophages, plasma cells, and fibroblasts (Fig. 527–3). Silica crystals are often present in these nodules. In a minority of patients, small nodules coalesce to form large masses that can compress and obliterate normal lung structures (so-called progressive massive fibrosis). These nodules occasionally cavitate in the absence of infection, but most often cavities result from infection with *Mycobacterium tuberculosis* and other mycobacteria. The appearance of accelerated silicosis is similar, but conglomerate nodules occur more commonly and giant cells may

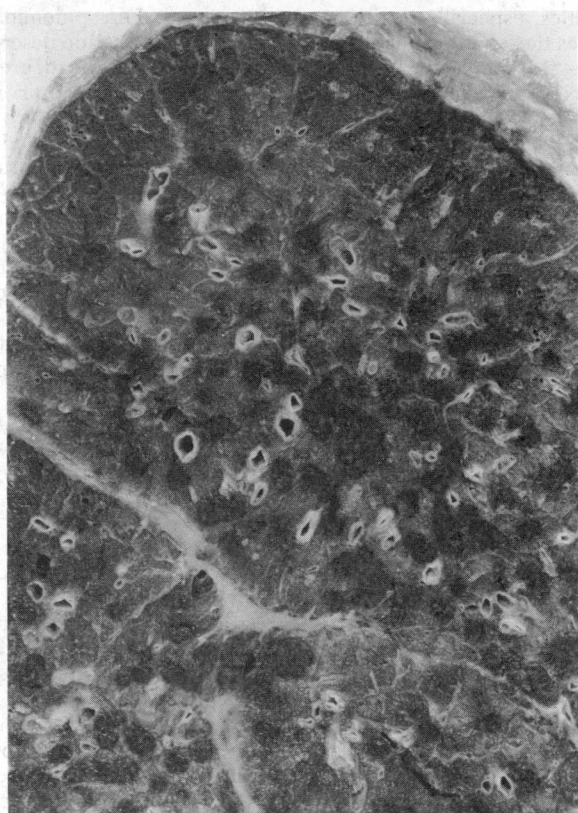

FIGURE 527–2. Close-up of the upper lobe of a slice of lung with marked simple silicosis. The rounded, sharply circumscribed black spots are silicotic nodules. The surrounding parenchyma is normal. (From Warnock ML, Kuwahara TJ, Wolery G: The relation of asbestos burden to asbestosis and lung cancer. Pathol Annu 18:109, 1983 [Part 2], reprinted with permission of Appleton-Century-Crofts, Norwalk, CT.)

be seen. Acute silicosis is characterized by an eosinophilic exudate that fills alveolar spaces and resembles alveolar proteinosis.

Tissue injury from silica is probably initiated by the interaction between silica crystals and alveolar macrophages and appears to involve disruption of phagolysosomes and release of lysosomal contents into the extracellular space. Macrophages stimulated by silica also secrete factors that are chemotactic for other macrophages and neutrophils and that stimulate fibroblasts to proliferate and lay down collagen.

CLINICAL MANIFESTATIONS. Chronic silicosis most commonly causes radiographic abnormalities without symptoms. When symptoms do develop, dyspnea is the most common, but it is usually severe only in patients with progressive massive fibrosis. Cough is commonly seen but is often attributable to chronic bronchitis in cigarette smokers or to superimposed infection. Patients with silicosis have an increased susceptibility to both tuberculous and nontuberculous mycobacterial infections; these should be suspected in affected workers who develop fever, weight loss, asymmetric upper lobe infiltrates, or cavitary lesions. Susceptibility to fungal infections is also increased. Chest pain and clubbing are not features of silicosis.

Chest radiographs usually show multiple small nodules that may be diffusely distributed but are often primarily in the upper lobes and are occasionally calcified. This pattern is called *simple silicosis.* Enlarged hilar lymph nodes may contain outer rims of calcium called *eggshell calcification.* In patients with progressive massive fibrosis, large masses are usually seen in the upper lobes, often symmetrically distributed around the hilar regions in a so-called angel's wing distribution. In these patients, compensatory emphysema is also common. Severe abnormalities in lung function are generally seen only in patients with conglomerate shadows who are said to have *complicated silicosis.* Because the airways and the pulmonary vascular bed are often distorted by these conglomerate masses, pulmonary function tests often reveal airway obstruction and a decrease in pulmonary diffusing capacity as well as the decrease in lung volumes commonly seen in patients with interstitial fibrosis.

Patients with rheumatoid arthritis who develop silicosis can present with multiple large pulmonary nodules that pathologically resemble extrapulmonary rheumatoid nodules. This presentation, called *Caplan's syndrome,* can also occur in workers with asbestosis or in coal workers' pneumoconiosis.

DIAGNOSIS. The diagnosis of silicosis is based on a history of significant occupational exposure to free silica and appropriate radiographic abnormalities. Pulmonary function tests are usually normal in patients with simple silicosis; they are not helpful in establishing the diagnosis. Pulmonary function tests are useful in evaluating and quantifying pulmonary impairment in symptomatic workers. In patients with simple silicosis, severe airflow obstruction is usually due to another coexisting disorder (e.g., bronchitis and/or emphysema) not caused by silica. However, recent evidence suggests that the adverse effects of cigarette smoking on lung function are probably exacerbated by exposure to silica. In accelerated or chronic silicosis, other causes of interstitial fibrosis should be considered in the differential diagnosis. In patients with progressive loss of lung function in whom the diagnosis is uncertain, lung biopsy should be performed to look for other treatable causes. Silica crystals can be seen as birefringent by plane polarizing microscopy, but this feature is not specific for free silica. In patients with mixed dust exposure, energy-dispersive x-ray analysis can identify silicon dioxide and other elements associated with silicates (e.g., calcium, magnesium, iron). Acute silicosis resembles other forms of alveolar proteinosis, but the history of massive silica exposure is usually obvious.

Antinuclear antibodies may be present in up to 40 per cent of patients with silicosis. This test is of no diagnostic value, however, since antibodies are also seen in a high percentage of exposed workers without silicosis. Rapid progression of conglomerate lesions, especially if this is unilateral, suggests coexisting mycobacterial infection or neoplasm and justifies aggressive efforts at diagnosis, as does the appearance of a new cavity. Some epide-

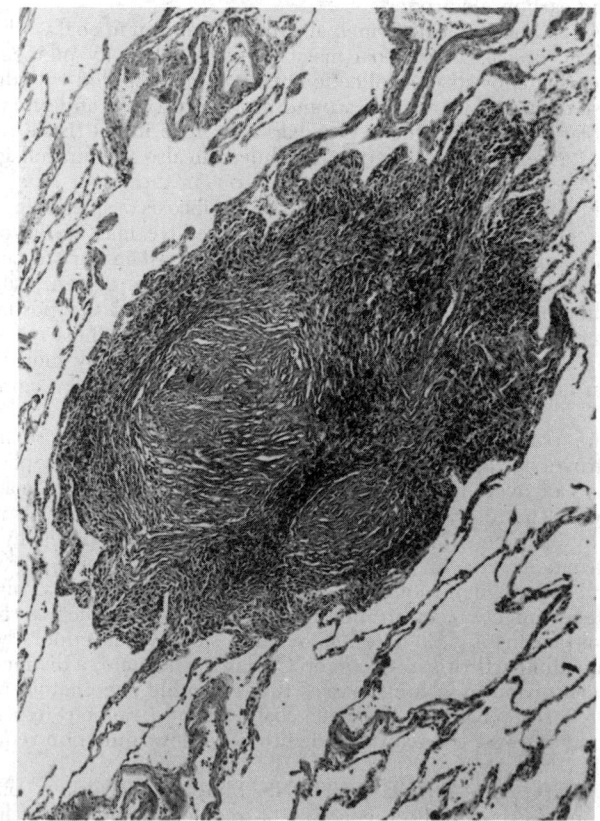

FIGURE 527–3. Light microscopic view of a typical silicotic nodule (original magnification, ×70). Note the whorled fibrous core. The surrounding alveoli are normal. (From Warnock ML, Kuwahara TJ, Wolery G: The relation of asbestos burden to asbestosis and lung cancer. Pathol Annu 18:109, 1983 [Part 2], reprinted with permission of Appleton-Century-Crofts, Norwalk, CT.)

miologic studies suggest that silica exposure increases the risk for pulmonary neoplasms, but most of these studies have involved workers exposed to other potential carcinogens, so the role of silica itself in pulmonary carcinogenesis remains controversial.

TREATMENT. There is no proven effective treatment for any form of silicosis. Patients with acute silicosis should probably be treated with sequential whole lung lavage, as are other patients with alveolar proteinosis. Mycobacterial infections should be treated with standard chemotherapy (Ch. 332). Patients with silicosis and a positive purified protein derivative (PPD) should receive a year of prophylactic therapy with isoniazid (300 mg daily).

The major hope for reducing the prevalence of silicosis lies with prevention. Industrial processes that generate respirable free silica should be enclosed or modified; dust containing silica should never be swept dry, and workers should always use personal respiratory protective devices for unavoidable short-term exposures. In many countries (not including the United States), sand is no longer allowed for use in abrasive blasting because of the large quantities of respirable silica produced. Such a ban should be instituted worldwide, since a number of acceptable replacements are available (e.g., steel grit and coal ash).

Davis GS: Pathogenesis of silicosis: Current concepts and hypothesis. Lung 164:139, 1986.

Silicosis and Silicate Disease Committee. Diseases associated with exposure to silica and nonfibrous silicate minerals. Arch Pathol Lab Med 112:673, 1988. *A recent consensus report focusing on the pathologic effects of silica.*

COAL WORKERS' PNEUMOCONIOSIS

DEFINITION. Coal workers' pneumoconiosis is the parenchymal lung disorder caused by inhalation of coal dust. A similar disorder occurs in workers exposed to graphite or carbon black. Coal dust inhalation also causes chronic bronchitis. These disorders occur primarily in coal miners but can occur in coal trimmers, graphite miners and millers, and workers involved in manufacturing carbon electrodes.

PATHOLOGY. The principal pathologic lesion in coal workers' pneumoconiosis is the coal macule, a small, heavily pigmented lesion that consists of a collection of macrophages filled with dust. These cells are distributed around terminal airways and often fill alveolar spaces, but there is remarkably little initial tissue reaction. Larger macules called coal nodules can also contain collagen. These lesions are usually more numerous in the upper lobes but can be found throughout the lungs. As in silicosis, a small minority of affected workers (~1%) develop progressive massive fibrosis. This complication appears to be related at least in part to heavy dust loads. Pathologically, large rubbery masses are seen, usually in the superior segments of the lower lobes and the posterior segments of the upper lobes. Microscopically, these masses resemble large coal nodules but contain considerably more collagen and are frequently associated with compensatory emphysema.

The pathogenesis of coal workers' pneumoconiosis remains controversial. The coal macules are probably produced by phagocytosis of overwhelming quantities of dust by air space macrophages. The interaction between coal dust and macrophages may not by itself be sufficient to explain the fibrosis and parenchymal destruction seen in patients with progressive massive fibrosis. Tissue injury may require concomitant exposure to silica, mycobacterial infection, or an immunologic abnormality such as rheumatoid arthritis. As noted above for silica, coal miners with rheumatoid arthritis can develop Caplan's syndrome, a distinctive pattern of multiple lung masses that resemble rheumatoid nodules. The mechanisms by which coal dust causes mucus hypersecretion (chronic bronchitis) and chronic airflow limitation require further investigation.

CLINICAL MANIFESTATIONS. Simple coal workers' pneumoconiosis most often consists of radiographic abnormalities without symptoms. Patients with complicated pneumoconiosis (progressive massive fibrosis) can develop progressive dyspnea, pulmonary hypertension, and respiratory failure. The risk of mycobacterial infection may be increased in patients with coal workers' pneumoconiosis, but not to the same extent as in patients with silicosis. Chest radiographs usually show small, irregular opacities, especially in the upper lung zones. For epidemiologic studies these can be quantified by the ILO classification described above. In simple coal workers' pneumoconiosis, the degree of profusion is well correlated with the dust burden, an observation that is not surprising, since radiographic abnormalities are primarily due to retained dust. In complicated pneumoconiosis, radiographs show large conglomerate shadows and compensatory emphysema.

Chronic sputum production and chronic airflow limitation are also complications of coal mining related to the quantity of dust exposure but not to radiographic abnormalities. Abnormalities in airflow tend to be mild in nonsmoking miners in the absence of complicated pneumoconiosis. In an individual coal miner who smokes, it is not possible to determine the relative contributions of coal dust and cigarette smoking to the development of chronic bronchitis and airway obstruction.

Pulmonary function tests in patients with simple coal workers' pneumoconiosis are usually normal. In patients with complicated pneumoconiosis, both airway obstruction (characterized by decreases in the FEV_1 and other tests of maximal flow) and lung restriction (characterized by a decrease in total lung capacity) can occur. In these patients, the diffusing capacity for carbon monoxide is often reduced as a result of obstruction or destruction of the pulmonary vascular bed. Some epidemiologic studies in coal miners have shown an increase in residual volume and a decrease in flow measured at low lung volumes in comparison to matched nonexposed control populations. These findings are consistent with mild airway obstruction caused by coal dust exposure.

DIAGNOSIS. The diagnosis of coal workers' pneumoconiosis is made on the basis of a history of exposure and appropriate radiographic abnormalities. In patients with large conglomerate shadows, mycobacterial infection needs to be excluded. Affected patients do not have an increased risk of lung cancer, but in smokers with unilateral enlarging masses, neoplasm must be excluded. The lesions of simple coal workers' pneumoconiosis do not generally progress or regress after the end of exposure, so a changing radiograph in a retired worker suggests another diagnosis.

TREATMENT AND PREVENTION. There is no effective treatment for coal workers' pneumoconiosis. Impending depletion of the world's oil reserves has stimulated an increased demand for coal, ensuring continued exposure to coal dust for years to come. Prevention of pneumoconiosis requires minimizing the airborne respirable dust concentration at each step in the extraction and processing of coal.

Heppleston AG: Prevalence and pathogenesis of pneumoconiosis in coal workers. Environ Health Perspect 78:159, 1988.

Disorders Caused by Asbestos

Inhaled asbestos is a more potent stimulus to tissue injury than is silica or coal. Furthermore, asbestos causes a broader range of clinical disorders besides pulmonary fibrosis: pleural fibrosis and effusion; mesothelioma of the pleura and peritoneum; and cancer of the lung, larynx, and gastrointestinal tract. The term *asbestosis* is usually reserved for the nonmalignant response of the lung parenchyma to inhaled asbestos fiber (pulmonary fibrosis).

OCCUPATIONAL EXPOSURE. Asbestos is not a single chemical entity, but rather a group of mineral silicates that have in common their fibrous nature and the potential to be woven. Worldwide use of asbestos increased dramatically throughout most of this century before beginning to decline in the late 1970's. Asbestos fibers have been widely used in ship building, construction, insulating, and automotive vehicle clutch and brake manufacturing because they are highly resistant to heat, acid, and chemical degradation. For the same reasons, asbestos has also been used in the manufacture of textiles and building supplies. In the past, the heaviest occupational exposures have occurred in miners, millers, shipyard workers, and insulation workers; but because of the diverse uses of asbestos, cases of asbestos-induced disease are seen among a wide variety of other occupations. As the use of asbestos in new construction has been nearly eliminated in the United States, continued exposure is likely to be due to demolition and renovation of buildings and ships containing asbestos. In developing countries, application of new asbestos continues to be widespread. Since most asbestos-induced diseases have a long latency, the prevalence of asbestos-induced diseases is not likely to fall for many years despite a marked decrease in exposure. Nonoccupational exposure can also cause disease. For instance, cases of mesothelioma and an increased prevalence of pleural thickening have been reported among household contacts of asbestos workers (presumably due to exposure to fibers brought home on work clothes).

PATHOLOGY AND PATHOGENESIS. *Pleural Disease.* Asbestos can cause localized or diffuse areas of acellular pleural fibrosis that are usually bilateral and primarily on the parietal pleura. Asbestos fibers are often found in the adjacent visceral pleura, suggesting that asbestos fibers that migrate out to the visceral pleural surface may injure the adjacent parietal pleura. Asbestos exposure can also cause benign exudative pleural effusions that usually contain a mixed population of inflammatory cells. The exudative lesion is nonspecific.

Pulmonary Fibrosis. Macroscopically, in advanced cases the lungs are small and stiff, and fibrous streaks are most prominent in the lower lobes and in subpleural locations. Honeycombing is occasionally seen (Fig. 527–4). Microscopically, asbestosis is indistinguishable from other causes of pulmonary fibrosis, except for the presence of asbestos fibers. A small percentage of asbestos fibers become coated with hemosiderin and form asbestos bodies that are visible under the light microscope. Identification of the more numerous uncoated fibers requires electron microscopy. The number of asbestos bodies recovered from dried lung correlates well with the total number of fibers (though there are several orders of magnitude more uncoated fibers). However, because asbestos bodies are not uniformly distributed throughout the lungs, examination of standard lung sections by light microscopy may not reveal asbestos bodies even from patients with a heavy asbestos burden and asbestosis. On the other hand, occasional asbestos bodies can be seen in urban dwellers without occupational exposure and are of little significance in the absence of associated pulmonary fibrosis.

In experimental animals exposed to asbestos, the earliest pathologic abnormality is an accumulation of inflammatory cells (especially macrophages) around asbestos fibers in the terminal

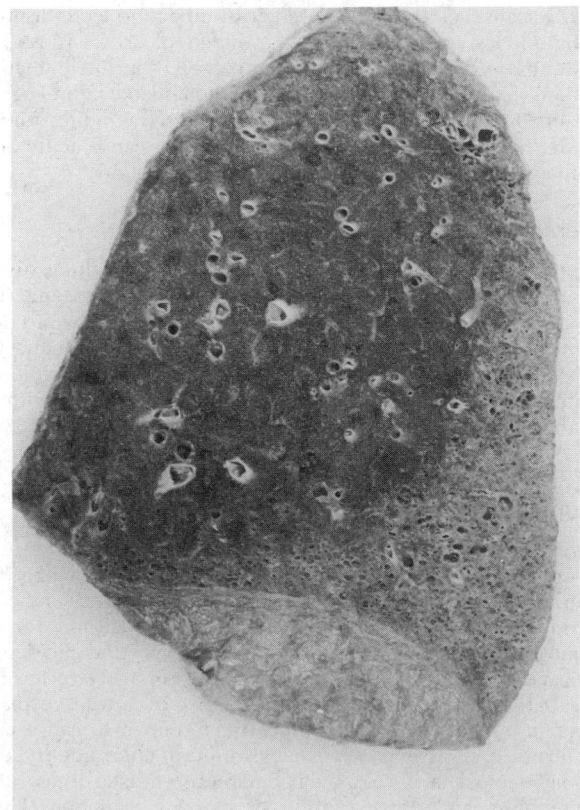

FIGURE 527–4. Slice of lower lobe from a patient with asbestosis. Note the thick pleural opacity at the base and the marked subpleural fibrosis with honeycombing. (From Warnock ML, Kuwahara TJ, Wolery G: The relation of asbestos burden to asbestosis and lung cancer. Pathol Annu 18:109, 1983 [Part 2], reprinted with permission of Appleton-Century-Crofts, Norwalk, CT.)

airways. Similar lesions are also common in asbestos-exposed workers and may explain why exposure to asbestos reduces airflow at low lung volumes.

Malignant pleural mesotheliomas are bulky, slow-growing tumors that spread by local extension to encase the lung and mediastinum. They vary histologically and can be difficult to distinguish from metastatic adenocarcinoma even in large specimens obtained by open pleural biopsy. Lung cancer can be of any cell type. Asbestos exposure and cigarette smoking act synergistically in causing lung cancer, so that heavily exposed smoking workers have a risk of lung cancer 30 to 90 times higher than that of unexposed nonsmokers (Ch. 68).

Asbestos fibers appear to cause tissue injury by stimulating alveolar macrophages to secrete cytotoxic materials, inflammatory cell chemoattractants, and at least one factor that stimulates fibroblast proliferation. Recent evidence suggests that reactive oxygen species are important in asbestos-induced lung injury. Because of their durability, individual fibers can repeatedly stimulate macrophages for many years without being degraded. This helps to explain the continued progression of asbestos-induced disease after exposure ceases and points out why the effective intensity of exposure depends on *time* from first exposure as well as total lung fiber burden. Nonetheless, the enormous variability in disease severity seen among individuals with equivalent exposure histories and lung fiber burdens suggests an important role for as yet uncharacterized host factors. One possibly important cofactor is cigarette smoking, which has been shown to increase the severity of radiographic abnormalities in workers exposed to asbestos.

CLINICAL MANIFESTATIONS. Pleural plaques are the most common manifestation of asbestos exposure. Patients with only pleural involvement are usually asymptomatic and have normal pulmonary function. Occasionally, patients with extensive pleural thickening develop extrapulmonary lung restriction that can cause dyspnea. The major significance of pleural plaques is that their appearance on a chest radiograph confirms a history of exposure. Diaphragmatic plaques are especially likely to calcify, and bilateral diaphragmatic calcification is almost always caused by asbestos exposure. Diffuse unilateral pleural thickening and/or pleuritic chest pain suggests the possibility of mesothelioma.

Asbestosis presents as do other forms of pulmonary fibrosis, with dyspnea that is initially most prominent with exertion and is often associated with cough. Bibasilar rales are a common finding, and clubbing can occur. The chest radiograph reveals linear and irregular opacities that are most prominent in the lower lung fields. Pleural thickening is often present but may not be radiographically apparent. As with other forms of pulmonary fibrosis, up to 10 per cent of patients with asbestos-induced fibrosis severe enough to cause lung restriction have normal chest radiographs. Progressive massive fibrosis is not seen. In patients with pulmonary fibrosis severe enough to cause dyspnea, pulmonary function tests usually show lung restriction (a symmetric reduction in all lung volumes) and a reduction in diffusing capacity. Flow-volume curves show reduced flow at low lung volumes, but marked airway obstruction, as manifested by a marked reduction in per cent of FEV_1, usually has other causes, such as cigarette smoking. In an asbestos-exposed smoker, a decrease in total lung capacity cannot be caused by smoking, but decreases in diffusing capacity and flow at low lung volume could be due to cigarettes, asbestos, or the combined effects of both.

DIAGNOSIS. The diagnosis of asbestos-induced pleural plaques is made on the basis of the typical bilateral appearance and a history of exposure. In approximately 80 per cent of patients with bilateral pleural plaques, asbestos exposure is responsible. Oblique radiographs increase the likelihood of detecting plaques, and CT is more sensitive than standard radiography and allows distinction between true plaques and subpleural fat. Since plaques themselves are rarely clinically significant, the considerable cost of these studies and the additional radiation exposure are difficult to justify, except for research purposes. The diagnosis of asbestos-induced pleural effusion depends on a history of exposure and exclusion of other causes of a pleural exudate.

Asbestosis is usually diagnosed on the basis of significant exposure, radiographic abnormalities, and pulmonary function studies showing lung restriction. Occasionally, in patients with early disease, radiographs or lung function studies may be normal, but exercise testing reveals abnormalities in pulmonary gas exchange. Lung biopsy should be performed only in patients with progressive disease to exclude causes of pulmonary fibrosis that might respond to treatment. If sufficient lung tissue is available (from open lung biopsy or autopsy), asbestos burden should be estimated by counting asbestos bodies from ashed tissue or asbestos fibers by electron probe analysis. In patients with stable lung function, lung biopsy should not be performed merely to establish asbestos exposure as the cause of lung fibrosis, since such a diagnosis does not lead to any specific therapy and all biopsy procedures are associated with some risk.

Asbestosis usually does not develop before 15 years after the first exposure to asbestos and usually requires several years of exposure. However, workers have been reported to develop the disease 15 to 30 years after periods of very heavy exposure as short as 6 months.

A diagnosis of asbestos-induced lung cancer is based on a history of heavy exposure that should ideally be confirmed by quantification of asbestos fiber burden from resected lung or autopsy specimens. Like pulmonary fibrosis, lung cancer does not develop within 15 years of first exposure and has its peak incidence within 25 to 40 years. The distribution of tumor cell types is the same as that seen in the general population. Epidemiologic evidence suggests that an increased incidence of lung cancer requires an intensity of asbestos exposure similar to that required to increase the incidence of pulmonary fibrosis. These data do not imply that both abnormalities would occur in the same individuals. Thus, lung cancer of any cell type in an individual with a well-documented history of heavy exposure can be reasonably considered to be due, at least in part, to asbestos exposure irrespective of coexistent pulmonary fibrosis.

TREATMENT AND PREVENTION. There is no proven effective treatment for asbestosis. The major strategy for prevention is worldwide elimination of new asbestos use and replacement with synthetic substitutes that appear to be considerably less toxic. Continuing exposure to asbestos currently in use needs to be minimized by use of engineering controls, personal protection, and public education. For prevention of lung cancer, individuals with past exposure should be strongly encouraged to stop smoking, since the risk of lung cancer falls dramatically (but is not eliminated) within a few years of smoking cessation.

American Thoracic Society, Medical Section of the American Lung Association: The diagnosis of nonmalignant diseases related to asbestos. Am Rev Respir Dis 143:363, 1990. *A concise review of the recommendations from a committee of experts in the evaluation of asbestos-related diseases.*

Becklake MR: Pneumoconiosis. *In* Murray JF, Nadel JA (ed.): Textbook of Respiratory Medicine. Philadelphia, W.B. Saunders Company, 1988, pp 1556–1592. *An excellent, comprehensive review of asbestos-induced diseases and other disorders induced by inorganic dusts.*

Beryllium Disease

Beryllium is a rare metal that can cause both acute and chronic disease. Acute beryllium disease results from intense exposure and resembles acute lung injury from other massive toxic exposures. Clinical manifestations include upper airway injury, bronchiolitis, and pulmonary edema. Mortality has been reported to be as high as 10 per cent. Chronic beryllium disease can follow acute disease but more often occurs without antecedent symptoms from months to years after first exposure. Because beryllium salts are absorbed through the respiratory tract and distributed throughout the body, exposure causes a systemic disease. Pathologically, chronic beryllium disease is characterized by noncaseating granulomas in lung, lymph nodes, liver, spleen, adrenal glands, and kidneys. Granulomas in the skin are thought to be due to direct exposure.

Before 1949, most cases of beryllium disease were due to the use of beryllium in fluorescent lights. Since such use was discontinued, most cases have occurred in the manufacturing of metal alloys and x-ray tubes and in the mining and milling of beryllium. The number of new cases has progressively fallen as industrial hygiene measures have been improved in these industries, but occasional cases continue to occur.

The diagnosis of chronic beryllium disease is made on the basis of a history of exposure and demonstration of granulomas on tissue biopsy. The lung pathology is nonspecific and indistinguishable from sarcoid and hypersensitivity pneumonitis (Ch. 67). Involvement of the uvea, salivary glands, or central nervous system and the presence of erythema nodosum favor sarcoid. Demonstration of beryllium in urine confirms exposure but does not correlate with disease. The disease is thought to be due to a cell-mediated immune response directed at beryllium-protein complexes. Lymphocyte transformation in response to beryllium has been demonstrated in vitro from peripheral blood lymphocytes and lung lymphocytes obtained by bronchoalveolar lavage from some patients with chronic beryllium disease. Transformation of blood lymphocytes is relatively insensitive, however, and can also be seen in exposed workers with no evidence of disease. The clinical course of chronic beryllium disease is quite variable. Most patients remain stable if exposure ceases, but the disease can remit or progress in some individuals. Treatment with corticosteroids has been recommended but has not been systematically studied.

Kriebel D, Brain JD, Sprince NL, et al.: The pulmonary toxicity of beryllium. Am Rev Respir Dis 137:464, 1988.

Newman LS, Kreiss K, King TE Jr, et al.: Pathologic and immunologic alterations in early stages of beryllium disease. Am Rev Respir Dis 139:1479, 1988.

Diseases Caused by Other Inorganic Dusts

Silicates other than asbestos can also cause pneumoconiosis. Kaolin, mica, and vermiculite, for example, cause radiographic abnormalities and pathologic lesions similar to those caused by coal dust. Talc inhalation causes pulmonary fibrosis with features of both asbestosis and silicosis, as well as foreign body granulomas. Pleural plaques have also been noted in workers exposed to talc, but they may be due to contamination of talc with asbestos. A severe granulomatous lung disease, sometimes associated with pulmonary hypertension, can occur in intravenous drug addicts from intravenous injection of talc. Synthetic vitreous fibers, such as fiberglass and glass wool, are physically similar to asbestos, but evidence to date suggests that they are considerably less toxic. Because of the long latency of fiber-induced disorders, continued close surveillance of the effects of use of these fibers is essential. As new technologies evolve, it is likely that new reactions to inorganic dusts will be recognized. For example, exposure to the dust of a variety of metals (including tungsten carbide, cobalt, titanium, and tantalum) may cause acute and/or chronic injury to the airways and lung parenchyma.

Hypersensitivity Pneumonitis

Hypersensitivity pneumonitis is a parenchymal lung disorder that usually results from occupational exposure to organic dusts. The disease is characterized clinically by recurrent episodes of cough, dyspnea, and signs of systemic illness (fever, leukocytosis, and myalgias). After long-term exposure to the responsible dust, affected workers can develop pulmonary fibrosis often with noncaseating granulomas in lung tissue. This disorder is discussed in detail in Ch. 59.

Occupational Lung Cancer

As the site of entry of most airborne carcinogens, the lung is the organ most often affected by occupational carcinogenesis. Definitive identification of an occupational agent as a lung carcinogen is made difficult by the long latency period for most carcinogens (20 to 40 years), the high background incidence of lung cancer, and the potent confounding effect of cigarette smoke. Thus, of the more than 100 agents suspected of causing respiratory cancer in animals, only a few have been shown to cause cancer in humans, e.g., arsenic, asbestos, cadmium, chloromethyl ether, chromates, coal tars, coke-oven emissions, mustard gas, nickel, and uranium and other sources of ionizing radiation. Chloromethyl ether appears to be especially likely to cause oat cell carcinoma, but most occupational carcinogens increase the risk for lung cancer of all common cell types. Prevention of occupational lung cancer requires minimizing exposure to suspected carcinogens *before* they are definitively shown to cause cancer in exposed workers.

528 Physical, Chemical, and Aspiration Injuries of the Lung

Claude A. Piantadosi

PHYSICAL AND CHEMICAL INJURIES OF THE LUNG

The lung has a large and delicate surface area that is protected from toxic substances in the environment by extensive defense mechanisms. Under normal conditions, inspired gas is fully humidified and warmed to body temperature, and all large particulate substances are cleared by the upper airways. These normal defenses are not adequate to handle exposure to many physical and chemical substances that cause lung injury. This chapter discusses lung disorders initiated by inhalation or aspiration of injurious chemicals or by exposure to potentially harmful physical environments.

Thermal Injuries and Smoke Inhalation

Approximately 130,000 patients per year require hospitalization in the United States for thermal injuries. After major burns, about one third of patients have pulmonary complications; these complications account for the majority of burn-related deaths. Thermal injury to the lung is associated with three groups of complications: (1) *immediate reaction*—direct thermal injury to upper airways, leading to upper airway obstruction, carbon monoxide poisoning, and smoke inhalation (potent bronchoconstrictors and edematogenic substances); (2) *adult respiratory distress syndrome* (ARDS) developing 24 to 48 hours after the thermal injury; and (3) *late-onset pulmonary complications*, which include pneumonia, atelectasis, thromboembolism, and chest wall restriction caused by circumferential thoracic burns.

The constituents of smoke are by-products of pyrolysis and incomplete combustion. Many of these products are potent mucosal irritants and bronchoconstrictors and contribute to both upper and lower lung lesions. Certain constituents of smoke have been identified consistently as contributors to respiratory injury. These are listed in Table 528–1. Smoke inhalation rarely causes thermal injury to the lung parenchyma; the large capacity of the upper airways to humidify and modify the temperatures of inhaled air protects the alveolar tissue from heat. Exceptions are steam burns and explosions in an enclosed space.

CLINICAL MANIFESTATIONS. The initial signs and symptoms of smoke inhalation are tachypnea, cough, dyspnea, wheezing, cyanosis, hoarseness, and stridor (an ominous sign). Facial burns may provide a clue to smoke inhalation and thermal injury to the upper airway. During the 12 to 48 hours immediately after the injury, the patient can manifest increasing hypoxemia, and lung compliance may decrease owing to noncardiogenic pulmonary edema. Roentgenograms of the chest may reveal a pattern of diffuse, patchy infiltrates. A major complication is infection, often caused by *Pseudomonas aeruginosa* or *Staphylococcus aureus*. The lung defenses against infection are compromised by thermal and chemical injury to the airway epithelium as well as by the presence of an endotracheal or tracheostomy tube. The pathway for infection is either by inhalation of airborne organisms or by hematogenous spread from cutaneous burns.

The ARDS may develop 24 to 48 hours after the initial injury. The causes of ARDS are controversial in burn patients, but possibilities include a chemical pneumonitis from constituents in smoke, a circulating burn toxin, disseminated intravascular coagulation, microembolism, and neurogenic pulmonary edema. The extent of surface thermal injury does not correlate with the degree of respiratory distress that occurs subsequently.

TREATMENT. The most immediate life-threatening complications in the patient presenting with major burns or with a history of smoke inhalation are upper airway obstruction and carbon monoxide intoxication. The patient should be closely observed for evidence of these complications. Laryngeal and tracheobronchial inflammation may be detected by fiberoptic bronchoscopy. Arterial blood gases should be measured and prompt intubation or tracheostomy performed if there is evidence of significant airway obstruction. Corticosteroids may be helpful to treat edema of the upper airways but must be used with caution, since infection is a major concern for managing both skin and pulmonary injury. Prophylactic antibiotics are of no value in preventing pneumonia and may predispose to infection with resistant organisms. Careful pulmonary toilet, humidification, and sterile suctioning should be used to reduce the risk of pneumonia. Serial bronchoscopy may be necessary to remove mucous plugs and thereby prevent segmental atelectasis and postobstructive infection.

Late-onset pulmonary burn complications—atelectasis, thromboembolism, and pneumonia—are discussed in Ch. 59, 65, and 292 to 295, respectively.

Haponik EF, Summer WR: Respiratory complications in burned patients: Pathogenesis and spectrum of inhalation injury. J Crit Care 2:49, 1987.
Haponik EF, Summer WR: Respiratory complications in burned patients: Diagnosis and management of inhalation injury. J Crit Care 2:121, 1987.

Carbon Monoxide Poisoning

Smoke inhalation is invariably accompanied by the uptake of carbon monoxide (CO) by the body. In some fires, CO exposure is complicated by cyanide poisoning from the combustion of plastic compounds. Carbon monoxide poisoning also is encountered frequently after exposure to automobile exhaust, and in the winter when victims are exposed to fumes from faulty furnaces. As a result, CO is the leading cause of accidental poisoning in the United States.

Carbon monoxide toxicity is a consequence of tissue hypoxia created by the displacement of oxygen from hemoglobin. Carbon monoxide competes with oxygen for binding at the iron-porphyrin centers of hemoglobin. These centers bind CO reversibly, but with an affinity more than 200 times greater than that for oxygen. The oxygen affinity of centers not occupied by CO is also increased in the presence of carboxyhemoglobin (HbCO). This HbCO-related increase in oxygen affinity shifts the oxyhemoglobin dissociation curve to the left and impairs the release of oxygen to the tissues. These two effects of CO on hemoglobin decrease the partial pressure of oxygen in the tissues. Tissue hypoxia has serious functional consequences for organ systems that require a continuous supply of oxygen, such as the brain and the heart. In addition, when tissue P_{O_2} is low, CO may bind more readily to intracellular hemoproteins such as myoglobin and cytochrome *c* oxidase, potentially inhibiting their functions.

CLINICAL MANIFESTATIONS. The clinical features of acute CO poisoning are diverse but most often related to the central nervous system. In normal, nonsmoking individuals, symptoms may appear when HbCO levels reach 10 per cent. Patients with chronic obstructive pulmonary disease (COPD) and coronary artery disease are more sensitive to the effects of HbCO. Smokers often maintain HbCO levels of 3 to 10 per cent, and they may tolerate slightly higher levels without symptoms. Common symptoms of CO poisoning include headache, nausea, vomiting, confusion, and visual disturbances. More severe CO poisoning can produce seizures, transient unconsciousness, coma, and death. Metabolic acidosis, pulmonary edema, and rhabdomyolysis may also accompany serious CO poisoning. The "classic" clinical findings of cherry red lips and nail beds are rare. The differential diagnosis includes drug overdoses, other poisonings (e.g. cyanide), and cerebrovascular accidents. The clinical diagnosis is confirmed by an elevated blood HbCO level measured by CO-oximetry. The severity of the clinical illness, however, may not correlate well with the HbCO level but may relate instead to the duration and extent of the exposure.

TABLE 528–1. TOXIC BY-PRODUCTS OF SMOKE IMPLICATED IN RESPIRATORY INJURY

Source	By-products
Cotton, paper, wood	Acrolein, CO, acetaldehyde
Petroleum products	Acrolein, CO, benzene
Polyvinyl chloride (PVC)	Hydrocyanic acid, CO, chlorine, phosgene
Nylon, silk, wool	Hydrocyanic acid, ammonia
Nitrocellulose	Oxides of nitrogen
Sulfur compounds	Sulfur dioxide

TREATMENT AND OUTCOME. Symptoms of mild CO poisoning generally subside within minutes to a few hours after removing the patient from the noxious environment. Patients with more severe forms of CO intoxication benefit from high inspired concentrations of oxygen to hasten the removal of CO from hemoglobin. In obtunded or comatose patients, 100 per cent oxygen should be administered via an endotracheal tube until the HbCO level is less than 5 per cent. Pure oxygen reduces the halftime for HbCO elimination from the body from approximately 240 minutes to 60 minutes. Patients with loss of consciousness or other neurologic impairment, cardiac symptoms or signs, or HbCO levels above 25 per cent should receive hyperbaric oxygen if it is readily available. Hyperbaric oxygen at 2.5 atmospheres absolute (ATA) reduces the HbCO halftime to approximately 30 minutes. Oxygen dissolved in plasma under hyperbaric pressure also bypasses the impairment of oxygen transport to tissues imposed by HbCO. As a result, potentially serious neurologic sequelae may be averted if the therapy can be instituted promptly. Adjunctive therapy, such as corticosteroids, hyperventilation, mannitol, and hypothermia, has been recommended for treatment of serious cases of CO intoxication, but benefit from these modalities is unproved.

Neurologic recovery in patients with mild to moderate CO poisoning is good. The prognosis after severe CO intoxication is variable and correlates with the extent and duration of the insult. Short-term memory impairment, depression, and syndromes related to lesions of the basal ganglia are well described. A syndrome of delayed neurologic deterioration occurs in approximately 3 per cent of victims of serious CO intoxication. Risk factors for the delayed syndrome include age over 40, prolonged exposure, and abnormalities of the brain on computed tomography (CT). Hyperbaric oxygen therapy has been reported to decrease the incidence of the delayed syndrome.

Piantadosi CA: Carbon monoxide intoxication. *In* Vincent JL (ed.): Update in Intensive Care and Emergency Medicine. Vol. 10. New York, Springer-Verlag, 1990, pp 460–471.

Other Toxic Inhaled Gases

A large number of gases and chemicals, to which exposures most frequently occur in an industrial setting, can cause acute and sometimes chronic injury to the respiratory system. A few agents cause an "asthma-like" reaction with cough, chest pain, and wheezing. Toluene di-isocyanate and other isocyanates (liberated as a gas during the manufacture of polyurethane foams), aluminum soldering flux, and platinum salts are typical examples. Reaginic and precipitating antibodies against platinum salts and soldering flux have been found in symptomatic individuals, suggesting an immunologic basis for the reaction. An allergic basis has not been demonstrated for the reaction to toluene di-isocyanate. The symptoms usually subside after removal from exposure; however, chronic lung injury may occur if the exposure is prolonged.

A number of highly irritating gases cause an *acute chemical pneumonitis*. Such gases include chlorine (used in the chemical and plastic industries and to disinfect water), ammonia (used in refrigeration), sulfur dioxide (used in paper manufacture and smelting of sulfide-containing ores), ozone (generated in welding and in photochemical smog), nitrogen dioxide (released from decomposed corn silage), and phosgene (used in production of aniline dyes).

An important injury of this type is *silo-filler's disease* (nitrogen dioxide). During the initial exposure, there may be no symptoms, there may be tracheobronchitis with cough and shortness of breath, or there may be the immediate onset of acute pulmonary edema. Signs of ocular and oropharyngeal mucous membrane irritation may be present. The symptoms can rapidly progress, but commonly the initial symptoms resolve and are followed by a period of minimal symptoms (cough) lasting up to 48 hours. Fever, myalgias, dyspnea, and progressive hypoxemia then occur, and the radiographic picture is that of pulmonary edema. These severe symptoms can resolve, only to recur 2 to 5 weeks later and lead to progressive pulmonary insufficiency with a picture of bronchiolitis obliterans. Treatment with corticosteroids (prednisone, 1 mg per kilogram per day) can dramatically improve the

acute illness. Bronchodilators, mechanical ventilation, and supplemental oxygen may be necessary. Since improvement after the initial exposure may be temporary, observation for a period of 48 hours is advisable.

The clinical response caused by each irritant gas varies but appears to be closely related to the degree of acute irritation it causes and to its water solubility. The less irritating gases, such as ozone and the oxides of nitrogen, phosgene, mercury, and nickel carbonyl, can be inhaled for prolonged periods and thereby cause injury throughout the respiratory system. Highly irritating and soluble gases, such as ammonia and hydrochloric acid, are less likely to be inhaled deeply and tend to result in immediate injury to the upper airways and have potential for obstruction secondary to mucosal edema. Less soluble substances, such as chlorine, cadmium, zinc chloride, osmium tetroxide, and vanadium, can cause injury to the entire tracheobronchial tree and generally do not produce upper airway obstruction as the initial presentation. Bronchiolitis and pulmonary edema are common, ultimately leading to bronchiolitis obliterans. Long-term consequences vary with the gas. Cadmium, for example, can cause diffuse emphysema and severe airway obstruction but only minimal fibrosis.

Different mechanisms are involved in the injury caused by irritant gases. Most of them cause injury by acting as a strong acid, a strong base, or an oxidant. Gases of chemicals that are strong acids or bases in water solution, such as hydrogen chloride, sulfuric acid, sulfur dioxide, and ammonia, tend to react more in the upper airways, where they change tissue pH and thereby cause cell damage.

Evans MJ: Oxidant gases. Environ Health Perspect 55:85, 1984. *A review of the effects of ozone, nitrogen dioxide, and oxygen on lung structures and the factors that can modulate the degree of damage.*

Pulmonary Oxygen Toxicity

Oxygen is toxic to the lungs when used in high concentrations for prolonged periods. This toxicity occurs clinically in patients in intensive care units who are on mechanical ventilators. The toxic effects of hyperoxia are believed to result from excessive generation of superoxide, an unstable free radical produced by the single electron reduction of oxygen. Superoxide is produced as a normal by-product of oxidative metabolism and scavenged by a protective enzyme, superoxide dismutase, that catalyzes its dismutation to hydrogen peroxide. If not scavenged by superoxide dismutase, this free radical can react with hydrogen peroxide to form hydroxyl radical (OH•), and free radical chain reactions can be initiated, resulting in the destruction of cell lipids and proteins (Fig. 528–1).

In the adult, the major site of oxygen injury is the pulmonary capillary endothelium. Pathologically, the lungs are atelectatic, congested, and edematous and have hyaline membranes. The most serious injury appears to be destruction of the capillary bed with resultant interstitial and alveolar edema, hypoxemia, and sometimes death. Alveolar epithelium is also injured, causing hyperplasia of type II cells. An acute tracheobronchitis also occurs, and histologic changes have been found in the ciliated epithelium and Clara cells in the small airways.

CLINICAL MANIFESTATIONS. Oxygen toxicity usually occurs in acutely ill patients who are receiving oxygen in high concentrations and mechanical ventilation for lung injuries that obscure the onset of pulmonary toxicity. Lung compliance progressively falls; the alveolar-arterial oxygen gradient gradually widens, and increasing concentrations of oxygen are needed to maintain adequate oxygenation of arterial blood. This cycle progresses to pulmonary edema, respiratory failure, and death.

The earliest symptoms of oxygen toxicity are those of acute tracheobronchitis. A dry, hacking cough and substernal pain may occur after 6 to 12 hours of breathing pure oxygen. Vital capacity decreases, and respiratory rate increases. The flow of tracheal mucus decreases after short exposures to excess oxygen, probably reflecting functional injury of airway epithelium. These patients are therefore more susceptible to mucus impaction and to infection caused by failure to clear inhaled pathogens adequately.

TREATMENT AND OUTCOME. The only proven therapy is prevention of the insult by judicious use of high oxygen concentrations. The physician often faces a dilemma in which increasing concentrations of oxygen are essential for immediate survival but eventually contribute to the demise of the patient. Alternative methods to enhance tissue oxygen delivery without using high inspired partial pressures of oxygen should be used whenever possible. These include positive end-expiratory pressure (PEEP), transfusion of packed red cells to raise the hematocrit to nearly normal levels, maintenance of cardiac output, and measures to decrease the tissue oxygen demand by reducing fever or agitation.

The safe maximal concentration of oxygen is not known. Many authors recommend 40 to 50 per cent oxygen as a safe limit because little injury has been demonstrated in normal animals or human volunteers breathing such concentrations for prolonged periods. The diseased lung, however, may be more susceptible to oxygen injury. A rational therapy is to use only enough oxygen to provide adequate arterial blood saturation, e.g., an Sa_{O_2} of 90 per cent. Corticosteroids have no benefit and may actually enhance the lung injury caused by hyperoxia. If the patient survives oxygen toxicity, some residual damage to the lung parenchyma may remain, with septal fibrosis replacing areas where the pulmonary capillary bed was destroyed by the hyperoxia.

Crapo JD: Morphologic changes in pulmonary oxygen toxicity. Annu Rev Physiol 48:721, 1986. *A detailed review of the time course and patterns of injury to the lung during exposure to hyperoxia.*

Jamieson D, Chance B, Cadenas E, et al.: The relationship of free radical production to hyperoxia. Annu Rev Physiol 48:703, 1986. *A review of the pathogenesis of hyperoxia-mediated cell injury.*

Radiation Lung Injury (See also Ch. 530)

The predominant factors determining the incidence of radiation pneumonitis are the total radiation dose, the number of fractions, and the duration of time over which the total dose is given. Some chemotherapeutic drugs may potentiate the damage from radiation. A total lung dose of less than 2000 rads generally is not associated with severe radiation pneumonitis, whereas a total dose in excess of 4000 rads, even if distributed over as many as 30 fractions, has virtually a 100 per cent risk of radiation pneumonitis.

The reaction of the lung to radiation injury can be divided into three phases. (1) An *acute phase*, occurring 1 to 2 months after radiation exposure, is characterized by vascular damage, congestion, edema, and mononuclear cell infiltration. Alveolar type II cells and alveolar macrophages are increased in number. (2) A *subacute phase* occurs 2 to 9 months later. The alveolar walls become infiltrated with mononuclear inflammatory cells and fibroblasts. (3) The *chronic* or *fibrotic phase* generally occurs more than 9 months after irradiation. Alveolar fibrosis and capillary sclerosis are its predominant histologic features.

CLINICAL MANIFESTATIONS. Signs of bronchial irritation, e.g., cough, may appear immediately after radiation therapy, followed shortly thereafter by esophagitis. Some patients may have no symptoms for 6 to 12 weeks. If large volumes of lung have been irradiated, or if high radiation doses have been given over short periods, the patient can develop dyspnea, tachypnea, and fever. These symptoms can be severe and will either progress to severe dyspnea and death or gradually subside, leaving varying degrees of respiratory impairment resulting from chronic lung fibrosis. Permanent fibrosis takes 6 to 24 months to evolve and then usually remains stable after 2 years if no further exposure occurs. Auscultation of the chest is usually normal, although rales, signs of consolidation, and pleural rubs may be found. Clubbing does not develop after radiation injury. Laboratory findings include a mild leukocytosis and an increased erythrocyte sedimentation rate. If the irradiated area is extensive, arterial hypoxemia may develop. Radiographic changes generally appear 1 to 3 months after treatment. The affected areas are generally demarcated by a "straight edge" defining the margins of the radiation portal and have a "ground-glass appearance"—a hazy increase in density with indistinct pulmonary markings. In the later phases of the radiation injury, fibrosis and contraction of the irradiated region are the predominant radiographic findings. Pulmonary function tests do not change until clinical symptoms appear, and then a restrictive ventilatory defect may be noted. Capillary sclerosis is associated with a decrease in blood flow to the affected region and a decrease in CO transfer capacity. Severe radiation injury is associated with a decrease in lung compliance and hypoxemia.

The diagnosis of acute radiation pneumonitis may be difficult to establish because of coincidental disease. The clinical picture is often complicated by the immunocompromised state of many of the patients, resulting in increased risk of bacterial or opportunistic pneumonias, e.g., that caused by *Pneumocystis carinii*, or by the signs and symptoms of the original neoplasm. Radiation pneumonitis has not been documented adequately in parts of the lung outside the radiation portal; however, a few patients have developed suspicious radiographic changes outside the field. Complications of radiation pneumonitis include small pleural effusions and, occasionally, spontaneous pneumothorax.

TREATMENT AND OUTCOME. The patient who develops radiation pneumonitis requires supportive care, including cough suppression, antipyretics, and supplemental oxygen for hypoxemia. Corticosteroids (prednisone, 1 mg per kilogram of body weight) have been advocated for treatment of severe cases of radiation pneumonitis, although there have been no controlled

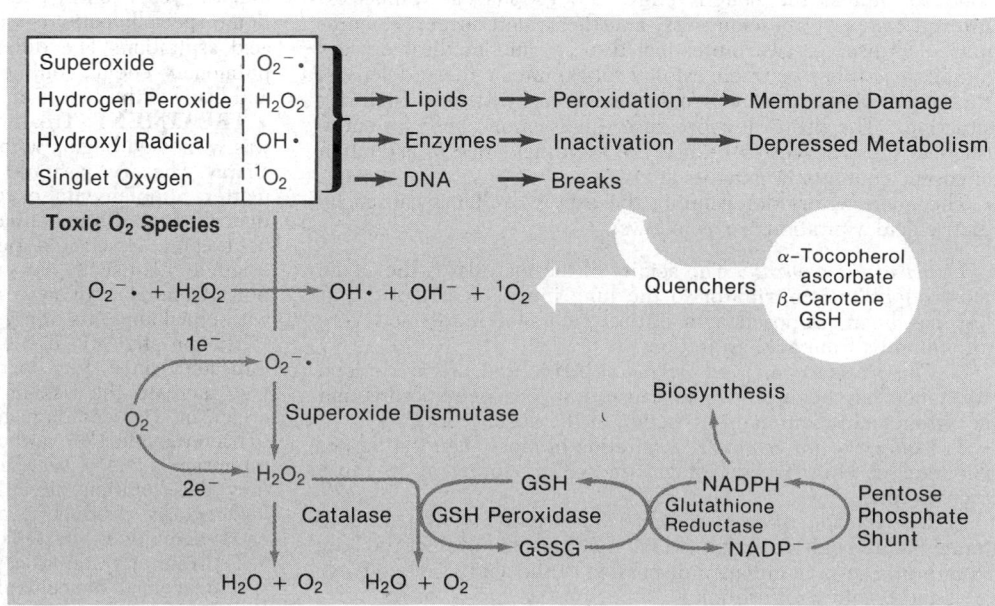

FIGURE 528–1. Toxic oxygen species and antioxidant defense systems. The incomplete reduction of oxygen produces superoxide and/or hydrogen peroxide. These species can react together in the presence of metal salts to form the hydroxyl radical and singlet oxygen. Free radical chain reactions can be initiated in lipid membranes, with enzymes and DNA also attacked by these reactive O_2 species. Quenchers interact with the oxygen species or with oxidized tissue components to block further tissue oxidation and to terminate free radical chain reactions. The antioxidant defense systems—superoxide dismutase, catalase, and glutathione peroxidase—function to detoxify superoxide and hydrogen peroxide, thus preventing the formation of other toxic O_2 species and the subsequent reactions with tissue. Glucose-6-phosphate dehydrogenase is the rate-limiting enzyme in the pentose phosphate shunt and thereby controls the availability of NADPH. This cofactor is essential both for the reduction of glutathione and for the biosynthetic pathways critical for repair processes. Net tissue injury represents the balance between the rate of production of partially reduced oxygen species, the rate at which these species are scavenged, and the rate of repair of any injury that occurs.

clinical trials. There is no evidence to support use of prophylactic corticosteroids, but their administration at the very onset of pneumonitis appears to be more effective than later therapy. On occasion, the response may be dramatic, with complete resolution of symptoms within 24 hours. Corticosteroids should be tapered carefully after achieving maximal clinical benefit. Pneumonitis has been reported occasionally after steroid withdrawal. No other effective therapeutic strategies are known. Antibiotic therapy should be reserved for patients in whom the clinical findings suggest infection. Since the lesion involves occlusion and thrombosis of many small blood vessels, anticoagulation has been tried, but there is no evidence of its effectiveness.

Gross NJ: The pathogenesis of radiation-induced lung damage. Lung 139:115, 1981. *A review of the biochemistry and cell biology of irradiated lung and how these factors relate to the clinical syndrome.*

Rosiello RA, Merrill WW: Radiation-induced lung injury. Clin Chest Med 11:65, 1990. *A summary of the clinical features of radiation-induced lung disease; with 51 references.*

ASPIRATION-RELATED INJURIES
Chemical Aspiration Pneumonitis

Injury to the respiratory system by aspiration can be categorized by the nature of the aspirate as (1) *infectious material*, (2) *chemical* or *inflammatory substances*, and (3) *inert material*. Contamination of the lungs by aspiration of oropharyngeal bacterial flora is discussed in Ch. 62. Aspiration of gastric acid is the most common example of chemical aspiration in adults; hydrocarbon aspiration occurs predominantly in children but is encountered occasionally in adults. Both of these injuries can cause fulminant illness. By contrast, lipids (mineral oil, vegetable and animal fats) most often provoke a chronic inflammatory reaction. Aspiration of inert material such as water causes injury (e.g., drowning), predominantly by asphyxia. Food particles can cause a fibrotic, granulomatous lesion or, if large enough to occlude the larynx or trachea, sudden death by asphyxiation ("café coronary").

GASTRIC ACID ASPIRATION

Aspiration pneumonitis refers to pulmonary injury caused by gastric acid. This condition is in contrast to "aspiration pneumonia," an infectious process caused by the contamination of the tracheobronchial tree by oropharyngeal flora. Aspiration of gastric acid can occur during vomiting or regurgitation, and in the latter instance the event may go unnoted—i.e., "silent aspiration." The normal protective mechanisms of the upper airway include epiglottic closure during deglutition, glottic closure on contact with solids or fluids, the cough reflex, and esophageal sphincters. Altered states of consciousness, anesthesia and surgery, neuromuscular disease, gastrointestinal disease, and medical devices (nasogastric tubes or tracheostomy tubes) impair these defenses. Protection of the airway is a major concern in these high-risk situations. The use of low-pressure, high-volume cuffs on endotracheal tubes serves to reduce the high incidence of aspiration of gastric contents in patients at risk.

The main factors determining the extent of illness caused by gastric acid aspiration are as follows:

1. *pH of the aspirate.* The acidity of the material is the single most important contributor to the lung injury. A pH of 2.5 or less has been proposed as a critical value for inducing severe pneumonitis from acid aspiration.

2. *The presence of food particles.* Aspiration of gastric food substance has been shown to cause a severe pneumonitis and peribronchial inflammatory reaction in the absence of acid.

3. *Volume of the aspirate.* Aspiration of more than 0.4 ml per kilogram of body weight of gastric acid is sufficient to cause pneumonitis.

4. *Distribution of the aspirate.* Many patients who aspirate immediately begin to cough, which may partially protect the lung from injury or may enhance dispersion of the acid over a greater area and create a diffuse injury.

After intratracheal instillation, acid is rapidly distributed in the lungs and can reach the pleura in 12 to 18 seconds. It is rapidly neutralized by bronchial secretions; in less than 30 minutes, the pH at the bronchial surface will have returned to normal. Acid causes chemical burns of the bronchi, bronchioles, and alveolar walls, with subsequent exudation of fluid into the lungs. Plasma volume may decrease by as much as 35 per cent in severe injury without fluid replacement, and cardiac output and systemic arterial blood pressure may fall. Pulmonary artery wedge pressure is normal or low, indicating a nonhydrostatic cause of the pulmonary edema. The characteristics of phospholipids in the alveolar surface lining layer (surfactant) are altered, causing increased surface forces and promoting early airway and alveolar closure. Lung compliance decreases secondary to the increase in interstitial fluids and the alteration of surface forces. These disturbances of airways, alveoli, and vascular elements cause profound imbalance of the normal ventilation-perfusion relationships. Increased intrapulmonary shunting is also common. As a result, hypoxemia is invariably present and usually severe.

CLINICAL MANIFESTATIONS. Some patients aspirate a large volume of gastric acid and almost immediately become apneic and hypotensive and die. More often, the patient survives the initial crisis but later develops a fulminant illness marked by dyspnea, cough, and frothy sputum. Alternatively, aspiration may be secondary to regurgitation and not accompanied by immediate coughing and agitation. After such silent aspiration, the patient may develop acute respiratory failure without an obvious reason for a precipitous deterioration in gas exchange. Within 1 to 5 hours after aspiration of gastric acid, tachypnea, rales, and rhonchi occur, and wheezing, cyanosis, cough, and hypotension may be present. Fever in the first 36 hours occurs in about 50 per cent of patients.

Laboratory tests are nonspecific. A moderate leukocytosis with left shift develops early. Arterial blood gases, the best variable to follow, show hypoxemia, and the arterial oxygen tension does not reach predicted levels after the patient has been breathing 100 per cent oxygen for several minutes, indicating increased intrapulmonary shunting of blood. The arterial Pco_2 may be slightly elevated, normal, or mildly reduced, and the pH will vary reciprocally. Abnormalities on chest roentgenograms are extremely variable, and no characteristic pattern is present. Radiographic abnormalities do not correlate with clinical outcome, although about 50 per cent of patients have changes consistent with pneumonitis. The acid is sometimes distributed preferentially to dependent areas, but usually the radiographic abnormalities are diffuse, presumably from enhanced dispersion of the acid during coughing. Pleural effusions and cavitation of infiltrates are not seen in uncomplicated cases. Bronchoscopic findings are diagnostic if food particles or other gastric contents are seen in the trachea or bronchi.

The diagnosis of aspiration pneumonitis begins with a high index of suspicion in patients with abrupt respiratory deterioration, especially patients with conditions that predispose to gastric acid aspiration. The differential diagnosis includes cardiogenic pulmonary edema, pulmonary embolism, bacterial pneumonia, and many of the causes of ARDS, such as sepsis and hypotension.

TREATMENT. Treatment of the individual whose aspiration was witnessed begins with prompt establishment of an adequate airway. The airway should be suctioned to remove any particulate matter. Supplemental oxygen is given to maintain a Pa_{O_2} of more than 60 torr. Bronchodilators (intravenous aminophylline) may be helpful. Associated pulmonary edema is noncardiogenic in origin and is usually associated with intravascular volume depletion. General supportive measures include fluid replacement with equal amounts of crystalloid and colloid solutions.

The prophylactic use of antibiotics for acid aspiration is not indicated, since they do not reduce morbidity or mortality and may increase the risk of subsequent infection with a resistant organism. The acid-damaged respiratory tract is more susceptible to bacterial infection, and up to one half of patients with significant aspiration develop bacterial pneumonia. Such patients undergo new deterioration after 2 or 3 days, with increasing fever, leukocytosis, production of purulent sputum, worsening hypoxemia, and new infiltrates on the chest radiograph.

The role of systemic corticosteroids in aspiration pneumonitis is controversial. No controlled human trials have been conducted. Early anecdotal reports supported their use, but more recent retrospective and prospective but uncontrolled series totaling approximately 250 patients have failed to show any decrease in morbidity or mortality.

Positive-pressure ventilation is helpful, particularly when it is initiated early after a major episode of aspiration. Arterial oxygen tensions improve, and mortality rates probably decrease with its use. Positive end-expiratory pressure to improve oxygenation has been beneficial in other forms of ARDS and is commonly used in the management of gastric acid aspiration. Caution should be used in applying PEEP, since it can increase extravascular water content in the acid-injured lung.

Aspiration pneumonitis carries a high mortality rate despite treatment, and because it largely occurs in a defined population at increased risk, efforts should be made at prevention. Elevation of the head of the bed will retard regurgitation. In intubated patients, placement of a nasogastric tube should be considered to keep the stomach decompressed. Aspiration may occur even in the presence of a cuffed endotracheal tube. Elective general anesthesia should be given with the stomach empty, after at least a 12-hour fast. Preoperatively, the pH of gastric contents can be raised by a single dose of an H_2 receptor blocker or by a single 10-ml oral dose of antacid given 2 to 4 hours before surgery.

OUTCOME. Mortality from aspiration pneumonitis is high, reaching 28 to 62 per cent of cases. Factors associated with highest mortality are age greater than 50 years, the early development of shock or apnea, severe and prolonged hypoxemia, very low pH of gastric contents at the time of aspiration, and the development of secondary bacterial pneumonia. Most patients survive the early moments but deteriorate over 12 to 24 hours. Some then show steady improvement, with radiographic resolution within a week. Others have a second episode of deterioration, an event that should suggest a new problem, such as bacterial infection, pulmonary embolism, heart failure, or another aspiration. Still others pursue a relentlessly worsening course to death. Few data exist regarding long-term clinical follow-up, but pulmonary fibrosis of varying degrees may occur in some of the survivors.

Bynum LJ, Pierce AK: Pulmonary aspiration of gastric contents. Am Rev Respir Dis 114:1129, 1976. *A retrospective analysis of the clinical features and outcome in 50 patients observed to aspirate gastric contents.*
Campbell JC, O'Donohue WJ Jr: Aspiration of gastric contents. Curr Pulmonol 8:163, 1987.

HYDROCARBON PNEUMONITIS

Hydrocarbon pneumonitis results from the direct toxic effects of volatile hydrocarbons on the respiratory epithelium and vasculature. It occurs in individuals who, having ingested the hydrocarbons, aspirate them into the respiratory tract. The problem occurs most often in children, particularly those below the age of 5 years. It is an uncommon problem in adults, occurring most often in industrial accidents, in patients attempting suicide, in siphoning of gasoline, and in uninformed alcoholics seeking an ethanol substitute.

Different hydrocarbons cause respiratory injury of varying extent, depending on the viscosity and volume of the aspirate. The lower the viscosity or the larger the volume, the worse the lesion. As lipid solvents, these compounds are directly toxic to respiratory tissues. The lungs of children dying of hydrocarbon pneumonitis demonstrate hemorrhage, pulmonary edema, atelectasis, hyaline membrane formation, and necrosis of airway epithelium and alveolar septa. These compounds also have systemic toxicity, and in fatal cases, degenerative changes have been seen in the liver and kidneys.

CLINICAL MANIFESTATIONS. Aspiration usually occurs at the time of hydrocarbon ingestion, although a history of vomiting after hydrocarbon ingestion is obtained in fewer than half the patients. Dyspnea, tachypnea, tachycardia, and high fever quickly ensue. Sputum may be bloody. Lethargy is common, but more severe disturbances of consciousness also occur, such as confusion, coma, and seizures. Auscultation is frequently normal, but rales and rhonchi may be present.

Laboratory tests give nonspecific results. A moderate leukocytosis with left shift is common. Arterial hypoxemia of various degrees develops owing to shunting and to ventilation-perfusion mismatching. The chest radiograph is particularly helpful, as infiltrates may occur within 20 to 30 minutes after aspiration of some types of hydrocarbons. The multiple, fluffy, ill-defined infiltrates favor dependent areas of the lungs. Some patients present a picture of bilateral perihilar infiltrates, a pulmonary edema pattern. Pleural effusions, pneumothorax, and pneumomediastinum occur but are uncommon. Pneumatoceles can form later, especially in children.

The differential diagnosis is that of respiratory distress of abrupt onset, frequently in a patient with an impaired sensorium at the time of presentation. The adult patient is often an alcoholic. Gastric acid aspiration, cardiogenic pulmonary edema, pulmonary embolism, and acute bacterial pneumonia can all manifest similarly. The correct diagnosis requires the history of hydrocarbon ingestion or aspiration. The diagnosis is also suggested by the odor of the patient's breath and by extensive radiographic abnormalities in a patient with a clear chest on auscultation.

TREATMENT. Emesis to remove ingested hydrocarbons is contraindicated. Gastric lavage by nasogastric tube may cause vomiting and should be performed only after placement of a cuffed endotracheal tube in the patient who has recently ingested a large volume of hydrocarbons. Supplemental oxygen should be given to maintain a Pa_{O_2} greater than 60 torr. Mechanical ventilation and PEEP may be necessary. No data support the routine use of antibiotics. The use of systemic corticosteroids (prednisone, 1 mg per kilogram per day) during the acute illness is supported by anecdotal reports of improvement after their use in children and adults.

OUTCOME. Hydrocarbon pneumonitis in adults is rare, so that estimates of morbidity and mortality are not available. In children, death occurs in about 10 per cent of cases, but most children have a prompt clinical recovery. Bronchiectasis, recurrent bronchitis, and/or pulmonary fibrosis ensues in an unknown portion of cases. After recovery, children frequently have normal chest examinations and radiographs, although pulmonary function abnormalities suggestive of small airway (<2-mm diameter) disease have been found in asymptomatic patients as late as 8 to 14 years after hydrocarbon pneumonitis.

Klein BL, Simon JE: Hydrocarbon poisonings. Pediatr Clin North Am 33:411, 1986. *A review showing that most ingestions can be managed by careful observation and respiratory support.*

LIPOID PNEUMONIA

Lipoid pneumonia is a chronic inflammatory reaction of the lungs that results from the aspiration of vegetable, animal, or (most commonly) mineral oils. This exogenous material differs greatly from the excessive accumulation of endogenous lipids in the lungs occurring in fat embolism, cholesterol pneumonitis, pulmonary alveolar proteinosis, and the lipid storage diseases.

The most frequently implicated agent is mineral oil used as a laxative and to reduce dysphagia, either in clear liquid form or as petroleum jelly. Mineral oil is bland and, when introduced into the pharynx, can enter the bronchial tree without eliciting the cough reflex. It also mechanically impedes the ciliary action of the airway epithelium. The risk of mineral oil aspiration is increased in debilitated or senile patients, in those having neurologic disease that interferes with deglutition, and in patients with esophageal disease. Mineral oil taken as nose drops to relieve nasal dryness has caused lipoid pneumonia and in earlier years was a frequent cause of the illness. Inhalation of mineral oil mist by airplane and automobile mechanics has also been implicated as a cause of the problem.

Mineral oils, which are relatively inert, cannot be hydrolyzed in the body and provoke a chronic inflammatory reaction that may not become clinically overt until years later. The fat is emulsified in the alveolar spaces, where macrophages accumulate and phagocytize it. Some macrophages disintegrate, releasing their lysosomal enzymes and fat. The alveolar septa become thickened and edematous, containing lymphocytes and lipid-laden macrophages. Oil droplets are seen in the pulmonary lymphatics and hilar nodes. Later, fibrosis develops, and the normal lung architecture is effaced. It is usual in a single specimen to find both the early inflammatory and the later fibrotic picture, in keeping with repetitive aspirations over many months or years. If nodular, the lesion may grossly resemble tumor and is called a paraffinoma.

CLINICAL MANIFESTATIONS AND TREATMENT. Most patients are asymptomatic, coming to the physician's attention because of an abnormal chest radiograph. When patients are symptomatic, cough and exertional dyspnea are the most frequent complaints. Chest pain (sometimes pleuritic), hemoptysis, fever (usually low grade), chills, night sweats, and weight loss may occur. The physical examination may be completely normal, or fever, tachypnea, dullness on percussion of the chest, bronchial or bronchovesicular breath sounds, rales, and rhonchi may be found. Clubbing and cor pulmonale are rare.

In mild lipoid pneumonia, arterial blood gas values may be normal with the patient at rest but may show hypoxemia after exercise. In more severe disease, resting hypoxemia, hypocapnia, and mild respiratory alkalosis develop. Pulmonary function testing reveals a restrictive ventilatory defect; static compliance of the lungs is decreased. The only specific laboratory finding is the presence in sputum or bronchoalveolar lavage of macrophages with clusters of vacuoles 5 to 50 μm in diameter that stain deep orange with Sudan IV and extracellular droplets that stain similarly.

Radiographically, the earliest abnormalities are air space infiltrates, unilateral or bilateral, localized or diffuse, but most often in the dependent portions of the right lung. Air bronchograms may be seen. Hilar adenopathy and pleural reaction are rare. As fibrosis develops, volume loss occurs and linear and nodular infiltrates appear. A solid lesion that closely resembles bronchogenic carcinoma may develop, and lipoid pneumonia may carry an increased risk for bronchoalveolar cell carcinoma..

The differential diagnosis is extensive, particularly in the late phase, when multiple other causes of pulmonary fibrosis must be considered. The key to the correct diagnosis before biopsy is the history of chronic oral or intranasal use of an oil- or a lipid-based product, or an occupational exposure to oil mists. The presence of lipid-laden macrophages in the sputum confirms the diagnosis.

Once the diagnosis has been made and the aspiration stopped, the subsequent course is variable. Some patients have no change in symptoms. Others improve in some or all parameters, whereas a few patients deteriorate, with worsening pulmonary function and cor pulmonale. Since the only way the lung can dispose of mineral oil is by expectoration, the patient should be instructed in coughing exercises to be performed many times each day for months. Expectorants have not been shown to help. Systemic corticosteroids are recommended by some on the basis of improvement seen in a few uncontrolled reports. The rationale has been that the cellular reaction, rather than the oil itself, is the destructive factor. Because of the well-recognized side effects of systemic corticosteroids, their use for lipoid pneumonia should be limited to those patients who have significant symptoms, and then for as brief a period as possible to "buy time" while decreasing the lipid burden by expectoration.

Blondal T, Hartvig P, Bengtsson A, et al.: An unnecessary case of paraffin oil pneumonia. Acta Med Scand 213:227, 1983. *The problems in diagnosis of mineral oil pneumonia are illustrated.*

Near-Drowning

Drowning accounts for about 9000 deaths annually in the United States, mostly in children and young adults. It is one of the three leading causes of accidental death. In adults, alcohol consumption and shallow water blackout during breath-hold diving are common aggravating factors. Pathophysiologically, drowning can be of two types: (1) "wet" drowning—initial laryngospasm but early relaxation and subsequent aspiration of copious amounts of fluid; the majority of drownings are of this sort: (2) "dry" drowning—asphyxiation secondary to intense glottic spasm that persists beyond the point of apnea, so that when the muscles relax, little or no water is aspirated; this accounts for 10 to 20 per cent of drownings. The immediate cause of death in many victims of drowning is cardiac arrhythmia. Victims who survive the initial episode frequently develop ARDS a few hours to a few days after the event (secondary drowning).

The most important consequences of near-drowning are attributed to asphyxia. Asphyxia results in severe hypoxemia, hypercarbia, and metabolic acidosis. The metabolic consequences of drowning in fresh water or salt water appear to differ little except for drowning in water with very high mineral content (e.g., the Dead Sea). In both cases, hypoxemia is caused by the occlusion of airways with water and particulate debris, by changes in surfactant activity, by direct injury to the alveolar septa, and by bronchospasm. Right-to-left shunting is markedly increased, and physiologic dead space is increased. Life-threatening electrolyte disturbances caused by water aspiration in humans are rare. Cardiac arrhythmias and central nervous system and renal insufficiency often occur after near-drowning. Brain anoxia is usually global anoxia, and if it is of sufficient duration and magnitude, it will lead to diffuse cerebral edema.

Autopsies of drowned persons demonstrate wet, heavy lungs with varying amounts of hemorrhage and edema and some disruption of alveolar walls. In about 70 per cent of victims, vomitus, sand, mud, and aquatic vegetation have been aspirated. Specimens from victims dying of secondary drowning show desquamation of alveolar epithelial cells, hemorrhage, hyaline membrane formation, acute inflammatory infiltrates, and foreign body reactions to particulate matter. Cerebral edema and diffuse neuronal injury are seen. Changes of acute tubular necrosis are found in the kidneys.

CLINICAL MANIFESTATIONS. The initial appearance of the patient can vary widely, from coma to agitated alertness. Cyanosis, coughing, and the production of frothy pink sputum are common. Tachypnea, tachycardia, and a low-grade fever in the first few hours are seen if the patient did not become hypothermic during submersion. Rales, rhonchi, and, less often, wheezes are heard. Neurologic signs vary and can fluctuate in any given patient but usually derive from diffuse cerebral dysfunction. Signs of associated trauma to the head and neck should be sought.

Laboratory studies reveal mild hypokalemia, hypernatremia, and hyperchloremia. A moderate leukocytosis may be present. Hematocrit and hemoglobin usually are normal at first measurement; in fresh water aspiration, the hematocrit may fall slightly in the first 24 hours owing to hemolysis. An isolated increase in serum free hemoglobin without a change in hematocrit is more common. Occasionally, the clinical picture of disseminated intravascular coagulation occurs in near-drowning. Arterial blood gas values, usually obtained after preliminary resuscitation, show severe hypoxemia and metabolic acidosis. The most common electrocardiographic changes are sinus tachycardia and nonspecific ST segment and T wave changes, which revert to normal within hours; however, other, more ominous abnormalities may occur—ventricular arrhythmias, complete heart block, or myocardial infarction. The chest radiograph may be normal initially despite severe respiratory disturbances. It often shows patchy infiltrates, and sometimes a classic pattern of pulmonary edema is seen.

TREATMENT. Treatment of the near-drowning victim begins with establishing an adequate airway and, if necessary, emergency cardiopulmonary resuscitation. Oxygen in high concentrations is necessary, since hypoxemia is present in essentially all victims. Even the patient who quickly becomes apparently normal should be hospitalized for 24 hours to watch for a subsequent clinical picture of ARDS. During transportation to a hospital, supplemental oxygen should be continued and precautions taken for potential head and neck injuries and other serious trauma.

In the hospital, therapy is dictated largely by the arterial blood gas values and the degree of respiratory failure. Continuous positive airway pressure or PEEP is particularly helpful for managing hypoxemia. Bronchospasm should be treated with nebulized β-agonists and intravenous theophylline. Patients with persistent localized atelectasis or localized wheezing should undergo bronchoscopy to exclude a foreign body as the etiology. Prophylactic antibiotics have not been shown to be beneficial, although many victims of near-drowning develop pneumonia, sometimes caused by unusual microorganisms. The use of corticosteroids for the pulmonary lesions of near-drowning remains controversial, and there have been no controlled prospective human studies to support their use. Animal models and retrospective studies in humans have failed to demonstrate any benefit.

The therapeutic approach to brain resuscitation after near-drowning is also controversial. If evidence of cerebral edema exists, intracranial pressure (ICP) monitoring may be useful to guide therapy. In the event of increased ICP, PEEP should be minimized, since it may increase ICP. Hyperventilation to maintain a Pa_{CO_2} of 25 to 30 torr decreases ICP at the expense of cerebral blood flow. Mannitol may decrease cerebral edema. It should be used to maintain the serum osmolarity near 300 mOsm per liter. Corticosteroids are used widely (e.g., dexamethasone, 10 mg given intravenously initially and then 4 to 6 mg given intravenously every 4 hours) but are not of proven benefit for the central nervous system injury. Seizures should be treated with anticonvulsants. Shivering or random, purposeless movements can increase ICP and should be aborted with muscle relaxants. If these maneuvers fail to lower ICP, then barbiturate coma can be undertaken for 24 to 48 hours.

OUTCOME. Outcome in near-drowning is best judged by the neurologic status, i.e., the presence or absence of coma. The shorter the interval between recovery from the water to first spontaneous gasp, the better the prognosis for recovery. The absence of spontaneous respiration after resuscitation from near-drowning is an ominous sign associated with severe neurologic sequelae. Permanent neurologic sequelae persist in about 20 per cent of comatose victims. Common sequelae include minimal brain dysfunction, spastic quadriplegia, extrapyramidal syndromes, optic and cerebral atrophy, and peripheral neuromuscular damage. Survival without neurologic damage is best in children who are hypothermic when recovered and may occur even after 40 minutes of submersion. Similar reports of survival after prolonged immersion in adults are very rare.

Hoff BH: Multisystem failure: A review with special references to drowning. Crit Care Med 7:310, 1979. *A complete review of the evaluation and care of the nearly drowned patient with attention to all critical organ systems.*

Redding JS: Drowning and near-drowning. Can the victim be saved? Postgrad Med 74:85, 1983. *A review of current therapy.*

DISORDERS CAUSED BY ALTERED BAROMETRIC PRESSURE

Significant alterations in environmental pressure are encountered by humans during ascent to altitude and during underwater diving. As altitude increases, barometric pressure falls from approximately 760 mm Hg at sea level to 380 mm Hg (0.5 ATA) at 18,000 feet. In seawater, the pressure of the water column increases by an amount equal to the barometric pressure for every 33 feet of depth. Hence at 33 feet of seawater, the absolute pressure is doubled (2 ATA). As a result, participants in activities such as mountaineering and scuba diving are often exposed to extremes of environmental pressure. Rapid pressure changes produce notable physiologic effects related to the behavior of atmospheric gases in the lungs and body tissues.

Diseases of High Altitudes

At high altitudes, the low barometric pressure causes physiologic effects due primarily to the decrease in the partial pressure of inspired oxygen. Physiologic changes begin to occur at 8000 to 10,000 feet. These changes become more apparent at altitudes above 10,000 feet owing to the shape of the oxygen-hemoglobin dissociation curve, which has a steep downslope below a P_{O_2} of approximately 60 mm Hg. A small drop in P_{O_2} below this level results in a relatively large decrease in arterial saturation. At 10,000 feet (3048 meters), the alveolar P_{O_2} is approximately 60 mm Hg, and some individuals manifest impairment of memory, judgment, and the ability to perform complex calculations. At 18,000 feet (5486 meters), the alveolar P_{O_2} is 40 mm Hg, and unacclimatized individuals may become unconscious after several hours.

Exposure to high altitude occurs most commonly in commercial aviation. In general, aircraft cabins are maintained at a pressure equal to or greater than that encountered at 8000 feet, so that supplemental oxygen is not required. Some patients with reduced cardiac reserve or with COPD may have difficulty tolerating even a small drop in arterial oxygen saturation and may require oxygen during flights. Aircraft regulations require that the flight crew receive supplemental oxygen when the cabin pressure drops below that at 10,000 feet and that passengers receive supplemental oxygen, should the cabin pressure drop below that at 15,000 feet.

ACUTE MOUNTAIN SICKNESS (AMS). Ascent to high altitude produces a wide spectrum of illness that depends on factors such as the absolute altitude, the rate of ascent, the length of stay, and individual susceptibility. Altitude illness may be classified into several syndromes, as shown in Table 528–2. The acute syndromes probably reflect a common pathophysiology initiated by a relatively abrupt lack of oxygen, although the precise mechanisms remain uncertain. The ventilatory response to hypoxia and poor physical conditioning may play a role in susceptible individuals. The most common malady is AMS, and self-limited symptoms of headache, anorexia, malaise, and disturbed sleep may appear within a few hours of arriving at altitudes above 8000 feet. Mild AMS may affect half of unacclimatized visitors to 14,000 feet. At altitudes above 9500 feet, AMS may be severe and followed sometimes by the more serious conditions of high-altitude pulmonary edema (HAPE) and high-altitude cerebral edema (HACE) (Table 528–2), which frequently coexist. High-altitude retinal hemorrhages (HARH) are prevalent above 14,000 feet and probably share a similar pathophysiology with cerebral edema. Retinal hemorrhages are not significant unless they produce visual symptoms; the latter circumstance usually indicates involvement of the macula and mandates immediate descent. The more serious forms of AMS are discussed below.

HIGH-ALTITUDE PULMONARY EDEMA (HAPE). Acute noncardiogenic pulmonary edema is a potentially fatal complication of rapid ascent to altitudes above 9500 feet. Symptoms begin after 6 to 36 hours at high altitude and may follow an episode of AMS. Dyspnea at rest, tachypnea, and crackles are characteristic features of HAPE. Cyanosis, orthopnea, and hemoptysis commonly develop in more advanced cases.

At autopsy, the lungs are typically heavy, congested, and edematous and have hyaline membranes in small airways and alveoli. The cause of hyaline membrane formation is not known; this is not a characteristic finding in death caused by other forms of hypoxia. Hemodynamic studies have shown elevated pulmonary artery pressure with normal pulmonary venous pressure. The pulmonary edema may be due to an increase in pulmonary capillary pressure in small regions of the pulmonary capillary bed or to increased permeability in lung capillaries.

HIGH-ALTITUDE CEREBRAL EDEMA (HACE). HACE is relatively uncommon, occurring in perhaps 1.5 per cent of individuals affected by AMS. Hypoxemia produces cerebral vasodilation and increased cerebral blood flow, which may lead to mild brain edema and produce the symptoms of AMS. Cerebral edema may also be aggravated by hypoxic inhibition of the adenosine triphosphate (ATP)–dependent sodium pump. By factors yet to be defined, the brain edema may progress and become life threatening. Signs and symptoms of HACE include severe, progressive headache, ataxia, confusion, anxiety, hallucinations, and coma. Papilledema and meningeal signs occur. Examination of the cerebrospinal fluid reveals high opening pressures and perhaps hemorrhage or leukocytosis. Pathologically, the pattern of cerebral edema appears to be heterogeneous, and focal areas of capillary damage, red cell sludging, and platelet aggregation are seen.

TREATMENT OF ACUTE HIGH-ALTITUDE DISEASE. The simplest approach to the prevention and treatment of acute

TABLE 528–2. HIGH-ALTITUDE SYNDROMES

Syndrome	Clinical Description
Acute mountain sickness (AMS)	Common, self-limited; characterized by headache, anorexia, and malaise after ascent to altitudes >8000 ft; "normal puna"
High-altitude pulmonary edema (HAPE)	Noncardiac pulmonary edema recognized by dyspnea and tachypnea at rest, cough, and bibasilar crackles; usually at altitudes >9500 ft; "pulmonary puna"
High-altitude cerebral edema (HACE)	Uncommon, severe central nervous system dysfunction following AMS, characterized by severe headache, memory loss, ataxia, hallucinations, and confusion; may progress to coma and death; "nervous puna"
High-altitude retinal hemorrhages (HARH)	Dilated retinal vessels and peripheral flame-shaped or dot hemorrhages; occasionally cause visual symptoms
Chronic mountain sickness (Monge's disease)	Cor pulmonale with minimal lung disease in long-term residents of high altitude

altitude illness is to ascend to altitude gradually and to descend when troubling symptoms appear. Gradual ascent allows time for the body's adaptive responses to be recruited. If possible, the rate of ascent should be limited to approximately 1000 feet per day between altitudes of 7000 and 10,000 feet. Slower ascent (500 feet per day) is recommended for altitudes above 10,000 feet. If slow ascent is impractical, prophylactic treatment with acetazolamide is effective for prevention of AMS. Acetazolamide increases renal bicarbonate excretion and lessens the degree of respiratory alkalosis. The recommended regimen is 250 mg every 8 hours the day before, during, and for 1 day after the ascent. Some authors use one half to one third of this amount of acetazolamide to avoid dehydration and potassium depletion. Other diuretics have not been proved to be effective, and in practice, liberal water intake appears to hasten bicarbonate excretion and prevent hemoconcentration. Dexamethasone (4 mg every 6 hours) has also been shown to reduce the incidence and early symptoms of AMS; however, it is not recommended widely because of potential side effects.

The management of AMS consists of rest, mild analgesics, alcohol avoidance, and adequate hydration. The symptoms usually abate within a few days. The definitive treatment for HAPE, HACE, and severe HARH is oxygen administration and descent to lower altitude. High-altitude pulmonary edema has been reported to improve dramatically with a descent of only a few thousand feet. If the descent is delayed, the combination of oxygen and PEEP or continuous positive airway pressure, or placing the victim in a pressurized bag or chamber, is effective.

CHRONIC MOUNTAIN SICKNESS (MONGE'S DISEASE). Chronic mountain sickness occurs in people living at high altitudes, usually at over 14,000 feet, for many years. These "highlanders" have a blunted respiratory drive in response to hypoxia and have a lower minute ventilation at high altitudes than do those who normally reside at lower altitudes. Chronic mountain sickness is characterized by an exaggerated response to hypoxia resulting in cor pulmonale. Physiologic responses include erythrocytosis with hemoglobin levels as high as 25 grams per deciliter, a decreased minute ventilation with an elevated P_{CO_2}, hypoxemia, and impaired sensitivity of the respiratory center to hypoxia. Clinical manifestations are similar to those of polycythemia rubra vera and include cyanosis, dyspnea, cough, palpitations, headache, giddiness, muscular weakness, pain in the extremities, sensory and motor changes, and episodic stupor. The only therapy is to move the patient to a lower altitude. Subacute forms of this illness, in which cyanosis and alveolar hypoventilation are absent, also occur. A similar syndrome, brisket disease, has been described in cattle.

Houston C: Altitude illness and pulmonary edema. Curr Pulmonol 7:227, 1986. *An excellent review of high-altitude disorders; with 82 references.*

Decompression Sickness

Variations in the ambient pressure outside the body must be reflected across the lungs by proportional changes in the partial pressures of various gases dissolved in the tissues of the body. This condition is a consequence of the physical behavior of gases and their interactions with solutions. Since the quantity of gas dissolved in tissue varies directly with atmospheric pressure, changes in gas concentrations in the body are most pronounced during diving with compressed air, when, in order for the diver to expand his or her lungs, the density of the breathing gas must be increased in proportion to the column of water around him or her. Nitrogen uptake is most important in this respect because it comprises 80 per cent of the atmosphere and, unlike oxygen, it is inert (not metabolized). Inert gases like nitrogen must be eliminated from the body after a decrease in ambient pressure, e.g., return from a compressed air dive or rapid ascent to high altitude. The process of inert gas elimination is called decompression.

During decompression, inert gas dissolved in the tissues may come out of physical solution if the fall in environmental pressure is too rapid. Bubbles of inert gas form within the tissues and venous blood and produce various clinical manifestations known as decompression sickness (DCS), or caisson disease. Decompression sickness, however, is not entirely explained by gas bubbles

TABLE 528–3. CLASSIFICATION OF DECOMPRESSION SICKNESS (DCS)

Organ System	Signs and Symptoms
Mild DCS (Type 1)	
Skin	Pruritus, mottling, urticaria
Musculoskeletal	Pain (bends) usually in the joints, numbness, edema
Serious DCS (Type 2)	
Central nervous system	
Cerebral	Loss of consciousness, ataxia, vertigo, aphasia, hemiparesis
Audiovestibular	Vertigo, nystagmus, auditory symptoms
Spinal cord	Back pain, paraparesis, bladder and bowel dysfunction
Cardiopulmonary	Cough, substernal pain, tachypnea, asphyxia (chokes)
Systemic	Extreme fatigue, hypovolemic shock

in blood and tissue, and not all bubbles cause symptoms. Bubbles produce a number of secondary manifestations attributed to surface activity at the interface between the bubble and the blood or tissue. These secondary effects, such as activation of complement, platelet aggregation, and release of vasoactive mediators, may lead to ischemia and some of the manifestations of DCS.

CLINICAL MANIFESTATIONS. Decompression sickness can occur during decompression after diving to more than 25 feet of seawater (1.75 ATA) or during rapid ascent from sea level to 18,000 feet (0.5 ATA). Decompression sickness is most commonly encountered in compressed air (or gas) divers after prolonged or repetitive dives or after severe exercise and in divers with excessive body fat, poor physical conditioning, and increasing age. The signs and symptoms of DCS usually appear within a few minutes to a few hours after the end of the dive. Clinically, DCS is classified as either mild (type 1) or serious (type 2). This distinction is somewhat arbitrary because both mild and serious manifestations of DCS occur simultaneously in about one third of patients. The common clinical features of DCS are outlined in Table 528–3.

TREATMENT AND OUTCOME. The first step in the treatment of DCS is the administration of high concentrations of oxygen by face mask. Prompt recompression in a hyperbaric chamber with 100 per cent oxygen usually relieves symptoms in a matter of minutes. Even mild symptoms of DCS, with the exception of skin manifestations, should be treated with recompression. If recompression therapy is delayed for more than a few hours, the illness is more difficult to treat. The rationale for recompression is based on (1) enhancing the dissolution of gas bubbles by compression and (2) lowering the concentration of inert gas in venous blood with oxygen, thus increasing the rate of removal of nitrogen from body tissues and bubbles. With prompt treatment, complete recovery is to be expected. If therapy is delayed for more than 24 hours, the outcome is less certain, although many patients, even those with serious neurologic disease, respond to recompression after delays of several days.

Pulmonary Barotrauma and Arterial Gas Embolism

Pulmonary barotrauma and arterial gas embolism (AGE) may occur in compressed air divers during ascent to the surface, particularly with failure to exhale normally. They are also encountered during explosive decompression at high altitude and in blast injury of the thorax. Under these circumstances, ambient hydrostatic or barometric pressure decreases rapidly, and gas within the lungs expands reciprocally according to Boyle's law. Under water near the surface, small decreases in depth result in large increases in gas volume. If the expanding gas is not allowed to escape, it may create a pressure gradient exceeding the compliance of lung tissue. This positive-pressure gradient between alveolar gas and the pulmonary interstitium may lead to alveolar disruption and pulmonary interstitial emphysema and then to soft tissue or mediastinal emphysema, pneumothorax, or pneumopericardium. This condition is known as pulmonary barotrauma. Free gas may also enter pulmonary venous blood and travel through the left side of the heart to the systemic circulation. Air can be embolized throughout the arterial system, including the cerebral, coronary, and renal arteries.

CLINICAL MANIFESTATIONS. The clinical manifestations of AGE usually occur within minutes after the diver surfaces. Signs and symptoms that suggest distribution of gas to the carotid arteries frequently develop. This condition leads to acute cerebral dysfunction characterized by severe headache, blindness, loss of consciousness, seizures, or paralysis. Depending on the amount of pulmonary barotrauma, the quantity of embolized gas may be very large. This serious complication of ascent can occur in compressed air diving after very brief exposures or at very shallow depths, when DCS is not a diagnostic consideration.

TREATMENT AND OUTCOME. Severe central nervous system deficits from AGE are more likely to be permanently disabling or lethal in the absence of adequate treatment than is DCS. Recompression therapy should commence within minutes if good neurologic recovery is to be ensured. The management is similar to that of DCS, but the magnitude, length, and number of recompression treatments are generally greater. If treatment is delayed more than 24 hours, the likelihood of benefit from recompression therapy is low.

529 Occupational Diseases of the Skin

Edward A. Emmett

Occupational skin diseases are a group of heterogeneous conditions that share a common occupational etiology. They account for about one half of reported occupational disease in the United States. Occupational contact dermatitis, the prototypical disorder, makes up about 95 per cent of all occupational skin diseases; infections, about 2.5 per cent; and a large number of different, infrequent diseases, the remainder. The relative frequency of each of these diseases in any location depends largely on the pattern of industrialization.

Almost all occupational skin disease is due to external contact with chemical, physical, and biologic agents. The cause is often multifactorial. In relatively few instances are systemically (rather than locally) absorbed agents responsible.

OCCUPATIONAL CONTACT DERMATITIS

DEFINITION. Occupational contact dermatitis is an erythematous or eczematous response of the skin as a result of local contact with one or more irritating, allergenic, or photosensitizing chemical agents.

ETIOLOGY. Many chemicals from a wide variety of classes—alkalies, acids, volatile organic solvents, metallic salts, organic prepolymers, and many others—are capable of inducing contact dermatitis. The cause is often multifactorial; in addition to one or more chemicals, friction, abrasion, changes in temperature and humidity, and ultraviolet (UV) radiation may play a role. Superinfection may occur. Severe and persistent occupational contact dermatitis, particularly from irritants, is more frequent in those with an atopic diathesis.

INCIDENCE AND PREVALENCE. Bureau of Labor Statistics reports put the incidence in the United States at about 0.9 per 1000 full-time workers per year; because of substantial underreporting, the true incidence is estimated to be from 10 to 50 times higher.

EPIDEMIOLOGY. The incidence of occupational contact dermatitis is generally highest in agriculture/forestry/fishing, followed by the manufacturing industries. The highest risks occur in poultry-dressing plants, meat-packing plants, fabrication of rubber products, leather tanning and finishing, manufacture of ophthalmic goods, plating and polishing, production of frozen fruits and vegetables, internal combustion engine manufacture, machining operations, and canning and curing of seafoods. Virtually no industry is immune.

PATHOGENESIS. Contact dermatitis may result from direct local irritation, cell-mediated immune reactions, or photosensitivity.

Direct local irritation may be immediate, as in irritation from strong acids or alkalies, or may be delayed and occur only after repeated or prolonged local application as cumulative insult dermatitis. The latter can occur from one or more relatively mildly irritating substances that are termed marginal irritants.

Allergic contact dermatitis occurs as a result of sensitization to specific haptens through a process of cell-mediated immunity. The hapten combines with protein in the skin to form a complete antigen that is processed and presented to T lymphocytes by epidermal Langerhans cells, specialized macrophages that form an intraepidermal network. Among the most frequent allergens are poison ivy or oak; rubber additives, particularly accelerators and antioxidants; monomers of plastics and resins, such as epoxies, acrylates, and di-isocyanates; nickel; chromium salts; paraphenylenediamine and derivatives; and formaldehyde. There are many more possible allergens. The number of substances reported to cause allergic contact dermatitis is very large.

Chemical photosensitivity results from the photochemical excitation of a UV-absorbing molecule with resultant tissue damage. In a photoirritant reaction there is direct damage to cellular components, for example, when psoralens irradiated with long UV bind covalently to DNA. Coal tar pitch, certain aromatic dyes, and UV absorbers used in printing processes also cause photoirritation. In the rarer photoallergic reaction, photochemical alteration of the inciting chemical either forms a hapten or leads to a hapten-protein combination in the skin; the subsequent steps are identical with those for allergic contact dermatitis.

A major factor in the human's resistance to environmental chemicals is the barrier provided by the outer stratum corneum layer of the epidermis. Damage to this barrier by trauma, inflammation, or skin disease or by altering barrier conditions, e.g., by occlusion, may play an important role in the development of contact dermatitis.

CLINICAL MANIFESTATIONS. The clinical presentation is dominated by dermatitis that is confined, at least initially, to the region of contact. The morphology varies according to the concentration and duration of the exposure, the pathogenesis, and individual constitutional differences. Acute irritant dermatitis is characterized by erythema, perhaps edema, papules and vesicles, or, in the more extreme instance, one or more large bullae filled with purulent fluid. Postinflammation hyperpigmentation and hypopigmentation may occur; necrosis may leave scars. The cause of acute irritant dermatitis is usually obvious because of the rapidity with which the reaction develops.

Cumulative insult dermatitis may develop only after a long period of contact. On the hands it tends to start under rings or watchbands and to be somewhat patchy in distribution. Individual susceptibility varies widely. Initially, drying and fissuring may be seen, with subsequent development of an eczematous response with papules and vesicles. Excoriations and lichenification are frequent if the process persists. Relapse may occur on relatively brief exposure to mild irritants, even when the dermatitis is clinically healed, especially if the epidermal barrier has not yet been fully re-established.

Allergic contact dermatitis most often presents as an acute or chronic eczematous reaction with erythema, papules, vesicles, scaling, and pruritus. Characteristically there is a latent period of at least 7 to 10 days before the development of dermatitis following first exposure to the allergen. Recurrence usually occurs 24 to 72 hours after an eliciting exposure. Certain allergens, e.g., epoxy resin monomers, have a tendency to produce severe acute reactions with significant edema.

Localization is important for diagnosis. Over 90 per cent of occupational contact dermatitis involves the hands, sometimes in conjunction with other sites. When the eruption is due to contact with objects or contaminated surfaces, the pattern of contact determines localization. Reaction to immersion of the hands in liquids generally involves the dorsum of the hands and palmar aspects of the wrists. Photosensitivity reactions on exposed sites may be distinguished from airborne contact dermatitis by the relative sparing of shaded areas, such as the eyelids or behind the ears.

DIAGNOSIS. A good occupational history is the cornerstone of diagnosis. It is most useful to get a description of the worker's daily activities, including nonoccupational activities, with particular attention to contact of the skin with chemicals. The localization of the eruption at its onset, initial appearance of lesions, nature of progression, and circumstances of remissions and recurrences help determine an occupational etiology. A personal or family history or both confirm the presence of atopy, in which there is increased susceptibility to irritants, changes in heat and humidity, and other factors. A complete examination of the skin helps rule out dermatoses other than contact dermatitis, including id reactions of the hands secondary to dermatophytosis of the feet. Allergic contact dermatitis is confirmed by diagnostic patch testing; photoallergy, by photopatch testing. Patch testing is relatively easy to perform, but the interpretation requires skill. There is no clinically useful confirmatory test for irritant contact dermatitis.

Other information may be necessary to make a precise diagnosis and formulate appropriate management. Toxicity information on industrial compounds can be obtained from Material Safety Data Sheets, which reveal the composition and properties of industrial materials. In the United States these are available to most employees and their physicians. A visit by the physician to the workplace allows the physician to view the work firsthand. If such a visit is made, opportunity for skin contact with hazardous agents should be explored, as well as the use of protective measures.

Epidemiologic surveys to establish the prevalence of dermatitis in workers at similar jobs and industrial hygiene surveys to characterize the nature and amount of chemical exposure may occasionally be helpful. Public health authorities, university centers for occupational and environmental health, and sometimes concerned employers may be able to assist in such investigations.

TREATMENT. Symptomatic treatment is similar to that for dermatitis of other types. Acute contact dermatitis is treated with cold wet dressings of Burow's solution. Systemic steroids in rapidly tapering doses are indicated in severe acute widespread disabling eruptions; topical steroids and emollients, for dry and chronic eczema. Superinfection requires appropriate systemic antibiotics. Antihistamines may be given for sedation and are mildly antipruritic. The patient should be given careful instruction to avoid casual exposures and should be alerted to the fact that even when the skin has apparently healed, the barrier may not have returned to normal. A temporary or permanent change of job tasks may be necessary. If a permanent job change is necessary, vocational rehabilitation should be considered. Some states require reporting of occupational diseases.

PROGNOSIS. The prognosis of occupational contact dermatitis is surprisingly poor, especially if effective treatment is not given early and if the dermatitis is prolonged. The reasons for this are not entirely clear; however, surveys have shown that a high percentage of individuals still have dermatitis several years later, in many cases despite a change of employment. Those with atopy appear to have the worst prognosis. In allergic contact dermatitis, the prognosis is dependent on the ease with which the allergen can be avoided.

PREVENTION. Preventive measures serve both to prevent recurrences and to halt the development of new disease. These include elimination of or substitution for strong irritants and sensitizers; education of workers regarding skin care; avoidance of overly harsh skin cleansers; prompt reporting and treatment of dermatitis; engineering controls to minimize skin contact with potential hazards; appropriate impervious protective clothing; good personal hygiene with rapid, effective removal of contaminants; and counseling of individuals with predisposing conditions, such as atopy, regarding career selection.

OTHER OCCUPATIONAL DERMATOSES

A relatively large number of other dermatoses can result from occupational exposure. In large part, management is dependent upon diagnostic recognition and on discontinuing further exposures, using measures outlined above.

Chemical burns result from corrosive agents that produce necrosis, ulceration, and subsequent scarring. Prompt removal

of these agents (such as strong acids, alkalies, phenol, alkyl metal compounds, and metal chlorides) from skin, eyes, and mucous membranes is essential. Water is generally best for removal. Quicklime, tin tetrachloride, and titanium tetrachloride should be removed with mineral oil. Specific antidotes are few; these include topical or injected calcium gluconate for hydrofluoric acid burns.

Urticaria may occur from local contact with or systemic absorption of agents that elicit an immediate hypersensitivity reaction or directly release histamine and other vasoactive substances.

Fiber glass dermatitis causes intense pruritus; there may be no visible changes, or it may be accompanied by excoriations, pinpoint petechial papules, or both. Microscopy of a cellophane tape stripping from the skin, which had been treated with 10 per cent potassium hydroxide, reveals the fibers.

Relatively deep indolent *ulcers* of skin and mucous membranes result from contact with arsenic, chromates, and lime.

Chemical acne and folliculitis may result from contact with greases and oils, coal tar pitch, creosote, and a number of cosmetics (acne cosmetica) and from ingestion of bromides, iodides, and isoniazid. These forms of acne typically commence with comedones or inflammatory papules.

Chloracne is due to halogenated aromatic compounds with specific molecular shape, including dioxin and related chlorinated aromatic hydrocarbons. The illness is characterized by small straw-colored cysts and comedones that first involve the malar crescent and behind the ear and may not spread beyond these areas. Inflammatory pustules, abscesses, and large cysts may be seen in severe cases. Chloracne is the first and most constant finding in chronic dioxin poisoning. More variable findings may include porphyrinuria, hyperpigmentation, hypertrichosis, central and peripheral nervous system effects, alteration of lipid metabolism, and mild hepatotoxicity. Experimentally observed effects include teratogenicity, immunosuppression, and tumor induction.

Cutaneous granulomas occur as slightly erythematous grouped flesh-colored papules, with or without inflammatory changes, from foreign body reactions at the site of contact with talc and silica or as an immunologic response to beryllium and zirconium.

Chemical leukoderma, which may mimic vitiligo but which is confined to the areas of skin contact, may result from a number of phenols and catechols, including hydroquinone, monobenzyl, and monomethyl ethers of hydroquinone (used as rubber additives) and *p*-tertiary butyl and related phenols (in disinfectants).

Basal and squamous cell carcinomas and keratoacanthomas result from prolonged exposures to UV radiation, ionizing radiation, polycyclic aromatic hydrocarbons (including coal tar pitches and related products), and arsenic. Exposures to arsenic may be associated with various internal malignant neoplasms.

Cutaneous T cell lymphoma (mycosis fungoides) may be more frequent in those who have worked in heavy industry or who have industrial chemical exposure, but the particular causal agents are uncertain.

INFECTIONS AND INFESTATIONS

The development of infections and infestations frequently depends on occupational factors, individual susceptibility, and the geographic distribution of the causal organism. Occupational associations include the following:

Viral. Herpes simplex (dentists, medical personnel), milkers' nodules and papular stomatitis (veterinarians, milk handlers), orf (farmers, shepherds, abattoir workers), viral warts (butchers), Rift Valley fever (shepherds).

Bacterial. Staphylococcal infections of hands (abattoir workers and butchers), erysipeloid (fish, fowl, rabbit, and pig handlers), anthrax (wool, hair, and hide handlers), tularemia (farmers), nontuberculous mycobacterial infections (aquarium workers and pet shop attendants). Bacterial and yeast infections and tinea versicolor are prominent where there is heat, humidity, and lack of hygiene.

Fungal. Dermatophyte infections are more frequent in farm workers, surveyors, zoo attendants, animal care technicians, and certain others. Particular examples include tinea verrucosum (farmers); infection due to *Trichophyton rubrum* (miners), *Microsporum canis* (pet shop workers), *Trichophyton violaceum* (wrestlers), and *Candida albicans* (those in wet work, particularly those in contact with sugar and fruit); sporotrichosis (mine workers); chromomycosis (agricultural workers); and actinomycosis (agricultural workers).

Protozoal. South American leishmaniasis (foresters).

Helminths. Creeping eruption (plumbers, gardeners, farm workers in the tropics), ankylostomiasis (miners), schistosomiasis and cercarial dermatitis (rice planters and canal workers).

In addition, bites and stings of arthropods and other creatures are common in those who work out of doors and in certain other occupations.

Adams RM: Occupational Skin Disease. New York, Grune & Stratton, 1983. *A comprehensive review of contact dermatitis and related conditions, with descriptions of skin diseases caused by a variety of agents and with detailed lists of agents encountered in various occupations.*

Maibach HI (ed.): Occupational and Industrial Dermatology. Chicago, Year Book Medical Publishers, 1987. *A multiauthor text that broadly covers occupational dermatoses and dermatotoxicology and describes the skin diseases caused by a number of specific agents.*

530 Radiation Injury

Theodore L. Phillips

DEFINITION. Radiation injury may be defined as any somatic or genetic disruption of function or form caused by electromagnetic waves or accelerated particles. Common sources of such injury include ultraviolet radiation from the sun and man-made sources; microwave radiation from radar, ovens, and other appliances; high-intensity ultrasound; and ionizing radiation from natural and man-made sources.

Ultraviolet radiation, produced by the sun, is largely absorbed by the atmosphere of the earth. It penetrates tissue poorly and so is a threat only to exposed body surfaces. Injury occurs through direct chemical effects in molecules with high ultraviolet absorbance. Ultrasound and microwaves exert their effects by generating heat during absorption.

Radiation with wavelengths shorter than that of light has an additional property: the ability to displace electrons from their normal orbits. As these electrons traverse tissue, they generate ions and free radicals, which then react with biologically important molecules, leading to cell death. High-energy rays have the ability to penetrate and cause severe biologic damage after deposition of small amounts of energy.

Ionizing radiation, both natural and man-made, is of two types—photons (or waves) and accelerated particles. Photons, called *gamma rays*, are given off in many types of nuclear decay. Man-made ionizing rays, called x-rays, occur when an electron is stopped in a dense material. Accelerated particles include protons from solar radiation, heavy nuclei in cosmic rays, and beta and alpha particles given up in nuclear decay. These particles are charged, and they cause direct ionization. Neutrons are given off in nuclear decay and cause damage through secondary reactions in tissue in which protons are produced.

Radiation dose is defined in terms of energy deposition. The basic unit is the *gray* (Gy), equal to 1 joule per kilogram. Radioactivity is defined in terms of the rate of decay; one disintegration per second is a becquerel (Bq) (Table 530–1).

Because radiations differ in the density of the ionization they cause, their biologic effects vary; densely ionizing radiations have profound biologic effects. Thus, a unit called the sievert (Sv) is used to express risk estimates in which a *quality factor* is applied to the absorbed dose. Additional weight may be applied, depending on the specific organ or organs irradiated.

Absorption of charged particles and their range in tissue are determined by their charge and mass. Particles with high charge and mass give up their energy rapidly and penetrate only short distances, unless they are of high energy. Photons are absorbed exponentially by electron or nuclear interactions. Because photons diverge as they leave the source, the dose decreases as the square of the distance from the source.

Injury from radiation may be either thermal or ionizing. Ionizing radiation injury expressed within a few hours or days is called *acute;* when expressed after months or years, it is called *delayed.*

ETIOLOGY. *Biology of Ultraviolet Radiation.* Ultraviolet light photons are capable of generating chemical changes in DNA and other molecules, the most important of which is the production of pyrimidine dimers. Although these dimers may be excised and the DNA repaired, if unrepaired, these lesions lead to reproductive cell death and desquamation after skin irradiation. Ultraviolet exposure also causes immediate effects, such as vasodilatation and erythema. The limited penetration and the absorption by melanin limit human injury to the superficial layers of the skin and the eye. Solar carcinogenesis in the skin and eye is a major problem.

Biology of Ionizing Radiations. When electrons traverse a cell, they cause the formation of ion pairs both in cell water and in the DNA. During such events, reactive radicals containing unpaired outer electrons are formed. These radicals react with DNA or occur in the DNA itself. A radical may be repaired by reduction by SH groups or fixed by oxidation or electron transfer. If a free radical persists, it leads to a break in the DNA strand. Single-strand breaks are generally repaired, but if two occur side by side, a double-strand break occurs. Unrepaired double-strand breaks lead to chromosome aberrations that are lethal.

Chromosome injury is expressed at the time of cell division, which causes most mammalian cells to die a mitotic death. Deletions and dicentric chromosomes lead to loss of genetic information at each cell division. Some cells may survive a few divisions but will be incapable of sustained reproduction. Intermitotic death occurs in some lymphocytes and gonadal cells, even after low radiation doses, but most cells will survive 10 to 30 Gy until mitosis occurs.

Dose-Response Relationships. The percentage of cells that survive after exposure to ionizing radiation decreases logarithmically with dose. There are two components to the injury, reparable and irreparable, so that most dose survival plots show a shallow slope at small doses and become steeper with increasing dose. Low-level effects are thus generally less than one would expect based on observations at high doses. Cells can repair radiation damage very effectively. Repair is primarily of single- and double-strand DNA breaks and requires only a few hours.

The radiation dose required to reduce survival in mammalian cells to 10 per cent is relatively uniform. The most sensitive cells require 1 Gy to reduce survival to 10 per cent and the most resistant, about 5 Gy. Changes in sensitivity by a factor of 3 occur under hypoxia and as cells traverse the mitotic cycle.

INCIDENCE AND PREVALENCE. *Background Radiation.* Both ionizing and ultraviolet radiations are ubiquitous in the universe because of the fusion processes in stars. Gamma rays, x-rays, and highly energetic particles are emitted by stars and by nuclear decay of isotopes produced by stellar processes. On the earth, radiation comes from isotopes in the earth, water, human body, and construction materials and from the sun and other sources in space. The dose of radiation that one receives from this natural radiation depends on the altitude and the geologic nature of the region. The average annual exposure is 3.6 millisieverts (mSv), about four fifths of which is natural radiation and two thirds of which is due to radon (Table 530–2).

TABLE 530–1. RADIATION DOSE SPECIFICATION

Type	Dose Unit	Definition
Radioactivity	Becquerel (Bq)	One disintegration/second
Absorbed dose	Gray (Gy)	Energy deposited in tissue (1 joule/kg)
Dose equivalent	Sievert (Sv)	Absorbed dose weighted for the quality (damaging effect) of the radiation
Effective dose equivalent	Sievert	Dose equivalent weighted for the sensitivity of the organs
Collective effective dose equivalent	Man sievert	Effective dose equivalent applied to a population

TABLE 530–2. AVERAGE ANNUAL EFFECTIVE DOSE EQUIVALENT OF IONIZING RADIATIONS TO A MEMBER OF THE U.S. POPULATION

Natural		Artificial	
Source	Dose (mSv*)	Source	Dose (mSv*)
Radon	2	Medical	0.53
Cosmic	0.27	Consumer products	0.10
Terrestrial	0.28	Occupational	<0.01
Internal	0.39	Nuclear power	<0.01
		Fallout	<0.01
Total natural	3.0	*Total artificial*	0.63

*MilliSieverts, including quality factor.

Medical Exposure. Shortly after the discovery of x-rays by Roentgen in 1895 and the subsequent discovery of radioactivity, the first medical injuries occurred. The early workers were unaware of the injurious properties of the rays until damage to hands, eyes, and bone marrow became evident. After World War II, the full hazards of radiation exposure were recognized, and exposures were strictly limited. Currently, injury of the acute and chronic types is rare after medical diagnostic exposure but is a side effect of radiation therapy.

Radiation is used in the treatment of 50 to 60 per cent of patients with malignancy; 300,000 to 400,000 patients are exposed annually. Although every precaution is taken to avoid clinically important delayed effects, acute reactions to radiation therapy are common. Since most tumors require doses for cure close to organ tolerance, the risk of injury is always present.

Rarely, injuries occur to medical workers or patients during machine malfunction or repair operations. Workers and patients, as well as the general public, are also exposed to low-level radiation either while obtaining diagnostic studies or while working in medical radiation environments. Permissible exposures have been reduced to 50 mSv for workers and 5 mSv for the public; less than half that exposure is highly recommended. These rules keep the additional medical exposure of the population as a whole to less than one-fifth that of the background level.

Industrial and Military Exposure. High-level radiation exposure to the largest populations occurred at the Hiroshima and Nagasaki fission weapon explosions in World War II. Although most casualties were due to blast and burns, 40 to 50 per cent of the survivors had radiation injury. Late effects have included several hundred cases of leukemia and other malignancies. Atomic weapons testing has led to the inadvertent exposure of 300 or more persons, about 25 per cent of whom show clinically detectable effects. The fallout from nuclear tests initially added about 0.02 mSv to the annual background radiation exposure, but this has now dropped to less than 0.01 mSv.

Radiation accidents can be divided into two groups, depending on whether they involve large groups of the population exposed to relatively low doses or a small number of individuals receiving high doses. In general, accidents involving large numbers of individuals are related to the dispersion of radioactive elements through large areas of environment. Although these accidents may have different causes, the source is extremely important in determining the nature of the radionuclides released.

Most radiation accidents that have occurred have originated in civilian installations. Two reactor accidents can be considered to have had essentially no human consequences, the accidents in the United Kingdom in 1957 (Windscale) and in the United States in 1979 (Three Mile Island). The Chernobyl accident in the Soviet Union in 1986, however, resulted in very extensive releases of radioactivity and contamination with significant doses to a large population in the vicinity of the reactor as well as large collective doses, i.e., small doses multiplied through a large population, in much of the Northern Hemisphere.

Secondary to an explosion and then fire in a graphite reactor of poor design, a cloud of effluent continuing 40 million Ci of iodine-131, 3 million Ci of cesium-137, and 50 million Ci of xenon radioisotopes was released. Thirty per cent of the material was deposited within a 30-km radius of the plant. The majority of the radiation dose to the exposed population came from cesium-137. To put things in perspective, 15 Ci of iodine-131 was released in the Three Mile Island incident.

Of 237 workers showing radiation sickness, 31 individuals died in the Chernobyl accident, 2 of whom were killed by the initial explosion and 29 of whom died of various combinations of thermal and radiation burns as well as gamma radiation injury. An estimated 50,000 Soviets received at least 0.5 Sv of exposure, and 4000 had an average of 2 Sv. The average dose in the United States was 0.002 mSv.

Accidents with sealed medical and industrial sources with high-energy gamma emissions have killed 28 persons. The most recent accident in Brazil involved improper disposal of a medical cesium source, leading to four deaths. In addition, nine persons have been killed in reactor criticality accidents.

Ingestion or inhalation of long-lived isotopes is also potentially injurious. About 5000 persons have been exposed to ingested radium, and at least 400 malignancies have occurred, with increased incidence in the sinuses and in bone. Inhalation of plutonium and other alpha emitters is a problem in the nuclear industry. Eleven deaths due to ingestion of radioactive isotopes other than radium have occurred.

EPIDEMIOLOGY. Radiation injury is not caused by a vector, and the source and nature of the exposure should be obvious. Persons may be exposed without awareness, and clinical symptoms must be identified before an exposure is suspected. In other cases, a psychologically deranged person may have access to radioactive materials and ingest them or expose himself or herself but deny the exposure.

It is important to determine the nature of the exposure and to reconstruct the dose distribution to predict the level of injury and the required treatment.

PATHOGENESIS. Cell Kinetics and Radiation Effects. Cells not subject to intermitotic death can live out their normal lifespan after irradiation, and their injury becomes apparent only because the dying cells cannot be replaced owing to mitotic death. Organs are made up of several populations of cells, some of which do not normally divide and persist for many years after a radiation exposure. Other cells, such as those in the renal tubules and the liver, are replaced slowly, and eventually depopulation occurs. The endothelial cells of the capillary system are slowly replaced. Radiation causes gradual loss of capillary patency, and the number of capillaries decreases.

Specific Tissue Radiobiology. The tissues of the body can be divided into those critical to life and those whose injury by radiation may cause morbidity but is not fatal. The critical tissues for survival are discussed below. *The doses quoted are single exposures to high-energy photons. Because of repair, doses two to four times higher are required for the same effect after fractionated exposures.*

Bone Marrow. Because of the short lifespan and rapid renewal of most peripheral blood and marrow cells, this organ shows the most dramatic clinical syndrome. Small lymphocytes die an intermitotic death, and depletion is seen in a few hours. The half-life of platelets and granulocytes is 1 week, and depletion is maximal at 3 weeks. The half-life of red cells is about 100 days. There is a dynamic balance between the declining numbers of mature cells and regeneration. The marrow regenerates after single whole-body exposures up to at least 6 Gy and may be repopulated by transplantation in some cases after doses up to 10 Gy.

Intestines. The mature surface and villus cells of the intestinal mucosa are replaced by the division of cells in the crypts that migrate up the villus. In contrast to this rapid renewal system, the muscular wall contains a slowly renewing capillary network. Doses as low as 1 Gy can reduce crypt cell survival to 50 per cent, but histopathologically detectable injury requires 10 Gy or more. After 15 Gy, the cell kill in the crypt is sufficient to cause complete loss of the villus and in some cases denudation, followed by repopulation. Higher local doses produce these acute changes but also lead to late fibrotic changes in the muscular layer and serosa caused by capillary injury.

Central Nervous System. The central nervous system has no rapid cell renewal systems, but the glial cells and the endothelial cells cycle slowly and can show injury. The neurons are not injured, except secondarily, at doses below 60 Gy. Large exposures of 50 to 500 Gy can produce acute functional changes and, at the highest doses, immediate death. After 15 Gy, changes begin in 4 to 5 months and persist in development over 1 to 2 years. Focal necrosis and calcification, demyelinization, and gliosis are seen, particularly in the white matter (see Ch. 162).

Skin. After exposure to between 3 and 9 Gy, the skin can show transient vasodilatation, cessation of mitosis in the basal layer, and thinning of the prickle cell layer. At doses above 20 Gy, denudation and ulceration occur before repopulation begins from either surviving basal cells or cells at the periphery of the exposed area. The cells of the hair follicles and sweat glands are often depleted and will not regenerate after 20 Gy. Late vascular damage can cause a second wave of ulceration.

Lung. In the lung, both the type II pneumocytes and the capillary cells, as well as the mucosal cells of the bronchial tree, regenerate slowly. About 90 days after a dose of 10 Gy, acute pneumonitis occurs, capillaries occlude, and endothelial cells are lost. This situation is preceded by depletion of surfactant and type II cells. Secondary influx of alveolar macrophages is seen. The acute phase is followed over the ensuing 9 months by replacement of the capillaries and alveoli by collagen. Acute pneumonitis is reversible only at the lowest doses, 6 to 10 Gy in a single exposure.

Heart. The cardiac muscle cells do not proliferate, so almost all radiation changes occur primarily in the endothelium of the capillaries. Four to 6 months after exposure of up to 15 Gy or more, the capillaries become occluded and show a dose-related reduction in number. This situation can lead to a secondary loss of muscle cells. The pericardium is also injured, with resulting effusion and fibrotic thickening.

Liver. The hepatocytes are normally replaced very slowly, but injury to the liver can induce a wave of cell division. The sinusoidal endothelium in the lobules is also continuously replaced. Six weeks after exposure to 10 Gy, central lobular occlusion occurs, and there is secondary hepatocyte loss and portal hypertension.

Kidney. After 10 Gy, the tubule cells are reduced in number and exhibit flattening in the tubule lining. Whole nephrons are lost over a period of 4 to 18 months after exposure. At the same time, many capillaries are occluded. At 1 year and beyond, damage in the glomerulus, with loss of foot processes and thickening of the basement membrane, can be seen. Secondary hypertension is common.

Gonads. In contrast to most other tissues during fractionated exposure, the gonads are quite sensitive to complete depopulation of the reproductive cells. Sterilization can occur after exposure to as little as 5 to 10 Gy, and prolonged hypospermia after even a smaller exposure. The hormone-secreting cells of the gonads are much more resistant, but, of course, ovarian hormone secretion is dependent on ovulation and is obliterated by sterilization.

CLINICAL MANIFESTATIONS. *Acute Whole-Body Exposures.* The classic acute whole-body radiation syndrome is usually seen after reactor accidents, after malfunction of large treatment or research accelerators or industrial radiation facilities, and after nuclear explosions. It is also seen after total-body irradiation for bone marrow transplantation and treatment of malignancy. In the subsequent discussion, doses quoted are for single exposures. *For fractionated exposures, doses two to four times higher are needed for the same effect because of repair.*

The initial symptoms are directly related to the radiation dose. After 2 Gy, about half the patients exhibit nausea and vomiting 2 to 6 hours after exposure. After 3 Gy, the incidence is 100 per cent. With doses above 3 Gy, three syndromes occur:

1. *The hematologic syndrome* occurs in patients who receive up to 10 or 12 Gy. At these doses, although the small intestine is affected, there is usually little or no diarrhea, and the bowel is not denuded. The chief effects are in the bone marrow, although patients who survive the acute phase can develop lung or kidney injury months to years later. In the hematologic syndrome, the patient experiences the prodromal symptoms of nausea and vomiting, and in the most serious cases these are often associated with malaise and weakness. These symptoms subside over the first 24 hours and may be followed by salivary gland swelling in some patients. If the dose has been less than 5 Gy, there will then be a quiescent period of 2 to 3 weeks. At that point, depopulation of the marrow and the resultant fall in granulocyte and platelet levels lead to infection and hemorrhage.

Purpura, petechiae, and fever are common. Skin erythema and desquamation can occur, particularly if there are local areas that have received higher doses. Temporary epilation occurs if the patient survives. If the dose is 3 Gy or below, recovery is the rule, and patients who have received doses up to 5 or 6 Gy can recover if they have medical support.

2. *The gastrointestinal syndrome* occurs at doses of 12 to 30 Gy. When the dose exceeds that needed to denude the small bowel, the gastrointestinal syndrome occurs before the hematologic syndrome and, since it is usually fatal, is the dominant manifestation. After initial symptoms similar to those of the hematologic syndrome, a brief asymptomatic period ensues, although malaise and diarrhea may be persistent. Five to 7 days after exposure, severe diarrhea and fluid loss occur, followed by infection with enteric bacteria. It is not possible to survive this syndrome after whole-body exposure, even with modern support techniques.

3. *The cardiovascular–central nervous system syndrome* occurs after very large doses and is uniformly fatal. After 20 to 50 Gy, the patient experiences immediate nausea, vomiting, and diarrhea. This condition is followed rapidly by ataxia, sweating, prostration, and shock. Huge doses, such as 300 to 500 Gy, can cause immediate death due to generalized central nervous system dysfunction.

Local or Regional Radiation Injury. The clinical syndromes following whole-body irradiation are all associated with acute effects that subside within 2 months of exposure. Local or regional exposures to very high doses may not be immediately fatal, and delayed effects can be seen. Local irradiation of the bone marrow does not usually produce a detectable clinical syndrome. The peripheral white and red cell counts are depressed, but more than half the marrow must be exposed to doses over 4 Gy before any clinical symptoms similar to those of the acute whole-body syndrome appear. Doses over 10 Gy in a single exposure or 25 Gy in a fractionated exposure produce prolonged aplasia of the marrow in the irradiated area. When the percentage of marrow irradiated is large, clinical symptoms of marrow hypoplasia will occur if additional radiation exposure, infection, or cytotoxic chemotherapy occurs. Abdominal irradiation can lead to signs and symptoms from the liver, kidney, and small bowel. The stomach and colon can be injured by doses of fractionated radiotherapy over 50 Gy. Radiation hepatopathy results in ascites, with other signs of portal hypertension 6 to 8 weeks after the exposure. Renal injury leads to proteinuria and edema 6 to 8 months later. Hypertension, occasionally severe, can be seen 1 to 10 years after exposure, as can renal failure. The acute small bowel or gastrointestinal syndrome can occur after abdominal exposure, but it is usually not fatal after local exposures. Delayed injury to the small bowel results in signs of intestinal obstruction, malabsorption, or diarrhea. Gastric irradiation produces signs of hypochlorhydria and at 15 Gy can lead to large greater curvature ulcers. Local irradiation of the central nervous system produces late signs. Whole-brain irradiation with 10 Gy in a single exposure causes edema with transient nausea and vomiting. Doses of 15 to 20 Gy can be fatal in 6 to 18 months, with generalized dementia. More focal irradiation can produce a mass lesion, with focal signs, headache, and vomiting. Injury to the skin results from local or regional exposures. This injury produces transient erythema the first day. After 3 weeks, erythema, dry desquamation, or moist desquamation can occur. Epidermolysis and chronic ulceration occur with single exposures over 25 Gy.

Thoracic irradiation can lead to symptoms due to either cardiac or pulmonary damage. Pulmonary damage is first seen 3 to 4 months after a single exposure or 6 weeks to 2 months after a fractionated exposure. The patient experiences fever, dyspnea, and cyanosis. If the acute phase is survived, chronic signs of pulmonary constriction and fibrosis will appear. Somewhat higher doses cause acute pericarditis, producing symptoms similar to those of a viral pericarditis, with fever, malaise, and some dyspnea 7 to 24 months after irradiation. Paradoxical pulse and cardiac tamponade can be seen with large pericardial effusions. Myocardial infarction and chronic myocarditis are sometimes seen.

Gonadal irradiation in the male rarely leads to symptoms. The patient becomes oligospermic after low doses and aspermic after higher doses about 6 weeks later. In the female, ovarian effects usually occur by the next menstrual cycle and result in amenorrhea, which is rarely reversible after doses of 5 Gy in single exposures or 20 Gy in fractionated exposures.

Systemic Exposure to Radionuclides. Systemic isotopes cause whole-body exposure and specific organ exposure, depending on the concentration of the isotope by the organ and the nature and energy of the radioactivity. Ingestion of iodine-131 leads to a whole-body exposure and high doses in the normal thyroid. There can be symptoms of nausea and vomiting, as well as the hematologic syndrome followed by hypothyroidism and pharyngitis. Plutonium concentrates in the pulmonary macrophages, causing local fibrosis and malignancy. For each isotope, it is necessary to know the distribution to predict the symptoms.

Delayed Effects of Low-Level Exposure. These effects are genetic and carcinogenic. If an exposure does not lead to sterilization, genetic damage can persist in the spermatogonia and oocytes. Experiments have shown point mutations in mice, but they have been difficult to prove in humans because of the background of about 10 per cent spontaneous abortions. The risk is estimated as being about one congenital abnormality per million live births per millisievert of exposure. The risk of carcinogenesis varies by organ and ranges from 70 to 1000 cases per sievert per million people exposed per year of follow-up.

DIAGNOSIS. It is essential that any facility likely to treat radiation injuries have a trained team on call. The physician should obtain as clear a history as possible about the exposure, including the nature of the radiation, the distance from the source, and any documentation such as monitors, badges, and witnesses. A preliminary estimate of the dose should be made from the history as well as from the symptoms. Malaise, nausea, and vomiting suggest an exposure over 1 Gy and occur in all patients who have been exposed to 3 Gy or more (Table 530–3). The physical examination should pay particular attention to the skin, conjunctivae, mucous membranes, and salivary glands. After high local doses, there may be acute erythema; 2 to 3 weeks after exposure, signs of infection or hemorrhage may be present.

Laboratory tests should include a complete blood count with differential. The total lymphocyte count directly reflects the whole-body dose within 24 hours. Elevation of the granulocyte count can occur transiently at 24 to 48 hours. If possible, a lymphocyte culture should be done by a cytogeneticist to determine the number of chromosome aberrations, which allows calculation of the dose received. Pulmonary function tests are useful after thoracic irradiation, as are lung scans and chest computed tomographs (CT's). Blood counts are essential 1 to 3 weeks after exposure to follow the pancytopenia and to direct therapy. In the gastrointestinal syndrome, there may be findings of dehydration and electrolyte imbalances.

Whole-Body Exposure. The total granulocyte count may rise transiently to 10,000 or more 24 to 48 hours after exposure, while the total lymphocyte count falls close to zero with doses of 3 Gy or more. The granulocyte count hits a nadir at 4 weeks and then returns toward normal at 8 weeks. The lymphocyte count may remain low for many years.

Local or Regional Exposure. Clinical findings after such exposure vary widely and reflect injury to the specific organ involved. Central nervous system damage will be reflected in an abnormal neurologic examination, with signs of edema and enhancing areas on the CT scan months to years after irradiation.

Radiation injury to the thorax is usually detected on the chest radiograph, although CT yields more accurate information on the volume of lung affected. Initially, areas of patchy or confluent pneumonitis conform to the shape of the exposed area. This condition progresses to stranded fibrosis and retraction. Cardiac injury may lead to transient electrocardiographic abnormalities, pericarditis with effusion detectable on ultrasound scans, and signs of myocardial ischemia.

Abdominal exposure leads to abnormal kidney and liver function test results. High doses to the pancreas can lead to diabetes and decreased pancreatic enzymes. Chronic diarrhea can occur owing to malabsorption and bile salt irritation.

Systemic Exposure to Radioisotopes. Large doses of gamma ray–emitting isotopes can cause symptoms and signs similar to those seen in the acute whole-body syndrome or local skin or mucosal injury. The most important diagnostic tests that must be obtained are radioactivity counts and spectroscopy to identify the isotope or isotopes, predict the dose, and localize the injury. Urine and blood samples should be obtained (and, if possible, a whole-body count in a suitable counter).

TREATMENT. Acute Whole-Body Exposure. The initial symptoms of whole-body exposure can be treated with antiemetics. The profound weakness seen at doses above 3 Gy can be reduced by a short course of intravenous corticosteroids. Further therapy is not needed for patients who have received 2 Gy or less. Above that, and up to 10 Gy, survival is possible with active medical management. Support similar to that used for the patient with pancytopenic leukemia is required, including reverse isolation or life island–type support. Trauma and burns complicate the situation and may dominate in terms of survival. Antibiotics should be used if the granulocyte count is below 1000 per microliter or if infection is present, in which case granulocyte transfusions should be used as well. Platelet transfusions should be given if the platelet count is below 10,000 per microliter. The diarrhea seen at doses below 10 Gy is usually mild but may require intravenous fluid and electrolyte replacement. Bone marrow transplantation may be a useful adjunct at doses of 5 Gy or more.

The experience after the Chernobyl accident, however, indicates that bone marrow transplantation in this kind of situation is only marginally effective. All the persons exposed to radiation doses at the level of 3 to 10 Gy or higher sustained significant trauma as well as thermal and superficial radiation burns. The effects of these injuries complicated the medical management. Bone marrow transplantation was used after Chernobyl in 13 patients, with 2 surviving. The donor marrow take was only transient in three patients who survived. Five died of burns, three of gastrointestinal damage, and three of pneumonitis, two of which were graft-versus-host related. Support with antibiotics, blood, platelets, and fluids seems the most effective treatment. Colony-stimulating factors and interleukins may be of great use in patients exposed to 6 to 10 Gy. Bone marrow transplantation can be considered for those exposed to 7 to 10 Gy if a good donor match is found.

Bone marrow samples and peripheral blood for tissue typing

TABLE 530–3. SYMPTOMS, THERAPY, AND PROGNOSIS AFTER RADIATION INJURY IN HUMANS

Dose range	0–1 Gy	1–2 Gy	2–6 Gy	6–10 Gy	10–20 Gy
Therapeutic needs	None	Observation	Specific treatment	Possible treatment	Palliative
Vomiting	None	5–50%	3 Gy = 100%	100%	100%
Time delay, nausea, and vomiting	—	3 hr	2 hr	1 hr	30 min
Main organ damaged	None	Lymphocytes	Bone marrow	Bone marrow	Small bowel
Symptoms and signs	—	Moderate leukopenia	Leukopenia, purpura, hemorrhage, epilation	Leukopenia, purpura, hemorrhage, epilation	Diarrhea, fever, electrolyte imbalance
Critical period	—	—	4–6 wk	4–6 wk	5–14 days
Therapy	Psycho-therapy	Observation	Transfusion of granulocytes, platelets; antibiotics	Transfusion; antibiotics; bone marrow transplant	Fluids and salts; possible bone marrow transplant
Prognosis	Excellent	Excellent	Guarded	Guarded	Poor
Lethality	None	None	0–80%	80–100%	100%
Time of death	—	—	2 mo	1–2 mo	2 wk
Cause of death	—	—	Infection, hemorrhage	Hemorrhage, infection	Enteritis, infection

should be obtained early, before depletion occurs. Techniques should be similar to those used for leukemia (Ch. 153). Exposures above 12 Gy (which will lead to the gastrointestinal or central nervous system syndrome) are uniformly fatal. Palliative support with fluids is indicated, as is the treatment of infection or hemorrhage.

Local or Regional Exposure. Skin reactions are the most common injury requiring treatment. Dry or moist desquamation occurs and can be ameliorated with cleansing, using an antibacterial soap. Crusts should be soaked off and the open areas dressed with petroleum jelly or bacitracin ointment. Large areas can benefit from temporary lanolin closed dressings, which should be changed daily, with the wound being washed before each redressing (Table 530–4).

The electrolyte imbalances seen with nausea and vomiting must be corrected. Radiation pneumonitis can be reversed at borderline doses with prednisone, 60 mg per day tapered the ensuing month. The acute symptoms of pericarditis can be relieved by aspirin or other anti-inflammatory agents. Cardiac tamponade should be treated by pericardiocentesis or a pericardial window. Delayed effects of doses of 20 Gy or more may require skin grafts, resection of necrotic bone, and other surgical procedures, including resection of necrotic brain tissue.

Systemic Exposure to Radionuclides. After the victim has been given urgent first aid and has been decontaminated, the dose and nature of the exposure should be determined, making use of a whole-body counter if possible. Large body burdens should be treated by specific methods designed to remove the isotope or to block uptake. After iodine exposure, stable iodine should be given as 5 drops of potassium iodide. One gram of soluble phosphate should be given to patients ingesting phosphorus-32. Radium ingestion can be treated with magnesium sulfate or epsom salts, 10 grams in 100 ml of water. Strontium exposure is treated with 100 ml of aluminum phosphate gel.

Pulmonary exposures to aerosols or dust can be treated by bronchial lavage, expectorants, or diethylenetriamine pentaacetic acid (DTPA) aerosol mist. DTPA products are available from the U.S. Department of Energy.

Gastrointestinal absorption can be reduced with mild laxatives. Sodium alginate and aluminum hydroxide gel may reduce strontium uptake. Certain heavier isotopes, including plutonium, americium, yttrium, lanthanum, cerium, scandium, and zinc, as well as other fission products can be partially removed from the body by DTPA. A dose of 0.5 to 1.0 gram should be given intravenously in 250 ml of normal saline.

PROGNOSIS. *Acute Radiation Syndromes.* Survival with little or no treatment other than good hygiene and treatment of infections can be expected after exposures to 3 Gy or less. Between 3 and 6 Gy, therapy with antibiotics, platelets, and granulocytes allows for a high survival rate. Leukemic patients show 80 per cent survival after 10 Gy of whole-body exposure at a dose rate of 4 Gy per hour when bone marrow transplantation is used. The use of all available methods may allow a high rate of survival after 5 Gy and some survival after acute exposures to 9 Gy.

The presence of traumatic and thermal injuries reduces the chances of survival across the whole range of radiation doses above 3 Gy. Of the 200 people receiving the highest doses at Chernobyl, 105 had received 1 to 2 Gy. All survived. Eight persons had higher doses but less than 6 Gy; seven survived. There were 25 patients thought to have received more than 6 Gy. Of these, 13 were given a bone marrow transplant, and 11 died. The other 12 did not undergo transplantation because of injuries (10), mismatch (1), or refusal (1) or because they were given fetal liver cells (6); all died. Thus, bone marrow transplantation in this group was less effective than that in patients undergoing transplantation for aplasia or leukemia.

Local Radiation Effects. Acute skin reactions usually heal completely. If the exposure has been over 20 Gy, late ulceration can be expected. Most delayed radiation injury is irreversible and slowly progressive as depopulation of stromal and capillary cells occurs.

Systemic Exposure. The prognosis depends on the whole-body radiation dose and the isotope. Large whole-body doses result in a prognosis similar to that for whole-body external exposure. Thyroid ablation occurs after 50 to 100 mCi of iodine-125, and bone marrow ablation occurs after smaller doses of phosphorus-32.

PREVENTION. Because radiation injury always has an irreversible component not subject to repair, prevention is essential. The largest exposure to the population is from the natural background and can be limited by careful selection of building materials and good ventilation of the home.

The next largest exposure is medical. This can be limited by careful selection of diagnostic tests. Optimal techniques and shielding of the gonads must be employed. Substitution of CT at some sites is helpful. The design of facilities must limit the exposure of public and monitored personnel to less than recommended levels. Proper training of workers using radiation is essential. Radiation treatment must be carried out by highly skilled specialists who limit the dose as much as possible to tumor areas.

Baramov A, Gale RP, Guskova A, et al.: Bone marrow transplantation after the Chernobyl nuclear accident. N Engl J Med 321:205, 1989. *A complete report on the attempts to treat persons exposed to high radiation doses at Chernobyl.*

Champlin RE, Kastenberg WE, Gale RP: Radiation accidents and nuclear energy: Medical consequences and therapy (clinical conference). Ann Intern Med 109:730, 1988. *A valuable general discussion of the handling of nuclear accidents.*

Hall EJ: Radiobiology for the Radiobiologist. 3rd ed. Philadelphia, J. B. Lippincott, 1988. *The best introductory text on the biologic effects of radiation for the medical worker.*

Health Effects of Exposures to Low Levels of Ionizing Radiation. Washington, D.C. BEIR V, National Academy Press, 1990. *The most up-to-date survey of health risks to populations from low-level radiation.*

Johns HE, Cunningham JR: The Physics of Radiology. 4th ed. Springfield, Ill., Charles C Thomas, 1983. *The most comprehensive text in the field of medical radiation physics.*

Nenot JC: Overview of the radiological accidents in the world, updated December 1989. Int J Radiat Biol 57:1073, 1990. *The most complete and most recent discussions of the world's major military, industrial, and medical accidents.*

TABLE 530–4. ORGAN DAMAGE, DYSFUNCTION, TREATMENT, AND PROGNOSIS AFTER IRRADIATION

Organ	Acute Lesion	Delayed Lesion	Clinical Signs	Treatment	Prognosis
Bone marrow	Pancytopenia	Vascular occlusion Myelofibrosis	Infection Hemorrhage	Antibiotics Transfusion	Good if percent of total marrow irradiation is small
Intestine	Flattened villi	Fibrosis, obstruction	Diarrhea	Fluid and electrolytes for acute symptoms Resection for obstruction	Good for acute Obstruction can be fatal
Central nervous system	Edema	Necrosis	Headache Focal neurologic	— Resection	Poor Fair
Skin	Desquamation	Ulcer, necrosis	Pain, oozing	Cleansing, ointments, graft	Good
Lung	Pneumonitis	Fibrosis	Cough, fever, cyanosis, dyspnea	Corticosteroids	Good at low dose Good if small volume
Heart	Pericarditis	Carditis	Fever dyspnea	Anti-inflammatory agents, pericardiocentesis	Fair
Liver	Central venous thrombosis	Fibrosis	Ascites	Diuretics	Fair
Kidney	Tubular degeneration	Fibrosis	Proteinuria Hypertension, renal failure	Dialysis Transplantation	Fair

Principles and general procedures for handling emergency and accidental exposures of workers. Ann ICRP 2:1, 1978. *Detailed instructions and useful references for physicians who may be required to deal with victims of accidental exposure.*

Protection against ionizing radiation from external sources used in medicine. Ann ICRP 9:1, 1982. *The basic international manual that sets dose limits, protection standards, and monitoring standards. Essential for anyone employing radiation equipment.*

Shapiro J: Radiation Protection: A Guide for Scientists and Physicians. 3rd ed. Cambridge, Mass., Harvard University Press, 1990. *The standard introductory text for all radiation workers.*

Sources, Effects and Risks of Ionizing Radiation. New York, United Nations Publications, 1988. *A detailed compendium of radiation units, dose assessments, and risk assessments, with a review of the present situation.*

531 Electrical Injury

Cleon W. Goodwin

DEFINITION AND PREVALENCE. Electrical injury manifests in a variety of forms, ranging from cardiopulmonary arrest and minimal tissue damage to devastating electrocution and vaporization of major body parts. Tissue damage is a direct consequence of thermal injury generated by the flow of electrical current. The extent of injury is proportional to current, voltage, duration of exposure, and whether the electricity is alternating current or direct current. Alternating current is more dangerous than direct current because it can produce tonic muscle contractions and the victim may be unable to release the source of electricity. Further, cardiac arrest and coma frequently accompany electrocution with alternating current, and these events are most likely to occur at current frequencies of 50 to 60 cycles per second. As frequency increases above 60 cycles per second, tissue damage and risk of cardiac arrest decrease. Tissue damage caused by line voltages less than 1000 volts arbitrarily is designated as low-voltage injury. High-tension electrical injury is caused by line voltages above 1000 volts.

Electricity causes injury by four mechanisms: direct contact, conduction, arc, and secondary ignition. Low-voltage electrical sources produce direct injury at the point of contact. Skin and subcutaneous tissue are involved most commonly, although occasionally muscle and bone beneath the cutaneous burn may be damaged. High-voltage current not only causes direct injury at the point of contact but also damages tissues that conduct the electricity through the body. Arc burns occur without actual contact of the body surface with the source of electricity. Very high voltages are required to produce charge transfer, and when arcing occurs, extremely high temperatures are produced. The duration of the arc is brief, and the "flash" injury produced is usually limited to the body surface. A variant of arc injury occurs when electrical current being conducted along a body part flashes directly to an adjacent body part; such injuries are frequently observed in the axilla and other flexion creases. Finally, burns occur when the electrical source ignites clothing and other flammable materials. Very deep flame burns may occur, especially if the patient is unconscious. The victim may not be able to verify whether direct contact has occurred, and patient evaluation and management must assume that diverse multisystem effects of electrical injury may be present.

In an adult, electrical burns are occupational hazards. However, in recent years, the increasing number of electrical injuries reflects the technologic sophistication of society. Sport parachuting and hot air ballooning and installation of home radio and television antennas have become common causes of electrical injuries. In urban environments, electric-powered mass transit conduits are one of the most common sources of such injuries. Household appliances cause most electrical injuries in children. Lightning injury affects all age groups, especially in rural areas. Electrical injuries comprise 1 to 5 per cent of burn center admissions and up to 15 per cent of deaths.

PATHOGENESIS. Meticulous laboratory investigations have verified that tissue damage associated with electrical injury occurs when electrical energy is converted to thermal energy. The resulting injury is a thermal burn that produces physiologic responses similar to those caused by other mechanisms of thermal injury. Skin represents the initial barrier to current flow and is an effective insulator to deeper tissues. After electrical contact and the onset of current flow, the skin undergoes coagulation necrosis and desiccates. With low-voltage injuries, the charred skin at the point of contact terminates current flow and limits the extent of injury. The skin surrounding the contact point may sustain an arc burn as the increase in skin resistance terminates current flow (Fig. 531–1). At high voltages (over 1000 volts) skin resistance initially is overcome, and current flow through deep tissue in the body is unimpeded. Except for bone, these internal tissues act as a volume conductor, offering little resistance to flow. Current flow is terminated when the tissue at the point of electrical contact desiccates and resistance increases markedly. At this point, electrical arcing frequently occurs. The charred tissue now acts as an electrical insulator. No further tissue damage is possible.

Deep tissue damage is related to the density of current flow through these tissues. Heat production and, hence, thermal injury depend on the density of current flow. In body parts with small cross-sectional areas, such as an extremity, current density is high, and tissue destruction is severe. In areas of large cross-sectional areas, such as the trunk, current density is reduced, and deep injuries are unusual. Superficial tissues cool faster than deep tissues. Because bone has high resistance to current flow, it heats to higher temperatures than does surrounding soft tissue. As a result, the most severely damaged soft tissues are usually muscle and nerves directly adjacent to the bone, a position almost impervious to clinical detection. The most severe cutaneous and deep injuries are adjacent to contact sites, and damage decreases with increasing distance from contact points.

The extent of tissue injury appears to be determined at the time of electrical contact. Progressive soft tissue injury probably does not occur in spite of the clinical observation that muscle that appears to be viable immediately after electrical injury becomes necrotic several days later. In addition, electrical energy may cause lesser degrees of damage without producing coagulation necrosis. This phenomenon may explain the transient abnormalities of visceral organ function that follow electrical injury. In the heart, this minor damage may have disastrous consequences. In electrically injured patients who experience fatal cardiac arrest, focal necrosis of the myocardium and the specialized tissue of the sinus and atrioventricular nodes and contraction band necrosis of smooth muscle cells of the coronary arteries are widespread.

CLINICAL MANIFESTATIONS. High-voltage electrical injuries commonly involve multiple organ systems and dictate treatment in specialized burn treatment centers with broad multidisciplinary capabilities. Many of the abnormalities produced by electrocution may not be reflected by the surface appearance of the electrical burn and may not manifest clinically until long after admission. Consequently, meticulous serial ex-

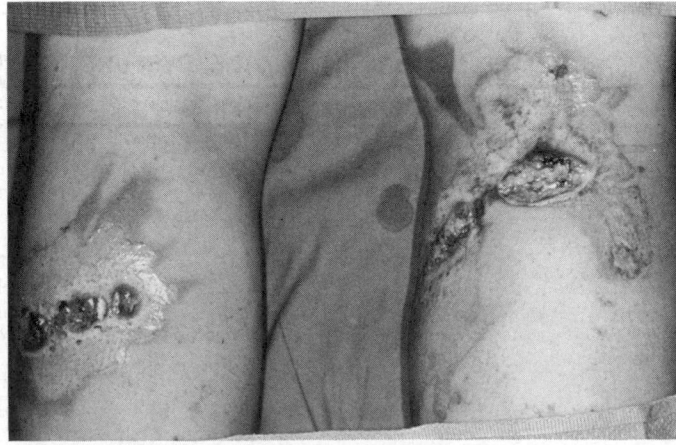

FIGURE 531–1. Charring of the skin of both calves indicates the points of contact with a high-voltage electrical current. These contact points are surrounded by full-thickness cutaneous burns caused by arcing of current. The extent of deep tissue destruction is often not related to the size of the cutaneous presentation of the injury.

aminations and documentation of electrically injured patients are necessary for both medical and legal assessment and for planning.

Cardiopulmonary Resuscitation. Cardiopulmonary arrest is common in patients with high-voltage electrical injuries, particularly lightning injury. Arrhythmias, conduction disturbances, and infarct patterns may be present on the admission electrocardiogram. Most arrhythmias are transitory, while conduction delays and infarct patterns are likely to be permanent. In those few patients who have undergone long-term cardiac function studies and angiography, these permanent electrocardiographic findings appear to represent no physiologic abnormalities.

Burn Wound. In patients who survive to be admitted to the hospital, the electrical burn itself becomes the major focus of treatment. Most high-voltage electrical injuries present with contact burns at the locations where the electrical current has entered or left the body. These contact burns typically are charred and excavated, and deeper anatomic structures may be visible in the depths of the wound. These contact areas are usually surrounded by less severe burns of variable depth. If ignition of clothing has occurred, the patient may have extensive cutaneous burns unrelated to the site of electrical contact.

Underlying injury to major muscle compartments is accompanied by edema formation, which may be accentuated by concomitant fluid resuscitation. When the tissue pressure beneath the muscle fascia increases, signs of vessel and nerve compression appear. Loss of sensation, pain, and decreased pulses indicate the presence of a compartment syndrome. Palpation often demonstrates tense muscle compartments, especially when the affected extremity is compared with an opposite unburned extremity. Even with good flow, the burned extremity may be cool to the touch and have no palpable pulse. Therefore, circulatory integrity is best judged by Doppler ultrasonography of distal pulses.

Acute Renal Failure. Acute renal failure presenting as early oliguria or anuria is not uncommon after electrical injury and is caused by two mechanisms. Gross underestimation of the extent of injury and of fluid resuscitation requirements rapidly leads to hypovolemia and oliguria. In many patients, the majority of severely damaged tissue is muscle that is hidden from view, and the need for fluid replacement may not be appreciated immediately. Second, necrotic muscle releases myoglobin, which is directly toxic to renal tubular cells. Hypovolemia potentiates the toxicity of myoglobin in the tubules unless high urine flow is maintained. Myoglobin causes the urine to appear reddish-brown. Deeply pigmented, concentrated urine typical of oliguric states may be mistaken for myoglobinuria. If uncertainty exists about the cause of urine pigments, a dipstick analysis will identify the heme nature of myoglobin. Visible myoglobinuria indicates massive acute muscle necrosis and impending renal failure. Life-threatening hyperkalemia may accompany massive muscle injury and myoglobinuria.

Nervous System. The electrical injury may involve both the central nervous system and the peripheral nervous system. A thorough neurologic examination on admission is essential, and because of the delayed presentation of neurologic complications, serial examinations should continue for several months. Both normal and abnormal function should be documented. Because extremities sustain the majority of direct electrical injuries, associated peripheral nerves are most often damaged at the time of contact. Such injuries are usually permanent and may determine the ultimate salvageability of the extremity. Some patients may also present with signs of peripheral neuropathy in locations anatomically distant from the sites of electrical injury. The mechanism responsible is not known, but fortunately these deficits usually are reversible. Motor involvement is more common than are sensory abnormalities. Several days to weeks following electrical injury, a syndrome of polyneuritis affecting nerves away from the sites of injury may occur. Associated deficits may only partially resolve. Immediate signs of spinal cord symptoms tend to be temporary and readily reversible. Spinal cord injuries of delayed onset are more often permanent or only partially reversible and manifest as transverse myelitis, ascending paralysis, hemiplegia, or related syndromes.

Fractures. Early evaluation should include assessment for skeletal trauma. Long-bone fractures frequently accompany falls, and fractures of the vertebral column may be produced by the tetanic contraction of the paraspinous muscle at the time of electrocution. Both types of fractures can be identified on appropriate roentgenograms.

Internal Organs. Electrical injuries to the major viscera most commonly occur when the body wall overlying an organ is in direct contact with the electrical current. Otherwise, the volume of the torso is large by comparison with the extremities and allows the electrical current to be distributed over a large cross-sectional area at relatively low resistance. As a result, direct injury to internal organs rarely occurs. Dysfunction of the liver, pancreas, and gut may occur during hospitalization but probably reflects the patient's underlying condition rather than the unique effects of electrical injury.

TREATMENT. Cardiopulmonary Resuscitation. Cardiopulmonary arrest is common following electrical injury, and resuscitative effort should be instituted immediately. Patients in whom cardiac arrest has occurred frequently respond to cardiopulmonary resuscitation, particularly after lightning injury. All patients should be placed on cardiac monitors or telemetry for 48 hours, and continued monitoring is needed only if arrhythmias persist. The choice of antiarrhythmic agents is dictated by the nature of the rhythm disturbance. All persistent electrocardiographic alterations should receive thorough cardiologic investigation once the acute electrical injury has healed.

Fluid Therapy. As with any other tissue injury, fluid loss into damaged tissue is one of the major physiologic derangements after electrical burns. Intravascular volume is replenished with lactated Ringer's solution sufficient to maintain a urinary output of 50 to 75 ml per hour. If the patient has grossly visible myoglobinuria, urinary output should be increased to 100 to 150 ml per hour by raising the fluid infusion rate. The increased urine production facilitates dilution of myoglobin and its washout from renal tubules. If myoglobinuria is severe or urinary output remains low in spite of an increased rate of fluid administration, mannitol, 12.5 grams, is added to each liter of lactated Ringer's solution. In such cases, the addition of sodium bicarbonate to the resuscitation solution alkalinizes the urine and increases the solubility of myoglobin.

Wound Management. Wound care involves treatment of both cutaneous and deep soft tissue injuries. Immediately after electrical injury, second- and third-degree cutaneous wounds are debrided, cleansed, and placed in topical antimicrobial burn creams. Sulfamylon (mafenide acetate) is preferred for electrical injuries because of its superior ability to penetrate injured tissue deeply and its anticlostridial and antibacterial properties. Tetanus prophylaxis is brought up to date. Prophylactic antibiotics have not been shown to decrease episodes of infection and are not used. Extremity muscle compartment pressures are monitored by physical palpation and by Doppler ultrasonography of major arterial pulses. Tissue manometry using needle-tipped transducers appears to reflect compartmental pressures, and measurements of over 30 to 40 torr are indications for surgical decompression. If the extremity has been injured by a circumferential third-degree burn, escharotomy is carried out. If the compartment symptom persists, fasciotomy involving all major compartments is performed (Fig. 531–2). Since blood loss may be difficult to control, fasciotomy should be carried out in an operating room. While fasciotomy may allow preservation of nutrient blood flow to potentially viable tissue, it is likely that the ultimate extent of tissue damage is determined at the time of electrical injury and that progression tissue loss seldom, if ever, occurs.

Dead tissue promotes infection, which may be life threatening, and definitive therapy of the electrical burn is directed toward the timely removal of necrotic tissue. At the present time, the amputation of electrically injured extremities is not automatic. The availability of several diagnostic tools may allow definition of viable and nonviable tissue in wounds whose surface appearance may not reflect deeper injuries. Technetium-99m pyrophosphate scintigraphy is the most common diagnostic technique employed for evaluation of injured extremities and provides useful results within the first 24 hours. Normal isotopic uptake reflects normal perfusion, while totally nonviable tissue exhibits no uptake. Areas of potentially reversible injury demonstrate increased isotope uptake, and serial scanning may be useful in determining the need for debridement. In extremities with intact flow of the major arteries, arteriography may be helpful. Truncation of flow

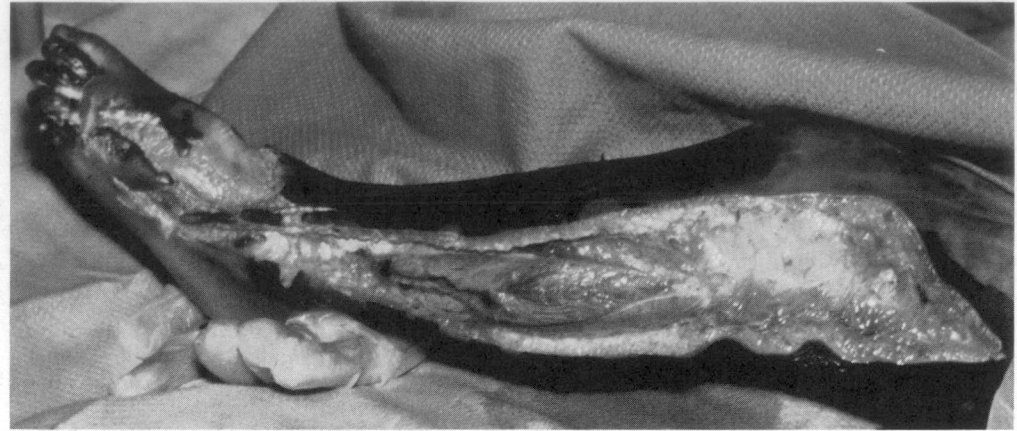

FIGURE 531–2. This severely burned lower extremity presented with no evidence of arterial circulation. Fasciotomy incisions were placed along the mid-medial and mid-lateral planes to decompress all muscle compartments. The incisional margins have separated because of massive edema in the proximal region of the incision. Necrotic muscle with overlying vessel thrombosis is seen distally. Following stabilization of the patient, exploration and debridement were carried out in the operating room.

to nutrient muscle branches indicates irreversible injury. Finally, the viability of deep tissue is determined most accurately by serial surgical exploration of the injured extremity.

The timing of surgical intervention and the extent of debridement are determined by the stability of the patient and the nature of the burn wound. Generally, initial exploration and debridement may commence at the end of the resuscitation phase, within 24 to 48 hours of injury. Distal portions of electrocuted extremities that are desiccated and mummified should be amputated. More proximally, it may be impossible to determine grossly the extent of deep tissue injury. These areas should be explored thoroughly, utilizing fasciotomy incisions if previously placed. All muscle groups should be inspected, especially those against bone. Only obviously necrotic tissue is removed, and every attempt should be made to salvage viable tissue. This approach requires daily wound examination and sequential operative debridements until all necrotic tissue is removed. Intervening complications, such as intractable hyperkalemia, severe myoglobinuria, or infection, may force abandonment of this sequential approach and require urgent amputation at a relatively high level. It is rarely advisable to proceed to early closure following amputation, and definitive closure of the debrided wound is carried out only when all necrotic tissue has been removed. Similarly, excision or grafting of full-thickness cutaneous burns may be delayed until this time. Long-term care requires multidisciplinary rehabilitation and prosthetics services.

LATE COMPLICATIONS. Patients sustaining electrical injuries may develop a number of apparently unrelated late complications that develop from a few months to several years after injury. As with cutaneous burns, more than half of electrically injured patients develop posttraumatic stress disorders, especially if a body part has been lost. Associated psychiatric symptoms respond well to psychotherapy and medication. Contractures require extensive rehabilitation care and reconstructive surgery. Cholelithiasis occurs with increased frequency in patients who have sustained electrical burns. Cataracts are particularly troublesome and occur in up to 6 per cent of electrically injured patients. The physical examination done on the admission of such patients should include a careful ophthalmologic evaluation to identify pre-existing cataracts. Although vision loss may be extensive, surgical correction is highly effective.

Amy BW, McManus WF, Goodwin CW Jr, et al.: Lightning injury with survival in five patients. JAMA 253:243, 1985. *The presentation and treatment of lightning injury are described, with emphasis on the primary role of first responder care.*

Baker MD, Chiaviello C: Household electric injuries in children. Am J Dis Child 143:59, 1989. *As with other forms of thermal injury, the household is the most common location of electrical injuries occurring in children. Similarly, most childhood electrical injuries can be prevented by utilization of inexpensive safety devices.*

Housinger TA, Green L, Shahangian S, et al.: A prospective study of myocardial damage in electrical injuries. J Trauma 25:122, 1985. *This report correlates serial electrocardiographic and cardiac enzyme determinations with radionuclide cardiac function studies in electrocuted patients. MB-creatine kinase values correlated poorly with other measurements of cardiac injury.*

Hunt JL, Mason AD Jr, Masterson TS, et al.: The pathophysiology of acute electric injury. J Trauma 16:335, 1976. *This classic experimental study demonstrates*

that electrical injury is caused by direct thermal damage to tissue. Further, the characteristic arteriographic findings of early occlusion of nutrient vessels to muscle and other tissues are related to subsequent necrosis.

Hunt JL, Sato RM, Baxter CR: Acute electric burns: Current diagnostic and therapeutic approaches to management. Arch Surg 115:434, 1980. *An excellent description of electrical injury in a large series of patients. The use of technetium-99m pyrophosphate scans was introduced by these authors, and its efficacy in defining injured and nonviable tissue is confirmed.*

James TN, Riddick LR, Embry JH: Cardiac abnormalities demonstrated postmortem in four cases of accidental electrocution and their potential significance relative to non-fatal electrical injuries of the heart. Am Heart J 120:143, 1990. *This report provides an exhaustive review of the effects of electricity on the heart and describes a detailed pathologic study of postmortem damage in young men presenting with fatal cardiac arrest.*

Saffle JR, Crandall A, Warden GD: Cataracts: A long-term complication of electrical injury. J Trauma 25:17, 1985. *Cataracts occur in 5 to 10 per cent of patients with electrical injury. This report emphasizes the importance of early ophthalmologic examination, documentation, and long-term follow-up in determining disability in such patients.*

532 Disorders Due to Heat and Cold

James P. Knochel

To maintain a normal body temperature requires that heat gain equal heat loss. Heat is produced by metabolism or gained from the environment. Thermoregulation is heavily dependent upon blood flow to cutaneous vessels. Cutaneous flow is regulated by hypothalamic centers. Vasoconstriction reduces and vasodilatation increases delivery of heated blood to the skin. Heat is exchanged between the skin and the environment by radiation, conduction, or convection. If heat loss is inadequate by these means, active sweating begins, and cooling occurs by vaporization of sweat. If heat gain is necessary, metabolic heat production rises by a voluntary increase of physical activity or involuntarily by shivering. Body heat thus produced is retained by cutaneous vasoconstriction. *Acclimatization*, a term defining critical cardiovascular, endocrine, exocrine, and other physiologic adaptations to heat stress, requires 1 to 2 weeks to develop. Such adaptations permit one to work comfortably and safely under conditions of heat stress that were previously intolerable.

DISORDERS DUE TO HEAT

HEAT CRAMPS. Workers who sweat profusely and consume water with inadequate salt may experience excruciating muscle cramps. They are more common in acclimatized, physically fit men who are able to sweat voluminously. The cramps tend to occur in muscles used while working and often do not appear until the person relaxes after work. Cooling the muscles during a cold shower may precipitate the attack. Cramps in the abdominal wall may suggest a perforated viscus. Mild hyponatremia is the rule. Severe cramps may cause modest rhabdomyolysis and elevations of muscle enzymes in serum (creatine phosphokinase, CK). Salted liquids orally or saline intravenously leads to rapid improvement. Heat cramps are preventable by replacement of sweat with a hypotonic salt solution (40 mmol per liter or 0.5 teaspoon of salt per liter) or merely by increasing dietary salt intake.

HEAT EXHAUSTION. Heat exhaustion is a common disorder occurring after sustained heat stress that causes water and/or salt depletion.

Dehydration sharply increases the risk of heat stroke. It occurs most often in the elderly, infirm, obtunded, or very young who are unable to communicate their thirst. It is also seen in active persons who take salt supplements without adequate water. Deliberate efforts should be made to ensure water intake by patients in nursing homes where summertime room temperatures are often too high. Hypernatremia of several days' duration may itself reduce secretion of antidiuretic hormone and recognition of thirst. Symptoms of heat exhaustion due to water loss include intense thirst, fatigue, paresthesias, weakness, anxiety, and impaired judgment. Signs may include dehydration, hyperventilation, tetany, agitation, hysteria, muscular incoordination, and psychotic behavior. Body temperature may rise to 38.9°C. Delirium, rising temperature, coma, and frank heatstroke may follow. Laboratory findings include hemoconcentration, hypernatremia, mild azotemia, and oliguria.

Salt depletion heat exhaustion occurs mainly in unacclimatized persons in whom losses of thermal sweat are replaced with water but not adequate salt. Dehydration, weight loss, and thirst are absent in the pure form. Sweating and urinary output remain normal. Symptoms include profound weakness, fatigue, severe headache, giddiness, and muscle cramps. In some patients, anorexia, myalgia, nausea, vomiting, and diarrhea may masquerade as a viral illness. Such patients appear haggard, with pale, clammy skin. Hypotension and tachycardia are common. Fever is notably absent.

Treatment of heat exhaustion should be individualized. Most patients can be treated with lightly salted fluids, rest, and elimination of heat stress. Hypernatremic dehydration should be treated with isotonic dextrose at a rate sufficient to reduce serum sodium about 2 mEq per liter per hour. It is seldom necessary to administer hypertonic salt solutions to patients with hyponatremic heat exhaustion.

HEATSTROKE. Heatstroke is a catastrophic illness requiring immediate treatment for survival. It is subdivided into two forms, classic and exertional (Table 532–1).

Classic heatstroke occurs especially in the poor, the elderly, infants, the chronically ill, alcoholics, patients with advanced heart disease, and the obese. Hot, humid weather usually precedes this disorder. Deaths due to heart disease increase sharply during heat waves because of demands placed upon the heart by heat stress. Certain medications also increase the propensity to develop heatstroke. These include drugs that impair sweating (anticholinergics, phenothiazines, beta blockers, antihistamines), diuretics, drugs that may increase heat production (amphetamines, cocaine, neuroleptics), and butyrophenone, which may depress thirst. Rarely, victims may recall a prodrome resembling heat exhaustion or cessation of sweating. Once sweating stops, body temperature mounts and collapse soon follows. Typical findings include central nervous system dysfunction, especially coma or bizarre behavior; hot, dry, flushed skin; and hyperpyrexia. Rectal temperature exceeds 40.6°C and may reach 44°C or more. Hypotension is common. It is probably due to redistribu-

tion of blood from the central to the peripheral circulation, since it often responds to cooling alone. Convulsive seizures, fasciculations, and muscle rigidity are absent until active cooling is under way.

Exertional heatstroke is more likely in laborers, farmers, military recruits, football players, long-distance runners, and those who work in boiler rooms or foundries. They display physical findings in the acute phase similar to those of classic heatstroke, with one common exception: About half of these patients continue to sweat. If this occurs, the skin may be deceptively cool despite a high core temperature.

Other major differences between classic and exertional heatstroke become apparent from laboratory measurements. In the classic form, respiratory alkalosis is usual. (Blood pH, P_{CO_2}, and P_{O_2} should be corrected for temperature; cf. Table 532–2.) Circulatory collapse may cause modest increases of lactate, a particularly ominous sign. In contrast, *lactic acidosis* is the rule in exertional heatstroke, may exceed 20 mol per liter, and is not a foreboding finding in this condition. Serum CK activity may be slightly increased in classic heatstroke (usually not greater than 1000 to 2000 IU per liter). However, clinically important rhabdomyolysis is rare unless the patient has a pre-existing myopathy. Major *rhabdomyolysis* and its associated complications, such as hyperkalemia, hyperphosphatemia, hypocalcemia out of proportion to hypoalbuminemia, hyperuricemia, and myoglobinuria, are almost invariable findings in exertional heatstroke. Both forms of heatstroke may be complicated by *hemorrhage* (resulting from *disseminated intravascular coagulation*, fibrinolysis, clotting factor deficiency due to hepatic injury, or *thrombocytopenia* due to bone marrow injury); *jaundice; acute renal failure; pancreatitis; brain damage; spinal cord infarction; peripheral neuropathy; myocardial necrosis and arrhythmias*; and pulmonary capillary damage with *adult respiratory distress syndrome*. Mounting evidence suggests that gut ischemia during exercise in the heat permits endotoxin absorption and production of tumor necrosis factor and interleukins. These substances may underlie the multiple systems organ failure (MSOF) syndrome seen in severe cases of heatstroke. Hypokalemia in heatstroke usually results

TABLE 532–1. MAJOR DIFFERENCES BETWEEN CLASSIC AND EXERTIONAL HEATSTROKE

	Classic	Exertional
Persons at risk	Infants, chronically ill, elderly	Laborers, soldiers, farmers, athletes
Skin	Usually hot, dry	Sweating may be present
Acid-base status	Respiratory alkalosis	Metabolic (lactic) acidosis
Rhabdomyolysis	Unusual	Major
Acute renal failure	Less than 5%	30% or more
Disseminated intravascular coagulation	Mild to moderate	Severe

TABLE 532–2. TEMPERATURE CORRECTION FACTORS FOR BLOOD pH AND GAS MEASUREMENTS

Patient's Temperature		pH	P_{CO_2}	P_{O_2}
°F	°C	(Add to observed values)		
110	43	−.09	+22%	+35%
109	42.5	−.08	+21%	+32%
108	42	−.07	+19%	+30%
107	41.5	−.07	+17%	+27%
106	41	−.06	+16%	+25%
105	40.5	−.05	+14%	+22%
104	40	−.04	+12%	+19%
103	39.5	−.04	+10%	+16%
102	39	−.03	+8%	+13%
101	38.5	−.02	+6%	+10%
100	38	−.01	+4%	+7%
98–99	37	None	None	None
97	36	+.01	−4%	−7%
96	35.5	+.02	−6%	−10%
95	35	+.03	−8%	−13%
94	34.5	+.04	−10%	−16%
93	34	+.04	−12%	−19%
91	33	+.06	−16%	−25%
90	32	+.07	−19%	−30%
88	31	+.09	−22%	−35%
86	30	+.10	−26%	−39%
84	29	+.12	−29%	−43%
82	28	+.13	−32%	−47%
81	27	+.15	−34%	−51%
79	26	+.16	−37%	−54%
77	25	+.18	−40%	−57%
75	24	+.19	−43%	−60%
73	23	+.21	−45%	−63%
72	22	+.22	−48%	−65%
70	21	+.24	−50%	−67%
68	20	+.25	−53%	−70%

from respiratory alkalosis, but it may represent potassium deficiency in those who have performed hard work in the heat for 1 or 2 weeks. Hypoglycemia may also occur.

Treatment of heatstroke is aimed at anticipation, prompt recognition, and rapid cooling. The importance of educating paramedical personnel, nurses, athletes, coaches, and trainers to prevent and accurately recognize heatstroke as well as to initiate immediate cooling cannot be overestimated. Common mistakes include administration of fluids to comatose patients or delay of cooling.

Proper emergency management includes removal from direct sunlight, removal of clothing, wetting the body surface, and fanning to move air and thereby promote vaporization. When such simple measures are undertaken on the spot, some victims awaken. Most require aggressive cooling in the hospital. A thermistor probe temperature device should be inserted high in the rectum to record core temperature. Tracheal intubation is advisable.

Conventional cooling techniques include immersion in ice water while the skin is rubbed briskly or placing the patient on a stretcher, rubbing the skin with ice bags while keeping the skin wet, and moving air over the skin to promote vaporization of the water. Rapid cooling by ice water immersion may cause cutaneous vasoconstriction, shivering, and convulsions. Immersion in cool water (11°C) may facilitate cooling with equal speed by avoiding cutaneous vasoconstriction. Ice water by gavage or enema is hazardous and may cause water intoxication.

Hypotension often responds to cooling alone, but if it persists, 0.5 liter of normal saline should be infused. Hypotension not responding to such quantities of saline suggests myocardial or capillary injury, and vasopressor support may be necessary. The stomach should be emptied, since vomiting and aspiration often occur during cooling. Cooling should be stopped when core temperature reaches 39°C to avoid progressive hypothermia.

Steroids are generally unnecessary. Hypokalemia and hypophosphatemia are very common in the acute phase but usually resolve quickly without treatment. Glucose may be necessary for hypoglycemia. Although lactic acidosis usually responds to volume expansion, if it persists in the absence of hypotension, 44 to 88 mEq of sodium bicarbonate may be helpful. Other complications described earlier should be anticipated, and appropriate measures taken as necessary.

MALIGNANT HYPERTHERMIA. This rare but serious disorder, representing an idiosyncratic reaction to general anesthesia, is discussed in Ch. 507.

MINOR DISORDERS RELATED TO HEAT STRESS. *Heat edema* is a transient, benign disorder that occurs during initial exposure to hot weather. It appears to result from aldosterone-mediated salt and water retention (a physiologic adaptation) and usually disappears spontaneously with continued heat exposure. It seldom, if ever, requires treatment. Diuretics should not be administered. *Miliaria* (heat rash) is caused by sweat gland occlusion. Its medical importance is enhanced, since it may impair sweat formation and evaporative heat loss.

Heat syncope is typified by simple fainting after prolonged standing in the heat. Salt and water losses induced by sweating and heat-induced vasodilatation of the superficial blood vessels contribute. When acclimatization occurs, the associated retention of salt and water corrects the problem. Besides syncope, findings usually include slight tachycardia and moist skin. Fever is absent. Recovery occurs rapidly if the patient is allowed to remain supine. Removal from the heat and administration of lightly salted liquids are helpful.

Hart GR, Anderson RJ, Crumpler CP, et al.: Epidemic classical heat stroke: Clinical characteristics and course of 28 patients. Medicine 61:189, 1982. *A detailed presentation of classic heatstroke, emphasizing the important roles of medications that impair heat loss and pre-existent disease in its pathogenesis. It also presents a detailed analysis of laboratory abnormalities commonly observed in this illness.*

Jones TS, Liang AP, Kilbourne EM, et al.: Morbidity and mortality associated with the July 1980 heat wave in St. Louis and Kansas City, Mo. JAMA 247:3327, 1982. *A report illustrating increased death rates during heat waves.*

Knochel JP: Catastrophic medical events with exhaustive exercise: "White collar rhabdomyolysis." Kidney Int 38:709, 1990.

Knochel JP, Reed G: Disorders of heat regulation. *In* Maxwell MH, Kleeman CR, Narins RG (eds.): Clinical Disorders of Fluid and Electrolyte Metabolism.

4th ed. New York, McGraw-Hill Book Company, 1986, pp 1197–1232. *A review of environmental heat illness, pharmacologic and endocrine hyperthermia, malignant hyperthermia, and hypothermic disorders.*

HYPOTHERMIA

Hypothermia, defined as a core temperature of less than 35°C, is a medical emergency that occurs in both temperate and cold environments. Its prompt recognition is critical to avoid serious morbidity or death. When body temperature declines, heat production increases by shivering, and heat loss is reduced by decreasing cutaneous blood flow. Reduction of core temperature decreases the rate of chemical reactions, so that cooling proceeds until a new equilibrium is established between the body and its environment.

As hypothermia develops, cerebral blood flow declines. The resulting fall in nutrient availability is offset by a reduction in brain metabolism. This fall in metabolic demand permits successful cerebral resuscitation of hypothermic patients even after prolonged periods of anoxia and circulatory arrest.

PATHOGENESIS. The causes of hypothermia seen in clinical practice are summarized in Table 532–3. Advanced age, disorders causing hypometabolism, central nervous system disease, malnutrition, a variety of drugs, and exposure commonly cause hypothermia. In elderly persons, hypothermia, hyperventilation, hypotension, and thrombocytopenia are common signs of bacteremia and sepsis.

CLINICAL MANIFESTATIONS. A decline in mental status, ataxia, tremulous speech, and hyperreflexia appear as temperature falls to about 32°C. At lower temperatures, hyporeflexia, stupor, dysarthria, and sluggish pupillary responses appear. Shivering usually stops below 32°C. Muscle rigidity becomes prominent. Established hypothermia reduces heart rate, blood pressure, peripheral vascular resistance, cardiac output, and central venous pressure. Creatine phosphokinase (MB isoenzyme) may increase with severe hypothermia without evidence of myocardial infarction, suggesting myocardial cellular damage. Atrial arrhythmias are usually benign. Ventricular ectopic beats may herald ventricular fibrillation, an imminent danger if core temperature becomes less than 28°C. Stimulation, such as urethral catheterization, movement, endotracheal intubation, and vascular catheterization, also predisposes to the development of this arrhythmia. Osborn waves, characterized by a widening of the base of the QRS complex and J point deflection, are the most characteristic ECG findings. They can be seen with hypothermia from any cause and do not herald the onset of ventricular fibrillation. Early tachypnea and respiratory alkalosis are replaced by progressive hypoventilation. Advancing hypothermia leads to carbon dioxide retention and respiratory acidosis. Shivering increases lactic acid production and hypoxia in muscles and may cause severe lactic acidosis.

In early hypothermia, hypokalemia may be caused by respiratory alkalosis. At lower temperatures, potassium becomes trapped inside cells despite acidosis and hypercarbia. During therapeutic rewarming, hyperkalemia may become important and contribute to arrhythmias.

TREATMENT. Significant hypothermia is a medical emergency. When it is suspected, an estimate of core temperature should be obtained by inserting a thermistor probe high into the rectum. Esophageal temperature probes are difficult to place

TABLE 532–3. CAUSES OF HYPOTHERMIA

Exposure plus:	
I. Central nervous system disease	III. Interference with muscle movement
Brain tumor, injury, seizure	
Cord transection	Paralysis, paresis
Hypoglycemia	Extremes of age
Thiamine deficiency	Drugs
Uremia	Alcohol
Hepatic failure	Phenothiazines
II. Interference with vasoconstriction	Hypothyroidism
Drugs	IV. Mixed causes
Alcohol	Starvation
Phenothiazines	Adrenal insufficiency
Sepsis	Hypothyroidism
Erythroderma	Hypopituitarism

Reproduced with permission from Fitzgerald FT, Jessop C: Accidental hypothermia: A report of 22 cases and review of the literature, *in* Stollerman GH, et al. (eds.): Advances in Internal Medicine, Volume 27. Copyright © 1982 by Year Book Medical Publishers, Inc., Chicago.

properly and may precipitate ventricular arrhythmias or fibrillation.

Airway patency must be ensured in comatose patients, and steps should be taken to prevent aspiration of gastric contents. A large intravenous catheter should be inserted, and thiamine and glucose given immediately in appropriate situations. Stimulation of the patient should be minimized to avoid precipitating ventricular fibrillation. Blood pressure, pulse, temperature, electrocardiogram, neurologic status, and urine output should be monitored frequently during rewarming.

A warming rate of about 0.5°C per hour is generally accepted as optimal. Most shivering patients spontaneously rewarm at a rate equal to or greater than this. *Passive* rewarming with blankets is ideal for hemodynamically stable, moderately hypothermic patients. This method allows a rise of 0.5 to 1°C per hour if the initial core temperature is greater than about 27°C. It is especially effective in patients with acute hypothermia who do not have underlying disease. *Active* rewarming becomes necessary in patients with severe hypothermia or cardiopulmonary arrest or both. This is especially important in patients with ventricular fibrillation or asystole because the hypothermic myocardium is resistant to mechanical or pharmacologic intervention until temperatures are above 28°C to 30°C. In such instances, warming by extracorporeal perfusion has been employed.

"Rewarming shock" and accentuated lactic acidosis have been most commonly encountered with active external rewarming techniques, i.e., heat applied to the surface of the body with hot water bottles or immersion in warm water. To avoid these problems, rapid rewarming of core blood has been attempted by several means in patients with severe hypothermia or cardiac arrest. Most patients with hypothermia tolerate warm intravenous fluids and heated oxygen. If rapid rewarming is required, peritoneal lavage with solutions warmed to about 40°C is effective.

Supportive measures may be very important. Because of the wide diversity of electrolyte derangements in hypothermic patients, no general recommendations can be made regarding fluid management other than warming the fluid to 37 to 40°C before administration. Plasma volume expanders may be given if the central venous pressure is low. Oxygen and bicarbonate should be given if serious metabolic acidosis exists. Subsequent metabolic alkalosis and its adverse effects on oxyhemoglobin dissociation, calcium, and ventricular irritability must be avoided. As patients are rewarmed, metabolic acidosis may worsen as lactate is washed out of previously hypoxic tissues. Recognition and treatment of this phenomenon are important to reduce the risk of ventricular fibrillation and cardiovascular collapse. Severe respiratory impairment with significant carbon dioxide retention should be treated with assisted ventilation. Ventilatory adjustments should be made with respect to reduced carbon dioxide production. Hypoglycemia should be suspected in any patient with hypothermia. Hyperglycemia should be treated only if severe and potentially life threatening. Vasopressors should be avoided if possible because of their ability to induce ventricular arrhythmias. Drugs with significant depressing effects on the myocardium, such as quinidine and propranolol, should be avoided. Thyroxine should be given only if significant hypothyroidism is suspected.

Burnet RW, Noonan DC: Calculations and correction factors used in determination of blood pH and blood gases. Clin Chem 20:1499, 1974.
Fitzgerald FR, Jessop C: Accidental hypothermia: A report of 22 cases and review of the literature. Adv Intern Med 27:127, 1982. Reuler JB: Hypothermia: Pathophysiology, clinical settings, and management. Ann Intern Med 89:519, 1978. *These two articles are excellent clinical reviews of hypothermia as seen in medical practice, with discussions of differential diagnosis, clinical manifestations, and treatment.*
Matz R: Hypothermia: Mechanisms and countermeasures. Hosp Pract 21:45, 1986. *This is a comprehensive presentation of the pathophysiology of hypothermia and its management.*

533 Trace Metal Poisoning

Donald B. Louria

Many trace elements, both metals and nonmetals, are capable of causing human disease. In some cases poisoning is a consequence of workplace exposure. In others the disease results from

use of prescription or nonprescription medicines or as an adverse effect of medical procedures such as hemodialysis or insertion of prosthetic devices. Occasionally trace element poisoning results from attempts at suicide or homicide.

Over the past few decades, increased awareness of the health consequences of industrial substances, more stringent federal and state regulations, and fear of lawsuits have resulted in a healthier workplace. However, the majority of the potentially exposed work force is employed by small industries that may not have plant physicians or insist on proper worker protection.

We know a great deal about overwhelming exposure that results in acute illness, but our knowledge of the subtle consequences of chronic, low-level trace element exposure is still grossly inadequate. This is well illustrated by lead exposure. Acute lead poisoning in children or adults is readily diagnosed, but we are only beginning to understand the consequences of increased body lead burdens in the absence of the anemia, colic, or clinically apparent encephalopathy.

The interrelationships between trace elements are also poorly understood. For example, copper smelter workers are exposed not only to copper but also to lead, zinc, arsenic, gold, silver, cadmium, and mercury; in these workers pneumonitis or other acute illnesses may result from two or more metals acting in concert. In other instances excesses or deficits of a trace element may act indirectly by inducing deficiency or toxicity of another trace element.

LEAD

ETIOLOGY. In the past lead poisoning was ascribed to pica (abnormal ingestion) among children living in dilapidated houses with peeling layers of lead-based paints. In the past two decades lead intoxication has occurred with increasing frequency in less socioeconomically deprived areas of the cities, as well as in more affluent suburbs. This may in part be related to environmental contamination from leaded gasoline; several studies relate environmental lead contamination to traffic density patterns. Contaminated soil is also a well-described source of lead.

In the United States, hundreds of occupations entail potentially significant exposure. It is estimated that more than 800,000 American workers have potentially significant lead exposure. Lead and other metal smelter workers or miners, welders, storage battery workers, and pottery makers are particularly heavily exposed. Workers in auto manufacturing, ship building, paint manufacture, and printing industries are also at substantial risk, as are house painters and those who repair old houses.

Lead-soldered kettles and cans and lead-glazed pottery can release lead when acidic fluids are stored or cooked in them; the latter appears to be a particularly worrisome problem in nursing homes and on psychiatric units. Demolition workers and those employed in firing ranges have become poisoned from intensive aerosol exposure. In the southern United States, moonshine whiskey is an important cause of poisoning. The stills are connected with lead solder, and old radiators containing lead are used as condensers; 20 to 90 per cent of moonshine samples contain lead in the potentially toxic range.

In past centuries lead was added to wine to sweeten it, a deception that was eventually made punishable by death. Recently, addition of lead to aphrodisiacs and various herbal and folk medicines has resulted in poisoning. Retained bullets can result in lead poisoning, especially if host metabolic changes favor lead mobilization or if a joint or bone is involved, since synovial fluid appears to be a good solvent for lead. The interval between lodging of the bullet and clinical evidence of lead poisoning has ranged from 2 days to 40 years. Lead poisoning has also occurred in adults who have eaten fowl and inadvertently ingested lead pellets that have lodged in the appendix. Children have been poisoned by swallowing lead household objects, such as lead curtain weights, that are then retained in the gastrointestinal tract for a prolonged time.

Gasoline sniffing for hedonistic purposes can produce lead poisoning; the organic tetraethyl lead appears to have a proclivity for the nervous system.

In a sense we are all lead poisoned; prior to the Industrial Revolution the total body burden of lead was about 2 mg, whereas currently in industrialized societies the whole body content is about 200 mg. One hundred fifty to 250 μg per day is ingested, 5 to 10 per cent of which is absorbed. In children the percentage is higher and absorption is facilitated by iron, calcium, magnesium, and perhaps zinc deficiency. Aerosol exposure is especially likely to result in poisoning, since approximately 40 per cent of inhaled lead is absorbed.

CLINICAL MANIFESTATIONS. The major toxic effects of lead are referable to the abdomen, the blood, and the nervous system.

Gastrointestinal Tract. The exact pathogenesis of lead colic remains uncertain; in part it appears to be due to a direct effect of lead on smooth muscle. The crampy, diffuse, often intractable abdominal pain may be accompanied by nausea, vomiting, anorexia, constipation, or occasionally diarrhea. The pain may be confined to the epigastric, periumbilical, or other areas of the abdomen and may simulate a variety of surgical and nonsurgical diseases. Lead-induced megacolon has been reported.

Blood. Lead interferes with a variety of red cell enzyme systems, including delta-aminolevulinic acid dehydratase and ferrochelatase. The former is needed for the conjugation of levulinic acid to form porphobilinogen; the latter facilitates the incorporation of iron into protoporphyrin IX (see Fig. 131–2). The red cell abnormalities include punctate basophilic stippling and clover leaf morphology. Anemia is frequent in severe acute lead poisoning and may be normocytic normochromic or microcytic hypochromic. An inherited deficiency in delta-aminolevulinic acid dehydratase can sensitize the individual to lead intoxication and result in the appearance of symptoms of acute lead poisoning at modest blood lead levels.

Nervous System. Either the brain or the peripheral nerves may be involved. The central nervous system (CNS) symptoms at first are vague and are often mistakenly disregarded. These manifestations include irritability, incoordination, memory lapses, labile affect, sleep disturbances, restlessness, listlessness, paranoia, headache, lethargy, and dizziness. In more serious cases manifestations include syncope-like attacks, disorientation, flaccidity, more intense headache, severe mental impairment, ataxia, vomiting, cranial nerve palsies, localized neurologic signs, psychosis, somnolence, seizures, blindness, and coma. Severe lead encephalopathy is not restricted to children. Occasionally the brain manifestations mimic a space-occupying lesion. The cerebrospinal fluid may be under increased pressure and may show an increased protein content, a modest pleocytosis (predominantly lymphocytic), and, rarely, diminished glucose levels. Papilledema has been reported, as have grayish deposits surrounding the optic disc and optic atrophy. Frank encephalopathy is an ominous prognostic sign in regard to both mortality and persistent brain damage. Most children who experience two or more bouts of clinically evident encephalopathy have neurologic residua.

The peripheral nerve involvement, seen more often in adults than in children, is almost always exclusively motor and involves muscle groups used extensively. Wrist drop and foot drop are seen most often; the former, depending on type of occupation, may be asymmetric, and there may be paresthesias.

The spinal cord may also be involved, manifestations having some similarity to those of amyotrophic lateral sclerosis.

Tetraethyl lead poisoning causes euphoria, nervousness, insomnia, hallucinations, convulsions, and sometimes frank psychosis.

There is increasing evidence of subtle brain damage in the absence of clinical evidence of encephalopathy. Inordinate body burdens of lead may result in mentation difficulties, emotional lability, deficits in intelligence and memory, impaired psychomotor and visual motor function, slowed nerve conduction, and behavioral aberrations in both children and adults, even in the absence of overt evidence of poisoning. These changes may occur at blood levels of 25 to 60 μg per deciliter (or even less in young children). Long-term effects of low-level exposure in childhood include poor performance in school.

Other Clinical Manifestations. In adults the kidneys are often involved (see Ch. 80), the characteristic lesion being interstitial nephritis; as the disease progresses, glomerular filtration rate falls. In children, Fanconi's syndrome, characterized by glycosuria, aminoaciduria, and phosphaturia, may occur transiently; and occasionally, asymptomatic renal failure supervenes. Lead

TABLE 533–1. POSITIVE SCREENING TESTS INDICATING UNDUE LEAD ABSORPTION

Whole-blood lead	Children	> 25 μg/dl
	Adults	> 40 μg/dl
Whole-blood erythrocyte protoporphyrin or zinc protoporphyrin	Children	> 35 μg/dl*
	Adults	> 50 μg/dl

*This value is unsettled.

poisoning appears to be responsible for some cases of renal failure associated with either gout or hypertension, and there is increasing suspicion based on epidemiologic studies that the level of systolic or diastolic blood pressure may be in part related to blood lead concentrations.

Polyarthralgias, mild hepatic dysfunction, and dysuria may occur. Occasionally arrhythmias and cardiomegaly have been reported, as have abnormalities of liver function. A gingival blue, blue-black, or gray line is found in up to 20 per cent of adult patients but is infrequent in children.

Lead readily crosses the placenta and is thought to be responsible for an increased incidence of spontaneous abortion and miscarriage. Some studies suggest lead poisoning may result in hypospermia and other sperm abnormalities. Teratogenic effects occur in lead-treated animals, but congenital abnormalities have not been convincingly documented in humans. Lead exposure may also result in transient chromosomal breakage. Placental transfer of lead stored in the maternal skeleton can reduce neonatal growth.

DIAGNOSIS. A high index of suspicion and a careful examination of the peripheral blood for basophilic stippling are mandatory. The interference with delta-aminolevulinic acid dehydratase results in marked increase in delta-aminolevulinic acid in the urine. Urinary coproporphyrin levels are also increased. Lead interferes with incorporation of iron into heme and zinc and then replaces the iron to form zinc protoporphyrin (ZPP). The latter or its hydrolysis product, erythrocyte protoporphyrin (EP), can be measured rapidly fluorometrically; both EP and ZPP are reliable indicators of lead poisoning. EP and ZPP elevations also occur in patients suffering from iron deficiency anemia or erythropoietic protoporphyria. Table 533–1 lists some indications of undue lead absorption.

Blood aminolevulinic acid dehydratase activity can also be measured directly. Blood lead levels are readily determined by atomic absorption spectrophotometry or anodic stripping voltometry. Specimens can be obtained by either venipuncture or finger stick; the latter technique is often difficult to interpret because of skin contamination. Urine lead concentrations can also be measured; if concentrations are normal, increased body burdens can still be detected by measuring urinary lead excretion after administration of calcium disodium edetate (Table 533–2). This test is particularly useful in assessing lead storage in bones.

Additional industrial exposure should not be permitted if blood levels exceed 40 μg per deciliter or if there is any increase in EP or ZPP.

More than 90 per cent of the body stores of lead are retained in bone, with a biologic half-life of several decades. Blood lead,

TABLE 533–2. CaNa₂ EDTA LEAD MOBILIZATION TEST

	Children	Adults
Normal premobilization test	< 100 μg/day	< 150 μg/day
	Normal	
Post-CaNa₂ EDTA, 50 mg/kg IM or IV or 500–1000 mg/m² (children); or 1 gm IM* × 2, 12 hours apart, or 1–2 gm IV (adults)	< 0.60 μg Pb/mg CaNa₂ EDTA† administered over 8- to 24-hour collection period	< 650 μg/day
	Increased Body Burden	
	> 0.60 μg Pb/mg CaNa₂ EDTA administered	> 650 μg/dl

*Procaine must be used with intramuscular injections.
†EDTA = edetate.

TABLE 533–3. LEVELS OF CHRONIC LEAD EXPOSURE BODY BURDENS IN ADULTS

Exposure	Blood Pb (μg/dl)	EDTA Test (μg Pb/day)	Tibial* [Pb] (μg/g)
1. Low ambient	< 25	< 600	< 20
2. Moderate (intermittent)	25–50	600–1000	20–40
3. High (industrial)	> 50	> 1000	> 40

*Wet weight. Determined by in vivo tibial KXRF.

on the other hand, has a biologic half-life of only a few weeks. Bone lead is therefore a better indicator of cumulative lead absorption. The bone lead concentration can be measured in vitro in biopsy samples or in vivo noninvasively using x-ray fluorescence (XRF). The relationship between blood lead (assuming relatively constant exposure), chelatable lead, and bone lead in adults is illustrated in Table 533–3.

TREATMENT. Three agents are used that form tight complexes with lead and thus promote its elimination from tissues (Table 533–4). Dimercaprol (British antilewisite, BAL) is given in oil intramuscularly; calcium disodium edetate (calcium versenate) can be given either intramuscularly or intravenously; and D-pencillamine is administered by mouth. Chelation should be undertaken only after careful consideration in those with milder evidence of poisoning, because each of the agents may be associated with significant adverse effects. Because most of the body lead is stored in the bones, clinical improvement and reduction in blood lead levels (or reduction in EP or ZPP) may be followed by increases in blood lead concentrations and clinical evidence of repoisoning owing to mobilization of lead from bone. In such cases chelating agents should again be administered. The newer, less toxic oral dimercaprol analogues dimercaptosuccinic acid and dimercaptopropanesulfonate may be effective.

Treatment is ordinarily successful in extra-CNS disease but is not predictably effective in patients with encephalopathy. Various degrees of mentation deficits may remain in both children and adults. Among adults the frequency of residual brain deficits is not clearly established.

Current acceptable blood concentrations of lead for children are 25 μg per deciliter, and permissible levels for adults are up to 40 μg per deciliter, including those industrially exposed (30 μg per deciliter or less is recommended for pregnant women); but there is mounting evidence that significant toxicity can occur at lower levels and that acceptable concentrations should be further reduced to 15 μg per deciliter or less for children and pregnant women and less than 30 μg per deciliter for adults. Blood lead levels have fallen in the United States (and some other countries) in the past 15 years, but millions of children and

TABLE 533–4. CHELATION REGIMENS

	Children*	Adults*	Duration
CaNa₂ EDTA	50 mg/kg/day IM† or IV, or 1500 mg/m²/24 hr (severe disease); 1000 mg/m²/day (mild-moderate intoxication)	1.0 gram IV in 5% dextrose twice daily, or 2.0 grams/day IM in divided doses; longer term, 1 gram IM 3× per week† until lead burden reduced to satisfactory levels	3 to 5 days
BAL	3 mg/kg/dose IM, or 300–450 mg/m²/24 hr IM	2.5 mg/kg/dose IM	3 to 5 days
	(Given in divided doses every 4 hr)		
Penicillamine	30 mg/kg/day PO	1.0–1.5 grams/day PO	Until blood lead and FEP‡ levels approach normal§

*CaNa₂ EDTA and BAL are ordinarily used together for symptomatic illness.
†Procaine must be used for IM injections of CaNa₂ EDTA.
‡FEP = free erythrocyte protoporphyrin.
§Must be monitored carefully, since toxicity occurs in up to 20% of cases.

adults are still exposed to potentially toxic levels that could be responsible for subtle mental changes, hyperactivity, aggressiveness, and antisocial behavior.

More than 20 years ago, the extraordinary scientist and philosopher Rene Dubos observed: "The problem is so well-defined, so neatly packaged with both causes and cures known, that if we don't eliminate this social crime, our society deserves all the disasters that have been forecast for it." Amen.

Agency for Toxic Substances and Disease Registry, Public Health Service, U.S. Department of Health and Human Services: The nature and extent of lead poisoning in children in the United States. A Report to Congress, 1988. *This is a comprehensive and authoritative review of the sources and implications of lead poisoning in childhood.*

Baker EL, White RF, Pothier LJ, et al.: Occupational lead neurotoxicity: Improvement in behavioral effects after reduction of exposure. Br J Indust Med 42:507, 1985. *This is one of a growing number of articles that together offer a reasonably persuasive argument that significant defects in brain function occur in lead-exposed persons who do not exhibit evidence of obvious poisoning and whose blood lead levels in the past would have been considered in the acceptable range. Thirty-one references.*

Batuman V, Landy E, Maesaka JK, et al.: Contribution of lead to hypertension with renal impairment. N Engl J Med 309:17, 1983. Batuman V, Maesaka JK, Haddad B, et al.: The role of lead in gout nephropathy. N Engl J Med 304:520, 1981. *These two articles present reasonably compelling evidence that renal dysfunction associated with either hypertension or gout may be related to lead intoxication in a small but important percentage of such cases.*

Landrigan PJ: Toxicity of lead at low dose. Br J Indust Med 46:593, 1989. *A brief but solid analysis. Fifty-nine references.*

Needleman HL: The persistent threat of lead: Medical and sociological issues. Curr Probl Pediatr 18:703, 1988. *Another good article on toxicity at "low levels," with a major focus on societal effects. One hundred ten references.*

Needleman HL, Schell A, Bellinger D, et al.: The long-term effects of exposure to low doses of lead in childhood. An 11 years follow-up report. N Engl J Med 322:83, 1990. *This important, although still controversial, article gives substantial support for the notion that subtle lead poisoning in childhood can result in significant pyschosocial defects later in life.*

Wedeen RP: *In vivo* XRF measurement of bone lead (editorial). Arch Environ Health 45:69, 1990. *A summary of currently available methods for assessing cumulative lead absorption.*

Whitfield CL, Ch'ien LT, Whitehead JD: Lead encephalopathy in adults. Am J Med 52:289, 1972. *Twenty-three adults exposed to moonshine developed encephalopathy, manifestations ranging from confusion to coma, seizures, and death. This article emphasizes that encephalopathy can be a major problem in adults. Chelation therapy appeared to be effective.*

MERCURY

ETIOLOGY. Mercury has been used for at least 2000 years. At present more than 60 occupations involve mercury exposure. These include chloralkali work; manufacture of pesticides, insecticides, and fungicides; manufacture of mercury-containing instruments, lamps, neon lights, batteries, paper, paint, dye, electrical equipment, and jewelry; and dentistry. The exposure in dental offices has diminished substantially in recent years.

In addition to occupational or industrial exposure, poisoning has resulted from inadvertent contamination of grains by mercury-containing pesticides as well as from accidental or intentional ingestion or injection of elemental mercury or mercury-containing compounds. In the past, mercury was administered medicinally as a component of cathartics, teething powders, and anthelmintics. Mercury compounds are now rarely used as diuretics.

CLINICAL MANIFESTATIONS AND TREATMENT. The biologic effects, tissue distribution, and toxicity of mercury depend on the form in which it is introduced into the body. Mercury possesses a strong affinity for sulfhydryl, amine, phosphoryl, and carboxyl groups and inactivates a wide variety of enzymes. Mercury poisoning can be conveniently divided into four categories.

Metallic Mercury. Elemental mercury is a liquid at environmental temperatures but vaporizes with agitation as well as gentle heating. Bulk mercury is used in dental amalgams; up to 10 per cent of dental offices have been found to have excessive mercury vapor levels; and accidental spillage has occurred occasionally in homes or offices. There is increasing concern about the potential health consequences from slow intraoral leakage of mercury from dental amalgams. The greatest exposure to metallic mercury is in industry. Additionally, many workers are potentially exposed because of the widespread use of mercury in electrical equipment. Heavy aerosol exposure to mercury produces chills, fever, cough, chest pain, and hemoptysis; roentgenograms show diffuse pulmonary infiltrates. Inhaled elemental mercury is readily absorbed from the alveoli; thereafter the target tissue is the brain. With mild exposure the manifestations are likely to be subtle and diagnosis is difficult. Insomnia, nervousness, mild tremor, impaired judgment and coordination, decreased mental efficiency, emotional lability, headache, fatigue, loss of sexual drive, and depression are early manifestations and are often mistakenly ascribed to psychogenic causes. These symptoms have been referred to as micromercurialism. Abdominal cramps, dermatitis, and diarrhea may also occur, and the victim may complain of a metallic taste. As the poisoning becomes more severe, persistent involuntary tremors of the extremities are noted. Thereafter, other signs of mercury poisoning may appear, including amblyopia, polyneuropathy, erythroderma, acrodynia, joint pains, swollen gums with a blue line around the teeth, sialorrhea, and paresthesias. The major manifestation of mercury vapor exposure may be renal damage, including the nephrotic syndrome.

Blood and urine levels may be unreliable, and clear evidence of poisoning may be documented only after administration of drugs that augment mercury excretion in the urine.

In most cases improvement occurs after removal from exposure or treatment with either dimercaprol (BAL) or N-acetyl penicillamine.

The effects of ingestion of even large amounts of metallic mercury range from no clinical disturbance to local gastrointestinal irritation to CNS damage. Aspiration of liquid mercury is also usually benign, although roentgenologic visualization of mercury globules may be evident for many years. After intravenous injection of mercury, there may be no abnormalities other than roentgenologic densities or an illness ranging from mild to lethal, with hepatic, renal, lung, and CNS dysfunction.

The wide range of clinical findings after elemental mercury exposure appears to relate in part to the rate of oxidation to mercuric salts and the rapidity of their subsequent excretion through the kidneys, saliva, and urine.

Inorganic Mercury. Exposure to $HgCl_2$ and Hg_2Cl_2 occurs primarily in industry and results from ingestion. $HgCl_2$ is far more toxic than Hg_2Cl_2. The major manifestations are renal and include proteinuria, granular casts in the urinary sediment, the nephrotic syndrome, and pyuria from tubular damage. In some cases severe oliguria, and even anuria, may occur. Additionally, diarrhea, abdominal pain, hepatic dysfunction, and lesser evidence of CNS disease may be found (micromercurialism). Rhabdomyolysis with striking muscle enzyme elevation and acrodynia have also been reported. In this type of mercury poisoning, BAL or penicillamine is usually effective.

Organomercurials with Rapid Metabolism to Inorganic Mercury. Included are phenyl and methoxyethyl mercury salts found in diuretics and fungicides. Toxicity is limited and usually renal.

Short-Chain Alkyl Mercury Compounds. Methyl mercury is far more toxic than ethyl or diethyl mercury; the latter produces primarily renal abnormalities.

Methyl mercury is well absorbed from the intestinal tract, is widely distributed in the body, and readily passes through the placenta into the fetus and also into breast milk. About 10 per cent localizes in the brain, and the ensuing damage is largely irreversible. Major epidemics have resulted from industrial contamination of water, with subsequent biotransformation of elemental and inorganic mercury into methyl mercury, followed by ingestion by fish and then by humans. Other epidemics have resulted from use of grains contaminated by organic mercurial pesticides or animal ingestion of seeds treated with mercury. The epidemics in the Minamata and Niigata regions of Japan and in Iraq, Guatemala, Pakistan, and the United States have resulted in a high death rate and an appalling amount of permanent brain damage. In addition to the milder symptoms listed under elemental mercury poisoning, CNS manifestations include severe paresthesias, dysarthria, ataxia, visual field constriction, hearing loss, blindness, microcephaly, spasticity, paralysis, and coma. Some of the children of methyl mercury–poisoned mothers show various degrees of cerebral palsy–like abnormalities and mental retardation, and some die.

Chang LW: Neurotoxic effects of mercury—a review. Environ Res 14:329, 1977. *A very useful review with good clinical-pathologic correlations.*

Elhassani SB: The many faces of methylmercury poisoning. J Toxicol Clin Toxicol 19:875, 1982–1983. *A very nice, thorough review with 133 references.*

Joselow MM, Louria DB, Browder AA: Mercurialism: Environmental and occupational aspects. Ann Intern Med 76:119, 1972. *A useful summary with 149 references.*

Magos L: Mercury and mercurials. Br Med Bull 31:241, 1975. *A concise, valuable summary of the clinical manifestations and tissue localization after exposure to different chemical forms of mercury.*

Scarlett JM, Gutenmann WH, Lisk DJ: A study of mercury in the hair of dentists and dental-related professionals in 1985 and subcohort comparison of 1972 and 1985 mercury hair levels. J Toxicol Environ Health 25:373, 1988. *Exposure, currently reduced in intensity, can apparently result either from inhalation or by a direct nose-brain pathway.*

ARSENIC

ETIOLOGY. Arsenic is ubiquitous in nature; it is present in the earth's crust in concentrations of 2 to 5 parts per billion. It is found in inordinately high concentrations in some well water. It is used in the glass, pigment, textile, tanning, and bronze-plating industries; in wood preservation; in a variety of metal alloys; in veterinary medicines; in some herbicides, insecticides, and rodenticides; in fire salts to produce multicolored flames; and by farmers and vintners. American industry uses about one half of the world's production of arsenic trioxide. Arsenic poisoning has also resulted from using certain herbal preparations, from the ingestion of illegal (moonshine) whiskey, from the burning of arsenate-treated wood, and from the administration of arsenic-containing prescription medicines.

Elemental arsenic is not toxic even if ingested in substantial amounts. There are three toxic forms of arsenic: pentavalent salts, trivalent salts, and arsine gas. The arsenic in the earth's crust and in most foods is in the pentavalent form. Trivalent arsenic, which is far more toxic, accumulates in the body more readily than the pentavalent form. Arsenic gas (arsine) is extraordinarily toxic; it is formed by the hydrolysis of metallic arsenide or by the action of acids or nascent hydrogen on arsenical compounds, especially in the refining of certain metals. Arsine is also manufactured for and used in the electronics industry. Arsine can be liberated in sewage plants, and in one small cluster of cases, eight children were poisoned while cleaning out a cattle dip in Australia.

CLINICAL MANIFESTATIONS. *Arsine gas* poisoning is usually overwhelming and frequently fatal. The onset of symptoms after exposure is usually between 1 and 12 hours. Fever, headache, muscle pains, nausea, vomiting, epigastric pain, dysuria, and explosive diarrhea characterize the acute episode. Because arsenic preferentially binds to red blood cells, hemolytic anemia and hemoglobinuria occur early, and red cell ghosts may be seen in the peripheral blood. There may also be cyanosis and profound hypoxia. Renal failure due to acute tubular necrosis (occasionally due to cortical necrosis) occurs in the first few days after onset of symptoms. This may be accompanied by shock and encephalopathy, characterized by agitation and disorientation. Both bone marrow depression and myocardial damage may occur. Those who do not die of intractable vascular collapse often develop subacute manifestations of arsenic poisoning, described below. Those who recover may develop chronic renal failure.

Arsenic Ingestion. Although arsine gas poisoning can be mimicked by arsenic ingestion, the latter is usually more insidious and less overwhelming. Cramping abdominal pain and diarrhea are characteristic. Other acute manifestations include nausea, vomiting, dysphagia, cyanosis, headache, hematuria, and weakness. Hyperesthesia, muscle cramps, conjunctivitis, syncope, excessive thirst, periorbital swelling, epistaxis, and tinnitus may also occur. The patient may complain of a metallic taste, and there may be a garlic odor to the breath, but the latter is not pathognomonic, since it also may be observed in selenium, tellurium, and phosphorus poisoning.

Leukopenia occurs frequently, but in some cases moderate leukocytosis is found and both monocytosis and eosinophilia have been described. Anemia and thrombocytopenia may supervene.

Shortly after the initial red cell binding, arsenic can be found in liver, spleen, heart, kidneys, brain, and intestinal tract. Skin, nails, and hair do not usually contain arsenic until 2 to 4 weeks after exposure, but occasionally hair accumulation can occur more rapidly.

Other manifestations that may occur in the first week include jaundice; hepatomegaly with hepatic enzyme abnormalities; electrocardiographic abnormalities; a cardiomyopathy that can be lethal; pericarditis; rhabdomyolysis; pulmonary edema; evidence of encephalopathy, including headache, irritability, confusion, delusions, and hallucinations; seizures; renal dysfunction; kidney failure with acute tubular necrosis; and respiratory muscle paralysis. Megaloblastic changes may be seen in the bone marrow. Optic neuritis with visual field constriction has been reported after pentavalent arsenic exposure.

The most prominent manifestation after the first week of illness is symmetric polyneuropathy. At first, sensory manifestations predominate, the patient complaining of a burning sensation in a stocking-glove distribution. Motor involvement follows almost immediately with diminished or absent reflexes and severe weakness. Occasionally the neuropathy is unilateral. Prolonged encephalopathy and/or psychosis has been reported in a few instances.

In cases of subacute poisoning, Aldrich-Mees lines (transverse white bands) may be seen in the nails; like the garlic odor, these may be seen in other trace element intoxications. Erythroderma and exfoliative dermatitis may also supervene.

Chronic exposure is associated with several abnormalities. The most characteristic of these are the cutaneous lesions, particularly hyperpigmentation (arsenic melanosis) and hyperkeratoses located primarily on the palms and soles. Alopecia and so-called raindrop depigmentation may also occur. In about 5 to 10 per cent of those chronically exposed, skin cancers appear after latent periods of 5 to more than 25 years; these tend to be multiple, are situated mainly on the trunk and upper extremities, and show either intraepithelial squamous cell (Bowen's disease) or basal cell morphology on histologic examination. In the United States the most frequent cause of such skin lesions in past years was the medicinal use of Fowler's solution, an inorganic trivalent arsenical. Currently most cases arise after occupational exposure, but a small number have been ascribed to chronic exposure to well water with high arsenic content.

Epidemiologic studies on gold ore and tin miners, vineyard workers, laborers in sheep-dip factories, and smelter workers show a clear increase in the incidence of squamous cell carcinoma of the lung, the risk of bronchogenic cancer correlating with the intensity and duration of arsenic trioxide exposure.

Several types of liver disease may occur; these include postnecrotic cirrhosis, hepatocellular carcinoma, and hemangioendothelioma. Additionally, portal fibrosis and/or sinusoidal collagenosis may be found, which can lead to a form of noncirrhotic portal hypertension with splenomegaly and esophageal varices but normal hepatic artery wedge pressure. Like the skin cancers, the liver abnormalities may occur many years after exposure to arsenic has been discontinued, and the exposure period can have been relatively brief.

Arsenic exposure is also thought to induce chromosomal aberrations, but the significance of these abnormalities is not clear.

In Taiwan, high concentrations in well water have been associated with peripheral vascular (blackfoot) disease and various cancers.

DIAGNOSIS. If the diagnosis is suspected, there is a qualitative urine test (Gutzeit test) employing sulfuric acid, zinc, and silver nitrate. Arsenic concentrations can be measured in blood, urine, hair, or nails by atomic absorption spectrophotometry or neutron activation techniques.

TREATMENT. The treatment of choice is dimercaprol (BAL), but it should be given within the first 24 hours after exposure. If the BAL is given later, it is less likely that improvement will be observed, and in most cases the peripheral neuropathy is refractory to treatment. Exchange transfusion or dialysis shortly after the onset of acute illness has also been reported to be beneficial. Penicillamine may also be useful, as may orally administered 2,3-dimercaptosuccinic acid.

The neuropathy and renal failure may slowly resolve completely, or there may be residual abnormalities that range from mild to severe.

Massey EW, Wold D, Heyman A: Homicidal intoxication. South Med J 77:848, 1984. *Four cases and a comprehensive review in four packed pages. Thirty-two references.*

Schoolmeester WL, White DR: Arsenic poisoning. South Med J 73:198, 1980. *A fine comprehensive review with 102 references. Includes 10 illustrative case reports.*

Wu MM, Kuo TL, Hwang YH, Chen CJ: Dose response relation between arsenic

concentration in well water and mortality from cancers and vascular diseases. Am J Epidemiol 130:1123, 1989. *A solid epidemiologic study. Fifty-three references.*

Zaloga GB, Deal J, Spurling T, et al.: Case report: Unusual manifestations of arsenic intoxication. Am J Med Sci 289:210, 1985. *The case (with facial palsy and pericarditis) is interesting, and the review is terrific. Twenty-eight references.*

TRACE ELEMENTS WHOSE TOXICITY IS IN LARGE PART ASSOCIATED WITH HEMODIALYSIS

ZINC. The normal adult body zinc content is 1.5 to 3.0 grams. Daily intake ranges from 5 to 35 mg. Zinc is bound to metallothioneins synthesized in the liver and kidney and is excreted by both the urine and the gastrointestinal tract. Particularly high concentrations are found in the uveal tract, choroid plexus, and prostate; substantial amounts are also found in bone, brain, skeletal muscles, and other tissues of the eye.

Zinc has a strong affinity for red cells and plasma proteins. Consequently, there is no loss across dialysis membranes; instead, blood zinc concentrations may increase markedly during hemodialysis. There appear to be two well-documented zinc sources: adhesive plaster (containing zinc oxide) used to prevent dialysis coils from unwinding and the water of the dialysis fluid. Even if water has an initially low zinc content, galvanized iron pipes or tanks may release substantial amounts. This can be prevented by using deionized or distilled water.

The manifestations of zinc toxicity do not necessarily correlate well with plasma or whole-blood zinc levels. Nausea, vomiting, anorexia, lethargy, irritability, weakness, abdominal pain, and anemia are the most frequent manifestations. The mechanisms responsible for the anemia are not well understood, but in many cases the anemia is microcytic and may be associated with copper deficiency. Zinc can decrease copper absorption in the gut and also promote urinary copper excretion. Fever may accompany zinc toxicity. Other manifestations may include diarrhea, muscle pain, lymphadenopathy, hyperamylasemia with or without pancreatitis, intestinal bleeding, thrombocytopenia, oliguria, hypotension, and renal failure with tubular necrosis. Injection of large amounts of zinc has resulted in death. Intestinal manifestations may supervene after either orally or parenterally induced zinc intoxication.

Welders, smelter workers, and solderers are exposed to aerosolized zinc and may experience zinc fume fever, characterized by chills, fever, myalgias, a metallic taste, cough, nausea, lethargy, and occasionally hemoptysis. There may be diffuse roentgenologic infiltrates and pulmonary dysfunction. Ordinarily all manifestations disappear rapidly after cessation of exposure. If more prolonged pulmonary dysfunction occurs, it is thought to result from the effects of other metals to which the workers are simultaneously exposed.

ALUMINUM. Aluminum-induced dialysis dementia is an often fatal disease. The tap water used during dialysis is often to blame. Some waters naturally contain high concentrations of aluminum. In other cases aluminum sulfate had been added to the community water supply to remove organic materials. In still other cases the dialysis fluid appeared to be less responsible than aluminum-containing gels administered by mouth to reduce phosphate levels. Indeed, if oral aluminum hydroxide is administered to nondialyzed patients suffering from renal failure, the encephalopathy syndrome can occasionally occur; young children appear to be particularly at risk. Dialysis encephalopathy occurs only after repeated dialyses, usually spanning at least several months. Peritoneal dialysis can also be complicated by encephalopathy. Use of parenteral nutrition solutions containing aluminum can also be followed by aluminum poisoning.

Early manifestations include malaise, memory loss, and a characteristic speech disturbance. As the disease progresses, dysarthria, asterixis, myoclonic twitches, dementia, somnolence, and seizures occur. The electroencephalogram shows slowing, together with bursts of delta activity and high-voltage, symmetric spikes. Among those who die, aluminum levels are markedly increased in the gray matter. The use of reverse osmosis or deionization treatment has markedly reduced the incidence of severe dialysis dementia, but there is increasing evidence of a mild form of encephalopathy in chronic dialysis patients, characterized by psychomotor dysfunction, memory defects, weakness, and mild myoclonus.

Other manifestations of aluminum intoxication include myalgias, proximal myopathy, and severe skeletal pain caused by profound osteodystrophy that is unresponsive to vitamin D and is followed by fractures. Aluminum is deposited at the calcified bone-osteoid junction, and bone formation is impaired (Ch. 234, 237). Aluminum also interferes with parathyroid function, and it may be associated with cardiomyopathy.

Aluminum toxicity is also characterized by a poorly understood microcytic anemia that may be related in part to aluminum binding to transferrin and interference with iron incorporation into heme.

Although frequently lethal, in some cases the encephalopathy has regressed after intake of oral aluminum is stopped or the aluminum content of the dialysis water is reduced or following renal transplantation. Treatment with deferoxamine (DFO), which complexes with aluminum, may be beneficial. Those suffering from uremia should avoid food additives and nonprescription drugs that contain substantial amounts of aluminum. Citrates may increase aluminum absorption, as may the H_2 receptor antagonist cimetidine. Those with uremia should also be wary of community water supplies with inordinately high concentrations of aluminum.

Serum aluminum levels often do not reflect body loads; intoxication may be documented by a DFO mobilization test. Although DFO treatment can be beneficial in both aluminum-induced encephalopathy and osteodystrophy, it can temporarily exacerbate the encephalopathy and can cause hearing and vision impairment, hypotension, and iron deficiency; it also has been associated with superinfection with Zygomycetes. DFO treatment appears to be less successful in parathyroidectomized persons. It has been suggested that Alzheimer's disease and amyotrophic lateral sclerosis may be related to brain aluminum deposition, but available data are unconvincing.

Those involved in aluminum processing or manufacturing, pottery or explosive making, or welding may be exposed to aluminum aerosols. Pulmonary granulomas, fibrosis, and in some cases postfibrosis emphysema may supervene. In bauxite smelters this is known as Shaver's disease. Those involved in aluminum smelting may develop wheezing, chest tightness, and evidence of airway obstruction (potroom asthma).

COPPER. Since the late 1960's, copper tubing in dialysis equipment has been known to release copper when exposed to acid water. Copper levels may also be inordinately high in the dialysis water if the water is supplied through copper plumbing. Copper is a potent red cell poison, damaging cell membranes and inhibiting a variety of red cell enzymes. Major manifestations of toxicity include hemolysis and gastrointestinal disturbances. Nausea, vomiting, diarrhea, abdominal pain, fever, chills, hemolytic anemia, jaundice, hemoglobinuria, and severe myalgias all occur frequently. Myoglobinemia, necrotizing pancreatitis, hepatic necrosis, and profound leukocytosis may also occur.

Copper poisoning during dialysis is fortunately readily avoidable, since copper is no longer a component of the tubing.

Copper poisoning may also occur after intentional or accidental ingestion. There may be a metallic taste, vomiting, and abdominal pain. In more severe cases, hematemesis, melena, hepatic necrosis, and shock supervene.

In Wilson's disease rapid increases in circulating copper concentrations may be followed by acute hemolytic anemia.

Those exposed to metallic copper industrially may develop transient pulmonary manifestations (metal fume fever) and, rarely, green hair. These disappear rapidly when exposure is stopped.

COBALT. Patients with renal failure may have elevated tissue cobalt levels. In some cases cobaltous chloride has been given by mouth to patients on maintenance hemodialysis to combat anemia. This has been associated with increased blood and myocardial cobalt levels and suggestive evidence of cardiomyopathy. Toxicity included nausea, vomiting, anorexia, tinnitus, peripheral neuropathy, goiter resulting from blockage of iodine uptake, neurogenic deafness, hyperlipidemia, optic atrophy, and renal tubular damage.

Cobalt was added to beer in the 1960's as a foam stabilizer. This resulted in cardiomyopathy, often accompanied by pericardial effusion. Mortality from heart failure or arrhythmias ranged from 5 to 47 per cent (see Ch. 50).

Persons exposed to cobalt industrially may also occasionally develop cardiomyopathy. Workers exposed to finely powdered cobalt may develop pulmonary interstitial fibrosis and cor pulmonale. Cobalt is often a component of alloys that are used in joint prostheses. Cases have been reported of joint pains, spontaneous dislocation of the prosthesis, and bone necrosis starting 9 months to 4 years postoperatively, apparently caused by a reaction to the cobalt in the alloy.

OTHER METALS. In one group of dialysis patients, *nickel* toxicity occurred when nickel leached from a stainless steel water heater tank into the dialysis fluid. Manifestations included nausea, vomiting, weakness, and headache. Symptoms developed within a few hours after dialysis and disappeared within 24 hours.

Tissue *tin* concentrations, especially in the liver, are increased in patients undergoing hemodialysis. However, tin levels are even higher in uremic patients who have not been dialyzed. No definite clinical disease has been associated with these increased body tin burdens.

Patients undergoing maintenance hemodialysis are often treated with *iron* for anemia. In such patients parenteral and occasionally oral iron administration may be followed by hemosiderosis and occasionally hemochromatosis. Serum ferritin concentrations exceed 500 ng per milliliter. A proximal myopathy has been described. The severity of the tissue iron overload and the likelihood of hemochromatosis may be related to the histocompatibility antigens A-3, B-7, and B-14. Iron overload has been complicated by porphyria cutanea tarda and by a variety of infections, including those due to species of *Yersinia* and *Vibrio* and to the yeast *Trichosporon cutaneum*. Treatment with deferoxamine may reduce the body iron burden.

Aggett PJ, Harrison JT: Current status of zinc in health and disease states. Arch Dis Child 54:909, 1979. *This is a superb review with 110 references. Only a small section is devoted to toxicity.*

Fosmire GJ: Zinc toxicity. Am J Clin Nutr 51:225, 1990. *A nice review; emphasizes problems inherent in self-administration of 50 to 300 mg a day for "health" purposes. Thirty-one references.*

Gruskin AB: Aluminum: A pediatric overview. Adv Pediatr 35:281, 1988. *A superb, comprehensive review with 255 references.*

O'Hare JA, Callaghan NM, Murnaghan DJ: Dialysis encephalopathy. Clinical, electroencephalographic and interventional aspects. Medicine 62:129, 1983. *A marvelous summary article and a careful analysis of 14 patients who developed encephalopathy 16 to 92 months after starting dialysis.*

Ott SM, Maloney NA, Klein GL, et al.: Aluminum is associated with low bone formation in patients receiving chronic parenteral nutrition. Ann Intern Med 98:910, 1983. *The toxicity of aluminum to bone is clearly shown in 14 patients receiving casein hydrolysate.*

Sandstead HH: Trace elements in uremia and hemodialysis. Am J Clin Nutr 33:1501, 1980. *A very good review article in which the author urges caution in ascribing the dialysis encephalopathy syndrome solely to aluminum.*

Sherrard DJ, Andress DL: Aluminum-related osteodystrophy. Adv Intern Med 34:307, 1989. *A very nice review with 81 references.*

Simon P, Allain P, Ang KS, et al.: Prevention and treatment of aluminum intoxication in chronic renal failure. Adv Nephrol 14:439, 1985. *This is as good a review as there is; with 179 references.*

Taylor A, Marks V: Cobalt: A review. J Hum Nutr 32:165, 1978. *A nice review with 73 references.*

Webster JD, Parker TF, Alfrey A, et al.: Acute nickel intoxication by dialysis. Ann Intern Med 92:631, 1980. *Nausea, vomiting, weakness, and headache were the predominant manifestations among 37 patients. Symptoms remitted 3 to 13 hours after dialysis was concluded.*

CADMIUM

ETIOLOGY. Over 10 million pounds of cadmium are used industrially every year in the United States. The metal is a component of alloys; it is used in the manufacture of electrical conductors and in electroplating; and it is present in ceramics, pigments, dental prosthetics, plastic stabilizers, and storage batteries. It is also a by-product of zinc smelting and is used in the photographic, rubber, motor, and aircraft industries. Smelters, metal-processing furnaces, and the burning of coal and oil are responsible for much of the cadmium in air.

CLINICAL MANIFESTATIONS. *Acute intoxication* by cadmium fumes produces a characteristic clinical picture. Four to 10 hours after exposure, dyspnea, cough, and substernal discomfort supervene, often accompanied by prominent myalgias, fatigue, headache, and vomiting. In more severe cases, wheezing, hemoptysis, and progressive dyspnea caused by pulmonary edema may occur and may be accompanied by hypotension and renal failure.

In most cases, the pulmonary manifestations resolve rapidly, but pulmonary function abnormalities may not disappear for months; in these cases vital capacity is reduced, and there is a restrictive defect. Occasionally pulmonary edema is lethal.

Ingestion of large amounts of cadmium results in nausea, vomiting, and abdominal pain, often accompanied by weakness, prostration, and myalgias. The onset of the gastroenteritis occurs one half to 5 hours after ingestion, and the condition lasts for less than 24 hours.

Chronic cadmium exposure by aerosol for at least 10 years has resulted in emphysema in a small number of cases. The emphysema is not accompanied by bronchitis and may appear many years after industrial exposure has stopped. Workers exposed for at least 10 years also may suffer olfactory nerve damage; in some cases this progresses to total anosmia. The most frequent long-term consequence of aerosol or oral exposure is proteinuria. After prolonged and heavy contact, cadmium urinary excretion continues for years and is associated with damage to the proximal tubule. The major urinary protein is a low molecular weight β_2 microglobulin. Urinary retinal-binding protein and N-acetyl-D-glucosaminidase levels also increase.

On occasion the proteinuria may be accompanied by glycosuria and aminoaciduria. Only infrequently is the proteinuria and tubular damage followed by progressive renal failure. An exception to the relatively benign course of the renal damage is the disease in Japan known as itai-itai (ouch-ouch), which affected almost exclusively multiparous women of ages 40 to 70 who lived in an area contaminated by industrial cadmium waste. Manifestations included striking back and joint pains, a waddly gait, osteomalacia, bone deformities, and fractures, all presumably secondary to cadmium-induced renal tubular damage.

Some studies on workers exposed to cadmium have suggested an increased risk of lung or prostatic carcinoma, but the data are not convincing.

Brenner I: Cadmium toxicity. World Rev Nutr Diet 32:165, 1978. *Interactions with calcium, zinc, copper, and selenium are emphasized. Additionally, there is a detailed analysis of the role of metallothioneins. Contains 183 references.*
Lauwery RR, Roels AA, Buchet JP, et al.: Investigations on the lung and kidney function of workers exposed to cadmium. Environ Health Perspect 28:137, 1979. *Three epidemiologic studies were conducted on more than 200 workers. The kidneys were affected to a much greater extent than the lungs. Both tubular and glomerular aberrations were found, mainly in persons with substantially increased blood and urine cadmium concentrations.*

NICKEL

ETIOLOGY. Nickel is used widely industrially in various alloys, iron shell casings, ball bearings, and heart and joint prostheses. It is also used in nickel plating; as a catalyst; in magnetic tapes, dyes, and paints; and in acrylic plastics. It is found in petroleum and coal, in diesel fuels, and in soil and air. Municipal incinerators may contribute to the ambient air nickel concentrations.

Nickel is a potent contact allergen; the most frequent adverse effect for humans is nickel dermatitis, which may be both persistent and severe. Serious systemic reactions have occurred in allergic persons from nickel-containing dental prostheses, jewelry, pacemakers, or even fluids given intravenously through a nickel-containing needle. Prosthetic joints and heart valves have failed because of a reaction to the nickel in the prosthesis. In cases of recalcitrant nickel dermatitis, restriction in dietary nickel may be helpful.

CLINICAL MANIFESTATIONS AND TREATMENT. By far, the most toxic of the nickel compounds is nickel carbonyl, created by a reaction between nickel and carbon monoxide. Industrial aerosol exposure is followed immediately by headache, drowsiness, substernal pain, nausea, and vomiting. This is followed by a latent period of 1 to 5 days, after which the victim experiences fever, chills, dyspnea, a feeling of chest tightness, cough that is sometimes productive of blood-tinged sputum, muscle pains, weakness, and fatigue. Hepatic enzyme concentrations may be considerably elevated. In severe cases cyanosis, progressive respiratory difficulties, and convulsions ensue, and death may follow in 4 to 23 days. At autopsy the lungs show hemorrhage, atelectasis, fibroblastic proliferation, and hyaline membrane formation. The treatment of choice is diethyl dithiocarbamate (Dithiocarb); dimercaprol (BAL) is an alternative but less effective therapeutic agent. Although overwhelming pneumonitis caused by nickel carbonyl is now rare, milder pulmonary

toxicity in occupations such as welding probably occurs quite commonly and goes unrecognized under the general rubric of metal fume fever. Nickel exposure may also be followed by Löffler's syndrome.

CARCINOGENESIS. Nickel is considered a potent respiratory tract carcinogen. Studies of nickel refinery workers have shown a fivefold increase in risk of lung cancer, a 150-fold increase in the risk of nasal cancer, and a substantially increased risk of larynx cancer. Those occupations most at risk among nickel workers are roasting, smelting, and electrolysis. Workers developing lung, laryngeal, and nasal cancers have usually been exposed for at least 10 years. Biopsies of nasal mucosa show potentially precancerous epithelial dysplasia in a substantial percentage of nickel workers. The cancer risk is so great that workers heavily exposed for over 10 years should probably have annual nasal mucosa biopsies as well as sputum cytologic studies and roentgenologic examinations every 4 to 6 months in an attempt at secondary prevention. The incidence of respiratory tract cancer in nickel workers is dependent on both the extent of nickel exposure and the effects of cocarcinogens, in particular, cigarette tobacco. Except for nickel miners and refinery workers, industrial nickel exposure has not been convincingly associated with increased risk of cancer.

Sunderman FW Jr: A review of the metabolism and toxicity of nickel. Ann Clin Lab Sci 7:377, 1977. *An excellent review by one of the world's leading authorities (with 177 references).*
Sunderman FW Sr: Efficacy of sodium diethyldithiocarbamate (Dithiocarb) in acute nickel carbonyl poisoning. Ann Clin Lab Sci 9:1, 1979. *The data presented strongly suggest that this is currently the agent of choice.*

OTHER TOXIC METALS

Thallium

ETIOLOGY AND PATHOGENESIS. Thallium is used in optical lenses, jewelry, low-temperature thermometers, semiconductors, luminescent tubes, dyes and pigments, scintillation counters, and fireworks. It forms a stainless alloy with silver and a corrosion-resistant alloy with lead and may be a by-product of lead and zinc production. In some areas it is still a component of rodenticides, pesticides, and insecticides. Thallium can enter the body through the respiratory tract, gastrointestinal tract, or skin. Like many other trace metals, thallium has a strong affinity for sulfhydryl groups and thus interferes with many enzyme systems. Additionally, it enters the cell, exchanging for intracellular potassium.

CLINICAL MANIFESTATIONS. Poisoning can be acute and overwhelming after suicidal ingestion, or it can be chronic and subtle. In acute poisoning, manifestations include nausea, vomiting, hematemesis, headache, lethargy, abdominal pain, diarrhea that may be bloody, insomnia, myalgias, muscle weakness, fever, hyperhidrosis, excessive thirst, confusion, delirium, seizures, coma, and respiratory failure. At least 10 per cent of acutely poisoned persons die.

Among those who survive at least a week or in those exposed to smaller amounts of thallium, the most predictable manifestations are a combined sensory and motor, often painful, peripheral neuropathy and alopecia. Although the head alopecia is total, the facial, axillary, and pubic hair is spared, as is the inner one third of the eyebrows. Motor manifestations may predominate, and the ascending, predominantly motor paralysis may mimic Guillain-Barré syndrome. The abdominal colic, nausea, and vomiting that occur frequently in both the acute and the subacute forms of thallium toxicity may so dominate the clinical picture that a diagnosis of acute appendicitis is made. Other manifestations of subacute intoxication include dementia, headache, fatigue, sleep disorders, intractable thirst, hallucinations, blindness caused by optic neuritis, impotence, amenorrhea, a blue discoloration of the gingivae, centrilobular hepatic necrosis, renal tubular necrosis, orthostatic hypotension, paralytic ileus, and myoclonic twitches. Multiple cranial nerves may be involved, but the eighth nerve is almost always spared. The electrocardiogram may show arrhythmias and changes similar to those associated with hypokalemia.

DIAGNOSIS. Thallium can be measured in blood and urine, but blood levels are often deceptively low even during clinically apparent poisoning. Since thallium is excreted in the urine, thallium determinations on 24-hour specimens are more reliable. A qualitative urine test is available. Urine is mixed with 0.4 per cent sodium bismuth in 20 per cent nitric acid and 10 per cent sodium iodide; if thallium is present, a red precipitate forms.

In some cases there is no history of occupational, environmental, or intentional exposure. Unexplained abdominal pain, neurologic abnormalities, and alopecia suggest the diagnosis.

TREATMENT. Treatment consists of hemodialysis, which can remove up to half the thallium body burden, potassium, forced diuresis, and administration of Prussian blue. Prussian blue, or activated charcoal given by mouth, absorbs thallium, so that fecal thallium concentrations increase. The half-life of thallium in the body is about 1 month, and repeated dialyses are usually needed. During potassium administration, thallium is displaced from its intracellular site, and this may cause transient exacerbations of clinical manifestations. Barbiturates may increase the severity of the disease, and their use should be avoided.

PROGNOSIS. As many as 30 per cent of those poisoned suffer some residual effects. The neuropathy may persist for many months before resolving, and some are left with variable amounts of dementia, neuropathy, ataxia, visual impairment, alopecia, and myoclonus.

Selenium

ETIOLOGY. Selenium is well absorbed from both the gastrointestinal tract and the lungs. The amount normally ingested varies markedly, depending on the local soil selenium content and on the geographic provenance of foods consumed. Grains, pork, kidney, seafoods, garlic, mushrooms, radishes, beef, egg yolk, and chicken frequently contain substantial amounts of selenium. The element is widely used in pigment, glass, electronics, ceramics, and steel industries.

CLINICAL MANIFESTATIONS. Both deficiency and toxicity syndromes are well described in animals. Deficiency, resulting from foraging on grains grown in soil deficient in selenium, produces white muscle disease, a diffuse, often severe myopathy. Excess caused by chronic ingestion of grains containing more than 10 parts per million of selenium results in two syndromes, alkali disease and the staggers. The former is milder and is characterized by anemia, emaciation, alopecia, and hoof deformity. The staggers is manifested by visual difficulties, anemia, liver cell degeneration, paralysis, and respiratory failure. In sheep, excessive selenium intake can produce severe cardiomyopathy.

In humans a *selenium deficiency syndrome* has not been clearly defined. However, in the Republic of China, diffuse cardiomyopathy (Keshan disease) has been associated with low soil and blood selenium levels, and the incidence of the disease apparently has been strikingly reduced by selenium supplementation.

Selenium toxicity syndromes in humans can be divided into acute and chronic poisoning. Subjects with inordinate exposure to selenium fumes experience one or more of the following: intestinal disturbances, giddiness, apathy, lassitude, pallor, nervousness, depression, hair and nail loss, a garlic odor to the breath, and a metallic taste. Sore throat, dyspnea, and cough may also be noted. Symptoms usually disappear after removal from the occupational exposure. Among those ingesting excessive selenium, the following symptoms and signs have been reported: nausea, vomiting, abdominal pain, diarrhea, anorexia, fatigue, sore throat, arthralgias, emotional lability, a metallic taste, a garlic odor to the breath, brittle nails, brittle hair, hair loss, a bronze color to the skin, hepatic dysfunction, and diffuse dermatitis. Increased selenium burdens may be associated with an increased prevalence of dental caries.

EPIDEMIOLOGY. A most impressive epidemic of chronic selenium intoxication was observed in China in the 1960's. Subacute and chronic selenium toxicity will likely be seen with an increasing frequency because selenium is being promoted as a nonprescription supplement. In experimental studies oral selenium in dosages of 0.1 to 2.0 parts per million diminishes the frequency of or delays the appearance of a variety of spontaneous or induced tumors. Some epidemiologic data suggest an inverse relationship between selenium blood levels and the incidence of certain cancers, particularly of the intestinal tract, but at present the evidence that increased selenium intake modifies or prevents human cancer is unpersuasive.

Manganese

Manganese toxicity occurs primarily in miners who have been exposed to manganese dioxide aerosols for prolonged periods. The manifestations, known as manganic madness, are limited to the CNS. The manganese is concentrated primarily in the basal ganglia and cerebellum, accounting for the extrapyramidal Parkinson-like facies, the rigidity, and the difficulty in walking. Other manifestations include compulsive behavior (including singing, dancing, fighting, and running), explosive and involuntary laughter, headache, muscular weakness, tremors, somnolence, dystonia, hypotonia, retropulsion and propulsion, dementia, speech disturbances, irritability, sialorrhea, impotence, hypersomnia, and memory defects. In some cases psychosis may be the dominant feature. There is no effective therapy. After removal from manganese exposure or following attempts to reduce the body manganese load by treatment with calcium versenate or L-dopa, the mental aberrations usually improve but the neurologic abnormalities persist. Manganese contamination of dialysates or manganese ingestion has been associated with abdominal pain, liver dysfunction, and evidence of pancreatitis.

Barium

Barium compounds are used in printing; in the production of paints, glass, paper, leather, soap, and rubber; in ceramics, plastic, steel, oil, textile, and dye industries; as fuel additives; and in insecticides, rodenticides, and depilatories. There are two major adverse effects. After accidental or intentional ingestion of large amounts, abdominal pain, vomiting, and increased peristalsis occur. If enough is absorbed, potassium is displaced intracellularly, resulting in profound hypokalemia, which in turn may produce flaccid paralysis, potentially dangerous cardiac arrhythmias, renal failure, and respiratory paralysis. Poisoning has also been described after barium chloride skin burn. Treatment consists of administration of potassium and forced diuresis to promote barium excretion. Severe allergic reaction has followed barium enema; whether this is due to the barium or preservatives is not clear.

The other adverse effect from contact with barium is a benign pneumoconiosis that may supervene after 1 or more years of aerosol exposure. Chest roentgenograms show extensive, very dense bilateral nodules up to 4 to 5 mm in diameter. There is no prominent fibrosis and no clinically significant disease; the nodules often regress after occupational exposure is stopped.

Boron

Borates are used in soaps, detergents, fertilizers, wood preservatives, fungicides, and fire-retardant paints. There are few reports of boron toxicity. Ingestion of boric acid or absorption from local application can result in nausea, vomiting, diarrhea, anemia, and seizures; a variety of skin eruptions characterized by intense erythema, desquamation, and exfoliation; and striking alopecia. In acute boric acid poisoning, forced diuresis and/or dialysis may be helpful. In addition, occupational aerosol exposure to diborane (B_2H_6) in high-energy fuels can produce acute pulmonary edema that resolves after the exposure is discontinued. Exposure to pentaborane or decaborane can produce headache, nausea, drowsiness, vertigo, coma, dementia, cortical blindness, deafness, seizures, muscle spasms, acidosis, and cardiac arrest. A subacute mild organic brain syndrome has also been observed.

Antimony

Industrial antimony toxicity is very rare, as is intentional ingestion or inadvertent poisoning from release of antimony from inexpensive enamelware. Manifestations of acute poisoning include nausea, abdominal pain, weakness, headache, vomiting, diarrhea, hematemesis, myalgias, liver function abnormalities, acute renal tubular dysfunction, electrolyte abnormalities, and circulatory collapse. Gaseous SbH_3 (stibine) is as toxic as arsine, producing CNS abnormalities and hemolysis. After antimonial injection for medicinal purposes, adverse effects include nausea, vomiting, cough, and muscle and joint pain. Hepatic dysfunction can occur, as can cardiac arrhythmias, including Adams-Stokes syndrome. Antimony is also considered one of the metals capable of causing metal fume fever. Treatment of oral ingestion consists of lavage, administration of activated charcoal, and administration of dimercaprol or the less toxic analogues dimercaptosuccinic acid or dimercaptopropanesulfonic acid.

Chromium

Chromium is used extensively in metal and galvanizing industries and in the manufacture of dyes, enamel, and paints. Hexavalent chromium exposure is associated with an increased incidence of lung and certain upper respiratory tract cancers. Additionally, chromium-exposed workers may show evidence of proximal renal tubule dysfunction and may suffer nasal septum perforations.

Molybdenum

In animals, molybdenum produces diarrhea, anemia, alopecia, diminished growth, and bone and joint abnormalities. No clearly defined molybdenum toxicity syndrome has been reported in humans.

Platinum

The major adverse effects observed in platinum workers are allergic pulmonary reactions, including bronchial asthma.

Plutonium

In experimental models, plutonium, because of its radioactivity, is a potent carcinogen. Workers have been generally well protected, but recent data suggest that occupational exposure may be a significant problem. Some still controversial epidemiologic studies have suggested that accidental community exposure has resulted in an increase in frequency of certain cancers and fetal malformations.

Tellurium

Used particularly in rubber, metallurgic, and electronics industries, tellurium can cause giddiness, headache, nausea, a metallic taste, and a garlic smell to the breath. In animals tellurium causes neuropathy, but this has not been convincingly demonstrated in humans.

Tin

Tin can be released into beverages or foods from tin cans; ingestion can produce nausea, vomiting, abdominal pain, and diarrhea. Such toxicity occurs infrequently. Additionally, there have been occasional reports of neurologic abnormalities following exposure to organic tin, including the triethyl, trimethyl, and triphenyl tins. These are used primarily in agriculture for their bactericidal, fungicidal, antiparasitic and molluscacidal properties. Manifestations include ataxic dysmetria, disorientation, seizures, nystagmus, impaired vision, hearing loss, headache, vertigo, paresthesias, intracranial hypertension, paresis, and polyneuropathy. Aerosol exposure to tin may result in stannosis, a mild pneumoconiosis in which there may be dense bilateral infiltrates but usually no pulmonary dysfunction.

Vanadium

Vanadium is used in alloys and in the steel and chemical industries. Its inhalation can result in neurasthenia, anorexia, vertigo, throat pain, nasal irritation (even nasal hemorrhage), and acute bronchitis characterized by a cough that is sometimes accompanied by a whoop. The nasal mucosa of vanadium-exposed workers shows vascular hyperemia and round cell infiltration. Recent studies also suggest that vanadium can interfere with heme synthesis.

Bencko V, Cikrt M: Manganese: A review of occupational and environmental toxicology. J Hyg Epidem Microbiol Immunol 28:139, 1984. *All you wanted to know about manganese and then some (77 references).*

Doig AT: Baritosis: A benign pneumoconiosis. Thorax 31:130, 1976. *Nine cases are described. Despite dense infiltrates, no significant clinical disease or physiologic abnormalities occurred.*

Lauwers LF, Roelants A, Rosseel PM, et al.: Oral antimony intoxications in man. Crit Care Med 18:324, 1990. *Four cases due to eating cake inadvertently spiked with antimony potassium tartrate; plus a nice review.*

Locatelli C, Minoia C, Tonini M, et al.: Human toxicology of boron with special reference to boric acid poisoning. Ital Med Lav 9:141, 1987. *It is difficult to find good reviews of boron toxicity. This is one of them; with 105 references.*

Nordberg GF: Factors influencing metabolism and toxicity of metals: A consensus report. Environ Health Persp 25:3, 1978. *This marvelous analysis covers the toxicity and interactions with other metals of arsenic, cadmium, lead, and mercury. Highly recommended. Contains 312 references.*

Silverman JJ, Hart RP, Garrettson LK, et al.: Post-traumatic stress disorders from pentaborane intoxication. JAMA 254:2603, 1985. *Fourteen persons exposed to B_5H_9 suffered neuropsychological deficits (33 references).*

Wainwright AP, Kox WJ, House IM, et al.: Clinical features and therapy of acute thallium poisoning. Q J Med 69:939, 1988. *A single case accompanied by an excellent discussion of clinical manifestations and treatment.*

Wilkinson GS, Tietjen GL, Wiggs LD, et al.: Mortality among plutonium and other radiation workers at a plutonium weapons facility. Am J Epidemiol 125:231, 1987. *Although confirmatory studies are needed, this very careful analysis of 5413 men suggests increased risks for several types of cancers.*

Wu RM, Chang YC, Chiu HC: Acute triphenyltin intoxication: A case report. J Neurol Neurosurg Psychiatry 53:356, 1990. *A brief report of a suicide attempt; with a useful literature review.*

Yang G, Wang S, Zhou R, et al.: Endemic selenium intoxication of humans in China. Am J Clin Nutr 37:872, 1983. *This is an excellent review of selenium intoxication based on a very significant epidemic in China. Selenium-laden vegetables and coal combined with a drought that reduced the rice crop were the major culprits. Seventeen references.*

PART XXVII
LABORATORY REFERENCE INTERVAL VALUES OF CLINICAL IMPORTANCE

534 Reference Intervals and Laboratory Values of Clinical Importance*

Ronald J. Elin

Reference intervals are valuable guidelines for the assessment of health and disease by the clinician, but they should not be used as absolute indicators of health and disease. For essentially every test, there is a significant overlap between the normal and diseased populations. Many factors may influence the determination of the reference interval. The method and mode of standardization are variables for the reference interval, particularly for immunologic and enzymatic tests. The selection of the "normal" population is also important, since factors such as age, sex, race, diet, personal habits (e.g., alcohol consumption, smoking), and exercise may influence the reference interval for a given analyte. Last, the statistics chosen to define the reference interval are also a factor. These multiple variables for the determination of the reference interval indicate why there are differences among institutions for the same analyte.

The values in this chapter are primarily for adults in the fasting state. Values for other groups, when included, are clearly identified. For convenience, this chapter is divided into the following three sections: clinical chemistry, toxicology, and serology; hematology and coagulation; and drugs—therapeutic and toxic. The list includes reference intervals for the most common tests used in the practice of internal medicine. For more information about the reference interval for a given test or a test not included in the list, I recommend *Clinical Guide to Laboratory Tests*, second edition, edited by Dr. Norbert W. Tietz. This book contains literature citations for most of the tests listed in this chapter.

All laboratory values are given in conventional and international units. If the value and units for a reference interval are the same for conventional and international units, the interval is listed only in the column for international units. The temperature for all enzyme assays listed in the chapter is 37°C. The pertinent prefixes denoting the decimal factors are listed.

---

*The material in this chapter was partially extracted from Tietz NW (ed.): Clinical Guide to Laboratory Tests. Philadelphia, W.B. Saunders Company, 1990. The material for the section on Therapeutic Drug Concentrations was partially extracted from Tietz NW: Textbook of Clinical Chemistry. Philadelphia, W.B. Saunders Company, 1986. The main contributors to this section of the book are NW Tietz and NM Logan. Other sources are listed under references for this chapter.

PREFIXES DENOTING DECIMAL FACTORS

Prefix	Symbol	Factor
mega	M	10^6
kilo	k	10^3
hecto	h	10^2
deka	da	10^1
deci	d	10^{-1}
centi	c	10^{-2}
milli	m	10^{-3}
micro	μ	10^{-6}
nano	n	10^{-9}
pico	p	10^{-12}
femto	f	10^{-15}

ABBREVIATIONS

AU	Arbitrary units
EU	Ehrlich unit
GD	General diagnostics
IFA	Immunofluorescent assay
IU	International unit (of hormone activity)
RIA	Radioimmunoassay
RID	Radial immunodiffusion
S	Substrate
U	International unit (of enzyme activity)

Beutler E: Hemolytic Anemia in Disorders of Red Cell Metabolism. New York, Plenum Publishing Company, 1978.

Brown SS, Mitchell FL, Young DS (eds.): Chemical Diagnosis of Disease. Amsterdam, Elsevier/North-Holland Biomedical Press, 1979.

Conn RB (ed.): Current Diagnosis. 7th ed. Philadelphia, W.B. Saunders Company, 1985.

Gilman AG, Rall TW, Nies AS, Taylor P (eds.): Goodman and Gilman's The Pharmacological Basis of Therapeutics. 8th ed. New York, Pergamon Press, 1990.

Henry JB (ed.): Clinical Diagnosis and Management by Laboratory Methods. 18th ed. Philadelphia, W.B. Saunders Company, 1991.

Hoeg JM, Gregg RE, Brewer HB: An approach to the management of hyperlipoproteinemia. JAMA 255:512, 1986.

Mabry C, Tietz NW: Tables of normal laboratory values. In Nelson WE, Vaughan VC, McKay JR, et al. (eds.): Nelson Textbook of Pediatrics. 23rd ed. Philadelphia, W.B. Saunders Company, 1983.

Miale JB: Laboratory Medicine: Hematology. 6th ed. St. Louis, The C.V. Mosby Company, 1982.

Tietz NW (ed.): Textbook of Clinical Chemistry. Philadelphia, W.B. Saunders Company, 1986.

Tietz NW, Blackburn RH (eds.): Reference Ranges and General Information. Clinical Laboratories, A.B. Chandler Medical Center, University of Kentucky, Lexington, Kentucky, 1984.

Tietz NW (ed.): Clinical Guide to Laboratory Tests. Philadelphia, W.B. Saunders Company, 1990.

Williams WJ, Beutler E, Erslev AJ, et al.: Hematology. 3rd ed. New York, McGraw-Hill Book Company, 1983.

CLINICAL CHEMISTRY, TOXICOLOGY, SEROLOGY

Test	Specimen	Reference Interval (Conventional Units)	Reference Interval (International Units)
Acetoacetate	Serum or plasma	Negative (<1 mg/dL)	Negative (<0.1 mmol/L)
Semiquantitative	(fluoride/oxalate)		
Acetone	Urine	Negative	Negative
Semiquantitative	Serum or plasma		
	(fluoride or oxalate)	Negative (<1.0 mg/dL)	Negative (<0.17 mmol/L)
Semiquantitative	Urine		Negative
Acid phosphatase	Serum		M: 2.5–11.7 U/L
(S:p-nitrophenylphosphate)			F: 0.3–9.2 U/L
Adrenocorticotropic	Plasma (heparin)	0800 h: 8–79 pg/mL	8–79 ng/L
hormone (ACTH)		1600 h: 7–30 pg/mL	7–30 ng/L
Alanine aminotransferase	Serum		8–20 U/L
(ALT, SGPT)			
Albumin			
Nephelometric, colorimetric	Serum	3.5–5.0 g/dL	35–50 g/L
Turbidimetric	CSF	15–45 mg/dL	150–450 mg/L
	Urine	<80 mg/d at rest	<80 mg/d
		<150 mg/d ambulatory	<150 mg/d
Aldolase	Serum		1.0–7.5 U/L
Aldosterone	Plasma (heparin EDTA)	Adult, average sodium diet	
	or serum	supine: 3–10 ng/dL	0.08–0.28 nmol/L
		upright: 5–30 ng/dL	0.14–0.83 nmol/L
Alkaline phosphatase	Serum		Adult (>18 y)
(S:4–NPP)			F: 42–98 U/L
			M: 53–128 U/L
δ-Aminolevulinic acid			
(δ-ALA)	Serum	15–23 μg/dL	1.1–8 μmol/L
	Urine	1.5–7.5 mg/d	11.4–57.2 μmol/d
Ammonia nitrogen	Serum or plasma		
Resin or enzymatic	(Na-heparin)	Adult 15–45 μg N/dL	11–32 μmol/L
	Urine, 24-h	140–1500 mg/d	10–107 mmol/d
Amylase	Serum		25–125 U/L
(S:Beckman, defined substrate)			
	Urine, timed specimen		1–17 U/h
Angiotensin I	Peripheral venous	11–88 pg/mL	11–88 ng/L
	plasma (EDTA)		
Angiotensin II	Plasma (EDTA)	10–60 pg/mL	10–60 ng/L
	Arterial blood		
α₁-Antitrypsin	Serum	78–200 mg/dL	0.78–2.00 g/L
(nephelometry)			
Anion gap	Plasma (heparin) or	7–14 mEq/L	7–14 mmol/L
[Na − (Cl⁻ + HCO₃⁻)]	serum		
Arsenic	Whole blood (heparin)	0.2–2.3 μg/dL	0.03–0.31 μmol/L
		Chronic poisoning: 10–50 μg/dL	1.33–6.65 μmol/L
		Acute poisoning: 60–93 μg/dL	7.98–12.37 μmol/L
	Urine, 24-h	5–50 μg/d	0.067–0.665 μmol/d
Ascorbic acid (see Vitamin C)			
Aspartate aminotransferase			
(AST, SGOT)	Serum		10–30 U/L
Base excess	Whole blood (heparin)	−2 to 3 mEq/L	−2 to 3 mmol/L
Bicarbonate	Serum	18–23 mEq/L	18–23 mmol/L
Bile acids, total	Serum, fasting	0.3–2.3 μg/mL	0.74–5.64 μmol/L
	Serum, 1-h postprandial	1.8–3.2 μg/mL	4.41–7.84 μmol/L
	Feces	120–225 mg/d	294–551 μmol/d
Bilirubin			
Total	Serum	0.2–1.0 mg/dL	3.4–17.1 μmol/L
	Urine	Negative	Negative
Conjugated (direct)	Serum	0–0.2 mg/dL	0–3.4 μmol/L
Calcium, ionized (iCa)	Serum	4.65–5.28 mg/dL	1.16–1.32 mmol/L
Calcium, total	Serum	8.4–10.2 mg/dL	2.10–2.55 mmol/L
	Urine, 24-h	100–300 mg/d	2.5–7.5 mmol/d
	CSF	4.2–5.4 mg/dL	1.05–1.35 mmol/L
Carbon dioxide,	Serum or plasma	23–29 mEq/L	23–29 mmol/L
total (TCO₂)	(heparin)		
Carcinoembryonic	Serum	Nonsmokers: <2.5 ng/mL	<2.5 μg/L
antigen (CEA)			
β-Carotene	Serum	10–85 μg/dL	0.19–1.58 μmol/L
Catecholamines, total	Urine, 24-h	<100 μg/d	<5.91 nmol/d
Ceruloplasmin (RID)	Serum	18–45 mg/dL	180–450 mg/L
Chloride	Serum or plasma	98–106 mEq/L	98–106 mmol/L
	(heparin)		
	CSF	118–132 mEq/L	118–132 mmol/L
	Urine, 24-h	110–250 mEq/d	110–250 mmol/d

Table continued on following page

CLINICAL CHEMISTRY, TOXICOLOGY, SEROLOGY *Continued*

Test	Specimen	Reference Interval (Conventional Units)	Reference Interval (International Units)
Cholesterol, total	Serum or plasma (EDTA)	Recommended: <200 mg/dL	<5.18 mmol/L
		Moderate risk: 200–239 mg/L	5.18–6.19 mmol/L
		High risk: ≥240 mg/dL	≥6.22 mmol/L
Chorionic gonadotropin, β-subunit (β-HCG)	Serum or plasma (EDTA)	M and nonpregnant F: <5.0 mU/mL	<5.0 IU/L
Complement			
Total hemolytic Complement activity	Plasma (EDTA)	75–160 U/mL	75–160 kU/L
Copper	Serum	M: 70–140 μg/dL	10.99–21.98 μmol/L
		F: 80–155 μg/dL	12.56–24.34 μmol/L
	Erythrocyte (heparin)	90–150 μg/dL	14.13–23.55 μmol/L
	Urine, 24-h	3–35 μg/d	0.047–0.55 μmol/d
Coproporphyrin	Urine, 24-h	34–234 μg/d	51–351 nmol/d
	Feces, 24-h	<30 μg/g dry wt	<45 nmol/g dry wt
Corticosteroid-binding globulin (CBG) (see Transcortin)		400–1200 μg/d	600–1800 nmol/d
Corticosterone	Serum	0800 h: 130–820 ng/dL	4–24 nmol/L
		1600 h: 60–220 ng/dL	2–6 nmol/L
Cortisol	Serum or plasma (heparin)	0800 h: 5–23 μg/dL	138–635 nmol/L
		1600 h: 3–15 μg/dL	82–413 nmol/L
		2000 h: ≤50% of 0800 h	Fraction of 0800 h: ≤0.50
Cortisol, free	Urine, 24-h	10–100 μg/d	27–276 nmol/d
C-Peptide	Serum	0.78–1.89 ng/mL	0.26–0.62 nmol/L
C-Reactive protein	Serum	68–8200 ng/mL	68–8200 μg/L
Creatine kinase (CK)	Serum		M: 38–174 U/L
			F: 26–140 U/L
Isoenzymes	Serum	Fraction 2 (MB) <4–6% of total (method-dependent)	Fraction of total: <0.04–0.06
Creatinine	Serum or plasma	M: 0.7–1.3 mg/dL	62–115 μmol/L
Jaffe, kinetic or enzymatic		F: 0.6–1.1 mg/dL	53–97 μmol/L
	Urine, 24-h	M: 14–26 mg/kg/d	124–230 μmol/kg/d
		F: 11–20 mg/kg/d	97–177 μmol/kg/d
Creatinine clearance (endogenous)	Serum or plasma, and urine	M: 90–139 mL/min/1.73 m²	0.87–1.34 mL/s/m²
		F: 80–125 mL/min/1.73 m²	0.77–1.20 mL/s/m²
Dehydroepiandrosterone serum (DHEA)	Serum	M: 1.8–12.5 ng/mL	6.2–43.3 nmol/L
		F: 1.3–9.8 ng/mL	4.5–34.0 nmol/L
Dehydroepiandrosterone sulfate (DHEA-S)	Serum	M: 1.7–6.7 μg/mL	4.6–18.2 μmol/L
		F: Premenopausal: 0.5–5.4 μg/mL	1.4–14.7 μmol/L
		Postmenopausal: 0.3–2.6 μg/mL	0.8–7.1 μmol/L
11-Deoxycortisol (compound S)	Serum	12–158 ng/dL	0.3–4.6 nmol/L
Estrogens, total	Serum	M: 20–80 pg/mL	20–80 ng/L
		F, cycle:	
		Follicular phase: 60–200 pg/mL	60–200 ng/L
		Luteal phase: 160–400 pg/mL	160–400 ng/L
		Postmenopausal: ≤130 pg/mL	≤130 ng/L
	Urine, 24-h		M: 15–40 μg/d
			F: Preovulation: 4–25 μg/d
			Ovulation: 28–100 μg/d
			Luteal peak: 22–80 μg/d
			Pregnancy, term: <45,000 μg/d
			Postmenopausal: <20 μg/d
Fat, fecal	Feces, 72-h		<7 g/d
			fat-free diet: <4 g/d
Fatty acids, nonesterified (free)	Serum or plasma (heparin)	8–25 mg/dL	0.28–0.89 mmol/L
Ferritin	Serum	M: 20–250 ng/mL	20–250 μg/L
		F: 10–120 ng/mL	10–120 μg/L
α₁-Fetoprotein	Serum	<10 ng/mL	<10 μg/L
Fibrinogen (see Hematology and Coagulation section)			
Folate	Serum	3–16 ng/mL	7–36 nmol/L
	Erythrocytes (EDTA)	130–628 ng/mL packed cells	294–1422 nmol/L packed cells
Follitropin (FSH)	Serum or plasma (heparin)	M: 4–25 mIU/mL	4–25 IU/L
		F: Follicular phase: 1–9 mU/mL	1–9 U/L
		Ovulatory peak: 6–26 mU/mL	6–26 U/L
		Luteal phase: 1–9 mU/mL	1–9 U/L
		Postmenopausal: 30–118 mU/mL	30–118 U/L
	Urine, 24-h		4–18 U/d
			3–12 U/d
Free thyroxine index (FT₄I)	Serum		4.2–13.0
Gastrin	Serum	<100 pg/mL	<100 ng/L

CLINICAL CHEMISTRY, TOXICOLOGY, SEROLOGY *Continued*

Test	Specimen	Reference Interval (Conventional Units)	Reference Interval (International Units)
Glucose	Serum	Adult: 70–105 mg/dL	3.9–5.8 mmol/L
		>60 y: 80–115 mg/dL	4.4–6.4 mmol/L
	Whole blood (heparin)	65–95 mg/dL	3.6–5.3 mmol/L
	CSF	40–70 mg/dL	2.2–3.9 mmol/L
Quantitative, enzymatic	Urine	<0.5 g/d	<2.8 mmol/d
Qualitative	Urine		Negative
Glucose, 2-h postprandial	Serum	<120 mg/dL	<6.7 mmol/L
Glucose tolerance test (GTT), oral	Serum		

	mg/dL		mmol/L	
	Normal	Diabetic	Normal	Diabetic
Fasting:	70–105	>140	3.9–5.8	>7.8
60 min:	120–170	≥200	6.7–9.4	≥11
90 min:	100–140	≥200	5.6–7.8	≥11
120 min:	70–120	≥140	3.9–6.7	≥7.8

Test	Specimen	Reference Interval (Conventional Units)	Reference Interval (International Units)
γ-Glutamyltransferase (GGT)	Serum		M: 9–50 U/L
			F: 8–40 U/L
Glycerol, free	Plasma	0.29–1.72 mg/dL	0.032—0.187 mmol/L
Growth hormone (HGH, somatotropin)	Serum or plasma (EDTA, heparin)	Adult, M: <2 ng/mL	<2 µg/L
		F: <10 ng/mL	<10 µg/L
		>60 y, M: 0.4–10 ng/mL	0.4–10 µg/L
		F: 1–14 ng/mL	1–14 µg/L
Haptoglobin (see Hematology and Coagulation section)			
HDL-cholesterol (HDLC) (5th percentile from Lipid Research Clinics)	Serum or plasma (EDTA)	M: >29 mg/dL	>0.75 mmol/L
		F: >35 mg/dL	>0.91 mmol/L
Hemoglobin A₁c (electrophoresis)	Whole blood (heparin, EDTA, or oxalate)	5.6–7.5% of total Hb	Fraction of Hb: 0.056–0.075
Homovanillic acid (HVA)	Urine, 24-h	1.4–8.8 mg/d	8–48 µmol/d
17-Hydroxycorticosteroids (17-OHCS)	Urine, 24-h	M: 3.0–10.0 mg/d	8.3–27.6 µmol/d
		F: 2.0–8.0 mg/d	5.5–22.1 µmol/d
5-Hydroxyindole acetic acid (5 HIAA)			
Qualitative	Fresh random urine		Negative
Quantitative	Urine, 24-h	2–6 mg/d	10.4–31.2 µmol/d
17-Hydroxyprogesterone (17-OHP)	Serum	M: 0.5–2.5 ng/mL	1.5–7.5 nmol/L
		F: Follicular: 0.2–1.0 ng/mL	0.6–3.0 nmol/L
		Luteal: 1.0–5.0 ng/mL	3.0–15.5 nmol/L
		Postmenopausal: ≤0.7 ng/mL	≤2.1 nmol/L
Immunoglobulin A (IgA)	Serum	40–350 mg/dL	400–3500 mg/L
Immunoglobulin D (IgD)	Serum	0–8 mg/dL	0–80 mg/L
Immunoglobulin E (IgE)	Serum	0–380 IU/mL	0–380 kIU/L
Immunoglobulin G (IgG)	Serum	650–1600 mg/dL	6.5–16 g/L
	CSF	0.5–5 mg/dL	5–50 mg/L
Immunoglobulin M (IgM)	Serum	55–300 mg/dL	550–3000 mg/L
Insulin (12-h fasting)	Serum	6–24 µIU/mL	42–167 pmol/L
Intrinsic factor (see Vitamin B₁₂)			
Iron	Serum	M: 65–175 µg/dL	11.6–31.3 µmol/L
		F: 50–170 µg/dL	9.0–30.4 µmol/L
Iron-binding capacity, total (TIBC)	Serum	250–450 µg/dL	44.8–80.6 µmol/L
Iron saturation	Serum	M: 20–50	Fraction of iron saturation: 0.20–0.5 (M)
		F: 15–50	0.15–0.5 (F)
17-Ketogenic steroids (17-KGS)	Urine, 24-h	M: 5–23 mg/d	17–80 µmol/d
		F: 3–15 mg/d	10–52 µmol/d
Ketone bodies			
Qualitative	Serum	Negative (0.5–3.0 mg/dL)	Negative (5–30 mg/L)
	Urine, random		Negative
17-Ketosteroids, total (17-KS)	Urine, 24-h	M: 18–30 y 9–22 mg/d	31–76 µmol/d
		>30 y 8–20 mg/d	28–70 µmol/d
		F: 6–15 mg/d	21–52 µmol/d
L-Lactate	Whole blood (heparin)	Venous: 4.5–19.8 mg/dL	0.5–2.2 mmol/L
		Arterial: 4.5–14.4 mg/dL	0.5–1.6 mmol/L
Lactate dehydrogenase (LDH)	Serum		208–378 U/L
LDH isoenzymes (Electrophoresis, agarose)	Serum	%	Fraction of total:
		Fraction 1: 18–33	0.18–0.33
		Fraction 2: 28–40	0.28–0.40
		Fraction 3: 18–30	0.18–0.30
		Fraction 4: 6–16	0.06–0.16
		Fraction 5: 2–13	0.02–0.13
Lead	Whole blood (heparin)	<40 µg/dL	<1.93 µmol/L
		Toxic: ≥100 µg/dL	≥4.83 µmol/L
	Urine, 24-h	<80 µg/L	<0.39 µmol/L

Table continued on following page

CLINICAL CHEMISTRY, TOXICOLOGY, SEROLOGY *Continued*

Test	Specimen	Reference Interval (Conventional Units)	Reference Interval (International Units)
Lipase (turbidimetric)	Serum		Adult: 10–140 U/L
			>60 y: 18–180 U/L
LDL-Cholesterol (LDLC)	Serum or plasma (EDTA)	Recommended: <130 mg/dL	<3.37 mmol/L
		Moderate risk: 130–159 mg/dL	3.37–4.12 mmol/L
		High risk: ≥160 mg/dL	≥4.14 mmol/L
Lutropin (LH)	Serum or plasma (heparin)	M: 1–8 mU/mL	1–8 U/L
		F: Follicular phase: 1–12 mU/mL	1–12 U/L
		Midcycle: 16–104 mU/mL	16–104 U/L
		Luteal: 1–12 mU/mL	1–12 U/L
		Postmenopausal: 16–66 mU/mL	16–66 U/L
	Urine		M: 9–23 U/d
			F: non-midcycle, 4–30 U/d
Lysozyme	Serum, plasma	0.4–1.3 mg/dL	4–13 mg/L
Magnesium	Serum	1.3–2.1 mEq/L	0.65–1.05 mmol/L
	Urine, 24-h	6.0–10.0 mEq/d	3.00–5.00 mmol/d
Mercury	Whole blood (EDTA)	<5.0 µg/dL	<0.25 µmol/L
	Urine, 24-h	<20 µg/L	<0.1 µmol/L
		Toxic: >150 µg/L	<0.75 µmol/L
Metanephrine, total	Urine, 24-h	0.05–1.20 µg/mg creatinine	0.03–0.69 mmol/mol creatinine
Myelin basic protein	CSF		<2.5 ng/mL
Myoglobin	Serum		M: 19–92 µg/L
			F: 12–76 µg/L
	Urine, random		Negative
Osmolality	Serum		275–295 mOsmol/kg
	Urine, random		50–1400 mOsmol/kg, depending on fluid intake
			After 12-h fluid restriction: >850 mOsmol/kg
	Urine, 24-h		~390–900 mOsmol/kg
Oxalate	Serum	1–2.4 µg/mL	11–27 µmol/L
		Ethylene glycol poisoning: >20 µg/mL	Ethylene glycol poisoning: >228 µmol/L
Oxygen (PO_2)	Whole blood, arterial (heparin)	83–100 mm Hg	11–14.4 kPa
Oxygen saturation	Whole blood, arterial (heparin)	95–98%	Fraction saturated: 0.95–0.98
pH (37°C)	Whole blood, arterial (heparin)		7.35–7.45
Phosphorus, inorganic	Serum	2.7–4.5 mg/dL	0.87–1.45 nmol/L
		>60 y, M: 2.3–3.7 mg/dL	0.74–1.2 nmol/L
		F: 2.8–4.1 mg/dL	0.90–1.3 nmol/L
	Urine, 24-h	0.4–1.3 g/d	13–42 mmol/d
Porphobilinogen (PBG)			
Quantitative	Urine, 24-h	0–2.0 mg/d	0–8.8 µmol/d
Qualitative	Urine, fresh random		Negative
Potassium	Serum	3.5–5.1 mEq/L	3.5–5.1 mmol/L
	Plasma (heparin)	3.5–4.5 mEq/L	3.5–4.5 mmol/L
	Urine, 24-h	25–125 mEq/d	25–125 mmol/d
Pregnanediol	Urine, 24-h	M: 0–1.9 mg/d	0–5.9 µmol/d
		F: Follicular: <2.6 mg/d	<8 µmol/d
		Luteal: 2.6–10.6 mg/d	8–33 µmol/d
		Postmenopausal: 0.2–1.0 mg/d	0.6–3.1 µmol/d
Progesterone	Serum	M: 0.13–0.97 ng/mL	0.4–3.1 nmol/L
		F: Follicular: 0.15–0.70 ng/mL	0.5–2.2 nmol/L
		Luteal: 2.0–25 ng/mL	6.4–79.5 nmol/L
Prolactin (hPRL)	Serum	0–20 ng/mL	0–20 µg/L
Protein			
Total	Serum	6.4–8.3 g/dL	64.0–83.0 g/L
Electrophoresis	Serum	Albumin: 3.5–5.0 g/dL	35–50 g/L
		α_1-Globulin: 0.1–0.3 g/dL	1–3 g/L
		α_2-Globulin: 0.6–1.0 g/dL	6–10 g/L
		β-Globulin: 0.7–1.1 g/dL	7–11 g/L
		γ-Globulin: 0.8–1.6 g/dL	8–16 g/L
Total	Urine, 24-h		50–80 mg/d at rest
Total	CSF	Lumbar: 15–45 mg/dL	150–450 mg/L
Protoporphyrin	Whole blood (heparin or EDTA)	17–77 µg/dL RBC	0.30–1.37 µmol/L RBC
	Feces, 24-h	≤60 µg/g dry wt or <1500 µg/d	≤0.11 mmol/kg dry wt or <2.67 µmol/d
Pyruvic acid	Whole blood (heparin)	0.3–0.9 mg/dL	0.03–0.10 mmol/L
Renin (normal diet)	Plasma (EDTA)	ng/mL/h ± 1 SE	µg/L/h ± 1 SE
		Supine: 1.6 ± 1.5	1.6 ± 1.5
		Standing: (4-h): 4.5 ± 2.9	4.5 ± 2.9

CLINICAL CHEMISTRY, TOXICOLOGY, SEROLOGY *Continued*

Test	Specimen	Reference Interval (Conventional Units)		Reference Interval (International Units)	
Riboflavin (see Vitamin B_2)					
Sediment	Urine, fresh, random			Hyaline: occasional (0–1) casts/hpf	
Casts				RBC: not seen	
				WBC: not seen	
				Tubular epithelial: not seen	
				Transitional and squamous epithelial: not seen	
Cells				RBC: 0–2/hpf	
				WBC: M: 0–3/hpf	
				F: 0–5/hpf	
				Epithelial: few	
				Bacteria:	
				Unspun: no organisms/oil immersion field	
				Spun: <20 organisms/hpf	
Sodium	Serum or plasma (heparin)	136–146 mEq/L		136–146 mmol/L	
	Urine, 24-h	40–220 mEq/d		40–220 mmol/d	
Specific gravity	Urine, random			1.002–1.030	
	Urine, 24-h			1.015–1.025	
			% of total		Fraction of total
Testosterone, free	Serum	M: 52–280 pg/mL	1.5–3.2	180.4–971.6 pmol/L	0.015–0.032
		F: 1.6–6.3 pg/mL	0.8–1.4	5.6–21.9 pmol/L	0.008–0.014
Testosterone, total	Serum	M: 300–1000 ng/dL		10.4–34.7 nmol/L	
		F: 20–75 ng/dL		0.69–2.6 nmol/L	
	Urine	20–50 y,			
		M: 50–135 μg/d		173–470 nmol/d	
		F: 2–12 μg/d		7–42 nmol/d	
		>50 y,			
		M: 40–60 μg/d		139–210 nmol/d	
		F: 2–8 μg/d		7–28 nmol/d	
Thiamine (see Vitamin B_1)	Serum				
Thyroglobulin (Tg)	Serum	3–42 ng/mL		3–42 μg/L	
Thyroglobulin antibodies	Serum			<1:10	
Thyroid microsomal antibodies	Serum			Nondetectable (hemagglutination) or <1:10 (IFA)	
Thyrotropin (hTSH)	Serum or plasma	2–10 μU/mL		2–10 mU/L	
Thyrotropin-releasing hormone	Plasma	5–60 pg/mL		5–60 ng/L	
Thyroxine, free (FT_4)	Serum	0.8–2.4 ng/dL		10–31 pmol/L	
Thyroxine (T_4), total	Serum	5–12 μg/dL		65–155 nmol/L	
		>60 y, M: 5.0–10.0 μg/dL		65–129 nmol/L	
		F: 5.5–10.5 μg/dL		71–135 nmol/L	
Thyroxine-binding globulin (TBG)	Serum	15.0–34.0 μg/mL		15.0–34.0 mg/L	
Thyroxine index, free (see Free thyroxine index)					
Transcortin	Serum	M: 18.8–25.2 mg/L		323–433 nmol/L	
		F: 14.9–22.9 mg/L		256–393 nmol/L	
Transferrin	Serum	200–400 mg/dL		2.0–4.0 g/L	
		>60 y: 180–380 mg/dL		1.80–3.80 g/L	
Triglycerides (TG)	Serum, after ≥12-hr fast	Recommended:			
		M: 40–160 mg/dL		0.45–1.81 mmol/L	
		F: 35–135 mg/dL		0.40–1.52 mmol/L	
Tri-iodothyronine, free	Serum	260–480 pg/dL		4.0–7.4 pmol/L	
Tri-iodothyronine, total (T_3)	Serum	100–200 ng/dL		1.54–3.08 mmol/L	
Tri-iodothyronine resin uptake test (T_3RU)	Serum	24–34%		24–34 AU (arbitrary units)	
Urea nitrogen	Serum or plasma	7–18 mg/dL		2.5–6.4 mmol/L	
	Urine	12–20 g/d		0.43–0.71 mol/d	
Urea nitrogen/creatinine ratio	Serum			12/1–20/1	
Uric acid (uricase)	Serum	M: 3.5–7.2 mg/dL		0.21–0.42 mmol/L	
		F: 2.6–6.0 mg/dL		0.15–0.35 mmol/L	
	Urine, 24-h	250–750 mg/d		1.48–4.43 mmol/d	
Urinary sediment (see Sediment)					
Urobilinogen	Urine, 2-h	0.1–0.8 EU		0.1–0.8 U	
	Urine, 24-h	0.5–4.0 EU		0.5–4.0 U	
	Feces	75–275 EU/100 g		750–2750 U/kg	
		75–400 EU/d		75–400 U/d	
		40–280 mg/d		67–473 μmol/d	
Uroporphyrin	Urine, 24-h	<50 μg/d		<60 nmol/d	
	Feces, 24-h specimen	10–40 μg/d		12–48 nmol/d	
	Erythrocytes (heparin or EDTA)			Negative	

Table continued on following page

CLINICAL CHEMISTRY, TOXICOLOGY, SEROLOGY *Continued*

Test	Specimen	Reference Interval (Conventional Units)	Reference Interval (International Units)
Vanillylmandelic acid (VMA)	Urine, 24-h	2–7 mg/d	10.1–35.4 μmol/d
Viscosity	Serum		1.10–1.22 centipoise
Vitamin A	Serum	30–80 μg/dL	1.05–2.8 μmol/L
Vitamin B₁ (Thiamine)	Serum	0–2 μg/dL	0–75 nmol/L
Vitamin B₂ (Riboflavin)	Serum	4–24 μg/dL	106–638 nmol/L
Vitamin B₆	Plasma (EDTA)	5–30 ng/mL	20–121 nmol/L
Vitamin B₁₂	Serum	100–700 pg/mL	74–516 pmol/L
Vitamin C	Plasma (oxalate, heparin, or EDTA)	0.5–1.5 mg/dL	28–85 μmol/L
Vitamin D₃, 1,25-dihydroxy	Serum	25–45 pg/mL	60–108 pmol/L
Vitamin D₃, 25-hydroxy	Plasma (heparin)	Summer: 15–80 ng/mL	37.4–200 nmol/L
		Winter: 14–42 ng/mL	34.9–105 nmol/L
Vitamin E	Serum	5.0–18.0 μg/mL	12–42 μmol/L
Zinc	Serum	70–150 μg/dL	10.7–22.9 μmol/L

HEMATOLOGY AND COAGULATION

Test	Specimen	Reference Interval (Conventional Units)	Reference Interval (International Units)
Activated partial thromboplastin time (APTT)	Whole blood (Na citrate)		25–35 sec
Bleeding time (BT)			
Ivy	Blood from skin		Normal: 2–7 min
			Borderline: 7–11 min
Simplate (G-D)			2.75–8 min
Blood volume	Whole blood (heparin)		M: 52–83 mL/kg
			F: 50–75 mL/kg
Bone marrow	Bone marrow aspirate	% (mean)	Number fraction (mean)
Differential count			
Myeloblasts		0.3–5.0 (2.0)	0.003–0.05 (0.02)
Promyelocytes		1.0–8.0 (5.0)	0.01–0.08 (0.05)
Myelocytes:			
Neutrophilic		5.0–19.0 (12.0)	0.05–0.19 (0.12)
Eosinophilic		0.5–3.0 (1.5)	0.005–0.03 (0.015)
Basophilic		0.0–0.5 (0.3)	0.00–0.005 (0.003)
Metamyelocytes		13.0–32.0 (22.0)	0.13–0.32 (0.22)
Polymorphonuclear neutrophils		7.0–3.0 (2.0)	0.07–0.30 (0.20)
Polymorphonuclear eosinophils		0.5–4.0 (2.0)	0.005–0.04 (0.02)
Polymorphonuclear basophils		0.0–0.7 (0.2)	0.0–0.007 (0.002)
Lymphocytes		3.0–17.0 (10.0)	0.03–0.17 (0.10)
Plasma cells		0.0–2.0 (0.4)	0.00–0.02 (0.004)
Monocytes		0.5–5.0 (2.0)	0.005–0.05 (0.02)
Reticulum cells		0.1–2.0 (0.2)	0.001–0.02 (0.002)
Megakaryocytes		0.03–3.0 (0.1)	0.0003–0.03 (0.001)
Pronormoblasts		1.0–8.0 (4.0)	0.01–0.08 (0.04)
Normoblasts		7.0–32.0 (18.0)	0.07–0.32 (0.18)
Clot lysis, 37°C	Whole clotted blood		48–72 h
Clot retraction screen	Whole blood (no anticoagulant)		Retraction begins at 1 h, maximum at 24 h
Clotting time, Lee-White, 37°C	Whole blood (no anticoagulant)		5–8 min
Differential count (see Bone marrow differential count or Leukocyte differential count)			
Eosinophil count	Whole blood (EDTA); capillary blood	50–400 cells/μL (mm³)	50–400 × 10⁶ cells/L
Erythrocyte count (RBC count)	Whole blood (EDTA)	millions of cells/μL (mm³)	× 10¹² cells/L
		M: 4.3–5.7	4.3–5.7
		F: 3.8–5.1	3.8–5.1
Erythrocyte sedimentation rate (ESR), Wintrobe			M: 0–15 mm/h
			F: 0–20 mm/h
Ferritin (see Chemistry section)			
Fibrin degradation products (Agglutination, Thrombo-Wellco test)	Whole blood: special tube containing thrombin and proteolytic inhibitor	<10 μg/mL	<10 mg/L
	Urine: 2 mL in special tube (see above)	<0.25 μg/mL	<0.25 mg/L
Fibrinogen	Plasma (Na citrate)	200–400 mg/dL	2.00–4.00 g/L
Glucose-6-phosphate dehydrogenase (G6PD) in erythrocytes	Whole blood (ACD, EDTA, or heparin)	12.1 ± 2.09 U/g Hb (1 SD)	0.78 ± 0.13 MU/mol Hb (1 SD)
Haptoglobin (Hp) RID	Serum; avoid hemolysis	26–185 mg/dL	260–1850 mg/L
Hematocrit (HCT, Hct)	Whole blood (EDTA)		
Calculated from MCV and RBC (electronic displacement or laser)		M: 39–49%	0.39–0.49 volume fraction
		F: 35–45%	0.35–0.45 volume fraction

HEMATOLOGY AND COAGULATION *Continued*

Test	Specimen	Reference Interval (Conventional Units)		Reference Interval (International Units)	
Hemoglobin (Hb)	Whole blood (EDTA)	M: 13.5–17.5 g/dL		2.09–2.71 mmol/L	
		F: 12.0–16.0 g/dL		1.86–2.48 mmol/L	
	Plasma (heparin, ACD)	<3 mg/dL		<0.47 µmol/L	
	Urine, fresh, random			Negative	
Hemoglobin electrophoresis	Whole blood (EDTA, citrate, or heparin)			Mass fraction	
		HbA >95%		HbA >0.95	
		HbA₂ 1.5–3.5%		HbA₂ 0.015–0.035	
		HbF <2%		HbF <0.02	
Leukocyte count (WBC count)	Whole blood (EDTA)	4.5–11.0 × 10³ cells/µL (mm³)		4.5–11.0 × 10⁹ cells/L	
	CSF	0.5 mononuclear cells/µgL		0.5 × 10⁶ cells/L	
Leukocyte	Whole blood (EDTA)	%	Cells/µL (mm³)	Number fraction	Cells × 10⁶/L
Differential count					
Myelocytes		0	0	0	0
Neutrophils—bands		3–5	150–400	0.03–0.05	150–400
Neutrophils—segmented		54–62	3000–5800	0.54–0.62	3000–5800
Lymphocytes		23–33	1500–3000	0.25–0.33	1500–3000
Monocytes		3–7	285–500	0.03–0.07	285–500
Eosinophils		1–3	50–250	0.01–0.03	50–250
Basophils		0–0.75	15–50	0–0.0075	15–50
Leukocyte					
Differential count	CSF	%		Number fraction	
Lymphocytes		62 ± 34		0.62 ± 0.324	
Monocytes (includes pia-arachnoid mesothelial cells)		36 ± 20		0.36 ± 0.20	
Neutrophils		2 ± 5		0.02 ± 0.05	
Histocytes				Rare	
Ependymal cells				Rare	
Eosinophils				Rare	
Mean corpuscular hemoglobin (MCH)	Whole blood (EDTA)	26–34 pg/cell		0.40–0.53 fmol/cell	
Mean corpuscular hemoglobin concentration (MCHC)	Whole blood (EDTA)	31–37% Hb/cell or gHb/dL RBC		4.81–5.74 mmol Hb/L RBC	
Mean corpuscular volume (MCV)	Whole blood (EDTA)			80–100 fL	
Methemoglobin (MetHb)	Whole blood (EDTA, heparin, or ACD)	0.06–0.24 g/dL		9.3–37.2 µmol/L	
Partial thromboplastin time (PTT)	Whole blood (Na citrate)			60–85 sec	
Plasma volume	Plasma (heparin)	M: 25–43 mL/kg		0.025–0.043 L/kg	
		F: 28–45 mL/kg		0.028–0.045 L/kg	
Platelet count (thrombocyte count)	Whole blood (EDTA)	150–450 × 10³/µL (mm³)		150–450 × 10⁹/L	
Prothrombin consumption	Whole blood (no anticoagulant)			>30 sec	
Prothrombin time, two-stage modified	Whole blood (Na citrate)			18–22 sec	
RBC count (see Erthyrocyte count)					
Red cell volume	Whole blood (heparin)	M: 20–36 mL/kg		M: 0.020–0.036 L/kg	
		F: 19–31 mL/kg		F: 0.019–0.031 L/kg	
Reticulocyte count	Whole blood (EDTA, heparin, or oxalate)	0.5–1.5% of erythrocytes		0.005–0.015 (number fraction)	
Sulfhemoglobin	Whole blood (EDTA, heparin, or ACD)	≤1.0% of total Hb		<0.010 of total Hb (mass fraction)	
Thrombin time	Whole blood (Na citrate)			Time of control ± 2S when control is 9–13 sec	
Thromboplastin time, activated (see Activated partial thromboplastin time [APTT])					

DRUGS—THERAPEUTIC AND TOXIC

Drug	Specimen	Reference Interval (Conventional Units)		Reference Interval (International Units)
Acetaminophen	Serum or plasma (hep or EDTA)	Therap:	10–30 µg/mL	66–199 µmol/L
		Toxic:	>200 µg/mL	>1324 µmol/L
Amikacin	Serum or plasma (EDTA)	Therap:		
		Peak	25–35 µg/mL	43–60 µmol/L
		Trough (severe infection):	4–8 µg/mL	6.8–13.7 µmol/L
		Toxic:		
		Peak	>35 µg/mL	>60 µmol/L
		Trough	>10 µg/mL	>17 µmol/L
ε-Aminocaproic acid	Serum or plasma (hep or EDTA); trough	Therap:	100–400 µg/mL	0.76–3.05 mmol/L
Amitriptyline	Serum or plasma (hep or EDTA); trough (>12 h after dose)	Therap:	120–250 ng/mL	433–903 nmol/L
		Toxic:	>500 ng/mL	>1805 nmol/L
Amobarbital	Serum	Therap:	1–5 µg/mL	4–22 µmol/L
		Toxic:	>10 µg/mL	>44 µmol/L
Amphetamine	Serum or plasma (hep or EDTA)	Therap:	20–30 ng/mL	148–222 nmol/L
		Toxic:	>200 ng/mL	>1480 nmol/L
Bromide	Serum	Therap:	750–1500 µg/mL	9.4–18.7 mmol/L
		Toxic:	>1250 µg/mL	>15.6 mmol/L

Table continued on following page

DRUGS—THERAPEUTIC AND TOXIC *Continued*

Drug	Specimen		Reference Interval (Conventional Units)	Reference Interval (International Units)
Caffeine	Serum or plasma (hep or EDTA)	Therap:	3–15 µg/mL	15–77 µmol/L
		Toxic:	>50 µg/mL	>258 µmol/L
Carbamazepine	Serum or plasma (hep or EDTA); trough	Therap:	4–12 µg/mL	17–51 µmol/L
		Toxic:	>15 µg/mL	>63 µmol/L
Carbenicillin	Serum or plasma	Therap:		Dependent on minimum inhibition concentration of specific organism
		Toxic:	>250 µg/mL	>660 µmol/L
Chloramphenicol	Serum or plasma (hep or EDTA); trough	Therap:	10–25 µg/L	31–77 µmol/L
		Toxic:	>25 µg/L	>77 µmol/L
Chlordiazepoxide	Serum or plasma (hep or EDTA); trough	Therap:	700–1000 ng/mL	2.34–3.34 µmol/L
		Toxic:	>5000 ng/mL	>16.7 µmol/L
Chlorpromazine	Serum or plasma (hep or EDTA); trough	Therap:	50–300 ng/mL	157–942 nmol/L
		Toxic:	>750 ng/mL	>2355 nmol/L
Cimetidine	Serum or plasma (hep or EDTA); trough	Therap:	0.5–1.2 µg/mL	2–5 µmol/L
Clonazepam	Serum or plasma (hep or EDTA; trough	Therap:	15–60 ng/mL	48–190 nmol/L
		Toxic:	>80 ng/mL	>254 nmol/L
Clonidine	Serum or plasma (hep or EDTA)	Therap:	1.0–2.0 ng/mL	4.4–8.7 nmol/L
Clorazepate	Serum or plasma (hep or EDTA)	As desmethyldiazepam:		
		Therap:	0.12–1.0 µg/mL	0.36–3.01 µmol/L
Cocaine	Serum or plasma (hep or EDTA); on ice	Therap:	100–500 ng/mL	330–1650 nmol/L
		Toxic:	>1000 ng/mL	>3300 nmol/L
Cyclosporine	Serum (12 h after dose)	Therap:	100–400 ng/mL	83–333 nmol/L
		Toxic:	>400 mg/mL	>333 µmol/L
Desipramine	Serum or plasma (hep or EDTA); trough (≥12 h after dose)	Therap:	75–300 ng/mL	281–1125 nmol/L
		Toxic:	>400 ng/mL	>1500 nmol/L
Diazepam	Serum or plasma (hep or EDTA); trough	Therap:	100–1000 ng/mL	0.35–3.51 µmol/L
		Toxic:	>5000 ng/mL	>17.55 µmol/L
Digitoxin	Serum or plasma (hep or EDTA) ≥6 h after dose	Therap:	20–35 ng/mL	24–46 nmol/L
		Toxic	>45 ng/mL	>59 nmol/L
Digoxin	Serum or plasma (hep or EDTA); trough (≥12 h after dose)	Therap:	0.8–1.5 mg/mL	1.1–1.9 nmol/L
		CHF: Arrhythmias:	1.5–2.0 ng/mL	1.9–2.6 nmol/L
		Toxic:	>2.5 ng/mL	>3.2 nmol/L
Diphenylhydantoin (see Phenytoin)				
Disopyramide	Serum or plasma (hep or EDTA); trough	Therap: Arrhythmias:		
		Atrial	2.8–3.2 µg/mL	8.3–9.4 µmol/L
		Ventricular	3.3–7.5 µg/mL	9.7–22 µmol/L
		Toxic:	>7 µg/mL	>20.7 µmol/L
Doxepin	Serum or plasma (hep or EDTA); trough (≥ 12 h after dose)	Therap:	30–150 ng/mL	107–537 nmol/L
		Toxic:	>500 ng/mL	>1790 nmol/L
Ethchlorvynol	Serum or plasma (hep or EDTA)	Therap:	2–8 µg/mL	14–55 µmol/L
		Toxic:	>20 µg/mL	>138 µmol/L
Ethosuximide	Serum or plasma (hep or EDTA); trough	Therap:	40–100 µg/mL	283–708 µmol/L
		Toxic:	>150 µg/mL	>1062 µmol/L
Fenoprofen	Plasma (EDTA)	Therap:	20–65 µg/mL	82–268 µmol/L
Flecainide	Serum or plasma (hep or EDTA); trough	Therap:	0.2–1.0 µg/mL	0.5–2.4 µmol/L
		Toxic:	>1.0 µg/mL	>2.4 µmol/L
Furosemide	Serum (30 min after dose)	Therap:	1–2 µg/mL	3–6 µmol/L
Gentamicin	Serum or plasma (EDTA)	Therap:		
		Peak (severe infection)	8–10 µg/mL	16.7–20.9 µmol/L
		Trough (severe infection)	2–4 µg/mL	4.2–8.4 µmol/L
		Toxic:		
		Peak	>10 µg/mL	>21 µmol/L
		Trough	>4 µg/mL	>8.4 µmol/L
Glutethimide	Serum	Therap:	2–6 µg/mL	9–28 µmol/L
		Toxic:	>5 µg/mL	>23 µmol/L
Imipramine	Serum or plasma (hep or EDTA); trough (≥12 h after dose)	Therap:	125–250 ng/mL	446–893 nmol/L
		Toxic:	>500 ng/mL	>1784 nmol/L
Isoniazid	Serum or plasma (hep or EDTA)	Therap:	1–7 µg/mL	7–51 µmol/L
		Toxic:	20–710 µg/mL	146–5176 µmol/L
Kanamycin	Serum or plasma (EDTA)	Therap:		
		Peak	25–35 µg/mL	52–72 µmol/L
		Trough (severe infection)	4–8 µg/mL	8–16 µmol/L
		Toxic:		
		Peak	>35 µg/mL	>72 µmol/L
		Trough	>10 µg/mL	>21 µmol/L
Lidocaine	Serum or plasma (hep or EDTA); ≥45 min following bolus dose	Therap:	1.5–6.0 µg/mL	6.4–26 µmol/L
		Toxic:		
		CNS or cardiovascular depression	6–8 µg/mL	26–34.2 µmol/L
		Seizures, obtundation, decreased cardiac output	>8 µg/mL	>34.2 µmol/L
Lithium	Serum or plasma (hep or EDTA); (>12 h after last dose)	Therap:	0.6–1.2 mEq/L	0.6–1.2 nmol/L
		Toxic:	>2 mEq/L	>2 mmol/L
Lorazepam	Serum or plasma (hep or EDTA)	Therap:	50–240 ng/mL	156–746 nmol/L
Meperidine	Serum or plasma (hep or EDTA)	Therap:	400–700 ng/mL	1620–2830 nmol/L
		Toxic:	>1 µg/mL	>4043 nmol/L
Meprobamate	Serum	Therap:	6–12 µg/mL	28–55 µmol/L
		Toxic:	>60 µg/mL	>275 µmol/L

DRUGS—THERAPEUTIC AND TOXIC *Continued*

Drug	Specimen	Reference Interval (Conventional Units)		Reference Interval (International Units)
Methadone	Serum or plasma (hep or EDTA)	Therap:	100–400 ng/mL	0.32–1.29 µmol/L
		Toxic:	>2000 ng/mL	>6.46 µmol/L
Methaqualone	Serum or plasma (hep or EDTA)	Therap:	2–3 µg/mL	8–12 µmol/L
		Toxic:	>10 µg/mL	>40 µmol/L
Methotrexate	Serum or plasma (hep or EDTA)	Therap:	variable	variable
		Toxic:		
		Low-dose therapy (1–2 wk)	>9.1 ng/mL	>20 nmol/L
		High-dose therapy (48 h)	>454 ng/mL	>1000 nmol/L
Methsuximide (*N*-desmethyl methsuximide)	Serum	Therap:	10–40 µg/mL	53–212 µmol/L
		Toxic:	>40 µg/mL	>212 µmol/L
Methyldopa	Plasma (EDTA)	Therap:	1–5 µg/mL	4.7–23.7 µmol/L
		Toxic:	>7 µg/mL	>33 µmol/L
Methyprylon	Serum	Therap:	8–10 µg/mL	43–55 µmol/L
		Toxic:	>50 µg/mL	>273 µmol/L
Mexiletine	Serum or plasma (hep or EDTA)	Therap:	0.7–2.0 µg/mL	3.9–11.2 µmol/L
		Toxic:	>2.0 µg/mL	>11.2 µmol/L
Morphine	Serum or plasma (hep or EDTA)	Therap:	10–80 ng/mL	35–280 nmol/L
		Toxic:	>200 ng/mL	>700 nmol/L
N-Acetylprocainamide	Serum or plasma (hep or EDTA); trough	Therap:	5–30 µg/mL	18–108 µmol/L
		Toxic:	>40 µg/mL	>144 µmol/L
Nitroprusside	Serum or plasma (EDTA)	As thiocyanate:		
		Therap:	6–29 µg/mL	103–499 µmol/L
Normethsuximide	Serum	Therap:	10–40 µg/mL	53–212 µmol/L
		Toxic:	>40 µg/mL	>212 µmol/L
Nortriptyline	Serum or plasma (hep or EDTA); trough (≥12 h after dose)	Therap:	50–150 ng/mL	190–570 nmol/L
		Toxic:	>500 ng/mL	>1900 nmol/L
Oxazepam	Serum or plasma (hep or EDTA)	Therap:	0.2–1.4 µg/mL	0.70–4.9 µmol/L
Paraquat	Whole blood (EDTA)	Toxic:	0.1–1.6 µg/mL	0.39–6.2 µmol/L
	Urine	Occup exp:	0.3 µg/mL	1.17 µmol/L
		Toxic:	0.9–64 µg/mL	3.50–249 µmol/L
Pentobarbital	Serum or plasma (hep or EDTA); trough	Therap:		
		Hypnotic	1–5 µg/mL	4–22 µmol/L
		Therap coma	20–50 µg/mL	88–221 µmol/L
		Toxic:	>10 µg/mL	>44 µmol/L
Phenacetin	Plasma (EDTA)	Therap:	1–30 µg/mL	6–167 µmol/L
		Toxic:	50–250 µg/mL	279–1395 µmol/L
Phencyclidine	Serum or plasma (hep or EDTA)	Toxic:	90–800 ng/mL	370–3288 nmol/L
Phenobarbital	Serum or plasma (hep or EDTA); trough	Therap:	15–40 µg/mL	65–170 µmol/L
		Toxic:		
		Slowness, ataxia, nystagmus	35–80 µg/mL	151–345 µmol/L
		Coma with reflexes	65–117 µg/mL	280–504 µmol/L
		Coma without reflexes	>100 µg/mL	>430 µmol/L
Phensuximide (both parent and *N*-desmethyl metabolites)	Serum or plasma (hep or EDTA)	Therap:	40–60µg/mL	228–324 µmol/L
Phenylbutazone	Plasma (EDTA)	Therap: (not well defined)	50–100 µg/mL	162–324 µmol/L
		Toxic:	>100 µg/mL	>324 µmol/L
Phenytoin	Serum or plasma (hep or EDTA); trough	Therap:	10–20 µg/mL	40–79 µmol/L
		Toxic:	>20 µg/mL	>79 µmol/L
Primidone	Serum or plasma (hep or EDTA); trough	Therap:	5–12 µg/mL	23–55 µmol/L
		Toxic:	>15 µg/mL	>69 µmol/L
Procainamide	Serum or plasma (hep or EDTA); trough	Therap:	4–10 µg/mL	17–42 µmol/L
		Toxic:	>10 µg/mL	>42 µmol/L
		Also consider effect of metabolite, *N*-acetylprocainamide		
Propoxyphene	Plasma (EDTA)	Therap:	0.1–0.4 µg/mL	0.3–1.2 µmol/L
		Toxic:	>0.5 µg/mL	>1.5 µmol/L
Propranolol	Serum or plasma (hep or EDTA); trough	Therap:	50–100 ng/mL	193–386 nmol/L
Protriptyline	Serum or plasma (hep or EDTA); trough (≥12 h after dose)	Therap:	70–250 ng/mL	266–950 nmol/L
		Toxic:	>500 ng/mL	>1900 nmol/L
Quinidine	Serum or plasma (hep or EDTA); trough	Therap:	2–5 µg/mL	6–15 µmol/L
		Toxic:	>6 µg/mL	>18 µmol/L
Salicylates	Serum or plasma (hep or EDTA); trough	Therap:	150–300 µg/mL	1086–2172 µmol/L
		Toxic:	>300 µg/mL	>2172 µmol/L
Secobarbital	Serum	Therap:	1–2 µg/mL	4.2–8.4 µmol/L
		Toxic:	>5 µg/mL	>21.0 µmol/L
Theophylline	Serum or plasma (hep or EDTA)	Therap:	8–20 µg/mL	44–111 µmol/L
		Toxic:	>20 µg/mL	>110 µmol/L
Thiocyanate	Serum or plasma (EDTA)			
		Nonsmoker:	1–4 µg/mL	17–69 µmol/L
		Smoker:	3–12 µg/mL	52–206 µmol/L
		Therap, after nitroprusside infusion:	6–29 µg/mL	103–499 µmol/L
	Urine	Nonsmoker:	1–4 mg/d	17–69 µmol/d
		Smoker:	7–17 mg/d	120–292 µmol/d
Thiopental	Serum or plasma (hep or EDTA); trough	Hypnotic:	1.0–5.0 µg/mL	4.1–20.7 µmol/L
		Coma:	30–100 µg/mL	124–413 µmol/L
		Anesthesia:	7–130 µg/mL	29–536 µmol/L
		Toxic conc:	>10 µg/mL	>41 µmol/L
Thioridazine	Serum or plasma (hep or EDTA)	Therap:	1.0–1.5 µg/mL	2.7–4.1 µmol/L
		Toxic:	>10 µg/mL	>27 µmol/L

Table continued on following page

DRUGS—THERAPEUTIC AND TOXIC *Continued*

Drug	Specimen	Reference Interval (Conventional Units)		Reference Interval (International Units)
Tobramycin	Serum or plasma (hep or EDTA)	Therap:		
		Peak (severe infection)	8–10 µg/mL	17–21 µmol/L
		Trough (severe infection)	<4 µg/mL	<9 µmol/L
		Toxic:		
		Peak	>10 µg/mL	>21 µmol/L
		Trough	>4 µg/mL	>9 µmol/L
Tocainide	Serum or plasma (hep or EDTA)	Therap:	4–10 µg/mL	21–52 µmol/L
Valproic acid	Serum or plasma (hep or EDTA); trough	Therap:	50–100 µg/mL	347–693 µmol/L
		Toxic:	>100 µg/mL	>693 µmol/L
Vancomycin	Serum or plasma (hep or EDTA); trough	Therap:	5–10 µg/mL	3–7 µmol/L
		Toxic: (not well established)	>80–100 µg/mL	>55–69 µmol/L
Verapamil	Serum or plasma (hep or EDTA)	Therap:	100–500 ng/mL	220–1100 nmol/L
Warfarin	Serum or plasma (hep or EDTA)	Therap:	1–10 µg/mL	3–32 µmol/L

INDEX

Note: Page numbers in **boldface** indicate major discussions; page numbers in *italics* indicate illustrations; page numbers followed by t refer to tables.

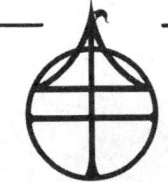